# Monograph sample

***Category* and *Indications*:** list the category of therapeutic use for the drug, the FDA- and HPB-approved indications, and additional indications that USP advisory panels consider to be medically accepted.

***Title section*:** tells the drug's VA classification codes, if it is a controlled substance in the U.S. or Canada, and what its commonly used brand and generic names are.

***Side/Adverse Effects*:** lists common and rare side effects of the drug, with presenting symptoms noted in parentheses, and tells whether the side effects require medical attention.

***General Dosing Information*:** provides general information, including effect on diet and nutrition and treatment of overdose.

***Precautions*:** explains significant clinical considerations, such as drug interactions, medical considerations, laboratory value alterations, recommended patient monitoring, use in pediatric or geriatric patients, cancer-causing potential, and special concerns relating to surgery and in dental practice.

***Pharmacology/Pharmacokinetics*:** provides information on pharmacologic actions and pharmacokinetics.

***Dosage forms*:** gives recommended dosages, prescribing limits, packaging and storage guidelines, and other specific information for each available dosage form.

***Patient Consultation*:** highlights details you may want to discuss with a patient. The most important information is marked with a chevron (»).

# Index guide

## General Index

The following excerpts are examples of the information included in the General Index:

**Drug Name**—Identifies drug by generic name, brand names (in *italics*), and other common names (not italicized).

> Acetaminophen [*Abenol; Aceta Elixir; Acetaminophen Uniserts; Aceta Tablets; Actamin; Actamin Extra; Actimol Chewable Tablets; Actimol Children's Suspension; Actimol Infants' Suspension; Actimol Junior Strength Caplets; Aminofen; Aminofen Max; Anacin-3; Anacin-3 Extra Strength; Apacet Capsules; Apacet Elixir; Apacet Extra Strength Caplets; Apacet Extra Strength Tablets; Apacet, Infants'; Apacet Regular Strength Tablets;* APAP; *Apo-Acetaminophen; Aspirin Free Anacin Maximum Strength Caplets; Aspirin Free Anacin Maxi-*

**Drug Manufacturer**—Identifies drug manufacturer and country for each brand name entry.

> cin B Lipid Complex (Systemic), §, 3092
> *Abenol*—SmithKline Beecham (Canada) brand of Acetaminophen (Systemic), 3

**Drug Effect**—Parenthetical modifiers identify a drug's effect (e.g., topical, otic, nasal, systemic).

> brand of Acetaminophen (Systemic), 3
> *Acetasol HC*—Barre (U.S.) brand of Hydrocortisone and Acetic Acid (Otic, 3047)

**Single Monograph Title**—"Drug Name" + "Drug Effect" = title of monograph.

> Abciximab [*c7E3 Fab; ReoPro*]
> (Systemic), 1
> Injection, 3

**Family Monograph Title**—If a monograph is a family monograph (i.e., covers more than one drug), the family title is listed.

> Acetaminophen and Salicylates (Systemic), 9
> Acetaminophen, Sodium Bicarbonate, and Citric

**Combination Listing**—Identifies combination products containing a designated component.

> Acetaminophen-containing Combinations, 8
> Acetaminophen and Salicylamide [*Duoprin*]
> See Acetaminophen and Salicylates (Sys-

**Page Number**—The first number identifies the first page of a monograph. Subsequent numbers refer to the Additional Products and Indications appendix and/or Orphan Drug and Biological Listing appendix. Numbers preceded by "MC" identify the page number of a pill image, if the dosage form is included in the Medicine Chart.

> *Accupril*—PD (U.S.) brand of Quinapril—**See Angiotensin-converting Enzyme (ACE) Inhibitors (Systemic)**, 166, MC-23
> *Accutane*—Roche (U.S.) brand of Isotretinoin (Systemic), 1770, MC-14
> *Accutane Roche*—Roche (Canada) brand of Isotretinoin (Systemic), 1770
> Acebutolol Hydrochloride [*Monitan; Sectral*]
> **See Beta-adrenergic Blocking Agents (Systemic)**, 568, 3027
> Capsules, 575, 3027
> Tablets, 575

**Dosage Forms**—Identifies available dosage forms and page numbers for dosing information.

> Acetaminophen, Aspirin, and Caffeine [*Duradyne; Excedrin Extra-Strength Caplets; Excedrin Extra-Strength Tablets; Goody's Extra Strength Tablets; Goody's Headache Powders*]
> (Systemic), 9
> Powders, Oral, 11
> Tablets USP, 11

## Indications Index

The following excerpts are examples of the information included in the Indications Index:

**Indication**—Lists indications identified in monographs, or in the Orphan Drug and Biological Listing appendix.
**Drug Name**—Identifies drugs used for indication.
**Definition**—Defines indication by prophylaxis, diagnosis, or treatment.

> Lymphomas, Hodgkin's (treatment)
> [Asparaginase (Systemic)], 465
> Bleomycin (Systemic), 597
> Carmustine (Systemic), 741
> Chlorambucil (Systemic), 784
> Cyclophosphamide (Systemic), 1100
> [Cytarabine (Systemic)][1], 1114
> Dacarbazine (Systemic)[1], 1119
> Doxorubicin (Systemic), 1282
> Epirubicin (Systemic)*, 3040
> [Etoposide (Systemic)], 1404
> Interleukin-3 Human, Recombinant (Systemic), 3109‡

VOLUME **I**

# Drug Information for the Health Care Professional

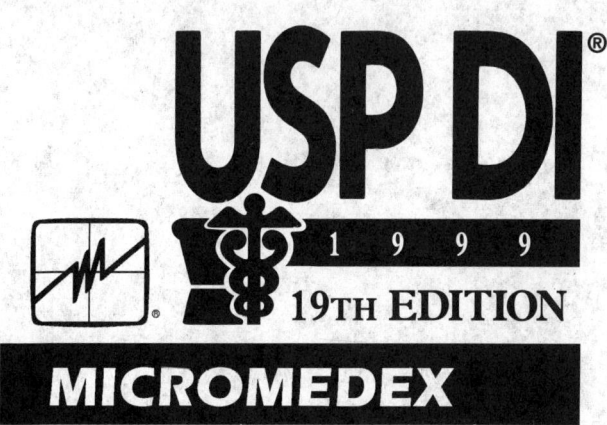

Content prepared by the United States Pharmacopeial Convention, Inc.

NOTICE AND WARNING

**Read the section, Description and Limitations of Information Included, of the "Preface" before consulting individual monographs.**

The inclusion in *USP Dispensing Information (USP DI)* of a monograph on any drug in respect to which patent or trademark rights may exist shall not be deemed, and is not intended as, a grant of, or authority to exercise, any right or privilege protected by such patent or trademark. All such rights and privileges are vested in the patent or trademark owner, and no other person may exercise the same without express permission, authority, or license secured from such patent or trademark owner.

The listing of selected brand names is intended only for ease of reference. The inclusion of a brand name does not mean the authors have any particular knowledge that the brand listed has properties different from other brands of the same drug, nor should it be interpreted as an endorsement. Similarly, the fact that a particular brand has not been included does not indicate that the product has been judged to be unsatisfactory or unacceptable.

Attention is called to the fact that all volumes of *USP Dispensing Information* are fully copyrighted: Volume I—*Drug Information for the Health Care Professional;* Volume II—*Advice for the Patient;* Volume III—*Approved Drug Products and Legal Requirements.*

For permission to copy or utilize limited excerpts of this text, address inquiries to Reprint Requests, Micromedex, Inc., 6200 S. Syracuse Way, Suite 300, Englewood, CO 80111.

Physicians, pharmacists, nurses, or other health practitioners are hereby given permission to reproduce a limited number of one or more pages of advice from the *Advice for the Patient* volume of *USP DI* but only when for direct distribution, without charge, to their patients or clients receiving the prescribed drug, provided that such reproduction shall include the copyright notice appearing on the pages from which it was copied.

This book is protected by copyright. No part of it may be reproduced, stored in a retrieval system, resold, redistributed, or transmitted in any form or by any means (electronic, mechanical, photocopying, recording, or otherwise) without the prior written permission from Micromedex, Inc., except as stated above.

© 1999 Micromedex, Inc., All Rights Reserved.
© 1980–1998 The United States Pharmacopeial Convention, Inc.

USP DI® is a registered trademark of The United States Pharmacopeial Convention, Inc. Used with permission.

Library of Congress Catalog Card Number  81-640842
ISBN  1-56363-322-1
ISSN  0740-4174

Printed by World Color Book Services, Taunton, Massachusetts 02780.

Distributed by Micromedex, Inc., 6200 S. Syracuse Way, Suite 300, Englewood, CO 80111.

# Contents

# USP DI—Volume I
## Drug Information for the Health Care Professional

Foreword .................................................................................................................................................. v
Preface .................................................................................................................................................... vii
USP People 1995–2000
    Officers and Board of Trustees ..................................................................................................... xv
    General Committee of Revision .................................................................................................... xv
    Executive Committee of Revision ................................................................................................. xvi
    Division of Information Development Executive Committee .................................................... xvi
    Division of Standards Development Executive Committee ....................................................... xvi
    Drug Nomenclature Committee .................................................................................................... xvi
    Division of Information Development Advisory Panels ............................................................ xvi
    Division of Information Development Additional Contributors ................................................ xx
    Headquarters Staff .......................................................................................................................... xxii
    Members of the United States Pharmacopeial Convention as of June, 1998 ........................... xxiii

Monographs ............................................................................................................................................ 1

Appendixes
       I:   Additional Products and Indications ............................................................................ 3009
      II:   Selected List of Drug-induced Effects ........................................................................ 3040
     III:   Therapeutic Guidelines .................................................................................................. 3044
    IV:   VA Medication Classification System
           Introduction ................................................................................................................ 3045
             Drug Listing by VA Code ..................................................................................... 3049
      V:   Poison Control Center Listing ...................................................................................... 3063
     VI:   Combination Cross-reference Listing ........................................................................... 3066
    VII:   The Medicine Chart ....................................................................................................... 3083
   VIII:   Orphan Drug and Biological Listing ........................................................................... 3127
     IX:   USP Practitioners' Reporting Network ....................................................................... 3172

Indications Index ................................................................................................................................. 3179

General Index ...................................................................................................................................... 3238

Ordering Information ........................................................................................................................... End

# Foreword

## INFORMATION: CLOSING ONE CHAPTER AND BEGINNING THE NEXT

In 1970 the United States Pharmacopeial Convention directed USP to lead the way in improving patient use of medicines by providing dispensing information that pharmacists and physicians could use to inform their patients about proper use. USP responded and published the first *USP Dispensing Information (USP DI)* for health care professionals in 1980. Included in that volume was a "Patient Consultation" section to provide guidance to the health care professional on what to tell a patient and corresponding lay language monographs (*Advice for the Patient*) that could be photocopied for patient use.

In an age when state pharmacy boards expressly directed pharmacists not to talk with their patients, USP members were almost heretical in asking that USP develop information to assist pharmacists in patient consultation. But, in 1970 the Convention perceived that current philosophies of practices of medicine and pharmacy needed to change and directed USP to provide the health care community with resources to stimulate and enable that change. The end result of the members' action 29 years ago has been that USP has helped motivate health care practitioners to counsel their patients, has helped empower consumers and patients to demand information about their medicines, and has stimulated the development and dissemination of drug and therapeutics information to assist the health care professional in making appropriate drug therapy decisions.

Having achieved the goal established by the 1970 Convention membership, USP has begun to close its chapter as a broad-based information developer and publisher and has started the process of opening a new chapter. For this to happen, it is necessary to define new strategies to answer the following questions: How can USP best use its volunteer experts and expertise to significantly impact public health? What unique contributions can USP make to health care practitioners and patients? What new needs for standards arise from emerging technologies and their uses? What standards should be applied to the quality and usefulness of information relating to products of health care technology? What must USP do, scientifically and fiscally, to ensure its ongoing capability to support its public health mission?

Although new strategies will be the focus of debate and action at the USP Quinquennial meeting in 2000, USP has already begun implementing selected strategies to increase contributions in the areas of professional and patient drug and therapeutics information that will carry a more vital USP into the 21st century. Based on findings and recommendations resulting from an intensive four-month study by the management consulting firm McKinsey & Company, the USP Board of Trustees has focused on strategic new directions relating to information, including:

- transition from being a broad-based supplier of drug and therapeutic information and products, to an organization focused on targeted initiatives that can significantly impact public health.
- seeking a partner to take over responsibility for the full USP DI database to help ensure its continuation.
- exploring collaborative opportunities that will enhance USP's ability to make significant and unique contributions to public health in areas that currently are not being adequately addressed, such as off-label use; pediatric drug use information; dietary supplement information; standards for useful patient information; compounded products information; veterinary information; radiopharmaceuticals information; drug utilization review; and outcomes/cost-effectiveness.

An information partner has been found and on September 17, 1998, the USP Board of Trustees (Board) entered into an agreement with The Thomson Corporation for the sale of the USP DI database and licensing of the USP DI trademark. We believe this agreement assures the continued involvement and influence of our expert advisory panelists in developing authoritative information for use by pharmacists, physicians, health care professionals, patients, and consumers, as evidenced by this 1999 edition of *USP DI*. We expect this agreement will expand dissemination of USP's authoritative information and maintain the role of USP's volunteer panelists in the development of the "value-added" knowledge needed by patients, practitioners, and other health care professionals in the interests of public health.

The agreement is being implemented through MICROMEDEX of Denver, Colorado, a Thomson Healthcare company recognized as a provider of comprehensive, evidence-based clinical knowledge databases for 25 years. USP will retain oversight of the USP DI database through the ongoing work of its Division of Information Development (DID) Executive Committee and more than 700 volunteer experts who serve on 35 therapeutic, practice, and special interest advisory panels. In addition, USP will retain approval rights for all USP DI trademarked products.

Specifically, the agreement pertains to *USP DI® Volume I, Drug Information for the Health Care Professional*; *USP DI® Volume II, Advice for the Patient®, Drug Information in Lay Language*; *USP DI Plus™* (the electronic version of the database); and *MedCoach®*. Portions of the USP DI database that are covered by the agreement include: drug information monographs, patient leaflet information, medicine chart images, dietary supplement information, therapeutic monographs, and veterinary information. Under a separate agreement, Thomson Healthcare will also exclusively license and market the print version of *USP DI® Volume III, Approved Drug Products and Legal Requirements*.

The new and renewed USP emphases will enable the organization to continue to ensure its leadership and change agent roles. In 1820, 11 physicians established USP as a major contributor to ensuring the safety and quality of drug products in the United States; today, those contributions benefit a worldwide audience. The first *Pharmacopeia of the United States of America* fulfilled, and today's *United States Pharmacopeia* and the *National Formulary (USP-NF)* continue to fulfill, the founders' vision. Equally important was the vision of USP's members from medicine, pharmacy, government, industry, and the consumer community who, in 1970, directed USP to respond to the need for health care professionals to consult with patients about their medicines. Today USP is recognized internationally as having established "the standard" for evidence-based, clinically relevant information for professionals and patients, and USP's leadership has helped spur the development of an entire drug information industry.

Few organizations can point to a history of public health contributions of almost 180 years. As it has often throughout its long and successful history, USP is once again shifting its focus in response to changes in the worlds of health care science, economics, and delivery. We look forward with great anticipation to continuing to serve as a catalyst for change, continuing to make a significant and unique public health impact, and remaining the source of quality standards and information for medicines that support health care professionals and patients.

Jerome A. Halperin
Executive Vice President-CEO

Rockville, Maryland
January 4, 1999

# Preface

Since 1820, the United States Pharmacopeia has set standards for the medications used by the American public. In establishing the Pharmacopeia, the founders were reacting to an unmet need of the professions and their patients—that is, the need for generally accepted procedures for the preparation of medications which would allow for confidence in their use.

The need for quality standards remains, and the work of USP in establishing those standards continues. However, additional needs regarding the use of medications have arisen, within both the health care provider and health care recipient populations. Some of these newly recognized needs relate to information sources. *USP DI* is one reaction to these previously unmet needs.

At the 1970 meeting of the Pharmacopeial Convention, a resolution to increase in the Pharmacopeia or in a companion volume the amount of information that would be useful to pharmacists and others was adopted. In response to this, the 1970-1975 Subcommittee on Posology and Related Information, under the chairmanship of John A. Owen, Jr., M.D., expanded the category and dose information and introduced in the *USP XIX* monographs of many dosage forms a section entitled Dispensing Information. This information served as a basic reminder or general guide to the pharmacist, who could vary or omit it in accordance with the best interests of the patient or the particular circumstances involved.

Continuing this development, the 1975-1980 Subcommittee, under the chairmanship of Harry C. Shirkey, R.Ph., M.D., greatly expanded the amount and kinds of information in the USP DI database, focusing on that believed to enhance the safe and effective use of a medication once it was prescribed. This included drug use information relating to dispensing, administration, monitoring, and patient consultation. The work of the Subcommittee resulted in the first edition (1980) of *USP DI*. From one book in 1980, it grew to two volumes in 1983, and three volumes in 1989.

*USP DI* is, and it always will be, a work in progress. The information is under constant revision. This nineteenth edition incorporates the experiences and comments generated by previous editions. New drug monographs and information have been added, and the existing text has been reviewed for changes and revised accordingly.

## Development of *USP DI*

The *USP DI* is a comprehensive collection of clinically relevant, established information about each drug. However, it is far more than that. It is a continuous collection of the current judgments of experts in the use of drugs. The information included is the result of a planned, organized, nationwide, evidence-based consensus-generating system (with worldwide input). This system has been designed to involve not only the experts but all interested parties through open public review and comment.

Using the parameters established by the USP Division of Information Development Executive Committee, staff develops draft monographs for each drug selected for inclusion in *USP DI*. These initial drafts are reviewed by the appropriate Advisory Panel(s) and other designated reviewers and are revised accordingly. Redrafted text may again be reviewed by Advisory Panel(s) as many times as necessary to achieve an initial consensus. Proposed monographs are then made available for general public review and comment. Announcement of availability is made in *USP DI Review*, made available on USP's homepage (www.usp.org) or in the *USP Standard* publication.

The comments generated by the public review process are fed back into the USP Advisory Panel system. If substantive changes result, the monograph is again listed in *USP DI Review* announcing additional proposed changes. The process is repeated as required to develop final consensus.

Of course, the consensus can change from one edition to the next, and users of *USP DI* are encouraged to submit comments at any time to:

USP
Division of Information Development
12601 Twinbrook Parkway
Rockville, Maryland 20852
Telephone: (301) 816-8351
Telefax: (301) 816-8374
E-mail: mlr@usp.org

## Organization of *USP DI*

*USP DI* comprises three distinct sections. The first volume, *Drug Information for the Health Care Professional*, includes the DI monographs arranged in alphabetic order. The Volume I general index includes established names, cross-references by brand names (both U.S. and Canadian), and older nonproprietary names. In addition, an indications index and appendixes presenting categories of use and other useful information are included. The second volume, *Advice for the Patient*, includes the lay language versions of the patient consultation guidelines found in Volume I. These lay language versions are intended to be used at the discretion of the health care provider as an aid to patient consultation if written information would be of benefit or if it is requested by the prescriber. Brand and generic names are cross-referenced in the index of *Advice for the Patient*. The third volume, *Approved Drug Products and Legal Requirements*, reproduces information from the Food and Drug Administration on therapeutic equivalence and other requirements relating to drug product selection. It includes USP and NF legal requirements for labeling, storage, packaging, and quality for drugs. It also contains those portions of the federal Controlled Substances Act Regulations, the Poison Prevention Packaging Act and Regulations, and the FD&C Act provisions relating to drugs for human use, and the Current Good Manufacturing Practice Regulations that are most relevant to the physician, pharmacist, nurse, and other health care professionals.

The individual Volume I monograph covers the basic information which is applicable to that substance when used for a specific area of effect (e.g., Systemic). Information that is unique for a specific dosage form of the base substance is then included under that specific dosage form heading. To illustrate this approach, assume that DRUG X is used for its systemic effects and its topical effects. Also assume that the drug is available in the following dosage forms: cream, injection, ointment, syrup, and tablet. The *USP DI* Volume I monographs for DRUG X would be organized as follows:

DRUG X (Systemic)
[General information applicable to Drug X's systemic use.]
    Drug X Syrup
    Drug X Tablets
    Drug X Injection
    [Specific information applicable to each of the systemic dosage forms.]

DRUG X (Topical)
[General information applicable to Drug X's topical use.]
    Drug X Cream
    Drug X Ointment
    [Specific information applicable to each of the topical dosage forms.]

Where appropriate, other major headings based on specific area of effect are used for Dental, Inhalation-Local, Intracavernosal, Mucosal-Local, Nasal-Local, Ophthalmic, Oral-Local, Otic, Parenteral-Local, Rectal-Local, Transdermal-Systemic, or Vaginal use.

Whenever feasible, monographs are grouped under family headings. This permits a sizable saving of space and also allows the practitioner to readily identify differences among agents of the same family. Significant differences are addressed in charts and in Summary of Differences sections.

The following headings and subheadings are employed, where appropriate, in organizing the information for each Volume I monograph:

Category
Indications
  General considerations
  Accepted
  Acceptance not established
  Unaccepted
Pharmacology/Pharmacokinetics
  Physicochemical characteristics
    Source
    Molecular weight
    pKa
    Solubility
    Partition coefficient
    Other characteristics
  Mechanism of action/Effect
  Other actions/effects
  Absorption
  Distribution
  Protein binding
  Biotransformation
  Half-life
  Onset of action
  Time to peak concentration
  Peak serum concentration
  Time to peak effect
  Duration of action
  Elimination
    In dialysis
Precautions to Consider
  Cross-sensitivity and/or related problems
  Carcinogenicity
  Tumorigenicity
  Mutagenicity
  Pregnancy/Reproduction
    Fertility
    Pregnancy
    Labor
    Delivery
    Postpartum
  Breast-feeding
  Pediatrics
  Adolescents
  Geriatrics
  Pharmacogenetics
  Dental
  Surgical
  Critical/Emergency care
  Drug interactions and/or related problems
  Laboratory value alterations
    With diagnostic test results
    With physiology/laboratory test values
  Medical considerations/Contraindications
  Patient monitoring
Side/Adverse Effects
  Those indicating need for medical attention
  Those indicating need for medical attention only if they continue or are bothersome
  Those not indicating need for medical attention
  Those indicating need for medical attention if they occur after medication is discontinued
Overdose
  Clinical effects of overdose
  Treatment of overdose
Patient Consultation
  Before using this medication
  Proper use of this medication
  Precautions while using this medication
  Side/adverse effects
General Dosing Information
  Diet/Nutrition
  Bioequivalence information
  Safety considerations for handling this medication
  For treatment of adverse effects
Dosage forms (each separate)
  Usual adult dose
  Usual adult prescribing limits
  Usual pediatric dose
  Usual pediatric prescribing limits
  Usual geriatric dose
  Strengths usually available
  Packaging and storage
  Preparation of dosage form
  Stability
  Incompatibilities
  Auxiliary labeling
  Caution
  Additional information
Selected Bibliography

**Description and Limitations of Information Included**

*USP DI* contains selected information and takes into account practice concerns. Selection is based on what is considered by the Committee of Revision and its Advisory Panels to be practical, clinically significant information needed to help assure that a drug is being safely and effectively used. It is meant to aid the health care professional and the patient in minimizing the risks and enhancing the benefits of the drugs used. Collectively, it is valuable in assessing the quality of care through drug utilization review programs. Ultimately, the information required is defined by the practice standards of medicine, pharmacy, nursing, dentistry, and the other health professions as well as by the information needs of the patient.

*USP DI* is not intended to be "full disclosure" information.

Readers are advised that the information in *USP DI* may contain statements that differ from those in the "full disclosure" information labeling approved or required by the United States or Canadian governments. On the other hand, readers should remember that FDA-approved full disclosure information can differ from brand to brand of the same generic drug product. It should not be inferred that the inclusion of information that is not in the approved labeling has been sought or agreed to by the manufacturer.

Selected brand names are included in the monographs as well as in the indexes of both volumes I and II for ease of reference purposes only. The inclusion of a brand name is not intended as an endorsement of a particular product. The omission of a particular brand name does not indicate that the article was judged to be inferior or inadequate. The inclusion of various brands in volumes I and II bears no relationship to and is not intended to affect any applicable brand interchange requirements.

The Veterans Administration medication classification codes (primary and secondary assignments) are included at the beginning of each monograph. See the VA Medication Classification System appendix in *USP DI* Volume I for a detailed description as well as a complete listing of primary and secondary classifications.

Where appropriate, controlled substance classifications are included at the beginning of the monograph. United States schedules include:

Schedule I—No legal medical use is recognized by the U.S. Controlled Substances Act. Use of Schedule I substances for research purposes is permitted with proper registration. Schedule I substances are not included in *USP DI*.
Examples: Heroin, LSD, peyote.

Schedule II—The most stringent classification for drugs recognized by the U.S. Controlled Substances Act as having a legitimate medical use; these drugs are characterized by a very high abuse potential and/or potential for severe physical and psychic dependency. Distribution and inventory are highly controlled; prescriptions are non-refillable. Emergency telephone orders for limited quantities of these drugs are authorized but the prescriber must provide a written, signed prescription order to the pharmacy within 72 hours. Examples: Amphetamines, anabolic steroids, meperidine, morphine, short-acting barbiturates.

Schedule III—Includes drugs having significant abuse potential, but to a lesser degree than Schedule II substances. Prescriptions can be refilled up to five times within six months after the date of issue if authorized by the prescriber. Telephone orders are permitted. Examples: Certain barbiturates not included in Schedule II, opiates in combination with other substances such as acetaminophen or aspirin.

Schedule IV—Includes drugs having a low abuse potential. Prescriptions can be refilled up to five times within six months after the date of issue if authorized by the prescriber. Telephone orders are permitted. Examples: Benzodiazepines, certain long-acting barbiturates, chloral hydrate, pentazocine, propoxyphene.

Schedule V—Includes products having the lowest abuse potential of the controlled substances. No limitations on refills other than those imposed by the prescriber. Some Schedule V products may be available without a prescription (for example, certain cough preparations and antidiarrheal preparations containing limited amounts of an opiate).

In addition to the federal Controlled Substances Act, most states have controlled substances acts similar to the federal requirements. In some instances, the state regulations may be more restrictive. These differences are not addressed in *USP DI* monographs.

Canadian controlled substance classifications (and the designations used in this publication) include:

Narcotics (N)—Includes products containing a narcotic. Within this broad classification, there are several levels of regulatory control. These levels range from strict controls for the most abusable of the substances (for example, single-entity narcotics; products containing a narcotic with one active non-narcotic ingredient; any preparation containing heroin, hydrocodone, or oxycodone) to lesser controls for preparations containing one narcotic and two active non-narcotic ingredients and exempt codeine preparations (those containing a limited amount of codeine plus two active non-narcotic ingredients).

Controlled Drugs (C)—Includes non-narcotic preparations with abuse potential. As with narcotics, different regulations apply depending on specific content. Examples: Amphetamines, barbiturates.

*Introductory Version Monographs*—Monographs on newly approved drugs based primarily on the manufacturer's package insert and reviewed by selected members of the appropriate USP DI Advisory Panels are now included in *USP DI Volume I* and *Volume II*. Introductory Version Monographs fill the immediate need for information until a full monograph for a given drug has been developed and assessed by the advisory panels.

**Category/Indications**—Statements of categories of use and indications are provided for each article.

The category of use indicates the area of therapeutic utility for which the drug was included and generally represents an application of the best known pharmacologic action of the article or its active ingredient. The statement is not intended to be all inclusive nor to indicate that the article may have no other activity or utility.

Indications of use stated in manufacturers' labeling and approved by the U.S. Food and Drug Administration (FDA) or Health Canada's Therapeutic Products Directorate are generally included, as well as additional off-label indications selected as appropriate by USP Advisory Panels. These two types of indications are included under an *Accepted* subheading. An *Unaccepted* indications section identifies uses of a drug that are considered by USP Advisory Panels to be inappropriate, obsolete, or unproven. For certain drugs whose place in therapy has not been determined and the use does not clearly fall into the "Accepted" or "Unaccepted" categorization, information is included under an *Acceptance not established* subheading.

A *General considerations* subsection is included in the Indications section for some drugs, such as antibiotics, to give the reader more complete information about the drug (e.g., the activity spectrum of antibiotics).

New uses for approved products that are not reflected in a product's labeling are often discovered after marketing. Before a pharmaceutical manufacturer may include any new indications in the labeling for a particular drug (and to promote the product for those uses), it must obtain the government's approval for the uses. Such approval requires the completion of adequate and well-controlled clinical trials to document the drug's safety and efficacy for the new uses. Since the clinical trials required for approval may take considerable time and effort, manufacturers, in some cases, may not seek or obtain approval for new uses since there may not be sufficient economic incentive for the product sponsor to perform the necessary research or to make application to the agency. In other cases, of course, the research may have been carried out by the manufacturer but the new proposed use found to be unsupported.

In an attempt to be of assistance to practitioners, USP Advisory Panels have been requested to include those off-label indications (i.e., not included in the labeling of *any* brand) which they believe represent reasonable, current prescribing practices based on their knowledge of the drug, the literature, and of current prescribing and utilization practices which practitioners should be prepared to address. In certain instances, particularly life-threatening diseases for which a definitive cure is not available (e.g., some cancers), off-label uses may be included as acceptable although experimental because other therapy is either unavailable or has been tried and has failed.

Medically accepted off-label indications are identified in the *Indications* section by brackets for the U.S. and a superscript 1 for Canada. The off-label indication may be followed by a brief explanatory statement.

The legality of the prescribing of approved drugs for uses not included in their official labeling is sometimes a cause for concern and confusion among practitioners. The appropriateness of prescribing or dispensing an approved drug for an off-label indication would ultimately be judged in accordance with normal legal principles governing professional activities such as negligence or strict liability in the event of a question of liability to an injured patient. In the U.S., the Federal Food, Drug, and Cosmetic Act does not prohibit practitioners from prescribing nor pharmacists from dispensing a drug product for a particular patient for an indication not contained in its approved labeling.

Another point of concern to practitioners relates to differences in approved labeled indications for different brands of the same generic drug product. Because of the legalities involved, it is possible for different manufactured products of the same generic product to have in their labeling different indications (as well as different precautions, side effects, dosage schedules, etc.). *USP DI* indications are not directed to a specific brand product unless a particular characteristic of a brand must be taken into account.

*Evidence ratings*—Evidence ratings based on study design and strength of endpoints are now being included in monographs to support the off-label use recommendations made by USP advisory panels. Once an off-label indication has been approved by the panel, the evidence rating supporting that use is placed in parentheses in Roman type (e.g., Evidence rating: IA) in the text after the paragraph that discusses the indication, or after each indication, if they are listed in a string within a statement. Ratings are assigned based on the following scheme:

Grade level (ranked in descending order of strength)—
**I:** Evidence from randomized, controlled trials or meta-analyses of a group of randomized, controlled trials.
**II.** Evidence from well-designed, internally controlled clinical trials without randomization, from cohort or case-controlled analytic studies, perferably from more than one center, from multiple time series, or from dramatic results in uncontrolled experiments.
**III:** Evidence from clinical trials with low power, preliminary reports of trials in progress, opinions of respected authorities on the basis of clinical experience, descriptive studies such as case reports or series, or reports of expert committees.

Strength of Endpoints (ranked in descending order of strength)—
**A.** Total Mortality (or overall survival from a defined point in time, such as the time of randomization).
**B.** Cause-Specific Mortality (or cause-specific mortality from a defined point in time).
**C.** Carefully Assessed Quality of Life (does not include reports of symptoms or toxicity).
**D.** Indirect Surrogates (includes disease-free survival, progression-free survival, tumor response rate).

**Pharmacology/Pharmacokinetics**—A brief statement of physicochemical characteristics and pharmacologic actions includes, whenever appropriate and available, source, molecular weight, pKa, solubility, partition coefficient, mechanism of action, actions other than the therapeutic actions, absorption, distribution in the body, protein-binding characteristics, biotransformation, half-life, onset of action, time to peak concentration, peak serum concentration, time to peak effect, duration of action, and elimination. The information is not intended to be inclusive. In some cases, protein binding is expressed in general terms with ranges as follows, rather than in terms of specific percentages:

Very high: >90%
High: 65–90%
Moderate: 35–64%
Low: 10–34%
Very low: <10%

**Precautions to Consider**—The precautions to consider in using a specific drug, as listed under this heading, are not intended to provide ''full disclosure'' information. Instead, precautions have been selected on the basis of their common or usual clinical significance to the population as a whole. It cannot be assumed that the omission of a precaution in *USP DI* means that such a precaution may not be of clinical significance for a specific patient. In many cases, there is a lack of scientifically valid information to support inclusion in *USP DI*. As in all aspects of medical care, risk-benefit considerations must be made on an individual basis, which may, in fact, supersede general precautions to the use of any medication.

*Cross-sensitivity and/or related problems*—Where known, potential for cross-sensitivity with other drugs is included.

*Carcinogenicity*—Where known, reference is made to the cancer-causing potential of a drug. Not all such precautions may necessarily be listed.

*Tumorigenicity*—Where known, reference is made to the tumor-causing potential of a drug. Not all such precautions may necessarily be listed.

*Mutagenicity*—Where known, reference is made to the mutagenic potential of a drug. Not all such precautions may necessarily be listed.

*Pregnancy/Reproduction*—Documented problems in humans with the use of a drug during pregnancy are included. Where appropriate, information is included on fertility, pregnancy, labor, delivery, and postpartum effects. In addition, reference is made to problems documented in animal studies even though the significance of such findings to humans may not be known. FDA-assigned pregnancy categories are included whenever available. These categories are:

A: Adequate and well-controlled studies have failed to demonstrate a risk to the fetus in the first trimester of pregnancy (and there is no evidence of risk in later trimesters).
B: Animal reproduction studies have failed to demonstrate a risk to the fetus and there are no adequate and well-controlled studies in pregnant women.
C: Animal reproduction studies have shown an adverse effect on the fetus and there are no adequate and well-controlled studies in humans, but potential benefits may warrant use of the drug in pregnant women despite potential risks.
D: There is positive evidence of human fetal risk based on adverse reaction data from investigational or marketing experience or studies in humans, but potential benefits may warrant use of the drug in pregnant women despite potential risks if the drug is needed in a life-threatening situation or for a serious disease for which safer drugs cannot be used or are ineffective.
X: Studies in animals or humans have demonstrated fetal abnormalities and/or there is positive evidence of human fetal risk based on adverse reaction data from investigational or marketing experience, and the risks involved in use of the drug in pregnant women clearly outweigh potential benefits.

*Breast-feeding*—Documented problems in humans associated with the use of a drug while breast-feeding are included. Where appropriate, reference is also made to problems documented in animal studies even though the significance of such findings to humans may not be known.

*Pediatrics*—Selected precautions relating to use of an agent in the pediatric patient are included. Not all precautions relevant to such use may necessarily be listed. If no information about the use of a drug in the pediatric patient is known, this is so stated.

*Adolescents*—Selected precautions relating to use of an agent in the adolescent patient are included. Not all precautions relevant to such use may necessarily be listed.

*Geriatrics*—Selected precautions relating to use of an agent in the geriatric patient are included. Not all precautions relevant to such use may necessarily be listed. If no information about the use of a drug in the geriatric patient is known, this is so stated.

*Pharmacogenetics*—Selected precautions relating to genetic factors and potential responses to drugs are included. Not all such potential effects may necessarily be listed.

*Dental*—Selected precautions relating to potential dental effects of an agent are included. Not all such potential effects may necessarily be listed.

*Surgical*—Selected precautions relating to potential effects of an agent on surgery are included. Not all precautions relevant to surgery may necessarily be listed.

*Critical/Emergency care*—Selected precautions relating to potential effects of an agent in a critical/emergency care situation are included. Not all such precautions may necessarily be listed.

*Drug interactions and/or related problems*—Drug and/or food interactions have been selected on the basis of their potential clinical significance. Those considered to have greater significance are identified with a chevron (») to the left of the drug entry. In some cases, an interaction appearing in one monograph may not be cross-referenced in the corresponding monograph. Since each monograph is finalized individually, such inconsistencies are constantly in the process of resolution in preparation for the next revision of the monograph.

*Laboratory value alterations*—This section includes effects of the drug on laboratory test values. No attempt has been made to provide a complete listing of effects on the normal or diseased body or interferences with other tests that may be required if proper diagnosis is to be expected. The information included in this section is broken down into two subsections:

- With diagnostic test results—Includes changes in laboratory test values caused by effects of the drug in the body or on the test materials or procedure that may produce inaccurate results (e.g., diagnostic tests for which the results may be false-positive or false-negative in patients receiving the drug).
- With physiology/laboratory test values—Includes changes in laboratory test values that may occur because of the physiologic effects of the drug (for example, increases or decreases in serum electrolytes).

Effects listed have been selected on the basis of potential clinical significance. The list is not necessarily inclusive.

*Medical considerations/Contraindications*—Some medical conditions, the presence of which may alter the decision to prescribe a drug for a given patient or may affect the dosage, are listed. As a general rule, the list is compiled from the approved labeling and covers precautions, warnings, and contraindications. Those conditions considered to be of greater importance are identified by a chevron (») to the left of the specific medical problem. Contraindications that are considered to be absolute, except under special circumstances, are listed first. Relative contraindications are included for those problems requiring risk-benefit consideration.

*Patient monitoring*—To exercise judgment in refilling prescriptions and to monitor continuing use of a medication, patient examinations that may be particularly important are listed. The list is not meant to be a complete listing of the check-ups a patient may require nor is it meant to imply that all check-ups listed are necessarily required for every patient taking the medication.

**Side/Adverse Effects**—Selected side effects are listed. Selection is based on seriousness (e.g., agranulocytosis), frequency of occurrence, effect on life style (e.g., drowsiness), and/or likelihood that a nonthreatening side effect might cause concern to the patient if he or she were not aware that the effect might occur (e.g., rapid pulse). Wherever possible, side effects are grouped according to reported incidence—i.e., incidence more frequent, incidence less frequent, or incidence rare; or by percentages, if available. Not all such side/adverse effects may necessarily be listed.

The side effects are listed by effect with presenting symptom(s) in parentheses.

**Overdose**—This section includes selected information on therapeutic and toxic concentrations of the drug, time to onset of overdose symptoms, clinical effects of overdose, and treatment of overdose.

**Patient Consultation**—Current medical practice embraces the belief that patient compliance and the effectiveness of therapy can be advanced in certain clinical situations if the prescriber provides, or asks the dispenser to provide, written drug use information of the type contained in *USP DI*. To help ensure patient understanding, the prescriber and dispenser should, in turn, translate the essence of this information in words suitable to the ability of the individual patient to understand.

Prior to providing oral consultation, health care professionals should apprise themselves of the entire monograph for the indicated medication. The patient consultation section is provided as a reminder, highlighting a limited, selected number of items peculiar to the medication for oral discussion and, in general, assumes more complete written information can be made available.

Suggested guidelines for patient consultation are listed. The statements marked with a chevron (») are considered to be of greatest importance. If written information is desired, the health care provider may refer to the corresponding lay language monograph in *Advice for the Patient*.

The information provided is intended to aid efforts to advance patient compliance and the effectiveness of the therapy selected by the prescriber. The information provided is not complete, but is intended to serve as a basic reminder or general guide to the health care provider who may vary or omit it in accordance with professional judgment taking into account the best interests of the patient, the request of the prescriber, or the particular circumstances involved. It is not intended as a substitute for professional judgment or to modify any legal requirements imposed on the dispenser. It serves also as a general reminder to the prescriber of the concerns of the dispenser in the dispenser-patient relationship.

Some drugs are not amenable to general rules since they may be prescribed for various purposes not necessarily known to the dispenser, to the person administering the drug, or to other physicians caring for the patient; also, the differences in their utilization might affect the advice to be given. However, where it is clear how a drug is being utilized, it may be helpful to reinforce the prescriber's instructions or to provide such additional advice as would assist the patient.

Occasionally, a dispenser or person administering a drug may have particular knowledge of problems peculiar to the patient that justifies giving exceptional instructions. The fact that *USP DI* makes no mention of such unusual or exceptional circumstances is not intended to limit or influence professional judgment in conveying to the patient information that is deemed to be correct and proper under the circumstances.

**General Dosing Information**—Dosing information of a general nature which may be applicable to the usual dispensing or administration situation and guidelines relating to diet/nutrition and bioequivalence are included, where appropriate. The information is meant to supplement the dosing information included under each specific dosage form and the two sets of information must be used together.

Information relating to safety considerations for handling a medication and the treatment of adverse effects is also included in this section.

**Dosage Forms**—The following information is listed separately for each dosage form, whenever appropriate:

*Summary of differences*—In family monographs, a summary of differences for each individual family member is included. Not all differences are necessarily included. The fact that this section does not include certain information does not necessarily indicate that the point in question does not occur with that particular family member. It may, instead, reflect a lack of information. Users of *USP DI* must exercise caution and not use the information included in family monographs as the sole basis of comparison between agents.

*Usual adult dose*—The usual adult dose given for each article is that which may ordinarily be expected to produce in adults with normal renal/hepatic function, following administration in the manner indicated, at such time intervals as may be specified, the diagnostic, therapeutic, prophylactic, or other effect for which the article is recognized. The usual adult dose is intended to serve only as a guide and it may be varied in the best interests of the patient and in accordance with the variables that affect the action of the drug. Where appropriate, information relating to dosing in a patient who has renal/hepatic function impairment is included.

The statements of dosage in the case of capsules and tablets are in terms of the content of active ingredient and rarely represent the total weight of the capsule contents or of the tablets.

In some instances, the dosage may be stated in terms of the pharmacologically active portion (moiety) of the molecule in order to permit the prescriber or dispenser to correlate the weight equivalent for salts, esters, or other chemical forms of the drug moiety. However, it is not to be inferred that all chemical forms in which the active moiety may be presented are therapeutically equivalent. Neither are different dosage forms administered by the same route always therapeutically equivalent, e.g., tablets vs. syrups or creams vs. ointments.

*Usual adult prescribing limits*—The usual adult prescribing limits subsection is intended primarily to guide the dispenser with respect to seeking confirmation of prescription orders calling for unusually small or large doses. In some cases, it may take into account some uses in addition to those implied in the statement of category. The time schedule and route of administration where given for the usual adult dose apply also to the usual adult prescribing limits unless otherwise specified.

The limits statement does not address the issue of toxicity levels but instead focuses on the generally accepted lower and/or upper ranges of dosage believed to be used in medical practice.

*Usual pediatric dose*—The usual pediatric dose generally given in the monograph is that which may ordinarily be expected to produce in infants and children with normal renal/hepatic function, following administration in the manner indicated, at such time intervals as may be designated, the diagnostic, therapeutic, or prophylactic effect for which the article is recognized. Where appropriate, information relating to dosing in a patient who has renal/hepatic function impairment is included.

The provision of the usual pediatric dose is not a recommendation or indication that the drug should be utilized in the pediatric patient, but is intended to serve only as a guide. It should be emphasized that metabolism and elimination of many drugs, including the "inactive" ingredients in the dosage forms, are markedly different in full-term newborn infants, and even more so in premature infants, from those in older children and adults.

*Usual pediatric prescribing limits*—The usual pediatric prescribing limits subsection is intended primarily to guide the dispenser with respect to seeking confirmation of prescription orders calling for unusually small or large doses. In some cases, it may take into account some uses in addition to those implied in the statement of category. The time schedule and route of administration where given for the usual pediatric dose apply also to the usual pediatric prescribing limits unless otherwise specified.

*Usual geriatric dose*—A usual geriatric dose statement is included if current knowledge allows. It is to be emphasized that metabolism and elimination of many drugs, including the "inactive" ingredients in the dosage forms, may be markedly different in the geriatric patient.

The provision of the usual geriatric dose is not a recommendation or indication that the drug should be utilized in the geriatric patient. It is intended to serve only as a guide and it may be varied in the best interests of the patient and in accordance with the variables that affect the action of the drug.

*Strength(s) usually available*—The statement on strengths usually available for a dosage form, given in the individual monograph, is not necessarily complete and is intended solely as information to physicians, pharmacists, nurses, and others concerned with the manner in which dosage forms are commercially supplied.

If a specific drug product is known to contain sulfites, large amounts of lactose, or other inactive ingredients known to cause allergic reactions in large numbers of patients, this information has been included for selected medications.

*Packaging and storage*—Information concerning packaging and storage of medications as applicable to the dispenser is provided in this section. The labeling of the brand product selected may contain additional or other packaging and storage information specific to that product.

The information included in this section is not intended to replace more definitive requirements that may be contained in the official *USP* monographs. For those dosage forms included in *USP*, compendial requirements for packaging and storage apply to the dispenser.

For those products not covered by *USP*, the packaging and storage recommendations found in *USP DI* are usually those recommended by the manufacturer(s).

*Preparation of dosage form*—Instructions on constitution and/or dilution of a dosage form for administration are included. Information on the extemporaneous preparation of certain drugs, for example, for pediatric use, is also included, where deemed appropriate.

*Stability*—Included is information concerning beyond-use dates for constituted solutions or suspensions, along with special stability problems associated with certain drug products (for example, nitroglycerin tablets). The labeling of the brand product selected may contain specific stability information which differs from that stated in *USP DI*.

*Incompatibilities*—Chemical and physical incompatibilities of certain admixtures (e.g., intravenous preparations) are included, where deemed appropriate.

*Auxiliary labeling*—Auxiliary information that is suggested for consideration of placement on the actual prescription container (in addition to the prescription labeling) in accordance with applicable practice requirements is specified in this section.

Recommended labeling that relates to physical properties of the product (e.g., "shake well" for suspensions) can be considered to be universally applicable.

Suggested labeling that relates to therapy (e.g., take on an empty stomach) and would be appropriate for most, but not necessarily all patients, must be considered on an individual basis by the dispenser.

*Caution*—Information on potential medication errors, where known, and steps to help minimize occurrence of such errors are included as appropriate.

*Additional information*—Additional information relating to the specific drug product is included if necessary, especially as this information relates to the act of dispensing the medication.

**Advice for the Patient (Volume II)**—*Advice for the Patient* (Volume II) presents in lay language the concepts listed in the Patient Consultation guidelines of Volume I. It is meant to reinforce the oral consultation and to be provided in written form at the discretion of the health care provider. In general, statements that warrant a chevron (») in Patient Consultation are printed in *italic* type for immediate notice in *Advice for the Patient*.

The information presented under the section entitled *Additional Information* includes information related to medically accepted off-label uses of the drug. This section is intended for use where the health care provider has knowledge that the medication has been prescribed for a particular purpose referred to therein. It is intended as an aid to providing individualized patient education and is not for use when providing the general population with information about the drug. Since the section may contain information which may be or seem to be contradictory or confusing to the patient receiving the drug for its labeled purposes, the health care provider should consider not including this section if photocopies of the information are given to patients routinely.

**Approved Drug Products and Legal Requirements (Volume III)**—The United States Pharmacopeial Convention is the publisher of the *United States Pharmacopeia* and the *National Formulary*. These texts are recognized as official compendia by the pharmacy and medical professions. They contain standards, specifications, and other requirements relating to drugs and other articles used in medical and pharmacy practice that may be enforceable under various statutes. These requirements are applicable not only when drugs are in the possession of the manufacturer, but at the practice level as well.

Although the standards continue to be applicable when drugs are dispensed or sold, it must also be recognized that most prescriptions today are filled with manufactured products and for the most part physicians and pharmacists no longer compound or analyze drug products. On the other hand, dispensers need to be aware of the quality attributes of products, their packaging and storage requirements, and the other applicable standards to which legal consequences may attach.

In recognition of this need, Volume III provides abstracts of *USP-NF* standards. Similarly, selected portions of the *USP-NF* General Notices and Chapters that are deemed to be especially relevant are reprinted in Volume III.

The incorporation of these official *USP-NF* materials into *USP DI* is for informational purposes only. Because of varying publication schedules, there may occasionally be a time difference between publication of revisions in the *USP-NF* and the appearance of these changes in *USP DI*. Readers are advised that only the standards as written in the *USP-NF* are regarded as official.

The *USP-NF* material included in *USP DI* is not intended to represent nor shall it be interpreted to be the equivalent of or a substitute for the official *United States Pharmacopeia* and/or *National Formulary*. In the event of any difference or discrepancy between the current official *USP* or *NF* standards and the information contained herein, the context and effect of the official compendia shall prevail.

Volume III also contains federal and state requirements relevant to the dispensing situation, including:

- the entire text of FDA's "Orange Book," *Approved Drug Products with Therapeutic Equivalence Evaluations;*
- separate listings of B-rated drugs from the FDA "Orange Book" and pre-1938 drugs ("grandfathered" drugs not included in the "Orange Book");
- selected portions of the federal Controlled Substance Act Regulations;
- the federal Food, Drug and Cosmetic Act requirements as they relate to human drugs, including the recent drug diversion and sampling amendments;
- FDA's Current Good Manufacturing Practice Regulations for Finished Pharmaceuticals.

### Appendixes

To help the user of *USP DI*, numerous appendixes have been included in both Volume I and Volume II.

**Volume I**—Volume I includes the following additional material as appendixes:

*Additional Products and Indications* (Appendix I)—Newly marketed and other products not included in the main text of *USP DI* are referenced in this appendix in order to provide as much useful information as possible. The information included has not gone through the USP DI review process and is based simply on the product's package insert.

*Selected List of Drug-induced Effects* (Appendix II)—A list of selected drug-induced side effects has been compiled for use primarily in conjunction with the drug interactions section of *USP DI* monographs. The listing of drugs is not meant to be inclusive.

*Therapeutic Guidelines* (Appendix III)—This appendix provides selected general therapeutic guidelines for the health care professional.

*VA Medication Classification System* (Appendix IV)—The Veterans Administration Medication Classification system was developed to provide a systematic and management approach to the classification of medications, investigational drugs, prosthetic items, and expendable supplies for hospital patients. Primary and secondary VA codes are included in each *USP DI* monograph and in this appendix. In addition, codes for new products are included in the Additional Products and Indications chart (Appendix I).

*Poison Control Center Listing* (Appendix V)—Includes a listing of certified regional U.S. poison control centers.

*Combination Cross-reference Listing* (Appendix VI)—This appendix provides a listing of the therapeutically active ingredients found in combination products included in the 1999 edition of *USP DI*, along with a cross-reference to the title of the monograph where the specific combination product can be found.

*The Medicine Chart* (Appendix VII)—The Medicine Chart presents photographs of many of the most frequently prescribed medicines in the United States. In general, commonly used brand names and a representative sampling of generic products have been included. Only solid oral dosage forms (tablets and capsules) have been included. Since color and size variations may exist and since product changes may have subsequently been adopted by a manufacturer, the chart should be used only as an initial guide, with verification of product identity being made before any further actions are taken.

*Orphan Drug and Biological Listing* (Appendix VIII)—As a service to users of the USP DI data base, this appendix reproduces the list of orphan drug and biological designations as issued by the U.S. Food and Drug Administration. This list includes the names of the substances, designated uses, and the names and addresses of sponsors. The information is inclusive for all orphan drug/biological designations made since the inception of the program. Some of these products have since been fully approved by the Food and Drug Administration and are currently being marketed. Others remain under investigation or are no longer being actively studied. The current status of each orphan drug/biological, where known, is included in the listing.

It should be noted that the names used in this listing for products that have not been approved for marketing may not be the established names approved by FDA for these products if they are eventually approved for marketing. Since these products are investigational, some may not have been reviewed for purposes of assigning the most appropriate name.

*The USP-Practitioners' Reporting Network* (Appendix IX)—To assist health care professionals in their responsibility to report reactions to or problems with medications, the appropriate reporting forms are reproduced in this appendix.

**Volume II**—As in Volume I, *The Medicine Chart* is included in Volume II in the front of the book. Also included are sections on General Information about Use of Medicines, Avoiding Medicine Mishaps, Getting the Most Out of Your Medicines, and About the Medicines You Are Taking.

In addition, Volume II includes:

*Additional Products and Uses* (Appendix I)—Newly marketed and other products not included in the main text of *USP DI* are referenced in this appendix in order to provide as much useful information as possible. The information included has not gone through the *USP DI* review process and is based simply on the product's package insert.

*Poison Control Center Listing* (Appendix II)—Includes a listing of certified regional U.S. poison control centers.

*USP People* (Appendix III)—This appendix lists USP Officers, Board of Trustees, Committees, Panels, and Members.

*Pictograms* (Appendix IV)—Visual images, or pictograms, which represent selected commonly used patients' directions are included in this appendix. The pictograms are intended to be used in a fashion that will reinforce other printed or oral instructions and as a reminder to patients as to the proper way to take or store their medication. They should not be used as the sole means of transferring information to the patient because of the potential for misinterpretation.

Although pictograms are copyrighted by the USPC, the USP has no objection to their use in accordance with the conditions described herein, provided the pictogram is accompanied by the indication of USP copyright ownership. USP assumes no responsibility for any misinterpretation or adverse results or effects resulting from the uses to which they may be put.

*Categories of Use* (Appendix V)—A listing of drugs by their category of use is included in this appendix only as a useful reference. It should not be used to make decisions concerning the appropriateness of therapy. In addition, the drugs included under each entry should not be considered interchangeable for any given patient since in many instances the drugs will differ significantly with regard to effectiveness, seriousness of side effects, and other critical considerations.

*Pregnancy Precaution Listing* (Appendix VI)—To assist the user of the *USP DI* database, this appendix provides a list of those *USP DI* monographs that have a specific precaution included as to use during pregnancy. Since the clinical significance of the precaution varies from drug to drug, the individual monograph should be consulted for additional information. The absence of a drug from the list is not meant to imply that the drug is necessarily known to be safe for use in pregnant patients.

*Breast-feeding Precaution Listing* (Appendix VII)—This appendix provides a list of those *USP DI* monographs that have a specific preaution included as to use of a drug while breast-feeding. Since the clinical significance of the precaution varies from drug to drug, the individual monograph should be consulted for additional information. The absence of a drug from the list is not meant to imply that the drug is necessarily known to be safe for use in women who are breast-feeding.

Volume II also includes a glossary of drug and medical terminology to help the consumer better understand the information presented in the *Advice for the Patient* monographs.

# USP PEOPLE 1995–2000

**OFFICERS**
*President:* Jane E. Henney, M.D., Albuquerque, NM
*Treasurer:* John T. Fay, Jr., Ph.D., San Clemente, CA
*Past President:* Mark Novitch, M.D., Washington, DC
*Secretary:* Jerome A. Halperin, Rockville, MD

**BOARD OF TRUSTEES**
Edwin D. Bransome, Jr., M.D., *Trustee, Medical Sciences*, Augusta, GA
William H. Campbell, Ph.D., *Trustee, Pharmaceutical Sciences*, Chapel Hill, NC
Jordan L. Cohen, Ph.D., *Trustee, Pharmaceutical Sciences*, Lexington, KY
Jean Paul Gagnon, Ph.D., *Trustee, At Large*, Kansas City, MO
Edward L. Langston, M.D., R.Ph., *Trustee, Medical Sciences*, Rock Island, IL
Joseph A. Mollica, Ph.D., *Trustee, At Large*, Princeton, NJ
Grace Powers Monaco, J.D., *Trustee, Public*, Burgess, VA
Edward Zalta, M.D., *Trustee, At Large*, Newport Beach, CA

**GENERAL COMMITTEE OF REVISION**
Loyd V. Allen, Jr., Ph.D., Edmond, OK
Thomas J. Ambrosio, Ph.D., Somerville, NJ
Ann B. Amerson, Pharm.D., Lexington, KY
Gordon L. Amidon, Ph.D., Ann Arbor, MI
Gregory E. Amidon, Ph.D., Kalamazoo, MI
Larry Augsburger, Ph.D., Baltimore, MD
Henry L. Avallone, Titusville, NJ
Leonard C. Bailey, Ph.D., Piscataway, NJ
Jorge R. Barrio, Ph.D., Los Angeles, CA
Gregory B. Bennett, Ph.D., Suffern, NY
Terrence F. Blaschke, M.D., Stanford, CA
Judy P. Boehlert, Ph.D., Park Ridge, NJ
James C. Boylan, Ph.D., Abbott Park, IL
R. Edward Branson, Ph.D., Brookville, MD
William H. Briner, Durham, NC
Harry G. Brittain, Ph.D., Maplewood, NJ
Paul M. Bummer, Ph.D., Lexington, KY
Stephen R. Byrn, Ph.D., West Lafayette, IN
Peter R. Byron, Ph.D., Richmond, VA
Ronald J. Callahan, Ph.D., Boston, MA
Herbert S. Carlin, D.Sc., Califon, NJ
Culley C. Carson III, M.D., Chapel Hill, NC
Lester Chafetz, Ph.D., Kansas City, MO
Yie W. Chien, Ph.D., Piscataway, NJ
Henry M. Chilton, Pharm.D., Winston-Salem, NC
Zak T. Chowhan, Ph.D., Hunt Valley, MD
Sebastian G. Ciancio, D.D.S., Buffalo, NY
Patricia E. Cole, Ph.D., M.D., Smithtown, NY
David S. Cooper, M.D., Baltimore, MD
Murray S. Cooper, Ph.D., Islamorada, FL
William A. Craig, M.D., Madison, WI
Stephanie Y. Crawford, Ph.D., Chicago, IL
Edward M. Croom, Jr., Ph.D., University, MS
Ian E. Davidson, Ph.D., M.B.A., Kansas City, MO
Leon Ellenbogen, Ph.D., Madison, NJ
Edward A. Fitzgerald, Ph.D., Rockville, MD
Everett Flanigan, Ph.D., Bradley, IL
Thomas S. Foster, Pharm.D., Lexington, KY
C. David Fox, Ph.D., Rouses Point, NY
Sylvan G. Frank, Ph.D., Columbus, OH
David O. Freedman, M.D., Birmingham, AL
Joseph F. Gallelli, Ph.D., Bethesda, MD
Barry D. Garfinkle, Ph.D., West Point, PA
Robert L. Garnick, Ph.D., South San Francisco, CA
John Christian Gillin, M.D., San Diego, CA
Douglas D. Glover, M.D., R.Ph., Morgantown, WV
Alan M. Goldberg, Ph.D., Baltimore, MD
Dennis K.J. Gorecki, Ph.D., Saskatoon, SK
Robert M. Guthrie, M.D., Columbus, OH
Samir A. Hanna, Ph.D., Lawrenceville, NJ
Stanley L. Hem, Ph.D., West Lafayette, IN

Evelyn V. Hess, M.D., M.A.C.P., M.A.C.R., Cincinnati, OH
Joy Hochstadt, Ph.D., New York, NY
Richard D. Johnson, Ph.D., Pharm D., Kansas City, MO
H. Thomas Karnes, Ph.D., Richmond, VA
David B. Katague, Ph.D., Rockville, MD
Rosalyn C. King, Pharm.D., M.P.H., Silver Spring, MD
Gordon L. Klein, M.D., M.P.H., Galveston, TX
Harvey G. Klein, M.D., Bethesda, MD
Joseph E. Knapp, Ph.D., Pittsburgh, PA
Michael S. Korczynski, Ph.D., Baltimore, MD
Helen F. Krause, M.D., Pittsburgh, PA
Paul Kucera, Ph.D., Warwick, NY
Pauline M. Lacroix, Nepean, ON
V. Cory Langston, D.V.M., Ph.D. Diplomate ACVCP, Mississippi State, MS
Thomas P. Layloff, Ph.D., St. Louis, MO
Patricia D. Leinbach, Ph.D., Rockville, MD
John W. Levchuk, Ph.D., Rockville, MD
Robert D. Lindeman, M.D., Albuquerque, NM
Charles H. Lochmüller, Ph.D., Durham, NC
Hugh E. Lockhart, Ph.D., East Lansing, MI
Edward G. Lovering, Ph.D., Nepean, ON
Catherine M. MacLeod, M.D., Waukegan, IL
Carol S. Marcus, Ph.D., M.D., Torrance, CA
Joan C. May, Ph.D., Rockville, MD
Michael Mayersohn, Ph.D., Tucson, AZ
Keith M. McErlane, Ph.D., Vancouver, BC
Thomas Medwick, Ph.D., Piscataway, NJ
Robert F. Morrissey, Ph.D., New Brunswick, NJ
Terry E. Munson, Fairfax, VA
Steven L. Nail, Ph.D., West Lafayette, IN
Harold S. Nelson, M.D., Denver, CO
David W. Newton, Ph.D., Winchester, VA
Sharon J. Northup, Ph.D., M.B.A., Deerfield, IL
Samuel W. Page, Ph.D., Washington, DC
Garnet E. Peck, Ph.D., West Lafayette, IN
Robert V. Petersen, Ph.D., Salt Lake City, UT
Rosemary C. Polomano, Ph.D., M.S.N., R.N., Pottstown, PA
Ronald E. Reid, Ph.D., Vancouver, BC
Thomas P. Reinders, Pharm.D., Richmond, VA
Christopher T. Rhodes, Ph.D., West Kingston, RI
Jim E. Riviere, D.V.M., Ph.D., Raleigh, NC
George A. Robertson, Ph.D., Frederick, MD
Joseph R. Robinson, Ph.D., Madison, WI
Lary A. Robinson, M.D., Tampa, FL
Harold N. Rode, Ph.D., Ottawa, ON
Dan M. Roden, M.D., Nashville, TN
David B. Roll, Ph.D., Salt Lake City, UT
Thomas W. Rosanske, Ph.D., Kansas City, MO
Theodore J. Roseman, Ph.D., Lincolnshire, IL
Peter C. Ruenitz, Ph.D., Athens, GA
Gordon D. Schiff, M.D., Chicago, IL
Paul L. Schiff, Jr., Ph.D., Pittsburgh, PA
Sally S. Seaver, Ph.D., Concord, MA
Ralph F. Shangraw, Ph.D., Baltimore, MD
Eli Shefter, Ph.D., La Jolla, CA
Eric B. Sheinin, Ph.D., Rockville, MD
Robert L. Siegle, M.D., San Antonio, TX
Edward B. Silberstein, M.D., Cincinnati, OH
Marilyn Dix Smith, Ph.D., Voorhess, NJ
E. John Staba, Ph.D., Minneapolis, MN
Thomas E. Starzl, M.D., Ph.D., Pittsburgh, PA
Robert S. Stern, M.D., Boston, MA
James T. Stewart, Ph.D., Athens, GA
Scott V.W. Sutton, Ph.D., Fort Worth, TX
Dennis P. Swanson, M.S., Pittsburgh, PA
Henry S.I. Tan, Ph.D., Cincinnati, OH
Thomas D. Thomson, Ph.D., V.M.D., Greenfield, IN
Clarence T. Ueda, Pharm D., Ph.D., Omaha, NE
Huib J.M. van de Donk, Ph.D., Bilthoven, The Netherlands
Stanley van den Noort, M.D., Irvine, CA
Joseph C. Veltri, Pharm.D., Salt Lake City, UT

xv

Robert E. Vestal, M.D., Boise, ID
Irving W. Wainer, Ph.D., Washington, D.C.
Philip D. Walson, M.D., Columbus, OH
Elliott T. Weisman, Philadelphia, PA
Paul F. White, Ph.D., M.D., Dallas, TX
Richard J. Whitley, M.D., Birmingham, AL
Robert J. Wolfangel, Ph.D., St. Louis, MO
Manfred E. Wolff, Ph.D., Laguna Beach, CA
Marie Linda A. Workman, Ph.D., R.N., Bay Village, OH
Wesley E. Workman, Ph.D., St. Charles, MO
Timothy J. Wozniak, Ph.D., Indianapolis, IN
Dale Eric Wurster, Ph.D., Iowa City, IA
John W. Yarbro, M.D., Columbia, MO
Lynn C. Yeoman, Ph.D., Houston, TX
Thom J. Zimmerman, M.D., Ph.D., Louisville, KY

### EXECUTIVE COMMITTEE OF REVISION
Jerome A. Halperin, *Chair*
Lester Chafetz, Ph.D.
Joseph F. Gallelli, Ph.D.
Gordon L. Klein, M.D., M.P.H.
Robert D. Lindeman, M.D.
Carol S. Marcus, Ph.D., M.D.
Joseph R. Robinson, Ph.D.

### DIVISION OF INFORMATION DEVELOPMENT EXECUTIVE COMMITTEE
Robert E. Vestal, M.D., *Chair*
Ann B. Amerson, Pharm.D.
James C. Boylan, Ph.D.
Herbert S. Carlin, D. Sc.
Culley C. Carson III, M.D.
Sebastian G. Ciancio, D.D.S.
Evelyn V. Hess, M.D., F.A.C.P., M.A.C.R.
V. Cory Langston, D.V.M., Ph.D. Diplomate ACVCP
Catherine M. MacLeod, M.D.
Rosemary C. Polomano, Ph.D., M.S.N., R.N.
Thomas P. Reinders, Pharm.D.
Dan M. Roden, M.D.
Gordon D. Schiff, M.D.
Robert S. Stern, M.D.
Joseph C. Veltri, Pharm.D.

### DIVISION OF STANDARDS DEVELOPMENT EXECUTIVE COMMITTEE
Thomas P. Layloff, Ph.D., *Chair*
Gregory E. Amidon, Ph.D.
Judy P. Boehlert, Ph.D.
James C. Boylan, Ph.D.
William H. Briner
Herbert S. Carlin, D.Sc.
Zak T. Chowhan, Ph.D.
Everett Flanigan, Ph.D.
Thomas S. Foster, Pharm.D.
Robert L. Garnick, Ph.D.
Dennis K.J. Gorecki, Ph.D.
Stanley L. Hem, Ph.D.
Joseph E. Knapp, Ph.D.
Paul Kucera, Ph.D.
Edward G. Lovering, Ph.D.
Thomas Medwick, Ph.D.
Sharon J. Northup, Ph.D., M.B.A.
Ralph F. Shangraw, Ph.D.
James T. Stewart, Ph.D.
Henry S.I. Tan, Ph.D.
Elliott T. Weisman

### DRUG NOMENCLATURE COMMITTEE
Herbert S. Carlin, D.Sc., *Chair*
Ann B. Amerson, Pharm.D.
Lester Chafetz, Ph.D.
Stephanie Y. Crawford, Ph.D.
Everett Flanigan, Ph.D.
Douglas D. Glover, M.D., R.Ph.
Richard D. Johnson, Ph.D., Pharm D.
Edward G. Lovering, Ph.D.
Rosemary C. Polomano, Ph.D., M.S.N., R.N.
Thomas P. Reinders, Pharm.D.
Eric B. Sheinin, Ph.D.
Thomas D. Thomson, Ph.D., V.M.D.
Philip D. Walson, M.D.

# DIVISION OF INFORMATION DEVELOPMENT ADVISORY PANELS

Members who serve as Chairs are listed first.

The information presented in this text represents an ongoing review of the drugs contained herein and represents a consensus of various viewpoints expressed. The individuals listed below have served on the USP Advisory Panels for the 1997–1998 revision period and have contributed to the development of the 1999 USP DI database. Such listing does not imply that these individuals have reviewed all of the material in this text or that they individually agree with all statements contained herein.

### Anesthesiology
Paul F. White, Ph.D., M.D., *Chair*, Dallas, TX; Charles J. Coté, M.D., Chicago, IL; Peter S.A. Glass, M.D., Durham, NC; Michele E. Gold, Ph.D., C.R.N.A., Beverly Hills, CA; Frederick J. Goldstein, Ph.D., Philadelphia, PA; Thomas K. Henthorn, M.D., Denver CO; Michael B. Howie, M.D., Columbus, OH; Robert J. Hudson, M.D., Winnipeg, Canada; Scott D. Kelley, M.D., San Francisco, CA; Susan K. Palmer, M.D., Aurora, CO; Carl E. Rosow, M.D., Ph.D., Boston, MA; Mark A. Schumacher, Ph.D., M.D., San Francisco, CA; Peter S. Sebel, Ph.D., Atlanta, GA; Mehernoor F. Watcha, M.D., Philadelphia, PA; Matthew B. Weinger, M.D., San Diego, CA; Richard B. Weiskopf, M.D., San Francisco, CA; David H. Wong, Pharm.D., M.D., Long Beach, CA

### Blood and Blood Products
Harvey G. Klein, M.D., *Chair*, Bethesda, MD; James P. AuBuchon, M.D., Lebanon, NH; Morris A. Blajchman, M.D., Hamilton, Ontario, Canada; Marcela Contreras, M.D., London, England; Alfred J. Grindon, M.D., Atlanta, GA; Douglas A. Kennedy, Ph.D., Ottawa, Ontario, Canada; Craig M. Kessler, M.D., Washington, DC; Jukka Koistinen, M.D., Ph.D., Helsinki, Finland; Volker Kretschmer, M.D., Ph.D., Marburg, Germany; Margot S. Kruskall, M.D., Boston, MA; Naomi L.C. Luban, M.D., Washington, DC; Jay E. Menitove, M.D., Kansas City, MO; Paul M. Ness, M.D., Baltimore, MD; Henk W. Reesink, M.D., Ph.D., Amsterdam, The Netherlands; William T. Sawyer, M.S., Chapel Hill, NC; Karen A. Skalla, RN, MSN, AOCN, Brownsville, VT; Ronald G. Strauss, M.D., Iowa City, IA

### Cardiovascular and Renal Drugs
Dan M. Roden, M.D., *Chair*, Nashville, TN; Jonathan Abrams, M.D., Albuquerque, NM; Joseph S. Alpert, M.D., Tucson, AZ; Jerry L. Bauman, Pharm.D., Chicago, IL; Ellen D. Burgess, M.D., Calgary, Alberta, Canada; James H. Chesebro, M.D., New York, NY; Moses Chow, Pharm.D., Hartford, CT; Joseph Cinanni, M.D., Ottawa, Ontario, Canada; Peter B. Corr, Ph.D., St. Louis, MO; David J. Driscoll, M.D., Rochester, MN; Dwain L. Eckberg, M.D., Richmond, VA; Andrew E. Epstein, M.D., Birmingham, AL; Arthur M. Feldman, M.D., Ph.D., Pittsburgh, PA; Michael P. Frenneaux, M.D., Wales, England; William H. Frishman, M.D., Valhalla, NY; Edward D. Frohlich, M.D., New Orleans, LA; Donald B. Hunninghake, M.D., Minneapolis, MN;

Joseph L. Izzo, Jr., M.D., Buffalo, NY; Norman M. Kaplan, M.D., Dallas, TX; Peter R. Kowey, M.D., Wynnewood, PA; Joseph Loscalzo, M.D., Ph.D., Boston, MA; Patrick A. McKee, M.D., Oklahoma City, OK; Juan Carlos Prieto, M.D., Santiago, Chile; Jane F. Schultz, R.N., M.S.N., Hayfield, MN; Alexander M.M. Shepherd, M.D., Ph.D., San Antonio, TX; Burton E. Sobel, M.D., Burlington, VT; Raymond L. Woosley, M.D., Ph.D., Washington, DC

**Children and Medicines (Ad Hoc)**
Janice M. Ozias, Ph.D., *Chair*, Austin, TX; Anna Birna Almarsdottir, Ph.D., Copenhagen, Denmark; Pilar Aramburuzabala, Ph.D., Segovia, Spain; Roger Bibace, Ph.D., Worcester, MA; Judith Igoe, RN, MS, FAAN, Denver, CO; Renée R. Jenkins, M.D., Washington, DC; Margo Kroshus, R.N., Rochester, MN; Colleen Lum Lung, R.N., MSN, CPNP, Littletown, CO; Carolyn H. Lund, R.N., San Francisco, CA; Robert O'Brien, Ph.D., Chevy Chase, MD; Robert H. Pantell, M.D., San Francisco, CA; Susan Schneider, M.P.H., Bethesda, MD; Bernard A. Sorofman, Ph.D., Iowa City, IA; Wayne A. Yankus, M.D., Midland Park, NJ

**Clinical Toxicology/Substance Abuse**
Joseph C. Veltri, Pharm.D., *Chair*, Salt Lake City, UT; Neal L. Benowitz, M.D., San Francisco, CA; Usoa E. Busto, Pharm.D., Toronto, Ontario, Canada; Timothy R. Dring, Woodbridge, NJ; David J. George, Ph.D., Madison, NJ; Edward P. Krenzelok, Pharm.D., Pittsburgh, PA; David C. Lewis, M.D., Providence, RI; Michael Montagne, Ph.D., Boston, MA; Claudio A. Naranjo, M.D., North York, Ontario, Canada; Edward J. Otten, M.D., Cincinnati, OH; Paul Pentel, M.D., Minneapolis, MN; Lorie G. Rice, San Francisco, CA; Elizabeth J. Scharman, Pharm.D., Charleston, WV; Michael W. Shannon, M.D., Boston, MA; Rose Ann G. Soloway, RN, MSEd, ABAT, Washington, DC; Anthony C. Tommasello, M.S., Baltimore, MD; Theodore G. Tong, Pharm.D., Tucson, AZ; Alison M. Trinkoff, ScD, RN, Baltimore, MD; William A. Watson, Pharm.D., San Antonio, TX; Julian White, M.D., North Adelaide, Australia

**Consumer Interest/Health Education**
Gordon D. Schiff, M.D., *Chair*, Chicago, IL; Michael J. Ackerman, Ph.D., Bethesda, MD; Frank J. Ascione, Pharm.D., Ph.D., Ann Arbor, MI; Roger Bibace, Ph.D., Worcester, MA; Allan H. Bruckheim, M.D., Harrison, NY; Mary E. Carman, Ottawa, Ontario, Canada; Margaret A. Charters, Ph.D., Syracuse, NY; Laura J. Cranston, Fairfax Station, VA; Jennifer Cross, San Francisco, CA; David A. Danielson, Roslindale, MA; Sandra M. Fabregas, R.Ph., San Juan, PR; Sophia Jones-Redmond, Chicago, IL; Louis H. Kompare, Franklin, TN; Margo Kroshus, R.N., Rochester, MN; Bruce L. Lambert, Ph.D., Chicago, IL; Arthur Levin, M.P.H., New York, NY; Roberto Lopez Linares, Lima, Peru; Janet M. Manuel, Halifax, Nova Scotia, Canada; Frederick S. Mayer, R.Ph., M.P.H., San Rafael, CA; Jacqueline D. McLeod, M.P.H., New York, NY; Charles Medawar, London, England; Nancy Milio, Ph.D., Chapel Hill, NC; Michael A. Moné, Frankfort, KY; Janet Ohene-Frempong, Philadelphia, PA; James C. Wohlleb, Little Rock, AR

**Critical Care Medicine**
Catherine M. MacLeod, M.D., *Chair*, Glen Elly, IL; Robert A. Balk, M.D., Chicago, IL; Philip S. Barie, M.D., New York, NY; Thomas P. Bleck, M.D., Charlottesville, VA; Eugene Y. Cheng, M.D., Milwaukee, WI; Susan S. Fish, Pharm.D., M.P.H., Boston, MA; Edgar R. Gonzalez, Pharm.D., Richmond, VA; Angela M. Hadbavny, Pharm.D., Pittsburgh, PA; John W. Hoyt, M.D., Pittsburgh, PA; Louis J. Ling, M.D., Minneapolis, MN; Sheldon A. Magder, M.D., Montreal, Quebec, Canada; Daniel A. Notterman, M.D., Princeton, NJ; Sharon D. Peters, M.D., St. John's, Newfoundland; Domenic A. Sica, M.D., Richmond, VA; George A. Skowronski, New South Wales, Australia

**Dentistry**
Sebastian G. Ciancio, D.D.S., *Chair*, Buffalo, NY; B. Ellen Byrne, D.D.S., Ph.D., Richmond, VA; Barbara R. Clark, Pharm.D., Kansas City, MO; Frederick Curro, D.M.D., Ph.D., Jersey City, NJ; Tommy W. Gage, D.D.S., Ph.D., Dallas, TX; Daniel A. Haas, D.D.S., Ph.D., Toronto, Ontario, Canada; Richard E. Hall, D.D.S., Ph.D., Buffalo, NY; John T. Hamilton, Ph.D., London, Ontario, Canada; Angelo J. Mariotti, D.D.S., Ph.D., Columbus, OH; Linda C. Niessen, D.M.D., Dallas, TX; Clarence L. Trummel, D.D.S., Farmington, CT; Joel M. Weaver II, D.D.S., Ph.D., Columbus, OH; Clifford W. Whall, Jr., Ph.D., Chicago, IL; Raymond P. White, Jr., D.D.S., Ph.D., Chapel Hill, NC; Richard L. Wynn, Ph.D., Baltimore, MD; John A. Yagiela, D.D.S., Ph.D., Los Angeles, CA

**Dermatology**
Robert S. Stern, M.D., *Chair*, Boston, MA; Beatrice B. Abrams, Ph.D., East Hanover, NJ; Richard D. Baughman, M.D., Lebanon, NH; Mary-Margaret Chren, M.D., San Francisco, CA; Diane M. Cooper, Ph.D., R.N., Bay Pines, FL; Ponciano D. Cruz, M.D., Dallas, TX; Vincent Falanga, M.D., Miami, FL; James J. Ferry, Ph.D., Kalamazoo, MI; Vincent C. Ho, M.D., Vancouver, British Columbia, Canada; Donald P. Lookingbill, M.D., Jacksonville, FL; Stuart Maddin, M.D., Vancouver, British Columbia, Canada; Milton Orkin, M.D., Minneapolis, MN; Amy S. Paller, M.D., Chicago, IL; Jean-Claude Roujeau, M.D., Creteil Cedex, France; Neil H. Shear, M.D., Toronto, Ontario, Canada; Celia A. Viets, M.D., Ottawa, Ontario, Canada; Dennis P. West, Ph.D., Chicago, IL

**Diagnostic Agents—Nonradioactive**
Robert L. Siegle, M.D., *Chair*, San Antonio, TX; Leonard M. Baum, R.Ph., Princeton, NJ; Martin J. K. Blomley, M.B., London, England; Robert C. Brasch, M.D., San Francisco, CA; Olivier Clement, M.D., Ph.D., Paris, France; Sachiko T. Cochran, M.D., Los Angeles, CA; Kathryn L. Grant, Pharm.D., Tucson, AZ; Kenneth D. Hopper, M.D., Hershey, PA; Fred T. Lee, Jr., M.D., Madison, WI; Robert F. Mattrey, M.D., San Diego, CA; James A. Nelson, M.D., Seattle, WA; Jovitas Skucas, M.D., Rochester, NY; Gerald L. Wolf, Ph.D., M.D., Charlestown, MA

**Drug Utilization Review**
Terrence F. Blaschke, M.D., *Chair*, Stanford, CA; David M. Angaran, R.Ph., Powell, OH; Edward P. Armstrong, Pharm.D., Tucson, AZ; Jim L. Blackburn, Pharm.D., Saskatoon, Saskatchewan, Canada; Catherine E. Burley, M.D., Fayetteville, GA; Patricia J. Byrns, M.D., Chicago, IL; Elizabeth A. Chrischilles, Ph.D., Iowa City, IA; Theodore M. Collins, R.Ph., Madison, WI; Robert P. Craig, Pharm.D., Scottsdale, AZ; W. Gary Erwin, Pharm.D., Radnor, PA; Stan N. Finklestein, M.D., Cambridge, MA; Catherine A. Harrington, Pharm.D., Ph.D., Fairfax, VA; Mark L. Horn, M.D., New York, NY; Judith K. Jones, M.D., Ph.D., Arlington, VA; Michael L. Kelly, R.Ph., Jackson, MS; Duane M. Kirking, Pharm.D., Ph.D., Ann Arbor, MI; Ann M. Koeniguer, R.Ph., Summerfield, NC; David Lee, M.D., Arlington, VA; Gary M. Levine, R.Ph., St. Louis, MO; Gladys Peachey, RN, MEd, MHSc, Dundas, Ontario, Canada; Eleanor M. Perfetto, Ph.D., Bethesda, MD; T. Donald Rucker, Ph.D., River Forest, IL; Daniel W. Saylak, D.O., Bryan, TX; Fredrica E. Smith, M.D., Los Alamos, NM; Brian L. Strom, M.D., M.P.H., Philadelphia, PA; Ilene H. Zuckerman, Pharm.D., Baltimore, MD

**Endocrinology**
David S. Cooper, M.D., *Chair*, Baltimore, MD; Robert L. Barbieri, M.D., Wellesley, MA; Stuart J. Brink, M.D., Waltham, MA; R. Keith Campbell, Pharm.D., Pullman, WA; Ernesto Canalis, M.D., Hartford, CT; Betty J. Dong, Pharm.D., San Francisco, CA; Shereen Ezzat, M.D., Toronto, Ontario, Canada; Lawrence A. Frohman, M.D., Chicago, IL; Steven R. Goldring, M.D., Boston, MA; Jerome M. Hershman, M.D., Los Angeles, CA; Robert G. Josse, M.B., Toronto, Ontario, Canada; Michael M. Kaplan, M.D., West Bloomfield, MI; Selna Kaplan, M.D., Ph.D., San Francisco, CA; Marvin E. Levin, M.D., Chesterfield, MO; Marvin M. Lipman, M.D., Scarsdale, NY; Daniel J. Marante, M.D., Miami, FL; Barbara J. Maschak-Carey, RN, Philadelphia, PA; Shlomo Melmed, M.D., Los Angeles, CA; Ronald P. Monsaert, M.D., Danville, PA; John E. Morley, M.B., B.Ch., St. Louis, MO; Paul Saenger, M.D., Bronx, NY; Mary Lee Vance, M.D., Charlottesville, VA; Leonard Wartofsky, M.D., Washington, DC

**Family Practice**
Robert M. Guthrie, M.D., *Chair*, Columbus, OH; John A. Brose, D.O., Athens, OH; Mark E. Clasen, M.D., Ph.D., Dayton, OH; Yves Gariepy, Ste-Foy, Quebec, Canada; Sloan Karver, M.D., Wyomissing, PA; Joseph A. Lieberman III, M.D., Wilmington, DE; Charles D. Ponte, Pharm.D., Morgantown, WV; John W. Robinson, M.D., Salt Lake City, UT; Jack M. Rosenberg, Pharm.D., Ph.D., Hillsdale, NJ; Jorge E. Sanchez, M.D., San Salvador, El Salvador; John E. Thornburg, D.O., Ph.D., East Lansing, MI; Richard A. Wherry, M.D., Dahlonega, GA; Theodore L. Yarboro, Sr., M.D., M.P.H., Sharon, PA

**Gastroenterology**
Gordon L. Klein, M.D., *Chair*, Galveston, TX; Karl E. Anderson, M.D., Galveston, TX; Paul Bass, Ph.D., Madison, WI; Adrian M. Di Bisceglie, M.D., St. Louis, MO; Jack A. DiPalma, M.D., Mobile, AL; Thomas Q. Garvey III, M.D., Potomac, MD; Flavio Habal, M.D., Ph.D., Toronto, Ontario, Canada; Eric G. Hassall, M.D., Vancouver,

British Columbia, Canada; Alan F. Hofmann, M.D., La Jolla, CA; Paul E. Hyman, M.D., Orange, CA; Agnes V. Klein, M.D., Ottawa, Ontario, Canada; James H. Lewis, M.D., Washington, DC; Bernard Mehl, D.P.S., New York, NY; Joel E. Richter, M.D., Cleveland, OH; William J. Snape, Jr., M.D., Long Beach, CA; C. Noel Williams, M.D., Halifax, Nova Scotia, Canada; Hyman J. Zimmerman, M.D., Bethesda, MD

**Geriatrics**
Robert E. Vestal, M.D., *Chair*, Boise, ID; Darrell R. Abernethy, M.D., Washington, DC; Mark H. Beers, M.D., West Point, PA; Robert A. Blouin, Pharm.D., Lexington, KY; S. George Carruthers, M.D., London, Ontario, Canada; Martin J. Connolly, M.D., Cheshire, England; Madeline Feinberg, Pharm.D., Silver Spring, MD; Jerry H. Gurwitz, M.D., Worcester, MA; Geri R. Hall, Ph.D., ARNP, CS, Fountain Hills, AZ; Martin D. Higbee, Pharm.D., Tucson, AZ; Brian B. Hoffman, M.D., Palo Alto, CA; Barbara A. Liu, M.D., North York, Canada, Ontario; Ann Miller, Morro Bay, CA; Paul A. Mitenko, M.D., Nanaimo, British Columbia, Canada; Janice B. Schwartz, M.D., Chicago, IL; Joanne G. Schwartzberg, M.D., Chicago, IL; William Simonson, Pharm.D., Portsmouth, VA; Daniel S. Sitar, Ph.D., Winnipeg, Manitoba, Canada; Alastair J.J. Wood, M.D., Nashville, TN; Carla Zeilmann, Pharm.D., St. Louis, MO

**Hematologic and Oncologic Disease**
John W. Yarbro, M.D., Ph.D., *Chair*, Columbia, MO; Joseph S. Bailes, M.D., Dallas, TX; Laurence H. Baker, D.O., Ann Arbor, MI; Edward Braud, M.D., Springfield, IL; Donald C. Doll, M.D., Columbia, MO; Ross C. Donehower, M.D., Baltimore, MD; Jan M. Ellerhorst-Ryan, R.N., Cincinnati, OH; Martha Harczy, M.D., Ottawa, Ontario, Canada; David T. Harris, M.D., Wynnewood, PA; Connie Henke Yarbro, R.N., Columbia, MO; Charles Hoppel, M.D., Cleveland, OH; B. J. Kennedy, M.D., Minneapolis, MN; Barnett S. Kramer, M.D., M.P.H., Bethesda, MD; Celeste Lindley, Pharm.D., Chapel Hill, NC; Michael J. Mastrangelo, M.D., Philadelphia, PA; Paulette Mehta, M.D., Gainesville, FL; Perry D. Nisen, M.D., Ph.D., Abbott Park, IL; David S. Rosenthal, M.D., Cambridge, MA; Roy L. Silverstein, M.D., New York, NY; Samuel G. Taylor, M.D., Chicago, IL; Raymond B. Weiss, M.D., Rockville, MD

**Infectious Disease Therapy**
William A. Craig, M.D., *Chair*, Madison, WI; P. Joan Chesney, M.D., Memphis, TN; C. Glenn Cobbs, M.D., Birmingham, AL; Courtney V. Fletcher, Pharm.D., Minneapolis, MN; Frederick G. Hayden, M.D., Charlottesville, VA; Carol A. Kauffman, M.D., Ann Arbor, MI; Marc LeBel, Pharm.D., Ste-Foy, Quebec, Canada; S. Ragnar Norrby, M.D., Ph.D., Lund, Sweden; Laszlo Palkonyay, M.D., Ottawa, Ontario, Canada; Douglas D. Richman, M.D., La Jolla, CA; Xavier Saez-Llorens, M.D., Miami, FL; Roy T. Steigbigel, M.D., Stony Brook, NY; Richard J. Whitley, M.D., Birmingham, AL

**International Health**
Rosalyn C. King, Pharm.D., M.P.H., *Chair*, Silver Spring, MD; Eugenie Brown, Pharm.D., Kingston, Jamaica; Laura Ceron, Pharm.D., Lima, Peru; Albin Chaves Matamoros, M.D., San Jose, Costa Rica; Gabriel Daniel, Washington, DC; Enrique Fefer, Ph.D., Rockville, MD; Peter H.M. Fontilus, Curacao, Netherlands Antilles; Reginald F. Gipson, M.D., M.P.H., Cairo, Egypt; Mariatou Tala Jallow, Pharm.D., Banjul, The Gambia; Mohan P. Joshi, M.D., Kathmandu, Nepal; David E. Kuhl, Pharm.D., Albuquerque, NM; Richard O. Laing, M.D., Boston, MA; Thomas Lapnet-Moustapha, Pharm.D., Yaounde, Cameroon; Denise Leclerc, Ph.D., Montreal, Quebec, Canada; Aissatou Lo, Dakar, Senegal; David Ofori-Adjei, M.D., Accra, Ghana; Dr. S. Ofosu-Amaah, Accra, Ghana; James Rankin, Arlington, VA; Dennis Ross-Degnan, Boston, MA; Budiono Santoso, M.D., Ph.D., Yogyakarta, Indonesia; Fela Viso Gurovich, Ph.D., Mexico City, Mexico; Krisantha Weerasuriya, M.D., Colombo, Sri Lanka; Albert I. Wertheimer, Ph.D., West Point, PA

**Medication Counseling Behavior Guidelines (Ad Hoc)**
Frank J. Ascione, Pharm.D., Ph.D., *Chair*, Ann Arbor, MI; John E. Arradondo, M.D., Nashville, TN; Candace Barnett, Atlanta, GA; Allan H. Bruckheim, M.D., Harrison, NY; Mark E. Clasen, M.D., Ph.D., Dayton, OH; Frederick Curro, D.M.D., Ph.D., Jersey City, NJ; Robin DiMatteo, Ph.D., Riverside, CA; Diane B. Ginsburg, Austin, TX; Denise Grimes, Jackson, MI; Richard Herrier, Tucson, AZ; Barry Kass, R.Ph., Boston, MA; Thomas Kellenberger, Pharm.D., Montvale, NJ; Alice Kimball, Darnestown, MD; Patricia A. Kramer, B.Sc., Bismarck, ND; Patricia Kummeth, Rochester, MN; Ken Leibowitz, Philadelphia,
PA; Colleen Lum Lung, R.N., MSN, CPNP, Littletown, CO; Louise Matte, B.Sc., B.Pharm., Montreal, Quebec, Canada; Amy Outlaw, Pharm.D., Stone Mountain, GA; Constance Pavlides, R.N., Rockville, MD; Scotti Russell, Richmond, VA; Lisa Tedesco, Ph.D., Ann Arbor, MI

**Neurology**
Stanley van den Noort, M.D., *Chair*, Irvine, CA; A. Leland Albright, M.D., Pittsburgh, PA; Elizabeth U. Blalock, M.D., Anaheim, CA; Mitchell F. Brin, M.D., New York, NY; Louis R. Caplan, M.D., Boston, MA; James C. Cloyd, Pharm.D., Minneapolis, MN; Mark J. Fisher, M.D., Los Angeles, CA; Kathleen M. Foley, M.D., New York, NY; Robert A. Gross, M.D., Ph.D., Rochester, NY; Stanley Hashimoto, M.D., Vancouver, British Columbia, Canada; William C. Koller, M.D., Ph.D., Kansas City, KS; Ilo E. Leppik, M.D., Minneapolis, MN; Ira T. Lott, M.D., Orange, CA; T.J. Murray, M.D., Halifax, Nova Scotia, Canada; Judith A. Paice, Ph.D., R.N., Chicago, IL; Richard D. Penn, M.D., Chicago, IL; Roger J. Porter, M.D., Philadelphia, PA; Neil H. Raskin, M.D., San Francisco, CA; James F. Toole, M.D., Winston-Salem, NC; Howard L. Weiner, M.D., Boston, MA

**Nursing Practice**
Rosemary C. Polomano, Ph.D., M.S.N., R.N., *Chair*, Pottstown, PA; Bonnie J. Adamson, R.N., London, Ontario, Canada; Ramona A. Benkert, M.S.N., R.N., Plymouth, MI; Mecca S. Cranley, Ph.D., R.N., Buffalo, NY; Linda Felver, Ph.D., R.N., Portland, OR; Hector Hugo Gonzalez, Ph.D., R.N., San Antonio, TX; Theodore L. Goodfriend, M.D., Madison, WI; Ada K. Jacox, R.N., Ph.D., Detroit, MI; Daisy M. Jones, R.N., Chicago, IL; Patricia Kummeth, Rochester, MN; Ida S. Martinson, Ph.D., R.N., Hung Hom, Hong Kong; Ginette A. Pepper, Ph.D., R.N., Denver, CO; Geraldine A. Peterson, M.A., R.N., Potomac, MD; Linda C. Pugh, Ph.D., R.N., Hershey, PA; Sharon S. Rising, M.S.N., Chesire, CT; April H. Vallerand, Ph.D., R.N., Manalapan, NJ

**Nutrition and Electrolytes**
Robert D. Lindeman, M.D., *Chair*, Albuquerque, NM; Jeffrey P. Baker, M.D., Toronto, Ontario, Canada; Connie W. Bales, Ph.D., R.D., Durham, NC; Dennis M. Bier, M.D., Houston, TX; Gladys Block, Ph.D., Berkeley, CA; Karim Anton Calis, Pharm.D., M.P.H., Rockville, MD; David F. Driscoll, Ph.D., Boston, MA; P.W.F. Fischer, Ph.D., Ottawa, Ontario, Canada; Dr. Nigel Gericke, Sun Valley, South Africa; Walter H. Glinsmann, M.D., Washington, DC; Helen A. Guthrie, Ph.D., State College, PA; John N. Hathcock, Ph.D., Washington, DC; Leslie M. Klevay, M.D., Grand Forks, ND; Linda S. Knox, Ph.D., R.N., Philadelphia, PA; Bonnie Liebman, M.S., Washington, DC; Sohrab Mobarhan, M.D., Maywood, IL; Robert M. Russell, M.D., Boston, MA; Harold H. Sandstead, M.D., Galveston, TX; Benjamin Torun, M.D., Ph.D., Miami, FL; Carlos A. Vaamonde, M.D., Miami, FL; Stanley Wallach, M.D., New York, NY

**Obstetrics and Gynecology**
Douglas D. Glover, M.D., *Chair*, Morgantown, WV; Rudi Ansbacher, M.D., Ann Arbor, MI; James E. Axelson, Ph.D., Aldergrove, British Columbia, Canada; Augusto Bondani, M.D., Ph.D., Mexico City, Mexico; Florence Comite, M.D., New Haven, CT; Marilynn C. Frederiksen, M.D., Chicago, IL; L. Wayne Hess, M.D., Columbia, MO; Art Jacknowitz, Pharm.D., Morgantown, WV; William J. Ledger, M.D., New York, NY; Andre-Marie Leroux, M.D., Ottawa, Ontario, Canada; William A. Nahhas, M.D., Dayton, OH; Warren N. Otterson, M.D., Bulverde, TX; Anne Pastuszak, Ph.D., Toronto, Ontario, Canada; Johanna F. Perlmutter, M.D., M.P.H., Boston, MA; Richard H. Reindollar, M.D., Boston, MA; Ronald J. Ruggiero, Pharm.D., San Francisco, CA; Pamela Shrock, Ph.D., Roslyn Harbor, NY; G. Millard Simmons, Jr., M.D., Morgantown, WV; Phillip G. Stubblefield, M.D., Boston, MA; Raul G. Toledo, M.D., San Salvador, El Salvador

**Ophthalmology**
Thom J. Zimmerman, M.D., *Chair*, Louisville, KY; Steven R. Abel, Pharm.D., Indianapolis, IN; Jules L. Baum, M.D., Wellesley Hills, MA; Lee R. Duffner, M.D., Golden Beach, FL; Forrest Ellis, M.D., Indianapolis, IN; David L. Epstein, M.D., Durham, NC; Robert Fechtner, M.D., Louisville, KY; Allan J. Flach, Pharm.D., M.D., Corte Madera, CA; Frederick T. Fraunfelder, M.D., Portland, OR; Gary N. Holland, M.D., Los Angeles, CA; David A. Lee, M.D., Los Angeles, CA; Vincent H.L. Lee, Ph.D., Los Angeles, CA; Joel S. Mindel, M.D., Ph.D., New York, NY; Steven M. Podos, M.D., New York, NY; Graham E. Trope, M.B., Ph.D., Toronto, Ontario, Canada; Roberto Warman, M.D., Miami, FL; Kirk R. Wilhelmus, M.D., Houston, TX

**Otorhinolaryngology**
Helen F. Krause, M.D., *Chair*, Pittsburgh, PA; Robert E. Brummett, Ph.D., Portland, OR; Linda J. Gardiner, M.D., Fort Myers, FL; Cedric F. Grigg, PhC, DBA, Victor, NY; Julianna Gulya, M.D., Bethesda, MD; James A. Hadley, M.D., Rochester, NY; David B. Hom, M.D., Minneapolis, MN; Donald C. Lanza, M.D., Philadelphia, PA; Richard L. Mabry, M.D., Dallas, TX; Scott C. Manning, M.D., Seattle, WA; Lawrence J. Marentette, M.D., Ann Arbor, MI; Robert A. Mickel, M.D., Ph.D., San Francisco, CA; Arnold M. Noyek, M.D., Toronto, Ontario, Canada; Randal A. Otto, M.D., San Antonio, TX; Leonard P. Rybak, M.D., Ph.D., Springfield, IL; Randal S. Weber, M.D., Philadelphia, PA

**Outcomes and Cost-Effectiveness (Ad Hoc)**
Elizabeth A. Chrischilles, Ph.D., *Co-chair*, Iowa City, IA; Stan N. Finklestein, M.D., *Co-chair*, Cambridge, MA; Jerome L. Avorn, M.D., Boston, MA; Lisa A. Bero, Ph.D., San Francisco, CA; Robert S. Epstein, M.D., Montvale, NJ; Steven F. Finder, M.D., M.B.A., San Antonio, TX; Deborah A. Freund, Ph.D., Bloomington, IN; Gordon H. Guyatt, M.D., Hamilton, Ontario, Canada; Abraham G. Hartzema, Pharm.D., Ph.D., Chapel Hill, NC; Joel W. Hay, Ph.D., Los Angeles, CA; Paul C. Langley, Ph.D., Denver, CO; Kathleen N. Lohr, Ph.D., Research Triangle Park, NC; Nicolaas Otten, Pharm.D., Ottawa, Ontario, Canada; A. David Paltiel, Ph.D., New Haven, CT; Eleanor M. Perfetto, Ph.D., Bethesda, MD; Kevin A. Schulman, M.D., M.B.A., Washington, DC; Kathleen A. Weis, Dr.P.H., NP, Rockville, MD

**Parasitic and Tropical Disease**
David O. Freedman, M.D., *Chair*, Birmingham, AL; Prof. Tomas D. Arias, Ph.D., Panama City, Panama; Michele Barry, M.D., New Haven, CT; Frank J. Bia, M.D., New Haven, CT; P. Das Gupta, M.D., New Delhi, India; Philip R. Fischer, M.D., Salt Lake City, UT; Eduardo Gotuzzo, M.D., Lima, Peru; M. Gail Hill, Ph.D., RN, CRNP, Birmingham, AL; Dennis D. Juranek, M.D., Atlanta, GA; Jay S. Keystone, M.D., Toronto, Ontario, Canada; Dennis E. Kyle, Ph.D., Washington, DC; Sornchai Looareesuwan, M.D., Bangkok, Thailand; Douglas W. MacPherson, M.D., Hamilton, Ontario, Canada; Philippa A. McDonald, M.D., Ottawa, Ontario, Canada; Richard Pearson, M.D., Charlottesville, VA; Peter D. Walzer, M.D., Cincinnati, OH; A. Clinton White, Jr., M.D., Houston, TX

**Pediatric Anesthesiology (Ad Hoc)**
Charles J. Coté, M.D., *Chair*, Chicago, IL; J. Michael Badgwell, M.D., Las Vegas, NV; Barbara W. Brandom, M.D., Pittsburgh, PA; Ryan Cook, M.D., Pittsburgh, PA; John J. Downes, M.D., Philadelphia, PA; Dennis M. Fisher, M.D., San Francisco, CA; John E. Forestner, M.D., Fort Worth, TX; Helen W. Karl, M.D., Seattle, WA; Harry G.G. Kingston, M.D., Portland, OR; Anne Marie Lynn, M.D., Seattle, WA; Robert J. Mamlok, M.D., Lubbock, TX; Mark Shriner, M.D., Philadelphia, PA; Victoria Simpson, M.D., Ph.D., Denver, CO; Mehernoor F. Watcha, M.D., Philadelphia, PA

**Pediatrics**
Philip D. Walson, M.D., *Chair*, Columbus, OH; Cheston M. Berlin, Jr., M.D., Hershey, PA; Nancy Jo Braden, M.D., Phoenix, AZ; George S. Goldstein, M.D., Elmsford, NY; Russell J. Hopp, D.O., Omaha, NE; Ralph E. Kauffman, M.D., Kansas City, MO; Joan M. Korth-Bradley, Pharm.D., Ph.D., Philadelphia, PA; Richard D. Leff, Pharm.D., Shawnee Mission, KS; Carolyn H. Lund, R.N., San Francisco, CA; Maureen C. Maguire, R.N., Baltimore, MD; Mark A. Riddle, M.D., Baltimore, MD; Emilio J. Sanz, M.D., Ph.D., Tenerife, Spain; Wayne Snodgrass, M.D., Galveston, TX; Stephen P. Spielberg, M.D., Ph.D., Raritan, NJ; Jose Teran, M.D., Quito, Ecuador; Robert M. Ward, M.D., Salt Lake City, UT; Sumner J. Yaffe, M.D., Bethesda, MD

**Pharmacy Practice**
Thomas P. Reinders, Pharm.D., *Chair*, Richmond, VA; Hannes Enlund, Ph.D., Kuopio, Finland; Donald J. Filibeck, Pharm.D., Dublin, OH; Ned E. Heltzer, M.S., Philadelphia, PA; Frederick Klein, Montvale, NJ; Calvin H. Knowlton, Ph.D., Lumberton, NJ; Patricia A. Kramer, B.Sc., Bismarck, ND; Diane Lamarre, Saint Lambert, Quebec, Canada; Shirley P. McKee, B.Sc., Houston, TX; Eucharia E. Nnadi-Okolo, Ph.D., Washington, DC; John E. Ogden, M.S., Burke, VA; Henry A. Palmer, Ph.D., Storrs, CT; Roger P. Potyk, Pharm.D., San Antonio, TX; Betsy L. Sleath, Ph.D., Chapel Hill, NC; William E. Smith, Pharm.D., Richmond, VA; Craig S. Stern, Pharm.D., Northridge, CA; Linda S. Tyler, Pharm.D., Salt Lake City, UT; John H. Vandel, R.Ph., Torrington, WY; Joan H. Veal, Rockville, MD; Mary Ann Wagner, Alexandria, VA; Glenn Y. Yokoyama, Pharm.D., Pasadena, CA

**Psychiatric Disease**
John Christian Gillin, M.D., *Chair*, San Diego, CA; Ross J. Baldessarini, M.D., Belmont, MA; R.H. Belmaker, M.D., Beersheva, Israel; Alex A. Cardoni, M.S. Pharm., Hartford, CT; Larry Ereshefsky, Pharm.D., San Antonio, TX; W. Edwin Fann, M.D., Houston, TX; Jan Fawcett, M.D., Chicago, IL; John Feighner, M.D., San Diego, CA; Burton J. Goldstein, M.D., Williams Island, FL; Clarice Gorenstein, Ph.D., Sao Paulo, Brazil; Paul Grof, M.D., Ottawa, Ontario, Canada; Russell T. Joffe, M.D., Hamilton, Ontario, Canada; Nancy E. Johnston, R.N., Thornhill, Ontario, Canada; Stephen R. Marder, M.D., Los Angeles, CA; Stuart A. Montgomery, M.D., London, England; Andrew A. Nierenberg, M.D., Boston, MA; Fred Quitkin, M.D., New York, NY; Ruth Robinson, Saskatoon, Saskatchewan, Canada; Matthew V. Rudorfer, M.D., Rockville, MD; Carl Salzman, M.D., Boston, MA; Colette F. Strnad, Ph.D., Ottawa, Ontario, Canada; Karen A. Theesen, Pharm.D., Omaha, NE; Thomas W. Uhde, M.D., Detroit, MI; George E. Woody, M.D., Philadelphia, PA

**Pulmonary Disease/Allergy**
Harold S. Nelson, M.D., *Chair*, Denver, CO; John A. Anderson, M.D., Detroit, MI; Emil J. Bardana, Jr., M.D., Portland, OR; I. Leonard Bernstein, M.D., Cincinnati, OH; Alexander G. Chuchalin, M.D., Ph.D., Moscow, Russia; Nicholas J. Gross, M.D., Hines, IL; Karen Huss, DNSc, R.N., Potomac, MD; Elliot Israel, M.D., Boston, MA; John W. Jenne, M.D., Sandia Park, NM; H. William Kelly, Pharm.D., Albuquerque, NM; James P. Kemp, M.D., San Diego, CA; Bennie C. McWilliams, Jr., M.D., Albuquerque, NM; Shirley Murphy, M.D., Chapel Hill, NC; Thomas F. Myers, M.D., Maywood, IL; Gary S. Rachelefsky, M.D., Los Angeles, CA; Joe Reisman, M.D., Toronto, Ontario, Canada; Robert E. Reisman, M.D., Williamsville, NY; Albert L. Sheffer, M.D., Boston, MA; Paul C. Stillwell, M.D., San Diego, CA; Stanley J. Szefler, M.D., Denver, CO; Virginia S. Taggart, M.P.H., Bethesda, MD; David G. Tinkleman, M.D., Denver, CO; John H. Toogood, M.D., London, Ontario, Canada; Martin D. Valentine, M.D., Baltimore, MD; Sally E. Wenzel, M.D., Denver, CO

**Radiopharmaceuticals**
Carol S. Marcus, Ph.D., M.D., *Chair*, Torrance, CA; J.D. Bernardy, J.D., Lexington, MA; Dik Blok, Pharm.D., Leiden, The Netherlands; Capt William H. Briner, Durham, NC; Janet F. Eary, M.D., Seattle, WA; David L. Gilday, M.D., Toronto, Ontario; Don Lyster, Ph.D., Vancouver, British Columbia, Canada; John G. McAfee, M.D., Chevy Chase, MD; James A. Ponto, M.S., Iowa City, IA; Mark H. Rotman, Pharm.D., M.S., Middletown, MD; Carl Seidel, M.S., Denton, TX; Barry A. Siegel, M.D., St. Louis, MO; Edward B. Silberstein, M.D., Cincinnati, OH; Roberta A. Strohl, RN, MN, Baltimore, MD; James B. Stubbs, Ph.D., Alpharetta, GA; Dennis P. Swanson, M.S., Pittsburgh, PA; Andrew T. Taylor, M.D., Atlanta, GA; Mathew L. Thakur, Ph.D., Philadelphia, PA; Ann Warbick-Cerone, Kanata, Ontario, Canada; John H. Waterman, MS, Arlington Heights, IL; Robert G. Wolfangel, Ph.D., St. Louis, MO

**Rheumatology-Clinical Immunology**
Evelyn V. Hess, M.D., *Chair*, Cincinnati, OH; Donato Alarcon-Segovia, M.D., Mexico City, Mexico; John Baum, M.D., Rochester, NY; David H. Campen, M.D., Santa Clara, CA; Paul Emery, M.D., Leeds, England; Daniel E. Furst, M.D., Seattle, WA; Jean G. Gispen, M.D., Oxford, MS; Esther Gonzales-Pares, M.D., San Juan, PR; Donna J. Hawley, R.N., Ed.D., Wichita, KS; Israeli A. Jaffe, M.D., New York, NY; Daniel J. Lovell, M.D., M.P.H., Cincinnati, OH; Walter P. Maksymowych, M.D., Edmonton, Alberta, Canada; Donald R. Miller, Pharm.D., Fargo, ND; Ivan G. Otterness, Ph.D., Groton, CT; Robert L. Rubin, Ph.D., La Jolla, CA; Lee S. Simon, M.D., Boston, MA; Daniel J. Stechschulte, M.D., Kansas City, KS; Michael E. Weinblatt, M.D., Boston, MA; Michael H. Weisman, M.D., San Diego, CA; William S. Wilke, M.D., Cleveland, OH; David E. Yocum, M.D., Tucson, AZ

**Surgical Drugs and Devices**
Lary A. Robinson, M.D., *Chair*, Tampa, FL; Kay A. Ball, M.S.A., R.N., Lewis Center, OH; Alan R. Dimick, M.D., Birmingham, AL; H. Kim Lyerly, M.D., Durham, NC; Henry J. Mann, Pharm.D., Minneapolis, MN; Joseph A. Moylan, M.D., Miami, FL; Ronald Lee Nichols, M.D.,

New Orleans, LA; Hiram C. Polk, Jr., M.D., Louisville, KY; Robert P. Rapp, Pharm.D., Lexington, KY; Ronald Rubin, M.D., West Newton, MA

**Therapeutic Information Management**
Ann B. Amerson, Pharm.D., *Chair*, Lexington, KY; Marie A. Abate, Pharm.D., Morgantown, WV; Wesley G. Byerly, Pharm.D., Winston-Salem, NC; Teresa Dowling, Pharm.D., Wilmington, DE; Thomas M. Gesell, Pharm.D., Morris Plains, NJ; Stephen R. Kaplan, M.D., Buffalo, NY; Ossy M.J. Kasilo, Ph.D., Harare, Zimbabwe; Aishah A. Latiff, Ph.D., Penang, Malaysia; Leslie A. Lenert, M.D., Stanford, CA; Dr. Hubert G.M. Leufkens, Utrecht, The Netherlands; M. Laurie Mashford, M.D., Victoria, Australia; Louise Matte, B.Sc., B.Pharm., Cap-Rouge, Quebec, Canada; Kurt A. Proctor, Ph.D., Alexandria, VA; Carol A. Romano, Ph.D., R.N., C., FAAN, Bethesda, MD; Cedric M. Smith, M.D., Buffalo, NY; Gary H. Smith, Pharm.D., Baltimore, MD; Dennis F. Thompson, Pharm.D., Oklahoma City, OK; William G. Troutman, Pharm.D., Albuquerque, NM; Gordon J. Vanscoy, Pharm.D., Irwin, PA; Valentin A. Vinogradov, M.D., Ph.D., Moscow, Russia; Lee A. Wanke, Seattle, WA; Antonio Carlos Zanini, M.D., Ph.D., Sao Paulo, Brazil

**Transplant Immunology**
Thomas E. Starzl, M.D., Ph.D., *Chair*, Pittsburgh, PA; Clyde F. Barker, M.D., Philadelphia, PA; Gilbert J. Burckart, Pharm.D., Pittsburgh, PA; Paul M. Colombani, M.D., Baltimore, MD; Allan P. Donner, Ph.D., London, Ontario, Canada; Robert A. Good, M.D., Ph.D., St. Petersburg, FL; Carl C. Groth, M.D., Ph.D., Huddinge, Sweden; John A. Hansen, M.D., Seattle, WA; Roger L. Jenkins, M.D., Boston, MA; John R. Lake, M.D., San Francisco, CA; Leonard Makowka, M.D., Ph.D., Los Angeles, CA; Suzanne V. McDiarmid, M.D., Los Angeles, CA; Ali Naji, M.D., Ph.D., Philadelphia, PA; David H. Sachs, M.D., Boston, MA; Joseph A. Tami, Pharm.D., Carlsbad, CA; Angus W. Thomson, Ph.D., Pittsburgh, PA; Raman Venkataramanan, Ph.D., Pittsburgh, PA; Professor Roger Williams, CBE, London, England

**Urology**
Culley C. Carson III, M.D., *Chair*, Chapel Hill, NC; John A. Belis, M.D., Hershey, PA; B.J. Reid Czarapata, CRNP, Rockville, MD; Sam D. Graham, Jr., M.D., Atlanta, GA; Mireille Gregoire, M.D., Quebec, Quebec, Canada; Wayne Hellstrom, M.D., New Orleans, LA; Joseph M. Khoury, M.D., Chapel Hill, NC; Marguerite C. Lippert, M.D., Charlottesville, VA; Michael G. Mawhinney, Ph.D., Morgantown, WV; Nelson Rodrigues Netto, Jr., M.D., Sao Paulo, Brazil; Mariano Rosello-Barbera, M.D., Palma de Mallorca, Spain; Randall G. Rowland, M.D., Ph.D., Lexington, KY; J. Patrick Spirnak, M.D., Cleveland, OH; William F. Tarry, M.D., Morgantown, WV; Chris M. Teigland, M.D., Charlotte, NC; Robert M. Weiss, M.D., New Haven, CT

**Veterinary Medicine**
V. Cory Langston, D.V.M., Ph.D., *Chair*, Mississippi State, MS; Michael D. Apley, D.V.M., Ph.D., Ames, IA; Gordon W. Brumbaugh, D.V.M., Ph.D., College Station, TX; Thomas J. Burkgren, D.V.M., M.B.A., Perry, IA; Cynthia T. Culmo, R.Ph., Austin, TX; Lloyd E. Davis, Ph.D., D.V.M., Champaign, IL; Patricia M. Dowling, D.V.M., M.S., Saskatoon, Saskatchewan, Canada; Stuart D. Forney, M.S., Fort Collins, CO; Antoinette D. Jernigan, D.V.M., Ph.D., Groton, CT; Mark G. Papich, D.V.M., Raleigh, NC; Thomas E. Powers, D.V.M., Ph.D., Columbus, OH; Jim E. Riviere, D.V.M., Ph.D., Raleigh, NC; Charles R. Short, D.V.M., Ph.D., Baton Rouge, LA; Hector Sumano Lopez, D.V.M., Ph.D., Mexico City, Mexico; Jeffrey R. Wilcke, D.V.M., Blacksburg, VA

# DIVISION OF INFORMATION DEVELOPMENT ADDITIONAL CONTRIBUTORS

The information presented in the USP DI database represents ongoing review and the consensus of various viewpoints expressed. In addition to the individuals listed below, many schools, associations, pharmaceutical companies, and governmental agencies have provided comment or otherwise contributed to the development of the 1999 USP DI database. Such listing does not imply that these individuals have reviewed all of the material in the database or that they individually agree with all statements contained herein.

David M. Aboulafia, M.D., Seattle, WA
Gary A. Abrams, M.D., Birmingham, AL
Lori J. Acuncius, Pharm.D., Hines, IL
Rodney Adam, M.D., Tucson, AZ
Peter C. Adamson, M.D., Bethesda, MD
David G. Addiss, M.D., Atlanta, GA
John Affronti, M.D., Durham, NC
Carmen Allegra, Bethesda, MD
Harunobu Amagase, Ph.D., Mission Viejo, CA
Jeffrey Anderson, M.D., Salt Lake City, UT
Stephen Anderson, M.D., Atlanta, GA
Frederick J. Angulo, DVM, Ph.D., Atlanta, GA
Dennis V.C. Awang, Ph.D., Ottawa, Ontario
Fred Ayers, M.D., Sutton, NE
Donna Bailey, MSN, Chapel Hill, NC
Patsy Barnett, Pharm.D., Birmingham, AL
Frank V. Beardell, M.D., Philadelphia, PA
Robert W. Beightol, Pharm.D, Roanoke, VA
Chandra P. Belani, M.D., Pittsburgh, PA
N.J. Benevenga, Madison, WI
William M. Bennett, M.D., Portland, OR
George Benson, M.D., Houston, TX
Stan Berlow, M.D., Madison, WI
Harlan Bigbee, D.V.M., Union, NJ
Mark Blumenthal, Austin, TX
Ernest C. Borden, M.D., Madison, WI
Samuel Bozzette, M.D., San Diego, CA
Wayne Bradley, R.Ph., MBA, Duluth, GA
Edwin D. Bransome, M.D., Augusta, GA
Lewis E. Braverman, M.D., Worcester, MA
Myron Brown, D.V.M., Shawnee Mission, KS

Bruce H. Brundage, M.D., Torrance, CA
Ronald Bukowski, M.D., Cleveland, OH
Thomas W. Burke, Houston, TX
Elizabeth Carilla, Castres, France
Bruce A. Chabner, M.D., Boston, MA
Jeffrey Chang, M.D., Davis, CA
Kyong-Mi Chang, M.D., La Jolla, CA
Terrence P. Clark, D.V.M., Ph.D., Auburn University, AL
Ronald I. Clyman, M.D., San Francisco, CA
Jay D. Coffman, M.D., Boston, MA
James W. Cooper, Pharm.D., Athens, GA
Larry J. Copeland, M.D., Columbus, OH
Clinton N. Corder, Ph.D., M.D., Oklahoma City, OK
Lawrence Corey, M.D., Seattle, WA
William T. Creasman, M.D., Charleston, SC
Professor M. Cruz, Tenerife, Spain
Philip E. Cryer, M.D., St. Louis, MO
Horace G. Cutler, Ph.D., Atlanta, GA
Thomas D. DeCillis, North Port, FL
D. Dionisio, M.D., Florence, Italy
Franco Di Silverio, M.D., Rome, Italy
Howard Druce, M.D., Madison, NJ
Brian O. L. Duke, M.D., Lancaster, England
Herbert L. Dupont, M.D., Houston, TX
Teena Eappen, R.Ph., Brooklyn, NY
Mark Edelstein, M.D., Ph.D., Detroit, MI
Lawrence H. Einhorn, M.D., Indianapolis, IN
Marc S. Ernstoff, M.D., Lebanon, NH
Bruce Ettinger, M.D., Oakland, CA
Jawed Fareed, M.D., Maywood, IL
Ronnie Fass, M.D., Tucson, AZ

Clara Fenger, D.V.M., Lexington, KY
Ruth Francis-Floyd, D.V.M., Gainesville, FL
William A. Gahl, M.D., Bethesda, MD
Jose P.B. Gallardo, R.Ph., Iowa City, IA
Robert Genco, D.D.S., Ph.D., Buffalo, NY
Welton M. Gersony, M.D., New York, NY
Mihai Gheorghiade, M.D., Chicago, IL
John Godwin, M.D., Maywood, IL
G. L. Goldberg, Bronx, NY
Stephen S. Gottlieb, M.D., Baltimore, MD
Maj. John D. Grabenstein, M.S., Chapel Hill, NC
David Y. Graham, M.D., Houston, TX
J. Richard Grayhill, M.D., San Antonio, TX
Gilman D. Grave, M.D., Bethesda, MD
David R. P. Guay, Pharm.D., St. Paul, MN
Rolf M. Gunnar, Berwyn, IL
Nortin M. Hadler, M.D., Chapel Hill, NC
Nina Han, Pharm.D., Chicago, IL
Prof. Dr. Gerhart Harrer, Salzburg, Austria
Gavin Hart, M.D., South Australia, Australia
H.M.C. Heick, M.D., Ph.D., Ottawa, Ontario
William J. Heinrich, P.D., M.S., Baltimore, MD
Christopher Hendel, M.S., Burlington, VT
S. Heptinstall, Nottingham, England
Michael A. Heymann, M.D., San Francisco, CA
Basil I. Hirschowitz, M.D., Birmingham, AL
William B. Hladik, III, M.S., Albuquerque, NM
M.E. Hoar, Springfield, MA
Patrick Hoffman, Ph.D., Hunt Valley, MD
Richard A. Holmes, M.D., St. Louis, MO
William Hopkins, Pharm.D., Atlanta, GA
William J. Hoskins, M.D., New York, NY
Peter J. Houghton, B.Pharm, Ph.D., London, England
Peter C. Hoyle, M.D., Ph.D., Frederick, MD
Wolf-Dietrich Hübner, M.D., Berlin, Germany
Suzy Huijghebaert, M.D., Brussels, Belgium
Robert Ignoffo, Pharm.D., San Francisco, CA
Jon I. Isenberg, M.D., San Diego, CA
Martin Jacobs, M.D., Dayton, OH
Robert R. Jacobson, M.D., Carville, LA
Norman Jaffee, M.D., Houston, TX
Cynda A. Johnson, M.D., Kansas City, KS
Jim Jones, Pharm.D., Columbus, OH
Barton Kamen, M.D., Dallas, TX
Sangeeta Kashyap, M.D., West Los Angeles, CA
John J. Kavanagh, M.D., Houston, TX
Charles Kilo, M.D., St. Louis, MO
Charles H. King, M.D., Cleveland, OH
A. Douglas Kinghorn, Ph.D., Chicago, IL
Joseph B. Kirsner, M.D., Chicago, IL
Thomas Kisker, M.D., Iowa City, IA
Vicki L. Kraus, R.N., Iowa City, IA
Susan E. Krown, M.D., New York, NY
Paul Kucera, Ph.D., Pearl River, NY
Paul B. Kuehn, Ph.D., Woodinville, WA
Thomas L. Kurt, M.D., Dallas, TX
Lynne Kushner, D.V.M., Mississippi State, MS
Richard A. Larson, M.D., Chicago, IL
Diane Lauver, R.N., Ph.D., Madison, WI
Larry Lawson, Springville, UT
Natalie Lazarowych, Ph.D., Toronto, Ontario
Mark Lebwohl, M.D., New York, NY
Harvey L. Levy, M.D., Boston, MA
Michael Lockshin, New York, NY
Franklin C. Lowe, M.D., New York, NY
Harvey Lui, M.D., Vancouver, B.C., Canada
David W. Lyter, M.D., M.P.H., Chicago, IL
Robert D. Madoff, M.D., St. Paul, MN
Howard I. Maibach, M.D., San Francisco, CA
Roger Maichel, West Lafayette, IN
B.K. Mandal, M.D., Manchester, England
Maurie Markman, M.D., Cleveland, OH
Keith Marks, M.D., Hershey, PA
David H. Martin, M.D., New Orleans, LA
Barry J. Materson, M.D., Miami, FL
James B. McAuley, M.D., Atlanta, GA
Norman L. McElroy, San Jose, CA

William P. McGuire, M.D., Atlanta, GA
Victor D. Menashe, M.D., Portland, OR
Franz H. Messerli, M.D., New Orleans, LA
Boyd E. Metzger, M.D., Chicago, IL
Garreth A. Moore, D.V.M., Pembroke, VA
Richard Moore, M.D., Baltimore, MD
Doris Hupfeld Moreno, Ph.D., Sao Paulo, Brazil
Marvin Moser, M.D., White Plains, NY
Richard B. Moss, M.D., Palo Alto, CA
Franco M. Muggia, M.D., New York, NY
James Nachman, M.D., Chicago, IL
Marguerite A. Neill, M.D., Pawtucket, RI
Robert Murphy, M.D., Chicago, IL
H.A.W. Neil, Oxford, England
D.W. Northfelt, M.D.,FACP, Palm Springs, CA
Cheryl Nunn-Thompson, Pharm.D., West Zundee, IL
Judith M. Ozbun, R.Ph., M.S., Fargo, ND
Ariel Pablos-Mendez, M.D., M.P.H., New York, NY
Samuel W. Page, Ph.D., Washington, DC
Robert C. Park, M.D., Silver Spring, MD
Asuncion Peiré, M.D., Tenerife, Spain
Peter L. Perrine, M.D., Seattle, WA
Bruce Petersen, M.D., Minneapolis, MN
Donald A. Podoloff, M.D., Houston, TX
Richard Powers, M.D., Oakland, CA
G.S. Rai, M.D., London, England
Lee B. Reichman, M.D., M.P.H., Newark, NJ
T.M.S. Reid, M.D., Aberdeen, England
Hans Reinemor, M.D., Salt Lake City, UT
Alfred J. Remillard, Pharm.D., Saskatoon, Saskatchewan
Joseph G. Reves, M.D., Durham, NC
Robert S. Rew, MS, ScD, Exton, PA
Shereif Rezkalla, M.D., Marshfield, WI
Stuart Rich, M.D., Chicago, IL
Karl Rickels, Philadelphia, PA
Matthew Riddle, Jr., M.D., Portland, OR
G.L. Ridgway, M.D. London, England
David Robertson, M.D., Nashville, TN
William J. Rodriguez, M.D., Ph.D., Washington, DC
David Roffman, Pharm.D., Baltimore, MD
D.S. Rosenblatt, London, Ontario
Lorri Rosenthal, Chattanooga, TN
Carl Rothenberg, Los Angeles, CA
Eric K. Rowinsky, M.D. San Antonio, TX
Lewis J. Rubin, M.D., Baltimore, MD
Gerald Salen, M.D., New York, NY
Evelyn Salerno, Pharm.D., Hialeah, FL
David Sarraf, M.D., West Los Angeles, CA
Fred Sattler, Los Angeles, CA
P. G. Satyaswaroop, Hershey, PA
Margretta A.R. Seashore, M.D., New Haven, CT
Saul Schaefer, M.D., Sacramento, CA
Anthony J. Schaeffer, Chicago, IL
Peter M. Schantz, M.D., Ph.D., Atlanta, GA
Alan F. Schatzberg, M.D., Stanford, CA
James M. Scheiman, M.D., Ann Harbor, MI
Paul L. Schiff, Jr., Ph.D., Pittsburgh, PA
Volker Schulz, M.D., Berlin, Germany
George S. Schuster, D.D.S., Ph.D., Augusta, GA
Charles F. Seifert, Pharm.D., Rapid City, SD
Jerry Shapiro, M.D., Vancouver, B.C., Canada
F.A. Shepherd, M.D., Toronto, Ontario
Patricia Simone, M.D., Atlanta, GA
Robert Simmons, D.V.M., Union, NJ
Irving Sivin, M.D., New York, NY
Michael Sly, M.D., Washington, DC
Geralynn B. Smith, Detroit, MI
Greta Snow, Pharm.D., Albuquerque, NM
Elliott M. Sogol, Ph.D., Research Triangle Park, NC
Roger Soloway, M.D., Galveston, TX
Joseph A. Sparano, M.D., Bronx, NY
Leon Speroff, M.D., Portland, OR
Stanley M. Spinola, M.D., Indianapolis, IN
Allen C. Steere, M.D., Boston, MA
John J. Stern, M.D., Philadelphia, PA
Irmin Sternlieb, M.D., San Diego, CA
David C. Stuhr, Denver, CO

Alan Sugar, M.D., Boston, MA
Linda Gore Sutherland, Pharm.D., Laramie, WY
R.S. Swerdloff, Torrance, CA
James T. Thigpen, M.D., Jackson, MS
Derek A. Ucleda, M.D., Salt Lake City, UT
Wulf Utian, M.D., Ph.D., Cleveland, OH
Michael Valentino, MHSA, R.Ph., Hines, IL
Akshay Vakharia, M.D., Dallas, TX
K.J. Varma, Ph.D., Union, NJ
Michael W. Varner, M.D., Salt Lake City, UT
J. Vesper, Berlin, Germany
Teresa J. Vietti, M.D., St. Louis, MO
Donald G. Vidt, M.D., Cleveland, OH
Nicolas J. Vogelzang, M.D., Western Springs, IL
Paul A. Volberding, M.D., San Francisco, CA
Ernst-Utrich Vorbach, M.D., Darmstadt, Germany

Anna Wald, M.D., M.P.H., Seattle, WA
William Warner, Ph.D., New York, NY
Gary Wasserman, M.D., Kansas City, MO
Miles M. Weinberger, M.D., Iowa City, IA
Timothy E. Welty, Pharm.D., Cincinnati, OH
Lisa Westing, King City, CA
Ray C. Williams, D.M.D., Chapel Hill, NC
Robert Willkens, M.D., Seattle, WA
Mary Wilson, M.D., Iowa City, IA
Naomi Winick, M.D., Dallas, TX
Robert Yarchoan, M.D., Bethesda, MD
Courtney Yen, Pharm.D., San Francisco, CA
John M. Zajecka, M.D., Chicago, IL
Jonathan M. Zenilman, M.D., Baltimore, MD
Mark Zetin, M.D., Orange, CA
Frederic J. Zucchero, M.A., R.Ph., Chesterfield, MO

# HEADQUARTERS STAFF

## DIVISION OF INFORMATION DEVELOPMENT
**Director:** Keith W. Johnson
**Assistant Director:** Georgie M. Cathey
**Manager, Strategic Planning and Patient Education Programs:** Stacy M. Hartranft
**Administrative Staff:** Maureen Rawson, Mayra L. Rios, Milagro M. Welter
**Senior Drug Information Specialists:** Ann Corken (*Supervisor and Nutrition Information Coordinator*), Nancy Lee Dashiell (*Supervisor*)
**Drug Information Specialists:** Nicoli R. Anderson, Susan Braun, Robin S. Isham-Schermerhorn, Jymeann King, Esther Klein, Denise S. Penn, Kathleen M. Phelan, Daniel W. Seyoum, Celia Sloan, Susan M. Sromek, Susanne Streety, Robyn C. Tyler, Ronald T. Wassel (*Supervisor*), Joyce P. Weaver
**Drug Utilization Review Program Director:** Thomas R. Fulda
**Medical Information Specialists:** Syed R. Ahmad, Joyce Carpenter, Rosaly Correa de Araujo, Jenny J. Tao, Lisa L. Wei
**Veterinary Drug Information Specialist:** Amy Neal
**Coordinator, USP Dictionary:** Jean R. Canada
**Computer/Database Applications:** Bernard G. Silverstein
**Consumer Information Development:** Diana M. Blais (*Manager*), Bandana Das (*Assistant*), Marilyn L. Foster (*Associate*), Lauren E. O'Connor (*Assistant*), Janet E. Schmidt (*Associate*)
**Translators:** Claudia Lopez-Muniz, Jamie A. Ramirez
**Editors:** Carol N. Hankin, Sakti P. Mukherjee, Doris Mullen, Toni Tyson, Deborah F. Zimmer
**Library Services:** Florence A. Hogan (*Manager*), Terri Rikhy (*Associate*), Madeleine Welsch (*Assistant*)
**International Programs:** Nancy L. Blum (*Coordinator*), Kirill A. Burimski (*Russia Project Coordinator*)
**Research Associate:** Marie C. Robie
**Consultants:** Barbara Bastow, Sandra Lee Boyer, Patricia J. Bush, Muriel Lippman, Angela M. Mayo, Marcelo Vernengo
**Medical Consultants:** William P. Baker, M.D., Ph.D.; Donald R. Bennett, M.D., Ph.D.; Carol Proudfit, Ph.D.; Joseph H. Smith, M.D.; Walter L. Way, M.D.
**Scholar in Residence:** James Blackburn, Saskatoon, Saskatchewan
**Student Interns:** Quynh-Van N. Duong, Virgina Commonwealth University, College of Pharmacy; Nate Wilkin, The Ohio State University, School of Medicine; Lee Yerkes, George Washington University School of Public Health
**Visiting Scholar:** Raul Cruzado Ubillus, National University of Trujillo, Peru

## USP ADMINISTRATIVE STAFF
**Executive Vice President-CEO:** Jerome A. Halperin
**Senior Vice President-COO:** John T. Fowler
**Senior Vice President and General Counsel:** Joseph G. Valentino
**Vice President for Policy and Strategic Planning:** Jacqueline L. Eng
**Director, Office of Personnel:** Arlene Bloom
**Director, Finance:** Abe Brauner
**Director, Fulfillment/Facilities:** Drew J. Lutz
**Legal:** Ken Alexander (*Associate Legal Counsel for Business Affairs*), Gail Bormel (*Associate Legal Counsel for Scientific Affairs*), Jennifer Devine (*Staff Attorney*)

## DIVISION OF STANDARDS DEVELOPMENT
**Vice President and Director:** Lee T. Grady
**Assistant Directors:** Charles H. Barnstein (*Revision*), Barbara B. Hubert (*DSD*)
**Senior Scientists:** Roger Dabbah, V. Srinivasan, William W. Wright
**Scientists:** Frank P. Barletta, W. Larry Paul, Todd L. Cecil
**Senior Scientific Associates:** Stephen H. Atwell, William E. Brown, Gabriel I. Giancaspro, Terry H. Mainprize, Claudia C. Okeke
**Manager, Standards Technical Editing:** Keith A. Seabaugh
**Senior Technical Editors:** Azra Medjedovic, Anna Marie Sibik, Melissa M. Smith
**Senior Translator:** Maria T. Gil-Montero
**Manager of Administrative Programs:** Anju K. Malhotra
**Program Director for Biological Sciences:** Gene Murano
**Support Staff:** Gerald L. Anderson, Angela M. Healey, Cecilia Luna, Nurilya U. Ivanov
**Drug Research and Testing Laboratory:** Richard F. Lindauer (*Director*)
**Reference Standards Operations:** Robert H. King (*Director*)
**Hazard Communications:** Linda Shear
**Consultants:** J. Joseph Belson, Martin Golden, Aubrey S. Outschoorn

## MARKETING
**Vice President:** Mark A. Sohasky
**Category Manager, MedMARx:** Joan April
**Category Manager, Drug Standards Publications:** Charlotte McKamy
**Outreach Program Manager:** Susan Williams
**Distribution Program Manager:** Mary Dougherty
**Assistant Category Manager, Latin American Marketing:** Claudia Cox
**Marketing Associate:** Matthew Valleskey
**Technical Support Specialist:** Jean Gallagher
**Marketing and Sales Assistant:** Gary Strackbein
**Marketing Assistant:** Barbara Wurth
**Office Assistant:** Daniel Janoski

## PRODUCTION SERVICES
**Production Manager, Information Products:** A. V. Precup
**Production Coordinators:** Susan J. Detwiler, Harriet S. Nathanson, Michael Spencer; Doreen Conrad and Michelle Wulffaert of Editech Services, Inc.
**Q/A Specialist/Proofreader:** Matthew Boyle
**Production Manager, Standards Products:** Sandra F. Boynton
**Senior Editorial Associates:** Jesusa D. Cordova, Margaret Kay
**Editorial Associate:** Ellen Elovitz
**Desktop Publishing Staff:** Susan L. Entwistle (*Supervisor/Applications Analyst*), Lauren Taylor Davis, Deborah James, M. T. Samahon, Donna Singh, Micheline Tranquille

**PRODUCT DEVELOPMENT**
**Manager Product Development:** Linda M. Guard
**Applications Analyst, SGML:** Laurie J. Manning
**Software Engineer:** Anthony M. Gray
**FOSI Development:** Deborah R. Connelly

**CREATIVE SERVICES**
**Senior Project Manager:** Derik Rice
**Project Manager:** Elayne Peterson
**Senior Designers:** Tia C. Morfessis, Randy White
**Designer:** Rodney Warren
**Production Coordinator:** Anna Schrock

**PRACTITIONER REPORTING PROGRAMS**
**Vice President, Practitioner Reporting Programs:** Diane D. Cousins
**Manager, Program Development:** Shawn C. Becker
**Manager, Program Operations:** Anne Paula Thompson
**Analyst Coder Specialist:** Rita F. Calnan
**Administrative Assistant:** Elida B. Amezquita
**Nurse Associate WATS:** M. Susan Zmuda
**Data Entry Specialist II:** Lata Rao
**Staff Assistant:** Lynn K. Murdock
**Program Assistant:** Patricia Floyd

# MEMBERS OF THE UNITED STATES PHARMACOPEIAL CONVENTION
### as of June, 1998

**U.S. Colleges and Schools of Medicine**

Albany Medical College, Albany, NY: Daniel S. Stein, M.D.
Allegheny University of Health Sciences, Philadelphia, PA: Edward J. Barbieri, Ph.D.
Boston University School of Medicine, Boston, MA: J. Worth Estes, M.D.
Brown University School of Medicine, Providence, RI: Edward Hawrot, Ph.D.
Case Western Reserve University School of Medicine, Cleveland, OH: Charles L. Hoppel, M.D.
Columbia University College of Physicians and Surgeons, New York, NY: Brian F. Hoffman, M.D.
Creighton University School of Medicine, Omaha, NE: Peter W. Abel, Ph.D.
Duke University Medical Center School of Medicine, Durham, NC: James C. McAllister III, M.S.
East Carolina University School of Medicine, Greenville, NC: Donald W. Barnes, Ph.D.
East Tennessee State University James H. Quillen College of Medicine, Johnson City, TN: Peter J. Rice, Ph.D.
Emory University School of Medicine, Atlanta, GA: Yung-Fong Sung, M.D.
Georgetown University School of Medicine, Washington, DC: Arthur Raines, Ph.D.
Harvard Medical School, Boston, MA: David E. Golan, M.D., Ph.D.
Howard University College of Medicine, Washington, DC: Robert E. Taylor, M.D., Ph.D.
Indiana University School of Medicine, Indianapolis, IN: D. Craig Brater, M.D.
Johns Hopkins University School of Medicine, Baltimore, MD: E. Robert Feroli, Pharm.D.
Loma Linda University School of Medicine, Loma Linda, CA: W. William Hughes, Ph.D.
Louisiana State University School of Medicine, New Orleans, LA: Paul L. Kirkendol, Ph.D.
Loyola University of Chicago Stritch School of Medicine, Maywood, IL: Stanley A. Lorens, Ph.D.
Marshall University School of Medicine, Huntington, WV: John L. Szarek, Ph.D.
Mayo Medical School, Rochester, MN: James J. Lipsky, M.D.
Medical College of Ohio, Toledo, OH: Robert D. Wilkerson, Ph.D.
Medical College of Pennsylvania and Hahnemann University School of Medicine, Philadelphia, PA: Edward J. Barbieri, Ph.D.
Medical College of Wisconsin, Milwaukee, WI: Garrett J. Gross, Ph.D.
Meharry Medical College School of Medicine, Nashville, TN: Dolores Shockley, Ph.D.
Michigan State University of Human Medicine, East Lansing, MI: John E. Thornberg, D.O., Ph.D.
Mount Sinai School of Medicine, New York, NY: Christopher P. Cardozo, M.D.
New York Medical College, Valhalla, NY: Mario A. Inchiosa, Jr., Ph.D.
Northwestern University Medical School, Chicago, IL: Marilynn C. Frederiksen, M.D.
Oregon Health Sciences University School of Medicine, Portland, OR: Hall Downes, M.D., Ph.D.
Ponce School of Medicine, Ponce, PR: Arthur L. Hupka, Ph.D.
Rush Medical College, Chicago, IL: Paul G. Pierpaoli, M.S.
St. Louis University Health Sciences Center School of Medicine, St. Louis, MO: Alvin H. Gold, Ph.D.
Stanford University School of Medicine, Stanford, CA: Leslie A. Lenert, M.D.
SUNY at Buffalo School of Medicine and Biomedical Sciences, Buffalo, NY: Cedric M. Smith, M.D.
SUNY Health Science Center at Syracuse, Syracuse, NY: Oliver M. Brown, Ph.D.
Temple University School of Medicine, Philadelphia, PA: Ronald J. Tallarida, Ph.D.
The Bowman Gray School of Medicine of Wake Forest University, Winston-Salem, NC: Jack W. Strandhoy, Ph.D.
The Medical College of Georgia School of Medicine, Augusta, GA: David W. Hawkins, Pharm.D.
The Ohio State University College of Medicine, Columbus, OH: Robert M. Guthrie, M.D.
The Pennsylvania State University College of Medicine, Hershey, PA: Cheston M. Berlin, Jr., M.D.
The University of Iowa College of Medicine, Iowa City, IA: John E. Kasik, M.D., Ph.D.
The University of Michigan Medical School, Ann Arbor, MI: Edward F. Domino, Ph.D.
The University of Mississippi Medical Center, Jackson, MS: George W. Moll, Jr., M.D., Ph.D.
Tufts University School of Medicine, Boston, MA: John M. Mazzullo, M.D.
Tulane University School of Medicine, New Orleans, LA: Floyd R. Domer, Ph.D.
Uniformed Services University of the Health Sciences, Bethesda, MD: Louis R. Cantilena, M.D., Ph.D.
University of Alabama School of Medicine, Birmingham, AL: Robert B. Diasio, M.D.
University of California, Davis School of Medicine, Davis, CA: Larry G. Stark, Ph.D.
University of California Los Angeles Center for Health Sciences School of Medicine, Los Angeles, CA: Marvin E. Ament, M.D.
University of California, San Diego School of Medicine, La Jolla, CA: Harold J. Simon, M.D., Ph.D.
University of California, San Francisco School of Medicine, San Francisco, CA: Mark A. Schumacher, Ph.D., M.D.
University of Chicago Pritzker School of Medicine, Chicago, IL: Patrick Horn, M.D.
University of Cincinnati College of Medicine, Cincinnati, OH: Leonard T. Sigell, Ph.D.
University of Colorado School of Medicine, Denver, CO: Alan S. Hollister, M.D., Ph.D.
University of Connecticut Health Center School of Medicine, Farmington, CT: Paul F. Davern, M.B.A.
University of Florida College of Medicine, Gainesville, FL: Lal C. Garg, Ph.D.
University of Hawaii John A. Burns School of Medicine, Honolulu, HI: Bert K.B. Lum, Ph.D., M.D.
University of Illinois at Chicago School of Medicine, Chicago, IL: Lawrence Isaac, Ph.D.
University of Kansas Medical Center School of Medicine, Kansas City, KS: Harold N. Godwin, M.S.
University of Louisville School of Medicine, Louisville, KY: Peter P. Rowell, Ph.D.
University of Massachusetts Medical School, Worcester, MA: Glenn R. Kershaw, M.D.
University of Medicine and Dentistry of New Jersey-New Jersey Medical School, Newark, NJ: Mohamed S. Abdel-Rahman, Ph.D.
University of Medicine and Dentistry of New Jersey-Robert Wood Johnson Medical School, New Brunswick, NJ: Richard D. Huhn, M.D.
University of Missouri-Columbia School of Medicine, Columbia, MO: John W. Yarbro, M.D.
University of Missouri-Kansas City School of Medicine, Kansas City, MO: Paul G. Cuddy, Pharm.D.
University of Nebraska College of Medicine, Omaha, NE: Manuchair Ebadi, Ph.D.
University of Nevada School of Medicine, Reno, NV: John Q. Adams, Pharm.D.
University of New Mexico School of Medicine, Albuquerque, NM: Jane E. Henney, M.D.
University of North Carolina School of Medicine, Chapel Hill, NC: Culley C. Carson, M.D.
University of North Dakota School of Medicine, Grand Forks, ND: David W. Hein, Ph.D.
University of Oklahoma College of Medicine, Oklahoma City, OK: Patrick A. McKee, M.D.
University of Pennsylvania School of Medicine, Philadelphia, PA: Marilyn E. Hess, Ph.D.
University of Rochester School of Medicine and Dentistry, Rochester, NY: Ira Shoulson, M.D.
University of South Florida College of Medicine, Tampa, FL: Joseph J. Krzanowski, Ph.D.
University of Tennessee, Memphis College of Medicine, Memphis, TN: Murray Heimberg, M.D., Ph.D.
University of Texas Health Science Center at San Antonio Medical School, San Antonio, TX: Alexander M.M. Shepherd, M.D., Ph.D.
University of Texas Houston Medical School, Houston, TX: Gary C. Rosenfeld, Ph.D.
University of Texas Southwestern Medical Center at Dallas, Dallas, TX: Paul F. White, Ph.D., M.D.
University of Washington School of Medicine, Seattle, WA: Georgiana K. Ellis, M.D.
Vanderbilt University School of Medicine, Nashville, TN: Dan M. Roden, M.D.

Virginia Commonwealth University/Medical College of Virginia School of Medicine, Richmond, VA: Aron H. Lichtman, Ph.D.
Wake Forest University School of Medicine, Wake Forest NC: Jack W. Strandhoy, Ph.D.
Wayne State University School of Medicine, Detroit, MI: Deborah G. May, M.D.
West Virginia University Robert C. Byrd Health Sciences Center, Morgantown, WV: Douglas D. Glover, M.D., R.Ph.
Wright State University School of Medicine, Dayton, OH: Robert L. Koerker, Ph.D.
Yale University School of Medicine, New Haven, CT: Florence Comite, M.D.

**State Medical Societies**
Alaska State Medical Association, Anchorage, AK: Keith M. Brownsberger, M.D.
California Medical Association, San Francisco, CA: Rene H. Bravo, M.D.
Connecticut State Medical Society, New Haven, CT: James E. O'Brien, M.D., Ph.D.
Florida Medical Association, Jacksonville, FL: Robert E. Windom, M.D.
Idaho Medical Association, Boise, ID: Lawrence L. Knight, M.D.
Illinois State Medical Society, Chicago, IL: Albino T. Bismonte, M.D.
Indiana State Medical Association, Indianapolis, IN: Daria Schooler, M.D., R.Ph.
Kansas Medical Society, Topeka, KS: James L. Early, M.D.
Kentucky Medical Association, Louisville, KY: Ellsworth C. Seeley, M.D.
Louisiana State Medical Society, Metairie, LA: Merlin H. Allen, M.D.
Massachusetts Medical Society, Waltham, MA: Errol Green, M.D.
Medical and Chirurgical Faculty of the State of Maryland, Baltimore, MD: David D. Collins, M.D.
Medical Association of Georgia, Atlanta, GA: Edwin D. Bransome, M.D.
Medical Association of the State of Alabama, Montgomery, AL: James R. Reed, M.D., Ph.D.
Medical Society of Delaware, Wilmington, DE: Michael J. Pasquale, M.D.
Medical Society of New Jersey, Lawrenceville, NJ: Joseph N. Micale, M.D.
Medical Society of the District of Columbia, Washington, DC: Kim A. Bullock, M.D.
Medical Society of the State of New York, Lake Success, NY: Richard Blum, M.D.
Medical Society of Virginia, Richmond, VA: Boyd M. Clements, M.D.
Michigan State Medical Society, East Lansing, MI: Douglas D. Notman, M.D.
Mississippi State Medical Association, Jackson, MS: William A. Causey, M.D.
Missouri State Medical Association, Jefferson City, MO: C.C. Swarens
Nebraska Medical Association, Lincoln, NE: Fred H. Ayers, M.D.
New Hampshire Medical Society, Concord, NH: Belinda L. Castor, M.D.
North Carolina Medical Society, Raleigh, NC: Don C. Chaplin, M.D.
North Dakota Medical Association, Bismarck, ND: William W. Barnes, M.D.
Ohio State Medical Association, Columbus, OH: Janet K. Bixel, M.D.
Oklahoma State Medical Association, Oklahoma City, OK: Clinton N. Corder, M.D., Ph.D.
Pennsylvania Medical Society, Harrisburg, PA: Benjamin Calesnick, M.D.
South Carolina Medical Association, Columbia, SC: Frank R. Ervin, M.D.
South Dakota State Medical Association, Sioux Falls, SD: Thomas C. Johnson, M.D.
State Medical Society of Wisconsin, Madison, WI: Melvin Rosen, M.D., Ph.D.
Tennessee Medical Association, Nashville, TN: John J. Ingram, M.D.
Texas Medical Association, Austin, TX: John E. Presley, M.D.
Utah Medical Association, Salt Lake City, UT: Douglas E. Rollins, M.D., Ph.D.
Washington State Medical Association, Seattle, WA: William O. Robertson, M.D.
West Virginia State Medical Association, Charleston, WV: Kevin W. Yingling, M.D., F.A.C.P., R.Ph.
Wyoming Medical Society, Inc., Cheyenne, WY: Wendy P. Curran

**U.S. Colleges and Schools of Pharmacy**
Albany College of Pharmacy, Albany, NY: Andra L. Stinchcomb, Ph.D.
Auburn University School of Pharmacy, Auburn, AL: Kenneth N. Barker, Ph.D.
Butler University College of Pharmacy and Health Sciences, Indianapolis, IN: Jayesh Vora, Ph.D.
Campbell University School of Pharmacy, Buies Creek, NC: Antoine Al-Achi, Ph.D.
Creighton University School of Pharmacy and Allied Health Professions, Omaha, NE: Kenneth R. Keefner, Ph.D.
Drake University College of Pharmacy and Health Sciences, Des Moines, IA: Sidney Finn, Ph.D.
Duquesne University School of Pharmacy, Pittsburgh, PA: Lawrence H. Block, Ph.D.
Ferris State University College of Pharmacy, Big Rapids, MI: Kenneth J. McMullen
Florida A&M University College of Pharmacy and Pharmaceutical Sciences, Tallahassee, FL: Seth Y. Ablordeppey, Ph.D.
Idaho State University College of Pharmacy, Pocatello, ID: Eugene I. Isaacson, Ph.D.
Long Island University Arnold & Marie Schwartz College of Pharmacy and Health Sciences, Brooklyn, NY: Jack Rosenberg, Pharm.D., Ph.D.
Massachusetts College of Pharmacy and Allied Health Sciences, Boston, MA: Sumner M. Robinson, Ph.D.
Medical University of South Carolina College of Pharmacy, Charleston, SC: Jaymin C. Shah, Ph.D.
Mercer University Southern School of Pharmacy, Atlanta, GA: J. Grady Strom, Jr., Ph.D.
Midwestern University Chicago College of Pharmacy, Downers Grove, IL: Mary W.L. Lee, Pharm.D.
North Dakota State University College of Pharmacy, Fargo, ND: Jagdish Singh, Ph.D.
Northeast Louisiana University School of Pharmacy, Monroe, LA: William M. Bourn, Ph.D.
Northeastern University School of Pharmacy, Boston, MA: Mehdi Boroujerdi, Ph.D.
NOVA Southeastern University College of Pharmacy, North Miami Beach, FL: William D. Hardigan, Ph.D.
Ohio Northern University College of Pharmacy, Ada, OH: Kimberly Broedel-Zaugg, Ph.D.
Oregon State University College of Pharmacy, Corvallis, OR: John H. Block, Ph.D.
Philadelphia College of Pharmacy and Science, Philadelphia, PA: Alfonso R. Gennaro, Ph.D.
Purdue University School of Pharmacy, West Lafayette, IN: Stephen R. Byrn, Ph.D.
Rutgers-The State University of New Jersey College of Pharmacy, Piscataway, NJ: Leonard C. Bailey, Ph.D.
Samford University School of Pharmacy, Birmingham, AL: Hilmer (Tony) A. McBride, Ph.D.
Shenandoah University School of Pharmacy, Winchester, VA: David W. Newton, Ph.D.
South Dakota State University College of Pharmacy, Brookings, SD: Chandradhar Dwivedi, Ph.D.
Southwestern Oklahoma State University School of Pharmacy, Weatherford, OK: Keith W. Reichmann, Ph.D.
St John's University College of Pharmacy and Allied Health Professions, Jamaica, NY: Thomas H. Wiser, Pharm.D.
St. Louis College of Pharmacy, St. Louis, MO: John W. Zuzack, Ph.D.
Temple University School of Pharmacy, Philadelphia, PA: Reza Fassihi, Ph.D.
Texas Southern University College of Pharmacy and Health Sciences, Houston, TX: William B. Harrell, Ph.D.
Texas Tech University School of Pharmacy, Amarillo, TX: Arthur A. Nelson, Ph.D.
The Ohio State University College of Pharmacy, Columbus, OH: Sylvan G. Frank, Ph.D.
The University of Arizona College of Pharmacy, Tucson, AZ: Michael Mayersohn, Ph.D.
The University of Georgia College of Pharmacy, Athens, GA: Stuart Feldman, Ph.D.
University at Buffalo School of Pharmacy, Buffalo, NY: Howard Forman, Pharm.D.
University of Arkansas for Medical Sciences College of Pharmacy, Little Rock, AR: Jonathan J. Wolfe, Ph.D.
University of California San Francisco, School of Pharmacy, San Francisco, CA: Emil T. Lin, Ph.D.
University of Cincinnati College of Pharmacy, Cincinnati, OH: Henry S.I. Tan, Ph.D.
University of Colorado School of Pharmacy, Denver, CO: Louis Diamond, Ph.D.
University of Connecticut School of Pharmacy, Storrs, CT: Michael C. Gerald, Ph.D.
University of Florida College of Pharmacy, Gainesville, FL: Michael A. Schwartz, Ph.D.
University of Houston College of Pharmacy, Houston, TX: Mustafa F. Lokhandwala, Ph.D.
University of Illinois College of Pharmacy, Chicago, IL: John F. Fitzloff, Ph.D.
University of Iowa College of Pharmacy, Iowa City, IA: Gilbert S. Banker, Ph.D.
University of Kansas School of Pharmacy, Lawrence, KS: John Stobaugh, Ph.D.
University of Kentucky College of Pharmacy, Lexington, KY: Paul M. Bummer, Ph.D.
University of Maryland at Baltimore School of Pharmacy, Baltimore, MD: Larry Augsburger, Ph.D.
University of Michigan School of Pharmacy, Ann Arbor, MI: Duane M. Kirking, Ph.D.
University of Minnesota College of Pharmacy, Minneapolis, MN: James C. Cloyd, Pharm.D.
University of Mississippi School of Pharmacy, University, MS: Alan B Jones, Ph.D.
University of Missouri-Kansas City School of Pharmacy, Kansas City, MO: William A. Watson, Pharm.D.
University of Montana School of Pharmacy and Allied Health Professions, Missoula, MT: Todd G. Cochran, Ph.D.
University of Nebraska College of Pharmacy, Omaha, NE: Clarence T. Ueda, Pharm D., Ph.D.
University of New Mexico College of Pharmacy, Albuquerque, NM: William M. Hadley, Ph.D.
University of North Carolina School of Pharmacy, Chapel Hill, NC: Richard J. Kowalsky, Pharm.D.
University of Oklahoma College of Pharmacy, Oklahoma City, OK: Loyd V. Allen, Jr., Ph.D.
University of Pittsburgh School of Pharmacy, Pittsburgh, PA: Dennis P. Swanson, M.S.
University of Puerto Rico, Medical Sciences Campus School of Pharmacy, San Juan, PR: Ilia I. Oquendo, Ph.D.
University of Rhode Island College of Pharmacy, Kingston, RI: Hossein Zia, Ph.D.
University of South Carolina College of Pharmacy, Columbia, SC: Bozena B. Michniak, Ph.D.
University of Southern California School of Pharmacy, Los Angeles, CA: Robert T. Koda, Pharm.D., Ph.D.
University of Tennessee College of Pharmacy, Memphis, TN: Dick R. Gourley, Pharm.D.
University of Texas College of Pharmacy, Austin, TX: James T. Doluisio, Ph.D.
University of the Pacific School of Pharmacy, Stockton, CA: Ravindra Vasavada, Ph.D.
University of Toledo College of Pharmacy, Toledo, OH: Paul W. Erhardt, Ph.D.
University of Utah College of Pharmacy, Salt Lake City, UT: David B. Roll, Ph.D.
University of Washington School of Pharmacy, Seattle, WA: Danny D. Shen, Ph.D.
University of Wisconsin School of Pharmacy, Madison, WI: Melvin H. Weinswig, Ph.D.
University of Wyoming School of Pharmacy, Laramie, WY: Kenneth F. Nelson, Ph.D.

Virginia Commonwealth University/Medical College of Virginia School of Pharmacy, Richmond, VA: Susanna Wu-Pong, Ph.D.
Washington State University College of Pharmacy, Pullman, WA: Mahmoud M. Abdel-Monem, Ph.D.
Wayne State University College of Pharmacy and Allied Health Professions, Detroit, MI: Craig K. Svenson, Pharm.D., Ph.D.
West Virginia University School of Pharmacy, Morgantown, WV: Arthur I. Jacknowitz, Pharm.D.
Western University of Health Sciences School of Pharmacy, Pomona, Ca: Krishna Kumar, Ph.D.
Wilkes University School of Pharmacy, Wilkes-Barre, PA: Arthur H. Kibbe, Ph.D.
Xavier University of Louisiana College of Pharmacy, New Orleans, LA: Merrill A. Patin, Pharm.D.

### State Pharmacy Associations
Alabama Pharmacy Association, Montgomery, AL: David L. Laven, R.Ph.
Alaska Pharmaceutical Association, Anchorage, AK: Barry D. Christensen, R.Ph.
Arizona Pharmacy Association, Tempe, AZ: Edward P. Armstrong, Ph.D.
Arkansas Pharmacists Association, Little Rock, AR: Leslee J. Falls, Pharm.D.
California Pharmacists Association, Sacramento, CA: R. David Lauper, Pharm.D.
Colegio de Farmaceuticos de Puerto Rico, San Juan, PR: Felix G. Mendez, R.Ph.
Colorado Pharmacists Association, Inc., Denver, CO: Thomas G. Arthur, R.Ph., M.S.A.
Connecticut Pharmacists Association, Rocky Hill, CT: Henry A. Palmer, Ph.D.
Delaware Pharmaceutical Society, Wilmington, DE: Kenneth Musto, Jr., R.Ph.
Florida Pharmacy Association, Tallahassee, FL: Michael A. Mone, B.S., J.D.
Georgia Pharmacy Association, Inc., Atlanta, GA: Larry L. Braden, R.Ph.
Hawaii Pharmaceutical Association, Honolulu, HI: Carolyn R. Otto, Pharm.D.
Illinois Pharmacists Association, Chicago, IL: Ronald Gottrich, R.Ph.
Iowa Pharmacists Association, Des Moines, IA: Lloyd E. Matheson, Ph.D.
Kansas Pharmacists Association, Topeka, KS: Ravi Gadi, Pharm.D., M.S.
Kentucky Pharmacists Association, Frankfort, KY: Robert L. Barnett, R.Ph.
Louisiana Pharmacists Association, Baton Rouge, LA: Christee G. Atwood
Maine Pharmacy Association, Bangor, ME: Stanley Stewart, R.Ph.
Maryland Pharmacists Association, Baltimore, MD: Matthew Shimoda, Pharm.D.
Massachusetts Pharmacists Association, Waltham, MA: Harold B. Sparr, R.Ph.
Michigan Pharmacists Association, Lansing, MI: Patrick L. McKercher, Ph.D.
Minnesota Pharmacists Association, St. Paul, MN: James K. Marttila, Pharm.D.
Mississippi Pharmacists Association, Jackson, MS: Dinah G. Jordan
Missouri Pharmacy Association, Jefferson City, MO: George L. Oestreich, R.Ph., M.P.A.
Montana State Pharmaceutical Association, Helena, MT: James Marmar, R.Ph.
Nebraska Pharmacists Association, Lincoln, NE: Leland C. Lucke
Nevada Pharmacists Association, Reno, NV: Herbert R. Bohner
New Hampshire Pharmacists Association, Concord, NH: Elizabeth A. Gower, R.Ph.
New Jersey Pharmacists Association, Robbinsville, NJ: Steven H. Zlotnick, Pharm.D.
North Dakota Pharmaceutical Association, Bismarck, ND: William J. Grosz, Sc.D.
Ohio Pharmacists Association, Dublin, OH: Amelia S. Bennett
Oklahoma Pharmaceutical Association, Oklahoma City, OK: Carl D. Lyons
Oregon State Pharmacists Association, Salem, OR: Charles F. Gress
Pennsylvania Pharmacists Association, Harrisburg, PA: Edward J. Bechtel, R.Ph.
Pharmaceutical Society of the State of New York, Albany, NY: Bruce Moden, R.Ph.
Rhode Island Pharmacists Association, Pawtucket, RI: Margot B. Kreplick, R.Ph.
South Carolina Pharmacy Association, Columbia, SC: James R. Bracewell
Tennessee Pharmacists Association, Nashville, TN: Roger L. Davis, Pharm.D.
Texas Pharmacy Association, Austin, TX: Eric H. Frankel, Pharm.D.
Utah Pharmaceutical Association, Orem, UT: C. Neil Jensen, R.Ph.
Vermont Pharmacists Association, Richmond, VT: Frederick H. Dobson III, Ph.D., R.Ph.
Virginia Pharmacy Association, Richmond, VA: Marianne R. Rollings, R.Ph.
Washington State Pharmacists Association, Renton, WA: Rodney D. Shafer, R.Ph.
Washington, D.C. Pharmaceutical Association, Washington, DC: James F. Harris, R.Ph.
Pharmacy Society of Wisconsin, Madison, WI: Judith E. Thompson, R.Ph., M.S.
Wyoming Pharmacists Association, Powell, WY: William H. Rathburn, R.Ph.

### National and State Professional and Scientific Organizations
Academy of Managed Care Pharmacy, Alexandria, VA: Darlene M. Mednick, R.Ph.
American Academy of Clinical Toxicology, Pittsburgh, PA: Edward P. Krenzclok, Pharm.D.
American Academy of Family Physicians, Washington, DC: Roger R. Tobias, M.D.
American Academy of Nurse Practitioners, Austin, TX: Jan Towers, Ph.D., NP-C
American Academy of Ophthalmology, San Francisco, CA: Joel S. Mindel, M.D., Ph.D.
American Academy of Pediatrics, Elk Grove Village, IL: Ralph E. Kauffman, M.D.
American Academy of Physician Assistants, Alexandria, VA: Greg P. Thomas, PA-C, M.P.H.
American Academy of Veterinary Pharmacology and Therapeutics, Mississippi State, MS: V. Cory Langston, D.V.M., Ph.D.; Diplomate, ACVCP
American Association of Colleges of Nursing, Washington, DC: Barbara A. Durand, Ed.D.
American Association of Colleges of Osteopathic Medicine, Chevy Chase, MD: Anthony J. Silvagni, D.O., Pharm.D.
American Association of Colleges of Pharmacy, Alexandria, Va: Richard P. Penna, Pharm.D.
American Association of Critical-Care Nurses, Aliso Viejo, CA: Barbara Johnston, Ph.D., R.N.
American Association of Dental Schools, Washington, DC: Gary E. Jeffers, D.M.D., M.S.
American Association of Pharmaceutical Scientists, Alexandria, Va: Richard A. Soltero, Ph.D.
American Association of Pharmacy Technicians, Inc., Greensboro, NC: Alice T. Foust
American Association of Poison Control Centers, Washington, DC: Toby L. Litovitz, M.D.
American Chemical Society, Washington, DC: Samuel M. Tuthill, Ph.D.
American College of Cardiology, Bethesda, MD: Bertram Pitt, M.D.
American College of Chest Physicians, Northbrook, IL: Irwin Ziment, M.D.
American College of Clinical Pharmacy, Kansas City, MO: Mary H.H. Ensom, Pharm.D.
American College of Obstetricians and Gynecologists, Washington, D.C.: Rudi Ansbacher, M.D.
American College of Radiology, Reston, Va: Bruce L. McClennan, M.D.
American College of Rheumatology, Atlanta, GA: Daniel E. Furst, M.D.
American Dental Association, Chicago, IL: Clifford W. Whall, Jr., Ph.D.
American Dietetic Association, Chicago, IL: Mary K. Russell, R.D., L.D.N., C.N.S.D.
American Geriatrics Society, New York, NY: Jerry Gurwitz, M.D.
American Medical Association, Chicago, IL: Joseph W. Cranston, Ph.D.
American Nurses Association, Inc. Washington, DC: Divina Grossman, Ph.D., R.N., ARNP, CS
American Optometric Association, St. Louis, MO: Jimmy D. Bartlett, O.D.
American Pharmaceutical Association, Washington, DC: Lowell J. Anderson
American Podiatric Medical Association, Bethesda, MD: Pamela J. Colman, DPM
American Psychiatric Association, Washington, DC: Deborah A. Zarin, M.D.
American Public Health Association, Washington, DC: J. Warren Salmon, Ph.D.
American Society for Clinical Pharmacology and Therapeutics, Norristown, PA: William J. Mroczek, M.D.
American Society for Parenteral and Enteral Nutrition, Silver Spring, MD: Jay Mirtallo, R.Ph.
American Society for Pharmacology and Experimental Therapeutics, Bethesda, MD: Kenneth L. Dretchen, Ph.D.
American Society for Quality Control, Milwaukee, WI: George L. Schorn, R.Ph.
American Society of Anesthesiologists, Park Ridge, IL: John R. Moyers, M.D.
American Society of Clinical Oncology, Alexandria, Va: Joseph S. Bailes, M.D.
American Society of Consultant Pharmacists, Alexandria, VA: Milton S. Moskowitz, R.Ph, FASCP
American Society of Health-System Pharmacists, Bethesda, MD: Charles E. Myers, M.S., M.B.A.
American Type Culture Collection, Rockville, MD: Raymond H. Cypess, D.V.M., Ph.D.
American Veterinary Medical Association, Schaumburg, IL: Jack W. Oliver, D.V.M., Ph.D.
AOAC International, Gaithersburg, MD: Thomas P. Layloff, Ph.D.
Association of American Veterinary Medical Colleges, Washington, DC: Curt J. Mann, D.V.M.
Drug Information Association, Ambler, PA: Judith Weissinger, Ph.D.
Federation of State Medical Boards, Euless, TX: Dale L. Austin, M.A.
Intravenous Nurses' Society, Cambridge, MA: Mary Alexander, CRNI
National Association of Boards of Pharmacy, Park Ridge, IL: Carmen A. Catizone, M.S., R.Ph.
National Community Pharmacists Association (formerly NARD), Alexandria, VA: Louis A. Mitchell, P.D.
National Pharmaceutical Association, Washington, DC: Barry Bleidt, Ph.D., Pharm.D., R.Ph.
Oncology Nursing Society, Pittsburgh, PA: Mary Garlick Roll, R.N., M.S.

### Governmental Bodies
Centers for Disease Control and Prevention, Atlanta, GA: John A. Becher
Department of Veterans Affairs Veterans Health Administration, Washington, DC: John E. Ogden
FDA Center for Biologics Evaluation and Research, Rockville, MD: Elaine C. Esber, M.D.
FDA Center for Devices and Radiological Health, Rockville, MD: Elizabeth D. Jacobson, Ph.D.
FDA Center for Drug Evaluation and Research, Rockville, MD: Roger L. Williams, M.D.
FDA Center for Veterinary Medicine, Rockville, MD: Richard H. Teske, D.V.M.
Health Canada, Tunney's Pasture, ON: Keith Bailey, D.Phil.
Health Care Financing Administration, Washington, DC: Grant Bagley, M.D.
Ministerio de Sanidad Y Consumo (Ministry of Health, Spain), Madrid, Spain: Federico Plaza, Farmaceutico
National Institute of Standards and Technology, Gaithersburg, MD: Thomas E. Gills
National Institutes of Health, Bethesda, MD: Joseph F. Gallelli, Ph.D.
Russian Center for Pharmaceutical and Medical Technical Information (PHARMEDINFO), Moscow, Russia: Galina Shashkova
Therapeutic Goods Administration of Australia, Woden, ACT: John Cable, Ph.D.
United States Agency for International Development, Washington, DC: Anthony Boni
United States Air Force, Andrews AFB, MD: James H. Young, BSPH/MSSM
United States Army Office of the Surgeon General, Falls Church, VA: Bruce A. Nelson, R.Ph.
United States Navy Bureau of Medicine and Surgery, Washington, DC: David R. Woker, R.Ph.

**Health Science and other Foreign Organizations and Pharmacopeias**
*Asociacion Farmaceutica Mexicana, A.C., Mexico, D.F.:* Jose Manuel Cardenas Gutierrez, O.F.B.
*Association of Faculties of Pharmacy of Canada, Vancouver, BC:* Dennis K.J. Gorecki, Ph.D.
*British Pharmacopoeia Commission, London, UK:* Robert C. Hutton, Ph.D.
*Canadian Association of University Schools of Nursing, Ottawa, ON:* Wendy McBride
*Canadian Nurses Association, Ottawa, ON:* Gladys Peachey, R.N., B.N., M.Ed., M.H.Sc.
*Canadian Pharmaceutical Association, Ottawa, ON:* Leroy C. Fevang, M.B.A.
*Committee on the Pharmacopeia of Japan, Tokyo, Japan:* Mitsuru Uchiyama, Ph.D.
*Department of the Quality of Medicines Council of Europe, Strasbourg, Cedex, France:* Agnes Artiges, Ph.D.
*Federation Internationale Pharmaceutique, Hague, The Netherlands:* Daan Crommelin, Ph.D.
*National Academy of Medicine (Academia Nacional de Medicina de Mexico), Colonia Doctores, Mex:* Fermin Valenzuela, M.D.
*Pan American Health Organization, Washington, DC:* Enrique Fefer, Ph.D.
*Permanent Commission of the Mexican United States Pharmacopeia, Mexico:* Q. Ma del Carmen Becerril, Chemist

**Consumer Organizations and Individuals Representing Public Interests**
*American Cancer Society, Atlanta, Ga:* Harmon J. Eyre, M.D.
*American Diabetes Association, Alexandria, VA:* Lawrence Blonde, M.D.
*American Heart Association, Dallas, TX:* Rodman D. Starke, M.D.
*Arthritis Foundation, Atlanta, GA:* Marianne H. Kaple, M.Ed.
*Asthma and Allergy Foundation of America, Washington, DC:* Mary E. Worstell, M.P.H.
*Center for Science in the Public Interest, Washington, DC:* Bonnie F. Liebman, M.S.
*Citizens for Public Action on Blood Pressure and Cholesterol, Inc., Bethesda, MD:* Gerald J. Wilson, M.A., M.B.A.
*Consumer's Union, Yonkers, NY:* Marvin M. Lipman, M.D.
*National Consumer's League, Washington, DC:* Brett M. Kay, M.P.P.
*National Organization for Rare Disorders, New Fairfield, CT:* Michael Langan

**Domestic, Foreign, and International Manufacturers, Trade, and Affiliated Associations**
*American Association of Health Plans, Washington, DC:* Clyde R. Cooper, Pharm.D.
*Animal Health Institute, Alexandria, Va:* Richard A. Carnevale, V.M.D.
*Council for Responsible Nutrition, Washington, DC:* V. Annette Dickinson, Ph.D.
*Generic Pharmaceutical Industry Association, Washington, DC:* Alice E. Till, Ph.D.
*Health Industry Manufacturers Association, Washington, DC:* Dee G. Simons, M.A.
*International Federation of Pharmaceutical Manufacturers Association, Geneva, Switzerland:* Richard Arnold, Ph.D.
*International Pharmaceutical Excipients Council, Wayne, NJ:* David R. Schoneker, M.S.
*Joint Commission on Accreditation of Healthcare Organizations, Oakbrook Terrace, IL:* Jerod M. Loeb, Ph.D.
*National Association of Pharmaceutical Manufacturers, Garden City, NY:* Loren R. Gelber, Ph.D.
*National Pharmaceutical Alliance, Alexandria, VA:* Gary L. Yingling, M.S., J.D.
*National Wholesale Druggists' Association, Reston, VA:* John M. Hammond
*Nonprescription Drug Manufacturers Association, Washington, DC:* R. William Soller, Ph.D.
*Nonprescription Drug Manufacturers Association of Canada, Ottawa, ON:* David S. Skinner
*Parenteral Drug Association, Bethesda, MD:* Russell E. Madsen, M.S.
*Pharmaceutical Research and Manufacturers of America, Washington, DC:* Maurice Q. Bectel, D.Sc.
*The Cosmetic, Toiletry and Fragrance Association, Washington, DC:* Gerald N. McEwen, Ph.D., J.D.
*The National Association of Chain Drug Stores, Alexandria, VA:* Leonard J. DeMino
*World Federation of Proprietary Medicine Manufacturers, London:* Jerome A. Reinstein, Ph.D.

**Members at Large**
Clement Bezold, Ph.D., Alexandria, VA
Lester Chafetz, Ph.D., Kansas City, MO
Thomas S. Foster, Pharm.D., Lexington, KY
Alan H. Kaplan, J.D., Washington, DC
Jay S. Keystone, M.D., Toronto, ON
Carol S. Marcus, Ph.D., M.D., Torrance, CA
Maurice L. Mashford, M.D., Parkville, Victoria
David Ofori-Adjei, M.D., FRCP, Accra, Ghana
Thomas F. Patton, Ph.D., St. Louis, MO
Gordon D. Schiff, M.D., Chicago, IL
Ralph F. Shangraw, Ph.D., Baltimore, MD
Robert E. Vestal, M.D., Boise, ID

**Ex Officio Members**
Donald R. Bennett, M.D., Ph.D., Downers Grove, IL
John V. Bergen, Ph.D., Wayne, PA
James C. Boylan, Ph.D., Abbott Park, IL
J. Richard Crout, M.D., Bethesda, MD
James T. Doluisio, Ph.D., Austin, TX
Arthur Hull Hayes, Jr., M.D., New Rochelle, NY

**Honorary Members**
George F. Archambault, Pharm.D., J.D., Bethesda, MD
William M. Heller, Ph.D., Stuart, FL
William J. Kinnard, Ph.D., Baltimore, MD
Frederick Mahaffey, Pharm.D., Bolivar, MO
Lloyd C. Miller, Ph.D., Escondidio, CA
John H. Moyer, M.D., D.Sc., Palmyra, PA
John A. Owen, Jr., M.D., Charlottesville, VA

**Committee Member(s)**
Eileen Hemphill, Washington, DC

# ABCIXIMAB  Systemic †

VA CLASSIFICATION (Primary/Secondary): BL170/CV900
Commonly used brand name(s): *ReoPro*.
Another commonly used name is c7E3 Fab.
Note: For a listing of dosage forms and brand names by country availability, see *Dosage Forms* section(s).

†Not commercially available in Canada.

## Category

Antithrombotic; monoclonal antibody (antithrombotic); platelet aggregation inhibitor.

## Indications

**Accepted**

Thrombosis, percutaneous coronary intervention–related (prophylaxis)—Abciximab is indicated as an adjunct to aspirin and heparin for the prevention of acute cardiac ischemic complications
• in patients undergoing percutaneous coronary intervention or
• in patients with unstable angina not responding to conventional medical therapy when percutaneous coronary intervention is planned within 24 hours.

## Pharmacology/Pharmacokinetics

**Physicochemical characteristics**
Source—Derived from the murine immunoglobulin $G_1$ monoclonal antibody, m7E3.
Molecular weight—Approximately 47,600 daltons.

**Mechanism of action/Effect**
Abciximab is a chimeric human-murine monoclonal antibody Fab (fragment antigen binding) fragment. It inhibits platelet aggregation by specifically binding to the glycoprotein GPIIb/IIIa receptor, the major surface receptor involved in the final common pathway for platelet aggregation. Inhibition of platelet aggregation occurs in a dose-dependent manner. Abciximab binding to the GPIIb/IIIa receptor prevents fibrinogen, von Willebrand factor, vitronectin, and other adhesive molecules from binding to the receptor, thereby inhibiting platelet aggregation. Abciximab is thought to block access of large molecules to the receptor by steric hindrance and/or conformational effects rather than interacting directly with the arginine-glycine-aspartic acid binding site of GPIIb/IIIa.

**Other actions/effects**
Abciximab may also bind to the vitronectin receptor and to the Mac-1 integrin receptor on activated monocytes. However, resulting clinical effects have not been identified.

**Half-life**
Cleared rapidly from plasma, with an initial phase half-life of less than 10 minutes and a second phase half-life of 30 minutes.

**Duration of action**
Platelet function generally recovers within 48 hours; however, low levels of GPIIb/IIIa receptor blockade are present for 15 days or more after discontinuation of the infusion.

**Elimination**
In general, Fab fragments are cleared more rapidly by the kidneys than are whole antibodies. Abciximab is probably catabolized in a manner similar to that of other natural proteins.

## Precautions to Consider

**Cross-sensitivity and/or related problems**
Patients with known sensitivity to murine monoclonal antibodies may also be sensitive to abciximab. Patients who develop human anti-chimeric antibody (HACA) titers after abciximab therapy may have allergic or hypersensitivity reactions when treated with other diagnostic or therapeutic monoclonal antibodies.

**Carcinogenicity**
Long-term studies evaluating the carcinogenic potential of abciximab have not been performed.

**Mutagenicity**
*In vitro* and *in vivo* mutagenicity studies have not demonstrated any mutagenic effect.

**Pregnancy/Reproduction**
Fertility—Studies evaluating abciximab's effect on fertility in male or female animals have not been done.
Pregnancy—Studies have not been done in humans.
Studies have not been done in animals.
FDA Pregnancy Category C.

**Breast-feeding**
It is not known whether abciximab is distributed into breast milk.

**Pediatrics**
No information is available on the relationship of age to the effects of abciximab in pediatric patients. Safety and efficacy have not been established.

**Geriatrics**
Early clinical data suggested there may be an increased risk of major bleeding in patients over 65 years of age. However, overall bleeding rates were reduced in the CAPTURE trial, and were reduced further in the EPILOG trial with modified dosing regimens and specific patient management techniques. Caution and attention to patient management are recommended.

**Drug interactions and/or related problems**
The following drug interactions and/or related problems have been selected on the basis of their potential clinical significance (possible mechanism in parentheses where appropriate)—not necessarily inclusive (» = major clinical significance):

Note: Combinations containing any of the following medications, depending on the amount present, may also interact with this medication.

» Anticoagulants, oral
 (administration within 7 days of abciximab is not recommended unless the prothrombin time is ≤ 1.2 times control because of the increased risk of bleeding)

Anti-inflammatory drugs, nonsteroidal or
Cefamandole or
Cefoperazone or
Cefotetan or
» Dipyridamole or
» Platelet aggregation inhibitors (see *Appendix II*) or
» Ticlopidine
 (concurrent use with abciximab may increase the risk of bleeding; caution is recommended during concurrent use)

» Dextran
 (concurrent or sequential use with abciximab may increase the risk of bleeding; concurrent use is not recommended)

» Thrombolytic agents
 (there are limited data evaluating the concurrent administration of abciximab with thrombolytic agents; because of the potential for bleeding, caution is recommended during concurrent or sequential use)

**Medical considerations/Contraindications**
The medical considerations/contraindications included have been selected on the basis of their potential clinical significance (reasons given in parentheses where appropriate)—not necessarily inclusive (» = major clinical significance).

*Except under special circumstances, this medication should not be used when the following medical problems exist:*

» Aneurysm, intracranial or
» Arteriovenous malformation, intracranial or
» Bleeding, active or
» Bleeding, gastrointestinal or genitourinary, recent (within 6 weeks) or
» Bleeding diathesis or
» Cerebrovascular accident (CVA), history of (within 2 years) or
» CVA with significant residual neurological deficit or
» Hypertension, severe, uncontrolled or
» Neoplasm, intracranial or
» Surgery, major, recent (within 6 weeks) or
» Thrombocytopenia (< 100,000 cells per microliter) or
» Trauma, major, recent (within 6 weeks) or
» Vasculitis, presumed or documented history of
 (increased risk of bleeding with abciximab)

*Risk-benefit should be considered when the following medical problems exist:*

» Age over 65 years or
» Gastrointestinal disease, history of or

» Weight < 75 kg
(increased risk of major bleeding with abciximab)
» Percutaneous coronary intervention, failed or
» Percutaneous coronary intervention, prolonged (lasting more than 70 minutes) or
» Percutaneous coronary intervention within 12 hours of the onset of symptoms of acute myocardial infarction
(increased risk of bleeding that may be additive to that of abciximab)
Sensitivity to abciximab or to murine proteins

**Patient monitoring**
The following may be especially important in patient monitoring (other tests may be warranted in some patients, depending on condition; » = major clinical significance):
» Activated clotting time (ACT)
(recommended during and following therapy; during percutaneous coronary intervention, the ACT should be maintained between 200 and 300 seconds; prior to arterial sheath removal, the ACT should be checked and should be ≤ 175 seconds before the sheath is removed)
» Activated partial thromboplastin time (APTT) and
» Prothrombin time (PT)
(recommended at baseline prior to initiation of abciximab therapy, during, and following therapy; when abciximab is initiated 18 to 24 hours before percutaneous coronary intervention, the APTT should be maintained between 60 and 85 seconds during the abciximab and heparin infusion period; if anticoagulation is continued following percutaneous coronary intervention, the APTT should be maintained between 60 and 85 seconds; prior to arterial sheath removal, the APTT should be checked and should be ≤ 50 seconds before the sheath is removed)
» Monitoring of potential bleeding sites
(careful attention to all potential bleeding sites, including catheter insertion sites, arterial and venous puncture sites, cutdown sites, needle puncture sites, and gastrointestinal, genitourinary, and retroperitoneal sites, is recommended)
» Platelet counts
(recommended at baseline prior to initiation of abciximab therapy, at 2 to 4 hours following the initial intravenous injection dose, and at 24 hours or prior to discharge, whichever is first. Additional platelet counts should be determined if a patient experiences an acute platelet decrease; if thrombocytopenia is verified, abciximab therapy should be discontinued immediately)

## Side/Adverse Effects

Note: Human anti-chimeric antibody (HACA) development may occur secondary to abciximab therapy. In the EPIC, EPILOG, and CAPTURE trials, positive HACA responses occurred in approximately 5.8% of the abciximab-treated patients. There was no excess hypersensitivity or allergic reactions related to abciximab treatment compared to placebo treatment. Patients who develop HACA titers may have allergic or hypersensitivity reactions when treated with other diagnostic or therapeutic monoclonal antibodies.

The following side/adverse effects have been selected on the basis of their potential clinical significance (possible signs and symptoms in parentheses where appropriate)—not necessarily inclusive:

**Those indicating need for medical attention**
Incidence more frequent
*Bleeding; hypotension*
Note: *Bleeding* was the most common complication of abciximab therapy in the EPIC trial in which heparin was used in a non–weight-adjusted, standard-dose regimen. Approximately 70% of abciximab-treated patients with *major bleeding* (intracranial hemorrhage or a decrease in hemoglobin concentration by more than 5 grams per dL) had bleeding at the arterial access site in the groin. An increased incidence of major bleeding from retroperitoneal, gastrointestinal, genitourinary, and other sites also occurred in abciximab-treated patients.

Bleeding rates were reduced in the CAPTURE trial, and were reduced further in the EPILOG trial with modified dosing regimens and specific patient management techniques (see *General Dosing Information*). In the EPILOG trial the incidence of *major bleeding* in patients treated with abciximab and low-dose, weight-adjusted heparin was not significantly different from that in patients receiving placebo.

If serious uncontrolled *bleeding* or the need for surgery occurs, abciximab should be discontinued. If platelet function does not return to normal, it may be partly restored with platelet transfusions.

Percutaneous coronary intervention within 12 hours of the onset of symptoms of acute myocardial infarction or prolonged or failed percutaneous coronary intervention may be associated in the angioplasty setting with an increased risk of *bleeding* that may be additive to that of abciximab.

*Hypotension* is often related to bleeding complications associated with abciximab.

Incidence less frequent
*Thrombocytopenia*
Note: In the EPIC trial, *thrombocytopenia* (< 100,000 platelets per microliter) and *severe thrombocytopenia* (< 50,000 platelets per microliter) occurred in 5.2% and 1.6%, respectively, of patients receiving an initial intravenous injection plus infusion of abciximab. The incidence of thrombocytopenia and requirement of platelet transfusions were lower in the subsequent CAPTURE and EPILOG trials.

Incidence rare
*Anemia; bradycardia; edema, peripheral; leukocytosis; pleural effusion or pleurisy; pneumonia*

**Those indicating need for medical attention only if they continue or are bothersome**
Incidence less frequent or rare
*Abnormal vision; confusion; hypesthesia; nausea; vomiting*

## General Dosing Information

The abciximab preparation for the initial intravenous injection should be administered with a syringe equipped with a sterile, nonpyrogenic, low–protein-binding 0.2- or 0.22-micrometer syringe filter. The abciximab preparation for continuous infusion should be filtered either upon its admixture using a sterile, nonpyrogenic, low–protein-binding 0.2- or 0.22-micrometer syringe filter, or upon its administration using an in-line, sterile, nonpyrogenic, low–protein-binding 0.2- or 0.22-micrometer filter.

Abciximab administration may result in human anti-chimeric antibody (HACA) formation. Therefore, readministration of abciximab may cause hypersensitivity reactions (including anaphylaxis), thrombocytopenia, or diminished benefit of abciximab. However, there are no data evaluating readministration of abciximab to patients who have developed a positive HACA response after its initial administration.

Hypersensitivity or anaphylaxis may occur at any time during abciximab administration.

**Patient management to reduce bleeding**
• Because of the risk of bleeding, arterial and venous punctures, intramuscular injections, and use of urinary catheters, nasotracheal tubes, nasogastric tubes, and automatic blood pressure cuffs should be minimized. Noncompressible sites, such as subclavian or jugular veins, should be avoided when obtaining intravenous access.
• If serious uncontrolled bleeding or the need for surgery occurs, abciximab should be discontinued. If platelet function does not return to normal, it may be partly restored with platelet transfusions.
• Since abciximab is associated with an increased bleeding rate, particularly at the site of arterial access for femoral sheath placement, care should be taken when attempting vascular access that only the anterior wall of the femoral artery is punctured, avoiding a Seldinger technique for obtaining sheath access. Femoral vein sheath placement is not recommended, unless needed. While the vascular sheath is in place, patients should be maintained on complete bed rest with the head of the bed placed at an angle of 30° or less and the affected limb kept in a straight position. Patients may be medicated for back or groin pain as necessary. Immediate discontinuation of heparin upon completion of the procedure and removal of the arterial sheath within 6 hours are strongly recommended, if the APTT is ≤ 50 seconds or the ACT is ≤ 175 seconds. In all cases, heparin should be discontinued at least 2 hours prior to arterial sheath removal. After the sheath is removed, pressure should be applied to the femoral artery for at least 30 minutes using either manual compression or a mechanical device for hemostasis. A pressure dressing should be applied following hemostasis and the patient maintained on bed rest for 6 to 8 hours following sheath removal or discontinuation of abciximab therapy, or 4 hours after heparin is discontinued, whichever is later. The pressure dressing should be removed prior to ambulation.
• The sheath insertion site and distal pulses of affected leg(s) should be checked frequently while the femoral artery sheath is in place and for 6 hours after the sheath is removed. Any hematoma should be measured and monitored for enlargement.

- Careful attention to all potential bleeding sites, including catheter insertion sites, arterial and venous puncture sites, cutdown sites, needle puncture sites, and gastrointestinal, genitourinary, and retroperitoneal sites, is recommended.

**Heparin anticoagulation**
Due to the high incidence of bleeding seen in the EPIC trial, the dosing regimens of concomitant heparin and the target levels for anticoagulation were successively varied in the CAPTURE and EPILOG trials. These modified dosing regimens, combined with other measures for patient management, were associated with reduced bleeding rates. For details of the anticoagulation regimens used in these trials, see the *ReoPro* package insert.

**For treatment of adverse effects**
Recommended treatment consists of the following
  For anaphylaxis
    • Stopping the infusion immediately.
    • Symptomatic and supportive treatment. Epinephrine, dopamine, theophylline, antihistamines, and corticosteroids should be readily available.
  For bleeding
    • Stopping the infusion immediately.
    • Symptomatic and supportive treatment.

## Parenteral Dosage Forms

### ABCIXIMAB INJECTION

**Usual adult dose**
Prophylaxis of percutaneous coronary intervention–related thrombosis—
  • In patients undergoing percutaneous coronary intervention:
    —Initial: Intravenous, 250 mcg (0.25 mg) per kg of body weight administered ten to sixty minutes prior to the start of percutaneous coronary intervention.
    —Maintenance: Intravenous infusion, 0.125 mcg per kg of body weight per minute (to a maximum of 10 mcg [0.01 mg] per minute) for twelve hours.
  • In patients with unstable angina not responding to conventional medical therapy when percutaneous coronary intervention is planned within 24 hours:
    —Initial: Intravenous, 250 mcg (0.25 mg) per kg of body weight.
    —Maintenance: Intravenous infusion, 10 mcg (0.01 mg) per minute for eighteen to twenty-four hours, concluding one hour after the percutaneous coronary intervention.

Note: Abciximab has been studied only with concomitant administration with heparin and aspirin.
The continuous infusion of abciximab should be stopped in cases of failed percutaneous coronary intervention, since there is no evidence for the efficacy of abciximab in that setting.
If serious bleeding that cannot be controlled by compression occurs, abciximab and heparin should be discontinued immediately.

**Usual pediatric dose**
Safety and efficacy have not been established.

**Strength(s) usually available**
U.S.—
  2 mg per mL (single-use 5-mL vials) (Rx) [*ReoPro* (buffered solution of 0.01 molar sodium phosphate; 0.15 molar sodium chloride; 0.001% polysorbate 80 in Water for Injection)].
Canada—
  Not commercially available.

**Packaging and storage**
Store at 2 to 8 °C (36 to 46 °F). Protect from freezing.

**Preparation of dosage form**
For the intravenous infusion solution, the necessary amount of abciximab should be added to an appropriate amount of 0.9% sodium chloride injection or 5% dextrose injection and infused at the calculated flow rate using a continuous infusion pump.

**Stability**
Discard any unused portion of the infusion solution.

**Incompatibilities**
Abciximab should be administered through a separate intravenous line. No other medications should be added to the infusion solution.

**Auxiliary labeling**
• Do not shake.

## Selected Bibliography

The EPILOG Investigators. Platelet glycoprotein IIb/IIIa receptor blockade and low dose heparin during percutaneous coronary revascularization. N Engl J Med 1997; 336: 1689-96.
The CAPTURE Investigators. Randomised placebo-controlled trial of abciximab before, during and after coronary intervention in refractory unstable angina: the CAPTURE study. Lancet 1997; 349: 1429-35.

Developed: 07/05/95
Interim revision: 02/20/98

---

# ACARBOSE   Systemic—INTRODUCTORY VERSION

VA CLASSIFICATION (Primary): HS504
Commonly used brand name(s): *Precose*.
Note: For a listing of dosage forms and brand names by country availability, see *Dosage Forms* section(s).

## Category
Antidiabetic agent.

## Indications

**Accepted**
Diabetes, type 2 (treatment)—Acarbose is indicated as adjunctive therapy to diet in the treatment of patients with type 2 diabetes (previously referred to as non–insulin-dependent diabetes mellitus [NIDDM]) whose blood glucose cannot be controlled by diet alone. It may be used as monotherapy or in combination with a sulfonylurea.

## Pharmacology/Pharmacokinetics

**Physicochemical characteristics**
Source—Acarbose is an oligosaccharide obtained from fermentation processes of the microorganism *Actinoplanes utahensis*.
Molecular weight—645.6.
pKa—5.1.

**Mechanism of action/Effect**
Acarbose lowers postprandial blood glucose concentrations in patients with diabetes by competitive, reversible inhibition of pancreatic alpha-amylase and membrane-bound intestinal alpha-glucoside hydrolases. These enzymes inhibit hydrolysis of complex starches to oligosaccharides in the lumen of the small intestine and hydrolysis of oligosaccharides, trisaccharides, and disaccharides to glucose and other monosaccharides in the brush border of the small intestine. Acarbose does not enhance insulin secretion and, when used as monotherapy, should not cause hypoglycemia.

**Other actions/effects**
Although the antihyperglycemic effect of acarbose is additive to that of sulfonylureas (which act via a different mechanism), acarbose decreases the insulinotropic and weight-increasing effects of sulfonylureas when used concurrently.
Acarbose does not inhibit lactase and would not be expected to cause lactose intolerance.

**Absorption**
Studies with radiolabeled acarbose indicate that less than 2% of an oral dose is absorbed in active form. Because the medication acts within the gastrointestinal tract, low systemic bioavailability is therapeutically desirable. However, approximately 35% of a dose is absorbed on a delayed basis, probably as metabolites formed in the gastrointestinal tract.

**Biotransformation**
Gastrointestinal, primarily by intestinal bacteria and, to a lesser extent, by digestive enzymes. At least 13 metabolites have been identified. One of these, formed by cleavage of a glucose molecule from acarbose, has alpha-glucosidase inhibitory activity. Other major metabolites are primarily sulfate, methyl, and glucuronide conjugates.

**Half-life**
Approximately 2 hours.

**Time to peak concentration**
In plasma:
  Acarbose: 1 hour.
  Metabolites: 14 to 24 hours.

**Elimination**
Fecal, as unabsorbed acarbose, approximately 51% of an oral dose within 96 hours.
Renal, approximately 34% of an oral dose as absorbed metabolites. Less than 2% of an oral dose is excreted in the urine as acarbose and its active metabolite.

## Precautions to Consider

### Carcinogenicity/Tumorigenicity
Up to 500 mg per kg of body weight (mg/kg) of acarbose administered orally to Sprague-Dawley rats for 104 weeks resulted in a significant increase in the incidence of renal adenomas and adenocarcinomas and benign Leydig cell tumors. The study was repeated with similar results. However, an increase in renal tumors did not occur in Sprague-Dawley rats when carbohydrate malnutrition was prevented by glucose supplementation or by administration of acarbose by daily postprandial gavage. Also, no evidence of tumorigenicity or carcinogenicity was found in two studies in Wistar rats receiving acarbose by postprandial gavage or two studies in hamsters given oral acarbose with or without glucose supplementation.

### Mutagenicity
No evidence of mutagenicity was noted in six *in vitro* and in three *in vivo* assays.

### Pregnancy/Reproduction
Fertility—Oral administration of acarbose to rats produced no impairment of fertility or overall reproductive capacity.

Pregnancy—Adequate and well-controlled studies have not been done in humans, and safety has not been established. Insulin is usually recommended for pregnant patients with diabetes.

Animal studies failed to show an adverse effect on the fetus in rats given up to 480 mg/kg (approximately 9 times the human exposure, based on blood concentrations) or in rabbits given up to 32 times the human dose (based on body surface area). In rabbit studies, high doses of acarbose caused a reduction in maternal weight gain, which may have been responsible for a slight increase in embryonic losses. However, no embryotoxicity occurred in rabbits given 160 mg/kg (corresponding to 10 times the human dose, based on body surface area).

FDA Pregnancy Category B.

### Breast-feeding
It is not known whether acarbose is distributed into human breast milk. In animal studies, administration of radiolabeled acarbose resulted in detection of a small quantity of radioactivity in the milk of lactating rats. Acarbose is not recommended for use by nursing women.

### Pediatrics
Safety and efficacy in pediatric patients have not been established.

### Geriatrics
In pharmacokinetic studies, maximum plasma concentrations of acarbose and the area under the acarbose concentration–time curve (AUC) were approximately 1.5 times higher in geriatric individuals than in younger adults, but the differences were not statistically significant.

### Drug interactions and/or related problems
The following drug interactions and/or related problems have been selected on the basis of their potential clinical significance (possible mechanism in parentheses where appropriate)—not necessarily inclusive (» = major clinical significance):

Note: Combinations containing any of the following medications, depending on the amount present, may also interact with this medication.

» Adsorbents, intestinal, such as activated charcoal or
» Digestive enzyme preparations containing carbohydrate-splitting enzymes, such as amylase or pancreatin
  (these medications may decrease the efficacy of acarbose; concurrent use is not recommended)

Antidiabetic agents, other
  (antihyperglycemic effects of acarbose are additive to those of other antidiabetic agents; although this effect is used for therapeutic benefit, the risk of hypoglycemia may be increased with concurrent use; a reduction in dosage of the other antidiabetic agent may be necessary)

Hyperglycemia-inducing medications, such as:
  Calcium channel blocking agents
  Corticosteroids
  Diuretics, especially thiazide diuretics
  Estrogens
  Estrogen and progestin–containing oral contraceptives
  Isoniazid
  Niacin
  Phenothiazines
  Phenytoin
  Sympathomimetic agents
  Thyroid hormones
    (these agents may cause loss of glycemic control; patients should be monitored for evidence of hyperglycemia and the dosage of the antidiabetic agent adjusted if necessary; also, patients receiving combined therapy with acarbose and another antidiabetic agent should be monitored for evidence of hypoglycemia after treatment with one of these agents is discontinued)

### Laboratory value alterations
The following have been selected on the basis of their potential clinical significance (possible effect in parentheses where appropriate)—not necessarily inclusive (» = major clinical significance):

With physiology/laboratory test values
  Bilirubin, serum
    (elevations have been reported rarely)

  Transaminases, serum
    (transaminase elevations occurred in 15% of acarbose-treated patients in clinical trials; in patients receiving a total of 150 to 300 mg of acarbose a day, elevations did not occur more often than in placebo controls, but elevations to more than three times the upper limit of normal occurred two to three times more often in patients receiving more than 300 mg per day than in placebo controls. The elevations were more common in female patients, reversible, and not associated with other evidence of liver injury. In postmarketing surveillance of more than 500,000 patients, 19 cases of transaminase elevations to 500 IU per L or higher have been reported, 12 of which were associated with jaundice. Of these 19 patients, 15 had been receiving total doses of 300 mg or more of acarbose per day, and 13 of the 16 patients for whom weights were reported weighed less than 60 kg. Hepatic abnormalities improved or resolved after treatment was discontinued in the 18 patients for whom follow-up information is available)

### Medical considerations/Contraindications
The medical considerations/contraindications included have been selected on the basis of their potential clinical significance (reasons given in parentheses where appropriate)—not necessarily inclusive (» = major clinical significance).

*Except under special circumstances, this medication should not be used when the following medical problems exist:*

» Diabetic ketoacidosis
» Hepatic cirrhosis
    (acarbose may cause transaminase elevations and, rarely, jaundice)

Intestinal disorders, including:
» Chronic conditions leading to marked disorders of absorption or digestion
» Conditions that would be affected adversely by increased intestinal gas formation
» Inflammatory or ulcerative intestinal disease
» Obstructive intestinal disease or predisposition to
» Renal function impairment, severe (serum creatinine higher than 2 mg/dL)
    (although long-term studies in patients with severe renal function impairment have not been done, use of acarbose is not recommended; pharmacokinetic studies have shown that plasma concentrations of acarbose increase in proportion to the degree of renal function impairment, with maximum concentrations being approximately five times higher and the area under the acarbose concentration–time curve [AUC] being approximately six times higher in patients with creatinine clearances of less than 25 mL per minute per 1.73 square meters of body surface area than in patients with normal renal function)

*Risk-benefit should be considered when the following medical problems exist:*

Fever or
Infection or
Surgery or
Trauma
  (these conditions may cause loss of glycemic control; temporary insulin therapy may be necessary)

Sensitivity to acarbose

### Patient monitoring

The following may be especially important in patient monitoring (other tests may be warranted in some patients, depending on condition; » = major clinical significance):

» Glucose concentrations, blood and/or urine
(monitoring essential as a guide to efficacy of treatment)

» Glycosylated hemoglobin determinations
(recommended at 3-month intervals for monitoring long-term glycemic control)

» Transaminase values
(monitoring recommended at 3-month intervals during the first year of treatment and periodically thereafter; a reduction of acarbose dosage or discontinuation of therapy may be necessary, especially if elevations persist)

## Side/Adverse Effects

The following side/adverse effects have been selected on the basis of their potential clinical significance (possible signs and symptoms in parentheses where appropriate)—not necessarily inclusive:

**Those indicating need for medical attention**
Incidence rare
*Jaundice* (yellow eyes or skin)

**Those indicating need for medical attention only if they continue or are bothersome**
Incidence more frequent
*Abdominal pain*—incidence 21%; *diarrhea*—incidence 33%; *flatulence* (bloated feeling or passing of gas)—incidence 77%

Note: These effects are related to the presence of undigested carbohydrates in the lower gastrointestinal tract, a result of acarbose's mechanism of action. In clinical trials, *abdominal pain* and *diarrhea* tended to return to pretreatment levels, and the frequency and severity of *flatulence* tended to abate, over time. Rarely, gastrointestinal effects may be severe enough to be confused with paralytic ileus.

## Overdose

For more information on the management of overdose or unintentional ingestion, **contact a Poison Control Center** (see *Poison Control Center Listing*).

**Clinical effects of overdose**
The most likely effects are increases in abdominal discomfort, diarrhea, and flatulence, which should subside without treatment. Hypoglycemia should not occur with an overdose of acarbose alone, but may occur if the patient is receiving combined therapy with other antidiabetic agents.

## Patient Consultation

As an aid to patient consultation, refer to *Advice for the Patient, Acarbose (Systemic)—Introductory Version*.
In providing consultation, consider emphasizing the following selected information (» = major clinical significance):

**Before using this medication**
» Conditions affecting use, especially:
  Sensitivity to acarbose
  Pregnancy—Insulin is usually recommended
  Breast-feeding—Use of acarbose is not recommended
  Other medications, especially digestive enzyme preparations, or intestinal adsorbents
  Other medical problems, especially diabetic ketoacidosis, hepatic cirrhosis, intestinal disorders, or renal function impairment

**Proper use of this medication**
» Importance of adherence to recommended regimens for diet, exercise, and glucose monitoring
» Taking medication at the beginning of each main meal
» Proper dosing
  Missed dose (if meal completed without having taken medication): Skipping missed dose; taking next dose with next meal; not doubling doses
» Proper storage

**Precautions while using this medication**
» Regular visits to physician to check progress
» *Carefully following special instructions of health care team*
  Discussing use of alcohol and tobacco
  Not taking other medications unless discussed with physician
  Getting counseling for family members to help them assist the diabetic patient; also, special counseling for pregnancy planning and contraception
  Making travel plans to include preparedness for diabetic emergencies and keeping meal times near the usual times with changing time zones
» Preparing for and understanding what to do in case of emergency; carrying medical history and current medication list and wearing medical identification
» Recognizing what brings on symptoms of hypoglycemia, such as using other antidiabetic medication; delaying or missing a meal; exercising more than usual; drinking significant amounts of alcohol; illness, including vomiting or diarrhea
» Recognizing symptoms of hypoglycemia: anxiety; behavior change similar to drunkenness; blurred vision; cold sweats; confusion; cool, pale skin; difficulty in concentrating; drowsiness; excessive hunger; fast heartbeat; headache; nausea; nervousness; nightmares; restless sleep; shakiness; slurred speech; and unusual tiredness or weakness
» Knowing what to do if symptoms of hypoglycemia occur, such as ingesting a source of dextrose (not sucrose) or, if severe, injecting glucagon
» Recognizing what brings on symptoms of hyperglycemia, such as not taking enough or skipping a dose of antidiabetic medication, overeating or not following meal plan, fever or infection, exercising less than usual
» Recognizing symptoms of hyperglycemia and ketoacidosis: blurred vision; drowsiness; dry mouth; flushed, dry skin; fruit-like breath odor; increased urination (frequency and volume); ketones in urine; loss of appetite; stomachache, nausea, or vomiting; tiredness; troubled breathing (rapid and deep); unconsciousness; unusual thirst
» Knowing what to do if symptoms of hyperglycemia occur, such as checking blood glucose and contacting a member of the health care team

**Side/adverse effects**
Signs of potential side effects, especially jaundice

## General Dosing Information

Dosage must be individualized on the basis of 1-hour postprandial blood glucose determinations and patient tolerance. The goal of treatment is to reduce postprandial plasma glucose concentrations and glycosylated hemoglobin concentrations to normal or near normal using the lowest effective dose of acarbose, alone or in conjunction with a sulfonylurea.

Starting treatment with a low dose that is increased gradually to the maximally effective dose is recommended to reduce gastrointestinal side effects as well as to facilitate identification of the lowest effective dose for the individual patient.

Acarbose is taken three times a day, at the beginning (with the first bite) of each main meal.

**For treatment of hypoglycemia**
Hypoglycemia should not occur as a result of acarbose monotherapy, but may occur during combined therapy with a sulfonylurea or insulin. Because acarbose inhibits hydrolysis of sucrose to glucose and fructose, sucrose is not recommended for treatment of mild to moderate hypoglycemia in acarbose-treated patients. A simple sugar, such as dextrose (glucose), should be ingested instead. Intravenous infusion of dextrose or administration of glucagon may be required for severe hypoglycemia.

## Oral Dosage Forms

### ACARBOSE TABLETS

**Usual adult dose**
Antidiabetic agent—
Oral, 25 mg three times a day, at the start of each main meal. Dosage may be adjusted, at four- to eight-week intervals, first to 50 mg three times a day, then, if necessary and appropriate, to 100 mg three times a day.

Note: If an increase in dosage to 100 mg three times a day fails to produce a further reduction in postprandial glucose concentration, consideration should be given to lowering the dose.

**Usual adult prescribing limits**
Antidiabetic agent—
Patients weighing 60 kg or less: 50 mg three times a day.
Patients weighing more than 60 kg: 100 mg three times a day.

**Usual pediatric dose**
Safety and efficacy have not been established.

**Usual geriatric dose**
Antidiabetic agent—
See *Usual adult dose*.

**Usual geriatric prescribing limits**
Antidiabetic agent—
See *Usual adult prescribing limits*.

**Strength(s) usually available**
U.S.—
  50 mg (Rx) [*Precose* (scored; starch; microcrystalline cellulose; magnesium stearate; colloidal silicon dioxide)].
  100 mg (Rx) [*Precose* (starch; microcrystalline cellulose; magnesium stearate; colloidal silicon dioxide)].

**Packaging and storage**
Store below 25 °C (77 °F), protected from moisture, unless otherwise directed by manufacturer.

Revised: 07/31/98

**ACEBUTOLOL**—See *Beta-adrenergic Blocking Agents (Systemic)*

# ACETAMINOPHEN  Systemic

INN:  Paracetamol
VA CLASSIFICATION (Primary/Secondary): CN103/CN850

Note:  For information on acetaminophen combinations that are used for antacid as well as analgesic effects, see *Acetaminophen, Sodium Bicarbonate, and Citric Acid (Systemic)*.

Commonly used brand name(s): *Abenol; Aceta Elixir; Aceta Tablets; Acetaminophen Uniserts; Actamin; Actamin Extra; Actamin Super; Actimol Chewable Tablets; Actimol Children's Suspension; Actimol Infants' Suspension; Actimol Junior Strength Caplets; Aminofen; Aminofen Max; Anacin-3; Anacin-3 Extra Strength; Apacet Capsules; Apacet Elixir; Apacet Extra Strength Caplets; Apacet Extra Strength Tablets; Apacet Regular Strength Tablets; Apacet, Infants'; Apo-Acetaminophen; Aspirin Free Anacin Maximum Strength Caplets; Aspirin Free Anacin Maximum Strength Gel Caplets; Aspirin Free Anacin Maximum Strength Tablets; Aspirin-Free Excedrin Caplets; Atasol Caplets; Atasol Drops; Atasol Forte Caplets; Atasol Forte Tablets; Atasol Oral Solution; Atasol Tablets; Banesin; Bayer Select Maximum Strength Headache Pain Relief Formula; Dapa; Dapa X-S; Datril Extra-Strength; Excedrin Caplets; Excedrin Extra Strength Caplets; Exdol; Exdol Strong; Feverall Junior Strength; Feverall Sprinkle Caps Junior Strength; Feverall Sprinkle Caps, Children's; Feverall, Children's; Feverall, Infants'; Genapap Children's Elixir; Genapap Children's Tablets; Genapap Extra Strength Caplets; Genapap Extra Strength Tablets; Genapap Regular Strength Tablets; Genapap, Infants'; Genebs Extra Strength Caplets; Genebs Regular Strength Tablets; Genebs X-Tra; Liquiprin Children's Elixir; Liquiprin Infants' Drops; Neopap; Oraphen-PD; Panadol; Panadol Extra Strength; Panadol Junior Strength Caplets; Panadol Maximum Strength Caplets; Panadol Maximum Strength Tablets; Panadol, Children's; Panadol, Infants'; Phenaphen Caplets; Redutemp; Robigesic; Rounox; Snaplets-FR; St. Joseph Aspirin-Free Fever Reducer for Children; Suppap-120; Suppap-325; Suppap-650; Tapanol Extra Strength Caplets; Tapanol Extra Strength Tablets; Tempra; Tempra Caplets; Tempra Chewable Tablets; Tempra D.S; Tempra Drops; Tempra Syrup; Tempra, Infants'; Tylenol Caplets; Tylenol Children's Chewable Tablets; Tylenol Children's Elixir; Tylenol Children's Suspension Liquid; Tylenol Drops; Tylenol Elixir; Tylenol Extra Strength Adult Liquid Pain Reliever; Tylenol Extra Strength Caplets; Tylenol Extra Strength Gelcaps; Tylenol Extra Strength Tablets; Tylenol Gelcaps; Tylenol Infants' Drops; Tylenol Infants' Suspension Drops; Tylenol Junior Strength Caplets; Tylenol Junior Strength Chewable Tablets; Tylenol Regular Strength Caplets; Tylenol Regular Strength Tablets; Tylenol Tablets; Valorin; Valorin Extra.*

Other commonly used names are APAP and paracetamol.

Note:  For a listing of dosage forms and brand names by country availability, see *Dosage Forms* section(s).

## Category
Analgesic; antipyretic.

## Indications

**Accepted**
Pain (treatment);
Pain, arthritic, mild (treatment); or
Fever (treatment)—Acetaminophen is indicated to relieve mild to moderate pain and reduce fever. It provides symptomatic relief only; additional therapy to treat the cause of the pain or fever should be instituted when necessary.

  Acetaminophen has minimal anti-inflammatory activity and does not relieve redness, swelling, or stiffness due to arthritis; it cannot be used in place of aspirin or other salicylates or other nonsteroidal anti-inflammatory drugs (NSAIDs) in the treatment of rheumatoid arthritis. However, it may be used to relieve pain due to mild osteoarthritis.

  Acetaminophen may be used when aspirin therapy is contraindicated or inadvisable, e.g., in patients receiving anticoagulants or uricosuric agents, patients with hemophilia or other bleeding problems, and those with upper gastrointestinal disease or intolerance or hypersensitivity to aspirin. However, chronic, high-dose acetaminophen therapy may require adjustment of anticoagulant dosage based on increased monitoring of prothrombin time in patients receiving a coumarin- or indandione-derivative anticoagulant.

Note:  The FDA has proposed that caffeine (present as an analgesic adjuvant in some products) be classified as a Category III ingredient (i.e., lacking documentation of efficacy) in OTC products containing acetaminophen as the sole analgesic/antipyretic agent.

## Pharmacology/Pharmacokinetics

**Physicochemical characteristics**
Molecular weight—151.16.

**Mechanism of action/Effect**
*For acetaminophen—*
  Analgesic:
    The mechanism of analgesic action has not been fully determined. Acetaminophen may act predominantly by inhibiting prostaglandin synthesis in the central nervous system (CNS) and, to a lesser extent, through a peripheral action by blocking pain-impulse generation. The peripheral action may also be due to inhibition of prostaglandin synthesis or to inhibition of the synthesis or actions of other substances that sensitize pain receptors to mechanical or chemical stimulation.
  Antipyretic:
    Acetaminophen probably produces antipyresis by acting centrally on the hypothalamic heat-regulating center to produce peripheral vasodilation resulting in increased blood flow through the skin, sweating, and heat loss. The central action probably involves inhibition of prostaglandin synthesis in the hypothalamus.
*For caffeine—*
  Caffeine is a mild CNS stimulant. Caffeine-induced constriction of cerebral blood vessels, which leads to a decrease in cerebral blood flow and in the oxygen tension of the brain, may contribute to relief of some types of headache.
  It has been suggested that the addition of caffeine to acetaminophen may provide a more rapid onset of action and/or enhanced pain relief with lower doses of the analgesic. However, the FDA has determined that studies performed to date have not demonstrated that caffeine is an effective analgesic adjuvant or that it does not interfere with acetaminophen's efficacy as an antipyretic.

**Absorption**
Oral—Rapid and almost complete; may be decreased if acetaminophen is taken following a high-carbohydrate meal.
Rectal—The rate and extent of absorption from the suppository dosage form may vary, depending on the composition of the base.

**Distribution**
In breast milk—Peak concentrations of 10 to 15 mcg per mL (66.2 to 99.3 micromoles/L) have been measured 1 to 2 hours following maternal ingestion of a single 650-mg dose. The half-life in breast milk is 1.35 to 3.5 hours.

**Protein binding**
Not significant with doses producing plasma concentrations below 60 mcg per mL (397.2 micromoles/L); may reach moderate levels with high or toxic doses.

**Biotransformation**
Approximately 90 to 95% of a dose is metabolized in the liver, primarily by conjugation with glucuronic acid, sulfuric acid, and cysteine. An intermediate metabolite, which may accumulate in overdosage after the primary metabolic pathways become saturated, is hepatotoxic and possibly nephrotoxic.

**Half-life**
1 to 4 hours; does not change with renal failure but may be prolonged in acute overdosage, in some forms of hepatic disease, in the elderly, and in the neonate; may be somewhat shortened in children.

**Time to peak concentration**
0.5 to 2 hours

**Peak plasma concentration**
5 to 20 mcg per mL (33.1 to 132.4 micromoles/L), with doses up to 650 mg.

**Time to peak effect**
1 to 3 hours

**Duration of action**
3 to 4 hours

**Elimination**
Renal, as metabolites, primarily conjugates; 3% of a dose may be excreted unchanged.
In dialysis—
  Hemodialysis: 120 mL per minute (for unmetabolized drug); metabolites are also cleared rapidly.
  Hemoperfusion: 200 mL per minute.
  Peritoneal dialysis: <10 mL per minute.

## Precautions to Consider

### Cross-sensitivity and/or related problems
Patients sensitive to aspirin may not be sensitive to acetaminophen; however, mild bronchospastic reactions with acetaminophen have been reported in some aspirin-sensitive asthmatics (less than 5% of those tested).

### Pregnancy/Reproduction
Fertility—Chronic toxicity studies in animals have shown that high doses of acetaminophen cause testicular atrophy and inhibition of spermatogenesis; the relevance of this finding to use in humans is not known.

Pregnancy—Problems in humans have not been documented. Although controlled studies have not been done, it has been shown that acetaminophen crosses the placenta.

### Breast-feeding
Problems in humans have not been documented. Although peak concentrations of 10 to 15 mcg per mL (66.2 to 99.3 micromoles/L) have been measured in breast milk 1 to 2 hours following maternal ingestion of a single 650-mg dose, neither acetaminophen nor its metabolites were detected in the urine of the nursing infants. The half-life in breast milk is 1.35 to 3.5 hours.

### Pediatrics
Studies performed to date have not demonstrated pediatrics-specific problems that would limit the usefulness of acetaminophen in children. However, some products intended for pediatric use contain aspartame, which is metabolized to phenylalanine, and must be used with caution, if at all, in children with phenylketonuria.

### Geriatrics
Appropriate studies performed to date have not demonstrated geriatrics-specific problems that would limit the usefulness of acetaminophen in the elderly.

### Drug interactions and/or related problems
The following drug interactions and/or related problems have been selected on the basis of their potential clinical significance (possible mechanism in parentheses where appropriate)—not necessarily inclusive (» = major clinical significance):

Note: Combinations containing any of the following medications, depending on the amount present, may also interact with this medication.

*For acetaminophen*
» Alcohol, especially chronic abuse of or
  Hepatic enzyme inducers (See *Appendix II*) or
  Hepatotoxic medications, other (See *Appendix II*)
    (risk of hepatotoxicity with single toxic doses or prolonged use of high doses of acetaminophen may be increased in alcoholics or in patients regularly taking other hepatotoxic medications or hepatic enzyme inducers)
    (chronic use of barbiturates [except butalbital] or primidone has been reported to decrease the therapeutic effects of acetaminophen, probably because of increased metabolism resulting from induction of hepatic microsomal enzyme activity; the possibility should be considered that similar effects may occur with other hepatic enzyme inducers)

Anticoagulants, coumarin- or indandione-derivative
  (concurrent chronic, high-dose administration of acetaminophen may increase the anticoagulant effect, possibly by decreasing hepatic synthesis of procoagulant factors; anticoagulant dosage adjustment based on increased monitoring of prothrombin time may be necessary when chronic, high-dose acetaminophen therapy is initiated or discontinued; however, this does not apply to occasional use, or to chronic use of doses below 2 grams per day, of acetaminophen)

Anti-inflammatory drugs, nonsteroidal (NSAIDs) or
Aspirin or other salicylates
  (prolonged concurrent use of acetaminophen and a salicylate is not recommended because recent evidence suggests that chronic, high-dose administration of the combined analgesics [1.35 grams daily, or cumulative ingestion of 1 kg annually, for 3 years or longer] significantly increases the risk of analgesic nephropathy, renal papillary necrosis, end-stage renal disease, and cancer of the kidney or urinary bladder; also, it is recommended that for short-term use, the combined dose of acetaminophen plus salicylate not exceed that recommended for acetaminophen or a salicylate given alone)
  (prolonged concurrent use of acetaminophen and NSAIDs other than aspirin may also increase the risk of adverse renal effects; it is recommended that patients be under close medical supervision while receiving such combined therapy)
  (diflunisal may increase the plasma concentration of acetaminophen by 50%, leading to increased risk of acetaminophen-induced hepatotoxicity)

*For formulations containing caffeine (in addition to those interactions listed above)*
CNS stimulation–producing medications, other (See *Appendix II*)
  (concurrent use with caffeine may result in excessive CNS stimulation, leading to unwanted effects such as nervousness, irritability, insomnia, or possibly convulsions or cardiac arrhythmias; close observation is recommended)

Lithium
  (caffeine increases urinary excretion of lithium, and may thereby reduce its therapeutic effect)

Monoamine oxidase (MAO) inhibitors, including furazolidone, procarbazine, and selegiline
  (the sympathomimetic side effects of caffeine may produce dangerous cardiac arrhythmias or severe hypertension when large doses of caffeine are used concurrently with MAO inhibitors)

### Laboratory value alterations
The following have been selected on the basis of their potential clinical significance (possible effect in parentheses where appropriate)—not necessarily inclusive (» = major clinical significance):

With diagnostic test results
  Glucose, blood, determinations
    (acetaminophen may cause falsely decreased values when the glucose oxidase/peroxidase method is used, but probably not when the hexokinase/glucose-6-phosphate dehydrogenase [G6PD] method is used)
    (values may be falsely increased when certain instruments are used in glucose analysis if high acetaminophen concentrations are present; instrument manufacturer's instruction manual should be consulted)

  5-Hydroxyindoleacetic acid (5-HIAA), serum, determinations
    (acetaminophen may cause false-positive results in qualitative screening tests using nitrosonaphthol reagent; the quantitative test is unaffected)

  Myocardial perfusion imaging, radionuclide, when adenosine or dipyridamole is used as an adjunct to the radiopharmaceutical
    (the caffeine in specific formulations may reverse the effects of adenosine or dipyridamole on myocardial blood flow, thereby interfering with test results; patients should be advised to avoid caffeine for 8 to 12 hours prior to the test)

  Pancreatic function test using bentiromide
    (administration of acetaminophen prior to the bentiromide test will invalidate test results because acetaminophen is also metabolized to an arylamine and will thus increase the apparent quantity of para-aminobenzoic acid [PABA] recovered; it is recommended that

# 8  Acetaminophen (Systemic)

acetaminophen be discontinued at least 3 days prior to administration of bentiromide)

Uric acid, serum, determinations
(acetaminophen may cause falsely increased values when the phosphotungstate uric acid test method is used)

With physiology/laboratory test values
Bilirubin concentrations, serum and
Lactate dehydrogenase activity, serum and
Prothrombin time and
Transaminase activity, serum
(may be increased, indicating hepatotoxicity, especially in alcoholics, patients taking other hepatic enzyme inducers, or patients with pre-existing hepatic disease, when single toxic doses [>8 to 10 grams] of acetaminophen are taken or prolonged use of lower doses [>3 to 5 grams a day])

**Medical considerations/Contraindications**
The medical considerations/contraindications included have been selected on the basis of their potential clinical significance (reasons given in parentheses where appropriate)—not necessarily inclusive (» = major clinical significance):

*Risk-benefit should be considered when the following medical problems exist:*

» Alcoholism, active or
» Hepatic disease or
» Viral hepatitis
(increased risk of hepatotoxicity)

Phenylketonuria
(products that contain aspartame, which is metabolized to phenylalanine, may be hazardous to patients with phenylketonuria, especially young children; caution is recommended)

Renal function impairment, severe
(risk of adverse renal effects may be increased with prolonged use of high doses; occasional use is acceptable)

Sensitivity to acetaminophen or aspirin
(increased risk of allergic reaction)

**Patient monitoring**
The following may be especially important in patient monitoring (other tests may be warranted in some patients, depending on condition; » = major clinical significance):

Hepatic function determinations
(may be required at periodic intervals during high-dose or long-term therapy, especially in patients with pre-existing hepatic disease)

## Side/Adverse Effects

The following side/adverse effects have been selected on the basis of their potential clinical significance (possible signs and symptoms in parentheses where appropriate)—not necessarily inclusive:

**Those indicating need for medical attention**
Incidence rare
*Agranulocytosis* (fever with or without chills; sores, ulcers or white spots on lips or in mouth; sore throat); *anemia* (unusual tiredness or weakness); *dermatitis, allergic* (skin rash, hives or itching); *hepatitis* (yellow eyes or skin); *renal colic* (pain, severe and/or sharp, in lower back and/or side)—with prolonged use of high doses in patients with severe renal function impairment; *renal failure* (sudden decrease in amount of urine); *sterile pyuria* (cloudy urine); *thrombocytopenia* (rarely, unusual bleeding or bruising; black, tarry stools; blood in urine or stools; pinpoint red spots on skin)—usually asymptomatic

Note: Acetaminophen-induced *renal function impairment* may be sufficiently severe to result in *uremia*, especially with prolonged use of high doses in patients with pre-existing renal impairment. Also, although a causal association has not been established, a retrospective study has suggested that long-term daily use of acetaminophen may be associated with an increased risk of *chronic renal failure* (analgesic nephropathy) in individuals without pre-existing renal function impairment.

## Overdose

For specific information on the agents used in the management of acetaminophen overdose, see:
• *Acetylcysteine (Systemic)* monograph; and/or
• *Charcoal, Activated (Oral-Local)* monograph.

For more information on the management of overdose or unintentional ingestion, **contact a Poison Control Center** (see *Poison Control Center Listing*).

**Clinical effects of overdose**
The following effects have been selected on the basis of their potential clinical significance (possible signs and symptoms in parentheses where appropriate)—not necessarily inclusive:

Acute
*Gastrointestinal upset* (diarrhea, loss of appetite, nausea or vomiting, stomach cramps or pain); *increased sweating*

Note: Although *gastrointestinal upset* and *increased sweating* often do not occur, they sometimes occur within 6 to 14 hours after ingestion of an overdose and persist for about 24 hours.

Chronic
*Hepatotoxicity* (pain, tenderness, and/or swelling in upper abdominal area)—may occur 2 to 4 days after the overdose is ingested

Note: The first indications of overdosage may be signs and symptoms of possible *liver damage* and abnormalities in liver function tests, which may not occur until 2 to 4 days after ingestion of the overdose. Maximal changes in liver function tests usually occur 3 to 5 days after ingestion of the overdose.

Overt *hepatic disease or failure* may occur 4 to 6 days after ingestion of the overdose. *Hepatic encephalopathy* (with mental changes, confusion, agitation, or stupor), *convulsions, respiratory depression, coma, cerebral edema, coagulation defects, gastrointestinal bleeding, disseminated intravascular coagulation, hypoglycemia, metabolic acidosis, cardiac arrhythmias,* and *cardiovascular collapse* may occur.

*Renal tubular necrosis* leading to *renal failure* (signs may include bloody or cloudy urine and sudden decrease in amount of urine) has also been reported in acetaminophen overdose, usually, but not exclusively, in conjunction with acetaminophen-induced *hepatotoxicity*.

**Treatment of overdose**
To decrease absorption—May include emptying the stomach via induction of emesis or gastric lavage.

Removing activated charcoal (if used) by gastric lavage may be advisable. Although activated charcoal is recommended in cases of mixed drug overdose, it may interfere with absorption of orally administered acetylcysteine (antidote used to protect against acetaminophen-induced hepatotoxicity) and decrease its efficacy.

To enhance elimination—Instituting hemodialysis or hemoperfusion to remove acetaminophen from the circulation may be beneficial if acetylcysteine administration cannot be instituted within 24 hours following ingestion of a massive acetaminophen overdose. However, the efficacy of such treatment in preventing acetaminophen-induced hepatotoxicity is not known.

Specific treatment—Use of acetylcysteine. *It is recommended that acetylcysteine administration be instituted as soon as possible after ingestion of an overdose has been reported,* without waiting for the results of plasma acetaminophen determinations or other laboratory tests. Acetylcysteine is most effective if treatment is started within 10 to 12 hours after ingestion of the overdose; however it may be of some benefit if treatment is started within 24 hours. See the package insert or *Acetylcysteine (Systemic)* monograph for specific dosing guidelines for use of this product.

Monitoring—May include determining plasma acetaminophen concentration at least 4 hours following ingestion of the overdose. Determinations performed prior to this time are not reliable for assessing potential hepatotoxicity. Initial plasma concentrations above 150 mcg per mL (993 micromoles/L) at 4 hours, 100 mcg per mL (662 micromoles/L) at 6 hours, 70 mcg per mL (463.4 micromoles/L) at 8 hours, 50 mcg per mL (331 micromoles/L) at 10 hours, 20 mcg per mL (132.4 micromoles/L) at 15 hours, 8 mcg per mL (53 micromoles/L) at 20 hours, or 3.5 mcg per mL (23.2 micromoles/L) at 24 hours postingestion indicate possible hepatotoxicity and the need for completing the full course of acetylcysteine treatment. If the initial determination indicates a plasma concentration below those listed at the times indicated, cessation of acetylcysteine therapy can be considered. However, some clinicians advise that more than one determination should be performed to ascertain peak absorption and half-life of acetaminophen prior to considering discontinuation of acetylcysteine.

Performing liver function tests (serum aspartate aminotransferase [AST; SGOT], serum alanine aminotransferase [ALT; SGPT], prothrombin time, and bilirubin) at 24-hour intervals for at least 96 hours postingestion if the plasma acetaminophen concentration indicates potential hepatotoxicity. If no abnormalities are detected within 96 hours, further determinations are not needed.

Monitoring renal and cardiac function and administering appropriate therapy as required.

Supportive care—May include maintaining fluid and electrolyte balance, correcting hypoglycemia, and administering vitamin $K_1$ (if prothrombin time ratio exceeds 1.5) and fresh frozen plasma or clotting factor concentrate (if prothrombin time ratio exceeds 3.0). Patients in whom intentional overdose is known or suspected should be referred for psychiatric consultation.

## Patient Consultation

As an aid to patient consultation, refer to *Advice for the Patient, Acetaminophen (Systemic)*.

In providing consultation, consider emphasizing the following selected information (» = major clinical significance):

**Before using this medication**
» Conditions affecting use, especially:
    Sensitivity to acetaminophen or aspirin
    Use in children—Aspartame-containing chewable tablets must be used with caution, if at all, in children with phenylketonuria
    Other medical problems, especially alcoholism (active), hepatic disease, or viral hepatitis

**Proper use of this medication**
» Importance of not taking more medication than the amount recommended because acetaminophen may cause kidney or liver damage with long-term use or greater-than-recommended doses
» Unless otherwise directed by physician, children should not receive more than 5 doses per day
» *Proper administration of:*
    Acetaminophen oral granules
    Acetaminophen oral powders
    Acetaminophen suppositories
» Proper dosing
» Proper storage

**Precautions while using this medication**
Regular visits to physician to check progress if long-term therapy is prescribed
Checking with physician because additional treatment may be needed:
    —if taking for pain, including arthritic pain, and pain persists for longer than 10 days for adults or 5 days for children, condition becomes worse, new symptoms occur, or the painful area is red or swollen
    —if taking for fever, and fever persists for longer than 3 days, condition becomes worse, or new symptoms occur
    —if taking for sore throat, and sore throat is severe, persists for longer than 2 days, or occurs together with or is followed by fever, headache, rash, nausea, or vomiting
» Risk of overdose if other medications containing acetaminophen are used
» Avoiding use of alcohol if taking more than an occasional 1 or 2 doses of this medication; increased risk of liver toxicity, especially in alcoholics, with high doses or prolonged use
Not using a salicylate or a nonsteroidal anti-inflammatory drug together with acetaminophen for more than a few days, unless directed by physician
Possible interference with some laboratory tests; preferably discussing use of the medication with physician in charge 3 to 4 days ahead of time; if this is not possible, informing physician in charge if acetaminophen taken within the past 3 or 4 days
Diabetics: Possible false results with blood glucose tests; checking with physician, nurse, or pharmacist if changes in test results noted
Not taking caffeine-containing formulations for 8 to 12 hours prior to adenosine- or dipyridamole-assisted myocardial perfusion imaging test
» Suspected overdose: Getting emergency help at once even if no symptoms apparent; symptoms of severe overdosage may be delayed, but treatment must be begun as soon as possible; treatment started 24 hours or more after the overdose may be ineffective in preventing liver damage or fatality

**Side/adverse effects**
Signs and symptoms of potential side effects, especially adverse renal effects, allergic dermatitis, hepatotoxicity, agranulocytosis, and thrombocytopenia

## General Dosing Information

The doses are based on the FDA's proposed labeling requirements for over-the-counter (OTC) internal analgesic, antipyretic, and antirheumatic products. The dosage unit of 80 mg (1.23 grains) is used for pediatric doses; the dosage unit of 325 mg (5 grains) is used for adult doses. The conversion factor of 1 grain equal to 65 mg is used. The doses recommended by manufacturers of individual products, and the strengths of individual products, may not conform to the recommended doses.

One retrospective study has suggested that long-term daily use of acetaminophen may be associated with an increased risk of chronic renal disease (analgesic nephropathy). The results of this study are not considered conclusive, and further investigation is required to establish a causal association. However, until more definitive information is available, prolonged daily administration of acetaminophen should probably be limited to patients who are receiving appropriate medical supervision.

## Oral Dosage Forms

### ACETAMINOPHEN CAPSULES USP

**Usual adult and adolescent dose**
Analgesic and
Antipyretic—
    Oral, 325 to 500 mg every three hours, 325 to 650 mg every four hours, or 650 mg to 1 gram every six hours as needed, while symptoms persist.

Note: For patient self-medication, it is recommended that a physician be consulted if pain is not relieved within ten days, fever within three days, or sore throat within two days.

**Usual adult prescribing limits**
For short-term therapy (up to ten days)—Up to 4 grams daily.
For long-term therapy—Up to 2.6 grams daily, unless chronic treatment with higher doses is prescribed and monitored by a physician.

**Usual pediatric dose**
Analgesic and
Antipyretic—
    Oral, 1.5 grams per square meter of body surface a day in divided doses; or for
    Infants up to 3 months of age—Oral, 40 mg every four hours as needed.
    Infants 4 to 12 months of age—Oral, 80 mg every four hours as needed.
    Children 1 to 2 years of age—Oral, 120 mg every four hours as needed.
    Children 2 to 4 years of age—Oral, 160 mg every four hours as needed, while symptoms persist.
    Children 4 to 6 years of age—Oral, 240 mg every four hours as needed, while symptoms persist.
    Children 6 to 9 years of age—Oral, 320 mg every four hours as needed, while symptoms persist.
    Children 9 to 11 years of age—Oral, 320 to 400 mg every four hours as needed, while symptoms persist.
    Children 11 to 12 years of age—Oral, 320 to 480 mg every four hours as needed, while symptoms persist.

Note: It is recommended that children up to 12 years of age receive no more than five doses in each twenty-four-hour period, unless otherwise directed by a physician, and that a physician be consulted if pain is not relieved within five days, fever within three days, or sore throat within two days.

Dosage recommendations for children younger than 2 years of age do not appear on OTC packaging.

Administration of an individual product to a pediatric patient depends upon ability to achieve suitable dosage for the age of the child. Liquid dosage forms (oral solution or suspension), granules, powders, or chewable tablets are usually used.

**Strength(s) usually available**
U.S.—
    325 mg (OTC) [GENERIC].
    500 mg (OTC) [*Apacet Capsules; Dapa X-S;* GENERIC].
Canada—
    Not commercially available.

**Packaging and storage**
Store below 40 °C (104 °F), preferably between 15 and 30 °C (59 and 86 °F), unless otherwise specified by manufacturer. Store in a tight container.

**Auxiliary labeling**
• Avoid alcoholic beverages.

### ACETAMINOPHEN ORAL GRANULES

**Usual adult and adolescent dose**
See *Acetaminophen Capsules USP*.

**Usual pediatric dose**
See *Acetaminophen Capsules USP*.

**Strength(s) usually available**
U.S.—
    80 mg (in individual packets) (OTC) [*Snaplets-FR*].
Canada—
    Not commercially available.

**Packaging and storage**
Store below 40 °C (104 °F), preferably between 15 and 30 °C (59 and 86 °F), unless otherwise specified by manufacturer.

**Preparation of dosage form**
Single dose—The contents of the packets are to be mixed with a small quantity of soft food, such as applesauce, ice cream, or jam immediately prior to ingestion.

### ACETAMINOPHEN ORAL POWDERS

**Usual adult and adolescent dose**
See *Acetaminophen Capsules USP*.

**Usual pediatric dose**
See *Acetaminophen Capsules USP*.

**Strength(s) usually available**
U.S.—
  80 mg (in capsules) (OTC) [*Feverall Sprinkle Caps, Children's*].
  160 mg (in capsules) (OTC) [*Feverall Sprinkle Caps Junior Strength*].
Canada—
  Not commercially available.

**Packaging and storage**
Store below 40 °C (104 °F), preferably between 15 and 30 °C (59 and 86 °F), unless otherwise specified by manufacturer.

**Preparation of dosage form**
Single dose—The capsules are not intended to be swallowed whole. They are to be opened and the contents sprinkled over a small quantity (< 5 mL) of water or other liquid immediately prior to ingestion. Alternatively, the contents of the capsules may be mixed with a small quantity of soft food, such as applesauce, ice cream, or jam, immediately prior to ingestion.

### ACETAMINOPHEN ORAL SOLUTION USP

**Usual adult and adolescent dose**
See *Acetaminophen Capsules USP*.

**Usual adult prescribing limits**
See *Acetaminophen Capsules USP*.

**Usual pediatric dose**
See *Acetaminophen Capsules USP*.

**Strength(s) usually available**
U.S.—
  100 mg per mL (80 mg per 0.8-mL dropperful) (OTC) [*Apacet, Infants'; Genapap, Infants'; Panadol, Infants'; St. Joseph Aspirin-Free Fever Reducer for Children; Tempra, Infants'; Tylenol Infants' Drops*; GENERIC].
  80 mg per 5 mL (OTC) [GENERIC].
  120 mg per 5 mL (OTC) [*Aceta Elixir* (alcohol 7%); *Oraphen-PD* (alcohol 5%); GENERIC].
  130 mg per 5 mL (OTC) [GENERIC].
  160 mg per 5 mL (OTC) [*Apacet Elixir; Genapap Children's Elixir; Liquiprin Children's Elixir; Panadol, Children's; St. Joseph Aspirin-Free Fever Reducer for Children; Tempra Syrup; Tylenol Children's Elixir* (sugar); GENERIC].
  Note: Also available generically in unit-dose cups containing 325 mg per 10.15 mL and 650 mg per 20.3 mL.
  500 mg per 15 mL (OTC) [*Tylenol Extra Strength Adult Liquid Pain Reliever* (alcohol 7%)].
Canada—
  80 mg per mL (OTC) [*Atasol Drops; Panadol; Tempra Drops* (alcohol 10%); *Tylenol Drops*; GENERIC].
  80 mg per 5 mL (OTC) [*Atasol Oral Solution; Panadol* (sodium); *Robigesic* (alcohol 8.5%); *Tempra Syrup*].
  160 mg per 5 mL (OTC) [*Tempra Syrup; Tylenol Elixir*; GENERIC].
Note: The strengths of specific products may not conform to some of the recommended pediatric dosages.

**Packaging and storage**
Store below 40 °C (104 °F), preferably between 15 and 30 °C (59 and 86 °F), unless otherwise specified by manufacturer. Store in a tight container. Protect from freezing.

**Auxiliary labeling**
• Avoid alcoholic beverages.

### ACETAMINOPHEN ORAL SUSPENSION USP

**Usual adult and adolescent dose**
See *Acetaminophen Capsules USP*.

**Usual pediatric dose**
See *Acetaminophen Capsules USP*.

**Strength(s) usually available**
U.S.—
  48 mg per mL (120 mg per 2.5-mL dropperful) (OTC) [*Liquiprin Infants' Drops*].
  100 mg per mL (80 mL per 0.8-mL dropperful) (OTC) [*Tylenol Infants' Suspension Drops*].
  160 mg per 5 mL (OTC) [*Tylenol Children's Suspension Liquid*].
Canada—
  80 mg per mL (OTC) [*Actimol Infants' Suspension*].
  80 mg per 5 mL (OTC) [*Actimol Children's Suspension*].

**Packaging and storage**
Store below 40 °C (104 °F), preferably between 15 and 30 °C (59 and 86 °F), unless otherwise specified by manufacturer. Store in a tight container. Protect from freezing.

**Auxiliary labeling**
• Shake well.

### ACETAMINOPHEN TABLETS USP

**Usual adult and adolescent dose**
See *Acetaminophen Capsules USP*.

**Usual adult prescribing limits**
See *Acetaminophen Capsules USP*.

**Usual pediatric dose**
See *Acetaminophen Capsules USP*.

**Strength(s) usually available**
U.S.—
  120 mg (OTC) [GENERIC].
  160 mg (OTC) [*Panadol Junior Strength Caplets; Tylenol Junior Strength Caplets* (scored)].
  325 mg (OTC) [*Aceta Tablets; Actamin; Aminofen; Apacet Regular Strength Tablets; Dapa; Genapap Regular Strength Tablets; Genebs Regular Strength Tablets; Phenaphen Caplets; Tylenol Regular Strength Caplets; Tylenol Regular Strength Tablets* (scored); *Valorin*; GENERIC].
  Note: In Canada, *Phenaphen* is available as capsules containing aspirin (ASA) and phenobarbital.
  500 mg (OTC) [*Aceta Tablets; Actamin Extra; Aminofen Max; Apacet Extra Strength Caplets; Apacet Extra Strength Tablets; Aspirin Free Anacin Maximum Strength Caplets; Aspirin Free Anacin Maximum Strength Gel Caplets; Aspirin Free Anacin Maximum Strength Tablets; Banesin; Datril Extra-Strength; Genapap Extra Strength Caplets; Genapap Extra Strength Tablets; Genebs Extra Strength Caplets; Genebs X-Tra; Panadol Maximum Strength Caplets; Panadol Maximum Strength Tablets; Redutemp; Tapanol Extra Strength Caplets; Tapanol Extra Strength Tablets; Tylenol Extra Strength Caplets; Tylenol Extra Strength Gelcaps; Tylenol Extra Strength Tablets; Valorin Extra*; GENERIC].
  650 mg (OTC) [GENERIC].
Canada—
  160 mg (OTC) [*Actimol Junior Strength Caplets* (scored); *Tempra Caplets; Tylenol Junior Strength Caplets*].
  325 mg (OTC) [*Anacin-3; Apo-Acetaminophen* (scored); *Atasol Caplets* (scored); *Atasol Tablets* (scored); *Exdol* (scored); *Panadol; Robigesic* (scored); *Rounox; Tylenol Caplets; Tylenol Tablets*; GENERIC].
  500 mg (OTC) [*Anacin-3 Extra Strength; Apo-Acetaminophen* (scored); *Atasol Forte Caplets; Atasol Forte Tablets* (scored); *Exdol Strong* (scored); *Panadol Extra Strength; Tylenol Caplets; Tylenol Gelcaps; Tylenol Tablets*; GENERIC].

**Packaging and storage**
Store below 40 °C (104 °F), preferably between 15 and 30 °C (59 and 86 °F), unless otherwise specified by manufacturer. Store in a tight container.

**Auxiliary labeling**
• Avoid alcoholic beverages.

### ACETAMINOPHEN TABLETS (CHEWABLE) USP

**Usual adult and adolescent dose**
See *Acetaminophen Capsules USP*.

**Usual pediatric dose**
See *Acetaminophen Capsules USP*.

**Strength(s) usually available**
U.S.—
  80 mg (OTC) [*Genapap Children's Tablets; Panadol, Children's* (scored); *St. Joseph Aspirin-Free Fever Reducer for Children; Tempra; Tylenol Children's Chewable Tablets* (scored); GENERIC].
  120 mg (OTC) [GENERIC].

160 mg (OTC) [*Tempra D.S* (scored); *Tylenol Junior Strength Chewable Tablets* (scored)].
Canada—
80 mg (OTC) [*Actimol Chewable Tablets*; *Panadol* (scored); *Tempra Chewable Tablets*; *Tylenol Children's Chewable Tablets* (scored); GENERIC].
160 mg (OTC) [*Tempra Chewable Tablets*].

### Packaging and storage
Store below 40 °C (104 °F), preferably between 15 and 30 °C (59 and 86 °F), unless otherwise specified by manufacturer. Store in a tight container.

### Auxiliary labeling
- Avoid alcoholic beverages.
- May be chewed.

## ACETAMINOPHEN AND CAFFEINE TABLETS USP

### Usual adult and adolescent dose
See *Acetaminophen Capsules USP*. Dosage is based on acetaminophen only.

### Usual adult prescribing limits
See *Acetaminophen Capsules USP*. Dosage is based on acetaminophen only.

### Usual pediatric dose
See *Acetaminophen Capsules USP*. Dosage is based on acetaminophen only.

### Strength(s) usually available
U.S.—
500 mg of acetaminophen and 65 mg of caffeine (OTC) [*Aspirin-Free Excedrin Caplets*; *Bayer Select Maximum Strength Headache Pain Relief Formula*].
500 mg of acetaminophen and 65.4 mg of caffeine (OTC) [*Actamin Super*].
Canada—
325 mg of acetaminophen and 65 mg of caffeine (OTC) [*Excedrin Caplets*].
500 mg of acetaminophen and 65 mg of caffeine (OTC) [*Excedrin Extra Strength Caplets*].
Note: In the U.S., *Excedrin* contains aspirin, in addition to acetaminophen and caffeine. See *Acetaminophen and Salicylates (Systemic)*. The U.S. product corresponding to the Canadian *Excedrin* formulation is *Aspirin-Free Excedrin*.

### Packaging and storage
Store below 40 °C (104 °F), preferably between 15 and 30 °C (59 and 86 °F), unless otherwise specified by manufacturer.

### Auxiliary labeling
- Avoid alcoholic beverages.

## Rectal Dosage Forms

## ACETAMINOPHEN SUPPOSITORIES USP

### Usual adult and adolescent dose
Analgesic and Antipyretic—
Rectal, 325 to 500 mg every three hours, 325 to 650 mg every four hours, or 650 mg to 1 gram every six hours as needed, while symptoms persist.

Note: For patient self-medication, it is recommended that a physician be consulted if pain is not relieved within ten days, fever within three days, or sore throat within two days.

### Usual adult prescribing limits
For short-term therapy (up to ten days)—Up to 4 grams daily.
For long-term therapy—Up to 2.6 grams daily, unless chronic treatment with higher doses is prescribed and monitored by a physician.

### Usual pediatric dose
Analgesic and Antipyretic—
Rectal, 1.5 grams per square meter of body surface a day in divided doses; or for
Children up to 2 years of age—Dosage must be individualized by physician.
Children 2 to 4 years of age—Rectal, 160 mg every four hours as needed, while symptoms persist.
Children 4 to 6 years of age—Rectal, 240 mg every four hours as needed, while symptoms persist.
Children 6 to 9 years of age—Rectal, 320 mg every four hours as needed, while symptoms persist.
Children 9 to 11 years of age—Rectal, 320 to 400 mg every four hours as needed, while symptoms persist.
Children 11 to 12 years of age—Rectal, 320 to 480 mg every four hours as needed, while symptoms persist.
Note: It is recommended that children up to 12 years of age receive no more than five doses in each twenty-four-hour period, unless otherwise directed by a physician, and that a physician be consulted if pain is not relieved within five days, fever within three days, or sore throat within two days.

### Strength(s) usually available
U.S.—
80 mg (OTC) [*Feverall, Infants'*].
120 mg (OTC) [*Acetaminophen Uniserts*; *Feverall, Children's*; *Neopap* (scored); *Suppap-120*; GENERIC].
300 mg (OTC) [GENERIC].
325 mg (OTC) [*Acetaminophen Uniserts*; *Feverall Junior Strength*; *Suppap-325*].
650 mg (OTC) [*Acetaminophen Uniserts*; *Suppap-650*; GENERIC].
Canada—
120 mg (OTC) [*Abenol*].
325 mg (OTC) [*Abenol*].
650 mg (OTC) [*Abenol*].
Note: The strengths of the specific products may not conform to the recommended pediatric doses.

### Packaging and storage
Store below 40 °C (104 °F), preferably between 15 and 30 °C (59 and 86 °F), in a well-closed container, unless otherwise specified by manufacturer. Protect from freezing.

### Auxiliary labeling
- Avoid alcoholic beverages.

Revised: 07/12/94

# ACETAMINOPHEN AND SALICYLATES  Systemic

This monograph includes information on the following: 1) Acetaminophen and Aspirin; 2) Acetaminophen, Aspirin, and Salicylamide; 3) Acetaminophen and Salicylamide.

INN: Acetaminophen—Paracetamol

VA CLASSIFICATION (Primary/Secondary): CN103/CN850

Commonly used brand name(s): *Buffets II*[1]; *Duoprin*[3]; *Duradyne*[1]; *Excedrin Extra-Strength Caplets*[1]; *Excedrin Extra-Strength Tablets*[1]; *Gelpirin*[1]; *Gemnisyn*[1]; *Goody's Extra Strength Tablets*[1]; *Goody's Headache Powders*[1]; *Presalin*[2]; *Rid-A-Pain Compound*[3]; *S-A-C*[3]; *Saleto*[2]; *Supac*[1]; *Tri-Pain Caplets*[2]; *Vanquish Caplets*[1].

NOTE: The *Acetaminophen and Salicylates (Systemic)* monograph is maintained on the USP DI electronic data base. For a printed copy of the most recent revision of the complete monograph, contact Micromedex, Inc. - Reprint Requests, 6200 S. Syracuse Way, Suite 300, Englewood, CO 80111; telephone (303) 486-6400; telefax (303) 486-6464; Email: USPDI@MDX.COM.

For information on the specific components of this combination, see the *USP DI* monographs for *Acetaminophen (Systemic)*, *Caffeine (Systemic)*, and *Salicylates (Systemic)*.

The information that follows is selectively abstracted from the complete monograph and is provided to facilitate drug use review and patient counseling.

Note: For a listing of dosage forms and brand names by country availability, see *Dosage Forms* section(s).

## Category
Analgesic; antipyretic.

## Indications

### Accepted
Pain (treatment)
Pain, arthritic, mild (treatment) or

Fever (treatment)—Acetaminophen and salicylate combinations are indicated to relieve mild to moderate pain and reduce fever. Salicylamide is less effective than acetaminophen or aspirin. These medications provide only symptomatic relief; additional therapy to treat the cause of the pain or fever should be instituted when necessary.

Acetaminophen and salicylate combinations are indicated to provide temporary relief of pain caused by mild inflammation or arthritis. Although acetaminophen may be effective in relieving pain caused by mild osteoarthritis, it has minimal anti-inflammatory activity. Salicylamide also has minimal anti-inflammatory activity. Therefore, efficacy in relieving pain caused by inflammation or arthritis may depend upon the quantity of aspirin present in the individual product.

Note: The FDA has proposed that salicylamide be classified as a Category III ingredient (i.e., lacking documentation of efficacy) in OTC analgesic/antipyretic products.

## Unaccepted

Acetaminophen and salicylate combinations are not recommended for the treatment of severe inflammation or severe arthritic pain, or for long-term treatment of chronic arthritis. Achieving and maintaining therapeutically effective salicylate plasma concentrations may require ingestion of undesirably large daily doses of other ingredients present in these formulations. Also, prolonged high-dose administration of these combinations is not recommended because of the risk of analgesic nephropathy.

## Patient Consultation

As an aid to patient consultation, refer to *Advice for the Patient, Acetaminophen and Salicylates (Systemic)*.

In providing consultation, consider emphasizing the following selected information (» = major clinical significance):

### Before using this medication
» Conditions affecting use, especially:
  Sensitivity to acetaminophen, aspirin, or nonsteroidal anti-inflammatory drugs (NSAIDs)
  Pregnancy—Not taking aspirin in third trimester unless prescribed by physician; high-dose chronic use or abuse of aspirin in third trimester may be hazardous to the mother as well as the fetus and/or neonate, causing heart problems in fetus or neonate and/or bleeding in mother, fetus, or neonate; high-dose chronic use or abuse may also prolong and complicate labor and delivery; large quantities of caffeine may cause arrhythmias and growth retardation in the fetus
  Use in children—Checking with physician before giving a salicylate to children with symptoms of acute febrile illness, especially influenza or varicella, because of the risk of Reye's syndrome; also, increased susceptibility to aspirin toxicity in children, especially with fever and dehydration
  Use in teenagers—Checking with physician before giving a salicylate to teenagers with symptoms of acute febrile illness, especially influenza or varicella, because of the risk of Reye's syndrome
  Use in the elderly—Increased risk of aspirin toxicity and of combination analgesic–induced adverse renal effects
  Other medications, especially anticoagulants, antidiabetic agents (oral), those cephalosporins that may cause hypoprothrombinemia, methotrexate, NSAIDs, platelet aggregation inhibitors, plicamycin, probenecid, sulfinpyrazone, and urinary alkalizers and, for buffered formulations, fluoroquinolone antibiotics, itraconazole, ketoconazole, and oral tetracyclines
  Other medical problems, especially alcoholism (active), coagulation or platelet function disorders, gastrointestinal problems such as ulceration or erosive gastritis (especially a bleeding ulcer), and hepatic disease or viral hepatitis

### Proper use of this medication
» Taking with food or a full glass (240 mL) of water to minimize gastrointestinal irritation
» Importance of not taking more medication than recommended on package label, unless otherwise directed by physician, because of risk of acetaminophen-induced liver damage with long-term use or greater-than-recommended doses, gastrointestinal toxicity with salicylates, and acetaminophen or salicylate overdose
» Importance of children not receiving more than 5 doses per day unless otherwise directed by physician
» Not taking for chronic or severe inflammatory or rheumatic conditions without first checking with physician because prolonged treatment may be necessary and medication may not be effective unless extremely high doses are taken
» Not taking combinations containing aspirin if a strong vinegar-like odor is present

» Proper dosing
» Proper storage

### Precautions while using this medication
» Regular visits to physician to check progress if long-term or high-dose therapy is prescribed
  Checking with physician because additional treatment may be needed:
    —if taking for pain or fever, and pain persists for longer than 10 days (5 days for children) or fever persists for longer than 3 days, if condition becomes worse, if new symptoms occur, or if the painful area is red or swollen
    —if taking for sore throat, and sore throat is severe, persists for longer than 2 days, or occurs together with or is followed by fever, headache, rash, nausea, or vomiting
  Not taking products containing aspirin for 5 days prior to any kind of surgery, unless otherwise directed by physician
» Caution if other medications containing acetaminophen, aspirin, or other salicylates (including diflunisal) are used
» Avoiding alcoholic beverages if taking more than an occasional 1 or 2 doses of these medications; alcohol consumption may increase risk of salicylate-induced gastrointestinal toxicity and acetaminophen-induced liver toxicity
  Not using an NSAID together with this medication for more than a few days, unless directed by physician or dentist
  Not taking buffered formulations within 6 hours before or 2 hours after ciprofloxacin or lomefloxacin, 8 hours before or 2 hours after enoxacin, 2 hours after itraconazole, 3 hours before or after ketoconazole, 2 hours before or after norfloxacin or ofloxacin, 3 to 4 hours before or after an oral tetracycline, or 1 to 2 hours before or after other oral medications
  Not taking a cellulose-containing laxative within 2 hours of aspirin-containing medications
  Possible interference with some laboratory tests; preferably discussing use of the medication with physician in charge 3 to 4 days ahead of time; if this is not possible, informing physician in charge if medication taken within the past 3 or 4 days
  Diabetics: Possible false results with blood and urine glucose tests; checking with physician, nurse, or pharmacist if changes in test results noted
  Not taking caffeine-containing formulations for 8 to 12 hours prior to adenosine- or dipyridamole-assisted myocardial perfusion imaging test
» Suspected overdose: Getting emergency help at once

### Side/adverse effects
Signs of potential side effects, especially allergic reactions, anemia, gastrointestinal toxicity, agranulocytosis, hepatotoxicity, renal failure, sterile pyuria, and thrombocytopenia.

---

## ACETAMINOPHEN AND ASPIRIN

## Oral Dosage Forms

### ACETAMINOPHEN AND ASPIRIN TABLETS USP

**Usual adult and adolescent dose**
Analgesic or
Antipyretic—
  Oral, up to a total of approximately 650 mg of acetaminophen and aspirin (combined) every four to six hours as needed, while symptoms persist.

Note: For patient self-medication, it is recommended that a physician be consulted if pain is not relieved within ten days, fever within three days, or sore throat within two days.

For geriatric patients, it may be advisable that acetaminophen and salicylate combinations not be used for longer than five days at a time, because such patients may be more susceptible to adverse renal effects.

**Usual adult prescribing limits**
For short-term therapy (up to ten days)—Up to a total of approximately 4 grams of acetaminophen and aspirin (combined) daily.
For long-term therapy—Up to a total of approximately 2.6 grams of acetaminophen and aspirin (combined) daily, unless chronic treatment with higher doses is prescribed and monitored by a physician.

**Usual pediatric dose**
Product of suitable strength not available.

**Usual geriatric dose**
See *Usual adult and adolescent dose*.

Note: Because geriatric patients may be more susceptible to adverse renal effects, it may be advisable that they not use acetaminophen and salicylate combinations for longer than five days at a time.

**Strength(s) usually available**
U.S.—
   325 mg of acetaminophen and 325 mg of aspirin (OTC) [*Gemnisyn*].
Canada—
   Not commercially available.

**Auxiliary labeling**
- Avoid alcoholic beverages.
- Take with food or a full glass of water.

### ACETAMINOPHEN, ASPIRIN, AND CAFFEINE ORAL POWDERS

**Usual adult and adolescent dose**
See *Acetaminophen and Aspirin Tablets USP*. Dosing is based only on the analgesic ingredients.

**Usual adult prescribing limits**
See *Acetaminophen and Aspirin Tablets USP*. Dosing is based only on the analgesic ingredients.

**Usual pediatric dose**
Product of suitable strength not available.

**Usual geriatric dose**
See *Acetaminophen and Aspirin Tablets USP*. Dosing is based only on the analgesic ingredients.

**Strength(s) usually available**
U.S.—
   260 mg of acetaminophen, 500 mg of aspirin, and 32.5 mg of caffeine (OTC) [*Goody's Headache Powders* (lactose)].
Canada—
   Not commercially available.

**Auxiliary labeling**
- Avoid alcoholic beverages.
- Take with a full glass of water or other liquid.

### ACETAMINOPHEN, ASPIRIN, AND CAFFEINE TABLETS USP

**Usual adult and adolescent dose**
See *Acetaminophen and Aspirin Tablets USP*. Dosing is based only on the analgesic ingredients.

**Usual adult prescribing limits**
See *Acetaminophen and Aspirin Tablets USP*. Dosing is based only on the analgesic ingredients.

**Usual pediatric dose**
Analgesic or
Antipyretic—
   Children up to 9 years of age: Product of suitable strength not available.
   Children 9 to 11 years of age: Oral, up to a total of approximately 400 mg of acetaminophen and aspirin (combined) every four hours as needed, while symptoms persist.
   Children 11 to 12 years of age: Oral, up to a total of approximately 480 mg of acetaminophen and aspirin (combined) every four hours as needed, while symptoms persist.
Note: Administration of a specific product to a pediatric patient depends upon ability to achieve suitable dosage for the age of the child.
   It is recommended that children up to 12 years of age receive no more than five doses in each twenty-four-hour period, unless otherwise directed by a physician, and that a physician be consulted if pain is not relieved within five days, fever within three days, or sore throat within two days.

**Usual geriatric dose**
See *Acetaminophen and Aspirin Tablets USP*. Dosing is based only on the analgesic ingredients.

**Strength(s) usually available**
U.S.—
   130 mg of acetaminophen, 260 mg of aspirin, and 16.25 mg of caffeine (OTC) [*Goody's Extra Strength Tablets*].
   180 mg of acetaminophen, 230 mg of aspirin, and 15 mg of caffeine (OTC) [*Duradyne*].
   250 mg of acetaminophen, 250 mg of aspirin, and 65 mg of caffeine (OTC) [*Excedrin Extra-Strength Caplets; Excedrin Extra-Strength Tablets*].
Canada—
   Not commercially available.
Note: In Canada, *Excedrin* contains only acetaminophen and caffeine. See *Acetaminophen (Systemic)*.

**Auxiliary labeling**
- Avoid alcoholic beverages.
- Take with food or a full glass of water.

### BUFFERED ACETAMINOPHEN, ASPIRIN, AND CAFFEINE TABLETS

**Usual adult and adolescent dose**
See *Acetaminophen and Aspirin Tablets USP*. Dosing is based only on the analgesic ingredients.

**Usual adult prescribing limits**
See *Acetaminophen and Aspirin Tablets USP*. Dosing is based only on the analgesic ingredients.

**Usual pediatric dose**
See *Acetaminophen, Aspirin, and Caffeine Tablets USP*. Dosing is based only on the analgesic ingredients.

**Usual geriatric dose**
See *Acetaminophen and Aspirin Tablets USP*. Dosing is based only on the analgesic ingredients.

**Strength(s) usually available**
U.S.—
   125 mg of acetaminophen, 240 mg of aspirin, 32 mg of caffeine, and buffering agents (OTC) [*Gelpirin*].
   160 mg of acetaminophen, 230 mg of aspirin, 33 mg of caffeine, and 60 mg of calcium gluconate (OTC) [*Supac* (scored)].
   162 mg of acetaminophen, 226.8 mg of aspirin, 32.4 mg of caffeine, and 50 mg of aluminum hydroxide (OTC) [*Buffets II*].
   194 mg of acetaminophen, 227 mg of aspirin, 33 mg of caffeine, 50 mg of magnesium hydroxide, and 25 mg of aluminum hydroxide (OTC) [*Vanquish Caplets*].
Canada—
   Not commercially available.

**Auxiliary labeling**
- Avoid alcoholic beverages.
- Take with food or a full glass of water.

---

## *ACETAMINOPHEN, ASPIRIN, AND SALICYLAMIDE*

## Oral Dosage Forms

### ACETAMINOPHEN, ASPIRIN, SALICYLAMIDE, AND CAFFEINE TABLETS

**Usual adult and adolescent dose**
Analgesic or
Antipyretic—
   Oral, up to a total of approximately 325 to 500 mg of acetaminophen, aspirin, and salicylamide (combined) every three hours, 325 to 650 mg of acetaminophen, aspirin, and salicylamide (combined) every four hours, or 650 mg to 1 gram of acetaminophen, aspirin, and salicylamide (combined) every six hours as needed, while symptoms persist.
Note: For patient self-medication, it is recommended that a physician be consulted if pain is not relieved within ten days, fever within three days, or sore throat within two days.
   For geriatric patients, it may be advisable that these medications not be used for longer than five days at a time, because such patients may be more susceptible to adverse renal effects.

**Usual adult prescribing limits**
For short-term therapy (up to ten days)—Up to a total of approximately 4 grams of acetaminophen, aspirin, and salicylamide (combined) daily.
For long-term therapy—Up to a total of approximately 2.6 grams of acetaminophen, aspirin, and salicylamide (combined) daily, unless chronic treatment with higher doses is prescribed and monitored by a physician.

**Usual pediatric dose**
Analgesic or
Antipyretic—
   Children up to 9 years of age: Product of suitable strength not available.
   Children 9 to 11 years of age: Oral, up to a total of approximately 320 to 400 mg of acetaminophen, aspirin, and salicylamide (combined) every four hours as needed, while symptoms persist.
   Children 11 to 12 years of age: Oral, up to a total of approximately 320 to 480 mg of acetaminophen, aspirin, and salicylamide (combined) every four hours as needed, while symptoms persist.
Note: Administration of a specific product to a pediatric patient depends upon ability to achieve suitable dosage for the age of the child.

It is recommended that children up to 12 years of age receive no more than five doses in each twenty-four-hour period, unless otherwise directed by a physician, and that a physician be consulted if pain is not relieved within five days, fever within three days, or sore throat within two days.

**Usual geriatric dose**
See *Usual adult and adolescent dose*.

Note: Because geriatric patients may be more susceptible to adverse renal effects, it may be advisable that they not use acetaminophen and salicylate combinations for longer than five days at a time.

**Strength(s) usually available**
U.S.—
115 mg of acetaminophen, 210 mg of aspirin, 65 mg of salicylamide, and 16 mg of caffeine (OTC) [*Saleto*].
162 mg of acetaminophen, 162 mg of aspirin, 162 mg of salicylamide, and 16.2 mg of caffeine (OTC) [*Tri-Pain Caplets*].
Canada—
Not commercially available.

**Auxiliary labeling**
- Avoid alcoholic beverages.
- Take with food or a full glass of water.
- May cause drowsiness.

### BUFFERED ACETAMINOPHEN, ASPIRIN, AND SALICYLAMIDE TABLETS

**Usual adult and adolescent dose**
See *Acetaminophen, Aspirin, Salicylamide, and Caffeine Tablets*. Dosing is based only on the analgesic ingredients.

**Usual adult prescribing limits**
See *Acetaminophen, Aspirin, Salicylamide, and Caffeine Tablets*. Dosing is based only on the analgesic ingredients.

**Usual pediatric dose**
Product of suitable strength not available.

**Usual geriatric dose**
See *Acetaminophen, Aspirin, Salicylamide, and Caffeine Tablets*. Dosing is based only on the analgesic ingredients.

**Strength(s) usually available**
U.S.—
120 mg of acetaminophen, 260 mg of aspirin, 120 mg of salicylamide, and 100 mg of aluminum hydroxide (OTC) [*Presalin*].
Canada—
Not commercially available.

**Auxiliary labeling**
- Avoid alcoholic beverages.
- Take with food or a full glass of water.
- May cause drowsiness.

---

## ACETAMINOPHEN AND SALICYLAMIDE

## Oral Dosage Forms

### ACETAMINOPHEN AND SALICYLAMIDE CAPSULES

**Usual adult and adolescent dose**
Analgesic
or Antipyretic—
Oral, 500 mg of acetaminophen and salicylamide (combined) every four hours, or 1 gram of acetaminophen and salicylamide (combined) every six hours as needed, while symptoms persist.

Note: For patient self-medication, it is recommended that a physician be consulted if pain is not relieved within ten days, fever within three days, or sore throat within two days.

For geriatric patients, it may be advisable that these medications not be used for longer than five days at a time, because such patients may be more susceptible to adverse renal effects.

**Usual adult prescribing limits**
For short-term therapy (up to ten days)—Up to a total of approximately 4 grams of acetaminophen and salicylamide (combined) daily.
For long-term therapy—Up to a total of approximately 2.6 grams of acetaminophen and salicylamide (combined) daily, unless chronic treatment with higher doses is prescribed and monitored by a physician.

**Usual pediatric dose**
Product of suitable strength not available.

**Usual geriatric dose**
See *Usual adult and adolescent dose*.

Note: Because geriatric patients may be more susceptible to adverse renal effects, it may be advisable that they not use acetaminophen and salicylate combinations for longer than five days at a time.

**Strength(s) usually available**
U.S.—
250 mg of acetaminophen and 250 mg of salicylamide (OTC) [*Duoprin*].
Canada—
Not commercially available.

**Auxiliary labeling**
- Avoid alcoholic beverages.
- Take with food or a full glass of water.
- May cause drowsiness.

### ACETAMINOPHEN, SALICYLAMIDE, AND CAFFEINE CAPSULES

**Usual adult and adolescent dose**
See *Acetaminophen and Salicylamide Capsules*. Dosing is based only on the analgesic ingredients.

**Usual adult prescribing limits**
See *Acetaminophen and Salicylamide Capsules*. Dosing is based only on the analgesic ingredients.

**Usual pediatric dose**
Analgesic or
Antipyretic—
Children up to 6 years of age: Product of suitable strength not available.
Children 6 to 9 years of age: Oral, up to a total of approximately 320 mg of acetaminophen and salicylamide (combined) every four hours as needed, while symptoms persist.
Children 9 to 11 years of age: Oral, up to a total of approximately 320 to 400 mg of acetaminophen and salicylamide (combined) every four hours as needed, while symptoms persist.
Children 11 to 12 years of age: Oral, up to a total of approximately 320 to 480 mg of acetaminophen and salicylamide (combined) every four hours as needed, while symptoms persist.

Note: Administration of a specific product to a pediatric patient depends upon ability to achieve suitable dosage for the age of the child.

It is recommended that children up to 12 years of age receive no more than five doses in each twenty-four-hour period, unless otherwise directed by a physician, and that a physician be consulted if pain is not relieved within five days, fever within three days, or sore throat within two days.

**Usual geriatric dose**
See *Acetaminophen and Salicylamide Capsules*. Dosing is based only on the analgesic ingredients.

**Strength(s) usually available**
U.S.—
226.8 mg of acetaminophen, 97.2 mg of salicylamide, and 32.4 mg of caffeine (OTC) [*Rid-A-Pain Compound*].
Canada—
Not commercially available.

**Auxiliary labeling**
- Avoid alcoholic beverages.
- Take with food or a full glass of water.
- May cause drowsiness.

### ACETAMINOPHEN, SALICYLAMIDE, AND CAFFEINE TABLETS

**Usual adult and adolescent dose**
See *Acetaminophen and Salicylamide Capsules*. Dosing is based only on the analgesic ingredients.

**Usual adult prescribing limits**
See *Acetaminophen and Salicylamide Capsules*. Dosing is based only on the analgesic ingredients.

**Usual pediatric dose**
Analgesic or
Antipyretic—
Children up to 9 years of age: Product of suitable strength not available.
Children 9 to 12 years of age: See *Acetaminophen and Salicylamide Capsules*. Dosing is based only on the analgesic ingredients.

**Usual geriatric dose**
See *Acetaminophen and Salicylamide Capsules*. Dosing is based only on the analgesic ingredients.

**Strength(s) usually available**
U.S.—
150 mg of acetaminophen, 230 mg of salicylamide, and 30 mg of caffeine (OTC) [*S-A-C*].

Canada—
Not commercially available.
**Auxiliary labeling**
• Avoid alcoholic beverages.

• Take with food or a full glass of water.
• May cause drowsiness.

Revised: 07/12/94

# ACETAMINOPHEN, SODIUM BICARBONATE, AND CITRIC ACID  Systemic

INN: Acetaminophen—Paracetamol
VA CLASSIFICATION (Primary): CN103
NOTE: The *Acetaminophen, Sodium Bicarbonate, and Citric Acid (Systemic)* monograph is maintained on the USP DI electronic data base. For a printed copy of the most recent revision of the complete monograph, contact Micromedex, Inc. - Reprint Requests, 6200 S. Syracuse Way, Suite 300, Englewood, CO 80111; telephone (303) 486-6400; telefax (303) 486-6464; Email: USPDI@MDX.COM.

For information on the specific components of this combination, see the *USP DI* monographs for *Acetaminophen (Systemic)*, *Sodium Bicarbonate (Systemic)*, and *Citrates (Systemic)*.

The information that follows is selectively abstracted from the complete monograph and is provided to facilitate drug use review and patient counseling.

Note: For a listing of dosage forms and brand names by country availability, see *Dosage Forms* section(s).

## Category
Analgesic-antacid.

## Indications
**Accepted**
Pain and upset stomach (treatment)—Acetaminophen, sodium bicarbonate, and citric acid combination is indicated for relief of mild to moderate pain, primarily when an upset stomach is also present. However, it is recommended that this medication be used only on an occasional or short-term basis; long-term use is not recommended because of the high sodium bicarbonate content.

## Patient Consultation
As an aid to patient consultation, refer to *Advice for the Patient, Acetaminophen, Sodium Bicarbonate, and Citric Acid (Systemic)*.
In providing consultation, consider emphasizing the following selected information (» = major clinical significance):

**Before using this medication**
» Conditions affecting use, especially:
  Allergic reaction to acetaminophen, aspirin, or sodium bicarbonate, history of
  Pregnancy—Acetaminophen crosses the placenta; sodium may cause edema and weight gain
  Use in the elderly—Because of the very high sodium content, use of this acetaminophen and antacid combination should preferably be limited to 5 days at a time, unless more prolonged therapy is prescribed and monitored by a physician
  Other medications, especially alcohol (especially chronic abuse of), mecamylamine, methenamine, oral ciprofloxacin, enoxacin, itraconazole, ketoconazole, lomefloxacin, norfloxacin, ofloxacin, and tetracyclines
  Other medical problems, especially alcoholism (active), symptoms of appendicitis or, hepatic disease or viral hepatitis, conditions in which sodium may be detrimental, and intestinal obstruction.

**Proper use of this medication**
» Following physician's or manufacturer's directions; not taking more medication than the amount recommended because acetaminophen may cause liver damage with long-term use or greater-than-recommended doses and because of the very high sodium content of this medication
  *Proper administration:*
  Dissolving granules in water prior to ingestion: Pouring measured dose into glass, then adding ½ glass (120 mL) cool water
  Drinking while solution is still effervescing, or after it has settled
  Drinking entire amount, then rinsing glass with a little more water and drinking that, to ensure receiving full dosage

» Proper dosing
  Missed dose (if on scheduled dosing): Taking as soon as possible; not taking if almost time for next dose; not doubling doses
» Proper storage

**Precautions while using this medication**
Regular visits to physician to check progress if long-term therapy is prescribed
Checking with physician, because additional treatment may be needed, if symptoms persist for longer than 10 days, condition becomes worse, new symptoms occur, or the painful area is red or swollen
» Not taking this medication within:
  —6 hours before or 2 hours after ciprofloxacin or lomefloxacin
  —8 hours before or 2 hours after enoxacin
  —2 hours after itraconazole
  —3 hours before or after ketoconazole
  —2 hours before or after norfloxacin or ofloxacin
  —3 to 4 hours before or after an oral tetracycline
  —1 or 2 hours before or after any other oral medication
» Caution if other medications containing acetaminophen or significant quantities of sodium are used
  Not using a salicylate or a nonsteroidal anti-inflammatory drug together with acetaminophen for longer than a few days, unless otherwise directed by physician
  If taking more than an occasional 1 or 2 doses of this medication:
» Avoiding alcoholic beverages; increased risk of liver toxicity, especially in alcoholics, with high doses or prolonged use of acetaminophen
» Avoiding large amounts of milk or milk products
  Possible need for sodium restriction
  Possible interference with some laboratory tests; preferably checking with laboratory 3 to 4 days ahead of time; if this is not possible, informing physician in charge if acetaminophen taken within the past 3 or 4 days
  Diabetics: Possible false results with blood glucose tests; checking with physician, nurse, or pharmacist if changes in test results noted
» Suspected overdose: Getting emergency help at once even if no symptoms apparent; symptoms of severe acetaminophen overdosage may be delayed, but treatment must be begun as soon as possible; treatment started 24 hours or more after the overdose may be ineffective in preventing liver damage or fatality

**Side/adverse effects**
Signs of potential side effects, especially edema, hypercalcemia associated with milk-alkali syndrome, increased blood pressure, metabolic alkalosis, agranulocytosis, anemia, allergic dermatitis, hepatitis, renal colic, renal failure, sterile pyuria, and thrombocytopenia

## Oral Dosage Forms

### ACETAMINOPHEN FOR EFFERVESCENT ORAL SOLUTION USP

**Usual adult and adolescent dose**
Analgesics-antacid—
Oral, 325 to 650 mg of acetaminophen every four hours as needed.

Note: It is recommended that a physician be consulted if symptoms are not relieved within ten days. However, geriatric patients should preferably not self-medicate with this product for longer than five days at a time, because of the very high sodium content.

**Usual pediatric dose**
Dosage has not been established.

**Strength(s) usually available**
U.S.—
325 mg of acetaminophen with 2.781 grams of sodium bicarbonate and 2.224 grams of citric acid per ¾-capful measured dose (OTC) [*Bromo-Seltzer* (sodium 761 mg [33.08 mmol] per 325-mg dose)].

**Preparation of dosage form**
The measured dose is to be dissolved in 120 mL of cool water just prior to administration.

**Auxiliary labeling**
- Avoid alcoholic beverages.
- Keep container tightly closed.

Revised: 07/12/94

---

**ACETAZOLAMIDE**—See *Carbonic Anhydrase Inhibitors (Systemic)*

---

**ACETOHEXAMIDE**—See *Antidiabetic Agents, Sulfonylurea (Systemic)*

---

**ACETOHYDROXAMIC ACID**—The *Acetohydroxamic Acid (Systemic)* monograph is not included in this published version of the USP DI database. Copies of the monograph are available on request from Micromedex, Inc. - Reprint Requests, 6200 S. Syracuse Way, Suite 300, Englewood, CO 80111; telephone (303) 486-6400; telefax (303) 486-6464; Email: USPDI@MDX.COM.

---

**ACETOPHENAZINE**—See *Phenothiazines (Systemic)*

---

**ACETYLCYSTEINE**—The *Acetylcysteine (Local)* monograph is not included in this published version of the USP DI database. Copies of the monograph are available on request from Micromedex, Inc. - Reprint Requests, 6200 S. Syracuse Way, Suite 300, Englewood, CO 80111; telephone (303) 486-6400; telefax (303) 486-6464; Email: USPDI@MDX.COM.

---

# ACETYLCYSTEINE  Systemic

JAN: *N*-Acetyl-L-Cysteine.
VA CLASSIFICATION (Primary/Secondary):
  Oral—RE400/AD900
  Parenteral—AD900

Commonly used brand name(s): *Mucomyst; Mucosil; Parvolex*.

Note: For a listing of dosage forms and brand names by country availability, see *Dosage Forms* section(s).

## Category
Antidote (to acetaminophen overdose).

## Indications
**Accepted**
Toxicity, acetaminophen (treatment)—Acetylcysteine is indicated in the treatment of acetaminophen overdose to protect against hepatotoxicity.

## Pharmacology/Pharmacokinetics
**Physicochemical characteristics**
Molecular weight—163.19.

**Mechanism of action/Effect**
Acetylcysteine may protect against acetaminophen overdose–induced hepatotoxicity by maintaining or restoring hepatic concentrations of glutathione. Glutathione is required to inactivate an intermediate metabolite of acetaminophen that is thought to be hepatotoxic. In acetaminophen overdose, excessive quantities of this metabolite are formed because the primary metabolic (glucuronide and sulfate conjugation) pathways become saturated. Acetylcysteine may act by reducing the metabolite to the parent compound and/or by providing sulfhydryl for conjugation of the metabolite. Experimental evidence also suggests that a sulfhydryl-containing compound such as acetylcysteine may also directly inactivate the metabolite.

**Biotransformation**
Deacetylated by the liver to cysteine and subsequently metabolized.

## Precautions to Consider
**Carcinogenicity**
Studies have not been done to determine the carcinogenic potential of acetylcysteine.

**Mutagenicity**
In the Ames test, both with and without metabolic activation, acetylcysteine was not shown to be mutagenic.

**Pregnancy/Reproduction**
Fertility—Reproductive studies performed in rats given oral doses of up to 1000 mg per kg of body weight (mg/kg) of acetylcysteine per day showed a slight reduction in fertility with doses of 500 or 1000 mg/kg per day (2.6 and 5.2 times the human dose, respectively). Studies in rabbits given up to 500 mg/kg per day (2.6 times the human dose) revealed no evidence of impaired fertility.

Pregnancy—Adequate and well-controlled studies in humans have not been done. However, several reports have indicated that use of acetylcysteine to treat acetaminophen overdose in pregnant women is safe and effective, and may prevent hepatotoxicity in the fetus as well as in the mother.

Studies in rabbits given oral doses of 500 mg/kg per day on Day 6 through Day 16 of gestation and in rabbits given 10% acetylcysteine plus 0.5% isoproterenol by inhalation for 30 or 35 minutes twice a day on Day 16 through Day 18 of gestation showed no evidence of teratogenicity or harm to the fetus. Also, studies in rats administered acetylcysteine and isoproterenol by inhalation showed no evidence of teratogenicity or harm to the fetus.

FDA Pregnancy Category B.

**Breast-feeding**
It is not known whether acetylcysteine is distributed into breast milk. However, problems in humans have not been documented.

**Pediatrics**
Appropriate studies on the relationship of age to the effects of acetylcysteine have not been performed in the pediatric population. However, no pediatrics-specific problems have been documented to date.

**Geriatrics**
No information is available on the relationship of age to the effects of acetylcysteine in geriatric patients being treated for acetaminophen overdose.

**Medical considerations/Contraindications**
The medical considerations/contraindications included have been selected on the basis of their potential clinical significance (reasons given in parentheses where appropriate)—not necessarily inclusive (» = major clinical significance).

*Risk-benefit should be considered when the following medical problems exist:*

Asthma, history of
  (risk of bronchospastic reactions—with intravenous administration)
Conditions predisposing to gastrointestinal hemorrhage, such as:
  Esophageal varices
  Peptic ulceration
    (acetylcysteine-induced vomiting may increase the risk of hemorrhage)
Sensitivity to acetylcysteine

## Side/Adverse Effects
The following side/adverse effects have been selected on the basis of their potential clinical significance (possible signs and symptoms in parentheses where appropriate)—not necessarily inclusive:

**Those indicating need for medical attention**
Incidence rare
  *Bronchospastic allergic reaction* (shortness of breath, troubled breathing, tightness in chest, or wheezing); *dermatitis, allergic* (skin rash or hives); *facial edema*

Note: *Bronchospasm* may also occur in conjunction with a generalized *anaphylactoid reaction*. These allergic reactions and *facial edema* have been reported only with intravenous administration.

**Those indicating need for medical attention only if they continue or are bothersome**
*Drowsiness; fever; nausea or vomiting*

## General Dosing Information

Because an injectable dosage form of acetylcysteine is not commercially available in the U.S., some emergency care practitioners have advocated that the oral solution be diluted and given by intravenous infusion when necessary. Oral administration is preferred because of the risk of bronchospastic or anaphylactoid reactions associated with intravenous administration of acetylcysteine. Also, the fact must be kept in mind that the oral solution available in the U.S., although sterile, is not required to be pyrogen-free.

Administration of acetylcysteine is only part of an overall regimen for the treatment of acetaminophen overdose. Other measures include emptying the stomach via induction of emesis or gastric lavage; monitoring plasma acetaminophen concentration, liver function, renal function, and fluid and electrolyte balance; and supportive treatment as described below. Administration of activated charcoal as part of the treatment regimen may be needed. Although its use has been recommended primarily in cases of mixed overdose, one study has shown that administration of activated charcoal plus acetylcysteine may be more effective than acetylcysteine alone in preventing hepatotoxicity after an acetaminophen overdose.

Acetylcysteine therapy should be initiated within 24 hours after ingestion of an acetaminophen overdose. If initiation of treatment will not be delayed beyond 10 to 12 hours after ingestion of the overdose, acetylcysteine therapy may be withheld until the results of plasma acetaminophen determinations are available. Otherwise, *an initial dose of acetylcysteine should be administered immediately*, without waiting for the results of acetaminophen determinations or other laboratory tests.

The plasma acetaminophen concentration should be determined not less than 4 hours following ingestion of the overdose. Concentrations determined prior to this time are not reliable for assessing potential hepatotoxicity. The following table shows plasma concentrations of acetaminophen that are potentially hepatotoxic if they are measured at the listed times after ingestion of a possible overdose. If the initial determination shows a higher concentration, a full course of acetylcysteine should be administered. If a lower plasma concentration is reported, initiation or continuation of acetylcysteine treatment is not necessary.

| Time after Ingestion of Overdose (hr) | Acetaminophen Concentration mcg/mL | micromoles/L |
|---|---|---|
| 4 | 150 | 993 |
| 6 | 100 | 662 |
| 8 | 70 | 463.4 |
| 10 | 50 | 331 |
| 15 | 20 | 132.4 |
| 20 | 8 | 53 |
| 24 | 3.5 | 23.2 |

Liver function tests (serum aspartate aminotransferase [AST; SGOT], serum alanine aminotransferase [ALT; SGPT], prothrombin time, and bilirubin) should be performed at 24-hour intervals for at least 96 hours postingestion if the plasma acetaminophen concentration indicates potential hepatotoxicity. If no abnormalities are detected within 96 hours, further determinations are not needed.

Renal and cardiac function should be monitored and appropriate therapy instituted if necessary.

Supportive treatment includes maintaining fluid and electrolyte balance, correcting hypoglycemia, and administering vitamin $K_1$ (if prothrombin time ratio exceeds 1.5) and fresh frozen plasma or clotting factor concentrate (if prothrombin time ratio exceeds 3).

Administration of diuretics and forced diuresis are not recommended.

Additional therapy to treat mixed overdose with other agents (i.e., naloxone for an opioid analgesic) may be needed, especially if symptoms of central nervous system (CNS) depression occur within a few hours after ingestion of the overdose.

Discontinuation of acetylcysteine therapy should be considered if generalized urticaria or other symptoms of an allergic reaction occur and cannot be controlled by other means.

**For oral dosage form only**
Acetylcysteine solution must be diluted prior to administration because of its unpleasant odor and its irritating or sclerosing properties. Dilution may also reduce the risk of vomiting. Also, the medication may be tolerated better if the diluted solution is administered well chilled (over ice, if necessary) and sipped from a covered container through a drinking straw. If necessary, an antiemetic may be used concurrently or acetylcysteine can be given via nasogastric tube.

## Oral Dosage Forms

Note: The dosage form administered orally is the same solution that is administered via inhalation as a mucolytic (see *Acetylcysteine [Local]*).

### ACETYLCYSTEINE SOLUTION USP

**Usual adult and adolescent dose**
Antidote (to acetaminophen overdose)—
  Oral, 140 mg per kg of body weight initially, followed by 70 mg per kg of body weight every four hours for seventeen additional doses.

Note: Any dose vomited within one hour of administration must be repeated. If necessary, an antiemetic may be given concurrently and/or acetylcysteine, diluted with water, may be given via nasogastric tube.

**Usual pediatric dose**
See *Usual adult and adolescent dose*.

**Strength(s) usually available**
U.S.—
  10% (100 mg per mL) (Rx) [*Mucomyst; Mucosil;* GENERIC].
  20% (200 mg per mL) (Rx) [*Mucomyst; Mucosil;* GENERIC].
Canada—
  20% (200 mg per mL) (Rx) [*Mucomyst*].

**Packaging and storage**
Store below 40 °C (104 °F), preferably between 15 and 30 °C (59 and 86 °F), unless otherwise specified by manufacturer. Keep container tightly closed. Protect from freezing.

**Preparation of dosage form**
For patients weighing up to 20 kg (usually children younger than 6 years of age)—Dilute each mL of acetylcysteine solution with 3 mL of cola or other soft drinks.

For patients weighing 20 kg or more—Dilute the required quantity of acetylcysteine solution with enough cola or other soft drinks to make a 5% solution. The following quantities of acetylcysteine (20% solution) and diluent are needed to prepare a 5% solution containing the required initial dose and subsequent doses for patients weighing up to 110 kg:

| Body weight (kg) | Acetylcysteine Grams | mL of 20% solution | mL of diluent | mL of 5% solution |
|---|---|---|---|---|
| **Loading dose** | | | | |
| 100–110 | 15 | 75 | 225 | 300 |
| 90–100 | 14 | 70 | 210 | 280 |
| 80–90 | 13 | 65 | 195 | 260 |
| 70–80 | 11 | 55 | 165 | 220 |
| 60–70 | 10 | 50 | 150 | 200 |
| 50–60 | 8 | 40 | 120 | 160 |
| 40–50 | 7 | 35 | 105 | 140 |
| 30–40 | 6 | 30 | 90 | 120 |
| 20–30 | 4 | 20 | 60 | 80 |
| **Maintenance dose** | | | | |
| 100–110 | 7.5 | 37 | 113 | 150 |
| 90–100 | 7.0 | 35 | 105 | 140 |
| 80–90 | 6.5 | 33 | 97 | 130 |
| 70–80 | 5.5 | 28 | 82 | 110 |
| 60–70 | 5.0 | 25 | 75 | 100 |
| 50–60 | 4.0 | 20 | 60 | 80 |
| 40–50 | 3.5 | 18 | 52 | 70 |
| 30–40 | 3.0 | 15 | 45 | 60 |
| 20–30 | 2.0 | 10 | 30 | 40 |

**Stability**
Because the solution contains no preservative, partially used vials should be refrigerated; opened vials should be discarded after 96 hours.
Diluted solutions should be freshly prepared and used within one hour.

**Incompatibilities**
Acetylcysteine reacts with certain metals, especially iron, nickel, and copper, and with rubber. Contact with these substances should be avoided.

# Acetylcysteine (Systemic)

Auxiliary labeling
- Store in refrigerator after opening.
- Discard opened vial after 96 hours.

## Parenteral Dosage Forms
### ACETYLCYSTEINE INJECTION
Usual adult and adolescent dose
Antidote (to acetaminophen overdose)—
    Intravenous, 300 mg per kg of body weight administered over twenty and one-fourth hours, divided as follows:
        Initial loading dose—150 mg per kg of body weight in up to 200 mL of 5% dextrose injection, administered over fifteen minutes.
        Second infusion—50 mg per kg of body weight in 500 mL of 5% dextrose injection, administered over four hours.
        Third infusion—100 mg per kg of body weight in 1000 mL of 5% dextrose injection, administered over the next sixteen hours.

Usual pediatric dose
See *Usual adult and adolescent dose*.

Note: The volumes and rates of infusion administered to children must be adjusted according to the medical circumstances and any restrictions in the volumes of parenteral fluids administered, as applicable to the individual patient.

Strength(s) usually available
U.S.—
    Not commercially available.
Canada—
    20% (200 mg per mL) (Rx) [*Mucomyst*; *Parvolex*].

Preparation of dosage form
Initial loading dose (to be administered over fifteen minutes)—
    Add the required quantity of acetylcysteine injection to the following quantities of 5% dextrose injection:
      For patients weighing 10 to 15 kg—40 mL.
      For patients weighing 15 to 20 kg—50 mL.
      For patients weighing 20 to 30 kg—75 mL.
      For patients weighing 30 to 40 kg—100 mL.
      For patients weighing 40 kg and over—200 mL.

Second infusion (to be administered over four hours)—
    Add the required quantity of acetylcysteine injection to 500 mL of 5% dextrose injection.
Third infusion (to be administered over sixteen hours)—
    Add the required quantity of acetylcysteine injection to 1 liter of 5% dextrose injection.
Note: The following quantities of acetylcysteine injection and 5% dextrose injection are needed for preparing initial and subsequent infusion solutions for administration to patients of various weights:

| Body weight (kg) | 20% Acetylcysteine (mL) First infusion/ 5% dextrose injection (mL) | Second infusion* | Third infusion† |
|---|---|---|---|
| 100–110 | 82.5/200 | 27.5 | 55 |
| 90–100 | 75/200 | 25 | 50 |
| 80–90 | 67.5/200 | 22.5 | 45 |
| 70–80 | 60/200 | 20 | 40 |
| 60–70 | 52.5/200 | 17.5 | 35 |
| 50–60 | 45/200 | 15 | 30 |
| 40–50 | 37.5/200 | 12.5 | 25 |
| 30–40 | 30/100 | 10 | 20 |
| 25–30 | 22.5/75 | 7.5 | 15 |
| 20–25 | 18.75/75 | 6.25 | 12.5 |
| 15–20 | 15/50 | 5 | 10 |
| 10–15 | 11.25/40 | 3.75 | 7.5 |

*Add to 500 mL of 5% dextrose injection.
†Add to 1000 mL of 5% dextrose injection.

### Incompatibilities
Acetylcysteine reacts with certain metals, especially iron, nickel, and copper, and with rubber. Contact with these substances should be avoided.

Revised: 07/29/94

---

# ACITRETIN  Systemic

VA CLASSIFICATION (Primary): DE801
Commonly used brand name(s): *Soriatane*.
Other commonly used names are 13-cis-acitretin, etretin, and isoetretin.
Note: For a listing of dosage forms and brand names by country availability, see *Dosage Forms* section(s).

## Category
Antipsoriatic (systemic); keratinization stabilizer (systemic).

## Indications
Note: Bracketed information in the *Indications* section refers to uses that are not included in U.S. product labeling.

### General considerations

Note: **FOR INFORMATION REGARDING PROBLEMS THAT HAVE OCCURRED DURING PREGNANCY SEE THE *PREGNANCY/REPRODUCTION* SECTION OF *PRECAUTIONS TO CONSIDER*.**

Since **acitretin is a teratogen in pregnant females** and can cause serious and severe side effects in both males and females, it should be prescribed only by physicians experienced in its use. It is not known if the concentration of acitretin in seminal fluid is sufficient to pose a risk to a fetus. Acitretin should not be used in females of childbearing potential, unless the patient is unresponsive to or intolerant of other treatments, and can accept routine clinical monitoring and the strict criteria for avoiding use of alcohol and preventing pregnancy before and after treatment is discontinued.

**FOR FEMALES OF CHILDBEARING POTENTIAL:**
- **The duration of teratogenic risk has not been determined. The minimum plasma concentration of acitretin and its active metabolite etretinate that is associated with teratogenicity is not known.** The sensitivity of tests to detect plasma concentrations of acitretin and its metabolites, 13-cis acitretin and etretinate, is inadequate. Also, testing for acitretin and its metabolites in plasma poorly predicts the presence or absence of these teratogens in subcutaneous tissue after acitretin treatment is stopped.
- **Use of acitretin is contraindicated in females of childbearing potential, unless all of the following criteria have been met:**
    —Patient shows severe, disfiguring, recalcitrant psoriasis or one of the accepted indications.
    —Patient understands treatment instructions and intends to follow them.
    —Patient is capable of complying with the mandatory contraceptive measures. Two effective forms of contraception should be used at least 1 month before therapy begins, during therapy, and for an undetermined amount of time following discontinuation of therapy, at least 2 years, according to Canadian labeling, or 3 years, according to U.S. labeling. A planned pregnancy should be discussed with the physician for a recommendation of timing.
    —Patient receives both verbal and written warnings of the hazards associated with pregnancy during and following acitretin therapy and she acknowledges in writing her responsibility to avoid pregnancy.
    —Patient is not pregnant, as concluded from a negative pregnancy test. The pregnancy test should be performed after normal menstrual cycles are achieved and within 1 week prior to initiation of acitretin therapy. If acitretin therapy is initiated, it should begin within the same week as the pregnancy test, on Day 2 or Day 3 of the menstrual period.

**For males and females**:
- During treatment and for 2 months after acitretin treatment discontinuation—*Patients should not drink alcohol-containing beverages* to avoid the prolonged effects of etretinate, an active metabolite of acitretin, that may accumulate from alcohol-induced transesterification. Alcohol is a major factor for inducing the conversion of acitretin to etretinate. It is not known what other substances may also induce this conversion.
- During treatment and for several years after acitretin treatment discontinuation—*Patients should not donate blood* intended for transfu-

sion purposes for 2 years, according to Canadian labeling, or for 3 years, according to U.S. labeling. Although the risk is small, a blood transfusion from such donors to pregnant women during their first trimester may expose the fetus to the medication.

**Accepted**

[Keratinization disorders (treatment)] such as: [Erythroderma, ichthyosiform][1]; [Ichthyosis, lamellar][1]; [Keratosis follicularis][1]—Acitretin is indicated to treat inherited disorders of keratinization, such as bullous or nonbullous ichthyosiform erythroderma, keratosis follicularis, and lamellar ichthyosis. Best results are obtained in treatment of keratosis follicularis (also called Darier's disease), severe recessive X-linked ichthyosis, and nonbullous congenital ichthyosis, such as erythrodermic or nonerythrodermic lamellar ichthyosis. Patients with bullous ichthyosiform erythroderma may experience improvement of their condition under less aggressive treatment with a low-dose regimen.

Psoriasis, severe (treatment)—Acitretin is indicated to treat symptoms of severe erythrodermic and generalized pustular psoriasis that involve more than 10% of the patient's body surface area, especially when psoriasis is physically, occupationally, or psychologically disabling. Acitretin is indicated for the treatment of localized palmoplantar pustulosis, but the localized condition is more recalcitrant to treatment than is generalized, severe psoriasis.

When treating severe plaque psoriasis, other therapies that have been added to a regimen of acitretin monotherapy after 1 or 2 months include ultraviolet B (UVB) light or psoralen plus ultraviolet A (UVA) light (PUVA), topical corticosteroids, or anthralin ointments.

**Acceptance not established**

There are published case reports of using the retinoids, acitretin or etretinate, in the treatment of *other disorders of keratinization*, including *cutaneous lichen planus*, *erythrokeratodermia variabilis*, *palmoplantar keratoses* (including *mal de Meleda* and *Papillon-Lefevre syndrome*), *pityriasis rubra pilaris*, and *Sjogren-Larsson syndrome*. Other studies are needed to evaluate fully acitretin's efficacy in the treatment of these conditions. Some children with *Netherton's syndrome* and *keratosis pilaris* experienced a worsening of their condition when treated with acitretin for several weeks; acitretin therapy was withdrawn.

Acitretin has been used in conjunction with interferon-alpha 2a to treat *cutaneous T-cell lymphoma* when there was no known internal organ involvement.

Small studies have been done using acitretin prophylactically in the treatment of *keratotic skin lesions* or *skin cancer*. Acitretin prevented development of new keratotic skin lesions in renal transplant patients who had a history of extensive keratotic skin lesions and/or recurrent squamous cell and basal cell carcinomas. Additional studies are needed.

Acitretin has been used as monotherapy in the treatment of *psoriasis associated with human immunodeficiency virus (HIV)* infection. Although acitretin does not appear to have immunosuppressive properties capable of worsening a compromised immune system, additional studies are needed to assess acitretin's immunosuppressive properties in HIV-positive patients.

**Unaccepted**

An *in vitro* study reported that acitretin was totally ineffective in the treatment of acute myelocytic leukemia.

Mild disorders of keratinization, including autosomal dominant ichthyosis vulgaris and mild recessive X-linked ichthyosis that can be controlled with topical medications generally should not be treated with acitretin because of risk-benefit issues. Also, acitretin treatment may cause skin erosions and exacerbate the epidermolytic form of palmoplantar keratoderma.

Acitretin is not efficacious and is not used to treat severe nodulocystic acne.

---

[1]Not included in Canadian product labeling.

## Pharmacology/Pharmacokinetics

Note: The length of time that etretinate (a metabolite of acitretin) remains in the blood has not been determined.

**Physicochemical characteristics**

Chemical group—Acitretin is considered a second-generation retinoid and a synthetic aromatic analog of vitamin A.
Molecular weight—326.44.
pKa—5.

**Mechanism of action/Effect**

The exact mechanism of action for acitretin is not known. One possible explanation is altered gene expression through nuclear retinoic acid receptors (RARs) and binding to DNA to cause transcription or transrepression changes in protein synthesis. Although acitretin binds to all three classes of RARs (alpha, beta, and gamma receptors), it binds selectively to beta and gamma receptors to modify gene expression.

Antipsoriatic—Studies suggest that acitretin affects immune response, epidermal proliferation, and glycoprotein synthesis in the skin. Specifically, acitretin helps to normalize cell differentiation and thin the cornified layer by directly reducing the keratinocytes' rate of proliferation. Acitretin's anti-inflammatory and antiproliferative actions in the skin decrease epidermal and dermal inflammation and reduce the scaling, erythema, and thickness of psoriatic lesions.

Keratolytic (systemic)—Acitretin is thought to interfere with the terminal differentiation of keratinocytes.

**Absorption**

The mean absolute bioavailability of acitretin is 59% (range, 36 to 95%). The dose absorbed is linear up to 50 mg a day, but may become non-proportional or nonlinear for doses greater than 50 mg a day. The rate and extent of acitretin absorption are doubled when 50 mg of acitretin is given with food when compared with the absorption of the same dose given under fasting conditions.

As judged from the area under the plasma concentration–time curve (AUC), the amount absorbed, corrected for body weight and dose, shows a six-fold systemic interindividual variation for the metabolite etretinate.

**Distribution**

The mean accumulation ratio is 1.2 for acitretin and 6.6 for the cis-metabolite. Acitretin has not been shown to accumulate in any particular organ; however, etretinate (an active metabolite) does accumulate in fat and, to a lesser degree, in the liver; lower tissue concentrations are found in the kidneys, brain, and testes. Five hours after acitretin administration, etretinate concentrations in the subcutaneous fat exceed those found in the plasma; however, accumulation does not occur. In one patient given acitretin orally, the concentration of etretinate in the adrenal glands exceeded that found in the fat tissue.

Patients receiving 30 mg of acitretin once a day for 30 days showed skin concentrations of acitretin that were 10 times higher than those observed in the plasma and 3 to 5 times higher than the skin concentrations of its metabolite, 13-cis acitretin. Concentrations of acitretin and 13-cis acitretin are higher in lesional skin than in uninvolved skin.

**Protein binding**

Acitretin and its metabolite etretinate are highly bound to plasma proteins ( 99%). Acitretin is primarily bound to albumin (91%) and etretinate is primarily bound to low-density lipoprotein (48%).

**Biotransformation**

Acitretin is metabolized to other active metabolites, including 13-cis acitretin and etretinate, following oral administration. No detectable etretinate was formed when a single dose of 100 mg of acitretin was administered without ingestion of alcohol, but the potential for its formation cannot be ruled out. Other metabolites are likely to occur.

The relative formation of the 13-cis acitretin does not change regardless of acitretin dose, dose formulation (capsules versus solution), and ingestion with or without food. Ingestion of alcohol increases the conversion of acitretin to etretinate (an active metabolite), even after discontinuation of treatment.

One crossover study of 10 healthy volunteers who took 100 mg of acitretin and 1.4 grams per kg of body weight of ethanol over approximately 3 hours showed a mean peak plasma concentration of 59 nanograms of etretinate per mL (range, 22 to 105 nanograms per mL), a concentration that is comparable to receiving a 5-mg dose of etretinate. In another study where protocol did not restrict patients from drinking alcohol, 57.5% of 240 patients taking 5 to 60 mg of acitretin a day for treatment of psoriasis had plasma etretinate concentrations of 5 to 62 nanograms per mL; 27% of patients showed a measurable trace of etretinate in their plasma.

**Half-life**

Elimination—
Acitretin: 49 hours (range, 33 to 96 hours; some studies have shown the upper limit of the half-life to be as high as 120 hours).
13-cis acitretin (active metabolite): 63 hours (range, 28 to 157 hours).
Etretinate (active metabolite): 120 days, mean (range, up to 168 days).

**Peak serum concentration**

Single dose of 50 mg acitretin—196 to 728 nanograms per mL.
At multiple doses of 10 to 50 mg acitretin a day—The dose-related trough steady-state plasma concentrations are between 6 and 25 nanograms per mL for acitretin; the serum concentration for the 13-cis metabolite is about five times higher than that of acitretin.

**Time to peak effect**

Single dose of 50 mg acitretin: 2 to 5 hours.
At doses of 10 to 50 mg acitretin a day, steady-state plasma concentrations are reached within 2 weeks.

**Elimination**
For acitretin or 13-cis acitretin conjugates, 34 to 54% renal and 16 to 53% fecal. No acitretin or 13-cis acitretin (active metabolite) was recovered in the urine.

If alcohol is taken during treatment with acitretin, more than 98% of etretinate would be eliminated after 2 years, assuming a mean half-life of 120 days. Using the upper limit of the half-life of 168 days, more than 98% of etretinate would be eliminated after 3 years. One woman who ingested alcohol sporadically during acitretin therapy showed detectable plasma and subcutaneous fat concentrations of etretinate 52 months after discontinuing acitretin treatment.

In dialysis—
 For patients taking a single 50-mg dose of acitretin, the mean AUC values of acitretin and 13-cis acitretin (active metabolite) were about 50% less in patients undergoing hemodialysis compared to patients without renal failure. No retinoids were detectable in the dialysate.

## Precautions to Consider

### Cross-sensitivity and/or related problems
Patients sensitive to isotretinoin, tretinoin, or vitamin A derivatives may be sensitive to this medication also, since acitretin is related to both retinoic acid and retinol (vitamin A). Also, allergy to parabens should be considered.

### Carcinogenicity
Male and female Wistar rats given acitretin in doses of 0.5, 1, or 2 mg per kg of body weight (mg/kg) a day for 104 weeks showed a greater incidence of non-neoplastic bone lesions compared to two control groups not given acitretin. Neoplastic lesions that developed in the endocrine and reproductive organs and the skin were consistent with those that developed in the control rats, and were not associated with use of acitretin.

### Mutagenicity
Acitretin is not mutagenic according to the following *in vitro* tests: Ames test, hamster HGPRT assay, unscheduled DNA synthesis in rat hepatocytes, induction of chromosomal aberrations in human lymphocytes, and mouse micronucleus assay.

### Pregnancy/Reproduction
The inability to detect plasma acitretin and its metabolite etretinate is a poor predictor of the absence of these teratogens in tissue after discontinuation of acitretin treatment.

Fertility—A small study of acitretin's effect in eight men showed no changes in sperm concentrations. However, for male patients taking acitretin, it is not known whether residual acitretin in seminal fluid during treatment or after treatment has been discontinued poses a risk to a fetus. The maximum acitretin concentration observed in human seminal fluid from systemic use of acitretin or etretinate was 12.5 nanograms per mL, which would transfer approximately 125 nanograms of acitretin per 10 mL of ejaculate. Of the four reported cases with known fetal outcomes in pregnant women whose male partner took acitretin, one infant was normal, two spontaneous abortions occurred, and one fetus had bilateral cystic hygromas and multiple cardiopulmonary malformations.

One study of dogs given doses of acitretin larger than 30 mg/kg per day for 1 year showed that a few of the dogs experienced spermatogenic arrest at 6 months of treatment, which improved by the end of the study.

Pregnancy—**Acitretin is teratogenic in humans and is contraindicated during pregnancy.** Unless abstinence is the chosen method, it is recommended that the patient use two forms of effective contraception to prevent pregnancy during treatment and for at least 2 years, according to Canadian labeling, or for at least 3 years, according to U.S. labeling, after acitretin has been discontinued.

**The duration of teratogenic risk is not known.** Teratogenic risk may continue longer if the mother has ingested alcoholic beverages during acitretin treatment. Whenever an unexpected pregnancy occurs during the time of teratogenic risk, the risk-benefit ratio of continuing the pregnancy must be considered. Major human fetal abnormalities associated with the use of acitretin or its metabolite etretinate include:
- Anophthalmia;
- Heart defects;
- Microcephalus; and
- Skeletal or connective tissue abnormalities, including absence of terminal phalanges, alterations of the skull and cervical vertebra, and malformations of hip, ankle, and forearm; facial dysmorphia; high palate; low-set ears; meningomyelocele; multiple synostoses; and syndactyly.

In one study of pregnant rats given acitretin in doses of 0 (control group), 0.3, 1, and 3 mg/kg a day, no drug-related parental mortality and no signs of parental toxicity were noted; however, in the 3 mg/kg group, fewer offspring survived (24% mortality compared to 8.8% for the control group). In addition, developmental tests showed hair growth, ear opening, auditory startle, pupillary contraction, and memory retention were affected. According to another study in rats, 7.5 mg/kg of acitretin per day was the highest dose that did not show teratogenic effects. Pregnant rats given 7.5 mg/kg of acitretin or higher produced fewer pups and, at doses greater than 7.5 mg/kg, their fetuses developed skeletal adverse effects, such as a cleft palate and abnormally shaped long bones.

In one study of pregnant mice given acitretin in doses of 0 (control group), 1, 3, and 10 mg/kg of acitretin per day, no drug-related maternal mortality and no signs of parental toxicity were noted. No teratogenic effects were seen in fetuses whose mothers received 1 mg/kg of acitretin per day. However, maternal doses of 3 and 10 mg/kg of acitretin per day caused fetal skeletal malformations (cervical, neural arches, and long bones) and soft tissue malformations (exencephaly, cleft palate, unilateral kidney agenesis, and enlarged renal pelvis).

In one study of pregnant rabbits given acitretin in doses of 0 (control group), 0.2, 0.6, and 2 mg/kg of acitretin per day, no drug-related parental mortality and no signs of parental toxicity were noted. No teratogenic effects were seen in fetuses whose mothers received 0.2 mg/kg of acitretin per day. However, maternal doses of 0.6 mg/kg of acitretin per day resulted in a low incidence of cleft palate and brain anomalies in fetuses. Maternal doses of 2 mg/kg of acitretin per day caused teratogenic effects in fetuses, including open eyes, ectrodactyly, spina bifida, ectopia of abdominal viscera, and bilateral apical deficiencies of the distal phalanges of forelimbs and hind limbs.

### Breast-feeding
It is not known if acitretin is distributed into human breast milk. Acitretin is not recommended for use in women who are breast-feeding. Breast-feeding is not recommended for an undetermined period, at least 2 or 3 years, after acitretin has been discontinued because of acitretin's potential to cause adverse effects in nursing infants.

### Pediatrics
Safety and efficacy have not been established. Acitretin is not routinely recommended for use in children because of its potential side/adverse effects, including skeletal hyperostosis and skeletal growth retardation resulting from premature epiphyseal closure and ossification of bones and tendons.

If acitretin is used in children with severe forms of keratinization unresponsive to alternative therapies, bone age should be evaluated before treatment initiation and annually during treatment. In children, radiographic studies to determine bone age, including radiographs (x-rays) of the knees, should be done before acitretin therapy is initiated, followed by annual monitoring of bone by scintigraphy (bone scans) and/or radiography. Special attention should be given to any child experiencing pain or limitation of motion.

### Geriatrics
Steady-state trough concentrations of acitretin for males 64 to 72 years of age were double compared with those for healthy males 24 to 32 years of age. Although the harmonic mean for the terminal half-life was similar at 53 and 54 hours in these age groups, the range was greater in older patients (37 to 96 hours compared with 39 to 70 hours in the younger adults), potentially making some older patients more sensitive to acitretin's effect.

### Dental
Acitretin can increase or decrease saliva production. Continuing dryness of the mouth may increase the risk of dental disease, including tooth decay, gum disease, and fungal infection. Having regular dental checkups and using artificial saliva or dissolving sugarless candy or ice in the mouth may help to reduce the incidence of dental problems.

### Drug interactions and/or related problems
The following drug interactions and/or related problems have been selected on the basis of their potential clinical significance (possible mechanism in parentheses where appropriate)—not necessarily inclusive (» = major clinical significance):

Note: Combinations containing any of the following medications, depending on the amount present, may also interact with this medication.

» Alcoholic beverages
 (concurrent use with acitretin causes increased metabolic conversion of acitretin to etretinate, which accumulates in the body. This increase in accumulation of etretinate increases the potential for teratogenicity in females using acitretin and for side/adverse effects in males and females, since etretinate is eliminated from the body much more slowly than acitretin)

» Cyclosporine
 (etretinate has been shown to inhibit the metabolism of cyclosporine and its metabolites by 33 to 45% via cytochrome P450 enzymes; acitretin may have a similar effect. Etretinate has been used thera-

peutically to reduce the needed dose of cyclosporine; however, some studies have failed to show a clear advantage to this use of etretinate)

Glyburide
(concurrent use may enhance glucose clearance as shown in three of seven healthy males; glyburide dose may need adjustment)

» Hepatotoxic medications, especially methotrexate
(concurrent use with acitretin may increase the risk of hepatoxicity, such as that seen when etretinate and methotrexate have been used together; concurrent use is not recommended)

» Hydantoin
(although not clinically proven, acitretin may potentially increase the free-fraction of hydantoins by causing protein-binding displacement of phenytoin or other hydantoins; changes of dose may be necessary)

Oral contraceptives, progestin-only
(contraceptive effect of progestins may be diminished with concurrent use of acitretin; it is not known if acitretin reduces the effect of other progestational contraceptives, such as implants or injections. Acitretin has not been shown to reduce the efficacy of estrogen and progestin oral contraceptives)

Retinoids, other, systemic, such as:
» Etretinate
» Isotretinoin
» Tretinoin, oral

Vitamin A and its derivatives, including vitamin supplements containing vitamin A or

Retinoids, topical, such as adapalene and tretinoin
(concurrent use of retinoids or doses of vitamin A larger than the minimum recommended daily allowance (RDA) increases risk of clinical symptoms resembling those of excessive vitamin A intake or toxicity, also called hypervitaminosis A)

Sensitivity to retinoids, vitamin A (also called retinol), or their derivatives

» Tetracycline, oral
(can increase intracranial pressure; concomitant use with acitretin is not recommended because of the combination's potential to exacerbate this effect)

## Laboratory value alterations

The following have been selected on the basis of their potential clinical significance (possible effect in parentheses where appropriate)—not necessarily inclusive (» = major clinical significance):

With physiology/laboratory test values
Alanine aminotransferase (ALT [SGPT]) and
Aspartate aminotransferase (AST [SGOT]) and
Lactate dehydrogenase (LDH)
(serum values increase in about 20 to 28% of patients taking acitretin; this effect is considered dose-related and may be transient)

Cholesterol, total, serum and
Triglyceride, serum
(increased serum total cholesterol concentrations occur in 9 to 33% of patients. Although triglyceride levels associated with pancreatitis are rare, hypertriglyceridemia occurs in about 66% of patients. These effects may be reversible upon reduction of dose or upon discontinuation of this medication)

High-density lipoprotein (HDL)
(decreased serum HDL concentrations occur in 30 to 40% of patients and are reversible upon dose reduction for many patients or upon discontinuation of this medication)

## Medical considerations/Contraindications

The medical considerations/contraindications included have been selected on the basis of their potential clinical significance (reasons given in parentheses where appropriate)—not necessarily inclusive (» = major clinical significance).

***Except under special circumstances, this medication should not be used when the following medical problems exist:***

» Allergy to parabens
» Hyperlipidemia, intractable, or history of or
» Pancreatitis
(66% of patients receiving acitretin in the clinical trials experienced an elevation in serum triglycerides, 9 to 33% of patients experienced elevated serum cholesterol, and 30 to 40% of patients developed a decrease in high-density lipoproteins; these trends reversed upon treatment discontinuation. If serum lipid levels cannot be controlled, acitretin treatment should be withdrawn to avoid increasing the patient's risk of cardiovascular disease and pancreatitis. Patients likely to develop intractable hyperlipidemia include those with diabetes mellitus, obesity, increased alcohol intake, or familial history of these conditions)

» Hypervitaminosis A, or history of or
» Hypersensitivity to etretinate, isotretinoin, tretinoin, or vitamin A and its derivatives
(these conditions may be exacerbated with use of acitretin)

***Risk-benefit should be considered when the following medical problems exist:***

Diabetes mellitus, type 1 or 2 or
Pancreatitis, history of
(acitretin may mildly increase or decrease glucose tolerance or increase serum lipid levels in these patients; pancreatitis may be exacerbated in patients with a history of pancreatitis; some patients with diabetes mellitus may require dose adjustment in their diabetes therapy regimens)

» Hepatic disease, severe or
» Renal disease, severe
(severe renal or hepatic function impairment can delay the elimination of acitretin and its metabolites, and, if a significant amount of drug accumulates, it potentially can make these conditions worse)
(a preliminary study of a single dose of 50 mg of acitretin in patients with end-stage renal failure showed that the pharmacokinetics of acitretin remain unaltered; however, there is concern that if acitretin is metabolized to etretinate, it may accumulate in fat tissues and prolong drug elimination)

## Patient monitoring

The following may be especially important in patient monitoring (other tests may be warranted in some patients, depending on condition; » = major clinical significance):

Bone-age determinations or
Bone radiography (x-rays), including x-rays of the knees
(recommended in children prior to therapy and yearly during therapy to determine effects on epiphyseal centers and as recommended by physician for older patients to evaluate the possibility of hyperostosis during long-term or recurrent courses of acitretin therapy. Some physicians recommend baseline evaluation for older patients if long-term therapy is anticipated and repeat bone tests only if patient becomes symptomatic)

» Contraceptive counseling and
» Pregnancy testing
(within 1 week before initiating treatment with acitretin, a negative pregnancy test should be obtained after a normal menstrual cycle has been established. Then acitretin treatment should be initiated on Day 2 or 3 of the menstrual cycle. Regularly testing for possible pregnancy is recommended, as well as counseling on importance of beginning contraception 1 month before treatment initiation and continuing the contraception counseling for as long as needed or appropriate; these measures should include patients with a history of infertility or tubal ligation)

» Hepatic function tests
(recommended before initiation, every 1 to 2 weeks during the first 2 months after treatment initiation, and then every 3 months during treatment or as clinically indicated. Weekly checking is recommended if liver test results are abnormal and medication should be withdrawn if results worsen. If liver test results do not return to normal after withdrawal of acitretin treatment, continued monitoring for at least 3 months is advised)

» Lipoprotein profile, serum
(determinations recommended in patients under fasting conditions prior to therapy and at 1- to 2-week intervals during therapy until the lipid response is established, usually within 4 to 8 weeks. Following consumption of alcohol, 36 hours should elapse before blood lipid determination)
(restricting dietary fat and alcohol intake and, when appropriate, lowering body weight are ways that patients can control significant serum concentration increases in triglycerides and decreases in high-density lipoproteins; discontinuation of retinoid should be considered if abnormal lipid or lipoprotein serum concentrations persist)

Monitoring etretinate concentrations, plasma
(some clinicians monitor plasma concentrations of etretinate, an active metabolite, to help assess patients taking acitretin and advise them in planning a future pregnancy; however, most studies have found that the absence of etretinate in plasma does not predict its absence in tissues and most clinicians do not monitor etretinate concentrations, even in cases of pregnancy)

Ophthalmologic examinations
(regular monitoring may be indicated since 29% of patients taking acitretin experience medication-related ophthalmic effects from acitretin; medication should be discontinued and neurological diagnosis and care considered for patients developing early symptoms of pseudotumor cerebri [benign intracranial hypertension], such as severe or continuing headache, nausea and vomiting, or blurred vision or other changes in vision. Also, medication should be discontinued and ophthalmologic examination should be done when any changes in vision occur)

## Side/Adverse Effects

The following side/adverse effects have been selected on the basis of their potential clinical significance (possible signs and symptoms in parentheses where appropriate)—not necessarily inclusive:

**Those indicating need for medical attention**
Incidence more frequent
*Arthralgia; hypertonia; myalgia; or spinal hyperostosis* (back pain; bone or joint pain; difficulty in moving or walking; stiff, painful muscles); *headache; nausea; vomiting*

Incidence less frequent
*Ophthalmologic effects, including blepharitis; conjunctivitis; eye irritation; photophobia; or other visual problems* (blurred vision; eye pain; loss of eyebrows or lashes; redness or swelling of the eyelid; redness of the eyes; sensitivity of eyes to light; watery eyes); *paronychia* (loosening of the fingernails; redness or soreness around fingernails)

Incidence rare
*Dermatologic effects, such as abnormal skin odor; dermatitis; or psoriasiform rash* (skin irritation or rash, including rash that looks like psoriasis); *fissuring; hypertrophy; infection; or ulceration of skin* (cracking of skin; redness of skin); *otitis externa* (itchy or painful ears); *paresthesia* (abnormal sensation of burning or stinging of skin); *pyogenic granuloma; or purpura* (small spots in skin where bleeding occurred); *hepatitis; jaundice; or pancreatitis* (abdominal pain; darkened urine; yellowing of the skin or eyes); *influenza-like symptoms; laryngitis; or pharyngitis* (coughing; hoarseness; trouble in speaking); *ophthalmologic effects, such as cortical, nuclear, and posterior subcapsular cataracts, pannus, or subepithelial corneal lesions* (eye pain; trouble in seeing); *decreased night vision* (decreased vision after sunset and before sunrise); *pseudotumor cerebri* (blurred or double vision; continuing severe headache, nausea, and vomiting); *or recurring stye* (sore on the edge of the eyelid); *vulvovaginitis* (thick, white, curd-like vaginal discharge; vaginal itching or irritation)—due to *Candida albicans*

**Those indicating need for medical attention only if they continue or are bothersome**
Incidence more frequent
*Alopecia* (loss of hair)—may be reversible after treatment discontinuation; *dermatologic effects, such as ceruminosis* (increased amount of ear wax); *chapped lips or cheilitis* (chapped, red, or swollen lips); *dry, irritated mucous membranes of nose or rhinitis* (dry or runny nose; nosebleeds); *pruritus* (itching skin); *scaling and peeling of eyelids, fingertips, palms, or soles of feet; and sticky skin; difficulty in wearing contact lenses; gingivitis or stomatitis* (irritation in mouth or swollen gums; mouth ulcers); *photosensitivity* (increased ability to sunburn); *xerophthalmia* (dryness of eyes)—23%; *unusual thirst*

Incidence less frequent
*Constipation; diarrhea; fatigue; increased sweating*

## Overdose

For more information on the management of overdose or unintentional ingestion, **contact a Poison Control Center** (see *Poison Control Center Listing*).

**Clinical effects of overdose**
The following effects have been selected on the basis of their potential clinical significance (possible signs and symptoms in parentheses where appropriate)—not necessarily inclusive:

Acute and/or chronic
*Drowsiness; intracranial pressure, elevated* (continuing severe headache, nausea, and vomiting); *irritability; itchy skin*

**Treatment of overdose**
Acute overdose with acitretin has not been reported, but symptoms are probably similar to those of vitamin A toxicity.

To decrease absorption—Evacuation of stomach should be considered within 2 hours of ingestion of acute overdose. Medication should be discontinued in patients with symptoms of overdose who were given therapeutic doses.

Monitoring—Monitor for increased intracranial pressure. Female patients of childbearing potential should have a pregnancy test at time of overdose and, if positive, teratogenic risk and continuance of pregnancy should be discussed.

Supportive care—Female patients of childbearing potential need to use an effective contraceptive method for 2 or 3 years after overdose. Patients in whom intentional overdose is confirmed or suspected should be referred for psychiatric consultation.

## Patient Consultation

As an aid to patient consultation, refer to *Advice for the Patient, Acitretin (Systemic)*.
In providing consultation, consider emphasizing the following selected information (» = major clinical significance):

**Before using this medication**
» Conditions affecting use, especially:
Sensitivity to acitretin, etretinate, isotretinoin, tretinoin, or vitamin A or its derivatives, or allergy to parabens
Pregnancy—Contraindicated for use during pregnancy; can cause birth defects of skeletal, heart, and connective tissue. Pregnancy is not recommended for at least 2 or 3 years after discontinuation of acitretin. Use of alcohol and alcohol products is prohibited; recommended waiting period may be longer if alcohol is consumed during treatment. Also, for women of childbearing potential, two effective forms of birth control should be used at least 1 month prior to initiating acitretin therapy, and continued for at least 2 to 3 years after acitretin therapy is stopped
Breast-feeding—Not recommended for use during breast-feeding; breast-feeding is not recommended for at least 2 or 3 years after discontinuing use of acitretin because of its potential adverse effects in nursing babies
Use in children—Use is not recommended, unless other medications fail and treatable condition is severe enough to be disabling; children may be more sensitive to medication; use warrants special monitoring for skeletal side effects, such as ossification of tendons and bones, to avoid premature long bone closure, short adult stature, hyperostosis, and limitation of motion
Use in the elderly—Geriatric patients may be more sensitive to medication since some patients, when compared to younger adults, may have higher acitretin serum concentrations resulting from slower elimination
Other medications, especially alcoholic beverages; cyclosporine; hepatotoxic medications, including methotrexate; hydantoin; progestin-only oral contraceptives; retinoids, other (systemic and topical); or tetracyclines
Other medical problems, especially hepatic disease, severe; hyperlipidemia (intractable); hypersensitivity to vitamin A or its derivatives; hypervitaminosis A; pancreatitis; or renal disease, severe

**Proper use of this medication**
» Reading accompanying patient information before using this medication
» Taking acitretin dose with a main meal or with a glass of milk
» For women—Special precautions are needed before beginning treatment to ensure that the patient is not pregnant, such as using an effective form of birth control for 30 days before initiating treatment, obtaining a negative pregnancy test after a normal menstrual period pattern has been established and within 1 week before initiating treatment, then starting medication on Day 2 or 3 of menstrual period. Women of reproductive age or potential are required to use two forms of contraception during treatment, beginning at least 1 month before initiation of treatment with acitretin. These women are required to continue contraception for an indeterminate time after medication is discontinued, for at least 2 years per Canadian labeling or for at least 3 years per U.S. labeling
» Proper dosing
Missed dose: Taking as soon as possible; not taking if almost time for next dose; not doubling doses.
» Proper storage

**Precautions while using this medication**
» Regular visits to physician to check progress during therapy and for up to 2 years after treatment is discontinued, especially in women wanting to become pregnant, children, and the elderly
» Checking with physician if skin condition does not improve within 8 to 12 weeks; expecting that skin irritation may occur or skin condition may worsen within the first several weeks of treatment but will lessen in severity with continued use

» Importance of not drinking alcoholic beverages or products containing alcohol during treatment and for 2 months after treatment discontinuation. Teratogenic risk may continue for longer periods of time if alcohol was consumed during acitretin treatment
» Importance of not donating blood for transfusion purposes during treatment and for at least 2 or 3 years after discontinuing treatment with acitretin as specified by physician
» Understanding that vision impairment can occur, including sudden night vision impairment, photophobia, blurred vision, or dryness of eyes. Vision problems can make driving a car or operating machinery dangerous

Checking with physician anytime vision problems occur; wearing contact lenses may be uncomfortable

Understanding that dental problems can occur resulting from dryness of mouth and may increase dental disease, including tooth decay, gum disease, and fungus infections; regular dental appointments are needed and use of sugarless candy or saliva substitute or melting ice in mouth may be necessary to lessen dental problems

Minimizing exposure of skin to wind, cold temperatures, and sunlight, including on cloudy days, to avoid sunburn, dryness, or irritation, especially during the first months of treatment. Also, not using artificial sunlight or sunlamp, unless directed otherwise by physician

Using sunscreen preparations (minimum sun protection factor [SPF] of 15) and wearing protective clothing over exposed areas and UV-blocking sunglasses when sunlight exposure cannot be avoided; avoiding direct sunlight between 10 a.m. and 3 p.m.; checking with physician at any time skin becomes too dry or irritated; choosing proper skin products to reduce skin dryness or irritation

Either checking with health care professional before using or avoiding use of topical acne or skin products containing a peeling agent (benzoyl peroxide, resorcinol, salicylic acid, or sulfur), irritating hair products (permanents or hair removal products), sun-sensitizing skin products (including products containing limes or spices), alcohol-containing skin products, or drying or abrasive skin products (some cosmetics, soaps, or skin cleansers)

Not using vitamin A or vitamin A–containing supplement in doses that exceed the minimum recommended daily allowances (RDA)

**Side/adverse effects**

Signs of potential side effects, especially arthralgia, hypertonia, myalgia, or spinal hyperostosis; headache; nausea; vomiting; ophthalmologic effects, including blepharitis, conjunctivitis, eye irritation, photophobia, or other visual problems; paronychia; dermatologic effects, such as abnormal skin odor, dermatitis or psoriasiform rash, fissuring, hypertrophy, infection, or ulceration of skin, otitis externa, paresthesia, pyogenic granuloma, or purpura; hepatitis, jaundice, or pancreatitis; influenza-like symptoms, laryngitis, or pharyngitis; ophthalmologic effects such as cortical, nuclear, and posterior subcapsular cataracts, pannus, or subepithelial corneal lesions, decreased night vision, pseudotumor cerebri, or recurring stye; and vulvovaginitis

## General Dosing Information

It is recommended that acitretin be prescribed only by physicians knowledgeable in the systemic use of retinoids. The product labeling includes a consent form for female patients of reproductive age or potential to read and sign after physician counseling.

Patients previously taking etretinate should continue to follow the contraception recommendations for etretinate.

There is a significant interpatient variation in absorption and metabolism of acitretin, of treatment efficacy, ability to tolerate treatment, and progress of psoriasis or keratinization condition. The dosage of acitretin should be individualized to achieve the maximal therapeutic response possible with a tolerable level of side effects.

Transient worsening of psoriasis commonly occurs on initiation of acitretin treatment. The full effect of acitretin may take 2 to 3 months, and its action can continue after treatment is discontinued. Treatment should be discontinued when psoriatic lesions are sufficiently resolved, and treatment reinstituted at initiation doses for relapses as needed.

Patients unresponsive to treatment with acitretin may be responsive to etretinate. When switching from etretinate to acitretin, a 20% reduction is recommended if the etretinate dose is greater than 0.75 mg per kg of body weight (mg/kg) a day or if side effects are dose-limiting. Otherwise the same dose can be used.

Other treatments that have been added to a patient's regimen after 1 or 2 months of acitretin monotherapy include ultraviolet B (UVB) light, PUVA (8-methoxypsoralen plus ultraviolet A [UVA] light), bath PUVA (trimethylpsoralen bath plus UVA), topical corticosteroids, or anthralin ointments. Dose reduction of acitretin may be required before beginning these other treatments.

**Diet/Nutrition**

Take with main meal of the day or with milk. Patient should follow a cholesterol-free diet for best results to lower serum cholesterol.

## Oral Dosage Forms

Note: Bracketed uses in the Dosage Forms section refer to categories of use and/or indications that are not included in U.S. product labeling.

### ACITRETIN TABLETS

**Usual adult dose**
Antipsoriatic (systemic)—
  Initial: Oral, 25 or 50 mg a day (or 0.5 mg per kg of body weight a day) as a single dose; dose may be increased up to 75 mg a day after four weeks, if needed and tolerated.
  Maintenance: Oral, 25 to 50 mg a day, increased if needed to 75 mg a day.
  Note: Lower doses of acitretin are used when initiating combination therapy in the treatment of severe plaque psoriasis.
[Keratinization stabilizer (systemic)]—
  Initial: Oral, 25 mg a day; dose may be increased up to 75 mg a day after four weeks, if needed and tolerated.
  Maintenance: Oral, 10 to 50 mg a day.

**Usual pediatric dose**
Antipsoriatic—
  Safety and efficacy have not been established.
[Keratinization stabilizer (systemic)]—
  Initial: Oral, 0.5 mg per kg of body weight once a day. May be increased to 1 mg per kg a day for limited periods of time as needed, not to exceed a total dose of 35 mg a day.
  Maintenance: Oral, 20 mg or lower once a day for prolonged treatment.

**Usual pediatric prescribing limits**
Oral, 35 mg a day.

**Usual geriatric dose**
See *Usual adult dose*.

**Strength(s) usually available**
U.S.—
  10 mg (Rx) [*Soriatane* (gelatin)].
  25 mg (Rx) [*Soriatane* (gelatin)].
Canada—
  10 mg (Rx) [*Soriatane* (gelatin)].
  25 mg (Rx) [*Soriatane* (gelatin)].

**Packaging and storage**
Store between 15 and 30 ºC (59 and 86 ºF), unless otherwise specified by manufacturer. Protect from light. Keep in a tightly closed container.

**Auxiliary labeling**
• Do not take this medication if you become pregnant.
• Take with food.
• Do not drink alcoholic beverages when taking this medication.
• Avoid prolonged or excessive exposure to sunlight.
• May cause dizziness or blurred vision.
• This medication may impair your ability to drive or operate machinery. Use care until you become familar with its effects.

**Note**
Include patient directions when dispensing.
Counsel female patients about using two forms of birth control 1 month before starting treatment, during treatment, and for at least 2 years, according to Canadian labeling, or for at least 3 years, according to U.S. labeling, after discontinuing treatment.
Counsel male and female patients:
  • Not to donate blood for transfusion during treatment and for at least 2 years, according to Canadian labeling, or for at least 3 years, according to U.S. labeling, after discontinuing treatment.
  • Not to drink alcoholic beverages during treatment and for at least 2 months after discontinuing treatment.
  • To be aware that sudden night vision inadequacies can occur, which can be hazardous when operating a vehicle.

## Selected Bibliography

Brindley CJ. Overview of recent clinical pharmacokinetic studies with acitretin (Ro 10-1670, Etretin). Dermatologica 1989; 178: 79-87.
Geiger JM, Czarnetzki BM. Acitretin (Ro 10-1670, Etretin): overall evaluation of clinical studies. Dermatologica 1988; 176: 182-90.

Developed: 4/24/98

**ACRIVASTINE**—See *Antihistamines (Systemic)*

# ACYCLOVIR Systemic

INN: Aciclovir
VA CLASSIFICATION (Primary): AM802
Commonly used brand name(s): *Avirax; Zovirax.*
Note: For a listing of dosage forms and brand names by country availability, see *Dosage Forms* section(s).

## Category
Antiviral (systemic).

## Indications
Note: Bracketed information in the *Indications* section refers to uses that are not included in U.S. product labeling.

### Accepted
Herpes genitalis, initial episode (treatment)—Oral acyclovir is indicated in the treatment of initial episodes of genital herpes infection in immunocompetent and immunocompromised patients. Parenteral acyclovir is indicated in the treatment of severe initial episodes of genital herpes infection in immunocompetent patients and in patients who are unable to take (or absorb) oral acyclovir.

Herpes genitalis, recurrent episodes (treatment)—Oral acyclovir is indicated in the treatment of frequently recurrent (≥ 6 episodes per year) or intermittent episodes of genital herpes infection in immunocompetent and immunocompromised patients.

Herpes simplex (treatment)—Parenteral [and oral][1] acyclovir are indicated in the treatment of initial and recurrent mucocutaneous herpes simplex (HSV-1 and HSV-2) infections in immunocompromised patients.

Herpes simplex encephalitis (treatment)[1]—Parenteral acyclovir is indicated in the treatment of herpes simplex encephalitis in immunocompetent patients.

Herpes zoster (treatment)—Oral acyclovir is indicated in the treatment of herpes zoster infections (shingles) caused by varicella-zoster virus (VZV) in any adult patient with herpes zoster. Therapy is most effective when started within 48 hours of the onset of rash. Parenteral acyclovir is indicated in the treatment of herpes zoster infections (shingles) caused by VZV in immunocompromised patients [and disseminated herpes zoster in immunocompetent patients][1].

Varicella (treatment)—Oral acyclovir is indicated in the treatment of varicella infections (chickenpox) in immunocompetent patients when started within 24 hours of the onset of a typical chickenpox rash. [Parenteral acyclovir is used in the treatment of varicella infections (chickenpox) caused by VZV in immunocompromised patients.][1]

Although acyclovir is indicated for the treatment of varicella infections in immunocompetent patients, the American Academy of Pediatrics does not recommend its use for the treatment of uncomplicated chickenpox in healthy children. It is recommended for certain groups at increased risk of severe varicella or its complications, such as otherwise healthy, nonpregnant persons 13 years of age or older; children older than 12 months of age with a chronic cutaneous or pulmonary disorder; and children receiving short, intermittent, or aerosolized courses of corticosteroids. If possible, steroids should be discontinued after known exposure to varicella.

[Herpes simplex (prophylaxis)][1]—Parenteral and oral acyclovir are used in the prophylaxis of herpes simplex virus (HSV) infections in patients who are immunocompromised, including transplant patients receiving immunosuppressant therapy, human immunodeficiency virus (HIV)-infected patients, and patients receiving chemotherapy.

[Herpes simplex virus, disseminated neonatal infection (treatment)][1]—Parenteral acyclovir is used in the treatment of disseminated HSV in neonates.

[Herpes zoster (prophylaxis)][1]—Oral acyclovir is used in the prophylaxis of herpes zoster infections (shingles) caused by VZV, after an initial period of treatment with parenteral acyclovir, in any immunocompromised patient, including transplant patients receiving immunosuppressant therapy, HIV-infected patients, and patients receiving chemotherapy.

[Herpes zoster ophthalmicus (treatment)][1]—Oral and parenteral acyclovir are indicated in the treatment of herpes zoster ophthalmicus.

Resistance of HSV and VZV to acyclovir has been reported to develop with prolonged treatment or repeated therapy in severely immunocompromised patients. Resistance may occasionally develop as quickly as within a few weeks. If lesions due to herpes simplex virus fail to respond to acyclovir therapy, especially with continued viral shedding, viral isolates should be tested for susceptibility to acyclovir.

[1]Not included in Canadian product labeling.

## Pharmacology/Pharmacokinetics

### Physicochemical characteristics
Molecular weight—Acyclovir: 225.21.
Acyclovir sodium: 247.19.
pH—Reconstituted acyclovir (50 mg per mL): Approximately 11.

### Mechanism of action/Effect
Acyclovir is converted to the nucleotide acyclovir monophosphate by the viral thymidine kinases of herpes simplex virus (HSV) and varicella-zoster virus (VZV). Acyclovir monophosphate is converted to the diphosphate by cellular guanylyl kinase and to the triphosphate by a number of cellular enzymes. Acyclovir triphosphate is incorporated into growing chains of viral DNA where it interferes with the DNA polymerase activity HSV and VZV; this results in termination of the DNA chain and inhibition of viral DNA replication.

### Absorption
Oral—Bioavailability 20% (range, 10 to 30%); decreases with increasing dose. Poorly absorbed from the gastrointestinal tract. Not significantly affected by food.

### Distribution
Widely distributed into tissues and body fluids, including brain, kidneys, lungs, liver, aqueous humor, tears, intestines, muscle, spleen, breast milk, uterus, vaginal mucosa, vaginal secretions, semen, amniotic fluid, cerebrospinal fluid (CSF), and herpetic vesicular fluid. Highest concentrations are found in kidneys, liver, and intestines. CSF concentrations are approximately 50% of plasma concentrations. Crosses the placenta, also.

Vol$_D$ (steady state)—
  Adults: Approximately 48 liters (L) per square meter of body surface area (m²) (range, 37 to 57 L per m²).
  Children and adolescents (1 to 18 years old): Approximately 45 L per m².
  Neonates (0 to 3 months old): Approximately 28 L per m² (range, 24 to 30 L per m²).
  End-stage renal disease: Approximately 41 L per m².

### Protein binding
Low (9 to 33%).

### Biotransformation
Hepatic; only major metabolite found in urine is 9-carboxymethoxymethylguanine, which accounts for approximately 9 to 14% of the dose. This metabolite has no known antiviral activity.

### Half-life
Elimination of parenteral acyclovir—
  Adults with normal renal function: Approximately 2.5 hours.
  Children (1 to 18 years old): Approximately 2.6 hours.
  Neonates (0 to 3 months old): Approximately 4 hours.
  Adults with renal function impairment:

| Creatinine clearance (mL/min)/(mL/sec) | Half-life (hr) |
|---|---|
| > 80/1.33 | 2.5 |
| 50–80/0.83–1.33 | 3 |
| 15–50/0.25–0.83 | 3.5 |
| Anuric | 19.5 |
| During hemodialysis | 5.7 |
| Continuous ambulatory peritoneal dialysis | 14–18 |

Oral acyclovir—
  2.5 to 3.3 hours.

### Time to peak serum concentration
Intravenous—End of infusion (approximately 1 hour).
Oral—1.7 hours.

**Mean peak serum concentration (steady-state)**
Oral—
  Adults:
    200 mg every 4 hours—0.83 mcg/mL (3.68 micromoles/L).
    400 mg every 4 hours—1.2 mcg/mL (5.3 micromoles/L).
    800 mg every 4 hours—1.6 mcg/mL (6.9 micromoles/L).
Intravenous—
  Adults:
    5 mg per kg (over 1 hour) every 8 hours—9.8 mcg/mL (43.5 micromoles/L).
    10 mg per kg (over 1 hour) every 8 hours—22.9 mcg/mL (101.7 micromoles/L).
  Children (1 to 18 years old):
    250 mg per m$^2$ (over 1 hour) every 8 hours—10.3 mcg/mL (45.8 micromoles/L).
    500 mg per m$^2$ (over 1 hour) every 8 hours—20.7 mcg/mL (91.9 micromoles/L).
  Neonates (0 to 3 months old):
    5 mg per kg (over 1 hour) every 8 hours—6.8 mcg/mL (30 micromoles/L).
    10 mg per kg (over 1 hour) every 8 hours—13.8 mcg/mL (61.2 micromoles/L).

**Elimination**
Renal—
  Excreted by both glomerular filtration and tubular secretion.
  Oral: Approximately 14% of total dose excreted unchanged in urine.
  Intravenous: Approximately 45 to 79% excreted unchanged in urine.
Fecal—
  Insignificant amounts (< 2%).
Lungs—
  Trace amounts in exhaled $CO_2$.
Dialysis—
  Hemodialysis: A single 6-hour period of hemodialysis reduces plasma acyclovir concentrations by approximately 60%.
  Peritoneal dialysis: Peritoneal dialysis does not substantially alter acyclovir clearance.

## Precautions to Consider

**Cross-sensitivity and/or related problems**
Patients allergic to ganciclovir may also be allergic to acyclovir because of the chemical similarity of the two medications.

**Tumorigenicity**
Lifetime bioassays in rats and mice given daily doses of up to 450 mg per kg of body weight (mg/kg) (up to two and six times, respectively, the recommended dose in humans) by gavage did not increase the incidence of tumors or shorten the latency of tumor formation. However, one of two *in vitro* cell transformation assays resulted in morphologically transformed cells that formed tumors when inoculated into immunosuppressed, syngeneic, weanling mice.

**Mutagenicity**
Acyclovir has been shown to be mutagenic in some *in vitro* cytogenetic assay systems (human lymphocytes and one mouse lymphoma cell line). However, acyclovir was not mutagenic in other *in vitro* cytogenetic assay systems (three Chinese hamster ovary cell lines and two mouse lymphoma cell lines) or in four microbial assays. Acyclovir was clastogenic in Chinese hamster cells at 380 to 760 times the human dose. No mutagenicity was reported in a dominant lethal study in mice (36 to 73 times the human dose).

**Pregnancy/Reproduction**
Fertility—Impairment of spermatogenesis, sperm motility, or morphology has not been documented in humans given the recommended doses of acyclovir.
High doses of parenteral acyclovir have caused testicular atrophy in rats and dogs. However, no testicular abnormalities were observed in dogs given intravenous acyclovir at doses of 50 mg/kg per day for 1 month (21 to 41 times the human dose) or in dogs given oral acyclovir at doses of 60 mg/kg per day for 1 year (6 to 12 times the human dose). Studies in mice given oral doses of 450 mg/kg per day or rats given subcutaneous doses of 25 mg/kg per day have shown that acyclovir does not impair fertility or reproduction. Studies in female rabbits given acyclovir subcutaneously subsequent to mating have shown a significant decrease in implantation efficiency, but no decrease in litter size, at doses of 50 mg/kg per day.
Pregnancy—Acyclovir crosses the placenta. Acyclovir has been used in all stages of pregnancy, and no adverse fetal effects have been reported. One small, controlled study found that pre-partum treatment of women with recurrent genital herpes helped prevent symptomatic recurrences and viral shedding at the time of delivery, reducing the risk of the infant being exposed to the virus. Also, a prospective epidemiological registry of acyclovir use in pregnant women reports that the rate of birth defects in 494 women exposed to systemic acyclovir during the first trimester of pregnancy approximates the rate found in the general population. However, the small size of the registry is insufficient to evaluate the risk of less common defects or to permit reliable and definitive conclusions regarding the safety of acyclovir use in pregnant women and their developing fetuses. Adequate and well-controlled studies in humans have not been done. During pregnancy, acyclovir should be used only if the potential benefit to the mother outweighs the potential risk to the fetus. Physicians are encouraged to register patients in the Acyclovir in Pregnancy Registry maintained by Glaxo Wellcome by calling (800) 722-9292, ext. 38465.
Acyclovir was not teratogenic in mice given oral doses of 450 mg/kg per day (9 to 18 times the human dose), rabbits given subcutaneous or intravenous doses of 50 mg/kg per day (11 to 22 times the human dose), or rats given subcutaneous doses of 50 mg/kg per day (16 to 106 times the human dose). However, in a nonstandard perinatal and postnatal study in rats given three subcutaneous doses of 100 mg/kg (63 to 125 times the human dose) on gestation day 10, fetal abnormalities, such as head and tail anomalies, and maternal toxicity were observed.
FDA Pregnancy Category B (oral acyclovir).
FDA Pregnancy Category C (parenteral acyclovir).

**Breast-feeding**
Acyclovir is distributed into breast milk at concentrations from 0.6 to 4.1 times the corresponding plasma concentration. These concentrations would potentially expose the nursing infant to a dose as high as 0.3 mg/kg per day. A very small amount of acyclovir has been measured in one nursing infant's urine; no toxicity was observed.

**Pediatrics**
Limited data are available about the use of oral acyclovir in children younger than 2 years of age. However, no unusual toxicity or pediatrics-specific problems have been observed in studies done in children using doses of up to 3000 mg per square meter of body surface area (mg/m$^2$) per day and 80 mg/kg per day. Intravenous acyclovir should be used with greater caution in neonates due to their age-related decrease in clearance. The half-life and clearance of intravenous acyclovir in children older than 1 year of age is similar to that seen in adults with normal renal function.

**Geriatrics**
Studies performed to date have not demonstrated geriatrics-specific problems that would limit the usefulness of acyclovir in the elderly. However, elderly patients are more likely to have an age-related decrease in renal function, which may require an adjustment of acyclovir dosage or dosing interval.

**Drug interactions and/or related problems**
The following drug interactions and/or related problems have been selected on the basis of their potential clinical significance (possible mechanism in parentheses where appropriate)—not necessarily inclusive (» = major clinical significance):

Note: Combinations containing any of the following medications, depending on the amount present, may also interact with this medication.

» Nephrotoxic medications, other (see *Appendix II*)
  (concurrent use with oral or parenteral acyclovir may increase the potential for nephrotoxicity, especially in the presence of renal function impairment)
Probenecid
  (may decrease renal tubular secretion of intravenous acyclovir when used concurrently, resulting in increased acyclovir serum and cerebrospinal fluid [CSF] concentrations, prolonged elimination half-life in the serum and CSF, and, potentially, increased toxicity)

**Laboratory value alterations**
The following have been selected on the basis of their potential clinical significance (possible effect in parentheses where appropriate)—not necessarily inclusive (» = major clinical significance):

With physiology/laboratory test values
» Blood urea nitrogen (BUN) and
» Creatinine, serum
  (concentrations may be increased because of renal tubular obstruction caused by intravenous acyclovir; no increase generally occurs with proper dosage and adequate hydration)

**Medical considerations/Contraindications**
The medical considerations/contraindications included have been selected on the basis of their potential clinical significance (reasons given in parentheses where appropriate)—not necessarily inclusive (» = major clinical significance).

***Risk-benefit should be considered when the following medical problems exist:***
» Dehydration or
» Renal function impairment, pre-existing
    (intravenous acyclovir may increase the potential for nephrotoxicity; it is recommended that acyclovir be administered in a reduced dosage to patients with impaired renal function)
  Hypersensitivity to acyclovir or ganciclovir
  Neurological abnormalities or
  Prior neurologic reactions to cytotoxic medications
    (intravenous acyclovir may increase the potential for neurologic side effects)

**Patient monitoring**
The following may be especially important in patient monitoring (other tests may be warranted in some patients, depending on condition; » = major clinical significance):
» Blood urea nitrogen (BUN) and
» Creatinine, serum
    (concentrations required prior to and during therapy since intravenous acyclovir may be nephrotoxic; if acyclovir is given by rapid intravenous injection or its urine solubility is exceeded, precipitation of acyclovir crystals may occur in renal tubules; renal tubular damage may occur and may progress to acute renal failure)

## Side/Adverse Effects

Note: Acute renal insufficiency may occur due to precipitation of acyclovir in the renal tubules. It is most likely to occur if acyclovir is given by rapid intravenous injection, concurrently with known nephrotoxic medications, to patients who are inadequately hydrated, or to patients with renal function impairment without appropriate dosage reduction. However, acute renal failure has also been reported in patients receiving oral acyclovir.

Neuropsychiatric toxicity has been associated with high plasma acyclovir concentrations—which may occur when high doses are used, or when patients with renal function impairment are not given an appropriately lowered dose. Neuropsychiatric toxicity may also be more likely to occur in immunocompromised patients and geriatric patients.

The following side/adverse effects have been selected on the basis of their potential clinical significance (possible signs and symptoms in parentheses where appropriate)—not necessarily inclusive:

**Those indicating need for medical attention**
Incidence more frequent
  *For parenteral acyclovir*
    ***Phlebitis or inflammation at the injection site*** (pain, swelling, or redness)
Incidence less frequent
  *For parenteral acyclovir—more common with rapid intravenous injection*
    ***Acute renal failure*** (abdominal pain; decreased frequency of urination or amount of urine; increased thirst; loss of appetite; nausea; vomiting; unusual tiredness or weakness)
Incidence rare
  *For parenteral acyclovir only*
    ***Encephalopathic changes*** (coma; confusion; hallucinations; seizures; tremors)

**Those indicating need for medical attention only if they continue or are bothersome**
Incidence more frequent—especially with high doses
  *For parenteral acyclovir*
    ***Gastrointestinal disturbances*** (loss of appetite; nausea or vomiting); ***lightheadedness***
Incidence less frequent—with long-term use or high doses
  *For oral acyclovir*
    ***Gastrointestinal disturbances*** (nausea or vomiting; diarrhea; abdominal pain); ***headache; lightheadedness***

## Overdose

For more information on the management of overdose or unintentional ingestion, **contact a Poison Control Center** (see *Poison Control Center Listing*).

**Clinical effects of overdose**
Patients have intentionally ingested overdoses of up to 20 grams of oral acyclovir with no unexpected adverse effects.

Overdosage of parenteral acyclovir (following administration of bolus injections or inappropriately high doses, or in patients whose fluid and electrolyte balance was not properly monitored) resulted in elevations in blood urea nitrogen and serum creatinine concentrations and subsequent renal failure. Lethargy, convulsions, and coma have been reported rarely.

**Treatment of overdose**
To enhance elimination—Sufficient urine flow should be maintained to prevent precipitation of acyclovir in renal tubules. The recommended urine output is 500 mL per gram of acyclovir infused. A 6-hour hemodialysis session results in a 60% decrease in plasma acyclovir concentration. Peritoneal dialysis may be significantly less efficient in removing acyclovir from the blood. In the event of acute renal failure and anuria, the patient may benefit from hemodialysis until renal function is restored.

Supportive care—Patients in whom intentional overdose is confirmed or suspected should be referred for psychiatric consultation.

## Patient Consultation

As an aid to patient consultation, refer to *Advice for the Patient, Acyclovir (Systemic)*.

In providing consultation, consider emphasizing the following selected information (» = major clinical significance):

**Before using this medication**
» Conditions affecting use, especially:
    Hypersensitivity to acyclovir or ganciclovir
    Pregnancy—Acyclovir crosses the placenta; acyclovir should be used only if the potential benefit to the mother outweighs the potential risk to the fetus
    Breast-feeding—Acyclovir is distributed into breast milk
    Use in children—Neonates have an age-related decrease in acyclovir clearance
    Other medications, especially nephrotoxic medications
    Other medical problems, especially dehydration or pre-existing renal function impairment

**Proper use of this medication**
  Supplying patient information about herpes simplex or varicella-zoster infections
» For treatment of herpes zoster (shingles) or recurrent herpes simplex infections, initiating use of the medication as soon as possible after symptoms of recurrence begin to appear
» For treatment of chickenpox (varicella), initiating use of oral acyclovir at the earliest sign or symptom; it is most effective when started within 24 hours of the onset of a typical chickenpox rash
  Capsules, tablets, and oral suspension may be taken with meals or on an empty stomach
  Taking with full glass of water
  Proper administration technique for oral liquids
» Compliance with full course of therapy; not using more often or for longer than prescribed
» Proper dosing
  Missed dose: Taking as soon as possible; not taking if almost time for next dose; not doubling doses
» Proper storage

**Precautions while using this medication**
  Checking with physician if no improvement within a few days
  Keeping affected areas as clean and dry as possible; wearing loose-fitting clothing to avoid irritation of lesions
» Use of acyclovir has not been shown to prevent the transmission of herpes simplex virus to sexual partners
» Herpes genitalis may be sexually transmitted even if partner is asymptomatic; sexual activity should be avoided if either partner has signs and symptoms of herpes genitalis; use of a condom may help prevent transmission of herpes; however, spermicidal jellies or diaphragms probably will not be adequately protective

**Side/adverse effects**
  Signs of potential side effects, especially phlebitis or inflammation at site of injection, acute renal failure, and encephalopathic changes

## General Dosing Information

Therapy should be initiated as soon as possible following the onset of signs and symptoms of herpes simplex or varicella zoster infections.

Because it may take longer for lesions to heal in immunocompromised patients (an average of 2 weeks of therapy for herpes simplex infections), the duration of therapy may need to be prolonged beyond the recommended number of days until the lesions are crusted over or epithelialized.

### For oral dosage forms only
Acyclovir capsules, tablets, and oral suspension may be taken with meals since absorption has not been shown to be significantly affected by food; however, they may be taken on an empty stomach.

Intermittent short-term treatment of recurrent herpes genitalis infections may be effective for some patients, especially when treatment is patient-initiated during the prodrome or first sign of lesion formation.

### For parenteral dosage forms only
Sterile acyclovir sodium should be administered by intravenous infusion only. It should not be administered topically, intramuscularly, orally, subcutaneously, or ophthalmically.

Intravenous infusions of acyclovir should be administered at a constant rate over at least a 1-hour period to avoid renal tubular obstruction. Rapid injection must be avoided since precipitation of acyclovir crystals in the tubules may occur and may result in renal function impairment.

Obese patients should be dosed based on ideal body weight.

Since maximum urinary concentrations of acyclovir are achieved within 2 hours, patients receiving intravenous infusions and high oral doses must be adequately hydrated during this period to prevent precipitation of acyclovir in renal tubules.

The dose of acyclovir should be adjusted so that a dose is repeated after hemodialysis, since each 6-hour hemodialysis period results in approximately a 60% reduction in acyclovir plasma concentrations.

### Bioequivalenence information
The capsule, oral suspension, and tablet dosage forms are bioequivalent.

### For treatment of adverse effects
Since there is no specific antidote, treatment of adverse effects should be symptomatic and supportive with possible utilization of the following:
- Adequate hydration to prevent precipitation of acyclovir in the renal tubules.
- Hemodialysis to aid in the removal of acyclovir from the blood, especially in patients with acute renal failure and anuria.

## Oral Dosage Forms

Note: Bracketed uses in the *Dosage Forms* section refer to categories of use and/or indications that are not included in U.S. product labeling.

### ACYCLOVIR CAPSULES

**Usual adult and adolescent dose**
Genital herpes infection—
Initial episode: Oral, 200 mg every four hours while awake, five times a day, for ten days.
Recurrent infections, intermittent therapy (< 6 episodes per year): Oral, 200 mg every four hours while awake, five times a day, for five days.
Recurrent infections, chronic suppressive therapy (≥ 6 episodes per year): Oral, 400 mg twice a day, or 200 mg three to five times a day, for up to twelve months.
[Herpes simplex, mucocutaneous (treatment)][1]—
Oral, 200 to 400 mg five times a day for ten days in immunocompromised patients.
[Herpes simplex, mucocutaneous (prophylaxis)][1]—
Oral, 400 mg every twelve hours.
Herpes zoster (shingles)—
Oral, 800 mg every four hours while awake, five times a day, for seven to ten days.
Varicella (chickenpox)—
Oral, 800 mg four times a day for five days. Treatment should be initiated at the earliest sign or symptom of chickenpox.

Note: Adults with acute or chronic renal impairment may require a reduction in dose as follows:

| Normal dosing regimen | Creatinine clearance (mL/min)/(mL/sec) | Adjusted dosing regimen |
|---|---|---|
| 200 mg every 4 hours, 5 times daily while awake | > 10/0.17 | 200 mg every 4 hours, 5 times daily while awake |
|  | 0–10/0–0.17 | 200 mg every 12 hours |
| 400 mg every 12 hours | > 10/0.17 | 400 mg every 12 hours |
|  | 0–10/0–0.17 | 200 mg every 12 hours |
| 800 mg every 4 hours, 5 times daily while awake | > 25/0.42 | 800 mg every 4 hours, 5 times daily while awake |
|  | 10–25/0.17–0.42 | 800 mg every 8 hours |
|  | 0–10/0–0.17 | 800 mg every 12 hours |

Hemodialysis patients: A dose should be administered after each dialysis session.

**Usual pediatric dose**
Varicella (chickenpox)—
Children 2 to 12 years of age, up to 40 kg of body weight: Oral, 20 mg per kg of body weight, up to 800 mg per dose, four times a day for five days. Treatment should be initiated at the earliest sign or symptom of chickenpox.
Children 2 to 12 years of age, 40 kg of body weight and over: See *Usual adult and adolescent dose*.
Children up to 2 years of age: Safety and efficacy have not been established. However, no unusual toxicity or pediatrics-specific problems have been observed in studies done in children given 3000 mg per square meter of body surface area per day or 80 mg per kg of body weight per day.

**Strength(s) usually available**
U.S.—
200 mg (Rx) [*Zovirax* (lactose; may contain one or more parabens); GENERIC].
Canada—
200 mg (Rx) [*Zovirax* (lactose; cornstarch; magnesium stearate; sodium lauryl sulfate)].

**Packaging and storage**
Store between 15 and 25 °C (59 and 77 °F), in a tight container. Protect from light and moisture.

**Auxiliary labeling**
- Continue medicine for full time of treatment.

### ACYCLOVIR ORAL SUSPENSION

**Usual adult and adolescent dose**
See *Acyclovir Capsules*.

**Usual pediatric dose**
See *Acyclovir Capsules*.

**Strength(s) usually available**
U.S.—
200 mg per 5 mL (Rx) [*Zovirax* (methylparaben 0.1%; propylparaben 0.02%; sorbitol)].
Canada—
200 mg per 5 mL (Rx) [*Zovirax* (methylparaben; propylparaben; sorbitol)].

**Packaging and storage**
Store between 15 and 25 °C (59 and 77 °F), in a tight container. Protect from light.

**Stability**
Suspension retains its potency for 24 months from date of manufacture. Does not require reconstitution or refrigeration.

**Auxiliary labeling**
- Continue medicine for full time of treatment.
- Shake well.
- Take with water.
- Beyond-use date.

**Note**
When dispensing, include a calibrated liquid-measuring device.

### ACYCLOVIR TABLETS

**Usual adult and adolescent dose**
See *Acyclovir Capsules*.

**Usual pediatric dose**
See *Acyclovir Capsules*.

**Strength(s) usually available**
U.S.—
400 mg (Rx) [*Zovirax*; GENERIC].
800 mg (Rx) [*Zovirax*; GENERIC].
Canada—
200 mg (Rx) [*Avirax* (scored; lactose); *Zovirax* (lactose)].
400 mg (Rx) [*Avirax* (scored); *Zovirax*].
800 mg (Rx) [*Avirax* (scored); *Zovirax* (scored)].

**Packaging and storage**
Store between 15 and 25 °C (59 and 77 °F), in a tight container. Protect from light.

**Auxiliary labeling**
- Continue medicine for full time of treatment.

## Parenteral Dosage Forms

Note: Bracketed uses in the *Dosage Forms* section refer to categories of use and/or indications that are not included in U.S. product labeling.
The dosing and strength of the dosage forms available are expressed in terms of acyclovir base.

# Acyclovir (Systemic)

**STERILE ACYCLOVIR SODIUM**

**Usual adult and adolescent dose**

Genital herpes infections, severe, initial episode—
  Intravenous infusion, 5 mg (base) per kg of body weight every eight hours for five days. Administer at a constant rate over at least a one-hour period.

Herpes simplex (HSV-1 and HSV-2) infections, mucocutaneous, in immunocompromised patients—
  Intravenous infusion, 5 to 10 mg (base) per kg of body weight every eight hours for seven to ten days. Administer at a constant rate over at least a one-hour period.

Herpes simplex encephalitis[1]—
  Intravenous infusion, 10 mg (base) per kg of body weight every eight hours for ten days. Administer at a constant rate over at least a one-hour period.

Herpes zoster, caused by varicella zoster virus, in immunocompromised patients—
  Intravenous infusion, 10 mg (base) per kg of body weight every eight hours for seven days. Administer at a constant rate over at least a one-hour period.

Note: Adults with acute or chronic renal impairment require a reduction in dose and/or dosing interval as follows:

| Creatinine clearance (mL/min)/(mL/sec) | Dose (base) | Dosing interval (hr) |
|---|---|---|
| > 50/0.83 | 100% | 8 |
| 25–50/0.42–0.83 | 100% | 12 |
| 10–25/0.17–0.42 | 100% | 24 |
| 0–10/0–0.17 | 50% | 24 |

Hemodialysis patients require administration of an additional dose following each hemodialysis session.

No additional dosing is required for peritoneal dialysis patients.

**Usual adult prescribing limits**

30 mg (base) per kg of body weight, or 1.5 grams per square meter of body surface, daily.

**Usual pediatric dose**

Genital herpes infections, severe, initial episode—
  Infants and children up to 12 years of age: Intravenous infusion, 250 mg (base) per square meter of body surface area every eight hours for five days. Administer at a constant rate over at least a one-hour period.
  Children 12 years of age and over: See *Usual adult and adolescent dose*.

Herpes simplex (HSV-1 and HSV-2) infections, mucocutaneous, in immunocompromised patients—
  Infants and children up to 12 years of age: Intravenous infusion, 250 mg (base) per square meter of body surface every eight hours for seven days. Administer at a constant rate over at least a one-hour period.
  Children 12 years of age and over: See *Usual adult and adolescent dose*.

Herpes simplex encephalitis[1]—
  Infants and children 6 months to 12 years of age: Intravenous infusion, 500 mg (base) per square meter of body surface area every eight hours for ten days. Administer at a constant rate over at least a one-hour period.

Herpes zoster, caused by varicella zoster virus, in immunocompromised patients—
  Children up to 12 years of age: Intravenous infusion, 500 mg (base) per square meter of body surface area every eight hours for seven days. Administer at a constant rate over at least a one-hour period.

[Disseminated HSV in neonates][1]—
  Intravenous infusion, 10 mg (base) per kg of body weight every eight hours for ten to fourteen days. Administer at a constant rate over at least a one-hour period.

**Strength(s) usually available**

U.S.—
  500 mg (base) (Rx) [*Zovirax*; GENERIC].
  1 gram (base) (Rx) [*Zovirax*; GENERIC].
Canada—
  500 mg (base) (Rx) [*Zovirax*].
  1 gram (base) (Rx) [*Zovirax*].

**Packaging and storage**

Prior to reconstitution, store between 15 and 25 °C (59 and 77 °F).

**Preparation of dosage form**

To prepare initial dilution for intravenous infusion, add 10 or 20 mL of sterile water for injection to each 500-mg or 1-gram vial, respectively, to provide a concentration of 50 mg per mL. **Do not use bacteriostatic water for injection containing benzyl alcohol or parabens**. To ensure complete dissolution, shake vial well until solution is clear. The resulting solution should be further diluted with a suitable diluent (standard electrolyte- and dextrose-containing solutions [see manufacturer's package insert]) to at least 100 mL. Final concentrations of 7 mg per mL or less are recommended. Higher concentrations (e.g., 10 mg per mL) may cause phlebitis or inflammation at the injection site upon inadvertent extravasation.

**Stability**

After reconstitution with sterile water for injection, solutions at concentrations of 50 mg per mL retain their potency for 12 hours at controlled room temperature (15 to 25 °C [59 to 77 °F]).

After further dilution with standard electrolyte- and dextrose-containing solutions for intravenous infusion, solutions retain their potency for 24 hours at controlled room temperature (15 to 25 °C [59 to 77 °F]).

Refrigeration of reconstituted solutions may result in the formation of a precipitate, which will redissolve when warmed to room temperature.

**Incompatibilities**

Sterile acyclovir sodium is incompatible with biological or colloidal solutions (e.g., blood products, protein-containing solutions).

Parabens are incompatible with sterile acyclovir sodium and may cause precipitation.

---

[1]Not included in Canadian product labeling.

## Selected Bibliography

Wagstaff AJ, Faulds D, Goa KL. Aciclovir. A reappraisal of its antiviral activity, pharmacokinetic properties, and therapeutic efficacy. Drugs 1994; 47(1): 153-205.

Whitley RJ, Gnann JW. Acyclovir: a decade later. N Engl J Med 1992; 327(11): 782-9.

---

Revised: 06/22/94
Interim revision: 04/20/98; 08/14/98

---

# ACYCLOVIR Topical

INN: Aciclovir
VA CLASSIFICATION (Primary): DE103
Commonly used brand name(s): *Zovirax*.
A commonly used name is acycloguanosine.
Note: For a listing of dosage forms and brand names by country availability, see *Dosage Forms* section(s).

## Category

Antiviral (topical).

## Indications

Note: Bracketed information in the *Indications* section refers to uses that are not included in U.S. product labeling.

**Accepted**

Herpes simplex (treatment)—Topical acyclovir is indicated in the treatment of limited non–life-threatening initial and recurrent mucocutaneous herpes simplex (HSV-1 and HSV-2) infections in immunocompromised patients; however, systemic acyclovir is more effective and may be preferred.

[Herpes zoster (treatment adjunct)]—Topical acyclovir is used as adjunctive therapy to improve cutaneous healing of localized herpes zoster in immunosuppressed persons being treated systemically with other treatment regimens for herpes zoster.

Resistance to acyclovir, although currently of minor clinical significance, has been reported to develop with prolonged treatment in immunocompromised patients. Resistance does not appear to be significant in patients with normal immune function.

**Unaccepted**

Herpes genitalis (treatment)—Although topical acyclovir is FDA approved for the treatment of *initial* herpes genitalis infections caused by herpes simplex virus (HSV), the Centers for Disease Control (CDC) and USP medical experts do not recommend it for use, because oral acyclovir is considerably more effective.

Topical acyclovir is not effective in the treatment of *recurrent* herpes genitalis or herpes febrilis (labialis) infections in nonimmunocompromised patients, although topical acyclovir may cause some reduction in the duration of viral shedding. Also, there is no evidence that topical acyclovir will prevent the transmission of herpes infection to others or that it will prevent recurrent infections in the absence of signs and symptoms of infection.

## Pharmacology/Pharmacokinetics

**Physicochemical characteristics**
Molecular weight—225.21.

**Mechanism of action/Effect**
Acyclovir is converted to acyclovir monophosphate, a nucleotide, by herpes simplex virus (HSV)-coded thymidine kinase. Acyclovir monophosphate is converted to the diphosphate by cellular guanylate kinase and to the triphosphate by a number of cellular enzymes. Acyclovir triphosphate interferes with HSV DNA polymerase and inhibits viral DNA replication. The triphosphate can be incorporated into growing chains of DNA by viral DNA polymerase, resulting in termination of the DNA chain. Since acyclovir is preferentially taken up and selectively converted to the active triphosphate form by HSV-infected cells, it is much less toxic to normal uninfected cells.

**Absorption**
Intact skin—Minimal; acyclovir not detected in blood or urine.
Diseased skin (herpes zoster)—Moderate; serum concentrations up to 0.28 mcg per mL have been reported in patients with normal renal function and up to 0.78 mcg per mL in patients with impaired renal function.

**Elimination**
Renal—Up to approximately 9% of the total daily dose may be excreted in the urine.

## Precautions to Consider

**Carcinogenicity**
Lifetime bioassays in rats and mice given daily doses of 50, 150, and 450 mg per kg of body weight (mg/kg) by gavage have not shown any evidence of carcinogenicity. However, *in vitro* cell transformation assays have given conflicting results, being positive at the highest dose used in one system. The resulting morphologically transformed cells induced tumors when inoculated into immunosuppressed, syngeneic, weanling mice, although results were negative in another animal system.

**Tumorigenicity**
Studies in rats and mice have not shown any statistically significant difference between the incidence of benign tumors produced in drug-treated animals and that produced in control animals.

**Mutagenicity**
No chromosomal damage was noted at maximum tolerated parenteral doses (100 mg/kg) in rats or Chinese hamsters. Higher doses (500 and 1000 mg/kg) were clastogenic in Chinese hamsters. No problems were reported in dominant lethal studies in mice. Also, there was no evidence of mutagenicity in 9 out of 11 microbial and mammalian cell assays. In 2 of the mammalian cell assays, a positive response for mutagenicity and chromosomal damage was noted, but only at concentrations at least 1000 times the usual plasma concentrations in humans following topical application.

**Pregnancy/Reproduction**
Fertility—Studies in mice given oral doses of up to 450 mg/kg per day have not shown that acyclovir impairs fertility or reproduction. Studies in female rabbits given acyclovir subcutaneously subsequent to mating have shown a significant decrease in implantation efficiency, but no decrease in litter size at doses of 50 mg/kg per day.
Pregnancy—Adequate and well-controlled studies in humans have not been done.
Studies done in rats and rabbits given subcutaneous doses of up to 50 mg/kg daily and in mice given oral doses of up to 450 mg/kg daily have not shown that acyclovir causes adverse effects on the fetus.
FDA Pregnancy Category C.

**Breast-feeding**
It is not known whether topical acyclovir is distributed into breast milk. However, acyclovir is unlikely to be distributed into breast milk in significant amounts following topical administration, since the total daily dose is small, even though absorption through diseased skin is moderate.

**Pediatrics**
Appropriate studies on the relationship of age to the effects of topical acyclovir have not been performed in the pediatric population. However, limited data are available about the use of oral acyclovir in the pediatric population, and no unusual toxicity or pediatrics-specific problems have been observed in studies done in children using doses of up to 3000 mg per square meter of body surface per day and 80 mg/kg per day.

**Geriatrics**
Appropriate studies on the relationship of age to the effects of topical acyclovir have not been performed in the geriatric population. However, no geriatrics-specific problems have been documented to date.

**Medical considerations/Contraindications**
The medical considerations/contraindications included have been selected on the basis of their potential clinical significance (reasons given in parentheses where appropriate)—not necessarily inclusive (» = major clinical significance).

*Risk-benefit should be considered when the following medical problem exists:*
Sensitivity to topical acyclovir

**Patient monitoring**
The following may be especially important in patient monitoring (other tests may be warranted in some patients, depending on condition; » = major clinical significance):
Papanicolaou (Pap) test
(although a clear association has not been shown to date, patients with genital herpes may be at increased risk of developing cervical cancer; Pap tests should be done at least once a year to detect early cervical changes)

## Side/Adverse Effects

The following side/adverse effects have been selected on the basis of their potential clinical significance (possible signs and symptoms in parentheses where appropriate)—not necessarily inclusive:

**Those indicating need for medical attention only if they continue or are bothersome**
Incidence more frequent—Approximately 28%
*Mild pain, burning, or stinging*

Incidence less frequent—Approximately 4%
*Pruritus* (itching)

Incidence rare—Approximately 0.3%
*Skin rash*

## Patient Consultation

As an aid to patient consultation, refer to *Advice for the Patient, Acyclovir (Topical)*.
In providing consultation, consider emphasizing the following selected information (» = major clinical significance):

**Proper use of this medication**
Reading patient information about herpes simplex infections
» Avoiding contact with eyes
» Using medication as soon as possible after symptoms of herpes begin to appear
» Proper administration technique
*To use*
Using a finger cot or rubber glove to prevent autoinoculation
Applying sufficient medication to cover affected areas; a 1.25-cm strip of ointment per 25 cm² of affected skin is usually sufficient
» Compliance with full course of therapy; not using more often or longer than prescribed
» Proper dosing
Missed dose: Applying as soon as possible; not applying if almost time for next dose
» Proper storage

**Precautions while using this medication**
» Women with herpes genitalis may be more likely to develop cervical cancer; annual or more frequent Pap tests may be required
Checking with physician if no improvement within 1 week
Keeping affected areas as clean and dry as possible; wearing loose-fitting clothing to avoid irritation of lesions
» Herpes genitalis may be sexually transmitted, even if sexual partner is asymptomatic; avoiding sexual activity if either partner has symptoms of herpes genitalis; use of condom may help prevent transmission of herpes; however, topical acyclovir or the use of spermicidal jellies or diaphragms will not prevent transmission of herpes to others

# Acyclovir (Topical)

## General Dosing Information

Use of topical antivirals may lead to skin sensitization, resulting in hypersensitivity reactions with subsequent topical or systemic use of the medication.

Topical acyclovir is for cutaneous use only; it should not be used in the eyes.

Therapy should be initiated as soon as possible following the onset of signs and symptoms of herpes infection.

A 1.25-cm (½-inch) strip of ointment should be applied per 25 cm² (4 inches²) of affected skin. A finger cot or rubber glove should be used to prevent autoinoculation of other body sites.

The recommended dose, frequency of application, and length of treatment should not be exceeded.

## Topical Dosage Forms

### ACYCLOVIR OINTMENT

**Usual adult and adolescent dose**
Antiviral—
 Topical, to the skin and mucous membranes, every three hours, six times a day, for seven days. Apply a sufficient quantity to cover all lesions adequately.

**Usual pediatric dose**
See *Usual adult and adolescent dose*.

**Strength(s) usually available**
U.S.—
 5% (Rx) [*Zovirax*].
Canada—
 5% (Rx) [*Zovirax*].

**Packaging and storage**
Store between 15 and 25 °C (59 and 78 °F) in a dry place, unless otherwise specified by manufacturer.

**Auxiliary labeling**
- For external use only.
- Do not use in the eye.
- Continue medicine for full time of treatment.

**Note**
Acyclovir ointment has a polyethylene glycol base.
Although herpes virus may theoretically persist for up to 24 hours on any fomite, it is unlikely that herpes infections can be transmitted via contaminated ointment tubes.

## Selected Bibliography

Pariser DM. Cutaneous viral infections: herpes simplex and varicella-zoster. Prim Care 1989 Sep;16(3): 577-89.

Revised: 01/15/92
Interim revision: 05/10/94

---

# ADAPALENE Topical

VA CLASSIFICATION (Primary): DE752
Commonly used brand name(s): *Differin*.
Note: For a listing of dosage forms and brand names by country availability, see *Dosage Forms* section(s).

## Category

Antiacne agent (topical).

## Indications

**Accepted**
*Acne vulgaris (treatment)*—Adapalene is indicated for the treatment of acne vulgaris. It is most effective for treating mild to moderate acne vulgaris.

## Pharmacology/Pharmacokinetics

**Physicochemical characteristics**
Chemical group—Synthetic retinoic acid analog; derivative of naphthoic acid.
Molecular weight—412.53.
Solubility—Slightly soluble in ethanol and insoluble in water.

**Mechanism of action/Effect**
The exact mechanism is not known. Adapalene exhibits some retinoic acid-like activity but it also has additional effects. It is thought that adapalene reduces important features of the pathology of acne vulgaris by normalizing the differentiation of follicular epithelial cells and keratinization to prevent microcomedone formation, similar to the mechanism of retinoic acid. Unlike retinoic acid, adapalene selectively binds to some nuclear retinoic acid receptors (RARs) and does not bind to cellular receptors called cytosolic retinoic acid binding proteins (CRABPs). It is hypothesized that by selectively binding to certain nuclear retinoic acid receptors and not others, adapalene enhances keratinocyte differentiation without inducing epidermal hyperplasia and severe irritation, such as is seen with retinoic acid. Also, adapalene may help reduce cell-mediated inflammation, an effect demonstrated by *in vitro* studies. Adapalene decreases formation of comedones and inflammatory and noninflammatory acne lesions.

**Absorption**
Low absorption through skin.

**Onset of action**
Although clinical response may be detected in 1 to 2 weeks, an optimal response is typically seen after 8 to 12 weeks.

**Elimination**
Fecal (biliary).

## Precautions to Consider

**Carcinogenicity/Tumorigenicity**
Adapalene was not found to be carcinogenic in mice administered topical doses of 0.3, 0.9, and 2.6 mg per kg of body weight (mg/kg) per day. Oral doses of 0.15, 0.5, and 1.5 mg/kg given to rats increased the incidence of follicular cell adenomas and carcinomas of the thyroid in female rats, and benign and malignant pheochromocytomas in the adrenal medulla in male rats.
Although no photocarcinogenicity studies were conducted with adapalene, other topical retinoids have shown increased risk of tumorigenicity in animals when they were exposed to sunlight or ultraviolet irradiation in the laboratory under certain circumstances but not in all test systems. The significance of these animal studies to humans is not known.

**Mutagenicity**
Adapalene was not found to be mutagenic or genotoxic in a series of *in vivo* and *in vitro* studies.

**Pregnancy/Reproduction**
*Pregnancy*—Adequate and well-controlled studies in humans have not been done. Although problems have not been reported with topical adapalene in the dose used for acne, it is recommended that pregnant women not use adapalene, based on data for other topical retinoids. As a general precaution, women of reproductive age may want contraception counseling before initiating treatment.
Teratologic studies of topical adapalene use in rats and rabbits are inconclusive. An increased number of ribs was seen in studies done in rats given topical doses of 0.6, 2, and 6 mg/kg a day (doses up to 150 times greater than the usual topical human dose); fetotoxicity was not seen in rats or rabbits at these doses. In oral doses of 25 mg/kg a day, adapalene is teratogenic in rats and rabbits.
FDA Pregnancy Category C.

**Breast-feeding**
It is not known whether adapalene is distributed into breast milk.

**Pediatrics**
No information is available on the relationship of age to the effects of adapalene in pediatric patients. Safety and efficacy in children up to 12 years of age have not been established.

**Geriatrics**
No information is available on the relationship of age to the effects of adapalene in geriatric patients. Acne vulgaris is not likely to occur in this age group.

**Drug interactions and/or related problems**
The following drug interactions and/or related problems have been selected on the basis of their potential clinical significance (possible mechanism in parentheses where appropriate)—not necessarily inclusive (» = major clinical significance):

Note: Combinations containing any of the following medications, depending on the amount present, may also interact with this medication.
    Acne products, topical, or topical products containing a peeling agent, such as
    Antibiotics, topical, such as
»     Clindamycin, topical
»     Erythromycin, topical
    Benzoyl peroxide
    Resorcinol
    Salicylic acid
    Sulfur or
    Alcohol-containing products or products containing strong drying agents, such as
    After-shave lotions
    Astringents
    Cosmetics or soaps with a strong drying effect
    Shaving creams or lotions
    Hair products, skin-irritating, such as hair permanents or hair removal products
    Products containing lime or spices, topical
    Soaps or skin cleansers, abrasive
    (concurrent use with adapalene may cause a cumulative irritating or drying effect resulting in irritation of the skin and/or sensitivity to the sun; if these effects occur, adapalene should be discontinued or initiation of treatment delayed until skin irritation has subsided)
    (use of benzoyl peroxide or topical antibiotics with adapalene on the same area of the skin at the same time is not recommended. A physical incompatibility between the medications or a change in pH may reduce adapalene's efficacy if used simultaneously. When used together for clinical effect, it is recommended that these medications be used at different times of the day, such as morning and night, to minimize possible skin irritation. If irritation results, the dose of adapalene may need to be reduced or temporarily discontinued until the skin is less sensitive)

### Medical considerations/Contraindications
The medical considerations/contraindications included have been selected on the basis of their potential clinical significance (reasons given in parentheses where appropriate)—not necessarily inclusive (» = major clinical significance).

*Risk-benefit should be considered when the following medical problems exist:*
    Dermatitis, seborrheicor
    Eczema
        (skin irritation may be increased)
    Sensitivity to adapalene or other ingredients of the formulation

## Side/Adverse Effects
The following side/adverse effects have been selected on the basis of their potential clinical significance (possible signs and symptoms in parentheses where appropriate)—not necessarily inclusive:

### Those indicating need for medical attention
Incidence more frequent
    **Burning sensation or stinging of skin; erythema** (redness of skin); **pruritus** (itching of skin); **scaling** (dryness and peeling of skin)
    Note: A *burning sensation or stinging of skin, erythema,* or *scaling* is commonly seen within the first 4 weeks of use and usually lessens over time. If these effects are severe, dosage frequency of adapalene should be reduced or the medication discontinued until the severe skin irritation subsides. Twenty percent of patients report transient burning and itching of skin upon application of adapalene.

### Those indicating need for medical attention only if they continue or are bothersome
Incidence rare
    *Acne flares* (worsening of acne)—1%
    Note: *Acne flares* are more commonly seen in the first month of treatment and decrease in frequency and severity thereafter.

## Patient Consultation
In providing consultation, consider emphasizing the following selected information (» = major clinical significance):

### Before using this medication
»   Conditions affecting use, especially:
    Sensitivity to adapalene or other ingredients of the formulation
    Pregnancy—Problems not reported for topical doses used for acne; however, adapalene use is not recommended during pregnancy; alerting physician if pregnant or trying to become pregnant while using this medication

### Proper use of this medication
»   Importance of not using more medication than amount prescribed
»   Not applying medication to windburned or sunburned skin or on open wounds
»   Avoiding contact with the eyes, lips, and mucous membranes of inner nose

*Proper administration*
»   Applying small amount to clean, dry skin; rubbing in gently and well; washing hands to remove medication afterwards
»   Continuing to use for the full time of treatment
»   Proper dosing
    Missed dose: Applying next dose at regularly scheduled time; not doubling doses
»   Proper storage

### Precautions while using this medication
    Possibility that acne may worsen during the first 3 weeks of therapy; not stopping medication unless irritation, dryness, or other symptoms become severe; checking with physician if improvement not seen by 8 to 12 weeks
    Avoiding application of any other topical products at the same time as adapalene, especially alcohol-containing products; abrasive or drying agents; sun-sensitizing agents, such as those containing lime or spices; antiacne topical agents, such as antibiotics or peeling agents; abrasive soaps or skin cleansers; or irritating hair products
    If using topical clindamycin, erythromycin, or benzoyl peroxide, applying at different times of the day (morning and evening)
    Alerting doctor if excessive skin irritation occurs or is bothersome; using moisturizers, creams, or lotions as necessary to reduce skin irritation or dryness
    Avoiding or minimizing exposure of treated areas to direct and artificial sunlight, wind, or extremely cold temperatures; using sunscreens or sunblocking agents of at least SPF 15 and protective clothing over treated areas

### Side/adverse effects
    Signs of potential side effects, especially burning sensation or stinging of skin; erythema; pruritus; and scaling

## General Dosing Information
Medication should not be applied to open wounds or windburned, sunburned, or otherwise irritated skin. If skin irritation occurs or is bothersome, adapalene should be discontinued until skin irritation subsides. Contact with the eyes, lips, and mucous membranes of inner nose should be avoided.

After applying a thin film of medication to skin, the medication should be rubbed in gently and well. Hands should be washed to remove any remaining medication.

Although temporary exacerbation of acne may occur during the first few weeks of use due to the action of adapalene on deep, previously unseen lesions, therapy should be continued.

Although clinical response may be detected in 1 to 2 weeks, treatment should be evaluated if no improvement is seen after 8 to 12 weeks.

## Topical Dosage Forms

### ADAPALENE GEL

#### Usual adult and adolescent dose
Acne vulgaris—
    Topical, to the involved areas of the skin, once a day as a thin film applied to clean, dry skin at least one hour before bedtime.

#### Usual pediatric dose
Acne vulgaris—
    Safety and efficacy have not been established.

#### Strength(s) usually available
U.S.—
    0.1% (Rx) [*Differin* (edetate disodium; methylparaben; propylene glycol; sodium hydroxide)].
Canada—
    0.1% (Rx) [*Differin* (edetate disodium; methylparaben; propylene glycol; sodium hydroxide)].

#### Packaging and storage
Store between 15 and 30 °C (59 and 86 °F).

#### Auxiliary labeling
• For external use only.

#### Note
Include patient instructions when dispensing.

## Selected Bibliography

Shalita A, Weiss JS, Chalker DK, et al. A comparison of the efficacy and safety of adapalene gel 0.1% and tretinoin gel 0.025% in the treatment of acne vulgaris: a multicenter trial. J Am Acad Dermatol 1996; 34: 482-5.

Developed: 06/02/97

---

# ADENOSINE    Systemic †

VA CLASSIFICATION (Primary/Secondary): CV300/DX900
Commonly used brand name(s): *Adenocard*.
Note: For a listing of dosage forms and brand names by country availability, see *Dosage Forms* section(s).

†Not commercially available in Canada.

## Category
Antiarrhythmic; diagnostic aid adjunct (ischemic heart disease).

## Indications
Note: Bracketed information in the *Indications* section refers to uses that are not included in U.S. product labeling.

### Accepted
Tachycardia, supraventricular, paroxysmal (treatment)—Adenosine is indicated for conversion to sinus rhythm of paroxysmal supraventricular tachycardia, including those due to atrioventricular (AV) node reentry and associated with accessory bypass tracts (Wolff-Parkinson-White syndrome), after appropriate vagal maneuvers (e.g., Valsalva maneuver) have been attempted.

[Myocardial perfusion imaging, radionuclide (adjunct)][1]; or
[Stress echocardiography (adjunct)][1]—Adenosine is used to induce coronary artery vasodilation in conjunction with myocardial perfusion imaging or two-dimensional echocardiography for the detection of perfusion defects or regional contraction abnormalities associated with coronary artery disease.

[1]Not included in Canadian product labeling.

## Pharmacology/Pharmacokinetics

### Mechanism of action/Effect
Antiarrhythmic—Slows impulse formation in the sinoatrial (SA) node, slows conduction time through the atrioventricular (AV) node, and can interrupt reentry pathways through the AV node. Adenosine depresses left ventricular function, but because of its short half-life, the effect is transient, allowing use in patients with existing poor left ventricular function.

Diagnostic aid—The precise mechanism of coronary vasodilation is not completely understood. However, it is speculated that adenosine may have a direct effect on smooth muscle receptors and may influence cellular calcium dynamics. Coronary vasodilation by adenosine contributes to the creation of heterogeneity of myocardial blood flow. The difference in coronary reserve in the vascular bed distal to a critical coronary stenosis versus that supplied by normal coronary arteries accounts for a significantly greater, 3- to 5-fold, increase in regional myocardial blood flow to normal epicardial vessels.

### Other actions/effects
Administration of doses larger than 12 mg by intravenous infusion decreases blood pressure by reducing peripheral vascular resistance. Physiologically, naturally occurring adenosine functions as an intermediate metabolite in a number of processes including regulation of coronary and systemic vascular tone, platelet function, lipolysis in fat cells, and intracardiac conduction.

### Biotransformation
Very rapid, by circulating enzymes in erythrocytes and vascular endothelial cells, by deamination, primarily to inactive inosine (further degraded to hypoxanthine and then to uric acid) and by phosphorylation to adenosine monophosphate (AMP).

### Half-life
Less than 10 seconds.

### Onset of action
Immediate.

### Elimination
Principal elimination routes are cellular uptake and metabolism. Metabolites excreted renally. The predominant final excretory metabolite is uric acid.

## Precautions to Consider

### Carcinogenicity
Studies have not been done.

### Mutagenicity
Mutagenicity tests in the Salmonella/mammalian microsome assay (Ames test) were negative. However, adenosine causes chromosomal alterations.

### Pregnancy/Reproduction
Fertility—In rats and mice, intraperitoneal administration of 50, 100, and 150 mg per kg of body weight (mg/kg) per day for 5 days caused decreased spermatogenesis and increased numbers of abnormal sperm.

Pregnancy—Studies have not been done in humans. Because adenosine occurs naturally in the body, problems are not expected. Scant reports of adenosine use in pregnant women have not revealed fetal or maternal sequelae.
Studies have not been done in animals.
FDA Pregnancy Category C.

### Breast-feeding
Because of rapid removal from circulation, adenosine is not expected to be distributed into breast milk.

### Pediatrics
Studies performed to date on adenosine's use as an antiarrhythmic have not demonstrated pediatrics-specific problems that would limit the usefulness of this medication in the pediatric population.

### Geriatrics
Appropriate studies on the relationship of age to the effects of adenosine have not been performed in the geriatric population. However, geriatrics-specific problems that would limit the usefulness of this medication in the elderly are not expected.

### Drug interactions and/or related problems
The following drug interactions and/or related problems have been selected on the basis of their potential clinical significance (possible mechanism in parentheses where appropriate)—not necessarily inclusive (» = major clinical significance):

Note: Combinations containing any of the following medications, depending on the amount present, may also interact with this medication.

Carbamazepine
(may increase heart block caused by adenosine)

Dipyridamole
(potentiates the effects of adenosine by inhibiting cellular uptake; dosage reduction is recommended)

Xanthines, especially caffeine and theophylline
(antagonize the effects of adenosine; larger doses of adenosine may be required or alternative therapy should be used)
(concurrent use with xanthines may invalidate test when adenosine is used as a diagnostic aid)

### Medical considerations/Contraindications
The medical considerations/contraindications included have been selected on the basis of their potential clinical significance (reasons given in parentheses where appropriate)—not necessarily inclusive (» = major clinical significance).

*Except under special circumstances, this medication should not be used when the following medical problem exists:*

» Atrioventricular (AV) block, pre-existing second or third degree without pacemaker
(risk of complete heart block)

*Risk-benefit should be considered when the following medical problems exist:*

Asthma
(although problems have not been reported with adenosine injection, inhaled adenosine has been reported to cause bronchoconstriction in asthmatic patients but not in normal individuals)

Sensitivity to adenosine

» Sick sinus syndrome
(sinus node recovery time prolonged; sinus bradycardia, sinus pause, or sinus arrest may occur)

**Patient monitoring**

The following may be especially important in patient monitoring (other tests may be warranted in some patients, depending on condition; » = major clinical significance):

» Blood pressure and
» Heart rate
(determinations recommended every 15 to 30 seconds for several minutes)
» Electrocardiogram (ECG)
(recommended to confirm efficacy of adenosine)

## Side/Adverse Effects

Note: Side/adverse effects are usually transient, generally lasting less than one minute. However, loss of consciousness and prolonged hypotension have been reported rarely.

The following side/adverse effects have been selected on the basis of their potential clinical significance (possible signs and symptoms in parentheses where appropriate)—not necessarily inclusive:

**Those indicating need for medical attention**
Incidence more frequent
*Arrhythmias, new, including premature ventricular contractions, atrial premature contractions, sinus bradycardia, sinus tachycardia, and skipped beats; chest, jaw, throat, or arm pain; dyspnea* (shortness of breath)
Note: *New arrhythmias* usually last only a few seconds.
Incidence rare
*Heart block, first-, second-, or third-degree*
Note: *Heart block* is usually of short duration and may occur more frequently in patients who receive a rapid intravenous dose of adenosine. Episodes of transient asystole have been reported.

**Those indicating need for medical attention only if they continue or are bothersome**
Incidence more frequent
*Flushing of face; headache*
Incidence less frequent
*Cough; dizziness or lightheadedness; nausea; numbness or tingling in arms*

## General Dosing Information

If high-level heart block occurs after one dose of adenosine, it is recommended that additional doses not be given. The effect usually resolves quickly because of adenosine's short duration of action.

Rapid intravenous administration of adenosine is recommended to achieve the desired negative chronotropic and dromotropic activity. Slow administration may result in an increase in heart rate in response to vasodilation.

**For treatment of adverse effects and/or overdose**

Because of adenosine's extremely short duration of action, adverse effects are usually self-limiting. Treatment of prolonged adverse effects should be individualized. Xanthines (e.g., caffeine, theophylline) are competitive antagonists of adenosine.

## Parenteral Dosage Forms

Note: Bracketed uses in the *Dosage Forms* section refer to categories of use and/or indications that are not included in U.S. product labeling.

**ADENOSINE INJECTION**

**Usual adult dose**
Antiarrhythmic—
Intravenous, rapid (over one to two seconds), 6 mg. If the first dose is not effective within one to two minutes, a rapid intravenous dose of 12 mg may be given, and repeated if necessary.

[Diagnostic aid adjunct][1]—
Intravenous, 140 mcg (0.14 mg) per kg of body weight per minute given for six minutes.

Note: In patients at increased risk for side/adverse effects, the dose may be titrated from 50 mcg (0.05 mg) per kg of body weight per minute up to 140 mcg (0.14 mg) per kg of body weight per minute at one-minute intervals. If side/adverse effects are severe, the infusion rate may be reduced to a more tolerable level. Doses of 75 and 100 mcg (0.075 and 0.1 mg) per kg of body weight per minute can adequately increase coronary blood flow.

Thallium injection should be given into a separate vein and is usually injected at the three- or four-minute mark of the adenosine infusion.

Note: To ensure that adenosine injection reaches the systemic circulation, it should be given directly into a vein or, if given into an intravenous line, be given as proximally as possible and followed by a rapid saline flush.

**Usual adult prescribing limits**
Up to 12 mg per dose.

**Usual pediatric dose**
Antiarrhythmic—
Intravenous, 50 mcg (0.05 mg) per kg of body weight. Dose may be increased in increments of 50 mcg (0.05 mg) per kg of body weight given every two minutes up to a maximum dose of 250 mcg (0.25 mg) per kg of body weight.

**Strength(s) usually available**
U.S.—
3 mg per mL (Rx) [*Adenocard*].
Canada—
Not commercially available.

**Packaging and storage**
Store between 15 and 30 °C (59 and 86 °F), unless otherwise specified by manufacturer. Do not refrigerate. Protect from freezing.

**Stability**
Because adenosine injection contains no preservatives, any unused portion should be discarded.

Crystallization may occur if adenosine injection is refrigerated. If that occurs, the crystals may be dissolved by warming the injection to room temperature. The solution must be clear before use.

---

[1]Not included in Canadian product labeling.

## Selected Bibliography

Parker RB, McCollam PL. Adenosine in the episodic treatment of paroxysmal supraventricular tachycardia. Clin Pharm 1990 Apr; 9: 261-71.

Gupta NC, Esterbrooks DJ, Hilleman DE, Mohiuddin SM. Comparison of adenosine and exercise thallium-201 single-photon emission computed tomography (SPECT) myocardial perfusion imaging. J Am Coll Cardiol 1992; 19: 248-57.

Rankin AC, Brooks R, Ruskin JN. Adenosine and the treatment of supraventricular tachycardia. Am J Med 1992; 92: 655-64.

---

Revised: 07/12/94

---

**ALATROFLOXACIN MESYLATE**—See *Trovafloxacin (Systemic)*

---

**ALBENDAZOLE**—The *Albendazole (Systemic)* monograph is not included in this published version of the USP DI database. Copies of the monograph are available on request from Micromedex, Inc. - Reprint Requests, 6200 S. Syracuse Way, Suite 300, Englewood, CO 80111; telephone (303) 486-6400; telefax (303) 486-6464; Email: USPDI@MDX.COM.

# ALBUMIN HUMAN Systemic

VA CLASSIFICATION (Primary): BL800

Commonly used brand name(s): *Albuminar-25; Albuminar-5; Albutein 25%; Albutein 5%; Buminate 25%; Buminate 5%; Plasbumin-25; Plasbumin-5.*

Note: For a listing of dosage forms and brand names by country availability, see *Dosage Forms* section(s).

## Category

Blood volume expander; antihyperbilirubinemic.

## Indications

### Accepted

Hypovolemia (treatment)—The 5 and 25% concentrations of albumin are indicated in the emergency treatment of hypovolemia with or without shock. Albumin restores intravascular volume and maintains cardiac output and colloid oncotic pressure. If blood loss is severe, a transfusion of whole blood or red blood cells may be indicated to restore the hemoglobin concentration and improve oxygen transport.

Hypoproteinemia (treatment)—The 5 and 25% concentrations of albumin are indicated in the treatment of hypoproteinemia caused by loss of plasma proteins. Loss of plasma proteins may occur through decreased absorption in gastrointestinal disorders, inadequate synthesis in chronic liver disease, or excessive urinary loss and increased catabolism in chronic kidney disease. This loss of protein leads to edema secondary to a fluid shift from the intravascular space to the interstitium and a compensatory increase in salt and water retention. Albumin serves to restore colloid oncotic pressure and, in conjunction with a diuretic, promote diuresis.

Burns, severe (treatment adjunct)—The 5 and 25% concentrations of albumin are indicated, in conjunction with large volumes of crystalloid injection, to maintain plasma volume and protein concentration and to prevent the intravascular hemoconcentration accompanying severe burns.

Hyperbilirubinemia, neonatal (treatment)—The 25% albumin injection is indicated in the treatment of hyperbilirubinemia whether or not it is associated with hemolytic disease. It may be used prior to or during an exchange transfusion to bind free bilirubin and to enhance its removal.

Respiratory distress syndrome, adult (ARDS) (treatment adjunct)—The 25% albumin injection may be indicated, in conjunction with diuretics, to correct the fluid volume overload associated with ARDS.

Cardiopulmonary bypass (treatment adjunct)—The 5 and 25% concentrations of albumin may be indicated as adjuncts to provide hemodilution in cardiopulmonary bypass procedures.

Ascites (treatment adjunct)[1]—The 5 and 25% concentrations of albumin may be used to maintain cardiovascular function following the removal of large volumes of ascitic fluid.

Nephrosis, acute (treatment adjunct) or
Nephrotic syndrome, acute (treatment adjunct)—The 25% albumin injection may be indicated as an adjunct in the control of edema in patients refractory to cyclophosphamide and corticosteroid therapy.

Hemodialysis—The 25% albumin injection may be used as an adjunct in patients who are undergoing long-term hemodialysis and are susceptible to shock and hypotension, or in dialysis patients who are hypervolemic and may not tolerate large volumes of crystalloid injection as treatment for shock or hypotension.

Pancreatitis (treatment adjunct) or
Intra-abdominal infections (treatment adjunct)—The 5 and 25% concentrations of albumin may be indicated, along with crystalloids, as fluid replacement in the treatment of shock associated with acute hemorrhagic pancreatitis or peritonitis when there is loss of fluid into the third space.

Liver failure, acute (treatment adjunct)—The 5 and 25% concentrations of albumin may be indicated as adjuncts in the treatment of acute liver failure to stabilize the circulation, maintain plasma colloid oncotic pressure, and bind excess bilirubin.

Red blood cell resuspension—Albumin may be indicated to provide sufficient volume and to prevent excessive hypoproteinemia during certain types of exchange transfusions or during the administration of large volumes of previously frozen or washed red blood cells.

[Plasmapheresis[1]]—The 5% concentration of albumin is indicated as volume or fluid replacement in large-volume plasma exchange, which is defined as more than 20 mL per kg in one session, or more than 20 mL per kg per week in repeated sessions.

### Unaccepted

Albumin has not been shown to be effective in the treatment of chronic cirrhosis or nephrosis.

Albumin does not contain all the essential amino acids and is, therefore, not an appropriate source of protein in the treatment of malnutrition. Given in excessive amounts, albumin may increase the catabolism of endogenous albumin.

[1]Not included in Canadian product labeling.

## Pharmacology/Pharmacokinetics

### Physicochemical characteristics

Source—Obtained from source blood, plasma, serum, or placentas of healthy human donorsby fractionation according to the Cohn cold ethanol process.

Albumin is heat pasteurized for 10 hours at 60 °C to inactivate human immunodeficiency virus (HIV) and hepatitis viruses; sodium caprylate and sodium acetyltryptophanate are added to prevent denaturation during this process.

Molecular weight—66,300 to 69,000.

pH—6.4 to 7.4.

### Mechanism of action/Effect

Blood volume expander—Albumin is an important regulator of the volume of circulating blood. It accounts for 70 to 80% of the colloid oncotic pressure of plasma. An infusion of albumin 5% is oncotically equivalent to an equal volume of human plasma and increases blood volume by an amount approximately equal to the volume of albumin infused; albumin 25% is oncotically equivalent to approximately 5 times the volume of human plasma and draws into the circulation an amount of fluid approximately 3.5 times the volume of albumin infused. Albumin provides a temporary increase in blood volume, which reduces hemoconcentration and blood viscosity.

Antihyperbilirubinemic—Albumin is a transport protein that reversibly binds both endogenous and exogenous substances including bilirubin, fatty acids, hormones, enzymes, drugs, dyes, and trace metals.

### Distribution

Albumin is distributed throughout the extracellular water; more than 60% is located in the extravascular fluid compartment.

### Half-life

Elimination—15 to 20 days.
Other—Intravascular: 24 hours.

### Onset of action

Blood volume expansion—With albumin 25% injection: 15 minutes, provided the patient is well hydrated.

### Duration of action

Dependent upon the initial blood volume of the patient. If blood volume is reduced, volume expansion persists for many hours; however, if blood volume is normal, the effect lasts a shorter time.

## Precautions to Consider

### Pregnancy/Reproduction

Pregnancy—Studies have not been done in humans.
Studies have not been done in animals.
FDA Pregnancy Category C.

### Breast-feeding

It is not known whether albumin is distributed into breast milk. However, problems in humans have not been documented.

### Pediatrics

Appropriate studies performed to date have not demonstrated pediatrics-specific problems that would limit the usefulness of albumin in children.

### Geriatrics

No information is available on the relationship of age to the effects of albumin in geriatric patients.

### Medical considerations/Contraindications

The medical considerations/contraindications included have been selected on the basis of their potential clinical significance (reasons given in parentheses where appropriate)—not necessarily inclusive (» = major clinical significance).

*Except under special circumstances, this medication should not be used when the following medical problems exist:*

» Anemia, severe or
» Cardiac failure or

» Hypervolemia or
» Pulmonary edema
(these medical problems may increase the risk of and/or be exacerbated by circulatory overload)

*Risk-benefit should be considered when the following medical problems exist:*

Hypertension or
Normal serum albumin concentrations
(increased plasma volume may lead to circulatory overload; hypertension may be exacerbated)

Renal function impairment
(aluminum, sometimes present as a contaminant in albumin injections, may accumulate, leading to anemia, dialysis encephalopathy, hypercalcemia, or vitamin D–refractory osteomalacia)

Sensitivity to albumin

### Patient monitoring

The following may be especially important in patient monitoring (other tests may be warranted in some patients, depending on condition; » = major clinical significance):

Aluminum concentrations, serum
(recommended in patients with renal function impairment, who are infused repeatedly with large volumes of albumin)

» Blood pressure measurements
(a rapid rise in blood pressure may reveal bleeding that was not apparent at the lower blood pressure)

Pulmonary wedge pressure determinations
(recommended to guard against circulatory overload)

## Side/Adverse Effects

The following side/adverse effects have been selected on the basis of their potential clinical significance (possible signs and symptoms in parentheses where appropriate)—not necessarily inclusive:

### Those indicating need for medical attention

Incidence less frequent
*Congestive heart failure*—especially in patients with compromised cardiovascular function; *decreased myocardial contractility; pulmonary edema; salt and water retention*

Note: These side effects are more likely to occur in patients given large volumes of crystalloids prior to the administration of albumin.

Incidence rare
*Changes in blood pressure, pulse, and respiration; chills; fever; increased salivation; nausea or vomiting; skin rash or hives; tachycardia*

## General Dosing Information

Albumin contains no blood group isoagglutinins and, therefore, may be given without regard to the blood group of the patient.

Albumin must be administered by intravenous infusion. It may be administered without dilution or diluted with 0.9% sodium chloride injection or 5% dextrose injection. **Sterile water for injection must not be used as a diluent for 25% albumin solutions as this results in a substantial reduction in osmolarity (tonicity), which increases the risks for potentially fatal hemolysis and acute renal failure, particularly when large volumes of the diluted solution are used in plasmapheresis.** It also may be administered with plasma, packed red blood cells, or whole blood; however, except when used as a red blood cell resuspension medium, albumin should not be added directly to any of these three components.

Note: Although 5% dextrose injection is considered an acceptable diluent, when it is used to dilute 25% albumin solutions and the resulting solution is used in the setting of plasma exchange or in conjunction with red blood cells, hemolysis might occur. Also, infusion of large volumes of the diluted solution can result in hyponatremia. Therefore, some clinicians recommend using only 0.9% sodium chloride injection as the diluting fluid except when there is concern about increasing the patient's sodium load and/or there is a need to maintain or restore the patient's blood glucose concentration.

Albumin may be administered at a rate of 1 to 2 mL per minute; however, the rate of infusion and the total volume of albumin administered ultimately must be guided by the hemodynamic response of the patient.

Patients with marked dehydration given 25% albumin injection require administration of additional fluids.

Transfusions of whole blood or packed red blood cells may be necessary following administration of large volumes of albumin to restore hemoglobin concentration and to prevent anemia.

## Parenteral Dosage Forms

### ALBUMIN HUMAN USP

**Usual adult dose**

Hypovolemia—
Intravenous infusion, 25 grams as a 5 or 25% injection, administered as rapidly as tolerated by the patient. If an adequate response is not achieved within fifteen to thirty minutes, an additional dose may be given.

Hypoproteinemia—
Intravenous infusion, 50 to 75 grams as a 25% injection, administered at a rate of 100 mL over thirty to forty minutes. For slow infusion, 50 grams in 300 mL of 10% dextrose injection, administered at a rate of 100 mL per hour.

Burns—
Therapy is usually begun with the administration of large volumes of crystalloid injection to maintain plasma volume. After 24 hours, albumin may be added at an initial dose of 25 grams, with the dose adjusted thereafter to maintain a plasma albumin concentration of 2.5 grams per 100 mL (25 grams/L), or a total serum protein concentration of 5.2 grams per 100 mL (52 grams/L).

Cardiopulmonary bypass—
Intravenous infusion, as a 5 or 25% injection, with crystalloid as a pump prime to achieve plasma albumin and hematocrit concentrations of 2.5 grams per 100 mL (25 grams/L) and 20%, respectively.

Nephrosis, acute or
Nephrotic syndrome, acute—
Intravenous infusion, 25 grams as a 25% injection, administered with an appropriate diuretic once a day for seven to ten days.

Hemodialysis—
Intravenous infusion, 25 grams as a 25% injection.

Red blood cell resuspension—
20 to 25 grams as a 25% injection, per liter of red blood cells.

**Usual adult prescribing limits**
Up to 2 grams per kg of body weight within twenty-four hours.

**Usual pediatric dose**

Hypovolemia—
Intravenous infusion, 2.5 to 12.5 grams, or 0.5 to 1 gram per kg of body weight, administered as rapidly as tolerated by the patient. If an adequate response is not achieved within fifteen to thirty minutes, an additional dose may be given.

Burns—
Therapy is usually begun with the administration of large volumes of crystalloid injection to maintain plasma volume. After 24 hours, albumin may be added at an initial dose of 25 grams, with the dose adjusted thereafter to maintain a plasma albumin concentration of 2 to 2.5 grams per 100 mL (20 to 25 grams/L), or a total serum protein concentration of 5.2 grams per 100 mL (52 grams/L).

Hyperbilirubinemia, neonatal—
Intravenous infusion, 1 gram per kg of body weight as a 25% injection, administered during, or one to two hours prior to, exchange transfusion.

**Strength(s) usually available**

U.S.—
5% in 50 mL (Rx) [*Albuminar-5* (sodium ion 130–160 mEq per L; potassium ion ≤ 1 mEq per L); *Plasbumin-5* [GENERIC (sodium ion 130–160 mEq per L)].

5% in 250 mL (Rx) [*Albuminar-5* (sodium ion 130–160 mEq per L; potassium ion ≤ 1 mEq per L); *Albutein 5%* (sodium ion 130–160 mEq per L); *Buminate 5%* (sodium ion 130–160 mEq per L); *Plasbumin-5* [GENERIC (sodium ion 130–160 mEq per L)].

5% in 500 mL (Rx) [*Albuminar-5* (sodium ion 130–160 mEq per L; potassium ion ≤ 1 mEq per L); *Albutein 5%* (sodium ion 130–160 mEq per L); *Buminate 5%* (sodium ion 130–160 mEq per L); *Plasbumin-5* [GENERIC (sodium ion 130–160 mEq per L)].

5% in 1000 mL (Rx) [*Albuminar-5* (sodium ion 130–160 mEq per L; potassium ion ≤ 1 mEq per L)].

25% in 20 mL (Rx) [*Albuminar-25* (sodium ion 130–160 mEq per L; potassium ion ≤ 1 mEq per L); *Albutein 25%* (sodium ion 130–160 mEq per L); *Buminate 25%* (sodium ion 130–160 mEq per L); *Plasbumin-25* [GENERIC (sodium ion 130–160 mEq per L)].

25% in 50 mL (Rx) [*Albuminar-25* (sodium ion 130–160 mEq per L; potassium ion ≤ 1 mEq per L); *Albutein 25%* (sodium ion 130–160 mEq per L); *Buminate 25%* (sodium ion 130–160 mEq per L); *Plasbumin-25* [GENERIC ( sodium ion 130–160 mEq per L)].

25% in 100 mL (Rx) [*Albuminar-25* (sodium ion 130–160 mEq per L; potassium ion ≤ 1 mEq per L); *Albutein 25%* (sodium ion 130–160 mEq per L); *Buminate 25%* (sodium ion 130–160 mEq per L); *Plasbumin-25* [GENERIC (sodium ion 130–160 mEq per L)].

# Albumin Human (Systemic)

Canada—
- 5% in 50 mL (Rx) [*Plasbumin-5*].
- 5% in 250 mL (Rx) [*Plasbumin-5*].
- 5% in 500 mL (Rx) [*Plasbumin-5*].
- 25% in 20 mL (Rx) [*Plasbumin-25*].
- 25% in 50 mL (Rx) [*Plasbumin-25*].
- 25% in 100 mL (Rx) [*Plasbumin-25*].

**Packaging and storage**
Store at 15 to 30 °C (59 to 86 °F), unless otherwise specified by manufacturer. Protect from freezing.

**Preparation of dosage form**
A 5% albumin solution may be prepared from the 25% solution by adding one volume of the 25% solution to four volumes of 0.9% sodium chloride injection or 5% dextrose injection. **Sterile water for injection must not be used as a diluent for 25% albumin solutions as this results in a substantial reduction in osmolarity (tonicity), which increases the risks for potentially fatal hemolysis and acute renal failure, particularly when large volumes of the diluted solution are used in plasmapheresis.**

Note: Although 5% dextrose injection is considered an acceptable diluent, when it is used to dilute 25% albumin solutions and the resulting solution is used in the setting of plasma exchange or in conjunction with red blood cells, hemolysis might occur. Also, infusion of large volumes of the diluted solution can result in hyponatremia. Therefore, some clinicians recommend using only 0.9% sodium chloride injection as the diluting fluid except when there is concern about increasing the patient's sodium load and/or there is a need to maintain or restore the patient's blood glucose concentration.

**Stability**
Should not be used if solution is turbid or contains a precipitate. Albumin contains no preservative and should be used within 4 hours after the vial is opened. Partially used vials should be discarded.

**Incompatibilities**
Albumin is incompatible with verapamil hydrochloride, alcohol-containing solutions, amino acid solutions, fat emulsions, and protein hydrolysates.

**Selected Bibliography**
Tullis JL. Albumin 1. Background and use. JAMA 1977; 237: 355-60.
Tullis JL. Albumin 2. Guidelines for clinical use. JAMA 1977; 237: 460-3.
Subcommittee of the Victorian Drug Usage Advisory Committee. Human albumin solutions: consensus statements for use in selected clinical situations. Med J Aust 1992; 157: 340-3.

Revised: 08/17/93
Interim revision: 07/28/98

---

**ALBUTEROL**—See *Bronchodilators, Adrenergic (Inhalation-Local)*; *Bronchodilators, Adrenergic (Systemic)*.

---

**ALCLOMETASONE**—See *Corticosteroids (Topical)*.

---

**ALCOHOL AND ACETONE**—The *Alcohol and Acetone (Topical)* monograph is not included in this published version of the USP DI database. Copies of the monograph are available on request from Micromedex, Inc. - Reprint Requests, 6200 S. Syracuse Way, Suite 300, Englewood, CO 80111; telephone (303) 486-6400; telefax (303) 486-6464; Email: USPDI@MDX.COM.

---

**ALCOHOL AND SULFUR**—The *Alcohol and Sulfur (Topical)* monograph is not included in this published version of the USP DI database. Copies of the monograph are available on request from Micromedex, Inc. - Reprint Requests, 6200 S. Syracuse Way, Suite 300, Englewood, CO 80111; telephone (303) 486-6400; telefax (303) 486-6464; Email: USPDI@MDX.COM.

---

# ALDESLEUKIN   Systemic †

VA CLASSIFICATION (Primary): AN900

Commonly used brand name(s): *Proleukin*.

Other commonly used names are interleukin-2, recombinant, and rIL-2.

Note: For a listing of dosage forms and brand names by country availability, see *Dosage Forms* section(s).

†Not commercially available in Canada.

## Category
Biological response modifier; antineoplastic.

## Indications

**Accepted**

Carcinoma, renal (treatment)—Aldesleukin is indicated for treatment of metastatic renal carcinoma in patients 18 years of age and older.

Melanoma, metastatic (treatment)—Aldesleukin is indicated for treatment of metastatic melanoma in patients 18 years of age and older.

Note: *Because of its potential life-threatening toxicities, USP DI Advisory Panels recommend that this medication be used only after careful consideration of risk-benefit.* It is recommended that aldesleukin be used only by qualified specialists who are fully aware of and equipped to monitor and treat the potential toxicities of this medication.

## Pharmacology/Pharmacokinetics

Note: Pharmacokinetics can be described by a 2-compartment model.

**Physicochemical characteristics**

Source—Synthetic. Produced by a recombinant DNA process involving genetically engineered *Escherichia coli* containing an analog of the human interleukin-2 gene. Genetic engineering techniques used to modify the human interleukin-2 gene result in an expression clone that encodes a modified human interleukin-2. Aldesleukin differs from naturally occurring interleukin-2 in that it is not glycosylated because it is derived from *Escherichia coli*, the molecule has no N-terminal alanine (the codon for this amino acid was deleted during the genetic engineering process), the molecule has serine substituted for cysteine at amino acid position 125 (this was accomplished by site-specific manipulation during the genetic engineering process), and the aggregation state of aldesleukin is likely to be different from that of native interleukin-2. The manufacturing process involves fermentation in a defined medium containing tetracycline hydrochloride; the presence of the antibiotic is not detectable in the final product.

Chemical group—Related to naturally occurring interleukins, which are lymphokines, a subgroup of the hormone-like glycoprotein growth factors also known as cytokines.

Molecular weight—Approximately 15,600 daltons.

**Mechanism of action/Effect**

Aldesleukin has been shown to possess the biological activity of human native interleukin-2. *In vitro* studies performed on human cell lines demonstrate the immunoregulatory properties of aldesleukin, including:
- Enhancement of lymphocyte mitogenesis and stimulation of long-term growth of human interleukin-2 dependent cell lines;
- Enhancement of lymphocyte toxicity;
- Induction of killer cell (lymphokine-activated killer [LAK] cells and natural killer [NK] cells) activity; and
- Induction of interferon-gamma production.

The *in vivo* administration of aldesleukin in select murine tumor models and in the clinic produces multiple immunological effects in a dose-dependent manner. These effects include activation of cellular immunity with profound lymphocytosis, eosinophilia, and thrombocytopenia, and the production of cytokines, including tumor necrosis factor, interleukin-1 and gamma interferon. *In vivo* experiments in murine tumor models have shown inhibition of tumor growth. However, the exact mechanism by which aldesleukin mediates its antitumor activity in animals and humans is unknown.

#### Other actions/effects
Aldesleukin causes a capillary leak syndrome (CLS) as a result of increased capillary permeability, leading to extravasation of plasma proteins and fluid into the extravascular space and contributing to loss of vascular resistance. Interleukin-2 has been reported to reversibly decrease serum cholesterol concentrations. Interleukin-2 has been reported to transiently decrease serum testosterone and dihydroepiandrosterone concentrations and to transiently increase plasma estradiol concentrations. It has also been reported to transiently increase adrenal secretion of ACTH and cortisol.

#### Distribution
Studies of intravenous aldesleukin in humans and sheep indicate that approximately 30% of the administered dose is distributed to the plasma initially. This is consistent with studies in rats that demonstrate a rapid and preferential uptake of approximately 70% of an administered dose into the liver, kidneys, and lungs.

#### Biotransformation
Renal. Greater than 80% of the amount of aldesleukin distributed to plasma, cleared from the circulation, and presented to the kidney is metabolized to amino acids in the cells lining the proximal convoluted tubules.

#### Half-life
Distribution—13 minutes.
Elimination—85 minutes.

#### Duration of action
Tumor regression may continue for up to 12 months following initiation of therapy.

#### Elimination
Renal. Cleared from the circulation by both glomerular filtration and peritubular extraction in the kidney. The dual mechanism for delivery of aldesleukin to the proximal tubule may account for the preservation of clearance in patients with rising serum creatinine values. The mean clearance rate in cancer patients is 268 mL per minute.

## Precautions to Consider

Note: In general, risks associated with aldesleukin therapy are dose- and schedule-related; toxicity of the high-dose regimen currently recommended is high.

#### Cross-sensitivity and/or related problems
Patients sensitive to *Escherichia coli*–derived proteins may also be sensitive to aldesleukin.

#### Carcinogenicity/Mutagenicity
Studies have not been done.

#### Pregnancy/Reproduction
Fertility—Studies have not been done. However, aldesleukin should not be administered to fertile persons of either sex not practicing effective contraception.

Pregnancy—Studies have not been done in humans. It is also not known whether aldesleukin can cause fetal harm when administered to a pregnant woman or can affect reproduction capacity. However, in view of the known adverse effects of aldesleukin, it should be given to a pregnant woman only with extreme caution; the potential benefit should be weighed against the risks associated with therapy.
Studies have not been done in animals.
FDA Pregnancy Category C.

#### Breast-feeding
It is not known whether aldesleukin is distributed into breast milk. However, because of the potential for serious adverse reactions in nursing infants from aldesleukin, a decision should be made whether to discontinue nursing or to discontinue treatment with aldesleukin, taking into account the importance of aldesleukin therapy to the mother.

#### Pediatrics
Safety and efficacy have not been established in children up to 18 years of age. Use is not recommended.

#### Geriatrics
Although appropriate studies on the relationship of age to the effects of aldesleukin have not been performed in the geriatric population, clinical trials have included elderly patients. There is some evidence that elderly patients do not tolerate aldesleukin's toxicity as well as younger patients. Cardiac status is of particular concern. In addition, elderly patients are more likely to have age-related renal function impairment, which may require caution in patients receiving aldesleukin.

#### Dental
The impairment of neutrophil function caused by aldesleukin may result in an increased incidence of microbial infection, delayed healing, and gingival bleeding. Dental work, whenever possible, should be completed prior to initiation of therapy or deferred until blood counts have returned to normal. Patients should be instructed in proper oral hygiene during treatment, including caution in use of regular toothbrushes, dental floss, and toothpicks.

Aldesleukin also commonly causes stomatitis, and less commonly causes glossitis, which may be associated with considerable discomfort.

### Drug interactions and/or related problems
The following drug interactions and/or related problems have been selected on the basis of their potential clinical significance (possible mechanism in parentheses where appropriate)—not necessarily inclusive (» = major clinical significance):

Note: Combinations containing any of the following medications, depending on the amount present, may also interact with this medication.

Blood dyscrasia–causing medications (see *Appendix II*)
(leukopenic and/or thrombocytopenic effects of aldesleukin may be increased with concurrent or recent therapy if these medications cause the same effects)

» Bone marrow depressants, other (see *Appendix II*) or
Radiation therapy
(additive bone marrow depression may occur)

» Cardiotoxic medications, other, including daunorubicin or doxorubicin
(concurrent use may result in increased cardiotoxicity)

Central nervous system (CNS) depressants
(concurrent use may result in increased CNS depression)

Contrast media, iodinated
(incidence of delayed [more than 1 hour after administration] reactions to intravenous iodinated contrast media [e.g., hypersensitivity, fever, skin rash, flu-like symptoms, joint pain, flushing, pruritus, emesis, hypotension, dizziness] may be increased in patients who have received interleukin-2; some symptoms may resemble a "recall" reaction to interleukin-2; supportive medical treatment may be necessary if symptoms are significant; there is some evidence that incidence of this reaction is reduced if contrast media administration is delayed until 6 weeks after interleukin-2 administration)

» Corticosteroids, glucocorticoid, systemic
(although glucocorticoids, especially dexamethasone, have been shown to reduce some adverse effects of aldesleukin, including fever, renal insufficiency, hyperbilirubinemia, confusion, and dyspnea, there is some evidence that concurrent use may reduce the antitumor efficacy of aldesleukin; therefore, it is generally recommended that dexamethasone be avoided, except in cases of life-threatening aldesleukin toxicity)

» Hepatotoxic medications, other (see *Appendix II*) or
» Nephrotoxic medications, other (see *Appendix II*)
(concurrent and/or sequential administration should be avoided since the potential for hepatotoxicity or nephrotoxicity may be increased, especially in the presence of hepatic or renal function impairment that may be caused by aldesleukin)

» Hypotension-producing medications, other (see *Appendix II*)
(concurrent use may result in increased hypotension)

### Laboratory value alterations
The following have been selected on the basis of their potential clinical significance (possible effect in parentheses where appropriate)—not necessarily inclusive (» = major clinical significance):

With physiology/laboratory test values
Alanine aminotransferase (ALT [SGPT]) values, serum and
Alkaline phosphatase values, serum and
Aspartate aminotransferase (AST [SGOT]) values, serum and
Bilirubin concentrations, serum and
Lactate dehydrogenase (LDH) values, serum
(increased in most patients)

Albumin and
Protein
(plasma concentrations may be decreased and urinary concentrations increased as a sign of renal toxicity)

Bicarbonate and
Calcium and
Magnesium and
Phosphate and
Potassium and
Sodium
(serum concentrations may be decreased but return to normal shortly after withdrawal of interleukin-2)

Blood urea nitrogen (BUN) and
Creatinine concentrations, serum
(dose-related increases commonly occur, indicating renal toxicity)

Creatine kinase (CK)
(serum concentrations may be increased with or without symptoms of cardiotoxicity and may be associated with nonischemic myocardial injury or myocarditis rather than myocardial ischemia or infarction)

Electrocardiogram (ECG) changes, including:
QRS voltage reductions
ST segment changes
T-wave changes
(may occur as signs of cardiotoxicity)

Left ventricular ejection fraction and
Left ventricular stroke work index
(frequently decreased in cardiotoxicity; these effects resemble septic shock)

Prothrombin time
(may be prolonged)

Uric acid
(concentrations in blood and urine may be increased, possibly as a result of catabolism of lymphokine-activated killer [LAK] cells and natural killer [NK] cells)

## Medical considerations/Contraindications

The medical considerations/contraindications included have been selected on the basis of their potential clinical significance (reasons given in parentheses where appropriate)—not necessarily inclusive (» = major clinical significance).

*Except under special circumstances, high-dose regimens of this medication should not be used when the following medical problems exist:*

» Cardiac function impairment, as determined by thallium stress test
» Organ allograft
(enhancement of cellular immune function by aldesleukin may increase the risk of allograft rejection)
» Pulmonary function impairment
» Because aldesleukin may exacerbate symptoms of clinically unrecognized or untreated central nervous system (CNS) metastases, generally treatment with aldesleukin should not begin until a patient has had thorough evaluation and treatment of CNS metastases, resulting in neurologic stability and a negative computed tomography (CT) scan.

*Risk-benefit should be considered when the following medical problems exist:*

Autoimmune disease, including autoimmune thyroiditis
(aldesleukin-associated hypothyroidism may be an autoimmune effect; autoimmune thyroiditis may be exacerbated)
» Bone marrow depression
» Cardiac function impairment, history of, even if function tests are normal
(may be exacerbated)
» Hepatic function impairment
(may be exacerbated)
Hypothyroidism, uncontrolled
(aldesleukin can cause hypothyroidism; no problems are anticipated in patients who are euthyroid as a result of thyroid hormone replacement therapy)
» Infection
(should be treated before initiation of aldesleukin therapy)
» Mental status impairment
(may be exacerbated)
Psoriasis
(may be exacerbated)
» Pulmonary function impairment, history of, even if function tests are normal
(may be exacerbated)
» Renal function impairment
(reduced elimination of aldesleukin, which may result in increased toxicity; impairment may be exacerbated by aldesleukin; patients with nephrectomy are eligible for high-dose aldesleukin therapy if their serum creatinine concentrations are less than or equal to 1.5 mg per deciliter)
» Seizure disorder, history of
(aldesleukin may cause seizures)
» Sensitivity to aldesleukin
» Caution should be used also in patients who have had previous cytotoxic drug therapy or radiation therapy.

## Patient monitoring

The following are especially important in patient monitoring (other tests may be warranted in some patients, depending on condition; » = major clinical significance):

» Body weight and
» Electrolytes, serum and
» Vital signs, including temperature, pulse, blood pressure, and respiratory rate
(recommended daily; if blood pressure decreases to less than 90 millimeters of mercury [mm Hg], constant cardiac rhythm monitoring, hourly vital signs, and central venous pressure [CVP] checks are recommended; if an abnormal complex or rhythm is seen, performance of an ECG and determination of cardiac enzymes are recommended)
» Cardiac function, including thallium stress test
(determination recommended prior to initiation of therapy; ejection fraction should be normal and wall function unimpaired; in patients with minor wall motion abnormalities of questionable significance suggested by the thallium stress test, a stress echocardiogram to document normal wall motion and exclude significant coronary disease may be useful; during treatment, cardiac function should be assessed daily by clinical examination and assessment of vital signs, adding ECG examination and creatine kinase [CK] evaluation for patients exhibiting signs or symptoms of chest pain, murmurs, gallops, irregular rhythm, or palpitations; a repeat thallium stress test is recommended if there is evidence of cardiac ischemia or congestive heart failure; use of a cardiac monitor is recommended if patients require pressor support)
» Hematocrit or hemoglobin and
» Leukocyte count, total and, if appropriate, differential and
» Platelet count
(determinations recommended prior to initiation of therapy and at periodic intervals during therapy; frequency varies according to clinical state, agent, dose, and other agents being used concurrently)
» Hepatic function and
» Renal function
(determinations recommended prior to initiation of therapy and daily during therapy)
» Pulmonary function, including arterial blood gases
(determination recommended prior to initiation of therapy; adequate pulmonary function, as defined by $FEV_1$ of greater than 2 liters or 75% or more of that predicted for height and age, should be present; during treatment, pulmonary function should be routinely monitored by clinical examination, assessment of vital signs, and pulse oximetry, adding arterial blood gas determination for patients exhibiting dyspnea or clinical signs of respiratory impairment [tachypnea or rales])
Thyroid function
(determinations recommended at periodic intervals during therapy)

## Side/Adverse Effects

Note: High-dose aldesleukin causes frequent, often serious, and sometimes fatal toxicity. Fatalities have occurred as a result of hepatic or renal failure, cardiac arrest, intestinal perforation, malignant hyperthermia, pulmonary edema, respiratory failure or arrest, pulmonary embolism, stroke, or severe depression leading to suicide.

Toxicity of aldesleukin is dose-related and schedule-dependent. Incidence of toxicity is probably increased in patients with a poor initial performance status.

Patient tolerance to interleukin-2 toxicity has been reported to decline with successive courses.

Most side/adverse effects are reversible within 2 or 3 days after aldesleukin is discontinued. However, permanent damage may result from myocardial infarction, bowel perforation or infarction, and gangrene.

Aldesleukin causes a dose-related capillary leak syndrome (CLS) as a result of increased capillary permeability, leading to extravasation of plasma proteins and fluid into the extravascular space and contributing to loss of vascular resistance. It is believed that hypotension and reduced organ perfusion that occur as a result of CLS are at least partially responsible for many of the toxicities of aldesleukin, including cardiac arrhythmias (supraventricular and ventricular), angina, myocardial infarction, respiratory insufficiency requiring intubation, gastrointestinal bleeding or infarction, renal insufficiency, and some mental status changes. The effects of CLS may be severe or fatal. CLS begins immediately after initiation of treatment, resulting initially, in most patients, in a decline in mean arterial blood pressure within 2 to 12 hours. Clinically significant hypotension (systolic blood pressure below 90 millimeters of mercury [mm Hg] or a 20 mm Hg decline from baseline systolic pressure) and hypoperfusion will occur with continued therapy. Protein and fluid extravasation will also cause edema and effusions; some patients may develop ascites or pleural effusions. Recovery from CLS begins soon after the end of aldesleukin therapy. Usually within a few hours, blood pressure rises, organ perfusion is restored, and resorption of extravasated fluid and protein begins.

In addition to CLS, other possible causes of interleukin-2 toxicity include growth of lymphocytes in visceral organs, which has been described in animal toxicology studies, and stimulation of secretion of other cytokines (e.g., tumor necrosis factor [TNF]) by cells of the immune system. For example, TNF and interleukin-1 secretion may be responsible for hemodynamic effects, which resemble septic shock.

Intravenous or subcutaneous aldesleukin administration frequently results in formation of low titers of non-neutralizing anti-interleukin-2 antibodies. Neutralizing antibodies have been detected in less than 1% of patients treated with aldesleukin. Evidence to date does not appear to indicate that antibody formation impairs response to aldesleukin.

It has been postulated that some toxicities (e.g., hypothyroidism, dermatologic effects) indicate a possible autoimmune effect of interleukin-2.

Hemodynamic and cardiac changes (e.g., peripheral vascular resistance, blood pressure, stroke index, left ventricular stroke volume, heart rate, ECG, creatine kinase) usually return to normal within a few days after interleukin-2 is discontinued.

The following side/adverse effects have been selected on the basis of their potential clinical significance (possible signs and symptoms in parentheses where appropriate)—not necessarily inclusive:

**Those indicating need for medical attention**
Incidence more frequent
*Anemia*—asymptomatic; *arrhythmias, especially sinus tachycardia* (fast or irregular heartbeat)—usually asymptomatic; *diarrhea; dizziness; edema, including peripheral edema with symptomatic nerve or vessel compression* (tingling of hands or feet); *eosinophilia; fever and/or chills; hepatotoxicity* (seen as changes on hepatic function tests that are attributable to severe cholestasis; yellow eyes and skin)—usually asymptomatic; *hypotension* (faintness)—usually asymptomatic; *hypothyroidism* (changes in menstrual periods; clumsiness; coldness; dry, puffy skin; headache; listlessness; muscle aches; sleepiness; tiredness; weakness; goiter [swelling in the front of the neck])—usually asymptomatic; *infection* (fever or chills); *leukopenia* (fever or chills; cough or hoarseness; lower back or side pain; painful or difficult urination)—usually asymptomatic; *lymphocytosis; nausea and vomiting; neuropsychiatric effects, including mental status changes* (agitation; confusion; mental depression; drowsiness; unusual tiredness); *pulmonary toxicity, including pulmonary congestion, pulmonary edema, pleural effusion* (shortness of breath); *renal toxicity, including oliguriaand anuria* (unusual decrease in urination); *stomatitis* (sores in mouth and on lips); *thrombocytopenia* (unusual bleeding or bruising; black, tarry stools; blood in urine or stools; pinpoint red spots on skin)—usually asymptomatic; *weight gain of 5 to 10 pounds or more*

Note: *Anemia* usually requires blood transfusions.

Supraventricular *arrhythmias* usually resolve after treatment has ended. Potentially fatal ventricular arrhythmias have been reported.

*Diarrhea* occurs in most patients. Severe diarrhea can lead to hypokalemia or acidosis.

*Dizziness* is a neurologic effect.

*Eosinophilia*, which can be pronounced, tends to occur near the end of therapy, during the first 5 days after treatment. Eosinophilic myocarditis has been reported.

*Fever, chills, rigors,* or *malaise* usually occurs within hours after administration.

*Hepatic* function tests usually return to normal within several days after treatment has ended.

Mean arterial pressure begins to decline within 2 to 12 hours after initiation of therapy, necessitating intravenous administration of fluids (to correct hypovolemia) and pressors (to maintain blood pressure and perfusion). *Hypotension* is accompanied by an increase in heart rate.

*Hypothyroidism* may require thyroid replacement therapy. A hyperthyroid phase may precede hypothyroidism. Thyroid function tests usually return to normal within a few days or weeks after therapy, although effects have been reported to persist for several months. In some patients, presence of antibodies to thyroglobulin suggests exacerbation or initiation of autoimmune thyroiditis.

Impaired neutrophil function (reduced chemotaxis) may also increase the risk of disseminated *infection*. Infection may include urinary tract, injection site, or central venous catheter tip infections, as well as bacterial endocarditis, phlebitis, or sepsis. Positive cultures may be found without symptomatic infection. Infections are usually gram-positive, although gram-negative infection has also been reported. Early signs and symptoms of sepsis (e.g., hypotension) may be masked by prophylactic medication for systemic effects.

*Mental status changes*, which appear after several days of treatment, may be signs of bacteremia or early bacterial sepsis, as well as cerebral edema or immune effects. Changes due solely to aldesleukin are usually reversible on withdrawal, although they may continue to progress for several days before recovery begins.

*Nausea and vomiting* occur in most patients.

*Oliguria* is accompanied by reversible prerenal azotemia (increased serum creatinine and BUN), hypoalbuminemia, and proteinuria. Fractional sodium excretion is also decreased. In a small percentage of patients, *renal toxicity* may require dialysis. Renal function tests usually return to normal within 7 to 30 days, although recovery may sometimes be prolonged or incomplete. Interstitial nephritis and glomerulonephritis have been reported.

*Stomatitis* may be severe enough to necessitate a liquid diet.

*Weight gain* may be 10% or more of pretreatment body weight. Reversal of weight gain may take up to 1 to 2 weeks after therapy, as patients diurese fluid.

Incidence less frequent
*Aphasia* (trouble in speaking); *ascites* (bloating and stomach pain); *exfoliative dermatitis* (blisters on skin); *gastrointestinal bleeding* (blood in stools; bloody vomit); *glossitis* (redness, swelling, and soreness of tongue); *intestinal ischemic necrosis or perforation* (bloody vomit; severe stomach pain); *myocardial ischemia or myocardial infarction* (chest pain); *pulmonary toxicity, including respiratory failure, tachypnea, and wheezing* (rapid breathing; severe shortness of breath); *sensory neurologic effects* (blurred or double vision; loss of taste)

Note: *Exfoliative dermatitis* can be fatal. Life-threatening bullous drug eruptions, resembling toxic epidermal necrolysis, have also been reported.

In a small percentage of patients, *gastrointestinal bleeding* may require surgery.

Frequency of *myocardial ischemia or infarction* can be reduced by careful patient screening before interleukin-2 treatment and monitoring during treatment.

Evidence of *pulmonary* infiltration may become apparent by the fourth day of therapy and usually resolves within a few weeks after therapy. Intubation may be required for *respiratory failure*.

*Vision* problems usually begin shortly after interleukin-2 administration and are reversible, although they may persist for several weeks.

Incidence rare
*Cardiovascular effects, other, including congestive heart failure, endocarditis, myocarditis, cardiomyopathy, gangrene, stroke, and thrombosis* (swelling of feet or lower legs; sudden weakness or inability to move); *coma; injection site reaction* (pain or redness at site of injection); *pericardial effusion; seizures*

**Those indicating need for medical attention only if they continue or are bothersome**
Incidence more frequent
*Dry skin; loss of appetite; macular erythema* (skin rash or redness with burning or itching, followed by peeling); *malaise* (unusual feeling of discomfort or illness); *weakness*

Note: *Macular erythema*, which seems to be an immunological effect, begins 2 to 3 days after initiation of treatment and usually begins to resolve, with desquamation, within 2 to 3 days after interleukin-2 is discontinued. Peeling of skin is most pronounced on palms and soles; skin appears normal within 2 to 3 weeks. It recurs with each cycle. Other dermatological effects, including angioedema, urticaria, and erythema nodosum, have also been reported.

Incidence less frequent
*Arthralgia or myalgia* (joint pain; muscle pain); *constipation; headache*

# Aldesleukin (Systemic)

## Overdose
For more information on the management of overdose or unintentional ingestion, **contact a Poison Control Center** (see *Poison Control Center Listing*).

### Treatment of overdose
Treatment consists of withdrawal of aldesleukin and supportive therapy. Life-threatening toxicities have been ameliorated by the intravenous administration of dexamethasone; however, this may result in loss of aldesleukin's therapeutic effect.

## Patient Consultation
As an aid to patient consultation, refer to *Advice for the Patient, Aldesleukin (Systemic)*.
In providing consultation, consider emphasizing the following selected information (» = major clinical significance):

### Before using this medication
» Conditions affecting use, especially:
    Sensitivity to aldesleukin
    Pregnancy—Use not recommended; advisability of using contraception; telling physician immediately if pregnancy is suspected
    Breast-feeding—Not recommended because of risk of serious side effects
    Other medications, especially other bone marrow depressants, other cardiotoxic medications, systemic glucocorticoids, other hepatotoxic medications, other hypotension-producing medications, other nephrotoxic medications, or other cytotoxic drug or radiation therapy
    Other medical problems, especially cardiac function impairment, organ allograft, pulmonary function impairment, hepatic function impairment, infection, mental status impairment, renal function impairment, or history of seizure disorder

### Proper use of this medication
» Proper dosing

### Precautions while using this medication
*Caution if impaired neutrophil function or thrombocytopenia occurs*
» Avoiding exposure to persons with infections, especially during periods of low blood counts; checking with physician immediately if fever or chills, cough or hoarseness, lower back or side pain, or painful or difficult urination occurs
» Checking with physician immediately if unusual bleeding or bruising; black, tarry stools; blood in urine or stools; or pinpoint red spots on skin occur
    Caution in use of regular toothbrush, dental floss, or toothpick; physician, dentist, or nurse may suggest alternatives; checking with physician before having dental work done
    Not touching eyes or inside of nose unless hands washed immediately before
    Using caution to avoid accidental cuts with use of sharp objects such as safety razor or fingernail or toenail cutters
    Avoiding contact sports or other situations where bruising or injury could occur

### Side/adverse effects
Importance of discussing possible life-threatening toxicity with physician
Signs of potential side effects, especially anemia, arrhythmias, diarrhea, dizziness, edema, fever and/or chills, eosinophilia, hepatotoxicity, hypotension, hypothyroidism, infection, leukopenia, lymphocytosis, nausea and vomiting, mental status changes, pericardial effusion, pulmonary toxicity, renal toxicity, stomatitis, thrombocytopenia, weight gain, ascites, aphasia, exfoliative dermatitis, gastrointestinal bleeding, glossitis, intestinal ischemic necrosis or perforation, myocardial ischemia or myocardial infarction, sensory neurological effects, other cardiovascular effects, injection site reaction, and seizures
Asymptomatic side effects, including anemia, cardiotoxicity, hepatotoxicity, hypotension, hypothyroidism, eosinophilia, leukopenia, renal toxicity, and thrombocytopenia
Physician or nurse can help in dealing with side effects

## General Dosing Information
Patients receiving aldesleukin should be under supervision of a physician experienced in cancer chemotherapy.

It is recommended that high-dose aldesleukin be administered in a tertiary care hospital setting, with an intensive care facility and specialists skilled in cardiopulmonary and intensive care medicine readily available.

Dosage of interleukin-2 is usually expressed in units of activity in promoting proliferation in a responsive cell line; conversion to Units from mg of protein varies somewhat, depending on the source of interleukin-2. In the literature, dosage of aldesleukin is expressed in terms of Cetus units; dosage of teceleukin, another form of recombinant interleukin-2, is expressed in Roche units or Nutley units. However, strength and dosage of commercially available aldesleukin are expressed in International Units (IU). Conversion to IU is as follows:
    1 Cetus Unit = 6 International Units.
    1 Roche Unit or Nutley Unit = 3 International Units.

In addition:
    18 million IU = 1.1 mg protein.

It is recommended that acetaminophen and a nonsteroidal anti-inflammatory drug (NSAID) such as indomethacin be administered prior to initiation of aldesleukin therapy, to reduce fever. The increased risk of nephrotoxicity with concurrent use of indomethacin must be kept in mind. Meperidine may be added to control the rigors associated with fever.

Ranitidine or cimetidine may be given for prophylaxis of gastrointestinal irritation and bleeding.

Dosage adjustment of high-dose aldesleukin in response to toxicity is accomplished by withholding the medication rather than by decreasing the dosage. Toxicity usually reverses promptly (within several hours) on withdrawal of aldesleukin. It is recommended that aldesleukin be held and restarted according to the following guidelines:
- Atrial fibrillation, supraventricular tachycardia, or bradycardia that requires treatment or is recurrent or persistent—Hold dose. Obtain ECG and cardiac enzymes. Subsequent doses may be given if patient is asymptomatic with full recovery to normal sinus rhythm.
- Systolic blood pressure less than 90 mm Hg with increasing requirement for pressors—Hold dose. Subsequent doses may be given if systolic blood pressure becomes greater than or equal to 90 mm Hg and stable, or requirements for pressors are improving.
- Any ECG change consistent with myocardial infarction or ischemia with or without chest pain; suspicion of cardiac ischemia—Hold dose. Subsequent doses may be given if patient is asymptomatic, myocardial infarction has been ruled out, or clinical suspicion of angina and/or myocarditis is low.
- Oxygen saturation of less than 90% with 2 liters $O_2$ by nasal prongs—Hold dose. Subsequent doses may be given if $O_2$ saturation becomes greater than or equal to 90% with 2 liters $O_2$ by nasal prongs.
- Mental status changes, including moderate confusion or agitation—Hold dose. Subsequent doses may be given if mental status changes are completely resolved.
- Sepsis syndrome, where patient is clinically unstable—Hold dose. Subsequent doses may be given if sepsis syndrome has resolved, patient is clinically stable, and infection is under treatment.
- Serum creatinine greater than or equal to 5 mg per deciliter or serum creatinine of any level in the presence of severe volume overload, acidosis, or hyperkalemia—Hold dose. Subsequent doses may be given if serum creatinine is less than 4 mg per deciliter and fluid and electrolyte status is stable.
- Signs of hepatic failure including encephalopathy, increasing ascites, liver pain, hypoglycemia—Discontinue all treatment for that course. Consider starting a new course of treatment at least 7 weeks after cessation of adverse event and hospital discharge if all signs of hepatic failure have resolved.
- Stool guaiac repeatedly greater than 3-4+—Hold dose. Subsequent doses may be given if stool guaiac is negative.
- Bullous dermatitis or marked worsening of pre-existing skin condition—Hold dose. Subsequent doses may be given upon resolution of all signs of bullous dermatitis. Avoid topical steroid therapy.

High-dose aldesleukin therapy should also be withheld for oliguria unresponsive to fluid replacement or diuretics and for respiratory distress.

It is recommended that aldesleukin be permanently discontinued in patients who experienced the following toxicities in an earlier course of therapy:
- Sustained ventricular tachycardia (5 beats or more)
- Cardiac rhythm disturbances not controlled or unresponsive to management
- Recurrent chest pain with ECG changes consistent with angina or myocardial infarction
- Pericardial tamponade
- Intubation required for more than 72 hours
- Renal function impairment requiring dialysis for more than 72 hours
- Coma or toxic psychosis lasting more than 48 hours
- Repetitive or difficult to control seizures
- Bowel ischemia/perforation
- Gastrointestinal bleeding requiring surgery

Special precautions are recommended in patients who develop thrombocytopenia as a result of administration of aldesleukin. These may include extreme care in performing invasive procedures; regular inspection of intravenous sites, skin (including perirectal area), and mucous membrane surfaces for signs of bleeding or bruising; limiting frequency of venipuncture and avoiding intramuscular injections; testing urine, emesis, stool, and secretions for occult blood; care in use of regular toothbrushes, dental floss, toothpicks, safety razors, and fingernail and toenail cutters; avoiding constipation; and using caution to prevent falls and other injuries. Such patients should avoid alcohol and aspirin intake because of the risk of gastrointestinal bleeding. Platelet transfusions may be required.

Patients should be observed carefully for signs of infection. Antibiotic support may be required. Because of the risk of infection, it is recommended that all patients with indwelling central lines receive antibiotic prophylaxis against *Staphylococcus aureus*, along with meticulous catheter care.

**For treatment of adverse effects**

Antiemetics and antidiarrheals may be given as needed to treat gastrointestinal effects. They usually are discontinued 12 hours after the last dose of aldesleukin.

Hydroxyzine or diphenhydramine and emollients may be used to prevent or control symptoms from pruritic rashes and are continued until resolution of pruritus. Some clinicians recommend that use of topical or systemic corticosteroids be avoided because of the risk of diminishing aldesleukin's therapeutic effect.

Supraventricular arrhythmias usually respond to conventional treatment (digoxin or verapamil).

Debilitating mental status changes may respond to low doses of haloperidol.

For capillary leak syndrome—

Capillary leak syndrome (CLS) is initially managed with careful monitoring of the patient's fluid and organ perfusion status by means of frequent determination of blood pressure and pulse and monitoring of organ function, including assessment of mental status and urine output. Hypovolemia is assessed by catheterization and central pressure monitoring. Because flexibility in fluid and pressor management is essential for maintaining organ perfusion and blood pressure, extreme caution is recommended in treating patients with fixed requirements for large volumes of fluid (e.g., patients with hypercalcemia).

Hypovolemia is managed by administration of intravenous fluids, either colloids or crystalloids, which are usually given when the central venous pressure (CVP) is below 3 to 4 mm Hg. Although correction of hypovolemia may require large volumes of fluids, caution is necessary because of the risk that unrestrained fluid administration may exacerbate problems associated with concomitant edema or effusions. A diuretic such as furosemide may be administered to reduce edema or pulmonary infiltration.

Management of edema, ascites, or pleural effusions depends on a careful balancing of the effects of fluid shifts so that neither the consequences of hypovolemia (e.g., impaired organ perfusion) nor the consequences of fluid accumulation (e.g., pulmonary edema) exceed the patient's tolerance.

Early administration of dopamine (1 to 5 mcg per kg of body weight [mcg/kg] per minute), before the onset of hypotension, may help maintain organ perfusion, particularly to the kidney, and preserve urine output. Weight and urine output should be carefully monitored. If this dose of dopamine fails to sustain organ perfusion and blood pressure, some clinicians increase the dose of dopamine to 6 to 10 mcg/kg per minute or add phenylephrine (1 to 5 mcg/kg per minute) to the lower dose of dopamine. However, prolonged use of pressors, either individually or in combination, at relatively high doses may be associated with cardiac rhythm disturbances.

If organ perfusion cannot be maintained (demonstrated by altered mental status, reduced urine output, reduction in blood pressure below 90 mm Hg, or onset of cardiac arrhythmias), it is recommended that subsequent doses of aldesleukin be withheld until recovery of organ perfusion and return of systolic pressure to above 90 mm Hg.

Once recovery from CLS begins and blood pressure has normalized, use of diuretics may hasten recovery in patients in whom there has been excessive weight gain or edema formation, particularly if associated with shortness of breath from pulmonary congestion.

Oxygen is administered if pulmonary function monitoring confirms that $P_aO_2$ is decreased.

For relief of anemia and to ensure maximal oxygen carrying capacity, administration of packed red cells may be used.

To resolve absolute thrombocytopenia and reduce the risk of gastrointestinal bleeding, platelet transfusions may be given.

## Parenteral Dosage Forms

### ALDESLEUKIN FOR INJECTION

**Usual adult dose**

Carcinoma, renal or
Melanoma, metastatic—
High dose therapy: Intravenous infusion (over fifteen minutes), 600,000 International Units (IU) per kg of body weight (0.037 mg per kg of body weight) every eight hours for a total of fourteen doses. Following nine days of rest, the schedule is repeated for another fourteen doses, for a maximum of twenty-eight doses per course.

Note: Although aldesleukin has been given in lower doses and by other routes (e.g., continuous intravenous infusion, subcutaneous) by some investigators to reduce toxicity, relative efficacy of these regimens compared to the high-dose regimen has not been established.

Although glass bottles and plastic (polyvinyl chloride) bags have been used in clinical trials with comparable results, the manufacturer recommends that plastic bags be used as the dilution container since experimental studies suggest that use of plastic containers results in more consistent drug delivery.

Use of in-line filters is not recommended during aldesleukin administration because of the risk of adsorption of aldesleukin to the filter.

If the aldesleukin solution has been refrigerated, it should be brought to room temperature before administration.

Each treatment period should be separated by a rest period of at least seven weeks from the date of hospital discharge.

Dose modification in response to toxicity is accomplished by holding or interrupting a dose rather than reducing the dose. Some toxicities necessitate permanent withdrawal of aldesleukin. For recommendations concerning toxicities requiring either permanent withdrawal or holding of a dose, see *General Dosing Information*.

**Usual pediatric dose**

Safety and efficacy have not been established.

**Size(s) usually available**

U.S.—
22 million IU (1.3 mg) (Rx) [*Proleukin* (mannitol; sodium dododecyl sulfate; monobasic sodium phosphate; dibasic sodium phosphate)].

Canada—
Not commercially available.

**Packaging and storage**

Store between 2 and 8 °C (36 and 46 °F), unless otherwise specified by the manufacturer. Protect from freezing.

**Preparation of dosage form**

Aldesleukin for injection is reconstituted for intravenous or subcutaneous administration by adding 1.2 mL of sterile water for injection to the vial (directing the diluent at the side of the vial and swirling the contents gently to avoid excess foaming), to produce a clear and colorless to slightly yellow solution containing 18 million Units (1.1 mg) per mL. The vial should not be shaken.

For administration by rapid intravenous infusion, the reconstituted solution is further diluted in 50 mL of 5% dextrose injection.

**Stability**

Reconstituted and diluted solutions should be stored in the refrigerator, since the product contains no preservative. Reconstituted solutions should be used within forty-eight hours. Any unused portion should be discarded.

**Incompatibilities**

Bacteriostatic water for injection or 0.9% sodium chloride injection should not be used for reconstitution because of increased aggregation.

**Auxiliary labeling**

- Do not shake.
- Do not freeze.

Revised: 09/30/97
Interim revision: 06/17/98

# ALENDRONATE Systemic

VA CLASSIFICATION (Primary/Secondary): HS301/HS303
Commonly used brand name(s): *Fosamax*.

Note: For a listing of dosage forms and brand names by country availability, see *Dosage Forms* section(s).

## Category
Bone resorption inhibitor.

## Indications

### Accepted

Osteoporosis, postmenopausal (treatment adjunct)—Alendronate is indicated for the treatment of osteoporosis in postmenopausal women, as confirmed by the finding of low bone mass (at least 2 standard deviations below the premenopausal mean) or by the presence or history of osteoporotic fracture. Alendronate should be used in conjunction with adequate intake of calcium (1 to 1.5 grams of elemental calcium a day) and vitamin D (400 to 800 Units a day) to aid in the prevention of progressive loss of bone mass.

Osteoporosis, postmenopausal (prophylaxis)—Alendronate is indicated for the prevention of osteoporosis in postmenopausal women who are at risk of developing osteoporosis and for whom the desired clinical outcome is to maintain bone mass and to reduce the risk of future fracture. Alendronate should be used in conjunction with adequate intake of calcium (1 to 1.5 grams of elemental calcium a day) and vitamin D (400 to 800 Units a day) to aid in the prevention of progressive loss of bone mass.

Paget's disease of bone (treatment)—Alendronate is indicated for the treatment of Paget's disease in patients with alkaline phosphatase concentrations at least two times the upper limit of normal, those who are symptomatic, or those at risk for future complications from the disease. Signs and symptoms of Paget's disease may include bone pain, deformity, and/or fractures; increased concentrations of *N*-telopeptide of type I collagen, serum alkaline phosphatase, and/or urinary hydroxyproline; neurologic disorders associated with skull lesions and spinal deformities; and elevated cardiac output and other vascular disorders associated with increased vascularity of bones.

## Pharmacology/Pharmacokinetics

### Physicochemical characteristics
Molecular weight—325.12.

### Mechanism of action/Effect
Animal studies indicate that alendronate shows preferential localization to sites of bone resorption where it inhibits osteoclast activity, but does not interfere with osteoclast recruitment or attachment. Studies in rats and mice showed that normal bone mass was formed on top of alendronate, thereby incorporating alendronate in the bone matrix. Alendronate is not pharmacologically active when incorporated; therefore, it must be administered continuously to suppress osteoclasts on newly formed resorption surfaces. Studies in baboons and rats indicate that alendronate treatment reduces bone turnover (i.e., the number of sites at which bone is remodeled). In addition, bone formation exceeds bone resorption at these remodeling sites, leading to increased bone mass. Data from long-term animal studies indicate that the bone formed during alendronate therapy is of normal quality.

### Absorption
Studies in humans showed that mean oral bioavailability in women was 0.7% for doses ranging from 5 to 40 mg when alendronate was administered after an overnight fast and 2 hours before a standardized breakfast. Oral bioavailability in men was 0.59% following administration of a 10-mg dose 2 hours before the first meal of the day. In postmenopausal women, bioavailability was decreased by approximately 40% when 10 mg of alendronate was given either 30 minutes or 1 hour before a standardized breakfast, when compared with dosing 2 hours before eating. Bioavailability was negligible when alendronate was administered with or up to 2 hours after a standardized breakfast. Concomitant administration with coffee or orange juice reduced bioavailability by approximately 60%.

### Distribution
Studies in male rats given an intravenous dose of 1 mg per kilogram of body weight (mg/kg) showed that alendronate was transiently distributed to soft tissue, but was then rapidly redistributed to bone or excreted in the urine.

$Vol_D$—At least 28 L in humans.

### Protein binding
High (approximately 78% in human plasma).

### Biotransformation
There is no evidence that alendronate is metabolized in humans or animals.

### Duration of action
In osteoporosis—Six weeks after a single 5-mg intravenous dose.
In Paget's disease of bone—Six months after a single 5-mg intravenous dose.

### Elimination
Renal; approximately 50% of an intravenous dose was excreted in urine within 72 hours, with little or none of the dose recovered in the feces. Following a single 10-mg intravenous dose, the renal clearance of alendronate was 71 mL per minute (mL/min); the systemic clearance did not exceed 200 mL/min. Plasma concentrations fell by more than 95% within 6 hours following intravenous alendronate administration.

## Precautions to Consider

### Carcinogenicity/Tumorigenicity
In a 92-week carcinogenicity study in mice given alendronate at doses of 1, 3, and 10 mg per kilogram of body weight (mg/kg) per day (males) or 1, 2, and 5 mg/kg per day (females) (0.5 to 4 times the 10-mg human dose based on body surface area), harderian gland (a retro-orbital gland not present in humans) adenomas were increased in high-dose females. In a 2-year carcinogenicity study in rats, parafollicular cell (thyroid) adenomas were increased in high-dose males at doses of 1 and 3.75 mg/kg (1 and 3 times the 10-mg human dose, respectively, based on body surface area).

### Mutagenicity
Alendronate was not genotoxic in the *in vitro* microbial mutagenesis assay with and without metabolic activation, in an *in vitro* mammalian cell mutagenesis assay, in an *in vitro* alkaline elution assay in rat hepatocytes, and in an *in vivo* chromosomal aberration assay in mice. However, in an *in vitro* chromosomal aberration assay in Chinese hamster ovary cells, alendronate was weakly positive at concentrations $\geq 5$ mmol in the presence of cytotoxicity.

### Pregnancy/Reproduction
Fertility—Studies in male and female rats given oral alendronate doses of up to 5 mg/kg per day (4 times the 10-mg human dose based on body surface area) found no effect on fertility.

Pregnancy—Adequate and well-controlled studies in humans have not been done.

Reproduction studies in rats given alendronate doses ranging from 1 to 10 mg/kg (1 to 9 times the 10-mg human dose based on body surface area) showed decreased postimplantation survival at 2 mg/kg per day and decreased body weight gain in normal pups at 1 mg/kg per day. Sites of incomplete fetal ossification of vertebrae (cervical, thoracic, and lumbar), skull, and sternebrae were statistically significantly increased in rats beginning at doses of 10 mg/kg per day. No similar fetal effects were seen when pregnant rabbits were treated at doses of up to 35 mg/kg per day (50 times the 10-mg human dose based on body surface area).

Both total and ionized calcium decreased in pregnant rats at doses of 15 mg/kg per day (13 times the 10-mg human dose based on body surface area), resulting in delays and failures of delivery. Protracted parturition due to maternal hypocalcemia occurred in rats at doses as low as 0.5 mg/kg per day (0.5 times the recommended human dose) when rats were treated from before mating through gestation. Maternotoxicity (late pregnancy deaths) occurred in the female rats treated with 15 mg/kg per day for varying periods of time, ranging from treatment only during premating to treatment only during early, middle, or late gestation; these deaths were decreased but not eliminated by cessation of treatment. Calcium supplementation, either in the drinking water or by minipump, did not ameliorate the hypocalcemia or prevent maternal and neonatal deaths due to delays in delivery; intravenous calcium supplementation prevented maternal, but not fetal, deaths.

FDA Pregnancy Category C.

### Breast-feeding
It is not known whether alendronate is distributed into human breast milk. Alendronate was distributed into the milk of rats after an intravenous dose.

### Pediatrics
No information is available on the relationship of age to the effects of alendronate in pediatric patients. Safety and efficacy have not been established.

**Geriatrics**
Appropriate studies performed to date have not demonstrated geriatrics-specific problems that would limit the usefulness of alendronate in the elderly.

**Drug interactions and/or related problems**
The following drug interactions and/or related problems have been selected on the basis of their potential clinical significance (possible mechanism in parentheses where appropriate)—not necessarily inclusive (» = major clinical significance):

Note: Combinations containing any of the following medications, depending on the amount present, may also interact with this medication.

Dietary supplements (including calcium) or
Food and beverages or
Medications, oral (including antacids)
(simultaneous use may interfere with the absorption of alendronate; patients should be advised to take alendronate at least 30 minutes before taking other medications, food, or beverages)

Ranitidine
(intravenous ranitidine was shown to double the bioavailability of oral alendronate; the clinical significance of this increased bioavailability is not known)

» Salicylates or salicylate-containing compounds
(an increased incidence of upper gastrointestinal adverse events was reported in individuals taking more than 10 mg of alendronate a day concurrently with salicylates or salicylate-containing compounds)

**Laboratory value alterations**
The following have been selected on the basis of their potential clinical significance (possible effect in parentheses where appropriate)—not necessarily inclusive (» = major clinical significance):

With physiology/laboratory test values
Calcium, serum, and
Phosphate, serum
(alendronate has been reported to cause a 2% reduction in serum calcium concentrations and a 4 to 6% reduction in serum phosphate concentrations in the first month after initiation of therapy; no further decreases have been observed during the 3-year duration of therapy)

**Medical considerations/Contraindications**
The medical considerations/contraindications included have been selected on the basis of their potential clinical significance (reasons given in parentheses where appropriate)—not necessarily inclusive (» = major clinical significance).

*Except under special circumstances, this medication should not be used when the following medical problems exist:*

» Gastrointestinal diseases such as duodenitis, dysphagia, symptomatic esophageal diseases, frequent heartburn, gastritis, gastroesophageal reflux disease, hiatal hernia, or ulcers
(alendronate may exacerbate these conditions)

» Renal function impairment when creatinine clearance is < 35 mL per minute (0.58 mL/sec)
(use is not recommended because elimination of alendronate may be reduced; greater accumulation of alendronate in the bone may be expected)

» Sensitivity to alendronate

*Risk-benefit should be considered when the following medical problems exist:*

Hypocalcemia or
Vitamin D deficiency
(alendronate may exacerbate these conditions; hypocalcemia and vitamin D deficiency should be corrected before alendronate therapy is begun)

**Patient monitoring**
The following may be especially important in patient monitoring (other tests may be warranted in some patients, depending on condition; » = major clinical significance):

For Paget's disease
Alkaline phosphatase, serum or
Hydroxyproline, urinary
(serum alkaline phosphatase determinations recommended every 3 to 6 months; urinary hydroxyproline determinations recommended every 6 to 12 months; values should decrease with treatment)

Calcium, serum
(determinations recommended every 3 to 4 months; values should increase with treatment)

N-telopeptide of type I collagen, urinary
(determinations recommended every 3 to 6 months; values should decrease with treatment)

For postmenopausal osteoporosis
Bone mineral density
(determinations recommended every 1 to 2 years to assess effectiveness of therapy; clinicians recommend monitoring hip, femur, or spine; values should increase with treatment)

Calcium, serum or
Creatinine, serum
(determinations recommended every 6 to 12 months; serum calcium values should increase with treatment)

## Side/Adverse Effects

The following side/adverse effects have been selected on the basis of their potential clinical significance (possible signs and symptoms in parentheses where appropriate)—not necessarily inclusive:

**Those indicating need for medical attention**
Incidence more frequent
*Abdominal pain*
Incidence less frequent
*Dysphagia* (difficulty swallowing); **heartburn; irritation, pain, or ulceration of the esophagus; muscle pain**

Note: There have been reports of severe *irritation, pain, or ulceration of the esophagus* in some patients. Presenting symptoms may include *dysphagia* and/or *heartburn*. Alendronate therapy should be discontinued if these symptoms develop.

Incidence rare
*Skin rash*

**Those indicating need for medical attention only if they continue or are bothersome**
Incidence less frequent
*Abdominal distension* (full or bloated feeling); **constipation; diarrhea; flatulence** (gas); **headache; nausea**

## Patient Consultation

As an aid to patient consultation, refer to *Advice for the Patient, Alendronate (Systemic)*.

In providing consultation, consider emphasizing the following selected information (» = major clinical significance):

**Before using this medication**
» Conditions affecting use, especially:
Sensitivity to alendronate
Pregnancy—Studies in animals showed decreased weight gain, incomplete fetal ossification, decreased survival of the fetus, and delays in delivery
Breast-feeding—Should not be given to nursing women because alendronate is distributed in milk of rats
Other medications, especially aspirin or compounds that contain aspirin
Other medical problems, especially gastrointestinal diseases or severe renal function impairment

**Proper use of this medication**
» Taking with 6 to 8 ounces of plain water on empty stomach, at least 30 minutes before first food, beverage, or medication of the day
» Not lying down for at least 30 minutes after taking alendronate
Possible need for calcium and vitamin D supplementation
» Proper dosing
Missed dose: Not taking later in the day; continuing usual schedule the next morning
» Proper storage

**Side/adverse effects**
Signs of potential adverse effects, especially abdominal pain; heartburn; dysphagia; irritation, pain, or ulceration of the esophagus; muscle pain; and skin rash

## General Dosing Information

To facilitate delivery of alendronate to the stomach and reduce esophageal irritation, patients should not lie down for at least 30 minutes after taking alendronate.

Safety of treatment for longer than 4 years has not been studied.

**Diet/Nutrition**
Alendronate should be taken with 6 to 8 ounces of plain water. Absorption of alendronate is best when taken in the morning, at least 30 minutes before the first food, beverage, or medication of the day. Food and beverages such as mineral water, coffee, tea, or juice will decrease the

## 44  Alendronate (Systemic)

absorption of alendronate. Waiting longer than 30 minutes will improve the absorption of alendronate.

Some patients may be instructed to take calcium or vitamin D supplements if their diet is inadequate. These supplements should be taken 30 minutes or longer after taking alendronate.

## Oral Dosage Forms

### ALENDRONATE TABLETS

**Usual adult dose**
Paget's disease of bone (treatment)—
  Oral, 40 mg once a day in the morning, at least thirty minutes before the first food, beverage, or medication. Treatment should continue for six months. Re-treatment may be considered for certain patients following a six-month post-treatment evaluation period.
Postmenopausal osteoporosis (treatment)—
  Oral, 10 mg once a day in the morning, at least thirty minutes before the first food, beverage, or medication. The dose should be taken with six to eight ounces of plain water.
Postmenopausal osteoporosis (prophylaxis)—
  Oral, 5 mg once a day in the morning, at least thirty minutes before the first food, beverage, or medication. The dose should be taken with six to eight ounces of plain water.

**Usual pediatric dose**
Safety and efficacy have not been established.

**Strength(s) usually available**
U.S.—
  5 mg (Rx) [*Fosamax* (lactose)].
  10 mg (Rx) [*Fosamax* (lactose)].
  40 mg (Rx) [*Fosamax* (lactose)].

Canada—
  10 mg (Rx) [*Fosamax* (lactose)].
  40 mg (Rx) [*Fosamax* (lactose)].

**Packaging and storage**
Store between 15 and 30 °C (59 and 86 °F), unless otherwise specified by manufacturer.

**Auxiliary labeling**
• Take on empty stomach.

Developed: 01/06/97
Interim revision: 03/24/98

---

## ALFACALCIDOL — See *Vitamin D and Analogs (Systemic)*

---

## ALFENTANIL — See *Fentanyl Derivatives (Systemic)*

---

## ALGLUCERASE — The *Alglucerase (Systemic)* monograph is not included in this published version of the USP DI database. Copies of the monograph are available on request from Micromedex, Inc. - Reprint Requests, 6200 S. Syracuse Way, Suite 300, Englewood, CO 80111; telephone (303) 486-6400; telefax (303) 486-6464; Email: USPDI@MDX.COM.

---

# ALLOPURINOL  Systemic

VA CLASSIFICATION (Primary/Secondary): MS400/GU900

Commonly used brand name(s): *Apo-Allopurinol*; *Lopurin*; *Purinol*; *Zyloprim*.

Note: For a listing of dosage forms and brand names by country availability, see *Dosage Forms* section(s).

## Category

Antihyperuricemic; antigout agent; antiurolithic (uric acid calculi; calcium oxalate calculi).

Note: Antihyperuricemic is the basic category; the other categories are specific categories of use.

## Indications

Note: Bracketed information in the *Indications* section refers to uses that are not included in U.S. product labeling.

### Accepted

Gouty arthritis, chronic (treatment)—Allopurinol is indicated for the long-term management of hyperuricemia associated with primary or secondary gout. The aim of allopurinol therapy is to reduce the number of acute gout attacks and decrease the risk of uric acid calculi and urate nephropathy in patients with chronic gout.

Allopurinol is recommended for patients in whom treatment with uricosuric antigout agents such as probenecid or sulfinpyrazone would be ineffective or inadvisable (e.g., patients who are hyperuricemic as a result of overproduction of urate, patients with extensive tophi or who are otherwise at risk for urate nephropathy, and patients with moderate to severe renal function impairment). Both allopurinol and the uricosuric antigout agents are effective in patients whose 24-hour renal excretion of uric acid is 800 mg (4.8 mmol) or less, i.e., individuals who are hyperuricemic as a result of underexcretion of uric acid. However, the uricosuric agents are less toxic than allopurinol and should be considered for use when appropriate.

Allopurinol has no anti-inflammatory activity and should not be used for the treatment of acute attacks of gouty arthritis. An anti-inflammatory agent, preferably a nonsteroidal anti-inflammatory drug (NSAID) or a corticosteroid (preferably via intrasynovial injection, when feasible), should be used to treat acute attacks. Also, initiation of antihyperuricemic therapy may lead to fluctuations in urate concentration that may result in prolongation of an acute attack or initiation of new attacks. The patient should be receiving appropriate anti-inflammatory therapy when allopurinol treatment is initiated.

Hyperuricemia (prophylaxis and treatment)—Allopurinol is indicated to control hyperuricemia secondary to blood dyscrasias, such as polycythemia vera or myeloid metaplasia, or their treatment. It is also indicated to prevent or treat hyperuricemia secondary to tumor lysis induced by cancer chemotherapy with cytotoxic antineoplastic agents or radiation therapy in patients with leukemias, lymphomas, or other neoplastic disease. [Allopurinol is also used to treat hyperuricemia secondary to the neoplastic disease itself.] Allopurinol prevents complications of hyperuricemia (e.g., acute uric acid nephropathy or renal calculi, tissue urate deposition, or gouty arthritis) in these patients. However, allopurinol may increase the toxicity of several antineoplastic agents, and some clinicians have questioned its routine administration during cancer chemotherapy.

[Allopurinol is also used to control hyperuricemia in patients with Lesch-Nyhan syndrome. However, it does not improve neurologic or behavioral abnormalities or affect the course of the disease in these patients.]

Nephropathy, uric acid (prophylaxis and treatment)—Allopurinol is indicated in the treatment of primary or secondary uric acid nephropathy (with or without accompanying symptoms of gouty arthritis) to prevent progression of the condition. However, this medicine will not reverse severe renal damage that has already occurred. Allopurinol is also indicated to prevent uric acid nephropathy in certain patients as described under *Hyperuricemia*, above.

Renal calculi, uric acid (prophylaxis)—Allopurinol is indicated to prevent recurrence of uric acid stone formation in patients with a history of recurrent uric acid calculi. It is also indicated to prevent uric acid calculi in certain other patients as described under *Hyperuricemia*, above.

Renal calculi, calcium oxalate, recurrence (prophylaxis)—Allopurinol is indicated to prevent recurrence of calcium stone formation in patients with a history of recurrent calcium oxalate calculi associated with hyperuricosuria (i.e., uric acid excretion > 800 mg [4.8 mmol] per day in males or 750 mg [4.5mmol] per day in females).

### Unaccepted

*Allopurinol is not recommended for treatment of asymptomatic hyperuricemia* associated with conditions or induced by medications other than those described above.

## Pharmacology/Pharmacokinetics

**Physicochemical characteristics**
Chemical group—A structural analog of hypoxanthine.
Molecular weight—136.11.
pKa—10.2.

### Mechanism of action/Effect
Allopurinol and its metabolite, oxipurinol (alloxanthine), decrease the production of uric acid by inhibiting the action of xanthine oxidase, the enzyme that converts hypoxanthine to xanthine and xanthine to uric acid. Also, allopurinol increases reutilization of hypoxanthine and xanthine for nucleotide and nucleic acid synthesis via an action involving the enzyme hypoxanthine-guanine phosphoribosyltransferase (HGPRTase). The resultant increase in nucleotide concentration leads to feedback inhibition of de novo purine synthesis. Allopurinol thereby decreases uric acid concentrations in both serum and urine.

By lowering both serum and urine concentrations of uric acid below its solubility limits, allopurinol prevents or decreases urate deposition, thereby preventing the occurrence or progression of both gouty arthritis and urate nephropathy. In patients with chronic gout, allopurinol may prevent or decrease tophi formation and chronic joint changes, promote resolution of existing urate crystals and deposits, and, after several months of therapy, reduce the frequency of acute gout attacks. Also, reductions in urine urate concentration prevent or decrease the formation of uric acid or calcium oxalate calculi.

### Other actions/effects
Allopurinol inhibits hepatic microsomal enzyme activity.

Allopurinol increases plasma and urine concentrations of xanthine and hypoxanthine. Although the concentrations of these oxypurines usually remain within their solubility limits, xanthine renal stones have been reported very rarely in patients with HGPRTase deficiency or very high pretreatment uric acid concentrations.

### Absorption
About 80 to 90% of a single 300-mg dose is absorbed from the gastrointestinal tract.

### Protein binding
Neither allopurinol nor its metabolite, oxipurinol, is bound to plasma proteins.

### Biotransformation
Primarily hepatic. About 70% of a dose is metabolized to the active metabolite, oxipurinol. One study indicates that allopurinol may also be taken up by, and metabolized in, red blood cells.

### Half-life
Allopurinol—1 to 3 hours
Oxipurinol—12 to 30 hours (average about 15 hours); may be greatly prolonged in patients with renal function impairment.

### Onset of action
A significant reduction of serum uric acid concentration usually occurs within 2 or 3 days.

Note: In some patients, especially those with severe tophaceous deposits or those who are underexcretors of uric acid, significant reduction of serum and urine uric acid concentrations may be substantially delayed, possibly because of mobilization of urate from existing tissue deposits.

### Time to peak serum concentration
Allopurinol—0.5 to 2 hours following a single 300-mg dose.
Oxipurinol—4.5 to 5 hours

### Peak serum concentration
Following a single 300-mg dose—
Allopurinol: About 2 to 3 mcg per mL (14.7 to 22.05 micromoles/L).
Oxipurinol: About 5 to 6.5 mcg per mL (32.85 to 42.7 micromoles/L); may be increased to 30 to 50 mcg per mL (197.1 to 328.5 micromoles/L) in patients with renal function impairment.

### Time to peak effect
Reduction of serum uric acid concentration to normal range—1 to 3 weeks.
Reduction of frequency of acute gout attacks—Several months of therapy may be required, even though the serum uric acid concentration returns to normal values, possibly because of mobilization and recrystallization of urate as serum concentrations fluctuate.

### Duration of action
The serum uric acid concentration usually returns to the pretreatment value 1 to 2 weeks after discontinuation of therapy.

### Elimination
Renal—Up to 10% of a dose is excreted as unchanged allopurinol and about 70% as oxipurinol.
Fecal—About 20% of a dose.
In dialysis—Both allopurinol and oxipurinol are dialyzable.

## Precautions to Consider

### Pregnancy/Reproduction
Fertility—No impairment of fertility was observed in rats or rabbits given up to 20 times the usual human dose.

Pregnancy—Although adequate and well-controlled studies in humans have not been done, 3 reports indicate no evidence of birth defects in offspring of women receiving allopurinol during pregnancy.

In a study in mice, administration of 100 mg of allopurinol per kg of body weight (mg/kg) intraperitoneally on Day 10 or Day 13 of gestation caused an increased number of fetal deaths; no such effect was seen with a dose of 50 mg/kg. In the same study, 50 or 100 mg/kg caused external fetal malformations when administered intraperitoneally on Day 10 of gestation and skeletal malformations when administered intraperitoneally on Day 13 of gestation. Whether these effects were due to maternal toxicity or a direct effect on the fetus has not been determined. However, other studies in rats and rabbits given up to 20 times the usual human dose have not shown that allopurinol affects the fetus adversely.

FDA Pregnancy Category C.

### Breast-feeding
Allopurinol and oxipurinol are distributed into breast milk. Whether this toxic medication may cause adverse effects in the nursing infant has not been determined. However, problems in humans have not been documented.

### Pediatrics
Appropriate studies performed to date have not demonstrated pediatrics-specific problems that would limit the usefulness of allopurinol in children. However, use of allopurinol in pediatric patients has been limited to children with certain rare inborn errors of purine metabolism or hyperuricemia secondary to a malignancy or cancer therapy.

### Geriatrics
No information is available on the relationship of age to the effects of allopurinol in geriatric patients. However, elderly patients are more likely to have age-related renal function impairment, which may require adjustment of the dose and/or dosing interval in patients receiving allopurinol.

### Drug interactions and/or related problems
The following drug interactions and/or related problems have been selected on the basis of their potential clinical significance (possible mechanism in parentheses where appropriate)—not necessarily inclusive (» = major clinical significance):

Note: Combinations containing any of the following medications, depending on the amount present, may also interact with this medication.

Acidifiers, urinary, such as:
 Ammonium chloride
 Ascorbic acid
 Potassium or sodium phosphate
  (urinary acidification by these medications may increase the possibility of allopurinol-induced xanthine kidney stone formation)

Alcohol or
Diazoxide or
Mecamylamine or
Pyrazinamide
 (these medications may increase serum uric acid concentrations; dosage adjustment of allopurinol may be necessary to control hyperuricemia and gout)

Amoxicillin or
Ampicillin or
Bacampicillin or
Hetacillin
 (concurrent use with allopurinol may significantly increase the possibility of skin rash; however, it has not been established that allopurinol, rather than the presence of hyperuricemia, is responsible for this effect)

» Anticoagulants, coumarin- or indandione-derivative
 (allopurinol may inhibit enzymatic metabolism of the anticoagulant, leading to potentiation of the anticoagulant effect; dosage adjustments based on increased monitoring of prothrombin time may be necessary during and after concurrent use)

Antineoplastics
 (rapidly cytolytic antineoplastic agents may increase serum uric acid concentrations; prophylactic administration of allopurinol may be indicated to prevent complications associated with antineoplastic agent–induced hyperuricemia; also, patients receiving allopurinol to treat pre-existing hyperuricemia or gout may require allopurinol dosage adjustment during and following concurrent therapy with one of these agents)

 (concurrent use of allopurinol with cyclophosphamide and possibly other antineoplastic agents may increase the potential for bone marrow depression; although studies of this possibility have reported conflicting results, it is recommended that patients receiving allo-

# Allopurinol (Systemic)

purinol concurrently with antineoplastic agents, especially cyclophosphamide, be carefully monitored)

» Azathioprine or
» Mercaptopurine

(allopurinol-induced inhibition of xanthine oxidase decreases metabolism of these medications and may potentiate therapeutic and toxic effects, especially bone marrow depression; the effect on azathioprine metabolism is especially critical in renal transplant patients because of the high risk of oxipurinol accumulation and consequent azathioprine toxicity if the transplanted kidney is rejected; if concurrent use is essential, it is recommended that azathioprine or mercaptopurine dosage be reduced to one-third to one-fourth of the usual dosage, that the patient be carefully monitored, and that subsequent dosage adjustments be based on patient response and evidence of toxicity)

(mercaptopurine may increase serum uric acid concentration in some patients; patients receiving allopurinol to treat pre-existing hyperuricemia or gout may require allopurinol dosage adjustment when mercaptopurine therapy is initiated or discontinued)

Chlorpropamide

(allopurinol may inhibit renal tubular secretion of chlorpropamide; patients receiving the medications concurrently should be monitored for possible increased hypoglycemic effect)

Dacarbazine

(dacarbazine inhibits xanthine oxidase and may cause additive hypouricemic effects when used concurrently with allopurinol)

Diuretics, thiazide

(caution and careful monitoring of the patient are advised when allopurinol and thiazide diuretics are used concurrently, especially in patients with known or possible renal function impairment, because severe hypersensitivity reactions to allopurinol may occur; although it has been suggested that compromised renal function, rather than the combination of medications, may be responsible for the adverse reactions, it has also been proposed that thiazide diuretics may increase serum oxipurinol concentrations by decreasing its renal excretion)

Probenecid

(probenecid increases urinary excretion of oxipurinol; however, the antihyperuricemic effects of the medications are additive, and increased therapeutic benefit has been reported with concurrent use)

Sulfinpyrazone

(the antihyperuricemic effects of allopurinol and sulfinpyrazone are additive; increased therapeutic benefit has been reported with concurrent use)

Vidarabine, systemic

(concurrent use with allopurinol may increase the risk of neurotoxicity and other side effects such as anemia, nausea, pain, and pruritus; caution is recommended if concurrent use is necessary)

Xanthines, such as:
  Aminophylline
  Oxtriphylline
  Theophylline

(concurrent use of large doses [600 mg per day] of allopurinol with the xanthines [except dyphylline] may decrease theophylline clearance, resulting in increased serum theophylline concentrations; when steady-state theophylline concentration is 13 mcg per mL [72.15 micromoles/L] or higher and 600 mg of allopurinol per day is required, serum theophylline concentrations should be monitored and theophylline dosage adjusted if necessary)

## Laboratory value alterations

The following have been selected on the basis of their potential clinical significance (possible effect in parentheses where appropriate)—not necessarily inclusive (» = major clinical significance):

With physiology/laboratory test values
  Alkaline phosphatase activity, serum and
  Bilirubin concentrations, serum and
  Transaminase activity, serum
    (may be increased, indicating hepatotoxicity, especially in patients with pre-existing hepatic or renal disease)
  Blood urea nitrogen (BUN) and
  Creatinine, serum
    (concentrations may be increased, indicating nephrotoxicity, especially in patients with pre-existing renal disease)

## Medical considerations/Contraindications

The medical considerations/contraindications included have been selected on the basis of their potential clinical significance (reasons given in parentheses where appropriate)—not necessarily inclusive (» = major clinical significance).

Risk-benefit should be considered when the following medical problems exist:

Renal function impairment or any illness that may predispose to a change in renal function, such as:
  Congestive heart disease
  Diabetes mellitus
  Hypertension
    (oxipurinol may accumulate; risk of severe allergic reactions and other adverse effects is increased; a reduction in dosage may be required)
    (risk of renal failure may be increased, especially when allopurinol is being used for hyperuricemia secondary to neoplastic disease or urate nephropathy; monitoring of renal function may be especially important when these conditions exist)

Sensitivity to allopurinol, history of

## Patient monitoring

The following may be especially important in patient monitoring (other tests may be warranted in some patients, depending on condition; » = major clinical significance):

Complete blood counts and
Hepatic function determinations and
Renal function determinations
  (recommended at periodic intervals during therapy, especially during the first few months)

» Uric acid, serum
  (monitoring may be required for proper dosing; the upper limit of normal is about 7 mg per 100 mL [416.36 micromoles/L] for males and postmenopausal females and about 6mg per 100 mL [356.88 micromoles/L] for premenopausal females but may vary, depending on the patient and laboratory methodology)

## Side/Adverse Effects

Note: Following initiation of allopurinol therapy for gouty arthritis, the most commonly encountered adverse effect is a temporary increase in the frequency of acute gout attacks. The occurrence of such reactions may be reduced by initiating therapy with a low dose that is gradually increased until the desired effect is obtained and by administration of prophylactic doses of colchicine or a nonsteroidal anti-inflammatory drug.

The following side/adverse effects have been selected on the basis of their potential clinical significance (possible signs and symptoms in parentheses where appropriate)—not necessarily inclusive:

### Those indicating need for medical attention

Incidence more frequent
  *Dermatitis, allergic* (skin rash, hives, or itching)
  Note: *Maculopapular skin rash* occurs most often; however, *eczematoid, exfoliative, urticarial, vesicular bullous,* or *purpuric lesions* and *lichen planus* have also been reported rarely.
  Very rarely, *skin rash* may be followed by more severe allergic reactions, usually in patients with renal function impairment and/or those receiving thiazide diuretics. *Generalized vasculitis, hepatotoxicity, and/or acute renal failure* may occur. Laboratory studies may indicate *eosinophilia* and *leukopenia* or *leukocytosis*. Several deaths have been attributed to these reactions.

Incidence rare
  *Agranulocytosis* (fever with or without chills; sores, ulcers, or white spots on lips or in mouth; sore throat); *anemia* (unusual tiredness and/or weakness); *angiitis [vasculitis], hypersensitivity* (chills, fever, and sore throat; muscle aches, pains, or weakness; shortness of breath, troubled breathing, tightness in chest, or wheezing; *aplastic anemia* (shortness of breath, troubled breathing, tightness in chest, and/or wheezing; sores, ulcers, or white spots on lips or in mouth; swollen and/or painful glands; unusual bleeding or bruising; unusual tiredness or weakness); *dermatitis, exfoliative* (possible prodrome of chills, fever, sore throat, muscle aches or pains, and/or nausea with or without vomiting; red, thickened, scaly skin); *erythema multiforme* (possible prodrome of chills, fever, sore throat, muscle aches or pains, and/or nausea with or without vomiting; sores, ulcers, or white spots in mouth or on lips; skin rash or sores, hives, and/or itching); *hepatotoxicity* (swelling in upper abdominal area; yellow eyes or skin); *hypersensitivity reaction, allopurinol-induced* (initially skin rash immediately preceding or concurrent with chills, fever, and sore throat; muscle aches or pains; and/or nausea with or without vomiting; followed by signs and symptoms of angiitis [vasculitis], hepatotoxicity, and/or acute renal failure); *loosening of fingernails; necrolysis, toxic epidermal* (possible prodrome of chills, fever, sore throat, muscle aches or pains, and/or nausea with or without vomiting; redness, tenderness, itching, burning, or peeling

of skin; red or irritated eyes); **neuritis, peripheral** (numbness, tingling, pain, or weakness in hands or feet); **renal calculus, xanthine** (blood in urine, difficult or painful urination, pain in lower back and/or side); **renal failure, acute** (sudden decrease in amount of urine; swelling of face, fingers, feet, and/or lower legs; weight gain, rapid); **Stevens-Johnson syndrome** (possible prodrome of chills, fever, sore throat, muscle aches and pains, and/or nausea with or without vomiting; sores, ulcers, or white spots in mouth or on lips; bleeding sores on lips); **thrombocytopenia** (usually asymptomatic; rarely, unusual bleeding or bruising; black, tarry stools; blood in urine or stools; pinpoint red spots on skin); **unexplained nosebleeds**

Note: Bone marrow depression has been reported to occur 6 weeks to 6 years after initiation of allopurinol therapy. Most of the affected patients were also receiving other medications with the potential for causing this reaction. However, bone marrow depression affecting one or more cell lines has rarely occurred in patients receiving allopurinol alone.

Hepatotoxicity may be hypersensitivity-mediated; hepatic necrosis, granulomatous hepatitis, and cholestatic jaundice have been reported.

Renal failure associated with allopurinol therapy has been reported in patients being treated for hyperuricemia secondary to neoplastic diseases or gouty nephropathy as well as in patients experiencing hypersensitivity reactions to the medication.

**Those indicating need for medical attention only if they continue or are bothersome**
Incidence less frequent or rare
*Diarrhea; drowsiness; headache; indigestion; nausea or vomiting without symptoms of skin rash, chills or fever, or muscle aches and pains; stomach pain; unusual hair loss*

## Overdose
For more information on the management of overdose or unintentional ingestion, **contact a Poison Control Center** (see *Poison Control Center Listing*).

**Treatment of overdose**
Immediate discontinuation of allopurinol.
To decrease absorption—Gastric lavage, if very large quantities have been ingested.
To enhance elimination—Although allopurinol and oxipurinol are dialyzable, the value of hemodialysis or peritoneal dialysis in the management of allopurinol overdose has not been established.
Monitoring—May include observing the patient and treating the observed symptoms.
Supportive care—Maintaining hydration. Patients in whom intentional overdose is known or suspected should be referred for psychiatric consultation.

## Patient Consultation
As an aid to patient consultation, refer to *Advice for the Patient, Allopurinol (Systemic)*.
In providing consultation, consider emphasizing the following selected information (» = major clinical significance):

**Before using this medication**
» Conditions affecting use, especially:
    Other medications, especially coumarin- or indandione-derivative anticoagulants, azathioprine, and mercaptopurine

**Proper use of this medication**
Taking after meals, if necessary, to minimize gastrointestinal irritation
» Compliance with therapy
    Importance of high fluid intake during therapy and compliance with therapy for alkalinization of urine, if prescribed, to help prevent kidney stones
    Several months of continuous therapy may be required for maximum effectiveness in patients with chronic gout
» Medication helps prevent, but does not relieve, acute gout attacks; need to continue taking allopurinol with medication prescribed for gout attacks
» Proper dosing
    Missed dose: Taking as soon as possible; not taking if almost time for next dose; not doubling doses
» Proper storage

**Precautions while using this medication**
Regular visits to physician to check progress during therapy; possible need for periodic blood tests to determine efficacy of therapy and/or occurrence of side effects

Avoiding large amounts of alcohol, which may increase uric acid concentrations and reduce effectiveness of medication
Possibility that vitamin C taken in large amounts may increase the potential for kidney stone formation
» Notifying physician immediately if skin rash occurs or if influenza-like symptoms (chills, fever, muscle aches and pains, or nausea or vomiting) occur concurrently with or shortly after skin rash; these symptoms may rarely indicate onset of severe hypersensitivity reaction
» Caution if drowsiness occurs

**Side/adverse effects**
Signs of potential adverse effects, especially allergic dermatitis, agranulocytosis, anemia, angiitis, aplastic anemia, exfoliative dermatitis, erythema multiforme, hepatotoxicity, hypersensitivity reaction, loosening of fingernails, toxic epidermal necrolysis, peripheral neuritis, renal caluli, renal failure, Stevens-Johnson syndrome, thrombocytopenia, and unexplained nosebleeds

## General Dosing Information
Allopurinol may be administered after meals to lessen gastrointestinal irritation.

An increase in the frequency of acute attacks of gouty arthritis may occur during the early months of allopurinol therapy. The risk of precipitating acute gout attacks may be reduced by initiating allopurinol therapy with a low dose, then gradually increasing dosage until the desired effect is obtained. Also, it is recommended that prophylactic doses of colchicine (or, if the patient cannot take colchicine, a nonsteroidal anti-inflammatory drug [NSAID]) be administered concurrently during the first 3 to 6 months of allopurinol therapy.

Acute attacks of gout may occur during allopurinol therapy, even with colchicine or NSAID prophylactic therapy. During an attack, allopurinol therapy should be continued at the same dose while an appropriate anti-inflammatory agent (preferably an NSAID or a corticosteroid [preferably via intrasynovial injection, when feasible]) is administered to relieve the attack. Because of the toxicity associated with therapeutic doses of colchicine, its use for treatment of an acute attack of gout should be reserved for patients in whom the preferred medications are contraindicated or ineffective.

The total daily dose may be administered in divided doses or as a single dose. Each single dose should not exceed 300 mg. Daily dosage requirements exceeding 300 mg should be administered in divided doses.

Monitoring of serum uric acid concentrations may be necessary for proper dosing.

To reduce the risk of xanthine calculi formation, and to help prevent renal precipitation of urates in patients receiving concomitant uricosuric agents, a high fluid intake (no less than 2.5 to 3 liters daily) and maintenance of a neutral, or preferably slightly alkaline, urine are recommended.

When uricosuric therapy is being changed to allopurinol therapy, the dose of the uricosuric agent should be reduced gradually over a period of several weeks and the dose of allopurinol increased gradually to the dose required for maintenance of normal serum uric acid concentrations.

It is recommended that allopurinol therapy be discontinued at once if a skin rash or any other sign of adverse reaction occurs. Skin rash may be followed by more severe hypersensitivity reactions. After a severe reaction, therapy should be discontinued permanently. However, after a mild reaction, it may be possible to reinstate therapy at a lower dosage (50 mg per day initially and increased very gradually) after the reaction has subsided. If skin rash recurs, therapy should be discontinued permanently.

**For treatment of adverse effects**
Hypersensitivity reactions—Administer glucocorticoids. Prolonged administration may be required after a severe reaction.

## Oral Dosage Forms

### ALLOPURINOL TABLETS USP
**Usual adult and adolescent dose**
Antigout agent—
    Initial—Oral, 100 mg once a day, to be increased by 100 mg per day at one-week intervals until the desired serum uric acid concentration is attained, not to exceed the maximum recommended dosage of 800 mg per day.
    Maintenance—Oral, 100 to 200 mg two or three times a day; or 300 mg as a single dose once a day. The usual maintenance dose is 200 to 300 mg per day in mild gout or 400 to 600 mg per day in moderately severe tophaceous gout.

## Allopurinol (Systemic)

Neoplastic disease therapy:—
    Initial—Oral, 600 to 800 mg per day starting twelve hours to three days (preferably two to three days) prior to initiation of chemotherapy or radiation therapy.
    Maintenance—Dosage should be based on serum uric acid determinations performed approximately forty-eight hours after initiation of allopurinol therapy and periodically thereafter. Allopurinol should be discontinued following the period of tumor regression.
Antiurolithic (uric acid calculi)—
    Oral, 100 to 200 mg one to four times a day; or 300 mg as a single dose once a day.
Antiurolithic (calcium oxalate calculi)—
    Oral, 200 to 300 mg a day as a single dose or in divided doses.
Note: Because oxipurinol is excreted primarily by the kidneys, accumulation may occur in patients with renal failure. Patients receiving dialysis may require usual therapeutic doses of allopurinol; however, in patients not receiving dialysis, it is recommended that the dosage be reduced as follows:

| Creatinine Clearance (mL/min) | Dose |
|---|---|
| 10 to 20 | 200 mg daily |
| 3 to 10 | no more than 100 mg daily |
| < 3 | 100 mg at intervals of more than 24 hours may be necessary |

    Some patients with renal function impairment may require even lower doses or longer intervals between doses. In some cases, 300 mg twice a week, or even less, may suffice.

**Usual adult prescribing limits**
300 mg per dose; 800 mg per day.

**Usual pediatric dose**
Antihyperuricemic, in neoplastic disease therapy—
    Children up to 6 years of age: Oral, 50 mg three times a day.
    Children 6 to 10 years of age: Oral, 100 mg three times a day; or 300 mg as a single dose once a day.
Note: Dosage adjustment may be necessary after approximately forty-eight hours of therapy, depending on the patient's response.

**Strength(s) usually available**
U.S.—
    100 mg (Rx) [*Lopurin* (scored); *Zyloprim* (scored); GENERIC].
    300 mg (Rx) [*Lopurin* (scored); *Zyloprim* (scored); GENERIC].
Canada—
    100 mg (Rx) [*Apo-Allopurinol* (scored); *Purinol* (scored); *Zyloprim* (scored)].
    200 mg (Rx) [*Apo-Allopurinol* (scored); *Purinol* (scored); *Zyloprim* (scored)].
    300 mg (Rx) [*Apo-Allopurinol* (scored); *Purinol* (scored); *Zyloprim* (scored)].

**Packaging and storage**
Store below 40 °C (104 °F), preferably between 15 and 25 °C (59 and 77 °F). Store in a well-closed container.

**Auxiliary labeling**
• Drink large amounts of fluids.

## Selected Bibliography

Ettinger B, Tang A, Citron JT, Livermore B, Williams T. Randomized trial of allopurinol in the prevention of calcium oxalate calculi. N Engl J Med 1986; 315: 1386-9.

Lupton GP, Odom RB. The allopurinol hypersensitivity syndrome. J Am Acad Dermatol 1979; 1: 365-74.

Revised: 08/25/94

---

## ALPHA$_1$-PROTEINASE INHIBITOR HUMAN—The *Alpha$_1$-proteinase Inhibitor, Human (Systemic)* monograph is not included in this published version of the USP DI database. Copies of the monograph are available on request from Micromedex, Inc. - Reprint Requests, 6200 S. Syracuse Way, Suite 300, Englewood, CO 80111; telephone (303) 486-6400; telefax (303) 486-6464; Email: USPDI@MDX.COM.

---

## ALPRAZOLAM—See *Benzodiazepines (Systemic)*

---

# ALPROSTADIL  Local

VA CLASSIFICATION (Primary/Secondary): HS200/CV500; GU900; DX900

Note: For information pertaining to the use of alprostadil for other indications, see *Alprostadil (Systemic)*. When using phentolamine or papaverine also, see *Phentolamine (Intracavernosal)* and *Papaverine (Intracavernosal)* monographs for additional information.

Commonly used brand name(s): *Caverject*; *Edex*; *Muse*; *Prostin VR*; *Prostin VR Pediatric*.

Other commonly used names are PGE$_1$ and prostaglandin E$_1$.

Note: For a listing of dosage forms and brand names by country availability, see *Dosage Forms* section(s).

## Category

Impotence therapy agent; diagnostic aid, erectile dysfunction; diagnostic aid, penile vasculature imaging.

## Indications

Note: Bracketed information in the *Indications* section refers to uses that are not included in U.S. product labeling.

**Accepted**
Erectile dysfunction (treatment)—Alprostadil for Injection and alprostadil intraurethral suppositories are indicated and [Alprostadil Injection USP][1] is used to facilitate erections in men with erectile dysfunction. [Low doses of a three-drug combination of alprostadil, papaverine, and phentolamine as an injection are sometimes used to achieve a synergistic action.][1] Erectile dysfunction that is medication-induced or caused by endocrine problems, such as hypogonadism or hyper- or hypothyroidism, should be evaluated and appropriately treated before alprostadil treatment is considered.

Erectile dysfunction (diagnosis) or
Penile vasculature imaging (diagnostic adjunct)—Alprostadil for Injection is indicated and [Alprostadil Injection USP][1] is used by intracavernosal injection as an aid in the evaluation of penile vasculature, alone or prior to angiography, cavernosography, or cavernosometry.

**Unaccepted**
Use of alprostadil to enhance erections in men who are not impotent is not recommended because of the risk of priapism and permanent damage to penile tissues.

[1]Not included in Canadian product labeling.

## Pharmacology/Pharmacokinetics

**Physicochemical characteristics**
Description: Suppository—Measures 1.4 millimeters (mm) in diameter and 3 mm or 6 mm in length and is located within the stem of its delivery device. A depressable button on the body of the device initiates the suppository's release from the stem.
Molecular weight—354.49.
pKa—6.3.

**Mechanism of action/Effect**
Alprostadil is a prostaglandin, specifically prostaglandin E$_1$, that is produced endogenously to relax vascular smooth muscle and cause vasodilation. The total prostaglandin concentration occurring naturally in human seminal fluid is 100 to 200 mg per mL and includes prostaglandins E$_1$ and E$_2$.

Impotence therapy agent—When administered by intracavernosal injection or as an intraurethral suppository, alprostadil acts locally to relax the trabecular smooth muscle of the corpora cavernosa and the cavernosal arteries. Swelling, elongation, and rigidity of the penis result when arterial blood rapidly flows into the corpus cavernosum to expand the lacunar spaces. The entrapped blood reduces the venous blood outflow as sinusoids compress against the tunica albuginea.

Adding papaverine and phentolamine to the alprostadil regimen synergistically increases arterial blood flow via separate mechanisms. Papaverine relaxes the sinusoid and the smooth muscle of the helicine arteries, while phentolamine relaxes arterial smooth muscle and blocks the alpha-adrenergic receptors that inhibit an erection.

### Absorption
Suppository—When inserted immediately after urination, residual urine in the urethra dissolves the urethral suppository. Within 10 minutes, alprostadil absorption occurs from the urethral lining, passing to the corpora cavernosa via the corpus spongiosum.

### Biotransformation
Local, rapid within the urethra, prostate, and corpus cavernosum; if any alprostadil is systemically absorbed, it is metabolized by a single pass through the lungs.

### Onset of action
5 to 10 minutes.

### Time to peak effect
Within 20 minutes.

### Duration of action
Injection—1 to 3 hours; dose-related.
Suppository—30 to 60 minutes.

## Precautions to Consider

### Carcinogenicity
Studies have not been done.

### Mutagenicity
Alprostadil is not mutagenic, according to results of the Ames test and alkaline elution assay.

### Pregnancy/Reproduction
Fertility—In an *in vitro* study of human sperm, an alprostadil concentration of 400 mcg/mL had no effect on sperm motility and viability.

Sperm number, motility, and morphology were not affected in a study of dogs given intraurethral doses greater than 3000 mcg a day for 13 weeks, a dose corresponding to 3.5 times the maximum recommended human dose (MRHD) when adjusted for body surface area.

Pregnancy—Adequate and well-controlled studies in humans have not been done. Despite lack of reported problems, males using the suppositories who have sexual intercourse with pregnant women should use condoms for barrier protection to prevent maternal and fetal exposure to alprostadil. Since alprostadil's effects in early pregnancy are unknown, couples should use adequate contraception if the female partner could become pregnant.

Studies of female animals indirectly exposed to the intraurethral suppository or intracavernosal injection by mating with male animals have not been done; however, direct intravaginal administration of 4000 mcg a day in pregnant rabbits (a dose corresponding to 12.5 times the MRHD) did not cause harmful effects in their fetuses. Other direct routes of administration to females using doses much larger than those used for erectile dysfunction have shown embryo and maternal toxicities in pregnant animals.

Suppository—FDA Pregnancy Category C.

Note: An FDA category has not been assigned for the injection dosage forms.

### Geriatrics
Studies in healthy men 56 years of age and older have shown results similar to those seen in younger patients, although some older men required slightly higher maintenance doses when arterial occlusive disease was present. Older patients are likely to differ from younger patients in the course and etiology of their erectile dysfunction.

### Drug interactions and/or related problems
The following drug interactions and/or related problems have been selected on the basis of their potential clinical significance (possible mechanism in parentheses where appropriate)—not necessarily inclusive (» = major clinical significance):

Note: Combinations containing any of the following medications, depending on the amount present, may also interact with this medication.

Sympathomimetic agents, alpha-adrenergic, especially epinephrine, metaraminol, and phenylephrine
(sympathomimetic agents reverse the vasodilating effect of alprostadil; phenylephrine and epinephrine may be used to treat priapism or overdose)

### Medical considerations/Contraindications
The medical considerations/contraindications included have been selected on the basis of their potential clinical significance (reasons given in parentheses where appropriate)—not necessarily inclusive (» = major clinical significance).

*Except under special circumstances, this medication should not be used when the following medical problems exist:*

» Abnormalities of the penis, such as
Anatomical deformity
Angulation of the penis
Cavernosal fibrosis
Hypospadia, severe
Peyronie's disease
Urethral stricture
(patients who have an anatomical deformity, angulation of the penis, cavernosal fibrosis, or Peyronie's disease are at increased risk of developing problems when using parenteral or intraurethral dosage forms of alprostadil)

(use of urethral suppositories is not recommended in patients with urethral stricture or severe hypospadia)

» Balanitis or
» Urethritis
(use of urethral suppositories is not recommended because infection or inflammation may worsen, and abrasions or minor bleeding from penis may be more likely to occur)

*Risk-benefit should be considered when the following medical problems exist:*

» Coagulation defects, severe
(risk of bleeding may be increased because alprostadil inhibits platelet aggregation; may be especially problematic when an improperly administered suppository or injection causes either a urethral abrasion or a contusion)

» Leukemia or
» Myeloma, multiple or
» Polycythemia or
» Priapism, history of or
» Sickle cell disease or
» Thrombocythemia
(increased risk of priapism, especially if hyperviscosity of blood or venous thrombosis results from these predisposing conditions)

Sensitivity to alprostadil

### Patient monitoring
The following may be especially important in patient monitoring (other tests may be warranted in some patients, depending on condition; » = major clinical significance):

Palpation of penis
(recommended at regular intervals by both the patient and the physician to check for developing fibrosis or curvature)

## Side/Adverse Effects

The following side/adverse effects have been selected on the basis of their potential clinical significance (possible signs and symptoms in parentheses where appropriate)—not necessarily inclusive:

### Those indicating need for medical attention
Incidence rare
*Hypotension* (faintness; lightheadedness)—incidence of 2%, more likely for injectable doses greater than 20 mcg; *prolonged erection* (erection continuing for 4 to 6 hours)—incidence of 0.3%; *priapism* (erection continuing for more than 6 hours with severe and continuing pain of the penis)—incidence of less than 0.1%; *testicular pain or edema* (swelling of testes)—incidence of less than 1% with use of injection and incidence of 5% with use of suppositories

Note: *Prolonged erection* can resolve spontaneously; at times it will require treatment, especially if *priapism* develops. Priapism usually is due to excessive dosage.

*For injection only*
*Fibrosis of penis* (curving of penis with pain during erection)—incidence 5.2%

Signs and symptoms of systemic absorption—associated with excessive doses
*Dizziness; faintness; hypertension, reflexive; prostatic disorders* (pelvic pain); *rapid pulse; respiratory infection* (flu-like symptoms)

### Those indicating need for medical attention only if they continue or are bothersome
Incidence more frequent
*Pain at site of administration; penile pain during erection*—incidences of 32% with use of suppository and 11% with use of injection

# Alprostadil (Local)

*For injection only*
   **Bleeding at injection site, transient**
*For suppositories only*
   **Bleeding or spotting from urethra**—incidence of 5%; **stinging of urethra**—incidence of 12%
   Note: When males used the suppository dosage form, 5.8% of female partners reported vaginal itching or stinging. These symptoms may partially result from an associated lack of recent sexual activity for these women.

Incidence rare
   *For injection only*
      **Ecchymosis or hematoma at site of injection** (bruising or localized blood clot in penis at site of injection)—incidence of 3%, usually due to incorrect injection technique

## Patient Consultation

As an aid to patient consultation, refer to *Advice for the Patient, Alprostadil (Local)* and, when also using papaverine and phentolamine, *Advice for the Patient, Phentolamine and Papaverine (Intracavernosal)*.

In providing consultation, consider emphasizing the following selected information (» = major clinical significance):

### Before using this medication
» Conditions affecting use, especially:
   Sensitivity to alprostadil
   Other medical problems, especially abnormalities of the penis, balanitis, severe coagulation defects, leukemia, multiple myeloma, polycythemia, history of priapism, sickle cell disease, thrombocythemia, or urethritis

### Proper use of this medication
» Reading patient package insert, although patient information may not be available for all products
*For injection dosage forms*
» Recognizing that different injection products have different mixing procedures
   *Proper preparation*
      Washing hands with soap and water; wiping tops of bottles but not needle with alcohol swab, then discarding the swab; attaching needle to the syringe if needed without taking the cap off needle
   *To mix*
      For *Caverject*—Adding plunger to the syringe; mixing alprostadil powder for injection with 1 mL of the diluent, Bacteriostatic Water for Injection USP, included in the packaging as a prefilled syringe or separate vial
      For *Edex*—Adding plunger to the syringe; mixing alprostadil powder for injection with 1.2 mL of the diluent, Sodium Chloride Injection USP, included in the packaging as a prefilled syringe
      For *Prostin VR* or *Prostin VR Pediatric*—Getting exact mixing instructions from the physician or pharmacist, and following them carefully if told to mix two solutions
   *Proper administration*
» Checking that final solution is clear before measuring dose; not using if injection is cloudy, colored, or contains solids
» Drawing the correct dose into syringe; removing air bubbles; rechecking dose
» After cleansing injection site with alcohol swab, giving injection by keeping needle at a 90-degree angle to the penis while inserting and injecting slowly over 5 to 10 seconds and directly into corpus cavernosum at sides or midshaft of penis; avoiding subcutaneous administration and injection into arteries or veins or injection at top or head of penis or at base of penis near the scrotum; if inadvertently injected subcutaneously (as evidenced by pain at injection site), stopping injection and withdrawing and repositioning needle
» After removing and recapping needle, applying gentle pressure at the injection site for 5 minutes to prevent bruising; massaging penis as directed by physician to distribute medication
» Varying site of injection
» Throwing away any unused mixture remaining in syringe; not reusing needles
*For suppository dosage forms*
   *Proper administration*
» Urinating just prior to insertion; residual urine in urethra helps to dissolve the suppository
   Removing delivery device and cap from applicator stem; inserting delivery stem into urethra after lengthening and stretching penis upward; withdrawing and reinserting delivery device if discomfort or pulling sensation is felt
   After depressing button to release suppository, holding delivery device still for 5 seconds, then rocking delivery device gently from side to side; after removing delivery device, inspecting the device for complete suppository release and, if needed, repeating process to insert any remaining suppository
   Rolling penis between hands for 10 seconds to distribute the suppository within the walls of the urethra; continuing motion for relief if stinging occurs
   Sitting, standing, or walking for 10 minutes while erection is developing to promote blood flow to the penis for a proper erection
*For injection and suppository dosage forms*
   Effect begins in about 5 to 10 minutes; attempting intercourse within 10 to 30 minutes after administration. Erection may continue after ejaculation
» Proper disposal
   For suppository delivery device—Replacing cap on device; placing in foil pouch; throwing away
   For syringes and needles from injection—Using plastic case with locking device that comes with some packaging, or using a heavy plastic container; cutting or breaking needle before disposing; alternatively, giving to a health care professional for disposal
» Proper dosing
» Proper storage

### Precautions while using this medication
» Not using medication with a penile implant unless advised by physician
» Compliance with therapy; importance of not exceeding prescribed dosage and frequency of use; risk of priapism, tissue ischemia, and permanent damage with overdose
» Telling physician immediately if erection persists longer than 4 hours or becomes painful
*For injection dosage forms*
   If bleeding occurs at injection site, applying pressure; checking with physician if bleeding persists
*For suppository dosage forms*
» Using a condom when having sexual intercourse with a pregnant female in order to protect the mother and fetus from exposure to alprostadil
» Using contraception when having sexual intercourse with a female of reproductive age

### Side/adverse effects
Signs of potential side effects, especially hypotension; prolonged erection; priapism; testicular pain or edema; fibrosis of penis (injection only)
Signs and symptoms of systemic absorption, usually resulting from excessive doses, including dizziness, faintness, reflexive hypertension, prostatic disorders, rapid pulse, or respiratory infection

## General Dosing Information

There is no information on administering alprostadil injections or suppositories to patients who also use a penile implant.

Patients receiving alprostadil should be under the supervision of a physician experienced in its use and familiar with proper management of prolonged erection and priapism. Medical personnel usually give the first dose(s) in a clinical setting, titrating the dose carefully according to guidelines. For all responses during the titration process, patient should remain under clinical supervision until complete detumescence occurs. Maintenance doses are usually self-administered.

Dosage adjustment should be made carefully, based on the degree and duration of tumescence achieved with the previous dose. In general, patients with neurogenic erectile dysfunction may be more sensitive to the effects of intracavernosal vasodilators, and may require lower doses.

### For injection dosage forms

In one clinical study of 579 patients having erectile dysfunction due to various etiologies, the doses after titration ranged between 5 and 20 mcg for 56% of patients; the mean maintenance dose was 17.8 mcg. In an uncontrolled self-injection study, the mean maintenance dose used after 6 months was 20.7 mcg. Specific to the cause of erectile dysfunction, mean maintenance doses of 12.4 mcg for psychogenic, 15.8 mcg for neurogenic, and 18.5 mcg for vasculogenic erectile dysfunction have been reported by the manufacturer. Other studies have shown similar results.

For treatment of erectile dysfunction, alprostadil is slowly injected (over 5 to 10 seconds) directly into the corpus cavernosum at the sides or midshaft of the penis. A characteristic give should be noticed as the needle penetrates the tunica albuginea and enters the corpus cavernosum. Proper injection technique is necessary to avoid injury. Alprostadil should not be injected into the urethra, arteries, veins, scrotum, upper- or bottom-most part of the penis (top or head of penis or area on the penile shaft near the scrotum), or into the dorsal area of the penis.

Injection sites should be alternated. After completion of the injection, pressure is applied to the injection site to prevent bleeding. The entire length of the corpus cavernosum on the side receiving the injection should be squeezed firmly to distribute the medication. To uniformly distribute the medication within both corpora cavernosa, the other side also can be squeezed.

A low-dose three-drug combination injection (alprostadil, papaverine, and phentolamine) may be more effective and, in some cases, less painful than alprostadil injected alone. A thorough evaluation of comparative studies is still needed. While the doses used in studies vary, an accepted strength is 17.6 mg papaverine, 0.6 mg phentolamine, and 5.9 mcg alprostadil per mL. The amount prescribed for self-injection is titrated according to individual response.

**For suppository dosage form**
In two placebo-controlled, parallel group studies of 1511 patients with erectile dysfunction, 996 patients (66%) completed the titration process; some patients could not complete the titration process because of accompanying penile pain. Of the 874 patients completing 3 months of treatment, doses for about 10, 20, 30, and 40% of patients were titrated to 125, 250, 500, and 1000 mcg, respectively.

Prior to inserting the intraurethral suppository, the patient should urinate; the residual urine remaining in the urethra will help dissolve the suppository.

The delivery device is inserted into the urethra with ease after the penis is first stretched lengthwise and pressed at top and bottom. After depressing a button to release the suppository into the urethra, the device is held upright and immobile for 5 seconds to help dissolve the suppository. Moving the device and the penis as a unit gently side to side helps to dissolve the suppository and enhances its release from the device. Whenever the patient feels an uncomfortable or pulling sensation, the delivery system should be removed and the procedure repeated if needed. Also, the procedure can be repeated to insert a partial suppository not fully dislodged from the device.

After the delivery device is withdrawn, the patient should roll his penis between his hands for 10 seconds to further distribute the suppository within the walls of the urethra and to ease any stinging sensation. Sitting, standing, or walking for 10 minutes while erection is developing promotes blood flow.

Use of contraception is recommended by the manufacturer if the patient engages in sexual intercourse with a female of reproductive age because potential effects on early pregnancy are not known. Using a condom is recommended when having sexual intercourse with a pregnant female; it provides a barrier and protects the mother and fetus from the effects of alprostadil.

**For treatment of prolonged erection or priapism**
A prolonged erection should be treated if it persists longer than 4 hours; priapism should be treated promptly. If tumescence is not reversed, interruption of blood flow may result in penile tissue ischemia and permanent tissue damage.

Treatment of adverse effects should be initiated by a physician trained in treating drug-induced tumescence. Depending on the severity, treatment may include:
- Application of ice packs to inner thigh, alternating between thighs, for no more than 10 minutes to shorten the duration of a prolonged erection.
- Aspiration of intracavernosal blood.
- Intracavernosal administration of an alpha-adrenergic agonist; phenylephrine is preferred to epinephrine. While monitoring blood pressure, an injection of 0.5 mg/mL *Phenylephrine Hydrochloride Injection USP* is given, followed by a second dose, if needed, in 15 minutes.
- Irrigation of the corpus cavernosum with 0.9% Sodium Chloride Irrigation USP or 20 mL of dilute solutions of phenylephrine (20 mg *Phenylephrine Hydrochloride Injection USP* in 500 mL of 0.9% Sodium Chloride Irrigation USP) or epinephrine (1 mL 1:1000 *Epinephrine Injection USP* in 1 liter of 0.9% Sodium Chloride Irrigation USP), using a 19-gauge needle to remove clotted blood.
- Surgery (rarely needed).

## Intraurethral Dosage Forms

### ALPROSTADIL SUPPOSITORIES
**Usual adult dose**
Impotence therapy agent—
  Initial: Intraurethral, 125 or 250 mcg a day, followed by dose adjustments in stepwise fashion on separate occasions as instructed by a physician.
  Maintenance: Intraurethral, an individual dose established by a physician is inserted by the patient between ten and thirty minutes before intercourse. Dosage adjustments require physician consultation. No more than two suppositories should be used within twenty-four hours.

**Strength(s) usually available**
U.S.—
  125 mcg (Rx) [*Muse* (polyethylene glycol)].
  250 mcg (Rx) [*Muse* (polyethylene glycol)].
  500 mcg (Rx) [*Muse* (polyethylene glycol)].
  1000 mcg (Rx) [*Muse* (polyethylene glycol)].
Canada—
  Not commercially available.
Note: The unit-dose packaging includes a suppository and delivery device; six unit-dose packages are contained in one box.

**Packaging and storage**
Store between 2 and 8 °C (36 and 46 °F), unless otherwise specified by manufacturer. Protect from freezing. May be stored between 15 and 30 °C (59 and 86 °F) for up to fourteen days.

**Auxiliary labeling**
- Refrigerate.
- Do not freeze.

**Note**
Include patient package insert (PPI) when dispensing.

## Parenteral Dosage Forms
Note: Bracketed information in the *Dosage Forms* section refers to uses that are not included in U.S. product labeling.

### ALPROSTADIL INJECTION USP
**Usual adult dose**
[Impotence therapy agent][1]—
For patients with erectile dysfunction of penile vasculogenic or mixed etiology—
  Initial—Intracavernosal, 2.5 mcg, followed by dosage adjustments as supervised by a physician according to patient response. The proper dose will produce a full erection that begins within five to twenty minutes, and lasts for no more than one hour. If an erection lasts longer than one hour, the dose should be reduced. Further dosing depends on whether the first dose produced a partial or no erectile response.
    For patients partially responding to the first dose, 7.5 mcg can be injected twenty-four hours or longer following the first dose. Until the proper dose is established, further doses scheduled on no more than two consecutive days (twenty-four hours apart) or three times a week can be increased by 5- to 10-mcg increments thereafter until an erection suitable for intercourse is achieved.
    For patients not responding to the first dose, 5 mcg more can be injected within the hour, resulting in a total daily dose of 7.5 mcg. Until proper dose is established, further doses scheduled on no more than two consecutive days (twenty-four hours apart) or three times a week can be increased by 5- to 10-mcg increments.
  Maintenance—Intracavernosal, an individual dose established by a physician is injected by the patient ten to thirty minutes before intended intercourse. Alprostadil should not be used more often than three times a week or on more than two consecutive days; at least twenty-four hours should elapse between doses. Dosing adjustments require physician-patient consultation.
  Note: For patients using a three-drug regimen, 0.25 mL (17.6 mg papaverine, 0.6 mg phentolamine, and 5.9 mcg alprostadil per mL) is the usual dose achieved after completing the titration process.
For patients with erectile dysfunction of psychogenic or neurogenic etiology—
  Initial—Intracavernosal, 1.25 mcg, followed by dosage adjustments as supervised by the physician according to patient response. The proper dose will produce a full erection that begins within five to twenty minutes, and lasts for no more than one hour. If an erection lasts longer than one hour, the dose should be reduced. Further dosing depends on whether the first dose produced a partial or no erectile response.
    For patients partially responding to the first dose, 2.5 mcg can be injected twenty-four hours or longer following the first dose. Until the proper dose is established, further doses scheduled on no more than two consecutive days (twenty-four hours apart) or three times a week can be increased by 5-mcg increments thereafter until an erection suitable for intercourse is achieved.
    For patients not responding to the first dose, 1.25 mcg more can be injected within the hour, resulting in a total daily dose of 2.5 mcg. Until proper dose is established, further doses scheduled on no more than two consecutive days (twenty-four hours apart) or three times a week can be increased by 5-mcg increments.

# Alprostadil (Local)

Maintenance—Intracavernosal, an individual dose established by a physician is injected by the patient ten to thirty minutes before intended intercourse. Alprostadil should not be used more often than three times a week or on more than two consecutive days; at least twenty-four hours should elapse between doses. Dosing adjustments require physician-patient consultation.

Note: For patients using a three-drug regimen, 0.12 mL (17.6 mg papaverine, 0.6 mg phentolamine, and 5.9 mcg alprostadil per mL) is the usual dose achieved after completing the titration process.

Diagnostic aid adjunct (penile vasculature imaging)[1] or
Diagnostic aid (erectile dysfunction)[1]—
Intracavernosal, the lowest single dose to cause an erection of firm rigidity.

Note: These patients are more likely to develop priapism that may require penile aspiration.

**Usual adult prescribing limits**
Impotence therapy agent—
60 mcg (0.06 mg) of alprostadil per dose.

**Strength(s) usually available**
U.S.—
500 mcg (0.5 mg) per mL (Rx) [*Prostin VR Pediatric* (dehydrated alcohol)].
Canada—
500 mcg (0.5 mg) per mL (Rx) [*Prostin VR* (dehydrated alcohol)].

Note: Distribution of *Prostin VR Pediatric* in the U.S. and *Prostin VR* in Canada is limited to acute-care facilities. As an alternative, compounding from bulk products is being done to make a multidose vial, single-use vials, or prefilled syringes; use of filters and preservatives should be considered as needed.

**Packaging and storage**
Store between 2 and 8 °C (36 and 46 °F), unless otherwise specified by manufacturer. Protect from freezing.

**Preparation of dosage form**
To prepare a solution of 20 mcg/mL of alprostadil, inject 1 mL of 500 mcg/mL Alprostadil Injection USP and 4 mL of 0.9% Sodium Chloride Injection USP into an empty vial to make a 100 mcg/mL alprostadil intermediate solution. After mixing, inject a 1-mL aliquot of 100 mcg/mL Alprostadil Injection USP into five 5-mL multidose vials. To make a 20 mcg/mL alprostadil solution, add 4 mL of 0.9% Sodium Chloride Injection USP to each vial. This multidose vial may be dispensed or separated into five 1-mL single-use vials or five 1-mL prefilled syringes. Other concentrations may be appropriate.

**Stability**
Stability after dilution is unknown.

**Auxiliary labeling**
- Refrigerate.
- Do not freeze.

## ALPROSTADIL FOR INJECTION

**Usual adult dose**
Impotence therapy agent or
Diagnostic aid adjunct (penile vasculature imaging) or
Diagnostic aid (erectile dysfunction)—
See *Alprostadil Injection USP*.

**Usual adult prescribing limits**
Impotence therapy agent—
See *Alprostadil Injection USP*.

**Size(s) usually available**
U.S.—
5 mcg (0.005 mg) (Rx) [*Caverject* (benzyl alcohol 8.4 mg; lactose 172 mg; sodium citrate 47 mg); *Edex* (alpha-cyclodextrin; lactose anhydrous 56.3 mg)].
10 mcg (0.01 mg) (Rx) [*Caverject* (benzyl alcohol 8.4 mg; lactose 172 mg; sodium citrate 47 mg); *Edex* (alpha-cyclodextrin; lactose anhydrous 56.3 mg)].
20 mcg (0.02 mg) (Rx) [*Caverject* (benzyl alcohol 8.4 mg; lactose 172 mg; sodium citrate 47 mg); *Edex* (alpha-cyclodextrin; lactose anhydrous 56.3 mg)].
40 mcg (0.04 mg) (Rx) [*Edex* (alpha-cyclodextrin; lactose anhydrous 56.3 mg)].
Canada—
10 mcg (0.01 mg) (Rx) [*Caverject* (benzyl alcohol 8.4 mg; lactose 172 mg; sodium citrate 47 mg)].
20 mcg (0.02 mg) (Rx) [*Caverject* (benzyl alcohol 8.4 mg; lactose 172 mg; sodium citrate 47 mg)].

Note: For the prefilled syringe—The 5-, 10-, and 20-mcg strengths of *Caverject* and all strengths of *Edex* include in their packaging a single-use vial containing sterile alprostadil powder, prefilled diluent syringe and needle (22-gauge, 1½-inch needle; or 27- or 30-gauge, ½-inch needle), separate syringe plunger, and alcohol swabs. Needle may or may not be attached to the syringe.

For the single-use vials—The 10- and 20-mcg strengths of *Caverject* include in their packaging a single-use vial containing sterile alprostadil powder, a vial of diluent, and a preassembled 3-cc, 27-gauge, ½-inch syringe.

For each product—Six unit-dose packages are contained in one box.

**Packaging and storage**
Store between 15 and 25 °C (59 and 77 °F). Protect from freezing.

**Preparation of dosage form**
Alprostadil for Injection is prepared by adding diluent to a vial of sterile alprostadil powder. The diluent is packaged as a prefilled syringe or in a separate vial. Solution is mixed, then drawn using the same syringe.
For *Caverject*: Add 1 mL of diluent (Bacteriostatic Water for Injection USP containing benzyl alcohol) to a vial of sterile alprostadil powder.
For *Edex*: Add 1.2 mL of diluent (Sodium Chloride Injection USP) to a vial of sterile alprostadil powder.

**Stability**
Stability of the medication after dilution is unknown. The manufacturer recommends that the reconstituted solution be used immediately.

**Auxiliary labeling**
- Store in a cool, dry place.
- Do not freeze.

**Note**
Include patient package insert (PPI) for Alprostadil for Injection when dispensing.

[1]Not included in Canadian product labeling.

## Selected Bibliography

Bernard F, Lue TF. Self-administration in the pharmacological treatment of impotence. Drugs 1990; 39(3): 394-8.

Bennett AH, Carpenter AJ, Barada JH. An improved vasoactive drug combination for a pharmacological erection program. J Urol 1991 Dec; 146: 1564-5.

Revised: 08/19/97

# ALPROSTADIL Systemic

VA CLASSIFICATION (Primary): HS200

Note: For information pertaining to use of alprostadil for diagnosis and treatment of impotence, see *Alprostadil (Intracavernosal)*.

Commonly used brand name(s): *Prostin VR*; *Prostin VR Pediatric*.

Other commonly used names are $PGE_1$ and prostaglandin $E_1$.

Note: For a listing of dosage forms and brand names by country availability, see *Dosage Forms* section(s).

## Category
Ductus arteriosus patency adjunct.

## Indications

Note: Bracketed information in the *Indications* section refers to uses that are not included in U.S. product labeling.

**Accepted**

Ductus arteriosus, patent (maintenance)—Alprostadil is indicated for palliative, not definitive, therapy in neonates born with various congenital heart defects, including pulmonary atresia, pulmonary stenosis, tricuspid atresia, tetralogy of Fallot, interruption of the aortic arch, coarctation of the aorta, transposition of the great vessels with or without other defects, [hypoplastic left heart syndrome][1], and [critical aortic valve stenosis][1]. The medication is used to maintain the patency of the ductus arteriosus (DA), thereby improving circulation and oxygenation until corrective or palliative surgery can be performed. Although alprostadil treatment is intended primarily as a short-term measure, long-term (up to several months) therapy may be needed, for example, when surgery must be delayed until a very small infant has grown sufficiently to undergo the procedure.

In infants with cyanotic congenital heart disease (for example, pulmonary atresia or stenosis, tricuspid atresia, tetralogy of Fallot, or transposition of the great vessels) in which there is a severe or complete obstruction to right ventricular outflow, patency of the DA is necessary to provide adequate pulmonary blood flow (and, therefore, an adequate oxygen supply) and to prevent or reverse acidemia. In infants with restricted pulmonary blood flow, the best results have generally been attained in patients with low pretreatment blood $PO_2$ who were 4 days old or less; little response was attained in patients with initial $PO_2$ values of 40 torr or more. In infants with acyanotic congenital heart disease (for example, with aortic arch anomalies such as aortic arch interruption or severe coarctation of the aorta) in which there is obstructed systemic outflow, partial or complete patency of the DA is necessary to provide adequate systemic blood flow and to prevent or reverse acidemia.

[1]Not included in Canadian product labeling.

## Pharmacology/Pharmacokinetics

### Physicochemical characteristics
Chemical group—Prostaglandins.
Molecular weight—354.49.
pKa—6.3.

### Mechanism of action/Effect
Alprostadil is one of a family of naturally occurring prostaglandins. It causes vasodilation by means of a direct effect on vascular and ductus arteriosus (DA) smooth muscle.

Ductus arteriosus (DA) patency maintenance—
By its effect on DA smooth muscle, alprostadil prevents or reverses the functional closure of the DA that occurs shortly after birth, which results in increased pulmonary or systemic blood flow in infants with impairment of this blood flow. A reduction in pulmonary vascular resistance has also been postulated, which may improve pulmonary perfusion in neonates in whom congenital heart disease is associated with increased pulmonary vascular resistance.

In cyanotic congenital heart disease, alprostadil's actions result in an increased oxygen supply to the tissues.

In infants with interrupted aortic arch or very severe aortic coarctation, alprostadil maintains distal aortic perfusion by permitting blood flow through the DA from the pulmonary artery to the aorta.In infants with aortic coarctation, alprostadil reduces aortic obstruction either by relaxing ductus tissue in the aortic wall or by increasing effective aortic diameter by dilating the DA. In infants with these aortic arch anomalies, systemic blood flow to the lower body is increased, improving tissue oxygen supply and renal perfusion.

### Other actions/effects
Alprostadil has been reported to inhibit macrophage activation, neutrophil chemotaxis, and release of oxygen radicals and lysosomal enzymes. Inhibition of neutrophil chemotaxis has the potential to impair defense mechanisms and increase the risk of bacterial infection.

Alprostadil inhibits coagulation by inhibiting platelet aggregation and possibly by inhibiting activation of factor X (by increasing the concentration of cyclic adenosine monophosphate [cAMP]). Alprostadil may also promote fibrinolysis by stimulating production of tissue plasminogen activator, which converts plasminogen to the fibrinolytic enzyme plasmin. Stimulation of cellular adenylate cyclase may initiate this effect.

Other effects of prostaglandins include stimulation of intestinal and uterine smooth muscle.

### Protein binding
High to very high (81 to 99%), depending on the method of measurement, to albumin.

### Biotransformation
Pulmonary. In patients with normal respiratory function, up to 80% of a dose may be metabolized in one pass through the lungs.

### Half-life
5 to 10 minutes (after a single dose), in healthy adults. Although the half-life in premature neonates has not been determined, a short half-life would be expected in these patients also.

### Time to peak effect
Acyanotic congenital heart disease—
Coarctation of the aorta: Usually about 3 hours (range, 15 minutes to 11 hours).

Interruption of aortic arch: Usually about 1.5 hours (range, 15 minutes to 4 hours).
Cyanotic congenital heart disease—
Approximately 30 minutes.

### Duration of action
Ductus arteriosus (DA) patency maintenance—As long as the infusion is continued; closure of the DA usually begins within 1 to 2 hours after the infusion is discontinued.

### Elimination
Renal (as metabolites); elimination is virtually complete within 24 hours after administration.

## Precautions to Consider

### Carcinogenicity
Studies have not been done.

### Mutagenicity
According to results of Ames and Alkaline Elution assays, alprostadil has no potential for mutagenicity.

### Drug interactions and/or related problems
The following drug interactions and/or related problems have been selected on the basis of their potential clinical significance (possible mechanism in parentheses where appropriate)—not necessarily inclusive (» = major clinical significance):

Note: In addition to the interactions listed below, the possibility should be considered that multiple effects leading to further impairment of blood clotting and/or increased risk of bleeding may occur if alprostadil is administered to a patient receiving any medication having a significant potential for causing hypoprothrombinemia, thrombocytopenia, or gastrointestinal ulceration or hemorrhage.

Anticoagulants, coumarin-derivative, or
Cefamandole or
Cefoperazone or
Cefotetan or
Heparin or
Moxalactam or
Platelet aggregation inhibitors, other (See *Appendix II*), or
Thrombolytic agents
(these medications may cause one or more interferences with blood clotting; concurrent use with alprostadil may increase the risk of bleeding)

Sympathomimetics, alpha-adrenergic, especially metaraminol, epinephrine, and phenylephrine
(these medications reverse the vasodilating effect of alprostadil)

Vasodilators, other
(concurrent use with alprostadil may increase the risk of vasodilation-associated side effects such as hypotension)

### Laboratory value alterations
The following have been selected on the basis of their potential clinical significance (possible effect in parentheses where appropriate)—not necessarily inclusive (» = major clinical significance):

With physiology/laboratory test values
Bilirubin concentrations
(may be increased—incidence less than 1%)
Calcium concentrations, serum
(may be decreased—incidence about 15%)
Glucose concentrations, blood
(may be decreased—incidence less than 1%)
Potassium concentrations, serum
(may be decreased or increased—incidence 1% or less)

### Medical considerations/Contraindications
The medical considerations/contraindications included have been selected on the basis of their potential clinical significance (reasons given in parentheses where appropriate)—not necessarily inclusive (» = major clinical significance).

*Except under special circumstances, this medication should not be used when the following medical problem exists:*

» Respiratory distress syndrome, neonatal
(closure of the ductus arteriosus [DA] is necessary to prevent overload of pulmonary circulation; a differential diagnosis between cyanotic heart disease [restricted pulmonary blood flow] and neonatal respiratory distress syndrome [hyaline membrane disease] is essential prior to administration)

## Alprostadil (Systemic)

*Risk-benefit should be considered when the following medical problems exist:*

Bleeding disorders
(increased risk of bleeding because alprostadil inhibits platelet aggregation and may promote fibrinolysis)

Conditions in which increased pulmonary blood flow may result in pulmonary edema

Sensitivity to alprostadil, history of

### Patient monitoring

The following may be especially important in patient monitoring (other tests may be warranted in some patients, depending on condition; » = major clinical significance):

*For all infants with congenital heart defects*

Blood gases (PO$_2$, PCO$_2$), arterial, measurement of
(recommended at intermittent intervals throughout the infusion)

Blood pH, arterial, measurement of
(recommended at frequent intervals during infusion)

Blood pressure, arterial, measurement of by umbilical artery catheter, auscultation, or Doppler transducer, and

Electrocardiogram (ECG) and

Heart rate, measurement of, and

Respiratory rate, measurement of, and

Temperature, rectal, measurement of, and

Respiratory status
(monitoring is recommended throughout therapy for maintaining neonatal ductus arteriosus patency; continuous monitoring is recommended initially, and may be continued throughout short-term therapy, but intermittent monitoring is usually sufficient when treatment is to be continued for an extended period after the patient's condition has stabilized)

Note: In infants with restricted pulmonary blood flow, efficacy of alprostadil may be determined by monitoring improvement in blood oxygenation. In infants with restricted systemic blood flow, improvement of systemic blood pressure and blood pH confirms efficacy.

*For infants with aortic arch anomalies (in addition to those listed above)*

Blood pressure, measured in descending aorta or lower extremity, and

Femoral pulse, palpation for, and

Renal output, measurement of
(recommended at periodic intervals during infusion to confirm efficacy)

## Side/Adverse Effects

Note: Cardiovascular side effects (especially cutaneous vasodilation) have been reported more frequently in infants with cyanotic lesions than in those with aortic lesions (possibly because the intra-aortic route [no longer recommended] was used more often in these patients).

Cardiovascular side effects are more frequent in infants weighing less than 2 kg or with infusions of greater than 48 hours' duration. Respiratory depression occurs more commonly in patients weighing less than 2 kg at birth and in cyanotic infants. Central nervous system (CNS) side effects are more frequent in neonates with preinfusion pH of 7.1 or less and with infusions of greater than 48 hours' duration.

Damage to the ductus, pulmonary artery, and aorta (weakening of the wall, leading to edema, laceration, and possible aneurysm) has been reported with long-term use.

The following side/adverse effects have been selected on the basis of their potential clinical significance (possible signs and symptoms in parentheses where appropriate)—not necessarily inclusive:

### Those indicating need for medical attention

Incidence more frequent

*Apnea*—incidence 10 to 12%; generally occurs within the first hour of infusion; the incidence is greatest in neonates weighing less than 2 kg at birth and is also increased if a rapid or large infusion is given initially (e.g., to purge the intravenous line); *fever*—incidence 14%, primarily a CNS effect, infection occurs in about 2% of patients; *flushing of face or arm*—incidence about 10%, especially with intra-arterial or intra-aortic administration, which is no longer recommended, may indicate misplacement of the catheter and introduction of alprostadil into the subclavian or carotid artery; *hypocalcemia*

Incidence less frequent

*Bradycardia*—incidence 7%; *diarrhea*—incidence 2%; *hypotension*—incidence 4%; *seizures*—incidence 4%; *tachycardia*—incidence 3%

Incidence rare—1% or less

*Anemia; anuria; bleeding; bradypnea, tachypnea, or bronchial wheezing; cardiac arrest; cerebral bleeding; congestive heart failure; cortical hyperostosis*—with long-term therapy, regresses after discontinuation of therapy; *disseminated intravascular coagulation; edema; gastric regurgitation; second degree heart block; hematuria; hypercapnia; hyperemia; hyperextension of the neck; ketotic hyperglycemia*—when given to an infant born to an insulin-dependent diabetic patient; *hyperirritability; hyperkalemia or hypokalemia; hypoglycemia; hypothermia; jitteriness; lethargy; peritonitis; respiratory distress, including respiratory depression; shock; spasm of right ventricle infundibulum; stiffness; supraventricular tachycardia; thrombocytopenia; ventricular fibrillation*

## Overdose

For more information on the management of overdose or unintentional ingestion, **contact a Poison Control Center** (see *Poison Control Center Listing*).

### Clinical effects of overdose

The following effects have been selected on the basis of their potential clinical significance (possible signs and symptoms in parentheses where appropriate)—not necessarily inclusive:

*Apnea; bradycardia; fever; flushing of skin; hypotension*

## General Dosing Information

Because of the risk of apnea, it is recommended that alprostadil be administered in an area with trained personnel and facilities necessary to provide pediatric intensive care. Respiratory support should be immediately available.

In patients with cyanotic heart defects, alprostadil is effective only if it is administered before permanent closure of the ductus arteriosus (DA) occurs. In normal-term infants, functional closure of the DA is usually complete within 10 to 15 hours after birth, and the DA is usually completely sealed off within 2 to 3 weeks. In clinical studies, the greatest response to alprostadil in patients with cyanotic heart defects was achieved in infants 4 days old or less. In infants with acyanotic heart defects, DA closure may be delayed, or the age of the patient and/or the extent of DA closure may be less critical. Beneficial responses to alprostadil may be achieved in infants up to 2 weeks of age, and occasionally in even older patients.

Because of its rapid metabolism, alprostadil must be diluted and administered by infusion. Use of a constant-rate infusion pump is recommended to avoid inadvertent rapid administration, because of the risk of apnea.

Alprostadil may be administered by intravenous infusion (peripheral or central) or intra-arterial infusion (through the pulmonary artery or an umbilical arterial catheter positioned at the level of the DA). The medication has also been administered via intra-aortic infusion, into the descending aorta adjacent to the DA. Theoretically, intra-aortic or intra-arterial administration should provide the greatest concentration to the DA and allow for rapid deactivation in the lungs, thereby reducing the risk of side effects. However, intra-arterial or intra-aortic administration has not proved more efficacious than intravenous administration, nor has it decreased the occurrence of side effects. Intravenous administration is now preferred for maintaining DA patency.

If fever or hypotension occurs, the rate of alprostadil infusion should be reduced

If a significant reduction of arterial blood pressure occurs, alprostadil should be discontinued immediately and appropriate treatment measures (e.g., volume replacement, administration of vasopressors) instituted. After the patient's blood pressure has stabilized, therapy may be reinstituted cautiously.

If apnea occurs, alprostadil should be discontinued or respiratory support instituted if continued use of alprostadil may be life saving.

If bradycardia occurs, alprostadil should be discontinued and appropriate medical treatment provided.

Flushing (peripheral arterial vasodilation) is usually the result of incorrect intra-arterial catheter placement and usually responds to repositioning of the catheter.

Alprostadil infusion may be continued during cardiac catheterization and may even facilitate the procedure.

Alprostadil infusion is usually continued until surgical repair is completed, usually within 24 to 48 hours after initiation of therapy, although it is sometimes continued postoperatively. Alprostadil should be administered for the shortest time and in the lowest dose that will produce the desired effect. However, long-term treatment may be required for some patients, especially very small infants who cannot undergo surgery until sufficient growth has taken place. The risks of long-term use (e.g., vascular damage, cortical proliferation of the long bones) must be weighed against the possible benefits. However, infants with severe cyanotic congenital heart disease have been treated for up to 3 months without adverse effects occurring.

## Parenteral Dosage Forms

### ALPROSTADIL INJECTION USP

**Usual pediatric dose**
Ductus arteriosus patency adjunct—
  Initial: Intravenous, into a large vein (preferred) or intra-arterial (via umbilical arterial catheter placed at the ductal opening),0.05 to 0.1 mcg per kg of body weight per minute. However, if the ductus arteriosus is nonrestrictive at the time of diagnosis, an initial dose as low as 0.01 mcg per kg of body weight per minute may be effective. The rate of infusion may gradually be increased to up to 0.4 mcg per kg of body weight per minute, if necessary, although doses higher than 0.1 mcg per kg of body weight per minute have not been shown to produce greater effects. After a satisfactory response is obtained, the rate of infusion may be reduced to the minimum level that will maintain the response. Dosage reduction is usually accomplished by progressively halving the previous dose, e.g., from 0.1 to 0.05 to 0.025 to 0.01 mcg per kg of body weight per minute.
  Maintenance: Intravenous, into a large vein (preferred) or intra-arterial (via umbilical arterial catheter placed at the ductal opening),infused at the minimum rate that will maintain the desired response. Doses as low as 0.002 mcg per kg of body weight per minute have been effective in some infants. However, maintenance dosage requirements may vary, and the infusion rate should be adjusted (increased or decreased) as necessary.

**Strength(s) usually available**
U.S.—
  500 mcg (0.5 mg) per mL (Rx) [*Prostin VR Pediatric* (in dehydrated alcohol)].
Canada—
  500 mcg (0.5 mg) per mL (Rx) [*Prostin VR* (in dehydrated alcohol)].

**Packaging and storage**
Store between 2 and 8 °C (36 and 46 °F), unless otherwise specified by manufacturer. Protect from freezing.

**Preparation of dosage form**
Alprostadil infusions are prepared by diluting 1 mL of the injection with a volume of 0.9% sodium chloride injection or 5% dextrose injection suitable for the pump delivery system available. For example, to provide 0.1 mcg per kg of body weight per minute, the following dilutions and infusion rates could be used:

| Amount of Diluent (mL) for each mL (500 mcg) of Alprostadil | Approximate Concentration of Resulting Solution (mcg/mL) | Infusion Rate (mL/min per kg of body weight) |
|---|---|---|
| 250 | 2 | 0.05 |
| 100 | 5 | 0.02 |
| 50 | 10 | 0.01 |
| 25 | 20 | 0.005 |

Caution: Use of diluents containing benzyl alcohol is not recommended for preparation of medications for use in neonates. A fatal toxic syndrome consisting of metabolic acidosis, CNS depression, respiratory problems, renal failure, hypotension, and possibly seizures and intracranial hemorrhages has been associated with this use.

**Stability**
Alprostadil infusions should be discarded 24 hours after they are prepared.

## Selected Bibliography

Roehl Sl, Townsend RJ. Alprostadil (Prostin VR Pediatric sterile solution, the Upjohn Company). Drug Intel Clin Pharm 1982 Nov; 16: 821-32.
Heymann MA, Clyman RI. Evaluation of alprostadil (prostaglandin E1) in the management of congenital heart disease in infancy. Pharmacotherapy 1982; 2: 148-55.
Bhatt V, Nahata MC. Pharmacologic management of patent ductus arteriosus. Clin Pharm 1989; 8: 17-33.

Revised: 04/09/92

---

**ALTEPLASE RECOMBINANT**—See *Thrombolytic Agents (Systemic)*

---

# ALTRETAMINE   Systemic

VA CLASSIFICATION (Primary): AN900

Commonly used brand name(s): *Hexalen*.

Another commonly used name is hexamethylmelamine.

Note: For a listing of dosage forms and brand names by country availability, see *Dosage Forms* section(s).

## Category
Antineoplastic.

## Indications

**Accepted**
Carcinoma, ovarian, epithelial (treatment)—Altretamine is indicated for use as a single agent in the palliative treatment of patients with persistent or recurrent epithelial ovarian cancer following first-line therapy with a cisplatin- and/or alkylating agent–based combination.

## Pharmacology/Pharmacokinetics

Note: Pharmacokinetic studies have been done in only a limited number of patients; figures below are based on a study in 11 patients.

**Physicochemical characteristics**
Source—Synthetic.
Chemical group—S-triazine derivative.

**Mechanism of action/Effect**
The exact mechanism of action is unknown. Although altretamine structurally resembles an alkylating agent, it has not been found to have alkylating activity *in vitro*. There is some evidence that it may inhibit DNA and RNA synthesis.

**Absorption**
Rapidly and well-absorbed following oral administration; however, because of rapid hepatic metabolism, peak plasma concentrations are variable.

**Distribution**
Because it is highly lipid-soluble, altretamine is distributed to tissues with a high lipid component (e.g., omentum and subcutaneous tissues).

**Protein binding**
Free fractions—
  Altretamine: 6%.
  Pentamethylmelamine: 25%.
  Tetramethylmelamine: 50%.

**Biotransformation**
Hepatic. Metabolism is required for activity. Altretamine undergoes rapid and extensive demethylation, catalyzed by cytochrome P450 enzymes.

**Half-life**
Elimination—Beta-phase: Range, 4.7 to 10.2 hours.

**Time to peak concentration**
Plasma—0.5 to 3 hours.

**Elimination**
Renal, less than 1% unchanged.

## Precautions to Consider

**Carcinogenicity**
Secondary malignancies are potential delayed effects of many antineoplastic agents, although it is not clear whether the effect is related to their mutagenic or immunosuppressive action. The effect of dose and duration of therapy is also unknown, although risk seems to increase with long-term use. Although information is limited, available data seem to indicate that the carcinogenic risk is greatest with the alkylating agents.
One case of acute myelocytic leukemia has been reported in a patient treated with altretamine.
Studies with altretamine in animals have not been done.

## Mutagenicity
Altretamine was weakly mutagenic in strain TA100 of *Salmonella typhimurium*.

## Pregnancy/Reproduction
*Fertility*—Gonadal suppression, resulting in amenorrhea or azoospermia, may occur in patients taking antineoplastic therapy, especially with the alkylating agents. In general, these effects appear to be related to dose and length of therapy and may be irreversible. Prediction of the degree of testicular or ovarian function impairment is complicated by the common use of combinations of several antineoplastics, which makes it difficult to assess the effects of individual agents.

No adverse effect on fertility was found in female rats when altretamine was administered from 14 days prior to breeding through the gestation period. Administration to male rats in doses of 120 mg per square meter of body surface per day for 60 days prior to mating resulted in testicular atrophy, reduced fertility, and a possible dominant lethal mutagenic effect; doses of 450 mg per square meter of body surface per day for 10 days caused decreased spermatogenesis, atrophy of testes, seminal vesicles, and ventral prostate.

*Pregnancy*—Studies have not been done in humans.

First trimester: It is usually recommended that use of antineoplastics, especially combination chemotherapy, be avoided whenever possible, especially during the first trimester. Although information is limited because of the relatively few instances of antineoplastic administration during pregnancy, the mutagenic, teratogenic, and carcinogenic potential of these medications must be considered.

Other hazards to the fetus include adverse reactions seen in adults.

In general, use of a contraceptive is recommended during cytotoxic drug therapy.

Altretamine is embryotoxic and teratogenic in rats and rabbits given 2 to 10 times the human dose.

FDA Pregnancy Category D.

## Breast-feeding
Although very little information is available regarding distribution of antineoplastic agents into breast milk, breast-feeding is not recommended during chemotherapy because of the potential risks to the infant (adverse effects, mutagenicity, carcinogenicity). It is not known whether altretamine or its metabolites are distributed into breast milk.

## Pediatrics
No information is available on the relationship of age to the effects of altretamine in pediatric patients. Safety and efficacy have not been established.

## Geriatrics
Although appropriate studies on the relationship of age to the effects of altretamine have not been performed in the geriatric population, clinical trials have included elderly patients and geriatrics-specific problems that would limit the usefulness of this medication in the elderly are not expected. However, elderly patients are more likely to have age-related renal function impairment, which may require caution in patients receiving altretamine.

## Dental
The bone marrow depressant effects of altretamine may result in an increased incidence of microbial infection, delayed healing, and gingival bleeding. Dental work, whenever possible, should be completed prior to initiation of therapy or deferred until blood counts have returned to normal. Patients should be instructed in proper oral hygiene during treatment, including caution in use of regular toothbrushes, dental floss, and toothpicks.

## Drug interactions and/or related problems
The following drug interactions and/or related problems have been selected on the basis of their potential clinical significance (possible mechanism in parentheses where appropriate)—not necessarily inclusive (» = major clinical significance):

Note: Combinations containing any of the following medications, depending on the amount present, may also interact with this medication.

Blood dyscrasia–causing medications (see *Appendix II*)
(leukopenic and/or thrombocytopenic effects of altretamine may be increased with concurrent or recent therapy if these medications cause the same effects; dosage adjustment of altretamine, if necessary, should be based on blood counts)

» Bone marrow depressants, other (see *Appendix II*) or
Radiation therapy
(additive bone marrow depression may occur; dosage reduction may be required when two or more bone marrow depressants, including radiation, are used concurrently or consecutively)

Cimetidine
(inhibition of the cytochrome-P450 enzyme system by cimetidine would be expected to cause a decrease in the hepatic metabolism of altretamine, which could result in delayed elimination and increased blood concentrations)

» Monoamine oxidase (MAO) inhibitors, including furazolidone, procarbazine, and selegiline
(concurrent use may result in severe orthostatic hypotension)

Vaccines, killed virus
(because normal defense mechanisms may be suppressed by altretamine therapy, the patient's antibody response to the vaccine may be decreased. The interval between discontinuation of medications that cause immunosuppression and restoration of the patient's ability to respond to the vaccine depends on the intensity and type of immunosuppression-causing medication used, the underlying disease, and other factors; estimates vary from 3 months to 1 year)

» Vaccines, live virus
(because normal defense mechanisms may be suppressed by altretamine therapy, concurrent use with a live virus vaccine may potentiate the replication of the vaccine virus, may increase the side/adverse effects of the vaccine virus, and/or may decrease the patient's antibody response to the vaccine; immunization of these patients should be undertaken only with extreme caution after careful review of the patient's hematologic status and only with the knowledge and consent of the physician managing the altretamine therapy. The interval between discontinuation of medications that cause immunosuppression and restoration of the patient's ability to respond to the vaccine depends on the intensity and type of immunosuppression-causing medication used, the underlying disease, and other factors; estimates vary from 3 months to 1 year. In addition, immunization with oral poliovirus vaccine should be postponed in persons in close contact with the patient, especially family members)

## Laboratory value alterations
The following have been selected on the basis of their potential clinical significance (possible effect in parentheses where appropriate)—not necessarily inclusive (» = major clinical significance):

With physiology/laboratory test values
Alkaline phosphatase
(increases in serum values have been reported)

Blood urea nitrogen (BUN) and
Creatinine concentrations, serum
(moderate increases have been reported)

## Medical considerations/Contraindications
The medical considerations/contraindications included have been selected on the basis of their potential clinical significance (reasons given in parentheses where appropriate)—not necessarily inclusive (» = major clinical significance).

***Risk-benefit should be considered when the following medical problems exist:***

» Bone marrow depression
(lower dosage may be necessary)

» Chickenpox, existing or recent (including recent exposure) or
» Herpes zoster
(risk of severe generalized disease)

» Infection

Hepatic function impairment, severe
(reduced activation or metabolism)

» Neurologic toxicity, severe

Renal function impairment
(reduced elimination)

» Sensitivity to altretamine

» Tumor cell infiltration of the bone marrow

» Caution should be used also in patients who have had previous cytotoxic drug therapy or radiation therapy.

## Patient monitoring
The following may be especially important in patient monitoring (other tests may be warranted in some patients, depending on condition; » = major clinical significance):

» Hematocrit or hemoglobin and
» Platelet count and
» Leukocyte count, total and, if appropriate, differential
(determinations recommended prior to initiation of therapy and at periodic intervals during therapy; frequency varies according to clinical state, agent, dose, and other agents being used concurrently)

» Neurologic examinations
(recommended at regular intervals during therapy)

## Side/Adverse Effects

Note: Many "side effects" of antineoplastic therapy are unavoidable and represent the medication's pharmacologic action. Some of these (for example, leukopenia and thrombocytopenia) are actually used as parameters to aid in individual dosage titration.

Toxicity is dose-related and cumulative.

Altretamine causes mild to moderate myelosuppression and neurotoxicity.

The following side/adverse effects have been selected on the basis of their potential clinical significance (possible signs and symptoms in parentheses where appropriate)—not necessarily inclusive:

### Those indicating need for medical attention
Incidence more frequent
*Anemia* (unusual tiredness)—usually asymptomatic; *leukopenia* (fever or chills; cough or hoarseness; lower back or side pain; painful or difficult urination)—usually asymptomatic; *neurotoxicity, including central nervous system (CNS) effects* (anxiety; clumsiness; confusion; dizziness; mental depression; weakness; seizures); *neurotoxicity, including peripheral neuropathy* (numbness in arms or legs); *thrombocytopenia* (unusual bleeding or bruising; black, tarry stools; blood in urine or stools; pinpoint red spots on skin)—usually asymptomatic

Note: In *leukopenia*, with intermittent dosing (e.g., 8 to 12 mg per kg of body weight [mg/kg] per day for 21 days), the nadir of leukocyte counts occurs at about 3 to 4 weeks, with recovery by 6 weeks; with continuous dosing, the nadir occurs at 6 to 8 weeks (median).

Incidence of *neurotoxicity* is greater with daily high-dose therapy than with intermittent moderate-dose therapy. Neurotoxicity is reversible on withdrawal of altretamine.

In *thrombocytopenia*, with intermittent dosing (e.g., 8 to 12 mg/kg per day for 21 days), the nadir of platelet counts occurs at about 3 to 4 weeks, with recovery by 6 weeks; with continuous dosing, the nadir occurs at 6 to 8 weeks (median).

Incidence rare
*Hepatotoxicity*—asymptomatic; *skin rash or itching*

### Those indicating need for medical attention only if they continue or are bothersome
Incidence more frequent
*Nausea and vomiting*

Note: *Nausea and vomiting* are usually mild to moderate, although they may be dose-limiting. The mechanism of the effect may be central because they usually do not occur until several days after initiation of treatment.

Incidence less frequent
*Diarrhea; loss of appetite; stomach cramps*

## Patient Consultation

As an aid to patient consultation, refer to *Advice for the Patient, Altretamine (Systemic)*.

In providing consultation, consider emphasizing the following selected information (» = major clinical significance):

### Before using this medication
» Conditions affecting use, especially:
Sensitivity to altretamine
Pregnancy—Use not recommended because of mutagenic, teratogenic, and carcinogenic potential; advisability of using contraception; telling physician immediately if pregnancy is suspected
Breast-feeding—Not recommended because of risk of serious side effects
Other medications, especially other bone marrow depressants, monoamine oxidase (MAO) inhibitors, or other cytotoxic drug or radiation therapy
Other medical problems, especially chickenpox, herpes zoster, other infections, or severe neurotoxicity

### Proper use of this medication
Frequency of nausea and vomiting; importance of continuing medication despite stomach upset; taking after meals to reduce stomach upset
» Proper dosing
Missed dose: Taking as soon as possible; however, if almost time for next dose, not taking missed dose; not doubling doses
» Proper storage

### Precautions while using this medication
» Importance of close monitoring by the physician

» Avoiding immunizations unless approved by physician; other persons in patient's household should avoid immunizations with oral poliovirus vaccine; avoiding other persons who have taken oral poliovirus vaccine or wearing a protective mask that covers nose and mouth

*Caution if bone marrow depression occurs*
» Avoiding exposure to persons with infections, especially during periods of low blood counts; checking with physician immediately if fever or chills, cough or hoarseness, lower back or side pain, or painful or difficult urination occur
» Checking with physician immediately if unusual bleeding or bruising; black, tarry stools; blood in urine or stools; or pinpoint red spots on skin occur
Caution in use of regular toothbrush, dental floss, or toothpick; physician, dentist, or nurse may suggest alternatives; checking with physician before having dental work done
Not touching eyes or inside of nose unless hands washed immediately before
Using caution to avoid accidental cuts with use of sharp objects such as safety razor or fingernail or toenail cutters
Avoiding contact sports or other situations where bruising or injury could occur

### Side/adverse effects
Signs of potential side effects, especially anemia, leukopenia, neurotoxicity, and thrombocytopenia
Physician or nurse can help in dealing with side effects

## General Dosing Information

Patients receiving altretamine should be under supervision of a physician experienced in cancer chemotherapy.

Dosage must be adjusted to meet the individual requirements of each patient, on the basis of clinical response and degree of bone marrow depression and neurotoxicity.

A variety of dosage schedules and regimens of altretamine, alone or in combination with other antitumor agents, are used. The prescriber may consult the medical literature as well as the manufacturer's literature in choosing a specific dosage.

Altretamine therapy should be temporarily withheld if any of the following occur:
Gastrointestinal intolerance unresponsive to symptomatic measures
Leukocyte count less than 2000 per cubic millimeter or granulocyte count less than 1000 per cubic millimeter
Platelet count less than 75,000 per cubic millimeter
Progressive neurotoxicity

After a period of at least 14 days, therapy may be reinitiated at a reduced dose of 200 mg per square meter of body surface per day.

If neurotoxicity continues even after dosage reduction, it is recommended that altretamine be discontinued.

Special precautions are recommended in patients who develop thrombocytopenia as a result of administration of altretamine. These may include extreme care in performing invasive procedures; regular inspection of intravenous sites, skin (including perirectal area), and mucous membrane surfaces for signs of bleeding or bruising; limiting frequency of venipuncture and avoiding intramuscular injections; testing urine, emesis, stool, and secretions for occult blood; care in use of regular toothbrushes, dental floss, toothpicks, safety razors, and fingernail and toenail cutters; avoiding constipation; and using caution to prevent falls and other injuries. Such patients should avoid alcohol and aspirin intake because of the risk of gastrointestinal bleeding. Platelet transfusions may be required.

Patients who develop leukopenia should be observed carefully for signs of infection. Antibiotic support may be required. In neutropenic patients who develop fever, broad-spectrum antibiotic coverage should be initiated empirically, pending bacterial cultures and appropriate diagnostic tests.

### Diet/Nutrition
It is recommended that altretamine be taken after meals to reduce nausea and vomiting.

## Oral Dosage Forms

### ALTRETAMINE CAPSULES
**Usual adult dose**
Carcinoma, ovarian, epithelial—
Oral, 260 mg per square meter of body surface per day, in four divided daily doses after meals and at bedtime, for either fourteen or twenty-one consecutive days in a twenty-eight–day cycle.

### Altretamine (Systemic)

Note: If excessive nausea and vomiting, leukopenia, thrombocytopenia, or neurotoxicity occur, it is recommended that altretamine be withheld for at least 14 days and then reinstituted at a dose of 200 mg per square meter of body surface per day.

**Usual pediatric dose**
Safety and efficacy have not been established.

**Strength(s) usually available**
U.S.—
  50 mg (Rx) [*Hexalen* (lactose)].
Canada—
  50 mg (Rx) [*Hexalen*].

**Packaging and storage**
Store below 40 °C (104 °F), preferably between 15 and 30 °C (59 and 86 °F), unless otherwise specified by manufacturer.

**Auxiliary labeling**
• Take after meals.

### Selected Bibliography
Hansen LA, Hughes TE. Altretamine. DICP Ann Pharmacother 1991; 24: 146-52.
Hellmann K, editor. Hexamethylmelamine. Cancer Treat Rev 1991 Mar; 18 (Suppl A): entire issue.

Revised: 07/23/92
Interim revision: 04/29/94; 09/26/97

---

## ALUMINUM CARBONATE, BASIC — See *Antacids (Oral-Local)*

## ALUMINUM HYDROXIDE — See *Antacids (Oral-Local)*

---

# AMANTADINE  Systemic

VA CLASSIFICATION (Primary/Secondary): AM809/AU350; CN900
Commonly used brand name(s): *Symadine*; *Symmetrel*.
Note: For a listing of dosage forms and brand names by country availability, see *Dosage Forms* section(s).

## Category
Antiviral (systemic); antidyskinetic; antifatigue, specifically in multiple sclerosis.

## Indications
Note: Bracketed information in the *Indications* section refers to uses that are not included in U.S. product labeling.

**Accepted**
Influenza A (prophylaxis and treatment)—Amantadine is indicated as a primary agent in the prophylaxis and treatment of respiratory tract infections caused by influenza A virus strains in high-risk patients (including those with pulmonary or cardiovascular disease, the elderly, and residents of nursing homes and other chronic care facilities who have chronic medical conditions), hospital ward contacts of high-risk patients, immunocompromised patients, those in critical public service positions (e.g., police, firefighters, medical personnel), in high-risk patients for whom the influenza vaccine is contraindicated, and patients with severe influenza A viral infections. It is effective against all strains of influenza A virus that have been tested to date, including Russian, Brazilian, Texan, London, and others. It may be given as chemoprophylaxis concurrently with inactivated influenza A virus vaccine until protective antibodies develop. However, it should be emphasized that vaccination of high-risk persons each year is the single most important measure for reducing the impact of influenza. No well-controlled studies have examined whether amantadine prevents complications of influenza A in high-risk persons.

Resistant strains of influenza A have been reported in patients receiving rimantadine; these resistant strains were also apparently transmitted to household contacts. Rimantadine has a similar chemical structure, spectrum of activity, and mechanism of action to amantadine, and drug-resistant strains of virus have cross-resistance to amantadine and rimantadine.

Extrapyramidal reactions, drug-induced (treatment) or
Parkinsonism (treatment)—Amantadine is indicated in the treatment of idiopathic parkinsonism (paralysis agitans; shaking palsy), postencephalitic parkinsonism, drug-induced extrapyramidal reactions, symptomatic parkinsonism following injury to the nervous system caused by carbon monoxide intoxication, and parkinsonism associated with cerebral arteriosclerosis in the elderly.

[Fatigue, multiple sclerosis–associated (treatment)][1]—Amantadine is used in the management of certain aspects of fatigue associated with multiple sclerosis, including lowered energy level, decreased sense of well-being, decreased perceived attention and memory, and diminished problem solving ability.

**Unaccepted**
Amantadine is not effective against other respiratory viral infections, including influenza B and parainfluenza.

[1]Not included in Canadian product labeling.

## Pharmacology/Pharmacokinetics

**Physicochemical characteristics**
Molecular weight—187.71.

**Mechanism of action/Effect**
Antiviral (systemic)—Not completely understood; amantadine appears to block the uncoating of influenza A virus and the release of viral nucleic acid into respiratory epithelial cells. May also affect early replicative phase of viruses that have already penetrated cells.
Antidyskinetic—Unknown; amantadine causes an increase in dopamine release in the animal brain. Probably increases release of dopamine and norepinephrine from central nerve terminals; also inhibits the reuptake of dopamine and norepinephrine.

**Absorption**
Rapidly and almost completely absorbed from gastrointestinal tract.

**Distribution**
Distributed to saliva, tear film, and nasal secretions; in animals, tissue (especially lung) concentrations higher than serum concentrations. Crosses the placenta and blood-brain barrier; excreted in breast milk. Cerebral spinal fluid concentrations were 52% of corresponding plasma concentrations in one patient.
Vol $_D$=—
  4.4 ± 0.2 liters per kg (normal renal function).
  5.1 ± 0.2 liters per kg (renal failure).

**Protein binding**
Normal renal function—Approximately 67%.
Hemodialysis patients—Approximately 59%.

**Biotransformation**
No appreciable metabolism. Small amounts of an acetyl metabolite identified.

**Half-life**
Normal renal function—11 to 15 hours.
Elderly patients—24 to 29 hours.
Renal function impairment, severe—7 to 10 days.
Hemodialysis—24 hours.

**Onset of action**
Antidyskinetic—Usually within 48 hours.

**Time to peak serum concentration**
2 to 4 hours (range, 1 to 8 hours); steady-state concentrations achieved within 2 to 3 days of daily administration.

**Peak serum concentration**
Approximately 0.3 mcg per mL; steady-state trough concentrations after 50, 200, and 300 mg per day are approximately 0.1, 0.3, and 0.6 mcg per mL, respectively. Plasma concentrations exceeding 1.0 mcg per mL are considered to be in the toxic range.

### Elimination
Renal; >90% excreted unchanged in urine by glomerular filtration and renal tubular secretion. Rate of excretion rapidly increased in acid urine.

In dialysis—Only small amounts (approximately 4%) removed from the blood by hemodialysis.

## Precautions to Consider

### Carcinogenicity
Long-term studies have not been done in animals.

### Mutagenicity
Studies have not been done.

### Pregnancy/Reproduction
Pregnancy—Amantadine crosses the placenta. However, adequate and well-controlled studies in humans have not been done.

Studies in animals have shown that amantadine is embryotoxic and teratogenic in rats at doses of 50 mg per kg of body weight (mg/kg) per day. No adverse effects were seen in rats at doses of 37 mg/kg per day.

FDA Pregnancy Category C.

### Breast-feeding
Amantadine is excreted in breast milk. However, the effects of amantadine in neonates and infants are not known.

### Pediatrics
Appropriate studies on the relationship of age to the effects of amantadine have not been performed in neonates and infants up to one year of age. However, use of amantadine in children older than 1 year of age has not been shown to cause any pediatrics-specific problems that would limit its usefulness in children.

### Geriatrics
Geriatric patients may exhibit increased sensitivity to the anticholinergic-like side effects of amantadine, including confusion. A dosage reduction of 50% (≤ 100 mg per day) appears to reduce the frequency of side effects without compromising antiviral prophylactic effectiveness. In addition, elderly patients are more likely to have an age-related decline in renal function, which may require a dosage reduction of greater than 50% in patients receiving amantadine, depending on the extent of renal dysfunction.

### Dental
Prolonged use of amantadine may decrease or inhibit salivary flow, thus contributing to the development of caries, periodontal disease, oral candidiasis, and discomfort.

### Drug interactions and/or related problems
The following drug interactions and/or related problems have been selected on the basis of their potential clinical significance (possible mechanism in parentheses where appropriate)—not necessarily inclusive (» = major clinical significance):

Note: Combinations containing any of the following medications, depending on the amount present, may also interact with this medication.

» Alcohol
(concurrent use with amantadine is not recommended since this may increase the potential for CNS effects such as dizziness, lightheadedness, orthostatic hypotension, or confusion)

» Anticholinergics (See *Appendix II*), or other medications with anticholinergic activity, or
Antidepressants, tricyclic, or
Antidyskinetics, other, or
Antihistamines or
Phenothiazines
(concurrent use with amantadine may potentiate the anticholinergic-like side effects, especially those of confusion, hallucinations, and nightmares; dosage adjustments of these medications or of amantadine may be necessary; also, patients should be advised to report occurrence of gastrointestinal problems promptly since paralytic ileus may occur with concurrent therapy)

Antidiarrheals, opioid- and anticholinergic-containing
(concurrent use with amantadine may potentiate the anticholinergic-like side effects; although significant interaction is unlikely with usual doses of opioid- and anticholinergic-containing antidiarrheals, significant interaction may occur if these medications are abused)

Carbidopa and levodopa combination or
Levodopa
(concurrent use with amantadine may result in increased efficacy of carbidopa and levodopa combination, and levodopa; however, concurrent use is not recommended if there is a history of psychosis)

» CNS stimulation–producing medications, other (See *Appendix II*)
(concurrent use with amantadine may result in additive CNS stimulation to excessive levels, which may cause unwanted effects such as nervousness, irritability, or insomnia, and possibly seizures or cardiac arrhythmias; close observation is recommended)

Hydrochlorothiazide and
Triamterene
(one or both of these drugs may reduce the renal clearance of amantadine, resulting in increased plasma concentrations and possible amantadine toxicity)

### Medical considerations/Contraindications
The medical considerations/contraindications included have been selected on the basis of their potential clinical significance (reasons given in parentheses where appropriate)—not necessarily inclusive (» = major clinical significance).

*Risk-benefit should be considered when the following medical problems exist:*

Eczematoid rash, recurrent, history of
» Edema, peripheral, or
» Heart failure, congestive
(amantadine may cause congestive heart failure and peripheral edema; presumed to be due to redistribution of fluid, not a gain of body water)

» Epilepsy, history of, or other seizure disorders
(amantadine may cause increased seizure activity; it may be necessary to reduce the dosage by 50% [≤ 100 mg per day]; this appears to reduce the frequency of side effects without compromising antiviral prophylactic effectiveness)

Hypersensitivity to amantadine

Psychosis or severe psychoneurosis
(anticholinergic-like side effects of amantadine may result in confusion, hallucinations, and nightmares; it may be necessary to reduce the dosage by 50% [≤ 100 mg per day]; this appears to reduce the frequency of side effects without compromising antiviral prophylactic effectiveness)

» Renal function impairment
(since amantadine is not metabolized and is excreted primarily in the urine, toxic concentrations may accumulate in patients with impaired renal function; it may be necessary to reduce the dosage by 50% [≤ 100 mg per day in such patients]; this appears to reduce the frequency of side effects without compromising antiviral prophylactic effectiveness)

## Side/Adverse Effects

Note: In controlled studies, side effects, including nausea, dizziness, insomnia, nervousness, and impaired concentration, were reported in 5 to 10% of young healthy adults taking the standard adult dosage of 200 mg per day. Side effects may diminish or cease after the first week of use. Serious, less frequent central nervous system (CNS) side effects, such as confusion or seizures, have usually only affected elderly patients, and patients with renal disease, seizure disorders, or altered mental/behavioral conditions. Reducing the dosage by 50% (≤ 100 mg per day) appears to reduce the frequency of side effects without compromising antiviral prophylactic effectiveness.

The following side/adverse effects have been selected on the basis of their potential clinical significance (possible signs and symptoms in parentheses where appropriate)—not necessarily inclusive:

### Those indicating need for medical attention
Incidence less frequent
*Anticholinergic-like effects* (blurred vision; confusion; difficult urination; hallucinations); *orthostatic hypotension* (fainting)

Incidence rare
*CNS toxicity* (impaired coordination; mental depression; seizures); *congestive heart failure* (swelling of feet or lower legs; unexplained shortness of breath)—usually only with chronic therapy; *corneal deposits* (irritation and swelling of the eye; decreased vision or any change in vision); *skin rash*

### Those indicating need for medical attention only if they continue or are bothersome
Incidence more frequent
*CNS toxicity* (difficulty concentrating; dizziness or lightheadedness; headache; insomnia; irritability; nervousness; nightmares); *gastrointestinal disturbances* (loss of appetite; nausea); *livedo reticularis* (purplish red, net-like, blotchy spots on skin)—usually only with chronic therapy

## 60  Amantadine (Systemic)

Incidence less frequent or rare
*Anticholinergic-like effects* (constipation; dry mouth, nose, and throat)—especially in elderly patients, patients receiving higher doses, and patients with renal dysfunction; *vomiting*

## Overdose
For more information on the management of overdose or unintentional ingestion, **contact a Poison Control Center** (See *Poison Control Center Listing*).

### Clinical effects of overdose
The following effects have been selected on the basis of their potential clinical significance (possible signs and symptoms in parentheses where appropriate)—not necessarily inclusive:

Symptoms of overdose
*Arrhythmias; pulmonary edema; status epilepticus; toxic psychosis* (hallucinations; aggressive and violent behavior)

### Treatment of overdose
There is no specific antidote for the treatment of amantadine overdose. Recommended treatment consists of the following:

To decrease absorption—

Gastric decontamination with activated charcoal; gastric lavage may be performed if the ingestion was very recent.

Vomiting should not be induced due to the risk of seizures after the overdose.

Supportive care—Supportive therapy. Patients in whom intentional overdose is known or suspected should be referred for psychiatric consultation.

## Patient Consultation
As an aid to patient consultation, refer to *Advice for the Patient, Amantadine (Systemic)*.
In providing consultation, consider emphasizing the following selected information (» = major clinical significance):

### Before using this medication
» Conditions affecting use, especially:
Hypersensitivity to amantadine
Pregnancy—Amantadine crosses the placenta
Breast-feeding—Amantadine is excreted in breast milk
Use in the elderly—Geriatric patients may exhibit increased sensitivity to the anticholinergic-like side effects of amantadine
Other medications, especially alcohol, anticholinergics or other medications with anticholinergic activity, or other CNS stimulation-producing medications
Other medical problems, especially congestive heart failure, peripheral edema, renal function impairment, seizure disorders, or a history of epilepsy

### Proper use of this medication
» Proper storage
» Proper dosing
Missed dose: Taking as soon as possible; not taking if almost time for next dose; not doubling doses
*For use as an antiviral*
Receiving a flu shot if have not already done so
» Taking before exposure or as soon as possible after exposure
» Compliance with full course of therapy
» Importance of not missing doses and taking at evenly spaced times
Proper administration technique for oral liquid
*For use as an antidyskinetic*
» Not taking more medication than the amount prescribed; not missing doses
May require up to 2 weeks for full benefit

### Precautions while using this medication
» Avoiding alcoholic beverages
» Caution if mental acuity or eyesight is impaired
Caution when getting up suddenly from a lying or sitting position
Possible dryness of mouth, nose, and throat; using sugarless candy or gum, ice, or saliva substitute for relief of dry mouth; checking with physician or dentist if dry mouth continues for more than 2 weeks
Possible appearance of livedo reticularis; gradual disappearance within 2 to 12 weeks after stopping medication
*For use as an antiviral*
Checking with physician if no improvement within a few days
*For use as an antidyskinetic*
» Resuming physical activities gradually as condition improves
Checking with physician if medication gradually loses its effectiveness
» Checking with physician before discontinuing medication; gradual dosage reduction may be necessary

### Side/adverse effects
Signs of potential side effects, especially anticholinergic-like effects, orthostatic hypotension, CNS toxicity, congestive heart failure, corneal deposits, and skin rash

## General Dosing Information
In controlled studies, side effects, including nausea, dizziness, insomnia, nervousness, and impaired concentration, were reported in 5 to 10% of young healthy adults taking the standard adult dosage of 200 mg per day. Data suggest that comparable protection may be provided by a daily prophylactic dosage of 100 mg, but with fewer side effects. No studies have been done comparing 100-mg and 200-mg doses for the treatment of influenza A infection.

Patients receiving doses exceeding 200 mg per day should be closely observed for signs of increased incidence of side effects or toxicity. Monitoring of such patients for blood pressure, pulse, respiration, and temperature should be considered, especially for a few days following the increase in dose. Patients with active seizure disorders may be at increased risk for seizures while receiving amantadine.

Changing from once-a-day to twice-a-day administration may eliminate or reduce the severity of side effects such as lightheadedness, insomnia, and nausea.

If possible, plasma concentrations should be monitored in patients with end-stage renal disease since a single dose may provide adequate concentrations for as long as 7 to 10 days.

### For use in the prophylaxis and treatment of influenza type A virus infection
Chemoprophylactic administration should be started in anticipation of contact with, or as soon as possible after exposure to, persons having influenza A virus infections. Administration should be continued for at least 10 days following exposure. In influenza epidemics, amantadine should be given daily during the epidemic (usually 6 to 8 weeks in most communities) or until active immunity can be expected from administration of inactivated influenza A virus vaccine. However, rimantadine, chemically similar to amantadine, has been reported to be ineffective when used prophylactically in household members while concurrently treating index cases for influenza A. This was apparently due to transmission of drug-resistant strains of the virus.

If administered concurrently with inactivated influenza A virus vaccine until protective antibodies develop, amantadine should be continued chemoprophylactically for 2 to 3 weeks after the vaccine has been administered. Amantadine may then be discontinued. However, since the vaccine is only 70 to 80% effective, more prolonged administration of amantadine may be beneficial in elderly or high-risk patients. If the vaccine is unavailable or contraindicated, amantadine should be administered for up to 90 days in cases of possible repeated or unknown exposure.

Treatment of the symptoms of influenza A virus infections should be started within 24 to 48 hours after their onset and should be continued for 48 hours after their disappearance. Cough may persist for several weeks.

### For use in the treatment of parkinsonism
Patients initially benefiting from the continuous administration of amantadine may experience a decline in effectiveness after a few months. Effectiveness may be restored by increasing the dose to 300 mg daily or temporarily discontinuing amantadine therapy for several weeks, and then resuming it.

Patients who have concurrent serious illnesses or are receiving high doses of other antiparkinsonian medications may be started on 100 mg of amantadine once a day. After one to several weeks, the dose may be increased to 100 mg two times a day, if necessary. If response is still not optimal, patients may benefit from a further increase to 400 mg daily in divided doses.

Concurrent administration of anticholinergic antiparkinsonian medications or levodopa with amantadine may provide additional benefit, including reduction in fluctuations in improvement occurring with levodopa alone. If dosage reductions of levodopa are required because of side effects, the benefit lost by the reduction may be restored by the concurrent administration of amantadine.

If carbidopa and levodopa combination or levodopa is initially being administered concurrently with amantadine, the dose of amantadine should be maintained at 100 mg one or two times a day while the dose of carbidopa and levodopa combination, or levodopa is gradually increased to provide optimal benefit.

Patients who have drug-induced extrapyramidal reactions may be started on 100 mg of amantadine two times a day. If response is not optimal, dose may be increased to 300 mg daily in divided doses.

When amantadine is to be discontinued, dosage should be reduced gradually in order to prevent a sudden increase in parkinsonian symptoms.

## Oral Dosage Forms

Note: Bracketed uses in the *Dosage Forms* section refer to categories of use and/or indications that are not included in U.S. product labeling.

### AMANTADINE HYDROCHLORIDE CAPSULES USP

**Usual adult and adolescent dose**
Antiviral (systemic)—
  Oral, 200 mg once a day; or 100 mg every twelve hours.
  Oral, 100 mg one or two times a day.
[Antifatigue, multiple sclerosis–associated][1]—
  Oral, 200 mg once a day; or 100 mg two times a day.

Note: Adults with impaired renal function may require a reduction in dose as noted below. Elderly patients, and patients with seizure disorders, or altered mental/behavioral conditions may require even further dose reductions.

| Creatinine Clearance (mL/min)/(mL/sec) | Dose |
| --- | --- |
| > 50/0.83 | See *Usual adult and adolescent dose* |
| 30–50/0.50–0.83 | 200 mg the first day, then 100 mg once a day |
| 15–29/0.25–0.48 | 200 mg the first day, then 100 mg every other day |
| < 15/0.25 | 200 mg once every 7 days |
| Hemodialysis patients | 200 mg once every 7 days |

**Usual adult prescribing limits**
Antiviral (systemic)—
  Up to 200 mg daily.
Antidyskinetic—
  Up to 400 mg daily.

**Usual pediatric dose**
Antiviral (systemic)—
  Neonates and infants up to 1 year of age: Dosage has not been established.
  Children 1 to 9 years of age: Oral, 1.5 to 3 mg per kg of body weight every eight hours; or 2.2 to 4.4 mg per kg of body weight every twelve hours. Maximum daily dose should not exceed 150 mg.
  Children 9 to 12 years of age: Oral, 100 mg every twelve hours.
  Children 12 years of age and over: See *Usual adult and adolescent dose*.

Note: For children 10 years of age or older weighing less than 45 kg of body weight, it may be advisable to use a dosage of 2.2 mg per kg of body weight every twelve hours.

Some references recommend doses as low as 1.5 mg per kg of body weight every twelve hours in children 1 to 9 years of age.

**Usual geriatric dose**
Antiviral (systemic)—
  Oral, 100 mg once a day.
Antidyskinetic—
  Oral, 100 mg once a day to start, titrating the dose to 100 mg two or three times a day.

Note: A daily dose of amantadine exceeding 100 mg should be used with caution in persons 65 years of age or older for influenza prophylaxis or treatment. If the patient has any renal function impairment, the dose should be reduced further.

**Strength(s) usually available**
U.S.—
  100 mg (Rx) [*Symadine*; *Symmetrel*; GENERIC].
Canada—
  100 mg (Rx) [*Symmetrel*].

**Packaging and storage**
Store below 40 °C (104 °F), preferably between 15 and 30 °C (59 and 86 °F), unless otherwise specified by manufacturer. Store in a tight container.

**Auxiliary labeling**
• May cause dizziness or blurred vision.
• Avoid alcoholic beverages.
• Continue medicine for full time of treatment (antiviral).

### AMANTADINE HYDROCHLORIDE SYRUP USP

**Usual adult and adolescent dose**
See *Amantadine Hydrochloride Capsules USP*.

**Usual adult prescribing limits**
See *Amantadine Hydrochloride Capsules USP*.

**Usual pediatric dose**
See *Amantadine Hydrochloride Capsules USP*.

**Usual geriatric dose**
See *Amantadine Hydrochloride Capsules USP*.

**Strength(s) usually available**
U.S.—
  50 mg per 5 mL (Rx) [*Symmetrel*; GENERIC].
Canada—
  50 mg per 5 mL (Rx) [*Symmetrel*].

**Packaging and storage**
Store below 40 °C (104 °F), preferably between 15 and 30 °C (59 and 86 °F), unless otherwise specified by manufacturer. Store in a tight container. Protect from freezing.

**Auxiliary labeling**
• May cause dizziness or blurred vision.
• Avoid alcoholic beverages.
• Continue medicine for full time of treatment (antiviral).

**Note**
When dispensing, include a calibrated liquid-measuring device for antiviral use.

---
[1] Not included in Canadian product labeling.

Revised: 02/23/93

---

**AMBENONIUM**—See *Antimyasthenics (Systemic)*

---

**AMCINONIDE**—See *Corticosteroids (Topical)*

---

# AMIFOSTINE  Systemic

VA CLASSIFICATION (Primary): AN700
Commonly used brand name(s): *Ethyol*.
Note: For a listing of dosage forms and brand names by country availability, see *Dosage Forms* section(s).

## Category
Antineoplastic adjunct; cytoprotective agent.

## Indications

### Accepted
Note: Bracketed information in the *Indications* section refers to uses that are not included in U.S. product labeling.

Nephrotoxicity, cisplatin-induced (prophylaxis)—Amifostine is indicated to reduce cumulative nephrotoxicity associated with cisplatin therapy in patients with advanced ovarian carcinoma, non–small cell lung carcinoma (NSCLC), or [advanced solid tumors of non–germ cell origin.]

[Bone marrow toxicity, antineoplastic agent–induced (prophylaxis)]—Amifostine is indicated to reduce acute and cumulative hematologic toxicities associated with a cisplatin and cyclophosphamide (CP) regimen in patients with advanced solid tumors of non–germ cell origin. [Amifostine is also indicated to decrease bone marrow toxicity during treatment with high-dose cisplatin alone for head and neck carcinoma (Evidence rating: IIIC), cyclophosphamide alone for malignant lymphoma (Evidence rating: IIIC), carboplatin for NSCLC (Evidence rating: IIIC), and carboplatin plus radiation therapy for head and neck carcinoma (Evidence rating: IIIC).][1]

[Neurotoxicity, cisplatin-induced (prophylaxis)][1]—Amifostine is also indicated to decrease the frequency or severity of cisplatin-induced peripheral neuropathy (Evidence rating: IC) and ototoxicity (Evidence rating: IC).

Note: Because some animal data indicate a possible interference with antitumorigenic efficacy, use of amifostine in patients with potentially curable malignancies is not recommended except in the context of a clinical study. However, amifostine did not interfere with the efficacy of a CP regimen for ovarian carcinoma, a cisplatin plus vinblastine regimen for non–small cell lung carcinoma, or any of the other treatments mentioned above.

[1]Not included in Canadian product labeling.

## Pharmacology/Pharmacokinetics

**Physicochemical characteristics**
Molecular weight—214.23.
Solubility—Freely soluble in water.

**Mechanism of action/Effect**
Amifostine is a prodrug that is metabolized by alkaline phosphatase to an active free thiol metabolite. The active thiol metabolite reduces cytotoxicity by binding to and detoxifying reactive metabolites of cisplatin and alkylating agents and by acting as a scavenger of free radicals that may develop in tissues exposed to cisplatin. These actions occur more readily in normal tissue than in tumors because of the greater phosphatase activity, higher pH, and better vascularity in normal tissue, resulting in selective protection of normal tissues.

**Distribution**
Measurable concentrations of the active free thiol metabolite have been found in bone marrow cells 5 to 8 minutes after intravenous administration.

**Biotransformation**
Amifostine is dephosphorylated by alkaline phosphatase in tissues primarily to the active free thiol metabolite and, subsequently, to a less active disulfide metabolite.

**Half-life**
Distribution—Less than 1 minute.
Elimination—Approximately 8 minutes.

**Elimination**
Primarily via rapid metabolism and uptake into tissues. Within 1 hour after infusion of 740 to 910 mg per square meter of body surface area (mg/m$^2$) over 15 minutes or rapid intravenous injection of 150 mg/m$^2$ over 10 seconds, urinary recovery of unchanged amifostine, the disulfide metabolite, and the thiol metabolite accounts for only 0.69%, 2.22%, and 2.64%, respectively, of the dose.

## Precautions to Consider

**Cross-sensitivity and/or related problems**
Patients sensitive to other aminothiol compounds also may be sensitive to amifostine.

**Carcinogenicity**
Long-term animal studies to evaluate the carcinogenic potential of amifostine have not been done. However, data from *in vitro* and *in vivo* studies indicate that amifostine may protect against the genotoxic effects of antineoplastic agents and the carcinogenic effects of radiation.

**Mutagenicity**
Amifostine demonstrated no mutagenic effects in the Ames test and in the mouse micronucleus test. However, the free thiol metabolite demonstrated mutagenic effects in the Ames test and in *in vitro* mouse studies. This metabolite demonstrated no mutagenic effects in the mouse micronucleus test and did not demonstrate clastogenicity in human lymphocytes. Data from *in vitro* and *in vivo* studies indicate that amifostine may protect against the mutagenic effects of chemotherapeutic agents.

**Pregnancy/Reproduction**
Pregnancy—Adequate and well-controlled studies in humans have not been done. However, the potential risks associated with the antineoplastic agent(s) that the patient will also be receiving must be considered. It is usually recommended that use of antineoplastics, especially combination chemotherapy, be avoided whenever possible, especially during the first trimester.
Amifostine is embryotoxic in rabbits at 60% of the recommended human dose based on body surface area. Amifostine also produces dose-dependent embryotoxicity, but not teratogenicity, in rats given doses higher than 200 mg per kg of body weight.
FDA Pregnancy Category C.

**Breast-feeding**
It is not known whether amifostine or its metabolites are distributed into breast milk. However, because of the potential risks associated with the antineoplastic agent(s) that the patient will also be receiving, breast-feeding is generally not recommended during treatment.

**Pediatrics**
Although there is limited experience with amifostine in pediatric patients, appropriate studies on the relationship of age to the effects of amifostine have not been performed in the pediatric population. Safety, efficacy, and dosage have not been established.

**Geriatrics**
Although there is limited experience with amifostine in patients older than 70 years of age, appropriate studies on the relationship of age to the effects of amifostine have not been performed in geriatric patients, and safety has not been established. However, elderly patients are more likely to have age-related cardiovascular and cerebrovascular conditions, which may require caution in patients receiving amifostine.

**Drug interactions and/or related problems**
The following drug interactions and/or related problems have been selected on the basis of their potential clinical significance (possible mechanism in parentheses where appropriate)—not necessarily inclusive (» = major clinical significance):

Note: Combinations containing any of the following medications, depending on the amount present, may also interact with this medication.

» Antihypertensives or
» Hypotension-producing medications, other (see *Appendix II*)
 (amifostine may temporarily produce hypotension; antihypertensive or other potentially hypotension-producing medications should be discontinued 24 hours prior to amifostine administration; patients receiving antihypertensive therapy that cannot be discontinued temporarily should not receive amifostine)

**Laboratory value alterations**
The following have been selected on the basis of their potential clinical significance (possible effect in parentheses where appropriate)—not necessarily inclusive (» = major clinical significance):

With physiology/laboratory test values
 Calcium, serum
  (concentrations may be decreased; however, clinically significant hypocalcemia is rare)

**Medical considerations/Contraindications**
The medical considerations/contraindications included have been selected on the basis of their potential clinical significance (reasons given in parentheses where appropriate)—not necessarily inclusive (» = major clinical significance):

*Risk-benefit should be considered when the following medical problems exist:*

Cardiovascular conditions, pre-existing, such as:
 Arrhythmias or
 Congestive heart failure or
 Ischemic heart disease
  (nausea, vomiting, and hypotension caused by amifostine may have serious consequences)

Cerebrovascular conditions, pre-existing, such as:
 Stroke, history of, or
 Transient ischemic attacks, history of
  (nausea, vomiting, and hypotension caused by amifostine may have serious consequences)

» Dehydration or
» Hypotension
  (amifostine may produce a temporary reduction in blood pressure; use of amifostine prior to correction of these conditions is not recommended)

Hypocalcemia, predisposition to
 (caution and careful monitoring of calcium concentrations are recommended in patients predisposed to hypocalcemia [e.g., patients with nephrotic syndrome])

» Sensitivity to aminothiol compounds

**Patient monitoring**
The following may be especially important in patient monitoring (other tests may be warranted in some patients, depending on condition; » = major clinical significance):

» Blood pressure determinations
  (recommended every 5 minutes during amifostine infusion)

Calcium, serum
 (recommended in patients at risk for developing hypocalcemia, e.g., those with nephrotic syndrome)

Fluid balance
 (monitoring recommended in patients receiving highly emetogenic chemotherapy)

## Side/Adverse Effects

The following side/adverse effects have been selected on the basis of their potential clinical significance (possible signs and symptoms in parentheses where appropriate)—not necessarily inclusive:

**Those indicating need for medical attention**
Incidence more frequent
   *Hypotension, asymptomatic*
   Note: *Hypotension* usually occurs 14 minutes after the start of the infusion and lasts 5 to 15 minutes (mean 6 minutes). Although usually asymptomatic, hypotension has rarely led to dizziness or fainting.
Incidence rare
   *Hypocalcemia* (burning or tingling sensation; muscle cramps)

**Those indicating need for medical attention only if they continue or are bothersome**
Incidence more frequent
   *Nausea and vomiting*
   Note: *Nausea* and *vomiting* may be severe. Administration of amifostine in addition to cisplatin plus cyclophosphamide increases the occurrence of nausea and vomiting on the day of infusion; in one clinical trial, the incidences of severe nausea and vomiting in amifostine-treated patients were almost double those in patients receiving only cisplatin plus cyclophosphamide. However, amifostine did not increase the occurrence of delayed cisplatin-induced nausea and vomiting.
Incidence less frequent or rare
   *Allergic reactions* (chills; skin rash; sneezing); *somnolence* (sleepiness, severe)

**Those not indicating need for medical attention**
Incidence less frequent or rare
   *Dizziness; feeling unusually warm or cold; flushing or redness of face or neck; hiccups*

## Overdose

For more information on the management of overdose, **contact a Poison Control Center** (see *Poison Control Center Listing*).

**Clinical effects of overdose**
Although overdose has not been reported, the most likely symptom of amifostine overdose is hypotension.

**Treatment of overdose**
Treatment of hypotension includes infusion of 0.9% sodium chloride injection along with supportive treatment.

## Patient Consultation

As an aid to patient consultation, refer to *Advice for the Patient, Amifostine (Systemic)*.
In providing consultation, consider emphasizing the following selected information (» = major clinical significance):

**Before using this medication**
» Conditions affecting use, especially:
   Sensitivity to aminothiol compounds
   Breast-feeding—Discontinuation of breast-feeding is recommended
   Other medications, especially antihypertensives or hypotension-producing medications
   Other medical problems, especially dehydration or hypotension

**Proper use of this medication**
» Proper dosing

**Side/adverse effects**
Signs of potential side effects, especially hypotension and hypocalcemia

## General Dosing Information

Amifostine should be administered as an intravenous infusion over a period of 15 minutes, beginning 30 minutes prior to chemotherapy. Longer infusion times are associated with a higher occurrence of side effects.

Because amifostine may cause severe nausea and vomiting, patients should receive antiemetic therapy that includes intravenous dexamethasone (20 mg) and a serotonin receptor antagonist before amifostine is administered. Other antiemetics may also be required, depending on the antineoplastic agents being given.

Because amifostine may cause temporary hypotension, patients should be adequately hydrated before it is administered. Patients should remain in the supine position, and their blood pressure should be monitored every 5 minutes during the infusion.

**For treatment of adverse effects**
If systolic blood pressure decreases significantly from baseline, it is recommended that the amifostine infusion be interrupted. A significant decrease is defined as:
• Baseline systolic blood pressure (mm Hg) < 100—A reduction of 20 mm Hg.
• Baseline systolic blood pressure (mm Hg) 100 to 119—A reduction of 25 mm Hg.
• Baseline systolic blood pressure (mm Hg) 120 to 139—A reduction of 30 mm Hg.
• Baseline systolic blood pressure (mm Hg) 140 to 179—A reduction of 40 mm Hg.
• Baseline systolic blood pressure (mm Hg) >180—A reduction of 50 mm Hg.

Patients who require an interruption in the amifostine infusion should be placed in the Trendelenburg position and given an intravenous infusion of 0.9% sodium chloride injection through a separate line. If blood pressure returns to normal within 5 minutes and the patient is asymptomatic, the infusion may be resumed and the full dose of amifostine administered. If the blood pressure does not return to normal, the amifostine dose for subsequent courses should be reduced.

If clinically significant hypocalcemia occurs, administration of calcium supplements may be necessary.

## Parenteral Dosage Forms

Note: Bracketed uses in the *Dosage Forms* section refer to indications that are not included in U.S. product labeling.

### AMIFOSTINE FOR INJECTION

**Usual adult dose**
Cisplatin-induced nephrotoxicity prophylaxis
[Antineoplastic agent-induced bone marrow toxicity prophylaxis]
[Cisplatin-induced neurotoxicity prophylaxis][1]—
   Intravenous infusion (over fifteen minutes), 910 mg per square meter of body surface area once a day, beginning thirty minutes prior to cisplatin chemotherapy.
Note: If systolic blood pressure decreases significantly from baseline, it is recommended that the amifostine infusion be interrupted. If blood pressure returns to normal within five minutes and the patient is asymptomatic, the infusion may be resumed and the full dose of amifostine administered. If blood pressure does not return to normal, the dose for subsequent courses should be reduced to 740 mg per square meter of body surface area.

**Usual adult prescribing limits**
Doses larger than 1300 mg per square meter of body surface area per day have not been studied.

**Usual pediatric dose**
Safety, efficacy, and dosage have not been established.

**Size(s) usually available**
U.S.—
   500 mg (anhydrous) single-dose vial (Rx) [*Ethyol*].
Canada—
   500 mg (anhydrous) single-dose vial (Rx) [*Ethyol*].

**Packaging and storage**
Store between 20 and 25 °C (68 and 77 °F).

**Preparation of dosage form**
Amifostine for injection is reconstituted by adding 9.7 mL of 0.9% sodium chloride injection, producing a solution containing 50 mg per mL. The injection should be further diluted with additional 0.9% sodium chloride injection for administration by intravenous infusion.

**Stability**
After reconstitution, the amifostine injection is stable for up to 5 hours at room temperature (25 °C [77 °F]) and for up to 24 hours in the refrigerator (2 to 8 °C [36 to 46 °F]). After further dilution to a concentration of between 5 and 40 mg per mL, the amifostine injection, when stored in a polyvinyl chloride (PVC) bag, is stable for up to 5 hours at room temperature and for up to 24 hours in the refrigerator. The reconstituted solution should not be used if it is turbid or contains a precipitate.

**Incompatibilities**
Amifostine for injection should not be mixed in solutions other than 0.9% sodium chloride injection or in 0.9% sodium chloride injections that contain other additives.

---

[1]Not included in Canadian product labeling.

Developed: 06/29/98

**AMIKACIN**—See *Aminoglycosides (Systemic)*

**AMILORIDE**—See *Diuretics, Potassium-sparing (Systemic)*

**AMINOBENZOATE POTASSIUM**—The *Aminobenzoate Potassium (Systemic)* monograph is not included in this published version of the USP DI database. Copies of the monograph are available on request from Micromedex, Inc. - Reprint Requests, 6200 S. Syracuse Way, Suite 300, Englewood, CO 80111; telephone (303) 486-6400; telefax (303) 486-6464; Email: USPDI@MDX.COM.

# AMINOCAPROIC ACID  Systemic

JAN: Epsilon-aminocaproic acid
VA CLASSIFICATION (Primary): BL116
Commonly used brand name(s): *Amicar*.
Note: For a listing of dosage forms and brand names by country availability, see *Dosage Forms* section(s).

## Category
Antifibrinolytic; antihemorrhagic.

## Indications
Note: Bracketed information in the *Indications* section refers to uses that are not included in U.S. product labeling.

**Accepted**
Hemorrhage, hyperfibrinolysis-induced (treatment)
Hemorrhage, postsurgical (prophylaxis and treatment)
[Hemorrhage, oral, in patients with hemophilia (treatment)] or
[Hemorrhage, following dental and oral surgery, in patients with hemophilia (prophylaxis and treatment)]—Aminocaproic acid is indicated for treatment of severe bleeding that may occur following heart surgery (with or without cardiac bypass procedures) and portacaval shunt, prostatectomy, or nephrectomy, and in association with hematologic disorders (such as aplastic anemia), abruptio placentae (with laboratory confirmation of hyperfibrinolysis), hepatic cirrhosis, neoplastic disease, and polycystic or neoplastic diseases of the genitourinary system.

[Aminocaproic acid is used in the management of hemophilic patients (i.e., patients with Factor VIII or Factor IX deficiency) who have oral mucosal bleeding, or are undergoing oral surgery, including tooth extractions or other dental surgical procedures. The medication prevents or decreases hemorrhaging in these patients and reduces the need for administration of clotting factors, particularly when desmopressin is also used.]

[Aminocaproic acid is also used to prevent intra- and postoperative hemorrhaging in patients with clotting defects other than hemophilia (including von Willebrand disease or deficiencies of factors other than Factor VIII or Factor IX).][1]

[Aminocaproic acid is used to treat severe hemorrhaging caused by thrombolytic agents (alteplase [tissue-type plasminogen activator, recombinant], anistreplase [anisoylated plasminogen-streptokinase activator complex], streptokinase, or urokinase). However, controlled studies to demonstrate its efficacy for this use have not been done in humans.][1]

[Hemorrhage, subarachnoid, recurrence (prophylaxis)]—Aminocaproic acid is used to prevent recurrence of subarachnoid hemorrhage, especially when surgery is delayed.

Note: In some patients receiving treatment for hemorrhaging, other emergency measures including transfusion of whole blood, fresh frozen plasma, specific clotting factors, or fibrinogen may be needed.

Aminocaproic acid is ineffective in bleeding caused by loss of vascular integrity; a definite clinical diagnosis or laboratory findings indicative of hyperfibrinolysis (hyperplasminemia) is essential prior to initiation of aminocaproic acid therapy. However, some conditions and laboratory findings suggestive of hyperfibrinolysis are also present in disseminated intravascular coagulation; differentiation between the two conditions is essential because aminocaproic acid may promote thrombus formation in patients with disseminated intravascular coagulation and must *not* be used unless heparin is administered concurrently. The following criteria may be useful in differential diagnosis:

| Test | Primary Hyperfibrinolysis Results | Disseminated Intravascular Coagulation Results |
|---|---|---|
| Platelet count* | Normal | Decreased |
| Protamine para-coagulation test | Negative | Positive |
| Euglobulin clot lysis time | Decreased | Normal |

*Following extracorporeal circulation (during cardiovascular surgery), decreased platelet count may not be useful for differentiating between primary hyperfibrinolysis and disseminated intravascular coagulation; the other criteria may be more useful in differential diagnosis in these patients.

[1]Not included in Canadian product labeling.

## Pharmacology/Pharmacokinetics

**Physicochemical characteristics**
Molecular weight—131.17.

**Mechanism of action/Effect**
Aminocaproic acid competitively inhibits activation of plasminogen, thereby reducing conversion of plasminogen to plasmin (fibrinolysin), an enzyme that degrades fibrin clots as well as fibrinogen and other plasma proteins including the procoagulant factors V and VIII. Aminocaproic acid also directly inhibits plasmin activity, but higher doses are required than are needed to reduce plasmin formation. *In vitro*, the antifibrinolytic potency of aminocaproic acid is approximately one-fifth to one-tenth that of tranexamic acid.

**Absorption**
Absorbed rapidly following oral administration.

**Protein binding**
Does not appear to bind to plasma protein.

**Time to peak concentration**
Within 2 hours following a single oral dose.

**Therapeutic plasma concentration**
For inhibition of systemic hyperfibrinolysis—130 mcg per mL (991 micromoles/L).
For prevention of recurrent subarachnoid hemorrhage—150 to 300 mcg per mL (1143 to 2287 micromoles/L).

**Elimination**
Renal. Excreted rapidly, mostly as unchanged drug.

## Precautions to Consider

**Pregnancy/Reproduction**
Fertility—Studies in rodents have suggested an adverse effect on fertility, consistent with aminocaproic acid's antifibrinolytic activity.

Pregnancy—Studies have not been done in humans.
Studies have not been done in animals.

Note: When aminocaproic acid is used topically as an oral rinse to control gingival bleeding in hemophilic patients during the first and second trimesters of pregnancy, the patient should be instructed not to swallow the syrup.

FDA Pregnancy Category C.

**Breast-feeding**
It is not known whether aminocaproic acid is distributed into breast milk. However, problems in humans have not been documented.

**Pediatrics**
Although studies on the relationship of age to the effects of aminocaproic acid have not been performed in the pediatric population, no pediatrics-specific problems attributed to aminocaproic acid have been documented to date. However, aminocaproic acid injections that contain benzyl alcohol should not be administered to premature neonates be-

cause the preservative has been associated with a fatal toxic syndrome consisting of metabolic acidosis, central nervous system (CNS) depression, respiratory problems, renal failure, hypotension, and possibly seizures and intracranial hemorrhages in these patients.

### Geriatrics
Although studies on the relationship of age to the effects of aminocaproic acid have not been performed in the geriatric population, no geriatrics-specific problems have been documented to date. However, elderly patients are more likely to have age-related renal function impairment, which may require dosage reduction in patients receiving aminocaproic acid.

### Drug interactions and/or related problems
The following drug interactions and/or related problems have been selected on the basis of their potential clinical significance (possible mechanism in parentheses where appropriate)—not necessarily inclusive (» = major clinical significance):

Note: Combinations containing any of the following medications, depending on the amount present, may also interact with this medication.

Anti-inhibitor coagulant complex or
Factor IX complex
  (although aminocaproic acid is often used in conjunction with clotting factor replacement for the perisurgical management of hemophilic patients, concurrent use may increase the risk of thrombotic complications; using aminocaproic acid as an oral rinse for oral surgical procedures and tooth extractions may minimize this complication; some hematologists recommend that administration of aminocaproic acid be delayed for 8 hours following injection of either of the clotting factor complexes)

Contraceptives, estrogen-containing, oral or
Estrogens
  (concurrent use with aminocaproic acid may increase the potential for thrombus formation)

Thrombolytic agents
  (the actions of aminocaproic acid and of thrombolytic agents [e.g., alteplase (tissue-type plasminogen activator, recombinant; tPA), anistreplase (anisoylated plasminogen-streptokinase activator complex; APSAC), streptokinase, or urokinase] are mutually antagonistic; although controlled studies to demonstrate its efficacy for this use have not been done in humans, aminocaproic acid may be useful in treating severe hemorrhage caused by a thrombolytic agent)

### Medical considerations/Contraindications
The medical considerations/contraindications included have been selected on the basis of their potential clinical significance (reasons given in parentheses where appropriate)—not necessarily inclusive (» = major clinical significance).

*Except under special circumstances, this medication should not be used when the following medical problem exists:*
» Intravascular clotting, active
  (risk of serious, even fatal, thrombus formation)

*Risk-benefit should be considered when the following medical problems exist:*
Cardiac disease
  (aminocaproic acid may cause hypotension and bradycardia, especially with rapid intravenous administration or if the patient is hypovolemic; also, endocardial hemorrhages and myocardial fat degeneration have been demonstrated in animals)

Hematuria of upper urinary tract origin
  (risk of intrarenal obstruction secondary to clot retention in the renal pelvis and ureters)

Hepatic disease
  (cause of bleeding may be more difficult to diagnose)

Renal disease
  (medication may accumulate; reduction in dosage may be required; also, aminocaproic acid has caused acute renal failure in a few patients and kidney concretions in animals)

Sensitivity to aminocaproic acid
Thrombosis, predisposition to, or history of
  (medication inhibits clot dissolution and may interfere with mechanisms for maintaining blood vessel patency)

## Side/Adverse Effects
Note: Patients receiving this medication must be monitored for signs of thromboembolic complications.

The following side/adverse effects have been selected on the basis of their potential clinical significance (possible signs and symptoms in parentheses where appropriate)—not necessarily inclusive:

### Those indicating need for medical attention
Incidence less frequent
  *Bladder obstruction caused by blood clot formation* (decreased urination); *decrease in blood pressure*—may reach hypotensive levels; *dizziness; headache; myopathy* (muscular pain or weakness, severe and continuing)—may be associated with necrosis of muscle fibers; *renal failure* (sudden decrease in amount of urine; swelling of face, fingers, feet, or lower legs; rapid weight gain); *ringing or buzzing in ears; skin rash; slow or irregular heartbeat*—after too-rapid intravenous administration; *stomach cramps; stuffy nose; thrombosis or thromboembolism* (pains in chest, groin, or legs [especially calves]; severe, sudden headache; sudden and unexplained shortness of breath, slurred speech, vision changes, and/or weakness or numbness in arm or leg; sudden loss of coordination)—signs and symptoms depend on site of thrombus formation or embolization; *unusual tiredness or weakness*—after too-rapid intravenous administration

Incidence rare
  *Rhabdomyolysis with myoglobinuria and renal failure*

### Those indicating need for medical attention only if they continue or are bothersome
Incidence less frequent
  *Diarrhea; dry ejaculation*—reported in hemophilia patients receiving the medication in conjunction with dental surgery; symptom has resolved within 24 to 48 hours after cessation of treatment in all cases reported to date; *nausea or vomiting; unusual menstrual discomfort*—caused by clotting of menstrual fluid; *unusual tiredness*—with long-term use; *watery eyes*

## Patient Consultation
As an aid to patient consultation, refer to *Advice for the Patient, Antifibrinolytic Agents (Systemic)*.

In providing consultation, consider emphasizing the following selected information (» = major clinical significance):

### Before using this medication
» Conditions affecting use, especially:
    Sensitivity to aminocaproic acid
    Other medical problems, especially active intravascular clotting

### Proper use of this medication
» Importance of not using more or less medication than the amount prescribed
» Proper dosing
    Missed dose: Taking as soon as possible, then returning to regular dosing schedule or doubling next dose
» Proper storage

### Side/adverse effects
Signs and symptoms of potential side effects, especially bladder obstruction caused by blood clot formation, decrease in blood pressure, dizziness, headache, myopathy, renal failure, ringing or buzzing in ears, skin rash, slow or irregular heartbeat, stomach cramps, stuffy nose, thrombosis or thromboembolism, unusual tiredness or weakness, and rhabdomyolysis with myoglobinuria and renal failure

## General Dosing Information
When aminocaproic acid is used during surgery, the bladder must first be freed of clots. Aminocaproic acid may accumulate in the clots and inhibit their dissolution.

A reduction in dosage may be required in patients with renal function impairment.

Aminocaproic acid therapy may be discontinued when there is evidence of cessation of bleeding or when laboratory determinations of fibrinolysis indicate that the medication is no longer required.

Aminocaproic acid syrup may be given as an oral rinse for the control of bleeding during dental and oral surgery in hemophilic patients.

### For parenteral dosage forms only
Intravenous injection of the undiluted aminocaproic acid solution is not recommended.

Rapid intravenous administration may induce hypotension or bradycardia and should be avoided.

To help minimize the possibility of thrombophlebitis, careful attention to the proper insertion of the needle and the fixing of its position is necessary before administration of this medication.

## Oral Dosage Forms

Note: Bracketed uses in the *Dosage Forms* section refer to categories of use and/or indications that are not included in U.S. product labeling.

### AMINOCAPROIC ACID SYRUP USP

**Usual adult dose**
Acute bleeding syndromes—
  Oral, 5 grams the first hour, followed by 1 or 1.25 grams per hour for approximately eight hours or until the desired response is obtained.
Note: Following prostatic surgery, a lower dose of 6 grams in the first twenty-four hours may be sufficient, since aminocaproic acid is concentrated in the urine. Also, the lower dosage may reduce the risk of clot formation and subsequent obstruction in the bladder.
[Prevention and treatment of oral hemorrhage, including hemorrhage following dental surgery, in hemophilic patients]—
  Oral, 75 mg per kg of body weight (up to 6 grams) immediately following surgery, then every six hours for seven to ten days.
  Oral rinse, 5 mL (1.25 grams) swished for thirty seconds four times a day for seven to ten days; small quantities may be swallowed, except when used during the first and second trimesters of pregnancy. In children or unconscious patients, the syrup may be applied with an applicator.
Note: When aminocaproic acid is used, a single factor VIII infusion of 40 International Units per kg of body weight, or coagulation factor IX infusion of 60 International Units per kg of body weight prior to surgery is often enough for normal hemostasis. However, because of an increased risk of thrombotic complications when aminocaproic acid and Factor IX or anti-inhibitor coagulant complex are administered concurrently, some hematologists recommend that aminocaproic acid not be administered within eight hours of these clotting factor concentrates.
[Hemorrhage, subarachnoid, recurrence]—
  To be administered following initial intravenous therapy: Oral, 36 grams per day (3 grams every two hours) until surgery is performed. If surgery is not performed, continue therapy with 3 grams every two hours for twenty-one days after the last bleeding episode. Dosage should then be reduced to 24 grams per day (2 grams every two hours) for three days, then to 12 grams per day (1 gram every two hours) for three days, prior to discontinuation of the medication.

**Usual adult prescribing limits**
[Hemorrhage, subarachnoid, recurrence]—36 grams per twenty-four hours.
Other indications—Up to 24 grams per twenty-four hours.

**Usual pediatric dose**
Acute bleeding syndromes—
  Oral, 100 mg per kg of body weight or 3 grams per square meter of body surface the first hour, followed by 33.3 mg per kg of body weight or 1 gram per square meter of body surface per hour, not to exceed 18 grams per square meter of body surface in twenty-four hours.
[Prevention and treatment of oral hemorrhage, including hemorrhage following dental surgery, in hemophilic patients]—
  See *Usual adult dose*.

**Strength(s) usually available**
U.S.—
  250 mg per mL (1.25 grams per 5 mL) (Rx) [*Amicar* (potassium sorbate 0.2%; sodium benzoate 0.1%; citric acid; flavorings; sodium saccharin; sorbitol)].
Canada—
  250 mg per mL (1.25 grams per 5 mL) (Rx) [*Amicar* (potassium sorbate 0.2%; sodium benzoate 0.1%)].

**Packaging and storage**
Store below 40 °C (104 °F), preferably between 15 and 30 °C (59 and 86 °F), unless otherwise specified by manufacturer. Store in a tight container. Protect from freezing.

### AMINOCAPROIC ACID TABLETS USP

**Usual adult dose**
See *Aminocaproic Acid Syrup USP*.

**Usual adult prescribing limits**
See *Aminocaproic Acid Syrup USP*.

**Usual pediatric dose**
See *Aminocaproic Acid Syrup USP*.

**Strength(s) usually available**
U.S.—
  500 mg (Rx) [*Amicar* (magnesium stearate; stearic acid; povidone)].
Canada—
  500 mg (Rx) [*Amicar*].

**Packaging and storage**
Store below 40 °C (104 °F), preferably between 15 and 30 °C (59 and 86 °F), unless otherwise specified by manufacturer. Store in a tight container.

## Parenteral Dosage Forms

Note: Bracketed uses in the *Dosage Forms* section refer to categories of use and/or indications that are not included in U.S. product labeling.

### AMINOCAPROIC ACID INJECTION USP

**Usual adult dose**
Acute bleeding syndromes—
  Intravenous infusion, initially 4 to 5 grams administered over a period of one hour, followed by continuous infusion at the rate of 1 gram per hour for approximately eight hours or until the desired response is obtained.
Note: Following prostatic surgery, a lower dose of 6 grams in the first twenty-four hours may be sufficient, since aminocaproic acid is concentrated in the urine. Also, the lower dosage may reduce the risk of clot formation and subsequent obstruction in the bladder.
[Prevention and treatment of oral hemorrhage, including hemorrhage following dental surgery, in hemophilic patients]—
  Intravenous infusion, 75 mg per kg of body weight (up to 6 grams) immediately following surgery, then every six hours for seven to ten days.
Note: When aminocaproic acid is used, a single factor VIII infusion of 40 International Units per kg of body weight or coagulation factor IX infusion of 60 International Units per kg of body weight prior to surgery is often enough for normal hemostasis. However, because of an increased risk of thrombotic complications when aminocaproic acid and Factor IX or anti-inhibitor coagulant complex are administered concurrently, some hematologists recommend that aminocaproic acid not be administered within eight hours of these clotting factor concentrates.
[Hemorrhage, subarachnoid, recurrence]—
  Intravenous infusion, 36 grams per day (18 grams in 400 mL of 5% dextrose injection infused over each twelve-hour period) for ten days. Therapy is continued using orally administered aminocaproic acid.

**Usual adult prescribing limits**
[Hemorrhage, subarachnoid, recurrence]—36 grams per twenty-four hours.
Other indications—Up to 24 grams per twenty-four hours.

**Usual pediatric dose**
Acute bleeding syndromes—
  Intravenous infusion, initially 100 mg per kg of body weight or 3 grams per square meter of body surface over a period of one hour, followed by continuous infusion at the rate of 33.3 mg per kg of body weight or 1 gram per square meter of body surface per hour, not to exceed 18 grams per square meter of body surface in twenty-four hours.
[Prevention and treatment of oral hemorrhage, including hemorrhage following dental surgery, in hemophilic patients]—
  See *Usual adult dose*.

**Strength(s) usually available**
U.S.—
  250 mg per mL (Rx) [*Amicar* (benzyl alcohol) [GENERIC (may contain benzyl alcohol—see labeling for individual product)].
Canada—
  250 mg per mL (Rx) [*Amicar* (benzyl alcohol)].

**Packaging and storage**
Store below 40 °C (104 °F), preferably between 15 and 30 °C (59 and 86 °F), unless otherwise specified by manufacturer. Protect from freezing.

**Preparation of dosage form**
For administration by slow intravenous infusion, the 250-mg-per-mL concentration must be diluted with a compatible intravenous vehicle such as sterile water for injection, 0.9% sodium chloride injection, 5% dextrose injection, or lactated Ringer's injection. However, dilution with sterile water for injection is not recommended when the medication is used in patients with subarachnoid hemorrhage.

Revised: 08/15/97

# AMINOGLUTETHIMIDE Systemic

VA CLASSIFICATION (Primary/Secondary): HS900/AN500
Commonly used brand name(s): *Cytadren*.

Note: For a listing of dosage forms and brand names by country availability, see *Dosage Forms* section(s).

## Category
Antiadrenal; antineoplastic.

## Indications
Note: Bracketed information in the *Indications* section refers to uses that are not included in U.S. product labeling.

**Accepted**

Cushing's syndrome (treatment)—Aminoglutethimide is indicated for temporary suppression of adrenal function in selected patients with Cushing's syndrome, including that associated with adrenal carcinoma and ectopic adrenocorticotropic hormone (ACTH)–producing tumors or adrenal hyperplasia.

[Carcinoma, breast (treatment)]—Aminoglutethimide is indicated to produce a "pharmacologic adrenalectomy" in the treatment of postmenopausal metastatic breast cancer, especially inoperable or recurrent breast cancer proven to be hormone-dependent, but resistant to therapy with tamoxifen.

[Carcinoma, prostatic (treatment)][1]—Aminoglutethimide is indicated for treatment of prostatic carcinoma unresponsive to hormonal or surgical therapy.

**Unaccepted**

Aminoglutethimide is no longer used as an anticonvulsant because of its adrenal suppressant effect.

---

[1]Not included in Canadian product labeling.

## Pharmacology/Pharmacokinetics

**Physicochemical characteristics**
Molecular weight—232.28.

**Mechanism of action/Effect**
Aminoglutethimide produces suppression of the adrenal cortex by inhibiting enzymatic conversion of cholesterol to pregnenolone, thus blocking synthesis of adrenal steroids; it may also affect other steps in the synthesis and metabolism of these steroids. A compensatory increase in secretion of adrenocorticotropic hormone (ACTH) by the pituitary occurs (except in patients with ACTH-independent adenomas or carcinomas), necessitating glucocorticoid administration to maintain aminoglutethimide's effect. Aminoglutethimide also inhibits estrogen production from androgens in peripheral tissues by blocking the aromatase enzyme. An additional mechanism in breast cancer, involving enhanced metabolism of estrone sulfate, has also been proposed.

**Other actions/effects**
Induces hepatic cytochrome P450 microsomal enzymes.

**Absorption**
Rapidly and completely absorbed from the gastrointestinal tract.

**Protein binding**
Low (20 to 25%).

**Biotransformation**
Hepatic; the major metabolite is *N*-acetylaminoglutethimide; there may be genetic variation among individuals in the rate of acetylation.

**Half-life**
12.5 hours; reduced to 7 hours after prolonged (2 to 32 weeks) treatment because aminoglutethimide induces hepatic enzymes and accelerates its own metabolism.

**Onset of action**
Suppression of adrenal function—3 to 5 days.

**Time to peak concentration**
1.5 hours.

**Duration of action**
Recovery of normal adrenal basal secretion and responsiveness to stress usually occurs within 72 hours after withdrawal of combined aminoglutethimide and hydrocortisone therapy; recovery may take longer after prolonged therapy (e.g., 1 year or longer).

**Elimination**
Renal, 34 to 54% unchanged.
In dialysis—Removable by hemodialysis.

## Precautions to Consider

**Cross-sensitivity and/or related problems**
Patients sensitive to glutethimide may be sensitive to aminoglutethimide also.

**Carcinogenicity/Mutagenicity**
Rats given doses of 10 to 60 mg per kg of body weight per day (mg/kg/day) developed benign and malignant tumors of the adrenal cortex, ovaries, thyroid, and urinary bladder.

**Pregnancy/Reproduction**
Fertility—Studies in female rats at doses equivalent to 0.5 and 1.25 times the maximum daily human dose found a decrease in fetal implantation.
Pregnancy—
Aminoglutethimide crosses the placenta and has been shown to cause pseudohermaphroditism in female infants whose mothers took concomitant anticonvulsants.
Aminoglutethimide has been shown to cause increased incidences of fetal death and teratogenic effects, including pseudohermaphroditism, in rats given up to three times the highest recommended human dose.
FDA Pregnancy Category D.

**Breast-feeding**
It is not known whether aminoglutethimide is distributed into breast milk. Problems in humans have not been documented; however, the manufacturer recommends discontinuing breast-feeding while receiving aminoglutethimide.

**Pediatrics**
Appropriate studies on the relationship of age to the effects of aminoglutethimide have not been performed in the pediatric population. However, aminoglutethimide was used for 3 days to 6½ months in nine pediatric patients 2 to 16 years of age with adrenal carcinoma, adrenal hyperplasia, or an ectopic adrenocorticotropic hormone–producing tumor. The effects of aminoglutethimide in these patients were difficult to assess because the patients were receiving combination therapy. Most of these patients showed decreases in plasma or urinary concentrations of steroids during therapy.

**Geriatrics**
Appropriate studies on the relationship of age to the effects of aminoglutethimide have not been performed in the geriatric population. However, the elderly may be more sensitive to the central nervous system (CNS) effects and more likely to become lethargic with this medication. In addition, elderly patients are more likely to have age-related renal function impairment, which may require caution in patients receiving aminoglutethimide.

**Drug interactions and/or related problems**
The following drug interactions and/or related problems have been selected on the basis of their potential clinical significance (possible mechanism in parentheses where appropriate)—not necessarily inclusive (» = major clinical significance):

Note: Combinations containing any of the following medications, depending on the amount present, may also interact with this medication.

Anticoagulants, coumarin-type or
Antidiabetic agents, sulfonylurea or
» Dexamethasone or
Digoxin or
Medroxyprogesterone or
Prednisone or
Prednisolone or
Theophylline
(effects may be reduced because of induction of hepatic microsomal enzymes by aminoglutethimide, resulting in accelerated clearance of these agents; if glucocorticoid therapy is necessary in a patient receiving aminoglutethimide, hydrocortisone is recommended; dosage adjustments of coumarin anticoagulants should be based on monitoring of coagulation times)

Corticotropin (ACTH)
(aminoglutethimide may inhibit the adrenal response to ACTH; this may interfere with the therapeutic response to ACTH)

CNS depression–producing medications (see *Appendix II*)
(additive CNS depression may occur)

Diuretics
(hyponatremia may occur)

**Laboratory value alterations**
The following have been selected on the basis of their potential clinical significance (possible effect in parentheses where appropriate)—not necessarily inclusive (» = major clinical significance):

With physiology/laboratory test values
  Aldosterone
    (urinary concentrations may be decreased, resulting in orthostatic hypotension and hyponatremia)
  Alkaline phosphatase values, serum and
  Aspartate aminotransferase (AST [SGOT] values, serum) and
  Bilirubin concentrations, serum
    (may be increased)
  Cortisol
    (plasma concentrations are decreased slowly in patients with adrenal hyperfunction and rapidly in patients with breast cancer and in otherwise healthy individuals)
  Sodium, serum
    (concentrations may be decreased)
  Thyroid-stimulating hormone (TSH)
    (serum concentrations may be increased as a reflex response to reduced serum thyroxine concentrations)
  Thyroxine
    (serum concentrations may be decreased; hypothyroidism is infrequent because of a reflex increase in TSH secretion)

**Medical considerations/Contraindications**
The medical considerations/contraindications included have been selected on the basis of their potential clinical significance (reasons given in parentheses where appropriate)—not necessarily inclusive (» = major clinical significance).

*Risk-benefit should be considered when the following medical problems exist:*
» Chickenpox, existing or recent (including recent exposure) or
» Herpes zoster
    (risk of severe generalized disease)
  Hepatic function impairment
    (reduced biotransformation)
  Hypothyroidism
    (aminoglutethimide may decrease serum thyroxine concentrations)
» Infection
    (reduced adrenal responsiveness may result in acute adrenocortical insufficiency; additional steroid supplementation may be necessary)
  Renal function impairment
    (reduced elimination)
» Sensitivity to aminoglutethimide or glutethimide

**Patient monitoring**
The following are especially important in patient monitoring (other tests may be warranted in some patients, depending on condition; » = major clinical significance):

  Alkaline phosphatase values, serum and
» Aspartate aminotransferase (AST [SGOT]) values, serum and
  Blood counts, complete and
» Thyroid function tests
    (recommended at periodic intervals; hematologic abnormalities are more likely to occur during the first 7 weeks of therapy with aminoglutethimide; the manufacturer recommends obtaining white blood cell and platelet counts at weeks 4, 8, and 12 after beginning therapy with aminoglutethimide; thereafter, blood counts are recommended as indicated by the clinical status and symptoms of the patient)
» Blood pressure determinations, recumbent and upright
    (recommended at periodic intervals to detect hypotension due to reduced aldosterone production)
» Electrolytes (sodium, potassium, chloride), serum
    (frequent measurements recommended)

*In adrenal disorders*
» Cortisol concentrations, 8 a.m. plasma or
» 17-Hydroxycorticosteroid concentrations, 24-hour urinary
    (recommended at periodic intervals to aid in assessing clinical response and determine if steroid supplement therapy is necessary)

*In prostatic carcinoma*
  Acid phosphatase concentrations, serum
    (recommended at periodic intervals to aid in assessing clinical response; concentrations should decrease)

## Side/Adverse Effects

Note: Most side effects decrease in incidence and severity after the first 2 to 6 weeks because of accelerated metabolism of the drug with continued use.

The following side/adverse effects have been selected on the basis of their potential clinical significance (possible signs and symptoms in parentheses where appropriate)—not necessarily inclusive:

**Those indicating need for medical attention**
Incidence more frequent
  *Drowsiness; measles-like skin rash or itching on face and/or palms of hands*
  Note: The *measles-like skin rash* is often accompanied by fever. It usually appears within 10 to 15 days after therapy is started and persists for 5 to 7 days; it is recommended that aminoglutethimide be withdrawn if mild to moderate skin rash persists for longer than 5 to 8 days or if skin rash is severe.
Incidence less frequent
  *Clumsiness; dizziness; fever; hypoglycemia* (dizziness); *hypotension, orthostatic or persistent* (chills; cold sweats; confusion; dizziness or lightheadedness, especially when getting up from a lying or sitting position; fast heartbeat; shakiness; slurred speech; unusual tiredness or weakness); *lethargy* (tiredness); *mental depression; nystagmus* (uncontrolled eye movements)
  Note: *CNS effects* usually are reduced within 2 to 6 weeks with continued treatment, although some may be severe enough to necessitate discontinuing treatment in some patients.
Incidence rare
  *Alveolitis* (coughing; shortness of breath)—possibly a hypersensitivity reaction; *hypersensitivity* (fever; yellow eyes or skin); *hypothyroidism and goiter* (neck tenderness or swelling); *leukopenia or agranulocytosis* (fever or chills; cough or hoarseness; lower back or side pain; painful or difficult urination)—usually asymptomatic; *thrombocytopenia* (unusual bleeding or bruising; black, tarry stools; blood in urine or stools; pinpoint red spots on skin)—usually asymptomatic
  Note: A rare *hypersensitivity* or drug reaction has been reported, consisting of cholestatic jaundice, fever, skin eruptions, increased aspartate aminotransferase (AST [SGOT]), and possibly eosinophilia.
    *Hypothyroidism and goiter* may occur with long-term use because aminoglutethimide blocks iodination of tyrosine.

**Those indicating need for medical attention only if they continue or are bothersome**
Incidence more frequent
  *Loss of appetite or nausea*
Incidence less frequent or rare
  *Headache; masculinization and hirsutism in females* (deepening of voice; increased hair growth; irregular menstrual periods); *myalgia* (muscle pain); *vomiting*

## Overdose

For specific information on the agents used in the management of aminoglutethimide overdose, see:
• *Corticosteroids—Glucocorticoid Effects (Systemic)* monograph; and/or
• *Sympathomimetic Agents—Cardiovascular Use (Parenteral-Systemic)* monograph.

For more information on the management of overdose or unintentional ingestion, **contact a Poison Control Center** (see *Poison Control Center Listing*).

**Clinical effects of overdose**
The following side/adverse effects have been selected on the basis of their potential clinical significance (possible signs and symptoms in parentheses where appropriate)—not necessarily inclusive:

Acute and chronic
  *Ataxia* (difficulty walking); *dizziness; hypotension* (dizziness); *lethargy* (tiredness and weakness); *respiratory depression* (slowed breathing); *weakness, extreme*

**Treatment of overdose**
To decrease absorption—Gastric lavage may decrease absorption of aminoglutethimide.

To enhance elimination—Dialysis may be used to enhance elimination if toxicity is severe.

Supportive care—Symptomatic, supportive treatment, including support of respiratory function, is recommended. If hypovolemia or hypotension occurs, intravenous norepinephrine plus rehydration may be used to support blood pressure.

Specific treatment—Intravenous hydrocortisone should be administered if glucocorticoid insufficiency develops. Fludrocortisone therapy may be instituted if mineralocorticoid insufficiency develops.

Note: No case of death due to aminoglutethimide overdose has been reported. A boy 10 years of age and a girl 16 years of age both survived after each consumed 10 grams of aminoglutethimide.

## Patient Consultation

As an aid to patient consultation, refer to *Advice for the Patient, Aminoglutethimide (Systemic)*.

In providing consultation, consider emphasizing the following selected information (» = major clinical significance):

**Before using this medication**
» Conditions affecting use, especially:
Sensitivity to aminoglutethimide or glutethimide
Pregnancy—Teratogenic in humans and animals
Breast-feeding—Although problems have not been reported, it is recommended that breast-feeding be discontinued
Use in the elderly—Lethargy may be more frequent
Other medications, especially dexamethasone
Other medical problems, especially chickenpox, herpes zoster, or infection

**Proper use of this medication**
» Importance of not taking more or less medication than the amount prescribed
» Possible nausea and vomiting; usually lessens with continued therapy; checking with physician before discontinuing medication
Checking with physician if vomiting occurs shortly after dose is taken
» Proper dosing
Missed dose: Taking as soon as possible if remembered within 2 to 4 hours; not taking if almost time for next dose; not doubling doses
» Proper storage

**Precautions while using this medication**
» Importance of close monitoring by physician
Carrying medical identification card or wearing bracelet stating that medication is being used
Caution if any kind of surgery (including dental surgery) or emergency treatment is required
» Checking with physician immediately if injury, infection, or other illness occurs, because of the risk of adrenal insufficiency; physician may prescribe steroid supplement
» Caution if drowsiness, dizziness, or hypotension occurs, especially if driving, using machines, or doing other things that require alertness

**Side/adverse effects**
Signs of potential side effects, especially drowsiness, measles-like skin rash or itching on face and/or palms of hands, clumsiness, dizziness, fever, hypoglycemia, hypotension, lethargy, mental depression, nystagmus, alveolitis, or hypothyroidism and goiter
Asymptomatic side effects, including leukopenia or agranulocytosis, and thrombocytopenia

## General Dosing Information

Patients receiving aminoglutethimide should be under the supervision of a physician experienced in cancer chemotherapy or a clinical endocrinologist.

Dosage must be adjusted to provide the desired level of adrenal suppression.

Patients should be monitored carefully during periods of stress such as surgery, trauma, or acute illness. Additional steroids may be required because adrenal suppression may prevent the normal response to stress. It is recommended that aminoglutethimide be temporarily withdrawn immediately following shock or severe trauma.

**For use as an antineoplastic**
Inhibition of the adrenal cortex by aminoglutethimide results in a reflex increase in secretion of adrenocorticotropic hormone (ACTH) by the pituitary (except in patients with ACTH-independent adenomas or carcinomas); therefore, replacement with a glucocorticoid (usually hydrocortisone) may be necessary to maintain the desired effect of aminoglutethimide by preventing adrenal cortical hypertrophy and renewed synthesis of steroids.

Replacement glucocorticoid therapy is usually required in patients with metastatic breast cancer.

Because of the rapid return of the adrenal cortex to normal responsiveness following withdrawal of aminoglutethimide and hydrocortisone, dosage tapering is usually not necessary.

**For treatment of adverse effects**
It is recommended that dosage be reduced if CNS side effects occur.

Mineralocorticoid replacement (such as fludrocortisone) may be necessary in 20 to 50% of patients because of reduction of aldosterone production caused by aminoglutethimide, which could lead to hyponatremia and orthostatic hypotension.

It is recommended that aminoglutethimide be withdrawn if mild to moderate skin rash persists for longer than 5 to 8 days or if skin rash is severe. Skin rash may respond to treatment with diphenhydramine and/or hydrocortisone. After a mild to moderate rash disappears, aminoglutethimide therapy may be restarted at a dose of 250 mg a day and gradually increased to the therapeutic dose.

Stevens-Johnson syndrome has been reported with the use of aminoglutethimide. Any rash appearing with the use of aminoglutethimide should be monitored closely. If an exfoliative rash occurs, aminoglutethimide should be discontinued.

## Oral Dosage Forms

Note: Bracketed uses in the *Dosage Forms* section refer to categories of use and/or indications that are not included in U.S. product labeling.

### AMINOGLUTETHIMIDE TABLETS USP

**Usual adult dose**
Antiadrenal—
Initial: Oral, 250 mg two or three times a day for approximately two weeks (to induce its metabolism and minimize CNS side effects).
Maintenance: Oral, 250 mg four times a day, preferably every six hours.
[Breast carcinoma] or
[Prostatic carcinoma][1]—
Initial: Oral, 125 mg two times a day for several days to one week, then two or three times a day for approximately two weeks (to induce metabolism and minimize CNS side effects), in combination with 100 mg of hydrocortisone in three divided doses for one to two weeks, then 40 mg of hydrocortisone a day (10 mg in the morning and at 5 p.m., and 20 mg at bedtime).
Maintenance: Oral, 250 mg four times a day, preferably every six hours, in combination with 40 mg of hydrocortisone a day (10 mg in the morning and at 5 p.m., and 20 mg at bedtime).

**Usual adult prescribing limits**
Cushing's syndrome—
2 grams a day.
[Breast carcinoma]—
2 grams a day.

**Usual pediatric dose**
Safety and efficacy have not been established.

**Usual geriatric dose**
See *Usual adult dose*.

**Strength(s) usually available**
U.S.—
250 mg (Rx) [*Cytadren* (double-scored)].
Canada—
250 mg (Rx) [*Cytadren* (scored)].

**Packaging and storage**
Store below 40 °C (104 °F), preferably between 15 and 30 °C (59 and 86 °F), unless otherwise specified by manufacturer. Store in a tight container. Protect from light.

[1]Not included in Canadian product labeling.

Revised: 09/30/97

---

# AMINOGLYCOSIDES Systemic

This monograph includes information on the following: 1) Amikacin; 2) Gentamicin; 3) Kanamycin†; 4) Neomycin†; 5) Netilmicin; 6) Streptomycin; 7) Tobramycin.

VA CLASSIFICATION (Primary/Secondary):
Amikacin—AM300
Gentamicin—AM300
Kanamycin—AM300
Neomycin—AM300
Netilmicin—AM300
Streptomycin—AM300/AM500
Tobramycin—AM300

Commonly used brand name(s): Amikin[1]; Cidomycin[2]; G-Mycin[2]; Garamycin[2]; Jenamicin[2]; Kantrex[3]; Nebcin[7]; Netromycin[5].

Note: For a listing of dosage forms and brand names by country availability, see *Dosage Forms* section(s).

[†]Not commercially available in Canada.

## Category

Antibacterial (systemic)—Amikacin; Gentamicin; Kanamycin; Netilmicin; Streptomycin; Tobramycin.
Antibacterial (antimycobacterial)—Streptomycin.

## Indications

### General considerations

Aminoglycosides are indicated in the treatment of serious systemic infections for which less toxic antibacterials are ineffective or contraindicated. The spectrum of aminoglycosides covers aerobic gram-negative bacilli, and some gram-positive organisms. They are not active against anaerobic organisms.

The antibacterial activity of aminoglycosides against different strains of organisms varies among institutions and regions. However, aminoglycosides are generally active against most Enterobacteriaceae, including *Escherichia coli*, *Proteus mirabilis*, indole-positive *Proteus*, *Citrobacter*, *Enterobacter*, *Klebsiella*, *Providencia*, and *Serratia* species. *Acinetobacter* and *Pseudomonas* species are also usually susceptible. Although tobramycin is more potent *in vitro* against *Pseudomonas aeruginosa*, and gentamicin is more potent *in vitro* against *Serratia* species, neither has been shown to be more clinically effective than other aminoglycosides if the organism is susceptible. Aminoglycosides are used concurrently with antipseudomonal penicillins or certain cephalosporins in the treatment of serious *Pseudomonas aeruginosa* infections.

Bacterial resistance to gentamicin and tobramycin is very similar, although a few organisms resistant to gentamicin remain susceptible to tobramycin. The antibacterial activity and resistance pattern of netilmicin is very similar to those of both gentamicin and tobramycin, although there are a few gentamicin- and tobramycin-resistant strains that remain susceptible to netilmicin.

Amikacin is similar to gentamicin, tobramycin, and netilmicin in its spectrum of activity; however, amikacin has the advantage of not being inactivated by the same enzymes that render other aminoglycosides inactive against resistant organisms. Therefore, amikacin may remain active against strains of *Pseudomonas aeruginosa* that are resistant to tobramycin and netilmicin. Kanamycin use has declined over the years due to the emergence of a large number of resistant organisms. However, because of its disuse, resistance has decreased in some areas.

Streptomycin is used primarily as an antitubercular and is active against *Mycobacterium tuberculosis* and *M. bovis*. It is also considered the drug of choice for the treatment of infections caused by *Francisella tularensis* and *Yersinia pestis*, and is often used to treat *Brucella* infections. Because many other gram-negative bacilli are resistant, streptomycin is rarely used to treat those organisms.

Aminoglycosides are also active against *Staphylococcus aureus*, but are rarely used as sole therapy since other, less toxic, antibiotics are available. Amikacin, gentamicin, netilmicin, or tobramycin, administered concurrently with a penicillin, is synergistic against certain susceptible strains of *Enterococcus faecalis*. Streptomycin has been used, in combination with penicillin or vancomycin, in the treatment of endocarditis caused by *Enterococcus faecalis* or *S. viridans*.

Aminoglycosides are indicated for the treatment of serious infections caused by, or strongly suspected to be caused by, susceptible gram-negative bacilli. Some aminoglycosides, such as amikacin, gentamicin, and tobramycin, may also be given as an aerosol nebulization. This is usually as an adjunct to parenteral therapy in patients with cystic fibrosis with acute exacerbations of pulmonary infections. Aminoglycosides are used to treat central nervous system (CNS) infections mainly in neonates due to better penetration across the blood-brain barrier in this age group; gentamicin may also be given intrathecally to treat CNS infections in adults. Aminoglycosides are also used in combination with other antibacterials for a possible synergistic effect.

### Accepted

Biliary tract infections (treatment)—Amikacin, gentamicin, kanamycin, netilmicin, and tobramycin are indicated in the treatment of biliary tract infections caused by susceptible organisms.

Bone and joint infections (treatment)—Amikacin, gentamicin, kanamycin, netilmicin, and tobramycin are indicated in the treatment of bone and joint infections caused by susceptible organisms.

Brucellosis (treatment)—Streptomycin is indicated in the treatment of brucellosis caused by *Brucella* species.

Central nervous system infections (including meningitis and ventriculitis) (treatment)—Amikacin, gentamicin, kanamycin, netilmicin, and tobramycin are indicated in the treatment of central nervous system infections caused by susceptible organisms.

Granuloma inguinale (treatment)—Streptomycin is indicated in the treatment of granuloma inguinale.

Intra-abdominal infections (including peritonitis) (treatment)—Amikacin, gentamicin, kanamycin, netilmicin, and tobramycin are indicated in the treatment of intra-abdominal infections caused by susceptible organisms.

Plague (treatment)—Streptomycin is indicated in the treatment of plague.

Pneumonia, gram-negative, bacterial (treatment)—Amikacin, gentamicin, kanamycin, netilmicin, and tobramycin are indicated in the treatment of bacterial, gram-negative pneumonia caused by susceptible organisms.

Septicemia, bacterial (treatment)—Amikacin, gentamicin, kanamycin, netilmicin, and tobramycin are indicated in the treatment of bacterial septicemia caused by susceptible organisms.

Skin and soft tissue infections (including burn wound infections) (treatment)—Amikacin, gentamicin, kanamycin, netilmicin, and tobramycin are indicated in the treatment of skin and soft tissue infections caused by susceptible organisms.

Tuberculosis (treatment)—Streptomycin is indicated in the treatment of tuberculosis.

Tularemia (treatment)—Streptomycin is indicated in the treatment of tularemia.

Urinary tract infections (recurrent complicated) (treatment)—Amikacin, gentamicin, kanamycin, netilmicin, and tobramycin are indicated in the treatment of recurrent complicated urinary tract infections caused by susceptible organisms.

Not all species or strains of a particular organism may be susceptible to a specific aminoglycoside.

### Unaccepted

Aminoglycosides are not indicated routinely in the treatment of staphylococcal infections since less toxic antibacterials are available.

Aminoglycosides are not routinely indicated in the initial treatment of uncomplicated urinary tract infections unless the organism is resistant to other less toxic antibacterials.

Parenteral neomycin has been replaced by safer and more effective agents. **Because of its potential toxicity, parenteral use of neomycin is not recommended for any indication.**

## Pharmacology/Pharmacokinetics

### Physicochemical characteristics

Molecular weight—
  Amikacin sulfate: 781.75.
  Kanamycin sulfate: 582.58.
  Netilmicin sulfate: 1441.54.
  Tobramycin sulfate: 1425.39.

### Mechanism of action/Effect

Actively transported across the bacterial cell membrane, irreversibly binds to one or more specific receptor proteins on the 30 S subunit of bacterial ribosomes, and interferes with an initiation complex between messenger RNA (mRNA) and the 30 S subunit. DNA may be misread, thus producing nonfunctional proteins; polyribosomes are split apart and are unable to synthesize protein. This results in accelerated aminoglycoside transport, increasing the disruption of bacterial cytoplasmic membranes, and eventual cell death.

Note: Aminoglycosides are bactericidal, while most other antibiotics that interfere with protein synthesis are bacteriostatic.

### Absorption

All aminoglycosides—
  Intramuscular: Rapidly and completely absorbed after intramuscular administration.
  Local; topical: May also be absorbed in significant amounts from body surfaces (except urinary bladder) following local irrigation or topical application. Intraperitoneal and intrapleural administration results in rapid absorption.
  Oral: Poorly absorbed from intact gastrointestinal tract after oral administration, but may accumulate in patients with renal failure.

**Distribution**
All aminoglycosides—
  Distributed to extracellular fluid, including serum, abscesses, ascitic, pericardial, pleural, synovial, lymphatic, and peritoneal fluids.
  High concentrations found in urine.
  Low concentrations found in bile, breast milk, aqueous humor, bronchial secretions, sputum, and cerebral spinal fluid (CSF). In adults, does not cross the blood-brain barrier (BBB) in therapeutically adequate concentrations. Small improvement in penetration with inflamed meninges. Higher levels are achieved in the CSF of newborns than in adults.
  Crosses the placenta.
  Also distributed to all body tissues, where aminoglycosides accumulate intracellularly.
  High concentrations found in highly perfused organs, such as the liver, lungs, and especially, the kidneys, where aminoglycosides accumulate in the renal cortex.
  Lower concentrations are seen in muscle, fat, and bone.
  $Vol_D$—
    Adults—0.26 L per kg (range, 0.20 to 0.40 L per kg).
    Children—0.2 to 0.4 L per kg.
    Neonates—
      < 1 week old, < 1500 grams: up to 0.68 L per kg.
      < 1 week old, > 1500 grams: up to 0.58 L per kg.
    Cystic fibrosis patients—0.30 to 0.39 L per kg.

**Protein binding**
All aminoglycosides—Low (0 to 10%).

**Biotransformation**
Not metabolized.

**Half-life**
All aminoglycosides—
  Distribution half-life:
    5 to 15 minutes.
  Elimination half-life:
    Adults—
      Normal renal function: 2 to 4 hours.
      Impaired renal function: Varies with degree of dysfunction; up to 100 hours.
      Cystic fibrosis patients: 1 to 2 hours.
      Burn patients and febrile patients: May have a shorter half-life than average due to increased clearance of the drug.
    Pediatrics—
      Neonates: 5 to 8 hours.
      Children: 2.5 to 4 hours.
  Terminal half-life:
    > 100 hours (release of intracellularly bound aminoglycoside).

**Time to peak concentration**
All aminoglycosides—
  Intramuscular: 0.5 to 1.5 hours.
  Intravenous (time to post-distributional peak level): 30 minutes after end of 30 minute infusion, or 15 minutes after end of 1 hour infusion.

**Time to peak bile concentration**
Kanamycin—Approximately 6 hours (intramuscular).

**Peak serum concentrations**
In adults with normal renal function—
  Amikacin:
    Intramuscular—7.5 mg per kg of body weight(mg/kg): 21 mcg per mL.
    Intravenous over 30 minutes—7.5 mg/kg: 38 mcg per mL.
  Gentamicin:
    Intramuscular or intravenous—1.5 mg/kg: 6 mcg per mL.
  Kanamycin:
    Intramuscular or intravenous—7.5 mg/kg: 22 mcg per mL.
  Netilmicin:
    Intramuscular—2 mg/kg: 5.5 mcg per mL.
    Intravenous over 30 minutes—2 mg/kg: 11.8 mcg per mL.
  Streptomycin:
    Intramuscular—1 gram: 25 to 50 mcg per mL.
  Tobramycin:
    Intramuscular or intravenous—1 mg/kg: 4 mcg per mL.

**Bile concentration**
Netilmicin—10% of serum concentrations; may vary up to 25% of serum concentrations with abnormal hepatic function.

**Elimination**
Renal; excreted unchanged by glomerular filtration. 70 to 95% of aminoglycoside dose recovered in urine over 24 hours. Small amount excreted in bile.

Hemodialysis—Each 4 to 6 hour hemodialysis period decreases plasma aminoglycoside concentrations by up to 50%.
Peritoneal dialysis—Less effective than hemodialysis. Removes approximately 25% of a dose in 48 to 72 hours.

## Precautions to Consider

**Cross-sensitivity and/or related problems**
Patients hypersensitive to one aminoglycoside may be hypersensitive to other aminoglycosides also.

**Carcinogenicity/Mutagenicity/Tumorigenicity**
*Amikacin and kanamycin*—Studies on the carcinogenic or mutagenic effects in humans have not been done.
*Netilmicin*—Lifetime carcinogenicity studies in mice and rats have not shown any netilmicin-related tumors. Mutagenicity studies in mice and rats have shown negative results.

**Pregnancy/Reproduction**
Fertility—*Amikacin:* Reproduction studies in rats and mice have not shown that amikacin causes impaired fertility.
*Gentamicin:* Reproduction studies in rats and rabbits have not shown that gentamicin causes impaired fertility.
*Kanamycin:* Studies in rats and rabbits have not shown that kanamycin causes impaired fertility.
*Netilmicin:* Reproduction studies in rats and rabbits given intramuscular and subcutaneous doses of netilmicin approximately 13 to 15 times the highest adult human dose have not shown that netilmicin impairs fertility or causes adverse effects on the fetus.

Pregnancy—All aminoglycosides cross the placenta, sometimes resulting in significant concentrations in the cord blood and/or amniotic fluid. Aminoglycosides may be nephrotoxic in the human fetus. In addition, some aminoglycosides (e.g., streptomycin, tobramycin) have been reported to cause total irreversible, bilateral congenital deafness in children whose mothers received aminoglycosides during pregnancy.
  *Amikacin:* Adequate and well-controlled studies in humans have not been done. Amikacin has not been shown to cause adverse effects on the fetus, even though peak fetal serum concentrations of amikacin average approximately 16% of peak maternal serum concentrations and amikacin may be concentrated in the fetal kidneys. However, since other aminoglycosides have been reported to cause deafness in the fetus, risk-benefit must be carefully considered when this medication is required in life-threatening situations or in serious diseases for which other medications cannot be used or are ineffective.
  FDA Pregnancy Category D.
  *Gentamicin:* Adequate and well-controlled studies in humans have not been done. Since other aminoglycosides have been reported to cause deafness in the fetus, risk-benefit must be carefully considered when this medication is required in life-threatening situations or in serious diseases for which other medications cannot be used or are ineffective.
  Studies in rats and rabbits have not shown that gentamicin causes adverse effects on the fetus.
  FDA Pregnancy Category C.
  *Kanamycin:* Fetal serum concentrations average approximately 16 to 50% of maternal serum concentrations. Adequate and well-controlled studies in humans have not been done.
  Studies in rats and rabbits have not shown that kanamycin is teratogenic. However, studies in rats and guinea pigs given doses of 200 mg/kg daily have shown that kanamycin causes hearing impairment in the fetus.
  FDA Pregnancy Category D.
  *Netilmicin:* Netilmicin has been detected in cord blood and in the human fetus. Therefore, risk-benefit must be carefully considered when this medication is required in life-threatening situations or in serious diseases for which other medications cannot be used or are ineffective.
  Studies in rats given netilmicin subcutaneously during pregnancy have not shown that netilmicin causes ototoxicity in the fetus.
  FDA Pregnancy Category D.
  *Streptomycin:* Adequate and well-controlled studies in humans have not been done. Fetal serum concentrations are usually less than 50% of maternal serum concentrations. Streptomycin has been shown to cause deafness in infants whose mothers received streptomycin during pregnancy. Therefore, risk-benefit must be carefully considered when this medication is required in life-threatening situations or in serious diseases for which other medications cannot be used or are ineffective.
  FDA Pregnancy Category D.

*Tobramycin:* Tobramycin concentrates in the fetal kidneys and has been shown to cause total irreversible bilateral congenital deafness in the human fetus. Therefore, risk-benefit must be carefully considered when this medication is required in life-threatening situations or in serious diseases for which other medications cannot be used or are ineffective.

FDA Pregnancy Category D.

### Breast-feeding

Aminoglycosides are excreted in breast milk in small but variable amounts (e.g., up to 18 mcg per mL for kanamycin). However, aminoglycosides are poorly absorbed from the gastrointestinal tract and problems in nursing infants have not been documented.

### Pediatrics

*All aminoglycosides*—CNS depression, characterized by stupor, flaccidity, coma, or deep respiratory depression, has been reported in very young infants receiving streptomycin at doses that exceeded the maximum recommended amount. However, all aminoglycosides have this potential to cause neuromuscular blockade.

*Amikacin, gentamicin, kanamycin, netilmicin, and tobramycin*—These aminoglycosides should be used with caution in premature infants and neonates because of these patients' immature renal capability, which may result in prolonged elimination half-life and aminoglycoside-induced toxicity. Dosage adjustments may be required in pediatric patients. See also *Patient monitoring* and *General Dosing Information*.

### Geriatrics

Because of their toxicity, aminoglycosides should be used with caution in elderly patients, only after less toxic alternatives have been considered and/or found ineffective. Elderly patients are more likely to have an age-related decrease in renal function. Recommended doses should not be exceeded, and the patient's renal function should be carefully monitored during therapy. Geriatric patients may require smaller daily doses of aminoglycosides in accordance with their increased age, decreased renal function, and, possibly, decreased weight. In addition, loss of hearing may result even in patients with normal renal function.

### Drug interactions and/or related problems

The following drug interactions and/or related problems have been selected on the basis of their potential clinical significance (possible mechanism in parentheses where appropriate)—not necessarily inclusive (» = major clinical significance):

Note: Combinations containing any of the following medications, depending on the amount present, may also interact with this medication.

» Aminoglycosides, 2 or more concurrently or
» Capreomycin

(concurrent and/or sequential use of 2 or more aminoglycosides by any route or concurrent use of capreomycin with aminoglycosides should be avoided since the potential for ototoxicity, nephrotoxicity, and neuromuscular blockade may be increased; hearing loss may occur and may progress to deafness even after discontinuation of the drug; loss of hearing may be reversible, but usually is permanent; neuromuscular blockade may result in skeletal muscle weakness and respiratory depression or paralysis [apnea]. Also, concurrent use of 2 or more aminoglycosides may result in reduced bacterial uptake of each one since the medications compete for the same uptake mechanism)

Antimyasthenics

(concurrent use of medications with neuromuscular blocking action may antagonize the effect of antimyasthenics on skeletal muscle; temporary dosage adjustments of antimyasthenics may be necessary to control symptoms of myasthenia gravis during and following use of medications with neuromuscular blocking action)

Beta-lactam antibiotics

(aminoglycosides can be inactivated by many beta-lactam antibiotics [cephalosporins, penicillins] *in vitro* and *in vivo* in patients with significant renal failure. Degradation depends on the concentration of the beta-lactam, storage time, and temperature)

Indomethacin, intravenous

(when aminoglycosides are administered concurrently with intravenous indomethacin in the premature neonate, renal clearance of aminoglycosides may be decreased, leading to increased plasma concentrations, elimination half-lives, and risk of aminoglycoside toxicity; dosage adjustment of aminoglycosides based on measurement of plasma concentrations and/or evidence of toxicity may also be required)

» Methoxyflurane or
» Polymyxins, parenteral

(concurrent and/or sequential use of these medications with aminoglycosides should be avoided since the potential for nephrotoxicity and/or neuromuscular blockade may be increased; neuromuscular blockade may result in skeletal muscle weakness and respiratory depression or paralysis [apnea]; caution is also recommended when methoxyflurane or polymyxins are used concurrently with aminoglycosides during surgery or in the postoperative period)

» Nephrotoxic medications, other (See *Appendix II*) or
» Ototoxic medications, other (See *Appendix II*)

(concurrent or sequential use of these medications with aminoglycosides may increase the potential for ototoxicity or nephrotoxicity; hearing loss may occur and may progress to deafness even after discontinuation of the drug and may be reversible, but usually is permanent; serial audiometric function determinations may be required with concurrent or sequential use of other ototoxic antibacterials; renal function determinations may be required)

(vancomycin and aminoglycosides must often be administered concurrently in the prophylaxis of bacterial endocarditis, in the treatment of endocarditis caused by streptococci and *Corynebacteria* species, in the treatment of resistant staphylococcal infections, or in penicillin-allergic patients; appropriate monitoring will help to reduce the risk of nephrotoxicity or ototoxicity; renal function determinations, serum aminoglycoside and vancomycin concentrations, dosage reductions, and/or dosage interval adjustments, or alternate antibacterials, may be required)

» Neuromuscular blocking agents or medications with neuromuscular blocking activity, other

(concurrent use of medications with neuromuscular blocking activity, including halogenated hydrocarbon inhalation anesthetics, opioid analgesics, and massive transfusions with citrate anticoagulated blood, with aminoglycosides should be carefully monitored since neuromuscular blockade may be enhanced, resulting in skeletal muscle weakness and respiratory depression or paralysis [apnea]; caution is recommended when these medications and aminoglycosides are used concurrently during surgery or in the postoperative period, especially if there is a possibility of incomplete reversal of neuromuscular blockade postoperatively; treatment with anticholinesterase agents or calcium salts may help reverse the blockade)

### Laboratory value alterations

The following have been selected on the basis of their potential clinical significance (possible effect in parentheses where appropriate)—not necessarily inclusive (» = major clinical significance):

With physiology/laboratory test values

Alanine aminotransferase (ALT [SGPT]), serum and
Alkaline phosphatase, serum and
Aspartate aminotransferase (AST [SGOT]), serum and
Bilirubin, serum and
Lactate dehydrogenase (LDH), serum
(values may be increased)

Blood urea nitrogen (BUN) and
Creatinine, serum
(concentrations may be increased)

Calcium, serum and
Magnesium, serum and
Potassium, serum and
Sodium, serum
(concentrations may be decreased)

### Medical considerations/Contraindications

The medical considerations/contraindications included have been selected on the basis of their potential clinical significance (reasons given in parentheses where appropriate)—not necessarily inclusive (» = major clinical significance).

*Risk-benefit should be considered when the following medical problems exist:*

» Botulism, infant or
» Myasthenia gravis or
» Parkinsonism

(aminoglycosides may cause neuromuscular blockade, resulting in further skeletal muscle weakness)

Dehydration or
» Renal function impairment

(possible increased risk of toxicity because of elevated serum concentrations; it is recommended that aminoglycosides be administered in a reduced dosage at a fixed interval, or in normal doses at prolonged intervals, to patients with impaired renal function)

» Eighth-cranial-nerve impairment

(aminoglycosides may cause auditory and vestibular toxicity)

» Previous allergic reaction to aminoglycosides
(hypersensitivity reaction to one aminoglycoside may contraindicate the use of other aminoglycosides due to known cross-sensitivity)

**Patient monitoring**

The following may be especially important in patient monitoring (other tests may be warranted in some patients, depending on condition; » = major clinical significance):

*For all aminoglycosides*

» Aminoglycoside concentrations, serum
(aminoglycoside levels should be monitored in all patients, especially neonates and the elderly, even without renal function impairment, to avoid potentially toxic concentrations from accumulation of the drug; peak levels should be drawn 30 minutes after a 30-minute aminoglycoside infusion, to allow for drug distribution, and trough levels, immediately prior to the next dose; see *General Dosing Information*)

» Audiograms and
» Renal function determinations and
» Vestibular function determinations
(may be required prior to, periodically during, and following treatment in patients with pre-existing renal or eighth-cranial-nerve impairment; twice-weekly or weekly audiometric testing to detect high-frequency hearing loss in patients old enough to be tested and daily renal function determinations may be required in patients on high-dose therapy or therapy continued for longer than 10 days, especially if renal function is changing; renal function determinations may be required to detect nephrotoxicity and to help prevent severe neurotoxic reactions; audiometric testing may also be required with concurrent or sequential administration of other ototoxic antibacterials; if renal, vestibular, or auditory function impairment occurs, reduction in dose or discontinuation of the aminoglycoside may be required)

» Urinalyses
(may be required prior to treatment and daily during treatment to detect albumin, casts, and cells in the urine, as well as decreased specific gravity)

*For streptomycin*

» Caloric stimulation tests
(may also be required prior to, periodically during, and following prolonged therapy to detect vestibular toxicity)

## Side/Adverse Effects

Note: Leg cramps, skin rash, fever, and seizures have been reported when gentamicin was administered concurrently by the systemic and intrathecal routes.

Neuromuscular blockade, respiratory paralysis, ototoxicity, and nephrotoxicity may occur following local irrigation and following topical application of aminoglycosides during surgery.

Because of its potential toxicity, use of parenteral neomycin is not recommended.

The following side/adverse effects have been selected on the basis of their potential clinical significance (possible signs and symptoms in parentheses where appropriate)—not necessarily inclusive:

**Those indicating need for medical attention**

Incidence more frequent
*Nephrotoxicity* (greatly increased or decreased frequency of urination or amount of urine; increased thirst; loss of appetite; nausea; vomiting); *neurotoxicity* (muscle twitching; numbness; seizures; tingling); *ototoxicity, auditory* (any loss of hearing; ringing or buzzing, or a feeling of fullness in the ears); *ototoxicity, vestibular* (clumsiness; dizziness; nausea; vomiting; unsteadiness); *peripheral neuritis* (burning of face or mouth; numbness; tingling)—streptomycin only

Incidence less frequent
*Hypersensitivity* (skin itching, redness, rash, or swelling); *optic neuritis* (any loss of vision)—streptomycin only

Incidence rare
*Neuromuscular blockade* (difficulty in breathing; drowsiness; weakness)

**Those indicating possible ototoxicity, vestibular toxicity, or nephrotoxicity and the need for medical attention if they occur and/or progress after medication is discontinued**

Any loss of hearing; clumsiness or unsteadiness; dizziness; greatly increased or decreased frequency of urination or amount of urine; increased thirst; loss of appetite; nausea or vomiting; ringing or buzzing or a feeling of fullness in the ears

## Overdose

For more information on the management of overdose or unintentional ingestion, **contact a Poison Control Center.** (See *Poison Control Center Listing.*)

**Treatment of overdose**

Specific treatment—

Hemodialysis or peritoneal dialysis to remove aminoglycosides from the blood of patients with impaired renal function.

Anticholinesterase agents, calcium salts, or mechanical respiratory assistance to treat neuromuscular blockade, resulting in prolonged skeletal muscle weakness and respiratory depression or paralysis (apnea), that may occur when two or more aminoglycosides are given concurrently.

Supportive care—Since there is no specific antidote, treatment of aminoglycoside overdose or toxic reactions should be symptomatic and supportive. Patients in whom intentional overdose is known or suspected should be referred for psychiatric consultation.

## Patient Consultation

As an aid to patient consultation, refer to *Advice for the Patient, Aminoglycosides (Systemic).*

In providing consultation, consider emphasizing the following selected information (» = major clinical significance):

**Before using this medication**

» Conditions affecting use, especially:
Hypersensitivity to aminoglycosides
Pregnancy—May be nephrotoxic in the fetus or cause irreversible deafness in children whose mothers received aminoglycosides during pregnancy
Use in children—Premature infants and neonates may be more susceptible to renal toxicity because of their immature renal capability
Use in the elderly—Geriatric patients may be at risk of renal toxicity because of an age-related decrease in renal function
Other medications, especially 2 or more aminoglycosides used together, capreomycin, other nephrotoxic or ototoxic medications, or other neuromuscular blocking agents
Other medical problems, especially eighth-cranial-nerve impairment, infant botulism, myasthenia gravis, parkinsonism, or renal function impairment

**Proper use of this medication**

» Importance of receiving medication for full course of therapy and on regular schedule
» Proper dosing

**Side/adverse effects**

Signs of potential side effects, especially hypersensitivity, optic neuritis, neuromuscular blockade, nephrotoxicity, neurotoxicity, auditory and vestibular ototoxicity, and peripheral neuritis, which are more likely to occur in children and the elderly

## General Dosing Information

Because of the low therapeutic index of aminoglycosides, it is best to base dosage calculations on ideal body weight (IBW) as follows:
IBW (males) = 50 kg + (2.3 kg × inches over 5 feet)
IBW (females) = 45 kg + (2.3 kg × inches over 5 feet)

Serum concentrations should be monitored, especially in neonates and the elderly, even without renal function impairment, and in patients with impaired renal function to ensure adequate concentrations and to avoid potentially toxic concentrations. Therapeutic concentrations are shown in the table below. Prolonged peak (post-distributional) concentrations (measured 15 to 30 minutes after injection) and trough concentrations (measured immediately prior to the next dose) greater than those shown below should be avoided.

| Drug | Therapeutic Concentration (mcg/mL) | Maximum Peak Concentration (mcg/mL) | Maximum Trough Concentration (mcg/mL) |
|---|---|---|---|
| Amikacin | 15–25 | 35 | 5 |
| Gentamicin | 4–10 | 10 | 2 |
| Kanamycin | 15–30 | 30–35 | 5 |
| Netilmicin | 6–12 | 16 | 2 |
| Streptomycin | — | 20–25 * | — |
| Tobramycin | 4–10 | 10 | 2 |

*In patients with renal damage. Peak concentrations greater than 50 mcg per mL are associated with increased risk of toxicity.

# Aminoglycosides (Systemic)

Because of their larger volume of distribution and reduced renal development, infants may require larger doses, given at less frequent intervals, for achievement of therapeutic serum concentrations. Cystic fibrosis patients and burn patients may also require larger doses, but because they eliminate the aminoglycoside faster than average, the dosing interval may need to be decreased too.

Serum concentrations should be used whenever possible to monitor aminoglycoside therapy. Creatinine clearance may be used to help monitor therapy, in conjunction with serum levels. Creatinine clearance (in mL per minute) may be calculated as follows:

Adult males: Creatinine clearance =
$[(140 - \text{age}) \times (\text{ideal body weight in kg})] / [72 \times \text{serum creatinine (mg per dL)}]$

Adult females: Creatinine clearance =
$[(140 - \text{age}) \times (\text{ideal body weight in kg})] / [72 \times \text{serum creatinine (mg per dL)}] \times 0.85$

Creatinine clearance may also be calculated in SI units (as mL per second) as follows:

Adult males: Creatinine clearance =
$[(140 - \text{age}) \times (\text{ideal body weight in kg})] / [50 \times \text{serum creatinine (micromoles per L)}]$

Adult females: Creatinine clearance =
$[(140 - \text{age}) \times (\text{ideal body weight in kg})] / [50 \times \text{serum creatinine (micromoles per L)}] \times 0.85$

The following dosing chart by Sarubbi and Hull (Ann Intern Med 1978; 89: 612-8) may be used to provide the clinician with an *initial* loading dose and maintenance dosage regimen in adult patients. *Further dosage adjustments should be individualized and based on peak and trough serum concentrations*, which should be drawn after the third maintenance dose.

1. Select loading dose based on the patient's ideal body weight (in mg per kg of body weight [mg/kg]) to provide peak serum concentration in the range listed below for the desired aminoglycoside.

| Aminoglycoside | Usual Loading Dose (mg/kg) | Expected Peak Serum Concentrations (mcg/mL) |
|---|---|---|
| Gentamicin Tobramycin | 1.5 to 2 | 4 to 10 |
| Amikacin Kanamycin | 5 to 7.5 | 15 to 30 |
| Netilmicin | 1.3 to 3.25 | 4 to 12 |

2. Select maintenance dose (as percentage of chosen loading dose) to maintain peak serum concentrations indicated above according to desired dosing interval and the patient's corrected creatinine clearance. This chart is not applicable to neonates and children.

| CrCl (mL/min)/ (mL/sec) | Half-life (hours) | 8 hours | 12 hours | 24 hours |
|---|---|---|---|---|
| 90/1.50 | 3.1 | 84% | — | — |
| 80/1.33 | 3.4 | 80 | 91% | — |
| 70/1.17 | 3.9 | 76 | 88 | — |
| 60/1.00 | 4.5 | 71 | 84 | — |
| 50/0.83 | 5.3 | 65 | 79 | — |
| 40/0.67 | 6.5 | 57 | 72 | 92% |
| 30/0.50 | 8.4 | 48 | 63 | 86 |
| 25/0.42 | 9.9 | 43 | 57 | 81 |
| 20/0.33 | 11.9 | 37 | 50 | 75 |
| 17/0.28 | 13.6 | 33 | 46 | 70 |
| 15/0.25 | 15.1 | 31 | 42 | 67 |
| 12/0.20 | 17.9 | 27 | 37 | 61 |
| 10*/0.17* | 20.4 | 24 | 34 | 56 |
| 7/0.12 | 25.9 | 19 | 28 | 47 |
| 5/0.08 | 31.5 | 16 | 23 | 41 |
| 2/0.03 | 46.8 | 11 | 16 | 30 |
| 0/0 | 69.3 | 8 | 11 | 21 |

*Dosing for patients with CrCl <10 mL/min (<0.17 mL/sec) should be assisted by measured serum levels.

After an initial full therapeutic loading dose, neonates or patients with impaired renal, vestibular, or auditory function may require (1) a reduction in the maintenance dose administered either (a) by administration of the usual dose at prolonged intervals or (b) by administration of reduced dose at fixed intervals or (2) discontinuation of the aminoglycoside. Since aminoglycosides are not metabolized and are excreted primarily in the urine, toxic concentrations may accumulate in patients with impaired renal function.

Because of the high concentrations of aminoglycosides in the urine and excretory system, patients should be well hydrated to prevent or minimize chemical irritation of the renal tubules. Therapeutic serum aminoglycoside levels are usually not needed to effectively treat urinary tract infections.

If a dose of this medication is missed, give it as soon as possible. However, if it is almost time for the next dose, skip the missed dose and go back to the regular dosing schedule. Do not double doses.

---

## AMIKACIN

## Additional Dosing Information

For initial dosing guidelines for patients with renal function impairment, see the Sarubbi and Hull nomogram in *General Dosing Information*.

Burn and certain other patients may require a dose of 5 to 7.5 mg per kg of body weight (mg/kg) every four to six hours because of the shorter half-life (1 to 1.5 hours) in these patients.

Amikacin sulfate injection may also be administered as an aerosol nebulization.

## Parenteral Dosage Forms

### AMIKACIN SULFATE INJECTION USP

**Usual adult and adolescent dose**
Antibacterial (systemic)—
  Intramuscular or intravenous infusion, 5 mg per kg of body weight every eight hours; or 7.5 mg per kg of body weight every twelve hours for seven to ten days.
Note: Urinary tract infections, bacterial (uncomplicated)—Intramuscular or intravenous infusion, 250 mg every twelve hours.
  Following hemodialysis, a supplemental dose of 3 to 5 mg per kg of body weight may be administered.

**Usual adult prescribing limits**
Up to 15 mg per kg of body weight daily, but not to exceed 1.5 grams daily for more than ten days.

**Usual pediatric dose**
Antibacterial (systemic):—
  Intramuscular or intravenous infusion:
    Premature neonates—
      Initially, 10 mg per kg of body weight, then 7.5 mg per kg of body weight every eighteen to twenty-four hours for seven to ten days.
    Neonates—
      Initially, 10 mg per kg of body weight, then 7.5 mg per kg of body weight every twelve hours for seven to ten days.
    Older infants and children—
      See *Usual adult and adolescent dose*.

**Strength(s) usually available**
U.S.—
  50 mg per mL (Rx) [*Amikin* (sodium bisulfite 0.13%); GENERIC].
  250 mg per mL (Rx) [*Amikin* (sodium bisulfite 0.66%); GENERIC].
Canada—
  250 mg per mL (Rx) [*Amikin* (sodium bisulfite 0.66%)].

**Packaging and storage**
Store below 40 °C (104 °F), preferably between 15 and 30 °C (59 and 86 °F), unless otherwise specified by manufacturer. Protect from freezing.

**Preparation of dosage form**
To prepare initial dilution for intravenous use, add the contents of each 500-mg vial to 100 to 200 mL of 0.9% sodium chloride injection, 5% dextrose injection, or other suitable diluent. The resulting solution should be administered slowly over a 30- to 60-minute period to help avoid neuromuscular blockade. Pediatric patients may require a proportionately smaller volume of diluent.

**Stability**
Intravenous infusions of amikacin retain their potency for 24 hours at room temperature at concentrations of 0.25 and 5 mg per mL in dextrose injection, dextrose and sodium chloride injection, 0.9% sodium chloride injection, lactated Ringer's injection, and other electrolyte-containing solutions (see manufacturer's package insert).

Intravenous infusions of amikacin retain their potency for 60 days at 4 °C (39 °F) at concentrations of 0.25 and 5 mg per mL in the above-listed diluents. When these solutions are then stored at 25 °C (77 °F), they retain their potency for 24 hours.

Intravenous infusions of amikacin retain their potency for 30 days when frozen at −15 °C (5 °F) at concentrations of 0.25 and 5 mg per mL in the above-listed diluents. When these solutions are thawed and stored at 25 °C (77 °F), they retain their potency for 24 hours.

Solutions may vary in color from colorless to light straw or very pale yellow; this variation does not affect their potency. Discard dark-colored solutions.

### Incompatibilities

Extemporaneous admixtures of beta-lactam antibacterials (penicillins and cephalosporins) and aminoglycosides may result in substantial mutual inactivation. If these groups of antibacterials are administered concurrently, they should be administered in separate sites. Do not mix them in the same intravenous bag or bottle.

Amikacin is incompatible with amphotericin B, cephalothin sodium, nitrofurantoin sodium, sulfadiazine sodium, and tetracyclines (in some solutions).

Since complexes form with a number of other drugs also, extemporaneous admixtures with Amikacin Sulfate Injection USP are not recommended.

### Additional information

Commercially available amikacin sulfate injection contains sodium bisulfite, an antioxidant, but no preservatives.

---

## GENTAMICIN

## Additional Dosing Information

Surgical, obstetrical, gynecological, or burn patients receiving gentamicin doses adjusted on the basis of serum concentrations may require less than the minimum recommended dose or greater than the maximum recommended dose of gentamicin because of wide interpatient variability. In patients receiving gentamicin intrathecally, CSF concentrations should also be monitored.

For initial dosing guidelines for patients with renal function impairment, see the Sarrubi and Hull nomogram in *General Dosing Information*.

Subcutaneous administration is not recommended and may be painful.

Commercially available gentamicin piggyback injections should be administered by intravenous infusion only.

Preservative-free gentamicin may also be administered directly into the subdural space, directly into the ventricles, or by means of an implanted reservoir.

Gentamicin sulfate injection may also be administered as an aerosol nebulization.

## Parenteral Dosage Forms

Note: The dosing and dosage forms available are expressed in terms of gentamicin base.

### GENTAMICIN SULFATE INJECTION USP

#### Usual adult and adolescent dose

Antibacterial (systemic)—
Intramuscular or intravenous infusion, 1 to 1.7 mg (base) per kg of body weight every eight hours for seven to ten days or more.
Note: Urinary tract infections, bacterial (uncomplicated)—Intramuscular or intravenous infusion:
Adults less than 60 kg of body weight—3 mg (base) per kg of body weight once a day; or 1.5 mg per kg of body weight every twelve hours.
Adults 60 kg of body weight and over—160 mg (base) once a day; or 80 mg every twelve hours.
Following hemodialysis, a supplemental dose of 1 to 1.7 mg (base) per kg of body weight may be administered, depending on the severity of the infection.
Intralumbar or intraventricular, 4 to 8 mg (base) once a day.

#### Usual adult prescribing limits

Up to 8 mg (base) per kg of body weight daily in severe, life-threatening infections.
Note: Doses up to 15 mg (base) per kg of body weight daily have been used in the treatment of intraocular infections.

#### Usual pediatric dose

Antibacterial (systemic)—
Intramuscular or intravenous infusion:
Premature or full-term neonates up to 1 week of age—
2.5 mg (base) per kg of body weight every twelve to twenty-four hours for seven to ten days or more.
Older neonates and infants—
2.5 mg (base) per kg of body weight every eight to sixteen hours for seven to ten days or more.
Children—
2 to 2.5 mg (base) per kg of body weight every eight hours for seven to ten days or more.
Note: The dosing interval of gentamicin in pediatric patients may vary from every four hours to every twenty-four hours, depending on the medical condition of the patient (cystic fibrosis, burns, renal dysfunction); serum levels must be monitored.
Following hemodialysis, a supplemental dose of 2 to 2.5 mg (base) per kg of body weight may be administered, depending on the severity of the infection.
Intralumbar or intraventricular:
Infants up to 3 months of age—
Dosage has not been established.
Infants and children 3 months of age and over—
1 to 2 mg (base) once a day.
Note: Doses up to 8 mg (base) daily have been used in infants with functioning ventricular shunts.

#### Strength(s) usually available

U.S.—
Intramuscular and intravenous:
10 mg per mL (base) (Rx) [*Garamycin* [GENERIC (sodium bisulfite 3.2 mg)].
40 mg per mL (base) (Rx) [*Garamycin; G-Mycin; Jenamicin* [GENERIC (sodium bisulfite 3.2 mg)].
Intrathecal:
2 mg per mL (base) (Rx) [*Garamycin*].
Canada—
Intramuscular and intravenous:
10 mg per mL (base) (Rx) [*Cidomycin* (sodium bisulfite 3.2 mg); *Garamycin* (sodium bisulfite)].
40 mg per mL (base) (Rx) [*Cidomycin* (sodium bisulfite 3.2 mg); *Garamycin* (sodium bisulfite)].

#### Packaging and storage

Store below 40 °C (104 °F), preferably between 15 and 30 °C (59 and 86 °F), unless otherwise specified by manufacturer. Protect from freezing.

#### Preparation of dosage form

Intravenous—To prepare initial dilution for intravenous use, add each dose to 50 to 200 mL of 0.9% sodium chloride injection or 5% dextrose injection to provide a concentration not exceeding 1 mg (base) per mL (0.1%). The resulting solution should be administered slowly over a 30- to 60-minute period to help decrease the chance of neuromuscular blockade. Pediatric patients may require a proportionately smaller volume of diluent.

Intralumbar and/or intraventricular (2 mg per mL)—To prepare initial dilution for intralumbar use, each dose should be drawn up into a 5- or 10-mL sterile syringe. Following lumbar puncture and the removal of a specimen of cerebrospinal fluid (CSF) for laboratory analysis, the syringe containing gentamicin is inserted into the hub of the spinal needle. A quantity of CSF equal to approximately 10% of the total estimated CSF volume is allowed to flow into the syringe and mix with the gentamicin. The resulting solution should be administered over a 3- to 5-minute period with the bevel of the spinal needle directed upward. Gentamicin may also be diluted with sodium chloride injection (without preservatives) if the CSF is grossly purulent or unobtainable. Since the 2-mg-per-mL concentration contains no preservatives, it should be used promptly after being opened; unused portions should be discarded.

#### Stability

Do not use if injection is discolored or contains a precipitate.

#### Incompatibilities

Extemporaneous admixtures of beta-lactam antibacterials (penicillins and cephalosporins) and aminoglycosides may result in substantial mutual inactivation. If these groups of antibacterials are administered concurrently, they should be administered in separate sites. Do not mix them in the same intravenous bag or bottle.

Since complexes form with a number of other drugs also, extemporaneous admixtures with Gentamicin Sulfate Injection USP are not recommended.

#### Additional information

Intrathecal gentamicin is commercially available as a preservative-free injection.

## GENTAMICIN SULFATE IN SODIUM CHLORIDE INJECTION

### Usual adult and adolescent dose
Antibacterial (systemic)—
  Intravenous infusion, 1 to 1.7 mg (base) per kg of body weight every eight hours for seven to ten days or more.
Note: Urinary tract infections, bacterial (uncomplicated)—Intravenous infusion:
  Adults less than 60 kg of body weight—3 mg (base) per kg of body weight once a day; or 1.5 mg per kg of body weight every twelve hours.
  Adults 60 kg of body weight and over—160 mg (base) once a day; or 80 mg every twelve hours.
  Following hemodialysis, a supplemental dose of 1 to 1.7 mg (base) per kg of body weight may be administered, depending on the severity of the infection.

### Usual adult prescribing limits
Up to 8 mg (base) per kg of body weight daily in severe, life-threatening infections.
Note: Doses up to 15 mg (base) per kg of body weight daily have been used in the treatment of intraocular infections.

### Usual pediatric dose
Antibacterial (systemic)—
  Intravenous infusion:
    Premature or full-term neonates up to 1 week of age—
      2.5 mg (base) per kg of body weight every twelve to twenty-four hours for seven to ten days or more.
    Older neonates and infants—
      2.5 mg (base) per kg of body weight every eight to sixteen hours for seven to ten days or more.
    Children—
      2 to 2.5 mg (base) per kg of body weight every eight hours for seven to ten days or more.
    Note: The dosing interval of gentamicin in pediatric patients may vary from every four hours to every twenty-four hours, depending on the medical conditions of the patient (cystic fibrosis, burns, renal dysfunction); serum levels must be monitored.
      Following hemodialysis, a supplemental dose of 2 to 2.5 mg (base) per kg of body weight may be administered, depending on the severity of the infection.

### Strength(s) usually available
U.S.—
  40 mg in 50 mL (base) (Rx) [GENERIC].
  40 mg in 100 mL (base) (Rx) [GENERIC].
  60 mg in 50 mL (base) (Rx) [GENERIC].
  60 mg in 100 mL (base) (Rx) [GENERIC].
  70 mg in 50 mL (base) (Rx) [GENERIC].
  80 mg in 50 mL (base) (Rx) [GENERIC].
  80 mg in 100 mL (base) (Rx) [GENERIC].
  90 mg in 100 mL (base) (Rx) [GENERIC].
  100 mg in 50 mL (base) (Rx) [GENERIC].
  100 mg in 100 mL (base) (Rx) [GENERIC].
  120 mg in 100 mL (base) (Rx) [GENERIC].
  160 mg in 100 mL (base) (Rx) [GENERIC].
  180 mg in 100 mL (base) (Rx) [GENERIC].
Canada—
  60 mg in 50 mL (base) (Rx) [GENERIC].
  70 mg in 50 mL (base) (Rx) [GENERIC].
  80 mg in 100 mL (base) (Rx) [GENERIC].

### Packaging and storage
Store between 2 and 30 °C (36 and 86 °F), unless otherwise specified by manufacturer. Protect from freezing.

### Preparation of dosage form
Commercially available gentamicin piggyback injections require no further dilution prior to administration (see manufacturer's labeling for instructions). Since these injections contain no preservatives, they should be used promptly after being opened; unused portions should be discarded.

### Stability
Do not use if injection is discolored or contains a precipitate.

### Incompatibilities
Extemporaneous admixtures of beta-lactam antibacterials (penicillins and cephalosporins) and aminoglycosides may result in substantial mutual inactivation. If these groups of antibacterials are administered concurrently, they should be administered in separate sites. Do not mix them in the same intravenous bag or bottle.

Since complexes form with a number of other drugs also, extemporaneous admixtures with gentamicin in sodium chloride injection are not recommended.

### Additional information
The sodium content is approximately 19.6 mEq (450 mg) per 50 mL. This must be considered in patients on a restricted sodium intake when calculating total daily sodium intake.

---

# KANAMYCIN

## Additional Dosing Information
For initial dosing guidelines for patients with renal function impairment, see the Sarubbi and Hull nomogram in *General Dosing Information*.
For intravenous use only:
  • Direct intravenous administration of undiluted kanamycin sulfate injection is not recommended because of the possibility of neuromuscular blockade.
For intramuscular use only:
  • Inject kanamycin sulfate injection deeply into the upper outer quadrant of the gluteal muscle.
For other routes:
  • Kanamycin sulfate injection may also be administered as an irrigation in a concentration of 0.25%.
  • Kanamycin sulfate injection may also be administered as an aerosol nebulization.
  • Kanamycin sulfate injection may also be administered intraperitoneally in a concentration of 2.5%.

## Parenteral Dosage Forms

### KANAMYCIN SULFATE INJECTION USP

#### Usual adult and adolescent dose
Antibacterial (systemic)—
  Inhalation treatment, 250 mg two to four times a day.
  Intramuscular, 3.75 mg per kg of body weight every six hours; 5 mg per kg of body weight every eight hours; or 7.5 mg per kg of body weight every twelve hours for seven to ten days.
  Intraperitoneal, 500 mg.
  Intravenous infusion, 5 mg per kg of body weight every eight hours; or 7.5 mg per kg of body weight every twelve hours for seven to ten days.

#### Usual adult prescribing limits
Up to 15 mg per kg of body weight daily, but not to exceed 1.5 grams daily.
Note: The total daily dose should take into account the amounts given by all routes, including intraperitoneal, inhalation, and irrigation. In intraocular infections, initial intramuscular doses of 2 grams, followed by 1 gram every twelve hours, have been used.

#### Usual pediatric dose
Antibacterial (systemic)—Intramuscular or intravenous infusion: See *Usual adult and adolescent dose*.
Note: Doses up to 30 mg per kg of body weight daily have been used in children.

#### Strength(s) usually available
U.S.—
  37.5 mg per mL (Rx) [*Kantrex*; GENERIC (sodium bisulfite 0.099%)].
  250 mg per mL (Rx) [*Kantrex*; GENERIC (sodium bisulfite 0.66%)].
  333.3 mg per mL (Rx) [*Kantrex*; GENERIC (sodium bisulfite 0.45%)].
Canada—
  Not commercially available.

#### Packaging and storage
Store below 40 °C (104 °F), preferably between 15 and 30 °C (59 and 86 °F), unless otherwise specified by manufacturer. Protect from freezing.

#### Preparation of dosage form
Intraperitoneal—To prepare dilution for intraperitoneal use, add the contents of each 500-mg vial to 20 mL of sterile water for injection. The resulting solution may be instilled postoperatively through a polyethylene catheter sutured into the wound at closure. To help prevent or minimize neuromuscular blockade, instillation of kanamycin should be postponed until the patient has fully recovered from the effects of anesthesia or neuromuscular blocking agents.
Intravenous—To prepare initial dilution for intravenous use, add the contents of each 500-mg vial to 100 to 200 mL or the contents of each 1-gram vial to 200 to 400 mL of 0.9% sodium chloride injection, 5% dextrose injection, or other suitable diluent. The resulting solution

should be administered over a 30- to 60-minute period. Pediatric patients may require a proportionately smaller volume of diluent.

**Stability**
Solutions may darken during storage; this darkening does not affect their potency.

**Incompatibilities**
Extemporaneous admixtures of beta-lactam antibacterials (penicillins and cephalosporins) and aminoglycosides may result in substantial mutual inactivation. If these groups of antibacterials are administered concurrently, they should be administered in separate sites. Do not mix them in the same intravenous bag or bottle.

Since complexes form with a number of other drugs also, extemporaneous admixtures with kanamycin sulfate injection are not recommended.

---

## NEOMYCIN

### STERILE NEOMYCIN SULFATE USP

Note: Parenteral neomycin has been replaced by safer and more effective agents. **Because of its potential toxicity, the parenteral use of neomycin is not recommended for any indication.**

**Size(s) usually available:**
U.S.—
  500 mg (Rx) [GENERIC].
Canada—
  Not commercially available.

---

## NETILMICIN

## Additional Dosing Information

Serum concentrations of netilmicin in febrile patients may be lower than in afebrile patients receiving the same dose because of shorter half-life. The half-life may also be shorter in anemic patients. However, when the body temperature returns to normal in febrile patients, serum concentrations may increase. Dosage adjustments are not usually necessary.

For initial dosing guidelines for patients with renal function impairment, see the Sarubbi and Hull nomogram in *General Dosing Information*.

In severely burned patients, serum concentrations of netilmicin may be lower than expected from a particular dose. Serum determinations are especially important in these patients for dosage adjustment.

## Parenteral Dosage Forms

Note: The dosing and dosage forms available are expressed in terms of netilmicin base.

### NETILMICIN SULFATE INJECTION USP

**Usual adult and adolescent dose**
Antibacterial (systemic)—
  Intramuscular or intravenous:
    Systemic infections (serious):
      1.3 to 2.2 mg (base) per kg of body weight every eight hours; or 2 to 3.25 mg (base) per kg of body weight every twelve hours for seven to fourteen days.
    Urinary tract infections, bacterial (complicated):
      1.5 to 2 mg (base) per kg of body weight every twelve hours for seven to fourteen days.
Note: Following hemodialysis, a supplemental dose of 1 mg (base) per kg of body weight may be administered.

**Usual adult prescribing limits**
Up to 7.5 mg (base) per kg of body weight daily.
Note: Doses up to 12 mg(base) per kg of body weight daily have been used in cystic fibrosis patients.

**Usual pediatric dose**
Antibacterial (systemic)—
  Intramuscular or intravenous:
    Neonates up to 6 weeks of age—
      2 to 3.25 mg (base) per kg of body weight every twelve hours for seven to fourteen days.
    Infants and children 6 weeks to 12 years of age—
      1.83 to 2.67 mg (base) per kg of body weight every eight hours; or 2.75 to 4 mg (base) per kg of body weight every twelve hours for seven to fourteen days.

**Strength(s) usually available**
U.S.—
  100 mg per mL (base) (Rx) [*Netromycin* (benzyl alcohol 10 mg, sodium metabisulfite 2.4 mg, sodium sulfite 0.8 mg)].

Canada—
  25 mg per mL (base) (Rx) [*Netromycin* (sodium metabisulfite 2.1 mg, sodium sulfite 1.2 mg)].
  50 mg per mL (base) (Rx) [*Netromycin* (sodium metabisulfite 2.1 mg, sodium sulfite 1.2 mg)].
  100 mg per mL (base) (Rx) [*Netromycin* (benzyl alcohol 10 mg, sodium metabisulfite 2.4 mg, sodium sulfite 0.8 mg)].

**Packaging and storage**
Store below 40 °C (104 °F), preferably between 15 and 30 °C (59 and 86 °F), unless otherwise specified by manufacturer. Protect from freezing.

**Preparation of dosage form**
To prepare initial dilution for intravenous use, each dose should be diluted in 50 to 200 mL of a suitable diluent (see manufacturer's package insert). The resulting solution should be administered slowly over a 30- to 60-minute period to help avoid neuromuscular blockade. Pediatric patients may require a proportionately smaller volume of diluent.

**Stability**
Intravenous infusions of netilmicin retain their potency for up to 72 hours at room temperature or when refrigerated and stored in glass containers at concentrations of 2.1 to 3 mg per mL in suitable diluents (see manufacturer's package insert).

**Incompatibilities**
Extemporaneous admixtures of beta-lactam antibacterials (penicillins and cephalosporins) and aminoglycosides may result in substantial mutual inactivation. If these groups of antibacterials are administered concurrently, they should be administered in separate sites. Do not mix them in the same intravenous bag or bottle.

---

## STREPTOMYCIN

## Summary of Differences

Indications: Used for the treatment of brucellosis, granuloma inguinale, plague, tuberculosis, and tularemia.
Pregnancy/Reproduction: Has been shown to cause deafness in humans.
Patient monitoring: Caloric stimulation tests may also be required.

## Additional Dosing Information

Tuberculosis therapy may have to be continued for 1 to 2 years, and may even be required for up to several years or indefinitely, although in some patients shorter treatment regimens may also be effective. However, streptomycin should be discontinued when toxicity or toxic symptoms appear or are impending, when organisms have become resistant, or when the full therapeutic effect has been achieved.

Injection sites should be alternated and concentrations greater than 500 mg per mL are not recommended.

## Parenteral Dosage Forms

Note: The dosing and dosage forms available are expressed in terms of streptomycin base.

### STREPTOMYCIN SULFATE INJECTION USP

**Usual adult and adolescent dose**
Antibacterial (antimycobacterial)—
  Tuberculosis:
    Intramuscular:
      In combination with other antimycobacterials, 1 gram (base) once a day. Dosage should be reduced to 1 gram two or three times a week as soon as clinically feasible.
Antibacterial (systemic)—
  Other infections:
    Intramuscular:
      In combination with other antibacterials, 250 mg to 1 gram (base) every six hours; or 500 mg to 2 grams every twelve hours.
Note: Plague—Intramuscular: 500 mg to 1 gram (base) every six hours; or 1 to 2 grams every twelve hours.
  Tularemia—Intramuscular: 250 to 500 mg (base) every six hours; or 500 mg to 1 gram every twelve hours for seven to ten days.

**Usual adult prescribing limits**
Tuberculosis—
  1 gram twice weekly to 2 grams (base) daily.
Other infections—
  Up to 4 grams (base) daily.

# Aminoglycosides (Systemic)

**Usual pediatric dose**
Antibacterial (antimycobacterial)—
  Tuberculosis:
    Intramuscular—
      In combination with other antimycobacterials, 20 mg (base) per kg of body weight once a day. Maximum dose per day should not exceed 1 gram.
Antibacterial (systemic)—
  Other infections:
    Intramuscular—
      In combination with other antibacterials, 5 to 10 mg (base) per kg of body weight every six hours; or 10 to 20 mg per kg of body weight every twelve hours.

**Usual geriatric dose**
Antibacterial (antimycobacterial)—
  Tuberculosis:
    Intramuscular—
      In combination with other antimycobacterials, 500 to 750 mg (base) once a day.

**Strength(s) usually available**
U.S.—
  Not commercially available.
Canada—
  500 mg per mL (base) (Rx) [GENERIC].

**Packaging and storage**
Store below 40 °C (104 °F), preferably between 15 and 30 °C (59 and 86 °F), unless otherwise specified by manufacturer. Protect from freezing.

**Stability**
Solutions may vary in color from colorless to yellow and may darken on exposure to light. This variation does not affect their potency.
Solutions should not be autoclaved since loss of potency may result.

## STERILE STREPTOMYCIN SULFATE USP

**Usual adult and adolescent dose**
Antibacterial (antimycobacterial)—
  Tuberculosis:
    Intramuscular:
      In combination with other antimycobacterials, 1 gram (base) once a day. Dosage should be reduced to 1 gram two or three times a week as soon as clinically feasible.
Antibacterial (systemic)—
  Other infections:
    Intramuscular:
      In combination with other antibacterials, 250 mg to 1 gram (base) every six hours; or 500 mg to 2 grams every twelve hours.
Note: Plague—Intramuscular: 500 mg to 1 gram (base) every six hours; or 1 to 2 grams every twelve hours.
      Tularemia—Intramuscular: 250 to 500 mg (base) every six hours; or 500 mg to 1 gram every twelve hours for seven to ten days.

**Usual adult prescribing limits**
Tuberculosis—
  1 gram twice weekly to 2 grams (base) daily.
Other infections—
  Up to 4 grams (base) daily.

**Usual pediatric dose**
Antibacterial (antimycobacterial)—
  Tuberculosis:
    Intramuscular—
      In combination with other antimycobacterials, 20 mg (base) per kg of body weight once a day. Maximum dose per day should not exceed 1 gram.
Antibacterial (systemic)—
  Other infections:
    Intramuscular—
      In combination with other antibacterials, 5 to 10 mg (base) per kg of body weight every six hours; or 10 to 20 mg per kg of body weight every twelve hours.

**Size(s) usually available:**
U.S.—
  1 gram (base) (Rx) [GENERIC].
Canada—
  Not commercially available.

**Packaging and storage**
Prior to reconstitution, store below 40 °C (104 °F), preferably between 15 and 30 °C (59 and 86 °F), unless otherwise specified by manufacturer.

**Preparation of dosage form**
To prepare initial dilution for intramuscular use, add 4.2 to 4.5 mL of 0.9% sodium chloride injection or sterile water for injection to each 1-gram vial, according to the manufacturer, to provide a concentration of 200 mg (base) per mL or 3.2 to 3.5 mL of diluent to provide a concentration of 250 mg per mL; and add 17 mL of diluent to each 5-gram vial to provide a concentration of 250 mg per mL or 6.5 mL of diluent to provide a concentration of 500 mg per mL.

**Stability**
After reconstitution, solutions retain their potency for 2 to 28 days at room temperature or for 14 days if refrigerated, depending on manufacturer.

---

## TOBRAMYCIN

### Summary of Differences
Pregnancy/Reproduction: Has been shown to cause deafness in humans.

### Additional Dosing Information
Commercially available tobramycin piggyback injections should be administered by intravenous infusion only.
Tobramycin sulfate injection may also be administered as an aerosol nebulization.

### Parenteral Dosage Forms
Note: The dosing and dosage forms available are expressed in terms of tobramycin base.

### TOBRAMYCIN SULFATE INJECTION USP

**Usual adult and adolescent dose**
Antibacterial (systemic)—
  Intramuscular or intravenous infusion, 0.75 mg to 1.25 mg (base) per kg of body weight every six hours; or 1 to 1.7 mg per kg of body weight every eight hours for seven to ten days or more.

**Usual adult prescribing limits**
Up to 8 mg (base) per kg of body weight daily in severe, life-threatening infections.

**Usual pediatric dose**
Antibacterial (systemic)—
  Intramuscular or intravenous infusion:
    Premature or full-term neonates up to 1 week of age—
      Up to 2 mg (base) per kg of body weight every twelve to twenty-four hours.
    Older infants and children—
      1.5 to 1.9 mg (base) per kg of body weight every six hours; or 2 to 2.5 mg per kg of body weight every eight to sixteen hours.
Note: The dosing interval of tobramycin in pediatric patients may vary from every four hours to every twenty-four hours, depending on the medical condition of the patient (cystic fibrosis, burns, renal dysfunction); serum levels must be monitored.

**Strength(s) usually available**
U.S.—
  10 mg per mL (base) (Rx) [Nebcin (sodium bisulfite 3.2 mg); GENERIC].
  20 mg per mL (base) (Rx) [GENERIC].
  40 mg per mL (base) (Rx) [Nebcin (sodium bisulfite 3.2 mg); GENERIC].
  60 mg per mL (base) (Rx) [GENERIC].
  80 mg per mL (base) (Rx) [GENERIC].
Canada—
  10 mg per mL (base) (Rx) [Nebcin (sodium bisulfite)].
  40 mg per mL (base) (Rx) [Nebcin (sodium bisulfite)].

**Packaging and storage**
Store below 40 °C (104 °F), preferably between 15 and 30 °C (59 and 86 °F), unless otherwise specified by manufacturer. Protect from freezing.

**Preparation of dosage form**
To prepare initial dilution for intravenous use, add each dose to 50 to 200 mL of 0.9% sodium chloride injection or 5% dextrose injection to provide a concentration not exceeding 1 mg (base) per mL (0.1%). The resulting solution should be administered slowly over a 30- to 60-minute period to avoid neuromuscular blockade. In addition, infusion periods of less than 20 minutes are not recommended since peak serum concentrations may exceed 12 mcg per mL. Pediatric patients may require a proportionately smaller volume of diluent.

### Incompatibilities
Extemporaneous admixtures of beta-lactam antibacterials (penicillins and cephalosporins) and aminoglycosides may result in substantial mutual inactivation. If these groups of antibacterials are administered concurrently, they should be administered in separate sites. Do not mix them in the same intravenous bag or bottle.

Since complexes form with a number of other drugs also, extemporaneous admixtures with tobramycin sulfate injection are not recommended.

### Additional information
Subcutaneous administration is not recommended and may be painful.

## STERILE TOBRAMYCIN SULFATE USP

### Usual adult and adolescent dose
Antibacterial (systemic)—
  Intravenous infusion, 0.75 mg to 1.25 mg (base) per kg of body weight every six hours; or 1 to 1.7 mg per kg of body weight every eight hours for seven to ten days or more.

### Usual adult prescribing limits
Up to 8 mg (base) per kg of body weight daily in severe, life-threatening infections.

### Usual pediatric dose
Antibacterial (systemic)—
  Intravenous infusion:
    Premature or full-term neonates up to 1 week of age—
      Up to 2 mg (base) per kg of body weight every twelve to twenty-four hours.
    Older infants and children—
      1.5 to 1.9 mg (base) per kg of body weight every six hours; or 2 to 2.5 mg per kg of body weight every eight to sixteen hours.
  Note: The dosing interval of tobramycin in pediatric patients may vary from every four hours to every twenty-four hours, depending on the medical condition of the patient (cystic fibrosis, burns, renal dysfunction); serum levels must be monitored.

### Size(s) usually available
U.S.—
  1.2 grams (base) (Rx) [*Nebcin;* GENERIC].
Canada—
  1.2 grams (base) (Rx) [*Nebcin*].

### Packaging and storage
Prior to reconstitution, store below 40 °C (104 °F), preferably between 15 and 30 °C (59 and 86 °F), unless otherwise specified by manufacturer.

### Preparation of dosage form
To prepare initial dilution for intravenous use, add 30 mL of sterile water for injection to each 1.2-gram vial to provide 40 mg (base) per mL. Withdraw each dose from the pharmacy bulk vial and add it to 50 to 200 mL of 0.9% sodium chloride injection or 5% dextrose injection to provide a final concentration not exceeding 1 mg per mL (0.1%). The resulting solution should be administered slowly over a 30- to 60-minute period to avoid neuromuscular blockade. In addition, infusion periods of less than 20 minutes are not recommended since peak serum concentrations may exceed 12 mcg per mL. Pediatric patients may require a proportionately smaller volume of diluent.

### Stability
After reconstitution, solutions retain their potency for 24 hours at room temperature or for 96 hours if refrigerated.

### Incompatibilities
Extemporaneous admixtures of beta-lactam antibacterials (penicillins and cephalosporins) and aminoglycosides may result in substantial mutual inactivation. If these groups of antibacterials are administered concurrently, they should be administered in separate sites. Do not mix them in the same intravenous bag or bottle.

Since complexes form with a number of other drugs also, extemporaneous admixtures with Sterile Tobramycin Sulfate USP are not recommended.

### Additional information
Sterile Tobramycin Sulfate USP is available only in a pharmacy bulk vial (multiple-dose) and is intended for use in the extemporaneous preparation of intravenous admixtures.

## TOBRAMYCIN SULFATE IN SODIUM CHLORIDE INJECTION

### Usual adult and adolescent dose
See *Tobramycin Sulfate Injection USP*.

### Usual adult prescribing limits
See *Tobramycin Sulfate Injection USP*.

### Usual pediatric dose
See *Tobramycin Sulfate Injection USP*.

### Strength(s) usually available
U.S.—
  60 mg in 50 mL (base) (Rx) [GENERIC].
  80 mg in 100 mL (base) (Rx) [GENERIC].
Canada—
  Not commercially available.

### Packaging and storage
Store between 2 and 30 °C (36 and 86 °F), unless otherwise specified by manufacturer. Protect from freezing.

### Preparation of dosage form
Commercially available tobramycin piggyback injections require no further dilution prior to administration (see manufacturer's labeling for instructions).

### Stability
Do not use if injection is discolored or contains a precipitate.

### Incompatibilities
Extemporaneous admixtures of beta-lactam antibacterials (penicillins and cephalosporins) and aminoglycosides may result in substantial mutual inactivation. If these groups of antibacterials are administered concurrently, they should be administered in separate sites. Do not mix them in the same intravenous bag or bottle.

Since complexes form with a number of other drugs also, extemporaneous admixtures with tobramycin in sodium chloride injection are not recommended.

### Additional information
The sodium content is approximately 19.6 mEq (450 mg) per 50 mL. This must be considered in patients on a restricted sodium intake when calculating total daily sodium intake.

Revised: 02/23/93
Interim revision: 04/24/95; 06/20/95

---

**AMINOPHYLLINE**—See *Bronchodilators, Theophylline (Systemic)*

---

**AMINOSALICYLATE SODIUM**—The *Aminosalicylate Sodium (Systemic)* monograph is not included in this published version of the USP DI database. Copies of the monograph are available on request from Micromedex, Inc. - Reprint Requests, 6200 S. Syracuse Way, Suite 300, Englewood, CO 80111; telephone (303) 486-6400; telefax (303) 486-6464; Email: USPDI@MDX.COM.

---

# AMIODARONE Systemic

VA CLASSIFICATION (Primary): CV300
Commonly used brand name(s): *Cordarone; Cordarone I.V.; Cordarone Intravenous.*
Note: For a listing of dosage forms and brand names by country availability, see *Dosage Forms* section(s).

## Category
Antiarrhythmic.

## Indications
Note: Bracketed information in the *Indications* section refers to uses that are not included in U.S. product labeling.

### Accepted
Arrhythmias, ventricular (prophylaxis and treatment)—Amiodarone in the oral dosage form is indicated only for the treatment of recurrent hemodynamically unstable ventricular tachycardia and recurrent ventricular fibrillation unresponsive to documented adequate doses of other available antiarrhythmic medications or when alternative agents cannot be tolerated. In patients for whom the oral form of amiodarone is in-

dicated, but who are unable to take oral medication, the intravenous form of amiodarone may be used.

Amiodarone in the intravenous dosage form is indicated for the initiation of treatment (acute treatment) and prophylaxis of frequently recurring ventricular fibrillation and hemodynamically unstable ventricular tachycardia in patients refractory to other therapy.

[Arrhythmias, supraventricular (prophylaxis and treatment)][1]—Amiodarone is used to suppress and prevent recurrence of supraventricular arrhythmias refractory to conventional treatment, especially when associated with Wolff-Parkinson-White (W-P-W) syndrome, including paroxysmal atrial fibrillation, atrial flutter, ectopic atrial tachycardia, and paroxysmal supraventricular tachycardia from both atrioventricular (AV) nodal re-entrant and AV re-entrant tachycardia in patients with W-P-W syndrome.

Note: Controlled clinical trials have not demonstrated that the use of amiodarone improves patient survival.

[1] Not included in Canadian product labeling.

## Pharmacology/Pharmacokinetics

### Physicochemical characteristics
Molecular weight—681.8.
pKa—5.6.
Other—Contains 37.3% iodine by weight; highly lipophilic.

### Mechanism of action/Effect
Amiodarone prolongs the action potential duration and the refractory period in all cardiac tissues (including the sinus node, atrium, atrioventricular [AV] node, and ventricle) by a direct action on the tissues, without significantly affecting the membrane potential. Amiodarone also decreases sinus node automaticity and junctional automaticity, prolongs AV conduction, and slows automaticity of spontaneously firing fibers in the Purkinje system. Refractoriness is prolonged and conduction is slowed in accessory pathway tissue in patients with Wolff-Parkinson-White (W-P-W) syndrome. Noncompetitive alpha- and beta-adrenergic receptor antagonism and calcium channel inhibition also occur and thyroid hormone metabolism is affected, but the relationship of these effects to the antiarrhythmic action of amiodarone is unknown. In the Vaughan Williams classification of antiarrhythmics, amiodarone is considered to be a predominantly class III agent, with some class I properties.

### Other actions/effects
Amiodarone has a mild negative inotropic effect that is more prominent with intravenous than with oral administration but that usually does not depress left ventricular function. Amiodarone causes coronary and peripheral vasodilation and, therefore, decreases peripheral vascular resistance (afterload) but only causes hypotension with large oral doses.

### Absorption
Slow and variable; about 20 to 55% of an oral dose is absorbed.

### Distribution
Volume of distribution is large and variable, a consequence of extensive accumulation in adipose tissue and highly perfused organs (liver, lung, spleen), and leads to slow achievement of steady-state and therapeutic plasma concentrations and prolonged elimination.

### Protein binding
Very high (96%).

### Biotransformation
Hepatic, extensive; one active metabolite (desethylamiodarone); possibly also by deiodination (a dose of 300 mg releases approximately 9 mg of elemental iodine).

### Half-life
Elimination (biphasic)—
  Initial:
    Amiodarone—2.5 to 10 days.
  Terminal:
    Amiodarone—26 to 107 days (mean 53 days; 40 to 55 days in most patients).
    Desethylamiodarone—Mean 61 days.

### Onset of antiarrhythmic action
2 to 3 days to 2 to 3 months, even with loading doses.

### Time to peak plasma concentration
3 to 7 hours.

### Therapeutic plasma concentration
1 to 2.5 mcg (0.001 to 0.0025 mg) per mL at steady-state (after 2 months of therapy). However, antiarrhythmic effect is difficult to predict by means of plasma concentrations, and toxicity may occur even at therapeutic concentrations.

### Elimination
Biliary.
In breast milk—About 25% of maternal dose is distributed into breast milk.
In dialysis—Not removable by hemodialysis.

## Precautions to Consider

### Carcinogenicity/Tumorigenicity
Studies in rats at doses one-half the maximum recommended human maintenance dose and greater found a dose-related increase in the incidence of thyroid follicular adenomas and/or carcinomas.

### Mutagenicity
Mutagenicity studies (Ames, micronucleus, and lysogenic tests) with amiodarone were negative.

### Pregnancy/Reproduction
Fertility—Studies in male and female rats at doses eight times the maximum recommended human maintenance dose found that amiodarone reduced fertility.

Pregnancy—Amiodarone crosses the placenta; neonatal plasma concentrations of amiodarone and desethylamiodarone are 10% and 25% of maternal plasma concentrations, respectively. Although studies in humans have not been done, some reports have indicated an absence of adverse effects when amiodarone was administered late in pregnancy. However, amiodarone can cause fetal harm when administered to pregnant women. Potential adverse effects include bradycardia and effects on thyroid status (iodine is known to cause fetal goiter, hypothyroidism, and mental retardation) in the neonate. There have been a small number of reports of congenital goiter/hypothyroidism and hyperthyroidism.

Studies in rats and one strain of mice at doses 18 times and one half the maximum recommended human maintenance dose, respectively, have shown that amiodarone is embryotoxic. Amiodarone was not embryotoxic in a second strain of mice or in rabbits at doses up to nine times the maximum recommended human maintenance dose.

FDA Pregnancy Category D.

Labor and delivery—Although studies in humans have not been done, studies in rodents found no adverse effects of amiodarone on duration of gestation or on parturition.

### Breast-feeding
Amiodarone is distributed into human breast milk. The infant receives approximately 25% of the maternal dose. Amiodarone has been shown to cause reduced viability and growth of offspring when used in lactating rats. Mothers should be advised to contact physician before nursing, since use by nursing mothers is not recommended.

### Pediatrics
Appropriate studies on the relationship of age to the effects of amiodarone have not been performed in the pediatric population. However, when amiodarone was used concurrently with digoxin, the interaction has been reported to be more acute in children than in adults. In addition, onset and duration of action of amiodarone may be shorter in pediatric patients.

### Geriatrics
Appropriate studies on the relationship of age to the effects of amiodarone have not been performed in the geriatric population. However, the elderly tend to be more sensitive to the effects of thyroid hormones and may also, therefore, be more sensitive to the effects of amiodarone on thyroid function. Thyroid function monitoring is particularly important in these patients. In addition, the elderly may experience an increased incidence of ataxia and other neurotoxic effects.

### Drug interactions and/or related problems
The following drug interactions and/or related problems have been selected on the basis of their potential clinical significance (possible mechanism in parentheses where appropriate)—not necessarily inclusive (» = major clinical significance):

Note: Because of its slow elimination, amiodarone may interact with other medications for weeks to months after it is discontinued.

Combinations containing any of the following medications, depending on the amount present, may also interact with this medication.

Anesthetics, inhalation
  (amiodarone may potentiate hypotension and atropine-resistant bradycardia)

» Antiarrhythmics, other
  (amiodarone may produce additive cardiac effects with other antiarrhythmics and increase the risk of tachyarrhythmias; amiodarone increases plasma concentrations of quinidine, procainamide, flecainide, and phenytoin; concurrent use of amiodarone with quinidine, disopyramide, procainamide, or mexiletine has been reported to result in a more prolonged QT interval and, rarely, *torsades de*

*pointes*, and therefore, concurrent use with all class I antiarrhythmics requires great caution; the doses of previously given antiarrhythmics should be reduced by 30 to 50% several days after initiation of amiodarone therapy and gradually withdrawn; if antiarrhythmic therapy is needed in addition to amiodarone, it should be initiated at one half the usual recommended dose)

» Anticoagulants, coumarin-derivative
(amiodarone inhibits metabolism and potentiates the anticoagulant effect, beginning as early as 4 to 6 days after initiation of amiodarone therapy and persisting as long as weeks or months after it is withdrawn; prothrombin times may double or triple, but effect is very erratic; it is recommended that the dose of anticoagulant be reduced by one third to one half and that prothrombin times be monitored closely)

Beta-adrenergic blocking agents or
Calcium channel blocking agents
(amiodarone may cause potentiation of bradycardia, sinus arrest, and atrioventricular [AV] block, especially in patients with underlying sinus function impairment. If this occurs, dosage reduction of amiodarone or the beta-blocking agent or calcium channel blocking agent is recommended; in some cases, amiodarone therapy may be continued after insertion of a pacemaker)

» Digitalis glycosides
(amiodarone increases serum concentrations of digoxin and probably other digitalis glycosides, possibly to toxic levels; when amiodarone therapy is initiated, the digitalis glycoside should be withdrawn or the dose reduced by 50%; if digitalis glycoside therapy is continued, serum concentrations should be carefully monitored; amiodarone and digitalis glycosides may also produce additive effects on sinoatrial [SA] and AV nodes)

Diuretics, loop or
Diuretics, thiazide or
Indapamide
(concurrent use of amiodarone with potassium-depleting diuretics may lead to an increased risk of arrhythmias associated with hypokalemia)

» Phenytoin
(amiodarone may increase plasma concentrations of phenytoin, resulting in increased effects and/or toxicity)

Photosensitizing medications, other
(concurrent use with amiodarone may cause additive photosensitizing effects)

Sodium iodide I 123 or
Sodium iodide I 131 or
Sodium pertechnetate Tc 99m
(thyroidal uptake may be inhibited by amiodarone)

**Laboratory value alterations**
The following have been selected on the basis of their potential clinical significance (possible effect in parentheses where appropriate)—not necessarily inclusive (» = major clinical significance):

With physiology/laboratory test values
Alanine aminotransferase (ALT [SGPT]) and
Alkaline phosphatase and
Aspartate aminotransferase (AST [SGOT])
(serum values are commonly increased; hepatotoxicity is rare)

Antinuclear antibody (ANA) titer concentration
(may be increased but usually not symptomatic; elevated concentrations may be associated with pulmonary toxicity)

Electrocardiogram (ECG) changes, such as:
PR prolongation and
QRS widening, slight and
QT prolongation and
T-wave amplitude reduction with T-wave widening and bifurcation and
U-wave development
(occur in most patients; QT prolongation may in some cases be associated with worsening of arrhythmias)

Thyroid function changes, such as
Free and total serum thyroxine ($T_4$) concentrations
(may be increased)

Free and total serum triiodothyronine ($T_3$) concentrations
(may be decreased)

Serum reverse $T_3$ ($rT_3$) concentrations
(may be increased)

Serum thyroid-stimulating hormone (TSH) concentrations
(may be increased initially; increase in TSH with continued amiodarone treatment, along with a decrease in $T_3$, is the determining sign of hypothyroidism)

Note: Amiodarone inhibits peripheral conversion of $T_4$ to $T_3$, leading to increased serum $T_4$ and $rT_3$ and a slight decrease in serum $T_3$.

Thyroid function abnormalities may persist for several weeks or months after withdrawal of amiodarone.

**Medical considerations/Contraindications**
The medical considerations/contraindications included have been selected on the basis of their potential clinical significance (reasons given in parentheses where appropriate)—not necessarily inclusive (» = major clinical significance).

*Except under special circumstances, this medication should not be used when the following medical problems exist:*

» Atrioventricular (AV) block, pre-existing 2nd or 3rd degree, without pacemaker
(risk of complete heart block)

» Bradycardic episodes resulting in syncope, unless controlled by pacemaker, or

» Sinus node function impairment, severe, causing marked sinus bradycardia, unless controlled by pacemaker
(amiodarone reduces sinus node automaticity and may cause atropine-resistant sinus bradycardia)

» Hypersensitivity to amiodarone

*Risk-benefit should be considered when the following medical problems exist:*

Congestive heart failure
(mild negative inotropic effect of amiodarone usually does not cause problems; hemodynamic deterioration may occur secondary to sympatholytic blockage of augmented sympathetic drive)

Hepatic function impairment
(reduced metabolism; lower doses may be required)

Hypokalemia
(amiodarone may be ineffective or arrhythmogenic; should be corrected prior to initiation of amiodarone therapy)

Thyroid function impairment, including goiter or nodules
(increased risk of hypothyroidism or hyperthyroidism)

Caution is recommended also during open-heart surgery in patients receiving amiodarone because of the risk of hypotension upon discontinuation of cardiopulmonary bypass.

**Patient monitoring**
The following may be especially important in patient monitoring (other tests may be warranted in some patients, depending on condition; » = major clinical significance):

» Alanine aminotransferase (ALT [SGPT]) and
» Alkaline phosphatase and
» Aspartate aminotransferase (AST [SGOT])
(serum value determinations recommended at regular intervals, especially in patients receiving high maintenance doses; dosage reduction of amiodarone is recommended if concentrations increase to three times normal or double in patients with elevated baseline concentrations, or if hepatomegaly occurs)

Auscultation of the chest
(recommended at periodic intervals; presence of rales, decreased breath sounds, or pleuritic friction rub may indicate pulmonary toxicity)

Bronchoscopy with lung biopsy
(may be useful if symptoms of pulmonary toxicity occur that cannot be diagnosed from a chest x-ray)

Chest x-ray
(recommended prior to initiation of therapy and at 3- to 6-month intervals during therapy to detect diffuse interstitial changes or alveolar infiltrates associated with pulmonary toxicity)

» ECG
(continuous Holter monitoring may assist in assessing efficacy and adjusting dosage; usefulness of programmed electrical stimulation in clinical management is controversial, although it may be useful for predicting efficacy of amiodarone)

Gallium radionuclide scan
(may be useful if symptoms of pulmonary toxicity occur that cannot be diagnosed from a chest x-ray; may show marked uptake in the lung)

Ophthalmologic examinations
(slit-lamp examinations recommended prior to initiation of therapy and if symptoms of ocular toxicity occur)

Plasma amiodarone determinations
(may be useful in dosage adjustment or to assess lack of response or unexpectedly severe toxicity, although correlation does not always occur, especially within first 2 months of therapy)

Pulmonary function determinations, including diffusion capacity and total lung capacity
(recommended prior to initiation of amiodarone therapy and if symptoms of pulmonary toxicity occur that cannot be diagnosed from a chest x-ray)

» Thyroid function determinations
(because amiodarone can cause either hypothyroidism or hyperthyroidism, it is recommended that thyroid function be monitored prior to initiation of and at periodic intervals during amiodarone therapy, especially in patients with a history of thyroid nodules, goiter, or other thyroid dysfunction and in patients who are elderly; interpretation of thyroid function tests in patients receiving amiodarone can be difficult because its effects are complex; a flat TSH response to protirelin will help confirm the presence of hyperthyroidism)

## Side/Adverse Effects

Note: Incidence of side/adverse effects is generally related to dose and duration of therapy. Side/adverse effects may occur even at therapeutic plasma amiodarone concentrations but are more common at concentrations over 2.5 mcg per mL and with continuous treatment for longer than 6 months.

Side/adverse effects may not appear until several days, weeks, or years after initiation of amiodarone therapy and may persist for several months after withdrawal.

Sinus bradycardia is symptomatic in only 2 to 4% of patients taking amiodarone. Sinus arrest and heart block occur rarely. Atrioventricular (AV) block occurs infrequently. New or exacerbated arrhythmias occur in 2 to 5% of patients and may include paroxysmal ventricular tachycardia, ventricular fibrillation, increased resistance to cardioversion, and *torsades de pointes*; they may be associated with marked QT prolongation. New or exacerbated arrhythmias may also be a sign of hyperthyroidism.

Amiodarone concentrations of > 3 mg per mL (mg/mL) in 5% Dextrose Injection USP (D$_5$W) have been associated with a high incidence of peripheral vein phlebitis; concentrations ≤ 2.5 mg/mL appear to be less irritating.

The following side/adverse effects have been selected on the basis of their potential clinical significance (possible signs and symptoms in parentheses where appropriate)—not necessarily inclusive:

### Those indicating need for medical attention
Incidence more frequent
*Hypotension* (dizziness, lightheadedness, or fainting); *neurotoxicity* (trouble in walking; numbness or tingling in fingers or toes; trembling or shaking of hands; unusual and uncontrolled movements of body; weakness of arms or legs); *photosensitivity, particularly to long-wave ultraviolet-A [UVA] light* (sensitivity of skin to sunlight); *pulmonary fibrosis or interstitial pneumonitis/alveolitis* (cough; painful breathing; shortness of breath; slight fever)

Note: *Neurotoxicity* is the most common adverse effect occurring with oral amiodarone therapy; it occurs in 20 to 40% of patients, especially during administration of loading doses; neurotoxicity may occur within 1 week to several months after initiation of therapy and may persist for more than a year after withdrawal.

*Hypotension* is the most common adverse effect occurring with intravenous amiodarone therapy. In clinical trials, hypotension occurred in 16% of patients treated with intravenous amiodarone. Clinically significant hypotension during infusion of amiodarone was seen most often in the first several hours of treatment and appeared to be related to the rate of infusion, rather than the dose. However, mean daily doses of above 2100 mg are associated with an increased risk of hypotension. Alteration in amiodarone therapy to alleviate hypotension was required in 3% of patients. Permanent discontinuation of amiodarone therapy because of hypotension was necessary in fewer than 2% of patients.

*Photosensitivity* may occur even through window glass and thin cotton clothing and is not dose-related. Use of protective clothing and a topical product that prevents sunburn is recommended, especially for patients with fair skin or with excessive sun exposure.

*Pulmonary fibrosis or interstitial pneumonitis/alveolitis* is clinically significant in up to 10 to 15% of patients, but abnormal diffusion capacity occurs in a much higher percentage; it may occur more frequently with doses of 400 mg per day and after several months of treatment but may also occur with small doses; usually reversible after withdrawal of amiodarone, with or without steroid treatment, but is fatal in about 10% of cases, especially when not diagnosed promptly; recurrence has been reported after withdrawal of several months of steroid therapy; often mistaken for but rarely related to congestive heart failure or pneumonic infection.

Incidence less frequent
*Arrhythmias, new or exacerbated* (fast or irregular heartbeat); *blue-gray coloring of skin on face, neck, and arms; congestive heart failure* (swelling of feet or lower legs); *hyperthyroidism* (nervousness; sensitivity to heat; sweating; trouble in sleeping; weight loss); *hypothyroidism* (coldness; dry, puffy skin; unusual tiredness; weight gain); *non-infectious epididymitis* (pain and swelling in scrotum); *ocular toxicity* (blurred vision or blue-green halos seen around objects; dry eyes; sensitivity of eyes to light); *including optic neuropathy and/or optic neuritis; sinus bradycardia* (slow heartbeat)

Note: *Blue-gray skin coloring* occurs with prolonged use, usually longer than 1 year, especially in patients with fair skin or with excessive sun exposure; slowly, and occasionally incompletely, reversible after withdrawal.

*Hyperthyroidism* occurs in about 2% of patients, although thyroid hormone concentration changes are common and may persist for several months after withdrawal of amiodarone. If signs of a new *arrhythmia* appear, hyperthyroidism should be considered. Amiodarone-associated hyperthyroidism may be followed by a transient period of hypothyroidism.

*Hypothyroidism* occurs in less than 10% of patients, although thyroid hormone concentration changes are common and may persist for several months after withdrawal of amiodarone.

*Optic neuropathy and/or optic neuritis*, usually resulting in visual impairment and sometimes progressing to permanent blindness, have been reported and may occur at any time during treatment with amiodarone. If symptoms of visual impairment, such as changes in visual acuity and decreases in peripheral vision, occur, a prompt ophthalmologic examination is recommended and amiodarone treatment should be re-evaluated. Regular ophthalmologic examinations that include funduscopy and slit-lamp procedures are recommended during treatment with amiodarone. Bilateral and symmetric asymptomatic corneal deposits appearing as yellow-brown pigmentation on slit-lamp examination occur in all patients after 6 months of treatment, but may appear sooner; symptomatic corneal deposits occur in up to 10% of patients; macular degeneration and decreased visual acuity are rare; corneal deposits are reversible after withdrawal of amiodarone, although it may take up to 7 months.

*Sinus bradycardia* usually responds to dosage reduction but may require a pacemaker; atropine-resistant.

Incidence rare
*Allergic reaction* (skin rash); *hepatitis* (yellow eyes or skin)

Note: *Allergic reaction* usually occurs within the first 2 weeks of therapy.

In *hepatitis*, hepatic enzymes are commonly elevated to several times normal within 2 months after initiation of therapy; deaths as a result of hepatic failure resembling alcoholic cirrhosis have occurred rarely.

### Those indicating need for medical attention only if they continue or are bothersome
Incidence more frequent—approximately 25%, especially during administration of high doses, as during loading
*Constipation; headache; loss of appetite*—may lead to severe weight loss; *nausea and vomiting*

Incidence less frequent
*Bitter or metallic taste; decreased sexual ability in males; decrease in sexual interest; dizziness* (central nervous system [CNS] effect; hypotension is rare); *flushing of face*

### Those indicating possible pulmonary toxicity and the need for medical attention if they occur after medication is discontinued
*Cough; fever, slight; painful breathing; shortness of breath*

## Overdose

For more information on the management of overdose or unintentional ingestion, **contact a Poison Control Center** (see *Poison Control Center Listing*).

**Treatment of overdose**

Decrease absorption—Recent oral ingestion may benefit from emesis and/or lavage.

Specific treatment—
Primarily supportive and symptomatic.
Monitoring of cardiac rhythm and blood pressure is important.
For bradycardia, a beta-adrenergic agonist or pacemaker may be indicated.
Hypotension may respond to positive inotropic and/or vasopressor agents.

## Patient Consultation

As an aid to patient consultation, refer to *Advice for the Patient, Amiodarone (Systemic)*.

In providing consultation, consider emphasizing the following selected information (» = major clinical significance):

**Before using this medication**
» Conditions affecting use, especially:
Hypersensitivity to amiodarone
Pregnancy—Potential risk of bradycardia and iodine toxicity in fetus
Breast-feeding—Distributed into breast milk
Use in children—Shorter onset and duration of action
Use in the elderly—Increased sensitivity to effects on thyroid function and increased incidence of ataxia and other neurotoxic effects
Other medications, especially other antiarrhythmics, coumarin-derivative anticoagulants, digitalis glycosides, or phenytoin
Other medical problems, especially pre-existing atrioventricular (AV) block without pacemaker, bradycardic episodes resulting in syncope (unless controlled by pacemaker), or severe sinus node function impairment causing marked bradycardia (unless controlled by pacemaker)

**Proper use of this medication**
» Compliance with therapy; taking as directed even if feeling well
» Proper dosing
Missed dose: Not taking at all; notifying physician if two or more doses in a row are missed; not doubling doses
» Proper storage

**Precautions while using this medication**
Regular visits to physician to check progress
Carrying medical identification card or bracelet
» Caution if any kind of surgery (including dental surgery) or emergency treatment is required
» Protecting skin from sunlight during and for several months following withdrawal of treatment; sunburns may occur even through window glass and thin cotton clothing; use of protective clothing and a topical product that prevents sunburn; checking with physician if severe sunburn occurs
Checking with physician if blue-gray discoloration of skin occurs
» Checking with physician if changes in vision, such as a decrease in peripheral vision or a decrease in clarity of vision, occur

**Side/adverse effects**
Signs and symptoms of potential side effects, especially hypotension; neurotoxicity; photosensitivity, particularly to long-wave ultraviolet-A (UVA) light; pulmonary fibrosis or interstitial pneumonitis/alveolitis; new or exacerbated arrhythmias; blue-gray coloring of skin on face, neck, and arms; congestive heart failure; hyperthyroidism; hypothyroidism; noninfectious epididymitis; ocular toxicity, including optic neuropathy and/or optic neuritis; sinus bradycardia; allergic reaction; and hepatitis

## General Dosing Information

Because of its delayed onset of action, difficulty in dosage adjustment, and potentially serious adverse effects, it is recommended that amiodarone administration be initiated in the hospital and that the patient remain in the hospital at least for the loading dose phase. Amiodarone should be administered only by physicians who are experienced in the treatment of life-threatening arrhythmias, are thoroughly familiar with the risks and benefits of amiodarone therapy, and have access to laboratory facilities equipped to adequately monitor the effectiveness and side effects of amiodarone therapy.

Dosage must be adjusted to meet the individual requirements of each patient, based on clinical response, appearance or severity of toxicity, and in some cases, plasma amiodarone concentrations.

**For treatment of adverse effects**
Recommended treatment consists of the following:
- Hypotension associated with intravenous amiodarone administration should be treated initially by slowing the infusion rate. Additional therapy, if needed, may include volume expansion and administration of vasopressor agents and/or positive inotropic agents.
- If hypothyroidism occurs, dosage reduction or withdrawal of amiodarone is recommended, along with addition of thyroid hormone supplementation.
- Hyperthyroidism, which may be associated with signs of new or breakthrough arrhythmias, should be treated by reducing the dose of or withdrawing amiodarone. Additional therapy may include the use of antithyroid drugs, beta adrenergic blocking agents, and/or temporary corticosteroid therapy. However, the effects of antithyroid drugs may be delayed due to substantial quantities of preformed thyroid hormones in the gland. Because amiodarone-induced hyperthyroidism is associated with low radioiodine uptake, radioactive iodine therapy is *contraindicated*. Thyroid surgery in this setting may be associated with a risk of inducing thyroid storm.
- If signs or symptoms of pulmonary toxicity occur, it is recommended that amiodarone therapy be withdrawn until the cause has been determined. If pulmonary toxicity is related to amiodarone, withdrawal of amiodarone is recommended. Usefulness of steroid therapy is controversial, but such therapy may be useful for severe toxicity.
- Nausea and vomiting may be relieved by reduction of dose or administration of amiodarone in divided doses.
- If epididymitis occurs, dosage reduction or withdrawal of amiodarone is recommended.

## Oral Dosage Forms

Note: Bracketed uses in the *Dosage Forms* section refer to categories of use and/or indications that are not included in U.S. product labeling.

### AMIODARONE HYDROCHLORIDE TABLETS

Note: Because amiodarone has a long terminal plasma elimination half-life, the time to reach steady-state would take several months if the drug were administered at usual doses; therefore, loading doses are necessary in order to ensure that an antiarrhythmic effect occurs within a reasonable period of time. The patient should be closely monitored during the loading phase of therapy, especially until the risk of recurrent ventricular tachycardia or fibrillation has subsided. Elimination of ventricular fibrillation and tachycardia, along with a reduction in complex and total ventricular ectopic beats, usually occurs within 1 to 3 weeks.

Because of the potential for interactions with other antiarrhythmic drugs, it is recommended that an attempt be made to gradually discontinue the administration of prior antiarrhythmic drugs upon starting amiodarone therapy.

**Usual adult dose**
Ventricular arrhythmias (ventricular fibrillation or hemodynamically unstable ventricular tachycardia)—
Loading: Oral, 800 mg to 1.6 grams per day for one to three weeks (or longer, if necessary) until an initial therapeutic response or side effects occur; may be given in divided doses with meals for doses greater than 1 gram per day or if gastrointestinal side effects occur. When adequate control is achieved or excessive side effects occur, the dose is reduced to 600 to 800 mg per day for one month and then decreased again to the lowest effective maintenance dose. The lowest effective maintenance dose should be used to prevent the occurrence of side effects.
Maintenance: Oral, approximately 400 mg per day, the dosage being increased or decreased as necessary. Higher maintenance doses (up to 600 mg per day) or lower maintenance doses may be required in some patients. The long-term maintenance dose should be determined according to the antiarrhythmic effect as assessed by symptoms, tolerance, and Holter recordings and/or programmed electrical stimulation. Amiodarone plasma concentration determinations may be helpful in evaluating nonresponsiveness or unexpectedly severe toxicity.
When dosage adjustments are necessary, patients should be closely monitored for an extended period of time because of the long and variable half-life of amiodarone and the difficulty of predicting the time required to attain a new steady-state amiodarone concentration.
[Supraventricular tachycardia][1]—
Loading: Oral, 600 to 800 mg per day for one weekor until an initial therapeutic response or side effects occur. When adequate control

is achieved or excessive side effects occur, the dose is reduced to 400 mg per day for three weeks.
Maintenance: Oral, 200 to 400 mg per day.

**Usual pediatric dose**
Ventricular arrhythmias
[Supraventricular arrhythmias][1]—
 Loading: Oral, 10 mg per kg of body weight per day or 800 mg per 1.72 square meters of body surface area per day for ten days or until an initial therapeutic response or side effects occur. When adequate control is achieved or excessive side effects occur, the dose is reduced to 5 mg per kg of body weight or 400 mg per 1.72 square meters of body surface area per day for several weeks and then decreased gradually to the lowest effective maintenance dose.
 Maintenance: Oral, 2.5 mg per kg of body weight per day or 200 mg per 1.72 square meters of body surface area per day.

**Strength(s) usually available**
U.S.—
 200 mg (Rx) [*Cordarone* (scored; lactose)].
Canada—
 200 mg (Rx) [*Cordarone* (scored; lactose)].

**Packaging and storage**
Store below 40 °C (104 °F), preferably between 15 and 30 °C (59 and 86 °F), unless otherwise specified by the manufacturer. Protect from light.

[1]Not included in Canadian product labeling.

## Parenteral Dosage Forms

Note: The surface properties of solutions containing injectable amiodarone are altered, reducing the solution drop size. This phenomenon may result in underdosing the patient by up to 30% if a drop counter infusion set is used; therefore, a volumetric infusion pump must be used to deliver amiodarone. Whenever possible, amiodarone should be administered through a central venous catheter dedicated to this purpose; an in-line filter should also be used during administration.

### AMIODARONE HYDROCHLORIDE INJECTION

Note: Amiodarone shows considerable interindividual variation in response; therefore, monitoring is necessary at dosage initiation, at dosage adjustments, and when switching to oral amiodarone therapy.

**Usual adult dose**
Ventricular arrhythmias (ventricular fibrillation or hemodynamically unstable ventricular tachycardia)—
 Note: The recommended starting dose of intravenous amiodarone is about 1000 mg over the first twenty-four hours.
 First twenty-four hours:
  Loading infusions (may be individualized for each patient)—
   First, rapid intravenous infusion:
    150 mg administered by rapid intravenous infusion over the first ten minutes (15 mg per minute).
   Next, slow intravenous infusion:
    360 mg administered by slow intravenous infusion over the next six hours (1 mg per minute).
  Maintenance infusion (decreasing the rate of the slow intravenous infusion):
   Intravenous infusion, 540 mg of amiodarone is delivered over the remaining eighteen hours (0.5 mg per minute).
 After the first twenty-four hours—
  The maintenance infusion rate of 0.5 mg per minute (720 mg per twenty-four hours) should be continued, using a concentration of 1 to 6 mg per mL (concentrations greater than 2 mg per mL should be administered via a central venous catheter). In the event of breakthrough episodes of ventricular fibrillation or hemodynamically unstable ventricular tachycardia, supplemental infusions of 150 mg may be administered. Such infusions should be administered over a period of ten minutes to minimize the potential for hypotension. The rate of the maintenance infusion may be increased to effectively achieve arrhythmia suppression.
 Intravenous amiodarone should be used for acute treatment until the patient's ventricular arrhythmias have been stabilized. Most patients will require therapy for forty-eight to ninety-six hours, and intravenous amiodarone may be safely administered for longer periods of time if necessary, although intravenous amiodarone is not intended for maintenance treatment. There has been limited experience in patients receiving intravenous amiodarone for longer than three weeks. Patients whose arrhythmias have been suppressed by intravenous amiodarone may be switched to oral amiodarone.

**Usual adult prescribing limits**
The initial infusion rate should not exceed 30 mg per minute. Infusions lasting longer than one hour should not exceed a concentration of 2 mg per mL unless a central venous catheter is used. Amiodarone concentrations of > 3 mg/mL in 5% Dextrose Injection USP (D$_5$W), have been associated with a high incidence of peripheral vein phlebitis; concentrations ≤ 2.5 mg/mL appear to be less irritating. In clinical trials, mean daily doses of above 2100 mg were associated with an increased risk of hypotension.
A maintenance infusion of up to 0.5 mg per minute of amiodarone can be cautiously continued for two to three weeks, regardless of the patient's age, renal function, or left ventricular function, but experience is limited in patients receiving intravenous amiodarone for longer than three weeks.

**Usual pediatric dose**
Safety and efficacy have not been established in patients younger than 18 years of age; use is not recommended.

**Strength(s) usually available**
U.S.—
 50 mg per mL (Rx) [*Cordarone I.V.*].
Canada—
 50 mg per mL (Rx) [*Cordarone Intravenous*].

**Packaging and storage**
Store at room temperature, between 15 and 25 °C (59 and 77 °F). Protect from light.
Note: Intravenous amiodarone does not need to be protected from light during administration.

**Preparation of dosage form**
To prepare the rapid intravenous infusion, add 3 mL of amiodarone (150 mg) to 100 mL of 5% Dextrose Injection USP (D$_5$W). The resulting concentration is 1.5 mg per mL.
To prepare the slow intravenous infusion, add 18 mL of amiodarone (900 mg) to 500 mL of 5% Dextrose Injection USP (D$_5$W). The resulting concentration is 1.8 mg per mL.

**Stability**
The dose administration schedule used in clinical trials was designed to take into consideration the adsorption of amiodarone to polyvinyl chloride (PVC) tubing. Because clinical trials were conducted using PVC tubing, its use is recommended for delivery of amiodarone. The recommended concentrations and infusion rates reflect those identified in clinical trials; it is important that these recommendations be followed closely. Amiodarone infusions exceeding 2 hours must be administered in glass or polyolefin bottles containing 5% Dextrose Injection USP (D$_5$W).
PVC container—
 Amiodarone is physically compatible; amiodarone loss is less than 10% at 2 hours in 5% Dextrose Injection USP (D$_5$W) at a concentration of 1 to 6 mg of amiodarone per mL.
Polyolefin or glass container—
 Amiodarone is physically compatible; no amiodarone loss occurs at 24 hours in 5% Dextrose Injection USP (D$_5$W) at a concentration of 1 to 6 mg of amiodarone per mL.

**Incompatibilities**
Amiodarone admixed with 5% Dextrose Injection USP (D$_5$W) to a concentration of 4 mg per mL is incompatible and forms a precipitate with aminophylline, cefamandole nafate, cefazolin sodium, and mezlocillin sodium. Amiodarone also forms a precipitate with sodium bicarbonate at a concentration of 3 mg per mL and with heparin sodium at an unknown concentration.

**Additional information**
Intravenous amiodarone is not intended for long-term (longer than 3 weeks) maintenance treatment; patients whose arrhythmias have been suppressed by intravenous amiodarone may be switched to oral amiodarone. The optimal dose to use when changing from intravenous to oral amiodarone will depend on the dose of intravenous amiodarone already administered, as well as the bioavailability of oral amiodarone. Clinical monitoring is recommended when patients, particularly the elderly, are changed to oral amiodarone therapy.

| Recommendations for oral dosage after intravenous infusion* ||
|---|---|
| Duration of intravenous amiodarone infusion (assuming a 720 mg per day infusion [0.5 mg per minute]) | Initial daily dose of oral amiodarone |
| < 1 week | 800 to 1600 mg |
| 1 to 3 weeks | 600 to 800 mg |
| > 3 weeks | 400 mg |

*Based on a comparable total body amount of amiodarone delivered by the intravenous and oral routes, based on 50% bioavailability of oral amiodarone.

## Selected Bibliography

Naccarelli GV, Romlemberger RL, Dougherty AH, et al. Amiodarone: pharmacology and antiarrhythmic and adverse effects. Pharmacother 1985 Nov/Dec; 5: 298-313.

Heger JJ, Prystowsky EN, Miles WM, et al. Clinical use and pharmacology of amiodarone. Med Clin North Am 1984 Sep; 68: 1339-66.

Focus on amiodarone. Drugs 1985; 29 Suppl 3.

Revised: 05/05/98

**AMITRIPTYLINE**—See *Antidepressants, Tricyclic (Systemic)*

# AMLEXANOX Mucosal-Local—INTRODUCTORY VERSION

VA CLASSIFICATION (Primary): OR900

Commonly used brand name(s): *Aphthasol*.

Note: For a listing of dosage forms and brand names by country availability, see *Dosage Forms* section(s).

## Category

Antiulcer agent (topical).

## Indications

**Accepted**

Stomatitis, aphthous (treatment)—Amlexanox is indicated for the treatment of aphthous stomatitis (aphthous ulcers) in people with normal immune systems.

## Pharmacology/Pharmacokinetics

**Physicochemical characteristics**

Chemical group—2-Amino-7-isopropyl-5-oxo-5*H*-[1]benzopyrano[2,3-*b*]pyridine-3-carboxylic acid.

Molecular weight—298.3.

**Mechanism of action/Effect**

The exact mechanism of action is unknown. *In vitro* studies show amlexanox to inhibit the formation and release of histamine and leukotrienes from mast cells, neutrophils, and mononuclear cells.

**Absorption**

The maximum serum concentration is approximately 120 nanograms per mL following oral application of 100 mg of amlexanox oral paste. Most of the systemic absorption of amlexanox is via the gastrointestinal tract, and the amount absorbed directly through the active ulcer is not a significant portion of the applied dose.

**Half-life**

Elimination—3.5 ± 1.1 hours.

**Elimination**

Renal—Up to 17% of the total dose may be excreted in the urine.

## Precautions to Consider

**Carcinogenicity**

Amlexanox was not found to be carcinogenic following oral administration to rats for 2 years and mice for 18 months.

**Mutagenicity**

*In vitro* and *in vivo* animal studies found no mutagenic potential of amlexanox.

**Pregnancy/Reproduction**

Fertility—Amlexanox did not significantly affect fertility of rats when it was administered at 200 times the estimated human daily dose on a mg per square meter of body surface area (mg/m²).

Pregnancy—Adequate and well-controlled studies in humans have not been done. Amlexanox was not found teratogenic when administered to rats and rabbits at doses 200 and 600 times, respectively, the estimated human daily dose on a mg/m² basis.

FDA Pregnancy Category B.

**Breast-feeding**

Amlexanox was found in the milk of lactating rats. Problems in humans have not been documented.

**Pediatrics**

Appropriate studies on the relationship of age to the effects of amlexanox have not been performed in the pediatric population. Safety and efficacy have not been established.

**Geriatrics**

No information is available on the relationship of age to the effects of amlexanox in geriatric patients.

**Medical considerations/Contraindications**

The medical considerations/contraindications included have been selected on the basis of their potential clinical significance (reasons given in parentheses where appropriate)—not necessarily inclusive (» = major clinical significance).

*Risk-benefit should be considered when the following medical problems exist:*

Sensitivity to amlexanox or other components of the formulation

Immune deficiency conditions in patients who are immunocompromised

(safety and efficacy have not been assessed)

## Side/Adverse Effects

The following side/adverse effects have been selected on the basis of their potential clinical significance (possible signs and symptoms in parentheses where appropriate)—not necessarily inclusive:

**Those indicating need for medical attention only if they continue or are bothersome**

Incidence less frequent

*Burning, stinging, or pain at application site*

Incidence rare

*Contact mucositis* (inflammation of mucous membranes); *diarrhea; nausea*

## Overdose

For more information on the management of overdose or unintentional ingestion, **contact a Poison Control Center** (see *Poison Control Center Listing*).

There are no reports of human ingestion overdose. Ingestion of a tube containing 5 grams of paste would result in systemic exposure below the maximum nontoxic dose of amlexanox in animals, and produce side effects such as diarrhea and vomiting.

## Patient Consultation

As an aid to patient consultation, refer to *Advice for the Patient, Amlexanox (Mucosal-Local)*—Introductory Version.

In providing consultation, consider emphasizing the following selected information (» = major clinical significance):

**Before using this medication**

» Conditions affecting use, especially:

Sensitivity to amlexanox or other components of the formulation

**Proper use of this medication**

Applying the paste as soon as symptoms occur

Applying a small amount of paste (approximately 1/4 inch), using gentle pressure, to each ulcer in the mouth

Washing hands immediately after applying paste

Using paste until ulcers are healed, but not longer than 10 days

Avoiding application in or near the eyes

» Proper dosing

Missed dose: Applying as soon as possible; not applying if almost time for the next dose

» Proper storage

## General Dosing Information

Apply as soon as possible after noticing the symptoms of an aphthous ulcer.

Amlexanox paste should be applied four times a day, preferably following oral hygiene after breakfast, lunch, dinner, and at bedtime.

# 86 Amlexanox (Mucosal-Local)—Introductory Version

Avoid contact with eyes.

Safety and efficacy have not been assessed in immunocompromised individuals.

## Topical Dosage Forms

### AMLEXANOX ORAL PASTE

**Usual adult dose**
Aphthous stomatitis—
Topical, to aphthous ulcers four times a day, until healed. Use is not recommended for longer than ten days.

**Usual pediatric dose**
Safety and efficacy have not been established.

**Strength(s) usually available**
U.S.—
5% (Rx) [*Aphthasol* (benzyl alcohol; gelatin; glyceryl monostearate; mineral oil; pectin; petrolatum; sodium carboxymethylcellulose)].

**Packaging and storage**
Store at controlled room temperature, preferably between 15 and 30 °C (59 and 86 °F).

**Auxiliary labeling**
• Avoid contact with eyes.

Developed: 1/26/98

---

# AMLODIPINE  Systemic †

VA CLASSIFICATION (Primary/Secondary): CV200/CV250; CV409
Commonly used brand name(s): *Norvasc*.

Note: For a listing of dosage forms and brand names by country availability, see *Dosage Forms* section(s).

†Not commercially available in Canada.

## Category
Antianginal; antihypertensive.

## Indications

**Accepted**

Angina, chronic stable (treatment)—Amlodipine is indicated for the treatment of chronic stable angina; it may be used alone or in combination with other antianginal agents.

Angina, vasospastic (treatment)—Amlodipine is indicated for the treatment of confirmed or suspected vasospastic angina. It may be used alone or in combination with other antianginal agents.

Hypertension (treatment)—Amlodipine is indicated for the treatment of hypertension; it may be used alone or in combination with other antihypertensive agents.

For additional information on initial therapeutic guidelines related to the treatment of hypertension, see *Appendix III*.

## Pharmacology/Pharmacokinetics

**Physicochemical characteristics**
Molecular weight—567.05.

**Mechanism of action/Effect**
Amlodipine is a dihydropyridine calcium channel blocking agent. Like the other dihydropyridine agents, amlodipine selectively inhibits calcium influx across cell membranes in cardiac and vascular smooth muscle, with a greater effect on vascular smooth muscle. Amlodipine is a peripheral arteriolar vasodilator; thus it reduces afterload.

**Other actions/effects**
Amlodipine exhibits negative inotropic effects *in vivo*, but appears to have no significant effect on the sinoatrial (SA) or atrioventricular (AV) node in humans.

**Absorption**
Slowly and almost completely absorbed from the gastrointestinal tract; absorption not affected by food. Bioavailability is approximately 60 to 65%.

**Distribution**
$Vol_D$—21 L per kg.

**Protein binding**
Very high (95 to 98%).

**Biotransformation**
Undergoes minimal presystemic metabolism. Amlodipine undergoes slow but extensive hepatic metabolism, producing metabolites lacking significant pharmacological activity.

**Half-life**
Elimination—Mean, 35 hours in healthy volunteers; may be prolonged to a mean of 48 hours in hypertensive patients, 65 hours in the elderly, and 60 hours in patients with hepatic function impairment. Not affected by renal function impairment.

**Time to peak concentration**
Single-dose—6 to 9 hours.

**Duration of action**
24 hours.

**Elimination**
Renal—59 to 62% (about 5% as unchanged amlodipine).
Biliary/fecal—20 to 25%.
In dialysis—Amlodipine is not removed by hemodialysis.

## Precautions to Consider

**Carcinogenicity**
No evidence of carcinogenicity was revealed in studies with rats and mice given amlodipine at dosages of 0.5, 1.25, and 2.5 mg per kg of body weight (mg/kg) per day for 2 years.

**Mutagenicity**
No evidence of mutagenicity was observed at the gene or chromosome level.

**Pregnancy/Reproduction**
Fertility—No impairment of fertility was observed in rats given amlodipine at doses 8 times the maximum recommended human dose prior to mating.

Pregnancy—Studies have not been done in humans.
No evidence of teratogenicity or other embryo/fetal toxicity was observed in rats or rabbits given up to 10 mg/kg during periods of major organogenesis. However, the number of intrauterine deaths increased about five-fold, and rat litter size was significantly decreased (by 50%).

FDA Pregnancy Category C.

Labor—Amlodipine has been shown to prolong the duration of labor in rats.

**Breast-feeding**
It is not known whether amlodipine is distributed into breast milk.

**Pediatrics**
No information is available on the relationship of age to the effects of amlodipine in pediatric patients. Safety and efficacy have not been established.

**Geriatrics**
The half-life of amlodipine may be increased in the elderly. These patients may be more sensitive to the hypotensive effects of amlodipine and may require a lower initial dose.

**Dental**
Gingival hyperplasia is a rare side effect that has been reported with amlodipine. It also has been reported with other calcium channel blocking agents, such as diltiazem, felodipine, verapamil, and, most commonly, nifedipine. It usually starts as gingivitis or gum inflammation in the first 1 to 9 months of treatment. Resolution of the hyperplasia and improvement of the clinical symptoms usually occur one to four weeks after discontinuation of therapy. A strictly enforced program of professional teeth cleaning combined with plaque control by the patient will minimize growth rate and severity of gingival enlargement. Periodontal surgery may be indicated in some cases, and should be followed by careful plaque control to inhibit recurrence of gum enlargement.

**Surgical**
Recent evidence suggests that withdrawal of antihypertensive therapy prior to surgery may be undesirable. However, the anesthesiologist must be aware of such therapy.

**Drug interactions and/or related problems**
The following drug interactions and/or related problems have been selected on the basis of their potential clinical significance (possible mechanism in parentheses where appropriate)—not necessarily inclusive (» = major clinical significance):

Note: Combinations containing any of the following medications, depending on the amount present, may also interact with this medication.

Anesthetics, hydrocarbon inhalation
(concurrent use with amlodipine may produce additive hypotension; although calcium channel blocking agents may be useful to prevent supraventricular tachycardias, hypertension, or coronary spasm during surgery, caution is recommended during use)

Anti-inflammatory drugs, nonsteroidal (NSAIDs), especially indomethacin
(NSAIDs may reduce the antihypertensive effects of amlodipine by inhibiting renal prostaglandin synthesis and/or causing sodium and fluid retention)

Beta-adrenergic blocking agents
(although reports of adverse effects resulting from concurrent use of amlodipine with the beta-adrenergic blocking agents are lacking, caution is recommended given the similarity of amlodipine to nifedipine; concurrent use of nifedipine with the beta-adrenergic blocking agents, although usually well-tolerated, may produce excessive hypotension and, in rare cases, may increase the possibility of congestive heart failure)

Estrogens
(estrogen-induced fluid retention may tend to increase blood pressure; the patient should be carefully monitored to confirm that the desired effect is being obtained)

Highly protein-bound medications, such as:
  Anticoagulants, coumarin- and indandione-derivative
  Anticonvulsants, hydantoin
  Anti-inflammatory drugs, nonsteroidal
  Quinine
  Salicylates
  Sulfinpyrazone
(caution is advised when these medications are used concurrently with amlodipine since amlodipine is highly protein bound; changes in serum concentrations of the free, unbound medications may occur)

Hypotension-producing medications, other (see *Appendix II*)
(antihypertensive effects may be potentiated when amlodipine is used concurrently with hypotension-producing medications; although some antihypertensive and/or diuretic combinations are frequently used for therapeutic advantage, when any of these medications are used concurrently, dosage adjustments may be necessary)

Lithium
(concurrent use with amlodipine potentially may result in neurotoxicity in the form of nausea, vomiting, diarrhea, ataxia, tremors, and/or tinnitus; caution is recommended)

Sympathomimetics
(concurrent use may reduce antihypertensive effects of amlodipine; the patient should be carefully monitored to confirm that the desired effect is being obtained)

### Medical considerations/Contraindications
The medical considerations/contraindications included have been selected on the basis of their potential clinical significance (reasons given in parentheses where appropriate)—not necessarily inclusive (» = major clinical significance):

*Except under special circumstances, this medication should not be used when the following medical problem exists:*
» Hypotension, severe
  (amlodipine may aggravate this condition)

*Risk-benefit should be considered when the following medical problems exist:*
  Aortic stenosis
  (increased risk of heart failure because of fixed impedance to flow across aortic valve)
  Congestive heart failure
  (amlodipine should be used with caution in patients with congestive heart failure because of the slight risk for negative inotropic effect)
  Hepatic function impairment
  (clearance of amlodipine may be reduced since it undergoes extensive hepatic metabolism; elimination half-life may be prolonged to 60 hours)
  Sensitivity to amlodipine

### Patient monitoring
The following may be especially important in patient monitoring (other tests may be warranted in some patients, depending on condition; » = major clinical significance):
» Blood pressure determinations and
» ECG readings and
» Heart rate determinations
  (recommended primarily during dosage titration or when dosage is increased from established maintenance dosage level; also recommended when other medications are added that affect cardiac conduction or blood pressure)
  (blood pressure determinations are recommended at periodic intervals to monitor efficacy and safety of amlodipine therapy; selected patients may be trained to perform blood pressure measurements at home and report the results at regular physician visits)

## Side/Adverse Effects
The following side/adverse effects have been selected on the basis of their potential clinical significance (possible signs and symptoms in parentheses where appropriate)—not necessarily inclusive:

### Those indicating need for medical attention
Incidence more frequent
  *Edema, peripheral* (swelling of ankles and feet)
Incidence less frequent
  *Dizziness; palpitations* (pounding heartbeat)
Incidence rare
  *Angina* (chest pain); *bradycardia* (slow heartbeat); *hypotension* (dizziness); *orthostatic hypotension* (dizziness or lightheadedness when getting up from a lying or sitting position)

### Those indicating need for medical attention only if they continue or are bothersome
Incidence more frequent
  *Flushing; headache*
Incidence less frequent
  *Fatigue* (unusual tiredness or weakness); *nausea*

## Patient Consultation
As an aid to patient consultation, refer to *Advice for the Patient, Amlodipine (Systemic)*.
In providing consultation, consider emphasizing the following selected information (» = major clinical significance):

### Before using this medication
» Conditions affecting use, especially:
  Use in the elderly—Half-life increased; increased sensitivity to hypotensive effects
  Dental—Risk of gingival hyperplasia
  Other medications
  Other medical problems, especially severe hypotension

### Proper use of this medication
» Compliance with therapy; importance of not taking more medication than amount prescribed
» Proper dosing
  Missed dose: Taking as soon as possible; not taking if almost time for next scheduled dose; not doubling doses
» Proper storage
*For use as an antihypertensive*
  Possible need for control of weight and diet, especially sodium intake
» Patient may not experience symptoms of hypertension; importance of taking medication even if feeling well
» Does not cure, but helps control hypertension; possible need for lifelong therapy; serious consequences of untreated hypertension

### Precautions while using this medication
  Regular visits to physician to check progress during therapy
  Checking with physician before discontinuing medication; gradual dosage reduction may be necessary
» Discussing exercise or physical exertion limits with physician; reduced occurrence of chest pain may tempt patient to be overactive
  Possible headache; checking with physician if continuing or severe
» Maintaining good dental hygiene and seeing dentist frequently for teeth cleaning to prevent tenderness, bleeding, and gum enlargement
*For use as an antihypertensive*
» Not taking other medications, especially nonprescription sympathomimetics, unless discussed with physician

# Amlodipine (Systemic)

### Side/adverse effects
Signs of potential side effects, especially peripheral edema, dizziness, palpitations, angina, bradycardia, hypotension, or orthostatic hypotension

## General Dosing Information
Concurrent administration of sublingual nitroglycerin or long-acting nitrates with amlodipine may produce an additive antianginal effect. Sublingual nitroglycerin may be used as needed to abort acute angina attacks during amlodipine therapy. Nitrate medication may be used during amlodipine therapy for angina prophylaxis.

Although no "rebound effect" has been reported upon discontinuation of amlodipine, a gradual decrease of dosage with physician supervision is recommended.

### For treatment of overdose or acute adverse effects
Recommended treatment consists of the following:
- Hypotension, symptomatic—Intravenous fluids, intravenous dopamine or dobutamine, calcium chloride, isoproterenol, metaraminol, or norepinephrine should be used as appropriate.
- Tachycardia, rapid ventricular rate in patients with antegrade conduction in atrial flutter fibrillation, and accessory pathway with Wolff-Parkinson-White or Lown-Ganong-Levine syndrome—Direct-current cardioversion, intravenous lidocaine, or intravenous procainamide. Intravenous fluids given by slow-drip.
- Bradycardia, rarely second or third degree atrioventricular (AV) block, with a few patients progressing to asystole—Intravenous atropine, isoproterenol, norepinephrine, or calcium chloride, or use of electronic cardiac pacemaker, as appropriate.

## Oral Dosage Forms

### AMLODIPINE BESYLATE TABLETS

**Usual adult dose**
Antianginal or antihypertensive—
Oral, 5 to 10 mg once a day.

Note: An initial antihypertensive dose of 2.5 mg is recommended for small, fragile, or elderly patients, patients with hepatic function impairment, or when adding amlodipine to other antihypertensive therapy.

An initial antianginal dose of 5 mg is recommended for the elderly and for patients with hepatic function impairment.

**Usual pediatric dose**
Safety and efficacy have not been established.

**Strength(s) usually available**
U.S.—
2.5 mg (Rx) [*Norvasc*].
5 mg (Rx) [*Norvasc*].
10 mg (Rx) [*Norvasc*].
Canada—
Not commercially available.

**Packaging and storage**
Store below 40 °C (104 °F), preferably between 15 and 30 °C (59 and 86 °F), in a tight, light-resistant container unless otherwise specified by manufacturer.

**Auxiliary labeling**
- Do not take other medicines without physician's advice.

## Selected Bibliography
Murdoch D, Heel RC. Amlodipine: a review of its pharmacodynamic and pharmacokinetic properties, and therapeutic use in cardiovascular disease. Drugs 1991; 41(3): 478-505.

The fifth report of the Joint National Committee on Detection, Evaluation, and Treatment of High Blood Pressure (JNC V). Arch Intern Med 1993; 153(2): 154-83.

Revised: 08/12/93

---

# AMLODIPINE AND BENAZEPRIL  Systemic—INTRODUCTORY VERSION

VA CLASSIFICATION (Primary): CV401
Commonly used brand name(s): *Lotrel*.
Note: For a listing of dosage forms and brand names by country availability, see *Dosage Forms* section(s).

## Category
Antihypertensive.

## Indications

**Accepted**
Hypertension (treatment)—The combination of amlodipine and benazepril is indicated for the treatment of hypertension. It is not indicated as initial treatment for hypertension.

## Pharmacology/Pharmacokinetics

**Physicochemical characteristics**
Molecular weight—Amlodipine besylate: 567.1.
Benazepril hydrochloride: 460.96.

**Mechanism of action/Effect**
Amlodipine is a dihydropyridine calcium channel blocking agent that inhibits the influx of calcium ions across cell membranes of vascular smooth muscle and in cardiac myocytes. Inhibition of the influx of calcium ions is selective, with a greater effect occurring in vascular smooth muscle cells than in cardiac myocytes. The direct action on vascular smooth muscle causes a reduction in peripheral vascular resistance and a reduction in blood pressure. Long-term treatment with amlodipine does not have a significant effect on heart rate or plasma catecholamine concentrations. In patients with normal ventricular function, amlodipine may cause a small increase in the cardiac index but it has no significant influence on the ratio of change of ventricular pressure to change in time (dP/dt) or on left ventricular end diastolic pressure or volume.

Benazepril is a nonsulfhydryl angiotensin-converting enzyme (ACE) inhibitor and a prodrug for benazeprilat, the active metabolite. Both benazepril and benazeprilat inhibit ACE. ACE catalyzes the conversion of angiotensin I to the vasoconstrictor angiotensin II. Angiotensin II normally stimulates secretion of aldosterone and inhibits the release of renin through a negative feedback mechanism. When ACE activity is inhibited, angiotensin II formation is decreased and the interruption of the negative feedback mechanism results in increased plasma renin concentrations. The reduction of angiotensin II formation also decreases aldosterone secretion and vasoconstriction. The decrease in aldosterone secretion causes a small increase in serum potassium concentrations. Suppression of the renin-angiotensin-aldosterone system is thought to be the primary mechanism through which ACE inhibitors lower blood pressure.

**Other actions/effects**
ACE is also known as kininase II, an enzyme that degrades bradykinin. Benazepril may increase concentrations of bradykinin, producing a therapeutic vasodilating effect.

**Absorption**
Amlodipine—64 to 90% absorbed.
Benazepril—Approximately 37% absorbed.

**Distribution**
Volume of distribution ($Vol_D$)—
Amlodipine: 21 L per kg (L/kg).
Benazeprilat: 0.7 L/kg, concentration-independent.

**Protein binding**
Amlodipine—Very high (93%).
Benazeprilat—Very high (slightly higher than amlodipine).

**Biotransformation**
Amlodipine—Extensively metabolized in the liver.
Benazepril—Almost completely converted, primarily in the liver, to its active metabolite, benazeprilat.

**Half-life**
Elimination—
Effective: Amlodipine—48 hours; may be increased to 56 hours in patients with hepatic function impairment.
Effective: Benazeprilat—10 to 11 hours.

**Time to peak concentration**
Amlodipine—6 to 12 hours.
Benazepril—0.5 to 2 hours.
Benazeprilat—1.5 to 4 hours.

**Elimination**
Amlodipine—Renal: Approximately 70%.
Benazepril—Primarily renal, but also biliary.
In dialysis—
Amlodipine: Not reported to be removable by hemodialysis.
Benazeprilat: Slightly removable by hemodialysis.

## Precautions to Consider

### Cross-sensitivity and/or related problems
Patients hypersensitive to other angiotensin-converting enzyme (ACE) inhibitors also may be hypersensitive to benazepril.

### Carcinogenicity
No evidence of carcinogenicity was found in rats or mice given amlodipine for 2 years at dietary doses of 0.5, 1.25, and 2.5 mg per kg of body weight (mg/kg) per day. For mice, the highest dose is approximately the maximum recommended human daily dose (MRHDD) on a mg per square meter of body surface area (mg/m$^2$) basis and is close to the maximum tolerated dose. For rats, this dose is approximately twice the MRHDD, on a mg/m$^2$ basis.

No evidence of carcinogenicity was found in rats or mice given benazepril for 104 weeks at doses of up to 150 mg/kg per day. This represents more than 100 times the MRHDD, based on body weight. Based on body surface area, this represents 18 and 9 times the MRHDD for rats and mice, respectively.

### Mutagenicity
Mutagenicity was not detected for amlodipine in studies at either the gene or chromosome level.

Mutagenicity was not detected for benazepril in the Ames test in bacteria, in an *in vitro* test for forward mutations in cultured mammalian cells, or in a nucleus anomaly test.

### Pregnancy/Reproduction
Fertility—No impairment of fertility was found in male or female rats treated with amlodipine 64 days and 14 days prior to mating, respectively, at doses of up to 10 mg/kg per day (eight times the MRHDD of 10 mg, on a mg/m$^2$ basis, assuming a 50-kg person).

Reproductive performance of male and female rats was not affected when given benazepril at doses of 50 to 500 mg/kg per day. This represents 38 to 375 times the MRHDD on a body weight basis and 6 to 61 times the MRHDD on a body surface area basis.

No impairment of fertility was found when amlodipine and benazepril combination was given to male and female rats. Amlodipine was administered at daily doses of up to 7.5 mg/kg and benazepril at daily doses of up to 15 mg/kg per day prior to mating and throughout gestation.

Pregnancy—ACE inhibitors can cause fetal and neonatal morbidity and mortality when administered to pregnant women during the second and third trimesters. Amlodipine and benazepril combination should be discontinued as soon as possible when pregnancy is detected unless no alternative therapy can be used. In the latter instance, serial ultrasound examinations should be performed to assess the intra-amniotic environment. If oligohydramnios is observed, amlodipine and benazepril combination should be discontinued unless it is considered lifesaving for the mother. Perinatal diagnostic tests, such as contraction-stress testing (CST), a nonstress test (NST), or biophysical profiling (BPP), also may be appropriate during the applicable week of pregnancy. Oligohydramnios may not be apparent until after the fetus has sustained irreversible damage.

Fetal exposure to ACE inhibitors during the second and third trimesters can cause hypotension, reversible or irreversible renal failure, anuria, neonatal skull hypoplasia, and death in the fetus or neonate. Maternal oligohydramnios, which may result from decreased fetal renal function, has been reported and is associated with fetal limb contractures, craniofacial deformation, and hypoplastic lung development. Other adverse effects that have been reported are prematurity, intrauterine growth retardation, and patent ductus arteriosus, although how these effects are related to exposure to ACE inhibitors is not clear. ACE inhibitor exposure, when limited to the first trimester, does not appear to be associated with these adverse effects.

Infants exposed *in utero* to ACE inhibitors should be observed closely for hypotension, oliguria, and hyperkalemia. Oliguria should be treated with support of blood pressure and renal perfusion. Dialysis or exchange transfusion may be necessary to reverse hypotension and/or substitute for disordered renal function.

Teratogenic effects were not observed in rabbits given daily combination doses of benazepril 1.5 mg/kg and amlodipine 0.75 mg/kg or in rats given daily combination doses of benazepril 50 mg/kg and amlodipine 25 mg/kg. These doses represent 0.97 and 24 times the maximum recommended human dose of the combination, respectively, on a mg/m$^2$ of body surface area basis, assuming a 50-kg woman.

FDA Pregnancy Category C (first trimester).

FDA Pregnancy Category D (second and third trimesters).

Labor—Dystocia was observed in rats given daily combination doses ranging from amlodipine 2.5 mg/kg and benazepril 5 mg/kg to amlodipine 25 mg/kg and benazepril 50 mg/kg. The 2.5 mg/kg per day dose of amlodipine is 3.6 times the amlodipine dose delivered, on a mg/m$^2$ basis, when the maximum recommended human dose of the combination is given to a 50-kg woman. The 5 mg/kg per day dose of benazepril represents approximately two times the benazepril dose delivered, on a mg/m$^2$ basis, when the maximum recommended dose of the combination is given to a 50-kg woman.

### Breast-feeding
It is not known whether amlodipine is distributed into breast milk. Benazepril and benazeprilat are distributed into breast milk. Less than 0.1% of the maternal benazepril dose appears in breast milk. It is recommended that breast-feeding be discontinued during administration of amlodipine and benazepril combination.

### Pediatrics
Appropriate studies on the relationship of age to the effects of amlodipine and benazepril combination have not been performed in the pediatric population. Safety and efficacy have not been established.

### Geriatrics
Use of amlodipine and benazepril combination in a limited number of patients 65 years of age and older (19% of patients in clinical studies) has not demonstrated geriatrics-specific problems that would limit the usefulness of this combination in the elderly. However, amlodipine clearance may be decreased, resulting in 35 to 70% increases in amlodipine peak plasma concentrations, elimination half-life, and area under the plasma concentration–time curve. Elderly patients also may be more sensitive to the drug effects than younger individuals.

### Pharmacogenetics
Black patients may benefit from a reduction in amlodipine-induced edema when benazepril is added to current amlodipine therapy, but an additional antihypertensive effect may not occur in these patients. Black patients have a higher incidence of ACE inhibitor–induced angioedema when compared with nonblack patients.

### Surgical
Patients receiving amlodipine and benazepril combination may experience excessive hypotension when undergoing a major surgery or anesthesia with agents that produce hypotension. If hypotension in these patients is thought to be the result of ACE inhibition, it can be corrected by volume expansion.

### Drug interactions and/or related problems
The following drug interactions and/or related problems have been selected on the basis of their potential clinical significance (possible mechanism in parentheses where appropriate)—not necessarily inclusive (» = major clinical significance):

Note: Combinations containing any of the following medications, depending on the amount present, may also interact with this medication.

» Diuretics
(concurrent use with ACE inhibitors may cause additive hypotension; the diuretic may need to be discontinued or salt intake cautiously increased prior to initiation of amlodipine and benazepril combination therapy)

» Diuretics, potassium-sparing or
» Potassium-containing salt substitutes or
» Potassium supplements
(concurrent use with ACE inhibitor therapy may increase the risk of hyperkalemia; serum potassium concentrations should be monitored appropriately)

Lithium
(concurrent use with an ACE inhibitor has resulted in increased serum lithium concentrations and symptoms of lithium toxicity; frequent monitoring of serum lithium concentrations is recommended)

### Laboratory value alterations
The following have been selected on the basis of their potential clinical significance (possible effect in parentheses where appropriate)—not necessarily inclusive (» = major clinical significance):

With physiology/laboratory test values
Bilirubin concentrations, serum and
Hepatic enzyme values
(increases have been reported; significant elevations in hepatic enzymes may be associated with ACE inhibitor–related hepatotoxicity)

Blood urea nitrogen (BUN) and
Creatinine, serum
(minor and transient increases in concentrations may occur, especially in patients concurrently receiving a diuretic or in patients with renal function impairment)

Potassium, serum
(concentrations may be slightly increased as a result of reduced circulating aldosterone concentrations)

Uric acid, serum
(increases in concentrations have been reported)

## Medical considerations/Contraindications
The medical considerations/contraindications included have been selected on the basis of their potential clinical significance (reasons given in parentheses where appropriate)—not necessarily inclusive (» = major clinical significance).

*Except under special circumstances, this medication should not be used when the following medical problem exists:*
» Hypersensitivity to benazepril, any other ACE inhibitor, or amlodipine

*Risk-benefit should be considered when the following medical problems exist:*

Aortic stenosis, severe
(increased risk of symptomatic hypotension with amlodipine-induced vasodilation)

Collagen-vascular disease, such as systemic lupus erythematosus (SLE) or scleroderma
(increased risk of developing neutropenia or agranulocytosis, especially if renal function is impaired)

» Congestive heart failure
(patients with or without renal function impairment may experience excessive hypotension as a result of ACE inhibitor therapy; excessive hypotension in these patients may be associated with oliguria, azotemia, acute renal failure, and/or death)

Coronary artery disease, severe, obstructive
(initiation or a dosage increase of calcium channel blocking agent therapy has resulted in an increase in the frequency, duration, and/or severity of angina or the development of acute myocardial infarction; the mechanism of this effect is not understood)

Dehydration (sodium or volume depletion due to excessive perspiration, vomiting, diarrhea, prolonged diuretic therapy, dialysis, or dietary salt restriction)
(increased risk of symptomatic hypotension with ACE inhibitor therapy)

Diabetes mellitus
(increased risk of hyperkalemia with ACE inhibitor therapy)

Dialysis with high-flux membranes or
Low-density lipoprotein apheresis with dextran sulfate absorption
(anaphylactoid reactions have been reported in patients undergoing these procedures while being treated with an ACE inhibitor)

Hepatic function impairment
(the plasma elimination half-life of amlodipine increases to 56 hours and the area under the plasma concentration–time curve for amlodipine may increase by 40 to 60% because of decreased hepatic clearance)

Hymenoptera venom desensitization treatment
(life-threatening anaphylactoid reactions have been reported in two patients undergoing desensitizing treatment with hymenoptera venom while receiving ACE inhibitors)

» Renal artery stenosis, bilateral or unilateral or
» Renal function impairment
(plasma concentration of benazeprilat may be increased due to decreased elimination; increased risk of developing neutropenia or agranulocytosis; increased risk of hyperkalemia; increases in blood urea nitrogen [BUN] and serum creatinine may occur, especially in patients who are pretreated with a diuretic; renal function should be monitored during the first few weeks of therapy; a dosage adjustment and/or discontinuation of the diuretic or of amlodipine and benazepril combination may be necessary)

## Patient monitoring
The following may be especially important in patient monitoring (other tests may be warranted in some patients, depending on condition; » = major clinical significance):

» Blood pressure measurements
(periodic monitoring is necessary for titration of dose according to the patient's response)

Renal function determinations
(monitoring may be necessary in renally impaired patients)

Leukocyte count determinations
(recommended for patients at risk of neutropenia or agranulocytosis, such as those with renal function impairment and/or a collagen-vascular disease)

Potassium, serum concentrations
(monitoring may be necessary in patients at risk of hyperkalemia, such as those with renal insufficiency, diabetes mellitus, or those concurrently taking potassium-sparing diuretics, potassium supplements, or potassium-containing salt substitutes)

## Side/Adverse Effects
The following side/adverse effects have been selected on the basis of their potential clinical significance (possible signs and symptoms in parentheses where appropriate)—not necessarily inclusive:

### Those indicating need for medical attention
Incidence less frequent
*Edema, dependent* (swelling of ankles, feet, and lower legs)—the incidence of amlodipine-associated edema is reduced when amlodipine is given in combination with benazepril; **hyperkalemia** (confusion; irregular heartbeat; nervousness; numbness or tingling in hands, feet, or lips; shortness of breath or difficulty breathing; weakness or heaviness of legs)—during clinical trials, hyperkalemia occurred in approximately 1.5% of patients; **hypotension** (dizziness, lightheadedness, or fainting)

Incidence rare
**Anemia, hemolytic** (bleeding gums; fatigue; nosebleeds; pale skin color); **angioedema** (sudden trouble in swallowing or breathing; swelling of face, mouth, hands, or feet; hoarseness); **hepatotoxicity** (yellow eyes or skin); **neutropenia or agranulocytosis** (chills; fever; sore throat)—occurs rarely in uncomplicated hypertension; occurs more frequently in patients with renal function impairment, especially if accompanied by a collagen-vascular disease; **pancreatitis** (abdominal pain and distention; fever; nausea; vomiting); **pemphigus** (blisters in the mouth followed by skin blisters on the trunk, scalp, or other areas); **Stevens-Johnson syndrome** (sudden onset of multiple skin lesions on the arms, feet, hands, legs, palms, mouth, and/or lips); **thrombocytopenia** (unusual bleeding or bruising)

Note: *Angioedema* is associated with ACE inhibitor therapy and may involve the face, extremities, lips, tongue, glottis, and larynx. Angioedema associated with laryngeal edema, resulting in airway obstruction, can be fatal. During clinical trials, angioedema occurred in 0.5% of patients taking benazepril alone. ACE inhibitor–associated angioedema occurs at a higher rate in black patients than in nonblack patients.

ACE inhibitor–associated *hepatotoxicity* occurs by a mechanism that is not understood, but is manifest as a syndrome of cholestatic jaundice, fulminant hepatic necrosis, and possibly death. Amlodipine and benazepril combination therapy should be discontinued in patients who develop jaundice or marked elevations of hepatic enzymes. Patients should receive appropriate medical follow-up.

### Those indicating need for medical attention only if they continue or are bothersome
Incidence less frequent
*Cough, dry and persistent; dizziness; flushing; palpitations* (heartbeat sensations); *somnolence* (sleepiness)

Note: *Cough* has been reported with ACE inhibitors and is thought to be due to increased plasma bradykinin concentrations as a result of kininase II inhibition. In clinical trials of benazepril, in combination with amlodipine and alone, the incidence of cough was 3.3% and 1.8%, respectively.

## Overdose
For specific information on the agents used in the management of amlodipine and benazepril combination overdose, see
• *Dopamine* and *Norepinephrine* in *Sympathomimetic Agents—Cardiovascular Use (Parenteral-Systemic)* monograph.

For more information on the management of overdose or unintentional ingestion, **contact a Poison Control Center** (see *Poison Control Center Listing*).

### Clinical effects of overdose
The following effects have been selected on the basis of their potential clinical significance (possible signs and symptoms in parentheses where appropriate)—not necessarily inclusive:

Acute and chronic
**Hypotension, severe** (dizziness; fainting; lightheadedness); **tachycardia** (rapid heartbeat)

### Treatment of overdose
Treatment is symptomatic and supportive. Calcium chloride and glucagon have been used to treat overdoses of other dihydropyridine calcium channel blocking agents, but their efficacy in the treatment of overdose is questionable.

For severe hypotension—Repletion of central fluid volume by placing the patient in a supine or Trendelenburg position and/or infusing normal saline. If necessary, vasopressors such as norepinephrine or high-dose dopamine may be used.

Monitoring—Patients should be monitored for possible pulmonary edema resulting from the return of peripheral vascular tone after dihydropyridine calcium channel blocking agent overdose.

Supportive care—Patients in whom intentional overdose is confirmed or suspected should be referred for psychiatric consultation.

## Patient Consultation

As an aid to patient consultation, refer to *Advice for the Patient, Amlodipine and Benazepril (Systemic)—Introductory Version*.

In providing consultation, consider emphasizing the following selected information (» = major clinical significance):

**Before using this medication**
» Conditions affecting use, especially:
  Hypersensitivity to benazepril, other angiotensin-converting enzyme (ACE) inhibitors, or amlodipine
  Pregnancy—ACE inhibitor–associated fetal and neonatal hypotension, skull hypoplasia, renal failure, and death reported in humans
  Breast-feeding—Less than 0.1% of the maternal dose of benazepril is distributed into breast milk; breast-feeding should be discontinued
  Use in the elderly—May be more sensitive to drug effects
  Other medications, especially diuretics, potassium-containing salt substitutes, potassium-sparing diuretics, or potassium supplements
  Other medical problems, especially congestive heart failure, renal artery stenosis, or renal function impairment

**Proper use of this medication**
» Compliance with therapy; taking medication at the same time each day to maintain the antihypertensive effect
» Proper dosing
  Missed dose: Taking as soon as possible; not taking if almost time for next scheduled dose; not doubling doses
» Proper storage

**Precautions while using this medication**
Regular visits to physician to check progress
Notifying physician immediately if pregnancy is suspected because of possibility of fetal or neonatal injury and/or death
Not taking other medications, especially potassium supplements or salt substitutes that contain potassium, without consulting physician
Caution when driving or doing other things requiring alertness because of possible dizziness, lightheadedness, and fainting due to symptomatic hypotension
Reporting any signs of infection (fever, sore throat, chills) to physician because of risk of neutropenia
Reporting any signs of facial or extremity swelling and/or difficulty in swallowing or breathing because of risk of angioedema
Checking with physician if severe nausea, vomiting, or diarrhea occurs and continues because of risk of dehydration, which may result in hypotension
Caution when exercising or during exposure to hot weather because of the risk of dehydration, which may result in hypotension
Telling physician you are taking this medication before undergoing any surgical procedure (including dental surgery) or emergency treatment

**Side/adverse effects**
Signs of potential side effects, especially dependent edema, hyperkalemia, hypotension, hemolytic anemia, angioedema, hepatotoxicity, neutropenia or agranulocytosis, pancreatitis, pemphigus, Stevens-Johnson syndrome, and thrombocytopenia

## General Dosing Information

Dosage must be adjusted to meet the individual requirements of each patient, on the basis of clinical response.

Combination amlodipine and benazepril therapy should be used only in patients who have failed to achieve the desired antihypertensive effect with one or the other medication as single-drug therapy, or have not been able to achieve the desired antihypertensive effect with amlodipine monotherapy without developing edema. For dosage ranges for the individual agents when given as single therapy, see
• *Amlodipine (Systemic)* monograph; and/or
• *Benazepril* in *Angiotensin-converting Enzyme (ACE) Inhibitors (Systemic)* monograph.

Black patients may benefit from a reduction in amlodipine-induced edema when benazepril is added to current amlodipine therapy, but additional antihypertensive effects may not occur in these patients.

Severe renal function impairment (creatinine clearance < 30 mL per minute) may increase the peak benazeprilat plasma concentrations and the time to steady state. Amlodipine and benazepril combination is not recommended in patients with a creatinine clearance of ≤ 30 mL per minute (serum creatinine > 3 mg per dL).

In patients with congestive heart failure, treatment should be initiated under close medical supervision. Patients who have heart failure should be followed closely for the first 2 weeks of treatment, at each increase in benazepril dosage, whenever a diuretic is added to the treatment, or when the dosage of a concurrently administered diuretic is increased.

**For treatment of adverse effects**
Recommended treatment consists of the following:
• Treatment of symptomatic hypotension involves placing the patient in a supine or Trendelenburg position and, if needed, administering normal saline intravenously.
• For treatment of ACE inhibitor–associated angioedema with swelling involving the tongue, glottis, or larynx, causing airway obstruction— Appropriate treatment, such as subcutaneous epinephrine, should be initiated immediately.

## Oral Dosage Form

### AMLODIPINE AND BENAZEPRIL HYDROCHLORIDE CAPSULES

**Usual adult dose**
Antihypertensive—
  Oral, 1 to 2 capsules a day, as determined by individual dosage titration with the component agents.

Note: The elimination half-life of amlodipine in patients with hepatic function impairment increases to 56 hours. The recommended initial dose of amlodipine as a component of combination therapy in these patients is 2.5 mg.
  The recommended initial dose of amlodipine as a component of combination therapy in small or frail patients is 2.5 mg.

**Usual adult prescribing limits**
5 mg of amlodipine and 20 mg of benazepril per day.

**Usual pediatric dose**
Safety and efficacy have not been established.

**Usual geriatric dose**
Antihypertensive—
  Oral, initially, 2.5 mg of amlodipine as a component of combination therapy.

**Strength(s) usually available**
U.S.—
  2.5 mg amlodipine and 10 mg benazepril (Rx) [*Lotrel*].
  5 mg amlodipine and 10 mg benazepril (Rx) [*Lotrel*].
  5 mg amlodipine and 20 mg benazepril (Rx) [*Lotrel*].

**Packaging and storage**
Store below 30 ºC (86 ºF). Protect from moisture and light.

**Auxiliary labeling**
• Do not take other medicines without your doctor's advice.

Developed: 10/17/97

# AMMONIA N 13 Systemic *†

VA CLASSIFICATION (Primary): DX201
Note: For a listing of dosage forms and brand names by country availability, see *Dosage Forms* section(s).

*Not commercially available in the U.S.
†Not commercially available in Canada.

## Category

Diagnostic aid, radioactive (cardiac disease; hepatic disease; cerebrovascular disease).

# Ammonia N 13 (Systemic)

## Indications

### Accepted

Note: Accepted indications for positron emitters, such as ammonia N 13 ($^{13}NH_3$), are still evolving. Ongoing studies are revealing new indications for these agents.

Cardiac imaging, positron emission tomographic—Positron emission tomography (PET) using $^{13}NH_3$ is used in studies of myocardial blood flow in various physiological and pathological states. PET-$^{13}NH_3$ is currently used for the following diagnostic studies:

Cardiac wall-motion abnormalities assessment—PET using $^{13}NH_3$ to assess the distribution of myocardial blood flow in conjunction with fludeoxyglucose F 18 to estimate myocardial metabolic viability in dysfunctional myocardial segments serves to predict, preoperatively, the presence of reversible regional wall-motion abnormalities, which is helpful in the selection of patients in whom revascularization may lead to improved ventricular function.

Coronary artery disease (diagnosis)—$^{13}NH_3$ myocardial PET performed at rest and during stress (either exercise or dipyridamole or adenosine infusion) is used to detect coronary artery disease (CAD) and to identify individual stenosed vessels.

Myocardial infarction (diagnosis) and

Myocardial perfusion imaging, positron emission tomographic—PET-$^{13}NH_3$ is used in myocardial perfusion imaging for the diagnosis and localization of myocardial infarction.

Ischemia, myocardial (diagnosis)—PET-$^{13}NH_3$ is used in patients with known or suspected CAD, to define the areas of the left ventricular myocardium that have become critically ischemic during acute coronary artery occlusion.

Cardiac bypass surgery assessment—PET-$^{13}NH_3$ is used before and after aortocoronary bypass surgery to help evaluate the effect of surgery on myocardial perfusion. Also, graft patency can be established with postoperative images.

Cardiac blood pool imaging, positron emission tomographic—Dynamic cardiac PET-$^{13}NH_3$ is used to obtain cardiac blood pool images, which permit the evaluation of size and configuration of ventricles and atria.

Liver imaging, positron emission tomographic—Carcinoma, hepatocellular (diagnosis): Dynamic PET-$^{13}NH_3$ is used for the detection of primary hepatocellular carcinoma (hepatoma).

Arterial blood flow, hepatic, regional, assessment: Dynamic PET-$^{13}NH_3$ is used to quantitate regional hepatic arterial blood flow to enhance understanding of various liver diseases.

Brain imaging, positron emission tomographic—Dynamic PET-$^{13}NH_3$ is used to locate and assess the extent of altered brain perfusion with cerebrovascular diseases.

## Physical Properties

### Nuclear Data

| Radionuclide (half-life) | Decay constant | Mode of decay | Principal emissions (keV) | Mean number of emissions/disintegration |
|---|---|---|---|---|
| N 13 (10 min) | 0.07 min$^{-1}$ | Positron decay | Gamma (annihilation) (511) | 2.0 |

## Pharmacology/Pharmacokinetics

### Mechanism of action/Effect

Cardiac imaging—
Based on myocardial tissue uptake of $^{13}NH_3$, which is related to regional myocardial blood flow. In the blood, more than 90% is in the form of ammonium ($^{13}NH_4$); however, at 3 to 5 minutes a significant percentage of the activity is present as [$^{13}N$]glutamine and urea. Although myocardial uptake was once thought to be the result of ammonium competition with potassium transport, it is now accepted that myocardial localization is due to diffusion across capillaries and cellular membranes as ammonia ($^{13}NH_3$). Retention in myocardial cells is the result of metabolism to glutamine. In myocardial infarct patients, the slow blood pool clearance and prolonged lung retention is apparently the result of a large pulmonary distribution volume.

Liver imaging—
Hepatocellular carcinoma: Accumulation in the hepatoma is not yet well understood. It is assumed that $^{13}NH_3$ accumulation in the tumors is governed by the capillary blood flow of the tumor and the extraction efficacy of the neoplastic tissues for $^{13}NH_3$. Localization of $^{13}NH_3$ in hepatoma is seen in early scans. As time progresses, the radioactivity accumulation in the rest of the liver continues to increase, making the recognition of the tumor difficult. The early accumulation of $^{13}NH_3$ in the hepatoma may be due to the greater relative perfusion to the hepatoma via the hepatic artery, while the main vascular supply to the liver is from the portal vein, which results in delayed and decreased delivery of the radiotracer.

Regional hepatic arterial blood flow assessment: High first-pass extraction of $^{13}NH_3$ by the liver allows assessment of hepatic arterial blood flow.

Brain imaging—
Based on the different patterns of accumulation of radioactivity in brain tissue, which reflect differences in regional cerebral perfusion. Ischemic lesions show as areas of low perfusion. Brain localization is probably due in part to diffusion across capillaries and cellular membranes as ammonia ($^{13}NH_3$).

### Distribution

$^{13}NH_3$, in equilibrium with $^{13}NH_4$, is transported in arterial blood and within a few minutes after injection is rapidly converted into metabolites (e.g., $^{13}N$-glutamine [amide]) by different organs of the body. The metabolites are mainly taken up by the liver, and to a lesser extent, by the myocardium.

### Biotransformation

$^{13}NH_3$ is metabolized principally to $^{13}N$-glutamine by glutamine synthetase in skeletal muscle, brain, liver, and other organs, and to $^{13}N$-urea by a five-enzyme step in the liver.

### Radiation dosimetry:

| Target organ | Estimated absorbed radiation dose* mGy/MBq | rad/mCi |
|---|---|---|
| Bladder wall | 0.0081 | 0.030 |
| Kidneys | 0.0046 | 0.017 |
| Brain | 0.0042 | 0.016 |
| Liver | 0.0040 | 0.015 |
| Spleen | 0.0025 | 0.0092 |
| Lungs | 0.0025 | 0.0092 |
| Adrenals | 0.0023 | 0.0085 |
| Heart | 0.0021 | 0.0077 |
| Pancreas | 0.0019 | 0.0070 |
| Uterus | 0.0019 | 0.0070 |
| Breast | 0.0018 | 0.0066 |
| Small intestine | 0.0018 | 0.0066 |
| Thyroid | 0.0017 | 0.0063 |
| Stomach wall | 0.0017 | 0.0063 |
| Bone surface | 0.0016 | 0.0059 |
| Other tissue | 0.0027 | 0.0099 |

Effective dose equivalent: 0.0027mSv/MBq (0.01 rem/mCi)

*For adults; intravenous injection.

### Elimination

Renal (10–20%).

## Precautions to Consider

### Pregnancy/Reproduction

Pregnancy—The possibility of pregnancy should be assessed in women of child-bearing potential. Clinical situations exist where the benefit to the patient and fetus from information derived from radiopharmaceutical use outweighs the risks from radiation exposure to the fetus. In this situation, the physician should use discretion and reduce the radiopharmaceutical dose to the lowest possible amount. However, the effects of radiation exposure to the embryo or fetus with the use of $^{13}NH_3$ are expected to be negligible due to $^{13}NH_3$'s rapid clearance from the blood and short physical half-life.

### Breast-feeding

It is not known whether $^{13}NH_3$ is excreted in breast milk; however, it is expected that some will be present. Temporary discontinuation of nursing for a period of 1 to 2 hours is considered adequate.

### Pediatrics

Although $^{13}NH_3$ is used in children, there have been no specific studies evaluating safety and efficacy. When used in children, the diagnostic benefit should be judged to outweigh the potential risk of radiation.

### Geriatrics

Diagnostic studies performed to date using $^{13}NH_3$ have not demonstrated geriatrics-specific problems that would limit the usefulness of $^{13}NH_3$ in the elderly.

**Drug interactions and/or related problems**
There are no known drug interactions and/or related problems associated with the use of $^{13}NH_3$.

**Laboratory value alterations**
The following have been selected on the basis of their potential clinical significance (possible effect in parentheses where appropriate)—not necessarily inclusive (» = major clinical significance):
There is no evidence of any alteration of laboratory test results associated with the use of $^{13}NH_3$.

**Medical considerations/Contraindications**
The medical considerations/contraindications included have been selected on the basis of their potential clinical significance (reasons given in parentheses where appropriate)—not necessarily inclusive (» = major clinical significance).
There is no information regarding medical problems that would present an increased risk or interfere with the use of $^{13}NH_3$.

## Side/Adverse Effects
There are no known side/adverse effects associated with the use of $^{13}NH_3$.

## Patient Consultation
As an aid to patient consultation, refer to *Advice for the Patient, Radiopharmaceuticals (Diagnostic)*.
In providing consultation, consider emphasizing the following selected information (» = major clinical significance):

**Description of use**
Action in the body: Concentration of radioactivity in heart, brain, and liver allows images to be obtained
Small amounts of radioactivity used in diagnosis; radiation received is low and considered safe

**Before having this test**
» Conditions affecting use, especially:
Pregnancy—Risk to fetus from radiation exposure as opposed to benefit derived from use should be considered
Breast-feeding—Risk to infant from radiation exposure; temporary discontinuation of breast-feeding for 1 to 2 hours recommended

**Preparation for this test**
Special preparatory instructions may be given; patient should inquire in advance

**Precautions after having test**
No special precautions

## General Dosing Information
Radiopharmaceuticals are to be administered only by or under the supervision of physicians who have had extensive training in the safe use and handling of radionuclides and who are approved by the appropriate regulatory agency or, outside the U.S., the appropriate authority.
Imaging is usually performed 3 minutes after injection of $^{13}NH_3$, or during administration if dynamic studies are performed.

**Safety considerations for handling this radiopharmaceutical**
Improper handling of this radiopharmaceutical may cause radioactive contamination. Guidelines for handling radioactive material have been prepared by scientific, professional, state, federal, and international bodies and are available to the specially qualified and authorized users who have access to radiopharmaceuticals.

## Parenteral Dosage Forms

### AMMONIA N 13 INJECTION USP
**Usual adult and adolescent dose**
Cardiac imaging—
Intravenous, 555 to 740 megabecquerels (15 to 20 millicuries).
Liver imaging—
Intravenous, 370 to 740 megabecquerels (10 to 20 millicuries).
Brain imaging—
Intravenous, 740 to 1480 megabecquerels (20 to 40 millicuries).

**Usual pediatric dose**
Dosage has not been established.
Note: Doses of 8 megabecquerels (0.22 millicuries) per kg of body weight have been used in pediatric patients.

**Usual geriatric dose**
See *Usual adult and adolescent dose*.

**Strength(s) usually available**
U.S.—
Prepared on-site at various clinical facilities.
Canada—
Prepared on-site at various clinical facilities.

**Packaging and storage**
Store below 40 °C (104 °F), preferably between 15 and 30 °C (59 and 86 °F). Protect from freezing.

**Note:**
Caution—Radioactive material.

## Selected Bibliography
Hayashi N, Tamaki N, Yonekura Y, et al. Imaging of the hepatocellular carcinoma using dynamic positron emission tomography with nitrogen-13 ammonia. J Nucl Med 1985; 26: 254-7.
Phelps ME, Mazziotta JC, Schelbert HR. Positron emission tomography and autoradiography. Raven Press, 1986: 593-5.
Schelbert HM, Wisenberg G, Phelps M, et al. Noninvasive assessment of coronary stenosis by myocardial imaging during pharmacologic coronary vasodilation. VI. Detection of coronary artery disease in man with intravenous [$^{13}NH_3$] ammonia and positron computed tomography. Am J Cardiol 1982; 49: 1197.
Tominaga T, Inoue O, Suzuki K, et al. Evaluation of $^{13}N$-amines as tracers. Nucl Med Biol 1987; 14(5): 485-90.

Revised: 07/08/92
Interim revision: 08/02/94

---

**AMMONIA SPIRIT, AROMATIC**—The *Ammonia Spirit, Aromatic (Inhalation-Systemic)* monograph is not included in this published version of the USP DI database. Copies of the monograph are available on request from Micromedex, Inc. - Reprint Requests, 6200 S. Syracuse Way, Suite 300, Englewood, CO 80111; telephone (303) 486-6400; telefax (303) 486-6464; Email: USPDI@MDX.COM.

---

**AMMONIATED MERCURY**—The *Ammoniated Mercury (Topical)* monograph is not included in this published version of the USP DI database. Copies of the monograph are available on request from Micromedex, Inc. - Reprint Requests, 6200 S. Syracuse Way, Suite 300, Englewood, CO 80111; telephone (303) 486-6400; telefax (303) 486-6464; Email: USPDI@MDX.COM.

---

**AMMONIUM MOLYBDATE**—See *Molybdenum Supplements (Systemic)*

---

**AMOBARBITAL**—See *Barbiturates (Systemic)*

---

**AMOXAPINE**—See *Antidepressants, Tricyclic (Systemic)*

---

**AMOXICILLIN**—See *Penicillins (Systemic)*

---

**AMPHETAMINE**—See *Amphetamines (Systemic)*

# AMPHETAMINES Systemic

This monograph includes information on the following: 1) Amphetamine†; 2) Amphetamine and Dextroamphetamine†; 3) Dextroamphetamine; 4) Methamphetamine†.

INN:
Amphetamine†—Amfetamine
Dextroamphetamine†—Dexamfetamine
Methamphetamine†—Metamfetamine

VA CLASSIFICATION (Primary): CN801

Note: Controlled substances in the U.S. and Canada as follows:

| Drug | U.S. | Canada |
| --- | --- | --- |
| Amphetamine | II | † |
| Dextroamphetamine | II | C |
| Methamphetamine | II | † |

Commonly used brand name(s): *Adderall*[2]; *Desoxyn*[4]; *Desoxyn Gradumet*[4]; *Dexedrine*[3]; *Dexedrine Spansule*[3]; *Dextrostat*[3].

Note: For a listing of dosage forms and brand names by country availability, see *Dosage Forms* section(s).

†Not commercially available in Canada.

## Category
Central nervous system (CNS) stimulant.

## Indications

Note: Bracketed information in the *Indications* section refers to uses that are not included in U.S. product labeling.

**Accepted**

Attention-deficit hyperactivity disorder (treatment)—Amphetamines are indicated as an integral part of a total treatment program that includes other remedial measures (psychological, educational, social) for a stabilizing effect in children [and adults][1] with attention-deficit hyperactivity disorder, characterized by moderate to severe distractibility, short attention span, hyperactivity, emotional lability, and impulsivity. Nonlocalizing neurological signs, learning disability, and abnormal electroencephalogram (EEG) may be present also. Amphetamines usually are not indicated when the above symptoms are associated with acute stress reactions.

Narcolepsy (treatment)—Amphetamine and dextroamphetamine are indicated in the treatment of well-established and proven narcolepsy.

**Unaccepted**

Due to their high potential for abuse, amphetamines are not recommended for use as appetite suppressants.

Amphetamines should not be used to combat fatigue or to replace rest in normal subjects.

[1]Not included in Canadian product labeling.

## Pharmacology/Pharmacokinetics

**Physicochemical characteristics**

Molecular weight—
Amphetamine sulfate: 368.49.
Dextroamphetamine sulfate: 368.49.
Methamphetamine hydrochloride: 185.70.

**Mechanism of action/Effect**

Amphetamines are sympathomimetic amines that increase motor activity and mental alertness, and diminish drowsiness and a sense of fatigue.

In attention-deficit hyperactivity disorder, amphetamines decrease motor restlessness and enhance the ability to pay attention.

The exact mechanism of action has not been established. However, in animals, amphetamines facilitate the action of dopamine and norepinephrine by blocking reuptake from the synapse, inhibit the action of monoamine oxidase (MAO), and facilitate the release of catecholamines. Increase in locomotor activity at relatively low doses and increase in stereotypic behavior with a concomitant decrease in activity at higher doses appear to be due to stimulation of mesocorticolimbic and nigrostriatal dopaminergic pathways. Dextroamphetamine may also stimulate inhibitory autoreceptors in the substantia nigra and ventral tegmentum.

Some studies support the theory that amphetamine exerts a dual effect on the striatal dopaminergic nerve terminal, thus explaining the paradoxical effects of amphetamines. Amphetamines may selectively facilitate the dopaminergic transmission by promoting the release of recently synthesized dopamine from a reserpine-resistant pool and, in addition, may inhibit the classical dopaminergic neurotransmission involving the calcium-dependent depolarization-evoked release of dopamine from reserpine-sensitive storage sites.

**Other actions/effects**

Peripheral actions include elevation of both diastolic and systolic blood pressure, and weak bronchodilator and respiratory stimulant actions.

**Biotransformation**

Hepatic.

**Half-life**

Amphetamine—
10 to 30 hours; dependent on urinary pH.
Dextroamphetamine—
10 to 12 hours in adults; 6 to 8 hours in children.
Methamphetamine—
4 to 5 hours; dependent on urinary pH.

**Elimination**

Renal; dependent on urinary pH. Excretion is accelerated in acidic urine and slowed in alkaline urine.

## Precautions to Consider

**Cross-sensitivity and/or related problems**

Patients sensitive to other sympathomimetics (for example, ephedrine, epinephrine, isoproterenol, metaproterenol, norepinephrine, phenylephrine, phenylpropanolamine, pseudoephedrine, terbutaline) may be sensitive to amphetamines also.

**Carcinogenicity/Mutagenicity**

Mutagenicity and long-term carcinogenicity studies in animals have not been done.

**Pregnancy/Reproduction**

Pregnancy—Although adequate and well-controlled studies in humans have not been done, use of amphetamines during early pregnancy may be associated with an increased risk of congenital malformations, especially in the cardiovascular system and biliary tract.

Reproduction studies in animals have suggested both an embryotoxic and a teratogenic potential when amphetamines were administered at high multiples of the human dose.

FDA Pregnancy Category C.

Delivery—Infants born to mothers dependent on amphetamines have an increased risk of premature delivery and low birth weight. These infants may experience symptoms of withdrawal, including agitation and significant drowsiness.

**Breast-feeding**

Amphetamines are distributed into breast milk. However, problems in nursing infants have not been documented.

**Pediatrics**

Data suggest that prolonged administration of amphetamines to children may inhibit growth. Careful monitoring during treatment is recommended.

Psychotic children may experience exacerbation of symptoms of behavior disturbance and thought disorder.

Amphetamines may provoke or exacerbate motor and vocal tics and Tourette's syndrome, necessitating clinical evaluation before administration of amphetamines.

**Geriatrics**

No information is available on the relationship of age to the effects of the amphetamines in geriatric patients.

**Drug interactions and/or related problems**

The following drug interactions and/or related problems have been selected on the basis of their potential clinical significance (possible mechanism in parentheses where appropriate)—not necessarily inclusive (» = major clinical significance):

Note: Combinations containing any of the following medications, depending on the amount present, may also interact with this medication.

Acidifiers, gastrointestinal, such as:
  Ascorbic acid
  Fruit juices
  Glutamic acid hydrochloride or
Acidifiers, urinary, such as:
  Ammonium chloride
  Sodium acid phosphate
  (concurrent use may decrease the effects of amphetamines as a result of decreased absorption and increased elimination)

Alkalizers, urinary, such as:
   Antacids, calcium- and/or magnesium-containing
   Carbonic anhydrase inhibitors
   Citrates
   Sodium bicarbonate
      (concurrent use may increase the effects of amphetamines as a result of decreased elimination caused by alkalinization of urine)
Anesthetics, inhalation
      (halothane and, to a much lesser extent, enflurane, isoflurane, and methoxyflurane, may sensitize the myocardium to the effects of sympathomimetics, including chronic use of amphetamines prior to anesthesia, so that the risk of severe ventricular arrhythmias is increased; sympathomimetics should be used with caution and in substantially reduced dosage in patients receiving these agents)
» Antidepressants, tricyclic
      (although tricyclic antidepressants may be used concurrently with amphetamines for therapeutic effect, concurrent use may potentiate cardiovascular effects due to the release of norepinephrine, possibly resulting in arrhythmias, tachycardia, or severe hypertension or hyperpyrexia; close monitoring is recommended and dosage adjustments may be necessary)
Antihypertensives or
Diuretics used as antihypertensives
      (hypotensive effects may be reduced when these medications are used concurrently with amphetamines; the patient should be carefully monitored to confirm that the desired effect is obtained)
» Beta-adrenergic blocking agents, including ophthalmics
      (concurrent use with amphetamines may result in unopposed alpha-adrenergic activity with a risk of hypertension and excessive bradycardia and possible heart block; risk may be less with labetalol because of its alpha-blocking activity)
» CNS stimulation–producing medications, other (see *Appendix II*)
      (additive CNS stimulation to excessive levels may result in nervousness, irritability, insomnia, or possibly seizures; close observation is recommended)
      (also, concurrent use of amphetamines with other sympathomimetics may increase cardiovascular effects of either medication)
      (in addition to possibly increasing CNS stimulation, concurrent use of norepinephrine with large doses of amphetamines may enhance the pressor response to norepinephrine; caution may also be warranted in patients receiving usual doses of amphetamines)
» Digitalis glycosides
      (concurrent use with amphetamines may cause additive effects, resulting in cardiac arrhythmias)
Ethosuximide or
Phenobarbital or
Phenytoin
      (concurrent use with amphetamines may cause a delay in the intestinal absorption of ethosuximide, phenobarbital, or phenytoin)
Haloperidol or
Loxapine or
Molindone or
Phenothiazines or
Pimozide or
Thioxanthenes
      (central stimulant effects of amphetamines may be inhibited because of alpha-adrenergic blockade by these agents; also, concurrent use with amphetamines may reduce the antipsychotic effects of these agents)
Levodopa
      (the risk of cardiac arrhythmias may be increased; dosage reduction of amphetamine is recommended)
Lithium
      (central stimulant effects of amphetamines may be antagonized by lithium)
» Meperidine
      (the analgesic effects of meperidine may be potentiated by amphetamines; however, concurrent use of meperidine is not recommended, as it may potentially result in hypotension, severe respiratory depression, coma, convulsions, hyperpyrexia, vascular collapse, and death in some patients due to the monoamine oxidase inhibition properties of amphetamines)
Metrizamide
      (intrathecal administration of metrizamide may increase the risk of seizures because of lowered seizure threshold; it is recommended that amphetamines be discontinued for at least 48 hours before and 24 hours after myelography)

» Monoamine oxidase (MAO) inhibitors, including furazolidone, procarbazine, and selegiline
      (concurrent use may prolong and intensify cardiac stimulant and vasopressor effects [including headache, cardiac arrhythmias, vomiting, sudden and severe hypertensive and hyperpyretic crises] of amphetamines because of the release of catecholamines that accumulate in intraneuronal storage sites during MAO inhibitor therapy; amphetamines should not be administered during or within 14 days following the administration of an MAO inhibitor)
Propoxyphene
      (overdosage of propoxyphene may potentiate central stimulant effects of amphetamines; fatal convulsions can occur)
» Thyroid hormones
      (the effects of either these medications or amphetamines may be increased; thyroid hormones enhance the risk of coronary insufficiency when amphetamines are administered to patients with coronary artery disease)

**Laboratory value alterations**
The following have been selected on the basis of their potential clinical significance (possible effect in parentheses where appropriate)—not necessarily inclusive (» = major clinical significance):
With diagnostic test results
   Urinary steroid determinations
      (may be altered, interfering with results of such tests as the metyrapone test)
With physiology/laboratory test values
   Plasma corticosteroid concentrations
      (may be increased, with greatest increase in evening)

**Medical considerations/Contraindications**
The medical considerations/contraindications included have been selected on the basis of their potential clinical significance (reasons given in parentheses where appropriate)—not necessarily inclusive (» = major clinical significance).

*Risk-benefit should be considered when the following medical problems exist:*
» Agitated states or
» Arteriosclerosis, advancedor
» Cardiovascular disease, symptomatic or
» Drug abuse or dependence, history of or
» Glaucoma or
» Hypertension or
» Hyperthyroidism or
   Psychoses, especially in children or
» Tourette's syndrome or other motor or vocal tics
      (increased risk of exacerbation)
   Sensitivity to amphetamines and other sympathomimetics

**Patient monitoring**
The following may be especially important in patient monitoring (other tests may be warranted in some patients, depending on condition; » = major clinical significance):
   Assessment of potential tolerance, dependence, or drug-seeking behavior and
   Blood pressure determinations and
   Cardiac rhythm determinations
      (recommended at periodic intervals during therapy)
   Monitoring of growth in children
      (recommended during therapy since data suggest that chronic administration of amphetamines may be associated with growth inhibition)
   Monitoring for motor and vocal tics
      (recommended during therapy)
   Reassessment of need for therapy for attention-deficit hyperactivity disorder in children
      (interruption of therapy at periodic intervals is recommended to determine if a recurrence of behavioral symptoms is sufficient to continue therapy)

## Side/Adverse Effects

Note: Psychological dependence and tolerance may occur with amphetamines following prolonged use or high doses.

The following side/adverse effects have been selected on the basis of their potential clinical significance (possible signs and symptoms in parentheses where appropriate)—not necessarily inclusive:

**Those indicating need for medical attention**
Incidence more frequent
   *Irregular heartbeat*

**Amphetamines (Systemic)**

Incidence rare
   *Allergic reaction* (skin rash or hives); *chest pain; CNS stimulation, severe,* or *Tourette's syndrome* (uncontrolled movements of the head, neck, arms, and legs); *hyperthermia* (extremely high body temperature)

With prolonged use or high doses
   *Cardiomyopathy* (chest discomfort or pain; difficulty in breathing; dizziness or feeling faint; irregular or pounding heartbeat; unusual tiredness or weakness); *increase in blood pressure; psychotic reactions or toxic psychoses* (mood or mental changes)

**Those indicating need for medical attention only if they continue or are bothersome**
Incidence more frequent
   *CNS stimulation* (false sense of well-being; irritability; nervousness; restlessness; trouble in sleeping)—drowsiness, fatigue, trembling, or mental depression may follow the stimulant effects

Incidence less frequent
   *Blurred vision; changes in sexual desire or decreased sexual ability; constipation; diarrhea; loss of appetite; nausea; stomach cramps or pain; weight loss; vomiting; dizziness; lightheadedness; headache; dryness of mouth or unpleasant taste; fast or pounding heartbeat; increased sweating*

**Those indicating possible withdrawal and the need for medical attention if they occur after medication is discontinued**
   *Mental depression; nausea; stomach cramps or pain; vomiting; trembling; unusual tiredness or weakness*

## Overdose

For specific information on the agents used in the management of amphetamine overdose, see:
   • *Barbiturates (Systemic)* monograph;
   • *Chlorpromazine* in *Phenothiazines (Systemic)* monograph; and/or
   • *Phentolamine (Systemic)* monograph.

For more information on the management of overdose or unintentional ingestion, **contact a Poison Control Center** (see *Poison Control Center Listing*).

**Treatment of overdose**
Since there is no specific antidote for overdosage with amphetamines, treatment is symptomatic and supportive.
   To decrease absorption—
      Induction of emesis and/or use of gastric lavage is primary.
      Use of saline cathartics to hasten evacuation of sustained-release dosage forms.
   To enhance elimination—
      Acidification of urine to increase amphetamine excretion. Acidification is contraindicated in presence of rhabdomyolysis, myoglobinuria, or hemoglobinemia, as renal failure may result.
      Forced diuresis if condition permits.
   Specific treatment—
      Barbiturate sedatives or chlorpromazine sometimes used to control excessive CNS stimulation.
      Intravenous phentolamine to control hypertension.
   Monitoring—
      Cardiovascular and respiratory monitoring.
   Supportive care—
      Protection of patient from self-injury by use of restraints if necessary.
      Intravenous fluids to control hypotension.
      Patients in whom intentional overdose is confirmed or suspected should be referred for psychiatric consultation.

## Patient Consultation

As an aid to patient consultation, refer to *Advice for the Patient, Amphetamines (Systemic)*.
In providing consultation, consider emphasizing the following selected information (» = major clinical significance):

### Before using this medication
» Conditions affecting use, especially:
   Sensitivity to amphetamines and other sympathomimetics
   Pregnancy—Increased risk of congenital malformations, especially in cardiovascular system and biliary tract; potential embryotoxic and teratogenic effects in animals given large doses; risk of premature delivery and low birth weight may be increased; newborn may experience withdrawal symptoms
   Breast-feeding—Not recommended since amphetamines are distributed into breast milk
   Use in children—May inhibit growth; may provoke motor and vocal tics and Tourette's syndrome; may exacerbate behavior problems and thought disorder in psychotic children
   Other medications, especially tricyclic antidepressants, beta-adrenergic blocking agents, digitalis glycosides, meperidine, monoamine oxidase inhibitors, other CNS stimulation–producing medications, or thyroid hormones
   Other medical problems, especially agitated states, advanced arteriosclerosis or symptomatic cardiovascular disease, history of drug dependence, glaucoma, hypertension, hyperthyroidism, or Tourette's syndrome or other tics

### Proper use of this medication
Taking the last dose of the day of the regular dosage form at least 6 hours before bedtime and the daily dose of the extended-release dosage form about 10 to 14 hours before bedtime to minimize the possibility of insomnia
Proper administration of extended-release dosage forms:
   Swallowing whole
   Not breaking, crushing, or chewing
» Importance of not taking more medication than the amount prescribed because of habit-forming potential
» Not increasing dose if medication becomes less effective after a few weeks; checking with physician
» Proper dosing
   Missed dose: If dosing schedule is—
      Once a day: Taking as soon as possible but not later than stated above; if remembered later, not taking until next day; not doubling doses
      Two or three times a day: Taking as soon as possible if remembered within an hour or so; not taking if remembered later; not doubling doses
» Proper storage

### Precautions while using this medication
Regular visits to physician to check progress during therapy
» Checking with physician before discontinuing medication after prolonged high-dose therapy; gradual dosage reduction may be necessary to avoid possibility of withdrawal symptoms
» Caution if dizziness or euphoria occurs; not driving, using machinery, or doing other activities that are potentially hazardous
   Caution if any laboratory tests required; possible interference with results of metyrapone test
» Suspected psychological or physical dependence; checking with physician

### Side/adverse effects
Signs of potential side effects, especially irregular heartbeat; allergic reaction; chest pain; tics or other signs of severe CNS stimulation; hyperthermia; cardiomyopathy; increased blood pressure; psychotic reactions
Potential unwanted effects during long-term use in children
Possibility of withdrawal effects, especially mental depression, nausea, stomach cramps or pain, vomiting, trembling, or unusual tiredness or weakness

## General Dosing Information

When the regular tablet dosage form of amphetamines is administered, the first dose should be taken on awakening, followed by 1 or 2 additional doses at intervals of 4 to 6 hours.

To reduce the possibility of insomnia, the last dose of the day of the regular dosage form should be administered at least 6 hours before bedtime, and the daily dose of the extended-release dosage form should be administered approximately 10 to 14 hours before bedtime.

The extended-release dosage form may be used for once-a-day dosing whenever it is feasible.

When symptoms of attention-deficit hyperactivity disorder are controlled in children, dosage reduction or interruption in therapy may be possible during the summer months and at other times when the child is under less stress; medication may be given on each of the 5 school days during the week, with medication-free weekends and school holidays.

Prolonged use of amphetamines may result in tolerance, extreme psychological dependence, or severe social disability.

When the medication is to be discontinued following prolonged high-dose administration, the dosage should be reduced gradually since abrupt withdrawal may result in extreme fatigue and mental depression.

---

## AMPHETAMINE

## Oral Dosage Forms

Note:  Bracketed uses in the *Dosage Forms* section refer to categories of use and/or indications that are not included in U.S. product labeling.

## AMPHETAMINE SULFATE TABLETS USP
**Usual adult dose**
[Attention-deficit hyperactivity disorder] or
Narcolepsy—
    Oral, 5 to 20 mg one to three times a day.

**Usual pediatric dose**
Attention-deficit hyperactivity disorder—
    Children younger than 3 years of age: Use is not recommended.
    Children 3 to 6 years of age: Oral, 2.5 mg once a day, the dosage being increased by 2.5 mg per day at one-week intervals until the desired response is obtained.
    Children 6 years of age and older: Oral, 5 mg one or two times a day, the dosage being increased by 5 mg per day at one-week intervals until the desired response is obtained.
Narcolepsy—
    Children younger than 6 years of age: Dosage has not been established.
    Children 6 to 12 years of age: Oral, 2.5 mg two times a day, the dosage being increased by 5 mg per day at one-week intervals until the desired response is obtained or until the adult dose is reached.
    Children 12 years of age and older: Oral, 5 mg two times a day, the dosage being increased by 10 mg per day at one-week intervals until the desired response is obtained or until the adult dose is reached.

**Strength(s) usually available**
U.S.—
    5 mg (Rx) [GENERIC].
    10 mg (Rx) [GENERIC].
Canada—
    Not commercially available.

**Packaging and storage**
Store below 40 °C (104 °F), preferably between 15 and 30 °C (59 and 86 °F), unless otherwise specified by manufacturer. Store in a well-closed container.

**Note**
Controlled substance in the U.S.

---

### AMPHETAMINE AND DEXTROAMPHETAMINE

## Oral Dosage Forms
### AMPHETAMINE ASPARTATE, AMPHETAMINE SULFATE, DEXTROAMPHETAMINE SACCHARATE, AND DEXTROAMPHETAMINE SULFATE TABLETS
**Usual adult dose**
Narcolepsy—
    Oral, 5 to 60 mg a day in divided doses.

**Usual pediatric dose**
Attention-deficit hyperactivity disorder—
    Children younger than 3 years of age: Use is not recommended.
    Children 3 to 6 years of age: Oral, initially 2.5 mg a day, the dosage being increased by 2.5 mg per day at one-week intervals until the desired response is obtained.
    Children 6 years of age and older: Oral, initially 5 mg one or two times a day, the dosage being increased by 5 mg per day at one-week intervals until the desired response is obtained.
Narcolepsy—
    Children younger than 6 years of age: Dosage has not been established.
    Children 6 to 12 years of age: Oral, initially 5 mg a day, the dosage being increased by 5 mg per day at one-week intervals until the desired response is obtained.
    Children 12 years of age and older: Oral, initially 10 mg a day, the dosage being increased by 10 mg per day at one-week intervals until the desired response is obtained.
Note: The usual pediatric dose rarely exceeds 40 mg a day.

**Strength(s) usually available**
U.S.—
    5 mg (1.25 mg each: amphetamine aspartate, amphetamine sulfate, dextroamphetamine saccharate, dextroamphetamine sulfate) (Rx) [*Adderall* (double scored; acacia; corn starch; FD&C Blue #1; lactose; magnesium stearate; sucrose)].
    10 mg (2.5 mg each: amphetamine aspartate, amphetamine sulfate, dextroamphetamine saccharate, dextroamphetamine sulfate) (Rx) [*Adderall* (double scored; acacia; corn starch; FD&C Blue #1; lactose; magnesium stearate; sucrose)].
    20 mg (5 mg each: amphetamine aspartate, amphetamine sulfate, dextroamphetamine saccharate, dextroamphetamine sulfate) (Rx) [*Adderall* (double scored; acacia; corn starch; FD&C Yellow #6; lactose; magnesium stearate; sucrose)].
    30 mg (7.5 mg each: amphetamine aspartate, amphetamine sulfate, dextroamphetamine saccharate, dextroamphetamine sulfate) (Rx) [*Adderall* (double scored; acacia; corn starch; FD&C Yellow #6; lactose; magnesium stearate; sucrose)].
Canada—
    Not commercially available.

**Packaging and storage**
Store between 15 and 30 °C (59 and 86 °F), unless otherwise specified by manufacturer. Store in a tight, light-resistant container.

**Note**
Controlled substance in the U.S.

**Additional information**
The 5 mg, 10 mg, 20 mg, and 30 mg tablets are equivalent to 3.13 mg, 6.3 mg, 12.5 mg, and 18.8 mg of amphetamine base, respectively.

---

### DEXTROAMPHETAMINE

## Oral Dosage Forms
Note: Bracketed uses in the *Dosage Forms* section refer to categories of use and/or indications that are not included in U.S. product labeling.

### DEXTROAMPHETAMINE SULFATE EXTENDED-RELEASE CAPSULES
Note: The extended-release dosage form should not be used for initiation of dosage, nor should it be used until the conventional titrated daily dosage is equal to or greater than the dosage provided in the extended-release dosage form.

**Usual adult dose**
[Attention-deficit hyperactivity disorder][1] or
Narcolepsy—
    Oral, 5 to 60 mg once a day, or in divided doses.

**Usual pediatric dose**
Attention-deficit hyperactivity disorder—
    Children younger than 3 years of age: Use is not recommended.
    Children 3 to 6 years of age: Oral, initially 2.5 mg once a day, the dosage being increased by 2.5 mg per day at one-week intervals until the desired response is obtained.
    Children 6 years of age and older: Oral, 5 mg once or twice a day, the dosage being increased by 5 mg a day at one-week intervals until the desired response is obtained.
Narcolepsy—
    Children younger than 3 years of age: Use is not recommended.
    Children 3 to 6 years of age: Dosage has not been established.
    Children 6 to 12 years of age: Oral, initially 5 mg once a day, the dosage being increased by 5 mg a day at one-week intervals until the desired response is obtained.
    Children 12 years of age and older: Oral, initially 10 mg once a day, the dosage being increased by 10 mg a day at one-week intervals until the desired response is obtained.
Note: The usual pediatric dose rarely exceeds 40 mg a day.

**Strength(s) usually available**
U.S.—
    5 mg (Rx) [*Dexedrine Spansule* (tartrazine)].
    10 mg (Rx) [*Dexedrine Spansule* (tartrazine)].
    15 mg (Rx) [*Dexedrine Spansule* (tartrazine)].
Canada—
    10 mg (Rx) [*Dexedrine Spansule* (tartrazine)].
    15 mg (Rx) [*Dexedrine Spansule* (tartrazine)].

**Packaging and storage**
Store between 15 and 30 °C (59 and 86 °F), in a tight, light-resistant container, unless otherwise specified by manufacturer.

**Auxiliary labeling**
• Swallow capsules whole.

**Note**
Controlled substance in both the U.S. and Canada.

### DEXTROAMPHETAMINE SULFATE TABLETS USP
**Usual adult dose**
[Attention-deficit hyperactivity disorder][1] or
Narcolepsy—
    Oral, 5 to 60 mg a day in divided doses as needed and tolerated.

**Usual pediatric dose**
Attention-deficit hyperactivity disorder—
  Children younger than 3 years of age: Use is not recommended.
  Children 3 to 6 years of age: Oral, 2.5 mg once a day, the dosage being increased by 2.5 mg a day at one-week intervals until the desired response is obtained.
  Children 6 years of age and older: Oral, 5 mg one or two times a day, the dosage being increased by 5 mg a day at one-week intervals until the desired response is obtained.
Narcolepsy—
  Children younger than 6 years of age: Dosage has not been established.
  Children 6 to 12 years of age: Oral, 5 mg a day, the dosage being increased by 5 mg a day at one-week intervals until the desired response is obtained or until the adult dose is reached.
  Children 12 years of age and older: Oral, 10 mg a day, the dosage being increased by 10 mg a day at one-week intervals until the desired response is obtained or until the adult dose is reached.
Note: The usual pediatric dose rarely exceeds 40 mg a day.

**Strength(s) usually available**
U.S.—
  5 mg (Rx) [*Dexedrine* (tartrazine); *Dextrostat*; GENERIC].
  10 mg (Rx) [GENERIC].
Canada—
  5 mg (Rx) [*Dexedrine* (tartrazine)].

**Packaging and storage**
Store below 40 °C (104 °F), preferably between 15 and 30 °C (59 and 86 °F), unless otherwise specified by manufacturer. Store in a tight container.

**Note**
Controlled substance in both the U.S. and Canada.

---

[1]Not included in Canadian product labeling.

---

## METHAMPHETAMINE

## Oral Dosage Forms

### METHAMPHETAMINE HYDROCHLORIDE TABLETS USP

**Usual pediatric dose**
Attention-deficit hyperactivity disorder—
  Children younger than 6 years of age: Use is not recommended.
  Children 6 years of age and older: Oral, 5 mg one or two times a day, the dosage being increased by 5 mg per day at one-week intervals until the desired response is obtained (usually 20 to 25 mg per day).

**Strength(s) usually available**
U.S.—
  5 mg (Rx) [*Desoxyn* (lactose)].
Canada—
  Not commercially available.

**Packaging and storage**
Store below 40 °C (104 °F), preferably between 15 and 30 °C (59 and 86 °F), in a well-closed container, unless otherwise specified by manufacturer.

**Note**
Controlled substance in the U.S.

### METHAMPHETAMINE HYDROCHLORIDE EXTENDED-RELEASE TABLETS

Note: The extended-release dosage form should not be used for initiation of dosage or until the conventional titrated daily dosage is equal to or greater than the dosage provided in the extended-release dosage form.

**Usual pediatric dose**
Attention-deficit hyperactivity disorder—
  Children younger than 6 years of age: Use is not recommended.
  Children 6 years of age and older: Oral, 20 to 25 mg once a day.

**Strength(s) usually available**
U.S.—
  5 mg (Rx) [*Desoxyn Gradumet*].
  10 mg (Rx) [*Desoxyn Gradumet*].
  15 mg (Rx) [*Desoxyn Gradumet* (tartrazine)].
Canada—
  Not commercially available.

**Packaging and storage**
Store below 40 °C (104 °F), preferably between 15 and 30 °C (59 and 86 °F), in a well-closed container, unless otherwise specified by manufacturer.

**Auxiliary labeling**
• Swallow tablets whole.
• Keep container tightly closed.

**Note**
Controlled substance in the U.S.

Revised: 08/18/94
Interim revision: 08/13/98

---

# AMPHOTERICIN B   Systemic

VA CLASSIFICATION (Primary/Secondary): AM700/AP109
Commonly used brand name(s): *Amphocin; Fungizone Intravenous*.
Note: For a listing of dosage forms and brand names by country availability, see *Dosage Forms* section(s).

## Category
Antifungal (systemic); antiprotozoal.

## Indications
Note: Bracketed information in the *Indications* section refers to uses that are not included in U.S. product labeling.

### Accepted
Aspergillosis (treatment)—Parenteral amphotericin B is indicated in the treatment of aspergillosis caused by *Aspergillus fumigatus*. [Intracavitary amphotericin B has also been used in the treatment of pulmonary aspergilloma with hemoptysis.]
Blastomycosis (treatment)—Parenteral amphotericin B is indicated in the treatment of North American blastomycosis caused by *Blastomyces dermatitidis*.
Candidiasis, disseminated (treatment)—Parenteral amphotericin B is indicated in the treatment of disseminated candidiasis caused by *Candida* species.
Coccidioidomycosis (treatment)—Parenteral amphotericin B is indicated in the treatment of coccidioidomycosis caused by *Coccidioides immitis*.
Cryptococcosis (treatment)—Parenteral amphotericin B is indicated in the treatment of cryptococcosis caused by *Cryptococcus neoformans*.
Endocarditis, fungal (treatment)—Parenteral amphotericin B is indicated in the treatment of fungal endocarditis.
Endophthalmitis, candidal (treatment)—Parenteral and intraocular administration of amphotericin B are used in the treatment of candidal endophthalmitis.
Histoplasmosis (treatment)—Parenteral amphotericin B is indicated in the treatment of histoplasmosis caused by *Histoplasma capsulatum*.
Intra-abdominal infections (treatment)—Parenteral and intraperitoneal administration of amphotericin B, with or without concurrent administration of other antifungal medications, are used for the treatment of intra-abdominal infections, including dialysis-related and non–dialysis-related peritonitis.
Leishmaniasis, American mucocutaneous (treatment)—Parenteral amphotericin B is indicated as an alternative agent in the treatment of American mucocutaneous leishmaniasis caused by *Leishmania braziliensis* and *L. mexicana*.
Meningitis, cryptococcal (treatment) or
Meningitis, cryptococcal (suppression) or
Meningitis, fungal, other (treatment)—Parenteral amphotericin B is indicated, with or without concurrent administration of flucytosine, in the treatment and suppression of cryptococcal meningitis caused by *Cryptococcus neoformans*.
  Parenteral amphotericin B is also indicated in the treatment of fungal meningitis caused by organisms such as *Coccidioides immitis*, *Candida* species, *Sporothrix schenckii*, and *Aspergillus* species.

Mucormycosis (treatment)—Parenteral amphotericin B is indicated in the treatment of mucormycosis (phycomycosis) caused by *Mucor, Rhizopus, Absidia, Entomophthora* and *Basidiobolus* organisms.

Septicemia, fungal (treatment)—Parenteral amphotericin B is indicated in the treatment of fungal septicemia.

Sporotrichosis, disseminated (treatment)—Parenteral amphotericin B is indicated in the treatment of disseminated sporotrichosis caused by *Sporothrix schenckii*.

Urinary tract infections, fungal (treatment)—Parenteral administration [and continuous bladder irrigation] of amphotericin B are indicated in the treatment of fungal (particularly *Candida* species) urinary tract infections.

[Meningoencephalitis, primary amebic (treatment)][1]—Parenteral amphotericin B is used in the treatment of primary amebic meningoencephalitis caused by *Naegleria* species.

[Paracoccidioidomycosis (treatment)][1]—Parenteral amphotericin B is used as a secondary agent in the treatment of paracoccidioidomycosis caused by *Paracoccidioides brasiliensis*.

Not all species or strains of a particular organism may be susceptible to amphotericin B. Because of its toxicity, amphotericin B is indicated primarily in patients with progressive, potentially fatal infections in whom the diagnosis is firmly established, preferably by positive culture or histologic study.

### Unaccepted
Amphotericin B is not indicated in the treatment of common, clinically inapparent fungal infections that show only positive skin or serologic tests.

Amphotericin B is not effective against bacteria, rickettsiae, or viruses.

[1]Not included in Canadian product labeling.

## Pharmacology/Pharmacokinetics
### Physicochemical characteristics
Molecular weight—924.09.

### Mechanism of action/Effect
Antifungal (systemic)—
Fungistatic in concentrations usually obtained clinically; however, in concentrations near the upper limits of tolerance, may be fungicidal. Probably acts by binding to sterols in the fungus cell membrane, producing a change in membrane permeability that allows loss of potassium and small molecules from the cell.

### Distribution
Distributed to lungs, liver, spleen, kidneys, adrenal glands, muscle, and other tissues (potentially therapeutic concentrations); reaches approximately two-thirds the concurrent plasma concentration in the fluids of inflamed pleura, peritoneum, synovium and aqueous humor; concentrations in cerebrospinal fluid (CSF) usually undetectable.

$Vol_D$—
Neonates: Variable (range, 1.5 to 9.4 L per kg).
Children: Variable (range, 0.4 to 8.3 L per kg).
Adults: Approximately 4 L per kg.

### Protein binding
Very high (90% or more).

### Biotransformation
Metabolic pathways unknown.

### Half-life
Elimination half-life—
Neonates: Variable (range, 18.8 to 62.5 hours).
Children: Variable (range, 5.5 to 40.3 hours).
Adults: Approximately 24 hours.
Terminal half-life—
Approximately 15 days.

### Peak plasma concentration
Approximately 0.5 to 2 mcg per mL, following repeated doses of approximately 0.5 mg per kg per day.

### Elimination
Renal— Very slow; 2 to 5% of a dose eliminated in biologically active form in urine; approximately 40% excreted over a 7-day period. May be detected in urine for at least 7 weeks after medication is discontinued.
Biliary—Minimal excretion of active form.
In dialysis—Poorly dialyzable.

## Precautions to Consider
### Carcinogenicity/Mutagenicity
Long-term studies in animals have not been done to evaluate the carcinogenic or mutagenic potential of amphotericin B.

### Pregnancy/Reproduction
Pregnancy—Amphotericin B crosses the placenta. Adequate and well-controlled studies in humans have not been done. However, no adverse fetal effects have been documented in numerous case reports where amphotericin B was used in all stages of pregnancy.

Studies in animals have not shown that amphotericin B causes adverse effects on the fetus.

FDA Pregnancy Category B.

### Breast-feeding
It is not known whether amphotericin B is excreted in breast milk. However, problems in humans have not been documented.

### Pediatrics
Appropriate studies on the relationship of age to the effects of amphotericin B have not been performed in the pediatric population. However, systemic fungal infections have been successfully treated in children and no pediatrics-specific problems have been documented to date.

### Geriatrics
No information is available on the relationship of age to the effects of amphotericin B in geriatric patients.

### Drug interactions and/or related problems
The following drug interactions and/or related problems have been selected on the basis of their potential clinical significance (possible mechanism in parentheses where appropriate)—not necessarily inclusive (» = major clinical significance):

Note: Combinations containing any of the following medications, depending on the amount present, may also interact with this medication.

Blood dyscrasia–causing medications (See *Appendix II*) or
» Bone marrow depressants (See *Appendix II*) or
» Radiation therapy
(concurrent use of these medications or radiation therapy with amphotericin B may increase the chance of anemia or other hematologic effects; dosage reduction may be required)

Carbonic anhydrase inhibitors or
» Corticotropin (ACTH), especially with chronic use or
» Corticosteroids, glucocorticoid, especially with significant mineralocorticoid activity or
» Corticosteroids, mineralocorticoid or
(concurrent use of these medications with parenteral amphotericin B may result in severe hypokalemia and should be undertaken with caution; patients should have serum potassium determinations at frequent intervals during concurrent therapy; cardiac function should also be monitored)

(concurrent use of corticotropin with parenteral amphotericin B may decrease adrenocortical responsiveness to corticotropin)

» Digitalis glycosides or
Neuromuscular blocking agents, nondepolarizing
(parenteral amphotericin B may induce hypokalemia, which may increase the potential for digitalis toxicity or enhance the blockade of nondepolarizing neuromuscular blocking agents)

(serum potassium determinations and correction of hypokalemia may be necessary prior to administration of nondepolarizing neuromuscular blocking agents or at frequent intervals during concurrent therapy with digitalis glycosides)

» Diuretics, potassium-depleting or
» Nephrotoxic medications, other (See *Appendix II*)
(concurrent use of diuretics and other nephrotoxic medications with amphotericin B may increase the potential for nephrotoxicity; dosage reduction or withdrawal of cyclosporine or amphotericin B may be necessary if renal impairment occurs. Concurrent use of diuretics with parenteral amphotericin B may also intensify electrolyte imbalance, particularly hypokalemia; frequent electrolyte determinations are necessary, and potassium supplementation may also be required)

Flucytosine
(concurrent use of amphotericin B and flucytosine may have additive or slightly synergistic effects; amphotericin B–induced renal dysfunction may decrease the clearance of flucytosine, which may result in increased flucytosine adverse effects, such as bone marrow toxicity. However, 2-drug therapy may allow the total daily dose of amphotericin B to be lowered, decreasing the risk of nephrotoxicity)

### Medical considerations/Contraindications
The medical considerations/contraindications included have been selected on the basis of their potential clinical significance (reasons given in parentheses where appropriate)—not necessarily inclusive (» = major clinical significance).

*Risk-benefit should be considered when the following medical problems exist:*

Hypersensitivity to amphotericin B
» Renal function impairment
(although amphotericin B is not renally excreted, it can be nephrotoxic and worsen any pre-existing renal function impairment)

**Patient monitoring**
The following may be especially important in patient monitoring (other tests may be warranted in some patients, depending on condition; » = major clinical significance):

» Blood urea nitrogen (BUN) and
» Creatinine, serum
(concentrations recommended every other day while dosage is being increased and then at least twice weekly thereafter during therapy; if the BUN and/or the serum creatinine increase to clinically significant concentrations, discontinuation of the medication may be necessary until renal function is improved)

Complete blood count (CBC) and
Platelet count
(recommended at weekly intervals during therapy)

Magnesium, serum and
» Potassium, serum
(concentrations recommended twice weekly during therapy)

## Side/Adverse Effects

Note: Since amphotericin B is frequently the only effective treatment for certain potentially fatal fungal infections, its life-saving benefits must be balanced against its potential for dangerous side/adverse effects.

Administration of an antipyretic, antihistamine, meperidine, and/or corticosteroid just prior to the amphotericin B infusion may decrease the fever and shaking chills that can be associated with amphotericin B administration.

The following side/adverse effects have been selected on the basis of their potential clinical significance (possible signs and symptoms in parentheses where appropriate)—not necessarily inclusive:

**Those indicating need for medical attention**
Incidence more frequent
*With intravenous infusion*
**Anemia** (unusual tiredness or weakness)—normocytic, normochromic; **hypokalemia** (irregular heartbeat; muscle cramps or pain; unusual tiredness or weakness); **infusion-related reaction** (fever and chills; nausea and vomiting; headache; hypotension); **renal function impairment** (increased or decreased urination); **thrombophlebitis** (pain at infusion site)

Incidence less frequent or rare
*With intravenous infusion*
**Blurred or double vision; cardiac arrhythmias** (irregular heartbeat)—usually with rapid infusion; **hypersensitivity** (skin rash; itching; shortness of breath; troubled breathing; wheezing; tightness in chest); **leukopenia** (sore throat and fever); **polyneuropathy** (numbness, tingling, pain, or weakness in hands or feet); **seizures; thrombocytopenia** (unusual bleeding or bruising)

*With intrathecal injection*
**Blurred vision or any change in vision; difficult urination; polyneuropathy** (numbness, tingling, pain, or weakness)

**Those indicating need for medical attention only if they continue or are bothersome**
Incidence more frequent
*With intravenous infusion*
**Gastrointestinal disturbance** (indigestion; loss of appetite; nausea; vomiting; diarrhea; stomach pain); **headache**

Incidence less frequent
*With intrathecal injection*
**Back, leg, or neck pain; dizziness or lightheadedness; headache; nausea or vomiting**

## Patient Consultation

As an aid to patient consultation, refer to *Advice for the Patient, Amphotericin B (Systemic).*

In providing consultation, consider emphasizing the following selected information (» = major clinical significance):

**Before using this medication**
» Conditions affecting use, especially:
Hypersensitivity to amphotericin B
Other medications, especially adrenocorticoids, corticotropin, other bone marrow depressants, digitalis glycosides, other nephrotoxic medications, potassium-depleting diuretics, or radiation therapy
Other medical problems, especially renal function impairment

**Side/adverse effects**
Signs of potential side effects, especially anemia, blurred or double vision, cardiac arrhythmias, difficult urination, hypersensitivity reactions, hypokalemia, infusion-related reaction, leukopenia, polyneuropathy, renal function impairment, seizures, thrombocytopenia, or thrombophlebitis

## General Dosing Information

Therapy interrupted for more than 7 days should be resumed by starting with the lowest dosage and gradually increasing to the desired dosage.

Therapy should be continued for a sufficient period of time to minimize the possibility of a relapse.

The intravenous administration of small doses of corticosteroids (i.e., ≤ 25 mg of hydrocortisone) just prior to or during intravenous infusion of amphotericin B may reduce the incidence of febrile reactions. Dosage and duration of concurrent corticosteroid therapy should be kept to a minimum. Also, acetaminophen, antihistamines, meperidine, and/or phenothiazines have been given empirically, just prior to the infusion, to decrease the nausea, fever, and chills associated with amphotericin B administration.

Amphotericin B should be infused over a period of 2 to 6 hours. In patients with normal renal function, rapid infusions of 1 to 2 hours have been used with infusion-related reactions similar to those associated with 4 to 6 hour infusions. However, rapid infusions have been associated with earlier infusion-related toxicity and more complaints of nausea and vomiting.

A cumulative dosage exceeding 4 grams may result in irreversible renal dysfunction.

Full dosage of amphotericin B is required even in patients with impaired renal function since the primary route of excretion is not renal. Patients should be observed closely if there is further loss of renal function. Nephrotoxicity may be decreased in sodium-depleted patients by salt loading prior to administration; however, routine prophylactic sodium loading is not recommended, especially in patients with underlying renal or cardiac disease.

Extravasation of the drug may cause severe local irritation.

To minimize local thrombophlebitis, which may occur with intravenous administration, heparin may be added to the amphotericin B infusion or the medication may be administered on alternate days. Administration on alternate days may also reduce the incidence of anorexia.

Alternate-day dosage should not exceed 1.5 mg per kg of body weight (mg/kg).

## Parenteral Dosage Forms

Note: The dosing and dosage forms available are expressed in terms of amphotericin B base.

### AMPHOTERICIN B FOR INJECTION USP

**Usual adult and adolescent dose**
Antifungal (systemic)—
Intracavitary instillation, initially 5 mg (base) in 10 to 20 mL of 5% dextrose injection administered over three to five minutes; then, 50 mg (base) of amphotericin B in 10 to 20 mL of 5% dextrose injection administered over three to five minutes each day. This is usually followed eight to twelve hours later by 20 mL of 5% N-acetylcysteine and overnight low-continuous wall suction.

Intrathecal, initially 0.01 to 0.1 mg (base) every forty-eight to seventy-two hours, the dosage being increased gradually to 0.5 mg as tolerated.

Intravenous infusion, initially 1 mg (base) as a test dose, administered in 20 to 50 mL of 5% dextrose injection over a period of ten to thirty minutes; the dosage may then be increased in 5- to 10-mg increments or more according to patient tolerance and severity of infection, up to a maximum of 50 mg per day, and administered over a period of two to six hours.

Note: In severely ill patients, some clinicians prefer to initiate therapy utilizing full dosage of amphotericin B.

Continuous bladder irrigation, 5 mg (base) of amphotericin B in 1000 mL of sterile water per day, administered at a rate of 40 mL per hour via a three-way catheter for five to ten days.

## Usual pediatric dose
**Antifungal (systemic)**—
Intravenous infusion, initially 0.25 mg (base) per kg of body weight per day, administered in 5% dextrose injection over a period of six hours, the dosage being increased gradually (usually by 0.125 to 0.25 mg per kg of body weight increments every day or every other day) as tolerated, up to a maximum of 1 mg per kg of body weight or 30 mg per square meter of body surface per day.

## Size(s) usually available
U.S.—
50 mg (base) (Rx) [*Amphocin; Fungizone Intravenous;* GENERIC].
Canada—
50 mg (base) (Rx) [*Fungizone Intravenous*].

## Packaging and storage
Prior to reconstitution, store between 2 and 8 °C (36 and 46 °F). Protect from light.

## Preparation of dosage form
To prepare initial dilution for intrathecal use or intravenous infusion, add 10 mL of sterile water for injection, without a bacteriostatic agent, to the vial containing 50 mg (base) of amphotericin B. For intrathecal use, the resulting solution containing 5 mg of amphotericin B per mL may be further diluted to a final concentration of 0.25 mg per mL by adding 1 mL (5 mg) of the solution to 19 mL of 5% dextrose injection with a pH above 4.2. Before injection, the dose is diluted with 5 to 30 mL of cerebrospinal fluid in the syringe. For intravenous infusion, the resulting solution containing 5 mg of amphotericin B per mL may be diluted to a final concentration of 0.1 mg per mL by adding 1 mL (5 mg) of the solution to 49 mL of 5% dextrose injection with a pH above 4.2.

The pH of the dextrose injection should be determined aseptically before the injection is used to dilute the 5-mg-per-mL concentration of the amphotericin B solution. If the pH is below 4.2, it should be adjusted. See the manufacturer's package insert for buffering procedure.

Amphotericin B should be reconstituted only with the diluents recommended, since solutions containing sodium chloride or a bacteriostatic agent (for example, benzyl alcohol) may cause precipitation of the medication.

## Stability
After reconstitution, concentrated solutions (5 mg per mL) in sterile water for injection retain their potency for 24 hours at room temperature, protected from light, or for 1 week if refrigerated. Diluted solutions for intravenous infusion (0.1 mg per mL or less) in 5% dextrose injection should be used promptly after dilution.

The manufacturer recommends that the intravenous infusion be protected from light during administration. However, this is probably not necessary, since it has been reported that the loss of drug potency is negligible when amphotericin B infusions are exposed to normal lighting conditions in a hospital.

Do not use if the initial concentrate or the infusion is cloudy or contains a precipitate or foreign matter.

## Incompatibilities
May be incompatible with sodium chloride or bacteriostatic agents such as benzyl alcohol.

## Additional information
Since the reconstituted preparation is a colloidal suspension, membrane filters in intravenous infusion lines may remove clinically significant amounts of the medication. If an in-line membrane filter is used, the mean pore diameter should be no less than 1 micron.

Revised: 02/23/93
Interim revision: 04/19/95

---

**AMPHOTERICIN B** — The *Amphotericin B (Topical)* monograph is not included in this published version of the USP DI database. Copies of the monograph are available on request from Micromedex, Inc. - Reprint Requests, 6200 S. Syracuse Way, Suite 300, Englewood, CO 80111; telephone (303) 486-6400; telefax (303) 486-6464; Email: USPDI@MDX.COM.

---

# AMPHOTERICIN B CHOLESTERYL COMPLEX   Systemic—INTRODUCTORY VERSION

VA CLASSIFICATION (Primary): AM700
Commonly used brand name(s): *Amphotec.*
Note: For a listing of dosage forms and brand names by country availability, see *Dosage Forms* section(s).

## Category
Antifungal (systemic).

## Indications

### General considerations
Amphotericin B cholesteryl complex is active *in vitro* against *Aspergillus* and *Candida* species, as well as against other fungi.

Fungal type variants with reduced susceptibility to amphotericin B have been isolated from several fungal species after serial passage in cell culture media containing amphotericin B, and from some patients receiving prolonged therapy with amphotericin B. Although the relevance of drug resistance to clinical outcome has not been established, fungal organisms that are resistant to amphotericin B may also be resistant to amphotericin B cholesteryl complex.

### Accepted
Aspergillosis (treatment)—Amphotericin B cholesteryl complex is indicated in the treatment of invasive aspergillosis in patients who are refractory to or intolerant of amphotericin B deoxycholate therapy.

## Pharmacology/Pharmacokinetics

### Physicochemical characteristics
Chemical group—Amphotericin B complexed with cholesteryl sulfate in a 1:1 molar ratio.
Molecular weight—Amphotericin B: 924.1.

### Mechanism of action/Effect
Amphotericin B binds primarily to ergosterol in cell membranes of sensitive fungi, causing leakage of intracellular contents and cell death due to changes in membrane permeability. Amphotericin B also binds to cholesterol in mammalian cell membranes; this action is believed to account for its toxicity in animals and humans.

### Distribution
Vol$_D$ (at steady state) of amphotericin B following administration of four doses of amphotericin B cholesteryl complex at a dose of—
3 mg per kg of body weight (mg/kg): 3.8 L per kg.
4 mg/kg: 4.1 L per kg.

### Half-life
Distribution of amphotericin B following administration of four doses of amphotericin B cholesteryl complex at a dose of—
3 mg/kg: 3.5 minutes.
4 mg/kg: 3.5 minutes.
Elimination of amphotericin B following administration of four doses of amphotericin B cholesteryl complex at a dose of—
3 mg/kg: 27.5 hours.
4 mg/kg: 28.2 hours.

### Peak plasma concentration
2.6 to 2.9 mcg per mL, following administration of 1 to 4 mg/kg per day for four days.

### Elimination
Amphotericin B cholesteryl complex is not dialyzable.

## Precautions to Consider

### Carcinogenicity
Long-term studies in animals have not been done to evaluate the carcinogenic potential of amphotericin B cholesteryl complex.

### Mutagenicity
No mutagenic effects were found *in vitro* in the *Salmonella* reverse mutation assay, the CHO cell chromosomal aberration assay, or the mouse lymphoma forward mutation assay, or *in vivo* in the mouse bone marrow micronucleus assay.

### Pregnancy/Reproduction
Fertility—Studies have not been done to evaluate the effects of amphotericin B cholesteryl complex on fertility. However, doses of up to 0.4 and 0.5 times the recommended human dose given to dogs and rats, re-

spectively, for up to 13 weeks did not affect ovarian or testicular histology.

Pregnancy—Adequate and well-controlled studies in humans have not been done.

Studies at doses of up to 0.4 and 1.1 times the recommended human dose given to rats and rabbits, respectively, showed no evidence of fetal harm.

FDA Pregnancy Category B.

### Breast-feeding

It is not known whether amphotericin B cholesteryl complex is distributed into breast milk. Because of the potential for serious adverse effects in nursing infants, a decision should be made to either stop breast-feeding or discontinue taking amphotericin B cholesteryl complex.

### Pediatrics

Ninety-seven pediatric patients have been treated with amphotericin B cholesteryl complex at daily doses similar to those in adults (on a mg per kg of body weight basis), and no unexpected adverse events have been reported.

### Geriatrics

Sixty-eight patients 65 years of age and older have been treated with amphotericin B cholesteryl complex, and no unexpected events have been reported.

### Drug interactions and/or related problems

The following drug interactions and/or related problems have been selected on the basis of their potential clinical significance (possible mechanism in parentheses where appropriate)—not necessarily inclusive (» = major clinical significance):

Note: Combinations containing any of the following medications, depending on the amount present, may also interact with this medication.

» Antineoplastic agents
(concurrent use with amphotericin B cholesteryl complex may enhance the potential for bronchospasm, hypotension, and renal toxicity; caution is required if these medications are to be used concurrently)

Clotrimazole or
Fluconazole or
Ketoconazole or
Miconazole or
Other imidazoles
(*in vitro* and *in vivo* animal studies have reported antagonism between amphotericin B and imidazole derivatives, such as ketoconazole and miconazole, that inhibit ergosterol synthesis; the clinical significance of these findings has not been determined)

» Corticosteroids or
» Corticotropin (ACTH)
(concurrent use with amphotericin B cholesteryl complex may potentiate hypokalemia, which may predispose the patient to cardiac dysfunction; cardiac function and serum electrolytes should be monitored)

Cyclosporine or
Tacrolimus
(adult and pediatric patients receiving amphotericin B cholesteryl complex with cyclosporine or tacrolimus had a 31% incidence of renal toxicity [a doubling or an increase of 1 mg per dL or more from baseline serum creatinine, or ≥ 50% decrease from baseline calculated creatinine clearance], compared with a 68% incidence of renal toxicity for patients receiving amphotericin B deoxycholate with cyclosporine or tacrolimus)

» Digitalis glycosides
(concurrent use with amphotericin B cholesteryl complex may induce hypokalemia and may potentiate digitalis toxicity; serum potassium concentrations should be monitored closely)

Flucytosine
(concurrent use with amphotericin B cholesteryl complex may increase the toxicity of flucytosine by possibly increasing its cellular uptake and/or impairing its renal excretion; caution should be used if flucytosine is to be used concurrently)

» Nephrotoxic medications (see *Appendix II*)
(concurrent use of amphotericin B cholesteryl complex with nephrotoxic medications, such as aminoglycosides or pentamidine, may potentiate medication-induced renal toxicity; caution is required if nephrotoxic medications are to be used concurrently, and renal function should be monitored frequently)

» Neuromuscular blocking agents, nondepolarizing
(amphotericin B may induce hypokalemia, which may enhance the activity of nondepolarizing neuromuscular blocking agents; serum potassium concentrations should be monitored closely)

### Laboratory value alterations

The following have been selected on the basis of their potential clinical significance (possible effect in parentheses where appropriate)—not necessarily inclusive (» = major clinical significance):

With diagnostic test results
Hepatic function tests
(values may be increased or decreased)

With physiology/laboratory test values
Alkaline phosphatase and
» Creatine kinase
(serum values may be increased)

Bilirubin and
Glucose, plasma
(concentrations may be increased)

Calcium and
Magnesium and
Potassium
(serum concentrations may be decreased)

### Medical considerations/Contraindications

The medical considerations/contraindications included have been selected on the basis of their potential clinical significance (reasons given in parentheses where appropriate)—not necessarily inclusive (» = major clinical significance).

*Risk-benefit should be considered when the following medical problem exists:*

» Hypersensitivity to amphotericin B cholesteryl complex

### Patient monitoring

The following may be especially important in patient monitoring (other tests may be warranted in some patients, depending on condition; » = major clinical significance):

Complete blood count (CBC)
(counts should be monitored as medically indicated)

Electrolytes, serum
(concentrations should be monitored as medically indicated)

Hepatic function tests and
Prothrombin time (PT) and
Renal function tests
(values should be monitored as medically indicated)

## Side/Adverse Effects

Note: Anaphylaxis has been reported with amphotericin B–containing medications.

Acute infusion-related reactions, including chills, fever, headache, hypotension, hypoxia, nausea, and tachypnea, usually occur 1 to 3 hours after intravenous infusion has been initiated. These reactions are usually more severe or more frequent with initial doses of amphotericin B cholesteryl complex and usually diminish with subsequent doses.

The following side/adverse effects have been selected on the basis of their potential clinical significance (possible signs and symptoms in parentheses where appropriate)—not necessarily inclusive:

### Those indicating need for medical attention

Incidence more frequent
***Infusion-related reaction*** (chills; fever; headache; hypoxia; nausea)

Incidence less frequent
***Dyspnea*** (difficulty in breathing); ***hypertension; hypotension*** (dizziness or fainting); ***tachycardia*** (increased heartbeat); ***thrombocytopenia*** (unusual bleeding or bruising)

Incidence rare
***Anaphylactic reaction*** (difficulty in breathing or swallowing; hives; itching, especially of feet or hands; reddening of skin, especially around ears; swelling of eyes, face, or inside of nose; unusual tiredness or weakness, sudden and severe)

### Those indicating need for medical attention only if they continue or are bothersome

Incidence less frequent
***Nausea; vomiting***

## Overdose

Amphotericin B deoxycholate overdose has been reported to result in cardiopulmonary arrest.

Amphotericin B cholesteryl complex is not dialyzable.

For more information on the management of overdose or unintentional ingestion, **contact a Poison Control Center** (see *Poison Control Center Listing*).

**Treatment of overdose**
Supportive care—Patients in whom intentional overdose is confirmed or suspected should be referred for psychiatric consultation.

## Patient Consultation

As an aid to patient consultation, refer to *Advice for the Patient, Amphotericin B Cholesteryl Complex (Systemic)—Introductory Version.*

In providing consultation, consider emphasizing the following selected information (» = major clinical significance):

**Before using this medication**
» Conditions affecting use, especially:
Sensitivity to amphotericin B cholesteryl complex
Other medications, especially antineoplastic agents, corticosteroids, corticotropin (ACTH), digitalis glycosides, nephrotoxic medications, or nondepolarizing neuromuscular blocking agents

**Side/adverse effects**
Signs of potential side effects, especially infusion-related reaction, dyspnea, hypertension, hypotension, tachycardia, thrombocytopenia, or anaphylactic reaction

## General Dosing Information

Intravenous infusion should be administered at a rate of 1 mg per kg of body weight per hour. A test dose immediately preceding the first dose is advisable when beginning all new courses of treatment. A small amount of the medication (e.g., 10 mL of the final preparation containing 1.6 to 8.3 mg) should be infused over 15 to 30 minutes, and the patient carefully observed for the next 30 minutes.

The infusion time may be shortened to a minimum of 2 hours for patients who show no evidence of intolerance or infusion-related reactions. If the patient experiences acute reactions or cannot tolerate the infusion volume, the infusion time may be extended.

**For treatment of adverse effects**
Recommended treatment consists of the following:
- For anaphylactic reaction
  —Immediately administer airway management, epinephrine, intravenous steroids, and oxygen as indicated.
  —For severe respiratory distress, immediately discontinue the infusion; the patient should not receive further infusions of amphotericin B cholesteryl complex.
- For infusion-related reaction
  —Reduce the rate of infusion and promptly administer antihistamines and corticosteroids.
  —In patients with a history of infusion-related reaction, pretreat the patients with antihistamines and corticosteroids.

## Parenteral Dosage Forms

### AMPHOTERICIN B CHOLESTERYL COMPLEX FOR INJECTION

Note: Rapid intravenous infusion should be avoided.

**Usual adult and adolescent dose**
Aspergillosis—
Intravenous infusion, 3 to 4 mg per kg of body weight, once a day.

**Usual pediatric dose**
See *Usual adult and adolescent dose.*

**Usual geriatric dose**
See *Usual adult and adolescent dose.*

**Strength(s) usually available**
U.S.—
50 mg (Rx) [*Amphotec* (lactose [950 mg])].
100 mg (Rx) [*Amphotec* (lactose [1900 mg])].

**Packaging and storage**
Prior to reconstitution, store between 15 and 30 °C (59 and 86 °F), unless otherwise specified by manufacturer.

After reconstitution with sterile water for injection, store between 2 and 8 °C (36 and 46 °F). Do not freeze. Use within 24 hours.

After further dilution with 5% dextrose for injection, store between 2 and 8 °C (36 and 46 °F). Do not freeze. Use within 24 hours. Discard any partially used vials.

**Preparation of dosage form**
Amphotericin B cholesteryl complex for injection should be reconstituted by the addition of sterile water for injection. Using a sterile syringe and a 20-gauge needle, rapidly add 10 or 20 mL of sterile water for injection to a 50-mg or 100-mg vial, respectively, to obtain a solution containing 5 mg of amphotericin B per mL. Shake gently by hand, rotating the vial until all solids have dissolved. The fluid may be clear or opalescent.

For infusion, further dilute the reconstituted solution to a final concentration of approximately 0.6 mg per mL (mg/mL) (range, 0.16 to 0.83 mg/mL) according to the following recommendations:

| Dose (mg) | Volume of reconstituted solution (mL) | Infusion bag size for 5% dextrose for injection (mL) |
|---|---|---|
| 10–35 | 2–7 | 50 |
| 35–70 | 7–14 | 100 |
| 70–175 | 14–35 | 250 |
| 175–350 | 35–70 | 500 |
| 350–1000 | 70–200 | 1000 |

**Stability**
After reconstitution in sterile water for injection, use within 24 hours.

**Incompatibilities**
The lyophilized powder should not be reconstituted with saline or dextrose solution, and the reconstituted liquid should not be admixed with saline or electrolytes. The use of any solution other than those recommended, or the presence of a bacteriostatic agent (e.g., benzyl alcohol) in the solution, may induce precipitation of amphotericin B cholesteryl complex.

The infusion admixture should not be mixed with other medications. If administered through an existing intravenous line, the line should be flushed with 5% dextrose for injection prior to infusion of amphotericin B cholesteryl complex. Alternatively, the admixture should be administered via a separate line.

The solution should not be filtered or used with an in-line filter.

**Additional information**
The solution should be visually inspected for particulate matter and discoloration prior to administration. The solution should not be used if a precipitate or foreign matter is present, or if the seal is not intact. Strict aseptic technique should always be observed since no preservatives are present in the lyophilized medication or in the solutions used for reconstitution and dilution.

Developed: 11/04/97
Interim revision: 04/28/98

---

# AMPHOTERICIN B LIPID COMPLEX        Systemic—INTRODUCTORY VERSION

VA CLASSIFICATION (Primary): AM700
Commonly used brand name(s): *ABELCET*.
Note: For a listing of dosage forms and brand names by country availability, see *Dosage Forms* section(s).

## Category

Antifungal (systemic).

## Indications

**Accepted**
Fungal infections, invasive (treatment)—Amphotericin B lipid complex is indicated in the treatment of invasive fungal infections in patients who are refractory to or intolerant of conventional amphotericin B therapy.

## Pharmacology/Pharmacokinetics

**Physicochemical characteristics**
Chemistry—A suspension of amphotericin B complexed with two phospholipids, L-alpha-dimyristoylphosphatidylcholine (DMPC) and L-al-

pha-dimyristoylphosphatidylglycerol (DMPG), in a 1:1 drug-to-lipid molar ratio.
Molecular weight—Amphotericin B: 924.1.

**Mechanism of action/Effect**
Amphotericin B acts by binding to sterols in the cell membrane of susceptible fungi, with a resultant change in the permeability of the membrane.

**Distribution**
High concentrations are found in the spleen, lung, and liver; also found in lymph node, kidney, heart, and brain tissues.
Apparent Vol$_D$—Approximately 131 L per kg.

**Biotransformation**
Metabolic pathways unknown.

**Half-life**
Terminal—Approximately 7.2 days.

**Peak plasma concentration**
After 5 mg per kg of body weight per day for 5 to 7 days—Approximately 1.7 micrograms per mL (1.8 micromoles per liter).

**Elimination**
Renal; approximately 0.9% is excreted in the urine over 24 hours after administration of the last dose.
In dialysis—Amphotericin B lipid complex is not hemodialyzable.

## Precautions to Consider

**Carcinogenicity**
Long-term studies in animals to evaluate the carcinogenic potential of amphotericin B lipid complex have not been done.

**Mutagenicity**
No mutagenic effects were found in the bacterial reverse mutation assay, mouse lymphoma forward mutation assay, chromosomal aberration assay in CHO cells, or the *in vivo* mouse micronucleus assay.

**Pregnancy/Reproduction**
Fertility—No impact on fertility was found in studies done in male and female rats at doses of up to 0.32 times the recommended human dose, based on body surface area.
Pregnancy—Adequate and well-controlled studies in humans have not been done.
Studies in rats and rabbits at doses of up to 0.64 times the recommended human dose, based on body surface area, revealed no harm to the fetus.
FDA Pregnancy Category B.

**Breast-feeding**
It is not known whether amphotericin B lipid complex is distributed into breast milk. Because of the potential for serious side effects in nursing infants, a decision should be made to either stop breast-feeding or discontinue taking amphotericin B lipid complex.

**Pediatrics**
One hundred eleven children 16 years of age and younger have been treated with amphotericin B lipid complex. No serious or unexpected adverse events have been reported.

**Geriatrics**
Forty-nine patients 65 years of age and older have been treated with amphotericin B lipid complex. No serious or unexpected adverse events have been reported.

**Drug interactions and/or related problems**
The following drug interactions and/or related problems have been selected on the basis of their potential clinical significance (possible mechanism in parentheses where appropriate)—not necessarily inclusive (» = major clinical significance):

Note: Combinations containing any of the following medications, depending on the amount present, may also interact with this medication.

Antifungals, azole
(azole antifungals have been reported to be antagonistic with amphotericin B in *in vitro* and *in vivo* animal studies)
Blood dyscrasia–causing medications (See *Appendix II*) or
» Bone marrow depressants (See *Appendix II*) or
» Radiation therapy
(concurrent use of these medications or radiation therapy with amphotericin B may increase the chance of renal toxicity, bronchospasm, and hypotension; these medications should be used with amphotericin B lipid complex with caution)
» Corticosteroids, glucocorticoid, especially with significant mineralocorticoid activity or
» Corticosteroids, mineralocorticoid or
» Corticotropin (ACTH), especially with long-term use
(concurrent use of these medications with amphotericin B lipid complex may result in hypokalemia, which could predispose the patient to cardiac arrhythmias; serum electrolytes and cardiac function should be monitored)
» Cyclosporin A or
» Nephrotoxic medications, other (See *Appendix II*)
(concurrent use of these medications may increase the chance for medication-induced renal toxicity; these medications should be used with amphotericin B lipid complex with caution)
» Digitalis glycosides or
Neuromuscular blocking agents, nondepolarizing
(amphotericin B may induce hypokalemia, which may increase the potential for digitalis toxicity or enhance the blockade of nondepolarizing neuromuscular blocking agents; serum potassium determinations and correction of hypokalemia may be necessary prior to administration of nondepolarizing neuromuscular blocking agents or at frequent intervals during concurrent therapy with digitalis glycosides)
Flucytosine
(concurrent use may increase flucytosine toxicity, possibly by increasing its cellular intake and/or impairing its renal excretion)
Zidovudine
(increased myelotoxicity and nephrotoxicity were seen in dogs that were administered either amphotericin B lipid complex at doses 0.16 or 0.5 times the recommended human dose or amphotericin B desoxycholate concurrently with zidovudine for 30 days; renal and hematologic functions should be monitored closely)

**Laboratory value alterations**
The following have been selected on the basis of their potential clinical significance (possible effect in parentheses where appropriate)—not necessarily inclusive (» = major clinical significance):

With physiology/laboratory test values
Alanine aminotransferase (ALT [SGPT]) and
Alkaline phosphatase and
Amylase and
Aspartate aminotransferase (AST [SGOT])
(serum values may be increased)
Blood urea nitrogen (BUN) and
Creatinine, serum and
Potassium, serum
(concentrations may be increased)
Calcium, serum and
Magnesium, serum
(concentrations may be decreased)

**Medical considerations/Contraindications**
The medical considerations/contraindications included have been selected on the basis of their potential clinical significance (reasons given in parentheses where appropriate)—not necessarily inclusive (» = major clinical significance).

*Except under special circumstances, this medication should not be used when the following medical problem exists:*
» Leukocyte transfusions
(acute pulmonary toxicity has been reported in patients receiving amphotericin B lipid complex and leukocyte transfusions; leukocyte transfusions and amphotericin B lipid complex should not be given concurrently)

*Risk-benefit should be considered when the following medical problems exist:*
Hypersensitivity to amphotericin B
» Renal function impairment
(amphotericin B lipid complex can produce dose-dependent nephrotoxicity; however, some patients with a serum creatinine above 2.5 mg per deciliter being treated for aspergillosis with amphotericin B lipid complex experienced a decline in serum creatinine during treatment)

**Patient monitoring**
The following may be especially important in patient monitoring (other tests may be warranted in some patients, depending on condition; » = major clinical significance):

Complete blood count (CBC)
(counts should be monitored frequently)

Creatinine, serum and
Magnesium, serum and

Potassium, serum
(concentrations should be monitored frequently)
Liver function tests
(values should be monitored frequently)

### Side/Adverse Effects

Note: One case of anaphylaxis has been reported.

Acute reactions, including fever and chills, may occur 1 to 2 hours after initiation of an infusion of amphotericin B lipid complex. These reactions are more likely to occur with the first few doses and generally diminish with subsequent doses. Amphotericin B lipid complex has rarely been associated with hypotension, bronchospasm, arrhythmias, and shock.

The following side/adverse effects have been selected on the basis of their potential clinical significance (possible signs and symptoms in parentheses where appropriate)—not necessarily inclusive:

**Those indicating need for medical attention**
Incidence more frequent
*Infusion-related reaction* (fever and chills; headache; nausea and vomiting)
Incidence less frequent
*Anemia* (unusual tiredness and weakness); *leukopenia* (sore throat and fever); *respiratory distress* (difficulty in breathing); *thrombocytopenia* (unusual bleeding or bruising)
Incidence rare
*Renal function impairment* (increased or decreased urination)

**Those indicating need for medical attention only if they continue or are bothersome**
Incidence more frequent
*Gastrointestinal disturbance* (diarrhea; loss of appetite; nausea; stomach pain; vomiting)

### Overdose

For more information on the management of overdose or unintentional ingestion, **contact a Poison Control Center** (see *Poison Control Center Listing*).

**Clinical effects of overdose**
Amphotericin B desoxycholate overdose has resulted in cardiopulmonary arrest. Fifteen patients have been reported to have received one or more doses of 7 to 13 mg per kg of body weight of amphotericin B lipid complex. None of these patients had a serious acute reaction. Amphotericin B lipid complex is not hemodialyzable.

**Treatment of overdose**
Supportive care—Patients in whom intentional overdose is confirmed or suspected should be referred for psychiatric consultation.

### Patient Consultation

As an aid to patient consultation, refer to *Advice for the Patient, Amphotericin B Lipid Complex (Systemic)—Introductory Version*.

In providing consultation, consider emphasizing the following selected information (» = major clinical significance):

**Before using this medication**
» Conditions affecting use, especially:
Hypersensitivity to amphotericin B
Breast-feeding—Not recommended, due to potential serious side effects in the nursing infant

Other medications, especially bone marrow depressants, corticosteroids, corticotropin, cyclosporin A, digitalis glycosides, other nephrotoxic medications, or radiation therapy
Other medical problems, especially leukocyte transfusions or renal function impairment

**Side/adverse effects**
Signs of potential side effects, especially infusion-related reactions, anemia, leukopenia, respiratory distress, thrombocytopenia, or renal function impairment

### General Dosing Information

Renal toxicity has been shown to be dose-dependent. There are no firm guidelines for adjusting the dose based on laboratory test results.

The infusion should be administered at a rate of 2.5 mg per kg of body weight per hour. If the infusion time exceeds 2 hours, the contents of the infusion bag should be shaken every 2 hours.

### Parenteral Dosage Forms

#### AMPHOTERICIN B LIPID COMPLEX INJECTION

**Usual adult and adolescent dose**
Fungal infections, invasive—Intravenous infusion, 5 mg per kg of body weight per day, administered at a rate of 2.5 mg per kg of body weight per hour.

**Usual pediatric dose**
See *Usual adult and adolescent dose*.

**Usual geriatric dose**
See *Usual adult and adolescent dose*.

**Size(s) usually available**
U.S.—
100 mg in 20 mL (Rx) [ABELCET (L-alpha-dimyristoylphosphatidylcholine [DMPC]; L-alpha-dimyristoylphosphatidylglycerol [DMPG])].

**Packaging and storage**
Prior to admixing, store between 2 and 8 °C (36 and 46 °F). Protect from light. Do not freeze.
After dilution with 5% dextrose injection, the admixture may be stored for up to 48 hours at 2 to 8 °C (36 to 46 °F) and an additional 6 hours at room temperature. Do not freeze.

**Preparation of dosage form**
The vial should be shaken gently until there is no evidence of any yellow sediment at the bottom. The appropriate dose of amphotericin B lipid complex should be withdrawn from the required number of vials into one or more 20-mL syringes using an 18-gauge needle. The needle is then replaced with the 5-micron filter needle supplied with each vial. Empty the contents of the syringe into a bag of 5% dextrose injection so that the final concentration is 1 mg per mL. For pediatric patients and patients with cardiovascular disease, the final infusion concentration may be 2 mg per mL. Before infusion, the bag should be shaken until the contents are thoroughly mixed.

**Incompatibilities**
Compatibility has not been established with sodium chloride injection or with other medications or electrolytes. An existing intravenous line should be flushed with 5% dextrose injection before infusion of amphotericin B lipid complex, or a separate infusion line should be used. **In-line filters should not be used.**

Developed: 05/28/96
Interim revision: 04/17/98

---

# AMPHOTERICIN B LIPOSOMAL COMPLEX Systemic—INTRODUCTORY VERSION

VA CLASSIFICATION (Primary/Secondary): AM700/AP109
Commonly used brand name(s): *AmBisome*.
Note: For a listing of dosage forms and brand names by country availability, see *Dosage Forms* section(s).

## Category
Antifungal (systemic); antiprotozoal.

## Indications

### General considerations
Amphotericin B liposomal complex is active *in vitro* and *in vivo* against *Aspergillus* and *Candida* species, *Blastomyces dermatitidis*, and *Cryptococcus neoformans*. *In vivo* activity has also been demonstrated against *Coccidioides immitis*, *Histoplasma capsulatum*, *Paracoccidioides brasiliensis*, *Leishmania donovani*, and *Leishmania infantum*.

Fungal variants with reduced susceptibility to amphotericin B have been isolated from several fungal species after serial passage in cell culture media containing amphotericin B, and from some patients receiving prolonged therapy with amphotericin B. Drug combination studies *in vitro* and *in vivo* suggest that imidazoles may induce resistance to amphotericin B. However, the clinical relevance of drug resistance has not been established.

### Accepted
Aspergillosis (treatment)
Candidiasis (treatment) or
Cryptococcosis (treatment)—Amphotericin B liposomal complex is indicated in the treatment of systemic fungal infections caused by *Aspergillus*, *Candida*, or *Cryptococcus* in patients refractory to or intolerant of amphotericin B deoxycholate.

Fungal infection, presumed, in febrile neutropenia (treatment)—Amphotericin B liposomal complex is indicated as empiric therapy for presumed fungal infection in patients with febrile neutropenia.

Leishmaniasis, visceral (treatment)—Amphotericin B liposomal complex is indicated in the treatment of visceral leishmaniasis.

## Pharmacology/Pharmacokinetics

Note: The pharmacokinetic profile of amphotericin B liposomal complex was determined in febrile neutropenic cancer and bone marrow transplant patients receiving 1- to 2-hour infusions of amphotericin B liposomal complex for 3 to 20 days.

### Physicochemical characteristics
Chemical group—Macrocyclic, polyene, antifungal antibiotic; amphotericin B liposomal complex drug delivery system contains amphotericin B intercalated into a single bilayer liposome consisting of alpha-tocopherol, distearoylphosphatidylglycerol, and hydrogenated soy phosphatidylcholine.
Molecular weight—Amphotericin B: 924.09.

### Mechanism of action/Effect
Amphotericin B binds primarily to ergosterol in cell membranes of sensitive fungi, causing changes in membrane permeability, which result in leakage of intracellular contents and cell death. Amphotericin B also binds to cholesterol in mammalian cell membranes, leading to cytotoxicity. Amphotericin B liposomal complex penetrates the cell wall of both extracellular and intracellular forms of susceptible fungi.

### Distribution
Vol$_D$ (steady-state) with a dose of—
1 mg per kg of body weight (mg/kg) per day: 0.14 ± 0.05 L per kg;
2.5 mg/kg per day: 0.16 ± 0.09 L per kg;
5 mg/kg per day: 0.1 ± 0.07 L per kg.

Steady-state concentrations are generally achieved within 4 days of dosing.

### Half-life
Distribution—
7 to 10 hours (mean) following a 24-hour period dosing interval.
Terminal elimination—
100 to 153 hours (mean) following up to 49 days after dosing; the long terminal elimination half-life is probably due to slow redistribution from tissues.

### Peak serum concentration
With a dose of—1 mg/kg per day: 12.2 ± 4.9 mcg/mL.
2.5 mg/kg per day: 31.4 ± 17.8 mcg/mL.
5 mg/kg per day: 83 ± 35.2 mcg/mL.

### Elimination
Excretion of amphotericin B liposomal complex has not been studied. The mean clearance at steady state is independent of dose.

## Precautions to Consider

### Carcinogenicity
Long-term studies in animals have not been done to evaluate the carcinogenic potential of amphotericin B liposomal complex.

### Mutagenicity
Amphotericin B liposomal complex has not been tested to determine its mutagenic potential.

### Pregnancy/Reproduction
Fertility—Amphotericin B liposomal complex does not affect fertility in rats.

Pregnancy—Adequate and well-controlled studies in humans have not been done. However, a small number of pregnant women have been successfully treated for systemic fungal infections with amphotericin B deoxycholate.

Female rats given doses of 10 and 15 mg per kg of body weight (mg/kg), equivalent to 1.6 and 2.4 mg/kg in humans based on body surface area considerations, exhibited an abnormal estrous cycle (prolonged diestrus) and decreased number of corpora lutea. There were no effects on male reproductive function. Amphotericin B liposomal complex is not teratogenic in rats or in rabbits. In rats, the maternal nontoxic dose was estimated to be 5 mg/kg (0.16 to 0.8 times the recommended human clinical dose range [1 to 5 mg/kg]), and in rabbits, 3 mg/kg (0.2 to 1 time the recommended human clinical dose range). Rabbits receiving doses equivalent to 0.5 to 2 times the recommended human dose of amphotericin B liposomal complex experienced a higher rate of spontaneous abortions than did control animals.

FDA Pregnancy Category B.

### Breast-feeding
It is not known whether amphotericin B liposomal complex is distributed into breast milk. Because of the potential for serious adverse effects in nursing infants, a decision should be made to either stop breast-feeding or discontinue taking amphotericin B liposomal complex.

### Pediatrics
The pharmacokinetics of amphotericin B liposomal complex have not been studied in pediatric patients. However, infants and children 1 month to 16 years of age have been successfully treated with amphotericin B liposomal complex. Studies in which pediatric patients were treated with amphotericin B or amphotericin B liposomal complex demonstrated no differences in safety or efficacy of amphotericin B liposomal complex compared with those in adults.

Safety and efficacy have not been established for infants up to 1 month of age.

### Geriatrics
The pharmacokinetics of amphotericin B liposomal complex have not been studied in geriatric patients. However, 71 patients, 65 years of age and older, have been treated with amphotericin B liposomal complex, and no adjustment in dose was necessary.

### Drug interactions and/or related problems
The following drug interactions and/or related problems have been selected on the basis of their potential clinical significance (possible mechanism in parentheses where appropriate)—not necessarily inclusive (» = major clinical significance):

Note: Combinations containing any of the following medications, depending on the amount present, may also interact with this medication.

» Antineoplastic agents
(concurrent use with amphotericin B liposomal complex may enhance the potential for bronchospasm, hypotension, and renal toxicity of these agents; caution should be used when these medications are administered concurrently with amphotericin B liposomal complex)

» Corticosteroids or
» Corticotropin (ACTH)
(concurrent use may potentiate hypokalemia, which may predispose the patient to cardiac dysfunction; cardiac function and serum electrolytes should be monitored)

» Digitalis glycosides
(amphotericin B may induce hypokalemia, which may potentiate digitalis toxicity when this medication is used concurrently with digitalis glycosides; serum potassium concentrations should be monitored closely)

Flucytosine
(concurrent use may increase the toxicity of flucytosine possibly by increasing its cellular uptake and/or impairing its renal excretion)

Imidazoles
(animal studies have suggested that imidazoles may induce fungal resistance to amphotericin B; caution should be used when administering these medications concurrently, especially in immunocompromised patients)

» Nephrotoxic medications, other (see *Appendix II*)
(concurrent use with nephrotoxic medications may potentiate medication-induced renal toxicity; caution should be exercised when these medications are used concurrently with amphotericin B liposomal complex, and renal function should be monitored frequently)

» Neuromuscular blocking agents, nondepolarizing
(amphotericin B may induce hypokalemia, which may enhance the activity of nondepolarizing neuromuscular blocking agents; serum potassium concentrations should be monitored closely)

### Laboratory value alterations
The following have been selected on the basis of their potential clinical significance (possible effect in parentheses where appropriate)—not necessarily inclusive (» = major clinical significance):

With physiology/laboratory test values
Alkaline phosphatase and
Creatine kinase (CK)
  (serum values may be increased)
Calcium and
Magnesium and
» Potassium
  (serum concentrations may be decreased)
Bilirubin, blood and
Blood urea nitrogen (BUN) and
Glucose, plasma
  (concentrations may be increased)

### Medical considerations/Contraindications
The medical considerations/contraindications included have been selected on the basis of their potential clinical significance (reasons given in parentheses where appropriate)—not necessarily inclusive (» = major clinical significance).

*Except under special circumstances, this medication should not be used when the following medical problems exist:*
» Hypersensitivity to amphotericin B liposomal complex
» Leukocyte transfusions
  (acute pulmonary toxicity has been reported in patients concurrently receiving intravenous amphotericin B and leukocyte transfusions)

*Risk-benefit should be considered when the following medical problem exists:*
Renal function impairment
  (amphotericin B may produce nephrotoxicity)

### Patient monitoring
The following may be especially important in patient monitoring (other tests may be warranted in some patients, depending on condition; » = major clinical significance):
» Electrolytes, serum
  (concentrations should be monitored)
Hematopoietic function tests and
Hepatic function tests and
Renal function tests
  (values should be monitored)

## Side/Adverse Effects
Note: There have been a few reports of back pain with or without chest tightness, chest pain, and flushing associated with administration of amphotericin B liposomal complex; on occasion these effects have been severe. These reactions developed within a few minutes after the start of infusion and disappeared rapidly when the infusion was stopped.

The following side/adverse effects have been selected on the basis of their potential clinical significance (possible signs and symptoms in parentheses where appropriate)—not necessarily inclusive:

### Those indicating need for medical attention
Incidence more frequent
  *Chills; fever; hypokalemia* (irregular heartbeat; muscle cramps or pain; unusual tiredness or weakness)
Incidence less frequent
  *Back pain; chest pain; dark urine; dyspnea* (difficulty in breathing); *infusion-related reaction* (chills; fever; headache); *yellowing of eyes or skin*
Incidence rare
  *Anaphylactic reaction* (difficulty in swallowing; hives; itching, especially of feet or hands; reddening of skin, especially around ears; swelling of eyes, face, or inside of nose; unusual tiredness or weakness, sudden and severe)

### Those indicating need for medical attention only if they continue or are bothersome
Incidence more frequent
  *Abdominal pain; diarrhea; headache; nausea; vomiting*
Incidence less frequent
  *Skin rash*

## Overdose
Repeated daily doses of up to 7.5 mg per kg of body weight have been administered in clinical trials with no reported dose-related toxicity.
For more information on the management of overdose or unintentional ingestion, **contact a Poison Control Center** (see *Poison Control Center Listing*).

### Treatment of overdose
In the case of overdose, administration should cease immediately.
Monitoring—Renal function should be monitored.
Supportive care—Treatment should be supportive and symptomatic. Patients in whom intentional overdose is confirmed or suspected should be referred for psychiatric consultation.

## Patient Consultation
As an aid to patient consultation, refer to *Advice for the Patient, Amphotericin B Liposomal Complex (Systemic)—Introductory Version.*
In providing consultation, consider emphasizing the following selected information (» = major clinical significance):

### Before using this medication
Conditions affecting use, especially:
  Hypersensitivity to amphotericin B liposomal complex
  Breast-feeding—It is recommended either to stop breast-feeding or to discontinue taking amphotericin B liposomal complex
  Other medications, especially antineoplastic agents, corticosteroids, corticotropin (ACTH), digitalis glycosides, other nephrotoxic medications, or nondepolarizing neuromuscular blocking agents
  Other medical problems, especially leukocyte transfusions

### Side/adverse effects
Signs of potential side effects, especially chills, fever, hypokalemia, back pain, chest pain, dark urine, dyspnea, infusion-related reaction, yellowing of eyes or skin, or anaphylactic reaction

## General Dosing Information
Intravenous infusion should be administered over a period of approximately 120 minutes. The infusion time may be reduced to approximately 60 minutes in patients in whom the treatment is well-tolerated. If the patient experiences discomfort during infusion, the duration of infusion may be increased.

## Parenteral Dosage Forms

### AMPHOTERICIN B LIPOSOMAL COMPLEX FOR INJECTION

#### Usual adult and adolescent dose
Aspergillosis or
Candidiasis or
Cryptococcosis—
  Intravenous infusion, 3 to 5 mg per kg of body weight per day.
Leishmaniasis, immunocompetent patients—
  Intravenous infusion, a three-week course of therapy consisting of 3 mg per kg of body weight per day for days one through five, on day fourteen and day twenty-one.
  Note: Patients who do not achieve parasitic clearance may require a repeat course of therapy.
Leishmaniasis, immunocompromised patients—
  Intravenous, a thirty-eight-day course of therapy consisting of 4 mg per kg of body weight per day for days one through five, on day ten, day seventeen, day twenty-four, day thirty-one, and day thirty-eight.
  Note: Patients who do not achieve parasitic clearance or who experience relapses should seek expert advice regarding further treatment.
Presumed fungal infections in patients with febrile neutropenia—
  Intravenous infusion, 3 mg per kg of body weight per day.

#### Usual pediatric dose
Infants and children 1 month to 12 years of age—See *Usual adult and adolescent dose*.
Infants up to 1 month of age—Safety and efficacy have not been established.

#### Usual geriatric dose
See *Usual adult and adolescent dose*.

#### Strength(s) usually available
U.S.—
  50 mg (Rx) [*AmBisome* (sucrose [900 mg])].

#### Packaging and storage
Prior to reconstitution, store between 2 and 8 °C (36 and 46 °F), unless otherwise specified by the manufacturer. Protect from freezing.

**Preparation of dosage form**
Add 12 mL of sterile water for injection (without a bacteriostatic agent) to each 50-mg vial to provide a concentration of 4 mg amphotericin B per mL. Immediately shake the vial vigorously for at least 30 seconds until all particulate matter is completely dispersed. Withdraw the appropriate volume of amphotericin B liposomal complex suspension and, using a 5-micron filter, dilute into 5% dextrose injection to provide a concentration of 1 to 2 mg per mL. Lower concentrations (0.2 to 0.5 mg per mL) may be appropriate for infants and small children to provide sufficient volume for infusion.

**Stability**
Once reconstituted with sterile water for injection, the suspension is stable for up to 24 hours at 2 to 8 °C (36 to 46 °F). Do not freeze.
Once diluted with 5% dextrose injection, infusion should begin within 6 hours.

**Incompatibilities**
To avoid possible precipitation, amphotericin B liposomal complex should not be reconstituted or admixed with saline or any solution containing a bacteriostatic agent.

The infusion admixture should not be mixed with other medications. If administered through an existing intravenous line, the line should be flushed with 5% dextrose injection prior to infusion of amphotericin B liposomal complex. Alternatively, the medications should be administered through separate lines.

An in-line membrane filter may be used for the intravenous infusion of amphotericin B liposomal complex provided the filter has a mean pore diameter of at least 1 micron.

Developed: 11/13/97
Interim revision: 03/26/98

---

**AMPICILLIN**—See *Penicillins (Systemic)*

---

# AMRINONE   Systemic

VA CLASSIFICATION (Primary/Secondary) (Primary): CV900
Commonly used brand name(s): *Inocor*.
Note: For a listing of dosage forms and brand names by country availability, see *Dosage Forms* section(s).

## Category
Cardiotonic.

## Indications

**Accepted**
Congestive heart failure (treatment)—Amrinone is indicated for the short-term management of congestive heart failure in patients who have not responded adequately to digitalis, diuretics, and/or vasodilators.

## Pharmacology/Pharmacokinetics

**Physicochemical characteristics**
Molecular weight—187.20.

**Mechanism of action/Effect**
Not precisely known; but seems to be peripheral vasodilation, reducing both preload and afterload, and possibly also direct stimulation of cardiac contractility (positive inotropic effect) as a result of phosphodiesterase inhibition.

**Other actions/effects**
Slightly increases atrioventricular (AV) conduction velocity.

**Protein binding**
Low to moderate (10 to 49%).

**Biotransformation**
Hepatic.

**Half-life**
Adults—
  Healthy volunteers: Approximately 3.6 hours.
  Congestive heart failure: Approximately 5.0 to 8.3 hours.
Neonates and infants—
  Less than 4 weeks: 12.7 to 22.2 hours.
  More than 4 weeks: 3.8 to 6.8 hours.

**Time to peak effect**
Within 10 minutes.

**Duration of action**
Dose-related—
  750 mcg (0.75 mg) per kg of body weight (mcg/kg): 30 minutes.
  3 mg per kg of body weight (mg/kg): 2 hours.

**Elimination**
Renal—About 63%, as unchanged drug (10 to 40%) and metabolites.
Fecal—About 18%.

## Precautions to Consider

**Cross-sensitivity and/or related problems**
Patients sensitive to bisulfites may also be sensitive to amrinone lactate injection, which contains sodium metabisulfite.

**Carcinogenicity**
A 2-year study in rats found no evidence of carcinogenicity.

**Mutagenicity**
Positive results were obtained in the mouse micronucleus test (at 7.5 to 10 times the maximum human dose) and in the Chinese hamster ovary chromosome aberration assay, indicating clastogenic potential and suppression of the number of polychromatic erythrocytes. However, negative results were obtained in the Ames Salmonella assay, mouse lymphoma study, and cultured human lymphocyte metaphase analysis.

**Pregnancy/Reproduction**
Pregnancy—Adequate and well-controlled studies in humans have not been done.
Studies in New Zealand white rabbits at oral doses of 16 and 50 mg per kg of body weight (mg/kg) have shown that amrinone causes fetal skeletal and gross external malformations. These effects did not occur in French Hy/Cr rabbits at oral doses of 32 mg/kg per day or in rats receiving intravenous doses approximately equivalent to the recommended daily human dose.
In mutagenicity studies, gestation levels in rats were slightly prolonged at doses of 50 and 100 mg/kg per day. At the higher dose, dystocia occurred in dams and the incidence of stillbirths, decreased litter size, and poor pup survival was increased.
FDA Pregnancy Category C.

**Breast-feeding**
It is not known whether amrinone is excreted in breast milk. However, problems in humans have not been documented.

**Pediatrics**
Studies and case reports of amrinone use for pulmonary hypertension, congestive heart failure, and postoperative low cardiac output in approximately 30 neonates and infants and 6 children up to 24 months of age have not demonstrated pediatrics-specific problems that would limit the usefulness of amrinone in pediatric patients.

**Geriatrics**
Although appropriate studies on the relationship of age to the effects of amrinone have not been performed in the geriatric population, no geriatrics-specific problems have been documented to date. However, elderly patients are more likely to have age-related renal function impairment, which may require adjustment of dosage in patients receiving amrinone.

**Laboratory value alterations**
The following have been selected on the basis of their potential clinical significance (possible effect in parentheses where appropriate)—not necessarily inclusive (» = major clinical significance):

With physiology/laboratory test values
  Blood pressure and
  Potassium concentrations, serum
    (may be decreased)
  Hepatic enzymes
    (serum concentrations may be increased)

**Medical considerations/Contraindications**
The medical considerations/contraindications included have been selected on the basis of their potential clinical significance (reasons given in parentheses where appropriate)—not necessarily inclusive (» = major clinical significance).

*Except under special circumstances, this medication should not be used when the following medical problems exist:*
- » Aortic or pulmonic valvular disease, severe
  (surgical relief of obstruction required)

*Risk-benefit should be considered when the following medical problems exist:*
- Hepatic function impairment
  (elimination reduced; dosage adjustment may be necessary)
- » Hypertrophic cardiomyopathy
  (amrinone may aggravate outflow tract obstruction)
- Renal function impairment
  (elimination reduced; dosage adjustment may be necessary)
- Sensitivity to amrinone

**Patient monitoring**
The following may be especially important in patient monitoring (other tests may be warranted in some patients, depending on condition; » = major clinical significance):
- » Blood pressure and
- » Heart rate
  (determinations at periodic intervals in patients receiving amrinone; amrinone infusion should be slowed or stopped in patients who develop an excessive fall in blood pressure)
- » Body weight
  (determinations recommended at periodic intervals to confirm efficacy of amrinone)
- Cardiac index and
- Central venous pressure and
- Pulmonary capillary wedge pressure
  (determinations recommended at periodic intervals to confirm efficacy of amrinone)
- Hepatic function determinations and
- Renal function determinations and
- Serum electrolyte, especially potassium, concentrations
  (recommended at periodic intervals in patients receiving amrinone; hypokalemia secondary to improved cardiac output and resultant diuresis may contribute to risk of arrhythmias)
  (dosage adjustment may be necessary in patients with existing or developing renal or hepatic function impairment)
- » Platelet counts
  (recommended prior to initiation and at periodic intervals during amrinone therapy. Dosage of amrinone may need to be reduced if thrombocytopenia occurs; in some cases, platelet levels stabilize with continuation at the same dose; any decision regarding a change in dosage should be based on monitoring of platelet counts; in some patients, withdrawal of amrinone may be necessary)

## Side/Adverse Effects

The following side/adverse effects have been selected on the basis of their potential clinical significance (possible signs and symptoms in parentheses where appropriate)—not necessarily inclusive:

**Those indicating need for medical attention**
Incidence less frequent
  *Arrhythmias* (irregular heartbeat); *hypotension* (dizziness)
Incidence rare
  *Burning at site of injection; chest pain; hepatotoxicity* (yellow eyes or skin); *thrombocytopenia* (unusual bleeding or bruising; black, tarry stools; blood in urine or stools; pinpoint red spots on skin)
  Note: *Thrombocytopenia* occurs in about 2.4% of patients but is rarely symptomatic; more common with high doses or prolonged treatment.

**Those indicating need for medical attention only if they continue or are bothersome**
Incidence less frequent or rare
  *Abdominal pain* (stomach pain); *fever; nausea or vomiting*

## Overdose

For more information on the management of overdose or unintentional ingestion, **contact a Poison Control Center** (see *Poison Contol Center Listing*).

**Treatment of overdose**
Treatment of overdose consists of general measures for circulatory support.

## General Dosing Information

Pretreatment with digitalis is recommended in patients with atrial flutter/fibrillation since amrinone may increase ventricular response rates because of its slight enhancement of atrioventricular (AV) conduction.
Patients who have received vigorous diuretic therapy may need cautiously liberalized fluid and electrolyte intake to ensure an adequate cardiac filling pressure for response to amrinone.
Caution is recommended to avoid extravasation of amrinone infusion.
Tachyphylaxis to the hemodynamic effects of amrinone occurs commonly, usually within 72 hours of initiation of therapy.

## Parenteral Dosage Forms

Note: The dosing and strengths of the dosage forms available are expressed in terms of amrinone base (not the lactate salt).

### AMRINONE LACTATE INJECTION

**Usual adult dose**
Initial—Intravenous, 750 mcg (0.75 mg) (base) per kg of body weight, undiluted, given slowly over 2 to 3 minutes; may be repeated after thirty minutes if necessary.
Maintenance—Intravenous infusion, 5 to 10 mcg (0.005 to 0.01 mg) (base) per kg of body weight per minute, the dosage being adjusted according to clinical response.

**Usual adult prescribing limits**
Up to 10 mg (base) per kg of body weight per day, although some patients have been given doses up to 18 mg per kg per day for short durations.

**Usual pediatric dose**
Neonates—
  Initial: Intravenous, 3.0 to 4.5 mg per kg of body weight in divided doses.
  Maintenance: Intravenous infusion, 3 mcg (0.003 mg) to 5 mcg (0.005 mg) per kg of body weight per minute.
Infants—
  Initial: Intravenous, 3.0 to 4.5 mg per kg of body weight in divided doses.
  Maintenance: Intravenous infusion, 10 mcg (0.01 mg) per kg of body weight per minute.

**Strength(s) usually available**
U.S.—
  5 mg (base) per mL (Rx) [*Inocor* (sodium metabisulphite)].
Canada—
  5 mg (base) per mL (Rx) [*Inocor* (sodium metabisulphite)].

**Packaging and storage**
Store below 40 °C (104 °F), preferably between 15 and 30 °C (59 and 86 °F), unless otherwise specified by manufacturer. Protect from light. Protect from freezing.

**Preparation of dosage form**
For administration by intravenous infusion, amrinone lactate injection may be diluted in 0.45% or 0.9% sodium chloride injection, to produce a solution containing 1 to 3 mg of amrinone (base) per mL.

**Stability**
Diluted solutions should be used within 24 hours.

**Incompatibilities**
Amrinone lactate injection should not be diluted with solutions containing dextrose since a chemical interaction occurs, developing slowly over 24 hours. However, amrinone lactate injection may be injected into running dextrose infusions through a Y-connector or directly into the tubing where preferable.
Furosemide should not be administered in intravenous lines containing amrinone, since an immediate precipitate is formed.

## Selected Bibliography

Bottorff MB, Rutledge DR, Pieper JA. Evaluation of intravenous amrinone: the first of a new class of positive inotropic agents with vasodilator properties. Pharmacotherapy 1985; 5(5): 227-37.
A symposium: amrinone. November 11, 1984, Miami, Florida. Am J Cardiol 1985 Jul 22; 56: 1B-42B.

Revised: 06/17/92

---

**AMYL NITRITE**—The *Amyl Nitrite (Systemic)* monograph is not included in this published version of the USP DI database. Copies of the monograph are available on request from Micromedex, Inc. - Reprint Requests, 6200 S. Syracuse Way, Suite 300, Englewood, CO 80111; telephone (303) 486-6400; telefax (303) 486-6464; Email: USPDI@MDX.COM.

# ANABOLIC STEROIDS  Systemic

This monograph includes information on the following: 1) Nandrolone; 2) Oxandrolone†; 3) Oxymetholone; 4) Stanozolol†.

VA CLASSIFICATION (Primary/Secondary):
Nandrolone—HS101/AN900; BL400
Oxandrolone—HS101
Oxymetholone—HS101/BL400; IM900
Stanozolol—HS101/BL400; IM900

Note: Controlled substance classification—
U.S.—Schedule III, Canada—C

Commonly used brand name(s): *Anadrol-50*[3]; *Anapolon 50*[3]; *Deca-Durabolin*[1]; *Durabolin*[1]; *Durabolin-50*[1]; *Hybolin Decanoate*[1]; *Hybolin-Improved*[1]; *Kabolin*[1]; *Oxandrin*[2]; *Winstrol*[4].

Note: For a listing of dosage forms and brand names by country availability, see *Dosage Forms* section(s).

†Not commercially available in Canada.

## Category

Note: All anabolic steroids are approximately equal in efficacy. Selection of a particular generic substance or dosage form is dependent upon the incidence of side effects, preferred route of administration, or the duration of action desired. Indications listed for individual generic products included are based on currently marketed product labeling.

Anabolic steroid—Nandrolone; Oxandrolone; Oxymetholone; Stanozolol.
Antianemic—Nandrolone; Oxymetholone; Stanozolol.
Antineoplastic—Nandrolone.
Antiangioedema (hereditary) agent—Oxymetholone; Stanozolol.

## Indications

Note: Bracketed information in the *Indications* section refers to uses that are not included in U.S. product labeling.

### Accepted

Catabolic or tissue-depleting processes (treatment)—[Nandrolone decanoate, stanozolol], and oxandrolone are indicated in conditions such as chronic infections, extensive surgery, [corticosteroid-induced myopathy, decubitus ulcers, burns], or severe trauma, which require reversal of catabolic processes or protein-sparing effects. These agents are adjuncts to, and not replacements for, conventional treatment of these disorders.

Anemia (treatment)—Nandrolone decanoate[1] is indicated for the treatment of anemia associated with renal insufficiency [and as adjuvant therapy for aplastic and sickle cell anemias]. Adequate iron intake is necessary for maximum therapeutic response.

[Nandrolone phenpropionate is indicated in the treatment of refractory deficient red cell production anemias. These may include aplastic anemia, myelofibrosis, myelosclerosis, agnogenic myeloid metaplasia, and hypoplastic anemias caused by malignancy or myelotoxic drugs. Anabolic steroid therapy should not replace other supportive measures.]

Oxymetholone is indicated in the treatment of bone marrow failure anemias and deficient red cell production anemias. Acquired and congenital aplastic anemias, myelofibrosis, and hypoplastic anemias due to myelotoxic medication often respond to oxymetholone. Oxymetholone should not replace other supportive measures such as transfusions; correction of iron, folic acid, vitamin $B_{12}$, or pyridoxine deficiency; antibacterial therapy; or the use of corticosteroids.

[Stanozolol is effective in raising hemoglobin concentrations in some cases of aplastic anemia (congenital or idiopathic).]

Carcinoma, breast (treatment)—Anabolic steroids such as [nandrolone decanoate][1] and nandrolone phenpropionate are indicated as treatment for palliation of inoperable metastatic breast cancer in postmenopausal women. However, anabolic steroids should be considered for use only after inadequate response to newer, less toxic medications such as tamoxifen in hormonally responsive breast cancer. Anabolic steroids have also been used to treat breast cancer in premenopausal women who have undergone oophorectomy and are considered to have a hormone-responsive tumor.

Angioedema, hereditary (prophylaxis)—Stanozolol and oxymetholone[1] are indicated in the prophylaxis of hereditary angioedema to decrease the frequency and severity of attacks.

Angioedema, hereditary (treatment)—[Stanozolol] and oxymetholone[1] are used in the treatment of hereditary angioedema.

[Antithrombin III deficiency (treatment)] or [Fibrinogen excess (treatment)]—Stanozolol is indicated in the treatment of conditions associated with decreased fibrinolytic activity due to antithrombin III deficiency or excess fibrinogen. These conditions may include cutaneous vasculitis, scleroderma of Raynaud's disease, vasculitis of Behcet's disease, and complications of deep vein thrombosis such as venous lipodermatosclerosis. Stanozolol is indicated in the prevention of recurrent venous thrombosis associated with antithrombin III deficiency. Stanozolol may be of benefit in patients susceptible to or with a history of thromboembolism for the treatment of vascular disorders associated with these forms of reduced fibrinolytic activity.

[Growth failure (treatment adjunct)]—Anabolic steroids may be used in children as an adjunct in the treatment of growth failure caused by pituitary growth hormone (GH) deficiency (pituitary dwarfism) or if the response to human growth hormone administration is inadequate.

[Turner's syndrome (treatment)]—Oxandrolone is used in the treatment of the short stature that accompanies Turner's syndrome (gonadal dysgenesis in females). Although the therapy is controversial, recent experimental reports seem to indicate that oxandrolone may be as effective as growth hormone and that oxandrolone may increase the efficacy of growth hormone therapy.

### Unaccepted

Anabolic steroids have been used for the treatment of symptoms associated with osteoporosis. However, this use has largely been discontinued because the questionable efficacy of these agents for this indication does not justify the risk of serious adverse effects.

Oxandrolone and oxymetholone have been used for the treatment of alcoholic hepatitis with encephalopathy. However, there is currently insufficient evidence to establish the efficacy of these agents for this indication.

Use of anabolic steroids by athletes is not recommended. Objective evidence is conflicting and inconclusive as to whether these medications significantly increase athletic performance by increasing muscle strength. Weight gains reported by athletes are due in part to fluid retention, which is a potentially hazardous side effect of anabolic steroid therapy. The risk of other unwanted effects, such as testicular atrophy and suppression of spermatogenesis in males; menstrual disturbances and virilization, such as deepening of voice, development of acne, and unnatural growth of body hair in females; peliosis hepatis or other hepatotoxicity; and hepatic cancer outweigh any possible benefit received from anabolic steroids and make their use in athletes inappropriate.

[1]Not included in Canadian product labeling.

## Pharmacology/Pharmacokinetics

### Physicochemical characteristics

Chemical group—
Anabolic steroids are synthetic derivatives of testosterone, and as such have androgenic properties. The deletion of the $CH_3$ group from the C-19 position results in reduction of its androgenic properties and retention of its anabolic, tissue-building properties. Since complete dissociation of anabolic and androgenic effects is not possible, many of the actions of anabolic steroids are similar to those of androgens.
The 17-alpha alkylated (oral methylated) anabolic steroids are oxandrolone, oxymetholone, and stanozolol.

Molecular weight—
Nandrolone decanoate: 428.66.
Nandrolone phenpropionate: 406.57.
Oxandrolone: 306.45.
Oxymetholone: 332.49.
Stanozolol: 328.50.

### Mechanism of action/Effect

Anabolic steroid—
Reverses catabolic processes and negative nitrogen balance by promoting protein anabolism and stimulating appetite if there is concurrently a proper intake of calories and proteins.

Antianemic—
Anemias due to bone marrow failure: Increases production and urinary excretion of erythropoietin.
Anemias due to deficient red cell production: Stimulates erythropoietin production and may have a direct action on bone marrow.
Anemias associated with renal disease: Increases hemoglobin and red blood cell volume.

Angioedema (hereditary) prophylactic—
Increases serum concentration of C1 esterase inhibitor and, as a result, C2 and C4 concentrations.

**Half-life**
Oxandrolone—
  Biphasic:
    1st phase—0.55 hours.
    2nd phase—9 hours.

**Time to peak serum concentration**
Nandrolone decanoate intramuscular—100-mg dose: 3 to 6 days.
Nandrolone phenpropionate intramuscular—100-mg dose: 1 to 2 days.

**Elimination**
Oxandrolone—Renal; small amount fecal.

## Precautions to Consider

**Carcinogenicity**
Hepatocellular carcinoma has been associated rarely with long-term, high-dose anabolic steroid therapy.

**Tumorigenicity**
Hepatic neoplasms have been associated rarely with long-term, high-dose anabolic steroid therapy.

**Mutagenicity**
For oxandrolone—Animal or *in vitro* mutagenicity studies have not been done.
For oxymetholone—Studies have not been done.
For stanozolol—Animal studies have not been done.

**Pregnancy/Reproduction**
Pregnancy—Anabolic steroids are not recommended for use during pregnancy, since studies in animals have shown that anabolic steroids cause masculinization of the fetus. Risk-benefit must be carefully considered.
For oxandrolone: Animal studies have also shown oxandrolone to cause embryotoxicity, fetotoxicity, and infertility, in addition to masculinization in offspring of animals receiving 9 times the human dose.
FDA Pregnancy Category X.

**Breast-feeding**
It is not known whether anabolic steroids are distributed into breast milk. Problems in humans have not been documented. However, anabolic steroids are rarely used by lactating women.

**Pediatrics**
Anabolic steroids should be used with caution in children and adolescents because of possible premature epiphyseal closure, precocious sexual development in males, and virilization in females. The epiphyseal maturation may be accelerated more rapidly than linear growth in children, and the effect may continue for 6 months after the medication has been discontinued.
For stanozolol—The safety and efficacy of stanozolol in children with hereditary angioedema have not been established. Attacks of hereditary angioedema may include symptoms such as life-threatening upper respiratory obstruction with or without severe gastrointestinal colic, but are generally infrequent in childhood. The risks from stanozolol therapy are substantially increased with long-term use. Therefore, long-term administration of stanozolol is generally not recommended in children, and should not be undertaken without consideration of risk-benefit involved and close follow-up for endocrine effects.

**Geriatrics**
Treatment of geriatric male patients with anabolic steroids may cause increased risk of prostatic hyperplasia or prostatic carcinoma.

**Drug interactions and/or related problems**
The following drug interactions and/or related problems have been selected on the basis of their potential clinical significance (possible mechanism in parentheses where appropriate)—not necessarily inclusive (» = major clinical significance):

Note: Combinations containing any of the following medications, depending on the amount present, may also interact with this medication.

» Anticoagulants, coumarin- or indandione-derivative or
  Anti-inflammatory analgesics, nonsteroidal or
  Salicylates, in therapeutic doses
    (anticoagulant effect may be increased during concurrent use with anabolic steroids, especially 17-alpha-alkylated compounds, because of decreased procoagulant factor concentration caused by alteration of procoagulant factor synthesis or catabolism and increased receptor affinity for the anticoagulant; anticoagulant dosage adjustment based on prothrombin time determinations may be required during and following concurrent use)

Antidiabetic agents, sulfonylurea or
Insulin
  (anabolic steroids may decrease blood glucose concentration; diabetic patients should be closely monitored for signs of hypoglycemia and dosage of hypoglycemic agent adjusted if necessary)
Corticosteroids, glucocorticoid, especially with significant mineralocorticoid activity or
Corticosteroids, mineralocorticoid or
Corticotropin, especially prolonged therapeutic use or
Sodium-containing medications or foods
  (concurrent use with anabolic steroids may increase the possibility of edema; in addition, concurrent use of glucocorticoids or corticotropin with anabolic steroids may promote development of severe acne)
» Hepatotoxic medications, other (see *Appendix II*)
  (concurrent use with anabolic steroids may result in an increased incidence of hepatotoxicity; patients, especially those on prolonged administration or those with a history of liver disease, should be carefully monitored)
Somatrem or
Somatropin
  (concurrent use of anabolic steroids with somatrem or somatropin may accelerate epiphyseal maturation)

**Laboratory value alterations**
The following have been selected on the basis of their potential clinical significance (possible effect in parentheses where appropriate)—not necessarily inclusive (» = major clinical significance):

With diagnostic test results
  Fasting blood sugar and
  Glucose tolerance test and
  Metyrapone test
    (may be altered)
  Thyroid function tests
    (radioactive iodine uptake and thyroxine-binding capacity [TBC] may be decreased; the decreased concentrations of thyroxine-binding globulin result in decreased total $T_3$ and $T_4$ serum concentrations and increased resin uptake of $T_3$ and $T_4$; altered tests usually persist for 2 to 3 weeks after stopping therapy)

With physiology/laboratory test values
  Alanine aminotransferase (ALT [SGPT]) and
  Alkaline phosphatase and
  Aspartate aminotransferase (AST [SGOT]) and
  Creatine kinase (CK)
    (values may be increased)
  Bilirubin, serum and
  Calcium, chloride, inorganic phosphates, potassium, and sodium, serum
    (concentrations may be increased)
  Clotting factors II, V, VII, and X
    (concentrations may be decreased)
  Creatine and creatinine excretion
    (may be increased; effect usually lasts up to 2 weeks after therapy is discontinued)
  Lipoproteins, high-density and
  Lipoproteins, low-density
    (high-density lipoprotein concentration may be lowered; low-density lipoprotein concentration may be elevated)
  Prothrombin time
    (may be increased)
  Serum lipid, especially triglyceride, concentrations and
  Urinary 17-ketosteroid (17-KS) excretion
    (may be decreased)

**Medical considerations/Contraindications**
The medical considerations/contraindications included have been selected on the basis of their potential clinical significance (reasons given in parentheses where appropriate)—not necessarily inclusive (» = major clinical significance).

*Except under special circumstances, these medications should not be used when the following medical problems exist:*
» Breast cancer, disseminated, in females with active hypercalcemia
» Breast cancer in males
» Hepatic function impairment, severe
» Hypercalcemia, active or history of
  (may be exacerbated or recurrence may result)

» Nephrosis or nephrotic phase of nephritis
» Prostate cancer
(tumor growth may be promoted)

*Risk-benefit should be considered when the following medical problems exist:*

Cardiac function impairment or
Hepatic function impairment or
Renal function impairment
(use of these medications may cause retention of sodium and water, resulting in edema, with or without congestive heart failure)
» Coronary artery disease, history of or
» Myocardial infarction, history of
(because of hypercholesterolemic effects of anabolic steroids)
Diabetes mellitus
(anabolic steroids may decrease blood sugar concentrations; insulin or oral hypoglycemic dosage may need to be adjusted)
Intolerance to anabolic steroids or androgens
Prostatic hyperplasia, benign
(further enlargement may occur)

**Patient monitoring**

The following may be especially important in patient monitoring (other tests may be warranted in some patients, depending on condition; » = major clinical significance):

Calcium
(measurement of serum concentrations recommended at regular intervals during anabolic steroid therapy in females with breast cancer)
» Cholesterol
(measurement of serum concentrations recommended at regular intervals during therapy because of possible decreased high-density lipoprotein and increased low-density lipoprotein, which may increase the risk of atherosclerosis)
Hematocrit value and
Hemoglobin concentration
(recommended periodically to detect polycythemia in patients taking high doses of anabolic steroids)
» Hepatic function determinations
(recommended at regular intervals during therapy because of possibility of hepatic dysfunction, peliosis hepatis, and liver cell tumors, especially with 17-alpha-alkylated compounds, which are more likely to cause hepatic dysfunction)
Iron concentrations, serum and
Total iron-binding capacity (TIBC) determinations
(recommended at regular intervals during therapy because of possible iron deficiency anemia manifested by low serum iron and decrease in percentage of transferrin saturation)
X-ray studies
(recommended at 6-month intervals in children and adolescents to monitor bone age in order to prevent the risk of compromising adult height)

## Side/Adverse Effects

Note: Peliosis hepatis and hepatic neoplasms, including hepatocellular carcinoma, have been associated with long-term, high-dose anabolic steroid therapy. These adverse reactions can be life-threatening or fatal.

The following side/adverse effects have been selected on the basis of their potential clinical significance (possible signs and symptoms in parentheses where appropriate)—not necessarily inclusive:

**Those indicating need for medical attention**

Incidence more frequent
*In females only*
**Virilism** (acne or oily skin; enlarging clitoris; hoarseness or deepening of voice; menstrual irregularities; unnatural hair growth or loss)

Note: *Enlarging clitoris, hoarseness or deepening of voice,* and *unnatural hair growth or loss* usually are not reversible even after prompt discontinuance of therapy. The concurrent use of estrogens will not prevent virilization in females.

*In prepubertal males only*
**Virilism** (acne; enlarging penis; increased frequency of erections; unnatural hair growth)

*In postpubertal males only*
**Bladder irritability** (frequent urge to urinate); **breast soreness**; **gynecomastia** (enlargement of breasts); **priapism** (frequent or continuing erections)

Incidence less frequent
*In both females and males*
**Anemia, iron deficiency** (loss of appetite; sore tongue); **edema** (swelling of feet or lower legs; rapid weight gain); **gastric irritation** (nausea; vomiting); **hepatic dysfunction** (yellow eyes or skin); **leukemia** (bone pain); **suppression of clotting factors** (unusual bleeding)
*In females only*
**Hypercalcemia** (mental depression; nausea; vomiting; unusual tiredness)
*In prepubertal males only*
**Unexplained darkening of skin**
*In geriatric males only*
**Prostatic carcinoma or prostatic hyperplasia** (difficult or frequent urination)

Incidence rare—with prolonged therapy
*In both females and males*
**Hepatic necrosis** (black, tarry stools; continuing feeling of discomfort; continuing headache; continuing unpleasant breath odor; vomiting of blood); **hepatocellular carcinoma** (abdominal or stomach pain; unexplained weight loss); **peliosis hepatis** (continuing loss of appetite; dark-colored urine; fever; hives; light-colored stools; nausea and vomiting; purple- or red-colored spots on body or inside the mouth or nose; sore throat)

**Those indicating need for medical attention only if they continue or are bothersome**

Incidence more frequent
*In males only*
Acne
Incidence less frequent
*In both females and males*
**Chills; decrease or increase in libido; diarrhea; feeling of abdominal or stomach fullness; muscle cramps; trouble in sleeping**
*In males only*
**Decreased sexual ability**

## Overdose

For more information on the management of overdose or unintentional ingestion, **contact a Poison Control Center** (see *Poison Control Center Listing*).

**Clinical effects of overdose**

The following effects have been selected on the basis of their potential clinical significance (possible signs and symptoms in parentheses where appropriate)—not necessarily inclusive:
**Hepatotoxicity**

**Treatment of overdose**

Treatment of overdose is symptomatic and supportive.

To decrease absorption—In acute oral overdose, decontamination includes induced emesis and/or gastric lavage.

Monitoring—Hepatic function.

Supportive care—Patients in whom intentional overdose is confirmed or suspected should be referred for psychiatric consultation.

## Patient Consultation

As an aid to patient consultation, refer to *Advice for the Patient, Anabolic Steroids (Systemic)*.

In providing consultation, consider emphasizing the following selected information (» = major clinical significance):

**Before using this medication**

» Conditions affecting use, especially:
Carcinogenicity—Hepatocellular carcinoma associated with long-term, high-dose therapy
Tumorigenicity—Hepatic neoplasms associated with long-term, high-dose therapy
Pregnancy—Not recommended during pregnancy because of possible masculinization of fetus
Use in children—Cautious use because of effects on growth and sexual development (precocious sexual development in males, virilization in females)
Use in the elderly—Increased risk of prostatic hyperplasia or prostatic carcinoma

Other medications, especially anticoagulants (coumarin- or indandione-derivatives) or hepatotoxic medications

Other medical problems, especially breast cancer, coronary artery disease, hepatic function impairment, hypercalcemia, myocardial infarction, nephrosis, nephrotic phase of nephritis, or prostatic cancer

**Proper use of this medication**
» Importance of not taking more medication than the amount prescribed; to do so may increase chance of side effects
» Importance of diet high in proteins and calories while taking this medication to achieve maximum therapeutic effect
» Proper dosing
Missed dose: If dosing schedule is—
Once daily: Taking as soon as possible; if not remembered until next day, not taking at all; not doubling doses
More than once daily: Taking as soon as possible; not taking if almost time for next dose; not doubling doses
» Proper storage

**Precautions while using this medication**
Regular visits to physician to check progress during therapy
Diabetics: May decrease blood sugar concentrations

**Side/adverse effects**
*Signs of potential side effects, especially:*
In females only—Virilism or hypercalcemia
In prepubertal males only—Virilism or unexplained darkening of skin
In postpubertal males only—Bladder irritability, breast soreness, gynecomastia, or priapism
In geriatric males only—Prostatic carcinoma or prostatic hyperplasia
In all patients, in addition to those side effects listed above—Anemia, iron deficiency; edema; gastric irritation; hepatic dysfunction, necrosis, or carcinoma; leukemia; suppression of clotting factors; or peliosis hepatis

## General Dosing Information
Many of the side/adverse effects of anabolic steroids are dose-related; therefore, patients should be placed on the lowest possible effective dose.

### Diet/Nutrition
A well-balanced diet that provides adequate proteins and calories should accompany all anabolic steroid therapy to achieve a maximum therapeutic effect.

---
### NANDROLONE
---

## Summary of Differences
Category:
Nandrolone decanoate—Antianemic.
Nandrolone phenpropionate—Antineoplastic.
Indications:
Nandrolone decanoate is indicated in the treatment of anemia associated with renal insufficiency.
Nandrolone phenpropionate is indicated in the treatment of metastatic breast cancer in women.

## Additional Dosing Information
See also *General Dosing Information.*

Nandrolone injections should be administered intramuscularly, preferably deep into the gluteal muscle.

When using nandrolone decanoate injection, an adequate iron intake is required for maximum response.

## Parenteral Dosage Forms
### NANDROLONE DECANOATE INJECTION USP
**Usual adult and adolescent dose**
Females—Intramuscular, 50 to 100 mg given at one- to four-week intervals.
Males—Intramuscular, 50 to 200 mg given at one- to four-week intervals.
Note: When given at three- to four-week intervals, therapy may be continued for up to 12 weeks. If necessary, cycle may be repeated if second course is preceded by a four-week rest period.
In the treatment of severe disease states, such as metastatic breast cancer and refractory anemias, a higher dose, based on therapeutic response and the benefit-to-risk ratio, may be required.

**Usual pediatric dose**
Children up to 2 years of age—Dosage has not been established.
Children 2 to 13 years of age—Intramuscular, 25 to 50 mg every three to four weeks.
Children 14 years of age and over—See *Usual adult and adolescent dose.*

**Strength(s) usually available**
U.S.—
50 mg per mL (Rx) [*Deca-Durabolin; Hybolin Decanoate; Kabolin;* GENERIC].
100 mg per mL (Rx) [*Deca-Durabolin; Hybolin Decanoate;* GENERIC].
200 mg per mL (Rx) [*Deca-Durabolin;* GENERIC].
Canada—
50 mg per mL (Rx) [*Deca-Durabolin* (benzyl alcohol 10%; sesame oil)].
100 mg per mL (Rx) [*Deca-Durabolin* (benzyl alcohol 10%; sesame oil)].

**Packaging and storage**
Store below 40 °C (104 °F), preferably between 15 and 30 °C (59 and 86 °F), unless otherwise specified by the manufacturer. Protect from light. Protect from freezing.

### NANDROLONE PHENPROPIONATE INJECTION USP
**Usual adult dose**
Intramuscular, 25 to 100 mg per week.
Note: Therapy may be continued for up to 12 weeks. If necessary, cycle may be repeated if second course is preceded by a four-week rest period.

**Usual pediatric dose**
Dosage has not been established.

**Strength(s) usually available**
U.S.—
25 mg per mL (Rx) [*Durabolin;* GENERIC].
50 mg per mL (Rx) [*Durabolin-50; Hybolin-Improved;* GENERIC].
Canada—
Not commercially available.

**Packaging and storage**
Store below 40 °C (104 °F), preferably between 15 and 30 °C (59 and 86 °F), unless otherwise specified by the manufacturer. Protect from light. Protect from freezing.

---
### OXANDROLONE
---

## Summary of Differences
Indications: Indicated in the treatment of catabolic or tissue-depleting processes.

## Additional Dosing Information
See also *General Dosing Information.*

In adults, 2 to 4 weeks of therapy are usually adequate. In both adults and children, therapy may be repeated intermittently as needed.

## Oral Dosage Forms
Note: Bracketed uses in the *Dosage Forms* section refer to categories of use and/or indications that are not included in U.S. product labeling.

### OXANDROLONE TABLETS USP
**Usual adult and adolescent dose**
Oral, 2.5 mg two to four times a day.
Note: The dosage may range from 2.5 to 20 mg per day.

**Usual pediatric dose**
Children—Oral, 250 mcg (0.25 mg) per kg of body weight per day.
[Turner's syndrome]—
Oral, 50 mcg to 125 mcg (0.05 to 0.125 mg) per kg of body weight per day. Generally, the patient should be started and maintained on the lowest effective dose to minimize the potential for adverse effects.

**Strength(s) usually available**
U.S.—
2.5 mg (Rx) [*Oxandrin* (scored; lactose)].
Canada—
Not commercially available.

**Packaging and storage**
Store below 40 °C (104 °F), preferably between 15 and 30 °C (59 and 86 °F), unless otherwise specified by the manufacturer. Store in a tight, light-resistant container.

## OXYMETHOLONE

### Summary of Differences
Category: Antianemic; angioedema (hereditary) agent.
Indications: Indicated in treatment of bone marrow failure anemias and in deficient red cell production anemias; also used in prophylaxis and treatment of hereditary angioedema.

### Additional Dosing Information
See also *General Dosing Information*.

Oxymetholone should be used for a minimum of 3 to 6 months, since a response is not always immediately observed.

Following remission of the anemia, some patients may be maintained without oxymetholone while others may be maintained on a low daily dose. Patients with congenital aplastic anemia usually require continued therapy with an appropriate maintenance dose.

### Oral Dosage Forms
**OXYMETHOLONE TABLETS USP**

**Usual adult and adolescent dose**
Oral, 1 to 5 mg per kg of body weight per day.

Note: The usual effective dose is 1 to 2 mg per kg of body weight a day, but higher doses may be required in some patients. Treatment of refractory anemias may require 3 to 6 months.

**Usual pediatric dose**
Premature infants and neonates—Oral, 175 mcg (0.175 mg) per kg of body weight or 5 mg per square meter of body surface area per day as a single dose.

Infants and children—See *Usual adult and adolescent dose*.

**Strength(s) usually available**
U.S.—
  50 mg (Rx) [*Anadrol-50* (scored)].
Canada—
  50 mg (Rx) [*Anapolon 50* (scored; lactose)].

**Packaging and storage**
Store below 40 °C (104 °F), preferably between 15 and 30 °C (59 and 86 °F), unless otherwise specified by the manufacturer. Store in a well-closed container.

## STANOZOLOL

### Summary of Differences
Category: Angioedema (hereditary) prophylactic.
Indications: Stanozolol is indicated in the prophylaxis of hereditary angioedema to decrease the frequency and severity of attacks and used in treatment of hereditary angioedema.

### Oral Dosage Forms
**STANOZOLOL TABLETS USP**

**Usual adult and adolescent dose**
Oral, 2 mg three times a day to 4 mg four times a day for 5 days, initially.

Note: A dose of 2 mg two times a day may be used in young women, who are particularly susceptible to the androgenic effects of stanozolol.

The dosage for continuous treatment of hereditary angioedema should be individualized according to patient response. After a favorable response is obtained, the dose should be decreased at intervals of 1 to 3 months to a maintenance dose of 2 mg a day; some patients may respond to a maintenance dose of 2 mg every other day. During the dose-reduction phase, close monitoring of patient response is indicated, especially if the patient has a history of upper respiratory tract involvement.

**Usual pediatric dose**
Children up to 6 years of age—Oral, 1 mg a day, to be administered only during an attack.
Children 6 to 12 years of age—Oral, up to 2 mg a day, to be administered only during an attack.

**Strength(s) usually available**
U.S.—
  2 mg (Rx) [*Winstrol* (scored; lactose)].
Canada—
  Not commercially available.

**Packaging and storage**
Store below 40 °C (104 °F), preferably between 15 and 30 °C (59 and 86 °F), unless otherwise specified by the manufacturer. Store in a tight, light-resistant container.

Revised: 06/20/92
Interim revision: 06/08/94; 06/23/97; 06/22/98

---

# ANAGRELIDE  Systemic—INTRODUCTORY VERSION

VA CLASSIFICATION (Primary): BL400
Commonly used brand name(s): *Agrylin*.
Note: For a listing of dosage forms and brand names by country availability, see *Dosage Forms* section(s).

## Category
Platelet count–reducing agent.

## Indications
**Accepted**
Thrombocythemia, essential (treatment)—Anagrelide is indicated for reduction of elevated platelet counts and of the risk of thrombosis, as well as for amelioration of symptoms, in patients with essential thrombocythemia.

Note: Decisions about whether or not to treat asymptomatic young adults with essential thrombocythemia should be made on an individual patient basis.

## Pharmacology/Pharmacokinetics
**Physicochemical characteristics**
Molecular weight—Anagrelide hydrochloride: 310.55.
Solubility—Very slightly soluble in water; sparingly soluble in dimethyl sulfoxide and in dimethylformamide.

**Mechanism of action/Effect**
The exact mechanism of action has not been established but it is thought to involve a dose-related reduction of platelet production through a decrease in megakaryocyte hypermaturation.

**Other actions/effects**
Anagrelide does not affect white cell counts or coagulation parameters at therapeutic doses and may have a small but clinically insignificant effect on red cell parameters. It inhibits platelet aggregation at doses higher than those necessary to reduce platelet counts. It inhibits cyclic adenosine monophosphate (cAMP)–phosphodiesterase, as well as adenosine diphosphate (ADP)–induced and collagen-induced platelet aggregation.

**Absorption**
Limited data indicate probable dose linearity between doses of 500 mcg (0.5 mg) and 2 mg. Bioavailability was found to be modestly reduced by an average of 13.8% when anagrelide was administered after food. However, this is considered not clinically significant.

**Biotransformation**
Extensive; less than 1% is recovered in the urine unchanged.

**Half-life**
Elimination—
  Plasma: 1.3 hours (at a dose of 0.5 mg while fasting).
Note: Plasma half-life was found to be increased (to 1.8 hours) when anagrelide was taken after food.

Steady-state plasma concentration measurements show no accumulation of anagrelide in plasma with repeated administration.

**Onset of action**
Platelet count response—Within 7 to 14 days at the proper dosage, which is usually between 1.5 and 3 mg per day.

**Time to peak concentration**
Plasma—Delayed by 2 hours when anagrelide is taken after food.

**Peak plasma concentration**
Reduced by an average of 45% when anagrelide is taken after food.

**Duration of action**
Increases in platelet counts are observed within 4 days following sudden withdrawal of anagrelide.

**Elimination**
Renal, more than 70% (less than 1% unchanged).

## Precautions to Consider

**Carcinogenicity**
Long-term studies in animals have not been done.

**Mutagenicity**
Anagrelide was not found to be mutagenic in the Ames test, the mouse lymphoma cell (L5178Y, TK$^{+/-}$) forward mutation test, the human lymphocyte chromosome aberration test, and the mouse micronucleus test.

**Pregnancy/Reproduction**
Fertility—Studies in male rats given oral doses of up to 240 mg per kg of body weight (mg/kg) per day (1440 mg per square meter of body surface area [mg/m$^2$] per day, which is 195 times the maximum recommended human dose [MRHD] based on body surface area), found no effect on fertility and reproduction. However, studies in female rats given oral doses of 60 mg/kg per day (360 mg/m$^2$ per day, which is 49 times the MRHD based on body surface area), or higher found disruption of implantation when anagrelide was administered during early pregnancy, and retarded or blocked parturition when anagrelide was administered in late pregnancy.

Pregnancy—Adequate and well-controlled studies in humans have not been done. However, five women became pregnant during treatment with 1 to 4 mg per day of anagrelide; the medication was stopped immediately when the pregnancy was discovered and the women delivered normal healthy babies.

Studies in pregnant rats given oral doses of up to 900 mg/kg per day (5400 mg/m$^2$ per day, which is 730 times the MRHD based on body surface area), and in pregnant rabbits given oral doses of up to 20 mg/kg per day (240 mg/m$^2$ per day, which is 32 times the MRHD based on body surface area), found no evidence of teratogenicity. Reproductive studies in female rats given oral doses of 60 mg/kg per day (360 mg/m$^2$ per day, which is 49 times the MRHD based on body surface area) or higher showed adverse effects on embryo/fetal survival; a perinatal and postnatal study at the same dose found deaths of nondelivering pregnant dams and their fully developed fetuses, and increased mortality in the pups born.

Because of the risks to the fetus, use of anagrelide is not recommended in women who are or who may become pregnant. Use of birth control is recommended during treatment with anagrelide. Patients who take the medication during pregnancy or who become pregnant during treatment with anagrelide should be advised of the risks to the fetus.

FDA Pregnancy Category C.

**Breast-feeding**
It is not known whether anagrelide is distributed into breast milk. However, because of the risk of serious adverse effects in the infant, a decision as to whether the medication should be discontinued or nursing should be discontinued should take into account the importance of the medication to the mother.

**Pediatrics**
Studies on the relationship of age to the effects of anagrelide have not been performed in the pediatric population. However, the medication has been administered successfully to eight patients ages 8 to 17 years (including three with essential thrombocythemia) at doses of 1 to 4 mg per day. Safety and efficacy in patients younger than 16 years of age have not been established.

**Adolescents**
Studies on the relationship of age to the effects of anagrelide have not been performed in the adolescent population. However, the medication has been administered successfully to eight patients ages 8 to 17 years (including three with essential thrombocythemia) at doses of 1 to 4 mg per day. Safety and efficacy in patients younger than 16 years of age have not been established.

**Laboratory value alterations**
The following have been selected on the basis of their potential clinical significance (possible effect in parentheses where appropriate)—not necessarily inclusive (» = major clinical significance):

With physiology/laboratory test values
Blood pressure
(standing blood pressure is reduced by an average of 22/15 mm Hg after a single 5-mg dose, usually causing dizziness; however, blood pressure changes are minimal following a 2-mg dose)
Hepatic enzymes
(may rarely be increased during therapy)

**Medical considerations/Contraindications**
The medical considerations/contraindications included have been selected on the basis of their potential clinical significance (reasons given in parentheses where appropriate)—not necessarily inclusive (» = major clinical significance).

*Risk-benefit should be considered when the following medical problems exist:*

» Cardiac disease, known or suspected
(because of its positive inotropic effects and cardiac side effects [vasodilation, tachycardia, palpitations, congestive heart failure], anagrelide should be used only after consideration of risk-benefit; a cardiovascular examination prior to initiation of therapy, as well as careful monitoring during therapy, is recommended)

» Hepatic function impairment
(risk-benefit should be considered before administering anagrelide to patients with hepatic function values [bilirubin, SGOT, or other hepatic function tests] more than 1.5 times the upper limit of normal; close monitoring for signs of hepatotoxicity is recommended during therapy)

» Renal function impairment
(risk-benefit should be considered before administering anagrelide to patients with renal insufficiency [serum creatinine of 2 mg per deciliter or more]; no dosage adjustment is required; close monitoring for signs of renal toxicity is recommended during therapy)

**Patient monitoring**
The following may be especially important in patient monitoring (other tests may be warranted in some patients, depending on condition; » = major clinical significance):

Alanine aminotransferase (ALT [SGPT]) values, serum and
Aspartate aminotransferase (AST [SGOT]) values, serum and
Blood urea nitrogen (BUN) concentrations and
Creatinine concentrations, serum and
Hemoglobin and
White blood cell counts
(monitoring is recommended while the platelet count is being lowered, which usually occurs during the first 2 weeks of therapy)

» Platelet counts
(determinations are recommended every 2 days during the first week of treatment and at least weekly after that until the maintenance dose is reached, in order to monitor the effect of anagrelide and prevent thrombocytopenia)

Signs and symptoms of cardiovascular effects
(therapeutic doses of anagrelide may cause cardiovascular effects, including vasodilation, tachycardia, palpitations, and congestive heart failure; close clinical supervision is recommended)

## Side/Adverse Effects

Note: Although most side/adverse effects reported have been mild and have decreased in frequency with continued therapy, serious cardiac, central nervous system (CNS), gastric, and pulmonary effects have occurred.

The following side/adverse effects have been selected on the basis of their potential clinical significance (possible signs and symptoms in parentheses where appropriate)—not necessarily inclusive:

**Those indicating need for medical attention**
Incidence more frequent (> 10%)
*Abdominal or stomach pain; asthenia* (weakness); *dizziness; palpitations; pulmonary infiltrates or pulmonary fibrosis* (shortness of breath)

Note: *Abdominal or stomach pain* may be a symptom of a gastric or duodenal ulcer or of pancreatitis.
*Dizziness* may be a symptom of hypotension.

Incidence less frequent (< 10%)
*Asthma, bronchitis, or pneumonia* (difficulty in breathing; shortness of breath); *cardiac toxicity, including congestive heart failure* (shortness of breath; swelling of feet or lower legs; unusual tiredness or weakness); *cardiomyopathy; cardiomegaly; complete heart block; atrial fibrillation* (rapid or irregular heartbeat); *myocardial infarction* (anxiety; cold sweating; increased heart rate; nausea or vomiting; severe pain or pressure in the chest and/or the jaw, neck, back, or arms; shortness of breath); *or pericarditis; cerebrovascular accident* (sudden severe headache or weakness); *blurred or double vision; dysuria* (painful or difficult urination); *hematuria* (blood in urine); *paresthesias* (numbness or tingling in hands or feet); *thrombocytopenia* (unusual bleeding or bruising); *vasodilation* (flushing; faintness)

Note: Renal abnormalities (including *dysuria* and *hematuria* occurred in approximately 2% of patients (10 of 551) in clinical trials. Of those, six experienced renal failure presumed to be drug-related.

## Anagrelide (Systemic)—Introductory Version

The other four were found to have pre-existing renal function impairment; no dosage adjustment was necessary and serum creatinine concentrations remained within normal limits.

*Thrombocytopenia* (platelet counts less than 100,000 per microliter) occurred in 35 of 551 patients in clinical trials; reductions below 50,000 per microliter occurred in 7 of 551 patients. Platelet counts recovered promptly after withdrawal of anagrelide.

**Those indicating need for medical attention only if they continue or are bothersome**
Incidence more frequent (> 10%)
*Diarrhea; dyspepsia* (heartburn); *flatulence* (gas or bloating of stomach); *headache; loss of appetite; malaise* (general feeling of discomfort or illness); *nausea; pain*

Incidence less frequent (< 10%)
*Aphthous stomatitis* (canker sore); *arthralgia* (joint pain); *back pain; confusion; constipation; fever or chills; insomnia* (trouble in sleeping); *leg cramps; mental depression; myalgia* (muscle pain); *nervousness; rhinitis* (stuffy or runny nose); *ringing in the ears; skin rash or itching; somnolence* (sleepiness); *unusual sensitivity to light; vomiting*

**Those not indicating need for medical attention**
Incidence less frequent or rare
*Alopecia* (loss of hair)

## Overdose

For more information on the management of overdose or unintentional ingestion, **contact a Poison Control Center** (see *Poison Control Center Listing*).

**Clinical effects of overdose**
The following effects have been selected on the basis of their potential clinical significance (possible signs and symptoms in parentheses where appropriate)—not necessarily inclusive:

Acute
*Cardiac toxicity; CNS toxicity; thrombocytopenia, which potentially can cause bleeding*
Note: There are no reports of overdosage with anagrelide in humans. In mice, rats, and monkeys, single oral doses of anagrelide hydrochloride of 2500, 1500, and 200 mg per kg of body weight, respectively, were not lethal.

**Treatment of overdose**
Close clinical supervision of the patient.
Monitoring—Platelet count, for thrombocytopenia.
Dosage should be decreased or anagrelide withdrawn, as appropriate, until the platelet count returns to normal.

## Patient Consultation

In providing consultation, consider emphasizing the following selected information (» = major clinical significance):

**Before using this medication**
» Conditions affecting use, especially:
Pregnancy—Use is not recommended; advisability of using contraception; telling physician immediately if pregnancy is suspected
Breast-feeding—Risk-benefit should be considered
Other medical problems, especially cardiac disease (known or suspected), hepatic function impairment, or renal function impairment

**Proper use of this medication**
» Proper dosing
» Proper storage

**Precautions while using this medication**
» Importance of close monitoring by the physician
» Notifying physician and/or getting emergency help immediately if signs and symptoms of a heart attack occur

**Side/adverse effects**
Signs of potential side effects, especially abdominal or stomach pain, asthenia, dizziness, palpitations, pulmonary infiltrates or pulmonary fibrosis, asthma, bronchitis, pneumonia, cardiac toxicity, cerebrovascular accident, blurred or double vision, dysuria, hematuria, paresthesias, thrombocytopenia, and vasodilation

## General Dosing Information

It is recommended that anagrelide therapy be initiated under close medical supervision.

Dosage reduction or withdrawal of anagrelide is recommended if thrombocytopenia occurs. Platelet counts usually recover promptly after withdrawal.

## Oral Dosage Forms

### ANAGRELIDE HYDROCHLORIDE CAPSULES

Note: Dose and strength are expressed in terms of anagrelide base.

**Usual adult dose**
Essential thrombocythemia—
Initial: Oral, 0.5 mg four times per day or 1 mg two times per day for at least one week. Dosage is then adjusted to the lowest effective dose that reduces and maintains platelet counts below 600,000 per microliter and ideally within the normal range.
Note: Dosage increases should not exceed 0.5 mg per day in any one week.
Single dosages should not exceed 2.5 mg per dose.

**Usual adult prescribing limits**
10 mg per day.

**Usual pediatric dose**
Safety and efficacy in patients younger than 16 years of age have not been established.

**Strength(s) usually available**
U.S.—
0.5 mg (base) (Rx) [*Agrylin* (lactose)].
1 mg (base) (Rx) [*Agrylin* (lactose)].

**Packaging and storage**
Store between 15 and 25 °C (59 and 77 °F). Protect from light.

Developed: 11/17/97
Interim revision: 07/23/98

# ANASTROZOLE Systemic—INTRODUCTORY VERSION

VA CLASSIFICATION (Primary): AN500
Commonly used brand name(s): *Arimidex*.
Note: For a listing of dosage forms and brand names by country availability, see *Dosage Forms* section(s).

## Category

Antineoplastic.

## Indications

**Accepted**
Carcinoma, breast (treatment)—Anastrozole is indicated for the treatment of advanced breast cancer in postmenopausal women whose disease has progressed despite previous tamoxifen therapy.
Note: Patients who have had no response to previous tamoxifen therapy and have estrogen-receptor-negative disease rarely respond to anastrozole.

## Pharmacology/Pharmacokinetics

**Physicochemical characteristics**
Molecular weight—293.4.
Solubility—Anastrozole is moderately soluble in water; freely soluble in acetone, ethanol, methanol, and tetrahydrofuran; and very soluble in acetonitrile.

**Mechanism of action/Effect**
Anastrozole is a nonsteroidal aromatase inhibitor that interferes with estradiol production in peripheral tissues. Adrenally generated androstenedione, the chief source of circulating estrogen in postmenopausal women, is converted by aromatase to estrone, which is further converted to estradiol. Growth of many breast cancer tumors containing estrogen receptors and aromatase can be promoted by estrogen.

**Absorption**
Well absorbed; the extent of absorption of anastrozole may be altered in the presence of food.

**Protein binding**
Moderate (40%).

**Biotransformation**
Hepatic; metabolized primarily by *N*-dealkylation, hydroxylation, and glucuronidation to inactive metabolites. Primary metabolite is an inactive triazole.

**Half-life**
Elimination—Approximately 50 hours.

**Onset of action**
A 70% reduction of serum estradiol usually occurs within 24 hours, with an 80% reduction in serum estradiol occurring after 14 days.

**Time to peak concentration**
Steady state concentrations are achieved after approximately 7 days.

**Duration of action**
Estrogen antagonism may persist for up to 6 days following the discontinuation of anastrozole.

**Elimination**
Primary route—Biliary: Approximately 85%.
Secondary route—Renal: Approximately 11% (about 10% unchanged and 60% as metabolites).

## Precautions to Consider

**Carcinogenicity**
Studies with anastrozole have not been done.

**Mutagenicity**
Anastrozole demonstrated no mutagenic effects in the Ames test, *Escherichia coli* bacterial test, Chinese hamster ovary-K1 mutation assay, an *in vitro* chromosomal aberration assay, and an *in vivo* micronucleus test in rats.

**Pregnancy/Reproduction**
Fertility—Adequate and well-controlled studies in humans have not been done.
Long-term studies in rats, at doses that produce a plasma concentration 19 times greater than that associated with the recommended human dose, have shown that anastrozole produces ovarian hypertrophy and follicular cysts. Studies in dogs have shown that anastrozole causes hyperplastic uteri at doses that produce a plasma concentration 22 times greater than that associated with the recommended human dose.
Pregnancy—Adequate and well-controlled studies in humans have not been done.
Studies in rats and rabbits, at 75% and 150% of the recommended human dose, respectively, have shown that anastrozole crosses the placenta.
Anastrozole is fetotoxic in rats, causing decreased fetal body weights and incomplete ossification, at doses that produce a plasma concentration 19 times greater than the plasma concentration associated with the recommended human dose. Studies in rats and rabbits during organogenesis, at 75% and 33% of the recommended human dose, respectively, have shown that anastrozole may cause increased implantation loss, increased resorption, and a decreased number of live fetuses. Anastrozole is not teratogenic in rats and rabbits at doses that produce plasma concentrations that are 19 and 3 times, respectively, greater than the plasma concentration associated with the recommended human dose. Studies in rabbits, at doses that produce a plasma concentration 16 times greater than the plasma concentration associated with the recommended human dose, have shown that anastrozole may cause pregnancy failure. Studies in rats, given 75% of the recommended human dose, have shown that anastrozole may cause an increase in placental weight.
FDA Pregnancy Category D.

**Breast-feeding**
It is not known whether anastrozole is distributed into breast milk. However, the manufacturer recommends that any decision regarding breast-feeding during anastrozole therapy should take into account the potential risk to the infant.

**Pediatrics**
No information is available on the relationship of age to the effects of anastrozole in pediatric patients. Safety and efficacy have not been established.

**Geriatrics**
Studies performed in approximately 188 postmenopausal women 65 years of age or older have not demonstrated geriatrics-specific problems that would limit the usefulness of anastrozole in the elderly.

**Laboratory value alterations**
The following have been selected on the basis of their potential clinical significance (possible effect in parentheses where appropriate)—not necessarily inclusive (» = major clinical significance):

With physiology/laboratory test values
    Alanine aminotransferase (ALT [SGPT]), serum and
    Alkaline phosphatase, serum and
    Aspartate aminotransferase (AST [SGOT]), serum and
    Gamma glutamyl transferase, serum
        (values may be increased, especially in patients with liver metastases)
    Cholesterol, serum, total and
    Low-density lipoprotein (LDL), serum
        (concentrations may be increased)

## Side/Adverse Effects

The following side/adverse effects have been selected on the basis of their potential clinical significance (possible signs and symptoms in parentheses where appropriate)—not necessarily inclusive:

**Those indicating need for medical attention**
Incidence more frequent
    *Chest pain; dyspnea* (shortness of breath); *edema, peripheral* (swelling of feet or lower legs)
Incidence less frequent
    *Anemia* (unusual tiredness or weakness); *hypertension* (dizziness, severe; continuing headache)—usually asymptomatic; *leukopenia, with or without infection* (fever or chills; cough or hoarseness; lower back or side pain; painful or difficult urination; sore throat)—usually asymptomatic; *thromboembolism* (sudden shortness of breath); *thrombophlebitis* (pain or tenderness in leg or foot; blue color in leg or foot; swelling of leg or foot); *vaginal hemorrhage* (heavy vaginal bleeding)

**Those indicating need for medical attention only if they continue or are bothersome**
Incidence more frequent
    *Asthenia* (weakness); *bone pain; cough; dizziness; dry mouth; flushing* (feeling of warmth; redness of face and neck); *gastrointestinal disturbances, including abdominal pain, diarrhea, nausea, or vomiting; headache; hot flashes; pelvic pain; skin rash; sweating*
Incidence less frequent
    *Arthralgia* (joint pain); *breast pain; myalgia* (muscle pain); *paresthesia* (numbness or tingling sensation of hands and feet); *pruritus* (itchy skin); *sinusitis or rhinitis* (stuffy nose); *vaginal dryness; weight gain*

**Those not indicating need for medical attention**
Incidence less frequent
    *Alopecia* (loss of hair)

## Overdose

For more information on the management of overdose or unintentional ingestion, **contact a Poison Control Center** (see *Poison Control Center Listing*).

**Clinical effects of overdose**
Studies in rats at doses that produce plasma concentrations 800 times greater than those associated with the recommended human dose have shown that anastrozole may cause severe stomach irritation.

**Treatment of overdose**
Treatment is essentially symptomatic and supportive and may consist of the following:
- Emptying the stomach via induction of emesis if patient is alert.
- Hemodialysis may be beneficial.

## Patient Consultation

As an aid to patient consultation, refer to *Advice for the Patient, Anastrozole (Systemic)—Introductory Version*.
In providing consultation, consider emphasizing the following selected information (» = major clinical significance):

**Before using taking this medication**
» Conditions affecting use, especially:
    Pregnancy—Use not recommended due to fetotoxic potential; telling physician immediately if pregnancy is suspected

**Proper use of this medication**
Importance of taking medication only as directed by physician; not taking more medication or more frequently than as ordered by physician
Importance of continuing medication even if nausea, vomiting, or diarrhea occurs
» Proper dosing
» Proper storage

**Precautions while using this medication**
Importance of close monitoring by physician

# Anastrozole (Systemic)—Introductory Version

### Side/adverse effects
Signs of potential side effects, especially chest pain; dyspnea; peripheral edema; anemia; hypertension; leukopenia, with or without infection; thromboembolism; thrombophlebitis; or vaginal hemorrhage
Possibility of hair loss

## General Dosing Information
Patients receiving anastrozole should be under supervision of a physician experienced in cancer chemotherapy.

Dosing adjustments are not necessary for patients with mild-to-moderate hepatic impairment because plasma concentrations of anastrozole in these patients remain within the limit found in patients with normal hepatic function. It is recommended, however, that these patients be monitored for adverse effects.

Anastrozole has no effect on cortisol or aldosterone secretion; therefore, glucocorticoid or mineralocorticoid replacement therapy is not required.

## Oral Dosage Forms

### ANASTROZOLE TABLETS

**Usual adult dose**
Carcinoma, breast—
   Oral, 1 mg once a day.

**Strength(s) usually available**
U.S.—
   1 mg (Rx) [*Arimidex* (lactose; magnesium stearate; hydroxypropylmethylcellulose; polyethylene glycol; povidone; sodium starch glycolate; titanium dioxide)].

**Packaging and storage**
Store between 20 and 25 °C (68 and 77 °F).

Developed: 2/26/97
Interim revision: 08/14/98

---

# ANDROGENS   Systemic

This monograph includes information on the following: 1) Fluoxymesterone; 2) Methyltestosterone; 3) Testosterone.
VA CLASSIFICATION (Primary/Secondary):
   Fluoxymesterone—HS101/AN900; BL400
   Methyltestosterone—HS101/AN900
   Testosterone—HS101/AN900
   Testosterone cypionate—HS101/AN900; BL400
   Testosterone enanthate—HS101/AN900; BL400
   Testosterone propionate—HS101/AN900
   Testosterone undecanoate—HS101

Note: Androgens are controlled substances in the U.S.—Schedule III

Commonly used brand name(s): *Andriol*[3]; *Andro L.A. 200*[3]; *Androderm*[3]; *Android*[3]; *Android-F*[1]; *Andronate 100*[3]; *Andronate 200*[3]; *Andropository 200*[3]; *Andryl 200*[3]; *Delatest*[3]; *Delatestryl*[3]; *Depo-Testosterone*[3]; *Depo-Testosterone Cypionate*[3]; *Depotest*[3]; *Everone 200*[3]; *Halotestin*[1]; *Malogen in Oil*[3]; *Metandren*[2]; *ORETON Methyl*[2]; *Scheinpharm Testone-Cyp*[3]; *T-Cypionate*[3]; *Testamone 100*[3]; *Testaqua*[3]; *Testex*[3]; *Testoderm*[3]; *Testoderm TTS*[3]; *Testoderm with Adhesives*[3]; *Testopel Pellets*[3]; *Testred*[2]; *Testred Cypionate 200*[3]; *Testrin-P.A*[3]; *Virilon*[2]; *Virilon IM*[3].

Note: For a listing of dosage forms and brand names by country availability, see *Dosage Forms* section(s).

## Category
Androgen—Fluoxymesterone; Methyltestosterone; Testosterone; Testosterone Undecanoate.
Antineoplastic—Fluoxymesterone; Methyltestosterone; Testosterone.
Antianemic—Fluoxymesterone; Testosterone Cypionate; Testosterone Enanthate.

## Indications
Note: Bracketed information in the *Indications* section refers to uses that are not included in U.S. product labeling.

### General considerations
Whenever long-term therapy is needed in men, testosterone or a testosterone ester is preferred over the oral methylated androgens (fluoxymesterone and methyltestosterone) because hepatotoxicity is less likely to occur.

### Accepted
Androgen deficiency, due to primary or secondary hypogonadism (treatment)—Androgens are primarily indicated in males as replacement therapy when congenital or acquired endogenous androgen absence or deficiency is associated with primary or secondary hypogonadism. Primary hypogonadism includes conditions such as: testicular failure due to cryptorchidism, bilateral torsion, orchitis, or vanishing testis syndrome; inborn errors in testosterone biosynthesis; or bilateral orchidectomy. Hypogonadotropic hypogonadism (secondary hypogonadism) conditions include gonadotropin-releasing hormone (GnRH) deficiency or pituitary-hypothalamic injury as a result of surgery, tumors, trauma, or radiation and are the most common forms of hypogonadism seen in older adults. Dosage adjustment is needed to accommodate individual clinical requirements for such life changes as induction of puberty, development of secondary sexual characteristics, impotence due to testicular failure, or infertility due to oligospermia.

Puberty, delayed male (treatment)—A 6-month-or-shorter course of an androgen is indicated for induction of puberty in patients with familial delayed puberty, a condition characterized by spontaneous, nonpathologic, late-onset puberty, if the patient does not respond to psychological treatment. Testosterone transdermal products are not presently indicated for treatment of delayed male puberty.

Carcinoma, breast (treatment)—Androgens are indicated as secondary or tertiary hormonal treatment for palliation of metastatic breast cancer in women who have been postmenopausal for 1 to 5 years or who are surgically menopausal, who have hormone receptor–positive tumors, or who have previously demonstrated a response to hormone therapy. Androgens have also been used in the treatment of metastatic breast cancer as a supplement to chemotherapy. Transdermal testosterone systems and subcutaneous implants are not indicated for these uses and should not be used by females.

[Anemia (treatment)][1]—Fluoxymesterone and testosterone cypionate or enanthate have been used to treat certain types of anemia, such as aplastic anemia, myelofibrosis, myelosclerosis, agnogenic myeloid metaplasia, and hypoplastic anemias caused by malignancy or myelotoxic drugs.

[Constitutional delay in growth (treatment)][1]—Androgens are used in the treatment of constitutional delay in growth. However, they are no longer considered the treatment of choice for most patients.

[Gender change, female-to-male][1]—Testosterone is used for the development and maintenance of secondary sexual characteristics in female-to-male transsexuals.

[Lichen sclerosus (treatment adjunct)][1]—Extemporaneously compounded topical testosterone is used for the treatment of itching resulting from lichen sclerosus.

[Microphallus (treatment)][1]—Intramuscular preparations of testosterone and testosterone esters, and extemporaneously compounded topical testosterone are used in the treatment of microphallus.

### Acceptance not established
Although testosterone cypionate and testosterone undecanoate are indicated in Canada for the following conditions if they are not due to primary or secondary hypogonadism, further studies are needed to define the role, safety, and efficacy of androgens to treat *male climacteric symptoms* and *male infertility due to oligospermia*. Further studies are also needed to assess androgens as adjunctive treatment for *male or female osteoporosis*.

### Unaccepted
Use of androgens to enhance athletic performance is illegal. Increases in muscle mass and muscle strength can be sufficient to enhance athletic performance. However, the risk of unwanted effects, such as suppression of spermatogenesis, testicular atrophy, menstrual disturbances, virilization in females, peliosis hepatis (hepatic parenchymal injury), hepatotoxicity, potential adverse effects on cardiovascular health, and development of hepatic cancer, counter athletic benefits received from androgens and make their use in athletes inappropriate. Furthermore, behavioral disturbances, including aggressive or violent behavior, have been reported with supraphysiological self-administered doses in athletes.

Androgens are not recommended for accelerating the healing of fractures or shortening the duration of postsurgical convalescence.

The use of androgens for the prevention of postpartum breast engorgement is not recommended. In most patients, postpartum breast engorgement is a benign, self-limiting condition that may respond to breast support and mild analgesics, such as acetaminophen and ibuprofen. Evidence supporting the efficacy of androgens for this indication is lacking.

[1]Not included in Canadian product labeling.

## Pharmacology/Pharmacokinetics

**Physicochemical characteristics**
Description—
  Testosterone implants are compressed crystalline testosterone, cylindrically shaped, measuring 3.2 millimeters (mm) in diameter and 8 to 9 mm in length.
  Two types of testosterone transdermal systems are available:
    Drug-in-adhesive matrix on film (matrix-type)—*Testoderm* contains three layers: a polyester liner that must be removed before using; an adhesive matrix containing testosterone; and the back outermost layer, a flexible polyurethane protective film with epoxy resin. *Testoderm with Adhesives* incorporates five additional adhesive strips onto the adhesive matrix of the drug film.
    Membrane-controlled drug reservoir (reservoir-type)—*Androderm* contains: a protective liner that must be removed before using; a disc, matted between adhesive layers, that protects the central drug reservoir and is removed before using; an adhesive layer; a membrane providing extended release of testosterone; a drug reservoir holding the testosterone, glycerin, and alcohol gelled with hydroxypropyl cellulose; and the back outermost layer, a polyester protective film. *Testoderm TTS* is similar but does not contain the protective disc.
  The matrix-type transdermal system is thinner than the reservoir-type.
Chemical group—
  Naturally occurring androgens include testosterone.
  Semi-synthetic androgens are testosterone cypionate, testosterone enanthate, and testosterone propionate.
  Synthetic androgens include fluoxymesterone and methyltestosterone.
  Oral methylated androgens (17-alpha-alkylated androgens) include fluoxymesterone and methyltestosterone.
Molecular weight—
  Fluoxymesterone: 336.45.
  Methyltestosterone: 302.46.
  Testosterone: 288.43.
  Testosterone cypionate: 412.62.
  Testosterone enanthate: 400.6.
  Testosterone propionate: 344.5.
  Testosterone undecanoate: 456.7.

**Mechanism of action/Effect**
  Endogenous plasma testosterone is maintained and regulated by gonadotropins within a normal range by a negative feedback system involving the hypothalamus and pituitary. Supraphysiologic doses of testosterone can effectively suppress the gonadotropins and spermatogenesis in eugonadal men.
  Androgens are highly lipid-soluble and enter cells of target tissues by passive diffusion. Testosterone or 5-alpha-dihydrotestosterone (DHT), a metabolite produced from testosterone by the enzyme 5-alpha-reductase, binds to an intracellular androgen receptor. The hormone receptor complex translocates into the nucleus and attaches to specific hormone receptor elements on the chromosome to initiate or suppress transcription and protein synthesis. Testosterone can produce estrogenic effects as a result of its conversion to estrogen.
Androgen deficiency—
  Physiologic concentrations of androgens stimulate spermatogenesis and male sexual maturity at puberty, and develop and maintain male secondary sexual characteristics. These effects include growth and maturation of the prostate, seminal vesicles, penis, and scrotum; male hair and muscle-to-fat body mass distribution; enlargement of the larynx; and thickening of vocal cords. Androgens increase linear bone growth and bone density, and, directly and indirectly, along with estrogen and growth factors, help fuse the epiphyseal growth centers. In adolescents, an increase in bone growth rate can also correspond to a disproportionate advancement of bone maturation.
Microphallus—
  Intramuscular administration of testosterone or testosterone esters or local application of testosterone propionate ointment may result in an increase in circulating serum concentrations of DHT, which is principally responsible for phallic growth.
Lichen sclerosus—
  The signs and symptoms of lichen sclerosus (vulvar itching, abnormal vulvar skin histology) may be the result of a deficiency of 5-alpha-reductase activity and subsequently reduced local DHT concentrations. Local application of testosterone propionate ointment may correct this deficiency in 5-alpha-reductase activity. Testosterone may cause a slight increase in local DHT concentrations, which may induce 5-alpha-reductase activity, and further increase local DHT concentrations.
Antianemic—
  Androgens stimulate the production of red blood cells by enhancing production of erythropoietic stimulating factors.

**Absorption**
Methyltestosterone—
  Absorbed from oral mucosa and gastrointestinal tract.
Testosterone—
  Matrix-type transdermal system: The patch must be applied to scrotal skin (5 to 30 times more permeable to testosterone than other skin sites) to produce an adequate testosterone serum concentration. A matrix transdermal system will not produce adequate serum testosterone concentrations if applied to nonscrotal skin. Serum testosterone concentrations reach a plateau at 3 to 4 weeks and, although testosterone is absorbed throughout a 24-hour period, concentrations do not simulate the circadian rhythm of endogenous testosterone in normal males. Interpatient variation in total plasma testosterone concentrations is high, approximately 35 to 49%; the average variation of concentration in a patient is approximately 30 to 41%.
  Reservoir-type transdermal system: Patients should avoid applying the reservoir-type patch to scrotal skin. The reservoir transdermal systems have similar sites of application, but manufacturers, depending on their clinical studies, recommend different sites and times for patch application. Since the reservoir patches show differences in time to peak effect, applying them either in the morning or at night, depending on the reservoir transdermal system and manufacturer instructions, achieves normal serum testosterone concentrations of circadian rhythm, peaking in the morning and decreasing throughout the rest of the day to plateau at night. Normal serum testosterone concentrations are reached during the first day of dosing, and drug accumulation does not occur with repeated applications. Intrapatient variation in total plasma testosterone concentrations is approximately 17%.
    For *Androderm*—Using two transdermal systems that deliver 2.5 mg of testosterone per day each, hypogonadal men absorb 4 to 5 mg of testosterone in 24 hours, and, if the patches are applied at 10 p.m. to the abdomen, back, thighs, or upper arms, concentrations simulate the circadian rhythm of endogenous testosterone in normal males. Similar results are expected with use of a single 5-mg patch. Hypogonadal men applying the patch to the chest or shin absorb 3 to 4 mg of testosterone in 24 hours.
    For *Testoderm TTS*—Studies of the three application sites (upper buttocks, arm, and back) showed that when a 5-mg patch was applied at 8 a.m., testosterone concentrations simulated the circadian rhythm of endogenous testosterone in normal males.
  Subcutaneous implant: Approximately one third of the testosterone dose is absorbed in the first month, one fourth in the second month, and one sixth in the third month. Absorption continues until the implant completely dissolves, which may take up to 6 months.

**Protein binding**
Testosterone—Very high (approximately 99%; 80% to sex hormone–binding globulin [SHBG], 19% to albumin, and 1% free). The metabolite DHT has greater affinity for SHBG than does testosterone.

**Biotransformation**
Hepatic.
Fluoxymesterone; methyltestosterone—Presence of 17-alpha alkyl group reduces susceptibility to hepatic enzyme degradation, which slows metabolism and allows oral administration.
Testosterone—Free testosterone is further converted into two of the major active metabolites, DHT and estradiol. Orally administered testosterone, but not testosterone undecanoate, undergoes nearly complete first-pass metabolism; both intramuscular and transdermal administration avoid first-pass metabolism.
  Oral: In first-pass metabolism, 90% of the oral testosterone dose is metabolized primarily to etiocholanolone, androsterone, and androstanediol, which are then conjugated. Unlike oral testosterone, oral testosterone undecanoate does not undergo hepatic first-pass metabolism.
  Injection: Testosterone esters (cypionate, enanthate, propionate) first undergo hydrolysis of the ester to the active form, free testosterone.
  Matrix-type transdermal systems: A threefold increase in DHT serum concentrations has been reported with the matrix-type testosterone

transdermal system applied to scrotal skin due to high conversion to DHT by 5-alpha-reductase in the scrotal tissue. Normal ranges of estradiol concentrations are produced; however, 3 of 72 male patients using the matrix patch experienced sporadic elevations of serum estradiol concentrations that were not associated with feminizing adverse effects.

Reservoir-type transdermal systems: The reservoir-type patch applied to nonscrotal skin produced normal DHT and estradiol serum concentrations.

## Half-life
The activity of testosterone in many tissues appears to be dependent on its reduction to DHT and the binding capacity of sex hormone–binding globulin (high in prepubertal children, declining through puberty and adulthood, and increasing again later in life).
Fluoxymesterone—Approximately 9.2 hours.
Methyltestosterone—2.5 to 3.5 hours.
Testosterone (intramuscular injection and matrix-type and reservoir-type transdermal systems)—10 to 100 minutes (plasma).
Testosterone cypionate (intramuscular)—Approximately 8 days.

## Time to peak concentration
Methyltestosterone—
  Tablets: 2 hours.
Testosterone undecanoate—
  Capsules: 4 to 5 hours.
Testosterone—
  Matrix-type transdermal systems: At steady state, approximately 2 to 4 hours after application.
  Reservoir-type transdermal systems:
    For *Androderm*: Approximately 6 to 10 hours after application. When the reservoir-type transdermal system was applied to the back, peak serum testosterone concentrations were achieved 6 to 12 hours after the application.
    For *Testoderm TTS*: At steady state, approximately 4 hours after application.

## Peak serum concentration
For testosterone transdermal systems—
  For matrix-type:
    Testosterone, serum concentration—593 nanograms of testosterone per deciliter (nanograms/dL) (20.6 nanomoles per liter [nanomoles/L]), mean serum concentration. At steady state (up to 3 weeks), approximately 60% of 30 hypogonadal males in a study had maximum testosterone serum concentrations reaching higher than 500 nanograms/dL (17.3 nanomoles/L, ranging from 11.5 to 44.9 nanomoles/L).
    DHT, serum concentration—Mean serum concentrations were elevated for the matrix-type transdermal system (range, 134 to 162 nanograms/dL [5.2 to 6.3 nanomoles/L] compared with the normal range of 30 to 85 nanograms/dL [1.2 to 3.3 nanomoles/L]). One 6-year study of hypogonadal men using scrotal transdermal systems reported normal serum testosterone concentrations from 306 to 1031 nanograms/dL (10.6 and 35.8 nanomoles/L) with the elevated DHT serum concentrations remaining stable.
    Estrogen, serum concentration—Serum concentrations of estrogen in patch users were normal. However, sporadic elevations above the normal range occurred in 3 of 72 patients using the matrix patch, but were not associated with feminizing side effects.
  For reservoir-type: Unlike the matrix-type system, which is placed on the scrotum, the reservoir-type system showed an average DHT and estrogen serum concentrations comparable to that of normal men.
    Testosterone, serum concentrations—
      For *Androderm*, beginning with a mean serum testosterone baseline of 76 nanograms/dL (2.6 nanomoles/L):
        2.5 mg patch—424 nanograms/dL (14.7 nanomoles/L), average peak serum concentration ($C_{avg}$).
        5 mg patch—584 nanograms/dL (20.2 nanomoles/L), $C_{avg}$; in another study of hypogonadal men (unknown baseline), 753 ± 276 nanograms/dL (26.1 nanomoles/L), mean peak serum concentration ($C_{max}$).
        7.5 mg patch—766 nanograms/dL (26.6 nanomoles/L), $C_{avg}$.
      For *Testoderm TTS*, beginning with a mean serum testosterone baseline of 150 nanograms/dL (5.2 nanomoles/L): 5 mg patch—366 nanograms/dL (12.7 nanomoles/L), $C_{avg}$; 462 to 499 nanograms/dL (16 to 17.3 nanomoles/L), mean $C_{max}$.

## Duration of action
Testosterone—Dependent upon the ester, dosage form, and route of administration.
  Injection: Enanthate and cypionate esters are longer acting than propionate ester and base.
  Oral: Undecanoate ester action continues for about 10 hours.
  Subcutaneous implants: Three to 4 months, but may continue for 6 months.
  Transdermal systems (matrix-type and reservoir-type): At 22 hours after application, serum testosterone concentration gradually falls to 60 to 80% of the peak serum concentration. On removal of the systems, testosterone serum concentration declines to baseline within 2 hours.

## Elimination
Generally renal excretion of metabolites. Approximately 90% of the administered dose is excreted in the urine, primarily as glucuronide or sulfated conjugates of the metabolites. Some fecal excretion due to enterohepatic circulation.
Fluoxymesterone—Less than 5% is excreted in urine as free steroid and glucuronide conjugate over a 24-hour period after oral doses of 20 to 200 mg.
Testosterone—Approximately 6% of dose is excreted in the feces.
Testosterone undecanoate—Approximately 77 to 93% of an orally administered dose is excreted in the urine and feces within 3 to 4 days.

# Precautions to Consider

## Carcinogenicity/Tumorigenicity
Hepatic neoplasms have been associated with long-term, high-dose androgen therapy in humans; some cases were irreversible after androgen withdrawal. This effect is more likely with oral methylated androgens.
It has been suggested that some strains of female mice injected with testosterone are at greater risk of hepatoma. When liver tumors were chemically induced in rats, testosterone increased the number of tumors and decreased tumor cell differentiation.
For testosterone—Studies in female mice given subcutaneous implants of testosterone showed an increase in cervical-uterine tumors. Some of these tumors metastasized. This effect was not seen in mice and rats given subcutaneous injections of testosterone or in rats given subcutaneous implants.

## Pregnancy/Reproduction
Fertility—In males, oligospermia, azoospermia, or reduced sperm function or ejaculatory volume resulting in possible infertility may occur during high-dose therapy with androgens if spermatogenesis is suppressed by a negative feedback mechanism. In females treated with androgens, amenorrhea may result, impairing fertility. In both females and males, fertility usually returns following cessation of therapy in females and dosage reduction or discontinuation in males.

Pregnancy—Androgens are contraindicated during pregnancy. Studies in humans have shown that androgens cause masculinization of the external genitalia of the female fetus, including clitoromegaly, abnormal vaginal development, and fusion of genital folds to form a scrotal-like structure. The degree of masculinization is dose-related.

FDA Pregnancy Category X.

## Breast-feeding
It is not known whether androgens are distributed into breast milk. Problems in humans have not been documented. However, androgens are rarely used by breast-feeding women and are not recommended. Potential adverse effects in infants include precocious sexual development in males and virilization of external genitalia in females.

## Pediatrics
Androgens should be used with caution in children and adolescents who are still growing because of possible premature epiphyseal closure in males and females, precocious sexual development in prepubertal males, or virilization in females. Skeletal maturation should be monitored at 6-month intervals by an x-ray of the hand and wrist. None of the *Testoderm* products have been evaluated in children up to 18 years of age. *Androderm* has not been evaluated in children up to 15 years of age.

## Geriatrics
Treatment of male patients 50 years of age and older with androgens should be preceded by a thorough examination of the prostate and baseline measurement of prostate-specific antigen serum concentration, since androgens may increase the risk of hyperplasia or may stimulate the growth of occult prostatic carcinoma. Periodic evaluation of prostate function also should be performed during the course of therapy.
For the testosterone transdermal system (reservoir-type)—No age-related differences in men up to 65 years of age were seen in clinical trials; however, absorption was 20% lower when the *Androderm* transdermal

system was applied to the backs of men between 66 and 79 years of age.

**Drug interactions and/or related problems**
The following drug interactions and/or related problems have been selected on the basis of their potential clinical significance (possible mechanism in parentheses where appropriate)—not necessarily inclusive (» = major clinical significance):

Note: Combinations containing any of the following medications, depending on the amount present, may also interact with this medication.

» Anticoagulants, coumarin- or indandione-derivative
(anticoagulant effect may be increased because of decreased procoagulant factor concentration caused by alteration of procoagulant factor synthesis or catabolism and increased receptor affinity for the anticoagulant; anticoagulant dosage adjustment may be required during and following concurrent use)

Antidiabetic agents, sulfonylurea or
Insulin
(androgens may increase or decrease blood glucose; doses of insulin or antidiabetic sulfonylurea medications may need to be adjusted, especially if hypoglycemia occurs)

Corticosteroids or
Corticotropin
(testosterone may contribute to the edema that can occur with administration of corticotropin or corticosteroids; caution is recommended during concomitant administration in patients who have special risks, such as patients who have cardiac or hepatic disease)

Cyclosporine
(methyltestosterone has been reported to increase plasma concentrations of cyclosporine and may increase the risk of nephrotoxicity; other androgens may have the same effect)

» Hepatotoxic medications, other (see *Appendix II*)
(may result in an increased incidence of hepatotoxicity; patients should be carefully monitored, especially those undergoing long-term therapy or those with a history of liver disease)

Human growth hormone (somatrem or somatropin)
(use of excessive doses of androgens in prepubertal males may accelerate epiphyseal maturation, although supplemental use of androgens may be necessary in patients with androgen deficiency to continue the growth response to human growth hormone)

Propranolol
(testosterone cypionate increases the clearance of propranolol; appropriate patient monitoring may be needed)

**Laboratory value alterations**
The following have been selected on the basis of their potential clinical significance (possible effect in parentheses where appropriate)—not necessarily inclusive (» = major clinical significance):

With diagnostic test results
Fasting blood sugar (FBS) and
Glucose tolerance test
(may be altered)

With physiology/laboratory test values
Alkaline phosphatase
(value may be increased)
Aspartate aminotransferase (AST [SGOT]), serum and
Calcium, chloride, inorganic phosphates, potassium, and sodium, serum and
17-Ketosteroid (17-KS), urine
(concentrations may be increased)
Bilirubin
(serum concentrations may be increased)
Clotting factors II, V, VII, and X
(may be suppressed)
Corticosteroid-binding globulin
(concentration may be decreased; free hormone concentration remains unchanged)
Creatinine
(serum concentrations may be increased; effect usually lasts up to 2 weeks after discontinuation of therapy)
Follicle-stimulating hormone (FSH) and
Luteinizing hormone (LH)
(serum concentrations may decrease)
(in one small study that used the testosterone transdermal system [reservoir-type], the LH and FSH serum concentrations decreased to normal within 6 to 12 months for 48% of the males with hypergonadotropic hypogonadism. For some men, the LH concentration may continue to be high despite normal testosterone concentrations)

Glucose
(blood concentrations may be increased or decreased, especially with pharmacologic doses or oral formulations; physiologic doses of androgens rarely cause hypoglycemia or hyperglycemia)

Hamster ova penetration test (HOPT) and
Spermatozoa count
(may be severely reduced at high doses)

Hematocrit and
Hemoglobin
(values may be increased with high-dose or long-term therapy)

High density lipoproteins (HDL)
(serum concentrations may be decreased, especially with pharmacologic doses and oral formulations)

Low density lipoproteins (LDL)
(serum concentrations may be increased, especially with pharmacologic doses and oral formulations; one study showed a slight reduction with testosterone)

Sex steroid–binding globulin
(concentration may be decreased; free hormone concentration remains unchanged)

Thyroxine-binding globulin
(may be decreased, resulting in decreased total $T_4$ serum concentrations and increased resin uptake of $T_3$ and $T_4$; free thyroid hormone levels remain unchanged, showing no clinical evidence of thyroid impairment)

**Medical considerations/Contraindications**
The medical considerations/contraindications included have been selected on the basis of their potential clinical significance (reasons given in parentheses where appropriate)—not necessarily inclusive (» = major clinical significance).

*Except under special circumstances, these medications should not be used when the following medical problems exist:*

» Breast cancer in males or
» Prostate cancer, known or suspected
(tumor growth may be promoted)

*Risk-benefit should be considered when the following medical problems exist:*

» Cardiac failure or
Cardiac function impairment or
» Cardiorenal disease, severe or
Edema or
Hepatic function impairment or
» Nephritis or
» Nephrosis or
Renal function impairment
(may cause fluid retention, resulting in edema with or without congestive heart failure; diuretics may be required before and during therapy)

Coronary artery disease or
» Myocardial infarction, history of
(may be worsened, due to hypercholesterolemic effects of androgens)

Diabetes mellitus
(use of androgens may increase or decrease blood glucose and produce an unfavorable profile of lipoprotein metabolism in patients without diabetes mellitus; a more exaggerated response can be expected in patients with diabetes mellitus, especially in obese patients. Effects may be greater for oral formulations or when pharmacologic doses of androgens are used. Doses of insulin or antidiabetic sulfonylurea medications may need to be adjusted, especially if hypoglycemia occurs. Physiologic doses of androgens rarely cause hypoglycemia or hyperglycemia)

» Hepatic function impairment
(biotransformation of androgens may be impaired, resulting in increased elimination half-life and increase in the incidence of gynecomastia)

» Hypercalcemia, due to metastatic breast cancer
(may be exacerbated)

» Prostatic hyperplasia, benign with urethral obstructive symptoms
(further enlargement may occur)

Sensitivity to anabolic steroids or androgens

**Patient monitoring**
The following may be especially important in patient monitoring (other tests may be warranted in some patients, depending on condition; » = major clinical significance):

Bone age determinations
(x-rays of hand and wrist are recommended every 6 months for children and growing adolescents to determine rate of bone maturation and effects on epiphyseal centers)

Cholesterol and/or
High density lipoproteins and
Low density lipoproteins
(serum profile determinations are recommended prior to initiation of therapy and, in some patients, at regular intervals during therapy)

Dihydrotestosterone, serum or
Testosterone, total, serum
(concentrations may be determined to ensure proper dosing; when done for *Testoderm* products, measurements are recommended after the patch has been used for 3 to 4 weeks and should be performed 2 to 4 hours after patch application)

Hematocrit determinations and
Hemoglobin
(recommended at regular intervals in patients receiving prolonged therapy or high doses of androgens to check for possible erythrocytosis)

Hepatic function determinations
(recommended at regular intervals during therapy, especially with oral methylated androgens)

Prostate-specific antigen and
Prostatic acid phosphatase
(recommended at regular intervals during therapy)

*For treatment of breast carcinoma*
Alkaline phosphatase, serum values and
Physical examination and
X-rays of known or suspected metastases
(recommended at regular intervals during therapy to monitor objective evidence of tumor response)

Calcium
(measurement of serum concentrations recommended at regular intervals in women with disseminated breast carcinoma)

*For gender change androgen therapy*
» Luteinizing hormone
(measurement of serum concentrations is recommended every 6 months to monitor success of therapy)
» Alanine aminotransferase (ALT [SGPT])
(measurement of serum values is recommended every 6 months to monitor for adverse effects)

## Side/Adverse Effects

Note: The side effects of testosterone enanthate and testosterone cypionate cannot be quickly reversed by discontinuing medication due to the long durations of action of these medications.

Replacement doses of androgens return the prostate to normal size and function for hypogonadal males. Although there is no evidence that exogenous androgens can induce development of prostate carcinoma, long-term androgen therapy or normal prostate activity carries a theoretical risk of prostatic hyperplasia or growth of occult prostatic carcinoma.

Behavioral disturbances, including aggressive or violent behavior, have been reported with self-administered supraphysiologic doses in athletes.

The following side/adverse effects have been selected on the basis of their potential clinical significance (possible signs and symptoms in parentheses where appropriate)—not necessarily inclusive:

**Those indicating need for medical attention**
Incidence more frequent
*In females only*
**Amenorrhea or oligomenorrhea** (absence of or unusual menstrual periods); **virilism** (acne; decreased breast size; enlarged clitoris; hoarseness or deepening of voice; male pattern baldness; oily skin; unnatural and excessive hair growth)
Note: *Virilism* may occur with usual systemic doses, as well as with excessive doses of topical testosterone. Hoarseness or deepening of voice and enlarged clitoris may not be reversible even after the medication has been discontinued. Virilism has also been reported in the female sexual partner of a male patient during his treatment with topical testosterone. The reservoir-type of testosterone transdermal system has a protective film that makes testosterone transfer between sexual partners unlikely.

*In males only*
**Bladder irritability or urinary tract infection** (frequent urge to urinate)—may be asymptomatic; **blistering of skin, local; breast soreness; erythema or pruritus, local** (itching of skin under skin patch, mild to severe; redness of skin under patch or at implant insertion site, mild to severe); **gynecomastia** (enlargement of breasts); **penile erections, frequent or continuing** (penile erections lasting up to 4 hours); **priapism** (painful erections lasting longer than 4 hours)—sign of excessive dosage

Note: *Blistering of skin* occurred as a single incident on one skin site in many patients; in most cases, it occurred when the reservoir-type of testosterone transdermal system was applied to skin over a bony prominence. This effect is less likely if such areas are avoided. It should be treated like a burn.
Medication should be discontinued and the patient given immediate medical attention if *priapism* occurs. If tumescence is not reversed, interruption of blood flow may result in penile tissue ischemia and permanent tissue damage.

*In prepubertal males only*
**Virilism** (acne; enlargement of penis; frequent or continuing erections; early growth of pubic hair)

Incidence less frequent
*In females and males*
**Edema** (rapid weight gain; swelling of feet or lower legs); **erythrocytosis or secondary polycythemia** (dizziness; flushing or redness of skin; headache, frequent or continuing; unusual bleeding; unusual tiredness)—in severe cases using oral or injection dosage forms; **gastrointestinal irritation** (nausea; vomiting); **headache; hepatic dysfunction, including cholestatic jaundice** (yellow eyes or skin; itching of skin)—more likely with the oral methylated androgens; **hypercalcemia** (confusion; constipation; increased thirst; mental depression; nausea; increased frequency of urination and quantity of urine; unusual tiredness; vomiting)—in females with breast cancer or immobilized patients

*In males only*
**Benign prostatic hyperplasia** (difficulty urinating); **burning sensation at transdermal application site**—incidence of 3%; **contact dermatitis, allergic** (itching and redness of skin, severe; skin rash, severe)—incidence of 4% with use of testosterone transdermal system (reservoir-type); **epididymitis, acute, nonspecific** (chills; pain in scrotum or groin); **induration, local** (hardening or thickening of skin under patch)—with use of testosterone transdermal system (reservoir-type); **pain at implant insertion site, continuing**—for subcutaneous implants

Incidence rare
*In females and males—more likely with oral or injection dosage forms, usually associated with long-term use or high doses*
**Hepatic necrosis** (abdominal or stomach pain, continuing; black, tarry stools; headache, continuing; malaise, continuing; unpleasant breath odor, continuing; vomiting of blood); **hepatocellular tumor** (pain or tenderness in upper abdomen; swelling of abdomen); **leukopenia** (fever; sore throat); **peliosis hepatis** (continuing loss of appetite; darkened urine; fever; hives; light-colored stools; nausea; purple or red spots on body or inside the mouth or nose; sore throat; vomiting)

**Those indicating need for medical attention only if they continue or are bothersome**
Incidence less frequent
*In females and males*
**Acne, mild; decrease or increase in libido; diarrhea; increase in pubic hair growth; infection, pain, redness or other irritation at site of injection**—for intramuscular injection only; **stomach pain; trouble in sleeping**

*In males only*
**Infection, pain, redness, swelling, sores or other skin irritation, local**—for transdermal systems; **testicular atrophy** (decrease in testicle size)—usually associated with high doses for oral or injection dosage forms

## Patient Consultation

As an aid to patient consultation, refer to *Advice for the Patient, Androgens (Systemic)*.
In providing consultation, consider emphasizing the following selected information (» = major clinical significance):

**Before using this medication**
» Conditions affecting use, especially:
Sensitivity to androgens or anabolic steroids
Carcinogenicity—Hepatocellular carcinoma is associated with long-term, high-dose therapy
Tumorigenicity—Hepatic neoplasms are associated with long-term, high-dose therapy
Fertility—May be severely impaired in males
Pregnancy—Contraindicated for use during pregnancy because of possible masculinization of female fetus
Breast-feeding—Not recommended
Use in children—Cautious use due to effects on growth and sexual development (precocious sexual development in males, virilization in females)
Use in the elderly—Increased risk of prostatic hyperplasia or occult prostatic carcinoma; not applying *Androderm* to the back in men over 65 years of age due to poor absorption at that location
Other medications, especially anticoagulants (coumarin- or indandione-derivative) or hepatotoxic medications
Other medical problems, especially breast cancer (male), cardiac failure, cardiorenal disease (severe), hepatic function impairment, hypercalcemia due to breast cancer, myocardial infarction (history of), nephritis, nephrosis, prostate cancer (known or suspected), or prostatic hyperplasia

**Proper use of this medication**
» Importance of not taking or using more medication than the amount prescribed
Understanding difference between the two types of testosterone patches; reading patient directions carefully before using the patch
Taking fluoxymesterone and methyltestosterone with food to minimize possible stomach upset

*Proper administration of testosterone transdermal systems*
For the matrix-type transdermal system—Applying to dry, clean, and hairless skin of scrotum; may be removed and reapplied after bathing, swimming, showering, or sexual activity
For the reservoir-type transdermal system—Applying *Androderm* to abdomen, back, thighs, or upper arms; rotating site. Applying *Testoderm TTS* to back, arms, or upper buttocks. Not applying the patches to the scrotum, chest, shin, bony prominences, or areas subject to prolonged pressure when sleeping or sitting. For *Androderm*, men older than 65 years of age should avoid applying patch to their backs. Not removing for showering, bathing, swimming, or sexual activity

» Proper dosing
Missed dose: For injection or oral dosage forms—Taking or using as soon as possible; not taking or using if almost time for next dose; not doubling doses
For transdermal patches—If dose is missed or patch falls off after being worn for 12 hours and cannot be reapplied, not using a new patch, returning to regular dosing schedule; not doubling doses

» Proper storage

**Precautions while using this medication**
Regular visits to physician to check progress during therapy
Diabetics: May alter blood sugar concentrations at high doses; minimal effect at physiologic doses
For testosterone transdermal system (matrix-type)—Checking with doctor if female sexual partner develops mild virilization when male partner uses the scrotal patch

**Side/adverse effects**
*Signs of potential side effects, especially:*
In females only—Amenorrhea, oligomenorrhea, or virilism
In males only—Bladder irritability or urinary tract infection; blistering of skin, local; breast soreness; erythema or pruritus of skin, mild to moderate, local; gynecomastia; penile erections, frequent or continuing; priapism; benign prostatic hyperplasia; burning sensation at transdermal application site; contact dermatitis, allergic; epididymitis, acute, nonspecific; induration, local; pain at implant insertion site, continuing
In prepubertal males only—Virilism
In all patients—Edema, erythrocytosis or secondary polycythemia, gastrointestinal irritation, headache, hepatic dysfunction, hepatic necrosis, hepatocellular tumor, hypercalcemia (in patients with breast cancer or immobilized patients), leukopenia, or peliosis hepatis

# General Dosing Information

The dosage and duration of therapy depend on the patient's age, sex, diagnosis, and response to therapy, and the appearance of adverse effects.

It is usually preferable to begin treatment for anemia and carcinoma with full therapeutic doses and to adjust later to individual requirements.

**For treatment of delayed puberty**
The dosage used in delayed puberty generally is in the lower range of the usual adult dose for androgen replacement therapy and is given for a limited duration, usually 3 to 6 months. The chronologic and skeletal ages should be considered, both in determining the initial dose and in adjusting the dose. After 3 to 6 months of therapy, the medication should be discontinued for 1 to 3 months and x-rays taken to determine the effect on bone growth or maturation.

Various dosage regimens have been used to induce pubertal changes in hypogonadal males. Some physicians prescribe a lower dose initially, gradually increase the dose as puberty progresses, and follow with a maintenance dose, which may be decreased. Other physicians use high initial doses to induce puberty, then decrease to an adjusting maintenance dose as puberty progresses.

Transdermal systems have not been investigated for this use.

**For treatment of breast cancer**
To determine whether there will be an objective response to antineoplastic therapy, treatment should be continued for at least 3 months, during which time a response to therapy is usually apparent. Therapy should be discontinued if the disease becomes progressive again. If clinical circumstances allow for an observation period, the patient should be observed for a period of improvement known as rebound regression.

Women should be checked for signs of virilization during androgen therapy. Some effects, such as voice changes or clitoromegaly, may not be reversible. A decision should be made by the patient and physician as to how much virilization will be tolerated as a result of androgen therapy. Alternatively, the drug should be discontinued or the dosage reduced. If virilization is to be prevented, medication must be discontinued when signs of mild virilization appear and before the process becomes irreversible.

Women with metastatic breast cancer should be followed closely because androgen therapy occasionally accelerates the disease. A shorter-acting androgen is preferred over one with prolonged activity, especially during the early stages of androgen therapy.

**For testosterone injection dosage form**
The suspension dosage form is absorbed relatively slowly; therefore, frequent injections may cause overdosage.

Testosterone cypionate or testosterone enanthate should not be used interchangeably with testosterone propionate or testosterone base because of different durations of action.

The intramuscular injections should be administered deeply into the gluteal muscle or the deltoid muscle in larger men. Injections should not be administered intravenously.

**For testosterone implant dosage form**
Insertion of testosterone implants requires a 15-minute procedure using local anesthesia. The number of implants inserted can vary according to patient need, diagnosis, and tolerance of testosterone. A good way to establish a proper testosterone dose for the implant is to assess patient response to a short-acting injectable form of testosterone. A 25-mg dose of testosterone propionate per week is equivalent to two 75-mg implants that last for 3 months.

The preferred application site is the lower abdomen, 5 cm away from the umbilicus; other sites used include the deltoid and gluteal muscles, and upper thigh. The clinician inserts and releases each implant into separate fan-like tracks using a trocar that is inserted into the 1-cm incision.

Afterwards, the patient should feel only minor discomfort and can apply pressure to stop minor bleeding at the incision site. Use of steri-strips covered by a water-resistant dressing for one week adequately closes and protects the incision without sutures. Postsurgical use of antibiotics is not needed.

The crystallized testosterone implants dissolve subcutaneously and rarely require removal. If needed, minor surgery to remove implants can rapidly terminate the effect of the medication.

**For testosterone transdermal system dosage forms**
There is a potential for transfer of testosterone from the matrix-type or scrotal transdermal system to the female sexual partner, resulting in mild virilization, such as changes in body hair distribution and increase in acne. The reservoir-type transdermal system includes a protective liner that makes transfer to a sexual partner unlikely.

The matrix-type transdermal system should be applied to clean, dry, and dry-shaved scrotal skin for optimal skin contact. Chemical depilatories should not be used.

The reservoir-type transdermal system should not be applied to scrotal skin. Instead, the abdomen, back, thighs, and upper arms are the optimal areas for application for *Androderm* and the arm, back, or upper buttocks for *Testoderm TTS*. Application areas for *Androderm* should be rotated, and a site should not be reused for 7 days. A patch added to or removed from the treatment regimen can change the testosterone concentrations by 27 to 37%. In addition, a 20% decrease in serum testosterone concentration was demonstrated in men over 65 years of age who applied *Androderm* to their backs.

**For treatment of adverse effects**
For all androgens
  For prolonged erection or priapism:
    A prolonged erection should be treated if it persists for longer than 4 hours; priapism should be treated promptly. If tumescence is not reversed, interruption of blood flow may result in penile tissue ischemia and permanent tissue damage.
    Treatment of adverse effects should be initiated by a physician trained in treating drug-induced tumescence. Depending on the severity, treatment may include:
    • Application of ice packs to inner thigh, alternating between thighs, for no more than 10 minutes to shorten the time of a prolonged erection.
    • Aspiration of intracavernosal blood.
    • Intracavernosal administration of an alpha-adrenergic agonist; phenylephrine is preferred over epinephrine. While monitoring blood pressure, an injection of 0.5 mg/mL Phenylephrine Hydrochloride Injection USP is given, followed by a second dose, if needed, in 15 minutes.
    • Irrigation of the corpus cavernosum with 0.9% Sodium Chloride Irrigation USP or 20 mL of dilute solutions of phenylephrine (20 mg Phenylephrine Hydrochloride Injection USP in 500 mL of 0.9% Sodium Chloride Irrigation USP) or epinephrine (1 mL 1:1000 Epinephrine Injection USP in 1 liter of 0.9% Sodium Chloride Irrigation USP) using a 19-gauge needle to remove clotted blood.
    • Surgery (rarely needed).
For testosterone transdermal system (reservoir-type)—
  For chemical-induced blistering—Symptomatic relief can be provided by administering a corticosteroid cream to relieve mild skin irritation underneath the patch. If burn-like blisters appear under the patch, use of patch should be discontinued and treatment of skin area should follow standard guidelines for treatment of burns.

---

## FLUOXYMESTERONE

## Summary of Differences
Indications: Also used as an antianemic.
Side/adverse effects: Methylated androgens are more likely to cause jaundice.

## Oral Dosage Forms
Note: Bracketed uses in the *Dosage Forms* section refer to categories of use and/or indications that are not included in U.S. product labeling.

### FLUOXYMESTERONE TABLETS USP
**Usual adult dose**
Androgen deficiency, due to primary or secondary hypogonadism—
  Oral, 5 mg one to four times a day. Replacement therapy is usually started at 10 mg per day, with subsequent adjustments as necessary.
Breast cancer in females—
  Oral, 10 to 40 mg per day in divided doses.
[Antianemic]¹—
  Oral, 20 to 50 mg per day, for minimum trial of two to six months.

**Usual pediatric dose**
Delayed puberty in males—
  Oral, 2.5 to 10 mg per day titrated to the lowest dose and to skeletal monitoring for a limited duration, usually four to six months.

**Strength(s) usually available**
U.S.—
  2 mg (Rx) [*Halotestin* (scored; lactose; sucrose; tartrazine)].
  5 mg (Rx) [*Halotestin* (scored; lactose; sucrose; tartrazine)].
  10 mg (Rx) [*Android-F* (scored); *Halotestin* (scored; lactose; sucrose; tartrazine); GENERIC (scored; may contain lactose and tartrazine)].
Canada—
  5 mg (Rx) [*Halotestin* (scored; tartrazine)].

**Packaging and storage**
Store below 40 °C (104 °F), preferably between 15 and 30 °C (59 and 86 °F), unless otherwise specified by manufacturer. Store in a well-closed container. Protect from light.

**Auxiliary labeling**
• Take with food.

¹Not included in Canadian product labeling.

---

## METHYLTESTOSTERONE

## Summary of Differences
Side/adverse effects: Methylated androgens are more likely to cause jaundice.

## Oral Dosage Forms
### METHYLTESTOSTERONE CAPSULES USP
**Usual adult dose**
Androgen deficiency, due to primary or secondary hypogonadism—
  Oral, 10 to 50 mg per day.
Breast cancer in females—
  Oral, 50 mg one to four times a day. After two to four weeks, dose may be decreased to 50 mg two times a day if response occurs.

**Usual pediatric dose**
Delayed puberty in males—
  Oral, 5 to 25 mg per day for a limited duration, usually four to six months.

**Strength(s) usually available**
U.S.—
  10 mg (Rx) [*Android; Testred; Virilon*].
Canada—
  Not commercially available.

**Packaging and storage**
Store below 40 °C (104 °F), preferably between 15 and 30 °C (59 and 86 °F), unless otherwise specified by manufacturer. Store in a well-closed container.

**Auxiliary labeling**
• Take with food.

### METHYLTESTOSTERONE TABLETS (Oral) USP
**Usual adult dose**
Androgen deficiency, due to primary or secondary hypogonadism or
Breast cancer in females—
  See *Methyltestosterone Capsules USP*.

**Usual pediatric dose**
Delayed puberty in males—
  See *Methyltestosterone Capsules USP*.

**Strength(s) usually available**
U.S.—
  10 mg (Rx) [*Android; ORETON Methyl* (lactose); GENERIC].
  25 mg (Rx) [*Android;* GENERIC].
Canada—
  10 mg (Rx) [*Metandren* (scored; lactose)].
  25 mg (Rx) [*Metandren* (scored; lactose)].

**Packaging and storage**
Store below 40 °C (104 °F), preferably between 15 and 30 °C (59 and 86 °F), unless otherwise specified by manufacturer. Store in a well-closed container.

**Auxiliary labeling**
• Take with food.

---

## TESTOSTERONE

## Summary of Differences
Indications: Testosterone cypionate and testosterone enanthate are used as antianemics and in androgen replacement in impotence or for male climacteric symptoms. Testosterone cypionate and testosterone enanthate are also used for female-to-male gender change. Intramuscular testosterone and testosterone esters, and extemporaneously compounded testosterone propionate ointments are used in the treatment of microphallus. Extemporaneously compounded testosterone propionate ointments are used in the treatment of lichen sclerosus.
Side/adverse effects: Side effects of the enanthate and cypionate forms cannot be quickly reversed because of the long duration of action of medication form and can include hives, infection, pain, redness, or irritation at site of injection.

## Oral Dosage Forms

### TESTOSTERONE UNDECANOATE CAPSULES

**Usual adult dose**
Androgen deficiency, due to primary or secondary hypogonadism—
  Oral, 120 to 160 mg divided into two doses a day with meals for two to three weeks. The dose may be decreased to 40 to 120 mg a day in divided doses, as appropriate, with meals.

**Usual pediatric dose**
Androgen deficiency, due to primary or secondary hypogonadism—
  Use and dose have not been established.

**Strength(s) usually available**
U.S.—
  Not commercially available.
Canada—
  40 mg (Rx) [*Andriol*].

**Packaging and storage**
Before dispensing, store between 2 and 8 °C (36 and 46 °F). Protect from freezing. Store in a well-closed container. Protect from light.
After dispensing, store between 15 and 25 °C (59 and 77 °F). Protect from light.

**Stability**
After the bottle is opened, capsules retain their potency for 90 days.

**Auxiliary labeling**
• Take with food.
• Beyond use date.

## Parenteral Dosage Forms

Note:  Bracketed uses in the *Dosage Forms* section refer to categories of use and/or indications that are not included in U.S. product labeling.

### TESTOSTERONE INJECTABLE SUSPENSION USP

Note:  Formerly known as Sterile Testosterone Suspension USP.

**Usual adult dose**
Androgen deficiency, due to primary or secondary hypogonadism—
  Intramuscular, 25 to 50 mg two or three times a week.
Breast cancer in females—
  Intramuscular, 50 to 100 mg three times a week.

**Usual pediatric dose**
Delayed puberty in males—
  Intramuscular, 100 mg (maximum) per month for a limited duration, usually four to six months.

**Strength(s) usually available**
U.S.—
  25 mg per mL (Rx) [GENERIC (may contain thimerosal)].
  50 mg per mL (Rx) [*Testaqua* (thimerosal); GENERIC (may contain thimerosal)].
  100 mg per mL (Rx) [*Testamone 100* (thimerosal); *Testaqua* (thimerosal); GENERIC (may contain thimerosal)].
Canada—
  Not commercially available.

**Packaging and storage**
Store below 40 °C (104 °F), preferably between 15 and 30 °C (59 and 86 °F), unless otherwise specified by manufacturer. Protect from freezing.

**Auxiliary labeling**
• Shake well.

### TESTOSTERONE CYPIONATE INJECTION USP

**Usual adult dose**
Androgen deficiency, due to primary or secondary hypogonadism—
  Intramuscular, 50 to 400 mg every two to four weeks.
Breast cancer in females—
  Intramuscular, 200 to 400 mg every two to four weeks.
[Gender change][1]—
  Intramuscular, 200 mg every two weeks. Occasional patients may require a higher dose to cause cessation of menses.

**Usual pediatric dose**
Delayed puberty in males—
  Intramuscular, 100 mg (maximum) per month for a limited duration, usually four to six months.

**Strength(s) usually available**
U.S.—
  100 mg per mL (Rx) [*Andronate 100* (benzyl alcohol); *Depotest* (benzyl alcohol); *Depo-Testosterone* (benzyl alcohol 9.45 mg per mL; benzyl benzoate 0.1 mL per mL; cottonseed oil); GENERIC (may contain benzyl alcohol and benzyl benzoate)].
  200 mg per mL (Rx) [*Andronate 200* (benzyl alcohol; benzyl benzoate); *Depotest* (benzyl alcohol; benzyl benzoate); *Depo-Testosterone* (benzyl alcohol 9.45 mg per mL; benzyl benzoate 0.2 mL per mL; cottonseed oil); *T-Cypionate*; *Testred Cypionate 200* (benzyl alcohol 0.9%; benzyl benzoate 20%); *Virilon IM*; GENERIC (may contain benzyl alcohol and benzyl benzoate)].
Canada—
  100 mg per mL (Rx) [*Depo-Testosterone Cypionate* (benzyl alcohol; benzyl benzoate; cottonseed oil); *Scheinpharm Testone-Cyp* (benzyl alcohol; cottonseed oil)].

**Packaging and storage**
Store below 40 °C (104 °F), preferably between 15 and 30 °C (59 and 86 °F), unless otherwise specified by manufacturer. Protect from light. Protect from freezing.

**Stability**
Crystals may form at low temperatures; warming and shaking the vial will redissolve any crystals.
Use of a wet needle or wet syringe may cause solution to cloud; however, potency of the medication will not be affected.

### TESTOSTERONE ENANTHATE INJECTION USP

**Usual adult dose**
Androgen deficiency, due to primary or secondary hypogonadism or
Breast cancer in females or
[Gender change][1]—
  See *Testosterone Cypionate Injection USP*.
[Antianemic][1]—
  Intramuscular, 400 mg a day for one week, then 400 mg one or two times a week. The maintenance dose is 200 to 400 mg every four weeks.

**Usual pediatric dose**
Delayed puberty in males—
  See *Testosterone Cypionate Injection USP*.
[Microphallus][1]—
  Intramuscular, 25 to 50 mg every month for 3 to 6 months.

**Strength(s) usually available**
U.S.—
  100 mg per mL (Rx) [*Delatest* (chlorobutanol); GENERIC (may contain benzyl alcohol)].
  200 mg per mL (Rx) [*Andro L.A. 200* (chlorobutanol 0.5%); *Andropository 200*; *Andryl 200* (chlorobutanol); *Delatestryl* (chlorobutanol 5 mg per mL); *Everone 200* (chlorobutanol); *Testrin-P.A* (chlorobutanol); GENERIC (may contain benzyl alcohol)].
Canada—
  200 mg per mL (Rx) [*Delatestryl* (chlorobutanol 0.5%)].

**Packaging and storage**
Store below 40 °C (104 °F), preferably between 15 and 30 °C (59 and 86 °F), unless otherwise specified by manufacturer. Protect from freezing.

**Stability**
Crystals may form at low temperatures; warming and shaking the vial will redissolve any crystals.
Use of a wet needle or wet syringe may cause solution to cloud; however, potency of the medication will not be affected.

### TESTOSTERONE PROPIONATE INJECTION USP

**Usual adult dose**
Androgen deficiency, due to primary or secondary hypogonadism or
Breast cancer in females—
  See *Testosterone Injectable Suspension USP*.

**Usual pediatric dose**
Delayed puberty in males—
  See *Testosterone Injectable Suspension USP*.

**Strength(s) usually available**
U.S.—
  100 mg per mL (Rx) [*Testex* (benzyl alcohol); GENERIC].
Canada—
  100 mg per mL (Rx) [*Malogen in Oil*].

**Packaging and storage**
Store below 40 °C (104 °F), preferably between 15 and 30 °C (59 and 86 °F), unless otherwise specified by manufacturer. Protect from freezing.

**Stability**
Crystals may form at low temperatures; warming and shaking the vial will redissolve any crystals.
Use of a wet needle or wet syringe may cause solution to cloud; however, potency of the medication will not be affected.

## Subcutaneous Dosage Forms

### TESTOSTERONE IMPLANTS

**Usual adult dose**
Androgen deficiency, due to primary or secondary hypogonadism—
   Subcutaneous, 150 to 450 mg every three to four months or, in some cases, as long as six months.

**Usual pediatric dose**
Puberty, delayed, male—
   Subcutaneous, dose to be determined by the physician. Low doses are used initially and increased gradually as puberty progresses.

**Strength(s) usually available**
U.S.—
   75 mg (Rx) [*Testopel Pellets*].
Canada—
   Not commercially available.

**Packaging and storage**
Store below 40 °C (104 °F), preferably between 15 and 30 °C (59 and 86 °F), unless otherwise specified by manufacturer.

## Topical Dosage Forms

Note: Bracketed uses in the *Dosage Forms* section refer to categories of use and/or indications that are not included in U.S. product labeling.

### TESTOSTERONE PROPIONATE OINTMENT

**Usual adult dose**
[Lichen sclerosus][1]—
   Initial, topical, to the vulva, as a 1 or 2% ointment, two times a day for six weeks or until relief of itching occurs. Dosage should be decreased to the minimum effective dose.

**Usual pediatric dose**
[Microphallus][1]—
   Topical, to the penis, as a 5% ointment, two times a day for three months.

**Strength(s) usually available**
U.S.—
   Not commercially available. Compounding required for prescription.
Canada—
   Not commercially available. Compounding required for prescription.

**Preparation of dosage form**
Formulations that have been used for the extemporaneous compounding of testosterone propionate ointments are as follows:
   For 15 grams of 2% testosterone propionate ointment—
   • 3 mL of 100-mg-per-mL testosterone propionate injection
   • 12 grams of white petrolatum.
   For 15 grams of 5% testosterone propionate ointment—
   • 7.5 mL of 100-mg-per-mL testosterone propionate injection
   • 7.5 grams of white petrolatum.

### TESTOSTERONE TRANSDERMAL SYSTEMS (Matrix-type)

**Usual adult dose**
Androgen deficiency, due to primary or secondary hypogonadism—
   Topical, one 6-mg transdermal dosage system (15 mg per sixty-centimeters-squared patch) applied to clean, dry and hairless skin of scrotum at approximately 8 a.m., every twenty-two to twenty-four hours. If scrotal area is inadequate, the smaller-sized 4-mg transdermal dosage system (10 mg per forty-centimeters-squared patch) should be used every twenty-two to twenty-four hours.

Note: Discontinue if desired response is not reached by six to eight weeks.

**Usual pediatric dose**
Children up to 18 years of age—Dosage has not been established.

**Strength(s) usually available**
U.S.—
   4 mg delivered per system per day (Rx) [*Testoderm*].
   6 mg delivered per system per day (Rx) [*Testoderm; Testoderm with Adhesives*].
Canada—
   Not commercially available.

**Packaging and storage**
Store between 15 and 30 °C (59 and 86 °F).

**Auxiliary labeling**
• For external use only.
• Apply patch to a clean, dry, hair-free area of the skin.

**Note**
The manufacturer's directions for the patient should be dispensed with the product.

Patients should be instructed to apply the patches to the scrotum.

### TESTOSTERONE TRANSDERMAL SYSTEMS (Reservoir-type)

**Usual adult dose**
Androgen deficiency, due to primary or secondary hypogonadism—
   Topical, 5 mg applied to clean, dry skin of the back, abdomen, upper arms, or thighs for *Androderm* at 10 p.m. and to the back, arms, or upper buttocks for *Testoderm TTS* at 8 a.m. every twenty-two to twenty-four hours. 2.5 mg may be used for nonvirilized patients or dose may be increased to 7.5 mg as appropriate.

Note: Patients should not apply the patches to the scrotum, bony prominences (deltoid region of the upper arm, the greater trochanter of the femur, and the ischial tuberosity), chest, or shin, or areas subject to prolonged pressure while sleeping or sitting.

**Usual pediatric dose**
Androgen deficiency, due to primary or secondary hypogonadism—
   For Androderm:
      Children up to 15 years of age—Use and dose have not been established.
      Children 15 years of age and older—See *Usual adult dose*.
   For Testoderm TTS:
      Children up to 18 years of age—Use and dose have not been established.

**Usual geriatric dose**
Androgen deficiency, due to primary or secondary hypogonadism—
   See *Usual adult dose*.

Note: Men over 65 years of age using *Androderm* should not apply the patch to their backs.

**Strength(s) usually available**
U.S.—
   2.5 mg delivered per system per day (Rx) [*Androderm*].
   5 mg delivered per system per day (Rx) [*Androderm; Testoderm TTS*].
Canada—
   Not commercially available.

**Packaging and storage**
For *Androderm*, store between 15 and 30 °C (59 and 86 °F). For *Testoderm TTS*, store below 25 °C (77 °F).

**Auxiliary labeling**
• For external use only.
• Apply patch to a clean, dry, hair-free area of the skin.

**Note**
The manufacturer's directions for the patient should be dispensed with the product.

[1] Not included in Canadian product labeling.

Revised: 06/24/98

# ANDROGENS AND ESTROGENS   Systemic

This monograph includes information on the following: 1) Diethylstilbestrol and Methyltestosterone; 2) Estrogens, Conjugated, and Methyltestosterone; 3) Estrogens, Esterified, and Methyltestosterone; 4) Fluoxymesterone and Ethinyl Estradiol; 5) Testosterone and Estradiol.

VA CLASSIFICATION (Primary/Secondary): HS950/GU900

NOTE: The *Androgens and Estrogens (Systemic)* monograph is maintained on the USP DI electronic data base. For a printed copy of the most recent revision of the complete monograph, contact Micromedex, Inc. - Reprint Requests, 6200 S. Syracuse Way, Suite 300, Englewood, CO 80111; telephone (303) 486-6400; telefax (303) 486-6464; Email: USPDI@MDX.COM.

For information on the specific components of this combination, see the *USP DI* monographs for *Androgens (Systemic)* and *Estrogens (Systemic)*.

The information that follows is selectively abstracted from the complete monograph and is provided to facilitate drug use review and patient counseling.

Note: For a listing of dosage forms and brand names by country availability, see *Dosage Forms* section(s).

## Category
Androgen-estrogen.

## Indications
**Unaccepted**
There is conflicting evidence and opinion as to whether the possible benefits of postmenopausal androgen pharmacologic or replacement therapy outweigh the risks of the frequently occurring virilizing side effects, adverse effects on serum cholesterol profile, or hepatotoxicity. Virilization may be somewhat reduced with the concomitant use of estrogens. However, because further data are needed regarding the efficacy of androgens in combination with estrogen and because side effects are frequent, the routine use of these products for any indication is not recommended.

## Patient Consultation
As an aid to patient consultation, refer to *Advice for the Patient, Androgens and Estrogens (Systemic)*.

In providing consultation, consider emphasizing the following selected information (» = major clinical significance):

**Before using this medication**
» Conditions affecting use, especially:
    Sensitivity to anabolic steroids, androgens, or estrogens
    Carcinogenicity/tumorigenicity—Hepatocellular carcinoma and neoplasms associated with long-term, high-dose androgen therapy; increased risk of endometrial cancer for patients with intact uteri when progestin is not used with estrogen; risk is decreased when a progestin is used with estrogen; continuous, long-term estrogen use in animal studies increased frequency of cancers of the breast, cervix, and liver
    Pregnancy—Androgens are not recommended for use during pregnancy, because of possible masculinization of female fetus; suggestion that use of some estrogens may be associated with congenital abnormalities
    Breast-feeding—Use is not recommended, because estrogens are distributed into breast milk and may have unpredictable effects; not known if androgens are distributed into breast milk; androgens could have adverse effects on the infant such as slowing or cessation of growth, precocious sexual development in males, or virilization in females
    Other medications, especially anticoagulants (coumarin- or indandione-derivatives), cyclosporine, or hepatotoxic medications
    Other medical problems, especially abnormal and undiagnosed vaginal bleeding; breast cancer; cardio-renal disease; cardiac failure; hepatic dysfunction or failure; history of myocardial infarction; nephrosis; nephritis; active thrombophlebitis or thromboembolic disorders

**Proper use of this medication**
    Reading patient package insert carefully
» Compliance with therapy
» Importance of not taking more medication than the amount prescribed
    Taking with or immediately after food to reduce nausea
» Proper dosing
    Missed dose: Taking as soon as possible; not taking if almost time for next dose; not doubling doses
» Proper storage

**Precautions while using this medication**
» Regular visits to physician at least every 6 to 12 months, or more often if so directed, to check progress
    Importance of mammography and regular self-breast examinations
    Possibility of dental problems, such as tenderness, swelling, or bleeding of gums; brushing and flossing teeth, massaging gums, and having dentist clean teeth regularly; checking with dentist if there are questions about care of teeth or gums or if tenderness, swelling, or bleeding of gums is noticed
    Diabetics: May alter blood glucose concentrations
» Stopping medication immediately and checking with physician if pregnancy is suspected
    Smoking while taking oral contraceptives containing estrogens can increase risk of cardiovascular side effects; not known whether elevated risk occurs with estrogen therapy
    Importance of not giving medication to anyone else

**Side/adverse effects**
    Withdrawal bleeding will occur in many postmenopausal patients placed on cyclic androgen and estrogen therapy with a progestin
    Signs of potential side effects, especially anaphylaxis, breast tumors, chorea, peripheral edema, erythrocytosis, gallbladder obstruction, hepatic necrosis, hepatitis, hepatocellular tumor, hepatic dysfunction, leukopenia, menstrual irregularities, peliosis hepatis, polycythemia, virilism

---
### DIETHYLSTILBESTROL AND METHYLTESTOSTERONE
---

## Oral Dosage Forms
### DIETHYLSTILBESTROL AND METHYLTESTOSTERONE TABLETS

**Usual adult dose**
Menopause, vasomotor symptoms of (treatment)—
    Initial dose: Oral, 250 mcg (0.25 mg) of diethylstilbestrol and 5 mg of methyltestosterone a day for twenty-one days, the dosage being repeated cyclically following seven days of no medication.
    Selected patients—Oral, 500 mcg (0.5 mg) of diethylstilbestrol and 10 mg of methyltestosterone a day for two weeks or less.
    Maintenance dosage: Oral, up to 125 mcg (0.125 mg) of diethylstilbestrol and 2.5 mg of methyltestosterone a day for twenty-one days, the dosage being repeated cyclically following seven days of no medication.

Note: To produce withdrawal bleeding, progesterone 5 mg per day may be given for the five days preceding the period of no medication of a cyclical schedule.

**Strength(s) usually available**
U.S.—
    250 mcg (0.25 mg) of diethylstilbestrol and 5 mg of methyltestosterone (Rx) [*Tylosterone* (scored; sucrose)].

---
### ESTROGENS, CONJUGATED, AND METHYLTESTOSTERONE
---

## Oral Dosage Forms
### CONJUGATED ESTROGENS AND METHYLTESTOSTERONE TABLETS

**Usual adult dose**
Menopause, vasomotor symptoms of (treatment)—
    Oral, 1.25 mg of conjugated estrogens and 10 mg of methyltestosterone a day for twenty-one days, the dosage being repeated cyclically following seven days of no medication.

**Strength(s) usually available**
U.S.—
    625 mcg (0.625 mg) of conjugated estrogens and 5 mg of methyltestosterone (Rx) [*Premarin with Methyltestosterone* (lactose; sucrose)].
    1.25 mg of conjugated estrogens and 10 mg of methyltestosterone (Rx) [*Premarin with Methyltestosterone* (lactose; sucrose)].
Canada—
    625 mcg (0.625 mg) of conjugated estrogens and 5 mg of methyltestosterone (Rx) [*Premarin with Methyltestosterone* (lactose; propylparaben; sucrose)].
    1.25 mg of conjugated estrogens and 10 mg of methyltestosterone (Rx) [*Premarin with Methyltestosterone* (lactose; sucrose; propylparaben)].

---
### ESTROGENS, ESTERIFIED, AND METHYLTESTOSTERONE
---

## Oral Dosage Forms
### ESTERIFIED ESTROGENS AND METHYLTESTOSTERONE TABLETS

**Usual adult dose**
Menopause, vasomotor symptoms of (treatment)—
    Oral, 625 mcg (0.625 mg) to 2.5 mg of esterified estrogens and 1.25 to 5 mg of methyltestosterone a day for twenty-one days, the dosage being repeated cyclically following seven days of no medication.

**Strength(s) usually available**
U.S.—
- 625 mcg (0.625 mg) of esterified estrogens and 1.25 mg of methyltestosterone (Rx) [*Estratest H.S* (lactose; methylparaben; propylparaben; sodium benzoate; sucrose)].
- 1.25 mg of esterified estrogens and 2.5 mg of methyltestosterone (Rx) [*Estratest* (lactose; methylparaben; propylparaben; sodium benzoate; sucrose)].

---

## *FLUOXYMESTERONE AND ETHINYL ESTRADIOL*

## Oral Dosage Forms

### FLUOXYMESTERONE AND ETHINYL ESTRADIOL TABLETS

**Usual adult dose**
Menopause, vasomotor symptoms of (treatment)—
  Oral, 1 to 2 mg of fluoxymesterone and 20 to 40 mcg (0.02 to 0.04 mg) ethinyl estradiol two times a day for twenty-one days, the dosage being repeated cyclically following seven days of no medication.

**Strength(s) usually available**
U.S.—
- 1 mg of fluoxymesterone and 20 mcg (0.02 mg) ethinyl estradiol (Rx) [*Halodrin* (scored; lactose; sucrose)].

---

## *TESTOSTERONE AND ESTRADIOL*

## Parenteral Dosage Forms

### TESTOSTERONE CYPIONATE AND ESTRADIOL CYPIONATE INJECTION

**Usual adult dose**
Menopause, vasomotor symptoms of (treatment)—
  Intramuscular, 50 mg of testosterone cypionate and 2 mg of estradiol cypionate every four weeks.

**Strength(s) usually available**
U.S.—
- 50 mg of testosterone cypionate and 2 mg of estradiol cypionate per mL (Rx) [*De-Comberol; depAndrogyn* (chlorobutanol; cottonseed oil); *Depo-Testadiol* (chlorobutanol anhydrous 5.4 mg per mL; cottonseed oil 874 mg per mL); *Depotestogen* (chlorobutanol; cottonseed oil); *Duo-Cyp* (chlorobutanol; cottonseed oil); *Duratestin* (chlorobutanol 0.5%; cottonseed oil); *Menoject-L.A* (chlorobutanol; cottonseed oil); *Tes Est Cyp* (chlorobutanol 0.5%; cottonseed oil); *Test-Estro Cypionate* (chlorobutanol; cottonseed oil); GENERIC].

**Additional information**
Medication should be injected deeply into the upper, outer quadrant of the gluteal muscle.

### TESTOSTERONE ENANTHATE AND ESTRADIOL VALERATE INJECTION

**Usual adult dose**
Menopause, vasomotor symptoms of (treatment)—
  Intramuscular, 90 mg of testosterone enanthate and 4 mg of estradiol valerate every four weeks.

**Strength(s) usually available**
U.S.—
- 90 mg of testosterone enanthate and 4 mg of estradiol valerate per mL (Rx) [*Andrest 90-4* (chlorobutanol 0.5%; sesame oil); *Andro-Estro 90-4* (chlorobutanol; sesame oil); *Androgyn L.A* (chlorobutanol 0.5%; sesame oil); *Deladumone* (chlorobutanol 5 mg per mL; sesame oil); *Delatestadiol* (chlorobutanol; sesame oil); *Duo-Gen L.A* (chlorobutanol; sesame oil); *Dura-Dumone 90/4* (chlorobutanol 0.5%; sesame oil); *OB* (chlorobutanol 0.5%; sesame oil); *Teev* (chlorobutanol; sesame oil); *Valertest No. 1* (chlorobutanol; sesame oil); GENERIC].
- 180 mg of testosterone enanthate and 8 mg of estradiol valerate per mL (Rx) [*Valertest No. 2* (benzyl alcohol; sesame oil); GENERIC].

Canada—
- 90 mg of testosterone enanthate and 4 mg of estradiol valerate per mL (Rx) [*Duogex L.A* (benzyl alcohol 2%)].
- 100 mg of testosterone enanthate and 6.5 mg of estradiol valerate per mL (Rx) [*Neo-Pause* (benzyl alcohol 2%; chlorobutanol 0.5%; sesame oil)].

### TESTOSTERONE ENANTHATE BENZILIC ACID HYDRAZONE, ESTRADIOL DIENANTHATE, AND ESTRADIOL BENZOATE INJECTION

**Usual adult dose**
Menopause, vasomotor symptoms of (treatment) or
Osteoporosis, estrogen deficiency–induced (treatment)—
  Intramuscular, 150 mg of testosterone enanthate benzilic acid hydrazone, 7.5 mg of estradiol dienanthate, and 1 mg of estradiol benzoate every four to eight weeks or less frequently.

**Usual adult prescribing limits**
Intramuscular, 150 mg testosterone enanthate benzilic acid hydrazone, 7.5 mg of estradiol dienanthate, and 1 mg of estradiol benzoate every four weeks

**Strength(s) usually available**
U.S.—
  Not commercially available.
Canada—
- 150 mg of testosterone enanthate benzilic acid hydrazone (69 mg base), 7.5 mg of estradiol dienanthate, and 1 mg of estradiol benzoate per mL (Rx) [*Climacteron* (benzoate alcohol 7.5%; benzyl benzoate)].

Revised: 06/30/92
Interim revision: 06/21/94

---

# ANESTHETICS  Mucosal-Local

This monograph includes information on the following: 1) Benzocaine; 2) Benzocaine, Butamben, and Tetracaine; 3) Dibucaine; 4) Dyclonine; 5) Lidocaine; 6) Pramoxine; 7) Tetracaine

Note: See also individual *Cocaine (Mucosal-Local)* monograph.

INN:
  Dibucaine—Cinchocaine
  Pramoxine—Pramocaine

BAN:
  Dibucaine—Cinchocaine
  Dyclonine—Dyclocaine
  Lidocaine—Lignocaine
  Tetracaine—Amethocaine

JAN:
  Benzocaine—Ethyl aminobenzoate

VA CLASSIFICATION (Primary/Secondary):

Note: Several of the dosage forms listed below are commercially available in more than one formulation. Because the vehicle into which a local anesthetic is incorporated may determine the appropriate usage and/or site(s) of application for a product, some of the VA classifications listed for a dosage form may apply only to specific formulations.

Benzocaine
  Dental paste—OR600
  Gel—NT300/GU900; OR600; RS900
  Lozenges—OR600
  Ointment—RS201/DE700; OR600; RS900
  Topical aerosol—DE700/NT300; OR600
  Topical solution—NT300/OR600
Benzocaine and Menthol
  Lozenges—OR600
Benzocaine and Phenol
  Gel—OR600
  Topical solution—OR600
Benzocaine, Butamben, and Tetracaine
  Gel—NT300/GU900; OR600; RS900
  Ointment—NT300/OR600
  Topical aerosol—NT300/OR600
  Topical solution—NT300/OR600
Dibucaine
  Ointment—RS201/DE700; RS900
Dyclonine
  Lozenges—OR600
  Topical solution—NT300/GU900; OR600; RS900

Lidocaine
    Ointment—NT300/DE700; OR600
    Oral topical solution—OR600
    Topical aerosol—NT300/OR600
Lidocaine Hydrochloride
    Jelly—NT300/GU900
    Oral topical solution—NT300/OR600
    Topical solution—NT300/OR600
    Topical spray solution—NT300
Pramoxine
    Aerosol foam—RS201/RS900
    Cream—RS201/DE700; RS900
    Ointment—RS201
Tetracaine
    Cream—RS201/DE700; RS900
    Topical aerosol—OR600
Tetracaine Hydrochloride
    Topical solution—NT300
Tetracaine and Menthol
    Ointment—RS201/DE700; RS900

Note: For information on local anesthetics applied topically to the skin to relieve minor dermatological conditions, see *Anesthetics (Topical)*.

For information on use of lidocaine hydrochloride by transtracheal injection to anesthetize the larynx and trachea, see *Anesthetics (Parenteral-Local)*.

Commonly used brand name(s): *Americaine*[1]; *Americaine Anesthetic Lubricant*[1]; *Americaine Hemorrhoidal*[1]; *Anbesol Baby Jel*[1]; *Anbesol Gel*[1]; *Anbesol Liquid*[1]; *Anbesol Maximum Strength Gel*[1]; *Anbesol Maximum Strength Liquid*[1]; *Anbesol Regular Strength Gel*[1]; *Anbesol Regular Strength Liquid*[1]; *Anbesol, Baby*[1]; *Anestacon Jelly*[5]; *Benzodent*[1]; *Cetacaine Topical Anesthetic*[2]; *Chloraseptic Lozenges*[1]; *Chloraseptic Lozenges Cherry Flavor*[1]; *Chloraseptic Lozenges, Children's*[1]; *Dent-Zel-Ite*[1]; *Dentapaine*[1]; *Dentocaine*[1]; *Dyclone*[4]; *Fleet Relief*[6]; *Hurricaine*[1]; *Num-Zit Gel*[1]; *Num-Zit Lotion*[1]; *Numzident*[1]; *Nupercainal*[3]; *Orabase, Baby*[1]; *Orabase-B with Benzocaine*[1]; *Orajel*[1]; *Orajel Extra Strength*[1]; *Orajel Liquid*[1]; *Orajel Maximum Strength*[1]; *Orajel Nighttime Formula, Baby*[1]; *Orajel, Baby*[1]; *Oratect Gel*[1]; *Pontocaine*[7]; *Pontocaine Cream*[7]; *Pontocaine Ointment*[7]; *ProctoFoam/non-steroid*[6]; *Rid-A-Pain*[1]; *SensoGARD Canker Sore Relief*[1]; *Spec-T Sore Throat Anesthetic*[1]; *Sucrets Maximum Strength*[4]; *Sucrets Regular Strength*[4]; *Sucrets, Children's*[4]; *Supracaine*[7]; *Topicaine*[1]; *Tronolane*[6]; *Tronothane*[6]; *Xylocaine*[5]; *Xylocaine Dental Ointment*[5]; *Xylocaine Endotracheal*[5]; *Xylocaine Viscous*[5]; *Zilactin-L*[5].

Some other commonly used names are:
    Amethocaine [Tetracaine]
    Butyl aminobenzoate [Butamben]
    Cinchocaine [Dibucaine]
    Dyclocaine [Dyclonine]
    Ethyl aminobenzoate [Benzocaine]
    Lignocaine [Lidocaine]
    Pramocaine [Pramoxine]

Note: For a listing of dosage forms and brand names by country availability, see *Dosage Forms* section(s).

# Category
Anesthetic (mucosal-local).

# Indications

Note: Bracketed information in the *Indications* section refers to uses that are not included in U.S. product labeling.

Gel, ointment, and topical solution dosage forms of benzocaine, ointment and topical solution dosage forms of lidocaine, and topical solution dosage forms of lidocaine hydrochloride are available in more than one formulation. The vehicles present in different formulations may determine the indication(s) for which the formulations are used. Therefore, some gel, ointment, or topical solution formulations that contain the same local anesthetic cannot be used interchangeably. For additional information regarding formulations and brand name products that may be used for specific indications, see the *Dosage Forms* section.

**Accepted**

Anesthesia, local—Indicated to provide topical anesthesia of accessible mucous membranes prior to examination, endoscopy or instrumentation, or other procedures involving the
  Esophagus—Benzocaine (gel and topical solution); benzocaine, butamben, and tetracaine; dyclonine (topical solution); lidocaine hydrochloride (4% topical solution, topical spray solution, and [oral topical solution]); and tetracaine hydrochloride (topical solution).
  Larynx—Benzocaine (gel and topical solution); benzocaine, butamben, and tetracaine; dyclonine (topical solution); lidocaine hydrochloride (4% topical solution and topical spray solution); and tetracaine hydrochloride (topical solution).
  Mouth (in dental procedures and oral surgery)—Benzocaine (gel, topical aerosol, and topical solution); benzocaine, butamben, and tetracaine; dyclonine (topical solution); lidocaine (ointment, topical aerosol, and oral topical solution); lidocaine hydrochloride (oral topical solution and 4% topical solution); and tetracaine (topical aerosol).
  Nasal cavity—Benzocaine (gel); benzocaine, butamben, and tetracaine; lidocaine hydrochloride (jelly and 4% topical solution); and tetracaine (topical solution).
  Pharynx or throat—Benzocaine (gel, topical aerosol, and topical solution); benzocaine, butamben, and tetracaine; dyclonine (topical solution); lidocaine (ointment and topical aerosol); lidocaine hydrochloride (jelly, oral topical solution, and topical spray solution); and tetracaine (topical solution).
  Rectum—Benzocaine (gel); benzocaine, butamben, and tetracaine (gel); and lidocaine hydrochloride (jelly).
  Respiratory tract or trachea—Benzocaine (gel, topical aerosol, and topical solution); benzocaine, butamben, and tetracaine; dyclonine (topical solution); lidocaine (ointment); lidocaine hydrochloride (jelly, [oral topical solution], and 4% and 10% topical solution); and tetracaine (topical solution).
  Urinary tract—Benzocaine (gel); dyclonine (topical solution); and lidocaine hydrochloride (jelly).
  Vagina—Benzocaine (gel); benzocaine, butamben, and tetracaine (gel); and dyclonine (topical solution).

Gag reflex suppression—Indicated to suppress the gag reflex and/or other laryngeal and esophageal reflexes to facilitate dental examination or procedures (including oral surgery), endoscopy, or intubation: Benzocaine (gel, topical aerosol, and topical solution); benzocaine, butamben, and tetracaine (topical aerosol); dyclonine (0.5% topical solution);[lidocaine (topical aerosol)]; lidocaine hydrochloride (oral topical solution and 10% topical solution); tetracaine (topical aerosol); and tetracaine hydrochloride (topical solution).

Anorectal disorders (treatment)—Indicated for the symptomatic relief of Hemorrhoids
  Inflammation, anorectal and
  Pain, anorectal—Benzocaine (ointment); dibucaine; pramoxine; tetracaine hydrochloride (cream); and tetracaine and menthol. These medications are effective when applied to the anal, perianal, or anorectal areas. However, they are not likely to relieve symptoms associated with conditions confined to the rectum, which lacks sensory nerve fibers.
  Pain, anogenital lesion–associated—Dyclonine (0.5% solution).
  Pain, anogenital, external and
  Pruritus, anogenital—Benzocaine (ointment); dibucaine; pramoxine (aerosol foam and cream); tetracaine hydrochloride (cream); tetracaine and menthol.

Oral cavity disorders (treatment); and Perioral lesions (treatment)—Indicated for relief of
  Canker sores or
  Cold sores or
  Fever blisters—Benzocaine (gel and topical solution); benzocaine and phenol (gel and topical solution); and lidocaine (2.5% topical solution).
  Pain, gingival or oral mucosal (i.e., pain caused by mouth or gum irritation, inflammation, lesions, or minor dental procedures)—Benzocaine (gel, dental paste, lozenges, and topical solution); dyclonine (lozenges and 0.5% topical solution); benzocaine and phenol (gel and topical solution); lidocaine (oral topical solution); and lidocaine hydrochloride (oral topical solution).
  Pain, dental prosthetic (i.e., pain or irritation caused by dentures or other dental or orthodontic appliances)—Benzocaine (dental paste, gel, ointment, and topical solution); benzocaine and phenol (gel and topical solution); and lidocaine (ointment).
  Pain, teething—Benzocaine (7.5% and 10% gel).
  Toothache—Benzocaine (10% and 20% gel and topical solution); and benzocaine and phenol (gel and topical solution).

Pain, esophageal (treatment)—Dyclonine (topical solution); and [lidocaine hydrochloride (oral topical solution)].

Pain, pharyngeal (treatment)—Benzocaine (lozenges); benzocaine and menthol (lozenges); dyclonine (lozenges); and lidocaine hydrochloride (oral topical solution).

Pain, vaginal (treatment)—Indicated to relieve pain following procedures such as episiotomy or perineorraphy: Benzocaine (topical aerosol and topical solution); and dyclonine (topical solution).

Urethritis (treatment)—Indicated to relieve or control pain: Lidocaine hydrochloride (jelly).

## Pharmacology/Pharmacokinetics

### Physicochemical characteristics
Chemical group—
  Amides: Dibucaine, lidocaine.
  Esters, aminobenzoic acid (para-aminobenzoic acid, PABA)–derivative: Benzocaine, butamben, tetracaine.
  Unclassified: Dyclonine, pramoxine.
Molecular weight—
  Benzocaine: 165.19.
  Butamben: 193.25.
  Dibucaine: 343.47.
  Dyclonine hydrochloride: 325.88.
  Lidocaine: 234.34.
  Lidocaine hydrochloride: 288.82.
  Pramoxine hydrochloride: 329.87.
  Tetracaine: 264.37.
  Tetracaine hydrochloride: 300.83.
pKa—
  Dibucaine: 8.8.
  Lidocaine: 7.9.
  Tetracaine: 8.2.

### Mechanism of action/Effect
Local anesthetics block both the initiation and conduction of nerve impulses by decreasing the neuronal membrane's permeability to sodium ions. This reversibly stabilizes the membrane and inhibits depolarization, resulting in the failure of a propagated action potential and subsequent conduction blockade.

### Other actions/effects
If substantial quantities of local anesthetics are absorbed through the mucosa, actions on the central nervous system (CNS) may cause CNS stimulation and/or CNS depression. Actions on the cardiovascular system may cause depression of cardiac conduction and excitability and, with some of these agents, peripheral vasodilation.

### Absorption
Except for benzocaine, which is minimally absorbed, these agents are readily absorbed through mucous membranes into the systemic circulation. The rate of absorption is influenced by the vascularity or rate of blood flow at the site of application, the total dosage (concentration and volume) administered, and the duration of exposure. Absorption from mucous membranes of the throat or respiratory tract may be especially rapid. Addition of a vasoconstrictor to the anesthetic may not reduce or slow absorption sufficiently to protect against systemic effects.

### Protein binding
Lidocaine—Concentration-dependent, to alpha 1-acid glycoprotein; usually about 60 to 80% at concentrations of 1 to 4 mcg per mL (4.3 to 17.2 micromoles per L).

### Biotransformation
Amides—
  Hepatic and some renal.
  Lidocaine: Xylidide metabolites are active and toxic, but less so than the parent compound.
Esters (PABA-derivative)—
  Hydrolyzed by plasma cholinesterases and, to a much lesser extent, by hepatic cholinesterases to PABA-containing metabolites.

### Onset of action
Benzocaine—About 1 minute.
Benzocaine, butamben, and tetracaine—About 30 seconds.
Dibucaine—Up to 15 minutes.
Dyclonine—Up to 10 minutes.
Lidocaine—Within 1 to 5 minutes, depending on formulation.
Pramoxine—3 to 5 minutes.
Tetracaine—3 to 10 minutes.

### Duration of action
Benzocaine—
  15 to 20 minutes.
Dibucaine—
  2 to 4 hours.
Dyclonine—
  Approximately 30 to 60 minutes.
Lidocaine—
  Approximately 30 to 60 minutes.
  Lidocaine oral topical solution: 15 to 20 minutes.
  Lidocaine topical aerosol: 10 to 15 minutes.
Tetracaine—
  Approximately 30 to 60 minutes.

### Elimination
Amides—
  Renal, primarily as metabolites.
  Lidocaine: Up to 10% of a dose may be excreted unchanged.
Esters—
  Renal, primarily as metabolites.

## Precautions to Consider

### Cross-sensitivity and/or related problems
Patients sensitive to one ester derivative (especially an aminobenzoic acid [para-aminobenzoic acid; PABA] derivative) may be sensitive to other ester derivatives also.
Patients sensitive to PABA, parabens, or paraphenylenediamine (a hair dye) may be sensitive to PABA-derivative local anesthetics also.
Patients sensitive to one amide derivative may rarely be sensitive to other amide derivatives also.
Cross-sensitivity between amide derivatives and ester derivatives, or between amides or esters and chemically unrelated local anesthetics (i.e., dyclonine or pramoxine), has not been reported. However, some lidocaine formulations and pramoxine cream contain parabens, to which cross-sensitivity with PABA-derivative local anesthetics may exist.

### Pregnancy/Reproduction
Fertility—
  *Dyclonine*—
    Studies have not been done.
  *Lidocaine*—
    Studies have not been done.
Pregnancy—
  *Benzocaine*—
    Studies in humans have not been done.
    Studies in animals have not been done.
    Benzocaine gel: FDA Pregnancy Category C.
  *Dyclonine*—
    Studies in humans have not been done.
    Studies in animals have not been done.
    Dyclonine topical solution: FDA Pregnancy Category C.
  *Lidocaine*—
    Adequate and well-controlled studies in humans have not been done.
    Studies in rats given up to 6.6 times the human dose have not shown evidence of teratogenicity or harm to the fetus.
    FDA Pregnancy Category B.
  *Other mucosal-local anesthetics*—
    Problems in humans have not been documented.

### Breast-feeding
*Lidocaine*—
  Distributed into breast milk in very small quantities that pose no risk to the infant.
*Other mucosal-local anesthetics*—
  Problems in humans have not been documented.

### Pediatrics
*Benzocaine*—
  Benzocaine should be used with caution in infants and young children because increased absorption may result in methemoglobinemia. Nonprescription teething products (i.e., 7.5% or 10% benzocaine gel) should not be used in infants younger than 4 months of age unless prescribed by a physician or dentist. Other nonprescription products that contain benzocaine for relief of dental pain, perioral lesions, or sore throat (e.g., gel, lozenges, ointment, or topical solution and combinations containing benzocaine with menthol or phenol) should not be used in children younger than 2 years of age unless prescribed by a physician or dentist.
*Other mucosal-local anesthetics*—
  Pediatric patients may be more susceptible to systemic toxicity with these medications. Nonprescription products that contain dyclonine or lidocaine for relief of sore throat or perioral lesions should not be used in children younger than 2 years of age unless prescribed by a physician or dentist. Dosage of other mucosal-local anesthetic formulations should be individualized, based on the child's age, weight, and physical condition.

### Geriatrics
Systemic toxicity may be more likely to occur in geriatric patients, who may require lower concentrations and/or lower total dosages of mucosal-local anesthetics, especially for endoscopic procedures.

**Drug interactions and/or related problems**
See also *Laboratory value alterations.*
The following drug interactions and/or related problems have been selected on the basis of their potential clinical significance (possible mechanism in parentheses where appropriate)—not necessarily inclusive (» = major clinical significance):

Note: Combinations containing any of the following medications, depending on the amount present, may also interact with this medication.

*For ester derivatives only*
Cholinesterase inhibitors
(metabolism of an ester-derivative local anesthetic may be inhibited, leading to increased risk of systemic toxicity, when it is administered to a patient receiving a cholinesterase inhibitor)
Sulfonamides
(metabolites of PABA-derivative local anesthetics may antagonize antibacterial activity of sulfonamides)

*For lidocaine only*
Antiarrhythmic agents, amide local anesthetic–derivative, other, such as:
  Mexiletine
  Tocainide or
  Lidocaine, systemic or parenteral-local
  (risk of cardiotoxicity associated with additive cardiac effects, and, with systemic or parenteral-local lidocaine, the risk of overdose, may be increased in patients receiving these medications when lidocaine is applied to the mucosa, especially if it is applied in large quantities, used repeatedly, used in the oral or pharyngeal area, or swallowed)
Beta-adrenergic blocking agents
(concurrent use may slow metabolism of lidocaine because of decreased hepatic blood flow, leading to increased risk of lidocaine toxicity, especially if lidocaine is applied to the mucosa in large quantities, used repeatedly, used in the oral or pharyngeal area, or swallowed)
Cimetidine
(cimetidine may inhibit hepatic metabolism of lidocaine, leading to increased risk of lidocaine toxicity, especially if lidocaine is applied to the mucosa in large quantities, used repeatedly, used in the oral or pharyngeal area, or swallowed)

**Laboratory value alterations**
The following have been selected on the basis of their potential clinical significance (possible effect in parentheses where appropriate)—not necessarily inclusive (» = major clinical significance):

With diagnostic test results
Cystoscopic procedures following pyelography
(dyclonine interferes with visualization by reacting with iodine-containing contrast agents, resulting in precipitation of iodine)
Pancreatic function determination using bentiromide
(administration of PABA-derivative anesthetics or lidocaine prior to the bentiromide test will invalidate test results [if the anesthetics are absorbed in sufficient quantity] since they are also metabolized to arylamines and will thus increase the apparent quantity of PABA recovered; discontinuation of these medications at least 3 days prior to the test is recommended)

**Medical considerations/Contraindications**
The medical considerations/contraindications included have been selected on the basis of their potential clinical significance (reasons given in parentheses where appropriate)—not necessarily inclusive (» = major clinical significance).

*Risk-benefit should be considered when the following medical problems exist:*
Hemorrhoids, bleeding—for rectal use
Local infection at area of treatment
(may alter pH at site of application, leading to decrease or loss of local anesthetic effect)
Sensitivity to the local anesthetic being considered for use and/or chemically related anesthetics or other compounds, history of
Traumatized mucosa, severe
(increased absorption of anesthetic, leading to increased risk of systemic toxicity)
Caution is also advised in pediatric, geriatric, acutely ill, or debilitated patients, who may be more susceptible to systemic toxicity with these medications.

## Side/Adverse Effects

Note: Adverse reactions are due to excessive dosage or rapid absorption, which produces high plasma concentrations, as well as to idiosyncrasy, hypersensitivity, or decreased patient tolerance.
Benzocaine and tetracaine are more likely to cause contact sensitization than are the other mucosal-local anesthetics. Also, tetracaine is more toxic than other mucosal-local anesthetics.

The following side/adverse effects have been selected on the basis of their potential clinical significance (possible signs and symptoms in parentheses where appropriate)—not necessarily inclusive:

**Those indicating need for medical attention**
Incidence less frequent
*Allergic contact dermatitis* (skin rash, redness, itching, or hives); *angioedema* (large, hive-like swellings on skin or in mouth or throat); *burning, stinging, swelling, or tenderness not present before therapy*
Incidence rare
*Urethritis* (blood in urine, increased frequency of urination, pain or burning during urination)—with urethral application

## Overdose

For specific information on the agents used in the management of an overdose, see:
• *Ascorbic Acid (Systemic)* monograph;
• *Benzodiazepines (Systemic)* monograph;
• *Methylene Blue (Systemic)* monograph; and/or
• *Sympathomimetic Agents—Cardiovascular Use (Parenteral-Systemic)* monograph.

For more information on the management of overdose or unintentional ingestion, **contact a Poison Control Center** (see *Poison Control Center Listing*).

**Clinical effects of overdose**
The following effects have been selected on the basis of their potential clinical significance (possible signs and symptoms in parentheses where appropriate)—not necessarily inclusive:

Acute and chronic effects
*Cardiovascular system depression* (increased sweating, low blood pressure, pale skin, slow or irregular heartbeat)—may lead to cardiac arrest; *CNS toxicity* (blurred or double vision; confusion; convulsions; dizziness or lightheadedness; drowsiness; feeling hot, cold, or numb; ringing or buzzing in ears; shivering or trembling; unusual anxiety, excitement, nervousness, or restlessness); *methemoglobinemia* (difficulty in breathing on exertion, dizziness, headache, tiredness, weakness)

Note: Stimulant and/or depressant manifestations of *CNS toxicity* may occur. CNS stimulation usually occurs first, followed by CNS depression. However, CNS stimulation may be transient or absent so that drowsiness may be the first symptom of toxicity in some patients. CNS depression may lead to unconsciousness and respiratory arrest.

**Treatment of overdose**
Specific treatment—
For circulatory depression—Administering a vasopressor and intravenous fluids.
For convulsions—Administering a benzodiazepine anticonvulsant, keeping in mind that intravenously administered benzodiazepines may cause respiratory and circulatory depression, especially when administered rapidly. Medications and equipment needed for support of respiration and for resuscitation must be immediately available.
For methemoglobinemia—Administering methylene blue (1 to 2 mg per kg of body weight, intravenously) and/or ascorbic acid (100 to 200 mg orally).
Supportive care—
Securing and maintaining a patent airway, administering 100% oxygen, and instituting assisted or controlled respiration as required. In some patients, endotracheal intubation may be required.

## Patient Consultation

As an aid to patient consultation, refer to *Advice for the Patient, Anesthetics (Dental)* and *Anesthetics (Rectal)*.
In providing consultation, consider emphasizing the following selected information (» = major clinical significance):

**Before using this medication**
» Conditions affecting use, especially:
Allergies to local anesthetics of the same chemical class, and, for ester derivatives only, aminobenzoic acid, parabens, or hair dye

## Anesthetics (Mucosal-Local)

Use in children—Caution recommended, especially with use of benzocaine or lidocaine in infants and young children
Use in the elderly—Increased risk of side effects

**Proper use of this medication**
Following physician's or dentist's instructions if prescribed
Following manufacturer's instructions if self-medicating
» Not using more, more often, or for a longer period of time than prescribed by physician or dentist or recommended on package label
» Checking with physician or dentist before using for problems other than those for which medication was prescribed or those stated on package label

*Proper administration technique*
*For lidocaine hydrochloride oral topical solution*
» Measuring dose accurately
Applying with cotton swab or swishing around in mouth (for mouth or gum conditions) or gargling (for throat conditions)
» Not swallowing unless specifically directed by physician or dentist
*For benzocaine film-forming gel*
Drying affected area with one of the swabs provided before applying
Applying gel to a second swab, then rolling the swab over the affected area
Keeping mouth open and dry for 30 to 60 seconds after applying, while film forms
Not removing film, which will slowly disintegrate over 6 hours
*For other nonprescription gel and solution dosage forms*
Applying to affected area(s) with a clean finger, a cotton-tipped applicator, or gauze
If using for pain caused by dental appliances, applying to sore area and, after relief is obtained, rinsing mouth before reinserting appliance; not applying directly to or using under appliance unless directed to do so by dentist
*For benzocaine dental paste*
Dabbing small amounts onto affected areas with cotton-tipped applicator; not rubbing or spreading, to prevent crumbling or grittiness
*For topical aerosol or spray dosage forms*
Using care not to inhale medication
Avoiding spraying back of throat or mouth unless specifically directed by physician or dentist
*For lozenges*
Dissolving slowly in mouth; not biting or chewing lozenges or swallowing them whole
*For rectal cream or ointment*
Reading patient directions
If applying externally: Cleansing area with mild soap and water or a cleansing wipe, rinsing thoroughly, and drying gently before applying
If inserting into anal canal: Using special applicator provided; lubricating applicator with a small amount of cream or ointment before inserting; washing reusable applicator after each use; discarding pre-filled disposable applicator
*For rectal aerosol foam*
Reading patient directions before use
Not inserting container into rectum; shaking container, attaching and filling the applicator provided, then detaching applicator from container prior to use
Applying a small amount of foam to lubricate the applicator before inserting
Taking applicator apart and washing thoroughly after each use
» Proper dosing
Missed dose (if prescribed for scheduled dosing)—Using as soon as possible; not using if almost time for next dose; not doubling doses of dental-local anesthetics
» Proper storage

**Precautions while using this medication**
» Contacting physician:
if using for sore throat and sore throat is severe, persists for more than 2 days, or is accompanied or followed by other symptoms such as fever, headache, rash, swelling, nausea, or vomiting
if using for hemorrhoids or other perianal conditions and condition does not improve within 7 days, bleeding occurs, or symptoms such as redness, irritation, swelling, or pain develop or worsen during treatment
» Contacting physician or dentist if using for perioral lesions and symptoms do not improve within 7 days, irritation or pain persists or worsens, or swelling, rash, or fever develops

» Contacting dentist:
as soon as possible to arrange an appointment if using to relieve toothache; medication is a temporary measure only
at regular intervals when medication used to relieve pain during adjustment of new dentures or other dental appliances
Not using benzocaine, lidocaine, or tetracaine for 72 hours prior to having pancreatic function test using bentiromide because of potential interference with test results

*For use in mouth or throat area*
» Not eating for one hour following use of medication because may impair swallowing, leading to risk of aspiration
» Not chewing gum or food while numbness persists because of risk of biting tongue or buccal mucosa

**Side/adverse effects**
Signs and symptoms of potential side effects, especially allergic contact dermatitis; angioedema; and burning, stinging, swelling, or tenderness not present before therapy

## General Dosing Information

The safety and effectiveness of local anesthetics, when they are used for examination or instrumentation procedures (especially those involving the esophagus, larynx, pharynx, respiratory tract, or urinary tract) depend upon proper dosage, correct administration technique, adequate precautions, and readiness for emergencies. *Resuscitative equipment, oxygen, and other required medications should be immediately available.*

The dosage of mucosal-local anesthetics, when they are used for examination or instrumentation procedures, depends on the technique of anesthesia, the area to be anesthetized, the vascularity of the tissues at the application site, and the patient's tolerance.

For use in examination or instrumentation procedures, the recommended adult doses are given as a guideline for use in the average adult. *The actual dosage and maximum dosage must be individualized,* based on the age, size, and physical status of the patient and the expected rate of systemic absorption from the administration site.

Depending on the area to be anesthetized, lower concentrations and/or lower total dosage may be required for pediatric, geriatric, acutely ill, or debilitated patients.

A standard textbook should be consulted for specific techniques and procedures applicable to the use of mucosal-local anesthetics for individual diagnostic and treatment procedures.

---
### BENZOCAINE
---

## Summary of Differences

Pharmacology/pharmacokinetics:
  Physicochemical characteristics—
    Benzocaine is a PABA derivative ester-type local anesthetic.
  Absorption—
    Minimally absorbed.
Precautions:
  Cross-sensitivity and/or related problems—
    May occur with other ester-type local anesthetics, especially other PABA derivatives, parabens, and paraphenylenediamine.
  Pediatrics—
    May cause methemoglobinemia in infants.
  Drug interactions and/or related problems—
    Cholinesterase inhibitors inhibit metabolism of benzocaine.
    May antagonize antibacterial activity of sulfonamides.
Side/adverse effects:
  More likely to cause contact sensitization than most other local anesthetics.
  See also *Side/Adverse Effects.*

## Dental Dosage Forms

Note: The gel, ointment, and topical solution dosage forms included in this section are specifically formulated for application only to the gingival or buccal mucosa or to perioral tissues. Gel and topical solution formulations that may be applied to other mucosal tissues (in addition to the gingival or buccal mucosa) are included in the *Topical Dosage Forms* section.

### BENZOCAINE GEL (DENTAL)

**Usual adult and adolescent dose**
Anesthetic, mucosal-local—Topical, as a 10 or 20% gel, applied to affected area(s) up to four times a day or as directed by a physician or dentist.

Note: The medication may be applied with cotton, a cotton swab, or a fingertip.

The gel should not be applied directly to, or used beneath, a dental appliance unless the patient is under the supervision of a dentist. Patients using this medication without the supervision of a dentist for relief of dental appliance pain should apply the medication directly to the affected gum area, wait until relief is obtained, and rinse the mouth before reinserting the appliance.

**Usual pediatric dose**
Anesthetic, mucosal-local—
  For teething pain:
    Infants up to 4 months of age—Dosage must be individualized by a physician or dentist.
    Infants and children 4 months to 2 years of age—Topical, as a 7.5 or 10% gel, applied to affected area(s) up to four times a day as needed or as directed by a physician or dentist.
    Children 2 years of age and older—Topical, as a 7.5% or stronger gel, applied to affected area(s) up to four times a day or as directed by a physician or dentist.
  For toothache:
    Children 2 years of age and older—See *Usual adult and adolescent dose*.

Note: Product may be applied with cotton, a cotton swab, or a fingertip.

**Strength(s) usually available**
U.S.—
  7.5% (OTC) [*Anbesol, Baby; Num-Zit Gel; Orabase, Baby; Orajel, Baby*].
  10% (OTC) [*Numzident; Orajel; Orajel Nighttime Formula, Baby; Rid-A-Pain*].
  20% (OTC) [*Anbesol Maximum Strength Gel* (alcohol 60%); *Orajel Maximum Strength; SensoGARD Canker Sore Relief*].
Canada—
  7.5% (OTC) [*Anbesol Baby Jel*].
  20% (OTC) [*Orajel Extra Strength; Topicaine*].

**Packaging and storage**
Store below 40 °C (104 °F), preferably between 15 and 30 °C (59 and 86 °F), unless otherwise specified by manufacturer. Protect from freezing.

## BENZOCAINE FILM-FORMING GEL

**Usual adult and adolescent dose**
Anesthetic, mucosal-local—Topical, as a 15% gel, applied with a cotton swab to affected area(s) up to four times a day or as directed by a physician or dentist. The area should be dried with a cotton swab prior to application.

**Usual pediatric dose**
Anesthetic, mucosal-local—
  Infants and children up to 2 years of age: Dosage must be individualized by a physician or dentist.
  Children 2 years of age and older: See *Usual adult and adolescent dose*.

Note: To ensure that this medication is applied correctly, children up to 12 years of age should apply it under the supervision of an adult.

**Strength(s) usually available**
U.S.—
  15% (OTC) [*Oratect Gel*].

**Packaging and storage**
Store below 40 °C (104 °F), preferably between 15 and 30 °C (59 and 86 °F), unless otherwise specified by manufacturer. Protect from freezing.

## BENZOCAINE LOZENGES

**Usual adult and adolescent dose**
Anesthetic, mucosal-local—Oral, one 10-mg lozenge to be dissolved slowly in the mouth. May be repeated at two-hour intervals as needed.

**Usual pediatric dose**
Anesthetic, mucosal-local—
  Children up to 2 years of age: Dosage must be individualized by a physician.
  Children 2 years of age and older: Oral, one 5-mg lozenge to be dissolved slowly in the mouth. May be repeated at two-hour intervals, if needed.

**Usual pediatric prescribing limits**
Not to exceed twelve 5-mg lozenges per day.

**Strength(s) usually available**
U.S.—
  5 mg (OTC) [*Chloraseptic Lozenges, Children's*].
  10 mg (OTC) [*Spec-T Sore Throat Anesthetic*].

**Packaging and storage**
Store below 40 °C (104 °F), preferably between 15 and 30 °C (59 and 86 °F), unless otherwise specified by manufacturer.

## BENZOCAINE OINTMENT (DENTAL) USP

**Usual adult and adolescent dose**
Anesthetic, mucosal-local—Topical, applied to cleaned and dried dentures up to four times a day.

**Usual pediatric dose**
Dosage has not been established.

**Strength(s) usually available**
U.S.—
  20% (OTC) [*Benzodent; Dentapaine*].

**Packaging and storage**
Store below 30 °C (86 °F). Store in a tight container. Protect from light. Protect from freezing.

## BENZOCAINE DENTAL PASTE

**Usual adult and adolescent dose**
Anesthetic, mucosal-local—Topical, applied to the affected area as needed.

**Usual pediatric dose**
Anesthetic, mucosal-local—
  Children up to 6 years of age: Dosage must be individualized by physician or dentist.
  Children 6 years of age and older: See *Usual adult and adolescent dose*.

**Strength(s) usually available**
U.S.—
  20% (OTC) [*Orabase-B with Benzocaine*].

**Packaging and storage**
Store below 40 °C (104 °F), preferably between 15 and 30 °C (59 and 86 °F), unless otherwise specified by manufacturer. Protect from freezing.

## BENZOCAINE TOPICAL SOLUTION (DENTAL) USP

**Usual adult and adolescent dose**
Anesthetic, mucosal-local—Topical, as a 20% solution, applied to affected area(s) up to four times a day or as directed by a physician or dentist.

Note: The medication may be applied with cotton, a cotton swab, or a fingertip.

**Usual pediatric dose**
Anesthetic, mucosal-local—
  Infants and children up to 2 years of age: Dosage must be individualized by a physician or dentist.
  Children 2 years of age and older: See *Usual adult and adolescent dose*.

**Strength(s) usually available**
U.S.—
  0.2% (OTC) [*Num-Zit Lotion* (alcohol 12.6%)].
  5% (OTC) [*Dent-Zel-Ite* (alcohol 81%)].
  20% (OTC) [*Anbesol Maximum Strength Liquid* (alcohol 60%)].
  Note: In Canada, *Anbesol Maximum Strength Liquid* also contains 0.45% of phenol. See *Benzocaine and Phenol Topical Solution*.
Canada—
  6.5% (OTC) [*Dentocaine*].
  7.5% (OTC) [*Orajel, Baby*].
  20% (OTC) [*Orajel Liquid*].

**Packaging and storage**
Store below 30 °C (86 °F). Store in a tight container. Protect from light. Protect from freezing.

## BENZOCAINE AND MENTHOL LOZENGES

**Usual adult and adolescent dose**
Anesthetic, mucosal-local—Oral, one lozenge dissolved slowly in the mouth every two hours as needed or as directed by a physician or dentist.

**Usual pediatric dose**
Anesthetic, mucosal-local—
  Children up to 2 years of age: Dosage must be individualized by a physician or dentist.
  Children 2 years of age and older: See *Usual adult and adolescent dose*.

**Strength(s) usually available**
U.S.—
  6 mg of benzocaine and 10 mg of menthol (OTC) [*Chloraseptic Lozenges*].
Canada—
  6 mg of benzocaine and 10 mg of menthol (OTC) [*Chloraseptic Lozenges Cherry Flavor*].

## Packaging and storage
Store below 40 °C (104 °F), preferably between 15 and 30 °C (59 and 86 °F), unless otherwise specified by manufacturer.

### BENZOCAINE AND PHENOL GEL

**Usual adult and adolescent dose**
Anesthetic, mucosal-local—Topical, applied to affected area(s) up to four times a day or as directed by a physician or dentist.

Note: The medication may be applied with cotton, a cotton swab, or a fingertip.

The gel should not be applied directly to, or used beneath, a dental appliance unless the patient is under the supervision of a dentist. Patients using this medication without the supervision of a dentist for relief of dental appliance pain should apply the medication directly to the affected gum area, wait until relief is obtained, and rinse the mouth before reinserting the appliance.

**Usual pediatric dose**
Anesthetic, mucosal-local—
  Infants and children up to 2 years of age: Dosage must be individualized by a physician or dentist.
  Children 2 years of age and older: See *Usual adult and adolescent dose*.

**Strength(s) usually available**
U.S.—
  6.3% of benzocaine and 0.5% of phenol (OTC) [*Anbesol Regular Strength Gel* (alcohol 70%)].
Canada—
  6.4% of benzocaine and 0.5% of phenol (OTC) [*Anbesol Gel* (alcohol)].

**Packaging and storage**
Store below 40 °C (104 °F), preferably between 15 and 30 °C (59 and 86 °F), unless otherwise specified by manufacturer. Protect from freezing.

### BENZOCAINE AND PHENOL TOPICAL SOLUTION

**Usual adult and adolescent dose**
Anesthetic, mucosal-local—Topical, applied to affected area(s) up to four times a day or as directed by a physician or dentist.

Note: The medication may be applied with cotton, a cotton swab, or a fingertip.

**Usual pediatric dose**
Anesthetic, mucosal-local—
  Infants and children up to 2 years of age: Dosage must be individualized by a physician or dentist.
  Children 2 years of age and older: See *Usual adult and adolescent dose*.

**Strength(s) usually available**
U.S.—
  6.3% of benzocaine and 0.5% of phenol (OTC) [*Anbesol Regular Strength Liquid* (alcohol 70%)].
Canada—
  6.5% of benzocaine and 0.45% of phenol (OTC) [*Anbesol Liquid* (alcohol)].
  20% of benzocaine and 0.45 % of phenol (OTC) [*Anbesol Maximum Strength Liquid* (alcohol)].

Note: In the U.S., *Anbesol Maximum Strength Liquid* does not contain phenol. See *Benzocaine Topical Solution USP (Dental)*.

**Packaging and storage**
Store below 40 °C (104 °F), preferably between 15 and 30 °C (59 and 86 °F), unless otherwise specified by manufacturer. Protect from freezing.

## Rectal Dosage Forms

### BENZOCAINE OINTMENT (RECTAL) USP

**Usual adult and adolescent dose**
Anesthetic, mucosal-local—Topical, applied to the perianal area up to six times a day after the area has been cleansed and dried. Medication should not be inserted into the rectum.

**Usual pediatric dose**
Dosage has not been established.

**Strength(s) usually available**
U.S.—
  20% (OTC) [*Americaine Hemorrhoidal*].

**Packaging and storage**
Store below 30 °C (86 °F). Store in a tight container. Protect from light. Protect from freezing.

## Topical Dosage Forms

### BENZOCAINE GEL

**Usual adult and adolescent dose**
Anesthetic, mucosal-local—
  Dental procedures: Topical, as a 20% gel, applied to area with a cotton applicator as needed.
  Other examination or instrumentation procedures: Topical, as a 20% gel, applied to area with a cotton applicator, or to instrument prior to insertion.

**Usual pediatric dose**
Dosage has not been established.

**Strength(s) usually available**
U.S.—
  20% (OTC) [*Americaine Anesthetic Lubricant; Hurricaine*].

**Packaging and storage**
Store below 40 °C (104 °F), preferably between 15 and 30 °C (59 and 86 °F), unless otherwise specified by manufacturer. Protect from freezing.

### BENZOCAINE TOPICAL AEROSOL USP

**Usual adult and adolescent dose**
Anesthetic, mucosal-local—Topical, as a 20% solution, sprayed on area for one second. May be repeated if necessary.

**Usual pediatric dose**
Dosage has not been established.

**Strength(s) usually available**
U.S.—
  20% (OTC) [*Americaine; Hurricaine*].

**Packaging and storage**
Store below 40 °C (104 °F), unless otherwise specified by manufacturer.

### BENZOCAINE TOPICAL SOLUTION USP

**Usual adult and adolescent dose**
Anesthetic, mucosal-local—Topical, as a 20% solution, applied to area with a cotton applicator as needed.

**Usual pediatric dose**
Dosage has not been established.

**Strength(s) usually available**
U.S.—
  20% (OTC) [*Hurricaine*].

**Packaging and storage**
Store below 30 °C (86 °F). Store in a tight container. Protect from light. Protect from freezing.

---

## BENZOCAINE, BUTAMBEN, AND TETRACAINE

## Summary of Differences
Pharmacology/pharmacokinetics:
  Physicochemical characteristics—
    Benzocaine, butamben, and tetracaine are all PABA-derivative ester-type local anesthetics.
Precautions:
  Cross-sensitivity and/or related problems—
    May occur with other ester-type local anesthetics, especially other PABA derivatives, parabens, and paraphenylenediamine.
  Drug interactions and/or related problems—
    Cholinesterase inhibitors inhibit metabolism of these local anesthetics.
    May antagonize antibacterial activity of sulfonamides.
Side/adverse effects:
  Benzocaine and tetracaine are more likely to cause contact sensitization than other local anesthetics.
  Tetracaine is more toxic than other mucosal-local anesthetics.
  See also *Side/Adverse Effects*.

## Additional Dosing Information
See also *General Dosing Information*.

In dentistry, this medication should not be used under dentures or cotton rolls, because retention under these materials may result in sloughing of tissue.

## Topical Dosage Forms

### BENZOCAINE, BUTAMBEN, AND TETRACAINE HYDROCHLORIDE GEL USP

**Usual adult and adolescent dose**
Anesthetic, mucosal-local—Topical, applied directly to desired area, or to instrument prior to insertion.

**Usual adult prescribing limits**
For the tetracaine component—20 mg.

**Usual pediatric dose**
Dosage has not been established.

**Strength(s) usually available**
U.S.—
  14% of benzocaine, 2% of butamben, and 2% of tetracaine hydrochloride (Rx) [*Cetacaine Topical Anesthetic*].

**Packaging and storage**
Store below 40 °C (104 °F), preferably between 15 and 30 °C (59 and 86 °F), unless otherwise specified by manufacturer. Protect from freezing.

### BENZOCAINE, BUTAMBEN, AND TETRACAINE HYDROCHLORIDE OINTMENT USP

**Usual adult and adolescent dose**
Anesthetic, mucosal-local—Topical, applied with a cotton pledget or directly to tissue.
  Note: Cotton pledget should not be held in position for extended periods of time, because of increased risk of local reactions to the anesthetics.

**Usual adult prescribing limits**
For the tetracaine component—20 mg.

**Usual pediatric dose**
Dosage has not been established.

**Strength(s) usually available**
U.S.—
  14% of benzocaine, 2% of butamben, and 2% of tetracaine hydrochloride (Rx) [*Cetacaine Topical Anesthetic*].

**Packaging and storage**
Store below 40 °C (104 °F), preferably between 15 and 30 °C (59 and 86 °F), unless otherwise specified by manufacturer. Protect from freezing.

### BENZOCAINE, BUTAMBEN, AND TETRACAINE HYDROCHLORIDE TOPICAL AEROSOL USP

**Usual adult and adolescent dose**
Anesthetic, mucosal-local—Topical, sprayed on desired area for approximately one second or less.

**Usual adult prescribing limits**
Duration of spray should not exceed two seconds.

**Usual pediatric dose**
Dosage has not been established.

**Strength(s) usually available**
U.S.—
  14% of benzocaine, 2% of butamben, and 2% of tetracaine hydrochloride (Rx) [*Cetacaine Topical Anesthetic*].

**Packaging and storage**
Store below 40 °C (104 °F), preferably between 15 and 30 °C (59 and 86 °F), unless otherwise specified by manufacturer.

**Auxiliary labeling**
• Shake well.

### BENZOCAINE, BUTAMBEN, AND TETRACAINE HYDROCHLORIDE TOPICAL SOLUTION USP

**Usual adult and adolescent dose**
Anesthetic, mucosal-local—Topical, applied with a cotton pledget or directly to tissue.
  Note: Cotton pledget should not be held in position for extended periods of time, because of increased risk of local reactions to the anesthetics.

**Usual adult prescribing limits**
For the tetracaine component—20 mg.

**Usual pediatric dose**
Dosage has not been established.

**Strength(s) usually available**
U.S.—
  14% of benzocaine, 2% of butamben, and 2% of tetracaine hydrochloride (Rx) [*Cetacaine Topical Anesthetic*].

**Packaging and storage**
Store below 40 °C (104 °F), preferably between 15 and 30 °C (59 and 86 °F), unless otherwise specified by manufacturer. Protect from freezing.

---

## DIBUCAINE

### Summary of Differences
Indications:
  Indicated for treatment of hemorrhoids and other anorectal disorders.
Pharmacology/pharmacokinetics:
  Physicochemical characteristics—
    Dibucaine is an amide-type local anesthetic.
Precautions:
  Cross-sensitivity and/or related problems—Rarely, may occur with other amide-type local anesthetics.
  Laboratory value alterations—No interference with pancreatic function test using bentiromide.

## Rectal Dosage Forms

### DIBUCAINE OINTMENT USP

**Usual adult and adolescent dose**
Anesthetic, mucosal-local—
  Rectal, a comfortable quantity, inserted three or four times a day, in the morning, in the evening, and after bowel movements; and/or
  Topical, to the perianal area three or four times a day, in the morning, in the evening, and after bowel movements.

**Usual pediatric dose**
Dosage has not been established.

**Strength(s) usually available**
U.S.—
  1% (OTC) [*Nupercainal* (acetone sodium bisulfite); GENERIC].
Canada—
  1% (OTC) [*Nupercainal* (bisulfite)].

**Packaging and storage**
Store below 40 °C (104 °F), preferably between 15 and 30 °C (59 and 86 °F), unless otherwise specified by manufacturer. Store in a collapsible tube or in a tight, light-resistant container. Protect from freezing.

---

## DYCLONINE

### Summary of Differences
Pharmacology/pharmacokinetics:
  Physicochemical characteristics—
    Dyclonine is neither an ester-type nor an amide-type local anesthetic.
Precautions:
  Cross-sensitivity and/or related problems—
    Does not occur with either ester-type or amide-type local anesthetics.
  Laboratory value alterations—
    May cause precipitation of iodine from contrast agents used in cystoscopic procedures following pyelography.
  No interference with pancreatic function test using bentiromide.

## Dental Dosage Forms

### DYCLONINE HYDROCHLORIDE LOZENGES

**Usual adult and adolescent dose**
Anesthetic, mucosal-local—Oral, one 2-mg or 3-mg lozenge to be dissolved slowly in the mouth. May be repeated at two-hour intervals, if needed.

**Usual pediatric dose**
Anesthetic, mucosal-local—
  Children up to 2 years of age: Dosage has not been established.
  Children 2 years of age and older: Oral, one 1.2-mg lozenge to be dissolved slowly in the mouth. May be repeated at two-hour intervals, if needed.

**Strength(s) usually available**
U.S.—
  1.2 mg (OTC) [*Sucrets, Children's*].
  2 mg (OTC) [*Sucrets Regular Strength*].
  3 mg (OTC) [*Sucrets Maximum Strength*].

**Packaging and storage**
Store below 40 °C (104 °F), preferably between 15 and 30 °C (59 and 86 °F), unless otherwise specified by manufacturer.

## Topical Dosage Forms

### DYCLONINE HYDROCHLORIDE TOPICAL SOLUTION USP

**Usual adult and adolescent dose**
Anesthetic, mucosal-local—
  Topical, 40 to 200 mg as a 0.5 or 1% solution; specifically: —
  For anogenital pain—
    Topical, as a 0.5% solution, applied with sponges or cotton pledgets.
  For dental procedures—
    Topical, as a 0.5% solution, used as a mouthwash or gargle and the excess expelled.
  For otorhinolaryngologic examinations—
    Topical, as a 0.5% solution, used as a spray or gargle.
  For perioral lesion pain—
    Topical, to the affected area(s), as a 0.5% solution, used as a rinse or swab.
  For vaginal pain—
    Topical, a 0.5 or 1% solution, applied as a wet compress or spray.
  For esophageal lesion pain—
    Oral, 25 to 150 mg (5 to 15 mL of a 0.5 or 1% solution).

**Usual adult prescribing limits**
Up to 300 mg (30 mL of a 1% solution) per examination, although this dose is rarely required. Adequate anesthesia is usually achieved with smaller quantities.

**Usual pediatric dose**
Dosage has not been established.

**Strength(s) usually available**
U.S.—
  0.5% (Rx) [*Dyclone*].
  1% (Rx) [*Dyclone*].

**Packaging and storage**
Store below 40 °C (104 °F), preferably between 15 and 30 °C (59 and 86 °F), unless otherwise specified by manufacturer. Store in a tight, light-resistant container. Protect from freezing.

---

## LIDOCAINE

### Summary of Differences
Pharmacology/pharmacokinetics:
  Physicochemical characteristics—Lidocaine is an amide-type local anesthetic.
  Protein binding—Concentration-dependent; 60 to 80% at nontoxic plasma concentrations.
Precautions:
  Cross-sensitivity and/or related problems—Rarely, may occur with other amide-type local anesthetics.
  Breast-feeding—Distributed into breast milk in very small quantities.
  Drug interactions and/or related problems—Also interacts with beta-adrenergic blocking agents, cimetidine, and amide local anesthetic–derivative antiarrhythmic agents.

## Dental Dosage Forms

Note: The topical solution formulations included in this section are specifically formulated for application only to gingival or buccal mucosa or to perioral tissues. Topical solution formulations that are applied to other mucosal tissues (in addition to the gingival or buccal mucosa) are included in the *Topical Dosage Forms* section.

### LIDOCAINE TOPICAL AEROSOL USP

**Usual adult and adolescent dose**
Anesthetic, mucosal-local—Topical, to gingival and oral mucous membranes, 20 mg (two metered sprays) per quadrant of gingiva and oral mucosa.

**Usual adult prescribing limits**
Not to exceed 30 mg of lidocaine (three metered sprays) per quadrant of gingiva and oral mucosa over a one-half-hour period or 200 mg (twenty metered sprays) in twenty-four hours.

**Usual pediatric dose**
Anesthetic, mucosal-local—Topical, to gingival and oral mucous membranes, up to a total of 3 mg per kg of body weight.

**Strength(s) usually available**
U.S.—
  10% (10 mg per metered spray) (Rx) [*Xylocaine*].
Canada—
  10% (10 mg per metered spray) (OTC) [*Xylocaine*].

**Packaging and storage**
Store below 40 °C (104 °F), preferably between 15 and 30 °C (59 and 86 °F), unless otherwise specified by manufacturer. Protect from freezing.

**Auxiliary labeling**
• Shake well.

### LIDOCAINE ORAL TOPICAL SOLUTION USP

**Usual adult and adolescent dose**
Anesthesia, mucosal-local—
  Dental procedures: Topical, 50 to 200 mg as a 5% solution, applied to the oral mucosa with a cotton applicator.
  Perioral lesions: Topical, as a 2.5% solution, applied to affected area(s) with a cotton swab every one or two hours for the first three days, then as needed.

**Usual adult prescribing limits**
Dental procedures—Not to exceed a total of 250 mg (5 mL of a 5% solution) for all quadrants in a three-hour period.

**Usual pediatric dose**
Anesthesia, mucosal-local—Dental procedures: Topical, the dosage being individualized, based on the child's age, weight, and physical condition up to a maximum of 4.5 mg per kg of body weight as 5% solution.

**Strength(s) usually available**
U.S.—
  2.5% (OTC) [*Zilactin-L*].
  5% (Rx) [*Xylocaine;* GENERIC].
Canada—
  5% (OTC) [*Xylocaine*].

**Packaging and storage**
Store below 40 °C (104 °F), preferably between 15 and 30 °C (59 and 86 °F), unless otherwise specified by manufacturer. Store in a tight container. Protect from freezing.

## Topical Dosage Forms

### LIDOCAINE OINTMENT USP

**Usual adult and adolescent dose**
Anesthetic, mucosal-local—
  Oral mucosa:
    Topical, as a 5% ointment, to previously dried oral mucosa.
    For use during fitting of new dentures—Apply to all denture surfaces that contact the mucosa, up to a maximum of 5 grams of ointment (250 mg of lidocaine) per single dose or 20 grams of ointment (1000 mg of lidocaine) per day.
    Note: The patient should be advised to consult the prescribing dentist at intervals not exceeding 48 hours throughout the fitting period.
  Oropharynx:
    Topical, as a 5% ointment, applied to desired area, or to instrument prior to insertion.

**Usual pediatric dose**
Anesthetic, mucosal-local—Topical, the dosage being individualized, based on the child's age, weight, and physical condition, up to a maximum of 4.5 mg per kg of body weight or 2.5 grams of ointment in a six-hour period.

**Strength(s) usually available**
U.S.—
  5% (Rx) [*Xylocaine;* GENERIC].
Canada—
  5% (OTC) [*Xylocaine Dental Ointment*].

**Packaging and storage**
Store below 40 °C (104 °F), preferably between 15 and 30 °C (59 and 86 °F), unless otherwise specified by manufacturer. Store in a tight container. Protect from freezing.

### LIDOCAINE HYDROCHLORIDE JELLY USP

**Usual adult and adolescent dose**
Anesthetic, mucosal-local—
  Esophagus, larynx, trachea:
    Topical, as a 2% jelly, applied to the outer surface of the instrument prior to insertion.
    Note: Care should be taken to avoid depositing any of the medication on the inner surface of an endoscope or other instrument. It may dry on the inner surface and leave a residue that may cause narrowing or, rarely, occlusion of the lumen.

Urinary tract:
Female—
Urethral, 3 to 5 mL, as a 2% jelly, several minutes prior to examination.
Note: Jelly may be deposited on a cotton swab and introduced into urethra.
Male—
Prior to catheterization: Urethral, 100 to 200 mg (5 to 10 mL) as a 2% jelly.
Prior to sounding or cystoscopy: Urethral, 600 mg (30 mL) to fill and dilate urethra. The medication is usually administered in two divided doses, with a penile clamp applied for several minutes between doses.

**Usual adult prescribing limits**
Not more than 600 mg (30 mL) in a twelve-hour period.

**Usual pediatric dose**
Anesthetic, mucosal-local—Topical, as a 2% jelly, dosage to be individualized, based on the child's age, weight, and physical condition, up to a maximum of 4.5 mg per kg of body weight.

**Strength(s) usually available**
U.S.—
2% (Rx) [*Anestacon Jelly; Xylocaine;* GENERIC].
Canada—
2% (OTC) [*Xylocaine*].

**Packaging and storage**
Store below 40 °C (104 °F), preferably between 15 and 30 °C (59 and 86 °F), unless otherwise specified by manufacturer. Store in a tight container. Protect from freezing.

### LIDOCAINE HYDROCHLORIDE ORAL TOPICAL SOLUTION USP

Note: Previous name—Lidocaine Hydrochloride Viscous Solution.

**Usual adult and adolescent dose**
Anesthetic, mucosal-local—
Oral cavity disorders: Topical, 300 mg (15 mL) swished around in the mouth, then expelled, or applied with a cotton-tipped applicator, every three hours as needed.
Pharyngeal pain: Topical, 300 mg (15 mL) used as a gargle every three hours as needed. May be swallowed if necessary.

**Usual adult prescribing limits**
Single dose—Not to exceed 4.5 mg per kg of body weight or 300 mg (15 mL). This dose should not be repeated more often than every three hours.
Multiple doses—Not to exceed 8 doses (2.4 grams or 120 mL) in twenty-four hours.

**Usual pediatric dose**
Anesthetic, mucosal-local—
Infants and children up to 3 years of age:
Topical, up to 1.25 mL of a 2% solution, applied to affected area(s) with a cotton-tipped applicator every three hours.
Note: It is recommended that the dosage be accurately measured and applied to the immediate area or specific lesion with a cotton-tipped applicator. The risk of systemic toxicity, especially convulsions, is increased if dosage is not carefully controlled and/or if the patient swallows significant quantities of the medication.
Children 3 years of age and older:
Topical, the dosage being individualized, based on the child's age, weight, and physical condition, up to a maximum of 4.5 mg per kg of body weight as 2% solution in a three-hour period.

**Strength(s) usually available**
U.S.—
2% (Rx) [*Xylocaine Viscous;* GENERIC].
Canada—
2% (OTC) [*Xylocaine Viscous*].

**Packaging and storage**
Store below 40 °C (104 °F), preferably between 15 and 30 °C (59 and 86 °F), unless otherwise specified by manufacturer. Store in a tight container. Protect from freezing.

### LIDOCAINE HYDROCHLORIDE TOPICAL SOLUTION USP

**Usual adult and adolescent dose**
Anesthetic, mucosal-local—Oral or nasal cavity or esophagus: Topical, as a 4% solution, 600 mcg (0.6 mg) to 3 mg per kg of body weight; or 40 to 200 mg (1 to 5 mL).

Note: May be applied as a spray, with cotton applicators or packs, or instilled directly into cavity.

**Usual adult prescribing limits**
For use in oral or nasal cavities or upper gastrointestinal tract—Not to exceed 4.5 mg per kg of body weight or 300 mg (7.5 mL of a 4% solution).

**Usual pediatric dose**
Dosage must be individualized by physician.

**Strength(s) usually available**
U.S.—
4% (Rx) [*Xylocaine;* GENERIC].
Canada—
4% (OTC) [*Xylocaine*].

**Packaging and storage**
Store below 40 °C (104 °F), preferably between 15 and 30 °C (59 and 86 °F), unless otherwise specified by manufacturer. Store in a tight container. Protect from freezing.

### LIDOCAINE HYDROCHLORIDE TOPICAL SPRAY SOLUTION

Note: The dosing and strength of this dosage form are expressed in terms of lidocaine base.

**Usual adult and adolescent dose**
Anesthetic, mucosal-local—Endoscopic procedures: Topical, up to 20 metered sprays (200 mg [base]) as a 10% (base) solution, sprayed onto the oropharyngeal or tracheal mucosa.

**Usual pediatric dose**
Anesthetic, mucosal-local—
Infants and children up to 3 years of age:
Use is not recommended; a less concentrated solution should be used instead.
Children 3 to 12 years of age:
Larynx or trachea—Topical, up to 1.5 mg (base) per kg of body weight.
Other mucosa—Topical, up to 3 mg (base) per kg of body weight.

**Strength(s) usually available**
U.S.—
Not commercially available.
Canada—
10% (base; 12 mg of lidocaine hydrochloride equivalent to 10 mg of lidocaine base per metered spray) (OTC) [*Xylocaine Endotracheal*].

**Packaging and storage**
Store below 40 °C (104 °F), preferably between 15 and 30 °C (59 and 86 °F), unless otherwise specified by manufacturer. Store in a tight container. Protect from freezing.

---

*PRAMOXINE*

---

## Summary of Differences

Indications:
Indicated for the treatment of hemorrhoids and other anorectal disorders.
Pharmacology/pharmacokinetics:
Physicochemical characteristics—
Pramoxine is neither an amide-type nor an ester-type local anesthetic.
Precautions:
Cross-sensitivity and/or related problems—Does not occur with either ester-type or amide-type local anesthetics.
Laboratory value alterations—No interference with pancreatic function test using bentiromide.

## Rectal Dosage Forms

### PRAMOXINE HYDROCHLORIDE AEROSOL FOAM

**Usual adult and adolescent dose**
Anesthetic, mucosal-local—
Rectal, one applicatorful two to three times a day; or
Topical, to the external anorectal area two to three times a day.

**Usual pediatric dose**
Dosage has not been established.

**Strength(s) usually available**
U.S.—
1% (OTC) [*ProctoFoam/non-steroid* (propylparaben)].

## Packaging and storage
Store below 40 °C (104 °F), preferably between 15 and 30 °C (59 and 86 °F), unless otherwise specified by manufacturer. Protect from freezing.

## Auxiliary labeling
- Shake well.
- For anorectal use only.

### PRAMOXINE HYDROCHLORIDE CREAM USP

**Usual adult and adolescent dose**
Anesthetic, mucosal-local—Topical, to the anorectal area, up to five times a day, after the area has been cleansed and dried.

**Usual pediatric dose**
Children up to 12 years of age—Dosage must be individualized by physician.

**Strength(s) usually available**
U.S.—
    1% (OTC) [*Tronolane; Tronothane*].
Canada—
    1% (OTC) [*Tronothane*].

**Packaging and storage**
Store below 40 °C (104 °F), preferably between 15 and 30 °C (59 and 86 °F), unless otherwise specified by manufacturer. Store in tight container. Protect from freezing.

### PRAMOXINE HYDROCHLORIDE OINTMENT

**Usual adult and adolescent dose**
Anesthetic, mucosal-local—
    Rectal, introduced into the rectum as a 1% ointment up to five times per day, in the morning, at night, and after bowel movements; or
    Topical, to the anorectal area as a 1% ointment up to five times a day.

**Usual pediatric dose**
Children up to 12 years of age—Dosage must be individualized by physician.

**Strength(s) usually available**
U.S.—
    1% (OTC) [*Fleet Relief*].

Note: Available in tubes and in pre-filled 4-mL disposable applicators.

**Packaging and storage**
Store below 40 °C (104 °F), preferably between 15 and 30 °C (59 and 86 °F), unless otherwise specified by manufacturer. Protect from freezing.

---

## TETRACAINE

## Summary of Differences
Pharmacology/pharmacokinetics:
    Physicochemical characteristics—
        Tetracaine is a PABA-derivative ester-type local anesthetic.
Precautions:
    Cross-sensitivity and/or related problems—
        May occur with other ester-type local anesthetics, especially other PABA derivatives, parabens, and paraphenylenediamine.
    Drug interactions and/or related problems—
        Cholinesterase inhibitors inhibit metabolism of tetracaine.
        May antagonize antibacterial activity of sulfonamides.
Side/adverse effects:
    More likely to cause contact sensitization than most other local anesthetics.
    More toxic than other mucosal-local anesthetics.
    See also *Side/Adverse Effects*.

## Dental Dosage Forms
### TETRACAINE TOPICAL AEROSOL

**Usual adult and adolescent dose**
Anesthetic, mucosal-local—Gingival and oral mucosa: Topical, 1.4 mg (two metered sprays).

**Usual adult prescribing limits**
Not to exceed 20 mg (approximately 28 metered sprays).

**Usual pediatric dose**
Dosage has not been established.

**Strength(s) usually available**
U.S.—
    Not commercially available.
Canada—
    700 mcg (0.7 mg) per metered spray (OTC) [*Supracaine*].

**Packaging and storage**
Store below 40 °C (104 °F), preferably between 15 and 30 °C (59 and 86 °F), unless otherwise specified by manufacturer. Protect from freezing.

**Auxiliary labeling**
- Shake well.

## Rectal Dosage Forms
### TETRACAINE HYDROCHLORIDE CREAM USP

Note: The dosing and strength of this dosage form are expressed in terms of tetracaine base.

**Usual adult and adolescent dose**
Anesthetic, mucosal-local—Rectal, introduced into rectum as a 1% (base) cream up to six times a day.

**Usual adult prescribing limits**
Not more than 28.35 grams in a twenty-four-hour period.

**Usual pediatric dose**
Dosage has not been established.

**Strength(s) usually available**
U.S.—
    1% (base) (OTC) [*Pontocaine Cream*].
Canada—
    Not commercially available.

**Packaging and storage**
Store below 40 °C (104 °F), preferably between 15 and 30 °C (59 and 86 °F), unless otherwise specified by manufacturer. Protect from freezing.

### TETRACAINE AND MENTHOL OINTMENT USP

**Usual adult and adolescent dose**
Anesthetic, mucosal-local—
    Rectal, introduced into rectum as a 0.5% ointment up to six times a day.
    Topical, applied as a 0.5% ointment spread with gauze or cotton, to anorectal area up to six times a day.

**Usual adult prescribing limits**
Not more than 28.35 grams in a twenty-four-hour period.

**Usual pediatric dose**
Dosage has not been established.

**Strength(s) usually available**
U.S.—
    0.5% of tetracaine and 0.5% of menthol (OTC) [*Pontocaine Ointment*].
Canada—
    Not commercially available.

**Packaging and storage**
Store below 40 °C (104 °F), preferably between 15 and 30 °C (59 and 86 °F), unless otherwise specified by manufacturer. Protect from freezing.

## Topical Dosage Forms
### TETRACAINE HYDROCHLORIDE TOPICAL SOLUTION USP

**Usual adult and adolescent dose**
Anesthetic, mucosal-local—Larynx, trachea, or esophagus—
    Topical, as a 0.25 or 0.5% solution prior to procedure; or
    Oral inhalation, as a nebulized 0.5% solution.

Note: 0.06 mL of 0.1% (1:1000) epinephrine may be added to each mL of tetracaine solution, to reduce absorption.

**Usual adult prescribing limits**
Not to exceed 20 mg.

**Usual pediatric dose**
Dosage has not been established.

**Strength(s) usually available**
U.S.—
    2% (Rx) [*Pontocaine*].
Canada—
    Not commercially available.

**Packaging and storage**
Store between 2 and 8 °C (36 and 46 °F), unless otherwise specified by manufacturer. Store in a tight, light-resistant container. Protect from freezing.

**Stability**
Do not use if solution is cloudy or discolored or contains crystals.

Revised: 09/01/94

*USP DI*  Anesthetics (Ophthalmic) 139

**ANESTHETICS**—The *Anesthetics (Ophthalmic)* monograph is not included in this published version of the USP DI database. Copies of the monograph are available on request from Micromedex, Inc. - Reprint Requests, 6200 S. Syracuse Way, Suite 300, Englewood, CO 80111; telephone (303) 486-6400; telefax (303) 486-6464; Email: USPDI@MDX.COM.

# ANESTHETICS Parenteral-Local

This monograph includes information on the following: 1) Articaine*; 2) Bupivacaine; 3) Chloroprocaine; 4) Etidocaine†; 5) Lidocaine; 6) Mepivacaine; 7) Prilocaine; 8) Procaine; 9) Tetracaine.

INN:  Lidocaine—Lignocaine

BAN:  Articaine—Carticaine

VA CLASSIFICATION (Primary): CN204

Commonly used brand name(s): *Astracaine 4%*[1]; *Astracaine 4% Forte*[1]; *Carbocaine*[6]; *Carbocaine with Neo-Cobefrin*[6]; *Citanest Forte*[7]; *Citanest Plain*[7]; *Dalcaine*[5]; *Dilocaine*[5]; *Duranest*[4]; *Duranest-MPF*[4]; *Isocaine*[6]; *Isocaine 2%*[6]; *Isocaine 3%*[6]; *L-Caine*[5]; *Lidoject-1*[5]; *Lidoject-2*[5]; *Marcaine*[2]; *Marcaine Spinal*[2]; *Nesacaine*[3]; *Nesacaine-CE*[3]; *Nesacaine-MPF*[3]; *Novocain*[8]; *Octocaine*[5]; *Octocaine-100*[5]; *Octocaine-50*[5]; *Polocaine*[6]; *Polocaine-MPF*[6]; *Pontocaine*[9]; *Sensorcaine*[2]; *Sensorcaine Forte*[2]; *Sensorcaine-MPF*[2]; *Sensorcaine-MPF Spinal*[2]; *Ultracaine D-S*[1]; *Ultracaine D-S Forte*[1]; *Xylocaine*[5]; *Xylocaine 5% Spinal*[5]; *Xylocaine Test Dose*[5]; *Xylocaine-MPF*[5]; *Xylocaine-MPF with Glucose*[5].

A commonly used name for lidocaine is lignocaine

Note:  For a listing of dosage forms and brand names by country availability, see *Dosage Forms* section(s).

*Not commercially available in U.S.
†Not commercially available in Canada.

## Category
Anesthetic (local).

## Indications
Note:  Bracketed information in the *Indications* section refers to uses that are not included in U.S. product labeling.

### General considerations
Parenteral-local anesthetics are generally used to provide local or regional anesthesia, analgesia, and varying degrees of motor blockade prior to surgical procedures, dental procedures, and obstetric delivery. They also may be used for other diagnostic or therapeutic purposes via routes of administration that are stated in product labeling.

Mixtures or combinations of local anesthetics are sometimes used to provide a rapid onset of action and a prolonged duration of action. However, the possibility of additive toxicity must be considered when such combinations are used.

Vasoconstrictors are added to local anesthetic injections to decrease the rate of local clearance of the local anesthetic. Local anesthetic injections containing a vasoconstrictor generally have the same indications as the corresponding local anesthetic injection without a vasoconstrictor. However, additional precautions pertinent to the use of a vasoconstrictor must be considered.

Dextrose is added to anesthetic solutions for subarachnoid administration to render the solution hyperbaric (heavier than cerebrospinal fluid [CSF]); the local anesthetic will exert its effect above or below the site of injection, depending upon the position of the patient during and immediately following the injection.

Local anesthetics may be combined with opioid analgesics for epidural administration for inducing postoperative analgesia. This combination may allow lower doses of both the local anesthetic and the opioid to be used as compared with either agent used alone, and may reduce the incidence of motor block, nausea, and urinary retention.

### Accepted
Central neural blocks—Caudal or lumbar epidural: Bupivacaine (with or without epinephrine), chloroprocaine, etidocaine (with or without epinephrine), lidocaine (with or without epinephrine), and mepivacaine are indicated. Only single-dose vials that do not contain an antimicrobial preservative should be used.

Subarachnoid: Bupivacaine and dextrose, lidocaine and dextrose, procaine[1], and tetracaine (with or without dextrose) are indicated. Commercially available products intended specifically for subarachnoid administration contain no antimicrobial preservatives. Solutions and diluents containing antimicrobial preservatives are not to be injected into the subarachnoid space and should not be used when preparing injections for administration via this route.

Dental infiltration or nerve block—[Articaine and epinephrine]; bupivacaine and epinephrine; chloroprocaine (with or without added epinephrine); etidocaine and epinephrine; lidocaine (with or without epinephrine); mepivacaine (with or without levonordefrin); prilocaine (with or without epinephrine) are indicated. Unless specifically contraindicated, a vasoconstrictor-containing solution is preferred.

Intravenous regional anesthesia (Bier block)[1]—[Chloroprocaine], lidocaine, and [mepivacaine] are indicated.

Local infiltration—Bupivacaine (with or without epinephrine), chloroprocaine, etidocaine (with or without epinephrine), lidocaine (with or without epinephrine), mepivacaine, and procaine are indicated.

Peripheral nerve block—Bupivacaine (with or without epinephrine), chloroprocaine, etidocaine (with or without epinephrine), lidocaine (with or without epinephrine), mepivacaine, and procaine are indicated.

Retrobulbar block: Bupivacaine, etidocaine, lidocaine, and [procaine][1] are indicated.

Sympathetic block—Bupivacaine (with or without epinephrine) and lidocaine (with or without epinephrine) are indicated.

Transtracheal—Lidocaine, [mepivacaine][1], and [tetracaine][1] are indicated.

### Unaccepted
For paracervical administration—Use of bupivacaine is not recommended for nonobstetrical procedures because of insufficient data concerning safety and dosage. Use of bupivacaine is not recommended in obstetrical procedures because such use has resulted in fetal bradycardia and death.

Solutions containing a vasoconstrictor should not be used for intravenous regional anesthesia (Bier block). Also, bupivacaine is not recommended for intravenous regional anesthesia.

For central neural block (peridural [lumbar or caudal epidural] or subarachnoid [spinal] administration)—Do not use solutions containing an antimicrobial preservative such as chlorobutanol or methylparaben.

Chloroprocaine and mepivacaine are not recommended for subarachnoid (spinal) administration.

[1]Not included in Canadian product labeling.

## Pharmacology/Pharmacokinetics
See *Table 1*, page 155.

### Physicochemical characteristics
Chemical group—
   Amides: Articaine, bupivacaine, etidocaine, lidocaine, mepivacaine, prilocaine.
   Esters, aminobenzoic acid (PABA)–derivative: Chloroprocaine, procaine, tetracaine.
Molecular weight—
   Articaine: 284.38.
   Bupivacaine hydrochloride: 342.91.
   Chloroprocaine hydrochloride: 307.22.
   Etidocaine: 276.42.
   Lidocaine hydrochloride: 288.82.
   Mepivacaine hydrochloride: 282.81.
   Prilocaine hydrochloride: 256.78.
   Procaine hydrochloride: 272.78.
   Tetracaine hydrochloride: 300.83.
pKa—
   See *Table 1* page 155.
Lipid solubility
   See *Table 1* page 155.

### Mechanism of action/Effect
Local anesthetics—
   Local anesthetics block both the initiation and conduction of nerve impulses by decreasing the neuronal membrane's permeability to sodium ions, perhaps by attaching to a site on the sodium channel. This reversibly stabilizes the membrane and inhibits depolarization,

resulting in the failure of a propagated action potential and subsequent conduction blockade.

The concentration of drug needed to block large nerve trunks is greater than that needed for smaller peripheral nerves.

Vasoconstrictors—
Act on alpha-adrenergic receptors in the vasculature of the skin, mucous membranes, conjunctiva, and viscera to produce vasoconstriction, thereby decreasing blood flow in the area of injection. The resultant reduction in the rate of local clearance of the local anesthetic prolongs the duration of action, lowers the peak serum concentration, decreases the risk of systemic toxicity, and increases the frequency of complete conduction blocks with low concentrations of the local anesthetic. Vasoconstrictors may also reduce bleeding when injected at the site of surgery.

## Other actions/effects

Local anesthetics—Actions on the central nervous system (CNS) may cause CNS stimulation and/or CNS depression. Actions on the cardiovascular system may cause depression of cardiac conduction and excitability and, with most of these agents, peripheral vasodilation.

Vasoconstrictors—Vasoconstrictors having beta-adrenergic activity (epinephrine, levonordefrin, and norepinephrine) may cause cardiac stimulation resulting in increased heart rate, contractility, conduction velocity, and irritability. Also, when used for obstetrical anesthesia, vasoconstrictors having beta-adrenergic activity may decrease the intensity of uterine contractions and prolong labor. Phenylephrine is also rarely used as a vasoconstrictor in conjunction with local anesthesia; it has only alpha-adrenergic activity and does not have these additional effects.

## Absorption

Complete systemic absorption. The rate of absorption is influenced by the site and route of administration (especially the vascularity or rate of blood flow at the injection site), total dosage (volume and concentration) administered, physical characteristics (such as degree of protein binding and lipid solubility) of the individual agent, and whether or not a vasoconstrictor is used concurrently.

## Biotransformation

Amides—
Hepatic.
Articaine: Inactivated by ester hydrolysis.
Lidocaine: Xylidide metabolites are active and toxic, but less so than the parent compound.
Prilocaine: May also be metabolized renally to some extent.

Esters—
PABA derivatives: Hydrolyzed primarily in the plasma and, to a much lesser extent, in the liver, by cholinesterases. Procaine is hydrolyzed to PABA. Chloroprocaine and tetracaine are hydrolyzed to PABA-containing compounds.

## Time to peak concentration

Usually 10 to 30 minutes. May occur 1 to 3 minutes after intravascular or transtracheal injection.

## Elimination

Renal, primarily as metabolites. For some of these agents, including lidocaine, mepivacaine, and tetracaine, renal excretion may follow biliary excretion into, and reabsorption from, the gastrointestinal tract.

Quantity of dose excreted unchanged—
Articaine: 2 to 5%.
Bupivacaine: 5%.
Etidocaine: Less than 10%.
Lidocaine: 10%.
Mepivacaine: 5 to 10%.
Procaine: Less than 2%.

# Precautions to Consider

## Cross-sensitivity and/or related problems

Patients sensitive to para-aminobenzoic acid (PABA) or parabens may be sensitive to procaine, chloroprocaine, or tetracaine also. They may also be sensitive to other local anesthetic solutions containing parabens as preservatives.

Patients sensitive to one ester-type local anesthetic may be sensitive to other ester-type local anesthetics also.

Patients sensitive to one amide-type local anesthetic may rarely be sensitive to other amide-type local anesthetics also.

Cross-sensitivity between ester-type local anesthetics and amide-type local anesthetics has not been reported.

## Pregnancy/Reproduction

Pregnancy—Local anesthetics cross the placenta by diffusion. The rate and degree of diffusion vary considerably among the various agents as determined by their rate of metabolism and physical characteristics such as plasma protein binding (reduced placental transfer with highly protein-bound agents), lipid solubility (greater placental transfer with highly lipid soluble agents), and degree of ionization (greater placental transfer with nonionized form of agent).

*All parenteral-local anesthetics*—Adequate and well-controlled prospective studies in humans have not been done. Retrospective studies of pregnant women receiving local anesthetics for emergency surgery early in pregnancy have not shown that local anesthetics cause birth defects.

*Articaine*—Studies of articaine in rats and rabbits using doses of up to 2.9 times the maximum recommended human dose (MRHD) have not shown adverse effects on the fetus.

*Bupivacaine*—Studies in rats and rabbits using doses 9 and 5 times the MRHD, respectively, have shown decreased survival in newborn rats and embryocidal effects in rabbits.

FDA Pregnancy Category C.

*Chloroprocaine, mepivacaine, and tetracaine*—Studies in animals have not been done.

FDA Pregnancy Category C.

*Etidocaine, lidocaine, and prilocaine*—Studies in rats or rabbits with etidocaine (using up to 1.7 times the MRHD), lidocaine (using up to 6.6 times the MRHD), or prilocaine (using 30 times the MRHD) have not shown adverse effects on the fetus.

FDA Pregnancy Category B.

*Procaine*—Studies in animals have not been done.

FDA Pregnancy Category C.

*Labor and delivery*—Epidural, subarachnoid, paracervical, or pudendal administration of a local anesthetic may produce changes in uterine contractility and/or maternal expulsive efforts. Paracervical block may shorten the first stage of labor and facilitate cervical dilation. However, epidural or subarachnoid administration of local anesthetics may prolong the second stage of labor by interfering with motor function or removing the patient's reflex urge to bear down. Use of a local anesthetic during delivery may increase the need for forceps-assisted delivery. Bupivacaine and etidocaine are not recommended for paracervical administration. Also, etidocaine may cause profound motor block; epidural administration of this agent is not recommended for normal vaginal delivery (although it may be used for cesarean section).

Maternal hypotension, caused by sympathetic nerve blockade resulting in vasodilation, may occur during regional anesthesia.

Maternal convulsions and cardiovascular collapse have been reported following paracervical administration of local anesthetics early in pregnancy (for elective abortion), suggesting rapid systemic absorption under these circumstances.

Maternal fatalities due to cardiac arrest have been reported following inadvertent intravascular injection of 0.75% bupivacaine during intended placement of an epidural block. Although the 0.75% strength is not recommended for epidural administration in obstetrics, lower concentrations of bupivacaine may be used.

Fetal bradycardia, possibly associated with fetal acidosis, has been reported in 20 to 30% of patients receiving amide-type local anesthetics via paracervical block. Fetal bradycardia without fetal acidosis also has been reported in 5 to 10% of patients receiving chloroprocaine via paracervical block. The risk of this complication may be increased if prematurity, postmaturity, toxemia of pregnancy, pre-existing fetal distress, or uteroplacental insufficiency is present. Risk-benefit must be considered when amide-type local anesthetics are considered for paracervical block in these conditions. Paracervical block with chloroprocaine is not recommended if prematurity, pre-existing fetal distress, or toxemia of pregnancy is present because its safety in these conditions has not been established. Monitoring of fetal heart rate is recommended during paracervical block.

*Postpartum*—Neonatal neurological disturbances such as diminished muscle strength and tone may occur for 1 to 2 days postpartum. Marked neonatal CNS depression has been reported following paracervical block. Also, inadvertent fetal intracranial injection during intended caudal, paracervical, or pudendal administration may cause neonatal depression and convulsions.

## Breast-feeding

It is not known whether most local anesthetics are distributed into breast milk. Bupivacaine is distributed into breast milk in small quantities. Lidocaine is distributed into breast milk. However, problems in humans have not been documented.

## Pediatrics

Although there is some evidence that systemic toxicity may be more likely to occur in pediatric patients, appropriate studies performed to date with mepivacaine have not demonstrated pediatrics-specific problems that would limit the use of the medication in children. Also, no information is available on the relationship of age to the effects of procainein pediatric patients. Although articaine is not approved for use in children younger than 4 years of age, a retrospective study of its use in patients younger than 4 years of age did not reveal any pediatrics-specific problems that would limit its use in children.

Infants up to 9 months of age have low plasma concentrations of alpha$_1$-acid glycoprotein (AAG). This results in an increased unbound fraction of bupivacaine and etidocaine, and may lead to systemic toxicity.

Reduced clearance of bupivacaine in pediatric patients may be more important than AAG concentrations in causing toxicity. Neonates may have total body clearance of bupivacaine only one third to one half the clearance of adults.

Appropriate studies performed to date have not demonstrated pediatrics-specific problems that would limit the usefulness of lidocaine in children.

### Geriatrics
Systemic toxicity may be more likely to occur in geriatric patients.

### Drug interactions and/or related problems
The following drug interactions and/or related problems have been selected on the basis of their potential clinical significance (possible mechanism in parentheses where appropriate)—not necessarily inclusive (» = major clinical significance):

Note: Combinations containing any of the following medications, depending on the amount present, may also interact with this medication.

*For all local anesthetics*
Anticoagulants, such as:
Ardeparin or
Dalteparin or
Danaparoid or
Enoxaparin or
Heparin or
Warfarin
(trauma to a blood vessel during peridural or subarachnoid administration of the local anesthetic may result in CNS or soft tissue hemorrhage in patients receiving anticoagulant therapy)

Antimyasthenics
(inhibition of neuronal transmission by local anesthetics may antagonize the effects of antimyasthenics on skeletal muscle, especially if large quantities of the anesthetic are rapidly absorbed; temporary dosage adjustment of antimyasthenics may be necessary to control symptoms of myasthenia gravis)

Beta-adrenergic blocking agents
(may slow metabolism of lidocaine by reducing hepatic blood flow, leading to increased risk of lidocaine toxicity)

Cimetidine
(cimetidine may inhibit hepatic metabolism of bupivacaine and lidocaine, leading to increased risk of toxicity)

» CNS depression–producing medications, including those commonly used as preanesthetic medication or for supplementation of local anesthesia (see *Appendix II* )
(concurrent use with a local anesthetic may result in additive depressant effects)

Disinfectant solutions containing heavy metals
(local anesthetics may cause release of heavy metal ions from these solutions, which, if injected along with the anesthetic, may cause severe local irritation, swelling, and edema; such solutions are not recommended for chemical disinfection of the container, and preventive measures are recommended if they are used for skin or mucous membrane disinfection prior to anesthetic administration)

Guanadrel or
Guanethidine or
Mecamylamine or
Trimethaphan
(the risk of severe hypotension and/or bradycardia may be increased if high levels of spinal or epidural anesthesia [i.e., sufficient to produce sympathetic blockade] are induced in patients receiving these ganglionic-blocking antihypertensive agents)

Halothane
(may increase the cardiotoxicity of bupivacaine)

Monoamine oxidase (MAO) inhibitors, including furazolidone, procarbazine, and selegiline
(concurrent use in patients receiving local anesthetics may increase the risk of hypotension; discontinuation of MAO inhibitors 10 days before elective surgery may be advisable if subarachnoid block anesthesia is planned)

Neuromuscular blocking agents
(inhibition of neuronal transmission by local anesthetics may enhance or prolong the action of neuromuscular blocking agents if large quantities of the anesthetic are rapidly absorbed)

Opioid (narcotic) analgesic anesthesia adjuncts
(alterations in respiration caused by high levels of spinal or peridural blockade may be additive to opioid analgesic–induced alterations in respiratory rate and alveolar ventilation)

(the vagal effects of alfentanil, fentanyl or sufentanil may also be more pronounced in patients with high levels of spinal or epidural anesthesia, and may lead to bradycardia and/or hypotension)

» Vasoconstrictors such as epinephrine, methoxamine, or phenylephrine
(use of methoxamine in combination with local anesthetics to prolong their action at local sites is not recommended, since methoxamine's extended effect may cause excessive restriction of circulation and lead to sloughing of tissue)

(other vasoconstrictors should be used cautiously and in carefully circumscribed quantities, if at all, with local anesthetics when anesthetizing areas with end arteries [such as the fingers, nose, toes, or penis] or with otherwise compromised blood supply; ischemia leading to gangrene may result)

*For ester-type local anesthetics (in addition to those interactions listed above as applying to all local anesthetics)*
Cholinesterase inhibitors such as:
Antimyasthenics
Cyclophosphamide
Demecarium
Echothiophate
Insecticides, neurotoxic, possibly including large quantities of topical malathion
Isoflurophate
Thiotepa
(concurrent use with an ester-type local anesthetic may inhibit the metabolism of the anesthetic leading to increased risk of toxicity)

Sulfonamides
(antibacterial activity may be antagonized by ester-type local anesthetics, which are metabolized to PABA or PABA derivatives)

*For concurrent use of sympathomimetic vasoconstrictors such as epinephrine, levonordefrin, norepinephrine, or phenylephrine (in addition to those interactions listed above and applicable to the specific local anesthetic)*

Note: The risk of a significant systemic effect resulting from an interaction between any of the following and a vasoconstrictor-containing local anesthetic solution depends on the total dose (volume and concentration) of vasoconstrictor administered and on factors affecting the rate of absorption of the vasoconstrictor (site and route of administration and potential for inadvertent intravascular administration).

Alpha-adrenergic blocking agents, such as
Labetalol
Phenoxybenzamine
Phentolamine
Prazosin
Tolazoline or
Other medications with alpha-adrenergic blocking action, such as
» Droperidol
» Haloperidol
Loxapine
» Phenothiazines
Thioxanthenes or
Vasodilators, rapidly acting, such as nitrates
(these medications may reduce the efficacy of the vasoconstrictor)

(in patients receiving epinephrine, levonordefrin, or norepinephrine, but not phenylephrine, alpha-adrenergic blockade may result in unopposed beta-adrenergic activity with a risk of severe hypotension and tachycardia)

(vasoconstrictors may also decrease the therapeutic effects of vasodilators, including the antianginal effects of nitrates)

» Anesthetics, hydrocarbon inhalation
(halothane and, to a much lesser extent, enflurane, isoflurane, or methoxyflurane may sensitize the heart to the effects of a sympathomimetic vasoconstrictor; concurrent use with a vasoconstrictor may cause dose-related cardiac arrhythmias)

» Antidepressants, tricyclic or
» Maprotiline
(concurrent use may potentiate the cardiovascular effects of the vasoconstrictor, possibly resulting in arrhythmias, tachycardia, or severe hypertension or hyperpyrexia)

## 142   Anesthetics (Parenteral-Local)

Antihypertensives
   (antihypertensive effects may be decreased by vasoconstrictors; monitoring of blood pressure is recommended)

» Beta-adrenergic blocking agents, including ophthalmic agents
   (concurrent use of nonselective beta-adrenergic blocking agents with a vasoconstrictor may result in unopposed alpha-adrenergic activity with a dose-dependent risk of hypertension and bradycardia with possible heart block)

CNS stimulation–producing medications, other, (see *Appendix II*), especially

» Cocaine, mucosal-local
   (concurrent use with a vasoconstrictor may result in excessive CNS stimulation, leading to nervousness, irritability, insomnia, and possibly convulsions or cardiac arrhythmias; close observation of the patient is recommended)

   (concurrent use of other sympathomimetics with vasoconstrictors also increases the risk of adverse cardiovascular effects; although vasoconstrictor-containing local anesthetic solutions are sometimes used in conjunction with low doses of cocaine for mucous membrane anesthesia, caution is recommended)

   (concurrent use of doxapram, mazindol, or methylphenidate with a vasoconstrictor may also increase the pressor effects of the vasoconstrictor; concurrent use may also increase the pressor effect of doxapram)

» Digitalis glycosides or
Levodopa
   (concurrent use with a vasoconstrictor may increase the risk of cardiac arrhythmias)

Ergot derivatives, including antimigraine agents and oxytocics
   (the vasoconstrictive effects of ergot derivatives may be additive to those of sympathomimetic vasoconstrictors; concurrent or sequential administration may cause severe, persistent hypertension; rarely, rupture of a cerebral blood vessel has occurred postpartum after an ergot-type oxytocic was administered within 3 to 4 hours following caudal block anesthesia with a vasoconstrictor)

Monoamine oxidase (MAO) inhibitors, including furazolidone, procarbazine, and selegiline
   (concurrent use may prolong and intensify cardiac stimulant and vasopressor effects of phenylephrine, possibly leading to headache, cardiac arrhythmias, and/or severe, sustained hypertension)

Rauwolfia alkaloids
   (in addition to possibly decreasing the antihypertensive effect of rauwolfia alkaloids, concurrent use may theoretically prolong the duration of action of the vasoconstrictor, by preventing uptake into storage granules; a "denervation supersensitivity" response is also possible; although problems with systemic vasoconstrictors have not been reported, a significant increase in blood pressure has been documented with administration of phenylephrine ophthalmic drops to patients taking reserpine; caution and close observation are recommended)

Ritodrine
   (concurrent use with epinephrine, levonordefrin, or norepinephrine may increase the effect of either medication and the risk of side effects)

Thyroid hormones
   (concurrent use with a sympathomimetic agent may increase the risk of coronary insufficiency in patients with coronary artery disease; dosage adjustment of the sympathomimetic is recommended, although the risk is reduced in euthyroid patients)

**Laboratory value alterations**
The following have been selected on the basis of their potential clinical significance (possible effect in parentheses where appropriate)—not necessarily inclusive (» = major clinical significance):

With diagnostic test results
   Pancreatic function determinations using bentiromide
     (administration of PABA-derivative local anesthetics or of lidocaine within 3 days before the bentiromide test may invalidate the test results because these anesthetics are metabolized to PABA or other arylamines and will therefore increase the true or apparent quantity of PABA recovered)

**Medical considerations/Contraindications**
The medical considerations/contraindications included have been selected on the basis of their potential clinical significance (reasons given in parentheses where appropriate)—not necessarily inclusive (» = major clinical significance).

Note:  A standard reference source should be consulted for more specific information concerning medical problems that may apply to specific local anesthetic procedures.

*Except under special circumstances, this medication should not be used when the following medical problems exist:*

*For prilocaine only*
» Methemoglobinemia
   (may be induced or exacerbated)

*For subarachnoid block*
» Complete heart block or
» Hemorrhage, severe or
» Hypotension, severe or
» Shock
   (may be exacerbated by cardiac depressant effects and vasodilation; also, metabolism of amides may be decreased because of reduced hepatic blood flow)

» Local infection at site of proposed lumbar puncture
   (lumbar puncture may spread infection into the arachnoid space; also, infection may alter pH at site of injection, resulting in decrease or loss of local anesthetic effect)

» Septicemia
   (decreased patient tolerance to CNS stimulant effects)

*Risk-benefit should be considered when the following medical problems exist:*

*For all local anesthetic usage*
Any condition in which hepatic blood flow may be decreased, such as:
Congestive heart failure or
Hepatic disease or impairment
   (increased risk of toxicity because of reduced clearance, especially with amides; a decrease in dosage and/or an increase in the interval between doses may be necessary, especially with lidocaine)

» Cardiovascular function impairment, especially heart block or shock
   (may be exacerbated by cardiac depressant effects)

» Drug sensitivity, history of, especially to the anesthetic being considered for use and chemically related anesthetics or other compounds
   (increased risk of hypersensitivity reactions)

» Inflammation and/or infection in region of injection
   (may alter pH at site of injection resulting in decrease or loss of anesthetic effect)

Plasma cholinesterase deficiency—for esters
   (increased risk of toxicity because of decreased metabolism)

Renal disease
   (anesthetic or metabolites may accumulate)

Caution is also recommended in very young, elderly, acutely ill, or debilitated patients, who may be more susceptible to systemic toxicity induced by local anesthetics.

*For paracervical administration in obstetrics*
Fetal distress, pre-existing or
Prematurity or
Postmaturity or
Toxemia of pregnancy or
Uteroplacental insufficiency, pre-existing
   (increased risk of fetal bradycardia and acidosis)

Note:  Use of chloroprocaine is not recommended if prematurity, pre-existing fetal distress, or toxemia of pregnancy is present because its safety in these conditions has not been established.

*For peridural (caudal or lumbar epidural) anesthesia*
Neurological disease, pre-existing

Septicemia
   (decreased patient tolerance to CNS stimulant effects)

Spinal deformity that may interfere with administration and/or effectiveness of local anesthetic

*For subarachnoid anesthesia*
Backache, chronic
   (may be exacerbated)

» CNS disease, pre-existing, attributable to infection, tumor or other causes

» Coagulation defects induced by anticoagulant therapy or hematologic disorders
   (trauma to a blood vessel during administration may result in uncontrollable CNS or soft tissue hemorrhage)

Headache, pre-existing, especially history of migraine
   (may be induced or exacerbated)

Hemorrhagic spinal fluid
   (risk of inadvertent intravascular administration)

Hypertension

Hypotension
   (may be exacerbated by cardiac depressant and vasodilating effects)

Paresthesias, persistent
Psychosis, hysteria or uncooperative patient
Spinal conditions or deformities that may interfere with administration and/or effectiveness of anesthetic

*For vasoconstrictor-containing preparations*
Asthma
(increased risk of anaphylactic or bronchospastic allergic-like reactions induced by the sulfites in commercially available solutions)
» Cardiac disease or arrhythmias or
Diabetes mellitus or
» Hyperthyroidism
(cardiac stimulant effects may be detrimental to patients with these conditions)
» Hypertension or
» Vascular disease, peripheral
(exaggerated vasoconstrictor response may occur, leading to increased risk of severe hypertension or ischemic injury or necrosis)

**Patient monitoring**
The following may be especially important in patient monitoring (other tests may be warranted in some patients, depending on condition; » = major clinical significance):
Cardiovascular status and
Respiratory status and
State of consciousness
(should be monitored after each local anesthetic injection to detect impending CNS and/or cardiovascular toxicity)
Fetal heart rate
(should be monitored during paracervical administration in obstetrics to detect fetal bradycardia)

## Side/Adverse Effects
Note: Adverse reactions are generally dose-related and may result from high plasma concentrations of anesthetic caused by inadvertent intravascular administration, excessive dosage, or rapid absorption from the injection site as well as reduced patient tolerance, idiosyncrasy, or hypersensitivity.

Adverse effects are also related to the specific local anesthetic used and the route and site of administration. Small doses of local anesthetics injected into the head and neck area (including retrobulbar, dental, and stellate ganglion blocks) or in the tracheobronchial area may produce adverse reactions similar to those caused by inadvertent intravascular injection of larger doses. Also, unintentional subarachnoid administration during intended performance of a peridural block or a nerve block near the vertebral column (especially in the head and neck area) may result in adverse effects that depend at least partially on the quantity of anesthetic administered subdurally.

Systemic reactions may occur rapidly or may be delayed for up to 30 minutes following administration.

The following side/adverse effects have been selected on the basis of their potential clinical significance (possible signs and symptoms in parentheses where appropriate)—not necessarily inclusive:

**Those indicating need for medical attention**
Incidence less frequent or rare
*Back pain; bradycardia* (dizziness); *cardiac arrhythmias* (irregular heartbeat); *chest pain*—may be sympathomimetic effect caused by vasoconstrictor added to local anesthetic, or may be caused by decreased perfusion resulting from hypotension; *dizziness; drowsiness; headache; hives* (raised red swellings on the skin, lips, tongue, or in the throat); *hypertension*—may be sympathomimetic effect caused by vasoconstrictor added to local anesthetic; *hypotension* (dizziness); *hypothermia* (shivering); *impotence* (loss of sexual function); *incontinence, fecal and/or urinary* (inability to hold bowel movement and/or urine)—may indicate *cauda equina syndrome*; *methemoglobinemia* (bluish lips and fingernails; breathing problems; dizziness; fatigue; headache; rapid heart rate; weakness); *nausea and/or vomiting; numbness or tingling of lips and mouth, prolonged*—may be caused when an anesthetic is used for dental anesthesia; *paralysis of legs*—may indicate *cauda equina syndrome*; *paresthesias* (tingling or "pins and needles" sensation )—may indicate *cauda equina syndrome*; *persistent anesthesia* (numbness); *pruritus* (itching); *respiratory paralysis* (inability to breath without assistance); *restlessness*—may be caused by vasoconstrictor added to local anesthetic; *seizures* (convulsions); *skin rash; tachycardia* (rapid heart rate)—may be caused by vasoconstrictor added to local anesthetic; *trismus of facial muscles* (difficulty in opening the mouth)—may occur when an anesthetic is used for dental anesthesia; *unconsciousness; vasodilation, peripheral* (dizziness)

Note: Anaphylactoid reactions, including shock, have been reported rarely. The effectiveness of a small test dose in predicting the risk of allergic reactions has not been determined.

Motor and sensory block extending higher on the trunk of the body than intended may occur following subarachnoid administration of local anesthetics. This may also occur following inadvertent subarachnoid administration during intended performance of a peridural block. Occasionally paralysis of chest wall muscles may result in *respiratory paralysis*.

Some patients receiving lidocaine for spinal anesthesia have developed neurologic complications following anesthesia. The neurologic complications usually are temporary *paresthesias* and *back pain (transient radicular irritation)*. However, persistant *paresthesia, paralysis of legs*, or impairment of bodily functions (e.g., *incontinence*) may indicate a serious neurologic complication, *cauda equina syndrome*. Uneven distribution of hyperbaric lidocaine following spinal administration may contribute to *cauda equina syndrome*. In cases of *transient radicular irritation*, symptoms resolve within a few days to a few weeks. However, neurotoxic effects may not resolve in cases of *cauda equina syndrome*. Other anesthetics may cause *cauda equina syndrome* also.

## Overdose
For specific information on the agents used in the management of a local anesthetic overdose, see:
- *Benzodiazepines (Systemic)* monograph;
- Ephedrine in *Sympathomimetic Agents—Cardiovascular Use (Parenteral-Systemic)*;
- Mephentermine in *Sympathomimetic Agents—Cardiovascular Use (Parenteral-Systemic)*;
- Metaraminol in *Sympathomimetic Agents—Cardiovascular Use (Parenteral-Systemic)*;
- *Methylene Blue (Systemic)* monograph;
- *Neuromuscular Blocking Agents (Systemic)* monograph; and/or
- Thiopental in *Anesthetics, Barbiturate (Systemic)* monograph.

For more information on the management of overdose or unintentional ingestion, **contact a Poison Control Center** (see *Poison Control Center Listing*).

**Clinical effects of overdose**
The following effects have been selected on the basis of their potential clinical significance (possible signs and symptoms in parentheses where appropriate)—not necessarily inclusive:
Acute
*Apnea; circulatory depression; methemoglobinemia; seizures*

**Treatment of overdose**
Specific treatment—
For circulatory depression: Administering a vasopressor and intravenous fluids is recommended. For maternal hypotension during obstetrical anesthesia, it is recommended that the patient be placed on her left side, if possible, to correct aortocaval compression by the gravid uterus. Delivery of the fetus may improve the response of the obstetric patient to cardiopulmonary resuscitation.
For seizures: Protect the patient and administer oxygen immediately. If seizures do not respond to respiratory support, administering a benzodiazepine such as diazepam or an ultrashort-acting barbiturate such as thiopental or thiamylal intravenously is recommended. The fact that these agents, especially the barbiturates, may cause circulatory depression when administered intravenously must be kept in mind. A neuromuscular blocking agent may also be used to decrease the muscular manifestations of persistent seizures if positive-pressure ventilation can be immediately provided. Hypoxia, hypercapnea, and acidosis can develop quickly following the onset of seizures.
For methemoglobinemia: If methemoglobinemia does not respond to administration of oxygen, administration of methylene blue is recommended.
Monitoring—Blood pressure, heart rate, neurologic status, and respiratory status should be monitored continuously.
Supportive care—Securing and maintaining a patent airway, administering oxygen, and instituting assisted or controlled respiration as required. In some patients, endotracheal intubation may be required.

## Patient Consultation

As an aid to patient consultation, refer to *Advice for the Patient, Anesthetics (Parenteral-Local)*.

In providing consultation, consider emphasizing the following selected information (» = major clinical significance):

### Before receiving this medication
» Conditions affecting use, especially:
  Allergies to the anesthetic considered for use, related anesthetics, other related compounds, and additives (methylparaben, sulfites)
  Pregnancy—Potential rare unwanted effects with obstetrical use
  Use in children—Increased risk of systemic toxicity
  Use in the elderly—Increased risk of systemic toxicity
  Other medications, especially nonselective beta-adrenergic blocking agents, CNS depression–producing medications, cocaine, digitalis glycosides, droperidol, haloperidol, hydrocarbon inhalation anesthetics, maprotiline, phenothiazines, tricyclic antidepressants, or vasoconstrictors such as epinephrine, methoxamine or phenylephrine
  Other medical problems, especially cardiac disease or arrhythmias, cardiovascular function impairment, coagulation defects, hypertension, hyperthyroidism, local infection at the site of injection or proposed lumbar puncture, methemoglobinemia, peripheral vascular disease, pre-existing CNS disease

### Proper use of this medication
  Proper dosing

### Precautions after receiving this medication
  Caution that injury may occur undetected while numbness persists in the affected area; using care to prevent injury, including not eating or chewing gum following dental anesthesia (to prevent biting trauma)

### Side/adverse effects
  Signs and/or symptoms of potential side effects, especially back pain, bradycardia, cardiac arrhythmias, chest pain, dizziness, drowsiness, headache, hives, hypertension, hypotension, hypothermia, impotence, incontinence (fecal and/or urinary), methemoglobinemia, nausea and/or vomiting, numbness or tingling of lips and mouth (prolonged), paralysis of legs, paresthesias, persistent anesthesia, pruritus, respiratory paralysis, restlessness, seizures, skin rash, tachycardia, trismus of facial muscles, vasodilation (peripheral)

## General Dosing Information

The safety and effectiveness of local anesthetics depend upon proper dosage, correct technique, adequate precautions, and readiness for emergencies. *Resuscitative equipment, oxygen, and other resuscitative drugs should be immediately available when any local anesthetic is used.*

A standard text should be consulted for specific techniques and procedures for administering local anesthetics.

The dosage of local anesthetics depends on the specific anesthetic procedure; vascularity of the tissues at or near the site of injection; specific nerve, plexus, or fiber to be blocked; type of surgery being performed (number of neuronal segments to be blocked, depth of anesthesia and degree of muscle relaxation required, and duration of anesthesia desired); and patient variables such as age and weight.

The recommended adult doses are given as a guideline for use in the average adult. *The actual dosage and maximum dosage must be individualized*, based on the age, size, and physical status of the patient and the expected rate of systemic absorption from the injection site. The lowest dosage (volume and concentration) that produces the desired results should be used.

Lower doses should be used for pediatric, geriatric, acutely ill, or debilitated patients and patients with cardiac or hepatic disease. Lower doses are also required for repeated injections (as for multiple nerve blocks or continuous catheter [intermittent] administration techniques), and for nerve blocks in highly vascular areas, in order to prevent excessively high plasma concentrations.

Local anesthetics may be administered as single injections or continuously or intermittently through an indwelling catheter. Fractional doses are especially recommended for peridural blocks.

Local anesthetics should be injected slowly, with frequent aspirations before and during the injection, to reduce the risk of inadvertent intravascular administration. Additional aspirations should be performed before and during each supplemental injection via an indwelling catheter. However, intravascular administration is possible even when aspiration for blood is negative. In one study, intravascular administration occurred despite negative results on aspiration in 20% of patients undergoing dental treatment.

For central neural blocks in obstetrical anesthesia, the anesthetic should not be injected during a strong uterine contraction or while the patient is bearing down because excessively high levels of anesthesia may result.

For peridural blocks, injection of a small test dose (usually 2 to 5 mL of solution, consult manufacturers' product information for details) is recommended so that the patient can be monitored for signs of inadvertent subarachnoid or intravascular administration. If clinical conditions permit, the use of a vasoconstrictor-containing solution is recommended because circulatory changes produced by a vasoconstrictor may indicate intravascular administration. The test dose should be repeated if a patient is moved in any manner that may cause displacement of the catheter.

For retrobulbar block, lack of corneal sensation should not be relied upon to determine readiness for surgery because lack of corneal sensation usually precedes clinically acceptable external ocular muscle akinesia.

The extent and degree of subarachnoid block depend on the position of the patient during and immediately after injection, dosage, specific gravity of the solution, volume of solution used, force of injection, and the level of puncture. Hyperbaric solutions (with dextrose added to render the solution heavier than cerebrospinal fluid [CSF]) are usually used for low spinal anesthesia. Isobaric solutions (having the same specific gravity as CSF) produce anesthesia at the level of intrathecal injection. Hypobaric solutions (diluted to have a lower specific gravity than CSF) are used to produce anesthesia of thoracic structures and for low spinal anesthesia. A standard text and/or manufacturers' product information may be consulted for details concerning dilution and positioning of patient during and following administration.

Vasoconstrictors decrease the rate of local clearance of the local anesthetic, thereby reducing the risk of systemic toxic reactions, prolonging the anesthetic effect, increasing the frequency of complete conduction blocks at low anesthetic concentrations, and permitting larger maximum single doses of anesthetic to be administered. Epinephrine 1:200,000 is the most commonly used vasoconstrictor for most purposes; levonordefrin, norepinephrine, and phenylephrine may also be used. In dentistry, epinephrine 1:50,000 to 1:200,000 and levonordefrin 1:20,000 are the most commonly used vasoconstrictors.

Solutions containing a vasoconstrictor should be used cautiously and in carefully circumscribed quantities, if at all, in tissues supplied by end arteries (such as the fingers, nose, toes, or penis) or having otherwise compromised blood supply; ischemia leading to gangrene may result. Also, a vasoconstrictor should not be injected repeatedly at the same site for dental procedures because reduced blood flow and increased oxygen consumption in the affected tissues may cause tissue anoxia, delayed healing, edema, or necrosis at the injection site.

Intravenous access should be obtained prior to the placement of major nerve blocks to permit the administration of emergency drugs during resuscitation if a serious adverse reaction occurs.

### For treatment of adverse effects
Recommended treatment consists of the following:
- For seizures—If seizures do not respond to respiratory support, administering a benzodiazepine such as diazepam (in 2.5-mg increments) or an ultrashort-acting barbiturate such as thiopental or thiamylal (in 50- to 100-mg increments) intravenously every 2 to 3 minutes is recommended. The fact that these agents, especially the barbiturates, may cause circulatory depression when administered intravenously must be kept in mind. A neuromuscular blocking agent may also be used to decrease the muscular manifestations of persistent seizures; artificial respiration is mandatory if such an agent is used.
- For methemoglobinemia—If methemoglobinemia does not respond to administration of oxygen, administration of methylene blue (intravenous, 1 to 2 mg per kg of body weight (mg/kg) as a 1% solution, over a 5-minute period) is recommended.

---

# ARTICAINE

## Summary of Differences

Indications:
  Indicated for dental infiltration or nerve block.
Note: Anesthesia of mandibular pulpal and lingual soft tissue and of maxillary palatal soft tissue with buccal infiltration of articaine is not effective in all patients who require the administration of articaine by nerve block technique. In a study in adults, there was no difference between prilocaine and articaine in providing successful anesthesia of mandibular pulpal and lingual soft tissue and of maxillary palatal soft tissue with buccal infiltration. After buccal infiltration of articaine, anesthesia was successful in 63% of cases for the mandibular pulp, 50% for mandibular lingual tissue, and 40% for

palatal tissue. The use of mandibular infiltration in pediatric patients for procedures in primary mandibular teeth has had mixed success, with one study showing results similar to those seen in adults.

Pharmacology/pharmacokinetics:
  Physicochemical characteristics—
    Chemical group: Amide-type local anesthetic with an ester linkage and a thiophene ring.
    Molecular weight: 284.38.
  Half-life—
    1.2 hours.
  Onset of action—
    Rapid.
  Duration of action—
    Intermediate (1 to 3 hours).

Precautions:
  Cross-sensitivity and/or related problems—
    May occur with other amide-type local anesthetics.
  Pediatrics—
    Although articaine is not approved for use in children younger than 4 years of age, a retrospective study of its use in 211 pediatric patients younger than 4 years of age did not reveal any pediatrics-specific problems that would limit its use in children.

## Additional Dosing Information

See *General Dosing Information*.

## Parenteral Dosage Forms

Note: Bracketed uses in the *Dosage Forms* section refer to categories of use and/or indications that are not included in U.S. product labeling.

### ARTICAINE HYDROCHLORIDE WITH EPINEPHRINE INJECTION

**Usual adult and adolescent dose**
[Dental infiltration anesthesia]—
  20 to 100 mg (0.5 to 2.5 mL) as a 4% solution.
[Dental nerve block anesthesia]—
  20 to 136 mg (0.5 to 3.4 mL) as a 4% solution.
[Oral surgery anesthesia]—
  40 to 204 mg (1 to 5.1 mL) as a 4% solution.

**Usual adult prescribing limits**
7 mg per kg of body weight.

**Usual pediatric dose**
Children younger than 4 years of age—Safety and efficacy have not been established.
Children 4 to 12 years of age—Dosage must be individualized, based on the age and weight of the patient.

**Usual pediatric prescribing limits**
Children 4 to 12 years of age—5 mg per kg of body weight.

**Strength(s) usually available**
U.S.—
  Not commercially available.
Canada—
  4% (40 mg per mL), with epinephrine 1:100,000 (Rx) [*Ultracaine D-S Forte* (sodium metabisulfite 0.5 mg per mL; methylparaben 1 mg per mL); *Astracaine 4% Forte* (sodium metabisulfite)].
  4% (40 mg per mL), with epinephrine 1:200,000 (Rx) [*Ultracaine D-S* (sodium metabisulfite 0.5 mg per mL; methylparaben 1 mg per mL); *Astracaine 4%* (sodium metabisulfite)].

**Packaging and storage**
Store below 25 °C (77 °F), unless otherwise specified by manufacturer. Protect from freezing. Protect from light.

---

## BUPIVACAINE

## Summary of Differences

Indications:
  Except as noted below, indicated (without epinephrine) for retrobulbar block; indicated (with or without epinephrine) for caudal or lumbar epidural block, local infiltration, peripheral nerve block, and sympathetic block; indicated (with epinephrine) for dental infiltration or nerve block; and indicated (with dextrose) for subarachnoid block.
  Paracervical administration not recommended.
  Not recommended for intravenous regional anesthesia (Bier block).

Pharmacology/pharmacokinetics:
  Physicochemical characteristics—
    Chemical group: Amide-type local anesthetic.
    Molecular weight: bupivacaine hydrochloride—342.91.
    pKa: 8.1.
    Lipid solubility: High.
  Protein binding—
    Very high.
  Half-life—
    3.5 hours (adults); 8.1 to 14 hours (neonates).
  Onset of action—
    Intermediate.
  Duration of action—
    Long (3 to 10 hours).
  Elimination—
    5% of a dose may be excreted unchanged.

Precautions:
  Cross-sensitivity and/or related problems—
    May occur rarely with other amide-type local anesthetics.
  Pregnancy—
    Embryocidal effects have been demonstrated in rats and rabbits.
  Breast-feeding—
    Distributed into breast milk.
  Pediatrics—
    Infants up to 9 months of age may have low plasma concentrations of alpha$_1$-acid glycoprotein (AAG). This results in an increased unbound fraction of bupivacaine, and may lead to systemic toxicity.
    Reduced clearance of bupivacaine in pediatric patients may be more important than AAG concentrations in causing toxicity. Neonates may have total body clearance of bupivacaine only one third to one half the clearance of adults.

Drug interactions and/or related problems:
  Interaction with cimetidine.
  Interaction with halothane.

Side/adverse effects:
  Prolonged cardiovascular depression and arrhythmias have been reported. The cardiotoxicity of bupivacaine may be increased if the patient experiences hypothermia, hyponatremia, hyperkalemia or myocardial ischemia. Concomitant use of halothane may cause increased cardiotoxicity of bupivacaine.

## Additional Dosing Information

See also *General Dosing Information*.

Bupivacaine 0.25% generally produces incomplete motor block and is used when muscle relaxation is not important. However, intercostal nerve block with this strength of bupivacaine may produce complete motor block for intra-abdominal surgery in some patients.

Bupivacaine 0.5% produces motor block and some muscle relaxation when used for caudal, epidural, or nerve block. With continuous catheter (intermittent) administration techniques, repeat doses increase the degree of motor block. The first repeat dose of 0.5% bupivacaine may produce complete motor block.

Bupivacaine 0.75% produces complete motor block and complete muscle relaxation. When used for epidural block, the 0.75% solution is intended for single-dose administration only; it should not be used for intermittent administration techniques.

Bupivacaine 0.75% is not recommended for epidural block in obstetrics because inadvertent intravascular injection has caused maternal cardiac arrest. However, lower concentrations may be used. When bupivacaine is used for epidural block in obstetrics, the dose of bupivacaine should be chosen to provide safe and adequate relief of pain without causing toxicity, prolonged hypotension, or loss of motor strength. The majority of obstetric patients will achieve analgesia with continuous epidural infusions of 0.0625 to 0.125% bupivacaine at 10 to 15 mL per hour. The addition of subarachnoid narcotics or epidural fentanyl (1 to 2 mcg per mL) or sufentanil (0.1 to 0.2 mcg per mL) usually will allow the use of a lower concentration or a lower infusion rate of bupivacaine. The use of the lowest possible concentration usually will reduce the risk of fetal or maternal toxicity while providing appropriate analgesia. However, in some patients where the goals are different, e.g., blood pressure control or the obliteration of any contraction sensation, higher concentrations may be required.

## Parenteral Dosage Forms

Note: Bracketed uses in the *Dosage Forms* section refer to categories of use and/or indications that are not included in U.S. product labeling.

### BUPIVACAINE HYDROCHLORIDE INJECTION USP

**Usual adult and adolescent dose**
Caudal anesthesia—
  Moderate motor block: 37.5 to 75 mg (15 to 30 mL) as a 0.25% solution, repeated once every three hours as needed.

Moderate to complete motor block: 75 to 150 mg (15 to 30 mL) as a 0.5% solution, repeated once every three hours as needed.

Epidural anesthesia—
Partial to moderate motor block: 25 to 50 mg (10 to 20 mL) as a 0.25% solution, repeated once every three hours as needed.
Moderate to complete motor block: 50 to 100 mg (10 to 20 mL) as a 0.5% solution, repeated once every three hours as needed.
Complete motor block: 75 to 150 mg (10 to 20 mL) as a 0.75% solution.

Epidural obstetric analgesia—
Continuous infusion, 6.25 to 18.75 mg per hour as a 0.0625 to 0.125% solution.

Local infiltration—
Single dose: 175 mg (70 mL) as a 0.25% solution.

Peripheral nerve block—
Moderate to complete motor block: 12.5 to 175 mg (5 to 70 mL) as a 0.25% solution; or 25 to 175 mg (5 to 37.5 mL) as a 0.5% solution. Dosage may be repeated every three hours if necessary.

Retrobulbar block—
15 to 30 mg (2 to 4 mL) as a 0.75% solution.

Sympathetic block—
50 to 125 mg (20 to 50 mL) as a 0.25% solution, repeated once every three hours as needed.

**Usual adult prescribing limits**
175 mg as a single dose or 400 mg per day.

**Usual pediatric dose**
Children weighing over 10 kg—
[Caudal analgesia, single dose]:
1 to 2.5 mg per kg of body weight as a 0.125 or 0.25% solution.
[Caudal analgesia, continuous infusion]:
0.2 to 0.4 mg per kg of body weight per hour as a 0.1, 0.125 or 0.25% solution, not to exceed 0.4 mg per kg of body weight per hour.
[Caudal or epidural anesthesia, single dose]:
1 to 2.5 mg per kg of body weight as a 0.125 or 0.25% solution.
[Caudal or epidural anesthesia, continuous infusion]:
0.2 to 0.4 mg per kg of body weight per hour as a 0.1, 0.125 or 0.25% solution, not to exceed 0.4 mg per kg of body weight per hour.
[Local infiltration]:
0.5 to 2.5 mg per kg of body weight as a 0.25 or 0.5% solution.
[Peripheral nerve block]:
0.3 to 2.5 mg per kg of body weight as a 0.25 or 0.5% solution.

Infants and children weighing up to 10 kg—
[Caudal analgesia, single dose]:
1 to 1.25 mg per kg of body weight as a 0.125 or 0.25% solution.
[Caudal analgesia, continuous infusion]:
0.1 to 0.2 mg per kg of body weight per hour as a 0.1, 0.125 or 0.25% solution, not to exceed 0.2 mg per kg of body weight per hour.
[Caudal or epidural anesthesia, single dose]:
1 to 1.25 mg per kg of body weight as a 0.125 or 0.25% solution.
[Caudal or epidural anesthesia, continuous infusion]:
0.1 to 0.2 mg per kg of body weight per hour as a 0.1, 0.125 or 0.25% solution, not to exceed 0.2 mg per kg of body weight per hour.
[Local infiltration]:
0.5 to 2.5 mg per kg of body weight as a 0.25 or 0.5% solution.
[Peripheral nerve block]:
0.3 to 2.5 mg per kg of body weight as a 0.25 or 0.5% solution.

Note: Bupivacaine is approved in the U.S. for use in patients older than 12 years of age. Bupivacaine is approved in Canada for use in patients older than 2 years of age.

**Usual pediatric prescribing limits**
[Local infiltration or]
[Peripheral nerve block]—
The usual maximum dose is 1 mL per kg of body weight of 0.25% bupivacaine. If bupivacaine 0.5% is used, the usual maximum is 0.5 mL per kg of body weight. The maximum dose to be used depends on the site of administration.

**Strength(s) usually available**
U.S.—
With preservative (methylparaben 1 mg per mL):
0.25% (2.5 mg per mL) (Rx) [*Marcaine; Sensorcaine;* GENERIC].
0.5% (5 mg per mL) (Rx) [*Marcaine; Sensorcaine;* GENERIC].
Without preservative:
0.25% (2.5 mg per mL) (Rx) [*Marcaine; Sensorcaine-MPF;* GENERIC].
0.5% (5 mg per mL) (Rx) [*Marcaine; Sensorcaine-MPF;* GENERIC].
0.75% (7.5 mg per mL) (Rx) [*Marcaine; Sensorcaine-MPF;* GENERIC].
Canada—
With preservative (methylparaben 1 mg per mL):
0.25% (2.5 mg per mL) (Rx) [*Marcaine*].
0.5% (5 mg per mL) (Rx) [*Marcaine*].
Without preservative:
0.25% (2.5 mg per mL) (Rx) [*Marcaine; Sensorcaine*].
0.5% (5 mg per mL) (Rx) [*Marcaine; Sensorcaine*].
0.75% (7.5 mg per mL) (Rx) [*Marcaine*].

**Packaging and storage**
Store below 40 °C (104 °F), preferably between 15 and 30 °C (59 and 86 °F), unless otherwise specified by manufacturer. Protect from freezing.

**Stability**
May be autoclaved.
For chemical disinfection of container surface, 91% isopropyl alcohol or 70% ethyl alcohol without denaturants is recommended; solutions containing heavy metals should not be used.
Unused portions of solutions without a preservative must be discarded.

# BUPIVACAINE HYDROCHLORIDE AND EPINEPHRINE INJECTION USP

**Usual adult and adolescent dose**
Dental—
For infiltration and nerve block in maxillary and mandibular area: 9 mg (1.8 mL) of bupivacaine hydrochloride as a 0.5% solution with epinephrine 1:200,000 per injection site. A second dose may be administered if necessary to produce adequate anesthesia after allowing up to 10 minutes for onset.
Other indications—
See *Bupivacaine Hydrochloride Injection USP*. Administration of epinephrine concurrently with the local anesthetic may permit use of doses somewhat larger than those listed.

**Usual adult prescribing limits**
In dentistry—
90 mg of bupivacaine hydrochloride per dental appointment.
Other indications—
225 mg as a single dose or 400 mg per day of bupivacaine hydrochloride.

**Usual pediatric dose**
See *Bupivacaine Hydrochloride Injection USP*.

**Strength(s) usually available**
U.S.—
With preservative (methylparaben 1 mg per mL):
0.25% (2.5 mg per mL), with epinephrine 1:200,000 (Rx) [*Marcaine* (sodium metabisulfite 0.5 mg per mL; edetate calcium disodium); *Sensorcaine* (sodium metabisulfite 0.5 mg per mL); GENERIC].
0.5% (5 mg per mL), with epinephrine 1:200,000 (Rx) [*Marcaine* (sodium metabisulfite 0.5 mg per mL; edetate calcium disodium); *Sensorcaine* (sodium metabisulfite 0.5 mg per mL); GENERIC].
Without preservative:
0.25% (2.5 mg per mL), with epinephrine 1:200,000 (Rx) [*Marcaine* (sodium metabisulfite 0.5 mg per mL; edetate calcium disodium); *Sensorcaine-MPF* (sodium metabisulfite 0.5 mg per mL; citric acid, anhydrous 0.2 mg per mL); GENERIC].
0.5% (5 mg per mL), with epinephrine 1:200,000 (Rx) [*Marcaine* (sodium metabisulfite 0.5 mg per mL; edetate calcium disodium); *Sensorcaine-MPF* (sodium metabisulfite 0.5 mg per mL; citric acid, anhydrous 0.2 mg per mL); GENERIC].
0.75% (7.5 mg per mL), with epinephrine 1:200,000 (Rx) [*Marcaine* (sodium metabisulfite 0.5 mg per mL; edetate calcium disodium); *Sensorcaine-MPF* (sodium metabisulfite 0.5 mg per mL; citric acid, anhydrous 0.2 mg per mL); GENERIC].
For dental use:
0.5% (5 mg per mL; 9 mg per 1.8-mL dental cartridge), with epinephrine 1:200,000 (Rx) [*Marcaine* (sodium metabisulfite 0.5 mg per mL; edetate calcium disodium)].
Canada—
Without preservative:
0.25% (2.5 mg per mL), with epinephrine 1:200,000 (Rx) [*Marcaine* (sodium bisulfite 0.5 mg per mL; edetate calcium disodium); *Sensorcaine* (sodium bisulfite 0.55 mg per mL; citric acid 0.2 mg per mL)].
0.5% (5 mg per mL), with epinephrine 1:200,000 (Rx) [*Marcaine* (sodium bisulfite 0.5 mg per mL; edetate calcium disodium); *Sensorcaine* (sodium bisulfite 0.55 mg per mL; citric acid 0.2 mg per mL)].

For dental use:
0.5% (5 mg per mL; 9 mg per 1.8-mL dental cartridge), with epinephrine 1:200,000 (Rx) [*Sensorcaine Forte* (sodium metabisulfite 0.55 mg per mL; citric acid 0.2 mg per mL)].

**Packaging and storage**
Store below 40 °C (104 °F), preferably between 15 and 30 °C (59 and 86 °F), unless otherwise specified by manufacturer. Protect from light. Protect from freezing.

**Stability**
On removal of doses from the vial, air is introduced, which slowly oxidizes the epinephrine causing discoloration of the solution and possible loss of potency. Do not use if solution is discolored or contains a precipitate.
Should not be autoclaved. For chemical disinfection of the container surface, 91% isopropyl alcohol or 70% ethyl alcohol without denaturants is recommended; solutions containing heavy metals are not recommended.
Unused portions of solutions without a preservative must be discarded.

## BUPIVACAINE HYDROCHLORIDE IN DEXTROSE INJECTION USP

**Usual adult dose**
Hyperbaric spinal anesthesia—
  Obstetrical anesthesia:
    Normal vaginal delivery—6 mg (0.8 mL) of bupivacaine hydrochloride as a 0.75% solution.
    Cesarean section—7.5 to 10.5 mg (1 to 1.4 mL) of bupivacaine hydrochloride as a 0.75% solution.
  Surgical anesthesia:
    Lower extremity and perineal procedures—7.5 mg (1 mL) of bupivacaine hydrochloride as a 0.75% solution.
    Lower abdominal procedures—12 mg (1.6 mL) of bupivacaine hydrochloride as a 0.75% solution.
    Upper abdominal surgery—15 mg (2 mL) in the horizontal position.

**Usual pediatric dose**
[Hyperbaric spinal anesthesia]—
  0.3 to 0.6 mg per kg of body weight as a 0.75% solution.

**Strength(s) usually available**
U.S.—
  Without preservative:
    0.75% (7.5 mg per mL), with dextrose 8.25% (82.5 mg per mL) (Rx) [*Marcaine Spinal; Sensorcaine-MPF Spinal;* GENERIC].
Canada—
  Without preservative:
    0.75% (7.5 mg per mL), with dextrose 8.25% (82.5 mg per mL) (Rx) [*Marcaine*].

**Packaging and storage**
Store below 40 °C (104 °F), preferably between 15 and 30 °C (59 and 86 °F), unless otherwise specified by manufacturer. Protect from freezing.

**Stability**
May be autoclaved once; with repeated autoclaving or prolonged storage, caramelization of the dextrose may occur, leading to discoloration. Discolored solutions should not be used.
Do not use if solution contains a precipitate.

---

## *CHLOROPROCAINE*

## Summary of Differences

Indications:
  Indicated for caudal or lumbar epidural block, dental infiltration or nerve block, local infiltration, peripheral nerve block, and intravenous regional anesthesia (Bier block).
  Not recommended for subarachnoid administration.
Pharmacology/pharmacokinetics:
  Physicochemical characteristics—
    Chemical group: Ester-type local anesthetic.
    Molecular weight: chloroprocaine hydrochloride—307.22.
    pKa: 9.
  Biotransformation—
    Metabolized to a PABA derivative.
  Half-life—
    19 to 26 seconds (adults); 41 to 45 seconds (neonates).
  Onset of action—
    Rapid.
  Duration of action—
    Short (30 to 60 minutes).

Precautions:
  Cross-sensitivity and/or related problems—
    May occur with PABA, parabens, or other ester-type local anesthetics.
  Pregnancy—
    Paracervical administration not recommended if prematurity, pre-existing fetal distress, or toxemia of pregnancy present, because safety in these conditions has not been established.
    May cause uterine artery constriction.
  Drug interactions and/or related problems—
    Interaction with cholinesterase inhibitors.
    Interaction with sulfonamides.
Side/adverse effects:
  May be especially likely to cause neuropathies.
  More likely than amide-type local anesthetics to cause hypersensitivity reactions.

## Additional Dosing Information

See also *General Dosing Information*.
Epinephrine 1:200,000 may be added to chloroprocaine *without* preservatives to prolong the duration of anesthetic effect.

## Parenteral Dosage Forms

### CHLOROPROCAINE HYDROCHLORIDE INJECTION USP

**Usual adult and adolescent dose**
Caudal anesthesia—
  300 to 500 mg (15 to 25 mL) as a 2% solution; or 450 to 750 mg (15 to 25 mL) as a 3% solution, repeated at forty- to sixty-minute intervals as needed.
Epidural anesthesia (lumbar and sacral regions)—
  40 to 50 mg (2 to 2.5 mL) as a 2% solution per segment; or 60 to 75 mg (2 to 2.5 mL) as a 3% solution per segment. The usual total dose is 300 to 750 mg (15 to 25 mL as a 2 or 3% solution). May be repeated at forty- to sixty-minute intervals using 40 to 120 mg (2 to 6 mL) less than original total dose as a 2% solution or 60 to 180 mg (2 to 6 mL) less than original total dose as a 3% solution.
Local infiltration—
  Depends on site to be infiltrated and extent of surgical procedure.
Nerve block—
  Brachial plexus:
    600 to 800 mg (30 to 40 mL) as a 2% solution.
  Digital:
    30 to 40 mg (3 to 4 mL) as a 1% solution.
  Infraorbital:
    10 to 20 mg (0.5 to 1 mL) as a 2% solution.
  Mandibular:
    40 to 60 mg (2 to 3 mL) as a 2% solution.
  Obstetrics:
    Paracervical block—30 mg (3 mL) as a 1% solution per each of four sites.
    Pudendal block—200 mg (10 mL) as a 2% solution per side.

**Usual adult prescribing limits**
Without epinephrine—
  800 mg per total dose.
With added epinephrine 1:200,000—
  1 gram per total dose.

**Usual pediatric dose**
Local infiltration—
  11 mg per kg of body weight as a 0.5 to 1% solution.
Nerve block—
  11 mg per kg of body weight as a 1 to 1.5% solution.
Note: Dosage must be individualized, based on the age and weight of the patient.

**Strength(s) usually available**
U.S.—
  With preservative (methylparaben 1 mg per mL):
    1% (10 mg per mL) (Rx) [*Nesacaine* (edetate disodium 0.11 mg per mL)].
    2% (20 mg per mL) (Rx) [*Nesacaine* (edetate disodium 0.11 mg per mL)].
  Without preservative:
    2% (20 mg per mL) (Rx) [*Nesacaine-MPF;* GENERIC].
    3% (30 mg per mL) (Rx) [*Nesacaine-MPF;* GENERIC].
Canada—
  Without preservative:
    2% (20 mg per mL) (Rx) [*Nesacaine-CE* (edetate calcium disodium; sodium bisulfite 0.7 mg per mL)].

3% (30 mg per mL) (Rx) [*Nesacaine-CE* (edetate calcium disodium; sodium bisulfite 0.7 mg per mL)].

**Packaging and storage**
Store below 40 °C (104 °F), preferably between 15 and 30 °C (59 and 86 °F), unless otherwise specified by manufacturer. Protect from freezing. Protect from light.

**Preparation of dosage form**
For administration to pediatric patients in concentrations lower than those commercially available—Dilute available concentrations with the quantity of 0.9% sodium chloride injection needed to obtain the required final concentration of local anesthetic solution.

**Stability**
May be autoclaved (prior to addition of epinephrine, if added).
Sterilization of vials with ethylene oxide is not recommended because absorption through the closure may occur.
Solutions may become discolored after prolonged exposure to light. Protection from direct sunlight is recommended. The solution should not be used if discoloration occurs.
Exposure to low temperatures may cause precipitation of chloroprocaine hydrochloride crystals. These crystals usually redissolve when the solution is returned to room temperature. Solutions containing undissolved material should not be used.
Unused portions of solutions without a preservative must be discarded.

---

## *ETIDOCAINE*

## Summary of Differences
Indications:
    Indicated (without epinephrine) for retrobulbar block; indicated (with or without epinephrine) for caudal or lumbar epidural block, local infiltration, and peripheral nerve block; and indicated (with epinephrine) for dental infiltration or nerve block.
Pharmacology/pharmacokinetics:
    Physicochemical characteristics—
        Chemical group: Amide-type local anesthetic.
        Molecular weight: 276.42.
        pKa: 7.74.
        Lipid solubility: High.
    Protein-binding—
        Very high.
    Half-life—
        2.5 hours (adults); 4 to 8 hours (neonates).
    Onset of action—
        Rapid.
    Duration of action—
        Long (3 to 10 hours).
Note: The addition of epinephrine does not prolong the duration of analgesia but allows maintenance of lower plasma concentrations of the anesthetic.
    Elimination—
        Less than 10% of a dose may be excreted unchanged.
Precautions:
    Cross-sensitivity and/or related problems—
        May occur rarely with other amide-type local anesthetics.
    Pregnancy—
        Studies in animals have not shown adverse effects on the fetus.
        Epidural administration not recommended for normal vaginal delivery.
        Not recommended for paracervical administration.
    Pediatrics—
        Infants up to 9 months of age may have low plasma concentrations of alpha$_1$-acid glycoprotein (AAG). This results in an increased unbound fraction of etidocaine, and may lead to systemic toxicity.

## Additional Dosing Information
Etidocaine produces a profound motor block after epidural administration. This may be useful for abdominal surgery, but profound motor block is usually not desirable for normal obstetric delivery.

## Parenteral Dosage Forms

### ETIDOCAINE HYDROCHLORIDE INJECTION
**Usual adult and adolescent dose**
See *Etidocaine Hydrochloride and Epinephrine Injection*. Doses somewhat smaller than those listed may be required when epinephrine is not used concurrently with the local anesthetic.

**Usual adult prescribing limits**
4 mg per kg of body weight or 300 mg per injection.

**Usual pediatric dose**
Dosage has not been established.

**Strength(s) usually available**
U.S.—
    Without preservative:
        1% (10 mg per mL) (Rx) [*Duranest-MPF*].
Canada—
    Not commercially available.

**Packaging and storage**
Store below 40 °C (104 °F), preferably between 15 and 30 °C (59 and 86 °F), unless otherwise specified by manufacturer. Protect from freezing.

**Stability**
May be autoclaved.
Unused portions of solutions must be discarded because they contain no preservative.

### ETIDOCAINE HYDROCHLORIDE AND EPINEPHRINE INJECTION
**Usual adult and adolescent dose**
Caudal anesthesia—
    50 to 150 mg (10 to 30 mL) of etidocaine hydrochloride as a 0.5% solution; or 100 to 300 mg (10 to 30 mL) of etidocaine hydrochloride as a 1% solution. Additional incremental doses may be administered at two- to three-hour intervals as needed.
Lumbar peridural anesthesia—
    Cesarean section or
    Intra-abdominal or pelvic surgery or
    Lower-limb surgery: 100 to 300 mg (10 to 30 mL) of etidocaine hydrochloride as a 1% solution; or 150 to 300 mg (10 to 20 mL) of etidocaine hydrochloride as a 1.5% solution. Additional incremental doses may be administered at two- to three-hour intervals as needed.
    Gynecological procedures: 50 to 150 mg (10 to 30 mL) of etidocaine hydrochloride as a 0.5% solution; or 50 to 200 mg (5 to 20 mL) of etidocaine hydrochloride as a 1% solution. Additional incremental doses may be administered at two- to three-hour intervals as needed.
Dental infiltration or nerve block—
    15 to 75 mg (1 to 5 mL) as a 1.5% solution.
Percutaneous infiltration—
    5 to 400 mg (1 to 80 mL) of etidocaine hydrochloride as a 0.5% solution.
Peripheral nerve block—
    25 to 400 mg (5 to 80 mL) of etidocaine hydrochloride as a 0.5% solution; or 50 to 400 mg (5 to 40 mL) of etidocaine hydrochloride as a 1% solution. Additional incremental doses may be administered at two- to three-hour intervals as needed.

**Usual adult prescribing limits**
5.5 mg per kg of body weight or 400 mg per injection of etidocaine hydrochloride with epinephrine 1:200,000.

**Usual pediatric dose**
Dosage has not been established.

**Strength(s) usually available**
U.S.—
    Without preservative:
        1% (10 mg per mL), with epinephrine 1:200,000 (Rx) [*Duranest-MPF* (sodium metabisulfite 0.5 mg per mL)].
        1.5% (15 mg per mL), with epinephrine 1:200,000 (Rx) [*Duranest-MPF* (sodium metabisulfite 0.5 mg per mL)].
    For dental use:
        1.5% (15 mg per mL; 27 mg per 1.8-mL dental cartridge), with epinephrine 1:200,000 (Rx) [*Duranest* (sodium metabisulfite 0.5 mg per mL)].
Canada—
    Not commercially available.

**Packaging and storage**
Store below 40 °C (104 °F), preferably between 15 and 30 °C (59 and 86 °F), unless otherwise specified by manufacturer. Protect from freezing. Protect from light.

**Stability**
Do not autoclave.
Do not use if solution is discolored.
Unused portions of solutions not containing a preservative must be discarded.

# LIDOCAINE

## Summary of Differences

Indications:
  Indicated (without epinephrine) for retrobulbar block, transtracheal anesthesia, and intravenous regional anesthesia (Bier block); indicated (with or without epinephrine) for caudal or lumbar epidural block, dental infiltration or nerve block, local infiltration, peripheral nerve block, and sympathetic block; and indicated (with dextrose) for subarachnoid block.
Pharmacology/pharmacokinetics:
  Physicochemical characteristics—
    Chemical group: Amide-type local anesthetic.
    Molecular weight: lidocaine hydrochloride—288.82.
    pKa: 7.9.
    Lipid solubility: Medium.
  Protein-binding—
    Moderate to high (60 to 90%), primarily to alpha$_1$-acid glycoprotein.
  Biotransformation—
    Xylidide metabolites are active and toxic, but less so than the parent compound.
  Half-life—
    1.5 to 2 hours (adults); 3.2 hours (neonates).
  Onset of action—
    Rapid.
  Duration of action—
    Intermediate (1 to 3 hours).
  Relative toxicity (compared to procaine)—
    2.
  Elimination—
    10% of a dose may be excreted unchanged.
Precautions:
  Cross-sensitivity and/or related problems—
    May occur rarely with other amide-type local anesthetics.
    Lidocaine and epinephrine injection contains sodium metabisulfite.
      Sodium metabisulfite can cause an anaphylactic reaction in some persons.
  Pregnancy—
    Studies in animals have not shown adverse effects on the fetus.
    May cause uterine artery constriction.
  Breast-feeding—
    Distributed into breast milk.
  Drug interactions and/or related problems—
    Interaction with beta-adrenergic blocking agents.
    Interaction with cimetidine.
Side/adverse effects:
  May be more likely than other local anesthetics to cause lumbosacral nerve root damage when used for spinal anesthesia.

## Additional Dosing Information

See also *General Dosing Information*.

Solutions containing epinephrine should be used when large doses are required.

A reduction in the dose of lidocaine, or an increase in the interval between doses, may be necessary in patients with decreased hepatic blood flow or hepatic function impairment.

For intravenous regional anesthesia, proper tourniquet technique is essential. Only the single-dose containers designated for intravenous regional anesthesia should be used. A vasoconstrictor should not be used.

Solutions containing dextrose are hyperbaric and are indicated for subarachnoid (spinal) anesthesia.

Some patients receiving lidocaine for spinal anesthesia have developed neurologic complications following anesthesia. The neurologic complications usually are temporary *paresthesias* and *back pain (transient radicular irritation)*. However, persistent *paresthesia*, *paralysis of legs*, or impairment of bodily functions (e.g., *incontinence*) may indicate a serious neurologic complication, *cauda equina syndrome*. Uneven distribution of hyperbaric lidocaine following spinal administration may contribute to *cauda equina syndrome*. In cases of *transient radicular irritation*, symptoms resolve within a few days to a few weeks. However, neurotoxic effects may not resolve in cases of *cauda equina syndrome*. Other anesthetics may cause *cauda equina syndrome* also. Diabetic patients and patients in lithotomy position may be at increased risk for cauda equina syndrome. Although not yet proven in clinical trials to decrease the incidence of cauda equina syndrome, it is recommended that hyperbaric 5% lidocaine be diluted with an equal volume of cerebrospinal fluid or preservative-free saline when it is used for spinal anesthesia. Alternatively, hyperbaric 2% lidocaine may be used for spinal anesthesia. The smallest dose necessary should be used. Spinal anesthesia should not be attempted again after failure of the first attempt. Lidocaine 5% with 7.5% glucose is not recommended for continuous spinal anesthesia.

## Parenteral Dosage Forms

Note:  Bracketed uses in the *Dosage Forms* section refer to categories of use and/or indications that are not included in U.S. product labeling.

### LIDOCAINE HYDROCHLORIDE INJECTION USP

**Usual adult and adolescent dose**
Caudal anesthesia—
  Obstetrical analgesia: 100 to 300 mg as a 0.5 to 1% solution.
  Surgical analgesia: 225 to 300 mg (15 to 20 mL) as a 1.5% solution.
  Note:  For continuous catheter (intermittent administration) techniques, the maximum dose should not be administered at intervals of less than 90 minutes.
Epidural anesthesia—
  Lumbar:
    Analgesia—250 to 300 mg (25 to 30 mL) as a 1% solution.
    Anesthesia—225 to 300 mg (15 to 20 mL) as a 1.5% solution; or 200 to 300 mg (10 to 15 mL) as a 2% solution.
  Thoracic: 200 to 300 mg (20 to 30 mL) as a 1% solution.
  Note:  Dosages given for epidural anesthesia are usual total doses; actual dosage must be based on the number of dermatomes to be anesthetized (2 to 3 mL of the indicated concentration per dermatome).
    For continuous catheter (intermittent administration) techniques, the maximum dose should not be administered at intervals of less than 90 minutes.
Infiltration—
  Intravenous regional: 50 to 300 mg (10 to 60 mL) as a 0.5% solution.
  Percutaneous: 5 to 300 mg (up to 60 mL as a 0.5% solution; up to 30 mL as a 1% solution).
Peripheral nerve block—
  Brachial: 225 to 300 mg (15 to 20 mL) as a 1.5% solution.
  Dental: 20 to 100 mg (1 to 5 mL) as a 2% solution.
  Intercostal: 30 mg (3 mL) as a 1% solution.
  Paracervical: 100 mg (10 mL) per side as a 1% solution; may be repeated if necessary at intervals of not less than 90 minutes.
  Paravertebral: 30 to 50 mg (3 to 5 mL) as a 1% solution.
  Pudendal: 100 mg (10 mL) per side as a 1% solution.
Retrobulbar—
  120 to 200 mg (3 to 5 mL) as a 4% solution.
Sympathetic nerve block—
  Cervical (stellate ganglion): 50 mg (5 mL) as a 1% solution.
  Lumbar: 50 to 100 mg (5 to 10 mL) as a 1% solution.
Transtracheal—
  80 to 120 mg (2 to 3 mL) as a 4% solution. In addition, topical administration of the 4% solution to the pharynx (as a spray) may be required to achieve complete analgesia. For combined use of injection and spray, it should rarely be necessary to administer more than 200 mg (5 mL) or 3 mg per kg of body weight.

**Usual adult prescribing limits**
Not to exceed 4.5 mg per kg of body weight or 300 mg per dose, except as noted below—
  Intravenous regional anesthesia: Do not exceed 4 mg per kg of body weight.

**Usual pediatric dose**
Local infiltration or
Nerve block—
  Up to 5 mg per kg of body weight as a 0.25 to 1% solution.
Intravenous regional anesthesia—
  Up to 3 mg per kg of body weight as a 0.25 to 0.5% solution.

**Usual pediatric prescribing limits**
5 mg per kg of body weight.

**Strength(s) usually available**
U.S.—
  With preservative (methylparaben 1 mg per mL):
    0.5% (5 mg per mL) (Rx) [*Xylocaine*; GENERIC].
    1% (10 mg per mL) (Rx) [*Dilocaine; L-Caine; Lidoject-1; Xylocaine*; GENERIC].
    2% (20 mg per mL) (Rx) [*Dilocaine; L-Caine; Lidoject-2; Xylocaine*; GENERIC].
  Without preservative:
    0.5% (5 mg per mL) (Rx) [*Xylocaine-MPF*].
    1% (10 mg per mL) (Rx) [*Xylocaine-MPF*; GENERIC].
    1.5% (15 mg per mL) (Rx) [*Xylocaine-MPF*; GENERIC].

2% (20 mg per mL) (Rx) [*Dalcaine; Xylocaine-MPF;* GENERIC].
4% (40 mg per mL) (Rx) [*Xylocaine-MPF;* GENERIC].
For dental use:
2% (20 mg per mL; 36 mg per 1.8-mL dental cartridge) (Rx) [*Xylocaine*].
Canada—
With preservative (methylparaben 1 mg per mL):
0.5% (5 mg per mL) (Rx) [*Xylocaine;* GENERIC].
1% (10 mg per mL) (Rx) [*Xylocaine;* GENERIC].
2% (20 mg per mL) (Rx) [*Xylocaine;* GENERIC].
Without preservative:
1% (10 mg per mL) (Rx) [*Xylocaine*].
1.5% (15 mg per mL) (Rx) [*Xylocaine;* GENERIC].
2% (20 mg per mL) (Rx) [*Xylocaine;* GENERIC].

**Packaging and storage**
Store below 40 °C (104 °F), preferably between 15 and 30 °C (59 and 86 °F), unless otherwise specified by manufacturer. Protect from freezing.

**Preparation of dosage form**
For administration to pediatric patients in concentrations lower than those commercially available—Dilute available concentrations with the quantity of 0.9% sodium chloride injection needed to obtain the required final concentration of local anesthetic solution.

**Stability**
May be autoclaved.
For chemical disinfection of the container surface, 91% isopropyl alcohol or 70% ethyl alcohol without denaturants is recommended; solutions containing heavy metals are not recommended.
Dental cartridges sealed with aluminum caps should not be kept in solutions made from antirust tablets or solutions containing quaternary ammonium salts such as benzalkonium chloride.
Unused portions of solutions without a preservative must be discarded.

## LIDOCAINE HYDROCHLORIDE AND DEXTROSE INJECTION USP

**Usual adult dose**
Obstetrical low spinal (saddle block) anesthesia—
Normal vaginal delivery: 9 to 15 mg (0.6 to 1 mL) of lidocaine hydrochloride as a 1.5% solution; or 50 mg (1 mL) of lidocaine hydrochloride as a 5% solutionto provide perineal anesthesia for about one hundred minutes and analgesia for about another forty minutes.
Cesarean section and deliveries requiring intrauterine manipulation: 75 mg (1.5 mL) of lidocaine hydrochloride as a 5% solution.
Surgical anesthesia
Abdominal—
75 to 100 mg (1.5 to 2 mL) of lidocaine hydrochloride as a 5% solution.

**Usual pediatric dose**
Spinal anesthesia—
Infants and children weighing up to 5 kg:
2.5 mg per kg of body weight.
Infants and children weighing 5 to 15 kg:
2 mg per kg of body weight.
Children weighing more than 15 kg:
1.5 mg per kg of body weight.

**Strength(s) usually available**
U.S.—
Without preservative:
1.5% (15 mg per mL), with dextrose 7.5% (75 mg per mL) (Rx) [*Xylocaine-MPF*].
5% (50 mg per mL), with dextrose 7.5% (75 mg per mL) (Rx) [*Xylocaine-MPF with Glucose;* GENERIC].
Canada—
Without preservative:
5% (50 mg per mL), with dextrose 7.5 % (75 mg per mL) (Rx) [*Xylocaine 5% Spinal*].

**Packaging and storage**
Store below 40 °C (104 °F), preferably between 15 and 30 °C (59 and 86 °F), unless otherwise specified by manufacturer. Protect from freezing.

**Stability**
May be autoclaved once; with repeated autoclaving or prolonged storage, caramelization of the dextrose may occur, leading to discoloration. Discolored solutions should not be used.
Do not use if solution contains a precipitate.
For chemical disinfection of the container surface, 91% isopropyl alcohol or 70% ethyl alcohol without a denaturant is recommended; solutions containing heavy metals are not recommended.
Unused portions of solutions must be discarded because they contain no preservative.

## LIDOCAINE HYDROCHLORIDE AND EPINEPHRINE INJECTION USP

**Usual adult and adolescent dose**
Dental anesthesia (for infiltration or nerve block)—
20 to 100 mg (1 to 5 mL) of lidocaine hydrochloride as a 2% solution with epinephrine 1:100,000 or 1:50,000.
Other indications—
See *Lidocaine Hydrochloride Injection USP*. Administration of epinephrine concurrently with the local anesthetic may permit use of doses somewhat larger than those listed.

**Usual adult prescribing limits**
Dental anesthesia—
7 mg per kg of body weight or 500 mg of lidocaine hydrochloride.
Note: A lower limit may apply for poor patient condition, or for some sites of administration. A higher limit may sometimes apply with the use of adjunct drugs. The utility of adjunct drugs to protect the patient from side effects varies depending on the drug and the side effect. For example, the use of benzodiazepines may help prevent seizures during the period of peak absorption of the anesthetic, but will not protect the patient from its cardiovascular toxicity.
Other indications—
7 mg of lidocaine hydrochloride per kg of body weight but not exceeding 500 mg as a single dose.

**Usual pediatric dose**
Dental anesthesia—
20 to 30 mg (1 to 1.5 mL) of lidocaine hydrochloride as a 2% solution with epinephrine 1:100,000.
Local infiltration or
Nerve block—
Up to 7 mg per kg of body weight, as a 0.25 to 1% solution.
Caudal epidural anesthesia—
Up to 7 mg per kg of body weight, as a 0.5 to 1% solution.

**Usual pediatric prescribing limits**
Dental anesthesia—
4 to 5 mg of lidocaine hydrochloride per kg of body weight or 100 to 150 mg as a single dose.
Local infiltration or
Nerve block or local infiltration—
7 mg of lidocaine hydrochloride per kg of body weight as a 0.25 to 1% solution with epinephrine 1:200,000.

**Strength(s) usually available**
U.S.—
With preservative (methylparaben 1 mg per mL):
0.5% (5 mg per mL), with epinephrine 1:200,000 (Rx) [*Xylocaine* (sodium metabisulfite 0.5 mg per mL)].
1% (10 mg per mL), with epinephrine 1:100,000 (Rx) [*Xylocaine* (sodium metabisulfite 0.5 mg per mL); GENERIC].
2% (20 mg per mL), with epinephrine 1:100,000 (Rx) [*Xylocaine* (sodium metabisulfite 0.5 mg per mL); GENERIC].
Without preservative:
1% (10 mg per mL), with epinephrine 1:100,000 (Rx) [GENERIC].
1% (10 mg per mL), with epinephrine 1:200,000 (Rx) [*Xylocaine-MPF* (sodium metabisulfite 0.5 mg per mL)].
1.5% (15 mg per mL), with epinephrine 1:200,000 (Rx) [*Xylocaine-MPF* (sodium metabisulfite 0.5 mg per mL)].
2% (20 mg per mL), with epinephrine 1:200,000 (Rx) [*Xylocaine-MPF* (sodium metabisulfite 0.5 mg per mL)].
For dental use:
2% (20 mg per mL; 36 mg per 1.8-mL dental cartridge), with epinephrine 1:100,000 (Rx) [*Octocaine* (sodium metabisulfite); *Xylocaine* (sodium metabisulfite 0.5 mg per mL)].
2% (20 mg per mL; 36 mg per 1.8-mL dental cartridge), with epinephrine 1:50,000 (Rx) [*Octocaine* (sodium metabisulfite); *Xylocaine* (sodium metabisulfite 0.5 mg per mL)].
Canada—
With preservative (methylparaben):
0.5% (5 mg per mL), with epinephrine 1:100,000 (Rx) [*Xylocaine* (sodium metabisulfite)].
1% (10 mg per mL), with epinephrine 1:200,000 (Rx) [*Xylocaine* (sodium metabisulfite)].
1% (10 mg per mL), with epinephrine 1:100,000 (Rx) [*Xylocaine* (sodium metabisulfite)].
2% (20 mg per mL), with epinephrine 1:100,000 (Rx) [*Xylocaine* (sodium metabisulfite)].
Without preservative:
0.5% (5 mg per mL), with epinephrine 1:200,000 (Rx) [*Xylocaine* (sodium metabisulfite)].

1.5% (15 mg per mL), with epinephrine 1:200,000 (Rx) [*Xylocaine* (sodium metabisulfite)]; *Xylocaine Test Dose* (sodium metabisulfite)].

2% (20 mg per mL), with epinephrine 1:200,000 (Rx) [*Xylocaine* (sodium metabisulfite)].

2% (20 mg per mL), with epinephrine 1:100,000 (Rx) [*Xylocaine* (sodium metabisulfite)].

For dental use:
2% (20 mg per mL; 36 mg per 1.8-mL dental cartridge), with epinephrine 1:100,000 (Rx) [*Octocaine-100* (sodium metabisulfite); *Xylocaine* (sodium metabisulfite)].

2% (20 mg per mL; 36 mg per 1.8-mL dental cartridge), with epinephrine 1:50,000 (Rx) [*Octocaine-50* (sodium metabisulfite); *Xylocaine* (sodium metabisulfite)].

**Packaging and storage**
Store below 40 °C (104 °F), preferably between 15 and 30 °C (59 and 86 °F), unless otherwise specified by manufacturer. Protect from freezing. Protect from light.

**Preparation of dosage form**
For administration to pediatric patients in concentrations lower than those commercially available—Dilute available concentrations with the quantity of 0.9% sodium chloride injection needed to obtain the required final concentration of local anesthetic solution.

**Stability**
Should not be autoclaved.
Do not use if solution is discolored or contains a precipitate.
For chemical disinfection of the container surface, 91% isopropyl alcohol or 70% ethyl alcohol without denaturants is recommended; solutions containing heavy metals are not recommended.
Dental cartridges sealed with aluminum caps should not be kept in solutions made from antirust tablets or solutions containing quaternary ammonium salts such as benzalkonium chloride.
Unused portions of solutions without a preservative must be discarded.

## MEPIVACAINE

## Summary of Differences
Indications:
Indicated for caudal or lumbar epidural block, local infiltration, intravenous regional anesthesia (Bier block), peripheral nerve block, and transtracheal anesthesia; and indicated (with or without levonordefrin) for dental infiltration or nerve block.
Not recommended for subarachnoid administration.
Pharmacology/pharmacokinetics:
Physicochemical characteristics—
Chemical group: Amide-type local anesthetic.
Molecular weight: mepivacaine hydrochloride—282.81.
pKa: 7.6.
Lipid solubility: Medium.
Protein-binding—
High.
Half-life—
1.9 to 3.2 hours (adults); 9 hours (neonates).
Onset of action—
Rapid to intermediate.
Duration of action—
Intermediate (1 to 3 hours).
Relative toxicity (compared to procaine)—
2.
Elimination—
5 to 10% of a dose may be excreted unchanged.
Precautions:
Cross-sensitivity and/or related problems—
May occur rarely with other amide-type local anesthetics.
Pediatrics—
Appropriate studies have not shown pediatrics-specific problems.

## Additional Dosing Information
See also *General Dosing Information*.
Mepivacaine 1, 1.5, and 2% are not intended for dental use.

## Parenteral Dosage Forms
### MEPIVACAINE HYDROCHLORIDE INJECTION USP
**Usual adult and adolescent dose**
Peripheral nerve block—
Brachial, cervical, intercostal, or pudendal: 50 to 400 mg (5 to 40 mL) as a 1% solution; or 100 to 400 mg (5 to 20 mL) as a 2% solution

Caudal and lumbar epidural block—
150 to 300 mg (15 to 30 mL) as a 1% solution; or 150 to 375 mg (10 to 25 mL) as a 1.5% solution; or 200 to 400 mg (10 to 20 mL) as a 2% solution.
Dental—
Single site in upper or lower jaw: 54 mg (1.8 mL) as a 3% solution.
Infiltration and nerve block of entire oral cavity—270 mg (9 mL) as a 3% solution.
Larger doses required for an extensive procedure should be calculated according to the patient's weight. Up to 6.6 mg per kg of body weight may be administered.
Local infiltration (other than in dentistry)—
Up to 400 mg (up to 40 mL) as a 0.5% or 1% solution.
Paracervical block—
Up to 100 mg (up to 10 mL) as a 1% solution per side; may be repeated if necessary in not less than 90 minutes.
Therapeutic block (management of pain)—
10 to 50 mg (1 to 5 mL) as a 1% solution; or 20 to 100 mg (1 to 5 mL) as a 2% solution.
Transvaginal (paracervical plus pudendal) block—
Up to 150 mg (up to 15 mL) as a 1% solution per side.

**Usual adult prescribing limits**
Dental—
6.6 mg per kg of body weight but not to exceed 400 mg per appointment.
Other indications—
7 mg per kg of body weight or 400 mg per procedure.
Note: Although doses of 550 mg have been administered without adverse effects, they are not recommended. If doses of 550 mg are needed, they should not be given at intervals of less than 1½ hours nor should more than 1 gram be given in 24 hours.

**Usual pediatric dose**
Up to 5 to 6 mg per kg of body weight.
Note: Dosage must be individualized based on the patient's age and weight. For local infiltration, concentrations of 0.2 to 0.5% are recommended for infants and children up to 3 years of age; concentrations of 0.5 to 1% are recommended for children over 3 years of age and weighing more than 13.65 kg. For nerve block in children, concentrations of 0.5 to 1% are recommended.
Maximum pediatric dosage in dentistry must be carefully calculated on the basis of the patient's weight but must not exceed 270 mg (9 mL) of the 3% solution.

**Strength(s) usually available**
U.S.—
With preservative (methylparaben 1 mg per mL):
1% (10 mg per mL) (Rx) [*Carbocaine; Polocaine;* GENERIC].
2% (20 mg per mL) (Rx) [*Carbocaine; Polocaine;* GENERIC].
Without preservative:
1% (10 mg per mL) (Rx) [*Carbocaine; Polocaine-MPF*].
1.5% (15 mg per mL) (Rx) [*Carbocaine; Polocaine-MPF*].
2% (20 mg per mL) (Rx) [*Carbocaine; Polocaine-MPF*].
For dental use:
3% (30 mg per mL; 54 mg per 1.8-mL dental cartridge) (Rx) [*Carbocaine; Isocaine; Polocaine;* GENERIC].
Canada—
With preservative (methylparaben 1 mg per mL):
1% (10 mg per mL) [*Carbocaine*].
Without preservative:
1% (10 mg per mL) [*Carbocaine*].
2% (20 mg per mL) [*Carbocaine*].
For dental use:
3% (30 mg per mL; 54 mg per 1.8-mL dental cartridge) [*Isocaine 3%; Polocaine*].

**Packaging and storage**
Store below 40 °C (104 °F), preferably between 15 and 30 °C (59 and 86 °F), unless otherwise specified by manufacturer. Protect from freezing.

**Preparation of dosage form**
For administration to pediatric patients in concentrations lower than those commercially available—Dilute available concentrations with the quantity of 0.9% sodium chloride injection needed to obtain the required final concentration of local anesthetic solution.

**Stability**
May be autoclaved (except for dental cartridges).
Dental cartridges sealed with aluminum caps should not be kept in solutions made from antirust tablets or solutions containing quaternary ammonium salts such as benzalkonium chloride.
Unused portions of solutions not containing a preservative must be discarded.

## MEPIVACAINE HYDROCHLORIDE AND LEVONORDEFRIN INJECTION USP

**Usual adult and adolescent dose**
Dental infiltration and nerve block—
  Single site: 36 mg (1.8 mL) of mepivacaine hydrochloride as a 2% solution with levonordefrin 1:20,000.
  Entire oral cavity: 180 mg (9 mL) of mepivacaine hydrochloride as a 2% solution with levonordefrin 1:20,000.
Note: Larger doses required for an extensive procedure should be calculated according to the patient's weight, and the injections spread out over time as required.

**Usual adult prescribing limits**
6.6 mg per kg of body weight but not to exceed 400 mg of mepivacaine hydrochloride per appointment.

**Usual pediatric dose**
Dental infiltration and nerve block—
  Must be individualized according to patient's weight.

**Usual pediatric prescribing limits**
Maximum dosage should be calculated on the basis of the patient's body weight, but should not exceed 6.6 mg per kg of body weight or 180 mg of mepivacaine hydrochloride as a 2% solution with levonordefrin 1:20,000.

**Strength(s) usually available**
U.S.—
  For dental use:
    2% (20 mg per mL; 36 mg per 1.8-mL dental cartridge), with levonordefrin 1:20,000 (Rx) [*Carbocaine with Neo-Cobefrin* (acetone sodium bisulfite 2 mg per mL); *Isocaine* (sodium bisulfite); *Polocaine* (sodium metabisulfite 0.5 mg per mL); GENERIC].
Canada—
  For dental use:
    2% (20 mg per mL; 36 mg per 1.8-mL dental cartridge), with levonordefrin 1:20,000 [*Isocaine 2%* (sodium bisulfite 1 mg per mL); *Polocaine* (sodium metabisulfite 0.5 mg per mL)].

**Packaging and storage**
Store below 40 °C (104 °F), preferably between 15 and 30 °C (59 and 86 °F), unless otherwise specified by manufacturer. Protect from freezing.

**Stability**
Do not autoclave dental cartridges.
Dental cartridges sealed with aluminum caps should not be kept in solutions made from antirust tablets or solutions containing quaternary ammonium salts such as benzalkonium chloride.
Unused portion of solution must be discarded.

---

## PRILOCAINE

## Summary of Differences
Indications:
  Indicated only for dental use.
Pharmacology/pharmacokinetics:
  Physicochemical characteristics—
    Chemical group: Amide-type local anesthetic.
    Molecular weight: prilocaine hydrochloride—256.78.
  pKa: 7.9.
  Lipid solubility: Medium.
  Protein-binding—
    Moderate.
  Biotransformation—
    Also metabolized by kidney and lung tissue.
  Half-life—
    1.6 hours.
  Onset of action—
    Rapid.
  Duration of action—
    Intermediate (1 to 3 hours).
  Relative toxicity (compared to procaine)—
    1.7.
Precautions:
  Cross-sensitivity and/or related problems—
    May occur rarely with other amide-type local anesthetics.
  Pregnancy—
    Studies in animals have not shown adverse effects on the fetus with doses of up to 30 times the maximum human dose.
Side/adverse effects:
  More likely than other local anesthetics to cause methemoglobinemia.

## Parenteral Dosage Forms

### PRILOCAINE HYDROCHLORIDE INJECTION USP

**Usual adult and adolescent dose**
Dental anesthesia—
  For local infiltration or nerve block: 40 to 80 mg (1 to 2 mL) as a 4% solution initially.

**Usual adult prescribing limits**
Dental—
  8 mg per kg of body weight, not to exceed 600 mg (15 mL) as a 4% solution within a two-hour period.

**Usual pediatric dose**
Dental—
  Children up to 10 years of age: Doses greater than 40 mg (1 mL) as a 4% solution per procedure are rarely needed.

**Strength(s) usually available**
U.S.—
  For dental use:
    4% (40 mg per mL; 72 mg per 1.8-mL dental cartridge) (Rx) [*Citanest Plain*].
Canada—
  For dental use:
    4% (40 mg per mL; 72 mg per 1.8-mL dental cartridge) [*Citanest Plain*].

**Packaging and storage**
Store below 40 °C (104 °F), preferably between 15 and 30 °C (59 and 86 °F), unless otherwise specified by manufacturer. Protect from freezing.

**Stability**
Dental cartridges should not be autoclaved.
For chemical disinfection of the container surface, 91% isopropyl alcohol or 70% ethyl alcohol without denaturants is recommended; solutions containing heavy metals are not recommended.
Dental cartridges are sealed with aluminum caps and therefore should not be kept in solutions made from antirust tablets or solutions containing quaternary ammonium salts such as benzalkonium chloride.

### PRILOCAINE AND EPINEPHRINE INJECTION USP

**Usual adult and adolescent dose**
Dental infiltration and nerve block—
  40 to 80 mg (1 to 2 mL) of prilocaine hydrochloride as a 4% solution with epinephrine 1:200,000 initially.

**Usual adult prescribing limits**
8 mg per kg of body weight, not to exceed 600 mg (15 mL) of prilocaine hydrochloride within a two-hour period.

**Usual pediatric dose**
Dental infiltration and nerve block in children up to 10 years of age—
  Doses greater than 40 mg (1 mL) of prilocaine hydrochloride as a 4% solution with epinephrine 1:200,000 are rarely needed.

**Strength(s) usually available**
U.S.—
  For dental use:
    4% (40 mg per mL; 72 mg per 1.8-mL dental cartridge), with epinephrine 1:200,000 (Rx) [*Citanest Forte* (sodium metabisulfite 0.5 mg per mL)].
Canada—
  For dental use:
    4% (40 mg per mL; 72 mg per 1.8-mL dental cartridge), with epinephrine 1:200,000 [*Citanest Forte* (sodium metabisulfite 0.5 mg per mL); GENERIC].

**Packaging and storage**
Store below 40 °C (104 °F), preferably between 15 and 30 °C (59 and 86 °F), unless otherwise specified by manufacturer. Protect from freezing. Protect from light.

**Stability**
Do not autoclave.
Do not use if solution is discolored.
For chemical disinfection of the container surface, 91% isopropyl alcohol or 70% ethyl alcohol without denaturants is recommended; solutions containing heavy metals are not recommended.
Dental cartridges are sealed with aluminum caps and therefore should not be kept in solutions made from antirust tablets or solutions containing quaternary ammonium salts such as benzalkonium chloride.
Unused portion of solution must be discarded.

## PROCAINE

### Summary of Differences
Indications:
  Indicated for subarachnoid block, local infiltration, peripheral nerve block, and retrobulbar block.
Pharmacology/pharmacokinetics:
  Physicochemical characteristics—
    Chemical group: An ester-type local anesthetic.
    Molecular weight: procaine hydrochloride—272.78.
    pKa: 8.9.
    Lipid solubility: Low.
  Protein-binding—
    Very low.
  Biotransformation—
    Metabolized to PABA. Hydrolyzed primarily in the plasma and, to a much lesser extent, in the liver, by cholinesterases.
  Half-life—
    30 to 50 seconds (adults); 54 to 114 seconds (neonates).
  Onset of action—
    Intermediate.
  Duration of action—
    Short (30 to 60 minutes).
  Relative toxicity—
    1. Procaine is the standard against which other local anesthetics are compared.
  Elimination—
    Less than 2% of a dose may be excreted unchanged.
Precautions:
  Cross-sensitivity and/or related problems—
    May occur with PABA, parabens, or other ester-type local anesthetics.
  Drug interactions and/or related problems—
    Interaction with cholinesterase inhibitors.
    Interaction with sulfonamides.
Side/adverse effects:
  More likely than amide-type local anesthetics to cause hypersensitivity reactions.

### Additional Dosing Information
See also *General Dosing Information*.

For peripheral nerve block, the 2% solution of procaine should be reserved for cases requiring a small volume of solution (up to 25 mL).

Epinephrine 1:200,000 or epinephrine 1:100,000 (0.5 to 1 mL of epinephrine 1:1000 per 100 mL of anesthetic solution) may be added to solutions of procaine hydrochloride for vasoconstrictive effect.

Procaine 10% is indicated for subarachnoid administration. The solution is to be diluted with 0.9% sodium chloride injection, sterile water for injection, CSF, or, for hyperbaric techniques, 10% dextrose injection. Consult a standard text or manufacturer's product information for details concerning dilution and injection sites.

### Parenteral Dosage Forms
Note:  Bracketed uses in the *Dosage Forms* section refer to categories of use and/or indications that are not included in U.S. product labeling.

#### PROCAINE HYDROCHLORIDE INJECTION USP

**Usual adult and adolescent dose**
Infiltration—
  350 to 600 mg as a 0.25 or 0.5% solution.
Peripheral nerve block—
  500 mg as a 0.5, 1, or 2% solution.
Subarachnoid—
  Perineum: 50 mg (0.5 mL) as a 10% solution diluted with an equal volume of diluent.
  Perineum and lower extremities: 100 mg (1 mL) as a 10% solution diluted with an equal volume of diluent.
  Up to costal margin: 200 mg (2 mL) as a 10% solution diluted with 1 mL of diluent.

**Usual adult prescribing limits**
Not to exceed 1 gram initially.

**Usual pediatric dose**
Up to 15 mg per kg of body weight of a 0.5% solution.

**Strength(s) usually available**
U.S.—
  With preservative (chlorobutanol 2.5 mg per mL):
    1% (Rx) [*Novocain* (acetone sodium bisulfite 2 mg per mL); GENERIC].
    2% (Rx) [*Novocain* (acetone sodium bisulfite 2 mg per mL); GENERIC].
  Without preservative:
    1% (Rx) [*Novocain* (acetone sodium bisulfite 2 mg per mL); GENERIC].
    10% (Rx) [*Novocain* (acetone sodium bisulfite 2 mg per mL)].
Canada—
  With preservative (chlorobutanol 2.5 mg per mL):
    2% [*Novocain* (acetone sodium bisulfite 2 mg per mL)].

**Packaging and storage**
Store below 40 °C (104 °F), preferably between 15 and 30 °C (59 and 86 °F), protected from light, unless otherwise specified by manufacturer. Protect from freezing.

**Preparation of dosage form**
For 0.25 or 0.5% concentrations for infiltration or nerve block—Dilute available concentration with enough sterile water for injection to provide the desired quantity and concentration of solution.

**Stability**
May be autoclaved (prior to addition of epinephrine, if added); however, repeated autoclaving is not recommended because of the increased likelihood of crystal formation. Autoclaving of the solution following dilution with dextrose injection may result in discoloration of the solution caused by caramelization of the dextrose.

Do not use if solution is cloudy or discolored or contains a precipitate.

For chemical disinfection of the container surface, 91% isopropyl alcohol or 70% ethyl alcohol without denaturants is recommended; solutions containing heavy metals are not recommended. Immersion of the container in antiseptic solution is not recommended.

Unused portions of solutions not containing a preservative must be discarded.

## TETRACAINE

### Summary of Differences
Indications:
  Indicated (with or without dextrose) for subarachnoid block; and indicated (without dextrose) for transtracheal anesthesia.
Pharmacology/pharmacokinetics:
  Physicochemical characteristics—
    Chemical group: Ester-type local anesthetic.
    Molecular weight: tetracaine hydrochloride—300.83.
    pKa: 8.2.
    Lipid solubility: High.
  Protein-binding—
    High.
  Biotransformation—
    Metabolized to a PABA derivative.
  Onset of action—
    Rapid.
  Duration of action—
    Intermediate to long (1 to 3 hours).
  Relative toxicity (compared to procaine)—
    10.
Precautions:
  Cross-sensitivity and/or related problems—
    May occur with PABA, parabens, or other ester-type local anesthetics.
  Drug interactions and/or related problems—
    Interaction with cholinesterase inhibitors.
    Interaction with sulfonamides.
Side/adverse effects:
  More likely than amide-type local anesthetics to cause hypersensitivity reactions.

### Additional Dosing Information
See also *General Dosing Information*.

Tetracaine hydrochloride injection 1% is isobaric. When used for isobaric spinal anesthesia, the solution is to be diluted with CSF prior to administration. Also, it may be diluted with 10% dextrose injection to provide a hyperbaric solution.

Isobaric or hyperbaric solutions prepared using sterile tetracaine hydrochloride are to be diluted with CSF prior to administration. A hypobaric solution may also be prepared using sterile tetracaine hydrochloride.

Consult a standard text and/or manufacturer's product information for preparation and administration techniques and for proper injection sites.

## Parenteral Dosage Forms

Note: Bracketed uses in the *Dosage Forms* section refer to categories of use and/or indications that are not included in U.S. product labeling.

### TETRACAINE HYDROCHLORIDE INJECTION USP

**Usual adult and adolescent dose**
Spinal anesthesia—
  Low spinal (saddle block) anesthesia for vaginal delivery: 2 to 5 mg (0.2 to 0.5 mL) as a 1% solution, to be diluted with 10% dextrose injection.
  Perineum: 5 mg (0.5 mL) as a 1% solution, to be diluted with CSF or 10% dextrose injection, depending upon technique used.
  Perineum and lower extremities: 10 mg (1 mL) as a 1% solution, to be diluted with CSF or 10% dextrose injection, depending upon technique used.
  Up to costal margin: 15 to 20 mg (1.5 to 2 mL) as a 1% solution diluted with CSF.
  Doses greater than 15 mg are rarely required.

**Usual pediatric dose**
[Spinal anesthesia][1]—
  Neonates and infants up to 3 months of age: 0.4 to 0.5 mg per kg of body weight.
  Infants and children 3 months to 2 years of age: 0.3 to 0.4 mg per kg of body weight.
  Children 2 years of age and older: 0.2 to 0.3 mg per kg of body weight.

**Strength(s) usually available**
U.S.—
  Without preservative:
    1% (10 mg per mL) (Rx) [*Pontocaine* (acetone sodium bisulfite 2 mg per mL)].
Canada—
  Not commercially available.

**Packaging and storage**
Store between 2 and 8 °C (36 and 46 °F). (Exception: Injections supplied as a component of spinal anesthesia trays may be stored at room temperature for 12 months.) Protect from light. Protect from freezing.

**Preparation of dosage form**
For isobaric techniques—Dilute with an equal volume of CSF.
For hyperbaric techniques—Dilute with an equal volume of 10% dextrose injection.

**Stability**
May be autoclaved once; repeated autoclaving is not recommended because of the increased likelihood of crystal formation. Unused autoclaved ampuls should be discarded.
Do not use if solution is cloudy or discolored or contains crystals prior to diluting with CSF.
Immersion of the container in an antiseptic solution is not recommended.
Unused portion of the solution must be discarded because it contains no preservative.

### STERILE TETRACAINE HYDROCHLORIDE USP

**Usual adult and adolescent dose**
Spinal anesthesia—
  Low spinal (saddle block) anesthesia for vaginal delivery: 2 to 5 mg.
  Perineum: 5 mg.
  Perineum and lower extremities: 10 mg.
  Up to costal margin: 15 to 20 mg.
  Doses exceeding 15 mg are rarely required.

**Usual pediatric dose**
[Spinal anesthesia][1]—
  *See Tetracaine Hydrochloride Injection USP*

**Size(s) usually available**
U.S.—
  Without preservative:
    20 mg (Rx) [*Pontocaine*].
Canada—
  Without preservative:
    20 mg [*Pontocaine*].

**Packaging and storage**
Prior to reconstitution, store below 40 °C (104 °F), preferably between 15 and 30 °C (59 and 86 °F), unless otherwise specified by manufacturer.

**Preparation of dosage form**
For isobaric techniques—Dissolve in CSF to give a concentration of 5 mg per mL.
For hyperbaric techniques—Dissolve 10 mg of sterile tetracaine hydrochloride in 1 mL of 10% dextrose injection. Dilute further with 1 mL of CSF to give a final concentration of 5 mg of tetracaine hydrochloride per mL and 5% of dextrose.
For hypobaric techniques—Dissolve the sterile tetracaine hydrochloride in enough sterile water for injection to provide a concentration of 1 mg per mL.

**Stability**
May be autoclaved. Autoclaving may cause the powder to undergo a change in appearance and to adhere to the sides of the ampul. This may slightly decrease the rate of dissolution of the powder but does not affect anesthetic potency.

### TETRACAINE HYDROCHLORIDE IN DEXTROSE INJECTION USP

**Usual adult and adolescent dose**
Obstetrical low spinal (saddle block) anesthesia—
  2 to 4 mg (1 to 2 mL) of tetracaine hydrochloride as a 0.2% solution.
Spinal anesthesia—
  Lower abdomen: 9 to 12 mg (3 to 4 mL) of tetracaine hydrochloride as a 0.3% solution.
  Perineal: 3 to 6 mg (1 to 2 mL) of tetracaine hydrochloride as a 0.3% solution.
  Upper abdomen: 15 mg (5 mL) of tetracaine hydrochloride as a 0.3% solution.

**Usual pediatric dose**
[Spinal anesthesia][1]—
  *See Tetracaine Hydrochloride Injection USP*

**Strength(s) usually available**
U.S.—
  Without preservative:
    0.2% of tetracaine hydrochloride (2 mg per mL) and 6% of dextrose (60 mg per mL) (Rx) [*Pontocaine*].
    0.3% of tetracaine hydrochloride (3 mg per mL) and 6% of dextrose (60 mg per mL) (Rx) [*Pontocaine*].
Canada—
  Not commercially available.

**Packaging and storage**
Store below 40 °C (104 °F), preferably between 15 and 30 °C (59 and 86 °F), protected from light. Protect from freezing.

**Stability**
May be autoclaved once; repeated autoclaving is not recommended because of the increased likelihood of crystal formation. Also, with repeated autoclaving, caramelization of the dextrose may occur, leading to discoloration. Unused autoclaved ampuls should be discarded.
Do not use if solution is cloudy or discolored or contains crystals.
Unused portions of solutions must be discarded because they contain no preservative.

---

[1]Not included in Canadian product labeling.

Revised: 07/30/98

## Table 1. Pharmacology/Pharmacokinetics—Anesthetics (Parenteral-Local)

| Drug | pKa | Lipid solubility (pH 7.4) | Protein binding | Half-life adult/neonate | Onset of action* | Duration of action† | Relative toxicity‡ |
|---|---|---|---|---|---|---|---|
| Articaine | 7.8 | High | Very high | 1.2 hr | Rapid | Intermediate | |
| Bupivacaine | 8.1 | High | Very high | 3.5 hr/8.1–14 hr | Intermediate to Slow | Long§ | |
| Chloroprocaine | 9 | | | 19–26 sec/41–45 sec | Rapid | Short | |
| Etidocaine | 7.74 | High | Very high | 2.5 hr/4–8 hr | Rapid | Long | |
| Lidocaine | 7.9 | Medium | Moderate to high | 1.5–2 hr/3.2 hr | Rapid# | Intermediate | 2 |
| Mepivacaine | 7.6 | Medium | High | 1.9–3.2 hr/9 hr | Rapid to intermediate# | Intermediate | 2 |
| Prilocaine | 7.9 | Medium | Moderate | 1.6 hr | Rapid | Intermediate | 1.7 |
| Procaine | 8.9 | Low | Very low | 30–50 sec/54–114 sec | Intermediate | Short | 1 |
| Tetracaine | 8.2 | High | High | | Rapid | Intermediate to long | 10 |

*Influenced by the site, route, and technique of administration; dosage (volume and concentration) administered; pH at injection site; physical characteristics, such as lipid solubility, molecular size, and pKa of the individual anesthetic; and individual patient.

†Short = 30 to 60 minutes; Intermediate = 1 to 3 hours; Long = 3 to 10 hours. Influenced by factors affecting rate of clearance from the injection site and individual patient.

‡As compared with procaine (the least toxic of these agents).

§Via nerve block, may produce analgesia for considerably longer than 10 hours.

#Adjustment of pH with 1 mEq (1 mmol) of sodium bicarbonate per 10 mL may increase the onset of conduction blocks (lidocaine hydrochloride injection, lidocaine and epinephrine injection, or mepivacaine hydrochloride injection).

# ANESTHETICS Topical

This monograph includes information on the following: 1) Benzocaine; 2) Benzocaine and Menthol; 3) Butamben; 4) Dibucaine; 5) Lidocaine; 6) Pramoxine; 7) Pramoxine and Menthol; 8) Tetracaine†; 9) Tetracaine and Menthol†

Note: See also individual *Lidocaine and Prilocaine (Topical)* monograph.

INN:
    Dibucaine—Cinchocaine
    Pramoxine—Pramocaine

BAN:
    Dibucaine—Cinchocaine
    Lidocaine—Lignocaine
    Tetracaine—Amethocaine

JAN:
    Benzocaine—Ethyl aminobenzoate

VA CLASSIFICATION (Primary/Secondary):

Note: Several of the dosage forms listed below are commercially available in more than one formulation. Because the vehicle into which a local anesthetic is incorporated may determine the appropriate usage and/or site(s) of application of a product, some of the VA classifications listed for a dosage form may apply only to specific formulations.

    Benzocaine
        Cream—DE700
        Ointment—RS201/DE700; RS900
        Topical Aerosol—DE700/NT300; OR600
        Topical Spray Solution—DE700
    Benzocaine and Menthol—DE700
    Butamben—DE700
    Dibucaine
        Cream—DE700
        Ointment—RS201/DE700; RS900
    Lidocaine
        Ointment 2.5%—DE700
        Ointment 5%—NT300/DE700; OR600
        Topical Spray Solution—DE700
    Lidocaine Hydrochloride
        Topical Aerosol—DE700
        Film-forming Gel—DE700
        Jelly—NT300/GU900; DE700
        Ointment—DE700
    Pramoxine
        Cream—RS201/DE700; RS900
        Lotion—DE700
    Pramoxine and Menthol
        Gel—DE700
        Lotion—DE700
    Tetracaine
        Cream—RS201/DE700; RE900
    Tetracaine and Menthol
        Ointment—RS201/DE700; RE900

Note: For information on local anesthetics applied topically to the oral, rectal, or other mucosa, see *Anesthetics (Mucosal-Local)*.

In Canada, *Nupercainal Cream* contains domiphen bromide in addition to dibucaine.

Commonly used brand name(s): *After Burn Double Strength Gel*[5]; *After Burn Double Strength Spray*[5]; *After Burn Gel*[5]; *After Burn Spray*[5]; *Almay Anti-itch Lotion*[6]; *Alphacaine*[5]; *Americaine Topical Anesthetic First Aid Ointment*[1]; *Americaine Topical Anesthetic Spray*[1]; *Butesin Picrate*[3]; *DermaFlex*[5]; *Dermoplast*[1]; *Endocaine*[1]; *Lagol*[1]; *Norwood Sunburn Spray*[5]; *Nupercainal Cream*[4]; *Nupercainal Ointment*[4]; *Pontocaine Cream*[8]; *Pontocaine Ointment*[8]; *Pramegel*[6]; *Prax*[6]; *Shield Burnasept Spray*[1]; *Tronothane*[6]; *Xylocaine*[5].

Other commonly used names are: Amethocaine [Tetracaine†], Butyl aminobenzoate [Butamben], Cinchocaine [Dibucaine], Ethyl aminobenzoate [Benzocaine], Lignocaine [Lidocaine], Pramocaine [Pramoxine].

Note: For a listing of dosage forms and brand names by country availability, see *Dosage Forms* section(s).

†Not commercially available in Canada.

## Category

Anesthetic, local.

## Indications

### Accepted

Skin disorders, minor (treatment)—Topical anesthetics are indicated to relieve pain, pruritus, and inflammation associated with minor skin disorders, including:
    Burns, minor, including sunburn.
    Bites (or stings), insect.
    Dermatitis, contact, including poison ivy, poison oak, or poison sumac.
    Wounds, minor, such as cuts and scratches.

## Pharmacology/Pharmacokinetics

### Physicochemical characteristics
Chemical group—
  Amides: Dibucaine, lidocaine.
  Esters, aminobenzoic acid (para-aminobenzoic acid, PABA)–derivative: Benzocaine, butamben, tetracaine.
  Unclassified: Pramoxine.
Molecular weight—
  Benzocaine: 165.19.
  Butamben picrate: 615.60.
  Dibucaine: 343.47.
  Lidocaine: 234.34.
  Lidocaine hydrochloride: 288.82.
  Pramoxine hydrochloride: 329.87.
  Tetracaine: 264.37.
  Tetracaine hydrochloride: 300.83.
pKa—
  Dibucaine: 8.8.
  Lidocaine: 7.9.
  Tetracaine: 8.2.

### Mechanism of action/Effect
Local anesthetics block both the initiation and conduction of nerve impulses by decreasing the neuronal membrane's permeability to sodium ions. This reversibly stabilizes the membrane and inhibits depolarization, resulting in the failure of a propagated action potential and subsequent conduction blockade.

### Other actions/effects
If significant quantities of topical anesthetics are absorbed, actions on the central nervous system (CNS) may lead to CNS stimulation and/or CNS depression. Actions on the cardiovascular system may cause depression of cardiac conduction and excitability, and possibly peripheral vasodilation.

### Absorption
Absorption is variable; dependent on specific drug and/or its specific salt. Benzocaine is minimally absorbed. In general, ionized forms(salts) of local anesthetics are not readily absorbed through intact skin. However, both nonionized (bases) and ionized forms of local anesthetics are readily absorbed through traumatized or abraded skin into the systemic circulation.

### Biotransformation
Amides—
  Hepatic and some renal.
  Lidocaine: Xylidide metabolites are active and toxic, but less so than the parent compound.
Esters, PABA-derivative—
  Hydrolyzed by plasma cholinesterases, and to a much lesser extent by hepatic cholinesterases, to PABA-containing metabolites.

### Onset of action
Dibucaine—Up to 15 minutes.
Pramoxine—3 to 5 minutes.
Tetracaine—Slow.

### Duration of action
Lidocaine—Approximately 45 minutes.
Tetracaine—Approximately 30 to 45 minutes.

### Elimination
Amides—
  Renal, primarily as metabolites.
  Lidocaine: Up to 10% of an absorbed dose may be excreted unchanged.
Esters—
  Renal, as metabolites.

## Precautions to Consider

### Cross-sensitivity and/or related problems
Patients sensitive to one ester-derivative (especially a PABA-derivative) local anesthetic may be sensitive to other ester derivatives also.
Patients sensitive to PABA, parabens, or paraphenylenediamine (a hair dye) may be sensitive to PABA-derivative topical anesthetics also.
Patients sensitive to one amide derivative may rarely be sensitive to other amide derivatives also.
Cross-sensitivity between amide derivatives and ester derivatives, or between amides or esters and the chemically unrelated pramoxine, has not been reported.

### Pregnancy/Reproduction
Pregnancy—Problems in humans with topical anesthetics have not been documented.

*Benzocaine, butamben, dibucaine, and pramoxine*—
  Studies in humans have not been done.
  Studies in animals have not been done.
*Lidocaine*—
  Adequate and well-controlled studies in humans have not been done.
  Studies in animals given up to 6.6 times the human dose have shown no adverse effects on the fetus.
  Lidocaine ointment 5%—FDA Pregnancy Category B.
*Tetracaine*—
  Studies in humans have not been done.
  Studies in animals have not been done.
  FDA Pregnancy Category C.

### Breast-feeding
Problems in humans have not been documented.

### Pediatrics
*Benzocaine*—Benzocaine should be used with caution in infants and young children because increased absorption through the skin (with excessive use) may result in methemoglobinemia. Benzocaine-containing topical formulations should not be used in children younger than 2 years of age unless prescribed by a physician.
*Other topical anesthetics*—No information is available on the relationship of age to the effects of these medications in pediatric patients following application to the skin. However, it is recommended that a physician be consulted before any topical local anesthetic is used in children younger than 2 years of age.

### Geriatrics
No information is available on the relationship of age to the effects of topical anesthetics in geriatric patients following application to the skin.

### Drug interactions and/or related problems
The following drug interactions and/or related problems have been selected on the basis of their potential clinical significance (possible mechanism in parentheses where appropriate)—not necessarily inclusive (» = major clinical significance):

Note: Combinations containing any of the following medications, depending on the amount present, may also interact with this medication.

*For ester derivatives*
  Cholinesterase inhibitors such as
    Antimyasthenics
    Cyclophosphamide
    Demecarium
    Echothiophate
    Insecticides, neurotoxic, possibly including large quantities of topical malathion
    Isoflurophate
    Thiotepa
      (these agents may inhibit metabolism of ester derivatives; absorption of significant quantities of ester derivatives in patients receiving a cholinesterase inhibitor may lead to increased risk of toxicity)
  Sulfonamides
    (metabolites of PABA-derivative topical anesthetics may antagonize antibacterial activity of sulfonamides, especially if the anesthetics are absorbed in significant quantities over prolonged periods of time)

*For lidocaine*
  Antiarrhythmic agents, amide local anesthetic–derivative, other, such as
    Mexiletine
    Tocainide or
  Lidocaine, systemic or parenteral-local
    (risk of cardiotoxicity associated with additive cardiac effects, and, with systemic or parenteral-local lidocaine, the risk of overdose, may be increased in patients receiving these medications if large quantities of topically applied lidocaine are absorbed)
  Beta-adrenergic blocking agents
    (concurrent use may slow metabolism of lidocaine because of decreased hepatic blood flow, leading to increased risk of lidocaine toxicity if large quantities are absorbed)
  Cimetidine
    (cimetidine inhibits hepatic metabolism of lidocaine; concurrent use may lead to lidocaine toxicity if large quantities are absorbed)

### Laboratory value alterations
The following have been selected on the basis of their potential clinical significance (possible effect in parentheses where appropriate)—not necessarily inclusive (» = major clinical significance):

With diagnostic test results
>   Pancreatic function determinations using bentiromide
>   (use of PABA-derivative topical anesthetics or lidocaine prior to the bentiromide test may invalidate test results since these medications are also metabolized to PABA or other arylamines and will thus increase the real or apparent quantity of PABA recovered; patients should be advised to discontinue use of these anesthetics 3 days prior to bentiromide administration)

### Medical considerations/Contraindications
The medical considerations/contraindications included have been selected on the basis of their potential clinical significance (reasons given in parentheses where appropriate)—not necessarily inclusive (» = major clinical significance).

*Risk-benefit should be considered when the following medical problems exist:*
>   Local infection at site of application
>   (infection may alter the pH at the treatment site, leading to decrease or loss of local anesthetic effect)
>   Sensitivity to the topical anesthetic being considered for use or to chemically related anesthetics and, for the ester derivatives, to PABA, parabens, or paraphenylenediamine, or
>   Sensitivity to other ingredients in the formulation
>   Skin disorders, severe or extensive, especially if skin is abraded or broken
>   (increased absorption of anesthetic)

## Side/Adverse Effects
Note: Adverse reactions are due to excessive dosage or rapid absorption, which produces high plasma concentrations, as well as to idiosyncrasy, hypersensitivity, or decreased patient tolerance.
>   Benzocaine and tetracaine are more likely to cause contact sensitization than are the other local anesthetics.

The following side/adverse effects have been selected on the basis of their potential clinical significance (possible signs and symptoms in parentheses where appropriate)—not necessarily inclusive:

**Those indicating need for medical attention**
Incidence less frequent
>   *Angioedema* (large, hive-like swellings on skin, mouth, or throat); *dermatitis, contact* (skin rash, redness, itching, or hives; burning, stinging, swelling, or tenderness not present before therapy)

## Overdose
For specific information on the agents used in the management of topical anesthetics overdose, see:
- *Ascorbic Acid (Systemic)* monograph;
- *Benzodiazepines (Systemic)* monograph;
- *Sympathomimetic Agents—Cardiovascular Use (Parenteral-Systemic)* monograph; and/or
- *Methylene Blue (Systemic)* monograph.

For more information on the management of overdose or unintentional ingestion, **contact a Poison Control Center** (see *Poison Control Center Listing*).

**Clinical effects of overdose**
The following effects have been selected on the basis of their potential clinical significance if excessive systemic absorption occurs (possible signs and symptoms in parentheses where appropriate)—not necessarily inclusive:
>   ***Cardiovascular system depression*** (low blood pressure; slow or irregular heartbeat; unusual paleness; increased sweating)—may lead to cardiac arrest; ***CNS toxicity*** (blurred or double vision; confusion; convulsions; dizziness or lightheadedness; drowsiness; feeling hot, cold, or numb; ringing or buzzing in the ears; shivering or trembling; unusual anxiety, excitement, nervousness, or restlessness); ***methemoglobinemia*** (difficulty in breathing on exertion; dizziness; headache; unusual tiredness or weakness)

Note: Stimulant and/or depressant manifestations of *CNS toxicity* may occur. CNS stimulation usually occurs first, followed by CNS depression. However, CNS stimulation may be transient or absent, so that drowsiness may be the first symptom of toxicity in some patients. CNS depression may lead to unconsciousness and respiratory arrest.

**Treatment of overdose**
Recommended treatment includes:
>   Specific treatment—
>   For methemoglobinemia—Administering methylene blue (1 to 2 mg per kg of body weight, intravenously) and/or ascorbic acid (100 to 200 mg orally).
>   For circulatory depression—Administration of a vasopressor and intravenous fluids is recommended.
>   For convulsions—Administering an anticonvulsant, usually a benzodiazepine, keeping in mind that benzodiazepines may cause respiratory and circulatory depression, especially when administered rapidly. Medications and equipment needed for support of respiration and for resuscitation must be immediately available.
>   Supportive Care—
>   For systemic reactions caused by excessive absorption—Securing and maintaining a patent airway, administering oxygen, and instituting assisted or controlled respiration as required. In some patients, endotracheal intubation may be required.

## Patient Consultation
As an aid to patient consultation, refer to *Advice for the Patient, Anesthetics (Topical)*.
In providing consultation, consider emphasizing the following selected information (» = major clinical significance):

**Before using this medication**
» Conditions affecting use, especially:
>   Sensitivity to local anesthetics of the same chemical class, and, for ester derivatives only, aminobenzoic acid, parabens, or hair dye
>   Use in children—Caution that excessive quantities of benzocaine may cause methemoglobinemia in children younger than 2 years of age; consulting physician before using any topical local anesthetic in children younger than 2 years of age

**Proper use of this medication**
>   Following physician's instructions if prescribed
>   Following manufacturer's instructions if self-medicating
» Not using on large areas, especially if skin broken or abraded, or for prolonged periods of time, without physician's advice
» Checking with physician before using for problems other than prescribed or recommended on package label, or if any suspicion of infection
» Not using products containing alcohol, which is flammable, near fire or open flame or while smoking; not smoking until area completely dry
» Using care not to get in eyes, mouth, or nose; if using topical aerosol or spray dosage forms, applying to face with hand or other suitable applicator
» Proper dosing
>   Missed dose (if on scheduled dosing): Applying as soon as possible; not applying if almost time for next dose
» Proper storage

*For butamben*
>   Butamben may permanently stain clothing and hair; covering area with a loose bandage after application to protect clothing and not allowing hair to come into contact with the medication

*For lidocaine film-forming gel*
>   Proper application technique: Drying area before applying; applying medication, then waiting 60 seconds until transparent film forms

**Precautions while using this medication**
» Taking precautions to prevent children from transferring medication to their mouths after application
»*Discontinuing use and checking with physician*
>   If condition does not improve within 7 days or worsens
>   If problem area becomes infected
>   If rash, irritation, or other symptoms not present before use occur
>   If medication is swallowed

**Side/adverse effects**
>   Signs and symptoms of potential side effects, especially angioedema, contact dermatitis, and overdose

## General Dosing Information
These medications should not be applied over large areas, or for prolonged periods of time, especially to broken or abraded skin, because of the increased risk of systemic absorption and toxicity.

Topical anesthetic–containing medications may be sprayed or applied directly to the affected area, or applied with a suitable applicator (for example, a sterile gauze pad or cotton swab).

## BENZOCAINE

### Summary of Differences
Physicochemical characteristics:
  An ester-type (PABA-derivative) local anesthetic.
Precautions:
  Cross-sensitivity and/or related problems—
    May occur with other ester-type anesthetics, especially other PABA derivatives, with PABA or parabens, and with paraphenylenediamine.
  Pediatrics—
    Excessive use may cause methemoglobinemia in infants and young children.
  Drug interactions and/or related problems—
    Cholinesterase inhibitors may inhibit metabolism of benzocaine.
    Benzocaine may antagonize antibacterial activity of sulfonamides.
Side/adverse effects:
  More likely to cause contact sensitization than most other topical anesthetics.
  See also *Side/Adverse Effects*.

### Topical Dosage Forms

#### BENZOCAINE CREAM USP
**Usual adult and adolescent dose**
Anesthetic, local—
  Topical, to the affected area three or four times a day as needed.
**Usual pediatric dose**
Anesthetic, local—
  Children up to 2 years of age: Dosage must be individualized by a physician.
  Children 2 years of age and older: See *Usual adult and adolescent dose*.
**Strength(s) usually available**
U.S.—
  5% (OTC) [GENERIC].
**Packaging and storage**
Store below 30 °C (86 °F). Store in a tight container. Protect from light. Protect from freezing.
**Auxiliary labeling**
• For external use only.

#### BENZOCAINE OINTMENT USP
**Usual adult and adolescent dose**
Anesthetic, local—
  Topical, to the affected area three or four times a day as needed.
**Usual pediatric dose**
Anesthetic, local—
  Children up to 2 years of age: Dosage must be individualized by a physician.
  Children 2 years of age and older: See *Usual adult and adolescent dose*.
**Strength(s) usually available**
U.S.—
  5% (OTC) [*Lagol*].
  20% (OTC) [*Americaine Topical Anesthetic First Aid Ointment*].
**Packaging and storage**
Store below 30 °C (86 °F). Store in a tight container. Protect from light. Protect from freezing.
**Auxiliary labeling**
• For external use only.

#### BENZOCAINE TOPICAL AEROSOL USP
**Usual adult and adolescent dose**
Anesthetic, local—
  Topical, sprayed on or applied to affected area three or four times a day as needed.
**Usual pediatric dose**
Anesthetic, local—
  Children up to 2 years of age: Dosage must be individualized by a physician.
  Children 2 years of age and older: See *Usual adult and adolescent dose*.
**Strength(s) usually available**
U.S.—
  20% (OTC) [*Americaine Topical Anesthetic Spray*].
**Packaging and storage**
Store below 40 °C (104 °F), preferably between 15 and 30 °C (59 and 86 °F), unless otherwise specified by manufacturer.
**Auxiliary labeling**
• Shake well.
• For external use only.

#### BENZOCAINE TOPICAL SPRAY SOLUTION
**Usual adult and adolescent dose**
Anesthetic, local—
  Topical, sprayed on or applied to affected area three or four times a day as needed.
**Usual pediatric dose**
Anesthetic, local—
  Children up to 2 years of age: Dosage must be individualized by a physician.
  Children 2 years of age and older: See *Usual adult and adolescent dose*.
**Strength(s) usually available**
Canada—
  2% (OTC) [*Shield Burnasept Spray*].
  20% (OTC) [*Endocaine*].
**Packaging and storage**
Store below 40 °C (104 °F), preferably between 15 and 30 °C (59 and 86 °F), unless otherwise specified by manufacturer.
**Auxiliary labeling**
• For external use only.

#### BENZOCAINE AND MENTHOL LOTION
**Usual adult and adolescent dose**
Anesthetic, local—
  Topical, to the affected area three or four times a day as needed.
**Usual pediatric dose**
Anesthetic, local—
  Children up to 2 years of age: Dosage must be individualized by a physician.
  Children 2 years of age and older: See *Usual adult and adolescent dose*.
**Strength(s) usually available**
U.S.—
  8% of benzocaine and 0.5% of menthol (OTC) [*Dermoplast* (methylparaben)].
**Packaging and storage**
Store below 30 °C (86 °F). Protect from freezing.
**Auxiliary labeling**
• For external use only.

#### BENZOCAINE AND MENTHOL TOPICAL AEROSOL
**Usual adult and adolescent dose**
Anesthetic, local—
  Topical, sprayed on or applied to affected area three or four times a day as needed.
**Usual pediatric dose**
Anesthetic, local—
  Children up to 2 years of age: Dosage must be individualized by a physician.
  Children 2 years of age and older: See *Usual adult and adolescent dose*.
**Strength(s) usually available**
U.S.—
  8% of benzocaine and 0.5% of menthol (OTC) [*Dermoplast* (methylparaben)].
Canada—
  4.5% of benzocaine and 0.5% of menthol (OTC) [*Dermoplast* (methylparaben; isopropyl alcohol)].
**Packaging and storage**
Store below 40 °C (104 °F), preferably between 15 and 30 °C (59 and 86 °F), unless otherwise specified by manufacturer.
**Auxiliary labeling**
• Shake well.
• For external use only.

## BUTAMBEN

### Summary of Differences
Physicochemical characteristics:
  Butamben is an ester-type (PABA-derivative) local anesthetic.

Precautions:
  Cross-sensitivity and/or related problems—
    May occur with other ester-type anesthetics, especially other PABA derivatives, with PABA or parabens, and with paraphenylenediamine.
  Drug interactions and/or related problems—
    Cholinesterase inhibitors may inhibit metabolism of butamben.
    Butamben may antagonize antibacterial activity of sulfonamides.

## Topical Dosage Forms
### BUTAMBEN PICRATE OINTMENT
**Usual adult and adolescent dose**
Anesthetic, local—
  Topical, to the skin, as a 1% ointment three or four times a day as needed.
Note: Area should be loosely bandaged to protect clothing from staining.
**Usual pediatric dose**
Dosage has not been established.
**Strength(s) usually available**
U.S.—
  1% (OTC) [*Butesin Picrate*].
**Packaging and storage**
Store below 25 °C (77 °F), unless otherwise specified by manufacturer. Protect from freezing.
**Auxiliary labeling**
• For external use only.

---
## DIBUCAINE
---

## Summary of Differences
Physicochemical characteristics:
  Dibucaine is an amide-type local anesthetic.
Precautions:
  Cross-sensitivity and/or related problems—Rarely, may occur with other amide-type local anesthetics.
  Laboratory value alterations—No interference with bentiromide test for pancreatic function.

## Topical Dosage Forms
### DIBUCAINE CREAM USP
**Usual adult and adolescent dose**
Anesthetic, local—
  Topical, to the skin, as a 0.5% cream three or four times a day as needed.
**Usual pediatric dose**
Anesthetic, local—
  Children up to 2 years of age: Dosage must be individualized by a physician.
  Children 2 years of age and older: See *Usual adult and adolescent dose*.
**Strength(s) usually available**
U.S.—
  0.5% (OTC) [*Nupercainal Cream* (acetone sodium bisulfite); GENERIC].
    Note: In Canada, *Nupercainal Cream* also contains domiphen bromide.
**Packaging and storage**
Store below 40 °C (104 °F), preferably between 15 and 30 °C (59 and 86 °F), unless otherwise specified by manufacturer. Store in a collapsible tube or a tight, light-resistant container. Protect from freezing.
**Auxiliary labeling**
• For external use only.

### DIBUCAINE OINTMENT USP
**Usual adult and adolescent dose**
Anesthetic, local—
  Topical, to the skin, as a 1% ointment three or four times a day as needed.
Note: Area may be lightly covered for protection.
**Usual adult prescribing limits**
Not more than 30 grams in a twenty-four-hour period.
**Usual pediatric dose**
Anesthetic, local—
  Children up to 2 years of age: Dosage must be individualized by a physician.
  Children 2 years of age and older: See *Usual adult and adolescent dose*.
**Usual pediatric prescribing limits**
Not more than 7.5 grams in a twenty-four-hour period.
**Strength(s) usually available**
U.S.—
  1% (OTC) [*Nupercainal Ointment*; GENERIC].
Canada—
  1% (OTC) [*Nupercainal Ointment*].
**Packaging and storage**
Store below 40 °C (104 °F), preferably between 15 and 30 °C (59 and 86 °F), unless otherwise specified by manufacturer. Store in a collapsible tube or in a tight, light-resistant container. Protect from freezing.
**Auxiliary labeling**
• For external use only.

---
## LIDOCAINE
---

## Summary of Differences
Physicochemical characteristics:
  Lidocaine is an amide-type local anesthetic.
Precautions:
  Cross-sensitivity and/or related problems—Rarely, may occur with other amide-type local anesthetics.
  Drug interactions—Possibility of toxicity in patients receiving local anesthetic–derivative antiarrhythmic agents, lidocaine via other routes of administration, beta-adrenergic blocking agents, or cimetidine if large quantities of topically administered lidocaine are absorbed.

## Topical Dosage Forms
### LIDOCAINE OINTMENT USP
**Usual adult and adolescent dose**
Anesthetic, local—
  Topical, as a 2.5% or 5% ointment, to the affected area three or four times a day as needed.
**Usual adult prescribing limits**
For the 5% ointment—Not more than 5 grams per single application or 20 grams per day.
**Usual pediatric dose**
Anesthetic, local—
  Dosage must be individualized, depending on the child's age, weight, and physical condition, up to a maximum of 4.5 mg per kg of body weight.
**Strength(s) usually available**
U.S.—
  2.5% (OTC) [*Xylocaine*].
  5% (Rx) [*Xylocaine*; GENERIC].
Canada—
  5% (OTC) [*Alphacaine; Xylocaine*].
**Packaging and storage**
Store below 40 °C (104 °F), preferably between 15 and 30 °C (59 and 86 °F), unless otherwise specified by manufacturer. Store in a tight container. Protect from freezing.
**Auxiliary labeling**
• For external use only.

### LIDOCAINE TOPICAL SPRAY SOLUTION
**Usual adult and adolescent dose**
Anesthetic, local—
  Topical, sprayed on or applied to affected area three or four times a day as needed.
**Usual pediatric dose**
Dosage has not been established.
**Strength(s) usually available**
Canada—
  2% (OTC) [*Norwood Sunburn Spray*].
**Packaging and storage**
Store below 40 °C (104 °F), preferably between 15 and 30 °C (59 and 86 °F), unless otherwise specified by manufacturer. Protect from freezing.
**Auxiliary labeling**
• For external use only.

## LIDOCAINE HYDROCHLORIDE TOPICAL AEROSOL

**Usual adult and adolescent dose**
Anesthetic, local—
   Topical, sprayed on or applied to the affected area three or four times a day as needed.

**Usual pediatric dose**
Dosage has not been established.

**Strength(s) usually available**
Canada—
   0.5% (OTC) [*After Burn Spray*].
   1% (OTC) [*After Burn Double Strength Spray*].

**Packaging and storage**
Store below 40 °C (104 °F), preferably between 15 and 30 °C (59 and 86 °F), unless otherwise specified by manufacturer. Protect from freezing.

**Auxiliary labeling**
• Shake well.
• For external use only.

## LIDOCAINE HYDROCHLORIDE FILM-FORMING GEL

**Usual adult and adolescent dose**
Anesthetic, local—
   Topical, applied to affected area three or four times a day as needed.

**Usual pediatric dose**
Dosage has not been established.

**Strength(s) usually available**
U.S.—
   2.5% (OTC) [*DermaFlex*].

**Packaging and storage**
Store below 40 °C (104 °F), preferably between 15 and 30 °C (59 and 86 °F), unless otherwise specified by manufacturer. Protect from freezing.

**Auxiliary labeling**
• For external use only.

## LIDOCAINE HYDROCHLORIDE JELLY USP

**Usual adult and adolescent dose**
Anesthetic, local—
   Topical, to the affected area three or four times a day as needed.

**Usual pediatric dose**
Dosage has not been established.

**Strength(s) usually available**
Canada—
   0.5% (OTC) [*After Burn Gel*].
   1% (OTC) [*After Burn Double Strength Gel*].

**Packaging and storage**
Store below 40 °C (104 °F), preferably between 15 and 30 °C (59 and 86 °F), unless otherwise specified by manufacturer. Protect from freezing.

**Auxiliary labeling**
• For external use only.

## LIDOCAINE HYDROCHLORIDE OINTMENT

**Usual adult and adolescent dose**
Anesthetic, local—
   Topical, as a 5% ointment, to the affected area three or four times a day as needed.

**Usual pediatric dose**
Anesthetic, local—
   Children up to 2 years of age: Dosage has not been established.
   Children 2 years of age and older: See *Usual adult and adolescent dose*.

**Strength(s) usually available**
U.S.—
   5% (Rx) [GENERIC].

**Packaging and storage**
Store below 40 °C (104 °F), preferably between 15 and 30 °C (59 and 86 °F), unless otherwise specified by manufacturer. Protect from freezing.

**Auxiliary labeling**
• For external use only.

---

# PRAMOXINE

## Summary of Differences

Physicochemical characteristics: Pramoxine is an unclassified (neither an amide-type nor an ester-type) local anesthetic.
Precautions: Diagnostic interference—No interference with bentiromide test for pancreatic function.

## Topical Dosage Forms

### PRAMOXINE HYDROCHLORIDE CREAM USP

**Usual adult and adolescent dose**
Anesthetic, local—
   Topical, as a 1% cream, every three to four hours as needed.

**Usual pediatric dose**
Anesthetic, local—
   Children up to 2 years of age: Dosage has not been established.
   Children 2 years of age and older: See *Usual adult and adolescent dose*.

**Strength(s) usually available**
U.S.—
   1% (OTC) [*Prax; Tronothane*].
Canada—
   1% (OTC) [*Tronothane*].

**Packaging and storage**
Store below 40 °C (104 °F), preferably between 15 and 30 °C (59 and 86 °F), unless otherwise specified by manufacturer. Store in tight container. Protect from freezing.

**Auxiliary labeling**
• For external use only.

### PRAMOXINE HYDROCHLORIDE LOTION

**Usual adult and adolescent dose**
Anesthetic, local—
   Topical, as a 1% lotion, every three or four hours as needed.

**Usual pediatric dose**
Anesthetic, local—
   Children up to 2 years of age: Dosage has not been established.
   Children 2 years of age and older: See *Usual adult and adolescent dose*.

**Strength(s) usually available**
U.S.—
   1% (OTC) [*Prax*].

**Packaging and storage**
Store below 40 °C (104 °F), preferably between 15 and 30 °C (59 and 86 °F), unless otherwise specified by manufacturer. Protect from freezing.

**Auxiliary labeling**
• For external use only.

### PRAMOXINE HYDROCHLORIDE AND MENTHOL GEL

**Usual adult and adolescent dose**
Anesthetic, local—
   Topical, applied to affected areas three or four times a day as needed.

**Usual pediatric dose**
Anesthetic, local—
   Children up to 2 years of age: Dosage has not been established.
   Children 2 years of age and older: See *Usual adult and adolescent dose*.

**Strength(s) usually available**
U.S.—
   1% of pramoxine hydrochloride and 0.5% of menthol (OTC) [*Pramegel*].
Canada—
   1% of pramoxine hydrochloride and 0.5% of menthol (OTC) [*Pramegel*].

**Packaging and storage**
Store below 40 °C (104 °F), preferably between 15 and 30 °C (59 and 86 °F), unless otherwise specified by manufacturer. Protect from freezing.

**Auxiliary labeling**
• For external use only.

### PRAMOXINE HYDROCHLORIDE AND MENTHOL LOTION

**Usual adult and adolescent dose**
Anesthetic, local—
   Topical, applied to affected areas three or four times a day as needed.

**Usual pediatric dose**
Anesthetic, local—
   Children up to 2 years of age: Dosage has not been established.
   Children 2 years of age and older: See *Usual adult and adolescent dose*.

**Strength(s) usually available**
U.S.—
   1% of pramoxine hydrochloride and 0.2% of menthol (OTC) [*Almay Anti-itch Lotion*].

USP DI              Anesthetics (Topical)    161

**Packaging and storage**
Store below 40 °C (104 °F), preferably between 15 and 30 °C (59 and 86 °F), unless otherwise specified by manufacturer. Protect from freezing.

**Auxiliary labeling**
- For external use only.

---

## TETRACAINE

## Summary of Differences
Physicochemical characteristics:
    An ester-type (PABA-derivative) local anesthetic.
Precautions:
    Cross-sensitivity and/or related problems—May occur with other ester-type anesthetics, especially other PABA derivatives, with PABA or parabens, and with paraphenylenediamine.
Drug interactions and/or related problems:
    Cholinesterase inhibitors may inhibit metabolism of tetracaine.
    Tetracaine may antagonize antibacterial activity of sulfonamides.
Side/adverse effects:
    More likely to cause contact sensitization than most other topical anesthetics.
    See also *Side/Adverse Effects*.

## Topical Dosage Forms

### TETRACAINE HYDROCHLORIDE CREAM USP

**Usual adult and adolescent dose**
Anesthetic, local—
    Topical, applied as a 1% cream to affected areas three or four times a day as needed.

**Usual adult prescribing limits**
Not more than 28.35 grams in a twenty-four-hour period.

**Usual pediatric dose**
Anesthetic, local—
    Children up to 2 years of age: Dosage must be individualized by a physician.
    Children 2 years of age and older: See *Usual adult and adolescent dose*.

**Usual pediatric prescribing limits**
Not more than 7 grams in a twenty-four-hour period.

**Strength(s) usually available**
U.S.—
    1% (OTC) [*Pontocaine Cream*].
Canada—
    Not commercially available.

**Packaging and storage**
Store below 40 °C (104 °F), preferably between 15 and 30 °C (59 and 86 °F), unless otherwise specified by manufacturer. Protect from freezing.

**Auxiliary labeling**
- For external use only.

### TETRACAINE AND MENTHOL OINTMENT USP

**Usual adult and adolescent dose**
Anesthetic, local—
    Topical, applied to affected area as a 0.5% ointment three or four times a day as needed.

**Usual adult prescribing limits**
Not more than 28.35 grams in a twenty-four-hour period.

**Usual pediatric dose**
Anesthetic, local—
    Children up to 2 years of age: Dosage must be individualized by a physician.
    Children 2 years of age and older: See *Usual adult and adolescent dose*.

**Usual pediatric prescribing limits**
Not more than 7 grams in a twenty-four-hour period.

**Strength(s) usually available**
U.S.—
    0.5% of tetracaine and 0.5% of menthol (OTC) [*Pontocaine Ointment*].
Canada—
    Not commercially available.

**Packaging and storage**
Store below 40 °C (104 °F), preferably between 15 and 30 °C (59 and 86 °F), unless otherwise specified by manufacturer. Protect from freezing.

**Auxiliary labeling**
- For external use only.

Revised: 08/29/94

---

# ANESTHETICS, BARBITURATE    Systemic

This monograph includes information on the following: 1) Methohexital; 2) Thiopental

BAN:
    Methohexital—Methohexitone
    Thiopental sodium—Thiopentone sodium

VA CLASSIFICATION (Primary): CN202

Note: Controlled substances in the U.S. and Canada as follows:

| Drug | U.S. | Canada |
|---|---|---|
| Methohexital | IV | G |
| Thiopental | III | G |

Commonly used brand name(s): *Brevital*[1]; *Brietal*[1]; *Pentothal*[2].

Other commonly used names are: Methohexitone, Thiopentone

Note: For a listing of dosage forms and brand names by country availability, see *Dosage Forms* section(s).

## Category
Anesthetic (general).

## Indications
Note: Bracketed information in the *Indications* section refers to uses that are not included in U.S. product labeling.

**Accepted**
Anesthesia, general—Methohexital and thiopental are indicated primarily for the induction of general anesthesia. They are also indicated for use alone as intravenous anesthesia for short (15-minute) surgical procedures with minimal painful stimuli; for supplementing other anesthetic agents; and to produce hypnosis during balanced anesthesia with other agents such as analgesics or muscle relaxants.

Barbiturate anesthetics may be administered in small doses and in combination with an opioid analgesic and nitrous oxide for maintenance of anesthesia in prolonged procedures.

Convulsions (treatment)—Thiopental for injection is indicated for short-term use in the control of convulsive states during or following inhalation anesthesia, local anesthesia, or other causes.

[Although parenteral thiopental has been reported to be effective in status epilepticus when used in low doses that do not depress the level of consciousness and has been used to induce general anesthesia in patients with prolonged status epilepticus who failed to respond to antiepileptic agents, including diazepam and phenytoin, these uses are controversial and further studies are needed.][1]

Hypertension, cerebral (treatment)[1]—Thiopental for injection may be indicated in the treatment of increased intracranial pressure if adequate ventilation is provided.It may be used to attenuate the increase in intracranial pressure during the use of volatile anesthetics. It may also be useful in the management of conditions associated with acutely increased intracranial pressure, such as Reye's syndrome, cerebral edema, and acute head injury.

Narcoanalysis[1]—Thiopental for injection is indicated for narcoanalysis in psychiatric disorders.

Anesthesia, basal or
Narcosis, basal—Thiopental rectal suspension may be indicated for basal anesthesia (preanesthetic sedation) or basal narcosis when administration via the rectal route is necessary, although absorption from the rectum may be unpredictable. Thiopental for rectal solution and methohexital for rectal solution also are used for basal anesthesia. Thiopental for rectal solution may be used for basal narcosis also. However, the barbiturate anesthetics generally have been superseded by other medications, such as diazepam, for sedation during short surgical operations, diagnostic procedures, or regional anesthesia.

[Hypoxia, cerebral (treatment)][1] or
[Ischemia, cerebral (treatment)][1]—Thiopental for injection is being used in high doses to protect the brain from hypoxia and ischemia following head injuries and other related conditions.

[1]Not included in Canadian product labeling.

## Pharmacology/Pharmacokinetics

### Physicochemical characteristics
Molecular weight—
 Methohexital sodium: 284.29.
 Thiopental sodium: 264.32.
pKa—
 Thiopental sodium: 7.4.
 Oil:water partition coefficient—Thiopental sodium: 580
 Note: Methohexital is also highly lipid-soluble, but its oil:water partition coefficient is lower than that of thiopental.

### Mechanism of action/Effect
Ultra short-acting barbiturate anesthetics depress the central nervous system (CNS) to produce hypnosis and anesthesia without analgesia.
 Anesthetic (general)—
  The exact mechanism by which barbiturate anesthetics produce general anesthesia is not completely understood. However, it has been proposed that they act by enhancing responses to gamma-aminobutyric acid (GABA), diminishing glutamate (GLU) responses, and directly depressing excitability by increasing membrane conductance (an effect reversed by the GABA antagonist picrotoxin), thereby producing a net decrease in neuronal excitability to provide anesthetic action.
  Although the mechanism of action of barbiturates as sedative-hypnotics has not been completely established, the barbiturates appear to act at the level of the thalamus where they inhibit ascending conduction in the reticular formation, thus interfering with the transmission of impulses to the cortex. Recent studies have suggested that the sedative-hypnotic effects of barbiturates may be related to their ability to enhance or mimic the inhibitory synaptic action of GABA.
  The mechanism of action of barbiturate anesthetics as anticonvulsants has not been completely established; however, in recent electrophysiological studies, barbiturate anesthetics (such as parenteral thiopental) that exert clinical anticonvulsant activity only at doses producing deep sedation or anesthesia have been shown to act by producing a GABA-like effect and enhancing postsynaptic inhibition responses to GABA.
  The mechanism by which thiopental reduces intracranial pressure and protects the brain from cerebral ischemia and hypoxia is not completely understood. However, it is related to thiopental's anesthetic action and results in increased cerebral vascular resistance with a decrease in cerebral blood flow and cerebral blood volume. Various mechanisms of action have been proposed, including a reduction of cerebral metabolic rate, a decrease in the functional activity of the brain, an inhibition of the brain stem neurogenic mechanism of vasoparalysis, a sealing effect on membranes, and a scavenging of free oxygen radicals.

### Other actions/effects
Barbiturate anesthetics are potent respiratory depressants; respiratory depression is dose-related and is potentiated by opioid premedication.
Laryngeal reflexes are depressed with deep levels of anesthesia.
Barbiturate anesthetics have little, if any, analgesic activity.
There is either a fall or no change in mean arterial blood pressure, the former being more pronounced in hypertensive or hypovolemic patients; a decrease in cardiac output; an increase in total calculated peripheral resistance; an increase or no change in heart rate; a considerable decrease in renal plasma flow; a decrease in intrathoracic blood volume; an increase in blood flow and volume in the extremities; a decrease or no change in the central, right atrial, and peripheral venous pressures; and a decrease in cerebral blood flow with a marked reduction in cerebrospinal fluid (CSF) pressure. Direct depression of cardiac contractility is dose-related.
Barbiturate anesthetics have no effect on uterine muscle tone.
Renal, hepatic, and gastrointestinal functions are depressed by barbiturate anesthetics, but the effects are rarely of clinical significance.

### Absorption
Thiopental rectal suspension—May be unpredictable.

### Distribution
Because of their high lipid solubility and low degree of ionization, barbiturate anesthetics rapidly cross the blood-brain barrier and are rapidly redistributed from the brain to other body tissues, first to highly perfused visceral organs (liver, kidneys, heart) and muscle, and later to fatty tissues.
When barbiturate anesthetics are administered repeatedly or by continuous infusion, accumulation in and slow release from lipoidal storage sites may result in prolonged anesthesia, somnolence, and respiratory and circulatory depression. Concentrations of thiopental in fatty tissues may be 6 to 12 times greater than in plasma. Because of methohexital's lower lipid solubility (and, consequently, lower concentrations in fatty tissues) and shorter elimination half-life, methohexital is less likely than thiopental to accumulate with repeated or continuous administration.
Barbiturate anesthetics rapidly cross the placenta and appear in cord blood. Also, after administration of large doses, thiopental is distributed into breast milk.
Volume of distribution at steady-state ($V_{DSS}$)—
 Methohexital: 1.9 to 2.2 L per kg of body weight (L/kg).
 Thiopental: 1.7 to 2.5 L/kg; may increase to 4.1 L/kg during pregnancy at term and to 7.9 L/kg in obese patients.

### Protein binding
Methohexital—High (3%).
Thiopental—High (72–86%).

### Biotransformation
Primarily hepatic; also, biotransformed to a small extent in other tissues, especially the kidneys and brain.
Methohexital is metabolized more rapidly than thiopental. Although most of thiopental's metabolites are inactive, about 3 to 5% of a dose is desulfurated to pentobarbital, which is cleared from the body much more slowly than thiopental. The significance of this metabolic pathway is relevant only in patients receiving large doses of thiopental.
When large quantities of thiopental are administered by continuous intravenous infusion over a prolonged period of time, progressively increasing saturation of hepatic metabolizing enzymes may occur, resulting in a rapid increase in the plasma concentration.

### Half-life
Distribution—Rapid.
 Methohexital:
  $5.6 \pm 2.7$ minutes.
 Thiopental:
  4.6 to 8.5 minutes.
Elimination—
 Methohexital:
  Adults—1.5 to 5 hours; increases with age.
 Thiopental:
  Adults—10 to 12 hours; increases with age. May be increased to 26.1 hours during pregnancy at term and to 27.85 hours in obese patients.
  Children—6.1 hours.
 Note: When low doses of thiopental (e.g., 5 mg per kg of body weight) are administered for induction of anesthesia, the elimination half-life is independent of plasma concentration.
  Administration of high doses of thiopental (e.g., 300 to 600 mg per kg of body weight) results in an increase in the elimination half-life.

### Onset of action
Rapid, due to the high lipid solubility of the barbiturate anesthetics.
 Anesthesia—
  Methohexital:
   Intravenous—Within 60 seconds.
   Rectal—Within 5 to 11 minutes.
  Thiopental:
   Intravenous—30 to 60 seconds.
   Rectal—Within 8 to 10 minutes.
 Note: After intravenous administration of induction doses of thiopental, muscle relaxation occurs about 30 seconds after unconsciousness is attained.
  After intravenous administration of induction doses of a barbiturate anesthetic, the depth of anesthesia may increase for up to 40 seconds and then decrease progressively until consciousness returns. This reflects rapid changes in the concentration of anesthetic at its sites of action in the brain and is a consequence of its initial distribution to the brain followed by subsequent redistribution to other tissues.
 Hypnosis—
  Thiopental (intravenous):
   Within 10 to 40 seconds.

**Time to peak concentration**
Intravenous administration—
  Brain: Methohexital or thiopental—Within 30 seconds.
  Muscles: Thiopental—15 to 30 minutes.
  Fat: Thiopental—Several hours.
Note: Very highly perfused tissues such as the brain, heart, liver, and kidneys achieve concentrations equal to peak plasma concentrations.

**Duration of action**
Intravenous administration—
  Methohexital: 5 to 7 minutes.
  Thiopental: 10 to 30 minutes.
Note: The brief duration of action is due to the rapid rate of redistribution and, to some extent, metabolism accompanied by a rapid fall in plasma concentration. Administration of large or repeated doses may substantially delay recovery.

**Elimination**
Renal; however, renal elimination is minimal because of extensive renal tubular reabsorption due to the high lipid solubility of barbiturate anesthetics.
  Clearance—
    In adults:
      Methohexital—9.3 to 12.1 mL/kg per minute.
      Thiopental—1.6 to 4.3 mL/kg per minute; may be increased during pregnancy at term to 286 mL per minute.
    Note: When thiopental is administered in large doses by continuous infusion over a prolonged period of time, the kinetics of elimination change from first-order to non-linear or zero-order kinetics. In low doses (e.g., 5 mg per kg of body weight) for induction of anesthesia, thiopental shows first-order kinetics and the rate of elimination is independent of plasma concentration. In higher doses (300 to 600 mg per kg of body weight) for more prolonged periods, it shows zero-order kinetics and the rate of elimination varies with the plasma concentration.

## Precautions to Consider

**Cross-sensitivity and/or related problems**
Patients sensitive to one barbiturate may be sensitive to other barbiturates also.

**Carcinogenicity/Mutagenicity**
Studies in animals have not been performed to determine the carcinogenic and mutagenic potential of methohexital or thiopental.

**Pregnancy/Reproduction**
Fertility—Studies in animals have not been performed to determine the effect of methohexital or thiopental on fertility.
Pregnancy—Use of barbiturate anesthetics during pregnancy may cause CNS depression in the fetus. Adequate and well-controlled studies in humans have not been done to determine whether barbiturate anesthetics are teratogenic.
  *Methohexital*—
    Methohexital crosses the placenta.
    Studies in pregnant rabbits and rats given methohexital up to 4 and 7 times the human dose, respectively, produced no evidence of teratogenicity and no fetal abnormalities.
    FDA Pregnancy Category B.
  *Thiopental*—
    Thiopental crosses the placenta. The concentration in cord vein blood is at its maximum 2 to 3 minutes after an intravenous dose is administered to the mother.
    Studies in animals have not been done.
    FDA Pregnancy Category C.

**Breast-feeding**
Problems in humans have not been documented. However, barbiturate anesthetics are distributed into breast milk; small amounts may appear in breast milk following administration of large doses to the nursing mother.

**Pediatrics**
Appropriate studies on the relationship of age to the effects of barbiturate anesthetics have not been performed in the pediatric population. However, no pediatrics-specific problems have been documented to date.

**Geriatrics**
Following administration of barbiturate anesthetics for short (outpatient) procedures, recovery of cognitive and psychomotor functions is generally slower in elderly patients than in younger adults. In addition, elderly patients are more likely to have age-related hepatic function impairment, which may require reduction of dosage in patients receiving barbiturate anesthetics, and age-related renal function impairment, which may prolong the effects of these medications.

**Drug interactions and/or related problems**
The following drug interactions and/or related problems have been selected on the basis of their potential clinical significance (possible mechanism in parentheses where appropriate)—not necessarily inclusive (» = major clinical significance):
Note: Combinations containing any of the following medications, depending on the amount present, may also interact with this medication.

» Alcohol or
» CNS depression–producing medications, other, including those commonly used for preanesthetic medication or induction or supplementation of anesthesia (See *Appendix II*)
  (concurrent administration may increase the CNS depressant, respiratory depressant, or hypotensive effects of barbiturate anesthetics as well as decreasing anesthetic requirements and prolonging recovery from anesthesia; dosage adjustments may be required)

Antihypertensives, especially diazoxide or ganglionic blockers such as guanadrel, guanethidine, mecamylamine, or trimethaphan or
Diuretics or
Hypotension-producing medications, other (See *Appendix II* )
  (concurrent use of these medications with barbiturate anesthetics may result in an additive hypotensive effect, which could be severe; dosage adjustments may be necessary; patients should be monitored for excessive fall in blood pressure during and following concurrent use)
  (concurrent use of antihypertensives with CNS depressant effects, such as clonidine, guanabenz, methyldopa, metyrosine, pargyline, and rauwolfia alkaloids, may increase the CNS depressant effects of barbiturate anesthetics)

Hypothermia-producing medications, other (See *Appendix II*)
  (concurrent use with barbiturate anesthetics may increase the risk of hypothermia)

Ketamine
  (concurrent use of ketamine, especially in high doses or when rapidly administered, with barbiturate anesthetics may increase the risk of hypotension and/or respiratory depression)

Magnesium sulfate, parenteral
  (concurrent use may increase the CNS depressant effects of barbiturate anesthetics)

Phenothiazines, especially promethazine
  (in addition to possibly increasing CNS depressant effects, concurrent use may potentiate the hypotensive and CNS excitatory effects of barbiturate anesthetics)

**Laboratory value alterations**
The following have been selected on the basis of their potential clinical significance (possible effect in parentheses where appropriate)—not necessarily inclusive (» = major clinical significance):
With diagnostic test results
  Sodium iodide I 123 and
  Sodium iodide I 131 and
  Sodium pertechnetate Tc 99m
    (thiopental may decrease thyroidal uptake of sodium iodide I 123 and I 131 and sodium pertechnetate Tc 99m)

**Medical considerations/Contraindications**
The medical considerations/contraindications included have been selected on the basis of their potential clinical significance (reasons given in parentheses where appropriate)—not necessarily inclusive (» = major clinical significance).

*Except under special circumstances, this medication should not be used when the following medical problems exist:*

*For parenteral and rectal administration*
» Porphyria, acute intermittent or variegata or history of
  (barbiturate anesthetics may aggravate symptoms by inducing enzymes responsible for porphyrin synthesis)

*For rectal administration*
» Inflammatory, ulcerative, bleeding or neoplastic lesions of the lower bowel
  (condition may be exacerbated)

*Risk-benefit should be considered when the following medical problems exist:*

Note: Dosage should be reduced and the medication administered slowly if barbiturate anesthetics are used in the presence of the following medical problems.

*For parenteral and rectal administration*
    Addison's disease or
    Anemia, severe or
    Hepatic function impairment or
    Myxedema or
    Renal function impairment
        (hypnotic effect may be prolonged or potentiated)
» Cardiovascular disease, severe or
» Congestive heart failure or
» Hypotension or shock
        (barbiturate anesthetics produce cardiovascular depressant effects; condition may be exacerbated)
    Myasthenia gravis or
    Neuromuscular disorders, other, such as muscular dystrophies and myotonias
        (respiratory depression may be prolonged; dosage should be carefully titrated)
» Respiratory disease involving dyspnea or obstruction, particularly status asthmaticus
        (barbiturate anesthetics produce respiratory depressant effects)
» Sensitivity to barbiturates
    Caution should be used also in debilitated patients because respiratory depression, apnea, or hypotension may be more likely to occur in these patients.

**Patient monitoring**
The following may be especially important in patient monitoring (other tests may be warranted in some patients, depending on condition; » = major clinical significance):
» Blood pressure and
» Body temperature and
» Cardiac/pulse rate and
» Electrocardiographic evaluation and
» Oxygenation and
» Respiratory and ventilatory status
    (it is recommended that the patient's blood and tissue oxygenation, ventilation, circulation, and body temperature be monitored continuously during anesthetic administration and as required during the recovery period)
Note: Various organizations, including medical specialty societies, and institutions have established standards for the pre-, intra-, and post-procedure care, evaluation, and monitoring of patients receiving various forms of anesthesia and/or sedation. The above recommendations represent the minimum standards established by the American Society of Anesthesiologists for monitoring the status of patients receiving general anesthesia. Individual patients may require additional monitoring.

*For thiopental only*
    Plasma thiopental concentrations
        (monitoring of plasma thiopental concentration is recommended if thiopental is administered by intravenous infusion over an extended period of time, such as in the treatment of increased intracranial pressure)

## Side/Adverse Effects

Note: Because barbiturate anesthetics are potent respiratory depressants, apnea may occur immediately after intravenous injection, especially in the presence of hypovolemia, cranial trauma, or opioid premedication.

    During induction of anesthesia or in lightly anesthetized patients, laryngeal spasm may be induced by a variety of stimuli such as surgical stimulation, the premature insertion of the laryngoscope blade or airway, and pharyngeal secretions.

    Excitatory phenomena such as involuntary muscle movements, coughing, and hiccups occur more frequently with methohexital than with thiopental.

    True anaphylaxis has been reported to occur with barbiturate anesthetics, but is rare.

    Overdosage may occur from too rapid or repeated injections. Too rapid injection may cause a severe drop in blood pressure, possibly to shock levels. Excessive or too rapid injections may result in respiratory difficulties such as laryngospasm and apnea. Repeated administration may also lead to accumulation of the barbiturate, resulting in substantial prolongation of the medication's effects.

    Impairment of psychomotor skills may occur following barbiturate anesthesia and may persist for varying lengths of time (usually about 24 hours), depending upon the anesthetic and/or combination of medications used and the total dosages administered. Possible adverse effects on the patient's ability to drive or perform other tasks requiring alertness and coordination should be kept in mind when a barbiturate anesthetic is administered for outpatient surgery.

The following side/adverse effects have been selected on the basis of their potential clinical significance (possible signs and symptoms in parentheses where appropriate)—not necessarily inclusive:

**Those indicating need for medical attention**
    *Allergic reaction, acute* (abdominal pain; anxiety or restlessness; skin rash, hives, itching, or redness; swelling of eyelids, face, or lips; unusually low blood pressure; wheezing or difficulty in breathing); *cardiac arrhythmias* (fast, slow, or irregular heartbeat); *circulatory depression* (unusually low blood pressure, severe or continuing); *excitatory phenomena* (coughing, difficulty in breathing, hiccups, muscle twitching or jerking)—occurring during induction of anesthesia or in light anesthesia; *respiratory depression* (shortness of breath, slow or irregular breathing, troubled breathing); *thrombophlebitis* (redness, swelling, or pain at injection site)

*With rectal administration only*
    *Cramping; diarrhea; rectal irritation or bleeding*

**Those occurring postsurgically and indicating need for medical attention**
Incidence rare
    *Emergence delirium* (anxiety; confusion; excitement; hallucinations; nervousness; restlessness); *immune hemolytic anemia with renal failure* (back, leg, or stomach pain; nausea, vomiting, or loss of appetite; unusual tiredness or weakness; fever; pale skin); *radial nerve palsy* (weakness of wrist and fingers)
    Note: *Immune hemolytic anemia with renal failure* and *radial nerve palsy* have occurred rarely with the use of thiopental.

**Those occurring postsurgically and indicating need for medical attention only if they continue**
Incidence more frequent
    *Increased sensitivity to cold, during recovery* (shivering or trembling)
Incidence less frequent or rare
    *Drowsiness, prolonged; headache; nausea or vomiting*

## Overdose

For more information on the management of overdose or unintentional ingestion, **contact a Poison Control Center** (see *PoisonControl Center Listing*).

The following effects have been selected on the basis of their potential clinical significance (possible signs and symptoms in parentheses where appropriate)—not necessarily inclusive:

**Acute effects**
    *CNS depression, severe; hypotension, severe; loss of peripheral vascular resistance; respiratory depression, severe, including apnea*
    Note: *Circulatory and respiratory depression* may result in *pulmonary edema* and/or *cardiorespiratory arrest*.

**Treatment of overdose**
Discontinuation of the anesthetic.

Specific treatment—If overdosage occurs with a rectal barbiturate anesthetic preparation, the contents of the rectum should be promptly evacuated; further dosing should be delayed until the effects of absorption of the initial dose can be determined.

Monitoring—Vital signs, blood gases, and serum electrolytes should be monitored.

Supportive care—Supportive measures such as establishing and maintaining a patent airway (by intubation if necessary), administering 100% oxygen with assisted ventilation if necessary. For hypotension—Intravenous fluids should be administered and the patients's legs raised. If a desirable increase in blood pressure is not obtained, vasopressor and/or inotropic drugs may be used as required.

## Patient Consultation

As an aid to patient consultation, refer to *Advice for the Patient, Anesthetics, General (Systemic)*.

In providing consultation, consider emphasizing the following selected information (» = major clinical significance):

**Before receiving this medication**
» Conditions affecting use, especially:
    Sensitivity to barbiturates
        Pregnancy—Crosses the placenta and may cause CNS depression in the fetus
    Other medications, especially other CNS depressants
    Other medical problems, especially acute intermittent or variegata porphyria (or history of); cardiovascular disease, severe; hypo-

tension or shock; respiratory disease involving dyspnea or obstruction (particularly status asthmaticus); and, for rectal administration only, inflammatory, ulcerative, bleeding, or neoplastic lesions of lower bowel

**Proper use of this medication**
Proper dosing

**Precautions after receiving this medication**
» Possibility of psychomotor impairment following use of anesthetics; for about 24 hours following anesthesia, using caution in driving or performing other tasks requiring alertness and coordination
» Avoiding use of alcohol or other CNS depressants within 24 hours following anesthesia except as directed by physician or dentist

## General Dosing Information

Barbiturate anesthetics should be administered only by individuals qualified in the use of general anesthetics. Appropriate resuscitative and endotracheal intubation equipment, oxygen, and medications for prevention and treatment of anesthetic emergencies must be immediately available. Airway patency must be maintained at all times.

Dosage of the barbiturate anesthetics must be individualized according to the desired depth of anesthesia, concomitant use of other medications and/or nitrous oxide, and the patient's physical condition, age, sex, and weight.

Young patients may require relatively larger doses than middle-aged or elderly patients. Prepuberty dose requirements are the same for both sexes, but adult females require smaller doses than adult males.

Care should be taken to avoid extravasation or intra-arterial injection of barbiturate anesthetics. Extravascular injection may cause pain, swelling, ulceration, and necrosis. Intra-arterial injection may produce arteritis, followed by vasospasm, edema, thrombosis, and gangrene of an extremity.

Repeated doses or continuous infusion of barbiturate anesthetics may cause cumulative effects, resulting in prolonged somnolence and respiratory and circulatory depression.

Caution is required if the patient requires a second anesthetic on the same day; a reduction in the dose of the intravenous barbiturate anesthetic may be required.

Although barbiturate anesthetics may be given in sufficient doses to produce deep surgical anesthesia in the presence of external stimulation such as surgical incision, these doses may also produce dangerous cardiovascular and respiratory depression.

Because the rapid distribution of barbiturate anesthetics out of the brain can result in light anesthesia characterized by reflex hyperactivity of the airway to stimulation (e.g., intubation, instrumentation, secretions), an adequate depth of anesthesia should be induced in patients predisposed to bronchospasm or with upper airway obstruction, when coughing and hiccupping are undesirable, and to avoid laryngospasm that may occur from direct or indirect stimulation.

To minimize mucous secretions, anticholinergics, such as atropine or glycopyrrolate, may be administered as premedication. In addition, an opiate may be administered to enhance the otherwise poor analgesic effects of the barbiturate anesthetic. The peak effects of the premedication should be attained shortly before induction of anesthesia. Also, muscle relaxants may be required and should be administered separately.

Tolerance has been reported following multiple use, as in burn patients.

Individuals tolerant to alcohol or barbiturates may require higher doses of barbiturate anesthetics.

**Treatment of adverse effects**
Recommended treatment for adverse effects of barbiturate anesthetics includes
• For laryngospasm—Positive pressure oxygen 100% should be administered; then, if necessary, a skeletal muscle relaxant may be administered; cricothyrotomy may be required in difficult cases.
• For extravasation—Procaine 1% may be administered locally to relieve pain and enhance vasodilation. Local application of heat may also help to increase local circulation and remove the infiltrate.
• For inadvertent intra-arterial injection—Treatment varies with the severity of symptoms. The injected barbiturate anesthetic should be diluted by removing the tourniquet and any restrictive garment. The needle should be left in place, if possible. A dilute solution of 1% procaine, 10 mL, may be injected into the artery to inhibit smooth muscle spasm. Sympathetic block of the brachial plexus or stellate ganglion should be performed, if necessary, to relieve pain and assist in opening collateral circulation. To prevent thrombus formation, heparinization should be instituted immediately, unless otherwise contraindicated. Local infiltration of an alpha-adrenergic blocking agent into the vasospastic area may be considered. Intraarterial injection of a glucocorticoid at the site of injury, followed by administration of systemic corticosteroids should be considered. Also, it has been reported that intra-arterial administration of urokinase may promote fibrinolysis even if administration is late in treatment. Postinjury arterial injection of vasodilators and/or arterial infusion of parenteral fluids are generally not useful in reducing the area of necrosis.
• For shivering—Treatment includes warming the patient with blankets, maintaining room temperature at 22 °C (72 °F), and administering chlorpromazine or methylphenidate.
• For thrombophlebitis—Treatment is symptomatic and may require rest and application of heat.

---

### *METHOHEXITAL*

## Summary of Differences

Pharmacology/pharmacokinetics:
  Physicochemical characteristics—Oil:water partition coefficient is lower than that of thiopental.
  Distribution—Does not concentrate in lipids to the same extent as thiopental; less likely than thiopental to accumulate with repeated or prolonged administration.
  Biotransformation—More rapid than thiopental.
  Half-life—Distribution and elimination half-lives are shorter than those of thiopental.
  Duration of action—Shorter than thiopental.
Side/adverse effects:
  Excitatory phenomena occur more frequently than with thiopental.

## Additional Dosing Information

See also *General Dosing Information*.

Methohexital is about 2 to 3 times more potent than thiopental.

Preanesthetic medication may be advisable with methohexital. Any preanesthetic medication may be used; however, the combination of an opioid and a belladonna derivative is preferable to the phenothiazines, which have been reported to potentiate the hypotensive and CNS excitatory effects of methohexital.

A 1% solution of methohexital is recommended for induction of anesthesia and for maintenance by intermittent injection. Higher concentrations greatly increase the incidence of muscular movements and irregularities in respiration and blood pressure.

## Parenteral Dosage Forms

### METHOHEXITAL SODIUM FOR INJECTION USP

**Usual adult dose**
Anesthesia, general—
  Induction:
    Dosage must be individualized by physician; however, as a general guideline—Intravenous, 1 to 2 mg per kg of body weight as required, administered cautiously.
  Maintenance:
    Dosage must be individualized by physician; however, as a general guideline—Intravenous (intermittent), 250 mcg (0.25 mg) to 1 mg per kg of body weight as required.
  Note: Some anesthesiologists prefer the continuous drip method of maintenance with a 0.2% solution, the rate of flow being individualized for each patient.

**Usual pediatric dose**
Anesthesia, general—
  Induction
    Dosage must be individualized by physician; however, as a general guideline—
    Intramuscular, 5 to 10 mg per kg of body weight as required.
    Intravenous, 1 to 2 mg per kg of body weight as required, administered cautiously.

**Size(s) usually available**
U.S.—
  500 mg (Rx) [*Brevital* (anhydrous sodium carbonate 30 mg)].
  2.5 grams (Rx) [*Brevital* (anhydrous sodium carbonate 150 mg)].
  5 grams (Rx) [*Brevital* (anhydrous sodium carbonate 300 mg)].
Canada—
  500 mg (Rx) [*Brietal* (anhydrous sodium carbonate)].
  2.5 grams (Rx) [*Brietal* (anhydrous sodium carbonate)].

**Packaging and storage**
Prior to reconstitution, store below 40 °C (104 °F), preferably between 15 and 30 °C (59 and 86 °F), unless otherwise specified by manufacturer.

**Preparation of dosage form**
Sterile water for injection, 5% dextrose injection, or 0.9% sodium chloride injection may be used as diluents. Bacteriostatic diluents and lactated Ringer's injection should not be used as diluents because they tend to cause precipitation.
For direct intravenous injection, sterile water for injection should be used as the diluent for preparation of a 1% methohexital sodium injection.
For more information on the preparation of a 1% methohexital injection, see the manufacturer's package insert.
For administration via intravenous infusion, a 0.2% injection is prepared by adding 500 mg of methohexital sodium to 250 mL of 5% dextrose injection or 0.9% sodium chloride injection; however, dextrose injections are sometimes sufficiently acid to cause precipitation. Sterile water for injection should not be used because of the resultant extreme hypotonicity, which will cause hemolysis.

**Stability**
Methohexital is stable in sterile water for injection at room temperature (25 °C [77 °F] or lower) for at least 6 weeks; solutions prepared with 5% dextrose injection or 0.9% sodium chloride injection are not stable for more than 24 hours.
Only clear injections should be used; if an injection becomes cloudy or a precipitate forms, the medication should be discarded.

**Incompatibilities**
Methohexital injections should not be mixed with acidic substances, such as atropine sulfate, metocurine iodide, and succinylcholine chloride, because precipitation will occur.
For additional information on the chemical compatibility of methohexital sodium with medications having a low (acid) pH, see the manufacturer's package insert.
Methohexital injections are incompatible with silicone and should not be allowed to come in contact with rubber stoppers or parts of disposable syringes that have been treated with silicone.
Methohexital sodium is incompatible with bacteriostatic diluents and with lactated Ringer's injection; precipitation will occur.

**Note**
Controlled substance in the U.S. and Canada.

## Rectal Dosage Forms
### METHOHEXITAL SODIUM FOR RECTAL SOLUTION
**Usual pediatric dose**
Anesthesia, basal—
  Rectal, 15 to 30 mg per kg of body weight as a 5 to 10% solution.
Note: For inactive or debilitated patients—Lower dosage is advisable.

**Size(s) usually available**
U.S.—
  Dosage form not commercially available. Compounding required for prescriptions.
Canada—
  Dosage form not commercially available. Compounding required for prescriptions.

**Packaging and storage**
Store below 40 °C (104 °F), preferably between 15 and 30 °C (59 and 86 °F), in a well-closed container. Protect from freezing.

**Preparation of dosage form**
To prepare a 5 to 10% methohexital rectal solution, dissolve an appropriate amount of methohexital sodium for injection in warm tap water.

**Stability**
If the solution becomes cloudy or a precipitate forms, the solution should be discarded.

**Incompatibilities**
Methohexital should not be mixed with acidic substances, such as atropine sulfate, metocurine iodide, and succinylcholine chloride, because precipitation will occur.
For additional information on the chemical compatibility of methohexital sodium with medications having a low (acid) pH, see the manufacturer's package insert for methohexital sodium for injection.
Methohexital solutions are incompatible with silicone and should not be allowed to come in contact with rubber stoppers or parts of disposable syringes that have been treated with silicone.
Methohexital sodium is incompatible with bacteriostatic diluents and with lactated Ringer's injection; precipitation will occur.

---

# THIOPENTAL

## Summary of Differences
Indications:
  Parenteral thiopental also indicated in the treatment of cerebral hypertension and for narcoanalysis in the treatment of psychiatric disorders; and is used in the treatment of cerebral ischemia and hypoxia.
Pharmacology/pharmacokinetics:
  Physicochemical characteristics—
    Oil:water partition coefficient is greater than that of methohexital.
  Distribution—
    Concentrates in fatty tissues to a greater extent than methohexital; risk of accumulation with repeated or prolonged administration is higher than with methohexital.
    Appears in breast milk following administration of large doses.
  Biotransformation—
    Less rapid than methohexital.
  Half-life—
    Distribution and elimination half-lives longer than those of methohexital.
  Duration of action—
    Greater than that of methohexital.
Patient monitoring:
  Monitoring of plasma concentrations is recommended if thiopental is administered by intravenous infusion over a prolonged period of time.

## Additional Dosing Information
See also *General Dosing Information*.
For parenteral dosage form only
  • A test dose of 25 to 75 mg (1 to 3 mL of a 2.5% solution) may be administered to determine tolerance or unusual sensitivity to thiopental; patient reaction should be observed for at least 60 seconds.
  • A 2 or 2.5% concentration of thiopental solution is used for intermittent intravenous administration.
  • A 3.4% concentration of thiopental in sterile water for injection is isotonic; concentrations less than 2% in sterile water for injection should not be used because they cause hemolysis.
For rectal suspension dosage form only
  • To assure easy extrusion of thiopental rectal suspension, instructions should be followed for filling the applicator and extruding a small amount before setting the stop device at the desired dose for rectal administration. Care should be taken not to use excessive pressure on the syringe plunger since this can cause the stop device to break or slip, which may result in an overdose.
  • A new applicator should be used for each repeat administration.
  • Unless there are unusual circumstances, such as fecal impaction, a cleansing enema is rarely required prior to administration of thiopental rectal suspension.

## Parenteral Dosage Forms
### THIOPENTAL SODIUM FOR INJECTION USP
**Usual adult dose**
Anesthesia, general—
  Induction:
    Dosage must be individualized by physician; however, as a general guideline—Intravenous, 50 to 100 mg (2 to 4 mL of a 2.5% solution) as required; or 3 to 5 mg per kg of body weight as a single dose.
  Maintenance:
    Dosage must be individualized by physician; however, as a general guideline—Intravenous (intermittent), 50 to 100 mg (2 to 4 mL of a 2.5% solution) as required.
    Note: When thiopental is used as the sole anesthetic agent, the desired level of anesthesia can be maintained by injection of small repeated doses as needed. Also, 0.2 to 0.4% solutions have been administered by continuous intravenous drip for maintenance.
Hypertension, cerebral[1]—
  Intravenous (intermittent), 1.5 to 3.5 mg per kg of body weight, repeated as required to reduce elevations of intracranial pressure.
  Note: Adequate ventilation must be provided.
Convulsions—
  Intravenous, 50 to 125 mg (2 to 5 mL of a 2.5% solution), administered as soon as possible after the convulsion begins.

Narcoanalysis[1]—
    Intravenous, as a 2.5% solution, administered at a rate of 100 mg per minute with the patient counting backwards from one hundred. Injection should be discontinued after counting becomes confused but before actual sleep is produced.
    Note: As alternative dosing, thiopental may be administered by rapid intravenous drip using a 0.2% concentration in 5% dextrose injection; however, the rate of administration should not exceed 50 mL per minute.

**Usual pediatric dose**
Anesthesia, general—
    Induction:
        Children up to 15 years of age—Dosage must be individualized by physician; however, as a general guideline: Intravenous, 3 to 5 mg per kg of body weight.
    Maintenance:
        Dosage must be individualized by physician; however, as a general guideline—Intravenous (intermittent), about 1 mg per kg of body weight as required.

**Size(s) usually available**
U.S.—
    250 mg (Rx) [*Pentothal;* GENERIC].
    400 mg (Rx) [*Pentothal;* GENERIC].
    500 mg (Rx) [*Pentothal;* GENERIC].
    1 gram (Rx) [*Pentothal*].
    2.5 grams (Rx) [*Pentothal;* GENERIC].
    5 grams (Rx) [*Pentothal;* GENERIC].
    10 grams (Rx) [GENERIC].
Canada—
    1 gram (Rx) [*Pentothal*].
    2.5 grams (Rx) [*Pentothal*].
    5 grams (Rx) [*Pentothal*].

**Packaging and storage**
Prior to reconstitution, store below 40 °C (104 °F), preferably between 15 and 30 °C (59 and 86 °F), unless otherwise specified by manufacturer.

**Preparation of dosage form**
Sterile water for injection, 0.9% sodium chloride injection, or 5% dextrose injection should be used as the diluent.
Sterile water for injection should not be used to prepare a 0.2 or 0.4% thiopental sodium injection for intravenous infusion because of the resultant extreme hypotonicity, which will cause hemolysis.
For more information on the preparation of thiopental injections, see the manufacturer's package insert.
Since Thiopental for Injection USP contains no added bacteriostatic agent, extreme care in preparation and handling should be used at all times to prevent the introduction of microbial contaminants.

**Stability**
Injections should be freshly prepared and used within 24 hours after reconstitution; discard unused portions after 24 hours.
Injections are most stable when prepared with sterile water for injection or 0.9% sodium chloride injection. They should be kept refrigerated and tightly stoppered.
Any factor or condition that tends to lower the pH of thiopental injections, such as diluents that are too acid or the absorption of carbon dioxide, which combines with water to form carbonic acid, will increase the possibility of precipitation of thiopental acid.
Sterilization by heating causes precipitation.
Injections containing a precipitate should not be administered.

**Incompatibilities**
Thiopental injections should not be mixed with succinylcholine, tubocurarine, or other medications that have an acid pH, because precipitation will occur.

**Note**
Controlled substance in the U.S. and Canada.

# Rectal Dosage Forms

## THIOPENTAL SODIUM FOR RECTAL SOLUTION

**Usual adult and adolescent dose**
Anesthesia, basal (preanesthetic sedation)—
    Rectal, 30 mg per kg of body weight.
Narcosis, basal—
    Normally active patients: Rectal, up to 9 mg per kg of body weight.
Note: For inactive or debilitated patients—Lower dosage is advisable.

**Usual adult prescribing limits**
Adults weighing 90 kg or more—
    Up to a total of 3 to 4 grams.

**Usual pediatric dose**
See *Usual adult and adolescent dose.*

**Strength(s) usually available**
U.S.—
    Dosage form not commercially available. Compounding required for prescriptions.
Canada—
    Dosage form not commercially available. Compounding required for prescriptions.

**Packaging and storage**
Store below 40 °C (104 °F), preferably between 15 and 30 °C (59 and 86 °F), in a well-closed container. Protect from freezing.

**Preparation of dosage form**
To prepare a thiopental rectal solution, dissolve an appropriate amount of thiopental sodium for injection in warm tap water.

**Stability**
Solutions should be freshly prepared and used within 24 hours after reconstitution; unused portions should be discarded after 24 hours.
Solutions are most stable when prepared with water or isotonic saline and kept refrigerated and tightly stoppered.
Any factor or condition that tends to lower the pH of thiopental solutions, such as diluents that are too acid or the absorption of carbon dioxide, which combines with water to form carbonic acid, will increase the possibility of precipitation of thiopental acid.
Sterilization by heating causes precipitation.
Solutions containing a precipitate should not be administered.

**Incompatibilities**
Thiopental solutions should not be mixed with succinylcholine, tubocurarine, or other medications that have an acid pH, because precipitation will occur.

## THIOPENTAL SODIUM RECTAL SUSPENSION

**Usual adult and adolescent dose**
Anesthesia, basal (preanesthetic sedation)—
    Rectal, 30 mg per kg of body weight.
Narcosis, basal—
    Normally active patients: Rectal, up to 9 mg per kg of body weight.
Note: For inactive or debilitated patients—Lower dosage is advisable.

**Usual adult prescribing limits**
Adults weighing 90 kg or more—
    Up to a total of 3 to 4 grams.

**Usual pediatric dose**
See *Usual adult and adolescent dose.*
Note: For children weighing 34 kg or more, a total dose of 1 to 1.5 grams should not be exceeded.
    For inactive or debilitated patients—Lower dosage is advisable.

**Strength(s) usually available**
U.S.—
    400 mg per gram (Rx) [*Pentothal* (mineral oil; dimethyldioctadecylammonium bentonite; anhydrous sodium carbonate 24 mg per gram)].

**Packaging and storage**
Store below 40 °C (104 °F), preferably between 15 and 30 °C (59 and 86 °F), unless otherwise specified by manufacturer. Protect from freezing.

**Stability**
Contains no bacteriostatic or antimicrobial agent. Intended only for one-time use.

**Auxiliary labeling**
• Shake well.

**Note**
Controlled substance in the U.S.

---

[1]Not included in Canadian product labeling.

Revised: 08/25/94

# ANESTHETICS, INHALATION Systemic

This monograph includes information on the following: 1) Enflurane; 2) Halothane; 3) Isoflurane; 4) Methoxyflurane; 5) Nitrous Oxide.

VA CLASSIFICATION (Primary): CN201

Commonly used brand name(s): *Ethrane*[1]; *Fluothane*[2]; *Forane*[3]; *Penthrane*[4]; *Somnothane*[2].

Note: For a listing of dosage forms and brand names by country availability, see *Dosage Forms* section(s).

## Category
Anesthetic (general).

## Indications
Note: Bracketed information in the *Indications* section refers to uses that are not included in U.S. product labeling.

### Accepted
Anesthesia, general—Enflurane, halothane, isoflurane, methoxyflurane, and nitrous oxide are indicated for the induction and maintenance of general anesthesia. However, inhalation anesthetic agents are rarely used alone; other medications are frequently administered to induce or supplement anesthesia.

Because of its weak anesthetic potency and muscle relaxant properties, nitrous oxide must be supplemented with another anesthetic or anesthesia adjunct (such as a barbiturate, benzodiazepine, opioid analgesic, or another inhalation anesthetic) and/or a neuromuscular blocking agent. Also, nitrous oxide is often administered concurrently with one of the other inhalation anesthetics to decrease the requirement for the more potent anesthetic.

[Enflurane][1], [isoflurane][1], methoxyflurane, and nitrous oxide are indicated in low doses to provide analgesia for procedures not requiring loss of consciousness.

Enflurane, [isoflurane][1], methoxyflurane, and nitrous oxide are indicated in low doses to provide analgesia for vaginal delivery.

For cesarean section: Enflurane, [halothane][1], [isoflurane][1], and [methoxyflurane][1] are indicated in low concentrations to supplement other general anesthetics during delivery by cesarean section.

### Unaccepted
Because of potential nephrotoxicity, administration of methoxyflurane in concentrations sufficient to produce muscle relaxation is not recommended; a neuromuscular blocking agent should be used concurrently if necessary. Also, it is recommended that methoxyflurane not be used during vascular surgery at or near renal blood vessels.

Halothane is not recommended for vaginal delivery unless uterine relaxation is required.

[1]Not included in Canadian product labeling.

## Pharmacology/Pharmacokinetics
See *Table 1*, page 173 and *Table 2*, page 174.

### Physicochemical characteristics
Molecular weight—
  Enflurane: 184.49.
  Halothane: 197.38.
  Isoflurane: 184.49.
  Methoxyflurane: 164.97.
  Nitrous oxide: 44.01.
Other Characteristics
  Blood-to-gas partition coefficient—
See *Table 1*, page 173.
  Oil-to-gas partition coefficient—
    See *Table 1*, page 173.

### Mechanism of action/Effect
The precise mechanism by which inhalation anesthetics produce loss of perception of sensations and unconsciousness is not known. Proposed mechanisms are based on the Meyer-Overton theory, which demonstrates the correlation between the potency of an anesthetic and its solubility in oil. Inhalation anesthetics may interfere with the physiological functioning of nerve cell membranes in the brain via an action at the lipid matrix of the membrane.

### Absorption
Inhalation anesthetics are rapidly absorbed into the circulation via the lungs.

## Precautions to Consider

### Carcinogenicity
For isoflurane: Although one study indicated that isoflurane may be carcinogenic, it is thought that exposure of the test animals to polybrominated biphenyls may have been responsible. Subsequent studies in which such exposure was avoided have not shown evidence of isoflurane-induced carcinogenicity.

For enflurane, halothane, methoxyflurane, and nitrous oxide: These anesthetics have not been shown to be carcinogenic.

### Tumorigenicity
For enflurane: Studies in mice have not shown evidence of tumorigenicity with enflurane.

### Mutagenicity
For halothane: *In vitro* testing (Ames test) has indicated that potential halothane metabolites (but not halothane itself) may be mutagenic.

For enflurane, isoflurane, methoxyflurane, and nitrous oxide: Mutagenic effects have not been observed with these inhalation anesthetics in the Ames test or the sister chromatid exchange test. However, statistically significant increases in sperm abnormalities have been observed in mice following 20 hours of exposure to 1.2% of enflurane.

### Pregnancy/Reproduction
Pregnancy—Inhalation anesthetics cross the placenta. Risk-benefit must be considered because studies (by retrospective survey) of operating room personnel chronically exposed to low concentrations of inhalation anesthetics indicate that pregnancies in female personnel and wives of male personnel may be subject to an increased incidence of spontaneous abortions, stillbirths, and possibly birth defects. However, the methods used in obtaining and interpreting the data in these studies have been questioned. Also, several animal studies (in which operating room conditions were simulated) have failed to show fetotoxic or teratogenic effects following chronic exposure of male and/or female animals to low concentrations of inhalation anesthetics prior to and/or during gestation.

First trimester: Administration of enflurane, halothane, or isoflurane early in pregnancy (for therapeutic abortion) has been reported to increase uterine bleeding. However, blood loss following enflurane administration was considered to be within acceptable limits.

For enflurane—Although studies in patients have not been done, some studies in rats and rabbits have not shown that enflurane causes adverse effects on the fetus. However, other studies in animals have shown that enflurane may be teratogenic.

FDA Pregnancy Category B.

For halothane—Although studies in patients have not been done, some animal studies have shown that halothane may be teratogenic.

For isoflurane—Although isoflurane has not been shown to cause fetal malformations in mice or rats, studies in mice receiving 7 MAC hours (the equivalent of 1 MAC [minimum alveolar concentration that prevents movement in 50% of subjects following a painful stimulus] administered for 7 hours) over a period of 10 days during gestation have indicated possible fetotoxicity as manifested by higher implantation losses and a significantly lower live birth index. Studies have not been done in patients.

For methoxyflurane—Although adequate and well-controlled studies in patients have not been done, some studies in animals have shown that methoxyflurane may be teratogenic. Also, studies in rats have indicated that exposure to doses equivalent to 67 hours of 0.2% methoxyflurane caused fetal growth retardation.

FDA Pregnancy Category C.

For nitrous oxide—Although problems in patients have not been documented, studies in rats have shown that nitrous oxide causes fetal death, growth retardation, and skeletal anomalies.

Labor and delivery—Enflurane, halothane, isoflurane, and methoxyflurane produce dose-dependent uterine relaxation, which may delay delivery and increase postpartum bleeding. Subanesthetic (analgesic) concentrations of enflurane, isoflurane, or methoxyflurane do not significantly decrease uterine contractions. Halothane is the most potent uterine relaxant; even low concentrations (< 0.5%) may decrease uterine contractions. Also, enflurane and halothane cause a dose-dependent decrease in the uterine response to oxytocics. Use of halothane during vaginal delivery is not recommended unless uterine relaxation is required (as for version or other intrauterine manipulations).

Although its safety in obstetrics has not been established by formal studies, isoflurane is used to provide obstetrical analgesia.

Postpartum—High concentrations of inhalation anesthetics administered during prolonged delivery may increase the risk of neonatal depression.

For methoxyflurane: Inorganic fluoride produced by methoxyflurane metabolism has been detected in cord blood in concentrations that are usually lower than, but sometimes equal to, the maternal blood concentration. The effect of inorganic fluoride on the neonate is not known; however, nephrotoxicity in the infant is thought to be unlikely following recommended doses of methoxyflurane.

**Breast-feeding**
Problems in humans have not been documented. However, halothane is distributed into breast milk.

**Pediatrics**
Studies performed to date have not demonstrated pediatrics-specific problems that would limit the usefulness of inhalation anesthetics in children. However, the minimum alveolar concentration (MAC) of inhalation anesthetics is higher in children than in adults. The MAC is highest in very young children and decreases as the age of the child increases.

**Geriatrics**
The MAC (minimum alveolar concentration) of an anesthetic is decreased in geriatric patients. Also, geriatric patients may be more susceptible to anesthetic-induced hypotension and circulatory depression and to methoxyflurane-induced nephrotoxicity; especially careful attention to dosage is recommended.

**Drug interactions and/or related problems**
See *Table 3*, page 175.

**Laboratory value alterations**
The following have been selected on the basis of their potential clinical significance (possible effect in parentheses where appropriate)—not necessarily inclusive (» = major clinical significance):

With physiology/laboratory test values
  Cerebrospinal fluid (CSF) pressure
    (anesthetics may increase CSF pressure)
  Liver function
    (abnormalities in liver function as shown by transient, mild increases in serum transaminase and/or lactate dehydrogenase activity may occur in the absence of hepatotoxicity; with enflurane, halothane, or methoxyflurane, significant abnormalities indicating hepatotoxicity may occur rarely)

**Medical considerations/Contraindications**
See *Table 4*, page 176.

**Patient monitoring**
The following may be especially important in patient monitoring (other tests may be warranted in some patients, depending on condition; » = major clinical significance):

*For all inhalation anesthetics*
  Blood pressure and
  Cardiac/pulse rate and
  Cardiac rhythm and
» Respiratory and ventilatory status
    (monitoring recommended during anesthetic administration)
  Body temperature
    (continuous monitoring advisable)

*For methoxyflurane*
» Renal function determinations
    (may be needed to detect possible nephrotoxicity if the patient's postoperative urine output is excessive)

## Side/Adverse Effects

Note: Hepatotoxicity ranging in severity from mild jaundice to hepatic necrosis has been reported following administration of enflurane, halothane, or methoxyflurane. Although a definite causal relationship has not been established, it has been proposed that a hypersensitivity reaction to the anesthetic may be involved. Hepatic damage has been reported much less frequently with enflurane or methoxyflurane than with halothane; however, the biochemical, clinical, and histologic features of the hepatotoxicity reported with each of these agents are similar. The risk of hepatotoxicity may be increased by intra- or postoperative hypoxia, repeated or sequential use of these agents, patient predisposition to hepatotoxicity, and patient history of hepatotoxicity not attributable to other causes following previous exposure to one of these anesthetics.

The risk of methoxyflurane-induced nephrotoxicity is related to the total dose (concentration and time) administered, degree of metabolism (which may be increased by hepatic enzyme induction), and patient predisposition to nephrotoxicity. Although polyuric renal failure has been most often reported, some patients have developed oliguric renal failure. Renal tubular necrosis may occur. Laboratory findings indicative of methoxyflurane-induced nephrotoxicity include elevations of blood sodium, blood urea nitrogen, blood creatinine, serum and urine fluoride, serum chloride, urine oxalic acid, and blood uric acid concentrations, and reductions of urine specific gravity and osmolality. Isolated cases of nephrotoxicity have also been reported with enflurane (following prolonged administration to patients with impaired renal function) and halothane; however, a definite causal relationship has not been established.

Impairment of psychomotor skills may occur following anesthesia and may persist for varying lengths of time, depending upon the anesthetic and/or combination of medications used and the total dosages administered. With halothane, it is thought that the impairment may be at least partially caused by bromide metabolites. Possible adverse effects on the patient's ability to drive or perform other tasks requiring alertness and coordination should be kept in mind when anesthesia is administered for outpatient surgery.

| The following side/adverse effects have been selected on the basis of their potential clinical significance (possible signs and symptoms in parentheses)—not necessarily inclusive:* | Legend: I=Enflurane II=Halothane III=Isoflurane IV=Methoxyflurane V=Nitrous Oxide |||||
|---|---|---|---|---|---|
|  | I | II | III | IV | V |
| Medical attention needed |  |  |  |  |  |
| *Bronchospasm* | R | X | U | R | U |
| *Cardiac arrhythmias*—Supraventricular arrhythmias and bradycardia are relatively common during induction of anesthesia and are not considered dangerous in patients with adequate cardiovascular function. Ventricular arrhythmias are rare in the absence of hypercapnea or hypoxia but may be more likely to occur with halothane. Other arrhythmias reported with halothane include nodal rhythm and atrioventricular dissociation. | R | R | R | R | R |
| *Circulatory depression* | R | R | R | R | R |
| *CNS excitation*—may lead to convulsions | R | X | X | X | X |
| *Emergence delirium, postanesthesia* | L | M | L | L | L |
| *Hepatotoxicity* (black or bloody vomit, severe or continuing headache, loss of appetite, severe or continuing nausea, pain in abdomen, yellow eyes or skin) | R | R | U | R | X |
| *Hypoxia*—with nitrous oxide, diffusion hypoxia may occur after discontinuation unless oxygen is administered | R | R | R | R | R |
| *Leukopenia*†—with prolonged use; may be first sign of reversible bone marrow depression | X | X | X | X | R |
| *Malignant hyperthermic crisis* | R | R | U | R | R |
| *Nephrotoxicity* (increased urination and rapid weight loss or decreased urination and rapid weight gain) | R | U | U | L | U |
| *Neurologic injury*†—with prolonged or repeated exposure | X | X | X | X | R |
| *Respiratory depression* | R | R | R | R | R |
| Medical attention needed only if continuing or bothersome |  |  |  |  |  |
| *Drowsiness, prolonged* | U | U | U | L | U |
| *Headache, mild* | U | R | L | R | U |
| *Nausea or vomiting, mild* | L | L | L | L | M |
| *Shivering or trembling* | M | M | M | L | L |

*Differences in frequency of occurrence may reflect either lack of clinical-use data or actual pharmacologic distinctions among agents. M=more frequent; L=less frequent; R=rare; U=unknown; X=does not occur.

†Operating room or dental office personnel may be at risk for this effect if they are chronically exposed to nitrous oxide because precautions to prevent contamination of the atmosphere in the room in which it is being used are not utilized or are inadequate.

## Overdose

For specific information on the agents used in the management of an inhalation anesthetic overdose, see:
- *Atropine* in *Anticholinergics/Antispasmodics (Systemic)* monograph; and/or
- *Sympathomimetic Agents—Cardiovascular Use (Parenteral-Systemic)* monograph.

For more information on the management of overdose, **contact a Poison Control Center** (see *Poison Control Center Listing*).

### Clinical effects of overdose

The following effects have been selected on the basis of their potential clinical significance (possible signs and symptoms in parentheses where appropriate)—not necessarily inclusive:

Acute
*Bradycardia; circulatory depression or hypotension, severe; respiratory depression*

### Specific treatment

For bradycardia—Administering atropine.

For circulatory depression or severe hypotension—Discontinuing or lightening anesthesia (if still being administered) and administering plasma and/or intravenous fluids. If surgical or postsurgical conditions permit, positioning the patient to improve venous return to the heart (i.e., in the Trendelenburg position) is recommended. If necessary, a vasopressor may be administered.

For respiratory depression—Decreasing anesthetic dosage (if still being administered), establishing a clear airway, and instituting assisted or controlled respiration with pure oxygen.

## Patient Consultation

As an aid to patient consultation, refer to *Advice for the Patient, Anesthetics, General (Systemic)*.

In providing consultation, consider emphasizing the following selected information (» = major clinical significance):

### Before receiving this medication
» Conditions affecting use, especially:
  Sensitivity to the anesthetic considered for use
  Pregnancy—Inhalation anesthetics cross the placenta; enflurane, halothane, and isoflurane may increase the risk of bleeding when used for first trimester abortion; hydrocarbon anesthetics used during labor and delivery may slow delivery, increase bleeding, and cause neonatal depression, depending on dosage
  Breast-feeding—Halothane passes into the breast milk
  Use in the elderly—Increased risk of adverse effects
  Any other medication, including use of "street" drugs
  Other medical problems

### Proper use of this medication
Proper dosing

### Precautions after receiving this medication
» Possibility of psychomotor impairment following use of anesthetics; using caution in driving or performing other tasks requiring alertness and coordination for about 24 hours postanesthesia
» Avoiding use of alcohol or central nervous system (CNS) depressants within 24 hours following anesthesia unless specifically prescribed or otherwise authorized by physician or dentist

### Side/adverse effects
Signs and symptoms of potential delayed side effects, especially hepatotoxicity and nephrotoxicity.

## General Dosing Information

Inhalation anesthetics are to be administered only by those individuals experienced in airway management and respiratory support. Equipment and personnel for support of ventilation must be immediately available.

The stated dosages are given as a guideline for use in the average adult. *The dosage of inhaled anesthetics must be individualized* according to surgical requirements; concurrent use of adjuvant medications and/or nitrous oxide; and patient variables, especially age, body temperature, and physical condition.

Anesthetic requirements are increased in very young children and decreased in geriatric patients.

Preanesthetic medications should be selected according to the needs of the individual patient and surgical requirements.

For patients who may be adversely affected by increases in intracranial pressure, measures (such as barbiturate administration or institution of hyperventilation) to reduce or abolish the increase produced by enflurane, halothane, isoflurane, or methoxyflurane should be carried out prior to or concurrently with administration of these agents. However, the fact that hyperventilation may increase the risk of enflurane-induced convulsive activity should be kept in mind.

Administration of inhalation anesthetics other than nitrous oxide to patients with known or suspected susceptibility to malignant hyperthermia should be avoided. Although prophylactic administration of dantrolene prior to anesthesia may prevent the occurrence of a malignant hyperthermic crisis during or shortly following surgery, this use of dantrolene is controversial and should be undertaken with caution. See *Dantrolene (Systemic)*.

An intravenous induction agent is often administered prior to an inhalation anesthetic to facilitate induction of anesthesia and prevent the transient initial CNS excitation that may occur with some of the inhaled anesthetics.

Enflurane, halothane, isoflurane, or methoxyflurane may be vaporized in a flow of oxygen or a nitrous oxide–oxygen mixture.

During maintenance of anesthesia, the concentration of inhaled anesthetic may be progressively decreased as necessary to prevent further increases in depth of anesthesia and/or hypotension.

Assisted or controlled respiration may be necessary, especially during deep levels of anesthesia, to control respiratory depression and/or respiratory acidosis.

Desiccation of carbon dioxide ($CO_2$) absorbents may occur, especially with the use of high flow-rates of gases. Some inhalation anesthetics (e.g., desflurane, enflurane and isoflurane) can react with desiccated $CO_2$ absorbents to produce carbon monoxide. This reaction may result in elevated levels of carboxyhemoglobin in some patients.

### For treatment of adverse effects

Recommended treatment includes:
- For cardiac arrhythmias—Determining whether the level of anesthesia is adequate for the given surgical stimulus and adjusting (deepening or lightening) the level of anesthesia accordingly or discontinuing anesthesia. Also, determining whether the arrhythmia is caused by hypercarbia, hypocarbia, or hypoxia and correcting as required.
- For malignant hyperthermic crisis—Discontinuing administration of possible triggering agents (such as potent inhalation anesthetics, succinylcholine, or stress), managing increased oxygen requirement, cooling the patient, and correcting fluid and electrolyte imbalances and metabolic acidosis. If necessary, administering dantroleneby continuous rapid intravenous push (at least 1 mg per kg of body weight [mg/kg] initially, continued until the symptoms subside or the maximum total dose of 10 mg/kg has been administered). Intravenous dantrolene administration may be repeated if symptoms recur. Dantrolene (4 to 8 mg/kg per day in four divided doses) may be administered orally or intravenously, with caution, for 1 to 3 days postoperatively to prevent recurrence of symptoms.
- For inadequate postoperative ventilation—Decreasing anesthetic dosage (if still being administered), establishing a clear airway, and instituting assisted or controlled respiration with oxygen.
- For emergence delirium—Administering small doses of an opioid (narcotic) analgesic.

---

## ENFLURANE

## Summary of Differences

Indications:
  Indicated in low concentrations to supplement other anesthetics for cesarean section.
  Also used in low doses to provide analgesia in obstetrics and for procedures not requiring loss of consciousness.
Pharmacology/pharmacokinetics:
  Minimum alveolar concentration (MAC)—
    In oxygen: 1.68%.
    In 70% nitrous oxide: 0.57%.
  Blood-to-gas partition coefficient (37 °C)—
    1.91
  Oil-to-gas partition coefficient (37 °C)—
    98.5
  Biotransformation—
    2.4% of dose metabolized.
  Elimination—
    Primary: 80% excreted unchanged by exhalation.
  Other actions/effects—
    Deeper levels of enflurane anesthesia, especially in the presence of hyperventilation, may produce convulsive activity in electroencephalogram (EEG).

Precautions:
 Mutagenicity—
  Studies in mice have shown that enflurane may cause sperm abnormalities.
 Pregnancy—
  May cause dose-dependent uterine relaxation (anesthetic doses).
  May cause dose-dependent decrease in uterine response to oxytocics.
 Drug interactions and/or related problems—
  Isoniazid and possibly other hydrazine-containing compounds may increase the formation of potentially nephrotoxic inorganic fluoride metabolite when used concurrently with enflurane.

## Additional Dosing Information

See also *General Dosing Information.*

When enflurane is used for induction of anesthesia, it is recommended that the concentration be increased slowly, i.e., by 0.5% every few breaths.

When assisted or controlled respiration is required, extreme hyperventilation should be avoided in order to minimize the risk of CNS excitation and convulsions.

Following enflurane administration, little or no postoperative analgesia is produced because of its short duration of action. Therefore, earlier administration of analgesics for pain relief may be necessary after enflurane than after other inhalation anesthetics.

## Inhalation Dosage Forms
### ENFLURANE USP

**Usual adult dose**
Anesthetic (general)—
 Surgical anesthesia:
  Induction—Dosage must be individualized.
  Maintenance—Inhalation, 0.5 to 3%.
 Supplemental obstetrical anesthesia (for cesarean section):
  Inhalation, 0.5 to 1%.
 For vaginal delivery in obstetrics:
  Inhalation, 0.25 to 1%.

**Usual adult prescribing limits**
For surgical anesthesia—
 Induction: The final concentration for induction should not exceed 4.5%.
 Maintenance: Maintenance concentration should not exceed 3%.

**Usual pediatric dose**
Dosage must be individualized.

**Product(s) usually available**
U.S.—
 [*Ēthrane*; GENERIC].
Canada—
 [*Ēthrane*].

**Packaging and storage**
Store below 40 °C (104 °F), preferably between 15 and 30 °C (59 and 86 °F), unless otherwise specified by manufacturer. Store in a tight, light-resistant container.

---
### HALOTHANE
---

## Summary of Differences

Indications:
 Also used in low concentrations to supplement other anesthetics for cesarean section.
 Not recommended for vaginal delivery unless uterine relaxation is required.
Pharmacology/pharmacokinetics:
 Minimum alveolar concentration (MAC)—
  In oxygen: 0.75%.
  In 70% nitrous oxide: 0.29%.
 Blood-to-gas partition coefficient (37 °C)—
  2.3
 Oil-to-gas partition coefficient (37 °C)—
  224
 Biotransformation—
  Up to 20% of dose metabolized.
 Elimination—
  Primary: 60 to 80% excreted unchanged by exhalation.
 Other actions/effects—
  Cardiovascular system: Heart/pulse rate decrease.
  Respiratory system secretions and salivation decrease.

Precautions::
 Mutagenicity—
  Potential halothane metabolites have been shown to be mutagenic in the Ames test.
 Pregnancy—
  May cause uterine relaxation even in low concentrations.
  May cause dose-dependent decrease in uterine response to oxytocics.
 Breast-feeding—
  Halothane is distributed into breast milk.
 Drug interactions and/or related problems—
  Halothane may prevent or reduce trimethaphan-induced tachycardia.
  Halothane greatly sensitizes the myocardium to the effects of sympathomimetics, especially catecholamines, so that the risk of severe ventricular arrhythmias is increased; sympathomimetics should be used with caution and in substantially reduced dosage in patients receiving halothane.
  Concurrent use of phenytoin may increase the risk of halothane hepatotoxicity; also, halothane-induced hepatic function impairment may increase the risk of phenytoin toxicity.
 Medical considerations/contraindications—
  Caution needed in cardiac arrhythmias since halothane may induce or exacerbate arrhythmias.
  In pheochromocytoma, there may be an increased risk of cardiac arrhythmias because the patient has high endogenous catecholamine concentrations.

## Inhalation Dosage Forms
### HALOTHANE USP

**Usual adult dose**
Anesthetic (general)—
 Induction:
  Dosage must be individualized.
 Maintenance:
  Inhalation, 0.5 to 1.5%.

**Usual pediatric dose**
Dosage must be individualized.

**Product(s) usually available**
U.S.—
 [*Fluothane*; GENERIC].
Canada—
 [*Fluothane*; *Somnothane*].
Other (U.K.)—
 [*Fluothane*].

**Packaging and storage**
Store below 40 °C (104 °F), preferably between 15 and 30 °C (59 and 86 °F), unless otherwise specified by manufacturer. Store in a tight, light-resistant container.

**Stability**
Stability of halothane is maintained by the addition of thymol and ammonia. Because the thymol does not vaporize along with the halothane, it accumulates in the vaporizer and may lead to a yellow discoloration of the remaining liquid or wick. Discolored solutions should be discarded and the vaporizer and wick cleaned by washing with diethyl ether. Complete removal of the diethyl ether is required to make certain that ether is not introduced into the system.

**Incompatibilities**
Halothane vapor, in the presence of moisture, reacts with aluminum, brass, and lead, but not copper.
Some plastics and rubber are soluble in halothane and will deteriorate rapidly in contact with halothane vapor or liquid.

---
### ISOFLURANE
---

## Summary of Differences

Indications:
 Also used in low doses to provide analgesia in obstetrics and for procedures not requiring loss of consciousness, and to supplement other anesthetics for cesarean section.
Pharmacology/pharmacokinetics:
 Minimum alveolar concentration (MAC)—
  In oxygen: 1.15%.
  In 70% nitrous oxide: 0.5%.
 Blood-to-gas partition coefficient (37 °C)—
  1.43

Oil-to-gas partition coefficient (37 °C)—
   97.8
Biotransformation—
   0.17% of dose metabolized.
Elimination—
   Primary: 95% excreted unchanged by exhalation.
Other actions/effects—
   Cardiac function: No decrease. Reduction in blood pressure is caused primarily by peripheral vasodilation rather than depression of cardiac function; however, recent evidence indicates that isoflurane decreases cardiac function and heart/pulse rate in infants.
   Heart/pulse rate: Increase.
Precautions:
   Pregnancy—
      Animal studies have indicated possible fetotoxicity.
      May cause uterine relaxation (anesthetic concentrations).
      Safety in obstetrics has not been established.

## Additional Dosing Information

See also *General Dosing Information*.

When isoflurane is used for induction of anesthesia, it is recommended that the concentration be increased slowly, i.e., by 0.1 to 0.25% every few breaths.

## Inhalation Dosage Forms

### ISOFLURANE USP

**Usual adult dose**
Anesthetic (general)—
   Induction:
      Inhalation, 1.5 to 3%.
   Maintenance:
      Inhalation, 1 to 3.5%.

**Usual pediatric dose**
Dosage must be individualized.

**Product(s) usually available:**
U.S.—
   [*Forane*].
Canada—
   [*Forane*].
Other (U.K.)—
   [*Forane*].

**Packaging and storage**
Store below 40 °C (104 °F), preferably between 15 and 30 °C (59 and 86 °F), unless otherwise specified by manufacturer. Store in a tight, light-resistant container.

---

## *METHOXYFLURANE*

## Summary of Differences

Indications:
   Administration of concentrations sufficient to provide muscle relaxation is not recommended.
   Not recommended for vascular surgery at or near the renal blood vessels.
   Also indicated in low doses to provide analgesia in obstetrics and for procedures not requiring loss of consciousness.
   Also used in low concentrations to supplement other anesthetics for cesarean section.
Pharmacology/pharmacokinetics:
   Minimum alveolar concentration (MAC)—
      In oxygen: 0.16%.
      In 70% nitrous oxide: 0.07%.
   Blood-to-gas partition coefficient (37 °C)—
      10 to 14
   Oil-to-gas partition coefficient (37 °C)—
      825 to 970
   Biotransformation—
      50% of dose metabolized.
      A substantial quantity of inorganic fluoride is formed; also metabolized to other potentially nephrotoxic substances.
   Time to onset of anesthesia—
      Slow.
   Time to change in depth of anesthesia when administered concentration is changed—
      Slow.
   Time to recovery from anesthesia—
      May be prolonged.
   Elimination—
      Primary: 35% excreted unchanged by exhalation.
   Other actions/effects—
      Respiratory system secretions do not increase.
Precautions:
   Pregnancy—
      May cause dose-dependent uterine relaxation.
   Drug interactions and/or related problems—
      Chronic use of hepatic enzyme–inducing agents may increase the formation of nephrotoxic metabolites, leading to increased risk of nephrotoxicity.
      Concurrent use of other nephrotoxic agents may increase the risk of severe nephrotoxicity.
   Medical considerations/contraindications—
      Caution needed in diabetes, uncontrolled or with polyuria or obesity; in renal function impairment or disease; or in toxemia of pregnancy, as methoxyflurane may increase the risk of nephrotoxicity.
   Patient monitoring—
      Monitoring of renal function may be needed to detect possible nephrotoxicity if patient's postoperative urine output is excessive.

## Additional Dosing Information

See also *General Dosing Information*.

A parenteral induction agent is recommended prior to administration of methoxyflurane.

Concurrent administration of at least 50% nitrous oxide is recommended, unless specifically contraindicated, to reduce the methoxyflurane requirement.

During long procedures, it is recommended that methoxyflurane be administered in decreasing concentrations because of the risk of nephrotoxicity. See manufacturer's prescribing information for an example of recommended concentrations at various times following initiation of methoxyflurane administration. Also, it is recommended that administration be limited to 4 hours or less.

Low doses of methoxyflurane may be self-administered using a hand-held inhaler. It is recommended that such use be limited to the briefest practical time and that the patient be under observation by trained personnel. The patient may be transferred to a conventional anesthesia machine if necessary. In obstetrics, methoxyflurane should not be self-administered until relief is necessary.

## Inhalation Dosage Forms

### METHOXYFLURANE USP

**Usual adult dose**
Anesthetic (general)—
   Inhalation, up to 2% administered with at least 50% nitrous oxide and oxygen initially, then decreased to the lowest effective concentration.
For obstetrics or procedures not requiring loss of consciousness—
   Inhalation, 0.3 to 0.8%, intermittently.
   Note: For patient self-administration, no more than a single 15-mL charge of liquid should be available to the patient.

**Usual adult prescribing limits**
For surgical anesthesia, administration should not exceed four hours of 0.25% methoxyflurane or two hours of 0.5% methoxyflurane or the equivalent total dosage.

**Usual pediatric dose**
Dosage must be individualized.

**Product(s) usually available:**
U.S.—
   [*Penthrane*].

**Packaging and storage**
Store below 40 °C (104 °F), preferably between 15 and 30 °C (59 and 86 °F). Store in a tight, light-resistant container. Protect from freezing.

**Stability**
Solutions of methoxyflurane contain an antioxidant, butylated hydroxytoluene, which may oxidize to a yellow pigment that progressively turns to brown. This substance may accumulate on the vaporizer wick. Diethyl ether may be used to clean the wick; complete removal of the diethyl ether is required to make certain that ether is not introduced into the system.

### Incompatibilities
Methoxyflurane is very soluble in rubber and in soda lime.
Polyvinyl chloride plastics are extracted by methoxyflurane; contact with such plastics should be avoided.

## NITROUS OXIDE

## Summary of Differences
Indications:
  Anesthetic potency relatively weak; usually must be supplemented with other agents.
  Often given concurrently with one of the more potent inhalation anesthetics to reduce the requirement for the other anesthetic.
  Also indicated in low doses to provide analgesia in obstetrics and for procedures not requiring loss of consciousness.
Pharmacology/pharmacokinetics:
  Minimum alveolar concentration (MAC) in oxygen—
    > 100%.
  Blood-to-gas partition coefficient (37 °C)—
    0.47
  Oil-to-gas partition coefficient (37 °C)—
    1.4
  Biotransformation—
    None of dose metabolized.
  Elimination—
    Primary: 100% excreted unchanged by exhalation.
  Other actions/effects:
    Blood pressure generally unchanged.
    Heart/pulse rate increases.
    Constriction of peripheral vasculature.
    No dose-related muscle relaxation.
Precautions:
  Pregnancy—
    Studies in animals have shown that nitrous oxide causes fetal death, growth retardation, and skeletal anomalies.
  Drug interactions and/or related problems—
    In addition to the increased central nervous system (CNS) depressant, respiratory depressant, and hypotensive effects that may occur when an anesthetic is used concurrently with any CNS depressant, concurrent use of high doses of fentanyl or its derivatives with nitrous oxide may decrease the heart rate and cardiac output. These effects may be more pronounced in patients with poor left ventricular function.
  Medical considerations/contraindications—
    Caution needed in the presence of air-enclosing cavities (such as pulmonary, renal, or occluded middle ear air cysts or air embolism), acute intestinal obstruction, or pneumothorax, or during or recently following the procedure of pneumoencephalography, as nitrous oxide may increase pressure within rigid-walled cavities or volume within nonrigid-walled cavities.

## Additional Dosing Information
See also *General Dosing Information*.

Nitrous oxide must be administered with at least 30% of oxygen to reduce the risk of hypoxia.

### For anesthesia
Premedication of the patient with an opioid analgesic or a barbiturate may be necessary in order to achieve induction of anesthesia.

Nitrous oxide may diffuse into the cuff of an endotracheal tube; periodic deflation of the endotracheal tube is recommended during administration.

The concentration administered during maintenance of anesthesia must be individualized, depending upon the condition of the patient and the type and quantity of supplemental medications administered.

When prolonged administration of nitrous oxide is discontinued, 100% oxygen should be administered briefly to reduce the risk of diffusion hypoxia.

## Inhalation Dosage Forms
### NITROUS OXIDE USP
**Usual adult dose**
Anesthetic (general)—
  Induction:
    Inhalation, 70% with 30% of oxygen.
  Maintenance:
    Inhalation, 30 to 70% with oxygen.
For obstetrics or procedures not requiring loss of consciousness—
  Inhalation, 25 to 50% with oxygen.

**Usual pediatric dose**
Dosage must be individualized.

**Product(s) usually available**
U.S.—
  [GENERIC].
Canada—
  [GENERIC].

**Packaging and storage**
Store below 40 °C (104 °F), preferably between 15 and 30 °C (59 and 86 °F), unless otherwise specified by manufacturer.

Revised: 06/29/90
Interim revision: 08/23/94; 08/20/97

---

### Table 1. Pharmacology/Pharmacokinetics

|  | Enflurane | Halothane | Isoflurane | Methoxyflurane | Nitrous Oxide |
|---|---|---|---|---|---|
| Minimum alveolar concentration (MAC)* | | | | | |
| In oxygen (%) | 1.68 | 0.75 | 1.15 | 0.16 | >100 |
| In 70% Nitrous Oxide (%) | 0.57 | 0.29 | 0.5 | 0.07 | — |
| Blood-to-Gas partition coefficient (37 °C)† | 1.91 | 2.3 | 1.43 | 10–14 | 0.47 |
| Oil-to-Gas partition coefficient (37 °C)‡ | 98.5 | 224 | 97.8 | 825–970 | 1.4 |
| Biotransformation§ | Hepatic | Hepatic | Hepatic | Hepatic | — |
| % of dose metabolized# | 2.4 | Up to 20 | 0.17 | 50 | 0 |
| Quantity of inorganic fluoride formed** | Small | Almost none | Very small | Substantial | — |
| Time to onset of anesthesia†† | Rapid | Rapid | Rapid | Slow | — |

  * MAC—The minimum alveolar concentration that prevents movement in 50% of patients subjected to a painful stimulus. Slightly higher concentrations may be required to ensure immobility in all patients. MAC decreases with increasing age (being highest in very young children), pregnancy, hypothermia, hypotension, and concurrent use of other CNS depressants. The MACs of individual inhaled anesthetics are additive.
  † Indicator of solubility in blood, which affects the rate at which the partial pressure of the anesthetic in the blood (and therefore in the brain) equilibrates with that in the alveoli. Low solubility results in rapid rates of induction, changes in depth of anesthesia, and recovery.
  ‡ Indicator of solubility in fatty tissues. High solubility increases both anesthetic potency and the rate of elimination of the agent from the body.
  § Via hepatic microsomal enzymes.
  # For enflurane, halothane, and methoxyflurane, the percentage metabolized may be increased by induction of hepatic enzymes.
  ** Indicator of nephrotoxic potential of agent. For enflurane, the quantity of inorganic fluoride produced is not increased by hepatic enzyme induction, but it may be increased by chronic isoniazid administration. Peak concentrations occur 4 to 12 hours postoperatively with enflurane and 2 to 4 days postoperatively with methoxyflurane. Methoxyflurane is also metabolized to other potentially nephrotoxic substances.
  †† Rapid=7 to 10 minutes; slow=20 to 30 minutes. The pungent odor of enflurane or isoflurane may cause breath-holding, coughing, or laryngospasm. This may limit the rate at which the administered concentration can be increased, resulting in a slightly longer induction time.
  ‡‡ Dependent on duration of anesthesia, administered concentration of anesthetic, and whether or not other CNS depressants are used. With isoflurane, administration for longer than 3 hours does not further prolong recovery time.
  §§ Primarily as metabolites. Small quantities of nitrous oxide may also be eliminated through the skin.

## Table 1. Pharmacology/Pharmacokinetics *(Continued)*

|  | Enflurane | Halothane | Isoflurane | Methoxyflurane | Nitrous Oxide |
|---|---|---|---|---|---|
| Time to change in depth of anesthesia when administered concentration changed | Rapid | Rapid | Rapid | Slow | — |
| Time to recovery from anesthesia‡‡ | Rapid | Rapid | Rapid | May be prolonged | Rapid |
| Elimination | | | | | |
| Primary—% excreted unchanged by exhalation | 80 | 60–80 | 95 | 35 | 100 |
| Secondary§§ | Renal | Renal | | Renal | |

* MAC—The minimum alveolar concentration that prevents movement in 50% of patients subjected to a painful stimulus. Slightly higher concentrations may be required to ensure immobility in all patients. MAC decreases with increasing age (being highest in very young children), pregnancy, hypothermia, hypotension, and concurrent use of other CNS depressants. The MACs of individual inhaled anesthetics are additive.

† Indicator of solubility in blood, which affects the rate at which the partial pressure of the anesthetic in the blood (and therefore in the brain) equilibrates with that in the alveoli. Low solubility results in rapid rates of induction, changes in depth of anesthesia, and recovery.

‡ Indicator of solubility in fatty tissues. High solubility increases both anesthetic potency and the rate of elimination of the agent from the body.

§ Via hepatic microsomal enzymes.

# For enflurane, halothane, and methoxyflurane, the percentage metabolized may be increased by induction of hepatic enzymes.

** Indicator of nephrotoxic potential of agent. For enflurane, the quantity of inorganic fluoride produced is not increased by hepatic enzyme induction, but it may be increased by chronic isoniazid administration. Peak concentrations occur 4 to 12 hours postoperatively with enflurane and 2 to 4 days postoperatively with methoxyflurane. Methoxyflurane is also metabolized to other potentially nephrotoxic substances.

†† Rapid=7 to 10 minutes; slow=20 to 30 minutes. The pungent odor of enflurane or isoflurane may cause breath-holding, coughing, or laryngospasm. This may limit the rate at which the administered concentration can be increased, resulting in a slightly longer induction time.

‡‡ Dependent on duration of anesthesia, administered concentration of anesthetic, and whether or not other CNS depressants are used. With isoflurane, administration for longer than 3 hours does not further prolong recovery time.

§§ Primarily as metabolites. Small quantities of nitrous oxide may also be eliminated through the skin.

## Table 2. Pharmacology/Pharmacokinetics

| Other actions/effects:<br>Action or Body System/Function Affected | Enflurane | Halothane | Isoflurane | Methoxyflurane | Nitrous Oxide |
|---|---|---|---|---|---|
| Analgesia (low concentrations) | Moderate | Relatively poor | | Good | Excellent |
| Brain | | | | | |
| Convulsive activity in electroencephalogram (EEG) | Yes* | No | No | No | No |
| Intracranial pressure† | Increase | Increase | Increase | Increase | May increase |
| Cardiovascular System | | | | | |
| Blood pressure‡ | Decrease | Decrease | Decrease | Decrease | Generally unchanged |
| Cardiac function | Decrease | Decrease | No decrease§ | Decrease | Slight decrease# |
| Circulation (high concentrations) | Depression | Depression | Depression | Depression | |
| Heart/pulse rate | May increase** | Decrease | Increase | May decrease | Increase |
| Peripheral vasculature | Dilation | Dilation | Dilation | | Constriction |
| Intraocular pressure†† | Significant decrease | Slight decrease | | | |
| Muscle relaxation (dose-dependent)‡‡ | Excellent | Moderate | Excellent | | None |
| Pharyngeal and laryngeal reflexes | Decrease | Decrease | Decrease | | |
| Renal function§§ | Decrease | Decrease | Decrease | Decrease | |
| Respiratory System | | | | | |
| Bronchi | Dilation | Dilation | | | |
| Respiration (dose-dependent)## | Depression | Depression | Depression | Depression | Depression |
| Secretions | May increase slightly | Decrease | May increase slightly | No increase | |
| Salivation | May increase slightly | Decrease | May increase slightly | | |

*EEG changes characterized by high voltage and fast frequency progressing through spike-dome complexes alternating with periods of electrical silence to frank seizure activity may occur during deeper levels of enflurane anesthesia, especially in the presence of hyperventilation.

†With enflurane, halothane, isoflurane (concentration 1.25 MAC), and methoxyflurane, may be caused by increased cerebral blood flow secondary to cerebral vasodilation. This effect may be eliminated by hyperventilation-induced hypocapnea or reduced by barbiturate administration.

‡Effect on blood pressure is dose-dependent and is a useful indication of depth of anesthesia. With enflurane or isoflurane, blood pressure may return to near preanesthetic values with surgical stimulation or stress.

§With isoflurane only, the reduction in blood pressure is caused primarily by peripheral vasodilation rather than depression of cardiac function. However, recent evidence indicates that isoflurane decreases cardiac function and heart/pulse rate in infants.

#Nitrous oxide may attenuate the cardiovascular effects of other inhaled anesthetics by reducing the requirement for the other anesthetic.

**With enflurane, the heart rate may be decreased if the preanesthetic heart rate is rapid; however, bradycardia usually does not occur.

††With 1% of enflurane or 0.5% of halothane, given with nitrous oxide and oxygen.

‡‡Enflurane or isoflurane may produce muscle relaxation sufficient for many types of surgery when used without a neuromuscular blocking agent.

§§Effect is dose-dependent; reduction in glomerular filtration rate, renal blood flow, and urine volume may reflect decreased mean arterial pressure.

##Respiratory depression may be partially reversed with surgical stimulation or stress.

## Table 3. Drug Interactions and/or Related Problems

The following drug interactions and/or related problems have been selected on the basis of their potential clinical significance (possible mechanism in parentheses where appropriate)—not necessarily inclusive (» = major clinical significance):

Note: Combinations containing any of the following medications, depending on the amount present, may also interact with this medication.

Legend:
I = Enflurane
II = Halothane
III = Isoflurane
IV = Methoxyflurane
V = Nitrous Oxide

| | I | II | III | IV | V |
|---|---|---|---|---|---|
| Alcohol, chronic ingestion (may increase anesthetic requirement) | ✓ | ✓ | ✓ | ✓ | ✓ |
| Alfentanil or Fentanyl or Sufentanil (in addition to the increased central nervous system [CNS] depressant, respiratory depressant, and hypotensive effects that may occur when an anesthetic is used concurrently with any CNS depressant, concurrent use of high doses of fentanyl or its derivatives with nitrous oxide may decrease heart rate and cardiac output; these effects may be more pronounced in patients with poor left ventricular function) | | | | | ✓ |
| » Aminoglycosides, systemic, or<br>» Capreomycin or<br>» Citrate-anticoagulated blood (massive transfusions) or<br>» Lincomycins, systemic, or<br>» Neuromuscular blocking agents, nondepolarizing, or<br>» Polymyxins, systemic<br>(caution should be used in concurrent administration with halogenated anesthetics, especially enflurane or isoflurane, because of the possibility of additive neuromuscular blockade; although increased or prolonged skeletal muscle weakness and respiratory depression or paralysis [apnea] may occur, clinical significance is minimal if the patient is being mechanically ventilated; however, dosage of nondepolarizing neuromuscular blocking agents should be decreased to 1/2 to 1/3 of the usual dose or as determined using a peripheral nerve stimulator; treatment with anticholinesterase agents or calcium salts may help reverse the blockade, but calcium salts are not recommended if tubocurarine has been given because they may potentiate, rather than reverse, its effects) | ✓ | ✓ | ✓ | ✓ | |
| Amiodarone (concurrent use with inhalation anesthetics may potentiate hypotension and increase the risk of atropine-resistant bradycardia) | ✓ | ✓ | ✓ | ✓ | ✓ |
| Anticoagulants, coumarin- or indandione-derivative (inhalation anesthetics have been reported to increase the effects of these anticoagulants; although clinical significance has not been determined, the possibility of increased anticoagulation during or shortly following concurrent use should be considered) | ✓ | ✓ | ✓ | ✓ | ✓ |
| Antihypertensive agents, especially diazoxide or ganglionic blockers such as guanadrel, guanethidine, mecamylamine, or trimethaphan, or<br>Chlorpromazine or<br>Diuretics or<br>Hypotension-producing medications, other (See *Appendix II*)<br>(hypotensive effects may be potentiated when these medications are used concurrently with inhalation anesthetics; patients should be monitored for excessive fall in blood pressure during and following concurrent use) | ✓ | ✓ | ✓ | ✓ | ✓ |
| (halothane may prevent or reduce trimethaphan-induced tachycardia) | | ✓ | | | |
| Antimyasthenics (antimyasthenics, especially neostigmine and pyridostigmine, may decrease neuromuscular blocking activity of halogenated hydrocarbon anesthetics; also, the neuromuscular blocking activity of these anesthetics, especially enflurane or isoflurane, may interfere with the efficacy of antimyasthenics so that temporary dosage adjustment may be required to control symptoms of myasthenia gravis postoperatively) | ✓ | ✓ | ✓ | | |
| Beta-adrenergic blocking agents, including ophthalmic betaxolol, levobunolol, or timolol (concurrent use with hydrocarbon inhalation anesthetics may result in prolonged severe hypotension because the beta-blockade reduces the ability of the heart to respond to beta-adrenergically mediated sympathetic reflex stimuli; if necessary to reverse the effects of beta-adrenergic blocking agents during surgery, agonists such as dobutamine, dopamine, isoproterenol, or norepinephrine may be used but should be administered with caution, especially in patients receiving halothane. Some clinicians recommend gradual withdrawal of beta-adrenergic blocking agents 48 hours prior to elective surgery; however, this recommendation is controversial) | ✓ | ✓ | ✓ | ✓ | |
| (it is recommended that high concentrations of halothane [3% or above] or other halogenated hydrocarbon anesthetics not be used when labetalol is used to produce controlled hypotension during surgery; possible additive effects may lead to excessive hypotension, large reduction in cardiac output, and increased central venous pressure) | ✓ | ✓ | ✓ | ✓ | |
| » Catecholamines such as dopamine, epinephrine, or norepinephrine, or<br>» Cocaine or<br>» Ephedrine or<br>» Levodopa or<br>» Metaraminol or<br>» Methoxamine or<br>Other sympathomimetic agents<br>(halothane greatly sensitizes the myocardium to the effects of sympathomimetics, especially catecholamines, so that the risk of severe ventricular arrhythmias is increased; sympathomimetics should be used with caution and in substantially reduced dosage in patients receiving halothane) | | ✓ | | | |
| (enflurane, isoflurane, or methoxyflurane may also cause some sensitization of the myocardium to the effects of sympathomimetics; caution is recommended during concurrent use) | ✓ | | ✓ | ✓ | |
| (levodopa increases endogenous dopamine concentration and should be discontinued 6 to 8 hours prior to anesthesia with these agents, especially halothane) | ✓ | ✓ | ✓ | ✓ | |

## Table 3. Drug Interactions and/or Related Problems *(Continued)*

The following drug interactions and/or related problems have been selected on the basis of their potential clinical significance (possible mechanism in parentheses where appropriate)—not necessarily inclusive (» = major clinical significance):

Note: Combinations containing any of the following medications, depending on the amount present, may also interact with this medication.

Legend:
I=Enflurane
II=Halothane
III=Isoflurane
IV=Methoxyflurane
V=Nitrous Oxide

| | I | II | III | IV | V |
|---|---|---|---|---|---|
| CNS depression–producing medications, other, including those commonly used for preanesthetic medication or induction or supplementation of anesthesia (see *Appendix II*) (concurrent administration may increase the CNS depressant, respiratory depressant, and hypotensive effects of inhalation anesthetics; decrease anesthetic requirement; and prolong recovery from anesthesia; careful attention to the dosage of each agent is required) | ✔ | ✔ | ✔ | ✔ | ✔ |
| Doxapram (doxapram may cause catecholamine release; it is recommended that initiation of doxapram therapy be delayed for at least 10 minutes following discontinuation of anesthetics known to sensitize the myocardium to catecholamines) | ✔ | ✔ | ✔ | ✔ | |
| Hepatic enzyme–inducing agents (see *Appendix II*) (chronic use of these medications prior to anesthesia may increase anesthetic metabolism leading to increased risk of hepatotoxicity) | ✔ | ✔ | | ✔ | |
| (chronic use of these medications prior to anesthesia may increase formation of nephrotoxic metabolites leading to increased risk of nephrotoxicity) | | | | ✔ | |
| Isoniazid and possibly other hydrazine-containing compounds (may increase formation of the potentially nephrotoxic inorganic fluoride metabolite when used concurrently with enflurane) | ✔ | | | | |
| Ketamine (volatile anesthetics may prolong elimination half-life of ketamine; recovery from anesthesia may be prolonged) | ✔ | ✔ | ✔ | ✔ | |
| Methyldopa (concurrent use with general anesthetics may decrease the anesthetic requirement) | ✔ | ✔ | ✔ | ✔ | ✔ |
| » Nephrotoxic agents, other (see *Appendix II*) (may increase the risk of severe nephrotoxicity if administered prior to, during, or following administration of methoxyflurane; concurrent or sequential use is generally not recommended) | | | | ✔ | |
| Nitrous oxide (concurrent administration with another inhalation anesthetic reduces the requirement for the other anesthetic and may therefore attenuate some of its cardiovascular effects) | ✔ | ✔ | ✔ | | |
| Oxytocics (enflurane [concentrations >1.5%], halothane [concentrations >1%], or possibly isoflurane produces a dose-dependent decrease in the uterine response to oxytocics and may abolish the response if sufficient concentrations [>3% of enflurane] are administered; uterine hemorrhage may result) | ✔ | ✔ | ✔ | | |
| Phenytoin (concurrent use may increase the risk of halothane hepatotoxicity; also, halothane-induced hepatic function impairment may increase the risk of phenytoin toxicity) | | ✔ | | | |
| Ritodrine, intravenous (concurrent use of halogenated hydrocarbon anesthetics may lead to potentiation of ritodrine's cardiovascular effects, especially cardiac arrhythmias or hypotension) | ✔ | ✔ | ✔ | ✔ | |
| Succinylcholine (concurrent use with halogenated hydrocarbon anesthetics may increase the risk of malignant hyperthermia; also, repeated concurrent use may increase the risk of bradycardia) | ✔ | ✔ | ✔ | ✔ | |
| (halogenated hydrocarbon anesthetics may potentiate succinylcholine-induced neuromuscular blockade but to a lesser extent than they potentiate the effects of nondepolarizing neuromuscular blocking agents) | ✔ | ✔ | ✔ | ✔ | |
| Xanthines (concurrent use with anesthetics, especially halothane, may increase the risk of cardiac arrhythmias) | ✔ | ✔ | ✔ | ✔ | ✔ |

## Table 4. Medical considerations/Contraindications

The medical considerations/contraindications included have been selected on the basis of their potential clinical significance (reasons given in parentheses where appropriate)—not necessarily inclusive (» = major clinical significance).

Legend:
I=Enflurane
II=Halothane
III=Isoflurane
IV=Methoxyflurane
V=Nitrous Oxide

| | I | II | III | IV | V |
|---|---|---|---|---|---|
| **Except under special circumstances, these medications should not be used when the following medical problem exists:** | | | | | |
| » Malignant hyperthermia, history of or suspected genetic predisposition to (risk of malignant hyperthermic crisis during or following anesthesia) | ✔ | ✔ | ✔ | ✔ | |

## Table 4. Medical considerations/Contraindications *(Continued)*

The medical considerations/contraindications included have been selected on the basis of their potential clinical significance (reasons given in parentheses where appropriate)—not necessarily inclusive (» = major clinical significance).

Legend:
I=Enflurane
II=Halothane
III=Isoflurane
IV=Methoxyflurane
V=Nitrous Oxide

| | I | II | III | IV | V |
|---|---|---|---|---|---|
| **Risk-benefit should be considered when the following medical problems exist:**<br>Air-enclosing cavities, such as pulmonary, renal, or occluded middle ear air cysts or air embolism, or<br>Intestinal obstruction, acute, or<br>Pneumoencephalography, during or recently following the procedure (pneumoencephalography), or<br>Pneumothorax<br>(may increase pressure within rigid-walled cavities or volume within nonrigid-walled cavities) | | | | | ✓ |
| Biliary tract disease or<br>» Hepatic function impairment or disease or<br>» Jaundice or acute hepatic damage, not attributable to other causes, following previous exposure to enflurane, halothane, or methoxyflurane<br>(increased risk of hepatotoxicity) | ✓ | ✓ | | ✓ | |
| Cardiac arrhythmias<br>(may be induced or exacerbated) | | ✓ | | | |
| Diabetes, uncontrolled or with polyuria or obesity, or<br>» Renal function impairment or disease or<br>» Toxemia of pregnancy<br>(increased risk of nephrotoxicity) | | | | ✓ | |
| Head injury or<br>Increased intracranial pressure, pre-existing, or<br>Intracranial lesions, space-occupying, or tumors<br>(may increase intracranial pressure) | ✓ | ✓ | ✓ | ✓ | ✓ |
| Myasthenia gravis<br>(muscle weakness may be increased because of neuromuscular blocking effects of anesthetics, especially enflurane and isoflurane) | ✓ | ✓ | ✓ | ✓ | |
| Pheochromocytoma<br>(increased risk of cardiac arrhythmias because patient has high endogenous catecholamine concentrations) | | ✓ | | | |
| Sensitivity to the anesthetic being considered for use, history of | ✓ | ✓ | ✓ | ✓ | ✓ |

# ANGIOTENSIN-CONVERTING ENZYME (ACE) INHIBITORS  Systemic

This monograph includes information on the following: 1) Benazepril†; 2) Captopril; 3) Enalapril; 4) Fosinopril†; 5) Lisinopril; 6) Quinapril†; 7) Ramipril†.

VA CLASSIFICATION (Primary/Secondary):
Benazepril—CV800/CV409; CV900
Captopril—CV800/CV409; CV900
Enalapril—CV800/CV409; CV900
Fosinopril—CV800/CV409; CV900
Lisinopril—CV800/CV409; CV900
Quinapril—CV800/CV409; CV900
Ramipril—CV800/CV409; CV900

Commonly used brand name(s): *Accupril*[6]; *Altace*[7]; *Capoten*[2]; *Lotensin*[1]; *Monopril*[4]; *Prinivil*[5]; *Vasotec*[3]; *Zestril*[5].

Note:  For a listing of dosage forms and brand names by country availability, see *Dosage Forms* section(s).

†Not commercially available in Canada.

## Category

Antihypertensive—Benazepril; Captopril; Enalapril; Fosinopril; Lisinopril; Quinapril; Ramipril.
Vasodilator, congestive heart failure—Benazepril; Captopril; Enalapril; Lisinopril; Quinapril; Ramipril.

## Indications

Note:  Bracketed information in the *Indications* section refers to uses that are not included in U.S. product labeling.

**Accepted**

Hypertension (treatment)—Angiotensin-converting enzyme (ACE) inhibitors are indicated, alone or in combination with a thiazide diuretic, in the treatment of hypertension.

[Captopril is also used for treatment of neonatal hypertension.][1]

ACE inhibitors are also used for [treatment of malignant, refractory, or accelerated hypertension][1], and for treatment of renovascular hypertension (except in patients with bilateral renal artery stenoses or renal artery stenosis in a solitary kidney—See *Medical considerations/contraindications*).

Congestive heart failure (treatment)—Captopril, enalapril, lisinopril, [benazepril], [quinapril], and [ramipril] are also indicated, in combination with diuretics and digitalis therapy, for treatment of congestive heart failure not responding to other measures.

[Captopril is used for the treatment of congestive heart failure secondary to ventricular left-to-right shunt not responding to standard therapy in infants and neonates.]

Left ventricular dysfunction, asymptomatic (treatment)[1]—Enalapril is indicated for the treatment of left ventricular dysfunction (ejection fraction ≤ 35%) in clinically stable patients who are asymptomatic. Enalapril has been shown to decrease the rate of development of overt heart failure and decrease the frequency of hospitalization secondary to heart failure.

Left ventricular dysfunction following myocardial infarction (treatment)[1]— Captopril is indicated following myocardial infarction in clinically stable patients with left ventricular dysfunction (ejection fraction ≤ 40%) to improve survival and decrease the incidence of overt heart failure and subsequent hospitalization for congestive heart failure.

Diabetic nephropathy (treatment)[1]—Captopril may be used in the treatment of nephropathy in patients with Type I insulin-dependent diabetes mellitus (IDDM). Captopril has been shown to slow the progression of diabetic nephropathy in normotensive and hypertensive IDDM patients with documented diabetic retinopathy, a serum creatinine concentration of ≤ 2.5 mg per deciliter, and urinary protein excretion of ≥ 500 mg in 24 hours. The greatest effect has been seen in those patients with poorer renal function at baseline (mean serum creatinine concentration ≥ 1.5 mg per deciliter).

# Angiotensin-converting Enzyme (ACE) Inhibitors (Systemic)

[Scleroderma, hypertension in (treatment)][1] or
[Scleroderma, renal crisis in (treatment)][1]—ACE inhibitors are also used for treatment of hypertension or renal crisis in scleroderma.

[1] Not included in Canadian product labeling.

## Pharmacology/Pharmacokinetics

### Physicochemical characteristics
Molecular weight—
  Benazepril hydrochloride: 460.96.
  Captopril: 217.28.
  Enalapril: 492.52.
  Enalaprilat (active metabolite): 384.43.
  Fosinopril sodium: 585.65.
  Lisinopril: 441.52.
  Quinapril hydrochloride: 474.98.
  Ramipril: 416.52.
pKa—
  Captopril: 3.7 and 9.8 (apparent).

### Mechanism of action/Effect
Benazepril—Benazeprilat (active metabolite)
Captopril—Not a prodrug
Enalapril—Enalaprilat (active metabolite)
Fosinopril—Fosinoprilat (active metabolite)
Lisinopril—Not a prodrug
Quinapril—Quinaprilat (active metabolite)
Ramipril—Ramiprilat (active metabolite)
Antihypertensive—Exact mechanism of antihypertensive action is unknown but is thought to be related to competitive inhibition of angiotensin I–converting enzyme (ACE) activity, resulting in a decreased rate of conversion of angiotensin I to angiotensin II, which is a potent vasoconstrictor. Decreased angiotensin II concentrations result in a secondary increase in plasma renin activity (PRA), through removal of the negative feedback of renin release, and a direct reduction in aldosterone secretion. ACE inhibitors may be less effective in control of blood pressures among hypertensives with low as compared to normal or high renin activity. ACE inhibitors reduce peripheral arterial resistance. In addition, a possible effect on the kallikrein-kinin system (interference with degradation and resulting increased concentrations of bradykinin) and an increase in prostaglandin synthesis have been suggested but not proven.
Vasodilator, congestive heart failure—Decrease in peripheral vascular (afterload) resistance, pulmonary capillary wedge pressure (preload), and pulmonary vascular resistance; and improved cardiac output and exercise tolerance.

### Other actions/effects
Captopril may reduce proteinuria in hypertensive patients with diabetic nephropathy. This effect may be due to the beneficial change in intrarenal hemodynamics (renal vasodilatation and reduced filtration pressure) produced by captopril resulting in decreased urinary protein excretion.

### Absorption
Benazepril—At least 37% absorbed from the gastrointestinal tract.
Captopril—Rapidly and at least 75% absorbed from the gastrointestinal tract. Absorption is reduced by 30 to 55% in the presence of food.
Enalapril—Approximately 60%; not affected by the presence of food.
Fosinopril—Slowly; about 36% absorbed from the gastrointestinal tract. Absorption rate may be decreased in presence of food, but extent of absorption is not affected.
Lisinopril—Approximately 25%, but widely variable between individuals (6 to 60%); not affected by the presence of food.
Quinapril—Approximately 60%; presence of food does not affect extent of absorption, but may increase the time to peak drug concentration. High-fat meals may moderately decrease absorption.
Ramipril—Rapidly and at least 50 to 60% absorbed from the gastrointestinal tract. Extent of absorption is not affected by the presence of food; however, the rate of absorption is reduced.

### Protein binding
Benazepril—Very high (96.7%).
Benazeprilat (active metabolite)—Very high (95.3%).
Captopril—Low (25 to 30%), primarily to albumin.
Enalaprilat—Moderate (50 to 60%).
Fosinoprilat (active metabolite)—Very high (97 to 98%).
Lisinopril—None.
Quinaprilat (active metabolite)—Very high (97%).
Ramipril—High (73%).
Ramiprilat (active metabolite)—High (56%).

### Biotransformation
Benazepril—Hepatic, to benazeprilat, the active metabolite.
Captopril—Hepatic.
Enalapril—Hepatic, by hydrolysis, to enalaprilat, the active metabolite.
Enalaprilat—None.
Fosinopril—Hepatic, gastrointestinal mucosa; by hydrolysis to fosinoprilat, the active metabolite.
Lisinopril—None.
Quinapril—Hepatic, gastrointestinal tract, extravascular tissue; by hydrolysis to quinaprilat, the active metabolite.
Ramipril—Hepatic.

### Half-life
Benazepril—0.6 hours.
Benazepril (active metabolite)—Effective accumulation half-life is 10 to 11 hours.
Captopril—Less than 3 hours; increased in renal failure (3.5 to 32 hours).
Enalaprilat—11 hours; increased in renal failure.
Fosinoprilat (active metabolite)—Effective accumulation half-life is approximately 11.5 hours.
Lisinopril—12 hours; increased in renal failure.
Quinapril—Approximately 1 to 2 hours.
Quinaprilat (active metabolite)—Effective accumulation half-life is approximately 3 hours.
Ramipril—5.1 hours.
Ramiprilat (active metabolite)—Effective accumulation half-life is 13 to 17 hours; increased in renal failure.

### Onset of action
Single dose—
  Benazepril: Within 1 hour.
  Captopril: 15 to 60 minutes.
  Enalapril: 1 hour.
  Enalaprilat (intravenous): 15 minutes.
  Fosinopril: Within 1 hour.
  Lisinopril: 1 hour.
  Quinapril: Within 1 hour.
  Ramipril: Within 1 to 2 hours.

### Time to peak serum concentration
Benazepril—0.5 to 1 hour.
Benazeprilat (active metabolite)—1 to 1.5 hours.
Captopril—30 to 90 minutes.
Enalapril—1 hour (3 to 4 hours for enalaprilat).
Enalaprilat (intravenous)—15 minutes.
Fosinoprilat (active metabolite)—2 to 4 hours.
Lisinopril—7 hours.
Quinapril—Within 1 hour.
Quinaprilat (active metabolite)—Within 2 hours.
Ramipril—Within 1 hour.
Ramiprilat (active metabolite)—3 hours.

### Time to peak effect
Single dose—
  Benazepril: 2 to 4 hours.
  Captopril: 60 to 90 minutes.
  Enalapril: 4 to 6 hours.
  Enalaprilat (intravenous): 1 to 4 hours.
  Fosinopril: 2 to 6 hours.
  Lisinopril: 6 hours.
  Quinapril: 2 to 4 hours.
  Ramipril: 4 to 6.5 hours.
Multiple doses—
  The full therapeutic effect may not be noticed until several weeks after initiation of oral therapy.

### Duration of action
Single-dose—
  Benazepril: Approximately 24 hours.
  Captopril: Approximately 6 to 12 hours; dose related.
  Enalapril: Approximately 24 hours.
  Enalaprilat (intravenous): Approximately 6 hours.
  Fosinopril: Approximately 24 hours.
  Lisinopril: Approximately 24 hours.
  Quinapril: Up to 24 hours; dose related.
  Ramipril: Approximately 24 hours.

### Elimination
Benazepril—
  Predominantly renal.
  Nonrenal (biliary): 11 to 12%.
  In dialysis: Benazeprilat is slightly removable by hemodialysis.
Captopril—
  Renal: More than 95%; 40 to 50% unchanged (may be less in patients with congestive heart failure); remainder as metabolites.
  In dialysis: Captopril is removable by hemodialysis.

Enalapril—
    Renal: 60% (20% as enalapril and 40% as enalaprilat).
    Fecal: 33% (6% as enalapril and 27% as enalaprilat).
    In dialysis: Enalaprilat is removable by hemodialysis, at the rate of 62 mL per minute, and by peritoneal dialysis.
Enalaprilat—
    Renal: 100% unchanged.
    In dialysis: Enalaprilat is removable by hemodialysis at the rate of 62 mL per minute.
Fosinopril—
    Renal: 44 to 50%.
    Fecal: 46 to 50%.
    In dialysis: Fosinopril is not well dialyzed. Fosinoprilat clearance by hemodialysis and peritoneal dialysis is approximately 2% and 7%, respectively, of urea clearance.
Lisinopril—
    Renal: 100% unchanged.
    In dialysis: Lisinopril is removable by hemodialysis.
Quinapril—
    Renal: 61% (56% as quinapril and quinaprilat).
    Fecal: 37%.
    In dialysis: Minimal effect on the elimination of quinapril and quinaprilat.
Ramipril—
    Renal: Approximately 60%.
    Fecal: Approximately 40%.
    In dialysis: It is not known whether ramipril or ramiprilat is removable by hemodialysis.

## Precautions to Consider

### Cross-sensitivity and/or related problems
Patients sensitive to one ACE inhibitor may also be sensitive to another.

### Carcinogenicity
*Benazepril*—Studies in mice and rats given doses of 150 mg per kg of body weight (mg/kg) per day (110 times the maximum recommended human dose by weight) for up to 2 years, revealed no evidence of carcinogenicity.
*Captopril*— Two-year studies in mice and rats at doses of 50 to 1350 mg/kg per day showed no evidence of carcinogenicity.
*Enalapril*—Studies in rats for 106 weeks and in mice for 94 weeks at doses up to 150 and 300 times the maximum daily human dose (based on a patient weight of 50 kg), respectively, found no evidence of tumorigenicity or carcinogenicity.
*Enalaprilat* (intravenous)—Studies have not been done. However, since actions of enalapril maleate are caused by enalaprilat, the active metabolite, the same information would be expected to apply.
*Fosinopril*—Studies in mice and rats given doses up to 400 mg/kg per day for up to 24 months, revealed no evidence of carcinogenicity. However, a slightly higher incidence of mesentery/omentum lipomas was found in male rats given the highest dose level (about 250 times the maximum human dose by weight).
*Lisinopril*—Studies in male and female rats for 105 weeks at doses up to 56 times the maximum recommended human daily dose (based on a patient weight of 50 kg) and in male and female mice for 92 weeks at doses up to 84 times the maximum recommended human daily dose (based on a patient weight of 50 kg) found no evidence of tumorigenicity.
*Quinapril*—Studies in mice and rats given doses up to 75 or 100 mg/kg per day (50 to 60 times the maximum recommended human daily dose by weight) for 104 weeks, revealed no evidence of carcinogenicity. However, female rats given the highest dose level had an increased incidence of mesenteric lymph node hemangiomas and skin/subcutaneous lipomas.
*Ramipril*—Studies in rats and mice given doses up to 500 mg/kg per day for 24 months and up to 1000 mg/kg per day for 18 months, respectively, revealed no evidence of tumorigenicity. Renal juxtaglomerular apparatus hypertrophy was found in mice, rats, dogs, and monkeys given doses greatly in excess of recommended human doses.

### Mutagenicity
*Benazepril*—No evidence of mutagenicity was found in tests including the Ames bacterial assay (with or without metabolic activation), an *in vitro* test for forward mutations in cultured mammalian cells, and a nucleus anomaly test.
*Enalapril* and *enalaprilat*—No evidence of mutagenicity was found in tests including the Ames bacterial assay with or without metabolic activation, rec-assay, reverse mutation assay with *E. coli*, sister chromatid exchange with cultured mammalian cells, the micronucleus test with mice, and in an *in vivo* cytogenic study using mouse bone marrow.
*Fosinopril*—No evidence of mutagenicity was found in tests including the Ames bacterial assay, the mouse lymphoma forward mutation assay, and a mitotic gene conversion assay. No evidence of genotoxicity was found in a mouse micronucleus test *in vivo* and a mouse bone marrow cytogenetic assay *in vivo*. An increased frequency of chromosomal aberrations was found in the Chinese hamster ovary cell cytogenetic assay at toxic cell concentrations tested without metabolic activation. However, this increase was not found at lower drug concentrations without metabolic activation or at any other concentration with metabolic activation.
*Lisinopril*—No evidence of mutagenicity was found in tests including the Ames bacterial assay with or without metabolic activation, forward mutation assay using Chinese hamster lung cells, *in vitro* alkaline elution rat hepatocyte assay, and chromosomal aberration studies *in vitro* in Chinese hamster ovary cells and *in vivo* in mouse bone marrow.
*Quinapril*—No evidence of mutagenicity was found in the Ames bacterial assay with or without metabolic activation.
*Ramipril*—No evidence of mutagenicity was found in tests including the Ames bacterial assay, the micronucleus test in mice, unscheduled DNA synthesis in a human cell line, and a forward gene-mutation assay in a Chinese hamster ovary cell line.

### Pregnancy/Reproduction
Fertility—*Benazepril:* No adverse effect on the reproductive performance of male and female rats was found.
*Captopril:* No impairment of fertility was found in rats.
*Enalapril:* No adverse effects on reproductive performance were found in male and female rats given 10 to 90 mg/kg per day of enalapril.
*Fosinopril:* No adverse reproductive effects were found in male and female rats given doses up to 60 mg/kg per day (about 38 times the maximum recommended human dose by weight). However, a slight increase in pairing time was observed in rats given a toxic dose of 240 mg/kg per day (150 times the maximum recommended human dose by weight).
*Lisinopril:* No adverse effects on reproductive performance were found in male and female rats given doses up to 300 mg/kg per day of lisinopril.
*Quinapril:* No adverse effects on fertility or reproduction were found in rats given doses up to 100 mg/kg per day (60 times the maximum daily human dose based on weight).
*Ramipril:* No impairment of fertility was found in rats given doses up to 500 mg/kg per day.
Pregnancy—In humans, ACE inhibitors can cause fetal and neonatal morbidity and mortality when administered to pregnant women.ACE inhibitors should be discontinued as soon as possible when pregnancy is detected.
ACE inhibitors cross the placenta.Fetal exposure to ACE inhibitors during the second and third trimesters can cause hypotension, renal failure, anuria, skull hypoplasia, and even death in the newborn. Maternal oligohydramnios has also been reported, probably reflecting decreasing fetal renal function.
Enalapril and lisinopril have been removed from neonatal circulation by peritoneal dialysis. Captopril is not removable by peritoneal dialysis. There are inadequate data concerning the effectiveness of hemodialysis and there is no information concerning use of exchange transfusion for removing captopril from general circulation. There has been no experience with hemodialysis, peritoneal dialysis, or exchange transfusion for removing benazepril, fosinopril, quinapril, or ramipril from neonatal circulation.
It is recommended that infants exposed in utero to ACE inhibitors be closely observed for hypotension, oliguria, and hyperkalemia. Oliguria should be treated with support of blood pressure and renal perfusion by administration of fluids and pressors as appropriate.
*Benazepril:* Studies in pregnant rats, mice, and rabbits at doses 300, 90, and more than 3 times, respectively, the maximum recommended human dose by weight, revealed no embryotoxic, fetotoxic, or teratogenic effects.
*Captopril:* Several cases of intrauterine growth retardation, fetal distress and hypotension, and one case of cranial malformation have been reported. Neonatal deaths have occurred in rats at up to 400 times the recommended human dose. Fetal deaths have occurred when rabbits were given 2 to 70 times the maximum recommended human dose and a low incidence of cranial malformations occurred in offspring. No teratogenicity has been noted in hamsters or rats.
*Enalapril:* Fetal toxicity (decrease in average fetal weight) has occurred in rats at doses of enalapril 2000 times the maximum daily human dose, and maternal and fetal toxicity has occurred in rabbits at doses almost double the maximum daily human dose. In some cases, saline supplementation prevented maternal and fetal toxicity. No teratogenicity has been noted in rabbits and neither fetal toxicity nor teratogenicity occurred in rats at doses up to 333 times the maximum daily human dose.
*Fosinopril:* Maternal toxicity was evident in pregnant rabbits given doses up to 40 mg/kg per day (about 50 times the maximum recommended human dose). Fosinopril at doses up to 40 mg/kg per day (about 50 times the maximum recommended human dose) was embryocidal in

rabbits, probably due to marked decreases in blood pressure secondary to ACE inhibition in this species. There was no evidence of teratogenicity in rabbits at any dosage level. Maternal toxicity was evident in pregnant rats at all dose levels tested up to 400 mg/kg per day (about 500 times the maximum recommended human dose). Furthermore, all dose levels produced slight reductions in placental weights and some degree of skeletal ossification. High doses resulted in reduced fetal body weight. Three similar orofacial malformations and one fetus with situs inversus occurred in animals given fosinopril. It is uncertain whether these anomalies were associated with drug treatment.

*Lisinopril:* Lisinopril was not teratogenic in mice given doses up to 625 times the maximum recommended human dose on days 6 to 15 of gestation; an increase in fetal resorptions occurred at doses of 62.5 times the maximum recommended human dose, but was prevented at doses of 625 times the maximum recommended human dose by saline supplementation. No fetotoxicity or teratogenicity occurred in rats given doses up to 188 times the maximum recommended human dose on days 6 to 17 of gestation, but an increased incidence of pup deaths and a lower average birth weight (both preventable by saline supplementation) occurred postpartum in rats given lisinopril on day 15 of gestation through day 21 postpartum. Lisinopril crosses the placenta in rats but has not been found in the fetus. Lisinopril did not cause teratogenicity in saline-supplemented rabbits given doses up to 1 mg/kg per day, but did cause fetotoxicity (increased fetal resorptions, increased incidence of incomplete ossification).

*Quinapril:* Quinapril at doses as high as 300 mg/kg per day (180 times the maximum daily human dose by weight) did not produce fetotoxic or teratogenic effects in rats, despite maternal toxicity at 150 mg/kg per day. However, reduced offspring body weight was observed at doses greater than 25 mg/kg per day, and changes in renal histology (juxtaglomerular cell hypertrophy, tubular/pelvic dilation, glomerulosclerosis) were seen in dams and offspring given 150 mg/kg per day when tested later in gestation and during lactation. Quinapril did not produce teratogenic effects in rabbits. However, in some rabbits maternal toxicity and embryotoxicity were observed at doses as low as 0.5 mg/kg per day (one time the recommended human dose) and 1.0 mg/kg per day.

*Ramipril:* Studies in rats, mice, monkeys, and rabbits at doses up to 2500 times (in rats and mice), more than 12 times, and more than 2 times, respectively, the maximum recommended human dose by weight, revealed an increased incidence of dilated renal pelvises in rat fetuses and retarded birth weights in mice. However, these studies did not show ramipril to produce terata or to affect fertility, reproductive performance, or pregnancy.

*For all ACE inhibitors:*

FDA Pregnancy Category C—First trimester.
FDA Pregnancy Category D—Second and third trimesters.

## Breast-feeding

*Benazepril*— Benazepril and benazeprilat are distributed into breast milk. A nursing infant would receive less than 0.1% of the mg/kg maternal dose of benazepril and benazeprilat.

*Captopril*— Captopril is distributed into breast milk; concentrations in breast milk are approximately 1% of maternal blood concentrations. However, problems in humans have not been documented.

*Enalapril*— It is not known whether enalapril is distributed into breast milk. However, problems in humans have not been documented.

*Fosinopril*— Fosinoprilat (active metabolite) is distributed into breast milk. Detectable levels of fosinoprilat in breast milk were found following ingestion of 20 mg per day for 3 days.

*Lisinopril*— It is not known whether lisinopril is distributed into human breast milk; it appears to distribute into the milk of lactating rats. However, problems in humans have not been documented.

*Quinapril*—It is not known whether quinapril or its metabolites are distributed into human breast milk; quinapril appears to distribute into the milk of lactating rats. However, problems in humans have not been documented.

*Ramipril*—A 10-mg dose of ramipril resulted in undetectable amounts of ramipril and its metabolites in breast milk. However, multiple doses may produce low milk concentrations.

## Pediatrics

Appropriate studies on the relationship of age to the effects of ACE inhibitors have not been done in the pediatric population. However, the use of ACE inhibitors in a limited number of neonates and infants has identified some potential pediatrics-specific problems. In neonates and infants, there is a risk of oliguria and neurologic abnormalities, possibly as a result of decreased renal and cerebral blood flow secondary to marked and prolonged reductions in blood pressure caused by ACE inhibitors; a lower initial dose and close monitoring are recommended.

## Geriatrics

ACE inhibitors are thought to be most effective in reducing blood pressure in patients with normal or high plasma renin activity. Since plasma renin activity appears to decline with increasing age, elderly individuals may be less sensitive to the hypotensive effects of ACE inhibitors. However, elevated serum ACE inhibitor concentrations resulting from age-related decline in renal function may compensate for the lower renin dependence. Pharmacokinetic studies with lisinopril, quinapril, and ramipril have revealed higher peak serum concentrations and area under the curve (AUC) in elderly patients given doses similar to those given to younger adults. The net result is that no significant differences in blood pressure response or side/adverse effects have been noted in elderly patients receiving ACE inhibitors. Nevertheless, some elderly patients may be more sensitive to the hypotensive effects of these medications and may require caution when receiving an ACE inhibitor.

## Drug interactions and/or related problems

The following drug interactions and/or related problems have been selected on the basis of their potential clinical significance (possible mechanism in parentheses where appropriate)—not necessarily inclusive (» = major clinical significance):

Note: Combinations containing any of the following medications, depending on the amount present, may also interact with this medication.

*For all ACE inhibitors*
» Alcohol or
» Diuretics or
  Hypotension-producing medications, other (See *Appendix II*)
  (concurrent use with ACE inhibitors may produce additive hypotensive effects)

  (antihypertensive agents that cause renin release or affect sympathetic activity have the greatest additive effect; concurrent use of captopril with beta-adrenergic blocking agents produces an increased but less than fully additive effect; although some antihypertensive and/or diuretic combinations may be used for therapeutic advantage, dosage adjustments may be necessary during concurrent use or when one drug is discontinued)

  (if significant systemic absorption of ophthalmic beta-blockers occurs, hypotensive effects of ACE inhibitors may be potentiated)

  (sudden and severe hypotension may occur within the first 1 to 5 hours after the initial dose of an ACE inhibitor, particularly in patients who are sodium- and volume-depleted as a result of diuretic therapy. Withdrawal of the diuretic or increase of salt intake approximately 1 week before start of captopril therapy or 2 to 3 days before start of benazepril enalapril, fosinopril, lisinopril, quinapril, or ramipril therapy, or initiating ACE inhibitor therapy in lower doses, will minimize the reaction; this reaction does not usually recur with subsequent doses, although caution in increasing doses is recommended; diuretics may be reinstituted as necessary)

  (risk of renal failure may be increased in patients who are sodium- and volume-depleted as a result of diuretic therapy)

  (ACE inhibitors may reduce the secondary aldosteronism and hypokalemia caused by diuretics)

Anti-inflammatory drugs, nonsteroidal (NSAIDs), especially indomethacin
  (concurrent use of these agents may reduce the antihypertensive effects of ACE inhibitors; indomethacin, and possibly other NSAIDs, may antagonize the antihypertensive effect by inhibiting renal prostaglandin synthesis and/or causing sodium and fluid retention; the patient should be carefully monitored to confirm that the desired effect is being obtained)

Blood from blood bank (may contain up to 30 mEq [mmol] of potassium per liter of plasma or up to 65 mEq [mmol] per liter of whole blood when stored for more than 10 days) or
Cyclosporine or
» Diuretics, potassium-sparing or
» Low-salt milk (may contain up to 60 mEq [mmol] of potassium per liter) or
» Potassium-containing medications or
» Potassium supplements or substances containing high concentrations of potassium or
» Salt substitutes (most contain substantial amounts of potassium)
  (concurrent administration with ACE inhibitors may result in hyperkalemia since reduction of aldosterone production induced by ACE inhibitors may lead to elevation of serum potassium; frequent determination of serum potassium concentrations is recommended if concurrent use of these agents is necessary; concurrent use is not recommended in patients with congestive heart failure)

Bone marrow depressants (See *Appendix II*)
(concurrent administration with an ACE inhibitor may result in an increased risk of development of potentially fatal neutropenia and/or agranulocytosis)

Estrogens
(estrogen-induced fluid retention may increase blood pressure; the patient should be carefully monitored to confirm that the desired effect is being obtained)

Lithium
(reversible increases in serum lithium concentrations and toxicity have been reported during concurrent use with ACE inhibitors; frequent monitoring of serum lithium concentrations is recommended during concurrent use)

Sympathomimetics
(concurrent use of these agents may reduce the antihypertensive effects of ACE inhibitors; the patient should be carefully monitored to confirm that the desired effect is being obtained)

*For quinapril only*
Tetracyclines or
Other drugs that interact with magnesium
(concurrent use of these agents with quinapril may reduce their absorption; absorption of tetracycline is reduced by approximately 28 to 37%, possibly due to the high magnesium content in Accupril brand of quinapril tablets)

**Laboratory value alterations**
The following have been selected on the basis of their potential clinical significance (possible effect in parentheses where appropriate)—not necessarily inclusive (» = major clinical significance):

With diagnostic test results
*For all ACE inhibitors*
Iodohippurate sodium I 123/I 131 renal imaging or
Technetium Tc 99m pentetate renal imaging
(in patients with renal artery stenosis, captopril [and probably all ACE inhibitors] may cause a reversible decrease in localization and excretion of iodohippurate I 123/I 131or technetium Tc 99m pentetate in the affected kidney; may cause confusion as to whether decreased renal function is drug-related)

*For captopril only*
Urinary acetone test
(captopril may produce false-positive results)

*For fosinopril only*
Digoxin levels
(fosinopril may cause a false low serum digoxin level with the Digi-Tab RIA Kit)

With physiology/laboratory test values
*For all ACE inhibitors*
Alkaline phosphatase, serum and
Bilirubin, serum and
Transaminases, serum
(concentration increases have been reported)

Antinuclear antibody (ANA) titer
(positive ANA has been reported)

Blood urea nitrogen (BUN) and
Creatinine, serum
(concentrations may be transiently increased, especially in patients with renal parenchymal and renovascular disease in patients who are volume- or sodium-depleted, in patients with renal artery stenosis, or after rapid reduction of long-standing or severe high blood pressure)

Hematocrit or
Hemoglobin
(may rarely be slightly decreased)

Potassium, serum
(concentrations may be slightly increased as a result of reduced circulating aldosterone concentrations and concomitant reduction in glomerular filtration rate [GFR], especially in patients with renal function impairment)

Sodium, serum
(concentrations may be slightly decreased, especially during initial therapy)

**Medical considerations/Contraindications**
The medical considerations/contraindications included have been selected on the basis of their potential clinical significance (reasons given in parentheses where appropriate)—not necessarily inclusive (» = major clinical significance).

*Risk-benefit should be considered when the following medical problems exist:*
*For all ACE inhibitors*
» Angioedema, history of, related to previous ACE inhibitor therapy or
» Hereditary angioedema or
» Idiopathic angioedema
(increased risk for development of ACE inhibitor–related angioedema)

Autoimmune disease, severe, especially systemic lupus erythematosus (SLE) or scleroderma
(increased risk for development of neutropenia or agranulocytosis)

Bone marrow depression
Cerebrovascular insufficiency or
Coronary insufficiency
(ischemia may be aggravated as a result of reduced blood pressure; cerebrovascular accident or myocardial infarction could be precipitated)

Diabetes mellitus
(increased risk of hyperkalemia)

» Hyperkalemia
» Renal artery stenosis, bilateral or in a solitary kidney or
» Renal transplant
(increased risk of renal function impairment)

» Renal function impairment
(decreased elimination of active ACE inhibitor [except fosinopril], resulting in higher plasma concentrations; increased risk of hyperkalemia, or, for captopril, proteinuria, neutropenia, and agranulocytosis. Patients with impaired renal function may require lower or less frequent doses and smaller increments in dose. However, dosage adjustment may not be necessary with fosinopril since total body drug clearance even in severe renal function impairment is not decreased significantly, possibly due to compensatory hepatobiliary elimination. If a diuretic is also required, a loop diuretic is recommended instead of a thiazide diuretic in patients with severe renal function impairment)

Sensitivity to the ACE inhibitor prescribed, or any other ACE inhibitor
» Caution is required also in patients on severe dietary sodium restriction or dialysis; these patients may be volume-depleted, and sudden reduction by the initial dose of ACE inhibitor in the angiotensin II levels that have been maintaining them at a near-normotensive state may result in sudden and severe hypotension. In addition, the risk of ACE inhibitor–induced renal failure may be increased in patients who are sodium- and volume-depleted, especially those with congestive heart failure.

*For benazepril, captopril, enalapril, fosinopril, quinapril, and ramipril (in addition to the above)*
Hepatic function impairment
(may reduce metabolism of captopril and may reduce conversion of prodrug to active moiety with benazepril, enalapril, fosinopril, quinapril, and ramipril)

**Patient monitoring**
The following may be especially important in patient monitoring (other tests may be warranted in some patients, depending on condition; » = major clinical significance):

» Blood pressure measurements
(recommended at periodic intervals in patients being treated for hypertension; selected patients may be trained to perform blood pressure measurements at home and report the results at regular physician visits)

Leukocyte count determinations, total and differential
(recommended prior to initiation of ACE inhibitor therapy and periodically thereafter; recommended every month for the first 3 to 6 months of therapy, and at periodic intervals thereafter for a period of up to 1 year in patients at increased risk for neutropenia [i.e., those with renal function impairment or collagen vascular disease] or receiving high doses; also recommended at the first sign of infection. It is recommended that ACE inhibitor therapy be withdrawn if neutropenia [neutrophil count less than 1000 per cubic millimeter $(1 \times 10^9/L)$] is confirmed)

Renal function determinations
(recommended at periodic intervals, especially in patients who are sodium- and volume-depleted as a result of diuretic therapy or who have severe congestive heart failure)

Urinary protein estimates by means of dip-stick on first morning urine
(recommended prior to initiation of therapy and at periodic intervals thereafter for up to 1 year in patients with renal function impairment or those receiving doses of captopril greater than 150 mg per day;

if excessive or increasing proteinuria occurs, it is recommended that ACE inhibitor therapy be re-evaluated)

## Side/Adverse Effects

Note: Proteinuria has occurred in about 1% of patients receiving greater than 150 mg of captopril per day. This adverse effect is thought to be due to the sulfhydryl moiety of captopril. However, whether this is a true causal relationship is unknown. Proteinuria usually occurs in patients with existing renal function impairment within 8 months of initiation of captopril therapy and usually reverses within 6 months even with continuation of therapy. Membranous glomerulopathy has been reported in some of these patients, especially with doses of captopril greater than 150 mg per day. Proteinuria has also been reported in patients receiving enalapril and lisinopril. Reported incidences range from 0% to 1.4% for enalapril and 0.7% for lisinopril.

There have been reports of reversible renal failure during ACE inhibitor therapy, especially in patients with bilateral renal artery stenoses or renal artery stenosis in a solitary kidney. There is also evidence that renal failure may be related to sodium and volume depletion from previous diuretic therapy or severe sodium restriction, especially in patients with congestive heart failure.

Hepatotoxicity has been reported rarely in patients receiving captopril, enalapril, and lisinopril. Cholestasis has been reported most frequently, although hepatic necrosis and hepatocellular injury have also been reported. The most common presenting symptoms are jaundice, pruritus, and abdominal tenderness. ACE inhibitor–associated hepatotoxicity is usually reversible upon discontinuation of therapy. Apparent cross-reactivity has been reported between captopril and enalapril and between lisinopril and enalapril.

The following side/adverse effects have been selected on the basis of their potential clinical significance (possible signs and symptoms in parentheses where appropriate)—not necessarily inclusive:

**Those indicating need for medical attention**
Incidence less frequent
*Hypotension* (dizziness, lightheadedness, or fainting)—especially following the initial dose in sodium- or volume-depleted patients or in patients receiving an ACE inhibitor for congestive heart failure; *skin rash, with or without itching, fever, or joint pain*

Note: Maculopapular or, rarely, urticarial rash usually occurs during the first 4 weeks of the therapy with captopril and usually disappears with dosage reduction or withdrawal, or administration of an antihistamine; between 7 and 10% of these patients may show eosinophilia and/or positive antinuclear antibody (ANA) titers. The reaction may also occur, less frequently, with the other ACE inhibitors.

Rarely, a persistent lichenoid or pemphigoid reaction, possibly with a photosensitive factor, has been reported with captopril.

Incidence rare
*Angioedema of the extremities, face, lips, mucous membranes, tongue, glottis, and/or larynx* (sudden trouble in swallowing or breathing; swelling of face, mouth, hands, or feet; hoarseness)—especially following the initial dose; *chest pain; hyperkalemia* (confusion; irregular heartbeat; nervousness; numbness or tingling in hands, feet, or lips; shortness of breath or difficult breathing; weakness or heaviness of legs); *neutropenia or agranulocytosis* (fever and chills); *pancreatitis* (abdominal pain; nausea; vomiting; abdominal distention; fever)

Note: *Angioedema* involving the tongue, glottis, or larynx may cause airway obstruction, which could be fatal.

*Chest pain* is usually associated with severe hypotension.

Incidence of *neutropenia or agranulocytosis* is much higher in patients with renal function impairment (0.2% for captopril) or collagen vascular disease (e.g., SLE or scleroderma) (3.7% for captopril). Neutropenia appears to be dose-related and may begin within 3 months after initiation of therapy, with the nadir of the leukocyte count occurring after 10 to 30 days and persisting about 2 weeks after withdrawal. Deaths from pancytopenia and sepsis have been reported with captopril in patients with and without autoimmune disease.

**Those indicating need for medical attention only if they continue or are bothersome**
Incidence more frequent
*Cough, dry, continuing; headache*

Note: *Cough* usually occurs within the first week of therapy (onset varies from 24 hours to several weeks after initiation), persists throughout therapy, and disappears within a few days after withdrawal of the ACE inhibitor. Characteristically the cough begins as a tickling sensation in the back of the throat leading to a dry, nonproductive, persistent cough; may be worse at night or in the supine position; onset can be paroxysmal and course may be episodic or intermittent; may occasionally lead to hoarseness or vomiting.

Incidence less frequent
*Diarrhea; dysgeusia* (loss of taste); *fatigue* (unusual tiredness); *nausea*

Note: *Loss of taste* is usually reversible after 2 to 3 months, even with continued treatment; may be associated with weight loss.

## Overdose

For more information on the management of overdose or unintentional ingestion, **contact a Poison Control Center** (see *Poison Control Center Listing*).

**Treatment of overdose**
Treatment of overdose consists of volume expansion for correction of hypotension. Captopril, enalaprilat, and lisinopril are removable by hemodialysis. Benazeprilat is slightly removable by hemodialysis.

## Patient Consultation

As an aid to patient consultation, refer to *Advice for the Patient, Angiotensin-converting Enzyme (ACE) Inhibitors*.

In providing consultation, consider emphasizing the following selected information (» = major clinical significance):

**Before using this medication**
» Conditions affecting use, especially:
    Sensitivity to any ACE inhibitor
    Pregnancy—ACE inhibitors cross the placenta; ACE inhibitor-associated fetal hypotension, oliguria, and death reported in humans; fetotoxicity found in animals
    Breast-feeding—Benazepril, captopril, and fosinopril are distributed into breast milk
    Other medications, especially alcohol, diuretics (particularly potassium-sparing), potassium-containing medications, or potassium supplements
    Other medical problems, especially angioedema related to previous ACE inhibitor therapy, hyperkalemia, renal artery stenosis, renal transplant, renal function impairment, or sodium and volume depletion
    Use of low-salt milk or salt substitutes

**Proper use of this medication**
Compliance with therapy; taking medication at the same time each day to maintain the therapeutic effect
» Proper dosing
Missed dose: Taking as soon as possible; not taking if almost time for next dose; not doubling doses
» Proper storage

*For captopril*
For best results, taking on an empty stomach 1 hour before meals

*For use as an antihypertensive*
Possible need for control of weight and diet, especially sodium intake; risks associated with sodium depletion; not taking salt substitutes or using low-salt milk unless approved by physician
» Patient may not experience symptoms of hypertension; importance of taking medication even if feeling well
» Does not cure, but helps control hypertension; possible need for lifelong therapy; checking with physician before discontinuing medication; serious consequences of untreated hypertension

**Precautions while using this medication**
Making regular visits to physician to check progress
Caution when driving or doing other things requiring alertness, because of possible dizziness, especially after initial dose of ACE inhibitor in patients taking diuretics
Checking with physician if severe nausea, vomiting, or diarrhea occurs and continues because of risk of dehydration, which may result in hypotension
Caution when exercising or during exposure to hot weather because of risk of dehydration (due to excessive perspiration), which may result in hypotension
Caution if any kind of surgery (including dental surgery) or emergency treatment is required

*For use as an antihypertensive*
» Not taking other medications, especially nonprescription sympathomimetics, unless discussed with physician

*For captopril and fosinopril*
Caution if any laboratory tests required; possible interference with test results

### Side/adverse effects
Signs of potential side effects, especially hypotension, skin rash (with or without itching, fever, or joint pain), angioedema, chest pain, neutropenia or agranulocytosis, pancreatitis, and hyperkalemia

## General Dosing Information
Dosage must be adjusted to meet the individual requirements of each patient, on the basis of clinical response.

The hypotensive effect of ACE inhibitors is about the same in both standing and supine positions.

Recent evidence suggests that withdrawal of antihypertensive therapy prior to surgery may be undesirable. However, the anesthesiologist must be aware of such therapy.

If increased blood urea nitrogen (BUN) and creatinine concentrations occur, reduction in dosage of the ACE inhibitor and/or withdrawal of the diuretic may be required. The possibility of renovascular hypertension should also be considered, especially in the presence of a solitary kidney, transplanted kidney, or bilateral renal artery stenosis.

Caution is recommended in initiating ACE inhibitor therapy for congestive heart failure in patients who have been receiving digitalis glycosides and/or diuretics. If the patient is sodium- and water-depleted, a lower initial dosage should be used.

If symptomatic hypotension occurs, dosage reduction of the ACE inhibitor or withdrawal of the ACE inhibitor or diuretic may be necessary.

### For treatment of adverse effects
For angioedema with swelling confined to the face, mucous membranes of the mouth, lips, and extremities, treatment other than withdrawal of the medication is usually not necessary, although antihistamines may relieve the symptoms.

Treatment of angioedema involving the tongue, glottis, or larynx may include the following:
- Withdrawal of the ACE inhibitor and hospitalization of the patient.
- Subcutaneous (or, rarely, intravenous) epinephrine.
- Intravenous diphenhydramine hydrochloride.
- Intravenous hydrocortisone.

---

## BENAZEPRIL

## Summary of Differences
Precautions:
Breast-feeding—Benazepril and benazeprilat are distributed into breast milk.

## Additional Dosing Information
See also *General Dosing Information*.

It is recommended that previous diuretic therapy be withdrawn 2 to 3 days before benazepril therapy is initiated, except in patients with accelerated or malignant hypertension or hypertension that is difficult to control. In these patients, benazepril therapy may be initiated immediately at a lower dose under careful medical supervision, and doses increased cautiously.

Benazepril is usually effective in once-daily dosing. However, if the antihypertensive effect is diminished before 24 hours, the total daily dose may be given as 2 divided doses.

## Oral Dosage Forms
Note: Bracketed uses in the *Dosage Forms* section refer to categories of use and/or indications that are not included in U.S. product labeling.

The dosing and strengths of the dosage forms available are expressed in terms of benazepril base (not the hydrochloride salt).

### BENAZEPRIL HYDROCHLORIDE TABLETS
**Usual adult dose**
Antihypertensive—
Initial: Oral, 10 mg (base) once a day.
Maintenance: Oral, 20 to 40 mg (base) once a day as a single dose or in two divided doses.

Note: An initial dose of 5 mg (base) should be used in patients who are sodium- and water-depleted as a result of prior diuretic therapy, patients continuing to receive diuretic therapy, or patients with renal failure (creatinine clearance less than 30 mL per minute per 1.73m$^2$). Such patients should be kept under medical supervision for at least two hours after this initial dose (and for an additional hour after blood pressure has stabilized), to watch for excessive hypotension.

[Vasodilator, congestive heart failure]—
Initial: Oral, 5 mg (base) once a day.
Maintenance: Oral, 5 to 10 mg (base) once a day.

**Usual adult prescribing limits**
Doses above 80 mg per day have not been evaluated.

**Usual pediatric dose**
Safety and efficacy have not been established.

**Strength(s) usually available**
U.S.—
5 mg (base) (Rx) [*Lotensin*].
10 mg (base) (Rx) [*Lotensin*].
20 mg (base) (Rx) [*Lotensin*].
40 mg (base) (Rx) [*Lotensin*].
Canada—
Not commercially available.

**Packaging and storage**
Store below 30 °C (86 °F), preferably between 15 and 30 °C (59 and 86 °F), unless otherwise specified by manufacturer. Store in a tight container.

**Auxiliary labeling**
- Do not take other medicines without your doctor's advice.

**Note**
Check refill frequency to determine compliance in hypertensive patients.

---

## CAPTOPRIL

## Summary of Differences
Indications:
Captopril is used for the treatment of neonatal hypertension and neonatal and infant congestive heart failure.
Pharmacology/pharmacokinetics:
Mechanism of action/Effect—Captopril is not a prodrug.
Duration of action—Single dose: 6 to 12 hours.
Precautions:
Breast-feeding—Captopril is distributed into breast milk.
Laboratory value alterations—May produce false-positive results in urinary acetone test.
Side/adverse effects:
Causes maculopapular or urticarial skin rash, sometimes with fever, joint pain, or elevated antinuclear antibody (ANA) titers.

## Additional Dosing Information
See also *General Dosing Information*.

It is recommended that previous antihypertensive therapy be withdrawn 1 week before captopril therapy is initiated, except in patients with accelerated or malignant hypertension or hypertension that is difficult to control. In these patients, captopril therapy may be initiated at the lowest dose immediately after previous therapy (except diuretics) is discontinued, under careful medical supervision, and the dosage increased every 24 hours or less until the medication is effective or the maximum dose is reached.

## Oral Dosage Forms
### CAPTOPRIL TABLETS USP

**Usual adult and adolescent dose**
Antihypertensive—
Initial: Oral, 12.5 mg two or three times a day, the dosage being increased if necessary after one or two weeks to 25 mg two or three times a day.
Left ventricular dysfunction following myocardial infarction—
Initial: Oral, a single dose of 6.25 mg. Then 12.5 mg three times a day, gradually increased to 25 mg three times a day over several days.
Maintenance: Oral, 50 mg three times a day.
Note: Captopril therapy may be initiated as early as three days following a myocardial infarction.
Diabetic nephropathy[1]—
Oral, 25 mg three times a day.
Vasodilator, congestive heart failure—
Initial: Oral, 12.5 mg two or three times a day, the dosage being increased gradually as necessary on a daily basis up to 50 mg two or three times a day. If further increases in dosage are needed, it is recommended that they be made after an interval of two weeks so that the full effects of captopril will be apparent.
Maintenance: Oral, 25 to 100 mg two or three times a day.

Note: An initial dose of 6.25 to 12.5 mg two or three times a day should be used in patients who are sodium- and water-depleted as a result of diuretic therapy, in patients continuing to receive diuretic therapy, or in patients with renal function impairment. Such patients should be kept under medical supervision for one hour after this initial dose, to watch for excessive hypotension.

Dosage increases in patients with significant renal function impairment should proceed slowly (one- to two-week intervals), and smaller increments should be used.

### Usual adult prescribing limits
450 mg per day.

### Usual pediatric dose
Newborns—
Initial: Oral, 10 mcg (0.01 mg) per kg of body weight two or three times a day, the dosage being adjusted as needed and tolerated.

Children—
Initial: Oral, 300 mcg (0.3 mg) per kg of body weight three times a day, the dosage being increased if necessary in increments of 300 mcg (0.3 mg) per kg of body weight at intervals of eight to twenty-four hours to the minimum effective dose.

Note: An initial dose of 150 mcg (0.15 mg) per kg of body weight three times a day should be used in patients who are sodium- and water-depleted as a result of diuretic therapy, in patients continuing to receive diuretic therapy, or in patients with renal function impairment.

### Strength(s) usually available
U.S.—
12.5 mg (Rx) [*Capoten* (scored)].
25 mg (Rx) [*Capoten* (scored)].
50 mg (Rx) [*Capoten* (scored)].
100 mg (Rx) [*Capoten* (scored)].
Canada—
12.5 mg (Rx) [*Capoten*].
25 mg (Rx) [*Capoten* (scored)].
50 mg (Rx) [*Capoten* (scored)].
100 mg (Rx) [*Capoten* (scored)].

### Packaging and storage
Store below 40 °C (104 °F), preferably between 15 and 30 °C (59 and 86 °F), in a tight container, unless otherwise specified by manufacturer.

### Preparation of dosage form
For patients who cannot take oral solids—Captopril oral solution may be prepared by crushing a 25-mg tablet, dissolving it in 25 or 100 mL of water, and shaking the solution well for at least 5 minutes. After the tablet has dissolved, the clear solution is poured off for administration and the remaining filler, which doesn't dissolve, is discarded. Because captopril is very unstable when dissolved in water, the solution should be used within one-half hour after preparation.

### Auxiliary labeling
• Take on an empty stomach, one hour before meals.
• Do not take other medicines without your doctor's advice.

### Note
Tablets may have a slight sulfurous odor.
Check refill frequency to determine compliance in hypertensive patients.

¹Not included in Canadian product labeling.

---

## ENALAPRIL

## Summary of Differences
Pharmacology/pharmacokinetics:
Onset of action—
Enalapril maleate: Oral—Single dose: 1 hour.
Enalaprilat: Intravenous—Single dose: 15 minutes.

## Additional Dosing Information
See also *General Dosing Information*.

It is recommended that previous diuretic therapy be withdrawn 2 to 3 days before enalapril therapy is initiated, except in patients with accelerated or malignant hypertension or hypertension that is difficult to control. In these patients, enalapril therapy may be initiated immediately at a lower dose under careful medical supervision, and increased cautiously.

Enalapril is usually effective in once-daily dosing. However, if the antihypertensive effect is diminished before 24 hours, the total daily dose may be given as 2 divided doses.

Hemodialysis reduces serum enalaprilat concentrations by approximately 35%.

## Oral Dosage Forms
### ENALAPRIL MALEATE TABLETS USP
#### Usual adult and adolescent dose
Antihypertensive—
Initial: Oral, 5 mg once a day, the dosage being adjusted after one or two weeks according to clinical response.
Maintenance: Oral, 10 to 40 mg per day, as a single dose or in two divided doses.

Note: An initial dose of 2.5 mg should be used in patients who are sodium- and water-depleted as a result of prior diuretic therapy, patients continuing to receive diuretic therapy, or patients with renal failure (creatinine clearance less than 30 mL per minute). Such patients should be kept under medical supervision for at least two hours after this initial dose (and for an additional hour after blood pressure has stabilized), to watch for excessive hypotension.

Vasodilator, congestive heart failure—
Initial: Oral, 2.5 mg once or twice a day, the dosage being adjusted after one or two weeks according to clinical response.
Maintenance: Oral, 5 to 20 mg per day, as a single dose or in two divided doses.

Left ventricular dysfunction, asymptomatic—
Oral, 2.5 mg two times a day titrated as tolerated up to a target dose of 20 mg a day in divided doses.

Note: Patients should be kept under medical supervision for at least two hours and until blood pressure has stabilized for an additional hour after the initial dose.

In patients with hyponatremia (serum sodium concentration less than 130 mEq per liter) or serum creatinine greater than 1.6 mg per deciliter, an initial dose of 2.5 mg once a day is recommended.

If possible, the dose of the diuretic should be reduced to decrease the likelihood of hypotension.

#### Usual adult prescribing limits
40 mg per day.

#### Usual pediatric dose
Safety and efficacy have not been established.

#### Strength(s) usually available
U.S.—
2.5 mg (Rx) [*Vasotec* (scored)].
5 mg (Rx) [*Vasotec* (scored)].
10 mg (Rx) [*Vasotec*].
20 mg (Rx) [*Vasotec*].
Canada—
2.5 mg (Rx) [*Vasotec*].
5 mg (Rx) [*Vasotec* (scored)].
10 mg (Rx) [*Vasotec*].
20 mg (Rx) [*Vasotec*].

#### Packaging and storage
Store below 40 °C (104 °F), preferably between 15 and 30 °C (59 and 86 °F), in a well-closed container, unless otherwise specified by manufacturer.

#### Auxiliary labeling
• Do not take other medicines without your doctor's advice.

#### Note
Check refill frequency to determine compliance in hypertensive patients.

## Parenteral Dosage Forms
### ENALAPRILAT INJECTION
#### Usual adult and adolescent dose
Antihypertensive—
Intravenous (over at least five minutes), 1.25 mg every six hours.

Note: An initial dose of 625 mcg (0.625 mg) should be used in patients who are sodium- and water-depleted as a result of prior diuretic therapy, patients continuing to receive diuretic therapy, or patients with renal failure (creatinine clearance less than or equal to 30 mL per minute). Such patients should be observed for one hour after this initial dose, to watch for excessive hypotension. If the clinical response is inadequate after one hour, the 625 mcg (0.625-mg) dose may be repeated, and therapy continued at a dose of 1.25 mg every six hours.

#### Usual pediatric dose
Safety and efficacy have not been established.

Note: Use of products containing benzyl alcohol is not recommended in neonates. A fatal toxic syndrome consisting of metabolic acidosis, CNS depression, respiratory problems, renal failure, hypotension, and possibly seizures and intracranial hemorrhages has been associated with this use.

**Strength(s) usually available**
U.S.—
 1.25 mg per mL (Rx) [*Vasotec* (benzyl alcohol)].
Canada—
 1.25 mg per mL (Rx) [*Vasotec* (benzyl alcohol)].

**Packaging and storage**
Store below 40 °C (104 °F), preferably between 15 and 30 °C (59 and 86 °F), unless otherwise specified by manufacturer.

**Preparation of dosage form**
Enalaprilat injection may be administered undiluted, or may be diluted with up to 50 mL of a compatible diluent.

**Stability**
Stable in compatible diluents (5% dextrose injection, 0.9% sodium chloride injection, 0.9% sodium chloride in 5% dextrose injection, 5% dextrose in lactated Ringer's injection) for 24 hours.

---

### FOSINOPRIL

## Summary of Differences
Precautions:
 Breast-feeding—Fosinoprilat (active metabolite) is distributed into breast milk.
 Medical considerations/contraindications—Dosage adjustment is not necessary in renal function impairment.
 Laboratory value alterations—May cause a false low serum digoxin level with the Digi-Tab RIA Kit.

## Additional Dosing Information
See also *General Dosing Information*.

It is recommended that previous diuretic therapy be withdrawn 2 to 3 days before fosinopril therapy is initiated, except in patients with accelerated or malignant hypertension or hypertension that is difficult to control. In these patients, fosinopril therapy may be initiated immediately at a lower dose under careful medical supervision (for at least 2 hours and until blood pressure has stabilized for at least an additional hour), and doses increased cautiously.

Fosinopril is usually effective in once-daily dosing. However, if the antihypertensive effect is diminished before 24 hours, the total daily dose may be given as 2 divided doses.

## Oral Dosage Forms
### FOSINOPRIL SODIUM TABLETS

**Usual adult dose**
Antihypertensive—
 Initial: Oral, 10 mg once a day, the dosage being adjusted according to clinical response.
 Maintenance: Oral, 20 to 40 mg once a day.

Note: In patients continuing to receive diuretic therapy, an initial fosinopril dose of 10 mg may be given with careful medical supervision for several hours and until blood pressure is stabilized.

**Usual adult prescribing limits**
80 mg per day.

**Usual pediatric dose**
Safety and efficacy have not been established.

**Strength(s) usually available**
U.S.—
 10 mg (Rx) [*Monopril*].
 20 mg (Rx) [*Monopril*].
Canada—
 Not commercially available.

**Packaging and storage**
Store below 30 °C (86 °F), preferably between 15 and 30 °C (59 and 86 °F), unless otherwise specified by manufacturer. Store in a tight container.

**Auxiliary labeling**
• Do not take other medicines without your doctor's advice.

**Note**
Check refill frequency to determine compliance in hypertensive patients.

---

### LISINOPRIL

## Summary of Differences
Pharmacology/pharmacokinetics:
 Mechanism of action/Effect—Lisinopril is not a prodrug.
 Protein binding—None.
 Biotransformation—None.

## Additional Dosing Information
See also *General Dosing Information*.

It is recommended that previous diuretic therapy be withdrawn 2 to 3 days before lisinopril therapy is initiated, except in patients with accelerated or malignant hypertension or hypertension that is difficult to control. In these patients, lisinopril therapy may be initiated immediately at a lower dose under careful medical supervision (for at least 2 hours and until blood pressure has stabilized for at least an additional hour), and increased cautiously.

Lisinopril is usually effective in once-daily dosing. However, if the antihypertensive effect is diminished before 24 hours, an increase in dosage may be necessary.

## Oral Dosage Forms
### LISINOPRIL TABLETS

**Usual adult and adolescent dose**
Antihypertensive—
 Initial: Oral, 10 mg once a day, the dosage being adjusted according to clinical response.
 Maintenance: Oral, 20 to 40 mg once a day.

Note: An initial dose of 5 mg should be used in patients who are sodium- and water-depleted as a result of prior diuretic therapy, patients continuing to receive diuretic therapy, or patients with renal failure (creatinine clearance less than or equal to 30 mL per minute). An initial dose of 2.5 mg should be used in patients with a creatinine clearance less than 10 mL per minute. Such patients should be kept under medical supervision for at least two hours after this initial dose (and for an additional hour after blood pressure has stabilized), to watch for excessive hypotension.

Vasodilator, congestive heart failure—
 Initial: Oral, 2.5 to 5 mg per day, the dosage being adjusted according to clinical response.
 Maintenance: Oral, 10 to 20 mg per day.

**Usual adult prescribing limits**
Doses up to 80 mg per day have been used but do not appear to have a greater effect.

**Usual pediatric dose**
Safety and efficacy have not been established.

**Strength(s) usually available**
U.S.—
 5 mg (Rx) [*Prinivil* (scored); *Zestril* (scored)].
 10 mg (Rx) [*Prinivil; Zestril*].
 20 mg (Rx) [*Prinivil; Zestril*].
 40 mg (Rx) [*Prinivil; Zestril*].
Canada—
 5 mg (Rx) [*Prinivil* (scored); *Zestril*].
 10 mg (Rx) [*Prinivil; Zestril*].
 20 mg (Rx) [*Prinivil; Zestril*].

**Packaging and storage**
Store below 40 °C (104 °F), preferably between 15 and 30 °C (59 and 86 °F), in a well-closed container, unless otherwise specified by manufacturer.

**Auxiliary labeling**
• Do not take other medicines without your doctor's advice.

**Note**
Check refill frequency to determine compliance in hypertensive patients.

---

### QUINAPRIL

## Summary of Differences
Precautions:
 Drug interactions and/or related problems—Quinapril may reduce absorption of tetracycline or other drugs that interact with magnesium, since quinapril has a high magnesium content.

## Additional Dosing Information
See also *General Dosing Information*.

It is recommended that previous diuretic therapy be withdrawn 2 to 3 days before quinapril therapy is initiated, except in patients with accelerated or malignant hypertension or hypertension that is difficult to control. In these patients, quinapril therapy may be initiated immediately at a lower dose under careful medical supervision (for at least 2 hours and until blood pressure has stabilized for at least an additional hour), and doses increased cautiously.

Quinapril is usually effective in once-daily dosing. However, if the antihypertensive effect is diminished before 24 hours, an increase in dosage may be necessary or the total daily dose may be given as 2 divided doses.

## Oral Dosage Forms

Note: Bracketed uses in the *Dosage Forms* section refer to categories of use and/or indications that are not included in U.S. product labeling.

The dosing and strengths of the dosage forms available are expressed in terms of quinapril base (not the hydrochloride salt).

### QUINAPRIL HYDROCHLORIDE TABLETS

**Usual adult dose**
Antihypertensive—
  Initial: Oral, 10 mg (base) once a day, the dosage being adjusted slowly (at 2-week intervals) and according to clinical response.
  Maintenance: Oral, 20 to 80 mg (base) once a day or divided into two equal doses.

Note: An initial dose of 5 mg should be used in patients who are sodium- and water-depleted as a result of prior diuretic therapy, patients continuing to receive diuretic therapy, or in patients with a creatinine clearance of 30 to 60 mL per minute. An initial dose of 2.5 mg should be used in patients with a creatinine clearance of 10 to 30 mL per minute. Such patients should be kept under medical supervision for at least two hours after this initial dose (and for an additional hour after blood pressure has stabilized), to watch for excessive hypotension.

There are insufficient data for a dosage recommendation in patients with a creatinine clearance less than 10 mL per minute.

[Vasodilator, congestive heart failure]—
  Initial: Oral, 2.5 mg (base) once a day.
  Maintenance: Oral, 5 to 40 mg once a day or divided into two equal doses.

**Usual pediatric dose**
Safety and efficacy have not been established.

**Strength(s) usually available**
U.S.—
  5 mg (Rx) [*Accupril* (scored)].
  10 mg (Rx) [*Accupril* (scored)].
  20 mg (Rx) [*Accupril* (scored)].
  40 mg (Rx) [*Accupril* (scored)].
Canada—
  Not commercially available.

**Packaging and storage**
Store below 40 °C (104 °F), preferably between 15 and 30 °C (59 and 86 °F), in a well-closed container, unless otherwise specified by manufacturer.

**Auxiliary labeling**
• Do not take other medicines without your doctor's advice.

**Note**
Check refill frequency to determine compliance in hypertensive patients.

---

### RAMIPRIL

## Additional Dosing Information
See also *General Dosing Information*.

It is recommended that previous diuretic therapy be withdrawn 2 to 3 days before ramipril therapy is initiated, except in patients with accelerated or malignant hypertension or hypertension that is difficult to control. In these patients, ramipril therapy may be initiated immediately at a lower dose under careful medical supervision (for at least 2 hours and until blood pressure has stabilized for at least an additional hour), and doses increased cautiously.

Ramipril is usually effective in once-daily dosing. However, if the antihypertensive effect is diminished before 24 hours, an increase in dosage may be necessary or the total daily dose may be given as 2 divided doses.

## Oral Dosage Forms

### RAMIPRIL CAPSULES
**Usual adult dose**
Antihypertensive—
  Initial: Oral, 2.5 mg once a day, the dosage being adjusted according to clinical response.
  Maintenance: Oral, 2.5 to 20 mg once a day or divided into two equal doses.

Note: An initial dose of 1.25 mg should be used in patients who are sodium- and water-depleted as a result of prior diuretic therapy, patients continuing to receive diuretic therapy, or in patients with a creatinine clearance less than 40 mL per minute per 1.73 m$^2$. Such patients should be kept under medical supervision for at least two hours after this initial dose (and for an additional hour after blood pressure has stabilized), to watch for excessive hypotension.

Dosage may be slowly titrated upward until adequate blood pressure control is achieved or to a maximum total daily dose of 5 mg.

**Usual pediatric dose**
Safety and efficacy have not been established.

**Strength(s) usually available**
U.S.—
  1.25 mg (Rx) [*Altace*].
  2.5 mg (Rx) [*Altace*].
  5 mg (Rx) [*Altace*].
  10 mg (Rx) [*Altace*].
Canada—
  Not commercially available.

**Packaging and storage**
Store below 40 °C (104 °F), preferably between 15 and 30 °C (59 and 86 °F), in a well-closed container, unless otherwise specified by manufacturer.

**Auxiliary labeling**
• Do not take other medicines without your doctor's advice.

**Note**
Check refill frequency to determine compliance in hypertensive patients.

## Selected Bibliography

**General**
Williams GH. Converting-enzyme inhibitors in the treatment of hypertension. N Engl J Med 1988 Dec 8; 1517-25.
Weber MA. Safety issues during antihypertenisve treatment with angiotensin converting enzyme inhibitors. Am J Med 1988; 84(suppl 4A): 16-23.
Massie BM. New trends in the use of angiotensin converting enzyme inhibitors in chronic heart failure. Am J Med 1988 Apr 15; 84(Suppl 4A): 36-46.

**For benazepril**
Balfour JA, Goa KL. Benazepril. A review of its pharmacodynamic and pharmacokinetic properties, and therapeutic efficacy in hypertension and congestive heart failure. Drugs 1991; 42(3): 511-39.

**For captopril**
Vidt DG, Bravo EL, Fouad FM. Captopril. N Engl J Med 1982 Jan 28; 306: 214-9.
Ram CVS. Captopril. Arch Intern Med 1982 May; 142: 914-6.

**For enalapril**
Cleary JD, Taylor JW. Enalapril: a new angiotensin converting enzyme inhibitor. Drug Intell Clin Pharm 1986 Mar; 20: 177-86.
Vlasses PH, Larijani GE, Conner DP, Ferguson RK. Enalapril, a nonsulfhydryl angiotensin-converting enzyme inhibitor. Clin Pharm 1985; 4: 27-40.

**For fosinopril**
Sica DA, Cutler RE, Parmer RJ, Ford NF. Comparison of the steady-state pharmacokinetics of fosinopril, lisinopril and enalapril in patients with chronic renal insufficiency. Clin Pharmacokinet 1991; 20(5): 420-7.
Oren S, Messerli FH, Grossman E, Garavaglia GE, Frohlich ED. Immediate and short-term cardiovascular effects of fosinopril, a new angiotensin-converting enzyme inhibitor, in patients with essential hypertension. J Am Coll Cardiol 1991; 17: 1183-7.

**For lisinopril**
Armayor GM, Lopez LM. Lisinopril: A new angiotensin-converting enzyme inhibitor. Drug Intell Clin Pharm 1988 May; 22: 365-72.
Lisinopril for hypertension. Med Lett Drugs Ther 1988 Apr 8; 30: 41-2.

Chase SL, Sutton JD. Lisinopril: A new angiotensin-converting enzyme inhibitor. Pharmacother 1989; 9(3): 120-30.

**For quinapril**
Cropp AB. Quinapril: A new second-generation ACE inhibitor. DICP 1991; 25: 499-504.

Wadworth AN, Brogden RN. Quinapril. A review of its pharmacologic properties, and therapeutic efficacy in cardiovascular disorders. Drugs 41(3): 378-99.

**For ramipril**
Todd PA, Benfield P. Ramipril. A review of its pharmacological properties and therapeutic efficacy in cardiovascular disorders. Drugs 1990; 39(1): 110-35.

Revised: 07/12/92
Interim revision: 08/04/93; 07/12/94; 08/12/98

---

# ANGIOTENSIN-CONVERTING ENZYME (ACE) INHIBITORS AND HYDROCHLOROTHIAZIDE   Systemic

This monograph includes information on the following: 1) Captopril and Hydrochlorothiazide†; 2) Enalapril and Hydrochlorothiazide; 3) Lisinopril and Hydrochlorothiazide.

VA CLASSIFICATION (Primary/Secondary): CV401/CV900

NOTE: The *Angiotensin-converting Enzyme (ACE) Inhibitors and Hydrochlorothiazide (Systemic)* monograph is maintained on the USP DI electronic data base. For a printed copy of the most recent revision of the complete monograph, contact Micromedex, Inc. - Reprint Requests, 6200 S. Syracuse Way, Suite 300, Englewood, CO 80111; telephone (303) 486-6400; telefax (303) 486-6464; Email: USPDI@MDX.COM.

For information on the specific components of this combination, see the *USP DI* monographs for *Angiotensin-converting Enzymes (ACE) Inhibitors (Systemic)* and *Diuretics, Thiazide (Systemic)*.

The information that follows is selectively abstracted from the complete monograph and is provided to facilitate drug use review and patient counseling.

Note: For a listing of dosage forms and brand names by country availability, see *Dosage Forms* section(s).

## Category

Antihypertensive; vasodilator, congestive heart failure.

## Indications

Note: Bracketed information in the *Indications* section refers to uses that are not included in U.S. product labeling.

**Accepted**

Hypertension (treatment)—The combination of captopril, enalapril, or lisinopril and hydrochlorothiazide is indicated in the treatment of hypertension.

Fixed-dosage combinations generally are not recommended for initial therapy, but are utilized in maintenance therapy after the required dose is established in order to increase convenience, economy, and patient compliance.

[Congestive heart failure (treatment)]—Captopril, enalapril, or lisinopril plus a diuretic, such as hydrochlorothiazide, and a digitalis glycoside are also used for treatment of severe congestive heart failure not responding to other measures.

## Patient Consultation

As an aid to patient consultation, refer to *Advice for the Patient, Angiotensin-converting Enzyme (ACE) Inhibitors and Hydrochlorothiazide (Systemic)*.

In providing consultation, consider emphasizing the following selected information (» = major clinical significance):

**Before using this medication**
» Conditions affecting use, especially:
  Sensitivity to any ACE inhibitor, thiazide diuretic, carbonic anhydrase inhibitor, or other sulfonamide-type medications
  Pregnancy—ACE inhibitor–associated fetal hypotension, oliguria, and death reported in humans; and fetotoxicity found in animals; hydrochlorothiazide may cause jaundice, thrombocytopenia, hypokalemia in infant
  Breast-feeding—Captopril and hydrochlorothiazide are distributed into breast milk
  Use in children—Caution if giving to infants with jaundice
  Use in the elderly—May be more sensitive to hypotensive and electrolyte effects
  Other medications, especially alcohol, cholestyramine, colestipol, diuretics (particularly potassium-sparing), potassium-containing medications, potassium supplements, low salt milk, salt substitutes, digitalis glycosides, lithium, cocaine, norepinephrine, or phenylephrine
  Other medical problems, especially angioedema related to previous ACE inhibitor therapy, hereditary angioedema, idiopathic angioedema, hyperkalemia, renal artery stenosis, renal transplant, renal function impairment, or sodium and volume depletion

**Proper use of this medication**
Compliance with therapy; taking medication at the same time each day to maintain the therapeutic effect
Diuretic effects of the medication and timing of doses to minimize inconvenience of diuresis
» Proper dosing
  Missed dose: Taking as soon as possible; not taking if almost time for next dose; not doubling doses
» Proper storage
*For captopril and hydrochlorothiazide*
  For best results, taking on an empty stomach 1 hour before meals
*For use as an antihypertensive*
  Possible need for control of weight and diet, especially sodium intake; risks associated with sodium depletion; not taking salt substitutes or using low-salt milk unless approved by physician
» Patient may not experience symptoms of hypertension; importance of taking medication even if feeling well
» Does not cure, but helps control hypertension; possible need for lifelong therapy; checking with physician before discontinuing medication; serious consequences of untreated hypertension

**Precautions while using this medication**
Making regular visits to physician to check progress
Caution when driving or doing other things requiring alertness, because of possible dizziness, especially with initial dose
To prevent dehydration and hypotension, checking with physician if severe nausea, vomiting, or diarrhea occurs and continues
Caution when exercising or during hot weather because of the risk of dehydration and hypotension due to reduced fluid volume
Caution if any kind of surgery (including dental surgery) or emergency treatment is required
Caution in using alcohol
Diabetics: May increase blood sugar levels
Possible photosensitivity; avoiding unprotected exposure to sun; using protective clothing and sun block product; avoiding use of sunlamp
Caution if any laboratory tests required; possible interference with test results
*For use as an antihypertensive*
» Not taking other medications, especially nonprescription sympathomimetics, unless discussed with physician

**Side/adverse effects**
Signs of potential side effects, especially hypotension, skin rash (with or without itching, fever, or joint pain), angioedema, chest pain, neutropenia or agranulocytosis, hyperuricemia or gout, cholecystitis or pancreatitis, thrombocytopenia, hepatic function impairment, and electrolyte imbalance

---

### *CAPTOPRIL AND HYDROCHLOROTHIAZIDE*

## Oral Dosage Forms

Note: Bracketed uses in the *Dosage Forms* section refer to categories of use and/or indications that are not included in U.S. product labeling.

### CAPTOPRIL AND HYDROCHLOROTHIAZIDE TABLETS

**Usual adult and adolescent dose**
Antihypertensive or
[Vasodilator, congestive heart failure]—

Oral, 1 tablet two or three times a day, as determined by individual titration with the component agents.

Note: Geriatric patients may be more sensitive to the effects of the usual adult dose.

**Usual pediatric dose**
Oral, as determined by individual titration with the component agents
Captopril: Oral, 300 mcg (0.3 mg) per kg of body weight three times a day, the dosage being increased if necessary in increments of 300 mcg (0.3 mg) per kg of body weight at intervals of eight to twenty-four hours to the minimum effective dose.
Hydrochlorothiazide: Oral, 1 to 2 mg per kg of body weight or 30 to 60 mg per square meter of body surface per day, as a single dose or in two divided daily doses, the dosage being adjusted according to response.

**Strength(s) usually available**
U.S.—
- 25 mg of captopril and 15 mg of hydrochlorothiazide (Rx) [*Capozide* (scored; lactose); GENERIC].
- 25 mg of captopril and 25 mg of hydrochlorothiazide (Rx) [*Capozide* (scored; lactose); GENERIC].
- 50 mg of captopril and 15 mg of hydrochlorothiazide (Rx) [*Capozide* (scored; lactose); GENERIC].
- 50 mg of captopril and 25 mg of hydrochlorothiazide (Rx) [*Capozide* (scored; lactose); GENERIC].

Canada—
- Not commercially available.

**Auxiliary labeling**
- Take on an empty stomach, 1 hour before meals.
- Avoid too much sun or use of sunlamp.
- Do not take other medicines without your doctor's advice.

---

## ENALAPRIL AND HYDROCHLOROTHIAZIDE

## Oral Dosage Forms

Note: Bracketed uses in the *Dosage Forms* section refer to categories of use and/or indications that are not included in U.S. product labeling.

### ENALAPRIL MALEATE AND HYDROCHLOROTHIAZIDE TABLETS

**Usual adult and adolescent dose**
Antihypertensive or
[Vasodilator, congestive heart failure]—
Oral, 1 tablet per day, as determined by individual titration with the component agents.

Note: Geriatric patients may be more sensitive to the effects of the usual adult dose.

**Usual pediatric dose**
Oral, as determined by individual titration with the component agents
Enalapril: Oral, initially 100 mcg (0.1 mg) per kg of body weight per day, the dosage being adjusted as needed and tolerated, up to a maximum of 500 mcg (0.5 mg) per kg of body weight per day.
Hydrochlorothiazide: Oral, 1 to 2 mg per kg of body weight or 30 to 60 mg per square meter of body surface per day, as a single dose or in two divided doses, the dosage being adjusted according to response.

**Strength(s) usually available**
U.S.—
- 5 mg of enalapril maleate and 12.5 mg of hydrochlorothiazide (Rx) [*Vaseretic* (lactose)].
- 10 mg of enalapril maleate and 25 mg of hydrochlorothiazide (Rx) [*Vaseretic* (lactose)].

Canada—
- 10 mg of enalapril maleate and 25 mg of hydrochlorothiazide (Rx) [*Vaseretic*].

**Auxiliary labeling**
- Avoid too much sun or use of sunlamp.
- Do not take other medicines without your doctor's advice.

---

## LISINOPRIL AND HYDROCHLOROTHIAZIDE

## Oral Dosage Forms

Note: Bracketed uses in the *Dosage Forms* section refer to categories of use and/or indications that are not included in U.S. product labeling.

### LISINOPRIL AND HYDROCHLOROTHIAZIDE TABLETS

**Usual adult and adolescent dose**
Antihypertensive or
[Vasodilator, congestive heart failure]—
Oral, 1 or 2 tablets once a day, as determined by individual titration with the component agents.

Note: Geriatric patients may be more sensitive to the effects of the usual adult dose.

**Usual pediatric dose**
Dosage has not been established.

**Strength(s) usually available**
U.S.—
- 10 mg of lisinopril and 12.5 mg of hydrochlorothiazide (Rx) [*Prinzide; Zestoretic*].
- 20 mg of lisinopril and 12.5 mg of hydrochlorothiazide (Rx) [*Prinzide; Zestoretic*].
- 20 mg of lisinopril and 25 mg of hydrochlorothiazide (Rx) [*Prinzide; Zestoretic*].

Canada—
- 10 mg of lisinopril and 12.5 mg of hydrochlorothiazide (Rx) [*Prinzide; Zestoretic*].
- 20 mg of lisinopril and 12.5 mg of hydrochlorothiazide (Rx) [*Prinzide; Zestoretic*].
- 20 mg of lisinopril and 25 mg of hydrochlorothiazide (Rx) [*Prinzide; Zestoretic*].

**Auxiliary labeling**
- Avoid too much sun or use of sunlamp.
- Do not take other medicines without your doctor's advice.

Revised: 07/28/92
Interim revision: 06/29/94; 08/12/98

---

**ANISINDIONE**—See *Anticoagulants (Systemic)*

---

**ANISOTROPINE**—See *Anticholinergics/Antispasmodics (Systemic)*

---

**ANISTREPLASE**—See *Thrombolytic Agents (Systemic)*

---

# ANTACIDS  Oral-Local

This monograph includes information on the following: 1) Alumina, Calcium Carbonate, and Sodium Bicarbonate*; 2) Alumina and Magnesia; 3) Alumina, Magnesia, Calcium Carbonate, and Simethicone†; 4) Alumina, Magnesia, and Magnesium Carbonate*; 5) Alumina, Magnesia, Magnesium Carbonate, and Simethicone*; 6) Alumina, Magnesia, and Simethicone; 7) Alumina, Magnesium Alginate, and Magnesium Carbonate*; 8) Alumina and Magnesium Carbonate†; 9) Alumina, Magnesium Carbonate, and Simethicone†; 10) Alumina, Magnesium Carbonate, and Sodium Bicarbonate†; 11) Alumina and Magnesium Trisilicate†; 12) Alumina, Magnesium Trisilicate, and Sodium Bicarbonate†; 13) Alumina and Simethicone†; 14) Alumina and Sodium Bicarbonate*; 15) Aluminum Carbonate, Basic†; 16) Aluminum Carbonate, Basic, and Simethicone†; 17) Aluminum Hydroxide; 18) Calcium Carbonate‡; 19) Calcium Carbonate and Magnesia; 20) Calcium Carbonate, Magnesia, and Simethicone; 21) Calcium Carbonate and Simethicone†; 22) Calcium and Magnesium Carbonates; 23) Magaldrate; 24) Magaldrate and Simethicone; 25) Magnesium Carbonate and Sodium Bicarbonate*; 26) Magnesium Hydroxide§; 27) Magnesium Oxide§†.

VA CLASSIFICATION (Primary/Secondary):
Alumina, Calcium Carbonate, and Sodium Bicarbonate—GA199
Alumina and Magnesia—GA103
Alumina, Magnesia, Calcium Carbonate, and Simethicone—GA199
Alumina, Magnesia, and Magnesium Carbonate—GA103
Alumina, Magnesia, Magnesium Carbonate, and Simethicone—GA199

Alumina, Magnesia, and Simethicone—GA199
Alumina, Magnesium Alginate, and Magnesium Carbonate—GA103
Alumina and Magnesium Carbonate—GA103
Alumina, Magnesium Carbonate, and Simethicone—GA199
Alumina, Magnesium Carbonate, and Sodium Bicarbonate—GA104
Alumina and Magnesium Trisilicate—GA103
Alumina, Magnesium Trisilicate, and Sodium Bicarbonate—GA104
Alumina and Simethicone—GA199
Alumina and Sodium Bicarbonate—GA199
Aluminum Carbonate, Basic—GA101/GU900
Aluminum Carbonate, Basic, and Simethicone—GA199
Aluminum Hydroxide—GA101/GA250; GU900
Calcium Carbonate—GA105/TN402
Calcium Carbonate and Magnesia—GA106
Calcium Carbonate, Magnesia, and Simethicone—GA199
Calcium Carbonate and Simethicone—GA199
Calcium and Magnesium Carbonates—GA106
Magaldrate—GA107
Magaldrate and Simethicone—GA199
Magnesium Carbonate and Sodium Bicarbonate—GA109
Magnesium Hydroxide—GA108/GA202; GU900
Magnesium Oxide—GA108/GA202

Note: For a listing of dosage forms and brand names by country availability, see *Dosage Forms* section(s).

*Not commercially available in U.S.
†Not commercially available in Canada.
‡See *Calcium Supplements (Systemic)* for systemic use of calcium carbonate in hypocalcemia
§See *Laxatives (Local)* for laxative use of magnesium hydroxide and magnesium oxide

## Category

Antacid—All drugs included in this monograph are used as antacids.
Antiurolithic (phosphate calculi)—Aluminum Carbonate; Aluminum Hydroxide.
Laxative, hyperosmotic, saline—Magnesium Hydroxide; Magnesium Oxide (see *Magnesium Hydroxide* and *Magnesium Oxide, Laxatives [Local]*).
Antihyperphosphatemic—Aluminum Carbonate; Aluminum Hydroxide; Calcium Carbonate (see *Calcium Carbonate, Calcium Supplements [Systemic]*).
Antihypocalcemic—Calcium Carbonate (see *Calcium Carbonate, Calcium Supplements [Systemic]*).
Antiurolithic (calcium calculi)—Magnesium Hydroxide.

## Indications

Note: Bracketed information in the *Indications* section refers to uses that are not included in U.S. product labeling.

### Accepted

Hyperacidity (treatment)
Ulcer, duodenal (treatment) or
Ulcer, gastric (treatment)—Antacids are indicated for relief of symptoms associated with hyperacidity (heartburn, acid indigestion, and sour stomach). In addition, antacids are used in hyperacidity associated with gastric and duodenal ulcers. However, there have been reports of increased gastrin levels and increased gastric secretion (acid rebound) associated with the use of antacids.

Some of the antacid combinations contain other ingredients that have no antacid properties. Simethicone, an antiflatulent, has been added as an aid in those conditions in which the retention of gas may be a problem; however, in the treatment of peptic ulcer diseases, the advantage of using antacid and simethicone combinations rather than antacids alone has not been clearly established.

Hypersecretory conditions, gastric (treatment adjunct)
Zollinger-Ellison syndrome (treatment adjunct)
Mastocytosis, systemic (treatment adjunct) or
Adenoma, multiple endocrine (treatment adjunct)—Antacids are indicated in conjunction with histamine H$_2$-receptor antagonists or omeprazole for transient symptomatic relief in the treatment of pathological gastric hypersecretion associated with Zollinger-Ellison syndrome (alone or as part of multiple endocrine neoplasia Type-I), systemic mastocytosis, and multiple endocrine adenoma.

Reflux, gastroesophageal (treatment)—Antacids are indicated in the symptomatic treatment of gastroesophageal reflux disease.

Stress-related mucosal damage (prophylaxis and treatment)—Antacids are indicated to prevent and treat upper gastrointestinal, stress-induced ulceration and bleeding, especially in intensive care patients.

[Hyperphosphatemia (treatment)][1]—Aluminum carbonate and aluminum hydroxide may be used in conjunction with a low-phosphate diet to reduce elevated phosphate levels and demineralization of bones in patients with renal insufficiency. However, use of aluminum-containing antacids as phosphate binders may lead to aluminum toxicity in patients with renal insufficiency. Other agents may be preferable for treating hyperphosphatemia in patients with renal insufficiency.

Hypocalcemia (treatment)—See *Calcium Carbonate, Calcium Supplements (Systemic)*.

[Aluminum hydroxide has been used in the treatment of neonatal hypocalcemia and diarrhea; however, it generally has been replaced by other agents. Aluminum carbonate and aluminum hydroxide have been used along with a low-phosphate diet to prevent formation of phosphatic (struvite) urinary stones; however, their use has been replaced by other agents. Magnesium hydroxide has been used to prevent recurrence of calcium stones; however, it has been replaced by other agents. Use of aluminum-containing antacids in young children and premature infants may lead to aluminum toxicity, especially in those patients with renal failure.][1]

### Unaccepted

Antacids have been used in patients undergoing anesthesia or during labor to lessen the danger from aspiration of gastric contents. However, the use of antacids to prevent acid aspiration has generally been replaced by the equally or more effective histamine H$_2$-receptor antagonists or citrate solutions.

[1] Not included in Canadian product labeling.

## Pharmacology/Pharmacokinetics

### Physicochemical characteristics

Molecular weight—
Aluminum hydroxide: 78.
Calcium carbonate: 100.09.
Magnesium hydroxide: 58.32.
Magnesium oxide: 40.30.
Sodium bicarbonate: 84.01.

### Mechanism of action/Effect

Antacid—These medications react chemically to neutralize or buffer existing quantities of stomach acid but have no direct effect on its output. This action results in increased pH value of stomach contents, thus providing relief of hyperacidity symptoms. Also, these medications reduce acid concentration within the lumen of the esophagus. This causes an increase in intra-esophageal pH and a decrease in pepsin activity.

Antiurolithic—Aluminum carbonate and aluminum hydroxide bind phosphate ions in the intestine to form insoluble aluminum phosphate, which is excreted in the feces. They thereby reduce phosphates in the urine and prevent formation of phosphatic (struvite) urinary stones. Magnesium hydroxide inhibits the precipitation of calcium oxalate and calcium phosphate, thus preventing the formation of calcium stones.

Antihyperphosphatemic—Aluminum carbonate and aluminum hydroxide reduce serum phosphate levels by binding with phosphate ions in the intestine to form insoluble aluminum phosphate, which passes through the intestinal tract unabsorbed.

Antihypocalcemic—Aluminum hydroxide may increase the release of calcium from bone as a result of the decreased serum phosphate levels.

Antidiarrheal—Aluminum hydroxide's constipating properties help decrease the fluidity of stools.

### Other actions/effects

Antacids may increase lower esophageal sphincter (LES) pressure. Aluminum-containing antacids have a cytoprotective effect on the gastric mucosa that may be associated with the stimulation of prostaglandin secretion, thus providing protection against mucosal necrosis and hemorrhage caused by corrosive agents, such as aspirin and ethanol.

### Absorption

Aluminum-containing—Small amounts of the aluminum in aluminum hydroxide are absorbed from the intestine.

Calcium-containing—Approximately 15% of the calcium in calcium carbonate is absorbed from the intestine in normal persons. The amount of calcium absorbed from the gastrointestinal tract is determined by hormonal factors, particularly parathyroid hormone, and vitamin D.

Magnesium-containing—Approximately 10% of the magnesium in magnesium hydroxide (magnesia) is absorbed from the intestine.

### Onset and duration of action

Onset of action is dependent upon the ability of the antacid to solubilize in the stomach and react with the hydrochloric acid. The poorly soluble antacids (e.g., magnesium trisilicate) will thus react more slowly with hydrochloric acid than will the more soluble ones. In most cases with slow-acting antacids, the onset of action is delayed and may not take place if gastric emptying is rapid.

Duration of action is determined primarily by gastric emptying time. Depending on the kind of antacid used, the duration of action in fasting patients may range from 20 to 60 minutes. However, when the antacid is given 1 hour after meals, the acid-neutralizing effect may be prolonged up to 3 hours.

The following table provides a relative comparison of onset and duration of action of different antacids.

| Antacid | Onset of action | Duration of action |
| --- | --- | --- |
| Aluminum Carbonate | Slow | Short |
| Aluminum Hydroxide | Slow | Prolonged * |
| Aluminum Phosphate | Slow | Short |
| Calcium Carbonate | Fast | Prolonged |
| Magaldrate | Intermediate | Prolonged |
| Magnesium Carbonate | Intermediate | Short |
| Magnesium Hydroxide | Fast | Short |
| Magnesium Oxide | Fast | Short |
| Magnesium Trisilicate | Slow | Prolonged † |
| Sodium Bicarbonate | Fast | Short |

*Absorptive properties of the gel prolong its duration of action
†If gastric emptying is rapid, stomach may empty before much of the acid is neutralized

### Elimination
Renal and fecal; 15 to 30% of the salts formed are absorbed and are then excreted by the kidneys.

## Precautions to Consider

### Pregnancy/Reproduction
Pregnancy—Antacids are generally considered safe as long as chronic high doses are avoided.

*Aluminum-, calcium-, or magnesium-containing antacids*—
Adequate and well-controlled studies in humans have not been done; however, there have been reports of antacids causing such adverse effects as hypercalcemia, hypomagnesemia, hypermagnesemia, and increased tendon reflexes in fetuses and/or neonates whose mothers were chronic users of aluminum-, calcium-, and/or magnesium-containing antacids, especially in high doses.
Studies have not been done in animals.

*Sodium bicarbonate–containing antacids*—
Problems in humans have not been documented; however, risk-benefit must be considered because sodium bicarbonate is absorbed systemically. Chronic use may lead to systemic alkalosis. The sodium load that is absorbed can also cause edema and weight gain.

### Breast-feeding
Problems in humans have not been documented; although some aluminum, calcium, and magnesium may be distributed into breast milk, the concentration is not great enough to produce an effect in the neonate.

### Pediatrics
Antacids should not be given to young children (up to 6 years of age) unless prescribed by a physician. Since children are not usually able to describe their symptoms precisely, proper diagnosis should precede the use of an antacid. This will avoid the complication of an existing condition (e.g., appendicitis) or the appearance of severe adverse effects.

Use of magnesium-containing antacids is contraindicated in very young children because there is a risk of hypermagnesemia, especially in dehydrated children or children with renal failure.

Use of aluminum-containing antacids is contraindicated in very young children because there is a risk of aluminum toxicity, especially in dehydrated infants and children or infants and children with renal failure.

### Geriatrics
Metabolic bone disease commonly seen in the elderly may be aggravated by the phosphorus depletion, hypercalciuria, and inhibition of absorption of intestinal fluoride caused by the chronic use of aluminum-containing antacids. Also, elderly patients are more likely to have age-related renal function impairment, which may lead to aluminum retention.

Although it is not known whether high intake of aluminum leads to Alzheimer's disease, the use of aluminum-containing antacids in Alzheimer's patients is not generally recommended. Research suggests that aluminum may contribute to the disease's development since it has been found to concentrate in neurofibrillary tangles in brain tissue.

### Drug interactions and/or related problems
See *Table 1*, page 191.

### Laboratory value alterations
See *Table 2*, page 193.

### Medical considerations/Contraindications
See *Table 3*, page 194.

### Patient monitoring
See *Table 4*, page 195.

## Side/Adverse Effects
See *Table 5*, page 196.

## Patient Consultation
See *Table 6*, page 196.

## General Dosing Information

### For antacid use
The dose of antacid needed to neutralize gastric acid varies among patients, depending on the amount of acid secreted and the buffering capacity of the particular preparation.

It is estimated that 99% of the gastric acid will be neutralized when a gastric pH of 3.3 is achieved.

The amount (in mEq) of 1 $N$ hydrochloric acid that can be titrated to pH 3.5 in 15 minutes by a certain dose of antacid is referred to as the neutralizing capacity of the antacid. Approximately 15 to 20 mEq of an aluminum- and magnesium-containing antacid are required to neutralize 1 mEq of gastric hydrochloric acid.

Patients with hypersecretory disorders (e.g., duodenal ulcer, Zollinger-Ellison syndrome, multiple endocrine adenomas, and systemic mastocytosis) may require 80 to 160 mEq of buffer at each dose for symptomatic relief; this is approximately 30 to 60 mL of most antacids. Only half of this dose is needed for patients with normal acid secretion.

The liquid dosage form of antacids is considered to be more effective than the solid or powder dosage form. In most cases, tablets must be thoroughly chewed before being swallowed; otherwise, they may not dissolve completely in the stomach before entering the small intestine.

The maximum recommended dosage should not be taken for more than 2 weeks, except under the advice or supervision of a physician.

Combinations of antacids containing aluminum and/or calcium compounds with magnesium salts may offer the advantage of balancing the constipating qualities of aluminum and/or calcium and the laxative qualities of magnesium.

### For use in peptic ulcer
In the treatment of peptic ulcer disease, to achieve adequate antacid effect in the stomach at the optimum time, most antacids are administered 1 and 3 hours after meals for prolonged acid-neutralizing effect and at bedtime. However, when taken at bedtime, their effect is not prolonged because of rapid gastric emptying. Additional doses of antacids may be administered to relieve the pain that may occur between the regularly scheduled doses.

Antacid therapy should be continued for at least 4 to 6 weeks after all symptoms have disappeared, since there is no correlation between disappearance of symptoms and actual healing of the ulcer.

*Aluminum hydroxide*—
In the treatment of peptic ulcer, 960 mg to 3.6 grams are given orally every one or two hours during waking hours, the dosage being adjusted as needed. For extremely severe symptoms of peptic ulcer (hospitalized patients), 2.6 to 4.8 grams diluted with two to three parts of water may be given intragastrically every thirty minutes for periods of twelve or more hours a day.

### For antihyperphosphatemic use
*Aluminum hydroxide*—
In adults, 1.9 to 4.8 grams of aluminum hydroxide are given orally three or four times a day in conjunction with dietary phosphate restriction. In children, a dose of 50 to 150 mg per kg of body weight is given in four to six divided doses in conjunction with dietary phosphate restriction.

### For antiurolithic use
*Aluminum carbonate*—
In the prevention of phosphate stones the equivalent of 1 to 3 grams of aluminum carbonate is given four times a day, one hour after meals and at bedtime.

## Oral Dosage Forms
See *Table 7*, page 198.

Revised: 08/15/95
Interim revision: 07/18/96

## Table 1. Drug Interactions and/or Related Problems

The following drug interactions and/or related problems have been selected on the basis of their potential clinical significance (possible mechanism in parentheses where appropriate)—not necessarily inclusive: (» = major clinical significance)

Note: Combinations containing any of the following medications, depending on the amount present, may also interact with this medication.

Only specific interactions between antacids and other oral medications have been identified in this monograph. However, because of antacids' ability to change gastric or urinary pH and to adsorb or form complexes with other drugs, the rate and/or extent of absorption of other medications may be increased or reduced when the medication is used concurrently with antacids. In general, patients should be advised not to take any other oral medications within 1 to 2 hours of antacids.

Legend:
I = Aluminum-containing
II = Calcium-containing
III = Magaldrate
IV = Magnesium-containing
V = Sodium Bicarbonate–containing

| | I | II | III | IV | V |
|---|---|---|---|---|---|
| Acidifiers, urinary, such as:<br>  Ammonium chloride<br>  Ascorbic acid<br>  Potassium or sodium phosphates<br>  Racemethionine<br>(antacids may alkalinize the urine and counteract the effect of urinary acidifiers; frequent use of antacids, especially in high doses, is best avoided by patients receiving therapy to acidify the urine) | ✔ | ✔ | ✔ | ✔ | ✔ |
| Amphetamines or<br>Quinidine<br>(urinary excretion may be inhibited when these medications are used concurrently with antacids in doses that cause the urine to become alkaline, possibly resulting in toxicity; dosage adjustment may be needed when therapy with these antacids is initiated or discontinued or if dosage is changed) | ✔ | ✔ | ✔ | ✔ | ✔ |
| Anticholinergics or other medications with anticholinergic activity (See *Appendix II*)<br>(concurrent use with antacids may decrease absorption, reducing the effectiveness of anticholinergics; doses of these medications should be spaced 1 hour apart from doses of antacids) | ✔ | ✔ | ✔ | ✔ | ✔ |
| (urinary excretion may be delayed by alkalinization of the urine, thus potentiating the side effects of the anticholinergic) | ✔ | ✔ | ✔ | ✔ | ✔ |
| Calcitonin or<br>Etidronate or<br>Gallium nitrate or<br>Pamidronate or<br>Plicamycin<br>(concurrent use with calcium carbonate may antagonize the effect of these medications in the treatment of hypercalcemia) | | ✔ | | | |
| Calcium-containing preparations<br>(concurrent and prolonged use with sodium bicarbonate may result in the milk-alkali syndrome) | | | | | ✔ |
| » Cellulose sodium phosphate<br>(concurrent use with calcium-containing antacids may decrease effectiveness of cellulose sodium phosphate in preventing hypercalciuria) | | ✔ | | | |
| (concurrent use with magnesium-containing antacids may result in binding of magnesium; patients should be advised not to take these medications within 1 hour of cellulose sodium phosphate) | | | ✔ | ✔ | |
| Chenodiol<br>(concurrent use with aluminum-containing antacids may result in binding of chenodiol, thus decreasing its absorption) | ✔ | | ✔ | | |
| Citrates<br>(concurrent use with antacids containing aluminum, calcium carbonates, magaldrate, or sodium bicarbonate may result in systemic alkalosis) | ✔ | ✔ | ✔ | | ✔ |
| (concurrent use of sodium citrate with sodium bicarbonate may promote the development of calcium stones in patients with uric acid stones, due to sodium ion opposition to the hypocalciuric effect of the alkaline load; may also cause hypernatremia) | | | | | ✔ |
| (concurrent use of aluminum-containing antacids and magaldrate with citrate salts can increase aluminum absorption, possibly resulting in acute aluminum toxicity, especially in patients with renal insufficiency) | ✔ | | ✔ | | |
| Digitalis glycosides<br>(concurrent use with aluminum- and magnesium-containing antacids may inhibit absorption, possibly decreasing plasma concentrations of digitalis glycosides; although actual clinical importance of this interaction has not been established, it is recommended that doses of antacids and digitalis glycosides be separated by several hours) | ✔ | | ✔ | ✔ | |
| Diuretics, potassium-depleting, such as bumetanide, ethacrynic acid, furosemide, indapamide, thiazide diuretics<br>(concurrent use of thiazide diuretics with large doses of calcium carbonate may result in hypercalcemia) | | ✔ | | | |
| Enteric-coated medications, such as bisacodyl<br>(concurrent administration of antacids with enteric-coated medications may cause the enteric coating to dissolve too rapidly, resulting in gastric or duodenal irritation) | ✔ | ✔ | ✔ | ✔ | ✔ |
| Ephedrine<br>(urine alkalinization induced by sodium bicarbonate may increase the half-life of ephedrine and prolong its duration of action, especially if the urine remains alkaline for several days or longer; dosage adjustment of ephedrine may be necessary) | | | | | ✔ |

## Table 1. Drug Interactions and/or Related Problems *(continued)*

The following drug interactions and/or related problems have been selected on the basis of their potential clinical significance (possible mechanism in parentheses where appropriate)—not necessarily inclusive: (» = major clinical significance)

Note: Combinations containing any of the following medications, depending on the amount present, may also interact with this medication.

Only specific interactions between antacids and other oral medications have been identified in this monograph. However, because of antacids' ability to change gastric or urinary pH and to adsorb or form complexes with other drugs, the rate and/or extent of absorption of other medications may be increased or reduced when the medication is used concurrently with antacids. In general, patients should be advised not to take any other oral medications within 1 to 2 hours of antacids.

Legend:
I = Aluminum-containing
II = Calcium-containing
III = Magaldrate
IV = Magnesium-containing
V = Sodium Bicarbonate–containing

| Interaction | I | II | III | IV | V |
|---|---|---|---|---|---|
| » Fluoroquinolones (alkalinization of the urine may reduce the solubility of ciprofloxacin and norfloxacin in the urine, especially when the urinary pH exceeds 7.0; if antacids and one of these medications are used concurrently, patients should be observed for signs of crystalluria and nephrotoxicity) | ✔ | ✔ | ✔ | ✔ | ✔ |
| (aluminum- and magnesium-containing antacids may reduce absorption of fluoroquinolones, resulting in lower serum and urine concentrations of these medications; therefore, concurrent use is not recommended; however, if aluminum- and magnesium-containing antacids must be used concurrently with these medications, it is recommended that enoxacin be taken at least 2 hours before or 8 hours after the antacid; ciprofloxacin and lomefloxacin should be taken at least 2 hours before or 6 hours after the antacid; and norfloxacin and ofloxacin should be taken at least 2 hours before or after the antacid) | ✔ | | ✔ | ✔ | |
| Folic acid (prolonged use of aluminum- and/or magnesium-containing antacids may decrease folic acid absorption by raising the pH of the small intestine; patients should be advised to take antacids at least 2 hours after folic acid) | ✔ | | ✔ | ✔ | |
| Histamine H$_2$-receptor antagonists (concurrent use with antacids may be indicated in the treatment of peptic ulcer to relieve pain; however, simultaneous administration of medium to high doses [80 mmol to 150 mmol] of antacids is not recommended since absorption of histamine H$_2$-receptor antagonists may be decreased; patients should be advised not to take any antacids within $^1/_2$ to 1 hour of histamine H$_2$-receptor antagonists) | ✔ | ✔ | ✔ | ✔ | ✔ |
| Iron preparations, oral (absorption may be decreased when these preparations are used concurrently with magnesium trisilicate or antacids containing carbonate; spacing the doses of the iron preparation as far as possible from doses of the antacid is recommended) | ✔ | ✔ | | ✔ | ✔ |
| » Isoniazid, oral (concurrent use with aluminum-containing antacids may delay and decrease absorption of oral isoniazid; concurrent use should be avoided or the patient should be advised to take oral isoniazid at least 1 hour before the antacid) | ✔ | | ✔ | | |
| » Ketoconazole (antacids may cause increased gastrointestinal pH; concurrent administration with antacids may result in a marked reduction in absorption of ketoconazole; patients should be advised to take antacids at least 3 hours after ketoconazole) | ✔ | ✔ | ✔ | ✔ | ✔ |
| Lithium (sodium bicarbonate enhances lithium excretion, possibly resulting in decreased efficacy; this may be partly due to the sodium content) | | | | | ✔ |
| Mexiletine (marked alkalinization of the urine caused by sodium bicarbonate may slow renal excretion of mexiletine) | | | | | ✔ |
| » Mecamylamine (alkalinization of the urine may slow excretion and prolong the effects of mecamylamine; concurrent use is not recommended) | ✔ | ✔ | ✔ | ✔ | ✔ |
| » Methenamine (concurrent use with antacids that cause the urine to become alkaline may reduce the effectiveness of methenamine by inhibiting its conversion to formaldehyde; concurrent use is not recommended) | ✔ | ✔ | ✔ | ✔ | ✔ |
| Milk or milk products (concurrent and prolonged use with calcium carbonate or sodium bicarbonate may result in the milk-alkali syndrome) | | ✔ | | | ✔ |
| Misoprostol (concurrent use with magnesium-containing antacids may aggravate misoprostol-induced diarrhea) | | | ✔ | ✔ | |
| Pancrelipase (concurrent administration of antacids may be required to prevent inactivation of pancrelipase [except enteric-coated dosage forms] by gastric pepsin and acid pH; however, calcium carbonate– and/or magnesium-containing antacids are not recommended since they may decrease the effectiveness of pancrelipase) | | ✔ | ✔ | ✔ | |
| Penicillamine (absorption may be reduced when penicillamine is administered concurrently with aluminum- or magnesium-containing antacids; although more studies are needed to establish the significance of this interaction, it is recommended that doses of antacids and penicillamine be separated by 2 hours) | ✔ | | ✔ | ✔ | |
| Phenothiazines, especially chlorpromazine, oral (absorption may be inhibited when these medications are used concurrently with aluminum- or magnesium-containing antacids; although more studies are needed to establish the significance of this interaction, simultaneous administration should be avoided) | ✔ | | ✔ | ✔ | |
| Phenytoin (concurrent use with aluminum-, magnesium-, and/or calcium carbonate–containing antacids may decrease absorption of phenytoin, thus reducing serum phenytoin concentrations; although more studies are needed to establish the significance of this interaction, it is recommended that doses of antacids and phenytoin be separated by about 2 to 3 hours) | ✔ | ✔ | ✔ | ✔ | |

## Table 1. Drug Interactions and/or Related Problems *(continued)*

The following drug interactions and/or related problems have been selected on the basis of their potential clinical significance (possible mechanism in parentheses where appropriate)—not necessarily inclusive: (» = major clinical significance)

Note: Combinations containing any of the following medications, depending on the amount present, may also interact with this medication.

Only specific interactions between antacids and other oral medications have been identified in this monograph. However, because of antacids' ability to change gastric or urinary pH and to adsorb or form complexes with other drugs, the rate and/or extent of absorption of other medications may be increased or reduced when the medication is used concurrently with antacids. In general, patients should be advised not to take any other oral medications within 1 to 2 hours of antacids.

Legend:
I = Aluminum-containing
II = Calcium-containing
III = Magaldrate
IV = Magnesium-containing
V = Sodium Bicarbonate-containing

| | I | II | III | IV | V |
|---|---|---|---|---|---|
| Phosphates, oral<br>(concurrent use with aluminum- or magnesium-containing antacids may bind the phosphate and prevent its absorption)<br>(concurrent use with calcium-containing antacids may increase potential of deposition of calcium in soft tissues if serum-ionized calcium is high) | ✓ | ✓ | ✓ | ✓ | |
| Quinine<br>(concurrent use with aluminum-containing antacids may decrease or delay the absorption of quinine) | ✓ | | ✓ | | |
| Salicylates<br>(alkalinization of the urine may increase renal salicylate excretion and lower serum salicylate levels; dosage adjustments of salicylates may be necessary when chronic high-dose antacid therapy is started or stopped, especially in patients receiving large doses of the salicylate, such as patients with rheumatoid arthritis or rheumatic fever) | ✓ | ✓ | ✓ | ✓ | ✓ |
| Sodium bicarbonate or Vitamin D<br>(concurrent and prolonged use with calcium carbonate may result in the milk-alkali syndrome) | | ✓ | | | |
| Sodium fluoride<br>(concurrent use with aluminum hydroxide may decrease absorption and increase fecal excretion of fluoride)<br>(calcium ions may complex with and inhibit absorption of fluoride) | ✓ | ✓ | ✓ | | |
| » Sodium polystyrene sulfonate resin (SPSR)<br>(neutralization of gastric acid may be impaired when SPSR is used concurrently with calcium- or magnesium-containing antacids, possibly resulting in systemic alkalosis; concurrent use is not recommended) | | ✓ | ✓ | ✓ | |
| Sucralfate<br>(concurrent use with antacids may be indicated in the treatment of duodenal ulcer to relieve pain; however, simultaneous administration is not recommended since antacids may interfere with binding of sucralfate to the mucosa; patients should be advised not to take any antacids within 1/2 hour before or after sucralfate; concurrent use with aluminum-containing antacids may cause aluminum toxicity in patients with chronic renal failure) | ✓ | ✓ | ✓ | ✓ | ✓ |
| » Tetracyclines, oral<br>(absorption may be decreased when oral tetracyclines are used concurrently with antacids because of possible formation of nonabsorbable complexes and/or increase in intragastric pH; patients should be advised not to take antacids within 3 to 4 hours of tetracyclines) | ✓ | ✓ | ✓ | ✓ | ✓ |
| Vitamin D, including calcifediol and calcitriol<br>(concurrent use with magnesium-containing antacids may result in hypermagnesemia, especially in patients with chronic renal failure)<br>(concurrent use with calcium-containing antacids may result in hypercalcemia) | | ✓ | ✓ | ✓ | |

## Table 2. Laboratory Value Alterations

The following have been selected on the basis of their potential clinical significance (possible effect in parentheses where appropriate)—not necessarily inclusive (» = major clinical significance):

Legend:
I = Aluminum-containing
II = Calcium-containing
III = Magaldrate
IV = Magnesium-containing
V = Sodium Bicarbonate-containing

| | I | II | III | IV | V |
|---|---|---|---|---|---|
| **With diagnostic test results**<br>» Gastric acid secretion test<br>(concurrent use of antacids may antagonize the effect of pentagastrin and histamine in the evaluation of gastric acid secretory function; administration of antacids is not recommended on the morning of the test) | ✓ | ✓ | ✓ | ✓ | ✓ |
| Meckel's diverticulum imaging<br>(prior administration of aluminum-containing antacids may decrease stomach and bladder uptake of sodium pertechnetate Tc 99m and thus interfere with Meckel's diverticulum evaluation) | ✓ | | ✓ | | |
| Reticuloendothelial cell imaging of liver, spleen, or bone marrow with technetium Tc 99m sulfur colloid<br>(high doses of aluminum-containing antacids may impair reticuloendothelial cell imaging due to the polyvalent cations that cause agglomeration of the individual colloidal particles, thus causing them to be trapped by the pulmonary capillary bed rather than by the reticuloendothelial cells of the liver, spleen, and bone marrow) | ✓ | | ✓ | | |
| Skeletal imaging<br>(prior administration of aluminum-containing antacids may result in liver uptake of technetium Tc 99m pyrophosphate due to the formation of submicroscopic precipitates) | ✓ | | ✓ | | |

## Table 2. Laboratory Value Alterations *(continued)*

| The following have been selected on the basis of their potential clinical significance (possible effect in parentheses where appropriate)—not necessarily inclusive (» = major clinical significance): | Legend:<br>I = Aluminum-containing<br>II = Calcium-containing<br>III = Magaldrate<br>IV = Magnesium-containing<br>V = Sodium Bicarbonate–containing ||||||
|---|---|---|---|---|---|
| | I | II | III | IV | V |
| **With physiology/laboratory test values** | | | | | |
|    Calcium, serum<br>      (concentrations may be increased with large doses) | | ✔ | | | |
|    Gastrin, serum<br>      (concentrations may be increased) | ✔ | ✔ | ✔ | ✔ | ✔ |
|    Phosphate, serum<br>      (concentrations may be decreased by excessive and prolonged use) | ✔ | ✔ | ✔ | | |
|    Systemic and urinary pH<br>      (may be increased) | ✔ | ✔ | ✔ | ✔ | ✔ |

## Table 3. Medical considerations/Contraindications

Note: A blank space usually signifies lack of information; it is not necessarily an indication that a given medical problem is of no concern. However, the pharmacologic similarity of these agents may suggest that if caution is required in particular medical problems for one agent, then it may be required for the others as well.

| The medical considerations/contraindications included have been selected on the basis of their potential clinical significance (reasons given in parentheses where appropriate)—not necessarily inclusive (» = major clinical significance). | Legend:<br>I = Aluminum-containing<br>II = Calcium-containing<br>III = Magaldrate<br>IV = Magnesium-containing<br>V = Sodium Bicarbonate–containing ||||||
|---|---|---|---|---|---|
| | I | II | III | IV | V |
| *Except under special circumstances, these medications should not be used when the following medical problems exist:* | | | | | |
| » Hypercalcemia<br>    (increased risk of exacerbation) | | ✔ | | | |
| » Intestinal obstruction | ✔ | ✔ | ✔ | ✔ | ✔ |
| » Renal function impairment, severe<br>    (increased risk of hypermagnesemia) | | | ✔ | ✔ | |
| *Risk-benefit should be considered when the following medical problems exist:* | | | | | |
| » Alzheimer's disease<br>    (may be exacerbated) | ✔ | | ✔ | | |
| » Appendicitis, or symptoms of<br>    (may complicate existing condition; laxative or constipating effects may increase danger of perforation or rupture) | ✔ | ✔ | ✔ | ✔ | ✔ |
|    Bleeding, gastrointestinal or rectal, undiagnosed<br>    (condition may be exacerbated) | ✔ | ✔ | ✔ | ✔ | ✔ |
|    Bone fractures | * | | * | | |
| » Cirrhosis of liver or<br>» Congestive heart failure or<br>» Edema or<br>» Toxemia of pregnancy<br>    (fluid retention may be increased; low-sodium antacids should be used) | †<br>†<br>†<br>† | †<br>†<br>†<br>† | | | ✔<br>✔<br>✔<br>✔ |
|    Colitis, ulcerative<br>    (may be aggravated by laxative effect of magnesium-containing antacids) | | | | ✔ | ✔ |
|    Colostomy or<br>   Diverticulitis or<br>» Ileostomy<br>    (increased risk of fluid or electrolyte imbalance) | | | ✔<br>✔<br>✔ | ✔<br>✔<br>✔ | |
| » Constipation or<br>» Fecal impaction<br>    (may be exacerbated) | ✔<br>✔ | ✔<br>✔ | | | |
|    Diarrhea, chronic<br>    (possible increased danger of phosphate depletion with aluminum-containing antacids)<br>    (possible increased laxative effect with magnesium-containing antacids) | ✔ | | ✔ | ✔ | |
| » Gastric outlet obstruction | ✔ | | ✔ | | |
| » Hemorrhoids<br>    (may be aggravated) | ✔ | ✔ | | | |

## Table 3. Medical considerations/Contraindications *(continued)*

Note: A blank space usually signifies lack of information; it is not necessarily an indication that a given medical problem is of no concern. However, the pharmacologic similarity of these agents may suggest that if caution is required in particular medical problems for one agent, then it may be required for the others as well.

| The medical considerations/contraindications included have been selected on the basis of their potential clinical significance (reasons given in parentheses where appropriate)—not necessarily inclusive (» = major clinical significance). | Legend:<br>I=Aluminum-containing<br>II=Calcium-containing<br>III=Magaldrate<br>IV=Magnesium-containing<br>V=Sodium Bicarbonate–containing | | | | |
|---|---|---|---|---|---|
| | I | II | III | IV | V |
| » Hypoparathyroidism<br>(calcium excretion may be decreased) | | ✔ | | | |
| » Hypophosphatemia | * | | * | | |
| » Renal function impairment<br>(possible increased risk of aluminum toxicity to brain tissue, bone, and parathyroid glands; possible onset of the neurological syndrome—dialysis dementia—in dialysis patients with long-term use of aluminum-containing antacids)<br>(possible increased danger of milk-alkali syndrome and hypercalcemia with calcium-containing antacids)<br>(possible increased danger of hypermagnesemia)<br>(may cause metabolic alkalosis) | ✔ | ✔ | ✔ | ‡ ‡ | ✔ |
| » Sarcoidosis<br>(increased risk of hypercalcemia or renal disease) | | ✔ | | | |
| Sensitivity to aluminum-, calcium-, magnesium-, simethicone-, or sodium bicarbonate–containing medications | ✔ | ✔ | ✔ | ✔ | ✔ |

*Aluminum hydroxide has the ability to form the insoluble complex of aluminum phosphate, which is excreted in the feces. This may lead to lowered serum phosphate concentrations and phosphorus mobilization from the bone. If phosphate depletion (e.g., malabsorption syndrome) is already present, osteomalacia, osteoporosis, and fracture may result, especially in patients with other bone disease. In such patients predisposed to phosphate depletion, other aluminum-containing antacids (except aluminum phosphate) will be of concern only in relation to their ability to form an aluminum phosphate complex

†Antacids containing more than 5 mEq (115 mg) of sodium per total daily dose should not be used without first checking with physician. The usual amount of sodium allowed in restricted diets is 3 grams or less per day

‡In patients with renal function impairment, use of antacids containing more than 50 mEq (608 mg) of magnesium per total daily dose should be carefully considered

## Table 4. Patient Monitoring

| The following may be especially important in patient monitoring (other tests may be warranted in some patients, depending on condition; » = major clinical significance): | Legend:<br>I=Aluminum-containing<br>II=Calcium-containing<br>III=Magaldrate<br>IV=Magnesium-containing<br>V=Sodium Bicarbonate–containing | | | | |
|---|---|---|---|---|---|
| | I | II | III | IV | V |
| Aluminum concentrations, serum<br>(determinations recommended at periodic intervals for patients with impaired renal function receiving aluminum-containing antacids, to prevent aluminum toxicity) | ✔ | | | | |
| Calcium concentrations, serum<br>(determinations recommended at periodic intervals for patients, especially those with impaired renal function, who are receiving chronic therapy with aluminum-containing antacids)<br>(recommended weekly when calcium-containing antacids are used in large doses) | ✔ | ✔ | ✔ | | |
| Phosphate concentrations, serum<br>(determinations recommended at periodic intervals for patients, especially those with impaired renal function, who are receiving chronic therapy with aluminum-containing antacids) | ✔ | | ✔ | | |
| Potassium concentrations, serum<br>(determinations recommended at periodic intervals for patients, especially those with impaired renal function, who are receiving antacids containing more than 25 mEq [925 mg] of potassium per daily dose) | ✔ | ✔ | ✔ | ✔ | ✔ |
| Renal function determinations<br>(recommended weekly in patients with renal function impairment, and whenever symptoms of hypercalcemia occur in patients receiving calcium-containing antacids in large doses)<br>(recommended at periodic intervals with long-term use of frequently repeated dosage) | ✔ | ✔ | ✔ | ✔ | ✔ |

## Table 5. Side/Adverse Effects*

The following side/adverse effects have been selected on the basis of their potential clinical significance (possible signs and symptoms in parentheses where appropriate)—not necessarily inclusive:

Legend:
I = Aluminum-containing
II = Calcium-containing
III = Magaldrate
IV = Magnesium-containing
V = Sodium Bicarbonate–containing

| | I | II | III | IV | V |
|---|---|---|---|---|---|
| **Medical attention needed** | | | | | |
| With long-term use in chronic renal failure in dialysis patients | | | | | |
| *Neurotoxicity* (mood or mental changes) | ✔ | | ✔ | | |
| With large doses | | | | | |
| *Fecal impaction* (continuing severe constipation) | ✔ | ✔ | | | |
| *Swelling of feet or lower legs* | | | | | ✔ |
| With large doses or in renal insufficiency | | | | | |
| *Metabolic alkalosis* (mood or mental changes; muscle pain or twitching; nervousness or restlessness; slow breathing; unpleasant taste; unusual tiredness or weakness) | | ✔ | | | ✔ |
| With long-term or prolonged use | | | | | |
| *Hypercalcemia associated with milk-alkali syndrome* (frequent urge to urinate; continuing headache; continuing loss of appetite; nausea or vomiting; unusual tiredness or weakness) | | † | | | ✔ |
| *Osteomalacia and osteoporosis due to phosphate depletion* (bone pain; swelling of wrists or ankles) | ✔ | | ‡ | | |
| With overuse or prolonged use | | | | | |
| *Renal calculi* (difficult or painful urination) | | ✔ | | § | |
| With prolonged use or large doses | | | | | |
| *Phosphorus depletion syndrome* (continuing feeling of discomfort; continuing loss of appetite; muscle weakness; unusual weight loss) | ✔ | | ✔ | | |
| With prolonged use or large doses and/or in renal disease | | | | | |
| *Hypermagnesemia or other electrolyte imbalance* (dizziness or lightheadedness; irregular heartbeat; mood or mental changes; unusual tiredness or weakness) | | | | ✔ | ✔ |
| **Medical attention needed only if continuing or bothersome** | | | | | |
| *Chalky taste* | M | M | M | M | U |
| *Constipation, mild* | M | L | U | U | U |
| *Diarrhea or laxative effect*—with overdose | U | U | U | M | U |
| *Increased thirst* | U | U | U | U | L |
| *Nausea or vomiting* | L | U | U | L | U |
| *Speckling or whitish discoloration of stools* (concentrations of fatty acid–salts of aluminum) | L | U | U | U | U |
| *Stomach cramps* | M | U | U | L | L |

*Differences in frequency of occurrence may reflect either lack of clinical-use data or actual pharmacologic distinctions among agents (although their pharmacologic similarity suggests that side effects occurring with one may occur with the others). M = more frequent; L = less frequent; R = rare; U = unknown

†May also occur with large doses and/or in chronic renal failure with calcium carbonate

‡Osteomalacia and osteoporosis have been reported after chronic ingestion of large doses of aluminum hydroxide–containing antacids. Since magaldrate is converted to aluminum and magnesium hydroxides *in vivo*, it is likely that osteomalacia and osteoporosis may occur with excessive use of magaldrate

§Chronic administration of magnesium trisilicate may infrequently produce silica renal stones.

## Table 6. Patient Consultation

As an aid to patient consultation, refer to *Advice for the Patient, Antacids (Oral)*.
In providing consultation, consider emphasizing the following selected information (» = major clinical significance):

Legend:
I = Aluminum-containing
II = Calcium-containing
III = Magaldrate
IV = Magnesium-containing
V = Sodium Bicarbonate–containing

| | I | II | III | IV | V |
|---|---|---|---|---|---|
| **Before using this medication** | | | | | |
| » Conditions affecting use, especially: | | | | | |
| Sensitivity to aluminum-, calcium-, magnesium-, simethicone-, or sodium bicarbonate–containing medication | ✔ | ✔ | ✔ | ✔ | ✔ |
| Pregnancy—Concern for fetus or neonate only with chronic high doses; sodium intake may cause edema and weight gain (for sodium-containing) | ✔ | ✔ | ✔ | ✔ | ✔ |
| Use in children—Not recommended for children up to 6 years of age; proper diagnosis required to avoid medical complications | ✔ | ✔ | ✔ | ✔ | ✔ |
| Use in the elderly— | | | | | |
| Possible aggravation of metabolic bone disease | ✔ | | | | |
| Possible exacerbation of Alzheimer's disease | ✔ | | | | |

USP DI                                                                                                      Antacids (Oral-Local)   197

### Table 6. Patient Consultation (continued)

As an aid to patient consultation, refer to *Advice for the Patient, Antacids (Oral)*.
In providing consultation, consider emphasizing the following selected information (» = major clinical significance):

Legend:
I = Aluminum-containing
II = Calcium-containing
III = Magaldrate
IV = Magnesium-containing
V = Sodium Bicarbonate–containing

| | I | II | III | IV | V |
|---|---|---|---|---|---|
| Other medications, especially: | | | | | |
|     Cellulose sodium phosphate | | ✓ | ✓ | ✓ | |
|     Fluoroquinolones | ✓ | ✓ | ✓ | ✓ | ✓ |
|     Isoniazid, oral | ✓ | | ✓ | | |
|     Ketoconazole | ✓ | ✓ | ✓ | ✓ | ✓ |
|     Mecamylamine | ✓ | ✓ | ✓ | ✓ | ✓ |
|     Methenamine | ✓ | ✓ | ✓ | ✓ | ✓ |
|     Sodium polystyrene sulfonate resin | | ✓ | ✓ | ✓ | |
|     Tetracyclines, oral | ✓ | ✓ | ✓ | ✓ | ✓ |
| Other medical problems, especially: | | | | | |
|     Alzheimer's disease | ✓ | | ✓ | | |
|     Appendicitis, symptoms of | ✓ | ✓ | ✓ | ✓ | ✓ |
|     Constipation or fecal impaction or intestinal obstruction | ✓ | ✓ | | | |
|     Edematous conditions | ✓ | ✓ | | | ✓ |
|     Hemorrhoids | ✓ | ✓ | | | |
|     Hypercalcemia | | ✓ | | | |
|     Hypoparathyroidism | | ✓ | | | |
|     Hypophosphatemia | ✓ | | | ✓ | |
|     Ileostomy | | | | ✓ | |
|     Renal function impairment | | | | ✓ | ✓ |
|     Sarcoidosis | | ✓ | | | |
| **Proper use of this medication** | | | | | |
|   Following physician's or manufacturer's instructions | ✓ | ✓ | ✓ | ✓ | ✓ |
| » Proper dosing | ✓ | ✓ | ✓ | ✓ | ✓ |
|   Missed dose: If on regular dosing schedule—Taking as soon as possible; not taking if almost time for next dose; not doubling doses | ✓ | ✓ | ✓ | ✓ | ✓ |
| » Proper storage | ✓ | ✓ | ✓ | ✓ | ✓ |
| *For chewable tablet dosage form* | | | | | |
|   Chewing tablets well before swallowing for faster results and maximum effectiveness | ✓ | ✓ | ✓ | ✓ | |
| *For use in treatment of ulcers* | | | | | |
| » Compliance with therapy | ✓ | ✓ | ✓ | ✓ | ✓ |
|   Taking 1 and 3 hours after meals and at bedtime for maximum effectiveness | ✓ | ✓ | ✓ | ✓ | ✓ |
| *For aluminum carbonate or aluminum hydroxide as an antiurolithic* | | | | | |
|   Drinking plenty of fluids for best results | ✓ | | | | |
| *For aluminum carbonate or aluminum hydroxide as an antihyperphosphatemic* | | | | | |
|   Possible need for low-phosphate diet | ✓ | | | | |
| **Precautions while using this medication** | | | | | |
|   Regular visits to physician to check progress of therapy if: | | | | | |
|     —taking large doses | | ✓ | | | |
|     —taking regularly for long period of time | ✓ | ✓ | ✓ | ✓ | ✓ |
| Possible interference with gastric acid secretion tests; need to inform physician of use of medication | ✓ | ✓ | ✓ | ✓ | ✓ |
| » Not taking this medication: | | | | | |
|     —if symptoms of appendicitis are present; checking with physician for proper diagnosis | ✓ | ✓ | ✓ | ✓ | ✓ |
|     —if symptoms of inflamed bowel are present | | | | ✓ | |
|     —within 1 to 2 hours of other oral medication | ✓ | ✓ | ✓ | ✓ | ✓ |
|     —with large amounts of milk or milk products | | ✓ | | | ✓ |
| Possible need for sodium restriction | ✓ | ✓ | | ✓ | ✓ |
| Possible interference with test using radiopharmaceutical; need to inform physician of using aluminum-containing antacid | ✓ | | ✓ | | |
| *For antacid use* | | | | | |
| » Not taking this medication for more than 2 weeks or if problem is recurring, unless otherwise directed by physician | ✓ | ✓ | ✓ | ✓ | ✓ |
| Alerting patients to laxative effect when taken too often or in large doses | | | | ✓ | ✓ |
| **Side/adverse effects** | | | | | |
| Signs of potential side effects, especially: | | | | | |
|     Neurotoxicity | ✓ | | ✓ | | |
|     Fecal impaction | ✓ | ✓ | | | |
|     Swelling of feet or lower legs | | | | | ✓ |
|     Metabolic alkalosis | | | ✓ | | ✓ |
|     Hypercalcemia | | ✓ | | | ✓ |
|     Osteomalacia and osteoporosis | ✓ | | | | |
|     Renal calculi | | ✓ | | | |
|     Phosphorus depletion syndrome | ✓ | | | ✓ | |
|     Hypermagnesemia | | | ✓ | ✓ | |

## Table 7. Oral Dosage Forms

**Note:** Content and acid neutralizing capacity per capsule, tablet, or 5 mL, unless otherwise stated. All products are available over-the-counter (OTC) in the U.S. and/or in Canada.

| Brand or generic name [availability] | Aluminum component | Calcium component | Magnesium component | Other ingredients | Acid neutralizing capacity | Other content information as per product label | Usual adult and adolescent dose prn † (maximum OTC dose/day) | Usual pediatric dose | Packaging, storage, and labeling § |
|---|---|---|---|---|---|---|---|---|---|
| *Advanced Formula Di-Gel* Tablets USP (Chewable) [U.S.] | | Calcium carbonate 280 mg | Magnesium hydroxide 128 mg | Simethicone 20 mg | 10 mEq | Sodium <5 mg | 2–4 tabs q 2 hr (24 tabs) | | b, g |
| *Alamag* Oral Suspension USP [U.S.] | Aluminum hydroxide (equiv. to dried gel) 225 mg | | Magnesium hydroxide 200 mg | | | Sodium <1.25 mg Sugar free | 10–20 mL (80 mL) | ‡ | b, c, d, e |
| *Alamag Plus* Oral Suspension USP [U.S.] | Aluminum hydroxide (equiv. to dried gel) 225 mg | | Magnesium hydroxide 200 mg | Simethicone 25 mg | | Sodium <5 mg Sugar free | 10–20 mL (80 mL) | | b, c, d, e |
| *Alenic Alka* Oral Suspension | Aluminum hydroxide 31.7 mg | | Magnesium carbonate 137 mg | Sodium alginate | | Sodium 13 mg | 15–30 mL (120 mL) | ‡ | b, c, d, e, h |
| *Chewable Tablets* | Aluminum hydroxide (dried gel) 80 mg | | Magnesium trisilicate 20 mg | Alginic acid, Sodium bicarbonate | | Sodium 18.4 mg | 2–4 tabs (16 tabs) | | a, g, h |
| *Alenic Alka Extra Strength* Tablets USP (Chewable) [U.S.] | Aluminum hydroxide 160 mg | | Magnesium carbonate 105 mg | Alginic acid, Sodium bicarbonate | | Sodium 29.9 mg | 2–4 tabs (16 tabs) | | b, g, h |
| *Alka-Mints* Tablets USP (Chewable) [U.S.] | | Calcium carbonate 850 mg | | | 15.9 mEq | Sodium <0.5 mg | 1–2 tabs (9 tabs) | | b, g |
| *Alkets* Tablets USP (Chewable) [U.S.] | | Calcium carbonate 500 mg | | | | Sodium ≦2 mg | 1–2 tabs (16 tabs) | | b, g |
| *Alkets Extra Strength* Tablets USP (Chewable) [U.S.] | | Calcium carbonate 750 mg | | | | Sodium ≦2 mg | 1–2 tabs (10 tabs) | | b, e, g |
| *Almacone* Oral Suspension [U.S.] | Aluminum hydroxide (equiv. to dried gel) 200 mg | | Magnesium hydroxide 200 mg | Simethicone 20 mg | 10 mEq | Sodium 0.75 mg | 5–10 mL (120 mL) | ‡ | b, c, d, e |
| Tablets USP (Chewable) [U.S.] | Aluminum hydroxide (dried gel) 200 mg | | Magnesium hydroxide 200 mg | Simethicone 20 mg | | | 1–2 tabs (24 tabs) | | b, g |
| *Almacone II* Oral Suspension USP [U.S.] | Aluminum hydroxide 400 mg | | Magnesium hydroxide 400 mg | Simethicone 40 mg | 20 mEq | Sodium 1.5 mg | 5–10 mL (60 mL) | ‡ | b, c, d, e |

## Table 7. Oral Dosage Forms (continued)

Note: Content and acid neutralizing capacity per capsule, tablet, or 5 mL, unless otherwise stated.
All products are available over-the-counter (OTC) in the U.S. and/or in Canada.

| Brand or generic name [availability] | Aluminum component | Calcium component | Magnesium component | Other ingredients | Acid neutralizing capacity | Other content information as per product label | Usual adult and adolescent dose prn † (maximum OTC dose/day) | Usual pediatric dose | Packaging, storage, and labeling § |
|---|---|---|---|---|---|---|---|---|---|
| *Almagel 200* Oral Suspension USP [Canada] | Aluminum hydroxide (equiv. to dried gel) 200 mg | | Magnesium hydroxide 200 mg | | | | 5–20 mL | | b, c, d, e |
| *AlternaGEL* Gel USP [U.S.] | Aluminum hydroxide (equiv. to dried gel) 600 mg | | | Simethicone | 16 mEq | Sodium <2.5 mg Sugar free | 5–10 mL (90 mL). See also *General Dosing Information* for other doses. | ‡ | b, c, d, e |
| *Alu-Cap* Capsules USP [U.S.] | Aluminum hydroxide (dried gel) 400 mg | | | | 8.5 mEq | | 3 caps (9 caps) | | a |
| *Aludrox* Oral Suspension USP [U.S.] | Aluminum hydroxide gel 307 mg | | Magnesium hydroxide 103 mg | Simethicone 5 mg | 12 mEq | Sodium 2 mg | 10 mL (60 mL) | ‡ | b, c, d, e |
| *Alugel* Gel USP [Canada] | Aluminum hydroxide gel 320 mg | | | | | | 10 mL (80 mL) | | b, c, d, e |
| Alumina and Magnesia* Oral Suspension USP [U.S.] | Aluminum hydroxide (equiv. to dried gel) 240 mg | | Magnesium hydroxide 210 mg | | 13.3 mEq | | 5–20 mL (80 mL) | | b, c, d, e |
| Oral Suspension USP [Canada] | Aluminum hydroxide (equiv. to dried gel) 225 mg | | Magnesium hydroxide 200 mg | | | Sugar free | 10–20 mL (80 mL) | | b, c, d, e |
| Alumina, Magnesia, and Simethicone* Oral Suspension USP [U.S.] | Aluminum hydroxide (equiv. to dried gel) 213 mg | | Magnesium hydroxide 200 mg | Simethicone 20 mg | 12.7 mEq | | 5–10 mL (120 mL) | | b, c, d, e |
| Oral Suspension USP [Canada] | Aluminum hydroxide (equiv. to dried gel) 225 mg | | Magnesium hydroxide 200 mg | Simethicone 25 mg | | Sugar free | 10–20 mL (80 mL) | | b, c, d, e |

*Specific formulations may vary among the different manufacturers; check product labeling
†In peptic ulcer disease, maximum therapeutic response may be obtained if taken 1 and 3 hours after meals and at bedtime. Severe symptoms may require more frequent dosing
‡Pediatric doses may range between 5 and 15 mL every 3 to 6 hours or 1 and 3 hours after meals and at bedtime, unless otherwise stated. However, these are general guidelines; proper diagnosis and dose individualization should precede the use of an antacid in a pediatric patient
§For appropriate *Packaging and storage* and *Label* information refer to designated letters as follows:
a—Store below 40 °C (104 °F), preferably between 15 and 30 °C (59 and 86 °F), in a well-closed container, unless otherwise specified by manufacturer.
b—Store below 40 °C (104 °F), preferably between 15 and 30 °C (59 and 86 °F), unless otherwise specified by manufacturer. Store in a tight container.
c—Protect from freezing.
d—Auxiliary labeling: • Shake well.
e—Auxiliary labeling: • Keep container tightly closed.
f—Auxiliary labeling: • May be chewed or swallowed whole.
g—Auxiliary labeling: • Chew tablets or wafers before swallowing.
h—Auxiliary labeling: • Follow with ½ to 1 glass of water or other liquid.
i—Auxiliary labeling: • May also be allowed to dissolve in mouth.

## Table 7. Oral Dosage Forms (continued)

Note: Content and acid neutralizing capacity per capsule, tablet, or 5 mL, unless otherwise stated. All products are available over-the-counter (OTC) in the U.S. and/or in Canada.

| Brand or generic name [availability] | Aluminum component | Calcium component | Magnesium component | Other ingredients | Acid neutralizing capacity | Other content information as per product label | Usual adult and adolescent dose prn† (maximum OTC dose/day) | Usual pediatric dose | Packaging, storage, and labeling § |
|---|---|---|---|---|---|---|---|---|---|
| Aluminum Hydroxide Gel* USP [U.S./Canada] | Aluminum hydroxide gel 320 mg<br>Aluminum hydroxide gel 450 mg<br>Aluminum hydroxide gel 600 mg<br>Aluminum hydroxide gel 675 mg | | | | | | 600 mg–1.2 grams. See also *General Dosing Information* for other doses. | ‡ | b, c, d, e |
| Aluminum Hydroxide Gel, Dried * Tablets USP [U.S./Canada] | Aluminum hydroxide (dried gel) 500 mg<br>Aluminum hydroxide (dried gel) 600 mg | | | | | | 600 mg–1.2 grams. See also *General Dosing Information* for other doses. | | a, g |
| *Alu-Tab* Tablets USP [U.S.] | Aluminum hydroxide (dried gel) 500 mg | | | | 10.6 mEq | | 3 tabs (9 tabs) | | a |
| Tablets USP [Canada] | Aluminum hydroxide (dried gel) 600 mg | | | | | Film-coated Tartrazine free | 1–2 tabs | | a |
| *Amitone* Tablets USP (Chewable) [U.S.] | | Calcium carbonate 350 mg | | | 7 mEq | Sodium <2 mg | 2 tabs (22 tabs) | | b, g |
| *Amphojel* Gel USP [U.S./Canada] | Aluminum hydroxide gel 320 mg | | | | 10 mEq | Sodium <2.3 mg (peppermint) | 10 mL (60 mL) | | b, c, d, e |
| Tablets USP [U.S./Canada] | Aluminum hydroxide (dried gel) 300 mg | | | | 8 mEq | Sodium 1.4 mg | 2 tabs (12 tabs) | | a, f, h |
| | Aluminum hydroxide (dried gel) 600 mg | | | | 16 mEq | Sodium 2.8 mg | 1 tab (6 tabs) | | a, g, h |

Table 7. Oral Dosage Forms (continued)

Note: Content and acid neutralizing capacity per capsule, tablet, or 5 mL, unless otherwise stated. All products are available over-the-counter (OTC) in the U.S. and/or in Canada.

| Brand or generic name [availability] | Aluminum component | Calcium component | Magnesium component | Other ingredients | Acid neutralizing capacity | Other content information as per product label | Usual adult and adolescent dose prn † (maximum OTC dose/day) | Usual pediatric dose | Packaging, storage, and labeling § |
|---|---|---|---|---|---|---|---|---|---|
| *Amphojel 500* Oral Suspension USP [Canada] | Aluminum hydroxide 500 mg | | Magnesium hydroxide 500 mg | | 37 mEq | Sodium 3 mg Tartrazine free Sugar free | 5–10 mL (40 mL) | ‡ | b, c, d, e |
| *Amphojel Plus* Oral Suspension USP [Canada] | Aluminum hydroxide 300 mg | | Magnesium hydroxide 300 mg | Simethicone 25 mg | | Sodium 7 mg Sugar free Tartrazine free | 5–10 mL (40 mL) | ‡ | b, c, d, e |
| Chewable Tablets [Canada] | | | Magnesium hydroxide 300 mg | Aluminum hydroxide and magnesium carbonate co-dried gel 300 mg, Simethicone 25 mg | | Sodium 10 mg Sugar free Tartrazine free | 1–2 tabs (8 tabs) | | a, g |
| *Antacid Gelcaps* Tablets USP [U.S.] | | Calcium carbonate 311 mg | Magnesium carbonate 232 mg | | | | 2–4 tabs (24 tabs) | | b |
| *Antacid Liquid* Oral Suspension USP [U.S.] | Aluminum hydroxide (equiv. to dried gel) 200 mg | | Magnesium hydroxide 200 mg | Simethicone 20 mg | | Sodium <1.25mg | 10–20 mL (120 mL) | | b, c, d, e |
| *Antacid Liquid Double strength* Oral Suspension USP [U.S.] | Aluminum hydroxide (equiv. to dried gel) 400 mg | | Magnesium hydroxide 400 mg | Simethicone 40 mg | | Sodium <1.25mg | 10–20 mL (60 mL) | | b, c, d, e |
| *Basaljel* Capsules [U.S.] | Dried basic aluminum carbonate gel equiv. to 500 mg of aluminum hydroxide or 608 mg of dried aluminum hydroxide gel | | | | 12 mEq | Sodium 2.76 mg | 2 caps q 2 hr (24 caps) See also *General Dosing Information* for other doses. | | a, h |

*Specific formulations may vary among the different manufacturers; check product labeling
†In peptic ulcer disease, maximum therapeutic response may be obtained if taken 1 and 3 hours after meals and at bedtime. Severe symptoms may require more frequent dosing
‡Pediatric doses may range between 5 and 15 mL every 3 to 6 hours or 1 and 3 hours after meals and at bedtime, unless otherwise stated. However, these are general guidelines; proper diagnosis and dose individualization should precede the use of an antacid in a pediatric patient
§For appropriate *Packaging and storage* and *Label* information refer to designated letters as follows:
a—Store below 40 °C (104 °F), preferably between 15 and 30 °C (59 and 86 °F), in a well-closed container, unless otherwise specified by manufacturer.
b—Store below 40 °C (104 °F), preferably between 15 and 30 °C (59 and 86 °F), unless otherwise specified by manufacturer. Store in a tight container.
c—Protect from freezing.
d—Auxiliary labeling: • Shake well.
e—Auxiliary labeling: • Keep container tightly closed.
f—Auxiliary labeling: • May be chewed or swallowed whole.
g—Auxiliary labeling: • Chew tablets or wafers before swallowing.
h—Auxiliary labeling: • Follow with ½ to 1 glass of water or other liquid.
i—Auxiliary labeling: • May also be allowed to dissolve in mouth.

202  Antacids (Oral-Local)  USP DI

Table 7. Oral Dosage Forms *(continued)*

Note: Content and acid neutralizing capacity per capsule, tablet, or 5 mL, unless otherwise stated.
All products are available over-the-counter (OTC) in the U.S. and/or in Canada.

| Brand or generic name [availability] | Aluminum component | Calcium component | Magnesium component | Other ingredients | Acid neutralizing capacity | Other content information as per product label | Usual adult and adolescent dose prn † (maximum OTC dose/day) | Usual pediatric dose | Packaging, storage, and labeling § |
|---|---|---|---|---|---|---|---|---|---|
| *Basaljel (continued)* Capsules [Canada] | Aluminum hydroxide (dried gel) 500 mg | | | | | Sodium <2 mg Tartrazine free | 2–3 caps (12 caps) | | a, h |
| Oral Suspension [U.S.] | Basic aluminum carbonate gel equiv. to 400 mg of aluminum hydroxide | | | Simethicone 5 mg | 11.5 mEq | Sodium 3 mg | 10 mL q 2 hr (120 mL) | ‡ | b, c, d, h |
| Tablets [U.S.] | Dried basic aluminum carbonate gel equiv. to 500 mg of aluminum hydroxide or 608 mg of dried aluminum hydroxide gel | | | | 12.5 mEq | Sodium 2.76 mg | 2 tabs q 2 hr (24 tabs) | | a, h |
| Calcium Carbonate* Oral Suspension USP [U.S.] | | Calcium carbonate 1250 mg | | | | | 5 mL | | b, c, e |
| Tablets USP [U.S.] | | Calcium carbonate 500 mg Calcium carbonate 600 mg Calcium carbonate 650 mg Calcium carbonate 1250 mg | | | | | 1–2 tabs See also *General Dosing Information* for other doses. | | b, h |
| Tablets USP (Chewable) [U.S.] | | Calcium carbonate 500 mg Calcium carbonate 750 mg | | | | | 1–2 tabs | | b, g |
| *Calglycine* Tablets USP (Chewable) [U.S.] | | Calcium carbonate 420 mg | | Glycine 150 mg | | Sugar free | 2 tabs (19 tabs) | | b, f, i |

USP DI  Antacids (Oral-Local) 203

Table 7. Oral Dosage Forms (continued)

Note: Content and acid neutralizing capacity per capsule, tablet, or 5 mL, unless otherwise stated. All products are available over-the-counter (OTC) in the U.S. and/or in Canada.

| Brand or generic name [availability] | Aluminum component | Calcium component | Magnesium component | Other ingredients | Acid neutralizing capacity | Other content information as per product label | Usual adult and adolescent dose prn † (maximum OTC dose/day) | Usual pediatric dose | Packaging, storage, and labeling § |
|---|---|---|---|---|---|---|---|---|---|
| *Chooz* Chewing Gum [U.S.] | | Calcium carbonate 500 mg | | | 10 mEq | Sodium <5 mg | 1–2 tabs q 2–4 hr (14 tabs) | 6–12 yrs: 1 tab q 2–4 hr (8 tabs) | a |
| *Dicarbosil* Tablets USP (Chewable) [U.S.] | | Calcium carbonate 500 mg | | | 10 mEq | Sodium <2 mg | 2 tabs (16 tabs) | | b, g, i |
| *Di-Gel* Oral Suspension USP [U.S.] | Aluminum hydroxide (dried gel) 200 mg | | Magnesium hydroxide 200 mg | Simethicone 20 mg | ≥9 mEq | Sodium ≤5 mg Sugar free | 10–20 mL q 2 hr (100 mL) | | b, c, d, e |
| *Diovol* Oral Suspension [Canada] | Aluminum hydroxide 165 mg | | Magnesium hydroxide 200 mg | Simethicone | 11.9 mEq | Alcohol 1% Sodium <1 mg Sugar free Tartrazine free | 10–20 mL (80 mL) | | b, c, d, e |
| Chewable Tablets [Canada] | | | Magnesium hydroxide 100 mg | Aluminum hydroxide and magnesium carbonate co-dried gel 300 mg | 10 mEq | Sodium 1 mg Sugar free Tartrazine free | 2–4 tabs (16 tabs) | | a, g |
| *Diovol Caplets* Tablets [Canada] | Aluminum hydroxide (equiv. to dried gel) 200 mg | | Magnesium hydroxide 200 mg | | | Sugar free Tartrazine free | 2–4 tabs (16 tabs) | | a |
| *Diovol Ex* Oral Suspension [Canada] | Aluminum hydroxide 494 mg | | Magnesium hydroxide 300 mg | | 25 mEq | Alcohol 1% Sodium <1 mg Sugar free Tartrazine free | 5–10 mL (40 mL) | ‡ | b, c, d, e |
| Tablets (Chewable) [Canada] | Aluminum hydroxide (equiv. to dried gel) 600 mg | | Magnesium hydroxide 300 mg | | 24.6 mEq | Sodium 1 mg Sugar free Tartrazine free | 1–2 tabs (8 tabs) | | b, g |

*Specific formulations may vary among the different manufacturers; check product labeling
†In peptic ulcer disease, maximum therapeutic response may be obtained if taken 1 and 3 hours after meals and at bedtime. Severe symptoms may require more frequent dosing
‡Pediatric doses may range between 5 and 15 mL every 3 to 6 hours or 1 and 3 hours after meals and at bedtime, unless otherwise stated. However, these are general guidelines; proper diagnosis and dose individualization should precede the use of an antacid in a pediatric patient
§For appropriate *Packaging and storage* and *Label* information refer to designated letters as follows:
 a–Store below 40 °C (104 °F), preferably between 15 and 30 °C (59 and 86 °F), in a well-closed container, unless otherwise specified by manufacturer.
 b–Store below 40 °C (104 °F), preferably between 15 and 30 °C (59 and 86 °F), unless otherwise specified by manufacturer. Store in a tight container.
 c–Protect from freezing.
   f–Auxiliary labeling: • May be chewed or swallowed whole.    h–Auxiliary labeling: • Follow with ½ to 1 glass of water or other liquid.
 d–Auxiliary labeling: • Shake well.    g–Auxiliary labeling: • Chew tablets or wafers before swallowing.    i–Auxiliary labeling: • May also be allowed to dissolve in mouth.
 e–Auxiliary labeling: • Keep container tightly closed.

## Table 7. Oral Dosage Forms (continued)

Note: Content and acid neutralizing capacity per capsule, tablet, or 5 mL, unless otherwise stated. All products are available over-the-counter (OTC) in the U.S. and/or in Canada.

| Brand or generic name [availability] | Aluminum component | Calcium component | Magnesium component | Other ingredients | Acid neutralizing capacity | Other content information as per product label | Usual adult and adolescent dose prn † (maximum OTC dose/day) | Usual pediatric dose | Packaging, storage, and labeling § |
|---|---|---|---|---|---|---|---|---|---|
| *Diovol Plus* Oral Suspension [Canada] | Aluminum hydroxide 165 mg | | Magnesium hydroxide 200 mg | Simethicone 25 mg | 11.9 mEq | Alcohol <1% Sodium <1 mg Sugar free Tartrazine free | 10–20 mL (80 mL) | ‡ | b, c, d, e |
| Chewable Tablets [Canada] | | | Magnesium hydroxide 100 mg | Aluminum hydroxide and magnesium carbonate co-dried gel 300 mg, Simethicone 25 mg | 10 mEq | Sodium 1 mg Sugar free Tartrazine free | 2–4 tabs (16 tabs) | | a, g, i |
| *Diovol Plus AF* Oral Suspension [Canada] | | Calcium carbonate 200 mg | Magnesium hydroxide 200 mg | Simethicone 25 mg | 9.8 mEq | Alcohol 1% Sodium 1 mg Sugar free Tartrazine free | 10–20 mL (80 mL) | | b, c, d |
| Chewable Tablets [Canada] | | Calcium carbonate 200 mg | Magnesium hydroxide 200 mg | Simethicone 25 mg | 10 mEq | Sodium 1 mg Sugar free Tartrazine free | 2–4 tabs (16 tabs) | | a, g |
| *Equilet* Tablets USP (Chewable) [U.S.] | | Calcium carbonate 500 mg | | | | Sodium 0.3 mg | 2 tabs | | b, g |
| *Foamicon* Tablets USP (Chewable) [U.S.] | Aluminum hydroxide 80 mg | | Magnesium trisilicate 20 mg | Alginic acid, Sodium bicarbonate | | Sodium 18.4 mg | 2–4 tabs (16 tabs) | | a, g, h |
| *Gasmas* Chewable Tablets [Canada] | | | Magnesium hydroxide 100 mg | Aluminum hydroxide and magnesium carbonate co-dried gel 300 mg, Simethicone 25 mg | | | 2 tabs | | a, g |
| *Gaviscon* Oral Suspension USP [U.S.] | Aluminum hydroxide 31.7 mg | | Magnesium carbonate 119.3 mg | Sodium alginate | 2.5–4.3 mEq | Sodium 13 mg | 15–30 mL (120 mL) | ‡ | b, c, d, e, h |
| Tablets USP (Chewable) [U.S.] | Aluminum hydroxide (dried gel) 80 mg | | Magnesium trisilicate 20 mg | Alginic acid, Sodium bicarbonate | 0.5 mEq | Sodium 18.4 mg | 2–4 tabs (16 tabs) | | a, g, h |
| *Gaviscon-2* Tablets USP (Chewable) [U.S.] | Aluminum hydroxide (dried gel) 160 mg | | Magnesium trisilicate 40 mg | Alginic acid, Sodium bicarbonate | 1 mEq | Sodium 36.8 mg | 1–2 tabs (8 tabs) | | a, g, h |

USP DI                                                                                                                                    Antacids (Oral-Local)    205

**Table 7. Oral Dosage Forms** *(continued)*

Note: Content and acid neutralizing capacity per capsule, tablet, or 5 mL, unless otherwise stated.
All products are available over-the-counter (OTC) in the U.S. and/or in Canada.

| Brand or generic name [availability] | Aluminum component | Calcium component | Magnesium component | Other ingredients | Acid neutralizing capacity | Other content information as per product label | Usual adult and adolescent dose prn † (maximum OTC dose/day) | Usual pediatric dose | Packaging, storage, and labeling § |
|---|---|---|---|---|---|---|---|---|---|
| *Gaviscon Acid Plus Gas Relief* Oral Suspension [Canada] | | Calcium carbonate 660 mg | Magnesium hydroxide 145 mg | Simethicone 30 mg | | | 10–20 mL (60 mL) | | b, d |
| Tablets USP (Chewable) [Canada] | | Calcium carbonate 585 mg | Magnesium hydroxide 120 mg | Simethicone 30 mg | | | 2–4 tabs (13 tabs) | | b, g |
| *Gaviscon Acid Relief* Oral Suspension [Canada] | | Calcium carbonate 660 mg | Magnesium hydroxide 145 mg | | | | 10–20 mL (60 mL) | | b, d |
| Tablets USP (Chewable) [Canada] | | Calcium carbonate 585 mg | Magnesium hydroxide 120 mg | | | | 2–4 tabs (13 tabs) | | b, g |
| *Gaviscon Extra Strength Acid Relief* Oral Suspension [Canada] | | Calcium carbonate 1 gram | Magnesium hydroxide 250 mg | | | | 10–15 mL (40 mL) | | b, d |
| *Gaviscon Extra Strength Relief Formula* Oral Suspension USP [U.S.] | Aluminum hydroxide 254 mg | | Magnesium carbonate 238 mg | Sodium alginate, Simethicone emulsion | 14.3 mEq | Sodium 20.7 mg | 10–20 mL (80 mL) | | b, c, d, e, h |
| Tablets USP (Chewable) [U.S.] | Aluminum hydroxide 160 mg | | Magnesium carbonate 105 mg | Alginic acid, Sodium bicarbonate | 5–7.5 mEq | Sodium 29.9 mg | 2–4 tabs (16 tabs) | | b, g, h |
| *Gaviscon Heartburn Relief* Oral Suspension USP [Canada] | Aluminum hydroxide (dried gel) 100 mg | | | Sodium alginate 250 mg | | Sodium 30 mg Alcohol free Sugar free Tartrazine free | 10–20 mL (100 mL) | | b, d, e |
| Oral Suspension [Canada] | | | Magnesium carbonate 100 mg | Sodium alginate 250 mg, Calcium carbonate, Sodium bicarbonate | | | 10–20 mL (100 mL) | | b, d |

\*Specific formulations may vary among the different manufacturers; check product labeling
†In peptic ulcer disease, maximum therapeutic response may be obtained if taken 1 and 3 hours after meals and at bedtime. Severe symptoms may require more frequent dosing
‡Pediatric doses may range between 5 and 15 mL every 3 to 6 hours or 1 and 3 hours after meals and at bedtime, unless otherwise stated. However, these are general guidelines; proper diagnosis and dose individualization should precede the use of an antacid in a pediatric patient
§For appropriate *Packaging and storage* and *Label* information refer to designated letters as follows:
  a–Store below 40 °C (104 °F), preferably between 15 and 30 °C (59 and 86 °F), in a well-closed container, unless otherwise specified by manufacturer.
  b–Store below 40 °C (104 °F), preferably between 15 and 30 °C (59 and 86 °F), unless otherwise specified by manufacturer. Store in a tight container.
  c–Protect from freezing.                                      f–Auxiliary labeling: • May be chewed or swallowed whole.         h–Auxiliary labeling: • Follow with ½ to 1 glass of water or other liquid.
  d–Auxiliary labeling: • Shake well.                           g–Auxiliary labeling: • Chew tablets or wafers before swallowing.  i–Auxiliary labeling: • May also be allowed to dissolve in mouth.
  e–Auxiliary labeling: • Keep container tightly closed.

# Antacids (Oral-Local)

## Table 7. Oral Dosage Forms (continued)

Note: Content and acid neutralizing capacity per capsule, tablet, or 5 mL, unless otherwise stated.
All products are available over-the-counter (OTC) in the U.S. and/or in Canada.

| Brand or generic name [availability] | Aluminum component | Calcium component | Magnesium component | Other ingredients | Acid neutralizing capacity | Other content information as per product label | Usual adult and adolescent dose prn † (maximum OTC dose/day) | Usual pediatric dose | Packaging, storage, and labeling § |
|---|---|---|---|---|---|---|---|---|---|
| Gaviscon Heartburn Relief (continued) Tablets USP (Chewable) [Canada] | Aluminum hydroxide (dried gel) 80 mg | | | Alginic acid 200 mg | | Sodium 22 mg Tartrazine free | 2–4 tabs (20 tabs) | | a, g |
| Chewable Tablets [Canada] | | | Magnesium carbonate 40 mg | Alginic acid 200 mg, Sodium bicarbonate | | | 2–4 tabs (20 tabs) | | a, g |
| Gaviscon Heartburn Relief Extra Strength Tablets USP (Chewable) [Canada] | Aluminum hydroxide (dried gel) 160 mg | | | Alginic acid 400 mg | | Tartrazine free | 2 tabs (10 tabs) | | a, g |
| Gelusil Oral Suspension USP [Canada] | Aluminum hydroxide (equiv. to dried gel) 200 mg | | Magnesium hydroxide 200 mg | Simethicone 25 mg | | Sodium 0.84 mg Sugar free Tartrazine free | 10–20 mL 4 times/day | | b, c, d, e |
| Tablets USP (Chewable) [U.S.] | Aluminum hydroxide 200 mg | | Magnesium hydroxide 200 mg | | 11 mEq | Sodium <5 mg | 2–4 tabs (12 tabs) | | b, g |
| Tablets USP (Chewable) [Canada] | Aluminum hydroxide (equiv. to dried gel) 200 mg | | Magnesium hydroxide 200 mg | | | Sodium 1.1 mg Tartrazine free | 2–4 tabs 4 times/day | | b, g |
| Gelusil Extra Strength Oral Suspension USP [Canada] | Aluminum hydroxide (equiv. to dried gel) 650 mg | | Magnesium hydroxide 350 mg | | | Sodium 1.4 mg Sugar free Tartrazine free | 10 mL 4 times/day | | b, c, d, e |
| Tablets USP (Chewable) [Canada] | Aluminum hydroxide (equiv. to dried gel) 400 mg | | Magnesium hydroxide 400 mg | | | Sodium 1.6 mg Tartrazine free | 2–4 tabs 4 times/day | | b, g, h |
| Genaton Oral Suspension USP [U.S.] | Aluminum hydroxide 31.7 mg | | Magnesium carbonate 137.3 mg | Sodium alginate | | Sodium 13 mg | 15–30 mL (120 mL) | | b, c, d, e, h |
| Tablets USP (Chewable) [U.S.] | Aluminum hydroxide 80 mg | | Magnesium trisilicate 20 mg | Alginic acid, Sodium bicarbonate | | Sodium 18.4 mg | 2–4 tabs (16 tabs) | | a, g, h |
| Genaton Extra Strength Tablets USP (Chewable) [U.S.] | Aluminum hydroxide 160 mg | | Magnesium carbonate 105 mg | Alginic acid, Sodium bicarbonate | | Sodium 35 mg | 2–4 tabs (16 tabs) | | b, e, g, h |
| Kudrox Double Strength Oral Suspension USP [U.S.] | Aluminum hydroxide 500 mg | | Magnesium hydroxide 450 mg | Simethicone 40 mg | 25 mEq | Sodium <5 mg | 10–20 mL (60 mL) | | b, c, d, e |

Table 7. Oral Dosage Forms (continued)

Note: Content and acid neutralizing capacity per capsule, tablet, or 5 mL, unless otherwise stated.
All products are available over-the-counter (OTC) in the U.S. and/or in Canada.

| Brand or generic name [availability] | Aluminum component | Calcium component | Magnesium component | Other ingredients | Acid neutralizing capacity | Other content information as per product label | Usual adult and adolescent dose prn † (maximum OTC dose/day) | Usual pediatric dose | Packaging, storage, and labeling § |
|---|---|---|---|---|---|---|---|---|---|
| *Life Antacid* Oral Suspension USP [Canada] | Aluminum hydroxide (dried gel) 228 mg | | Magnesium hydroxide 200 mg | | | Sugar free | 10–20 mL (80 mL) | | b, c, d, e |
| *Life Antacid Plus* Oral Suspension USP [Canada] | Aluminum hydroxide (dried gel) 228 mg | | Magnesium hydroxide 200 mg | Simethicone 25 mg | | Sugar free | 10–20 mL (80 mL) | | b, c, d, e |
| Tablets USP (Chewable) [Canada] | Aluminum hydroxide (dried gel) 200 mg | | Magnesium hydroxide 200 mg | Simethicone 25 mg | | | 1–4 tabs | | b, g |
| *Losopan* Oral Suspension USP [U.S.] | | | | Magaldrate 540 mg | | Sodium <5 mg | 5–10 mL (90 mL) | | b, c, d, e |
| *Losopan Plus* Oral Suspension USP [U.S.] | | | | Magaldrate 540 mg, Simethicone 40 mg | | Sodium <5 mg | 5–10 mL (90 mL) | | b, c, d, e |
| *Lowsium Plus* Oral Suspension USP [U.S.] | | | | Magaldrate 540 mg, Simethicone 40 mg | | Sodium <5 mg | 5–10 mL (90 mL) | ‡ | b, c, d, e |
| *Maalox* Oral Suspension USP [U.S.] | Aluminum hydroxide (equiv. to dried gel) 225 mg | | Magnesium hydroxide 200 mg | | 13.3 mEq | Sodium <1.5 mg Sugar free | 10–20 mL (80 mL) | ‡ | b, c, d |
| Oral Suspension USP [Canada] | Aluminum hydroxide (equiv. to dried gel) 225 mg | | Magnesium hydroxide 200 mg | | 13.3 mEq | Sodium 0.92 mg Sugar free Tartrazine free | 10–20 mL (80 mL) | ‡ | b, c, d |
| Original Tablets USP (Chewable) [U.S.] | Aluminum hydroxide (dried gel) 200 mg | | Magnesium hydroxide 200 mg | | 9.7 mEq | Sodium 0.7 mg Sugar free | 2–4 tabs (16 tabs) | | b, e, g |

*Specific formulations may vary among the different manufacturers; check product labeling
†In peptic ulcer disease, maximum therapeutic response may be obtained if taken 1 and 3 hours after meals and at bedtime. Severe symptoms may require more frequent dosing
‡Pediatric doses may range between 5 and 15 mL every 3 to 6 hours or 1 and 3 hours after meals and at bedtime, unless otherwise stated. However, these are general guidelines; proper diagnosis and dose individualization should precede the use of an antacid in a pediatric patient
§For appropriate *Packaging and storage* and *Label* information refer to designated letters as follows:
  a–Store below 40 °C (104 °F), preferably between 15 and 30 °C (59 and 86 °F), in a well-closed container, unless otherwise specified by manufacturer.
  b–Store below 40 °C (104 °F), preferably between 15 and 30 °C (59 and 86 °F), unless otherwise specified by manufacturer. Store in a tight container.
  c–Protect from freezing.
  d–Auxiliary labeling: • Shake well.
  e–Auxiliary labeling: • Keep container tightly closed.
  f–Auxiliary labeling: • May be chewed or swallowed whole.
  g–Auxiliary labeling: • Chew tablets or wafers before swallowing.
  h–Auxiliary labeling: • Follow with ½ to 1 glass of water or other liquid.
  i–Auxiliary labeling: • May also be allowed to dissolve in mouth.

# Antacids (Oral-Local)

## Table 7. Oral Dosage Forms (continued)

Note: Content and acid neutralizing capacity per capsule, tablet, or 5 mL, unless otherwise stated. All products are available over-the-counter (OTC) in the U.S. and/or in Canada.

| Brand or generic name [availability] | Aluminum component | Calcium component | Magnesium component | Other ingredients | Acid neutralizing capacity | Other content information as per product label | Usual adult and adolescent dose prn† (maximum OTC dose/day) | Usual pediatric dose | Packaging, storage, and labeling § |
|---|---|---|---|---|---|---|---|---|---|
| *Maalox (continued)* Tablets USP (Chewable) [Canada] | Aluminum hydroxide (equiv. to dried gel) 400 mg | | Magnesium hydroxide 400 mg | | | Sodium 0.93 mg Tartrazine free | 1–2 tabs (8 tabs) | | b, g, h |
| *Maalox Antacid Caplets* Tablets USP [U.S./Canada] | | Calcium carbonate 311 mg | Magnesium carbonate 232 mg | | | | 2–4 tabs (24 tabs) | | b |
| *Maalox Heartburn Relief Formula* Oral Suspension [U.S.] | | | Magnesium carbonate 175 mg | Aluminum hydroxide-magnesium carbonate co-dried gel 140 mg | 8.5 mEq | Sodium <1.5 mg Tartrazine | 10–20 mL (80 mL) | | b, c, d, e |
| *Maalox HRF* Oral Suspension [Canada] | | | Magnesium carbonate 175 mg | Aluminum hydroxide-magnesium carbonate codried gel 140 mg | | Sodium <5 mg Sugar free Tartrazine free | 10–20 mL (80 mL) | | b, c, d |
| Tablets (Chewable) [Canada] | | | Magnesium alginate 250 mg, Magnesium carbonate 160 mg | Aluminum hydroxide-magnesium carbonate codried gel 180 mg | | Sodium <3 mg Tartrazine free | 2–4 tabs (16 tabs) | | a, g, h |
| *Maalox Plus* Oral Suspension USP [Canada] | Aluminum hydroxide (equiv. to dried gel) 225 mg | | Magnesium hydroxide 200 mg | Simethicone 25 mg | 13.35 mEq | Sodium 0.92 mg Sugar free Tartrazine free | 10–20 mL (80 mL) | | b, c, d, e |
| Tablets USP (Chewable) [U.S.] | Aluminum hydroxide (equiv. to dried gel) 200 mg | | Magnesium hydroxide 200 mg | Simethicone 25 mg | 10.65 mEq | Sodium ≦1 mg | 1–4 tabs (16 tabs) | | b, g |
| Tablets USP (Chewable) [Canada] | Aluminum hydroxide (equiv. to dried gel) 200 mg | | Magnesium hydroxide 200 mg | Simethicone 25 mg | | Sodium 1 mg (lemon) 0.94 mg (mint) Tartrazine free | 2–4 tabs (16 tabs) | | a, g, h |
| *Maalox Plus, Extra Strength* Oral Suspension USP [U.S.] | Aluminum hydroxide (equiv. to dried gel) 500 mg | | Magnesium hydroxide 450 mg | Simethicone 40 mg | 26.1 mEq | Sodium <1 mg Sugar free | 10–20 mL (60 mL) | | b, c, d, e |
| Oral Suspension USP [Canada] | Aluminum hydroxide (equiv. to dried gel) 500 mg | | Magnesium hydroxide 450 mg | Simethicone 40 mg | | Sodium 1.2 mg Sugar free Tartrazine free | 10–20 mL (60 mL) | | b, c, d, e |

Table 7. Oral Dosage Forms (continued)

Note: Content and acid neutralizing capacity per capsule, tablet, or 5 mL, unless otherwise stated. All products are available over-the-counter (OTC) in the U.S. and/or in Canada.

| Brand or generic name [availability] | Aluminum component | Calcium component | Magnesium component | Other ingredients | Acid neutralizing capacity | Other content information as per product label | Usual adult and adolescent dose prn ‡ (maximum OTC dose/day) | Usual pediatric dose | Packaging, storage, and labeling § |
|---|---|---|---|---|---|---|---|---|---|
| *Maalox Plus, Extra Strength (continued)* Tablets USP (Chewable) [U.S./Canada] | Aluminum hydroxide (dried gel) 350 mg | | Magnesium hydroxide 350 mg | Simethicone 30 mg | 16.7 mEq | Sodium 1.4 mg Sugar 0.72 gram | 1–3 tabs (12 tabs) | | b, g |
| *Maalox TC* Oral Suspension USP [U.S.] | Aluminum hydroxide (equiv. to dried gel) 600 mg | | Magnesium hydroxide 300 mg | | 27.2 mEq | Sodium <1 mg Sugar free | 5–10 mL (40 mL) | | b, c, d, e |
| Oral Suspension USP [Canada] | Aluminum hydroxide (equiv. to dried gel) 600 mg | | Magnesium hydroxide 300 mg | | | Sodium 0.95 mg Sugar free Tartrazine free | 5–10 mL (40 mL) | | b, c, d, e |
| Tablets USP (Chewable) [Canada] | Aluminum hydroxide (dried gel) 600 mg | | Magnesium hydroxide 300 mg | | 28 mEq | Sodium 0.98 mg Tartrazine free | 1–2 tabs (8 tabs) | | b, g |
| *Magaldrate* Oral Suspension USP [U.S.] | | | | Magaldrate 540 mg | | Sodium free Sugar free Dye free | 5–10 mL (100 mL) | ‡ | b, c, d |
| *Magaldrate and Simethicone* Oral Suspension USP [U.S.] | | | | Magaldrate 540 mg, Simethicone 20 mg | | | 5–10 mL (100 mL) | ‡ | b, c, d, e |
| *Magnalox* Oral Suspension USP [U.S.] | Aluminum hydroxide (equiv. to dried gel) 225 mg | | Magnesium hydroxide 200 mg | Simethicone | | Sugar free | 10–20 mL (80 mL) | | b, c, d, e |
| *Magnalox Plus* Oral Suspension USP [U.S.] | Aluminum hydroxide (equiv. to dried gel) 500 mg | | Magnesium hydroxide 450 mg | Simethicone 40 mg | | | 10–20 mL (60 mL) | | b, c, d, e |
| *Magnesium Hydroxide* Magnesia Tablets USP (Chewable) [Canada] | | | Magnesium hydroxide 385 mg | | | Sugar free | 2–4 tabs (16 tabs) | | b, f, h |

*Specific formulations may vary among the different manufacturers; check product labeling
†In peptic ulcer disease, maximum therapeutic response may be obtained if taken 1 and 3 hours after meals and at bedtime. Severe symptoms may require more frequent dosing
‡Pediatric doses may range between 5 and 15 mL every 3 to 6 hours or 1 and 3 hours after meals and at bedtime, unless otherwise stated. However, these are general guidelines; proper diagnosis and dose individualization should precede the use of an antacid in a pediatric patient
§For appropriate *Packaging and storage* and *Label* information refer to designated letters as follows:
 a–Store below 40 °C (104 °F), preferably between 15 and 30 °C (59 and 86 °F), in a well-closed container, unless otherwise specified by manufacturer.
 b–Store below 40 °C (104 °F), preferably between 15 and 30 °C (59 and 86 °F), unless otherwise specified by manufacturer. Store in a tight container.
 c–Protect from freezing.
 d–Auxiliary labeling: • Shake well.
 e–Auxiliary labeling: • Keep container tightly closed.
 f–Auxiliary labeling: • May be chewed or swallowed whole.
 g–Auxiliary labeling: • Chew tablets or wafers before swallowing.
 h–Auxiliary labeling: • Follow with ½ to 1 glass of water or other liquid.
 i–Auxiliary labeling: • May also be allowed to dissolve in mouth.

## Table 7. Oral Dosage Forms (continued)

Note: Content and acid neutralizing capacity per capsule, tablet, or 5 mL, unless otherwise stated.
All products are available over-the-counter (OTC) in the U.S. and/or in Canada.

| Brand or generic name [availability] | Aluminum component | Calcium component | Magnesium component | Other ingredients | Acid neutralizing capacity | Other content information as per product label | Usual adult and adolescent dose prn † (maximum OTC dose/day) | Usual pediatric dose | Packaging, storage, and labeling § |
|---|---|---|---|---|---|---|---|---|---|
| Milk of Magnesia USP* [U.S.] | | | Magnesium hydroxide 400 mg | | 14 mEq | | 5–15 mL (60 mL) | ‡ | b, c, d, e |
| Milk of Magnesia USP* [Canada] | | | Magnesium hydroxide 440 mg | | | Sugar free | 10–20 mL | | b, c, d, e |
| Mag-Ox 400 Tablets USP [U.S.] | | | Magnesium oxide 400 mg | | 20 mEq | | 1–2 tabs/day (2 tabs) | | a |
| Mallamint Tablets USP (Chewable) [U.S.] | | Calcium carbonate 420 mg | | | | Sodium <0.1 mg Sugar free | 2 tabs | | a, g |
| Maox 420 Tablets USP [U.S.] | | | Magnesium oxide 420 mg | | 21 mEq | Tartrazine | 1 tab/day | | a |
| Marblen Oral Suspension [U.S.] | | Calcium carbonate 520 mg | Magnesium carbonate 400 mg | | 18 mEq | Sugar free | 5–10 mL (60 mL) | | c, d, e |
| Tablets USP [U.S.] | | Calcium carbonate 520 mg | Magnesium carbonate 400 mg | | 18 mEq | Sugar free | 1–2 tabs (12 tabs) | | g, i |
| Mi-Acid Oral Suspension USP [U.S.] | Aluminum hydroxide (equiv. to dried gel) 200 mg | | Magnesium hydroxide 200 mg | Simethicone 20 mg | | Sodium <5 mg | 10–20 mL (120 mL) | ‡ | b, c, d, e |
| Tablets USP [U.S.] | | Calcium carbonate 311 mg | Magnesium carbonate 232 mg | Simethicone 40 mg | | | 2–4 tabs (24 tabs) | | a |
| Mi-Acid Double Strength Oral Suspension USP [U.S.] | Aluminum hydroxide (equiv. to dried gel) 400 mg | | Magnesium hydroxide 400 mg | | | Sodium <5 mg | 10–20 mL (60 mL) | | b, c, d, e |
| Mintox Oral Suspension USP [U.S.] | Aluminum hydroxide (equiv. to dried gel) 225 mg | | Magnesium hydroxide 200 mg | | | Sodium 1.38 mg | 10–20 mL (80 mL) | ‡ | b, c, d, e |
| Tablets USP (Chewable) [U.S.] | Aluminum hydroxide 200 mg | | Magnesium hydroxide 200 mg | | | | 2 tabs | | a, g |

Table 7. Oral Dosage Forms (continued)

Note: Content and acid neutralizing capacity per capsule, tablet, or 5 mL, unless otherwise stated. All products are available over-the-counter (OTC) in the U.S. and/or in Canada.

| Brand or generic name [availability] | Aluminum component | Calcium component | Magnesium component | Other ingredients | Acid neutralizing capacity | Other content information as per product label | Usual adult and adolescent dose prn † (maximum OTC dose/day) | Usual pediatric dose | Packaging, storage, and labeling § |
|---|---|---|---|---|---|---|---|---|---|
| *Mintox Extra Strength* Oral Suspension USP [U.S.] | Aluminum hydroxide (equiv. to dried gel) 500 mg | | Magnesium hydroxide 450 mg | Simethicone 40 mg | | Sodium <5 mg | 10–20 mL (60 mL) | | b, c, d, e |
| Tablets USP (Chewable) [U.S.] | Aluminum hydroxide 200 mg | | Magnesium hydroxide 200 mg | Simethicone 25 mg | | | 1–2 tabs | | b, g |
| *Mygel* Oral Suspension USP [U.S.] | Aluminum hydroxide (equiv. to dried gel) 200 mg | | Magnesium hydroxide 200 mg | Simethicone 20 mg | | Sodium 1.38 mg | 10–20 mL (120 mL) | ‡ | b, c, d, e |
| *Mygel II* Oral Suspension USP [U.S.] | Aluminum hydroxide (equiv. to dried gel) 400 mg | | Magnesium hydroxide 400 mg | Simethicone 40 mg | | Sodium 1.3 mg | 10–20 mL (60 mL) | ‡ | b, c, d, e |
| *Mylanta* Lozenges [U.S.] | | Calcium carbonate 600 mg | | | 11.4 mEq | | 1–2 lozenges (12 lozenges) | | a |
| Oral Suspension USP [U.S.] | Aluminum hydroxide (equiv. to dried gel) 200 mg | | Magnesium hydroxide 200 mg | Simethicone 20 mg | 12.7 mEq | Sodium 0.68 mg Sugar free | 10–20 mL (120 mL) | ‡ | b, c, d, e |
| Oral Suspension USP [Canada] | Aluminum hydroxide (equiv. to dried gel) 200 mg | | Magnesium hydroxide 200 mg | Simethicone 20 mg | | Sodium 3.2 mg Sugar free Tartrazine free | 10–20 mL 4 times/day | | b, c, d, e |
| Tablets USP (Chewable) [U.S.] | | Calcium carbonate 350 mg | Magnesium hydroxide 150 mg | | 12 mEq | Sodium 0.3 mg | 2–4 tabs (20 tabs) | | b, g |
| Tablets USP (Chewable) [Canada] | Aluminum hydroxide (dried gel) 200 mg | | Magnesium hydroxide 200 mg | Simethicone 20 mg | | Sodium 0.9 mg Tartrazine free | 2–4 tabs 4 times/day | | a, g, i |

*Specific formulations may vary among the different manufacturers; check product labeling

†In peptic ulcer disease, maximum therapeutic response may be obtained if taken 1 and 3 hours after meals and at bedtime. Severe symptoms may require more frequent dosing

‡Pediatric doses may range between 5 and 15 mL every 3 to 6 hours or 1 and 3 hours after meals and at bedtime, unless otherwise stated. However, these are general guidelines; proper diagnosis and dose individualization should precede the use of an antacid in a pediatric patient

§For appropriate *Packaging and storage* and *Label* information refer to designated letters as follows:
  a—Store below 40 °C (104 °F), preferably between 15 and 30 °C (59 and 86 °F), in a well-closed container, unless otherwise specified by manufacturer.
  b—Store below 40 °C (104 °F), preferably between 15 and 30 °C (59 and 86 °F), unless otherwise specified by manufacturer. Store in a tight container.
  c—Protect from freezing.
  d—Auxiliary labeling: • Shake well.
  e—Auxiliary labeling: • Keep container tightly closed.
  f—Auxiliary labeling: • May be chewed or swallowed whole.
  g—Auxiliary labeling: • Chew tablets or wafers before swallowing.
  h—Auxiliary labeling: • Follow with ½ to 1 glass of water or other liquid.
  i—Auxiliary labeling: • May also be allowed to dissolve in mouth.

## Table 7. Oral Dosage Forms (continued)

Note: Content and acid neutralizing capacity per capsule, tablet, or 5 mL, unless otherwise stated. All products are available over-the-counter (OTC) in the U.S. and/or in Canada.

| Brand or generic name [availability] | Aluminum component | Calcium component | Magnesium component | Other ingredients | Acid neutralizing capacity | Other content information as per product label | Usual adult and adolescent dose prn † (maximum OTC dose/day) | Usual pediatric dose | Packaging, storage, and labeling § |
|---|---|---|---|---|---|---|---|---|---|
| *Mylanta Double Strength* Oral Suspension USP [U.S.] | Aluminum hydroxide 400 mg | | Magnesium hydroxide 400 mg | Simethicone 40 mg | 25.4 mEq | Sodium 1.14 mg Sugar free | 10–20 mL (60 mL) | ‡ | b, c, d, e |
| Tablets USP (Chewable) [U.S.] | | Calcium carbonate 700 mg | Magnesium hydroxide 300 mg | | 24 mEq | Sodium 0.6 mg | 2–4 tabs (10 tabs) | | b, g |
| Tablets USP (Chewable) [Canada] | Aluminum hydroxide (equiv. to dried gel) 400 mg | | Magnesium hydroxide 400 mg | Simethicone 30 mg | | Sodium 1.5 mg Tartrazine free | 2–4 tabs 4 times/day | | b, g |
| *Mylanta Double Strength Plain* Oral Suspension USP [Canada] | Aluminum hydroxide (equiv. to dried gel) 400 mg | | Magnesium hydroxide 400 mg | | | Sodium 10 mg Sugar free Tartrazine free | 5–10 mL 4 times/day | | b, c, d, e |
| *Mylanta Extra Strength* Oral Suspension USP [Canada] | Aluminum hydroxide (equiv. to dried gel) 650 mg | | Magnesium hydroxide 350 mg | Simethicone 30 mg | | Sodium 1.8 mg Sugar free Tartrazine free | 5–10 mL 4 times/day | | b, c, d, e |
| *Mylanta Gelcaps* Tablets [U.S.] | | Calcium carbonate 550 mg | Magnesium hydroxide 125 mg | | 11.5 mEq | Benzyl alcohol, Sodium 2.5 mg | 2–4 tabs (24 tabs) | | a |
| *Nephrox* Oral Suspension [U.S.] | Aluminum hydroxide gel 320 mg | | | Mineral oil 10% | 9 mEq | Sugar free | 10 mL (60 mL) | | c, d, e |
| *Neutralca-S* Oral Suspension USP [Canada] | Aluminum hydroxide (equiv. to dried gel) 200 mg | | Magnesium hydroxide 200 mg | | | Sodium 0.6 mg Sugar free | 5–15 mL | ‡ | b, c, d |
| Tablets USP (Chewable) [Canada] | Aluminum hydroxide (dried gel) 400 mg | | Magnesium hydroxide 400 mg | | | Sodium 1.01 mg Scored | 1–2 tabs | | b, g |
| *Phillips'* Magnesia Tablets USP (Chewable) [Canada] | | | Magnesium hydroxide 311 mg | | | Low sodium Sucrose 195 mg | 2–4 tabs (16 tabs) | 7–14 yrs: 1 tab (4 tabs) | b, e, g |
| Milk of Magnesia USP [U.S.] | | | Magnesium hydroxide 400 mg | | | | 5–15 mL (60 mL) | | b, c, d, e |
| Milk of Magnesia USP [Canada] | | | Magnesium hydroxide 400 mg | | | Alcohol free Sodium <2.2 mg Sugar free (plain and mint) | 5–15 mL (60 mL) | 1–12 yrs: 1–10 mL | b, c, d, e |

USP DI  Antacids (Oral-Local) 213

## Table 7. Oral Dosage Forms (continued)

Note: Content and acid neutralizing capacity per capsule, tablet, or 5 mL, unless otherwise stated. All products are available over-the-counter (OTC) in the U.S. and/or in Canada.

| Brand or generic name [availability] | Aluminum component | Calcium component | Magnesium component | Other ingredients | Acid neutralizing capacity | Other content information as per product label | Usual adult and adolescent dose prn † (maximum OTC dose/day) | Usual pediatric dose | Packaging, storage, and labeling § |
|---|---|---|---|---|---|---|---|---|---|
| *Phillips' Chewable Magnesia Tablets USP* (Chewable) [U.S.] | | | Magnesium hydroxide 311 mg | | | | 2–4 tabs (16 tabs) | 7–14 yrs: 1 tab (4 tabs) | b, g |
| *Phillips' Concentrated Double-strength Milk of Magnesia USP* [U.S.] | | | Magnesium hydroxide 800 mg | | | Sugar free | 2.5–7.5 mL (30 mL) | | b, c, d, e |
| *PMS Alumina, Magnesia, and Simethicone* Oral suspension USP [Canada] | Aluminum hydroxide 200 mg | | Magnesium hydroxide 200 mg | Simethicone 25 mg | | | 10–20 mL 4 times/day (80 mL) | | b, c, d, e |
| *Rafton* Oral Suspension [Canada] | Aluminum hydroxide 100 mg | | | Calcium carbonate, Sodium bicarbonate, Sodium alginate 250 mg | | Alcohol free Sodium 30 mg Sugar free Tartrazine free | 10–20 mL 1–4 times/day (80 mL) | | b, c, d, e, h |
| Chewable tablets [Canada] | Aluminum hydroxide (equiv. to dried gel) 80 mg | | | Alginic acid 200 mg, Sodium bicarbonate | | Sodium 22 mg Sucrose 1.2 grams Tartrazine free | 2–4 tabs 1–4 times/day (16 tabs) | | a, g, h |
| *Riopan* Oral Suspension USP [U.S.] | | | | Magaldrate 540 mg | 15 mEq | Sodium <0.3 mg | 5–10 mL (80 mL) | ‡ | b, c, d, e |
| Oral Suspension USP [Canada] | | | | Magaldrate 480 mg | | Alcohol free Sodium <0.7 mg Sugar free Tartrazine free | 10–20 mL | ‡ | b, c, d, e |
| Tablets USP (Chewable) [Canada] | | | | Magaldrate 480 mg | | Sodium 0.7 mg Tartrazine free | 1–4 tabs | | a, g |

*Specific formulations may vary among the different manufacturers; check product labeling
†In peptic ulcer disease, maximum therapeutic response may be obtained if taken 1 and 3 hours after meals and at bedtime. Severe symptoms may require more frequent dosing
‡Pediatric doses may range between 5 and 15 mL every 3 to 6 hours or 1 and 3 hours after meals and at bedtime, unless otherwise stated. However, these are general guidelines; proper diagnosis and dose individualization should precede the use of an antacid in a pediatric patient
§For appropriate *Packaging and storage* and *Label* information refer to designated letters as follows:
 a–Store below 40 °C (104 °F), preferably between 15 and 30 °C (59 and 86 °F), in a well-closed container, unless otherwise specified by manufacturer.
 b–Store below 40 °C (104 °F), preferably between 15 and 30 °C (59 and 86 °F), unless otherwise specified by manufacturer. Store in a tight container.
 c–Protect from freezing.
 d–Auxiliary labeling: • Shake well.
 e–Auxiliary labeling: • Keep container tightly closed.
 f–Auxiliary labeling: • May be chewed or swallowed whole.
 g–Auxiliary labeling: • Chew tablets or wafers before swallowing.
 h–Auxiliary labeling: • Follow with ½ to 1 glass of water or other liquid.
 i–Auxiliary labeling: • May also be allowed to dissolve in mouth.

## Table 7. Oral Dosage Forms (continued)

Note: Content and acid neutralizing capacity per capsule, tablet, or 5 mL, unless otherwise stated.
All products are available over-the-counter (OTC) in the U.S. and/or in Canada.

| Brand or generic name [availability] | Aluminum component | Calcium component | Magnesium component | Other ingredients | Acid neutralizing capacity | Other content information as per product label | Usual adult and adolescent dose prn † (maximum OTC dose/day) | Usual pediatric dose | Packaging, storage, and labeling § |
|---|---|---|---|---|---|---|---|---|---|
| *Riopan Extra Strength* Oral Suspension USP [Canada] | | | | Magaldrate 1080 mg | | Alcohol free Sodium 0.3 mg Sugar free Tartrazine free | 5–10 mL | | b, c, d, e |
| *Riopan Plus* Oral Suspension USP [U.S.] | | | | Magaldrate 540 mg, Simethicone 40 mg | 15 mEq | Sodium <0.3 mg | 5–10 mL (60 mL) | ‡ | b, c, d, e |
| Oral Suspension USP [Canada] | | | | Magaldrate 480 mg, Simethicone 20 mg | 13.5 mEq | Alcohol free Sodium 0.7 mg Sugar free Tartrazine free | 10–20 mL | | b, c, d, e |
| Tablets USP (Chewable) [U.S./Canada] | | | | Magaldrate 480 mg, Simethicone 20 mg | 13.5 mEq | Sodium 0.1 mg | 2–4 tabs (25 tabs) | | b, g |
| *Riopan Plus Double Strength* Oral Suspension USP [U.S.] | | | | Magaldrate 1080 mg, Simethicone 40 mg | | Sodium ≤0.3 mg | 5–10 mL (60 mL) | ‡ | b, c, d, e |
| Tablets USP (Chewable) [U.S.] | | | | Magaldrate 1080 mg, Simethicone 20 mg | 30 mEq | Sodium ≤0.5 mg | 2–4 tabs (25 tabs) | | b, g |
| *Riopan Plus Extra Strength* Oral Suspension USP [Canada] | | | | Magaldrate 1080 mg, Simethicone 30 mg | | Sodium 0.3 mg Sugar free Tartrazine free | 5–10 mL | | b, c, d, e |
| *Rolaids* Tablets USP (Chewable) [U.S.] | | Calcium carbonate 550 mg | Magnesium hydroxide 110 mg | | 14.8 mEq | Sodium <0.1 mg | 1–4 tabs (12 tabs) | | b, g |
| Tablets USP (Chewable) [Canada] | | Calcium carbonate 317 mg | Magnesium hydroxide 64 mg | | | Sodium <1 mg Tartrazine free | 1–2 tabs (12 tabs) | | b, g |
| *Rolaids Extra Strength* Tablets USP (Chewable) [Canada] | | Calcium carbonate 750 mg | Magnesium hydroxide 64 mg | | | Sodium <1 mg Tartrazine free | 1–2 tabs (10 tabs) | | b, g |
| *Rulox* Oral Suspension USP [U.S.] | Aluminum hydroxide (equiv. to dried gel) 225 mg | | Magnesium hydroxide 200 mg | | 12 mEq | Sodium <1 mg | 10–20 mL (80 mL) | ‡ | b, c, d, e |

## Table 7. Oral Dosage Forms (continued)

Note: Content and acid neutralizing capacity per capsule, tablet, or 5 mL, unless otherwise stated. All products are available over-the-counter (OTC) in the U.S. and/or in Canada.

| Brand or generic name [availability] | Aluminum component | Calcium component | Magnesium component | Other ingredients | Acid neutralizing capacity | Other content information as per product label | Usual adult and adolescent dose prn † (maximum OTC dose/day) | Usual pediatric dose | Packaging, storage, and labeling § |
|---|---|---|---|---|---|---|---|---|---|
| *Rulox No. 1* Tablets USP (Chewable) [U.S.] | Aluminum hydroxide (dried gel) 200 mg | | Magnesium hydroxide 200 mg | | | | 1–2 tabs (16 tabs) | | b, e, g, h |
| *Rulox No. 2* Tablets USP (Chewable) [U.S.] | Aluminum hydroxide (dried gel) 400 mg | | Magnesium hydroxide 400 mg | | | | 1–2 tabs (8 tabs) | | b, e, g, h |
| *Rulox Plus* Oral Suspension USP [U.S.] | Aluminum hydroxide (equiv. to dried gel) 500 mg | | Magnesium hydroxide 450 mg | Simethicone 40 mg | | | 10–20 mL (80 mL) | | b, c, d, e |
| *Simaal Gel* Oral Suspension USP [U.S.] | Aluminum hydroxide (equiv. to dried gel) 200 mg | | Magnesium hydroxide 200 mg | Simethicone 20 mg | | Sodium 1.4 mg Sugar free | 10–20 mL (120 mL) | | b, c, d, e |
| *Simaal 2 Gel* Oral Suspension USP [U.S.] | Aluminum hydroxide (equiv. to dried gel) 400 mg | | Magnesium hydroxide 400 mg | Simethicone 40 mg | | Sodium 1.84 mg Sugar free | 10–20 mL (60 mL) | ‡ | b, c, d, e |
| *Tempo* Tablets USP (Chewable) [U.S.] | Aluminum hydroxide 133 mg | Calcium carbonate 414 mg | Magnesium hydroxide 81 mg | Simethicone 20 mg | 14 mEq | Sodium 3 mg | 1 tab (12 tabs) | | b, g |
| *Titralac* Tablets USP (Chewable) [U.S.] | | Calcium carbonate 420 mg | | Glycine 183 mg | 7.5 mEq | Sodium 1.1 mg Sugar free | 2 tabs (19 tabs) | | b, f, i |
| *Titralac Extra Strength* Tablets USP (Chewable) [U.S.] | | Calcium carbonate 750 mg | | Glycine 321 mg | | Sodium 1.1 mg Sugar free | 1–2 tabs (10 tabs) | | b, f, h, i |
| *Titralac Plus* Oral Suspension [U.S.] | | Calcium carbonate 500 mg | | Simethicone 20 mg | | Sodium 2.5 mg Sugar free | 10 mL (80 mL) | | b, c, d |

*Specific formulations may vary among the different manufacturers; check product labeling
†In peptic ulcer disease, maximum therapeutic response may be obtained if taken 1 and 3 hours after meals and at bedtime. Severe symptoms may require more frequent dosing
‡Pediatric doses may range between 5 and 15 mL every 3 to 6 hours or 1 and 3 hours after meals and at bedtime, unless otherwise stated. However, these are general guidelines; proper diagnosis and dose individualization should precede the use of an antacid in a pediatric patient
§For appropriate *Packaging and storage* and *Label* information refer to designated letters as follows:
  a– Store below 40 °C (104 °F), preferably between 15 and 30 °C (59 and 86 °F), in a well-closed container, unless otherwise specified by manufacturer.
  b– Store below 40 °C (104 °F), preferably between 15 and 30 °C (59 and 86 °F), unless otherwise specified by manufacturer. Store in a tight container.
  c– Protect from freezing.
  d– Auxiliary labeling: • Shake well.
  e– Auxiliary labeling: • Keep container tightly closed.
  f– Auxiliary labeling: • May be chewed or swallowed whole.
  g– Auxiliary labeling: • Chew tablets or wafers before swallowing.
  h– Auxiliary labeling: • Follow with ½ to 1 glass of water or other liquid.
  i– Auxiliary labeling: • May also be allowed to dissolve in mouth.

# Table 7. Oral Dosage Forms (continued)

Note: Content and acid neutralizing capacity per capsule, tablet, or 5 mL, unless otherwise stated.
All products are available over-the-counter (OTC) in the U.S. and/or in Canada.

| Brand or generic name [availability] | Aluminum component | Calcium component | Magnesium component | Other ingredients | Acid neutralizing capacity | Other content information as per product label | Usual adult and adolescent dose prn † (maximum OTC dose/day) | Usual pediatric dose | Packaging, storage, and labeling § |
|---|---|---|---|---|---|---|---|---|---|
| *Titralac Plus (continued)* Chewable Tablets [U.S.] | | Calcium carbonate 420 mg | | Glycine 173 mg Simethicone 21 mg | | Sodium 1.1 mg Sugar free | 2 tabs (19 tabs) | | b, f, i |
| *Trial* Tablets USP (Chewable) [Canada] | | Calcium carbonate 420 mg | | | | | 1–2 tabs (18 tabs) | | a, g |
| *Tums* Tablets USP (Chewable) [U.S.] | | Calcium carbonate 500 mg | | | 10 mEq | Sodium <2 mg | 2–4 tabs (16 tabs) | | b, g, i |
| Tablets USP (Chewable) [Canada] | | Calcium carbonate 500 mg | | | 10 mEq | Sodium <2 mg | 1–2 tabs (16 tabs) | | b, g |
| *Tums Anti-gas/Antacid* Chewable Tablets [U.S.] | | Calcium carbonate 500 mg | | Simethicone 20 mg | 10 mEq | Sodium ≤2 mg | 1–2 tabs (16 tabs) | | a, g |
| *Tums E-X* Tablets USP (Chewable) [U.S.] | | Calcium carbonate 750 mg | | | 15 mEq | Sodium <2 mg | 2–4 tabs (10 tabs) | | b, g |
| *Tums Extra Strength* Tablets USP (Chewable) [Canada] | | Calcium carbonate 750 mg | | | 15 mEq | Sodium <2 mg | 1–2 tabs (10 tabs) | | b, g |
| *Tums Ultra* Tablets USP (Chewable) [U.S.] | | Calcium carbonate 1 gram | | | 20 mEq | Sodium ≤4 mg | 2–3 tabs (8 tabs) | | b, g |
| *Tums Ultra* Tablets USP (Chewable) [Canada] | | Calcium carbonate 1 gram | | | 20 mEq | Sodium ≤4 mg | 1–2 tabs (8 tabs) | | b, g |

USP DI    Antacids (Oral-Local)    217

## Table 7. Oral Dosage Forms (continued)

Note: Content and acid neutralizing capacity per capsule, tablet, or 5 mL, unless otherwise stated.
All products are available over-the-counter (OTC) in the U.S. and/or in Canada.

| Brand or generic name [availability] | Aluminum component | Calcium component | Magnesium component | Other ingredients | Acid neutralizing capacity | Other content information as per product label | Usual adult and adolescent dose prn † (maximum OTC dose/day) | Usual pediatric dose | Packaging, storage, and labeling § |
|---|---|---|---|---|---|---|---|---|---|
| *Univol* Oral Suspension [Canada] | Aluminum hydroxide 165 mg | | Magnesium hydroxide 200 mg | | | Alcohol 1% Sodium 1 mg Sugar free Tartrazine free | 10–20 mL (80 mL) | | b, c, d, e |
| *Uro-Mag* Capsules USP [U.S.] | | | Magnesium oxide 140 mg | | 7 mEq | | 3–4 caps/daily | | a |

*Specific formulations may vary among the different manufacturers; check product labeling
†In peptic ulcer disease, maximum therapeutic response may be obtained if taken 1 and 3 hours after meals and at bedtime. Severe symptoms may require more frequent dosing
‡Pediatric doses may range between 5 and 15 mL every 3 to 6 hours or 1 and 3 hours after meals and at bedtime, unless otherwise stated. However, these are general guidelines; proper diagnosis and dose individualization should precede the use of an antacid in a pediatric patient
§For appropriate *Packaging and storage* and *Label* information refer to designated letters as follows:
  a–Store below 40 °C (104 °F), preferably between 15 and 30 °C (59 and 86 °F), in a well-closed container, unless otherwise specified by manufacturer.
  b–Store below 40 °C (104 °F), preferably between 15 and 30 °C (59 and 86 °F), unless otherwise specified by manufacturer. Store in a tight container.
  c–Protect from freezing.
  d–Auxiliary labeling: • Shake well.  f–Auxiliary labeling: • May be chewed or swallowed whole.  h–Auxiliary labeling: • Follow with ½ to 1 glass of water or other liquid.
  e–Auxiliary labeling: • Keep container tightly closed.  g–Auxiliary labeling: • Chew tablets or wafers before swallowing.  i–Auxiliary labeling: • May also be allowed to dissolve in mouth.

# ANTHRALIN Topical

INN: Dithranol
BAN: Dithranol
VA CLASSIFICATION (Primary/Secondary): DE802/DE900
Commonly used brand name(s): *Anthraforte 1; Anthraforte 2; Anthranol 0.1; Anthranol 0.2; Anthranol 0.4; Anthrascalp; Dritho-Scalp; Drithocreme; Drithocreme HP; Micanol.*

Note: For a listing of dosage forms and brand names by country availability, see *Dosage Forms* section(s).

## Category
Antipsoriatic (topical); hair growth stimulant, alopecia areata (topical).

## Indications

### Accepted
**Psoriasis (treatment)**—Anthralin is indicated in the topical treatment of quiescent or chronic psoriasis of the skin and scalp.

### Acceptance not established
Anthralin has been used in patients for the topical treatment of *alopecia areata* after other treatments were unsuccessful. The best results were achieved in patients who recently had acquired alopecia areata; 0.5% anthralin cream produced a low rate of cosmetically acceptable results. Study results evaluating the use of anthralin are preliminary and larger studies are required. (Evidence rating: C-3.)

### Unaccepted
Anthralin should not be used on acutely inflamed psoriatic eruptions.

## Pharmacology/Pharmacokinetics

### Physicochemical characteristics
Molecular weight—226.23.

### Mechanism of action/Effect
**Antipsoriatic**—The mechanism of action of anthralin is not known. Anthralin restores the normal rate of epidermal cell proliferation and keratinization by reducing the mitotic activity of the hyperplastic epidermis of psoriasis. *In vitro* studies show that anthralin prolongs the prophase of mitosis for keratinocytes and leukocytes; *in vivo* studies show that anthralin inhibits DNA synthesis and may increase the release of reactive oxygen species, upsetting oxidative metabolic processes.

**Hair growth stimulant**—Although its mechanism is not known, anthralin does not have direct follicular stimulating effects. Anthralin's hair growth properties may be due to its irritant properties and its ability to cause a nonallergenic inflammatory dermatitis.

### Absorption
The amount of anthralin absorbed through the skin has not been fully determined; however, absorption appears to be low. Anthralin penetrates damaged skin and psoriatic lesions faster and to a greater extent than normal skin, possibly because of greater blood flow to the lesions or a poor barrier junction of psoriatic skin.

### Elimination
Two studies found evidence of anthralin metabolites (mainly danthron) in the urine. However, a later study using a detection limit of 20 mcg per mL found no evidence of excretion of anthraquinones in the urine. In addition, other studies have found no evidence of systemic toxicity, even in patients with renal disease.

## Precautions to Consider

### Carcinogenicity/Tumorigenicity
Some long-term studies in mice have shown anthralin to be tumorigenic to mouse skin; the carcinogenic potential has not been evaluated. Tumorigenic and carcinogenic effects of anthralin have not been reported in humans.

### Pregnancy/Reproduction
Pregnancy—Anthralin may be systemically absorbed.
Studies have not been done in humans.
Studies have not been done in animals.
FDA Pregnancy Category C.

### Breast-feeding
It is not known whether anthralin is distributed into breast milk, and problems in humans have not been documented. However, anthralin may be systemically absorbed.

### Pediatrics
Appropriate studies on the relationship of age to the effects of anthralin have not been performed in the pediatric population. Safety and efficacy have not been established.

### Geriatrics
Appropriate studies on the relationship of age to the effects of anthralin have not been performed in the geriatric population. However, no geriatrics-specific problems have been documented to date.

### Medical considerations/Contraindications
The medical considerations/contraindications included have been selected on the basis of their potential clinical significance (reasons given in parentheses where appropriate)—not necessarily inclusive (» = major clinical significance).

*Risk-benefit should be considered when the following medical problems exist:*

» Acute eruptions or presence of inflammation of skin, including folliculitis

Allergy to components of formulation, such as parabens

Sensitivity to anthralin or to components of formulation, such as salicylic acid
(transient irritation of uninvolved skin surrounding the psoriatic lesions occurs frequently and may be occasionally severe; medication should be discontinued if a sensitivity skin reaction or excessive irritation occurs. Some formulations contain 2 to 3% salicylic acid, a keratolytic, to serve as an antioxidant. Rarely, anthralin may cause allergic contact dermatitis)

## Side/Adverse Effects
Note: Severe conjunctivitis may occur if this medication comes into contact with the eye.

The following side/adverse effects have been selected on the basis of their potential clinical significance (possible signs and symptoms in parentheses where appropriate)—not necessarily inclusive:

### Those indicating need for medical attention
Incidence more frequent
**Redness or other skin irritation not present before therapy**—including treated and uninvolved skin
Incidence rare
*Allergic reaction* (skin rash)

## Patient Consultation
As an aid to patient consultation, refer to *Advice for the Patient, Anthralin (Topical)*.
In providing consultation, consider emphasizing the following selected information (» = major clinical significance):

### Before using this medication
» Conditions affecting use, especially:
   Sensitivity to anthralin or to components of formulation, such as salicylic acid, or allergy to components of formulation, such as parabens
   Other medical problems, especially acute eruptions or presence of inflammation of skin, including folliculitis

### Proper use of this medication
» Avoiding contact with the eyes and mucous membranes
» Not applying medication to blistered, raw, or oozing areas of skin or scalp
» Not using medication on face or sex organs or in the folds and creases of the skin; checking with physician if necessary
» Using medication only as directed; importance of not using more medication than the amount prescribed
Knowing correct method of administration; checking with physician if necessary

*Proper administration*
If irritation of normal skin occurs, applying petrolatum around affected areas before applying anthralin
Applying a thin layer to only the affected areas; rubbing in well
Washing hands immediately after application
*For short contact anthralin therapy*
Allowing medication to remain on affected area for 10 to 30 minutes or as prescribed by physician; then bathing, if applied to the skin, or shampooing, if applied to the scalp, to remove medication

*For patients using the cream for overnight treatment*
  If the skin is being treated—Removing cream from skin by bathing the next morning
  If the scalp is being treated—Shampooing to remove scales and any previous application, then drying and parting hair before application; checking with physician to see when cream should be removed

*For patients using the ointment for overnight treatment*
  If the skin is being treated—Removing ointment from skin with warm liquid petrolatum the next morning, then bathing
  If the scalp is being treated—Removing from scalp by shampooing the next morning

» Proper dosing
  Missed dose: Applying as soon as possible; not applying if almost time for next dose; not doubling doses
» Proper storage

**Precautions while using this medication**
» Staining may occur on contact with this medication, especially to skin, hair, fingernails, clothing, bed linens, or bathtub or shower; staining of skin or hair wears off several weeks after medication is discontinued
  Minimizing or preventing possible staining from anthralin by:
    • Wearing plastic gloves to prevent staining of hands
    • Checking with physician to see if plastic cap may be worn to prevent staining of pillow if medication is applied to scalp at night
    • Removing any medication on surface of bathtub or shower by rinsing with cool to lukewarm water immediately after bathing or showering, then washing with a household cleanser to remove any remaining deposit of medication on bathtub or shower stall

**Side/adverse effects**
  Anthralin has been shown to cause tumors in animals. However, there have been no reports of anthralin causing tumors in humans
  Signs of potential side effects, especially redness or other skin irritation not present before therapy (for both treated and uninvolved skin) or allergic reaction

## General Dosing Information

Anthralin's skin-irritating properties increase with its concentration. The optimal period of contact will vary according to the strength used and the patient's response or tolerance to anthralin therapy. A short contact time and the initial use of a low concentration are recommended, with subsequent increase in contact time and/or concentration only as necessary.

One criterion for determining the optimal concentration for use is the occurrence of erythema on normal skin adjacent to the lesions. When erythema occurs, the dosage, frequency of application, and/or duration of treatment should be reduced. Any time severe skin irritation or edema of treated or untreated skin occurs, patients should notify their physicians, and anthralin dosage adjustment or treatment discontinuation should be considered.

Anthralin should be carefully applied directly to psoriatic skin lesions to avoid exposing uninvolved skin. Unintentionally applied medication should be washed off, especially residue collected behind ears when anthralin is applied to the scalp. Contact with the eyes and mucous membranes should be avoided. It is recommended that anthralin not be applied to:
• acute psoriatic lesions;
• blistered, raw, or oozing areas of skin or scalp;
• genitalia;
• facial skin, for most formulations;
• intertriginous skin areas; or
• folds or creases of skin.

In the treatment of psoriasis, two types of anthralin therapy are being used:
  Conventional therapy—Anthralin cream or ointment is applied once (sometimes twice) a day to dry skin or scalp, preferably at night, and allowed to remain on the affected area overnight, then removed by bathing or shampooing the next morning or before the next application.
  Short contact anthralin therapy (S.C.A.T.)—Anthralin 0.1 to 1% cream or ointment is applied once a day to dry skin or scalp and allowed to remain on the affected area for only 10 to 30 minutes or as prescribed by physician, then removed by bathing, if applied to skin, or by shampooing, if applied to scalp.

Some products require that a metal cover on tube be pierced at initial use by inverting the cap. Formulations used on the scalp may contain a black applicator that can be screwed onto the tube.

Many surfaces stain on contact with anthralin, including skin, hair, fingernails, clothing, bed linens, bathtubs, and showers. It may take several weeks after medication is discontinued to remove the stains from treated skin or hair. Patients can be instructed in ways to limit the contact of medication from unintended surfaces or areas. Suggestions include:
• using plastic gloves for application; otherwise, washing hands thoroughly after using the medication.
• pretreating the uninvolved skin around psoriatic lesions with a protective film of petrolatum or other suitable emollient.
• immediately removing medication from inanimate surfaces, such as bathtubs or shower stalls, by rinsing surfaces with cool to lukewarm water and then washing with household cleansers.
• wearing plastic caps during sleep, if appropriate, to protect bed linens for patients applying anthralin to scalp before bedtime.

Long-term use of topical corticosteroids may destabilize psoriasis and, on their withdrawal, result in a rebound effect; it is recommended by the manufacturer that corticosteroids be discontinued for 1 week before initiating treatment with anthralin. Using petrolatum or another appropriate emollient during this 1-week interval may be useful for the patient. Some clinicians have not found a rebound effect in such treated patients.

## Topical Dosage Forms

### ANTHRALIN CREAM USP

**Usual adult and adolescent dose**
Psoriasis—
  Conventional therapy: Topical, to dry, affected skin, once a day, preferably at night. Wash medication off at the end of the contact time.
  Short contact therapy: Topical, to dry, affected skin, once a day for ten to thirty minutes or as prescribed by physician. Wash medication off at the end of the contact time. Strengths of 1% or higher are generally used for short contact therapy and cream may be preferred for scalp administration.

**Usual pediatric dose**
Safety and efficacy have not been established.

**Usual geriatric dose**
See *Usual adult and adolescent dose*.

**Strength(s) usually available**
U.S.—
  0.1% (Rx) [*Drithocreme* (ascorbic acid; cetostearyl alcohol; chlorocresol; petrolatum; salicylic acid; sodium lauryl sulfate; water)].
  0.25% (Rx) [*Drithocreme* (ascorbic acid; cetostearyl alcohol; chlorocresol; petrolatum; salicylic acid; sodium lauryl sulfate; water); *Dritho-Scalp* (ascorbic acid; cetostearyl alcohol; chlorocresol; petrolatum; salicylic acid; sodium lauryl sulfate; water)].
  0.5% (Rx) [*Drithocreme* (ascorbic acid; cetostearyl alcohol; chlorocresol; petrolatum; salicylic acid; sodium lauryl sulfate; water); *Dritho-Scalp* (ascorbic acid; cetostearyl alcohol; chlorocresol; petrolatum; salicylic acid; sodium lauryl sulfate; water)].
  1% (Rx) [*Drithocreme HP* (ascorbic acid; cetostearyl alcohol; chlorocresol; petrolatum; salicylic acid; sodium lauryl sulfate; water); *Micanol* (citric acid; glyceryl monolaurate; glyceryl monomyristate; sodium hydroxide; water)].
Canada—
  0.1% (Rx) [*Anthranol 0.1* (vanishing cream base)].
  0.2% (Rx) [*Anthranol 0.2* (vanishing cream base)].
  0.4% (Rx) [*Anthranol 0.4* (vanishing cream base); *Anthrascalp* (bisulfite; parabens; vanishing cream base)].

**Packaging and storage**
Store between 8 and 15 °C (46 and 59 °F), unless otherwise specified by manufacturer. Store in a tight container. Protect from light. Protect from freezing.

**Auxiliary labeling**
• For external use only.

### ANTHRALIN OINTMENT USP

**Usual adult and adolescent dose**
Psoriasis—
  Conventional therapy: Topical, to the dry, affected skin, once a day or as directed by physician. Wash medication off at the end of the contact time.
  Short contact therapy: See *Anthralin Cream USP*. Strengths of 1% or higher are generally used for short contact therapy.

**Usual pediatric dose**
See *Anthralin Cream USP*.

### Usual geriatric dose
See *Usual adult and adolescent dose*.

### Strength(s) usually available
U.S.—
  Not commercially available.
Canada—
  1% (Rx) [*Anthraforte 1* (petrolatum)].
  2% (Rx) [*Anthraforte 2* (petrolatum)].

### Packaging and storage
Store between 8 and 15 °C (46 and 59 °F), unless otherwise specified by manufacturer. Store in a tight container. Protect from light. Protect from freezing.

### Auxiliary labeling
- For external use only.

Revised: 06/30/98

# ANTIANDROGENS, NONSTEROIDAL Systemic

This monograph includes information on the following: 1) Bicalutamide; 2) Flutamide; 3) Nilutamide.
VA CLASSIFICATION (Primary): AN900
Note: For a listing of dosage forms and brand names by country availability, see *Dosage Forms* section(s).

## Category
Antineoplastic.

## Indications
Note: Bracketed information in the *Indications* section refers to uses that are not included in U.S. product labeling.

All of the nonsteroidal antiandrogens have similar pharmacologic actions; however, clinical uses among specific agents may vary because of availability of specific testing, differences in side effects, and/or availability of clinical-use data.

### Accepted
Carcinoma, prostatic (treatment)—Nonsteroidal antiandrogens are indicated, in conjunction with testosterone-lowering measures, such as administration of a luteinizing hormone–releasing hormone (LHRH) analog (e.g., goserelin or leuprolide) or surgical castration (bilateral orchiectomy), for the treatment of prostatic carcinoma. Specifically:
*Bicalutamide* is indicated, in combination with an LHRH analog or [bilateral orchiectomy], for the treatment of locally advanced (stage $B_2$ or C) or metastatic (stage $D_2$) prostatic carcinoma.
*Flutamide* is indicated, in combination with an LHRH analog or [bilateral orchiectomy], for the treatment of locally advanced (stage $B_2$ or C) or metastatic (stage $D_2$) prostatic carcinoma.
*Nilutamide* is indicated, in conjunction with bilateral orchiectomy [or an LHRH analog][1] (Evidence rating: IIID), for the treatment of metastatic (stage $D_2$) prostatic carcinoma.

### Acceptance not established
Flutamide is being studied, alone and in combination with other medications with antiandrogenic activity, for the treatment of hirsutism. Flutamide seems to be effective for treating idiopathic hirsutism (Evidence rating: III) as well as hirsutism due to polycystic ovary syndrome (PCOS) (Evidence rating: III), and data from a limited number of patients indicate that flutamide also relieves associated skin conditions (i.e., acne and seborrhea) (Evidence rating: III). However, its place in the treatment of hirsutism has not been established because of concerns about safety; severe hepatotoxicity has occurred during treatment. At least three comparative studies have found other antiandrogenic medications to be equally effective, and other studies have shown that reversal of flutamide's beneficial effects begins within a few months after treatment is discontinued. Until the benefits and risks of treatment have been better defined, especially with long-term or repeated use, flutamide should be considered only for severe cases unresponsive to other therapy and used in the lowest effective dosage. Also, flutamide must be used in conjunction with adequate contraception and should not be used during breast-feeding because of the potential risks (feminization of a male fetus and adverse developmental or toxic effects in nursing infants).

### Unaccepted
Use of flutamide for benign prostatic hyperplasia (BPH) is not recommended because of limited efficacy and the risk of adverse effects, including severe, potentially fatal, hepatotoxicity.

Flutamide has been studied, and found ineffective, for treatment of hepatocellular carcinoma (Evidence rating: IA) or ovarian carcinoma (Evidence rating: IIID).

[1] Not included in Canadian product labeling.

## Pharmacology/Pharmacokinetics

### Physicochemical characteristics
Molecular weight—
  Bicalutamide: 430.38.
  Flutamide: 276.22.
  Nilutamide: 317.23.
pKa—
  Bicalutamide: Approximately 12.
Other characteristics
  Bicalutamide is a racemate. The *R*-enantiomer is responsible for almost all of the medication's activity. The *S*-enantiomer is virtually inactive.

### Mechanism of action/Effect
Nonsteroidal antiandrogens bind to cytosol androgen receptors and competitively inhibit the uptake and/or binding of androgens in target tissues, thereby interfering with the actions of androgens at the cellular level. Prostatic carcinoma is androgen-sensitive; ablation of endogenous androgen activity inhibits tumor growth and causes tumor regression. The antiandrogenic effect of these medications complements medical or surgical treatments (luteinizing hormone–releasing hormone [LHRH] analog therapy or bilateral orchiectomy) that result in inhibition or cessation of testicular (but not adrenal) androgen production.

When administered in conjunction with an LHRH analog, nonsteroidal antiandrogens inhibit the temporary surge in plasma testosterone concentration and the resultant "flare" reaction that may occur, prior to the sustained decrease in testosterone production, when monotherapy with an LHRH analog is initiated.

### Other actions/effects
When administered alone, nonsteroidal antiandrogens inhibit the negative feedback response to testosterone by the hypothalamus. In patients who have not undergone surgical castration, this effect results in increased serum concentrations of testosterone and, consequently, of estrogen. Concurrent administration of an LHRH analog inhibits the stimulant effect of the nonsteroidal antiandrogen(but not the suppressant effect of the LHRH analog) on the serum testosterone concentration.

Nilutamide inhibits hepatic cytochrome P450 enzymes.

Bicalutamide has been shown to induce hepatic enzymes in animal studies, but enzyme induction has not been detected in humans receiving up to 150 mg per day(three times the recommended daily dose).

### Absorption
Bicalutamide—Extensive; the rate and extent of absorption are not affected by concurrent administration with food.
Flutamide—Rapid and complete.
Nilutamide—Rapid and complete; not affected by concurrent administration with food.

### Protein binding
Bicalutamide—Very high (96%).
Flutamide—Very high (94 to 96% for flutamide; 92 to 94% for the active alpha-hydroxylated metabolite hydroxyflutamide at steady-state).
Nilutamide—Moderate (84%), to plasma proteins; low, to erythrocytes. Binding studies confirm linear pharmacokinetics.

### Biotransformation
Bicalutamide—Hepatic; extensive. Metabolism is stereospecific. The active *R*-enantiomer is metabolized primarily by oxidation to an inactive metabolite, which, in turn, undergoes glucuronidation. The inactive *S*-enantiomer is metabolized primarily by glucuronidation. The *S*-enantiomer is cleared more rapidly than the *R*-enantiomer.
Flutamide—Hepatic; rapid and extensive. At least six metabolites have been identified. The major metabolite found in plasma is a biologically active alpha-hydroxy derivative, hydroxyflutamide. Another metabolite is 4-nitro-3-fluoro-methylaniline, which may cause aniline toxicity (e.g., cholestatic jaundice, hemolytic anemia, methemoglobinemia) in susceptible individuals.

Nilutamide—Hepatic; extensive. Five metabolites have been identified. *In vitro*, one of the metabolites showed 25 to 50% of the activity of the parent compound; the activity of the D-isomer of this metabolite was equal to or greater than that of the L-isomer.

**Half-life**
Elimination—
Bicalutamide: 5.8 days to 1 week (for the active *R*-enantiomer). Values are significantly prolonged in patients with severe hepatic function impairment, but not in patients with mild to moderate hepatic disease.
Flutamide: The half-life of the active metabolite hydroxyflutamide is approximately 6 hours. Values are prolonged in geriatric patients to approximately 8 hours following administration of a single dose and approximately 9.6 hours at steady-state, and are slightly prolonged in patients with chronic renal function impairment (creatinine clearance < 29 mL/min).
In geriatric patients, the half-life of the parent compound, flutamide, is approximately 7.8 hours at steady-state.
Nilutamide: Mean, 39 to 59.1 hours (most values between 41 and 49 hours) after a single dose of 100 to 300 mg. Although the pharmacokinetics of nilutamide's metabolites have not been investigated fully, the half-life of at least one metabolite is known to be longer than that of the parent compound (59 to 126 hours).

**Time to peak concentration**
Bicalutamide—For the active *R*-enantiomer: Mean, 31.3 hours.
Flutamide—In geriatric volunteers: 1.9 and 2.7 hours for flutamide and hydroxyflutamide, respectively, after administration of a single dose; 1.3 and 1.9 hours for flutamide and hydroxyflutamide, respectively, at steady-state.

**Peak serum concentration**
Bicalutamide—For the active *R*-enantiomer: 0.768 mcg per mL (mcg/mL).
Flutamide—In geriatric volunteers, following a single dose: 25 nanograms per mL (nanograms/mL) for flutamide and 894 nanograms/mL for hydroxyflutamide. Maximum concentrations and the area under the flutamide plasma concentration–time curve (AUC) are not altered in patients with chronic renal function impairment, but the effect of hepatic function impairment is unknown.

**Time to steady-state concentration**
Flutamide—In geriatric patients receiving 250 mg three times a day, steady-state concentrations of flutamide and hydroxyflutamide are approached after the fourth dose.
Nilutamide—In patients receiving 150 mg twice a day, steady-state conditions are reached in 2 to 4 weeks.

**Steady-state plasma concentration**
Bicalutamide—Mean, approximately 9 mcg/mL (approximately 99% of which is the active *R*-enantiomer) following administration of 50 mg per day.
Flutamide—For the active metabolite hydroxyflutamide: Mean minimum and maximum concentrations are approximately 673 and 1629 nanograms/mL, respectively.
Nilutamide—Steady-state values for the area under the nilutamide plasma concentration–time curve for 12 hours after dosing ($AUC_{0-12}$) are approximately 110% higher than single-dose values, which, together with *in vitro* metabolism data, suggests metabolic enzyme inhibition.

**Elimination**
Bicalutamide—Renal and fecal (34% and 43% of a dose, respectively, within 9 days), as glucuronide derivatives. The rate of elimination is not significantly affected by renal function impairment.
Flutamide—Primarily renal; only 4.2% of a dose is eliminated in the feces within 72 hours.
Nilutamide—Renal, 62% of a dose (< 2% as unchanged nilutamide) within 120 hours after administration of a single dose. Small quantities (1.4 to 7% of a dose) are eliminated in the feces.
In dialysis—
Because all of the nonsteroidal antiandrogens are extensively bound to plasma proteins, significant quantities are not likely to be removed from the circulation by dialysis.

# Precautions to Consider

## Carcinogenicity/Tumorigenicity
Bicalutamide—Oral carcinogenicity studies in male and female rats and mice given 5, 15, or 75 mg per kg of body weight (mg/kg) per day for 2 years showed target organ effects attributable to bicalutamide's antiandrogenic activity. Testicular benign interstitial (Leydig) cell tumors occurred in male rats at all dose levels, which provided concentrations equivalent to or higher than two thirds of the human therapeutic concentration (the concentration achieved by administering 50 mg per day to a 70-kg patient). Uterine adenocarcinomas occurred in female rats given 75 mg/kg per day (which produced concentrations equivalent to 1.5 times the human therapeutic concentration). Also, a small increase in the incidence of hepatocellular carcinoma occurred in male mice given 75 mg/kg per day (which produced concentrations equivalent to four times the human therapeutic concentration), and an increased incidence of benign thyroid follicular cell adenomas occurred in rats given 5 mg/kg per day (which produced concentrations equivalent to two thirds of the human therapeutic concentration) or more. These neoplastic changes were progressions of nonneoplastic changes related to hepatic enzyme induction (which has been observed in animal toxicity studies, but not in humans receiving up to 150 mg per day). There were no tumorigenic effects suggestive of genotoxic carcinogenesis. Leydig cell hyperplasia has not been observed in humans receiving bicalutamide.
Flutamide—Although a causal relationship has not been established, malignant breast tumors have been reported in two men receiving flutamide therapy. In animal carcinogenicity studies, testicular interstitial cell adenomas and mammary adenomas, adenocarcinomas, and fibroadenomas developed in male rats given daily oral doses of 10, 30, and 50 mg/kg per day (which produced maximum concentrations equivalent to one, two to three, and four times, respectively, the concentration produced in humans by therapeutic doses).
Nilutamide—In an 18-month study, benign Leydig cell tumors occurred in 35% of male rats given 45 mg/kg per day (which produced area under the nilutamide plasma concentration–time curve [AUC] values equivalent to one or two times the values achieved in humans receiving therapeutic doses). This effect is attributable to elevated luteinizing hormone (LH) concentrations resulting from loss of feedback inhibition, which does not occur in castrated men receiving the medication. Nilutamide had no other effect on the incidence, size, or time of onset of spontaneous tumor development in animals.

## Mutagenicity
Bicalutamide—No evidence of genotoxic activity was found in several *in vitro* and *in vivo* tests (including yeast gene conversion, Ames, *E. coli*, CHO/HGPRT, human lymphocyte cytogenetic, mouse micronucleus, and rat bone marrow cytogenetic tests).
Flutamide—No evidence of mutagenicity was found in the Ames *Salmonella*/microsome mutagenesis assay or in the dominant lethal test in rats.
Nilutamide—No evidence of mutagenicity was found in a variety of *in vitro* and *in vivo* tests, including the Ames test, mouse micronucleus test, and two chromosomal aberration studies.

## Pregnancy/Reproduction
Note: The effect on fertility and reproduction of other treatments used concurrently with the nonsteroidal antiandrogen, i.e., luteinizing hormone–releasing hormone (LHRH) analog therapy or bilateral orchiectomy, must be considered.

Fertility—
*Bicalutamide*: May inhibit spermatogenesis. Long-term effects on male fertility have not been studied in humans. In male rats given 250 mg/kg per day (which produced concentrations equivalent to two times the human therapeutic concentration), the precoital interval and time to successful mating were increased in the first pairing, but no effects on fertility after successful mating were seen. Observed effects were reversed by 7 weeks after the end of an 11-week treatment period. There were no effects on female rats given 10, 50, or 250 mg/kg per day (which produced concentrations equivalent to two thirds, one, and two times the human therapeutic concentration, respectively).
*Flutamide*: Flutamide monotherapy caused decreased sperm counts in a 6-week study in humans. In animal studies, flutamide had no effect on the estrous cycle and caused no interference with the mating behavior of female and male rats given 25 or 75 mg/kg per day prior to mating. Although males treated with 150 mg/kg per day (30 times the minimum effective antiandrogenic dose) failed to mate, mating behavior returned to normal after the medication was discontinued. Conception rates were decreased at all dosage levels. Also, suppression of spermatogenesis occurred in rats given approximately 3, 8, or 17 times the human dose for 52 weeks and in dogs given 1.4, 2.3, and 3.7 times the human dose for 78 weeks.
*Nilutamide*: Studies in male and female rats showed no effect on reproductive function with doses as high as 45 mg/kg per day (which produced AUC values one to two times those achieved in humans receiving therapeutic doses).

Pregnancy—There are currently no indications in U.S. or Canadian product labeling for use of any of the nonsteroidal antiandrogens in female patients. However, if a nonsteroidal antiandrogen is given to a female of child-bearing potential (e.g., administration of flutamide for hirsutism), it must be used in conjunction with adequate contraception because of the risk of causing feminization of a male fetus.
*Bicalutamide*—
Animal studies revealed no adverse effects on the female offspring of rats given 10, 50, or 250 mg/kg per day (which produced

concentrations equivalent to two thirds, one, and two times the human therapeutic concentration, respectively). However, reduced anogenital distance and feminization leading to hypospadias and impotence occurred in the male offspring. No other teratogenic effects were found in rabbits receiving up to 200 mg/kg per day or in rats receiving up to 250 mg/kg per day (which produced concentrations equivalent to approximately one third and two times the human therapeutic concentration, respectively).

FDA Pregnancy Category X.

*Flutamide*—
Studies in rats given 30, 100, or 200 mg/kg per day (3, 9, and 19 times the human dose, respectively) found a decrease in 24-hour survival of offspring. In addition, at the two higher doses, feminization of male offspring and a slight increase in minor variations in the development of the sternebrae and vertebrae occurred. Studies in rabbits at a dose of 15 mg/kg per day (1.4 times the human dose) found a decreased survival rate in offspring.

FDA Pregnancy Category D.

*Nilutamide*—
Studies in humans have not been done. Studies in rats given up to 45 mg/kg per day (which produced AUC values one to two times the values produced in humans by therapeutic doses) showed no lethal, teratogenic, or growth-suppressive effects.

FDA Pregnancy Category C.

## Breast-feeding

There are currently no indications in U.S. or Canadian product labeling for use of any of the nonsteroidal antiandrogens in female patients. It is not known whether any of these medications is distributed into breast milk. However, it is recommended that breast-feeding be avoided by any woman who might be receiving a nonsteroidal antiandrogen (e.g., flutamide therapy for hirsutism) because of the potential risks to the infant (adverse developmental and toxic effects).

## Pediatrics

Studies with the nonsteroidal antiandrogens have not been done in pediatric patients. Safety and efficacy have not been established. Possible adverse effects on the sexual development of young males must be considered.

## Geriatrics

Appropriate studies performed to date have not demonstrated geriatrics-specific problems that would limit the use of any of the nonsteroidal antiandrogens in geriatric patients.
*Bicalutamide*: Pharmacokinetic studies in patients receiving up to 150 mg of bicalutamide per day have shown that steady-state concentrations of total bicalutamide and its active enantiomer are not significantly different in geriatric patients than in younger adults.
*Flutamide*: Although the elimination half-life of flutamide and its active metabolite hydroxyflutamide are increased in the elderly, no adjustment of dosage on the basis of age is needed.

## Pharmacogenetics

*Nilutamide*: A significantly higher incidence of interstitial pneumonitis (17% versus 2% in the overall patient population) and a higher frequency of increased transaminase values occurred in a small study performed in Japan. There were no significant differences in the pharmacokinetics of nilutamide in these patients, compared with Caucasian patients, that might account for this finding. Caution in the treatment of Asian patients is recommended.

## Drug interactions and/or related problems

The following drug interactions and/or related problems have been selected on the basis of their potential clinical significance (possible mechanism in parentheses where appropriate)—not necessarily inclusive (» = major clinical significance):

Note: Combinations containing any of the following medications, depending on the amount present, may also interact with this medication.

*For flutamide and nilutamide only*
» Anticoagulants, coumarin-derivative
(caution and increased monitoring of prothrombin time [PT] or International Normalized Ratio [INR] are recommended if treatment with flutamide or nilutamide is initiated in a patient stabilized on a coumarin-derivative anticoagulant. Increases in PT have occurred after flutamide therapy was started in patients receiving long-term warfarin treatment. Also, inhibition of hepatic cytochrome P450 [CYP 450] isoenzymes by nilutamide, which may interfere with anticoagulant metabolism, may result in increased anticoagulant activity during concurrent use. Adjustment of anticoagulant dosage may be necessary)

*For nilutamide only (in addition to the interaction listed above)*
» Alcohol
(alcohol intolerance, characterized by symptoms of facial flushing, malaise, and hypotension, has been reported in approximately 5% of patients treated with nilutamide; patients who experience such reactions should be advised to avoid further alcohol consumption during nilutamide therapy)

» Medications with narrow therapeutic margins that are metabolized by hepatic CYP 450 isoenzymes, such as:
Phenytoin
Theophylline
(inhibition of hepatic CYP 450 isoenzymes by nilutamide may result in delayed elimination, increased elimination half-life, and increased risk of toxicity of medications that are metabolized by these enzymes; dosage reduction, especially of medications with narrow therapeutic margins, may be necessary during concurrent use)

## Laboratory value alterations

The following have been selected on the basis of their potential clinical significance (possible effect in parentheses where appropriate)—not necessarily inclusive (» = major clinical significance):

With physiology/laboratory test values
» Alanine aminotransferase (ALT [SGPT]), serum, and
» Aspartate aminotransferase (AST [SGOT]), serum
(may be increased; rarely, may indicate hepatitis or jaundice)

Alkaline phosphatase, serum
(may be increased)

Bilirubin, serum or
Blood urea nitrogen (BUN) or
Creatinine, serum
(concentrations may be increased)

Estradiol, plasma or
Testosterone, plasma
(concentrations may be increased if a nonsteroidal antiandrogen is administered without an LHRH analog to a patient who has not undergone bilateral orchiectomy)

Glucose, blood
(concentrations may be increased, possibly to hyperglycemic levels, with bicalutamide or nilutamide)

Hemoglobin values or
White blood cell count
(may be decreased)

## Medical considerations/Contraindications

The medical considerations/contraindications included have been selected on the basis of their potential clinical significance (reasons given in parentheses where appropriate)—not necessarily inclusive (» = major clinical significance).

*Except under special circumstances, this medication should not be used when the following medical problems exist:*

*For nilutamide only*
» Hepatic function impairment
(use of nilutamide is not recommended because the medication has been reported to cause substantial hepatotoxicity, which may have particularly serious consequences in patients with pre-existing hepatic function impairment)

» Respiratory impairment, severe
(use of nilutamide is not recommended because the medication has caused interstitial pneumonitis in clinical trials; the frequency of occurrence was substantially higher in Japanese patients than in the overall patient population)

*Risk-benefit should be considered when the following medical problems exist:*

*For all nonsteroidal antiandrogens*
» Hypersensitivity to the nonsteroidal antiandrogen considered for use, history of

*For bicalutamide only (in addition to the medical problem listed above for all nonsteroidal antiandrogens)*
» Hepatic function impairment, moderate to severe
(metabolism of bicalutamide may be delayed, resulting in prolonged elimination half-life and increased risk of toxicity)

*For flutamide only (in addition to the medical problem listed above for all nonsteroidal antiandrogens)*
Conditions predisposing to aniline toxicity, such as:
Glucose-6–phosphate dehydrogenase (G6PD) deficiency or
Hemoglobin M disease or
Tobacco smoking

(increased risk of toxicity associated with aniline exposure, such as methemoglobinemia, hemolytic anemia, and cholestatic jaundice [one metabolite of flutamide is a methylaniline derivative])

» Hepatic function impairment
(use of flutamide should be carefully considered, especially in patients with moderate or severe hepatic function impairment, because it may cause severe hepatotoxicity, which may have particularly serious consequences in patients with pre-existing hepatic function impairment)

**Patient monitoring**

The following may be especially important in patient monitoring (other tests may be warranted in some patients, depending on condition; » = major clinical significance):

*For all nonsteroidal antiandrogens*
» Hepatic function tests
(determinations recommended prior to nilutamide therapy because nilutamide should not be used in patients with pre-existing hepatic function abnormalities)
(recommended periodically during therapy with flutamide, recommended every 3 months during treatment with nilutamide, and should be considered during long-term use of bicalutamide, because of the possibility of transaminase elevations and hepatotoxicity during treatment. Treatment should be discontinued immediately if there is laboratory evidence of hepatic injury [e.g., transaminase values higher than two or three times the upper limit of normal] in the absence of hepatic metastases, or if clinical signs and symptoms of hepatotoxicity [e.g., jaundice, pruritus, dark urine, fatigue, persistent anorexia, abdominal pain or upper right quadrant tenderness, unexplained "flu-like" symptoms, unexplained gastrointestinal symptoms] occur. Hepatotoxicity is usually reversible after discontinuation of therapy, but hepatotoxicity-related deaths have been reported, rarely, in patients receiving flutamide or nilutamide)

Prostate specific antigen (PSA), serum
(may be helpful in assessing response to treatment; the patient should be re-evaluated for disease progression if values rise during therapy)

*For flutamide only (in addition to the tests listed above for all nonsteroidal antiandrogens)*
Methemoglobin concentrations
(monitoring recommended in patients susceptible to aniline toxicity)

*For nilutamide only (in addition to the tests listed above for all nonsteroidal antiandrogens)*
Chest radiograph
(recommended prior to initiation of therapy and at the first sign of new or increasing dyspnea or other indication of possible pneumonitis; if there are findings suggestive of interstitial pneumonitis, nilutamide should be discontinued)

Pulmonary function studies, including diffusing capacity of the lung for carbon monoxide (DL$_{CO}$)
(recommended if a chest radiograph performed to evaluate onset or worsening of dyspnea is normal; if DL$_{CO}$ is significantly decreased and/or a restrictive pattern is observed, nilutamide should be discontinued)

## Side/Adverse Effects

Note: The side/adverse effects listed below for bicalutamide and for flutamide were reported during concurrent use of the antiandrogen with a luteinizing hormone–releasing hormone (LHRH) analog. For flutamide, the reported effects occurred in long-term studies in patients with Stage D$_2$ prostatic carcinoma. In a relatively short-term study in which the medications were given in conjunction with radiation therapy for Stage B$_2$ or Stage C disease, the reported adverse effects (i.e., diarrhea, cystitis, rectal bleeding, proctitis, hematuria) were not significantly different or more frequent than with radiation therapy alone. The side/adverse effects listed below for nilutamide were reported in two separate studies in which the medication was used in conjunction with bilateral orchiectomy or with an LHRH analog. Many adverse effects occurred exclusively or significantly more often with the nilutamide plus LHRH analog regimen; only the higher frequency of occurrence is reported below. Placebo-controlled clinical trials with flutamide or nilutamide showed that many of the adverse effects, especially those related to low androgen activity (i.e., hot flashes, impotence, loss of libido, gynecomastia) may occur with an LHRH analog or bilateral orchiectomy alone.

In addition to the side/adverse effects listed below, urogenital effects including hematuria, urinary tract infections, and dysuria or urinary retention have been reported during treatment with these medications. Such symptoms commonly occur in men with prostatic tumors and may improve, as a result of tumor regression, during successful antiandrogen therapy.

| The following side/adverse effects have been selected on the basis of their potential clinical significance (possible signs and symptoms in parentheses where appropriate)—not necessarily inclusive:* | Legend:<br>I=Bicalutamide<br>II=Flutamide<br>III=Nilutamide | | |
|---|---|---|---|
| | I | II | III |
| **Medical attention needed** | | | |
| *Anemia*† (unusual tiredness or weakness)—usually asymptomatic | L | L | L |
| *Dyspnea* (shortness of breath or difficult breathing) | L | U | L |
| *Edema* (swelling of face, fingers, feet, or lower legs) | L | L | M |
| *Fever* | L | U | L |
| *Gastrointestinal or rectal bleeding* (bloody or black, tarry stools) | L | U | R |
| *Hepatitis or jaundice, including cholestatic jaundice*‡ (dark urine; "flu-like" symptoms; gastrointestinal upset; loss of appetite; nausea or vomiting; pain or tenderness in upper right area of abdomen; unusual tiredness; yellow eyes or skin) | R | R | R |
| *Hypertension*—usually asymptomatic | L | R | L |
| *Infection, including pulmonary or upper respiratory tract infection*§ (cough or hoarseness; fever; runny nose; shortness of breath, troubled breathing, tightness in chest, or wheezing; sneezing; sore throat) | M | U | M |
| *Itching of skin* | L | R | L |
| *Leukopenia* (cough or hoarseness; fever or chills; lower back or side pain; painful or difficult urination)—usually asymptomatic | U | L | U |
| *Mental depression* | L | R | L |
| *Methemoglobinemia* (bluish-colored lips, fingernails, or palms of hands; dizziness, severe, or fainting; feeling of severe pressure in head; shortness of breath; weak and fast heartbeat)—usually asymptomatic | U | U# | U |
| *Neuromuscular symptoms or neuropathy* (numbness, tingling, pain, or muscle weakness in hands, arms, feet, or legs) | L | L | U |
| *Pulmonary disorder*** (chest pain; cough; shortness of breath or troubled breathing) | L | R | L |
| *Skin rash* | L | L†† | L |
| *Thrombocytopenia* (black, tarry stools; blood in urine or stools; pinpoint red spots on skin; unusual bleeding or bruising) | U | R | U |
| **Medical attention needed only if continuing or bothersome** | | | |
| *Alcohol intolerance* (dizziness or lightheadedness; feeling faint; flushing of face; general feeling of illness) | U | U | L |
| *Bloated feeling, gas, or indigestion* | L | U# | L |
| *Chills* | L | U | U |
| *Confusion* | L | R | U |
| *Constipation* | M | U# | M |
| *Decrease in or loss of appetite* | L | L | M |
| *Diarrhea*‡‡ | M | M | L |
| *Dizziness* | L | R | M |
| *Drowsiness* | L | R | R |
| *Dryness of mouth* | L | L | L |
| *Flu-like syndrome* (fever; headache; muscle or joint pain; tiredness) | L | U | L |
| *Gynecomastia* (pain or tenderness in breasts; swelling of breasts) | L | L | M |
| *Headache* | L | R | M |
| *Impaired adaptation of eyes to dark* (delay in seeing clearly when going from light to dark areas)—effect may last from seconds to minutes | U | U | M |
| *Impotence or decrease in sexual desire* | L | M | M |
| *Nausea* | M | M | M |
| *Nervousness* | L | R | L |

The following side/adverse effects have been selected on the basis of their potential clinical significance (possible signs and symptoms in parentheses where appropriate)—not necessarily inclusive:*

Legend:
I = Bicalutamide
II = Flutamide
III = Nilutamide

| | I | II | III |
|---|---|---|---|
| *Trouble in sleeping* | L | R | M |
| *Visual disturbances, including chromatopsia* (change in color vision) *and impaired adaptation or increased sensitivity to light* | U | U | L |
| *Vomiting* | L | L | L |
| *Weakness* | M | R | M |
| **Medical attention not needed** | | | |
| *Hot flashes* (feeling of warmth; flushing; sudden sweating) | M | M | M |
| *Urine discoloration* (amber or yellow-green urine coloration)—attributed to presence of flutamide or its metabolites | U | U# | U |

*Differences in frequency of occurrence may reflect either lack of clinical-use data or actual pharmacologic distinctions among agents. M = more frequent (10% or higher); L = less frequent (> 1% to < 10%); R = rare (1% or lower); U = unknown.

†Hypochromic anemia and iron deficiency anemia have been reported with bicalutamide. In addition to unspecified anemia(s), there have been postmarketing reports of hemolytic anemia and macrocytic anemia with flutamide, and, although a causal relationship has not been established, of aplastic anemia with nilutamide.

‡Hepatotoxicity, especially when detected by hepatic function test abnormalities before symptoms occur, usually resolves when therapy is withdrawn. However, progression to hepatic encephalopathy and hepatic necrosis has been reported with flutamide, and fatalities have been reported with flutamide and nilutamide.

§Bronchitis, pneumonia, sepsis, and other unspecified infections have been reported during bicalutamide therapy, and upper respiratory tract infections and pneumonia have been reported during nilutamide therapy.

#Has been reported, generally postmarketing; actual frequency of occurrence unknown.

**Interstitial pneumonitis has been reported with nilutamide, unspecified pulmonary symptoms have been reported with flutamide, and other unspecified lung disorder(s) have been reported with bicalutamide and nilutamide. Signs of nilutamide-associated interstitial pneumonitis, including interstitial or alveolo-interstitial changes in the chest radiograph, usually occur within the first 3 months of nilutamide therapy and are usually reversible upon discontinuation of therapy.

††There also have been reports of photosensitivity-associated erythema, ulceration, bullous eruptions, and epidermal necrolysis during flutamide therapy.

‡‡In a clinical trial comparing the efficacy and toxicity of bicalutamide and flutamide, each in conjunction with an LHRH agonist, severe diarrhea resulting in discontinuation of therapy occurred substantially more often with flutamide than with bicalutamide.

## Overdose

For more information on the management of overdose or unintentional ingestion, **contact a Poison Control Center** (see *Poison Control Center Listing*).

Bicalutamide: A single dose that would result in potentially life-threatening symptoms has not been established. Doses as high as 200 mg per day (four times the usual daily dose) were well tolerated in clinical trials. Also, bicalutamide showed low acute toxicity in animal studies. It has been estimated that doses in excess of 2000 mg per kg of body weight (mg/kg) would be required to produce significant mortality in mice and rats.

Flutamide: A single dose that would result in potentially life-threatening symptoms has not been established. Doses as high as 1500 mg per day (two times the usual daily dose), given for up to 36 weeks in clinical trials, caused gynecomastia, breast tenderness, and increased hepatic enzyme concentrations, all of which have been reported with usual adult doses. Signs of acute overdosage in animal studies included hypoactivity, piloerection, ataxia, lacrimation, anorexia, emesis, methemoglobinemia, tranquilization, and slow respiration.

In chronic toxicity studies in beagle dogs, flutamide caused cardiac lesions, including chronic myxomatous degeneration, intra-atrial fibrosis, myocardial acidophilic degeneration, vasculitis, and perivasculitis, in 2 of 10 animals given 25 mg/kg per day for 78 weeks and in 3 of 16 animals given 40 mg/kg per day for 2 to 4 years. These doses produced hydroxyflutamide concentrations 1- to 12-fold higher than those present in humans receiving therapeutic doses.

Nilutamide: There has been one report of massive overdosage, in which a 79-year-old man ingested 13 grams of nilutamide (43 times the maximum recommended dose). Although gastric lavage was performed and active charcoal was given orally, plasma nilutamide concentrations peaked at six times the usual therapeutic range, and concentrations 3.5 times the usual therapeutic range were present 72 hours after ingestion. Symptoms were limited to moderate vomiting and diarrhea during the first 12 hours, and the patient recovered. In repeated-dose tolerance studies, doses of 600 and 900 mg per day (up to three to six times the usual daily dose), administered to nine and four patients, respectively, caused nausea, vomiting, malaise, headache, and dizziness, but no major toxicity, although hepatic enzyme concentrations were increased transiently in one patient.

In chronic toxicity studies in beagle dogs, fatalities related to hepatotoxicity occurred in 100% of the animals given 60 mg/kg per day for 1 month; 70% and 20% of the animals given 30 or 20 mg/kg per day, respectively, for 6 months; and 50%, 33%, and 8% of the animals given 12, 6, or 3 mg/kg per day, respectively, for 1 year. Hepatocellular swelling and vacuolization were found in the affected animals. However, hepatotoxicity was not consistently associated with elevated hepatic enzyme concentrations.

In chronic toxicity studies in rats, administration of 45 mg/kg per day of nilutamide for 18 months caused lung pathology (granulomatous inflammation and chronic alveolitis).

**Treatment of overdose**

There is no specific antidote to overdose with these agents. Vomiting may be induced if the patient is alert and does not vomit spontaneously. Dialysis is not likely to remove significant quantities of these medications from the body because of extensive protein binding. General supportive care, including frequent monitoring of vital signs and close observation of the patient, is recommended, with treatment of observed symptoms as warranted.

Patients in whom intentional overdose is confirmed or suspected should be referred for psychiatric consultation.

## Patient Consultation

As an aid to patient consultation, refer to *Advice for the Patient, Antiandrogens, Nonsteroidal (Systemic)*.

In providing consultation, consider emphasizing the following selected information (» = major clinical significance):

**Before using this medication**
» Conditions affecting use, especially:
  Sensitivity to the nonsteroidal antiandrogen considered for use
  Fertility—Nonsteroidal antiandrogens, and other treatments used concurrently for prostatic carcinoma, may decrease sperm count and impair fertility
  Pregnancy—Adequate contraception essential if being given to a woman of child-bearing potential because of the risk of causing feminization of a male fetus
  Breast-feeding—Not recommended because of the potential for causing adverse developmental and toxic effects in the infant
  Pharmacogenetics—For nilutamide only: Caution in Asian patients because of increased risk of interstitial pneumonitis
  Other medications, especially coumarin-derivative anticoagulants (for flutamide and nilutamide), and, for nilutamide only, alcohol and medications with narrow therapeutic margins metabolized by hepatic cytochrome P450 isoenzymes (e.g., phenytoin, theophylline)
  Other medical problems, especially hepatic function impairment and, for nilutamide only, respiratory impairment

**Proper use of this medication**
» Importance of not using more or less medication than the amount prescribed
» Taking medication at the same time each day
  Bicalutamide and nilutamide may be taken with or without food
» Importance of following physician's instructions for concurrent use of LHRH analog (if patient has not undergone bilateral orchiectomy)
» Importance of continuing medication despite side effects
  Checking with physician if vomiting occurs shortly after dose is taken
» Proper dosing
  Missed dose: Taking as soon as possible; not taking if not remembered until next day (bicalutamide or nilutamide) or almost time for next dose (flutamide); not doubling doses
» Proper storage

**Precautions while using this medication**
» Importance of regular visits to physician to monitor progress
» Checking with physician immediately if symptoms of hepatotoxicity occur

*For nilutamide only*
» Checking with physician immediately if shortness of breath occurs or worsens

- » Possible ocular effects, including delay in visual adaptation from light to dark (which may persist for several seconds to several minutes), delayed adaptation from dark to light, and increased sensitivity of eyes to light; using caution when driving, especially after entering or emerging from tunnels; tinted glasses may alleviate these effects
- » Avoiding further alcohol ingestion if symptoms of alcohol intolerance (facial flushing, malaise, hypotension) occur

**Side/adverse effects**
  Signs of potential side effects, especially anemia, dyspnea or other symptoms of a pulmonary disorder, edema, fever or other sign of infection (bicalutamide, nilutamide), gastrointestinal or rectal bleeding (bicalutamide, nilutamide), hepatitis or jaundice, hypertension, itching of skin, leukopenia (flutamide), mental depression, methemoglobinemia (flutamide), neuromuscular symptoms or neuropathy (bicalutamide, flutamide), skin rash, and thrombocytopenia (flutamide)

## General Dosing Information

Patients taking a nonsteroidal antiandrogen should be under supervision of a physician experienced in cancer chemotherapy.

---
### BICALUTAMIDE
---

## Summary of Differences

Indications:
  Indicated, in conjunction with medical or surgical castration, for treatment of advanced or metastatic prostatic carcinoma.
Pharmacology/pharmacokinetics:
  Physicochemical characteristics—A racemate; only the R-enantiomer is active.
  Other actions/effects—Induction of hepatic enzymes has been demonstrated in animal studies, but not in humans receiving up to 150 mg per day (three times the recommended daily dose).
  Protein binding—Very high (96%).
  Biotransformation—Stereospecific; the inactive S-enantiomer is cleared more rapidly than the active R-enantiomer.
  Half-life (elimination)—5.8 days to 1 week for the active R-enantiomer.
  Time to peak concentration—31.3 hours for the active R-enantiomer.
  Peak serum concentration—0.768 mcg per mL for the active R-enantiomer.
  Steady-state plasma concentration (dose of 50 mg per day)—9 mcg per mL, approximately 99% of which is the active R-enantiomer.
  Elimination—Renal and fecal, as glucuronide derivatives. The rate of elimination is not significantly affected by renal function impairment.
Precautions to consider:
  Medical considerations/contraindications—Risk-benefit should be considered in patients with moderate to severe hepatic function impairment.
  Patient monitoring—Periodic assessment of hepatic function should be considered during long-term use.
Side/adverse effects:
  Hypochromic and iron deficiency anemia have been reported.
  Bronchitis, pneumonia, sepsis, other unspecified infections, and other unspecified lung disorders have been reported.

## Additional Dosing Information

Treatment with bicalutamide should be initiated at the same time as treatment with a luteinizing hormone–releasing hormone (LHRH) analog or surgical castration.

Bicalutamide should be taken at the same time every day (usually in the morning or evening).

No dosage adjustment is needed in patients with renal function impairment or mild hepatic function impairment.

Bicalutamide may be taken with food or on an empty stomach.

## Oral Dosage Forms

### BICALUTAMIDE TABLETS

**Usual adult dose**
Carcinoma, prostatic—
  Oral, 50 mg once a day, in the morning or evening. The medication is to be used concurrently with an LHRH analog or after surgical castration.

**Usual pediatric dose**
Safety, efficacy, and dosage have not been established.

**Usual geriatric dose**
See *Usual adult dose*.

**Strength(s) usually available**
U.S.—
  50 mg (Rx) [*Casodex* (lactose)].
Canada—
  50 mg (Rx) [*Casodex* (lactose)].

**Packaging and storage**
Store between 15 and 30 °C (59 and 86 °F).

---
### FLUTAMIDE
---

## Summary of Differences

Indications:
  Indicated, in conjunction with medical or surgical castration, for treatment of advanced or metastatic prostatic carcinoma.
Pharmacology/pharmacokinetics:
  Protein binding—Very high (94 to 96% for flutamide, 92 to 94% for the active metabolite).
  Biotransformation—Major metabolite hydroxyflutamide is active antiandrogenic substance; another metabolite is an aniline derivative that may cause aniline toxicity.
  Half-life (elimination)—For hydroxyflutamide, approximately 6 hours; may be prolonged in geriatric patients and in patients with chronic renal function impairment.
  Time to peak concentration (in geriatric volunteers)—For hydroxyflutamide, 2.7 and 1.9 hours after administration of a single dose and at steady-state, respectively. For flutamide, 1.9 and 1.3 hours after administration of a single dose and at steady-state, respectively.
  Peak serum concentration (geriatric volunteers, following a single dose)—25 and 894 nanograms per mL for flutamide and hydroxyflutamide, respectively; not affected by chronic renal function impairment.
  Time to steady-state concentration (administration three times a day)—Steady-state conditions approached after the fourth dose.
  Steady-state concentration (hydroxyflutamide)—Mean minimum and maximum concentrations are approximately 673 and 1629 nanograms per mL, respectively.
  Elimination—Primarily renal; small quantities eliminated in the feces.
Precautions to consider:
  Pregnancy—Decreased survival rates and minor variations in development of sternebrae and vertebrae demonstrated in animal studies.
  Drug interactions and/or related problems—Increase in prothrombin time reported in patients receiving concurrent therapy with coumarin-derivative anticoagulant.
  Medical considerations/contraindications—Caution also recommended in conditions predisposing to aniline toxicity.
  Patient monitoring—Periodic assessment of hepatic function (all patients) and methemoglobin concentrations (patients at risk for aniline toxicity) recommended.
Side/adverse effects:
  Hepatotoxicity progressing to hepatic encephalopathy, hepatic necrosis, and fatalities has been reported.
  Hemolytic anemia, macrocytic anemia, leukopenia, methemoglobinemia, and thrombocytopenia have been reported.
  Unspecified pulmonary symptoms and photosensitivity-associated erythema, ulcerations, bullous eruptions, and epidermal necrolysis have also been reported.
  More likely than bicalutamide to cause severe diarrhea requiring discontinuation of treatment.

## Additional Dosing Information

When flutamide is used for the treatment of Stage $B_2$ or Stage C carcinoma, treatment should begin simultaneously with, or 24 hours prior to, initiation of LHRH analog therapy. Treatment with both agents should commence 8 weeks prior to, and continue throughout, radiation therapy. When flutamide is used in conjunction with an LHRH analog for treatment of metastatic (Stage $D_2$) carcinoma, therapy should begin simultaneously with, or 24 hours prior to, initiation of LHRH analog therapy. Treatment should continue until disease progression is documented.

## Oral Dosage Forms

### FLUTAMIDE CAPSULES USP

**Usual adult dose**
Carcinoma, prostatic—
  Oral, 250 mg every eight hours.

**Usual pediatric dose**
Dosage has not been established.

**Usual geriatric dose**
See *Usual adult dose.*

**Strength(s) usually available**
U.S.—
  125 mg (Rx) [*Eulexin* (lactose)].
Canada—
  Not commercially available.

**Packaging and storage**
Store below 40 °C (104 °F), preferably between 15 and 30 °C (59 and 86 °F). Store in a well-closed, light-resistant container.

### FLUTAMIDE TABLETS
**Usual adult dose**
See *Flutamide Capsules USP.*

**Usual pediatric dose**
Dosage has not been established.

**Usual geriatric dose**
See *Flutamide Capsules USP.*

**Strength(s) usually available**
U.S.—
  Not commercially available.
Canada—
  250 mg (Rx) [*Euflex* (scored; lactose)].

**Packaging and storage**
Store below 40 °C (104 °F), preferably between 15 and 30 °C (59 and 86 °F), in a well-closed container, unless otherwise specified by the manufacturer.

---

## NILUTAMIDE

## Summary of Differences
Indications:
  Indicated, in conjunction with surgical or medical castration, for treatment of metastatic prostatic carcinoma. Should be used only in patients with normal hepatic function.
Pharmacology/pharmacokinetics:
  Other actions/effects—Inhibits hepatic cytochrome P450 (CYP 450) isoenzymes.
  Protein binding—Moderate (84%), to plasma proteins; low, to erythrocytes.
  Biotransformation—One metabolite has 25 to 50% of the antiandrogenic activity of the parent compound.
  Half-life (elimination)—Mean, 39 to 59.1 hours (mostly between 41 and 49 hours).
  Time to steady-state concentration (doses of 150 mg twice a day)—2 to 4 weeks.
  Elimination—Primarily renal; small quantities eliminated in the feces.
Precautions to consider:
  Pharmacogenetics—Caution in administration to Asian patients recommended; increased risk of interstitial pneumonitis has been demonstrated in Japanese patients.
  Drug interactions and/or related problems—Caution also required with medications with narrow therapeutic margins that are metabolized by hepatic CYP 450 isoenzymes (e.g., coumarin-derivative anticoagulants, phenytoin, theophylline); also, has caused alcohol intolerance in some patients.
  Medical considerations/contraindications—Use in patients with hepatic function impairment or severe respiratory impairment not recommended.
  Patient monitoring—Hepatic function should be assessed prior to initiation of treatment and every 3 months during therapy.

Side/adverse effects:
  Fatality associated with hepatotoxicity has been reported.
  Pneumonia, upper respiratory tract infections, and interstitial pneumonitis and other unspecified lung disorders have been reported.
  Visual disturbances, including impaired adaptation of eyes to dark or light, chromatopsia, and ocular photosensitivity have been reported.

## Additional Dosing Information
For maximum benefit, it is recommended that nilutamide therapy be initiated on the same day as or the day after surgical castration.

Nilutamide may be taken with food or on an empty stomach.

At the first sign of dyspnea or worsening of pre-existing dyspnea, it is recommended that nilutamide be withheld and a chest radiograph obtained. If signs of interstitial pneumonitis are seen, it is recommended that nilutamide therapy be discontinued. If the chest radiograph is normal, pulmonary function tests including $DL_{CO}$ (diffusing capacity of the lung for carbon monoxide) are recommended. A significant decrease in $DL_{CO}$ and/or a restrictive pattern observed on pulmonary function testing is cause for discontinuing nilutamide therapy. If neither chest radiograph nor pulmonary function test findings confirm interstitial pneumonitis, nilutamide treatment may be reinstituted with close monitoring of pulmonary symptoms.

At the first sign or symptom of hepatotoxicity, nilutamide should be withheld and appropriate laboratory testing performed. If serum transaminases exceed three times the upper limit of normal, nilutamide therapy should be discontinued immediately.

## Oral Dosage Forms
### NILUTAMIDE TABLETS
**Usual adult dose**
Carcinoma, prostatic—
  Oral, 300 mg once a day for thirty days, then 150 mg once a day thereafter.
  Note: If the patient is unable to tolerate the 300-mg dose, the lower dose may be instituted earlier.

**Usual pediatric dose**
Safety and efficacy have not been established.

**Usual geriatric dose**
See *Usual adult dose.*

**Strength(s) usually available**
U.S.—
  50 mg (Rx) [*Nilandron* (lactose)].
Canada—
  50 mg (Rx) [*Anandron* (lactose)].

**Packaging and storage**
Store between 15 and 30 °C (59 and 86 °F), protected from light.

**Auxiliary labeling**
• Protect from light.

## Selected Bibliography
Smith JA Jr, Janknegt RA, Abbou CC, et al. Effect of androgen deprivation therapy on local symptoms and tumour progression in men with metastatic carcinoma of the prostate. Eur Urol 1997; 31 Suppl 3: 25-9.
Schellhammer PF, Sharifi R, Block NL, et al. Clinical benefits of bicalutamide compared with flutamide in combined androgen blockade for patients with advanced prostatic carcinoma: final report of a double-blind, randomized, multicenter trial. Urology 1997; 50: 330-6.

Developed: 06/22/98
Interim revision: 08/13/98

---

# ANTICHOLINERGICS/ANTISPASMODICS Systemic

This monograph includes information on the following: 1) Anisotropine†; 2) Atropine; 3) Belladonna†; 4) Clidinium†; 5) Dicyclomine; 6) Glycopyrrolate; 7) Homatropine†; 8) Hyoscyamine; 9) Mepenzolate†; 10) Methantheline†; 11) Methscopolamine*†; 12) Pirenzepine*; 13) Propantheline; 14) Scopolamine.
INN:
  Anisotropine—Octatropine
  Dicyclomine—Dicycloverine
  Glycopyrrolate—Glycopyrronium Bromide
  Methantheline—Methanthelinium
  Methscopolamine—Hyoscine Methobromide

VA CLASSIFICATION (Primary/Secondary):
Anisotropine—AU350/GA801
Atropine
  Oral—AU350/GA801; GU201; AD900
  Parenteral—AU350/GA801; CV300; GU201; AD900
Belladonna—AU350/GA801
Clidinium—AU350/GA801
Dicyclomine—AU350/GA801
Glycopyrrolate
  Oral—AU350/GA801; GA250
  Parenteral—AU350/GA801; CV300; GA250; AD900

Homatropine—AU350/GA801
Hyoscyamine
    Oral—AU350/GA801; GU201
    Parenteral—AU350/GA801; GU201; CV300; AD900
Mepenzolate—AU350/GA801
Methantheline—AU350/GA801; GU201
Methscopolamine—AU350/GA801
Pirenzepine—AU350/GA801
Propantheline—AU350
Scopolamine
    Oral—AU350/GA801; CN550; GA650; GU201
    Parenteral—AU350/GA801; CV300; CN206; CN550; GA650
    Rectal—AU350
    Transdermal—CN550

Commonly used brand name(s): *A-Spas S/L*[8]; *Anaspaz*[8]; *Banthine*[10]; *Bentyl*[5]; *Bentylol*[5]; *Buscopan*[14]; *Cantil*[9]; *Cystospaz*[8]; *Cystospaz-M*[8]; *Donnamar*[8]; *ED-SPAZ*[8]; *Formulex*[5]; *Gastrosed*[8]; *Gastrozepin*[12]; *Homapin*[7]; *Levbid*[8]; *Levsin*[8]; *Levsin/SL*[8]; *Levsinex Timecaps*[8]; *Pro-Banthine*[13]; *Propanthel*[13]; *Quarzan*[4]; *Robinul*[6]; *Robinul Forte*[6]; *Spasmoban*[5]; *Symax SL*[8]; *Symax SR*[8]; *Transderm-Scop*[14]; *Transderm-V*[14].

Other commonly used names are: Dicycloverine [Dicyclomine], Glycopyrronium bromide [Glycopyrrolate], Hyoscine hydrobromide [Scopolamine], Hyoscine methobromide [Methscopolamine*[†]], Methanthelinium [Methantheline[†]], Octatropine [Anisotropine[†]].

Note: For a listing of dosage forms and brand names by country availability, see *Dosage Forms* section(s).

*Not commercially available in U.S.
[†]Not commercially available in Canada.

## Category

Note: All of these medications have anticholinergic and, to some extent, antispasmodic actions; however, the labeled indications for specific agents may vary because of minor differences in potency and/or receptor selectivity. **In general, there is a lack of specific testing and/or clinical-use data to support the indication of anticholinergics/antispasmodics in most conditions.**

Anticholinergic—Anisotropine; Atropine; Belladonna; Clidinium; Dicyclomine; Glycopyrrolate; Homatropine; Hyoscyamine; Mepenzolate; Methantheline; Methscopolamine; Pirenzepine; Propantheline; Scopolamine.
Antispasmodic, gastrointestinal—Dicyclomine; Scopolamine Butylbromide.
Antidysmenorrheal—Belladonna; Scopolamine Butylbromide.
Antiarrhythmic—Atropine (parenteral only); Glycopyrrolate (parenteral only); Hyoscyamine (parenteral only); Scopolamine (parenteral only).
Antidote (to cholinesterase inhibitors)—Atropine; Hyoscyamine (parenteral only).
Antidote (to muscarine)—Atropine; Hyoscyamine (parenteral only).
Antidote (to organophosphate pesticides)—Atropine.
Antispasmodic, urinary—Atropine; Scopolamine.
Cholinergic adjunct (curariform block)—Atropine (parenteral only); Glycopyrrolate (parenteral only); Hyoscyamine (parenteral only).
Anesthesia adjunct—Scopolamine (parenteral only).
Antiemetic—Scopolamine.
Antivertigo agent—Belladonna; Scopolamine.
Antidiarrheal—Glycopyrrolate.

## Indications

Note: Bracketed information in the *Indications* section refers to uses that are not included in U.S. product labeling.

### Accepted

Ulcer, peptic (treatment adjunct)—All anticholinergics included in this monograph, except dicyclomine and scopolamine hydrobromide, are FDA approved in conjunction with antacids or histamine H$_2$-receptor antagonists in the treatment of peptic ulcer, to reduce further gastric acid secretion and delay gastric emptying. However, the use of most anticholinergics as treatment adjunct in peptic ulcer has been replaced by the use of more effective agents. Results with anticholinergics usually are inconsistent and transient and require high doses, which result in significant side effects. Atropine, belladonna, clidinium, hyoscyamine, pirenzepine, and propantheline taken orally may be used rarely. Intravenous use of hyoscyamine may be indicated for prompt relief of pain in the treatment of both the moderately severe and the severe peptic ulcer. Anisotropine, glycopyrrolate, homatropine, mepenzolate, methantheline, and methscopolamine are generally no longer used for this indication.

Bowel syndrome, irritable (treatment)—Atropine, belladonna, [clidinium], dicyclomine, [glycopyrrolate], hyoscyamine, [propantheline], and [scopolamine] are indicated in the treatment of irritable bowel syndrome, mainly in patients in whom other therapy, such as sedation and/or change in diet, has failed. However, results usually are inconsistent and transient and require high doses, which result in significant side effects. Anisotropine, mepenzolate, methantheline, methscopolamine, and pirenzepine are generally no longer used for this indication.

Urologic disorders, symptoms of (treatment)—Oral hyoscyamine is indicated to control hypermotility in cystitis. However, results of anticholinergic treatment usually are inconsistent and transient and require high doses, which result in significant side effects. Atropine and scopolamine butylbromide are generally no longer used for this indication.

Urinary incontinence (treatment)—[Propantheline][1] is used in the treatment of uninhibited hypertonic neurogenic bladder to increase bladder capacity by reducing amplitude and frequency of bladder contractions. Atropine and methantheline are generally no longer used for this indication.

Hypersecretory conditions, gastric, in anesthesia (prophylaxis)—Parenteral glycopyrrolate is indicated as preanesthetic medication to reduce gastric acid secretion.

Salivation and respiratory tract secretions, excessive, in anesthesia (prophylaxis)—Oral and parenteral atropine and the parenteral forms of glycopyrrolate and scopolamine[1] are indicated as antisialagogue preanesthetic medications to prevent or reduce salivation and respiratory tract secretions. Parenteral hyoscyamine is no longer used for these indications.

Arrhythmias, succinylcholine-induced (prophylaxis) or
Arrhythmias, surgical procedure–induced (prophylaxis)—The parenteral form of atropine is indicated as adjunct to anesthesia to prevent reflex bradycardia, sinus arrest, and hypotension induced by succinylcholine during intubation of the trachea or produced by certain surgical manipulations. Parenteral scopolamine is generally no longer used for these indications.

Arrhythmias, cardiac (treatment) or
Bradycardia, sinus (treatment)—Parenteral atropine is indicated to reduce severe sinus bradycardia and syncope associated with hyperactive carotid sinus reflex; and to lessen the degree of atrioventricular heart block in Type I atrioventricular (AV) conduction deficits. It is also used to treat ventricular asystole. Parenteral atropine also is indicated as an antidote for sinus bradycardia resulting from the improper administration of a choline ester medication. Parenteral hyoscyamine is generally no longer used for these indications.

Arrhythmias, in anesthesia (treatment) or
Arrhythmias, in surgery (treatment)—The parenteral form of atropine is indicated to restore cardiac rate and arterial pressure when increased vagal activity has reduced pulse rate and cardiac action. Parenteral glycopyrrolate is indicated to block cardiac vagal inhibitory reflexes during induction of anesthesia and intubation. Parenteral glycopyrrolate is also indicated intraoperatively to counteract drug-induced or vagal traction reflexes with the associated arrhythmias. Parenteral hyoscyamine and parenteral scopolamine are generally no longer used for these indications.

Toxicity, cholinesterase inhibitor (prophylaxis)—The parenteral forms of atropine and glycopyrrolateare indicated for administration prior to or concurrently with neostigmine or pyridostigmine during reversal of nondepolarizing neuromuscular blockade to protect against the muscarinic effects of these drugs, such as bradycardia and excessive secretions. Parenteral hyoscyamine is generally no longer used for this indication.

Toxicity, cholinesterase inhibitor (treatment)
Toxicity, muscarine (treatment) or
Toxicity, organophosphate pesticide (treatment)—Oral and parenteral atropine are indicated in the treatment of poisoning from cholinesterase inhibitors such as neostigmine, pilocarpine, physostigmine, and methacholine, and in the treatment of the rapid type of mushroom (muscarine) poisoning. Atropine is also indicated in the treatment of poisoning caused by pesticides that are organophosphate cholinesterase inhibitors, chemical warfare, and "nerve" gases. Parenteral hyoscyamine is generally no longer used for these indications.

Anesthesia, general, adjunct—Parenteral administration of scopolamine[1], in combination with morphine or meperidine, is indicated in preanesthesia to reduce excitement and produce amnesia. Scopolamine may also be used for opioid-induced respiratory depression. Parenteral scopolamine[1] is also indicated in conjunction with analgesics in cardiopulmonary bypass patients who cannot be deeply anesthetized because of the risk of severe hypotension or circulatory collapse.

**228** Anticholinergics/Antispasmodics (Systemic)

Motion sickness (prophylaxis and treatment)—Transdermal scopolamine is indicated for prophylaxis of nausea and vomiting associated with motion sickness.

Pneumonitis, aspiration (prophylaxis)—Parenteral glycopyrrolate may provide some protection against aspiration of gastric contents during anesthesia.

[Salivation, excessive, postsurgical (prophylaxis)][1] or
[Salivation, excessive, medical condition–related (prophylaxis)][1]—Transdermal scopolamine is used for short-term control of drooling in postsurgical patients and in patients with goiter or other medical conditions in whom excessive salivation becomes a social problem.

[Salivation, excessive, in dental procedures (prophylaxis)][1]—The oral forms of atropine, glycopyrrolate, methantheline, and propantheline are used to control excessive salivation that interferes with dental procedures. Belladonna is generally no longer used for this indication.

Anticholinergics/antispasmodics listed below are FDA (U.S.) and HPB (Canada) approved for the following indications; however, they generally have been replaced by more effective agents—
- Biliary tract disorders (treatment adjunct)—Atropine, hyoscyamine, and scopolamine butylbromide.
- Radiography, gastrointestinal, adjunct—Parenteral atropine and parenteral hyoscyamine.
- Dysmenorrhea (treatment)—Belladonna and scopolamine butylbromide.
- Enuresis, nocturnal (treatment)—Belladonna and scopolamine butylbromide.
- Rhinitis, allergic, severe (treatment)—Oral hyoscyamine.

Anticholinergics/antispasmodics listed below have been used for the following indications; however, they generally have been replaced by more effective agents—
- [Diarrhea (treatment)][1]—Glycopyrrolate.
- [Parkinsonism (treatment)][1]—Oral atropine, belladonna, parenteral hyoscyamine, oral hyoscyamine and scopolamine combination, and oral scopolamine.

### Unaccepted
Hyoscyamine elixir and oral solution have been used in the treatment of infant colic. However, there is no conclusive evidence of effectiveness for this use.

---
[1] Not included in Canadian product labeling.

## Pharmacology/Pharmacokinetics

### Physicochemical characteristics
Chemical group—
   Tertiary amines: Atropine, belladonna, hyoscyamine, and scopolamine.
   Quaternary ammonium compounds: Anisotropine, clidinium, glycopyrrolate, homatropine, mepenzolate, methantheline, methscopolamine, and propantheline.
Molecular weight—
   Anisotropine methylbromide: 362.35.
   Atropine: 289.37.
   Clidinium bromide: 432.36.
   Dicyclomine hydrochloride: 345.95.
   Glycopyrrolate: 398.34.
   Homatropine methylbromide: 370.29.
   Hyoscyamine: 289.37.
   Hyoscyamine sulfate: 712.85.
   Mepenzolate bromide: 420.35.
   Methantheline bromide: 420.35.
   Methscopolamine bromide: 398.30.
   Pirenzepine: 351.41.
   Propantheline bromide: 448.40.
   Scopolamine hydrobromide: 438.31.
pKa—
   Atropine: 9.8.
   Dicyclomine: 9.0.
   Scopolamine: 7.55–7.81.

### Mechanism of action/Effect
Anticholinergic—The naturally occurring belladonna alkaloids, semisynthetic derivatives, quaternary ammonium compounds, and, to a lesser extent, the synthetic tertiary amines inhibit the muscarinic actions of acetylcholine on structures innervated by postganglionic cholinergic nerves as well as on smooth muscles that respond to acetylcholine but lack cholinergic innervation. These postganglionic receptor sites are present in the autonomic effector cells of the smooth muscle, cardiac muscle, sinoatrial and atrioventricular nodes, and exocrine glands. Depending on the dose, anticholinergics may reduce the motility and secretory activity of the gastrointestinal system, and the tone of the ureter and urinary bladder and may have a slight relaxant action on the bile ducts and gallbladder. In general, the smaller doses of anticholinergics inhibit salivary and bronchial secretions, sweating, and accommodation; cause dilatation of the pupil; and increase the heart rate. Larger doses are required to decrease motility of the gastrointestinal and urinary tracts and to inhibit gastric acid secretion.

Antispasmodic, gastrointestinal—Unproven. A local and direct action on smooth muscle, to reduce tone and motility of the gastrointestinal tract, has been suggested to explain the apparent gastrointestinal antispasmodic effect of the synthetic tertiary amine compounds.

Antidysmenorrheal—Effectiveness in relieving dysmenorrhea is due to spasmolytic action.

Antiarrhythmic—Inhibition of muscarinic actions of acetylcholine at postganglionic receptor sites present in the autonomic effector cells of the cardiac muscle, and sinoatrial and atrioventricular nodes.

Antidote (to cholinesterase inhibitors; to muscarine; to organophosphate pesticides)—Atropine and hyoscyamine antagonize the actions of cholinesterase inhibitors at muscarinic receptor sites, including increased tracheobronchial and salivary secretion, bronchoconstriction, autonomic ganglionic stimulation, and, to a moderate extent, central actions.

Cholinergic adjunct (curariform block)—Atropine and hyoscyamine antagonize the actions, such as vagal and secretory enhancing effects, of cholinesterase inhibitors used in the treatment of nondepolarizing neuromuscular blockade.

Anesthesia adjunct—Scopolamine depresses the cerebral cortex; in large doses and in conjunction with analgesics, produces loss of memory.

Antiemetic—Belladonna and scopolamine act primarily by reducing the excitability of the labyrinthine receptors and by depressing conduction in the vestibular cerebellar pathway.

Antivertigo—The exact mechanism by which belladonna and scopolamine exert their antimotion sickness and antivertigo effects is unknown; however, they probably act either on the cortex or more peripherally on the maculae of the utricle and saccule.

Antidiarrheal—Glycopyrrolate may reduce the activity of the gastrocolic reflex and the excessive peristaltic activity of both the small and large bowels.

### Other actions/effects
Natural tertiary amines—
  Atropine: Stimulates or depresses the central nervous system (CNS), depending on the dose; and has a more prolonged and potent action than the other belladonna alkaloids on the heart, intestine, and bronchial muscle.
  Belladonna alkaloids: In parkinsonism, selectively depress certain central motor mechanisms in the CNS, controlling muscle tone and movement.
  Hyoscyamine: Has actions similar to those of atropine, but is more potent in both its central and peripheral effects.
  Scopolamine: Has peripheral action similar to that of atropine but, in contrast to atropine, is depressant to the CNS at therapeutic doses; it does not stimulate the medullary centers and therefore does not increase respiration or elevate blood pressure. Scopolamine has a more potent action than atropine on the sphincter muscle of the iris and the ciliary muscle of the lens, and on the secretory glands such as salivary, bronchial, and sweat glands.

Quaternary ammonium compounds, semisynthetic and synthetic—
  In contrast to atropine and scopolamine, effects of these medications on the CNS are negligible. These medications are also less likely to affect the pupil or ciliary muscle of the eye. Ganglionic blockade is attributed to some increased effects of the high dosage range, and toxic doses produce neuromuscular blockade.

Synthetic tertiary amines—
  These medications produce less prominent CNS effects than do the natural tertiary amines.

### Absorption
Tertiary amines—Rapidly absorbed from gastrointestinal tract; also enter the circulation through the mucosal surfaces of the body.

Quaternary ammonium compounds—Gastrointestinal absorption is poor and irregular. Total absorption after an oral dose is about 10 to 25%.

### Distribution
Exact distribution of anticholinergics has not been fully determined. However, tertiary amines appear to be distributed throughout the entire body and readily cross the blood-brain barrier, while quaternary ammonium compounds exhibit minimal passage across the blood-brain barrier and into the eye.

Atropine, belladonna, and hyoscyamine are distributed into breast milk.

### Protein binding
Atropine—Moderate.
Hyoscyamine—Moderate.
Scopolamine hydrobromide—Low.

**Biotransformation**
Most anticholinergics—Hepatic, by enzymatic hydrolysis.

**Half-life**
Elimination—
   Atropine: 2.5 hours.
   Dicyclomine hydrochloride: 1.8 hours (initial phase) and 9 to 10 hours (secondary phase).
   Glycopyrrolate: 1.7 hours (range 0.6–4.6 hours).
   Hyoscyamine: 3.5 hours.
   Pirenzepine—10 to 12 hours.
   Propantheline bromide—1.6 (mean) hours.
   Scopolamine—8 hours.

**Time to peak effect**
Glycopyrrolate—Intramuscular: 30 to 45 minutes.

| Drug | Onset of Action | Duration of Action | Elimination (% excreted unchanged) |
|---|---|---|---|
| Anisotropine methylbromide | | | * |
| Atropine | | Oral: 4–6 hr Parenteral: Brief | Renal (30–50) |
| Belladonna | 1–2 hr | 4 hr | Renal (30–50 of atropine and 1 of scopolamine) |
| Clidinium bromide | 1 hr | Up to 3 hr | * |
| Dicyclomine hydrochloride | | | * |
| Glycopyrrolate | IM or SC: 15–30 min IV: 1 min | Antisialagogue: Up to 7 hr Vagal blocking effect: 2–3 hr | Renal |
| Homatropine | | | * |
| Hyoscyamine sulfate | Oral: 20–30 min Parenteral: 2–3 min | 4–6 hr | Renal (majority) |
| Mepenzolate bromide | | | Renal (3–22) |
| Methantheline bromide | | | * |
| Methscopolamine bromide | 1 hr | 6–8 hr | * |
| Pirenzepine hydrochloride | | | Renal/hepatic (80–90) |
| Propantheline bromide | | 6 hr | Renal (<6) |
| Scopolamine | | Transdermal: Up to 72 hr | Renal |
| Scopolamine hydrobromide | Antisialagogue— Oral: 30–60 min Parenteral: 30 min | Oral: 4–6 hr Parenteral: 4 hr | Renal (1 of oral dose) (3.4 of SC dose) |

*Assumed to be renal/fecal.

## Precautions to Consider

### Cross-sensitivity and/or related problems
For all anticholinergics—Patients sensitive to one belladonna alkaloid or derivative may be sensitive to the other belladonna alkaloids or derivatives also.

### Pregnancy/Reproduction
Pregnancy—
   *For anistropine methylbromide—*
      Problems in humans have not been documented.
      FDA pregnancy category not currently included in product labeling.
   *For atropine—*
      Atropine crosses the placenta. Well-controlled studies in humans have not been done. Intravenous administration of atropine during pregnancy or near term may produce tachycardia in the fetus.
      Studies in mice have not shown that atropine given in doses of 50 mg per kg of body weight (mg/kg) has adverse effects on the fetus.
      FDA Pregnancy Category C.
   *For belladonna—*
      Belladonna crosses the placenta. Studies with belladonna have not been done in either animals or humans.
      FDA Pregnancy Category C.
   *For clidinium—*
      Adequate and well-controlled studies in humans have not been done.
      Reproduction studies in rats have not shown that clidinium has adverse effects on the fetus.
      FDA pregnancy category not currently included in product labeling.
   *For dicyclomine—*
      Dicyclomine has been associated in several isolated cases with human malformations; however, in retrospective studies there has been no evidence of dicyclomine having any untoward effect on the embryo.
      FDA pregnancy category not currently included in product labeling.
   *For glycopyrrolate—*
      Controlled studies in humans have not been done.
      Studies in rats and rabbits have not shown that glycopyrrolate causes teratogenic effects. However, studies in rats have shown that rates of conception and of survival at weaning decreased in a dose-related manner with glycopyrrolate. Studies in dogs with high doses of glycopyrrolate suggest that this may be caused by a decrease in seminal secretion.
      FDA Pregnancy Category B.
   *For hyoscyamine—*
      Hyoscyamine crosses the placenta. Studies with hyoscyamine have not been done in either animals or humans. Intravenous administration of hyoscyamine during pregnancy, especially near term, may produce tachycardia in the fetus.
      FDA Pregnancy Category C.
   *For mepenzolate—*
      Adequate and well-controlled studies in humans have not been done.
      Reproduction studies in rats and rabbits have not shown that mepenzolate has adverse effects on the fetus.
      FDA pregnancy category not currently included in product labeling.
   *For propantheline—*
      Studies have not been done in either animals or humans.
      FDA Pregnancy Category C.
   *For scopolamine—*
      Scopolamine crosses the placenta. Studies with scopolamine have not been done in either animals or humans.
      FDA Pregnancy Category C.
Labor—For scopolamine: Parenteral administration of scopolamine before the onset of labor may cause CNS depression in the neonate and may contribute to neonatal hemorrhage due to reduction in vitamin K–dependent clotting factors in the neonate.

### Breast-feeding
For all anticholinergics—Anticholinergics may inhibit lactation.
For atropine, belladonna, and hyoscyamine—These drugs are distributed into breast milk. Although amounts have not been quantified, the chronic use of these medications should be avoided during nursing since infants are usually very sensitive to the effects of anticholinergics.
For dicyclomine—Although a causal relationship has not been established, the use of dicyclomine in nursing mothers is not recommended, since respiratory distress has been reported in infants less than 3 months of age who ingested dicyclomine directly (not through breast milk).
For quaternary ammonium compounds—It is unlikely that these drugs are excreted in breast milk since they are incompletely absorbed from the gastrointestinal tract and have poor lipid solubility.

### Pediatrics
*For all anticholinergics—*
   Infants and young children are especially susceptible to the toxic effects of anticholinergics.
   Close supervision is recommended for infants and children with spastic paralysis or brain damage since an increased response to anticholinergics has been reported in these patients and dosage adjustments are often required.

When anticholinergics are given to children where the environmental temperature is high, there is risk of a rapid increase in body temperature because of these medications' suppression of sweat gland activity.

A paradoxical reaction characterized by hyperexcitability may occur in children taking large doses of anticholinergics.

*For dicyclomine—*
Respiratory symptoms, such as difficulty in breathing, shortness of breath, respiratory collapse and apnea; as well as seizures, syncope, asphyxia, pulse rate fluctuations, muscular hypotonia, and coma have been reported in some infants, 3 months old and under, with the use of dicyclomine syrup. These side effects occurred within minutes of ingestion and lasted 20 to 30 minutes. They are believed to have been caused by local irritation and/or aspiration rather than by a direct pharmacologic action.

*For hyoscyamine—*
Hyoscyamine sulfate injection contains benzyl alcohol as a preservative and should not be used in newborn and immature infants. The use of benzyl alcohol in neonates has been associated with a fatal toxic syndrome consisting of metabolic acidosis and CNS, respiratory, circulatory, and renal function impairment.

## Geriatrics

Geriatric patients may respond to usual doses of anticholinergics with excitement, agitation, drowsiness, or confusion.

Geriatric patients are especially susceptible to the anticholinergic side effects, such as constipation, dryness of mouth, and urinary retention (especially in males). If these side effects occur and continue or are severe, medication should probably be discontinued.

Caution is also recommended when anticholinergics are given to geriatric patients, because of the danger of precipitating undiagnosed glaucoma.

Memory may become severely impaired in geriatric patients, especially those who already have memory problems, with the continued use of anticholinergics since these drugs block the actions of acetylcholine, which is responsible for many functions of the brain, including memory functions.

## Dental

Prolonged use of anticholinergics may decrease or inhibit salivary flow, thus contributing to the development of caries, periodontal disease, oral candidiasis, and discomfort.

## Drug interactions and/or related problems

The following drug interactions and/or related problems have been selected on the basis of their potential clinical significance (possible mechanism in parentheses where appropriate)—not necessarily inclusive (» = major clinical significance):

Note: Combinations containing any of the following medications, depending on the amount present, may also interact with this medication.

Only specific interactions between anticholinergics and other oral medications have been identified in this monograph. However, because of decreased gastrointestinal motility and delayed gastric emptying, absorption of other oral medications may be decreased during concurrent use with anticholinergics.

*For all anticholinergics*
Alkalizers, urinary, such as:
Antacids, calcium- and/or magnesium-containing
Carbonic anhydrase inhibitors
Citrates
Sodium bicarbonate
(urinary excretion of anticholinergics may be delayed by alkalinization of the urine, thus potentiating the anticholinergics' therapeutic and/or side effects)

» Antacids or
» Antidiarrheals, adsorbent
(simultaneous use of these medications may reduce absorption of anticholinergics, resulting in decreased therapeutic effectiveness; doses of these medications should be spaced 2 or 3 hours apart from doses of anticholinergics)

» Anticholinergics or other medications with anticholinergic activity, other (see *Appendix II*)
(concurrent use with anticholinergics may intensify anticholinergic effects; patients should be advised to report occurrence of gastrointestinal problems promptly since paralytic ileus may occur with concurrent therapy)

Antimyasthenics
(concurrent use with anticholinergics may further reduce intestinal motility; therefore, caution is recommended; although atropine may be used to reduce or prevent the muscarinic effects of antimyasthenics, routine concurrent use is not recommended since the muscarinic effects may be the first signs of antimyasthenic overdose, and masking such effects with atropine may prevent early recognition of cholinergic crisis)

» Cyclopropane
(concurrent intravenous administration of anticholinergics with cyclopropane anesthesia may result in ventricular arrhythmias; however, if the anticholinergic used is glycopyrrolate, the risk is reduced if glycopyrrolate is given in increments of 100 mcg [0.1 mg] or less)

Haloperidol
(antipsychotic effectiveness of haloperidol may be decreased in schizophrenic patients)

» Ketoconazole
(anticholinergics may increase gastrointestinal pH, possibly resulting in a marked reduction in ketoconazole absorption during concurrent use with anticholinergics; patients should be advised to take these medications at least 2 hours after ketoconazole)

Metoclopramide
(concurrent use with anticholinergics may antagonize metoclopramide's effects on gastrointestinal motility)

Opioid (narcotic) analgesics
(concurrent use with anticholinergics may result in increased risk of severe constipation, which may lead to paralytic ileus, and/or urinary retention)

» Potassium chloride, especially wax-matrix preparations
(concurrent use with anticholinergics may increase severity of potassium chloride–induced gastrointestinal lesions)

*For scopolamine (in addition to interactions listed above)*
» CNS depression–producing medications, other (see *Appendix II*)
(concurrent use may potentiate the effects of either these medications or scopolamine, resulting in additive sedation)

Lorazepam, parenteral
(concurrent use of scopolamine and parenteral lorazepam is reported to have no added beneficial effect and their combined effect may increase the incidence of sedation, hallucination, and irritational behavior)

## Laboratory value alterations

The following have been selected on the basis of their potential clinical significance (possible effect in parentheses where appropriate)—not necessarily inclusive (» = major clinical significance):

With diagnostic test results
*For all anticholinergics*
» Gastric acid secretion test
(concurrent use of anticholinergics may antagonize the effect of pentagastrin and histamine in the evaluation of gastric acid secretory function; administration of anticholinergics is not recommended during the 24 hours preceding the test)

Radionuclide gastric emptying studies
(use of anticholinergics may result in delayed gastric emptying)

*For atropine (in addition to those listed for all anticholinergics)*
» Phenolsulfonphthalein (PSP) excretion test
(atropine utilizes the same tubular mechanism of excretion as PSP resulting in decreased urinary excretion of PSP; concurrent use of atropine is not recommended in patients receiving PSP excretion test)

*For scopolamine (in addition to those listed for all anticholinergics)*
Neuroradiological tests
(residual cycloplegia and mydriasis following use of transdermal disk of scopolamine may affect results of neuroradiological tests for intracranial neoplasm, subdural hematoma, or aneurysm)

With physiology/laboratory test values
*For glycopyrrolate*
Serum uric acid
(may be decreased in patients with hyperuricemia or gout)

## Medical considerations/Contraindications

The medical considerations/contraindications included have been selected on the basis of their potential clinical significance (reasons given in parentheses where appropriate)—not necessarily inclusive (» = major clinical significance).

### Risk-benefit should be considered when the following medical problems exist:

Brain damage, in children
(CNS effects may be exacerbated)

» Cardiac disease, especially cardiac arrhythmias, congestive heart failure, coronary artery disease, and mitral stenosis
(increase in heart rate may be undesirable)

Down's syndrome
(abnormal increase in pupillary dilation and acceleration of heart rate may occur)
» Esophagitis, reflux
(decrease in esophageal and gastric motility and relaxation of lower esophageal sphincter may promote gastric retention by delaying gastric emptying and may increase gastroesophageal reflux through an incompetent sphincter)
Fever
(may be increased through suppression of sweat gland activity)
» Gastrointestinal tract obstructive disease as in achalasia and pyloroduodenal stenosis
(decrease in motility and tone may occur, resulting in obstruction and gastric retention)
» Glaucoma, angle-closure, or predisposition to
(mydriatic effect resulting in increased intraocular pressure may precipitate an acute attack of angle-closure glaucoma)
» Glaucoma, open-angle
(mydriatic effect may cause a slight increase in intraocular pressure; glaucoma therapy may need to be adjusted)
» Hemorrhage, acute, with unstable cardiovascular status
(increase in heart rate may be undesirable)
Hepatic function impairment
(decreased metabolism of anticholinergic)
» Hernia, hiatal, associated with reflux esophagitis
(anticholinergics may aggravate condition)
Hypertension
(may be aggravated)
Hyperthyroidism
(characterized by tachycardia, which may be increased)
» Intestinal atony in the elderly or debilitated patient or
» Paralytic ileus
(anticholinergic use may result in obstruction)
Lung disease, chronic, especially in infants, small children, and debilitated patients
(reduction in bronchial secretion can lead to inspissation and formation of bronchial plugs)
» Myasthenia gravis
(condition may be aggravated because of inhibition of acetylcholine action)
Neuropathy, autonomic
(urinary retention and cycloplegia may be aggravated)
» Prostatic hypertrophy, nonobstructive or
» Urinary retention, or predisposition to or
» Uropathy, obstructive, such as bladder neck obstruction due to prostatic hypertrophy
(urinary retention may be precipitated or aggravated)
» Pyloric obstruction
(may be aggravated)
Renal function impairment
(decreased excretion may increase the risk of side effects)
Sensitivity to any belladonna alkaloids or derivatives
Spastic paralysis, in children
(response to anticholinergics may be increased)
» Tachycardia
(may be increased)
Toxemia of pregnancy
(hypertension may be aggravated)
» Ulcerative colitis
(large anticholinergic doses may suppress intestinal motility, possibly causing paralytic ileus; also, use may precipitate or aggravate the serious complication, toxic megacolon)
Xerostomia
(prolonged use may further reduce limited salivary flow)
Caution in use is also recommended in patients over 40 years of age because of the danger of precipitating undiagnosed glaucoma.

**Patient monitoring**
The following may be especially important in patient monitoring (other tests may be warranted in some patients, depending on condition; » = major clinical significance):
Intraocular pressure determinations
(recommended at periodic intervals, as these medications may increase the intraocular pressure by producing mydriasis)

## Side/Adverse Effects
Note: When anticholinergics are given to patients, especially children, where the environmental temperature is high, there is risk of a rapid increase in body temperature because of suppression of sweat gland activity.

Infants, patients with Down's syndrome, and children with spastic paralysis or brain damage may show an increased response to anticholinergics, thus increasing the potential for side effects.

Geriatric or debilitated patients may respond to usual doses of anticholinergics with excitement, agitation, drowsiness, or confusion.

Following use of the transdermal disk of scopolamine, a dilated and fixed pupil has been reported on the side where the disk was worn. This condition usually resolves spontaneously within a few days, but may persist for up to 2 weeks after the disk has been removed and thus may be mistaken for a sign of intracranial neoplasm, subdural hematoma, or aneurysm. To avoid extensive neuroradiological tests, instillation of 1% pilocarpine solution is recommended as an aid in the diagnosis of non-neurogenic dilation of the pupil.

See *Table 1, page 241.*

## Overdose
For specific information on the agents used in the management of overdose with anticholinergics/antispasmodics, see:
• *Benzodiazepines (Systemic)* monograph;
• *Charcoal, Activated (Oral-Local)* monograph;
• *Chloral Hydrate (Systemic)* monograph;
• *Neostigmine Methylsulfate* in *Antimyasthenics (Systemic)* monograph;
• *Norepinephrine Bitartrate* or *Metaraminol Bitartrate* in *Sympathomimetic Agents—Cardiovascular Use (Parenteral-Systemic)* monograph;
• *Physostigmine Salicylate (Systemic)* monograph; and/or
• *Thiopental* in *Anesthetics, Barbiturate (Systemic)* monograph.

For more information on the management of overdose or unintentional ingestion, **contact a Poison Control Center** (see *Poison Control Center Listing*).

**Clinical effects of overdose**
The following effects have been selected on the basis of their potential clinical significance (possible signs and symptoms in parentheses where appropriate)—not necessarily inclusive:
*Blurred vision, continuing, or changes in near vision; clumsiness or unsteadiness; confusion; difficulty in breathing*—may lead to respiratory paralysis with quaternary ammonium compounds because of curare-like effects; *dizziness; drowsiness, severe; dryness of mouth, nose, or throat, severe; fast heartbeat; fever; hallucinations; muscle weakness, severe*—may lead to respiratory paralysis with quaternary ammonium compounds because of curare-like effects; *seizures; slurred speech; tiredness, severe*—may lead to respiratory paralysis with quaternary ammonium compounds because of curare-like effects; *unusual excitement, nervousness, restlessness, or irritability; unusual warmth, dryness, and flushing of skin*

**Treatment of overdose**
Recommended treatment for anticholinergic overdose includes the following:
To decrease absorption—
Emesis or gastric lavage with 4% tannic acid solution.
Administration of an aqueous slurry of activated charcoal.
Specific treatment—
To reverse severe anticholinergic symptoms, slow, intravenous administration of physostigmine in doses of 0.5 to 2 mg (0.5 to 1 mg in children, up to a total dose of 2 mg), at a rate not to exceed 1 mg per minute; may be given in repeated doses of 1 to 4 mg as needed, up to a total dose of 5 mg in adults.
Or, neostigmine methylsulfate administered intramuscularly in doses of 0.5 to 1 mg, repeated every 2 to 3 hours; or intravenously in doses of 0.5 to 2 mg, repeated as needed.
To control excitement or delirium, administration of small doses of a short-acting barbiturate (100 mg thiopental sodium) or benzodiazepines, or rectal infusion of 2% solution of chloral hydrate.
To restore blood pressure, infusion of norepinephrine bitartrate or metaraminol.
Supportive care—
Artificial respiration with oxygen if needed for respiratory depression.
Adequate hydration.
Symptomatic treatment as necessary.
Patients in whom intentional overdose is confirmed or suspected should be referred for psychiatric consultation.

## Patient Consultation

As an aid to patient consultation, refer to *Advice for the Patient, Anticholinergics/Antispasmodics (Systemic)*.

In providing consultation, consider emphasizing the following selected information (» = major clinical significance):

### Before using this medication
» Conditions affecting use, especially:
Sensitivity to any of the belladonna alkaloids or derivatives
Breast-feeding—Excreted in breast milk (except for quaternary ammonium compounds); possible inhibition of lactation
Use in children—Increased susceptibility to toxic effects of anticholinergics; increased response in infants and children with spastic paralysis or brain damage; risk of increased body temperature in hot weather; hyperexcitability (paradoxical reaction) with large doses; increased risk of respiratory depression and collapse (with dicyclomine)
Use in the elderly—Increased susceptibility to mental and other toxic effects of anticholinergics; danger of precipitating undiagnosed glaucoma; possible impairment of memory
Dental—Possible development of dental problems because of decreased salivary flow
Other medications, especially other anticholinergics, antacids, antidiarrheals, cyclopropane, ketoconazole, CNS depressants (with scopolamine), and potassium chloride
Other medical problems, especially cardiac disease, glaucoma, hemorrhage, hiatal hernia, intestinal atony or paralytic ileus, myasthenia gravis, obstruction in gastrointestinal or urinary tract, prostatic hypertrophy, reflux esophagitis, tachycardia, and ulcerative colitis

### Proper use of this medication
*For oral dosage forms*
Taking medication 30 minutes to 1 hour before meals
*For rectal dosage forms*
Proper administration technique
*For transdermal scopolamine*
Reading patient directions
Washing and drying hands thoroughly before and after application
Applying to hairless, intact area of skin behind ear; not applying over cuts or irritations
» Importance of not taking more medication than the amount prescribed
Missed dose: Taking as soon as possible; not taking if almost time for next dose; not doubling doses
» Proper dosing
» Proper storage

### Precautions while using this medication
» Suspected overdose: Getting emergency help at once
» Caution during exercise or hot weather; overheating may result in heat stroke
» Possible increased sensitivity of eyes to light
Caution about abrupt withdrawal
» Caution if blurred vision occurs
» Possible dizziness or drowsiness; caution when driving or doing things requiring alertness
Possible dizziness or lightheadedness; caution when getting up suddenly from a lying or sitting position
Possible dryness of mouth; using sugarless candy or gum, ice or saliva substitute for relief; checking with physician or dentist if dry mouth continues for more than 2 weeks
*For scopolamine*
» Avoiding use of alcohol or other CNS depressants
*For oral dosage forms*
Avoiding use of antacids and antidiarrheal medications within 2 or 3 hours of taking this medication

### Side/adverse effects
Signs of potential side effects, especially allergic reaction, confusion, increased intraocular pressure, orthostatic hypotension (especially with high doses of quaternary ammonium compounds)

## General Dosing Information

Tolerance to some of the adverse reactions may develop following continued use and/or smaller doses of anticholinergics, but effectiveness may also be reduced.

Dosage adjustments are often required for infants, patients with Down's syndrome, children with brain damage or spasticity, since an increased responsiveness to anticholinergics has been reported in these patients.

Geriatric and debilitated patients may respond to usual doses with excitement, agitation, drowsiness, or confusion; lower doses may be required in these patients.

Anticholinergics should not be withdrawn abruptly since withdrawal-like symptoms may occur. Vomiting, malaise, sweating, transient dizziness, and salivation have been reported after sudden withdrawal of large doses of scopolamine.

If scopolamine is used as antisialagogue preanesthetic medication in minor surgical procedures that do not require more than a few hours' stay in the hospital, the patient should be alerted at time of discharge about scopolamine's lingering detrimental effects on memory and motor tasks.

High dosage of quaternary ammonium compounds should not be given continuously for prolonged periods, since ganglionic and skeletal neuromuscular transmission may be blocked. Stimulation of the CNS and a curare-like action may result.

### For oral dosage forms only
Administration of anticholinergics 30 minutes to 1 hour before meals is recommended to maximize absorption.

### For parenteral dosage forms only
Atropine, hyoscyamine, and scopolamine may be administered by intramuscular, subcutaneous, or intravenous injection.

Glycopyrrolate may be administered by intramuscular or intravenous injection.

After parenteral administration a temporary feeling of lightheadedness and local irritation may occur.

### For transdermal dosage forms only
Transdermal application delivers reduced doses of scopolamine, which are large enough to be effective but small enough to eliminate most of the adverse effects, except drowsiness and cycloplegia.

---

## *ANISOTROPINE*

## Oral Dosage Forms

### ANISOTROPINE METHYLBROMIDE TABLETS

**Usual adult and adolescent dose**
Anticholinergic—
Oral, 50 mg three times a day, the dosage being adjusted as needed and tolerated.

Note: Geriatric patients may be more sensitive to the effects of the usual adult dose.

**Usual pediatric dose**
Dosage has not been established.

**Strength(s) usually available**
U.S.—
50 mg (Rx) [GENERIC].
Canada—
Not commercially available.

**Packaging and storage**
Store between 15 and 30 °C (59 and 86 °F), unless otherwise specified by manufacturer.

**Auxiliary labeling**
• May cause blurred vision.

---

## *ATROPINE*

## Summary of Differences

Category:
Also an antidote (to cholinesterase inhibitors; to organophosphate pesticides; to muscarine) and a urinary antispasmodic. Parenteral atropine is used as an antiarrhythmic and cholinergic adjunct (curariform block).
Indications:
Also indicated for biliary tract disorders and duodenography. In preanesthesia and dental anesthesia, indicated as antisialagogue.
Pharmacology/pharmacokinetics:
Protein binding—Moderate.
Half-life (elimination)—2.5 hours.
Duration of action—Oral, 4 to 6 hours; parenteral, brief.
Elimination—Renal; 30 to 50% excreted unchanged.
Precautions:
Pregnancy—Intravenous administration may produce tachycardia in fetus.
Laboratory value alterations—May decrease excretion of phenolsulfonphthalein (PSP) during PSP excretion test.

## Additional Dosing Information
See also *General Dosing Information*.

Doses of 0.5 to 1 mg of atropine are mildly stimulating to the CNS. Larger doses may produce mental disturbances; very large doses have depressant effect.

The fatal dose of atropine in children may be as low as 10 mg.

## Oral Dosage Forms
### ATROPINE SULFATE TABLETS USP
**Usual adult and adolescent dose**
Anticholinergic—
  Oral, 300 mcg (0.3 mg) to 1.2 mg every four to six hours.
Prophylaxis of excessive salivation and respiratory tract secretions, in anesthesia—
  Oral, 2 mg.
Note: Geriatric patients may be more sensitive to the effects of the usual adult dose.

**Usual pediatric dose**
Anticholinergic—
  Oral, 10 mcg (0.01 mg) per kg of body weight, not to exceed 400 mcg (0.4 mg), or 300 mcg (0.3 mg) per square meter of body surface, every four to six hours.

**Strength(s) usually available**
U.S.—
  400 mcg (0.4 mg) (Rx) [GENERIC].
Canada—
  Not commercially available.

**Packaging and storage**
Store below 40 °C (104 °F), preferably between 15 and 30 °C (59 and 86 °F), in a well-closed container, unless otherwise specified by manufacturer.

**Auxiliary labeling**
- May cause blurred vision.

### ATROPINE SULFATE SOLUBLE TABLETS
**Usual adult and adolescent dose**
Anticholinergic—
  Oral, 300 mcg (0.3 mg) to 1.2 mg every four to six hours.
Prophylaxis of excessive salivation and respiratory tract secretions, in anesthesia—
  Oral, 2 mg.
Note: Geriatric patients may be more sensitive to the effects of the usual adult dose.

**Usual pediatric dose**
Anticholinergic—
  Oral, 10 mcg (0.01 mg) per kg of body weight, not to exceed 400 mcg (0.4 mg), or 300 mcg (0.3 mg) per square meter of body surface, every four to six hours.

**Strength(s) usually available**
U.S.—
  400 mcg (0.4 mg) (Rx) [GENERIC].
  600 mcg (0.6 mg) (Rx) [GENERIC].
Canada—
  Not commercially available.

**Packaging and storage**
Store below 40 °C (104 °F), preferably between 15 and 30 °C (59 and 86 °F), in a well-closed container, unless otherwise specified by manufacturer.

**Auxiliary labeling**
- May cause blurred vision.

## Parenteral Dosage Forms
### ATROPINE SULFATE INJECTION USP
**Usual adult and adolescent dose**
Anticholinergic—
  Intramuscular, intravenous, or subcutaneous, 400 to 600 mcg (0.4 to 0.6 mg) every four to six hours.
  Gastrointestinal radiography—
    Intramuscular, 1 mg.
  Prophylaxis of excessive salivation and respiratory tract secretions, in anesthesia—
    Intramuscular, 200 to 600 mcg (0.2 to 0.6 mg) one-half to one hour before surgery.
Antiarrhythmic—
  Intravenous, 400 mcg (0.4 mg) to 1 mg every one to two hours as needed, up to a maximum of 2 mg.
Cholinergic adjunct (curariform block)—
  Intravenous, 600 mcg (0.6 mg) to 1.2 mg administered a few minutes before or concurrently with 500 mcg (0.5 mg) to 2 mg of neostigmine methylsulfate, using separate syringes.
Antidote (to cholinesterase inhibitors)—
  Intravenous, 2 to 4 mg initially, then 2 mg repeated every five to ten minutes until muscarinic symptoms disappear or signs of atropine toxicity appear.
Antidote (to muscarine in mushroom poisoning)—
  Intramuscular or intravenous, 1 to 2 mg every hour until respiratory effects subside.
Antidote (to organophosphate pesticides)—
  Intramuscular or intravenous, 1 to 2 mg, repeated in twenty to thirty minutes as soon as cyanosis has cleared. Continue dosage until definite improvement occurs and is maintained, sometimes for two days or more.
Note: Geriatric patients may be more sensitive to the effects of the usual adult dose.

**Usual pediatric dose**
Anticholinergic—
  Subcutaneous, 10 mcg (0.01 mg) per kg of body weight, not to exceed 400 mcg (0.4 mg), or 300 mcg (0.3 mg) per square meter of body surface, every four to six hours.
Prophylaxis of excessive salivation and respiratory tract secretions, in anesthesia or
Prophylaxis of succinylcholine- or surgical procedure–induced arrhythmias—
  Subcutaneous:
    Children weighing up to 3 kg: 100 mcg (0.1 mg).
    Children weighing 7 to 9 kg: 200 mcg (0.2 mg).
    Children weighing 12 to 16 kg: 300 mcg (0.3 mg).
    Children weighing 20 to 27 kg: 400 mcg (0.4 mg).
    Children weighing 32 kg: 500 mcg (0.5 mg).
    Children weighing 41 kg: 600 mcg (0.6 mg).
Antiarrhythmic—
  Intravenous, 10 to 30 mcg (0.01 to 0.03 mg) per kg of body weight.
Antidote (to cholinesterase inhibitors)—
  Intravenous or intramuscular, 1 mg initially, then 0.5 to 1 mg every five to ten minutes until muscarinic symptoms disappear or signs of atropine toxicity appear.

**Strength(s) usually available**
U.S.—
  50 mcg (0.05 mg) per mL (Rx) [GENERIC].
  100 mcg (0.1 mg) per mL (Rx) [GENERIC].
  300 mcg (0.3 mg) per mL (Rx) [GENERIC].
  400 mcg (0.4 mg) per mL (Rx) [GENERIC].
  500 mcg (0.5 mg) per mL (Rx) [GENERIC].
  800 mcg (0.8 mg) per mL (Rx) [GENERIC].
  1 mg per mL (Rx) [GENERIC].
Canada—
  400 mcg (0.4 mg) per mL (Rx) [GENERIC].
  600 mcg (0.6 mg) per mL (Rx) [GENERIC].

**Packaging and storage**
Store below 40 °C (104 °F), preferably between 15 and 30 °C (59 and 86 °F), unless otherwise specified by manufacturer. Protect from freezing.

**Additional information**
The intravenous injection of atropine should be administered *slowly*.

---

## BELLADONNA

## Summary of Differences
Category:
  Also an antidysmenorrheal and antivertigo agent.
Indications:
  Also indicated in nocturnal enuresis. In dental procedures, may be used as antisialagogue.
Pharmacology/pharmacokinetics:
  Onset of action—1 to 2 hours.
  Duration of action—4 hours.
  Elimination—Renal; 30 to 50% of atropine and 1% of scopolamine excreted unchanged.

## Oral Dosage Forms
### BELLADONNA TINCTURE USP

**Usual adult and adolescent dose**
Anticholinergic—
  Oral, 180 to 300 mcg (0.18 to 0.3 mg) three or four times a day, thirty minutes to one hour before meals and at bedtime, the dosage being adjusted as needed and tolerated.

Note: Geriatric patients may be more sensitive to the effects of the usual adult dose.

**Usual pediatric dose**
Anticholinergic—
  Oral, 9 mcg (0.009 mg) per kg of body weight or 240 mcg (0.24 mg) per square meter of body surface a day, in three or four divided doses.

**Strength(s) usually available**
U.S.—
  300 mcg (0.3 mg) per mL (Rx) [GENERIC].

Note: Belladonna tincture contains 300 mcg (0.3 mg) of belladonna alkaloids (principally hyoscyamine and atropine) per mL.

Canada—
  Not commercially available.

**Packaging and storage**
Store below 40 °C (104 °F), preferably between 15 and 30 °C (59 and 86 °F), unless otherwise specified by manufacturer. Store in a tight, light-resistant container. Protect from freezing.

**Auxiliary labeling**
- May cause blurred vision.
- Keep container tightly closed.

---

## CLIDINIUM

### Summary of Differences
Pharmacology/pharmacokinetics:
  Onset of action—1 hour.
  Duration of action—Up to 3 hours.

### Oral Dosage Forms
### CLIDINIUM BROMIDE CAPSULES USP

**Usual adult and adolescent dose**
Anticholinergic—
  Oral, 2.5 to 5 mg three or four times a day, before meals and at bedtime, the dosage being adjusted as needed and tolerated.

Note: Geriatric or debilitated patients—Oral, 2.5 mg three times a day before meals.

**Usual pediatric dose**
Dosage has not been established.

**Strength(s) usually available**
U.S.—
  2.5 mg (Rx) [*Quarzan*].
  5 mg (Rx) [*Quarzan*].
Canada—
  Not commercially available.

**Packaging and storage**
Store below 40 °C (104 °F), preferably between 15 and 30 °C (59 and 86 °F), unless otherwise specified by manufacturer. Store in a tight, light-resistant container.

**Auxiliary labeling**
- May cause blurred vision.

---

## DICYCLOMINE

### Summary of Differences
Category:
  Also gastrointestinal antispasmodic.
Indications:
  Not indicated for peptic ulcer.
Pharmacology/pharmacokinetics:
  Half-life (elimination)—1.8 hours (initial phase) and 9 to 10 hours (secondary phase).

Precautions:
  Pediatrics—Respiratory symptoms, seizures, syncope, asphyxia, pulse rate fluctuations, muscular hypotonia, and coma reported with the use of the syrup in some infants 3 months old and under.

### Oral Dosage Forms
### DICYCLOMINE HYDROCHLORIDE CAPSULES USP

**Usual adult and adolescent dose**
Antispasmodic, gastrointestinal: Irritable bowel syndrome—
  Oral, 10 to 20 mg three or four times a day, the dosage being adjusted as needed and tolerated.

Note: Geriatric patients may be more sensitive to the effects of the usual adult dose.

**Usual adult prescribing limits**
Up to 160 mg daily.

**Usual pediatric dose**
Antispasmodic, gastrointestinal—
  Children up to 6 years of age: Product not suitable for pediatric administration. See *Dicyclomine Hydrochloride Syrup USP*.
  Children 6 years of age and over: Oral, 10 mg three or four times a day, the dosage being adjusted as needed and tolerated.

**Strength(s) usually available**
U.S.—
  10 mg (Rx) [*Bentyl;* GENERIC].
  20 mg (Rx) [GENERIC].
Canada—
  10 mg (Rx) [*Formulex*].

**Packaging and storage**
Store below 40 °C (104 °F), preferably between 15 and 30 °C (59 and 86 °F), unless otherwise specified by manufacturer. Store in a well-closed container.

**Auxiliary labeling**
- May cause blurred vision.

### DICYCLOMINE HYDROCHLORIDE SYRUP USP

**Usual adult and adolescent dose**
Antispasmodic, gastrointestinal: Irritable bowel syndrome—
  Oral, 10 to 20 mg three or four times a day, the dosage being adjusted as needed and tolerated.

Note: Geriatric patients may be more sensitive to the effects of the usual adult dose.

**Usual adult prescribing limits**
Up to 160 mg daily.

**Usual pediatric dose**
Antispasmodic, gastrointestinal—
  Children up to 6 months of age: Use is not recommended.
  Children 6 months to 2 years of age: Oral, 5 to 10 mg three or four times a day, the dosage being adjusted as needed and tolerated.
  Children 2 years of age and over: Oral, 10 mg three or four times a day, the dosage being adjusted as needed and tolerated.

**Strength(s) usually available**
U.S.—
  10 mg per 5 mL (Rx) [*Bentyl;* GENERIC].
Canada—
  10 mg per 5 mL (Rx) [*Bentylol*].

**Packaging and storage**
Store below 40 °C (104 °F), preferably between 15 and 30 °C (59 and 86 °F), unless otherwise specified by manufacturer. Store in a tight container. Protect from freezing.

**Auxiliary labeling**
- May cause blurred vision.

### DICYCLOMINE HYDROCHLORIDE TABLETS USP

**Usual adult and adolescent dose**
Antispasmodic, gastrointestinal: Irritable bowel syndrome—
  Oral, 10 to 20 mg three or four times a day, the dosage being adjusted as needed and tolerated.

Note: Geriatric patients may be more sensitive to the effects of the usual adult dose.

**Usual adult prescribing limits**
Up to 160 mg daily.

**Usual pediatric dose**
Antispasmodic, gastrointestinal—
  Children up to 6 years of age: Product not suitable for pediatric administration. See *Dicyclomine Hydrochloride Syrup USP*.

Children 6 years of age and over: Oral, 10 mg three or four times a day, the dosage being adjusted as needed and tolerated.

**Strength(s) usually available**
U.S.—
  20 mg (Rx) [*Bentyl;* GENERIC].
Canada—
  10 mg (Rx) [*Bentylol*].
  20 mg (Rx) [*Bentylol; Spasmoban*].

**Packaging and storage**
Store below 40 °C (104 °F), preferably between 15 and 30 °C (59 and 86 °F), unless otherwise specified by manufacturer. Store in a well-closed container.

**Auxiliary labeling**
• May cause blurred vision.

### DICYCLOMINE HYDROCHLORIDE EXTENDED-RELEASE TABLETS

**Usual adult and adolescent dose**
Antispasmodic, gastrointestinal—
  Oral, 30 mg two times a day.

Note: Geriatric patients may be more sensitive to the effects of the usual adult dose.

**Usual pediatric dose**
Antispasmodic, gastrointestinal—
  Product not suitable for pediatric administration. See *Dicyclomine Hydrochloride Syrup USP*.

**Strength(s) usually available**
U.S.—
  Not commercially available.
Canada—
  Not commercially available.

**Packaging and storage**
Store below 40 °C (104 °F), preferably between 15 and 30 °C (59 and 86 °F), unless otherwise specified by manufacturer. Store in a tight container.

**Auxiliary labeling**
• May cause blurred vision.

## Parenteral Dosage Forms
### DICYCLOMINE HYDROCHLORIDE INJECTION USP

**Usual adult and adolescent dose**
Antispasmodic, gastrointestinal: Irritable bowel syndrome—
  Intramuscular, 20 mg every four to six hours, the dosage being adjusted as needed and tolerated.

Note: Not for intravenous use.
  Geriatric patients may be more sensitive to the effects of the usual adult dose.

**Usual pediatric dose**
Dosage has not been established.

**Strength(s) usually available**
U.S.—
  10 mg per mL (Rx) [*Bentyl;* GENERIC].
Canada—
  Not commercially available.

**Packaging and storage**
Store below 40 °C (104 °F), preferably between 15 and 30 °C (59 and 86 °F), unless otherwise specified by manufacturer. Protect from freezing.

---

## GLYCOPYRROLATE

### Summary of Differences
Category:
  Also, an [antidiarrheal]. Parenteral glycopyrrolate is used as an antiarrhythmic and cholinergic adjunct (curariform block).
Indications:
  Indicated as antisialagogue in preanesthesia. Also, indicated as antiarrhythmic in preanesthesia, anesthesia, and surgery. In addition, indicated to prevent aspiration pneumonitis during anesthesia. May be used as antidiarrheal and for cholinesterase inhibitor toxicity.
Pharmacology/pharmacokinetics:
  Half-life (elimination)—1.7 hours (range 0.6–4.6 hours).
  Onset of action—15 to 30 minutes with intramuscular or subcutaneous administration; 1 minute with intravenous administration.
  Duration of action—Antisialagogue effect up to 7 hours; vagal blocking effect 2 to 3 hours.
Precautions:
  Pregnancy—Rates of conception and survival at weaning decreased in studies with rats.
  Laboratory value alterations—Serum uric acid may be decreased in patients with hyperuricemia or gout.

## Oral Dosage Forms
### GLYCOPYRROLATE TABLETS USP

**Usual adult and adolescent dose**
Anticholinergic: Peptic ulcer—
  Oral, initially 1 to 2 mg two or three times a day and occasionally 2 mg at bedtime, then 1 mg two times a day, the dosage being adjusted as needed and tolerated.

Note: Geriatric patients may be more sensitive to the effects of the usual adult dose.

**Usual adult prescribing limits**
Up to 8 mg daily.

**Usual pediatric dose**
Dosage has not been established.

**Strength(s) usually available**
U.S.—
  1 mg (Rx) [*Robinul;* GENERIC].
  2 mg (Rx) [*Robinul Forte;* GENERIC].
Canada—
  1 mg (Rx) [*Robinul*].
  2 mg (Rx) [*Robinul Forte*].

**Packaging and storage**
Store below 40 °C (104 °F), preferably between 15 and 30 °C (59 and 86 °F), unless otherwise specified by manufacturer. Store in a tight container.

**Auxiliary labeling**
• May cause blurred vision.

## Parenteral Dosage Forms
### GLYCOPYRROLATE INJECTION USP

**Usual adult and adolescent dose**
Anticholinergic—
  Peptic ulcer:
    Intramuscular or intravenous, 100 to 200 mcg (0.1 to 0.2 mg), the dosage being repeated, if necessary, at four-hour intervals up to a maximum of four times a day.
  Prophylaxis of excessive salivation and respiratory tract secretions, in anesthesia and
  Prophylaxis of gastric hypersecretory conditions, in anesthesia:
    Intramuscular, 4.4 mcg (0.0044 mg) per kg of body weight one-half to one hour before induction of anesthesia or at the time the preanesthetic narcotic and/or sedative are administered.
Antiarrhythmic, in anesthesia or
Antiarrhythmic, in surgery—
  Intravenous, 100 mcg (0.1 mg), the dosage being repeated if necessary at two- to three-minute intervals.
Cholinergic adjunct (curariform block)—
  Intravenous, 200 mcg (0.2 mg) for each 1 mg of neostigmine or 5 mg of pyridostigmine given simultaneously; may be mixed in the same syringe.

Note: Geriatric patients may be more sensitive to the effects of the usual adult dose.

**Usual pediatric dose**
Anticholinergic—
  Peptic ulcer:
    Dosage has not been established.
  Prophylaxis of excessive salivation and respiratory tract secretions, in anesthesia and
  Prophylaxis of gastric hypersecretory conditions, in anesthesia:
    Intramuscular, 4.4 to 8.8 mcg (0.0044 to 0.0088 mg) per kg of body weight one-half to one hour before induction of anesthesia or at the time the preanesthetic narcotic and/or sedative are administered.
Antiarrhythmics, in anesthesia or
Antiarrhythmic, in surgery—
  Intravenous, 4.4 mcg (0.0044 mg) per kg of body weight up to a maximum of 100 mcg (0.1 mg), the dosage being repeated, if necessary, at two- to three-minute intervals.

Cholinergic adjunct (curariform block)—
Intravenous, 200 mcg (0.2 mg) for each 1 mg of neostigmine or 5 mg of pyridostigmine given simultaneously; may be mixed in the same syringe.

**Strength(s) usually available**
U.S.—
200 mcg (0.2 mg) per mL (Rx) [*Robinul*; GENERIC].
Canada—
200 mcg (0.2 mg) per mL (Rx) [*Robinul*].

**Packaging and storage**
Store below 40 °C (104 °F), preferably between 15 and 30 °C (59 and 86 °F), unless otherwise specified by manufacturer.

**Preparation of dosage form**
Glycopyrrolate may be mixed and administered with glucose 5 or 10% in water or saline, meperidine injection, morphine sulfate, fentanyl plus droperidol injection, hydroxyzine injection, neostigmine injection, or pyridostigmine injection.

**Stability**
Stability of glycopyrrolate may be affected at a pH higher than 6. A pH above 6 will result when glycopyrrolate is mixed with dexamethasone sodium phosphate or a buffered solution of lactated Ringer's solution.

**Incompatibilities**
Chloramphenicol, diazepam, dimenhydrinate, methohexital sodium, pentobarbital sodium, secobarbital sodium, thiopental sodium, and sodium bicarbonate are *not* suitable for mixing in the same syringe with glycopyrrolate since a gas or a precipitate may result.

---
## HOMATROPINE
---

## Oral Dosage Forms
### HOMATROPINE METHYLBROMIDE TABLETS USP

**Usual adult and adolescent dose**
Anticholinergic—
Oral, 5 to 10 mg three or four times a day, the dosage being adjusted as needed and tolerated.

Note: Geriatric patients may be more sensitive to the effects of the usual adult dose.

**Usual pediatric dose**
Dosage has not been established.

**Strength(s) usually available**
U.S.—
5 mg (Rx) [*Homapin*].
10 mg (Rx) [*Homapin*].
Canada—
Not commercially available.

**Packaging and storage**
Store below 40 °C (104 °F), preferably between 15 and 30 °C (59 and 86 °F), unless otherwise specified by manufacturer. Store in a tight, light-resistant container.

**Auxiliary labeling**
• May cause blurred vision.

---
## HYOSCYAMINE
---

## Summary of Differences
Category:
Parenteral hyoscyamine is also an antiarrhythmic, antidote (to cholinesterase inhibitors and to muscarine), and a cholinergic adjunct (curariform block).
Indications:
Also indicated for biliary disorders, cystitis, duodenography, and acute rhinitis. In preanesthesia, indicated as antisialagogue and also as antiarrhythmic during anesthesia and surgery.
Pharmacology/pharmacokinetics:
Protein binding—Moderate.
Half-life (elimination)—3.5 hours.
Onset of action—20 to 30 minutes with oral administration of hyoscyamine sulfate; 2 to 3 minutes with parenteral administration.
Duration of action—4 to 6 hours.
Elimination—Renal; majority of drug excreted unchanged.
Precautions:
Pregnancy—Intravenous administration may produce tachycardia in fetus.
Side/adverse effects:
Constipation has been reported less often with hyoscyamine.

**Additional Dosing Information**
See also *General Dosing Information*.
Hyoscyamine is effective at half the dosage of atropine.
In dehydrated patients, such as those with diarrhea and vomiting, treatment with hyoscyamine should be initiated at a lower dosage.

## Oral Dosage Forms
### HYOSCYAMINE TABLETS USP

**Usual adult and adolescent dose**
Anticholinergic—
Oral, 125 to 500 mcg (0.125 to 0.5 mg) three or four times a day, thirty minutes to one hour before meals and at bedtime, the dosage being adjusted as needed and tolerated.

Note: Geriatric patients may be more sensitive to the effects of the usual adult dose.

**Usual pediatric dose**
Dosage must be individualized by physician.

**Strength(s) usually available**
U.S.—
150 mcg (0.15 mg) (Rx) [*Cystospaz*].
Canada—
Not commercially available.

**Packaging and storage**
Store below 40 °C (104 °F), preferably between 15 and 30 °C (59 and 86 °F), unless otherwise specified by manufacturer. Store in a well-closed, light-resistant container.

**Auxiliary labeling**
• May cause blurred vision.

### HYOSCYAMINE SULFATE EXTENDED-RELEASE CAPSULES

**Usual adult and adolescent dose**
Anticholinergic—
Oral, 375 mcg (0.375 mg) two times a day, in the morning and at bedtime, the dosage being increased, if necessary, to obtain the desired response.

Note: Geriatric patients may be more sensitive to the effects of the usual adult dose.

**Usual pediatric dose**
Anticholinergic—
Children up to 12 years of age: Use is not recommended.
Children 12 years of age and over: See *Usual adult and adolescent dose*.

**Strength(s) usually available**
U.S.—
375 mcg (0.375 mg) (Rx) [*Cystospaz-M*; *Levsinex Timecaps*; *Symax SR*; GENERIC].
Canada—
Not commercially available.

**Packaging and storage**
Store below 40 °C (104 °F), preferably between 15 and 30 °C (59 and 86 °F), in a tight, light-resistant container, unless otherwise specified by manufacturer.

**Auxiliary labeling**
• Swallow capsules whole.
• May cause blurred vision.

### HYOSCYAMINE SULFATE EXTENDED-RELEASE TABLETS

**Usual adult and adolescent dose**
Anticholinergic—
Oral, 375 mcg (0.375 mg) to 750 mcg (0.75 mg) every twelve hours, not to exceed four tablets in twenty-four hours. Tablets may be broken for dosage titration.

**Usual pediatric dose**
Anticholinergic—
Children up to 12 years of age: Use is not recommended.
Children 12 years of age and over: See *Usual adult and adolescent dose*.

**Strength(s) usually available**
U.S.—
375 mcg (0.375 mg) (Rx) [*Levbid* (scored)].

Canada—
Not commercially available.

**Packaging and storage**
Store below 40 °C (104 °F), preferably between 15 and 30 °C (59 and 86 °F), in a tight, light-resistant container, unless otherwise specified by manufacturer.

**Auxiliary labeling**
- May cause blurred vision.

## HYOSCYAMINE SULFATE ELIXIR USP

**Usual adult and adolescent dose**
Anticholinergic—
Oral, 125 to 250 mcg (0.125 to 0.25 mg) every four to six hours, the dosage being adjusted as needed and tolerated.

Note: Geriatric patients may be more sensitive to the effects of the usual adult dose.

**Usual pediatric dose**
Anticholinergic—
Oral, the following doses every four hours as needed:
Children weighing 2.3 to 3.3 kg—12.5 mcg (0.0125 mg).
Children weighing 3.4 to 4.4 kg—15.6 mcg (0.0156 mg).
Children weighing 4.5 to 6.7 kg—18.8 mcg (0.0188 mg).
Children weighing 6.8 to 9 kg—25 mcg (0.025 mg).
Children weighing 9.1 to 13.5 kg—31.3 mcg (0.0313 mg).
Children weighing 13.6 to 22.6 kg—63 mcg (0.063 mg).
Children weighing 22.7 to 33 kg—94 to 125 mcg (0.094 to 0.125 mg).
Children weighing 34 to 36 kg—125 to 187 mcg (0.125 to 0.187 mg).

**Strength(s) usually available**
U.S.—
125 mcg (0.125 mg) per 5 mL (Rx) [*Levsin*].
Canada—
Not commercially available.

**Packaging and storage**
Store between 15 and 30 °C (59 and 86 °F), unless otherwise specified by manufacturer. Store in a tight, light-resistant container. Protect from freezing.

**Auxiliary labeling**
- May cause blurred vision.
- Keep container tightly closed.

## HYOSCYAMINE SULFATE ORAL SOLUTION USP

**Usual adult and adolescent dose**
Anticholinergic—
Oral, 125 to 250 mcg (0.125 to 0.25 mg) every four to six hours, the dosage being adjusted as needed and tolerated.

Note: Geriatric patients may be more sensitive to the effects of the usual adult dose.

**Usual pediatric dose**
Anticholinergic—
Oral, the following doses every four hours as needed:
Children weighing 2.3 to 3.3 kg—12.5 mcg (0.0125 mg).
Children weighing 3.4 to 4.4 kg—15.6 mcg (0.0156 mg).
Children weighing 4.5 to 6.7 kg—18.8 mcg (0.0188 mg).
Children weighing 6.8 to 9 kg—25 mcg (0.025 mg).
Children weighing 9.1 to 13.5 kg—31.3 mcg (0.0313 mg).
Children weighing 13.6 to 22.6 kg—63 mcg (0.063 mg).
Children weighing 22.7 to 33 kg—94 to 125 mcg (0.094 to 0.125 mg).
Children weighing 34 to 36 kg—125 to 187 mcg (0.125 to 0.187 mg).

**Strength(s) usually available**
U.S.—
125 mcg (0.125 mg) per mL (Rx) [*Gastrosed; Levsin* (alcohol 5%)].
Canada—
125 mg (0.125 mg) per mL (Rx) [*Levsin* (alcohol 5%)].
Note: 1 mL = approximately 28 drops (may vary with dropper).

**Packaging and storage**
Store below 40 °C (104 °F), preferably between 15 and 30 °C (59 and 86 °F), unless otherwise specified by manufacturer. Store in a tight, light-resistant container. Protect from freezing.

**Auxiliary labeling**
- May cause blurred vision.
- Keep container tightly closed.

**Note**
Dispense in dropper bottle.

## HYOSCYAMINE SULFATE TABLETS USP

**Usual adult and adolescent dose**
Anticholinergic—
Oral or sublingual, 125 to 500 mcg (0.125 to 0.5 mg) three or four times a day, thirty minutes to one hour before meals and at bedtime, the dosage being adjusted as needed and tolerated.

Note: Geriatric patients may be more sensitive to the effects of the usual adult dose.

**Usual pediatric dose**
Anticholinergic—
Children weighing up to 22.7 kg—Product not suitable for pediatric administration. See *Hyoscyamine Sulfate Oral Solution USP*.
Children weighing 22.7 to 33 kg—Oral, 94 to 125 mcg (0.094 to 0.125 mg).
Children weighing 34 to 36 kg—Oral, 125 to 187 mcg (0.125 to 0.187 mg).

**Strength(s) usually available**
U.S.—
125 mcg (0.125 mg) (Rx) [*Anaspaz; A-Spas S/L; Donnamar; ED-SPAZ; Gastrosed; Levsin; Levsin/SL; Symax SL;* GENERIC].
Canada—
125 mg (0.125 mg) (Rx) [*Levsin*].

**Packaging and storage**
Store below 40 °C (104 °F), preferably between 15 and 30 °C (59 and 86 °F), unless otherwise specified by manufacturer. Store in a tight, light-resistant container.

**Auxiliary labeling**
- May be chewed, swallowed whole, or allowed to dissolve under the tongue.
- May cause blurred vision.

# Parenteral Dosage Forms

## HYOSCYAMINE SULFATE INJECTION USP

**Usual adult and adolescent dose**
Anticholinergic—
Intramuscular, intravenous, or subcutaneous, 250 to 500 mcg (0.25 to 0.5 mg) every four to six hours.
Gastrointestinal radiography—
Intramuscular, intravenous, or subcutaneous, 250 to 500 mcg (0.25 to 0.5 mg) five to ten minutes prior to the diagnostic procedure.
Peptic ulcer—
Initial: Intravenous, 250 to 500 mcg (0.25 to 0.5 mg).
Maintenance: Intramuscular or subcutaneous, 250 to 500 mcg (0.25 to 0.5 mg) every six hours until all pain has ceased.
Prophylaxis of excessive salivation and respiratory tract secretions, in anesthesia—
Intramuscular, intravenous, or subcutaneous, 500 mcg (0.5 mg); or 5 mcg (0.005 mg) per kg of body weight thirty to sixty minutes before induction of anesthesia.
Antiarrhythmic—
Intravenous, 125 mcg (0.125 mg), repeated as needed.
Cholinergic adjunct (curariform block)—
Intravenous, 200 mcg (0.2 mg) for each 1 mg of neostigmine or the equivalent dose of physostigmine or pyridostigmine.

Note: Geriatric patients may be more sensitive to the effects of the usual adult dose.

**Usual pediatric dose**
Anticholinergic—
Prophylaxis of excessive salivation and respiratory tract secretions, in anesthesia:
Children up to 2 years of age—Use is not recommended.
Children 2 years of age and over—Intramuscular, intravenous, or subcutaneous, 5 mcg (0.005 mg) per kg of body weight thirty to sixty minutes before induction of anesthesia.

Note: Hyoscyamine sulfate injection that contains benzyl alcohol as a preservative should not be used in newborn and immature infants. The use of benzyl alcohol in neonates has been associated with a fatal toxic syndrome consisting of metabolic acidosis and CNS, respiratory, circulatory, and renal function impairment.

**Strength(s) usually available**
U.S.—
500 mcg (0.5 mg) per mL (Rx) [*Levsin* (benzyl alcohol 1.5%)].
Canada—
Not commercially available.

## MEPENZOLATE

### Summary of Differences
Pharmacology/pharmacokinetics:
  Elimination—Renal; 3 to 22% excreted unchanged.
Precautions:
  Pregnancy—Reproduction studies in rats and rabbits have not shown adverse effects on fetus.

### Oral Dosage Forms
**MEPENZOLATE BROMIDE TABLETS**

**Usual adult and adolescent dose**
Anticholinergic—
  Oral, 25 to 50 mg four times a day with meals and at bedtime, the dosage being adjusted as needed and tolerated.
Note: Geriatric patients may be more sensitive to the effects of the usual adult dose.

**Usual pediatric dose**
Dosage has not been established.

**Strength(s) usually available**
U.S.—
  25 mg (Rx) [*Cantil*].
Canada—
  Not commercially available.

**Packaging and storage**
Store below 40 °C (104 °F), preferably between 15 and 30 °C (59 and 86 °F), unless otherwise specified by manufacturer. Store in a well-closed container.

**Auxiliary labeling**
• May cause blurred vision.

## METHANTHELINE

### Summary of Differences
Indications:
  Also indicated for urinary incontinence.

### Oral Dosage Forms
**METHANTHELINE BROMIDE TABLETS**

**Usual adult and adolescent dose**
Anticholinergic—
  Oral, 50 to 100 mg every six hours, the dosage being adjusted as needed and tolerated.
Note: Geriatric patients may be more sensitive to the effects of the usual adult dose.

**Usual pediatric dose**
Anticholinergic—
  Children up to 1 month of age: Oral, 12.5 mg two times a day, the dosage being increased to three times a day if needed and tolerated.
  Children 1 month to 1 year of age: Oral, 12.5 mg four times a day, the dosage being increased to 25 mg four times a day if needed and tolerated.
  Children 1 year of age and over: Oral, 12.5 to 50 mg four times a day, the dosage being adjusted as needed and tolerated.

**Strength(s) usually available**
U.S.—
  50 mg (Rx) [*Banthine* (scored)].
Canada—
  Not commercially available.

**Packaging and storage**
Store below 40 °C (104 °F), preferably between 15 and 30 °C (59 and 86 °F), unless otherwise specified by manufacturer. Store in a well-closed container.

**Auxiliary labeling**
• May cause blurred vision.

## METHSCOPOLAMINE

### Summary of Differences
Pharmacology/pharmacokinetics:
  Onset of action—1 hour.
  Duration of action—6 to 8 hours.

### Oral Dosage Forms
**METHSCOPOLAMINE BROMIDE TABLETS**

**Usual adult and adolescent dose**
Anticholinergic—
  Oral, 2.5 mg four times a day, one-half hour before meals and 2.5 to 5 mg at bedtime.
  For severe symptoms: Oral, initially 5 mg four times a day, one-half hour before meals and at bedtime, the dosage being increased, if necessary, to obtain the desired response.
Note: Geriatric patients may be more sensitive to the effects of the usual adult dose.

**Usual pediatric dose**
Anticholinergic—
  Oral, 200 mcg (0.2 mg) per kg of body weight or 6 mg per square meter of body surface a day (in four divided doses, before meals and at bedtime).

**Strength(s) usually available**
U.S.—
  Not commercially available.
Canada—
  Not commercially available.

**Packaging and storage**
Store between 15 and 30 °C (59 and 86 °F), unless otherwise specified by manufacturer. Store in a tight container.

**Auxiliary labeling**
• May cause blurred vision.

## PIRENZEPINE

### Summary of Differences
Pharmacology/pharmacokinetics:
  Half-life (elimination)—10 to 12 hours.
  Elimination—Renal and hepatic; 80 to 90% of drug excreted unchanged.

### Oral Dosage Forms
**PIRENZEPINE HYDROCHLORIDE TABLETS**

**Usual adult and adolescent dose**
Anticholinergic—
  Oral, 50 mg two times a day, in the morning and at bedtime, the dosage being increased to three times a day, if needed and tolerated.
Note: Geriatric patients may be more sensitive to the effects of the usual adult dose.

**Usual pediatric dose**
Dosage has not been established.

**Strength(s) usually available**
U.S.—
  Not commercially available.
Canada—
  50 mg (Rx) [*Gastrozepin*].

**Packaging and storage**
Store below 40 °C (104 °F), preferably between 15 and 30 °C (59 and 86 °F), unless otherwise specified by manufacturer.

**Auxiliary labeling**
• May cause blurred vision.

## PROPANTHELINE

### Summary of Differences
Indications:
  Also used for duodenography and urinary incontinence.

Pharmacology/pharmacokinetics:
    Half-life (elimination)—1.6 (mean) hours.
    Duration of action—6 hours.
    Elimination—Renal; less than 6% of drug excreted unchanged.

## Oral Dosage Forms
### PROPANTHELINE BROMIDE TABLETS USP
**Usual adult and adolescent dose**
Anticholinergic—
    Oral, 15 mg three times a day, one-half hour before meals, and 30 mg at bedtime, the dosage being adjusted as needed and tolerated.
Note: Patients of less than average body weight may require only 7.5 mg three or four times a day.

**Usual adult prescribing limits**
Up to 120 mg daily.

**Usual pediatric dose**
Anticholinergic—
    Oral, 375 mcg (0.375 mg) per kg of body weight or 10 mg per square meter of body surface four times a day, the dosage being adjusted as needed and tolerated.
Note: Pediatric administration is limited by the available dosage form. The tablets are not suitable for subdivision.

**Usual geriatric dose**
Oral, 7.5 mg three or four times a day.

**Strength(s) usually available**
U.S.—
    7.5 mg (Rx) [*Pro-Banthine*].
    15 mg (Rx) [*Pro-Banthine*; GENERIC].
Canada—
    7.5 mg (Rx) [*Pro-Banthine*].
    15 mg (Rx) [*Pro-Banthine; Propanthel*].

**Packaging and storage**
Store below 40 °C (104 °F), preferably between 15 and 30 °C (59 and 86 °F), unless otherwise specified by manufacturer. Store in a well-closed container.

**Auxiliary labeling**
• May cause blurred vision.

---

## SCOPOLAMINE

## Summary of Differences
Category:
    Also a gastrointestinal antispasmodic, antidysmenorrheal, urinary antispasmodic, antiemetic, and antivertigo agent. Parenteral scopolamine is used as an antiarrhythmic and anesthesia adjunct.
Indications—
    Indicated in preanesthesia as antisialagogue. Also indicated for biliary tract disorders, nocturnal enuresis, and excessive salivation. Not indicated for peptic ulcer.
Pharmacology/pharmacokinetics:
    Protein binding—
        Scopolamine hydrobromide: Low.
    Half-life (elimination)—
        8 hours.
    Onset of action—
        Oral scopolamine hydrobromide:
            30 to 60 minutes (antisialagogue effect).
        Parenteral scopolamine hydrobromide:
            30 minutes (antisialagogue effect).
    Duration of action—
        Scopolamine hydrobromide:
            Oral—4 to 6 hours.
            Parenteral—4 hours.
        Scoolamine Transdermal:
            Up to 72 hours.
    Elimination—
        Renal; 1% of oral dose excreted unchanged, and 3.4% of subcutaneous dose excreted unchanged.
Precautions:
    Pregnancy—
        Parenteral administration before onset of labor may cause CNS depression and hemorrhage in neonate.
    Drug interactions and/or related problems—
        Additive sedation with other CNS depressants.

Laboratory value alterations—
    Residual cycloplegia and mydriasis with transdermal dosage form may affect results of neuroradiological tests for intracranial neoplasm, subdural hematoma, or cerebral aneurysm.
Side/adverse effects:
    Scopolamine has been reported to cause paradoxical reaction (trouble in sleeping). Anxiety, irritability, nightmares, and trouble in sleeping may indicate rebound reduction in rapid eye movement (REM) time. Drowsiness and a false sense of well being are more common also.

## Additional Dosing Information
See also *General Dosing Information*.

In the presence of pain, scopolamine may act as a stimulant, often producing delirium, if used without morphine or meperidine.

Cardiac rate is much slower with low doses of scopolamine (0.1 to 0.2 mg) than with average clinical doses of atropine. With higher doses, a short-lived cardioacceleration occurs followed within 30 minutes by a return to the normal rate.

## Oral Dosage Forms
### SCOPOLAMINE BUTYLBROMIDE TABLETS
**Usual adult and adolescent dose**
Anticholinergic or
Antispasmodic, gastrointestinal or
Antidysmenorrheal—
    Oral, 10 to 20 mg three or four times a day, the dosage being adjusted as needed and tolerated.
Note: Geriatric patients may be more sensitive to the effects of the usual adult dose.

**Usual pediatric dose**
Dosage has not been established.

**Strength(s) usually available**
U.S.—
    Not commercially available.
Canada—
    10 mg (Rx) [*Buscopan*].

**Packaging and storage**
Store below 40 °C (104 °F), preferably between 15 and 30 °C (59 and 86 °F), in a well-closed container, unless otherwise specified by manufacturer.

**Auxiliary labeling**
• May cause drowsiness or blurred vision.
• Avoid alcoholic beverages.

## Parenteral Dosage Forms
### SCOPOLAMINE BUTYLBROMIDE INJECTION
**Usual adult and adolescent dose**
Anticholinergic or
Antispasmodic, gastrointestinal—
    Intramuscular, intravenous, or subcutaneous, 10 to 20 mg three or four times a day, the dosage being adjusted as needed and tolerated.

**Usual pediatric dose**
Dosage has not been established.

**Strength(s) usually available**
U.S.—
    Not commercially available.
Canada—
    20 mg per mL (Rx) [*Buscopan*].

**Packaging and storage**
Store below 40 °C (104 °F), preferably between 15 and 30 °C (59 and 86 °F), unless otherwise specified by manufacturer. Protect from freezing.

### SCOPOLAMINE HYDROBROMIDE INJECTION USP
**Usual adult and adolescent dose**
Anticholinergic—
    Intramuscular, intravenous, or subcutaneous, 300 to 600 mcg (0.3 to 0.6 mg) as a single dose.
Prophylaxis of excessive salivation and respiratory tract secretions, in anesthesia:
    Intramuscular, 200 to 600 mcg (0.2 to 0.6 mg) one-half to one hour before induction of anesthesia.
Antiemetic—
    Intramuscular, intravenous, or subcutaneous, 300 to 600 mcg (0.3 to 0.6 mg) as a single dose.

Anesthesia adjunct—
    Sedation-hypnosis:
        Intramuscular, intravenous, or subcutaneous, 600 mcg (0.6 mg) three or four times a day.
    Amnesia:
        Intramuscular, intravenous, or subcutaneous, 320 to 650 mcg (0.32 to 0.65 mg).
Note: Geriatric patients may be more sensitive to the effects of the usual adult dose.

**Usual pediatric dose**
Anticholinergic or
Antiemetic—
    Intramuscular, intravenous, or subcutaneous, 6 mcg (0.006 mg) per kg of body weight or 200 mcg (0.2 mg) per square meter of body surface, as a single dose.
Prophylaxis of excessive salivation and respiratory tract secretions, in anesthesia—
    Intramuscular, administered forty-five minutes to one hour before induction of anesthesia for:
    Children up to 4 months of age—Use is not recommended.
    Children 4 to 7 months of age—100 mcg (0.1 mg).
    Children 7 months to 3 years of age—150 mcg (0.15 mg).
    Children 3 to 8 years of age—200 mcg (0.2 mg).
    Children 8 to 12 years of age—300 mcg (0.3 mg).

**Strength(s) usually available**
U.S.—
    300 mcg (0.3 mg) per mL (Rx) [GENERIC].
    400 mcg (0.4 mg) per mL (Rx) [GENERIC].
    500 mcg (0.5 mg) per mL (Rx) [GENERIC].
    600 mcg (0.6 mg) per mL (Rx) [GENERIC].
    860 mcg (0.86 mg) per mL (Rx) [GENERIC].
    1 mg per mL (Rx) [GENERIC].
Canada—
    Not commercially available.

**Packaging and storage**
Store below 40 °C (104 °F), preferably between 15 and 30 °C (59 and 86 °F), unless otherwise specified by manufacturer. Store in a light-resistant container. Protect from freezing.

**Preparation of dosage form**
When given intravenously, scopolamine should be diluted with sterile water for injection before administration.

# Rectal Dosage Forms
## SCOPOLAMINE BUTYLBROMIDE SUPPOSITORIES
**Usual adult and adolescent dose**
Anticholinergic or
Antispasmodic, gastrointestinal or
Antidysmenorrheal—
    Rectal, 10 mg three or four times a day, the dosage being adjusted as needed and tolerated.
Note: Geriatric patients may be more sensitive to the effects of the usual adult dose.

**Usual pediatric dose**
Dosage has not been established.

**Strength(s) usually available**
U.S.—
    Not commercially available.
Canada—
    10 mg (Rx) [Buscopan].

**Packaging and storage**
Store below 40 °C (104 °F), preferably between 15 and 30 °C (59 and 86 °F), unless otherwise specified by manufacturer.

**Auxiliary labeling**
• May cause drowsiness or blurred vision.

**Note**
Include patient instructions when dispensing.

# Transdermal Dosage Forms
## SCOPOLAMINE TRANSDERMAL SYSTEM
**Usual adult and adolescent dose**
Antiemetic or
Antivertigo agent—
    Topical, to the postauricular skin, 1 transdermal system delivering 500 mcg (0.5 mg) over a period of three days, applied at least four hours before antiemetic effect is required.
Note: Canadian brand product delivers 1 mg over a period of three days and should be applied approximately twelve hours before the antiemetic effect is required.
    Geriatric patients may be more sensitive to the effects of the usual adult dose.

**Usual pediatric dose**
Use is not recommended.

**Strength(s) usually available**
U.S.—
    1.5 mg (Rx) [Transderm-Scop].
Canada—
    1.5 mg (Rx) [Transderm-V].

**Packaging and storage**
Store below 40 °C (104 °F), preferably between 15 and 30 °C (59 and 86 °F), unless otherwise specified by manufacturer.

**Auxiliary labeling**
• May cause drowsiness or blurred vision.

**Note**
Include patient instructions when dispensing.

Revised: 01/29/92
Interim revision: 09/09/94; 07/19/95; 02/24/98

# Table 1. Side/Adverse Effects*

The following side/adverse effects have been selected on the basis of their potential clinical significance (possible signs and symptoms in parentheses where appropriate)—not necessarily inclusive:

Legend:
I=Anisotropine
II=Atropine
III=Belladonna
IV=Clidinium
V=Dicyclomine
VI=Glycopyrrolate
VII=Homatropine
VIII=Hyoscyamine
IX=Mepenzolate
X=Methantheline
XI=Methscopolamine
XII=Pirenzepine
XIII=Propantheline
XIV=Scopolamine

M=more frequent; L=less frequent; R=rare; U=unknown.

| | I | II | III | IV | V | VI | VII | VIII | IX | X | XI | XII | XIII | XIV |
|---|---|---|---|---|---|---|---|---|---|---|---|---|---|---|
| **Medical attention needed** | | | | | | | | | | | | | | |
| Allergic reaction (skin rash or hives) | R | R | R | R | R | R | R | R | R | R | R | R | R | R |
| Confusion# | R | R | R | R | R | R | R | R | R | R | R | R | R | R |
| Increased intraocular pressure (eye pain)† | R | R | R | R | R | R | R | R | R | R | R | R | R | R |
| Orthostatic hypotension (dizziness, feeling faint, or continuing lightheadedness) | § | R | R | § | R | § | § | R | § | § | § | R | § | R |
| **Medical attention needed only if continuing or bothersome** | | | | | | | | | | | | | | |
| Bloated feeling | R | R | R | R | R | R | R | R | R | R | R | R | R | R |
| Constipation | M | M | M | M | M | M | M | L | L | M | M | M | M | M |
| Decreased flow of breast milk | L | L | L | L | L | L | L | L | L | L | L | L | L | L |
| Decreased salivary secretion (difficulty in swallowing) | L | L | L | L | L | L | L | L | L | L | L | L | L | L |
| Decreased sweating | M | M | M | M | M | M | M | M | M | M | M | M | M | M |
| Difficult urination** | R | R | R | R | R | R | R | R | R | R | R | R | R | R |
| Difficulty in accommodation of the eye (blurred vision)† | R | L | L | L | L | L | R | L | R | L | R | L | R | L |
| Drowsiness††† | R | R | R | R | R | R | R | R | R | R | R | R | R | M |
| Dryness of mouth, nose, throat, or skin | M | M | M | M | M | M | M | M | M | M | M | M | M | M |
| False sense of well-being | U | U | U | U | U | U | U | U | U | U | U | U | U | R |
| Headache | R | R | R | R | R | R | R | R | R | R | R | R | R | R |
| Lightheadedness, temporary—with parenteral administration | U | U | U | U | R | R | U | R | U | U | U | R | U | R |
| Loss of memory‡‡ | U | U | U | U | R | R | U | R | U | U | U | R | U | R |
| Mydriatic effect (increased sensitivity of eyes to light)† | R | L | L | R | L | L | R | L | R | R | R | L | R | L |
| Nausea or vomiting | R | R | R | R | R | R | R | R | R | R | R | R | R | R |
| Paradoxical reaction (trouble in sleeping) | U | U | U | U | U | U | U | U | U | U | U | U | U | R |
| Redness or other signs of irritation at injection site | U | M | U | U | M | M | R | M | U | U | U | R | U | M |
| Unusual tiredness or weakness | R | R | R | R | R | R | R | R | R | R | R | R | R | R |

*Differences in frequency of occurrence may reflect either lack of clinical-use data or actual pharmacologic distinctions among agents (although their pharmacologic similarity suggests that side effects occurring with one may occur with the others). M=more frequent; L=less frequent; R=rare; U=unknown.
†Quaternary ammonium compounds are fully ionized in the pH range of body fluids and possess reduced lipid solubility. Therefore, they penetrate cellular barriers less effectively and only pass across the blood-brain barrier or into the eye with difficulty. Central and ocular effects are negligible and/or less likely to occur with quaternary ammonium compounds.
‡With quaternary ammonium compounds, difficulty in breathing, severe muscle weakness, and severe tiredness may occur because of the compounds' curare-like effects; these effects may lead to respiratory paralysis.
§Orthostatic hypotension, due to ganglion-blocking activity, is more likely to occur with high doses of quaternary ammonium compounds.
#Confusion may occur more frequently in geriatric patients.
**Difficult urination is more likely to occur in older men and may require medical attention in patients with symptoms of prostatism.
††More frequent with high doses of anticholinergics, but a common side effect with therapeutic doses of oral or parenteral scopolamine.
‡‡Scopolamine, administered parenterally as preanesthetic medication and/or given in large doses, may have a temporary but detrimental effect on memory. In geriatric patients, especially those who already have memory problems, the continued use of any anticholinergic may severely impair memory.
§§May indicate rebound reduction in rapid eye movement (REM) time.

## Table 1. Side/Adverse Effects (continued)*

The following side/adverse effects have been selected on the basis of their potential clinical significance (possible signs and symptoms in parentheses where appropriate)—not necessarily inclusive:

Legend:
I = Anisotropine
II = Atropine
III = Belladonna
IV = Clidinium
V = Dicyclomine
VI = Glycopyrrolate
VII = Homatropine
VIII = Hyoscyamine
IX = Mepenzolate
X = Methantheline
XI = Methscopolamine
XII = Pirenzepine
XIII = Propantheline
XIV = Scopolamine

| | I | II | III | IV | V | VI | VII | VIII | IX | X | XI | XII | XIII | XIV |
|---|---|---|---|---|---|---|---|---|---|---|---|---|---|---|
| **Medical attention needed if they occur after scopolamine is discontinued** | | | | | | | | | | | | | | |
| *Anxiety* | U | U | U | U | U | U | U | U | U | U | U | U | U | §§ |
| *Irritability* | U | U | U | U | U | U | U | U | U | U | U | U | U | §§ |
| *Nightmares* | U | U | U | U | U | U | U | U | U | U | U | U | U | §§ |
| *Trouble in sleeping* | U | U | U | U | U | U | U | U | U | U | U | U | U | §§ |

*Differences in frequency of occurrence may reflect either lack of clinical-use data or actual pharmacologic distinctions among agents (although their pharmacologic similarity suggests that side effects occurring with one may occur with the others). M = more frequent; L = less frequent; R = rare; U = unknown.

†Quaternary ammonium compounds are fully ionized in the pH range of body fluids and possess reduced lipid solubility. Therefore, they penetrate cellular barriers less effectively and only pass across the blood-brain barrier or into the eye with difficulty. Central and ocular effects are negligible and/or less likely to occur with quaternary ammonium compounds.

‡With quaternary ammonium compounds, difficulty in breathing, severe muscle weakness, and severe tiredness may occur because of the compounds' curare-like effects; these effects may lead to respiratory paralysis.

§Orthostatic hypotension, due to ganglion-blocking activity, is more likely to occur with high doses of quaternary ammonium compounds.

#Confusion may occur more frequently in geriatric patients.

**Difficult urination is more likely to occur in older men and may require medical attention in patients with symptoms of prostatism.

††More frequent with high doses of anticholinergics, but a common side effect with therapeutic doses of oral or parenteral scopolamine.

‡‡Scopolamine, administered parenterally as preanesthetic medication and/or given in large doses, may have a temporary but detrimental effect on memory. In geriatric patients, especially those who already have memory problems, the continued use of any anticholinergic may severely impair memory.

§§May indicate rebound reduction in rapid eye movement (REM) time.

# ANTICOAGULANTS Systemic

This monograph includes information on the following: 1) Anisindione†; 2) Dicumarol†; 3) Warfarin

Note: See also individual *Heparin (Systemic)* and *Antithrombin III (Systemic)* monographs.

INN: Dicumarol†—Dicoumarol

VA CLASSIFICATION (Primary): BL100

Commonly used brand name(s): *Coumadin*³; *Miradon*¹; *Panwarfin*³; *Sofarin*³; *Warfilone*³.

¹Not included in Canadian product labeling.

## Category
Anticoagulant.

## Indications

Note: Bracketed information in the *Indications* section refers to uses that are not included in U.S. product labeling.

Note: Several of the indications for coumarin- or indandione-derivative anticoagulant therapy are identical to those for thrombolytic (alteplase [tissue-type plasminogen activator, recombinant; tPA], anistreplase [anisoylated plasminogen-streptokinase activator complex; APSAC] streptokinase, or urokinase) and/or heparin therapy. Thrombolytic agents are used primarily to lyse obstructive thrombi and restore blood flow in a recently occluded blood vessel, whereas anticoagulants are used primarily to prevent thrombus formation and extension of existing thrombi. For treatment of acute deep venous thrombosis and acute pulmonary embolism, a thrombolytic agent may be the treatment of choice; however, the selection of thrombolytic therapy or anticoagulant therapy as opposed to other forms of treatment, including vascular surgery, must be based on determination of the severity of thrombotic disease and assessment of patient condition and history.

Because the therapeutic effects of coumarin- or indandione-derivative anticoagulants may not occur until after several days of therapy, heparin is the agent of choice when an immediate anticoagulant effect is required. A coumarin or indandione derivative is usually administered when an immediate anticoagulant effect is not necessary or when long-term anticoagulation is required following initial thrombolytic and/or heparin therapy.

### Accepted

Thrombosis, deep venous (prophylaxis and treatment) or
Thromboembolism, pulmonary (prophylaxis and treatment)—Anticoagulants are indicated in the treatment of patients with recent deep vein thrombosis or thrombophlebitis to prevent extension and embolization of the thrombus and to reduce the risk of pulmonary embolism or recurrent thrombus formation. In acute pulmonary embolism or venous thrombosis, anticoagulants are indicated following initial thrombolytic and/or heparin therapy to decrease the risk of extension, recurrence, or death.

Anticoagulants are indicated for prophylaxis of venous thrombosis and pulmonary embolism postoperatively or in high-risk patients, such as those with a history of thromboembolism or those requiring prolonged immobilization. However, subcutaneous administration of low-dose heparin is more commonly used to prevent postsurgical thromboembolic complications.

Thromboembolism (prophylaxis)—Anticoagulants are indicated [or used] for prophylaxis of thromboembolism associated with:

Chronic atrial fibrillation—Anticoagulants may prevent the formation of mural thrombi in the heart, which may lead to systemic thromboembolism in patients with chronic atrial fibrillation, especially those with rheumatic mitral stenosis, prosthetic heart valves, left atrial enlargement, or cardiomyopathy. In these patients, anticoagulants may decrease the risk of arterial embolism, pulmonary embolism, or subsequent stroke.

Myocardial infarction—Anticoagulants are indicated as adjunctive therapy to reduce the risk of systemic thromboembolic complications following acute myocardial infarction (especially an anterior wall myocardial infarction or a large apical infarction), primarily in high-risk patients such as those with shock, congestive heart failure, prolonged arrhythmias (especially atrial fibrillation), previous myocardial infarction, or history of thromboembolism.

[Cardioversion of chronic atrial fibrillation, electric or pharmacologic]—Anticoagulants are used to reduce the risk of postconversion emboli.

[Prosthetic heart valves]—Anticoagulants are used to reduce the risk of thromboembolic complications in patients with certain types of prosthetic heart valves. The effectiveness of these agents may be increased by concurrent use of a platelet aggregation inhibitor such as dipyridamole. Aspirin is also sometimes used concurrently with anticoagulants for this purpose; however, the risk of hemorrhage is increased.

[Thromboembolism, cerebral, recurrence (prophylaxis)]—Anticoagulants are used to reduce the risk of recurrence of cerebral embolism in patients with recent cerebral embolism, especially when the source of the embolism is thought to be the heart. The possibility that cerebral hemorrhage may be present must be ruled out before anticoagulant therapy is initiated. Although administration of an anticoagulant too soon after a cerebral embolism may increase the risk of cerebral hemorrhage, recent studies have indicated that the risk of early recurrence may be greater than the risk of anticoagulant therapy.

[Myocardial reinfarction (prophylaxis)]—Long-term use of anticoagulants following myocardial infarction to prevent reinfarction remains controversial; many clinicians report that recurrence of acute attacks and/or risk of death may not be reduced by such therapy. A few studies have indicated that long-term anticoagulation may reduce the risk of recurrent myocardial infarction and of nonhemorrhagic cerebrovascular accidents in patients older than 60 years of age. However, aspirin is also effective, and is more commonly used, for this purpose.

[Ischemic attacks, transient, in females and males (treatment)]—Warfarin has been used as an adjunct in the treatment of patients with transient ischemic attacks. It may reduce the incidence of repeat attacks and/or subsequent stroke, especially during the first few months of therapy. However, the risk of death may not be decreased. FDA has classified warfarin as being possibly effective for this indication; this classification requires the submission of adequate and well-controlled studies in order to provide substantial evidence of effectiveness. Platelet aggregation inhibitors (especially aspirin) are more commonly being used for this indication.

[Anticoagulants have also been used to reduce the risk of thrombosis and/or occlusion of the aortocoronary bypass following coronary bypass surgery. However, their efficacy has not been proven and platelet aggregation inhibitors are now being administered for this purpose.]

## Pharmacology/Pharmacokinetics

### Physicochemical characteristics
Chemical group—
  Coumarin derivatives: Dicumarol, warfarin.
  Indandione derivative: Anisindione.
Molecular weight—
  Anisindione: 252.27.
  Dicumarol: 336.30.
  Warfarin sodium: 330.31.

### Mechanism of action/Effect
Both coumarin and indandione derivatives are indirect-acting anticoagulants (act only *in vivo*); they prevent the formation of active procoagulation factors II, VII, IX, and X in the liver by inhibiting the vitamin K–mediated gamma-carboxylation of precursor proteins. Full therapeutic action is delayed until circulating coagulation factors are removed by normal catabolism, which occurs at different rates for each factor. Although prothrombin time (PT) may be prolonged when factor VII (which has the shortest half-life) is depleted, it is believed that peak antithrombotic effects are not achieved until all four factors are removed. These agents have no direct thrombolytic effect, although they may limit extension of existing thrombi.

### Absorption
Anisindione and warfarin are well absorbed from the gastrointestinal tract. The rate, but not the extent, of warfarin absorption is decreased by food. Dicumarol is slowly and incompletely absorbed from the gastrointestinal tract.

### Protein binding
Very high (99%); to albumin.

### Biotransformation
Hepatic.

## Elimination
Via hepatic metabolism, followed by renal excretion of metabolites; following enterohepatic circulation.

| Drug | Half-life* | Onset of Action† (days) | Duration of Action‡ (days) |
|---|---|---|---|
| Anisindione | 3–5 days | 2–3 | 1–3 |
| Dicumarol | 1–4 days§ | 1–5 | 2–10 |
| Warfarin# | 1.5–2.5 days** | 0.5–3 | 2–5 |

*Subject to intra- and inter-patient variation.

†As determined by effect on PT; may reflect early depletion of factor VII rather than peak antithrombotic effects. Also, may reflect use of initial loading doses, which is currently not recommended.

‡Time after discontinuation of therapy for prothrombin activity to return to the pretreatment value.

§Dose-dependent.

#For oral, intramuscular, or intravenous administration.

**Mean is approximately 50 hours.

## Precautions to Consider

### Pregnancy/Reproduction

Pregnancy—Coumarin- and indandione-derivative anticoagulants cross the placenta and are not recommended during pregnancy. Congenital malformations and other adverse effects on fetal development, including severe nasal hypoplasia, stippling of bones, optic atrophy, microcephaly, and growth and mental retardation have been reported in infants born to mothers taking these agents during pregnancy. This is especially critical during the first trimester. However, many clinicians recommend that these agents not be used at all during pregnancy because facial anomalies in the infant have occurred following maternal use in the third trimester. Also, fetal or neonatal hemorrhage, fetal death in utero, and increased risk of maternal hemorrhage during the second and third trimesters have been reported. However, other clinicians state that these agents may be used for brief periods in the second and third trimesters.

Women of childbearing potential should be informed of the risks of becoming pregnant while receiving a coumarin or indandione derivative and advised to use an effective (nonhormonal) method of birth control throughout therapy. Patients who wish to become pregnant during therapy should first discuss their plans with the prescriber. Also, patients should be instructed to contact the prescribing physician immediately if they suspect that they are pregnant. Some clinicians recommend that, if a woman becomes pregnant during coumarin or indandione anticoagulant therapy, termination of the pregnancy be considered.

If an anticoagulant is required during pregnancy, heparin may be preferred because it does not cross the placenta. A patient receiving a coumarin or indandione derivative who wishes to become pregnant should preferably be changed to heparin therapy prior to conception.

Labor and delivery—If a coumarin or indandione derivative is used during the third trimester, it should be discontinued after the 37th week of gestation, and heparin substituted if maternal anticoagulation is required, to reduce the risk of fetal hemorrhage during labor and of neonatal hemorrhage following delivery. Anticoagulants also increase the risk of maternal hemorrhage during or following delivery.

Postpartum—Anticoagulants may increase the risk of maternal hemorrhage if administered in the postpartum period.

### Breast-feeding

Warfarin is distributed into breast milk in extremely small quantities, if at all, and is not considered hazardous to the nursing infant. With other anticoagulants, there is a possibility of significant quantities being distributed into breast milk; the nursing infant should be monitored for evidence of hypoprothrombinemia and vitamin K administered if necessary.

### Pediatrics

Infants, especially neonates, may be more susceptible to the effects of anticoagulants because of vitamin K deficiency.

### Geriatrics

Geriatric patients may be more susceptible to the effects of anticoagulants, resulting in increased risk of hemorrhage, possibly because of the presence of advanced vascular disease resulting in altered homeostatic mechanisms, hepatic function impairment resulting in decreased procoagulant factor synthesis or anticoagulant metabolism, or renal function impairment. Lower maintenance doses than those usually recommended for adults may be required for these patients.

### Dental

Bleeding from gingival tissue may be a sign of anticoagulant overdose.

Anticoagulant therapy increases the risk of localized hemorrhage during and following oral surgical procedures. Consultation with the prescribing physician may be advisable prior to oral surgery, to determine whether a temporary dosage reduction or withdrawal of anticoagulant therapy is feasible. Also, local measures to minimize bleeding should be used at the time of surgery.

### Drug interactions and/or related problems

All interactions between coumarin or indandione derivatives and other medications have not been identified. Also, several medications may interact with anticoagulant therapy by more than one mechanism; in several cases, both increased anticoagulation and decreased anticoagulation have been reported for the same interacting medication. Therefore, the net effect of some concurrently used medications on anticoagulant therapy may be unpredictable. In addition, control of anticoagulant therapy may be more difficult to achieve if an interacting medication is used intermittently rather than chronically.

Because of the possible serious consequences of interference with anticoagulant therapy, increased monitoring of the prothrombin time (PT) is recommended when *any* medication is added to or withdrawn from the regimen of a patient stabilized on a coumarin or indandione derivative, or if the dosage of a concurrently used medication is changed. Anticoagulant dosage must be adjusted as necessary to prevent hemorrhage or loss of effect. Also, substantial alteration of initial anticoagulant dosage may be necessary when anticoagulant therapy is initiated in a patient receiving a medication known to cause significant alteration of anticoagulant effect.

See *Table 1*, page 249.

### Laboratory value alterations

The following have been selected on the basis of their potential clinical significance (possible effect in parentheses where appropriate)—not necessarily inclusive (» = major clinical significance):

With diagnostic test results
  Urinalysis
    (tests based on color changes may be interfered with because alkaline urine may turn orange following administration of anisindione; acidification of the urine eliminates this color)

### Medical considerations/Contraindications

The medical considerations/contraindications included have been selected on the basis of their potential clinical significance (reasons given in parentheses where appropriate)—not necessarily inclusive (» = major clinical significance).

*Except under special circumstances, these medications should not be used when the following medical problems exist:*

» Abortion, threatened or incomplete or
» Aneurysm, cerebral or dissecting aorta or
» Bleeding, active or
» Cerebrovascular hemorrhage, confirmed or suspected or
» Neurosurgery, recent or contemplated or
» Ophthalmic surgery, recent or contemplated or
» Surgery, major, other, especially if resulting in large open surfaces
    (increased risk of uncontrollable hemorrhage)
    Note: Although anticoagulants are generally contraindicated following major surgery, they may be required following orthopedic (hip) surgery to reduce the risk of thromboembolism.

» Blood dyscrasias, hemorrhagic, such as thrombocytopenia or
» Hemophilia or
» Hemorrhagic tendency, other
    (increased risk of hemorrhage)
» Hypertension, severe uncontrolled
    (increased risk of cerebral hemorrhage)

» Pericardial effusion or
» Pericarditis
   (increased risk of severe hemorrhagic pericardial effusions and pericardial tamponade)

*Risk-benefit should be considered when the following medical problems exist:*

Allergic or anaphylactic disorders, severe
Any condition in which increased risk of hemorrhage is present, such as:
» Childbirth, recent
» Diabetes, severe
   Gastrointestinal ulceration, history of
   Intrauterine contraceptive device, use of
   Radiation therapy, recent
   Renal function impairment, mild to moderate
» Renal function impairment, severe
» Trauma, severe, especially to the central nervous system (CNS)
   Tuberculosis, active
» Ulceration or other lesions of the gastrointestinal, respiratory, or urinary tract, active
» Vasculitis, severe
Any condition that may reduce the effectiveness of the anticoagulant, such as:
   Edema
   Hypercholesterolemia
   Hyperlipidemia
   Hypothyroidism
Any condition that may directly or indirectly increase the patient's response to the anticoagulant leading to increased risk of bleeding, such as:
   Biliary obstruction
» Carcinoma, visceral
   Collagen disease
   Congestive heart failure
   Diarrhea, prolonged
   Dietary insufficiency, prolonged
   Fever
   Hepatic function impairment, mild to moderate
» Hepatic function impairment, severe, or cirrhosis
   Hepatitis, infectious
   Hyperthyroidism
   Pancreatic disorders
   Sprue
   Steatorrhea
» Vitamin C deficiency
» Vitamin K deficiency
Any condition that may result in reduced compliance by unsupervised outpatients, such as:
   Alcoholism (active)
   Emotional instability
   Psychosis
   Senility
   Uncooperative patient
Any medical or dental procedure or condition in which the risk of bleeding or hemorrhage is present, such as:
» Anesthesia, regional or lumbar block
   Catheters, indwelling
   Drainage tubes in any orifice or wound
» Spinal puncture
» Endocarditis, subacute bacterial
   (increased risk of hemorrhage into infarcted area)
   Hypertension, mild to moderate
» Polyarthritis
   Protein C deficiency, known or suspected, or any other condition predisposing to tissue necrosis
   (increased risk of anticoagulant-induced tissue necrosis, although patients with protein C deficiency may require long-term anticoagulant therapy to prevent recurrent thrombus formation; administration of heparin during the first 5 to 7 days of coumarin or indandione anticoagulant therapy may reduce the risk of tissue necrosis)
   Sensitivity to the anticoagulant prescribed, history of
   Caution in use is also recommended in geriatric or very young patients, and in severely debilitated patients, who may be more sensitive to the effects of anticoagulants.

**Patient monitoring**

The following may be especially important in patient monitoring (other tests may be warranted in some patients, depending on condition; » = major clinical significance):

*For all anticoagulants*
» Prothrombin time determinations
   (recommended prior to initiation of therapy, at 24-hour intervals while maintenance dosage is being established, then once or twice weekly for the following 3 to 4 weeks, then at 1- to 4-week intervals for the duration of treatment)
   Stool tests for occult blood loss and
   Urine tests for hematuria
   (recommended at periodic intervals during therapy)

*For anisindione*
   Hematopoietic function determinations and
   Hepatic function determinations and
   Renal function determinations and
   Urine tests for proteinuria
   (may be advisable at periodic intervals during anisindione therapy because of the increased risk of nephrotoxicity, hepatotoxicity, and blood dyscrasias associated with phenindione [an anticoagulant chemically related to anisindione that is no longer available])

## Side/Adverse Effects

Note: The occurrence of gastrointestinal hemorrhage during anticoagulant therapy, especially if the prothrombin time (PT) is within the therapeutic range, may indicate the presence of an underlying occult lesion such as a tumor or ulcer.

Hemorrhagic necrosis (bleeding into the skin and subcutaneous tissue with resultant necrosis, vasculitis, and thrombosis) has been reported to occur rarely during anticoagulant therapy. This complication occurs more frequently in females than in males; the fatty tissues of the abdomen, breasts, buttocks, and thighs are most often affected. Tissue necrosis may be more likely to occur in patients with protein C deficiency. Concurrent use of heparin during the first 5 to 7 days of anticoagulant therapy may decrease the risk of tissue necrosis.

Adrenal hemorrhage resulting in acute adrenal insufficiency has been reported to occur rarely during anticoagulant therapy. Diagnosis may be difficult because the initial symptoms (abdominal pain, apprehension, diarrhea, dizziness or fainting, headache, loss of appetite, nausea or vomiting, and weakness) are nonspecific and variable. If acute adrenal insufficiency is suspected, anticoagulant therapy must be discontinued and high-dose adrenocorticoid therapy (preferably with hydrocortisone, since other glucocorticoids may not provide sufficient sodium retention) instituted immediately. Delay of treatment while laboratory confirmation of the diagnosis is awaited may prove fatal for the patient. It has been proposed that abdominal computerized axial tomographic (CAT) scanning may be of use in diagnosing this condition more rapidly.

| The following side/adverse effects have been selected on the basis of their potential clinical significance (possible signs and symptoms in parentheses where appropriate)—not necessarily inclusive:* | Legend: I=Anisindione II=Dicumarol III=Warfarin | | |
|---|---|---|---|
| | I | II | III |
| **Medical attention needed** | | | |
| *Adrenal insufficiency, acute* (diarrhea, nausea with or without vomiting, stomach cramps or pain) | R | R | R |
| *Agranulocytosis or* | U† | R | R |
| *Leukopenia* (chills, fever, sore throat, unusual tiredness or weakness) | U† | L | L |
| *Dermatitis, allergic* (skin rash, hives, and/or itching) | L | R | R |
| *Diarrhea* | U† | M | L |
| *Hepatotoxicity* (dark urine, yellow eyes or skin) | U† | R | R |
| *Nausea or vomiting* | U† | L | L |
| *"Purple toes" syndrome* (blue or purple toes, pain in toes) | U | R | R |
| *Renal damage with resultant edema and proteinuria* (bloody or cloudy urine; difficult or painful urination; sudden decrease in amount of urine; swelling of face, feet and/or lower legs) | U† | R | R |
| *Sores, ulcers, or white spots in mouth or throat* | U† | R | R |
| *Stomach cramps or pain* | U† | L | L |
| **Medical attention needed only if continuing or bothersome** | | | |
| *Bloated stomach or gas* | U | M | U |

The following side/adverse effects have been selected on the basis of their potential clinical significance (possible signs and symptoms in parentheses where appropriate)—not necessarily inclusive:*

Legend:
I = Anisindione
II = Dicumarol
III = Warfarin

| | I | II | III |
|---|---|---|---|
| *Loss of appetite* | U | L | U |
| *Paralysis of accommodation* (blurred vision or other vision problems) | U† | U | U |
| *Unusual hair loss* | U† | L | L |

*Differences in frequency of occurrence may reflect either lack of clinical-use data or actual pharmacologic distinctions among agents. M=more frequent; L=less frequent; R=rare; U=unknown.

†Although not documented with anisindione, these effects have been reported with phenindione, an indandione derivative that is no longer commercially available. Other adverse effects or abnormalities reported with phenindione include aplastic anemia, eosinophilia, leukocytosis, thrombocytopenia, atypical mononuclear cells, red cell aplasia, presence of leukocyte agglutinins, and exfoliative dermatitis. Because anisindione is chemically related to phenindione, these side effects should be considered potential side effects of anisindione also.

**Signs and symptoms of hemorrhage indicating need for medical attention**
*Bleeding from gums when brushing teeth; unexplained bruising or purplish areas on skin; unexplained nosebleeds; unusually heavy bleeding or oozing from cuts or wounds; unusually heavy or unexpected menstrual bleeding*
  Note: With anisindione, the possibility exists that unusual bruising or bleeding may also indicate thrombocytopenia.

**Signs and symptoms of internal bleeding indicating need for medical attention**
*Abdominal pain or swelling; back pain or backaches; blood in urine; bloody or black tarry stools; constipation caused by hemorrhage-induced paralytic ileus or intestinal obstruction; coughing up blood; dizziness; headache, severe or continuing; joint pain, stiffness, or swelling; vomiting blood or material that looks like coffee grounds*

## Overdose

For specific information on the agents used in the management of anticoagulant overdose, see the *Vitamin K (Systemic)* monograph.

For more information on the management of overdose or unintentional ingestion, **contact a Poison Control Center** (see *Poison Control Center Listing*).

**Clinical effects of overdose**
The following effects have been selected on the basis of their potential clinical significance (possible signs and symptoms in parentheses where appropriate)—not necessarily inclusive:

Early signs of overdose
*Bleeding from gums when brushing teeth; unexplained bruising or purplish areas on skin; unexplained nosebleeds; unusually heavy bleeding or oozing from cuts or wounds; unusually heavy or unexpected menstrual bleeding*
  Note: With anisindione, the possibility exists that unusual bruising or bleeding may also indicate thrombocytopenia.

Signs and symptoms of internal bleeding
*Abdominal pain or swelling; back pain or backaches; blood in urine; bloody or black tarry stools; constipation caused by hemorrhage-induced paralytic ileus or intestinal obstruction; coughing up blood; dizziness; headache, severe or continuing; joint pain, stiffness, or swelling; vomiting blood or material that looks like coffee grounds*

**Treatment of overdose**
Recommended treatment of anticoagulant overdose includes withdrawing the medication temporarily if excessive prolongation of PT or minor bleeding occurs.
  Specific treatment—
    Administering vitamin K$_1$ orally or intravenously (1 to 5 mg for mild overdosage; 20 to 40 mg for more severe overdosage) if necessary. However, the fact that vitamin K$_1$ may interfere with subsequent anticoagulant therapy must be kept in mind.
    Transfusing fresh frozen plasma (1 to 1.5 liters may be required) or prothrombin complex (about 1500 Units), in addition to administering vitamin K$_1$, if needed in severe cases. Although whole blood may be given if blood loss has been extensive, transfusion of whole blood will not elevate procoagulant factor concentrations sufficiently to eliminate the need for administration of plasma or prothrombin complex.

## Patient Consultation

As an aid to patient consultation, refer to *Advice for the Patient, Anticoagulants (Systemic)*.

In providing consultation, consider emphasizing the following selected information (» = major clinical significance):

**Before using this medication**
» Conditions affecting use, especially:
    Sensitivity to the anticoagulant considered for therapy
    Pregnancy—Not becoming pregnant during therapy without first discussing plans with physician, or informing physician immediately if any suspicion of pregnancy; these medications should not be used during the first trimester because of their teratogenic effects or after the 37th week of pregnancy because of the risk of fetal and neonatal bleeding
    Use in children—Infants, especially neonates, are especially sensitive to effects because of vitamin K deficiency
    Use in the elderly—Increased risk of bleeding
    Other medications
    Other medical problems, especially bleeding or clotting defects, or history of; recent surgery or childbirth; diabetes mellitus; severe renal or hepatic function impairment; active gastrointestinal, respiratory, or urinary tract ulceration; malignancy; recent spinal puncture; subacute bacterial endocarditis; or polyarthritis

**Proper use of this medication**
» Taking medication only as directed
» Regular prothrombin-time tests and regular visits to physician or clinic to check progress
» Proper dosing
    Missed dose: Taking as soon as possible; not taking if not remembered until next day; not doubling doses; keeping a record of doses taken to avoid mistakes; keeping record of missed doses to give physician
» Proper storage

**Precautions while using this medication**
» Need for patient to inform all physicians, dentists, and pharmacists that this medication is being used
» Not taking or discontinuing any other medication, including salicylates or any other over-the-counter (OTC) medications, without physician's permission
» Carrying identification indicating use of an anticoagulant
    Not engaging in activities that may lead to injuries
    Using care in activities that may cause a cut or bleeding (such as shaving)
    Minimizing alcohol consumption; i.e., not consuming more than an occasional drink or two
    Eating a normal, balanced diet; not changing dietary habits, taking vitamins, or using nutritional supplements without first seeking professional advice because of possible alteration of anticoagulant effect by substantial changes in intake of Vitamin K (present in some multiple vitamins and nutritional supplements as well as foods, including green, leafy vegetables [such as broccoli, cabbage, collard greens, kale, lettuce, spinach], and, to a lesser extent, meats and dairy products)
    Checking with physician if unable to eat for several days or if continuing gastric upset, diarrhea, or fever occurs
    Caution following cessation of therapy while body is recovering blood-clotting abilities

**Side/adverse effects**
» Checking with physician immediately if any symptoms of bleeding occur
    Checking with physician if anisindione turns urine orange
    Signs and symptoms of potential side effects, especially bleeding, agranulocytosis, renal damage, hepatotoxicity, and "purple toes" syndrome

## General Dosing Information

Patient compliance is essential to the safe use of these medications. The patient must be responsible and willing to carry out the demands that accompany the use of anticoagulants.

Dosage of anticoagulants must be individualized and adjusted according to prothrombin-time (PT) determinations. Determinations of clotting time, bleeding time, or anticoagulant plasma concentration are not effective measures for monitoring anticoagulant therapy. It is recommended that PT determinations be performed prior to initiation of therapy, at 24-hour intervals while maintenance dosage is being established, then once or twice weekly for the following 3 to 4 weeks, then at 1- to 4-week intervals for the duration of treatment.

PT is often reported by listing the value in seconds along with the control value in seconds. Alternately, PT may be reported as the ratio of the prolonged (therapeutic) value to the control value. In the past, the therapeutic value was considered to be 1½ to 2½ times the control value. Because the tissue thromboplastins currently used in the U.S. for PT determinations are less sensitive than those previously used, the therapeutic value for most patients is now considered to be 1.3 to 1.5 times the control value. However, when an especially high risk of thromboembolism exists (e.g., in patients with a history of recurrent systemic embolism or patients with mechanical heart valves), maintaining the PT at 1.5 to 2 times the control value may be necessary. Tissue thromboplastins currently used in North America for PT determinations are not identical to, and are less sensitive than, thromboplastins used in other countries. In 1983, the World Health Organization introduced a standardized system of reporting PT values that provides a common basis for communicating PT results and interpreting therapeutic ranges. This system is based on the determination of an International Normalized Ratio (INR), which is derived from calibrations of commercial thromboplastin reagents against the International Reference Preparation, a sensitive human brain thromboplastin. With the rabbit brain thromboplastins currently commercially available in North America, PT values of 1.3 to 1.5 times the control value are equivalent to INR values of 2 to 3 times the control value and PT values of 1.5 to 2 times the control value are equivalent to INR values of 3 to 4.5 times the control value. For other thromboplastins, the INR can be calculated using the International Sensitivity Index (available from the manufacturer) as a calibration factor.

Levels of anticoagulation (in terms of the desired PT and INR) that are recommended for specific indications by a panel assembled for the Second American College of Chest Physicians Conference on Antithrombotic Therapy are:

For prevention of venous thromboembolism and pulmonary embolism in high-risk surgical patients when low-dose heparin is ineffective (e.g., surgery for fractured hip, other [elective] hip surgery, or knee reconstruction) or when heparin is contraindicated for any reason—
Surgery for fractured hip: PT 1.3 to 1.5 (INR 2.0 to 3.0) times the control value.
Elective hip surgery: PT 1.3 to 1.5 (INR 2.0 to 3.0) times the control value.

For treatment of acute deep venous thrombosis of the popliteal and more proximal vessels or pulmonary embolism (following initial thrombolytic and/or heparin therapy)—PT 1.3 to 1.5 (INR 2.0 to 3.0) times the control value. The oral anticoagulant should be administered concurrently with heparin for at least four to five days, after which heparin can be discontinued (provided that prothrombin time determinations indicate an adequate response to the oral anticoagulant). Treatment with the oral anticoagulant should be continued for at least three months (indefinitely if recurrent venous thrombosis or continuing risk factors [e.g., antithrombin III deficiency, protein C or protein S deficiency, malignancy] exist).

For treatment of isolated symptomatic calf-vein thrombosis—PT 1.3 to 1.5 (INR 2.0 to 3.0) times the control value. Therapy should be continued for three months.

For prevention of cardiogenic systemic or cerebral embolism (either a first episode or a recurrence) in patients with the following risk factors—
Mitral valve disease with documented systemic embolism: PT 1.5 to 2.0 (INR 3.0 to 4.5) times the control value. If embolism recurs, dipyridamole (225 to 400 mg per day) should be considered for addition to the regimen. Therapy should be continued at that level of anticoagulation for at least one year after an embolism occurs, after which dosage may be reduced to provide a PT of 1.3 to 1.5 (INR 2.0 to 3.0) times the control value. Long-term therapy is recommended.
Mitral valve disease and associated chronic or paroxysmal atrial fibrillation: PT 1.3 to 1.5 (INR 2.0 to 3.0) times the control value. Long-term therapy is recommended.
Mitral valve disease, when the left atrial diameter is >5.5 cm (but normal sinus rhythm is present): PT 1.3 to 1.5 (INR 2.0 to 3.0) times the control value. Long-term therapy is recommended.
Mitral valve prolapse associated with documented, unexplained transient ischemic attacks unresponsive to a sufficient trial of aspirin therapy: PT 1.3 to 1.5 (INR 2.0 to 3.0) times the control value. Long-term therapy is recommended.
Mitral valve prolapse and documented systemic embolism: PT 1.5 to 2.0 (INR 3.0 to 4.5) times the control value. Therapy should be continued at that level of anticoagulation for at least one year after an embolism occurs, after which dosage may be reduced to provide a PT of 1.3 to 1.5 (INR 2.0 to 3.0) times the control value. Long-term therapy is recommended.
Mitral valve prolapse associated with chronic or paroxysmal atrial fibrillation: PT 1.3 to 1.5 (INR 2.0 to 3.0) times the control value. Long-term therapy is recommended.
Mitral annular calcification complicated by systemic thromboembolism: PT 1.5 to 2.0 (INR 3.0 to 4.5) times the control value. Therapy should be continued at that level of anticoagulation for at least one year after an embolism occurs, after which dosage may be reduced to provide a PT of 1.3 to 1.5 (INR 2.0 to 3.0) times the control value. Long-term therapy is recommended.
Mitral annular calcification associated with atrial fibrillation: PT 1.3 to 1.5 (INR 2.0 to 3.0) times the control value. Long-term therapy is recommended.
Mechanical prosthetic heart valves: PT 1.5 to 2.0 (INR 3.0 to 4.5) times the control value. Dipyridamole (400 mg per day) may be added to the regimen (optional, although it is strongly recommended if an embolism occurs despite adequate anticoagulation). If the recommended level of anticoagulation is contraindicated or not tolerated, a lower dose that provides a PT of 1.3 to 1.5 (INR 2.0 to 3.0) times control should be administered concurrently with dipyridamole (400 mg per day). Long-term therapy is recommended.
Bioprosthetic mitral heart valves: PT 1.3 to 1.5 (INR 2.0 to 3.0) times the control value for three months following insertion. However, if there is a history of systemic embolism, evidence of a left atrial thrombus, or atrial fibrillation, dosage sufficient to prolong the PT to 1.5 to 2.0 (INR 3.0 to 4.5) times the control value should be administered for three months, followed by long-term therapy at a reduced dosage that provides a PT of 1.3 to 1.5 (INR 2.0 to 3.0) times the control value.
Atrial fibrillation and systemic embolism: PT 1.5 to 2 (INR 3.0 to 4.5) times the control value. Therapy should be continued at that level of anticoagulation for one year after an embolism occurs, after which dosage may be reduced to provide a PT of 1.3 to 1.5 (INR 2.0 to 3.0) times the control value. Long-term therapy is recommended.
Atrial fibrillation associated with dilated and hypertrophic cardiomyopathy: PT 1.3 to 1.5 (INR 2.0 to 3.0) times the control value. Long-term therapy is recommended.
Atrial fibrillation associated with congestive heart failure: Long-term anticoagulation providing a PT of 1.3 to 1.5 (INR 2.0 to 3.0) times the control value should be considered.
Atrial fibrillation associated with coronary artery disease, hypertension, congenital heart disease, or other forms of nonvalvular heart disease: Although conclusive evidence indicating that anticoagulation is required in these circumstances is lacking, anticoagulation (PT 1.3 to 1.5 [INR 2.0 to 3.0] times the control value) should be considered for young patients who are not at increased risk of hemorrhagic complications.
Atrial fibrillation associated with thyrotoxic heart disease: PT 1.3 to 1.5 (INR 2.0 to 3.0) times the control value. Treatment should be continued for four weeks after sinus rhythm and a euthyroid state have been restored.
Atrial fibrillation, idiopathic: Long-term anticoagulation is not needed for young patients. However, for patients 60 years of age or older, long-term anticoagulation (PT 1.3 to 1.5 [INR 2.0 to 3.0] times the control value) should be considered on an individual basis.
Cardioversion (elective) of atrial fibrillation: PT 1.3 to 1.5 (INR 2.0 to 3.0) times the control value. Therapy should be started three weeks before elective cardioversion and continued until normal sinus rhythm has been maintained for at least four weeks. Anticoagulation is not needed for cardioversion of atrial fibrillation of only one or two days' duration, or for cardioversion of atrial flutter or supraventricular tachycardia, unless other risk factors for systemic embolism exist.
Anterior transmural myocardial infarction (following initial thrombolytic and/or heparin therapy): PT 1.3 to 1.5 (INR 2.0 to 3.0) times the control value. Therapy is generally continued for three months.
Acute myocardial infarction with atrial fibrillation, history of previous systemic or pulmonary embolism or venous thromboembolism, persistently decreased left ventricular function, or chronic congestive heart failure (following initial thrombolytic and/or heparin therapy): PT 1.3 to 1.5 (INR 2.0 to 3.0) times the control value for at least three months. Long-term anticoagulation may not reduce the risk of recurrent acute myocardial infarction, but is recommended if a risk factor for systemic or pulmonary embolism is still present after three months of therapy.

For prevention of recurrent cardiogenic brain emboli (following initial heparin therapy)—Anticoagulant therapy should be initiated only if the patient is not hypertensive and a computerized tomographic (CT) scan performed 24 hours or longer following the onset of the stroke shows no evidence of hemorrhagic transformation. If severe hypertension is present, or the embolic stroke is large, there is a risk of late hemorrhagic transformation; anticoagulant therapy should be delayed for several days. If hemorrhagic transformation is documented, anticoagulant therapy should be postponed for at least 8 to 10 days. Initially, the oral anticoagulant should be administered in dosage sufficient to provide a PT of 1.5 to 2.0 (INR 3.0 to 4.5) times the control value. Therapy should be continued at that level of anticoagulation for one year after the embolism, after which dosage may be reduced to provide a PT of 1.3 to 1.5 (INR 2.0 to 3.0) times the control value. Long-term therapy is recommended.

For prevention of recurrent arterial thrombi or emboli—PT 1.5 to 2.0 (INR 3.0 to 4.5) times the control value. If no thrombus or embolism has recurred after one year of therapy, dosage may be reduced to provide a PT of 1.3 to 1.5 (INR 2.0 to 3.0) times the control value.

Increased monitoring of the PT is recommended when any new medication, including nonprescription medication, is added to or withdrawn from the regimen of a patient stabilized on a coumarin or indandione derivative, or when the dosage of a concurrently used medication is changed. Anticoagulant dosage must be adjusted as necessary to prevent hemorrhage or loss of effect. Also, substantial alteration of initial anticoagulant dosage may be necessary when anticoagulant therapy is initiated in a patient receiving a medication known to cause significant alteration of anticoagulant effect.

Lower doses may be required for geriatric patients because enhanced anticoagulant effect may occur.

Decreased sensitivity to the effects of anticoagulants may be evident during initiation of therapy in patients with edema, hyperlipidemia, hypercholesterolemia, or hypothyroidism. Loss of anticoagulant effect may occur if any of these conditions develop during therapy. Correction of these problems will increase or restore the effectiveness of the anticoagulant.

Some patients also exhibit resistance to anticoagulant therapy because of genetic variations in the vitamin K receptor site or because of an increased rate of anticoagulant metabolism and excretion. Doses much higher than those usually recommended may be required to achieve successful anticoagulation in these patients. Some patients resistant to therapy with a coumarin derivative may respond to the indandione derivative anisindione.

Increased anticoagulant effect may occur in a previously stabilized patient if prolonged fever occurs during therapy.

When anticoagulant therapy is initiated with heparin and continued with a coumarin or indandione derivative, it is recommended that both agents be given concurrently until PT determinations indicate an adequate response to the coumarin or indandione derivative. However, the fact that heparin may prolong the PT must be kept in mind. Full therapeutic doses given by subcutaneous administration or as a single intravenous injection may prolong the PT considerably because of the high concentrations of heparin in the blood, whereas therapeutic doses of heparin given by continuous intravenous infusion or low (prophylactic) doses of heparin administered subcutaneously usually do not increase the PT by more than a few seconds. To minimize problems in interpreting PT test results, draw blood for the PT test just prior to, or at least 5 hours after, a single intravenous dose or 24 hours following subcutaneous administration of a full therapeutic dose of heparin. Also, the fact that reduction in PT may reflect early depletion of factor VII rather than peak antithrombotic effects of coumarin or indandione derivatives must be kept in mind. Some clinicians recommend continuation of heparin therapy for up to 5 to 7 days after initiation of therapy with a coumarin or indandione derivative to ensure that peak antithrombogenic activity has been reached.

Manufacturers' dosage recommendations may include administration of an initial loading dose that is to be gradually reduced to the maintenance dose indicated by PT determinations. Many clinicians recommend that large loading doses of these medications be avoided because of the increased risk of hemorrhage and because a more rapid anticoagulant effect can be achieved with heparin.

It is recommended that therapy with these medications be discontinued if there is any suspicion that anticoagulant-induced tissue necrosis is developing. Anticoagulant therapy may be continued with heparin, if necessary.

**Diet/Nutrition**
Loss of anticoagulant effect may occur in a previously stabilized patient if intake of vitamin K from dietary sources (green leafy vegetables such as broccoli, cabbage, collard greens, kale, lettuce, or spinach and, to a lesser extent, dairy products or meats) or vitamin K–containing multiple vitamins or nutritional supplements is increased during therapy.

Increased anticoagulant effect may occur in a previously stabilized patient if prolonged malnutrition or vitamin C deficiency develops, or if diarrhea, other illness, or changes in diet resulting in decreased intake or absorption of vitamin K occur during therapy.

## ANISINDIONE†

## Summary of Differences
Physicochemical characteristics:
    Indandione-derivative anticoagulant.
Pharmacology/pharmacokinetics:
    See *Pharmacology/Pharmacokinetics*.
Precautions:
    Drug interactions and/or related problems—Concurrent use with heparin does not lead to severe factor IX deficiency.
    Laboratory value alterations—Alkaline urine may turn orange.
    Patient monitoring—Monitoring of hematopoietic function, hepatic function, renal function, and urine protein may also be necessary.
Side/adverse effects:
    See *Side/Adverse Effects*.

## Oral Dosage Forms
### ANISINDIONE TABLETS
**Usual adult and adolescent dose**
Oral, 25 to 250 mg a day, as indicated by prothrombin-time determinations.

**Usual pediatric dose**
Dosage has not been established.

**Strength(s) usually available**
U.S.—
    50 mg (Rx) [*Miradon*].
Canada—
    Not commercially available.

**Packaging and storage**
Store below 40 °C (104 °F), preferably between 15 and 30 °C (59 and 86 °F), in a well-closed container, unless otherwise specified by manufacturer.

**Auxiliary labeling**
• Do not take other medicines without advice from your doctor.

## DICUMAROL

## Summary of Differences
Physicochemical characteristics: Coumarin-derivative anticoagulant.
Pharmacology/pharmacokinetics: See *Pharmacology/Pharmacokinetics*.
Side/adverse effects: See *Side/Adverse Effects*.

## Oral Dosage Forms
### DICUMAROL TABLETS USP
**Usual adult and adolescent dose**
Oral, 25 to 200 mg a day, as indicated by prothrombin-time determinations.

**Usual pediatric dose**
Dosage has not been established.

**Strength(s) usually available**
U.S.—
    25 mg (Rx) [GENERIC].
Canada—
    Not commercially available.

**Packaging and storage**
Store below 40 °C (104 °F), preferably between 15 and 30 °C (59 and 86 °F). Store in a well-closed container.

**Auxiliary labeling**
• Do not take other medicines without advice from your doctor.

## WARFARIN

## Summary of Differences
Indications: Also used for treatment of transient ischemic attacks in females and males.
Physicochemical characteristics: Coumarin-derivative anticoagulant.
Pharmacology/pharmacokinetics: See *Pharmacology/Pharmacokinetics*.
Side/adverse effects: See *Side/Adverse Effects*.

## Oral Dosage Forms

### WARFARIN SODIUM TABLETS USP

**Usual adult and adolescent dose**
Oral, 10 to 15 mg a day for two to four days, then 2 to 10 mg a day, as indicated by prothrombin-time determinations.

**Usual pediatric dose**
Dosage has not been established.

**Strength(s) usually available**
U.S.—
- 1 mg (Rx) [*Coumadin*].
- 2 mg (Rx) [*Coumadin* (scored; lactose); *Panwarfin* (lactose); *Sofarin* (scored; lactose); GENERIC].
- 2.5 mg (Rx) [*Coumadin* (scored; lactose); *Panwarfin* (lactose); *Sofarin* (scored; lactose); GENERIC].
- 4 mg (Rx) [*Coumadin* (scored; lactose)].
- 5 mg (Rx) [*Coumadin* (scored; lactose); *Panwarfin* (lactose); *Sofarin* (scored; lactose); GENERIC].
- 7.5 mg (Rx) [*Coumadin* (scored; lactose); *Panwarfin* (scored; lactose; tartrazine); GENERIC].
- 10 mg (Rx) [*Coumadin* (scored; lactose); *Panwarfin* (scored; lactose); GENERIC].

Canada—
- 2 mg (Rx) [*Coumadin* (scored; lactose)].
- 2.5 mg (Rx) [*Coumadin* (scored; lactose)].
- 4 mg (Rx) [*Coumadin* (scored; lactose)].
- 5 mg (Rx) [*Coumadin* (scored; lactose); *Warfilone* (scored; tartrazine)].
- 10 mg (Rx) [*Coumadin* (scored; lactose)].

**Packaging and storage**
Store below 40 °C (104 °F), preferably between 15 and 30 °C (59 and 86 °F), unless otherwise specified by manufacturer. Store in a tight, light-resistant container.

**Auxiliary labeling**
- Do not take other medicines without advice from your doctor.

## Parenteral Dosage Forms

### WARFARIN SODIUM FOR INJECTION USP

**Usual adult and adolescent dose**
Intramuscular or intravenous, 10 to 15 mg a day for two to four days, then 2 to 10 mg a day, as indicated by prothrombin-time determinations.

**Usual pediatric dose**
Dosage has not been established.

**Size(s) usually available**
U.S.—
- 50 mg (Rx) [*Coumadin* (thimerosal)].

Canada—
- Not commercially available.

**Packaging and storage**
Store below 40 °C (104 °F), preferably between 15 and 30 °C (59 and 86 °F), unless otherwise specified by manufacturer. Protect from light.

**Preparation of dosage form**
Warfarin sodium for injection is reconstituted by adding 2 mL of sterile water for injection to the vial containing 50 mg of warfarin sodium to provide a solution containing 25 mg of warfarin sodium per mL.

**Stability**
Administer immediately after reconstitution.
Discard any unused solution.

Revised: June 1990
Interim revision: 07/28/94

## Table 1. Drug Interactions and/or Related Problems

The following drug interactions and/or related problems have been selected on the basis of their potential clinical significance (possible mechanism in parentheses where appropriate)—not necessarily inclusive (» = major clinical significance).

Note: In addition to the listed interactions, the possibility should be considered that the risk of hemorrhage may be increased by concurrent use of any medication that may inhibit platelet aggregation or cause hypoprothrombinemia, thrombocytopenia, or gastrointestinal ulceration.

Combinations containing any of the following medications, depending on the amount present, may also interact with this medication.

| | Drug | Effect on Anticoagulant Activity | Mechanism* | Other Effects† | Additional Information |
|---|---|---|---|---|---|
| | Acetaminophen (chronic high-dose usage) | Increase | A | | Does not apply to occasional use or chronic use of less than 2 grams per day of acetaminophen |
| | Alcohol (acute intoxication) (chronic abuse) | Increase Decrease | B C | | Other acute effects of alcohol on the liver may also be involved However, increased activity possible in advanced hepatic cirrhosis |
| » | Allopurinol | Increase | B | | |
| | Aminosalicylates | Increase | A | | |
| » | Amiodarone | Increase | B | | Potentiation reported to occur in 4 to 6 days after initiation of amiodarone therapy and to persist up to 4 months following discontinuation of amiodarone |
| » | Anabolic steroids | Increase | D, E | | Especially with 17-alpha-alkylated compounds |

*Mechanisms leading to increase or decrease in anticoagulant activity as shown by measurement of prothrombin time: (A) Decreased hepatic synthesis of procoagulant factors. (B) Inhibition of enzymatic metabolism of anticoagulant. (C) Accelerated metabolism of anticoagulant secondary to stimulation of hepatic microsomal enzyme activity. (D) Alteration of procoagulant factor synthesis or catabolism. (E) Increased receptor affinity for anticoagulant. (F) Decreased absorption of anticoagulant from gastrointestinal tract. (G) Decreased vitamin K synthesis secondary to alterations in intestinal flora. (H) Displacement of anticoagulant from protein-binding sites. (I) Increased metabolism of anticoagulant. (J) Interference with enterohepatic circulation of anticoagulant. (K) Decreased vitamin K absorption or synthesis. (L) Increased hepatic synthesis of procoagulant factors. (M) Reduction of plasma volume leading to concentration of procoagulant factors in the blood; diuretic-induced improvement of hepatic congestion may lead to improved hepatic function resulting in increased procoagulant factor synthesis. (N) Severe factor IX deficiency (with coumarin derivatives only). (O) Increased prothrombin synthesis or activation.

†Effects resulting in increased risk of hemorrhage in patients receiving anticoagulants; cannot be shown by measurement of prothrombin time: (a) Inhibition of platelet aggregation. (b) Potential occurrence of gastrointestinal ulceration or hemorrhage during therapy. (c) Adverse effect on vascular integrity. (d) Interference with platelet formation. (e) Anticoagulant activity of heparin. (f) Thrombolytic activity may lead to hemorrhage.

‡Clinical significance has not been determined.

## Table 1. Drug Interactions and/or Related Problems *(continued)*

The following drug interactions and/or related problems have been selected on the basis of their potential clinical significance (possible mechanism in parentheses where appropriate)—not necessarily inclusive (» = major clinical significance).

Note: In addition to the listed interactions, the possibility should be considered that the risk of hemorrhage may be increased by concurrent use of any medication that may inhibit platelet aggregation or cause hypoprothrombinemia, thrombocytopenia, or gastrointestinal ulceration.

Combinations containing any of the following medications, depending on the amount present, may also interact with this medication.

| Drug | Effect on Anticoagulant Activity | Mechanism* | Other Effects† | Additional Information |
|---|---|---|---|---|
| » Androgens | Increase | D, E | | |
| Anesthetics, inhalation‡ | Increase | Unknown | | |
| Antacids | Decrease | F | | May be avoided if medications given several hours apart |
| Antibiotics‡ | Increase | G | | Significant potentiation very rare if dietary intake of vitamin K adequate |
| | | | | See also separate table entries for azlocillin, carbenicillin, cefamandole, cefoperazone, chloramphenicol, erythromycins, mezlocillin, piperacillin, rifampin, and ticarcillin |
| » Antidiabetic agents, oral | Increase | H | | Initial effect |
| | Decrease | I | | With continued concurrent use |
| | | | | Hepatic metabolism of antidiabetic agent may be decreased, leading to increased plasma concentration and half-life, hypoglycemic effect, and risk of toxicity of antidiabetic agent, especially with dicumarol |
| Ascorbic acid | Decrease | | | With large doses of ascorbic acid |
| » Aspirin | Increase | A (with large doses), H | a, b | Decreased platelet aggregation may occur with single doses as low as 40 mg |
| » Azlocillin | | | a | |
| » Barbiturates | Decrease | C | | |
| Bromelains | Increase | Unknown | | |
| » Carbamazepine | Decrease | C | | |
| » Carbenicillin (parenteral) | | | a | |
| » Cefamandole | Increase | D | a | |
| » Cefoperazone | Increase | D | a | |
| » Chloral hydrate | Increase | H | | Initial effect, usually during first 2 weeks of concurrent use; with continued concurrent use, anticoagulant activity may return to baseline level or be decreased |
| » Chloramphenicol | Increase | B | | |
| Chlorinated insecticides‡ | Decrease | C | | |
| Chlorobutanol‡ | Decrease | Unknown | | |
| » Cholestyramine | Decrease | F | | May be avoided if medications given 6 hours apart |
| | Decrease | J | | Not avoided if medications given 6 hours apart |
| | Increase | K | | |
| Chymotrypsin‡ | Increase | Unknown | | |
| » Cimetidine | Increase | B | | |
| Cinchophen | Increase | Unknown | | |
| » Clofibrate | Increase | D, H | | Other mechanisms may also be involved |
| Colchicine | | | b | May also cause thrombocytopenia (with chronic use) and coagulation defects including disseminated intravascular coagulation (with overdose) |
| » Colestipol | Decrease | F | | May be avoided if medications given 6 hours apart |
| | Increase | K | | Not avoided if medications given 6 hours apart |
| » Contraceptives, oral | Decrease | L | | |
| | Increase | Unknown | | |
| Corticotropin | Increase | Unknown | b, c | |
| | Decrease | Unknown | | |
| Cyclophosphamide | Increase | A | d | |
| | Decrease | Unknown | | |
| » Danazol | Increase | A | | |
| » Dextran | | | a | |
| » Dextrothyroxine | Increase | D, E | | Effect may depend on thyroid status of patient |
| Diazoxide | Increase | H | | |

## Table 1. Drug Interactions and/or Related Problems *(continued)*

The following drug interactions and/or related problems have been selected on the basis of their potential clinical significance (possible mechanism in parentheses where appropriate)—not necessarily inclusive (» = major clinical significance).

Note: In addition to the listed interactions, the possibility should be considered that the risk of hemorrhage may be increased by concurrent use of any medication that may inhibit platelet aggregation or cause hypoprothrombinemia, thrombocytopenia, or gastrointestinal ulceration.

Combinations containing any of the following medications, depending on the amount present, may also interact with this medication.

| Drug | Effect on Anticoagulant Activity | Mechanism* | Other Effects† | Additional Information |
|---|---|---|---|---|
| » Diflunisal | Increase | H | a, b | Decreased platelet aggregation occurs only with greater-than-recommended daily doses |
| » Dipyridamole | | | a | With doses greater than 400 mg per day |
| Disopyramide‡ | Decrease / Increase | Unknown / Unknown | | |
| » Disulfiram | Increase | B | | May also act in the liver to increase directly the hypopro-thrombinemia-inducing activity of coumarin derivatives |
| Diuretics‡ | Decrease | M | | See also separate table entry for ethacrynic acid |
| Divalproex | | | a | |
| » Erythromycins | Increase | B | | |
| » Estramustine | Decrease | L | | |
| » Estrogens | Decrease | L | | |
| Ethacrynic acid‡ | Increase | H | b | |
| » Ethchlorvynol | Decrease | C | | |
| » Fenoprofen | Increase | H | a, b | |
| » Gemfibrozil | Increase | Unknown | | |
| Glucagon‡ | Increase | Unknown | | Potentiation reported only with doses >25 mg per day for 2 or more days; however, these doses are rarely if ever used |
| Glucocorticoids | Increase / Decrease | Unknown / Unknown | b, c | |
| » Glutethimide | Decrease | C | | |
| » Griseofulvin | Decrease | C | | |
| Haloperidol‡ | Decrease / Increase | C / Unknown | | |
| Heparin | Increase | N | e | May prolong prothrombin time used to monitor therapy, especially when given as an intravenous bolus or if full therapeutic doses given subcutaneously; to minimize problems, draw blood for test just prior to, or at least 5 hours after, the intravenous bolus dose or 24 hours after subcutaneous injection of a full therapeutic dose |
| Ibuprofen | | | a, b | |
| » Indomethacin | Increase | H | a, b | |
| Influenza vaccine | Increase | B | | |
| Isoniazid | Increase | B | | |
| Ketoconazole | Increase | Unknown | | |
| Ketoprofen | | | a, b | |
| Laxatives, bulk-forming | Decrease | F | | May be avoided if medications given several hours apart |
| Meclofenamate | Increase | H | b | |
| » Mefenamic acid | Increase | H | b | |

*Mechanisms leading to increase or decrease in anticoagulant activity as shown by measurement of prothrombin time: (A) Decreased hepatic synthesis of procoagulant factors. (B) Inhibition of enzymatic metabolism of anticoagulant. (C) Accelerated metabolism of anticoagulant secondary to stimulation of hepatic microsomal enzyme activity. (D) Alteration of procoagulant factor synthesis or catabolism. (E) Increased receptor affinity for anticoagulant. (F) Decreased absorption of anticoagulant from gastrointestinal tract. (G) Decreased vitamin K synthesis secondary to alterations in intestinal flora. (H) Displacement of anticoagulant from protein-binding sites. (I) Increased metabolism of anticoagulant. (J) Interference with enterohepatic circulation of anticoagulant. (K) Decreased vitamin K absorption or synthesis. (L) Increased hepatic synthesis of procoagulant factors. (M) Reduction of plasma volume leading to concentration of procoagulant factors in the blood; diuretic-induced improvement of hepatic congestion may lead to improved hepatic function resulting in increased procoagulant factor synthesis. (N) Severe factor IX deficiency (with coumarin derivatives only). (O) Increased prothrombin synthesis or activation.

†Effects resulting in increased risk of hemorrhage in patients receiving anticoagulants; cannot be shown by measurement of prothrombin time: (a) Inhibition of platelet aggregation. (b) Potential occurrence of gastrointestinal ulceration or hemorrhage during therapy. (c) Adverse effect on vascular integrity. (d) Interference with platelet formation. (e) Anticoagulant activity of heparin. (f) Thrombolytic activity may lead to hemorrhage.

‡Clinical significance has not been determined.

## Table 1. Drug Interactions and/or Related Problems (continued)

The following drug interactions and/or related problems have been selected on the basis of their potential clinical significance (possible mechanism in parentheses where appropriate)—not necessarily inclusive (» = major clinical significance).

Note: In addition to the listed interactions, the possibility should be considered that the risk of hemorrhage may be increased by concurrent use of any medication that may inhibit platelet aggregation or cause hypoprothrombinemia, thrombocytopenia, or gastrointestinal ulceration.

Combinations containing any of the following medications, depending on the amount present, may also interact with this medication.

| Drug | Effect on Anticoagulant Activity | Mechanism* | Other Effects† | Additional Information |
|---|---|---|---|---|
| Meperidine | Increase | Unknown | | |
| Mercaptopurine | Increase<br>Decrease | A<br>O | d | |
| » Methimazole | Increase | A | | Effect may also depend upon dosage and subsequent thyroid status of patient |
| Methotrexate | Increase | A | d | |
| Methyldopa | Increase | Unknown | | |
| Methylphenidate | Increase | B | | |
| » Metronidazole | Increase | B | | |
| » Mezlocillin | | | a | |
| Miconazole | Increase | Unknown | | |
| Mineral oil | Decrease<br>Increase | F<br>K | | May be avoided if medications given 6 hours apart<br>Not avoided if medications given 6 hours apart |
| Monoamine oxidase (MAO) inhibitors‡ | Increase | Unknown | | |
| » Nalidixic acid | Increase | H | | |
| Naproxen | | | a, b | |
| Nifedipine | Increase | H | | Nifedipine may also be displaced from protein-binding sites, leading to increased plasma concentrations of free [unbound] medication and risk of toxicity |
| » Phenylbutazone | Increase | B, H | a, b | |
| » Phenytoin, and possibly other hydantoin-type anticonvulsants | Increase<br><br>Decrease | H<br><br>C | | Initial effect<br><br>With continued concurrent use<br>Hepatic metabolism of hydantoin anticonvulsants, especially phenytoin, may be decreased, leading to increased anticonvulsant plasma concentration, half-life, and risk of toxicity, especially with dicumarol |
| » Piperacillin | | | a | |
| Piroxicam | | | a, b | Possibility that anticoagulant activity may be increased because of displacement from protein-binding sites should be considered; however, has not been demonstrated |
| » Plicamycin | Increase | A | d | |
| » Primidone | Decrease | C | | Effect caused by barbiturate metabolite |
| Propoxyphene‡ | Increase | Unknown | | |
| » Propylthiouracil | Increase | A | | Effect may also depend upon dosage and subsequent thyroid status of patient |
| » Quinidine | Increase | D, E | | |
| Quinine | Increase | A | | |
| Radioactive compounds | Increase | Unknown | | |
| » Rifampin | Decrease | C | | |
| » Salicylates | Increase | A (with large doses), H | b | See also separate table entries for aspirin and diflunisal |
| » Streptokinase | | | f | Concurrent use not recommended; however, sequential use may be indicated |
| » Sulfinpyrazone | Increase | B, H | a, b | Biphasic response, with decreased anticoagulation occurring following initial potentiation, reported in one patient; reason for this unclear since other reports indicate only potentiation of anticoagulant effect |
| » Sulfonamides | Increase | B, H | | |
| » Sulindac | Increase | H | a, b | |
| Testolactone | Increase | | | |

## Table 1. Drug Interactions and/or Related Problems *(continued)*

The following drug interactions and/or related problems have been selected on the basis of their potential clinical significance (possible mechanism in parentheses where appropriate)—not necessarily inclusive (» = major clinical significance).

Note: In addition to the listed interactions, the possibility should be considered that the risk of hemorrhage may be increased by concurrent use of any medication that may inhibit platelet aggregation or cause hypoprothrombinemia, thrombocytopenia, or gastrointestinal ulceration.

Combinations containing any of the following medications, depending on the amount present, may also interact with this medication.

| Drug | Effect on Anticoagulant Activity | Mechanism* | Other Effects† | Additional Information |
|---|---|---|---|---|
| » Thyroid hormones | Increase | D, E | | Effect may depend upon dosage and subsequent thyroid status of patient |
| » Ticarcillin | | | a | |
| Tobacco smoking | Decrease | C | | Thrombogenic potential of tobacco smoking should also be considered |
| Tolmetin | | | a, b | |
| Tricyclic antidepressants‡ | Increase | B | | Especially with amitriptyline or nortriptyline |
| » Urokinase | | | f | Concurrent use not recommended; however, sequential use may be indicated |
| Valproic acid | Increase | A | a | |
| Verapamil | Increase | H | | Verapamil may also be displaced from protein-binding sites, leading to increased plasma concentrations of free [unbound] medication and risk of toxicity |
| Vitamin A | Increase | Unknown | | With high doses of vitamin |
| Vitamin E‡ | Increase | Unknown | | With high doses of vitamin |
| » Vitamin K | Decrease | L | | |

*Mechanisms leading to increase or decrease in anticoagulant activity as shown by measurement of prothrombin time: (A) Decreased hepatic synthesis of procoagulant factors. (B) Inhibition of enzymatic metabolism of anticoagulant. (C) Accelerated metabolism of anticoagulant secondary to stimulation of hepatic microsomal enzyme activity. (D) Alteration of procoagulant factor synthesis or catabolism. (E) Increased receptor affinity for anticoagulant. (F) Decreased absorption of anticoagulant from gastrointestinal tract. (G) Decreased vitamin K synthesis secondary to alterations in intestinal flora. (H) Displacement of anticoagulant from protein-binding sites. (I) Increased metabolism of anticoagulant. (J) Interference with enterohepatic circulation of anticoagulant. (K) Decreased vitamin K absorption or synthesis. (L) Increased hepatic synthesis of procoagulant factors. (M) Reduction of plasma volume leading to concentration of procoagulant factors in the blood; diuretic-induced improvement of hepatic congestion may lead to improved hepatic function resulting in increased procoagulant factor synthesis. (N) Severe factor IX deficiency (with coumarin derivatives only). (O) Increased prothrombin synthesis or activation.

†Effects resulting in increased risk of hemorrhage in patients receiving anticoagulants; cannot be shown by measurement of prothrombin time: (a) Inhibition of platelet aggregation. (b) Potential occurrence of gastrointestinal ulceration or hemorrhage during therapy. (c) Adverse effect on vascular integrity. (d) Interference with platelet formation. (e) Anticoagulant activity of heparin. (f) Thrombolytic activity may lead to hemorrhage.

‡Clinical significance has not been determined.

**ANTICONVULSANTS, DIONE**—The *Anticonvulsants, Dione (Systemic)* monograph is not included in this published version of the USP DI database. Copies of the monograph are available on request from Micromedex, Inc. - Reprint Requests, 6200 S. Syracuse Way, Suite 300, Englewood, CO 80111; telephone (303) 486-6400; telefax (303) 486-6464; Email: USPDI@MDX.COM.

# ANTICONVULSANTS, HYDANTOIN Systemic

This monograph includes information on the following: 1) Ethotoin†; 2) Fosphenytoin†; 3) Mephenytoin†; 4) Phenytoin

BAN:
Mephenytoin—Methoin

VA CLASSIFICATION (Primary/Secondary):
Ethotoin—CN400
Fosphenytoin—CN400
Mephenytoin—CN400
Phenytoin—CN400/CV300; MS200

Commonly used brand name(s): *Cerebyx*[2]; *Dilantin*[4]; *Dilantin Infatabs*[4]; *Dilantin Kapseals*[4]; *Dilantin-125*[4]; *Dilantin-30*[4]; *Mesantoin*[3]; *Peganone*[1]; *Phenytex*[4].

Another commonly used name for phenytoin is diphenylhydantoin.

Note: For a listing of dosage forms and brand names by country availability, see *Dosage Forms* section(s).

†Not commercially available in Canada.

## Category

Anticonvulsant—Ethotoin; Fosphenytoin; Mephenytoin; Phenytoin.
Antiarrhythmic—Phenytoin.
Antineuralgic (trigeminal neuralgia)—Phenytoin.
Skeletal muscle relaxant—Phenytoin.

## Indications

Note: Bracketed information in the *Indications* section refers to uses that are not included in U.S. product labeling.

**Accepted**

Epilepsy (treatment)—Hydantoin anticonvulsants are indicated in the suppression and control of tonic-clonic (grand mal) and simple or complex partial (psychomotor or temporal lobe) seizures.

Ethotoin may be administered as a second-line agent when seizures have not been adequately controlled by the primary anticonvulsants and before proceeding to more toxic anticonvulsants.

Mephenytoin also is used in the treatment of simple partial (focal and Jacksonian) seizures in patients who have not responded to less toxic anticonvulsants.

Status epilepticus (treatment)—Parenteral fosphenytoin and phenytoin are both indicated for the control of tonic-clonic type status epilepticus. Although parenteral benzodiazepines are often used initially for rapid control of status epilepticus, both fosphenytoin and phenytoin are indicated for sustained control of seizure activity.

Seizures in neurosurgery (prophylaxis and treatment)—Fosphenytoin and phenytoin are both indicated for the prevention and treatment of seizures during and following neurosurgery.

[Arrhythmias, digitalis-induced (treatment)][1]—Phenytoin is used in the correction of atrial and ventricular arrhythmias, especially those caused by digitalis glycoside toxicity.

[Choreoathetosis, paroxysmal (treatment)][1]—Phenytoin may be effective in treating paroxysmal choreoathetosis, especially the kinesigenic type. This condition, which is considered a form of reflex epilepsy, is characterized by tonic, dystonic, or choreoathetoid contortions of the extremities, trunk, or face, which are usually precipitated by the patient's initiation of sudden voluntary movement.

[Neuralgia, trigeminal (treatment)][1]—Phenytoin is used alone or with other anticonvulsants to control paroxysmal pain in some patients with trigeminal neuralgia (tic douloureux). Carbamazepine is considered the first-line agent, effectively relieving pain in about 66% of patients. However, since phenytoin relieves pain during long-term use in approximately 20% of patients, it may be used alone in some patients or added to carbamazepine therapy when symptoms persist.

[Neuromyotonia (treatment)][1]
[Myotonia congenita (treatment)][1] or
[Myotonic muscular dystrophy (treatment)][1]—Phenytoin is effective in some patients as a muscle relaxant in the treatment of muscle hyperirritability, characterized by delayed relaxation of muscle after voluntary or mechanically induced contraction and by a state of continuous muscle contraction at rest. Neuromyotonia includes continuous muscle fiber activity syndrome, Isaac's syndrome, and "stiff man" syndrome.

[Toxicity, tricyclic antidepressant (treatment adjunct)][1]—Intravenous phenytoin loading has been used to treat quinidine-like conduction defects, bradyarrhythmias, or heart block, in tricyclic antidepressant overdose. Although its use has been supplanted by other agents, in some instances it remains a therapeutic option.

### Unaccepted

Hydantoin anticonvulsants are *not* indicated in the treatment of absence (petit mal) seizures, or as first-line treatment of febrile, hypoglycemic, or other metabolic seizures. When tonic-clonic (grand mal) seizures coexist with absence seizures, combined therapy may be necessary.

Although phenytoin has been used in patients with recessive dystrophic epidermolysis bullosa for the treatment of blistering and erosions of the skin that may result from even minor trauma or injury, it is no longer considered preferred therapy.

---

[1]Not included in Canadian product labeling.

## Pharmacology/Pharmacokinetics

### Physicochemical characteristics

Molecular weight—
    Ethotoin: 204.23.
    Fosphenytoin sodium: 406.24.
    Mephenytoin: 218.26.
    Phenytoin: 252.27.
    Phenytoin sodium: 274.26.

pKa—
    Phenytoin: 8.06 to 8.33.

pH
    Fosphenytoin sodium injection: 8.6 to 9.
    Phenytoin sodium injection: 12.

    Note: Fosphenytoin is a water-soluble prodrug that is rapidly converted to phenytoin following parenteral administration.

### Mechanism of action/Effect

Anticonvulsant—The mechanism of action is not completely known, but is thought to involve stabilization of neuronal membranes at the cell body, axon, and synapse and limitation of the spread of neuronal or seizure activity. In neurons, phenytoin decreases sodium and calcium ion influx by prolonging voltage-dependent channel inactivation time during generation of nerve impulses. Phenytoin blocks the voltage-dependent sodium channels of neurons and inhibits the calcium flux across neuronal membranes, thus helping to stabilize neurons. It also decreases synaptic transmission, and decreases post-tetanic potentiation at the synapse. Phenytoin enhances the sodium-potassium ATPase activity of neurons and/or glial cells. It also influences second messenger systems by inhibiting calcium-calmodulin protein phosphorylation and possibly altering cyclic nucleotide production or metabolism.

Antiarrhythmic—Phenytoin may act to normalize influx of sodium and calcium to cardiac Purkinje fibers. Abnormal ventricular automaticity and membrane responsiveness are decreased. Also, phenytoin shortens the refractory period, and therefore shortens the QT interval and the duration of the action potential.

Antineuralgic—Exact mechanism is unknown. Phenytoin may act in the central nervous system (CNS) to decrease synaptic transmission or to decrease summation of temporal stimulation leading to neuronal discharge (antikindling). Phenytoin raises the threshold of facial pain and shortens the duration of attacks by diminishing self-maintenance of excitation and repetitive firing.

Skeletal muscle relaxant—Phenytoin's mechanism of action as a muscle relaxant is thought to be similar to its anticonvulsant action. In movement disorders, the membrane-stabilizing effect reduces abnormal sustained repetitive firing and potentiation of nerve and muscle cells.

### Other actions/effects

Therapy with phenytoin significantly increases the amounts and activities of some CYP P450 isoenzymes, the uridine diphosphate glucuronosyltransferase (UDPGT) system, and epoxide hydrolase enzymes, thus enhancing the metabolism of many other drugs. Also, phenytoin may compete with drugs metabolized by the same CYP isoenzymes (CYP2C9 and CYP2C19), thus decreasing the metabolic clearance of those agents.

### Absorption

Ethotoin—
    Rapid.
Fosphenytoin—
    Intravenous: Immediate.
    Intramuscular: Rapid and complete.
Note: Bioavailability from either the intravenous or intramuscular route is essentially 100%.
Mephenytoin—
    Rapid.
Phenytoin—
    Oral: Slow and variable among products; poor in neonates.
    Intravenous: Immediate.
    Intramuscular: Very slow, but complete (92%).

### Distribution

Fosphenytoin—Most likely distributed in humans to heart, kidneys, small intestine, liver, lungs, and spleen, where it is hydrolyzed by phosphatases to phenytoin. Predominately distributed in the central (plasma) compartment. The volume of distribution (Vol$_D$) ranges from 4.3 to 10.8 liters, and increases with increasing dose and administration rate of fosphenytoin.

Phenytoin—Distributed into cerebrospinal fluid, saliva, semen, gastrointestinal fluids, bile, and breast milk; also crosses the placenta, with fetal serum concentrations equal to those of the mother.

### Protein binding

Fosphenytoin—Very high (95 to 99%); degree of binding is saturable, with the result that the percent bound decreases as the total plasma fosphenytoin concentration increases.

Phenytoin—Very high (90% or more); may be lower in neonates (84%) and in hyperbilirubinemic infants (80%); also altered in patients with hypoalbuminemia (< 37 mg per dL), uremia, or acute trauma, and in pregnant patients.

    Note: Fosphenytoin has a high affinity for phenytoin protein binding sites; before its conversion to phenytoin, it binds to these sites, retarding the binding of newly formed phenytoin, thus increasing free (unbound) phenytoin concentrations. In the absence of fosphenytoin, approximately 12% of total plasma phenytoin exists in the free (unbound) state over the clinically relevant concentration range. With the administration of fosphenytoin, total free (unbound) phenytoin plasma concentrations may increase up to 30% during the period required for the conversion of fosphenytoin to phenytoin (approximately 30 to 60 minutes postinfusion).

    In patients with renal or hepatic function impairment or hypoalbuminemia, fosphenytoin conversion to phenytoin may be increased without a similar increase in the clearance of phenytoin, potentially leading to an increased incidence of adverse effects.

### Biotransformation

Hepatic via microsomal oxidative enzymes of the P450 system, specifically the CYP2 family of isozymes; rate increased in younger children, in pregnant women, in women during menses, and in patients with acute trauma; rate decreases with advancing age.

Mephenytoin has an active metabolite, nirvanol (5-ethyl-5-phenylhydantoin). The metabolism of mephenytoin is genetically determined. Patients who are slow metabolizers of mephenytoin are at risk of increased adverse effects; Oriental and black populations are more likely than white populations to be slow metabolizers of mephenytoin.

The major inactive metabolite of phenytoin is 5-(*p*-hydroxyphenyl)-5-phenylhydantoin (HPPH). Phenytoin also may be metabolized slowly in a small number of individuals due to genetic predisposition, which may cause limited enzyme availability and lack of induction.

Fosphenytoin undergoes rapid hydrolysis to phenytoin. *In vivo*, 1.5 mg of fosphenytoin sodium injection liberates 1 mg of phenytoin sodium; thus, 75 mg of fosphenytoin sodium is essentially equivalent to 50 mg of phenytoin sodium. Conversion of fosphenytoin also yields two additional metabolites, phosphate and formaldehyde. Formaldehyde is subsequently converted to formate, which in turn is metabolized via a folate-dependent mechanism. Biological effects from the production of phosphate and formaldehyde generally occur only at doses exceeding usual clinical doses of fosphenytoin. Phosphatase enzymes probably play a major role in the conversion of fosphenytoin to phenytoin.

**Half-life**
Ethotoin—3 to 9 hours.
Fosphenytoin—The conversion half-life to phenytoin ranges from 8 to 15 minutes. This value is independent of dose, infusion rate, or plasma concentrations of either fosphenytoin or phenytoin. The elimination half-life of fosphenytoin after intravenous or intramuscular injection also is independent of dose.
Mephenytoin—About 7 hours, but for active metabolite, nirvanol, about 95 to 144 hours.
Phenytoin—Because phenytoin exhibits saturable, zero-order, or dose-dependent pharmacokinetics, the apparent half-life of phenytoin changes with dose and serum concentration. This is due to the saturation of the enzyme system responsible for metabolizing phenytoin, which occurs at therapeutic concentrations of the drug. Thus, a constant amount of drug is metabolized (capacity-limited metabolism), and small increases in dose may cause disproportionately large increases in serum concentrations and apparent half-life, possibly causing unexpected toxicity.

**Time to peak concentration**
Fosphenytoin—
  Intravenous: 6 minutes (average) after administration.
  Intramuscular: 36 minutes (average) after administration; one dose administered in more than one injection resulted in an increase in time to peak concentration.
Mephenytoin—
  45 minutes to 4 hours.
  Nirvanol: 16 to 36 hours.
Phenytoin (tablets or oral suspension)—
  1½ to 3 hours.
Phenytoin sodium—
  Extended capsules: 4 to 12 hours.
  Prompt capsules: 1½ to 3 hours.

**Therapeutic serum concentration**
Ethotoin—
  15 to 50 mcg per mL (74 to 245 micromoles per L).
Mephenytoin—
  25 to 40 mcg per mL (115 to 183 micromoles per L) (in combination with nirvanol).
Phenytoin—
  10 to 20 mcg per mL (40 to 80 micromoles per L). Steady-state serum concentration is usually achieved in 5 to 10 days with daily oral dosage of 300 mg. Serum concentrations of 20 to 40 mcg per mL (80 to 159 micromoles per L) usually produce symptoms of toxicity; > 40 mcg per mL (159 micromoles per L) usually produce severe toxicity. The serum concentrations of phenytoin needed for efficacy may be influenced by seizure type. Higher concentrations (23 mcg per mL [91 micromoles per L] or greater) may be needed to control simple or complex partial seizures, with or without tonic-clonic seizures, or status epilepticus than are necessary for control of tonic-clonic seizures alone (10 to 20 mcg per mL [40 to 80 micromoles per L]). Occasionally, a patient may have seizure control with serum phenytoin concentrations of 6 to 9 mcg per mL (24 to 36 micromoles per L). Effective treatment, therefore, should be guided by clinical response, not drug serum concentrations. In patients who have hypoalbuminemia and/or renal failure, or who are taking other medications that displace phenytoin from binding sites, hydantoin serum concentrations of 5 to 10 mcg per mL (20 to 40 micromoles per L) may be adequate. For cardiac arrhythmias, plasma concentrations of 10 to 18 mcg per mL (40 to 71 micromoles per L) have been reported to be effective.
  Therapeutic concentrations of free (unbound) phenytoin, which are frequently monitored in patients with altered protein binding (e.g., in neonates and in patients with renal failure, hypoalbuminemia, or acute trauma), usually fall in the range of 0.8 to 2 mcg per mL (3 to 8 micromoles per L).

Note: The pharmacokinetic parameters of phenytoin derived from fosphenytoin administered by intravenous or intramuscular injection do not differ from those values for trough concentrations or area under the plasma concentration–time curve (AUC) of orally administered equivalent doses of phenytoin.

**Elimination**
Ethotoin, mephenytoin, and phenytoin—Primarily renal as metabolites; also in feces. Very little phenytoin is excreted in the feces; most is excreted in the bile as metabolites that are reabsorbed in the intestine and excreted in the urine. Phenytoin excretion is enhanced by alkaline urine.

Fosphenytoin—Not excreted in urine. Phenytoin derived from fosphenytoin is excreted in the urine, primarily as metabolites; little unchanged phenytoin (about 1 to 5% of the fosphenytoin dose) is recovered in the urine.

## Precautions to Consider

**Cross-sensitivity and/or related problems**
Patients sensitive to one hydantoin anticonvulsant may be sensitive to other hydantoin anticonvulsants also. In addition, cross-sensitivity to structurally similar compounds, such as barbiturates, succinimides, and oxazolidinediones, may occur.

**Tumorigenicity**
Phenytoin: There have been isolated reports of malignancies, including neuroblastoma, in children whose mothers received phenytoin during pregnancy.

**Mutagenicity**
Fosphenytoin: Structural chromosome aberration frequency in cultured V79 Chinese hamster lung cells was increased by exposure to fosphenytoin in the presence of metabolic activation. No evidence of mutagenicity of fosphenytoin was observed in bacteria (Ames test) or Chinese hamster lung cells in vitro. No evidence of clastogenic activity of fosphenytoin was observed in the in vivo mouse bone marrow micronucleus test.

**Pregnancy/Reproduction**
Pregnancy—Hydantoin anticonvulsants cross the placenta; risk-benefit must be considered, although a definite cause and effect relationship has not been established between the hydantoins and teratogenic effects. Reports in recent years indicate a higher incidence of congenital abnormalities in children whose mothers used anticonvulsant medication during pregnancy, although most epileptic mothers have delivered normal infants. Reported abnormalities include cleft lip, cleft palate, heart malformations, and the "fetal hydantoin syndrome" (also known as the "fetal anticonvulsant syndrome" and characterized by prenatal growth deficiency, microcephaly, craniofacial abnormalities, hypoplasia of the fingernails, and mental deficiency associated with intrauterine development during therapy). Medication has not been definitively proven to be the cause of "fetal hydantoin syndrome". The reports, to date, relate primarily to the more widely used anticonvulsants, phenytoin and phenobarbital. Pending availability of more precise information, this risk-benefit consideration of anticonvulsant use during pregnancy is extended to the entire family of anticonvulsant medications.

Ethotoin, phenytoin—FDA Pregnancy Category C.
Fosphenytoin—FDA Pregnancy Category D.
Mephenytoin—FDA pregnancy category not included in product labeling.
Because of altered absorption and protein binding and/or increased metabolic clearance of hydantoin anticonvulsants during pregnancy, pregnant women receiving these medications may experience an increased incidence of seizures. Serum hydantoin concentrations must be monitored and doses increased accordingly. A gradual resumption of the patient's usual dosage may be necessary after delivery. However, some patients may experience a rapid reduction in maternal hepatic phenytoin metabolism at time of delivery, requiring the dosage to be reduced within 12 hours postpartum.

Delivery—Exposure to hydantoins prior to delivery may lead to an increased risk of life-threatening hemorrhage (related to decreased concentrations of vitamin K–dependent clotting factors) in the neonate, usually within 24 hours of birth. Hydantoins may also produce a deficiency of vitamin K in the mother, causing increased maternal bleeding during delivery. Risk of maternal and infant bleeding may be reduced by administering vitamin K to the mother during delivery and to the neonate, intramuscularly or subcutaneously, immediately after birth.

**Breast-feeding**
Ethotoin and phenytoin are distributed into breast milk; significant amounts may be ingested by the infant. Information is not available for mephenytoin.

**Pediatrics**
Children and young adults are more susceptible to gingival hyperplasia than older adults. See Dental section.
Some reports suggest that children may experience decreased school performance during long-term treatment with hydantoin anticonvulsants, especially at high therapeutic or toxic concentrations.
Coarsening of facial features and excessive body hair growth may be more pronounced in young patients.
Other anticonvulsants less likely to cause problems should be considered first.
Fosphenytoin: Limited pharmacokinetic data in children older than 5 years of age suggest that the conversion of fosphenytoin to phenytoin occurs

in a manner similar to that in adults. However, the safety of fosphenytoin in children has not been established.

**Geriatrics**
Geriatric patients tend to metabolize hydantoins slowly, thereby increasing the possibility of the medication reaching toxic serum concentrations. Also, serum albumin may be low in older patients, causing a decrease in protein binding of phenytoin. Lower dosage and subsequent adjustments may be required. The rate of administration of intravenous dosage should be no more than 25 mg per minute, and possibly as low as 5 to 10 mg per minute.

**Pharmacogenetics**
The metabolism of mephenytoin is genetically determined. Patients who are slow metabolizers of mephenytoin are at risk of increased adverse effects; Oriental and black populations are more likely than white populations to be slow metabolizers of mephenytoin.

Phenytoin also may be metabolized slowly in a small number of individuals due to genetic predisposition, which may cause limited enzyme availability and lack of induction.

**Dental**
Gingival hyperplasia, a common complication of phenytoin or mephenytoin therapy, usually starts during the first 6 months of treatment as gingivitis or gum inflammation. The incidence is higher in patients up to 23 years of age than in older patients, and severe gingival hyperplasia is less likely to occur with dosage under 500 mg per day. Anterior tissue overgrowth may be greater than posterior overgrowth, creating esthetic and psychological problems for the young patient. A strictly enforced program of teeth cleaning by a professional, combined with plaque control by the patient, if begun within 10 days of initiation of hydantoin anticonvulsant therapy, will minimize growth rate and severity of gingival enlargement. Periodontal surgery may be indicated, and should be followed by careful plaque control to inhibit recurrence of gum enlargement. If gingival hyperplasia cannot be controlled by standard dental procedures, ethotoin may be substituted for phenytoin, without loss of seizure control, usually at doses four to six times greater than those of phenytoin.

In addition, the leukopenic effects of hydantoin anticonvulsants may result in an increased incidence of microbial infection, delayed healing, and gingival bleeding. If leukopenia occurs, dental work should be deferred until blood counts have returned to normal. Patient instruction in proper oral hygiene should include caution in use of regular toothbrushes, dental floss, and toothpicks.

**Drug interactions and/or related problems**
The following drug interactions and/or related problems have been selected on the basis of their potential clinical significance (possible mechanism in parentheses where appropriate)—not necessarily inclusive (» = major clinical significance):

Note: Possible interactions of hydantoin anticonvulsants, particularly phenytoin, with medications known to be metabolized by the hepatic cytochrome P450 enzyme system should be considered. Phenytoin therapy significantly increases the amounts and activities of some CYP isoenzymes, the uridine diphosphate glucuronosyltransferase (UDPGT) system, and epoxide hydrolase enzymes, thus enhancing the metabolism of many other drugs. Also, phenytoin may compete with drugs metabolized by the same CYP isoenzymes (CYP2C9 and CYP2C19), thus decreasing the metabolic clearance of those agents. Metabolism of phenytoin is particularly susceptible to inhibition by other medications using the P450 enzyme system, due to phenytoin's potentially saturable metabolism.

In addition, other highly protein-bound medications may displace phenytoin from its serum protein binding sites, increasing serum concentrations of free (unbound) phenytoin and increasing the risk of toxicity.

The possibility of significant interactions with hepatic enzyme inducers, hepatic enzyme inhibitors, and medications metabolized by the hepatic P450 isoenzyme system, other than those listed below, should be considered and the patient should be carefully monitored during and following concurrent use.

Combinations containing any of the following medications, depending on the amount present, may also interact with this medication.

Acetaminophen
(risk of hepatotoxicity from a single toxic dose or prolonged use of acetaminophen may be increased and therapeutic efficacy may be decreased in patients regularly taking other hepatic enzyme–inducing agents such as phenytoin)

» Alcohol or
» CNS depression–producing medications (see *Appendix II*)
(CNS depression may be enhanced)
(chronic use of alcohol may decrease the serum concentrations and effectiveness of hydantoins; concurrent use of hydantoin anticonvulsants with acute alcohol intake may increase serum hydantoin concentrations)

» Amiodarone
(concurrent use with phenytoin and possibly with other hydantoin anticonvulsants may increase plasma concentrations of the hydantoin, resulting in increased effects and/or toxicity)

» Antacids, aluminum and/or magnesium–containing and calcium carbonate–containing
(concurrent use may decrease the bioavailability of phenytoin; doses of antacids and phenytoin should be separated by about 2 to 3 hours)

» Anticoagulants, coumarin- or indandione-derivative or
» Chloramphenicol or
» Cimetidine or
» Disulfiram or
Influenza virus vaccine or
» Isoniazid or
Methylphenidate or
Metronidazole or
» Phenylbutazone or
Ranitidine or
Salicylates or
» Sulfonamides or
Trazodone or
Trimethoprim
(serum phenytoin concentrations may be increased because of inhibition of its metabolism by these agents, resulting in increased effects and/or toxicity of phenytoin; dosage adjustments may be necessary)

(in addition, the anticoagulant effect of coumarin- or indandione-derivative anticoagulants may be increased initially, but decreased with continued concurrent use)

(phenylbutazone and salicylates also may displace phenytoin from protein binding sites, resulting in increased free [unbound] phenytoin concentrations)

(trimethoprim may increase the half-life of phenytoin by up to 50%, and decrease its clearance by 30% through inhibition of metabolism of phenytoin)

Anticonvulsants, succinimide
(induction of hepatic microsomal enzyme activity may result in decreased serum concentrations of either succinimide or hydantoin anticonvulsants; careful monitoring is suggested, especially when any anticonvulsant is added to or withdrawn from an existing regimen)

» Corticosteroids, glucocorticoid or
Cyclosporine or
Digitalis glycosides or
Disopyramide or
Doxycycline or
Furosemide or
Levodopa or
Mexiletine or
Quinidine
(therapeutic effects of these medications may be decreased because of increased metabolism and decreased plasma concentrations, which may result from hydantoin anticonvulsants' induction of hepatic microsomal enzymes; dosage adjustments of these medications may be necessary)

Antidepressants, tricyclic or
Bupropion or
Clozapine or
Haloperidol or
Loxapine or
Maprotiline or
Molindone or
Monoamine oxidase (MAO) inhibitors, including furazolidone, procarbazine, and selegiline or
Phenothiazines or
Pimozide or
Thioxanthenes
(these medications may lower the seizure threshold and decrease the anticonvulsant effects of hydantoin anticonvulsants; CNS depression may be enhanced; dosage adjustment of the hydantoin anticonvulsant may be necessary)

(concurrent use of phenytoin with tricyclic antidepressants may lower serum concentrations of the antidepressant; dosage increases of the tricyclic antidepressant may be required to produce improvement of the depressed state)

(concurrent use of phenytoin with haloperidol may result in significant reductions in haloperidol serum concentrations)

(molindone contains calcium ions, which interfere with the absorption of phenytoin; patients should be advised to take phenytoin and molindone one to three hours apart)

(concurrent use of phenothiazines may inhibit phenytoin metabolism, leading to phenytoin intoxication)

Antidiabetic agents, oral or
Insulin
(hydantoin anticonvulsants may increase serum glucose concentrations and the possibility of hyperglycemia; dosage adjustment of either or both medications may be necessary)

(tolbutamide may displace phenytoin from protein binding sites, resulting in increased plasma phenytoin concentrations)

» Antifungals, azole, including:
» Fluconazole or
» Itraconazole or
» Ketoconazole or
» Miconazole
(concurrent use of any azole antifungal with phenytoin may decrease the metabolism of phenytoin, resulting in increased plasma phenytoin concentrations; a 75% increase in the area under the plasma concentration–time curve [AUC] of phenytoin was found in volunteers given 200 mg of fluconazole per day; concurrent use has also been reported to decrease the plasma concentration of azole antifungals, which may lead to clinical failure or relapse of the fungal infection; response to both medications should be closely monitored)

Antineoplastic agents, such as:
Bleomycin
Carmustine (BCNU)
Cisplatin
Dacarbazine
Doxorubicin
Ifosfamide
Methotrexate
Vinblastine
(increased metabolism of phenytoin may occur, although other factors such as reduced absorption secondary to chemotherapy-induced gastrointestinal toxicity and concomitant administration of steroids and antacids may contribute to this effect)

(phenytoin may induce the metabolism of ifosfamide to its alkylating metabolites, resulting in increased toxicity)

Barbiturates or
Primidone
(phenytoin and phenobarbital interact reciprocally through multiple mechanisms; concurrent use may produce variable and unpredictable effects; close monitoring of the patient is advised)

(metabolism of primidone to phenobarbital may be increased by phenytoin)

» Calcium
(when used as an excipient in phenytoin capsules, calcium sulfate can decrease phenytoin absorption by as much as 20%)

(concurrent use of phenytoin with calcium supplements or any tablets or capsules that contain calcium sulfate as an excipient may result in formation of nonabsorbable complexes, thereby decreasing the bioavailability of both calcium and phenytoin; patients should be advised to take these medications 1 to 3 hours apart)

Calcium channel blocking agents, including:
Diltiazem or
Nifedipine or
Verapamil
(caution is advised when these medications are used concurrently with phenytoin because of their ability to displace phenytoin from its protein binding sites, increasing serum free [unbound] phenytoin concentrations)

(phenytoin also may induce the metabolism of these medications, causing decreased efficacy)

Carbamazepine
(carbamazepine has complex and variable effects on phenytoin; it may increase or decrease the clearance of phenytoin; in most patients, phenytoin metabolism is inhibited and plasma concentrations may increase significantly, resulting in phenytoin toxicity, which can be mistaken for carbamazepine toxicity. In addition, phenytoin may reduce plasma carbamazepine concentrations, mainly by increasing CYP enzymes; in many cases, plasma concentrations of carbamazepine's active metabolite do not change, but the ratio of metabolite to parent drug concentration increases, with a higher contribution of carbamazepine-10,11-epoxide to the overall clinical effects. Monitoring of plasma concentrations is recommended as a guide to dosage, especially when either medication is added to or withdrawn from an existing regimen)

Carbonic anhydrase inhibitors
(osteopenia induced by hydantoin anticonvulsants may be enhanced; it is recommended that patients receiving concurrent therapy be monitored for early signs of osteopenia and that the carbonic anhydrase inhibitor be discontinued and appropriate treatment initiated if necessary)

Chlordiazepoxide or
Clonazepam or
Diazepam
(chlordiazepoxide and diazepam may cause increased plasma concentrations of phenytoin due to inhibition of its metabolism; phenytoin may increase the clearance of clonazepam and diazepam, decreasing their efficacy; careful monitoring is recommended, since the clinical significance of this interaction is controversial)

» Contraceptives, estrogen-containing, oral or
» Contraceptives, progestin-containing, oral, injection, or subdermal implants
(concurrent use of hydantoin anticonvulsants with estrogen- or progestin-containing contraceptives may result in breakthrough bleeding and contraceptive failure due to the increased rate of hepatic enzyme metabolism of steroids induced by hydantoins; phenytoin has also been shown to increase sex hormone–binding globulin [SHBG], which may lower the amount of free progestin available for biological action and contribute to the lowered effectiveness of the oral contraceptive)

» Diazoxide, oral
(concurrent use with hydantoin anticonvulsants may decrease the efficacy of phenytoin and the hyperglycemic effect of diazoxide and is not recommended)

Dopamine
(use of intravenous phenytoin in patients maintained on dopamine may produce sudden hypotension and bradycardia; this reaction is considered to be dose-rate dependent; if anticonvulsant therapy is necessary during administration of dopamine, an alternative to phenytoin should be considered)

Enteral feeding solutions
(concurrent use with phenytoin may decrease absorption of phenytoin, possibly necessitating an increase in dosage; some clinicians recommend that at least 2 hours should elapse between feeding and phenytoin administration; if phenytoin suspension or capsule contents are administered via nasogastric tubing, flushing the tube with 2 to 4 ounces of water before and after administration has been suggested; phenytoin serum concentrations should be carefully monitored during concurrent therapy)

» Estrogens or
» Progestins
(therapeutic effects of these medications may be decreased because of increased metabolism and decreased plasma concentrations, which may result from induction of hepatic microsomal enzymes by hydantoin anticonvulsants; phenytoin plasma concentrations may also be increased; dosage adjustments of these medications may be necessary)

» Felbamate
(felbamate is a competitive inhibitor of phenytoin metabolism; when felbamate is added to a phenytoin regimen, a decrease of approximately 20 to 33% of the phenytoin dose is necessary; phenytoin also induces the metabolism of felbamate)

» Fluoxetine
(concurrent use of fluoxetine with phenytoin has been reported to cause elevated plasma phenytoin concentrations, resulting in symptoms of toxicity; caution and close monitoring are suggested)

Folic acid or
Leucovorin
(although hydantoin anticonvulsants deplete the body of folate stores, supplementation with folic acid may result in lowered serum hydantoin concentrations and possible loss of seizure control; therefore, an increase in hydantoin dosage may be necessary in patients who receive folate supplementation)

(because leucovorin is a reduced form of folic acid, large doses may counteract the anticonvulsant effects of hydantoin anticonvulsants)

Halothane (and possibly enflurane or methoxyflurane)
(chronic use of hydantoin anticonvulsants prior to anesthesia may increase metabolism of anesthetic, leading to increased risk of hep-

atotoxicity, and may result in increased phenytoin concentrations, leading to increased risk of hydantoin toxicity)

Lamotrigine
(effects of lamotrigine may be reduced because of phenytoin's ability to induce the metabolism [specifically, the UDPGT-dependent glucuronidation] of lamotrigine)

Levothyroxine
(concurrent use with phenytoin may reduce serum protein binding of levothyroxine and reduce total serum thyroxine [$T_4$] by 15 to 25%; however, most patients remain euthyroid, and dosage of thyroid hormone does not need to be altered)

» Lidocaine or
Propranolol and probably other beta-adrenergic blocking agents
(concurrent use with intravenous phenytoin may produce additive cardiac depressant effects; hydantoin anticonvulsants may also increase hepatic enzyme metabolism of lidocaine, reducing its concentration)
(in addition, propranolol may inhibit the metabolism of phenytoin, increasing the risk of adverse effects)

» Methadone
(long-term use of phenytoin may increase metabolism of methadone, probably by induction of hepatic microsomal enzyme activity, and may precipitate withdrawal symptoms in patients being treated for opioid dependence; methadone dosage adjustments may be necessary when phenytoin therapy is initiated or discontinued)

Omeprazole
(inhibition of the cytochrome P450 enzyme system by omeprazole, especially at higher doses, may cause a decrease in the hepatic metabolism of phenytoin; delayed elimination and increased serum concentrations may result, with considerable interpatient variability)

Paroxetine
(concomitant administration with phenytoin may decrease the systemic availability of either agent; also, both medications may exhibit nonlinear pharmacokinetic properties; no initial dosage adjustments are recommended, but subsequent titration should be based on clinical effects)

» Phenacemide
(risk of additive toxicity when phenacemide is used concurrently with hydantoin anticonvulsants; concurrent use of phenacemide with ethotoin has been reported to cause paranoid symptoms; extreme caution is recommended during concurrent use of these medications)

Praziquantel
(one small, single-dose, controlled study found that epileptic patients taking phenytoin had significantly lower plasma concentrations of praziquantel [24% of the control group]; this effect is thought to be due to induction of the cytochrome P450 microsomal enzyme system by phenytoin; patients on phenytoin may require a larger dose of praziquantel)

» Rifampin
(concurrent use with phenytoin may stimulate the hepatic metabolism of phenytoin, increasing its elimination and thus counteracting its anticonvulsant effect; careful monitoring of serum hydantoin concentrations and dosage adjustments may be necessary)

» Streptozocin
(phenytoin may protect pancreatic beta cells from the toxic effects of streptozocin, thus reducing streptozocin's therapeutic effects; concurrent use is not recommended)

» Sucralfate
(concurrent use of sucralfate may decrease the absorption of hydantoin anticonvulsants)

Ticlopidine
(several cases of elevated phenytoin plasma concentrations with associated somnolence and lethargy have been reported following ticlopidine administration)

» Valproic acid
(valproic acid may displace phenytoin from protein-binding sites and may inhibit the metabolism of phenytoin; phenytoin, through enzyme induction, may lower valproate concentrations; there may be an increased risk of liver toxicity, especially in infants; close monitoring of the patient is required since variable serum phenytoin concentrations have resulted; monitoring of free [unbound] phenytoin concentrations as well as total plasma phenytoin concentrations is advised by some clinicians; dosage of phenytoin should be adjusted as required by clinical situation; caution is advised also for use with other hydantoin anticonvulsants)

Vitamin D
(hydantoin anticonvulsants may reduce effect of vitamin D by accelerating metabolism through hepatic microsomal enzyme induction; patients on long-term anticonvulsant therapy may require vitamin D supplementation to prevent osteomalacia, although rickets is rare)

Xanthines, such as:
Aminophylline
Caffeine
Oxtriphylline
» Theophylline
(concurrent use may stimulate hepatic metabolism of theophylline [and possibly other xanthines except dyphylline], resulting in increased theophylline clearance, especially if plasma phenytoin concentrations are in the usual therapeutic range for at least 5 days; also, simultaneous use with theophylline may inhibit phenytoin absorption, resulting in decreased serum phenytoin concentrations; serum concentrations of phenytoin and theophylline should be monitored during concurrent therapy; dosage adjustments of both phenytoin and theophylline may be necessary)

**Laboratory value alterations**
The following have been selected on the basis of their potential clinical significance (possible effect in parentheses where appropriate)—not necessarily inclusive (» = major clinical significance):

With diagnostic test results
Dexamethasone test or
Metyrapone test
(results may be inaccurate because of increased dexamethasone or metyrapone metabolism resulting from enzyme induction; dexamethasone or metyrapone doses may need to be increased)

Gallium citrate Ga 67 imaging
(phenytoin may stimulate a benign alteration in lymphoid tissue, which may result in a Ga 67 scintigram similar to that seen in patients with malignant melanoma)

Schilling test
(phenytoin in combination with other anticonvulsant medications may cause a reversible malabsorption of vitamin $B_{12}$)

Thyroid function tests
(free, circulating thyroxine [$FT_4$] and total thyroxine [$T_4$] concentrations are decreased by phenytoin therapy, mainly due to enhanced conversion to triiodothyronine [$T_3$]; however, $T_3$ and thyroid stimulating hormone [TSH] concentrations generally remain unchanged, and most patients remain euthyroid)

With physiology/laboratory test values
Alkaline phosphatase and
Gamma-glutamyl transpeptidase (GGT)
(values may be increased)

Glucose, serum
(concentrations may be increased)

**Medical considerations/Contraindications**
The medical considerations/contraindications included have been selected on the basis of their potential clinical significance (reasons given in parentheses where appropriate)—not necessarily inclusive (» = major clinical significance).

*Except under special circumstances, this medication should not be used when the following medical problem exists:*

» Cardiac function impairment, such as Adams-Stokes syndrome, second- and third-degree AV block, sino-atrial block, and sinus bradycardia
(parenteral phenytoin administration may affect ventricular automaticity and result in ventricular arrhythmias)

*Risk-benefit should be considered when the following medical problems exist:*

Alcoholism, active
(serum phenytoin concentrations may be decreased)

» Blood dyscrasias
(risk of serious infections may be increased)

Cardiovascular disease
(intravenous phenytoin administration may result in atrial and ventricular conduction depression, ventricular fibrillation, or reduced cardiac output, especially in the elderly or seriously ill patients; phenytoin should be administered at a rate of no more than 25 mg per minute, and if necessary, at a slow rate of 5 to 10 mg per minute)

Diabetes mellitus
(hyperglycemia may be potentiated)

Fever or febrile illness—temperature > 38.2 °C (101 °F) for more than 24 hours
   (serum concentrations of hydantoin anticonvulsants may be decreased because of induction of hepatic oxidative enzymes during fever)
» Hepatic function impairment
   (metabolism of hydantoin anticonvulsants may be reduced, thereby increasing the possibility of toxic serum concentrations; alterations in protein binding are also likely, due to a secondary decrease in albumin concentrations)
» Porphyria
   (risk of exacerbation)
» Renal function impairment
   (excretion and protein binding may be altered)
» Sensitivity to hydantoin anticonvulsants, or to structurally similar compounds such as barbiturates, succinimides, and oxazolidinediones
   Systemic lupus erythematosus
   (risk of exacerbation)
   Thyroid function impairment
   (free, circulating thyroxine [$FT_4$] and total thyroxine [$T_4$] concentrations are decreased by phenytoin therapy; patients usually remain euthyroid)

**Patient monitoring**
The following may be especially important in patient monitoring (other tests may be warranted in some patients, depending on condition; » = major clinical significance):
   Albumin concentrations, serum and
   Calcium concentrations, serum and
» Complete blood cell and platelet counts and
» Hepatic function determinations
   (some or all may be required at periodic intervals during therapy depending on individual needs of the patient; however, these determinations may be necessary only during early weeks or months of treatment)
» Blood pressure determinations and
» Cardiac function and
» Respiratory function
   (patients receiving fosphenytoin or phenytoin intravenously should be carefully monitored; hypotension may occur; severe cardiovascular reactions [including atrial and ventricular conduction depression and ventricular fibrillation] and fatalities have occurred following intravenous administration of phenytoin; severe complications occur most commonly in elderly or seriously ill patients)
» Dental examinations
   (recommended at 3-month intervals for teeth cleaning and reinforcement of patient's plaque control for inhibition of gingival hyperplasia)
» Electroencephalograms (EEGs) and
» Hydantoin concentrations, serum
   (in patients maintained at steady-state hydantoin concentrations with well-controlled seizures, routine screening usually is not needed; however, in newly diagnosed patients or in those with poorly controlled seizures, periodic monitoring, possibly with video recording of seizures, and medical and physical reassessment may prevent neurotoxicity and facilitate dosage titration)
   (when monitoring hydantoin serum concentrations, all blood samples should be drawn at standardized times within the dosing schedule, preferably just before a dose is administered [except for fosphenytoin]; since the hepatic metabolism of phenytoin is saturable, a small increment in dose, at higher doses, will produce a disproportionate and unpredictable increase in serum concentrations to the upper therapeutic ranges, and can lead to clinical toxicity. After administration of fosphenytoin, phenytoin concentrations should not be measured until conversion to phenytoin is essentially complete [i.e., 2 hours after the end of an intravenous infusion or 4 hours after an intramuscular injection]. Prior to complete conversion of fosphenytoin to phenytoin, commonly used immunoanalytical techniques [such as TDx®/TDxFLx® (fluorescence polarization) and Emit® 2000 (enzyme multiplied)] may significantly overestimate plasma phenytoin concentrations because of cross-reactivity with fosphenytoin. The error is dependent on plasma concentrations of phenytoin and fosphenytoin, which are influenced by the dose, route, and rate of administration of fosphenytoin, the time of sampling relative to dosing, and the analytical method. Chromatographic assay methods accurately quantitate phenytoin concentrations in biological fluids in the presence of fosphenytoin. Prior to complete conversion, blood samples for phenytoin monitoring should be collected in tubes containing EDTA as an anticoagulant to minimize *ex vivo* conversion of fosphenytoin to phenytoin. However, even with specific assay methods, phenytoin concentrations measured before conversion of fosphenytoin is complete will not accurately reflect phenytoin concentrations ultimately achieved)
   (free [unbound] hydantoin serum concentrations should be monitored in patients with altered protein binding of phenytoin [e.g., neonates, and patients with renal failure, hypoalbuminemia, or acute trauma] and in patients experiencing adverse reactions who have phenytoin concentrations within the therapeutic or target range)
   (because of altered metabolism and protein binding, and/or increased metabolic clearance of hydantoin anticonvulsants during pregnancy, monthly measurements of serum hydantoin concentrations are recommended to assess the need for an increase in dosage; weekly measurements are recommended during the postpartum period to ascertain adequate reduction of dosage; some patients may have a significant decrease in hydantoin metabolism at time of delivery; therefore, serum hydantoin concentrations should be followed closely during the immediate postpartum period [within 12 hours])
   Folate concentrations, serum
   (recommended periodically because of increased folate requirements of patients on long-term phenytoin therapy)
   Phosphate concentrations in patients with renal insufficiency receiving fosphenytoin
   (these patients may be prone to phosphate intoxication; the phosphate load from administration of fosphenytoin is 0.0037 millimoles of phosphate per mg of phenytoin sodium equivalents [PE])
   Physical examination, with special attention to lymph glands and skin
   (all cases of lymphadenopathy or skin rash should be monitored for an extended period because of possible phenytoin hypersensitivity syndrome with lymphadenopathy or pseudolymphoma; should these problems occur, every effort should be made to achieve seizure control using alternative anticonvulsants)
   Thyroid function determinations
   (recommended during the first few months of therapy to detect symptoms of hypothyroidism, which may be unmasked by hydantoins; when a patient receiving phenytoin is suspected of having hypothyroidism, $T_3$ and thyroid-stimulating hormone [TSH] concentrations should be measured rather than $T_4$ and free $T_4$ index [FTI], since the latter are both typically depressed in patients receiving phenytoin)
Note: Even after patients have been stabilized on a maintenance dose, it is important that they have periodic examinations during therapy since phenytoin (and possibly other hydantoins) may deplete body stores of folic acid and vitamin D, possibly resulting in megaloblastic anemia or osteomalacia.

## Side/Adverse Effects
Note: Although not all of these side effects have been attributed specifically to each hydantoin anticonvulsant, a potential exists for their occurrence during the use of any hydantoin.
The following side/adverse effects have been selected on the basis of their potential clinical significance (possible signs and symptoms in parentheses where appropriate)—not necessarily inclusive:

### Those indicating need for medical attention
Incidence more frequent
   ***CNS toxicity, including ataxia*** (clumsiness or unsteadiness); ***confusion; nystagmus*** (uncontrolled back-and-forth and/or rolling eye movements); ***slurred speech or stuttering; trembling of hands; and unusual excitement, nervousness, or irritability; gingival hyperplasia*** (bleeding, tender, or enlarged gums)—higher incidence in children and young adults; incidence in all age groups rare with ethotoin; ***lupus erythematosus, phenytoin hypersensitivity syndrome, Stevens-Johnson syndrome, or toxic epidermal necrolysis*** (fever; muscle pain; skin rash; sore throat)
Note: *CNS toxicity* usually occurs with long-term use, but may be dose-related.
   *Phenytoin hypersensitivity syndrome* may be manifested in many ways. Fever, rash, and lymphadenopathy frequently occur together, and may be part of more than one hypersensitivity syndrome. Skin rash is the most frequent hypersensitivity reaction; licheniform or maculopapular or morbilliform rash, often pruritic, may present simply or may be prodromal of more serious dermatological reactions such as *Stevens-Johnson syndrome* or *toxic epidermal necrolysis*. Lymphoid syndromes (including lymphoid hyperplasia, pseudolymphomas, and pseudo-pseudolymphomas) occur less commonly and are generally re-

versible upon discontinuation of phenytoin. Phenytoin-induced hepatitis and hepatic necrosis are other major hypersensitivity reactions, as is eosinophilia, which occurs commonly. Less commonly occurring syndromes include polyarteritis, polymyositis, or systemic *lupus erythematosus;* disseminated intravascular coagulopathy, serum sickness, and renal failure may also occur.

Rash usually appears in the first 2 weeks of treatment; *hypersensitivity syndrome* usually occurs 3 to 8 weeks after, but may occur as long as 12 weeks after initiation of phenytoin therapy. The syndrome may be life-threatening, but early intervention may prevent renal failure, severe rhabdomyolysis, or hepatic necrosis. Other factors, such as a positive family history for phenytoin hypersensitivity reactions or concomitant administration of cranial radiation therapy, may increase the risk of hypersensitivity syndrome occurring.

Incidence rare
*Blood dyscrasias, including agranulocytosis* (chills; fever; sore throat; unusual tiredness or weakness); *leukopenia* (fever; chills; sore throat); *pancytopenia* (nosebleeds or other unusual bleeding or bruising); *and thrombocytopenia* (fever; sore throat; unusual bleeding or bruising); *cholestatic jaundice or hepatitis* (dark urine; light gray–colored stools; loss of appetite and weight; severe stomach pain; yellow eyes or skin; skin rash or itching; dizziness; nausea or vomiting; joint pain; unusual tiredness or weakness); *choreoathetoid movements, transient* (restlessness or agitation; uncontrolled jerking or twisting movements of hands, arms, or legs; uncontrolled movements of lips, tongue, or cheeks); *cognitive impairment* (defects in intelligence, short-term memory, learning ability, and attention); *periarteritis nodosa* (abdominal pain; soreness of muscles; unusual tiredness or weakness; fever with or without chills; headache; loss of appetite and weight); *Peyronie's disease* (pain of penis on erection); *pulmonary infiltrates or fibrosis* (fever; troubled or quick, shallow breathing; unusual tiredness or weakness; loss of appetite and weight; chest discomfort); *vitamin D and/or calcium imbalance* (frequent bone fractures; bone malformations; slowed growth)

Note: Many cases of mephenytoin-induced *blood dyscrasias* occur in patients given mephenytoin for a second time after a period of abstinence.

*Choreoathetoid movements* may be due to rapid administration of intravenous phenytoin for status epilepticus; the effect usually lasts 24 to 48 hours after discontinuation of phenytoin and may resolve spontaneously; it is unrelated to serum hydantoin toxicity or duration of use.

With chronic use
*Peripheral polyneuropathy, predominantly sensory* (numbness, tingling, or pain in hands or feet)—with phenytoin

With parenteral use only
Note: Both phenytoin and fosphenytoin may cause hypotension and cardiovascular collapse and/or CNS depression when administered rapidly by the intravenous route, although hypotension and cardiac sequelae are less likely with fosphenytoin. Cardiovascular collapse following rapid intravenous infusion of phenytoin may be primarily attributable to its propylene glycol vehicle. The rate of intravenous infusion of phenytoin should not exceed 50 mg per minute; the rate of fosphenytoin infusions should not exceed 150 mg phenytoin sodium equivalents (PE) per minute. The incidence of cardiovascular effects may be higher in patients who are hypoxic or who have ischemic heart disease.

*Phenytoin*
*Burning pain or irritation at injection site*—rarely with necrosis and sloughing
Note: Fosphenytoin also may be associated with *irritation at injection site,* but usually to a lesser degree, due to its water-solubility and its more favorable pH.

*Fosphenytoin*
*Paresthesias and pruritus* (burning; tingling; pain; or itching)—occurring most commonly in groin areas, but also in face, scalp, head, and neck areas, in lower back, buttocks, and abdominal areas
Note: *Paresthesias and pruritus* may be severe; occurrence and intensity can often be lessened by slowing or temporarily stopping the intravenous infusion. Most alert patients who received intravenous fosphenytoin doses of 15 mg PE per kg or greater at a rate of 150 mg PE per minute experienced some degree of discomfort. Most effects resolved within 10 minutes following completion of the infusion; however, some patients experienced sensory disturbances for hours. The pharmacologic basis for these effects is not known, but similar symptoms have been reported with other phosphate ester drugs that deliver phosphate loads. These sensory disturbances are seen more frequently following intravenous than intramuscular injections of fosphenytoin.

**Those indicating need for medical attention only if they continue or are bothersome**
Incidence more frequent
*Constipation; mild dizziness; mild drowsiness; nausea and vomiting*
Incidence less frequent
*Diarrhea*—with ethotoin; *enlargement of facial features, including thickening of lips, widening of nasal tip, and protrusion of jaw; gynecomastia* (swelling of breasts)—in males; *headache; hypertrichosis* (unusual and excessive hair growth on body and face)—primarily with phenytoin; *insomnia* (trouble in sleeping); *muscle twitching*

## Overdose

For specific information on the agents used in the management of hydantoin anticonvulsant overdose, see the *Charcoal, Activated (Oral-Local)* monograph.

For more information on the management of overdose or unintentional ingestion, **contact a Poison Control Center** (see *Poison Control Center Listing*).

**Clinical effects of overdose**
The following effects have been selected on the basis of their potential clinical significance (possible signs and symptoms in parentheses where appropriate)—not necessarily inclusive:
*Ataxia* (clumsiness or unsteadiness); *or staggering walk; blurred or double vision; severe confusion; severe dizziness or drowsiness; dysarthria* (stuttering); *or slurred speech; hyperreflexia; nausea and vomiting; nystagmus* (continuous, uncontrolled back-and-forth and/or rolling eye movements); *seizures; tremor; unusual tiredness or weakness*

Note: The lethal dose of phenytoin in adults is estimated to be 2 to 5 grams. The lethal dose in children is unknown.

The formate and phosphate metabolites of fosphenytoin may contribute to toxicity. Formate toxicity is associated with severe anion-gap metabolic acidosis. Large increases in phosphate concentrations may cause hypocalcemia with paresthesias, muscle spasms, and seizures.

**Treatment of overdose**
Since there is no specific antidote for overdose with hydantoin anticonvulsants, treatment is symptomatic and supportive.

To decrease absorption—Induction of emesis or gastric lavage. Multiple oral doses of activated charcoal and cathartic may shorten the duration of symptoms.

To enhance elimination—Forced fluid diuresis, peritoneal dialysis, exchange transfusions, hemodialysis, and plasmapheresis are ineffective; there is little renal elimination and a danger of fluid overload.

Monitoring—If an overdose of fosphenytoin is suspected, ionized free calcium concentrations should be monitored as a sign of phosphate toxicity.

Supportive care—Oxygen, vasopressors, and assisted ventilation may be necessary for CNS, respiratory, or cardiovascular depression. Patients in whom intentional overdose is confirmed or suspected should be referred for psychiatric consultation.

Following recovery, careful evaluation of blood-forming organs is advisable.

## Patient Consultation

As an aid to patient consultation, refer to *Advice for the Patient, Anticonvulsants, Hydantoin (Systemic).*

In providing consultation, consider emphasizing the following selected information (» = major clinical significance):

**Before using this medication**
» Conditions affecting use, especially:
Sensitivity to hydantoin anticonvulsants or to structurally similar compounds, such as barbiturates, succinimides, and oxazolidinediones
Pregnancy—Hydantoin anticonvulsants cross the placenta; risk-benefit should be considered because of possibility of increased birth defects; seizures may increase during pregnancy with need for dose increase; bleeding problems may occur in mother during delivery and in baby immediately after delivery

Breast-feeding—Ethotoin and phenytoin distributed into breast milk

Use in children—Bleeding, tender, and enlarged gums more common in children; unusual and excessive hair growth, more noticeable in young girls; decreased performance in school (cognitive impairment) may occur with long-term use of high doses

Use in the elderly—Side effects more likely to occur in the elderly; hydantoin anticonvulsants metabolized more slowly in elderly, possibly leading to toxicity

Dental—Gingival hyperplasia may appear; good dental hygiene and visits to dentist every 3 months for cleaning recommended; agranulocytosis or thrombocytopenia may cause gingival bleeding, slowed healing, and infections

Other medications, especially alcohol, amiodarone, antacids, anticoagulants, azole antifungals, calcium-containing medicine, chloramphenicol, cimetidine, CNS depressants, corticosteroids, diazoxide, disulfiram, estrogen- or progestin-containing contraceptives, estrogens, felbamate, fluoxetine, isoniazid, lidocaine, methadone, phenacemide, phenylbutazone, progestins, rifampin, streptozocin, sucralfate, sulfonamides, theophylline, or valproic acid

Other medical problems, especially blood dyscrasias, cardiac function impairment, hepatic function impairment, history of hydantoin hypersensitivity, porphyria, or renal function impairment

**Proper use of this medication**
*Proper administration*
For liquid dosage forms—Shaking well; using an accurate measuring device, such as a specially marked measuring spoon, a plastic syringe, or a small graduated cup
For chewable tablet dosage form—Chewing or crushing tablets or swallowing them whole
For capsule dosage form—Swallowing capsule whole
Taking with food to reduce gastrointestinal irritation
» Compliance with therapy; taking every day exactly as directed
» Proper dosing
» Missed dose: If dosing schedule is—
One dose a day: Taking as soon as possible unless next day, then continuing on schedule; not doubling doses
Several doses a day: Taking as soon as possible unless within 4 hours of next scheduled dose, then continuing on regular schedule; not doubling doses
Checking with doctor if doses are missed for 2 or more days in a row
» Proper storage

**Precautions while using this medication**
» Regular visits to physician to check progress of therapy
» Not taking other medication without physician's advice
» Avoiding the use of alcoholic beverages and other CNS depressants while taking this medicine
Not taking within 2 to 3 hours of taking antacids or medication for diarrhea
Not changing brands or dosage forms of phenytoin without checking with physician or pharmacist
» Checking with physician before discontinuing medication; gradual dosage reduction is usually needed to maintain seizure control
Carrying medical identification card or bracelet during therapy
Diabetic patients: Checking blood or urine sugar concentrations
Caution if any laboratory tests required; possible interference with test results of dexamethasone, metyrapone, or Schilling tests, thyroid function tests, or gallium citrate Ga 67 imaging
» Caution if any kind of surgery, dental treatment, or emergency treatment is required
» Caution when driving, using machines, or doing other jobs requiring alertness
» Using different or additional means of birth control than estrogen- or progestin-containing contraceptives
*For phenytoin or mephenytoin only*
» Maintaining good dental hygiene and seeing dentist every 3 months for teeth cleaning, to prevent tenderness, bleeding, and enlargement of gums

**Side/adverse effects**
Increased incidence of gingival hyperplasia in children and young adults taking phenytoin or mephenytoin
Unusual and excessive hair growth more noticeable in young girls
Signs of potential side effects, especially CNS toxicity, lupus erythematosus, phenytoin hypersensitivity syndrome, Stevens-Johnson syndrome, toxic epidermal necrolysis, blood dyscrasias, cholestatic jaundice, hepatitis, transient choreoathetoid movements, cognitive impairment, periarteritis nodosa, Peyronie's disease, pulmonary infiltrates or fibrosis, or vitamin D and/or calcium imbalance

## General Dosing Information

Dosage must be individualized. Monitoring of serum phenytoin concentrations is recommended because of the great variation of response among patients to the hydantoin anticonvulsants and because of the relatively narrow therapeutic serum concentration range.

Geriatric patients, seriously ill patients, or patients with impaired hepatic function may require lower initial dosage with subsequent adjustments, because of slow hydantoin metabolism or decreased protein binding. If phenytoin is administered intravenously, the rate must be slowed to not more than 25 mg a minute, and possibly to as low as 5 to 10 mg a minute.

When patients are transferred from hydantoins to other anticonvulsant medication or vice versa, there should be a gradual (over a period of a few weeks) increase in the dosage of the added medication and a gradual decrease in the dosage of the medication to be discontinued. When an enzyme-inducing medication is added to or removed from a regimen, the metabolism of the other medications will be altered. In most patients, changes in enzyme induction may occur over a period of weeks.

When single-drug anticonvulsant therapy is to be discontinued in patients with seizure disorders, dosage should be reduced gradually over a period of 6 to 12 months to prevent possible recurrence of seizures. Abrupt withdrawal may lead to status epilepticus.

**Diet/Nutrition**
Oral hydantoin anticonvulsants may be taken with or immediately after meals to lessen gastric irritation. However, the medication should always be taken at the same time in relation to meals to ensure consistent absorption.

Patients on long-term hydantoin therapy may have increased folic acid requirements. However, increased hydantoin dosages may be necessary in patients who receive folate supplementation because such supplementation may result in decreased serum hydantoin concentrations and possible loss of seizure control.

Patients on long-term hydantoin therapy may also require vitamin D supplementation, especially those patients taking high doses of phenytoin, those with low dietary intake of vitamin D, those with limited sun exposure, and those with reduced levels of physical activity.

**For treatment of adverse effects**
Intolerance or allergic reactions—Hydantoin anticonvulsants should be discontinued immediately. Effects are usually observed within 9 to 14 days after start of therapy. If rash is morbilliform (measles-like) or scarlatiniform (scarlet fever–like), therapy may be restarted after the rash has completely disappeared, but should be discontinued if the rash reappears. If rash is exfoliative, purpuric, bullous, or if lupus erythematosus or Stevens-Johnson syndrome is suspected, hydantoin therapy should not be resumed. Attempts should be made to differentiate lymph gland enlargement from other lymph node pathology. The patient should be monitored closely for an extended length of time, and alternative (nonhydantoin) anticonvulsant therapy initiated.

CNS or cerebellar toxicity—Dosage reduction or discontinuation of hydantoin anticonvulsant may improve or reverse effects. Cerebellar toxicity may occur after long-term administration, usually at serum concentrations above 30 mcg. However, CNS toxicity has also been reported at lower serum concentrations, due to free fraction variability.

Gingival or gum enlargement—Consultation with dentist; following recommendations for care to reduce effects.

---

### ETHOTOIN

## Summary of Differences
Pharmacology/pharmacokinetics:
Half-life—
3 to 9 hours.
Side/adverse effects:
Diarrhea has been reported.
Drowsiness and sedation are dose related and quite common.
Gum hyperplasia is rare; ethotoin is sometimes substituted for phenytoin therapy when gingival hyperplasia is a problem.
Incidence of ataxia is rare.
Incidence of hypertrichosis is lower than with other hydantoin anticonvulsants.

## Additional Dosing Information
See also *General Dosing Information*.
Ethotoin may be substituted for phenytoin without loss of seizure control for improvement of gum hyperplasia, or other side effects, during anticonvulsant therapy. Ethotoin doses are usually four to six times greater than those of phenytoin.

## Oral Dosage Forms
### ETHOTOIN TABLETS USP

**Usual adult and adolescent dose**
Anticonvulsant—
   Oral, 500 mg to 1 gram the first day, usually divided into four to six doses, the dosage being gradually increased over several days until seizure control is obtained.

Note: Maintenance dosage of less than 2 grams a day has been found to be ineffective in most adults.
   Debilitated patients may require a lower initial dosage.

**Usual adult prescribing limits**
Up to 3 grams a day.

**Usual pediatric dose**
Anticonvulsant—
   Oral, up to 750 mg a day initially, on the basis of age and weight, the dosage being adjusted as needed and tolerated until seizure control is obtained.

Note: A total daily dose of 3 grams may be required for some patients.

**Usual geriatric dose**
See *Usual adult and adolescent dose*. However, geriatric patients may require a lower initial dosage.

**Strength(s) usually available**
U.S.—
   250 mg (Rx) [*Peganone* (scored; lactose)].
   500 mg (Rx) [*Peganone* (scored; lactose)].
Canada—
   Not commercially available.

**Packaging and storage**
Store below 40 °C (104 °F), preferably between 15 and 30 °C (59 and 86 °F), unless otherwise specified by manufacturer. Store in a tight container.

**Auxiliary labeling**
• May cause drowsiness.
• Avoid alcoholic beverages.

---

## FOSPHENYTOIN

## Summary of Differences

Physicochemical characteristics: Fosphenytoin is a water-soluble prodrug that is rapidly converted to phenytoin following parenteral administration.

Pharmacology/pharmacokinetics: Fosphenytoin has no intrinsic pharmacologic activity before its conversion to phenytoin. After conversion, the pharmacologic and toxicologic effects are essentially the same as those of phenytoin. For each millimole of fosphenytoin administered, one millimole of phenytoin is produced. This means that 1.5 mg of fosphenytoin liberates 1 mg of phenytoin, or that 75 mg of fosphenytoin sodium is essentially equivalent to 50 mg of phenytoin sodium. To avoid performing molecular weight–based adjustments when converting between fosphenytoin sodium and phenytoin sodium, the amount and concentration of fosphenytoin is expressed in terms of phenytoin sodium equivalents (PE). Fosphenytoin should always be prescribed and dispensed in phenytoin sodium equivalents (PE).

Pharmacokinetics of fosphenytoin following intravenous administration are complex; when used in an emergent setting, such as status epilepticus, differences in the rate of availability of phenytoin could be critical. Therefore, studies have empirically determined infusion rates for fosphenytoin that produce the rate and extent of systemic phenytoin availability similar to that obtained from a phenytoin sodium infusion of 50 mg per minute.

Side/adverse effects: The incidence of adverse reactions following intravenous administration of fosphenytoin tends to increase with dose and infusion rate. Doses of 15 mg PE per kg of body weight administered at 150 mg PE per minute may cause transient pruritus, tinnitus, nystagmus, somnolence, and ataxia to occur two to three times more often than do lower doses or slower administration rates.

## Additional Dosing Information

See also *General Dosing Information*.

Dosing of fosphenytoin sodium injection is always expressed in terms of phenytoin sodium equivalents (PE).

**Bioequivalenece information**
*In vivo*, 1.5 mg of fosphenytoin sodium injection liberates 1 mg of phenytoin sodium; thus, 75 mg of fosphenytoin sodium is essentially equivalent to 50 mg of phenytoin sodium.

## Parenteral Dosing Forms
### FOSPHENYTOIN SODIUM INJECTION

Note: Dosing for fosphenytoin sodium injection is expressed in terms of phenytoin sodium equivalents (PE).
   During intravenous infusion of fosphenytoin, continuous monitoring of the patient's electrocardiogram (ECG), blood pressure, and respiration is essential.
   Intramuscular fosphenytoin doses of 20 to 30 mL have been safely administered as a single intramuscular injection, with little or no local irritation reported.

**Usual adult and adolescent dose**
Anticonvulsant in status epilepticus—
   Loading: Intravenous, 15 to 20 mg phenytoin sodium equivalents (PE) per kg of body weight, administered at a rate of 100 to 150 mg PE per minute. The infusion rate should not exceed 150 mg PE per minute.
   Maintenance: Intravenous or intramuscular, initially 4 to 6 mg PE per kg of body weight per day.

Note: Because the effect of fosphenytoin is not immediate, other measures including concomitant administration of a benzodiazepine will usually be necessary in status epilepticus.

Anticonvulsant for nonemergent conditions—
   Loading: Intravenous or intramuscular, 10 to 20 mg phenytoin sodium equivalents (PE) per kg of body weight.
   Maintenance: Initially 4 to 6 mg PE per kg of body weight per day.

As substitute for oral phenytoin therapy—
   The same total daily dose and frequency as phenytoin sodium has been administered. Since fosphenytoin is 100% bioavailable by both intravenous and intramuscular routes, either route may be used. However, the intramuscular route obviates the need for monitoring and the equipment necessary for intravenous infusion. Since phenytoin sodium delayed-release capsules are approximately 90% bioavailable, plasma concentrations of phenytoin may increase modestly when parenteral fosphenytoin is substituted. Clinical response and therapeutic plasma phenytoin concentrations should be used to guide fosphenytoin therapy after 3 to 5 days.

**Usual pediatric dose**
Anticonvulsant in status epilepticus—
   Loading: Intravenous, 15 to 20 mg phenytoin sodium equivalents (PE) per kg of body weight, administered at up to 3 mg PE per kg of body weight per minute.
   Maintenance: Intravenous or intramuscular, initially 4 to 6 mg PE per kg of body weight.

**Usual geriatric dose**
Anticonvulsant in status epilepticus—
   Loading: Intravenous, 14 mg phenytoin sodium equivalents (PE) per kg of body weight.

Note: In patients who require phosphate restriction, such as those with severe renal function impairment, the contribution of fosphenytoin of 0.0037 millimole of phosphate per mg phenytoin sodium equivalent (PE) must be considered.

**Strength(s) usually available**
U.S.—
   75 mg per mL, equivalent to 50 mg of phenytoin sodium per mL (Rx) [*Cerebyx* (Tromethamine USP (TRIS); Hydrochloric acid NF; Sodium hydroxide NF; Water for injection USP)].
Canada—
   Not commercially available.

**Packaging and storage**
Store between 2 and 8 °C (36 to 46 °F), unless otherwise specified by manufacturer. Do not store at room temperature for more than 48 hours.

**Preparation of dosage form**
Prior to intravenous administration, fosphenytoin sodium must be diluted in 5% dextrose injection or 0.9% sodium chloride injection to a concentration of 1.5 to 25 mg phenytoin sodium equivalents (PE) per mL.

**Stability**
Unopened vials should be refrigerated; however, unopened vials will remain stable for 48 hours at room temperature. Vials that develop particulate matter should not be used.
Once diluted for intravenous administration, fosphenytoin sodium solutions are stable for 8 hours at room temperature and 24 hours under refrigeration.

**Additional information**
Fosphenytoin sodium injection is buffered to a pH of 8.6 to 9.

## MEPHENYTOIN

### Summary of Differences
Pharmacology/pharmacokinetics: Half-life is approximately 7 hours but averages 95 to 144 hours for the active metabolite, nirvanol.
Side/adverse effects: Drowsiness and sedation are dose related and quite common.

### Additional Dosing Information
See also *General Dosing Information*.
Mephenytoin usually is used only after safer anticonvulsants have been tried and have proven unsatisfactory.

### Oral Dosage Forms
#### MEPHENYTOIN TABLETS USP
**Usual adult and adolescent dose**
Anticonvulsant—
  Oral, 50 to 100 mg once a day, the dosage being increased by an additional 50 to 100 mg a day at one-week intervals until seizure control is obtained.
Note: Debilitated patients may require a lower initial dosage.

**Usual adult prescribing limits**
1.2 grams a day.

**Usual pediatric dose**
Anticonvulsant—
  Oral, 25 to 50 mg a day, the dosage being increased by an additional 25 to 50 mg a day at one-week intervals until seizure control is obtained.

**Usual pediatric prescribing limits**
400 mg a day.
Note: Dose may be divided and should be based on severity of seizures, age, and serum concentrations.

**Usual geriatric dose**
See *Usual adult and adolescent dose*. However, geriatric patients may require a lower initial dosage.

**Strength(s) usually available**
U.S.—
  100 mg (Rx) [*Mesantoin* (scored; lactose; sucrose)].
Canada—
  Not commercially available.

**Packaging and storage**
Store below 40 °C (104 °F), preferably between 15 and 30 °C (59 and 86 °F), unless otherwise specified by manufacturer. Store in a well-closed container.

**Auxiliary labeling**
- May cause drowsiness.
- Avoid alcoholic beverages.

## PHENYTOIN

### Summary of Differences
Category: Also used as an antiarrhythmic, for ventricular arrhythmias, especially when arrhythmia is digitalis-induced or caused by tricyclic antidepressant toxicity; as an antineuralgic in trigeminal neuralgia; and as a muscle relaxant in certain movement disorders.
Pharmacology/pharmacokinetics: Because phenytoin exhibits saturable, zero-order, or dose-dependent pharmacokinetics, the apparent half-life of phenytoin changes with dose and serum concentration.
Side/adverse effects: Incidence of hypertrichosis is more frequent than with other hydantoin anticonvulsants.

### Additional Dosing Information
See also *General Dosing Information*.

**For oral dosage forms**
Extended Phenytoin Sodium Capsules USP is the only dosage form used for once-a-day dosing, and then, only after patients have been stabilized on a divided dosage, generally 300 to 400mg a day.
Phenytoin oral suspension is generally not recommended for once-a-day dosing because it is not an extended-release dosage form. The suspension may be adequate for more frequent dosing, if vigorously shaken to avoid inadequate dispersal of phenytoin throughout the vehicle.

**For parenteral dosage forms**
Intravenous phenytoin sodium should be administered by direct intravenous injection into a large vein through a large-gauge needle or intravenous catheter at a rate not to exceed 50 mg a minute. Faster rates of administration may result in hypotension, cardiovascular collapse, or CNS depression, related to the propylene glycol diluent.
Intravenous administration should be monitored by cardiac function and blood pressure readings.
To minimize local venous irritation from intravenous injection of phenytoin, each dose must be followed by 0.9% sodium chloride injection through the same in-place needle or catheter. Extravasation should be avoided, as phenytoin injection is caustic to tissues because of its high alkalinity (pH = 12), and possibly also because of the propylene glycol in the vehicle. Soft tissue injury ranging from irritation to extensive necrosis and sloughing has been reported even when extravasation has not occurred.
Some clinicians suggest that, to prevent serious local inflammatory reactions, intermittent phenytoin infusion may be desirable and that such an infusion can be made feasible if all of the following criteria are met:
- Phenytoin injection is admixed only with no more than 50 mL of 0.9% sodium chloride injection.
- The final concentration of phenytoin is between 1 and 10 mg per mL.
- Admixture is done *immediately* before beginning the infusion.
- Infusion is completed within 1 hour.
- All tubing is flushed with 0.9% sodium chloride injection before and after infusion.
- A 0.45- to 0.22-micron filter is placed on the line.

When phenytoin injection is administered by infusion, the maximum rate of infusion is 50 mg a minute. However, for patients who may develop hypotension, who are on a sympathomimetic medication, who have cardiovascular disease, or who are older than 65 years of age, the maximum rate of infusion should be 25 mg a minute and possibly as low as 5 to 10 mg a minute. Vigilant ECG monitoring of cardiovascular status throughout the duration of infusion is required.
For rapid control of seizures, concomitant administration of an intravenous benzodiazepineor a short-acting barbiturate may be necessary because of the slow rate of administration necessary for phenytoin injection.
Because of the delayed absorption of intramuscularly administered phenytoin and the high degree of local irritation from the alkaline solution, the intramuscular route of administration is not recommended when the intravenous or oral route is available.
Intramuscular administration is not recommended for treatment of status epilepticus since serum concentrations in the therapeutic range cannot be readily achieved for up to 24 hours. Erratic absorption is partly caused by tissue precipitation of phenytoin. Muscle necrosis has also been reported.
Intramuscular administration during neurosurgery, for patients stabilized on oral phenytoin, requires a dose 50% greater than the oral dosage used to maintain serum concentrations. When a patient is returned to the oral route, dosage should be reduced by 50% of the original oral dosage for 1 week to compensate for the sustained release of medication from prior intramuscular injections.
If the need for intramuscular administration continues for more than 1 week, alternative routes such as gastric intubation should be considered.

**Bioequivalenence information**
For oral dosage forms only—
  The prescribing physician should be consulted before a prescription is changed from one phenytoin dosage form to another because of possible differences in bioavailability, due to varying amounts of calcium sulfate excipient or amount of phenytoin acid contained in the product. Phenytoin dosage forms based on phenytoin acid (oral suspension and chewable tablets) contain 8% more drug on a mg-per-mg basis than those based on phenytoin sodium. Phenytoin intoxication has been reported following weight-for-weight substitution of phenytoin acid for phenytoin sodium.
  The prescribing physician should be consulted before a product is dispensed that is different from that currently taken by the patient, or from that originally prescribed. Bioavailability may vary enough among oral phenytoin sodium products of different manufacturers to result in either a loss of seizure control or a toxic blood concentration.

## Oral Dosage Forms

Note: Bracketed uses in the *Dosage Forms* section refer to categories of use and/or indications that are not included in U.S. product labeling.

### PHENYTOIN ORAL SUSPENSION USP

Note: Phenytoin Oral Suspension USP is not an extended phenytoin product and is not intended for once-a-day dosage.

**Usual adult and adolescent dose**
Anticonvulsant—
  Oral, initially 125 mg three times a day, the dosage being adjusted at seven- to ten-day intervals as needed and tolerated.

Note: For seriously ill or debilitated patients, or patients with impaired hepatic function, the total dose is often reduced.

**Usual pediatric dose**
Anticonvulsant—
  Initial: Oral, 5 mg per kg of body weight a day, divided into two or three doses, the dosage being adjusted as needed and tolerated.
  Maintenance: Oral, 4 to 8 mg per kg of body weight or 250 mg per square meter of body surface area a day, divided into two or three doses.

**Usual geriatric dose**
Anticonvulsant—
  Oral, initially 3 mg per kg of body weight a day, in divided doses, the dosage being adjusted according to serum hydantoin concentrations and the patient's response.

**Strength(s) usually available**
U.S.—
  125 mg per 5 mL (Rx) [*Dilantin-125* (sucrose); GENERIC].
Canada—
  30 mg per 5 mL (Rx) [*Dilantin-30*].
  125 mg per 5 mL (Rx) [*Dilantin-125*].

**Packaging and storage**
Store below 40 °C (104 °F), preferably between 15 and 30 °C (59 and 86 °F), unless otherwise specified by manufacturer. Store in a tight container. Protect from freezing.

**Auxiliary labeling**
• Shake well.
• Protect from freezing.
• Avoid alcoholic beverages.

**Note:**
Remind patient to shake bottle well before removing each dose.
Advise patient to use an accurate measuring spoon, plastic syringe, or graduated measuring cup.

**Additional information**
May contain 0.6% alcohol.

### PHENYTOIN TABLETS (CHEWABLE) USP

Note: Phenytoin chewable tablets are not intended for once-a-day dosage as they may be too promptly bioavailable. Once-a-day use of phenytoin chewable tablets may result in toxic serum concentrations of phenytoin.

**Usual adult and adolescent dose**
Anticonvulsant—
  Oral, initially 100 to 125 mg three times a day, the dosage being adjusted at seven- to ten-day intervals as needed and tolerated.

Note: For seriously ill or debilitated patients, or patients with impaired hepatic function, the total dose is often reduced.

**Usual pediatric dose**
Anticonvulsant—
  Initial: Oral, 5 mg per kg of body weight a day, divided into two or three doses, the dosage being adjusted as needed and tolerated.
  Maintenance: Oral, 4 to 8 mg per kg of body weight or 250 mg per square meter of body surface area a day, divided into two or three doses.

**Usual geriatric dose**
Anticonvulsant—
  Oral, initially 3 mg per kg of body weight a day, in divided doses, the dosage being adjusted according to serum hydantoin concentrations and the patient's response.

**Strength(s) usually available**
U.S.—
  50 mg (Rx) [*Dilantin Infatabs* (saccharin; sucrose)].
Canada—
  50 mg (Rx) [*Dilantin Infatabs*].

Note: One 100-mg capsule of phenytoin sodium contains 92% phenytoin and is therefore not equivalent to two 50-mg phenytoin chewable tablets containing 100% phenytoin.

**Packaging and storage**
Store below 40 °C (104 °F), preferably between 15 and 30 °C (59 and 86 °F), unless otherwise specified by manufacturer. Store in a well-closed container.

**Auxiliary labeling**
• May be chewed or crushed.
• Avoid alcoholic beverages.

### EXTENDED PHENYTOIN SODIUM CAPSULES USP

Note: Only phenytoin sodium capsules labeled "Extended" are to be used for once-a-day dosage. Once-a-day use of capsules labeled "Prompt" may result in toxic serum phenytoin concentrations.

**Usual adult and adolescent dose**
Anticonvulsant—
  Oral, initially 100 mg three times a day, the dosage being adjusted at seven- to ten-day intervals as needed and tolerated. When established, the daily maintenance dosage may be given on a once-a-day basis in accordance with patient tolerance.

Note: An oral loading dose of 1 gram may be given, the dose being divided as follows: Initially 400 mg, then 300 mg after two hours, followed by an additional 300 mg in two hours; normal maintenance dosing is started twenty-four hours after the loading dose. Alternatively, some clinicians recommend an oral loading dose of 20 mg per kg of body weight, divided into three to four doses and administered at two-hour intervals.

Patients with a history of renal or liver disease should not receive a loading dose. Use of this regimen should be limited to patients in a clinic or hospital setting where phenytoin serum concentrations can be closely monitored.

Once-a-day dosage should be considered only for adult patients whose condition has been stabilized by divided doses of extended phenytoin sodium capsules given as 100 mg three times a day. This single 300-mg daily dosage has the advantage of convenience and improved compliance.

For seriously ill patients or for debilitated patients or patients with impaired hepatic function, the total dose is often reduced.

[Antineuralgic][1]—
  Oral, 200 to 600 mg a day, in divided doses, the dose being adjusted as needed and tolerated.
[Skeletal muscle relaxant][1]—
  Oral, up to 300 to 600 mg a day, as needed and tolerated.

**Usual pediatric dose**
Anticonvulsant—
  Initial: Oral, 5 mg per kg of body weight a day, divided into two or three doses, the dosage then being adjusted as needed and tolerated.
  Maintenance: Oral, 4 to 8 mg per kg of body weight or 250 mg per square meter of body surface area a day, divided into two or three doses.

**Usual geriatric dose**
Anticonvulsant—
  Oral, initially 3 mg per kg of body weight a day, in divided doses, the dosage being adjusted according to serum hydantoin concentrations and the patient's response.

Note: For geriatric patients, the total dose is often reduced.

**Strength(s) usually available**
U.S.—
  30 mg (Rx) [*Dilantin Kapseals* (lactose; sucrose); GENERIC].
  100 mg (Rx) [*Dilantin Kapseals* (lactose; sucrose); *Phenytex*; GENERIC].
Canada—
  30 mg (Rx) [*Dilantin* (lactose)].
  100 mg (Rx) [*Dilantin* (lactose)].

Note: One 100-mg capsule of phenytoin sodium contains 92% phenytoin and is therefore not equivalent to two 50-mg phenytoin chewable tablets containing 100% phenytoin.

**Packaging and storage**
Store below 40 °C (104 °F), preferably between 15 and 30 °C (59 and 86 °F), unless otherwise specified by manufacturer. Store in a tight container.

**Auxiliary labeling**
• Avoid alcoholic beverages.

**Additional information**
The sodium content of phenytoin sodium is 0.35 mEq (8 mg) per 100-mg capsule.

### PROMPT PHENYTOIN SODIUM CAPSULES USP

Note: Phenytoin sodium capsules labeled "Prompt" are not intended for once-a-day dosage because the phenytoin may be too promptly bioavailable and may cause toxic serum concentrations of phenytoin.

**Usual adult and adolescent dose**
Anticonvulsant—
  Oral, 100 mg three times a day, the dosage being adjusted at seven- to ten-day intervals as needed and tolerated.
Note: For seriously ill patients, debilitated patients, or patients with impaired hepatic function, the total dose is often reduced.

**Usual pediatric dose**
Anticonvulsant—
  Initial: Oral, 5 mg per kg of body weight a day, divided into two or three doses, the dosage then being adjusted as needed and tolerated.
  Maintenance: Oral, 4 to 8 mg per kg of body weight or 250 mg per square meter of body surface area a day, divided into two or three doses in accordance with patient tolerance.

**Usual geriatric dose**
Anticonvulsant—
  Oral, initially 3 mg per kg of body weight a day, in divided doses, the dosage being adjusted according to serum hydantoin concentrations and the patient's response.
Note: For geriatric patients, the total dose is often reduced.

**Strength(s) usually available**
U.S.—
  30 mg (Rx) [GENERIC].
  100 mg (Rx) [GENERIC].
Canada—
  Not commercially available.
Note: One 100-mg capsule of phenytoin sodium contains 92% phenytoin and is therefore not equivalent to two 50-mg phenytoin chewable tablets containing 100% phenytoin.

**Packaging and storage**
Store below 40 °C (104 °F), preferably between 15 and 30 °C (59 and 86 °F), unless otherwise specified by manufacturer. Store in a tight container.

**Auxiliary labeling**
• Avoid alcoholic beverages.

**Additional information**
The sodium content of phenytoin sodium is 0.35 mEq (8 mg) per 100-mg capsule.

## Parenteral Dosage Forms

Note: Bracketed uses in the *Dosage Forms* section refer to categories of use and/or indictions that are not included in U.S. product labeling.

### PHENYTOIN SODIUM INJECTION USP

**Usual adult and adolescent dose**
Anticonvulsant in status epilepticus—
  Initial:
    Intravenous, direct, 15 to 20 mg per kg of body weight, administered at a rate not to exceed 50 mg a minute.
    Note: For obese patients, the loading dose should be calculated on the basis of ideal body weight plus 1.33 times the excess weight over ideal weight, since phenytoin preferentially distributes into fat.
  Maintenance:
    Intravenous, direct, 100 mg every six to eight hours, at a rate not to exceed 50 mg a minute.
    Note: Maintenance therapy, intravenously, 100 mg every six to eight hours, or orally, 5 mg per kg of body weight a day, divided into two to four doses, should begin about twelve to twenty-four hours after a loading dose is given.

[Antiarrhythmic][1]—
  Intravenous, direct, 50 to 100 mg every ten to fifteen minutes as needed and tolerated to stop arrhythmia, but not to exceed a total dose of 15 mg per kg of body weight, administered slowly at a rate no greater than 50 mg a minute.
Note: For geriatric or seriously ill patients or for debilitated patients or patients with impaired hepatic function, the total dose is often reduced and the rate of intravenous administration slowed to 25 mg a minute, possibly as low as 5 to 10 mg a minute, to lessen the possibility of side effects.
  During intravenous infusion of phenytoin, continuous monitoring of the patient's electrocardiogram (ECG), blood pressure, and respiration is essential.
  Although the manufacturers recommend that phenytoin not be added to intravenous infusions, some clinicians routinely use such infusions. If phenytoin is administered by infusion, the rate of administration should not exceed 50 mg per minute; some investigators have suggested rates of 20 to 40 mg per minute.

**Usual pediatric dose**
Anticonvulsant in status epilepticus—
  Intravenous, direct, 15 to 20 mg per kg of body weight, or 250 mg per square meter of body surface area, administered at a rate of 1mg per kg of body weight per minute, not to exceed 50 mg a minute.

**Usual geriatric dose**
See *Usual adult and adolescent dose*.

**Strength(s) usually available**
U.S.—
  50 mg per mL (Rx) [*Dilantin* (alcohol 10%); GENERIC].
Canada—
  50 mg per mL (Rx) [*Dilantin* (alcohol 10%); GENERIC].

**Packaging and storage**
Store between 15 and 30 °C (59 and 86 °F). Protect from freezing.

**Stability**
A slight yellowing of the solution will not affect its potency. After being refrigerated, solution may form a precipitate that usually dissolves after being warmed to room temperature; however, do not use if the solution is not clear.

**Incompatibilities**
The manufacturers recommend that parenteral phenytoin sodium not be added to intravenous infusions or mixed with other medication because precipitation of phenytoin may occur. However, some clinicians routinely use infusion solutions of phenytoin in 0.9% sodium chloride in concentrations of 1 to 10 mg of phenytoin per mL, provided the infusion is started immediately after preparation and is completed within 1 hour; the admixture must be carefully observed for signs of precipitation, and use of a 0.45- to 0.22-micron in-line filter is recommended; in addition, flushing of all tubing with 0.9% sodium chloride injection before and after infusion of phenytoin is recommended.

**Additional information**
The sodium content of phenytoin sodium injection is approximately 0.2 mEq (4.5 mg) per mL.

---

[1] Not included in Canadian product labeling.

## Selected Bibliography

Levy RH, Mattson RH, Meldrum BS, editors. Antiepileptic drugs. 4th ed. New York: Raven Press; 1995. p. 45-6, 64-77, 315-57, 711, 813-4.
Boucher BA. Fosphenytoin: a novel phenytoin prodrug. Pharmacotherapy 1996; 16(5): 777-91.

Revised: 08/12/97

---

**ANTICONVULSANTS, SUCCINAMIDE**—The *Anticonvulsants, Succinamide (Systemic)* monograph is not included in this published version of the USP DI database. Copies of the monograph are available on request from Micromedex, Inc. - Reprint Requests, 6200 S. Syracuse Way, Suite 300, Englewood, CO 80111; telephone (303) 486-6400; telefax (303) 486-6464; Email: USPDI@MDX.COM.

# ANTIDEPRESSANTS, MONOAMINE OXIDASE (MAO) INHIBITOR Systemic

This monograph includes information on the following: 1) Phenelzine; 2) Tranylcypromine.

VA CLASSIFICATION (Primary/Secondary): CN602/CN900

Commonly used brand name(s): *Nardil*[1]; *Parnate*[2].

Note: This monograph does not cover other MAO inhibitors, such as furazolidone and procarbazine, which are not used as antidepressants, and selegiline, which has its own monograph.

Note: For a listing of dosage forms and brand names by country availability, see *Dosage Forms* section(s).

## Category

Antidepressant; antipanic agent; headache (vascular; tension) prophylactic.

## Indications

Note: Bracketed information in the *Indications* section refers to uses that are not included in U.S. product labeling.

### Accepted

Depression, mental (treatment)—Phenelzine is effective in the treatment of patients with major depression with or without melancholia, or with atypical, nonendogenous depression, or depressive neurosis. These patients often have mixed anxiety and depression with phobic or hypochondriacal features. Phenelzine is more often used as a second-line antidepressant in patients who have failed to respond to other antidepressants. Nevertheless, many clinicians may consider phenelzine the first choice for treatment of certain dysphorias and minor periodic or chronic depressions (dysthymic disorders).

Tranylcypromine is indicated for treatment of major depression [with or] without melancholia in closely supervised adult patients not responding to or unable to tolerate other antidepressants. [It is also used to treat the depressed phase of bipolar disorder and depressive neurosis of moderate to severe intensity.]

[Panic disorder (treatment)][1]—Phenelzine and, to a lesser extent, tranylcypromine are used in conjunction with psychotherapy and behavioral therapy in the treatment of panic disorder, with or without agoraphobia.

[Headache, vascular (prophylaxis)][1] or

[Headache, tension (prophylaxis)][1]—Monoamine oxidase inhibitors are used in the prophylaxis of vascular headaches (including migraine), tension-type headaches, and mixed headache syndrome. However, due to potentially severe side effects, these agents are not considered first-line therapy.

[1]Not included in Canadian product labeling.

## Pharmacology/Pharmacokinetics

### Physicochemical characteristics

Molecular weight—
  Phenelzine sulfate: 234.27.
  Tranylcypromine sulfate: 364.46.

### Mechanism of action/Effect

The exact mechanism of antidepressant effect is unknown; however, it is established that the activity of the enzyme monoamine oxidase (MAO) is inhibited. MAO subtypes A and B are involved in the metabolism of serotonin and catecholamine neurotransmitters such as epinephrine, norepinephrine, and dopamine. Phenelzine and tranylcypromine, as nonselective MAO inhibitors, bind irreversibly to monoamine oxidase–A (MAO-A) and monoamine oxidase–B (MAO-B). The reduced MAO activity results in an increased concentration of these neurotransmitters in storage sites throughout the central nervous system (CNS) and sympathetic nervous system. This increased availability of one or more monoamines has been thought to be the basis for the antidepressant activity of MAO inhibitors. The effects of the nonselective MAO inhibitors phenelzine and tranylcypromine lead to downregulation (desensitization) of alpha$_2$- or beta-adrenergic and serotonin receptors. It is thought that changes in receptor characteristics produced by chronic administration of MAO inhibitors correlate better with antidepressant action than does the increased activity of the neuron secondary to increased neurotransmitter concentrations, and may also account for the delay of 2 to 4 weeks in therapeutic response.

### Other actions/effects

MAO inhibitors exhibit a hypotensive effect, which varies with the specific agent; the hypotensive mechanism of action is probably mediated through central inhibition of vasomotor centers, or it may be due to chronic accumulation of the false neurotransmitter octopamine in adrenergic terminals.

MAO inhibitors prevent the inactivation of tyramine by hepatic and gastrointestinal monoamine oxidase. Circulating tyramine releases norepinephrine from the sympathetic nerve terminals and produces a sudden increase in blood pressure.

### Absorption

Well absorbed from the gastrointestinal tract.

### Biotransformation

Hepatic; rapid; by oxidation; possible active metabolites.

### Onset of action

As early as 7 to 10 days with appropriate dosage in some patients, but may take up to 4 to 8 weeks to achieve full therapeutic effect.

### Time to peak plasma concentration

Phenelzine—2 to 4 hours after oral dose.
Tranylcypromine—1 to 3.5 hours.

### Duration of action

At least 10 days for MAO activity to be recovered because of irreversible binding.

### Elimination

Renal, as metabolites.

## Precautions to Consider

### Tumorigenicity

Phenelzine, like other hydrazine derivatives, has been reported in an uncontrolled lifetime study to induce pulmonary and vascular tumors in mice.

### Pregnancy/Reproduction

Pregnancy—Tranylcypromine (and probably phenelzine) crosses the placenta. A limited study in humans reported an increased risk of fetal malformations when these medications were administered in the first trimester.

Animal studies have shown that MAO inhibitors, in doses much higher than the maximum recommended human dose (MRHD), cause hyperexcitability and a reduced rate of growth in the neonate.

For phenelzine: FDA Pregnancy Category C.

For tranylcypromine: FDA pregnancy category not currently included in product labeling.

### Breast-feeding

Tranylcypromine is distributed into human breast milk; it is not known whether phenelzine is distributed into human breast milk. Problems in humans have not been documented.

### Pediatrics

Appropriate studies on the relationship of age to the effects of MAO inhibitors have not been performed in children younger than 16 years of age. Safety and efficacy have not been established. Animal studies have shown that these medications may cause growth retardation in the young.

### Geriatrics

Experience with the use of MAO inhibitors in the elderly is relatively limited. However, there have been reports that phenelzine is safe and effective in the treatment of elderly depressed patients with a history of atypical depression or depressive neurosis. MAO inhibitors may also be useful for anergic or apathetic retarded depressions. The potential for increased vascular accidents (especially in the event of sudden hypertensive episodes), increased sensitivity to hypotensive effects, and reduced metabolic capacity discourages the first-time use of MAO inhibitors in patients over 60 years of age. When an MAO inhibitor is prescribed for an elderly patient, the patient's history of depression, ability to comply with prescribing instructions, and any potential drug interactions must also be considered.

### Drug interactions and/or related problems

The following drug interactions and/or related problems have been selected on the basis of their potential clinical significance (possible mechanism in parentheses where appropriate)—not necessarily inclusive (» = major clinical significance):

Note: Combinations containing any of the following medications, depending on the amount present, may also interact with this medication.

» Alcohol or
» CNS depression–producing medications, other, (see *Appendix II*)
  (concurrent use with MAO inhibitors may increase CNS depressant effects)
  (also, possible tyramine content in some alcoholic beverages, especially beer, wine, or ale, may induce hypertensive reactions)
  (in addition to additive CNS depressant effects caused by some antihypertensives such as clonidine, guanabenz, methyldopa, metyrosine, and pargyline, postural hypotension may be aggravated)
» Anesthetics, local, with epinephrine or levonordefrin or
» Cocaine
  (concurrent use with MAO inhibitors may cause severe hypertension due to sympathomimetic effects)
  (cocaine should not be administered during or within 14 days following administration of an MAO inhibitor; phenelzine also inhibits cholinesterase activity and may reduce or slow cocaine metabolism, thereby increasing the risk of cocaine toxicity)

Anesthetics, spinal
  (use of MAO inhibitors in patients receiving local anesthetics via subarachnoid block may increase the risk of hypotension; discontinuation of MAO inhibitors 10 days before elective surgery may be advisable; however, to avoid interruption of antidepressant therapy, patients receiving long-term MAO inhibition may undergo surgery without discontinuation of the MAO inhibitor; dosages of the anesthetic must be adjusted carefully)

Anticholinergics or other medications with anticholinergic activity (see *Appendix II*) or
Antidyskinetic agents or
Antihistamines
  (concurrent use with MAO inhibitors may intensify the anticholinergic effects of these medications because of secondary anticholinergic activities of MAO inhibitors)
  (also, concurrent use with MAO inhibitors may block detoxification of anticholinergics, thus potentiating their action; patients should be advised to report occurrence of gastrointestinal problems promptly since paralytic ileus may occur with concurrent therapy)
  (concurrent use with MAO inhibitors may also prolong and intensify the CNS depressant and anticholinergic effects of antihistamines; concurrent use is not recommended)

Anticoagulants, coumarin- or indandione-derivative
  (concurrent use may increase anticoagulant activity; although the mechanism of action and clinical significance are unknown, caution is recommended)

Anticonvulsants
  (in addition to increasing CNS depressant effects, concurrent use with MAO inhibitors may cause a change in the pattern of epileptiform seizures; dosage adjustment of anticonvulsant may be necessary)

» Antidepressants, tricyclic or
» Fluoxetine or
» Paroxetine or
» Sertraline or
» Trazodone
  (a potentially lethal hyperserotonergic state known as the serotonin syndrome may occur as the result of combining serotonergic agents [such as amitriptyline, clomipramine, doxepin, or imipramine; fluoxetine, paroxetine, or sertraline; or trazodone] with MAO inhibitors. The syndrome may be manifested by mental status changes [confusion, hypomania], restlessness, myoclonus, hyperreflexia, diaphoresis, shivering, tremor, diarrhea, incoordination, and/or fever. If recognized early, the syndrome usually resolves quickly upon withdrawal of the offending agents)
  (in addition to increased anticholinergic effects, concurrent use of tricyclic antidepressants with MAO inhibitors has resulted in an increased risk of hyperpyretic episodes, hypertensive crises, severe convulsions, and death; however, recent studies have shown that some tricyclic antidepressants can be used concurrently with MAO inhibitors for refractory depression with no adverse effects if both medications are initiated simultaneously at lower than usual doses and the doses raised gradually, or if the MAO inhibitor is gradually added to the tricyclic, also at low doses; tricyclics should not be added to an established MAO inhibitor regimen; clomipramine, desipramine, imipramine, nortriptyline, and protriptyline are not recommended for use in such a regimen; careful monitoring for side effects of either medication is necessary)
  (concurrent use of fluoxetine with MAO inhibitors may result in confusion, agitation, restlessness, and gastrointestinal symptoms, or possibly hyperpyretic episodes, severe convulsions, and hypertensive crises. Based on experience with tricyclic antidepressants, at least 14 days should elapse between discontinuation of an MAO inhibitor and initiation of fluoxetine. However, because of the long half-lives of fluoxetine and its active metabolite, at least 5 weeks [approximately 5 half-lives of norfluoxetine] should elapse between discontinuation of fluoxetine and initiation of therapy with an MAO inhibitor. Administration of an MAO inhibitor within 5 weeks of discontinuation of fluoxetine may increase the risk of serious events. While a causal relationship to fluoxetine has not been established, death has been reported following the initiation of an MAO inhibitor shortly after fluoxetine administration was stopped)

» Antidiabetic agents, oral or
» Insulin
  (hypoglycemic effects may be enhanced by MAO inhibitors; reduction in dosage of hypoglycemic medication may be necessary during and after concurrent therapy)

Beta-adrenergic blocking agents
  (a few cases of significant bradycardia have been reported in elderly patients receiving a beta-adrenergic blocking agent concurrently with phenelzine; monitoring of pulse rate during concurrent administration has been recommended)

Bromocriptine
  (concurrent use may increase serum prolactin concentrations and interfere with effects of bromocriptine; dosage adjustment of bromocriptine may be necessary)

» Bupropion
  (concurrent use of MAO inhibitors with bupropion may increase the risk of acute bupropion toxicity and is contraindicated; a medication-free interval of at least 2 weeks should elapse between discontinuation of the MAO inhibitor and initiation of bupropion therapy)

» Buspirone
  (concurrent use with MAO inhibitors is not recommended because elevation of blood pressure may occur; at least 10 days should elapse between discontinuation of one medication and initiation of the other)

» Caffeine-containing medications
  (concurrent use of excessive amounts of caffeine, consumed in coffee, tea, cola, chocolate, or "stay awake" products, with MAO inhibitors may produce dangerous cardiac arrhythmias or severe hypertension because of sympathomimetic side effects of caffeine)

» Carbamazepine or
» Cyclobenzaprine or
» Maprotiline or
» Monoamine oxidase (MAO) inhibitors, other, including furazolidone, procarbazine, or selegiline
  (concurrent use with MAO inhibitors has resulted in hyperpyretic crises, hypertensive crises, severe convulsions, and death; a medication-free interval of at least 2 weeks should elapse between discontinuation of one medication and initiation of another; for patients switching from one MAO inhibitor to another, an interval of 2 weeks is recommended)
  (in addition, MAO inhibitors cause a change in the pattern of epileptiform seizures in patients receiving carbamazepine as an anticonvulsant)

» Dextromethorphan
  (concurrent use with MAO inhibitors may cause excitation, hypertension, and hyperpyrexia)

Diuretics
  (concurrent use with MAO inhibitors may result in an increased hypotensive effect)

» Doxapram
  (concurrent use may increase the pressor effects of either doxapram or the MAO inhibitor)

» Guanadrel or
» Guanethidine or
» Rauwolfia alkaloids
  (concurrent use with these agents may result in moderate to severe hypertension due to release of catecholamines; withdrawal of MAO inhibitor at least 1 week prior to initiation of therapy with these agents is recommended)
  (when an MAO inhibitor is added to existing therapy with a rauwolfia alkaloid, serious potentiation of CNS depressant effects may result; however, if a rauwolfia alkaloid is added to an MAO inhibitor regimen, CNS excitation and hypertension may result from release of excessive amounts of accumulated norepinephrine and serotonin)

Haloperidol or
Loxapine or
Molindone or
Phenothiazines or
Pimozide or
Thioxanthenes
   (concurrent use may prolong and intensify the sedative, hypotensive, and anticholinergic effects of either these medications or MAO inhibitors)

» Levodopa
   (concurrent use with MAO inhibitors is not recommended, as the combination may result in sudden moderate to severe hypertensive crisis; it is recommended that MAO inhibitors be discontinued for 2 to 4 weeks prior to initiation of levodopa therapy)

» Meperidine, and possibly other opioid (narcotic) analgesics
   (concurrent use with MAO inhibitors may produce immediate excitation, sweating, rigidity, and severe hypertension; in some patients, hypotension, severe respiratory depression, coma, convulsions, hyperpyrexia, vascular collapse, and death may occur; reactions may be due to accumulation of serotonin resulting from MAO inhibition; avoidance of meperidine use within 2 to 3 weeks following MAO inhibition is recommended; other opioid analgesics such as morphine are not likely to cause such severe reactions and may be used cautiously in reduced dosage in patients receiving MAO inhibitors; however, it is recommended that a small test dose [¼ of the usual dose] or several small incremental test doses over a period of several hours should first be administered to permit observation of any adverse effects; caution is also recommended in the use of alfentanil, fentanyl, or sufentanil as an adjunct to anesthesia if the patient has received an MAO inhibitor within 14 days; although the risk of a significant interaction has been questioned, the use of a small test dose is advised to detect any possible interaction)

» Methyldopa
   (may cause hyperexcitability in patients receiving an MAO inhibitor; also headache, severe hypertension, and hallucinations have been reported with concurrent use)

» Methylphenidate
   (concurrent use with MAO inhibitors may potentiate the CNS stimulant effects of methylphenidate, possibly resulting in a hypertensive crisis; methylphenidate should not be administered during or within 14 days following the administration of MAO inhibitors)

Metrizamide
   (concurrent use with MAO inhibitors may lower the seizure threshold and increase the risk of seizures; MAO inhibitors should be discontinued at least 48 hours before myelography and should not be resumed for at least 24 hours after procedure)

Phenylephrine, nasal or ophthalmic
   (if significant systemic absorption of nasal or ophthalmic phenylephrine occurs, concurrent use with MAO inhibitors may potentiate the pressor effect of phenylephrine; nasal or ophthalmic phenylephrine should not be administered during or within 14 days following the administration of an MAO inhibitor)

Succinylcholine
   (concurrent use with phenelzine may decrease plasma concentrations or activity of pseudocholinesterase, the enzyme that metabolizes succinylcholine, thereby enhancing the neuromuscular blockade of succinylcholine and possibly resulting in prolonged respiratory depression or apnea)

» Sympathomimetics
   (concurrent use with MAO inhibitors may prolong and intensify cardiac stimulant and vasopressor effects [including headache, cardiac arrhythmias, vomiting, sudden and severe hypertensive and hyperpyretic crises] of these medications because of release of catecholamines that accumulate in intraneuronal storage sites during MAO inhibitor therapy; these medications should not be administered during or within 14 days following the administration of an MAO inhibitor)

» Tryptophan
   (concurrent use with MAO inhibitors may cause hyperreflexia, shivering, hyperventilation, hyperthermia, mania or hypomania, and disorientation or confusion; if tryptophan is added to an MAO inhibitor regimen, especially tranylcypromine, it should be started in low dosages and the dose titrated upwards gradually with close monitoring of mental status and blood pressure)

» Tyramine- or other high pressor amine–containing foods and beverages, such as aged cheese; fava or broad bean pods; yeast/protein extracts; smoked or pickled meats, poultry, or fish; fermented sausage (bologna, pepperoni, salami, summer sausage) or other fermented meat; sauerkraut; any overripe fruit; beer; reduced-alcohol and alcohol-free beer and wine; red and white wines; sherry; and liqueurs
   (concurrent use with MAO inhibitors may cause sudden and severe hypertensive reactions; reactions are usually limited to a few hours and easily treated with rapidly acting hypotensive agents [such as labetolol, nifedipine, or if necessary in severe cases refractory to other agents, phentolamine]; severity depends on amount of tyramine ingested, rate of gastric emptying, and length of interval between dose of MAO inhibitor and ingestion of tyramine; when MAO inhibitors are discontinued, dietary restrictions must continue for at least 2 weeks; other tyramine- or high pressor amine–containing foods, such as yogurt, sour cream, cream cheese, cottage cheese, chocolate, and soy sauce, if eaten when fresh and in moderation, are considered unlikely to cause serious problems)

**Medical considerations/Contraindications**
The medical considerations/contraindications included have been selected on the basis of their potential clinical significance (reasons given in parentheses where appropriate)—not necessarily inclusive (» = major clinical significance).

*Except under special circumstances, this medication should not be used when the following medical problems exist:*
» Alcoholism, active
» Congestive heart failure
» Hepatic function impairment, severe
   (hepatic precoma may be precipitated in patients with cirrhosis, who are extremely sensitive to effects of MAO inhibitors)
» Pheochromocytoma
   (pressor substances secreted by such tumors may alter blood pressure during therapy with MAO inhibitors)
» Renal function impairment, severe
   (cumulative effects of MAO inhibitors may occur because of reduced renal excretion)
Sensitivity to any MAO inhibitor, including furazolidone, procarbazine, or selegiline

*Risk-benefit should be considered when the following medical problems exist:*
Asthma or bronchitis
   (medications used in the treatment of these conditions may interact with MAO inhibitors)
Bipolar disorder
   (switch from depressive to manic phase may occur)
» Cardiac arrhythmias
» Cardiovascular disease or coronary insufficiency or
Cerebrovascular disease
   (ischemia may be aggravated as a result of reduced blood pressure; however, in patients with serious heart block or a conduction disturbance, an MAO inhibitor may be preferred to a tricyclic antidepressant because of significant slowing of resting pulse [heart rate] or shortening of the PR and QT intervals, and a significant decrease in blood pressure)
Diabetes mellitus
   (insulin or oral hypoglycemic requirements may be altered)
Epilepsy
   (pattern of epileptiform seizures may be changed)
» Headaches, severe or frequent
   (headache as a first sign of hypertensive reaction during therapy may be masked)
» Hepatic function impairment
   (hepatic precoma may be precipitated in patients with cirrhosis, who are extremely sensitive to effects of MAO inhibitors)
» Hypertension
   (use of MAO inhibitors is not recommended in patients on multiple-drug therapy since hypotensive effects may be potentiated; hypertensive crises resulting from dietary lapses may be more severe in hypertensive patients)
Hyperthyroidism
   (sensitivity to pressor amines may be increased)
Parkinson's disease
   (may be aggravated)
» Renal function impairment
   (cumulative effects may occur)
» Schizophrenia
   (MAO inhibitors may aggravate psychosis and/or cause excessive stimulation in schizophrenic patients)

» Suicidal tendencies
(patients may continue to exhibit suicidal tendencies because significant improvement may not occur for several weeks after initiation of therapy with MAO inhibitors)

» Caution is required also in patients who have undergone sympathectomy; these patients may be more sensitive to the hypotensive effects of MAO inhibitors.

**Patient monitoring**

The following may be especially important in patient monitoring (other tests may be warranted in some patients, depending on condition; » = major clinical significance):

» Blood pressure measurements
(careful and frequent monitoring is recommended because of the variety of factors that may produce dangerous alterations in pressure during therapy)

Hepatic function determinations
(although rare, drug-induced hepatitis has occurred with MAO inhibitor therapy)

## Side/Adverse Effects

The following side/adverse effects have been selected on the basis of their potential clinical significance (possible signs and symptoms in parentheses where appropriate)—not necessarily inclusive:

**Those indicating need for medical attention**
Incidence more frequent
*Orthostatic hypotension, severe* (dizziness or lightheadedness, especially when getting up from a lying or sitting position)
Note: Falling or fainting may result. *Orthostatic hypotension* occurs in hypertensive as well as normal and hypotensive patients. Reduction in the dosage of MAO inhibitor may be required to bring blood pressure up to pretreatment levels.

Incidence less frequent
*Diarrhea; peripheral edema* (swelling of feet and lower legs); *sympathetic stimulation* (fast or pounding heartbeat; unusual excitement or nervousness)
Note: *Edema* may subside spontaneously within a week. However, if edema persists, electrolytes should be monitored to rule out syndrome of inappropriate antidiuretic hormone secretion (SIADH).

Incidence rare
*Hepatitis* (dark urine; skin rash; yellow eyes or skin); *leukopenia* (fever; sore throat); *parkinsonian syndrome* (slurred speech; staggering gait)
Note: A potentially lethal hyperserotonergic state known as the serotonin syndrome may occur, typically as the result of combining serotonergic agents (such as amitriptyline, clomipramine, doxepin, or imipramine; fluoxetine, paroxetine, or sertraline; or trazodone) with MAO inhibitors. The syndrome may be manifested by mental status changes (confusion, hypomania), restlessness, myoclonus, hyperreflexia, diaphoresis, shivering, tremor, diarrhea, incoordination, and fever. If recognized early, the syndrome usually resolves quickly upon withdrawal of the offending agents.

Symptoms of hypertensive crisis
*Severe chest pain; enlarged pupils; fast or slow heartbeat; severe headache; increased sensitivity of eyes to light; increased sweating, possibly with fever or cold, clammy skin; nausea or vomiting; stiff or sore neck*
Note: Intracranial bleeding (sometimes fatal in outcome) has occurred in association with *hypertensive crisis*.
*Palpitation or frequent headaches* may be prodromal signs of a hypertensive reaction.

**Those indicating need for medical attention only if they continue or are bothersome**
Incidence more frequent
*Anticholinergic effect or syndrome of inappropriate antidiuretic hormone secretion [SIADH]* (decreased urine output); *blurred vision; CNS stimulation* (muscle twitching during sleep; restlessness or agitation; trouble in sleeping)—more likely with tranylcypromine; *decreased sexual ability; drowsiness*—more likely with phenelzine; *mild headache without increase in blood pressure; increased appetite and weight gain, related to carbohydrate craving; increased sweating; orthostatic hypotension, mild* (dizziness or lightheadedness; tiredness and weakness); *shakiness or trembling; weakness*

Note: *Decreased sexual ability* may include anorgasmia in males and females; ejaculatory disorders; and, less commonly, impotence in males.

Incidence less frequent or rare
*Anorexia* (decreased appetite); *chills; constipation; dryness of mouth*

## Overdose

For specific information on the agents used in the management of monoamine oxidase (MAO) inhibitor antidepressant overdose, see:
• *Charcoal, Activated (Oral-Local)* monograph;
• *Dantrolene (Systemic)* monograph; and/or
• *Diazepam* in *Benzodiazepines (Systemic)* monograph.

For more information on the management of overdose or unintentional ingestion, **contact a Poison Control Center** (see *Poison Control Center Listing*).

**Clinical effects of overdose**
The following effects have been selected on the basis of their potential clinical significance (possible signs and symptoms in parentheses where appropriate)—not necessarily inclusive:
*Severe anxiety; confusion; convulsions; cool, clammy skin; severe dizziness; severe drowsiness; fast and irregular pulse; fever; hallucinations; severe headache; high or low blood pressure; hyperactive reflexes; muscle stiffness; respiratory depression or failure* (troubled breathing); *slowed reflexes; sweating; severe trouble in sleeping; unusual irritability*

**Treatment of overdose**
Note: *Symptoms of overdose* may be absent or minimal for nearly 12 hours after ingestion, and develop slowly thereafter, reaching a maximum in 24 to 48 hours. Immediate hospitalization with close monitoring of patient is essential during this period. Death has resulted.

To decrease absorption—
Induction of vomiting or gastric lavage with protected airway followed by instillation of charcoal slurry in early overdose.

To enhance elimination—
In tranylcypromine overdose, acidification of urine to pH of 5.
Hemodialysis may be beneficial but is of unproven value.

Specific treatment—
Treatment of signs and symptoms of CNS stimulation with diazepam, administered intravenously and slowly. Phenothiazines should not be used because of additive hypotensive effects.
Treatment of hypotension and vascular collapse with intravenous fluids and a dilute pressor agent.
Close monitoring of body temperature, and vigorous treatment of hyperpyrexia with antipyretics and a cooling blanket. Maintenance of fluid and electrolyte balance is essential.
Reduction of symptoms of hypermetabolic state (coma, respiratory failure, hyperpyrexia, tachycardia, muscular rigidity, tremor, and hyperreflexia) with intravenous dantrolene sodium at 2.5 mg per kg of body weight (mg/kg) a day in divided doses, with careful monitoring for signs of hepatotoxicity and pleural or pericardial effusions.

Monitoring—
Close monitoring of body temperature.

Supportive care—
Support of respiration by management of the airway, and mechanical ventilation with the use of supplemental oxygen, as required.
Patients in whom intentional overdose is known or suspected should be referred for psychiatric consultation.

Note: Pathophysiologic effects of massive overdose may persist for several days; recovery from mild overdose may take 3 to 4 days.

## Patient Consultation

As an aid to patient consultation, refer to *Advice for the Patient, Antidepressants, Monoamine Oxidase (MAO) Inhibitor (Systemic)*.
In providing consultation, consider emphasizing the following selected information (» = major clinical significance):

**Before using this medication**
» Conditions affecting use, especially:
Sensitivity to any MAO inhibitor, including furazolidone or procarbazine
Pregnancy—MAO inhibitors cross placenta; no appropriate human studies done; animal studies have shown hyperexcitability and reduced growth rate in neonates
Breast-feeding—Not known if distributed into human breast milk; animal studies have shown distribution into milk
Use in the elderly—Increased sensitivity to hypotensive effects
Other medications, especially CNS depressants, tricyclic antidepressants, oral antidiabetic agents, insulin, bupropion, buspi-

rone, caffeine in high doses, carbamazepine, cyclobenzaprine, cocaine, maprotiline, dextromethorphan, fluoxetine, paroxetine, or sertraline, trazodone, guanadrel, guanethidine, rauwolfia alkaloids, levodopa, meperidine, methyldopa, methylphenidate, sympathomimetics, tryptophan, or foods and beverages containing tyramine
- Other medical problems, especially alcoholism (active), congestive heart failure, hepatic function impairment, pheochromocytoma, renal function impairment, cardiac arrhythmias, cardiovascular disease, coronary insufficiency, severe or frequent headaches, hypertension, schizophrenia, or suicidal tendencies

## Proper use of this medication
» May require up to 3 or 4 weeks of therapy to obtain signs of improvement; regular visits to physician, especially during first few months of therapy, to check progress of therapy and to check for unwanted effects
» Taking exactly as directed by physician
» Importance of not taking more medication than the amount prescribed
» Proper dosing
 Missed dose: Taking as soon as possible within 2 hours of next dose; going back to regular dosing schedule; not doubling doses
» Proper storage

## Precautions while using this medication
» Avoiding tyramine-containing foods, alcoholic beverages, and large quantities of caffeine-containing beverages, over-the-counter cold and cough medicines, and other medications, unless prescribed; having list of such for reference
» Checking with hospital emergency room or physician if symptoms of hypertensive crisis develop
» Checking with physician before discontinuing medication; gradual reduction may be needed to prevent withdrawal effects
» Dizziness may occur; caution when getting up suddenly from a lying or sitting position
» Drowsiness and blurred vision may occur; caution when driving or doing things requiring alertness or clear vision
» Caution if any kind of surgery, dental treatment, or emergency treatment is required
 Carrying medical identification card
» Patients with angina: Not increasing physical activities without consulting physician
 Diabetic patients: Carefully checking urine or blood sugar; results may be lowered by this medication
» Obeying rules of caution for 14 days after discontinuing medication

### Side/adverse effects
» Signs of potential side effects, especially symptoms of hypertensive crisis, severe orthostatic hypotension, diarrhea, peripheral edema, sympathetic stimulation, hepatitis, leukopenia, or parkinsonian syndrome

## General Dosing Information

This medication is usually used for closely supervised patients who have not responded to other antidepressant therapy.

Patient response to these agents is variable, and patients not responsive to one MAO inhibitor may be treated successfully with another.

Potentially suicidal patients should not have access to large quantities of this medication since depressed patients, particularly those who use alcohol excessively, may continue to exhibit suicidal tendencies until significant improvement occurs.

It has been recommended that therapy with an MAO inhibitor be withdrawn gradually at least 10 to 14 days prior to surgery; however, to avoid interruption of antidepressant therapy, patients receiving long-term MAO inhibition may undergo surgery without discontinuation of the MAO inhibitor. Reduction of opioid (narcotic) analgesic or other premedication dosage to ¼ of the usual dose is recommended, along with careful adjustment of anesthetic dosage. Avoidance of meperidine or cocaine use within 2 to 3 weeks following MAO inhibition is recommended.

Because insomnia or other sleep disturbances may be produced by their psychomotor-stimulating effect, these medications are usually not given in the evening.

After dosage is stopped, the effects of these medications may persist for up to 2 weeks (time required for regeneration of monoamine oxidase). During this period, food and drug contraindications must be observed.

### Diet/Nutrition
Foods and beverages containing tyramine or other high pressor amines, such as aged cheese; fava or broad bean pods; yeast/protein extracts; smoked or pickled meats, poultry, or fish; fermented sausage (bologna, pepperoni, salami, summer sausage) or other fermented meat; sauerkraut; any overripe fruit; beer; reduced-alcohol and alcohol-free beer and wine; red and white wines; sherry; and liqueurs, when used concurrently with MAO inhibitors, may cause sudden and severe hypertensive reactions. The reactions are usually limited to a few hours and are easily treated with rapidly acting hypotensive agents (such as labetalol, nifedipine, or if necessary in severe cases refractory to other agents, phentolamine). The severity depends on the amount of tyramine ingested, rate of gastric emptying, and length of the interval between the dose of MAO inhibitor and ingestion of tyramine. When MAO inhibitors are discontinued, dietary restrictions must continue for at least 2 weeks. Other foods, such as yogurt, sour cream, cream cheese, cottage cheese, chocolate, and soy sauce, if eaten when fresh and in moderation, are considered unlikely to cause serious problems.

### For treatment of hypertensive crisis
Recommended treatment includes:
- Discontinuing MAO inhibitor.
- Lowering blood pressure immediately with intravenous administration of 5 mg of phentolamine, with care being taken to inject slowly, to prevent excessive hypotensive effect. Alternatively, some clinicians prefer to use labetalol (intravenously or orally), reserving phentolamine for severe or non-responding cases.
- Reducing fever by external cooling.

---

## PHENELZINE

## Additional Dosing Information

See also *General Dosing Information*.

The initial dosage should be increased gradually, depending on patient tolerance. Rapid dosage increases can cause early hypotensive effects and may result in patient noncompliance. A more conservative increase usually avoids this. At least 4 weeks at a given dosage may be necessary for some patients to achieve improvement and significant MAO inhibition.

## Oral Dosage Forms

Note: Bracketed uses in the *Dosage Forms* section refer to categories of use and/or indications that are not included in U.S. product labeling.

### PHENELZINE SULFATE TABLETS USP

**Usual adult dose**
Antidepressant—
 Initial: Oral, 1 mg per kg of body weight a day.
 Maintenance: Oral, 45 mg a day.
[Antipanic agent][1]—
 Oral, initially 15 mg every morning for the first four days, the dosage being increased gradually over two weeks as needed and tolerated, up to 15 mg three or four times a day.

**Usual adult prescribing limits**
90 mg per day.

**Usual pediatric dose**
Children younger than 16 years of age—Safety and efficacy have not been established.

**Usual geriatric dose**
Antidepressant—
 Oral, initially 0.8 to 1 mg per kg of body weight a day in divided doses, the dosage being gradually increased as needed and tolerated, up to a maximum of 60 mg a day.

Note: Elderly patients are often started on 15 mg in the morning and require a more gradual titration of dose than other adults, to minimize the adverse effects, especially hypotension.

**Strength(s) usually available**
U.S.—
 15 mg (Rx) [*Nardil* (acacia; calcium carbonate; carnauba wax; corn starch; FD&C Yellow No. 6; gelatin; kaolin; magnesium stearate; mannitol; pharmaceutical glaze; povidone; sucrose; talc; white wax; white wheat flour)].
Canada—
 15 mg (Rx) [*Nardil*].

**Packaging and storage**
Store between 15 and 30 °C (59 and 86 °F). Store in a tight container. Protect from heat and light.

**Auxiliary labeling**
- Avoid alcoholic beverages.
- May cause drowsiness.

**Note**
Depressed patients with suicidal tendencies, particularly those who use alcohol excessively, should not have access to large quantities of MAO inhibitors.

[1]Not included in Canadian product labeling.

---

### TRANYLCYPROMINE

## Summary of Differences
Side/adverse effects: May produce more CNS stimulation than other MAO inhibitors.

## Additional Dosing Information
See also *General Dosing Information*.

Dosage should be individualized. If there are no signs of improvement after up to 2 weeks on the usual effective dosage of 30 mg a day, the dosage may be increased by 10 mg a day at intervals of 1 to 3 weeks, up to a maximum of 60 mg a day.

When electroconvulsive therapy is being administered concurrently, 10 mg twice a day can usually be given during the series, the dose being reduced to 10 mg a day for maintenance therapy.

Gradual withdrawal from tranylcypromine is recommended, to avoid recurrence of original symptoms, which may reappear if medication is withdrawn prematurely.

## Oral Dosage Forms
Note: Bracketed uses in the *Dosage Forms* section refer to categories of use and/or indications that are not included in U.S. product labeling.

### TRANYLCYPROMINE SULFATE TABLETS

**Usual adult dose**
Antidepressant—
  Initial: Oral, 30 mg a day in divided doses. If there are no signs of improvement after two weeks, the dosage may be increased by 10 mg a day at intervals of one to three weeks, up to a maximum of 60 mg a day.
  Maintenance: Oral, 10 to 40 mg a day.

[Antipanic agent][1]—
  Oral, initially 10 mg in the morning for the first four days, the dosage being increased gradually over two weeks as needed and tolerated, up to 20 to 30 mg a day.

**Usual adult prescribing limits**
60 mg per day.

**Usual pediatric dose**
Children younger than 16 years of age—Safety and efficacy have not been established.

**Usual geriatric dose**
Antidepressant—
  Oral, initially 2.5 to 5 mg a day, the dosage being increased gradually in increments of 2.5 to 5 mg every three to four days, up to a maximum of 45 mg a day.

**Strength(s) usually available**
U.S.—
  10 mg (Rx) [*Parnate* (acacia; calcium sulfate; cellulose; ethylcellulose; FD&C Red No. 3; FD&C Yellow No. 6; gelatin; iron oxide; magnesium stearate; starch; sucrose)].
Canada—
  10 mg (Rx) [*Parnate* (gluten; sodium <1 mmol [0.003 mg]; sucrose)].

**Packaging and storage**
Store below 40 °C (104 °F), preferably between 15 and 30 °C (59 and 86 °F), unless otherwise specified by manufacturer. Store in a well-closed, light-resistant container.

**Auxiliary labeling**
- Avoid alcoholic beverages.
- May cause drowsiness.

**Note**
Depressed patients with suicidal tendencies, particularly those who use alcohol excessively, should not have access to large quantities of MAO inhibitors.

[1]Not included in Canadian product labeling.

Revised: 05/23/94
Interim revision: 11/5/96; 08/07/98

---

# ANTIDEPRESSANTS, TRICYCLIC  Systemic

This monograph includes information on the following: 1) Amitriptyline; 2) Amoxapine; 3) Clomipramine; 4) Desipramine; 5) Doxepin; 6) Imipramine; 7) Nortriptyline; 8) Protriptyline; 9) Trimipramine.

VA CLASSIFICATION (Primary/Secondary):
  Amitriptyline—CN601/GU900; CN103; GA309; CN900
  Amoxapine—CN601
  Clomipramine—CN601/CN900; CN103
  Desipramine—CN601/CN103; CN900
  Doxepin—CN601/CN900; DE890; CN103; GA309
  Imipramine—CN601/GU900; CN900; CN103
  Nortriptyline—CN601/CN103; CN900
  Protriptyline—CN601/CN900
  Trimipramine—CN601/GA309; CN103

Commonly used brand name(s): *Anafranil*[3]; *Apo-Amitriptyline*[1]; *Apo-Imipramine*[6]; *Apo-Trimip*[9]; *Asendin*[2]; *Aventyl*[7]; *Elavil*[1]; *Endep*[1]; *Impril*[6]; *Levate*[1]; *Norfranil*[6]; *Norpramin*[4]; *Novo-Doxepin*[5]; *Novo-Tripramine*[9]; *Novopramine*[6]; *Novotriptyn*[1]; *Pamelor*[7]; *Pertofrane*[4]; *Rhotrimine*[9]; *Sinequan*[5]; *Surmontil*[9]; *Tipramine*[6]; *Tofranil*[6]; *Tofranil-PM*[6]; *Triadapin*[5]; *Triptil*[8]; *Vivactil*[8].

Note: For a listing of dosage forms and brand names by country availability, see *Dosage Forms* section(s).

## Category
Note: All of the tricyclic antidepressants have similar pharmacologic actions; however, clinical uses among specific agents may vary because of actual pharmacokinetic differences, availability of specific testing, differences in side effects, and/or availability of clinical-use data.

Antidepressant— Amitriptyline; Amoxapine; Clomipramine; Desipramine; Doxepin; Imipramine; Nortriptyline; Protriptyline; Trimipramine.

Antienuretic—Amitriptyline; Imipramine Hydrochloride.
Antiobsessive-compulsive agent—Clomipramine.
Antipanic agent—Clomipramine; Desipramine; Doxepin; Imipramine; Nortriptyline.
Antineuralgic—Amitriptyline; Clomipramine; Desipramine; Doxepin; Imipramine; Nortriptyline; Trimipramine.
Antiulcer agent—Amitriptyline; Doxepin; Trimipramine.
Antinarcolepsy adjunct—Imipramine; Protriptyline.
Anticataplectic—Clomipramine; Desipramine; Imipramine; Protriptyline.
Antibulimic—Amitriptyline; Clomipramine; Desipramine; Imipramine.
Antipruritic—Doxepin.

## Indications
Note: Bracketed information in the *Indications* section refers to uses that are not included in U.S. product labeling.

### Accepted
Depression, mental (treatment)—Amitriptyline, amoxapine, [clomipramine], desipramine, doxepin, imipramine, nortriptyline, protriptyline, and trimipramine are indicated for the relief of symptoms of major depressive episodes; bipolar disorder, depressed type; dysthymia; and atypical depressions. Some conditions associated with or accompanied by depression that are treated with tricyclic antidepressants include alcoholism, organic disease such as stroke or Parkinson's disease, and agitation or anxiety.

Enuresis (treatment adjunct)—Imipramine hydrochloride, but not pamoate, and [amitriptyline] are indicated as aids in the temporary treatment of nocturnal enuresis in children 6 years of age or older, after possible organic causes have been excluded by appropriate tests.

Obsessive-compulsive disorder (treatment)—Clomipramine is used to relieve symptoms of obsessive-compulsive disorders, independent of concomitant depression.

[Panic disorder (treatment)][1]—Tricyclic antidepressants, especially clomipramine, desipramine, doxepin, imipramine, and nortriptyline are used in conjunction with psychotherapy and behavior therapy to block the recurrence of panic attacks, with or without phobias. Imipramine's antipanic effect does not appear to be correlated with presence of depressive symptoms.

[Pain, neurogenic (treatment)][1]—Tricyclic antidepressants, especially amitriptyline, clomipramine, desipramine, doxepin, imipramine, nortriptyline, and trimipramine are used in patients with normal or depressed mood for the management of chronic, severe pain as in cancer; migraine and chronic, daily muscle-contraction headaches; rheumatic disorders; atypical facial pain; post-herpetic neuralgia; post-traumatic neuropathy; and diabetic or other peripheral neuropathy.

[Attention deficit hyperactivity disorder (treatment)][1]—Desipramine, imipramine, and protriptyline are used to relieve the symptoms of attention deficit hyperactivity disorder in some children over 6 years of age and in young adults. Tricyclic antidepressants may be more useful than stimulants when the patient has become withdrawn and depressed.

[Headache (prophylaxis)][1]—Tricyclic antidepressants are used in the prophylaxis of vascular headache (including migraine) and mixed headache syndrome.

[Ulcer, peptic (treatment)][1]—Although amitriptyline, doxepin, and trimipramine are effective in the treatment of peptic ulcer disease and in relieving nocturnal ulcer pain, their use has been largely supplanted by histamine $H_2$-receptor antagonists, omeprazole, and sucralfate.

[Narcolepsy/cataplexy syndrome (treatment)][1] or
[Narcolepsy/cataplexy syndrome (treatment adjunct)][1]—Tricyclic antidepressants, especially clomipramine, desipramine, imipramine, and protriptyline, are used to treat cataplexy associated with narcolepsy, with little or no effect on narcoleptic sleep attacks. Imipramine may be used in combination with amphetamines or methylphenidate when a patient requires treatment for both cataplexy and sleep attacks. Patients with sleep disorders such as hypersomnia or impaired morning arousal may benefit by the use of protriptyline.

[Bulimia nervosa (treatment)][1]—Amitriptyline, clomipramine, desipramine, and imipramine have been shown to be effective in controlling the binge eating and subsequent purging of bulimia nervosa.

[Cocaine withdrawal (treatment)][1]—Desipramine and imipramine are used to reduce craving and/or prevent depression upon withdrawal of cocaine.

[Urinary incontinence (treatment)][1]—Imipramine is used for the treatment of stress and urge incontinence.

[Pruritus (treatment)][1]—Doxepin is used in treatment of pruritus in idiopathic cold urticaria.

[1]Not included in Canadian product labeling.

## Pharmacology/Pharmacokinetics
See *Table 1*, page 283.
**Physicochemical characteristics**
Molecular weight—
  Amitriptyline hydrochloride: 313.87.
  Amoxapine: 313.79.
  Clomipramine hydrochloride: 351.32.
  Desipramine hydrochloride: 302.85.
  Doxepin hydrochloride: 315.84.
  Imipramine hydrochloride: 316.87.
  Imipramine pamoate: 949.2.
  Nortriptyline hydrochloride: 299.84.
  Protriptyline hydrochloride: 299.84.
  Trimipramine maleate: 410.51.
pKa—
  Amitriptyline: 9.4.
  Amoxapine: 7.6.
  Clomipramine: 9.5.
  Desipramine: 1.5 and 10.2.
  Doxepin: 9.0.
  Imipramine: 9.5.
  Nortriptyline: 9.7.
  Trimipramine: 8.0.

## Mechanism of action/Effect
Antidepressant—
  Although the exact mechanism of action in the treatment of depression is unclear, tricyclic antidepressants have been thought to increase the synaptic concentration of norepinephrine (levarterenol; NE) and/or serotonin (5-hydroxytryptamine; 5-HT) in the central nervous system (CNS). One theory suggests that these neurotransmitters are increased through inhibition of their reuptake by the presynaptic neuronal membrane.

  Amoxapine, desipramine, trimipramine, nortriptyline, and probably protriptyline mainly inhibit the reuptake of norepinephrine. Amitriptyline and clomipramine appear to be more potent than other tricyclics in blocking serotonin, although, through their metabolites, they become powerful inhibitors of norepinephrine reuptake also. Clomipramine's effectiveness in the treatment of obsessive-compulsive disorder may be related to the inhibition of serotonin reuptake. Imipramine inhibits reuptake of norepinephrine and serotonin equally. Doxepin is a moderate inhibitor of norepinephrine and a weak inhibitor of serotonin.

  Recent research has shown that after long-term treatment with antidepressants, changes in postsynaptic beta-adrenergic receptor sensitivity and increased responsiveness of the adrenergic and serotonergic systems to physiologic and environmental stimuli contribute to the mechanism of action. Antidepressants may produce a downregulation (desensitization) of alpha$_2$- or beta-adrenergic and serotonin receptors, equilibrating the noradrenergic system, and thus correcting the dysregulated monoamine output of depressed patients. Receptor changes resulting from chronic administration of tricyclic antidepressants appear to correlate better with antidepressant action than does the synaptic reuptake blockade of neurotransmitters, and may also account for the delay of 2 to 4 weeks in therapeutic response.

  Amoxapine, as a metabolite of the neuroleptic, loxapine, also has a potent postsynaptic dopamine-blocking effect. This may account for the extrapyramidal side effects and increases in serum prolactin concentrations seen with amoxapine. Amoxapine is metabolized to 7-hydroxyamoxapine, also a potent dopamine-blocking agent.

Antienuretic—
  The exact antienuretic action of imipramine hydrochloride has not been established. It is thought to be associated with the anticholinergic effects of imipramine.

Antiobsessional agent—
  The exact antiobsessional action of clomipramine has not been established. It is thought to be associated with clomipramine's inhibition of serotonin reuptake and compensatory down regulation of serotonin receptor subtypes.

Antianxiety agent—
  In panic disorders, studies suggest an impaired function of the autonomic nervous system that causes an excessive release of norepinephrine from the locus ceruleus. Tricyclic antidepressants are thought to decrease the firing rate of the locus ceruleus by regulating the alpha$_2$- and beta-adrenergic receptor functions and norepinephrine turnover.

Antineuralgic—
  The exact mechanism by which tricyclic antidepressants relieve chronic pain is also unknown. Some studies support the theory that pain relief results when depression is relieved. However, other studies have found that pain may be ameliorated without a significant change in depression. Analgesic activity may be effected by the changing concentrations of central monoamines, especially serotonin, and by the direct or indirect effect of tricyclic antidepressants on the endogenous opioid systems.

Antiulcer agent—
  In peptic ulcer disease, tricyclic antidepressants are effective in relieving pain and aid in complete healing because of their histamine$_2$-receptor blocking property on the parietal cells, and their sedative and anticholinergic effects.

Antibulimic—
  In bulimia nervosa, the mechanism of action is unclear, although it may be similar to that in depression. Evidence shows there is a distinct antibulimic effect in patients without depression and in depressed patients whose bulimia was relieved without a concomitant relief of depression.

Urinary incontinence—
  The exact mechanism by which imipramine enhances urinary continence has not been established but may include anticholinergic activity, resulting in increased bladder capacity; direct beta-adrenergic stimulation; alpha-adrenergic agonist activity, resulting in increased sphincter tone; and central blockade of serotonin uptake.

## Other actions/effects
Tricyclic antidepressants also produce prominent peripheral and central anticholinergic effects due to their potent and high binding affinity for muscarinic receptors; sedative effects due to strong binding affinity for histamine $H_1$-receptors (although the central actions of histamine are poorly understood, increased cholinoceptive activity in the brain has been associated with clinical depression); and orthostatic hypotension due to alpha blockade. In addition, tricyclic antidepressants are Class 1A antiarrhythmic agents which, like quinidine, moderately slow ven-

tricular conduction in therapeutic doses, and in overdose may cause severe conduction block and occasional ventricular arrhythmia.

**Absorption**
Rapidly and well absorbed after oral administration.

**Protein binding**
Very highly protein bound (90% or more) in plasma and tissues.

**Biotransformation**
Exclusively hepatic, with first-pass effect.

**Onset of action**
Antidepressant—2 to 3 weeks.

**Elimination**
As metabolites, primarily renal, over several days; poorly dialyzable because of high protein binding.

## Precautions to Consider

### Cross-sensitivity and/or related problems
Patients sensitive to one tricyclic antidepressant may be sensitive to other tricyclic antidepressants, and possibly to carbamazepine, maprotiline, and trazodone, also.

### Carcinogenicity/Mutagenicity
Amitriptyline—In one study with rats, no evidence of increase in incidence of any tumor was found. However, amitriptyline has not been adequately studied in animals to permit an evaluation of its carcinogenic potential. No evidence of mutagenicity was found in rats tested with the Ames salmonella test.

Amoxapine—Pancreatic islet cell hyperplasia occurred in rats, with slightly increased incidence at doses 5 to 10 times the human dose.

### Pregnancy/Reproduction
Pregnancy—
*For amitriptyline*—
Adequate and well-controlled studies in pregnant women have not been done.
Animal studies have shown amitriptyline to cause teratogenic effects when used in doses many times the human dose.
FDA Pregnancy Category C.

*For amoxapine*—
Adequate and well-controlled studies in pregnant women have not been done.
Animal studies have shown amoxapine to cause embryotoxic effects in doses approximating the human dose and fetotoxic effects such as intrauterine death, stillbirth, decreased birth weight, and decreased postnatal (0 to 4 days) survival at doses many times the human dose.
FDA Pregnancy Category C.

*For clomipramine, desipramine, and nortriptyline*—
Adequate and well-controlled studies in pregnant women have not been done.
Animal reproduction studies have been inconclusive.
FDA Pregnancy Category C.

*For doxepin*—
Adequate and well-controlled studies in pregnant women have not been done.
Animal studies have shown no evidence of teratogenic effects at doses up to 25 mg per kg of body weight (mg/kg) per day for 8 to 9 months and no changes in litter size, number of live births, or lactation. However, a decreased rate of conception was observed when male rats were given 25 mg/kg per day for prolonged periods.

*For imipramine*—
Adequate and well-controlled studies in pregnant women have not been done. However, there have been clinical reports of congenital malformations associated with the use of imipramine.
Animal reproduction studies have been inconclusive.

*For protriptyline*—
Adequate and well-controlled studies in pregnant women have not been done.
Animal reproduction studies have shown that protriptyline causes no apparent adverse effects at doses 10 times greater than recommended human doses.

*For trimipramine*—
Adequate and well-controlled studies in pregnant women have not been done.
Animal studies have shown trimipramine to cause embryotoxicity and major anomalies at 20 times the human dose.
FDA Pregnancy Category C.

Delivery—For all tricyclic antidepressants: There have been reports of cardiac problems, irritability, respiratory distress, muscle spasms, seizures, and urinary retention in infants whose mothers received tricyclic antidepressants immediately prior to delivery.

### Breast-feeding
Tricyclic antidepressants have been found in small amounts in breast milk in an approximate milk to plasma ratio of 0.4:1.5. Doxepin has been reported to cause sedation and respiratory depression in the nursing infant.

### Pediatrics
Although tricyclic antidepressants are generally not recommended for depression in children under 12 years of age, some, especially amitriptyline, desipramine, imipramine, and nortriptyline, are used in children over the age of 6 years for recognized major depressive illness. However, the effectiveness of tricyclic antidepressants in the treatment of depression in children and adolescents has not been definitively established. Amitriptyline and imipramine are also used for treatment of enuresis in children 6 years of age or older. Clomipramine is used for the treatment of obsessive-compulsive disorder in children 10 years of age or older. Imipramine, desipramine, and protriptyline are being used in the treatment of attention deficit hyperactivity disorder in children over 6 years of age and adolescents. However, deaths have been reported in children treated with desipramine for hyperactivity.

Children are more sensitive than adults to acute overdosage, which should be considered serious and potentially fatal. Increasing the dose in children increases the risk of adverse effects, such as alterations in electrocardiogram (ECG) patterns, nervousness, sleep disorders, tiredness, hypertension in some children, or mild gastrointestinal problems, without necessarily enhancing the therapeutic effect. Adolescent patients may require reduced dosage because they are also prone to exhibit increased dose sensitivity.

### Geriatrics
Elderly patients often require lower dosage and more gradual dose increases to avoid toxicity, because of slower metabolic rates and/or excretion and an increased ratio of fat to lean tissue. The elderly also exhibit increased sensitivity to anticholinergic effects, such as urinary retention (especially in older men with prostatic hypertrophy), anticholinergic delirium, and increased sedative and hypotensive effects. Increased anxiety may result from these adverse effects, possibly leading to unnecessary dose increases. If cardiovascular disease is present, the risk of conduction defects, arrhythmias, tachycardia, stroke, congestive heart failure, or myocardial infarction is increased.

### Dental
The peripheral anticholinergic effects of tricyclic antidepressants may decrease or inhibit salivary flow, especially in middle-aged or elderly patients, thus contributing to the development of caries, periodontal disease, oral candidiasis, and discomfort.

The blood dyscrasia–causing effects of tricyclic antidepressants, although rare, may be life-threatening. The result may be an increased incidence of microbial infection, delayed healing, and gingival bleeding. If agranulocytosis, leukopenia, or thrombocytopenia occurs, dental work should be deferred until blood counts have returned to normal. Patient instruction in proper oral hygiene should include caution in use of regular toothbrushes, dental floss, and toothpicks.

Extrapyramidal reactions that may be induced by amoxapine will result in increased motor activity of the head, face, and neck. Occlusal adjustments, bite registrations, and treatment for bruxism may be made less reliable.

### Drug interactions and/or related problems
The following drug interactions and/or related problems have been selected on the basis of their potential clinical significance (possible mechanism in parentheses where appropriate)—not necessarily inclusive (» = major clinical significance):

Note: Combinations containing any of the following medications, depending on the amount present, may also interact with this medication.

Although not all of the following interactions have been reported for every tricyclic antidepressant, the potential for their occurrence exists and should be considered.

» Alcohol or
» CNS depression–producing medications, other (See *Appendix II*)
(concurrent use with tricyclic antidepressants may result in serious potentiation of CNS depression, respiratory depression, and hypotensive effects; caution is recommended, and dosage of one or both agents should be reduced)

(in addition, tricyclics may increase the effects of alcohol, especially during first few days of tricyclic antidepressant treatment; in patients who use alcohol excessively, tricyclics may increase the danger inherent in any suicide attempt)

Amantadine or
Anticholinergics or other medications with anticholinergic activity (See *Appendix II*) or
Antidyskinetics or
Antihistamines
 (concurrent use with tricyclic antidepressants may intensify anticholinergic effects, especially mental confusion, hallucinations, and nightmares, because of secondary anticholinergic activities of tricyclic antidepressants)
 (concurrent use may potentiate the CNS depressant effects of either antihistamines or tricyclic antidepressants)
 (concurrent use with tricyclic antidepressants may block detoxification of atropine and related compounds; patients should be advised to report occurrence of gastrointestinal problems promptly since paralytic ileus may occur with concurrent therapy)

Anticoagulants, coumarin- or indandione-derivative
 (concurrent use with tricyclic antidepressants, especially amitriptyline or nortriptyline, may increase anticoagulant activity, possibly by inhibiting enzymatic metabolism of the anticoagulant)

Anticonvulsants
 (tricyclic antidepressants may enhance CNS depression, lower the seizure threshold when taken in high doses, and decrease the effects of the anticonvulsant medication; dosage adjustment of the anticonvulsant may be necessary to control seizures; monitoring of serum concentrations of both medications may be necessary to detect possible interaction; concurrent use of phenytoin with desipramine may lower serum concentrations of desipramine; dosage increases of desipramine above maximum recommended doses may be required to produce clinical improvement in depression)

» Antithyroid agents
 (concurrent use with tricyclic antidepressants may increase the risk of agranulocytosis)

Barbiturates or
Carbamazepine
 (plasma concentrations and therapeutic effects of tricyclic antidepressants may be decreased during concurrent use with barbiturates, especially phenobarbital, or carbamazepine because of increased metabolism resulting from induction of hepatic microsomal enzymes)

Bupropion or
Clozapine or
Cyclobenzaprine or
Haloperidol or
Loxapine or
Maprotiline or
Molindone or
» Phenothiazines or
Thioxanthenes
 (the sedative and anticholinergic effects of either these medications or tricyclic antidepressants may be prolonged and intensified; these medications may increase the risk of seizures by lowering the seizure threshold and should be added or withdrawn with caution; psychotic depressions respond well to a combination of tricyclic antidepressant and antipsychotic agent, but both medications must be initially administered at lower doses and are increased only as clinically indicated)
 (concurrent use of phenothiazines may increase serum concentrations of tricyclic antidepressants, especially desipramine and imipramine, due to inhibition of metabolism; conversely, tricyclics may inhibit phenothiazine metabolism; also, the risk of neuroleptic malignant syndrome [NMS] may be increased)

» Cimetidine
 (cimetidine may inhibit tricyclic metabolism and increase plasma concentrations, leading to toxicity; lowering the dose of the tricyclic antidepressant by 20 to 30% may be necessary when cimetidine is given concurrently; patient should be closely observed for sedation, anticholinergic effects, and orthostatic hypotension)

» Clonidine or
» Guanadrel or
» Guanethidine
 (concurrent use may decrease the hypotensive effects of these medications)
 (concurrent use of clonidine with tricyclic antidepressants may result in potentiation of CNS depressant effects)

Cocaine
 (concurrent use with tricyclic antidepressants may increase the risk of cardiac arrhythmias; if use of cocaine is necessary in patients receiving tricyclics, it is recommended that the cocaine be administered with caution, in reduced dosage, and in conjunction with electrocardiographic monitoring)

Contraceptives, oral, estrogen-containing or
Estramustine or
Estrogens
 (concurrent use of imipramine and possibly other tricyclic antidepressants by chronic long-term users of oral contraceptives or estrogens may increase the bioavailability of imipramine because of inhibition of hepatic enzyme metabolism; this may result in toxicity, obscuring therapeutic effects and worsening depression; may be dose-related, with lower doses of estrogens having less effect on enzyme inhibition than larger doses; dosage adjustments of the tricyclic may be necessary)

Corticosteroids, glucocorticoid
 (tricyclic antidepressants do not relieve, and may exacerbate, corticosteroid-induced mental depression)

Disulfiram or
Ethchlorvynol
 (concurrent use with tricyclics, especially amitriptyline, may result in transient delirium)
 (also, CNS depressant effects may be increased when ethchlorvynol is used concurrently with tricyclic antidepressants)

Electroconvulsive therapy
 (although electroconvulsive therapy may be used in conjunction with tricyclic antidepressants, caution should be used as hazards may be increased)

» Extrapyramidal reaction–causing medications, other (See *Appendix II*)
 (concurrent use with amoxapine and possibly other tricyclic antidepressants may increase the severity and frequency of extrapyramidal effects)

Fluoxetine
 (concurrent use with tricyclic antidepressants has produced increased plasma concentrations of the tricyclic antidepressant, possibly due to inhibition of tricyclic antidepressant metabolism; some clinicians recommend dosage reductions for tricyclic antidepressants of about 50% if used concurrently with fluoxetine)

Methylphenidate
 (serum concentrations of tricyclic antidepressants, especially desipramine and imipramine, may be increased due to inhibition of metabolism when methylphenidate is used concurrently; also, concurrent use may antagonize the effects of methylphenidate)

» Metrizamide
 (administration of intrathecal metrizamide may lower the seizure threshold and increase the risk of seizures in patients taking tricyclic antidepressants; it is recommended that tricyclic antidepressants be discontinued for at least 48 hours before and at least 24 hours after myelography)

» Monoamine oxidase (MAO) inhibitors, including furazolidone, procarbazine, and selegiline
 (concurrent use with tricyclic antidepressants has resulted in an increased incidence of hyperpyretic episodes, severe convulsions, hypertensive crises, and death; however, recent studies have shown that concurrent use of some tricyclic antidepressants with MAO inhibitors can be used for refractory depression with no adverse effects if both medications are initiated simultaneously at lower than usual doses, with doses being raised gradually thereafter, or if the MAO inhibitor is gradually added to the tricyclic, also at low doses; a tricyclic should not be added to an existing MAO inhibitor regimen; the tricyclic antidepressants most commonly used in this combined therapy are amitriptyline, doxepin, and trimipramine; imipramine, desipramine, nortriptyline, protriptyline, and clomipramine are not recommended for use in such a regimen because of potential excessive stimulation)

Naphazoline, ophthalmic or
Oxymetazoline, nasal or ophthalmic or
Phenylephrine, nasal or ophthalmic or
Xylometazoline, nasal
 (if significant systemic absorption occurs, concurrent use with tricyclic antidepressants may potentiate pressor effects of these medications)

Pimozide
 (concurrent use with tricyclic antidepressants may potentiate cardiac arrhythmias, which are seen on ECG as prolongation of the QT interval)

Probucol
 (additive QT interval prolongation may increase risk of ventricular tachycardia)

» Sympathomimetics
  (concurrent use with tricyclic antidepressants may potentiate cardiovascular effects possibly resulting in arrhythmias, tachycardia, or severe hypertension or hyperpyrexia; phentolamine can control the adverse reaction)
  (significant systemic absorption of ophthalmic epinephrine may also potentiate cardiovascular effects; also, local anesthetics with vasoconstrictors should be avoided or a minimal amount of the vasoconstrictor should be used with the local anesthetic)
  (concurrent use with tricyclic antidepressants may decrease the pressor effect of ephedrine and mephentermine)

Thyroid hormones
  (concurrent use with tricyclic antidepressants may increase the therapeutic and toxic effects of both medications, possibly due to increased receptor sensitivity to catecholamines; toxic effects include cardiac arrhythmias and CNS stimulation)

**Laboratory value alterations**
The following have been selected on the basis of their potential clinical significance (possible effect in parentheses where appropriate)—not necessarily inclusive (» = major clinical significance):

With diagnostic test results
  ECG
    (changes include prolonged PR intervals, widened QRS complexes, and inverted or flattened T-waves)
  Metyrapone test
    (amitriptyline may decrease the response to metyrapone)

With physiology/laboratory test values
  Blood sugar concentrations
    (may be increased or decreased)

**Medical considerations/Contraindications**
The medical considerations/contraindications included have been selected on the basis of their potential clinical significance (reasons given in parentheses where appropriate)—not necessarily inclusive (» = major clinical significance).

Note: This medication should *not* be used during the acute recovery period following a myocardial infarction.

*Risk-benefit should be considered when the following medical problems exist:*
» Alcoholism, active
    (CNS depression may be potentiated)
» Asthma
    (may be aggravated)
» Bipolar disorder
    (swing to hypomanic or manic phase may be accelerated and reversible rapid cycling between mania and depression may be induced by antidepressants in some patients; tricyclic antidepressant may have to be discontinued and lithium considered for a sustained remission)
» Blood disorders
    (may be potentiated)
» Cardiovascular disorders, especially in children and the elderly
    (increased risk of arrhythmias, heart block, congestive heart failure, myocardial infarction, or stroke)
» Gastrointestinal disorders
    (risk of paralytic ileus)
  Genitourinary disease
    (may be masked by the use of imipramine for enuresis in children)
» Glaucoma, narrow-angle, predisposition to or
» Increased intraocular pressure
    (may be aggravated)
» Hepatic function impairment
    (metabolism of tricyclic may be altered)
» Hyperthyroidism
    (risk of cardiovascular toxicity)
» Prostatic hypertrophy
    (risk of urinary retention)
» Renal function impairment
    (excretion of tricyclic may be altered)
» Schizophrenia
    (psychosis may be activated)
» Seizure disorders
    (seizure threshold may be lowered)
» Sensitivity to tricyclic antidepressants, carbamazepine, maprotiline, or trazodone

» Urinary retention
    (may be aggravated)

**Patient monitoring**
The following may be especially important in patient monitoring (other tests may be warranted in some patients, depending on condition; » = major clinical significance):

Blood cell counts (usually during extended therapy and in patients with sore throat or fever) and
Blood pressure and pulse measurements and
Glaucoma tests and
Hepatic function determinations and
Renal function determinations
  (may be required at periodic intervals during therapy to detect development of adverse effects that may not be evident to the patient)
Cardiac function monitoring
  (ECG may be required in the elderly, in children, and in patients with existing cardiac disease, or in patients receiving antiarrhythmics such as quinidine, procainamide, or disopyramide, before initiation of therapy as a baseline and at periodic intervals thereafter)
  (for children taking imipramine for enuresis who are not responding to standard doses, ECG may be required before dosage is increased)
Careful supervision of depressed patients with suicidal tendencies
  (recommended especially during early weeks of treatment; hospitalization may be required as a protective measure)
Dental examination
  (recommended at least twice yearly)
Plasma tricyclic determinations
  (recommended for patients who fail to respond to treatment, when there are increased side effects, when patient is at high risk, when there is doubt about patient compliance, or as a means of maximizing the response; optimum sampling time is immediately before the first morning dose or a minimum of 8 hours after a dose; See *Table 1* for therapeutic plasma concentration ranges)

*For amoxapine (in addition to the above)*
Careful observation for early signs of tardive dyskinesia
  (recommended at periodic intervals, especially in the elderly; if early symptoms of tardive dyskinesia appear, amoxapine should be discontinued)

## Side/Adverse Effects
Note: Although not all of these side effects have been attributed specifically to each tricyclic antidepressant, a potential exists for their occurrence during the use of any tricyclic antidepressant.

The following side/adverse effects have been selected on the basis of their potential clinical significance (possible signs and symptoms in parentheses where appropriate)—not necessarily inclusive:

**Those indicating need for medical attention**
Incidence less frequent
  *For all tricyclic antidepressants*
    **Anticholinergic effects** (blurred vision; confusion; delirium or hallucinations; constipation, especially in the elderly, possibly resulting in paralytic ileus; difficult urination; eye pain due to aggravation of glaucoma); **fast, slow, or irregular heartbeat; fine-muscle tremors, especially in arms, hands, head, and tongue** (shakiness); **hypotension** (fainting); **nervousness or restlessness; Parkinsonian syndrome** (difficulty in speaking or swallowing; loss of balance control; mask-like face; shuffling walk; slowed movements; stiffness of arms and legs; trembling and shaking of fingers and hands); **sexual function impairment**—more common with amoxapine and clomipramine

  *For amoxapine only (in addition to the above)*
    **Tardive dyskinesia** (lip smacking or puckering; puffing of cheeks; rapid or worm-like movements of tongue; uncontrolled chewing movements; uncontrolled movements of the arms or legs)

Incidence rare
  *For all tricyclic antidepressants*
    **Agranulocytosis or other blood dyscrasias** (red or brownish spots on skin; sore throat and fever; unusual bleeding or bruising); **allergic reaction** (increased sensitivity to sunlight; skin rash and itching; swelling of face and tongue); **alopecia** (hair loss); **anxiety; breast enlargement in both males and females**—more common with amoxapine; **cholestatic jaundice** (yellow eyes or skin); **galactorrhea** (inappropriate secretion of milk)—in females; **seizures**—more common with clomipramine; **syndrome of inappropriate secretion of antidiuretic hormone [SIADH]** (irritability; muscle twitching; weakness); **testicular swelling**—more common with amoxapine; **tinnitus** (ringing, buzzing, or other unexplained noises

**276**  Antidepressants, Tricyclic (Systemic)

in the ears); *trouble with teeth or gums*—more common with clomipramine

For amoxapine only (in addition to the above)
**Neuroleptic malignant syndrome (NMS)** (convulsions; difficult or fast breathing; fast heartbeat or irregular pulse; fever; high or low [irregular] blood pressure; increased sweating; loss of bladder control; severe muscle stiffness; unusually pale skin; unusual tiredness or weakness)

  Note: May occur after prolonged treatment or after combined treatment with *tricyclic antidepressants* and *neuroleptics*.

**Those indicating need for medical attention only if they continue or are bothersome**
Incidence more frequent
  *Drowsiness; dryness of mouth; headache; increased appetite*—may include craving for sweets; *nausea; orthostatic hypotension* (dizziness); *tiredness or weakness, mild; unpleasant taste; weight gain*
Incidence less frequent
  *Diarrhea; excessive sweating; heartburn; trouble in sleeping*—more common with protriptyline, especially when taken late in the day; *vomiting*

**Those indicating possible withdrawal and the need for medical attention if they occur after medication is discontinued**
Occurring upon abrupt withdrawal, due to cholinergic rebound
  For all tricyclic antidepressants
    *Headache; nausea, vomiting, or diarrhea; trouble in sleeping, with vivid dreams; unusual excitement*
Occurring with gradual withdrawal after long-term treatment
  For all tricyclic antidepressants
    *Irritability; restlessness; trouble in sleeping, with vivid dreams*
  For amoxapine only (in addition to the above)
    *Tardive dyskinesia, withdrawal-emergent* (lip smacking or puckering; puffing of cheeks; rapid or worm-like movements of tongue; uncontrolled chewing movements; uncontrolled movements of the arms and legs)

## Overdose
For specific information on the agents used in the management of tricyclic antidepressant overdose, see:
- *Anesthetics, Inhalation (Systemic)* monograph;
- *Charcoal, Activated (Oral-Local)* monograph;
- *Diazepam* in *Benzodiazepines (Systemic)* monograph;
- *Digitalis Glycosides (Systemic)* monograph;
- *Lidocaine (Systemic)* monograph;
- *Paraldehyde (Systemic)* monograph;
- *Phenytoin* in *Anticonvulsants, Hydantoin (Systemic)* monograph;
- *Physostigmine (Systemic)* monograph;
- *Propranolol* in *Beta-adrenergic Blocking Agents (Systemic)* monograph; and/or
- *Sodium Bicarbonate (Systemic)* monograph.

For more information on the management of overdose or unintentional ingestion, **contact a Poison Control Center** (see *Poison Control Center Listing*).

**Clinical effects of overdose**
The following effects have been selected on the basis of their potential clinical significance (possible signs and symptoms in parentheses where appropriate)—not necessarily inclusive:
Acute
  *Confusion; convulsions*—more severe and refractory with amoxapine; *disturbed concentration; drowsiness, severe; enlarged pupils; fast, slow, or irregular heartbeat; fever; hallucinations; restlessness and agitation; shortness of breath or troubled breathing; unusual tiredness or weakness, severe; vomiting*

**Treatment of overdose**
Treatment is essentially symptomatic and supportive, possibly including:
  To decrease absorption—
    Emptying stomach with gastric lavage.
  To enhance elimination—
    Administering activated charcoal slurry repeatedly, followed by a stimulant cathartic.
  Specific treatment—
    Digitalizing cautiously for congestive heart failure.
    Controlling cardiac arrhythmias with lidocaine or by alkalinizing blood to pH 7.4 to 7.5 with intravenous sodium bicarbonate. Arrhythmias refractory to lidocaine and sodium bicarbonate may be managed with slow intravenous infusion of phenytoin while monitoring ECG. Propranolol is also effective but should be used with caution because of its negative inotropic and hypotensive effects. Quinidine and procainamide should be avoided.
    For all tricyclics except amoxapine: Although routine use is not recommended, administering physostigmine salicylate, 1 to 3 mg (adults) by slow intravenous infusion over 2 to 3 minutes, may help reverse severe anticholinergic effects (myoclonic seizures, severe hallucinations, hypertension, and ventricular arrhythmias). For children, start with 0.5 mg and repeat dosage at 5 minute intervals to determine the minimum effective dose, not exceeding 2 mg per dose. Because of the short duration of action of physostigmine, dosage may need to be repeated at 30- to 60-minute intervals, especially if life-threatening symptoms occur. Routine administration of physostigmine is not recommended because of its toxicity. When used in tricyclic antidepressant overdose, it may cause bronchospasm, increased respiratory secretions, muscle weakness, bradycardia, hypotension, and may itself cause seizures. Physostigmine should be reserved for patients in coma with respiratory depression, uncontrollable seizures, severe hypertension, or serious cardiac arrhythmias. Physostigmine is contraindicated in amoxapine overdose because it may increase seizure activity.
    Administering anticonvulsants such as diazepam, paraldehyde, phenytoin, or an inhalation anesthetic to control convulsions. Seizures may be especially severe and refractory with amoxapine overdose and may lead to acute tubular necrosis and rhabdomyolysis.
  Monitoring—
    Monitoring cardiovascular function (ECG) for not less than 5 days.
  Supportive care—
    Maintaining respiratory and cardiac function.
    Maintaining body temperature.
    Using standard measures to manage circulatory shock and metabolic acidosis.
    Patients in whom intentional overdose is known or suspected should be referred for psychiatric consultation.
- Note: Hemodialysis, peritoneal dialysis, exchange transfusions, and forced diuresis of tricyclic antidepressants have not been successful because of their high protein binding and rapid fixation in tissues.

## Patient Consultation
As an aid to patient consultation, refer to *Advice for the Patient, Antidepressants, Tricyclic (Systemic)*.
In providing consultation, consider emphasizing the following selected information (» = major clinical significance):

**Before using this medication**
» Conditions affecting use, especially:
    Sensitivity to tricyclic antidepressants, maprotiline, or trazodone
    Pregnancy—Clinical reports of fetal malformations with imipramine; animal studies have shown some tricyclics to cause embryotoxic or fetotoxic effects, and decreased rate of conception; when tricyclics taken by mother immediately before delivery, clinical reports of newborns suffering from muscle spasms, and heart, breathing, and urinary problems
    Breast-feeding—Pass into breast milk and may cause drowsiness in nursing baby
    Use in children—Children and adolescents more sensitive to effects, requiring lower doses; may cause nervousness, sleeping problems, tiredness, mild stomach upset; generally not recommended for depression in children
    Use in the elderly—Elderly more sensitive to effects; lower doses and more gradual increases required
    Dental—Decreased salivary flow contributes to caries, periodontal disease, candidiasis, and discomfort; blood dyscrasias may cause increased infections, delayed healing, and gingival bleeding; increased extrapyramidal motor activity of head, face, and neck with amoxapine may cause difficulty with occlusal and other procedures
    Other medications, especially CNS depressants, antithyroid agents, cimetidine, clonidine, guanadrel, guanethidine, phenothiazines, extrapyramidal reaction–causing medications, MAO inhibitors, metrizamide, or sympathomimetics
    Other medical problems, especially alcoholism (active), asthma, bipolar disorder, blood disorders, cardiovascular disorders, gastrointestinal disorders, glaucoma or increased intraocular pressure, hepatic function impairment, hyperthyroidism, prostatic hypertrophy, renal function impairment, schizophrenia, seizure disorders, or urinary retention

**Proper use of this medication**
Taking with food to reduce gastrointestinal irritation
» Compliance with therapy; not taking more or less medicine than prescribed
» May require from 1 to 6 weeks of therapy to obtain antidepressant effects

*Proper administration of doxepin oral solution*
Using dropper provided by manufacturer for accurate measurement
Diluting medication in one-half glass of recommended beverage (water, milk, or fruit juice, but not grape juice or carbonated beverages) immediately before use
Not preparing or storing bulk solutions
» Proper dosing
Missed dose: If dosing schedule is—
More than one dose a day: Taking as soon as possible unless almost time for next dose; not doubling doses
One dose at bedtime: Not taking in morning because of side effects; checking with physician
» Proper storage

**Precautions while using this medication**
Regular visits to physician to check progress of therapy
» Avoiding the use of alcoholic beverages; not taking other medication unless prescribed by physician
» Possible drowsiness; caution when driving or doing things requiring alertness
» Possible dizziness or lightheadedness; caution when getting up suddenly from a lying or sitting position
» Possible dryness of mouth; using sugarless gum or candy, ice, or saliva substitute for relief; checking with physician or dentist if dry mouth continues for more than 2 weeks
» Possible skin photosensitivity; avoiding unprotected exposure to sun; using protective clothing; using a sun block product that includes protection against both UVA-caused photosensitivity reactions and UVB-caused sunburn reactions; avoiding use of sunlamp, tanning bed, or tanning booth
Caution if any laboratory tests required; possible interference with results of metyrapone test.
» Caution if any kind of surgery, dental treatment, or emergency treatment is required
» Checking with physician before discontinuing medicine; gradual dosage reduction may be needed to avoid worsening of condition or withdrawal symptoms
» Observing precautions for 3 to 7 days after stopping medication
*For protriptyline*
Possibility of sleep interference if taken late in the day

**Side/adverse effects**
Signs of potential side effects, especially anticholinergic effects; hypotension; fast, slow, or irregular heartbeat; Parkinsonian syndrome; nervousness or restlessness; sexual function impairment; shakiness or tremors; neuroleptic malignant syndrome (NMS) or tardive dyskinesia (with amoxapine only); anxiety; breast enlargement in males and females; galactorrhea; testicular swelling; alopecia; allergic reactions; blood dyscrasias; cholestatic jaundice; seizures; SIADH; tinnitus; or trouble with teeth or gums

# General Dosing Information

Dosage of tricyclic antidepressants must be individualized for each patient by titration.

Plasma concentrations of tricyclic antidepressants, in general, vary greatly among patients. However, nortriptyline appears to have a well-defined "therapeutic window" at 50 to 150 nanograms per mL of plasma. Other therapeutic plasma concentration ranges that are generally accepted include desipramine, 150 to 250 nanograms per mL, and imipramine, 200 to 250 nanograms per mL. See *Table 1*.

Although a sedative action may occur following the initial dose (with the possible exception of protriptyline), 1 to 6 weeks of therapy may be required before the desired antidepressant response is obtained.

Maintenance therapy of the sedating tricyclic antidepressants is usually given as a single dose at bedtime. A divided dose may be preferred, however, for protriptyline, and for all tricyclic antidepressants in geriatric or cardiovascular patients, or in adolescents or children. Maintenance is often continued for 6 months to 1 year. Recent data suggest that some patients with recurrent depression may benefit from prolonged maintenance treatment at the full (acute treatment) daily dose.

A trial of four to six weeks at the upper therapeutic dose range may be considered an adequate antidepressant trial, after which alternate therapy should be considered.

The single daily dose at bedtime is useful when side effects such as excessive drowsiness or dizziness might be bothersome or dangerous during working hours. An exception to bedtime dosage is protriptyline, which if taken late in the day may cause insomnia or nightmares in some patients. Therefore, protriptyline is often given in divided doses with the last daily dose in the afternoon.

Withdrawal symptoms, such as headache, malaise, nausea or vomiting, and vivid dreams, may occur if high or prolonged dosage is abruptly discontinued. Also, patients with a history of only unipolar depression may experience a fast-cycling bipolar disorder (manic-depressive illness) with mania or hypomania. Although this has not been reported with all of the tricyclics, a gradual reduction in dosage over a 1- to 2-month period is recommended when any of these medications is to be discontinued.

Potentially suicidal patients should not have access to large quantities of these medications since depressed patients, particularly those who may use alcohol excessively, may continue to exhibit suicidal tendencies until significant improvement occurs. Some clinicians recommend that not more than the equivalent of 1 gram of amitriptyline be dispensed to such patients at any one time. However, most clinicians agree that the judgment must be made according to each patient's individual condition.

The condition of depressed patients with bipolar disorder may sometimes change to the manic phase during tricyclic antidepressant therapy, although such change has not been reported with every tricyclic antidepressant.

**Diet/Nutrition**
Oral doses may be taken with or immediately after food to lessen gastric irritation.
The requirements for riboflavin may be increased in patients receiving amitriptyline or imipramine.

**For treatment of adverse effects**
Neuroleptic malignant syndrome (NMS) (for amoxapine only)—
Treatment is essentially symptomatic and supportive and includes
 • *Discontinuing amoxapine immediately*.
 • Hyperthermia: Administering antipyretics (aspirin or acetaminophen); using cooling blanket.
 • Dehydration: Restoring fluids and electrolytes.
 • Cardiovascular instability: Monitoring blood pressure and cardiac rhythm closely.
 • Hypoxia: Administering oxygen; considering airway insertion and assisted ventilation.
 • Muscle rigidity: Dantrolene sodium may be administered (100 to 300 mg a day in divided doses; 0.75 to 1 mg per kg, intravenously, every 6 hours, increased up to 3 mg per kg every 6 hours as needed).
Parkinsonism—
In most cases, mild effects may be reversed by dosage reduction. Administration of antiparkinsonism drugs such as benztropine, diphenhydramine, or trihexyphenidyl may reverse severe reactions.
Secretion of inappropriate antidiuretic hormone syndrome (SIADH)—
Recommended treatment includes
 • *Discontinuing tricyclic antidepressant*.
 • If urgent treatment is required, administering several hundred milliliters of 5% sodium chloride intravenously over several hours while monitoring serum sodium concentration and the symptoms, and watching for fluid overload.
 • After initial phase, or for less urgent treatment, restricting water intake to 1000 mL a day.
 • Monitoring serum electrolytes for several days.
Tardive dyskinesia (for amoxapine only)—
No known effective treatment. Dosage of the tricyclic should be lowered or medication gradually discontinued at earliest signs of tardive dyskinesia, to prevent irreversible effects.

## AMITRIPTYLINE

# Summary of Differences

Indications:
Also used to manage some types of chronic, severe, neurogenic pain, and to treat bulimia and peptic ulcer disease.
Pharmacology/pharmacokinetics:
Effects—
Anticholinergic: High.
Sedative: High.
Orthostatic hypotension: Moderate to high.

## Oral Dosage Forms

Note: Bracketed uses in the *Dosage Forms* section refer to categories of use and/or indications that are not included in U.S. product labeling.

### AMITRIPTYLINE HYDROCHLORIDE TABLETS USP

**Usual adult dose**
Antidepressant—
   Oral, initially 25 mg two to four times a day, the dosage being adjusted gradually as needed and tolerated.

**Usual adult prescribing limits**
Outpatients—Up to 150 mg a day.
Hospitalized patients—Up to 300 mg a day.
Geriatric patients—Up to 100 mg a day.

**Usual pediatric dose**
Antidepressant—
   Children 6 to 12 years of age: Oral, 10 to 30 mg, or 1 to 5 mg per kg of body weight, a day in two divided doses.
   Adolescents: Oral, initially 10 mg three times a day and 20 mg at bedtime, the dosage being adjusted as needed and tolerated, up to a maximum of 100 mg a day in divided doses or as a single dose at bedtime.
[Enuresis]—
   Children up to 6 years of age: Oral, 10 mg a day as a single dose at bedtime.
   Children over 6 years of age: Oral, initially 10 mg a day as a single dose at bedtime, the dose being increased as needed and tolerated up to a maximum of 25 mg.

**Usual geriatric dose**
Antidepressant—
   Oral, initially 25 mg at bedtime, the dosage being adjusted as needed and tolerated, up to 10 mg three times a day and 20 mg at bedtime.

**Strength(s) usually available**
U.S.—
   10 mg (Rx) [*Elavil; Endep* (scored); GENERIC].
   25 mg (Rx) [*Elavil; Endep* (scored); GENERIC].
   50 mg (Rx) [*Elavil; Endep* (scored); GENERIC].
   75 mg (Rx) [*Elavil; Endep* (scored); GENERIC].
   100 mg (Rx) [*Elavil; Endep* (scored); GENERIC].
   150 mg (Rx) [*Elavil; Endep* (scored); GENERIC].
Canada—
   10 mg (Rx) [*Apo-Amitriptyline; Elavil; Novotriptyn*].
   25 mg (Rx) [*Apo-Amitriptyline; Elavil; Novotriptyn;* GENERIC].
   50 mg (Rx) [*Apo-Amitriptyline; Elavil; Novotriptyn*].
   75 mg (Rx) [*Apo-Amitriptyline; Elavil; Levate*].

**Packaging and storage**
Store below 40 °C (104 °F), preferably between 15 and 30 °C (59 and 86 °F), unless otherwise specified by manufacturer. Store in a well-closed container.

**Auxiliary labeling**
• May cause drowsiness.
• Avoid alcoholic beverages.

### AMITRIPTYLINE PAMOATE SYRUP

**Usual adult dose**
Antidepressant—
   Oral, initially 25 mg (base) two to four times a day, the dosage being adjusted gradually as needed and tolerated.

**Usual pediatric dose**
Antidepressant—
   Children 6 to 12 years of age: Oral, 10 to 30 mg (base), or 1 to 5 mg per kg of body weight, a day in two divided doses.
   Adolescents: Oral, initially 10 mg (base) three times a day and 20 mg at bedtime, the dosage being adjusted as needed and tolerated, up to a maximum of 100 mg a day, in divided doses or as a single dose at bedtime.
[Enuresis]—
   Children up to 6 years of age: Oral, 10 mg (base) a day as a single dose at bedtime.
   Children over 6 years of age: Oral, initially 10 mg (base) a day as a single dose at bedtime, the dose being increased as needed and tolerated up to a maximum of 25 mg.

**Usual geriatric dose**
Antidepressant—
   Oral, initially 10 mg (base) three times a day and 20 mg at bedtime, the dosage being adjusted as needed and tolerated, up to a maximum of 100 mg a day, in divided doses or as a single dose at bedtime.

**Strength(s) usually available**
U.S.—
   Not commercially available.
Canada—
   10 mg (base) per 5 mL (Rx) [*Elavil* (methyl- and propylparaben)].

**Packaging and storage**
Store below 40 °C (104 °F), preferably between 15 and 30 °C (59 and 86 °F), in a well-closed container, unless otherwise specified by manufacturer.

**Auxiliary labeling**
• May cause drowsiness.
• Avoid alcoholic beverages.

## Parenteral Dosage Forms

### AMITRIPTYLINE HYDROCHLORIDE INJECTION USP

**Usual adult dose**
Antidepressant—
   Intramuscular, 20 to 30 mg four times a day.

**Usual pediatric dose**
Antidepressant—
   Children up to 12 years of age: Dosage has not been established.

**Strength(s) usually available**
U.S.—
   10 mg per mL (Rx) [*Elavil* (dextrose; methylparaben; propylparaben); GENERIC].
Canada—
   Not commercially available.

**Packaging and storage**
Store below 40 °C (104 °F), preferably between 15 and 30 °C (59 and 86 °F), unless otherwise specified by manufacturer. Protect from freezing.

---

### *AMOXAPINE*

## Summary of Differences
Pharmacology/pharmacokinetics:
   Effects—
      Anticholinergic: Moderate.
      Sedative: Low to moderate.
      Orthostatic hypotension: Low.
   Onset of action—
      Antidepressant: Within 1 to 2 weeks.
Side/adverse effects:
   Neuroleptic malignant syndrome, parkinsonian reactions and tardive dyskinesia may occur. Sexual function impairment, breast enlargement in both males and females, testicular swelling, and severe, refractory seizures on acute overdose are all more frequent with amoxapine than with other tricyclic antidepressants.

## Oral Dosage Forms

### AMOXAPINE TABLETS USP

**Usual adult dose**
Antidepressant—
   Oral, initially 50 mg two or three times a day, the dosage being increased to 100 mg two or three times a day within the first week of treatment as needed and tolerated.

Note: Increases above 300 mg a day should be made with caution and only if 300 mg a day has been ineffective during a trial period of at least two weeks.

**Usual adult prescribing limits**
Hospitalized patients—Up to 600 mg a day in divided doses.

**Usual pediatric dose**
Children up to 16 years of age—Dosage has not been established.

**Usual geriatric dose**
Antidepressant—
   Oral, initially 25 mg two or three times a day, the dosage being increased, if tolerated, to 50 mg two or three times a day within the first week.

**Strength(s) usually available**
U.S.—
   25 mg (Rx) [*Asendin* (scored); GENERIC].
   50 mg (Rx) [*Asendin* (scored); GENERIC].
   100 mg (Rx) [*Asendin* (scored); GENERIC].
   150 mg (Rx) [*Asendin* (scored); GENERIC].

USP DI

Canada—
- 25 mg (Rx) [*Asendin* (scored)].
- 50 mg (Rx) [*Asendin* (scored)].
- 100 mg (Rx) [*Asendin* (scored)].
- 150 mg (Rx) [*Asendin* (scored)].

**Packaging and storage**
Store below 40 °C (104 °F), preferably between 15 and 30 °C (59 and 86 °F), in a well-closed container, unless otherwise specified by manufacturer.

**Auxiliary labeling**
- May cause drowsiness.
- Avoid alcoholic beverages.

## CLOMIPRAMINE

## Summary of Differences
Indications:
  Also used to treat obsessive-compulsive disorder, panic disorder, bulimia nervosa, cataplexy associated with narcolepsy, and to manage some types of chronic, severe, neurogenic pain.
Pharmacology/pharmacokinetics:
  Effects—
    Anticholinergic: High.
    Sedative: Moderate.
    Orthostatic hypotension: Moderate.
Precautions:
  Drug interactions and/or related problems—
    Not recommended for concurrent use with monoamine oxidase inhibitors.
Side/adverse effects:
  Sexual function impairment, seizures, and nausea and vomiting may occur more frequently with clomipramine than with other tricyclic antidepressants.

## Additional Dosing Information
See also *General Dosing Information*.
Clomipramine should be given in divided doses with meals during initial titration to minimize gastrointestinal side effects; after titration, the total daily dose may be given at bedtime to minimize daytime sedation.

## Oral Dosage Forms
Note: Bracketed uses in the *Dosage Forms* section refer to categories of use and/or indications that are not included in U.S. product labeling.

### CLOMIPRAMINE HYDROCHLORIDE CAPSULES
**Usual adult dose**
[Antidepressant]—
  Oral, initially 25 mg three times a day, the dosage being adjusted as needed and tolerated.
Antiobsessional agent—
  Oral, initially 25 mg once a day, the dosage being gradually increased to 100 mg during the first two weeks. The dosage may be further increased over the next several weeks, up to a maximum of 250 mg a day.

**Usual adult prescribing limits**
Outpatients: Up to 250 mg a day.
Hospitalized patients: Up to 300 mg a day.

**Usual pediatric dose**
[Antidepressant]—
  Children up to 12 years of age: Dosage has not been established.
  Adolescents: Oral, 20 to 30 mg a day, the dosage being increased by 10 mg at 4 or 5 day intervals as needed and tolerated.
Antiobsessional agent—
  Children up to 10 years of age: Dosage has not been established.
  Children 10 years of age and over, and adolescents: Oral, initially 25 mg once a day, the dose being increased as needed and tolerated up to 100 mg a day or 3 mg per kg of body weight, whichever is less. The dosage may be further increased up to a maximum of 200 mg a day or 3 mg per kg of body weight, whichever is less.
Note: The strengths of the specific products may not conform to the recommended pediatric doses.

**Usual geriatric dose**
Oral, 20 to 30 mg a day, the dosage being increased as needed and tolerated.
Note: The strengths of the specific products may not conform to the recommended geriatric doses.

Antidepressants, Tricyclic (Systemic)  279

**Strength(s) usually available**
U.S.—
  25 mg (Rx) [*Anafranil* (methylparaben; propylparaben); GENERIC].
  50 mg (Rx) [*Anafranil* (methylparaben; propylparaben); GENERIC].
  75 mg (Rx) [*Anafranil* (methylparaben; propylparaben); GENERIC].
Canada—
  Not commercially available.

**Packaging and storage**
Store below 40 °C (104 °F), preferably between 15 and 30 °C (59 and 86 °F), in a tight, light-resistant container, unless otherwise specified by manufacturer.

**Auxiliary labeling**
- May cause drowsiness.
- Avoid alcoholic beverages.

### CLOMIPRAMINE HYDROCHLORIDE TABLETS
**Usual adult dose**
See *Clomipramine Hydrochloride Capsules*.

**Usual adult prescribing limits**
See *Clomipramine Hydrochloride Capsules*.

**Usual pediatric dose**
See *Clomipramine Hydrochloride Capsules*.

**Usual geriatric dose**
See *Clomipramine Hydrochloride Capsules*.

**Strength(s) usually available**
U.S.—
  Not commercially available.
Canada—
  10 mg (Rx) [*Anafranil* (lactose)].
  25 mg (Rx) [*Anafranil* (lactose)].
  50 mg (Rx) [*Anafranil* (lactose)].

**Packaging and storage**
Store below 40 °C (104 °F), preferably between 15 and 30 °C (59 and 86 °F), in a tight, light-resistant container, unless otherwise specified by manufacturer.

**Auxiliary labeling**
- May cause drowsiness.
- Avoid alcoholic beverages.

## DESIPRAMINE

## Summary of Differences
Indications:
  Also used to manage some types of chronic, severe, neurogenic pain; to reduce craving and/or prevent depression upon withdrawal of cocaine; to control binge eating and purging in bulimia; and to treat cataplexy associated with narcolepsy; and is being used to relieve the symptoms of attention deficit hyperactivity disorder in children over 6 years of age and in adolescents.
Pharmacology/pharmacokinetics:
  Effects—
    Anticholinergic: Low.
    Sedative: Low.
    Orthostatic hypotension: Moderate.
Precautions:
  Drug interactions and/or related problems—
    Not recommended for concurrent use with monoamine oxidase inhibitors.
    Concurrent use of phenytoin with desipramine may lower serum concentrations of desipramine; dosage increases above maximum recommended doses of desipramine may be necessary for clinical improvement of depression.

## Oral Dosage Forms
### DESIPRAMINE HYDROCHLORIDE TABLETS USP
**Usual adult dose**
Antidepressant—
  Oral, 100 to 200 mg a day in divided doses or as a single dose, the dosage being adjusted as needed and tolerated.

**Usual adult prescribing limits**
Up to 300 mg a day.
Note: Geriatric patients—Up to 150 mg a day.

**Usual pediatric dose**
Antidepressant—
  Children 6 to 12 years of age: Oral, 10 to 30 mg, or 1 to 5 mg per kg of body weight, a day in divided doses.
  Adolescents: Oral, 25 to 50 mg a day in divided doses, the dosage being adjusted as needed and tolerated, up to a maximum of 100 mg a day.

**Usual geriatric dose**
Antidepressant—
  Oral, 25 to 50 mg a day in divided doses, the dosage being adjusted as needed and tolerated, up to a maximum of 150 mg a day.

**Strength(s) usually available**
U.S.—
  10 mg (Rx) [*Norpramin*; GENERIC].
  25 mg (Rx) [*Norpramin*; GENERIC].
  50 mg (Rx) [*Norpramin*; GENERIC].
  75 mg (Rx) [*Norpramin*; GENERIC].
  100 mg (Rx) [*Norpramin*; GENERIC].
  150 mg (Rx) [*Norpramin*; GENERIC].
Canada—
  10 mg (Rx) [*Norpramin* (sucrose; mannitol; corn starch)].
  25 mg (Rx) [*Norpramin*; *Pertofrane*; GENERIC].
  50 mg (Rx) [*Norpramin*; *Pertofrane*; GENERIC].
  75 mg (Rx) [*Norpramin*; GENERIC].
  100 mg (Rx) [*Norpramin*].

**Packaging and storage**
Store below 40 °C (104 °F), preferably between 15 and 30 °C (59 and 86 °F), unless otherwise specified by manufacturer. Store in a tight container.

**Auxiliary labeling**
- May cause drowsiness.
- Avoid alcoholic beverages.

---

## DOXEPIN

## Summary of Differences
Indications:
  Also used in treatment of some types of chronic, severe neurogenic pain; peptic ulcer disease; and pruritus in idiopathic cold urticaria.
Pharmacology/pharmacokinetics:
  Effects—
    Anticholinergic: High.
    Sedative: High.
    Orthostatic hypotension: High.

## Additional Dosing Information
See also *General Dosing Information*.
Patients with mild symptomology or emotional symptoms accompanying organic disease may be controlled on doses as low as 25 to 50 mg a day.
The once-a-day dosage maximum is 150 mg, which may be given at bedtime.

## Oral Dosage Forms
Note: Bracketed uses in the *Dosage Forms* section refer to categories of use and/or indications that are not included in U.S. product labeling.

### DOXEPIN HYDROCHLORIDE CAPSULES USP
**Usual adult dose**
Antidepressant—
  Oral, initially 25 mg (base) three times a day, the dosage being adjusted gradually as needed and tolerated.
[Antipruritic][1]—
  Oral, initially 10 mg (base) at bedtime, the dosage being increased gradually up to 25 mg, as needed and tolerated.

**Usual adult prescribing limits**
Outpatients: Up to 150 mg (base) a day.
Hospitalized patients: Up to 300 mg (base) a day.

**Usual pediatric dose**
Antidepressant—
  Children up to 12 years of age: Dosage has not been established.

**Usual geriatric dose**
Antidepressant—
  Oral, initially 25 to 50 mg (base) a day, the dosage being adjusted gradually as needed and tolerated.

**Strength(s) usually available**
U.S.—
  10 mg (base) (Rx) [*Sinequan*; GENERIC].
  25 mg (base) (Rx) [*Sinequan*; GENERIC].
  50 mg (base) (Rx) [*Sinequan*; GENERIC].
  75 mg (base) (Rx) [*Sinequan*; GENERIC].
  100 mg (base) (Rx) [*Sinequan*; GENERIC].
  150 mg (base) (Rx) [*Sinequan*; GENERIC].
Canada—
  10 mg (base) (Rx) [*Sinequan*; *Triadapin*].
  25 mg (base) (Rx) [*Novo-Doxepin*; *Sinequan*; *Triadapin*].
  50 mg (base) (Rx) [*Novo-Doxepin*; *Sinequan*; *Triadapin*].
  75 mg (base) (Rx) [*Novo-Doxepin*; *Sinequan*; *Triadapin*].
  100 mg (base) (Rx) [*Novo-Doxepin*; *Sinequan*; *Triadapin*].
  150 mg (base) (Rx) [*Novo-Doxepin*; *Sinequan*].

**Packaging and storage**
Store between 15 and 30 °C (59 and 86 °F), unless otherwise specified by manufacturer. Store in a well-closed container.

**Auxiliary labeling**
- May cause drowsiness.
- Avoid alcoholic beverages.

**Note:**
The 150-mg capsule is intended for maintenance therapy only, and not for initiation of therapy.

### DOXEPIN HYDROCHLORIDE ORAL SOLUTION USP
**Usual adult dose**
See *Doxepin Hydrochloride Capsules USP*.

**Usual adult prescribing limits**
See *Doxepin Hydrochloride Capsules USP*.

**Usual pediatric dose**
See *Doxepin Hydrochloride Capsules USP*.

**Strength(s) usually available**
U.S.—
  10 mg (base) per mL (Rx) [*Sinequan*; GENERIC].
Canada—
  Not commercially available.

**Packaging and storage**
Store between 15 and 30 °C (59 and 86 °F), unless otherwise specified by manufacturer. Store in a tight, light-resistant container.

**Incompatibilities**
Oral solution may be incompatible with many carbonated beverages and with grape juice.

**Auxiliary labeling**
- May cause drowsiness.
- Avoid alcoholic beverages.
- Must be diluted before taking.

**Note:**
When dispensing, include the manufacturer-provided graduated dropper.

[1]Not included in Canadian product labeling.

---

## IMIPRAMINE

## Summary of Differences
Indications:
  Imipramine hydrochloride (but not pamoate) is indicated in treatment of childhood enuresis.
  Imipramine is also used to manage some types of chronic, severe, neurogenic pain; to reduce craving and/or prevent depression upon cocaine withdrawal; to relieve symptoms of attention deficit hyperactivity disorder in children over 6 years of age and in adolescents; as a treatment adjunct with amphetamines or methylphenidate in cataplexy associated with narcolepsy; to block the recurrence of panic attacks, with or without phobias; in the treatment of stress and urge incontinence; and to control binge eating and purging in bulimia.
Pharmacology/pharmacokinetics:
  Effects—
    Anticholinergic: Moderate.
    Sedative: Moderate.
    Orthostatic hypotension: High.
Precautions:
  Drug interactions and/or related problems—
    Not recommended for concurrent use with monoamine oxidase inhibitors.

## Additional Dosing Information
See also *General Dosing Information*.
**For oral dosage forms only**
In enuretic children, a daily dose exceeding 75 mg does not normally increase results. The usual pediatric prescribing limits are 2.5 mg per kg of body weight (mg/kg) a day.

For early-night bedwetters, the dosage may be more effective when one-half of the dose is given at mid-afternoon and one-half at bedtime.

A gradual decrease in dosage is less likely to cause relapse than an abrupt discontinuation.

Younger children should not be allowed to self-administer imipramine because of their increased sensitivity to side effects, especially cardiovascular effects and acute overdosage (plasma concentrations over 225 nanograms per mL), which are potentially fatal.

A medication-free interval after adequate therapeutic trial should be considered for children. However, dosage should be decreased gradually to prevent relapse. Children who have relapsed may not respond when treatment is reinitiated.

**For parenteral dosage forms only**
Used only for initiating therapy in patients who are not able or are unwilling to take oral medication. Oral dosage forms should replace the parenteral as soon as possible.

## Oral Dosage Forms
Note: Bracketed uses in the *Dosage Forms* section refer to categories of use and/or indications that are not included in U.S. product labeling.

### IMIPRAMINE HYDROCHLORIDE TABLETS USP
**Usual adult dose**
Antidepressant—
   Oral, 25 to 50 mg three or four times a day, the dosage being adjusted as needed and tolerated.
[Urinary incontinence][1]—
   Oral, 10 to 50 mg a day, the dosage being adjusted as needed and tolerated, to a maximum of 150 mg a day.

**Usual adult prescribing limits**
Outpatients: Up to 200 mg a day.
Hospitalized patients: Up to 300 mg a day.
Geriatric patients: Up to 100 mg a day.

**Usual pediatric dose**
Antidepressant—
   Children up to 6 years of age: Use is not recommended.
   Children 6 to 12 years of age: Oral, 10 to 30 mg a day in two divided doses.
   Adolescents: Oral, 25 to 50 mg a day in divided doses, the dosage being adjusted as needed and tolerated, up to 100 mg a day.
Antienuretic—
   Oral, 25 mg once a day, one hour before bedtime. If a satisfactory response is not obtained within one week, the dosage may be increased to 50 mg nightly in children under 12 years of age and to 75 mg nightly in children 12 or over.

**Usual geriatric dose**
Antidepressant—
   Oral, initially 25 mg at bedtime, the dosage being adjusted as needed and tolerated, up to 100 mg a day in divided doses.

**Strength(s) usually available**
U.S.—
   10 mg (Rx) [*Tipramine; Tofranil;* GENERIC].
   25 mg (Rx) [*Norfranil; Tipramine; Tofranil;* GENERIC].
   50 mg (Rx) [*Norfranil; Tipramine; Tofranil;* GENERIC].
Canada—
   10 mg (Rx) [*Apo-Imipramine; Novopramine; Tofranil*].
   25 mg (Rx) [*Apo-Imipramine; Novopramine; Tofranil*].
   50 mg (Rx) [*Apo-Imipramine; Novopramine; Tofranil*].
   75 mg (Rx) [*Apo-Imipramine* (scored); *Impril; Tofranil*].

**Packaging and storage**
Store between 15 and 30 °C (59 and 86 °F), unless otherwise specified by manufacturer. Store in a tight container.

**Auxiliary labeling**
• May cause drowsiness.
• Avoid alcoholic beverages.

### IMIPRAMINE PAMOATE CAPSULES
**Usual adult dose**
Antidepressant—
   Oral, initially 75 mg a day, usually given at bedtime, the dosage being adjusted as needed and tolerated.

Note: The dose level at which optimum response is usually obtained is 150 mg a day, usually given at bedtime.

**Usual adult prescribing limits**
Outpatients: Up to 200 mg a day.
Hospitalized patients: Up to 300 mg a day.

**Usual pediatric dose**
Antidepressant—
   Children up to 12 years of age: Use is not recommended.

**Strength(s) usually available**
U.S.—
   75 mg (Rx) [*Tofranil-PM*].
   100 mg (Rx) [*Tofranil-PM*].
   125 mg (Rx) [*Tofranil-PM*].
   150 mg (Rx) [*Tofranil-PM*].
   Note: The above strengths of imipramine pamoate are equivalent to the same strengths of imipramine hydrochloride.
Canada—
   Not commercially available.

**Packaging and storage**
Store between 15 and 30 °C (59 and 86 °F), in a tight container, unless otherwise specified by manufacturer.

**Auxiliary labeling**
• May cause drowsiness.
• Avoid alcoholic beverages.

## Parenteral Dosage Forms
### IMIPRAMINE HYDROCHLORIDE INJECTION USP
**Usual adult dose**
Antidepressant—
   Intramuscular, up to 100 mg a day in divided doses.

**Usual adult prescribing limits**
Up to 300 mg a day.

**Usual pediatric dose**
Antidepressant—
   Children up to 12 years of age: Use is not recommended.

**Strength(s) usually available**
U.S.—
   12.5 mg per mL (Rx) [*Tofranil* (ascorbic acid 1 mg; sodium bisulfite 0.5 mg; anhydrous sodium sulfite 0.5 mg)].
Canada—
   Not commercially available.

**Packaging and storage**
Store below 40 °C (104 °F), preferably between 15 and 30 °C (59 and 86 °F), unless otherwise specified by manufacturer. Protect from freezing.

**Auxiliary labeling**
• For intramuscular use only.

---

[1]Not included in Canadian product labeling.

---

## NORTRIPTYLINE

## Summary of Differences
Indications:
   Also used to manage some types of chronic, severe, neurogenic pain and in the treatment of panic disorder.
Pharmacology/pharmacokinetics:
   Effects—
      Anticholinergic: Low.
      Sedative: Moderate.
      Orthostatic hypotension: Low.

## Oral Dosage Forms
### NORTRIPTYLINE HYDROCHLORIDE CAPSULES USP
**Usual adult dose**
Antidepressant—
   Oral, 25 mg (base) three or four times a day, the dosage being adjusted as needed and tolerated.

**Usual adult prescribing limits**
Up to 150 mg (base) a day.

**Usual pediatric dose**
Antidepressant—
   Children 6 to 12 years of age: Oral, 10 to 20 mg (base), or 1 to 3 mg per kg of body weight, a day in divided doses.

Adolescents: Oral, 25 to 50 mg, or 1 to 3 mg per kg of body weight, a day in divided doses, the dosage being adjusted as needed and tolerated.

**Usual geriatric dose**
Oral, 30 to 50 mg a day in divided doses, the dosage being adjusted as needed and tolerated.

**Strength(s) usually available**
U.S.—
 10 mg (base) (Rx) [*Aventyl; Pamelor;* GENERIC].
 25 mg (base) (Rx) [*Aventyl; Pamelor;* GENERIC].
 50 mg (base) (Rx) [*Pamelor;* GENERIC].
 75 mg (base) (Rx) [*Pamelor;* GENERIC].
Canada—
 10 mg (base) (Rx) [*Aventyl*].
 25 mg (base) (Rx) [*Aventyl*].

**Packaging and storage**
Store between 15 and 30 °C (59 and 86 °F), unless otherwise specified by manufacturer. Store in a tight container.

**Auxiliary labeling**
• May cause drowsiness.
• Avoid alcoholic beverages.

### NORTRIPTYLINE HYDROCHLORIDE ORAL SOLUTION USP

**Usual adult dose**
See *Nortriptyline Hydrochloride Capsules USP*.

**Usual pediatric dose**
See *Nortriptyline Hydrochloride Capsules USP*.

**Strength(s) usually available**
U.S.—
 10 mg (base) per 5 mL (Rx) [*Aventyl* (alcohol 4%); *Pamelor* (alcohol 4%)].
Canada—
 Not commercially available.

**Packaging and storage**
Store below 40 °C (104 °F), preferably between 15 and 30 °C (59 and 86 °F), unless otherwise specified by manufacturer. Store in a tight, light-resistant container. Protect from freezing.

**Auxiliary labeling**
• May cause drowsiness.
• Avoid alcoholic beverages.

## PROTRIPTYLINE

### Summary of Differences

Indications:
 Also used in the treatment of narcolepsy, as an adjunct with amphetamines or methylphenidate in the treatment of cataplexy associated with narcolepsy, in sleep disorders such as hypersomnia or impaired morning arousal, and may be used to relieve symptoms of attention deficit hyperactivity disorder in some children over 6 years of age and in adolescents.
Pharmacology/pharmacokinetics:
 Effects—
  Anticholinergic: Moderate.
  Sedative: Very low.
  Orthostatic hypotension: Low.

### Additional Dosing Information

See also *General Dosing Information*.

When dosage increases of protriptyline are indicated, the increase should be made in the morning. This drug often has a psychic-energizing action and usually not the sedative action exhibited by other tricyclics, although it may intensify the sedative effect of other medications.

Protriptyline is often given in divided doses with the last daily dose in the afternoon to avoid insomnia or nightmares when given to some patients before bedtime.

When protriptyline is used in narcolepsy, 15 to 20 mg given in a single daily dose at bedtime may relieve symptoms of arousal difficulty and daytime sleepiness.

### Oral Dosage Forms

Note: Bracketed uses in the *Dosage Forms* section refer to categories of use and/or indications that are not included in U.S. product labeling.

### PROTRIPTYLINE HYDROCHLORIDE TABLETS USP

**Usual adult dose**
Antidepressant—
 Oral, initially 5 to 10 mg three or four times a day, the dosage being adjusted as needed and tolerated.
[Anticataplectic][1]—
 Oral, 15 to 20 mg a day at bedtime.

**Usual adult prescribing limits**
Up to 60 mg a day.

**Usual pediatric dose**
Antidepressant—
 Children up to 12 years of age: Dosage has not been established.
 Adolescents: Oral, initially 5 mg three times a day, the dosage being adjusted as needed and tolerated.

**Usual geriatric dose**
Antidepressant—
 Oral, initially 5 mg three times a day, the dosage being adjusted as needed and tolerated.
Note: When the daily dose for geriatric patients exceeds 20 mg, the cardiovascular response should be closely monitored.

**Strength(s) usually available**
U.S.—
 5 mg (Rx) [*Vivactil* (lactose); GENERIC].
 10 mg (Rx) [*Vivactil* (lactose); GENERIC].
Canada—
 10 mg (Rx) [*Triptil*].

**Packaging and storage**
Store between 15 and 30 °C (59 and 86 °F), unless otherwise specified by manufacturer. Store in a tight container.

**Auxiliary labeling**
• May cause drowsiness.
• Avoid alcoholic beverages.

[1]Not included in Canadian product labeling.

## TRIMIPRAMINE

### Summary of Differences

Indications:
 Also used in treatment of peptic ulcer disease and in the management of some types of chronic, severe, neurogenic pain.
Pharmacology/pharmacokinetics:
 Effects—
  Anticholinergic: High.
  Sedative: High.
  Orthostatic hypotension: Moderate.

### Additional Dosing Information

See also *General Dosing Information*.

For patient compliance and convenience of therapy for outpatients, the total daily dosage may be given at bedtime.

Following remission, maintenance therapy should continue for about 3 months at the lowest dose necessary to maintain remission.

In resistant cases of depression in adults in which dosage exceeds 2.5 mg per kg of body weight (mg/kg) a day, the ECG should be monitored during initiation of therapy and at appropriate intervals during stabilization of dose.

### Oral Dosage Forms

Note: The dosing and strengths of the dosage forms available are expressed in terms of trimipramine base (not the maleate).

### TRIMIPRAMINE MALEATE CAPSULES

**Usual adult dose**
Antidepressant—
 Outpatients:
  Initial—Oral, 75 mg (base) a day in divided doses, the dosage being adjusted gradually to 150 mg a day as needed and tolerated, up to a maximum of 200 mg a day.
  Maintenance—Oral, 50 to 150 mg (base) a day.
 Hospitalized patients:
  Oral, initially 100 mg (base) a day in divided doses, the dosage being increased gradually in a few days to 200 mg a day, up to 250 to 300 mg a day in two to three weeks.

**Usual pediatric dose**
Antidepressant—
Children up to 12 years of age: Dosage has not been established.
Adolescents: Oral, initially 50 mg (base) a day in divided doses, the dosage being adjusted as needed and tolerated, up to a maximum of 100 mg a day.

**Usual geriatric dose**
Oral, initially 50 mg (base) a day in divided doses, the dosage being adjusted as needed and tolerated, up to a maximum of 100 mg a day.

**Strength(s) usually available**
U.S.—
25 mg (base) (Rx) [*Surmontil;* GENERIC].
50 mg (base) (Rx) [*Surmontil;* GENERIC].
100 mg (base) (Rx) [*Surmontil;* GENERIC].
Canada—
75 mg (base) (Rx) [*Apo-Trimip; Rhotrimine; Surmontil*].

**Packaging and storage**
Store between 15 and 30 °C (59 and 86 °F), in a tight container, unless otherwise specified by manufacturer.

**Auxiliary labeling**
• May cause drowsiness.
• Avoid alcoholic beverages.

## TRIMIPRAMINE MALEATE TABLETS

**Usual adult dose**
See *Trimipramine Maleate Capsules*.

**Usual pediatric dose**
See *Trimipramine Maleate Capsules*.

**Usual geriatric dose**
Antidepressant—
Oral, initially 25 to 50 mg (base) a day in divided doses, the dosage being increased by 25 mg a week, up to a maximum of 150 mg a day.

**Strength(s) usually available**
U.S.—
Not commercially available.
Canada—
12.5 mg (base) (Rx) [*Apo-Trimip; Rhotrimine; Surmontil*].
25 mg (base) (Rx) [*Apo-Trimip; Novo-Tripramine; Rhotrimine; Surmontil*].
50 mg (base) (Rx) [*Apo-Trimip; Novo-Tripramine; Rhotrimine; Surmontil*].
100 mg (base) (Rx) [*Apo-Trimip; Novo-Tripramine; Rhotrimine; Surmontil*].

**Packaging and storage**
Store between 15 and 30 °C (59 and 86 °F), in a tight container, unless otherwise specified by manufacturer.

**Auxiliary labeling**
• May cause drowsiness.
• Avoid alcoholic beverages.

Revised: 05/22/92
Interim revision: 06/1/92; 03/01/93; 04/29/94; 08/08/97

## Table 1. Pharmacology/Pharmacokinetics

| Drug | Anticholinergic Effects* | Sedation* | Orthostatic Hypotension* | Active Metabolites | Protein Binding (%) | Volume of Distribution (L/Kg) | Half-life (hours) | Therapeutic Plasma Concentration (ng/mL)† |
|---|---|---|---|---|---|---|---|---|
| Amitriptyline | High | High | Moderate to high | Nortriptyline 10-Hydroxyamitriptyline | 95 | 12–18 | 10–26 | |
| Amoxapine | Moderate | Low to moderate | Low | 7- and 8-Hydroxyamoxapine | 92 | N.A.‡ | 8–30 | |
| Clomipramine | High | Moderate | Moderate | Desmethylclomipramine | 96–97 | 12 | 21–31 | |
| Desipramine | Low | Low | Moderate | 2-Hydroxydesipramine | 90–92 | 17–42 | 12–27 | 125–300 |
| Doxepin | High | High | High | Desmethyldoxepin | N.A.‡ | 12–28 | 11–23 | |
| Imipramine | Moderate | Moderate | High | Desipramine 2-Hydroxydesipramine | 89–95 | 15–31 | 11–25 | 150–300§ |
| Nortriptyline | Low | Moderate | Low | 10-Hydroxynortriptyline | 92 | 14–22 | 18–44 | 50–150** |
| Protriptyline | Moderate | Very low | Low | N.A.‡ | 92 | 22 | 67–89 | |
| Trimipramine | High | High | Moderate | N.A.‡ | N.A.‡ | N.A.‡ | 9–11 | |

*Relative effects among tricyclic antidepressants only.
†Although various values have been reported, there is little consensus about therapeutic plasma concentrations, except for desipramine, imipramine, and nortriptyline. Steady-state plasma levels exhibit marked interindividual variations due to genetic factors (e.g., hepatic metabolism) and physiochemical properties of the medication (e.g., lipid solubility).
‡Not available.
§Includes metabolites.
**Denotes therapeutic window, outside of which effects are lessened.

# ANTIDIABETIC AGENTS, SULFONYLUREA  Systemic

This monograph includes information on the following: 1) Acetohexamide; 2) Chlorpropamide; 3) Gliclazide*; 4) Glipizide†; 5) Glyburide; 6) Tolazamide†; 7) Tolbutamide.

INN:
Glyburide—Glibenclamide
BAN:
Glyburide—Glibenclamide
JAN:
Glyburide—Glibenclamide
VA CLASSIFICATION (Primary/Secondary):
Acetohexamide—HS521
Chlorpropamide—HS521/CV900
Gliclazide—HS521
Glipizide—HS521
Glyburide—HS521
Tolazamide—HS521
Tolbutamide—HS521

Commonly used brand name(s): *Albert Glyburide*[5]; *Apo-Chlorpropamide*[2]; *Apo-Glyburide*[5]; *Apo-Tolbutamide*[7]; *DiaBeta*[5]; *Diabinese*[2]; *Diamicron*[3]; *Dimelor*[1]; *Dymelor*[1]; *Euglucon*[5]; *Gen-Glybe*[5]; *Glucotrol*[4]; *Glucotrol XL*[4]; *Glynase PresTab*[5]; *Micronase*[5]; *Mobenol*[7]; *Novo-Butamide*[7]; *Novo-Glyburide*[5]; *Novo-Propamide*[2]; *Nu-Glyburide*[5]; *Orinase*[7]; *Tol-Tab*[7]; *Tolinase*[6].

Another commonly used name for glyburide is glibenclamide.

Note: For a listing of dosage forms and brand names by country availability, see *Dosage Forms* section(s).

*Not commercially available in U.S.
†Not commercially available in Canada.

## Category
Antidiabetic—Acetohexamide; Chlorpropamide; Gliclazide; Glipizide; Glyburide; Tolazamide; Tolbutamide.
Antidiuretic—Chlorpropamide.

## Indications
Note: Bracketed information in the *Indications* section refers to uses that are not included in U.S. product labeling.

### Accepted
Diabetes mellitus (treatment), including
　Diabetes mellitus, non–insulin-dependent (NIDDM)—Sulfonylureas are indicated as adjunctive therapy to diet and exercise in the treatment and control of certain patients with NIDDM (Type II diabetes; previously known as adult-onset diabetes, maturity-onset diabetes, ketosis-resistant diabetes, or stable diabetes), which occurs in individuals who produce or secrete insufficient quantities of endogenous insulin or who have developed resistance to endogenous insulin. An attempt to control diabetes through changes in diet and level of physical activity is usually first-line management before beginning pharmacologic treatment. Those patients not responding adequately to diet alone or those patients requiring diet plus insulin, especially if they require 40 USP Units or less of insulin a day, may be candidates for therapy with a sulfonylurea as monotherapy or combination therapy.
　Diabetes mellitus, other, associated with certain conditions or syndromes, such as:
- Endocrine disease, including endocrine overactivity due to Cushing's syndrome, hyperthyroidism, pheochromocytoma, somatostatinoma, or aldosteronoma; or endocrine underactivity due to hypoparathyroidism-hypocalcemia, type I isolated growth hormone deficiency, or multitropic pituitary deficiency or
- Genetic syndromes, including, inborn errors of metabolism, such as glycogen-storage disease type I, or insulin-resistant syndromes, such as muscular dystrophies, late onset proximal myopathy, or Huntington's chorea.
- Sulfonylureas may be used in conditions causing diabetes mellitus induced by hormones, medications, or chemicals in patients who have functioning pancreatic beta cells when the diabetes cannot be controlled by diet or exercise.

Combination use of insulin and sulfonylurea agents in insulin-dependent diabetes mellitus (IDDM) patients is controversial because many studies have indicated that sulfonylureas are not effective in the treatment of these patients.

Short-term administration of a sulfonylurea or insulin for transient loss of blood glucose control may be sufficient for NIDDM patients normally well-controlled with diet. Switching to another sulfonylurea agent may be beneficial if one particular sulfonylurea does not optimally control the diabetes mellitus; however, use of a sulfonylurea should be discontinued if satisfactory reduction of blood glucose concentration is not achieved.

The effectiveness of sulfonylureas in controlling blood glucose can decrease over time. If maximum doses of a sulfonylurea fail to control blood glucose, switching to another sulfonylurea or adding metformin to a sulfonylurea treatment regimen may be beneficial in increasing glycemic control and lipoprotein metabolism, and to help avoid initiation of insulin therapy. This is especially successful in NIDDM patients poorly controlled by insulin alone, in short-term diabetics, or in patients who are 120 to 160% over ideal baseline body weight but who are not excessively insulin-resistant. Alternatively, low-dose insulin in conjunction with sulfonylureas can help to avoid using large doses of insulin, especially for obese NIDDM patients; however, complications, such as weight gain, the effects of hyperinsulinemia, and an increased risk of hypoglycemia need to be considered. Some nonobese NIDDM patients experiencing secondary sulfonylurea failure may be best treated with insulin. A sulfonylurea should be discontinued anytime it fails to contribute to the lowering of plasma glucose in a patient for whom compliance with proper diet and sulfonylurea dosing has been determined to be adequate.

[Diabetes insipidus, central, partial (treatment)][1]—Chlorpropamide is also used as secondary therapy in selected patients to treat partial central diabetes insipidus. Used as an antidiuretic, chlorpropamide has successfully reduced polyuria in about 50% of such treated patients. Chlorpropamide may be used alone or in combination with another agent such as carbamazepine or clofibrate so that the dose of both can be reduced and side effects minimized. Nasal or subcutaneous desmopressin is considered the primary treatment for diabetes insipidus.

### Unaccepted
Sulfonylureas are not effective in the treatment of insulin-dependent diabetes mellitus (IDDM; Type I diabetes).

Chlorpropamide is not effective in the treatment of nephrogenic diabetes insipidus.

---
[1] Not included in Canadian product labeling.

## Pharmacology/Pharmacokinetics
See *Table 1*, page 296.

### Physicochemical characteristics
Chemical group—
　Sulfonylurea.
　　First generation: Acetohexamide, chlorpropamide, tolazamide, tolbutamide.
　　Second generation: Gliclazide, glipizide, glyburide.
Molecular weight—
　Acetohexamide: 324.4.
　Chlorpropamide: 276.75.
　Gliclazide: 323.42.
　Glipizide: 445.55.
　Glyburide: 494.01.
　Tolazamide: 311.41.
　Tolbutamide: 270.35.
pKa—
　Chlorpropamide: 4.8.
　Gliclazide: 5.98.
　Glipizide: 5.9.
　Glyburide: 5.3.
　Tolazamide: 3.5, 5.7.
　Tolbutamide: 5.3.

### Mechanism of action/Effect
Antidiabetic—
　Sulfonylureas lower blood glucose in NIDDM by directly stimulating the acute release of insulin from functioning beta cells of pancreatic islet tissue by an unknown process that involves a sulfonylurea receptor on the beta cell. Sulfonylureas inhibit the ATP-potassium channels on the beta cell membrane and potassium efflux, which results in depolarization and calcium influx, calcium-calmodulin binding, kinase activation, and release of insulin-containing granules by exocytosis, an effect similar to that of glucose. Insulin is a hormone that lowers blood glucose and controls the storage and metabolism of carbohydrates, proteins, and fats. Therefore, sulfonylureas are effective only in patients whose pancreata are capable of producing insulin.
　With chronic sulfonylurea treatment, insulin production is not increased and may return to pretreatment values, but insulin efficacy continues and is thought to involve extrapancreatic mechanisms to increase insulin sensitivity in target tissues, such as liver, muscle, and fat as well as in other cells, such as monocytes and erythrocytes. This can result in a decrease in hepatic glycogenolysis and gluconeogenesis. It is unclear if the sulfonylurea's extrapancreatic actions that increase insulin's efficacy are direct or indirect effects, but it is clear that the mechanism of action is not due to a direct sulfonylurea action on the insulin receptor. Because this peripheral effect is not apparent in IDDM patients, it suggests that this may not be the clinically significant mechanism for NIDDM patients either. However, it is clear that tissues of sulfonylurea-treated NIDDM patients become more responsive to lower levels of endogenous insulin. Primary failure of sulfonylurea therapy may occur if the ability of beta cells to function is severely impaired. In addition to stimulating insulin secretion through the beta-cell sulfonylurea receptor, gliclazide may have a direct effect on intracellular calcium transport that specifically improves the biphasic response of the beta cell to a meal, that is, the immediate first phase of insulin release as well as the normally delayed second phase.

Antidiuretic—
　Chlorpropamide seems to potentiate the effect of minimal levels of antidiuretic hormone present in patients with partial central diabetes insipidus.

### Other actions/effects
Acetohexamide and its more potent major metabolite, hydroxyhexamide, have uricosuric properties. Gliclazide, at therapeutic doses, reduces platelet adhesiveness and aggregation by inhibition of arachidonic acid release and thromboxane synthesis, increased production of $PGI_2$, and release of plasminogen activator, which increases fibrinolysis. It is also thought that gliclazide and glyburide have protective activity against

cardiac arrhythmias because they can stabilize potassium and calcium concentrations by inhibition of the sodium-potassium-ATPase pump transport system. Tolbutamide and chlorpropamide decrease free water clearance while glyburide, glipizide, and tolazamide produce a mild diuresis effect by enhancement of renal free water clearance. In contrast to glyburide, tolazamide and tolbutamide increase hexose uptake in adipocytes and myocytes. Sulfonylureas directly increase the secretion of pancreatic and gastric somatostatin and do not seem to have a direct effect on glucagon.

**Absorption**
Rapidly and well absorbed but may have wide inter- and intra-individual variability. By impairing gastric motility and gastric emptying, hyperglycemia may significantly delay sulfonylurea absorption; glipizide plasma concentration has been shown to be reduced by 50% with plasma glucose concentrations over 198 mg/dL (11 millimoles/L).

*Chlorpropamide*—Food delays absorption of chlorpropamide.

*Gliclazide*—Food delays absorption of gliclazide up to 187 minutes; may be best taken 30 minutes before or with a meal.

*Glipizide*—Food delays absorption of immediate release glipizide by 40 minutes; therefore, it is recommended that glipizide be taken 30 minutes before a meal. While food had no effect on the lag time of absorption (3 to 4 hours) for extended release glipizide, administration of glipizide to normal males before a meal high in fat showed a 40% increase in the time to peak serum concentrations; area-under-the-time curve (AUC) was not affected.

*Glyburide*—Bioavailability of nonmicronized glyburide is lowest when given with a high fat diet compared to fasting or a high carbohydrate diet. Micronized glyburide is more consistent in its bioavailability and in its time to reach peak serum concentrations with regard to all meal types than is the nonmicronized formulation. Also, micronized glyburide is better absorbed and is effective at a lower dose than is nonmicronized glyburide.

*Tolbutamide*—Absorption is unaltered if taken with food but is increased with high pH.

## Precautions to Consider

### Cross-sensitivity and/or related problems
Patients sensitive to one of the sulfonylureas may be sensitive to the others also; cross-sensitivity to other sulfonamide- or thiazide-type medications may also occur.

### Carcinogenicity
*Acetohexamide*—Long-term studies in rats and mice showed no evidence of carcinogenicity.

*Chlorpropamide*—Chronic toxicity studies in dogs treated for 6, 13, and 20 months with doses of chlorpropamide greater than 20 times the human dose showed no histological or pathological abnormalities.

*Gliclazide*—Specific carcinogenicity studies have not been done in animals; however, long-term toxicity studies have not shown any evidence of drug-related carcinogenicity.

*Glipizide*—Large dose studies using up to 75 times the maximum human dose in rats and in mice for 20 and 18 months, respectively, showed no evidence of drug-related carcinogenicity.

*Glyburide*—An 18-month study in rats given doses of up to 300 mg per kg of body weight (mg/kg) a day and a 2-year oncogenicity study in mice showed no evidence of drug-related carcinogenicity.

*Tolazamide*—A 103-week study in rats and mice at both low and high doses showed no evidence of carcinogenicity.

*Tolbutamide*—A 78-week study in male and female rats and mice showed no evidence of carcinogenicity.

### Mutagenicity
*Acetohexamide*—Sister chromatid exchange testing showed no evidence of mutagenicity.

*Chlorpropamide*—The micronucleus test in one strain of Swiss mice given chlorpropamide doses of 200, 400, 800, and 1600 mg/kg (32 times greater than the therapeutic adult dose) showed no evidence of mutagenicity; however, 3 strains of mice showed positive results when evaluated using the *Salmonella*/microsome test. The results are questionable because negative results were also shown in rats and Chinese hamsters. Although an increase in chromosomal breakage has not been observed in treated mammals, Chinese hamsters, rats, or mice, the sister chromatin exchange showed a positive reaction with Chinese hamsters *in vivo* and *in vitro*; however, spontaneous breakage in this study was not even doubled in extremely high doses. It is difficult to assign a cause-and-effect to the slightly positive results in these animal studies.

*Gliclazide*—The Ames test, human lymphocyte test, and micronucleus test did not reveal mutagenicity.

*Glipizide*—Bacterial and *in vivo* mutagenicity testing showed no evidence of mutagenicity.

*Glyburide*—Testing with the Ames test, DNA damage/alkaline elution assay, and the micronucleus test (at doses 60 to 240 times the average human therapeutic dose) showed no evidence of mutagenicity.

*Tolbutamide*—The Ames test and the micronucleus test in mice (at doses of 500 mg/kg) showed no evidence of mutagenicity.

### Pregnancy/Reproduction
Fertility—
*Acetohexamide, tolazamide, tolbutamide*—
Studies in humans have not been done.
Studies in animals have not been done.

*Chlorpropamide*—
Studies in humans have not been done.
Studies in rats treated with high doses of chlorpropamide (125 mg/kg) for 6 to 12 months showed varying degrees of spermatogenesis suppression.

*Gliclazide*—
Studies in humans have not been done.
Studies in female rats and the first generation offspring of treated male and female rats showed no evidence of impaired fertility.

*Glipizide*—
Studies in humans have not been done.
Studies in male and female rats given 75 times the maximum human dose showed no evidence of impaired fertility.

*Glyburide*—
Studies in humans have not been done.
Studies in rats and rabbits given 500 times the human dose have not shown evidence of impaired fertility.

Pregnancy—Chlorpropamide crosses the placenta; glyburide does not significantly cross the placenta, and it is not known whether other sulfonylureas cross the placenta. Use of insulin rather than sulfonylurea antidiabetic agents during pregnancy allows for the maintenance of blood glucose concentrations that are as close to normal as possible. Abnormal blood glucose levels have been associated with a higher incidence of congenital abnormalities during early pregnancy, and with increased perinatal morbidity and mortality later in pregnancy. Adequate and well-controlled studies in humans have not been done to determine whether sulfonylureas are teratogenic. It remains possible that sulfonylureas cause congenital malformations if they cross the placenta, but current data leave unresolved the issue of whether the abnormalities are due to poor glucose control or to sulfonylurea treatment. Generally, sulfonylureas are not recommended during pregnancy. In the rare case that sulfonylureas are used during pregnancy, they should be discontinued to allow an interval before delivery appropriate for the particular sulfonylurea being used because of the risk that they will cause insulin release and hypoglycemia in the neonate at delivery.

*Acetohexamide*—
Adequate and well-controlled studies in humans have not been done.
Acetohexamide has been shown to be teratogenic in animal studies when large doses were administered.
FDA Pregnancy Category C.

*Chlorpropamide*—
Chlorpropamide crosses the placenta. Adequate and well-controlled studies have not been done in humans. Low doses (250 mg a day or less) of chlorpropamide have been used in pregnant women without adverse effects. The manufacturer recommends discontinuing chlorpropamide at least one month before expected delivery date.

Using an *in vitro* method and whole embryo mouse culture, one study compared the difference between growth in embryos bathed in hypoglycemic and euglycemic chlorpropamide-treated rat serums. The teratologic evaluation of the treated early somite mouse embryos showed malformations and growth retardation at doses similar to human therapeutic concentrations, which suggested that the teratogenicity was due to chlorpropamide and not to hypoglycemia; untreated mouse embryos showed normal development.

FDA Pregnancy Category C.

*Gliclazide*—
Studies in humans have not been done. Gliclazide is not recommended for use during pregnancy.
No teratogenic effects were found in studies of mice and rabbits. Embryotoxicity was not seen in studies of rats. However, a significant decrease in offspring viability at 48 hours was seen when pregnant females were treated up to delivery. It is unclear how this relates or if it applies to humans.

*Glipizide*—
Studies in humans have not been done. Glipizide should be discontinued at least 1 month before the expected delivery date.

Studies in rats have shown glipizide to be fetotoxic at all doses from 5 to 50 mg/kg; the fetotoxicity is thought to be due to the pharmacologic hypoglycemic effect during the perinatal period. No teratogenic effects were found in studies in rats and rabbits.

FDA Pregnancy Category C.

*Glyburide*—
Glyburide does not significantly cross the placenta according to an *in vitro* study using human placentas. Studies in humans have not been done. Use should be discontinued at least 2 weeks before the expected delivery date.

Studies in rats and rabbits given up to 500 times the human dose have produced no evidence of teratogenicity.

FDA Pregnancy Category B *(Micronase, Glynase)*.

FDA Pregnancy Category C *(Diabeta)*.

*Tolazamide*—
Studies in humans have not been done. Use should be discontinued at least 2 weeks before the expected delivery date.

Studies in rats given 10 times the human dose have shown tolazamide to cause reduced litter sizes. No teratogenic effects were found. High doses of 100 mg/kg a day also produced reduced litter sizes and increased perinatal mortality in pups.

FDA Pregnancy Category C.

*Tolbutamide*—
Studies in humans have not been done. Use should be discontinued at least 2 weeks before the expected delivery date.

Studies in rats given doses of tolbutamide that were 25 to 100 times greater than the human dose have shown teratogenic effects, such as ocular and bone abnormalities, and increased mortality in the offspring. Repeat studies in rabbits showed no teratogenic effects.

FDA Pregnancy Category C.

Delivery—Prolonged severe hypoglycemia lasting from 4 to 10 days has been reported in neonates born to mothers who were receiving a sulfonylurea antidiabetic agent at the time of delivery. This effect has been reported more frequently with those agents with longer half-lives, such as chlorpropamide. If sulfonylureas are used during pregnancy, they should be discontinued according to the manufacturer's labeling.

**Breast-feeding**
Chlorpropamide and tolbutamide are distributed into breast milk and potentially may cause hypoglycemia in the infant. It is not known if acetohexamide, gliclazide, glipizide, glyburide, or tolazamide is distributed into breast milk.

*Chlorpropamide*: Chlorpropamide has been found to be distributed into breast milk at a concentration of 5 mcg per mL after 5 hours for a single 500-mg dose (after 5 hours, blood concentration for a single dose of 250 mg chlorpropamide is 30 mcg per mL); therefore, its use during breast-feeding is not recommended. Its effect on the nursing infant is not known.

*Tolbutamide*: Tolbutamide was distributed into breast milk at a concentration averaging 3 and 18 mcg per mL in two patients taking 500 mg twice a day (milk: plasma ratio of 0.09 and 0.4, respectively). The effect on the nursing infants is not known. The American Academy of Pediatrics considers tolbutamide to be compatible with breast-feeding.

**Pediatrics**
Oral antidiabetic agents are not effective in insulin-dependent (juvenile-onset; type I) diabetes. Because type II diabetes occurs rarely in this age group, very little or no published pediatrics-specific information is available. Safety and efficacy have not been established.

**Geriatrics**
In general, no overall difference in safety or efficacy was apparent in persons over 65 years of age when compared to persons younger than 65 years of age taking sulfonylureas for diabetes mellitus. Lower doses are used initially because of possible increased sensitivity to these agents due to age-related metabolism and excretion changes; the steady state concentration of extended-release glipizide has been delayed for 1 or 2 days in elderly patients. The risk of adverse reactions is relatively low when other factors for toxicity, including liver and kidney disease and known drug interactions, are considered. Special counseling with emphasis on hydration, diet, and exercise may be necessary because of the greater risk of hypoglycemia in this age group. Special instruction to recognize hypoglycemia may be needed because early warning adrenergic symptoms of hypoglycemia (such as sweating, weakness, tachycardia, and nervousness) are absent in many patients. Hypoglycemia manifests as neurological symptoms (such as headache, irritability, mental confusion, unusual tiredness, and drowsiness) and may be more prolonged and severe in the elderly. Combining antidiabetic agents (sulfonylureas with metformin or insulin) or using long-acting sulfonylureas, such as chlorpropamide and glyburide, is most often associated with hypoglycemia in elderly patients and is not generally recommended; shorter acting sulfonylureas cause fewer problems. Also, instructions may be needed to help the patient monitor urine or blood glucose if visual problems are present.

Geriatric patients may be more likely to develop a reversible SIADH (syndrome of inappropriate antidiuretic hormone) from the use of chlorpropamide. The incidence of SIADH is rare and occurs with greater incidence when thiazides are taken concurrently with chlorpropamide than when chlorpropamide is taken alone (10% versus 3%, respectively). In one study, women over 70 years of age were affected 10 times more often than women under 60 years of age when thiazides were used concurrently with chlorpropamide. It is not thought to be a gender-oriented effect. SIADH has been rarely reported with tolbutamide.

**Drug interactions and/or related problems**
The following drug interactions and/or related problems have been selected on the basis of their potential clinical significance (possible mechanism in parentheses where appropriate)—not necessarily inclusive (» = major clinical significance):

Note: Combinations containing any of the following medications, depending on the amount present, may also interact with this medication.

There is an increased chance of hypoglycemia occurring if more than one hypoglycemia-causing agent is used concurrently with sulfonylureas. If the need exists to administer any medications that may affect metabolic or glycemic control of diabetes mellitus, blood glucose concentrations should be monitored by the patient or health care professional. This is particularly important when any medication is added or removed from an established drug regimen. Subsequent adjustments in diet or antidiabetic agent dosage or both may be necessary; these adjustments may differ depending on the severity of the diabetes.

» Alcohol
(a disulfiram-like reaction, which is characterized primarily by flushing of the face, neck, and arms, may occur with any of the sulfonylureas when alcohol is ingested concurrently, but has not been reported with glipizide; risk is lowest with tolbutamide and glyburide, and highest with chlorpropamide for which it has occurred 12 hours after a single 250-mg dose of chlorpropamide and 40 mL of 18% alcohol)

(the risk of hypoglycemia may be increased or prolonged when moderate or large amounts of alcohol have been consumed concurrently with sulfonylurea antidiabetic agents use; small amounts of alcohol taken with meals do not usually result in hypoglycemia)

Allopurinol
(increased risk of hypoglycemia due to inhibition of renal tubular secretion of chlorpropamide; closer monitoring required)

Angiotensin-converting enzyme agents, such as:
  Captopril or
  Enalapril
(the mechanism of enhanced hypoglycemia that occurs rarely is unknown; concurrent use need not be avoided and may be used advantageously in the treatment of diabetes mellitus; however, the dosage of the sulfonylurea may need to be modified in some patients)

» Anticoagulants, coumarin- or indandione-derivative
(the mechanism is not completely known; however, mutual interactions of both agents have increased their anticoagulant and hypoglycemic effects. A hypoglycemic effect may be partially due to the decrease in hepatic metabolism of sulfonylureas caused by anticoagulants, which can prolong the half-life of the sulfonylureas two- to three-fold. An increased protein binding displacement of anticoagulants by sulfonylureas has increased prothrombin times, but because metabolism of dicumarol is increased and can result in up to a 50% reduced half-life, an increase, decrease, or no effect on coagulation may result. Although these effects have been reported specifically for chlorpropamide, tolbutamide, and dicumarol, concurrent use of all sulfonylurea antidiabetic agents with anticoagulants should be well-monitored and dosage adjustments of both agents may be required)

(glipizide and glyburide have lower plasma concentrations and exhibit only nonionic plasma protein binding; therefore, they may be less susceptible to displacement from plasma proteins by other medications that exhibit ionic binding to plasma proteins; studies have not been done and caution is still warranted)

» Antifungal, azoles, systemic, such as:
  Miconazole
  Fluconazole
(severe hypoglycemia has been reported shortly after concurrent use of tolbutamide, glyburide, and glipizide with these oral azole antifungal agents. In one study, glipizide and fluconazole increased the

area-under-the-time curve [AUC] of glipizide 56.9% [range, 35–81%]. Also, hypoglycemia has been reported for gliclazide taken concurrently with miconazole, but not with fluconazole)

Appetite suppressants
(when appetite suppressants and a concurrent dietary regimen are used, blood glucose concentrations may be altered in diabetic patients; dosage adjustment of antidiabetic agent may be necessary during and after therapy)

» Asparaginase or
» Corticosteroids or
» Diuretics, thiazide or
» Lithium
(these medications have intrinisic hyperglycemic activity in both diabetics and nondiabetics; dosage of the sulfonylurea may need to be modified during and after treatment. Some studies of lithium have reported hypoglycemia)

(concurrent treatment using thiazides with chlorpropamide, and more rarely with tolbutamide, may increase the chance of hyponatremia and hypo-osmolality, especially in patients over 70 years of age)

Barbiturates
(chlorpropamide may prolong the effect of barbiturates and barbiturates may prolong the effect of gliclazide; other sulfonylureas may also exhibit these effects; dosage adjustment of the sulfonylurea or the barbiturate may be necessary)

» Beta-adrenergic blocking agents, including ophthalmics, if significant absorption occurs
(beta-adrenergic blocking agents may decrease the hypoglycemic effects of sulfonylureas to some extent by inhibition of insulin secretion, modification of carbohydrate metabolism, and increased peripheral insulin resistance, leading to hyperglycemia; an adjustment in dose may be required. Other mechanisms that control the normal physiological response to a fall in blood glucose may be affected also, such as a blocked catecholamine mediated response to hypoglycemia [glycogenolysis and mobilization of glucose], thereby prolonging the time it takes to achieve euglycemia and increasing the risk of a severe hypoglycemic reaction. Selective beta$_1$-adrenergic blocking agents [such as, acebutolol, atenolol, betaxolol, bisoprolol, and metoprolol] exhibit the above actions to a lesser extent; however, any of the agents can blunt some of the symptoms of developing hypoglycemia, such as increased heart rate or tremors [increased sweating and blood pressure may not be altered], making detection of this complication more difficult)

» Cimetidine or
» Ranitidine
(these agents, in therapeutic doses, can significantly decrease the postprandial rise in blood glucose and increase the hypoglycemic effects of glipizide, gliclazide, and glyburide in diabetics; also, cimetidine has decreased tolbutamide's elimination and increased absorption of tolbutamide and glyburide; ranitidine did not affect glyburide's area-under-the-time curve [AUC]; close monitoring for dose adjustments of sulfonylureas may be needed when these agents are added or withdrawn)

» Ciprofloxacin
(use of glyburide with ciprofloxacin has caused hypoglycemia; since the mechanism is not understood, similar effects with other sulfonylurea antidiabetic agents should be considered when these medications are used together)

» Cyclosporine
(glipizide may significantly increase the plasma concentration of cyclosporine by reducing its metabolism; dose reduction of cyclosporine may be necessary; similar effects may be possible with other sulfonylureas)

» Guanethidine or
» Monoamine oxidase (MAO) inhibitors, including furazolidone, procarbazine, and selegiline or
» Quinidine or
» Quinine or
» Salicylates, in large doses
(these medications have intrinsic hypoglycemic activity in both diabetics and nondiabetics, possibly severe with quinine, quinidine, or salicylates in high doses but is unlikely with low doses of salicylates. Also, salicylates may interfere with chlorpropamide's renal excretion. Salicylate dose may need to be reduced)

Hemolytics, other (See *Appendix II*)
(concurrent use may increase the incidence of sulfonylurea-induced hemolysis through a possible additive effect; reported cases of hemolysis effects have rarely occurred with chlorpropamide or tolbutamide and have not been reported with other sulfonylureas)

Hepatic enzyme inducers, such as:
Rifabutin
Rifampin
(metabolism of sulfonylureas may be increased due to stimulation of hepatic microsomal enzymes; dosage adjustments may be necessary during and after concurrent treatment)

(drug interaction data for rifabutin are not available; it is structurally related to rifampin but appears to be a less potent enzyme inducer of the hepatic cytochrome P-450 system than is rifampin. It is recommended that patients taking rifabutin concurrently with sulfonylurea antidiabetic agents be monitored since the significance of possible drug interactions is not known)

Hepatic enzyme inhibitors, such as:
» Chloramphenicol
(metabolism of sulfonylureas may be decreased due to inhibition of hepatic microsomal enzymes; dosage adjustments may be necessary during and after concurrent use)

(also, chlorpropamide's half-life has increased up to 146 hours; this may be partially due to interference by chloramphenicol with renal excretion of chlorpropamide)

Highly protein-bound medications such as:
Anti-inflammatory drugs, nonsteroidal (NSAIDs), such as phenylbutazone
Clofibrate
Probenecid
Sulfinpyrazone
Sulfonamides
(these medications enhance the hypoglycemic effects of sulfonylureas when given concurrently; the mechanism is unknown but may be due to displacement of sulfonylureas from protein binding sites and alterations in their renal excretion; concurrent use need not be avoided; however, the dosage of the sulfonylurea may need to be modified in some patients)

(clofibrate also shows intrinsic hypoglycemic effects by causing increased insulin sensitivity and has been used advantageously in the treatment of diabetes mellitus; also, clofibrate has intrinsic antidiuretic effects that have been used to treat diabetes insipidus; this effect may be lessened with concurrent use of glyburide or increased with concurrent use of chlorpropamide or tolbutamide)

(sulfinpyrazone and phenylbutazone have been shown to inhibit the hepatic metabolism of tolbutamide; they also inhibit the renal excretion of acetohexamide but not of glyburide; the effect on other sulfonylureas by NSAIDs [other than ibuprofen, naproxen, sulindac, and tolmetin, which do not affect sulfonylureas] is not known)

(NSAIDs inhibit synthesis of prostaglandin E, which inhibits endogenous insulin secretion; this increases basal insulin secretion, the response to a glucose load, and the hypoglycemic effect of insulin secretion; dosage adjustment of each medicine used may be necessary following chronic use of NSAIDs)

(glipizide and glyburide have lower plasma concentrations and exhibit nonionic plasma protein binding only; therefore, these sulfonylureas may be less susceptible to displacement from plasma proteins by other medications that exhibit ionic binding to plasma proteins)

Hyperglycemia-causing agents, such as:
Calcium channel blockers
Clonidine
Danazol
Dextrothyroxine
Diazoxide, parenteral
Estrogen
Estrogen–progestin-containing oral contraceptives
Furosemide
Glucagon
Growth hormone
Hydantoin anticonvulsants
Isoniazid
Morphine
Nicotinic acid
Phenothiazines, such as chlorpromazine
Sympathomimetics, such as beta-adrenergic agents or epinephrine
Thyroid hormones
(these medications may change many factors that affect the metabolic control of glucose concentrations and, unless the changes can be controlled with diet, may necessitate an increased sulfonylurea dose and regular monitoring)

(hyperglycemic effects have resulted with doses greater than 100 mg of chlorpromazine; other phenothiazines or lower doses of chlorpromazine have not had this effect. However, caution may be warranted for concurrent use of phenothiazines with sulfonylureas)

(isoniazid usually causes hyperglycemia, but hypoglycemia has occurred in some diabetics taking tolbutamide; a decrease in dose of tolbutamide is then warranted)

(beta-adrenergic agonists increase risk of hyperglycemia by increasing glycogenolysis. If given during pregnancy, these agents may cause hypoglycemia in the fetus, independent of maternal blood glucose concentrations, by causing a depletion of fetal glycogen stores; sulfonylurea dose adjustment may be necessary if these agents are given together during pregnancy)

Hypoglycemia-causing agents, such as:
Anabolic steroids
Androgens
Bromocriptine
Disopyramide
Pyridoxine
Tetracycline
Theophylline
(these medications may change metabolic control of glucose concentrations and, unless the changes can be controlled with diet, may necessitate a decreased sulfonylurea dose; patients susceptible to hypoglycemia should be closely monitored)

Insulin
(sulfonylurea agents chronically stimulate the pancreatic beta cell to release insulin and increase receptor and tissue sensitivity to insulin; although concurrent use of the medications with insulin may increase the hypoglycemic response, the effect may be unpredictable)

(although the combination has been used to treat a select group of diabetic patients whose condition is not well-controlled with either agent alone, many studies have shown there is generally no additional benefit from using oral agents for the treatment of IDDM)

» Octreotide
(octreotide suppresses pancreatic insulin and counterregulatory hormones, such as glucagon and growth hormone, and delays or lowers glucose absorption from the gastrointestinal tract; depending on the dose, concurrent use with sulfonylureas may cause hypo- or hyperglycemia so that dose adjustment of the sulfonylurea may be needed; octreotide has been used beneficially for sulfonylurea overdose or insulinomas)

» Pentamidine
(pentamidine has a toxic effect on pancreatic beta cells resulting in a biphasic effect on glucose concentration, i.e., initial insulin release and hypoglycemia followed by hypoinsulinemia and hyperglycemia with continued use of pentamidine; dose alterations and continued use of sulfonylureas should be considered)

**Laboratory value alterations**
The following have been selected on the basis of their potential clinical significance (possible effect in parentheses where appropriate)—not necessarily inclusive (» = major clinical significance):

With diagnostic test results
Blood urea nitrogen (BUN)
(acetohexamide produces a reaction with diacetyl and falsely elevates results of this test)

Creatinine, serum
(acetohexamide has significantly increased the creatinine concentration for some laboratory tests by as much as 2.2 or 3.3 mg/dL and as little as 0.3 mg/dL for others)

Protein, total, serum
(tolbutamide interferes with sulfosalicylic acid test by causing turbidity)

» Sodium iodide I 123 or
» Sodium iodide I 131
(tolbutamide may decrease thyroidal uptake of I 123 or I 131; withdrawal of tolbutamide 1 week or longer before reactive iodine uptake test is necessary to prevent interference)

With physiology/laboratory test values
Alanine aminotransferase, serum (ALT [SGPT]) or
Alkaline phosphatase, serum or
Aspartate aminotransferase (AST [SGOT]) or
Lactate dehydrogenase (LDH)
(values may be mildly increased, usually not associated with clinical symptoms, and may be due to the sulfonylurea or to the underlying diabetes; however, hepatitis or cholestatic jaundice is caused rarely by sulfonylureas and should be considered with high values)

Bile, urine or
Bilirubin, urine
(concentrations may be mildly increased and usually do not present with clinical symptoms; however, hepatitis or cholestatic jaundice is caused rarely by sulfonylureas and should be considered with high values)

C-peptide, serum
(increased concentration for the first three months of sulfonylurea treatment; can return to pretreatment values long-term [18 months in one study])

Osmolality, urine or
Sodium, serum
(may be decreased with acetohexamide, gliclazide, glipizide, glyburide, or tolazamide because of their slight diuretic effect)
(chlorpropamide increases osmolality because of its antidiuretic effect and has caused dilutional hyponatremia)
(sodium may also decrease in response to hyperglycemia; each 100 mg/dL (5.51 mmol/L) increase in blood glucose decreases serum sodium by 1.6 mEq/L)

Uric acid, serum
(serum concentrations are considerably reduced by use of acetohexamide due to its mild uricosuric effect)

Urine collection, 24-hour
(quantity is mildly increased due to normal slight diuretic response by acetohexamide, gliclazide, glipizide, glyburide, or tolazamide)
(decreased with chlorpropamide due to its antidiuretic effect)

*For gliclazide*
Factors VIII, XI
(concentrations may be decreased with gliclazide)
Tissue plasminogen activator
(concentrations may be increased with gliclazide)

**Medical considerations/Contraindications**
The medical considerations/contraindications included have been selected on the basis of their potential clinical significance (reasons given in parentheses where appropriate)—not necessarily inclusive (» = major clinical significance).

*Except under special circumstances, this medication should not be used when the following medical problems exist:*

For all oral sulfonylurea antidiabetic agents
» Acidosis, significant or
» Burns, severe or
» Diabetic coma or
» Diabetic ketoacidosis, with or without coma or
» Hyperosmolar nonketotic coma or
» Surgery, major or
» Trauma, severe or
» Any other condition that causes severe blood glucose fluctuations or
» Any other condition in which insulin needs change rapidly
(fluctuations in blood glucose levels associated with certain disease states are more closely controlled by titration of insulin dosing, possibly on a short-term basis, rather than with oral antidiabetic agents, such as sulfonylureas)

*Risk-benefit should be considered when the following medical problems exist:*

For all oral sulfonylurea antidiabetic agents
Allergy to oral antidiabetic agents, sulfonamides, or thiazide-type diuretics
» Diarrhea, severe or
» Gastroparesis or
» Intestinal obstruction or
» Vomiting, prolonged or
» Other conditions causing delayed food absorption
(delayed stomach emptying or intestinal movement or vomiting may require modification of a sulfonylurea dose or a change to insulin therapy)
» Hepatic disease
(sulfonylureas that are extensively metabolized in the liver should not be used when there is hepatic impairment; hypoglycemia that develops may be more severe when these sulfonylureas are being used)

» Hyperglycemia-causing conditions, such as:
  Female hormone changes or
  Fever, high or
  Hyperadrenalism, not optimally controlled or
  Infection, severe or
  Psychological stress
    (these conditions, by increasing blood glucose, may increase the need for more frequent glucose monitoring and for a permanent or temporary dose increase for sulfonylureas or a change to insulin if blood glucose is uncontrolled)

» Hyperthyroidism, not optimally controlled
    (hyperthyroidism aggravates diabetes mellitus by increasing plasma glycogen concentrations and glucose absorption, and by impairing glucose tolerance; thyroid hormone has dose-dependent biphasic effects on glycogenolysis and glycogeneogenesis; hyperthyroidism can make glycemic control difficult until the patient is euthyroid; patients with this condition may require an increased dose of the sulfonylurea until euthyroidism is achieved)

» Hypoglycemia-causing conditions, such as:
  Adrenal insufficiency, not optimally controlled or
  Debilitated physical condition or
  Malnourishment or
  Pituitary insufficiency, not optimally controlled
    (these conditions, which inherently predispose patients to the risk of developing hypoglycemia, increase the patient's risk of developing severe hypoglycemia with concurrent treatment of sulfonylurea antidiabetic agents; reduced sulfonylurea dose or more frequent monitoring may be required for patients with these conditions)

  Hypothyroidism, not optimally controlled
    (sulfonylurea metabolism may be reduced with hypothyroidism and may mildly aggravate this underlying condition, which already exhibits reduced glucose absorption and altered glucose and lipoprotein metabolism [tolbutamide has goitrogenic properties]; low doses of a sulfonylurea may be needed when hypothyroid conditions exist and an increase in sulfonylurea dosing may be required when initiating thyroid treatment; euglycemic control may be difficult until the patient is euthyroid)

» Renal function impairment
    (use of sulfonylureas increases the risk of possibly prolonged hypoglycemia with renal function impairment)
    (the elimination half-lives of all the sulfonylureas are increased with renal function impairment, especially where tubular involvement predominates or if azotemia is present, and less so if the glomerular filtration rate is mildly reduced; sulfonylureas with longer half-lives, such as acetohexamide and chlorpropamide, are not recommended since renal excretion is important in the elimination of chlorpropamide and the active metabolite of acetohexamide [hydroxyhexamide]; weakly active metabolites of tolazamide and glyburide may also accumulate, particularly in those patients with a creatinine clearance of less than 30 mL/min [0.5 mL/sec]; sulfonylureas with shorter half-lives, such as gliclazide, glipizide, or tolbutamide, should present fewer problems but should be used cautiously in renal impairment)

*For chlorpropamide or tolbutamide*
» Congestive heart failure
    (fluid retention, caused rarely by chlorpropamide and even less often by tolbutamide, may result in hyponatremia and precipitate congestive heart failure in the elderly when other risk factors for congestive heart failure are present)

**Patient monitoring**
The following may be especially important in patient monitoring (other tests may be warranted in some patients, depending on condition; » = major clinical significance):

» Blood glucose determinations
    (blood or plasma glucose reflects the current degree of metabolic control and should be routinely self-monitored by the patient at home and by the physician [every 3 months or more often when patient is not stabilized] to confirm that blood glucose concentration is maintained within agreed upon targets by the selected diet and dosing regimen; this is particularly important during dosage adjustments. Self-monitoring of blood glucose by the patient may require testing multiple times during the day or once to several times a week)
    (caution in interpreting blood glucose concentrations is needed because normal whole blood glucose values are approximately 15% lower than plasma glucose values; it is also laboratory and method specific. Normal fasting whole blood glucose for adults of all ages is 65 to 95 mg/dL [3.6 to 5.3 mmol/L]. Normal fasting serum glucose is 70 to 105 mg/dL [3.9 to 5.8 mmol/L] for adults younger than 60 years of age and 80 to 115 mg/dL [4.4 to 6.4 mmol/L] for adults 60 years of age and older. For pregnant diabetic women, a normal fasting serum glucose is less than 105 mg/dL [5.8 mmol/L] and a fasting whole blood glucose is less than 120 mg/dL [6.7 mmol/L]. Goals of conventional sulfonylurea antidiabetic therapy are based on the absence of symptoms of hyper- and hypoglycemia)
    (capillary blood glucose measurement provides important information when done properly, but caution is warranted because of potential errors in technique and readings; it has been suggested that the values be relied upon only if the reported glucose concentration for stable diabetics is between 75 mg/dL and 325 mg/dL [4.12 mmol/L and 17.88 mmol/L, respectively])

» Complete blood count (CBC)
    (leukopenia, agranulocytosis, thrombocytopenia, and hemolytic and aplastic anemias have rarely occurred with sulfonylureas)

  Glucose, urine or
  Ketones, urine
    (if blood glucose concentrations exceed 200 mg/dL [11.1 mmol/L], monitoring of urine for the presence of glucose and ketones may be necessary; normalization of glucose in the urine generally lags quantitatively behind serum glucose concentrations; test methods are generally capable of detecting serum glucose concentrations greater than 180 mg/dL [10 mmol/L])

» Glycosylated hemoglobin (hemoglobin $A_{1c}$) determinations
    (hemoglobin $A_{1c}$ values [normal whole blood hemoglobin $A_{1c}$ is approximately 4 to 6% of total hemoglobin; specific values are laboratory-dependent] reflect the metabolic control over the preceding 3 months, but assessment of this parameter does not eliminate the need for daily blood glucose monitoring. Hemoglobin $A_{1c}$ may be falsely elevated in unstable diabetics when the intermediate precursor is elevated [i.e., in alcoholism] and falsely lowered in conditions of shortened red blood cell lifespan [i.e., in anemia and acute or chronic blood loss] or in patients with hemoglobinopathies [i.e., sickle cell])

  Osmolarity determinations, plasma or
  Sodium concentrations, serum
    (may be necessary with use of chlorpropamide or tolbutamide, especially for the elderly or when thiazides are being taken concurrently)

  pH measurements, serum or
  Potassium concentrations, serum
    (determinations may be important if patient is hypoglycemic and ketoacidotic)

## Side/Adverse Effects

Note: It has been suggested by some studies, including the University Group Diabetes Program (UGDP), that certain sulfonylurea antidiabetic agents increased cardiovascular mortality in diabetic patients, a population that already has a greater risk of cardiovascular disease and mortality when blood glucose is not controlled. Other studies have not reached a similar conclusion and have in fact suggested that control of elevated blood glucose with sulfonylurea antidiabetic agents may lessen the danger of cardiovascular disease and mortality. Despite questions regarding the interpretation of the results and the adequacy of the experimental design, the findings of the UGDP study provide an adequate basis for caution, especially for certain high risk patients with coronary artery disease, congestive heart failure, or angina pectoris. If sulfonylurea treatment is necessary, glyburide or gliclazide may be the preferred sulfonylureas for use in patients at risk for conditions causing cardiac hypoxia. The patient should be informed of the potential risks and advantages of sulfonylurea antidiabetic agents and of alternative modes of therapy.

The following side/adverse effects have been selected on the basis of their potential clinical significance (possible signs and symptoms in parentheses where appropriate)—not necessarily inclusive:

### Those indicating need for medical attention
Incidence more frequent
  *Hypoglycemia—mild, including nocturnal hypoglycemia* (anxiety; behavior change, similar to drunkenness; blurred vision; cold sweats; confusion; cool pale skin; difficulty in concentrating; drowsiness; excessive hunger; fast heartbeat; headache; nausea; nervousness; nightmares; restless sleep; shakiness; slurred speech; unusual tiredness or weakness); *weight gain*

Note: Predisposing factors related to diet, exercise, age, or concurrent use of other hypoglycemia-causing drugs (including insulin) increase the chances of hypoglycemic episodes occurring. The occurrence of a recent episode of *hypoglycemia* may lessen the symptoms of a second episode. In the elderly, *hypoglycemia* symptoms are variable and harder to identify. Furthermore, *nocturnal hypoglycemia* may be asymptomatic in 33% or more of affected patients. Hypoglycemic episodes are experienced by 20% of the patients taking sulfonylureas every 6 months (6% experiencing monthly episodes).

*Weight gain* is greater with combination use of insulin and sulfonylureas than with sulfonylurea therapy alone. Gliclazide alone, or metformin in combination with sulfonylureas, usually results in less weight gain than other sulfonylureas and has exhibited a weight loss effect.

Incidence less frequent
**Erythema multiforme or exfoliative dermatitis** (peeling of skin; skin redness, itching, or rash); **hypoglycemia—severe** (convulsions or coma)

*For chlorpropamide or, rarely, tolbutamide*
**Dilutional hyponatremia, hypo-osmolality, or syndrome of inappropriate antidiuretic hormone (SIADH)** (depression; dizziness; headache; lethargy; nausea; swelling or puffiness of face, ankles, or hands with occasional progression to seizures, coma, or stupor)

Note: The incidence of *severe hypoglycemia* episodes is 0.22 episodes per 1000 patient-years. It occurs more often with long-acting sulfonylureas, such as chlorpropamide or glyburide, when other predisposing factors or conditions are present, and can be relapsing and prolonged; glyburide results in a higher fatality rate than does chlorpropamide.

Incidence rare
**Anemia, aplastic or hemolytic** (continuing and unexplained tiredness or weakness, headache, shortness of breath brought on by exercise); **blood dyscrasias, specifically, agranulocytosis, leukopenia, pancytopenia** (fever and sore throat; pale skin; unusual bleeding or bruising; unusual tiredness, or weakness); **cholestasis, cholestatic jaundice, hepatic function impairment, hepatic porphyria, hepatitis, or porphyria cutanea tarda** (dark urine; fluid-filled skin blisters; itching of the skin; light-colored stools; sensitivity to the sun; skin thinness; yellow eyes or skin); **eosinophilia** (chills; increased sweating; general feeling of ill health; increased production of sputum; shortness of breath; chest pain; blood in sputum); **thrombocytopenia** (unusual bleeding or bruising)

Note: Sulfonylurea-induced *blood dyscrasias and dermatologic conditions* generally occur within the initial six weeks of therapy and are thought to be hypersensitivity reactions.

**Those indicating need for medical attention only if they continue or are bothersome**
Incidence more frequent
**Changes in sensation of taste; dizziness; drowsiness; gastrointestinal disturbances** (constipation; diarrhea; flatulence; heartburn; loss of or increase in appetite; nausea; stomach fullness; vomiting); **headache; polyuria** (increased volume of urine and frequency of urination)

Incidence less frequent or rare
**Photosensitivity** (increased sensitivity of skin to sunlight)

## Patient Consultation

As an aid to patient consultation, refer to *Advice for the Patient, Antidiabetic Agents, Sulfonylurea (Systemic)*.
In providing consultation, consider emphasizing the following selected information (» = major clinical significance):

**Before using this medication**
» Conditions affecting use, especially:
Allergy to sulfonylurea antidiabetic agents, sulfonamides, or thiazides
Pregnancy—Chlorpropamide crosses the placenta. Should not be used during pregnancy, especially when insulin is available. In the rare cases that a sulfonylurea is used, chlorpropamide and glipizide should be discontinued at least 1 month before delivery date and other sulfonylureas stopped at least 2 weeks before delivery date. Importance of controlling and monitoring blood glucose concentrations before, during, and after pregnancy by adjusting antidiabetic agent dosing in order to help prevent maternal and fetal problems, including fetal macrosomnia, anomalies, and hyperglycemia
Breast-feeding—Chlorpropamide and tolbutamide are distributed into breast milk, and their effect on breast-fed infants is not known; some physicians believe that tolbutamide is compatible with breast-feeding; it is not known if other sulfonylureas are distributed into breast milk
Use in children—Safety and efficacy have not been established. Published information is not available for this age group as NIDDM rarely occurs

Use in the elderly—May be more susceptible to hypoglycemia, especially when treated with glyburide and chlorpropamide, or when other hypoglycemia-causing agents are concurrently being prescribed along with sulfonylureas; also, the elderly have higher risk of developing hyponatremia or a reversible syndrome of inappropriate antidiuretic hormone when treated with chlorpropamide

Other medications, especially alcohol; asparaginase; azole antifungals; beta-adrenergic blocking agents; chloramphenicol; cimetidine; ciprofloxacin; corticosteroids; coumarin- or indandione- derivative anticoagulants; cyclosporine; guanethidine; lithium; MAO inhibitors including furazolidone, procarbazine, and selegiline; octreotide; pentamidine; quinidine; quinine; ranitidine; salicylates, large doses; or thiazide diuretics

Other medical problems, especially conditions causing delayed food absorption including gastroparesis, intestinal obstruction, prolonged vomiting, or severe diarrhea; conditions that cause severe blood glucose fluctuations or rapidly change insulin needs including diabetic coma, diabetic ketoacidosis, hyperosmolar nonketotic coma, major surgery, severe burns, severe trauma, or significant acidosis; hyperglycemia-causing conditions including female hormone changes, high fever, not optimally controlled hyperadrenalism, psychological stress, or severe infection; hypoglycemia-causing conditions including hepatic disease, debilitated physical condition, malnourishment, not optimally controlled adrenal or pituitary insufficiency or hyperthyroidism; renal function impairment; in addition, for chlorpropamide or tolbutamide, congestive heart failure

**Proper use of this medication**
» Compliance with therapy, including not taking more or less medication than directed; alternative dosing or therapy changes for modifications in diet, exercise, and sick day management
» Proper dosing
Missed dose: Taking as soon as possible; not taking if almost time for next dose; not doubling doses
» Proper storage

**Precautions while using this medication**
Regular visits to physician to check progress
» *Carefully following special instructions of health care team*
Discussing use of alcohol and tobacco
Not taking other medications unless discussed with physician
Getting counseling for family to help assist diabetic; also, special counseling for pregnancy planning and contraception
Making travel plans to include preparedness for diabetic emergencies and keeping meal times near the usual times with changing time zones
Wearing sunscreen and protective clothing to protect against sunburn and photosensitivity
» Preparing for and understanding what to do in case of an emergency by carrying medical history and current drug list, wearing medical identification, keeping nonexpired glucagon kit and needles and quick-acting sugar close by
» Recognizing what brings on symptoms of hypoglycemia, such as delaying or missing a meal, exercising more than usual, drinking significant amounts of alcohol, taking certain medicines, using too much antidiabetic medication, such as insulin or sulfonylurea, being sick, including vomiting or diarrhea
» Knowing what to do if symptoms of hypoglycemia occur, such as using glucagon, eating glucose tablets or gel, corn syrup, honey, or sugar cubes, or drinking fruit juice, nondiet soft drink, or dissolved sugar in water; also, eating small snack, such as crackers or half sandwich, when scheduled meal is longer than 1 hour away; not eating foods high in fat, such as chocolate, since fat slows gastric emptying
» Recognizing symptoms of hyperglycemia and ketoacidosis: blurred vision; drowsiness; dry mouth; flushed, dry skin; fruit-like breath odor; increased urination (frequency and volume); ketones in urine; loss of appetite; somnolence (sleepiness); stomachache, nausea, or vomiting; tiredness; troubled breathing (rapid and deep); unconsciousness; unusual thirst
» Recognizing what brings on symptoms of hyperglycemia, such as fever or infection; not taking enough insulin; skipping an insulin dose; exercising less than usual; taking certain medicines; overeating or not following meal plan
» Knowing what to do if symptoms of hyperglycemia occur, such as checking blood glucose and contacting a member of the health care team

**Side/adverse effects**
Signs of potential side effects, especially mild or severe hypoglycemia; weight gain; erythema multiforme or exfoliative dermatitis; aplastic or hemolytic anemia; blood dyscrasias; cholestasis; cholestatic jaun-

dice; hepatic function impairment; hepatic porphyria; hepatitis; or porphyria cutanea tarda; eosinophilia; thrombocytopenia; in addition, for chlorpropamide only—dilutional hyponatremia, hypo-osmolality, or syndrome of inappropriate antidiuretic hormone (SIADH)

## General Dosing Information

There is little evidence that one sulfonylurea is more effective in lowering blood glucose than another, especially between first and second generation sulfonylureas. Some pharmacokinetic differences between sulfonylureas may result in small qualitative and temporal differences that may make one medication more suitable in a certain situation. For instance, glyburide and gliclazide exert a better effect on fasting blood glucose than does glipizide (possibly due to glyburide's longer duration of action and effect on hepatic glucose suppression), which results in lowered nocturnal and morning blood glucose; glipizide has greater postprandial insulin release and lower postprandial blood glucose levels. Overall, the resulting blood glucose level reduction is similar between sulfonylureas.

Conservative initial and maintenance doses may be required in patients with medical problems that make them more sensitive to effects of sulfonylureas.

Secondary failure of oral antidiabetic therapy may occur in certain patients. This may be due to increasing severity of diabetes or to diminished responsiveness to the medication.

When adding a sulfonylurea to an insulin regimen that is poorly controlled with insulin alone, the insulin dose at times may be reduced 25 to 50%.

When adding a sulfonylurea to maximum doses of metformin or metformin to maximum doses of a sulfonylurea, even if primary or secondary failure of a sulfonylurea has occurred, the new medication should be added gradually and titrated to the lowest effective dose. Both agents should be discontinued and insulin should be initiated if the patient does not respond to maximum doses within 3 months (or less, depending on clinician's decision). No transition time is needed when transferring between sulfonylureas, metformin, or insulin, except with chlorpropamide, which may require a 2-week transition because of chlorpropamide's prolonged duration of action.

### Diet/Nutrition

Absorption of chlorpropamide or glipizide may be delayed if the medication is ingested with food, and should be taken 30 minutes before a meal. Gliclazide may be taken 30 minutes before a meal or with a meal but not after a meal. Furthermore, nonmicronized glyburide should not be taken with a diet high in fat; nonmicronized glyburide does not have any other dietary restrictions.

### For treatment of adverse effects and/or overdose

Recommended treatment consists of the following:

For mild to moderate hypoglycemia—
- Treating with immediate ingestion of a source of sugar, such as glucose gel, glucose tablets, fruit juice, corn syrup, non-diet soft drinks, honey, sugar cubes, or table sugar dissolved in water. A frequently used source of sugar is a glassful of orange juice.
- Documenting blood glucose and rechecking in 15 minutes.
- Counseling patient to seek medical assistance promptly.
- Closely monitoring for at least 3 to 5 days patients who develop hypoglycemia during use of chlorpropamide.

For severe hypoglycemia or acute overdose, including coma

Note: Glucose administration is the basis for treatment of hypoglycemia; however, an exposure to sudden or excessive hyperglycemia caused by an injection of hypertonic glucose solution may further stimulate the sulfonylurea-primed pancreas to release more insulin, worsening the hypoglycemia.

- Counseling patient to obtain emergency medical assistance immediately
- Immediately treating with 50 mL of 50% dextrose given intravenously to stabilize the patient. Then, administering a continuous infusion of 5 to 10% dextrose in water to maintain slight hyperglycemia (approximately 100 mg/dL blood glucose concentration) for up to 12 days. The intravenous glucose therapy should not be terminated suddenly. A central venous line for long-term use (24 to 48 hours) in cases of chlorpropamide overdose may be required. (Oral glucose cannot be relied upon to maintain euglycemia because 60% of an oral glucose dose is stored as hepatic glycogen with only 15% left for brain utilization and 15% for insulin-dependent tissues even though 75% of oral glucose is absorbed after 150 to 180 minutes.)
- Glucagon, 1 to 2 mg administered intramuscularly, is useful for fast onset of action to mobilize hepatic glucose stores but may be ineffective or variable in its effect if glycogen stores are depleted and must follow the use of glucose.

- Diazoxide therapy (200 mg orally every 4 hours or 300 mg intravenously over a 30-minute period every 4 hours) can be used for nonresponders to glucose therapy or for patients in a coma as an aid to glucose infusion to reduce hypoglycemia; patient should be monitored for sodium concentration and for hypotension.
- Emesis can be induced with ipecac syrup if sulfonylurea overdose is recent (within the past 30 minutes) if patient is alert, has an intact gag reflex, and is not obtunded or convulsing. Otherwise, gastric lavage after endotracheal tube placement is required.
- Gastric removal by administration of repeated doses of oral activated charcoal with appropriate cathartic, although the usefulness of this has not been established.
- Alkalinization of urine with sodium bicarbonate to pH of 8 can eliminate 80% of chlorpropamide over 24 hours, but is not useful with other sulfonylureas. Caution with concurrent use with diazoxide treatment because of possible significant sodium retention.
- Monitoring vital signs, arterial blood gases, blood glucose, and serum electrolytes (especially calcium, potassium, and sodium) as required. Initially, blood glucose concentrations should be monitored as frequently as every 1 to 3 hours. Blood urea nitrogen and serum creatinine concentrations should also be obtained.
- Cerebral edema—Managing with mannitol and dexamethasone.
- Hypokalemia—Managing with potassium supplements.
- Hospitalization for 6 to 91 hours (mean, 24 hours), because the hypoglycemia may be recurrent and prolonged; for chlorpropamide this period may be extended to 3 to 5 days or longer.
- Other supportive measures should also be employed as needed.

---

### ACETOHEXAMIDE

## Summary of Differences

Pharmacology/pharmacokinetics:
  Protein binding—Very high, ionic.
  Serum half-life—Parent 1.3 hours; metabolite 6 hours.
  Duration of action—8 to 24 hours.
  Active metabolite.
Precautions:
  Laboratory value alterations—Reduces serum uric acid concentration.
  Medical considerations/contraindications—Not recommended for use in patients with renal function impairment.

## Additional Dosing Information

See also *General Dosing Information*.

When patients are transferred to acetohexamide from another oral antidiabetic medication (with the exception of chlorpropamide), no transition period is required. When transferring patients from chlorpropamide, caution should be exercised during the first 1 to 2 weeks because of the prolonged retention of chlorpropamide in the body.

During conversion from insulin therapy to acetohexamide therapy, no gradual dosage adjustment usually is required for patients using less than 20 USP Units of insulin daily. For patients using 20 or more USP Units daily, a 25 to 30% reduction in insulin every day or every second day with gradual dosage adjustment is advisable. Hospitalization for some patients on a higher insulin dosage may be required for uneventful conversion.

## Oral Dosage Forms

### ACETOHEXAMIDE TABLETS USP

**Usual adult dose**
Antidiabetic—
  Initial: Oral, 250 mg once a day, the dosage being increased by 250 or 500 mg every 5 to 7 days as needed.
  Maintenance: Oral, 250 to 1000 mg once a day before breakfast or 1000 to 1500 mg divided into two doses taken before breakfast and evening meals.

**Usual adult prescribing limits**
Up to 1.5 grams daily.

**Usual pediatric dose**
Safety and efficacy have not been established.

**Usual geriatric dose**
See *Usual adult dose*.

Note: If an elderly patient tends toward hypoglycemia during the first 24 hours after an initial dose of 250 mg at breakfast, the dose should be reduced or the medication discontinued.

## Antidiabetic Agents, Sulfonylurea (Systemic)

**Strength(s) usually available**
U.S.—
250 mg (Rx) [*Dymelor* (scored); GENERIC].
500 mg (Rx) [*Dymelor* (scored); GENERIC].
Canada—
500 mg (Rx) [*Dimelor* (scored)].

**Packaging and storage**
Store below 40 °C (104 °F), preferably between 15 and 30 °C (59 and 86 °F), unless otherwise specified by manufacturer. Store in a well-closed container.

**Auxiliary labeling**
- Avoid alcoholic beverages.
- Do not take other medicines without advice from your doctor.
- Avoid too much sun.

## CHLORPROPAMIDE

## Summary of Differences

Indications:
  Also used in the treatment of central diabetes insipidus.
Pharmacology/pharmacokinetics:
  Other actions/effects—Antidiuretic effect.
  Protein binding—Very high, ionic.
  Half-life, serum—36 hours.
Precautions:
  Pregnancy—Crosses the placenta.
  Breast-feeding—Distributed into breast milk.
  Geriatrics—Use is generally avoided.
  Drug interactions and/or related problems—Risk of disulfiram-like reaction with alcohol is higher with chlorpropamide than with other sulfonylureas.
  Medical considerations/contraindications—Not recommended for use in patients with renal function impairment or congestive heart failure.
Side/adverse effects:
  Potential for serious adverse effects (e.g., prolonged hypoglycemia and severe hyponatremia) because of prolonged action of chlorpropamide, especially with predisposed individuals.

## Additional Dosing Information

See also *General Dosing Information*.

When patients are transferred to chlorpropamide from another sulfonylurea, no transition period is required. When transferring patients from chlorpropamide, caution should be exercised during the first 1 to 2 weeks because of the prolonged retention of chlorpropamide in the body.

During conversion from insulin therapy to chlorpropamide therapy, no gradual dosage adjustment usually is required for patients using less than 40 Units of insulin daily. For patients using 40 Units or more daily, a 50% reduction in insulin in the first few days is advisable. Hospitalization for some patients on a higher insulin dosage may be required for uneventful conversion.

## Oral Dosage Forms

Note: Bracketed uses in the *Dosage Forms* section refer to categories of use and/or indications that are not included in U.S. product labeling.

### CHLORPROPAMIDE TABLETS USP

**Usual adult dose**
Antidiabetic—
  Initial: Oral, 250 mg once a day, the dosage being changed by 50 to 125 mg every three to five days if needed.
  Maintenance: Oral, 100 to 500 mg a day as a single dose.
[Antidiuretic][1]—
  Oral, 100 to 250 mg as a single dose daily, the dosage being adjusted at two- or three-day intervals as needed and tolerated.
Note: Occasionally, divided doses are administered, usually twice a day before the morning and evening meals, to improve gastrointestinal tolerance.

**Usual adult prescribing limits**
Antidiabetic—
  Oral, up to 750 mg per day.
[Antidiuretic][1]—
  Oral, up to 500 mg per day.

**Usual pediatric dose**
Safety and efficacy have not been established.

**Usual geriatric dose**
Antidiabetic—
  Oral, initially, 100 to 125 mg once a day, the dosage being increased by 50 to 125 mg at three- to five-day intervals as needed.

**Strength(s) usually available**
U.S.—
100 mg (Rx) [*Diabinese* (scored); GENERIC (may be scored)].
250 mg (Rx) [*Diabinese* (scored); GENERIC (may be scored)].
Canada—
100 mg (Rx) [*Apo-Chlorpropamide* (scored); *Diabinese* (scored) [GENERIC].
250 mg (Rx) [*Apo-Chlorpropamide* (scored); *Diabinese* (scored); *Novo-Propamide* (scored) [GENERIC].

**Packaging and storage**
Store below 40 °C (104 °F), preferably between 15 and 30 °C (59 and 86 °F), unless otherwise specified by manufacturer. Store in a well-closed container.

**Auxiliary labeling**
- Avoid alcoholic beverages.
- Do not take other medicines without advice from your doctor.
- Avoid too much sun.

[1]Not included in Canadian product labeling.

## GLICLAZIDE

## Summary of Differences

Pharmacology/pharmacokinetics:
  Other actions/effects—Protective activity for some cardiac arrhythmias; also, reduces platelet adhesiveness and aggregation and has fibrinolytic activity.
  Protein binding—Very high, non-ionic.
  Serum half-life—Approximately 10.4 hours.
  Duration of action—Approximately 24 hours.
Precautions:
  Drug interactions and/or related problems—Displacement from plasma proteins by other medications is less likely.
  Medical considerations/contraindications—May be preferred for those patients with moderate renal function impairment; should not be used with severe renal failure.
Side/adverse effects:
  Less weight gain when compared to other sulfonylureas.

## Additional Dosing Information

See also *General Dosing Information*.

When patients are transferred to gliclazide from another oral antidiabetic medication (with the exception of chlorpropamide), no transition period is required. When transferring patients from chlorpropamide, caution should be exercised during the first 1 to 2 weeks because of the prolonged retention of chlorpropamide in the body.

During conversion from insulin therapy to gliclazide therapy, no gradual dosage adjustment usually is required for patients using less than 20 USP Units of insulin daily. For patients using 20 or more USP Units daily, a 25 to 30% reduction in insulin every day or every second day with gradual dosage adjustment is advisable. Hospitalization for some patients on a higher insulin dosage may be required for uneventful conversion.

## Oral Dosage Forms

### GLICLAZIDE TABLETS

**Usual adult dose**
Antidiabetic—
  Initial: Oral, 160 mg two times a day with meals.
  Maintenance: Oral, 80 to 320 mg a day with meals.

**Usual adult prescribing limits**
Oral, up to 320 mg daily.

**Usual pediatric dose**
Safety and efficacy have not been established.

**Usual geriatric dose**
See *Usual adult dose*.

**Strength(s) usually available**
U.S.—
  Not commercially available.
Canada—
  80 mg (Rx) [*Diamicron* (quad-scored)].

USP DI                                                        Antidiabetic Agents, Sulfonylurea (Systemic)   293

**Packaging and storage**
Store below 40 °C (104 °F), preferably between 15 and 30 °C (59 and 86 °F), in a well-closed container, unless otherwise specified by manufacturer.

**Auxiliary labeling**
- Avoid alcoholic beverages.
- Do not take other medicines without advice from your doctor.
- Avoid too much sun.

---

## GLIPIZIDE

### Summary of Differences
Pharmacology/pharmacokinetics:
  Other actions/effects—Has mild diuretic effect.
  Protein binding—Very high, non-ionic.
  Serum half-life—2 to 4 hours.
  Duration of action—12 to 24 hours.
Precautions:
  Drug interactions and/or related problems—
    Displacement from plasma proteins by other medications is less likely than with ionic sulfonylureas.

### Additional Dosing Information
See also *General Dosing Information*.

When patients are transferred to glipizide from another oral antidiabetic medication (with the exception of chlorpropamide), no transition period is required. When transferring patients from chlorpropamide, caution should be exercised during the first 1 to 2 weeks because of the prolonged retention of chlorpropamide in the body.

During conversion from insulin therapy to glipizide therapy, no gradual dosage adjustment usually is required for patients using less than 20 USP Units of insulin daily. For patients using 20 or more USP Units daily, a 50% reduction of insulin the first day, with gradual dosage adjustments of glipizide as needed, is desirable. Hospitalization for some patients on a higher insulin dosage may be required for uneventful conversion.

## Oral Dosage Forms

### GLIPIZIDE EXTENDED-RELEASE TABLETS
**Usual adult dose**
Antidiabetic—
  Initial: Oral, 5 mg once daily with breakfast; dosage is increased by 5 mg based on resulting hemoglobin $A_{1c}$ measurements taken three months later or, less commonly, based on two or more consecutive fasting blood glucose measurements taken seven days apart.
  Maintenance: Oral, 5 to 10 mg once a day with breakfast.
Note: In most cases, if no improvement of hemoglobin $A_{1c}$ is noted after three months of use of a higher dose, the previous dose should be resumed.

**Usual adult prescribing limits**
Up to 20 mg once a day.

**Usual pediatric dose**
Safety and efficacy have not been established.

**Usual geriatric dose**
See *Usual adult dose*.
Note: When adjusting the dose in the elderly, consider that steady-state levels for glipizide extended-release may be delayed by approximately one or two days as compared to other age groups.

**Strength(s) usually available**
U.S.—
  5 mg (Rx) [*Glucotrol XL*].
  10 mg (Rx) [*Glucotrol XL*].
  Note: Although similar in appearance to a conventional tablet, *Glucotrol XL* actually is a specially formulated gastrointestinal system (GITS) consisting of a semipermeable membrane surrounding an osmotically active drug core, which is designed to release glipizide at a constant rate over twenty-four hours; following drug release, the system is eliminated in the feces as an insoluble shell.
Canada—
  Not commercially available.

**Packaging and storage**
Store below 40 °C (104 °F), preferably between 15 and 30 °C (59 and 86 °F), in a tight container, unless otherwise specified by manufacturer.

**Auxiliary labeling**
- Avoid alcoholic beverages.
- Do not take other medicines without advice from your doctor.
- Avoid too much sun.

### GLIPIZIDE TABLETS USP
**Usual adult dose**
Antidiabetic—
  Initial: Oral, 5 mg once a day thirty minutes before breakfast, with dosage being changed by 2.5 to 5 mg every several days as needed.
  Maintenance: Oral, up to 40 mg a day thirty minutes before meals. Single daily doses are adequate with 15 mg or less but may be divided when necessary, while larger doses should be divided into two doses a day and taken thirty minutes before meals.

**Usual adult prescribing limits**
Oral, up to 40 mg daily.

**Usual pediatric dose**
Safety and efficacy have not been established.

**Usual geriatric dose**
Antidiabetic—
  Initial: Oral, 2.5 mg per day thirty minutes before breakfast, with dosage being changed by 2.5 to 5 mg every several days as needed.
  Maintenance: Oral, See *Usual adult dose*.

**Strength(s) usually available**
U.S.—
  5 mg (Rx) [*Glucotrol* (scored); GENERIC (may be scored)].
  10 mg (Rx) [*Glucotrol* (scored); GENERIC (may be scored)].
Canada—
  Not commercially available.

**Packaging and storage**
Store below 40 °C (104 °F), preferably between 15 and 30 °C (59 and 86 °F), unless otherwise specified by manufacturer. Store in a tight container.

**Auxiliary labeling**
- Avoid alcoholic beverages.
- Do not take other medicines without advice from your doctor.
- Avoid too much sun.
- Take this medication on an empty stomach, 30 minutes before meals.

---

## GLYBURIDE

### Summary of Differences
Pharmacology/pharmacokinetics:
  Other actions/effects—
    Protective activity for some cardiac arrhythmias; also, has mild diuretic activity.
  Protein binding—
    Very high, nonionic.
  Half-life—
    10 hours.
  Duration of action—
    24 hours.
  Elimination—
    Biliary: 50%.
    Renal: 50%.
Precautions:
  Geriatrics—
    Use is generally avoided.
  Drug interactions and/or related problems—
    Disulfiram-type reaction with concurrent alcohol use less likely with glyburide than with other antidiabetics. Also, displacement from plasma proteins by other medications is less likely.
Side/adverse effects:
  Fatal hypoglycemia occurs more often with glyburide than with chlorpropamide; potential for serious adverse effect because of prolonged action of glyburide, especially with predisposed individuals.

### Additional Dosing Information
See also *General Dosing Information*.

When patients are transferred to glyburide from another oral antidiabetic medication (with the exception of chlorpropamide), no transition period is required. When transferring patients from chlorpropamide, caution should be exercised during the first 1 to 2 weeks because of the prolonged retention of chlorpropamide in the body and subsequent overlapping of drug effects that could cause hypoglycemia.

During conversion from insulin therapy to glyburide therapy, no gradual dosage adjustment usually is required for patients using less than 40

## Antidiabetic Agents, Sulfonylurea (Systemic)

USP Units of insulin daily. Patients requiring more than 40 USP Units should receive a 50% reduction of insulin the first day with initiation of 3 mg of micronized glyburide or 5 mg of nonmicronized glyburide as a single dose and gradual dosage adjustments of glyburide as needed. Hospitalization for some patients on a higher insulin dosage may be required for uneventful conversion.

**Bioequivalenence information**
Micronized glyburide cannot be substituted for nonmicronized glyburide. Bioavailability studies have demonstrated that micronized glyburide is not bioequivalent to glyburide (nonmicronized); retitration is necessary if patients are transferred.

Micronized glyburide has an AB rating but may not be deemed bioequivalent according to some state formularies when the scored tablet is divided.

Glyburide (nonmicronized) has a BX rating and is not substitutable. However, some specific products are manufactured under the same new drug application (NDA) and may be deemed bioequivalent by some state formularies:
- Upjohn's product, *Micronase*, and Greenstone's generic glyburide (nonmicronized) are manufactured at Upjohn under the same NDA; Greenstone's generic product is distributed by Geneva and Greenstone.
- Hoescht-Roussel produces *DiaBeta* and its own generic, which is distributed by Copley, under the same NDA.

The products manufactured under one NDA cannot be substituted for those products produced under the other NDA; the products are not bioequivalent nor substitutable. The FDA Orange Book will list an NDA only once with the original manufacturer that applied for the product; hence, the Orange Book does not address multiple manufacturers under one NDA. Pharmacists should verify the regulations and formularies of their state or verify with the physician before substituting a BX-rated product under one NDA for a similar product under another.

## Oral Dosage Forms

### GLYBURIDE TABLETS

Note: Glyburide (nonmicronized) has an FDA BX rating denoting that data are insufficient to determine therapeutic equivalence. However, glyburide produced and distributed by the U.S. manufacturer Hoescht-Roussel and also distributed by Copley may be substitutable by some state pharmacy formularies because they use the same new drug application (NDA). Similarly, glyburide distributed by the U.S. manufacturers Greenstone and Upjohn share the same NDA. As long as glyburide holds a BX rating, substitution of products of different NDAs is not permissible without the physician's permission.

In contrast, glyburide (micronized) has an AB rating, denoting that bioequivalence for many state formularies has been resolved; however, some state formularies have deemed the AB-rated generic nonsubstitutable if a scored tablet is divided. State formularies should be checked before substitution is made with this type of product.

**Usual adult dose**
Antidiabetic—
   Initial: Oral, 2.5 to 5 mg once a day with breakfast or the first main meal, with dosage changes being made by no more than 2.5 mg at weekly intervals if needed. Patients more sensitive to hypoglycemia may need 1.25 mg a day.
   Maintenance: Oral, 1.25 to 20 mg a day, of which doses up to 10 mg are usually taken as a single dose with breakfast or the first main meal, while doses over 10 mg are usually divided into two daily doses with meals.

**Usual adult prescribing limits**
Oral, up to 20 mg daily.

**Usual pediatric dose**
Safety and efficacy have not been established.

**Usual geriatric dose**
Antidiabetic—
   Initial: Oral, 1.25 to 2.5 mg a day with breakfast, with dosage changes being made by no more than 2.5 mg at weekly intervals if needed.
   Maintenance: See *Usual adult dose*.
   Note: This dose should also be used in patients with medical problems that make them more sensitive to the effects of glyburide.

**Strength(s) usually available**
U.S.—
   1.25 mg (Rx) [*DiaBeta* (scored); *Micronase* (scored); GENERIC (may be scored)].
   2.5 mg (Rx) [*DiaBeta* (scored); *Micronase* (scored); GENERIC (may be scored)].
   5 mg (Rx) [*DiaBeta* (scored); *Micronase* (scored); GENERIC (may be scored)].
Canada—
   2.5 mg (Rx) [*Albert Glyburide* (scored); *Apo-Glyburide* (scored); *DiaBeta* (scored); *Euglucon* (scored); *Gen-Glybe* (scored); *Novo-Glyburide* (scored); *Nu-Glyburide* (scored)].
   5 mg (Rx) [*Albert Glyburide* (scored); *Apo-Glyburide* (scored); *DiaBeta* (scored); *Euglucon* (scored); *Gen-Glybe* (scored); *Novo-Glyburide* (scored); *Nu-Glyburide* (scored)].

**Packaging and storage**
Store below 40 °C (104 °F), preferably between 15 and 30 °C (59 and 86 °F), in a well-closed container, unless otherwise specified by manufacturer.

**Auxiliary labeling**
- Avoid alcoholic beverages.
- Do not take other medicines without advice from your doctor.
- Avoid too much sun.

### GLYBURIDE TABLETS (MICRONIZED)

Note: Micronized glyburide has an AB rating. However, some state formularies may not consider certain generic products bioequivalent when scored tablets are divided; state formularies should be checked before substituting one product for another.

Micronized glyburide cannot be substituted for nonmicronized glyburide. Bioavailability studies have demonstrated that micronized glyburide is not bioequivalent to glyburide (nonmicronized); retitration is necessary if patients are transferred.

**Usual adult dose**
Antidiabetic—
   Initial: Oral, 1.5 to 3 mg once a day with breakfast or the first main meal. Some patients sensitive to glyburide's effects may need to be started on 0.75 mg a day. Dose titration should be made with changes of no more than 1.5 mg at weekly increments.
   Maintenance: Oral, 0.75 to 12 mg a day; doses up to 6 mg are usually taken as a single dose with breakfast or the first main meal, while doses over 6 mg are usually taken as divided doses with meals.

**Usual adult prescribing limits**
Oral, up to 12 mg daily.

**Usual pediatric dose**
Safety and efficacy have not been established.

**Usual geriatric dose**
Antidiabetic—
   Initial: Oral, 0.75 to 3 mg per day with breakfast or the first main meal, with dosage being changed by no more than 1.5 mg at weekly increments.
   Maintenance: See *Usual adult dose*.

**Strength(s) usually available**
U.S.—
   1.5 mg (Rx) [*Glynase PresTab* (scored); GENERIC (may be scored)].
   3 mg (Rx) [*Glynase PresTab* (scored); GENERIC (may be scored)].
   6 mg (Rx) [*Glynase PresTab* (scored)].
   Note: *Glynase PresTab* is formulated to divide easily in even halves by pressing gently on the scored area of the tablet.
Canada—
   Not commercially available.

**Packaging and storage**
Store below 40 °C (104 °F), preferably between 15 and 30 °C (59 and 86 °F), in a well-closed container, unless otherwise specified by manufacturer.

**Auxiliary labeling**
- Avoid alcoholic beverages.
- Do not take other medicines without advice from your doctor.
- Avoid too much sun.

## TOLAZAMIDE

## Summary of Differences

Pharmacology/pharmacokinetics:
   Other actions/effects—Has mild diuretic activity.
   Protein binding—Very high, ionic.
   Serum half-life—7 hours.
   Duration of action—10 or 20 hours.
Precautions:
   Drug interactions and/or related problems—Displacement from plasma proteins by other medications is more likely than with non-ionic sulfonylureas.

Medical considerations/contraindications—Tolazamide may accumulate in patients with creatinine clearance less than 30 mL per minute (0.5 mL/sec).

## Additional Dosing Information
See also *General Dosing Information*.

When patients are transferred to tolazamide from another oral antidiabetic medication (with the exception of chlorpropamide), no transition period is required. When transferring patients from chlorpropamide, caution should be exercised during the first 1 to 2 weeks because of the prolonged retention of chlorpropamide in the body.

During conversion from insulin therapy to tolazamide therapy, no gradual dosage adjustment usually is required for patients using less than 40 USP Units of insulin daily. For patients requiring 40 or more USP Units daily, a 50% reduction of insulin the first few days with gradual dosage adjustment of tolazamide as needed is advisable. Hospitalization for some patients on a higher insulin dosage may be required for uneventful conversion.

## Oral Dosage Forms
### TOLAZAMIDE TABLETS USP
**Usual adult dose**
Antidiabetic—
  Initial: Oral, 100 to 250 mg once a day with breakfast or the first main meal, with dosage being changed by 100 to 250 mg at weekly intervals as needed.
  Maintenance: Oral, 250 to 500 mg a day with breakfast or the first main meal; some patients may need less (100 mg a day) or more (up to 1000 mg a day). Doses greater than 500 mg should be divided and given two times a day with meals.

**Usual adult prescribing limits**
Oral, up to 1 gram daily.

**Usual pediatric dose**
Safety and efficacy have not been established.

**Usual geriatric dose**
Antidiabetic—
  Initial: Oral, 100 mg once a day in the morning with breakfast or the first main meal, with the dose being changed by 100 to 250 mg at weekly intervals as needed.
  Maintenance: See *Usual adult dose*.
Note: Lower initial doses may also be required in patients with medical problems that make them more sensitive to the effects of tolazamide.

**Strength(s) usually available**
U.S.—
  100 mg (Rx) [*Tolinase* (scored); GENERIC (may be scored)].
  250 mg (Rx) [*Tolinase* (scored); GENERIC (may be scored)].
  500 mg (Rx) [*Tolinase* (scored); GENERIC (may be scored)].
Canada—
  Not commercially available.

**Packaging and storage**
Store below 40 °C (104 °F), preferably between 15 and 30 °C (59 and 86 °F), unless otherwise specified by manufacturer. Store in a tight container.

**Auxiliary labeling**
- Avoid alcoholic beverages.
- Do not take other medicines without advice from your doctor.
- Avoid too much sun.

---

## TOLBUTAMIDE

## Summary of Differences
Pharmacology/pharmacokinetics:
  Other actions/effects—
    Has mild antidiuretic activity.
  Protein binding—
    Very high, ionic.
  Serum half-life—
    4.5 to 6.5 hours.
  Duration of action—
    6 to 12 hours.

Precautions:
  Drug interactions and/or related problems—
    Disulfiram-type reaction with concurrent alcohol use less likely with tolbutamide than with other antidiabetics. Also, displacement from plasma proteins by other medications is more likely than with non-ionic sulfonylureas.
    Metabolism of tolbutamide inhibited by sulfinpyrazone and phenylbutazone.
  Laboratory value alterations—
    Tolbutamide interferes with thyroidal uptake of I 123 and I 131.
  Medical considerations/contraindications—
    May be preferred for those patients with moderate renal function impairment, but should be discontinued with renal failure.

## Additional Dosing Information
See also *General Dosing Information*.

When patients are transferred to tolbutamide from another oral antidiabetic medication (with the exception of chlorpropamide), no transition period is required. When transferring patients from chlorpropamide, caution should be exercised during the first 1 to 2 weeks because of the prolonged retention of chlorpropamide in the body.

During conversion from insulin therapy to tolbutamide therapy, no gradual dosage adjustment usually is required for patients using less than 20 USP Units of insulin daily. Patients using 20 to 40 USP Units require a 30 to 50% reduction in insulin the first day with gradual dosage adjustment as needed. Patients requiring more than 40 USP Units should receive a 20% reduction of insulin the first day with gradual dosage adjustment of tolbutamide as needed. Hospitalization for some patients on a higher insulin dosage may be required for uneventful conversion.

## Oral Dosage Forms
### TOLBUTAMIDE TABLETS USP
**Usual adult dose**
Antidiabetic—
  Initial: Oral, 1000 to 2000 mg a day as single morning or divided doses.
  Maintenance: Oral, 250 to 2000 mg a day as single morning or divided doses.
Note: Lower initial doses may also be required in patients with medical problems that make them more sensitive to the effects of tolbutamide.

**Usual adult prescribing limits**
Oral, up to 3000 mg a day.

**Usual pediatric dose**
Safety and efficacy have not been established.

**Usual geriatric dose**
Lower initial dose may be required. See *Usual adult dose*.
Note: Lower initial doses may also be required in patients with medical problems that make them more sensitive to the effects of tolbutamide.

**Strength(s) usually available**
U.S.—
  500 mg (Rx) [*Orinase* (scored); *Tol-Tab;* GENERIC (may be scored)].
Canada—
  500 mg (Rx) [*Apo-Tolbutamide* (scored); *Mobenol* (scored); *Novo-Butamide* (scored); *Orinase* (scored) [GENERIC].
  1000 mg (Rx) [*Orinase* (scored)].

**Packaging and storage**
Store below 40 °C (104 °F), preferably between 15 and 30 °C (59 and 86 °F), unless otherwise specified by manufacturer. Store in a well-closed container.

**Auxiliary labeling**
- Avoid alcoholic beverages.
- Do not take other medicines without advice from your doctor.
- Avoid too much sun.

Revised: 08/03/95

## Table 1. Pharmacology/Pharmacokinetics

| Drug | $V_D$ (L/kg) | Protein* binding (%) | Biotransformation (%) | Elimination half-life (hrs) | Time to peak (hrs) | Peak serum concentration — Concentration per mL | Peak serum concentration — Dose (mg) | Duration of Action (hrs) | Elimination (%) |
|---|---|---|---|---|---|---|---|---|---|
| Acetohexamide Hydroxyhexamide‡ (metabolite) | 0.21 | Very high, 65–90; Ionic | Hepatic, mainly; erythrocytes | 1.3 † 4.6–6 | 1.5–2 2–6 | 47 mcg 60 mcg | 1000 | 8–24 | Renal: 71 Fecal: 15 |
| Chlorpropamide | 0.09–0.27 | Very high, >90; Ionic | Hepatic | 36 § (range, 24–48) | 2–4 | N/A | N/A | 24–72 | Renal: In 96 hours: Unchanged— 6–20 Active and inactive metabolites |
| Gliclazide | 0.2 | Very high, 94; Nonionic | Hepatic | 10.4 | 4–6 | 5 mcg | 3 | 24 | Renal: Unchanged— <1 Metabolites, conjugates— 60–70 Fecal: Metabolites, conjugates—10–20 |
| Glipizide | 0.14–0.16 | Very high, 99; Nonionic | Hepatic (no first-pass) | 2–4 | | N/A | N/A | | Renal: Unchanged— <10 Metabolites, inactive, and conjugates— 80 Fecal: 10 |
| immediate release | | | | | 1–3 | | | 12–24 | |
| extended release | | | | | 6–12 | | | 24 | |
| Glyburide | 0.14–0.16 | Very high, 99; Nonionic | Hepatic | | | | | 24 | Renal: 50 Metabolites, active—2 weak, short-lived Biliary: 50 |
| Nonmicronized | | | | 6–10 # | 3.4–4.5 | 87.5 nanograms | 5 | | |
| Micronized | | | | 4 # | 2.3–3.5 | 97.2 nanograms | 3 | | |
| Tolazamide ** | N/A | Very high, 94; Ionic | Hepatic | 7 | 3–4 | N/A | | 10–20 | Renal: 85 †† Metabolites, major—5 metabolites (potency 0–70%) Fecal: 7 |
| Tolbutamide ** | 0.10 | Very high, 96; Ionic | Hepatic | 4.5–6.5 | 3–4 | N/A | | 6–12 | Renal: 100 Metabolites, inactive—75% |

*Primarily to albumin.
†Renal impairment prolongs acetohexamide half-life to 30 hours.
‡A primary metabolite for acetohexamide, hydroxyhexamide, accounts for 47–60% of dose and is 2.5 times more potent than parent.
§A randomized crossover study of five phases conducted over a 2 to 3 week period demonstrated that the half-life of chlorpropamide can be affected by the pH of the urine; half-life is 69 ± 26 hours with acidic urine (pH 4.7 to 5.5) and 13 ± 3 hours with basic urine (pH 7.1 to 8.2).
#Micronized glyburide allows greater solubility, faster absorption and, therefore, faster elimination; it is not bioequivalent to nonmicronized glyburide; micronized glyburide's area under the curve (AUC) is 568 ng•hr/mL and nonmicronized glyburide's AUC is 746 ng•hr/mL.
**Tolazamide is approximately 5–6.7 times more potent than tolbutamide and equal in its potency to chlorpropamide on a milligram per milligram basis.
††The majority of a single dose of tolazamide is eliminated in urine within 24 hours and elimination is complete after 5 days. Less active metabolites include carboxytolazamide, hydroxytolazamide, and p-toulene sulfonamide.

# ANTIDYSKINETICS Systemic

This monograph includes information on the following: 1) Benztropine; 2) Biperiden; 3) Ethopropazine; 4) Procyclidine; 5) Trihexyphenidyl.

INN:
   Benztropine—Benzatropine
   Ethopropazine—Profenamine

BAN:
   Benztropine—Benzatropine
   Trihexyphenidyl—Benzhexol

VA CLASSIFICATION (Primary): AU350

Commonly used brand name(s): *Akineton*[2]; *Apo-Benztropine*[1]; *Apo-Trihex*[5]; *Artane*[5]; *Artane Sequels*[5]; *Cogentin*[1]; *Kemadrin*[4]; *PMS Benztropine*[1]; *PMS Procyclidine*[4]; *PMS Trihexyphenidyl*[5]; *Parsidol*[3]; *Parsitan*[3]; *Procyclid*[4]; *Procyclid].*[4]; *Trihexane*[5]; *Trihexy*[5].

Note: For a listing of dosage forms and brand names by country availability, see *Dosage Forms* section(s).

## Category
Antidyskinetic.

## Indications
Note: Bracketed information in the *Indications* section refers to uses that are not included in U.S. product labeling.

**Accepted**

Parkinsonism (treatment)—Antidyskinetics are indicated in the treatment of mild cases of postencephalitic, arteriosclerotic, or idiopathic parkinsonism(paralysis agitans) in patients in whom anticholinergic therapy is not contraindicated. Antidyskinetics also are indicated as adjuncts to more potent medications to maximize improvement of symptoms. Procyclidine usually produces a more beneficial effect in conditions of rigidity than in those of tremor.

Extrapyramidal reactions, drug-induced (treatment)—Antidyskinetics are indicated in the control of extrapyramidal disorders(except tardive dyskinesia) due to central nervous system (CNS) drugs such as reserpine, phenothiazines, dibenzoxazepines, thioxanthenes, and butyrophenones. However, concomitant therapy with antipsychotics is not recommended beyond 3 months because extrapyramidal symptoms resulting from antipsychotic therapy usually resolve in 3 to 6 months and because prolonged, routine use of antidyskinetics with antipsychotics may predispose patients to the more serious neurological condition, tardive dyskinesia.

[Athetosis, congenital (treatment)][1]or
[Degeneration, hepatolenticular (treatment)][1]—Ethopropazine is used for the symptomatic treatment of hepatolenticular degeneration and congenital athetosis.

[1]Not included in Canadian product labeling.

## Pharmacology/Pharmacokinetics

**Physicochemical characteristics**

Molecular weight—
   Benztropine mesylate: 403.54.
   Biperiden hydrochloride: 347.93.
   Biperiden lactate: 401.54.
   Ethopropazine hydrochloride: 348.93.
   Procyclidine hydrochloride: 323.91.
   Trihexyphenidyl hydrochloride: 337.93.

**Mechanism of action/Effect**

Specific mode of action is unknown, but it is thought that these agents partially block central (striatal) cholinergic receptors, thereby helping to balance cholinergic and dopaminergic activity in the basal ganglia; salivation may be decreased, and smooth muscle may be relaxed. Drug-induced extrapyramidal symptoms and those due to parkinsonism may be relieved, but tardive dyskinesia is not alleviatedand may be aggravated by anticholinergic effects.

**Other actions/effects**

Benztropine and ethopropazine also have a slight antihistaminic and local anesthetic effect. Biperiden may have a slight effect on the cardiovascular and respiratory systems. Procyclidine and trihexyphenidyl have a direct antispasmodic effect on smooth muscle. In small doses trihexyphenidyl depresses the CNS, but larger doses may cause cerebral excitation.

**Absorption**

Well-absorbed from gastrointestinal tract.

**Onset of action**

Benztropine—
   Oral: 1 to 2 hours.
   Intramuscular or intravenous: Within a few minutes.
Biperiden—
   Intramuscular: Average of 10 to 30 minutes.
   Intravenous: Within a few minutes.
Trihexyphenidyl—
   Oral: 1 hour.

**Duration of action**

Benztropine—Oral, intramuscular, or intravenous: 24 hours.
Biperiden—Intravenous: 1 to 8 hours.
Ethopropazine—Oral: 4 hours.
Procyclidine—Oral: 4 hours.
Trihexyphenidyl—Oral: 6 to 12 hours.

## Precautions to Consider

**Pregnancy/Reproduction**

Pregnancy—Problems in humans have not been documented with benztropine, ethopropazine, procyclidine, or trihexyphenidyl.
For biperiden—Studies have not been done with biperiden in humans. Studies have not been done in animals.
FDA Pregnancy Category C.

**Breast-feeding**

It is not known whether antidyskinetics are distributed into breast milk. However, antidyskinetics may inhibit lactation.

**Pediatrics**

No information is available on the relationship of age to the effects of antidyskinetics in pediatric patients. However, it is known that pediatric patients exhibit increased sensitivity to other medications with anticholinergic properties.

**Geriatrics**

Chronic use of antidyskinetics may predispose geriatric patients to glaucoma.
Geriatric patients, especially those with arteriosclerotic changes, may respond to the usual doses of antidyskinetics, ethopropazine and procyclidine in particular, with mental confusion, disorientation, agitation, hallucinations, and psychotic-like symptoms.
Memory may become severely impaired in geriatric patients, especially those who already have memory problems, with the continued use of antidyskinetics since these drugs block the action of acetylcholine, which is responsible for many functions of the brain, including memory functions.

**Dental**

Prolonged use of antidyskinetics may decrease or inhibit salivary flow, thus contributing to the development of caries, periodontal disease, oral candidiasis, and discomfort.

**Drug interactions and/or related problems**

The following drug interactions and/or related problems have been selected on the basis of their potential clinical significance (possible mechanism in parentheses where appropriate)—not necessarily inclusive (» = major clinical significance):

Note: Combinations containing any of the following medications, depending on the amount present, may also interact with this medication.

» Alcohol or
» CNS depression–producing medications (See *Appendix II* )
   (concurrent use with antidyskinetics may cause increased sedative effects)

Amantadine or
» Anticholinergics or other medications with anticholinergic action (See *Appendix II*) or
Monoamine oxidase (MAO) inhibitors, including furazolidone, procarbazine, and selegiline
   (concurrent use may intensify anticholinergic effects of antidyskinetics because of the secondary anticholinergic activities of these medications; patients should be advised to report occurrence of gastrointestinal problems, fever, or heat intolerancepromptly since paralytic ileus, hyperthermia, or heat stroke may occur with concurrent therapy)

Antidiarrheals, adsorbent
   (simultaneous administration may reduce therapeutic effects of antidyskinetics because of particle adsorption; to avoid this effect, patients should be advised to allow at least 1 or 2 hours between doses of the different medications)

Carbidopa and levodopa or
Levodopa
(concurrent use of these medications with benztropine, procyclidine, or trihexyphenidyl may result in increased efficacy of levodopa; however, concurrent use is not recommended if there is a history of psychosis)

Chlorpromazine
(concurrent use of chlorpromazine with antidyskinetics may increase metabolism of chlorpromazine, resulting in decreased plasma concentration because of reduction in gastrointestinal motility)

**Medical considerations/Contraindications**
The medical considerations/contraindications included have been selected on the basis of their potential clinical significance (reasons given in parentheses where appropriate)—not necessarily inclusive (» = major clinical significance).

*Risk-benefit should be considered when the following medical problems exist:*

Cardiac arrhythmias
(increased risk of tachycardia)

» Cardiovascular instability
(increased risk of cardiac arrhythmias)

» Dyskinesia, tardive
(may be aggravated)

Extrapyramidal reactions, such as those resulting from phenothiazines or reserpine, in patients with mental disorders
(mental symptoms may be intensified, precipitating toxic psychosis)

» Glaucoma, angle-closure, or predisposition to
(mydriatic effect resulting in increased intraocular pressure may precipitate an acute attack of angle-closure glaucoma)

» Glaucoma, open-angle
(mydriatic effect may cause a slight increase in intraocular pressure; glaucoma therapy may need to be adjusted)

Hepatic function impairment
(metabolism may be altered)

Hypertension
(may be aggravated)

» Intestinal obstruction, complete, partial or history of
(decreased motility and tone may aggravate or precipitate obstruction)

» Myasthenia gravis
(condition may be aggravated because of inhibition of acetylcholine action)

Prostatic hypertrophy, moderate to severe or
» Urinary retention
(anticholinergic effect of antidyskinetics may precipitate or aggravate urinary retention)

Renal function impairment
(decreased elimination may increase risk of side effects)

Sensitivity to antidyskinetics (history of)

**Patient monitoring**
The following may be especially important in patient monitoring (other tests may be warranted in some patients, depending on condition; » = major clinical significance):

Intraocular pressure determinations
(recommended at periodic intervals during therapy, especially in patients with angle-closure and open-angle glaucoma)

## Side/Adverse Effects

Note: Anticholinergic side effects that may occur with antidyskinetics are rarely severe and either disappear as therapy is continued, or diminish when the dose is reduced.

Anhidrosis and subsequent hyperthermia may occur with antidyskinetics when patients, especially geriatric, chronically ill, and alcoholic, are exposed to high environmental temperatures.

Ethopropazine is a phenothiazine derivative. Although the likelihood of ethopropazine causing such side effects as changes in vision, jaundice, rare hematologic reactions, and electrocardiogram (ECG) abnormalities associated with phenothiazines seems to be minimal, the possibility exists.

The following side/adverse effects have been selected on the basis of their potential clinical significance (possible signs and symptoms in parentheses where appropriate)—not necessarily inclusive:

**Those indicating need for medical attention**
Incidence rare
*Allergic reaction* (skin rash); *confusion*—more frequent in the elderly or with high doses; *increased intraocular pressure* (eye pain)

**Those indicating need for medical attention only if they continue or are bothersome**
Incidence more frequent
*Anticholinergic effects, mild* (blurred vision; constipation; decreased sweating; difficult or painful urination, especially in older men; drowsiness; dryness of mouth, nose, or throat; increased sensitivity of eyes to light; nausea or vomiting).

Incidence less frequent or rare
*False sense of well-being*—especially in the elderly or with high doses; *headache; loss of memory*—especially in the elderly; *muscle cramps; nervousness; numbness or weakness in hands or feet; orthostatic hypotension* (dizziness or lightheadedness when getting up from a lying or sitting position); *soreness of mouth and tongue; stomach upset or pain; unusual excitement*—more frequent with high doses of trihexyphenidyl

**Those indicating possible withdrawal symptoms and the need for medical attention if they occur after discontinuation of long-term therapy**
*Anxiety; extrapyramidal symptoms, recurrence or worsening of* (difficulty in speaking or swallowing; loss of balance control; mask-like face; muscle spasms, especially of face, neck, and back; restlessness or desire to keep moving; shuffling walk; stiffness of arms or legs; trembling and shaking of hands and fingers; twisting movements of body)—especially after abrupt withdrawal of antidyskinetic medication; may require reinstatement of the antidyskinetic; *fast heartbeat; orthostatic hypotension* (dizziness or lightheadedness when getting up from a lying or sitting position); *trouble in sleeping*

## Overdose

For specific information on the agents used in the management of antidyskinetics, see:
*Barbiturates (Systemic)* monograph;
*Diazepam* in *Benzodiazepines (Systemic)* monograph;
*Physostigmine Salicylate (Systemic)* monograph; and/or
*Pilocarpine (Ophthalmic)* monograph.

For more information on the management of overdose or unintentional ingestion, **contact a Poison Control Center** (see *Poison Control Center Listing*).

**Clinical effects of overdose**
The following effects have been selected on the basis of their potential clinical significance (possible signs and symptoms in parentheses where appropriate)—not necessarily inclusive:
*Anticholinergic effects, severe* (clumsiness or unsteadiness; severe drowsiness; severe dryness of mouth, nose, or throat; fast heartbeat; shortness of breath or troubled breathing; warmth, dryness, and flushing of skin); *CNS depression* (severe drowsiness); *CNS stimulation* (hallucinations, seizures, trouble in sleeping); *toxic psychoses* (mood or mental changes)—especially in patients with mental illness being treated with neuroleptic drugs

**Treatment of overdose**
Recommended treatment for overdose with antidyskinetics includes the following:
To decrease absorption—
Emesis or gastric lavage, except in precomatose, convulsive, or psychotic states.
Specific treatment—
Intramuscular or *slow* intravenous administration of 1 to 2 mg of physostigmine salicylate, repeated after 2 hours if needed (0.5 mg initially in children, repeated at five-minute intervals, up to a maximum of 2 mg), to reverse the cardiovascular and CNS toxic effects.
Administration of small doses of diazepam or a short-acting barbiturate to manage excitement.
Administration of pilocarpine 0.5%, to counteract mydriasis.
Supportive care—
Respiratory assistance and symptomatic support.
Patients in whom intentional overdose is confirmed or suspected should be referred for psychiatric consultation.

## Patient Consultation

As an aid to patient consultation, refer to *Advice for the Patient, Antidyskinetics (Systemic)*.

In providing consultation, consider emphasizing the following selected information (» = major clinical significance):

**Before using this medication**
» Conditions affecting use, especially:
Sensitivity to antidyskinetics (history of)
Breast-feeding—May inhibit lactation

Use in children—Increased susceptibility to anticholinergic effects
Use in the elderly—Predisposition to glaucoma with chronic use; increased risk of mental confusion and other psychotic-like symptoms; impairment of memory
Dental—Decrease or inhibition of salivary flow
Other medications, especially other anticholinergics and CNS depressants
Other medical problems, especially cardiovascular instability, tardive dyskinesia, glaucoma, intestinal obstruction, myasthenia gravis, or urinary retention

**Proper use of this medication**
» Importance of not taking more medication than the amount prescribed
Taking with food to relieve gastric irritation
» Proper dosing
Missed dose: Taking as soon as possible; not taking if within 2 hours of next dose; not doubling doses
» Proper storage

**Precautions while using this medication**
Regular visits to physician to check progress during prolonged therapy; eye examination may also be needed
» Checking with physician before discontinuing medication; gradual dosage reduction may be necessary
» Avoiding use of alcohol or other CNS depressants
Avoiding use of antidiarrheal medications within 1 or 2 hours of taking this medication
Suspected overdose: Getting emergency help at once
Possible increased eye sensitivity to bright light
» Caution if drowsiness or blurred vision occurs
Caution when getting up suddenly from a lying or sitting position
» Caution during exercise and hot weather
Possible dryness of mouth; using sugarless gum or candy, ice, or saliva substitute for relief; checking with physician or dentist if dry mouth continues for more than 2 weeks

**Side/adverse effects**
Signs of potential side effects, especially allergic reaction, confusion, increased intraocular pressure, anticholinergic effects, or CNS depression or stimulation

## General Dosing Information

**For oral dosage forms only**
Therapy should be initiated with a low dose because of cumulative action, and dosage should be increased gradually at 5- or 6-day intervals.
Titrated dosage is necessary to achieve the individual required therapeutic level, especially for geriatric patients, who tend to be more sensitive to anticholinergic effects, and patients receiving other medications.
During therapy, necessary dosage adjustments of antidyskinetic or other medication used concurrently should be made gradually to maintain proper control of the patient's condition.
Postencephalitic and younger parkinsonism patients often require and tolerate higher dosages than idiopathic, arteriosclerotic, or geriatric parkinsonism patients.
A drug-abuse potential exists with these medications as they may cause euphoria and hallucinations at higher dosages.
When an antidyskinetic is to be discontinued, dosage should be reduced gradually to prevent a sudden increase in adverse symptoms.

**Diet/Nutrition**
Antidyskinetics may be taken with or immediately after meals to lessen gastric irritation.

---

### BENZTROPINE

## Summary of Differences

Pharmacology/pharmacokinetics:
Other actions/effects—
Has slight antihistaminic and local anesthetic effect.
Onset of action—
Oral: 1 to 2 hours.
Intramuscular or intravenous: Within a few minutes.
Duration of action—
Oral, intramuscular, or intravenous: 24 hours.
Precautions:
Drug interactions and/or related problems—
May increase efficacy of levodopa if used concurrently; however, concurrent use not recommended if there is history of psychosis.

## Additional Dosing Information

A single daily oral dose of benztropine at bedtime often provides maximum benefit for the patient because of the long duration of effect.

## Oral Dosage Forms

### BENZTROPINE MESYLATE TABLETS USP

**Usual adult and adolescent dose**
Parkinsonism—
Oral, 1 to 2 mg a day, the dosage being adjusted as needed and tolerated.
Note: Idiopathic parkinsonism—Therapy may be initiated in some patients with a single oral daily dose of 500 mcg (0.5 mg) to 1 mg at bedtime.
Postencephalitic parkinsonism—Therapy may be initiated in most patients with 2 mg a day, given once a day or in divided doses.
Drug-induced extrapyramidal reactions—
Oral, 1 to 4 mg one or two times a day. Or, 1 to 2 mg two or three times a day if drug-induced extrapyramidal reactions develop soon after initiation of treatment with neuroleptic drugs.

**Usual adult prescribing limits**
Up to 6 mg daily.

**Usual pediatric dose**
Parkinsonism or drug-induced extrapyramidal reactions—
Children up to 3 years of age: Use is not recommended.
Children 3 years of age and over: Dosage must be individualized by physician.

**Usual geriatric dose**
See *Usual adult and adolescent dose*.
Note: Geriatric patients may be more sensitive to the effects of the usual adult dose.

**Strength(s) usually available**
U.S.—
500 mcg (0.5 mg) (Rx) [*Cogentin* (scored); GENERIC].
1 mg (Rx) [*Cogentin* (scored); GENERIC].
2 mg (Rx) [*Cogentin* (scored); GENERIC].
Canada—
500 mcg (0.5 mg) (Rx) [*PMS Benztropine*].
1 mg (Rx) [*PMS Benztropine* (scored)].
2 mg (Rx) [*Apo-Benztropine* (double-scored); *Cogentin* (scored; lactose); *PMS Benztropine* (scored); GENERIC].

**Packaging and storage**
Store below 40 °C (104 °F), preferably between 15 and 30 °C (59 and 86 °F), in a well-closed container, unless otherwise specified by manufacturer.

**Auxiliary labeling**
• May cause drowsiness.
• Avoid alcoholic beverages.

## Parenteral Dosage Forms

### BENZTROPINE MESYLATE INJECTION USP

**Usual adult and adolescent dose**
Parkinsonism—
Intramuscular or intravenous, 1 to 2 mg a day, the dosage being adjusted as needed and tolerated.
Drug-induced extrapyramidal reactions—
Intramuscular or intravenous, 1 to 4 mg one or two times a day.

**Usual adult prescribing limits**
Up to 6 mg daily.

**Usual pediatric dose**
Parkinsonism or drug-induced extrapyramidal reactions—
Children up to 3 years of age: Use is not recommended.
Children 3 years of age and over: Dosage must be individualized by physician.

**Usual geriatric dose**
See *Usual adult and adolescent dose*.
Note: Geriatric patients may be more sensitive to the effects of the usual adult dose.

**Strength(s) usually available**
U.S.—
1 mg per mL (Rx) [*Cogentin* (sodium chloride 9 mg/mL)].
Canada—
1 mg per mL (Rx) [*Cogentin* (sodium chloride 9 mg/mL); GENERIC].

**Packaging and storage**
Store below 40 °C (104 °F), preferably between 15 and 30 °C (59 and 86 °F), unless otherwise specified by manufacturer. Protect from freezing.

## BIPERIDEN

### Summary of Differences
Pharmacology/pharmacokinetics:
   Other actions/effects—
      Slight cardiovascular and respiratory effects.
Side/adverse effects:
   Has slight effect on cardiovascular and respiratory systems.

## Oral Dosage Forms
### BIPERIDEN HYDROCHLORIDE TABLETS USP

**Usual adult and adolescent dose**
Parkinsonism—
   Oral, 2 mg three or four times a day, the dosage being adjusted as needed and tolerated.
Drug-induced extrapyramidal reactions—
   Oral, 2 mg one to three times a day.

**Usual adult prescribing limits**
Parkinsonism—
   Up to 16 mg daily.

**Usual pediatric dose**
Safety and efficacy have not been established.

**Usual geriatric dose**
See *Usual adult and adolescent dose*.

Note: Geriatric patients may be more sensitive to the effects of the usual adult dose.

**Strength(s) usually available**
U.S.—
   2 mg (Rx) [*Akineton* (scored; corn syrup; lactose; magnesium stearate; potato starch; talc)].
Canada—
   2 mg (Rx) [*Akineton*].

**Packaging and storage**
Store below 40 °C (104 °F), preferably between 15 and 30 °C (59 and 86 °F), unless otherwise specified by manufacturer. Store in a tight container.

**Auxiliary labeling**
- May cause drowsiness.
- Avoid alcoholic beverages.
- Keep container tightly closed.

## Parenteral Dosage Forms
### BIPERIDEN LACTATE INJECTION USP

**Usual adult and adolescent dose**
Drug-induced extrapyramidal reactions—
   Intramuscular or slow intravenous, 2 mg repeated at half-hour intervals as needed and tolerated up to a total of four doses a day.

**Usual pediatric dose**
Drug-induced extrapyramidal reactions—
   Intramuscular, initially 40 mcg (0.04 mg) per kg of body weight, or 1.2 mg per square meter of body surface; dose may be repeated at half-hour intervals if necessary, up to four doses a day.

**Usual geriatric dose**
See *Usual adult and adolescent dose*.

Note: Geriatric patients may be more sensitive to the effects of the usual adult dose.

**Strength(s) usually available**
U.S.—
   5 mg per mL (Rx) [*Akineton* (1.4% sodium lactate)].
Canada—
   Not commercially available.

**Packaging and storage**
Store below 40 °C (104 °F), preferably between 15 and 30 °C (59 and 86 °F), unless otherwise specified by manufacturer. Protect from light. Protect from freezing.

## ETHOPROPAZINE

### Summary of Differences
Indications:
   Also used for the symptomatic treatment of hepatolenticular degeneration and congenital athetosis.
Pharmacology/pharmacokinetics:
   Other actions/effects—
      Has slight antihistaminic and local anesthetic effect.
   Duration of action—
      Oral: 4 hours.
Side/adverse effects:
   May possess phenothiazine side effects, especially in high dosages.

## Oral Dosage Forms
### ETHOPROPAZINE HYDROCHLORIDE TABLETS USP

**Usual adult and adolescent dose**
Parkinsonism and
Drug-induced extrapyramidal reactions—
   Oral, 50 mg one or two times a day, the dosage being increased as needed and tolerated. In severe cases, the dose may be increased gradually to a total of 500 to 600 mg a day.

**Usual pediatric dose**
Dosage has not been established.

**Usual geriatric dose**
See *Usual adult and adolescent dose*.

Note: Geriatric patients may be more sensitive to the effects of the usual adult dose.

**Strength(s) usually available**
U.S.—
   10 mg (Rx) [*Parsidol*].
   50 mg (Rx) [*Parsidol* (scored)].
Canada—
   50 mg (Rx) [*Parsitan* (scored)].

**Packaging and storage**
Store below 40 °C (104 °F), preferably between 15 and 30 °C (59 and 86 °F), in a well-closed container, unless otherwise specified by manufacturer. Protect from light.

**Auxiliary labeling**
- May cause drowsiness.
- Avoid alcoholic beverages.

## PROCYCLIDINE

### Summary of Differences
Pharmacology/pharmacokinetics:
   Other actions/effects—
      Direct antispasmodic effect on smooth muscle.
   Duration of action—
      Oral: 4 hours.
Precautions:
   Drug interactions and/or related problems—
      May increase efficacy of levodopa if used concurrently; however, concurrent use not recommended if there is history of psychosis.
General dosing information:
   Provides more beneficial effect in conditions of rigidity than in those of tremor.

## Oral Dosage Forms
### PROCYCLIDINE HYDROCHLORIDE ELIXIR

**Usual adult and adolescent dose**
Parkinsonism—
   Oral, initially 2.5 mg three times a day after meals. If tolerated, the dosage may be gradually increased to 5 mg three times a day and, occasionally, 5 mg at bedtime.

Note: For patients being transferred from other therapy, 2.5 mg three times a day may be substituted for all or part of the original medication. The dose of procyclidine may be increased while the original medication is decreased until a level of maximum benefit is reached.

Drug-induced extrapyramidal reactions—
   Oral, initially 2.5 mg three times a day, the dosage being increased in 2.5-mg increments per day as needed and tolerated.

**Usual pediatric dose**
Dosage has not been established.

**Usual geriatric dose**
See *Usual adult and adolescent dose*.

Note: Geriatric patients may be more sensitive to the effects of the usual adult dose.

**Strength(s) usually available**
U.S.—
   Not commercially available.

Canada—
   2.5 mg per 5 mL (Rx) [*Kemadrin* (alcohol 10%); *PMS Procyclidine* (spearmint-flavored); *Procyclid*].].

**Packaging and storage**
Store below 40 °C (104 °F), preferably between 15 and 30 °C (59 and 86 °F), unless otherwise specified by manufacturer. Store in a tight container. Protect from freezing.

**Auxiliary labeling**
• May cause drowsiness.
• Avoid alcoholic beverages.
• Keep container tightly closed.

## PROCYCLIDINE HYDROCHLORIDE TABLETS USP

**Usual adult and adolescent dose**
See *Procyclidine Hydrochloride Elixir*.

**Usual pediatric dose**
See *Procyclidine Hydrochloride Elixir*.

**Usual geriatric dose**
See *Procyclidine Hydrochloride Elixir*.

**Strength(s) usually available**
U.S.—
   5 mg (Rx) [*Kemadrin* (scored)].
Canada—
   2.5 mg (Rx) [*PMS Procyclidine* (scored)].
   5 mg (Rx) [*Kemadrin* (scored); *PMS Procyclidine* (scored); *Procyclid* (scored)].

**Packaging and storage**
Store below 40 °C (104 °F), preferably between 15 and 30 °C (59 and 86 °F), unless otherwise specified by manufacturer. Store in a tight container.

**Auxiliary labeling**
• May cause drowsiness.
• Avoid alcoholic beverages.
• Keep container tightly closed.

---

### TRIHEXYPHENIDYL

## Summary of Differences
Pharmacology/pharmacokinetics:
   Other actions/effects—
      Direct antispasmodic effect on smooth muscle; small doses depress CNS; larger doses may cause cerebral excitation.
   Onset of action—
      Oral: 1 hour.
   Duration of action—
      Oral: 6 to 12 hours.
Precautions:
   Drug interactions and/or related problems—
      May increase efficacy of levodopa if used concurrently; however, concurrent use not recommended if there is history of psychosis.
Side/adverse effects:
   Unusual excitement (with high doses).

## Oral Dosage Forms

### TRIHEXYPHENIDYL HYDROCHLORIDE EXTENDED-RELEASE CAPSULES USP

**Usual adult and adolescent dose**
Parkinsonism—
   Oral, 5 mg a day after breakfast with an additional 5 mg taken twelve hours later as needed.
Note: This dosage form is usually utilized only after the patient has been stabilized on the conventional dosage forms.

**Usual adult prescribing limits**
Up to 15 mg daily.

**Usual pediatric dose**
Dosage has not been established.

**Usual geriatric dose**
See *Usual adult and adolescent dose*.
Note: Geriatric patients may be more sensitive to the effects of the usual adult dose.

**Strength(s) usually available**
U.S.—
   5 mg (Rx) [*Artane Sequels*].
Canada—
   5 mg (Rx) [*Artane Sequels*].

**Packaging and storage**
Store below 40 °C (104 °F), preferably between 15 and 30 °C (59 and 86 °F), in a tight container, unless otherwise specified by manufacturer.

**Auxiliary labeling**
• May cause drowsiness.
• Avoid alcoholic beverages.

### TRIHEXYPHENIDYL HYDROCHLORIDE ELIXIR USP

**Usual adult and adolescent dose**
Parkinsonism—
   Oral, 1 to 2 mg the first day, the dosage being increased by an additional 2 mg at three- to five-day intervals until the desired response is obtained or until the total dose per day reaches 6 to 10 mg, usually divided into three doses taken at mealtimes.
Note: Postencephalitic parkinsonism—A total dose of 12 to 15 mg per day may be required.
Drug-induced extrapyramidal reactions—
   Oral, initially 1 mg a day, the dosage being increased as needed and tolerated or until the total daily dose reaches 5 to 15 mg.

**Usual adult prescribing limits**
Up to 15 mg daily.

**Usual pediatric dose**
Dosage has not been established.

**Usual geriatric dose**
See *Usual adult and adolescent dose*.
Note: Geriatric patients may be more sensitive to the effects of the usual adult dose.

**Strength(s) usually available**
U.S.—
   2 mg per 5 mL (Rx) [*Artane* (lime-mint flavored); GENERIC].
Canada—
   2 mg per 5 mL (Rx) [*Artane* (lime flavored); *PMS Trihexyphenidyl*].

**Packaging and storage**
Store below 40 °C (104 °F), preferably between 15 and 30 °C (59 and 86 °F), unless otherwise specified by manufacturer. Store in a tight container. Protect from freezing.

**Auxiliary labeling**
• May cause drowsiness.
• Avoid alcoholic beverages.
• Keep container tightly closed.

### TRIHEXYPHENIDYL HYDROCHLORIDE TABLETS USP

**Usual adult and adolescent dose**
See *Trihexyphenidyl Hydrochloride Elixir USP*.

**Usual adult prescribing limits**
See *Trihexyphenidyl Hydrochloride Elixir USP*.

**Usual pediatric dose**
See *Trihexyphenidyl Hydrochloride Elixir USP*.

**Usual geriatric dose**
See *Trihexyphenidyl Hydrochloride Elixir USP*.

**Strength(s) usually available**
U.S.—
   2 mg (Rx) [*Artane* (scored); *Trihexane*; *Trihexy*; GENERIC].
   5 mg (Rx) [*Artane* (scored); *Trihexane*; *Trihexy*; GENERIC].
Canada—
   2 mg (Rx) [*Apo-Trihex* (scored, sodium <1 mmol (0.113 mg)/2 mg); *Artane* (scored); *PMS Trihexyphenidyl* (sodium <1 mmol (0.113 mg)/2 mg)].
   5 mg (Rx) [*Apo-Trihex* (scored, sodium <1 mmol (0.188 mg)/5 mg); *Artane* (scored); *PMS Trihexyphenidyl* (sodium <1 mmol (0.188 mg)/5 mg)].

**Packaging and storage**
Store below 40 °C (104 °F), preferably between 15 and 30 °C (59 and 86 °F), unless otherwise specified by manufacturer. Store in a tight container.

**Auxiliary labeling**
• May cause drowsiness.
• Avoid alcoholic beverages.
• Keep container tightly closed.

Revised: 05/11/93

# ANTIFUNGALS, AZOLE  Systemic

This monograph includes information on the following: 1) Fluconazole; 2) Itraconazole; 3) Ketoconazole.
VA CLASSIFICATION (Primary/Secondary):
Fluconazole—AM700
Itraconazole—AM700
Ketoconazole—AM700/HS900; AN900

Commonly used brand name(s): *Diflucan*[1]; *Diflucan-150*[1]; *Nizoral*[3]; *Sporanox*[2].

Note: For a listing of dosage forms and brand names by country availability, see *Dosage Forms* section(s).

## Category

Antiadrenal; antineoplastic (systemic)—Ketoconazole.
Antifungal (systemic)—Fluconazole; Itraconazole; Ketoconazole.

## Indications

Note: Bracketed information in the *Indications* section refers to uses that are not included in U.S. product labeling.

### Accepted

Aspergillosis (treatment)—Itraconazole is indicated in the treatment of aspergillosis caused by *Aspergillus* species in patients who are intolerant of or refractory to amphotericin B therapy.

Blastomycosis (treatment)—Itraconazole is indicated for the treatment of pulmonary and extrapulmonary blastomycosis caused by *Blastomyces dermatiditis* in immunocompromised and nonimmunocompromised patients. Ketoconazole[1] is also indicated in the treatment of blastomycosis.

Candidiasis (prophylaxis)—Fluconazole is indicated for the prophylaxis of candidiasis in patients undergoing bone marrow transplant who receive cytotoxic chemotherapy and/or radiation therapy.

Candidiasis, esophageal (treatment) or
Candidiasis, oropharyngeal (treatment)—Fluconazole, itraconazole, and ketoconazole are indicated for the treatment of esophageal and oropharyngeal candidiasis (thrush) caused by *Candida* species.

Candidiasis, disseminated (treatment)—Fluconazole and ketoconazole are indicated for the treatment of serious infections, including peritonitis, pneumonia, and urinary tract infections, caused by susceptible *Candida* species.

Candidiasis, mucocutaneous, chronic (treatment)—[Fluconazole][1], [itraconazole][1], and ketoconazole are indicated in the treatment of severe, chronic extensive mucocutaneous candidiasis caused by *Candida* species.

Candidiasis, vulvovaginal (treatment)—Fluconazole, [itraconazole][1], and [ketoconazole][1] are indicated in the treatment of vulvovaginal candidiasis caused by *Candida* species.

Chromomycosis (treatment)—[Itraconazole] and ketoconazole are indicated as secondary agents in the treatment of chromomycosis caused by *Cladosporium carrioni*, *Exophiala dermatitidis*, *Fonsecaea pedrosi*, *Fonsecaea compactum*, *Phialophora verrucosa*, *Rhinocladiella aquaspersa*, and *Rhinocladiella cerophilum*.

Coccidioidomycosis (treatment)—[Fluconazole][1] and [itraconazole][1] are indicated in the treatment of pulmonary and disseminated coccidioidomycosis caused by *Coccidioides immitis*. Ketoconazole is indicated as a secondary agent in the treatment of severe coccidioidomycosis.

Histoplasmosis (treatment)—Itraconazole is indicated for the treatment of histoplasmosis, including chronic cavitary pulmonary disease and disseminated disease caused by *Histoplasma capsulatum*, in immunocompromised and nonimmunocompromised patients. Ketoconazole is also indicated in the treatment of pulmonary and disseminated histoplasmosis caused by *H. capsulatum*.

Meningitis, cryptococcal (treatment) or
Meningitis, cryptococcal (suppression)—Fluconazole is indicated for the treatment and suppression of cryptococcal meningitis. [Itraconazole][1] is indicated as an alternative agent as suppressive, maintenance therapy for cryptococcal meningitis.

Preliminary studies indicate that amphotericin B plus flucytosine are more efficacious than fluconazole in the primary treatment of cryptococcal meningitis in patients with acquired immunodeficiency syndrome (AIDS), although there was a greater incidence of toxicity with this combination. Another study found that amphotericin B alone was superior to fluconazole in the treatment of acute cryptococcal meningitis; however, fluconazole was better tolerated for maintenance therapy.

Onychomycosis (treatment)—[Fluconazole], itraconazole[1], and [ketoconazole] are indicated in nonimmunocompromised patients for the treatment of onychomycosis caused by *Trichophyton* species and *Candida* species.

Paracoccidioidomycosis (treatment)—[Itraconazole] and ketoconazole are indicated in the treatment of paracoccidioidomycosis caused by *Paracoccidioides brasiliensis*.

Pityriasis versicolor (treatment)
Tinea corporis (treatment)
Tinea cruris (treatment) or
Tinea pedis (treatment)—Ketoconazole is indicated in the treatment of recalcitrant or very severe disfiguring or disabling pityriasis versicolor, tinea corporis, tinea cruris, and tinea pedis infections unresponsive to griseofulvin, or in patients allergic to or unable to tolerate griseofulvin. [Fluconazole][1] and [itraconazole] are used in the treatment of tinea corporis (ringworm of the body), tinea cruris (ringworm of the groin; jock itch), and tinea pedis (ringworm of the foot; athlete's foot).

[Carcinoma, prostatic (treatment)][1]—High-dose ketoconazole is indicated as a secondary antiandrogen agent in the treatment of advanced prostatic carcinoma.

[Cryptococcosis (treatment)][1]—Fluconazole and itraconazole are indicated in the treatment of extrameningeal cryptococcosis caused by *Cryptococcus neoformans*.

[Cushing's syndrome (treatment)][1]—High-dose ketoconazole is indicated as a secondary agent in the treatment of Cushing's syndrome.

[Hirsutism (treatment)][1]—Ketoconazole is indicated as an alternative (third or fourth line) agent in the treatment of hirsutism (*Evidence rating: III*). Ketoconazole has been shown to lower androgen levels and to decrease hair growth with long-term (> 6 months) use in hirsute women. However, some medical experts state that the potential benefits of treating hirsutism with ketoconazole do not outweigh the potential risks (including serious hepatotoxicity) because other less toxic agents are available.

[Histoplasmosis (suppression)][1]—Itraconazole is indicated for the suppression of disseminated histoplasmosis caused by *Histoplasma capsulatum*, in immunocompromised patients.

[Leishmaniasis, cutaneous (treatment)][1]—Itraconazole and ketoconazole are indicated for the treatment of cutaneous leishmaniasis.

[Paronychia (treatment)][1]—Itraconazole and ketoconazole are indicated in the treatment of fungal paronychia.

[Pneumonia, fungal (treatment)][1]—Fluconazole, itraconazole, and ketoconazole are indicated in the treatment of fungal pneumonia.

[Septicemia, fungal (treatment)][1]—Fluconazole, itraconazole, and ketoconazole are indicated in the treatment of fungal septicemia.

[Sporotrichosis, disseminated (treatment)]—Itraconazole and ketoconazole[1] are indicated in the treatment of disseminated sporotrichosis.

[Tinea barbae (treatment)] or
[Tinea capitis (treatment)][1]—Systemic ketoconazole is indicated, in combination with topical imidazoles, in the treatment of griseofulvin-resistant tinea barbae (ringworm of the beard) and tinea capitis (ringworm of the scalp).

[Tinea manuum (treatment)][1]—Fluconazole and itraconazole are indicated in the treatment of tinea manuum (ringworm of the hand).

Fluconazole is approved for the treatment of systemic candidal infections and is an appropriate, less toxic alternative to amphotericin B.

Fluconazole has been shown to be efficacious *in vivo* in the treatment of animals infected with candidiasis, cryptococcosis, histoplasmosis, coccidioidosis, blastomycosis, aspergillosis, and paracoccidioidosis. The *in vitro* susceptibility testing of fluconazole is affected by composition of the culture medium, pH, inoculum size, incubation temperature, and time. Because of this, published *in vitro* minimum inhibitory concentration (MIC) data vary widely, and a correlation between this and *in vivo* clinical efficacy cannot reliably be made.

### Unaccepted

Ketoconazole is not effective in the treatment of fungal meningitis because it penetrates poorly into the cerebrospinal fluid (CSF). Also, it is not effective against *Aspergillus* or *Zygomycetes* (agents of mucormycosis) or in mycetoma.

---

[1]Not included in Canadian product labeling.

## Pharmacology/Pharmacokinetics

See *Table 1*, and *Table 2*, page 309–310.

**Physicochemical characteristics**
Molecular weight—
 Fluconazole: 306.28.
 Itraconazole: 705.65.
 Ketoconazole: 531.44.
Chemical class
 Fluconazole: Triazole derivative.
 Itraconazole: Triazole derivative.
 Ketoconazole: Imidazole derivative.

**Mechanism of action/Effect**
Fungistatic; may be fungicidal, depending on concentration; azole antifungals interfere with cytochrome P450 enzyme activity, which is necessary for the demethylation of 14-alpha-methylsterols to ergosterol. Ergosterol, the principal sterol in the fungal cell membrane, becomes depleted. This damages the cell membrane, producing alterations in membrane functions and permeability. In *Candida albicans*, azole antifungals inhibit transformation of blastospores into invasive mycelial form.

**Other actions/effects**
High-dose ketoconazole therapy can interfere with the conversion of lanosterol to cholesterol, a major precursor of several hormones. It has been shown to suppress corticosteroid secretion and lower serum testosterone concentrations, which return to baseline values when ketoconazole is discontinued. Adrenocorticotropic hormone (ACTH)–induced serum corticosteroid concentrations and serum testosterone concentrations may be decreased by doses of 800 mg of ketoconazole daily; serum testosterone concentrations are abolished by doses of 1.6 grams of ketoconazole daily, leading to reduced libido and impotence, but return to baseline values when ketoconazole is discontinued.

Compared to ketoconazole, fluconazole and itraconazole have a very weak, noncompetitive inhibitory effect on the liver cytochrome P450 enzyme system, while maintaining a high affinity for fungal cytochrome P450 enzyme activity.

Fluconazole and itraconazole have not been reported to have antiandrogenic activity at currently used doses. Itraconazole has not affected cortisol metabolism in patients treated with clinically recommended doses; however, a decrease in cortisol synthesis was observed in a patient receiving high-dose itraconazole therapy (600 mg a day).

**Distribution**
Fluconazole—Fluconazole is widely distributed throughout the body, with good penetration into the cerebrospinal fluid (CSF) (ranging from 52 to 85% in patients with fungal meningitis), the eye, and peritoneal fluid.
Itraconazole—Highly lipophilic; extensively distributed to tissues, concentrating in fatty tissues, the omentum, the liver, and the kidneys. Aqueous fluids, such as the CSF, aqueous humor, and saliva, contain negligible concentrations of itraconazole. Itraconazole also does not distribute into peritoneal dialysate effluent. Exudates, such as pus, may have up to 3.5 times the simultaneous plasma concentration; tissues that are prone to fungal invasion, such as skin, lung tissue, and the female genital tract, have several times the plasma concentration.
Ketoconazole—Well distributed; distributed to inflamed joint fluid, saliva, bile, urine, breast milk, sebum, cerumen, feces, tendons, skin and soft tissues, and testes (small amounts); crosses the placenta; crosses the blood-brain barrier poorly; only negligible amounts reach the CSF. Although concentrations of 2.2 to 3 mcg per mL have been reported in the CSF with corresponding serum concentrations of 9 to 12 mcg per mL, most studies indicate that CSF concentrations 1 mcg per mL are rare, regardless of dose.

## Precautions to Consider

**Cross-sensitivity and/or related problems**
Patients allergic to one azole antifungal agent (fluconazole, itraconazole, ketoconazole) may also be allergic to the other antifungals in this family.

**Carcinogenicity/Tumorigenicity**
*Fluconazole*—Studies in rats and mice treated with oral doses of 2.5 to 10 mg per kg of body weight (mg/kg) per day (2 to 7 times the recommended human dose) for 24 months showed no carcinogenic potential. Male rats treated with 5 to 10 mg/kg per day had an increased incidence of hepatocellular adenomas.
*Itraconazole*—No evidence of carcinogenicity was found in mice given oral doses of up to 80 mg/kg per day, or approximately 10 times the maximum recommended human dose (MRHD), for 23 months. Male rats given 3 times the MRHD had a slightly increased incidence of soft tissue sarcoma. These sarcomas may have been a consequence of hypercholesterolemia, which is caused by chronic itraconazole administration in rats, but did not occur in dogs or humans. Female rats who were given 6.25 times the MRHD had an increased incidence of squamous cell carcinoma in the lung, compared to the untreated group, although the increase in this study was not statistically significant.
*Ketoconazole*—Long-term feeding studies in Swiss albino mice and in Wistar rats have not shown evidence of oncogenesis.

**Mutagenicity**
*Fluconazole*—Mutagenicity tests for fluconazole (with and without metabolic activation) in four strains of *Salmonella typhimurium* and in the mouse lymphoma L5178Y system were negative. Cytogenetic studies *in vivo* and *in vitro* showed no evidence of chromosomal mutations.
*Itraconazole*—Itraconazole produced no mutagenic effects when assayed in appropriate bacterial, non-mammalian and mammalian test systems.
*Ketoconazole*—Dominant lethal mutation tests have not shown mutation in any stage of germ cell development in male and female mice given single, oral doses of ketoconazole as high as 80 mg/kg. In addition, the Ames/*Salmonella* microsomal activator tests have not shown evidence of mutagenicity.

**Pregnancy/Reproduction**
Fertility—*Fluconazole*: Fertility was not affected in male or female rats treated with oral daily doses of 5 to 20 mg/kg or parenteral doses of 5, 25, or 75 mg/kg, although the onset of parturition was slightly delayed with oral doses of 20 mg/kg.
*Itraconazole*: Itraconazole did not affect the fertility of male or female rats treated with oral doses of up to 5 times the MRHD, although parental toxicity was present at this dosage level.
*Ketoconazole*: Ketoconazole has been shown to decrease or abolish serum testosterone concentrations when used in high doses (e.g., 800 mg to 1.6 grams daily). Ketoconazole has also been shown to cause menstrual irregularities, oligospermia, azoospermia, impotence, and decreased male libido.

Pregnancy—
 *Fluconazole*: Studies in humans have not been done.
 Maternal weight gain was impaired in pregnant rabbits administered oral fluconazole at doses ranging from 5 to 75 mg/kg per day. Abortions occurred at 75 mg/kg (20 to 60 times the recommended human dose); no adverse fetal effects were detected. Pregnant rats administered oral fluconazole showed impaired maternal weight gain and increased placental weight at 25 mg/kg. A slight increase in the number of stillborn pups and a decrease in neonatal survival were also seen at these doses. Supernumerary ribs, renal pelvis dilation, and delays in ossification were observed at doses of 25 mg/kg and higher. In rats, death of embryos and fetal abnormalities, including wavy ribs, cleft palate, and abnormal craniofacial ossification, occurred at doses ranging from 80 to 320 mg/kg (approximately 20 to 60 times the recommended human dose). These effects are consistent with the inhibition of estrogen synthesis in rats and may be a result of known effects of lowered estrogen on pregnancy, organogenesis, and parturition; this effect has not been observed in women treated with fluconazole.
 FDA Pregnancy Category C.
 *Itraconazole*: Adequate and well-controlled studies in humans have not been done.
 Studies in rats found that itraconazole causes a dose-related increase in maternal toxicity, embryotoxicity, and teratogenicity, consisting of major skeletal defects, at doses approximately 5 to 20 times the MRHD. Studies in mice also found that itraconazole causes a dose-related increase in maternal toxicity, embryotoxicity, and teratogenicity, consisting of encephaloceles and/or macroglossia, at doses approximately 10 times the MRHD.
 FDA Pregnancy Category C.
 *Ketoconazole*: Ketoconazole crosses the placenta. Adequate and well-controlled studies in humans have not been done.
 Studies in rats given doses of 80 mg/kg per day (10 times the MRHD) have shown ketoconazole to be teratogenic, causing syndactyly and oligodactyly. Ketoconazole has also been shown to be embryotoxic in rats given doses greater than 80 mg/kg during the first trimester.
 FDA Pregnancy Category C.

Labor—*Fluconazole*: Dystocia and prolongation of parturition were observed in a few pregnant rats given 20 and 40 mg/kg of intravenous fluconazole.
*Ketoconazole*: Ketoconazole has also been shown to cause dystocia in rats given doses greater than 10 mg/kg (greater than 1.25 times the MRHD) during the third trimester.

**Breast-feeding**
*Fluconazole*—Fluconazole is distributed into breast milk at concentrations similar to those in plasma.
*Itraconazole*—Itraconazole is distributed into breast milk.
*Ketoconazole*—Ketoconazole is distributed into breast milk.

**Pediatrics**
*Fluconazole*—Use of fluconazole in children 6 months of age and older with fungal infections is supported by evidence from adequate and well-

controlled studies in adults, with additional data from pediatric pharmacokinetics studies and controlled clinical trials in pediatric patients. Appropriate studies on the relationship of age to the effects of fluconazole have not been performed in children up to 6 months of age; safety and efficacy have not been established. However, a small number of patients from 1 day to 6 months of age have been treated safely with fluconazole.

*Itraconazole*—Appropriate studies on the relationship of age to the effects of itraconazole have not been performed in the pediatric population. Safety and efficacy have not been established. However, a small number of patients from 3 to 16 years of age have been treated with itraconazole capsules, 100 mg per day, for systemic fungal infections, and no serious adverse effects have been reported. Also, a small number of patients from 6 months to 12 years of age have been treated with itraconazole oral solution, 5 mg/kg per day, for systemic fungal infections, and no serious, unexpected adverse events have been reported.

*Ketoconazole*—Several cases of hepatitis have been reported in children who have taken ketoconazole. Appropriate studies on the relationship of age to the effects of ketoconazole have not been performed in children up to 2 years of age. However, no pediatrics-specific problems have been documented to date in children over 2 years of age.

**Geriatrics**
No information is available on the relationship of age to the effects of azole antifungals in geriatric patients. However, elderly patients are more likely to have an age-related decrease in renal function, which may require an adjustment in dosage or dosing interval in patients receiving fluconazole.

**Drug interactions and/or related problems**
The following drug interactions and/or related problems have been selected on the basis of their potential clinical significance (possible mechanism in parentheses where appropriate)—not necessarily inclusive (» = major clinical significance):

Note: Combinations containing any of the following medications, depending on the amount present, may also interact with this medication.

» Alcohol or
» Hepatotoxic medications, other (see *Appendix II*)
   (concurrent use with ketoconazole may result in an increased incidence of hepatotoxicity; patients, especially those on prolonged administration or those with a history of liver disease, should be monitored carefully and should be advised to avoid alcoholic beverages and other hepatotoxins)
   (concurrent ingestion of alcohol with ketoconazole has been reported to result in a disulfiram-like reaction, characterized by facial flushing; other symptoms may include difficult breathing, slight fever, and tightness of the chest; these effects subsided spontaneously within 24 hours with no lasting ill effects)

» Antacids or
» Anticholinergics/antispasmodics or
» Histamine H$_2$-receptor antagonists or
» Omeprazole or
» Sucralfate
   (these medications increase gastrointestinal pH; this may result in a marked reduction in absorption of itraconazole and ketoconazole; ketoconazole depends on stomach acid for dissolution and subsequent absorption; patients should be advised to take these medications at least 2 hours after taking itraconazole or ketoconazole)

» Antidiabetic agents, oral
   (concurrent use of fluconazole or itraconazole with tolbutamide, chlorpropamide, glyburide, or glipizide has increased the plasma concentrations of these sulfonylurea agents; hypoglycemia has been noted; blood glucose concentrations should be monitored, and the dose of the oral hypoglycemic agent may need to be reduced)

» Astemizole or
» Terfenadine
   (concurrent use of these medications with itraconazole or ketoconazole is **contraindicated**; concurrent use of these antihistamines with itraconazole or ketoconazole may result in elevated plasma concentrations of astemizole or terfenadine by inhibiting the cytochrome P450 enzyme metabolic pathways; this has led to cardiac arrhythmias, including ventricular tachycardia and torsades de pointes, and death; in a small study, fluconazole was given with terfenadine and a small pharmacokinetic interaction was found; although no change in cardiac repolarization or accumulation of parent terfenadine was found, concurrent use of terfenadine with fluconazole at doses of 400 mg or greater per day is **contraindicated**)

» Carbamazepine
   (concurrent use may decrease itraconazole plasma concentrations, leading to treatment failure or clinical relapse)

» Cisapride
   (concurrent use of cisapride with oral itraconazole or oral ketoconazole is **contraindicated**; concurrent use of cisapride with these antifungals may inhibit the cytochrome P450 enzyme metabolic pathways, resulting in elevated plasma concentrations of cisapride; this has led to ventricular arrhythmias, including torsades de pointes, in patients taking cisapride and oral ketoconazole)

» Cyclosporine
   (itraconazole, ketoconazole, and high doses of fluconazole have been reported to inhibit the metabolism of cyclosporine; this may increase the plasma concentration of cyclosporine to potentially toxic levels; a few studies have not found a significant interaction between fluconazole and cyclosporine; however, plasma cyclosporine concentrations should be monitored carefully in patients receiving any of the azole antifungals; the dose of cyclosporine may need to be reduced; it is currently recommended that the dose of cyclosporine be reduced by 50% when itraconazole is started)

» Didanosine (ddI)
   (didanosine contains a buffer that increases gastrointestinal pH in order to increase its absorption; itraconazole and ketoconazole require an acidic environment for their optimal absorption; concurrent administration may result in a marked reduction in absorption of any of these medications; itraconazole and ketoconazole should be administered at least 2 hours before or 2 hours after didanosine is given)

» Digoxin
   (itraconazole and ketoconazole may increase serum digoxin concentrations, leading to toxicity; digoxin concentrations should be monitored)

Hydrochlorothiazide
   (concurrent use of fluconazole with hydrochlorothiazide 50 mg for 10 days in volunteers resulted in a 41% increase in peak plasma concentration, and a 43% increase in the area under the plasma concentration–time curve [AUC] of fluconazole; this is thought to be due to a mean decrease of approximately 20% in the renal clearance of fluconazole)

» Indinavir
   (concurrent use of ketoconazole with indinavir increases the AUC for indinavir by 68 ± 48%; a dose reduction of indinavir to 600 mg every 8 hours is recommended)

» Isoniazid or
» Rifampin
   (concurrent use of rifampin may increase the metabolism of fluconazole, itraconazole, and ketoconazole, lowering their plasma concentrations; this may lead to clinical failure or relapse; concurrent use of isoniazid with ketoconazole has also been reported to decrease serum concentrations of ketoconazole; isoniazid or rifampin should be used with caution when given concurrently with azole antifungals)

» Lovastatin or
» Simvastatin
   (itraconazole inhibits the metabolism of lovastatin, resulting in significantly elevated plasma concentrations of lovastatin or lovastatic acid, which have been associated with rhabdomyolysis; use of 3-hydroxy-3-methylglutaryl coenzyme A (HMG-CoA) reductase inhibitors that are metabolized by the cytochrome P450 enzyme system, such as lovastatin and simvastatin, should be temporarily discontinued during itraconazole therapy)

» Midazolam or
» Triazolam
   (concurrent use with itraconazole or ketoconazole elevates the plasma concentration of oral midazolam or triazolam, which may potentiate and prolong their hypnotic and sedative effects; oral midazolam and triazolam should not be used in patients treated with itraconazole or ketoconazole)

» Phenytoin
   (concurrent use with any azole antifungal may decrease the metabolism of phenytoin, resulting in increased plasma phenytoin concentrations; a 75% increase in the AUC of phenytoin was found in volunteers given 200 mg of fluconazole per day; concurrent use has also been reported to decrease the plasma concentration of azole antifungals, which may lead to treatment failure or relapse of the fungal infection; response to both medications should be monitored closely)

Rifabutin
   (pharmacokinetic studies with fluconazole and rifabutin show that fluconazole appears to increase the serum concentration of rifabutin; however, this is not thought to have clinical significance, and rifa-

butin dosing does not need to be modified in patients receiving fluconazole)

Theophylline
(fluconazole has been found to increase serum theophylline concentrations by approximately 13%, which may lead to toxicity; theophylline concentrations should be monitored)

» Warfarin
(anticoagulant effects may be increased when warfarin is used concurrently with any azole antifungal, resulting in an increase in prothrombin time [PT]; PT must be monitored carefully in patients receiving warfarin and azole antifungals)

**Laboratory value alterations**
The following have been selected on the basis of their potential clinical significance (possible effect in parentheses where appropriate)—not necessarily inclusive (» = major clinical significance):

With physiology/laboratory test values
» Alanine aminotransferase (ALT [SGPT]) and
» Alkaline phosphatase and
» Aspartate aminotransferase (AST [SGOT]) and
» Bilirubin
(serum values may be elevated)

» Potassium, serum
(hypokalemia has occurred in approximately 2 to 6% of patients treated with itraconazole, and has resulted in ventricular fibrillation, especially at higher doses)

» Corticosteroid concentrations, serum, adrenocorticotropic hormone (ACTH)-induced and
» Testosterone concentrations, serum
(ACTH-induced serum corticosteroid concentrations and serum testosterone concentrations may be decreased by doses of 800 mg of ketoconazole daily; serum testosterone concentrations are abolished by doses of 1.6 grams of ketoconazole daily, but return to baseline values when ketoconazole is discontinued)

**Medical considerations/Contraindications**
The medical considerations/Contraindications included have been selected on the basis of their potential clinical significance (reasons given in parentheses where appropriate)—not necessarily inclusive (» = major clinical significance).

*Except under special circumstances, this medication should not be used when the following medical problem exists:*
» Hypersensitivity to azole antifungals

*Risk-benefit should be considered when the following medical problems exist:*
» Achlorhydria or
» Hypochlorhydria
(may cause marked reduction in absorption of itraconazole and ketoconazole; patients with acquired immunodeficiency syndrome [AIDS] may have reduced itraconazole and ketoconazole absorption due to hypochlorhydria)

» Alcoholism, active or in remission or
» Hepatic function impairment
(azole antifungals are metabolized in the liver and may, infrequently, be hepatotoxic; azole antifungals, especially ketoconazole, should be used with caution in patients with liver function impairment or a history of alcoholism)

(ketoconazole has also been reported to cause a disulfiram-like reaction to alcohol, characterized by flushing, rash, peripheral edema, nausea, and headache; symptoms resolved within a few hours)

» Renal function impairment
(because fluconazole is excreted through the kidneys, a reduction in dosage, or increase in dosing interval, is recommended in patients with renal function impairment)

**Patient monitoring**
The following may be especially important in patient monitoring (other tests may be warranted in some patients, depending on condition; » = major clinical significance):

Blood urea nitrogen or
Creatinine concentration, serum
(blood urea nitrogen or serum creatinine concentrations should be monitored as clinically indicated in patients taking fluconazole since patients with renal function impairment will require an adjustment in dosage)

» Hepatic function determinations
(liver function tests are recommended prior to treatment, monthly for 3 to 4 months after treatment is started, and periodically thereafter during treatment in patients receiving ketoconazole; elevated serum enzyme values may occur without clinical hepatitis; however, ketoconazole should be discontinued if even minor abnormalities in enzyme values persist or worsen, or if they are accompanied by symptoms of hepatotoxicity; mild, transient increase in transaminases may occur with fluconazole and itraconazole therapy, and may, on rare occasion, progress to hepatotoxicity; liver function tests should be monitored periodically during treatment; fluconazole and itraconazole should be discontinued if abnormal enzyme values persist or worsen, or if they are accompanied by symptoms of hepatotoxicity)

» Potassium, serum
(hypokalemia has occurred in patients treated with itraconazole, and has been associated with ventricular fibrillation)

## Side/Adverse Effects

Note: In patients taking ketoconazole, hepatotoxicity, consisting primarily of hepatocellular damage or mixed hepatocellular and cholestatic changes, has been reported in approximately 1 in 10,000 exposed patients. It is usually, but not always, reversible upon discontinuation of ketoconazole, and fatalities have been reported rarely. It is considered to be an idiosyncratic reaction and can occur at any time during therapy. Females and patients over the age of 40 may be predisposed to hepatotoxicity. Several cases of hepatitis have also been reported in children.

High-dose ketoconazole therapy has also been shown to suppress corticosteroid secretion. In addition, ketoconazole has been shown to lower serum testosterone concentrations at doses of 800 mg per day, and abolish concentrations at 1600 mg per day; these concentrations return to baseline values when ketoconazole is discontinued.

The overall incidence of side effects with fluconazole has been reported to be higher in human immunodeficiency virus (HIV)-infected patients (21%) than in those being treated with fluconazole who were not infected with HIV (13%); however, many patients in these studies were also receiving other medications known to be hepatotoxic or associated with exfoliative skin disorders, making a direct causal association with fluconazole difficult.

The following side/adverse effects have been selected on the basis of their potential clinical significance (possible signs and symptoms in parentheses where appropriate)—not necessarily inclusive:

**Those indicating need for medical attention**
Incidence less frequent
*Hypersensitivity* (fever and chills; skin rash or itching)

Incidence rare
*Agranulocytosis* (fever and sore throat)—for fluconazole; *exfoliative skin disorders, including Stevens-Johnson syndrome* (reddening, blistering, peeling, or loosening of skin and mucous membranes)—for fluconazole; *hepatotoxicity* (dark or amber urine; loss of appetite; pale stools; stomach pain; unusual tiredness or weakness; yellow eyes or skin); *thrombocytopenia* (unusual bleeding or bruising)—for fluconazole

**Those indicating need for medical attention only if they continue or are bothersome**
Incidence less frequent
*Central nervous system (CNS) effects* (dizziness; drowsiness; headache); *gastrointestinal disturbances* (abdominal pain; constipation; diarrhea; loss of appetite; nausea; vomiting)

Incidence rare—for ketoconazole
*Gynecomastia* (enlargement of the breasts in males); *impotence* (decreased sexual ability in males); *menstrual irregularities; photophobia* (increased sensitivity of the eyes to light)

Note: *Gynecomastia* and *impotence* are due to inhibition of testosterone and adrenal steroid synthesis.

## Patient Consultation

As an aid to patient consultation, refer to *Advice for the Patient, Antifungals, Azole (Systemic).*

In providing consultation, consider emphasizing the following selected information (» = major clinical significance):

**Before using this medication**
» Conditions affecting use, especially:
Hypersensitivity to azole antifungals
Fertility—High doses of ketoconazole have been shown to cause menstrual irregularities, oligospermia, azoospermia, and impotence
Pregnancy—High doses of azole antifungals may cause maternal toxicity, embryotoxicity, and teratogenicity in animals

**306** Antifungals, Azole (Systemic)

Contraindicated medications—Astemizole (with itraconazole or ketoconazole), cisapride (with oral itraconazole or oral ketoconazole), and terfenadine (with fluconazole ≥ 400 mg per day, itraconazole, or ketoconazole).

Other medications, especially alcohol, antacids, anticholinergics/antispasmodics, oral antidiabetic agents, carbamazepine, cyclosporine, didanosine, digoxin, hepatotoxic medications, histamine H$_2$-receptor antagonists, indinavir, isoniazid, lovastatin, midazolam, omeprazole, phenytoin, rifampin, simvastatin, sucralfate, triazolam, or warfarin

Other medical problems, especially achlorhydria, alcoholism, hepatic function impairment, hypochlorhydria, or renal function impairment

## Proper use of this medication
» Taking itraconazole capsules and ketoconazole with food to increase absorption
» Taking itraconazole oral solution on an empty stomach to increase absorption

Proper administration technique for oral liquids
Proper administration technique in achlorhydria
» Compliance with full course of therapy
» Importance of not missing doses and taking at evenly spaced times
» Proper dosing
Missed dose: Taking as soon as possible; not taking if almost time for next dose; not doubling doses
» Proper storage

## Precautions while using this medication
Checking with physician if no improvement within a few days
» Not taking oral itraconazole or oral ketoconazole with terfenadine, cisapride, or astemizole, and not taking ≥ 400 mg per day of fluconazole with terfenadine; concurrent use may cause cardiac arrhythmias
» Avoiding intake of alcoholic beverages or other alcohol-containing preparations while taking ketoconazole because of increased risk of hepatotoxicity
» Avoiding use of antacids and other medications that increase gastrointestinal pH while taking itraconazole or ketoconazole; concurrent use may decrease the absorption of itraconazole or ketoconazole
Possible photophobic reactions when taking ketoconazole; wearing sunglasses and avoiding bright light to minimize potential eye discomfort

## Side/adverse effects
Agranulocytosis, exfoliative skin disorders, hepatotoxicity, and thrombocytopenia

---

### FLUCONAZOLE

## Summary of Differences
Indications:
Also indicated for the treatment of vulvovaginal candidiasis.
Pharmacology/pharmacokinetics:
Good penetration into the cerebrospinal fluid; 80% of an administered dose is eliminated as unchanged drug in the urine.
Precautions:
Medical considerations/contraindications—Dose may need to be adjusted in patients with renal function impairment.
Drug interactions and/or related problems—Use with oral antidiabetic agents has increased the plasma concentration of these sulfonylurea agents, leading to hypoglycemia. At fluconazole doses of 400 mg per day or greater, concurrent use with terfenadine is contraindicated and may increase the risk of cardiac arrhythmias, including torsades de pointes.
Side/adverse effects:
Increased risk of exfoliative skin disorders, including Stevens-Johnson syndrome, agranulocytosis, and thrombocytopenia.

## Additional Dosing Information
Because oral fluconazole is almost completely bioavailable, the daily oral dose is the same as the intravenous dose.

Intravenous fluconazole should be administered at a maximum rate of approximately 200 mg per hour by continuous infusion.

The dose of fluconazole and the length of treatment should be based on the site of infection and the individual response to therapy. Treatment should be continued until clinical parameters and laboratory tests indicate that active fungal infection has subsided. Acquired immunodeficiency syndrome (AIDS) patients with cryptococcal meningitis or recurrent oropharyngeal candidiasis require maintenance therapy to prevent relapse.

Patients undergoing bone marrow transplantion in whom severe granulocytopenia is anticipated should start fluconazole prophylaxis several days before the anticipated onset of neutropenia, and continue treatment for seven days after the neutrophil count rises above 1000 cells per mm$^3$.

Adults with impaired renal function require an adjustment in dose as follows:

| Creatinine clearance (mL/min)/(mL/sec) | Percent of recommended dose |
|---|---|
| > 50/0.83 | 100 |
| 11–50/0.18–0.83 | 50 |
| Hemodialysis patients | 100 after each dialysis |

On dialysis days, the dose of fluconazole should be administered after hemodialysis has been performed since a single 3-hour dialysis period will reduce plasma fluconazole concentrations by approximately 50%.

## Oral Dosage Forms
### FLUCONAZOLE CAPSULES
**Usual adult dose**
Candidiasis, vulvovaginal—
Oral, 150 mg as a single dose.

**Usual pediatric dose**
Safety and efficacy have not been established for children up to 18 years of age.

**Strength(s) usually available**
U.S.—
Not commercially available.
Canada—
150 mg (Rx) [*Diflucan-150* (lactose)].

**Packaging and storage**
Store between 15 and 30 °C (59 and 86 °F).

### FLUCONAZOLE FOR ORAL SUSPENSION
**Usual adult and adolescent dose**
Candidiasis (prophylaxis)—
Oral, 400 mg once a day.
Candidiasis, disseminated—
Oral, 400 mg on the first day, then 200 mg once a day for at least four weeks and for at least two weeks following the resolution of symptoms.
Candidiasis, esophageal—
Oral, 200 mg on the first day, then 100 mg once a day for at least three weeks and for at least two weeks following the resolution of symptoms. Doses of up to 400 mg once a day may be used depending on clinical response.
Candidiasis, oropharyngeal—
Oral, 200 mg on the first day, then 100 mg once a day for at least two weeks.
Candidiasis, vulvovaginal—
Oral, 150 mg as a single dose.
Meningitis, cryptococcal (treatment)—
Oral, 400 mg once a day until a clear clinical response is seen, then 200 to 400 mg once a day for at least ten to twelve weeks after the cerebrospinal fluid becomes culture-negative.
Note: Some clinicians prefer a loading dose of 400 mg two times a day for two days, then 400 mg a day for at least ten to twelve weeks after the cerebrospinal fluid becomes culture-negative.
Meningitis, cryptococcal (suppressive therapy)—
Oral, 200 mg once a day.

**Usual pediatric dose**
Candidiasis, esophageal—
Infants and children 6 months of age and older: Oral, 3 mg per kg of body weight once a day for at least three weeks, and for at least two weeks following resolution of symptoms.
Infants up to 6 months of age: Dosage has not been established.
Candidiasis, oropharyngeal—
Infants and children 6 months of age and older: Oral, 3 mg per kg of body weight once a day for at least two weeks.
Infants up to 6 months of age: Dosage has not been established.
Meningitis, cryptococcal (treatment)—
Infants and children 6 months of age and older: Oral, 6 to 12 mg per kg of body weight once a day for at least ten to twelve weeks after the cerebrospinal fluid becomes culture-negative.
Infants up to 6 months of age: Dosage has not been established.

Meningitis, cryptococcal (suppressive therapy)—
  Infants and children 6 months of age and older: Oral, 6 mg per kg of body weight once a day.
  Infants up to 6 months of age: Dosage has not been established.

Note: Patients with acute infections should be given a loading dose equal to twice the daily dose, not to exceed 12 mg per kg of body weight, on the first day of treatment.

**Usual pediatric prescribing limits**
600 mg per day.

**Strength(s) usually available**
U.S.—
  10 mg per mL (when reconstituted according to manufacturer's instructions) (Rx) [*Diflucan* (sodium benzoate; sucrose)].
  40 mg per mL (when reconstituted according to manufacturer's instructions) (Rx) [*Diflucan* (sodium benzoate; sucrose)].
Canada—
  10 mg per mL (when reconstituted according to manufacturer's instructions) (Rx) [*Diflucan* (sodium benzoate; sucrose)].
  40 mg per mL (when reconstituted according to manufacturer's instructions) (Rx) [*Diflucan* (sodium benzoate; sucrose)].

**Packaging and storage**
Store between 5 and 30 °C (41 and 86 °F) in a well-closed container. Protect from freezing.

**Stability**
After reconstitution, suspensions retain their potency for 14 days.

**Auxiliary labeling**
• Shake well.
• Continue medicine for full time of treatment.
• Beyond-use date.

**Note**
When dispensing, include a calibrated liquid-measuring device.

## FLUCONAZOLE TABLETS

**Usual adult and adolescent dose**
See *Fluconazole for Oral Suspension*.

**Usual pediatric dose**
See *Fluconazole for Oral Suspension*.

**Strength(s) usually available**
U.S.—
  50 mg (Rx) [*Diflucan*].
  100 mg (Rx) [*Diflucan*].
  150 mg (Rx) [*Diflucan*].
  200 mg (Rx) [*Diflucan*].
Canada—
  50 mg (Rx) [*Diflucan*].
  100 mg (Rx) [*Diflucan*].
  200 mg (Rx) [*Diflucan*].

**Packaging and storage**
Store below 40 °C (104 °F), preferably between 15 and 30 °C (59 and 86 °F), in a well-closed container.

**Auxiliary labeling**
• Continue for full time of treatment.

# Parenteral Dosage Forms

## FLUCONAZOLE INJECTION

**Usual adult and adolescent dose**
Candidiasis (prophylaxis)—
  Intravenous, 400 mg once a day.
Candidiasis, disseminated—
  Intravenous, 400 mg on the first day, then 200 mg once a day for at least four weeks and for at least two weeks following the resolution of symptoms.
Candidiasis, esophageal—
  Intravenous, 200 mg on the first day, then 100 mg once a day for at least three weeks and for at least two weeks following the resolution of symptoms. Doses of up to 400 mg once a day may be used depending on clinical response.
Candidiasis, oropharyngeal—
  Intravenous, 200 mg on the first day, then 100 mg once a day for at least two weeks.
Meningitis, cryptococcal (treatment)—
  Intravenous, 400 mg once a day until a clear clinical response is seen, then 200 to 400 mg once a day for at least ten to twelve weeks after the cerebrospinal fluid becomes culture-negative. The patient should be switched to fluconazole tablets when oral therapy can be administered.

Note: Some clinicians prefer a loading dose of 400 mg two times a day for two days, then 400 mg a day for at least ten to twelve weeks after the cerebrospinal fluid becomes culture-negative.

Meningitis, cryptococcal (suppressive therapy)—
  Intravenous, 200 mg once a day.

**Usual pediatric dose**
Candidiasis, esophageal—
  Infants and children 6 months of age and older: Intravenous, 3 mg per kg of body weight once a day for at least three weeks, and for at least two weeks following resolution of symptoms.
  Infants up to 6 months of age: Dosage has not been established.
Candidiasis, oropharyngeal—
  Infants and children 6 months of age and older: Intravenous, 3 mg per kg of body weight once a day for at least two weeks.
  Infants up to 6 months of age: Dosage has not been established.
Meningitis, cryptococcal (treatment)—
  Infants and children 6 months of age and older: Intravenous, 6 to 12 mg per kg of body weight once a day for at least ten to twelve weeks after the cerebrospinal fluid becomes culture-negative.
  Infants up to 6 months of age: Dosage has not been established.
Meningitis, cryptococcal (suppressive therapy)—
  Infants and children 6 months of age and older: Intravenous, 6 mg per kg of body weight once a day.
  Infants up to 6 months of age: Dosage has not been established.

Note: Patients with acute infections should be given a loading dose equal to twice the daily dose, not to exceed 12 mg per kg of body weight, on the first day of treatment.

**Usual pediatric prescribing limits**
600 mg per day.

**Strength(s) usually available**
U.S.—
  200 mg in 100 mL (Rx) [*Diflucan* (56 mg dextrose per mL)].
  200 mg in 100 mL (Rx) [*Diflucan* (9 mg sodium chloride per mL)].
  400 mg in 200 mL (Rx) [*Diflucan* (56 mg dextrose per mL)].
  400 mg in 200 mL (Rx) [*Diflucan* (9 mg sodium chloride per mL)].
Canada—
  200 mg in 100 mL (Rx) [*Diflucan* (9 mg sodium chloride per mL)].
  400 mg in 200 mL (Rx) [*Diflucan* (9 mg sodium chloride per mL)].

**Packaging and storage**
Store below 40 °C (104 °F), preferably between 15 and 30 °C (59 and 86 °F). Protect from freezing.

**Incompatibilities**
Intravenous admixtures of fluconazole and other medications are not recommended.

---

### ITRACONAZOLE

## Summary of Differences
Precautions:
  Drug interactions and/or related problems—
    Antacids, anticholinergics/antispasmodics, histamine $H_2$-receptor antagonists, omeprazole, or sucralfate will increase the pH of the stomach and decrease the absorption of itraconazole.
    Use with astemizole, cisapride, or terfenadine is contraindicated and may increase the risk of cardiac arrhythmias, including torsades de pointes.
    Didanosine contains a buffer to increase its absorption; this will decrease the absorption of itraconazole since itraconazole needs an acidic environment.
    Use with oral antidiabetic agents has increased the plasma concentration of these sulfonylurea agents, leading to hypoglycemia.
    Use with carbamazepine may decrease itraconazole plasma concentrations, leading to treatment failure or relapse.
    Itraconazole may increase digoxin concentrations, leading to digoxin toxicity.
    Use with lovastatin or simvastatin may increase the plasma concentrations of these cholesterol-lowering agents and may increase the risk of rhabdomyolysis.
    Use with midazolam or triazolam may potentiate the hypnotic and sedative effects of these benzodiazepines.
  Medical considerations/contraindications—
    Achlorhydria or hypochlorhydria will decrease the absorption of itraconazole.

## Additional Dosing Information
Itraconazole capsules and itraconazole oral solution are not bioequivalent; the two dosage forms should not be used interchangeably.

The dose of itraconazole and the length of treatment should be based on the site of infection and the individual response to therapy. Treatment may be continued for weeks or months until clinical parameters and laboratory tests indicate that active fungal infection has subsided.

Because patients with acquired immunodeficiency syndrome (AIDS) may have reduced absorption of itraconazole due to hypochlorhydria, they may require higher doses to achieve a clinical response.

Although studies did not provide for a loading dose, in life-threatening situations, a loading dose of 200 mg three times a day (600 mg per day) for the first 3 days is recommended, based on pharmacokinetic data.

Doses above 200 mg per day should be given in two divided doses.

**Diet/Nutrition**

Itraconazole capsules should be taken with food to increase absorption of the medication.

Itraconazole oral solution should be taken on an empty stomach to increase absorption of the medication.

## Oral Dosage Forms

Note: Bracketed uses in the *Dosage Forms* section refer to categories of use and/or indications that are not included in U.S. product labeling.

### ITRACONAZOLE CAPSULES

**Usual adult and adolescent dose**
Aspergillosis—
  Oral, 200 mg one or two times a day with meals for at least three months.
Blastomycosis or
Histoplasmosis (treatment)—
  Oral, 200 mg once a day with meals. The dose may be increased by 100 mg, up to a maximum of 400 mg a day, if there is no obvious improvement or if there is evidence of progressive fungal disease.
[Candidiasis, esophageal] or
[Candidiasis, oropharyngeal]—
  Oral, 100 to 200 mg once a day with a meal for fourteen days; the dose for AIDS and neutropenic patients is increased to 200 mg for four weeks.
[Candidiasis, vulvovaginal][1]—
  Oral, 200 mg once a day with a meal for three days.
[Chromomycosis]—
  Oral, 100 to 200 mg once a day with a meal for three to six months.
[Coccidioidomycosis][1]—
  Oral, 200 mg two times a day with meals for six weeks.
[Cryptococcosis (treatment)][1] or
[Meningitis, cryptococcal (suppression)][1]—
  Oral, 200 mg two times a day with meals.
[Histoplasmosis (suppression)][1]—
  Oral, 200 mg two times a day with meals.
Onychomycosis[1]—
  Fingernails only: Oral, 200 mg two times a day with meals for one week; this treatment is suspended for three weeks, then resumed for one week.
  Toenails with or without fingernail involvement: Oral, 200 mg once a day with meals for twelve consecutive weeks.
[Paracoccidioidomycosis]—
  Oral, 100 mg once a day with a meal for six months.
[Sporotrichosis]—
  Oral, 100 mg once a day with a meal for three months.
[Tinea corporis]or
[Tinea cruris]—
  Oral, 100 mg once a day with a meal for fifteen days.
[Tinea manuum][1] or
[Tinea pedis]—
  Oral, 100 mg once a day with a meal for thirty days.

**Usual pediatric dose**
Safety and efficacy have not been established. However, a small number of patients 3 to 16 years of age have been treated with itraconazole capsules, 100 mg per day, for systemic fungal infections, and no serious adverse effects have been reported.

**Strength(s) usually available**
U.S.—
  100 mg (Rx) [*Sporanox* (sucrose)].
Canada—
  100 mg (Rx) [*Sporanox* (sugar spheres NF)].

**Packaging and storage**
Store below 40 °C (104 °F), preferably between 15 and 30 °C (59 and 86 °F), in a well-closed container.

**Auxiliary labeling**
- Take with food.
- Continue medicine for full time of treatment.

### ITRACONAZOLE ORAL SOLUTION

**Usual adult and adolescent dose**
Candidiasis, esophageal—
  Oral, 100 mg once a day for a minimum of three weeks; treatment should continue for two weeks after resolution of symptoms.
Candidiasis, oropharyngeal—
  Oral, 200 mg once a day for seven to fourteen days.
Note: For patients unresponsive or refractory to treatment with fluconazole, 100 mg two times a day for two to four weeks.

**Usual pediatric dose**
Safety and efficacy have not been established. However, a small number of patients 6 months to 12 years of age have been treated with itraconazole oral solution, 5 mg per kg per day, for systemic fungal infections, and no unexpected serious adverse effects have been reported.

U.S.—
  100 mg per 10 mL (Rx) [*Sporanox* (hydroxypropyl-beta-cyclodextrin [400 mg per mL]; sodium saccharin)].
Canada—
  Not commerically available.

**Packaging and storage**
Store at or below 25 °C (77 °F). Protect from freezing.

**Proper use of dosage form**
Itraconazole oral solution should be vigorously swished in the mouth, 10 mL at a time, for several seconds and swallowed.

**Auxiliary labeling**
- Take on an empty stomach.

---

[1]Not included in Canadian product labeling.

---

## KETOCONAZOLE

## Summary of Differences

Pharmacology/pharmacokinetics:
  Ketoconazole has been shown to suppress corticosteroid secretion and lower serum testosterone concentrations.
  Ketoconazole penetrates poorly into the cerebrospinal fluid.
Precautions:
  Pregnancy/reproduction—
    Ketoconazole may cause menstrual irregularities, oligospermia, azoospermia, impotence, and decreased male libido.
  Drug interactions and/or related problems—
    Alcohol and hepatotoxic medications may increase the risk of hepatotoxicity.
    Antacids, anticholinergics/antispasmodics, histamine $H_2$-receptor antagonists, omeprazole, or sucralfate will increase the pH of the stomach and decrease the absorption of ketoconazole.
    Use with astemizole, cisapride, or terfenadine is contraindicated and may increase the risk of cardiac arrhythmias, including torsades de pointes.
    Didanosine contains a buffer to increase its absorption, which will decrease the absorption of ketoconazole.
    Ketoconazole may increase digoxin concentrations, leading to digoxin toxicity.
    Ketoconazole may increase plasma concentrations of indinavir; a dose reduction of indinavir is recommended.
    Use with midazolam or triazolam may potentiate the hypnotic and sedative effects of these benzodiazepines.
  Medical considerations/contraindications—
    Achlorhydria or hypochlorhydria will decrease the absorption of ketoconazole.
Side/adverse effects:
  Increased risk of hepatotoxicity and of side effects due to inhibition of testosterone and corticosteroid synthesis, such as menstrual irregularities, oligospermia, azoospermia, impotence, and decreased male libido.

## Additional Dosing Information

In patients with achlorhydria or hypochlorhydria, higher serum concentrations may be achieved by taking the medication with an acidic drink. Ketoconazole may be dissolved in cola or seltzer water and swallowed, or the medication may be taken with a glass of cola or seltzer water. An alternative is to dissolve each tablet in 4 mL of 0.2 N hydrochloric acid. Patients may further dilute the resulting mixture in a small amount of water and should be instructed to drink it through a plastic or glass straw to avoid contact with the teeth. This should be followed by one-half glass (120 mL) of water, which is swished around in the mouth and swallowed.

Therapy should be continued for at least 1 to 2 weeks in candidiasis (3 to 5 days in vaginal candidiasis); for 1 to 8 weeks in dermatomycoses caused by yeasts or dermatophytes, and mycoses of hair and scalp; for 3 months to 1 year in paracoccidioidomycosis; and for 6 months or longer in other systemic mycoses. Chronic mucocutaneous candidiasis following a remission usually requires indefinite maintenance treatment to prevent relapse.

**Diet/Nutrition**
Ketoconazole may be taken with a meal or snack to minimize nausea or vomiting and to promote absorption.

## Oral Dosage Forms

Note: Bracketed uses in the *Dosage Forms* section refer to categories of use and/or indications that are not included in U.S. product labeling.

### KETOCONAZOLE ORAL SUSPENSION

**Usual adult and adolescent dose**
[Candidiasis, vulvovaginal][1]—
  Oral, 200 to 400 mg once a day for five days.
[Carcinoma, prostatic][1]—
  Oral, 400 mg three times a day.
[Cushing's syndrome][1]—
  Oral, 600 mg to 1.2 grams a day.
[Paronychia][1]—
  Oral, 200 to 400 mg once a day.
Pityriasis versicolor—
  Oral, 200 mg once a day for five to ten days.
[Pneumonia, fungal][1] or
[Septicemia, fungal][1]—
  Oral, 400 mg to 1 gram once a day.
For all other antifungal indications—
  Oral, 200 to 400 mg once a day.

**Usual adult prescribing limits**
Antifungal—
  1 gram a day.
[Antiadrenal; antineoplastic][1]—
  1.2 grams a day

**Usual pediatric dose**
[Candidiasis, vulvovaginal][1]—
  Children 2 years of age and older: Oral, 5 to 10 mg per kg of body weight once a day for five days.
  Infants and children up to 2 years of age: Dosage has not been established.
[Paronychia][1] or
[Pneumonia, fungal][1] or
[Septicemia, fungal][1]—
  Children 2 years of age and older: Oral, 5 to 10 mg per kg of body weight once a day.
  Infants and children up to 2 years of age: Dosage has not been established.
For all other antifungal indications—
  Children 2 years of age and older: Oral, 3.3 to 6.6 mg per kg of body weight once a day.
  Infants and children up to 2 years of age: Dosage has not been established.

**Strength(s) usually available**
U.S.—
  Not commercially available.
Canada—
  100 mg per 5 mL (Rx) [*Nizoral* (sodium [< 0.55 mg per mL]; sodium benzoate; sucrose)].

**Packaging and storage**
Store below 40 °C (104 °F), preferably between 15 and 30 °C (59 and 86 °F), in a well-closed container. Protect from freezing.

**Auxiliary labeling**
• Shake well.
• Take with food.
• Avoid alcoholic beverages.
• May cause dizziness or drowsiness.
• Continue medicine for full time of treatment (antifungal only).

### KETOCONAZOLE TABLETS USP

**Usual adult and adolescent dose**
See *Ketoconazole Oral Suspension*.

**Usual adult prescribing limits**
See *Ketoconazole Oral Suspension*.

**Usual pediatric dose**
See *Ketoconazole Oral Suspension*.

**Strength(s) usually available**
U.S.—
  200 mg (Rx) [*Nizoral* (scored; lactose)].
Canada—
  200 mg (Rx) [*Nizoral* (scored; lactose)].

**Packaging and storage**
Store below 40 °C (104 °F), preferably between 15 and 30 °C (59 and 86 °F). Store in a well-closed container.

**Auxiliary labeling**
• Take with food.
• Avoid alcoholic beverages.
• May cause dizziness or drowsiness.
• Continue medicine for full time of treatment (antifungal only).

[1]Not included in Canadian product labeling.

Revised: 05/20/94
Interim revision: 11/14/94; 04/18/95; 08/14/97; 08/03/98

## Table 1. Pharmacology/Pharmacokinetics*

| Drug | Route of administration* | Bioavailability (%) | Vol$_D$ | CSF/Serum concentrations (%) | Protein binding (%) | Metabolism |
|---|---|---|---|---|---|---|
| Fluconazole | IV, PO | 90 (fasting) | 0.7-1 L/kg | 54-85 (patients with meningitis) | 11 | Hepatic† |
| Itraconazole | PO, capsules | 40-55 (fasting) 90-100 (with food) | 796 L | < 10 | 99 | Hepatic‡ |
| | PO, oral solution | 90-100 (fasting) 55 (with food) | 796 L | | 99 | Hepatic‡ |
| Ketoconazole | PO | 75 (with food) | 0.36 L/kg | < 10 | 99 | Hepatic |

*IV = intravenous; PO = oral; Vol$_D$ = apparent volume of distribution; CSF = cerebrospinal fluid; L/kg = liters per kilogram.
†Fluconazole is primarily excreted by the kidneys; however, a small amount of the drug undergoes hepatic metabolization.
‡Itraconazole is extensively metabolized by the liver, with more than 30 identifiable inactive metabolites. The major metabolite, hydroxyitraconazole, has antifungal activity.

## Table 2. Pharmacology/Pharmacokinetics

| Drug | Half-life (hr) Normal renal function | Half-life (hr) Impaired renal function | Time to peak serum concentration (hr) | Peak serum concentration after dose mcg/mL | Peak serum concentration after dose Dose | Renal excretion (% unchanged) | Biliary excretion |
|---|---|---|---|---|---|---|---|
| Fluconazole | 30 (adults) 14-20 (children) | 98-125 | 1-2 | 4.5-8 | 100 mg | > 80 | Yes; small amount |
| Itraconazole (capsules) | 21 (single dose) 64 (steady state) | | 3-4 | 0.132* 0.234* | 100 mg (with food) 200 mg (with food) | 0.03 | 3-18% |
| Itraconazole (oral solution) | 39 (steady state) 37 (steady state) | | 2.5 4.4 | 1.96* 1.43* | 200 mg (fasting) 200 mg (with food) | 0.03 | |
| Ketoconazole | 8 | | 1-4 | 3.5 | 200 mg (with food) | 2-4 | Yes; primary route of elimination |

*The plasma concentrations reported were measured by high performance liquid chromatography (HPLC), specific for itraconazole. When itraconazole in plasma is measured by a bioassay, values reported are approximately 3.3 times higher than those detected by HPLC due to the presence of the bioactive metabolite, hydroxyitraconazole.

# ANTIFUNGALS, AZOLE   Vaginal

This monograph includes information on the following: 1) Butoconazole†; 2) Clotrimazole; 3) Econazole*; 4) Miconazole; 5) Terconazole; 6) Tioconazole.

VA CLASSIFICATION (Primary): GU302

Commonly used brand name(s): *Canesten 1-Day Cream Combi-Pak[2]; Canesten 1-Day Therapy[2]; Canesten 3-Day Therapy[2]; Canesten 6-Day Therapy[2]; Canesten Combi-Pak 1-Day Therapy[2]; Canesten Combi-Pak 3-Day Therapy[2]; Clotrimaderm[2]; Ecostatin Vaginal Ovules[3]; FemCare[2]; Femizol-M[4]; Femstat 3[1]; Gyne-Lotrimin[2]; Gyne-Lotrimin Combination Pack[2]; Gyne-Lotrimin3[2]; Gyne-Lotrimin3 Combination Pack[2]; GyneCure[6]; GyneCure Ovules[6]; GyneCure Vaginal Ointment Tandempak[6]; GyneCure Vaginal Ovules Tandempak[6]; Miconazole-7[4]; Micozole[4]; Monazole 7[4]; Monistat 1[6]; Monistat 3[4]; Monistat 3 Combination Pack[4]; Monistat 3 Dual-Pak[4]; Monistat 3 Vaginal Ovules[4]; Monistat 5 Tampon[4]; Monistat 7[4]; Monistat 7 Combination Pack[4]; Monistat 7 Dual-Pak[4]; Monistat 7 Vaginal Suppositories[4]; Mycelex Twin Pack[2]; Mycelex-7[2]; Mycelex-G[2]; Myclo-Gyne[4]; Novo-Miconazole Vaginal Ovules[4]; Terazol 3[5]; Terazol 3 Dual-Pak[5]; Terazol 3 Vaginal Ovules[5]; Terazol 7[5]; Vagistat-1[6]*.

Note:   For a listing of dosage forms and brand names by country availability, see *Dosage Forms* section(s).

*Not commercially available in U.S.
†Not commercially available in Canada.

## Category

Antifungal (vaginal).

## Indications

### Accepted

**Candidiasis, vulvovaginal (treatment)**—Vaginal azoles are indicated in the local treatment of vulvovaginal candidiasis caused by *Candida albicans* and other species of *Candida* in pregnant (second and third trimesters only) and nonpregnant women. It is recommended that nonpregnant women self-medicate with nonprescription antifungal vaginal medications only if they have been diagnosed previously with vulvovaginal candidiasis and have the same symptoms. If symptoms recur within 2 months, women should seek professional medical care. Pregnant women treating vulvovaginal candidiasis with antifungal vaginal agents should use at least a 7-day treatment regimen and seek their physician's advice before using medication in the first trimester.

Not all species or strains of a particular organism may be susceptible to a specific vaginal azole.

### Unaccepted

Vaginal azoles are not effective in the treatment of vulvovaginitis caused by other common pathogens such as *Trichomonas vaginalis*.

## Pharmacology/Pharmacokinetics

### Physicochemical characteristics

Chemical group—
   Imidazoles: Butoconazole, clotrimazole, econazole nitrate, miconazole nitrate, tioconazole.
   Triazole: Terconazole.

Molecular weight—
   Butoconazole nitrate: 474.80.
   Clotrimazole: 344.85.
   Econazole nitrate: 444.70.
   Miconazole nitrate: 479.15.
   Terconazole: 532.47.
   Tioconazole: 387.72.

### Mechanism of action/Effect

Fungistatic; may be fungicidal, depending on concentration; exact mechanism of action is unknown. Azoles inhibit biosynthesis of ergosterol or other sterols, damaging the fungal cell membrane and altering its permeability. As a result, loss of essential intracellular elements may occur.

Azoles also inhibit biosynthesis of triglycerides and phospholipids by fungi. In addition, azoles inhibit oxidative and peroxidative enzyme activity, resulting in intracellular buildup of toxic concentrations of hydrogen peroxide, which may contribute to deterioration of subcellular organelles and cellular necrosis. In *Candida albicans*, azoles inhibit transformation of blastospores into invasive mycelial form.

Terconazole—Triazoles are more slowly metabolized than imidazoles. Triazoles also affect sterol synthesis to a lesser degree.

### Absorption

Butoconazole—Approximately 5.5% absorbed systemically following intravaginal administration.

Clotrimazole—3 to 10% estimated to be absorbed following intravaginal administration.

Econazole; miconazole; tioconazole—Small amounts absorbed systemically following intravaginal administration.

Terconazole—Approximately 5 to 8% absorbed in hysterectomized patients and approximately 12 to 16% absorbed in nonhysterectomized patients with tubal ligations.

### Biotransformation

Clotrimazole—Rapidly metabolized to inactive metabolites.

## Precautions to Consider

### Carcinogenicity

*Butoconazole; miconazole; terconazole; tioconazole*—Long-term studies in animals have not been done.

*Clotrimazole*—Long-term studies of intravaginal clotrimazole in animals have not been done. However, a long-term study of oral clotrimazole in Wistar strains of rats has not shown that clotrimazole is carcinogenic.

*Terconazole*—Studies have not been done.

**Mutagenicity**
*Butoconazole*—Butoconazole has not been shown to be mutagenic in studies in appropriate indicator microorganisms.
*Terconazole*—Terconazole has not been shown to be mutagenic in studies for induction of microbial point mutations (Ames test), induction of cellular transformation, chromosomal breaks (micronucleus test), or in studies for dominant lethal mutations in mouse germ cells.
*Tioconazole*—No mutagenic or cytogenic effects were observed.

**Pregnancy/Reproduction**
Fertility—*Butoconazole*: Studies in rabbits or rats, given oral doses of up to 30 or 100 mg per kg of body weight (mg/kg) daily, respectively, have not shown that butoconazole causes impaired fertility.
*Terconazole*: Terconazole, given orally in doses of up to 40 mg/kg daily, has not been shown to cause impairment of fertility in female rats.

Pregnancy—Pregnant women treating vulvovaginal candidiasis with antifungal vaginal agents should use at least a 7-day treatment regimen. A decision to use antifungal vaginal agents during the first trimester should be based on risk-benefit status and on advice of the physician.
*Butoconazole*: Adequate and well-controlled studies in humans have not been done during the first trimester. Clinical studies in over 200 pregnant women, given butoconazole intravaginally for 3 or 6 days during the second and third trimesters, have not shown that butoconazole causes adverse effects on the fetus. Follow-up reports on infants born to these women have not shown that butoconazole causes any adverse effects.
Studies in rats, given intravaginal doses of 6 mg/kg daily (three to seven times the usual human dose) during organogenesis, have shown that butoconazole causes an increase in resorption rate and a decrease in litter size. Butoconazole was not shown to be teratogenic.
Studies in rats, given oral doses of up to 50 mg/kg daily throughout organogenesis, have not shown that butoconazole causes adverse effects on the fetus. The administration of oral doses of 100, 300, or 750 mg/kg daily has resulted in adverse effects (abdominal wall defects, cleft palate) on the fetus, although maternal stress was evident at these higher dosages.
Studies in rabbits, given oral doses (e.g., 150 mg/kg) that caused maternal stress, have not shown that butoconazole causes adverse effects on the fetus.
FDA Pregnancy Category C.
*Clotrimazole*: Adequate and well-controlled studies in humans have not been done during the first trimester. Reports on up to 177 pregnant females given clotrimazole intravaginally during the second and third trimesters have not shown that clotrimazole causes adverse effects on the fetus. Follow-up reports on 71 infants born to these females have not shown that clotrimazole causes any adverse effects.
Studies in rats, given repeated intravaginal doses of up to 100 mg/kg daily, have not shown that clotrimazole causes adverse effects on the fetus.
Studies in rats and mice, given repeated oral doses of 50 to 120 mg/kg, have shown that clotrimazole causes embryotoxicity (possibly secondary to maternal toxicity), impairment of mating, decreased litter size and number of viable young, and decreased survival to weaning. Studies in mice, rabbits, and rats, given oral doses of up to 200, 180, and 100 mg/kg, respectively, have not shown that clotrimazole is teratogenic.
FDA Pregnancy Category B.
*Econazole*: Adequate and well-controlled studies have not been performed in humans.
*Miconazole*: Clinical studies in over 500 pregnant females given miconazole intravaginally for 14 days have not shown that miconazole causes adverse effects on the fetus. Follow-up reports on infants born to these women have not shown that miconazole causes any adverse effects.
Miconazole crosses the placenta in animals. Studies in animals have shown that miconazole, given in oral doses of 80 mg/kg, causes embryotoxicity and fetotoxicity. Studies in rats have shown that miconazole, given orally, causes prolonged gestation, although this was not shown in studies using rabbits.
FDA Pregnancy Category B.
*Terconazole*: At oral doses less than or equal to 10 mg/kg, no embryotoxicity was seen in rats. Studies in rats given terconazole orally in doses of 10 mg/kg daily have shown that terconazole causes delayed fetal ossification. In studies in rats given 20 to 40 mg/kg orally during organogenesis, terconazole was shown to cause embryotoxicity (e.g., decreased litter size and number of viable young, reduced fetal weight, delayed ossification, and increased incidence of skeletal abnormalities). The skeletal changes observed (delayed ossification, short wavy ribs) were felt to be secondary to maternal toxicity or stress, which was evident from reduced body weight gain during most of the organogenesis period.
Terconazole has not been shown to be teratogenic in rats given oral doses of up to 40 mg/kg daily or given subcutaneous doses of up to 20 mg/kg daily, or in rabbits given doses of 20 mg/kg daily.
FDA Pregnancy Category C.
*Tioconazole*: Adequate and well-controlled studies have not been performed in humans.
In limited and uncontrolled clinical use in about 20 patients, a single dose administered at varying stages of pregnancy did not appear to interfere with normal progress of the pregnancy and delivery. However, 1-day treatment may not be effective in pregnant patients and is not recommended.
In studies in rats, adverse effects on parturition and/or fetal development were observed during local and systemic use.
FDA Pregnancy Category C.

Labor—Vaginal azoles have been shown to cause dystocia in rats when given through parturition.
*Butoconazole*: Butoconazole has not been shown to cause dystocia in rabbits given oral doses of up to 100 mg/kg.
*Terconazole*: Terconazole has not been shown to adversely affect parturition in rats given up to 40 mg/kg orally per day during pregnancy, up through 3 weeks of lactation.

**Breast-feeding**
It is not known whether vaginal azoles are distributed into breast milk. However, problems in humans have not been documented.

**Pediatrics**
No information is available on the relationship of age to the effects of vaginal azoles in pediatric patients. Safety and efficacy have not been established in children up to 12 years of age.

**Geriatrics**
Appropriate studies on the relationship of age to the effects of vaginal azoles have not been performed in the geriatric population. However, no geriatrics-specific problems have been documented to date.

**Medical considerations/Contraindications**
The medical considerations/contraindications included have been selected on the basis of their potential clinical significance (reasons given in parentheses where appropriate)—not necessarily inclusive (» = major clinical significance).

*Risk-benefit should be considered when the following medical problem exists:*
    Allergy to azoles

## Side/Adverse Effects
The following side/adverse effects have been selected on the basis of their potential clinical significance (possible signs and symptoms in parentheses where appropriate)—not necessarily inclusive:

**Those indicating need for medical attention**
Incidence less frequent
    *Vaginal burning, itching, discharge, or other irritation not present before therapy*
Incidence rare
    *Hypersensitivity* (skin rash or hives)

**Those indicating need for medical attention only if they continue or are bothersome**
Incidence less frequent or rare
    *Abdominal or stomach cramps or pain; burning or irritation of penis of sexual partner; headache*

## Patient Consultation
As an aid to patient consultation, refer to *Advice for the Patient, Antifungals, Azole (Vaginal)*.
In providing consultation, consider emphasizing the following selected information (» = major clinical significance):

**Before using this medication**
» Conditions affecting use, especially:
    Allergy to azoles
        Pregnancy—Some animal studies have shown that vaginal azoles may be embryotoxic or fetotoxic; however, problems have not been documented in humans. Use of at least a 7-day treatment regimen is recommended for pregnant patients in the second and third trimesters instead of regimens of shorter duration; use of the medication in the first trimester should be based on risk-benefit status and on the advice of a physician
        Labor—Vaginal azoles have been shown in some studies to cause dystocia when given through labor

**Proper use of this medication**
Reading patient instructions before using medication
Using at bedtime, unless otherwise directed by physician; retaining miconazole vaginal tampons overnight and removing them the following morning
Checking with physician before using applicator if pregnant
Using cream, which is packaged with some of the vaginal suppositories or tablets, by applying it externally to genitalia to treat genital itching
» Compliance with full course of therapy, even if menstruation begins
» Proper dosing
Missed dose: Inserting as soon as possible; not inserting if almost time for next dose
» Proper storage

**Precautions while using this medication**
Checking with physician if no improvement within 3 days, if symptoms do not disappear within 7 days, or if symptoms worsen during use of 1-, 3-, and 7-day treatment regimens; also, checking with physician if symptoms return within 2 months or if exposure to human immunodeficiency virus (HIV) occurs
Protecting clothing because of possible soiling with vaginal azoles; avoiding the use of unmedicated tampons
»*Using hygienic measures to cure infection and prevent reinfection*
Wearing cotton panties instead of synthetic underclothes
Wearing only freshly washed underclothes
» Routine treatment of sexual partner is unnecessary unless male partner is experiencing symptoms of local itching or skin irritation of the penis
» Understanding that some vaginal products may contain oils that damage latex; avoiding concurrent use of latex products, such as condoms, diaphragms, and cervical caps, during treatment and for 3 days after discontinuing medication
» Checking with doctor before douching between doses to obtain recommendation for use and advice for proper procedure

**Side/adverse effects**
Signs of potential side effects, especially vaginal burning, itching, discharge, or other irritation not present before therapy, and hypersensitivity

## General Dosing Information

Diagnosis of first-time users of vaginal azole antifungal agents should be made by physicians. Patients should consult a physician if symptoms return within 2 months or if exposure to HIV occurs. Recurring yeast infections may be a sign of other conditions, such as diabetes or impaired immune function. Recurring conditions or severe local vaginal infections may benefit from vaginal treatments of longer duration, such as 10 to 14 days, or from the use of appropriate oral medications instead.

If there is no response to therapy, the course of therapy may be repeated after other pathogens have been ruled out by potassium hydroxide (KOH) smears and cultures.

If sensitization or irritation occurs, treatment with vaginal azoles should be discontinued.

It is recommended that the patient wait 3 days after treatment with azole antifungal agents to resume using latex barrier devices such as condoms or diaphragms. The vehicles for some vaginal azole products contain lipid-based components. It is likely that many of these products affect the performance of latex contraceptive devices, such as cervical caps, condoms, or diaphragms.

Unmedicated tampons may absorb vaginal creams, ointments, or suppositories and are not recommended for use concurrently with vaginal azole antifungal agents.

**For tioconazole ointment**
Symptomatic relief following one dose of tioconazole ointment may take up to 7 days to achieve.

---
### BUTOCONAZOLE
---

## Vaginal Dosage Forms

### BUTOCONAZOLE NITRATE CREAM (VAGINAL) USP

**Usual adult and adolescent dose**
Antifungal (vaginal)—
Nonpregnant patients: Intravaginal, 100 mg (1 applicatorful of a 2% cream) once a day at bedtime for three days. May be repeated for an additional three days if needed.
Pregnant patients (second and third trimesters only): Intravaginal, 100 mg (1 applicatorful of a 2% cream) once a day at bedtime for six days.

**Usual pediatric dose**
Children up to 12 years of age: Safety and efficacy have not been established.

**Strength(s) usually available**
U.S.—
2% (100 mg per applicatorful) (OTC) [*Femstat 3*].
Note: Packaging may include either three prefilled applicators or three cardboard applicators plus tube of cream.
Canada—
Not commercially available.

**Packaging and storage**
Store below 40 °C (104 °F), preferably between 15 and 30 °C (59 and 86 °F), unless otherwise specified by manufacturer. Store in a tight container. Protect from freezing.

**Auxiliary labeling**
• For vaginal use only.
• Continue medicine for full time of treatment.

**Note**
Include patient instructions when dispensing.

### BUTOCONAZOLE NITRATE VAGINAL SUPPOSITORIES

**Usual adult and adolescent dose**
Antifungal (vaginal)—
Nonpregnant patients: Intravaginal, 100 mg once a day at bedtime for three days. May be repeated for an additional three days if needed.

**Usual pediatric dose**
Children up to 12 years of age: Safety and efficacy have not been established.

**Strength(s) usually available**
U.S.—
Not commercially available.
Canada—
Not commercially available.

**Packaging and storage**
Store below 40 °C (104 °F), preferably between 15 and 30 °C (59 and 86 °F), unless otherwise specified by manufacturer. Store in a well-closed container.

**Auxiliary labeling**
• For vaginal use only.
• Continue medicine for full time of treatment.

**Note**
Include patient instructions when dispensing.

---
### CLOTRIMAZOLE
---

## Vaginal Dosage Forms

### CLOTRIMAZOLE CREAM (VAGINAL) USP

**Usual adult and adolescent dose**
Antifungal (vaginal)—
Intravaginal, 50 mg (1 applicatorful of a 1% vaginal cream) once a day, preferably at bedtime, for six to fourteen consecutive days; or
Intravaginal, 100 mg (1 applicatorful of a 2% vaginal cream) once a day, preferably at bedtime, for three days; or
Intravaginal, 500 mg (1 applicatorful of a 10% vaginal cream) as a single dose, preferably at bedtime.

**Usual pediatric dose**
Children up to 12 years of age: Safety and efficacy have not been established.

**Strength(s) usually available**
U.S.—
1% (50 mg per applicatorful) (OTC) [*FemCare; Gyne-Lotrimin; Mycelex-7;* GENERIC].
Canada—
1% (50 mg per applicatorful) (OTC) [*Canesten 6-Day Therapy; Clotrimaderm; Myclo-Gyne*].
2% (100 mg per applicatorful) (OTC) [*Canesten 3-Day Therapy; Clotrimaderm*].
10% (500 mg per applicatorful) (OTC) [*Canesten 1-Day Therapy; Canesten 1-Day Cream Combi-Pak*].
Note: Many of these products are packaged with one reusable vaginal applicator or more than one single-use vaginal applicator, or as prefilled vaginal applicators.

Combi-paks also contain a small tube of 1% clotrimazole cream for external application to genitals for treatment of itching.

**Packaging and storage**
Store between 2 and 30 °C (36 and 86 °F). Store in a collapsible tube or in a tight container.

**Auxiliary labeling**
- For vaginal use only.
- Continue medicine for full time of treatment.

**Note**
Include patient instructions when dispensing.

### CLOTRIMAZOLE VAGINAL TABLETS USP

**Usual adult and adolescent dose**
Antifungal (vaginal)—
  Nonpregnant patients: Intravaginal, 500 mg as a single dose, preferably at bedtime; 200 mg once a day, preferably at bedtime, for three consecutive days; or 100 mg once a day, preferably at bedtime, for six or seven consecutive days.
  Pregnant patients: Intravaginal, 100 mg once a day, preferably at bedtime, for seven consecutive days.
Note: The three-day regimen is not effective in pregnant women.
  In severe vulvovaginal candidiasis, single-dose treatment with clotrimazole 500-mg vaginal tablets may not be effective. Longer treatment with the 100- or 200-mg vaginal tablets or vaginal cream is recommended.

**Usual pediatric dose**
Children up to 12 years of age: Safety and efficacy have not been established.

**Strength(s) usually available**
U.S.—
  100 mg (OTC) [*FemCare; Gyne-Lotrimin; Gyne-Lotrimin Combination Pack; Mycelex-7;* GENERIC].
  200 mg (OTC) [*Gyne-Lotrimin3; Gyne-Lotrimin3 Combination Pack*].
  500 mg (Rx) [*Mycelex-G; Mycelex Twin Pack*].
Canada—
  100 mg (OTC) [*Myclo-Gyne*].
  200 mg (OTC) [*Canesten Combi-Pak 3-Day Therapy*].
  500 mg (OTC) [*Canesten Combi-Pak 1-Day Therapy*].
Note: Twin and combination packs and combi-paks also contain a small tube of 1% clotrimazole cream for external application to genitals for treatment of itching.

**Packaging and storage**
Store below 40 °C (104 °F), preferably between 15 and 30 °C (59 and 86 °F), unless otherwise specified by manufacturer. Store in a well-closed container.

**Auxiliary labeling**
- For vaginal use only.
- Continue medicine for full time of treatment.

**Note**
Include patient instructions when dispensing.

---
## ECONAZOLE
---

## Vaginal Dosage Forms

### ECONAZOLE NITRATE VAGINAL SUPPOSITORIES

**Usual adult and adolescent dose**
Antifungal (vaginal)—
  Intravaginal, 150 mg once a day at bedtime for three days. May be repeated if needed.

**Usual pediatric dose**
Children up to 12 years of age: Safety and efficacy have not been established.

**Strength(s) usually available**
U.S.—
  Not commercially available.
Canada—
  150 mg (Rx) [*Ecostatin Vaginal Ovules*].

**Packaging and storage**
Store below 30 °C (86 °F), in a well-closed container, unless otherwise specified by manufacturer.

**Auxiliary labeling**
- For vaginal use only.
- Continue medicine for full time of treatment.

**Note**
Include patient instructions when dispensing.

---
## MICONAZOLE
---

## Vaginal Dosage Forms

### MICONAZOLE NITRATE VAGINAL CREAM

**Usual adult and adolescent dose**
Antifungal (vaginal)—
  Intravaginal, 20 mg (one applicatorful) once a day at bedtime for seven days. May be repeated if needed.

**Usual pediatric dose**
Children up to 12 years of age: Safety and efficacy have not been established.

**Strength(s) usually available**
U.S.—
  2% (OTC) [*Femizol-M; Miconazole-7; Monistat 7;* GENERIC].
Canada—
  2% (OTC) [*Micozole; Monazole 7; Monistat 7*].
Note: Many of these products are packaged with one reusable vaginal applicator or more than one single-use vaginal applicator, or as prefilled vaginal applicators.

**Packaging and storage**
Store below 40 °C (104 °F), preferably between 15 and 30 °C (59 and 86 °F), unless otherwise specified by manufacturer. Store in a tight container. Protect from freezing.

**Auxiliary labeling**
- For vaginal use only.
- Continue medicine for full time of treatment.

**Note**
Include patient instructions when dispensing.

### MICONAZOLE NITRATE VAGINAL SUPPOSITORIES USP

**Usual adult and adolescent dose**
Antifungal (vaginal)—
  Intravaginal, 100 mg once a day at bedtime for seven days. May be repeated for seven days if needed; or
  Intravaginal, 200 or 400 mg once a day at bedtime for three days. May be repeated if needed.

**Usual pediatric dose**
Children up to 12 years of age: Safety and efficacy have not been established.

**Strength(s) usually available**
U.S.—
  100 mg (OTC) [*Monistat 7; Monistat 7 Combination Pack;* GENERIC].
  200 mg (OTC) [*Monistat 3 Combination Pack*].
  200 mg (Rx) [*Monistat 3*].
Canada—
  100 mg (OTC) [*Monistat 7 Vaginal Suppositories; Monistat 7 Dual-Pak*].
  400 mg (OTC) [*Monistat 3 Vaginal Ovules; Monistat 3 Dual-Pak; Novo-Miconazole Vaginal Ovules*].
Note: Dual-paks and combination packs also contain a small tube of 2% miconazole cream for external application to genitals for treatment of itching.

**Packaging and storage**
Store between 15 and 30 °C (59 and 86 °F). Store in a tight container.

**Auxiliary labeling**
- For vaginal use only.
- Continue medicine for full time of treatment.

**Note**
Include patient instructions when dispensing.

### MICONAZOLE NITRATE VAGINAL TAMPONS

**Usual adult and adolescent dose**
Antifungal (vaginal)—
  Intravaginal, 100 mg (1 tampon) once a day at bedtime for five consecutive days; retain vaginally overnight and remove tampon the following morning.

**Usual pediatric dose**
Children up to 12 years of age: Safety and efficacy have not been established.

**Strength(s) usually available**
U.S.—
  5% (Rx) [*Monistat 5 Tampon*].
  Note: Available in California only.
Canada—
  Not commercially available.

**Packaging and storage**
Store below 40 °C (104 °F), preferably between 15 and 30 °C (59 and 86 °F), in a well-closed container, unless otherwise specified by manufacturer.

**Auxiliary labeling**
• For vaginal use only.
• Continue medicine for full time of treatment.

**Note**
Include patient instructions when dispensing.

---
### TERCONAZOLE
---

## Vaginal Dosage Forms

### TERCONAZOLE VAGINAL CREAM

**Usual adult and adolescent dose**
Antifungal (vaginal)—
  Intravaginal, 20 mg (1 applicatorful of a 0.4% cream) once a day at bedtime for seven days; or
  Intravaginal, 40 mg (1 applicatorful of a 0.8% cream) once a day at bedtime for three days.

**Usual pediatric dose**
Children up to 12 years of age: Safety and efficacy have not been established.

**Strength(s) usually available**
U.S.—
  0.4% (20 mg per applicatorful) (Rx) [*Terazol 7*].
  0.8% (40 mg per applicatorful) (Rx) [*Terazol 3*].
Canada—
  0.4% (20 mg per applicatorful) (Rx) [*Terazol 7*].
  0.8% (40 mg per applicatorful) (Rx) [*Terazol 3*].

**Packaging and storage**
Store below 40 °C (104 °F), preferably between 15 and 30 °C (59 and 86 °F), in a well-closed container, unless otherwise specified by manufacturer. Protect from freezing.

**Auxiliary labeling**
• For vaginal use only.
• Continue medicine for full time of treatment.

**Note**
Include patient instructions when dispensing.

### TERCONAZOLE VAGINAL SUPPOSITORIES

**Usual adult and adolescent dose**
Antifungal (vaginal)—
  Intravaginal, 80 mg once a day at bedtime for three days.

**Usual pediatric dose**
Children up to 12 years of age: Safety and efficacy have not been established.

**Strength(s) usually available**
U.S.—
  80 mg (Rx) [*Terazol 3*].
Canada—
  80 mg (Rx) [*Terazol 3 Dual-Pak; Terazol 3 Vaginal Ovules*].
Note: Dual-paks also contain a small tube of 0.8% terconazole cream for external application to genitals for treatment of itching.

**Packaging and storage**
Store below 40 °C (104 °F), preferably between 15 and 30 °C (59 and 86 °F), in a well-closed container, unless otherwise specified by manufacturer.

**Auxiliary labeling**
• For vaginal use only.
• Continue medicine for full time of treatment.

**Note**
Include patient instructions when dispensing.

---
### TIOCONAZOLE
---

## Vaginal Dosage Forms

### TIOCONAZOLE VAGINAL OINTMENT

**Usual adult and adolescent dose**
Antifungal (vaginal)—
  Intravaginal, 300 mg (1 applicatorful of a 6.5% vaginal ointment) as a single dose, preferably at bedtime.
Note: Limited data suggest that a second dose one or two weeks later may be effective for those patients with residual symptoms after one dose.

**Usual pediatric dose**
Children up to 12 years of age: Safety and efficacy have not been established.

**Strength(s) usually available**
U.S.—
  6.5% (OTC) [*Monistat 1; Vagistat-1*].
Canada—
  6.5% (OTC) [*GyneCure; GyneCure Vaginal Ointment Tandempak*].
Note: Tandempaks also contain a small tube of 1% tioconazole cream for external application to genitals for treatment of itching.

**Packaging and storage**
Store below 40 °C (104 °F), preferably between 15 and 30 °C (59 and 86 °F), in a well-closed container, unless otherwise specified by manufacturer.

**Auxiliary labeling**
• For vaginal use only.

### TIOCONAZOLE VAGINAL SUPPOSITORIES

**Usual adult and adolescent dose**
Antifungal (vaginal)—
  Intravaginal, 300 mg, as a single dose, preferably at bedtime.
Note: Limited data suggest that a second dose one or two weeks later may be effective for those patients with residual symptoms after one dose.

**Usual pediatric dose**
Children up to 12 years of age: Safety and efficacy have not been established.

**Strength(s) usually available**
U.S.—
  Not commercially available.
Canada—
  300 mg (OTC) [*GyneCure Ovules; GyneCure Vaginal Ovules Tandempak*].
Note: Tandempaks also contain a small tube of 1% tioconazole cream for external application to genitals for treatment of itching.

**Packaging and storage**
Store below 40 °C (104 °F), preferably between 15 and 30 °C (59 and 86 °F), in a well-closed container, unless otherwise specified by manufacturer.

**Auxiliary labeling**
• For vaginal use only.

**Note**
Include patient instructions when dispensing.

## Selected Bibliography
Doering PL, Santiago TM. Drugs for treatment of vulvovaginal candidiasis: comparative efficacy of agents and regimens [review]. Drug Intell Clin Pharm 1990; 24: 1078-83.

Revised: 08/10/98

# ANTIGLAUCOMA AGENTS, CHOLINERGIC, LONG-ACTING  Ophthalmic

This monograph includes information on the following: 1) Demecarium; 2) Echothiophate; 3) Isoflurophate.

INN: Echothiophate—Ecothiopate Iodide

VA CLASSIFICATION (Primary/Secondary): OP180/OP900; DX900

Commonly used brand name(s): *Floropryl*[3]; *Humorsol*[1]; *Phospholine Iodide*[2].

Other commonly used names are: DFP [Isoflurophate] Difluorophate [Isoflurophate] Dyflos [Isoflurophate]

Note: For a listing of dosage forms and brand names by country availability, see *Dosage Forms* section(s).

## Category
Antiglaucoma agent (ophthalmic); cyclostimulant (accommodative esotropia); diagnostic aid (accommodative esotropia).

## Indications

**Accepted**

Glaucoma (treatment)—Demecarium, echothiophate, and isoflurophate, which are long-acting cholinesterase inhibitors, are potent miotics. Because of their toxicity, they should be reserved for use in patients with open-angle glaucoma or other chronic glaucomas not satisfactorily controlled with the short-acting miotics and other agents.

Glaucoma, open-angle (treatment): Demecarium, echothiophate, and isoflurophate are indicated in the treatment of chronic open-angle glaucoma.

Glaucoma, angle-closure, *after* iridectomy (treatment): Demecarium, echothiophate, and isoflurophate are indicated in the treatment of subacute or chronic angle-closure glaucoma following iridectomy if continued drug therapy is required and short-acting miotics and other agents are inadequate. Long-acting cholinesterase inhibitors are usually not recommended for use in angle-closure glaucoma *prior* to iridectomy, because they may increase the pupillary block. However, echothiophate may be indicated in subacute or chronic angle-closure glaucoma when surgery is refused or contraindicated in the informed patient who understands the increased risk of pupillary block.

Glaucoma, secondary (treatment): Echothiophate is indicated in the treatment of certain nonuveitic secondary types of glaucoma, especially glaucoma following cataract surgery.

Esotropia, accommodative (diagnosis) or

Esotropia, accommodative (treatment)—Demecarium, echothiophate, and isoflurophate are indicated in the diagnosis of accommodative esotropia. Demecarium and isoflurophate are indicated in the treatment of accommodative esotropia uncomplicated by anisometropia. Echothiophate may be indicated in the treatment of concomitant esotropias with a significant accommodative component.

## Pharmacology/Pharmacokinetics

**Physicochemical characteristics**

Molecular weight—
 Demecarium bromide: 716.60.
 Echothiophate iodide: 383.22.
 Isoflurophate: 184.15.

**Mechanism of action/Effect**

Demecarium, echothiophate, and isoflurophate are indirect-acting parasympathomimetic agents, which are also known as cholinesterase inhibitors and anticholinesterases. Cholinesterase inhibitors prolong the effect of acetylcholine, which is released at the neuroeffector junction of parasympathetic postganglion nerves, by inactivating the cholinesterases that break it down. Echothiophate and isoflurophate primarily inactivate pseudocholinesterase and incompletely inactivate acetylcholinesterase, whereas demecarium inactivates both pseudocholinesterase and acetylcholinesterase. In the eye, this causes constriction of the iris sphincter muscle (causing miosis) and the ciliary muscle (affecting the accommodation reflex and causing a spasm of the focus to near vision). The outflow of the aqueous humor is facilitated, which leads to a reduction in intraocular pressure. Of the 2 actions, the effect on the accommodation reflex is the more transient and generally disappears before termination of the miosis.

Antiglaucoma agent (ophthalmic)—Cholinesterase inhibitors reduce intraocular pressure in both types of primary glaucoma (i.e., angle-closure glaucoma and open-angle glaucoma) primarily by lowering the resistance to the outflow of the aqueous humor. In angle-closure glaucoma, the abnormal contact between the peripheral iris and the peripheral cornea blocks the access of the anterior chamber of aqueous humor to the trabecular meshwork. In open-angle glaucoma, the block is between the trabecular meshwork and the canal of Schlemm. Effects on the volumes of the various intraocular vascular beds (e.g., those of the iris and the ciliary body) and on the rate of secretion of the aqueous humor into the posterior chamber may contribute secondarily to the lowering of pressure. Contraction of the ciliary muscle may act to increase tone and alignment of the trabecular meshwork, which improves outflow of aqueous humor through the meshwork to the canal of Schlemm. The longitudinal ciliary muscle is the major component; the iris sphincter is notrelevant in open-angle glaucoma, but its contraction may improve (or worsen) angle-closure glaucoma. In angle-closure glaucoma, the outflow of the aqueous humor is facilitated by the drug-induced contraction of the iris sphincter muscle. This contraction prevents the iris from blocking the entrance to the trabecular space at the canal of Schlemm by lessening pupillary block. However, extreme miosis may actually increase pupillary block, thus worsening angle-closure glaucoma prior to iridectomy. In open-angle glaucoma, although there is no physical obstruction at the entrance to the trabecular space, the trabeculae, which are a meshwork of small-diameter pores, increase their resistance and lose their permeability.

Cyclostimulant (accommodative esotropia)—Cholinesterase inhibitors reduce the amount of convergence associated with a given amount of accommodation, thereby reducing the degree of esotropia.

Diagnostic aid (accommodative esotropia)—See *Cyclostimulant (accommodative esotropia)* above. An accommodative factor is demonstrated if the eyes become better aligned.

**Onset of action**

Miosis—Less than 1 hour.

Reduction in intraocular pressure—Within 4 hours.

**Time to peak effect**

Miosis—Within 2 hours.

Reduction in intraocular pressure—Within 24 hours.

**Duration of action**

Miosis—Up to 1 month.

Reduction in intraocular pressure—Up to 1 month, but usually 24 to 48 hours.

## Precautions to Consider

**Carcinogenicity/Mutagenicity**

Studies have not been done for demecarium, echothiophate, and isoflurophate.

**Pregnancy/Reproduction**

Fertility—Studies have not been done for demecarium, echothiophate, and isoflurophate.

Pregnancy—

 *Demecarium and isoflurophate*—
  Use of demecarium and isoflurophate is not recommended during pregnancy, because of the toxicity of cholinesterase inhibitors in general. If pregnancy occurs while one of these medications is being administered, the patients should be advised of the potential hazard to the fetus.

  FDA Pregnancy Category X.

 *Echothiophate*—
  Studies have not been done in humans. However, this ophthalmic medication may be systemically absorbed and should be administered to pregnant women only if clearly needed.
  Studies have not been done in animals.

  FDA Pregnancy Category C.

Note: Although the FDA Pregnancy Categories are different for the above medications, some experts think that all three medications should be rated the same, namely, category X.

**Breast-feeding**

Problems in humans have not been documented; however, these ophthalmic medications may be systemically absorbed. Because of the toxicity of cholinesterase inhibitors in general, and the potential for serious adverse reactions in the nursing infant, some clinicians believe that a decision should be made whether to discontinue nursing or discontinue the medication. Other clinicians believe that the concentration of medication in breast milk would be so minute that it would not present a problem.

**Pediatrics**

The iris cysts at the pupil margins that may occur following prolonged use of these medications occur frequently in children. The most common systemic effects, especially in children, are *nausea, vomiting, diarrhea,* and *stomach cramps* or *pain*. No other information is available on whether the risk of adverse effects is increased in children, except that one drop of medication will result in a greater systemic dose per kg of body weight in a child than in an adult. Because of the toxicity of these medications, they should be used with caution, after less toxic alternatives have been considered and/or found ineffective. Recommended doses should not be exceeded, and the patient should be carefully monitored during therapy.

### Geriatrics
No information is available on whether the risk of adverse effects from long-acting cholinergic antiglaucoma agents is increased in the elderly. However, because of the toxicity of these medications, they should be used with caution, after less toxic alternatives have been considered and/or found ineffective. Recommended doses should not be exceeded, and the patient should be carefully monitored during therapy.

### Drug interactions and/or related problems
The following drug interactions and/or related problems have been selected on the basis of their potential clinical significance (possible mechanism in parentheses where appropriate)—not necessarily inclusive (» = major clinical significance):

Note: Combinations containing any of the following medications, depending on the amount present, may also interact with this medication.

*For echothiophate or isoflurophate only*
  Physostigmine, ophthalmic
    (use of this medication prior to echothiophate or isoflurophate may partially block the effects of the latter medications and shorten their duration of action. Echothiophate and isoflurophate primarily inactivate pseudocholinesterase and incompletely inactivate acetylcholinesterase, whereas physostigmine and demecarium inactivate both pseudocholinesterase and acetylcholinesterase. Prior use of physostigmine inactivates the available acetylcholinesterase, thereby rendering it inaccessible to the incomplete inactivation by echothiophate or isoflurophate. This effect does not occur when physostigmine is given prior to demecarium, because both medications inactivate acetylcholinesterase, thereby producing an additive effect)

*For demecarium, echothiophate, or isoflurophate*
  Anesthetics, mucosal-local, ester-derivative, such as benzocaine, butacaine, butamben, and tetracaine or
  Anesthetics, parenteral-local, ester-derivative, such as chloroprocaine, procaine, propoxycaine, and tetracaine
    (concurrent use with demecarium, echothiophate, or isoflurophate may inhibit the metabolism of these anesthetics leading to prolonged anesthetic effect and increased risk of toxicity)
» Anticholinergics or other medications with anticholinergic activity (See *Appendix II*) or
» Antimyasthenics (See *Appendix II*) or
» Cholinesterase inhibitors, other, possibly including topical malathion
    (concurrent use of these medications with demecarium, echothiophate, or isoflurophate is not recommended except under strict medical supervision, because of the possibility of additive toxicity; caution may also be warranted with topical application of malathion if excessive quantities of it are used)
  Belladonna alkaloids, ophthalmic or
  Cyclopentolate or
  Tropicamide
    (concurrent use of these parasympatholytics may antagonize the antiglaucoma and miotic actions of demecarium, echothiophate, or isoflurophate; however, tropicamide is expected to have little effect, since it is so short acting)
  Carbamate- or organophosphate-type insecticides or pesticides
    (exposure of patients using demecarium, echothiophate, or isoflurophate to these preparations may increase the possibility of systemic effects due to absorption of the insecticide or pesticide through the respiratory tract or skin; patients should be advised to protect themselves from contact with such insecticides or pesticides during therapy with demecarium, echothiophate, or isoflurophate)
  Cocaine
    (inhibition of cholinesterase activity by demecarium, echothiophate, or isoflurophate reduces or slows cocaine metabolism, thereby increasing and/or prolonging cocaine's effects and increasing the risk of toxicity; cholinesterase inhibition may persist for weeks or months after demecarium, echothiophate, or isoflurophate has been discontinued)
  Corticosteroids, ophthalmic
    (chronic or intensive use of ophthalmic corticosteroids may increase intraocular pressure and decrease the efficacy of the antiglaucoma agents)
  Edrophonium
    (caution is recommended in administering edrophonium to patients with symptoms of myasthenic weakness who are also using demecarium, echothiophate, or isoflurophate; symptoms of cholinergic crisis [overdosage] may be similar to those occurring with myasthenic crisis [underdosage] and the patient's condition may be worsened by use of edrophonium)
» Succinylcholine
    (demecarium, echothiophate, or isoflurophate may decrease plasma concentrations or activity of pseudocholinesterase, the enzyme that metabolizes succinylcholine, thereby enhancing the neuromuscular blockade of succinylcholine when it is used concurrently; cardiovascular collapse may occur; in addition, increased or prolonged respiratory depression or paralysis [apnea] may occur, which is of minor clinical significance while the patient is being mechanically ventilated; however, caution and careful monitoring of the patient are recommended during and following concurrent or sequential use, especially if there is a possibility of incomplete reversal of neuromuscular blockade postoperatively; the effects of this interaction may persist for several weeks or months after demecarium, echothiophate, or isoflurophate has been discontinued)

### Medical considerations/Contraindications
The medical considerations/contraindications included have been selected on the basis of their potential clinical significance (reasons given in parentheses where appropriate)—not necessarily inclusive (» = major clinical significance).

*Risk-benefit should be considered when the following medical problems exist:*
  Asthma, bronchial
    (systemic absorption of medication may precipitate an attack)
  Bradycardia and hypotension, pronounced
  Down's syndrome (mongolism)
    (echothiophate, and possibly demecarium or isoflurophate, may cause hyperactivity in these children)
  Epilepsy
  Gastrointestinal disturbances, spastic
  Glaucoma, angle-closure, or predisposition to
    (medication may increase the narrowing of the angle)
» Glaucoma associated with iridocyclitis
    (medication may aggravate the inflammatory process and lead to the development of posterior synechiae)
  Hypertension, systemic
  Hyperthyroidism
  Iritis, quiescent or history of
    (medication may aggravate the inflammatory process)
  Myasthenia gravis
  Myocardial infarction, recent
  Parkinsonism
  Peptic ulcer
» Retinal detachment, predisposition to or history of
    (may result from drug-induced spasm of accommodation)
  Sensitivity to the long-acting cholinergic antiglaucoma agent prescribed
  Surgery, intraocular
    (intraocular surgery performed during the action of these medications may be complicated by severe uveitis that is very difficult to manage; it is recommended that elective intraocular surgery not be performed until the full duration of action of these medications has elapsed)
  Urinary tract obstruction
» Uveitis, active or
  Uveitis, quiescent or history of
    (medication may predispose the patient to the development of posterior synechiae)
  Vagotonia, marked

### Patient monitoring
The following may be especially important in patient monitoring (other tests may be warranted in some patients, depending on condition; » = major clinical significance):
  Gonioscopy
    (recommended prior to, and soon after, initiation of therapy)
  Intraocular pressure determinations
    (recommended at periodic intervals during therapy)
  Ophthalmologic examinations
    (recommended at periodic intervals for patients on prolonged ther-

apy, since formation of iris cysts [especially in children], conjunctival thickening, obstruction of nasolacrimal canals, retinal detachment, and lens opacities may occur; also, the condition of the optic nerve should be monitored in patients with glaucoma)

## Side/Adverse Effects

Note: Lens opacities and cataracts may occur following prolonged use of echothiophate, isoflurophate, and possibly demecarium. While there is strong evidence implicating the phosphorylating medications, echothiophate and isofluorophate, there is little or no similar evidence implicating the carbamylating medication, demecarium. If lens opacities occur, they may regress if therapy is discontinued early in their development; however, once cataracts are established, they often continue developing despite cessation of therapy. The incidence of cataracts appears to be directly related to the age of the patient and the concentration, frequency, and duration of the medication.

Retinal detachment has been reported in a few patients during the use of ophthalmic long-acting cholinergic antiglaucoma agents, such as demecarium, echothiophate, or isoflurophate.

Repeated administration of demecarium, echothiophate, or isoflurophate may cause depression of the concentration of cholinesterase in the serum and erythrocytes, resulting in systemic effects.

Iris cysts, conjunctival thickening, and obstruction of nasolacrimal canals may occur following prolonged use of demecarium, echothiophate, or isoflurophate. If iris cysts occur and treatment with demecarium, echothiophate, or isoflurophate is continued, the cysts may enlarge and obscure the vision. In addition, rarely, the cysts may rupture or break free of the iris into the aqueous humor. The cysts usually decrease in size following discontinuation of the medication.

Activation of latent iritis or uveitis may occur following use of demecarium, echothiophate, or isoflurophate.

A paradoxical increase in intraocular pressure may occur following use of demecarium, echothiophate, or isoflurophate. This may be alleviated by the use of a sympathomimetic, such as phenylephrine.

The following side/adverse effects have been selected on the basis of their potential clinical significance (possible signs and symptoms in parentheses where appropriate)—not necessarily inclusive:

### Those indicating need for medical attention
Incidence rare
*Burning, redness, stinging, or other irritation of eyes; eye pain; retinal detachment* (veil or curtain appearing across part of vision)

Symptoms of systemic absorption
*Bradycardia* (slow or irregular heartbeat); *bronchospasm* (shortness of breath, tightness in chest, or wheezing); *hypotension, severe* (unusual tiredness or weakness); *increased sweating; loss of bladder control; muscle weakness; nausea, vomiting, diarrhea, or stomach cramps or pain; watering of mouth*

Note: The most common systemic effects, especially in children, are *nausea, vomiting, diarrhea,* and *stomach cramps* or *pain.*

Systemic absorption is rare with isoflurophate because systemic absorption from ointment bases is minimal and the isoflurophate that is absorbed is hydrolyzed in the circulation almost immediately.

### Those indicating need for medical attention only if they continue or are bothersome
*Accommodative myopia* (blurred vision or change in near or distance vision); *browache; headache; miosis* (difficulty in seeing at night or in dim light); *twitching of eyelids; watering of eyes*

## Overdose

For specific information on the agents used in the management of ophthalmic long-acting cholinergic antiglaucoma agents overdose, see:
• *Atropine* in *Anticholinergics/Antispasmodics (Systemic)* monograph; and/or
• *Diazepam* in *Benzodiazepines (Systemic)* monograph.

For more information on the management of overdose or unintentional ingestion, **contact a Poison Control Center** (see *Poison Control Center Listing*).

### Treatment of overdose
Atropine sulfate injection is used as an antidote to the systemic cholinergic effects of demecarium, echothiophate, or isoflurophate.
*For adults*—Intravenous, 2 to 4 mg initially, then 2 mg repeated every five to ten minutes until cholinergic symptoms disappear or signs of atropine toxicity appear.
*For children*—Intravenous or intramuscular, 1 mg initially, then 0.5 to 1 mg every five to ten minutes until cholinergic symptoms disappear or signs of atropine toxicity appear.

Intravenous pralidoxime chloride (dose of 25 mg per kg of body weight [mg/kg]) may be used as an adjunct to atropine therapy to reverse the muscle paralysis caused by nicotinic effects of demecarium, echothiophate, or isoflurophate.

A short-acting barbiturate or diazepam may be administered for convulsions not controlled by atropine; however, the dosage of the barbiturate should be adjusted to avoid central respiratory depression.

Artificial respiration and maintenance of a clear airway are indicated for severe weakness or paralysis of muscles of respiration.

## Patient Consultation

As an aid to patient consultation, refer to *Advice for the Patient, Antiglaucoma Agents, Cholinergic, Long-acting (Ophthalmic)*.

In providing consultation, consider emphasizing the following selected information (» = major clinical significance):

### Before using this medication
» Conditions affecting use, especially:
  Sensitivity to demecarium, echothiophate, or isoflurophate
  Pregnancy—Because of the toxicity of cholinesterase inhibitors in general, these medications are not recommended during pregnancy
  Breast-feeding—Medications may be absorbed into the body and are not recommended during breast-feeding, since they may cause adverse effects in nursing infants; a decision should be made whether to discontinue nursing or discontinue the medication
  Use in children—The iris cysts that may occur following prolonged use of these medications occur frequently in children
  Other medications, especially antimyasthenics; anticholinergics or other medications with anticholinergic activity; or other cholinesterase inhibitors, possibly including topical malathion
  Recent exposure to pesticides or insecticides
  Other medical problems, especially glaucoma associated with iridocyclitis, predisposition to or history of retinal detachment, or active uveitis

### Proper use of this medication
Proper administration technique for ophthalmic solution; removing excess solution around eye with clean tissue, being careful not to touch eye; washing hands immediately after application to avoid possible systemic absorption; not touching applicator tip to any surface; keeping container tightly closed

Proper administration technique for ophthalmic ointment; washing hands immediately after application to avoid possible systemic absorption; not washing tip of ointment tube or allowing it to touch moist surface, since medication loses efficacy when exposed to moisture; not touching applicator tip to any surface, wiping tip of ointment tube with clean tissue; keeping container tightly closed; applying at bedtime, since ointment causes blurred vision after administration

» Importance of not using more medication than the amount prescribed
» Proper dosing
   **Missed dose**
   If dosing schedule is—
     Every other day: Applying as soon as possible if remembered same day; if not remembered until the next day, applying it at that time, then skipping a day; not doubling doses
     Once a day: Applying as soon as possible; if not remembered until next day, skipping missed dose and going back to regular dosing schedule; not doubling doses
     More than once a day: Applying as soon as possible; if almost time for next dose, skipping missed dose and going back to regular dosing schedule; not doubling doses

» Proper storage

### Precautions while using this medication
Regular visits to physician during therapy to check eye pressure and, for patients on prolonged therapy, to examine eyes
» Caution if any kind of surgery is required
» Caution in exposure to carbamate- or organophosphate-type insecticides or pesticides during therapy
» Making sure vision is clear before driving, using machines, or doing anything else that could be dangerous if not able to see well; caution because of possibility of decreased night vision, blurred vision or change in near or distance vision, or blurred vision for short time if using ointment

### Side/adverse effects
Signs of potential side effects, especially burning, redness, stinging, or other symptoms of systemic absorption; irritation of the eyes; eye pain; and retinal detachment

# General Dosing Information

To reduce the inconvenience of post-medication miosis, the daily dose or one of the daily doses of the medication may be administered at bedtime.

A stronger concentration may be required to produce adequate miosis and reduction in intraocular pressure in eyes with hazel or brown irides than in eyes with blue or light-colored irides because miotics are less effective in heavily pigmented eyes.

To reduce the incidence of iris cyst formation, the frequency of administration should be minimal in all patients, especially in children. In addition, the simultaneous administration of 2.5 to 10% ophthalmic phenylephrine with demecarium, echothiophate, or isoflurophate may prevent iris cyst formation. However, phenylephrine will not prevent iris cysts if the phenylephrine is administered several hours before or after demecarium, echothiophate, or isoflurophate. The 2.5% concentration of phenylephrine appears to be as effective as the 10% concentration and causes less burning upon administration.

Concurrent use of demecarium, echothiophate, or isoflurophate with epinephrine, a beta-adrenergic blocking agent, and/or a carbonic anhydrase inhibitor results in additive effects, thereby providing better control of glaucoma. A reduced dose of demecarium, echothiophate, or isoflurophate may be possible. A dosage reduction of the miotic medication (i.e., demecarium, echothiophate, or isoflurophate) results in the patient experiencing less miosis and/or accommodative block. In addition, concomitant administration of 2.5 to 10% ophthalmic phenylephrine or 1 to 2% ophthalmic epinephrine may improve the visual acuity of some patients by dilating the miotic eye without increasing the intraocular pressure.

Tolerance to demecarium, echothiophate, or isoflurophate may develop with prolonged use. Effectiveness may be restored by changing to another miotic for a short time and then resuming the original medication.

Following long-term use of these medications, dilation of blood vessels and resulting greater permeability will increase postoperative inflammation and may increase the risk of hyphema during ophthalmic surgery; therefore, demecarium, echothiophate, or isoflurophate should be discontinued 2 to 3 weeks before eye surgery.

**For the solution dosage forms only**

Although some manufacturers recommend a dose of 2 drops of an ophthalmic solution at appropriate intervals, the conjunctival sac will usually hold only 1 drop. In addition, because of the potency of these medications and the possibility of systemic absorption, the smallest dose possible should be administered.

To avoid excessive systemic absorption, patient should press finger to the lacrimal sac during and for 1 or 2 minutes following instillation of medication.

---

## DEMECARIUM

# Summary of Differences

Precautions: Drug interactions and/or related problems—Physostigmine not listed as a precaution.

# Ophthalmic Dosage Forms

## DEMECARIUM BROMIDE OPHTHALMIC SOLUTION USP

### Usual adult and adolescent dose
Antiglaucoma agent (ophthalmic)—
 Topical, to the conjunctiva, 1 drop of a 0.125 or 0.25% solution one or two times a day.
Cyclostimulant (accommodative esotropia)—
 Topical, to the conjunctiva, 1 drop of a 0.125 or 0.25% solution once a day for two to three weeks, then 1 drop every two days for three to four weeks, at which time the patient's status should be reevaluated. Thereafter, 1 drop one or two times a week to once every two days, depending on the patient's condition.

Note: In the treatment of esotropia uncomplicated by anisometropia, the patient's condition should be evaluated every four to twelve weeks. It is recommended that therapy be discontinued after four months if a dosage of 1 drop every two days is still required to control condition.

Diagnostic aid (accommodative esotropia)—
 Topical, to the conjunctiva, 1 drop of a 0.125 or 0.25% solution once a day for two weeks, then 1 drop every two days for two to three weeks.

### Usual pediatric dose
Antiglaucoma agent (ophthalmic)
Cyclostimulant (accommodative esotropia) or
Diagnostic aid (accommodative esotropia)—
 For infants and young children: Use is not recommended.
 Older children: See *Usual adult and adolescent dose*.

Note: Clinicians differ as to the age at which children may receive this medication, their recommendations ranging from 12 months to 15 years. Other clinicians feel that the lower end of the adult dose range, administered less frequently, may be used for infants and children.

### Strength(s) usually available
U.S.—
 0.125% (Rx) [*Humorsol* (benzalkonium chloride 1:5000; sodium chloride)].
 0.25% (Rx) [*Humorsol* (benzalkonium chloride 1:5000; sodium chloride)].

### Packaging and storage
Store below 40 °C (104 °F), preferably between 15 and 30 °C (59 and 86 °F), unless otherwise specified by manufacturer. Store in a tight, light-resistant container. Protect from freezing.

### Auxiliary labeling
- For the eye.
- Keep container tightly closed.

---

## ECHOTHIOPHATE

# Ophthalmic Dosage Forms

## ECHOTHIOPHATE IODIDE FOR OPHTHALMIC SOLUTION USP

### Usual adult and adolescent dose
Antiglaucoma agent (ophthalmic)—
 Topical, to the conjunctiva, 1 drop of a 0.03 to 0.25% solution one or two times a day.
Cyclostimulant (accommodative esotropia)—
 Topical, to the conjunctiva, 1 drop of a 0.03 to 0.125% solution once a day or every two days.
Diagnostic aid (accommodative esotropia)—
 Topical, to the conjunctiva, 1 drop of a 0.125% solution once a day at bedtime for two to three weeks.

### Usual pediatric dose
Antiglaucoma agent (ophthalmic)
Cyclostimulant (accommodative esotropia) or
Diagnostic aid (accommodative esotropia)—
 For infants and young children: Use is not recommended.
 Older children: See *Usual adult and adolescent dose*.

Note: Clinicians differ as to the age at which children may receive this medication, their recommendations ranging from 12 months to 15 years, with 2 years being the most recommended age. Other clinicians feel that the lower end of the adult dose range, administered less frequently, may be used for infants and children.

### Strength(s) usually available
U.S.—
 0.03% (equivalent to 1.5 mg per 5 mL of sterile diluent) (Rx) [*Phospholine Iodide* (in powder—potassium acetate; in powder—sodium hydroxide; in powder—acetic acid; in diluent—chlorobutanol 0.55%; in diluent—mannitol; in diluent—boric acid; in diluent—sodium phosphate)].
 0.06% (equivalent to 3 mg per 5 mL of sterile diluent) (Rx) [*Phospholine Iodide* (in powder—potassium acetate; in powder—sodium hydroxide; in powder—acetic acid; in diluent—chlorobutanol 0.55%; in diluent—mannitol; in diluent—boric acid; in diluent—sodium phosphate)].
 0.125% (equivalent to 6.25 mg per 5 mL of sterile diluent) (Rx) [*Phospholine Iodide* (in powder—potassium acetate; in powder—sodium hydroxide; in powder—acetic acid; in diluent—chlorobutanol 0.55%; in diluent—mannitol; in diluent—boric acid; in diluent—sodium phosphate)].
 0.25% (equivalent to 12.5 mg per 5 mL of sterile diluent) (Rx) [*Phospholine Iodide* (in powder—potassium acetate; in powder—sodium hydroxide; in powder—acetic acid; in diluent—chlorobutanol 0.55%; in diluent—mannitol; in diluent—boric acid; in diluent—sodium phosphate)].
Canada—
 0.06% (equivalent to 3 mg per 5 mL of sterile diluent) (Rx) [*Phospholine Iodide* (in powder—potassium acetate; in powder—sodium hydroxide; in powder—acetic acid; in diluent—chlorobutanol 0.5%; in diluent—mannitol; in diluent—hydrochloric acid; in diluent—sodium phosphate)].

0.125% (equivalent to 6.25 mg per 5 mL of sterile diluent) (Rx) [*Phospholine Iodide* (in powder—potassium acetate; in powder—sodium hydroxide; in powder—acetic acid; in diluent—chlorobutanol 0.5%; in diluent—mannitol; in diluent—hydrochloric acid; in diluent—sodium phosphate)].

0.25% (equivalent to 12.5 mg per 5 mL of sterile diluent) (Rx) [*Phospholine Iodide* (in powder—potassium acetate; in powder—sodium hydroxide; in powder—acetic acid; in diluent—chlorobutanol 0.5%; in diluent—mannitol; in diluent—hydrochloric acid; in diluent—sodium phosphate)].

**Packaging and storage**
Prior to reconstitution, store between 15 and 30 °C (59 and 86 °F), in a tight container. Protect the reconstituted solution from freezing.

**Preparation of dosage form**
For reconstitution of echothiophate iodide powder, use only the diluent supplied by the manufacturer to provide for optimum stability. Use aseptic technique.

**Stability**
Reconstituted solution is stable for about 3 to 4 weeks at room temperature or for 3 to 6 months if refrigerated, depending on the manufacturer.

**Auxiliary labeling**
- For the eye.
- Beyond-use date.
- Keep container tightly closed.

---

## ISOFLUROPHATE

## Ophthalmic Dosage Forms

### ISOFLUROPHATE OPHTHALMIC OINTMENT USP

**Usual adult and adolescent dose**
Antiglaucoma agent (ophthalmic)—
   Topical, to the conjunctiva, a thin strip (approximately 0.5 cm) of a 0.025% ointment once every three days to three times a day.
Cyclostimulant (accommodative esotropia)—
   Topical, to the conjunctiva, a thin strip (approximately 0.5 cm) of a 0.025% ointment once a day at bedtime for two weeks, then once a week to once every two days, depending on the patient's condition, for two months.

Note: In the treatment of esotropia uncomplicated by anisometropia, it is recommended that therapy be discontinued if the patient's condition cannot be maintained on a dosage interval of at least every two days.

Diagnostic aid (accommodative esotropia)—
   Topical, to the conjunctiva, a thin strip (approximately 0.5 cm) of a 0.025% ointment once a day at bedtime for two weeks.

**Usual pediatric dose**
Antiglaucoma agent (ophthalmic)
Cyclostimulant (accommodative esotropia) or
Diagnostic aid (accommodative esotropia)—
   For infants and young children: Use is not recommended.
   Older children: See *Usual adult and adolescent dose*.

Note: Clinicians differ as to the age at which children may receive this medication, their recommendations ranging from 12 months to 15 years, with 2 years being the most recommended age. Other clinicians feel that the lower end of the adult dose range, administered less frequently, may be used for infants and children.

**Strength(s) usually available**
U.S.—
   0.025% (Rx) [*Floropryl* (polyethylene mineral oil gel)].

**Packaging and storage**
Store below 40 °C (104 °F), preferably between 15 and 30 °C (59 and 86 °F), unless otherwise specified by manufacturer. Protect from freezing.

**Stability**
Isoflurophate hydrolyzes in the presence of water to form hydrofluoric acid and becomes inactivated.

**Auxiliary labeling**
- For the eye.
- Keep container tightly closed.

## Selected Bibliography
Havener, WH. Ocular pharmacology. 5th ed. St. Louis: Mosby, 1983: 261-418, 635-72.
Pavan-Langston D, editor. Manual of ocular diagnosis and therapy. 2nd ed. Boston: Little, Brown, 1985: 201-29.

Revised: 06/21/94

---

# ANTIHEMOPHILIC FACTOR   Systemic

VA CLASSIFICATION (Primary): BL150
Commonly used brand name(s): *Alphanate; Bioclate; Helixate; Hemofil M; Humate-P; Hyate:C; Koate-HP; Kogenate; Monoclate-P; Recombinate*.

Other commonly used names are AHF and factor VIII.

Note: For a listing of dosage forms and brand names by country availability, see *Dosage Forms* section(s).

## Category
Antihemorrhagic.

## Indications
Note: Bracketed information in the *Indications* section refers to uses that are not included in U.S. product labeling.

**Accepted**
Hemophilia A, hemorrhagic complications of (prophylaxis and treatment)—Antihemophilic factor (AHF) is indicated for the control and prevention of bleeding, including bleeding during and following surgical procedures, in patients with hemophilia A (classical hemophilia). Human AHF is not likely to be effective in patients with acquired inhibitor antibodies to human AHF when the antibody concentration exceeds 5 to 10 Bethesda Units (BU) per mL. Alternative treatment modalities available to these patients include anti-inhibitor coagulant complex concentrates, factor IX complex concentrates, and porcine AHF.

Hemorrhagic complications in patients with factor VIII inhibitors (prophylaxis and treatment)—AHF (Porcine) is indicated for the control and prevention of bleeding, including bleeding during and following surgical procedures, in hemophilic patients with antibodies to human factor VIII, and in previously non-hemophilic patients with spontaneously acquired antibodies to human factor VIII. AHF (Porcine) is used in patients with anti–human factor VIII antibody concentrations between 10 and 50 BU per mL, or more than 50 BU per mL if the anti–porcine factor VIII antibody concentration is less than 15 to 20 BU per mL, provided that *in vitro* testing has demonstrated lack of cross-reactivity with the factor VIII antibody. Patients with antibody concentrations beyond these ranges are not likely to receive any therapeutic benefit from this product.

von Willebrand disease (treatment)
Hypofibrinogenemia (treatment) or
Factor XIII deficiency (treatment)—Cryoprecipitated AHF is indicated in the treatment of type I, type II, and type III (severe) von Willebrand disease and for the replacement of fibrinogen and factor XIII.

[Coagulation, disseminated intravascular (treatment adjunct)][1] or
[Kasabach-Merritt syndrome (treatment adjunct)][1]—Cryoprecipitated AHF may be used as a source of fibrinogen in the treatment of disseminated intravascular coagulation. It may be given in conjunction with fresh frozen plasma and platelet concentrates, which replace other clotting factors and platelets, respectively. Heparin may be added to this regimen, although such use is controversial, to inhibit the formation of thrombin and microthrombi and to reduce the inappropriate activation and consumption of clotting factors and platelets.

Cryoprecipitated AHF may be used as a source of fibrinogen in the treatment of Kasabach-Merritt syndrome. It may be used in conjunction with aminocaproic acid and thrombin, which inhibit fibrinolysis and promote thrombosis in, and subsequent shrinkage of, the tumor.

**Unaccepted**
AHF products other than the cryoprecipitated AHF do not contain sufficient quantities of von Willebrand factor, and therefore are not indicated, in the treatment of von Willebrand disease.

---

[1]Not included in Canadian product labeling.

## Pharmacology/Pharmacokinetics

### Physicochemical characteristics

Source—Antihemophilic factor (AHF) is obtained from pooled human plasma or purified porcine plasma, or produced by recombinant DNA technology.

Almost all of the plasma-derived AHF products currently available are sterile, nonpyrogenic, high-purity concentrates purified by gel permeation chromatography, ion exchange chromatography, or immunoaffinity chromatography utilizing murine monoclonal antibodies to factor VIII or von Willebrand factor (vWf). The purified concentrates contain 50 to 150 times as much AHF as an equal volume of fresh plasma. Some products contain albumin as a stabilizer, and monoclonal purified products contain trace amounts of mouse protein. *Humate-P* is an intermediate-purity product and contains small amounts of foreign proteins, including vWf. However, this product is not indicated for use in the treatment of von Willebrand disease.

AHF (Porcine) is a sterile, high-purity, freeze-dried concentrate that also contains platelet aggregating factor, the equivalent of porcine vWf, at a concentration of 1 porcine vWf unit for at least 5 units of porcine factor VIII.

Human recombinant AHF (rAHF) is a sterile, nonpyrogenic concentrate with biologic activity comparable to that of plasma-derived AHF. rAHF contains albumin as a stabilizer and trace amounts of mouse, hamster, and bovine proteins. vWf is co-expressed with rAHF in the production of *Recombinate*, and helps to stabilize it; however, it is present in such minute quantities that it offers no therapeutic benefit to patients with von Willebrand disease.

Cryoprecipitated AHF is a sterile, frozen concentrate of human AHF obtained from the plasma of 1 unit of whole blood or from 1 or more units of single-donor fresh frozen plasma.

### Mechanism of action/Effect

Antihemophilic Factor (AHF), or factor VIII, is an endogenous glycoprotein necessary for blood clotting and hemostasis. It is a cofactor necessary for factor IX to activate factor X in the intrinsic pathway. In hemophilia A (classical hemophilia), there is a deficiency of this clotting factor. The average normal plasma activity of factor VIII is designated as 100%, and a factor VIII concentration of 25% of normal is required for hemostasis. Patients with severe hemophilia have a factor VIII concentration of less than 1% of normal and frequently experience bleeding even in the absence of trauma. Patients with a factor VIII concentration between 1 and 5% (moderate hemophilia) experience less bleeding, and patients with a factor VIII concentration greater than 5% (mild hemophilia) usually experience bleeding only after obvious trauma. The administration of AHF temporarily replaces the missing clotting factor to correct or prevent bleeding episodes.

### Half-life

Distribution—2.4 to 8 hours.

Elimination—8.4 to 19.3 hours. However, the half-life may be significantly reduced in the presence of inhibitor antibodies, or during active consumption of clotting factors.

### Time to peak concentration

There is conflicting information regarding the time to achieve peak concentration; values have ranged from 10 minutes to 2 hours after intravenous administration.

### Time to peak effect

1 to 2 hours after intravenous administration.

## Precautions to Consider

### Cross-sensitivity and/or related problems

Patients with a history of allergies, especially those who are allergic to pork or pork products, may be allergic to this medication also.

### Carcinogenicity

The carcinogenic potential of antihemophilic factor has not been investigated.

### Mutagenicity

Recombinant antihemophilic factor (rAHF) does not induce reverse mutations, chromosomal aberrations, or an increase in micronuclei in bone marrow polychromatic erythrocytes at doses considerably exceeding plasma concentrations of rAHF *in vitro*, and at doses 10 to 40 times the maximum clinical dose *in vivo*.

### Pregnancy/Reproduction

Pregnancy—Studies have not been done in humans.
Studies have not been done in animals.
FDA Pregnancy Category C.

### Breast-feeding

It is not known whether antihemophilic factor is distributed into breast milk. However, problems in humans have not been documented.

### Pediatrics

Appropriate studies performed to date have not demonstrated pediatrics-specific problems that would limit the usefulness of antihemophilic factor in children.

### Geriatrics

Appropriate studies performed to date have not demonstrated geriatrics-specific problems that would limit the usefulness of antihemophilic factor in the elderly.

### Medical considerations/Contraindications

The medical considerations/contraindications included have been selected on the basis of their potential clinical significance (reasons given in parentheses where appropriate)—not necessarily inclusive (» = major clinical significance).

*Risk-benefit should be considered when the following medical problems exist:*

Sensitivity to mouse, hamster, or bovine protein
  (risk of allergic reaction to these proteins, which may be present in monoclonal antibody–derived and recombinant AHF products)

Sensitivity to antihemophilic factor

### Patient monitoring

The following may be especially important in patient monitoring (other tests may be warranted in some patients, depending on condition; » = major clinical significance):

» Antibody determinations
  (recommended periodically to detect the development and concentration of antibodies to factor VIII, and to predict whether or not a patient is likely to respond to AHF therapy. Patients with antibody concentrations lower than 10 Bethesda Units [BU] per mL may be given larger amounts of AHF to complex with and thereby inactivate the antibodies. However, patients with antibody concentrations greater than 10 BU per mL are not likely to respond, even to very large amounts of AHF, and therefore must be treated with alternative modalities; (see the Hemophilia therapeutic monograph for information about the treatment of patients with inhibitor antibodies.)

Direct Coombs' test and
Hematocrit determinations
  (recommended when large volumes and/or frequent doses are administered, to detect the onset of progressive anemia; some products contain red blood cell anti-A and anti-B isoantibodies, which may precipitate intravascular hemolysis in patients with blood types A, B, or AB)

» Plasma factor VIII determinations
  (recommended periodically to assure that adequate factor VIII concentrations have been achieved and are maintained)

Platelet count
  (recommended during the administration of AHF [Porcine] to detect thrombocytopenia)

Pulse rate determinations
  (recommended before and during administration; if a significant increase in pulse rate occurs, the infusion should be slowed or halted until the pulse rate returns to normal)

## Side/Adverse Effects

Note: To reduce the risk of *transmission of viruses* by blood and blood components, potential blood donors are screened, and donor blood is tested and must be found negative for antibodies to human immunodeficiency virus (HIV), hepatitis B surface antigen, antibody to hepatitis B core antigen, and antibody to hepatitis C (non-A, non-B) virus. The concentration of alanine aminotransferase (ALT) also must be within normal limits. However, these precautions are not totally effective in eliminating viral infectivity. To further reduce the risk, plasma-derived AHF concentrates, with the exception of the cryoprecipitated product, undergo viral inactivation procedures. The inactivation methods currently employed are treatment with an organic solvent/detergent combination (tri-*n*-butyl-phosphate [TNBP] and polysorbate-80 [Tween-80], sodium cholate, or Triton X-100) with or without heat treatment, vapor treatment, or nanofiltration; pasteurization by heating at 60 °C (140 °F) for 10 hours in an aqueous solution; vapor heating; dry heating at 80 °C (176 °F) for 72 hours; sodium thiocyanate plus ultrafiltration; and immunoaffinity purification. These processes effectively inactivate lipid-enveloped viruses such as HIV; hepatitis B virus; and hepatitis C virus. Hepatitis A and human parvovirus B19 are nonlipid-enveloped viruses and have been reported in patients receiving solvent/detergent-treated AHF. However, it is not known if these cases were caused by the concentrate, the water used in processing, or by other sources. Also, unknown viruses and prions, such as the agent that causes Creutzfeldt-Jakob disease (CJD), may not be eliminated by current inactivation and purification methods and could be transmitted. There is no evidence, however, of CJD transmission through any transfused blood component, and it remains only a theoretical concern. AHF (Porcine) is screened for porcine viruses; there have been no reports of transmission of hepatitis or HIV associated with its use. Recombinant AHF carries a very slight risk of transmission of viruses; however, there have been no cases of viral infection attributed to this product.

Unlike the intermediate-purity AHF concentrates, the high-purity concentrates currently available contain virtually no contaminating proteins. The many foreign proteins and alloantigens contained in the intermediate-purity concentrates have been reported to cause *downmodulation of immune function*, primarily by inhibiting phagocytic function of monocytes and macrophages and by inhibiting secretion of interleukin-2. Studies have not shown downmodulation of immune function with high-purity concentrates; there is minimal evidence that the highly purified concentrates may stabilize the immune function of HIV-positive hemophiliacs. However, other studies have shown conflicting results.

The development of *inhibitor antibodies*, which neutralize the procoagulant activity of factor VIII, is a complication associated with the use of AHF. The incidence of antibody development is between 15 and 35% in patients with hemophilia A. Inhibitor antibodies have been reported after treatment with both plasma-derived factor VIII concentrates and recombinant factor VIII, but it is unclear if the incidence differs among the various AHF products. The antibody concentration begins to increase 4 to 7 days after AHF exposure and peaks in 2 to 3 weeks. The risk of developing an antibody is greatest in patients with severe disease, and most often in those younger than 5 years of age. Antibodies also may develop spontaneously in postpartum women, patients with autoimmune disorders or cancer, or otherwise healthy older adults. [See the Hemophilia therapeutic monograph for information about the treatment of patients with inhibitor antibodies.]

The following side/adverse effects have been selected on the basis of their potential clinical significance (possible signs and symptoms in parentheses where appropriate)—not necessarily inclusive:

### Those indicating need for medical attention
Incidence less frequent
*Anaphylaxis or other allergic reaction to AHF, or to mouse, hamster, or bovine protein* (changes in facial skin color; fast or irregular breathing; puffiness or swelling of the eyelids or around the eyes; shortness of breath, troubled breathing, tightness in chest, and/or wheezing; skin rash, hives, and/or itching)—may include anaphylactic shock with sudden, severe decrease in blood pressure and collapse; *hemolytic anemia* (unusual tiredness or weakness)—primarily associated with the use of large volumes of low- or intermediate-purity factor VIII preparations in patients with group A, B, or AB red blood cell antigens; *thrombosis* (tenderness, pain, swelling, warmth, skin discoloration, and prominent superficial veins over affected area)

Incidence rare
*Allergic reaction to albumin* (chills; fever; hives; nausea); *hyperfibrinogenemia; thrombocytopenia* (unusual bleeding or bruising)—for AHF (Porcine) only
Note: Chills and fever also may occur independently of an *allergic reaction to albumin* (incidence less frequent).

### Those indicating need for medical attention only if they continue or are bothersome
Incidence less frequent
*Burning, stinging, or inflammation at injection site* (swelling); *dizziness or lightheadedness; dry mouth; fatigue* (unusual tiredness or weakness); *flushing* (redness of face); *headache; nausea or vomiting; nosebleed; skin rash; unpleasant taste*

## Patient Consultation
As an aid to patient consultation, refer to *Advice for the Patient, Antihemophilic Factor (Systemic)*.
In providing consultation, consider emphasizing the following selected information (» = major clinical significance):

### Before using this medication
» Conditions affecting use, especially:
Sensitivity to antihemophilic factor or to mouse, hamster, or bovine protein

### Proper use of this medication
» Proper preparation of medication: bringing dry concentrate and diluent to room temperature before reconstitution; when reconstituting, directing stream of diluent against side of vial of concentrate to avoid foaming of contents; gently swirling vial to dissolve contents; not shaking hard

» Administering within 1 or 3 hours of reconstitution, according to the individual manufacturer's instructions
» Use of plastic disposable syringe and filter needle; safe handling and disposal of syringe and needle
Proper dosing
Missed dose: Contacting physician as soon as possible for instructions; if physician is unavailable, using usual dose as soon as it is remembered
» Proper storage

### Precautions while using this medication
Need for patients newly diagnosed with hemophilia to receive hepatitis A and hepatitis B vaccines
» Need to carry identification stating condition and treatment
» Notifying physician if medication seems less effective than usual; this may indicate the development of antibodies to factor VIII

### Side/adverse effects
Signs of potential side effects, especially allergic reactions, hemolytic anemia, thrombosis, hyperfibrinogenemia, or thrombocytopenia

## General Dosing Information
### Choice of product
The types of factor VIII products currently available include:
- recombinant factor VIII (rFVIII), produced in cultured hamster cell lines that have been transfected with a gene for human FVIII, and stabilized in human albumin (*Bioclate, Helixate, Kogenate, Recombinate*);
- immunoaffinity-purified (ultrahigh purity) FVIII, derived from human plasma (*Hemofil M; Monoclate P;* Antihemophilic Factor, Method M);
- intermediate- and high-purity FVIII, derived from human plasma (*Alphanate, Humate-P, Koate-HP*);
- porcine FVIII (*Hyate:C*), reserved for patients with inhibitors to human factor VIII.

In general, it is recommended that previously untreated patients and those who are HIV-negative receive recombinant factor VIII. For HIV-positive patients, some studies have shown that the use of immunoaffinity-purified or recombinant products may preserve cellular immunity better than products of intermediate purity. However, other studies have shown conflicting results.

Random-donor cryoprecipitated antihemophilic factor is not recommended as a treatment alternative for hemophilia A because the product does not undergo a viral attenuation process. Appropriately screened, single-donor cryoprecipitate (such as from desmopressin-treated fathers of hemophilic children) has been used as an inexpensive alternative to the use of factor VIII concentrates for the management of hemophilia in small children.

It is important to verify the existence of a factor VIII deficiency before administering antihemophilic factor (AHF).

AHF is recommended for intravenous use only.

AHF should be administered via plastic disposable syringes because it tends to adhere to the ground-glass surface of all glass syringes.

AHF should be filtered before administration.

AHF may be administered as a continuous intravenous infusion via a minipump or syringe pump for severe, life-threatening bleeding, or following surgery. When administered this way, the addition of heparin, 1 to 5 USP Units per mL of concentrate, may be considered if problems with local thrombophlebitis occur at the injection site.

Long-term prophylactic therapy for severe hemophilia, in which factor replacement is given several times a week to maintain the factor level above 1%, has been used extensively in Europe. The goal is to convert severe hemophilia to a mild or moderate form of the disease to prevent spontaneous bleeding and preserve joint function.

Because AHF (Porcine) is a foreign-species protein, there is a slight risk of an anaphylactic or other allergic reaction. Pretreatment with hydrocortisone and/or an antihistamine may minimize or prevent these reactions.

Antifibrinolytic therapy is useful adjunctive therapy in hemophilic patients with oral or mucous membrane bleeding, particularly that which occurs during dental and oral surgery. It prevents or controls bleeding, thus reducing the need for replacement therapy. Aminocaproic acid may be given orally or intravenously at a dose of 75 mg per kg of body weight (up to 6 grams) immediately after surgery, then every six hours for seven to ten days. Or, tranexamic acid may be given as a single dose of 25 mg per kg of body weight orally or 10 mg per kg of body weight intravenously two hours before surgery, followed, after surgery, by 25 mg per kg of body weight orally every six to eight hours for seven to ten days. When antifibrinolytic agents are used in this manner, a single factor VIII infusion of 40 International Units per kg of body weight prior to surgery is often enough for normal hemostasis. These agents can also be given as an oral rinse (5 mL of aminocaproic acid syrup, or 10 mL of a 5% tranexamic acid solution four times a day for seven to ten days).

## Parenteral Dosage Forms

### ANTIHEMOPHILIC FACTOR (HUMAN) USP

Note: Each vial of AHF is labeled with the AHF activity expressed in International Units (IU) per vial. This potency assignment is referenced to the World Health Organization International Standard. One IU of factor VIII activity is approximately equal to the AHF activity of 1 mL of fresh plasma, and increases the plasma concentration of factor VIII by 2%. The specific factor VIII activity ranges from 2 to over 3000 AHF IU per mg of total protein, after discounting the human albumin used to stabilize these products.

Although the dose of AHF must be individualized for each patient based on patient weight, circulating antibody concentration, type of hemorrhage, and desired plasma factor VIII concentration, the following formulas may be used as guides in determining dosage:

Desired AHF increase (% of normal) = ([Dose AHF(IU)]/[Body weight (kg)]) × 2

Dose AHF (IU) = Body weight (kg) × Desired AHF increase × 0.5

*Hemofil M* and *Alphanate* may be administered at a rate not exceeding 10 mL per minute; *Monoclate-P* and *Humate-P* may be administered at a rate of 2 or 4 mL per minute, respectively; and the entire dose of *Koate-HP* may be administered over five to ten minutes. However, the rate at which AHF is administered should be guided by the comfort of the patient.

### Usual adult and adolescent dose

Prophylaxis of spontaneous hemorrhage—
  Intravenous, 25 to 40 IU per kg of body weight, administered three times per week, maintaining the trough factor level above 1% between doses.

Treatment of hemorrhage—
  Schedules for administration of clotting factor concentrates are based on the severity of the bleeding diathesis. Currently, there is no consensus among practitioners regarding the optimal dose of factor replacement therapy for the treatment of the various types of bleeding, and the optimal therapeutic level for control of such bleeding remains debatable. The doses in Table 1 should be considered only as a guideline, since recommendations may vary from one hemophilia center to another. Doses and duration of treatment may be adjusted according to the patient's condition.
  See *Table 1*, page 324.

Control of perisurgical hemostasis—
Dental and oral surgery—
  Intravenous, 40 IU per kg of body weight prior to surgery. A single dose is often sufficient for normal hemostasis when an antifibrinolytic agent, such as aminocaproic acid or tranexamic acid, is used as adjunctive treatment.

Other surgical procedures—
  Intravenous, 50 IU per kg of body weight to obtain a plasma factor VIII level of 100%, which must be confirmed prior to surgery. Subsequent doses equal to half the initial dose are given every eight to twelve hours to maintain that plasma level for the first few days after surgery. As an alternative to the intermittent dosing of replacement factor, continuous infusion of factor VIII may be given following surgery at a dose of 3 IU per kg of body weight per hour via a minipump or syringe pump. The dose can then be tapered to maintain a plasma factor level 30% for the following one to two weeks. Major orthopedic surgery may require several weeks of replacement therapy.

### Usual pediatric dose
See *Usual adult and adolescent dose*.

### Size(s) usually available
U.S.—
  250 IU with 2.5 mL sterile water for injection provided as diluent (Rx) [*Monoclate-P* (sodium ion 300 to 450 mmol per liter; calcium chloride 2 to 5 mmol per liter; albumin human 1 to 2%; mouse protein < 50 nanograms per 100 IU)].
  250 IU with 5 mL sterile water for injection provided as diluent (Rx) [*Koate-HP* (heparin ≤ 5 units per mL; calcium chloride ≤ 3 mmol; aluminum ≤ 1 part per million (ppm); albumin human ≤ 10 mg per mL)].
  250 IU with 10 mL sterile water for injection provided as diluent (Rx) [*Alphanate* (albumin human 0.05 to 1 gram per 100 mL; calcium ≤ 10 mmol per L; heparin ≤ 2 Units per mL; sodium ≤ 10 mEq); *Hemofil M* (albumin human 12.5 mg per mL; mouse protein ≤ 0.1 nanogram); *Humate-P* (sodium citrate 14 to 28 mg per 100 IU; sodium chloride 8 to 16 mg per 100 IU; albumin human 16 to 24 mg per 100 IU; other proteins 4 to 20 mg per 100 IU); GENERIC].
  500 IU with 5 mL sterile water for injection provided as diluent (Rx) [*Koate-HP* (heparin ≤ 5 units per mL; calcium chloride ≤ 3 mmol; aluminum ≤ 1 ppm; albumin human ≤ 10 mg per mL); *Monoclate-P* (sodium ion 300 to 450 mmol per liter; calcium chloride 2 to 5 mmol per liter; albumin human 1 to 2%; mouse protein < 50 nanograms per 100 IU)].
  500 IU with 10 mL sterile water for injection provided as diluent (Rx) [*Alphanate* (albumin human 0.05 to 1 gram per 100 mL; calcium ≤ 10 mmol per L; heparin ≤ 2 Units per mL; sodium ≤ 10 mEq); *Hemofil M* (albumin human 12.5 mg per mL; mouse protein ≤ 0.1 nanogram); GENERIC].
  500 IU with 20 mL sterile water for injection provided as diluent (Rx) [*Humate-P* (sodium citrate 14 to 28 mg per 100 IU; sodium chloride 8 to 16 mg per 100 IU; albumin human 16 to 24 mg per 100 IU; other proteins 4 to 20 mg per 100 IU)].
  1000 IU with 10 mL sterile water for injection provided as diluent (Rx) [*Alphanate* (albumin human 0.05 to 1 gram per 100 mL; calcium ≤ 10 mmol per L; heparin ≤ 2 Units per mL; sodium ≤ 10 mEq); *Hemofil M* (albumin human 12.5 mg per mL; mouse protein ≤ 0.1 nanogram); *Koate-HP* (heparin ≤ 5 units per mL; calcium chloride ≤ 3 mmol); aluminum ≤ 1 ppm; albumin human ≤ 10 mg per mL); *Monoclate-P* (sodium ion 300 to 450 mmol per liter; calcium chloride 2 to 5 mmol per liter; albumin human 1 to 2%; mouse protein < 50 nanograms per 100 IU); GENERIC].
  1000 IU with 30 mL sterile water for injection provided as diluent (Rx) [*Humate-P* (sodium citrate 14 to 28 mg per 100 IU; sodium chloride 8 to 16 mg per 100 IU; albumin human 16 to 24 mg per 100 IU; other proteins 4 to 20 mg per 100 IU)].
  1500 IU with 10 mL sterile water for injection provided as diluent (Rx) [*Alphanate* (albumin human 0.05 to 1 gram per 100 mL; calcium ≤ 10 mmol per L; heparin ≤ 2 Units per mL; sodium ≤ 10 mEq); *Koate-HP* (heparin ≤ 5 units per mL; calcium chloride ≤ 3 mmol; aluminum ≤ 1 ppm; albumin human ≤ 10 mg per mL)].

Canada—
  250 IU with 5 mL sterile water for injection provided as diluent (Rx) [*Koate-HP* (heparin ≤ 5 units per mL; calcium chloride ≤ 3 mmol; aluminum ≤ 1 ppm; albumin human ≤ 10 mg per mL); GENERIC].
  250 IU with 10 mL sterile water for injection provided as diluent (Rx) [*Hemofil M* (albumin human 12.5 mg per mL; mouse protein ≤ 0.1 nanogram)].
  500 IU with 5 mL sterile water for injection provided as diluent (Rx) [*Koate-HP* (heparin ≤ 5 units per mL; calcium chloride ≤ 3 mmol; aluminum ≤ 1 ppm; albumin human ≤ 10 mg per mL); GENERIC].
  500 IU with 10 mL sterile water for injection provided as diluent (Rx) [*Hemofil M* (albumin human 12.5 mg per mL; mouse protein ≤ 0.1 nanogram)].
  1000 IU with 10 mL sterile water for injection provided as diluent (Rx) [*Hemofil M* (albumin human 12.5 mg per mL; mouse protein ≤ 0.1 nanogram); *Koate-HP* (heparin ≤ 5 units per mL; calcium chloride ≤ 3 mmol; aluminum ≤ 1 ppm; albumin human ≤ 10 mg per mL); GENERIC].
  1500 IU with 10 mL sterile water for injection provided as diluent (Rx) [*Koate-HP* (heparin ≤ 5 units per mL; calcium chloride ≤ 3 mmol; aluminum ≤ 1 ppm; albumin human ≤ 10 mg per mL); GENERIC].

### Packaging and storage
The dry concentrates are preferably stored between 2 and 8 °C (36 and 46 °F). However, some products may be stored at temperatures not exceeding 30 °C (86 °F) for 2 months (*Alphanate*) or 25 °C (77 °F) for 6 months (*Koate-HP*, *Monoclate-P*, *Humate-P*), according to the individual manufacturer's instructions. The solutions should not be refrigerated after reconstitution. The diluent should be protected from freezing.

### Preparation of dosage form
The diluent and dry concentrate should be brought to room temperature, approximately 25 °C (77 °F), prior to reconstitution. They may be removed from the refrigerator and allowed to sit just until they reach room temperature, or in an urgent situation, they may be placed in a warm water bath, 30 to 37 °C (86 to 96 °F). The reconstituted solution should not be shaken, since excessive shaking will cause foaming. The reconstituted solution should be at approximately room temperature at the time of administration.

### Stability
Administration should begin within 1 or 3 hours after reconstitution, according to the individual manufacturer's instructions. Partially used vials should be discarded. For use as a continuous infusion, studies have shown reconstituted AHF remains stable for extended periods.

### Incompatibilities
It is recommended that AHF, after reconstitution with the provided diluent, be administered through a separate line, by itself, and without mixing with other intravenous fluids or medications. However, when administered as a continuous intravenous infusion, the addition of heparin, 1 to 5 USP Units per mL of concentrate, may be considered if problems with local thrombophlebitis occur at the injection site, without affecting stability.

## ANTIHEMOPHILIC FACTOR (PORCINE)
Note: The specific activity of AHF (Porcine) is more than 15 porcine units per mg of protein.

*Hyate:C* must be tested *in vitro*, prior to administration, to demonstrate that it will not cross-react with anti-human factor VIII antibodies.

The dose of AHF (Porcine) must be individualized for each patient based on patient weight, circulating antibody concentration, type of hemorrhage, and desired plasma factor VIII concentration.

*Hyate:C* should be administered at a rate of not more than 2 to 5 mL per minute.

### Usual adult and adolescent dose
Hemorrhagic complications in patients with factor VIII inhibitors (prophylaxis and treatment)—
Intravenous, initially, 50 to 100 International Units (IU) per kg of body weight. Further doses are titrated according to the patient's clinical response and by monitoring the patient's factor VIII response.

### Usual pediatric dose
See *Usual adult and adolescent dose*.

### Size(s) usually available
U.S.—
 400 to 700 Porcine Units (Rx) [*Hyate:C* (sodium ion ≤ 200 mmol per liter; citrate ion ≤ 55 mmol per liter)].
Canada—
 400 to 700 Porcine Units (Rx) [*Hyate:C* (sodium ion ≤ 200 mmol per liter; citrate ion ≤ 55 mmol per liter)].

### Packaging and storage
The dry concentrate should be stored between −20 and −15 °C (−4 and +5 °F).

### Preparation of dosage form
The dry concentrate should be warmed to 20 to 37 °C (68 to 96 °F) prior to reconstitution. It may be removed from the refrigerator and allowed to sit just until it reaches room temperature or, in an urgent situation, it may be placed in a warm water bath, 20 to 37 °C (68 to 96 °F). The dry concentrate should then be dissolved with 20 mL of sterile water for injection. The vial should be shaken gently until the concentrate is dissolved, taking care to prevent foaming.

### Stability
Administration should begin within 3 hours after reconstitution. Partially used vials should be discarded.

### Incompatibilities
It is recommended that AHF (Porcine), after reconstitution, be administered through a separate line, by itself, and without mixing with other intravenous fluids or medications.

## ANTIHEMOPHILIC FACTOR (RECOMBINANT)
Note: Each vial of AHF is labeled with the AHF activity expressed in International Units (IU) per vial. This potency assignment is referenced to the World Health Organization International Standard. One IU of factor VIII activity is approximately equal to the AHF activity of 1 mL of fresh plasma, and increases the plasma concentration of factor VIII by 2%. The following formulas may be used as guides in determining dosage:

Desired AHF increase (% of normal) = ([Dose AHF(IU)]/[Body weight (kg)]) × 2

Dose AHF (IU) = Body weight (kg) × Desired AHF increase × 0.5

*Kogenate* may be administered over five to ten minutes, and *Recombinate* at a rate of up to 10 mL per minute. However, the rate at which recombinant AHF is administered should be guided by the comfort of the patient.

### Usual adult and adolescent dose
See *Antihemophilic Factor USP (Human)*.

### Usual pediatric dose
See *Antihemophilic Factor USP (Human)*.

### Size(s) usually available
U.S.—
 250 IU with 2.5 mL sterile water for injection provided as diluent (Rx) [*Helixate; Kogenate* (calcium chloride 2 to 5 mmol; sodium 100 to 130 mEq per liter; chloride 100 to 130 mEq per liter; albumin human 4 to 10 mg per mL; mouse protein ≤ 0.03 nanogram per IU; hamster protein ≤ 0.04 nanogram per IU)].
 250 IU with 10 mL sterile water for injection provided as diluent (Rx) [*Bioclate; Recombinate* (albumin human 12.5 mg per mL; sodium 180 mEq per liter; calcium 200 mcg per mL; von Willebrand factor ≤ 2 nanograms per IU; mouse protein ≤ 0.1 nanogram per IU; hamster and bovine proteins ≤ 1 nanogram per IU)].
 500 IU with 5 mL sterile water for injection provided as diluent (Rx) [*Helixate; Kogenate* (calcium chloride 2 to 5 mmol; sodium 100 to 130 mEq per liter; chloride 100 to 130 mEq per liter; albumin human 4 to 10 mg per mL; mouse protein ≤ 0.03 nanogram per IU; hamster protein ≤ 0.04 nanogram per IU)].
 500 IU with 10 mL sterile water for injection provided as diluent (Rx) [*Bioclate; Recombinate* (albumin human 12.5 mg per mL; sodium 180 mEq per liter; calcium 200 mcg per mL; von Willebrand factor ≤ 2 nanograms per IU; mouse protein ≤ 0.1 nanogram per IU; hamster and bovine proteins ≤ 1 nanogram per IU)].
 1000 IU with 10 mL sterile water for injection provided as diluent (Rx) [*Helixate; Kogenate* (calcium chloride 2 to 5 mmol; sodium 100 to 130 mEq per liter; chloride 100 to 130 mEq per liter; albumin human 4 to 10 mg per mL; mouse protein ≤ 0.03 nanogram per IU; hamster protein ≤ 0.04 nanogram per IU); *Bioclate; Recombinate* (albumin human 12.5 mg per mL; sodium 180 mEq per liter; calcium 200 mcg per mL; von Willebrand factor ≤ 2 nanograms per IU; mouse protein ≤ 0.1 nanogram per IU; hamster and bovine proteins ≤ 1 nanogram per IU)].

Canada—
 250 IU with 2.5 mL sterile water for injection provided as diluent (Rx) [*Kogenate* (calcium chloride 2 to 5 mmol; sodium 100 to 130 mEq per liter; chloride 100 to 130 mEq per liter; albumin human 4 to 10 mg per mL; mouse protein ≤ 0.03 nanogram per IU; hamster protein ≤ 0.04 nanogram per IU)].
 250 IU with 10 mL sterile water for injection provided as diluent (Rx) [*Recombinate* (albumin human 12.5 mg per mL; sodium 180 mEq per liter; calcium 200 mcg per mL; von Willebrand factor ≤ 2 nanograms per IU; mouse protein ≤ 0.1 nanogram per IU; hamster and bovine proteins ≤ 1 nanogram per IU)].
 500 IU with 5 mL sterile water for injection provided as diluent (Rx) [*Kogenate* (calcium chloride 2 to 5 mmol; sodium 100 to 130 mEq per liter; chloride 100 to 130 mEq per liter; albumin human 4 to 10 mg per mL; mouse protein ≤ 0.03 nanogram per IU; hamster protein ≤ 0.04 nanogram per IU)].
 500 IU with 10 mL sterile water for injection provided as diluent (Rx) [*Recombinate* (albumin human 12.5 mg per mL; sodium 180 mEq per liter; calcium 200 mcg per mL; von Willebrand factor ≤ 2 nanograms per IU; mouse protein ≤ 0.1 nanogram per IU; hamster and bovine proteins ≤ 1 nanogram per IU)].
 1000 IU with 10 mL sterile water for injection provided as diluent (Rx) [*Kogenate* (calcium chloride 2 to 5 mmol; sodium 100 to 130 mEq per liter; chloride 100 to 130 mEq per liter; albumin human 4 to 10 mg per mL; mouse protein ≤ 0.03 nanogram per IU; hamster protein ≤ 0.04 nanogram per IU); *Recombinate* (albumin human 12.5 mg per mL; sodium 180 mEq per liter; calcium 200 mcg per mL; von Willebrand factor ≤ 2 nanograms per IU; mouse protein ≤ 0.1 nanogram per IU; hamster and bovine proteins ≤ 1 nanogram per IU)].

### Packaging and storage
The dry concentrates are preferably stored between 2 and 8 °C (36 and 46 °F). However, *Kogenate* may be stored at temperatures not exceeding 25 °C (77 °F) for 3 months. The solution should not be refrigerated after reconstitution. The diluent should be protected from freezing.

### Preparation of dosage form
The diluent and dry concentrate should be brought to room temperature, approximately 25 °C (77 °F), prior to reconstitution. They may be removed from the refrigerator and allowed to sit just until they reach room temperature or, in an urgent situation, they may be placed in a warm water bath, 30 to 37 °C (86 to 96 °F). The reconstituted solution should not be shaken, since excessive shaking will cause foaming. The reconstituted solution should be at approximately room temperature at the time of administration.

### Stability
Administration should begin within 3 hours after reconstitution. Partially used vials should be discarded. For use as a continuous infusion, studies have shown reconstituted recombinant AHF remains stable for extended periods.

### Incompatibilities
It is recommended that recombinant AHF, after reconstitution with the provided diluent, be administered through a separate line, by itself, and

without mixing with other intravenous fluids or medications. However, when administered as a continuous intravenous infusion, the addition of heparin, 1 to 5 USP Units per mL of concentrate, may be considered if problems with local thrombophlebitis occur at the injection site, without affecting stability.

## CRYOPRECIPITATED ANTIHEMOPHILIC FACTOR USP

Note: Random-donor cryoprecipitated antihemophilic factor is not recommended as a treatment alternative for hemophilia A because the product does not undergo a viral attenuation process. Appropriately screened, single-donor cryoprecipitate (such as from desmopressin-treated fathers of hemophilic children) has been used as an inexpensive alternative to the use of factor VIII concentrates for the management of hemophilia in small children.

Cryoprecipitated AHF is blood group–specific; ABO-compatible material is preferred when large amounts of this component are infused, to avoid hemolysis.

Each bag of cryoprecipitated AHF contains a minimum of 80 IU of factor VIII. The following formula may be used as a guide in determining dosage:

Number of bags required = [Body weight (kg) × Desired AHF increase (% normal) × 0.5]/[Average IU cryoprecipitate per bag (minimum 80)]

### Usual adult and adolescent dose

Hemophilia A—
Intravenous, initially, a loading dose to achieve the desired plasma factor VIII concentration, administered at a rate of 10 mL per minute, followed by a smaller maintenance dose every eight to twelve hours. To maintain hemostasis after surgery, it may be necessary to continue therapy for ten days or more.

von Willebrand disease—
Intravenous, 1 bag per 10 kg of body weight, administered every eight to twelve hours for several days.

Hypofibrinogenemia—
Intravenous, a quantity sufficient to raise the plasma fibrinogen concentration to 50 mg per 100 mL for minor bleeding, or to 100 mg per 100 mL for surgery. Each bag of cryoprecipitated AHF can be expected to raise the fibrinogen concentration 4 to 7 mg per 100 mL.

Disseminated intravascular coagulation—
Intravenous, 1 to 2 bags of cryoprecipitate per liter of patient's plasma.

Kasabach-Merritt syndrome—
Intravenous, a quantity sufficient to raise the plasma fibrinogen concentration to 100 mg per 100 mL.

### Usual pediatric dose
See *Usual adult and adolescent dose*.

### Strength(s) usually available
U.S.—
80 IU (Rx) [GENERIC (Available only through approved blood banks; fibrinogen ≥ 150 mg per 15 mL plasma; von Willebrand factor; factor XIII; fibronectin)].

Canada—
80 IU (Rx) [GENERIC (Available only through approved blood banks; fibrinogen ≥ 150 mg; von Willebrand factor)].

### Packaging and storage
The concentrate should be stored at −18 °C (−0.4 °F). It may be stored for up to 1 year from the date of collection of source material. The solution should not be refrozen after thawing.

### Preparation of dosage form
The frozen concentrate should be thawed in a water bath at 30 to 37 °C (86 to 98.6 °F) for up to 15 minutes. The reconstituted solution should be maintained at room temperature and administered as soon as possible, but no more than 6 hours after thawing, or 4 hours after the container is entered. For pooling, the precipitate in each concentrate may be mixed with 10 to 15 mL of 0.9% sodium chloride injection. Cryoprecipitated AHF, Pooled, usually requires no extra diluent.

### Stability
Should not be used if container shows evidence of breakage or if thawing occurred during storage.

### Incompatibilities
It is recommended that cryoprecipitated AHF be administered through a separate line, by itself, and without mixing with other intravenous fluids (with the exception of 0.9% sodium chloride injection) or medications.

## Selected Bibliography

Lusher JM. Considerations for current and future management of haemophilia and its complications. Haemophilia 1995; 1: 2-10.
DiMichele D. Hemophilia 1996: new approaches to an old disease. Pediatr Clin North Am 1996; 43: 709-36.

Revised: 08/15/97

---

Table 1. General Factor Replacement Guidelines for the Treatment of Bleeding in Hemophilia

| Indication | Initial minimum desired factor level (%) | Factor VIII dose* (IU/kg) | Duration (days) |
|---|---|---|---|
| Severe epistaxis | 20–30 | 10–15 | 1–2 |
| Oral mucosal bleeding† | 20–30 | 10–15 | 1–2 |
| Hemarthrosis | 30–50 | 15–25 | 1–2 |
| Hematoma | 30–50 | 15–25 | 1–2 |
| Persistent hematuria‡ | 30–50 | 15–25 | 1–2 |
| Gastrointestinal bleeding | 30–50 | 15–25 | at least 1–2 days after bleeding stops |
| Retroperitoneal bleeding | 30–50 | 15–25 | at least 3 |
| Trauma without signs of bleeding | 40–50 | 20–25 | 2–3 |
| Tongue/retropharyngeal bleeding† | 40–50 | 20–25 | 3–4 |
| Trauma with bleeding§ | 100 | 50 | 10–14 |
| Intracranial bleeding§ | 100 | 50 | 10–14 |

*Dosing intervals are based on a half-life for Factor VIII of 8 to 12 hours (2 to 3 doses/day). Maintenance doses of one half the initial dose may be given at these intervals. The frequency depends on the severity of bleeding, with more frequent dosing for serious bleeding.
†In addition to antifibrinolytics.
‡Painless spontaneous hematuria usually requires no treatment. Increased oral or intravenous fluids are necessary to maintain renal output.
§Continuous factor infusion may be administered. Following the initial loading dose, a continuous infusion at a dose of 3 IU/kg per hour is given. Subsequent doses are adjusted according to the plasma factor levels.

# ANTIHISTAMINES  Systemic

This monograph includes information on the following: 1) Acrivastine#†; 2) Astemizole; 3) Azatadine; 4) Bromodiphenhydramine‡; 5) Brompheniramine; 6) Carbinoxamine‡; 7) Cetirizine; 8) Chlorpheniramine; 9) Clemastine; 10) Cyproheptadine; 11) Dexchlorpheniramine; 12) Dimenhydrinate; 13) Diphenhydramine; 14) Diphenylpyraline§*; 15) Doxylamine†; 16) Hydroxyzine; 17) Loratadine; 18) Phenindamine†; 19) Pyrilamine#†; 20) Terfenadine*; 21) Tripelennamine; 22) Triprolidine#†

Note: Products listed in this monograph contain single-entity antihistamines. For products containing antihistamines in combination with other medications, refer to *Antihistamines and Decongestants (Systemic)*, *Antihistamines, Decongestants, and Analgesics (Systemic)*, and *Cough/Cold Combinations (Systemic)*.

Note: Products containing terfenadine were withdrawn from the U.S. market by the Food and Drug Administration in February 1998.

INN:
  Bromodiphenhydramine—Bromazine
  Chlorpheniramine—Chlorphenamine
  Pyrilamine†—Mepyramine

VA CLASSIFICATION (Primary/Secondary):
  Acrivastine—AH109
  Astemizole—AH102
  Azatadine—AH109
  Bromodiphenhydramine—AH109
  Brompheniramine—AH109
  Carbinoxamine—AH109
  Cetirizine—AH109
  Chlorpheniramine—AH109
  Clemastine—AH109
  Cyproheptadine—AH109
  Dexchlorpheniramine—AH109
  Dimenhydrinate—AH109/CN550
  Diphenhydramine
    Oral—AH109/AU350; CN309; CN550; RE302
    Parenteral—CN204
  Diphenylpyraline—AH109
  Doxylamine—AH109/CN309
  Hydroxyzine—AH109/CN309
  Loratadine—AH102
  Phenindamine—AH109
  Pyrilamine—AH109
  Terfenadine—AH102
  Tripelennamine—AH109
  Triprolidine—AH109

Commonly used brand name(s): *Aller-Chlor*[8]; *Aller-med*[13]; *AllerMax Caplets*[13]; *Allerdryl*[13]; *Apo-Dimenhydrinate*[12]; *Apo-Hydroxyzine*[16]; *Apo-Terfenadine*[20]; *Atarax*[16]; *Banophen*[13]; *Banophen Caplets*[13]; *Benadryl*[13]; *Benadryl Allergy*[13]; *Bromphen*[5]; *Calm X*[12]; *Chlo-Amine*[8]; *Chlor-Trimeton*[8]; *Chlor-Trimeton Allergy*[8]; *Chlor-Trimeton Repetabs*[8]; *Chlor-Tripolon*[8]; *Chlorate*[8]; *Claritin*[17]; *Claritin RediTabs*[17]; *Compoz*[13]; *Contac 12 Hour Allergy*[9]; *Dexchlor*[11]; *Dimetane*[5]; *Dimetapp Allergy Liqui-Gels*[5]; *Dinate*[12]; *Diphen Cough*[13]; *Diphenhist*[13]; *Diphenhist Captabs*[13]; *Dormarex 2*[13]; *Dramamine*[12]; *Dramanate*[12]; *Gen-Allerate*[8]; *Genahist*[13]; *Gravol*[12]; *Gravol Filmkote*[12]; *Gravol I/M*[12]; *Gravol I/V*[12]; *Gravol L/A*[12]; *Gravol Liquid*[12]; *Hismanal*[2]; *Hydrate*[12]; *Hyrexin*[13]; *Hyzine-50*[16]; *Multipax*[16]; *Nasahist B*[5]; *Nervine Nighttime Sleep-Aid*[13]; *Nolahist*[18]; *Novo-Hydroxyzin*[16]; *Novo-Pheniram*[8]; *Novo-Terfenadine*[20]; *Nytol Quick-Caps*[13]; *Nytol QuickGels*[13]; *Optimine*[3]; *PBZ*[21]; *PBZ-SR*[21]; *PMS-Cyproheptadine*[10]; *PMS-Dimenhydrinate*[12]; *PediaCare Allergy Formula*[8]; *Pelamine*[21]; *Periactin*[10]; *Phenetron*[8]; *Polaramine*[11]; *Polaramine Repetabs*[11]; *Pyribenzamine*[21]; *Reactine*[7]; *Seldane*[20]; *Seldane Caplets*[20]; *Siladryl*[13]; *Sleep-Eze D*[13]; *Sleep-Eze D Extra Strength*[13]; *Sleep-eze D Extra Strength*[13]; *Sominex*[13]; *Tavist*[9]; *Tavist-1*[9]; *Telachlor*[8]; *Teldrin*[8]; *Traveltabs*[12]; *Triptone Caplets*[12]; *Twilite Caplets*[13]; *Unisom Nighttime Sleep Aid*[15]; *Unisom SleepGels Maximum Strength*[13]; *Vistaril*[16]; *Zyrtec*[7].

Note: For a listing of dosage forms and brand names by country availability, see *Dosage Forms* section(s).

*Not commercially available in U.S.
†Not commercially available in Canada.
‡Not available in the U.S. or Canada as a single entity; however, it is available in combination products.
§Not available in the U.S. or Canada as a single entity; however, it is available in Canada in combination products.
#Not available in the U.S. as a single entity; however, it is available in the U.S. in a combination product.

## Category

Antihistaminic (H₁-receptor)—Acrivastine; Astemizole; Azatadine; Bromodiphenhydramine; Brompheniramine; Carbinoxamine; Cetirizine; Chlorpheniramine; Clemastine; Cyproheptadine; Dexchlorpheniramine; Dimenhydrinate; Diphenhydramine; Diphenylpyraline; Doxylamine; Hydroxyzine; Loratadine; Phenindamine; Pyrilamine; Terfenadine; Tripelennamine; Triprolidine.
Antianxiety agent—Hydroxyzine.
Antidyskinetic—Diphenhydramine.
Antiemetic—Dimenhydrinate; Diphenhydramine; Hydroxyzine (parenteral).
Antitussive—Diphenhydramine Elixir.
Antivertigo agent—Dimenhydrinate; Diphenhydramine.
Sedative-hypnotic—Diphenhydramine; Doxylamine; Hydroxyzine.
Appetite stimulant—Cyproheptadine.
Vascular headache suppressant—Cyproheptadine.
Antiasthmatic—Astemizole; Cetirizine; Loratadine; Terfenadine.

## Indications

Note: Bracketed information in the *Indications* section refers to uses that are not included in U.S. product labeling.

### Accepted

Rhinitis, perennial and seasonal allergic or vasomotor (prophylaxis and treatment) or
Conjunctivitis, allergic (prophylaxis and treatment)—Antihistamines are indicated in the prophylactic and symptomatic treatment of perennial and seasonal allergic rhinitis, vasomotor rhinitis, and allergic conjunctivitis due to inhalant allergens and foods.

Pruritus (treatment)
Urticaria (treatment)
Angioedema (treatment)
Dermatographism (treatment) or
Transfusion reactions, urticarial (treatment)—Antihistamines are indicated for the symptomatic treatment of pruritus associated with allergic reactions and of mild, uncomplicated allergic skin manifestations of urticaria and angioedema, in dermatographism, and in urticaria associated with transfusions. Cyproheptadine may be particularly useful for cold urticaria. [Antihistamines are also used in the treatment of pruritus associated with pityriasis rosea.][1]

Sneezing (treatment) or
Rhinorrhea (treatment)—Antihistamines are indicated for the relief of sneezing and rhinorrhea associated with the common cold. However, controlled clinical studies have not demonstrated that antihistamines are significantly more effective than placebo in relieving cold symptoms. Non-sedating (i.e., second-generation) antihistamines are unlikely to be useful in the treatment of the common cold symptoms since they do not have clinically significant anticholinergic effects (e.g., drying effects on nasal mucosa).

Anaphylactic or anaphylactoid reactions (treatment adjunct)—Antihistamines are indicated as adjunctive therapy to epinephrine and other standard measures for anaphylactic reactions after the acute manifestations have been controlled, and to ameliorate the allergic reactions to blood or plasma.

Anxiety (treatment) and
Tension, psychosis-related (treatment)—Hydroxyzine is indicated for the relief of anxiety and tension associated with psychoneurosis and as an adjunct in organic disease states in which anxiety is manifested. The effectiveness of hydroxyzine as an antianxiety agent for long-term use (for example, more than 4 months) has not been assessed by systematic clinical studies.

Alcohol withdrawal (treatment)—Parenteral hydroxyzine is indicated in the acute or chronic alcoholic with anxiety withdrawal symptoms.

Parkinsonism (treatment)[1] or
Extrapyramidal reactions, drug-induced (treatment)[1]—Diphenhydramine is indicated for the symptomatic treatment of parkinsonism and drug-induced extrapyramidal reactions in elderly patients unable to tolerate more potent antidyskinetic medications, for mild cases of parkinsonism in other age groups and, in combination with centrally acting anticholinergic agents, for other cases of parkinsonism.

Cough (treatment)—Diphenhydramine hydrochloride syrup is currently indicated as a non-narcotic cough suppressant for control of cough due to colds or allergy.

# Antihistamines (Systemic)

Motion sickness (prophylaxis and treatment) or
Vertigo (treatment)—Dimenhydrinate and diphenhydramine are indicated for the prevention and treatment of the nausea, vomiting, dizziness, or vertigo of motion sickness.

Nausea or vomiting (prophylaxis and treatment)—Parenteral hydroxyzine is indicated for the control of nausea and vomiting, excluding nausea and vomiting of pregnancy.

Sedation—Diphenhydramine and hydroxyzine are indicated for their sedative and hypnotic effects and as preoperative medications.

Insomnia (treatment)—Diphenhydramine and doxylamine are indicated as nighttime sleep aids to help reduce the time to fall asleep in patients having difficulty falling asleep.

Analgesia adjunct, during surgery
Anesthesia, general, adjunct or
Anesthesia, local, adjunct—Parenteral hydroxyzine is useful as pre- and postoperative, and pre- and postpartum adjunctive medication to allow reduction in narcotic dosage, and to control anxiety and emesis.

[Appetite, lack of (treatment)]—Cyproheptadine is used as an appetite stimulant, in adults and children.

[Headache, vascular (treatment)]—Cyproheptadine is used for treatment of vascular headaches, such as migraine and histamine cephalalgia.

[Asthma, bronchial (treatment adjunct)][1]—Astemizole, cetirizine, loratadine, and terfenadine are used as adjunctive treatment to asthma medications to reduce symptoms and improve bronchodilation in patients with mild atopic asthma.

## Unaccepted

Cyproheptadine has been used in the treatment of Cushing's disease because of its pronounced antiserotonin properties, which may decrease corticotropin release. Cyproheptadine may also provide antidiarrheal action against intestinal hypermotility associated with the excessive production of serotonin in patients with carcinoid tumors, and in some other conditions involving the release of serotonin. However, there is no conclusive evidence of effectiveness for these uses.

[1] Not included in Canadian product labeling.

## Pharmacology/Pharmacokinetics

### Physicochemical characteristics

Chemical group—
  Ethanolamine derivatives: Bromodiphenhydramine; Carbinoxamine; Clemastine; Dimenhydrinate (chlorotheophylline salt of diphenhydramine); Diphenhydramine; Doxylamine.
  Ethylenediamine derivatives: Pyrilamine; Tripelennamine.
  Piperidine derivatives: Astemizole; Azatadine; Cyproheptadine; Diphenylpyraline; Loratadine; Phenindamine; Terfenadine.
  Piperazine derivative: Cetirizine (metabolite of hydroxyzine); Hydroxyzine.
  Propylamine derivatives (alkylamines): Acrivastine; Brompheniramine; Chlorpheniramine; Dexchlorpheniramine; Triprolidine.

Molecular weight—
  Astemizole: 458.58.
  Azatadine maleate: 522.56.
  Bromodiphenhydramine hydrochloride: 370.72.
  Brompheniramine maleate: 435.32.
  Carbinoxamine maleate: 406.87.
  Cetirizine hydrochloride: 461.82.
  Chlorpheniramine maleate: 390.87.
  Clemastine fumarate: 459.97.
  Cyproheptadine hydrochloride: 350.89.
  Dexchlorpheniramine maleate: 390.87.
  Dimenhydrinate: 469.97.
  Diphenhydramine hydrochloride: 291.82.
  Diphenylpyraline hydrochloride: 317.86.
  Doxylamine succinate: 388.46.
  Hydroxyzine hydrochloride: 447.83.
  Hydroxyzine pamoate: 763.29.
  Loratadine: 382.89.
  Phenindamine tartrate: 411.45.
  Pyrilamine maleate: 401.46.
  Terfenadine: 471.69.
  Tripelennamine citrate: 447.49.
  Tripelennamine hydrochloride: 291.82.
  Triprolidine hydrochloride: 332.87.

pKa—
  Azatadine maleate: 9.3.
  Brompheniramine maleate: 3.59 and 9.12.
  Carbinoxamine maleate: 8.1.
  Chlorpheniramine maleate: 9.2.
  Cyproheptadine hydrochloride: 9.3.
  Diphenhydramine hydrochloride: 9.
  Doxylamine succinate: 5.8 and 9.3.
  Hydroxyzine hydrochloride: 2.6 and 7.
  Tripelennamine: 3.9 and 9.
  Triprolidine hydrochloride: 3.6 and 9.3.

### Mechanism of action/Effect

Antihistaminic ($H_1$-receptor)—Antihistamines used in the treatment of allergy act by competing with histamine for $H_1$-receptor sites on effector cells. They thereby prevent, but do not reverse, responses mediated by histamine alone. Antihistamines antagonize, in varying degrees, most of the pharmacological effects of histamine, including urticaria and pruritus. Also, the anticholinergic actions of most antihistamines provide a drying effect on the nasal mucosa.

Antianxiety agent—Hydroxyzine's sedative action may be due to a suppression of activity in certain key regions of the subcortical area of the central nervous system (CNS). It is not a cortical depressant.

Antidyskinetic—The actions of diphenhydramine in parkinsonism and in drug-induced dyskinesias appear to be related to a central inhibition of the actions of acetylcholine, which are mediated via muscarinic receptors (anticholinergic action), and to its sedative effects.

Antiemetic; antivertigo agent—The mechanism by which some antihistamines exert their antiemetic, anti–motion sickness, and antivertigo effects is not precisely known but may be related to their central anticholinergic actions. They diminish vestibular stimulation and depress labyrinthine function. An action on the medullary chemoreceptive trigger zone may also be involved in the antiemetic effect.

Antitussive—Diphenhydramine suppresses the cough reflex by a direct effect on the cough center in the medulla of the brain.

Sedative-hypnotic—Most antihistamines cross the blood-brain barrier and produce sedation due to inhibition of histamine $N$-methyltransferase and blockage of central histaminergic receptors. Antagonism of other central nervous system receptor sites, such as those for serotonin, acetylcholine, and alpha-adrenergic stimulation, may also be involved. Central depression is not significant with astemizole, cetirizine (low doses), loratadine, or terfenadine because they do not readily cross the blood-brain barrier. Also, they bind preferentially to peripheral $H_1$-receptors rather than to central nervous system $H_1$-receptors.

Appetite stimulant—Cyproheptadine competes with serotonin for receptor sites, thus blocking the responses to serotonin in vascular, intestinal, and other smooth muscles. It is possible that by altering serotonin activity in the appetite center of the hypothalamus, cyproheptadine stimulates appetite.

Vascular headache suppressant—Cyproheptadine's vascular headache suppressant effect is probably due to its antiserotonin action.

Antiasthmatic—Astemizole, cetirizine, loratadine, and terfenadine have been shown to cause mild bronchodilation and also to block histamine-induced bronchoconstriction in asthmatic patients. Also, astemizole, loratadine, and terfenadine have been shown to diminish exercise-induced bronchospasm and hyperventilation-induced bronchospasm. Cetirizine has not been shown to be uniformly effective in preventing allergen- or exercise-induced bronchoconstriction; however, due to its inhibition of late-phase eosinophil recruitment after local allergen challenge, it has been shown to be more effective, in higher doses, than other antihistamines in reducing the symptoms of pollen-induced asthma.

### Other actions/effects

Anticholinergic—Antihistamines prevent responses to acetylcholine that are mediated via muscarinic receptors. The ethanolamine derivatives may show greater anticholinergic activity than the other classes of antihistamines. Astemizole, loratadine, and terfenadine have no significant anticholinergic activity; cetirizine has minimal anticholinergic activity.

Anesthetic, local, dental—Antihistamines are structurally related to local anesthetics and have local anesthetic activity. Local anesthetics prevent the initiation and transmission of nerve impulses by decreasing the permeability of the nerve cell membrane to sodium ions. This action decreases the rate of depolarization of the membrane and prevents the generation of the action potential.

### Absorption

Well absorbed after oral administration.

Note: Ingestion of food may enhance the absorption of loratadine by 40% and of its active metabolite by 15%; however, it may decrease the absorption of astemizole by 60%.

Food may delay the rate, but not the extent of cetirizine absorption.

In one study involving patients 66 to 78 years of age the extent of absorption and peak plasma levels of loratadine and its metabolite were significantly higher (55%) than those in studies with younger patients.

**Protein binding**
Astemizole—96%.
Cetirizine—93%.
Chlorpheniramine—72%.
Diphenhydramine—98 or 99%.
Loratadine—97% (at concentrations of 2.5 to 100 ng/mL). Descarboethoxyloratadine (active metabolite): 73 to 77% (at concentrations of 0.5 to 100 ng/mL).
Terfenadine—97%.

**Biotransformation**
Hepatic (cytochrome P-450 system); some renal. Of the second-generation antihistamines, astemizole, loratadine, and terfenadine are metabolized by the hepatic cytochrome P-450 system and have active metabolites; however, cetirizine is minimally metabolized and excreted unchanged primarily through the kidneys.

**Half-life**
Elimination—
   Acrivastine—1.5 to 3.5 hours.
   Astemizole (plus hydroxylated metabolites)—Multiple doses, biphasic with an initial half-life of 7 to 9 days (with plasma concentrations being reduced by 75% within this phase) and a terminal half-life of about 19 days.
   Azatadine—12 hours.
   Brompheniramine—25 hours.
   Carbinoxamine—10 to 20 hours.
   Cetirizine—8 hours (range, 6.5 to 10 hours).
      In dialysis patients: 20 hours.
      In children: 4.1 to 6 hours.
   Chlorpheniramine—14 to 25 hours.
   Diphenhydramine—1 to 4 hours.
   Hydroxyzine—20 to 25 hours.
   Loratadine—3 to 20 hours (mean, 8.4 hours). Descarbethoxyloratadine (active metabolite): 8.8 to 92 hours (mean, 28 hours).
   Terfenadine—8.5 hours. Acid metabolite of terfenadine: Biphasic with an initial mean plasma half-life of 3.5 hours followed by a mean plasma half-life of 6 hours.
   Triprolidine—3 to 3.3 hours.
Note: In children, cetirizine, chlorpheniramine, hydroxyzine, and terfenadine have been found to have shorter elimination half-life values.

**Onset of action**
Oral—
   Most first-generation antihistamines: 15 to 60 minutes.
   Acrivastine: 0.5 hour.
   Astemizole: < 24 hours (depending on initial severity of symptoms, the maximum effect may not occur until the second or third day).
   Cetirizine: Histamine skin wheal studies— 1 and 0.5 hours following 5 and 10 mg doses, respectively.
   Loratadine: Histamine skin wheal studies—1 to 3 hours.
   Terfenadine: Histamine skin wheal studies—1 to 2 hours.
Parenteral—
   Dimenhydrinate: Intramuscular, 20 to 30 minutes.
Rectal—
   Dimenhydrinate: 30 to 45 minutes.

**Time to peak concentration**
Oral—
   Acrivastine—0.8 to 1.7 hours.
   Astemizole—Within 1 hour.
   Azatadine—4 hours.
   Brompheniramine—2 to 5 hours.
   Cetirizine—1 hour.
   Chlorpheniramine—2 to 6 hours.
   Clemastine—2 to 4 hours.
   Diphenhydramine—1 to 4 hours.
   Loratadine—1.3 hours. Descarbethoxyloratadine (active metabolite)—2.5 hours.
   Terfenadine—2 hours.
   Triprolidine—2 hours.

**Time to peak effect**
Oral—
   Astemizole: 9 to 12 days.
   Brompheniramine: 3 to 9 hours.
   Chlorpheniramine: 6 hours.
   Clemastine: 5 to 7 hours.
   Loratadine: Histamine skin wheal studies—8 to 12 hours.
   Terfenadine: Histamine skin wheal studies—3 to 4 hours.
   Triprolidine: 2 to 3 hours.

**Duration of action**
Ethanolamine derivatives—
   6 to 8 hours.
      Clemastine: 12 hours.
      Dimenhydrinate: 3 to 6 hours.
Ethylenediamine derivatives—
   Pyrilamine: 8 hours.
   Tripelennamine: 4 to 6 hours.
Piperazine derivatives—
   4 to 6 hours.
      Cetirizine: Up to 24 hours.
Piperidine derivatives—
   Astemizole: Depending on the length of therapy, skin test suppression may last for several weeks after discontinuation of astemizole.
   Azatadine: 12 hours.
   Cyproheptadine: 8 hours.
   Diphenylpyraline: 12 hours.
   Loratadine: Histamine skin wheal studies—At least 24 hours.
   Phenindamine: 4 to 6 hours.
   Terfenadine: Histamine skin wheal studies—Over 12 hours.
Propylamine derivatives—
   4 to 8 hours.
      Acrivastine: 6 to 8 hours.

**Elimination**
Renal (primarily fecal with astemizole and terfenadine). Most of the antihistamines studied (except cetirizine) are excreted as metabolites within 24 hours.
Cetirizine—
   Approximately 60% of the total dose administered is excreted unchanged in urine within 24 hours; about 10% is excreted in feces.
Loratadine—
   Approximately 80% of the total dose administered is excreted equally in urine and feces in the form of metabolic products after 10 days. Twenty-seven percent of the total dose is excreted in the urine in the conjugated form within 24 hours.
Terfenadine—
   Sixty percent of the dose is eliminated in the feces (50% as acid metabolite, 2% unchanged terfenadine, and the remainder as unidentified metabolites). Approximately 40% of the total dose is excreted renally (40% as acid metabolite, 30% dealkyl metabolite, and 30% unidentified metabolites).

## Precautions to Consider

### Cross-sensitivity and/or related problems
Patients sensitive to one of the antihistamines may be sensitive to others.

### Carcinogenicity/Tumorigenicity/Mutagenicity
Long-term animal studies to evaluate carcinogenic, tumorigenic, or mutagenic potential of most antihistamines have not been performed.
   *Loratadine*—
      In carcinogenicity studies, AUC data demonstrated that the exposure of mice given loratadine 40 mg/kg was 3.6 (loratadine) and 18 (active metabolite) times higher than that for a human given 10 mg/day. Exposure of rats given 25 mg/kg was 28 (loratadine) and 67 (active metabolite) times higher than that for a human given 10 mg/day. Male mice given 40 mg/kg had a significantly higher incidence of hepatocellular tumors (combined adenomas and carcinomas) than concurrent controls. In rats, a significantly higher incidence of hepatocellular tumors (combined adenomas and carcinomas) was observed in males given 10 mg/kg and males and females given 25 mg/kg. The clinical significance of these findings during long-term use of loratadine is not known.
   *Terfenadine*—
      Studies in mice and rats have not shown evidence of tumorigenicity when terfenadine was given in oral doses approximately 5 and 10 times the maximum recommended human daily dose on a mg per square meter of body surface area basis, respectively. Microbial and micronucleus test assays with terfenadine have not shown evidence of mutagenesis.

### Pregnancy/Reproduction
Pregnancy—Animal studies have suggested that meclizine and cyclizine, chemically related to antihistamines, might have a teratogenic potential.
   *Astemizole*—
      Adequate and well-controlled studies in humans have not been done. However, on the basis of 6 times the terminal half-life of astemizole, metabolites may remain in the body as long as 4 months after dosing has stopped.
      Studies in rats showed embryocidal effects accompanied by maternal toxicity at doses 100 times the recommended human dose.

However, at doses 50 times the recommended human dose, embryotoxicity or maternal toxicity has not been observed in rats or rabbits.

FDA Pregnancy Category C.

*Azatadine, brompheniramine, chlorpheniramine, clemastine, cyproheptadine, dexchlorpheniramine, dimenhydrinate, and loratadine—*
Well-controlled studies with azatadine, brompheniramine, chlorpheniramine, clemastine, cyproheptadine, dexchlorpheniramine, dimenhydrinate, and loratadine in humans have not been done. Studies in animals have not shown that these medicines cause adverse effects on the fetus.

FDA Pregnancy Category B.

*Cetirizine—*
Adequate and well-controlled studies in humans have not been done. Cetirizine was not teratogenic in mice, rats, and rabbits.

FDA Pregnancy Category B.

*Diphenhydramine—*
Adequate and well-controlled studies in humans have not been done.
Studies in rats and rabbits at doses up to 5 times the human dose have revealed no evidence of impaired fertility or harm to the fetus.

FDA Pregnancy Category B.

*Doxylamine—*
The Food and Drug Administration has stated that human epidemiologic data have not produced convincing evidence that the doxylamine and pyridoxine combination, a medication previously prescribed to treat nausea and vomiting during pregnancy, causes diaphragmatic hernias or other birth defects.

FDA Pregnancy Category B.

*Hydroxyzine—*
Adequate and well-controlled studies in humans have not been done. However, hydroxyzine is not recommended for use in the early months of pregnancy since studies in rats have shown that it causes fetal abnormalities when given in doses substantially above the human therapeutic range.

FDA Pregnancy Category C.

*Terfenadine—*
Adequate and well-controlled studies in humans have not been done.

FDA Pregnancy Category C.

*Tripelennamine—*
Adequate and well-controlled studies in humans have not been done. However, there is no evidence linking the use of tripelennamine with congenital defects.
Limited animal reproduction studies have not shown that tripelennamine causes adverse effects in the fetus.

FDA Pregnancy Category B.

*Triprolidine—*
Adequate and well-controlled studies in humans have not been done. However, there is no evidence linking the use of triprolidine with congenital defects.
Studies in animals have shown no evidence of adverse effects in the fetus.

FDA Pregnancy Category C.

**Breast-feeding**
First-generation antihistamines may inhibit lactation because of their anticholinergic actions.

Small amounts of antihistamines are distributed into breast milk; use is not recommended in nursing mothers because of the risk of adverse effects, such as unusual excitement or irritability, in infants.

*Astemizole—*
It is not known whether astemizole is distributed into human breast milk. Astemizole is distributed into the milk of dogs. However, problems in humans have not been documented.

*Cetirizine—*
The extent of distribution into human breast milk is unknown. Studies in dogs indicated that approximately 3% of the dose is distributed into milk.

*Loratadine—*
Loratadine and its metabolite descarboethoxyloratadine are distributed into breast milk, achieving concentrations equivalent to plasma levels. In one study, approximately 0.03% of the administered dose was distributed into breast milk over 48 hours after maternal ingestion of a single oral dose of 40 mg.

*Terfenadine—*
A small amount of terfenadine metabolite is distributed into breast milk.

**Pediatrics**
Use is not recommended in newborn or premature infants because this age group has an increased susceptibility to anticholinergic side effects, such as central nervous system (CNS) excitation, and an increased tendency toward convulsions.

A paradoxical reaction characterized by hyperexcitability may occur in children taking antihistamines.

*Astemizole, cetirizine, loratadine, and terfenadine—*
Although adequate and well-controlled studies have not been done in the pediatric population, astemizole, loratadine, and terfenadine are not likely, and cetirizine is less likely than first-generation antihistamines, to cause anticholinergic or significant CNS effects in children.

**Geriatrics**
Dizziness, sedation, confusion, and hypotension may be more likely to occur in geriatric patients taking antihistamines.

A paradoxical reaction characterized by hyperexcitability may occur in geriatric patients taking antihistamines.

Geriatric patients are especially susceptible to the anticholinergic side effects, such as dryness of mouth and urinary retention (especially in males), of the antihistamines. If these side effects occur and continue or are severe, medication should probably be discontinued.

*Astemizole, cetirizine, loratadine, and terfenadine—*
Astemizole, loratadine, and terfenadine are not likely, and cetirizine is less likely than first-generation antihistamines, to cause anticholinergic or significant CNS effects in geriatric patients. However, because elderly patients are more likely to have age-related renal function impairment, cetirizine and loratadine may accumulate and cause anticholinergic or CNS effects when given in such patients at the usual adult dose.

**Dental**
Prolonged use of antihistamines (except astemizole, cetirizine, loratadine, or terfenadine) may decrease or inhibit salivary flow, thus contributing to the development of caries, periodontal disease, oral candidiasis, and discomfort.

**Drug interactions and/or related problems**
The following drug interactions and/or related problems have been selected on the basis of their potential clinical significance (possible mechanism in parentheses where appropriate)—not necessarily inclusive (» = major clinical significance):

Note: It is not likely that astemizole, cetirizine, loratadine, or terfenadine will interact with most of the following medications because they lack significant anticholinergic and CNS actions. However, cetirizine and loratadine have been shown to cause dose-related CNS effects (e.g., sedation); and cetirizine has minimal anticholinergic effects.

Combinations containing any of the following medications, depending on the amount present, may also interact with this medication.

» Alcohol or
» CNS depression–producing medications, other (see *Appendix II*)
(concurrent use may potentiate the CNS depressant effects of either these medications or antihistamines; also, concurrent use of maprotiline or tricyclic antidepressants may potentiate the anticholinergic effects of either antihistamines or these medications)

» Anticholinergics or other medications with anticholinergic activity (see *Appendix II*)
(anticholinergic effects may be potentiated when these medications are used concurrently with antihistamines; patients should be advised to report occurrence of gastrointestinal problems promptly since paralytic ileus may occur with concurrent therapy)

Apomorphine
(prior administration of dimenhydrinate, diphenhydramine, doxylamine, or hydroxyzine may decrease the emetic response to apomorphine in the treatment of poisoning)

Azithromycin
» Clarithromycin

- » Erythromycin or
- » Troleandomycin
    (concurrent use of erythromycin with astemizole or terfenadine has been reported to increase the risk of cardiotoxic effects [prolongation of the QT interval, torsades de pointes, and other ventricular arrhythmias])

    (concurrent use of terfenadine with clarithromycin, erythromycin, or troleandomycin is **contraindicated**; pending further evaluation, concurrent use of terfenadine and azithromycin is not recommended)

    (concurrent use of astemizole with clarithromycin, erythromycin, or troleandomycin is **contraindicated**; pending further evaluation, concurrent use of astemizole with other macrolide antibiotics, such as azithromycin, is not recommended)

    Fluconazole
- » Itraconazole
- » Ketoconazole
    Metronidazole
    Miconazole or
    Other potent inhibitors of the cytochrome P450 enzyme system
    (concurrent use of ketoconazole or itraconazole with astemizole or terfenadine is **contraindicated**; concurrent use of these medications may increase plasma levels of astemizole, loratadine, and terfenadine, because of inhibition of the P450 metabolic pathways by these antifungals; increased plasma levels of astemizole and terfenadine may result in cardiotoxic effects [prolongation of the QT interval, torsades de pointes, and other ventricular arrhythmias]; there are no reports to date of serious ventricular arrhythmias associated with increased plasma levels of loratadine)

    (due to the chemical similarity of fluconazole, metronidazole, and miconazole to ketoconazole, caution also is recommended with concurrent use of these other imidazole antifungals and terfenadine, and concurrent use of these other imidazole antifungals and astemizole is not recommended; also, concurrent use of other potent inhibitors of the cytochrome P450 enzyme system with astemizole is not recommended)

- » Grapefruit juice
    (concurrent use with astemizole or terfenadine may inhibit the metabolism of these medications, leading to increased plasma concentrations; prolonged QT intervals have been reported when grapefruit juice is administered concurrently with terfenadine; concurrent use with astemizole or terfenadine is not recommended)

- » Human immunodeficiency virus (HIV) protease inhibitors, such as:
    Indinavir
    Nelfinavir
    Ritonavir
    Saquinavir or
- » Serotonin reuptake inhibitors, such as:
    Fluoxetine
    Fluvoxamine
    Nefazodone
    Paroxetine
    Sertraline
    (fluvoxamine, nefazodone, ritonavir, and sertraline have been shown to inhibit the metabolism of terfenadine *in vitro*; however, the clinical significance of these findings has not been established; pending further evaluation, concurrent use of terfenadine with HIV protease inhibitors or serotonin reuptake inhibitors is not recommended)

    (concurrent use of astemizole with HIV protease inhibitors or serotonin reuptake inhibitors is not recommended)

- » Medications causing QT interval prolongation, such as:
    Antidepressants, tricyclic
    Calcium channel blocking agents, especially bepridil
    Cisapride
    Disopyramide
    Maprotiline
    Phenothiazines
    Pimozide
    Procainamide
    Quinidine
    Sparfloxacin
    (concurrent use of these medications with astemizole or terfenadine may increase risk of cardiac arrhythmias, which are seen on electrocardiogram [ECG] as prolongation of the QT interval)

- » Mibefradil
    (concurrent use with astemizole or terfenadine has been reported to cause an increase in the plasma concentrations of astemizole or terfenadine and to prolong the QT interval; concurrent use is **contraindicated**)

- » Monoamine oxidase (MAO) inhibitors, including furazolidone and procarbazine
    (concurrent use of MAO inhibitors with antihistamines may prolong and intensify the anticholinergic and CNS depressant effects of antihistamines; concurrent use is not recommended)

    Ototoxic medications (see *Appendix II*)
    (concurrent use with antihistamines may mask the symptoms of ototoxicity such as tinnitus, dizziness, or vertigo)

    Photosensitizing medications, other
    (concurrent use of these medications with antihistamines may cause additive photosensitizing effects)

- » Quinine
    (concurrent use of a single 430-mg dose of quinine with astemizole has been reported to increase plasma concentrations of astemizole and its metabolite, desmethylastemizole, resulting in prolongation of the electrocardiographic QT interval; concurrent use is **contraindicated**)

- » Zileuton
    (although concurrent use with terfenadine has been reported to increase plasma concentrations of terfenadine, this increase was not associated with a significant prolongation of the QT interval; pending further evaluation, concurrent use is not recommended)

    (concurrent use with astemizole is not recommended)

**Laboratory value alterations**
The following have been selected on the basis of their potential clinical significance (possible effect in parentheses where appropriate)—not necessarily inclusive (» = major clinical significance):

With diagnostic test results
*For all antihistamines*
  Skin tests using allergen extracts
    (antihistamines may inhibit the cutaneous histamine response, thus producing false-negative results; it is recommended that antihistamines be discontinued at least 72 hours before testing begins [at least 4 weeks with astemizole and 1 week with loratadine and terfenadine])

*For hydroxyzine (in addition to those listed for all antihistamines)*
  Urine 17-hydroxycorticosteroid determinations
    (false increases have been reported with concurrent use of hydroxyzine)

With physiology/laboratory test values
*For cyproheptadine*
  Amylase and
  Prolactin
    (serum concentrations may be increased when cyproheptadine is administered with thyrotropin-releasing hormone)

**Medical considerations/Contraindications**
The medical considerations/contraindications included have been selected on the basis of their potential clinical significance (reasons given in parentheses where appropriate)—not necessarily inclusive (» = major clinical significance).

***Except under special circumstances, this medication should not be used when the following medical problems exist:***
- » Hepatic function impairment
    (increased plasma concentrations of astemizole or terfenadine may result, increasing the risk of cardiac arrhythmias or QT prolongation)
- » QT interval prolongation, history of
    (increased risk of astemizole- or terfenadine-induced arrhythmias)

***Risk-benefit should be considered when the following medical problems exist:***
- » Bladder neck obstruction or
- » Prostatic hypertrophy, symptomatic or
- » Urinary retention, predisposition to
    (anticholinergic effects may precipitate or aggravate urinary retention)
- » Glaucoma, angle-closure, or predisposition to
    (anticholinergic mydriatic effect resulting in increased intraocular pressure may precipitate an attack of angle-closure glaucoma)
  Glaucoma, open-angle
    (anticholinergic mydriatic effect may cause a slight increase in intraocular pressure; glaucoma therapy may need to be adjusted)

» Hypokalemia
(potassium deficiency, especially from use of diuretics, should be corrected before initiation of therapy with astemizole or terfenadine because of risk of ventricular arrhythmias)

Sensitivity to the antihistamine used

Caution is recommended when dimenhydrinate, diphenhydramine, or hydroxyzine is used, since their antiemetic action may impede diagnosis of such conditions as appendicitis and obscure signs of toxicity from overdosage of other drugs.

## Side/Adverse Effects

The following side/adverse effects have been selected on the basis of their potential clinical significance (possible signs and symptoms in parentheses where appropriate)—not necessarily inclusive:

### Those indicating need for medical attention
Incidence less frequent or rare
*Blood dyscrasias* (sore throat; fever; unusual bleeding or bruising; unusual tiredness or weakness); *cardiac arrhythmias* (fast or irregular heartbeat)—with high doses of astemizole or terfenadine

Note: Prolonged QT intervals and ventricular arrhythmias (torsades de pointes or fibrillation), accompanied by syncope and cardiac arrest, have been reported in association with high doses and/or overdose of astemizole and terfenadine. Severe ventricular arrhythmias have been reported with ingestion of 360 mg or more of terfenadine, and with overdoses greater than 200 mg of astemizole. There have been rare cases of this effect occurring with doses as low as 20 to 30 mg of astemizole a day, and in some patients, with possible potentiating circumstances (e.g., concurrent use of medications that prolong the QT interval), taking 10 mg daily. Small increases in QT interval have been observed in clinical trials in patients with rhinitis, but otherwise healthy, given terfenadine in doses of 60 mg two times a day. At a dose of 300 mg two times a day, a mean increase in the QT interval of 10% was observed.

### Those indicating need for medical attention only if they continue or are bothersome
Incidence more frequent—less frequent with cetirizine; rare with astemizole, loratadine, and terfenadine
*Drowsiness; thickening of mucus*

Note: In general, sedative effects are more pronounced with the ethanolamine derivatives (except clemastine) and less pronounced with the propylamine (alkylamine) derivatives.

Tolerance to central effects may develop quickly with some antihistamines, so that sedation is no longer troublesome after a few days.

Incidence of sedation may increase when the recommended doses of astemizole, cetirizine, loratadine, or terfenadine are exceeded.

Incidence less frequent or rare
*Blurred vision or any change in vision; confusion; difficult or painful urination; dizziness; dryness of mouth, nose, or throat; increased appetite or weight gain*—with astemizole, cetirizine, cyproheptadine, loratadine, and terfenadine only; *increased sweating; loss of appetite*—except with astemizole, cetirizine, cyproheptadine, loratadine, and terfenadine; *paradoxical reaction* (nightmares; unusual excitement, nervousness, restlessness, or irritability); *photosensitivity* (increased sensitivity of skin to sun); *ringing or buzzing in ears; skin rash; stomach upset or pain*—more frequent with the ethylenediamine derivatives; *tachycardia* (fast heartbeat)

Note: Confusion; difficult or painful urination; drowsiness; dizziness; and dryness of mouth, nose, or throat are more likely to occur in the elderly.

Nightmares, unusual excitement, nervousness, restlessness, or irritability is more likely to occur in children and elderly patients.

## Overdose

For more information on the management of overdose or unintentional ingestion, **contact a Poison Control Center** (see *Poison Control Center Listing*).

### Clinical effects of overdose
Symptoms of overdose
*Anticholinergic effects* (clumsiness or unsteadiness; severe drowsiness; severe dryness of mouth, nose, or throat; flushing or redness of face; shortness of breath or troubled breathing); *cardiac arrhythmias* (fast or irregular heartbeat)—especially with astemizole or terfenadine; *CNS depression* (severe drowsiness); *CNS stimulation* (hallucinations, seizures, trouble in sleeping); *hypotension* (feeling faint)

Note: Anticholinergic and CNS stimulant effects are more likely to occur in children with overdose. Hypotension may also occur in the elderly at usual doses.

Anticholinergic and CNS effects may be less likely to occur with astemizole, cetirizine, loratadine, or terfenadine than with the first-generation antihistamines.

### Treatment of overdose
Since there is no specific antidote for overdose with antihistamines, treatment is symptomatic and supportive.
To decrease absorption—
Induction of emesis (syrup of ipecac recommended); however, precaution against aspiration is necessary, especially in infants and children.
Gastric lavage (isotonic or 0.45% sodium chloride solution) if patient is unable to vomit within 3 hours of ingestion.
To enhance elimination—
Saline cathartics (milk of magnesia) are sometimes used.
Specific treatment—
Vasopressors to treat hypotension; however, epinephrine should not be used since it may further lower blood pressure.
Oxygen and intravenous fluids.
Precaution against use of stimulants (analeptic agents) because they may cause seizures.

## Patient Consultation

As an aid to patient consultation, refer to *Advice for the Patient, Antihistamines (Systemic)*.
In providing consultation, consider emphasizing the following selected information (» = major clinical significance):

### Before using this medication
» Conditions affecting use, especially:
Sensitivity to any antihistamine
Pregnancy—Not taking during early months of pregnancy because of fetal abnormalities in studies in animals (for hydroxyzine only); risk-benefit should be considered because of fetal abnormalities in studies in animals with doses above the human therapeutic range (for astemizole and terfenadine only)
Breast-feeding—Use not recommended; may cause unusual excitement or irritability in nursing infant
Use in children—Increased susceptibility to anticholinergic side effects in newborn or premature infants; hyperexcitability (paradoxical reaction) may occur in children
Use in the elderly—Increased susceptibility to anticholinergic side effects; hyperexcitability (paradoxical reaction) may occur
Dental—Increased risk of dental problems because of decrease or inhibition of salivary flow
**Contraindicated medications**—Erythromycin and other macrolide antibiotics (with astemizole and terfenadine), itraconazole and ketoconazole (with astemizole and terfenadine), mibefradil (with astemizole and terfenadine), and quinine (with astemizole)
Other medications, especially alcohol or other CNS depressants; anticholinergics; calcium channel blocking agents, cisapride, disopyramide, HIV protease inhibitors, maprotiline, phenothiazines, pimozide, procainamide, quinidine, serotonin reuptake inhibitors, sparfloxacin, tricyclic antidepressants, and zileuton (with astemizole and terfenadine); or MAO inhibitors
Other medical problems, especially angle-closure glaucoma, hepatic function impairment (with astemizole or terfenadine only), hypokalemia (with astemizole or terfenadine only), prostatic hypertrophy, or urinary retention

### Proper use of this medication
» Importance of not taking more medication than the amount recommended
» Proper dosing
Missed dose: If on scheduled dosing regimen—Using as soon as possible; not using if almost time for next dose; not doubling doses
» Proper storage

*For oral dosage forms*
Taking with food, water, or milk to minimize gastric irritation; taking astemizole on an empty stomach to minimize absorption problems
Swallowing extended-release dosage forms whole

*For injection dosage forms*
Knowing correct administration technique for self-administration; checking with physician if necessary

*For rectal dosage forms*
  Proper administration technique
*For dimenhydrinate and diphenhydramine when used as antivertigo agent*
  Taking at least 30 minutes (preferably 1 to 2 hours) before traveling

**Precautions while using this medication**
  Possible interference with skin tests using allergens; need to inform physician if using medication
  May mask ototoxic effects of large doses of salicylates
» Not taking erythromycin or other macrolide antibiotics, itraconazole, ketoconazole, or mibefradil while taking astemizole or terfenadine, and not taking quinine with astemizole
» Avoiding use of alcohol or other CNS depressants
» Caution if drowsiness occurs
  Possible dryness of mouth; using sugarless gum or candy, ice, or saliva substitute for relief; checking with physician or dentist if dry mouth continues for more than 2 weeks
» Not taking astemizole or terfenadine with grapefruit juice
*For dimenhydrinate, diphenhydramine, or hydroxyzine*
  Need to inform physician of use: Possible interference with diagnosis of appendicitis; may mask signs of toxicity from overdosage of other drugs
*For diphenhydramine and doxylamine when used in the treatment of insomnia*
» Not using concurrently with other sedatives or tranquilizers

**Side/adverse effects**
  Signs of potential side effects, especially blood dyscrasias and cardiac arrhythmias (with astemizole and terfenadine only)

## General Dosing Information

**For oral dosage forms only**
Most antihistamines may be taken with food, water, or milk to lessen gastric irritation. Astemizole should be taken on an empty stomach since food may decrease absorption.

**Diet/Nutrition**
Although administration of a single 430-mg dose of quinine has been reported to elevate the plasma concentration of astemizole and desmethylastemizole, resulting in prolongation of the electrocardiographic QT interval, ingestion of small amounts of quinine, such as that found in beverages containing quinine (up to 80 mg per day or about 32 ounces of tonic water), has not been shown to have a clinically or statistically significant effect on the QT interval.

**For parenteral dosage forms only**
Intramuscular injections should be administered deeply into the muscle.
Intravenous injections should be administered slowly, preferably with the patient in a recumbent position.
  *For hydroxyzine—*
    Administration should be by deep intramuscular injection into a large muscle mass, preferably the upper outer quadrant of the buttock or the mid-lateral thigh.
    Intramuscular injections should not be made into the lower or mid-third of the upper arm.
    When used preoperatively or prepartum, narcotic requirements may be decreased as much as 50%.

---

## ASTEMIZOLE

### Summary of Differences
Indications:
  Used as treatment adjunct in asthma.
Pharmacology/pharmacokinetics:
  Chemical group—Piperidine derivative.
  Other actions/effects—No significant anticholinergic activity. Mild bronchodilator.
  Absorption—Decreased absorption with ingestion of food.
  Protein binding—96%.
  Half-life—With multiple doses: 7 to 9 days (initial); 19 days (terminal).
  Onset of action—< 24 hours; effect may not occur until day 2 or 3, depending on initial severity of symptoms.
  Time to peak concentration—Within 1 hour.
  Time to peak effect—9 to 12 days.
  Duration of action—Up to several weeks.
  Elimination—Primarily fecal.
Precautions:
  Drug interactions and/or related problems—Possible cardiotoxic effects with erythromycin and other macrolide antibiotics, itraconazole, or ketoconazole, or with medications causing QT interval prolongation.
  Medical considerations/contraindications—Possible cardiotoxic effects with hepatic function impairment, history of QT interval prolongation, or with hypokalemia.
Side/adverse effects:
  Sedative and anticholinergic effects less likely. Cardiac arrhythmias with high doses or overdose. May cause increased appetite and weight gain.

## Oral Dosage Forms

Note: Bracketed uses in the *Dosage Forms* section refer to categories of use and/or indications that are not included in U.S. product labeling.

### ASTEMIZOLE ORAL SUSPENSION

**Usual adult and adolescent dose**
Antihistaminic (H$_1$-receptor)—
  Oral, 10 mg once a day.

**Usual pediatric dose**
Antihistaminic (H$_1$-receptor)—
  Children up to 6 years of age: Oral, 2 mg per 10 kg of body weight once a day.
  Children 6 to 12 years of age: Oral, 5 mg once a day.
  Children 12 years of age and over: See *Usual adult and adolescent dose*.

**Usual geriatric dose**
See *Usual adult and adolescent dose*.

Note: Geriatric patients may be more sensitive to the effects of the usual adult dose.

**Strength(s) usually available**
U.S.—
  Not commercially available.
Canada—
  2 mg per mL (OTC) [*Hismanal* (alcohol 5%)].

**Packaging and storage**
Store below 40 °C (104 °F), preferably between 15 and 30 °C (59 and 86 °F), in a well-closed container, unless otherwise specified by manufacturer. Protect from freezing.

**Auxiliary labeling**
• Shake well.
• Take on empty stomach.

### ASTEMIZOLE TABLETS

**Usual adult and adolescent dose**
See *Astemizole Oral Suspension*.

**Usual pediatric dose**
[Antihistaminic (H$_1$-receptor)]—
  Children 6 to 12 years of age: Oral, 5 mg once a day.
  Children 12 years of age and over: Oral, 10 mg once a day.

**Usual geriatric dose**
See *Astemizole Oral Suspension*.

Note: Geriatric patients may be more sensitive to the effects of the usual adult dose.

**Strength(s) usually available**
U.S.—
  10 mg (Rx) [*Hismanal* (scored)].
Canada—
  10 mg (OTC) [*Hismanal* (scored)].

**Packaging and storage**
Store below 40 °C (104 °F), preferably between 15 and 30 °C (59 and 86 °F), unless otherwise specified by manufacturer.

**Auxiliary labeling**
• Take on empty stomach.

---

## AZATADINE

### Summary of Differences
Pharmacology/pharmacokinetics:
  Chemical group—Piperidine derivative.
  pKa—9.3.
  Half-life—12 hours.
  Time to peak concentration—4 hours.
  Duration of action—12 hours.

## Oral Dosage Forms
### AZATADINE MALEATE TABLETS USP

**Usual adult and adolescent dose**
Antihistaminic (H₁-receptor)—
   Oral, 1 to 2 mg every eight to twelve hours as needed.

**Usual pediatric dose**
Antihistaminic (H₁-receptor)—
   Children up to 12 years of age: Use is not recommended.
   Children 12 years of age and over: Oral, 500 mcg (0.5 mg) to 1 mg two times a day as needed.

**Usual geriatric dose**
See *Usual adult and adolescent dose*.

Note: Geriatric patients may be more sensitive to the effects of the usual adult dose.

**Strength(s) usually available**
U.S.—
   1 mg (Rx) [*Optimine* (scored)].
Canada—
   1 mg (Rx) [*Optimine* (scored)].

**Packaging and storage**
Store below 40 °C (104 °F), preferably between 15 and 30 °C (59 and 86 °F), unless otherwise specified by manufacturer. Store in a well-closed container.

**Auxiliary labeling**
- May cause drowsiness.
- Avoid alcoholic beverages.

---

## BROMPHENIRAMINE

### Summary of Differences
Pharmacology/pharmacokinetics:
   Chemical group—Propylamine derivative.
   pKa—3.59 and 9.12.
   Half-life—25 hours.
   Time to peak concentration—2 to 5 hours.
   Time to peak effect—3 to 9 hours.
   Duration of action—4 to 8 hours.
Side/adverse effects:
   Sedative effects less pronounced.

## Oral Dosage Forms
### BROMPHENIRAMINE MALEATE CAPSULES

**Usual adult and adolescent dose**
Antihistaminic (H₁-receptor)—
   Oral, 4 mg every four to six hours as needed.

**Usual adult prescribing limits**
Up to 24 mg daily.

**Usual pediatric dose**
Antihistaminic (H₁-receptor)—
   Children younger than 12 years of age: See *Brompheniramine Maleate Elixir USP*.
   Children 12 years of age and over: Oral, 4 mg every four to six hours as needed.

Note: The available strength of the capsule may not conform to some of the recommended pediatric dosages.

**Usual geriatric dose**
See *Usual adult and adolescent dose*.

Note: Geriatric patients may be more sensitive to the effects of the usual adult dose.

**Strength(s) usually available**
U.S.—
   4 mg (Rx) [*Dimetapp Allergy Liqui-Gels*].
Canada—
   Not commercially available.

**Packaging and storage**
Store between 15 and 30 °C (59 and 86 °F), unless otherwise specified by manufacturer. Protect from freezing.

**Auxiliary labeling**
- May cause drowsiness.
- Avoid alcoholic beverages.

### BROMPHENIRAMINE MALEATE ELIXIR USP

**Usual adult and adolescent dose**
See *Brompheniramine Maleate Capsules*.

**Usual adult prescribing limits**
See *Brompheniramine Maleate Capsules*.

**Usual pediatric dose**
Antihistaminic (H₁-receptor)—
   Oral, 500 mcg (0.5 mg) per kg of body weight or 15 mg per square meter of body surface per day, in three or four divided doses, as needed; or for
   Children 2 to 6 years of age: Oral, 1 mg every four to six hours as needed.
   Children 6 to 12 years of age: Oral, 2 mg every four to six hours as needed.
   Children 12 years of age and over: Oral, 4 mg every four to six hours as needed.

Note: Premature and full-term neonates—Use is not recommended.

**Usual geriatric dose**
See *Brompheniramine Maleate Capsules*.

Note: Geriatric patients may be more sensitive to the effects of the usual adult dose.

**Strength(s) usually available**
U.S.—
   2 mg per 5 mL (Rx/OTC) [*Bromphen;* GENERIC].
   2 mg per 5 mL (OTC) [GENERIC].
Canada—
   2 mg per 5 mL (OTC) [*Dimetane* (alcohol 3%)].

**Packaging and storage**
Store below 40 °C (104 °F), preferably between 15 and 30 °C (59 and 86 °F), unless otherwise specified by manufacturer. Store in a well-closed, light-resistant container. Protect from freezing.

**Auxiliary labeling**
- May cause drowsiness.
- Avoid alcoholic beverages.
- Keep container tightly closed.

### BROMPHENIRAMINE MALEATE TABLETS USP

**Usual adult and adolescent dose**
See *Brompheniramine Maleate Capsules*.

**Usual pediatric dose**
See *Brompheniramine Maleate Elixir USP*.

Note: The available strength of the tablet may not conform to some of the recommended pediatric dosages.

**Usual geriatric dose**
See *Brompheniramine Maleate Capsules*.

Note: Geriatric patients may be more sensitive to the effects of the usual adult dose.

**Strength(s) usually available**
U.S.—
   Not commercially available.
Canada—
   4 mg (OTC) [*Dimetane*].

**Packaging and storage**
Store below 40 °C (104 °F), preferably between 15 and 30 °C (59 and 86 °F), unless otherwise specified by manufacturer. Store in a tight container.

**Auxiliary labeling**
- May cause drowsiness.
- Avoid alcoholic beverages.

## Parenteral Dosage Forms
### BROMPHENIRAMINE MALEATE INJECTION USP

**Usual adult and adolescent dose**
Antihistaminic (H₁-receptor)—
   Intramuscular, intravenous, or subcutaneous, 10 mg every eight to twelve hours as needed.

**Usual adult prescribing limits**
Up to 40 mg daily.

**Usual pediatric dose**
Antihistaminic (H₁-receptor)—
   Children up to 12 years of age: Intramuscular, intravenous, or subcutaneous, 125 mcg (0.125 mg) per kg of body weight or 3.75 mg per square meter of body surface three or four times a day as needed.

Note: Premature and full-term neonates—Use is not recommended.

USP DI

Usual geriatric dose
See *Usual adult and adolescent dose*.

Note: Geriatric patients may be more sensitive to the effects of the usual adult dose.

Strength(s) usually available
U.S.—
  10 mg per mL (Rx) [*Nasahist B;* GENERIC].
Canada—
  Not commercially available.

Packaging and storage
Store below 40 °C (104 °F), preferably between 15 and 30 °C (59 and 86 °F), unless otherwise specified by manufacturer. Protect from light. Protect from freezing.

Stability
Crystallization may occur if cooled below 0 °C (32 °F); but on warming to 30 °C (86 °F), the crystals will redissolve.

Additional information
The period of protection provided by a single dose ranges from three to twelve hours.

---

## CETIRIZINE

### Summary of Differences
Indications:
  Used as treatment adjunct in asthma.
Pharmacology/pharmacokinetics:
  Chemical group—Hydroxyzine metabolite.
  Absorption—Decreased absorption rate, but not extent, with food.
  Protein binding—93%.
  Half-life—8 hours.
  Time to peak concentration—1 hour.
Side/adverse effects:
  Minimal anticholinergic effects; dose-related sedation.

### Oral Dosage Forms

#### CETIRIZINE HYDROCHLORIDE SYRUP

Usual adult and adolescent dose
Antihistaminic ($H_1$-receptor)—
  Oral, 5 to 10 mg once a day.

Note: In patients with reduced creatinine clearance (< 31 mL per min) and with hepatic impairment, a dose of 5 mg once a day is recommended.

Usual adult prescribing limits
10 mg a day.

Usual pediatric dose
Antihistaminic ($H_1$-receptor)[1]—
  Children up to 2 years of age: Safety and efficacy have not been established.
  Children 2 to 6 years of age: Oral, 2.5 mg once a day. The dosage may be increased to a maximum daily dose of 5 mg, given as 5 mg once a day or 2.5 mg every 12 hours.
  Children 6 years of age and older: Oral, 5 or 10 mg once a day.

Note: The dosage should be decreased in patients who have reduced renal function (creatinine clearance of 11–31 mL per minute) or hepatic function impairment. In patients up to 6 years of age with renal or hepatic dysfunction, cetirizine use is not recommended. For children 6 years of age and older, the lower dosage of 5 mg once a day should be used.

Usual geriatric dose
See *Usual adult and adolescent dose*.

Strength(s) usually available
U.S.—
  5 mg per 5 mL (Rx) [*Zyrtec* (alcohol and dye free)].
Canada—
  Not commercially available.

Packaging and storage
Store between 15 and 30 °C (59 and 86 °F), in a tight container, unless otherwise specified by the manufacturer.

Auxiliary labeling
• May cause drowsiness.
• Avoid alcoholic beverages.

Antihistamines (Systemic) 333

#### CETIRIZINE HYDROCHLORIDE TABLETS

Usual adult and adolescent dose
Antihistaminic ($H_1$-receptor)—
  See *Cetirizine Syrup*.

Usual pediatric dose
Antihistaminic ($H_1$-receptor)—
  See *Cetirizine Syrup*.

Usual geriatric dose
See *Cetirizine Syrup*.

Strength(s) usually available
U.S.—
  5 mg (Rx) [*Zyrtec* (dye free)].
  10 mg (Rx) [*Zyrtec* (dye free)].
Canada—
  10 mg (OTC) [*Reactine; Zyrtec*].

Packaging and storage
Store between 15 and 30 °C (59 and 86 °F), in a well-closed container, unless otherwise specified by manufacturer.

Auxiliary labeling
• May cause drowsiness.
• Avoid alcoholic beverages.

[1] Not included in Canadian product labeling.

---

## CHLORPHENIRAMINE

### Summary of Differences
Pharmacology/pharmacokinetics:
  Chemical group—Propylamine derivative.
  pKa—9.2.
  Protein binding—72%.
  Half-life—14 to 25 hours.
  Time to peak concentration—2 to 6 hours.
  Time to peak effect—6 hours.
  Duration of action—4 to 8 hours.
Side/adverse effects:
  Sedative effects less pronounced.

### Oral Dosage Forms

#### CHLORPHENIRAMINE MALEATE EXTENDED-RELEASE CAPSULES USP

Usual adult and adolescent dose
Antihistaminic ($H_1$-receptor)—
  Oral, 8 or 12 mg every eight to twelve hours as needed.

Usual pediatric dose
Antihistaminic ($H_1$-receptor)—
  Children up to 12 years of age: Use is not recommended.
  Children 12 years of age and over: Oral, 8 mg every twelve hours as needed.

Usual geriatric dose
See *Usual adult and adolescent dose*.

Note: Geriatric patients may be more sensitive to the effects of the usual adult dose.

Strength(s) usually available
U.S.—
  8 mg (Rx) [*Telachlor;* GENERIC].
  8 mg (OTC) [GENERIC].
  12 mg (Rx) [*Telachlor;* GENERIC].
  12 mg (OTC) [*Teldrin;* GENERIC].
Canada—
  Not commercially available.

Packaging and storage
Store below 40 °C (104 °F), preferably between 15 and 30 °C (59 and 86 °F), unless otherwise specified by manufacturer. Store in a tight container.

Auxiliary labeling
• Swallow capsules whole.
• May cause drowsiness.
• Avoid alcoholic beverages.

#### CHLORPHENIRAMINE MALEATE SYRUP USP

Usual adult and adolescent dose
Antihistaminic ($H_1$-receptor)—
  Oral, 4 mg every four to six hours as needed.

Usual adult prescribing limits
Up to 24 mg daily.

### Usual pediatric dose
Antihistaminic (H$_1$-receptor)—
> Oral, 87.5 mcg (0.0875 mg) per kg of body weight or 2.5 mg per square meter of body surface every six hours as needed; or for
> Children up to 6 years of age: Use is not recommended.
> Children 6 to 12 years of age: Oral, 2 mg three or four times a day as needed, not to exceed 12 mg per day.

### Usual geriatric dose
See *Usual adult and adolescent dose.*

Note: Geriatric patients may be more sensitive to the effects of the usual adult dose.

### Strength(s) usually available
U.S.—
- 1 mg per 5 mL (OTC) [*PediaCare Allergy Formula*].
- 2 mg per 5 mL (OTC) [*Aller-Chlor* (alcohol 7%); *Chlor-Trimeton* (alcohol 5%); GENERIC].

Canada—
- 2.5 mg per 5 mL (OTC) [*Chlor-Tripolon* (alcohol 7%)].

### Packaging and storage
Store below 40 °C (104 °F), preferably between 15 and 30 °C (59 and 86 °F), unless otherwise specified by manufacturer. Store in a tight, light-resistant container. Protect from freezing.

### Auxiliary labeling
- May cause drowsiness.
- Avoid alcoholic beverages.

## CHLORPHENIRAMINE MALEATE TABLETS USP

### Usual adult and adolescent dose
See *Chlorpheniramine Maleate Syrup USP.*

### Usual pediatric dose
See *Chlorpheniramine Maleate Syrup USP.*

### Usual geriatric dose
See *Chlorpheniramine Maleate Syrup USP.*

Note: Geriatric patients may be more sensitive to the effects of the usual adult dose.

### Strength(s) usually available
U.S.—
- 4 mg (Rx) [*Phenetron* (scored); GENERIC].
- 4 mg (OTC) [*Aller-Chlor; Chlorate; Chlor-Trimeton* (scored); *Chlor-Trimeton Allergy; Gen-Allerate;* GENERIC].

Canada—
- 4 mg (OTC) [*Chlor-Tripolon* (scored); *Novo-Pheniram* (scored)].

### Packaging and storage
Store below 40 °C (104 °F), preferably between 15 and 30 °C (59 and 86 °F), unless otherwise specified by manufacturer. Store in a tight container.

### Auxiliary labeling
- May cause drowsiness.
- Avoid alcoholic beverages.

## CHLORPHENIRAMINE MALEATE TABLETS USP (CHEWABLE)

### Usual adult and adolescent dose
See *Chlorpheniramine Maleate Syrup USP.*

### Usual pediatric dose
See *Chlorpheniramine Maleate Syrup USP.*

### Usual geriatric dose
See *Chlorpheniramine Maleate Syrup USP.*

Note: Geriatric patients may be more sensitive to the effects of the usual adult dose.

### Strength(s) usually available
U.S.—
- 2 mg (OTC) [*Chlo-Amine*].

Canada—
Not commercially available.

### Packaging and storage
Store below 40 °C (104 °F), preferably between 15 and 30 °C (59 and 86 °F), unless otherwise specified by manufacturer. Store in a tight container.

### Auxiliary labeling
- Chew before swallowing.
- May cause drowsiness.
- Avoid alcoholic beverages.

## CHLORPHENIRAMINE MALEATE EXTENDED-RELEASE TABLETS

### Usual adult and adolescent dose
See *Chlorpheniramine Maleate Extended-release Capsules USP.*

### Usual pediatric dose
See *Chlorpheniramine Maleate Extended-release Capsules USP.*

### Usual geriatric dose
See *Chlorpheniramine Maleate Extended-release Capsules USP.*

Note: Geriatric patients may be more sensitive to the effects of the usual adult dose.

### Strength(s) usually available
U.S.—
- 8 mg (Rx) [*Phenetron;* GENERIC].
- 8 mg (OTC) [*Chlor-Trimeton Repetabs;* GENERIC].
- 12 mg (Rx) [*Phenetron* (sugar-coated); GENERIC].
- 12 mg (OTC) [*Chlor-Trimeton Repetabs* (sugar-coated); GENERIC].

Canada—
- 12 mg (OTC) [*Chlor-Tripolon*].

### Packaging and storage
Store below 40 °C (104 °F), preferably between 15 and 30 °C (59 and 86 °F), in a well-closed container, unless otherwise specified by manufacturer.

### Auxiliary labeling
- Swallow tablets whole.
- May cause drowsiness.
- Avoid alcoholic beverages.

# Parenteral Dosage Forms

## CHLORPHENIRAMINE MALEATE INJECTION USP

### Usual adult and adolescent dose
Antihistaminic (H$_1$-receptor)—
> Intramuscular, intravenous, or subcutaneous, 5 to 40 mg administered as a single dose as needed.

### Usual adult prescribing limits
Up to 40 mg daily.

### Usual pediatric dose
Antihistaminic (H$_1$-receptor)—
> Subcutaneous, 87.5 mcg (0.0875 mg) per kg of body weight or 2.5 mg per square meter of body surface every six hours as needed.

Note: Premature and full-term neonates—Use is not recommended.

### Usual geriatric dose
See *Usual adult and adolescent dose.*

Note: Geriatric patients may be more sensitive to the effects of the usual adult dose.

### Strength(s) usually available
U.S.—
- 10 mg per mL (Rx) [GENERIC].

Canada—
- 10 mg per mL (Rx) [*Chlor-Tripolon*].

### Packaging and storage
Store below 40 °C (104 °F), preferably between 15 and 30 °C (59 and 86 °F), unless otherwise specified by manufacturer. Protect from light. Protect from freezing.

### Additional information
The 10-mg-per-mL solution may be administered intravenously, intramuscularly, or subcutaneously.

---

# CLEMASTINE

## Summary of Differences
Pharmacology/pharmacokinetics:
> Chemical group—Ethanolamine derivative.
> Other actions/effects—Greater anticholinergic activity.
> Time to peak concentration—2 to 4 hours.
> Time to peak effect—5 to 7 hours.
> Duration of action—12 hours.

Side/adverse effects:
> Sedative effects not as pronounced.

## Oral Dosage Forms

### CLEMASTINE FUMARATE SYRUP

**Usual adult and adolescent dose**
Antihistaminic (H$_1$-receptor)—
  Oral, 1.34 mg two times a day or 2.68 mg one to three times a day as needed.
Note: Clemastine is indicated for dermatologic conditions at the 2.68-mg dosage level only.

**Usual adult prescribing limits**
Up to 8.04 mg daily.

**Usual pediatric dose**
Antihistaminic (H$_1$-receptor)—
  Children up to 6 years of age: Dosage has not been established.
  Children 6 to 12 years of age: Oral, 670 mcg (0.67 mg) to 1.34 mg two times a day, not to exceed 4.02 mg per day.
Note: Clemastine is indicated for dermatologic conditions at the 1.34-mg dosage level only.

**Usual geriatric dose**
See *Usual adult and adolescent dose*.
Note: Geriatric patients may be more sensitive to the effects of the usual adult dose.

**Strength(s) usually available**
U.S.—
  0.67 mg per 5 mL (Rx) [*Tavist* (alcohol 5.5%); GENERIC].
Canada—
  0.67 mg per 5 mL (OTC) [*Tavist* (alcohol 6.1%)].

**Packaging and storage**
Store below 25 °C (77 °F), preferably between 15 and 25 °C (59 and 77 °F), in a well-closed container, unless otherwise specified by manufacturer. Protect from freezing.

**Auxiliary labeling**
- May cause drowsiness.
- Avoid alcoholic beverages.

### CLEMASTINE FUMARATE TABLETS USP

**Usual adult and adolescent dose**
See *Clemastine Fumarate Syrup*.
Note: Clemastine is indicated for dermatologic conditions at the 2.68-mg dosage level only.

**Usual pediatric dose**
See *Clemastine Fumarate Syrup*.
Note: Clemastine is indicated for dermatologic conditions at the 1.34-mg dosage level only.

**Usual geriatric dose**
See *Clemastine Fumarate Syrup*.
Note: Geriatric patients may be more sensitive to the effects of the usual adult dose.

**Strength(s) usually available**
U.S.—
  1.34 mg (OTC) [*Contac 12 Hour Allergy*; *Tavist-1* (scored); GENERIC].
  2.68 mg (Rx) [*Tavist* (scored); GENERIC].
Canada—
  1 mg (base) (OTC) [*Tavist* (scored)].

**Packaging and storage**
Store between 15 and 30 °C (59 and 86 °F), unless otherwise specified by manufacturer. Store in a tight, light-resistant container.

**Auxiliary labeling**
- May cause drowsiness.
- Avoid alcoholic beverages.

---

## CYPROHEPTADINE

## Summary of Differences

Indications:
  Also indicated in cold urticaria and used as an appetite stimulant in adults and children.
Pharmacology/pharmacokinetics:
  Chemical group—Piperidine derivative.
  pKa—9.3.
  Other actions/effects—Serotonin antagonist.
  Duration of action—8 hours.
Precautions:
  Laboratory value alterations—
    May increase serum amylase and serum prolactin concentrations when administered with thyrotropin-releasing hormone.
Side/adverse effects:
  May cause increased appetite and weight gain.

## Oral Dosage Forms

Note: Bracketed uses in the *Dosage Forms* section refer to categories of use and/or indications that are not included in U.S. product labeling.

### CYPROHEPTADINE HYDROCHLORIDE SYRUP USP

**Usual adult and adolescent dose**
Antihistaminic (H$_1$-receptor)—
  Oral, initially 4 mg every eight hours, the dosage being increased as needed. For most patients the therapeutic range is 4 to 20 mg a day. However, doses up to 32 mg a day have been used occasionally.
[Appetite stimulant]—
  Oral, 4 mg three times a day with meals.
Note: Treatment period to promote weight gain should not exceed six months.
[Vascular headache suppressant]—
  Initial: Oral, 4 mg at the start of the attack, repeated after thirty minutes if necessary.
  Maintenance: Oral, 4 mg every four to six hours.

**Usual adult prescribing limits**
500 mcg (0.5 mg) per kg of body weight daily.

**Usual pediatric dose**
Antihistaminic (H$_1$-receptor)—
  Oral, 125 mcg (0.125 mg) per kg of body weight or 4 mg per square meter of body surface, every eight to twelve hours as needed or for
  Children 2 to 6 years of age: Oral, 2 mg every eight to twelve hours as needed, not to exceed 12 mg per day.
  Children 6 to 14 years of age: Oral, 4 mg every eight to twelve hours as needed, not to exceed 16 mg per day.
[Appetite stimulant]—
  Children 2 to 6 years of age: Oral, initially 2 mg two or three times a day with meals. The dosage may be increased, if necessary, but not to exceed 8 mg a day.
  Children 6 to 14 years of age: Oral, initially 2 mg three or four times a day with meals. The usual maintenance dose is 4 mg two or three times a day. The dosage may be increased, if necessary, but not to exceed 16 mg a day.
Note: Premature and full-term neonates—Use is not recommended.
Treatment period to promote weight gain should not exceed 3 months.

**Usual geriatric dose**
See *Usual adult and adolescent dose*.
Note: Geriatric patients may be more sensitive to the effects of the usual adult dose.

**Strength(s) usually available**
U.S.—
  2 mg per 5 mL (Rx) [*Periactin* (alcohol 5%); GENERIC].
Canada—
  2 mg per 5 mL (OTC) [*Periactin* (alcohol 5%)].

**Packaging and storage**
Store below 40 °C (104 °F), preferably between 15 and 30 °C (59 and 86 °F), unless otherwise specified by manufacturer. Store in a tight container. Protect from freezing.

**Auxiliary labeling**
- May cause drowsiness.
- Avoid alcoholic beverages.

### CYPROHEPTADINE HYDROCHLORIDE TABLETS USP

**Usual adult and adolescent dose**
See *Cyproheptadine Hydrochloride Syrup USP*.

**Usual adult prescribing limits**
See *Cyproheptadine Hydrochloride Syrup USP*.

**Usual pediatric dose**
See *Cyproheptadine Hydrochloride Syrup USP*.

**Usual geriatric dose**
See *Cyproheptadine Hydrochloride Syrup USP*.
Note: Geriatric patients may be more sensitive to the effects of the usual adult dose.

## Antihistamines (Systemic)

**Strength(s) usually available**
U.S.—
  4 mg (Rx) [*Periactin* (scored); GENERIC].
Canada—
  4 mg (OTC) [*Periactin* (scored); *PMS-Cyproheptadine*].

**Packaging and storage**
Store below 40 °C (104 °F), preferably between 15 and 30 °C (59 and 86 °F), unless otherwise specified by manufacturer. Store in a well-closed container.

**Auxiliary labeling**
- May cause drowsiness.
- Avoid alcoholic beverages.

---

### DEXCHLORPHENIRAMINE

## Summary of Differences
Pharmacology/pharmacokinetics:
  Chemical group—Propylamine derivative.
  Duration of action—4 to 8 hours.
Side/adverse effects:
  Sedative effects less pronounced.

## Oral Dosage Forms

### DEXCHLORPHENIRAMINE MALEATE SYRUP USP

**Usual adult and adolescent dose**
Antihistaminic ($H_1$-receptor)—
  Oral, 2 mg every four to six hours as needed.

**Usual pediatric dose**
Antihistaminic ($H_1$-receptor)—
  Children up to 12 years of age: Oral, 150 mcg (0.15 mg) per kg of body weight or 4.5 mg per square meter of body surface per day, in four divided doses or for
  Children 2 to 5 years of age: Oral, 500 mcg (0.5 mg) every four to six hours as needed.
  Children 5 to 12 years of age: Oral, 1 mg every four to six hours as needed.

Note: Premature and full-term neonates—Use is not recommended.

**Usual geriatric dose**
See *Usual adult and adolescent dose*.

Note: Geriatric patients may be more sensitive to the effects of the usual adult dose.

**Strength(s) usually available**
U.S.—
  2 mg per 5 mL (Rx) [*Polaramine* (alcohol 6%)].
Canada—
  2 mg per 5 mL (OTC) [*Polaramine* (alcohol 5%)].

**Packaging and storage**
Store below 40 °C (104 °F), preferably between 15 and 30 °C (59 and 86 °F), unless otherwise specified by manufacturer. Store in a tight container. Protect from light. Protect from freezing.

**Auxiliary labeling**
- May cause drowsiness.
- Avoid alcoholic beverages.

### DEXCHLORPHENIRAMINE MALEATE TABLETS USP

**Usual adult and adolescent dose**
See *Dexchlorpheniramine Maleate Syrup USP*.

**Usual pediatric dose**
See *Dexchlorpheniramine Maleate Syrup USP*.

**Usual geriatric dose**
See *Dexchlorpheniramine Maleate Syrup USP*.

Note: Geriatric patients may be more sensitive to the effects of the usual adult dose.

**Strength(s) usually available**
U.S.—
  2 mg (Rx) [*Polaramine*].
Canada—
  2 mg (OTC) [*Polaramine*].

**Packaging and storage**
Store below 40 °C (104 °F), preferably between 15 and 30 °C (59 and 86 °F), unless otherwise specified by manufacturer. Store in a tight container.

**Auxiliary labeling**
- May cause drowsiness.
- Avoid alcoholic beverages.

### DEXCHLORPHENIRAMINE MALEATE EXTENDED-RELEASE TABLETS

**Usual adult and adolescent dose**
Antihistaminic ($H_1$-receptor)—
  Oral, 4 or 6 mg every eight to twelve hours as needed.

**Usual pediatric dose**
Use is not recommended.

**Usual geriatric dose**
See *Usual adult and adolescent dose*.

Note: Geriatric patients may be more sensitive to the effects of the usual adult dose.

**Strength(s) usually available**
U.S.—
  4 mg (Rx) [*Dexchlor; Polaramine Repetabs* (sugar-coated); GENERIC].
  6 mg (Rx) [*Dexchlor; Polaramine Repetabs* (sugar-coated); GENERIC].
Canada—
  6 mg (OTC) [*Polaramine Repetabs*].

**Packaging and storage**
Store below 40 °C (104 °F), preferably between 15 and 30 °C (59 and 86 °F), in a well-closed container, unless otherwise specified by manufacturer.

**Auxiliary labeling**
- Swallow tablets whole.
- May cause drowsiness.
- Avoid alcoholic beverages.

---

### DIMENHYDRINATE

## Summary of Differences
Category:
  Also indicated as an antiemetic and antivertigo agent.
Pharmacology/pharmacokinetics:
  Chemical group—Ethanolamine derivative.
  Other actions/effects—Greater anticholinergic activity.
  Duration of action—3 to 6 hours.
Precautions:
  Drug interactions and/or related problems—May decrease emetic response to apomorphine.
  Medical considerations/contraindications—May impede diagnosis of appendicitis; may obscure signs of overdose.
Side/adverse effects:
  Sedative effects more pronounced.

## Additional Dosing Information
See also *General Dosing Information*.
When dimenhydrinate is used for prophylaxis of motion sickness, it should be taken at least 30 minutes, and preferably 1 or 2 hours, before exposure to conditions that may precipitate motion sickness.
For parenteral dosage form only
- Do not administer intra-arterially.

## Oral Dosage Forms

### DIMENHYDRINATE EXTENDED-RELEASE CAPSULES

**Usual adult and adolescent dose**
Antiemetic or
Antivertigo agent—
  Oral, 1 capsule every twelve hours.

**Usual pediatric dose**
Use is not recommended.

**Usual geriatric dose**
See *Usual adult and adolescent dose*.

Note: Geriatric patients may be more sensitive to the effects of the usual adult dose.

**Strength(s) usually available**
U.S.—
  Not commercially available.
Canada—
  75 mg (25 mg for immediate release and 50 mg for extended release) (OTC) [*Gravol L/A*].

## DIMENHYDRINATE ORAL SOLUTION

**Usual adult and adolescent dose**
Antiemetic or
Antivertigo agent—
  Oral, 50 to 100 mg every four to six hours.

**Usual adult prescribing limits**
400 mg per 24 hours.

**Usual pediatric dose**
Antiemetic or
Antivertigo agent—
  Children 2 to 6 years of age: Oral, 12.5 to 25 mg every six to eight hours as needed, not to exceed 75 mg per day.
  Children 6 to 12 years of age: Oral, 25 to 50 mg every six to eight hours as needed, not to exceed 150 mg per day.

Note: Premature and full-term neonates—Use is not recommended.

**Usual geriatric dose**
See *Usual adult and adolescent dose*.

Note: Geriatric patients may be more sensitive to the effects of the usual adult dose.

**Strength(s) usually available**
U.S.—
  12.5 mg per 5 mL (OTC) [GENERIC].
Canada—
  15 mg per 5 mL (OTC) [*Gravol Liquid* (alcohol-free)].

**Packaging and storage**
Store below 40 °C (104 °F), preferably between 15 and 30 °C (59 and 86 °F), unless otherwise specified by manufacturer. Store in a well-closed container.

**Auxiliary labeling**
• May cause drowsiness.
• Avoid alcoholic beverages.

## DIMENHYDRINATE SYRUP USP

**Usual adult and adolescent dose**
See *Dimenhydrinate Oral Solution*.

**Usual adult prescribing limits**
See *Dimenhydrinate Oral Solution*.

**Usual pediatric dose**
See *Dimenhydrinate Oral Solution*.

Note: Premature and full-term neonates—Use is not recommended.

**Usual geriatric dose**
See *Dimenhydrinate Oral Solution*.

Note: Geriatric patients may be more sensitive to the effects of the usual adult dose.

**Strength(s) usually available**
U.S.—
  12.5 mg per 5 mL (OTC) [*Dramamine*; GENERIC].
Canada—
  15 mg per 5 mL (OTC) [*PMS-Dimenhydrinate*].

**Packaging and storage**
Store below 40 °C (104 °F), preferably between 15 and 30 °C (59 and 86 °F), unless otherwise specified by manufacturer. Store in a tight container. Protect from freezing.

**Auxiliary labeling**
• May cause drowsiness.
• Avoid alcoholic beverages.

## DIMENHYDRINATE TABLETS USP

**Usual adult and adolescent dose**
See *Dimenhydrinate Oral Solution*.

**Usual adult prescribing limits**
See *Dimenhydrinate Oral Solution*.

**Usual pediatric dose**
See *Dimenhydrinate Oral Solution*.

Note: Premature and full-term neonates—Use is not recommended.

**Usual geriatric dose**
See *Dimenhydrinate Oral Solution*.

Note: Geriatric patients may be more sensitive to the effects of the usual adult dose.

**Strength(s) usually available**
U.S.—
  50 mg (OTC) [*Calm X* (scored); *Dramamine* (scored); *Triptone Caplets*; GENERIC].
Canada—
  15 mg (OTC) [*Gravol Filmkote*].
  25 mg (OTC) [*Gravol Filmkote* (Junior Strength)].
  50 mg (OTC) [*Apo-Dimenhydrinate*; *Gravol Filmkote*; *PMS-Dimenhydrinate*; *Traveltabs*].

**Packaging and storage**
Store below 40 °C (104 °F), preferably between 15 and 30 °C (59 and 86 °F), unless otherwise specified by manufacturer. Store in a well-closed container.

**Auxiliary labeling**
• May cause drowsiness.
• Avoid alcoholic beverages.

## DIMENHYDRINATE TABLETS (CHEWABLE) USP

**Usual adult and adolescent dose**
See *Dimenhydrinate Oral Solution*.

**Usual adult prescribing limits**
See *Dimenhydrinate Oral Solution*.

**Usual pediatric dose**
See *Dimenhydrinate Oral Solution*.

Note: Premature and full-term neonates—Use is not recommended.

**Usual geriatric dose**
See *Dimenhydrinate Oral Solution*.

Note: Geriatric patients may be more sensitive to the effects of the usual adult dose.

**Strength(s) usually available**
U.S.—
  50 mg (OTC) [*Dramamine* (scored)].
Canada—
  15 mg (OTC) [*Gravol*].
  50 mg (OTC) [*Gravol*].

**Packaging and storage**
Store below 40 °C (104 °F), preferably between 15 and 30 °C (59 and 86 °F), unless otherwise specified by manufacturer. Store in a well-closed container.

**Auxiliary labeling**
• May cause drowsiness.
• Avoid alcoholic beverages.

# Parenteral Dosage Forms

## DIMENHYDRINATE INJECTION USP

**Usual adult and adolescent dose**
Antiemetic or
Antivertigo agent—
  Intramuscular, 50 mg repeated every four hours as needed.
  Intravenous, 50 mg in 10 mL of 0.9% sodium chloride injection, administered slowly over a period of at least two minutes, repeated every four hours as needed.

**Usual pediatric dose**
Antiemetic or
Antivertigo agent—
  Intramuscular, 1.25 mg per kg of body weight or 37.5 mg per square meter of body surface, every six hours as needed, not to exceed 300 mg per day.
  Intravenous, 1.25 mg per kg of body weight or 37.5 mg per square meter of body surface, in 10 mL of 0.9% sodium chloride injection, administered slowly over a period of at least two minutes, every six hours as needed, not to exceed 300 mg per day.

Note: Premature and full-term neonates—Use is not recommended.

**Usual geriatric dose**
See *Usual adult and adolescent dose*.

Note: Geriatric patients may be more sensitive to the effects of the usual adult dose.

**Strength(s) usually available**
U.S.—
  50 mg per mL (Rx) [*Dinate*; *Dramanate*; *Hydrate*; GENERIC].

Canada—
- 10 mg per mL (Rx) [*Gravol I/V* (for intravenous administration only; ethyl alcohol)].
- 50 mg per mL (Rx) [*Gravol I/M* (for intramuscular administration; methylparaben; propylene glycol; propylparaben)].

Note: The 50-mg-per-mL concentration is intended for intramuscular use. To use this concentration for intravenous administration, the solution must be further diluted at a ratio of at least 1:10 (10 mL of diluent for each 1 mL of dimenhydrinate) with a compatible intravenous solution, such as sterile saline or 5% dextrose in water.

**Packaging and storage**
Store below 40 °C (104 °F), preferably between 15 and 30 °C (59 and 86 °F), unless otherwise specified by manufacturer. Protect from freezing.

## Rectal Dosage Forms
### DIMENHYDRINATE SUPPOSITORIES

**Usual adult and adolescent dose**
Antiemetic or
Antivertigo agent—
    Rectal, 50 to 100 mg every six to eight hours as needed.

**Usual pediatric dose**
Antiemetic or
Antivertigo agent—
    Children up to 6 years of age: Dosage has not been established.
    Children 6 to 8 years of age: Rectal, 12.5 to 25 mg every eight to twelve hours as needed.
    Children 8 to 12 years of age: Rectal, 25 to 50 mg every eight to twelve hours as needed.
    Children 12 years of age and over: Rectal, 50 mg every eight to twelve hours as needed.

**Usual geriatric dose**
See *Usual adult and adolescent dose*.

Note: Geriatric patients may be more sensitive to the effects of the usual adult dose.

**Strength(s) usually available**
U.S.—
    Not commercially available.
Canada—
    25 mg (OTC) [*Gravol*].

**Packaging and storage**
Store between 8 and 15 °C (46 and 59 °F), in a well-closed container, unless otherwise specified by manufacturer.

**Auxiliary labeling**
- May cause drowsiness.
- Avoid alcoholic beverages.

**Note**
When dispensing, include patient instructions.

---

## DIPHENHYDRAMINE

## Summary of Differences
Category:
    Also indicated as an antidyskinetic, antiemetic, antitussive (syrup only), antivertigo agent, and a sedative-hypnotic.
Pharmacology/pharmacokinetics:
    Chemical group—Ethanolamine derivative.
    pKa—9.
    Other actions/effects—Greater anticholinergic activity.
    Protein binding—98 to 99%.
    Half-life—1 to 4 hours.
    Time to peak concentration—1 to 4 hours.
    Duration of action—6 to 8 hours.
Precautions:
    Drug interactions and/or related problems—May decrease emetic response to apomorphine.
    Medical considerations/contraindications—May impede diagnosis of appendicitis; may obscure signs of overdose.
Side/adverse effects:
    Sedative effects more pronounced.

## Additional Dosing Information
See also *General Dosing Information*.

When diphenhydramine is used for prophylaxis of motion sickness, it should be taken at least 30 minutes, and preferably 1 or 2 hours, before exposure to conditions that may precipitate motion sickness.

## Oral Dosage Forms
### DIPHENHYDRAMINE HYDROCHLORIDE CAPSULES USP

**Usual adult and adolescent dose**
Antihistaminic ($H_1$-receptor)—
    Oral, 25 to 50 mg every four to six hours as needed.
Antidyskinetic[1]—
    For idiopathic and postencephalitic parkinsonism: Oral, 25 mg three times a day initially, the dose then being gradually increased to 50 mg four times a day if needed.
Antiemetic or
Antivertigo agent—
    Oral, 25 to 50 mg every four to six hours as needed.
Sedative-hypnotic—
    Oral, 50 mg twenty to thirty minutes before bedtime if needed.

**Usual adult prescribing limits**
Up to 300 mg daily.

**Usual pediatric dose**
Antihistaminic ($H_1$-receptor)—
    Children up to 6 years of age: Oral, 6.25 to 12.5 mg every four to six hours.
    Children 6 to 12 years of age: Oral, 12.5 to 25 mg every four to six hours, not to exceed 150 mg per day.
Antiemetic or
Antivertigo agent—
    Oral, 1 to 1.5 mg per kg of body weight every four to six hours as needed, not to exceed 300 mg per day.

Note: The available strength of the capsule may not conform to some of the recommended pediatric dosages.

**Usual geriatric dose**
See *Usual adult and adolescent dose*.

Note: Geriatric patients may be more sensitive to the effects of the usual adult dose.

**Strength(s) usually available**
U.S.—
    25 mg (Rx) [GENERIC].
    25 mg (OTC) [*Banophen; Benadryl Allergy; Genahist; Nytol Quick-Caps;* GENERIC].
    50 mg (Rx) [GENERIC].
    50 mg (OTC) [*Nytol QuickGels; Sleep-eze D Extra Strength; Unisom SleepGels Maximum Strength;* GENERIC].
Canada—
    25 mg (Rx) [*Allerdryl*].
    25 mg (OTC) [*Benadryl*].
    50 mg (Rx) [*Allerdryl*].
    50 mg (OTC) [*Benadryl*].

**Packaging and storage**
Store below 40 °C (104 °F), preferably between 15 and 30 °C (59 and 86 °F), unless otherwise specified by manufacturer. Store in a tight container.

**Auxiliary labeling**
- May cause drowsiness.
- Avoid alcoholic beverages.

### DIPHENHYDRAMINE HYDROCHLORIDE ELIXIR USP

**Usual adult and adolescent dose**
See *Diphenhydramine Hydrochloride Capsules USP*.

**Usual adult prescribing limits**
See *Diphenhydramine Hydrochloride Capsules USP*.

**Usual pediatric dose**
Antihistaminic ($H_1$-receptor)—
    Oral, 1.25 mg per kg of body weight or 37.5 mg per square meter of body surface, every four to six hours, not to exceed 300 mg a day
    or for
    Children weighing up to 9.1 kg: Oral, 6.25 to 12.5 mg every four to six hours.
    Children weighing 9.1 kg and over: Oral, 12.5 to 25 mg every four to six hours.
Antiemetic or
Antivertigo agent—
    Oral, 1 to 1.5 mg per kg of body weight every four to six hours as needed, not to exceed 300 mg per day.
Antitussive—
    Children up to 2 years of age: Dosage must be individualized by physician.

Children 2 to 6 years of age: Oral, 6.25 mg every four to six hours as needed, not to exceed 25 mg per day.
Children 6 to 12 years of age: Oral, 12.5 mg every four to six hours as needed, not to exceed 75 mg per day.

Note: Premature and full-term neonates—Use is not recommended.

**Usual geriatric dose**
See *Usual adult and adolescent dose*.

Note: Geriatric patients may be more sensitive to the effects of the usual adult dose.

**Strength(s) usually available**
U.S.—
  12.5 mg per 5 mL (Rx) [GENERIC].
  12.5 mg per 5 mL (OTC) [*Diphen Cough* (alcohol 5%); *Diphenhist*; *Genahist* (alcohol 14%); *Siladryl* (alcohol 5.6%); GENERIC].
Canada—
  12.5 mg per 5 mL (OTC) [*Benadryl* (alcohol 14%)].

**Packaging and storage**
Store below 40 °C (104 °F), preferably between 15 and 30 °C (59 and 86 °F), unless otherwise specified by manufacturer. Store in a tight container. Protect from light. Protect from freezing.

**Auxiliary labeling**
- May cause drowsiness.
- Avoid alcoholic beverages.
- Keep container tightly closed.

### DIPHENHYDRAMINE HYDROCHLORIDE TABLETS

**Usual adult and adolescent dose**
See *Diphenhydramine Hydrochloride Capsules USP*.

**Usual adult prescribing limits**
See *Diphenhydramine Hydrochloride Capsules USP*.

**Usual pediatric dose**
See *Diphenhydramine Hydrochloride Elixir USP*.

**Usual geriatric dose**
See *Diphenhydramine Hydrochloride Capsules USP*.

Note: Geriatric patients may be more sensitive to the effects of the usual adult dose.

**Strength(s) usually available**
U.S.—
  25 mg (Rx) [GENERIC].
  25 mg (OTC) [*Aller-med; Banophen Caplets; Benadryl; Diphenhist Captabs; Nervine Nighttime Sleep-Aid; Sleep-Eze D; Sominex*].
  50 mg (Rx) [GENERIC].
  50 mg (OTC) [*AllerMax Caplets; Compoz; Dormarex 2; Sleep-Eze D Extra Strength; Twilite Caplets*].
Canada—
  Not commercially available.

**Packaging and storage**
Store below 40 °C (104 °F), preferably between 15 and 30 °C (59 and 86 °F), in a well-closed container, unless otherwise specified by manufacturer.

**Auxiliary labeling**
- May cause drowsiness.
- Avoid alcoholic beverages.

## Parenteral Dosage Forms

### DIPHENHYDRAMINE HYDROCHLORIDE INJECTION USP

**Usual adult and adolescent dose**
Antihistaminic (H$_1$-receptor) or
Antidyskinetic[1]—
  Intramuscular or intravenous, 10 to 50 mg.
Antiemetic or
Antivertigo agent—
  Intramuscular or intravenous, 10 mg initially, may be increased to 20 to 50 mg every two to three hours.

**Usual adult prescribing limits**
Up to 100 mg per dose or 400 mg daily.

**Usual pediatric dose**
Antihistaminic (H$_1$-receptor) or
Antidyskinetic—
  Intramuscular, 1.25 mg per kg of body weight or 37.5 mg per square meter of body surface, four times a day, not to exceed 300 mg per day.
Antiemetic or
Antivertigo agent—
  Intramuscular, 1 to 1.5 mg per kg of body weight every six hours, not to exceed 300 mg per day.

Note: Premature and full-term neonates—Use is not recommended.

**Usual geriatric dose**
See *Usual adult and adolescent dose*.

Note: Geriatric patients may be more sensitive to the effects of the usual adult dose.

**Strength(s) usually available**
U.S.—
  10 mg per mL (Rx) [GENERIC].
  50 mg per mL (Rx) [*Benadryl; Hyrexin;* GENERIC].
Canada—
  50 mg per mL (Rx) [*Benadryl* [GENERIC].

**Packaging and storage**
Store below 40 °C (104 °F), preferably between 15 and 30 °C (59 and 86 °F), unless otherwise specified by manufacturer. Protect from light. Protect from freezing.

[1]Not included in Canadian product labeling.

---

## DOXYLAMINE

### Summary of Differences
Category:
  Also indicated as a sedative-hypnotic.
Pharmacology/pharmacokinetics:
  Chemical group—Ethanolamine derivative.
  pKa—5.8 and 9.3.
  Other actions/effects—Greater anticholinergic activity.
  Duration of action—6 to 8 hours.
Precautions:
  Drug interactions and/or related problems—
    May decrease emetic response to apomorphine.
Side/adverse effects:
  Sedative effects more pronounced.

## Oral Dosage Forms

### DOXYLAMINE SUCCINATE TABLETS USP

**Usual adult and adolescent dose**
Antihistaminic (H$_1$-receptor)—
  Oral, 12.5 to 25 mg every four to six hours as needed.
Sedative-hypnotic—
  Oral, 25 mg thirty minutes before bedtime if needed.

**Usual adult prescribing limits**
Up to 150 mg daily.

**Usual pediatric dose**
Antihistaminic (H$_1$-receptor)—
  Children up to 6 years of age: Use is not recommended.
  Children 6 to 12 years of age: Oral, 6.25 to 12.5 mg every four to six hours as needed.
Sedative-hypnotic—
  Use is not recommended.

**Usual geriatric dose**
See *Usual adult and adolescent dose*.

Note: Geriatric patients may be more sensitive to the effects of the usual adult dose.

**Strength(s) usually available**
U.S.—
  25 mg (OTC) [*Unisom Nighttime Sleep Aid* (scored)].
Canada—
  Not commercially available.

**Packaging and storage**
Store below 40 °C (104 °F), preferably between 15 and 30 °C (59 and 86 °F), unless otherwise specified by manufacturer. Store in a well-closed container. Protect from light.

**Auxiliary labeling**
- May cause drowsiness.
- Avoid alcoholic beverages.

# HYDROXYZINE

## Summary of Differences

Category:
  Also indicated in the treatment of anxiety and psychosis-related tension; antiemetic agent and sedative-hypnotic.

Pharmacology/pharmacokinetics:
  Chemical group—Piperazine derivative.
  pKa—Hydroxyzine hydrochloride: 2.6 and 7.
  Half-life (elimination)—20 to 25 hours.
  Duration of action—4 to 6 hours.

Precautions:
  Pregnancy—Not taking during early months of pregnancy because of fetal abnormalities in studies in animals.
  Drug interactions and/or related problems—May decrease emetic response to apomorphine.
  Laboratory value alterations—False increases in urine 17-hydroxycorticosteroid determinations.
  Medical considerations/contraindications—May impede diagnosis of appendicitis; may obscure signs of overdose.

## Oral Dosage Forms

### HYDROXYZINE HYDROCHLORIDE CAPSULES

**Usual adult and adolescent dose**
Antianxiety agent or
Sedative-hypnotic—
  Oral, 50 to 100 mg as a single dose.
Antihistaminic (H$_1$-receptor) or
Antiemetic—
  Oral, 25 to 100 mg three or four times a day as needed.

**Usual pediatric dose**
Antianxiety agent or
Sedative-hypnotic—
  Oral, 600 mcg (0.6 mg) per kg of body weight as a single dose.
Antihistaminic (H$_1$-receptor) or
Antiemetic—
  Oral, 500 mcg (0.5 mg) per kg of body weight or 15 mg per square meter of body surface every six hours as needed; or for
  Children up to 6 years of age: Oral, 30 to 50 mg a day in divided doses, or 12.5 mg every six hours as needed.
  Children 6 to 12 years of age: Oral, 50 to 100 mg a day in divided doses, or 12.5 to 25 mg every six hours as needed.

**Usual geriatric dose**
See *Usual adult and adolescent dose*.

Note: Geriatric patients may be more sensitive to the effects of the usual adult dose.

**Strength(s) usually available**
U.S.—
  Not commercially available.
Canada—
  10 mg (Rx) [*Apo-Hydroxyzine; Atarax; Multipax; Novo-Hydroxyzin*].
  25 mg (Rx) [*Apo-Hydroxyzine; Atarax; Multipax; Novo-Hydroxyzin*].
  50 mg (Rx) [*Apo-Hydroxyzine; Atarax; Multipax; Novo-Hydroxyzin*].

**Packaging and storage**
Store below 40 °C (104 °F), preferably between 15 and 30 °C (59 and 86 °F), unless otherwise specified by manufacturer.

**Auxiliary labeling**
• May cause drowsiness.
• Avoid alcoholic beverages.

### HYDROXYZINE HYDROCHLORIDE SYRUP USP

**Usual adult and adolescent dose**
See *Hydroxyzine Hydrochloride Capsules*.

**Usual pediatric dose**
See *Hydroxyzine Hydrochloride Capsules*.

**Usual geriatric dose**
See *Hydroxyzine Hydrochloride Capsules*.

Note: Geriatric patients may be more sensitive to the effects of the usual adult dose.

**Strength(s) usually available**
U.S.—
  10 mg per 5 mL (Rx) [*Atarax* (alcohol 0.5%); GENERIC].
Canada—
  10 mg per 5 mL (Rx) [*Atarax*].

**Packaging and storage**
Store below 40 °C (104 °F), preferably between 15 and 30 °C (59 and 86 °F), unless otherwise specified by manufacturer. Store in a tight, light-resistant container. Protect from freezing.

**Auxiliary labeling**
• May cause drowsiness.
• Avoid alcoholic beverages.

### HYDROXYZINE HYDROCHLORIDE TABLETS USP

**Usual adult and adolescent dose**
See *Hydroxyzine Hydrochloride Capsules*.

**Usual pediatric dose**
See *Hydroxyzine Hydrochloride Capsules*.

**Usual geriatric dose**
See *Hydroxyzine Hydrochloride Capsules*.

Note: Geriatric patients may be more sensitive to the effects of the usual adult dose.

**Strength(s) usually available**
U.S.—
  10 mg (Rx) [*Atarax*; GENERIC].
  25 mg (Rx) [*Atarax*; GENERIC].
  50 mg (Rx) [*Atarax*; GENERIC].
  100 mg (Rx) [*Atarax*; GENERIC].
Canada—
  Not commercially available.

**Packaging and storage**
Store below 40 °C (104 °F), preferably between 15 and 30 °C (59 and 86 °F), unless otherwise specified by manufacturer. Store in a tight container.

**Auxiliary labeling**
• May cause drowsiness.
• Avoid alcoholic beverages.

### HYDROXYZINE PAMOATE CAPSULES USP

**Usual adult and adolescent dose**
Antianxiety agent or
Sedative-hypnotic—
  Oral, 50 to 100 mg as a single dose.
Antihistaminic (H$_1$-receptor) or
Antiemetic—
  Oral, 25 to 100 mg three to four times a day as needed.

**Usual pediatric dose**
Antianxiety agent or
Sedative-hypnotic—
  Oral, 600 mcg (0.6 mg) per kg of body weight as a single dose.
Antihistaminic (H$_1$-receptor) or
Antiemetic—
  Oral, 500 mcg (0.5 mg) per kg of body weight or 15 mg per square meter of body surface every six hours as needed; or for
  Children 6 years of age and over: Oral, 12.5 to 25 mg every six hours as needed.

**Usual geriatric dose**
See *Usual adult and adolescent dose*.

Note: Geriatric patients may be more sensitive to the effects of the usual adult dose.

**Strength(s) usually available**
U.S.—
  The equivalent of hydroxyzine hydrochloride:
    25 mg (Rx) [*Vistaril* [GENERIC].
    50 mg (Rx) [*Vistaril* [GENERIC].
    100 mg (Rx) [*Vistaril* [GENERIC].
Canada—
  Not commercially available.

**Packaging and storage**
Store below 40 °C (104 °F), preferably between 15 and 30 °C (59 and 86 °F), in a well-closed container, unless otherwise specified by manufacturer.

**Auxiliary labeling**
• May cause drowsiness.
• Avoid alcoholic beverages.

### HYDROXYZINE PAMOATE ORAL SUSPENSION USP

**Usual adult and adolescent dose**
See *Hydroxyzine Pamoate Capsules USP*.

**Usual pediatric dose**
Antianxiety agent or
Sedative-hypnotic—
  Oral, 600 mcg (0.6 mg) per kg of body weight as a single dose.
Antihistaminic (H$_1$-receptor) or
Antiemetic—
  Oral, 500 mcg (0.5 mg) per kg of body weight or 15 mg per square meter of body surface every six hours as needed; or for
  Children up to 6 years of age: Oral, 12.5 mg every six hours as needed.
  Children 6 years of age and over: Oral, 12.5 to 25 mg every six hours as needed.

**Usual geriatric dose**
See *Hydroxyzine Pamoate Capsules USP*.
Note: Geriatric patients may be more sensitive to the effects of the usual adult dose.

**Strength(s) usually available**
U.S.—
  The equivalent of hydroxyzine hydrochloride:
    25 mg per 5 mL (Rx) [*Vistaril*].
Canada—
  Not commercially available.

**Packaging and storage**
Store below 40 °C (104 °F), preferably between 15 and 30 °C (59 and 86 °F), unless otherwise specified by manufacturer. Store in a tight, light-resistant container. Protect from freezing.

**Auxiliary labeling**
• Shake well.
• May cause drowsiness.
• Avoid alcoholic beverages.

## Parenteral Dosage Forms
### HYDROXYZINE HYDROCHLORIDE INJECTION USP

**Usual adult and adolescent dose**
Antianxiety agent—
  Intramuscular, 50 to 100 mg, repeated as needed every four to six hours.
Sedative-hypnotic—
  Intramuscular, 50 mg as a single dose.
  Adjunct to narcotic medication: Intramuscular, 25 to 100 mg.
Antiemetic—
  Intramuscular, 25 to 100 mg.

**Usual pediatric dose**
Adjunct to narcotic medication or
Antiemetic—
  Intramuscular, 1 mg per kg of body weight, or 30 mg per square meter of body surface, as a single dose.

**Usual geriatric dose**
See *Usual adult and adolescent dose*.
Note: Geriatric patients may be more sensitive to the effects of the usual adult dose.

**Strength(s) usually available**
U.S.—
  25 mg per mL (Rx) [*Vistaril;* GENERIC].
  50 mg per mL (Rx) [*Hyzine-50; Vistaril;* GENERIC].
Canada—
  50 mg per mL (Rx) [*Atarax* [GENERIC].

**Packaging and storage**
Store below 40 °C (104 °F), preferably between 15 and 30 °C (59 and 86 °F), unless otherwise specified by manufacturer. Protect from light. Protect from freezing.

---

## LORATADINE

## Summary of Differences
Indications:
  Used as treatment adjunct in asthma.
Pharmacology/pharmacokinetics:
  Chemical group—Piperidine derivative.
  Other actions/effects—No significant anticholinergic activity. Mild bronchodilator.
  Protein binding—97%.
  Half-life—3 to 20 hours.
  Onset of action—Histamine skin wheal studies—1 to 3 hours.
  Time to peak concentration—1 to 2 hours.
  Time to peak effect—Histamine skin wheal studies—8 to 12 hours.
  Duration of action—Histamine skin wheal studies—At least 24 hours.

Side/adverse effects:
  Anticholinergic effects not likely; dose-related sedation.

## Oral Dosage Forms
### LORATADINE SYRUP

**Usual adult and adolescent dose**
Antihistaminic (H$_1$-receptor)—Oral, 10 mg once a day.
Note: In patients with hepatic failure or decreased renal function (creatinine clearance < 30 mL per minute), the initial dose should be 10 mg every other day.

**Usual pediatric dose**
Antihistaminic (H$_1$-receptor)—
  Children 2 to 6 years of age: Oral, 5 mg once a day.
  Children 6 years of age and over: See *Usual adult and adolescent dose*.

**Usual geriatric dose**
See *Usual adult and adolescent dose*.

**Strength(s) usually available**
U.S.—
  5 mg per 5 mL (Rx) [*Claritin*].
Canada—
  5 mg per 5 mL (OTC) [*Claritin*].

**Packaging and storage**
Store between 2 and 30 °C (36 and 86 °F), in a well-closed container, unless otherwise specified by manufacturer.

### LORATADINE TABLETS

**Usual adult and adolescent dose**
See *Loratadine Syrup*.

**Usual pediatric dose**
See *Loratadine Syrup*.

**Usual geriatric dose**
See *Loratadine Syrup*.

**Strength(s) usually available**
U.S.—
  10 mg (Rx) [*Claritin* (scored); *Claritin RediTabs* (rapidly-disintegrating)].
Canada—
  10 mg (OTC) [*Claritin* (scored)].

**Packaging and storage**
Store below 40 °C (104 °F), preferably between 15 and 30 °C (59 and 86 °F), in a well-closed container, unless otherwise specified by manufacturer.

---

## PHENINDAMINE

## Summary of Differences
Pharmacology/pharmacokinetics:
  Chemical group—Piperidine derivative.
  Duration of action—4 to 6 hours.

## Oral Dosage Forms
### PHENINDAMINE TARTRATE TABLETS

**Usual adult and adolescent dose**
Antihistaminic (H$_1$-receptor)—
  Oral, 25 mg every four to six hours as needed.

**Usual adult prescribing limits**
Up to 150 mg daily.

**Usual pediatric dose**
Antihistaminic (H$_1$-receptor)—
  Children up to 6 years of age: Dosage must be individualized by physician.
  Children 6 to 12 years of age: Oral, 12.5 mg every four to six hours as needed, not to exceed 75 mg per day.
  Children 12 years of age and over: See *Usual adult and adolescent dose*.

**Usual geriatric dose**
See *Usual adult and adolescent dose*.
Note: Geriatric patients may be more sensitive to the effects of the usual adult dose.

**Strength(s) usually available**
U.S.—
  25 mg (OTC) [*Nolahist* (scored)].

## 342  Antihistamines (Systemic)

Canada—
  Not commercially available.

**Packaging and storage**
Store below 40 °C (104 °F), preferably between 15 and 30 °C (59 and 86 °F), in a well-closed container, unless otherwise specified by manufacturer.

**Auxiliary labeling**
- May cause drowsiness.
- Avoid alcoholic beverages.

---

### TERFENADINE

## Summary of Differences
Indications:
  Used as treatment adjunct in asthma.
Pharmacology/pharmacokinetics:
  Chemical group—Piperidine derivative.
  Other actions/effects—No significant anticholinergic activity. Mild bronchodilator.
  Protein binding—97%.
  Half-life—8.5 hours.
  Onset of action—Histamine skin wheal studies—1 to 2 hours.
  Time to peak concentration—2 hours.
  Time to peak effect—Histamine skin wheal studies—3 to 4 hours.
  Duration of action—Histamine skin wheal studies—Over 12 hours.
  Elimination—Primarily fecal.
Precautions:
  Pregnancy—Risk-benefit should be considered because of fetal abnormalities in studies in animals with doses above the human therapeutic range.
  Drug interactions and/or related problems—Possible cardiotoxic effects with erythromycin and other macrolide antibiotics, grapefruit juice, HIV protease inhibitors, itraconazole, ketoconazole, medications causing QT interval prolongation, mibefradil, serotonin reuptake inhibitors, or zileuton.
  Medical considerations/contraindications—Possible cardiotoxic effects with hepatic function impairment, history of QT interval prolongation, or with hypokalemia.
Side/adverse effects:
  Sedative and anticholinergic side effects less likely. Cardiac arrhythmias with high doses or overdose. May cause increased appetite and weight gain.

## Oral Dosage Forms
Note: Bracketed uses in the *Dosage Forms* section refer to categories of use and/or indications that are not included in U.S. product labeling.

### TERFENADINE ORAL SUSPENSION
**Usual adult and adolescent dose**
Antihistaminic ($H_1$-receptor)—
  Oral, 60 mg every twelve hours, [or 120 mg once a day], as needed.

**Usual pediatric dose**
Antihistaminic ($H_1$-receptor)—
  Children 3 to 7 years of age: Oral, 15 mg every twelve hours as needed.
  Children 7 to 12 years of age: Oral, 30 mg every twelve hours as needed.

Note: Premature and full-term neonates—Use is not recommended.

**Usual geriatric dose**
See *Usual adult and adolescent dose*.

Note: Geriatric patients may be more sensitive to the effects of the usual adult dose.

**Strength(s) usually available**
U.S.—
  Not commercially available.
Canada—
  6 mg per mL (OTC) [*Seldane*].

**Packaging and storage**
Store below 40 °C (104 °F), preferably between 15 and 30 °C (59 and 86 °F), unless otherwise specified by manufacturer. Store in a well-closed container, unless otherwise specified by manufacturer. Protect from freezing.

**Auxiliary labeling**
- Shake well.

### TERFENADINE TABLETS USP
**Usual adult and adolescent dose**
See *Terfenadine Oral Suspension*.

**Usual pediatric dose**
The available strength of the tablet does not conform to the recommended pediatric dosages for this age group. See *Terfenadine Oral Suspension*.

**Usual geriatric dose**
See *Terfenadine Oral Suspension*.

Note: Geriatric patients may be more sensitive to the effects of the usual adult dose.

**Strength(s) usually available**
U.S.—
  Not commercially available.
  Note: Withdrawn from the U.S. market by the Food and Drug Administration in February 1998.
Canada—
  60 mg (OTC) [*Apo-Terfenadine; Novo-Terfenadine; Seldane*].
  120 mg (OTC) [*Apo-Terfenadine; Seldane Caplets*].

**Packaging and storage**
Store below 40 °C (104 °F), preferably between 15 and 30 °C (59 and 86 °F), in a tight container, unless otherwise specified by manufacturer.

---

### TRIPELENNAMINE

## Summary of Differences
Pharmacology/pharmacokinetics:
  Chemical group—Ethylenediamine derivative.
  pKa—3.9 and 9.
  Duration of action—4 to 6 hours.
Side/adverse effects:
  Gastrointestinal effects more pronounced.

## Oral Dosage Forms

### TRIPELENNAMINE CITRATE ELIXIR USP
**Usual adult and adolescent dose**
Antihistaminic ($H_1$-receptor)—
  Oral, the equivalent of tripelennamine hydrochloride: 25 to 50 mg every four to six hours as needed.

**Usual adult prescribing limits**
Up to the equivalent of 600 mg of tripelennamine hydrochloride daily.

**Usual pediatric dose**
Antihistaminic ($H_1$-receptor)—
  Oral, the equivalent of tripelennamine hydrochloride, 1.25 mg per kg of body weight or 37.5 mg per square meter of body surface every six hours as needed, not to exceed 300 mg per day.

Note: Premature and full-term neonates—Use is not recommended.

**Usual geriatric dose**
See *Usual adult and adolescent dose*.

Note: Geriatric patients may be more sensitive to the effects of the usual adult dose.

**Strength(s) usually available**
U.S.—
  37.5 mg of tripelennamine citrate (equivalent to 25 mg of tripelennamine hydrochloride) per 5 mL (Rx) [*PBZ (alcohol 12%)*].
Canada—
  Not commercially available.

**Packaging and storage**
Store below 40 °C (104 °F), preferably between 15 and 30 °C (59 and 86 °F), unless otherwise specified by manufacturer. Store in a tight, light-resistant container. Protect from freezing.

**Auxiliary labeling**
- May cause drowsiness.
- Avoid alcoholic beverages.
- Keep container tightly closed.

### TRIPELENNAMINE HYDROCHLORIDE TABLETS USP
**Usual adult and adolescent dose**
Antihistaminic ($H_1$-receptor)—Oral, 25 to 50 mg every four to six hours as needed.

**Usual adult prescribing limits**
Up to 600 mg daily.

**Usual pediatric dose**
Antihistaminic ($H_1$-receptor)—Oral, 1.25 mg per kg of body weight or 37.5 mg per square meter of body surface every six hours as needed, not to exceed 300 mg per day.

Note: Premature and full-term neonates—Use is not recommended.

*USP DI*     Antihistamines (Systemic)   343

**Usual geriatric dose**
See *Usual adult and adolescent dose*.

Note: Geriatric patients may be more sensitive to the effects of the usual adult dose.

**Strength(s) usually available**
U.S.—
    25 mg (Rx) [*PBZ* (scored)].
    50 mg (Rx) [*PBZ* (scored); *Pelamine* (scored); GENERIC].
Canada—
    50 mg (OTC) [*Pyribenzamine* (scored)].

**Packaging and storage**
Store below 40 °C (104 °F), preferably between 15 and 30 °C (59 and 86 °F), unless otherwise specified by manufacturer. Store in a well-closed container.

**Auxiliary labeling**
- May cause drowsiness.
- Avoid alcoholic beverages.

## TRIPELENNAMINE HYDROCHLORIDE EXTENDED-RELEASE TABLETS

**Usual adult and adolescent dose**
Antihistaminic (H$_1$-receptor)—Oral, 100 mg every eight to twelve hours as needed.

**Usual adult prescribing limits**
Up to 600 mg daily.

**Usual pediatric dose**
Use is not recommended.

**Usual geriatric dose**
See *Usual adult and adolescent dose*.

Note: Geriatric patients may be more sensitive to the effects of the usual adult dose.

**Strength(s) usually available**
U.S.—
    100 mg (Rx) [*PBZ-SR*].
Canada—
    Not commercially available.

**Packaging and storage**
Store below 40 °C (104 °F), preferably between 15 and 30 °C (59 and 86 °F), in a well-closed container, unless otherwise specified by manufacturer. Protect from light.

**Auxiliary labeling**
- Swallow tablets whole.
- May cause drowsiness.
- Avoid alcoholic beverages.

Revised: 07/26/94
Interim revision: 07/10/96; 09/29/97; 12/31/97; 03/02/98; 07/29/98

# ANTIHISTAMINES AND DECONGESTANTS   Systemic

This monograph includes information on the following: 1) Acrivastine and Pseudoephedrine; 2) Azatadine and Pseudoephedrine; 3) Brompheniramine and Phenylephrine; 4) Brompheniramine, Phenylephrine, and Phenylpropanolamine; 5) Brompheniramine and Phenylpropanolamine; 6) Brompheniramine and Pseudoephedrine; 7) Carbinoxamine and Pseudoephedrine; 8) Chlorpheniramine, Phenindamine, and Phenylpropanolamine; 9) Chlorpheniramine and Phenylephrine; 10) Chlorpheniramine, Phenylephrine, and Phenylpropanolamine; 11) Chlorpheniramine and Phenylpropanolamine; 12) Chlorpheniramine, Phenyltoloxamine, and Phenylephrine; 13) Chlorpheniramine, Phenyltoloxamine, Phenylephrine, and Phenylpropanolamine; 14) Chlorpheniramine and Pseudoephedrine; 15) Chlorpheniramine, Pyrilamine, and Phenylephrine; 16) Chlorpheniramine, Pyrilamine, Phenylephrine, and Phenylpropanolamine; 17) Clemastine and Phenylpropanolamine; 18) Dexbrompheniramine and Pseudoephedrine; 19) Diphenhydramine and Pseudoephedrine; 20) Loratadine and Pseudoephedrine; 21) Pheniramine and Phenylephrine; 22) Pheniramine, Phenyltoloxamine, Pyrilamine, and Phenylpropanolamine; 23) Pheniramine, Pyrilamine, and Phenylpropanolamine; 24) Promethazine and Phenylephrine; 25) Terfenadine and Pseudoephedrine; 26) Triprolidine and Pseudoephedrine

Note: Products containing terfenadine and pseudoephedrine were withdrawn from the U.S. market by the Food and Drug Administration in February 1998.

INN: Chlorpheniramine—Chlorphenamine
VA CLASSIFICATION (Primary/Secondary) (Primary): RE501

**NOTE:** The *Antihistamines and Decongestants (Systemic)* monograph is maintained on the USP DI electronic data base. For a printed copy of the most recent revision of the complete monograph, contact Micromedex, Inc. - Reprint Requests, 6200 S. Syracuse Way, Suite 300, Englewood, CO 80111; telephone (303) 486-6400; telefax (303) 486-6464; Email: USPDI@MDX.COM.

For information on the specific components of this combination, see the *USP DI* monographs for *Antihistamines (Systemic)*, *Phenylephrine (Systemic)*, *Phenylpropanolamine (Systemic)*, and *Pseudoephedrine (Systemic)*, and *Sympathominetic Agents—Cardiovascular Use (Systemic)*.

The information that follows is selectively abstracted from the complete monograph and is provided to facilitate drug use review and patient counseling.

Note: For a listing of dosage forms and brand names by country availability, see *Dosage Forms* section(s).

## Category
Antihistaminic (H$_1$-receptor)-decongestant.

## Indications

**Accepted**
Congestion, nasal (treatment);
Sneezing (treatment); and
Rhinorrhea (treatment)—Antihistamine and decongestant combinations are indicated for the temporary relief of nasal and sinus congestion, sneezing, and rhinorrhea associated with the common cold and allergic rhinitis.

The therapeutic effectiveness of oral phenylephrine as a nasal decongestant has been questioned, especially at the usual oral dose.

## Patient Consultation
As an aid to patient consultation, refer to *Advice for the Patient, Antihistamines and Decongestants (Systemic)*.

In providing consultation, consider emphasizing the following selected information (» = major clinical significance):

**Before using this medication**
» Conditions affecting use, especially:
    Sensitivity to any of the antihistamines or sympathomimetic amines
    Pregnancy—Concern for the fetus and/or newborn infant only with high doses and long-term therapy; psychiatric disorders more likely with use of phenylpropanolamine in postpartum women
    Breast-feeding—Antihistamines may cause excitement or irritability in nursing infants; high risk for infants from sympathomimetic amines
    Use in children—Increased susceptibility to anticholinergic effects of antihistamines and to vasopressor effects of sympathomimetic amines; psychiatric disorders more likely with use of phenylpropanolamine in children under 6 years of age; hyperexcitability (paradoxical reaction) may occur
    Use in the elderly—Anticholinergic and CNS stimulant effects more likely to occur
    Contraindicated medications (with the terfenadine-containing combination only)—Erythromycin and other macrolide antibiotics, itraconazole, ketoconazole, and mibefradil
    Other medications, especially anticholinergics; CNS depressants or stimulants; cisapride (with the terfenadine-containing combination only); HIV protease inhibitors (with the terfenadine-containing combination only); medicine for high blood pressure or depression; serotonin reuptake inhibitors (with the terfenadine-containing combination only); sparfloxacin (with the terfenadine-containing combination only); or zileuton (with the terfenadine-containing combination only)

Other medical problems, especially cardiovascular disease, diabetes, hepatic function impairment, hypertension, hyperthyroidism, prostatic hypertrophy, or renal function impairment

**Proper use of this medication**
» Importance of not taking more medication than the amount recommended
  Taking with food, water, or milk to minimize gastric irritation
  Swallowing extended-release dosage form whole
» Proper dosing
  Missed dose: If on scheduled dosing regimen—Taking as soon as possible; not taking if almost time for next dose; not doubling doses
» Proper storage

**Precautions while using this medication**
  Caution if skin tests using allergens required; possible interference with test results
  May mask ototoxic effects of large doses of salicylates
» Not taking erythromycin or other macrolide antibiotics, itraconazole, ketoconazole, or mibefradil while taking the terfenadine-containing combination
» Avoiding use of alcohol or other CNS depressants
» Caution if drowsiness or dizziness occurs

» Caution if taking phenylpropanolamine-containing appetite suppressants
» Possible insomnia; taking the medication a few hours before bedtime
  Possible dryness of mouth; using sugarless gum or candy, ice, or saliva substitute for relief; checking with dentist if dry mouth continues for more than 2 weeks.
» Not taking terfenadine-containing combination with grapefruit juice

*For promethazine*
  Possible interference with diagnosis of intestinal obstruction, brain tumor, or overdosage of toxic drugs; need to inform physician of use

**Side/adverse effects**
  Signs of potential side effects, especially blood dyscrasias, cardiac arrhythmias, psychotic episodes, and tightness in chest

## Oral Dosage Forms

See *Table 1*, page 344.

---

Revised: 07/19/94
Interim revision: 07/25/95; 08/28/96; 09/29/97; 12/29/97; 08/13/98

## Table 1. Oral Dosage Forms

Note: Content per capsule, tablet, or 5 mL, unless otherwise stated.

| Brand or generic name [availability] | Antihistamines | Decongestants | Other content information as per product label | Usual adult and adolescent dose* prn | Usual pediatric dose prn | Packaging, storage, and auxiliary labeling† |
|---|---|---|---|---|---|---|
| *Actagen* Syrup USP (OTC) [U.S.] | Triprolidine HCl 1.25 mg | Pseudoephedrine HCl 30 mg | | 10 mL q 4–6 hr (max 40 mL/day) | 6–12 yrs: 5 mL q 4–6 hr | b, e, f, g |
| Tablets USP (OTC) [U.S.] | Triprolidine HCl 2.5 mg | Pseudoephedrine HCl 60 mg | | 1 tab q 4–6 hr (max 4 tabs/day) | | b, f |
| *Actifed* Syrup USP (OTC) [Canada] | Triprolidine HCl 1.25 mg | Pseudoephedrine HCl 30 mg | Alcohol free | 10 mL q 4–6 hr (max 4 doses/day) | 4 mos–2 yrs: 1.25 mL, 2–4 yrs: 2.5 mL, 4–6 yrs: 3.75 mL, 6–12 yrs: 5 mL, q 4–6 hr (max 4 doses/day) | b, e, f, g |
| Tablets USP (OTC) [U.S./Canada] | Triprolidine HCl 2.5 mg | Pseudoephedrine HCl 60 mg | | 1 tab q 4–6 hr (max 4 tabs/day) | 6–12 yrs: ½ tab q 4–6 hr (max 4 doses/day) | b, f, g |
| *Actifed Allergy Nighttime Caplets* Tablets (OTC) [U.S.] | Diphenhydramine HCl 25 mg | Pseudoephedrine HCl 30 mg | Available in a dual package that also contains *Actifed Allergy Daytime Caplets* | 2 tabs hs, or 2 tabs q 4–6 hr (max 8 total Day and Nighttime tabs/day) | Not recommended | b, f, g |
| *Alcomed* Oral Solution (OTC) [U.S.] | Brompheniramine maleate 2 mg | Phenylpropanolamine HCl 12.5 mg | Alcohol free Dye free Sugar free | 10 mL q 4 hr (max 60 mL/day) | 6–12 yrs: 5 mL q 4 hr (max 30 mL/day) | b, g |
| *Alcomed 2-60* Tablets (OTC) [U.S.] | Dexbrompheniramine maleate 2 mg | Pseudoephedrine HCl 60 mg | Dye free | 1 tab q 4–6 hr (max 4 tabs/day) | 6–12 yrs: ½ tab 4–6 hr (max 2 tabs/day) | b, g |
| *Allent* Extended-release Capsules (Rx) [U.S.] | Brompheniramine maleate 12 mg | Pseudoephedrine HCl 120 mg | Dye free | 1 cap q 12 hr | | a, g |
| *Allercon* Tablets USP (OTC) [U.S.] | Triprolidine HCl 2.5 mg | Pseudoephedrine HCl 60 mg | | 1 tab q 4–6 hr (max 4 tabs/day) | | b, f, g |
| *Allerest Maximum Strength* Tablets (OTC) [U.S.] | Chlorpheniramine maleate 2 mg | Pseudoephedrine HCl 30 mg | | 2 tabs q 4–6 hr (max 8 tabs/day) | 6–12 yrs: 1 tab q 4–6 hr (max 4 tabs/day) | a |
| *Allerfrim* Syrup USP (OTC) [U.S.] | Triprolidine HCl 1.25 mg | Pseudoephedrine HCl 30 mg | | 10 mL q 4–6 hr (max 40 mL/day) | | b, e, f, g |
| Tablets USP (OTC) [U.S.] | Triprolidine HCl 2.5 mg | Pseudoephedrine HCl 60 mg | Scored | 1 tab q 4–6 hr (max 4 tabs/day) | | a, f, g |

## Table 1. Oral Dosage Forms *(continued)*

Note: Content per capsule, tablet, or 5 mL, unless otherwise stated.

| Brand or generic name [availability] | Antihistamines | Decongestants | Other content information as per product label | Usual adult and adolescent dose* prn | Usual pediatric dose prn | Packaging, storage, and auxiliary labeling† |
|---|---|---|---|---|---|---|
| *Allerphed* Syrup USP (OTC) [U.S.] | Triprolidine HCl 1.25 mg | Pseudoephedrine HCl 30 mg | | 10 mL q 4–6 hr (max 40 mL/day) | 6–12 yrs: 5 mL q 4–6 hr | b, e, f, g |
| *Amilon* Extended-release Tablets (Rx) [U.S.] | Chlorpheniramine maleate 4 mg, Phenindamine tartrate 24 mg | Phenylpropanolamine HCl 50 mg | | 1 tab q 8 hr (mild cases q 10–12 hr) | | b, f, g |
| *Anamine* Syrup (Rx) [U.S.] | Chlorpheniramine maleate 2 mg | Pseudoephedrine HCl 30 mg | Alcohol free Sugar free Dye free | 10 mL q 4–6 hr | | a, e, g |
| *Anamine T.D.* Extended-release Capsules (Rx) [U.S.] | Chlorpheniramine maleate 8 mg | Pseudoephedrine HCl 120 mg | | 1 cap q 8–12 hr | | a, g |
| *Andec* Tablets (Rx) [U.S.] | Carbinoxamine maleate 4 mg | Pseudoephedrine HCl 60 mg | | 1 tab q 6 hr | >6 yrs: 1 tab 6 hr | a, g |
| *Andec-TR* Extended-release Tablets (Rx) [U.S.] | Carbinoxamine maleate 8 mg | Pseudoephedrine HCl 120 mg | | 1 tab q 12 hr | | a, g |
| *Aprodrine* Syrup USP (OTC) [U.S.] | Triprolidine HCl 1.25 mg | Pseudoephedrine HCl 30 mg | | 10 mL q 4–6 hr (max 40 mL/day) | 6–12 yrs: 5 mL q 4–6 hr | b, e, f, g |
| Tablets USP (OTC) [U.S.] | Triprolidine HCl 2.5 mg | Pseudoephedrine HCl 60 mg | Scored | 1 tab q 4–6 hr (max 4 tabs/day) | 6–12 yrs: ½ tab q 4–6 hr | b, f, g |
| *A.R.M. Maximum Strength Caplets* Tablets (OTC) [U.S.] | Chlorpheniramine maleate 4 mg | Phenylpropanolamine HCl 25 mg | | 1 tab q 4–6 hr | 6–12 yrs: ½ tab q 4–6 hr | b, g |
| *Atrofed* Tablets USP (OTC) [U.S.] | Triprolidine HCl 2.5 mg | Pseudoephedrine HCl 60 mg | | 1 tab q 4–6 hr | 6–12 yrs: ½ tab q 4–6 hr | b, f, g |
| *Atrohist Pediatric* Extended-release Capsules (Rx) [U.S.] | Chlorpheniramine maleate 4 mg | Pseudoephedrine HCl 60 mg | | 2 caps q 12 hr | 6–12 yrs: 1 cap q 12 hr | b, g |
| *Atrohist Pediatric Suspension Dye Free* Oral Suspension (Rx) [U.S.] | Chlorpheniramine tannate 2 mg, Pyrilamine tannate 12.5 mg | Phenylephrine tannate 5 mg | | Intended for pediatric use | 2–6 yrs: 2.5–5 mL, 6–12 yrs: 5–10 mL, q 12 hr | a, e, g, i |
| *Banophen* Capsules USP (OTC) [U.S.] | Diphenhydramine HCl 25 mg | Pseudoephedrine HCl 60 mg | | 1 cap q 4–6 hr (max 4 caps/day) | | b, g |

*Geriatric patients may be more sensitive to the effects of the usual adult dose.

†For appropriate *Packaging and storage* and *Auxiliary labeling* information refer to designated letters as follows:

   a—Store below 40 °C (104 °F), preferably between 15 and 30 °C (59 and 86 °F), in a tight container, unless otherwise specified by manufacturer.
   b—Store between 15 and 30 °C (59 and 86 °F), in a tight container, unless otherwise specified by manufacturer.
   c—Store between 2 and 30 °C (36 and 86 °F), in a tight container, unless otherwise specified by manufacturer.
   d—Store below 25 °C (77 °F), in a tight container, unless otherwise specified by manufacturer.
   e—Protect from freezing.
   f—Protect from light.
   g—Auxiliary labeling:
      May cause drowsiness.
      Avoid alcoholic beverages.
   h—Auxiliary labeling: • May be chewed.
   i—Auxiliary labeling: • Shake well.
   j—Color may change over time from pink to peach. This does not reflect any change in quality or potency of tablets.

## Table 1. Oral Dosage Forms (continued)

Note: Content per capsule, tablet, or 5 mL, unless otherwise stated.

| Brand or generic name [availability] | Antihistamines | Decongestants | Other content information as per product label | Usual adult and adolescent dose* prn | Usual pediatric dose prn | Packaging, storage, and auxiliary labeling† |
|---|---|---|---|---|---|---|
| *Benadryl Allergy Decongestant Liquid Medication* Oral Solution (OTC) [U.S.] | Diphenhydramine HCl 12.5 mg | Pseudoephedrine HCl 30 mg | Alcohol free Sugar free | 10 mL q 4–6 hr (max 40 mL/day) | 6–12 yrs: 5 mL q 4–6 hr (max 20 mL/day) | c, e, g |
| Tablets (OTC) [U.S./Canada] | Diphenhydramine HCl 25 mg | Pseudoephedrine HCl 60 mg | | 1 tab q 4–6 hr (max 4 tabs/day) | | b, g |
| *Biohist-LA* Extended-release Tablets (Rx) [U.S.] | Carbinoxamine maleate 8 mg | Pseudoephedrine HCl 120 mg | Dye free Lactose Scored | 1 tab q 12 hr | | a, g |
| *Brexin L.A.* Extended-release Capsules (Rx) [U.S.] | Chlorpheniramine maleate 8 mg | Pseudoephedrine HCl 120 mg | | 1 cap q 12 hr | | b, g |
| *Brofed Liquid* Oral Solution (Rx) [U.S.] | Brompheniramine maleate 4 mg | Pseudoephedrine HCl 30 mg | | 10 mL q 8 hr (max 3 doses/day) | 2–6 yrs: 2.5 mL, 6–12 yrs: 5 mL, q 8 hr (max 3 doses/day) | a, e, f, g |
| *Bromadrine PD* Extended-release Capsules (Rx) [U.S.] | Brompheniramine maleate 6 mg | Pseudoephedrine HCl 60 mg | | 1–2 caps q 12 hr | 6–12 yrs: 1 cap q 12 hr | b, g |
| *Bromadrine TR* Extended-release Capsules (Rx) [U.S.] | Brompheniramine maleate 12 mg | Pseudoephedrine HCl 120 mg | | 1 cap q 12 hr | | b, g |
| *Bromaline* Elixir (OTC) [U.S.] | Brompheniramine maleate 2 mg | Phenylpropanolamine HCl 12.5 mg | Alcohol 2.3% | 10 mL q 4–6 hr | | a, e, g |
| *Bromanate* Elixir (OTC) [U.S.] | Brompheniramine maleate 2 mg | Phenylpropanolamine HCl 12.5 mg | Alcohol free Sugar free | 10 mL q 4–6 hr | | a, e, g |
| *Bromatapp* Extended-release Tablets (Rx) (OTC) [U.S.] | Brompheniramine maleate 12 mg | Phenylpropanolamine HCl 75 mg | | 1 tab q 12 hr | | a, g |
| *Bromfed* Extended-release Capsules (Rx) [U.S.] | Brompheniramine maleate 12 mg | Pseudoephedrine HCl 120 mg | | 1 cap q 12 hr | | a, g |
| Syrup (OTC) [U.S.] | Brompheniramine maleate 2 mg | Pseudoephedrine HCl 30 mg | Alcohol free | 10 mL q 4–6 hr (max 40 mL/day) | 6–12 yrs: 5 mL q 4–6 hr (max 20 mL/day) | b, e, f, g |
| Tablets (Rx) [U.S.] | Brompheniramine maleate 4 mg | Pseudoephedrine HCl 60 mg | Scored | 1 tab q 4 hr (max 6 tabs/day) | 6–12 yrs: ½ tab 4 hr (max 3 tabs/day) | a, g |
| *Bromfed-PD* Extended-release Capsules (Rx) [U.S.] | Brompheniramine maleate 6 mg | Pseudoephedrine HCl 60 mg | | 1–2 caps q 12 hr | 6–12 yrs: 1 cap q 12 hr | b, g |
| *Bromfenex* Extended-release Capsules (Rx) [U.S.] | Brompheniramine maleate 12 mg | Pseudoephedrine HCl 120 mg | | 1 cap q 12 hr | | a, g |
| *Bromfenex PD* Extended-release Capsules (Rx) [U.S.] | Brompheniramine maleate 6 mg | Pseudoephedrine HCl 60 mg | | 1–2 caps q 12 hr | 6–12 yrs: 1 cap q 12 hr | a, g |
| *Bromophen T.D.* Extended-release Tablets (Rx) [U.S.] | Brompheniramine maleate 12 mg | Phenylephrine HCl 15 mg, Phenylpropanolamine HCl 15 mg | Sugar coated | 1 tab q 8–12 hr | | b, f, g |
| Brompheniramine Maleate and Phenylpropanolamine HCl Elixir (OTC) [U.S.] | Brompheniramine maleate 2 mg | Phenylpropanolamine HCl 12.5 mg | | 10 mL q 4–6 hr | | a, e, g |

## Table 1. Oral Dosage Forms (continued)

Note: Content per capsule, tablet, or 5 mL, unless otherwise stated.

| Brand or generic name [availability] | Antihistamines | Decongestants | Other content information as per product label | Usual adult and adolescent dose* prn | Usual pediatric dose prn | Packaging, storage, and auxiliary labeling† |
|---|---|---|---|---|---|---|
| Brompheniramine Maleate and Pseudoephedrine HCl Extended-release Capsules (Rx) [U.S.] | Brompheniramine maleate 6 mg | Pseudoephedrine HCl 60 mg | | 1–2 caps q 12 hr | 6–12 yrs: 1 cap q 12 hr | a, g |
| | Brompheniramine maleate 12 mg | Pseudoephedrine HCl 120 mg | | 1 cap q 12 hr | | a, g |
| Syrup (Rx) [U.S.] | Brompheniramine maleate 2 mg | Pseudoephedrine HCl 30 mg | | 10 mL q 4–6 hr | 6–12 yrs: 5 mL q 4–6 hr | b, e, f, g |
| *Brompheril* Extended-release Tablets (OTC) [U.S.] | Dexbrompheniramine maleate 6 mg | Pseudoephedrine sulfate 120 mg | | 1 tab q 12 hr | | a, g |
| *Carbiset* Tablets (Rx) [U.S.] | Carbinoxamine maleate 4 mg | Pseudoephedrine HCl 60 mg | Dye free | 1 tab q 6 hr | 6–12 yrs: 1 tab q 6 hr | a, g |
| *Carbiset-TR* Extended-release Tablets (Rx) [U.S.] | Carbinoxamine maleate 8 mg | Pseudoephedrine HCl 120 mg | Dye free | 1 tab q 12 hr | | a, g |
| *Carbodec* Syrup (Rx) [U.S.] | Carbinoxamine maleate 4 mg | Pseudoephedrine HCl 60 mg | | 5 mL q 6 hr | 18 mos–6 yrs: 2.5 mL, 6–12 yrs: 5 mL, q 6 hr | a, e, g |
| Tablets (Rx) [U.S.] | Carbinoxamine maleate 4 mg | Pseudoephedrine HCl 60 mg | | 1 tab q 6 hr | | a, g |
| *Carbodec TR* Extended-release Tablets (Rx) [U.S.] | Carbinoxamine maleate 8 mg | Pseudoephedrine HCl 120 mg | Film coated | 1 tab q 12 hr | | a, g |
| *Cardec* Syrup (Rx) [U.S.] | Carbinoxamine maleate 4 mg | Pseudoephedrine HCl 60 mg | | 5 mL q 6 hr | 18 mos–6 yrs: 2.5 mL, 6–12 yrs: 5 mL, q 6 hr | a, e, g |
| Tablets (Rx) [U.S.] | Carbinoxamine maleate 4 mg | Pseudoephedrine HCl 60 mg | | 1 tab q 6 hr | 6–12 yrs: 1 tab 6 hr | a, g |
| Extended-release Tablets (Rx) [U.S.] | Carbinoxamine maleate 8 mg | Pseudoephedrine HCl 120 mg | | 1 tab q 12 hr | | a, g |
| *Cardec-S* Syrup (Rx) [U.S.] | Carbinoxamine maleate 4 mg | Pseudoephedrine HCl 60 mg | | 5 mL q 6 hr | 18 mos–6 yrs: 2.5 mL, 6–12 yrs: 5 mL, q 6 hr | a, e, g |
| *Cenafed Plus* Tablets USP (OTC) [U.S.] | Triprolidine HCl 2.5 mg | Pseudoephedrine HCl 60 mg | | 1 tab q 4–6 hr (max 4 tabs/day) | | b, f, g |
| *Chemdec* Oral Solution (Rx) [U.S.] | Carbinoxamine maleate 4 mg | Pseudoephedrine HCl 60 mg | Alcohol free Sugar free | 5 mL q 6 hr | 18 mos–6 yrs: 2.5 mL, 6–12 yrs: 5 mL, q 6 hr | a, e, g |
| *C-Hist-SR* Extended-release Capsules (Rx) [U.S.] | Chlorpheniramine maleate 4 mg, Phenyltoloxamine citrate 50 mg | Phenylephrine HCl 20 mg | | 1 cap q 8–12 hr | | a, g |

*Geriatric patients may be more sensitive to the effects of the usual adult dose.

†For appropriate *Packaging and storage* and *Auxiliary labeling* information refer to designated letters as follows:
 a—Store below 40 °C (104 °F), preferably between 15 and 30 °C (59 and 86 °F), in a tight container, unless otherwise specified by manufacturer.
 b—Store between 15 and 30 °C (59 and 86 °F), in a tight container, unless otherwise specified by manufacturer.
 c—Store between 2 and 30 °C (36 and 86 °F), in a tight container, unless otherwise specified by manufacturer.
 d—Store below 25 °C (77 °F), in a tight container, unless otherwise specified by manufacturer.
 e—Protect from freezing.
 f—Protect from light.
 g—Auxiliary labeling:
  May cause drowsiness.
  Avoid alcoholic beverages.
 h—Auxiliary labeling: • May be chewed.
 i—Auxiliary labeling: • Shake well.
 j—Color may change over time from pink to peach. This does not reflect any change in quality or potency of tablets.

## Table 1. Oral Dosage Forms (continued)

Note: Content per capsule, tablet, or 5 mL, unless otherwise stated.

| Brand or generic name [availability] | Antihistamines | Decongestants | Other content information as per product label | Usual adult and adolescent dose* prn | Usual pediatric dose prn | Packaging, storage, and auxiliary labeling† |
|---|---|---|---|---|---|---|
| *Chlorafed* Oral Solution (OTC) [U.S.] | Chlorpheniramine maleate 2 mg | Pseudoephedrine HCl 30 mg | Alcohol free Sugar free Dye free | 10 mL q 4–6 hr (max 40 mL/day) | | a, e, g |
| *Chlorafed H.S. Timecelles* Extended-release Capsules (Rx) [U.S.] | Chlorpheniramine maleate 4 mg | Pseudoephedrine HCl 60 mg | Dye free | 2 caps q 12 hr | | a, g |
| *Chlorafed Timecelles* Extended-release Capsules (Rx) [U.S.] | Chlorpheniramine maleate 8 mg | Pseudoephedrine HCl 120 mg | Dye free | 1 cap q 12 hr | | a, g |
| *Chlordrine S.R.* Extended-release Capsules (Rx) [U.S.] | Chlorpheniramine maleate 8 mg | Pseudoephedrine HCl 120 mg | | 1 cap q 12 hr | | a, g |
| *Chlorfed* Extended-release Capsules (Rx) [U.S.] | Chlorpheniramine maleate 8 mg | Pseudoephedrine HCl 120 mg | | 1 cap q 12 hr | | a, g |
| *Chlorfed II* Tablets (Rx) [U.S.] | Chlorpheniramine maleate 4 mg | Pseudoephedrine HCl 60 mg | | 1 tab q 4–6 hr | | a, g |
| *Chlorphedrine SR* Extended-release Capsules (Rx) [U.S.] | Chlorpheniramine maleate 8 mg | Pseudoephedrine HCl 120 mg | | 1 cap q 12 hr | | a, g |
| Chlorpheniramine Maleate and Phenyl-propanolamine HCl Extended-release Capsules (Rx) [U.S.] | Chlorpheniramine maleate 12 mg | Phenylpropanolamine HCl 75 mg | | 1 cap q 12 hr | | a, g |
| Chlorpheniramine Maleate and Pseudoephedrine HCl Extended-release Capsules (Rx) [U.S.] | Chlorpheniramine maleate 8 mg | Pseudoephedrine HCl 120 mg | | 1 cap q 12 hr | | a, g |
| *Chlor-Rest* Tablets (OTC) [U.S.] | Chlorpheniramine maleate 2 mg | Phenylpropanolamine HCl 18.7 mg | | 2 tabs q 4 hr (max 8 tabs/day) | | a, g |
| *Chlortox* Extended-release Capsules (Rx) [U.S.] | Chlorpheniramine maleate 4 mg, Phenyltoloxamine citrate 50 mg | Phenylephrine HCl 20 mg | | 1 cap q 8–12 hr | | a, g |
| *Chlor-Trimeton 4 Hour Relief* Tablets (OTC) [U.S.] | Chlorpheniramine maleate 4 mg | Pseudoephedrine sulfate 60 mg | Lactose | 1 tab q 4–6 hr (max 4 tabs/day) | 6–12 yrs: ½ tab q 4–6 hr (max 2 tabs/day) | c, g |
| *Chlor-Trimeton 12 Hour Relief* Extended-release Tablets (OTC) [U.S.] | Chlorpheniramine maleate 8 mg | Pseudoephedrine sulfate 120 mg | Lactose | 1 tab q 12 hr (max 2 tabs/day) | | c, g |
| *Chlor-Trimeton Allergy-D 12 Hour* Extended-release Tablets (OTC) [U.S.] | Chlorpheniramine maleate 8 mg | Pseudoephedrine sulfate 120 mg | Lactose | 1 tab q 12 hr (max 2 tabs/day) | | c, g |
| *Chlor-Tripolon Decongestant* Syrup (OTC) [Canada] | Chlorpheniramine maleate 2 mg | Phenylpropanolamine HCl 12.5 mg | Alcohol 7%, Tartrazine free | 5–10 mL q 6–8 hr | 6–12 yrs: 2.5–5 mL q 6–8 hr | a, e, g |

## Table 1. Oral Dosage Forms (continued)

Note: Content per capsule, tablet, or 5 mL, unless otherwise stated.

| Brand or generic name [availability] | Antihistamines | Decongestants | Other content information as per product label | Usual adult and adolescent dose* prn | Usual pediatric dose prn | Packaging, storage, and auxiliary labeling† |
|---|---|---|---|---|---|---|
| *Chlor-Tripolon N.D.* Extended-release Tablets (OTC) [Canada] | Loratadine 5 mg | Pseudoephedrine sulfate 120 mg | Tartrazine free | 1 tab q 12 hr | | d |
| *Claritin-D 12 Hour* Extended-release Tablets (Rx) [U.S.] | Loratadine 5 mg | Pseudoephedrine sulfate 120 mg | | 1 tab q 12 hr (In renal function impairment [creatinine clearance <30 mL/min]: 1 tab q 24 hr) | | d |
| *Claritin-D 24 Hour* Extended-release Tablets (Rx) [U.S.] | Loratadine 10 mg | Pseudoephedrine sulfate 240 mg | | 1 tab q 24 hr (In renal function impairment [creatinine clearance <30 mL/min]: 1 tab q 48 hr) | | d |
| *Claritin Extra* Extended-release Tablets (OTC) [Canada] | Loratadine 5 mg | Pseudoephedrine sulfate 120 mg | | 1 tab q 12 hr | | a |
| *Codimal–L.A.* Extended-release Capsules (Rx) [U.S.] | Chlorpheniramine maleate 8 mg | Pseudoephedrine HCl 120 mg | | 1 cap q 12 hr | | a, g |
| *Codimal–L.A. Half* Extended-release Capsules (Rx) [U.S.] | Chlorpheniramine maleate 4 mg | Pseudoephedrine HCl 60 mg | | 2 caps q 12 hr | 6–12 yrs: 1 cap q 12 hr | a, g |
| *Cold and Allergy* Elixir (OTC) [U.S.] | Brompheniramine maleate 2 mg | Phenylpropanolamine HCl 12.5 mg | Alcohol free | 10 mL q 4–6 hr (max 60 mL/day) | 6–12 yrs: 5 mL, q 4–6 hr (max 30 mL/day) | b, e, g |
| *Cold-Gest Cold* Extended-release Capsules (OTC) [U.S.] | Chlorpheniramine maleate 8 mg | Phenylpropanolamine HCl 75 mg | | 1 cap q 12 hr | | a, g |
| *Colfed-A* Extended-release Capsules (Rx) [U.S.] | Chlorpheniramine maleate 8 mg | Pseudoephedrine HCl 120 mg | | 1 cap q 12 hr | | a, g |
| *Comhist* Tablets (Rx) [U.S.] | Chlorpheniramine maleate 2 mg, Phenyltoloxamine citrate 25 mg | Phenylephrine HCl 10 mg | Scored | 1–2 tabs q 8 hr | | a, g |
| *Comhist LA* Extended-release Capsules (Rx) [U.S.] | Chlorpheniramine maleate 4 mg, Phenyltoloxamine citrate 50 mg | Phenylephrine HCl 20 mg | | 1 cap q 8–12 hr | Not recommended | a, g |

*Geriatric patients may be more sensitive to the effects of the usual adult dose.

†For appropriate *Packaging and storage* and *Auxiliary labeling* information refer to designated letters as follows:
   a—Store below 40 °C (104 °F), preferably between 15 and 30 °C (59 and 86 °F), in a tight container, unless otherwise specified by manufacturer.
   b—Store between 15 and 30 °C (59 and 86 °F), in a tight container, unless otherwise specified by manufacturer.
   c—Store between 2 and 30 °C (36 and 86 °F), in a tight container, unless otherwise specified by manufacturer.
   d—Store below 25 °C (77 °F), in a tight container, unless otherwise specified by manufacturer.
   e—Protect from freezing.
   f—Protect from light.
   g—Auxiliary labeling:
      May cause drowsiness.
      Avoid alcoholic beverages.
   h—Auxiliary labeling: • May be chewed.
   i—Auxiliary labeling: • Shake well.
   j—Color may change over time from pink to peach. This does not reflect any change in quality or potency of tablets.

## Table 1. Oral Dosage Forms (continued)

Note: Content per capsule, tablet, or 5 mL, unless otherwise stated.

| Brand or generic name [availability] | Antihistamines | Decongestants | Other content information as per product label | Usual adult and adolescent dose* prn | Usual pediatric dose prn | Packaging, storage, and auxiliary labeling† |
|---|---|---|---|---|---|---|
| *Contac 12-Hour* Extended-release Capsules (OTC) [U.S.] | Chlorpheniramine maleate 8 mg | Phenylpropanolamine HCl 75 mg | | 1 cap q 12 hr (max 2 caps/day) | | b, g |
| *Contac Maximum Strength 12-Hour Caplets* Extended-release Tablets (OTC) [U.S.] | Chlorpheniramine maleate 12 mg | Phenylpropanolamine HCl 75 mg | | 1 tab q 12 hr (max 2 tabs/day) | | b, g |
| *Cophene No. 2* Extended-release Capsules (Rx) [U.S.] | Chlorpheniramine maleate 12 mg | Pseudoephedrine HCl 120 mg | | 1 cap q 12 hr | | a, g |
| *Co-Pyronil 2* Capsules (OTC) [U.S.] | Chlorpheniramine maleate 4 mg | Pseudoephedrine HCl 60 mg | | 1 cap q 6 hr | | a, g |
| *Coricidin D Long Acting* Extended-release Tablets (OTC) [Canada] | Chlorpheniramine maleate 8 mg | Phenylpropanolamine HCl 50 mg | Tartrazine free | 1 tab q 12 hr | | a |
| *Corsym* Extended-release Oral Suspension (OTC) [Canada] | Equivalent of 4 mg of chlorpheniramine maleate (as polistirex) | Equivalent of 37.5 mg of phenylpropanolamine HCl (as polistirex) | Alcohol free Tartrazine free | 10 mL q 12 hr (max 20 mL/day) | 2–5 yrs: 2.5 mL, 6–12 yrs: 5 mL, q 12 hr (max 2 doses/day) | a, e, i |
| *CP Oral* Oral Solution (Rx) [U.S.] | Carbinoxamine maleate 2 mg/mL | Pseudoephedrine HCl 25 mg/mL | Intended for pediatric use | | 1–3 mos: ¼ mL, 3–6 mos: ½ mL, 6–9 mos: ¾ mL, 9–18 mos: 1 mL, q 6 hr | a, e |
| *Dallergy Jr.* Extended-release Capsules (Rx) [U.S.] | Brompheniramine maleate 6 mg | Pseudoephedrine HCl 60 mg | | 2 caps q 12 hr (max 2 doses/day) | 6–12 yrs: 1 cap q 12 hr (max 2 doses/day) | a, g |
| *Deconamine* Syrup (Rx) [U.S.] | Chlorpheniramine maleate 2 mg | Pseudoephedrine HCl 30 mg | Alcohol free Dye free | 5–10 mL q 6–8 hr | 2–6 yrs: 2.5 mL, 6–12 yrs: 2.5–5 mL, q 6–8 hr | b, g |
| Tablets (Rx) [U.S.] | Chlorpheniramine maleate 4 mg | Pseudoephedrine HCl 60 mg | Dye free Scored | 1 tab q 6–8 hr | Not recommended See *Deconamine Syrup* and *Chewable Tablets* | b, g |
| Chewable Tablets (Rx) [U.S.] | Chlorpheniramine maleate 1 mg | Pseudoephedrine HCl 15 mg | Dye free Scored | 2–4 tabs q 6–8 hr | 2–6 yrs: 1 tab, 6–12 yrs: 1–2 tabs, q 6–8 hr | b, g, h |
| *Deconamine SR* Extended-release Capsules (Rx) [U.S.] | Chlorpheniramine maleate 8 mg | Pseudoephedrine HCl 120 mg | | 1 cap q 12 hr | Not recommended See *Deconamine Syrup* and *Chewable Tablets* | b, g |
| *Decongestabs* Extended-release Tablets (Rx) [U.S.] | Chlorpheniramine maleate 5 mg, Phenyltoloxamine citrate 15 mg | Phenylephrine HCl 10 mg, Phenylpropanolamine HCl 40 mg | | 1 tab q 8 hr | | a, g |
| *Deconomed SR* Extended-release Capsules (Rx) [U.S.] | Chlorpheniramine maleate 8 mg | Pseudoephedrine HCl 120 mg | | 1 cap q 12 hr | | a, f, g |
| *Delhistine D* Elixir (Rx) [U.S.] | Pheniramine maleate 4 mg, Phenyltoloxamine citrate 4 mg, Pyrilamine maleate 4 mg | Phenylpropanolamine HCl 12.5 mg | Alcohol 4% | 10 mL q 4 hr | 2–6 yrs: 2.5 mL, 6–12 yrs: 5 mL, q 4 hr | a, e, f, g |

## Table 1. Oral Dosage Forms (continued)

Note: Content per capsule, tablet, or 5 mL, unless otherwise stated.

| Brand or generic name [availability] | Antihistamines | Decongestants | Other content information as per product label | Usual adult and adolescent dose* prn | Usual pediatric dose prn | Packaging, storage, and auxiliary labeling† |
|---|---|---|---|---|---|---|
| *Demazin* Syrup (OTC) [U.S.] | Chlorpheniramine maleate 2 mg | Phenylpropanolamine HCl 12.5 mg | | 10 mL q 4–6 hr (max 60 mL/day) | 6–11 yrs: 5 mL q 4–6 hr (max 30 mL/day) | b, g |
| *Demazin Repetabs* Extended-release Tablets (OTC) [U.S.] | Chlorpheniramine maleate 4 mg | Phenylpropanolamine HCl 25 mg | Sugar coated | 2 tabs q 8 hr (max 6 tabs/day) | 6–11 yrs: 1 tab 8 hr (max 3 tabs/day) | c, g |
| *Dexaphen SA* Extended-release Tablets (Rx) [U.S.] | Dexbrompheniramine maleate 6 mg | Pseudoephedrine sulfate 120 mg | | 1 tab q 12 hr | | a, g |
| *Dexophed* Extended-release Tablets (Rx) [U.S.] | Dexbrompheniramine maleate 6 mg | Pseudoephedrine sulfate 120 mg | | 1 tab q 12 hr | | a, g |
| *Dimaphen* Elixir (OTC) [U.S.] | Brompheniramine maleate 2 mg | Phenylpropanolamine HCl 12.5 mg | Alcohol 2.3% | 10 mL q 4 hr | | a, e, g |
| Tablets (OTC) [U.S.] | Brompheniramine maleate 4 mg | Phenylpropanolamine HCl 25 mg | | 1 tab q 4 hr | | a, g |
| *Dimaphen S.A.* Extended-release Tablets (OTC) [U.S.] | Brompheniramine maleate 12 mg | Phenylpropanolamine HCl 75 mg | | 1 tab q 12 hr | | a, g |
| *Dimetane Decongestant* Elixir (OTC) [U.S.] | Brompheniramine maleate 2 mg | Phenylephrine HCl 5 mg | Alcohol 2.3% Sorbitol | 10 mL q 4 hr | 6–12 yrs: 5 mL q 4 hr | a, e, g |
| *Dimetane Decongestant Caplets* Tablets (OTC) [U.S.] | Brompheniramine maleate 4 mg | Phenylephrine HCl 10 mg | Scored | 1 tab q 4 hr | 6–12 yrs: ½ tab 4 hr | b, g |
| *Dimetapp* Elixir (OTC) [U.S.] | Brompheniramine maleate 2 mg | Phenylpropanolamine HCl 12.5 mg | Alcohol free | 10 mL q 4 hr (max 60 mL/day) | 6–12 yrs: 5 mL q 4 hr (max 30 mL/day) | b, e, g |
| Elixir (OTC) [Canada] | Brompheniramine maleate 4 mg | Phenylephrine HCl 5 mg, Phenylpropanolamine HCl 5 mg | Alcohol 2.3% Sorbitol | 5–10 mL q 6–8 hr | 1–6 mos: 1.25 mL, 7–24 mos: 2.5 mL, 2–4 yrs: 3.75 mL, 4–12 yrs: 5 mL, q 6–8 hr | b, e, g |
| Tablets (OTC) [Canada] | Brompheniramine maleate 4 mg | Phenylephrine HCl 5 mg, Phenylpropanolamine HCl 5 mg | Scored | 1–2 tabs q 6–8 hr | 2–4 yrs: ½ tab, 4–12 yrs: 1 tab, q 6–8 hr | b, g |
| *Dimetapp Chewables* Chewable Tablets (OTC) [Canada] | Brompheniramine maleate 1 mg | Phenylpropanolamine HCl 6.25 mg | Scored | Intended for pediatric use | 2–6 yrs: 1 tab, 6–12 yrs: 2 tabs, q 4 hr | a, g, h |
| *Dimetapp Clear* Oral Solution (OTC) [Canada] | Brompheniramine maleate 2 mg | Phenylpropanolamine HCl 12.5 mg | Alcohol free Sorbitol | 10 mL q 4–6 hr (max 60 mL/day) | 2–6 yrs: 2.5 mL, 6–12 yrs: 5 mL, q 4–6 hr | b, e, g |
| *Dimetapp Cold and Allergy* Chewable Tablets (OTC) [U.S.] | Brompheniramine maleate 1 mg | Phenylpropanolamine HCl 6.25 mg | Phenylalanine 8 mg Scored | Intended for pediatric use | 6–12 yrs: 2 tabs q 4 hr (max 12 tabs/day) | a, g, h |

*Geriatric patients may be more sensitive to the effects of the usual adult dose.

†For appropriate *Packaging and storage* and *Auxiliary labeling* information refer to designated letters as follows:
  a—Store below 40 °C (104 °F), preferably between 15 and 30 °C (59 and 86 °F), in a tight container, unless otherwise specified by manufacturer.
  b—Store between 15 and 30 °C (59 and 86 °F), in a tight container, unless otherwise specified by manufacturer.
  c—Store between 2 and 30 °C (36 and 86 °F), in a tight container, unless otherwise specified by manufacturer.
  d—Store below 25 °C (77 °F), in a tight container, unless otherwise specified by manufacturer.
  e—Protect from freezing.
  f—Protect from light.
  g—Auxiliary labeling:
    May cause drowsiness.
    Avoid alcoholic beverages.
  h—Auxiliary labeling: • May be chewed.
  i—Auxiliary labeling: • Shake well.
  j—Color may change over time from pink to peach. This does not reflect any change in quality or potency of tablets.

## Table 1. Oral Dosage Forms (continued)

Note: Content per capsule, tablet, or 5 mL, unless otherwise stated.

| Brand or generic name [availability] | Antihistamines | Decongestants | Other content information as per product label | Usual adult and adolescent dose* prn | Usual pediatric dose prn | Packaging, storage, and auxiliary labeling† |
|---|---|---|---|---|---|---|
| *Dimetapp Cold & Allergy Quick Dissolve* Tablets (OTC) [U.S.] | Brompheniramine maleate 1 mg | Phenylpropanolamine HCl 6.25 mg | Phenylalanine 2.1 mg | Intended for pediatric use | 6–12 yrs: 2 tabs q 4 hr (max 6 doses/day) | a, g |
| *Dimetapp Extentabs* Extended-release Tablets (OTC) [U.S.] | Brompheniramine maleate 12 mg | Phenylpropanolamine HCl 75 mg | Sugar coated | 1 tab q 12 hr (max 2 tabs/day) | | b, g |
| Extended-release Tablets (OTC) [Canada] | Brompheniramine maleate 12 mg | Phenylephrine HCl 15 mg, Phenylpropanolamine HCl 15 mg | Sugar coated | 1 tab q 12 hr | | b, g |
| *Dimetapp 4-Hour* Tablets (OTC) [U.S.] | Brompheniramine maleate 4 mg | Phenylpropanolamine HCl 25 mg | | 1 tab q 4 hr (max 6 doses/day) | 6–12 yrs: 1/2 tab 4 hr (max 6 doses/day) | a, g |
| *Dimetapp Liqui-Fills* Capsules (OTC) [Canada] | Brompheniramine maleate 4 mg | Phenylpropanolamine HCl 25 mg | | 1 cap q 4 hr (max 6 caps/day) | Not recommended | a, g |
| *Dimetapp Oral Infant Drops* Oral Solution (OTC) [Canada] | Brompheniramine maleate 2 mg/mL | Phenylephrine HCl 2.5 mg/mL, Phenylpropanolamine HCl 2.5 mg/mL | Alcohol 2.3% | Intended for pediatric use | 5 kg: 0.5 mL, 7.5 kg: 0.75 mL, 10 kg: 1 mL, >10 kg: 1.5 mL, q 6–8 hr | b, e, g |
| *Disobrom* Extended-release Tablets (Rx) [U.S.] | Dexbrompheniramine maleate 6 mg | Pseudoephedrine sulfate 120 mg | | 1 tab q 12 hr | | a, g |
| *Disophrol Chronotabs* Extended-release Tablets (OTC) [U.S.] | Dexbrompheniramine maleate 6 mg | Pseudoephedrine sulfate 120 mg | Sugar coated | 1 tab q 12 hr (max 2 tabs/day) | | c, g |
| *Dorcol Children's Cold Formula* Oral Solution (OTC) [U.S.] | Chlorpheniramine maleate 1 mg | Pseudoephedrine HCl 15 mg | Alcohol free Sorbitol | Intended for pediatric use | 3–12 mos: 2 drops/kg of body weight, 1–2 yrs: 5 drops/kg of body weight, 2–6 yrs: 5 mL, 6–12 yrs: 10 mL, q 4–6 hr | a, e, g |
| *Drixomed* Extended-release Tablets (OTC) [U.S.] | Dexbrompheniramine maleate 6 mg | Pseudoephedrine sulfate 120 mg | | 1 tab q 12 hr (max 2 tabs/day) | | c, f, g |
| *Drixoral* Extended-release Tablets (OTC) [Canada] | Dexbrompheniramine maleate 6 mg | Pseudoephedrine sulfate 120 mg | Sugar coated | 1 tab q 8–12 hr | | c, g |
| *Drixoral Cold and Allergy* Extended-release Tablets (OTC) [U.S.] | Dexbrompheniramine maleate 6 mg | Pseudoephedrine sulfate 120 mg | Lactose | 1 tab q 12 hr (max 2 tabs/day) | | c, g |
| *Drixoral Night* Tablets (OTC) [Canada] | Dexbrompheniramine maleate 2 mg | Pseudoephedrine sulfate 60 mg | Tartrazine free Available in a dual package that also contains *Drixoral N.D.* | 1 tab hs | | a, g |
| *Drixtab* Tablets (OTC) [Canada] | Dexbrompheniramine maleate 2 mg | Pseudoephedrine sulfate 60 mg | Tartrazine free | 1 tab q 6–8 hr | 6–12 yrs: 1/2 tab q 6–8 hr | a, g |

## Table 1. Oral Dosage Forms *(continued)*

Note: Content per capsule, tablet, or 5 mL, unless otherwise stated.

| Brand or generic name [availability] | Antihistamines | Decongestants | Other content information as per product label | Usual adult and adolescent dose* prn | Usual pediatric dose prn | Packaging, storage, and auxiliary labeling† |
|---|---|---|---|---|---|---|
| *Drize* Extended-release Capsules (Rx) [U.S.] | Chlorpheniramine maleate 12 mg | Phenylpropanolamine HCl 75 mg | Dye free | 1 cap q 12 hr | | a, g |
| *Duralex* Extended-release Capsules (Rx) [U.S.] | Chlorpheniramine maleate 8 mg | Pseudoephedrine HCl 120 mg | | 1 cap q 12 hr | | a, g |
| *Dura-Tap PD* Extended-release Capsules (Rx) [U.S.] | Chlorpheniramine maleate 4 mg | Pseudoephedrine HCl 60 mg | | 2 caps q 12 hr | 6–12 yrs: 1 cap q 12 hr | b, g |
| *Dura-Vent/A* Extended-release Capsules (Rx) [U.S.] | Chlorpheniramine maleate 10 mg | Phenylpropanolamine HCl 75 mg | | 1 cap q 12 hr | | b, g |
| *Ed A-Hist* Oral Solution (Rx) [U.S.] | Chlorpheniramine maleate 4 mg | Phenylephrine HCl 10 mg | Alcohol 5% | 5 mL q 6–8 hr | 2–5 yrs: 1.25 mL, 6–12 yrs: 2.5 mL, q 6–8 hr | a, f, g |
| Extended-release Tablets (Rx) [U.S.] | Chlorpheniramine maleate 8 mg | Phenylephrine HCl 20 mg | | 1 tab q 12 hr | | a, g |
| *Endafed* Extended-release Capsules (Rx) [U.S.] | Brompheniramine maleate 12 mg | Pseudoephedrine HCl 120 mg | | 1 cap q 12 hr | | a, g |
| *E.N.T* Extended-release Tablets (Rx) [U.S.] | Brompheniramine maleate 12 mg | Phenylpropanolamine HCl 75 mg | | 1 tab q 12 hr | | a, g |
| *Fedahist* Tablets (OTC) [U.S.] | Chlorpheniramine maleate 4 mg | Pseudoephedrine HCl 60 mg | Scored | 1 tab q 4–6 hr (max 4 tabs/day) | 6–12 yrs: ½ tab q 4–6 hr (max 2 tabs/day) | b, g |
| *Fedahist Gyrocaps* Extended-release Capsules (Rx) [U.S.] | Chlorpheniramine maleate 10 mg | Pseudoephedrine HCl 65 mg | | 1 cap q 12 hr (max 2 caps/day) | Not recommended | b, g |
| *Fedahist Timecaps* Extended-release Capsules (Rx) [U.S.] | Chlorpheniramine maleate 8 mg | Pseudoephedrine HCl 120 mg | | 1 cap q 12 hr (max 2 caps/day) | Not recommended | b, g |
| *Genac* Tablets USP (OTC) [U.S.] | Triprolidine HCl 2.5 mg | Pseudoephedrine HCl 60 mg | | 1 tab q 4–6 hr (max 4 tabs/day) | | b, f |
| *Genamin* Syrup (OTC) [U.S.] | Chlorpheniramine maleate 1 mg | Phenylpropanolamine HCl 6.25 mg | Alcohol free | 20 mL q 4–6 hr (max 120 mL/day) | 6–12 yrs: 10 mL q 4–6 hr (max 60 mL/day) | c, e, g |
| *Genatap* Elixir (OTC) [U.S.] | Brompheniramine maleate 2 mg | Phenylpropanolamine HCl 12.5 mg | Alcohol free Saccharin Sorbitol | 10 mL q 4 hr | | a, e, g |
| *Gencold* Extended-release Capsules (OTC) [U.S.] | Chlorpheniramine maleate 8 mg | Phenylpropanolamine HCl 75 mg | | 1 cap q 12 hr | | a, g |
| *Hayfebrol* Oral Solution (OTC) [U.S.] | Chlorpheniramine maleate 2 mg | Pseudoephedrine HCl 30 mg | Alcohol free Sugar free Dye free | 10 mL q 6 hr | 2–6 yrs: 2.5 mL, 6–12 yrs: 5 mL, q 6 hr | a, e, g |

*Geriatric patients may be more sensitive to the effects of the usual adult dose.

†For appropriate *Packaging and storage* and *Auxiliary labeling* information refer to designated letters as follows:
    a—Store below 40 °C (104 °F), preferably between 15 and 30 °C (59 and 86 °F), in a tight container, unless otherwise specified by manufacturer.
    b—Store between 15 and 30 °C (59 and 86 °F), in a tight container, unless otherwise specified by manufacturer.
    c—Store between 2 and 30 °C (36 and 86 °F), in a tight container, unless otherwise specified by manufacturer.
    d—Store below 25 °C (77 °F), in a tight container, unless otherwise specified by manufacturer.
    e—Protect from freezing.
    f—Protect from light.
    g—Auxiliary labeling:
        May cause drowsiness.
        Avoid alcoholic beverages.
    h—Auxiliary labeling: • May be chewed.
    i—Auxiliary labeling: • Shake well.
    j—Color may change over time from pink to peach. This does not reflect any change in quality or potency of tablets.

## Table 1. Oral Dosage Forms *(continued)*

Note: Content per capsule, tablet, or 5 mL, unless otherwise stated.

| Brand or generic name [availability] | Antihistamines | Decongestants | Other content information as per product label | Usual adult and adolescent dose* prn | Usual pediatric dose prn | Packaging, storage, and auxiliary labeling† |
|---|---|---|---|---|---|---|
| *Histalet* Syrup (Rx) [U.S.] | Chlorpheniramine maleate 3 mg | Pseudoephedrine HCl 45 mg | Alcohol free | 10 mL q 6 hr (max 4 doses/day) | 2–6 yrs: 2.5 mL, 6–12 yrs: 5 mL, q 6 hr (max 4 doses/day) | b, e, g |
| *Histalet Forte* Tablets (Rx) [U.S.] | Chlorpheniramine maleate 4 mg, Pyrilamine maleate 25 mg | Phenylephrine HCl 10 mg, Phenylpropanolamine HCl 50 mg | Scored | 1 tab q 8–12 hr (max 2 tabs/day) | 6–12 yrs: 1/2 tab q 8–12 hr (max 1 tab/day) | b, f, g |
| *Histatab Plus* Tablets (OTC) [U.S.] | Chlorpheniramine maleate 2 mg | Phenylephrine HCl 5 mg | | 2 tabs initially, then 1 tab q 4 hr | | a, g |
| *Histatan* Tablets (Rx) [U.S.] | Chlorpheniramine tannate 8 mg, Pyrilamine tannate 25 mg | Phenylephrine tannate 25 mg | | 1 tab q 12 hr | | a, g |
| *Hista-Vadrin* Tablets (Rx) [U.S.] | Chlorpheniramine maleate 6 mg | Phenylephrine HCl 5 mg, Phenylpropanolamine HCl 40 mg | | 1 tab q 6 hr | | a, g |
| *Histor-D* Syrup (Rx) [U.S.] | Chlorpheniramine maleate 2 mg | Phenylephrine HCl 5 mg | Alcohol 2% | 5–10 mL q 4–6 hr | | a, e, g |
| *Iofed* Extended-release Capsules (Rx) [U.S.] | Brompheniramine maleate 12 mg | Pseudoephedrine HCl 120 mg | | 1 cap q 12 hr | | a, f, g |
| *Iofed PD* Extended-release Capsules (Rx) [U.S.] | Brompheniramine maleate 6 mg | Pseudoephedrine HCl 60 mg | | 1–2 caps q 12 hr | 6–12 yrs: 1 cap q 12 hr | a, f, g |
| *Iohist-D* Elixir (Rx) [U.S.] | Pheniramine maleate 4 mg, Phenyltoloxamine citrate 4 mg, Pyrilamine maleate 4 mg | Phenylpropanolamine HCl 12.5 mg | Alcohol 4% | 10 mL q 4 hr | 2–6 yrs: 2.5 mL, 6–12 yrs: 5 mL, q 4 hr | a, e, f, g |
| *Klerist-D* Extended-release Capsules (Rx) [U.S.] | Chlorpheniramine maleate 8 mg | Pseudoephedrine HCl 120 mg | Dye free | 1 cap q 12 hr | | a, g |
| Tablets (Rx) [U.S.] | Chlorpheniramine maleate 4 mg | Pseudoephedrine HCl 60 mg | Dye free | 1 tab q 6–8 hr | | b, g |
| *Kronofed-A Jr. Kronocaps* Extended-release Capsules (Rx) [U.S.] | Chlorpheniramine maleate 4 mg | Pseudoephedrine HCl 60 mg | Dye free | 1–2 caps q 12 hr | 6–12 yrs: 1 cap q 12 hr | a, g |
| *Kronofed-A Kronocaps* Extended-release Capsules (Rx) [U.S.] | Chlorpheniramine maleate 8 mg | Pseudoephedrine HCl 120 mg | Dye free | 1 cap q 12 hr | | a, g |
| *Linhist-L.A.* Extended-release Capsules (Rx) [U.S.] | Chlorpheniramine maleate 4 mg, Phenyltoloxamine citrate 50 mg | Phenylephrine HCl 20 mg | | 1 cap q 8–12 hr | | a, g |
| *Liqui-Histine-D* Elixir (Rx) [U.S.] | Pheniramine maleate 4 mg, Phenyltoloxamine citrate 4 mg, Pyrilamine maleate 4 mg | Phenylpropanolamine HCl 12.5 mg | Alcohol 4% | 10 mL q 4 hr | 2–6 yrs: 2.5 mL, 6–12 yrs: 5 mL, q 4 hr | a, e, f, g |
| *Liqui-Minic Infant Drops* Oral Solution (Rx) [U.S.] | Pheniramine maleate 10 mg/mL, Pyrilamine maleate 10 mg/mL | Phenylpropanolamine HCl 20 mg/mL | | Intended for pediatric use | 1.1 drop/kg (1 drop/2 lb) body weight q 6 hr | a, e |

## Table 1. Oral Dosage Forms (continued)

Note: Content per capsule, tablet, or 5 mL, unless otherwise stated.

| Brand or generic name [availability] | Antihistamines | Decongestants | Other content information as per product label | Usual adult and adolescent dose* prn | Usual pediatric dose prn | Packaging, storage, and auxiliary labeling† |
|---|---|---|---|---|---|---|
| *Lodrane LD* Extended-release Capsules (Rx) [U.S.] | Brompheniramine maleate 6 mg | Pseudoephedrine HCl 60 mg | Dye free | 1–2 caps q 12 hr | | a, g |
| *Lodrane Liquid* Oral Solution (Rx) [U.S.] | Brompheniramine maleate 4 mg | Pseudoephedrine HCl 60 mg | Dye free Sugar free Alcohol free | | 2–6 yrs: 1.25 mL 6–12 yrs: 2.5 mL ≥12 yrs: 5 mL q 4–6 hr | b, e, g |
| *Med-Hist* Extended-release Capsules (Rx) [U.S.] | Chlorpheniramine maleate 8 mg | Pseudoephedrine HCl 120 mg | | 1 cap q 12 hr | | a, g |
| *Metahistine D* Elixir (Rx) [U.S.] | Pheniramine maleate 4 mg, Phenyltoloxamine citrate 4 mg, Pyrilamine maleate 4 mg | Phenylpropanolamine HCl 12.5 mg | Alcohol 4% | 10 mL q 4 hr | 2–6 yrs: 2.5 mL, 6–12 yrs: 5 mL, q 4 hr | a, e, f, g |
| *M-Hist* Extended-release Capsules (Rx) [U.S.] | Brompheniramine maleate 12 mg | Pseudoephedrine HCl 120 mg | | 1 cap q 12 hr | | a, g |
| *Mooredec* Extended-release Tablets (Rx) [U.S.] | Carbinoxamine maleate 8 mg | Pseudoephedrine HCl 120 mg | | 1 tab q 12 hr | | a, g |
| *Myphetapp* Elixir (OTC) [U.S.] | Brompheniramine maleate 2 mg | Phenylpropanolamine HCl 12.5 mg | Alcohol 2.3% | 10 mL q 4 hr | | a, e, g |
| *Nalda-Relief Pediatric Drops* Oral Solution (Rx) [U.S.] | Chlorpheniramine maleate 0.5 mg/mL, Phenyltoloxamine citrate 2 mg/mL | Phenylephrine HCl 1.25 mg/mL, Phenylpropanolamine HCl 5 mg/mL | | Intended for pediatric use | 3–6 mos: ¼ mL, 6–12 mos: ½ mL, 1–6 yrs: 1 mL, q 3–4 hr | a, e, g |
| *Naldecon* Syrup (Rx) [U.S.] | Chlorpheniramine maleate 2.5 mg, Phenyltoloxamine citrate 7.5 mg | Phenylephrine HCl 5 mg, Phenylpropanolamine HCl 20 mg | Sorbitol | 5 mL q 3–4 hr (max 20 mL/day) | 6–12 yrs: 2.5 mL q 3–4 hr | a, e, g |
| Extended-release Tablets (Rx) [U.S.] | Chlorpheniramine maleate 5 mg, Phenyltoloxamine citrate 15 mg | Phenylephrine HCl 10 mg, Phenylpropanolamine HCl 40 mg | Scored | 1 tab q 8 hr | 6–12 yrs: ½ tab q 8 hr | a, g |
| *Naldecon Pediatric Drops* Oral Solution (Rx) [U.S.] | Chlorpheniramine maleate 0.5 mg/mL, Phenyltoloxamine citrate 2 mg/mL | Phenylephrine HCl 1.25 mg/mL, Phenylpropanolamine HCl 5 mg/mL | Sorbitol | Intended for pediatric use | 3–6 mos: ¼ mL, 6–12 mos: ½ mL, 1–6 yrs: 1 mL, q 3–4 hr | a, e, g |
| *Naldecon Pediatric Syrup* Syrup (Rx) [U.S.] | Chlorpheniramine maleate 0.5 mg, Phenyltoloxamine citrate 2 mg | Phenylephrine HCl 1.25 mg, Phenylpropanolamine HCl 5 mg | | Intended for pediatric use | 6–12 mos: 2.5 mL, 1–6 yrs: 5 mL, 6–12 yrs: 10 mL, q 3–4 hr | a, e, g |
| *Naldelate* Syrup (Rx) [U.S.] | Chlorpheniramine maleate 2.5 mg, Phenyltoloxamine citrate 7.5 mg | Phenylephrine HCl 5 mg, Phenylpropanolamine HCl 20 mg | | 5 mL q 3–4 hr (max 20 mL/day) | 6–12 yrs: 2.5 mL q 4 hr | a, e, g |

*Geriatric patients may be more sensitive to the effects of the usual adult dose.

†For appropriate *Packaging and storage* and *Auxiliary labeling* information refer to designated letters as follows:
  a—Store below 40 °C (104 °F), preferably between 15 and 30 °C (59 and 86 °F), in a tight container, unless otherwise specified by manufacturer.
  b—Store between 15 and 30 °C (59 and 86 °F), in a tight container, unless otherwise specified by manufacturer.
  c—Store between 2 and 30 °C (36 and 86 °F), in a tight container, unless otherwise specified by manufacturer.
  d—Store below 25 °C (77 °F), in a tight container, unless otherwise specified by manufacturer.
  e—Protect from freezing.
  f—Protect from light.
  g—Auxiliary labeling:
    May cause drowsiness.
    Avoid alcoholic beverages.
  h—Auxiliary labeling: • May be chewed.
  i—Auxiliary labeling: • Shake well.
  j—Color may change over time from pink to peach. This does not reflect any change in quality or potency of tablets.

## Table 1. Oral Dosage Forms *(continued)*

Note: Content per capsule, tablet, or 5 mL, unless otherwise stated.

| Brand or generic name [availability] | Antihistamines | Decongestants | Other content information as per product label | Usual adult and adolescent dose* prn | Usual pediatric dose prn | Packaging, storage, and auxiliary labeling† |
|---|---|---|---|---|---|---|
| *Naldelate Pediatric Drops* Oral Solution (Rx) [U.S.] | Chlorpheniramine maleate 0.5 mg/mL, Phenyltoloxamine citrate 2 mg/mL | Phenylephrine HCl 1.25 mg/mL, Phenylpropanolamine HCl 5 mg/mL | | Intended for pediatric use | 3–6 mos: ¼ mL, 6–12 mos: ½ mL, 1–6 yrs: 1 mL, q 3–4 hr | a, e, g |
| *Naldelate Pediatric Syrup* Syrup (Rx) [U.S.] | Chlorpheniramine maleate 0.5 mg, Phenyltoloxamine citrate 2 mg | Phenylephrine HCl 1.25 mg, Phenylpropanolamine HCl 5 mg | | Intended for pediatric use | 6–12 mos: 2.5 mL, 1–6 yrs: 5 mL, 6–12 yrs: 10 mL, q 3–4 hr | a, e, g |
| *Nalex-A* Extended-release Tablets (Rx) [U.S.] | Chlorpheniramine maleate 4 mg, Phenyltoloxamine citrate 40 mg | Phenylephrine HCl 20 mg | Lactose Scored | ½–1 tab q 8–12 hr | 6–12 yrs: ½ tab q 8–12 hr | a, f, g |
| *Nalfed* Extended-release Capsules (Rx) [U.S.] | Brompheniramine maleate 12 mg | Pseudoephedrine HCl 120 mg | | 1 cap q 12 hr | | a, g |
| *Nalfed-PD* Extended-release Capsules (Rx) [U.S.] | Brompheniramine maleate 6 mg | Pseudoephedrine HCl 60 mg | | 1–2 caps q 12 hr | 6–12 yrs: 1 cap q 12 hr | b, g |
| *Nalgest* Syrup (Rx) [U.S.] | Chlorpheniramine maleate 2.5 mg, Phenyltoloxamine citrate 7.5 mg | Phenylephrine HCl 5 mg, Phenylpropanolamine HCl 20 mg | Alcohol free Sugar free | 5 mL q 3–4 hr (max 20 mL/day) | 6–12 yrs: 2.5 mL q 3–4 hr | a, e, g |
| Extended-release Tablets (Rx) [U.S.] | Chlorpheniramine maleate 5 mg, Phenyltoloxamine citrate 15 mg | Phenylephrine HCl 10 mg, Phenylpropanolamine HCl 40 mg | | 1 tab q 8 hr | | a, g |
| *Nalgest Pediatric* Oral Solution (Rx) [U.S.] | Chlorpheniramine maleate 0.5 mg/mL, Phenyltoloxamine citrate 2 mg/mL | Phenylephrine HCl 1.25 mg/mL, Phenylpropanolamine HCl 5 mg/mL | Sorbitol | Intended for pediatric use | 3–6 mos: 0.25 mL, 6–12 mos: 0.5 mL, 1–6 yrs: 1 mL, q 3–4 hr | a, e, g |
| Syrup (Rx) [U.S.] | Chlorpheniramine maleate 0.5 mg, Phenyltoloxamine citrate 2 mg | Phenylephrine HCl 1.25 mg, Phenylpropanolamine HCl 5 mg | Sorbitol | Intended for pediatric use | 6–12 mos: 2.5 mL q 3–4 hr (max 10 mL/day), 1–6 yrs: 5 mL q 3–4 hr (max 20 mL/day), 6–12 yrs: 10 mL q 3–4 hr (max 40 mL/day) | a, e, g |
| *Nalphen* Syrup (Rx) [U.S.] | Chlorpheniramine maleate 2.5 mg, Phenyltoloxamine citrate 7.5 mg | Phenylephrine HCl 5 mg, Phenylpropanolamine HCl 20 mg | | 5 mL q 3–4 hr | 6–12 yrs: 2.5 mL q 3–4 hr | a, e, g |
| *Nalphen Pediatric* Oral Solution (Rx) [U.S.] | Chlorpheniramine maleate 0.5 mg/mL, Phenyltoloxamine citrate 2 mg/mL | Phenylephrine HCl 1.25 mg/mL, Phenylpropanolamine HCl 5 mg/mL | | Intended for pediatric use | 3–6 mos: ¼ mL, 6–12 mos: ½ mL, 1–6 yrs: 1 mL, q 3–4 hr | a, e, g |
| Syrup (Rx) [U.S.] | Chlorpheniramine maleate 0.5 mg, Phenyltoloxamine citrate 2 mg | Phenylephrine HCl 1.25 mg, Phenylpropanolamine HCl 5 mg | | Intended for pediatric use | 6–12 mos: 2.5 mL, 1–6 yrs: 5 mL, 6–12 yrs: 10 mL, q 3–4 hr | a, e, g |
| *ND Clear T.D.* Extended-release Capsules (Rx) [U.S.] | Chlorpheniramine maleate 8 mg | Pseudoephedrine HCl 120 mg | Dye free | 1 cap q 12 hr | | a, g |
| *Neo Citran A* for Oral Solution (OTC) [Canada] | Pheniramine maleate 20 mg/pouch | Phenylephrine HCl 10 mg/pouch | Vitamin C 50 mg/pouch | 1 pouch dissolved in 225 mL of hot water q 3–4 hr | | a, g |
| *Nolamine* Extended-release Tablets (Rx) [U.S.] | Chlorpheniramine maleate 4 mg, Phenindamine tartrate 24 mg | Phenylpropanolamine HCl 50 mg | | 1 tab q 8 hr (mild cases q 8–12 hr) | | b, f, g |

## Table 1. Oral Dosage Forms *(continued)*

Note: Content per capsule, tablet, or 5 mL, unless otherwise stated.

| Brand or generic name [availability] | Antihistamines | Decongestants | Other content information as per product label | Usual adult and adolescent dose* prn | Usual pediatric dose prn | Packaging, storage, and auxiliary labeling† |
|---|---|---|---|---|---|---|
| *Novafed A* Extended-release Capsules (Rx) [U.S.] | Chlorpheniramine maleate 8 mg | Pseudoephedrine HCl 120 mg | | 1 cap q 12 hr | | b, g |
| *Novahistex* Extended-release Capsules (OTC) [Canada] | Chlorpheniramine maleate 8 mg | Pseudoephedrine HCl 120 mg | | 1 cap q 12 hr | | a, g |
| *Novahistine* Elixir (OTC) [U.S.] | Chlorpheniramine maleate 2 mg | Phenylephrine HCl 5 mg | Alcohol 5% Sugar free Sorbitol | 10 mL q 4 hr (max 60 mL/day) | 6–12 yrs: 5 mL q 4 hr (max 30 mL/day) | a, e, g |
| *Ornade* Oral Solution (OTC) [Canada] | Chlorpheniramine maleate 1.5 mg | Phenylpropanolamine HCl 15 mg | Alcohol 3.8% Sugar free | 5–10 mL q 6–8 hr | 1–5 yrs: 2.5 mL, 6–12 yrs: 5 mL, q 6–8 hr | a, e, g |
| *Ornade-A.F.* Extended-release Capsules (OTC) [Canada] | Chlorpheniramine maleate 12 mg | Phenylpropanolamine HCl 75 mg | | 1 cap q 12 hr | Not recommended | a, g |
| Oral Solution (OTC) [Canada] | Chlorpheniramine maleate 2.5 mg | Phenylpropanolamine HCl 15 mg | Alcohol 3.8% Sugar free | 5–10 mL q 6–8 hr | 1–5 yrs: 2.5 mL, 6–12 yrs: 5 mL, q 6–8 hr | a, e, g |
| *Ornade Spansules* Extended-release Capsules (Rx) [U.S.] | Chlorpheniramine maleate 12 mg | Phenylpropanolamine HCl 75 mg | | 1 cap q 12 hr | Not recommended | b, f, g |
| Extended-release Capsules (OTC) [Canada] | Chlorpheniramine maleate 8 mg | Phenylpropanolamine HCl 75 mg | | 1 cap q 12 hr | | b, g |
| *PediaCare Cold-Allergy* Chewable Tablets (OTC) [U.S.] | Chlorpheniramine maleate 1 mg | Pseudoephedrine HCl 15 mg | Phenylalanine 8 mg Scored | Intended for pediatric use | 2–3 yrs: 1 tab, 4–5 yrs: 1½ tabs, 6–8 yrs: 2 tabs, 9–10 yrs: 2½ tabs, 11 yrs: 3 tabs, q 4–6 hr | a, g, h |
| *PediaCare Cold Formula* Oral Solution (OTC) [U.S.] | Chlorpheniramine maleate 1 mg | Pseudoephedrine HCl 15 mg | Alcohol free Saccharin free | Intended for pediatric use | 6–11 yrs: 10 mL q 4–6 hr | b, e, g |
| *Phenergan VC* Syrup (Rx) [U.S.] | Promethazine HCl 6.25 mg | Phenylephrine HCl 5 mg | Alcohol 7% Saccharin | 5 mL q 4–6 hr (max 30 mL/day) | 2–6 yrs: 1.25–2.5 mL, 6–12 yrs: 2.5–5 mL, q 4–6 hr | d, e, f, g |
| *Pherazine VC* Syrup (Rx) [U.S.] | Promethazine HCl 6.25 mg | Phenylephrine HCl 5 mg | Alcohol 7% | 5 mL q 4–6 hr | 2–6 yrs: 1.25–2.5 mL, 6–12 yrs: 2.5–5 mL, q 4–6 hr | d, e, f, g |

*Geriatric patients may be more sensitive to the effects of the usual adult dose.

†For appropriate *Packaging and storage* and *Auxiliary labeling* information refer to designated letters as follows:
   a—Store below 40 °C (104 °F), preferably between 15 and 30 °C (59 and 86 °F), in a tight container, unless otherwise specified by manufacturer.
   b—Store between 15 and 30 °C (59 and 86 °F), in a tight container, unless otherwise specified by manufacturer.
   c—Store between 2 and 30 °C (36 and 86 °F), in a tight container, unless otherwise specified by manufacturer.
   d—Store below 25 °C (77 °F), in a tight container, unless otherwise specified by manufacturer.
   e—Protect from freezing.
   f—Protect from light.
   g—Auxiliary labeling:
       May cause drowsiness.
       Avoid alcoholic beverages.
   h—Auxiliary labeling: • May be chewed.
   i—Auxiliary labeling: • Shake well.
   j—Color may change over time from pink to peach. This does not reflect any change in quality or potency of tablets.

## Table 1. Oral Dosage Forms *(continued)*

Note: Content per capsule, tablet, or 5 mL, unless otherwise stated.

| Brand or generic name [availability] | Antihistamines | Decongestants | Other content information as per product label | Usual adult and adolescent dose* prn | Usual pediatric dose prn | Packaging, storage, and auxiliary labeling† |
|---|---|---|---|---|---|---|
| *Poly D* Elixir (Rx) [U.S.] | Pheniramine maleate 4 mg, Phenyltoloxamine citrate 4 mg, Pyrilamine maleate 4 mg | Phenylpropanolamine HCl 12.5 mg | Alcohol 4% | 10 mL q 4 hr | 2–6 yrs: 2.5 mL, 6–12 yrs: 5 mL, q 4 hr | a, e, f, g |
| *Poly-D* Elixir (Rx) [U.S.] | Pheniramine maleate 4 mg, Phenyltoloxamine citrate 4 mg, Pyrilamine maleate 4 mg | Phenylpropanolamine HCl 12.5 mg | Alcohol 4% | 10 mL q 4 hr | 2–6 yrs: 2.5 mL, 6–12 yrs: 5 mL, q 4 hr | a, e, f, g |
| *Poly Hist Forte* Tablets (Rx) [U.S.] | Chlorpheniramine maleate 4 mg, Pyrilamine maleate 25 mg | Phenylephrine HCl 10 mg, Phenylpropanolamine HCl 50 mg | | 1 tab q 8–12 hr | 6–12 yrs: ½ tab q 8–12 hr | b, f, g |
| *Poly-Histine-D* Extended-release Capsules (Rx) [U.S.] | Pheniramine maleate 16 mg, Phenyltoloxamine citrate 16 mg, Pyrilamine maleate 16 mg | Phenylpropanolamine HCl 50 mg | | 1 cap q 8–12 hr | | a, g |
| Elixir (Rx) [U.S.] | Pheniramine maleate 4 mg, Phenyltoloxamine citrate 4 mg, Pyrilamine maleate 4 mg | Phenylpropanolamine HCl 12.5 mg | Alcohol 4% | 10 mL q 4 hr | 2–6 yrs: 2.5 mL, 6–12 yrs: 5 mL, q 4 hr | a, e, g |
| *Poly-Histine-D Ped* Extended-release Capsules (Rx) [U.S.] | Pheniramine maleate 8 mg, Phenyltoloxamine citrate 8 mg, Pyrilamine maleate 8 mg | Phenylpropanolamine HCl 25 mg | | Intended for pediatric use | 6–12 yrs: 1 cap q 8–12 hr | a, g |
| Promethazine HCl and Phenylephrine HCl Syrup (Rx) [U.S.] | Promethazine HCl 6.25 mg | Phenylephrine HCl 5 mg | Alcohol 7% | 5 mL q 4–6 hr | 2–6 yrs: 1.25–2.5 mL, 6–12 yrs: 2.5–5 mL, q 4–6 hr | d, e, f, g |
| *Promethazine VC* Syrup (Rx) [U.S.] | Promethazine HCl 6.25 mg | Phenylephrine HCl 5 mg | | 5 mL q 4–6 hr (max 20 mL/day) | 2–6 yrs: 1.25–2.5 mL, 6–12 yrs: 2.5–5 mL, q 4–6 hr | d, e, f, g |
| *Prometh VC Plain* Syrup (Rx) [U.S.] | Promethazine HCl 6.25 mg | Phenylephrine HCl 5 mg | Alcohol 7% | 5 mL q 4–6 hr (max 20 mL/day) | 2–6 yrs: 1.25–2.5 mL, 6–12 yrs: 2.5–5 mL, q 4–6 hr | d, e, f, g |
| *Prop-a-Hist* Extended-release Tablets (Rx) [U.S.] | Chlorpheniramine maleate 5 mg, Phenyltoloxamine citrate 15 mg | Phenylephrine HCl 10 mg, Phenylpropanolamine HCl 40 mg | | 1 tab q 8 hr | | a, g |
| *Pseudo-Chlor* Extended-release Capsules (Rx) [U.S.] | Chlorpheniramine maleate 8 mg | Pseudoephedrine HCl 120 mg | | 1 cap q 12 hr | | a, g |
| *Pseudo-gest Plus* Tablets (OTC) [U.S.] | Chlorpheniramine maleate 4 mg | Pseudoephedrine HCl 60 mg | Scored | 1 tab q 4–6 hr (max 4 tabs/day) | | a, g |
| *Q-Hist LA* Extended-release Capsules (Rx) [U.S.] | Chlorpheniramine maleate 4 mg, Phenyltoloxamine citrate 50 mg | Phenylephrine HCl 20 mg | | 1 cap q 8–12 hr | | a, g |

## Table 1. Oral Dosage Forms *(continued)*

Note: Content per capsule, tablet, or 5 mL, unless otherwise stated.

| Brand or generic name [availability] | Antihistamines | Decongestants | Other content information as per product label | Usual adult and adolescent dose* prn | Usual pediatric dose prn | Packaging, storage, and auxiliary labeling† |
|---|---|---|---|---|---|---|
| *Resaid S.R.* Extended-release Capsules (Rx) [U.S.] | Chlorpheniramine maleate 12 mg | Phenylpropanolamine HCl 75 mg | | 1 cap q 12 hr | | b, f, g |
| *Rescon* Extended-release Capsules (Rx) [U.S.] | Chlorpheniramine maleate 12 mg | Pseudoephedrine HCl 120 mg | | 1 cap q 12 hr | | a, g |
| Oral Solution (OTC) [U.S.] | Chlorpheniramine maleate 2 mg | Phenylpropanolamine HCl 12.5 mg | Alcohol free Sugar free | 10 mL q 4 hr (max 40 mL/day) | | a, e, g |
| *Rescon-ED* Extended-release Capsules (Rx) [U.S.] | Chlorpheniramine maleate 8 mg | Pseudoephedrine HCl 120 mg | | 1 cap q 12 hr | | a, g |
| *Rescon JR* Extended-release Capsules (Rx) [U.S.] | Chlorpheniramine maleate 4 mg | Pseudoephedrine HCl 60 mg | Dye free | Intended for pediatric use | 6–12 yrs: 1 cap q 12 hr | a, g |
| *Respahist* Extended-release Capsules (Rx) [U.S.] | Brompheniramine maleate 6 mg | Pseudoephedrine HCl 60 mg | Dye free | 1–2 caps q 12 hr | 6–12 yrs: 1 cap q 12 hr | a, f, g |
| *Rhinatate* Tablets (Rx) [U.S.] | Chlorpheniramine tannate 8 mg, Pyrilamine tannate 25 mg | Phenylephrine tannate 25 mg | | 1–2 tabs q 12 hr | | a, g |
| *Rhinolar-EX* Extended-release Capsules (Rx) [U.S.] | Chlorpheniramine maleate 8 mg | Phenylpropanolamine HCl 75 mg | Dye free | 1 cap q 12 hr | | a, g |
| *Rhinolar-EX 12* Extended-release Capsules (Rx) [U.S.] | Chlorpheniramine maleate 12 mg | Phenylpropanolamine HCl 75 mg | Dye free | 1 cap q 12 hr | | a, g |
| *Rhinosyn* Oral Solution (OTC) [U.S.] | Chlorpheniramine maleate 4 mg | Pseudoephedrine HCl 60 mg | Alcohol 0.45% | 5 mL q 4 hr | | a, e, g |
| *Rhinosyn-PD* Oral Solution (OTC) [U.S.] | Chlorpheniramine maleate 2 mg | Pseudoephedrine HCl 30 mg | Alcohol 1.2% | 10 mL q 4 hr | | a, e, g |
| *Ricobid* Tablets (Rx) [U.S.] | Chlorpheniramine tannate 8 mg | Phenylephrine tannate 25 mg | | 1–2 tabs q 12 hr | | a, g |
| *Ricobid Pediatric* Oral Suspension (Rx) [U.S.] | Chlorpheniramine tannate 4 mg | Phenylephrine tannate 5 mg | Alcohol free Sugar free | Intended for pediatric use | 2–6 yrs: 2.5–5 mL, 6–12 yrs: 5–10 mL, q 12 hr | a, e, g, i |
| *Rinade B.I.D.* Extended-release Capsules (Rx) [U.S.] | Chlorpheniramine maleate 8 mg | Pseudoephedrine HCl 120 mg | Dye free | 1 cap q 12 hr | | a, g |

\*Geriatric patients may be more sensitive to the effects of the usual adult dose.

†For appropriate *Packaging and storage* and *Auxiliary labeling* information refer to designated letters as follows:
- a—Store below 40 °C (104 °F), preferably between 15 and 30 °C (59 and 86 °F), in a tight container, unless otherwise specified by manufacturer.
- b—Store between 15 and 30 °C (59 and 86 °F), in a tight container, unless otherwise specified by manufacturer.
- c—Store between 2 and 30 °C (36 and 86 °F), in a tight container, unless otherwise specified by manufacturer.
- d—Store below 25 °C (77 °F), in a tight container, unless otherwise specified by manufacturer.
- e—Protect from freezing.
- f—Protect from light.
- g—Auxiliary labeling:
    May cause drowsiness.
    Avoid alcoholic beverages.
- h—Auxiliary labeling: • May be chewed.
- i—Auxiliary labeling: • Shake well.
- j—Color may change over time from pink to peach. This does not reflect any change in quality or potency of tablets.

## Table 1. Oral Dosage Forms *(continued)*

Note: Content per capsule, tablet, or 5 mL, unless otherwise stated.

| Brand or generic name [availability] | Antihistamines | Decongestants | Other content information as per product label | Usual adult and adolescent dose* prn | Usual pediatric dose prn | Packaging, storage, and auxiliary labeling† |
|---|---|---|---|---|---|---|
| *Rolatuss Plain* Oral Solution (OTC) [U.S.] | Chlorpheniramine maleate 2 mg | Phenylephrine HCl 5 mg | Alcohol 5% | 10 mL q 4–6 hr | | a, e, g |
| *Rondamine* Syrup (Rx) [U.S.] | Carbinoxamine maleate 4 mg | Pseudoephedrine HCl 60 mg | | 5 mL q 6 hr | 18 mos–6 yrs: 2.5 mL, 6–12 yrs: 5 mL, q 6 hr | a, e, g |
| Tablets (Rx) [U.S.] | Carbinoxamine maleate 4 mg | Pseudoephedrine HCl 60 mg | | 1 tab q 6 hr | 6–12 yrs: 1 tab q 6 hr | a, g |
| Extended-release Tablets (Rx) [U.S.] | Carbinoxamine maleate 8 mg | Pseudoephedrine HCl 120 mg | | 1 tab q 12 hr | | a, g |
| *Rondec* Syrup (Rx) [U.S.] | Carbinoxamine maleate 4 mg | Pseudoephedrine HCl 60 mg | Alcohol free Sugar Free | 5 mL q 6 hr | 18 mos–6 yrs: 2.5 mL, 6–12 yrs: 5 mL, q 6 hr | a, e, g |
| Tablets (Rx) [U.S.] | Carbinoxamine maleate 4 mg | Pseudoephedrine HCl 60 mg | Film coated | 1 tab q 6 hr | 6–12 yrs: 1 tab q 6 hr | a, g |
| *Rondec Chewable* Chewable Tablets (Rx) [U.S.] | Brompheniramine maleate 4 mg | Pseudoephedrine HCl 60 mg | Aspartame | 1 tab q 4 hr (max 6 tabs/day) | 6–12 yrs: 1/2 tab 4 hr (max 6 doses [3 tabs]/day) | a, g, j |
| *Rondec Drops* Oral Solution (Rx) [U.S.] | Carbinoxamine maleate 2 mg/mL | Pseudoephedrine HCl 25 mg/mL | Alcohol free | Intended for pediatric use | 1–3 mos: 1/4 mL, 3–6 mos: 1/2 mL, 6–9 mos: 3/4 mL, 9–18 mos: 1 mL, q 6 hr | a, e, g |
| *Rondec-TR* Extended-release Tablets (Rx) [U.S.] | Carbinoxamine maleate 8 mg | Pseudoephedrine HCl 120 mg | Film coated | 1 tab q 12 hr | | a, g |
| *R-Tannamine* Tablets (Rx) [U.S.] | Chlorpheniramine tannate 8 mg, Pyrilamine tannate 25 mg | Phenylephrine tannate 25 mg | | 1–2 tabs q 12 hr | | a, g |
| *R-Tannamine Pediatric* Oral Suspension (Rx) [U.S.] | Chlorpheniramine tannate 2 mg, Pyrilamine tannate 12.5 mg | Phenylephrine tannate 5 mg | | Intended for pediatric use | 2–6 yrs: 2.5–5 mL, 6–12 yrs: 5–10 mL, q 12 hr | a, e, g, i |
| *R-Tannate* Tablets (Rx) [U.S.] | Chlorpheniramine tannate 8 mg, Pyrilamine tannate 25 mg | Phenylephrine tannate 25 mg | | 1–2 tabs q 12 hr | | a, g |
| *R-Tannate Pediatric* Oral Suspension (Rx) [U.S.] | Chlorpheniramine tannate 2 mg, Pyrilamine tannate 12.5 mg | Phenylephrine tannate 5 mg | | Intended for pediatric use | 2–6 yrs: 2.5–5 mL, 6–12 yrs: 5–10 mL, q 12 hr | a, e, g, i |
| *Ru-Tuss* Oral Solution (OTC) [U.S.] | Chlorpheniramine maleate 2 mg | Phenylephrine HCl 5 mg | Alcohol 5% | 10 mL q 4–6 hr | | a, e, g |
| *Ryna* Oral Solution (OTC) [U.S.] | Chlorpheniramine maleate 2 mg | Pseudoephedrine HCl 30 mg | Alcohol free Dye free Sugar free Sorbitol | 10 mL q 6 hr (max 40 mL/day) | 6–12 yrs: 5 mL q 6 hr (max 20 mL/day) | a, e, g |
| *Rynatan* Tablets (Rx) [U.S.] | Chlorpheniramine tannate 8 mg, Pyrilamine tannate 25 mg | Phenylephrine tannate 25 mg | Scored | 1–2 tabs q 12 hr | | a, g |
| *Rynatan Pediatric* Oral Suspension (Rx) [U.S.] | Chlorpheniramine tannate 2 mg, Pyrilamine tannate 12.5 mg | Phenylephrine tannate 5 mg | | Intended for pediatric use | 2–6 yrs: 2.5–5 mL, 6–12 yrs: 5–10 mL, q 12 hr | a, e, g, i |

## Table 1. Oral Dosage Forms *(continued)*

Note: Content per capsule, tablet, or 5 mL, unless otherwise stated.

| Brand or generic name [availability] | Antihistamines | Decongestants | Other content information as per product label | Usual adult and adolescent dose* prn | Usual pediatric dose prn | Packaging, storage, and auxiliary labeling† |
|---|---|---|---|---|---|---|
| *Rynatan-S Pediatric* Oral Suspension (Rx) [U.S.] | Chlorpheniramine tannate 2 mg, Pyrilamine tannate 12.5 mg | Phenylephrine tannate 5 mg | | Intended for pediatric use | 2–6 yrs: 2.5–5 mL, 6–12 yrs: 5–10 mL, q 12 hr | a, e, g, i |
| *Seldane-D* Extended-release Tablets (Rx) [U.S.] Note: Withdrawn from U.S. market by FDA in 2/98. | Terfenadine 60 mg | Pseudoephedrine HCl 120 mg (10 mg immediate-release outer core; 110 mg extended-release core) | | 1 tab q 12 hr | | b |
| *Semprex-D* Capsules (Rx) [U.S.] | Acrivastine 8 mg | Pseudoephedrine HCl 60 mg | | 1 cap q 4–6 hr (max 4 caps/day) | | a, f, g |
| *Shellcap* Extended-release Capsules (Rx) [U.S.] | Brompheniramine maleate 12 mg | Pseudoephedrine HCl 120 mg | | 1 cap q 12 hr | | a, g |
| *Shellcap PD* Extended-release Capsules (Rx) [U.S.] | Brompheniramine maleate 6 mg | Pseudoephedrine HCl 60 mg | | 1–2 caps q 12 hr | 6–12 yrs: 1 cap q 12 hr | a, g |
| *Silafed* Syrup (OTC) [U.S.] | Triprolidine HCl 1.25 mg | Pseudoephedrine HCl 30 mg | | 10 mL q 4–6 hr (max 40 mL/day) | 6–12 yrs: 5 mL q 4–6 hr (max 20 mL/day) | b, f, g |
| *Silaminic* Syrup (OTC) [U.S.] | Chlorpheniramine maleate 2 mg | Phenylpropanolamine HCl 12.5 mg | Alcohol free | 10 mL q 4 hr (max 60 mL/day) | 6–12 yrs: 5 mL q 4 hr (max 30 mL/day) | b, g |
| *Sinucon* Syrup (Rx) [U.S.] | Chlorpheniramine maleate 2.5 mg, Phenyltoloxamine citrate 7.5 mg | Phenylephrine HCl 5 mg, Phenylpropanolamine HCl 20 mg | | 5 mL q 3–4 hr | 6–12 yrs: 2.5 mL q 3–4 hr | a, e, g |
| *Sinucon Pediatric Drops* Oral Solution (Rx) [U.S.] | Chlorpheniramine maleate 0.5 mg/mL, Phenyltoloxamine citrate 2 mg/mL | Phenylephrine HCl 1.25 mg/mL, Phenylpropanolamine HCl 5 mg/mL | | Intended for pediatric use | 3–6 mos: ¼ mL, 6–12 mos: ½ mL, 1–6 yrs: 1 mL, q 3–4 hr | a, e, g |
| *Sinucon Pediatric Syrup* Syrup (Rx) [U.S.] | Chlorpheniramine maleate 0.5 mg, Phenyltoloxamine citrate 2 mg | Phenylephrine HCl 1.25 mg, Phenylpropanolamine HCl 5 mg | | Intended for pediatric use | 6–12 mos: 2.5 mL, 1–6 yrs: 5 mL, 6–12 yrs: 10 mL, q 3–4 hr | a, e, g |
| *Sudafed Plus* Tablets (OTC) [U.S.] | Chlorpheniramine maleate 4 mg | Pseudoephedrine HCl 60 mg | Scored | 1 tab q 4–6 hr (max 4 tabs/day) | 6–12 yrs: ½ tab q 4–6 hr (max 4 doses/day) | b, f, g |
| *Tamine S.R.* Extended-release Tablets (Rx) [U.S.] | Brompheniramine maleate 12 mg | Phenylephrine HCl 15 mg, Phenylpropanolamine HCl 15 mg | Sugar coated | 1 tab q 8–12 hr | | b, f, g |
| *Tanafed* Oral Suspension (Rx) [U.S.] | Chlorpheniramine tannate 4.5 mg | Pseudoephedrine tannate 75 mg | | 10–20 mL q 12 hr | 2–6 yrs: 2.5–5 mL (max 10 mL/day), 6–12 yrs: 5–10 mL (max 20 mL/day), q 12 hr | b, e, f, g, i |

*Geriatric patients may be more sensitive to the effects of the usual adult dose.

†For appropriate *Packaging and storage* and *Auxiliary labeling* information refer to designated letters as follows:
    a—Store below 40 °C (104 °F), preferably between 15 and 30 °C (59 and 86 °F), in a tight container, unless otherwise specified by manufacturer.
    b—Store between 15 and 30 °C (59 and 86 °F), in a tight container, unless otherwise specified by manufacturer.
    c—Store between 2 and 30 °C (36 and 86 °F), in a tight container, unless otherwise specified by manufacturer.
    d—Store below 25 °C (77 °F), in a tight container, unless otherwise specified by manufacturer.
    e—Protect from freezing.
    f—Protect from light.
    g—Auxiliary labeling:
        May cause drowsiness.
        Avoid alcoholic beverages.
    h—Auxiliary labeling: • May be chewed.
    i—Auxiliary labeling: • Shake well.
    j—Color may change over time from pink to peach. This does not reflect any change in quality or potency of tablets.

## Table 1. Oral Dosage Forms *(continued)*

Note: Content per capsule, tablet, or 5 mL, unless otherwise stated.

| Brand or generic name [availability] | Antihistamines | Decongestants | Other content information as per product label | Usual adult and adolescent dose* prn | Usual pediatric dose prn | Packaging, storage, and auxiliary labeling† |
|---|---|---|---|---|---|---|
| *Tanoral* Tablets (Rx) [U.S.] | Chlorpheniramine tannate 8 mg, Pyrilamine tannate 25 mg | Phenylephrine tannate 25 mg | | 1–2 tabs q 12 hr | | a, g |
| *Tavist-D* Extended-release Tablets (OTC) [U.S.] | Clemastine fumarate 1.34 mg (immediate release) | Phenylpropanolamine HCl 75 mg | Film coated | 1 tab q 12 hr (max 2 tabs/day) | | a, g |
| Extended-release Tablets (OTC) [Canada] | Clemastine hydrogen fumarate 1.34 mg (immediate release) | Phenylpropanolamine HCl 75 mg | Film coated | 1 tab q 12 hr (max 2 tabs/day) | | a, g |
| *Teldrin 12 Hour Allergy Relief* Extended-release Capsules (OTC) [U.S.] | Chlorpheniramine maleate 8 mg | Phenylpropanolamine HCl 75 mg | | 1 cap q 12 hr (max 2 caps/day) | | b, g |
| *Temazin Cold* Syrup (OTC) [U.S.] | Chlorpheniramine maleate 2 mg | Phenylpropanolamine HCl 12.5 mg | | 10 mL q 4 hr (max 40 mL/day) | | a, e, g |
| *Touro A&H* Extended-release Capsules (Rx) [U.S.] | Brompheniramine maleate 6 mg | Pseudoephedrine HCl 60 mg | | 1–2 caps q 12 hr | 6–12 yrs: 1 cap q 12 hr | a, g |
| *Triaminic* Syrup (OTC) [U.S.] | Chlorpheniramine maleate 1 mg | Phenylpropanolamine HCl 6.25 mg | Alcohol free | 20 mL q 4 hr (max 120 mL/day) | 3–12 mos: 1.25 mL, 12–24 mos: 2.5 mL, 2–6 yrs: 5 mL, 6–12 yrs: 10 mL, q 4 hr | a, e, g |
| Syrup (OTC) [Canada] | Chlorpheniramine maleate 2 mg | Phenylpropanolamine HCl 12.5 mg | Alcohol free Tartrazine free | 10 mL q 4 hr | 2–5 yrs: 2.5 mL 6–12 yrs: 5 mL, q 4 hr | a, e, g |
| Extended-release Tablets (OTC) [Canada] | Pheniramine maleate 25 mg, Pyrilamine maleate 25 mg | Phenylpropanolamine HCl 50 mg | Tartrazine free | 1 tab q 8 hr | | a, g |
| *Triaminic-12* Extended-release Tablets (OTC) [U.S.] | Chlorpheniramine maleate 12 mg | Phenylpropanolamine HCl 75 mg | | 1 tab q 12 hr (max 2 tabs/day) | | a, g |
| *Triaminic Allergy* Tablets (OTC) [U.S.] | Chlorpheniramine maleate 4 mg | Phenylpropanolamine HCl 25 mg | Scored | 1 tab q 4 hr (max 6 tabs/day) | 6–12 yrs: ½ tab q 4 hr (max 3 tabs/day) | a, g |
| *Triaminic Chewables* Chewable Tablets (OTC) [U.S.] | Chlorpheniramine maleate 0.5 mg | Phenylpropanolamine HCl 6.25 mg | | Intended for pediatric use | 2–6 yrs: 1 tab, 6–12 yrs: 2 tabs, q 4 hr | a, g, h |
| *Triaminic Cold* Syrup (OTC) [U.S.] | Chlorpheniramine maleate 2 mg | Phenylpropanolamine HCl 12.5 mg | Alcohol free Sorbitol | 10 mL q 4 hr | 3–12 mos: 1 drop/kg of body weight, 1–2 yrs: 3 drops/kg of body weight, 2–6 yrs: 2.5 mL, 6–12 yrs: 5 mL, q 4 hr | b, e, g |
| Tablets (OTC) [U.S.] | Chlorpheniramine maleate 2 mg | Phenylpropanolamine HCl 12.5 mg | | 2 tabs q 4 hrs (max 12 tabs/day) | 6–12 yrs: 1 tab q 4 hr (max 6 tabs/day) | a, g |
| *Triaminic Oral Infant Drops* Oral Solution (Rx) [U.S.] | Pheniramine maleate 10 mg/mL, Pyrilamine maleate 10 mg/mL | Phenylpropanolamine HCl 20 mg/mL | | Intended for pediatric use | 1.1 drop/kg (1 drop/2 lb) body weight q 6 hr | a, e, g |

## Table 1. Oral Dosage Forms *(continued)*

Note: Content per capsule, tablet, or 5 mL, unless otherwise stated.

| Brand or generic name [availability] | Antihistamines | Decongestants | Other content information as per product label | Usual adult and adolescent dose* prn | Usual pediatric dose prn | Packaging, storage, and auxiliary labeling† |
|---|---|---|---|---|---|---|
| *Triaminic TR* Extended-release Tablets (Rx) [U.S.] | Pheniramine maleate 25 mg, Pyrilamine maleate 25 mg | Phenylpropanolamine HCl 50 mg | Film coated | 1 tab q 8–12 hr | | a, g |
| *Trihist-D* Elixir (Rx) [U.S.] | Pheniramine maleate 4 mg, Phenyltoloxamine citrate 4 mg, Pyrilamine maleate 4 mg | Phenylpropanolamine HCl 12.5 mg | Alcohol 4% | 10 mL q 4 hr | 2–6 yrs: 2.5 mL, 6–12 yrs: 5 mL, q 4 hr | a, e, f, g |
| *Trinalin Repetabs* Extended-release Tablets (Rx) [U.S./Canada] | Azatadine maleate 1 mg | Pseudoephedrine sulfate 120 mg | Sugar coated | 1 tab q 12 hr | Not recommended | c, g |
| *Tri-Nefrin Extra Strength* Tablets (OTC) [U.S.] | Chlorpheniramine maleate 4 mg | Phenylpropanolamine HCl 25 mg | Lactose | 1 tab q 4 hr (max 6 tabs/day) | 6–12 yrs: ½ tab q 4 hr (max 3 tabs/day) | a, g |
| *Triofed* Syrup USP (OTC) [U.S.] | Triprolidine HCl 1.25 mg | Pseudoephedrine HCl 30 mg | | 10 mL q 4–6 hr (max 40 mL/day) | 6–12 yrs: 5 mL q 4–6 hr | b, e, f, g |
| *Triotann* Tablets (Rx) [U.S.] | Chlorpheniramine tannate 8 mg, Pyrilamine tannate 25 mg | Phenylephrine tannate 25 mg | | 1–2 tabs q 12 hr | | a, g |
| *Triotann Pediatric* Oral Suspension (Rx) [U.S.] | Chlorpheniramine tannate 2 mg, Pyrilamine tannate 12.5 mg | Phenylephrine tannate 5 mg | | Intended for pediatric use | 2–6 yrs: 2.5–5 mL, 6–12 yrs: 5–10 mL, q 12 hr | a, e, g, i |
| *Triotann-S Pediatric* Oral Suspension (Rx) [U.S.] | Chlorpheniramine tannate 2 mg, Pyrilamine tannate 12.5 mg | Phenylephrine tannate 5 mg | | Intended for pediatric use | 2–6 yrs: 2.5–5 mL, 6–12 yrs: 5–10 mL, q 12 hr | a, e, g, i |
| *Tri-Phen-Chlor* Syrup (Rx) [U.S.] | Chlorpheniramine maleate 2.5 mg, Phenyltoloxamine citrate 7.5 mg | Phenylephrine HCl 5 mg, Phenylpropanolamine HCl 20 mg | | 5 mL q 4 hr (max 20 mL/day) | 6–12 yrs: 2.5 mL q 4 hr | a, e, g |
| *Tri-Phen-Chlor Pediatric* Oral Solution (Rx) [U.S.] | Chlorpheniramine maleate 0.5 mg/mL, Phenyltoloxamine citrate 2 mg/mL | Phenylephrine HCl 1.25 mg/mL, Phenylpropanolamine HCl 5 mg/mL | | Intended for pediatric use | 3–6 mos: 0.25 mL, 6–12 mos: 0.5 mL, 1–6 yrs: 1 mL, q 3–4 hr | a, e, g |
| Syrup (Rx) [U.S.] | Chlorpheniramine maleate 0.5 mg, Phenyltoloxamine citrate 2 mg | Phenylephrine HCl 1.25 mg, Phenylpropanolamine HCl 5 mg | Sorbitol | Intended for pediatric use | 6–12 mos: 2.5 mL, 1–6 yrs: 5 mL, 6–12 yrs: 10 mL, q 3–4 hr (max 4 doses/day) | a, e, g, i |
| *Tri-Phen-Chlor T.R.* Extended-release Tablets (Rx) [U.S.] | Chlorpheniramine maleate 5 mg, Phenyltoloxamine citrate 15 mg | Phenylephrine HCl 10 mg, Phenylpropanolamine HCl 40 mg | | 1 tab q 8 hr | 6–12 yrs: ½ tab q 8 hr | a, g |

\*Geriatric patients may be more sensitive to the effects of the usual adult dose.

†For appropriate *Packaging and storage* and *Auxiliary labeling* information refer to designated letters as follows:
- a—Store below 40 °C (104 °F), preferably between 15 and 30 °C (59 and 86 °F), in a tight container, unless otherwise specified by manufacturer.
- b—Store between 15 and 30 °C (59 and 86 °F), in a tight container, unless otherwise specified by manufacturer.
- c—Store between 2 and 30 °C (36 and 86 °F), in a tight container, unless otherwise specified by manufacturer.
- d—Store below 25 °C (77 °F), in a tight container, unless otherwise specified by manufacturer.
- e—Protect from freezing.
- f—Protect from light.
- g—Auxiliary labeling:
    - May cause drowsiness.
    - Avoid alcoholic beverages.
- h—Auxiliary labeling: • May be chewed.
- i—Auxiliary labeling: • Shake well.
- j—Color may change over time from pink to peach. This does not reflect any change in quality or potency of tablets.

## Table 1. Oral Dosage Forms (continued)

Note: Content per capsule, tablet, or 5 mL, unless otherwise stated.

| Brand or generic name [availability] | Antihistamines | Decongestants | Other content information as per product label | Usual adult and adolescent dose* prn | Usual pediatric dose prn | Packaging, storage, and auxiliary labeling† |
|---|---|---|---|---|---|---|
| *Tri-Phen-Mine Pediatric Drops* Oral Solution (Rx) [U.S.] | Chlorpheniramine maleate 0.5 mg/mL, Phenyltoloxamine citrate 2 mg/mL | Phenylephrine HCl 1.25 mg/mL, Phenylpropanolamine HCl 5 mg/mL | Alcohol free Sugar free | Intended for pediatric use | 3–6 mos: 0.25 mL, 6–12 mos: 0.5 mL, 1–6 yrs: 1 mL, q 3–4 hr (max 4 doses/day) | a, e, g |
| *Tri-Phen-Mine Pediatric Syrup* Syrup (Rx) [U.S.] | Chlorpheniramine maleate 0.5 mg, Phenyltoloxamine citrate 2 mg | Phenylephrine HCl 1.25 mg, Phenylpropanolamine HCl 5 mg | Alcohol free Sugar free | Intended for pediatric use | 6–12 mos: 2.5 mL, 1–6 yrs: 5 mL, 6–12 yrs: 10 mL, q 3–4 hr (max 4 doses/day) | a, e, g, i |
| *Tri-Phen-Mine S.R.* Extended-release Tablets (Rx) [U.S.] | Chlorpheniramine maleate 5 mg, Phenyltoloxamine citrate 15 mg | Phenylephrine HCl 10 mg, Phenylpropanolamine HCl 40 mg | Scored | 1 tab q 8 hr | 6–12 yrs: ½ tab q 8 hr | a, g |
| *Triphenyl* Syrup (OTC) [U.S.] | Chlorpheniramine maleate 1 mg | Phenylpropanolamine HCl 6.25 mg | Alcohol free | 20 mL q 4 hr | | a, e, g |
| *Triposed* Syrup USP (OTC) [U.S.] | Triprolidine HCl 1.25 mg | Pseudoephedrine HCl 30 mg | | 10 mL q 4–6 hr (max 40 mL/day) | 6–12 yrs: 5 mL q 4–6 hr | b, e, f, g |
| Triprolidine HCl and Pseudoephedrine HCl Syrup USP (Rx) (OTC) [U.S.] | Triprolidine HCl 1.25 mg | Pseudoephedrine HCl 30 mg | | 10 mL q 4–6 hr (max 40 mL/day) | 6–12 yrs: 5 mL q 4–6 hr | b, e, f, g |
| Tablets USP (Rx) (OTC) [U.S.] | Triprolidine HCl 2.5 mg | Pseudoephedrine HCl 60 mg | | 1 tab q 4–6 hr | 6–12 yrs: ½ tab 4–6 hr | b, f, g |
| *Tritan* Tablets (Rx) [U.S.] | Chlorpheniramine tannate 8 mg, Pyrilamine tannate 25 mg | Phenylephrine tannate 25 mg | Lactose Scored | 1–2 tabs q 12 hr | | a, g |
| *Tri-Tannate* Tablets (Rx) [U.S.] | Chlorpheniramine tannate 8 mg, Pyrilamine tannate 25 mg | Phenylephrine tannate 25 mg | | 1–2 tabs q 12 hr | | a, g |
| *Tri-Tannate Pediatric* Oral Suspension (Rx) [U.S.] | Chlorpheniramine tannate 2 mg, Pyrilamine tannate 12.5 mg | Phenylephrine tannate 5 mg | | Intended for pediatric use | 2–6 yrs: 2.5–5 mL, 6–12 yrs: 5–10 mL, q 12 hr | a, e, g, i |
| *ULTRAbrom* Extended-release Capsules (Rx) [U.S.] | Brompheniramine maleate 12 mg | Pseudoephedrine HCl 120 mg | | 1 cap q 12 hr | | a, g |
| *ULTRAbrom PD* Extended-release Capsules (Rx) [U.S.] | Brompheniramine maleate 6 mg | Pseudoephedrine HCl 60 mg | | 1–2 caps q 12 hr | 6–12 yrs: 1 cap q 12 hr | a, g |
| *Uni-Decon* Extended-release Tablets (Rx) [U.S.] | Chlorpheniramine maleate 5 mg, Phenyltoloxamine citrate 15 mg | Phenylephrine HCl 10 mg, Phenylpropanolamine HCl 40 mg | | 1 tab q 8 hr | | a, g |
| *Uni-Multihist D* Elixir (Rx) [U.S.] | Pheniramine maleate 4 mg, Phenyltoloxamine citrate 4 mg, Pyrilamine maleate 4 mg | Phenylpropanolamine HCl 12.5 mg | Alcohol 4% | 10 mL q 4 hr | 2–6 yrs: 2.5 mL, 6–12 yrs: 5 mL, q 4 hr | a, e, f, g |

## Table 1. Oral Dosage Forms (continued)

Note: Content per capsule, tablet, or 5 mL, unless otherwise stated.

| Brand or generic name [availability] | Antihistamines | Decongestants | Other content information as per product label | Usual adult and adolescent dose* prn | Usual pediatric dose prn | Packaging, storage, and auxiliary labeling† |
|---|---|---|---|---|---|---|
| *Vanex Forte Caplets* Extended-release Tablets (Rx) [U.S.] | Chlorpheniramine maleate 4 mg, Pyrilamine maleate 25 mg | Phenylephrine HCl 10 mg, Phenylpropanolamine HCl 50 mg | Scored Film coated | 1 tab q 12 hr | 6–12 yrs: ½ tab 12 hr | a, g |
| *Vasofrinic* Oral Solution (OTC) [Canada] | Chlorpheniramine maleate 2 mg | Pseudoephedrine HCl 30 mg | | 5–10 mL q 6–8 hr | 2–6 yrs: 2.5 mL, 6–12 yrs: 5 mL, q 6–8 hr | b, e, g |
| *Vicks Children's DayQuil Allergy Relief* Oral Solution (OTC) [U.S.] | Chlorpheniramine maleate 0.67 mg | Pseudoephedrine HCl 10 mg | Alcohol free | Intended for pediatric use | 6–11 yrs: 15 mL q 6 hr (max 60 mL/day) | a, e, g |
| *Vicks DayQuil 4 Hour Allergy Relief* Tablets (OTC) [U.S.] | Brompheniramine maleate 4 mg | Phenylpropanolamine HCl 25 mg | | 1 tab q 4 hr (max 6 tabs/day) | 6–12 yrs: ½ tab q 4 hr | b, g |
| *Vicks DayQuil 12 Hour Allergy Relief* Extended-release Tablets (OTC) [U.S.] | Brompheniramine maleate 12 mg | Phenylpropanolamine HCl 75 mg | | 1 tab q 12 hr (max 2 tabs/day) | | b, g |
| *West-Decon* Extended-release Tablets (Rx) [U.S.] | Chlorpheniramine maleate 5 mg, Phenyltoloxamine citrate 15 mg | Phenylephrine HCl 10 mg, Phenylpropanolamine HCl 40 mg | | 1 tab q 8 hr | | a, g |

*Geriatric patients may be more sensitive to the effects of the usual adult dose.

†For appropriate *Packaging and storage* and *Auxiliary labeling* information refer to designated letters as follows:
    a—Store below 40 °C (104 °F), preferably between 15 and 30 °C (59 and 86 °F), in a tight container, unless otherwise specified by manufacturer.
    b—Store between 15 and 30 °C (59 and 86 °F), in a tight container, unless otherwise specified by manufacturer.
    c—Store between 2 and 30 °C (36 and 86 °F), in a tight container, unless otherwise specified by manufacturer.
    d—Store below 25 °C (77 °F), in a tight container, unless otherwise specified by manufacturer.
    e—Protect from freezing.
    f—Protect from light.
    g—Auxiliary labeling:
        May cause drowsiness.
        Avoid alcoholic beverages.
    h—Auxiliary labeling: • May be chewed.
    i—Auxiliary labeling: • Shake well.
    j—Color may change over time from pink to peach. This does not reflect any change in quality or potency of tablets.

# ANTIHISTAMINES, DECONGESTANTS, AND ANALGESICS   Systemic

This monograph includes information on the following: 1) Brompheniramine, Phenylpropanolamine, and Acetaminophen; 2) Brompheniramine, Pseudoephedrine, and Acetaminophen; 3) Chlorpheniramine, Phenylephrine, and Acetaminophen; 4) Chlorpheniramine, Phenylpropanolamine, and Acetaminophen; 5) Chlorpheniramine, Phenylpropanolamine, Acetaminophen, and Caffeine; 6) Chlorpheniramine, Phenylpropanolamine, and Aspirin; 7) Chlorpheniramine, Phenyltoloxamine, Phenylpropanolamine, and Acetaminophen; 8) Chlorpheniramine, Pseudoephedrine, and Acetaminophen; 9) Chlorpheniramine, Pyrilamine, Phenylephrine, and Acetaminophen; 10) Chlorpheniramine, Pyrilamine, Phenylephrine, Phenylpropanolamine, and Acetaminophen; 11) Dexbrompheniramine, Pseudoephedrine, and Acetaminophen; 12) Diphenhydramine, Phenylpropanolamine, and Aspirin; 13) Diphenhydramine, Pseudoephedrine, and Acetaminophen; 14) Diphenylpyraline, Phenylpropanolamine, Acetaminophen, and Caffeine; 15) Pheniramine, Phenylephrine, and Acetaminophen; 16) Pheniramine, Phenylephrine, Sodium Salicylate, and Caffeine; 17) Pheniramine, Pyrilamine, Phenylpropanolamine, Acetaminophen, and Caffeine; 18) Phenyltoloxamine, Phenylpropanolamine, and Acetaminophen; 19) Pyrilamine, Phenylephrine, Aspirin, and Caffeine; 20) Pyrilamine, Phenylpropanolamine, Acetaminophen, and Caffeine; 21) Triprolidine, Pseudoephedrine, and Acetaminophen.

VA CLASSIFICATION (Primary): RE599

NOTE: The *Antihistamines, Decongestants, and Analgesics (Systemic)* monograph is maintained on the USP DI electronic data base. For a printed copy of the most recent revision of the complete monograph, contact Micromedex, Inc. - Reprint Requests, 6200 S. Syracuse Way, Suite 300, Englewood, CO 80111; telephone (303) 486-6400; telefax (303) 486-6464; Email: USPDI@MDX.COM.

For information on the specific components of this combination, see the *USP DI* monographs for *Acetaminophen (Systemic)*, *Antihistamines (Systemic)*, *Caffeine (Systemic)*, *Phenylpropanolamine (Systemic)*, *Pseudoephedrine (Systemic)*, *Salicylates (Systemic)*, and *Sympathomimetic Agents—Cardiovascular Use (Parenteral-Systemic)*.

The information that follows is selectively abstracted from the complete monograph and is provided to facilitate drug use review and patient counseling.

Note: For a listing of dosage forms and brand names by country availability, see *Dosage Forms* section(s).

## Category
Antihistaminic ($H_1$-receptor)-decongestant-analgesic.

## Indications
### Accepted
Cold symptoms (treatment);
Congestion, nasal (treatment); and
Congestion, sinus (treatment)—Antihistamine, decongestant, and analgesic combinations are indicated for the temporary relief of nasal and sinus congestion and headaches, pains, and general discomfort due to colds, flu, or allergies. The antihistamine in these combinations may provide added relief of nasal congestion, rhinorrhea, and sneezing. It may also serve as an adjunct because of its anticholinergic drying effects.

The therapeutic effectiveness of oral phenylephrine as a nasal decongestant has been questioned, especially at the usual oral dose.

## Patient Consultation
As an aid to patient consultation, refer to *Advice for the Patient, Antihistamines, Decongestants, and Analgesics (Systemic)*.
In providing consultation, consider emphasizing the following selected information (» = major clinical significance):

### Before using this medication
» Conditions affecting use, especially:
   Sensitivity to any of the medications in the combination being taken
   Pregnancy—Concern for the fetus and/or newborn infant only with high doses and long-term therapy; psychiatric disorders more likely with use of phenylpropanolamine in postpartum women; use of aspirin-containing combinations not recommended during third trimester
   Breast-feeding—Antihistamines may cause excitement or irritability in nursing infant; high risk for infants from sympathomimetic amines; also, concern with high doses and chronic use because of high salicylate intake by infant
   Use in children—Increased susceptibility to anticholinergic effects of antihistamines and to vasopressor effects of sympathomimetic amines; psychiatric disorders more likely with use of phenylpropanolamine in children under 6 years of age; hyperexcitability (paradoxical reaction) may occur; also, increased susceptibility to toxic effects of salicylates, especially if fever and dehydration present; possible association between aspirin usage and Reye's syndrome
   Use in adolescents—Possible association between aspirin usage and Reye's syndrome
   Use in the elderly—Anticholinergic and CNS stimulant effects more likely to occur; increased susceptibility to toxic effects of salicylates
   Other medications, especially anticholinergics, medicine for high blood pressure or depression, or CNS depressants or stimulants
   Other medical problems, especially alcoholism, cardiovascular disease, diabetes, gastritis or peptic ulcer (with salicylate-containing), hypertension, hyperthyroidism, or prostatic hypertrophy

### Proper use of this medication
» Importance of not taking more medication than the amount recommended
   Taking with food, water, or milk to minimize gastric irritation
   Swallowing extended-release dosage form whole
» Not taking combinations containing aspirin if a strong vinegar-like odor is present
» Proper dosing
   Missed dose: If on scheduled dosing regimen—Taking as soon as possible; not taking if almost time for next dose; not doubling doses
» Proper storage

### Precautions while using this medication
Caution if skin tests using allergens required; possible interference with test results
Checking with physician if symptoms persist or become worse, or if high fever is present
» Avoiding alcoholic beverages or other CNS depressants while taking these medications; also, alcohol consumption may increase risk of salicylate-induced gastrointestinal toxicity and acetaminophen-induced liver toxicity
» Caution if drowsiness or dizziness occurs
» Possible insomnia; taking the medication a few hours before bedtime
» Caution if taking phenylpropanolamine-containing appetite suppressants
   Need to inform physician or dentist of use of medication if any kind of surgery (including dental surgery) or emergency treatment is required
   Possible dryness of mouth; using sugarless gum or candy, ice, or saliva substitute for relief; checking with dentist if dry mouth continues for more than 2 weeks
» Caution if other medications containing acetaminophen, aspirin, or other salicylates (including diflunisal) are used
» Suspected overdose: Getting emergency help at once
   Not taking products containing aspirin for 5 days prior to any kind of surgery, unless otherwise directed by physician
   Diabetics: Aspirin present in some combination formulations may cause false urine sugar test results with prolonged use of 8 or more 325-mg (5-grain) doses per day

### Side/adverse effects
Signs of potential side effects, especially allergic reactions, anticholinergic effects, blood dyscrasias, jaundice (with acetaminophen-containing), and signs of gastrointestinal irritation or bleeding (with salicylate-containing)

## Oral Dosage Forms
See *Table 1*, page 367.

Revised: 08/30/94
Interim revision: 07/18/95; 05/30/96

## Table 1. Oral Dosage Forms

Note: Content per capsule, tablet, or 5 mL, unless otherwise stated.

| Brand or generic name [availability] | Antihistamines | Decongestants | Analgesics | Other content information as per product label | Usual adult and adolescent dose* (prn) | Usual pediatric dose (prn) | Packaging, storage, and auxiliary labeling† |
|---|---|---|---|---|---|---|---|
| *Aclophen* Extended-release Tablets (Rx) [U.S.] | Chlorphenirmine maleate 8 mg | Phenylephrine HCl 40 mg | Acetaminophen 500 mg | Dye-free | 1 tab q 8 hr | | a, d |
| *Actifed Cold & Sinus* Tablets (OTC) [U.S.] | Triprolidine HCl 1.25 mg | Pseudoephedrine HCl 30 mg | Acetaminophen 500 mg | | 2 tabs q 6 hr (max 8 tabs/day) | Not recommended | a, d |
| *Actifed Cold & Sinus* Caplets Tablets (OTC) [U.S.] | Triprolidine HCl 1.25 mg | Pseudoephedrine HCl 30 mg | Acetaminophen 500 mg | | 2 tabs q 6 hr (max 8 tabs/day) | Not recommended | a, d |
| *Actifed Plus Extra Strength Caplets* Tablets (OTC) [Canada] | Triprolidine HCl 2.5 mg | Pseudoephedrine HCl 60 mg | Acetaminophen 500 mg | Scored | 1 tab q 4–6 hr (max 4 tabs/day) | | a, d |
| *Actifed Sinus Nighttime* Tablets (OTC) [U.S.] | Diphenhydramine HCl 25 mg | Pseudoephedrine HCl 30 mg | Acetaminophen 500 mg | In dual package that also contains *Actifed Sinus Daytime Tablets* | 2 tabs hs or 2 tabs q 6 hr (max 8 tabs/day) | Not recommended | a, d |
| *Actifed Sinus Nighttime Caplets* Tablets (OTC) [U.S.] | Diphenhydramine HCl 25 mg | Pseudoephedrine HCl 30 mg | Acetaminophen 500 mg | In dual package that also contains *Actifed Sinus Daytime Caplets* | 2 tabs hs or 2 tabs q 6 hr (max 8 tabs/day) | Not recommended | a, d |
| *Alka-Seltzer Plus Allergy Medicine Liqui-Gels* Capsules (OTC) [U.S.] | Chlorpheniramine maleate 2 mg | Pseudoephedrine HCl 30 mg | Acetaminophen 250 mg | | 2 caps q 4 hr (max 8 caps/day) | 6–12 yrs: 1 cap q 4 hr (max 4 caps/day) | a, d |
| *Alka-Seltzer Plus Cold Medicine Effervescent Tablets* (OTC) [U.S./Canada] | Chlorpheniramine maleate 2 mg | Phenylpropanolamine bitartrate 24.08 mg | Aspirin 325 mg | Sodium 506 mg | 2 tabs q 4 hr dissolved in 120 mL water (max 8 tabs/day) | | a, d |
| *Alka-Seltzer Plus Cold Medicine Liqui-Gels* Capsules (OTC) [U.S.] | Chlorpheniramine maleate 2 mg | Pseudoephedrine HCl 30 mg | Acetaminophen 250 mg | | 2 caps q 4 hr (max 8 caps/day) | 6–12 yrs: 1 cap q 4 hr (max 4 caps/day) | a, d |
| *Allerest Sinus Pain Formula Caplets* Tablets (OTC) [U.S.] | Chlorpheniramine maleate 2 mg | Pseudoephedrine HCl 30 mg | Acetaminophen 500 mg | | 2 tabs q 6 hr (max 8 tabs/day) | | a |
| *Alumadrine* Tablets (Rx) [U.S.] | Chlorpheniramine maleate 4 mg | Phenylpropanolamine HCl 25 mg | Acetaminophen 500 mg | Scored | 1 tab q 4 hr (max 6 tabs/day) | | a, d |
| *BC Multi Symptom Cold Powder* for Oral Solution (OTC) [U.S.] | Chlorpheniramine maleate 4 mg per packet | Phenylpropanolamine HCl 25 mg per packet | Aspirin 650 mg per packet | Lactose | 1 packet dissolved in water q 4 hr (max 4 doses/day) | | a, d |

*Geriatric patients may be more sensitive to the effects of usual adult dose.

†For appropriate *Packaging and storage* and *Auxiliary labeling* information refer to designated letters as follows:
 a—Store below 40 °C (104 °F), preferably between 15 and 30 °C (59 and 86 °F), in a tight container, unless otherwise specified by manufacturer.
 b—Store between 2 and 30 °C (36 and 86 °F), in a well-closed container, unless otherwise specified by manufacturer.
 c—Protect from freezing.
 d—Auxiliary labeling: • May cause drowsiness. • Avoid alcoholic beverages.
 e—Auxiliary labeling: • Shake well.

## Table 1. Oral Dosage Forms *(continued)*

Note: Content per capsule, tablet, or 5 mL, unless otherwise stated.

| Brand or generic name [availability] | Antihistamines | Decongestants | Analgesics | Other content information as per product label | Usual adult and adolescent dose* (prn) | Usual pediatric dose (prn) | Packaging, storage, and auxiliary labeling† |
|---|---|---|---|---|---|---|---|
| *Benadryl Allergy/Cold* Tablets (OTC) [U.S.] | Diphenhydramine HCl 12.5 mg | Pseudoephedrine HCl 30 mg | Acetaminophen 500 mg | | 2 tabs q 6 hr (max 8 tabs/day) | Not recommended | a, d |
| *Benadryl Allergy/ Sinus Headache Caplets* Tablets (OTC) [U.S.] | Diphenhydramine HCl 12.5 mg | Pseudoephedrine HCl 30 mg | Acetaminophen 500 mg | | 2 tabs q 6 hr (max 8 tabs/day) | | a, d |
| *BQ Cold* Tablets (OTC) [U.S.] | Chlorpheniramine maleate 2 mg | Phenylpropanol-amine HCl 12.5 mg | Acetaminophen 325 mg | | 2 tabs q 4 hr | | a, d |
| *Children's Tylenol Cold Multi-Symptom* Oral Solution (OTC) [U.S.] | Chlorpheniramine maleate 1 mg | Pseudoephedrine HCl 15 mg | Acetaminophen 160 mg | Sorbitol Alcohol free | Intended for pediatric use | 2–5 yrs: 5 mL, 6–11 yrs: 10 mL, q 4–6 hr (max 4 doses/day) | a, c, d |
| Chewable Tablets (OTC) [U.S.] | Chlorpheniramine maleate 0.5 mg | Pseudoephedrine HCl 7.5 mg | Acetaminophen 80 mg | Phenylalanine 4 mg Scored | Intended for pediatric use | 2–5 yrs: 2 tabs, 6–11 yrs: 4 tabs, q 4–6 hr (max 4 doses/day) | a, d |
| *Chlor-Trimeton Allergy-Sinus Caplets* Tablets (OTC) [U.S.] | Chlorpheniramine maleate 2 mg | Phenylpropanol-amine HCl 12.5 mg | Acetaminophen 500 mg | | 2 tabs q 6 hr | | b, d |
| *Codimal* Capsules (OTC) [U.S.] | Chlorpheniramine maleate 2 mg | Pseudoephedrine HCl 30 mg | Acetaminophen 325 mg | | 2 caps or tabs q 4–6 hr | 6–12 yrs: 1 cap or tab q 4–6 hr | a, d |
| Tablets (OTC) [U.S.] | | | | Scored, coated | | | |
| *Co-Hist* Tablets (OTC) [U.S.] | Chlorpheniramine maleate 2 mg | Pseudoephedrine HCl 30 mg | Acetaminophen 325 mg | Sodium metabisulfite | 2 tabs q 6 hr (max 8 tabs/day) | | a, d |
| *Comtrex Allergy-Sinus* Tablets (OTC) [U.S.] | Chlorpheniramine maleate 2 mg | Pseudoephedrine HCl 30 mg | Acetaminophen 500 mg | Coated | 2 tabs q 6 hr (max 8 tabs/day) | | a, d |
| *Comtrex Allergy-Sinus Caplets* Tablets (OTC) [U.S.] | Chlorpheniramine maleate 2 mg | Pseudoephedrine HCl 30 mg | Acetaminophen 500 mg | Coated | 2 tabs q 6 hr (max 8 tabs/day) | | a, d |
| *Congestant D* Tablets (OTC) [U.S.] | Chlorpheniramine maleate 2 mg | Phenylpropanol-amine HCl 12.5 mg | Acetaminophen 325 mg | | 2 tabs q 4 hr | | a, d |
| *Contac Allergy/ Sinus Night Caplets* Tablets (OTC) [U.S.] | Diphenhydramine HCl 50 mg | Pseudoephedrine HCl 60 mg | Acetaminophen 650 mg | In dual package that also contains *Contac Allergy/Sinus Day Caplets* | 1 tab q 6 hr (max 4 tabs/day of any combination of Day or Night Caplets) | | a, d |
| *Contac Cold/Flu Night Caplets* Tablets (OTC) [U.S.] | Diphenhydramine HCl 50 mg | Pseudoephedrine HCl 60 mg | Acetaminophen 650 mg | In dual package that also contains *Contac Cold/Flu Day Caplets* | 1 tab q 6 hr (max 4 tabs/day) | | a, d |

## Table 1. Oral Dosage Forms (continued)

Note: Content per capsule, tablet, or 5 mL, unless otherwise stated.

| Brand or generic name [availability] | Antihistamines | Decongestants | Analgesics | Other content information as per product label | Usual adult and adolescent dose* (prn) | Usual pediatric dose (prn) | Packaging, storage, and auxiliary labeling† |
|---|---|---|---|---|---|---|---|
| *Coricidin D* Tablets (OTC) [Canada] | Chlorpheniramine maleate 2 mg | Phenylpropanolamine HCl 12.5 mg | Aspirin 325 mg | Coated Tartrazine-free | 2 tabs q 4 hr (max 8 tabs/day) | 10–14 yrs: 1 tab q 4 hr | b, d |
| Tablets (OTC) [U.S.] | Chlorpheniramine maleate 2 mg | Phenylpropanolamine HCl 12.5 mg | Acetaminophen 325 mg | | 2 tabs q 4 hr (max 12 tabs/day) | 6–11 yrs: 1 tab q 4 hr (max 5 tabs/day) | b, d |
| *Covangesic* Tablets (OTC) [U.S.] | Chlorpheniramine maleate 2 mg, Pyrilamine maleate 12.5 mg | Phenylephrine HCl 7.5 mg, Phenylpropanolamine HCl 12.5 mg | Acetaminophen 275 mg | Tartrazine | 1 tab q 4–6 hr (max 4 tabs/day) | | a, d |
| *Dapacin Cold* Capsules (OTC) [U.S.] | Chlorpheniramine maleate 2 mg | Phenylpropanolamine HCl 12.5 mg | Acetaminophen 325 mg | | 1–2 caps q 6–8 hr | | a, d |
| *Dimetapp Allergy Sinus Caplets* Tablets (OTC) [U.S.] | Brompheniramine maleate 2 mg | Phenylpropanolamine HCl 12.5 mg | Acetaminophen 500 mg | Coated | 2 tabs q 6 hr (max 8 tabs/day) | | a, d |
| *Dimetapp Cold & Fever Suspension* Oral Suspension (OTC) [U.S.] | Brompheniramine maleate 1 mg | Pseudoephedrine HCl 15 mg | Acetaminophen 160 mg | | Intended for pediatric use | 6–11 mos: 2.5 mL, 12–23 mos: 5 mL, q 6–8 hr (max 4 doses/day); 2–6 yrs: 5 mL, 6–12 yrs: 10 mL, q 4 hr | a, c, d, e |
| *Dristan* Capsules (OTC) [Canada] | Chlorpheniramine maleate 2 mg | Phenylephrine HCl 5 mg | Acetaminophen 325 mg | | 2 caps or tabs q 4 hr (max 8 caps or tabs/day) | 6–12 yrs: 1 cap or tab q 4 hr (max 4 caps or tabs/day) | a, d |
| Tablets (OTC) [Canada] | | | | | | | |
| *Dristan Cold Maximum Strength Caplets* Tablets (OTC) [U.S.] | Brompheniramine maleate 2 mg | Pseudoephedrine HCl 30 mg | Acetaminophen 500 mg | | 2 tabs q 6 hr | | a, d |
| *Dristan Cold Multi-Symptom Formula* Tablets (OTC) [U.S.] | Chlorpheniramine maleate 2 mg | Phenylephrine HCl 5 mg | Acetaminophen 325 mg | | 2 tabs q 4 hr | | a, d |
| *Dristan Extra Strength Caplets* Tablets (OTC) [Canada] | Chlorpheniramine maleate 2 mg | Phenylephrine HCl 5 mg | Acetaminophen 500 mg | | 2 tabs q 4–6 hr (max 8 tabs/day) | | a, d |
| *Dristan Formula P* Tablets (OTC) [Canada] | Pyrilamine maleate 12.5 mg | Phenylephrine HCl 5 mg | Aspirin 325 mg | Caffeine 16 mg Tartrazine-free | 2 tabs q 4 hr | 10–14 yrs: 1 tab q 4 hr | a, d |

*Geriatric patients may be more sensitive to the effects of usual adult dose.

†For appropriate *Packaging and storage* and *Auxiliary labeling* information refer to designated letters as follows:
  a—Store below 40 °C (104 °F), preferably between 15 and 30 °C (59 and 86 °F), in a tight container, unless otherwise specified by manufacturer.
  b—Store between 2 and 30 °C (36 and 86 °F), in a well-closed container, unless otherwise specified by manufacturer.
  c—Protect from freezing.
  d—Auxiliary labeling: • May cause drowsiness. • Avoid alcoholic beverages.
  e—Auxiliary labeling: • Shake well.

## Table 1. Oral Dosage Forms (continued)

Note: Content per capsule, tablet, or 5 mL, unless otherwise stated.

| Brand or generic name [availability] | Antihistamines | Decongestants | Analgesics | Other content information as per product label | Usual adult and adolescent dose* (prn) | Usual pediatric dose (prn) | Packaging, storage, and auxiliary labeling† |
|---|---|---|---|---|---|---|---|
| *Drixoral Allergy-Sinus* Extended-release Tablets (OTC) [U.S.] | Dexbrompheniramine maleate 3 mg | Pseudoephedrine sulfate 60 mg | Acetaminophen 500 mg | | 2 tabs q 12 hr | | b, d |
| *Drixoral Cold and Flu* Extended-release Tablets (OTC) [U.S.] | Dexbrompheniramine maleate 3 mg | Pseudoephedrine sulfate 60 mg | Acetaminophen 500 mg | | 2 tabs q 12 hr | | b, d |
| *Duadacin* Capsules (OTC) [U.S.] | Chlorpheniramine maleate 2 mg | Phenylpropanolamine HCl 12.5 mg | Acetaminophen 325 mg | | 2 caps q 4 hr | | a, d |
| *Gendecon* Tablets (OTC) [U.S.] | Chlorpheniramine maleate 2 mg | Phenylephrine HCl 5 mg | Acetaminophen 325 mg | | 2 tabs q 4 hr | | a, d |
| *Histagesic Modified* Tablets (OTC) [U.S.] | Chlorpheniramine maleate 4 mg | Phenylephrine HCl 10 mg | Acetaminophen 324 mg | | 1 tab q 4 hr | | a, d |
| *Histosal* Tablets (OTC) [U.S.] | Pyrilamine maleate 12.5 mg | Phenylpropanolamine HCl 20 mg | Acetaminophen 324 mg | Caffeine 30 mg | 1–2 tabs q 4 hr (max 8 tabs/day) | | a, d |
| *Kolephrin Caplets* Tablets (OTC) [U.S.] | Chlorpheniramine maleate 2 mg | Pseudoephedrine HCl 30 mg | Acetaminophen 325 mg | | 2 tabs q 4–6 hr (max 8 tabs/day) | 6–12 yrs: 1 tab q 4–6 hr (max 4 tabs/day) | a, d |
| *ND-Gesic* Tablets (OTC) [U.S.] | Chlorpheniramine maleate 2 mg, Pyrilamine maleate 12.5 mg | Phenylephrine HCl 5 mg | Acetaminophen 300 mg | Sugar coated | 2 tabs q 6 hr | | a, d |
| *Neo Citran Colds and Flu* for Oral Solution (OTC) [Canada] | Pheniramine maleate 20 mg per pouch | Phenylephrine HCl 10 mg per pouch | Acetaminophen 325 mg per pouch | Vitamin C 50 mg per pouch | 1 pouch dissolved in 8 oz of hot water q 3–4 hr | | a, d |
| *Neo Citran Colds and Flu Calorie Reduced* for Oral Solution (OTC) [Canada] | Pheniramine maleate 20 mg per pouch | Phenylephrine HCl 10 mg per pouch | Acetaminophen 325 mg per pouch | Vitamin C 50 mg per pouch | 1 pouch dissolved in 8 oz of hot water q 3–4 hr | | a, d |
| *Neo Citran Extra Strength Colds and Flu* for Oral Solution (OTC) [Canada] | Pheniramine maleate 20 mg per pouch | Phenylephrine HCl 10 mg per pouch | Acetaminophen 500 mg per pouch | Vitamin C 50 mg per pouch | 1 pouch dissolved in 8 oz of hot water q 3–4 hr | | a, d |
| *Night-Time Effervescent Cold* Effervescent Tablets (OTC) [U.S.] | Diphenhydramine citrate 38.3 mg | Phenylpropanolamine HCl 15 mg | Aspirin 325 mg | | 2 tabs dissolved in 120 mL water q 4–6 hr (max 8 tabs/day) | | a, d |
| *Norel Plus* Capsules (Rx) [U.S.] | Chlorpheniramine maleate 4 mg, Phenyltoloxamine dihydrogen citrate 25 mg | Phenylpropanolamine HCl 25 mg | Acetaminophen 325 mg | | 1 cap q 3–4 hr (max 6 caps/day) | | a, d |

## Table 1. Oral Dosage Forms (continued)

Note: Content per capsule, tablet, or 5 mL, unless otherwise stated.

| Brand or generic name [availability] | Antihistamines | Decongestants | Analgesics | Other content information as per product label | Usual adult and adolescent dose* (prn) | Usual pediatric dose (prn) | Packaging, storage, and auxiliary labeling† |
|---|---|---|---|---|---|---|---|
| *Oradrine-2* Tablets (OTC) [Canada] | Diphenylpyraline HCl 2 mg | Phenylpropanolamine HCl 25 mg | Acetaminophen 325 mg | Caffeine 32.4 mg | 1 tab q 4 hr | | a, d |
| *Phenate T.D.* Extended-release Tablets (Rx) [U.S.] | Chlorpheniramine maleate 4 mg | Phenylpropanolamine HCl 40 mg | Acetaminophen 325 mg | | 1 tab q 6–8 hr | | a, d |
| *Pyrroxate Caplets* Tablets (OTC) [U.S.] | Chlorpheniramine maleate 4 mg | Phenylpropanolamine HCl 25 mg | Acetaminophen 650 mg | | 1 tab q 4 hr (max 6 tabs/day) | Not recommended | a, d |
| *Scot-Tussin Original 5-Action Cold Formula* Oral Solution (OTC) [U.S.] | Pheniramine maleate 13.3 mg | Phenylephrine HCl 4.2 mg | Sodium salicylate 83.3 mg | Caffeine citrate 25 mg; Sodium citrate 83.3 mg; Alcohol free; With or without sugar | 5 mL q 3–4 hr (max 20 mL/day) | 6–12 yrs: 2.5 mL q 3–4 hr | a, c, d |
| *Simplet* Tablets (OTC) [U.S.] | Chlorpheniramine maleate 4 mg | Pseudoephedrine HCl 60 mg | Acetaminophen 650 mg | | 1 tab q 6–8 hr (max 4 tabs/day) | | a, d |
| *Sinapils* Tablets (OTC) [U.S.] | Chlorpheniramine maleate 2 mg | Phenylpropanolamine HCl 12.5 mg | Acetaminophen 325 mg | Caffeine 32.5 mg | 2 tabs q 4–6 hr (max 12 tabs/day) | 6–12 yrs: 1 tab q 4–6 hr (max 6 tabs/day) | a, d |
| *Sinarest* Tablets (OTC) [U.S.] | Chlorpheniramine maleate 2 mg | Pseudoephedrine HCl 30 mg | Acetaminophen 325 mg | | 2 tabs q 4–6 hr (max 8 tabs/day) | 6–12 yrs: 1 tab q 4–6 hr (max 4 tabs/day) | a |
| *Sinarest Extra Strength Caplets* Tablets (OTC) [U.S.] | Chlorpheniramine maleate 2 mg | Pseudoephedrine HCl 30 mg | Acetaminophen 500 mg | | 2 tabs q 6 hr (max 8 tabs/day) | | a |
| *Sine-Off Sinus Medicine Caplets* Tablets (OTC) [U.S.] | Chlorpheniramine maleate 2 mg | Pseudoephedrine HCl 30 mg | Acetaminophen 500 mg | | 2 tabs q 6 hr (max 8 tabs/day) | | a, d |
| *Singlet for Adults* Tablets (OTC) [U.S.] | Chlorpheniramine maleate 4 mg | Pseudoephedrine HCl 60 mg | Acetaminophen 650 mg | | 1 tab q 6–8 hr (max 4 tabs/day) | | a, d |
| *Sinulin* Tablets (OTC) [U.S.] | Chlorpheniramine maleate 4 mg | Phenylpropanolamine HCl 25 mg | Acetaminophen 650 mg | Scored | 1 tab q 4–6 hr (max 6 tabs/day) | | a, d |
| *Sinus Headache & Congestion* Tablets (OTC) [U.S.] | Chlorpheniramine maleate 2 mg | Pseudoephedrine HCl 30 mg | Acetaminophen 325 mg | | 2 tabs q 6 hr (max 8 tabs/day) | | a, d |
| *Sinutab Extra Strength Caplets* Tablets (OTC) [Canada] | Chlorpheniramine maleate 2 mg | Pseudoephedrine HCl 30 mg | Acetaminophen 500 mg | | 1–2 tabs q 4–6 hr (max 8 tabs/day) | | a, d |

*Geriatric patients may be more sensitive to the effects of usual adult dose.

†For appropriate *Packaging and storage* and *Auxiliary labeling* information refer to designated letters as follows:
  a—Store below 40 °C (104 °F), preferably between 15 and 30 °C (59 and 86 °F), in a tight container, unless otherwise specified by manufacturer.
  b—Store between 2 and 30 °C (36 and 86 °F), in a well-closed container, unless otherwise specified by manufacturer.
  c—Protect from freezing.
  d—Auxiliary labeling: • May cause drowsiness. • Avoid alcoholic beverages.
  e—Auxiliary labeling: • Shake well.

## Table 1. Oral Dosage Forms (continued)

Note: Content per capsule, tablet, or 5 mL, unless otherwise stated.

| Brand or generic name [availability] | Antihistamines | Decongestants | Analgesics | Other content information as per product label | Usual adult and adolescent dose* (prn) | Usual pediatric dose (prn) | Packaging, storage, and auxiliary labeling† |
|---|---|---|---|---|---|---|---|
| *Sinutab Regular Caplets* Tablets (OTC) [Canada] | Chlorpheniramine maleate 2 mg | Pseudoephedrine HCl 30 mg | Acetaminophen 325 mg | Scored | 2 tabs q 4–6 hr (max 8 tabs/day) | 6–12 yrs: 1 tab q 4–6 hr (max 4 tabs/day) | a, d |
| *Sinutab SA* Extended-release Tablets (OTC) [Canada] | Phenyltoloxamine citrate 66 mg | Phenylpropanolamine HCl 100 mg | Acetaminophen 600 mg | Scored | 1 tab q 12 hr (max 2 tabs/day) | 10–14 yrs: ½ tab q 12 hr (max 1 tab/day) | a, d |
| *Sinutab Sinus Allergy Maximum Strength* Tablets (OTC) [U.S.] | Chlorpheniramine maleate 2 mg | Pseudoephedrine HCl 30 mg | Acetaminophen 500 mg | | 2 tabs q 6 hr (max 8 tabs/day) | | a, d |
| *Sinutab Sinus Allergy Maximum Strength Caplets* Tablets (OTC) [U.S.] | Chlorpheniramine maleate 2 mg | Pseudoephedrine HCl 30 mg | Acetaminophen 500 mg | | 2 tabs q 6 hr (max 8 tabs/day) | | a, d |
| *TheraFlu/Flu and Cold Medicine* for Oral Solution (OTC) [U.S.] | Chlorpheniramine maleate 4 mg per packet | Pseudoephedrine HCl 60 mg per packet | Acetaminophen 650 mg per packet | | 1 packet dissolved in 6-oz of hot water q 4 hr (max 4 doses/day) | | a, d |
| *TheraFlu/Flu and Cold Medicine for Sore Throat* for Oral Solution (OTC) [U.S.] | Chlorpheniramine maleate 4 mg per packet | Pseudoephedrine HCl 60 mg per packet | Acetaminophen 1000 mg per packet | | 1 packet dissolved in 6-oz of hot water q 6 hr (max 4 doses/day) | Not recommended | a, d |
| *Triaminicin* Tablets (OTC) [Canada] | Pheniramine maleate 12.5 mg, Pyrilamine maleate 12.5 mg | Phenylpropanolamine HCl 25 mg | Acetaminophen 325 mg | Caffeine 30 mg Tartrazine-free | 1 tab q 8 hr | | a, d |
| *Triaminicin Cold, Allergy, Sinus* Tablets (OTC) [U.S.] | Chlorpheniramine maleate 4 mg | Phenylpropanolamine HCl 25 mg | Acetaminophen 650 mg | | 1 tab q 4 hr (max 6 tabs/day) | Not recommended | a, d |
| *Tylenol Allergy Sinus Medication Extra Strength Caplets* Tablets (OTC) [Canada] | Chlorpheniramine maleate 2 mg | Pseudoephedrine HCl 30 mg | Acetaminophen 500 mg | Film-coated; Tartrazine-free | 2 tabs q 6 hr (max 8 tabs/day) | | a, d |
| *Tylenol Allergy Sinus Medication Maximum Strength Caplets* Tablets (OTC) [U.S.] | Chlorpheniramine maleate 2 mg | Pseudoephedrine HCl 30 mg | Acetaminophen 500 mg | | 2 tabs q 6 hr (max 8 tabs/day) | Not recommended | a, d |
| *Tylenol Allergy Sinus Medication Maximum Strength Gelcaps* Tablets (OTC) [U.S.] | Chlorpheniramine maleate 2 mg | Pseudoephedrine HCl 30 mg | Acetaminophen 500 mg | | 2 tabs q 6 hr (max 8 tabs/day) | Not recommended | a, d |
| *Tylenol Allergy Sinus Medication Maximum Strength Geltabs* Tablets (OTC) [U.S.] | Chlorpheniramine maleate 2 mg | Pseudoephedrine HCl 30 mg | Acetaminophen 500 mg | | 2 tabs q 6 hr (max 8 tabs/day) | Not recommended | a, d |

### Table 1. Oral Dosage Forms *(continued)*
Note: Content per capsule, tablet, or 5 mL, unless otherwise stated.

| Brand or generic name [availability] | Antihistamines | Decongestants | Analgesics | Other content information as per product label | Usual adult and adolescent dose* (prn) | Usual pediatric dose (prn) | Packaging, storage, and auxiliary labeling† |
|---|---|---|---|---|---|---|---|
| *Tylenol Allergy Sinus Night Time Medicine Maximum Strength Caplets* Tablets (OTC) [U.S.] | Diphenhydramine HCl 25 mg | Pseudoephedrine HCl 30 mg | Acetaminophen 500 mg | | 2 tabs hs | Not recommended | a, d |
| *Tylenol Cold Medication Children's* Oral Solution (OTC) [Canada] | Chlorpheniramine maleate 1 mg | Pseudoephedrine HCl 15 mg | Acetaminophen 160 mg | Sorbitol; Alcohol-free | Intended for pediatric use | 2–5 yrs: 5 mL, 6–12 yrs: 10 mL, q 4–6 hr (max 4 doses/day) | a, c, d |
| Chewable Tablets (OTC) [Canada] | Chlorpheniramine maleate 0.5 mg | Pseudoephedrine HCl 7.5 mg | Acetaminophen 80 mg | Phenylalanine; Scored | Intended for pediatric use | 2–5 yrs: 2 tabs, 6–12 yrs: 4 tabs, q 4–6 hr (max 4 doses/day) | a, d |
| *Tylenol Flu Medication Extra Strength Gelcaps* Tablets (OTC) [Canada] | Diphenhydramine HCl 25 mg | Pseudoephedrine HCl 30 mg | Acetaminophen 500 mg | | 1–2 tabs q 6 hr (max 8 tabs/day) | | a, d |
| *Tylenol Flu NightTime Hot Medication Maximum Strength* for Oral Solution (OTC) [U.S.] | Diphenhydramine HCl 50 mg per packet | Pseudoephedrine HCl 60 mg per packet | Acetaminophen 1000 mg per packet | | 1 packet dissolved in 6-oz of hot water q 6 hr (max 4 doses/day) | Not recommended | a, d |
| *Tylenol Flu NightTime Medication Maximum Strength Gelcaps* Tablets (OTC) [U.S.] | Diphenhydramine HCl 25 mg | Pseudoephedrine HCl 30 mg | Acetaminophen 500 mg | | 2 tabs hs may repeat q 6 hr (max 8 tabs/day) | Not recommended | a, d |

*Geriatric patients may be more sensitive to the effects of usual adult dose.
†For appropriate *Packaging and storage* and *Auxiliary labeling* information refer to designated letters as follows:
  a—Store below 40 °C (104 °F), preferably between 15 and 30 °C (59 and 86 °F), in a tight container, unless otherwise specified by manufacturer.
  b—Store between 2 and 30 °C (36 and 86 °F), in a well-closed container, unless otherwise specified by manufacturer.
  c—Protect from freezing.
  d—Auxiliary labeling: • May cause drowsiness. • Avoid alcoholic beverages.
  e—Auxiliary labeling: • Shake well.

# ANTIHISTAMINES, DECONGESTANTS, AND ANTICHOLINERGICS   Systemic

This monograph includes information on the following: 1) Chlorpheniramine, Phenylephrine, and Methscopolamine; 2) Chlorpheniramine, Phenylephrine, Phenylpropanolamine, Atropine, Hyoscyamine, and Scopolamine; 3) Chlorpheniramine, Phenylpropanolamine, and Methscopolamine; 4) Chlorpheniramine, Pseudoephedrine, and Methscopolamine.

VA CLASSIFICATION (Primary): RE599

**NOTE:** The *Antihistamines, Decongestants, and Anticholinergics (Systemic)* monograph is maintained on the USP DI electronic data base. For a printed copy of the most recent revision of the complete monograph, contact Micromedex, Inc. - Reprint Requests, 6200 S. Syracuse Way, Suite 300, Englewood, CO 80111; telephone (303) 486-6400; telefax (303) 486-6464; Email: USPDI@MDX.COM.

For information on the specific components of this combination, see the USP DI monographs for *Anticholinergics/Antispasmodics (Systemic), Antihistamines (Systemic), Phenylpropanolamine (Systemic), Pseudoephedrine (Systemic),* and *Sympathomimetic Agents—Cardiovascular Use (Systemic).*

The information that follows is selectively abstracted from the complete monograph and is provided to facilitate drug use review and patient counseling.

Note: For a listing of dosage forms and brand names by country availability, see *Dosage Forms* section(s).

## Category

Antihistaminic ($H_1$-receptor)-decongestant-anticholinergic.

## Indications

**Accepted**
Congestion, nasal (treatment)
Cold symptoms (treatment) and
Rhinitis, perennial and seasonal allergic or vasomotor (treatment)—Antihistamine, decongestant, and anticholinergic combinations are indicated

in the symptomatic treatment of allergic rhinitis, sinusitis, and the common cold.

The therapeutic effectiveness of oral phenylephrine as a nasal decongestant has been questioned, especially at the usual oral dose.

## Patient Consultation

As an aid to patient consultation, refer to *Advice for the Patient, Antihistamines, Decongestants, and Anticholinergics (Systemic)*.
In providing consultation, consider emphasizing the following selected information (» = major clinical significance):

### Before using this medication
» Conditions affecting use, especially:
   Sensitivity to any of the medications in the combination being taken
   Pregnancy—Postpartum women are particularly susceptible to psychiatric disorders that may be caused by phenylpropanolamine; in animal studies, pseudoephedrine caused reduced average weight, length, and rate of skeletal ossification in the fetus
   Breast-feeding—Antihistamines may cause excitement or irritability in nursing infant; high risk to infants from sympathomimetic amines; possible inhibition of lactation
   Use in children—Increased susceptibility to anticholinergic effects and to vasopressor effects; children under 6 years of age may be particularly susceptible to psychiatric disorders that may be caused by phenylpropanolamine; hyperexcitability (paradoxical reaction) may occur; increased response to anticholinergics in infants and children with spastic paralysis or brain damage; caution should be used in infants, especially newborn and premature infants, because of higher-than-usual risk of side/adverse effects of pseudoephedrine
   Use in the elderly—Anticholinergic and CNS stimulant effects more likely to occur in older patients; danger of precipitating undiagnosed glaucoma; possible impairment of memory
   Dental—Possible development of dental problems because of decreased salivary flow
   Other medications, especially alcohol, other anticholinergics, beta-adrenergic blocking agents, CNS depressants or stimulants, cocaine, digitalis glycosides, medicine for high blood pressure or depression, monoamine oxidase (MAO) inhibitors, and potassium chloride
   Other medical problems, especially cardiovascular disease, diabetes mellitus, hemorrhage, severe hypertension, hyperthyroidism, myasthenia gravis, obstruction in gastrointestinal or urinary tract, prostatic hypertrophy, tachycardia, urinary retention, and xerostomia

### Proper use of this medication
» Importance of not taking more medication than the amount recommended
   Taking with food, water, or milk to minimize gastric irritation
   Swallowing extended-release dosage form whole
» Proper dosing
   Missed dose: Taking as soon as possible; not taking if almost time for next dose; not doubling doses
» Proper storage

### Precautions while using this medication
   Checking with physician if symptoms persist or become worse, or if high fever is present
   Caution if skin tests using allergens required; possible interference with test results
» Caution during exercise or hot weather; overheating may result in heat stroke
» Possible increased sensitivity of eyes to light
» Caution if blurred vision occurs
» Caution if drowsiness or dizziness occurs
» Possible insomnia; taking the medication a few hours before bedtime
» Caution if taking phenylpropanolamine-containing appetite suppressants
   Need to inform physician or dentist of use of medication if any kind of surgery (including dental surgery or emergency treatment) is required
   Possible dryness of mouth; using sugarless gum or candy, ice, or saliva substitute for relief; checking with dentist if dry mouth continues for more than 2 weeks
» Suspected overdose: Getting emergency help at once

### Side/adverse effects
Signs of potential side effects, especially allergic reactions, severe anticholinergic effects, blood dyscrasias, CNS stimulation, severe drowsiness, hypertension, psychotic episodes, tightness in chest, convulsions, irregular or slow heartbeat, and shortness of breath or troubled breathing

## Oral Dosage Forms

See *Table 1*, page 374.

Revised: 07/19/94
Interim revision: 09/16/96

## Table 1. Oral Dosage Forms

Note: Content per capsule, tablet, or 5 mL, unless otherwise stated.

| Brand or generic name [availability] | Antihistamines | Decongestants | Anticholinergics | Other information | Usual adult and adolescent dose* (prn) | Usual pediatric dose (prn) | Packaging, storage, and auxiliary labeling† |
|---|---|---|---|---|---|---|---|
| *AH-chew* Chewable Tablets (Rx) [U.S.] | Chlorpheniramine maleate 2 mg | Phenylephrine HCl 10 mg | Methscopolamine nitrate 1.25 mg | Scored | 1–2 tabs q 4 hr | 6–12 yrs: 1 tab q 4 hr | a, c, d |
| *Atrohist Plus* Extended-release Tablets (Rx) [U.S.] | Chlorpheniramine maleate 8 mg | Phenylephrine HCl 25 mg, Phenylpropanolamine HCl 50 mg | Atropine sulfate 0.04 mg, Hyoscyamine sulfate 0.19 mg, Scopolamine HBr 0.01 mg | Scored | 1 tab q 12 hr (max 2 tabs/day) | Not recommended | a, d |
| *D.A. Chewable* Chewable Tablets (Rx) [U.S.] | Chlorpheniramine maleate 2 mg | Phenylephrine HCl 10 mg | Methscopolamine nitrate 1.25 mg | Scored | 1–2 tabs q 4 hr | 6–12 yrs: 1 tab q 4 hr | a, c, d |
| *Dallergy* Syrup (Rx) [U.S.] | Chlorpheniramine maleate 2 mg | Phenylephrine HCl 10 mg | Methscopolamine nitrate 0.625 mg | | 10 mL q 4–6 hr | 6–12 yrs: 5 mL q 4–6 hr | a, b, d |
| Tablets (Rx) [U.S.] | Chlorpheniramine maleate 4 mg | Phenylephrine HCl 10 mg | Methscopolamine nitrate 1.25 mg | Scored | 1 tab q 4–6 hr | 6–12 yrs: ½ tab q 4–6 hr | a, d |

## Table 1. Oral Dosage Forms (continued)

Note: Content per capsule, tablet, or 5 mL, unless otherwise stated.

| Brand or generic name [availability] | Antihistamines | Decongestants | Anticholinergics | Other information | Usual adult and adolescent dose* (prn) | Usual pediatric dose (prn) | Packaging, storage, and auxiliary labeling† |
|---|---|---|---|---|---|---|---|
| *Dallergy Caplets* Extended-release Tablets (Rx) [U.S.] | Chlorpheniramine maleate 8 mg | Phenylephrine HCl 20 mg | Methscopolamine nitrate 2.5 mg | Scored | 1 tab q 12 hr | 6–12 yrs: ½ tab q 12 hr | a, d |
| *Deconhist* Extended-release Tablets (Rx) [U.S.] | Chlorpheniramine maleate 8 mg | Phenylephrine HCl 25 mg, Phenylpropanolamine HCl 50 mg | Atropine sulfate 0.04 mg, Hyoscyamine sulfate 0.19 mg, Scopolamine HBr 0.01 mg | | 1 tab q 12 hr (max 2 tabs/day) | Not recommended | a, d |
| *Dura-Vent/DA* Extended-release Tablets (Rx) [U.S.] | Chlorpheniramine maleate 8 mg | Phenylephrine HCl 20 mg | Methscopolamine nitrate 2.5 mg | Scored | 1 tab q 12 hr | 6–12 yrs: ½ tab q 12 hr | a, d |
| *Extendryl* Syrup (Rx) [U.S.] | Chlorpheniramine maleate 2 mg | Phenylephrine HCl 10 mg | Methscopolamine nitrate 1.25 mg | | 10 mL q 4 hr | 6–12 yrs: 5 mL q 4 hr | a, b, d |
| Chewable Tablets (Rx) [U.S.] | Chlorpheniramine maleate 2 mg | Phenylephrine HCl 10 mg | Methscopolamine nitrate 1.25 mg | | 2 tabs q 4 hr | 6–12 yrs: 1 tab q 4 hr | a, c, d |
| *Extendryl JR* Extended-release Capsules (Rx) [U.S.] | Chlorpheniramine maleate 4 mg | Phenylephrine HCl 10 mg | Methscopolamine nitrate 1.25 mg | | Intended for pediatric patients | 6–12 yrs: 1 cap q 12 hr | a, d |
| *Extendryl SR* Extended-release Capsules (Rx) [U.S.] | Chlorpheniramine maleate 8 mg | Phenylephrine HCl 20 mg | Methscopolamine nitrate 2.5 mg | | 1 cap q 12 hr | | a, d |
| *Mescolor* Extended-release Tablets (Rx) [U.S.] | Chlorpheniramine maleate 8 mg | Pseudoephedrine HCl 120 mg | Methscopolamine nitrate 2.5 mg | Scored Dye free | 1 tab q 12 hr (max 2 tabs/day) | 6–12 yrs: ½ tab q 12 hr (max 1 tab/day) | a, d |
| *OMNIhist L.A.* Extended-release Tablets (Rx) [U.S.] | Chlorpheniramine maleate 8 mg | Phenylephrine HCl 20 mg | Methscopolamine nitrate 2.5 mg | Scored | 1 tab q 12 hr | 6–12 yrs: ½ tab q 12 hr | a, d |
| *Pannaz* Extended-release Tablets (Rx) [U.S.] | Chlorpheniramine maleate 8 mg | Phenylpropanolamine HCl 75 mg | Methscopolamine nitrate 2.5 mg | Dye free | 1 tab q 12 hr (max 2 tabs/day) | 5–12 yrs: ½ tab q 12 hr (max 1 tab/day) | a, d |
| *Phenahist-TR* Extended-release Tablets (Rx) [U.S.] | Chlorpheniramine maleate 8 mg | Phenylephrine HCl 25 mg, Phenylpropanolamine HCl 50 mg | Atropine sulfate 0.04 mg, Hyoscyamine sulfate 0.19 mg, Scopolamine HBr 0.01 mg | | 1 tab q 12 hr | | a, d |

*Geriatric patients may be more sensitive to the effects of usual adult dose.
†For appropriate *Packaging and storage* and *Auxiliary labeling* information refer to designated letters as follows:
   a—Store below 40 °C (104 °F), preferably between 15 and 30 °C (59 and 86 °F), in a tight container, unless otherwise specified by manufacturer.
   b—Protect from freezing.
   c—May be chewed.
   d—Auxiliary labeling: • May cause drowsiness. • Avoid alcoholic beverages.

## Table 1. Oral Dosage Forms (continued)

Note: Content per capsule, tablet, or 5 mL, unless otherwise stated.

| Brand or generic name [availability] | Antihistamines | Decongestants | Anticholinergics | Other information | Usual adult and adolescent dose* (prn) | Usual pediatric dose (prn) | Packaging, storage, and auxiliary labeling† |
|---|---|---|---|---|---|---|---|
| *Phenchlor S.H.A.* Extended-release Tablets (Rx) [U.S.] | Chlorpheniramine maleate 8 mg | Phenylephrine HCl 25 mg, Phenylpropanolamine HCl 50 mg | Atropine sulfate 0.04 mg, Hyoscyamine sulfate 0.19 mg, Scopolamine HBr 0.01 mg | | 1 tab q 12 hr | Not recommended | a, d |
| *Pre-Hist-D* Extended-release Tablets (Rx) [U.S.] | Chlorpheniramine maleate 8 mg | Phenylephrine HCl 20 mg | Methscopolamine nitrate 2.5 mg | Scored | 1 tab q 12 hr (max 2 tabs/day) | 6–12 yrs: ½ tab q 12 hr (max 1 tab/day) | a, d |
| *Pro-Tuss* Extended-release Tablets (Rx) [U.S.] | Chlorpheniramine maleate 8 mg | Phenylephrine HCl 25 mg, Phenylpropanolamine HCl 50 mg | Atropine sulfate 0.04 mg, Hyoscyamine sulfate 0.19 mg, Scopolamine HBr 0.01 mg | | 1 tab q 12 hr (max 2 tabs/day) | Not recommended | a, d |
| *Q-Tuss* Extended-release Tablets (Rx) [U.S.] | Chlorpheniramine maleate 8 mg | Phenylephrine HCl 25 mg, Phenylpropanolamine HCl 50 mg | Atropine sulfate 0.04 mg, Hyoscyamine sulfate 0.19 mg, Scopolamine HBr 0.01 mg | | 1 tab q 12 hr (max 2 tabs/day) | Not recommended | a, d |
| *Rolatuss SR* Extended-release Tablets (Rx) [U.S.] | Chlorpheniramine maleate 8 mg | Phenylephrine HCl 25 mg, Phenylpropanolamine HCl 50 mg | Atropine sulfate 0.04 mg, Hyoscyamine sulfate 0.19 mg, Scopolamine HBr 0.01 mg | | 1 tab q 12 hr (max 2 tabs/day) | Not recommended | a, d |
| *Ru-Tab* Extended-release Tablets (Rx) [U.S.] | Chlorpheniramine maleate 8 mg | Phenylephrine HCl 25 mg, Phenylpropanolamine HCl 50 mg | Atropine sulfate 0.04 mg, Hyoscyamine sulfate 0.19 mg, Scopolamine HBr 0.01 mg | | 1 tab q 12 hr (max 2 tabs/day) | Not recommended | a, d |
| *Ru-Tuss* Extended-release Tablets (Rx) [U.S.] | Chlorpheniramine maleate 8 mg | Phenylephrine HCl 25 mg, Phenylpropanolamine HCl 50 mg | Atropine sulfate 0.04 mg, Hyoscyamine sulfate 0.19 mg, Scopolamine HBr 0.01 mg | Scored | 1 tab q 12 hr | Not recommended | a, d |
| *Stahist* Extended-release Tablets (Rx) [U.S.] | Chlorpheniramine maleate 8 mg | Phenylephrine HCl 25 mg Phenylpropanolamine HCl 50 mg | Atropine sulfate 0.04 mg, Hyoscyamine sulfate 0.19 mg, Scopolamine HBr 0.01 mg | Scored Dye free | 1 tab q 12 hr | | a, d |

### Table 1. Oral Dosage Forms (continued)

Note: Content per capsule, tablet, or 5 mL, unless otherwise stated.

| Brand or generic name [availability] | Antihistamines | Decongestants | Anticholinergics | Other information | Usual adult and adolescent dose* (prn) | Usual pediatric dose (prn) | Packaging, storage, and auxiliary labeling† |
|---|---|---|---|---|---|---|---|
| Tuss Delay Extended-release Tablets (Rx) [U.S.] | Chlorpheniramine maleate 8 mg | Phenylephrine HCl 25 mg, Phenylpropanolamine HCl 50 mg | Atropine sulfate 0.04 mg, Hyoscyamine sulfate 0.19 mg, Scopolamine HBr 0.01 mg | | 1 tab q 12 hr (max 2 tabs/day) | Not recommended | a, d |

*Geriatric patients may be more sensitive to the effects of usual adult dose.
†For appropriate *Packaging and storage* and *Auxiliary labeling* information refer to designated letters as follows:
  a—Store below 40 °C (104 °F), preferably between 15 and 30 °C (59 and 86 °F), in a tight container, unless otherwise specified by manufacturer.
  b—Protect from freezing.
  c—May be chewed.
  d—Auxiliary labeling: • May cause drowsiness. • Avoid alcoholic beverages.

# ANTIHISTAMINES, PHENOTHIAZINE-DERIVATIVE  Systemic

This monograph includes information on the following: 1) Methdilazine†; 2) Promethazine; 3) Trimeprazine.

INN: Trimeprazine—Alimemazine

VA CLASSIFICATION (Primary/Secondary):
  Methdilazine—AH101
  Promethazine—AH101/CN309; GA700
  Trimeprazine—AH101

Commonly used brand name(s): *Anergan 25*[2]; *Anergan 50*[2]; *Antinaus 50*[2]; *Histantil*[2]; *Panectyl*[3]; *Pentazine*[2]; *Phenazine 25*[2]; *Phenazine 50*[2]; *Phencen-50*[2]; *Phenergan*[2]; *Phenergan Fortis*[2]; *Phenergan Plain*[2]; *Phenerzine*[2]; *Phenoject-50*[2]; *Pro-50*[2]; *Pro-Med 50*[2]; *Promacot*[2]; *Promet*[2]; *Prorex-25*[2]; *Prorex-50*[2]; *Prothazine*[2]; *Prothazine Plain*[2]; *Shogan*[2]; *Tacaryl*[1]; *Temaril*[3]; *V-Gan-25*[2]; *V-Gan-50*[2].

Note: For a listing of dosage forms and brand names by country availability, see *Dosage Forms* section(s).

†Not commercially available in Canada.

## Category

Antihistaminic (H₁-receptor)—Methdilazine; Promethazine; Trimeprazine.
Antiemetic—Promethazine.
Antivertigo agent—Promethazine.
Sedative-hypnotic—Promethazine; Trimeprazine.

## Indications

Note: Bracketed information in the *Indications* section refers to uses that are not included in U.S. product labeling.

**Accepted**

Rhinitis, perennial and seasonal allergic or vasomotor (treatment) or
Conjunctivitis, allergic (treatment)—Antihistamines are indicated in the symptomatic treatment of perennial and seasonal allergic rhinitis, vasomotor rhinitis, and allergic conjunctivitis due to inhalant allergens and foods.

Pruritus (treatment)
Urticaria (treatment)
Angioedema (treatment)
Dermatographism (treatment) or
Transfusion reactions, urticarial (treatment)—Antihistamines are indicated for the symptomatic treatment of pruritus associated with allergic reactions and of mild, uncomplicated allergic skin manifestations of urticaria and angioedema, in dermatographism, and in urticaria associated with transfusions. Methdilazine is also indicated in the treatment of pruritus associated with pityriasis rosea.

Sneezing (treatment) or
Rhinorrhea (treatment)—Antihistamines are indicated for the relief of sneezing and rhinorrhea associated with the common cold. However, controlled clinical studies have not demonstrated that antihistamines are significantly more effective than placebo in relieving cold symptoms.

Anaphylactic or anaphylactoid reactions (treatment adjunct)—Antihistamines are indicated as adjunctive therapy to epinephrine and other standard measures for anaphylactic reactions after the acute manifestations have been controlled, and to ameliorate the allergic reactions to blood or plasma.

Motion sickness (prophylaxis and treatment) or
Vertigo (treatment)—Promethazine is indicated for the prevention and treatment of the nausea, vomiting, dizziness, or vertigo of motion sickness.

Nausea or vomiting (prophylaxis and treatment)—Promethazine is indicated in the control of nausea and vomiting associated with certain types of anesthesia and surgery.

Sedation—Promethazine and [trimeprazine][1] are indicated for their sedative and hypnotic effects and as adjuncts to preoperative and postoperative medication.

Pain, postoperative (treatment adjunct)—Promethazine is indicated as an adjunct to analgesics for control of postoperative pain.

Analgesia adjunct, during surgery
Anesthesia, general, adjunct or
Anesthesia, local, adjunct—Intravenous administration of promethazine is indicated in special surgical situations (such as repeated bronchoscopy, ophthalmic surgery, and poor-risk patients) in combination with reduced amounts of meperidine or other narcotic analgesics as an adjunct to anesthesia and analgesia.

[1]Not included in Canadian product labeling.

## Pharmacology/Pharmacokinetics

**Physicochemical characteristics**
Chemical group—
  Phenothiazine derivatives.
Molecular weight—
  Methdilazine hydrochloride: 332.89.
  Promethazine hydrochloride: 320.88.
  Trimeprazine tartrate: 746.98.
pKa—
  Promethazine: 9.1.

**Mechanism of action/Effect**

Antihistaminic (H₁-receptor)—Antihistamines used in the treatment of allergy act by competing with histamine for H₁-receptor sites on effector cells. They thereby prevent, but do not reverse, responses mediated by histamine alone. Antihistamines antagonize, in varying degrees, most of the pharmacological effects of histamine, including urticaria and pruritus. In addition, the anticholinergic actions of most antihistamines provide a drying effect on the nasal and oral mucosa.

Antiemetic; antivertigo—The mechanism by which some antihistamines exert their antiemetic, anti-motion sickness, and antivertigo effects is not precisely known but may be related to their central anticholinergic actions. They diminish vestibular stimulation and depress labyrinthine function. Activity on the medullary chemoreceptive trigger zone may also be involved in the antiemetic effect.

Sedative-hypnotic—Most antihistamines cross the blood-brain barrier and produce sedation due to inhibition of histamine N-methyltransferase and blockage of central histaminergic receptors. Antagonism of other central nervous system receptor sites, such as those for serotonin, acetylcholine, and alpha-adrenergic stimulation, may also be involved. Phenothiazines are thought to cause indirect reduction of stimuli to the brain stem reticular system.

**Other actions/effects**
Anticholinergic—Antihistamines prevent responses to acetylcholine that are mediated via muscarinic receptors.
Antiemetic—Methdilazine and trimeprazine also possess antiemetic properties. However, only promethazine is labeled for this indication.

**Absorption**
Well absorbed after oral administration.

**Protein binding**
Promethazine—High (65–90%).

**Biotransformation**
Hepatic; some renal.

**Half-life**
Elimination—Promethazine: 7 to 14 hours.

**Onset of action**
Oral—
  15 to 60 minutes.
Parenteral—
  Promethazine:
    Intramuscular—20 minutes.
    Intravenous—3 to 5 minutes.
Rectal—
  Promethazine:
    20 minutes.

**Duration of action**
Methdilazine—6 to 12 hours.
Promethazine—4 to 6 hours; may persist for up to 12 hours.
Trimeprazine—3 to 6 hours.

**Elimination**
Renal. Most of the antihistamines studied are excreted as metabolites within 24 hours.

## Precautions to Consider

**Cross-sensitivity and/or related problems**
Patients sensitive to other phenothiazines may be sensitive to methdilazine, promethazine, and trimeprazine also.

**Carcinogenicity/Tumorigenicity/Mutagenicity**
Long-term animal studies to evaluate the carcinogenic, tumorigenic, or mutagenic potential of most antihistamines have not been performed.

**Pregnancy/Reproduction**
Pregnancy—Phenothiazines have been reported to cause jaundice and extrapyramidal symptoms in infants whose mothers received these medications during pregnancy.
  *For promethazine—*
    Adequate and well-controlled studies in humans have not been done. However, promethazine taken within 2 weeks prior to delivery may inhibit platelet aggregation in the newborn.
    Studies in rats with doses 2.1 to 4.2 times the maximum recommended human daily dose have not shown that promethazine causes adverse effects on fetal development.
    FDA Pregnancy Category C.

**Breast-feeding**
Small amounts of antihistamines may be distributed into breast milk; use is not recommended in nursing mothers because of the risk of adverse effects, such as unusual excitement or irritability, in infants.
Antihistamines may inhibit lactation because of their anticholinergic actions.
Some studies have indicated that the use of promethazine in children up to 2 years of age may be associated with the sudden infant death syndrome (SIDS) and an increase in sleep apnea, thus possibly increasing the risk to the nursing infant. Therefore, the use of phenothiazine-derivative antihistamines by nursing mothers should be discouraged until more studies have been performed to confirm the potential risk to the nursing infant.

**Pediatrics**
Use is not recommended in newborn or premature infants because this age group has an increased susceptibility to anticholinergic side effects, such as central nervous system (CNS) excitation, and an increased tendency toward convulsions.
A paradoxical reaction characterized by hyperexcitability may occur in children taking antihistamines.
The use of phenothiazine-derivative antihistamines is not recommended in infants up to 3 months of age, because of the possible absence or deficiency of detoxifying enzyme and inefficient renal function usually noted in this age group. Also, increased susceptibility to dystonias has been reported in newborn or premature infants, acutely ill or dehydrated children, and children with acute infections who have received phenothiazine medication.
Some studies have associated the use of promethazine with sudden infant death syndrome (SIDS) and with an increase in infant sleep apnea. Until more studies have been performed to confirm this potential risk, phenothiazine derivatives should not be used in children up to 2 years of age.
In children with signs and symptoms suggestive of Reye's syndrome, phenothiazine-derivative antihistamines should not be used since the extrapyramidal symptoms that may occur, especially after parenteral administration of large doses, may be confused with the CNS signs of this syndrome, thus making diagnosis difficult.

**Adolescents**
In adolescents with signs and symptoms suggestive of Reye's syndrome, phenothiazine-derivative antihistamines should not be used since the extrapyramidal symptoms that may occur, especially after parenteral administration of large doses, may be confused with the CNS signs of this syndrome, thus making diagnosis difficult.

**Geriatrics**
Dizziness, sedation, confusion, and hypotension may be more likely to occur in geriatric patients taking antihistamines.
A paradoxical reaction characterized by hyperexcitability may occur in geriatric patients taking antihistamines.
Geriatric patients are especially susceptible to the anticholinergic side effects, such as dryness of the mouth and urinary retention (especially in males), of the antihistamines. If these side effects occur and continue or are severe, the medication should probably be discontinued.
Extrapyramidal signs, especially parkinsonism, akathisia, and persistent dyskinesia, may also be more likely to occur in geriatric patients, especially at the higher doses or with parenteral administration.

**Dental**
Prolonged use of antihistamines may decrease or inhibit salivary flow, especially in middle-aged or elderly patients, thus contributing to the development of caries, periodontal disease, oral candidiasis, and discomfort.
Involuntary orofacial muscle movement may result from extrapyramidal effects. These involuntary movements may result in occlusal adjustments, bite registrations, and treatment for bruxism being less reliable.

**Drug interactions and/or related problems**
The following drug interactions and/or related problems have been selected on the basis of their potential clinical significance (possible mechanism in parentheses where appropriate)—not necessarily inclusive (» = major clinical significance):

Note:  Combination products containing any of the following medications, depending on the amount present, may also interact with this medication.

» Alcohol or
» CNS depression–producing medications, other (See *Appendix II*)
  (concurrent use may potentiate the CNS depressant effects of either these medications or antihistamines; also, concurrent use of maprotiline or tricyclic antidepressants may potentiate the anticholinergic effects of either antihistamines or these medications)

Amphetamines
  (concurrent use may decrease stimulant effects of amphetamines since phenothiazine derivatives produce alpha-adrenergic blockade)

» Anticholinergics or other medications with anticholinergic activity (See *Appendix II*)
  (anticholinergic effects may be potentiated when these medications are used concurrently with antihistamines; patients should be advised to report occurrence of gastrointestinal problems promptly since paralytic ileus may occur with concurrent therapy)

Anticonvulsants, including barbiturates
  (phenothiazine derivatives may lower the convulsion threshold; dosage adjustment of anticonvulsant medications may be necessary; potentiation of anticonvulsant effects does not occur)

Appetite suppressants
  (concurrent use with phenothiazine derivatives may antagonize the anorectic effect of appetite suppressants)

Beta-adrenergic blocking agents, especially propranolol
(concurrent use with phenothiazine derivatives may result in increased plasma concentration of each medication because of inhibition of metabolism; this may result in additive hypotensive effects, irreversible retinopathy, cardiac arrhythmias, and tardive dyskinesia)

Bromocriptine
(concurrent use may increase serum prolactin concentrations and interfere with effects of bromocriptine; dosage adjustments of bromocriptine may be necessary)

Dopamine
(concurrent use may antagonize peripheral vasoconstriction produced by high doses of dopamine because of the alpha-adrenergic blocking action of phenothiazine derivatives)

Ephedrine or
Metaraminol or
Methoxamine
(alpha-adrenergic blocking action of phenothiazine derivatives may decrease the pressor response to these medications when used concurrently)

» Epinephrine
(alpha-adrenergic effects of epinephrine may be blocked when it is used concurrently with phenothiazine derivatives, possibly resulting in severe hypotension and tachycardia)

» Extrapyramidal reaction–causing medications, other (See *Appendix II*)
(concurrent use with phenothiazine derivatives may increase the severity and frequency of extrapyramidal effects)

Guanadrel or
Guanethidine
(neuronal uptake of these medications may be inhibited when they are used concurrently with phenothiazine derivatives, causing a decrease of their antihypertensive effect)

Hepatotoxic medications, other (See *Appendix II*)
(concurrent use of phenothiazine derivatives with other hepatotoxic medications may increase the potential for hepatotoxicity; patients, especially those on prolonged therapy or with a history of liver disease, should be carefully monitored)

Hypotension-producing medications, other (See *Appendix II*)
(concurrent use with phenothiazine derivatives may produce additive hypotensive effects)

» Levodopa
(antiparkinsonian effects of levodopa may be inhibited when used concurrently with phenothiazine derivatives because of blockade of dopamine receptors in the brain; levodopa has not been shown to be effective in phenothiazine-induced parkinsonism)

» Metrizamide, intrathecal
(concurrent use with phenothiazine derivatives may lower the seizure threshold; phenothiazine derivatives should be discontinued at least 48 hours before, and not resumed for at least 24 hours following, myelography)

» Monoamine oxidase (MAO) inhibitors, including furazolidone, procarbazine, and selegiline
(concurrent use of MAO inhibitors with antihistamines in general may prolong and intensify the anticholinergic and CNS depressant effects of antihistamines; concurrent use of MAO inhibitors with phenothiazine-derivative antihistamines may increase the risk of hypotension and extrapyramidal reactions; concurrent use is not recommended)

Ototoxic medications (See *Appendix II*)
(concurrent use with antihistamines may mask the symptoms of ototoxicity such as tinnitus, dizziness, or vertigo)

Quinidine
(concurrent use with phenothiazine-derivative antihistamines may result in additive cardiac effects)

Riboflavin
(requirements for riboflavin may be increased in patients receiving phenothiazine-derivative antihistamines)

## Laboratory value alterations

The following have been selected on the basis of their potential clinical significance (possible effect in parentheses where appropriate)—not necessarily inclusive (» = major clinical significance):

With diagnostic test results
Glucose tolerance test
(an increase in glucose tolerance has been reported in patients receiving phenothiazine-derivative antihistamines)

Immunologic urine pregnancy tests
(may produce false-positive or false-negative results in patients receiving phenothiazine-derivative antihistamines, depending on the test used)

Skin tests using allergen extracts
(antihistamines may inhibit the cutaneous histamine response, thus producing false-negative results; it is recommended that antihistamines be discontinued at least 72 hours before testing begins)

## Medical considerations/Contraindications

The medical considerations/contraindications included have been selected on the basis of their potential clinical significance (reasons given in parentheses where appropriate)—not necessarily inclusive (» = major clinical significance).

*Risk-benefit should be considered when the following medical problems exist:*

» Bladder neck obstruction or
» Prostatic hypertrophy, symptomatic or
» Urinary retention, predisposition to
(anticholinergic effects may precipitate or aggravate urinary retention)

Bone marrow depression
(increased risk of leukopenia and agranulocytosis)

Cardiovascular disease
(increased risk of transient hypotension)

» Coma
(may be exacerbated)

Epilepsy
(parenteral administration of promethazine may increase severity of seizures)

» Glaucoma, angle-closure or predisposition to
(mydriatic effect resulting in increased intraocular pressure may precipitate an attack of angle-closure glaucoma)

Glaucoma, open-angle
(mydriatic effect may cause a slight increase in intraocular pressure; glaucoma therapy may need to be adjusted)

Hepatic function impairment
(metabolism may be decreased; higher serum concentrations may increase sensitivity to CNS effects)

» Jaundice
(may be exacerbated with parenteral administration of promethazine)

Reye's syndrome
(extrapyramidal symptoms that may be produced by parenteral administration of promethazine may be confused with CNS signs of Reye's syndrome)

Sensitivity to the antihistamine used

Caution is recommended when phenothiazine-derivative antihistamines are used, since their antiemetic action may impede diagnosis of such conditions as appendicitis and obscure signs of toxicity from overdosage of other drugs.

## Side/Adverse Effects

The following side/adverse effects have been selected on the basis of their potential clinical significance (possible signs and symptoms in parentheses where appropriate)—not necessarily inclusive:

### Those indicating need for medical attention
Incidence less frequent or rare
*Blood dyscrasias* (sore throat; fever; unusual bleeding or bruising; unusual tiredness or weakness)

### Those indicating need for medical attention only if they continue or are bothersome
Incidence more frequent
*Drowsiness; thickening of mucus*

Note: Sedative effects are more pronounced with promethazine and less pronounced with trimeprazine and methdilazine, in that order.

Incidence less frequent or rare
*Blurred vision or any change in vision; burning or stinging of rectum*—for promethazine rectal dosage form only; *confusion; difficult or painful urination; dizziness; dryness of mouth, nose, or throat; hypotension* (feeling faint); *increased sweating; loss of appetite; paradoxical reaction* (nightmares; unusual excitement, nervousness, restlessness, or irritability); *photosensitivity* (increased sensitivity of skin to sun); *ringing or buzzing in ears; skin rash; tachycardia* (fast heartbeat)

Note: *Confusion; difficult or painful urination; dizziness; drowsiness; and dryness of mouth, nose, or throat* are more likely to occur in the elderly.

*Nightmares, unusual excitement, nervousness, restlessness, or irritability* are more likely to occur in children and elderly patients.

## Overdose

For specific information on the agents used in the management of phenothiazine-derivative antihistamines overdose, see:
- *Antidyskinetics (Systemic)* monograph;
- *Antihistamines (Systemic)* monograph;
- *Barbiturates (Systemic)* monograph; and/or
- *Ipecac (Oral-local)* monograph.

For more information on the management of overdose or unintentional ingestion, **contact a Poison Control Center** (see *Poison Control Center Listing*).

### Clinical effects of overdose
The following effects have been selected on the basis of their potential clinical significance (possible signs and symptoms in parentheses where appropriate)—not necessarily inclusive:

Acute and chronic
**Anticholinergic effects** (clumsiness or unsteadiness; severe drowsiness; severe dryness of mouth, nose, or throat; flushing or redness of face; shortness of breath or troubled breathing); **CNS depression** (severe drowsiness); **CNS stimulation** (hallucinations; seizures; trouble in sleeping); **extrapyramidal effects** (muscle spasms, especially of neck and back; restlessness; shuffling walk; tic-like [jerky] movements of head and face; trembling and shaking of hands); **hypotension, severe** (feeling faint)

Note: *Anticholinergic* and *CNS stimulant* effects are more likely to occur in children with overdose. *Hypotension* may also occur in the elderly at usual doses.

### Treatment of overdose
Since there is no specific antidote for overdose with antihistamines, treatment is symptomatic and supportive with possible utilization of the following:

To decrease absorption—
Induction of emesis (syrup of ipecac recommended); however, precaution against aspiration is necessary, especially in infants and children.
Gastric lavage (isotonic or 0.45% sodium chloride solution) if patient is unable to vomit within 3 hours of ingestion.

To enhance elimination—
Saline cathartics (milk of magnesia) are sometimes used.

Specific treatment—
Vasopressors to treat hypotension; however, epinephrine should not be used since it may further lower blood pressure.
Anticholinergic antiparkinson agents, diphenhydramine, or barbiturates, to control extrapyramidal reactions.
Precaution against use of stimulants (analeptic agents) because they may cause seizures.

Supportive care—
Oxygen and intravenous fluids.

## Patient Consultation

As an aid to patient consultation, refer to *Advice for the Patient, Antihistamines, Phenothiazine-derivative (Systemic)*.

In providing consultation, consider emphasizing the following selected information (» = major clinical significance):

### Before using this medication
» Conditions affecting use, especially:
Sensitivity to the antihistamine used or to phenothiazine medications
Pregnancy—Not taking during the 2 weeks before delivery, to avoid possible inhibition of platelet aggregation in newborn; also, jaundice and extrapyramidal effects may occur in infant
Breast-feeding—Use not recommended; may cause unusual excitement or irritability in nursing infant; possible association with sudden infant death syndrome (SIDS) and sleep apnea
Use in children—Increased susceptibility to anticholinergic side effects in newborn or premature infants; hyperexcitability (paradoxical reaction) may occur in children; possible association with sudden infant death syndrome (SIDS) and sleep apnea; diagnosis of Reye's syndrome may be obscured if extrapyramidal effects occur
Use in adolescents—Diagnosis of Reye's syndrome may be obscured if extrapyramidal effects occur
Use in the elderly—Increased susceptibility to CNS and anticholinergic side effects; hyperexcitability (paradoxical reaction) may occur; extrapyramidal symptoms more likely to occur
Dental—Increased risk of dental problems with prolonged use because of decrease or inhibition of salivary flow; involuntary orofacial muscle movements may result from extrapyramidal effects
Other medications, especially alcohol or other CNS depressants, anticholinergics, epinephrine, extrapyramidal reaction-causing medications, levodopa, MAO inhibitors, or metrizamide (intrathecal)
Other medical problems, especially angle-closure glaucoma (or predisposition to), bladder neck obstruction, prostatic hypertrophy, or urinary retention; jaundice (for parenteral promethazine)

### Proper use of this medication
» Importance of not taking more medication than the amount recommended
» Proper dosing
Missed dose: If on scheduled dosing regimen—Using as soon as possible; not using if almost time for next dose; not doubling doses
» Proper storage

*For oral dosage forms*
Taking with food, water, or milk to minimize gastric irritation
Swallowing extended-release dosage forms whole

*For injection dosage forms*
Knowing correct administration technique for self-administration; checking with physician if necessary

*For rectal dosage forms*
Proper administration technique

*For promethazine when used to prevent motion sickness*
Taking 30 minutes to 1 hour before traveling

### Precautions while using this medication
Possible interference with skin tests using allergens; need to inform physician of using medication
May mask ototoxic effects of large doses of salicylates
» Avoiding use of alcohol or other CNS depressants
» Caution if drowsiness occurs
Possible dryness of mouth; using sugarless gum or candy, ice, or saliva substitute for relief; checking with physician or dentist if dry mouth continues for more than 2 weeks
Need to inform physician of use: Possible interference with diagnosis of appendicitis; may mask signs of toxicity from overdosage of other drugs

### Side/adverse effects
Signs of potential side effects, especially blood dyscrasias

## General Dosing Information

### For oral dosage forms only
Most antihistamines may be taken with food, water, or milk to lessen gastric irritation.

### For parenteral dosage forms only
*For promethazine—*
The preferred route of administration is by deep intramuscular injection. Although intravenous administration is well tolerated, promethazine should not be administered in concentrations greater than 25 mg per mL and at a rate in excess of 25 mg per minute. Rapid intravenous administration of promethazine may produce a transient fall in blood pressure.
Intra-arterial administration is not recommended because of the possibility of severe arteriospasm and resultant gangrene; also, subcutaneous administration is not recommended, since chemical irritation has been noted and necrotic lesions have resulted on rare occasions.

---

## METHDILAZINE

## Summary of Differences

Indications: Used in the treatment of pruritus associated with pityriasis rosea.
Pharmacology/pharmacokinetics: Duration of action—6 to 12 hours.
Side/adverse effects: Least sedative effects.

## Oral Dosage Forms

### METHDILAZINE HYDROCHLORIDE SYRUP USP

**Usual adult and adolescent dose**
Antihistaminic ($H_1$-receptor)—
 Oral, 8 mg every six to twelve hours as needed.

**Usual pediatric dose**
Antihistaminic ($H_1$-receptor)—
 Children up to 3 years of age: Use is not recommended.
 Children 3 to 12 years of age: Oral, 4 mg every six to twelve hours as needed.

**Usual geriatric dose**
See *Usual adult and adolescent dose*.
Note: Geriatric patients may be more sensitive to the effects of the usual adult dose.

**Strength(s) usually available**
U.S.—
 4 mg per 5 mL (Rx) [*Tacaryl* (alcohol 7.37%)].
Canada—
 Not commercially available.

**Packaging and storage**
Store below 40 °C (104 °F), preferably between 15 and 30 °C (59 and 86 °F), unless otherwise specified by manufacturer. Store in a tight, light-resistant container. Protect from freezing.

**Auxiliary labeling**
• May cause drowsiness.
• Avoid alcoholic beverages.

### METHDILAZINE HYDROCHLORIDE TABLETS USP

**Usual adult and adolescent dose**
See *Methdilazine Hydrochloride Syrup USP*.

**Usual pediatric dose**
See *Methdilazine Hydrochloride Syrup USP*.

**Usual geriatric dose**
See *Usual adult and adolescent dose*.
Note: Geriatric patients may be more sensitive to the effects of the usual adult dose.

**Strength(s) usually available**
U.S.—
 8 mg (Rx) [*Tacaryl* (scored)].
Canada—
 Not commercially available.

**Packaging and storage**
Store below 40 °C (104 °F), preferably between 15 and 30 °C (59 and 86 °F), unless otherwise specified by manufacturer. Store in a tight, light-resistant container.

**Auxiliary labeling**
• May cause drowsiness.
• Avoid alcoholic beverages.

### METHDILAZINE HYDROCHLORIDE TABLETS (CHEWABLE) USP

**Usual adult and adolescent dose**
See *Methdilazine Hydrochloride Syrup USP*.

**Usual pediatric dose**
See *Methdilazine Hydrochloride Syrup USP*.

**Usual geriatric dose**
See *Usual adult and adolescent dose*.
Note: Geriatric patients may be more sensitive to the effects of the usual adult dose.

**Strength(s) usually available**
U.S.—
 4 mg (Rx) [*Tacaryl*].
Canada—
 Not commercially available.

**Packaging and storage**
Store below 40 °C (104 °F), preferably between 15 and 30 °C (59 and 86 °F), unless otherwise specified by manufacturer. Store in a tight, light-resistant container.

**Auxiliary labeling**
• May cause drowsiness.
• Avoid alcoholic beverages.

---

## PROMETHAZINE

## Summary of Differences

Pharmacology/pharmacokinetics: Duration of action—Usually 4 to 6 hours.
Precautions: Medical considerations/contraindications—Caution needed in epilepsy, jaundice, and Reye's syndrome (with parenteral administration).
Side/adverse effects: Most pronounced sedative effects.

## Oral Dosage Forms

### PROMETHAZINE HYDROCHLORIDE SYRUP USP

**Usual adult and adolescent dose**
Antihistaminic ($H_1$-receptor)—
 Oral, 10 to 12.5 mg four times a day before meals and at bedtime; or 25 mg at bedtime as needed.
Antiemetic—
 Oral, 25 mg initially, then 10 to 25 mg every four to six hours as needed.
Antivertigo agent—
 Oral, 25 mg two times a day as needed.
 Note: For motion sickness, the initial 25-mg dose should be taken one-half to one hour before travel, and the dose repeated eight to twelve hours later, if necessary.
Sedative-hypnotic—
 Oral, 25 to 50 mg for nighttime, presurgical, postsurgical, or obstetrical sedation.
 Note: A 50-mg dose (with an equal amount of meperidine and an appropriate dose of an atropine-like drug) is used the night before surgery to relieve apprehension and produce sleep.

**Usual adult prescribing limits**
Up to 150 mg daily.

**Usual pediatric dose**
Children up to 2 years of age—
 Use is not recommended.
Children 2 years of age and older:
 Antihistaminic ($H_1$-receptor)—
  Oral, 125 mcg (0.125 mg) per kg of body weight or 3.75 mg per square meter of body surface every four to six hours, or 500 mcg per kg of body weight or 15 mg per square meter of body surface at bedtime as needed; or 5 to 12.5 mg three times a day or 25 mg at bedtime as needed.
 Antiemetic—
  Oral, 250 to 500 mcg (0.25 to 0.5 mg) per kg of body weight or 7.5 to 15 mg per square meter of body surface every four to six hours as needed; or 10 to 25 mg every four to six hours as needed.
 Antivertigo agent—
  Oral, 500 mcg (0.5 mg) per kg of body weight or 15 mg per square meter of body surface every twelve hours as needed; or 10 to 25 mg two times a day as needed.
 Sedative-hypnotic—
  Oral, 500 mcg (0.5 mg) to 1 mg per kg of body weight or 15 to 30 mg per square meter of body surface as needed; or 10 to 25 mg as needed.
Note: For preoperative sedation, children require doses of 1.1 mg per kg of body weight in combination with an equal dose of meperidine and the appropriate dose of an atropine-like drug.
 For postoperative sedation, 10 to 25 mg may be used.

**Usual geriatric dose**
See *Usual adult and adolescent dose*.
Note: Geriatric patients may be more sensitive to the effects of the usual adult dose.

**Strength(s) usually available**
U.S.—
 6.25 mg per 5 mL (Rx) [*Pentazine; Phenergan Plain* (alcohol 7%); *Prothazine Plain* (alcohol 7%); GENERIC].
 25 mg per 5 mL (Rx) [*Phenergan Fortis* (alcohol 1.5%); GENERIC].
Canada—
 10 mg per 5 mL (OTC) [*Phenergan* (alcohol 3%)].

**Packaging and storage**
Store below 40 °C (104 °F), preferably between 15 and 30 °C (59 and 86 °F), unless otherwise specified by manufacturer. Store in a tight, light-resistant container. Protect from freezing.

**Auxiliary labeling**
- May cause drowsiness.
- Avoid alcoholic beverages.

## PROMETHAZINE HYDROCHLORIDE TABLETS USP

**Usual adult and adolescent dose**
See *Promethazine Hydrochloride Syrup USP*.

**Usual adult prescribing limits**
Up to 150 mg daily.

**Usual pediatric dose**
See *Promethazine Hydrochloride Syrup USP*.

**Usual geriatric dose**
See *Usual adult and adolescent dose*.

Note: Geriatric patients may be more sensitive to the effects of the usual adult dose.

**Strength(s) usually available**
U.S.—
  12.5 mg (Rx) [*Phenergan* (scored); GENERIC].
  25 mg (Rx) [*Phenergan* (scored); *Promacot;* GENERIC].
  50 mg (Rx) [*Phenergan;* GENERIC].
Canada—
  10 mg (OTC) [*Phenergan* (scored)].
  25 mg (OTC) [*Histantil* (film coated); *Phenergan* (film coated)].
  50 mg (OTC) [*Histantil* (film coated); *Phenergan* (scored)].

**Packaging and storage**
Store below 40 °C (104 °F), preferably between 15 and 30 °C (59 and 86 °F), unless otherwise specified by manufacturer. Store in a tight, light-resistant container.

**Auxiliary labeling**
- May cause drowsiness.
- Avoid alcoholic beverages.

## Parenteral Dosage Forms
### PROMETHAZINE HYDROCHLORIDE INJECTION USP

**Usual adult and adolescent dose**
Antihistaminic (H$_1$-receptor)—
  Intramuscular or intravenous, 25 mg; may be repeated within two hours if necessary.
Antiemetic—
  Intramuscular or intravenous, 12.5 to 25 mg every four hours as needed.
Sedative-hypnotic—
  Intramuscular or intravenous, 25 to 50 mg for nighttime, presurgical, postsurgical, or obstetrical sedation.

  Note: For preoperative and postoperative sedation, 25 to 50 mg of promethazine may be combined with appropriately reduced doses of analgesics and anticholinergics.

  For obstetrical sedation, in the early stages of labor, 50 mg of promethazine will provide sedation and relief of apprehension. After labor is definitely established, 25 to 75 mg of promethazine may be administered with an appropriately reduced dose of an opioid analgesic, and may be repeated once or twice every four hours during the course of a normal labor.

**Usual adult prescribing limits**
Up to 150 mg daily.

**Usual pediatric dose**
Children up to 2 years of age—
  Use is not recommended.
Children 2 years of age and older:
  Antihistaminic (H$_1$-receptor)—
    Intramuscular, 125 mcg (0.125 mg) per kg of body weight or 3.75 mg per square meter of body surface every four to six hours or 500 mcg (0.5 mg) per kg of body weight or 15 mg per square meter of body surface at bedtime as needed; or 6.25 to 12.5 mg three times a day or 25 mg at bedtime as needed.
  Antiemetic—
    Intramuscular, 250 to 500 mcg (0.25 to 0.5 mg) per kg of body weight or 7.5 to 15 mg per square meter of body surface every four to six hours as needed; or 12.5 to 25 mg every four to six hours as needed.
  Sedative-hypnotic—
    Intramuscular, 500 mcg (0.5 mg) to 1 mg per kg of body weight as needed; or 12.5 to 25 mg as needed.

  Note: For preoperative sedation, children require doses of 1.1 mg per kg of body weight in combination with an equal dose of meperidine and the appropriate dose of an atropine-like drug.

  For postoperative sedation, 12.5 to 25 mg may be used.

**Usual geriatric dose**
See *Usual adult and adolescent dose*.

Note: Geriatric patients may be more sensitive to the effects of the usual adult dose.

**Strength(s) usually available**
U.S.—
  25 mg per mL (Rx) [*Anergan 25; Phenazine 25; Phenergan; Prorex-25; Prothazine; Shogan; V-Gan-25;* GENERIC].
  50 mg per mL (Rx) [*Anergan 50; Antinaus 50; Pentazine; Phenazine 50; Phencen-50; Phenergan; Phenerzine; Phenoject-50; Pro-50; Promacot; Pro-Med 50; Promet; Prorex-50; Prothazine; Shogan; V-Gan-50;* GENERIC].
Canada—
  25 mg (base) per mL (Rx) [*Phenergan;* GENERIC].

**Packaging and storage**
Store below 40 °C (104 °F), preferably between 15 and 30 °C (59 and 86 °F), unless otherwise specified by manufacturer. Protect from light. Protect from freezing.

**Stability**
Do not use if discolored or if a precipitate is present.

## Rectal Dosage Forms
### PROMETHAZINE HYDROCHLORIDE SUPPOSITORIES USP

**Usual adult and adolescent dose**
Antihistaminic (H$_1$-receptor)—
  Rectal, 25 mg; may be repeated in two hours if necessary.
Antiemetic—
  Rectal, 25 mg initially, then 12.5 to 25 mg every four to six hours as needed.
Antivertigo agent—
  Rectal, 25 mg two times a day as needed.
Sedative-hypnotic—
  Rectal, 25 to 50 mg for nighttime, presurgical, postsurgical, or obstetrical sedation.

  Note: A 50-mg dose (with an equal amount of meperidine and an appropriate dose of an atropine-like drug) is used the night before surgery to relieve apprehension and produce sleep.

**Usual adult prescribing limits**
Up to 150 mg daily.

**Usual pediatric dose**
Children up to 2 years of age—
  Use is not recommended.
Children 2 years of age and older:
  Antihistaminic (H$_1$-receptor)—
    Rectal, 125 mcg (0.125 mg) per kg of body weight or 3.75 mg per square meter of body surface every four to six hours, or 500 mcg (0.5 mg) per kg of body weight or 15 mg per square meter of body surface at bedtime as needed; or 6.25 to 12.5 mg three times a day or 25 mg at bedtime as needed.
  Antiemetic—
    Rectal, 250 to 500 mcg (0.25 to 0.5 mg) per kg of body weight or 7.5 to 15 mg per square meter of body surface every four to six hours as needed; or 12.5 to 25 mg every four to six hours as needed.
  Antivertigo agent—
    Rectal, 500 mcg (0.5 mg) per kg of body weight or 15 mg per square meter of body surface every twelve hours as needed; or 12.5 to 25 mg two times a day as needed.
  Sedative-hypnotic—
    Rectal, 500 mcg (0.5 mg) to 1 mg per kg of body weight or 15 to 30 mg per square meter of body surface as needed; or 12.5 to 25 mg as needed.

  Note: For preoperative sedation, children require doses of 1.1 mg per kg of body weight in combination with an equal dose of meperidine and the appropriate dose of an atropine-like drug.

  For postoperative sedation, 12.5 to 25 mg may be used.

**Usual geriatric dose**
See *Usual adult and adolescent dose*.

Note: Geriatric patients may be more sensitive to the effects of the usual adult dose.

**Strength(s) usually available**
U.S.—
  12.5 mg (Rx) [*Phenergan*].
  25 mg (Rx) [*Phenergan*].
  50 mg (Rx) [*Phenergan;* GENERIC].

## TRIMEPRAZINE

## Summary of Differences
Pharmacology/pharmacokinetics: Duration of action—3 to 6 hours.

## Oral Dosage Forms
Note: The dosing and strengths of the dosage forms available are expressed in terms of trimeprazine base (not the tartrate salt).

### TRIMEPRAZINE TARTRATE EXTENDED-RELEASE CAPSULES

**Usual adult and adolescent dose**
Antihistaminic ($H_1$-receptor)—
  Oral, 5 mg (base) every twelve hours as needed.

**Usual pediatric dose**
Antihistaminic ($H_1$-receptor)—
  Children up to 6 years of age: Use is not recommended.
  Children 6 years of age and over: Oral, 5 mg (base) once a day as needed.

**Usual geriatric dose**
See *Usual adult and adolescent dose.*
Note: Geriatric patients may be more sensitive to the effects of the usual adult dose.

**Strength(s) usually available**
U.S.—
  5 mg (base) (Rx) [*Temaril*].
Canada—
  Not commercially available.

**Packaging and storage**
Store below 40 °C (104 °F), preferably between 15 and 30 °C (59 and 86 °F), in a well-closed container, unless otherwise specified by manufacturer.

**Auxiliary labeling**
• May cause drowsiness.
• Avoid alcoholic beverages.

### TRIMEPRAZINE TARTRATE SYRUP USP

**Usual adult and adolescent dose**
Antihistaminic ($H_1$-receptor)—
  Oral, 2.5 mg (base) four times a day as needed.

**Usual pediatric dose**
Antihistaminic ($H_1$-receptor)—
  Children up to 2 years of age: Use is not recommended.
  Children 2 to 3 years of age: Oral, 1.25 mg (base) at bedtime or three times a day as needed.
  Children 3 years of age and over: Oral, 2.5 mg (base) at bedtime or three times a day as needed.

**Usual geriatric dose**
See *Usual adult and adolescent dose.*
Note: Geriatric patients may be more sensitive to the effects of the usual adult dose.

**Strength(s) usually available**
U.S.—
  2.5 mg (base) per 5 mL (Rx) [*Temaril* (alcohol 5.7%); GENERIC].
Canada—
  2.5 mg (base) per 5 mL (Rx) [*Panectyl* (alcohol 0.6%)].

**Packaging and storage**
Store below 40 °C (104 °F), preferably between 15 and 30 °C (59 and 86 °F), unless otherwise specified by manufacturer. Store in a tight, light-resistant container. Protect from freezing.

**Auxiliary labeling**
• May cause drowsiness.
• Avoid alcoholic beverages.

### TRIMEPRAZINE TARTRATE TABLETS USP

**Usual adult and adolescent dose**
Antihistaminic ($H_1$-receptor)—
  Oral, 2.5 mg (base) four times a day as needed.

**Usual pediatric dose**
Antihistaminic ($H_1$-receptor)—
  Children up to 2 years of age: Use is not recommended.
  Children 2 to 3 years of age: The available strength of the tablet may not conform to the recommended pediatric dosage. See *Trimeprazine Tartrate Syrup USP.*
  Children 3 years of age and over: Oral, 2.5 mg (base) at bedtime or three times a day as needed.

**Usual geriatric dose**
See *Usual adult and adolescent dose.*
Note: Geriatric patients may be more sensitive to the effects of the usual adult dose.

**Strength(s) usually available**
U.S.—
  2.5 mg (base) (Rx) [*Temaril*].
Canada—
  2.5 mg (base) (Rx) [*Panectyl*].
  5 mg (base) (Rx) [*Panectyl*].

**Packaging and storage**
Store below 40 °C (104 °F), preferably between 15 and 30 °C (59 and 86 °F), unless otherwise specified by manufacturer. Store in a well-closed, light-resistant container.

**Auxiliary labeling**
• May cause drowsiness.
• Avoid alcoholic beverages.

## Selected Bibliography
Simons FE, Simons KJ: $H_1$-receptor antagonist treatment of chronic rhinitis. J Allergy Clin Immunol 1988; 81: 975-80.
Simons FE, Simons KJ, Chung M, Yeh J. The comparative pharmacokinetics of $H_1$-receptor antagonists. Ann Allergy 1987 Dec; 59: 20-4.

Revised: 07/26/94

---

Canada—
  Not commercially available.

**Packaging and storage**
Store between 2 and 8 °C (36 and 46 °F), in a tight, light-resistant container, unless otherwise specified by manufacturer.

**Auxiliary labeling**
• May cause drowsiness.
• Avoid alcoholic beverages.

**Note**
Include patient instructions when dispensing.
Explain administration technique.

---

# ANTI-INFLAMMATORY DRUGS, NONSTEROIDAL Ophthalmic

This monograph includes information on the following: 1) Diclofenac; 2) Flurbiprofen; 3) Indomethacin*; 4) Suprofen†.
INN: Indomethacin—Indometacin
VA CLASSIFICATION (Primary/Secondary):
  Diclofenac—OP302/OP900
  Flurbiprofen—OP900/OP302
  Indomethacin—OP900/OP302
  Suprofen—OP900
Commonly used brand name(s): *Indocid*[3]; *Ocufen*[2]; *Profenal*[4]; *Voltaren Ophtha*[1]; *Voltaren Ophthalmic*[1].
Another commonly used name for indomethacin* is indometacin.

Note: For a listing of dosage forms and brand names by country availability, see *Dosage Forms* section(s).

*Not commercially available in U.S.
†Not commercially available in Canada.

## Category
Prostaglandin synthesis inhibitor, ophthalmic—Diclofenac; Flurbiprofen; Indomethacin; Suprofen.
Anti-inflammatory, nonsteroidal, ophthalmic—Diclofenac; Flurbiprofen; Indomethacin.
Miosis inhibitor, in ophthalmic surgery—Diclofenac; Flurbiprofen; Indomethacin; Suprofen.

# Anti-inflammatory Drugs, Nonsteroidal (Ophthalmic)

## Indications

Note: Bracketed information in the *Indications* section refers to uses that are not included in U.S. product labeling.

### Accepted

Inflammation, ocular (treatment)—Diclofenac is indicated to reduce postoperative inflammation following cataract surgery. [Diclofenac is also indicated in the treatment of conjunctivitis, keratoconjunctivitis, corneal ulcers, and posttraumatic inflammation of the cornea and conjunctiva, provided that these conditions are not associated with an ocular infection.] [Flurbiprofen] and indomethacin[1] are indicated to reduce inflammation of the anterior segment of the eye following ocular surgery or laser trabeculoplasty. However, flurbiprofen and indomethacin have produced inconsistent results in clinical studies and may not produce clinically significant reductions in postprocedure inflammation. In one study, these nonsteroidal anti-inflammatory drugs (NSAIDs) reduced conjunctival injection, but not the anterior chamber reaction, following argon laser trabeculoplasty.

Ophthalmic NSAIDs may be administered concurrently with an ophthalmic corticosteroid, if necessary. There is some evidence of a synergistic or additive effect when the two types of medication are used together.

Miosis, during ophthalmic surgery (prophylaxis)—[Diclofenac], flurbiprofen, indomethacin, and suprofen are indicated to inhibit intraoperative miosis, which may occur in response to surgical trauma despite preoperative establishment of mydriasis. These NSAIDs may facilitate cataract extraction and lens implantation. However, published clinical studies have shown small and variable effects on pupil size, and some investigators have reported flurbiprofen to be ineffective. Also, studies demonstrating that ophthalmic NSAIDs produce clinically significant inhibition of miosis in surgical procedures other than cataract surgery have not been published.

Use of ophthalmic NSAIDs to inhibit miosis during surgery does not eliminate the need for mydriatic agents prior to and during surgery.

Edema, cystoid macular, following cataract surgery (prophylaxis and treatment)—[Diclofenac] and indomethacin are indicated to reduce the occurrence and severity of cystoid macular edema following cataract surgery. These agents are usually used concurrently with an ophthalmic corticosteroid; clinical studies indicate that concurrent use of both types of medication provides a synergistic effect.

There is insufficient evidence to determine whether flurbiprofen or suprofen is effective in reducing cystoid macular edema following cataract surgery.

Photophobia, following incisional refractive surgery—Diclofenac is indicated for the treatment of photophobia in patients who have undergone incisional refractive surgery.

---

[1]Not included in Canadian product labeling.

## Pharmacology/Pharmacokinetics

### Physicochemical characteristics

Chemical group—
Anti-inflammatory drug, nonsteroidal (NSAID)—
  Indoleacetic acid derivative—Indomethacin.
  Phenylacetic acid derivative—Diclofenac.
  Propionic acid derivatives—Flurbiprofen, suprofen.
Molecular weight—
  Diclofenac sodium: 318.13.
  Flurbiprofen sodium: 302.28.
  Indomethacin: 357.79.
  Suprofen: 260.31.

### Mechanism of action/Effect

Ophthalmic NSAIDs inhibit the activity of the enzyme cyclo-oxygenase in ocular tissues, resulting in decreased formation of precursors of prostaglandins from arachidonic acid and subsequent inhibition of prostaglandin synthesis. These medications do not inhibit the actions of prostaglandins. Studies in animals have shown that trauma to the anterior segment of the eye, especially the iris, increases endogenous prostaglandin synthesis; that endogenous prostaglandins produce constriction of the iris sphincter independently of cholinergic mechanisms; and that endogenous prostaglandins may contribute to the development of intraocular inflammation by causing disruption of the blood–aqueous humor barrier, vasodilatation, increased vascular permeability, and leukocytosis. It is proposed that inhibition of prostaglandin synthesis in ocular tissues by ophthalmic NSAIDs decreases these effects, thereby reducing the severity of intraoperative miosis, signs and symptoms of postoperative inflammation, and postoperative cystoid macular edema (which may occur, independently of inflammation, because of prostaglandin-induced alterations in vascular permeability). Diclofenac and indomethacin have been shown to stabilize, or speed postoperative re-establishment of, the blood–aqueous humor barrier. However, the clinical consequences (benefit or harm) of this action in the treatment of postoperative inflammation have not been determined. Also, studies of flurbiprofen's or indomethacin's efficacy in reducing ocular inflammation following ophthalmic procedures have produced conflicting results. It is proposed that the anti-inflammatory activity of these medications may be limited, possibly because they do not inhibit the formation or activity of mediators of inflammation in the eye other than prostaglandins.

### Other actions/effects

Clinical studies indicate that perioperative use of ophthalmic NSAIDs does not significantly affect intraocular pressure.

Ophthalmic NSAIDs may increase the risk of bleeding in ocular tissues following ophthalmic procedures; postoperative bleeding, including hyphema, has been documented with flurbiprofen.

Studies in animals have shown that ophthalmic flurbiprofen may delay wound healing following certain types of surgery. Diclofenac also may slow or delay healing postoperatively. However, ophthalmic suprofen did not delay wound healing in a study in animals.

The anti-inflammatory activity of ophthalmic NSAIDs may mask the onset and/or progression of ocular infections.

### Absorption

Diclofenac—Studies suggest that limited, if any, systemic absorption occurs after a single application of up to 16 drops of a 0.1% solution.

Flurbiprofen—Flurbiprofen penetrates the cornea; significant systemic absorption may occur. In one study, 74% of the quantity of flurbiprofen applied to the conjunctiva appeared in the systemic circulation.

Indomethacin—The medication has not been detected in serum after ophthalmic administration. However, the possibility of significant systemic absorption must be considered, because a bronchospastic reaction has been reported in one asthmatic patient following ophthalmic administration of the medication.

Suprofen—No data regarding the extent of systemic absorption following ophthalmic application are available.

## Precautions to Consider

### Cross-sensitivity and/or related problems

Patients sensitive to aspirin or other systemically administered nonsteroidal anti-inflammatory drugs (NSAIDs) may be sensitive to ophthalmic NSAIDs also.

### Carcinogenicity

*Diclofenac*—No evidence of carcinogenicity was found in long-term studies in rats or mice receiving up to 2 mg per kg of body weight (mg/kg) per day orally.

*Flurbiprofen*—No evidence of carcinogenicity was found in a 24-month study in rats receiving up to 4 mg/kg per day, a second 24-month study in rats receiving 12 mg/kg per day for 32 weeks followed by 5 mg/kg per day thereafter, or an 80-week study in mice receiving up to 12 mg/kg per day orally.

*Indomethacin*—No evidence of carcinogenicity was found in long-term studies in rats or mice receiving up to 1.5 mg/kg per day orally.

*Suprofen*—No evidence of carcinogenicity was found in long-term studies in rats or mice receiving up to 40 mg/kg per day orally.

### Tumorigenicity

*Diclofenac*—A slight increase in the occurrence of benign mammary fibroadenomas was found in female rats, but the increase was not significant for this common rat tumor. No other evidence of tumorigenicity was found in rats receiving up to 2 mg/kg per day orally.

*Flurbiprofen*—No evidence of tumorigenicity was found in a 2-year study in rats receiving up to 12 mg/kg per day for 32 weeks, followed by up to 5 mg/kg per day orally for the remainder of the study period.

*Indomethacin*—No evidence of tumorigenicity was found in an 81-week study in rats receiving up to 1 mg/kg per day orally.

*Suprofen*—An increased incidence of benign hepatomas occurred in female mice receiving 40 mg/kg per day and in male mice receiving 2 mg/kg per day or more orally.

### Mutagenicity

*Diclofenac*—No mutagenic activity was found in *in vitro* tests using mammalian cells or bacteria (with or without microsomal activation) or in various *in vivo* tests.

*Flurbiprofen*—Long-term mutagenicity studies have not been performed.

*Indomethacin*—No mutagenic activity was found in *in vitro* tests (Ames test or *E. coli*, with or without metabolic activation) or in *in vivo* tests (host-mediated assay, sex-linked recessive lethals in *Drosophila*, and micronucleus test in mice).

*Suprofen*—No mutagenic activity was found in the Ames, micronucleus, and dominant lethal tests.

## Pregnancy/Reproduction

*Fertility*—*Diclofenac*: No impairment of fertility was found in reproduction studies in rats receiving up to 4 mg/kg per day orally.

*Flurbiprofen*: No impairment of fertility was found in reproduction studies in rats receiving up to 4 mg/kg per day orally.

*Indomethacin*: No impairment of fertility was found in a 2-generation reproduction study in rats or in a 2-litter reproduction study in rats receiving up to 0.5 mg/kg per day orally.

*Suprofen*: No impairment of fertility was found in reproduction studies in rats receiving up to 40 mg/kg per day. However, a slight reduction in fertility was found in rats receiving 80 mg/kg per day orally. Testicular atrophy and hypoplasia occurred in a 6-month study in dogs receiving 80 mg/kg per day and a 12-month study in rats receiving 40 mg/kg per day orally.

*Pregnancy*—Adequate and well-controlled studies with ophthalmic NSAIDs have not been performed in pregnant women. However, use of ophthalmic NSAIDs late in pregnancy is not recommended because oral NSAIDs caused premature closure of the ductus arteriosus in animal studies.

*First trimester*
Diclofenac:
Diclofenac readily crosses the placenta.
No teratogenicity occurred in reproduction studies in mice receiving up to 20 mg/kg per day orally and in rats and rabbits receiving up to 10 mg/kg per day orally. However, maternal toxicity and embryotoxicity (reduced fetal weights and growth, reduced fetal survival) occurred in studies in rats receiving 2 or 4 mg/kg per day. Also, increases in resorption rates, decreased fetal weight, abnormal skeletal findings, and definite embryotoxicity occurred in studies in rabbits receiving 5 or 10 mg/kg per day orally.
FDA Pregnancy Category B.

Flurbiprofen:
Flurbiprofen crosses the placenta.
No teratogenicity occurred in reproduction studies in mice receiving up to 12 mg/kg per day, rats receiving up to 25 mg/kg per day, or rabbits receiving up to 7.5 mg/kg per day, orally. However, studies in rats have shown doses of 0.4 mg/kg per day or higher to be embryotoxic or embryocidal (causing reduced weight or slower fetal growth, increased stillbirths, and decreased pup survival). Also, stillbirths, retained fetuses, and/or fetal distress occurred in studies in rats receiving as little as 0.2 mg/kg per day. In addition, fetotoxicity related to maternal toxicity (gastrointestinal ulceration, retardation of weight gain, intrauterine hemorrhage, and maternal deaths) occurred in rats receiving 25 mg/kg per day from Days 1 through 20 of pregnancy. With lower doses (0.2, 0.675, or 2.25 mg/kg per day), such effects did not occur when the medication was discontinued on Day 17 of pregnancy. Maternal deaths due to gastrointestinal ulceration also occurred in rabbits receiving the medication.
FDA Pregnancy Category C.

Indomethacin:
Indomethacin crosses the placenta.
Studies in rats and mice have shown that indomethacin in doses of 4 mg/kg per day orally causes retarded ossification secondary to decreased average fetal weight. In other studies in mice, higher doses (5 to 15 mg/kg per day orally) caused maternal toxicity and death, increased fetal resorptions, and fetal malformations. Doses lower than 4 mg/kg per day produced no adverse effects in these studies.

Suprofen:
Studies in rats receiving 40 mg/kg or more per day, and rabbits receiving 80 mg/kg or more per day, orally have shown that suprofen causes an increased incidence of fetal resorption associated with maternal toxicity. In rats receiving 2.5 mg/kg or more per day orally, there was an increase in stillbirths and a decrease in pup survival.
FDA Pregnancy Category C.

*Third trimester*
Diclofenac:
Studies in animals have shown that maternally toxic doses, administered orally, are associated with prolonged gestation and dystocia.

Flurbiprofen:
Studies in rats have shown that administration of 0.4 mg/kg or more per day orally causes prolonged gestation and delayed parturition.

Indomethacin:
Studies in rats and mice have shown that administration of 4 mg/kg per day orally during the last 3 days of gestation is associated with an increased incidence of neuronal necrosis in the diencephalon and some maternal and fetal deaths. Indomethacin also caused a slight delay in the onset of parturition in rats, but not in rabbits.

Suprofen:
Studies in rats have shown that suprofen causes a delay in parturition.

## Breast-feeding

Although it is not known whether NSAIDs are distributed into breast milk after ophthalmic administration, it is known that orally administered diclofenac, indomethacin, and suprofen are distributed into human breast milk. It is not known whether orally administered flurbiprofen is distributed into breast milk. However, problems in humans have not been documented with any of these medications.

## Pediatrics

Appropriate studies on the relationship of age to the effects of ophthalmic NSAIDs have not been performed in the pediatric population. Safety and efficacy have not been established.

## Geriatrics

Studies performed to date have not demonstrated geriatrics-specific problems that would limit the usefulness of ophthalmic NSAIDs in the elderly.

## Drug interactions and/or related problems

The following drug interactions and/or related problems have been selected on the basis of their potential clinical significance (possible mechanism in parentheses where appropriate)—not necessarily inclusive (» = major clinical significance):

Note: Combinations containing any of the following medications, depending on the amount present, may also interact with this medication.

Acetylcholine chloride or
Carbachol
(these medications may be less effective when administered after an ophthalmic NSAID has been used to inhibit miosis during ocular surgery; although the pharmacologic basis for the interaction has not been established, it has been suggested that NSAID-induced maintenance of a larger pupillary diameter during surgery, and the possibility that the duration of action of the NSAID may exceed that of acetylcholine chloride, may account for the apparent reduction in the ability of acetylcholine chloride to reverse mydriasis postoperatively)

Any medication that may interfere with blood clotting or prolong bleeding time, such as:
Anticoagulants, coumarin- or indandione-derivative or
Heparin or
Platelet aggregation inhibitors
(concurrent use with ophthalmic NSAIDs, which may also increase the bleeding tendency, may increase the risk of postoperative ocular bleeding)

Epinephrine (ophthalmic) and possibly other antiglaucoma agents
(the possibility should be considered that ophthalmic flurbiprofen may decrease the intraocular pressure–lowering effects of these medications; however, in one study, administration of ophthalmic flurbiprofen [1 drop every 10 minutes for 4 doses] had no effect on the intraocular pressure–lowering effect of 1% apraclonidine or 0.5% timolol)

## Medical considerations/Contraindications

The medical considerations/contraindications included have been selected on the basis of their potential clinical significance (reasons given in parentheses where appropriate)—not necessarily inclusive (» = major clinical significance).

### Risk-benefit should be considered when the following medical problems exist:

» Allergic reaction, such as anaphylaxis, bronchospasm, angioedema, allergic rhinitis, or urticaria, to aspirin or other systemic NSAIDs, history of
(possibility of cross-sensitivity)

Epithelial herpes simplex keratitis, active
(in one study in rabbits, ophthalmic flurbiprofen exacerbated herpes simplex keratitis [i.e., increased ulceration and conjunctivitis] and delayed healing; however, in another study in rabbits, neither flurbiprofen nor diclofenac exacerbated or prolonged acute herpes keratitis or prolonged viral shedding; although the risk of exacerbation or delayed healing of active epithelial herpes simplex keratitis in

humans has not been determined, it is recommended that ophthalmic NSAIDs be administered with caution and in conjunction with an antiviral agent)

(suprofen is contraindicated in patients with active herpes simplex keratitis)

Epithelial herpes simplex keratitis, history of
(close monitoring of the patient following flurbiprofen administration is recommended because the risk of reactivation has not been determined)
(close monitoring of the patient following suprofen administration is recommended)

Hemophilia or other bleeding problems or coagulation defects or
Prolonged bleeding time
(increased risk of bleeding)

» Sensitivity to the ophthalmic NSAID considered for use

Soft contact lenses, use of
(wearing hydrogel soft contact lenses while using diclofenac is contraindicated because ocular irritation, such as redness and burning of the eye, may occur)

## Side/Adverse Effects

Note: Oral administration of suprofen has caused acute flank pain and renal insufficiency, possibly manifestations of acute uric acid nephropathy. This reaction has occurred after ingestion of as few as 1 or 2 doses of 200 mg, > 25 times more than the total quantity of suprofen that would be administered over 2 days with recommended ophthalmic doses. The risk of such a reaction occurring after ophthalmic administration is unknown.

Keratitis, elevated intraocular pressure, corneal edema, chemosis, and anterior chamber reaction have also been reported with various ophthalmic nonsteroidal anti-inflammatory drugs (NSAIDs). Since these effects frequently occur following some types of ophthalmic procedures, a causal relationship has not been established.

The following side/adverse effects have been selected on the basis of their potential clinical significance (possible signs and symptoms in parentheses where appropriate)—not necessarily inclusive:

### Those indicating need for medical attention
Incidence less frequent or rare
*For diclofenac*
**Allergic reaction** (itching; tearing)—in a patient hypersensitive to systemic NSAIDs; **corneal opacity** (blurred vision or other change in vision); **discharge, ocular** (sticky or matted eyelashes); **facial edema** (swelling of face); **fever or chills; iritis** (throbbing pain; tearing; sensitivity to light); **nausea or vomiting; pain**

*For flurbiprofen*
**Bleeding in eye; redness in eye**—not resulting from surgery and not present before use; **fibrosis**

*For indomethacin*
**Bronchospastic allergic reaction** (shortness of breath; troubled breathing; tightness in chest; wheezing)—reported in an asthmatic patient; **corneal epithelial defects, including corneal abrasion and punctate keratitis; redness in eye**—not resulting from surgery and not present before use; **striate keratopathy**

*For suprofen*
**Iritis** (throbbing pain; tearing; sensitivity to light); **punctate epithelial staining**

Note: *Eye pain* and *photophobia* have also been reported independently of iritis.

### Those indicating need for medical attention only if they continue or are bothersome
Incidence more frequent
**Dry eye; irritation, ocular** (burning; stinging; itching; mild discomfort)
Incidence less frequent or rare
**Asthenia** (unusual weakness); **headache; insomnia; miosis** (smaller pupils [black part of eye]); **mydriasis** (bigger pupils [black part of eye]); **rhinitis** (runny or stuffy nose)

## Overdose

For more information on the management of overdose or unintentional ingestion, **contact a Poison Control Center** (see *Poison Control Center Listing*).

### Treatment of overdose
Recommended treatment in case of accidental ingestion consists of drinking large quantities of fluids, to dilute the medication.

## Patient Consultation

As an aid to patient consultation, refer to *Advice for the Patient, Anti-inflammatory Drugs, Nonsteroidal (Ophthalmic)*.

In providing consultation, consider emphasizing the following selected information (» = major clinical significance):

### Before using this medication
» Conditions affecting use, especially:
Sensitivity to aspirin or other systemic nonsteroidal anti-inflammatory drugs (NSAIDs), or to the ophthalmic NSAID considered for use
Pregnancy—Diclofenac, flurbiprofen, and indomethacin known to cross the placenta when administered systemically
Breast-feeding—Indomethacin and suprofen known to be distributed into breast milk after oral administration

### Proper use of this medication
Proper administration technique
Preventing contamination: Not touching dropper or applicator tip to any surface and keeping container tightly closed
» Importance of not using more medication than the amount prescribed
» Checking with physician before using medication for future eye problems
» Proper dosing
Missed dose: Using as soon as possible; not using if almost time for next dose
» Proper storage

### Precautions while using this medication
» For diclofenac: Not wearing soft contact lenses during treatment

### Side/adverse effects
Signs of potential side effects, especially allergic reaction; corneal opacity; ocular discharge; facial edema; fever or chills; iritis; nausea or vomiting; pain, bleeding or redness in the eye; fibrosis; bronchospastic allergic reaction; corneal epithelial defects, including corneal abrasion, and punctate keratitis; striate keratopathy; and punctate epithelial staining.

## General Dosing Information

When an ophthalmic nonsteroidal anti-inflammatory drug (NSAID) is used to prevent or reduce postoperative inflammation and/or cystoid macular edema, therapy should be started prior to the procedure. Ophthalmic NSAIDs are more effective in inhibiting the development of these complications than in treating them after they have fully developed.

---

### DICLOFENAC

## Additional Dosing Information

It is recommended that patients not wear hydrogel soft contact lenses during diclofenac therapy. Ocular irritation manifested by redness and burning has occurred in patients wearing this type of contact lens while using the medication.

## Ophthalmic Dosage Forms

Note: Bracketed uses in the *Dosage Forms* section refer to categories of use and/or indications that are not included in U.S. product labeling.

### DICLOFENAC SODIUM OPHTHALMIC SOLUTION

**Usual adult dose**

Anti-inflammatory, nonsteroidal, ophthalmic—
Treatment of inflammation following cataract surgery: Topical, to the conjunctiva, 1 drop in the affected eye four times a day, starting twenty-four hours postoperatively and continuing for the first two postoperative weeks. In some patients, treatment has been continued for six weeks or longer.

[Treatment of conjunctivitis, keratoconjunctivitis, corneal ulcers, or post-traumatic inflammation]: Topical, to the conjunctiva, 1 drop in the affected eye four to five times a day, depending on the severity of the disease.

[Miosis inhibitor, in ophthalmic surgery] and
[Prostaglandin synthesis inhibitor, ophthalmic]—
Prevention or reduction of intraoperative miosis and postoperative cystoid macular edema: Topical, to the conjunctiva, 1 drop in the affected eye, applied up to five times during the three hours prior to surgery; fifteen minutes, thirty minutes, and forty-five minutes postoperatively; then three to five times a day for as long as needed.

Photophobia, in incisional refractive surgery—
Topical, to the conjunctiva, 1 drop in the affected eye within one hour prior to surgery, then 1 drop within fifteen minutes after surgery, then 1 drop four times a day beginning four to six hours after surgery and continuing for up to three days as needed.

**Usual pediatric dose**
Safety and efficacy have not been established.

**Strength(s) usually available**
U.S.—
  0.1% (1 mg per mL) (Rx) [*Voltaren Ophthalmic* (boric acid; edetate disodium 1 mg per mL; polyoxyl 35 castor oil; sorbic acid 2 mg per mL; tromethamine)].
Canada—
  0.1% (1 mg per mL) (Rx) [*Voltaren Ophtha* (boric acid; cremophor EL; edetate disodium; sorbic acid; tromethamine [TRIS])].

**Packaging and storage**
Store between 15 and 30 °C (59 and 86 °F), protected from light and from freezing, unless otherwise directed by manufacturer.

**Auxiliary labeling**
• For the eye.

**Note**
Dispense in original unopened container.

---

### FLURBIPROFEN

## Ophthalmic Dosage Forms
Note: Bracketed uses in the *Dosage Forms* section refer to categories of use and/or indications that are not included in U.S. product labeling.

**FLURBIPROFEN SODIUM OPHTHALMIC SOLUTION USP**

**Usual adult dose**
Miosis inhibitor, in ophthalmic surgery—
  Topical, to the conjunctiva, 1 drop every thirty minutes, beginning two hours prior to surgery, for a total of 4 drops.
[Anti-inflammatory, nonsteroidal, ophthalmic]—
  Treatment of inflammation following ophthalmic surgery or laser trabeculoplasty: Topical, to the conjunctiva, 1 drop every four hours for one to three weeks.

**Usual pediatric dose**
Safety and efficacy have not been established.

**Strength(s) usually available**
U.S.—
  0.03% (Rx) [*Ocufen* (polyvinyl alcohol 1.4%; edetate disodium; thimerosal 0.005%; potassium chloride; sodium chloride; sodium citrate; citric acid; hydrochloric acid and/or sodium hydroxide)].
Canada—
  0.03% (Rx) [*Ocufen* (citric acid; edetate disodium; hydrochloric acid and/or sodium hydroxide; polyvinyl alcohol; potassium chloride; sodium chloride; sodium citrate; thimerosal)].

**Packaging and storage**
Store below 40 °C (104 °F), preferably between 15 and 30 °C (59 and 86 °F), unless otherwise specified by manufacturer. Store in a tight container. Protect from light.

**Auxiliary labeling**
• For the eye.

**Note**
Dispense in original unopened container.

---

### INDOMETHACIN

## Additional Dosing Information
Because an ophthalmic dosage form of indomethacin is not commercially available in the U.S., ophthalmic preparations are being compounded extemporaneously in some pharmacies. Eye injuries resulting from *Pseudomonas* contamination have occurred following use of such preparations. Pharmacists are advised **not** to use the contents of commercially available indomethacin capsules in the preparation of ophthalmic indomethacin solutions or suspensions, because of a lack of data on stability, concentration, and possible effects of excipients. Also, the sterility of compounded preparations must be assured.

## Ophthalmic Dosage Forms
**INDOMETHACIN OPHTHALMIC SUSPENSION**

**Usual adult dose**
Prostaglandin synthesis inhibitor, ophthalmic and
Miosis inhibitor, in cataract surgery—
  Prevention or reduction of intraoperative miosis and postoperative cystoid macular edema: Topical, to the conjunctiva, 1 drop four times a day on the day prior to surgery, 1 drop forty-five minutes before surgery, then 1 drop four times a day for ten to twelve weeks postoperativelyor as long as needed.

**Usual pediatric dose**
Safety and efficacy have not been established.

**Strength(s) usually available**
U.S.—
  Not commercially available.
Canada—
  1% (10 mg per mL) (Rx) [*Indocid* (lecithin; sodium bisulfite; sodium chloride; polysorbate 80; hydroxyethylcellulose; sorbitol; disodium edetate; benzalkonium chloride solution 0.02%; benzyl alcohol 0.25%; phenylethyl alcohol 0.25%)].

**Packaging and storage**
Store between 15 and 30 °C (59 and 86 °F), protected from light and from freezing, unless otherwise specified by manufacturer.

**Auxiliary labeling**
• For the eye.
• Shake well before using.

**Note**
Dispense in original unopened container.

---

### SUPROFEN

## Ophthalmic Dosage Forms
**SUPROFEN OPHTHALMIC SOLUTION USP**

**Usual adult dose**
Miosis inhibitor, in ophthalmic surgery—
  Topical, to the conjunctiva, 2 drops three, two, and one hour prior to surgery. If desired, 2 drops may be applied every four hours while the patient is awake on the day prior to surgery.

**Usual pediatric dose**
Safety and efficacy have not been established.

**Strength(s) usually available**
U.S.—
  1% (10 mg per mL) (Rx) [*Profenal* (thimerosal 0.005%; caffeine 2%; edetate disodium; dibasic sodium phosphate; monobasic sodium phosphate; sodium chloride; sodium hydroxide and/or hydrochloric acid)].
Canada—
  Not commercially available.

**Packaging and storage**
Store below 40 °C (104 °F), preferably between 15 and 30 °C (59 and 86 °F), protected from freezing, unless otherwise directed by manufacturer.

**Auxiliary labeling**
• For the eye.

**Note**
Dispense in original unopened container.

## Selected Bibliography
Keates RH, McGowan KA. Clinical trial of flurbiprofen to maintain pupillary dilation during cataract surgery. Ann Ophthalmol 1984; 16: 919-21.
Heinrichs DA, Leith AB. Effect of flurbiprofen on the maintenance of pupillary dilation during cataract surgery. Can J Ophthalmol 1990; 25: 239-42.
Stark WJ, Fagadau WR, Stewart RH, et al. Reduction of pupillary constriction during cataract surgery using suprofen. Arch Ophthalmol 1986; 104: 364-6.
Flach AJ. Cyclo-oxygenase inhibitors in ophthalmology. Surv Ophthalmol 1992; 36: 259-84.

Revised: 08/14/98

# ANTI-INFLAMMATORY DRUGS, NONSTEROIDAL   Systemic

This monograph includes information on the following: 1) Diclofenac; 2) Diflunisal; 3) Etodolac†; 4) Fenoprofen; 5) Floctafenine*; 6) Flurbiprofen; 7) Ibuprofen; 8) Indomethacin; 9) Ketoprofen; 10) Meclofenamate†; 11) Mefenamic Acid; 12) Nabumetone; 13) Naproxen; 14) Oxaprozin†; 15) Phenylbutazone; 16) Piroxicam; 17) Sulindac; 18) Tenoxicam*; 19) Tiaprofenic Acid*; 20) Tolmetin

Note: See also individual *Ketorolac (Systemic)* monograph.

See also *Indomethacin (Systemic—For Patent Ductus Arteriosus)*.

See also *Anti-inflammatory Agents, Nonsteroidal (Ophthalmic)* for information on ophthalmic use of diclofenac, flurbiprofen, and indomethacin.

See also *Salicylates (Systemic)* for information on aspirin and other salicylates.

INN:
Etodolac†—Etodolic acid.
Indomethacin†—Indometacin.
Meclofenamate†—Meclofenamic acid.

BAN:
Meclofenamate†—Meclofenamic acid.

JAN:
Indomethacin†—Indometacin.

VA CLASSIFICATION (Primary/Secondary):
Diclofenac—MS102/CN104; MS400; CN105
Diflunisal—MS102/CN104; MS400; CN105
Etodolac—MS102/CN104; MS400; CN105
Fenoprofen—MS102/CN104; MS400; CN105
Floctafenine—CN104/CN105; MS400
Flurbiprofen—MS102
Ibuprofen—MS102/CN104; CN850; MS400; CN105
Indomethacin—MS102/MS400; CN850; CN105; CV900
Ketoprofen—MS102/CN104; MS400; CN105
Meclofenamate—MS102/CN104; CN105
Mefenamic Acid—CN104/CN105
Nabumetone—MS102
Naproxen—MS102/CN104; CN850; MS400; CN105
Oxaprozin—MS102
Phenylbutazone—MS102/MS400
Piroxicam—MS102/MS400
Sulindac—MS102/MS400
Tenoxicam—MS102
Tiaprofenic Acid—MS102
Tolmetin—MS102

Commonly used brand name(s): *Actiprofen Caplets*[7]; *Actron*[9]; *Advil*[7]; *Advil Caplets*[7]; *Advil, Children's*[7]; *Albert Tiafen*[19]; *Aleve*[13]; *Alka Butazolidin*[15]; *Anaprox*[13]; *Anaprox DS*[13]; *Ansaid*[6]; *Apo-Diclo*[1]; *Apo-Diflunisal*[2]; *Apo-Flurbiprofen*[6]; *Apo-Ibuprofen*[7]; *Apo-Indomethacin*[8]; *Apo-Keto*[9]; *Apo-Keto-E*[9]; *Apo-Napro-Na*[13]; *Apo-Napro-Na DS*[13]; *Apo-Naproxen*[13]; *Apo-Phenylbutazone*[15]; *Apo-Piroxicam*[16]; *Apo-Sulin*[17]; *Bayer Select Ibuprofen Pain Relief Formula Caplets*[7]; *Butazolidin*[15]; *Cataflam*[1]; *Clinoril*[17]; *Cotylbutazone*[15]; *Cramp End*[7]; *Daypro*[14]; *Dolgesic*[7]; *Dolobid*[2]; *EC-Naprosyn*[13]; *Excedrin IB*[7]; *Excedrin IB Caplets*[7]; *Feldene*[16]; *Froben*[6]; *Froben SR*[6]; *Genpril*[7]; *Genpril Caplets*[7]; *Haltran*[7]; *Ibifon 600 Caplets*[7]; *Ibren*[7]; *Ibu*[7]; *Ibu-200*[7]; *Ibu-4*[7]; *Ibu-6*[7]; *Ibu-8*[7]; *Ibu-Tab*[7]; *Ibu-Tab*[7]; *Ibuprin*[7]; *Ibuprohm*[7]; *Ibuprohm Caplets*[7]; *Idarac*[5]; *Indocid*[8]; *Indocid SR*[8]; *Indocin*[8]; *Indocin SR*[8]; *Lodine*[3]; *Meclomen*[10]; *Medipren*[7]; *Medipren Caplets*[7]; *Midol IB*[7]; *Mobiflex*[18]; *Motrin*[7]; *Motrin*[7]; *Motrin Chewables*[7]; *Motrin, Children's*[7]; *Motrin, Children's Oral Drops*[7]; *Motrin, Junior Strength Caplets*[7]; *Motrin-IB*[7]; *Motrin-IB Caplets*[7]; *Nalfon*[4]; *Nalfon 200*[4]; *Naprosyn*[13]; *Naprosyn*[13]; *Naprosyn-E*[13]; *Naprosyn-SR*[13]; *Naxen*[13]; *Naxen*[13]; *Novo-Difenac*[1]; *Novo-Difenac SR*[1]; *Novo-Diflunisal*[2]; *Novo-Flurprofen*[6]; *Novo-Keto-EC*[9]; *Novo-Methacin*[8]; *Novo-Naprox*[13]; *Novo-Naprox Sodium*[13]; *Novo-Naprox Sodium DS*[13]; *Novo-Pirocam*[16]; *Novo-Profen*[7]; *Novo-Profen*[7]; *Novo-Sundac*[17]; *Novo-Tolmetin*[20]; *Nu-Diclo*[1]; *Nu-Flurbiprofen*[6]; *Nu-Ibuprofen*[7]; *Nu-Indo*[8]; *Nu-Naprox*[13]; *Nu-Pirox*[16]; *Nuprin*[7]; *Nuprin Caplets*[7]; *Orudis*[9]; *Orudis KT*[9]; *Orudis-E*[9]; *Orudis-SR*[9]; *Oruvail*[9]; *PMS-Piroxicam*[16]; *Pamprin-IB*[7]; *Ponstan*[11]; *Ponstel*[11]; *Q-Profen*[7]; *Relafen*[12]; *Rhodis*[9]; *Rhodis-EC*[9]; *Rufen*[7]; *Surgam*[19]; *Surgam SR*[19]; *Synflex*[13]; *Synflex DS*[13]; *Tolectin 200*[20]; *Tolectin 400*[20]; *Tolectin 600*[20]; *Tolectin DS*[20]; *Trendar*[7]; *Voltaren*[1]; *Voltaren Rapide*[1]; *Voltaren SR*[1].

Other commonly used names are Etodolic acid [Etodolac†]; Indometacin [Indomethacin]; Meclofenamic acid [Meclofenamate†].

Note: For a listing of dosage forms and brand names by country availability, see *Dosage Forms* section(s).

*Not commercially available in U.S.
†Not commercially available in Canada.

## Category

Note: All of these medications have analgesic, antipyretic, and anti-inflammatory actions; however, indications for specific agents may vary because of lack of specific testing and/or clinical-use data as well as the toxicity of the individual nonsteroidal anti-inflammatory drug (NSAID). **Clinically, most of these agents are used to treat a variety of painful and/or inflammatory conditions, both rheumatic and nonrheumatic, even though the specific uses are not listed in U.S. or Canadian product labeling.**

Antirheumatic (nonsteroidal anti-inflammatory)—Diclofenac; Diflunisal; Etodolac; Fenoprofen; Flurbiprofen; Ibuprofen; Indomethacin; Ketoprofen; Meclofenamate; Nabumetone; Naproxen; Oxaprozin; Phenylbutazone; Piroxicam; Sulindac; Tenoxicam; Tiaprofenic Acid; Tolmetin.

Analgesic—Diclofenac; Diflunisal; Etodolac; Fenoprofen; Floctafenine; Ibuprofen; Ketoprofen; Meclofenamate; Mefenamic Acid; Naproxen.

Antigout agent—Diclofenac; Diflunisal; Etodolac; Fenoprofen; Floctafenine; Ibuprofen; Indomethacin; Ketoprofen; Naproxen; Phenylbutazone; Piroxicam; Sulindac.

Anti-inflammatory (nonsteroidal)—Flurbiprofen; Indomethacin; Naproxen; Sulindac; Tenoxicam.

Antipyretic—Ibuprofen; Indomethacin; Naproxen.

Antidysmenorrheal—Diclofenac; Flurbiprofen; Ibuprofen; Indomethacin; Ketoprofen; Meclofenamate; Mefenamic Acid; Naproxen; Piroxicam.

Vascular headache prophylactic—Fenoprofen; Ibuprofen; Indomethacin; Mefenamic Acid; Naproxen.

Vascular headache suppressant—Diclofenac; Diflunisal; Etodolac; Fenoprofen; Floctafenine; Ibuprofen; Indomethacin; Ketoprofen; Meclofenamate; Mefenamic Acid; Naproxen.

Prostaglandin synthesis inhibitor, renal (Bartter's syndrome)—Indomethacin.

## Indications

Note: Bracketed information in the Indications section refers to uses that are not included in U.S. product labeling.

### Accepted

Rheumatic disease (treatment), such as
  Arthritis, rheumatoid—Diclofenac, diflunisal, fenoprofen, flurbiprofen, ibuprofen, indomethacin, ketoprofen, meclofenamate, nabumetone, naproxen, oxaprozin, phenylbutazone[1], piroxicam, sulindac, tenoxicam, tiaprofenic acid, and tolmetin are indicated for the treatment of acute or chronic rheumatoid arthritis.
  Osteoarthritis—Diclofenac, diflunisal, etodolac, fenoprofen, flurbiprofen, ibuprofen, indomethacin, ketoprofen, meclofenamate, nabumetone, naproxen, oxaprozin, phenylbutazone[1], piroxicam, sulindac, tenoxicam, tiaprofenic acid, and tolmetin are indicated for relief of acute or chronic osteoarthritis.
  Ankylosing spondylitis—Diclofenac[1], [diflunisal][1], [fenoprofen][1], [flurbiprofen], [ibuprofen][1], indomethacin, [ketoprofen], naproxen, phenylbutazone, [piroxicam], sulindac, tenoxicam, and [tolmetin] are indicated for relief of acute or chronic ankylosing spondylitis.
  Arthritis, juvenile—Ibuprofen, indomethacin[1], naproxen, and tolmetin are indicated for relief of acute or chronic juvenile arthritis.
  [Arthritis, psoriatic][1]—Diflunisal, fenoprofen, ibuprofen, indomethacin, ketoprofen, meclofenamate, phenylbutazone, and tolmetin are used in the treatment of psoriatic arthritis.
  [Reiter's disease][1]—Indomethacin is used in the treatment of Reiter's disease.
  [Rheumatic complications associated with Paget's disease of bone][1]—Indomethacin is used in the treatment of this condition.
  Although NSAIDs may be required for relief of [rheumatic complications occurring in association with systemic lupus erythematosus (SLE)][1], extreme caution is recommended because patients with

SLE may be predisposed toward NSAID-induced central nervous system (CNS) and/or renal toxicity. Several NSAIDs, including ibuprofen, sulindac, and tolmetin, have been shown to cause serious adverse effects, including aseptic meningitis, in patients with SLE. In addition, ibuprofen (although a causal relationship has not been established), meclofenamate, and phenylbutazone have rarely been reported to cause an SLE-like syndrome and/or to exacerbate pre-existing SLE.

NSAIDs do not affect the progressive course of some forms of rheumatic disease. Some patients with rheumatoid arthritis may need additional treatment.

Pain (treatment)—Diclofenac, diflunisal, etodolac, fenoprofen[1], floctafenine, ibuprofen, ketoprofen, meclofenamate, mefenamic acid, and naproxen are indicated for relief of mild to moderate pain, especially when anti-inflammatory actions may also be desired, e.g., following dental, obstetric, or orthopedic surgery, and for relief of musculoskeletal pain due to soft tissue athletic injuries (strains or sprains). Only immediate-release dosage forms are recommended for relief of acute pain because of their more rapid onset of action relative to delayed-release or extended-release dosage forms.

Mefenamic acid is indicated for relief of mild to moderate pain when therapy will not exceed 1 week.

Those NSAIDs indicated for relief of pain are also recommended for relief of mild to moderate bone pain caused by metastatic neoplastic disease. However, careful patient selection is necessary, especially in patients receiving chemotherapy, because of the potential gastrointestinal or renal toxicity and the platelet aggregation–inhibiting actions of these medications.

Gouty arthritis, acute (treatment) or
[Calcium pyrophosphate deposition disease, acute (treatment)][1]—[Diclofenac][1], [diflunisal][1], [etodolac], [fenoprofen][1], floctafenine[1], [ibuprofen][1], indomethacin, [ketoprofen][1], [meclofenamate], [mefenamic acid][1], naproxen[1], phenylbutazone, [piroxicam][1], and sulindac are indicated [or used] for relief of the pain and inflammation of acute gouty arthritis and [acute calcium pyrophosphate deposition disease (pseudogout; chondrocalcinosis articularis; synovitis, crystal-induced)][1]. Only immediate-release dosage forms are recommended for relief of acute attacks because of their more rapid onset of action relative to delayed-release or extended-release dosage forms.

[Long-term prophylactic use of an NSAID may decrease the incidence or severity of recurrent acute gout attacks, especially during the early months of antihyperuricemic therapy. The NSAIDs do not correct hyperuricemia (although diclofenac, diflunisal, etodolac, oxaprozin, and phenylbutazone have some uricosuric activity) and do not eliminate the need for administration of an antihyperuricemic agent for the long-term management of chronic gout. Colchicine is the recommended agent for preventing acute gout attacks because, in low (prophylactic) doses, it is less toxic for long-term use than NSAIDs. NSAIDs (other than phenylbutazone, which is *not recommended for long-term treatment*) should be used only for patients unable to tolerate even prophylactic doses of colchicine.]

Inflammation, nonrheumatic (treatment)—Most of the NSAIDs are indicated [or used] in the treatment of painful nonrheumatic inflammatory conditions, such as:
  Athletic injuries
  Bursitis
  Capsulitis
  Synovitis
  Tendinitis or
  Tenosynovitis—[Flurbiprofen is indicated for relief of bursitis, tendinitis, and soft tissue injuries.] Indomethacin[1] and sulindac are indicated for treatment of bursitis and/or tendinitis of the shoulder. Naproxen is indicated for treatment of bursitis and/or tendinitis of any joint. Tenoxicam is indicated for treatment of tendinitis, bursitis, and periarthritis of the shoulders or hips. [Other NSAIDs, especially those approved by U.S. and/or Canadian regulatory agencies for relief of pain, are also used in the treatment of these and other painful inflammatory conditions.][1]

Fever (treatment)—Ibuprofen and naproxen[1] are indicated for reduction of fever.

[Fever, due to malignancy (treatment)][1]—Indomethacin (rapidly acting dosage forms only) is used to reduce fever in patients with Hodgkin's disease, other lymphomas, and hepatic metastases of solid tumors. Indomethacin should be used only after aspirin and acetaminophen have proven ineffective. If antipyretic therapy at an adequate dosage is not effective within 48 hours, indomethacin should be discontinued.

Dysmenorrhea (treatment)—Diclofenac, [flurbiprofen], ibuprofen, [indomethacin][1], ketoprofen, meclofenamate, mefenamic acid, naproxen, and [piroxicam] are indicated for relief of the pain and other symptoms of primary dysmenorrhea. [Other NSAIDs that have been approved by U.S. and/or Canadian regulatory agencies for relief of pain are also used to relieve dysmenorrhea.][1] Only immediate-release dosage forms are recommended for relief of dysmenorrhea because of their more rapid onset of action relative to delayed-release or extended-release dosage forms.

[Because of the high incidence of adverse effects with effective doses of indomethacin, it is recommended that indomethacin be used only for severe primary dysmenorrhea unresponsive to other, less toxic, NSAIDs.]

Hypermenorrhea (treatment)—Meclofenamate is indicated for treatment of idiopathic excessive menstrual bleeding. The absence of an underlying pathologic condition should be verified before meclofenamate therapy is instituted. [NSAIDs that are used for relief of dysmenorrhea (see *Dysmenorrhea*, above) may also decrease excessive menstrual blood loss caused by an intrauterine device in addition to relieving other symptoms.][1]

[Headache, vascular (prophylaxis)][1] or
[Headache, vascular (treatment)][1]—Diclofenac, diflunisal, etodolac, fenoprofen, floctafenine, ibuprofen, indomethacin, ketoprofen, meclofenamate, mefenamic acid, and naproxen are used to relieve (when taken at the first sign of onset) migraine headache or other vascular headaches. Fenoprofen, ibuprofen, indomethacin, and naproxen are also used chronically to prevent recurrence of such headaches. Fenoprofen, ibuprofen, indomethacin, mefenamic acid, and naproxen may also be taken prior to and during menstruation to prevent migraine associated with menstruation.

[Bartter's syndrome (treatment)][1]—Indomethacin is used in the treatment of Bartter's syndrome. However, its use in this condition has been associated with adverse effects, including pseudotumor cerebri. Because long-term therapy is required, it has been suggested that other, less toxic, NSAIDs may be suitable alternatives to indomethacin.

[Pericarditis][1]—Indomethacin (rapidly acting dosage forms only) is used to relieve pain, fever, and inflammation associated with pericarditis.

**Unaccepted**
Except in the treatment of ankylosing spondylitis, for which it is a treatment of choice, and Bartter's syndrome, indomethacin is not recommended as initial therapy because of its potential for causing severe side effects. Also, although indomethacin, like other NSAIDs, has analgesic and antipyretic activity, it should not be used indiscriminately (because of its toxicity) to relieve pain or reduce fever.

**Phenylbutazone is not recommended as initial therapy for any indication.** Because of its potential for causing severe side effects, including agranulocytosis and aplastic anemia, it should be used only after less toxic treatments (including other, less toxic, NSAIDs) have been found ineffective. In many countries, phenylbutazone is approved only for treatment of severe ankylosing spondylitis unresponsive to other NSAIDs. Use of phenylbutazone to relieve the pain and inflammation of acute painful shoulder (i.e., peritendinitis, capsulitis, or bursitis of that joint) is no longer FDA-approved. It is strongly recommended that use of phenylbutazone be restricted to short-term treatment of severe flares of rheumatic disease, gout, or calcium pyrophosphate deposition disease.

---

[1]Not included in Canadian product labeling.

## Pharmacology/Pharmacokinetics
See *Table 1*, page 420, and *Table 2*, page 423.

**Physicochemical characteristics**
Chemical group—
  Fenamate derivatives: Meclofenamate, mefenamic acid.
  Indoleacetic acid derivative: Indomethacin. Indomethacin is chemically related to the pyrroleacetic acid derivatives sulindac and tolmetin and to the pyranoindoleacetic acid derivative etodolac.
  Naphthylalkanone derivative: Nabumetone.
  Oxicam derivative: Piroxicam, tenoxicam.
  Phenylacetic acid derivative: Diclofenac.
  Propionic acid derivatives: Fenoprofen, flurbiprofen, ibuprofen, ketoprofen, naproxen, oxaprozin, tiaprofenic acid.
  Pyranoindoleacetic acid: Etodolac. This medication is chemically related to the indoleacetic acid derivative indomethacin and to the pyrroleacetic acid derivatives sulindac and tolmetin.
  Pyrazole derivative: Phenylbutazone.
  Pyrroleacetic acid derivatives: Sulindac, tolmetin. These medications are chemically related to the indoleacetic acid derivative indomethacin and to the pyranoindoleacetic acid derivative etodolac.
  Salicylic acid derivative: Diflunisal. However, diflunisal is not metabolized to salicylic acid *in vivo*.

Molecular weight—
  Diclofenac potassium: 334.24.
  Diclofenac sodium: 318.13.
  Diflunisal: 250.2.
  Etodolac: 287.36.
  Fenoprofen calcium: 558.64.
  Floctafenine: 406.36.
  Flurbiprofen: 244.26.
  Ibuprofen: 206.28.
  Indomethacin: 357.79.
  Ketoprofen: 254.28.
  Meclofenamate sodium: 336.15.
  Mefenamic acid: 241.29.
  Nabumetone: 228.29 Active nabumetone metabolite 6-methoxy-2-naphthylacetic acid (6-MNA)—216.25.
  Naproxen: 230.26.
  Naproxen sodium: 252.24.
  Oxaprozin: 293.32.
  Phenylbutazone: 308.38.
  Piroxicam: 331.35.
  Sulindac: 356.41.
  Tenoxicam: 337.37.
  Tiaprofenic acid: 260.31.
  Tolmetin sodium: 315.3.
Other characteristics
  Ketoprofen: Highly lipophilic.
  Oxaprozin: Lipophilic.
pKa—
  Diclofenac potassium: 4.0.
  Diclofenac sodium: 4.0.
  Diflunisal: 3.3.
  Etodolac: 4.65.
  Fenoprofen calcium: 4.5 (25 °C).
  Flurbiprofen: 4.22.
  Ibuprofen: 4.43.
  Indomethacin: 4.5.
  Ketoprofen: 5.94 (in methanol:water [3:1]).
  Mefenamic acid: 4.2.
  Naproxen: 4.2.
  Oxaprozin: 4.3.
  Piroxicam: 1.8 and 5.1.
  Tiaprofenic acid: 3.0.
  Tolmetin sodium: 3.5.
  Note: 6-MNA, the active metabolite of nabumetone, but not nabumetone itself, is acidic. Other NSAIDs not listed above are also acidic.

## Mechanism of action/Effect

Nonsteroidal anti-inflammatory drugs (NSAIDs) inhibit the activity of the enzyme cyclo-oxygenase, resulting in decreased formation of precursors of prostaglandins and thromboxanes from arachidonic acid. Also, meclofenamate and mefenamic acid have been shown to inhibit competitively the actions of prostaglandins. Although the resultant decrease in prostaglandin synthesis and activity in various tissues may be responsible for many of the therapeutic (and adverse) effects of NSAIDs, other actions may also contribute significantly to the therapeutic effects of these medications.

Antirheumatic (nonsteroidal anti-inflammatory)—
  Act via analgesic and anti-inflammatory mechanisms; the therapeutic effects are not due to pituitary-adrenal stimulation. These medications do not affect the progressive course of rheumatoid arthritis.

Analgesic—
  May block pain impulse generation via a peripheral action that may involve reduction of the activity of prostaglandins, and possibly inhibition of the synthesis or actions of other substances that sensitize pain receptors to mechanical or chemical stimulation. The antibradykinin activity of ketoprofen may also be involved in relief of pain, because bradykinin has been shown to act together with prostaglandins to cause pain.

Antigout agent—
  Act via analgesic and anti-inflammatory mechanisms; do not correct hyperuricemia.

Anti-inflammatory (nonsteroidal)—
  Exact mechanisms have not been determined. NSAIDs may act peripherally in inflamed tissue, probably by reducing prostaglandin activity in these tissues and possibly by inhibiting the synthesis and/or actions of other local mediators of the inflammatory response. Inhibition of leukocyte migration, inhibition of the release and/or actions of lysosomal enzymes, and actions on other cellular and immunological processes in mesenchymal and connective tissue may be involved. Indomethacin has been shown to inhibit phosphodiesterase, with a resultant increase in intracellular cyclic adenosine monophosphate (cAMP) concentration. Ketoprofen has been shown to inhibit leukotriene synthesis, inhibit bradykinin activity, and stabilize lysosomal membranes.

Antipyretic—
  Probably produce antipyresis by acting centrally on the hypothalamic heat-regulating center to produce peripheral vasodilation, resulting in increased blood flow through the skin, sweating, and heat loss. The central action probably involves reduction of prostaglandin activity in the hypothalamus.

Antidysmenorrheal—
  By inhibiting the synthesis and activity of intrauterine prostaglandins (which are thought to be responsible for the pain and other symptoms of primary dysmenorrhea), NSAIDs decrease uterine contractility and uterine pressure, increase uterine perfusion, and relieve ischemic as well as spasmodic pain. The antibradykinin activity of ketoprofen may also be involved in relief of dysmenorrhea, because bradykinin has been shown to induce uterine contractions and to act together with prostaglandins to cause pain. Also, NSAIDs may relieve to some extent extrauterine symptoms (such as headache, nausea, and vomiting) that may be associated with excessive prostaglandin production.

Vascular headache prophylactic and suppressant—
  Analgesic actions may be involved in relief of headache. Also, by reducing prostaglandin activity, NSAIDs may directly prevent or relieve certain types of headache thought to be caused by prostaglandin-induced dilation or constriction of cerebral blood vessels.

Prostaglandin synthesis inhibitor, renal—
  Inhibition of renal prostaglandin synthesis probably is responsible for indomethacin's beneficial effect in patients with Bartter's syndrome, which is thought to be caused by excessive production of renal prostaglandins.

## Other actions/effects

Most of the NSAIDs inhibit platelet aggregation. However, their antiplatelet effect, unlike that of aspirin, is reversible. Single doses of 4 to 10 mg of flurbiprofen inhibit platelet aggregation. Oxaprozin is as potent as aspirin in inhibiting platelet aggregation induced by epinephrine or collagen *in vitro*. With diflunisal, the effect is clinically significant only with greater-than-recommended daily doses. Also, usual doses of diclofenac, meclofenamate, mefenamic acid, or nabumetone (as determined after administration of 1000 mg per day for 7 to 10 days) may not significantly alter platelet aggregability. Recovery of platelet function may occur within 1 day after discontinuation of diclofenac, diflunisal, flurbiprofen, ibuprofen, indomethacin, or sulindac; 2 days after discontinuation of tolmetin; 4 days after discontinuation of naproxen; or 2 weeks following discontinuation of slowly eliminated agents such as oxaprozin or piroxicam.

Diclofenac, diflunisal, etodolac, oxaprozin, and phenylbutazone also have uricosuric activity.

Phenylbutazone also induces hepatic microsomal enzyme activity.

Studies have demonstrated that IgM rheumatoid factor production (which may be partially mediated by prostaglandins) may be decreased (but not totally inhibited) during NSAID therapy. However, because these medications do not affect the progressive course of rheumatoid arthritis, the clinical significance of this effect has not been determined.

It has been proposed that the gastrointestinal toxicity of NSAIDs may be caused primarily by reduction of the synthesis and activity of prostaglandins (which exert a protective effect on the gastrointestinal mucosa) because upper gastrointestinal toxicity has been reported following rectal or parenteral administration of some of these medications. However, when administered orally, some of these acidic medications probably also exert a direct irritant or erosive effect on the mucosa. Because nabumetone is a nonacidic prodrug, and the active metabolite 6-MNA is not formed until after absorption, the risk of serious upper gastrointestinal tract toxicity may be lower with nabumetone than with other NSAIDs. Also, in one study, gastric and duodenal prostaglandin concentrations were not altered by 4 weeks of administration of therapeutic doses of etodolac.

The renal toxicity associated with NSAIDs (i.e., decreased renal perfusion, sodium and fluid retention, and decreased renal function) may be caused by inhibition of renal prostaglandins, which are directly involved in the maintenance of renal hemodynamics and sodium and fluid balance. Renal prostaglandins are especially important in maintaining renal function in the presence of generalized vasoconstriction or volume depletion. Sulindac is a prodrug; its sulfide metabolite is the active substance. Because this active metabolite is not excreted via the kidneys, renal toxicity may be less likely with sulindac than with other NSAIDs. However, there have been reports of renal toxicity associated with sulindac therapy. Etodolac has been shown to decrease some measures of renal function, with maximum effects occurring within 1.5 to 2.5 hours after a dose. However, with administration of up to 500 mg every 12 hours, recovery of renal function occurred prior to administration of the next dose, even in patients with pre-existing mild to moderate renal function impairment (creatinine clearances ranging from 20 to 88 mL per minute). Whether more frequent administration of etodolac may cause cumulative effects on renal function has not been determined.

The analgesic, antipyretic, and anti-inflammatory effects of NSAIDs may mask symptoms of the onset and/or progression of an infection.

**Therapeutic effect**
When these medications are used in the treatment of arthritis, their analgesic actions may produce some relief of pain within the first day or two. Significant relief of other symptoms of inflammation usually occurs within a few days to a week; however, in severe cases, 2 weeks or more of continuous use may be required.

| Drug and Indication | Onset of Action | Peak Effect | Duration of Action |
|---|---|---|---|
| Diclofenac Tablets Pain | 30 min | | Up to 8 hr |
| Diflunisal Pain | 1 hr | 2–3 hr | 8–12 hr |
| Etodolac Pain 200 mg 400 mg | 30 min | 1–2 hr | 4–5 hr 5–6 hr, but 8–12 hr in some patients |
| Ibuprofen Fever 5 mg/kg 10 mg/kg Pain | 0.5 hr | 2-4 hr | 6 hr 8 hr or more 4–6 hr |
| Indomethacin Gout Heat, tenderness Swelling | 2–4 hr | 2–3 days 3–5 days | |
| Meclofenamate Pain | 1 hr | | 4–6 hr |
| Naproxen Gout Pain | 1 hr | 1–2 days 2–4 hr | Up to 7 hr |
| Piroxicam Gout | 2–4 hr | 3–5 days | 24 hr |

**Synovial fluid concentrations**
Studies with several of the NSAIDs have shown that these medications enter the synovial fluid and that, several hours after administration of a single dose, synovial fluid concentrations equal or exceed the simultaneously measured plasma concentration. In addition, there is some evidence that ketoprofen, oxaprozin, and possibly other NSAIDs, may accumulate in synovial fluid when administered chronically.

| Drug and Dose | Time to Peak (hr) | Peak (mcg/mL) | Half-life* (hr) |
|---|---|---|---|
| Diclofenac | 3† | 0.28† | Up to 6 |
| Etodolac‡ | 2.7–3.7 | Total 2.6 Free (unbound) 44–84 nanograms/mL | 6.5–7 |
| Flurbiprofen 100 mg† | 5.2 | 4.4 | 4.6 |
| Indomethacin 50 mg | 2 | 0.69 | |
| Ketoprofen 50 mg 100 mg | 2 | 0.7–0.9 0.7–0.9 | |
| Nabumetone 1000 mg | ±8 | 20§; 35# | |
| Tenoxicam 40 mg | 10 | 1.82 | |

| Drug and Dose | Time to Peak (hr) | Peak (mcg/mL) | Half-life* (hr) |
|---|---|---|---|
| Tiaprofenic Acid Tablets 200 mg† 300 mg† | 4 4 | 5.3 7.7 | |
| Extended-release Capsules | 8 | | 8.6 |
| Tolmetin 400 mg† | 2 | 5.6 | 6.9 |

*Elimination.
†Determined at steady-state, after administration of a single dose in patients receiving chronic therapy (for diclofenac—50 mg 3 times a day; for flurbiprofen—100 mg twice a day; for tiaprofenic acid—200 mg 3 times a day for 7 days or 300 mg twice a day for 7 days; for tolmetin—400 mg 4 times a day for 7 days).
‡Determined at steady-state.
§Single dose; simultaneous plasma concentration 36 mcg/mL.
#Multiple doses (1000 mg every 12 hours on the first day, then 1000 mg per day for 3 days); simultaneous plasma concentration 41 mcg/mL.

## Precautions to Consider

**Cross-sensitivity and/or related problems**
Patients sensitive to one of the nonsteroidal anti-inflammatory drugs (NSAIDs), including aspirin, ketorolac, and NSAIDs no longer commercially available (such as oxyphenbutazone, suprofen, and zomepirac) may be sensitive to any of the other NSAIDs also.

NSAIDs may cause bronchoconstriction or anaphylaxis in aspirin-sensitive asthmatics, especially those with aspirin-induced nasal polyps, asthma, and other allergic reactions (the "aspirin triad").

Patients with bronchospastic reactions to aspirin may be desensitized to this effect by administration of initially small and gradually increasing doses of aspirin. Desensitization must be carried out by physicians who are experienced with the technique, in a facility having personnel, equipment, and medications immediately available for treatment of any adverse reaction to the medication (especially anaphylaxis or severe bronchospasm). Desensitization to aspirin also desensitizes the patient to other NSAIDs. However, unless aspirin or another NSAID is then administered on a daily basis, sensitivity to these medications redevelops within a few days.

**Carcinogenicity**
Diclofenac—
  No oncogenic potential was demonstrated with diclofenac sodium in a 2-year carcinogenicity study in male mice given up to 0.3 mg per kg of body weight(mg/kg) (0.9 mg per square meter of body surface area [mg/m $^2$]) per day or in female mice given up to 1 mg/kg (3 mg/m $^2$) per day.
Diflunisal—
  No effect on the incidence or type of neoplasia was found in a 105-week study in rats given up to 40 mg/kg per day (approximately 1.3 times the maximum recommended human dose [MRHD]) or in long-term studies in mice given up to 80 mg/kg per day (approximately 2.7 times the MRHD).
Etodolac—
  No carcinogenicity was demonstrated in mice or rats receiving up to 15 mg/kg per day (corresponding to 45 mg/m $^2$ for mice and 89 mg/m $^2$ for rats) for 2 years or 18 months, respectively.
Floctafenine—
  No effect on the incidence of neoplasia was found in studies in CD-1 mice receiving up to 240 mg/kg per day.
Flurbiprofen—
  No evidence of carcinogenicity was found in an 80-week study in mice receiving up to 14 mg/kg per day or in a 2-year study in rats receiving up to 12 mg/kg per day for 32 weeks, then up to 5 mg/kg per day thereafter.
Indomethacin—
  No evidence of carcinogenicity was found in studies in mice receiving up to 1.5 mg/kg per day for 62 to 88 weeks or in studies in rats receiving up to 1.5 mg/kg per day for 73 to 110 weeks.
  Leukemia has been reported in a few patients receiving indomethacin; however, a causal relationship has not been established.
Ketoprofen—
  No evidence of carcinogenicity was found in studies in mice receiving up to 32 mg/kg (96 mg/m $^2$) per day (approximately 0.5 times the MRHD based on body surface area).

Meclofenamate—
No evidence of carcinogenicity was found in an 18-month study in rats.
Naproxen—
No evidence of carcinogenicity was found in a 24-month study in rats.
Oxaprozin—
An increased incidence of hepatic adenomas and carcinomas occurred in 2-year studies in male CD mice, but not in female CD mice or in rats, given oxaprozin. The significance of this species-specific finding is not known.
Phenylbutazone—
Leukemia has been reported in a few patients receiving phenylbutazone; however, a causal relationship has not been established.
Long-term studies in animals have not been done to determine whether phenylbutazone has carcinogenic activity.
Tenoxicam—
No evidence of carcinogenicity was found in an 80-week study in mice receiving up to 5 mg/kg per day or in a 104-week study in rats receiving up to 6 mg/kg per day.
Tiaprofenic acid—
No evidence of carcinogenicity was found in an 80-week study in mice receiving up to 30 mg/kg per day or in a 104-week study in rats receiving up to 30 mg/kg per day.
Tolmetin—
No evidence of carcinogenicity was found in an 18-month study in mice receiving up to 50 mg/kg per day or in a 24-month study in rats receiving up to 75 mg/kg per day.

**Tumorigenicity**
Diclofenac—
No tumorigenicity was demonstrated in studies in rats receiving up to 2 mg/kg per day (approximately the recommended human dose). Although there was a slight increase in benign mammary fibroadenomas in female rats given 0.5 mg/kg (3 mg/m$^2$) per day, the increase was not significant.
Flurbiprofen—
No tumorigenicity was demonstrated in a 2-year study in rats receiving up to 12 mg/kg per day for 32 weeks, then up to 5 mg/kg per day.
Indomethacin—
No tumorigenicity was demonstrated in an 81-week study in rats receiving up to 1 mg/kg per day.
Ketoprofen—
No tumorigenicity was demonstrated in studies in rats receiving 6 mg/kg (36 mg/m$^2$) per day for 81 weeks or lower doses for 104 weeks.
Nabumetone—
No tumorigenicity was demonstrated in 2-year studies in mice and rats.

**Mutagenicity**
Diclofenac—
No mutagenic activity was demonstrated in *in vitro* tests using mammalian cells or bacteria (with or without microsomal activation) or in *in vivo* tests, including dominant lethal and male germinal epithelial chromosomal studies in mice and nucleus anomaly and chromosomal aberration studies in Chinese hamsters.
Diflunisal—
No mutagenic activity was demonstrated in the dominant lethal assay, Ames microbial mutagen test, or V-79 Chinese hamster lung cell assay.
Etodolac—
No mutagenic activity was demonstrated in *in vitro* tests performed with *Salmonella typhimurium* and mouse lymphoma cells or in an *in vivo* mouse micronucleus test. However, in the *in vitro* human peripheral lymphocyte test, concentrations of 50 to 200 mcg per mL (mcg/mL) of etodolac produced an increase in the number of gaps (3 to 5.3% unstained regions in the chromatid without dislocation, compared with 2% in controls).
Indomethacin—
No mutagenic activity was demonstrated in *in vitro* tests (Ames test or *E. coli*, with or without metabolic activation) or in *in vivo* tests (host-mediated assay, sex-linked recessive lethals in *Drosophila*, and micronucleus test in mice).
Ketoprofen—
No mutagenic activity was demonstrated in the Ames test.
Nabumetone—
No mutagenic activity was demonstrated in the Ames test or in the mouse micronucleus test *in vivo*. However, chromosomal aberrations occurred in lymphocytes exposed *in vitro* to nabumetone or its active metabolite 6-methoxy-2-naphthylacetic acid (6-MNA) at concentrations of 80 mcg/mL (369.6 micromoles/L) or higher.
Oxaprozin—
No mutagenic activity was demonstrated in the Ames test, forward mutation testing in yeast and Chinese hamster ovary cells, DNA repair testing in Chinese hamster ovary cells, micronucleus testing in mouse bone marrow, chromosomal aberration testing in human lymphocytes, or cell transformation testing in mouse fibroblasts.
Phenylbutazone—
No mutagenic activity was demonstrated in tests in mice, Chinese hamsters, or rats given up to 33 times the maximum daily human dose, or in bacteria or fungi. However, *in vitro* tests using Chinese hamster fibroblast cells have shown that phenylbutazone concentrations exceeding 860 mg/L produce chromosome abnormalities. Although an increased incidence of chromosome anomalies has been reported in cultured leukocyte cells from patients receiving therapeutic doses of the medication, other similar studies in humans and in horses have yielded inconclusive or negative results.
Piroxicam—
No mutagenic activity was demonstrated (test systems used not specified).
Tenoxicam—
No mutagenic activity was demonstrated in studies in 3 bacterial systems and 4 eukaryotic test systems.
Tiaprofenic acid—
No mutagenic activity was demonstrated in the Ames test or in the micronucleus test in mice.
Tolmetin—
No mutagenic activity was demonstrated in the Ames test.

**Pregnancy/Reproduction**
Fertility—
Diclofenac—
No impairment of fertility was demonstrated in reproduction studies in rats receiving up to 4 mg/kg (24 mg/m$^2$) per day.
Diflunisal—
No impairment of fertility was demonstrated in reproduction studies in rats receiving up to 50 mg/kg per day.
Etodolac—
A reduction in the implantation of fertilized eggs was demonstrated in reproduction studies in rats receiving 8 mg/kg per day, but no impairment of fertility was demonstrated in male or female rats receiving up to 16 mg/kg (94 mg/m$^2$) per day.
Floctafenine—
No impairment of fertility was demonstrated in reproduction studies in rats receiving up to 160 mg/kg per day.
Flurbiprofen—
No impairment of fertility was demonstrated in reproduction studies in rats receiving 2.25 mg/kg per day.
Indomethacin—
No impairment of fertility was demonstrated in a 2-generation reproduction study in mice or in a 2-litter reproduction study in rats receiving up to 0.5 mg/kg per day.
Ketoprofen—
No impairment of fertility was demonstrated in reproduction studies in male rats receiving up to 9 mg/kg (54 mg/m$^2$) per day. However, a decrease in the number of implantation sites was demonstrated in female rats receiving 6 or 9 mg/kg (36 or 54 mg/m$^2$) per day. In other studies, high doses of ketoprofen caused abnormal spermatogenesis or inhibition of spermatogenesis in rats and dogs, and decreased testicular weight in dogs and baboons.
Mefenamic acid—
Impairment of fertility was demonstrated in reproduction studies in rats receiving 10 times the human dose.
Nabumetone—
No impairment of fertility was demonstrated in male or female rats receiving 320 mg/kg (1888 mg/m$^2$) per day.
Naproxen—
No impairment of fertility was demonstrated in mice, rats, or rabbits receiving up to 6 times the human dose.
Oxaprozin—
No impairment of fertility was demonstrated in male or female rats receiving up to 200 mg/kg (1180 mg per square meter of body surface area [mg/m$^2$]) per day. For comparison, the usual human dose is about 17 mg/kg (629 mg/m$^2$) per day. However, testicular degeneration occurred in beagle dogs given 37.5 mg/kg (750 mg/m$^2$) or more per day for 42 days or longer. This finding did not occur in other species, and the clinical relevance to humans is unknown.
Phenylbutazone—
No impairment of fertility was demonstrated in reproduction studies in mice, Chinese hamsters, and rats receiving up to 33 times the maximum daily human dose.
Piroxicam and tolmetin—
No impairment of fertility was demonstrated in animal reproduction studies.

*Tenoxicam—*
No impairment of fertility was demonstrated in male rats receiving up to 8 mg per day for at least 63 days prior to mating. Administration of 8 mg per day, but not lower doses, to female rats from 14 days prior to, to 7 days after, mating resulted in a significant decrease in the number of corpora lutea and implantations, resulting in fewer live fetuses.

*Tiaprofenic—*
No impairment of fertility was demonstrated in reproduction studies in female or male rats receiving up to 20 mg/kg per day. However, an increased number of pre- and post-implantation losses was demonstrated in studies in female rats receiving 20 mg/kg per day, and a decrease in the number of implantation sites was demonstrated in studies in rabbits receiving 75 mg/kg per day.

Pregnancy—
First trimester
Diclofenac:
Adequate and well-controlled studies in humans have not been done.
Diclofenac crosses the placenta in mice and rats. Studies in rats receiving 2 or 4 mg/kg per day have shown that diclofenac is embryotoxic (causing low birth weight, a slightly decreased growth rate, and failure to survive, especially with the higher dose). Also, in studies in rabbits receiving 5 or 10 mg/kg per day, diclofenac caused increases in the resorption rates, decreased fetal weights, abnormal skeletal findings, and definite embryotoxicity with the higher dose. However, no teratogenicity was demonstrated in reproduction studies in rabbits receiving up to 10 mg/kg (80 mg/m$^2$) per day, in mice receiving up to 20 mg/kg (60 mg/m$^2$) per day, or in rats receiving up to 10 mg/kg (60 mg/m$^2$) per day.
FDA Pregnancy Category B.
Diflunisal:
Adequate and well-controlled studies in humans have not been done.
Studies in animals have shown that diflunisal is teratogenic in rabbits (causing fetal vertebral and rib malformations at doses ranging from 40 to 50 mg/kg per day) but not in mice (in doses of 45 mg/kg per day) or rats (in doses of 100 mg/kg per day). Diflunisal also caused maternotoxicity and embryotoxicity (increased fetal resorptions) in rabbits receiving 60 mg/kg per day (2 times the maximum human dose).
FDA Pregnancy Category C.
Etodolac:
Adequate and well-controlled studies in humans have not been done.
Isolated alterations of limb development, including polydactyly (extra digits), oligodactyly (missing digits), syndactyly (digits attached by webbing), and unossified phalanges, occurred in rats receiving 2 to 14 mg/kg per day. Also, oligodactyly and synostosis of metatarsals occurred in rabbits receiving 2 to 14 mg/kg per day. However, the frequency and dosage group distribution in initial and repeated studies did not establish a clear drug- or dose-response relationship.
FDA Pregnancy Category C.
Fenoprofen, ibuprofen, naproxen, and tolmetin:
Adequate and well-controlled studies in humans have not been done.
Studies in animals have not shown that these agents cause adverse effects on fetal development. Naproxen was studied in mice, rats, and rabbits receiving up to 6 times the human dose. Tolmetin was studied in rats and rabbits receiving up to 50 mg/kg (1.5 times the maximum human dose).
Naproxen: FDA Pregnancy Category B.
Tolmetin: FDA Pregnancy Category C.
Floctafenine:
Studies in mice receiving up to 320 mg/kg per day, rats receiving up to 240 mg/kg per day, and rabbits receiving up to 160 mg/kg per day have not shown that floctafenine is teratogenic. However, embryotoxicity (increased fetal losses in mice, decreased fetal weight in rats, and increased fetal losses in rabbits) was demonstrated with these high doses (but not at lower dosage levels).
Flurbiprofen:
Although adequate and well-controlled studies in humans have not been done, it has been shown that flurbiprofen crosses the placenta.
Studies in mice receiving up to 12 mg/kg per day, rats receiving up to 25 mg/kg per day, and rabbits receiving up to 7.5 mg/kg per day have not shown evidence of teratogenicity. However, studies in rats have shown doses of 0.4 mg/kg per day or higher to be embryocidal (causing reduced weight or slower fetal growth, increased stillbirths, and decreased pup survival). Also, stillbirths, retained fetuses, and/or fetal distress occurred in studies in rats receiving as little as 0.2 mg/kg per day. In addition, fetotoxicity related to maternal toxicity (gastrointestinal ulceration, retardation of weight gain, intrauterine hemorrhage, and maternal deaths) occurred in rats receiving 25 mg/kg per day from Days 1 through 20 of pregnancy. With lower doses (0.2, 0.675, or 2.25 mg/kg per day), such effects did not occur when the medication was discontinued on Day 17 of pregnancy. Maternal deaths due to gastrointestinal ulceration also occurred in rabbits receiving the medication.
FDA Pregnancy Category B.
Indomethacin:
Although studies in humans have not been done, it has been shown that indomethacin crosses the placenta.
Studies in rats and mice have shown that indomethacin (at a dosage of 4 mg/kg per day) causes decreased average fetal weight and retarded ossification. In other studies in mice, higher doses (5 to 15 mg/kg per day) caused maternal toxicity and death, increased fetal resorptions, and fetal malformations.
Ketoprofen:
Adequate and well-controlled studies in humans have not been done.
Studies in animals have not shown evidence of teratogenicity or embryotoxicity in mice receiving up to 12 mg/kg (36 mg/m$^2$) per day or in rats receiving up to 9 mg/kg (54 mg/m$^2$) per day. In studies in rabbits, maternally toxic doses were embryotoxic but not teratogenic.
FDA Pregnancy Category B.
Meclofenamate:
Adequate and well-controlled studies in humans have not been done.
Animal studies have shown meclofenamate to cause fetotoxicity, minor skeletal malformations (e.g., supernumerary ribs), and delayed ossification, but no major teratogenicity.
Mefenamic acid:
Although adequate and well-controlled studies in humans have not been done, it has been demonstrated that mefenamic acid metabolites readily cross the placenta.
Mefenamic acid caused increases in the number of resorptions in rabbits receiving 2.5 times the human dose and decreases in survival to weaning (possibly due to maternal neglect) in rats receiving 10 times the human dose. Although no fetal abnormalities were reported in these studies or in studies in dogs receiving up to 10 times the human dose, it has been recommended that mefenamic acid not be used during pregnancy.
FDA Pregnancy Category C.
Nabumetone:
Adequate and well-controlled studies in humans have not been done.
Nabumetone did not cause teratogenicity in rats receiving up to 400 mg/kg (2360 mg/m$^2$) per day or in rabbits receiving up to 300 mg/kg (3540 mg/m$^2$) per day. However, fetotoxicity (post-implantation losses) occurred in rats receiving 100 mg/kg (590 mg/m$^2$) per day or more. These doses are equivalent to the maximum recommended human dose of nabumetone.
FDA Pregnancy Category C.
Oxaprozin:
Adequate and well-controlled studies in humans have not been done.
Fetal malformations occurred infrequently in rabbits receiving 7.5 to 30 mg/kg per day (doses within the usual human dose range). However, no teratogenicity occurred in mice or rats receiving 50 to 200 mg/kg (225 to 900 mg/m$^2$) per day.
FDA Pregnancy Category C.
Phenylbutazone:
Adequate and well-controlled studies in humans have not been done.
Although studies in rats and rabbits have not shown that phenylbutazone (in doses up to 16 times the maximum daily human dose) is teratogenic, slightly reduced litter sizes were demonstrated in both species.
FDA Pregnancy Category C.

Piroxicam:
: Studies in humans have not been done.
: Studies in animals have not shown that piroxicam causes teratogenic effects in doses up to 10 mg/kg per day.

Sulindac:
: Studies in humans have not been done.
: Animal studies have shown that sulindac (at dosage levels of 20 and 40 mg/kg per day—2.5 and 5 times the MRHD) causes decreased average fetal weight and an increased number of deaths (observed on the first day of the postpartum period). Also, some studies in rabbits have shown a low incidence of visceral and skeletal malformations with sulindac. However, these effects did not occur in repeat studies using the same or higher dosages.

Tenoxicam:
: Studies in mice receiving up to 8 mg/kg per day from Day 6 to Day 15 of gestation did not show tenoxicam to adversely affect the fetuses or neonates. Teratogenic effects did not occur in offspring of rats receiving up to 12 mg/kg per day from Day 7 to Day 17 of gestation. However, a higher mortality rate associated with panperitonitis, gastric lesions characteristic of NSAIDs, and uterine hemorrhage occurred in dams receiving 8 or 12 mg/kg, but not 4 mg/kg or less, per day. Tenoxicam was embryotoxic (causing increased resorptions), but not teratogenic, in rabbits receiving 32 mg/kg, but not 16 mg/kg or less, per day from Day 6 to Day 18 of gestation.

Tiaprofenic acid:
: Tiaprofenic acid crosses the placenta.
: Studies in mice receiving up to 100 mg/kg per day have not shown that the medication is teratogenic. However, an increase in the fetal loss rate was demonstrated in studies in mice receiving 100 mg/kg per day, rats receiving 10 or 25 (but not 5) mg/kg per day, and rabbits receiving 75 (but not 25 or 50) mg/kg per day.

*Second and third trimesters*

All NSAIDs:
: Although studies in humans have not been done with NSAIDs other than indomethacin, use of NSAIDs during the second half of pregnancy is not recommended because of possible adverse effects on the fetus, such as premature closure of the ductus arteriosus, which may lead to persistent pulmonary hypertension in the newborn. Studies in full-term pregnant rats have shown that diclofenac, fenoprofen, flurbiprofen, ibuprofen, indomethacin, ketoprofen, mefenamic acid, naproxen, and tolmetin have a strong constrictive effect on the fetal ductus arteriosus, whereas floctafenine, phenylbutazone, piroxicam, sulindac, and tiaprofenic acid have a moderate constrictive effect.

: Animal studies have also shown that administration of NSAIDs during late pregnancy may cause prolonged gestation, dystocia, and delayed parturition, possibly because of decreased uterine contractility resulting from inhibition of uterine prostaglandins. Decreases in pup survival rates also have been reported. Studies with piroxicam and nabumetone (at a dose of 320 mg/kg per day) have indicated that dystocia may cause an increased mortality rate in both offspring and dams, and a study with tenoxicam showed a dose-dependent prolongation of gestation and decrease in neonatal viability with doses ranging between 0.5 and 2 mg/kg per day. Also, delayed and prolonged parturition was associated with decreased pup survival in studies with etodolac and with an increased number of stillbirths in studies with flurbiprofen and tiaprofenic acid. Administration of indomethacin to rats and mice during the last 3 days of gestation increased the incidence of neuronal necrosis in the diencephalon and caused maternal and fetal deaths. Administration of oxaprozin to rats during late pregnancy resulted in decreased pup survival, and administration of 3.5 times the maximum human daily dose of phenylbutazone to rats during late pregnancy and lactation resulted in an increased number of stillbirths and reduced survival of offspring. Studies in animals have also shown that administration of piroxicam during the third trimester may increase the risk of maternal gastrointestinal tract toxicity.

Indomethacin:
: In addition to the adverse effects in animal studies described above, administration of indomethacin to pregnant women during the third trimester has caused closure of the ductus arteriosus, inhibition of platelet function resulting in bleeding, renal function impairment or failure with oligohydramnios, gastrointestinal bleeding or perforation, and myocardial degenerative changes in the fetus.

**Breast-feeding**

Problems in humans have not been documented with most of the NSAIDs.

*Diclofenac—*
: Diclofenac is distributed into breast milk. In one study, long-term use of 150 mg per day produced concentrations of 100 nanograms per gram in the breast milk. An infant of 4 to 5 kg consuming one liter per day would therefore ingest approximately 0.03 mg/kg per day.

*Diflunisal—*
: Diflunisal is distributed into breast milk. Concentrations may reach 2 to 7% of the maternal plasma concentration.

*Etodolac, floctafenine, and tiaprofenic acid—*
: It is not known whether these medications are distributed into breast milk.

*Fenoprofen and mefenamic acid—*
: Fenoprofen and mefenamic acid are distributed into breast milk in very small quantities.

*Flurbiprofen—*
: Flurbiprofen is distributed into breast milk in very small quantities. In one study, the peak concentration of 0.09 mcg/mL occurred 3 hours following a single 100-mg dose. A maximum of 0.07% of the dose appeared in breast milk within 24 hours after administration. A nursing infant whose mother is taking 200 mg per day could receive approximately 0.1 mg of flurbiprofen per day.

*Ibuprofen—*
: Studies in humans have failed to detect ibuprofen in breast milk using methodology capable of detecting the medication in a concentration of 1 mcg/mL. The maternal dosage was 400 mg four times a day.

*Indomethacin—*
: Indomethacin is distributed into breast milk. Risk-benefit must be considered because convulsions were reported in one breast-fed infant whose mother received 200 mg of indomethacin per day, of which 0.5 to 2 mg per day was distributed into the breast milk.

*Ketoprofen—*
: It is not known whether ketoprofen is distributed into human breast milk; however, in animal studies, the concentration in the milk of lactating dogs was 4 to 5% of the maternal plasma concentration. In other studies, no adverse effect on perinatal development was observed in offspring of rats receiving 9 mg/kg (54 mg/m$^2$) per day, corresponding to 1.5 times the MRHD based on weight or 0.3 times the MRHD based on body surface area.

*Meclofenamate—*
: Trace amounts of meclofenamate are distributed into breast milk. Use of meclofenamate in nursing mothers is not recommended because animal studies have shown meclofenamate to interfere with normal development of the young before weaning.

*Nabumetone—*
: It is not known whether nabumetone or its metabolites are distributed into human breast milk. Problems in humans have not been documented. However, 6-MNA is distributed into the milk of lactating rats in concentrations approximately equal to those in plasma.

*Naproxen—*
: Naproxen is distributed into breast milk; concentrations may reach 1% of the maternal plasma concentration. The peak concentration in breast milk occurs 4 hours after a dose.

*Oxaprozin—*
: It is not known whether oxaprozin is distributed into human breast milk. However, it is distributed into the milk of lactating rats.

*Phenylbutazone—*
: Phenylbutazone is distributed into breast milk; use by nursing mothers may cause severe adverse effects, including blood dyscrasias, in the infant.

*Piroxicam—*
: Piroxicam is distributed into breast milk; concentrations may reach 1 to 3% of the maternal plasma concentration. Also, use of piroxicam by nursing mothers is not recommended because studies in rats have shown that piroxicam causes a dose-dependent inhibition of lactation.

*Sulindac—*
: It is not known whether sulindac is distributed into human breast milk, but it is distributed into the milk of lactating rats.

*Tolmetin—*
: Tolmetin is distributed into breast milk. In one study, an average concentration of 0.075 mcg/mL was measured, with the peak concentration occurring 1 hour following administration to the mother. The half-life in breast milk was 1.5 hours.

## Pediatrics
*Ibuprofen—*
Appropriate studies performed to date have not demonstrated pediatrics-specific problems that would limit the usefulness of ibuprofen in children 6 months of age or older. Safety and efficacy in infants younger than 6 months of age have not been established.

*Indomethacin—*
Although appropriate studies have not been done in the pediatric population, no pediatrics-specific problems have been documented to date (with the immediate-release capsule or oral suspension dosage form; the extended-release dosage form is not recommended for pediatric patients). However, because of indomethacin's toxicity, it is recommended that its use be limited to patients unresponsive to (or intolerant of) other antirheumatic agents, that the patient be carefully monitored (especially for the presence of infection), and that the recommended pediatric doses not be exceeded.

*Naproxen—*
Studies in children 2 years of age and older with juvenile arthritis have shown higher incidences of naproxen-induced skin rash and increased bleeding time as compared with adults. Studies in children younger than 2 years of age have not been done.

*Oxaprozin—*
Although a study with oxaprozin has been conducted in patients 3 to 16 years of age, controlled studies have not been published. Preliminary evidence indicates that, although the risk of overt hepatotoxicity appears to be minimal, elevated aspartate aminotransferase (AST [SGOT]) values during oxaprozin therapy may occur more often in patients treated for juvenile arthritis than in patients treated for other forms of arthritic disease. Safety and efficacy in pediatric patients have not been established.

*Phenylbutazone—*
Because of phenylbutazone's toxicity, use in children younger than 15 years of age is not recommended.

*Tolmetin—*
Appropriate studies performed to date have not demonstrated pediatrics-specific problems that would limit the usefulness of tolmetin in children 2 years of age or older. Studies in children younger than 2 years of age have not been done.

*Other NSAIDs—*
No information is available on the relationship of age to the effects of these medications in pediatric patients. Safety, efficacy, and appropriate dosages have not been established.

## Geriatrics
*All NSAIDs—*
Whether geriatric patients are at increased risk of serious gastrointestinal toxicity during NSAID therapy has not been established. However, NSAID-induced gastrointestinal ulceration and/or bleeding may be more likely to cause serious consequences, including fatalities, in geriatric patients than in younger adults. In addition, elderly patients are more likely to have age-related renal function impairment, which may increase the risk of NSAID-induced hepatic or renal toxicity and may also require dosage reduction to prevent accumulation of the medication. Some clinicians recommend that geriatric patients, especially those 70 years of age or older, be given one-half of the usual adult dose initially. Also, careful monitoring of the patient is recommended.

*Etodolac—*
Studies performed to date with 200 mg of etodolac twice a day have not shown differences in the pharmacokinetics of the medication in geriatric patients compared with younger adults. Also, studies with 600 mg of etodolac per day have not shown differences in the side effects profile of etodolac in geriatric patients compared with younger adults.

*Flurbiprofen—*
Studies have shown that the peak plasma concentration of flurbiprofen may be increased in females 74 to 94 years of age, but not in males 66 to 90 years of age.

*Indomethacin—*
In addition to the increased risks of therapy with any NSAID as described above, geriatric patients are more likely to develop adverse CNS effects, especially confusion, while taking indomethacin.

*Ketoprofen—*
Studies have shown that protein binding and clearance of ketoprofen may be reduced, leading to increased and prolonged serum concentration and elimination half-life.

*Nabumetone—*
Studies in geriatric patients have not shown differences in the efficacy or safety of nabumetone compared with younger adults. However, plasma concentrations of 6-MNA are higher in geriatric patients, and interpatient variability in the pharmacokinetic parameters for 6-MNA is greater in geriatric patients than in younger adults.

*Naproxen—*
Studies have shown that the unbound (free) fraction of naproxen, but not the total plasma concentration, may be increased in geriatric patients. The steady-state concentration of unbound naproxen may be almost doubled in geriatric patients as compared with younger adults.

*Oxaprozin—*
Studies have not demonstrated a need for adjustment of initial oxaprozin dosage in elderly patients on the basis of pharmacokinetic considerations.

The relationship of age to the risk of adverse effects in patients receiving oxaprozin has been examined using data from 3 studies in patients with rheumatoid arthritis and 1 study in patients with osteoarthritis. The data indicate that oxaprozin is more likely to cause a potentially significant decrease in renal function, adverse gastrointestinal effects, or a significant decrease in hemoglobin concentration in patients older than 60 years of age than in younger adults. Although it has also been reported, with other NSAIDs, that geriatric patients seem to be more susceptible to NSAID-induced hepatotoxicity, there were no significant age-related differences in measures of hepatic function in the 4 studies with oxaprozin.

*Phenylbutazone—*
In patients 60 years of age and over, therapy should be limited to short periods (not to exceed 1 week if possible) because of the high risk of severe, possibly fatal, toxic reactions. Specifically, the risk of aplastic anemia and agranulocytosis is increased in elderly patients.

*Piroxicam—*
Studies in geriatric patients have shown a tendency toward increased elimination half-life and steady-state plasma concentration in these patients, especially elderly females.

*Tenoxicam—*
The risk of hyperkalemia may be increased in elderly patients.

*Tiaprofenic acid—*
The risk of adverse renal effects reflected by hyperkalemia and/or an increase in blood urea nitrogen (BUN) may be increased in elderly patients; an increase in BUN occurred in 11.8% of elderly patients, but only 2.5% of all patients, in clinical trials.

## Dental
NSAIDs may cause soreness, irritation, or ulceration of the oral mucosa.
Most of the NSAIDs may rarely cause leukopenia and/or thrombocytopenia, which may result in an increased incidence of microbial infection, delayed healing, and gingival bleeding. If leukopenia or thrombocytopenia occurs, dental work should be deferred until blood counts have returned to normal, and patients should be instructed in proper oral hygiene, including caution in use of regular toothbrushes, dental floss, and toothpicks.

## Surgical
Caution is recommended in patients who require surgery. Most NSAIDs inhibit platelet aggregation and may prolong bleeding time, which may increase intra- and postoperative bleeding. The risk may be lower with usual doses of diclofenac, diflunisal, meclofenamate, mefenamic acid, or nabumetone, which may not significantly alter platelet aggregability (although mefenamic acid–induced hypoprothrombinemia, if present, could be hazardous to the patient). Recovery of platelet function may occur within 1 day after discontinuation of diclofenac, diflunisal, flurbiprofen, ibuprofen, indomethacin, or sulindac; 2 days after discontinuation of tolmetin; 4 days after discontinuation of naproxen; or 2 weeks following discontinuation of slowly eliminated agents such as oxaprozin or piroxicam. Consideration should be given to discontinuing NSAID treatment for an appropriate length of time prior to elective surgery, depending on the potency and duration of effect of the individual agent on platelet aggregability. In particular, it is recommended that treatment with oxaprozin, which is as potent as aspirin in inhibiting platelet aggregation, be discontinued 1 to 2 weeks prior to elective surgery.

## Drug interactions and/or related problems
The following drug interactions and/or related problems have been selected on the basis of their potential clinical significance (possible mechanism in parentheses where appropriate)—not necessarily inclusive (» = major clinical significance):

Note: Combinations containing any of the following medications, depending on the amount present, may also interact with this medication.

In addition to the interactions listed below, the possibility should be considered that additive or multiple effects leading to impaired blood clotting and/or increased risk of bleeding may occur if any NSAID is used concurrently with any medication having a significant potential for causing hypoprothrombinemia, thrombocytopenia, or gastrointestinal ulceration or hemorrhage.

For all NSAIDs

Note: All of the following interactions have not been documented with every NSAID. However, they have been reported with several of these medications and should be considered potential precautions to the use of any NSAID, especially with chronic administration.

Acetaminophen
(prolonged concurrent use of acetaminophen with an NSAID may increase the risk of adverse renal effects; it is recommended that patients be under close medical supervision while receiving such combined therapy)
(concurrent use with diflunisal may also increase the risk of acetaminophen-induced hepatotoxicity because diflunisal may increase the acetaminophen plasma concentration by 50%)

Alcohol or
Corticosteroids, glucocorticoid or
Corticotropin (chronic therapeutic use) or
Potassium supplements
(concurrent use with an NSAID may increase the risk of gastrointestinal side effects, including ulceration or hemorrhage; however, concurrent use with a glucocorticoid or corticotropin in the treatment of arthritis may provide additional therapeutic benefit and permit reduction of glucocorticoid or corticotropin dosage)

» Anticoagulants, coumarin- or indandione-derivative or
» Heparin or
» Thrombolytic agents, such as:
  Alteplase
  Anistreplase
  Streptokinase
  Urokinase
(inhibition of platelet aggregation by NSAIDs, and the possibility of NSAID-induced gastrointestinal ulceration or bleeding, may be hazardous to patients receiving anticoagulant or thrombolytic therapy; although nabumetone may be less likely than other NSAIDs to increase the risk of bleeding because it may be less likely to cause gastrointestinal ulceration or hemorrhage and because it has minimal, if any, platelet aggregation–inhibiting activity, caution is recommended; also, with usual doses, diclofenac, diflunisal, meclofenamate, and mefenamic acid may be less likely than other NSAIDs to significantly alter platelet aggregability)
(diflunisal, etodolac, fenoprofen, floctafenine, flurbiprofen, indomethacin, meclofenamate, mefenamic acid, phenylbutazone, piroxicam, sulindac, tiaprofenic acid, and tolmetin have been reported to potentiate the effects of coumarin- or indandione-derivative anticoagulants; the effect of floctafenine on coagulation test results becomes apparent only after 2 weeks of concurrent use; potentiation may result from displacement of the anticoagulant from protein-binding sites and, with phenylbutazone, from inhibition of the metabolism of the anticoagulant; concurrent use of phenylbutazone with an anticoagulant is not recommended; if another NSAID is used concurrently, coagulation tests should be monitored and anticoagulant dosage adjustments made, if necessary, when NSAID therapy is initiated or discontinued)

Antidiabetic agents, oral or
Insulin
(NSAIDs may increase the hypoglycemic effect of these medications because prostaglandins are directly involved in regulatory mechanisms of glucose metabolism and possibly because of displacement of the oral antidiabetics from serum proteins; dosage adjustments of the antidiabetic agent may be necessary; glipizide and glyburide, due to their nonionic binding characteristics, may not be affected as much as the other oral antidiabetic agents; however, caution with concurrent use is recommended)
(diclofenac has also been reported to decrease the effects of these medications, leading to hyperglycemia)

Antihypertensives or
Diuretics, especially
» Triamterene
(increased monitoring of the response to an antihypertensive agent may be advisable when any NSAID is used concurrently because flurbiprofen, indomethacin, ibuprofen, naproxen, oxaprozin, and piroxicam have been shown to reduce or reverse the effects of antihypertensives, possibly by inhibiting renal prostaglandin synthesis and/or by causing sodium and fluid retention)
(NSAIDs may decrease the diuretic, natriuretic, and antihypertensive effects of diuretics, probably by inhibiting renal prostaglandin synthesis; flurbiprofen has also been shown to interfere with furosemide-induced kaliuresis; however, diflunisal does not decrease the diuretic effect of furosemide)
(indomethacin may block the increase in plasma renin activity [PRA] induced by bumetanide, furosemide, or indapamide)
(concurrent use of an NSAID and a diuretic may increase the risk of renal failure secondary to a decrease in renal blood flow caused by inhibition of renal prostaglandin synthesis; specifically, concurrent use of triamterene and indomethacin is not recommended because this combination has caused renal function impairment [azotemia and reduced creatinine clearance] and a few cases of renal failure requiring hemodialysis)
(concurrent use of a potassium-sparing diuretic with indomethacin or diclofenac, and possibly other NSAIDs, may increase the risk of hyperkalemia)
(diflunisal significantly increases the plasma concentration of hydrochlorothiazide and decreases the hyperuricemic effect of hydrochlorothiazide or furosemide)

» Aspirin or
NSAIDs, two or more concurrently, especially
» Diflunisal and indomethacin concurrently or
Salicylates other than aspirin and diflunisal
(concurrent use of two or more NSAIDs, including aspirin, is not recommended; concurrent therapy may increase the risk of gastrointestinal toxicity, including ulceration or hemorrhage, without providing additional symptomatic relief; specifically, concurrent use of diflunisal and indomethacin has resulted in fatal gastrointestinal hemorrhage)
(concurrent use of aspirin with other NSAIDs may also increase the risk of bleeding at sites other than the gastrointestinal tract because of additive inhibition of platelet aggregation)
(concurrent administration of two or more NSAIDs may alter the pharmacokinetic profile of at least one of the medications, which may alter the therapeutic effect and/or increase the risk of adverse effects; specifically, aspirin decreases protein binding of ketoprofen and etodolac [but does not alter etodolac clearance], increases plasma clearance of ketoprofen, interferes with the formation and excretion of ketoprofen conjugates, decreases concentrations of the active sulfide metabolite of sulindac, and decreases the bioavailability of diclofenac, diflunisal, fenoprofen, flurbiprofen [by 50%], ibuprofen [by 50% in multiple-dose studies], indomethacin [by 20%], meclofenamate, piroxicam [by 20%], a single dose of tenoxicam [by 20%], and tolmetin. Also, diflunisal decreases the renal clearance of indomethacin, resulting in significantly increased indomethacin plasma concentrations, and decreases the concentration of the active sulfide metabolite of sulindac by 33%. Although studies to determine whether phenylbutazone alters etodolac clearance have not been done, phenylbutazone has been shown in vitro to decrease the protein binding of etodolac, leading to an 80% increase in the concentration of unbound etodolac))

Bone marrow depressants (See Appendix II)
(leukopenic and/or thrombocytopenic effects of these medications may be increased with concurrent or recent therapy if an NSAID causes the same effects; dosage adjustment of the bone marrow depressant, if necessary, should be based on blood counts)

» Cefamandole or
» Cefoperazone or
» Cefotetan or
» Plicamycin or
» Valproic acid
(these medications may cause hypoprothrombinemia; in addition, plicamycin or valproic acid may inhibit platelet aggregation; concurrent use with an NSAID may increase the risk of bleeding because of additive interferences with platelet function and/or the potential occurrence of NSAID-induced gastrointestinal ulceration or hemorrhage)

Colchicine
(concurrent use with an NSAID may increase the risk of gastrointestinal ulceration or hemorrhage, and concurrent use with phenylbutazone may also increase the risk of adverse hematologic effects)
(inhibition of platelet aggregation by NSAIDs, added to colchicine's effects on blood clotting mechanisms [colchicine may cause thrombocytopenia with chronic use and clotting defects, including disseminated intravascular coagulation, with overdose], may increase the risk of bleeding at sites other than the gastrointestinal tract)

» Cyclosporine or
Gold compounds or
Nephrotoxic medications, other (See Appendix II)
(inhibition of renal prostaglandin activity by NSAIDs may increase the plasma concentration of cyclosporine and/or the risk of cyclo-

sporine-induced nephrotoxicity; patients should be carefully monitored during concurrent use)

(the risk of adverse renal effects may also be increased when an NSAID is used concurrently with other nephrotoxic medications, possibly including gold compounds [although NSAIDs and gold compounds are commonly used concurrently in the treatment of arthritis])

Digitalis glycosides

(diclofenac and ibuprofen have been shown to increase serum digoxin concentrations, and indomethacin has increased digitalis concentrations in neonates being treated for patent ductus arteriosus; the possibility should be considered that some of the other NSAIDs may also increase digoxin concentrations, leading to an increased risk of digitalis toxicity; increased monitoring and dosage adjustments of the digitalis glycoside may be necessary during and following concurrent NSAID therapy; however, studies have failed to show that flurbiprofen, ketoprofen, piroxicam, or tenoxicam increases digoxin concentrations, and phenylbutazone may decrease digitalis concentrations [see individual *For phenylbutazone* listing, below])

» Lithium

(diclofenac, ibuprofen, indomethacin, naproxen, and piroxicam have been reported to increase the steady-state concentration of lithium, possibly by decreasing its renal clearance; with indomethacin, the steady-state lithium concentration was increased by up to 50%; other NSAIDs may have a similar effect; increased monitoring of lithium concentrations is recommended during and following concurrent use)

» Methotrexate

(concurrent use with phenylbutazone may increase the risk of agranulocytosis or bone marrow depression and is not recommended)

(NSAIDs may decrease protein binding and/or renal elimination of methotrexate, resulting in increased and prolonged methotrexate plasma concentrations and an increased risk of toxicity, especially during high-dose methotrexate infusion therapy; indomethacin has caused toxicity with intermediate-dose methotrexate infusions; fatalities have been reported; it is recommended that NSAID therapy be withheld for varying periods of time, depending on the elimination half-life of the individual NSAID [12 to 24 hours for agents with a short elimination half-life to up to 10 or 12 days for agents with a very long elimination half-life] prior to administration of a high-dose methotrexate infusion [for indomethacin, an intermediate- or high-dose methotrexate infusion]; also, NSAID therapy should not be resumed following the infusion until the methotrexate plasma concentration has decreased to a nontoxic level, usually at least 12 hours)

(severe, sometimes fatal, methotrexate toxicity has also been reported when NSAIDs were used concurrently with low to moderate doses of methotrexate, including doses commonly used in the treatment of rheumatoid arthritis or psoriasis; caution in concurrent use is recommended, with dosage of methotrexate being adjusted as determined by monitoring the plasma methotrexate concentration and/or adequacy of the patient's renal function)

Photosensitizing medications, other

(concurrent use with photosensitizing NSAIDs may cause additive photosensitizing effects)

Platelet aggregation inhibitors, other (See *Appendix II*)

(concurrent use with an NSAID may increase the risk of bleeding because of additive inhibition of platelet aggregation, as well as the potential for NSAID-induced gastrointestinal ulceration or hemorrhage)

(concurrent use of sulfinpyrazone with NSAIDs may also increase the risk of gastrointestinal ulceration or hemorrhage)

» Probenecid

(concurrent use of probenecid with ketoprofen is not recommended; probenecid decreases ketoprofen's renal clearance [by approximately 66%] and protein binding [by 28%], and inhibits formation and renal clearance of ketoprofen conjugates, leading to greatly increased ketoprofen plasma concentration and risk of toxicity)

(probenecid has also been shown to decrease renal and biliary clearance of indomethacin, and to increase plasma concentrations of indomethacin and naproxen, leading to increased risk of toxicity and possibly to increased effectiveness of the NSAID; if concurrent use is necessary, it is recommended that these NSAIDs be administered in reduced dosage and that increases in dosage be made slowly and in small increments)

(probenecid may also decrease excretion and increase serum concentrations of other NSAIDs, possibly enhancing effectiveness and/or increasing the potential for toxicity; a decrease in dosage of the NSAID may be necessary if adverse effects occur)

(probenecid may increase the plasma concentration of sulindac and its sulfone metabolite, and slightly decrease the plasma concentration of the active sulfide metabolite)

*For diflunisal (in addition those listed for all NSAIDs)*
Antacids

(concurrent chronic use may significantly decrease the plasma concentration of diflunisal)

*For fenoprofen (in addition to those listed for all NSAIDs)*
Antacids

(concurrent chronic use may significantly decrease the plasma concentration of fenoprofen)

Phenobarbital

(phenobarbital may increase metabolism of fenoprofen by inducing hepatic microsomal enzymes, leading to a decrease in the elimination half-life of fenoprofen; fenoprofen dosage adjustment may be required)

*For indomethacin (in addition to those listed for all NSAIDs)*
Aminoglycosides

(administration of indomethacin to neonates being treated for a patent ductus has decreased the renal clearance and increased the plasma concentration of concurrently administered aminoglycoside antibiotics; although not documented, similar effects may occur in other patients, leading to increased risk of toxicity; adjustment of aminoglycoside dosage may be required)

» Zidovudine

(indomethacin may competitively inhibit hepatic glucuronidation and decrease the clearance of zidovudine, possibly leading to potentiation of zidovudine toxicity; indomethacin toxicity may also be increased; concurrent use of the two medications should be avoided)

*For phenylbutazone (in addition to those listed for all NSAIDs)*

Note: Phenylbutazone induces hepatic microsomal enzymes and is itself metabolized by the same enzymes. It has been reported to increase the metabolism of several medications metabolized by hepatic microsomal enzymes and to decrease the metabolism of others. Although not documented, it has been proposed that, in some cases, phenylbutazone may compete with other medications for the enzymes.

Alcohol

(concurrent use of alcohol with phenylbutazone may increase the potential for impairment of psychomotor skills)

Anticonvulsants, hydantoin, especially

» Phenytoin

(phenylbutazone may displace hydantoin anticonvulsants from their protein-binding sites and inhibit their metabolism, possibly leading to increased elimination half-life and toxicity; hydantoin dosage adjustment, based on monitoring of plasma concentrations and/or observed signs of toxicity, may be required)

Barbiturates or
Cortisone

(phenylbutazone may decrease the efficacy of these medications by inducing hepatic microsomal enzymes and increasing their metabolism; the possibility should be considered that corticosteroids other than cortisone may be similarly affected)

Cholestyramine

(cholestyramine may decrease absorption of phenylbutazone; administration of phenylbutazone 1 hour before or 4 to 6 hours after cholestyramine may decrease the risk of impaired absorption and of toxicity resulting from sudden increases in absorption and serum concentration of phenylbutazone if cholestyramine therapy is discontinued)

Contraceptives, estrogen-containing, oral

(concurrent long-term use with phenylbutazone may result in reduced contraceptive reliability and increased incidence of breakthrough bleeding)

Dermatitis-causing medications, especially
Chloroquine
Hydroxychloroquine

(concurrent use with phenylbutazone may increase the risk of severe dermatologic reactions)

» Digitalis glycosides, possibly excepting digoxin

(phenylbutazone may increase the hepatic metabolism of digitalis, leading to a decrease in digitalis serum concentration; digitalis glycoside dosage adjustment may be necessary during and following concurrent use)

Hepatic enzyme inducers, other (See *Appendix II*)
(hepatic enzyme inducers may increase phenylbutazone metabolism and decrease its half-life)
Methylphenidate
(methylphenidate may inhibit metabolism of phenylbutazone, leading to increased plasma concentrations and toxicity; dosage adjustments may be necessary)
» Penicillamine
(concurrent use with phenylbutazone may increase the risk of serious hematologic and/or renal adverse effects)
Sulfonamides
(sulfonamides may displace phenylbutazone from its protein binding sites and potentiate its effects; phenylbutazone has also been reported to potentiate the effects of sulfonamides)
Other medications, oral, especially:
» Ciprofloxacin
» Enoxacin
» Itraconazole
» Ketoconazole
» Lomefloxacin
» Norfloxacin
» Ofloxacin
» Tetracyclines, oral
(antacids present in buffered phenylbutazone formulations may decrease absorption of many other orally administered medications by forming nonabsorbable complexes and/or increasing intragastric pH; if used concurrently, buffered phenylbutazone should be taken at least 6 hours before or 2 hours after ciprofloxacin or lomefloxacin, 8 hours before or 2 hours after enoxacin, 2 hours after itraconazole, 3 hours before or after ketoconazole, 2 hours before or after norfloxacin or ofloxacin, 1 to 3 hours before or after tetracycline, and at least 1 to 2 hours before or after other orally administered medications)

*For sulindac (in addition to those listed for all NSAIDs)*
Antacids
(concurrent chronic use may significantly decrease the plasma concentration of sulindac)
Dimethyl sulfoxide (DMSO)
(topical application of DMSO to arthritic joints [not recommended because safety and efficacy are unproven] by patients receiving sulindac has been reported to cause peripheral neuropathy and to decrease the plasma concentration of sulindac's active metabolite, thereby decreasing its efficacy)

*For tenoxicam (in addition to those listed for all NSAIDs)*
Cholestyramine
(cholestyramine decreased the average half-life of an intravenous dose of tenoxicam from 67.4 to 31.9 hours and increased the apparent clearance of tenoxicam by 105%)

*For tiaprofenic acid (in addition to those listed for all NSAIDs)*
Anticonvulsants, hydantoin, especially
» Phenytoin
(tiaprofenic acid may displace hydantoin anticonvulsants from their protein-binding sites, which may lead to an increase in the concentration of the unbound fraction and to toxicity; hydantoin dosage adjustment, based on monitoring of plasma concentrations and/or observed signs of toxicity, may be required)

## Laboratory value alterations
The following have been selected on the basis of their potential clinical significance (possible effect in parentheses where appropriate)—not necessarily inclusive (» = major clinical significance):
With diagnostic test results
*For diflunisal*
Salicylate concentrations, serum
(diflunisal may produce falsely elevated serum salicylate values determined via the Abbott TDx fluorescence polarization immunoassay, the Trinder colorimetric assay, or the Du Pont *aca* method, despite the fact that diflunisal is not metabolized to salicylate *in vivo*)

*For etodolac*
Bilirubin, urine, determinations
(phenolic metabolites of etodolac may cause false-positive test results)
Ketones, urine, determinations
(false-positive test results may occur with dipstick method of determination)

*For fenoprofen*
Triiodothyronine ($T_3$) determinations
(fenoprofen may interfere with total and free $T_3$ determinations in the Amerlex-M kit assay; thyroid stimulating hormone, total thyroxine, and thyrotropin releasing hormone test responses are not affected)

*For indomethacin*
Dexamethasone suppression test for endogenous depression
(indomethacin may produce false-negative test results [i.e., no indication of endogenous depression] because plasma cortisol concentration is reduced to a greater extent than with dexamethasone alone)
5-Hydroxyindoleacetic acid (5-HIAA), urinary, determinations
(false 5-HIAA concentration values may be measured via the Goldenberg modification of Undenfriend's method because indomethacin metabolites are structurally similar to 5-HIAA)

*For ketoprofen*
Albumin, urine, determinations and
Bile salts, urine, determinations and
17-Ketosteroid (17-KS), urine, determinations and
17-Hydroxycorticosteroid (17-OHCS), urine, determinations
(ketoprofen metabolites in urine may interfere with test procedures that rely on acid precipitation as an end point or on color reactions of carbonyl groups; no interference occurs in tests for urinary protein using commercially available dye-impregnated test strips)

*For mefenamic acid*
Bile, urinary, determinations
(false-positive test results may occur when the diazo tablet test is used; the Harrison test is not affected)

*For naproxen*
5-HIAA, urine, determinations
(naproxen may interfere with some assays)
Steroid, urine, determinations
(17-ketogenic steroid concentrations may be falsely increased by naproxen when *m*-dinitrobenzene reagent is used; although 17-hydroxycorticosteroid measurements are not significantly altered when the Porter-Silber test is used, naproxen therapy should be discontinued 72 hours before adrenal function tests are performed)

*For phenylbutazone*
Thyroid function tests
(phenylbutazone may decrease 24-hour $^{131}$I thyroidal uptake [effect lasts about 14 days] or increase resin or red cell $T_3$ uptake)

*For tolmetin*
Protein, urine, determinations
(the metabolites of tolmetin in urine produce false-positive tests for urine protein when the sulfosalicylic acid method is used; no interference occurs in tests for urine protein when commercially available dye-impregnated reagent strips are used)

With physiology/laboratory test values
Bleeding time
(may be prolonged by most NSAIDs [with ketoprofen, by 3 to 4 minutes above baseline values] because of suppressed platelet aggregation; effects may persist for less than 1 day [flurbiprofen, ibuprofen, indomethacin, sulindac], 2 days [tolmetin], 4 days [naproxen], or 2 weeks [oxaprozin and piroxicam] following discontinuation of therapy)
(effects on platelet aggregation and bleeding time appear minimal with usual doses of diclofenac, meclofenamate, or mefenamic acid, up to 1000 mg twice a day of diflunisal, or up to 1000 mg per day of nabumetone)

Glucose concentrations
(decrease in blood glucose concentration has been reported with ibuprofen, indomethacin, and piroxicam)
(increase in blood glucose concentration has been reported with indomethacin, phenylbutazone, piroxicam, and sulindac)
(increase in urine glucose concentration has also been reported with indomethacin)

Hematocrit or
Hemoglobin
(values may be decreased, possibly because of gastrointestinal bleeding or microbleeding and/or hemodilution caused by fluid retention)

Leukocyte count and
Platelet count
(may be decreased)

Liver function tests, including:
  Alkaline phosphatase, serum and
  Lactate dehydrogenase (LDH), serum and
  Transaminases, serum
    (values may be increased; liver function test abnormalities may return to normal despite continued use; however, if significant abnormalities occur, clinical signs and symptoms consistent with liver disease develop, or systemic manifestations such as eosinophilia or rash occur, the medication should be discontinued)
    (the incidence of significantly increased transaminase values is higher with diclofenac than with other NSAIDs; in clinical trials with diclofenac, elevations to more than 3 times the upper limit of normal occurred with overall rates of 2% in patients treated for 2 months and 4% in patients treated for 2 to 6 months; values in excess of 8 times the upper limit of normal occurred in approximately 1% of the patients)
Plasma renin activity (PRA)
  (indomethacin has been reported to decrease PRA and to block the increase in PRA usually produced by bumetanide, furosemide, or indapamide)
Potassium, serum, concentrations
  (may be increased)
Protein, urine (including albumin) concentrations
  (increases have been reported with diclofenac, diflunisal, indomethacin, phenylbutazone, piroxicam, sulindac, tenoxicam, and tolmetin)
Renal function tests, including:
  Blood urea nitrogen (BUN)
  Creatinine, serum
  Electrolyte, blood and urine, concentrations
  Urine volume
    (NSAIDs may decrease renal function, resulting in increased BUN, serum creatinine, and serum electrolyte concentrations and in decreased urine volume and urine electrolyte concentrations; however, in some cases, water retention may exceed that of sodium, resulting in dilutional hyponatremia)
Uric acid concentrations
  (serum concentrations may be decreased and urine concentrations increased by diclofenac, diflunisal, etodolac, oxaprozin, and phenylbutazone; in clinical trials with etodolac, the serum concentration was usually decreased by 1 to 2 mg per 100 mL [59 to 118 micromoles/L] after 4 weeks of therapy with 600 to 1000 mg per day and the reduction was maintained during the study period)

*For mefenamic acid only*
Prothrombin time
  (may be prolonged)

## Medical considerations/Contraindications
The medical considerations/contraindications included have been selected on the basis of their potential clinical significance (reasons given in parentheses where appropriate)—not necessarily inclusive (» = major clinical significance).

*Except under special circumstances, this medication should not be used when the following medical problems exist:*
*For all NSAIDs*
» Allergic reaction, severe, such as anaphylaxis or angioedema, induced by aspirin or other NSAIDs, history of or
» Nasal polyps associated with bronchospasm, aspirin-induced
  (high risk of severe allergic reactions because of cross-sensitivity)
*For diclofenac (in addition to those listed for all NSAIDs)*
» Blood dyscrasias, active or history of or
» Bone marrow depression
  (diclofenac may induce or exacerbate these conditions)
*For phenylbutazone (in addition to those listed for all NSAIDs)*
» Blood dyscrasias, active or history of or
» Bone marrow depression
  (phenylbutazone may induce or exacerbate these conditions)
» Cardiac disease, severe or
» Cardiac failure, incipient or
» Cardiopulmonary disease, severe
  (sodium and fluid retention caused by phenylbutazone may increase plasma volume and the risk of edema, acute pulmonary edema, and cardiac decompensation)
» Hepatic disease, severe or
» Renal disease, severe
  (increased phenylbutazone blood concentrations and potential for toxicity may result from decreased clearance; also, potential for adverse renal effects may be increased in the presence of pre-existing severe hepatic or renal disease)
» Peptic ulcer disease, active
  (may be exacerbated; increased risk of perforation and/or bleeding)

*Risk-benefit should be considered when the following medical problems exist:*
*For all NSAIDs*
Allergic reaction, mild, such as allergic rhinitis, urticaria, or skin rash, induced by aspirin or other NSAIDs, history of
  (possibility of cross-sensitivity)
Anemia or
Asthma
  (may be exacerbated)
Conditions predisposing to and/or exacerbated by fluid retention, such as:
  Compromised cardiac function
  Congestive heart disease
  Edema, pre-existing
  Hypertension
  Renal function impairment or failure
    (NSAIDs may cause fluid retention and edema)
Conditions predisposing to gastrointestinal toxicity, such as:
  Alcoholism, active
» Inflammatory or ulcerative disease of the upper or lower gastrointestinal tract, including Crohn's disease, diverticulitis, peptic ulcer disease, or ulcerative colitis, active or history of
  Tobacco use, or recent history of
    (NSAIDs should preferably not be given to patients with active peptic ulcer disease or gastrointestinal bleeding; if NSAID administration is considered essential, an antiulcer regimen should be administered concurrently)
    (caution and close supervision are also recommended for other patients in whom there is a significant risk of gastrointestinal toxicity; misoprostol or sucralfate should be considered as prophylaxis for those at high risk)
Congestive heart failure or
Diabetes mellitus or
Edema, pre-existing or
Extracellular volume depletion or
Sepsis
  (increased risk of renal failure)
» Hemophilia or other bleeding problems including coagulation or platelet function disorders
  (increased risk of bleeding because most NSAIDs inhibit platelet aggregation and may cause gastrointestinal ulceration or hemorrhage; although the risk of these problems is lower with nabumetone than with most other NSAIDs, caution is recommended)
Hepatic cirrhosis or
Hepatic function impairment
  (risk of renal failure is increased in patients with hepatic function impairment)
  (most NSAIDs are metabolized hepatically; impairment of metabolism may be particularly problematic for nabumetone, since metabolism to the active metabolite 6-MNA may be decreased sufficiently to reduce efficacy)
  (although stable hepatic cirrhosis does not alter the clearance of etodolac, the possibility should be considered that unstable hepatic disease or severe hepatic function impairment may do so)
  (hepatic function impairment, especially if associated with chronic alcoholic cirrhosis, produces variability in ketoprofen pharmacokinetics and reduces ketoprofen protein binding; the concentration of unbound ketoprofen may be doubled; caution and careful monitoring are recommended; also, only immediate-release ketoprofen dosage forms should be used if the patient's serum albumin is lower than 3.5 grams per deciliter)
  (hepatic cirrhosis, especially if associated with chronic alcoholism, increases the concentration of unbound naproxen, even though the total plasma concentration may be decreased; the lowest effective dose should be administered and the patient carefully monitored)
  (although the clearance of oxaprozin is not altered by well-compensated hepatic cirrhosis, caution is recommended in patients with severe hepatic function impairment)
  (biotransformation of sulindac to the active sulfide metabolite is slowed; however, biliary elimination of the metabolite is greatly decreased, leading to increased and prolonged plasma concentrations and increased risk of toxicity; the patient should be carefully monitored and dosage adjusted as necessary)

Renal function impairment
(increased risk of hyperkalemia and of adverse renal effects, including acute renal failure; especially careful monitoring of the patient is recommended)

(NSAIDs and/or their metabolites are excreted primarily via the kidneys; a reduction in dosage may be required to prevent accumulation)

(etodolac has not been shown to increase the risk of renal toxicity, and the pharmacokinetic profile of etodolac is not altered, when up to 500 mg of etodolac is administered every 12 hours to patients with mild to moderate renal function impairment; however, the possibility of renal toxicity associated with a reduction of renal prostaglandin synthesis leading to a decrease in renal blood flow cannot be discounted; caution and monitoring of patients considered to be at risk are recommended)

(although less than 1% of the active 6-MNA metabolite of nabumetone is eliminated in the urine unchanged, and increased concentrations of 6-MNA were not measured after administration of a single dose, caution is recommended in patients with renal function impairment because the extent to which metabolites may accumulate and cause adverse effects has not been determined)

(in end-stage renal disease, conversion of sulindac to its active metabolite is decreased)

» Renal function impairment
(the risk of toxicity associated with accumulation of the NSAID and/or the risk of adverse renal effects may be higher with diflunisal, fenoprofen, indomethacin, and piroxicam than with other NSAIDs; individualization of dosage and especially careful monitoring of the patient are recommended)

» Stomatitis
(may be induced by NSAIDs; this symptom of possible NSAID-induced blood dyscrasias may be masked by pre-existing stomatitis)

Systemic lupus erythematosus (SLE)
(patient may be predisposed to NSAID-induced central nervous system and/or renal adverse effects)

» Caution is also recommended in geriatric patients, who may be more likely to develop adverse hepatic or renal effects with these medications and in whom gastrointestinal ulceration or bleeding is more likely to cause serious consequences, including fatalities.

Caution is also recommended when an NSAID, especially fenoprofen, is used in patients who developed genitourinary tract problems such as dysuria, cystitis, hematuria, nephritis, or nephrotic syndrome during treatment with another NSAID.

The sodium content of diclofenac sodium, meclofenamate sodium, naproxen sodium, naproxen oral suspension, and tolmetin sodium should be considered when selecting an NSAID for patients who must restrict their sodium intake.

*For diclofenac (in addition to those listed for all NSAIDs)*
Porphyria, hepatic
(diclofenac may precipitate an acute attack)

*For indomethacin (in addition to those listed for all NSAIDs)*
Epilepsy or
» Mental depression or other psychiatric disturbances or
Parkinsonism
(indomethacin may aggravate these conditions)

*For mefenamic acid (in addition to those listed for all NSAIDs)*
» Hypoprothrombinemia, when prothrombin activity is 10 to 20% of normal
(increased risk of bleeding, since mefenamic acid may further increase the prothrombin time)

*For phenylbutazone (in addition to those listed for all NSAIDs)*
» Polymyalgia rheumatica or
» Temporal arteritis
(phenylbutazone may aggravate these conditions)

*For sulindac (in addition to those listed for all NSAIDs)*
» Renal calculus or history of
(renal calculi containing sulindac metabolites have occurred, rarely, in patients receiving sulindac; it is recommended that the medication be used with caution, and in conjunction with adequate fluid intake, in patients who may be predisposed to calculus formation)

*For rectal administration (in addition to those listed as applying to oral use of the NSAIDs with rectal dosage forms)*
» Bleeding, rectal or anal, active or recent history of or
» Hemorrhoids or
» Lesions, inflammatory, of anus or rectum or
» Proctitis or recent history of
(may be exacerbated or reactivated)

**Patient monitoring**
The following may be especially important in patient monitoring (other tests may be warranted in some patients, depending on condition; » = major clinical significance):

Blood urea nitrogen (BUN) determinations or
Creatinine concentrations, serum and/or
Potassium concentrations, serum
(monitoring may be required at periodic intervals during therapy, especially in patients with documented hepatic or renal function impairment, other patients known or suspected to be at risk for renal function impairment, and/or those taking diuretics concurrently; also, may be required if signs of possible renal toxicity, such as substantial increases in blood pressure, fluid retention, or rapid weight gain occur)

Complete physical examinations, including urinalyses
(recommended prior to and at regular frequent intervals during phenylbutazone therapy)

Hematocrit determinations and/or
Hemoglobin determinations and/or
Stool tests for occult blood loss
(may be performed at one- to six-month intervals to detect blood loss during prolonged therapy, depending on the individual patient's risk of developing gastrointestinal toxicity; however, these tests [unlike endoscopy, which is not recommended on a routine basis] are not capable of detecting ulcerations that are developing asymptomatically or of predicting whether severe gastrointestinal bleeding is likely to occur)

» Hematologic determinations
(recommended prior to initiation of phenylbutazone therapy and at regular intervals of 3 to 4 weeks during therapy for patients receiving the medication for periods longer than 1 week)

(although routine monitoring is not necessary during therapy with other NSAIDs, appropriate testing should be performed if symptoms of blood dyscrasias occur)

Liver function tests, especially determination of transaminase (AST [SGOT]; ALT [SGPT]) values
(may be required at periodic intervals during indomethacin therapy; also, it is recommended that hepatic function tests be performed within eight weeks following initiation of diclofenac therapy and periodically thereafter)

(may also be required at periodic intervals during therapy with other NSAIDs if the patient is known or suspected to be at increased risk of developing hepatic adverse effects)

(although routine monitoring is not necessary for most patients during therapy with NSAIDs other than diclofenac or indomethacin, appropriate tests should be performed if signs and/or symptoms of hepatotoxicity occur)

Ophthalmologic examinations
(may be required if vision problems such as blurred vision occur during therapy)

Upper gastrointestinal diagnostic tests
(recommended for patients with persistent or severe dyspepsia or other signs of possible gastrointestinal toxicity)

## Side/Adverse Effects

See *Table 3*, page 425.

Note: *Hypersensitivity reactions* with these medications may be similar to those reported for aspirin, i.e., *rhinosinusitis/asthma* or *angioedema/urticaria*. *Anaphylaxis* has also been reported, both in aspirin-sensitive patients and in those without known hypersensitivity to any of these agents. The risk of anaphylaxis, characterized by respiratory distress, circulatory collapse, and angioedema and/or urticaria with or without pruritus, may be increased when previously discontinued therapy with one of these medications is reinstituted. Although anaphylaxis occurs rarely with these agents, several reports have indicated a higher incidence of anaphylactic reactions with tolmetin than with the others.

Other *hypersensitivity reactions* affecting multiple body systems have also been reported with several of the NSAIDs. A hypersensitivity syndrome consisting of fever and chills, skin rashes or other cutaneous manifestations, hepatotoxicity, renal toxicity (including renal failure), leukopenia, thrombocytopenia, eosinophilia, inflamed glands or lymph nodes, and arthralgias has been reported rarely with diflunisal and with sulindac. Fever, skin rashes, and arthralgias have also preceded fenoprofen-induced renal toxicity. In addition, a syndrome of fever and chills, nausea, vomiting, and abdominal pain has been reported with ibuprofen, and a serum sickness– or influenza-like syndrome that may consist of troubled breathing, arthralgias, fever and chills, fatigue, pruritus, and/or skin rash or other cutaneous manifestations, has been reported with ibuprofen (although a positive causal relationship has not been established), meclofenamate, phenylbutazone, piroxicam, and tolmetin.

The antipyretic, analgesic, and anti-inflammatory actions of NSAIDs may mask symptoms of the occurrence or worsening of infections. *Reactivation of latent pulmonary tuberculosis* has been reported in a few patients receiving indomethacin.

Two cases of *biliary obstruction* associated with sulindac therapy have been reported. The obstruction was caused in each case by the presence in the common bile duct of a "sludge" of crystals containing a sulindac metabolite.

*Metabolic acidosis* and *respiratory alkalosis* have also been reported rarely (incidences < 1%) with phenylbutazone.

Patients 40 years of age and older may be more susceptible to the toxic effects of phenylbutazone. In patients 60 years of age and older, there is an increased risk of severe, possibly fatal, toxic reactions.

Phenylbutazone-induced *agranulocytosis* may occur with a rapid onset, especially in relatively young patients. *Aplastic anemia* may occur more frequently in patients receiving prolonged therapy, especially older female patients. Both *agranulocytosis* and *aplastic anemia* are more likely to occur in geriatric patients.

Because diflunisal is a salicylic acid derivative, the possibility that it may be associated with the development of *Reye's syndrome* in children, teenagers, or young adults with acute febrile illnesses, especially influenza or varicella, should be kept in mind.

## Overdose

For specific information on the agents used in the mangement of anti-inflammatory agents, nonsteroidal overdose, see:
- *Diazepam* in *Benzodiazepines (Systemic)* monograph;
- *Dopamine* or *Dobutamine* in *Sympathomimetic Agents—Cardiovascular Use (Parenteral-Systemic)* monograph; and/or
- *Vitamin K₁—Phytonadione* in *Vitamin K (Systemic)* monograph.

For more information on the management of overdose or unintentional ingestion, **contact a Poison Control Center** (see *Poison Control Center Listing*).

### Clinical effects of overdose

The following effects have been selected on the basis of their potential clinical significance (possible signs and symptoms in parentheses where appropriate)—not necessarily inclusive:

Acute and chronic
For phenylbutazone
> ***Bluish color of fingernails, lips, or skin; convulsions, especially in children; difficulty in hearing or ringing or buzzing in the ears; dizziness or lightheadedness; hallucinations; headache, severe and continuing; increase or decrease in blood pressure; mood or mental changes; nausea, vomiting, or stomach pain, severe; periorbital edema*** (swelling around the eyes); ***shortness of breath, troubled breathing, or unusually slow, fast, or irregular breathing; swelling of face, hands, feet, or lower legs***

> Note: The lowest fatal doses reported for phenylbutazone are 14 grams (in an adult) and 2 grams (in a 3-year-old child). The highest doses reported to have been survived are 40 grams (in a young adult) and 5 grams (in a 3-year-old child).
>
> Laboratory findings in overdose may reveal respiratory or metabolic acidosis or alkalosis, other electrolyte disturbances, impaired hepatic or renal function, and abnormalities of formed blood elements.
>
> Late manifestations of massive overdosage may occur 2 to 7 days following ingestion and may include hepatomegaly, jaundice, electrocardiographic abnormalities, blood dyscrasias, and ulceration of the buccal or gastrointestinal mucosa.

For other NSAIDs
> Note: The symptoms of overdose of most of the other NSAIDs have not been described as completely as for phenylbutazone. Reported symptoms have generally reflected the gastrointestinal, renal, and CNS toxicities of these medications. Following overdosage with a propionic acid derivative or indomethacin, patients may remain asymptomatic or experience only relatively mild *CNS effects* (e.g., lethargy, drowsiness) or *gastrointestinal symptoms* (e.g., abdominal pain, nausea, vomiting). However, more serious effects, such as *gastrointestinal hemorrhage, acute renal failure, convulsions,* and *coma* have been reported with these, as well as other, NSAIDs. *Convulsions* may be especially likely to occur following mefenamic acid overdose. Also, *hypoprothrombinemia* has been reported following overdose of several NSAIDs.

### Treatment of overdose

To decrease absorption—Emptying the stomach via induction of emesis (in alert patients only) or gastric lavage. However, syrup of ipecac may induce symptoms similar to those of NSAID toxicity, which may complicate diagnosis, and is therefore not recommended for induction of emesis.

Administering activated charcoal. The efficacy of activated charcoal in decreasing absorption of these medications when given more than 2 hours (6 hours for piroxicam) following ingestion of the overdose has not been determined. However, there is some evidence that repeated administration of activated charcoal may interrupt enterohepatic circulation and/or bind any of the medication that has diffused from the circulation into the intestine, thereby increasing nonrenal excretion.

To enhance elimination—Administering antacids or other urinary alkalizers may increase diflunisal or sulindac excretion. Antacids may also relieve adverse gastrointestinal effects.

Inducing diuresis may be helpful in overdosage with fenoprofen, ibuprofen, or tolmetin; however, furosemide does not lower fenoprofen blood concentration.

Hemodialysis may be necessary to treat renal failure, but cannot be relied upon to decrease plasma concentrations of most NSAIDs because of their high degree of protein binding. Studies have shown that diclofenac and ketoprofen are dialyzable, but that diflunisal, etodolac, ibuprofen, indomethacin, and oxaprozin are not.

Specific treatment—

For severe hypotension plasma:

Use of volume expanders

For convulsions:

Diazepam or other appropriate benzodiazepine anticonvulsants. See the package insert or *Diazepam* in *Benzodiazepines (Systemic)* for specific dosing guidelines for use of this product.

For hypoprothrombinemia:

Use of Vitamin K₁. See the package insert or *Vitamin K₁—Phytonadione* in *Vitamin K (Systemic)* for specific dosing guidelines for use of this product.

For prevention or reversal of early indications of, renal failure:

Use of dopamine plus dobutamine intravenously. See the package insert or *Dopamine* or *Dobutamine* in *Sympathomimetic Agents—Cardiovascular Use (Parenteral-Systemic)* for specific dosing guidelines for use of this product.

Instituting symptomatic and other supportive treatment as necessary. Certain adverse effects of NSAIDs, including nephritis or nephrotic syndrome, thrombocytopenia, hemolytic anemia, and severe cutaneous or other hypersensitivity reactions, may respond to glucocorticoid administration.

Monitoring—The possibility must be considered that gastrointestinal ulceration or hemorrhage, and phenylbutazone-induced blood dyscrasias, may occur several days after ingestion of an overdose. Patients being discharged after initial treatment should be informed of possible presenting symptoms and advised to seek immediate treatment if they occur.

Supportive care—Monitoring and supporting vital functions. If respiratory support is required following phenylbutazone overdose, respiratory stimulants should not be used. Patients in whom intentional overdose is known or suspected should be referred for psychiatric consultation.

## Patient Consultation

As an aid to patient consultation, refer to *Advice for the Patient, Anti-inflammatory Drugs, Nonsteroidal (Systemic).*

In providing consultation, consider emphasizing the following selected information (» = major clinical significance):

### Before using this medication

» Conditions affecting use, especially:
  Allergies to aspirin or any of the nonsteroidal anti-inflammatory drugs (NSAIDs)
  Pregnancy—Use of an NSAID during second half of pregnancy not recommended because of potential adverse effect on fetal blood flow and possible prolongation of pregnancy, dystocia, and difficult and/or delayed delivery
  Breast-feeding—*For indomethacin:* Has caused convulsions in a nursing infant
    *For meclofenamate and piroxicam:* These NSAIDs have caused adverse effects in animal studies

*For phenylbutazone:* May cause blood dyscrasias or other adverse effects in the infant

Use in children—*For indomethacin:* Because of toxicity, should be used with caution and only in patients unresponsive to less toxic NSAIDs

*For naproxen:* Skin rash more common in pediatric patients

*For phenylbutazone:* Because of toxicity, not recommended in children < 15 years of age

Use in the elderly—Increased risk of toxicity; initial dosage should be reduced and patients carefully monitored

Other medications, especially—

*For all NSAIDs:* Anticoagulants, aspirin, cephalosporins that may induce hypoprothrombinemia, cyclosporine, lithium, methotrexate, plicamycin, probenecid, triamterene, and valproic acid

*For indomethacin (in addition to those applying to all NSAIDs):* Zidovudine

*For phenylbutazone (in addition to those applying to all NSAIDs):* Digitalis, penicillamine, and phenytoin

*For buffered phenylbutazone (in addition to those applying to all NSAIDs and to phenylbutazone):* Ciprofloxacin, enoxacin, itraconazole, ketoconazole, lomefloxacin, norfloxacin, ofloxacin, and oral tetracyclines

*For tiaprofenic acid (in addition to those applying to all NSAIDs):* Phenytoin

Other medical problems, especially—

*For all NSAIDs:* Blood dyscrasias, bone marrow depression, cardiac or cardiopulmonary disease or predisposition to, clotting defects, hepatic disease, peptic ulcer or other inflammatory or ulcerative gastrointestinal tract disease or predisposition to, renal disease or predisposition to, and stomatitis

*For indomethacin (in addition to those applying to all NSAIDs):* Epilepsy, mental illness, and parkinsonism

*For phenylbutazone (in addition to those applying to all NSAIDs):* Polymyalgia rheumatica and temporal arteritis

*For sulindac (in addition to those applying to all NSAIDs):* Renal calculus or history of

*For rectal dosage forms (in addition to those applying to oral use of the NSAIDs with rectal dosage forms):* Anal or rectal bleeding, hemorrhoids, inflammatory lesions of anus or rectum, and proctitis or recent history of

**Proper use of this medication**
*For all NSAIDs*
» Not taking more medication than prescribed or recommended on OTC package label
» For use in arthritis—Compliance with therapy; noticeable improvement in condition usually requires a few days to a week of treatment (but up to 2 weeks, and sometimes even longer, in severe cases) and maximum effectiveness may require several weeks of treatment
» Proper dosing
  Missed dose (scheduled dosing): If dosing schedule is—
    Once or twice a day: Taking as soon as possible if remembered within one or two hours after dose should have been taken; skipping dose if not remembered until later
    More than twice a day: Taking as soon as possible; not taking if almost time for next dose; not doubling doses
» Proper storage

*For all capsule and tablet dosage forms*
  Taking with a full glass of water and not lying down for 15 to 30 minutes after taking

*For indomethacin, mefenamic acid, phenylbutazone, and piroxicam*
» Taking oral dosage forms with meals or antacids (a magnesium-and aluminum-containing antacid may be preferred) to reduce gastrointestinal irritation

*For flurbiprofen extended-release tablets, nabumetone, and naproxen extended-release tablets*
  Taking with food or antacids (a magnesium- and aluminum-containing antacid may be preferred) to reduce gastrointestinal irritation; taking with food also increases absorption

*For immediate-release and extended-release oral dosage forms of NSAIDs not listed above*
  Taking with food or antacids (a magnesium- and aluminum-containing antacid may be preferred) to reduce gastrointestinal irritation, although when used for acute conditions (e.g., pain, gout, fever, or dysmenorrhea) the first 1 or 2 doses may be taken on an empty stomach to speed the onset of action

*For oral suspensions*
  Not mixing suspension with an antacid or other liquid prior to use

*For delayed-release (enteric-coated) or extended-release dosage forms, diflunisal tablets, and all phenylbutazone tablet formulations*
  Swallowing whole; not breaking, chewing or crushing before swallowing

*For all suppository dosage forms*
  Proper administration technique

*For indomethacin suppositories*
  Retaining in rectum for 1 full hour to ensure maximum absorption

*For nonprescription use of ibuprofen or naproxen*
» Reading patient information sheet provided in package

*For phenylbutazone*
» Taking for prescribed indications only; not taking to relieve other aches and pains

*For mefenamic acid*
» Not taking longer than 7 days at a time unless otherwise directed by physician

**Precautions while using this medication**
» Regular visits to physician during prolonged therapy
» Possibility that use of alcohol may increase the risk of ulceration and, with phenylbutazone, depressant effects
  Not taking 2 or more NSAIDs, including ketorolac, concurrently, and not taking acetaminophen or aspirin or other salicylates for more than a few days while receiving NSAID therapy, unless concurrent use is prescribed by, and patient remains under the care of, a physician or dentist
  Caution if any surgery is required because of possible enhanced bleeding (although may be less of a problem with diclofenac, diflunisal, meclofenamate, mefenamic acid, and nabumetone)
  Caution if confusion, dizziness or lightheadedness, drowsiness, or vision problems occur
» Possibility of photosensitivity
  Possibility of gastrointestinal ulceration and bleeding
» Notifying physician immediately if influenza-like symptoms(chills, fever, or muscle aches and pains) occur shortly prior to or together with a skin rash; rarely, these symptoms may indicate a serious reaction to the medication
  Possibility of anaphylaxis

*For buffered phenylbutazone*
» Not taking within:
  —6 hours before or 2 hours after ciprofloxacin or lomefloxacin
  —8 hours before or 2 hours after enoxacin
  —2 hours after itraconazole
  —3 hours before or after ketoconazole
  —2 hours before or after norfloxacin or ofloxacin
  —1 to 3 hours before or after an oral tetracycline

*For mefenamic acid*
  Discontinuing use and checking with physician if severe diarrhea occurs

*For nonprescription use of ibuprofen or naproxen*
  Checking with health care professional if symptoms do not improve or if they worsen, if using for fever and fever lasts more than 3 days or returns, or if painful area is red or swollen

**Side/adverse effects**
» Stopping medication and obtaining emergency treatment if symptoms of any of the following occur:

*For all NSAIDs*
  Anaphylaxis, angioedema, or bronchospasm

» Stopping medication and checking with physician immediately if symptoms of the following occur:

*For all NSAIDs*
  Spitting up blood, unexplained nosebleeds, chest pain, convulsions, fainting, gastrointestinal ulceration or bleeding, and blood dyscrasias

*For mefenamic acid (in addition to those applying to all NSAIDs)*
  Diarrhea

*For phenylbutazone (in addition to those applying to all NSAIDs)*
  Edema

Signs and symptoms of other potential side effects, especially:

*For all NSAIDs*
  Dysarthria, hallucinations, aseptic meningitis, migraine, mood or mental changes, peripheral neuropathy, syncope, or other central nervous system effects; dermatitis (allergic or exfoliative), Stevens-Johnson syndrome, or other dermatologic effects; colitis, dysphagia, esophagitis, gastritis, gastroenteritis, or other digestive system effects; crystalluria, urinary tract irritation or infection, or other genitourinary effects; anemia or hypocoagulation; hepatitis; angiitis, fever, allergic rhinitis, or other hypersensitivity reactions not listed previously; loosening or splitting of fingernails; lymphadenopathy;

vision problems, conjunctivitis, or other ocular effects; stomatitis, glossitis, or other oral/perioral effects; hearing problems or tinnitus; pancreatitis; and edema, hyperkalemia, polyuria, renal impairment or failure, or other renal effects

*For indomethacin (in addition to those applying to all NSAIDs)*
  Headache (severe), especially in the morning

Possibility that the following may occur many days or weeks after medication is discontinued:

*For phenylbutazone*
  Blood dyscrasias

## General Dosing Information

The sodium content of diclofenac sodium, meclofenamate sodium, naproxen sodium, naproxen oral suspension, and tolmetin sodium should be considered when selecting a nonsteroidal anti-inflammatory drug (NSAID) for patients who must restrict their sodium intake. Also, the sucrose content of ibuprofen and naproxen suspensions must be considered when selecting an NSAID for patients who must restrict their sucrose intake.

Patients who do not respond to one NSAID may respond to another. In responsive patients, partial symptomatic relief of arthritic symptoms usually occurs within 1 or 2 weeks, although maximum effectiveness may occur only after several weeks of therapy.

A reduction of initial dosage, possibly as low as one-half the usual adult dose, is recommended for geriatric patients, especially those 70 years of age or older. However, if the reduced dose fails to produce an adequate clinical response and the medication is well tolerated, dosage may be increased as required and tolerated.

A reduction of dosage may also be required to prevent accumulation of NSAIDs and/or their metabolites (some of which may be unstable and may be hydrolyzed to the parent compound when their excretion is delayed) in patients with renal function impairment.

Long-term use of NSAIDs in doses that approach or exceed maximum dosage recommendations should be considered only if the clinical benefit is increased sufficiently to offset the higher risk of gastrointestinal toxicity or other adverse effects.

Indomethacin, mefenamic acid, phenylbutazone, and piroxicam should be administered immediately after meals or with food or antacids to reduce gastrointestinal irritation. Flurbiprofen extended-release capsules, nabumetone, or naproxen extended-release tablets should also be taken with food to increase absorption as well as reduce gastrointestinal irritation. The other NSAIDs (except for delayed-release [enteric-coated] and rectal dosage forms) are also preferably taken after meals or with food or antacids to reduce gastrointestinal irritation, especially during chronic use; however, for faster absorption when a rapid initial effect is required (as for analgesic or antipyretic use), the first 1 or 2 doses may be taken 30 minutes before meals or at least 2 hours after meals. If an antacid is taken concurrently, an aluminum and magnesium–containing formulation may be preferred, since studies have shown that this formulation does not adversely affect absorption of most NSAIDs (See *Table 1*, page 420).

It is recommended that solid oral dosage forms of NSAIDs be taken with a full glass (240 mL) of water and that the patient remain in an upright position for 15 to 30 minutes after administration. These measures may reduce the risk of tablets or capsules becoming lodged in the esophagus, which has been reported to cause prolonged esophageal irritation and difficulty in swallowing in some patients receiving these medications.

In the treatment of primary dysmenorrhea, maximum benefit is achieved by initiating NSAID therapy as rapidly as possible after the onset of menses. Prophylactic therapy (i.e., starting NSAID administration a few days prior to the expected onset of the menstrual period) has not been found to provide additional therapeutic benefit.

Concurrent use of an NSAID with an opioid analgesic provides additive analgesia and may permit lower doses of the opioid analgesic to be utilized.

The analgesic activity of non-opioid analgesics is subject to a ceiling effect. Therefore, administration of an NSAID in higher-than-recommended analgesic doses may not provide additional therapeutic benefit in the treatment of pain not associated with inflammation.

In the treatment of arthritis, most of these agents have been shown to provide additional symptomatic relief when administered concurrently with gold compounds or glucocorticoids. NSAIDs may permit reduction of glucocorticoid dosage; however, reductions of glucocorticoid dosage, especially following long-term use, should be gradual to avoid symptoms associated with adrenal insufficiency or other manifestations of too-sudden withdrawal.

---

## DICLOFENAC

## Summary of Differences

Indications:
  Indicated for rheumatoid arthritis, osteoarthritis, and ankylosing spondylitis. Immediate-release tablets only indicated for pain and primary dysmenorrhea, and may also be used to relieve acute attacks of gout or calcium pyrophosphate deposition disease (pseudogout) and pain associated with nonrheumatic inflammatory conditions or vascular headaches.

Pharmacology/pharmacokinetics:
  Physicochemical characteristics—Chemical group: A phenylacetic acid derivative.
  Other actions/effects—
    With usual doses, has lesser effect on platelet aggregation than most NSAIDs.
    Also has uricosuric activity.
  Biotransformation—Almost 50% of a dose eliminated via first-pass metabolism.
  Half-life—Elimination: 1.2–2 hours.
  Onset of action—Pain: Tablets—30 minutes.
  Duration of action—Pain: Tablets—Up to 8 hours.

Precautions:
  Pregnancy/reproduction—Embryotoxicity and other adverse effects, but not teratogenicity, demonstrated in animal studies.
  Surgical—With recommended doses may be less likely than most other NSAIDs to increase perisurgical bleeding.
  Drug interactions and/or related problems—
    Also, reported to increase digoxin plasma concentrations.
    Also, concurrent use with potassium-sparing diuretics may cause hyperkalemia.
    Also, reported to decrease effects of antidiabetic agents or insulin.
  Laboratory value alterations—
    With usual doses is less likely than most other NSAIDs to increase bleeding time significantly.
    Higher incidence of transaminase values being elevated to > 3 times the upper limit of normal than with other NSAIDs.
    Also, may decrease plasma concentration and increase urine concentration of uric acid.
  Medical considerations/contraindications—
    Not recommended for patients with blood dyscrasias (or history of) or bone marrow depression.
    Caution also required in patients with hepatic porphyria; may precipitate an acute attack.
    Caution with diclofenac sodium–containing dosage forms in patients who must restrict their sodium intake.
  Patient monitoring—Routine liver function tests recommended.

Side/adverse effects:
  See *Table 3*, page 425.

## Additional Dosing Information

See also *General Dosing Information*.

Diclofenac therapy should be discontinued if gastrointestinal bleeding or ulceration occurs.

**For oral dosage forms only**

The delayed-release tablets and the extended-release tablets are to be swallowed whole, not crushed or chewed.

## Oral Dosage Forms

### DICLOFENAC POTASSIUM TABLETS

**Usual adult dose**
Analgesic and
Antidysmenorrheal—
  Oral, 50 mg three times a day as needed. If necessary, 100 mg may be administered for the first dose only.
Rheumatoid arthritis—
  Oral, 150 to 200 mg per day in three or four divided doses, initially. After a satisfactory response has been obtained, dosage should be reduced to the minimum dose that provides continuing control of symptoms, usually 75 to 100 mg a day in three divided doses.
Osteoarthritis—
  Oral, 100 to 150 mg per day in two or three divided doses, initially. After a satisfactory response has been obtained, dosage should be reduced to the minimum dose that provides continuing control of symptoms.

Ankylosing spondylitis[1]:—
    Oral, 100 to 125 mg a day in four or five divided doses, initially. After a satisfactory response has been obtained, dosage should be reduced to the minimum dose that provides continuing control of symptoms.

**Usual adult prescribing limits**
Analgesic and
Antidysmenorrheal—
    Up to 200 mg on the first day, then 150 mg per day thereafter.
Rheumatoid arthritis—
    225 mg per day.
Osteoarthritis—
    150 mg per day; higher doses have not been studied.

**Usual pediatric dose**
Safety and efficacy have not been established.

**Strength(s) usually available**
U.S.—
    25 mg (Rx) [*Cataflam* (calcium phosphate; colloidal silicon dioxide; iron oxides; magnesium stearate; microcrystalline cellulose; polyethylene glycol; povidone; sodium starch glycolate; starch; sucrose; talc; titanium dioxide)].
    50 mg (Rx) [*Cataflam* (calcium phosphate; colloidal silicon dioxide; iron oxides; magnesium stearate; microcrystalline cellulose; polyethylene glycol; povidone; sodium starch glycolate; starch; sucrose; talc; titanium dioxide)].
Canada—
    50 mg [*Voltaren Rapide* (carnauba wax; cellulose; colloidal silicon dioxide; corn starch; ferric oxide; magnesium stearate; polyethylene glycol; povidone; sodium carboxymethyl starch; sucrose; talc; titanium dioxide; tribasic calcium phosphate; white ink)].

**Packaging and storage**
Store below 30 °C (86 °F), in a tight container, unless otherwise directed by manufacturer. Protect from moisture.

**Auxiliary labeling**
- Take with food.
- Take with a full glass of water.
- Avoid alcoholic beverages.

### DICLOFENAC SODIUM DELAYED-RELEASE TABLETS

**Usual adult dose**
Analgesic
and Antidysmenorrheal—
    The delayed-release formulation is not recommended. See *Diclofenac Potassium Tablets*, which should be used for these indications.
Antirheumatic (nonsteroidal anti-inflammatory)—
    See *Diclofenac Potassium Tablets*.

**Usual pediatric dose**
Safety and efficacy have not been established.

**Strength(s) usually available**
U.S.—
    25 mg (Rx) [*Voltaren* (hydroxypropyl methylcellulose; iron oxide; lactose; magnesium stearate; methacrylic acid copolymer; microcrystalline cellulose; polyethylene glycol; povidone; propylene glycol; sodium hydroxide; sodium starch glycolate; talc; titanium dioxide; D&C Yellow #10 Aluminum Lake)].
    50 mg (Rx) [*Voltaren* (hydroxypropyl methylcellulose; iron oxide; lactose; magnesium stearate; methacrylic acid copolymer; microcrystalline cellulose; polyethylene glycol; povidone; propylene glycol; sodium hydroxide; sodium starch glycolate; talc; titanium dioxide; FD&C Blue #1 Aluminum Lake)].
    75 mg (Rx) [*Voltaren* (hydroxypropyl methylcellulose; iron oxide; lactose; magnesium stearate; methacrylic acid copolymer ; microcrystalline cellulose; polyethylene glycol; povidone; propylene glycol; sodium hydroxide; sodium starch glycolate; talc; titanium dioxide)].
Canada—
    25 mg (Rx) [*Apo-Diclo* (sodium <1 mmol [1.81 mg]); *Novo-Difenac*; *Nu-Diclo* (sodium <1 mmol); *Voltaren* (lactose; sodium < 1 mmol [2.03 mg])].
    50 mg (Rx) [*Apo-Diclo* (sodium <1 mmol [3.62 mg]); ; *Novo-Difenac*; *Nu-Diclo* (sodium <1 mmol); *Voltaren* (lactose; sodium < 1 mmol [4.06 mg])].

**Packaging and storage**
Store below 30 °C (86 °F), in a tight container, unless otherwise specified by manufacturer. Protect from moisture.

**Auxiliary labeling**
- Swallow tablets whole.
- Take with a full glass of water.
- Avoid alcoholic beverages.

### DICLOFENAC SODIUM EXTENDED-RELEASE TABLETS

**Usual adult dose**
Antirheumatic (nonsteroidal anti-inflammatory)—
    Oral, 75 or 100 mg once a day, in the morning or evening, or 75 mg two times a day, in the morning and evening.
Note: The extended-release dosage form is not intended as initial therapy; the daily maintenance dose should be determined using an immediate- or delayed-release formulation. The extended-release dosage form may then be used, if desired, provided that the required dose can be achieved with the available strengths.

**Usual pediatric dose**
Safety and efficacy have not been established.

**Strength(s) usually available**
U.S.—
    Not commercially available.
Canada—
    75 mg (Rx) [*Voltaren SR* (sodium < 1 mmol [6.1 mg])].
    100 mg (Rx) [*Novo-Difenac SR*; *Voltaren SR* (sodium < 1 mmol [8.13 mg])].

**Packaging and storage**
Store below 40 °C (104 °F), preferably between 15 and 30 °C (59 and 86 °F), unless otherwise specified by manufacturer.

**Auxiliary labeling**
- Take with food.
- Swallow tablets whole.
- Take with a full glass of water.
- Avoid alcoholic beverages.

## Rectal Dosage Forms

### DICLOFENAC SODIUM SUPPOSITORIES

**Usual adult dose**
Antirheumatic (nonsteroidal anti-inflammatory)—
    Rectal, 50 or 100 mg, as a substitute for the last oral dose of the day.

**Usual adult prescribing limits**
Total daily dosage (oral and rectal) should not exceed 150 mg.

**Usual pediatric dose**
Safety and efficacy have not been established.

**Strength(s) usually available**
U.S.—
    Not commercially available.
Canada—
    50 mg (Rx) [*Voltaren* (sodium < 1 mmol [4.06 mg])].
    100 mg (Rx) [*Voltaren* (sodium < 1 mmol [8.13 mg])].

**Packaging and storage**
Store below 40 °C (104 °F), preferably between 15 and 30 °C (59 and 86 °F), unless otherwise specified by manufacturer.

**Auxiliary labeling**
- Avoid alcoholic beverages.
- For rectal use.

---

[1]Not included in Canadian product labeling.

---

## *DIFLUNISAL*

## Summary of Differences

Indications:
    Indicated for rheumatoid arthritis, osteoarthritis, ankylosing spondylitis, and psoriatic arthritis, and pain. May also be used to relieve acute attacks of gout or calcium pyrophosphate deposition disease (pseudogout), dysmenorrhea, and pain associated with nonrheumatic inflammatory conditions or vascular headaches.
Pharmacology/pharmacokinetics:
    Physicochemical characteristics—Chemical group: A salicylate derivative, although not metabolized to salicylate *in vivo*.
    Other actions/effects—
    Platelet aggregation inhibition significant only with greater-than-recommended doses.
    Also has uricosuric activity.
    Half-life—Elimination: 8–12 hours; greatly prolonged by renal function impairment.
    Onset of action—Pain: 1 hour.
    Duration of action—Pain: 8–12 hours.

Precautions:
   Pregnancy/reproduction—Embryotoxic and teratogenic effects demonstrated in rabbits, but not found to be teratogenic in mice.
   Surgical—With recommended doses may be less likely than most other NSAIDs to increase perisurgical bleeding.
   Drug interactions and/or related problems—
   Also, may increase risk of acetaminophen-induced hepatotoxicity.
   Also, chronic concurrent use of antacids significantly decreases diflunisal plasma concentration.
   Diflunisal also increases plasma concentration of hydrochlorothiazide and decreases hyperuricemic effect of hydrochlorothiazide or furosemide, but has not been shown to decrease furosemide-induced diuresis.
   Laboratory value alterations—
   Interference with salicylate determinations; may cause falsely elevated salicylate values.
   With usual doses is less likely than most other NSAIDs to increase bleeding time significantly.
   May decrease plasma concentrations and increase urine concentrations of uric acid.
   Medical considerations/contraindications—Higher risk than with most other NSAIDs in patients with renal function impairment.
Side/adverse effects:
   Reported to cause a characteristic hypersensitivity syndrome.
   Possibility of Reye's syndrome in children and adolescents with acute febrile illness should be considered (as with other salicylates).
   See also *Table 3*, page 425.

## Additional Dosing Information
See also *General Dosing Information*.

Administration of a 1-gram initial loading dose is recommended to provide faster onset of analgesic action, shorter time to peak analgesic effect, and greater peak analgesic action. For long-term use, the initial loading dose decreases the time needed to reach steady-state plasma concentrations; if a loading dose is not administered, 2 to 3 days may be required to evaluate changes in treatment regimens.

In patients with impaired renal function, especially if renal function is decreased to ½ the normal value or below, a reduction in dosage and/or an increase in the dosing interval may be necessary to prevent diflunisal accumulation.

Tablets are to be swallowed whole, not crushed or chewed.

Because diflunisal is not hydrolyzed to salicylic acid *in vivo*, serum salicylate concentration cannot be used as a guide to dosage or potential toxicity during therapy.

## Oral Dosage Forms
### DIFLUNISAL TABLETS USP
**Usual adult dose**
Rheumatoid arthritis or
Osteoarthritis—
   Oral, 250 to 500 mg two times a day; dosage may be increased or decreased according to patient response.
Analgesic—
   Oral, 1 gram initially, followed by 500 mg every eight to twelve hours as needed.
   Note: For some patients, 500 mg initially followed by 250 mg every eight to twelve hours may be appropriate, depending on the severity of pain or the age, weight, or response of the patient.

**Usual adult prescribing limits**
Up to 1.5 grams daily.

**Usual pediatric dose**
Dosage has not been established.

**Strength(s) usually available**
U.S.—
   250 mg (Rx) [*Dolobid;* GENERIC].
   500 mg (Rx) [*Dolobid;* GENERIC (talc; titanium dioxide)].
Canada—
   250 mg (Rx) [*Apo-Diflunisal; Dolobid; Novo-Diflunisal*].
   500 mg (Rx) [*Apo-Diflunisal; Dolobid; Novo-Diflunisal*].

**Packaging and storage**
Store below 40 °C (104 °F), preferably between 15 and 30 °C (59 and 86 °F). Store in a well-closed container.

**Auxiliary labeling**
• Take with food.
• Swallow tablets whole.
• Take with a full glass of water.
• Avoid alcoholic beverages.

---
## ETODOLAC

## Summary of Differences
Indications:
   Indicated for treatment of osteoarthritis and for pain. May also be used to relieve acute attacks of gout or calcium pyrophosphate deposition disease (pseudogout), dysmenorrhea, and pain associated with non-rheumatic inflammatory conditions or vascular headaches.
Pharmacology:
   Physicochemical characteristics—Chemical group: A pyranoindole-acetic acid derivative.
   Other actions/effects—Also has uricosuric activity.
   Decreases renal function, but with administration of up to 500 mg every 12 hours recovery occurs prior to administration of next dose.
   Half-life—Elimination:
   Single dose—6–7 hours.
   At steady-state—7.3±4 hours.
   Onset of action—Pain: 30 minutes.
   Time to peak effect—Pain: 1–2 hours.
   Duration of action—Pain:
   200-mg single dose—4–5 hours.
   400-mg single dose—Generally 5–6 hours; up to 8–12 hours in some patients.
Precautions:
   Pregnancy/reproduction—Alterations of limb development demonstrated in animal studies, but drug- or dose-response relationship not established.
   Geriatrics—No differences relative to younger adults in pharmacokinetic profile with 200 mg twice a day or in side effects profile with 600 mg per day.
   Laboratory value alterations—May cause false-positive test results in urinary bilirubin and urinary ketone determinations.
   Decrease in serum uric acid concentration may be expected.
   Medical considerations/contraindications: Significant problems have not been demonstrated in patients with mild to moderate renal function impairment receiving up to 500 mg every 12 hours.
Side/adverse effects:
   See *Table 3*, page 425.

## Oral Dosage Forms
### ETODOLAC CAPSULES
**Usual adult dose**
Antirheumatic (nonsteroidal anti-inflammatory)—
   Oral, 400 mg two or three times a day or 300 mg three or four times a day, initially. After a satisfactory response has been obtained, dosage should be individualized according to patient tolerance and response. Most patients are maintained on 600 to 1200 mg per day. However, as little as 200 mg two times a day has been effective in some patients.
   Note: Although doses of up to 1 gram per day have been effective when administered in two divided doses (500 mg every twelve hours), administration on a three-dose-a-day schedule may provide greater benefit.
Analgesic—
   Oral, 400 mg initially, then 200 to 400 mg every six to eight hours as needed. If a 400-mg dose fails to provide eight hours of analgesia, a regimen of 300 mg every six hours may be effective.

**Usual adult prescribing limits**
Patients weighing less than 60 kg—20 mg per kg of body weight per day.
Patients weighing 60 kg or more—1.2 grams per day.

**Usual pediatric dose**
Safety and efficacy have not been established.

**Usual geriatric dose**
See *Usual adult dose*.

**Strength(s) usually available**
U.S.—
   200 mg (Rx) [*Lodine* (cellulose; gelatin; iron oxides; lactose; magnesium stearate; povidone; sodium lauryl sulfate; sodium starch glycolate; titanium dioxide)].
   300 mg (Rx) [*Lodine* (cellulose; gelatin ; iron oxides; lactose; magnesium stearate; povidone; sodium lauryl sulfate; sodium starch glycolate; titanium dioxide)].
Canada—
   Not commercially available.

**Packaging and storage**
Store below 40 °C (104 °F), preferably between 15 and 30 °C (59 and 86 °F), unless otherwise specified by manufacturer.

### Auxiliary labeling
- Take with food.
- Take with a full glass of water.
- Avoid alcoholic beverages.

## ETODOLAC TABLETS

**Usual adult dose**
See *Etodolac Capsules*.

**Usual adult prescribing limits**
See *Etodolac Capsules*.

**Usual pediatric dose**
Safety and efficacy have not been established.

**Usual geriatric dose**
See *Etodolac Capsules*.

**Strength(s) usually available**
U.S.—
   400 mg (Rx) [*Lodine* (cellulose; FD&C Yellow #10; FD&C Blue #2; FD&C Yellow #6; hydroxypropyl methylcellulose; lactose; magnesium stearate; polyethylene glycol; polysorbate 80; povidone; sodium starch glycolate; titanium dioxide)].
Canada—
   Not commercially available.

**Packaging and storage**
Store below 40 °C (104 °F), preferably between 15 and 30 °C (59 and 86 °F), unless otherwise specified by manufacturer.

**Auxiliary labeling**
- Take with food.
- Take with a full glass of water.
- Avoid alcoholic beverages.

---

## FENOPROFEN

## Summary of Differences
Indications:
   Indicated for rheumatoid arthritis, osteoarthritis, ankylosing spondylitis, and psoriatic arthritis; pain; and acute attacks of gout or calcium pyrophosphate deposition disease (pseudogout). May also be used to relieve dysmenorrhea and pain associated with nonrheumatic inflammatory conditions or vascular headaches. Also used for vascular headache prophylaxis.
Pharmacology/pharmacokinetics:
   Physicochemical characteristics—Chemical group: A propionic acid derivative.
   Half-life—Elimination: 3 hours.
Precautions:
   Pregnancy/reproduction—No teratogenic or other adverse effects demonstrated in animal studies.
   Drug interactions and/or related problems—Concurrent chronic use with antacids significantly decreases fenoprofen plasma concentration.
   Also, phenobarbital may increase metabolism and decrease half-life of fenoprofen.
   Laboratory value alterations—Interference with triiodothyronine ($T_3$) determinations using the Amerlex-M kit assay.
   Medical considerations/contraindications—Higher risk than with most other NSAIDs in patients with renal function impairment.
Side/adverse effects:
   See *Table 3*, page 425.

## Additional Dosing Information
See also *General Dosing Information*.

In the treatment of arthritis, improvement in condition may occur within a few days, but 2 to 3 weeks of continuous use on a regular basis may be required for maximum effectiveness.

## Oral Dosage Forms
Note: Bracketed uses in the *Dosage Forms* section refer to categories of use and/or indications that are not included in U.S. product labeling. The dosing and strengths of the available dosage forms are expressed in terms of the free acid (not the calcium salt).

## FENOPROFEN CALCIUM CAPSULES USP

**Usual adult dose**
Antirheumatic (nonsteroidal anti-inflammatory)—
   Oral, 300 to 600 mg (free acid), depending on the severity of the symptoms, three or four times a day, then adjusted as needed.
   Note: Higher doses generally are required in rheumatoid arthritis than in osteoarthritis.
Analgesic[1] or
[Antidysmenorrheal][1]—
   Oral, 200 mg (free acid) every four to six hours as needed.

**Usual adult prescribing limits**
Antirheumatic (nonsteroidal anti-inflammatory)—
   Up to 3.2 grams (free acid) daily.

**Usual pediatric dose**
Safety and dosage have not been established.

**Strength(s) usually available**
U.S.—
   200 mg (free acid) (Rx) [*Nalfon 200;* GENERIC].
   300 mg (free acid) (Rx) [*Nalfon;* GENERIC].
Canada—
   300 mg (free acid) (Rx) [*Nalfon*].

**Packaging and storage**
Store below 40 °C (104 °F), preferably between 15 and 30 °C (59 and 86 °F). Store in a well-closed container.

**Auxiliary labeling**
- Take with food.
- Take with a full glass of water.
- May cause drowsiness.
- Avoid alcoholic beverages.

## FENOPROFEN CALCIUM TABLETS USP

**Usual adult dose**
See *Fenoprofen Calcium Capsules USP*.

**Usual adult prescribing limits**
See *Fenoprofen Calcium Capsules USP*.

**Usual pediatric dose**
Safety and dosage have not been established.

**Strength(s) usually available**
U.S.—
   600 mg (free acid) (Rx) [*Nalfon* (scored); GENERIC].
Canada—
   600 mg (free acid) (Rx) [*Nalfon*].

**Packaging and storage**
Store below 40 °C (104 °F), preferably between 15 and 30 °C (59 and 86 °F). Store in a well-closed container.

**Auxiliary labeling**
- Take with food.
- Take with a full glass of water.
- May cause drowsiness.
- Avoid alcoholic beverages.

[1]Not included in Canadian product labeling.

---

## FLOCTAFENINE

## Summary of Differences
Indications:
   Indicated for relief of pain. May also be used to relieve acute attacks of gout or calcium pyrophosphate deposition disease (pseudogout), dysmenorrhea, and pain associated with nonrheumatic inflammatory conditions or vascular headaches.
Precautions:
   Pregnancy/reproduction—Embryotoxicity but not teratogenicity demonstrated in animal studies.
   Drug interactions and/or related problems—Floctafenine-induced increase in effect of coumarin- or indandione-derivative anticoagulants may not become apparent until after 2 weeks of concurrent use.
Side/adverse effects:
   See *Table 3*, page 425.

## Additional Dosing Information
See also *General Dosing Information*.

Because the safety and efficacy of floctafenine for long-term administration has not been established, this medication is recommended for short-term use only.

## Oral Dosage Forms
### FLOCTAFENINE TABLETS
**Usual adult dose**
Analgesic—
　Oral, 200 to 400 mg every six to eight hours, as needed.

**Usual adult prescribing limits**
Dosage should not exceed 1.2 grams per day.

**Usual pediatric dose**
Use is not recommended.

**Strength(s) usually available**
U.S.—
　Not commercially available.
Canada—
　200 mg (Rx) [*Idarac* (corn starch)].
　400 mg (Rx) [*Idarac* (corn starch)].

**Packaging and storage**
Store below 40 °C (104 °F), preferably between 15 and 30 °C (59 and 86 °F), unless otherwise specified by manufacturer. Protect from light.

**Auxiliary labeling**
• Take with food.
• Take with a full glass of water.
• May cause drowsiness.
• Avoid alcoholic beverages.

---
### FLURBIPROFEN
---

## Summary of Differences
Indications:
　Indicated for rheumatoid arthritis, osteoarthritis, ankylosing spondylitis, bursitis, tendinitis, soft tissue injuries, and dysmenorrhea.
Pharmacology/pharmacokinetics:
　Physicochemical characteristics—Chemical group: A propionic acid derivative.
　Half-life—Elimination: 5.7 hours.
　Peak plasma concentration—Extended-release capsules: Increased by food.
Precautions:
　Pregnancy/reproduction—Embryocidal and fetotoxic, but not teratogenic, effects demonstrated in animal studies.
　Geriatrics—Peak plasma concentrations increased in elderly females.
　Drug interactions and/or related problems—Studies failed to show that flurbiprofen increases digoxin plasma concentrations.
Side/adverse effects:
　See *Table 3*, page 425.

## Oral Dosage Forms
Note:　Bracketed uses in the *Dosage Forms* section refer to categories of use and/or indications that are not included in U.S. product labeling.

### FLURBIPROFEN EXTENDED-RELEASE CAPSULES
**Usual adult dose**
Antirheumatic (nonsteroidal anti-inflammatory)—
　Oral, 200 mg once a day in the evening.

Note:　The extended-release dosage form is not intended as initial therapy; the daily maintenance dose should be determined using the immediate-release formulation. The extended-release dosage form may then be used, if desired, provided that the required dose can be achieved with the available strength.

**Usual pediatric dose**
Safety and efficacy have not been established.

**Strength(s) usually available**
U.S.—
　Not commercially available.
Canada—
　200 mg (Rx) [*Froben SR*].

**Packaging and storage**
Store below 40 °C (104 °F), preferably between 15 and 30 °C (59 and 86 °F), unless otherwise specified by manufacturer.

**Auxiliary labeling**
• Take with food.
• Swallow capsules whole.
• Take with a full glass of water.
• Avoid alcoholic beverages.

### FLURBIPROFEN TABLETS USP
**Usual adult dose**
Rheumatoid arthritis or
Osteoarthritis—
　Oral, 200 to 300 mg a day in two to four divided doses, initially. Dosage may then be individualized according to the severity of the disease and patient response.
　[Ankylosing spondylitis]—
　　Oral, 200 mg a day in four divided doses, initially, although some patients may require 250 to 300 mg a day.
Note:　After a satisfactory response has been obtained, dosage should be decreased to the lowest dose that provides continuing control of symptoms.
[Antidysmenorrheal]—
　Oral, 50 mg four times a day.
[Anti-inflammatory (nonsteroidal)]—
　Oral, 50 mg every four to six hours as needed.

**Usual adult prescribing limits**
The maximum recommended single dose is 100 mg. Total daily dosage should not exceed 300 mg. This maximum dose is recommended for short-term use only, i.e., for initiation of therapy or for treating acute exacerbations of symptoms; it should not be used as a maintenance dose.

**Usual pediatric dose**
Safety and efficacy have not been established.

**Strength(s) usually available**
U.S.—
　50 mg (Rx) [*Ansaid* (lactose); GENERIC].
　100 mg (Rx) [*Ansaid* (lactose); GENERIC].
Canada—
　50 mg (Rx) [*Ansaid; Apo-Flurbiprofen; Froben; Novo-Flurprofen; Nu-Flurbiprofen;* GENERIC].
　100 mg (Rx) [*Ansaid; Apo-Flurbiprofen; Froben; Novo-Flurprofen; Nu-Flurbiprofen;* GENERIC].

**Packaging and storage**
Store below 40 °C (104 °F), preferably between 15 and 30 °C (59 and 86 °F), unless otherwise specified by manufacturer.

**Auxiliary labeling**
• Take with food.
• Take with a full glass of water.
• Avoid alcoholic beverages.

---
### IBUPROFEN
---

## Summary of Differences
Indications:
　Indicated for rheumatoid arthritis, osteoarthritis, juvenile arthritis, and psoriatic arthritis; pain; gouty arthritis or calcium pyrophosphate deposition disease (pseudogout); fever; and dysmenorrhea. May also be used for prophylaxis and treatment of vascular headaches.
Pharmacology/pharmacokinetics:
　Physicochemical characteristics—Chemical group: A propionic acid derivative.
　Half-life—Elimination: 1.8–2 hours.
　Onset of action—Pain: 0.5 hour.
　Time to peak effect—Fever: 2–4 hours.
　Duration of action—
　Fever:
　　5-mg/kg dose—6 hours.
　　10-mg/kg dose—8 hours or more.
　Pain: 4–6 hours.
Precautions:
　Pregnancy/reproduction—Teratogenic effects in animals have not been shown.
　Breast-feeding—Methodology capable of detecting 1 mcg/mL failed to show that ibuprofen is distributed into breast milk.
　Pediatrics—Studied in children 6 months of age and older; pediatrics-specific problems have not been demonstrated.
　Drug interactions and/or related problems—Also, reported to increase digoxin plasma concentrations.

Laboratory value alterations—Also, may decrease blood glucose concentrations.

Side/adverse effects:
Reported to cause a characteristic hypersensitivity syndrome.
Reported to cause a serum sickness– or influenza-like syndrome.
See also *Table 3*, page 425.

## Additional Dosing Information
See also *General Dosing Information*.

In the treatment of arthritis, improvement in condition may occur within 7 days, but 1 to 2 weeks of continuous use on a regular basis may be required for maximum effectiveness.

## Oral Dosage Forms

### IBUPROFEN ORAL SUSPENSION

**Usual adult and adolescent dose**
Antirheumatic (nonsteroidal anti-inflammatory)—
   Oral, 1200 to 3200 mg a day in three or four divided doses. After a satisfactory response has been obtained, dosage should be reduced to the lowest maintenance dose that provides continuing control of symptoms.
   Note: Higher doses generally are required in rheumatoid arthritis than in osteoarthritis.
Analgesic (mild to moderate pain)
Antipyretic or
Antidysmenorrheal—
   Oral, 200 to 400 mg every four to six hours as needed.

**Usual adult prescribing limits**
Antirheumatic (nonsteroidal anti-inflammatory)—
   Up to 3600 mg per day. The maximum dosage should be used only if the clinical benefit is increased sufficiently to offset the higher risk of adverse effects.
Analgesic
Antipyretic; or
Antidysmenorrheal—
   For patient self-medication (over-the-counter use): Not to exceed 1200 mg per day.

**Usual pediatric dose**
Antirheumatic (nonsteroidal anti-inflammatory)—
   Infants up to 6 months of age: Safety and efficacy have not been established.
   Children 6 months to 12 years of age: Oral, initially 30 to 40 mg per kg of body weight a day in three or four divided doses, although 20 mg per kg of body weight per day may be sufficient for patients with mild disease. After a satisfactory response has been achieved, dosage should be reduced to the lowest dose needed to control disease activity.
Antipyretic—
   Infants up to 6 months of age: Safety and efficacy have not been established.
   Children 6 months to 12 years of age: Oral, 5 mg per kg of body weight for fevers less than 39.17 °C (102.5 °F) and 10 mg per kg of body weight for higher fevers. Dosage may be repeated, if necessary, at intervals of 4 to 6 hours or more.

**Usual pediatric prescribing limits**
Antirheumatic—
   Oral, 50 mg per kg of body weight per day.
Antipyretic—
   Oral, 40 mg per kg of body weight per day.

**Strength(s) usually available**
U.S.—
   40 mg per mL (OTC) [*Motrin, Children's Oral Drops*].
   40 mg per mL (Rx) [*Motrin, Children's Oral Drops*].
   100 mg per 5 mL (OTC) [*Advil, Children's* (sucrose; cellulose gum; citric acid; disodium EDTA; FD&C Red #40; glycerin; microcrystalline cellulose; polysorbate 80; sodium benzoate; sorbitol; xanthan gum)].
   100 mg per 5 mL (Rx) [*Advil, Children's* (sucrose; cellulose gum; citric acid; disodium EDTA; FD&C Red #40; glycerin; microcrystalline cellulose; polysorbate 80; sodium benzoate; sorbitol; xanthan gum)].
   100 mg per 5 mL (OTC) [*Motrin, Children's* (sucrose; citric acid; glycerin; polysorbate 80; sodium benzoate; starch; xanthan gum; yellow #10; red #40)].
   100 mg per 5 mL (Rx) [*Motrin, Children's* (sucrose; citric acid; glycerin; polysorbate 80; sodium benzoate; starch; xanthan gum; yellow #10; red #40)].

Canada—
   Not commercially available.

**Packaging and storage**
Store between 15 and 30 °C (59 to 86 °F). Protect from freezing.

**Auxiliary labeling**
• Take with food or antacids.
• Shake well.
• Avoid alcoholic beverages.

### IBUPROFEN TABLETS USP

**Usual adult and adolescent dose**
See *Ibuprofen Oral Suspension*.

**Usual adult prescribing limits**
See *Ibuprofen Oral Suspension*.

**Usual pediatric dose**
See *Ibuprofen Oral Suspension*.

**Usual pediatric prescribing limits**
See *Ibuprofen Oral Suspension*.

**Strength(s) usually available**
U.S.—
   100 mg (Rx) [*Motrin, Junior Strength Caplets*].
   100 mg (OTC) [*Motrin, Junior Strength Caplets*].
   200 mg (OTC) [*Advil; Advil Caplets; Bayer Select Ibuprofen Pain Relief Formula Caplets; Cramp End; Excedrin IB; Excedrin IB Caplets; Genpril; Genpril Caplets; Haltran; Ibu-200; Ibuprin; Ibuprohm; Ibuprohm Caplets; Ibu-Tab; Medipren; Medipren Caplets; Midol IB; Motrin-IB; Motrin-IB Caplets; Nuprin; Nuprin Caplets; Pamprin-IB; Q-Profen; Trendar;* GENERIC].
   300 mg (Rx) [*Motrin;* GENERIC].
   400 mg (Rx) [*Dolgesic; Ibu; Ibu-4; Ibuprohm; Ibu-Tab; Motrin; Rufen;* GENERIC].
   600 mg (Rx) [*Ibifon 600 Caplets; Ibren; Ibu; Ibu-6; Ibu-Tab; Motrin; Rufen;* GENERIC].
   800 mg (Rx) [*Ibu; Ibu-8; Ibu-Tab; Motrin; Rufen;* GENERIC].
Canada—
   200 mg (OTC) [*Actiprofen Caplets; Advil; Advil Caplets; Apo-Ibuprofen; Medipren Caplets; Motrin-IB; Motrin-IB Caplets; Novo-Profen;* GENERIC].
   300 mg (Rx) [*Apo-Ibuprofen; Motrin; Novo-Profen; Nu-Ibuprofen;* GENERIC].
   400 mg (Rx) [*Apo-Ibuprofen; Motrin; Novo-Profen; Nu-Ibuprofen;* GENERIC].
   600 mg (Rx) [*Apo-Ibuprofen; Motrin; Novo-Profen; Nu-Ibuprofen;* GENERIC].

**Packaging and storage**
Store between 15 and 30 °C (59 and 86 °F), in a light-resistant container, unless otherwise specified by manufacturer. Store in a well-closed container.

**Auxiliary labeling**
• Take with food.
• Take with a full glass of water.
• May cause drowsiness.
• Avoid alcoholic beverages.

### IBUPROFEN TABLETS (CHEWABLE)

**Usual adult and adolescent dose**
See *Ibuprofen Oral Suspension*.

**Usual adult prescribing limits**
See *Ibuprofen Oral Suspension*.

**Usual pediatric dose**
See *Ibuprofen Oral Suspension*.

**Usual pediatric prescribing limits**
See *Ibuprofen Oral Suspension*.

**Strength(s) usually available**
U.S.—
   50 mg (Rx) [*Motrin Chewables*].
   100 mg (Rx) [*Motrin Chewables*].
Canada—
   Not commercially available.

**Packaging and storage**
Store between 15 and 30 °C (59 and 86 °F), in a well-closed, light-resistant container, unless otherwise specified by manufacturer.

**Auxiliary labeling**
• Take with food.
• Take with a full glass of water.
• May cause drowsiness.
• Avoid alcoholic beverages.

## INDOMETHACIN

### Summary of Differences

Indications:
  Indicated for rheumatoid arthritis, osteoarthritis, ankylosing spondylitis, juvenile arthritis, psoriatric arthritis, Reiter's disease, and rheumatic complications associated with Paget's disease of bone; acute gouty arthritis and calcium pyrophosphate deposition disease (pseudogout); bursitis and tendinitis; fever associated with malignancy; dysmenorrhea; prevention and treatment of vascular headaches; Bartter's disease; and pericarditis.
  Drug of first choice in ankylosing spondylitis; for other indications (except Bartter's syndrome), recommended only for patients unresponsive to less toxic NSAIDs or, in the case of fever, to other antipyretic agents.
Pharmacology/pharmacokinetics:
  Physicochemical characteristics—Chemical group: An indoleacetic acid derivative.
  Absorption—Oral: Capsules and oral suspension—90% of a dose absorbed within 4 hours.
  Extended-release capsules—90% of a dose absorbed within 12 hours.
  Rectal: 80 to 90% of a dose absorbed; incomplete absorption may result from failure to retain suppository in rectum for a full hour.
  Half-life—Elimination: Average, about 4.5 hours; subject to substantial intersubject variability, possibly because of differences in enterohepatic circulation and subsequent reabsorption.
  Onset of action—Gout: 2–4 hours.
  Time to peak effect—Gout (capsules or oral suspension): 2–3 days for relief of heat and tenderness; 3–5 days for relief of swelling.
Precautions:
  Pregnancy/reproduction—
    First trimester: Crosses the placenta; fetotoxic, teratogenic, and other adverse effects demonstrated in animal studies.
    Third trimester: Has caused closure of the ductus arteriosus, inhibition of platelet function resulting in bleeding, renal function impairment or failure with oligohydramnios, gastrointestinal bleeding or perforation, and myocardial degenerative changes in fetuses when given to pregnant women during the third trimester.
  Breast-feeding—Distributed into breast milk; one report of convulsions in a breast-fed infant exposed to the medication.
  Pediatrics—Recommended only for pediatric patients who are unresponsive to or intolerant of less toxic agents. Only immediate-release oral dosage forms should be used. Also, recommended doses should not be exceeded and the patient carefully monitored.
  Geriatrics—Also, increased risk of adverse CNS effects, especially confusion.
  Drug interactions and/or related problems—
  Also, concurrent use with potassium-sparing diuretics may cause hyperkalemia.
  Also, may block the increase in plasma renin activity induced by bumetanide, furosemide, or indapamide.
  Also, concurrent use with zidovudine not recommended; toxicity of either or both of the medications may be increased.
  Caution also recommended with aminoglycosides and digitalis glycosides; indomethacin has caused increased plasma concentrations of these medications in infants.
  Laboratory value alterations—Also, may cause false-negative test results with dexamethasone suppression test for endogenous depression and one test for urinary 5-hydroxyindoleacetic acid (5-HIAA).
  Also, may increase or decrease blood glucose concentrations.
  Medical considerations/contraindications—
  Higher risk than with most other NSAIDs in patients with renal function impairment.
  Also, may aggravate epilepsy, mental depression or other mental disturbances, or parkinsonism.
  Patient monitoring—Routine monitoring of liver function recommended.
Side/adverse effects:
  See *Table 3*, page 425.

### Additional Dosing Information

See also *General Dosing Information*.

Indomethacin should be administered in the lowest dose that provides symptomatic relief. Doses greater than 150 to 200 mg per day may increase the risk of adverse effects without providing additional clinical benefit. If therapy is to be continued after the acute phase of the disease has been controlled, periodic attempts should be made to reduce the dose to the lowest dose providing continuing control of symptoms.

If minor adverse effects occur, dosage should be reduced and the patient carefully monitored. If severe side effects occur, therapy should be discontinued.

**For oral dosage forms only**

Oral dosage forms of indomethacin should always be administered after meals or with food or an antacid to reduce gastrointestinal irritation. However, the oral suspension should not be mixed with an antacid or other liquid prior to use.

To facilitate dosage adjustment and assessment of patient tolerance of the medication, it is recommended that an immediate-release, rather than the extended-release, dosage form be used for initiation of therapy or to increase the daily dose. If the extended-release dosage form is used for initial therapy, or to increase the daily dose, careful observation of the patient is recommended.

**For rectal dosage form only**

To ensure maximum absorption, the suppository should be retained for at least one full hour after insertion.

### Oral Dosage Forms

Note: Bracketed uses in the *Dosage Forms* section refer to categories of use and/or indications that are not included in U.S. product labeling.

#### INDOMETHACIN CAPSULES USP

**Usual adult dose**

Antirheumatic (nonsteroidal anti-inflammatory)—
  Oral, initially 25 or 50 mg two to four times a day; if well tolerated, the dosage per day may be increased by 25 or 50 mg at weekly intervals until a satisfactory response is obtained or up to a maximum dose of 200 mg per day. After a satisfactory response has been achieved, dosage should be reduced to the lowest dose that provides continuing control of symptoms.
  Note: In acute flare-ups of rheumatoid arthritis, dosage may be increased by 25 or 50 mg daily, as needed and tolerated.
    For those arthritic patients who have persistent night pain and/or morning stiffness, up to 100 mg of the total daily dose may be given at bedtime. Lower bedtime doses may not provide adequate symptomatic relief.
    A daily dose of less than 75 mg may not be effective in active inflammatory disease.
    A daily dose of more than 150 to 200 mg may increase the risk of adverse effects without providing additional clinical benefit.
Antigout agent—
  Oral, 100 mg initially, then 50 mg three times a day until pain is relieved, with the dosage then being reduced until medication is discontinued.
Anti-inflammatory (nonsteroidal)[1]—
  75 to 150 mg per day in three or four divided doses.
  Note: When used to treat conditions not requiring chronic therapy, such as acute bursitis or tendinitis of the shoulder, indomethacin should be discontinued when symptoms of inflammation have been controlled for several days. The usual length of treatment is 7 to 14 days.
[Antipyretic][1]—
  Oral, 25 or 50 mg three or four times a day.

**Usual adult prescribing limits**
Oral, 200 mg a day.

**Usual pediatric dose**
Antirheumatic (nonsteroidal anti-inflammatory)—
  Oral, 1.5 to 2.5 mg per kg of body weight per day, administered in three or four divided doses, up to a maximum of 4 mg per kg of body weight per day or 150 to 200 mg per day, whichever is less. After a satisfactory response has been obtained, dosage should be reduced to the lowest dose that provides continuing control of symptoms.

**Strength(s) usually available**
U.S.—
  25 mg (Rx) [*Indocin* (lactose); GENERIC].
  50 mg (Rx) [*Indocin* (lactose); GENERIC].
Canada—
  25 mg (Rx) [*Apo-Indomethacin; Indocid* (lactose); *Novo-Methacin; Nu-Indo*].
  50 mg (Rx) [*Apo-Indomethacin; Indocid* (lactose); *Novo-Methacin; Nu-Indo*].

**Packaging and storage**
Store below 40 °C (104 °F), preferably between 15 and 30 °C (59 and 86 °F). Store in a well-closed container.

**Auxiliary labeling**
- Take with food or antacids.
- Take with a full glass of water.
- Avoid alcoholic beverages.

## INDOMETHACIN EXTENDED-RELEASE CAPSULES USP

**Usual adult dose**
Antirheumatic (nonsteroidal anti-inflammatory)—
Oral, 75 mg once a day, in the morning or at bedtime; may be increased to 75 mg two times a day if necessary.

Note: It is generally recommended that the daily maintenance dose be determined using the immediate-release formulation. The extended-release dosage form may then be used, if desired, provided that the required dose can be achieved with the available strength.

Careful observation of the patient for signs of intolerance is recommended if the extended-release capsule is used for initiating indomethacin therapy or for increasing the daily dose. Initiation of therapy with one extended-release capsule daily provides the maximum initial dose recommended by the manufacturer. Use of the extended-release capsule to increase the dose provides a greater-than-recommended increase in daily dosage.

**Usual pediatric dose**
Dosage has not been established.

**Strength(s) usually available**
U.S.—
75 mg (Rx) [*Indocin SR* (sugar); GENERIC].
Canada—
75 mg (Rx) [*Indocid SR* (sucrose)].

**Packaging and storage**
Store below 40 °C (104 °F), preferably between 15 and 30 °C (59 and 86 °F), unless otherwise specified by manufacturer. Store in a well-closed container.

**Auxiliary labeling**
- Take with food or antacids.
- Take with a full glass of water.
- Avoid alcoholic beverages.

**Additional information**
The extended-release capsules are designed to release 25 mg of indomethacin immediately and the remaining 50 mg over a 12-hour period.

## INDOMETHACIN ORAL SUSPENSION USP

**Usual adult dose**
See *Indomethacin Capsules USP*.

**Usual adult prescribing limits**
See *Indomethacin Capsules USP*.

**Usual pediatric dose**
See *Indomethacin Capsules USP*.

**Strength(s) usually available**
U.S.—
25 mg per 5 mL (Rx) [*Indocin* (alcohol 1%); GENERIC].
Canada—
Not commercially available.

**Packaging and storage**
Store below 30 °C (86 °F). Store in a tight, light-resistant container. Protect from freezing.

**Incompatibilities**
Indomethacin is unstable in an alkaline medium and should not be mixed with antacids or other liquids having an alkaline pH.

**Auxiliary labeling**
- Take with food or antacids.
- Shake well.
- Avoid alcoholic beverages.

# Rectal Dosage Forms

## INDOMETHACIN SUPPOSITORIES USP

**Usual adult dose**
Antirheumatic (nonsteroidal anti-inflammatory)
Anti-inflammatory (nonsteroidal)[1]
Antigout agent or
[Antipyretic][1]—
Rectal, 50 mg up to four times a day.

Note: A daily dose of less than 75 mg may not be effective in active inflammatory disease.

For those arthritic patients who have persistent night pain and/or morning stiffness, up to 100 mg of the total daily dose may be given at bedtime. Lower bedtime doses may not provide adequate symptomatic relief.

A daily dose of more than 150 to 200 mg may increase the risk of adverse effects without providing additional clinical benefit.

**Usual adult prescribing limits**
Rectal or combined oral and rectal, 200 mg per day.

**Usual pediatric dose**
Antirheumatic (nonsteroidal anti-inflammatory)—
Rectal, 1.5 to 2.5 mg per kg of body weight per day, administered in 3 or 4 divided doses, up to a maximum of 4 mg per kg of body weight or 150 to 200 mg per day, whichever is less.

**Strength(s) usually available**
U.S.—
50 mg (Rx) [*Indocin* (butylated hydroxyanisole; butylated hydroxytoluene; edetic acid; glycerin; polyethylene glycol 3350; polyethylene glycol 8000; sodium chloride)].
Canada—
50 mg (Rx) [*Indocid*].
100 mg (Rx) [*Indocid*].

**Packaging and storage**
Store below 40 °C (104 °F), preferably between 15 and 30 °C (59 and 86 °F), unless otherwise specified by manufacturer. Store in a well-closed container. Protect from freezing.

**Auxiliary labeling**
- For rectal use.
- Avoid alcoholic beverages.

[1] Not included in Canadian product labeling.

---

## KETOPROFEN

## Summary of Differences

Indications:
Indicated for rheumatoid arthritis, osteoarthritis, ankylosing spondylitis, and psoriatic arthritis; pain; acute gouty arthritis and calcium pyrophosphate deposition disease (pseudogout); and dysmenorrhea. May also be used to relieve pain associated with nonrheumatic inflammatory disorders or vascular headaches.

Pharmacology/pharmacokinetics:
Physicochemical characteristics—Chemical group: A propionic acid derivative.
Half-life—Elimination:
Capsules—1.6 hours; increased by 26% in geriatric patients; also increased by renal function impairment.
Extended-release capsules—About 5.4 hours; higher value (relative to immediate-release capsules) represents prolonged absorption; increased by 54% in geriatric patients.
Extended-release tablets—About 3–4 hours; higher value (relative to immediate-release capsules) represents prolonged absorption.
Elimination—Dialyzable.

Precautions:
Pregnancy/reproduction—Fertility: Decreased number of implantation sites in female rats (but no effect on fertility in male rats); high doses caused abnormal spermatogenesis or impaired spermatogenesis in rats and dogs and decreased testicular weight in dogs and baboons.
First trimester: No teratogenicity demonstrated in animal studies; in rabbits, maternally toxic doses shown to be embryotoxic.
Geriatrics—Protein binding and clearance reduced in elderly people, leading to increased plasma concentration and prolonged half-life.

Drug interactions and/or related problems—
Probenecid may greatly increase ketoprofen plasma concentration and the risk of toxicity; concurrent use not recommended.
Studies failed to show that ketoprofen increases digoxin plasma concentration.
Laboratory value alterations—Interference with determinations of urinary albumin, bile salts, 17-ketosteroids, and 17-hydroxycorticosteroids via test procedures that rely on acid precipitation or on color reaction of carbonyl groups as an end point.

Side/adverse effects:
See *Table 3*, page 425.

## Oral Dosage Forms
### KETOPROFEN CAPSULES
**Usual adult dose**
Antirheumatic (nonsteroidal anti-inflammatory)—
  Oral, 150 to 300 mg a day in three or four divided doses, usually 75 mg three times a day or 50 mg four times a day, initially, then adjusted according to patient response.
Analgesic or
Antidysmenorrheal—
  Oral, 25 to 50 mg every six to eight hours as needed. Dosage may be increased if necessary, but single doses higher than 75 mg have not been shown to provide additional analgesia. In the treatment of dysmenorrhea, 75-mg doses may be more effective than lower doses.
Note: In patients with renal function impairment, a 33 to 50% reduction of dosage is recommended.
  The analgesic dosage for self-medication with ketoprofen using the over-the-counter product is 12.5 mg every four to six hours.

**Usual adult prescribing limits**
Oral, 300 mg a day in three or four divided doses.
Note: Risk/benefit must be considered when the maximum dose is prescribed because the incidence of gastrointestinal effects and headache is increased with administration of 300 mg per day (as compared with 200 mg per day).

**Usual pediatric dose**
Safety and efficacy have not been established.

**Strength(s) usually available**
U.S.—
  25 mg (Rx) [*Orudis* (lactose); GENERIC].
  50 mg (Rx) [*Orudis* (lactose); GENERIC].
  75 mg (Rx) [*Orudis* (lactose); GENERIC].
Canada—
  50 mg (Rx) [*Apo-Keto; Orudis; Rhodis*].

**Packaging and storage**
Store below 40 °C (104 °F), preferably between 15 and 30 °C (59 and 86 °F), in a tight container, unless otherwise specified by manufacturer.

**Auxiliary labeling**
• Take with food.
• Take with a full glass of water.
• Avoid alcoholic beverages.

### KETOPROFEN EXTENDED-RELEASE CAPSULES
**Usual adult dose**
Antirheumatic (nonsteroidal anti-inflammatory)—
  Oral, 150 or 200 mg once a day, in the morning or evening. Elderly or debilitated patients may require lower doses.
Note: The extended-release dosage form is not intended as initial therapy; the daily maintenance dose should be determined using an immediate- or delayed-release formulation. The extended-release dosage form may then be used, if desired, provided that the required dose can be achieved with the available strength(s).

**Usual pediatric dose**
Safety and efficacy have not been established.

**Strength(s) usually available**
U.S.—
  100 mg (Rx) [*Oruvail*].
  150 mg (Rx) [*Oruvail*].
  200 mg (Rx) [*Oruvail*].
Canada—
  150 mg (Rx) [*Oruvail*].
  200 mg (Rx) [*Oruvail*].

**Packaging and storage**
Store below 40 °C (104 °F), preferably between 15 and 30 °C (59 and 86 °F), in a well-closed container, unless otherwise specified by manufacturer.

**Auxiliary labeling**
• Swallow capsule whole.
• Take with a full glass of water.
• Avoid alcoholic beverages.

**Note**
The extended-release capsule is formulated with delayed-release as well as extended-release characteristics. Dissolution of the contents of the capsules (coated pellets) does not occur until the medication reaches the alkaline pH of the small intestine.

### KETOPROFEN DELAYED-RELEASE TABLETS
**Usual adult dose**
See *Ketoprofen Capsules*.

**Usual adult prescribing limits**
See *Ketoprofen Capsules*.

**Usual pediatric dose**
Safety and efficacy have not been established.

**Strength(s) usually available**
U.S.—
  Not commercially available.
Canada—
  50 mg (Rx) [*Apo-Keto-E; Novo-Keto-EC; Orudis-E; Rhodis-EC*].
  100 mg (Rx) [*Apo-Keto-E; Novo-Keto-EC; Orudis-E; Rhodis-EC*].

**Packaging and storage**
Store below 40 °C (104 °F), preferably between 15 and 30 °C (59 and 86 °F), in a well-closed container, unless otherwise specified by manufacturer.

**Auxiliary labeling**
• Take with a full glass of water.
• Swallow tablets whole.
• Avoid alcoholic beverages.

### KETOPROFEN EXTENDED-RELEASE TABLETS
**Usual adult dose**
See *Ketoprofen Extended-release Capsules*.

**Usual pediatric dose**
Safety and efficacy have not been established.

**Strength(s) usually available**
U.S.—
  Not commercially available.
Canada—
  200 mg (Rx) [*Orudis-SR;* GENERIC].

**Packaging and storage**
Store below 40 °C (104 °F), preferably between 15 and 30 °C (59 and 86 °F), in a well-closed container, unless otherwise specified by manufacturer.

**Auxiliary labeling**
• Take with food.
• Take with a full glass of water.
• Swallow tablets whole.
• Avoid alcoholic beverages.

### KETOPROFEN TABLETS
**Usual adult dose**
See *Ketoprofen Capsules*.

**Usual adult prescribing limits**
See *Ketoprofen Capsules*.

**Usual pediatric dose**
Safety and efficacy have not been established.
U.S.—
  12.5 mg (OTC) [*Orudis KT* (tartrazine)].
  12.5 mg (OTC) [*Actron* (lactose)].
Canada—
  Not commercially available.

**Packaging and storage**
Store below 40 °C (104 °F), preferably between 15 and 30 °C (59 and 86 °F), in a well-closed container, unless otherwise specified by manufacturer.

**Auxiliary labeling**
• Take with a full glass of water.
• Avoid alcoholic beverages.

## Rectal Dosage Forms
### KETOPROFEN SUPPOSITORIES
**Usual adult dose**
Antirheumatic (nonsteroidal anti-inflammatory)—
  Rectal, 50 or 100 mg two times a day, in the morning and evening; or 50 or 100 mg in the evening in conjunction with oral administration during the day.

**Usual adult prescribing limits**
Rectal or combined oral and rectal, 300 mg a day.

### Usual pediatric dose
Safety and efficacy have not been established.

### Strength(s) usually available
U.S.—
  Not commercially available.
Canada—
  50 mg (Rx) [*Orudis*].
  100 mg (Rx) [*Orudis; Rhodis*].

### Packaging and storage
Store below 30 °C (86 °F), in a well-closed container, unless otherwise specified by manufacturer. Protect from freezing.

### Auxiliary labeling
- For rectal use.
- Avoid alcoholic beverages.

---

## MECLOFENAMATE

## Summary of Differences
Indications:
  Indicated for rheumatoid arthritis, osteoarthritis, psoriatic arthritis, pain, dysmenorrhea, and idiopathic hypermenorrhea. May also be used to relieve acute attacks of gout or calcium pyrophosphate deposition disease (pseudogout) and pain associated with nonrheumatic inflammatory conditions or vascular headaches.
Pharmacology/pharmacokinetics:
  Physicochemical characteristics—Chemical group: A fenamate derivative.
  Other actions/effects—With usual doses has lesser effect on platelet aggregation than most other NSAIDs.
  Biotransformation—Hydroxymethyl metabolite has anti-inflammatory activity.
  Half-life—Elimination:
    Single dose—2 hours.
    Multiple doses—3.3 hours.
  Onset of action—Pain: 1 hour.
  Duration of action—Pain: 4–6 hours.
Precautions:
  Pregnancy/reproduction—Fetotoxicity and developmental abnormalities have been demonstrated in animals.
  Breast-feeding—Use not recommended because animal studies have shown this agent to interfere with normal development of the young before weaning.
  Surgical—With recommended doses may be less likely than most other NSAIDs to increase perisurgical bleeding.
  Laboratory value alterations—With usual doses may be less likely than most other NSAIDs to increase bleeding time significantly.
  Medical considerations/contraindications—Caution in patients on a sodium-restricted diet.
Side/adverse effects:
  Reported to cause a serum sickness or influenza-like syndrome.
  See also *Table 3*, page 425.

## Additional Dosing Information
See also *General Dosing Information*.

Improvement in condition may occur within a few days, but 2 to 3 weeks of continuous use on a regular basis may be required for maximum effectiveness.

Gastrointestinal side effects may respond to a reduction in dosage; however, if severe adverse reactions occur, therapy should be discontinued.

## Oral Dosage Forms
Note: The dosing and strengths of the available dosage form are expressed in terms of meclofenamic acid (not the sodium salt).

### MECLOFENAMATE SODIUM CAPSULES USP
#### Usual adult dose
Antirheumatic (nonsteroidal anti-inflammatory)—
  Oral, 200 mg (meclofenamic acid) a day, in three or four divided doses, initially. Dosage may be increased to up to 400 mg a day if necessary. After a satisfactory response has been obtained, dosage should be reduced to the lowest maintenance dose that provides continuing control of symptoms.
Analgesic—
  Oral, 50 mg (meclofenamic acid) every four to six hours. If necessary, dosage may be increased to 100 mg every four to six hours.
Antidysmenorrheal and
Antihypermenorrheal—
  Oral, 100 mg (meclofenamic acid) three times a day for up to six days.

#### Usual adult prescribing limits
Antirheumatic (nonsteroidal anti-inflammatory)
and analgesic—
  Up to 400 mg daily.

#### Usual pediatric dose
Children up to 14 years of age—Safety and efficacy have not been established.

#### Strength(s) usually available
U.S.—
  50 mg (meclofenamic acid) (Rx) [*Meclomen* (lactose); GENERIC].
  100 mg (meclofenamic acid) (Rx) [*Meclomen* (lactose); GENERIC].
Canada—
  Not commercially available.

#### Packaging and storage
Store between 15 and 30 °C (59 and 86 °F), unless otherwise specified by manufacturer. Store in a tight, light-resistant container.

#### Auxiliary labeling
- Take with food.
- Take with a full glass of water.
- Avoid alcoholic beverages.

---

## MEFENAMIC ACID

## Summary of Differences
Indications:
  Indicated for short-term use (7 days or less) to relieve pain and dysmenorrhea. May also be used for acute attacks of gout or calcium pyrophosphate deposition disease (pseudogout), for pain associated with nonrheumatic inflammatory conditions or vascular headaches, and to prevent migraines associated with menstruation.
Pharmacology/pharmacokinetics:
  Physicochemical characteristics— Chemical group: A fenamate derivative.
  Other actions/effects—With usual doses has lesser effect on platelet aggregation than most other NSAIDs.
  Half-life—Elimination: 2 hours
Precautions:
  Pregnancy/reproduction—
  Fertility: Decreased fertility demonstrated in rodents.
  Pregnancy: Increased number of resorptions and decreased survival to weaning demonstrated in rodents.
  Surgical—With usual doses may be less likely than other NSAIDs to inhibit platelet aggregation significantly, but has been reported to cause hypoprothrombinemia, which may increase the risk of perisurgical bleeding.
  Laboratory value alterations—
  Interference with urinary bile determinations via the diazo tablet test.
  With usual doses is less likely than most other NSAIDs to increase bleeding time significantly because of lesser effect on platelet aggregation; however, may prolong prothrombin time.
  Medical considerations/contraindications—Also, may exacerbate pre-existing hypoprothrombinemia.
Side/adverse effects:
  See *Table 3*, page 425.

## Additional Dosing Information
See also *General Dosing Information*.

It is recommended that mefenamic acid therapy be discontinued promptly if diarrhea or a skin rash develops. Patients who develop diarrhea during mefenamic acid therapy are usually unable to tolerate the drug thereafter.

Mefenamic acid should not be used for more than 7 days at a time.

## Oral Dosage Forms
### MEFENAMIC ACID CAPSULES USP
#### Usual adult dose
Analgesic or
Antidysmenorrheal—
  Oral, 500 mg initially, followed by 250 mg every six hours as needed.
Note: It is recommended that mefenamic acid be used for no longer than 7 days at a time.

#### Usual pediatric dose
Children up to 14 years of age—Safety and efficacy have not been established.

**Strength(s) usually available**
U.S.—
    250 mg (Rx) [*Ponstel* (lactose; sodium benzoate)].
Canada—
    250 mg (Rx) [*Ponstan* (lactose)].

**Packaging and storage**
Store below 40 °C (104 °F), preferably between 15 and 30 °C (59 and 86 °F). Store in a tight container.

**Auxiliary labeling**
- Take with food.
- Take with a full glass of water.
- May cause drowsiness.
- Avoid alcoholic beverages.

---

## NABUMETONE

## Summary of Differences
Indications:
    Indicated for rheumatoid arthritis and osteoarthritis.
Pharmacology/pharmacokinetics:
    Physicochemical characteristics—
    Chemical group: A naphthylalkanone derivative.
    Other characteristics:
    Nabumetone (prodrug)—Nonacidic.
    6-MNA (active metabolite)—Acidic.
    Other actions/effects—With usual doses has lesser effect on platelet aggregation than most other NSAIDs.
    Absorption—Rate and extent increased by food or milk.
    Biotransformation—Metabolite 6-MNA, not nabumetone itself, is active substance.
    Half-life (plasma)—Elimination: 6-MNA—23±3.7 hours; increased in geriatric patients to 30±8.1 hours (although values as high as 74 hours have been reported) and to 39 hours in patients with renal function impairment (creatinine clearance < 30 mL/minute/1.73 cubic meters of body surface area).
    Time to peak plasma concentration—6-MNA, at steady-state: Decreased by food; significantly delayed by hepatic cirrhosis.
    Peak plasma concentration—6-MNA: Increased by food; may be increased in geriatric patients and substantially decreased in patients with hepatic cirrhosis.
    Elimination—6-MNA: Significantly delayed by moderately severe renal function impairment (creatinine clearance < 30 mL/minute/1.73 cubic meters of body surface area).
Precautions:
    Mutagenicity—Induced chromosomal aberrations in lymphocytes.
    Pregnancy/reproduction—Fetotoxicity but not teratogenicity demonstrated in rats.
    Geriatrics—Higher plasma concentrations and greater interpatient variability in pharmacokinetics of 6-MNA in geriatric patients.
    Surgical—In doses up to 1000 mg per day may be less likely than other NSAIDs to increase perisurgical bleeding.
    Drug interactions and/or related problems—May be less likely than other NSAIDs to cause problems in patients receiving anticoagulant or thrombolytic therapy.
    Medical considerations/contraindications—Hepatic function impairment may decrease biotransformation to active metabolite sufficiently to decrease efficacy.
Side/adverse effects:
    Lower incidence of peptic ulceration and bleeding than with other NSAIDs.
    See also *Table 3*, page 425.

## Oral Dosage Forms
### NABUMETONE TABLETS
**Usual adult dose**
Antirheumatic (nonsteroidal anti-inflammatory)—
    Oral, initially 1000 mg a day, as a single dose (usually at night) or in two divided doses (in the morning and evening). Dosage may be increased, if necessary, to 1500 mg or 2000 mg a day in two divided doses. After a satisfactory response has been obtained, dosage should be individualized according to patient tolerance and response. The lowest dose that provides continuing control of symptoms should be used for maintenance.

**Usual adult prescribing limits**
Doses larger than 2000 mg a day have not been studied and are not recommended.

**Usual pediatric dose**
Safety and efficacy have not been established

**Usual geriatric dose**
See *Usual adult dose*.

**Strength(s) usually available**
U.S.—
    500 mg (Rx) [*Relafen*].
    750 mg (Rx) [*Relafen*].
Canada—
    500 mg (Rx) [*Relafen*].

**Packaging and storage**
Store between 15 and 30 °C (59 and 86 °F), in a well-closed container, unless otherwise specified by manufacturer.

**Auxiliary labeling**
- Take with food.
- Take with a full glass of water.
- Avoid alcoholic beverages.

---

## NAPROXEN

## Summary of Differences
Indications:
    Indicated for rheumatoid arthritis, osteoarthritis, ankylosing spondylitis, and juvenile arthritis; pain; acute attacks of gout and calcium pyrophosphate deposition disease (pseudogout); bursitis and tendinitis; fever; and dysmenorrhea; and for prophylaxis and treatment of vascular headaches.
Pharmacology/pharmacokinetics:
    Physicochemical characteristics—Chemical group: A propionic acid derivative.
    Absorption—May be increased by sodium bicarbonate.
    Half-life—Elimination: 13 hours
    Onset of action—Naproxen sodium: Pain—1 hour.
    Time to peak plasma concentration—Extended-release tablets: Decreased by food.
    Peak plasma concentration—Extended-release tablets: Increased by food.
    Time to peak effect—Gout: 1–2 days.
    Pain: 2–4 hours.
    Duration of action—Pain: Up to 7 hours.
Precautions:
    Pregnancy/reproduction—Teratogenic effects in animals have not been shown.
    Pediatrics—Higher risk of skin rash and increases in bleeding time than in adults receiving the medication.
    Laboratory value alterations—Interference with some assays for urinary 5-hydroxyindoleacetic acid (5-HIAA) and urinary 17-ketogenic steroids.
    Medical considerations/contraindications—Caution with naproxen sodium and naproxen oral suspension for patients who must restrict their sodium intake.
Side/adverse effects:
    See *Table 3*, page 425.

## Additional Dosing Information
See also *General Dosing Information*.

In arthritis, improvement in condition may occur within 2 weeks, but 2 to 4 weeks of continuous use on a regular basis may be required for maximum effectiveness.

Naproxen should be administered in the lowest effective dose to geriatric patients, patients with hepatic function impairment, or patients with renal function impairment (especially if creatinine clearance is < 20 mL per minute).

## Oral Dosage Forms
### NAPROXEN ORAL SUSPENSION
**Usual adult dose**
Antirheumatic (nonsteroidal anti-inflammatory)—
    Oral, 250, 375, or 500 mg two times a day, morning and evening.
    Note: During long-term administration, dosage may be adjusted according to patient response; lower doses may suffice.
        For acute exacerbations of rheumatic disease, dosage may be increased to up to 1.5 grams per day for limited periods. Use of this high dose requires that the clinical benefit be increased sufficiently to offset the potential increased risk of adverse effects.

Anti-inflammatory (nonsteroidal)
Analgesic (mild to moderate pain) and
Antidysmenorrheal—
   Oral, 500 mg initially, then 250 mg every six to eight hours as needed.
Antigout agent[1]—
   Oral, 750 mg initially, then 250 mg every eight hours until the attack has subsided.

**Usual adult prescribing limits**
For mild to moderate pain and dysmenorrhea—
   Up to a total dose of 1.25 grams daily.

**Usual pediatric dose**
Antirheumatic (nonsteroidal anti-inflammatory)—
   Oral, 10 mg per kg of body weight per day, given in two divided doses.

**Strength(s) usually available**
U.S.—
   125 mg per 5 mL (Rx) [*Naprosyn* (fumaric acid; imitation orange flavor; imitation pineapple flavor; magnesium aluminum silicate; methylparaben; sodium 8 mg [<1 mmol] per mL; sorbitol; sucrose)].
Canada—
   125 mg per 5 mL (Rx) [*Naprosyn*].

**Packaging and storage**
Store below 40 °C (104 °F), preferably between 15 and 30 °C (59 and 86 °F), in a well-closed, light-resistant container, unless otherwise specified by manufacturer. Protect from freezing.

**Auxiliary labeling**
• Take with food.
• Shake well.
• Avoid alcoholic beverages.

## NAPROXEN TABLETS USP

**Usual adult dose**
See *Naproxen Oral Suspension*.

**Usual adult prescribing limits**
See *Naproxen Oral Suspension*.

**Usual pediatric dose**
See *Naproxen Oral Suspension*.

**Strength(s) usually available**
U.S.—
   250 mg (Rx) [*Naprosyn*; GENERIC].
   375 mg (Rx) [*Naprosyn*; GENERIC].
   500 mg (Rx) [*Naprosyn*; GENERIC].
Canada—
   125 mg (Rx) [*Apo-Naproxen*; *Naprosyn* (lactose); *Naxen* (lactose); *Novo-Naprox*; *Nu-Naprox*].
   250 mg (Rx) [*Apo-Naproxen*; *Naprosyn* (lactose); *Naxen* (lactose); *Novo-Naprox*; *Nu-Naprox*].
   375 mg (Rx) [*Apo-Naproxen* (scored); *Naprosyn* (scored; lactose); *Naxen* (scored; lactose); *Novo-Naprox* (scored); *Nu-Naprox* (scored)].
   500 mg (Rx) [*Apo-Naproxen* (scored); *Naprosyn* (scored; lactose); *Naxen* (scored; lactose); *Novo-Naprox* (scored); *Nu-Naprox* (scored)].

**Packaging and storage**
Store between 15 and 30 °C (59 and 86 °F). Store in a well-closed container.

**Auxiliary labeling**
• Take with food.
• Take with a full glass of water.
• May cause drowsiness.
• Avoid alcoholic beverages.

## NAPROXEN DELAYED-RELEASE TABLETS

**Usual adult dose**
See *Naproxen Oral Suspension*.

**Usual adult prescribing limits**
See *Naproxen Oral Suspension*.

**Usual pediatric dose**
See *Naproxen Oral Suspension*.

**Strength(s) usually available**
U.S.—
   375 mg (Rx) [*EC-Naprosyn* (croscarmellose sodium; povidone; magnesium stearate; methacrylic acid copolymer; talc; triethyl citrate; sodium hydroxide; simethicone emulsion)].
   500 mg (Rx) [*EC-Naprosyn* (croscarmellose sodium; povidone; magnesium stearate; methacrylic acid copolymer; talc; triethyl citrate; sodium hydroxide; simethicone emulsion)].

Canada—
   250 mg (Rx) [*Naprosyn-E*].
   375 mg (Rx) [*Naprosyn-E*].
   500 mg (Rx) [*Naprosyn-E*].

**Packaging and storage**
Store between 15 and 30 °C (59 and 86 °F), unless otherwise directed by manufacturer.

**Auxiliary labeling**
• Swallow tablets whole.
• Take with a full glass of water.
• Avoid alcoholic beverages.

## NAPROXEN EXTENDED-RELEASE TABLETS

**Usual adult dose**
Antirheumatic (nonsteroidal anti-inflammatory)—
   Oral, 750 mg once a day in the morning or evening.

Note:  The extended-release dosage form is not intended as initial therapy; the daily maintenance dose should be determined using an immediate- or delayed-release formulation. The extended-release dosage form may then be used, if desired, provided that the required dose can be achieved with the available strength.

**Usual pediatric dose**
Pediatric strength not available.

**Strength(s) usually available**
U.S.—
   Not commercially available.
Canada—
   750 mg (Rx) [*Naprosyn-SR*].

**Packaging and storage**
Store between 15 and 30 °C (59 and 86 °F), in a well-closed container, unless otherwise specified by manufacturer.

**Auxiliary labeling**
• Take with food.
• Take with a full glass of water.
• Swallow tablets whole.
• May cause drowsiness.
• Avoid alcoholic beverages.

## NAPROXEN SODIUM TABLETS USP

**Usual adult dose**
Antirheumatic (nonsteroidal anti-inflammatory)—
   Oral, 275 or 550 mg two times a day, morning and evening; or 275 mg in the morning and 550 mg in the evening.

Note:  During long-term administration, dosage may be adjusted according to patient response; lower doses may suffice.

   If necessary, dosage may be increased to up to 1650 mg per day for short periods. The use of this higher dose requires that the clinical benefit be increased sufficiently to offset the potential increased risk.

Anti-inflammatory (nonsteroidal) or
Analgesic (mild to moderate pain)—
   Oral, 550 mg initially, then 275 mg every six to eight hours as needed.
Antigout agent[1]—
   Oral, 825 mg initially, then 275 mg every eight hours until the attack has subsided.
Antidysmenorrheal—
   Oral, 550 mg initially, then 275 mg every six to eight hours as needed.

Note:  For patient self-medication (over-the-counter use) for pain, fever, or dysmenorrhea—Patients 12 years of age and older: Oral, 220 mg every eight to twelve hours while symptoms persist, or

   Oral, 440 mg for the first dose only, followed by 220 mg twelve hours later and every eight to twelve hours thereafter as needed.

**Usual adult prescribing limits**
For mild to moderate pain and dysmenorrhea—
   Up to a total dose of 1375 mg daily.

Note:  For patient self-medication (over-the-counter use) for pain, fever, or dysmenorrhea—Not to exceed 2 tablets (220 mg each) in twenty-four hours for patients 65 years of age or older or 3 tablets in twenty-four hours for patients 12 to 65 years of age.

**Usual pediatric dose**
Pediatric strength not available. It is recommended that naproxen oral suspension or tablets be administered instead.

**Strength(s) usually available**
U.S.—
- 220 mg (equivalent to 200 mg of naproxen, with 20 mg of sodium) (OTC) [*Aleve* (magnesium stearate; microcrystalline cellulose; povidone; talc; Opadry YS-1-4215)].
- 275 mg (equivalent to 250 mg of naproxen, with 25 mg [approximately 1.1 mmol] of sodium) (Rx) [*Anaprox* (lactose); GENERIC].
- 550 mg (equivalent to 500 mg of naproxen, with 50 mg [approximately 2.2 mmol] of sodium) (Rx) [*Anaprox DS;* GENERIC].

Canada—
- 275 mg (equivalent to 250 mg of naproxen, with 25 mg [approximately 1.1 mmol] of sodium) (Rx) [*Anaprox* (lactose); *Apo-Napro-Na; Novo-Naprox Sodium; Synflex*].
- 550 mg (equivalent to 500 mg of naproxen, with 50 mg [approximately 2.2 mmol] of sodium) (Rx) [*Anaprox DS; Apo-Napro-Na DS; Novo-Naprox Sodium DS; Synflex DS*].

**Packaging and storage**
Store between 15 and 30 °C (59 and 86 °F). Store in a well-closed container.

**Auxiliary labeling**
- Take with food.
- Take with a full glass of water.
- May cause drowsiness.
- Avoid alcoholic beverages.

## Rectal Dosage Forms
### NAPROXEN SUPPOSITORIES
**Usual adult dose**
Antirheumatic (nonsteroidal anti-inflammatory)—
  Rectal, 500 mg at bedtime, administered in conjunction with oral administration during the day.

**Usual adult prescribing limits**
Total daily dose administered orally and rectally should not exceed 1.5 grams a day. The 1.5-gram daily dose is recommended only for short-term administration during acute exacerbations of rheumatic disease. Also, use of this high dose requires that the additional clinical benefit be sufficient to offset the potential increased risk of adverse effects.

**Usual pediatric dose**
Dosage has not been established.

**Strength(s) usually available**
U.S.—
  Not commercially available.
Canada—
  500 mg (Rx) [*Naprosyn; Naxen*].

**Packaging and storage**
Store below 40 °C (104 °F), preferably between 15 and 30 °C (59 and 86 °F), unless otherwise specified by manufacturer. Protect from freezing.

**Auxiliary labeling**
- For rectal use.
- Avoid alcoholic beverages.

---
¹Not included in Canadian product labeling.

---

## OXAPROZIN

## Summary of Differences
Indications:
  Indicated for rheumatoid arthritis and osteoarthritis.
Pharmacology/pharmacokinetics:
  Physicochemical characteristics—Chemical group: A proprionic acid derivative.
  Other actions/effects—
  Is as potent as aspirin as an inhibitor of platelet aggregation.
  Also has uricosuric activity.
  Half-life—Elimination
    600 mg per day—25 hours
    1200 mg per day—21 hours
  Peak plasma concentration—Accumulates with chronic dosing.
Precautions:
  Carcinogenicity—Increased hepatic adenomas and carcinomas in male CD mice, but not in female CD mice or in rats.
  Pregnancy/reproduction—Caused fetal malformations in rabbits with doses within the usual human therapeutic range, but not in mice or rats.
  Pediatrics—Preliminary studies done in patients 3 to 16 years of age; elevated aspartate aminotransferase values occurred more frequently in patients treated for juvenile arthritis than for other forms of arthritis.
  Geriatrics—Dosage adjustment not needed on basis of pharmacokinetic considerations. Studies showed increased occurrence of impaired renal function and of decreased hemoglobin concentration, but not of changes in hepatic function, in patients 60 years of age and older compared to younger adults.
  Surgical—Recommended that oxaprozin be discontinued 1 to 2 weeks before elective surgery; may be more likely than most other NSAIDs to increase risk of perisurgical bleeding because of potent and prolonged inhibitory effect on platelet aggregation.
  Laboratory value alterations—Also, may decrease plasma concentrations and increase urine concentrations of uric acid.
Side/adverse effects:
  See *Table 3,* page 425.

## Oral Dosage Forms
### OXAPROZIN TABLETS
**Usual adult dose**
Rheumatoid arthritis—
  Oral, 1200 mg per day, initially, then adjusted according to patient tolerance and response.
Osteoarthritis—
  Oral, 1200 mg per day, initially, although a lower dose of 600 mg per day may be sufficient for mild disease or for patients of low body weight.

Note: Initial dosage must be individualized according to the severity of disease and patient variables such as body weight and renal function.

A single 1200-mg or 1800-mg loading dose may be administered to patients with normal renal function if necessary to speed the onset of action.

An initial dose of 600 mg per day is recommended for patients with renal function impairment. If this dose is well tolerated, higher doses may be administered if needed.

Doses of up to 1200 mg per day are usually administered once a day, but patients who are unable to tolerate a single dose of this size may tolerate divided doses.

Very severe arthritis may require doses higher than 1200 mg per day, which should be administered in two or three divided doses. It is recommended that these higher doses be reserved for patients weighing more than 50 kg who have normal hepatic and renal function and a low risk of peptic ulceration and who have not experienced adverse effects with lower doses.

After a beneficial response has been achieved, dosage should be reduced to the lowest dose that provides continuing control of symptoms.

**Usual adult prescribing limits**
Oral, 1800 mg per day or 26 mg per kg of body weight per day, whichever is lower, in two or three divided doses.

**Usual pediatric dose**
Safety and efficacy in children have not been established. However, one preliminary study in children 3 to 16 years of age used a starting dose of 10 mg per kg of body weight. The dose was increased to 20 mg per kg of body weight if necessary.

**Strength(s) usually available**
U.S.—
  600 mg (Rx) [*Daypro* (scored)].
Canada—
  Not commercially available.

**Packaging and storage**
Store below 30 °C (86 °F), preferably between 15 and 30 °C (59 and 86 °F), in a tight, light-resistant container, unless otherwise specified by manufacturer.

Note: Protect unit-dose packages from light.

**Auxiliary labeling**
- Take with food.
- Take with a full glass of water.
- Avoid alcoholic beverages.

## PHENYLBUTAZONE

### Summary of Differences
Indications:
  Recommended only for short-term treatment of severe arthritic conditions, gout, or calcium pyrophosphate deposition disease (pseudogout) in patients unresponsive to less toxic NSAIDs. Not recommended as initial therapy for any indication.
Pharmacology/pharmacokinetics:
  Physicochemical characteristics—Chemical group: A pyrazole derivative.
  Other actions/effects—Also induces hepatic microsomal enzyme activity.
  Also has uricosuric activity.
  Biotransformation—Metabolized via hepatic microsomal enzymes. Metabolite oxyphenbutazone is active.
  Half-life—Elimination: 54–99 (average, 77) hours; increased to 105 hours in geriatric patients.
Precautions:
  Mutagenicity—High concentrations induced chromosome abnormalities in Chinese hamster fibroblast cells *in vitro*.
  Pregnancy/reproduction—Fetotoxicity, but not teratogenicity, demonstrated in animal studies.
  Breast-feeding—Distributed into breast milk; may cause blood dyscrasias or other adverse effects in nursing infants.
  Pediatrics—Use in children up to 15 years of age not recommended.
  Geriatrics—Also, increased risk of blood dyscrasias. Recommended that duration of treatment be limited to 1 week in patients 60 years of age and older.
  Drug interactions and/or related problems—
  Concurrent use with alcohol may also impair psychomotor skills.
  Higher risk of bleeding with coumarin- or indandione-derivative anticoagulants than with other NSAIDs because phenylbutazone inhibits the anticoagulant's metabolism; concurrent use not recommended.
  Also, increased risk of toxicity with hydantoin anticonvulsants because phenylbutazone may displace them from protein-binding sites and inhibit their metabolism.
  Also, by inducing hepatic microsomal enzymes, phenylbutazone may decrease effects of barbiturates, cortisone and possibly other corticosteroids, estrogen-containing oral contraceptives, and digitalis glycosides.
  Also, increased risk of severe dermatologic reactions with other dermatitis-causing medications.
  Also, cholestyramine may decrease absorption of phenylbutazone; recommend administering phenylbutazone 1 hour before or 4 to 6 hours after cholestyramine.
  Also, increased risk of adverse hematologic effects if used concurrently with colchicine.
  Also, other hepatic enzyme inducers may increase phenylbutazone metabolism and decrease its half-life.
  Concurrent use with methotrexate may also increase risk of agranulocytosis or bone marrow depression.
  Also, methylphenidate may inhibit phenylbutazone metabolism, leading to increased plasma concentration and risk of toxicity.
  Also, concurrent use with penicillamine may increase risk of serious hematologic and/or renal adverse effects.
  Also, concurrent use with sulfonamides may potentiate effects of either or both medications.
  Also, antacids in buffered formulations may interfere with absorption of many other medications.
  Laboratory value alterations—Interference with thyroid function tests, specifically, decreases 24-hour $^{131}$I thyroidal uptake and increases resin or red cell triiodothyronine ($T_3$) uptake.
  Also, may decrease blood glucose concentrations.
  Also, may decrease plasma concentrations and increase urine concentrations of uric acid.
  Medical considerations/contraindications—Also, not recommended in patients with blood dyscrasias (or history of), bone marrow depression, severe cardiac or cardiopulmonary disease or cardiac failure, severe hepatic or renal disease, or active peptic ulcer disease.
  Also, may aggravate polymyalgia rheumatica or temporal arteritis.
  Patient monitoring—Complete physical examinations, including urinalyses, and hematologic examinations recommended at regular intervals.
Side/adverse effects:
  Higher risk of blood dyscrasias than with other NSAIDs, especially in geriatric patients.
  Reported to cause a serum sickness– or influenza-like syndrome.
  Blood dyscrasias may occur days or weeks after medication is discontinued.
  See also *Table 3*, page 425.

### Additional Dosing Information
See also *General Dosing Information*.

Because of its toxicity, phenylbutazone should be used in the minimum effective dosage and for the shortest possible time.

In geriatric patients, therapy should be limited to short periods, preferably not to exceed 1 week, because of the high risk of severe, possibly fatal, toxic reactions.

Phenylbutazone is generally better tolerated when administered with food to lessen gastric irritation.

If therapy is not effective within 1 week, the medication should be discontinued.

Edema may be dose-related and may be prevented in some patients by reducing the dosage.

### Oral Dosage Forms
Note: Bracketed uses in the *Dosage Forms* section refer to categories of use and/or indications that are not included in U.S. product labeling.

#### PHENYLBUTAZONE CAPSULES USP
**Usual adult dose**
Rheumatoid arthritis[1] or
Osteoarthritis, acute attacks[1] or
Ankylosing spondylitis
[Psoriatic arthritis]—
  Oral, 300 to 600 mg a day in three or four divided doses.
Antigout agent—
  Oral, initially 400 mg as a single dose; then 100 mg every four hours for approximately four days or until a satisfactory response is obtained, with the duration of therapy not exceeding one week.
  Note: Some clinicians use a dose of 200 mg every four hours for approximately four days or until a satisfactory response is obtained, with the duration of therapy not exceeding two weeks.

**Usual pediatric dose**
Children up to 15 years of age—Use is not recommended.

**Strength(s) usually available**
U.S.—
  100 mg (Rx) [*Cotylbutazone;* GENERIC].
Canada—
  Not commercially available.

**Packaging and storage**
Store below 40 °C (104 °F), preferably between 15 and 30 °C (59 and 86 °F), unless otherwise specified by manufacturer. Store in a tight container.

**Auxiliary labeling**
• Take with food.
• Take with a full glass of water.
• Avoid alcoholic beverages.

#### PHENYLBUTAZONE TABLETS USP
**Usual adult dose**
See *Phenylbutazone Capsules USP*.

**Usual pediatric dose**
Children up to 15 years of age—Use is not recommended.

**Strength(s) usually available**
U.S.—
  100 mg (Rx) [GENERIC].
Canada—
  100 mg (Rx) [*Apo-Phenylbutazone; Butazolidin*].

**Packaging and storage**
Store below 40 °C (104 °F), preferably between 15 and 30 °C (59 and 86 °F), unless otherwise specified by manufacturer. Store in a tight container.

**Auxiliary labeling**
• Take with food.
• Swallow tablets whole.
• Take with a full glass of water.
• Avoid alcoholic beverages.

#### PHENYLBUTAZONE TABLETS BUFFERED
**Usual adult dose**
See *Phenylbutazone Capsules USP*.

**Usual pediatric dose**
Children up to 15 years of age—Use is not recommended.

**Strength(s) usually available**
U.S.—
  Not commercially available.
Canada—
  100 mg of phenylbutazone, with 150 mg of magnesium trisilicate and 100 mg of dried aluminum hydroxide gel (Rx) [*Alka Butazolidin*].

**Packaging and storage**
Store below 40 °C (104 °F), preferably between 15 and 30 °C (59 and 86 °F), in a tight container, unless otherwise specified by manufacturer.

**Auxiliary labeling**
- Take with food.
- Swallow tablets whole.
- Take with a full glass of water.
- Avoid alcoholic beverages.

[1]Not included in Canadian product labeling.

---

## PIROXICAM

## Summary of Differences
Indications:
  Indicated for rheumatoid arthritis, osteoarthritis, ankylosing spondylitis, acute attacks of gout or calcium pyrophosphate deposition disease (pseudogout), and dysmenorrhea.
Pharmacology/pharmacokinetics:
  Physicochemical characteristics—Chemical group: An oxicam derivative.
  Half-life—Elimination: 50 hours, although values ranging from 14 to 158 hours have been reported. Increased in patients with renal function impairment. May also be increased in elderly patients, especially females.
  Onset of action—Gout: 2–4 hours.
  Peak effect time—Gout: 3–5 days.
  Duration of action—Gout: 24 hours.
Precautions:
  Pregnancy/reproduction—Teratogenic effects not demonstrated in animal studies.
  Breast-feeding—Distributed into breast milk; use by breast-feeding mothers not recommended because piroxicam inhibits lactation in animals.
  Geriatrics—Tendency toward increased half-life and steady-state concentrations, especially in females.
  Drug interactions and/or related problems—Studies failed to show that piroxicam increases digoxin plasma concentrations.
  Laboratory value alterations—Also, may increase or decrease blood glucose concentrations.
  Medical considerations/contraindications—Higher risk than with most other NSAIDs in patients with renal function impairment.
Side/adverse effects:
  Reported to cause a serum sickness– or influenza-like syndrome.
  See also *Table 3*, page 425.

## Additional Dosing Information
See also *General Dosing Information*.

Because steady-state plasma concentrations are not reached for 7 to 12 days following initiation of therapy, the effectiveness of therapy with piroxicam should not be assessed for 2 weeks.

## Oral Dosage Forms
Note: Bracketed uses in the *Dosage Forms* section refer to categories of use and/or indications that are not included in U.S. product labeling.

### PIROXICAM CAPSULES USP
**Usual adult dose**
Antirheumatic (nonsteroidal anti-inflammatory)—
  Oral, 20 mg once a day or 10 mg two times a day.
[Antidysmenorrheal]—
  Oral, 40 mg at the onset of symptoms on the first day only, then 20 mg once a day thereafter if necessary.

**Usual pediatric dose**
Dosage has not been established.

**Strength(s) usually available**
U.S.—
  10 mg (Rx) [*Feldene* (lactose); GENERIC].
  20 mg (Rx) [*Feldene* (lactose); GENERIC].
Canada—
  10 mg (Rx) [*Apo-Piroxicam*; *Feldene* (lactose); *Novo-Pirocam*; *Nu-Pirox*; *PMS-Piroxicam*].
  20 mg (Rx) [*Apo-Piroxicam*; *Feldene* (lactose); *Novo-Pirocam*; *Nu-Pirox*; *PMS-Piroxicam*].

**Packaging and storage**
Store below 30 °C (86 °F). Store in a tight, light-resistant container.

**Auxiliary labeling**
- Take after meals.
- Take with a full glass of water.
- Avoid alcoholic beverages.

## Rectal Dosage Forms
### PIROXICAM SUPPOSITORIES
**Usual adult dose**
Antirheumatic (nonsteroidal anti-inflammatory)—
  Rectal, 20 mg once a day or 10 mg two times a day.

**Usual adult prescribing limits**
Rectal or combined oral and rectal—20 mg a day.

**Usual pediatric dose**
Dosage has not been established.

**Strength(s) usually available**
U.S.—
  Not commercially available.
Canada—
  10 mg (Rx) [*Feldene*].
  20 mg (Rx) [*Feldene*].

**Packaging and storage**
Store below 40 °C (104 °F), preferably between 15 and 30 °C (59 and 86 °F), unless otherwise specified by manufacturer. Protect from freezing.

**Auxiliary labeling**
- For rectal use.
- Avoid alcoholic beverages.

---

## SULINDAC

## Summary of Differences
Indications:
  Indicated for rheumatoid arthritis, osteoarthritis, ankylosing spondylitis, acute attacks of gout or calcium pyrophosphate deposition disease (pseudogout), bursitis, and tendinitis.
Pharmacology/pharmacokinetics:
  Physicochemical characteristics—Chemical group: A pyrroleacetic acid derivative.
  Biotransformation—Hepatic; sulfide metabolite, not sulindac itself, is active substance.
  Half-life—Elimination:
  Sulindac—7.8 hours
  Sulindac sulfide—16.4 hours
  Time to peak plasma concentration—Sulindac sulfide: Substantially delayed in patients with alcoholic hepatic disease.
  Elimination: Less than 1% of a sulindac dose excreted via the kidneys as the active sulfide metabolite.
Precautions:
  Pregnancy/reproduction—Fetotoxicity, and, in some studies, a low incidence of teratogenicity, have been demonstrated in animals.
  Drug interactions and/or related problems—
  Concurrent chronic use of antacids significantly decreases sulindac plasma concentration.
  Decreased concentration of active sulfide metabolite of sulindac and peripheral neuropathy reported with concurrent (topical) use of dimethyl sulfoxide.
  Laboratory value alterations—Also, may increase blood glucose concentrations.
  Medical considerations/contraindications—
  Hepatic function impairment may slow metabolism to, but also decrease biliary elimination of, the active sulfide metabolite; net result is increased and prolonged plasma concentration and higher risk of toxicity.
  Also, caution and adequate fluid intake recommended for patients with renal calculi (or history of) because renal calculi containing sulindac metabolites have occurred in a few patients.
Side/adverse effects:
  May be less likely than most other NSAIDs to cause renal toxicity.
  Reported to cause biliary obstruction.
  Reported to cause a characteristic hypersensitivity syndrome.
  See also *Table 3*, page 425.

## Additional Dosing Information

See also *General Dosing Information*.

In the treatment of arthritis, improvement in condition may occur within 7 days, but 2 to 3 weeks of continuous use on a regular basis may be required for maximum effectiveness.

Patients with impaired renal function may require lower doses.

Therapy for 7 days in acute gouty arthritis and for 7 to 14 days in acute painful shoulder is usually sufficient.

## Oral Dosage Forms
### SULINDAC TABLETS USP

**Usual adult dose**
Antirheumatic (nonsteroidal anti-inflammatory)—
   Oral, 150 or 200 mg two times a day; may be increased or decreased, depending on patient response.

   Note: Although some patients have received doses higher than 400 mg per day, such doses have not been fully evaluated and are not recommended.

Antigout agent—
   Oral, 200 mg two times a day; dosage to be decreased according to patient response.

Anti-inflammatory (acute painful shoulder)—
   Oral, 200 mg two times a day; dosage to be decreased according to patient response.

**Usual pediatric dose**
Safety and efficacy have not been established.

**Strength(s) usually available**
U.S.—
   150 mg (Rx) [*Clinoril*; GENERIC].
   200 mg (Rx) [*Clinoril* (scored); GENERIC (may be scored)].
Canada—
   150 mg (Rx) [*Apo-Sulin* (scored); *Clinoril*; *Novo-Sundac* (scored)].
   200 mg (Rx) [*Apo-Sulin* (scored); *Clinoril* (scored); *Novo-Sundac* (scored)].

**Packaging and storage**
Store below 40 °C (104 °F), preferably between 15 and 30 °C (59 and 86 °F). Store in a well-closed container.

**Auxiliary labeling**
- Take with food.
- Take with a full glass of water.
- Avoid alcoholic beverages.

---
## TENOXICAM
---

## Summary of Differences

Indications:
   Indicated for rheumatoid arthritis, osteoarthritis, ankylosing spondylitis, bursitis, tendinitis, and periarthritis.
Pharmacology/pharmacokinetics:
   Physicochemical characteristics—Chemical group: An oxicam derivative.
   Half-life—Elimination: $72 \pm 26$ (range, 32–110) hours.
Precautions:
   Pregnancy/reproduction—
   Fertility: Decreased number of corpora lutea and implantations in female rats, but no impairment of fertility in male rats, demonstrated in animal studies.
   First trimester: Maternotoxicity (panperitonitis, gastric lesions, and uterine hemorrhage) and embryotoxicity, but not teratogenicity, demonstrated in animal studies.
   Geriatrics—Also, risk of hyperkalemia may be increased in geriatric patients.
   Drug interactions and/or related problems—
   Studies failed to show that tenoxicam increases digoxin concentrations. Also, cholestyramine administered in conjunction with intravenously administered tenoxicam shown to decrease half-life of tenoxicam from 67.4 to 31.9 hours and increase tenoxicam clearance by 105%.
Side/adverse effects:
   See *Table 3*, page 425.

## Oral Dosage Forms
### TENOXICAM TABLETS

**Usual adult dose**
Antirheumatic (nonsteroidal anti-inflammatory)
and Anti-inflammatory (nonsteroidal)—
   Oral, 20 mg once a day, at the same time each day. For some patients, 10 mg once a day may be sufficient. The smallest effective dose should be used.

**Usual adult prescribing limits**
20 mg per day. Higher doses may increase the risk of adverse effects without providing a significantly greater therapeutic response.

**Usual pediatric dose**
Children up to 16 years of age—Dosage has not been established.

**Strength(s) usually available**
U.S.—
   Not commercially available.
Canada—
   20 mg (Rx) [*Mobiflex* (scored; corn starch; hydroxypropyl methylcellulose; iron oxide; lactose; magnesium stearate; talc; titanium dioxide)].

**Packaging and storage**
Store between 15 and 30 °C (59 and 86 °F), unless otherwise specified by manufacturer.

**Auxiliary labeling**
- Take with food.
- Take with a full glass of water.
- Avoid alcoholic beverages.

---
## TIAPROFENIC ACID
---

## Summary of Differences

Indications:
   Indicated for rheumatoid arthritis and osteoarthritis.
Pharmacology/pharmacokinetics:
   Physicochemical characteristics—Chemical group: A propionic acid derivative.
   Half-life—Elimination
   Single dose—Tablets: 1.7 hours; increased to 2.5 hours in geriatric patients.
   At steady-state—Extended-release capsules (600 mg once a day): 4.2 hours.
Precautions:
   Pregnancy/reproduction—
   Fertility: Decreased number of implantation sites in female rabbits, but no effect on fertility in male or female rats.
   First trimester:
   Crosses the placenta.
   Fetotoxicity, but not teratogenicity, demonstrated in animal studies.
   Geriatrics—Substantially higher frequency of hyperkalemia and/or increased blood urea nitrogen documented in studies.
   Drug interactions and/or related problems—Also, may displace hydantoin anticonvulsants from their protein-binding sites, possibly leading to increased hydantoin half-life and toxicity.
Side/adverse effects:
   See *Table 3*, page 425.

## Oral Dosage Forms
### TIAPROFENIC ACID EXTENDED-RELEASE CAPSULES

**Usual adult dose**
Antirheumatic (nonsteroidal anti-inflammatory)—
   Oral, 600 mg once a day, at the same time each day.

**Usual pediatric dose**
Safety and efficacy have not been established.

**Strength(s) usually available**
U.S.—
   Not commercially available.
Canada—
   300 mg (Rx) [*Surgam SR*].

**Packaging and storage**
Store below 40 °C (104 °F), preferably between 15 and 30 °C (59 and 86 °F), unless otherwise specified by manufacturer.

## Auxiliary labeling
- Take with food.
- Swallow capsules whole.
- Take with a full glass of water.
- Avoid alcoholic beverages.

### TIAPROFENIC ACID TABLETS

**Usual adult dose**
Rheumatoid arthritis—
  Oral, 600 mg a day in two or three divided doses.
Osteoarthritis—
  Oral, 600 mg a day in two or three divided doses, initially. After a satisfactory response has been obtained, dosage may be reduced. Some patients may be maintained on 300 mg a day in divided doses.

**Usual adult prescribing limits**
600 mg a day.

**Usual pediatric dose**
Safety and efficacy have not been established.

**Strength(s) usually available**
U.S.—
  Not commercially available.
Canada—
  200 mg (Rx) [*Albert Tiafen* (scored); *Surgam* (scored)].
  300 mg (Rx) [*Albert Tiafen* (scored); *Surgam* (scored)].

**Packaging and storage**
Store below 40 °C (104 °F), preferably between 15 and 30 °C (59 and 86 °F), unless otherwise specified by manufacturer.

**Auxiliary labeling**
- Take with food.
- Take with a full glass of water.
- Avoid alcoholic beverages.

---

## TOLMETIN

## Summary of Differences
Indications:
  Indicated for rheumatoid arthritis, osteoarthritis, ankylosing spondylitis, juvenile arthritis, and psoriatic arthritis.
Pharmacology/pharmacokinetics:
  Physicochemical characteristics—Chemical group: A pyrroleacetic acid derivative.
  Absorption—Extent decreased by food and milk.
  Half-life—Elimination: 5 hours
Precautions:
  Pregnancy/reproduction—No teratogenicity or other adverse effects on fetal development demonstrated in animal studies.
  Pediatrics—Studied in pediatric patients 2 years of age and older; no pediatrics-specific problems documented.
  Laboratory value alterations—Interference with sulfosalicylic acid test method for urinary protein.
  Medical considerations/contraindications—Caution in patients who must restrict their sodium intake.
Side/adverse effects:
  Higher incidence of anaphylactic reactions than with other NSAIDs.
  Reported to cause a serum sickness- or influenza-like syndrome.
  See also *Table 3*, page 425.

## Additional Dosing Information
See also *General Dosing Information*.

Improvement in condition may occur within 7 days, but 1 to 2 weeks of continuous use on a regular basis may be required for maximum effectiveness.

## Oral Dosage Forms
Note: The dosing and strengths of the available dosage forms are expressed in terms of the free acid (not the sodium salt).

### TOLMETIN SODIUM CAPSULES USP

**Usual adult dose**
Antirheumatic (nonsteroidal anti-inflammatory)—
  Initial: Oral, 400 mg (free acid) three times a day, preferably including a dose in the morning and a dose at bedtime.
  Maintenance: Rheumatoid arthritis—
    Oral, 600 mg to 1.8 grams (free acid) a day in three or four divided doses.
  Osteoarthritis—
    Oral, 600 mg to 1.6 grams (free acid) a day in three or four divided doses.

**Usual adult prescribing limits**
Up to 2 grams (free acid) daily for rheumatoid arthritis or 1.6 grams (free acid) daily for osteoarthritis.

**Usual pediatric dose**
Antirheumatic (nonsteroidal anti-inflammatory)—
  Children up to 2 years of age: Dosage has not been established.
  Children 2 years of age and over: Initial—Oral, 20 mg (free acid) per kg of body weight a day in three or four divided doses.
  Maintenance—Oral, 15 to 30 mg (free acid) per kg of body weight a day in divided doses.

Note: Doses higher than 30 mg (free acid) per kg of body weight per day have not been studied and therefore are not recommended.

**Strength(s) usually available**
U.S.—
  400 mg (free acid, with 36 mg [1.568 mmol] of sodium) (Rx) [*Tolectin DS*; GENERIC].
Canada—
  400 mg (free acid, with 36 mg [1.568 mmol] of sodium) (Rx) [*Novo-Tolmetin*; *Tolectin 400*].

**Packaging and storage**
Store below 40 °C (104 °F), preferably between 15 and 30 °C (59 and 86 °F). Store in a tight container.

**Auxiliary labeling**
- Take with food.
- Take with a full glass of water.
- Avoid alcoholic beverages.

### TOLMETIN SODIUM TABLETS USP

**Usual adult dose**
See *Tolmetin Sodium Capsules USP*.

**Usual adult prescribing limits**
See *Tolmetin Sodium Capsules USP*.

**Usual pediatric dose**
See *Tolmetin Sodium Capsules USP*.

**Strength(s) usually available**
U.S.—
  200 mg (free acid, with 18 mg [0.784 mmol] of sodium) (Rx) [*Tolectin 200* (scored); GENERIC].
  600 mg (free acid, with 54 mg [2.352 mmol] of sodium) (Rx) [*Tolectin 600*; GENERIC].
Canada—
  200 mg (free acid, with 18 mg [0.784 mmol] of sodium) (Rx) [*Tolectin 200* (scored)].
  600 mg (free acid, with 54 mg [2.352 mmol] of sodium) (Rx) [*Tolectin 600*].

**Packaging and storage**
Store between 15 and 30 °C (59 and 86 °F). Store in a well-closed container.

**Auxiliary labeling**
- Take with food.
- Take with a full glass of water.
- Avoid alcoholic beverages.

Revised: 09/13/94
Interim revision: 07/24/96

## Table 1. Pharmacology/Pharmacokinetics

| Drug and Route | Absorption: Rate (Factors that decrease) | Absorption: Extent (Factors that decrease) | % Protein-Binding* (Factors that decrease) | Plasma Concentration: Time to Peak (hr) [dose in mg] | Plasma Concentration: Peak (mcg/mL) [dose in mg] | Time to Steady-State (days) [dose in mg/doses per day] | Steady-State (mcg/mL) [dose in mg/doses per day] |
|---|---|---|---|---|---|---|---|
| **Diclofenac** Oral | | | >99 | | | | |
| Tablets | Rapid (food) | Complete | | 1, range 0.33–2†; up to 3.6‡ | | | |
| Delayed-release Tablets | Rapid (food) | Complete | | 2, range 0.25–4†; 6‡ | 0.7–1.1 [25] 1.5–1.6 [50]† 2 [75] Decreased 40% by food | | |
| Extended-release Tablets | | | | 4 | | | |
| Rectal | Rapid | | | 0.5–2 | | | |
| **Diflunisal** Oral | Rapid (food) | Complete | >99 | 2–3 | 41 [250] 87 [500] 124 [1000] | | 56 [250/2] 190 [500/2] |
| **Etodolac** Oral | Rapid (food)§ | Extensive | >99 | 1.3, range 0.8–1.8†; 2.2–5.6‡ [200–600]; Steady-state 1.7±1.3 | 10–46 [200–600] Decreased 50% by food and 15–20% by antacids | | 16.5–19 [200/2] |
| **Fenoprofen** Oral | Rapid (food, milk)§ | | 99 | 1–2 [600]† Increased by food | 50 [600]† Decreased by food | | |
| **Floctafenine** Oral | Rapid (food) | | | 1–2 | | Within 3 | |
| **Flurbiprofen** Oral | | | 99 | | | | |
| Tablets | Rapid (food) | | | 1.5; range 0.5–4 | 5–6; 8.7 # [50] 10–15 [100]** Decreased by food | | 5–6 [50/3] |
| Extended-release Capsules | | | | 5.5†; 8.3‡ | 8.56 Increased by food | 2–3 [200/1] | 10.78 [200/1] |
| **Ibuprofen** Oral | Rapid (food)§ | | 99 | 1.2–2.1 | 22–27 [200] 23–45 [400] 42–57 [600]†† 56–66 [800] Decreased up to 30% by food | | |
| **Indomethacin** Oral | | | 99 | | | | |
| Capsules; Oral Suspension | Rapid (food, antacids [Al- and/or Mg-containing]) | Complete; 90% in 4 hr | | 0.5–2 [25] | 0.8–2.5 [25] 2.5–4 [50] | | 1.4 [25/3] 2.8 [50/3] |
| Extended-release Capsules | | 90% in 12 hr | | 2–4.25 [75] | 1.5–3 [75] | | 1.4 [75/1] |
| Rectal | Rapid | 80–90‡‡ | | | | | |
| **Ketoprofen** | | | 99 (hepatic cirrhosis, advanced age) | | | <1 | |
| Oral Capsules | Rapid (food, milk)§ | Complete | | 0.5–2 [50] average 1.1† average 2‡ | 4.1 [50]†# 2.4 [50]‡# | | |

## Table 1. Pharmacology/Pharmacokinetics (continued)

| Drug and Route | Absorption Rate (Factors that decrease) | Absorption Extent (Factors that decrease) | % Protein-Binding* (Factors that decrease) | Plasma Concentration Time to Peak (hr) [dose in mg] | Plasma Concentration Peak (mcg/mL) [dose in mg] | Time to Steady-State (days) [dose in mg/ doses per day] | Steady-State (mcg/mL) [dose in mg/ doses per day] |
|---|---|---|---|---|---|---|---|
| Ketoprofen (continued) Oral (continued) Extended-release Capsules | Slow | Almost complete | | 6–7†; 8–9‡ | 3.1±1.2†; 3.4±1.3‡ [200] | | |
| Delayed-release Tablets | Delayed by ±1.5 hr | | | 1.5–4 [50] | | | |
| Extended-release Tablets | | | | 5.5–8 | Decreased 20% by high-fat meal | | |
| Rectal§§ | | | | 0.5–2 | | | |
| Meclofenamate Oral | Rapid (food)§ | Complete (food) | >99 | 0.5–2 | 8–9 [100] | | 4.8, range 1.8-7.2 [100/3] Decreased by food |
| Mefenamic Acid Oral | Rapid | | | 2.5 [250] 1–2 [500] 2–4 [1000] | 3.6 [250] 3.5 [500] 10 [1000] | 2 [1000/4] | 20 [1000/4] |
| Nabumetone (prodrug) Oral 6-methoxy-2-naph-thylacetic acid (6-MNA) (active substance) | Increased by food, milk§ | Increased by food, milk§ | >99 | Steady-state 3, range 1–12 [1000]##; 2.5, range 1–8 [2000] Decreased by food | 24 [500]‡ 22–23†; 36–38 ‡# [1000]*** 64 [2000] | 3 [500/2 or 1000/1] | 18.5[500/2]; trough 33, peak 52 [1000/1]# |
| Naproxen Oral Tablets; Oral Suspension | Rapid (food, antacids [Al- and Mg-containing])††† | Complete | >99 (hepatic cirrhosis, advanced age) | Naproxen: 2–4 [750] Sodium salt: 1–2 [825] | 46.6 [375] 63.1 [500]‡‡‡ 90 [750] | 2–2.5 (500/2) | 55 [500/2] |
| Delayed-release Tablets | | | | 4.2-4.5 Decreased by antacids Increased by high-fat meal | 47.9 [375] 58.2 [2×250] 60.7 [500]§§§ | | |
| Extended-release Tablets | | | | 9.7†; 7.7‡ [1000] | 63.1†; 86.1‡ [1000] | | |

*To albumin.
†Taken on an empty stomach.
‡Taken with food.
§Absorption not affected by antacids, specifically: For fenoprofen, ibuprofen, ketoprofen, meclofenamate, piroxicam, sulindac, tolmetin—Aluminum- and magnesium-containing; For tiaprofenic acid—Aluminum-containing.
#May be increased in geriatric patients (For flurbiprofen, geriatric females only).
**Decreased by 40% in patients with end-stage renal disease undergoing continuous ambulatory peritoneal dialysis.
††Decrease to 37 mcg/mL demonstrated in obese patients, probably because volume of distribution increased.
‡‡Failure to retain suppository in rectum for one full hour may be responsible for incomplete absorption.
§§Bioavailability 73–93% of that achieved with oral administration.
##Mean 8 hours in patients with hepatic cirrhosis. Not significantly different in geriatric patients than in younger adults.
***Administration of a second 1000-mg dose 12 hours after an initial 1000-mg dose produced peak concentrations of ±71 mcg/mL. Peak concentrations are significantly decreased (to as low as 18 mcg/mL) in patients with hepatic cirrhosis.
†††May be increased by concurrent administration of sodium bicarbonate.
‡‡‡Similar values reported with administration of 500-mg tablets to adults and with administration of 5 mg/kg of oral suspension to children 5 to 16 years of age with juvenile arthritis.
§§§Increased to 70.7 mcg/mL by concurrent administration with antacid.
###May be increased to 2 to 3 weeks if elimination half-life is greatly prolonged.
****May be increased if elimination half-life is greatly prolonged and/or renal function is impaired.
††††May be increased to 4 to 7 hours in patients with alcoholic hepatic disease.

## Table 1. Pharmacology/Pharmacokinetics (continued)

| Drug and Route | Absorption Rate (Factors that decrease) | Absorption Extent (Factors that decrease) | % Protein-Binding* (Factors that decrease) | Time to Peak (hr) [dose in mg] | Peak (mcg/mL) [dose in mg] | Time to Steady-State (days) [dose in mg/doses per day] | Steady-State (mcg/mL) [dose in mg/doses per day] |
|---|---|---|---|---|---|---|---|
| Oxaprozin Oral | Relatively slow§ (food–slight effect) | | ±99.9 (renal impairment, congestive heart failure, hepatic cirrhosis) | 3–5 | 70–80 [1200] | 4–7 | 98–230 [600/1 or 1200/1] Accumulates with chronic dosing |
| Phenylbutazone Oral | Rapid | | 98 | 2–2.5 | 43 [300] | | Phenylbutazone: up to 172 Oxyphenbutazone: up to 86 |
| Piroxicam Oral | (food)§ | | | 3–5 [20] | 1.5–2 [20] | 7–12 [20/1]### | 3–8 [20/1]**** |
| Rectal | | | | 10 [20] | | | |
| Sulindac (prodrug) Oral | (food)§ | 90% | | 2† 3–4‡ | 1–2 [200] | | |
| Sulindac sulfide (active substance) | | | | 1.7†††† | | 4–5 [200/2] | 4 [200/2] |
| Tenoxicam Oral | (food)§ | Extensive§ | 98–99 | 1.25, range 0.5–6† | 1.46–3.31† [20] | | |
| Tiaprofenic Acid Oral Tablets | Rapid (food)§ | | 98 | 0.5–1.5† Up to 2‡ | 26 [200] 50 [300] | Within 1 [200/3] | |
| Extended-release Capsules | | | | Steady-state 4–8 [600/1] | | | |
| Tolmetin Oral | Rapid (food)§ | Almost complete (food, milk) | >99 | 0.5–1 | 40 [400]† 20 [400]‡ | | |

*To albumin.
†Taken on an empty stomach.
‡Taken with food.
§Absorption not affected by antacids, specifically: For fenoprofen, ibuprofen, ketoprofen, meclofenamate, piroxicam, sulindac, tolmetin—Aluminum- and magnesium-containing; For tiaprofenic acid—Aluminum-containing.
#May be increased in geriatric patients (For flurbiprofen, geriatric females only).
**Decreased by 40% in patients with end-stage renal disease undergoing continuous ambulatory peritoneal dialysis.
††Decrease to 37 mcg/mL demonstrated in obese patients, probably because volume of distribution increased.
‡‡Failure to retain suppository in rectum for one full hour may be responsible for incomplete absorption.
§§Bioavailability 73–93% of that achieved with oral administration.
##Mean 8 hours in patients with hepatic cirrhosis. Not significantly different in geriatric patients than in younger adults.
***Administration of a second 1000-mg dose 12 hours after an initial 1000-mg dose produced peak concentrations of ±71 mcg/mL. Peak concentrations are significantly decreased (to as low as 18 mcg/mL) in patients with hepatic cirrhosis.
†††May be increased by concurrent administration of sodium bicarbonate.
‡‡‡Similar values reported with administration of 500-mg tablets to adults and with administration of 5 mg/kg of oral suspension to children 5 to 16 years of age with juvenile arthritis.
§§§Increased to 70.7 mcg/mL by concurrent administration with antacid.
###May be increased to 2 to 3 weeks if elimination half-life is greatly prolonged.
****May be increased if elimination half-life is greatly prolonged and/or renal function is impaired.
††††May be increased to 4 to 7 hours in patients with alcoholic hepatic disease.

## Table 2. Pharmacology/Pharmacokinetics

| Drug | Biotransformation | Half-Life Distribution (hr) | Half-Life Elimination (hr) | Renal Elimination % of Dose | Renal Elimination % Unchanged | Biliary/Fecal Elimination % of Dose | Biliary/Fecal Elimination % Unchanged |
|---|---|---|---|---|---|---|---|
| Diclofenac* | Hepatic; almost 50% eliminated via first-pass metabolism† | | 1.2–2 | 40–65 | Little or none | 35 | Little or none |
| Diflunisal‡ | | | 8–12<br>22 (GFR 10–50)§#<br>60 (GFR 2–10)§#<br>115 (GFR <2)§# | 80–95 in 72–96 hr<br>53 in 72 hr (GFR 10–50)§<br>9.5 in 72 hr (GFR 2–10)§<br>2.7 in 72 hr (GFR <2)§ | <5 | Little or none | |
| Etodolac‡ | Hepatic, extensive. No significant first-pass metabolism | 0.71±0.5, at steady-state | Single dose 6–7; Steady-state 7.3±4 | 72; 60% in 24 h | <1 | 16 | |
| Fenoprofen | Hepatic | | 3 | 90 in 24 hr | | | |
| Floctafenine | Hepatic; rapid | 1 | 8 | 40** | | 60** | |
| Flurbiprofen | | 3 | 5.7, range 2–12 | 88–98; 73 within 48 hr | 20–25 | | |
| Ibuprofen‡ | Hepatic | | 1.8–2 | 100 in 24 hr | <1 | | |
| Indomethacin‡ | Hepatic | 1 | 2.6–11.2 (average 4.5)†† | 60 | 10–20 | 33‡‡ | 1.5 |
| Ketoprofen* | Primarily hepatic; glucuronide conjugation may also occur in other tissues§§ | 0.33 | Capsules 1.6; Extended-release Capsules 5.4±2.2; Extended-release Tablets 3–4## | 80 in 24 hr | Up to 10 | *** | |
| Meclofenamate | ††† | | 2 (single dose)<br>3.3 (multiple doses) | 66 | Little or none | 33 | |
| Mefenamic Acid | Hepatic | | 2 | 67 | | Up to 25 | |

*Dialyzable.
†Some metabolites may be active.
‡Not dialyzable.
§In patients with renal function impairment. GFR=glomerular filtration rate in mL per minute, when specified.
#Reason for prolonged half-life is unclear because only small amounts are excreted unchanged. It has been proposed that biliary excretion of metabolites with subsequent hydrolysis to, and reabsorption of, the parent compound may occur in renal failure. Alternatively, slower renal excretion may permit hydrolysis of an unstable metabolite to the parent compound.
**Excretion (renal plus biliary/fecal) complete within 24 hours.
††Subject to large interindividual variation, possibly because of differences in enterohepatic circulation and subsequent reabsorption.
‡‡Undergoes extensive enterohepatic circulation.
§§Acyl-glucuronide conjugate is unstable; in patients with renal function impairment, this conjugate may accumulate and be deconjugated to the parent compound.
##Higher values for the extended-release dosage forms reflect prolonged absorption. In geriatric patients, values for the capsules and the extended-release capsules are prolonged by 26% and 54%, respectively. Also, values for the capsules may be prolonged to 3 hours in patients with mild renal function impairment and to 5 to 9 hours in patients with moderate to severe renal function impairment.
***Enterohepatic recirculation has been proposed to account for elimination of the other 40% of the dose; however, studies to confirm this possibility have not been done.
†††Hydroxymethyl metabolite has anti-inflammatory activity approximately 20% of that of the parent compound.
‡‡‡In geriatric patients, in whom values are especially subject to substantial interpatient variability; values as high as 74 hours have been measured. Also, increased to about 39 hours in patients with creatinine clearances <30 mL/minute/1.73 cubic meters of body surface area), but not in patients with lesser degrees of renal function impairment or in patients receiving hemodialysis.
§§§In patients with moderately severe renal function impairment (creatinine clearances 10–30 mL/min/1.73 cubic meters of body surface area).
###Several studies reported terminal elimination half-life values of 50 to 60 hours. However, these lower "accumulation" half-life values are recommended for use in clinical practice, e.g., for estimating time to reach steady-state, determining appropriate dosing intervals, and determining intervals for dosage adjustment.
****In geriatric patients.
††††Average; usual range 30 to 60 hours, but values ranging from 14 to 158 hours have been reported. Half-life may be especially prolonged in patients with renal function impairment.

Table 2. Pharmacology/Pharmacokinetics (continued)

| Drug | Biotransformation | Half-Life Distribution (hr) | Half-Life Elimination (hr) | Renal Elimination % of Dose | Renal Elimination % Unchanged | Biliary/Fecal Elimination % of Dose | Biliary/Fecal Elimination % Unchanged |
|---|---|---|---|---|---|---|---|
| Nabumetone | Hepatic, with extensive first-pass metabolism. 35–38% of a 1000-mg dose metabolized to the active substance 6-MNA, which is further metabolized hepatically; bioavailability of 6-MNA decreased in patients with severe hepatic function impairment | | 6-MNA: 23±3.7; 30±8.1‡‡‡ | 6-MNA: 80; 75 in 48 hr; complete in 168 hr; 32.5 in 96 hr§§§ | 6-MNA: <1 | | |
| Naproxen | Hepatic | | 13 | 95 | | | |
| Oxaprozin‡ | Hepatic, 65% via microsomal oxidation followed by glucuronic acid conjugation and 35% via direct glucuronic acid conjugation | | Steady-state (mg/day) 25 (600) 21 (1200)### | 65%, as glucuronide metabolites | Very small amounts | 35%, as glucuronide metabolites | Very small amounts |
| Phenylbutazone | Slow, via hepatic microsomal enzymes | | 54–99 (average 77) 105**** | 61–75; may remain in body 7–10 days after last dose | Trace amounts | 25–27 | <5 |
| Oxyphenbutazone (active metabolite) | | | | 4 | | | |
| Piroxicam | Hepatic | | 50†††† | 66 | <5 | 33 | |
| Sulindac | Hepatic; sulfide metabolite, not sulindac itself, is active | | 7.8 | 50 | | ‡‡ | |
| Sulindac sulfide | | | 16.4 | <1 | | 25‡‡ | |
| Tenoxicam | | | 72±28 (range, 32–110) | 66 | <0.5 | 17 | |
| Tiaprofenic Acid | | | Tablets 1.7; 2.5**** Extended-release Capsules (at steady-state) 4.2 | 60 | 90 | 40 | |
| Tolmetin | Hepatic | 1–2 | 5 | 100 in 24 hr | Up to 17 | | |

*Dialyzable.
†Some metabolites may be active.
‡Not dialyzable.
§In patients with renal function impairment. GFR=glomerular filtration rate in mL per minute, when specified.
#Reason for prolonged half-life is unclear because only small amounts are excreted unchanged. It has been proposed that biliary excretion of metabolites with subsequent hydrolysis to, and reabsorption of, the parent compound may occur in renal failure. Alternatively, slower renal excretion may permit hydrolysis of an unstable metabolite to the parent compound.
**Excretion (renal plus biliary/fecal) complete within 24 hours.
††Subject to large interindividual variation, possibly because of differences in enterohepatic circulation and subsequent reabsorption.
‡‡Undergoes extensive enterohepatic circulation.
§§Acyl-glucuronide conjugate is unstable; in patients with renal function impairment, this conjugate may accumulate and be deconjugated to the parent compound.
##Higher values for the extended-release dosage forms reflect prolonged absorption. In geriatric patients, values for the capsules and the extended-release capsules are prolonged by 26% and 54%, respectively. Also, values for the capsules may be prolonged to 3 hours in patients with mild renal function impairment and to 5 to 9 hours in patients with moderate to severe renal function impairment.
***Enterohepatic recirculation has been proposed to account for elimination of the other 40% of the dose; however, studies to confirm this possibility have not been done.
†††Hydroxymethyl metabolite has anti-inflammatory activity approximately 20% of that of the parent compound.
‡‡‡In geriatric patients, in whom values are especially subject to substantial interpatient variability; values as high as 74 hours have been measured. Also, increased to about 39 hours in patients with creatinine clearances <30 mL/minute/1.73 cubic meters of body surface area), but not in patients with lesser degrees of renal function impairment or in patients receiving hemodialysis.
§§§In patients with moderately severe renal function impairment (creatinine clearances 10–30 mL/min/1.73 cubic meters of body surface area).
###Several studies reported terminal elimination half-life values of 50 to 60 hours. However, these lower "accumulation" half-life values are recommended for use in clinical practice, e.g., for estimating time to reach steady-state, determining appropriate dosing intervals, and determining intervals for dosage adjustment.
****In geriatric patients.
††††Average; usual range 30 to 60 hours, but values ranging from 14 to 158 hours have been reported. Half-life may be especially prolonged in patients with renal function impairment.

# Table 3. Side/Adverse Effects*

**Legend:**
I = Diclofenac
II = Diflunisal
III = Etodolac
IV = Fenoprofen
V = Floctafenine
VI = Flurbiprofen
VII = Ibuprofen
VIII = Indomethacin
IX = Ketoprofen
X = Meclofenamate
XI = Mefenamic Acid
XII = Nabumetone
XIII = Naproxen
XIV = Oxaprozin
XV = Phenylbutazone
XVI = Piroxicam
XVII = Sulindac
XVIII = Tenoxicam
XIX = Tiaprofenic Acid
XX = Tolmetin

| | I | II | III | IV | V | VI | VII | VIII | IX | X | XI | XII | XIII | XIV | XV | XVI | XVII | XVIII | XIX | XX |
|---|---|---|---|---|---|---|---|---|---|---|---|---|---|---|---|---|---|---|---|---|
| **Medical attention needed** | | | | | | | | | | | | | | | | | | | | |
| **Cardiovascular effects** | | | | | | | | | | | | | | | | | | | | |
| Note: Many of these cardiovascular effects may occur secondary to NSAID-induced renal function impairment. | | | | | | | | | | | | | | | | | | | | |
| Angina pectoris or exacerbation of (chest pain) | L | U | U | U | L | R† | U | U | U | U | U | R† | U | U | U | R | U | U | R | U |
| Bleeding, other than gastrointestinal, including: | | | | | | | | | | | | | | | | | | | | |
| Hemoptysis (spitting blood) | U | U | U | U | U | U | U | U | R | U | U | U | U | U | U | U | U | U | U | U |
| Nosebleeds, unexplained | R | U | U | U | U | R | R† | R | R | U | U | U | U | U | U | R | U | R | L | R |
| Cardiac arrhythmias | L | U | R† | R† | U | R† | R† | R | R† | U | U | R† | U | U | U | U | R† | U | U | U |
| Chest pain | R† | R† | U | U | U | R | U | R | U | U | U | R | U | U | U | U | U | U | R | L |
| Congestive heart failure or exacerbation of (chest pain; shortness of breath; troubled breathing, tightness in chest, and/or wheezing; decrease in amount of urine; swelling of face, fingers, feet, or lower legs; unusual tiredness; weight gain) | R | R | R | U | R | R | U | R | R | U | U | U | U | U | U | R | U | U | R | R |
| Edema, pulmonary (shortness of breath, troubled breathing, tightness in chest, and/or wheezing) | U | U | U | R† | U | U | U | R | U | U | U | U | U | U | U | U | U | U | U | U |
| Increased blood pressure—may reach hypertensive levels | R | R | R | R | U | R | U | R | R | U | U | R† | U | R | R | R | U | R | R | M |
| Pericarditis (chest pain; fever with or without chills; shortness of breath, troubled breathing, and/or tightness in chest) | U | U | U | U | U | R | U | U | U | U | U | U | U | U | R | U | U | U | U | U |
| **Central nervous system effects** | | | | | | | | | | | | | | | | | | | | |
| Confusion | U | R | U | U | L | R | U | R | R | U | U | R | U | L | R | R† | U | R | U | U |
| Convulsions | R† | U | U | R† | U | U | U | U | U | U | U | U | U | U | U | U | R | U | R | U |
| Dysarthria (trouble in speaking) | U | U | U | U | U | U | U | U | U | U | U | U | U | U | U | U | U | U | U | U |
| Forgetfulness | R† | U | U | U | U | L | U | R | U | U | U | U | U | U | U | U | U | U | U | U |
| Hallucinations | U | R | U | U | U | U | R† | R | R† | U | U | U | U | U | U | R† | U | U | U | U |
| Headache, severe, especially in the morning | U | U | U | U | U | U | U | M§ | U | U | U | U | U | U | U | U | U | U | U | U |
| Meningitis, aseptic (severe headache, drowsiness, confusion, stiff neck and/or back, general feeling of illness, nausea) | R | U | U | U | U | R | U | U | U | U | U | U | R† | U | U | U | U | U | R | R |

*Differences in frequency of occurrence may reflect either lack of clinical-use data or actual pharmacologic distinctions among agents (although their pharmacologic similarity suggests that side effects occurring with one may occur with the others). M=more frequent (3–9%); L=less frequent (1–3%); R=rare (<1%); U=unknown; unless otherwise specified.
†Has been reported, but a causal relationship has not been established.
‡Has been reported, but actual frequency of occurrence unknown.
§Frequency of occurrence 10% or higher.
#Serious gastrointestinal effects, including ulceration, perforation, and/or bleeding, may occur at any time, with or without warning signs and/or symptoms, during chronic therapy with nonsteroidal anti-inflammatory drugs (NSAIDs). The risk of NSAID-induced gastrointestinal toxicity may increase with the duration of therapy as well as with dosage. In clinical trials with nabumetone, peptic ulceration occurred in approximately 0.3%, 0.5%, and 0.8% of patients treated for 6 months, 1 year, and 2 years, respectively. In clinical trials with other NSAIDs, upper gastrointestinal tract ulceration, bleeding, or perforation occurred in approximately 1% of patients treated for 3 to 6 months and in approximately 2 to 4% of patients treated for 1 year. Risk factors that may increase the risk of NSAID-induced gastrointestinal toxicity, other than those associated with an increased risk of peptic ulcer disease in any patient, have not been identified.
**See also Dermatologic effects, Hematologic effects, Hepatic effects, and Renal effects for signs and symptoms of many of the reported components of this syndrome.
††Diarrhea occurring during mefenamic acid therapy requires medical attention.

## Table 3. Side/Adverse Effects* (continued)

Legend:
I = Diclofenac
II = Diflunisal
III = Etodolac
IV = Fenoprofen
V = Floctafenine
VI = Flurbiprofen
VII = Ibuprofen
VIII = Indomethacin
IX = Ketoprofen
X = Meclofenamate
XI = Mefenamic Acid
XII = Nabumetone
XIII = Naproxen
XIV = Oxaprozin
XV = Phenylbutazone
XVI = Piroxicam
XVII = Sulindac
XVIII = Tenoxicam
XIX = Tiaprofenic Acid
XX = Tolmetin

| | I | II | III | IV | V | VI | VII | VIII | IX | X | XI | XII | XIII | XIV | XV | XVI | XVII | XVIII | XIX | XX |
|---|---|---|---|---|---|---|---|---|---|---|---|---|---|---|---|---|---|---|---|---|
| **Migraine** (headache, severe and throbbing, sometimes with nausea or vomiting) | U | | | U | U | | | U | R | U | U | U | U | | | U | U | U | U | U |
| **Mood or mental changes, including:** | | | | | | | | | | | | | | | | | | | | |
| Disorientation | U | R | R | R | U | U | U | R | U | U | U | R | U | U | U | U | U | U | R | U |
| Feeling of depersonalization or muzziness | U | U | R | R† | U | U | U | U | U | U | U | U | U | U | R | U | U | U | U | U |
| Mental depression | R | R | L | R | U | L | L | L | L | L | ‡ | R | L | L | R | R | L | R | L | L |
| Psychotic reaction | R† | U | U | U | U | U | U | R | U | U | U | U | U | U | U | U | R | U | U | U |
| **Neuropathy, peripheral** (numbness, tingling, pain, or weakness in hands or feet) | R† | R† | U | U | U | U | R† | R | U | R† | U | U | R† | U | R† | R† | R | U | R | U |
| **Syncope** (fainting) | U | R† | R | U | U | U | U | R | U | U | U | R† | U | | | U | R | U | U | U |
| **Dermatologic effects** | | | | | | | | | | | | | | | | | | | | |
| **Dermatitis, allergic** | | | | | | | | | | | | | | | | | | | | |
| (bullous eruption/blisters) | R | U | R | R | U | U | R | U | R | U | U | R | U | U | U | R | U | U | U | U |
| (eczema) | U | U | R | R | R | R | R | R | U | U | U | U | U | R | R | U | U | U | R | R |
| (hives) | R | R | R | R | L | L | R | R | R | L | ‡ | R | M | R | R | R | R | R | U | R |
| (itching) | L | R | L | M | L | R | L | R | L | L | ‡ | M | R† | R | L | L | L | L | M | L |
| (skin rash) | L | M | L | M | L | L | M | R | L | M | L | L | M | M | L | L | M | L | L | L |
| **Dermatitis, exfoliative** (fever with or without chills; red, thickened, or scaly skin; swollen and/or painful glands; unusual bruising) | R† | R | U | R† | U | R | R | R | R | R | U | U | U | U | U | R | R | U | U | U |
| **Desquamation** (peeling of skin) | U | U | R† | U | U | U | U | U | U | U | U | U | U | U | U | R | U | U | U | U |
| **Erythema** (reddening of skin) or other skin discoloration | U | U | U | U | U | U | U | U | R | R | U | R | R | U | R | U | R | U | R | |
| **Erythema multiforme** (fever with or without chills; muscle cramps or pain; skin rash; sores, ulcers, or white spots on lips or in mouth) | R | R | U | R† | U | U | U | R | U | R | U | R† | R† | U | R | R | R | R | U | R |
| **Erythema nodosum** (fever with or without chills; skin rash) | U | R | U | U | U | U | U | R | U | R† | U | U | U | | R | R | U | U | U | U |
| **Photosensitivity reactions resembling porphyria cutanea tarda and epidermyolysis bullosa** (blistering, scarring, darkening or lightening of skin color) | U | U | U | U | U | | U | U | U | U | U | U | R† | U | R† | U | U | U | U | U |
| **Stevens-Johnson syndrome** (bleeding or crusting sores on lips; chest pain; fever with or without chills; muscle cramps or pain; skin rash; sores, ulcers, or white spots in mouth; sore throat) | R | R | U | R† | U | U | R | R | U | U | U | U | R† | U | R | R | R | U | U | U |
| **Toxic epidermal necrolysis** (redness, tenderness, itching, burning, or peeling of skin; sore throat; fever with or without chills) | U | R | R | U | U | | R† | R | U | U | U | R | R† | U | R | R | R | U | U | R |

Table 3. Side/Adverse Effects* *(continued)*

Legend:
I = Diclofenac
II = Diflunisal
III = Etodolac
IV = Fenoprofen
V = Floctafenine
VI = Flurbiprofen
VII = Ibuprofen
VIII = Indomethacin
IX = Ketoprofen
X = Meclofenamate
XI = Mefenamic Acid
XII = Nabumetone
XIII = Naproxen
XIV = Oxaprozin
XV = Phenylbutazone
XVI = Piroxicam
XVII = Sulindac
XVIII = Tenoxicam
XIX = Tiaprofenic Acid
XX = Tolmetin

| | I | II | III | IV | V | VI | VII | VIII | IX | X | XI | XII | XIII | XIV | XV | XVI | XVII | XVIII | XIX | XX |
|---|---|---|---|---|---|---|---|---|---|---|---|---|---|---|---|---|---|---|---|---|
| **Digestive system effects** | | | | | | | | | | | | | | | | | | | | |
| Abdominal distention (swelling of abdomen) | L | U | U | U | U | U | U | R | U | U | — | — | U | R | R | U | U | R | U | U |
| Bleeding from rectum—with rectal dosage forms | ‡ | — | — | — | — | — | — | R | M | — | — | — | R | — | — | L | — | — | — | — |
| Colitis or exacerbation of or Enterocolitis or | R | U | R† | U | U | U | U | R | U | R | — | — | R | — | R | U | R | U | R | U |
| | U | — | — | U | — | — | — | R | U | — | — | — | U | — | U | U | U | U | R | U |
| Regional enteritis or exacerbation of (abdominal pain, cramping, or discomfort; bloody stools; diarrhea) | U | — | — | U | U | U | U | R | U | — | — | — | U | — | R | U | U | U | U | U |
| Dysphagia (difficulty in swallowing) | U | U | U | U | U | U | U | U | U | U | — | R | U | — | U | U | U | R | U | U |
| Esophagitis (burning feeling in throat or chest, difficulty in swallowing) | U | U | R† | U | U | U | U | U | U | U | — | — | U | — | U | U | U | U | U | U |
| Gastritis (burning feeling in chest or stomach, indigestion, tenderness in stomach area) | U | R | L | R | U | R | R | U | U | R | — | L | L | R | R | U | R | — | R | L |
| Gastroenteritis (severe abdominal pain, diarrhea, loss of appetite, nausea, weakness) | U | — | — | U | U | U | U | R | U | U | — | — | U | — | R | U | R | U | U | U |
| Gastrointestinal bleeding or hemorrhage—reported independently of gastrointestinal ulceration or perforation, including melena (bloody stools) and hematemesis (vomiting blood or material that looks like coffee grounds)** | R | R | L | R | M | L | R | R | R | R | — | — | R | — | R | R | R | R | R | R |
| Gastrointestinal perforation# and/or Gastrointestinal ulceration#, including esophageal, gastric, or peptic ulceration, multiple gastrointestinal ulcerations, and perforation of pre-existing sigmoid lesions, e.g., diverticula, carcinoma (severe pain, cramping, or burning; bloody or black, tarry stools; vomiting of blood or material that looks like coffee grounds; severe and continuing nausea, heartburn, and/or indigestion)# | U | R | U | R | M | L | R | R | R | R | — | — | R | — | R | R | R | U | U | R |
| | L | R | L | R | M | R | R | R | R | L | — | — | R | — | R | R | R | R | R | L |

Note: *Intestinal ulceration* may lead to stenosis and obstruction. Also, paralytic ileus has been reported with meclofenamate, but a causal relationship has not been established.

*Differences in frequency of occurrence may reflect either lack of clinical-use data or actual pharmacologic distinctions among agents (although their pharmacologic similarity suggests that side effects occurring with one may occur with the others). M=more frequent (3–9%); L=less frequent (1–3%); R=rare (<1%); U=unknown; unless otherwise specified.
†Has been reported, but a causal relationship has not been established.
‡Has been reported, but actual frequency of occurrence unknown.
§Frequency of occurrence 10% or higher.
#Serious gastrointestinal effects, including ulceration, perforation, and/or bleeding, may occur at any time, with or without warning signs and/or symptoms, during chronic therapy with nonsteroidal anti-inflammatory drugs (NSAIDs). The risk of NSAID-induced gastrointestinal toxicity may increase with the duration of therapy as well as with dosage. In clinical trials with nabumetone, peptic ulceration occurred in approximately 0.3%, 0.5%, and 0.8% of patients treated for 6 months, 1 year, and 2 years, respectively. In clinical trials with other NSAIDs, upper gastrointestinal tract ulceration, bleeding, or perforation occurred in approximately 1% of patients treated for 3 to 6 months and in approximately 2 to 4% of patients treated for 1 year. Risk factors that may increase the risk of NSAID-induced gastrointestinal toxicity, other than those associated with an increased risk of peptic ulcer disease in any patient, have not been identified.
**See also Dermatologic effects; Hematologic effects; Hepatic effects; and Renal effects for signs and symptoms of many of the reported components of this syndrome.
††Diarrhea occurring during mefenamic acid therapy requires medical attention.

Table 3. Side/Adverse Effects* (continued)

Legend:
I = Diclofenac
II = Diflunisal
III = Etodolac
IV = Fenoprofen
V = Floctafenine
VI = Flurbiprofen
VII = Ibuprofen
VIII = Indomethacin
IX = Ketoprofen
X = Meclofenamate
XI = Mefenamic Acid
XII = Nabumetone
XIII = Naproxen
XIV = Oxaprozin
XV = Phenylbutazone
XVI = Piroxicam
XVII = Sulindac
XVIII = Tenoxicam
XIX = Tiaprofenic Acid
XX = Tolmetin

| | I | II | III | IV | V | VI | VII | VIII | IX | X | XI | XII | XIII | XIV | XV | XVI | XVII | XVIII | XIX | XX |
|---|---|---|---|---|---|---|---|---|---|---|---|---|---|---|---|---|---|---|---|---|
| **Genitourinary effects** | | | | | | | | | | | | | | | | | | | | |
| Bladder pain | U | U | U | U | U | U | U | U | U | U | U | U | U | U | U | U | U | U | R | U |
| Bleeding from vagina, unexplained, unexpected, and/or unusually heavy menstrual | R† | U | R† | U | U | U | R† | R | R | U | U | U | R | R | U | R | R | U | R | U |
| Blood in urine | R† | U | R† | R | M | R | R | R | R | U | ‡ | U | R | R | R | R | R | R | U | R |
| Crystalluria, renal calculi, or ureteral obstruction (blood in urine; difficult, burning, or painful urination; severe pain in lower back, side, or abdomen)—with phenylbutazone, may be composed of uric acid crystals and with sulindac, may be composed of sulindac metabolites | U | U | R† | U | U | U | U | U | U | U | U | U | U | U | U | U | R | U | U | U |
| Cystitis or | R | R | R† | R | M | R | R | R† | L | U | R | U | R | U | U | R† | U | R | R | R |
| Urethritis or | U | U | U | U | M | U | U | U | U | U | U | U | U | U | U | U | U | U | U | U |
| Urinary tract infection (bloody or cloudy urine; difficult, burning, or painful urination; frequent urge to urinate) | U | U | U | U | U | M | U | U | U | U | U | U | U | U | U | U | U | U | L | L |
| Dysuria (burning, painful, or difficult urination) | U | U | U | U | M | U | U | U | R | U | R | U | U | U | U | R† | R | R | R | R |
| Frequent urge to urinate | R† | R | L | L | U | U | R | U | U | U | U | U | U | U | U | U | U | R | R | U |
| Incontinence (loss of bladder control) | U | U | U | U | U | R | U | U | U | U | U | R | U | U | U | U | U | U | U | U |
| Proteinuria (cloudy urine) | R | R | U | U | U | U | U | R | U | U | U | U | U | U | U | R | R | R | U | R |
| Strong-smelling urine | U | U | U | U | M | U | U | U | U | U | U | U | U | U | U | U | U | U | U | U |
| **Hematologic effects** | | | | | | | | | | | | | | | | | | | | |
| Agranulocytosis [granulocytopenia] (fever with or without chills; sores, ulcers, or white spots on lips or in mouth; sore throat) | R | R | U | R | U | R | R | R | R | R | R | R | R | U | R | U | R | R | U | R |
| Anemia (unusual tiredness or weakness)—may be associated with gastrointestinal bleeding or microbleeding or with hemodilution caused by fluid retention | R | U | R | U | U | R | R | R | R | R | L | R | U | U | U | U | U | L | L | R |
| Aplastic anemia [pancytopenia] (shortness of breath, troubled breathing, tightness in chest, and/or wheezing; sores, ulcers, or white spots on lips or in mouth; sore throat) | U | U | U | U | U | U | R | R | U | U | R | U | R† | U | R | R | R | R | U | R |
| Bone marrow depression—signs and symptoms are listed under the individual entries for Aplastic anemia and Thrombocytopenia | U | U | U | U | U | U | U | R | U | U | U | R | U | U | R | R | U | U | U | U |
| Disseminated intravascular coagulation | U | U | U | U | M | U | U | R | U | R | U | U | U | U | R | R | U | U | R | U |
| Ecchymosis/bruising | R† | U | U | R | U | R | U | U | U | R | U | U | L | R | U | L | U | U | R | U |
| Eosinophilia | U | U | U | U | M | U | U | U | U | R | ‡ | U | R† | U | R | R† | R | U | U | U |
| Hemolytic anemia (troubled breathing, exertional; unusual tiredness or weakness) | R | R | U | R | U | R | U | R | R | R | R | U | U | U | R | R† | U | U | U | U |

USP DI — Anti-inflammatory Drugs, Nonsteroidal (Systemic) 429

Table 3. Side/Adverse Effects* (continued)

Legend:
I = Diclofenac
II = Diflunisal
III = Etodolac
IV = Fenoprofen
V = Floctafenine
VI = Flurbiprofen
VII = Ibuprofen
VIII = Indomethacin
IX = Ketoprofen
X = Meclofenamate
XI = Mefenamic Acid
XII = Nabumetone
XIII = Naproxen
XIV = Oxaprozin
XV = Phenylbutazone
XVI = Piroxicam
XVII = Sulindac
XVIII = Tenoxicam
XIX = Tiaprofenic Acid
XX = Tolmetin

| | I | II | III | IV | V | VI | VII | VIII | IX | X | XI | XII | XIII | XIV | XV | XVI | XVII | XVIII | XIX | XX |
|---|---|---|---|---|---|---|---|---|---|---|---|---|---|---|---|---|---|---|---|---|
| **Hypocoagulability** (bleeding from cuts or scratches that lasts longer than usual) | U | U | U | U | U | U | U | U | R | U | R | U | U | U | U | U | U | U | U | U |
| **Leukopenia [neutropenia]** (usually asymptomatic; rarely, fever or chills, cough or hoarseness, lower back or side pain, painful or difficult urination) | R | U | R† | U | U | R | R | R | U | R | R | U | R | R | R | L | R | R | R | U |
| **Petechia** (pinpoint red spots on skin) | U | U | | | U | U | R† | R | U | U | | U | U | U | R | R | U | R | U | U |
| **Purpura** (bruises and/or red spots on skin) — may be associated with thrombocytopenia | | | | | | | | | | | | | | | | | | | | |
| **Thrombocytopenia with or without purpura** (usually asymptomatic; rarely, unusual bleeding or bruising; black, tarry stools; blood in urine or stools; pinpoint red spots on skin) | R | R | R | R | U | R | R | R | R | R | R | | R | R | R | R | R | R | U | R |
| **Hepatic effects, including:** | | | | | | | | | | | | | | | | | | | | |
| Cholestatic hepatitis or jaundice (dark urine; fever; itching; light-colored stools; pain, tenderness, and/or swelling in upper abdominal area; skin rash; swollen glands) | U | | | U | U | U | R | U | U | U | U | | U | U | R | U | R | | U | U |
| **Hepatitis or jaundice, toxic** (loss of appetite, nausea, vomiting, yellow eyes or skin, swelling in upper abdominal area) | R | R | R | R | U | R | R | R | R | R | R | | R | R | R | R | R | U | U | R |
| **Hypersensitivity reactions** See also Dermatologic effects | | | | | | | | | | | | | | | | | | | | |
| Anaphylaxis or anaphylactoid reactions (changes in facial skin color; skin rash, hives, and/or itching; fast or irregular breathing; puffiness or swelling of the eyelids or around the eyes; shortness of breath, troubled breathing, tightness in chest, and/or wheezing) — may include anaphylactic shock with sudden, severe decrease in blood pressure and collapse | | | | | | | | | | | | | | | | | | | | |
| **Angiitis [vasculitis]** (muscle pain, cramps, and/or weakness; shortness of breath, troubled breathing, tightness in chest, and/or wheezing; skin rash; spitting blood; unusual tiredness or weakness) | U | R | U | U | U | R | R† | R | U | U | U | | R† | U | R | R | R | | U | R |

*Differences in frequency of occurrence may reflect either lack of clinical-use data or actual pharmacologic distinctions among agents (although their pharmacologic similarity suggests that side effects occurring with one may occur with the others). M = more frequent (3–9%); L = less frequent (1–3%); R = rare (<1%); U = unknown; unless otherwise specified.
†Has been reported, but a causal relationship has not been established.
‡Has been reported, but actual frequency of occurrence unknown.
§Frequency of occurrence 10% or higher.
#Serious gastrointestinal effects, including ulceration, perforation, and/or bleeding, may occur at any time, with or without warning signs and/or symptoms, during chronic therapy with nonsteroidal anti-inflammatory drugs (NSAIDs). The risk of NSAID-induced gastrointestinal toxicity may increase with the duration of therapy as well as with dosage. In clinical trials with nabumetone, peptic ulceration occurred in approximately 0.3%, 0.5%, and 0.8% of patients treated for 6 months, 1 year, and 2 years, respectively. In clinical trials with other NSAIDs, upper gastrointestinal tract ulceration, bleeding, or perforation occurred in approximately 1% of patients treated for 3 to 6 months and in approximately 2 to 4% of patients treated for 1 year. Risk factors that may increase the risk of NSAID-induced gastrointestinal toxicity, other than those associated with an increased risk of peptic ulcer disease in any patient, have not been identified.
**See also Dermatologic effects, Hematologic effects, Hepatic effects, and Renal effects for signs and symptoms of many of the reported components of this syndrome.
††Diarrhea occurring during mefenamic acid therapy requires medical attention.

## Table 3. Side/Adverse Effects* (continued)

Legend:
I = Diclofenac
II = Diflunisal
III = Etodolac
IV = Fenoprofen
V = Floctafenine
VI = Flurbiprofen
VII = Ibuprofen
VIII = Indomethacin
IX = Ketoprofen
X = Meclofenamate
XI = Mefenamic Acid
XII = Nabumetone
XIII = Naproxen
XIV = Oxaprozin
XV = Phenylbutazone
XVI = Piroxicam
XVII = Sulindac
XVIII = Tenoxicam
XIX = Tiaprofenic Acid
XX = Tolmetin

| | I | II | III | IV | V | VI | VII | VIII | IX | X | XI | XII | XIII | XIV | XV | XVI | XVII | XVIII | XIX | XX |
|---|---|---|---|---|---|---|---|---|---|---|---|---|---|---|---|---|---|---|---|---|
| *Angioedema* (large, hive-like swellings on face, eyelids, mouth, lips, and/or tongue) | R | R | R | R | R | R | R† | R | U | U | U | R | R† | U | R | R | R | R | R | U |
| *Bronchospastic allergic reactions* (shortness of breath, troubled breathing, tightness in chest, and/or wheezing) | R | R | R | U | U | R | R | R | R | U | U | R† | U | U | R | R | R | R | U | U |
| *Fever with or without chills* | U | U | L | R† | U | R | U | R | U | U | U | R† | R | U | R | R | R | U | R | R |
| *Hypersensitivity syndrome, multisystemic, diflunisal-induced, including dermatologic reactions; hematologic effects including eosinophilia, leukopenia, thrombocytopenia, and disseminated intravascular coagulation; jaundice; renal impairment or failure; and nonspecific signs and symptoms* (disorientation, fever and chills, general feeling of illness or discomfort, loss of appetite, muscle and/or joint pain, swollen and/or painful glands)** | — | R | — | — | — | — | — | — | — | — | — | — | — | — | — | — | — | — | — | — |
| *Hypersensitivity syndrome, multisystemic, sulindac-induced, including dermatologic reactions; conjunctivitis; hepatic failure and jaundice; pancreatitis; pneumonitis with or without pleural effusions* (difficulty in breathing, coughing, tightness in chest, wheezing); *hematologic effects including leukopenia, leukocytosis, eosinophilia, disseminated intravascular coagulation, and anemia; renal impairment or failure; and nonspecific signs and symptoms* (chest pain, fast heartbeat, fever and chills, flushing, general feeling of illness or discomfort, low blood pressure, muscle and/or joint pain, sweating, tiredness)** | — | — | — | — | — | — | — | — | — | — | — | — | — | — | — | — | R | — | — | — |
| *Laryngeal edema* (shortness of breath or troubled breathing) | R | U | U | U | U | U | U | U | R | U | U | U | R | U | U | U | U | U | U | U |
| *Loeffler syndrome [eosinophilic pneumonitis]* (chest pain; fever with or without chills; shortness of breath, troubled breathing, tightness in chest, and/or wheezing; unusual weakness) | U | U | U | R† | U | U | U | U | U | U | U | U | U | U | U | U | U | U | R | U |
| *Rhinitis, allergic* (unexplained runny nose or sneezing) | U | U | U | U | L | R | R | U | R | R | U | U | R | R | R | U | U | U | U | R |
| *Serum sickness-like reaction* (fever with or without chills; muscle cramps, pain, and/or weakness; skin rash, hives, and/or itching; shortness of breath, troubled breathing, tightness in chest, and/or wheezing; swollen and/or painful glands) | U | — | — | — | — | — | R† | — | — | — | — | — | — | — | R | — | — | — | — | R |
| *Systemic lupus erythematosus [SLE]-like syndrome* (bloody or cloudy urine; chest pain; fever with or without chills; shortness of breath, troubled breathing, tightness in chest, and/or wheezing; skin rash, hives, and/or itching; sudden decrease in amount of urine; swelling of face, fingers, feet, and/or lower legs; swollen and/or painful glands; unusual weakness; rapid weight gain) | U | U | U | U | U | U | U | U | U | R | U | U | U | U | R | U | U | U | U | U |

Table 3. Side/Adverse Effects* (continued)

Legend:
I = Diclofenac
II = Diflunisal
III = Etodolac
IV = Fenoprofen
V = Floctafenine
VI = Flurbiprofen
VII = Ibuprofen
VIII = Indomethacin
IX = Ketoprofen
X = Meclofenamate
XI = Mefenamic Acid
XII = Nabumetone
XIII = Naproxen
XIV = Oxaprozin
XV = Phenylbutazone
XVI = Piroxicam
XVII = Sulindac
XVIII = Tenoxicam
XIX = Tiaprofenic Acid
XX = Tolmetin

| | I | II | III | IV | V | VI | VII | VIII | IX | X | XI | XII | XIII | XIV | XV | XVI | XVII | XVIII | XIX | XX |
|---|---|---|---|---|---|---|---|---|---|---|---|---|---|---|---|---|---|---|---|---|
| Loosening or splitting of fingernails or other nail disorder | U | | | U | | | | | R | U | | | U | U | U | R† | U | | R | U |
| Lymphadenopathy (swollen and/or painful glands) | U | U | R | R† | U | R† | U | R | U | U | U | | U | U | U | U | U | U | U | R |
| Muscle cramps or pain—not present before treatment and not related to condition being treated | U | R† | U | M | | | | R | | | | | R | | R | | U | U | U | M |
| **Ocular effects** | | | | | | | | | | | | | | | | | | | | |
| Amblyopia, toxic, or | R† | U | | | U | U | R | U | U | U | | | U | | R† | U | U | | U | U |
| Corneal opacity or | U | U | | | U | U | U | U | U | U | | | U | | U | U | U | | U | U |
| Retinal or macular disturbances (blurred vision or other vision change) | U | U | | | U | U | R† | R | U | R† | | | U | | R† | R† | R† | | U | R† |
| Blurred or double vision or any change in vision | R | R | L | L | L | R | R | R | L | R† | ‡ | | L | R | R† | R | R | L | R | U |
| Conjunctivitis (eye pain, redness, irritation, and/or swelling) | U | U | R† | R† | U | R† | R† | U | R† | R† | ‡ | | U | R | U | U | U | R | R | U |
| Corneal deposits | U | U | | | U | U | U | R | U | U | | | U | | R | U | U | | U | U |
| Dry, irritated, or swollen eyes | U | U | | | U | U | R | R | R | R† | ‡ | | U | U | U | U | U | | R | U |
| Eye pain | U | U | | | U | U | R | R | R | U | | | U | U | U | R | U | | U | U |
| Palpebral edema (swollen eyelids) | U | U | | | U | U | U | U | U | U | | | U | U | U | U | U | U | R | U |
| Retinal hemorrhage (red eyes) | R† | U | | | R† | U | R† | U | R | U | | | U | | R† | U | U | | R | U |
| Scotomata (change in vision) | R | U | | | U | U | U | R | R | U | | | R | U | R† | L | U | | R | U |
| **Oral/perioral effects** | | | | | | | | | | | | | | | | | | | | |
| Gingival ulceration or | U | U | | R† | U | U | R | R | L | L | L | R† | U | L | U | U | U | L | U | R |
| Stomatitis, aphthous (sores, ulcers, or white spots on lips or in mouth) | R | R | R | L | R | R† | R | R | L | R | L | | R† | R | R | L | R | R | L | R |
| Glossitis (irritated tongue) | U | U | | | U | U | U | U | U | U | U | U | U | U | U | U | R | U | U | U |
| Swelling of lips and tongue | U | U | | | U | U | U | R | U | U | U | R† | U | U | U | R† | U | U | R | U |
| **Otic effects** | | | | | | | | | | | | | | | | | | | | |
| Decreased hearing or any change in hearing | R | L | | L | L | R† | U | R | R | U | U | L | R† | R | L | L | R | R | R | R |
| Ringing or buzzing in ears | L | L | | L | L | U | R† | L | L | L | L | U | R | L | U | M | L | L | L | L |

*Differences in frequency of occurrence may reflect either lack of clinical-use data or actual pharmacologic distinctions among agents (although their pharmacologic similarity suggests that side effects occurring with one may occur with the others). M=more frequent (3–9%); L=less frequent (1–3%); R=rare (<1%); U=unknown; unless otherwise specified.
†Has been reported, but a causal relationship has not been established.
‡Has been reported, but actual frequency of occurrence unknown.
§Frequency of occurrence 10% or higher.
#Serious gastrointestinal effects, including ulceration, perforation, and/or bleeding, may occur at any time, with or without warning signs and/or symptoms, during chronic therapy with nonsteroidal anti-inflammatory drugs (NSAIDs). The risk of NSAID-induced gastrointestinal toxicity may increase with the duration of therapy as well as with dosage. In clinical trials with nabumetone, peptic ulceration occurred in approximately 0.3%, 0.5%, and 0.8% of patients treated for 6 months, 1 year, and 2 years, respectively. In clinical trials with other NSAIDs, upper gastrointestinal tract ulceration, bleeding, or perforation occurred in approximately 1% of patients treated for 3 to 6 months and in approximately 2 to 4% of patients treated for 1 year. Risk factors that may increase the risk of NSAID-induced gastrointestinal toxicity, other than those associated with an increased risk of peptic ulcer disease in any patient, have not been identified.
**See also Dermatologic effects, Hematologic effects, Hepatic effects, and Renal effects for signs and symptoms of many of the reported components of this syndrome.
††Diarrhea occurring during mefenamic acid therapy requires medical attention.

## Table 3. Side/Adverse Effects* (continued)

Legend:
I = Diclofenac
II = Diflunisal
III = Etodolac
IV = Fenoprofen
V = Floctafenine
VI = Flurbiprofen
VII = Ibuprofen
VIII = Indomethacin
IX = Ketoprofen
X = Meclofenamate
XI = Mefenamic Acid
XII = Nabumetone
XIII = Naproxen
XIV = Oxaprozin
XV = Phenylbutazone
XVI = Piroxicam
XVII = Sulindac
XVIII = Tenoxicam
XIX = Tiaprofenic Acid
XX = Tolmetin

| | I | II | III | IV | V | VI | VII | VIII | IX | X | XI | XII | XIII | XIV | XV | XVI | XVII | XVIII | XIX | XX |
|---|---|---|---|---|---|---|---|---|---|---|---|---|---|---|---|---|---|---|---|---|
| *Pancreatitis* (abdominal pain, fever with or without chills, swelling and/or tenderness in upper abdominal or stomach area) | R | U | U | R† | U | U | R | R | R† | U | R | R† | U | | R† | R† | R | U | U | U |
| **Renal effects** | | | | | | | | | | | | | | | | | | | | |
| *Fluid retention/edema* (increased blood pressure; decrease in amount of urine; swelling of face, fingers, feet, and/or lower legs; rapid weight gain) | M | R | R | M | M | M | M | M | M | U | U | M | M | R | M | L | L | L | L | M |
| *Glomerulitis or glomerulonephritis* | U | U | | U | U | U | U | U | U | U | U | U | U | U | R | R | U | U | U | U |
| *Hyperkalemia* (difficulty in speaking, low blood pressure, slow or irregular heartbeat, troubled breathing, severe weakness in arms or legs) | | | R† | | | R† | | R | | | | | | | | R | | U | L | U |
| *Interstitial nephritis* (bloody or cloudy urine; increased blood pressure; sudden decrease in amount of urine; swelling of face, fingers, feet, and/or lower legs; rapid weight gain)—may be hypersensitivity-mediated | R | R | | R | U | U | R | U | R | U | U | U | R | R | U | R | R | U | R | R |
| *Nephrosis* (sudden decrease in amount of urine; swelling of face, fingers, feet, and/or lower legs; rapid weight gain) | U | U | | R | U | U | R | U | U | U | U | U | U | U | U | U | U | U | U | U |
| *Nephrotic syndrome* (cloudy urine, swelling of face) | R | R† | | R | U | R† | U | R | R | U | U | R† | U | U | U | U | R | U | U | R |
| *Oliguria/anuria* (cessation of urination)—reported independently of renal impairment or failure | R | U | | R | U | U | R | U | U | U | U | R† | U | R† | R | U | R | U | U | U |
| *Polyuria* (sudden, large increase in frequency and quantity of urine) | U | U | | U | L | U | R | U | U | U | U | R | U | U | U | U | U | U | U | U |
| *Renal impairment or failure* (increased blood pressure; shortness of breath, troubled breathing, tightness in chest, and/or wheezing; sudden decrease in amount of urine; swelling of face, fingers, feet, and/or lower legs; continuing thirst; unusual tiredness or weakness; weight gain) | R | R† | R† | M | L | U | R | R | R | R | R | U | R | U | U | R | R | U | U | R |
| *Renal papillary or tubular necrosis* | R | R† | | U | L | R† | R | R | R | U | R | R | M | U | U | R† | R | R | R | R |
| *Shortness of breath or troubled breathing* | | | | U | L | L | L | M | R | U | ‡ | R | L | U | U | R† | U | U | R | U |
| *Thirst, continuing* | U | U | | U | U | L | U | U | R | R | ‡ | U | L | U | U | U | R | U | U | U |
| **Medical attention needed only if continuing or bothersome** | | | | | | | | | | | | | | | | | | | | |
| **Cardiovascular effects** | | | | | | | | | | | | | | | | | | | | |
| *Fast heartbeat* | R† | U | U | L | L | L | R† | R | R | U | U | U | U | U | U | U | U | R | U | U |
| *Flushing or hot flashes* | R† | L | U | L | L | L | L | R | U | U | ‡ | L | U | U | U | U | R | R | L | R |
| *Increased sweating* | R† | R | U | U | L | L | U | L | L | L | ‡ | R† | L | U | L | R | R | R | R | R |
| *Pounding heartbeat* | R† | R† | R | M | M | R† | R | R | R† | R† | R | R† | R† | R† | R | R† | R | R | R | R |
| **Central nervous system effects** | | | | | | | | | | | | | | | | | | | | |
| *Anxiety* | U | U | U | M | U | L | U | U | U | U | U | R | U | U | U | U | U | U | U | U |
| *Dizziness* | L | L | M | M | M | M | M | M | M | M | ‡ | M | M | U | R | L | M | M | M | M |
| *Drowsiness* | R | L | R | M | M | M | R | L | L | U | ‡ | L | M | L | R | L | R | U | L | L |

## Table 3. Side/Adverse Effects* (continued)

Legend:
I = Diclofenac
II = Diflunisal
III = Etodolac
IV = Fenoprofen
V = Floctafenine
VI = Flurbiprofen
VII = Ibuprofen
VIII = Indomethacin
IX = Ketoprofen
X = Meclofenamate
XI = Mefenamic Acid
XII = Nabumetone
XIII = Naproxen
XIV = Oxaprozin
XV = Phenylbutazone
XVI = Piroxicam
XVII = Sulindac
XVIII = Tenoxicam
XIX = Tiaprofenic Acid
XX = Tolmetin

| | I | II | III | IV | V | VI | VII | VIII | IX | X | XI | XII | XIII | XIV | XV | XVI | XVII | XVIII | XIX | XX |
|---|---|---|---|---|---|---|---|---|---|---|---|---|---|---|---|---|---|---|---|---|
| **Headache, mild to moderate** | M | M | M | M | M | M | L | M§ | M | M | ‡ | M | M | U | R | L | L | M | M | M |
| **Lightheadedness/vertigo** | U | R | U | U | U | M | U | L | R | U | U | R | L | L | U | L | R | R | R | U |
| **Nervousness or irritability** | R | R | L | M | M | M | L | R | M | U | ‡ | L | U | R† | U | R | L | R | U | L |
| **Trembling or twitching** | R† | U | U | L | U | L | L | U | U | U | ‡ | R | U | L | L | U | U | U | L | U |
| **Trouble in sleeping** | R | L | R | L | M | L | R | R | R† | R† | ‡ | L | R | L | U | R | R | R | R | L |
| **Unusual weakness with no other signs or symptoms** | R | L | M | M | U | M | U | R | U | R† | U | R | R | M | R | R† | R | R | R | M |
| **Dermatologic effects** | | | | | | | | | | | | | | | | | | | | |
| Photosensitive or photoallergic dermatologic reaction (severe sunburn; skin rash, redness, itching, and/or discoloration after exposure to sunlight) | R | R | R† | U | R | R | R† | R | R | U | U | R | R | R | R | R | M§ | R | U | U |
| **Gastrointestinal effects** | | | | | | | | | | | | | | | | | | | | |
| Abdominal cramps, pain, or discomfort, mild to moderate | M | M | M | M | M | M | M | M | M | M | M | M§ | M | L | M | M | M§ | U | M | M |
| Bitter taste or other taste change | R | U | U | R† | U | L | L | U | R† | R† | U | R | U | R† | U | U | R | U | U | U |
| Bloated feeling or gas | L | L | M | L | R | L | L | R | M | M | L | M | U | L | R | L | L | L | L | M |
| Constipation | M | L | L | M | M | L | L | L | M | L | L | M | M | M | R | L | M | L | L | L |
| Decreased appetite or loss of appetite | R | R | R | L | L | L | L | R | L | L | ‡ | U | U | M | R | L | L | L | R | R |
| Diarrhea | M | M | M | M | M | M | L | L | M | M§ | M†† | M§ | L | M | R | L | M | R | R | M |
| Epigastric pain or discomfort (stomach pain or discomfort, mild to moderate) | U | U | U | U | U | M | M | U | U | U | ‡ | U | U | U | U | M | U | L | L | U |
| Heartburn | U | M | U | M§ | M | M | L | M | M§ | M | L | M§ | M | L | U | U | U | L | M | U |
| Indigestion | M | M | M | M | M | M | L | M§ | M | L | L | M | L | L | M | L | L | M | M§ | M |
| Nausea | M | M | M | M | M | M | M | M | M | M§ | M | M | M | M | M | M | M | L | M | M§ |
| Rectal irritation—with rectal dosage forms | ‡ | — | — | — | — | — | — | R | — | — | — | — | — | — | — | ‡ | — | — | — | — |
| Vomiting | R | L | R | L | L | L | L | L | L | L | U | L | L | L | R | L | L | R | M | M |

*Differences in frequency of occurrence may reflect either lack of clinical-use data or actual pharmacologic distinctions among agents (although their pharmacologic similarity suggests that side effects occurring with one may occur with the others). M=more frequent (3–9%); L= less frequent (1–3%); R= rare (<1%); U=unknown; unless otherwise specified.
†Has been reported, but a causal relationship has not been established.
‡Has been reported, but actual frequency of occurrence unknown.
§Frequency of occurrence 10% or higher.
#Serious gastrointestinal effects, including ulceration, perforation, and/or bleeding, may occur at any time, with or without warning signs and/or symptoms, during chronic therapy with nonsteroidal anti-inflammatory drugs (NSAIDs). The risk of NSAID-induced gastrointestinal toxicity may increase with the duration of therapy as well as with dosage. In clinical trials with nabumetone, peptic ulceration occurred in approximately 0.3%, 0.5%, and 0.8% of patients treated for 6 months, 1 year, and 2 years, respectively. In clinical trials with other NSAIDs, upper gastrointestinal tract ulceration, bleeding, or perforation occurred in approximately 1% of patients treated for 3 to 6 months and in approximately 2 to 4% of patients treated for 1 year. Risk factors that may increase the risk of NSAID-induced gastrointestinal toxicity, other than those associated with an increased risk of peptic ulcer disease in any patient, have not been identified.
**See also Dermatologic effects, Hematologic effects, Hepatic effects, and Renal effects for signs and symptoms of many of the reported components of this syndrome.
††Diarrhea occurring during mefenamic acid therapy requires medical attention.

Table 3. Side/Adverse Effects* (continued)

Legend:
I = Diclofenac
II = Diflunisal
III = Etodolac
IV = Fenoprofen
V = Floctafenine
VI = Flurbiprofen
VII = Ibuprofen
VIII = Indomethacin
IX = Ketoprofen
X = Meclofenamate
XI = Mefenamic Acid
XII = Nabumetone
XIII = Naproxen
XIV = Oxaprozin
XV = Phenylbutazone
XVI = Piroxicam
XVII = Sulindac
XVIII = Tenoxicam
XIX = Tiaprofenic Acid
XX = Tolmetin

| | I | II | III | IV | V | VI | VII | VIII | IX | X | XI | XII | XIII | XIV | XV | XVI | XVII | XVIII | XIX | XX |
|---|---|---|---|---|---|---|---|---|---|---|---|---|---|---|---|---|---|---|---|---|
| **General feeling of discomfort or illness** | R | U | U | L | U | L | U | L | L | R† | U | R | R | R | U | L | U | R | U | U |
| **Irritation, dryness, or soreness of mouth** | R | L | R | L | L | R† | R | R | R | L | U | L | U | U | U | R | R | R | L | R |
| **Muscle weakness** | U | U | U | U | U | U | U | R | U | U | U | U | R | U | U | U | R | R | U | L |
| **Photophobia** (increased sensitivity of eyes to light) | U | U | R | U | U | U | U | U | U | U | U | U | U | U | U | U | U | U | U | U |
| **Weight loss, unexplained** | R† | U | U | U | U | U | U | U | R | U | U | U | U | R | U | U | U | U | U | M |

*Differences in frequency of occurrence may reflect either lack of clinical-use data or actual pharmacologic distinctions among agents (although their pharmacologic similarity suggests that side effects occurring with one may occur with the others). M=more frequent (3–9%); L=less frequent (1–3%); R=rare (<1%); U=unknown; unless otherwise specified.
†Has been reported, but a causal relationship has not been established.
‡Has been reported, but actual frequency of occurrence unknown.
§Frequency of occurrence 10% or higher.
#Serious gastrointestinal effects, including ulceration, perforation, and/or bleeding, may occur at any time, with or without warning signs and/or symptoms, during chronic therapy with nonsteroidal anti-inflammatory drugs (NSAIDs). The risk of NSAID-induced gastrointestinal toxicity may increase with the duration of therapy as well as with dosage. In clinical trials with nabumetone, peptic ulceration occurred in approximately 0.3%, 0.5%, and 0.8% of patients treated for 6 months, 1 year, and 2 years, respectively. In clinical trials with other NSAIDs, upper gastrointestinal tract ulceration, bleeding, or perforation occurred in approximately 1% of patients treated for 3 to 6 months and in approximately 2 to 4% of patients treated for 1 year. Risk factors that may increase the risk of NSAID-induced gastrointestinal toxicity, other than those associated with an increased risk of peptic ulcer disease in any patient, have not been identified.
**See also Dermatologic effects, Hematologic effects, Hepatic effects, and Renal effects for signs and symptoms of many of the reported components of this syndrome.
††Diarrhea occurring during mefenamic acid therapy requires medical attention.

# ANTI-INHIBITOR COAGULANT COMPLEX Systemic

VA CLASSIFICATION (Primary): BL150
Commonly used brand name(s): *Autoplex T; FEIBA VH*.
Another commonly used name is activated prothrombin complex concentrate (APCC).
Note: For a listing of dosage forms and brand names by country availability, see *Dosage Forms* section(s).

## Category
Antihemorrhagic.

## Indications

### General considerations
The anti-inhibitor coagulant complex (AICC) concentrates and the factor IX complex concentrates (prothrombin complex concentrates [PCCs]) are used in the treatment of hemorrhagic disorders associated with inhibitors (alloantibodies or autoantibodies) to specific coagulation factors. The use of AICC and PCCs is also referred to as bypass therapy, as the products are thought to bypass the need for factors VIII or IX for clot formation. The AICC concentrates are essentially PCCs that have undergone an *in vitro* activation during manufacturing, resulting in an increased content of activated and precursor vitamin K–dependent clotting factors.

In general, AICC or PCC concentrates are used in patients with high factor VIII inhibitor titers ( 10 Bethesda units [BU]) and who are classified as high responders (individuals in whom administration of factor VIII results in a marked increase in the inhibitor level). Single doses of either agent are effective in treating bleeding episodes in these patients in about 50% of the cases. Double-blind studies comparing activated PCCs to their nonactivated counterparts have shown activated PCCs to be not significantly different to only marginally more effective than nonactivated PCCs. For more information on the treatment of patients with factor inhibitors, see the *Hemophilia* monograph.

### Accepted
Hemorrhagic complications in hemophilic patients with factor VIII or factor IX inhibitors (prophylaxis and treatment)—AICC is indicated for use in hemophilic patients with inhibitors who are bleeding or are to undergo surgery.

Hemorrhagic complications in non-hemophilic patients with acquired inhibitors (prophylaxis and treatment)—AICC has been used in a few non-hemophilic patients with acquired inhibitors to factors VIII, XI, and XII.

### Unaccepted
AICC is not to be used for the treatment of bleeding episodes in patients with coagulation factor deficiencies who do not have inhibitors.

## Pharmacology/Pharmacokinetics

### Physicochemical characteristics
Source—Anti-inhibitor coagulant complex (AICC) is a sterile, dried concentrate prepared from pooled human Source Plasma and/or Plasma. The product is heat-treated as a method of viral inactivation. *Autoplex T* is dry-heated for 144 hours at 60 °C (140 °F), while *FEIBA VH* undergoes vapor-heating for 10 hours at 60 °C (140 °F) with an excess pressure of 190 ± 20 millibars, followed by 1 hour at 80 °C (176 °F) with an excess pressure of 370 ± 30 millibars.

Composition—AICC contains variable amounts of activated and precursor vitamin K–dependent clotting factors (factors II, VII, IX, and X). Traces of factors of the kinin generating system are also present. In addition, there are variable amounts of factor VIII coagulant antigen (FVIIIC:Ag), which may result in an anamnestic response to the product. AICC is standardized by its ability to correct the clotting time of factor VIII–deficient plasma or factor VIII inhibitor plasma.

### Mechanism of action/Effect
The exact mechanism of action of AICC is unknown, although it may be related to one or more of the active clotting factors and their ability to bypass the factor VIII inhibitor. *In vitro* experiments suggest the possibility of a factor Xa–like substance; or a complex of FVIIIC: Ag, factor IXa, and phospholipid as the active principle, which is only minimally inhibited by an inhibitor.

## Precautions to Consider

### Pregnancy/Reproduction
Pregnancy—Studies have not been done in humans.
Studies have not been done in animals.
FDA Pregnancy Category C.

### Breast-feeding
It is not known whether the proteins present in coagulation factor concentrates are distributed into breast milk. However, distribution into breast milk would be highly unlikely because of the large size of the protein molecules.

### Pediatrics
Studies performed in which patients as young as 3 years of age were included have not demonstrated pediatrics-specific problems that would limit the usefulness of anti-inhibitor coagulant complex (AICC) in children. However, premature infants and neonates may be at increased risk for developing thrombotic complications, and may experience higher morbidity and mortality associated with hepatitis acquired from contaminated concentrates.

### Geriatrics
Appropriate studies on the relationship of age to the effects of AICC have not been performed in the geriatric population. However, geriatrics-specific problems that would limit the usefulness of this medication in the elderly are not expected.

### Dental
AICC has been used successfully in patients with inhibitors who have had bleeding in the oral cavity (both surgical and nonsurgical in origin). Antifibrinolytic agents, such as aminocaproic acid and tranexamic acid, are used commonly in conjunction with clotting factor replacement to control excessive bleeding in hemophilic patients undergoing tooth extractions or experiencing other oral bleeding. However, care should be taken, as systemic use of antifibrinolytic agents may potentiate the thrombogenic effects of the concentrate. Using the antifibrinolytic agent as an oral rinse, or delaying its use for 8 to 12 hours after administration of AICC, may minimize this complication.

### Surgical
AICC has been used successfully for the control of hemostasis in patients with inhibitors who are undergoing surgical procedures. However, it should be used cautiously, as the risk of thrombotic complications is increased in surgical patients who receive large, repeated doses of factor IX complex or who have significant hepatic dysfunction.

### Drug interactions and/or related problems
The following drug interactions and/or related problems have been selected on the basis of their potential clinical significance (possible mechanism in parentheses where appropriate)—not necessarily inclusive (» = major clinical significance):

Note: Combinations containing any of the following medications, depending on the amount present, may also interact with this medication.

Aminocaproic acid or
Tranexamic acid
(although these antifibrinolytic agents are used commonly in conjunction with clotting factor replacement to control excessive bleeding in hemophilic patients undergoing tooth extractions or experiencing other oral bleeding, systemic use of antifibrinolytic agents may potentiate the thrombogenic effects of the concentrate; using the antifibrinolytic agent as an oral rinse, or delaying its use for 8 to 12 hours after administration of AICC, may minimize this complication)

### Medical considerations/Contraindications
The medical considerations/contraindications included have been selected on the basis of their potential clinical significance (reasons given in parentheses where appropriate)—not necessarily inclusive (» = major clinical significance).

*Except under special circumstances, this medication should not be used when the following medical problems exist:*
» Disseminated intravascular coagulation (DIC) or
» Hyperfibrinolytic states or
» Thromboembolism, history of
(risk of thrombotic complications)

**Risk-benefit should be considered when the following medical problems exist:**
- Crush injuries or
- Hepatic function impairment, severe or
- Surgery
  (risk of thrombotic complications)
- Sensitivity to anti-inhibitor coagulant complex

**Patient monitoring**

The following may be especially important in patient monitoring (other tests may be warranted in some patients, depending on condition; » = major clinical significance):

Note: Laboratory tests to monitor the effectiveness of factor replacement, such as the activated partial thromboplastin time (APTT), do not correlate with clinical improvement; therefore, response should be based on the patient's condition. Attempts to normalize laboratory values by increasing the dose of anti-inhibitor coagulant complex may result in DIC.

Coagulation tests, such as
- Activated partial thromboplastin time (APTT)
- D-dimer
- Fibrin/fibrinogen degradation products (FDPs)
- Fibrinogen concentration
- Prothrombin time (PT)
- Thrombin time (TT) and
- Platelet count
  (used to confirm the presence of DIC following the occurrence of clinical signs of intravascular coagulation; severe DIC is indicated by absolute decreases in fibrinogen and platelet count, the presence of FDPs, an increased D-dimer, and significantly prolonged APTT, PT, and TT)

» Observation for signs and symptoms of allergic reactions

» Symptoms of thrombotic complications, such as chest pain, cough, and respiratory distress and

» Vital signs, such as blood pressure, pulse, and respiratory rate
  (changes in blood pressure, pulse rate, and respiration, along with chest pain and cough, may be indicative of intravascular coagulation; also, hypotension may occur following infusion)

## Side/Adverse Effects

Note: Anti-inhibitor coagulant complex (AICC) is prepared from pooled human plasma, which may contain the causative agents of *hepatitis*, *human immunodeficiency virus (HIV) infection*, and other *viral diseases*. Improved donor screening and treatment of concentrates with viral inactivation procedures have greatly reduced the risk of transmission of HIV infection or hepatitis. However, the risk of virus transmission cannot be totally eliminated and, therefore, some patients may develop these viral infections.

*Anamnestic responses* with a rise in factor VIII inhibitor titers have been observed in up to 20% of cases following treatment with AICC. These responses are more likely to occur in patients who have a low inhibitor titer at the time of treatment and have a marked increase in inhibitor level following factor VIII exposure, and in those patients treated with AICC over several days.

The following side/adverse effects have been selected on the basis of their potential clinical significance (possible signs and symptoms in parentheses where appropriate)—not necessarily inclusive:

**Those indicating need for medical attention**

Incidence more frequent

*Disseminated intravascular coagulation (DIC)* (cyanosis [bluish coloring], especially of the hands and feet; ecchymoses at injection sites [large, nonelevated blue or purplish patches in the skin]; persistent bleeding or oozing from puncture sites or mucous membranes [bowel, mouth, nose, or urinary bladder]); *myocardial infarction* (anxiety; cold sweating; dizziness, lightheadedness, or fainting; increased heart rate; nausea or vomiting; severe pain or pressure in the chest and/or the jaw, neck, back, or arms; shortness of breath); *thrombosis or thromboembolism* (pain in chest, groin, or legs [especially calves]; rapid breathing; severe, sudden headache; sudden and unexplained shortness of breath; slurred speech, vision changes, and/or weakness or numbness in arm or legs; sudden loss of coordination)—depending on site of thrombus formation or embolization

Note: The risk of *thrombotic complications*, *DIC*, and *myocardial infarction* is increased with the use of large, repetitive doses, especially following orthopedic surgical procedures, crush injuries, or for large, intramuscular hemorrhages. Significant hepatic function impairment also increases the risk.

Incidence less frequent

*Allergic reaction* (changes in facial skin color; chills; fast or irregular breathing; fever; puffiness or swelling of the eyelids or around the eyes; shortness of breath, troubled breathing, tightness in chest, and/or wheezing; skin rash, hives, and/or itching)—may include anaphylactic shock with sudden, severe decrease in blood pressure and collapse; *hypotension* (feeling faint; lightheadedness)—occurs with too rapid an injection rate; also, with *Autoplex T*, may occur if the infusion is done later than 1 hour following reconstitution; *injection reaction* (changes in blood pressure or pulse rate; flushing [redness of face]; headache)—occurs with too rapid an injection rate

## General Dosing Information

Before initiating treatment with anti-inhibitor coagulant complex (AICC), it is essential to demonstrate the presence of circulating inhibitors to one or more coagulation factors.

AICC is administered by intravenous injection through a syringe, or as an intravenous drip infusion.

**For treatment of adverse effects**

Recommended treatment consists of the following:
- Hypotension and injection reactions (particularly, headache)—Stop the infusion to allow the symptoms to disappear; the infusion may be resumed at a slower rate in all but the most reactive individuals.
- Allergic reactions—The administration of AICC should be discontinued and the patient should be treated as appropriate with antihistamines and corticosteroids.

## Parenteral Dosage Forms

### ANTI-INHIBITOR COAGULANT COMPLEX

Note: A unit of *FEIBA VH* is expressed as factor VIII inhibitor bypassing activity and *is not* equivalent to a unit of *Autoplex T*, which is expressed as factor VIII correctional units. However, the recommended dose is the same, regardless of the product used.

*Autoplex T should be infused initially at a rate of 2 mL per minute. If this infusion rate is well tolerated, the rate may be gradually increased to 10 mL per minute. For FEIBA VH, the maximum infusion rate must not exceed 2 units per kilogram of body weight (units/kg) per minute. For a patient weighing 75 kg, this corresponds to an infusion rate of 2.5 to 7.5 mL per minute, depending on the number of units per vial.*

**Usual adult and adolescent dose**

Prevention and control of bleeding in patients with inhibitors to one or more coagulation factors—
Intravenous, 75 units per kg of body weight. A single dose may be sufficient, but additional doses, six or twelve hours apart, may be given depending on the patient's clinical response.

**Usual adult and adolescent prescribing limits**

Single doses greater than 100 units per kg, and daily doses greater than 200 units per kg are not recommended. Higher doses and/or prolonged administration increase the risk of the development of thrombotic complications.

**Usual pediatric dose**

See *Usual adult and adolescent dose*.

**Usual pediatric prescribing limits**

See *Usual adult and adolescent prescribing limits*.

**Strength(s) usually available**

U.S.—
Each bottle is labeled with the number of units it contains, with sterile water for injection provided as diluent (Rx) [*Autoplex T* (heparin ≤ 2 USP units per mL; sodium 177 ± 15 mEq per liter); *FEIBA VH* (sodium 183 mEq per liter)].

Canada—
Each bottle is labeled with the number of units it contains, with sterile water for injection provided as diluent (Rx) [*FEIBA VH* (sodium 183 mEq per liter)].

**Packaging and storage**

Store the dried concentrates between 2 and 8 °C (36 and 46 °F). The solution should not be refrigerated after reconstitution. The diluent should be protected from freezing.

**Preparation of dosage form**
The diluent and dry concentrate should be brought to room temperature prior to reconstitution. The solution should be gently swirled, not shaken, until all of the concentrate is dissolved. The reconstituted solution should be approximately at room temperature at the time of administration.

Note: Some clinicians recommend adding heparin to the reconstituted concentrate (5 to 10 USP units per mL) as a way to prevent thrombotic complications when anti-inhibitor coagulant complex is used in high, repeated doses.

**Stability**
Administration should begin as soon as practical following reconstitution; however, it must be completed within 1 hour for *Autoplex T*, and within 3 hours for *FEIBA VH*.

## Selected Bibliography
Lusher JM. Use of prothrombin complex concentrates in management of bleeding in hemophiliacs with inhibitors—benefits and limitations. Semin Hematol 1994; 2 Suppl 4: 49-52.

Roberts HR. Hemophiliacs with inhibitors: therapeutic options [editorial]. N Engl J Med 1981; 305: 757-8.

Developed: 03/24/98

# ANTIMYASTHENICS Systemic

This monograph includes information on the following: 1) Ambenonium†; 2) Neostigmine; 3) Pyridostigmine.

VA CLASSIFICATION (Primary): AU300

Commonly used brand name(s): *Mestinon*[3]; *Mestinon Timespans*[3]; *Mestinon-SR*[3]; *Mytelase Caplets*[1]; *Prostigmin*[2]; *Regonol*[3].

Note: For a listing of dosage forms and brand names by country availability, see *Dosage Forms* section(s).

†Not commercially available in Canada.

## Category

Note: Cholinergic (cholinesterase inhibitor) is the basic category; the other categories are specific categories of use.

Cholinergic (cholinesterase inhibitor)—Ambenonium; Neostigmine; Pyridostigmine;

Antimyasthenic—Ambenonium; Neostigmine; Pyridostigmine;

Antidote (to nondepolarizing neuromuscular block)—Neostigmine (parenteral only); Pyridostigmine (parenteral only);

Diagnostic aid (myasthenia gravis)—Neostigmine (parenteral only).

## Indications

Note: Bracketed information in the *Indications* section refers to uses that are not included in U.S. product labeling.

**Accepted**

Myasthenia gravis (treatment)—Ambenonium, neostigmine, and pyridostigmine are indicated in the treatment of myasthenia gravis. Ambenonium is used less commonly than neostigmine or pyridostigmine but may be preferred in patients hypersensitive to the bromide ion. Oral neostigmine or pyridostigmine is most useful in prolonged therapy where no difficulty in swallowing is present. In acute myasthenic crisis where difficulty in breathing and swallowing is present, the parenteral dosage form should be used and the patient transferred to the oral dosage form as soon as tolerated.

In the treatment of myasthenia gravis, other treatment (such as respiratory therapy and control of secondary infection) must be administered concurrently with the antimyasthenic.

Ileus, gastrointestinal, postoperative (prophylaxis and treatment); or

Urinary retention, postoperative (prophylaxis and treatment)—Parenteral neostigmine is indicated in the treatment of postoperative nonobstructive urinary retention. Although it is not commonly used, parenteral neostigmine may also be indicated for the prevention and treatment of postoperative gastrointestinal ileus and prevention of postoperative urinary retention.

Neuromuscular blockade, nondepolarizing (treatment)—Parenteral neostigmine and pyridostigmine are indicated as antidotes to tubocurarine and other nondepolarizing neuromuscular blocking agents.

[Myasthenia gravis (diagnosis)][1]—Parenteral neostigmine has been used as a diagnostic test for myasthenia gravis. Although edrophonium is usually considered the agent of first choice because of its rapid onset and brief duration of action, neostigmine is sometimes used to confirm the edrophonium response.

**Unaccepted**

Although parenteral neostigmine has been used as a screening test for pregnancy and in the treatment of delayed menstruation, these uses of neostigmine are obsolete.

[1]Not included in Canadian product labeling.

## Pharmacology/Pharmacokinetics
See *Table 1*, page 442.

**Physicochemical characteristics**
Molecular weight—
 Neostigmine bromide: 303.20.
 Neostigmine methylsulfate: 334.39.
 Pyridostigmine bromide: 261.12.
Other characteristics—
 Neostigmine methylsulfate injection: pH approximately 5.9.
 Pyridostigmine bromide injection: pH approximately 5.0.

**Mechanism of action/Effect**
Cholinergic (cholinesterase inhibitor)—
 Antimyasthenics inhibit destruction of acetylcholine by acetylcholinesterase, thereby facilitating transmission of impulses across the myoneural junction. Cholinergic responses produced are miosis, bradycardia, increased tonus of intestinal and skeletal muscle, constriction of bronchi and ureters, and stimulation of secretion by salivary and sweat glands. In addition, these medications have a direct cholinomimetic effect on skeletal muscle. Neostigmine may also act on autonomic ganglion cells and neurons of the central nervous system (CNS).

Neostigmine prevents or relieves postoperative distention by stimulating gastric motility and increasing gastric tone, which probably represents a combination of actions at the ganglion cells of Auerbach's plexus and at the muscle fibers as a result of the preservation of acetylcholine released by the cholinergic preganglionic and postganglionic fibers, respectively.

Neostigmine prevents or relieves urinary retention by increasing the tone of the detrusor muscle of the urinary bladder to produce contractions strong enough to initiate micturition.

Antimyasthenic—
 Muscle strength and response to repetitive nerve stimulation is increased as a result of these medications enhancing the peak effect and prolonging the duration of action of acetylcholine at the motor end plate.

Antidote (to nondepolarizing neuromuscular block)—
 Since nondepolarizing neuromuscular blocking agents combine reversibly with the receptors, preventing access of acetylcholine, antagonism can be overcome by increasing the amount of agonist at the receptors; therefore, muscle paralysis induced by nondepolarizing neuromuscular blocking agents is reversed by neostigmine or pyridostigmine, which increases concentration of acetylcholine at the receptors.

Diagnostic aid (myasthenia gravis)—
 By prolonging the duration of action of acetylcholine at the motor end plate, neostigmine increases muscle strength in patients with myasthenia gravis, whereas patients with other disorders develop either no increase in muscle strength or even a slight weakness and possibly fasciculations.

**Absorption**
Oral—Poorly absorbed from the gastrointestinal tract.
Parenteral—Intramuscular: Neostigmine is rapidly absorbed.

## Precautions to Consider

**Cross-sensitivity and/or related problems**
Patients sensitive to bromides may be sensitive to neostigmine (oral) or pyridostigmine also.

## Pregnancy/Reproduction

Pregnancy—Problems with cholinesterase inhibitors in the human fetus have not been documented; however, transient muscular weakness has occurred in about 20% of infants born to mothers who received these medications during pregnancy.

For neostigmine: Studies with neostigmine have not been done in either animals or humans.

FDA Pregnancy Category C.

Labor and delivery—Anticholinesterase agents may cause uterine irritability and induce premature labor when given intravenously to pregnant women near term.

## Breast-feeding

Pyridostigmine is distributed into breast milk in concentrations of 36 to 113% of maternal plasma concentrations. It is not known whether ambenonium and neostigmine are distributed into breast milk. However, problems in humans have not been documented.

## Pediatrics

Appropriate studies on the relationship of age to the effects of cholinesterase inhibitors have not been performed in the pediatric population. However, no pediatrics-specific problems have been documented to date.

## Geriatrics

Extensive studies with cholinesterase inhibitors have not been performed in the geriatric population. However, in one study in which 14 out of 32 adult patients were over 60 years of age, the duration of antagonism of neuromuscular blockade by neostigmine and pyridostigmine in the elderly group was prolonged compared to younger patients.

## Drug interactions and/or related problems

The following drug interactions and/or related problems have been selected on the basis of their potential clinical significance (possible mechanism in parentheses where appropriate)—not necessarily inclusive (» = major clinical significance):

Note: Combinations containing any of the following medications, depending on the amount present, may also interact with this medication.

Aminoglycosides, systemic or
Anesthetics, hydrocarbon inhalation, such as:
   Chloroform
   Cyclopropane
   Enflurane
   Halothane
   Methoxyflurane
   Trichloroethylene or
Anesthetics, parenteral-local, large doses or
Capreomycin or
Lidocaine, intravenous or
Lincomycins or
Polymyxins, such as colistimethate, colistin, and polymyxin B or
Quinine
   (neuromuscular blocking action of these medications may antagonize the effect of antimyasthenics on skeletal muscle; temporary dosage adjustments of antimyasthenics may be necessary to control symptoms of myasthenia gravis during and following concurrent use)
   (antimyasthenics, especially in large doses, may decrease the neuromuscular blocking activity of these medications)

Anesthetics, local, ester-derivative
   (antimyasthenic agent–induced inhibition of plasma cholinesterase activity reduces the metabolism of these anesthetics, leading to increased risk of toxicity; it is recommended that local anesthetics that are not ester derivatives be used instead)

Anticholinergic agents, especially atropine and related compounds
   (atropine may be used to reduce or prevent the muscarinic effects of antimyasthenics; however, routine concurrent use is not recommended since the muscarinic effects may be the first signs of overdose and masking them with atropine may prevent early recognition of cholinergic crisis)
   (concurrent use of anticholinergics with antimyasthenics may further reduce intestinal motility; therefore, caution is recommended)

» Cholinesterase inhibitors, other, including demecarium, echothiophate, and isoflurophate, and possibly topical malathion
   (concurrent use of other cholinesterase inhibitors with antimyasthenics is not recommended except under strict medical supervision because of the possibility of additive toxicity; caution may also be warranted with topical application of malathion if excessive quantities are used)

Edrophonium
   (caution is recommended in administering edrophonium to patients with symptoms of myasthenic weakness who are also receiving antimyasthenics, since symptoms of cholinergic crisis [overdosage] may be similar to those occurring with myasthenic crisis [underdosage] and the patient's condition may be worsened by use of edrophonium)

» Guanadrel or
» Guanethidine or
» Mecamylamine or
» Trimethaphan
   (these ganglionic-blocking medications may antagonize the effects of antimyasthenics when used concurrently, leading to increased muscle weakness, respiratory weakness, and/or difficulty in swallowing; the possibility should be considered that the antihypertensive effects of the ganglionic-blocking medication may also be decreased during concurrent use)

Neuromuscular blocking agents
   (phase I block of depolarizing neuromuscular blocking agents such as succinylcholine may be prolonged when used concurrently with neostigmine or pyridostigmine; however, if a depolarizing neuromuscular blocking agent has been used over a prolonged period of time and the depolarization block has changed to a nondepolarization block, neostigmine or pyridostigmine may reverse the nondepolarization block)
   (effects of nondepolarizing neuromuscular blocking agents are antagonized by parenteral neostigmine or pyridostigmine; this interaction may be used to therapeutic advantage to reverse muscle relaxation following surgery)
   (neuromuscular blockade antagonizes the effect of antimyasthenics on skeletal muscle; temporary dosage adjustments of antimyasthenics may be required to control symptoms of myasthenia gravis following use of a neuromuscular blocking agent)

» Procainamide or
Quinidine
   (neuromuscular blocking activity and/or secondary anticholinergic effects of these medications may antagonize the action of antimyasthenics; caution is recommended during concurrent use in patients with myasthenia gravis)

## Medical considerations/Contraindications

The medical considerations/contraindications included have been selected on the basis of their potential clinical significance (reasons given in parentheses where appropriate)—not necessarily inclusive (» = major clinical significance):

***Risk-benefit should be considered when the following medical problems exist:***

Asthma, bronchial
   (increase in bronchial secretions and other respiratory effects of antimyasthenics may aggravate condition)

Atelectasis, postoperative, or
Pneumonia
   (may be exacerbated)

Cardiac dysrhythmias, especially bradycardia and atrioventricular (AV) block
   (increased risk of cardiac arrhythmias)

» Intestinal or urinary tract obstruction, mechanical
   (may be exacerbated)

Sensitivity to any of these medications or to bromides

» Urinary tract infections
   (increase in urinary bladder muscle tone may aggravate symptoms)

» Caution is also recommended in the postsurgical patient because antimyasthenics may exacerbate respiratory problems caused by postoperative pain, sedation, retained secretions, or atelectasis. In the myasthenic patient, if a postoperative respiratory problem cannot be attributed to myasthenia gravis alone, mechanical ventilation is recommended.

## Side/Adverse Effects

Note: Most common adverse reactions to cholinesterase inhibitors are caused by excessive cholinergic stimulation. These include both muscarinic and nicotinic effects.

Ambenonium produces fewer muscarinic side/adverse effects than neostigmine but more than pyridostigmine.

Neostigmine produces more severe muscarinic side effects than ambenonium or pyridostigmine.

Pyridostigmine may produce a significantly lower degree and incidence of bradycardia, salivation, and gastrointestinal stimulation than neostigmine.

The following side/adverse effects have been selected on the basis of their potential clinical significance (possible signs and symptoms in parentheses where appropriate)—not necessarily inclusive:

**Those indicating need for medical attention**
Incidence rare
*Sensitivity to bromide ion of neostigmine or pyridostigmine* (skin rash); *thrombophlebitis* ( redness, swelling, or pain at injection site)— for pyridostigmine injection only

**Those indicating need for medical attention only if they continue or are bothersome**
Incidence more frequent
*Muscarinic effects* (diarrhea; increased sweating; increased watering of mouth; nausea or vomiting; stomach cramps or pain)

Incidence less frequent
*Muscarinic effects* (frequent urge to urinate; increase in bronchial secretions; unusually small pupils; unusual watering of eyes)

# Overdose

For specific information on the agents used in the management of antimyasthenics overdose, see: Atropine in *Anticholinergics/Antispasmodics (Systemic)* monograph.

For more information on the management of overdose or unintentional ingestion, **contact a Poison Control Center** (see *Poison Control Center Listing*).

**Clinical effects of overdose**
The following effects have been selected on the basis of their potential clinical signifiance (possible signs and symptoms in parentheses where appropriate)—not necessarily inclusive:

Acute and chronic
*CNS effects* (clumsiness or unsteadiness; confusion; difficulty in breathing; seizures; slurred speech; unusual irritability, nervousness, restlessness, or fear); *muscarinic effects* (blurred vision; severe diarrhea; excessive increase in bronchial secretions or salivation; severe vomiting; shortness of breath; troubled breathing; wheezing, or tightness in chest; slow heartbeat; severe stomach cramps or pain; unusual tiredness or weakness); *nicotinic effects* (increasing muscle weakness or paralysis, especially in the arms, neck, shoulders, and tongue; muscle cramps or twitching)

Note: *Breathing problems* may also be caused by atelectasis.

*Unusual tiredness or weakness* may also be caused by hypokalemia resulting from severe diarrhea and vomiting.

In the myasthenic patient, *increased muscle weakness* may be caused by underdosage or resistance instead of by overdosage.

Note: Overdosage may induce cholinergic crisis, which is characterized by nicotinic effects in addition to intensified muscarinic effects.

In patients with myasthenia gravis or in the postoperative patient, cholinergic crisis may be difficult to distinguish from myasthenic crisis on a symptomatic basis because the principal symptom common to both is generalized muscle weakness. The time of onset of weakness may help determine whether the crisis is caused by overdosage or underdosage (or resistance). Weakness beginning about 1 hour after administration of antimyasthenic is probably overdosage while that occurring 3 or more hours after administration is probably underdosage or resistance.

If a differential diagnosis cannot be made on the basis of signs and symptoms, edrophonium may be used to distinguish cholinergic crisis from myasthenic crisis; however, caution is recommended because edrophonium will cause increased oropharyngeal secretions and further weakness in muscles of respiration in a cholinergic crisis. This may be especially critical in the postoperative patient.

**Treatment of overdose**
Recommended treatment for cholinergic crisis—
Prompt discontinuation of antimyasthenic.
Specific treatment—Use of intavenous atropine sulfate to counteract muscarinic effects.
Supportive care—May include establishment of endotracheal tube, if necessary.

# Patient Consultation

As an aid to patient consultation, refer to *Advice for the Patient, Antimyasthenics (Systemic).*

In providing consultation, consider emphasizing the following selected information (»= major clinical significance):

**Before using this medication**
» Conditions affecting use, especially:
Sensitivity to antimyasthenics or to bromides
Pregnancy—Possible transient muscle weakness in newborns whose mothers received antimyasthenics during pregnancy
Use in the elderly—In one study in a limited number of patients, duration of antagonism of neuromuscular blockade by neostigmine and pyridostigmine was prolonged
Other medications, especially other cholinesterase inhibitors, guanadrel, guanethidine, mecamylamine, procainamide, or trimethaphan
Other medical problems, especially intestinal or urinary tract blockage or, urinary tract infection

**Proper use of this medication**
Taking with food or milk to decrease possibility of side effects
» Importance of not taking more medication than the amount prescribed
For use in myasthenia gravis: Keeping daily record of dosing and effects on condition during initial therapy
Missed dose: Taking as soon as possible; not taking if almost time for next dose; not doubling doses
» Proper dosing
» Proper storage

**Side/adverse effects**
Signs of potential side effects, especially thrombophlebitis at injection site (for pyridostigmine only), and sensitivity

# General Dosing Information

In myasthenia gravis, the dosage must be individualized according to the severity of the disease and the response of the patient.

To assist the physician in arranging an optimum therapeutic regimen in the treatment of myasthenia gravis, patients should keep a daily record of their condition.

Therapy in myasthenia gravis is frequently required day and night. Larger portions of the total daily dose may be taken at times of greater fatigue such as in the afternoons or at mealtimes.

Following prolonged therapy, myasthenic patients may become refractory to these medications. Responsiveness may be restored, especially when the resistance may have been caused by overdosage, by reducing the dosage or discontinuing the medication for a few days.

**For parenteral dosage forms only**
Patients should be closely observed for cholinergic reactions, especially when neostigmine or pyridostigmine is administered intravenously.

Atropine injection and antishock medication should always be readily available because of the possibility of hypersensitivity reactions.

When large doses of parenteral neostigmine or pyridostigmine are administered, as during reversal of muscle relaxants, prior or concurrent administration of atropine injection is recommended to counteract the muscarinic side effects.

**Diet/Nutrition**
Administration of oral forms of these medications with food or milk may decrease the muscarinic side effects by slowing down absorption of the medication and reducing serum peaks.

---

## *AMBENONIUM*

# Summary of Differences

Pharmacology/pharmacokinetics:
Has longer duration of action than neostigmine or pyridostigmine.
Side/adverse effects:
Produces fewer muscarinic side effects than neostigmine, but more than pyridostigmine.

# Oral Dosage Forms

## AMBENONIUM CHLORIDE TABLETS

**Usual adult and adolescent dose**
Antimyasthenic—
Oral, initially 5 mg three or four times a day, the dosage being adjusted as required at intervals of one to two days to avoid accumulation of medication and overdosage.

Note: When doses of more than 200 mg per day are administered, the patient should be closely observed for cholinergic reactions.

**Usual pediatric dose**
Antimyasthenic—
Oral, initially 300 mcg (0.3 mg) per kg of body weight or 10 mg per square meter of body surface per day (divided into three or four

440    Antimyasthenics (Systemic)

doses), the dosage being increased, if necessary, to 1.5 mg per kg of body weight or 50 mg per square meter of body surface per day (divided into three or four doses).

**Usual geriatric dose**
See *Usual adult and adolescent dose*.

**Strength(s) usually available**
U.S.—
  10 mg (Rx) [*Mytelase Caplets* (scored; acacia; dibasic calcium phosphate; gelatin; lactose; magnesium stearate; starch; and sucrose)].
Canada—
  Not commercially available.

**Packaging and storage**
Store below 40 °C (104 °F), preferably between 15 and 30 °C (59 and 86 °F), unless otherwise specified by manufacturer. Store in a tight container.

---

### NEOSTIGMINE

## Summary of Differences
Category: Parenteral neostigmine:
  Also indicated as an antidote (to nondepolarizing neuromuscular block) and a diagnostic aid (myasthenia gravis).
Indications: Parenteral neostigmine:
  Also indicated in the treatment of postoperative nonobstructive urinary retention.
  May also be indicated for prevention and treatment of postoperative gastrointestinal ileus and prevention of postoperative urinary retention.
Pharmacology/pharmacokinetics:
  Has shorter duration of action than ambenonium.
Precautions: Cross-sensitivity and/or related problems:
  Oral neostigmine contains bromide ion to which some patients may be sensitive.
Side/adverse effects:
  Produces more severe muscarinic side effects than ambenonium or pyridostigmine.

## Additional Dosing Information
See also *General Dosing Information*.
Generally, 15 mg of neostigmine bromide administered orally is equivalent to 500 mcg (0.5 mg) of neostigmine methylsulfate administered parenterally.

*For oral dosage forms only*
• Neostigmine is poorly absorbed from the gastrointestinal tract following oral administration; therefore, much larger doses are required for oral than for parenteral use.
• Large oral doses should be avoided in conditions where there may be an increased absorption rate from the intestinal tract, in order to avoid possible toxicity.

*For parenteral dosage forms only: When used as an antidote to nondepolarizing neuromuscular block*
• It is recommended that the exact dose required be titrated, using a peripheral nerve stimulator device.
• Unless tachycardia is present, atropine (0.6 to 1 mg) should be administered concomitantly or several minutes before neostigmine to prevent bradycardia.
• In the presence of bradycardia, the pulse rate should be increased to about 80 per minute with atropine prior to administration of neostigmine.

*When used as a diagnostic aid (myasthenia gravis)*
• Significant improvement of muscle weakness occurring within several minutes to 1 hour following administration of neostigmine usually indicates myasthenia gravis. However, diagnosis also should include clinical and electromyographic (EMG) evaluation.

## Oral Dosage Forms
### NEOSTIGMINE BROMIDE TABLETS USP
**Usual adult and adolescent dose**
Antimyasthenic—
  Initial—Oral, 15 mg every three to four hours, the dose and frequency of administration being adjusted as necessary.
  Maintenance—Oral, 150 mg administered over a twenty-four-hour period, the intervals between doses being determined by response of the patient.
  Note: The twenty-four-hour maintenance dose is highly variable among individuals.

**Usual pediatric dose**
Antimyasthenic—
  Oral, 2 mg per kg of body weight or 60 mg per square meter of body surface per day, divided into six to eight doses.

**Usual geriatric dose**
See *Usual adult and adolescent dose*.

**Strength(s) usually available**
U.S.—
  15 mg (Rx) [*Prostigmin* (scored; lactose); GENERIC].
Canada—
  15 mg (Rx) [*Prostigmin* (scored; lactose)].

**Packaging and storage**
Store below 40 °C (104 °F), preferably between 15 and 30 °C (59 and 86 °F), unless otherwise specified by manufacturer. Store in a tight container.

## Parenteral Dosage Forms
Note: Bracketed uses in the Dosage Forms section refer to categories of use and/or indications that are not included in U.S. product labeling.

### NEOSTIGMINE METHYLSULFATE INJECTION USP
**Usual adult and adolescent dose**
Antimyasthenic—
  Intramuscular or subcutaneous, 500 mcg (0.5); subsequent doses should be based on the patient's response.
Antidote (to nondepolarizing neuromuscular block)—
  Intravenous, 500 mcg (0.5) to 2 mg administered slowly, repeated as required up to a total dose of 5 mg.
  Note: Subsequent doses may be less than 500 mcg (0.5mg).
    When neostigmine is administered intravenously, it is recommended that 600 mcg (0.6) to 1.2 mg of atropine sulfate be administered intravenously prior to or concurrently with neostigmine to counteract its muscarinic side effects.
Diagnostic aid (myasthenia gravis)[1]—
  Intramuscular or subcutaneous, 1.5 mg administered simultaneously with 600 mcg (0.6 mg) of atropine
  Note: Significant improvement of muscle weakness occurring within several minutes to one hour indicates myasthenia gravis.
Prevention of postoperative distention or urinary retention—
  Intramuscular or subcutaneous, 250 mcg (0.25 mg) immediately following surgery, repeated every four to six hours for two or three days.
Treatment of postoperative distention—
  Intramuscular or subcutaneous, 500 mcg (0.5 mg) as needed.
Treatment of urinary retention—
  Intramuscular or subcutaneous, 500 mcg (0.5 mg); dose repeated every three hours for at least five doses after patient has voided or the bladder has been emptied.
  Note: If urination does not occur within one hour following the initial 500-mcg (0.5-mg) dose, the patient should be catheterized.

**Usual pediatric dose**
Antimyasthenic—
  Intramuscular or subcutaneous, 10 to 40 mcg (0.01 to 0.04 mg) per kg of body weight every two to three hours.
  Note: A dose of 10 mcg (0.01 mg) of atropine per kg of body weight may be administered intramuscularly or subcutaneously with each dose or with alternate doses of neostigmine to counteract the muscarinic side effects.
Antidote (to nondepolarizing neuromuscular block)—
  Intravenous, 40 mcg (0.04 mg) per kg of body weight administered with 20 mcg (0.02 mg) of atropine per kg of body weight.
[Diagnostic aid (myasthenia gravis)][1]—
  Intramuscular, 40 mcg (0.04 mg) per kg of body weight or 1 mg per square meter of body surface per dose.
  Intravenous, 20 mcg (0.02 mg) per kg of body weight or 500 mcg (0.5 mg) per square meter of body surface.

**Usual geriatric dose**
See *Usual adult and adolescent dose*.

**Strength(s) usually available**
U.S.—
  0.25 mg per mL (1:4000) (Rx) [*Prostigmin* (parabens 0.2% [methyl and propyl]; sodium hydroxide); GENERIC].
  0.5 mg per mL (1:2000) (Rx) [*Prostigmin* (parabens 0.2% [methyl and propyl]; sodium hydroxide—in 1-ml ampuls; phenol 0.45%; sodium acetate 0.02%; acetic acid; sodium hydroxide—in 10-mL vials); GENERIC].

1 mg per mL (1:1000) (Rx) [*Prostigmin* (phenol 0.45%; sodium acetate 0.02%; acetic acid; sodium hydroxide); GENERIC].

Canada—
0.5 mg per mL (1:2000) (Rx) [*Prostigmin* (methylparaben 1.8 mg; propylparaben 0.2 mg; sodium <0.01 mmol/mL—in 1–mL ampuls; phenol 0.45% ; sodium acetate; acetic acid; sodium <0.01 mmol/mL—in 10-mL vials)].

1 mg per mL (1:1000) (Rx) [*Prostigmin* (phenol 0.45%; sodium acetate; acetic acid ; sodium hydroxide; sodium <0.01 mmol/mL))].

2.5 mg per mL (1:400) (Rx) [*Prostigmin* (phenol 0.4%,; sodium chloride; sodium hydroxide; sodium <0.01 mmol/mL)].

**Packaging and storage**
Store below 40 °C (104 °F), preferably between 15 and 30 °C (59 and 86 °F), unless otherwise specified by manufacturer. Protect from freezing. Protect from light.

---

[1]Not included in Canadian product labeling.

---

## PYRIDOSTIGMINE

## Summary of Differences
Category:
  Parenteral pyridostigmine also indicated as an antidote (to nondepolarizing neuromuscular block).
Pharmacology/pharmacokinetics:
  Generally has shorter duration of action than ambenonium and a slower onset and longer duration of action than neostigmine.
Precautions:
  Cross-sensitivity and/or related problems—Contains bromide ion to which some patients may be sensitive.
Side/adverse effects:
  May produce a significantly lower degree and incidence of bradycardia, salivation, and gastrointestinal stimulation than neostigmine.

## Additional Dosing Information
See also *General Dosing Information*.
For oral dosage forms only:
- The syrup dosage form may be preferred for use in children and "brittle" myasthenic patients who require fractions of 60-mg doses. Also, the syrup is more easily swallowed, especially in the morning, by patients with bulbar involvement.
- It has been reported that the extended-release dosage form may pass intact through the gastrointestinal tract in patients with increased gastrointestinal activity or diarrhea. Use of other oral dosage forms may be required temporarily for continued control of symptoms.

## Oral Dosage Forms
### PYRIDOSTIGMINE BROMIDE SYRUP USP
**Usual adult and adolescent dose**
Antimyasthenic—
  Initial—Oral, 30 to 60 mg every three to four hours, the dosage being adjusted as required.
  Maintenance—Oral, 600 mg (range 60 mg to 1.5 grams) per day.

**Usual pediatric dose**
Antimyasthenic—
  Oral, 7 mg per kg of body weight or 200 mg per square meter of body surface per day, divided into five or six doses.

**Usual geriatric dose**
See *Usual adult and adolescent dose*.

**Strength(s) usually available**
U.S.—
  60 mg per 5 mL (Rx) [*Mestinon* (alcohol 5%; glycerin; lactic acid; sodium benzoate; sorbitol; sucrose; FD&C Red No. 40; FD&C Blue No. 1; flavors; water)].
Canada—
  Not commercially available.

**Packaging and storage**
Store below 40 °C (104 °F), preferably between 15 and 30 °C (59 and 86 °F), unless otherwise specified by manufacturer. Store in a tight, light-resistant container. Protect from freezing.

### PYRIDOSTIGMINE BROMIDE TABLETS USP
**Usual adult and adolescent dose**
See *Pyridostigmine Bromide Syrup USP*.

**Usual pediatric dose**
See *Pyridostigmine Bromide Syrup USP*.

**Usual geriatric dose**
See *Pyridostigmine Bromide Syrup USP*.

**Strength(s) usually available**
U.S.—
  60 mg (Rx) [*Mestinon* (scored; lactose; silicon dioxide; stearic acid)].
Canada—
  60 mg (Rx) [*Mestinon* (scored; lactose 272 mg)].

**Packaging and storage**
Store below 40 °C (104 °F), preferably between 15 and 30 °C (59 and 86 °F), unless otherwise specified by manufacturer. Store in a tight container.

### PYRIDOSTIGMINE BROMIDE EXTENDED-RELEASE TABLETS
**Usual adult and adolescent dose**
Antimyasthenic—
  Oral, 180 to 540 mg one or two times a day, with at least six hours between doses.
Note: For optimum control of symptoms, it may be necessary to administer the more rapidly acting regular tablet or syrup dosage form concurrently with extended-release therapy.
   Extended-release preparations may increase the risk of cholinergic crisis and, therefore, are usually not recommended.

**Usual pediatric dose**
Dosage has not been established.

**Usual geriatric dose**
See *Usual adult and adolescent dose*.

**Strength(s) usually available**
U.S.—
  180 mg (Rx) [*Mestinon Timespans* (carnauba wax; corn-derived proteins; magnesium stearate; silica gel; tribasic calcium phosphate)].
Canada—
  180 mg (Rx) [*Mestinon-SR* (scored)].

**Packaging and storage**
Store below 40 °C (104 °F), preferably between 15 and 30 °C (59 and 86 °F), in a well-closed container, unless otherwise specified by manufacturer.

**Auxiliary labeling**
- Swallow tablets whole.

## Parenteral Dosage Forms
### PYRIDOSTIGMINE BROMIDE INJECTION USP
**Usual adult and adolescent dose**
Antimyasthenic—
  Intramuscular or intravenous, 2 mg (approximately one-thirtieth of the usual oral dose ) every two to three hours.
Antidote (to nondepolarizing neuromuscular block)—
  Intravenous, 10 to 20 mg.
Note: Prior to administration of pyridostigmine, it is recommended that 600 mcg (0.6 mg) to 1.2 mg of atropine sulfate be given intravenously to counteract the muscarinic effects.

**Usual pediatric dose**
Antimyasthenic—
  Neonates of myasthenic mothers—Intramuscular, 50 to 150 mcg (0.05 to 0.15 mg) per kg of body weight every four to six hours.

**Usual geriatric dose**
See *Usual adult and adolescent dose*.

**Strength(s) usually available**
U.S.—
  5 mg per mL (Rx) [*Mestinon* (parabens 0.2% [methyl and propyl]; sodium citrate 0.02%; citric acid; sodium hydroxide); *Regonol* (benzyl alcohol 1%)].
Canada—
  5 mg per mL (Rx) [*Regonol* (parabens 0.2% [methyl and propyl]; sodium citrate 0.02%; citric acid; sodium hydroxide)].

**Packaging and storage**
Store below 40 °C (104 °F), preferably between 15 and 30 °C (59 and 86 °F), unless otherwise specified by manufacturer. Protect from light. Protect from freezing.

---

Revised: 09/30/91
Interim revision: 07/18/94

## Table 1. Pharmacology/Pharmacokinetics

| Drug | Oral Bioavailability | Volume of Distribution $V_D$ (L/kg) | Protein Binding | Biotrans-formation | Half-life Distribution (min) | Half-life Elimination (min) | Onset of Action (min) | Time to Peak Plasma Concentration (hr) | Peak Plasma Concentration (mcg/mL) | Peak Effect (min) | Duration of Action (hr) | Elimination (% excreted unchanged) | Clearance (L/hr/kg) |
|---|---|---|---|---|---|---|---|---|---|---|---|---|---|
| Ambenonium | | | | | | | 20–30 | | | | 3–8 | | |
| Neostigmine | | | Low (15–25%) | Plasma; hepatic | | | | | | | | Renal (about 50) | |
| Oral | 1–2% | 0.74±0.2 | | | 3.6±1.2 | 77.4±48 | 45–75*‡ | 1–2 | 1–5† | 30 | 3–6 | | 0.55±0.14 |
| Parenteral | | 0.37–1.08 | | | 5.4 | 24–79.2 | 20–30 | 0.5 | | | 2–4 | | 0.24–1.0 |
| Intramuscular | | | | | | | 4–8 | | | | 2–4 | | |
| Intravenous | | | | | | | | | | | | | |
| Pyridostigmine | | | Not bound | Plasma; hepatic | | | | | | | | Renal | |
| Oral | 10–20% | | | | | | | | | | | | |
| Syrup, Tablets | | | | | | | 30–45 | 1–2 | 40–60§ | 60–120 | 3–6 | | |
| Extended-release Tablets | | | | | | | 30–60 | | | | 6–12 | | |
| Parenteral | | 1.03–1.76 | | | | 63–112 | <15 | | | | 2–4 | | 0.52–1.0 |
| Intramuscular | | | | | | | | | | | | | |
| Intravenous | | | | | 7.2–8.4 | | 2–5 | | | | 2–4 | | |

*Peristaltic activity begins in 2 to 4 hours.
†Following a single 30-mg oral dose.
‡Peristaltic activity begins in 10 to 30 minutes.
§Following a single 60-mg oral dose.

# ANTIPYRINE AND BENZOCAINE Otic

INN: Antipyrine—Phenazone.
BAN: Antipyrine—Phenazone.
JAN: Benzocaine—Ethyl aminobenzoate.
VA CLASSIFICATION (Primary/Secondary): OT400/OT300
Commonly used brand name(s): *A/B Otic; Allergen; Analgesic Otic; Antiben; Auralgan; Aurodex; Auroto; Dolotic; Ear Drops; Earache Drops; Otocalm.*

Note: For a listing of dosage forms and brand names by country availability, see *Dosage Forms* section(s).

## Category
Analgesic-anesthetic (otic); cerumen removal adjunct.

## Indications
**Unaccepted**
Antipyrine and benzocaine otic combination has been used to relieve pain and inflammation in the congestive and serous stages of acute otitis media and to facilitate removal of cerumen from the wall of the ear canal. However, it is no longer recommended for these purposes, because of questionable effectiveness and because benzocaine frequently causes contact dermatitis.

## Pharmacology/Pharmacokinetics
**Physicochemical characteristics**
Chemical group—
  Antipyrine: A pyrazolone derivative.
  Benzocaine: An aminobenzoic acid (para-aminobenzoic acid; PABA) derivative.
Molecular weight—
  Antipyrine: 188.23.
  Benzocaine: 165.19.
  Glycerin: 92.09.

**Mechanism of action/Effect**
Both antipyrine and benzocaine are employed for their analgesic/local anesthetic effects. The anhydrous glycerin vehicle is hygroscopic and may provide a decongestant action.

## Precautions to Consider
**Cross-sensitivity and/or related problems**
Patients sensitive to benzocaine or other ester-derivative anesthetics may be sensitive to this medication also.

**Carcinogenicity/Mutagenicity**
Studies have not been done.

**Pregnancy/Reproduction**
Pregnancy—Studies in humans have not been done. However, problems have not been documented.
Studies in animals have not been done.
FDA Pregnancy Category C.

**Breast-feeding**
It is not known whether this medication is distributed into breast milk. However, problems in humans have not been documented.

**Pediatrics**
The risk of benzocaine-induced methemoglobinemia may be increased in infants, especially infants up to 3 months of age. However, pediatrics-specific problems that would limit the usefulness of antipyrine and benzocaine combination in older children are not expected.

**Geriatrics**
Appropriate studies on the relationship of age to the effects of antipyrine and benzocaine combination have not been performed in the geriatric population. However, no geriatrics-specific problems have been documented to date.

**Medical considerations/Contraindications**
The medical considerations/contraindications included have been selected on the basis of their potential clinical significance (reasons given in parentheses where appropriate)—not necessarily inclusive (» = major clinical significance).

*Risk-benefit should be considered when the following medical problems exist:*
  Sensitivity to antipyrine or benzocaine
  Spontaneous perforation of or drainage through the eardrum membrane (increased risk of otorrhea and irritation)

## Side/Adverse Effects
The following side/adverse effects have been selected on the basis of their potential clinical significance (possible signs and symptoms in parentheses where appropriate)—not necessarily inclusive:

**Those indicating need for medical attention only if they continue or are bothersome**
  Allergic reaction, local (itching, burning, redness, or oozing sores in the ear)

## Patient Consultation
As an aid to patient consultation, refer to *Advice for the Patient, Antipyrine and Benzocaine (Otic).*

In providing consultation, consider emphasizing the following selected information (» = major clinical significance):

**Before using this medication**
» Conditions affecting use, especially:
    Sensitivity to benzocaine or antipyrine
    Use in children—Risk of methemoglobinemia in infants

**Proper use of this medication**
*Proper administration technique*
    May warm medication to body temperature (37 °C or 98.6 °F) by holding bottle in hand for a few minutes before using
    Slowly fill ear canal while lying on side or tilting head with affected ear facing up
    Keep ear facing up for 5 minutes or, for patients who cannot stay still that long, for at least 1 or 2 minutes
    A cotton plug moistened with medication may be gently placed at the ear opening for no longer than 5 to 10 minutes to ensure retention
    For cerumen removal, the ear canal should be irrigated with warm water after the medication has been used for 2 or 3 days
    Preventing contamination of ear drops by not touching dropper to any surface including ear
» Not rinsing dropper after use; keeping container tightly closed
    Missed dose: Using as soon as possible; not using if almost time for next dose
» Proper dosing
» Proper storage

**Side/adverse effects**
    Discontinuing treatment if signs and symptoms of local allergic reaction occur

## General Dosing Information
This medication may be warmed to body temperature (37 °C or 98.6 °F) by holding the bottle in the hand for a few minutes prior to using.

The medication should be instilled with the affected ear facing up. Several minutes after the medication has been instilled the patient should gently place a cotton plug moistened with a little medication at the ear opening for no longer than 5 to 10 minutes to ensure retention.

When the medication is used to facilitate removal of cerumen, the ear canal should be irrigated with warm water, preferably by the physician, after the medication has been used for 2 or 3 days.

Treatment should be discontinued immediately if any sign of hypersensitivity or irritation occurs.

## Otic Dosage Forms

### ANTIPYRINE AND BENZOCAINE OTIC SOLUTION USP
**Usual adult and adolescent dose**
Analgesic-anesthetic, otic—
  Topical, to the ear canal, a sufficient quantity to fill the ear canal every one to two hours until relief is obtained.
Cerumen removal adjunct[1]—
  Topical, to the ear canal, a sufficient quantity to fill the ear canal three times a day for two or three days. After two or three days the ear canal should be irrigated with warm water.

**Usual pediatric dose**
See *Usual adult and adolescent dose.*

**Strength(s) usually available**
U.S.—
  54 mg of antipyrine and 14 mg of benzocaine, dissolved in anhydrous glycerin to make 1 mL (Rx) [*A/B Otic; Allergen; Analgesic Otic* (-

oxyquinoline sulfate); *Antiben; Auralgan* (oxyquinoline sulfate); *Aurodex; Auroto* (oxyquinoline sulfate); *Dolotic; Ear Drops* (oxyquinoline sulfate); *Otocalm* [GENERIC].

Canada—
54 mg of antipyrine and 14 mg of benzocaine, dissolved in anhydrous glycerin to make 1 mL (OTC) [*Auralgan*].

90 mg of antipyrine and 14 mg of benzocaine, dissolved in anhydrous glycerin to make 1 mL (OTC) [*Earache Drops*].

**Packaging and storage**
Store below 40 °C (104 °F), preferably between 15 and 30 °C (59 and 86 °F), unless otherwise specified by manufacturer. Store in a tight, light-resistant container. Protect from freezing.

Note: The solution congeals at 0 °C (32 °F) but returns to liquid state at room temperature. Therapeutic qualities are not affected.

**Auxiliary labeling**
- For the ear.
- Keep container tightly closed.

[1]Not included in Canadian product labeling.

Revised: 07/14/95

# ANTITHROMBIN III   Systemic†

VA CLASSIFICATION (Primary): BL119

Commonly used brand name(s): *ATnativ; Thrombate III*.

Other commonly used names are ATIII and heparin cofactor I.

Note: For a listing of dosage forms and brand names by country availability, see *Dosage Forms* section(s).

†Not commercially available in Canada.

## Category
Anticoagulant; antithrombotic.

## Indications
Note: Bracketed information in the *Indications* section refers to uses that are not included in U.S. product labeling.

**Accepted**

Thromboembolism associated with hereditary antithrombin III deficiency (prophylaxis)—Antithrombin III is indicated as prophylaxis against the development of thrombotic complications in patients with hereditary antithrombin III deficiency in situations in which the risk of thromboembolism is increased, such as surgery, delivery (including spontaneous or induced abortion), [pregnancy], [trauma], and [prolonged ( 24 hours) immobilization]. Heparin enhances the effects of antithrombin III (and vice versa) and may be given concurrently, using a full-dose, adjusted-dose, or low-dose heparin regimen as determined by the clinical circumstances.

Although long-term prophylaxis may be required in patients with hereditary antithrombin III deficiency, antithrombin III is usually not used, whether or not a high-risk situation, such as those listed above, exists. A coumarin- or indandione-derivative anticoagulant is usually used for this purpose. However, these anticoagulants should not be administered during the first trimester of pregnancy, and some clinicians recommend that they not be used at all during pregnancy. Heparin is usually used instead, but may be ineffective when concentrations of endogenous antithrombin III are low. Long-term prophylactic use of antithrombin III may therefore be required if heparin alone fails to produce adequate anticoagulation.

Thromboembolism associated with hereditary antithrombin III deficiency (treatment adjunct)—Antithrombin III is indicated as an adjunct to heparin therapy for the treatment of thromboembolism in patients with hereditary antithrombin III deficiency.

[The safety and efficacy of antithrombin III as an adjunct to heparin for the treatment of thromboembolism associated with acquired antithrombin III deficiency have not been established. However, use of antithrombin III may be considered for individual patients in whom heparin alone is ineffective.]

## Pharmacology/Pharmacokinetics

**Physicochemical characteristics**
Source—Pooled human plasma.
Chemical group—An alpha-2-globulin.
Molecular weight—58,000 daltons.
Description—A glycoprotein consisting of 425 amino acids in a single polypeptide chain cross-linked by three disulfide bridges.
pH (after reconstitution with 10 mL of sterile water for injection)—6.5–7.5

**Mechanism of action/Effect**
Antithrombin III, which is synthesized in the liver and endothelial cells, is an endogenous inhibitor of blood coagulation, providing approximately 75% of the antithrombin activity of the blood. It combines in a 1:1 molar ratio with the activated serine proteases of the intrinsic coagulation pathway (primarily thrombin [factor IIa] and factor Xa, and, to a lesser extent, factors IXa, XIa, and XIIa) to form inactive complexes. The active binding center is at the $Arg_{384}$–$Ser_{385}$ peptide bond. Hereditary antithrombin III deficiency has been shown to increase the risk of thromboembolism in some individuals; initial episodes in these patients have occurred most often between 15 and 30 years of age. Administration of exogenous antithrombin III corrects the deficiency, thus normalizing the patient's coagulation-inhibiting capability and inhibiting formation of thromboemboli.

Note: Antithrombin III also has lysine binding sites to which heparin binds in a 1:1 molar ratio. Formation of the antithrombin III–heparin complex produces a conformational change in the antithrombin III molecule that results in more rapid binding with and inactivation of the clotting factors than can be achieved by antithrombin III alone. Because heparin produces its anticoagulant effect only through its cofactors (the primary cofactor being antithrombin III), the efficacy of heparin is substantially reduced in antithrombin III deficiency. A reduction in the plasma activity of antithrombin III to 70% of the normal value may decrease the efficacy of heparin to 45%, and a reduction to 50% of the normal antithrombin III value may decrease the efficacy of heparin to 20%, of that achieved in the presence of normal antithrombin III activity. Administration of antithrombin III augments or restores the efficacy of heparin.

**Other actions/effects**
Antithrombin III also inactivates the fibrinolytic enzyme plasmin, but to a lesser extent than it inactivates the clotting factors.

**Distribution**
Antithrombin III is removed from the blood by binding to the epithelium and by redistribution into the extravascular compartment.
Antithrombin III–clotting factor complexes are removed rapidly from the circulation by binding to a specific receptor present on hepatocytes.

**Half-life**
Elimination—2 to 3 days; may be decreased by concurrent use of heparin, following surgery, and in patients with disseminated intravascular coagulation.

**Therapeutic plasma concentration**
Therapeutic benefit requires an antithrombin III activity of 80% or more of the normal value, which ranges between 100 and 200 mcg per mL (100 to 200 mg per L) in individuals 3 months of age and older.

Note: Plasma antithrombin III activity in patients with a hereditary deficiency is generally 25 to 60% of that present in normal adult plasma.

Plasma antithrombin III activity is normally reduced in neonates. Healthy, full-term neonates exhibit 40 to 85% of the antithrombin III activity present in normal adults; gradual increases occur until adult values are reached, generally at about 3 months of age. Antithrombin III activity is even lower in premature neonates.

## Precautions to Consider

**Pregnancy/Reproduction**

Note: Transmission of hereditary antithrombin III deficiency is autosomal-dominant; a deficiency state may occur in the child if either parent is affected. Homozygous fetuses often do not survive (depending on the specific type of antithrombin III deficiency). Patients with hereditary antithrombin III deficiency should be counseled about the potential risk to a child. Also, female patients with diagnosed hereditary antithrombin III deficiency and their spouses should be informed of the very high risk of thrombosis in antithrombin III–deficient women during pregnancy and delivery.

Pregnancy—Antithrombin III is effective in preventing thrombotic complications during pregnancy in women with hereditary antithrombin III deficiency, including women with a prior history of thrombosis, and women who are heparin-resistant. Studies in pregnant women have not shown that antithrombin III increases the risk of fetal abnormalities when administered during the third trimester of pregnancy. Antithrombin III has also been administered to a few women during the first 2 trimesters of pregnancy. No adverse effects on the fetus attributable to antithrombin III were reported.

Studies have not been done in animals.

FDA Pregnancy Category C.

Labor and delivery—Administration of a coumarin- or indandione-derivative anticoagulant or heparin during pregnancy increases the risk of hemorrhage during and following delivery; heparin should be discontinued 12 hours, and coumarin- or indandione-derivative anticoagulants several days, prior to delivery or therapeutic abortion. Antithrombin III therapy, when instituted or continued after another anticoagulant has been discontinued, is effective in preventing thromboembolic complications during and following delivery or therapeutic abortion, even in women who had previously had such complications. Such use of antithrombin III has not been reported to cause problems in the neonate.

**Breast-feeding**
Problems in nursing infants have not been reported. Distribution of antithrombin III into breast milk is highly unlikely because of antithrombin III's large molecule size.

**Pediatrics**
Appropriate studies on the relationship of age to the effects of antithrombin III have not been performed in the pediatric population. However, the medication has been administered to a limited number of neonates and children.

Because hereditary antithrombin III deficiency is transmitted in an autosomal-dominant manner, neonates born to a parent with hereditary antithrombin III deficiency should be tested at birth. Fatal thromboemboli have occurred in these neonates. However, even healthy, full-term neonates normally have low antithrombin III activity (compared to adults), and antithrombin III activity is even further reduced in preterm infants (especially if they are ill with respiratory distress syndrome, necrotizing enterocolitis, sepsis, or disseminated intravascular coagulation). Therefore, identification of infants at risk for thrombotic complications associated with hereditary antithrombin III deficiency may be difficult, and the advice of an expert should be sought before any prophylactic measure, including antithrombin III administration, is instituted.

**Geriatrics**
Appropriate studies on the relationship of age to the effects of antithrombin III have not been performed in the geriatric population. However, no geriatrics-specific problems have been documented to date.

**Drug interactions and/or related problems**
The following drug interactions and/or related problems have been selected on the basis of their potential clinical significance (possible mechanism in parentheses where appropriate)—not necessarily inclusive (» = major clinical significance):

Heparin
(concurrent administration of heparin and antithrombin III increases the anticoagulant effect of both medications, and usually decreases heparin dosage requirements, because antithrombin III is the primary cofactor required for heparin to exert an anticoagulant effect; in some patients [especially patients in whom disseminated intravascular coagulation caused by multiple trauma has produced an acquired antithrombin III deficiency] concurrent use may also increase the risk of bleeding, even with very low doses of heparin)

(heparin decreases the half-life of antithrombin III)

**Patient monitoring**
The following may be especially important in patient monitoring (other tests may be warranted in some patients, depending on condition; » = major clinical significance):

Antithrombin III activity
(monitoring is essential as a guide to dosage requirements and patient response; for patients with hereditary antithrombin III deficiency, it is recommended that determinations be performed twice a day until the dosage requirement has stabilized, after which determinations may be performed once daily, immediately prior to a dose; however, under certain circumstances, more frequent determinations may be needed)

Note: Antithrombin III may be measured quantitatively, using immunoassays, or qualitatively, using procedures that determine functional activity (e.g., measurement of the thrombin-inhibiting or factor Xa–inhibiting ability of the blood). Functional assays are preferred because, in some forms of antithrombin III deficiency, functional antithrombin III activity may be decreased despite normal immunologic (quantitative) test results.

## Side/Adverse Effects

Note: All products derived from human blood or plasma have the potential to transmit viral diseases, including acquired immunodeficiency syndrome (AIDS) and non-A, non-B hepatitis. Plasma used for preparation of antithrombin III for injection has been tested and found nonreactive for hepatitis B surface antigen and for antibody to the human immunodeficiency virus (HIV). In addition, prior to freeze-drying, the product is heat-treated (60 °C for not less than 10 hours). These measures may not be completely effective in eliminating the risk of viral transmission, but no documented cases of hepatitis resulting from administration of antithrombin III to patients with hereditary deficiencies have been reported to date.

Diuretic and vasodilatory effects leading to a fall in blood pressure were reported in 2 of 65 patients receiving antithrombin III for an acquired deficiency caused by severe disseminated intravascular coagulation. In addition, dyspnea and increased blood pressure occurred in one patient who received the medication at a too-rapid rate of administration (1500 IU in 5 minutes).

Chest pain or tightness, fever, hematoma, hives, oozing, and shortness of breath were also reported in a small number of patients. However, it was not clearly indicated that the symptoms were caused by the medication and were not related to the disease states of the patients. If these side/adverse effects should occur secondary to the infusion of antithrombin III, they may be abated by slowing or temporarily discontinuing the infusion.

## General Dosing Information

The potency of antithrombin III is expressed in international units (IU) and is determined using a standard calibrated against a World Health Organization (WHO) antithrombin III reference standard. One IU is equivalent to the quantity of endogenous antithrombin III present in 1 mL of normal human plasma.

## Parenteral Dosage Forms

### ANTITHROMBIN III (HUMAN) FOR INJECTION

**Usual adult and adolescent dose**
Thromboembolism associated with hereditary antithrombin III deficiency—
Intravenous, administered at a rate of 50 to 100 IU (not to exceed 100 IU) per minute:
Initial—A sufficient quantity to increase the antithrombin III activity, determined 30 minutes after administration, to 120% of the normal activity.
Maintenance—A sufficient quantity to increase the antithrombin III activity to 80% or more of the normal activity. Maintenance doses are generally administered at twenty-four-hour intervals.

Note: Initial dosage is calculated according to the following formula, based on an anticipated 1% increase in plasma antithrombin III (ATIII) activity for each 1 IU per kg of body weight:

Dose = [desired ATIII activity (as % of normal) − baseline ATIII activity (as % of normal)] × body weight (in kg) ÷ 1%.

Maintenance dosage is also calculated using the formula shown above for calculating initial dosage, but the actual increase in ATIII activity (in %) produced by 1 IU per kg of body weight, determined 30 minutes after administration of the initial dose, should be substituted for the 1% (the divisor) in the formula.

Increasing the antithrombin III activity to 120% (rather than 100%) of the normal value with the initial dose prolongs the interval before a second dose is required. However, dosage requirements may be increased in some patients. More frequent monitoring of antithrombin III activity may be required, with the dosage and frequency of administration being adjusted accordingly.

The duration of therapy depends on the indication for antithrombin III administration, the patient's condition and history, and the judgment of the physician. Treatment is usually continued for 2 to 8 days. In some circumstances (e.g., during pregnancy), more prolonged administration may be needed. Also, when treatment is given in conjunction with surgery or during prolonged immobilization, it is recommended that antithrombin III therapy be continued until the patient is fully mobilized.

**Usual pediatric dose**
See *Usual adult and adolescent dose*. The target percentage of normal human antithrombin III activity to be achieved for pediatric patients, is the same as for other patients.

**Size(s) usually available**
U.S.—
  500 IU (Rx) [*ATnativ* (human albumin 100 mg; sodium chloride 90 mg); *Thrombate III* (sodium chloride 110 to 210 mEq per L; alanine 0.075 to 0.125M; heparin ≤0.004 USP units per IU antithrombin III)].
  1000 IU (Rx) [*Thrombate III* (sodium chloride 110 to 210 mEq per L; alanine 0.075 to 0.125M; heparin ≤0.004 USP units per IU antithrombin III)].
Canada—
  Not commercially available.

**Packaging and storage**
Store at 2 to 8 °C (36 and 46 °F), unless otherwise specified by manufacturer.

**Preparation of dosage form**
Antithrombin III for injection is reconstituted using 10 mL of sterile water for injection (provided by the manufacturer) or an alternate solution, such as 0.9% sodium chloride injection or 5% dextrose injection. Do not shake the vial while reconstituting. The solution should then be brought to room temperature before administration. If desired, the reconstituted injection may be further diluted, using the same diluent.

Caution—Use of diluents containing benzyl alcohol is not recommended for preparation of medications for use in neonates. A fatal toxic syndrome consisting of metabolic acidosis, CNS depression, respiratory problems, renal failure, hypotension, and possibly seizures and intracranial hemorrhages has been associated with this use.

**Stability**
After reconstitution, the solution must be used within 3 hours.
Because antithrombin III for injection contains no preservative, any unused solution should be discarded.

**Selected Bibliography**
Rosenberg RD, editor. Role of antithrombin III in coagulation disorders: state-of-the-art review. Am J Med 1989; 87 (3B Suppl): 1S-67S.
Vinazzer H. Clinical use of antithrombin III concentrates. Vox Sang 1987; 53: 193-8.

Revised: 02/23/94

---

# ANTITHYROID AGENTS   Systemic

This monograph includes information on the following: 1) Methimazole; 2) Propylthiouracil.
INN: Methimazole—Thiamazole
VA CLASSIFICATION (Primary): HS852
Commonly used brand name(s): *Propyl-Thyracil*[2]; *Tapazole*[1].
Note:  For a listing of dosage forms and brand names by country availability, see *Dosage Forms* section(s).

## Category
Antihyperthyroid agent.

## Indications
**Accepted**
Hyperthyroidism (treatment)—Methimazole and propylthiouracil are indicated in the treatment of hyperthyroidism, including prior to surgery or radiotherapy, and as adjuncts in the treatment of thyrotoxicosis or thyroid storm. Propylthiouracil may be preferred over methimazole for use in thyroid storm, since propylthiouracil inhibits peripheral conversion of thyroxine [$T_4$] to triiodothyronine [$T_3$].

Further studies are needed to establish the safety and efficacy of using propylthiouracil for the treatment of alcoholic liver disease.

**Unaccepted**
Efficacy of antithyroid medications has been inconsistent in the treatment of angina pectoris. These agents are probably useful for this purpose only in hyperthyroid patients with angina pectoris.

Antithyroid medications are not effective in the treatment of thyrotoxicosis resulting from exogenous thyroid hormone overdosage.

## Pharmacology/Pharmacokinetics
**Physicochemical characteristics**
Chemical group—
  Methimazole and propylthiouracil are thioamide derivatives.
Molecular weight—
  Methimazole: 114.16.
  Propylthiouracil: 170.23.
pKa—
  Propylthiouracil: 7.8.

**Mechanism of action/Effect**
Inhibit synthesis of thyroid hormone within the thyroid gland by serving as substrates for thyroid peroxidase, which catalyzes the incorporation of oxidized iodide into tyrosine residues in thyroglobulin molecules and couples iodotyrosines. This diverts iodine from the synthesis of thyroid hormones. Antithyroid agents do not interfere with the actions of exogenous thyroid hormone or inhibit the release of thyroid hormones. Therefore, stores of thyroid hormones must be depleted before clinical effects will be apparent. Antithyroid agents may also have moderating effects on the underlying immunologic abnormalities in hyperthyroidism due to Graves' disease (toxic diffuse goiter), but evidence on this point reported to date is inconclusive.

Propylthiouracil—
  Additionally, inhibits peripheral conversion of $T_4$ to $T_3$, which may theoretically make it more effective in the treatment of thyroid storm.

**Absorption**
Rapid.
  Methimazole—
    Oral: Bioavailability 93%. Absorption may be unpredictably affected by food.
    Rectal: In one study in healthy subjects, absorption of extemporaneously compounded 60-mg rectal suppositories was similar to that of oral tablets.
  Propylthiouracil—
    Oral: Bioavailability 65 to 75%.
    Rectal: In one study in healthy subjects, absorption of extemporaneously compounded 100-mg rectal suppositories was slower and less extensive than that of oral tablets (AUC$_{0 \text{ to } 8h}$: 23.77 ± 1.24 mcg•hr/mL [oral], 6.16 ± 2.07 mcg•hr/mL [rectal]).

**Distribution**
Both methimazole and propylthiouracil are actively concentrated by the thyroid.
Methimazole—Volume of distribution is approximately 0.6 liter per kilogram (L/kg) of body weight.
Propylthiouracil—Volume of distribution is approximately 0.4 L/kg of body weight.

**Protein binding**
Methimazole—Not significant.
Propylthiouracil—High (80%), primarily to albumin.

**Biotransformation**
Primarily hepatic; active metabolites of either compound have not been demonstrated.
Propylthiouracil—Primarily undergoes glucuronidation. Approximately 33% of an orally administered dose is metabolized by a first-pass effect.

**Half-life**
Methimazole—5 to 6 hours.
Propylthiouracil—1 to 2 hours.

**Onset of action**
Methimazole—In one study, substantial reductions in mean serum thyroxine and triiodothyronine concentrations were seen after 5 days of methimazole therapy at 40 mg per day.

**Time to peak serum concentration**
Methimazole—
  Oral/Rectal:
    Approximately 30 to 60 minutes (occurrence of peak blood concentrations, after administration of a 60-mg rectal suppository or a 60-mg oral dose to healthy subjects).
Propylthiouracil—
  Oral:
    1.99 ± 0.26 hours (after administration of a 100-mg dose to healthy subjects).

Rectal:
    Solution—Approximately 3 hours (after administration of a 400-mg rectal dose of propylthiouracil in an aqueous solution of sodium phosphates to a patient with thyroid storm).
    Suppository—4.72 ± 0.96 hours (after administration of a 100-mg suppository to healthy subjects).

**Peak serum concentration**
Methimazole—
  Oral:
    1.184 ± 0.12 mcg/mL (blood concentrations, after administration of a 60-mg dose to healthy subjects).
  Rectal:
    1.163 ± 0.15 mcg/mL (blood concentrations, after administration of a 60-mg suppository to healthy subjects).
Propylthiouracil—
  Oral:
    7.12 ± 0.48 mcg/mL (after administration of a 100-mg dose to healthy subjects).
  Rectal:
    Solution—3.1 mcg/mL (approximate, after administration of a 400-mg rectal dose of propylthiouracil in an aqueous solution of sodium phosphates to a patient with thyroid storm).
    Suppository—1.2 ± 0.31 mcg/mL (after administration of a 100-mg rectal suppository to healthy subjects).

**Time to peak effect**
Methimazole—7 weeks (average) to normalize serum $T_3$ and $T_4$ concentrations with use of 30 mg per day. In one study, 4 weeks (approximate) to normalize serum $T_3$ and $T_4$ concentrations with use of 40 mg per day.
Propylthiouracil—17 weeks (average) to normalize serum $T_3$ and $T_4$ concentrations with use of 300 mg per day.

**Elimination**
Methimazole—
  Less than 10% is excreted in the urine unchanged. Total body clearance is approximately 10 L per hour.
Propylthiouracil—
  Less than 1% is excreted in the urine unchanged. Total body clearance is approximately 7 L per hour.
  In dialysis: Elimination and pharmacokinetics are not significantly altered in hemodialysis. In one patient undergoing hemodialysis, 5% of a 200-mg oral dose was removed by 3 hours of hemodialysis; elimination rate was not significantly altered. Peak serum concentration was decreased (from 7.9 to 4.9 mcg/mL), although it remained within an approximate therapeutic range.

## Precautions to Consider

### Cross-sensitivity and/or related problems
Cross-sensitivity may occur frequently (in about 50% of patients) between antithyroid thioamide medications.

If a persistent or severe reaction necessitates withdrawal of one agent, therapy may be switched to the other, although there is a risk of cross-reactivity occurring. However, if agranulocytosis, thrombocytopenia, or hepatic dysfunction occurs, substitution with another thioamide is not recommended.

### Carcinogenicity/Mutagenicity
Methimazole—Studies have not been done in either animals or humans.
Propylthiouracil—Thyroid hyperplasia and carcinoma have occurred in laboratory animals treated with propylthiouracil for longer than 1 year. Similar effects are seen with continuous thyroid suppression with various antithyroid agents, dietary iodine deficiency, subtotal thyroidectomy, and ectopic thyrotropin-secreting pituitary tumors. Pituitary adenomas have also occurred.

### Pregnancy/Reproduction
Pregnancy—Methimazole and propylthiouracil cross the placenta and can cause fetal hypothyroidism and goiter. However, the possible risks of adverse effects due to antithyroid agents must be weighed against the risks of possible adverse effects due to continuing hyperthyroidism during pregnancy. Propylthiouracil is considered by some clinicians as the agent of choice for women who require antithyroid medications during pregnancy. Propylthiouracil crosses the placenta less readily than methimazole, and the use of methimazole during pregnancy has been associated with several cases of scalp defects (aplasia cutis) in the infant. The reduced placental transfer of propylthiouracil is presumably due to its high level of serum protein binding and high level of ionization at a pH of 7.4.

The actual risk of fetal death, goiter, hypothyroidism, or certain congenital abnormalities with administration of antithyroid agents appears to be low, especially if maternal doses are low (for example, less than 100 to 150 mg of propylthiouracil or an equivalent dose of methimazole per day). Fetal goiters induced by antithyroid agents are generally not as large as iodide-induced fetal goiters and have not usually been reported to be obstructive. Fetal hypothyroidism and goiter usually occur when the antithyroid agents are used close to term, since the fetal thyroid does not begin to produce thyroid hormones until the 11th or 12th week of gestation. In long-term follow-up of some children exposed *in utero* to maternal therapeutic doses of propylthiouracil, gross abnormalities in development or diminished intellectual performance have not been observed.

It is recommended that antithyroid medication be prescribed at the lowest effective dose to maintain maternal thyroid function within the upper-normal range for normal pregnant women, especially during the last trimester, to reduce the risk of fetal and maternal hypothyroidism and goiter. Thyroid hyperfunction may diminish as pregnancy progresses, allowing a reduction in antithyroid dosage and, in some cases, withdrawal of antithyroid therapy 2 to 3 months before delivery. However, thyroid function may vary and dosing should be based on frequent and careful monitoring. Hyperthyroidism may recur soon after delivery. Because radioactive iodine is absolutely contraindicated during pregnancy, thyroidectomy may be very rarely required in refractory cases of hyperthyroidism or in patients who are noncompliant with the use of antithyroid medications.

Thyroid hormones are minimally transferred across the placenta and therefore have little protective effect on the fetus. They may also mask signs of remission of hyperthyroidism, resulting in fetal and maternal exposure to unnecessarily high doses of antithyroid agents. For these reasons, adjunctive treatment with thyroid hormones is not recommended during pregnancy.

Several case reports have been published in which antithyroid agents were given to a euthyroid mother of a hyperthyroid fetus. Fetal heart rate monitoring and ultrasound examinations were used to monitor fetal response. Fetal tachycardia was reduced and the infants were euthyroid at delivery. However, further data are needed regarding this form of therapy for fetal hyperthyroidism.

FDA Pregnancy Category D.

### Breast-feeding
Small amounts of methimazole and propylthiouracil are distributed into breast milk. However, the use of average maintenance doses of these agents is not generally considered an absolute contraindication to breast-feeding, although serial monitoring of thyroid function (by measurement of serum thyrotropin and thyroxine concentrations) of the infant is advisable. Propylthiouracil is generally preferred over methimazole during lactation because methimazole is distributed into breast milk more readily (approximately ten-fold), presumably due to its insignificant level of protein binding and ionization. Maternal serum and breast milk concentrations of methimazole are nearly equal. However, some clinicians feel that small doses of methimazole (e.g., ≤ 10–15 mg per day) do not pose a significant risk to the infant if thyroid function is monitored frequently.

There is a theoretical risk of causing hypothyroidism and/or agranulocytosis in the infant with high maternal doses of antithyroid agents. Termination of breast-feeding may be necessary prior to initiation of high-dose therapy.

### Pediatrics
Antithyroid agents are frequently used to treat hyperthyroidism in children. Children seem to respond to antithyroid agents as well as do adults. Pharmacokinetic studies conducted in children also did not reveal any differences unique to the pediatric population.

Caution is necessary in interpreting results of thyroid function tests in neonates, because serum concentrations of thyroid hormones are higher at birth than those of healthy children or adults and begin to fall to normal in the first week of life.

### Adolescents
Antithyroid agents are frequently used to treat hyperthyroidism in adolescents. Adolescents seem to respond to antithyroid agents as well as do adults. Pharmacokinetic studies conducted in adolescents did not reveal any differences unique to the adolescent population.

### Geriatrics
One study showed that agranulocytosis is more likely to occur in patients older than 40 years of age or in patients taking more than 40 mg of methimazole per day.

In one pharmacokinetic study, no significant differences were found for geriatric patients in certain pharmacokinetic parameters (e.g., Vd, Vd beta, Vd at steady state, area under the curve, and clearance). Rate of absorption was decreased (approximately one-third that of younger subjects) though there are no data regarding the clinical significance of this finding.

Geriatric patients with severe cardiac disease should be given antithyroid agents and/or beta-adrenergic blocking agents, such as propranolol, for 4 to 6 weeks prior to treatment with radioiodine to help reduce possible exacerbation of heart disease by radiation-induced thyroiditis. Antithyroid drugs must be discontinued at least 3 to 4 days prior to radioiodine treatment and should not be readministered until 1 week after treatment. However, a beta-adrenergic blocking agent may be used throughout the treatment period if needed.

### Dental
The bone marrow depressant effects of antithyroid agents may result in an increased incidence of microbial infection, delayed healing, and gingival bleeding. If leukopenia or thrombocytopenia occurs, dental work should be deferred until blood counts have returned to normal, and patients should be instructed in proper oral hygiene, including caution in use of regular toothbrushes, dental floss, and toothpicks.

### Drug interactions and/or related problems
The following drug interactions and/or related problems have been selected on the basis of their potential clinical significance (possible mechanism in parentheses where appropriate)—not necessarily inclusive (» = major clinical significance):

Note: Combinations containing any of the following medications, depending on the amount present, may also interact with this medication.

Aminophylline or
Oxtriphylline or
Theophylline
(hyperthyroid patients have exhibited increased metabolic clearance of aminophylline and theophylline, which returned to normal as the patients became euthyroid; decreased dose of aminophylline, oxtriphylline, or theophylline may be necessary as patients become euthyroid)

» Amiodarone or
» Iodinated glycerol or
» Iodine or
» Potassium iodide
(iodide or iodine excess may decrease response to antithyroid agents, requiring an increase in dosage or longer duration of therapy with antithyroid agents; amiodarone contains 37% iodine by weight, and therefore its use significantly increases iodine intake; iodine deficiency may increase response to antithyroid agents, requiring a decrease in dosage or shorter duration of therapy with antithyroid agents)

» Anticoagulants, coumarin- or indandione-derivative
(as thyroid and metabolic status of patient decreases toward normal, response to oral anticoagulants may decrease; however, if thioamide-induced hypoprothrombinemia occurs, anticoagulant effect may be enhanced; adjustment of oral anticoagulant dosage on the basis of prothrombin time is recommended)

» Digitalis glycosides
(serum concentrations of digoxin and digitoxin have been reported to increase as the thyroid and metabolic status of patients taking antithyroid agents decreased; reduction in dosage of any digitalis glycoside may be necessary as patients become euthyroid)

» Sodium iodide I 131
(antithyroid agents may decrease thyroidal uptake of I 131; a rebound increase in uptake may occur up to 5 days after sudden withdrawal of the antithyroid agent)

### Laboratory value alterations
The following have been selected on the basis of their potential clinical significance (possible effect in parentheses where appropriate)—not necessarily inclusive (» = major clinical significance):

With diagnostic test results
» Sodium iodide I 123 or
» Sodium iodide I 131 or
» Sodium pertechnetate Tc 99m
(antithyroid agents may decrease thyroidal uptake of I 123, I 131, or pertechnetate; withdrawal of the antithyroid agent 5 days or more before radioactive iodine uptake tests is necessary to prevent interference)

With physiology/laboratory test values
Alanine aminotransferase (ALT [SGPT]), serum concentrations and
Alkaline phosphatase, serum concentrations and
Aspartate aminotransferase (AST [SGOT]), serum concentrations and
Bilirubin, serum concentrations and
Lactate dehydrogenase (LDH), serum concentrations and
Prothrombin time (PT)
(may be increased; may indicate hepatotoxicity and be associated with splenomegaly)

### Medical considerations/Contraindications
The medical considerations/contraindications included have been selected on the basis of their potential clinical significance (reasons given in parentheses where appropriate)—not necessarily inclusive (» = major clinical significance).

*Except under special circumstances, this medication should not be used when the following medical problem exists:*

» Severe adverse reaction or severe allergic reaction to either methimazole or propylthiouracil, or history of

*Risk-benefit should be considered when the following medical problem exists:*

» Hepatic function impairment
(elimination half-life may be prolonged, in proportion to the degree of hepatic insufficiency)

### Patient monitoring
The following may be especially important in patient monitoring (other tests may be warranted in some patients, depending on condition; » = major clinical significance):

Leukocyte count, total and differential
(determinations recommended prior to initiation of treatment and if infection occurs)

» Free thyroxine ($T_4$), by direct assay and/or
» Thyrotropin (TSH) by sensitive radioimmunoassay and/or

Total thyroxine ($T_4$), either by competitive protein-binding assay or by radioimmunoassay and/or

Total triiodothyronine ($T_3$) by radioimmunoassay
(determination of serum concentrations is recommended prior to initiation of therapy, at monthly intervals during initial therapy, then every 2 to 3 months; some clinicians recommend at least yearly follow-up for life in patients successfully treated with antithyroid medications; in patients treated with these agents who do not undergo thyroid ablation with sodium iodide I 131 or surgery, the risk of subsequent hypothyroidism is related to immunogenic thyroid disease itself, and not the medication; recurrence of hyperthyroidism is common)

## Side/Adverse Effects

Note: Incidence of most adverse reactions is dose-related; most side effects occur within the first 4 to 8 weeks.

The following side/adverse effects have been selected on the basis of their potential clinical significance (possible signs and symptoms in parentheses where appropriate)—not necessarily inclusive:

### Those indicating need for medical attention
Incidence more frequent
*Fever, mild and transient; leukopenia* (continuing or severe fever or chills, throat infection, cough, mouth sores, or hoarseness)—usually asymptomatic; *skin rash or itching*

Note: Mild *leukopenias* occur more frequently in patients (12% of adults and 25% of children) treated with antithyroid agents. Also, approximately 10% of untreated hyperthyroid patients have leukocyte levels below 4000 per cubic millimeter.

Incidence of *skin rash or itching* is 3 to 5%. Usually consists of maculopapular eruptions. An allergic reaction occurs less frequently and may disappear spontaneously with continued treatment; appears to be dose-related. Skin rash may also be a sign of vasculitis.

Incidence less frequent
*Agranulocytosis* (continuing or severe fever or chills, throat infection, cough, mouth sores, or hoarseness); *arthralgias or arthritis or vasculitis* (pain, swelling, or redness in joints)—usually with propylthiouracil; *lupus-like syndrome* (fever or chills; general feeling of discomfort or illness or weakness)—usually with propylthiouracil; *peripheral neuropathy* (numbness or tingling of fingers, toes, or face)

Note: *Agranulocytosis* (incidence 0.4%) usually occurs during the first 3 months of therapy. May occur less predictably and with lower doses of propylthiouracil. Deaths due to agranulocytosis have been reported.

Incidence rare
*Aplastic anemia* (continuing or severe fever or chills, throat infection, cough, mouth sores, or hoarseness); *hypoprothrombinemia (for propylthiouracil); or thrombocytopenia* (rarely, increase in bleeding or bruising; black, tarry stools; blood in urine or stools; pinpoint red spots on skin)—usually asymptomatic; *cholestatic jaundice* (yellow eyes or skin)—for methimazole; *hepatic necrosis* (yellow eyes or skin)—primarily with propylthiouracil; *interstitial pneumonitis* (cough or short-

ness of breath)—with propylthiouracil; *lymphadenopathy* (swollen lymph nodes); *sialadenopathy* (swollen salivary glands); *nephritis (for methimazole) or renal vasculitis (usually with propylthiouracil)* (backache; increase or decrease in urination; swelling of feet or lower legs)

> Note: *Jaundice* may persist for up to 10 weeks after drug discontinuance. Fatal *hepatic necrosis* has been reported with both agents.

**Those indicating need for medical attention only if they continue or are bothersome**
Incidence less frequent
> *Dizziness; loss of taste*—for methimazole; *nausea or vomiting; stomach pain*

## Overdose

For more information on the management of overdose or unintentional ingestion, **contact a Poison Control Center** (see *Poison Control Center Listing*).

**Clinical effects of overdose (hypothyroidism)**
The following effects have been selected on the basis of their potential clinical significance (possible signs and symptoms in parentheses where appropriate)—not necessarily inclusive:
*Changes in menstrual periods; coldness; constipation; dry, puffy skin; goiter* (swelling in the front of the neck); *headache; listlessness or sleepiness; muscle aches; nausea or vomiting, severe; unusual tiredness or weakness; weight gain, unusual*

> Note: *Hypothyroidism* may be an unavoidable long-term sequela to hyperthyroidism.

## Patient Consultation

As an aid to patient consultation, refer to *Advice for the Patient, Antithyroid Agents (Systemic)*.
In providing consultation, consider emphasizing the following selected information (» = major clinical significance):

**Before using this medication**
» Conditions affecting use, especially:
  Allergies to any thioamide
  Pregnancy—May be used but careful monitoring is necessary
  Breast-feeding—Distributed into breast milk, although propylthiouracil is distributed in much lesser amounts; may continue breast-feeding with low doses and monitoring of infant
  Other medications, especially iodides, coumarin- or indandione-derivative anticoagulants, amiodarone, digitalis glycosides, or radioiodide
  Other medical problems, especially hepatic function impairment

**Proper use of this medication**
» Importance of not taking more or less medication than the amount prescribed
» Importance of not missing doses and, if taking more than one dose per day, of taking at evenly spaced intervals
  Taking methimazole at same time in relation to meals every day
» Proper dosing
  Missed dose: Taking as soon as possible; taking both doses together if almost time for next dose; checking with physician if more than one dose is missed
» Proper storage

**Precautions while using this medication**
» Importance of close monitoring by the physician
» Checking with physician before discontinuing medication
» Caution if any kind of surgery (including dental surgery) or emergency treatment is required, because of the risk of thyroid storm
» Checking with physician immediately if injury, infection, or other illness occurs, because of the risk of thyroid storm
  Caution if any laboratory tests required; possible interference with test results

**Side/adverse effects**
  Signs of potential side effects, especially fever, skin rash or itching, bone marrow depression, hepatic dysfunction, lupus-like syndrome, arthralgias, arthritis, nephritis (for methimazole), vasculitis, pneumonitis, lymphadenopathy, sialadenopathy, hypoprothrombinemia (for propylthiouracil), or peripheral neuropathy

## General Dosing Information

Dosage must be adjusted to meet the individual requirements of each patient, on the basis of clinical response and results of thyroid function tests.

In some patients, once- or twice-a-day therapy may be associated with a decreased incidence of side effects and improved compliance, although divided daily doses may be more effective. If divided daily doses are given, they should be administered at evenly spaced intervals throughout the day. Methimazole has a longer duration of action and therefore may frequently be more effective than propylthiouracil in once-daily dosing.

Confirmation of remission may be by sensitive TSH assay, trial withdrawal of the medication, protirelin test, thyroid suppression test, or thyroid-stimulating immunoglobulin (TSI) titer.

Duration of treatment necessary to produce a prolonged remission varies from 6 months to several years, with an average duration of 1 to 2 years. Control of hyperthyroidism with medication is sometimes followed by a spontaneous remission. Premature withdrawal may result in exacerbation of hyperthyroidism, although some clinicians feel that treatment may be withdrawn as soon as a euthyroid state is obtained (usually within 4 to 5 months), with no problems of rebound.

Iodide is usually added to thioamide antithyroid therapy for 7 to 10 days prior to surgery to reduce the vascularity of the thyroid gland, thereby decreasing subsequent blood loss during surgery.

If an antithyroid agent is being used in severely hyperthyroid patients to improve their thyroid state prior to radioactive iodine therapy, the antithyroid medication must be discontinued 2 to 4 days before treatment to prevent impairment of radioactive iodine uptake. Antithyroid treatment may be resumed, if desired, 3 to 7 days after radioactive iodine treatment to hasten return to euthyroidism, until effects of the iodine are apparent.

**Diet/Nutrition**
Food may inconsistently alter the bioavailability of methimazole. It is recommended that methimazole be taken at the same time in relation to meals every day.

**For treatment of adverse effects**
Reduction in dosage or temporary withdrawal of antithyroid medication may be recommended if signs and symptoms of hypothyroidism occur. Some clinicians recommend adjunctive thyroid therapy (except during pregnancy) to prevent development of hypothyroidism. However, hypothyroidism may be an unavoidable long-term sequela to hyperthyroidism.

It is recommended that antithyroid therapy be discontinued promptly and supportive measures initiated if signs and symptoms of agranulocytosis, aplastic anemia, hepatic dysfunction, lupus-like syndrome, severe skin rash, swelling of cervical lymph nodes, or vasculitis occur. If laboratory examinations show only a mild leukopenia, periodic blood count monitoring without withdrawal or reduction in dosage may be sufficient. Mild reactions may not require withdrawal, although they may precede more serious reactions. Leukocyte production usually returns to normal within 1 to 2 weeks after withdrawal.

---

### METHIMAZOLE

## Summary of Differences

General dosing information: May be more suitable for once-daily administration.

## Oral Dosage Forms

**METHIMAZOLE TABLETS USP**

**Usual adult and adolescent dose**
Hyperthyroidism—
  Initial:
    Mild hyperthyroidism—Oral, 15 mg a day as one daily dose or as two divided daily doses for six to eight weeks until the patient becomes euthyroid.
    Moderately severe hyperthyroidism—Oral, 30 to 40 mg a day as one daily dose or as two divided daily doses for six to eight weeks until the patient becomes euthyroid.
    Severe hyperthyroidism—Oral, 60 mg a day as one daily dose or as two divided daily doses for six to eight weeks until the patient becomes euthyroid.
  Maintenance:
    Oral, 5 to 30 mg a day in one daily dose or as two divided daily doses.
  Thyrotoxic crisis:
    Oral, 15 to 20 mg every four hours during the first day, as an adjunct to other measures.

**Usual pediatric dose**
Hyperthyroidism—
  Initial: Oral, 400 mcg (0.4 mg) per kg of body weight a day as one daily dose or as two divided daily doses.

Maintenance: Oral, 200 mcg (0.2 mg) per kg of body weight a day as one daily dose or as two divided daily doses.

**Strength(s) usually available**
U.S.—
 5 mg (Rx) [*Tapazole* (scored; lactose)].
 10 mg (Rx) [*Tapazole* (scored; lactose)].
Canada—
 5 mg (Rx) [*Tapazole* (scored)].

**Packaging and storage**
Store below 40 °C (104 °F), preferably between 15 and 30 °C (59 and 86 °F), unless otherwise specified by manufacturer. Store in a well-closed, light-resistant container.

**Auxiliary labeling**
- Take at the same time in relation to meals every day.

## Rectal Dosage Forms
### METHIMAZOLE SUPPOSITORIES

**Usual adult and adolescent dose**
Hyperthyroidism—
 Initial: Thyrotoxic crisis—Rectal, 15 to 20 mg every four hours during the first day, as an adjunct to other measures, with the dosage being adjusted according to patient response.

**Usual pediatric dose**
Hyperthyroidism—
 Initial: Thyrotoxic crisis—Rectal, 400 mcg (0.4 mg) per kg of body weight a day as one daily dose or as two divided daily doses.

**Strength(s) usually available**
U.S.—
 Not commercially available. Compounding required for prescription.
Canada—
 Not commercially available. Compounding required for prescription.

**Packaging and storage**
Store between 2 and 8 °C (36 and 46 °F). Store in a well-closed container. Protect from freezing.

**Preparation of dosage form**
A formulation that has been used for the extemporaneous compounding of methimazole suppositories is as follows:
- 1200 mg methimazole dissolved in 12 mL of distilled water
- 2 drops of Span 80
- Cocoa butter (warmed to 37 °C [98.6 °F]) of sufficient quantity to make 20 suppositories containing 60 mg methimazole each.

**Auxiliary labeling**
- Refrigerate.
- For rectal use only.

**Note**
Use of methimazole suppositories is generally reserved for treatment of thyrotoxic emergencies, in patients who are unable to tolerate oral medications. The efficacy of chronic rectal dosing with extemporaneously compounded formulations has not been established.

---

## PROPYLTHIOURACIL

## Summary of Differences
Precautions:
 Pregnancy—May be preferred to methimazole, due to lower rate of placental transfer.
 Breast-feeding—May be preferred to methimazole, due to a lower rate of distribution into breast milk.
Side/adverse effects:
 Agranulocytosis may be less predictable, because it is usually not dose-related.

## Oral Dosage Forms
### PROPYLTHIOURACIL TABLETS USP

**Usual adult and adolescent dose**
Hyperthyroidism—
 Initial:
  Oral, 300 to 900 mg a day as one to four divided daily doses until the patient becomes euthyroid.
  Note: Patients with severe hyperthyroidism may occasionally require up to 1.2 grams a day.
 Maintenance:
  Oral, 50 to 600 mg a day as one to four divided daily doses.
 Thyrotoxic crisis:
  Oral, 200 to 400 mg every four hours during the first day, as an adjunct to other measures, the dosage then being decreased as the crisis subsides.

**Usual pediatric dose**
Hyperthyroidism—
 Initial:
  Children 6 to 10 years of age—Oral, 50 to 150 mg a day as one to four divided daily doses.
  Children 10 years of age and over—Oral, 50 to 300 mg a day as one to four divided daily doses.
 Maintenance:
  Oral, determined by response.
 Neonatal thyrotoxicosis:
  Oral, 10 mg per kg of body weight a day in divided daily doses.

**Strength(s) usually available**
U.S.—
 50 mg (Rx) [GENERIC].
Canada—
 50 mg (Rx) [*Propyl-Thyracil* (scored)].
 100 mg (Rx) [*Propyl-Thyracil* (scored)].

**Packaging and storage**
Store below 40 °C (104 °F), preferably between 15 and 30 °C (59 and 86 °F), unless otherwise specified by manufacturer. Store in a well-closed container.

**Auxiliary labeling**
- Take at the same time in relation to meals every day.

## Rectal Dosage Forms
### PROPYLTHIOURACIL ENEMA

**Usual adult and adolescent dose**
Hyperthyroidism—
 Initial: Thyrotoxic crisis—Rectal, 200 to 400 mg every four hours during the first day, as an adjunct to other measures, with the dosage being adjusted according to patient response.

**Usual pediatric dose**
Hyperthyroidism—Initial: Thyrotoxic crisis—
 Children 6 to 10 years of age: Rectal, 50 to 150 mg a day as one to four divided daily doses, with the dosage being adjusted according to patient response.
 Children 10 years of age and over: Rectal, 50 to 300 mg a day as one to four divided daily doses, with the dosage being adjusted according to patient response.
 Neonatal thyrotoxicosis: Rectal, 10 mg per kg of body weight a day in divided daily doses, with the dosage being adjusted according to patient response.

**Strength(s) usually available**
U.S.—
 Not commercially available. Compounding required for prescription.
Canada—
 Not commercially available. Compounding required for prescription.

**Packaging and storage**
Store between 2 and 8 °C (36 and 46 °F). Store in a well-closed container. Protect from freezing.

**Preparation of dosage form**
A formulation that has been used for the extemporaneous compounding of propylthiouracil enemas is as follows:
- 400 mg propylthiouracil (8-50 mg tablets)
- 60 mL aqueous sodium phosphates solution (*Fleet's Phospho-Soda*, pH 4.4 to 5.4).

**Auxiliary labeling**
- For rectal use only.

**Note**
Use of propylthiouracil enema is generally reserved for treatment of thyrotoxic emergencies, in patients who are unable to tolerate oral medications. The efficacy of chronic rectal dosing with extemporaneously compounded formulations has not been established.

### PROPYLTHIOURACIL SUPPOSITORIES

**Usual adult and adolescent dose**
Hyperthyroidism—
 Initial: Thyrotoxic crisis—Rectal, 200 to 400 mg every four hours during the first day, as an adjunct to other measures, with the dosage being adjusted according to patient response.

## Usual pediatric dose

Hyperthyroidism—Initial: Thyrotoxic crisis—

Children 6 to 10 years of age: Rectal, 50 to 150 mg a day as one to four divided daily doses, with the dosage being adjusted according to patient response.

Children 10 years of age and over: Rectal, 50 to 300 mg a day as one to four divided daily doses, with the dosage being adjusted according to patient response.

Neonatal thyrotoxicosis: Rectal, 10 mg per kg of body weight a day in divided daily doses, with the dosage being adjusted according to patient response.

## Strength(s) usually available

U.S.—
  Not commercially available. Compounding required for prescription.
Canada—
  Not commercially available. Compounding required for prescription.

## Packaging and storage

Store between 2 and 8 °C (36 and 46 °F). Store in a well-closed container. Protect from freezing.

## Preparation of dosage form

A formulation that has been used for the extemporaneous compounding of propylthiouracil suppositories is as follows:
- 400 mg propylthiouracil (8-50 mg tablets) in
- Hardfat (Witepsol H15), of sufficient quantity to make 4 suppositories containing 100 mg each.

## Auxiliary labeling

- For rectal use only.

## Note

Use of propylthiouracil suppositories is generally reserved for treatment of thyrotoxic emergencies, in patients who are unable to tolerate oral medications. The efficacy of chronic rectal dosing with extemporaneously compounded formulations has not been established.

## Selected Bibliography

Cooper DS. Antithyroid drugs. N Engl J Med 1984; 311(21): 1353-62.
Cooper DS. Which antithyroid drug? Am J Med 1986; 80(6): 1165-8.
Stockigt JR, Topliss DJ. Hyperthyroidism: current drug therapy. Drugs 1989; 37: 375-81.

Revised: 04/21/92
Interim revision: 06/03/94

---

**ANTIVENIN, CHIRONEX FLECKERI**—The *Antivenin, Chironex Fleckeri (Systemic)* monograph is not included in this published version of the USP DI database. Copies of the monograph are available on request from Micromedex, Inc. - Reprint Requests, 6200 S. Syracuse Way, Suite 300, Englewood, CO 80111; telephone (303) 486-6400; telefax (303) 486-6464; Email: USPDI@MDX.COM.

**ANTIVENIN, CROTALIDAE POLYVALENT**—The *Antivenin, Crotalidae, Polyvalent (Systemic)* monograph is not included in this published version of the USP DI database. Copies of the monograph are available on request from Micromedex, Inc. - Reprint Requests, 6200 S. Syracuse Way, Suite 300, Englewood, CO 80111; telephone (303) 486-6400; telefax (303) 486-6464; Email: USPDI@MDX.COM.

**ANTIVENIN, ENHYDRINA SCHISTOSA**—The *Antivenin, Enhydrina Schistosa (Systemic)* monograph is not included in this published version of the USP DI database. Copies of the monograph are available on request from Micromedex, Inc. - Reprint Requests, 6200 S. Syracuse Way, Suite 300, Englewood, CO 80111; telephone (303) 486-6400; telefax (303) 486-6464; Email: USPDI@MDX.COM.

**ANTIVENIN, LATRODECTUS MACTANS**—The *Antivenin, Latrodectus Mactans (Systemic)* monograph is not included in this published version of the USP DI database. Copies of the monograph are available on request from Micromedex, Inc. - Reprint Requests, 6200 S. Syracuse Way, Suite 300, Englewood, CO 80111; telephone (303) 486-6400; telefax (303) 486-6464; Email: USPDI@MDX.COM.

**ANTIVENIN, MICRURUS FULVIUS**—The *Antivenin, Micrurus Fulvius (Systemic)* monograph is not included in this published version of the USP DI database. Copies of the monograph are available on request from Micromedex, Inc. - Reprint Requests, 6200 S. Syracuse Way, Suite 300, Englewood, CO 80111; telephone (303) 486-6400; telefax (303) 486-6464; Email: USPDI@MDX.COM.

**ANTIVENIN, NOTECHIS SCUTATUS**—The *Antivenin, Notechis Scutatus (Systemic)* monograph is not included in this published version of the USP DI database. Copies of the monograph are available on request from Micromedex, Inc. - Reprint Requests, 6200 S. Syracuse Way, Suite 300, Englewood, CO 80111; telephone (303) 486-6400; telefax (303) 486-6464; Email: USPDI@MDX.COM.

**ANTIVENIN, PSEUDONAJA TEXTILIS**—The *Antivenin, Pseudonaja Textilis (Systemic)* monograph is not included in this published version of the USP DI database. Copies of the monograph are available on request from Micromedex, Inc. - Reprint Requests, 6200 S. Syracuse Way, Suite 300, Englewood, CO 80111; telephone (303) 486-6400; telefax (303) 486-6464; Email: USPDI@MDX.COM.

**APOMORPHINE**—The *Apomorphine (Systemic)* monograph is not included in this published version of the USP DI database. Copies of the monograph are available on request from Micromedex, Inc. - Reprint Requests, 6200 S. Syracuse Way, Suite 300, Englewood, CO 80111; telephone (303) 486-6400; telefax (303) 486-6464; Email: USPDI@MDX.COM.

# APPETITE SUPPRESSANTS Systemic

This monograph includes information on the following: 1) Benzphetamine†; 2) Diethylpropion; 3) Fenfluramine*†; 4) Mazindol; 5) Phendimetrazine†; 6) Phentermine.

Note: **Use of fenfluramine or its dextrostereoisomer, dexfenfluramine, as a single agent or in combination with phentermine, has been associated with valvular heart disease. Because of the seriousness of this adverse effect, fenfluramine and dexfenfluramine were withdrawn from the market in September of 1997.**

INN:
- Benzphetamine—Benzfetamine
- Diethylpropion—Amfepramone

VA CLASSIFICATION (Primary):
- Benzphetamine—GA751
- Diethylpropion—GA751
- Fenfluramine—GA751
- Mazindol—GA751
- Phendimetrazine—GA751
- Phentermine—GA751

Note: Controlled substances in the U.S. and Canada as follows:

| Drug | U.S. | Canada |
|---|---|---|
| Benzphetamine | III | † |
| Diethylpropion | IV | C |
| Fenfluramine | IV | † |
| Mazindol | IV | |
| Phendimetrazine | III | † |
| Phentermine | IV | C |

Commonly used brand name(s): *Adipex-P*[6]; *Adipost*[5]; *Anorex SR*[5]; *Appecon*[5]; *Bontril PDM*[5]; *Bontril Slow-Release*[5]; *Didrex*[1]; *Fastin*[6]; *Ionamin*[6]; *Mazanor*[4]; *Melfiat-105 Unicelles*[5]; *OBY-CAP*[6]; *Obalan*[5]; *Obe-Nix*[6]; *Obezine*[5]; *PT 105*[5]; *Panshape M*[6]; *Parzine*[5]; *Phendiet*[5]; *Phendiet-105*[5]; *Phendimet*[5]; *Phentercot*[5]; *Phentride*[6]; *Plegine*[5]; *Prelu-2*[5]; *Rexigen Forte*[5]; *Sanorex*[4]; *T-Diet*[4]; *Tenuate*[2]; *Tenuate Dospan*[2]; *Tepanil Ten-Tab*[2]; *Teramine*[6]; *Wehless*[5]; *Wehless-105 Timecelles*[5]; *Zantryl*[6].

Note: For a listing of dosage forms and brand names by country availability, see *Dosage Forms* section(s).

*Not commercially available in the U.S.
†Not commercially available in Canada.

## Category
Appetite suppressant.

## Indications
Note: Bracketed information in the *Indications* section refers to uses that are not included in U.S. product labeling.

### Accepted
Obesity, exogenous (treatment)—Benzphetamine, diethylpropion, mazindol, phendimetrazine, and phentermine are indicated in the management of exogenous obesity for short-term use (a few weeks) in conjunction with a regimen of weight reduction based on caloric restriction, exercise, and behavior modification. The limited usefulness of these agents should be measured against risk factors inherent in their use.

### Unaccepted
Fenfluramine has been used as an appetite suppressant in the treatment of exogenous obesity and has been used off-label in the treatment of infantile autism. However, use of fenfluramine, as a single agent or in combination with phentermine, has been associated with valvular heart disease. Because of the seriousness of this adverse effect, fenfluramine was withdrawn from the market in September of 1997.

## Pharmacology/Pharmacokinetics

### Physicochemical characteristics
Molecular weight—
- Benzphetamine hydrochloride: 275.82.
- Diethylpropion hydrochloride: 241.76.
- Fenfluramine hydrochloride: 267.72.
- Mazindol: 284.74.
- Phendimetrazine tartrate: 341.36.
- Phentermine: 149.24.
- Phentermine hydrochloride: 185.70.

### Mechanism of action/Effect
Although the mechanism of action of the appetite suppressants has not been completely established, they are sympathomimetic amines and have pharmacological effects similar to those of amphetamines, including central nervous system (CNS) stimulation and elevation of blood pressure. Tachyphylaxis or tolerance to appetite suppression has been shown to develop. It is believed that the main effect of these medications is on the appetite control center in the hypothalamus and that hunger is decreased by alteration of the chemical control of nerve impulse transmission.

Fenfluramine differs from the other appetite suppressants in that it is more likely to produce CNS depression instead of stimulation, and, often, a decrease in blood pressure. Its main CNS action is probably through serotonin metabolism instead of dopamine and norepinephrine metabolism.

Mazindol differs by lacking the phenethylamine structure of the other appetite suppressants. It appears to inhibit neuronal uptake of norepinephrine and synaptically released dopamine.

It has not been established that the action of these medications in treating obesity is primarily suppression of appetite. Other CNS actions and/or metabolic effects may be involved.

### Biotransformation
Hepatic.

| Drug | Half-life (hr) | Duration of Action (hr) | Elimination |
|---|---|---|---|
| Benzphetamine | 6–12 | | |
| Diethylpropion | 4–6 | | Renal |
|   Tablets | | 4 | |
|   Extended-release Tablets | | 12 | |
| Fenfluramine | 11–30 | 4–6 | Renal |
| Mazindol | 10 | 8–15 | Renal |
| Phendimetrazine | 5–12.5 | 4 | |
| Phentermine | 19–24 | | Renal |
|   Capsules, Tablets (8 mg) | | 4 | |
|   Capsules (30 mg), Tablets (37.5 mg), or Resin Capsules | | 12–14 | |

## Precautions to Consider

### Cross-sensitivity and/or related problems
Patients sensitive to other sympathomimetics (for example, amphetamines, ephedrine, epinephrine, isoproterenol, metaproterenol, norepinephrine, phenylephrine, phenylpropanolamine, pseudoephedrine, terbutaline) may be sensitive to this medication also.

### Carcinogenicity/Mutagenicity
Studies have not been done.

### Pregnancy/Reproduction
Pregnancy—
*Benzphetamine*—
- Benzphetamine is contraindicated during pregnancy because it may cause harm to the fetus. If pregnancy occurs during therapy, the patient should be informed of the risk to the fetus.
- Studies in mammals have shown amphetamines to be teratogenic and embryotoxic when given in high multiples of the human dose.

FDA Pregnancy Category X.

*Diethylpropion*—
- Adequate and well controlled studies in humans have not been done. Abuse of diethylpropion during pregnancy may result in withdrawal symptoms in the neonate since diethylpropion and its active metabolites are believed to cross the placenta.
- Studies in rats given up to 9 times the human dose have shown no evidence of impaired fertility or harm to the fetus.

FDA Pregnancy Category B.

*Fenfluramine*—
- Studies in humans have not been done.
- Studies in animals have shown that fenfluramine is potentially embryotoxic and reduces conception rate when given in doses 20 times the human dose.

FDA Pregnancy Category C.

*Mazindol*—
Reproduction studies in animals have shown that mazindol increases neonatal mortality and possibly increases the incidence of rib anomalies when given in relatively high doses.

FDA pregnancy category not currently included in product labeling.

*Phendimetrazine*—
Problems with phendimetrazine in humans have not been documented.

FDA pregnancy category not currently included in product labeling.

*Phentermine*—
Problems with phentermine in humans have not been documented.

FDA pregnancy category not currently included in product labeling.

**Breast-feeding**
Diethylpropion and its metabolites and benzphetamine are distributed into breast milk. It is not known if the other appetite suppressants are distributed into breast milk and problems in nursing infants have not been documented.

**Pediatrics**
Appetite suppressants are not recommended for use in children up to 12 years of age, because appropriate studies have not been performed in the pediatric population.

**Geriatrics**
No information is available on the relationship of age to the effects of the appetite suppressants in geriatric patients.

**Dental**
Appetite suppressants may decrease or inhibit salivary flow, especially in middle-aged or elderly patients, thus contributing to the development of caries, periodontal disease, oral candidiasis, and discomfort.

The leukopenic and thrombocytopenic effects of diethylpropion, although rarely reported, may result in an increased incidence of microbial infection, delayed healing, and gingival bleeding. If leukopenia or thrombocytopenia occurs, dental work should be deferred until blood counts have returned to normal. Patient instruction in proper oral hygiene should include caution in use of regular toothbrushes, dental floss, and toothpicks.

**Drug interactions and/or related problems**
See *Table 1*, page 457.

**Medical considerations/Contraindications**
See *Table 2*, page 458.

**Patient monitoring**
The following may be especially important in patient monitoring (other tests may be warranted in some patients, depending on condition; » = major clinical significance):

» Cardiac evaluations
(recommended to detect cardiopulmonary disease in patients who are receiving appetite suppressants in combination or for long-term treatment; heart murmur usually is detectable before more severe symptoms of valvular heart disease develop)

## Side/Adverse Effects

Note: An epidemiologic study found an increased risk of primary pulmonary hypertension in patients who had used anorexigenic medications, primarily fenfluramine and its dextrostereoisomer, dexfenfluramine, within the previous year or for longer than 3 months. The risk of primary pulmonary hypertension associated with long-term appetite suppressant use (> 3 months) is estimated to be 23 to 46 cases per million persons exposed per year. This condition has a 4-year survival rate of about 55%. Appetite suppressant treatment should be discontinued in any patient who develops unexplained dyspnea, angina pectoris, syncope, or lower extremity edema. These patients should be evaluated for pulmonary hypertension and valvular heart disease.

Abnormalities in the mitral, aortic, and/or tricuspid valves have been reported in patients receiving the combination of phentermine and fenfluramine for 1 to 28 months as well as in patients receiving either fenfluramine or its dextrostereoisomer, dexfenfluramine, as monotherapy. The histopathological abnormalities of the involved heart valves resemble those seen in carcinoid syndrome or ergotamine toxicity. Heart murmur usually is detectable before more severe symptoms develop. Also, abnormal valve function, primarily aortic regurgitation, was found in about 30% of 291 asymptomatic patients receiving either fenfluramine or dexfenfluramine in combination with phentermine who were given echocardiographic evaluations.

The following side/adverse effects have been selected on the basis of their potential clinical significance (possible signs and symptoms in parentheses where appropriate)—not necessarily inclusive:

**Those indicating need for medical attention**
Incidence more frequent
*Elevated blood pressure*—rare with fenfluramine; *valvular heart disease* (decreased ability to exercise; swelling of feet or lower legs; trouble in breathing)—may be asymptomatic

Note: *Valvular heart disease* has been reported with use of fenfluramine or its dextrostereoisomer, dexfenfluramine, either as a single agent or in combination with phentermine. Among asymptomatic patients receiving either fenfluramine or dexfenfluramine in combination with phentermine who were tested, about 30% had abnormal valve findings in echocardiographic evaluations.

Incidence less frequent or rare
*Allergic reaction* (skin rash or hives); *blood dyscrasias* (sore throat and fever; unusual bleeding or bruising)—with diethylpropion; *confusion or mental depression; psychotic episodes; primary pulmonary hypertension* (chest pain; decreased ability to exercise; fainting; swelling of feet or lower legs; trouble in breathing)—usually with fenfluramine or its dextrostereoisomer, dexfenfluramine

**Those indicating need for medical attention only if they continue or are bothersome**
Incidence more frequent
*CNS stimulation* (false sense of well-being or mild euphoria; irritability; nervousness or restlessness; trouble in sleeping)

Note: Drowsiness, fatigue, or mental depression may follow the stimulant effects.

Incidence less frequent or rare
*Blurred vision; changes in libido* (changes in sexual desire); *constipation; clumsiness or unsteadiness*—with fenfluramine; *diarrhea; difficulty in talking*—with fenfluramine; *dizziness or lightheadedness; drowsiness; dryness of mouth; dysuria* (difficult or painful urination); *fast, pounding, or irregular heartbeat; headache; impotence* (decreased sexual ability); *increased sweating; nausea or vomiting; nightmares*—with fenfluramine; *polyuria or urinary frequency* (frequent urge to urinate or increased urination); *stomach cramps or pain; unpleasant taste; unusual tiredness or weakness*—with fenfluramine

**Those indicating possible withdrawal and/or the need for medical attention if they occur after medication is discontinued**
*Mental depression; nausea or vomiting; stomach cramps or pain; trembling; trouble in sleeping or nightmares; unusual tiredness or weakness*

## Overdose

For specific information on the agents used in the management of appetite suppressant overdose, see:
- *Barbiturates (Systemic)* monograph;
- *Beta-adrenergic Blocking Agents (Systemic)* monograph;
- *Charcoal, Activated (Oral-Local)* monograph;
- *Chlorpromazine* in *Phenothiazines (Systemic)* monograph;
- *Diazepam* in *Benzodiazepines (Systemic)* monograph;
- *Haloperidol (Systemic)* monograph;
- *Lidocaine (Systemic)* monograph;
- *Nitrates (Systemic)* monograph; and/or
- *Phentolamine (Systemic)* monograph.

For more information on the management of overdose or unintentional ingestion, **contact a Poison Control Center** (see *Poison Control Center Listing*).

**Clinical effects of overdose**
The following effects have been selected on the basis of their potential clinical significance (possible signs and symptoms in parentheses where appropriate)—not necessarily inclusive:
*Abdominal or stomach cramps; arrhythmias* (irregular heartbeat); *confusion; diarrhea, severe; fast breathing; fever; hostility with assaultiveness; hallucinations* (seeing, hearing, or feeling things that are not there); *irregular blood pressure; nausea or vomiting, severe; panic state; restlessness; tremor*

Note: Hyperpyrexia, rhabdomyolysis, cardiovascular effects such as arrhythmias, hypertension or hypotension, and circulatory collapse may occur. Convulsions and coma usually precede death.

Diarrhea, hostility, hallucinations, irregular blood pressure, panic state, rhabdomyolysis, and cardiovascular effects have not been reported for fenfluramine.

## Treatment of overdose
Since there is no specific antidote for overdosage with appetite suppressants, treatment is symptomatic and supportive with possible utilization of the following:
To decrease absorption—
Induction of emesis and/or use of gastric lavage followed by the administration of activated charcoal is primary (fenfluramine overdose may produce early unconsciousness; drug-induced emesis is not recommended for fenfluramine).
To enhance elimination—
Acidification of urine and forced diuresis are recommended.
Specific treatment—
Barbiturate sedatives or chlorpromazine (or haloperidol to lessen anticholinergic effects) are sometimes used to control excessive CNS stimulation. (Diazepam or phenobarbital may be used to control convulsions or muscular hyperactivity associated with fenfluramine overdosage. Caution necessary with use of CNS depressants and fenfluramine because of possible additive CNS depressant effects.)
Intravenous phentolamine or nitrites to control hypertension.
Intravenous lidocaine for cardiac arrhythmias.
Beta-blocker for control of tachycardia.
Monitoring—
Monitor cardiovascular and respiratory functions.
Supportive care—
Intravenous fluids for hypotension control.
Mechanical respirator, when necessary.
Protect patient from self-injury by use of restraints if necessary.
Patients in whom intentional overdose is known or suspected should be referred for psychiatric consultation.

## Patient Consultation
As an aid to patient consultation, refer to *Advice for the Patient, Appetite Suppressants (Systemic)*.
In providing consultation, consider emphasizing the following selected information (» = major clinical significance):

### Before using this medication
» Conditions affecting use, especially:
Sensitivity to appetite suppressants or other sympathomimetics
Pregnancy—Benzphetamine is contraindicated in human pregnancy (FDA Category X); in animal studies, fenfluramine was shown to be embryotoxic and to reduce rate of conception; mazindol was shown to increase the incidence of neonatal mortality and possibly to increase the incidence of rib anomalies when given in relatively high doses
Breast-feeding—Benzphetamine and diethylpropion are distributed into breast milk
Use in children—Not recommended for appetite suppression in children up to 12 years of age
Other medications, especially alcohol, other appetite suppressants, MAO inhibitors, other CNS stimulants (with all appetite suppressants except fenfluramine), or CNS depressants (with fenfluramine)
Other medical problems, especially agitated states, alcoholism, advanced arteriosclerosis, symptomatic cardiovascular disease including arrhythmias, cerebral ischemia, history of drug abuse or dependence, glaucoma, hypertension, hyperthyroidism, psychosis, or uremia

### Proper use of this medication
Taking the last dose of the regular dosage form for each day about 4 to 6 hours before bedtime (does not apply to fenfluramine)
» Importance of not taking more medication than the amount prescribed, because of habit-forming potential
» Not increasing dose if medication is not effective after a few weeks; checking with physician
» Proper dosing
» Proper storage
*For extended-release and long-acting dosage forms only*
Proper administration: Swallowing whole; not breaking, crushing, or chewing
Taking the daily dose about 10 to 14 hours before bedtime to minimize the possibility of insomnia (does not apply to fenfluramine)
*For mazindol*
1-mg tablet—Taking last dose 4 to 6 hours before bedtime
2-mg tablet—Taking once-a-day dose 10 to 14 hours before bedtime

### Precautions while using this medication
Regular visits to physician to check progress during therapy
Possible dryness of mouth; using sugarless candy or gum, ice, or saliva substitute for relief; checking with physician or dentist if dry mouth continues for more than 2 weeks
» Caution if dizziness, drowsiness, lightheadedness, or elated mood or euphoria occurs; not driving or using machines or doing other things that require alertness
» Caution if any kind of surgery, dental treatment, or emergency treatment is required
» Importance of reporting chest pain, decreased exercise tolerance, fainting, swelling of feet or lower legs, or trouble in breathing to physician immediately
» Suspected physical or psychological dependence: checking with physician
» Not increasing dosage if tolerance develops; checking with physician
Diabetic patients: Insulin or oral antidiabetic–agent requirements may be altered
» Checking with physician before discontinuing medication after prolonged high-dose therapy; gradual dosage reduction may be necessary to avoid possibility of withdrawal symptoms
*For fenfluramine*
» Avoiding the use of alcoholic beverages or other CNS depressants

### Side/adverse effects
Symptoms of potential side effects, especially elevated blood pressure, valvular heart disease (reported with fenfluramine or its dextrostereoisomer, dexfenfluramine, either as a single agent or in combination with phentermine), allergic reaction, blood dyscrasias (with diethylpropion), confusion or mental depression, psychotic episodes, or primary pulmonary hypertension (usually with fenfluramine or dexfenfluramine)

## General Dosing Information
The dosage of appetite suppressants should be individualized to obtain an adequate response with the lowest effective dose.

To reduce the possibility of insomnia caused by appetite suppressants (except fenfluramine), the last dose of the regular dosage form for each day should be administered approximately 4 to 6 hours before bedtime and the daily dose of the extended-release or long-acting dosage form should be administered approximately 10 to 14 hours before bedtime.

Appetite suppressants are recommended for short-term use only, since tolerance to the anorectic effect may develop in a few weeks.

If tolerance to the anorectic effect develops, the medication should be discontinued. The dosage should not be increased in an attempt to increase the effect.

Patients should report decreased exercise tolerance to physician immediately, as this may be an early symptom of primary pulmonary hypertension or a symptom of valvular heart disease. Also, any chest pain, fainting, swelling of feet or lower legs, or trouble in breathing should be reported to physician immediately, and appetite suppressant treatment should be discontinued.

Prolonged use, especially of larger-than-usual therapeutic doses, may result in mental or physical dependence.

When the medication is to be discontinued following prolonged high-dose administration, the dosage should be reduced gradually in order to avoid the possibility of a rebound increase in appetite and to decrease withdrawal symptoms.

---

### BENZPHETAMINE

## Summary of Differences
Precautions:
Pregnancy/reproduction—FDA Pregnancy Category X.
Drug interactions and/or related problems—Caution is needed with concomitant use of urinary acidifiers and alkalizers with benzphetamine.

## Additional Dosing Information
See also *General Dosing Information*.
If a single daily dose is administered, it is preferably given either mid-morning or mid-afternoon, depending on the patient's eating habits.

## Oral Dosage Forms

### BENZPHETAMINE HYDROCHLORIDE TABLETS

**Usual adult dose**
Appetite suppressant—
　Oral, initially 25 to 50 mg once a day in midmorning or midafternoon, the dosage being increased as needed and tolerated.

**Usual adult prescribing limits**
Up to 150 mg a day.

**Usual pediatric dose**
Children up to 12 years of age—Use is not recommended.

**Strength(s) usually available**
U.S.—
　50 mg (Rx) [*Didrex* (scored; lactose; sorbitol)].
Canada—
　Not commercially available.

**Packaging and storage**
Store between 15 and 30 °C (59 and 86 °F), in a tight container, unless otherwise specified by manufacturer.

**Note**
Controlled substance in the U.S.

---

## DIETHYLPROPION

## Summary of Differences

Precautions:
　Medical considerations/contraindications—Caution also needed in epilepsy.

## Oral Dosage Forms

### DIETHYLPROPION HYDROCHLORIDE TABLETS USP

**Usual adult dose**
Appetite suppressant—
　Oral, 25 mg three times a day, one hour before meals. Alternatively, a dose may be taken in mid-evening, if desired, to overcome night hunger.

**Usual pediatric dose**
Children up to 12 years of age—Use is not recommended.

**Strength(s) usually available**
U.S.—
　25 mg (Rx) [*Tenuate* (lactose); GENERIC].
Canada—
　25 mg (Rx) [*Tenuate* (tartrazine)].

**Packaging and storage**
Store below 40 °C (104 °F), preferably between 15 and 30 °C (59 and 86 °F), unless otherwise specified by manufacturer. Store in a well-closed container.

**Note**
Controlled substance in both the U.S. and Canada.

### DIETHYLPROPION HYDROCHLORIDE EXTENDED-RELEASE TABLETS

**Usual adult dose**
Appetite suppressant—
　Oral, 75 mg once a day at mid-morning.

**Usual pediatric dose**
Children up to 12 years of age—Use is not recommended.

**Strength(s) usually available**
U.S.—
　75 mg (Rx) [*Tenuate Dospan; Tepanil Ten-Tab;* GENERIC].
Canada—
　75 mg (Rx) [*Tenuate Dospan*].

**Packaging and storage**
Store below 40 °C (104 °F), preferably between 15 and 30 °C (59 and 86 °F), in a well-closed container, unless otherwise specified by manufacturer.

**Auxiliary labeling**
• Swallow tablets whole.

**Note**
Controlled substance in both the U.S. and Canada.

---

## FENFLURAMINE

## Summary of Differences

Indications:
　Also has been used for treatment of infantile autism.
Pharmacology/pharmacokinetics:
　More likely to produce CNS depression instead of CNS stimulation.
Precautions:
　Pregnancy—
　　Animal reproduction studies have suggested an embryotoxic potential.
　Drug interactions and/or related problems—
　　Hypotensive effects of antihypertensives may be increased with concurrent use of fenfluramine.
　　Enhanced CNS depressant effects may result from concurrent use of fenfluramine and CNS depression–producing medications.
　　No additive effects with CNS stimulation–producing medications or thyroid hormones.
　　No potential interaction with phenothiazines.
　Medical considerations/contraindications—
　　Not contraindicated in agitated states, advanced arteriosclerosis, or hyperthyroidism.
　　Caution needed in patients with history of mental depression.
Side/adverse effects:
　Elevated blood pressure is rare with fenfluramine.
　Primary pulmonary hypertension may occur rarely.
　Valvular heart disease has been reported with use of fenfluramine either as a single agent or in combination with phentermine.
　CNS depressant side effects, such as drowsiness, occur more frequently than with other appetite suppressants.

## Additional Dosing Information

See also *General Dosing Information*.
Fenfluramine has an onset of action of 1 to 2 hours.

## Oral Dosage Forms

### FENFLURAMINE HYDROCHLORIDE EXTENDED-RELEASE CAPSULES

**Usual adult dose**
Appetite suppressant—
　Oral, initially 60 mg once a day, the dosage being increased to 120 mg per day as needed and tolerated.

**Usual adult prescribing limits**
Up to 120 mg a day.

**Usual pediatric dose**
Appetite suppressant—
　Children up to 12 years of age: Use is not recommended.

**Strength(s) usually available**
U.S.—
　Not commercially available.
Canada—
　Not commercially available.

Note: Because of the seriousness of the valvular heart disease associated with the use of fenfluramine, the medication was withdrawn from the market in September of 1997.

**Packaging and storage**
Store below 40 °C (104 °F), preferably between 15 and 30 °C (59 and 86 °F), in a well-closed container, unless otherwise specified by manufacturer.

**Auxiliary labeling**
• Swallow capsules whole.

**Note**
Controlled substance in the U.S.

### FENFLURAMINE HYDROCHLORIDE TABLETS

**Usual adult dose**
Appetite suppressant—
　Oral, initially 20 mg three times a day thirty minutes to one hour before meals, the dosage being increased by 20 mg per day at one-week intervals, if necessary, up to a maximum of 40 mg three times a day.

Note: If the initial dosage is not well tolerated, the dosage may be reduced to 20 mg twice daily and thereafter increased gradually in order to minimize side effects.

**Usual adult prescribing limits**
Up to 120 mg a day.

**Usual pediatric dose**
Appetite suppressant—
  Children up to 12 years of age: Use is not recommended.

**Strength(s) usually available**
U.S.—
  Not commercially available.
Canada—
  Not commercially available.

Note: Because of the seriousness of the valvular heart disease associated with the use of fenfluramine, the medication was withdrawn from the market in September of 1997.

**Packaging and storage**
Store below 40 °C (104 °F), preferably between 15 and 30 °C (59 and 86 °F), in a well-closed container, unless otherwise specified by manufacturer.

**Note**
Controlled substance in the U.S.

## MAZINDOL

## Summary of Differences
Precautions:
  Pregnancy—
    Animal studies have suggested a teratogenic potential with high doses.
  Drug interactions and/or related problems—
    Effects of vasopressors may be potentiated when used concomitantly with mazindol.
  Medical considerations/contraindications—
    Contraindicated in cerebral ischemia, psychosis, and uremia.
    Not contraindicated in advanced arteriosclerosis or hyperthyroidism.

## Oral Dosage Forms

### MAZINDOL TABLETS USP

**Usual adult dose**
Appetite suppressant—
  Oral, initially, 1 mg once daily one hour before the first meal of the day, the dosage being increased to 1 mg three times a day one hour before meals; or 2 mg once a day one hour before lunch.

**Usual pediatric dose**
Children up to 12 years of age—Use is not recommended.

**Strength(s) usually available**
U.S.—
  1 mg (Rx) [*Mazanor* (scored; lactose); *Sanorex* (lactose)].
  2 mg (Rx) [*Sanorex* (scored; lactose)].
Canada—
  1 mg (Rx) [*Sanorex* (corn starch; lactose)].
  2 mg (Rx) [*Sanorex* (scored; corn starch; lactose; tartrazine)].

**Packaging and storage**
Store below 25 °C (77 °F), unless otherwise specified by manufacturer. Store in a tight container.

**Note**
Controlled substance in the U.S.

## PHENDIMETRAZINE

## Oral Dosage Forms

### PHENDIMETRAZINE TARTRATE CAPSULES USP

**Usual adult dose**
Appetite suppressant—
  Oral, 35 mg two or three times a day one hour before meals.

**Usual adult prescribing limits**
70 mg three times a day.

**Usual pediatric dose**
Children up to 12 years of age—Use is not recommended.

**Strength(s) usually available**
U.S.—
  35 mg (Rx) [*Obalan; Phendiet; Wehless;* GENERIC].
Canada—
  Not commercially available.

**Packaging and storage**
Store below 40 °C (104 °F), preferably between 15 and 30 °C (59 and 86 °F), unless otherwise specified by manufacturer. Store in a tight container.

**Note**
Controlled substance in the U.S.

### PHENDIMETRAZINE TARTRATE EXTENDED-RELEASE CAPSULES

**Usual adult dose**
Appetite suppressant—
  Oral, 105 mg once a day, thirty to sixty minutes before the morning meal.

**Usual pediatric dose**
Children up to 12 years of age—Use is not recommended.

**Strength(s) usually available**
U.S.—
  105 mg (Rx) [*Adipost; Anorex SR; Appecon; Bontril Slow-Release; Melfiat-105 Unicelles; Phendiet-105; Prelu-2; PT 105; Rexigen Forte; Wehless-105 Timecelles;* GENERIC].
Canada—
  Not commercially available.

**Packaging and storage**
Store below 40 °C (104 °F), preferably between 15 and 30 °C (59 and 86 °F), in a well-closed container, unless otherwise specified by manufacturer.

**Auxiliary labeling**
• Swallow capsules whole.

**Note**
Controlled substance in the U.S.

### PHENDIMETRAZINE TARTRATE TABLETS USP

**Usual adult dose**
Appetite suppressant—
  Oral, 17.5 to 35 mg two or three times a day one hour before meals.

**Usual adult prescribing limits**
70 mg three times a day.

**Usual pediatric dose**
Children up to 12 years of age—Use is not recommended.

**Strength(s) usually available**
U.S.—
  35 mg (Rx) [*Bontril PDM* (scored); *Obalan; Obezine; Parzine; Phendiet; Phendimet; Plegine* (scored); GENERIC].
Canada—
  Not commercially available.

**Packaging and storage**
Store below 40 °C (104 °F), preferably between 15 and 30 °C (59 and 86 °F), unless otherwise specified by manufacturer. Store in a well-closed container.

**Note**
Controlled substance in the U.S.

### PHENDIMETRAZINE TARTRATE EXTENDED-RELEASE TABLETS

**Usual adult dose**
See *Phendimetrazine Tartrate Extended-Release Capsules*.

**Usual pediatric dose**
See *Phendimetrazine Tartrate Extended-Release Capsules*.

**Strength(s) usually available**
U.S.—
  105 mg (Rx) [GENERIC].
Canada—
  Not commercially available.

**Packaging and storage**
Store below 40 °C (104 °F), preferably between 15 and 30 °C (59 and 86 °F), in a well-closed container, unless otherwise specified by manufacturer.

**Auxiliary labeling**
• Swallow capsules whole.

**Note**
Controlled substance in the U.S.

## PHENTERMINE

### Summary of Differences
Side/adverse effects:
  Valvular heart disease has been reported with use of phentermine in combination with fenfluramine or its dextrostereoisomer, dexfenfluramine.

## Oral Dosage Forms

### PHENTERMINE HYDROCHLORIDE CAPSULES USP

**Usual adult dose**
Appetite suppressant—
  Oral, 15 to 37.5 mg (base) once a day before breakfast, or one to two hours after breakfast.

**Usual pediatric dose**
Children up to 12 years of age—Use is not recommended.

**Strength(s) usually available**
U.S.—
  15 mg (base) (Rx) [*Phentride;* GENERIC].
  18.75 mg (base) (Rx) [*Phentercot;* GENERIC].
  30 mg (base) (Rx) [*Fastin; Obe-Nix; OBY-CAP; Phentercot; Phentride; T-Diet; Teramine; Zantryl;* GENERIC].
  37.5 mg (base) (Rx) [*Adipex-P; Obe-Nix; Phentercot; Phentride;* GENERIC].
Canada—
  30 mg (base) (Rx) [*Fastin*].

**Packaging and storage**
Store below 40 °C (104 °F), preferably between 15 and 30 °C (59 and 86 °F), unless otherwise specified by manufacturer. Store in a tight container.

**Note**
Controlled substance in both the U.S. and Canada.

### PHENTERMINE HYDROCHLORIDE TABLETS USP

**Usual adult dose**
Appetite suppressant—
  Oral, 15 to 37.5 mg (base) a day, as a single dose before breakfast or one to two hours after breakfast, or in divided doses one half hour before meals.

**Usual pediatric dose**
Children up to 12 years of age—Use is not recommended.

**Strength(s) usually available**
U.S.—
  8 mg (base) (Rx) [*Phentercot; Phentride; Teramine;* GENERIC].
  30 mg (base) (Rx) [*Phentride;* GENERIC].
  37.5 mg (base) (Rx) [*Adipex-P* (scored); *Panshape M; Phentercot;* GENERIC].
Canada—
  Not commercially available.

**Packaging and storage**
Store below 40 °C (104 °F), preferably between 15 and 30 °C (59 and 86 °F), unless otherwise specified by manufacturer. Store in a tight container.

**Note**
Controlled substance in the U.S.

### PHENTERMINE RESIN CAPSULES

**Usual adult dose**
Appetite suppressant—
  Oral, 15 or 30 mg once a day before breakfast.

**Usual pediatric dose**
Children up to 12 years of age—Use is not recommended.

**Strength(s) usually available**
U.S.—
  15 mg (Rx) [*Ionamin;* GENERIC].
  30 mg (Rx) [*Ionamin;* GENERIC].
Canada—
  15 mg (Rx) [*Ionamin*].
  30 mg (Rx) [*Ionamin*].

**Packaging and storage**
Store between 15 and 30 °C (59 and 86 °F), in a tight container, unless otherwise specified by manufacturer.

**Auxiliary labeling**
• Swallow capsules whole.
• Take in the morning.

**Note**
Controlled substance in both the U.S. and Canada.

Revised: 08/29/94
Interim revision: 06/30/95; 08/19/97; 09/23/97

## Table 1. Drug Interactions and/or Related Problems

The following drug interactions and/or related problems have been selected on the basis of their potential clinical significance (possible mechanism in parentheses where appropriate)—not necessarily inclusive (» = major clinical significance):

Note: Combinations containing any of the following medications, depending on the amount present, may also interact with this medication.

Legend:
I = Benzphetamine
II = Diethylpropion
III = Fenfluramine
IV = Mazindol
V = Phendimetrazine
VI = Phentermine

| | I | II | III | IV | V | VI |
|---|---|---|---|---|---|---|
| Acidifiers, urinary, such as:<br>  Ammonium chloride<br>  Ascorbic acid<br>  Potassium or sodium phosphates<br>  (concurrent use with benzphetamine may decrease serum concentrations and increase excretion of benzphetamine) | ✔ | | | | | |
| » Alcohol<br>  (concurrent use with appetite suppressants is not recommended since this may increase the potential for CNS effects such as dizziness, lightheadedness, fainting, confusion, or drowsiness [with fenfluramine]) | ✔ | ✔ | ✔ | ✔ | ✔ | ✔ |
| Alkalizers, urinary, such as:<br>  Antacids, calcium- and/or magnesium-containing<br>  Carbonic anhydrase inhibitors<br>  Citrates<br>  Sodium bicarbonate<br>  (concurrent use with benzphetamine may increase serum concentrations and decrease excretion of benzphetamine) | ✔ | | | | | |
| Anesthetics, hydrocarbon inhalation, especially halothane<br>  (chronic use of appetite suppressants prior to anesthesia may result in cardiac arrhythmias because these anesthetics sensitize the myocardium to the effects of sympathomimetics) | ✔ | ✔ | ✔ | ✔ | ✔ | ✔ |

## Table 1. Drug Interactions and/or Related Problems (continued)

| The following drug interactions and/or related problems have been selected on the basis of their potential clinical significance (possible mechanism in parentheses where appropriate)—not necessarily inclusive (» = major clinical significance):<br>Note: Combinations containing any of the following medications, depending on the amount present, may also interact with this medication. | Legend:<br>**I**=Benzphetamine **IV**=Mazindol<br>**II**=Diethylpropion **V**=Phendimetrazine<br>**III**=Fenfluramine **VI**=Phentermine |||||||
|---|:---:|:---:|:---:|:---:|:---:|:---:|
| | **I** | **II** | **III** | **IV** | **V** | **VI** |
| Antidiabetic agents, oral or<br>Insulin<br>    (when appetite suppressants and the concurrent dietary regimen are used in the treatment of obesity, blood glucose concentrations may be altered in patients with diabetes mellitus; dosage adjustment of the hypoglycemic agent may be necessary during and after concurrent therapy) | ✓ | ✓ | ✓ | ✓ | ✓ | ✓ |
| Antihypertensives, especially clonidine, guanadrel, guanethidine, methyldopa, or rauwolfia alkaloids<br>    (hypotensive effects may be increased when used concurrently with fenfluramine) | | | | ✓ | | |
|     (hypotensive effects may be decreased when these medications are used concurrently with appetite suppressants because of displacement from and inhibition of uptake by adrenergic neurons) | ✓ | ✓ | | ✓ | ✓ | ✓ |
| » Appetite suppressants, other, including amphetamines<br>    (valvular heart disease has been reported in patients receiving fenfluramine or its dextrostereoisomer, dexfenfluramine, either as a single agent or in combination with phentermine; abnormal valve function, primarily aortic regurgitation, was found in about 30% of 291 asymptomatic patients receiving either dexfenfluramine or fenfluramine in combination with phentermine who were given echocardiographic evaluations; combined use of appetite suppressants is not recommended) | ✓ | ✓ | ✓ | ✓ | ✓ | ✓ |
| » CNS depression–producing medications, other (see *Appendix II*)<br>    (concurrent use may increase the CNS depressant effects of either these medications or fenfluramine) | | | ✓ | | | |
| » CNS stimulation–producing medications, other (see *Appendix II*) or<br>Thyroid hormones<br>    (concurrent use may increase the CNS stimulant effects of either these medications or appetite suppressants) | ✓ | ✓ | ✓ | ✓ | ✓ | ✓ |
| » Monoamine oxidase (MAO) inhibitors, including furazolidone, procarbazine, and selegiline<br>    (concurrent use may potentiate the sympathomimetic effects of appetite suppressants, possibly resulting in a hypertensive crisis; appetite suppressants should not be administered during or within 14 days following the administration of MAO inhibitors) | ✓ | ✓ | ✓ | ✓ | ✓ | ✓ |
| Phenothiazines, especially chlorpromazine<br>    (concurrent use may antagonize the anorectic effect of appetite suppressants) | ✓ | ✓ | | ✓ | ✓ | ✓ |
| Vasopressors<br>    (effects may be potentiated when vasopressors are used concurrently with mazindol; if necessary to administer a press or amine agent to a patient who has recently received mazindol, initiating pressor therapy in reduced dosage and monitoring of blood pressure at frequent intervals are recommended) | | | | ✓ | | |

## Table 2. Medical considerations/Contraindications*

| The medical considerations/contraindications included have been selected on the basis of their potential clinical significance (reasons given in parentheses where appropriate)—not necessarily inclusive (» = major clinical significance). | Legend:<br>**I**=Benzphetamine **IV**=Mazindol<br>**II**=Diethylpropion **V**=Phendimetrazine<br>**III**=Fenfluramine **VI**=Phentermine |||||||
|---|:---:|:---:|:---:|:---:|:---:|:---:|
| | **I** | **II** | **III** | **IV** | **V** | **VI** |
| ***Except under special circumstances, this medicine should not be used when the following medical problems exist:*** | | | | | | |
| »   Agitated states or | ✓ | ✓ | | ✓ | ✓ | ✓ |
| »   Arteriosclerosis, advanced or | ✓ | ✓ | | | ✓ | ✓ |
| »   Cardiovascular disease, symptomatic, including arrhythmias or | ✓ | | ✓ | ✓ | ✓ | ✓ |
| »   Cerebral ischemia or | | | | ✓ | | |
| »   Glaucoma or | ✓ | ✓ | ✓ | ✓ | ✓ | ✓ |
| »   Hypertension, moderate to severe or | ✓ | ✓ | ✓ | ✓ | ✓ | ✓ |
| »   Hyperthyroidism or | ✓ | ✓ | | | ✓ | ✓ |
| »   Psychosis<br>    (condition may be exacerbated) | | | | ✓ | | |
| »   Alcoholism, active or in remission or | ✓ | ✓ | ✓ | | ✓ | ✓ |
| »   Drug abuse or dependence, history of<br>    (dependence on appetite suppressants may develop) | ✓ | ✓ | | ✓ | ✓ | ✓ |
| »   Uremia<br>    (excretion of appetite suppressants may be altered) | | | | ✓ | | |
| ***Risk-benefit should be considered when the following medical problems exist:*** | | | | | | |
| Cardiovascular disease, symptomatic, including arrhythmias or | | ✓ | | | | |
| Depression, mental, history of or | | | ✓ | | | |
| Hypertension, mild or | ✓ | ✓ | ✓ | ✓ | ✓ | ✓ |

## Table 2. Medical considerations/Contraindications (continued)*

The medical considerations/contraindications included have been selected on the basis of their potential clinical significance (reasons given in parentheses where appropriate)—not necessarily inclusive (» = major clinical significance).

Legend:
I = Benzphetamine
II = Diethylpropion
III = Fenfluramine
IV = Mazindol
V = Phendimetrazine
VI = Phentermine

| | I | II | III | IV | V | VI |
|---|---|---|---|---|---|---|
| Psychosis, especially schizophrenia (condition may be exacerbated) | ✓ | ✓ | ✓ | | ✓ | ✓ |
| Diabetes mellitus (use of appetite suppressants and concomitant dietary restrictions may change the amount of insulin or oral antidiabetic agents needed) | ✓ | ✓ | ✓ | ✓ | ✓ | ✓ |
| Epilepsy (increased risk of seizures) | | | ✓ | | | |
| Sensitivity to appetite suppressants or other sympathomimetics | ✓ | ✓ | ✓ | ✓ | ✓ | ✓ |

*Fenfluramine differs from the other appetite suppressants in that it is more likely to produce CNS depression instead of CNS stimulation

# APRACLONIDINE  Ophthalmic

VA CLASSIFICATION (Primary): OP114
Commonly used brand name(s): *Iopidine*.
Other commonly used names are aplonidine and p-aminoclonidine.
Note: For a listing of dosage forms and brand names by country availability, see *Dosage Forms* section(s).

## Category
Antiglaucoma agent (ophthalmic); antihypertensive, ocular.

## Indications

### Accepted
Glaucoma, open angle (treatment)—Apraclonidine 0.5% is indicated for short-term adjunctive therapy in patients who are on maximally tolerated doses of other medications intended to reduce intraocular pressure (IOP) and who need additional IOP reduction. Patients who already receive two aqueous suppressing medications (e.g., a beta-adrenergic blocking agent and a carbonic anhydrase inhibitor) may not derive additional IOP reduction from the addition of apraclonidine to their treatment regimen, since apraclonidine is also an aqueous-suppressing medication.

Hypertension, ocular (prophylaxis and treatment)—Apraclonidine 1% is indicated to control or prevent postsurgical elevations in intraocular pressure that occur in patients after argon laser trabeculoplasty, argon laser iridotomy, or Nd:YAG laser posterior capsulotomy.

## Pharmacology/Pharmacokinetics

**Physicochemical characteristics**
Molecular weight—281.57.
pKa—9.22.
Other characteristics—The pH of apraclonidine hydrochloride ophthalmic solution is 4.4 to 7.8

**Mechanism of action/Effect**
Apraclonidine is a relatively selective alpha$_2$ adrenergic agonist. When instilled into the eye, apraclonidine ophthalmic solution reduces elevated, as well as normal, intraocular pressure. Aqueous fluorophotometry studies demonstrate that the predominant mechanism of action of ophthalmic apraclonidine is the reduction of aqueous humor flow via stimulation of the alpha-adrenergic system.

**Other actions/effects**
Apraclonidine does not have significant membrane stabilizing (local anesthetic) activity. In addition, ophthalmic apraclonidine has minimal effect on cardiovascular parameters.

**Half-life**
For 0.5% apraclonidine—8 hours.

**Onset of action**
Usually within one hour.

**Peak serum concentration**
For 0.5% apraclonidine—0.9 nanograms per mL.

**Time to peak effect**
Usually three to five hours after application of a single dose.

## Precautions to Consider

**Cross-sensitivity and/or related problems**
Patients sensitive to clonidine may be sensitive to apraclonidine also.

**Carcinogenicity**
Rats and mice administered oral apraclonidine for 2 years in doses of 1 and 0.6 mg per kg of body weight (mg/kg), respectively, did not have any significant change in tumor incidence or type.

**Mutagenicity**
Apraclonidine was not shown to be mutagenic in an *in vivo* mouse micronucleus assay and a series of *in vitro* mutagenicity tests, including the Ames test, a mouse lymphoma forward mutation assay, a chromosome aberration assay in cultured Chinese hamster ovary (CHO) cells, a sister chromatid exchange assay in CHO cells, and a cell transformation assay.

**Pregnancy/Reproduction**
Fertility—Studies on reproduction and fertility in male and female rats given 0.5 mg/kg of apraclonidine have not shown adverse effects on fertility.

Pregnancy—Adequate and well-controlled studies have not been done in humans.

Apraclonidine has been shown to have an embryocidal effect on rabbits that were given 3 mg/kg apraclonidine orally. Dose-related maternal toxicity was observed in pregnant rats given 0.3 mg/kg apraclonidine.

FDA Pregnancy Category C.

**Breast-feeding**
It is not known whether ophthalmic apraclonidine is distributed into breast milk. However, problems in humans have not been documented. It is recommended that patients do not breast-feed on the day on which 1% apraclonidine is administered.

**Pediatrics**
Appropriate studies on the relationship of age to the effects of apraclonidine have not been performed in the pediatric population. Safety and efficacy have not been established.

**Geriatrics**
No information is available on the relationship of age to the effects of apraclonidine in geriatric patients.

**Drug interactions and/or related problems**
The following drug interactions and/or related problems have been selected on the basis of their potential clinical significance (possible mechanism in parentheses where appropriate)—not necessarily inclusive (» = major clinical significance):

Note: Combinations containing any of the following medications, depending on the amount present, may also interact with this medication.

Monoamine oxidase (MAO) inhibitors, including furazolidone, procarbazine, and selegiline
(some clinicians believe that apraclonidine should not be used during or within 14 days following administration of MAO inhibitors, because the antihypertensive effects of either apraclonidine or the MAO inhibitor may be potentiated by concurrent use; however, this is controversial)

### Medical considerations/Contraindications

The medical considerations/contraindications included have been selected on the basis of their potential clinical significance (reasons given in parentheses where appropriate)—not necessarily inclusive (» = major clinical significance).

*Risk-benefit should be considered when the following medical problems exist:*

» Cardiovascular disease, severe, including hypertension or
Cerebrovascular disease or
Coronary insufficiency or
Myocardial infarction, recent or
Raynaud's disease or
Thromboangiitis obliterans
(in clinical studies, the total usual adult dose of 2 drops of 1% and short-term three-times-a-day use of 0.5% ophthalmic apraclonidine had minimal effect on heart rate and blood pressure. However, since there is a possibility of systemic absorption and because apraclonidine is a potent medication, caution should be used when administering 0.5 or 1% apraclonidine to patients who have severe cardiovascular disease, including hypertension, and when administering 0.5% apraclonidine to patients with other cardiovascular diseases)

Depression
(use of apraclonidine 0.5% has been infrequently associated with depression; caution is recommended when apraclonidine is used in patients with depression)

Exaggerated response to medications that reduce intraocular pressure
(patients who exhibit an exaggerated response to medications that reduce intraocular pressure should be closely monitored during treatment with apraclonidine, since apraclonidine is a potent depressor of intraocular pressure)

Hepatic function impairment
(since a structurally related medication, clonidine, is partly metabolized in the liver, monitoring of cardiovascular parameters in patients with liver function impairment who are using apraclonidine 0.5% is recommended)

Renal function impairment
(since a structurally related medication, clonidine, undergoes a significant increase in half-life in patients with severe renal impairment, monitoring of cardiovascular parameters in patients with renal function impairment who are using apraclonidine 0.5% is recommended)

Sensitivity to apraclonidine

Vasovagal attack, history of
(the possibility of a vasovagal attack occurring during laser surgery should be considered; caution should be used when administering 1% apraclonidine to patients with a history of this medical problem)

### Patient monitoring

The following may be especially important in patient monitoring (other tests may be warranted in some patients, depending on condition; » = major clinical significance):

Ophthalmology examinations
(patients using 0.5% apraclonidine should have frequent followup examinations to check intraocular pressure, and their visual fields should be monitored periodically)

## Side/Adverse Effects

Note: Ophthalmic apraclonidine 0.5% used three times a day is systemically absorbed; the 2 drops of ophthalmic apraclonidine 1% used during laser surgery may also be systemically absorbed, but it may not be as likely to cause systemic side/adverse effects as is the 0.5% dosage.

The following side/adverse effects have been selected on the basis of their potential clinical significance (possible signs and symptoms in parentheses where appropriate)—not necessarily inclusive:

**Those indicating need for medical attention**
Incidence more frequent
*For 0.5% ophthalmic apraclonidine*
**Allergic reaction** (redness of eye; itching of eye; tearing of eye)

Incidence less frequent or rare
*For 0.5% ophthalmic apraclonidine*
**Abnormal coordination** (clumsiness or unsteadiness); **arrhythmia** (irregular heartbeat); **asthma** (wheezing or troubled breathing); **blepharitis**; **blepharoconjunctivitis**; **conjunctivitis** (redness of eye, eyelid, or inner lining of eyelid); **blurred vision or change in vision**; **chest pain**; **contact dermatitis** (rash around eyes); **corneal erosion**; **corneal infiltrate**; **foreign body sensation**; **keratitis**; **ker-atopathy** (eye redness, irritation, or pain); **depression**; **dizziness**; **dyspnea** (troubled breathing); **edema of eye, eyelid, or conjunctiva** (swelling of eye, eyelid, or inner lining of eyelid); **eye discharge**; **facial edema** (swelling of face); **lid retraction** (raising of upper eyelid); **paresthesia** (numbness or tingling in fingers or toes); **peripheral edema** (swelling of hands or feet)

*For 1% ophthalmic apraclonidine*
**Allergic reaction** (redness of eye or inner lining of eyelid, swelling of eyelid, or watering of eye); **arrhythmia** (irregular heartbeat); **ocular inflammation or injection** (redness of eye)

**Those indicating need for medical attention only if they continue or are bothersome**
Incidence more frequent
*For 0.5% ophthalmic apraclonidine*
**Dryness of mouth**; **eye discomfort**

*For 1% ophthalmic apraclonidine*
**Conjunctival blanching** (paleness of eye or inner lining of eyelid); **lid retraction** (raising of upper eyelid); **mydriasis** (increase in size of pupil of eye)

Incidence less frequent or rare
*For 0.5% ophthalmic apraclonidine*
**Asthenia** (tiredness or weakness); **conjunctival blanching** (paleness of eye or inner lining of eyelid); **constipation**; **corneal staining** (discoloration of white part of eye); **crusting or scales on eyelid or corner of eye**; **dry nose or eyes**; **headache**; **insomnia** (trouble in sleeping); **malaise** (general feeling of discomfort or illness); **myalgia** (muscle aches); **nausea**; **nervousness**; **parosmia or taste perversion** (change in taste or smell); **pharyngitis** (sore throat); **photophobia** (increased sensitivity of eyes to light); **rhinitis** (runny nose); **somnolence** (drowsiness or sleepiness)

*For 1% ophthalmic apraclonidine*
**Nasal decongestion** (runny nose)

## Overdose

No information is available regarding overdosage of apraclonidine in humans.

## Patient Consultation

As an aid to patient consultation, refer to *Advice for the Patient, Apraclonidine (Ophthalmic)*.

In providing consultation, consider emphasizing the following selected information (» = major clinical significance):

### Before using this medication

» Conditions affecting use, especially:
Sensitivity to apraclonidine or clonidine
Pregnancy—Fetal death occurred after the administration of large oral doses of apraclonidine in rabbit studies
Breast-feeding—It may be necessary to stop breast-feeding during the day of surgery
Other medical problems, especially severe cardiovascular disease, including hypertension

### Proper use of this medication

Waiting at least 10 minutes between instillation of two different ophthalmic solutions
Proper administration technique; using a second drop if necessary; not touching applicator tip to any surface; keeping container tightly closed
» Importance of not using more medication than the amount prescribed
» Regular visits to physician to check eye pressure during therapy
» Proper dosing
Missed dose: Using as soon as possible; not using if almost time for next dose; using next dose at regularly scheduled time; not doubling doses
» Proper storage

### Precautions while using this medication

» Medication may cause dizziness or drowsiness; using caution when driving, using machines, or doing anything else requiring alertness
Possible photophobia; wearing sunglasses or avoiding bright light

### Side/adverse effects

*Signs of potential side effects, especially*
For 0.5% ophthalmic apraclonidine
Allergic reaction, abnormal coordination, arrhythmia, asthma, blepharitis, blepharoconjunctivitis, conjunctivitis, blurred vision or change in vision, chest pain, contact dermatitis, corneal erosion, corneal infiltrate, foreign body sensation, keratitis, keratopathy, depression, dizziness, dyspnea, edema of eye, eyelid, or conjunctiva,

eye discharge, facial edema, lid retraction, paresthesia, or peripheral edema

For 1% ophthalmic apraclonidine
Allergic reaction, arrhythmia, or ocular inflammation or injection

## General Dosing Information

The intraocular pressure (IOP) lowering efficacy of 0.5% ophthalmic apraclonidine diminishes over time and the benefit for most patients is less than one month.

When instilling two different ophthalmic solutions, patient should wait at least 10 minutes between instillations to avoid a "wash-out" effect.

If hypersensitivity develops, therapy with ophthalmic apraclonidine should be discontinued.

## Ophthalmic Dosage Forms

### APRACLONIDINE HYDROCHLORIDE OPHTHALMIC SOLUTION

**Usual adult and adolescent dose**
Open angle glaucoma—
Topical, to the conjunctiva, 1 drop of 0.5% solution in each eye two or three times a day.
Ocular hypertension—
Topical, to the conjunctiva, 1 drop of 1% solution in the affected eye one hour before initiating anterior segment laser surgery and 1 drop in the same eye immediately upon completion of the laser surgical procedure.

**Usual pediatric dose**
Safety and efficacy have not been established.

**Usual geriatric dose**
See *Usual adult and adolescent dose*.

**Strength(s) usually available**
U.S.—
0.5% (base) (Rx) [*Iopidine* (benzalkonium chloride 0.01%)].
1% (base) (Rx) [*Iopidine* (benzalkonium chloride 0.01%)].

Canada—
0.5% (base) (Rx) [*Iopidine* (benzalkonium chloride 0.01%)].
1% (base) (Rx) [*Iopidine* (benzalkonium chloride 0.01%)].

Note: Each mL of the 0.5% solution contains 5.75 mg of apraclonidine HCl equivalent to 5 mg of apraclonidine base.

Each mL of the 1% solution contains 11.5 mg of apraclonidine hydrochloride equivalent to 10 mg of apraclonidine base.

**Packaging and storage**
For the 0.5% solution—Store between 2 and 27 °C (36 and 80 °F), unless otherwise specified by manufacturer. Protect from freezing and light.
For the 1% solution—Store below 40 °C (104 °F), preferably between 15 and 30 °C (59 and 86 °F), unless otherwise specified by manufacturer. Protect from freezing and light.

**Auxiliary labeling**
• For the eye.
• Protect from light.
• Do not freeze.

## Selected Bibliography

Robin AL. Short-term effects of unilateral 1% apraclonidine therapy. Arch Ophthalmol 1988 Jul; 106(7): 912-5.
Pollack IP, et al. Prevention of the rise in intraocular pressure following neodymium-YAG posterior capsulotomy using topical 1% apraclonidine. Arch Ophthalmol 1988 Jun; 106(6): 754-7.

Revised: 06/21/94
Interim revision: 07/03/95

---

## APROBARBITAL — See *Barbiturates (Systemic)*

---

# APROTININ  Systemic

VA CLASSIFICATION (Primary): BL116
Commonly used brand name(s): *Trasylol*.
Note: For a listing of dosage forms and brand names by country availability, see *Dosage Forms* section(s).

## Category

Antifibrinolytic; antihemorrhagic; proteinase inhibitor.

## Indications

**Accepted**

Hemorrhage, coronary artery bypass graft surgery–associated (prophylaxis)[1]—Aprotinin is indicated to reduce perioperative blood loss and the need for blood transfusion in patients undergoing cardiopulmonary bypass in the course of repeat coronary artery bypass graft (CABG) surgery. It is also indicated, in selected cases, in first CABG procedures when the risk of bleeding is especially high (e.g., impaired hemostasis due to platelet aggregation inhibitor therapy or other coagulopathy) or when transfusion is unavailable or unacceptable. However, when aprotinin is being considered for use in a first CABG procedure, the risk of renal function impairment and the risk of anaphylaxis should a second procedure be needed must be taken into account.

**Acceptance not established**

Aprotinin has also been studied for use in the reduction of bleeding and transfusion requirements in other types of surgery including *orthotopic liver transplantation, total hip replacement, colorectal surgery, peripheral vascular surgery,* and *heart and heart-lung transplantation*. Study results evaluating the use of aprotinin for these indications are preliminary. Further studies are required to assess aprotinin's efficacy in these indications.

The use of aprotinin to control bleeding in *emergency cardiac surgery after thrombolysis* with alteplase, streptokinase, or urokinase has been reported. Although aprotinin may be effective in preventing severe hemorrhage in this setting, controlled studies to verify its efficacy and safety have not been done.

A few studies have evaluated the use of aprotinin in *pediatric patients* undergoing cardiac surgery. However, dosages and dosing regimens varied widely and the results have not been uniform. These studies have generally shown aprotinin to be less than beneficial in terms of reducing blood loss and the need for transfusions. Further studies are necessary to define the role of aprotinin in pediatric cardiac surgery.

**Unaccepted**

Aprotinin was originally introduced for the treatment of acute pancreatitis because of its proteinase inhibiting property. However, most studies have failed to show any benefit from this use.

Use of aprotinin for the treatment of subcutaneous insulin resistance syndrome has been described in a limited number of case reports from the early 1980s. However, no recent reports are available supporting such use, possibly due to concern for its safety during long-term use.

[1]Not included in Canadian product labeling.

## Pharmacology/Pharmacokinetics

**Physicochemical characteristics**
Source—Isolated from bovine lung.
Molecular weight—6511.57.

**Mechanism of action/Effect**

Aprotinin is a proteinase inhibitor. The exact mechanism by which it reduces bleeding is unclear; however, it has been shown to have a number of effects on the coagulation system.

Patients undergoing cardiopulmonary bypass (CPB) develop adverse changes in their blood components, blood cells, and specific proteins involved in coagulation, which increase the risk of serious postoperative bleeding. Platelet function impairment is considered to be the main hemostatic defect during CPB. There is evidence that aprotinin preserves platelet function; however, the mechanism by which this occurs is uncertain. In addition, aprotinin directly prevents fibrinolysis by inhibiting plasmin and kallikrein. It also inhibits the early phase of the intrinsic clotting cascade (contact phase) by inhibiting kallikrein, which in turn inhibits activation of factor XII.

**Distribution**

Rapidly distributed into the total extracellular space following intravenous injection, leading to a rapid initial decrease in plasma aprotinin concentration. Aprotinin is actively reabsorbed and accumulated by the proximal tubules in the kidney.

**Biotransformation**
Slowly degraded by lysosomal activity in the kidney.

**Half-life**
Elimination—
  Initial, following the distribution phase: Approximately 150 minutes.
  Terminal, occuring beyond 5 hours after administration: Approximately 10 hours.

**Steady-state plasma concentration**
Average steady-state intraoperative plasma concentrations were 250 Kallikrein Inhibitor Units per mL (KIU/mL) in cardiac surgery patients receiving a dosage regimen of 2 million KIU as an intravenous loading dose, 2 million KIU added to the pump prime fluid, and 500,000 KIU per hour as a continuous intravenous infusion during the procedure. Average steady-state intraoperative plasma concentrations were 137 KIU/mL after administration of half of the above regimen.

**Therapeutic plasma concentration**
For plasma kallikrein inhibition—Approximately 200 KIU/mL.
For plasmin inhibition—Approximately 50 KIU/mL.

**Elimination**
Renal; almost entirely as inactive metabolites.

## Precautions to Consider

**Carcinogenicity**
Long-term animal studies to evaluate the carcinogenic potential of aprotinin have not been performed.

**Mutagenicity**
Results of microbial *in vitro* tests using *Salmonella typhimurium* and *Bacillus subtilis* have shown no mutagenic effect of aprotinin.

**Pregnancy/Reproduction**
Fertility—Studies in rats given intravenous doses up to 2.4 times the human dose on a mg per kg of body weight (mg/kg) basis (0.37 times the human dose on a mg per square meter of body surface area [mg/m$^2$] basis) for 11 days, and in rabbits given intravenous doses up to 1.2 times the human dose on a mg/kg basis (0.36 times the human dose on a mg/m$^2$ basis) for 13 days have revealed no evidence of impaired fertility.

Pregnancy—Adequate and well-controlled studies in pregnant women have not been done.

Studies in rats given intravenous doses up to 2.4 times the human dose on a mg/kg basis (0.37 times the human dose on a mg/m$^2$ basis) for 11 days, and in rabbits given intravenous doses up to 1.2 times the human dose on a mg/kg basis (0.36 times the human dose on a mg/m$^2$ basis) for 13 days have revealed no evidence of harm to the fetus.

FDA Pregnancy Category B.

**Breast-feeding**
There are no available studies on the distribution of aprotinin into breast milk. However, since aprotinin is not absorbed after oral administration, there would be no effect on a nursing infant even if the breast milk did contain any of the medication.

**Pediatrics**
Safety and efficacy have not been established.
A few studies have evaluated the use of aprotinin in pediatric patients undergoing cardiac surgery. Results of these studies have not been uniform, but they have generally shown aprotinin to be less than beneficial in terms of reducing blood loss and the need for transfusions. Further studies are necessary to define the role of aprotinin in pediatric cardiac surgery.

**Geriatrics**
Clinical trials of aprotinin in cardiac surgery have been conducted mainly in older patients, and geriatrics-specific problems that would limit the usefulness of this medication in the elderly have not been evident. However, retrospective data from patients undergoing surgery of the thoracic aorta, using deep hypothermic circulatory arrest, revealed an increase in renal function impairment and failure, and of myocardial infarction and death, in a subset of patients 65 years of age or older who received high-dose aprotinin. The incidence of these complications in the patients receiving aprotinin far exceeded that in a previous group of age-matched patients who underwent similar operations but did not receive aprotinin. The investigators suggest that profound hypothermia with low blood flow or circulatory arrest may be a predisposing factor for significant adverse effects, particularly in patients older than 65 years of age. However, no data to confirm these findings is available from prospective studies involving large numbers of patients. Caution should be used when administering aprotinin during deep hypothermic circulatory arrest, especially in patients over the age of 65.

**Drug interactions and/or related problems**
The following drug interactions and/or related problems have been selected on the basis of their potential clinical significance (possible mechanism in parentheses where appropriate)—not necessarily inclusive (» = major clinical significance):

Note: Combinations containing any of the following medications, depending on the amount present, may also interact with this medication.

Angiotensin-converting enzyme (ACE) inhibitors
  (in a pharmacologic study evaluating the role of kinins in the antihypertensive effect of ACE inhibition, an intravenous infusion of aprotinin blocked the acute hypotensive effect of a 100-mg dose of captopril in 9 study patients with untreated hypertension; the clinical significance of this interaction is uncertain)

» Thrombolytic agents, such as:
  Alteplase
  Anistreplase
  Streptokinase
  Urokinase
  (the actions of antifibrinolytic agents and of thrombolytic agents are mutually antagonistic; although aprotinin may be effective in preventing severe hemorrhage in patients who have received a thrombolytic agent prior to cardiac surgery, controlled studies to verify its efficacy and safety for this use have not been done)

**Laboratory value alterations**
The following have been selected on the basis of their potential clinical significance (possible effect in parentheses where appropriate)—not necessarily inclusive (» = major clinical significance):

With diagnostic test results
» Activated clotting time (ACT) and
  Partial thromboplastin time (PTT)
  (aprotinin causes marked elevations in the ACT and PTT by inhibiting foreign surface contact–activation of the intrinsic clotting system, a method used in these tests; these elevations persist following surgery due to circulating concentrations of aprotinin)
  (aprotinin significantly prolongs the ACT as measured by the Hemochron® method, which utilizes a celite contact activator [used to monitor the adequacy of heparinization during cardiopulmonary bypass]; this is an artifactual prolongation of this particular test value and does not indicate excessive anticoagulation or a need to decrease heparin dosage)

With physiology/laboratory test values
  Creatine kinase (CK), serum
  (aprotinin may increase serum CK with increased MB fractions; however, the clinical significance of this effect is not known)

  Creatinine, serum
  (aprotinin may transiently increase serum creatinine concentrations, but this effect is generally not severe; during clinical use, aprotinin has had no clinically significant effect on serum creatinine or renal function)

  Transaminases, serum
  (may be increased; in controlled studies in the U.S., the percentage of subjects developing an elevation of alanine aminotransferase [ALT] greater than 1.8 times the upper limit of normal was higher in the aprotinin-treated group, but only in those patients undergoing repeat coronary artery bypass graft surgery, suggesting an indirect effect possibly related to the risk of repeated surgery; however, the etiology and clinical significance of this effect are uncertain)

**Medical considerations/Contraindications**
The medical considerations/contraindications included have been selected on the basis of their potential clinical significance (reasons given in parentheses where appropriate)—not necessarily inclusive (» = major clinical significance).

*Except under special circumstances, this medication should not be used when the following medical problem exists:*
» Allergy to aprotinin

*Risk-benefit should be considered when the following medical problems exist:*

  Allergies, multiple, history of or
» Previous aprotinin therapy
  (there is an increased risk of allergic reactions; a case of fatal anaphylactic shock following re-exposure to aprotinin has been reported; it is important to verify any previous aprotinin exposure, and all patients should first receive a test dose to assess the potential for allergic reactions)

» Caution is also required in patients undergoing deep hypothermic circulatory arrest, especially those older than 65 years of age, as increases in renal failure and fatalities have been reported in patients receiving aprotinin in this setting in connection with surgery of the aortic arch.

**Patient monitoring**
The following may be especially important in patient monitoring (other tests may be warranted in some patients, depending on condition; » = major clinical significance):

» Observation for signs and symptoms of anaphylaxis

## Side/Adverse Effects

Note: Patients undergoing deep hypothermic circulatory arrest in connection with surgery of the aortic arch may be predisposed to significant adverse effects including renal failure and fatality, particularly patients older than 65 years of age. These effects appear to be attributable to *disseminated intravascular coagulation*, possibly caused by the combination of high-dose aprotinin and profound hypothermia with low blood flow or circulatory arrest.

A trend toward increased incidences of *vein graft closure* and *myocardial infarction* was found in pooled data of U.S. studies in aprotinin-treated patients undergoing cardiopulmonary bypass. However, the differences in the incidence rates were not statistically significant. Two studies that investigated graft occlusion rates showed no statistically significant difference in patency between treatment and placebo groups, although the number of patients was small. It has been suggested that the patients in the early studies were inadequately anticoagulated with heparin because the effect of aprotinin on the activated clotting time (ACT) in the presence of heparin was not fully taken into consideration. Current evidence suggests that aprotinin has no clinically significant effect on graft thrombosis.

The following side/adverse effects have been selected on the basis of their potential clinical significance (possible signs and symptoms in parentheses where appropriate)—not necessarily inclusive:

**Those indicating need for medical attention**
Incidence rare (1% or less)
*Allergic reaction* (skin eruptions, itching, dyspnea, nausea, tachycardia, hypotension, and bronchospasm); *anaphylaxis, including shock with circulatory failure*

Note: A case of fatal *anaphylactic shock* following aprotinin re-exposure has been reported. It is important to verify any previous aprotinin exposure, and a test dose should be given to all patients to assess the potential for allergic reactions.

## General Dosing Information

Because of the increased risk of allergic reactions upon re-exposure to aprotinin, it is important to document the use of aprotinin in the patient's medical records and to ascertain any previous use of aprotinin.

Administration of aprotinin includes a 1-mL test dose, a loading dose, a dose to be added to the priming fluid of the cardiopulmonary bypass circuit ("pump prime" dose), and a constant infusion dose.

All intravenous doses of aprotinin should be administered through a central venous line. *No other medication should be administered through the same line.*

All patients should first receive a *test dose* to assess the potential for allergic reactions. The test dose (1 mL) should be administered intravenously at least 10 minutes prior to the loading dose.

Particular caution is needed when administering aprotinin (even test doses) to patients who have received it previously because of the risk of anaphylaxis. In *re-exposure cases*, after a successful test dose, prophylactic intravenous administration of an $H_1$-histamine antagonist (e.g., diphenhydramine) is recommended shortly before the loading dose of aprotinin.

Patients who experience any allergic reaction to the test dose of aprotinin should not receive further administration of the medication. Even after the uneventful administration of the test dose, the full therapeutic dose may cause anaphylaxis. In addition, anaphylaxis can occur in patients with no prior exposure to aprotinin. In the event of an anaphylactic reaction, the infusion should be stopped immediately and emergency treatment for anaphylaxis should begin. Patients with a history of allergies to medications or other agents may be at greater risk of developing an allergic reaction.

The loading dose of aprotinin should be given intravenously after induction of anesthesia but prior to sternotomy. The dose should be given with patients in the supine position and administered over a 20- to 30-minute period as rapid administration can cause a transient fall in blood pressure.

Either of 2 dosing regimens can be utilized, a high-dose regimen (Regimen A), or a low-dose regimen (Regimen B). The low-dose regimen is exactly one-half of the high-dose regimen. The high-dose regimen was used in the original studies in an effort to achieve plasma concentrations of aprotinin necessary to inhibit plasmin and plasma kallikrein. Interest in use of lower doses has arisen from a desire to find the most cost-effective regimen and, possibly, to reduce the potential for side effects. However, results of studies utilizing low-dose aprotinin have been equivocal, with variable effects on transfusion requirements.

No pharmacokinetic data is available from patients with pre-existing hepatic disease or renal insufficiency. Age and impaired renal function do not change aprotinin pharmacokinetics enough to warrant dosage adjustments.

**For treatment of adverse effects**
Anaphylaxis or other severe allergic reactions require immediate emergency treatment, which consists of the following:
- Parenteral epinephrine.
- Oxygen.
- Parenteral antihistamines.
- Intravenous corticosteroids.
- Airway management (including intubation).

**During cardiopulmonary bypass (CPB) with heparin**
Aprotinin prolongs the activated clotting time (ACT) as measured by the Hemochron® method, which utilizes a celite contact activator. Therefore, the standard method of monitoring heparinization by keeping the ACT above 400 to 450 seconds may lead to inadequate anticoagulation and the potential for coagulation through the extrinsic clotting system. Some investigators suggest maintaining the ACT above 750 seconds. Others propose utilizing tests not affected by aprotinin, such as high-dose thromboplastin time (HiPT) and high-dose thrombin time (HiTT), or kaolin-based activated coagulation time (AKT). However, the safety and efficacy of these alternative methods must be confirmed by further study. In any event, reduction of heparin dose is not recommended during CPB, as adequate heparin concentrations are needed to prevent clotting through the extrinsic system. Standard doses of heparin should be used during CPB; however, additional heparin may be administered based on the duration of CPB and patient weight, or the results of monitoring heparin concentrations using a heparin-protamine titration. Whole blood measurements of heparin are not affected by aprotinin and correlate well with plasma anti-Xa heparin measurements, making the automated protamine titration assay acceptable for monitoring of heparin concentrations in patients treated with aprotinin.

## Parenteral Dosage Forms

Note: The following doses are given in Kallikrein Inhibitor Units (KIU). The strength of commercially available aprotinin injection is labeled in KIU per mL.

### APROTININ INJECTION

**Usual adult dose**
Hemorrhage, coronary artery bypass graft surgery–associated (prophylaxis)[1]—
High-dose regimen—
Test dose—Intravenous, 10,000 KIU (1 mL).
Initial dose—Intravenous, 2,000,000 KIU (200 mL).
Maintenance dose—Intravenous infusion, 500,000 KIU per hour (50 mL per hour).
"Pump prime" dose—Added to the priming fluid, 2,000,000 KIU (200 mL).
Low-dose regimen—
Test dose—Intravenous, 10,000 KIU (1 mL).
Initial dose—Intravenous, 1,000,000 KIU (100 mL).
Maintenance dose—Intravenous infusion, 250,000 KIU per hour (25 mL per hour).
"Pump prime" dose—Added to the priming fluid, 1,000,000 KIU (100 mL).

Note: The test dose should be administered intravenously at least ten minutes prior to the initial dose. The initial dose is given slowly over twenty to thirty minutes with the patient in the supine position after induction of anesthesia but prior to sternotomy. Following the initial dose, the maintenance dose is given by constant infusion until surgery is complete and the patient leaves the operating room. The "pump prime" dose is added to the priming fluid of the cardiopulmonary bypass circuit, by replacement of an aliquot of the priming fluid, prior to initiation of cardiopulmonary bypass.

464    Aprotinin (Systemic)

**Usual adult prescribing limits**
Total doses of more than 7,000,000 KIU have not been studied in controlled trials.

**Usual pediatric dose**
Safety and efficacy have not been established.

Note: A few studies have evaluated the use of aprotinin in pediatric patients undergoing cardiac surgery. However, dosages and dosing regimens varied widely and the results have not been uniform. These studies have generally shown aprotinin to be less than beneficial in terms of reducing blood loss and the need for transfusions. Further studies are necessary to define the role of aprotinin in pediatric cardiac surgery.

**Strength(s) usually available**
U.S.—
  10,000 KIU per mL (100- and 200-mL vials) (Rx) [*Trasylol*].
Canada—
  10,000 KIU per mL (50-mL vials) (Rx) [*Trasylol*].

**Packaging and storage**
Store between 2 and 25 °C (36 and 77 °F). Protect from freezing.

**Stability**
Aprotinin is stable when stored in sealed vials at room temperature. The medication should not be used if a precipitate or particulate matter is present or if the contents are cloudy. Once a vial has been opened, it should be used immediately. Any unused portion should be discarded.

**Incompatibilities**
Aprotinin is incompatible *in vitro* with corticosteroids, heparin, tetracyclines, and nutrient solutions containing amino acids or fat emulsions. If aprotinin is to be given concomitantly with another medication, each medication should be administered separately through a different venous line or catheter. **No other medication should be administered through the same intravenous line with aprotinin.**

[1]Not included in Canadian product labeling.

## Selected Bibliography
Davis R, Whittington R. Aprotinin: a review of its pharmacology and therapeutic efficacy in reducing blood loss associated with cardiac surgery. Drugs 1995; 49: 954-83.
Lemmer JH, Stanford W, Bonney SL, et al. Aprotinin for coronary bypass operations: efficacy, safety, and influence on early saphenous vein graft patency. A multicenter, randomized, double-blind, placebo-controlled study. J Thorac Cardiovasc Surg 1994; 107: 543-53.
Royston D. High-dose aprotinin therapy: a review of the first five years' experience. J Cardiothorac Vasc Anesth 1992; 6: 76-100.

Developed: 08/17/95

---

# ARBUTAMINE    Systemic—INTRODUCTORY VERSION

VA CLASSIFICATION (Primary/Secondary): AU100/CV053
Commonly used brand name(s): *GenESA*.
Note: For a listing of dosage forms and brand names by country availability, see *Dosage Forms* section(s).

## Category
Diagnostic aid, coronary artery disease.

## Indications
**Accepted**
Coronary artery disease (CAD) (diagnosis)—Arbutamine, administered through a closed-loop, computer-controlled drug-delivery system, is indicated to elicit acute cardiovascular responses, similar to those produced by exercise, in order to aid in diagnosing the presence or absence of CAD in patients who cannot exercise adequately. Arbutamine must not be administered without the use of the approved computer-controlled device. Cardiac stress testing with arbutamine always must be performed under the direct supervision of a physician, and cardiac emergency equipment and supplies, such as a defibrillator and intravenous beta-adrenergic blocking agents, must be available.

## Pharmacology/Pharmacokinetics
**Physicochemical characteristics**
Chemical group—Catecholamine.
Molecular weight—353.85.

**Mechanism of action/Effect**
Arbutamine is a synthetic catecholamine with positive chronotropic and inotropic properties. The chronotropic (increase in heart rate [HR]) and inotropic (increase in force of contraction) effects of arbutamine serve to mimic exercise by increasing cardiac work (producing stress) and provoke myocardial ischemia in patients with compromised coronary arteries. The increase in HR caused by arbutamine is thought to limit regional subendocardial perfusion, thereby limiting tissue oxygenation. In functional assays, arbutamine is more selective for beta-adrenergic receptors than for alpha-adrenergic receptors. The beta-agonist activity of arbutamine provides cardiac stress by increasing HR, cardiac contractility, and systolic blood pressure. The degree of hypotension that occurs for a given chronotropic activity is less with arbutamine than, for example, with isoproterenol because alpha receptor activity is retained.

**Distribution**
Volume of distribution (Vol$_D$)—0.74 liters per kg (L/kg).

**Protein binding**
Moderate (approximately 58%).

**Biotransformation**
Arbutamine is primarily metabolized to methoxyarbutamine. Another possible metabolite is ketoarbutamine. The metabolites of arbutamine appear to have a longer half-life and less pharmacological activity than arbutamine.

**Half-life**
Elimination—
  Approximately 8 minutes.

**Elimination**
Renal—84%.
Fecal—9%.
  In dialysis—
    Arbutamine is rapidly eliminated and in cases of overdose, peritoneal or hemodialysis may not be required.

## Precautions to Consider
**Carcinogenicity**
No carcinogenicity tests have been performed with arbutamine.

**Mutagenicity**
Arbutamine was not found to be genotoxic in the Ames microbial mutagen test with or without S9 mix, nor in the mouse micronucleus test. However, arbutamine was found to be genotoxic in the human lymphocyte chromosomal aberration assay (> 66 mcg per mL [mcg/mL]) and in the mouse lymphoma cell assay (> 39 mcg/mL).

**Pregnancy/Reproduction**
Fertility—Adequate and well-controlled studies in humans to determine the effect of arbutamine on fertility have not been done.

Pregnancy—Although no adequate and well-controlled studies in pregnant women have been done, reproduction studies performed in rats and rabbits given intravenous doses of arbutamine of up to 0.9 and 0.36 mg per kg of body weight (mg/kg) per day, respectively, revealed no evidence of harm to the fetus. These doses represent 4 and 12 times, respectively, the maximum recommended human dose (MRHD) on a mg per square meter of body surface area (mg/m$^2$) basis.

FDA Pregnancy Category B.

**Breast-feeding**
Problems in humans have not been documented.

**Pediatrics**
No information is available on the relationship of age to the effects of arbutamine in pediatric patients. Safety and efficacy have not been established.

**Geriatrics**
No information is available on the relationship of age to the effects of arbutamine in geriatric patients.

### Drug interactions and/or related problems
The following drug interactions and/or related problems have been selected on the basis of their potential clinical significance (possible mechanism in parentheses where appropriate)—not necessarily inclusive (» = major clinical significance):

Note: Combinations containing any of the following medications, depending on the amount present, may also interact with this medication.

» Beta-adrenergic blocking agents
(concurrent use may blunt the response to arbutamine; beta-adrenergic blocking agents should be withdrawn at least 48 hours before conducting an arbutamine-mediated stress test)

» Antiarrhythmic agents, class I, such as:
» Flecainide or
» Lidocaine or
» Quinidine
(concurrent use with arbutamine may have a proarrhythmic effect and is not recommended)

» Antidepressants, tricyclic or
» Atropine or other anticholinergic agents or
» Digitalis glycosides
(concurrent use with arbutamine may produce additive inotropic and/or chronotropic effects)

### Laboratory value alterations
The following have been selected on the basis of their potential clinical significance (possible effect in parentheses where appropriate)—not necessarily inclusive (» = major clinical significance):

With physiology/laboratory test values
Potassium, serum
(transient decreases have occurred, but hypokalemia is rare)

### Medical considerations/Contraindications
The medical considerations/contraindications included have been selected on the basis of their potential clinical significance (reasons given in parentheses where appropriate)—not necessarily inclusive (» = major clinical significance):

*Except under special circumstances, this medication should not be used when the following medical problems exist:*

» Congestive heart failure, New York Heart Association (NYHA) class III or IV or
» Hypertrophic subaortic stenosis, idiopathic or
» Ventricular tachycardia, recurrent sustained, history of
(the inotropic and/or chronotropic effects of arbutamine in these patients may worsen the existing condition or, in the case of a history of recurrent sustained ventricular tachycardia, may precipitate ventricular arrhythmias)

» Cardiac pacemaker, implanted or
» Cardioverter/defibrillator, automated, present
» Hypersensitivity to arbutamine

*Risk-benefit should be considered when the following medical problems exist:*

Angina, unstable or
Cardiac transplant or
Cerebrovascular accident, history of or
Glaucoma, narrow-angle or
Hypertension, uncontrolled or
Hyperthyroidism, uncontrolled or
Left ventricular outflow obstruction, mechanical, such as
Aortic stenosis, valvular, severe or
Peripheral vascular disorder resulting in cerebral or aortic aneurysm, history of
(the inotropic and chronotropic effects of arbutamine may exacerbate the existing condition and its use in these patients is not recommended)

Arrhythmias, supraventricular or ventricular, sustained, history of
(use of arbutamine in these patients is not recommended because it may precipitate the arrhythmia)

Myocardial infarction, recent (within 30 days)
(use of arbutamine in these patients has not been evaluated)

Sensitivity to sulfites
(arbutamine injection contains sodium metabisulfite, which may cause allergic- or anaphylactic-type reactions and life-threatening or less severe asthmatic episodes in individuals who are sensitive to sulfites; sensitivity to sulfites is more common in asthmatic patients than in nonasthmatic patients)

### Patient monitoring
The following may be especially important in patient monitoring (other tests may be warranted in some patients, depending on condition; » = major clinical significance):

» Blood pressure, systolic
(monitored continuously by the computerized drug-delivery device; arbutamine may cause rapid increases or paradoxical decreases in systolic blood pressure)

» Electrocardiogram (ECG)
(continuous monitoring is recommended; although the device provides monitoring capabilities, it is not designed to detect arrhythmias and a diagnostic-quality ECG machine also must be used; arbutamine infusion has been associated with a transient increase in the corrected QT interval [QTc], as measured from the surface ECG; however, this effect does not appear to be associated with an increased incidence of arrhythmias)

» Heart rate (HR)
(the HR response of the patient is measured by the device; the HR slope [rate of rise] and target HR are chosen by the physician and are based on the desired duration of the test and the desired rate of HR rise; following the completion of the test after the HR target has been reached or after a total of 10 mcg per kg of body weight [mcg/kg] of arbutamine has been administered, the patient's HR should be monitored until it has returned to an acceptable level; in clinical trials, after termination of the infusion, HR decreased by 50% within 13 to 16 minutes. Arbutamine may cause rapid increases or paradoxical decreases in HR; it is possible that upon the occurrence of an arrhythmia, the device may record an inaccurate heart rate)

## Side/Adverse Effects
Note: Supraventricular and ventricular arrhythmias, most commonly, isolated premature ventricular and atrial contractions, have occurred with administration of arbutamine. In clinical trials, most of the arrhythmias that occurred were self-limiting and all arrhythmias resolved without further effects. Although the overall incidence of serious adverse events was low (0.5%), 10 *serious* adverse events occurred: three episodes of ventricular fibrillation, one episode of sustained ventricular tachycardia, three episodes of atrial fibrillation, one event of myocardial infarction, and two cases of severe angina. Two of the three cases of ventricular fibrillation occurred after the delivery device had detected a plateau in heart rate (HR) response and had terminated the arbutamine infusion, but the physician restarted the infusion. No deaths occurred.

Arbutamine may cause rapid increases or paradoxical decreases in heart rate and systolic blood pressure.

Arbutamine injection contains sodium metabisulfite, which may cause allergic-type reactions, including anaphylactic symptoms and life-threatening or less severe asthmatic episodes in certain individuals.

The following side/adverse effects have been selected on the basis of their potential clinical significance (possible signs and symptoms in parentheses where appropriate)—not necessarily inclusive:

### Those indicating need for medical attention
Note: Many side/adverse effects are similar to those of arbutamine toxicity. See *Clinical effects of overdose* section.

Incidence more frequent
*Angina pectoris* (chest pain, severe)—incidence 12%; *cardiac arrhythmias, ventricular and supraventricular*—incidence 12%; *headache*—incidence 9%; *hypotension* (dizziness, lightheadedness, or fainting)—incidence 6%; *tremor*—incidence 15%

Incidence less frequent
*Anxiety; chest pain*—incidence 4%; *dizziness*—incidence 4%; *dry mouth; dyspnea* (difficult or labored breathing)—incidence 4%; *fatigue* (unusual tiredness); *flushing or hot flushes* (redness of face)—incidence 3%; *hypoesthesia* (decreased touch sensation); *nausea*—incidence 3%; *pain, nonspecific; palpitations* (heartbeat sensations)—incidence 4%; *paresthesia* (burning or tingling skin sensation); *sweating, increased; taste perversion* (change in sense of taste)

Incidence rare
*Hypertension; myocardial ischemia; skin rash; ST segment depression*

## Overdose

For specific information on the agents used in the management of arbutamine overdose, see:
- *Esmolol (Systemic)* monograph; and/or
- *Metoprolol* or *Propranolol* in *Beta-adrenergic Blocking Agents (Systemic)* monograph; and/or
- *Nitroglycerin* or *Isosorbide Dinitrate* in *Nitrates (Systemic)* monograph.

For more information on the management of overdose or unintentional ingestion, **contact a Poison Control Center** (see *Poison Control Center Listing*).

### Clinical effects of overdose

The following effects have been selected on the basis of their potential clinical significance (possible signs and symptoms in parentheses where appropriate)—not necessarily inclusive:

Acute

***Angina pectoris; anxiety; dizziness; flushing or hot flushes; headache; hypertension; hypotension; myocardial infarction; nausea; paresthesia; ST segment abnormalities; sweating, increased; tachyarrhythmias; tremor; ventricular fibrillation***

### Treatment of overdose

The maximum total dose of arbutamine permitted by the drug delivery device is 10 mcg per kg of body weight (mcg/kg). Arbutamine is metabolized and eliminated rapidly; therefore, an overdosage should be of short duration and forced diuresis, peritoneal dialysis, hemodialysis, or charcoal hemoperfusion is unlikely to be required. If arbutamine is ingested, absorption from the mouth and gastrointestinal tract may be unpredictable.

Initial treatment—Arbutamine should be discontinued and an airway established to ensure adequate oxygenation and ventilation.

Specific treatment—Severe signs or symptoms, such as angina, tachyarrhythmias, ST segment abnormalities, or hypotension, may be treated with an intravenous beta-adrenergic blocking agent, such as esmolol, metoprolol, or propranolol. Other treatment, such as sublingual nitrates, should be used if appropriate and necessary.

## General Dosing Information

Arbutamine is intended for direct intravenous infusion only with the approved drug delivery device. The device has a single-channel electrocardiogram (ECG) (R wave) detector, a noninvasive blood pressure monitor, computer software (closed-loop algorithm) that controls drug delivery, an intravenous syringe pump, display functions, and an operator key pad. ECG, heart rate (HR), blood pressure, and dosing information are displayed continuously. The device uses visual and auditory alerts and alarms to warn of conditions that may require attention and can stop drug delivery if a potential safety hazard is detected.

The drug delivery device is not designed to detect arrhythmias, and appropriate monitoring equipment, such as a diagnostic-quality ECG machine, must be used during a patient test.

### For treatment of adverse effects

Recommended treatment consists of the following:
- If any arrhythmia occurs that is of clinical concern, administration of arbutamine should be stopped immediately and appropriate therapy administered, if necessary.

## Parenteral Dosage Forms

### ARBUTAMINE HYDROCHLORIDE INJECTION

Note: Refer to the manufacturer's labeling for complete operating instructions and directions for use of the drug delivery system for administration of arbutamine.

### Usual adult dose

Diagnostic aid, coronary artery disease (CAD)—
Intravenous infusion, up to a maximum of 10 mcg per kg of body weight as administered by the drug delivery device.

Drug delivery by the device—
The delivery device, using a closed-loop algorithm, individualizes the dosing regimen of arbutamine according to the heart rate (HR) response of the patient. Initially, the device administers a small dose of arbutamine (0.1 mcg per kg of body weight [mcg/kg] per minute for one minute) and measures the patient's HR response. The device calculates the difference between the desired and actual HR response, and maintains or modifies, as necessary, the infusion rate. The physician conducting the test may manually interrupt the delivery of arbutamine at any time, if clinically appropriate. The infusion of arbutamine may be restarted by the operator if the condition resulting in the interruption of infusion has been corrected, a diagnostic end point has not been reached, and it is considered safe and appropriate to do so.

Heart rate selection and monitoring—
The physician selects the desired rate of HR rise (HR slope) and the maximum HR to be achieved (HR target) for each patient test:

HR slope:
Low (four beats per minute per minute [bpm/min]), medium (eight bpm/min), or high (twelve bpm/min) (or any value from four to twelve bpm/min may be selected), based upon the desired duration of the test and the rate of HR rise that is determined by the physician to be most appropriate. Clinical data, obtained using an HR slope of eight bpm/min, support the use of a medium slope in a majority of patients.

HR target:
Estimated by the device as 85% of (220 − age), or adjusted manually by the operator.

The device has a feature ("Hold HR") that allows the HR to be maintained at an approximate level for up to five minutes. The maximal HR response to arbutamine, determined by a flattening or plateau of the HR response to increasing doses of arbutamine ("HR saturation"), is an end point of the stress test. If such a flattening or plateau is detected when the HR is ≤ forty bpm above the baseline level, restart of the infusion is allowed by the device. If the HR is > forty bpm above baseline and an "HR saturation" alarm occurs, restart of the arbutamine infusion is prevented by the device because any further clinically significant increases in HR are unlikely to occur following restart and there is a potential risk for serious cardiac arrhythmias.

Termination of the infusion—
The infusion of arbutamine should be terminated when a diagnostic end point (e.g., ST segment deviation on ECG) has been reached, if clinically significant symptoms or arrhythmias occur, or if clinically appropriate for any other reason. The device will stop drug delivery when the HR target has been reached or after a total 10 mcg/kg of arbutamine has been delivered. Following completion of the infusion, the patient should be monitored (using the device or other means), until HR and blood pressure have returned to acceptable levels.

### Usual adult prescribing limits

The maximum infusion rate delivered by the device is 0.8 mcg per kg of body weight per minute (mcg/kg/min) and the maximum total dose permitted by the device is 10 mcg/kg.

### Usual pediatric dose

Diagnostic aid, CAD—
Safety and efficacy have not been established.

### Strength(s) usually available

U.S.—
0.05 mg per mL (Rx) [*GenESA* (20 mL prefilled syringe. Each syringe contains 1 mg of arbutamine hydrochloride)].

### Packaging and storage

Store between 2 and 8 °C (36 and 46 °F). Protect from light. Protect from freezing.

### Preparation of dosage form

Arbutamine must be administered from the prefilled syringe and must not be diluted or transferred to another syringe.

### Stability

Arbutamine injection should be inspected visually for particulate matter and discoloration prior to administration.

Developed: 04/26/98

# ARDEPARIN Systemic—INTRODUCTORY VERSION

VA CLASSIFICATION (Primary): BL111
Commonly used brand name(s): *Normiflo*.
Note: For a listing of dosage forms and brand names by country availability, see *Dosage Forms* section(s).

## Category
Anticoagulant; antithrombotic.
Note: Ardeparin is one of a group of substances known as low molecular weight heparins (LMWHs).

## Indications
**Accepted**
Thromboembolism, pulmonary (prophylaxis) and
Thrombosis, deep venous (prophylaxis)—Ardeparin is indicated for prevention of deep vein thrombosis, which may result in pulmonary embolism, following knee replacement surgery.

## Pharmacology/Pharmacokinetics
Note: Because plasma concentrations cannot be measured directly, the pharmacokinetic and pharmacodynamic properties of ardeparin are evaluated on the basis of changes in plasma serine protease activity that are considered important in hemostasis and are affected by ardeparin.

**Physicochemical characteristics**
Source—Isolated from porcine intestinal mucosa.
Molecular weight—Average: 6000 daltons.
pH—4.5 to 7.

**Mechanism of action/Effect**
Ardeparin acts at multiple sites in the normal coagulation system to inhibit reactions that lead to the clotting of blood and the formation of fibrin clots both *in vitro* and *in vivo*. Ardeparin inhibits thrombosis by binding to antithrombin III and accelerating its activity, thus inactivating factor Xa and thrombin. Ardeparin also inhibits thrombin by binding to heparin cofactor II. At recommended dosages, ardeparin has no effect on prothrombin time (PT) assays and may or may not prolong the activated partial thromboplastin time (APTT).
Note: Ardeparin has a higher ratio of anti-factor Xa to anti-factor IIa activity (about 2:1) than does unfractionated heparin (about 1:1 or less).

**Absorption**
Well-absorbed after subcutaneous administration, with a mean bioavailability of 92% based on anti-factor Xa activity.
Note: Ardeparin pharmacokinetics fit a one-compartment pharmacokinetic model with apparent first-order absorption. Dose proportionality is slightly nonlinear; each doubling of the dose produces an anti-factor Xa area under the plasma concentration–time curve (AUC) that is about 25% higher than would be expected with linear dose proportionality, although anti-factor IIa activity over the same dose range does exhibit linear dose proportionality.

**Half-life**
Elimination—
 Anti-factor Xa activity: Average, 3.3 hours following a single intravenous dose.
 Anti-factor IIa activity: Average, 1.2 hours following a single intravenous dose.

**Time to peak concentration**
Mean peak plasma anti-factor Xa activity—2.7 hours after a single subcutaneous dose of 30 to 100 units per kg of body weight (units/kg).
Mean plasma anti-factor IIa activity—3 hours after a single subcutaneous dose of 100 units/kg.

**Peak plasma concentration**
Mean peak plasma anti-factor Xa activity—0.09 to 0.32 units per mL (units/mL) after 30 to 100 anti-factor Xa units/kg single doses.
Mean plasma anti-factor IIa activity—Barely detectable after 30 anti-factor Xa units/kg and 0.07 units/mL after 100 anti-factor Xa units/kg single doses.
Note: Peak anti-factor Xa plasma concentrations of ardeparin after single subcutaneous doses of 60 mg (5400 anti-factor Xa units) were about twice as high as those after subcutaneous doses of 60 mg (9600 anti-factor Xa units) of heparin.

**Elimination**
Renal.
 In dialysis—
  Ardeparin does not appear to be removable by hemodialysis.

## Precautions to Consider

**Cross-sensitivity and/or related problems**
Patients sensitive to heparin or to pork products may be sensitive to ardeparin also.

**Carcinogenicity**
Long-term studies in animals have not been done.

**Mutagenicity**
Ardeparin was not found to be mutagenic in *in vitro* tests including the Ames test, the Chinese hamster ovarian cell (CHO/HGPRT) forward mutation test, or in *in vivo* tests including the mouse micronucleus test and the rat bone marrow cell chromosome aberration test.

**Pregnancy/Reproduction**
Fertility—Studies in male rats at subcutaneous doses of up to 3180 anti-factor Xa units per kg of body weight (units/kg) per day (19,080 anti-factor Xa units per square meter of body surface area [units/m$^2$] per day, approximately five times the recommended human dose based on body surface area) and in female rats at subcutaneous doses of up to 1590 units/kg per day (9540 units/m$^2$ per day, approximately three times the recommended human dose based on body surface area) found no evidence of impairment of fertility or of reproductive performance.
Pregnancy—Adequate and well-controlled studies in humans have not been done.
Studies in pregnant rats at subcutaneous doses of up to 1590 units/kg per day (9540 units/m$^2$ per day, approximately three times the recommended human dose based on body surface area) and in pregnant rabbits at subcutaneous doses of up to 3180 units/kg per day (34,980 units/m$^2$ per day, approximately 10 times the recommended human dose based on body surface area) found no evidence of teratogenicity. However, ardeparin was found to be teratogenic (scoliosis) in rats at intravenous doses of 4240 units/kg per day (25,440 units/m$^2$ per day, approximately seven times the recommended human dose based on body surface area) and was also teratogenic (interventricular septal defects, stenosis of the aortic arch and pulmonary trunk, and fused sternebrae) in rabbits at intravenous doses of 3744 units/kg per day and above (41,184 units/m$^2$ per day, approximately 11 times the recommended human dose based on body surface area).
FDA Pregnancy Category C.

**Breast-feeding**
It is not known whether ardeparin is distributed into breast milk. However, problems in humans have not been documented.

**Pediatrics**
Appropriate studies on the relationship of age to the effects of ardeparin have not been performed in the pediatric population. Safety and efficacy have not been established.

**Geriatrics**
Studies performed in patients up to 92 years of age have not demonstrated geriatrics-specific problems that would limit the usefulness of ardeparin in the elderly.
Based on results of pharmacokinetic studies in 934 patients in two large-scale clinical trials, age and gender do not need to be considered in dosing ardeparin.

**Drug interactions and/or related problems**
The following drug interactions and/or related problems have been selected on the basis of their potential clinical significance (possible mechanism in parentheses where appropriate)—not necessarily inclusive (» = major clinical significance):
Note: Combinations containing any of the following medications, depending on the amount present, may also interact with this medication.
 Anticoagulants, coumarin- or indandione-derivative or
 Platelet aggregation inhibitors such as:
  Anti-inflammatory drugs, nonsteroidal (NSAIDs)
  Aspirin
   (increased risk of bleeding)

**Laboratory value alterations**
The following have been selected on the basis of their potential clinical significance (possible effect in parentheses where appropriate)—not necessarily inclusive (» = major clinical significance):

## Ardeparin (Systemic)—Introductory Version

With physiology/laboratory test values
Alanine aminotransferase (ALT [SGPT]), serum and
Aspartate aminotransferase (AST [SGOT]), serum
(increases in values to as high as three times the upper limit of normal have been reported in both normal subjects and patients given ardeparin; these effects are similar to those seen with heparin and other low molecular weight heparins; these increases are usually fully reversible and are rarely associated with increases in serum bilirubin concentrations; however, because of the importance of aminotransferase determinations in the differential diagnosis of myocardial infarction, hepatic disease, and pulmonary embolism, elevations should be interpreted with caution)

Triglycerides
(paradoxical increases in serum concentrations have been reported, even though ardeparin is known to increase lipoprotein lipase activity)

Note: At normal doses, ardeparin has no effect on prothrombin time (PT). There is no effect on, or only a slight prolongation (usually less than 50 seconds) of, activated partial thromboplastin time (APTT).

### Medical considerations/Contraindications

The medical considerations/contraindications included have been selected on the basis of their potential clinical significance (reasons given in parentheses where appropriate)—not necessarily inclusive (» = major clinical significance).

*Except under special circumstances, this medication should not be used when the following medical problems exist:*

» Bleeding, major, active
(may be exacerbated)
» Hypertension, severe, uncontrolled
(increased risk of cerebral hemorrhage)
» Stroke, hemorrhagic
(increased risk of uncontrollable hemorrhage)
» Thrombocytopenia associated with positive *in vitro* tests for antiplatelet antibody in the presence of ardeparin or
» Thrombocytopenia, heparin-induced, history of
(risk of recurrence)

*Risk-benefit should be considered when the following medical problems exist:*

Any medical procedure or condition in which the risk of bleeding or hemorrhage is present, such as:
» Anesthesia, epidural or spinal
(risk of epidural or spinal hematoma, which can result in long-term or permanent paralysis; this risk is increased with the use of indwelling epidural catheters or by the concomitant use of medications that affect hemostasis, such as nonsteroidal anti-inflammatory drugs, platelet inhibitors, or other anticoagulants; the risk also may be increased by traumatic or repeated epidural or spinal puncture)
» Blood dyscrasias, hemorrhagic, congenital or acquired
» Endocarditis, bacterial
» Hepatic function impairment, severe
» Renal function impairment, severe
» Retinopathy, diabetic or hypertensive
» Surgery, especially brain, spinal, or ophthalmologic
» Ulceration, other lesions, or recent bleeding of the gastrointestinal tract, active
Sensitivity to ardeparin, heparin, methylparaben, pork products, propylparaben, or sulfites

### Patient monitoring

The following may be especially important in patient monitoring (other tests may be warranted in some patients, depending on condition; » = major clinical significance):

Note: Routine monitoring of coagulation parameters (activated partial thromboplastin time [APTT]) is not necessary.

» Blood counts, complete (CBC), including
Hematocrit
Platelet count
(recommended during treatment to detect occult bleeding or any degree of thrombocytopenia)
Blood pressure measurement
(recommended periodically during therapy; an unexplained drop in blood pressure may signal occult bleeding)
» Neurologic status
(frequent monitoring for signs and symptoms of neurological impairment is recommended; if neurologic compromise is noted, urgent treatment is necessary)
Stool tests for occult blood
(should be performed at regular intervals during therapy)
Urinalysis
(recommended during treatment to detect occult bleeding)

### Side/Adverse Effects

The following side/adverse effects have been selected on the basis of their potential clinical significance (possible signs and symptoms in parentheses where appropriate)—not necessarily inclusive:

**Those indicating need for medical attention**
Incidence less frequent
*Anemia; fever; hematoma at injection site* (deep, dark purple bruise, pain, or swelling at place of injection); *hemorrhage* (bleeding gums; coughing up blood; difficulty in breathing or swallowing; dizziness; headache; increased menstrual flow or vaginal bleeding; nosebleeds; paralysis; prolonged bleeding from cuts; red or dark brown urine; red or black, tarry stools; shortness of breath; unexplained pain, swelling, or discomfort, especially in the chest, abdomen, joints, or muscles; unusual bruising; vomiting of blood or coffee ground–like material; weakness)

Incidence rare
*Allergic reaction* (fever; skin rash, hives, or itching); *epidural or spinal hematoma* (back pain; bowel/bladder dysfunction; leg weakness; numbness; paralysis; paresthesias)—back pain is not a typical presentation but some patients may experience this symptom; *thrombocytopenia* (bleeding from mucous membranes; rash consisting of pinpoint, purple-red spots, often beginning on the legs; unusual bruising)

Note: If an *epidural or spinal hematoma* is suspected, urgent intervention is necessary.

**Those indicating need for medical attention only if they continue or are bothersome**
Incidence less frequent
*Nausea; pain at injection site; vomiting*

### Overdose

For specific information on the agent used in the management of ardeparin overdose, see the *Protamine (Systemic)* monograph.

For more information on the management of overdose or unintentional ingestion, **contact a Poison Control Center** (see *Poison Control Center Listing*).

**Clinical effects of overdose**
The following effects have been selected on the basis of their potential clinical significance (possible signs and symptoms in parentheses where appropriate)—not necessarily inclusive:

Acute
*Hemorrhage*
Note: Bleeding at the surgical site or at venipuncture sites may be the first sign of *bleeding complications*. Other signs may include epistaxis, hematuria, or blood in stools. Easy bruising or petechiae may be seen before frank bleeding.

**Treatment of overdose**
Most bleeding can be controlled by discontinuing ardeparin, applying pressure to the site, if possible, and replacing volume and hemostatic blood elements (e.g., fresh frozen plasma, platelets) as required.

Specific treatment—
Protamine sulfate may be administered if the above is ineffective or if a known ardeparin overdosage has occurred in a bleeding patient. A dose of 1 mg of protamine sulfate neutralizes approximately 100 anti-factor Xa units of ardeparin. The anti-factor IIa activity of intravenously administered ardeparin is completely neutralized within 10 minutes following an intravenous infusion dose of equal weight protamine sulfate (about 1 mg protamine sulfate for each 100 anti-factor Xa units of administered ardeparin). The anti-factor Xa and clot-based anti-factor Xa assay activities of ardeparin are reduced by about 75% within 10 minutes and are almost completely neutralized within 30 minutes after protamine sulfate administration. If protamine sulfate is given and bleeding persists, approximately 2 hours after the dose of protamine, blood should be withdrawn and residual anti-factor Xa levels determined. Additional protamine sulfate may be administered if clinically important bleeding persists or if anti-factor Xa levels remain higher than desired.

Protamine sulfate should be administered with great care to avoid an overdose. Severe hypotensive and anaphylactoid reactions, possibly fatal, may occur with protamine sulfate. It should be administered only when resuscitation techniques and treatment of anaphylactic shock are readily available.

## Patient Consultation

As an aid to patient consultation, refer to *Advice for the Patient, Ardeparin (Systemic)—Introductory Version.*

In providing consultation, consider emphasizing the following selected information (» = major clinical significance):

**Before using this medication**
» Conditions affecting use, especially:
   Sensitivity to ardeparin, heparin, methylparaben, pork products, propylparaben, or sulfites
   Other medical problems, especially bacterial endocarditis; bleeding; diabetic or hypertensive retinopathy; hemorrhagic blood dyscrasias; severe hepatic function impairment; severe renal function impairment; severe, uncontrolled hypertension; stroke; surgery; thrombocytopenia; or ulcers or other lesions of the gastrointestinal tract

**Proper use of this medication**
» Proper dosing

**Precautions while using this medication**
» Need to inform all health care providers of use of medication
» Notifying physician immediately if signs and symptoms of bleeding or epidural/spinal hematoma occur

**Side/adverse effects**
Signs of potential side effects, especially anemia, fever, hematoma at injection site, hemorrhage, allergic reaction, epidural or spinal hematoma, and thrombocytopenia

## General Dosing Information

Ardeparin cannot be used interchangeably (unit for unit) with heparin sodium or other low molecular weight heparins.

Ardeparin should be administered subcutaneously. Intramuscular injection is not recommended because of the possibility of hematoma at the injection site. Ardeparin is not intended for intravenous administration.

Injection technique: The patient should be sitting or lying down during injection. It may be given by deep (intra-fat) injection into the abdomen (avoiding the navel), the anterior aspect of the thighs, or the outer aspect of the upper arms; the site should be rotated with each injection. A skin fold, held between the thumb and forefinger, must be lifted, and the entire length of the needle inserted into the fold at a 45- to 90-degree angle. The plunger of the needle should be drawn back before the medication is injected to ensure that the needle is not in the intravascular space. To reduce bruising, the injection site should not be rubbed after the injection is completed.

Subcutaneous dosing is calculated according to body weight because, in early clinical trials, plasma anti-factor Xa activity after fixed doses was found to be lower in patients of greater body weight; dosing according to body weight produces relatively constant anti-factor Xa activity.

Because of the lack of correlation between renal function and bleeding rates and because ardeparin clearance was not reduced to a greater extent in patients with severe renal function impairment than in those with mild to moderate impairment, dosage adjustment does not appear to be necessary in patients with renal disease.

Close observation for possible bleeding is recommended if ardeparin is administered during or immediately after diagnostic lumbar puncture, epidural anesthesia, or spinal anesthesia.

If thromboembolism develops in spite of ardeparin prophylactic therapy, it is recommended that ardeparin be withdrawn and appropriate therapy initiated.

## Parenteral Dosage Forms

### ARDEPARIN SODIUM INJECTION

**Usual adult dose**
Thromboembolism, pulmonary (prophylaxis) and
Thrombosis, deep venous (prophylaxis)—
   Subcutaneous (by deep [intra-fat] injection), 50 anti-factor Xa units per kg of body weight every twelve hours following knee replacement surgery. Treatment should be initiated in the evening of the day of surgery or the following morning, and should continue for up to fourteen days or until the patient is fully ambulatory, whichever is shorter.

**Usual pediatric dose**
Safety and efficacy have not been established.

**Strength(s) usually available**
U.S.—
   5000 anti-factor Xa units per 0.5 mL (in a single-use sterile cartridge-needle unit) (Rx) [*Normiflo* (glycerin; methylparaben; sodium metabisulfite; propylparaben; sodium hydroxide [to adjust pH]; water for injection)].
   10,000 anti-factor Xa units per 0.5 mL (in a single-use sterile cartridge-needle unit) (Rx) [*Normiflo* (glycerin; methylparaben; sodium metabisulfite; propylparaben; sodium hydroxide [to adjust pH]; water for injection)].

**Packaging and storage**
Store between 15 and 25 °C (59 and 77 °F).

**Preparation of dosage form**
To calculate the volume (in mL) for a 50 anti-factor Xa units per kg (units/kg) subcutaneous dose, one of the following formulas may be used, depending on the strength used:
• For patients weighing up to 100 kg (220 pounds) (using the 5000 anti-factor Xa units per 0.5 mL strength)—Patient's body weight (kg) x 0.005 mL per kg.
• For patients weighing more than 100 kg (220 pounds) (using the 10,000 anti-factor Xa units per 0.5 mL strength)—Patient's body weight (kg) x 0.0025 mL per kg.

Note: The manufacturer provides detailed information in the labeling in tabular form regarding the volume of ardeparin sodium injection to be administered for a range of patient weights.

**Incompatibilities**
Mixing of ardeparin sodium injection with other injections or infusions is not recommended.

Developed: 11/17/97
Interim revision: 07/10/98

---

# ASCORBIC ACID  Systemic

This monograph includes information on the following: 1) Ascorbic Acid; 2) Sodium Ascorbate†.

VA CLASSIFICATION (Primary/Secondary):
   Ascorbic acid—VT400/AD900; DX900
   Sodium Ascorbate—VT400/AD900

Commonly used brand name(s): *Apo-C*[1]; *Ascorbicap*[1]; *Cebid Timecelles*[1]; *Cecon*[1]; *Cecore 500*[1]; *Cee-500*[1]; *Cemill*[1]; *Cenolate*[2]; *Cetane*[1]; *Cevi-Bid*[1]; *Flavorcee*[1]; *Mega-C/A Plus*[1]; *Ortho/CS*[2]; *Sunkist*[1].

Another commonly used name is vitamin C.

Note: For a listing of dosage forms and brand names by country availability, see *Dosage Forms* section(s).

†Not commercially available in Canada.

## Category

Note: Ascorbic acid (vitamin C) is a water-soluble vitamin.

Nutritional supplement (vitamin)—Ascorbic Acid; Sodium Ascorbate.
Diagnostic aid adjunct (red blood cell disease)—Ascorbic Acid Injection.
Deferoxamine adjunct (chronic iron overdose)—Ascorbic Acid; Sodium Ascorbate.
Methemoglobinemia (idiopathic) therapy adjunct—Ascorbic Acid.

## Indications

Note: Bracketed information in the *Indications* section refers to uses that are not included in U.S. product labeling.

**Accepted**

Vitamin C deficiency (prophylaxis and treatment)—Ascorbic acid and sodium ascorbate are indicated for prevention and treatment of ascorbic acid deficiency states. Ascorbic acid deficiency may occur as a result of inadequate nutrition but does not occur in healthy individuals receiving an adequate balanced diet. For prophylaxis of ascorbic acid deficiency, dietary improvement rather than supplementation is advisable. For treatment of vitamin C deficiency, supplementation is preferred.

Deficiency of ascorbic acid may lead to scurvy.

Requirements may be increased and/or supplementation may be necessary in the following persons or conditions (based on documented ascorbic acid deficiency):
AIDS (acquired immune deficiency syndrome)
Alcoholism
Burns
Cancer
Exposure to cold temperatures, prolonged
Fever, prolonged
Gastrectomy
Hemodialysis, chronic
Hyperthyroidism
Infants receiving unfortified formulas
Infection, continuing
Intestinal diseases—diarrhea, prolonged; ileal resection
Peptic ulcer
Smokers
Stress, continuing
Surgery
Trauma, continuing
Tuberculosis

Some unusual diets (e.g., reducing diets that drastically restrict food selection) may not supply minimum daily requirements for ascorbic acid. Supplementation is necessary in patients receiving total parenteral nutrition (TPN) or undergoing rapid weight loss or in those with malnutrition, because of inadequate dietary intake.

Recommended intakes for all vitamins and most minerals are increased during pregnancy. Many physicians recommend that pregnant women receive multivitamin and mineral supplements, especially those pregnant women who do not consume an adequate diet and those in high-risk categories (i.e., women carrying more than one fetus, heavy cigarette smokers, and alcohol and drug abusers). Taking excessive amounts of a multivitamin and mineral supplement may be harmful to the mother and/or fetus and should be avoided.

Recommended intakes for all vitamins and most minerals are increased during breast-feeding.

Red blood cells, labeling of, adjunct—Ascorbic acid injection is used as a reducing agent in the preparation of sodium chromate Cr 51 injection for the *in vitro* labeling of red blood cells.

[Toxicity, iron, chronic (treatment adjunct)][1]—Ascorbic acid or sodium ascorbate has been used to increase iron excretion by improving chelation during deferoxamine therapy.

Ascorbic acid has been used as treatment adjunct for idiopathic methemoglobinemia; however, its use has generally been replaced by more effective agents.

**Acceptance not established**
There are insufficient data to show that ascorbic acid may reduce the risk of *cardiovascular disease* and certain types of *cancer*.

**Unaccepted**
A potential role for ascorbic acid in the treatment of cancer has not been proven. Ascorbic acid is not useful for treatment of pyorrhea or gingival infections, hemorrhagic states, hematuria, retinal hemorrhages, immune system dysfunction, or mental depression not related to ascorbic acid deficiency. Ascorbic acid has not been proven effective for treatment of dental caries, anemia, acne, asthma, infertility, aging, atherosclerosis, peptic ulcer, tuberculosis, schizophrenia, dysentery, collagen disorders, fractures, skin ulcers, hay fever, or drug toxicity, nor for prevention of vascular thrombosis or the common cold.

---

[1]Not included in Canadian product labeling.

## Pharmacology/Pharmacokinetics

### Physicochemical characteristics
Molecular weight—
Ascorbic acid: 176.13.
Sodium ascorbate: 198.11.
pKa—
4.2 and 11.6.

### Mechanism of action/Effect
Nutritional supplement (vitamin)—Ascorbic acid is necessary for collagen formation and tissue repair in the body and may be involved in some oxidation-reduction reactions. It is also involved in metabolism of phenylalanine, tyrosine, folic acid, norepinephrine, histamine, iron, and some drug enzyme systems; utilization of carbohydrates; synthesis of lipids, proteins, and carnitine; immune function; hydroxylation of serotonin; and preservation of blood vessel integrity. In addition, ascorbic acid enhances the absorption of nonheme iron.

Diagnostic aid adjunct (red blood cell disease)—Ascorbic acid reduces unbound dianionic chromium 51 to the anionic state, which does not penetrate red blood cells, thereby terminating the *in vitro* labeling of red blood cells.

Deferoxamine adjunct (chronic iron overdose)—Complex interaction; vitamin C given orally in small doses (150 to 250 mg per day) may improve the chelating action of deferoxamine and increase the amount of iron excreted.

### Absorption
Readily absorbed from gastrointestinal tract (jejunum); may be reduced with large doses.

### Protein binding
Low (25%).

### Storage
Ascorbic acid is taken up by all cells of the body. The highest concentrations are found in glandular tissues, leukocytes, the liver, and the lens of the eye. The body stores up to approximately 1500 mg of ascorbic acid with intake of the recommended daily amount, and 2500 mg with an intake of 200 mg a day.

### Biotransformation
Hepatic.

### Elimination
Renal, very little as unchanged vitamin and metabolites except with high doses; urinary excretion increases with plasma concentrations of greater than 1.4 mg per 100 mL.
In dialysis—Removable by hemodialysis.

## Precautions to Consider

### Pregnancy/Reproduction
Pregnancy—Studies have not been done in humans. Problems in humans have not been documented with intake of normal daily recommended amounts. Ascorbic acid crosses the placenta. Ingestion of large quantities of ascorbic acid daily throughout pregnancy may possibly harm the fetus.
Studies have not been done in animals.
FDA Pregnancy Category C (parenteral ascorbic acid).

### Breast-feeding
Problems in humans have not been documented with intake of normal daily recommended amounts. Ascorbic acid is distributed into breast milk.

### Pediatrics
Problems in pediatrics have not been documented with intake of normal daily recommended amounts.

### Geriatrics
Problems in geriatrics have not been documented with intake of normal daily recommended amounts.

### Dental
Excessive use of chewable ascorbic acid tablets has been reported to cause breakdown of tooth enamel.

### Drug interactions and/or related problems
The following drug interactions and/or related problems have been selected on the basis of their potential clinical significance (possible mechanism in parentheses where appropriate)—not necessarily inclusive (» = major clinical significance):

Note: Combinations containing any of the following medications, depending on the amount present, may also interact with this medication.

Large doses of ascorbic acid (but not sodium ascorbate) may lower urinary pH and cause renal tubular reabsorption of acidic medications with concurrent administration; alkaline medications may exhibit decreased reabsorption.

Anticoagulants, coumarin- or indandione-derivative
(doses of 10 grams or more a day of ascorbic acid have been reported to impair gastrointestinal absorption of the anticoagulant)

Cellulose sodium phosphate
(concurrent use may result in metabolism of ascorbic acid to oxalate)

» Deferoxamine
(concurrent use with ascorbic acid may enhance tissue iron toxicity, especially in the heart, causing cardiac decompensation; therefore, this regimen should be used with caution in older patients; the need for ascorbic acid supplementation should be completely documented by measurements of iron excretion before and after supplements, and the oral dose of ascorbic acid should be given an hour or two after the deferoxamine infusion has been initiated when adequate concentrations of deferoxamine have been achieved)

Disulfiram
(concurrent use with ascorbic acid, especially with chronic use or high doses, may interfere with the disulfiram-alcohol interaction)

**Laboratory value alterations**
The following have been selected on the basis of their potential clinical significance (possible effect in parentheses where appropriate)—not necessarily inclusive (» = major clinical significance):

Note: Because ascorbic acid is a strong reducing agent, it interferes with laboratory tests based on oxidation-reduction reactions.

With diagnostic test results
Glucose determinations, urine, by cupric sulfate (Benedict's) reagent
(concentration may be falsely increased)
Glucose determinations, urine, by glucose oxidase (*Tes-Tape*) method
(concentration may be falsely decreased)
Lactate dehydrogenase (LDH) and
Transaminase, hepatic
(serum concentrations as measured by auto-analyzer may be decreased with doses of ascorbic acid greater than 200 mg a day)
Occult blood in stool
(large doses may cause false-negative results)

With physiology/laboratory test values
Bilirubin
(serum concentrations may be elevated)
pH, urine
(may be decreased by large doses of ascorbic acid, but not by sodium ascorbate)
Uric acid and
Oxalate, urine
(concentrations may be increased in patients receiving large doses of ascorbic acid)

**Medical considerations/Contraindications**
The medical considerations/contraindications included have been selected on the basis of their potential clinical significance (reasons given in parentheses where appropriate)—not necessarily inclusive (» = major clinical significance).

*Risk-benefit should be considered when the following medical problems exist:*

Diabetes mellitus
(possible interference with glucose determinations by very high doses of ascorbic acid)
Glucose-6-phosphate dehydrogenase (G6PD) deficiency
(high doses of ascorbic acid may cause hemolytic anemia)
Hemochromatosis or
Sideroblastic anemia or
Thalassemia
(high doses of ascorbic acid may increase iron absorption)
Hyperoxaluria or oxalosis or
Renal stones, history of
(risk of hyperoxaluria and possible precipitation of oxalate stones in urinary tract after high doses of ascorbic acid)
Sensitivity to ascorbic acid or sodium ascorbate

**Patient monitoring**
The following may be especially important in patient monitoring (other tests may be warranted in some patients, depending on condition; » = major clinical significance):

Ascorbic acid determinations, buffy coat, plasma, or serum
(recommended to determine ascorbic acid deficiency; buffy coat levels are used to determine ascorbic acid stores)

## Side/Adverse Effects

Note: Withdrawal scurvy may occur after prolonged administration of 2 to 3 grams per day.

The following side/adverse effects have been selected on the basis of their potential clinical significance (possible signs and symptoms in parentheses where appropriate)—not necessarily inclusive:

Those indicating need for medical attention
Incidence dose-related
*Kidney stones, oxalate* (side or lower back pain)
Note: Occasionally, prolonged doses of ascorbic acid in excess of 1 g per day have been reported to cause an increase in urinary oxalate, which may cause precipitation of oxalate stones in the urinary tract in patients with renal disease, especially those on hemodialysis, or in patients with a history of renal stones. However, studies have not found an increase in urinary oxalate formation with high doses of ascorbic acid.

Those indicating need for medical attention only if they continue or are bothersome
Incidence less frequent or rare
*Dizziness or faintness*—with rapid intravenous administration
With high doses
*Diarrhea*—with oral doses greater than 1 gram per day; *flushing or redness of skin; headache; increase in urination, mild*—with doses greater than 600 mg per day; *nausea or vomiting; stomach cramps*

## Patient Consultation

As an aid to patient consultation, refer to *Advice for the Patient, Ascorbic Acid (Vitamin C) (Systemic)*.

In providing consultation, consider emphasizing the following selected information (» = major clinical significance):

**Description of use**
Description should include function in the body, signs of deficiency, conditions that may cause deficiency, and unproven uses

**Importance of diet**
Importance of proper nutrition; supplement may be needed because of inadequate dietary intake
Food sources of ascorbic acid; effects of processing
Not using vitamins as substitute for balanced diet
Recommended daily intake for ascorbic acid

**Before using this dietary supplement**
» Conditions affecting use, especially:
Pregnancy—Crosses placenta; large quantities during pregnancy may be harmful to the fetus
Breast-feeding—Distributed into breast milk
Dental—Breakdown of enamel has been reported with excessive use of chewable tablets
Other medications, especially deferoxamine

**Proper use of this dietary supplement**
» Proper dosing
Missed dose: No cause for concern because of length of time necessary for depletion; remembering to take as directed
Proper administration of oral solution:
Taking by mouth even though it comes in dropper bottle
May be dropped directly into the mouth or mixed with cereal, fruit juice, or other food
» Proper storage

**Precautions while using this dietary supplement**
Ascorbic acid not stored; excessive amounts excreted in urine; very high doses may interfere with glucose determinations and diagnostic tests for occult blood in stool

**Side/adverse effects**
Signs of potential side effects, especially increase in urinary oxalate and possible precipitation of oxalate kidney stones

## General Dosing Information

**For parenteral dosage forms**
The intramuscular route is usually preferred because ascorbic acid is absorbed and utilized more efficiently with this method of administration.

**Diet/Nutrition**
Recommended dietary intakes for ascorbic acid are defined differently worldwide.
For U.S.—
The Recommended Dietary Allowances (RDAs) for vitamins and minerals are determined by the Food and Nutrition Board of the National Research Council and are intended to provide adequate nutrition in most healthy persons under usual environmental stresses. In addition, a different designation may be used by the FDA for food and dietary supplement labeling purposes, as with Daily Value (DV). DVs replace the previous labeling terminology United States Recommended Daily Allowances (USRDAs).

For Canada—
Recommended Nutrient Intakes (RNIs) for vitamins, minerals, and protein are determined by Health and Welfare in Canada and provide recommended amounts of a specific nutrient while minimizing the risk of chronic diseases.

Daily recommended intakes for ascorbic acid are generally defined as follows:

| Persons | U.S. (mg) | Canada (mg) |
|---|---|---|
| Infants and children | | |
| Birth to 3 years of age | 30–40 | 20 |
| 4 to 6 years of age | 45 | 25 |
| 7 to 10 years of age | 45 | 25 |
| Adolescent and adult males | 50–60 | 25–40 |
| Adolescent and adult females | 50–60 | 25–30 |
| Pregnant females | 70 | 30–40 |
| Breast-feeding females | 90–95 | 55 |
| Smokers | 100 | 45–60 |

These are usually provided by nutritionally adequate diets.

Best dietary sources of ascorbic acid include citrus fruits (oranges, lemons, grapefruit), green vegetables (peppers, broccoli, cabbage), tomatoes, and potatoes. Gradual loss of ascorbic acid occurs in fresh foods with storage, but not when frozen (except over prolonged periods). Ascorbic acid in foods is rapidly destroyed by exposure to air (oxygen), drying, salting, and ordinary cooking (30 to 50%, especially in copper pots). Mincing of fresh vegetables and mashing of potatoes also reduces the ascorbic acid content.

## ASCORBIC ACID

## Oral Dosage Forms

### ASCORBIC ACID EXTENDED-RELEASE CAPSULES

**Usual adult and adolescent dose**
Deficiency (prophylaxis)—
Oral, amount based on normal daily recommended intakes:

| Persons | U.S. (mg) | Canada (mg) |
|---|---|---|
| Adolescent and adult males | 50–60 | 25–40 |
| Adolescent and adult females | 50–60 | 25–30 |
| Pregnant females | 70 | 30–40 |
| Breast-feeding females | 90–95 | 55 |
| Smokers | 100 | 45–60 |

Deficiency (treatment)—
Treatment dose is individualized by prescriber based on severity of deficiency. The following dosage has been established: Scurvy—Oral, 500 mg a day for at least 2 weeks.

**Usual pediatric dose**
Dosage form not appropriate for pediatric patients.

**Strength(s) usually available**
U.S.—
500 mg (OTC) [*Ascorbicap* (tartrazine); *Cebid Timecelles; Cetane; Cevi-Bid;* GENERIC].
Canada—
Not commercially available.

Note: The strength of these ascorbic acid preparations may exceed the dosage range recommended by USP DI Advisory Panels based on the amount necessary to meet normal nutritional needs.

**Packaging and storage**
Store below 40 °C (104 °F), preferably between 15 and 30 °C (59 and 86 °F), in a tight container, unless otherwise specified by manufacturer. Protect from light.

### ASCORBIC ACID ORAL SOLUTION USP

**Usual adult and adolescent dose**
See *Ascorbic Acid Extended-release Capsules*.

**Usual pediatric dose**
Deficiency (prophylaxis)—
Oral, amount based on intake of normal daily recommended intakes:

| Persons | U.S. (mg) | Canada (mg) |
|---|---|---|
| Infants and children | | |
| Birth to 3 years of age | 30–40 | 20 |
| 4 to 6 years of age | 45 | 25 |
| 7 to 10 years of age | 45 | 25 |

Deficiency (treatment)—
Treatment dose is individualized by prescriber based on severity of deficiency. The following dosage has been established: Scurvy—Oral, 100 to 300 mg a day for at least 2 weeks.

**Strength(s) usually available**
U.S.—
50 mg per mL (OTC) [GENERIC].
100 mg per mL (OTC) [*Cecon*].
Canada—
Not commercially available.

Note: The strength of these ascorbic acid preparations may exceed the dosage range recommended by USP DI Advisory Panels based on the amount necessary to meet normal nutritional needs.

**Packaging and storage**
Store below 40 °C (104 °F), preferably between 15 and 30 °C (59 and 86 °F), unless otherwise specified by manufacturer. Store in a tight, light-resistant container. Protect from freezing.

### ASCORBIC ACID SYRUP

**Usual adult and adolescent dose**
See *Ascorbic Acid Extended-release Capsules*.

**Usual pediatric dose**
See *Ascorbic Acid Oral Solution USP*.

**Strength(s) usually available**
U.S.—
250 mg per 5 mL (OTC) [GENERIC].
500 mg per 5 mL (OTC) [GENERIC].
Canada—
Not commercially available.

Note: Some strengths of these ascorbic acid preparations may exceed the dosage range recommended by USP DI Advisory Panels based on the amount necessary to meet normal nutritional needs.

**Packaging and storage**
Store below 40 °C (104 °F), preferably between 15 and 30 °C (59 and 86 °F), in a tight container, unless otherwise specified by manufacturer. Protect from light. Protect from freezing.

### ASCORBIC ACID TABLETS USP

**Usual adult and adolescent dose**
See *Ascorbic Acid Extended-release Capsules*.

**Usual pediatric dose**
See *Ascorbic Acid Oral Solution USP*.

**Strength(s) usually available**
U.S.—
25 mg (OTC) [GENERIC].
50 mg (OTC) [GENERIC].
100 mg (OTC) [GENERIC].
125 mg (OTC) [GENERIC].
250 mg (OTC) [GENERIC].
500 mg (OTC) [*Sunkist;* GENERIC].
1 gram (OTC) [GENERIC].
1.5 grams (OTC) [GENERIC].
Canada—
100 mg (OTC) [*Apo-C* (scored)].
250 mg (OTC) [*Apo-C* (scored)].
500 mg (OTC) [*Apo-C*].
1 gram (OTC) [*Apo-C;* GENERIC].

Note: Some strengths of these ascorbic acid preparations may exceed the dosage range recommended by USP DI Advisory Panels based on the amount necessary to meet normal nutritional needs.

**Packaging and storage**
Store below 40 °C (104 °F), preferably between 15 and 30 °C (59 and 86 °F), unless otherwise specified by manufacturer. Store in a tight, light-resistant container.

### ASCORBIC ACID TABLETS (CHEWABLE) USP

**Usual adult and adolescent dose**
See *Ascorbic Acid Extended-release Capsules*.

**Usual pediatric dose**
See *Ascorbic Acid Oral Solution USP*.

**Strength(s) usually available**
U.S.—
   60 mg (OTC) [*Sunkist;* GENERIC].
   100 mg (OTC) [*Flavorcee;* GENERIC].
   250 mg (OTC) [*Flavorcee; Sunkist;* GENERIC].
   500 mg (OTC) [*Flavorcee; Sunkist;* GENERIC].
   1 gram (OTC) [GENERIC].
Canada—
   60 mg (OTC) [GENERIC].
   250 mg (OTC) [GENERIC].
   500 mg (OTC) [GENERIC].

Note: Some chewable ascorbic acid tablets may also contain sodium ascorbate.
      Some strengths of these ascorbic acid preparations may exceed the dosage range recommended by USP DI Advisory Panels based on the amount necessary to meet normal nutritional needs.

**Packaging and storage**
Store below 40 °C (104 °F), preferably between 15 and 30 °C (59 and 86 °F), unless otherwise specified by manufacturer. Store in a tight, light-resistant container.

### ASCORBIC ACID TABLETS (EFFERVESCENT) USP

**Usual adult and adolescent dose**
See *Ascorbic Acid Extended-release Capsules*.

**Usual pediatric dose**
See *Ascorbic Acid Oral Solution USP*.

**Strength(s) usually available**
U.S.—
   1 gram (OTC) [GENERIC].
Canada—
   Not commercially available.

**Packaging and storage**
Store below 40 °C (104 °F), preferably between 15 and 30 °C (59 and 86 °F), unless otherwise specified by manufacturer. Store in a tight, light-resistant container.

**Preparation of dosage form**
Ascorbic acid effervescent tablets should be dissolved in a glass of water immediately prior to ingestion.

### ASCORBIC ACID EXTENDED-RELEASE TABLETS

**Usual adult and adolescent dose**
See *Ascorbic Acid Extended-release Capsules*.

**Usual pediatric dose**
Dosage form not appropriate for pediatric patients.

**Strength(s) usually available**
U.S.—
   500 mg (OTC) [*Cemill;* GENERIC].
   1 gram (OTC) [*Cemill;* GENERIC].
   1.5 gram (OTC) [GENERIC].
Canada—
   500 mg (OTC) [GENERIC].

Note: Some strengths of these ascorbic acid preparations may exceed the dosage range recommended by USP DI Advisory Panels based on the amount necessary to meet normal nutritional needs.

**Packaging and storage**
Store below 40 °C (104 °F), preferably between 15 and 30 °C (59 and 86 °F), in a tight container, unless otherwise specified by manufacturer. Protect from light.

## Parenteral Dosage Forms

### ASCORBIC ACID INJECTION USP

**Usual adult and adolescent dose**
Deficiency (prophylaxis)—
   Intravenous infusion, as part of total parenteral nutrition solutions, the specific amount determined by individual patient need.
Deficiency (treatment)—
   Intravenous infusion, as part of total parenteral nutrition solutions, the specific amount determined by individual patient need.
   Intramuscular, 100 to 500 mg a day for at least 2 weeks.
Diagnostic aid adjunct (red blood cell disease)—
   For use in labeling of red blood cells, 100 mg of ascorbic acid injection injected into the vial of sodium chromate Cr 51 injection.

**Usual pediatric dose**
Deficiency(prophylaxis)—
   Intravenous infusion, as part of total parenteral nutrition solutions, the specific amount determined by individual patient need.
Deficiency (treatment)—
   Intravenous infusion, as part of total parenteral nutrition solutions, the specific amount determined by individual patient need.
   Intramuscular, 100 to 300 mg a day for at least 2 weeks.

**Strength(s) usually available**
U.S.—
   222 mg per mL (Rx) [GENERIC].
   250 mg per mL (Rx) [GENERIC].
   500 mg per mL (Rx) [*Cecore 500; Cee-500; Mega-C/A Plus;* GENERIC].
Canada—
   Not commercially available.

**Packaging and storage**
Store below 40 °C (104 °F), preferably between 15 and 30 °C (59 and 86 °F), unless otherwise specified by manufacturer. Store in a light-resistant container. Protect from freezing.

**Stability**
Ascorbic acid is oxidized rapidly, especially in the presence of catalyzing metal ions such as copper. Loss of ascorbic acid is greatest from admixtures stored in plastic containers, especially for longer than 48 hours. Exposure to light causes degradation of ascorbic acid; however, the slight color that develops during storage does not impair therapeutic activity. Some clinicians recommend that total parenteral nutrition solutions that contain ascorbic acid should be protected from light.

**Incompatibilities**
Ascorbic acid injection is physically incompatible with aminophylline, bleomycin, cefazolin sodium, cephapirin, chlordiazepoxide, conjugated estrogen, dextran, doxapram hydrochloride, erythromycin lactobionate, methicillin sodium, nafcillin sodium, penicillin G potassium, phytonadione, sodium bicarbonate, and warfarin.

---

## SODIUM ASCORBATE

## Parenteral Dosage Form

### SODIUM ASCORBATE INJECTION

**Usual adult and adolescent dose**
See *Ascorbic Acid Injection USP*.

**Usual pediatric dose**
See *Ascorbic Acid Injection USP*.

**Strength(s) usually available**
U.S.—
   250 mg (222 mg ascorbic acid) per mL (Rx) [*Ortho/CS;* GENERIC].
   562.5 mg (500 mg ascorbic acid) per mL (Rx) [*Cenolate* (0.5% sodium hydrosulfate)].
Canada—
   Not commercially available.

**Packaging and storage**
Store below 40 °C (104 °F), preferably between 15 and 30 °C (59 and 86 °F), protected from light, unless otherwise specified by manufacturer. Protect from freezing.

## 474 Ascorbic Acid (Systemic)

**Stability**

Ascorbic acid is oxidized rapidly, especially in the presence of catalyzing metal ions such as copper. Loss of ascorbic acid is greatest from admixtures stored in plastic containers, especially for longer than 48 hours. Exposure to light causes degradation of ascorbic acid; however, the slight color that develops during storage does not impair therapeutic activity. Some clinicians recommend that total parenteral nutrition solutions that contain ascorbic acid should be protected from light.

**Incompatibilities**

Ascorbic acid injection is physically incompatible with aminophylline, bleomycin, cefazolin sodium, cephapirin, chlordiazepoxide, conjugated estrogen, dextran, doxapram hydrochloride, erythromycin lactobionate, methicillin sodium, nafcillin sodium, penicillin G potassium, phytonadione, sodium bicarbonate, and warfarin.

**Additional information**

Each gram of sodium ascorbate contains approximately 5 mEq of sodium.

Revised: 05/01/95

---

# ASPARAGINASE   Systemic

VA CLASSIFICATION (Primary): AN900.

Commonly used brand name(s): *Elspar; Kidrolase*.

Another commonly used name is colaspase.

Note:  For a listing of dosage forms and brand names by country availability, see *Dosage Forms* section(s).

## Category

Antineoplastic.

## Indications

Note:  Bracketed information in the *Indications* section refers to uses that are not included in U.S. product labeling.

**Accepted**

Leukemia, acute lymphocytic (treatment)—Asparaginase is indicated, in combination with other agents, for induction of remissions in acute lymphocytic leukemia (primarily in pediatric patients). It is recommended that asparaginase not be used as part of a maintenance regimen because of the rapid development of resistance (as cells develop the capability to synthesize asparagine) to the medication.

[Lymphomas, non-Hodgkin's (treatment)]—Asparaginase is used for treatment of lymphosarcoma and reticulum cell sarcoma (reticulosarcoma).

## Pharmacology/Pharmacokinetics

**Physicochemical characteristics**

Source—Asparaginase is a high molecular weight enzyme obtained commercially from *Escherichia coli*.

**Mechanism of action/Effect**

Asparaginase breaks down extracellular asparagine, which is required for cell survival, to aspartic acid and ammonia. Normal cells are capable of synthesizing their own asparagine but certain malignant cells are not. Asparaginase interferes with protein synthesis and also with DNA and RNA synthesis, and appears to be cell cycle–specific for the $G_1$ phase of cell division. Cell death then results from fragmentation of the cell into membrane-bound particles that are eliminated by phagocytosis.

**Other actions/effects**

Has immunosuppressant activity in animals.

**Distribution**

Crosses the blood-brain barrier to only a limited extent; cerebrospinal fluid concentrations are less than 1% of concurrent plasma concentrations; slow sequestration by the reticuloendothelial system.

**Half-life**

Intramuscular—39 to 49 hours.
Intravenous—8 to 30 hours.

**Onset of action**

Blood concentrations of asparagine fall to undetectable levels almost immediately after administration of asparaginase. Normal or below-normal leukocyte counts are noted frequently within the first several days after treatment with asparaginase is started.

**Time to peak plasma concentration**

After intramuscular administration—14 to 24 hours.

**Duration of action**

Concentrations of asparagine in the blood remain low for 7 to 10 days after discontinuation of therapy with asparaginase.

**Elimination**

Unknown; only trace amounts appear in the urine following intravenous administration.

## Precautions to Consider

**Cross-sensitivity and/or related problems**

In one study, cross-sensitivity between commercially available asparaginase and one product for investigational use derived from *Erwinia carotovora* was reported in 22.6% of patients. Allergic reactions included urticaria, tachypnea, wheezing, shortness of breath, pruritus, and tachycardia.

**Carcinogenicity**

Secondary malignancies are potential delayed effects of many antineoplastic agents, although it is not clear whether the effect is related to their mutagenic or immunosuppressive action. The effect of dose and duration of therapy is also unknown, although risk seems to increase with long-term use. Although information is limited, available data seem to indicate that the carcinogenic risk is greatest with the alkylating agents.

Intraperitoneal administration of 2500 Units of asparaginase per kg of body weight per day for 4 days reportedly caused a small increase in pulmonary adenomas in newborn Swiss mice.

**Mutagenicity**

Asparaginase was not found to be mutagenic at concentrations of 152 to 909 international units (IU) per plate in the Ames microbial mutagen test with or without metabolic activation.

**Pregnancy/Reproduction**

Pregnancy—Adequate and well-controlled studies in humans have not been done.

First trimester: It usually is recommended that use of antineoplastics, especially combination chemotherapy, be avoided whenever possible, especially during the first trimester. Although information is limited because of the relatively few instances of antineoplastic administration during pregnancy, the teratogenic and carcinogenic potential of these medications must be considered.

Other hazards to the fetus include adverse reactions seen in adults.

In general, use of a contraceptive is recommended during cytotoxic drug therapy.

Studies in mice and rats have shown that asparaginase, given in doses of greater than 1000 IU per kg of body weight (the recommended human dose), retards the weight gain of mothers and fetuses and causes resorptions, gross abnormalities, and skeletal abnormalities. Dose-dependent embryotoxicity and gross abnormalities also have been reported with intravenous administration of 50 or 100 IU of asparaginase per kg of body weight to pregnant rabbits on days 8 and 9 of gestation.

FDA Pregnancy Category C.

**Breast-feeding**

It is not known whether asparaginase is distributed into breast milk. Although very little information is available regarding distribution of antineoplastic agents into breast milk, breast-feeding is not recommended while asparaginase is being administered because of the risks to the infant (adverse effects, carcinogenicity).

**Pediatrics**

Appropriate studies performed to date have not demonstrated pediatrics-specific problems that would limit the usefulness of asparaginase in children. In fact, incidence of toxicity appears to be lower in pediatric patients than in adult patients.

**Geriatrics**

No information is available on the relationship of age to the effects of asparaginase in geriatric patients.

**Dental**

Asparaginase may cause stomatitis associated with considerable discomfort.

**Drug interactions and/or related problems**

The following drug interactions and/or related problems have been selected on the basis of their potential clinical significance (possible mechanism in parentheses where appropriate)—not necessarily inclusive (» = major clinical significance):

Note: Combinations containing any of the following medications, depending on the amount present, may also interact with this medication.

Allopurinol or
Colchicine or
» Probenecid or
» Sulfinpyrazone
(asparaginase may raise the concentration of blood uric acid; dosage adjustment of antigout agents may be necessary to control hyperuricemia and gout; allopurinol may be preferred to prevent or reverse asparaginase-induced hyperuricemia because of risk of uric acid nephropathy with uricosuric antigout agents)

Antidiabetic agents, sulfonylurea or
Insulin
(asparaginase may alter blood glucose concentrations; for adult-onset diabetics, dosage adjustment of hypoglycemic medications may be necessary during and after asparaginase therapy)

Corticosteroids, glucocorticoid, especially prednisone or
» Vincristine
(concurrent use may enhance the hyperglycemic effect of asparaginase and may increase the risk of neuropathy and disturbances in erythropoiesis; toxicity appears to be less pronounced when asparaginase is administered after vincristine and prednisone rather than before or with these medications)

Immunosuppressant medications, other, such as:
Azathioprine
Chlorambucil
Cyclophosphamide
Cyclosporine
Mercaptopurine
Muromonab-CD3 or
Radiation therapy
(concurrent use with asparaginase may increase the total effects of these medications and radiation therapy; dosage reduction may be required)

» Methotrexate
(asparaginase may block the effects of methotrexate by inhibiting cell replication; this inhibition of methotrexate's action appears to correlate with suppression of asparagine concentrations. Some studies indicate that administration of asparaginase 9 to 10 days before or within 24 hours after methotrexate administration does not produce this inhibition of antineoplastic effect and may reduce the gastrointestinal and hematological effects of methotrexate)

Vaccines, killed virus
(because normal defense mechanisms may be suppressed by asparaginase therapy, the patient's antibody response to the vaccine may be decreased. The interval between discontinuation of medications that cause immunosuppression and restoration of the patient's ability to respond to the vaccine depends on the intensity and type of immunosuppression-causing medication used, the underlying disease, and other factors; estimates vary from 3 months to 1 year)

» Vaccines, live virus
(because normal defense mechanisms may be suppressed by asparaginase therapy, concurrent use with a live virus vaccine may potentiate the replication of the vaccine virus, may increase the side/adverse effects of the vaccine virus, and/or may decrease the patient's antibody response to the vaccine; immunization of these patients should be undertaken only with extreme caution after careful review of the patient's hematologic status and only with the knowledge and consent of the physician managing the asparaginase therapy. The interval between discontinuation of medications that cause immunosuppression and restoration of the patient's ability to respond to the vaccine depends on the intensity and type of immunosuppression-causing medication used, the underlying disease, and other factors; estimates vary from 3 months to 1 year. Patients with leukemia in remission should not receive live virus vaccine until at least 3 months after their last chemotherapy. In addition, immunization with oral poliovirus vaccine should be postponed in persons in close contact with the patient, especially family members)

**Laboratory value alterations**

The following have been selected on the basis of their potential clinical significance (possible effect in parentheses where appropriate)—not necessarily inclusive (» = major clinical significance):

With diagnostic test results
Thyroid function tests
(results may be altered because asparaginase decreases serum thyroxine-binding globulin concentrations within 2 days after the first dose; concentrations return to normal within 4 weeks of the last dose of asparaginase)

With physiology/laboratory test values
Ammonia concentrations, blood and
Blood urea nitrogen (BUN) concentrations
(may be increased because of breakdown of asparagine)
Cholesterol
(serum concentrations may be reversibly decreased; increases and decreases of total lipids have occurred)

**Medical considerations/Contraindications**

The medical considerations/contraindications included have been selected on the basis of their potential clinical significance (reasons given in parentheses where appropriate)—not necessarily inclusive (» = major clinical significance).

*Except under special circumstances, this medication should not be used when the following medical problems exist:*

» Pancreatitis, or history of
(potentially fatal acute hemorrhagic pancreatitis has been associated with asparaginase treatment)
» Previous allergic reaction to asparaginase

*Risk-benefit should be considered when the following medical problems exist:*

» Chickenpox, existing or recent (including recent exposure) or
» Herpes zoster
(risk of severe generalized disease)
Diabetes mellitus
(asparaginase may increase blood glucose concentrations)
Gout, history of or
Urate renal stones, history of
(asparaginase may increase serum uric acid concentrations)
» Hepatic function impairment
(may be increased by asparaginase)
» Infection
(immunosuppressive effects)
» Caution should be used also in patients who have had previous cytotoxic drug therapy and radiation therapy.

**Patient monitoring**

The following may be especially important in patient monitoring (other tests may be warranted in some patients, depending on condition; » = major clinical significance):

» Amylase concentrations, serum and
Bone marrow aspiration studies and
» Central nervous system (CNS) function, clinical and
» Coagulation tests, plasma and
Glucose concentrations, blood and
Hepatic function and
Peripheral blood count and
Renal function and
Uric acid concentrations, serum
(recommended at the initiation of therapy and at frequent intervals during therapy)

## Side/Adverse Effects

Note: Incidence of toxicity appears to be greater in adult patients than in pediatric patients.

The following side/adverse effects have been selected on the basis of their potential clinical significance (possible signs and symptoms in parentheses where appropriate)—not necessarily inclusive:

**Those indicating need for medical attention**
Incidence more frequent
*Allergic reaction* (trouble in breathing; joint pain; puffy face; skin rash or itching); *decrease in blood clotting factors* (unusual bleeding or bruising)—usually asymptomatic; *hepatotoxicity, including fatty changes*—asymptomatic; *pancreatitis* (severe stomach pain with nausea and vomiting)

Note: *Allergic reactions* occur frequently and may be severe or even fatal. The risk is increased with repeated doses, but may occur on initial administration, including during desensitization.

An *allergic reaction* to a therapeutic dose may occur even after a negative reaction to the intradermal skin test. Rarely, an anaphylactic reaction to the intradermal skin test itself may occur.

*Anaphylaxis* may be less common after intramuscular than after intravenous administration in children with advanced leukemia (although incidence of mild allergic reactions may be increased), or when asparaginase is given in combination with immunosuppressive agents.

The most common and most marked *decreases in blood clotting factors* occur in fibrinogen and factors V and VIII, with a variable decrease in factors VII and IX. Bleeding is rare, but intracranial hemorrhage and fatal bleeding have been reported. A compensatory increase in fibrinolytic activity has also occurred.

*Hepatotoxicity* usually occurs within 2 weeks of start of treatment.

Incidence less frequent
*CNS effects, reversible* (confusion; drowsiness; hallucinations; mental depression; nervousness; unusual tiredness); *hyperglycemia* (frequent urination; unusual thirst); *hyperuricemia or uric acid nephropathy* (lower back or side pain; swelling of feet or lower legs); *hypoalbuminemia or renal failure* (swelling of feet or lower legs); *stomatitis* (sores in mouth and on lips)

Note: *CNS effects* occur mostly in adults, in whom incidence may be as high as 30 to 60%; they usually occur within the first day of treatment and subside 1 to 3 days after asparaginase is withdrawn.

*Hyperglycemia* resembles hyperosmolar, nonketotic hyperglycemia. It usually responds to withdrawal of asparaginase and appropriate treatment, but may occasionally be fatal.

*Hyperuricemia or uric acid nephropathy* occurs most commonly during initial treatment of patients with leukemia or lymphoma, as a result of rapid cell breakdown leading to elevated serum uric acid concentrations.

Azotemia, usually pre-renal, occurs frequently. Fatal *renal insufficiency* has been reported.

Incidence rare
*Hyperthermia* (fever or chills); *immunosuppression* (infection); *intracranial hemorrhage or thrombosis* (severe headache; inability to move arm or leg); *leg vein thrombosis* (pain in lower legs); *leukopenia*

Note: *Leukopenia* may be marked but bone marrow depression is transient.

*Hyperthermia* may be fatal.

**Those indicating need for medical attention only if they continue or are bothersome**
Incidence more frequent
*Hyperammonemia* (mild headache; loss of appetite; nausea or vomiting; stomach cramps; weight loss)

**Those indicating the need for medical attention if they occur after medication is discontinued**
*Intracranial hemorrhage or thrombosis* (severe headache; inability to move arm or leg); *pancreatitis* (severe stomach pain with nausea and vomiting)

## Patient Consultation

As an aid to patient consultation, refer to *Advice for the Patient, Asparaginase (Systemic)*.

In providing consultation, consider emphasizing the following selected information (» = major clinical significance):

### Before using this medication
» Conditions affecting use, especially:
    Sensitivity to asparaginase
    Pregnancy—Embryotoxicity and abnormalities reported in animals; advisability of using contraception; telling physician immediately if pregnancy is suspected
    Breast-feeding—Not recommended because of risk of serious side effects
    Other medications, especially probenecid, sulfinpyrazone, or previous cytotoxic drug or radiation therapy
    Other medical problems, especially chickenpox, herpes zoster, pancreatitis, hepatic function impairment, or infection

### Proper use of this medication
Caution with combination therapy; taking each medication at the right time
Importance of ample fluid intake and subsequent increase in urine output to aid in excretion of uric acid
Possible nausea, vomiting, and loss of appetite; importance of continuing medication despite stomach upset
» Proper dosing

### Precautions while using this medication
» Importance of close monitoring by physician
» Avoiding immunizations unless approved by physician; other persons in patient's household should avoid immunizations with oral poliovirus vaccine; avoiding persons who have taken oral poliovirus vaccine or wearing a protective mask that covers nose and mouth
Caution if thyroid function test required; possible interference with test results

### Side/adverse effects
Importance of discussing possible adverse effects, including cancer, with physician
Signs of potential side effects, especially allergic reaction, decrease in blood clotting factors, hepatotoxicity, pancreatitis, CNS effects, hyperglycemia, hyperuricemia or uric acid nephropathy, hypoalbuminemia or renal failure, stomatitis, hyperthermia, immunosuppression, intracranial hemorrhage or thrombosis, leg vein thrombosis, and leukopenia
Asymptomatic side effects, including hepatotoxicity
Physician or nurse can help in dealing with side effects

## General Dosing Information

It is recommended that asparaginase be administered to patients only in a hospital setting under the supervision of a physician experienced in cancer chemotherapy. It is also recommended that equipment and medications (including epinephrine, diphenhydramine, oxygen, and intravenous steroids) necessary for treatment of a possible anaphylactic reaction be immediately available during each administration of asparaginase.

A variety of dosage schedules and regimens of asparaginase, alone or in combination with other antitumor agents, are used. The prescriber may consult the medical literature as well as the manufacturer's literature in choosing a specific dosage.

Dosage must be adjusted to meet the individual requirements of each patient, on the basis of clinical response and appearance or severity of toxicity.

Although the intradermal skin test has not been found entirely reliable in predicting allergic reactions to asparaginase, it is recommended that this test be performed prior to the initial administration of asparaginase and when a week or more has passed between doses. The test solution is prepared by adding 5 mL of sterile water for injection or 0.9% sodium chloride injection to the 10,000–International Unit (IU) vial of asparaginase, shaking to dissolve, and withdrawing 0.1 mL of the resulting solution (2000 IU per mL) and injecting it into another vial containing 9.9 mL of diluent to produce a test solution containing approximately 20 IU per mL. An intradermal injection of 0.1 mL (about 2 IU) is administered and the site observed for 1 hour for the appearance of a wheal or erythema, which indicates a positive reaction.

It is recommended that a desensitization method of administration of the first dose be utilized in patients who have had a positive reaction to the intradermal skin test and on re-treatment of a patient with asparaginase. A recommended schedule begins with the intravenous administration of 1 IU and doubles the dosage every 10 minutes, provided no allergic reaction has occurred, until the accumulated total dosage equals the dosage for that day.

It is recommended that when asparaginase is administered intravenously, it be given over a period of not less than 30 minutes through the side arm of an already running infusion of 0.9% sodium chloride injection or 5% dextrose injection. Asparaginase should not be infused through a filter. However, if gelatinous fiber-like particles develop on standing, reconstituted asparaginase may be filtered through a 5-micron filter during administration without loss in potency. Use of a 0.2-micron filter may result in a loss of potency.

No more than 2 mL of asparaginase solution should be injected at a single intramuscular injection site.

Development of uric acid nephropathy in patients with leukemia or lymphoma may be prevented by adequate oral hydration and, in some cases, administration of allopurinol. Alkalinization of urine may be necessary if serum uric acid concentrations are elevated.

If pancreatitis occurs, it is recommended that asparaginase therapy be permanently discontinued.

### Safety considerations for handling this medication
There is limited but increasing evidence and concern that personnel involved in preparation and administration of parenteral antineoplastics may be at some risk because of the potential mutagenicity, teratogenicity, and/or carcinogenicity of these agents, although the actual risk is

unknown. USP advisory panels recommend cautious handling both in preparation and disposal of antineoplastic agents. Precautions that have been suggested include:
- Use of a biological containment cabinet during reconstitution and dilution of parenteral medications and wearing of disposable surgical gloves and masks.
- Use of proper technique to prevent contamination of the medication, work area, and operator during transfer between containers (including proper training of personnel in this technique).
- Cautious and proper disposal of needles, syringes, vials, ampuls, and unused medication.

A number of medical centers have developed detailed guidelines for handling of antineoplastic agents.

**Combination chemotherapy**
Asparaginase may be used in combination with other agents in various regimens. As a result, incidence and/or severity of side effects may be altered and different dosages (usually reduced) may be used.

## Parenteral Dosage Forms

### ASPARAGINASE FOR INJECTION

**Usual adult dose**
Acute lymphocytic leukemia—
  Induction: Intravenous, 200 IU per kg of body weight a day for twenty-eight days.
Note: Because use of asparaginase in adults is primarily investigational at this time, the prescriber should consult the medical literature in choosing a specific dosage.

**Usual pediatric dose**
Acute lymphocytic leukemia—
  Intramuscular, 6000 IU per square meter of body surface on days 4, 7, 10, 13, 16, 19, 22, 25, and 28 of the treatment period, in combination with vincristine and prednisone or
  Intravenous, 1000 IU per kg of body weight per day for ten days beginning on day 22 of the treatment period, in combination with vincristine and prednisone.
Note: Many dosage regimens of asparaginase are in use at this time. A review of all of them is impossible in this space. Consultation of current medical literature is recommended. Use of asparaginase as the sole induction agent generally is not recommended unless combination therapy is considered inappropriate.

**Strength(s) usually available**
U.S.—
  10,000 IU (Rx) [*Elspar* (mannitol 80 mg)].
Canada—
  10,000 IU (Rx) [*Kidrolase*].

**Packaging and storage**
Store between 2 and 8 °C (36 and 46 °F).

**Preparation of dosage form**
Caution: Asparaginase is a contact irritant, and both the powder and solution should be handled with care to prevent inhalation of dust or vapors or contact with skin or mucous membranes (especially eyes). If accidental contact occurs, the affected area should be flushed with water for at least 15 minutes.
*Elspar* is reconstituted for intravenous use by adding 5 mL of sterile water for injection or 0.9% sodium chloride injection to a vial containing 10,000 IU of asparaginase and shaking to dissolve the medication. (Caution: Overly vigorous shaking may cause foaming and difficulty in withdrawing the contents of the vial.) Only a clear solution should be used. The resulting colorless solution, containing 2000 IU of asparaginase per mL, may be used for direct intravenous administration within 8 hours of reconstitution, provided the solution remains clear, or may be further diluted with 0.9% sodium chloride injection or 5% dextrose injection for administration by intravenous infusion. The infusion solution may also be used within 8 hours, provided it remains clear.
*Elspar* is reconstituted for intramuscular use by adding 2 mL of 0.9% sodium chloride injection to the 10,000-IU vial. The resulting solution should be used within 8 hours provided it remains clear.
If gelatinous fiber-like particles develop on standing, reconstituted *Elspar* may be filtered through a 5-micron filter during administration without loss in potency. Use of a 0.2-micron filter may result in a loss of potency.
*Kidrolase* is reconstituted for intramuscular or intravenous use by adding 4 mL of sterile water for injection to a vial containing 10,000 IU of asparaginase and rotating gently to dissolve the medication. (Caution: Rotate gently; do not shake.) The resulting solution may be further diluted with 0.9% sodium chloride injection or isotonic glucose solution for administration by intravenous infusion.

**Stability**
*Elspar*—Contains no preservative. Unused, reconstituted solution should be stored at 2 to 8 °C (36 to 46 °F) and discarded after 8 hours or sooner if it becomes cloudy.
*Kidrolase*—Unused, reconstituted solution may be stored at 2 to 8 °C (36 to 46 °F) for 14 days.

Revised: 09/26/97

---

**ASPIRIN** — See *Salicylates (Systemic)*

---

**ASPIRIN, BUFFERED** — See *Salicylates (Systemic)*

---

# ASPIRIN, SODIUM BICARBONATE, AND CITRIC ACID  Systemic

VA CLASSIFICATION (Primary/Secondary): CN103/BL160
NOTE: The *Aspirin, Sodium Bicarbonate, and Citric Acid (Systemic)* monograph is maintained on the USP DI electronic data base. For a printed copy of the most recent revision of the complete monograph, contact Micromedex, Inc. - Reprint Requests, 6200 S. Syracuse Way, Suite 300, Englewood, CO 80111; telephone (303) 486-6400; telefax (303) 486-6464; Email: USPDI@MDX.COM.
  For information on the specific components of this combination, see the *USP DI* monographs for *Salicylates (Systemic)*, *Sodium Bicarbonate (Systemic)*, and *Citrates (Systemic)*.
  The information that follows is selectively abstracted from the complete monograph and is provided to facilitate drug use review and patient counseling.
Commonly used brand name(s): *Alka-Seltzer Effervescent Pain Reliever and Antacid*; *Flavored Alka-Seltzer Effervescent Pain Reliever and Antacid*.
Note: For a listing of dosage forms and brand names by country availability, see *Dosage Forms* section(s).

## Category
Analgesic-antacid; platelet aggregation inhibitor.

## Indications
Note: Bracketed information in the *Indications* section refers to uses that are not included in U.S. product labeling.

**Accepted**
Pain and upset stomach (treatment)—Aspirin, sodium bicarbonate, and citric acid combination is indicated to relieve pain, especially when an upset stomach is also present. However, this medication is not recommended for long-term, high-dose use because of the high sodium bicarbonate content.
Platelet aggregation (prophylaxis)[1]— Aspirin, sodium bicarbonate, and citric acid combination is indicated to provide the platelet aggregation–inhibiting action of aspirin in the following:
  Ischemic attacks, transient, in males (prophylaxis);
  Thromboembolism, cerebral (prophylaxis); or
  [Thromboembolism, cerebral, recurrence (prophylaxis)]—Aspirin is indicated in the treatment of men who have had transient brain ischemia due to fibrin platelet emboli, to reduce the recurrence of transient ischemic attacks (TIAs) and the risk of stroke and death.
  [Aspirin is also used in the treatment of women with transient brain ischemia due to fibrin platelet emboli. However, its efficacy in preventing stroke and death in female patients has not been established].

[Aspirin is also indicated in the treatment of patients with documented, unexplained TIAs associated with mitral valve prolapse. However, if TIAs continue to occur after an adequate trial of aspirin therapy, aspirin should be discontinued and an oral anticoagulant administered instead].

[Aspirin is also indicated to prevent initial or recurrent cerebrovascular embolism, TIAs, and stroke following carotid endarterectomy].

[Aspirin is indicated in the treatment of patients who have had a completed thrombotic stroke, to prevent a recurrence].

Myocardial infarction (prophylaxis); or

Myocardial reinfarction (prophylaxis)—Aspirin is indicated to prevent myocardial infarction in patients with unstable angina pectoris and to prevent recurrence of myocardial infarction in patients with a history of myocardial infarction.

In one study, aspirin significantly reduced the rate of reocclusion, reinfarction, stroke, and death when a single dose was administered within a few hours after the onset of symptoms of acute myocardial infarction and daily thereafter. The benefit of early treatment with aspirin was additive to that of streptokinase. Therefore, it is recommended that aspirin therapy be initiated as soon as possible after the onset of symptoms, even if the patient is receiving thrombolytic therapy.

[One study has shown that aspirin may also prevent myocardial infarction in individuals who have no history of unstable angina pectoris or myocardial infarction. However, an increased incidence of hemorrhagic stroke was reported in subjects receiving aspirin. Also, the incidence of myocardial infarction, although higher in the placebo group than in the aspirin group, was low in both groups. Therefore, use of aspirin for this purpose remains controversial; whether aspirin's benefit outweighs its risk in apparently healthy individuals has not been established. However, aspirin may be indicated for prevention of an initial myocardial infarction in selected patients, especially those who may be at risk because of the presence of chronic stable coronary artery disease (as shown by exertional or episodic angina pectoris, abnormal coronary arteriogram, or positive stress test) and/or other risk factors.]

[Thromboembolism (prophylaxis)]—Aspirin is used in low doses to decrease the risk of thromboembolism following orthopedic (hip) surgery (especially total hip replacement) and in patients with arteriovenous shunts.

Platelet aggregation inhibitors, although not as consistently effective as an anticoagulant or an anticoagulant plus dipyridamole, may provide some protection against the development of thromboembolic complications in patients with mechanical prosthetic heart valves. Therefore, administration of aspirin, alone or in combination with dipyridamole, may be considered if anticoagulant therapy is contraindicated for these patients. Patients with bioprosthetic cardiac valves who are in normal sinus rhythm generally do not require prolonged antithrombotic therapy, but long-term aspirin administration may be considered on an individual basis.

Aspirin is also indicated, alone or in combination with dipyridamole, to reduce the risk of thrombosis and/or reocclusion of saphenous vein aortocoronary bypass grafts following coronary bypass surgery.

Aspirin is also indicated, alone or in combination with dipyridamole, to reduce the risk of thrombosis and/or reocclusion of prosthetic or saphenous vein femoral popliteal bypass grafts.

Because the patient may be at risk for thromboembolic complications, including myocardial infarction and stroke, long-term aspirin therapy may also be indicated for maintaining patency following coronary or peripheral vascular angioplasty and for treating patients with peripheral vascular insufficiency caused by arteriosclerosis.

Prolonged antithrombotic therapy is generally not needed to maintain vessel patency following vascular reconstruction procedures in high-flow, low-resistance arteries larger than 6 mm in diameter. However, long-term aspirin therapy may be indicated, because patients requiring such procedures may be at risk for other thrombotic complications.

---

[1]Not included in Canadian product labeling.

## Patient Consultation

As an aid to patient consultation, refer to *Advice for the Patient, Aspirin, Sodium Bicarbonate, and Citric Acid (Systemic)*.

In providing consultation, consider emphasizing the following selected information (» = major clinical significance):

### Before using this medication
» Conditions affecting use, especially:

Sensitivity to aspirin, nonsteroidal anti-inflammatory drugs (NSAIDs), or sodium bicarbonate

Pregnancy—Not taking aspirin in third trimester unless prescribed by physician; high-dose, chronic use or abuse of aspirin in third trimester may be hazardous to the mother as well as the fetus and/or neonate, causing heart problems in fetus or neonate and/or bleeding in mother, fetus, or neonate; high-dose, chronic use or abuse may also prolong and complicate labor and delivery; sodium may cause edema and weight gain

Use in children—Checking with physician before giving to children with symptoms of acute febrile illness, especially influenza or varicella, because of the risk of Reye's syndrome; also, increased susceptibility to aspirin toxicity in children, especially with fever and dehydration

Use in teenagers—Checking with physician before giving to teenagers with symptoms of acute febrile illness, especially influenza or varicella, because of the risk of Reye's syndrome

Use in the elderly—Increased risk of aspirin toxicity; also, because of the very high sodium content, use should preferably be limited to 5 days at a time, unless more prolonged therapy is prescribed and monitored by a physician

Other medications, especially anticoagulants, oral antidiabetic agents, oral imidazole antifungals, mecamylamine, methenamine, methotrexate, NSAIDs, platelet aggregation inhibitors, those cephalosporins that may cause hypoprothrombinemia, probenecid, sulfinpyrazone, oral tetracyclines, and vancomycin

Other medical problems, especially symptoms of appendicitis, coagulation or platelet function disorders, conditions in which sodium may be detrimental, gastrointestinal problems such as ulceration or erosive gastritis (especially a bleeding ulcer) or gastrointestinal obstruction, and renal function impairment

### Proper use of this medication
» Importance of not taking more medication than recommended on package label, unless otherwise directed by physician, because of risk of aspirin- or sodium bicarbonate–induced adverse effects

Proper administration:

Taking in liquid form only; not ingesting tablets or tablet fragments

Preparing liquid: Placing 1 or 2 tablets in glass, then adding ½ glass (120 mL) cool water

Checking for complete tablet dissolution before drinking; drinking while solution is still effervescing, or after it has settled

Drinking entire amount, then rinsing glass with a little more water and drinking that, to ensure receiving full dosage

» Proper dosing

Missed dose (if on scheduled dosing): Taking as soon as possible; not taking if almost time for next dose; not doubling doses

» Proper storage

### Precautions while using this medication
» Regular visits to physician to check progress if long-term or high-dose therapy is prescribed

Checking with physician if symptoms persist for longer than 10 days for adults or 5 days for children, condition becomes worse, new symptoms occur, or the painful area is red or swollen

» Not taking this medication within:

—6 hours before or 2 hours after ciprofloxacin or lomefloxacin
—8 hours before or 2 hours after enoxacin
—2 hours after itraconazole
—3 hours before or after ketoconazole
—2 hours before or after norfloxacin or ofloxacin
—3 to 4 hours before or after an oral tetracycline
—1 or 2 hours before or after any other oral medication

Not taking a cellulose-containing laxative within 2 hours of taking aspirin

» Possibility of overdose if other medications containing aspirin or other salicylates (including diflunisal) or significant quantities of sodium are used

Not taking aspirin for 5 days prior to any kind of surgery, unless otherwise directed by physician

» If taking aspirin as a platelet aggregation inhibitor:

Taking only the amount prescribed; checking with physician to determine whether an alternative medication, rather than additional aspirin, should be used to relieve pain, fever, arthritis

Not discontinuing therapy without first checking with the prescriber

Not using an NSAID together with this medication for more than a few days, unless otherwise directed by physician

*USP DI*

If taking more than an occasional 1 or 2 doses of this medication:
» Avoiding alcoholic beverages, because of the increased risk of aspirin-induced gastrointestinal toxicity
» Avoiding large amounts of milk or milk products
  Possible need for sodium restriction
  Caution if any laboratory tests required; possible interference with test results
  Diabetics: Aspirin may cause false urine sugar test results with prolonged use of 8 or more 325-mg (5-grain) doses per day
» Suspected overdose: Getting emergency help at once

### Side/adverse effects

Signs of potential side effects, especially edema, hypercalcemia associated with milk-alkali syndrome, increased blood pressure, metabolic alkalosis, anaphylaxis, anemia, bronchospastic allergic reaction, allergic dermatitis, and gastrointestinal ulceration or bleeding

## Oral Dosage Forms

### ASPIRIN EFFERVESCENT TABLETS FOR ORAL SOLUTION USP

#### Usual adult and adolescent dose

Analgesic/antacid—
  Oral, 325 to 500 mg of aspirin every three hours, 325 to 650 mg of aspirin every four hours, or 650 mg to 1 gram of aspirin every six hours as needed, while symptoms persist.

  Note: It is recommended that the total daily dose of aspirin not exceed 4 grams, and that a physician be consulted if symptoms are not relieved within ten days.

Platelet aggregation inhibitor[1]—
  Oral, 325 mg of aspirin a day.

  Note: Optimal dosage has not been established. Doses lower than 325 mg of aspirin a day are often utilized, since there is evidence that 160 mg of aspirin every twenty-four hours may effectively inhibit platelet aggregation while minimizing the risk of aspirin-induced side effects. Doses higher than 325 mg of aspirin a day are also recommended for specific indications responsive to platelet aggregation inhibition. However, because of its high sodium bicarbonate content, this formulation is not recommended for long-term therapy with doses higher than 325 mg of aspirin a day.

#### Usual adult prescribing limits

Geriatric patients—Oral, up to 4 regular-strength or extra-strength tablets a day. Limiting the duration of treatment to five days may be advisable, unless longer treatment is prescribed and monitored by a physician.

Nongeriatric adults—Oral, up to 8 regular-strength unflavored tablets, 6 regular-strength flavored tablets, or 7 extra-strength tablets a day. A physician should be consulted if symptoms are not relieved within ten days.

  Note: The lower maximum daily dosage recommended for the flavored regular-strength formulation, which contains more citric acid per tablet than the unflavored regular-strength formulation, is dictated by the FDA-mandated twenty-four-hour dosing limit for citric acid in OTC products.

#### Usual pediatric dose

Analgesic/antacid—
  Children up to 3 years of age: Dosage must be individualized by physician.

  Children 3 to 5 years of age: Oral, 167 mg of aspirin (one-half of a regular-strength tablet) every four to six hours as needed, while symptoms persist.

  Children 6 to 12 years of age: Oral, 325 mg (one regular-strength tablet) every four to six hours as needed, while symptoms persist.

  Note: It is recommended that children up to 12 years of age receive no more than five doses in each twenty-four-hour period, unless otherwise directed by a physician, and that a physician be consulted if symptoms are not relieved within five days.

#### Strength(s) usually available

Note: When dissolved in water, aspirin effervescent tablets for oral solution provide aspirin in the form of sodium acetylsalicylate.

U.S.—
  Regular-strength:
    325 mg of aspirin, with 1.916 grams of sodium bicarbonate and 1 gram of citric acid (OTC) [*Alka-Seltzer Effervescent Pain Reliever and Antacid* (sodium 567 mg [24.65 mmol] per tablet)].
    325 mg of aspirin, with 1.71 grams of sodium bicarbonate and 1.22 grams of citric acid (OTC) [*Flavored Alka-Seltzer Effervescent Pain Reliever and Antacid* (sodium 506 mg [22 mmol] per tablet)].
  Extra-strength:
    500 mg of aspirin, with 1.985 grams of sodium bicarbonate and 1 gram of citric acid (OTC) [*Alka-Seltzer Effervescent Pain Reliever and Antacid* (sodium 588 mg [25.56 mmol] per tablet)].

Canada—
  Regular strength:
    325 mg of ASA, with 1.916 grams of sodium bicarbonate and 1 gram of citric acid (OTC) [*Alka-Seltzer Effervescent Pain Reliever and Antacid* (sodium 567 mg [24.65 mmol] per tablet)].
    325 mg of ASA, with 1.71 grams of sodium bicarbonate and 1.22 grams of citric acid (OTC) [*Flavored Alka-Seltzer Effervescent Pain Reliever and Antacid* (sodium 506 mg [22 mmol] per tablet)].

  Note: *Aspirin* is a brand name in Canada; acetylsalicylic acid is the generic name. ASA, a commonly used designation for aspirin (or acetylsalicylic acid) in both the U.S. and Canada, is the term used in Canadian product labeling.

#### Auxiliary labeling

• Keep container tightly closed.

---

[1]Not included in Canadian product labeling.

Revised: 08/29/94

---

## ASTEMIZOLE — See *Antihistamines (Systemic)*

## ATENOLOL — See *Beta-adrenergic Blocking Agents (Systemic)*

---

# ATORVASTATIN Systemic—INTRODUCTORY VERSION

VA CLASSIFICATION (Primary): CV601

Commonly used brand name(s): *Lipitor*.

Note: For a listing of dosage forms and brand names by country availability, see *Dosage Forms* section(s).

## Category

Antihyperlipidemic; HMG-CoA reductase inhibitor.

## Indications

### Accepted

Hyperlipidemia (treatment)—Atorvastatin is indicated as an adjunct to diet to reduce elevated total cholesterol (total-C), low-density lipoprotein cholesterol (LDL-C), apolipoprotein B (apo B), and triglyceride (TG) concentrations in patients with primary hypercholesterolemia (heterozygous familial and nonfamilial) and mixed dyslipidemia (Fredrickson Types IIa and IIb).

Atorvastatin is also indicated to reduce total-C and LDL-C in patients with homozygous familial hypercholesterolemia as an adjunct to other lipid-lowering treatments, such as low-density lipoprotein apheresis, or if such treatments are unavailable.

## Pharmacology/Pharmacokinetics

### Physicochemical characteristics

Molecular weight—1209.42.

### Mechanism of action/Effect

3-hydroxy-3-methylglutaryl coenzyme A (HMG-CoA) reductase inhibitors competitively inhibit the enzyme that catalyzes the conversion of HMG-CoA to mevalonate, the rate-limiting step in cholesterol biosynthesis. The primary site of action of HMG-CoA reductase inhibitors is the liver, which is the principal site of cholesterol synthesis and low-density lipoprotein clearance. Cholesterol and triglycerides circulate in the bloodstream as part of lipoprotein complexes. These complexes are composed of high-density lipoprotein (HDL), intermediate-density lipoprotein (IDL), low-density lipoprotein (LDL), and very-low-density lipoprotein (VLDL). In the liver, triglycerides (TG) and cholesterol are incorporated into VLDL, which is released into the plasma for transport to the peripheral tissues. LDL is formed from VLDL and is catabolized primarily through the LDL receptor. Elevated plasma concentrations of total cholesterol (total-C), LDL-cholesterol (LDL-C), and apoliproprotein B (apo B) promote human atherosclerosis and are risk factors for developing cardiovascular disease. Increased plasma concentrations of HDL-C are associated with decreased cardiovascular risk. Atorvastatin lowers plasma cholesterol and lipoprotein concentrations by inhibiting HMG-CoA reductase and cholesterol synthesis in the liver and by increasing the number of hepatic LDL receptors on the cell surface to enhance uptake and catabolism of LDL. Atorvastatin also reduces LDL production and the number of LDL particles. Atorvastatin reduces total-C, LDL-C, and apo B in patients with homozygous and heterozygous familial hypercholesterolemia (FH), nonfamilial forms of hypercholesterolemia, and mixed dyslipidemia. Atorvastatin also reduces VLDL-C and TG and produces variable increases in HDL-C and apolipoprotein A-1.

**Absorption**
Atorvastatin is rapidly absorbed, the extent of absorption increasing in proportion to the dose. The absolute bioavailability of atorvastatin is approximately 12%. Atorvastatin has a low systemic availability due to pre-systemic clearance in the gastrointestinal mucosa and/or hepatic first-pass metabolism. Food decreases the rate and extent of absorption by approximately 25% and 9%, respectively; although, LDL-C reduction is similar when atorvastatin is given with or without food. The concentration of atorvastatin in plasma ($C_{max}$) and the area under the plasma concentration–time curve (AUC) are lower by approximately 30% following evening administration when compared with morning administration. However, LDL-C reduction is the same, regardless of the time of day of administration.

**Distribution**
Mean volume of distribution ($Vol_D$)—Approximately 565 L.

**Protein binding**
Very high ($\geq 98\%$).

**Biotransformation**
Atorvastatin undergoes extensive hepatic and/or extra-hepatic metabolism to form ortho- and parahydroxylated derivatives and various beta-oxidation products. It does not appear to undergo enterohepatic recirculation. Atorvastatin and its ortho- and parahydroxylated metabolites were found to have equal inhibitory effects on HMG-CoA reductase *in vitro*. The active metabolites are responsible for approximately 70% of the inhibition of HMG-CoA reductase. Studies *in vitro* suggest that atorvastatin is metabolized by the cytochrome P450 3A4 isozyme.

**Half-life**
Elimination—
  Approximately 14 hours.

**Time to peak concentration**
1 to 2 hours.

**Elimination**
Primarily fecal (biliary).
Renal: $< 2\%$.
  In dialysis—
    Although studies have not been performed, atorvastatin is not expected to be removed significantly by hemodialysis because of its extensive binding to plasma proteins.

## Precautions to Consider

**Carcinogenicity**
In a 2-year study in mice, doses of 100, 200, or 400 mg per kg (mg/kg) of body weight per day resulted in a marked increase in liver adenomas in male mice given high doses and liver carcinomas in female mice given high doses. These events occurred at area under the plasma concentration–time curve ($AUC_{[0-24]}$) values of approximately six times the mean human plasma drug exposure after an 80-mg oral dose.
In a 2-year study in rats, doses of 10, 30, and 100 mg/kg per day resulted in rare muscle tumors. Rhabdomyosarcoma occurred in one female rat given high doses and fibrosarcoma occurred in another female rat given high doses. The high dose represents an $AUC_{(0-24)}$ value of approximately 16 times the mean human plasma drug exposure after an 80-mg oral dose.

**Mutagenicity**
No evidence of mutagenicity or clastogenicity was found in *in vitro* tests, with and without metabolic activation, including the Ames test with *Salmonella typhimurium* and *Escherichia coli*, the HGPRT forward mutation assay in Chinese hamster lung cells, the chromosomal aberration assay in Chinese hamster lung cells, or in the *in vivo* mouse micronucleus test.

**Pregnancy/Reproduction**
Fertility—No changes in fertility were observed in studies in rats given doses of up to 175 mg/kg (15 times the human exposure) of atorvastatin. In 2 of 10 rats given 100 mg/kg per day for 3 months (16 times the human exposure at the 80-mg dose), aplasia and aspermia in the epididymis resulted. Testis weights were significantly decreased with 30 and 100 mg/kg doses and epididymal weight was lower at 100 mg/kg. Doses of 100 mg/kg per day given to male rats for 11 weeks prior to mating resulted in decreases in sperm motility and spermatid head concentration and increases in the number of abnormal sperm. No adverse effects were observed on semen parameters or in reproductive organ histopathology in dogs given doses of 10, 40, or 120 mg/kg for 2 years.

Pregnancy—Atorvastatin therapy is *contraindicated* in pregnant women because it decreases cholesterol synthesis and possibly the synthesis of other biologically active substances, such as steroids and cell membranes, that are derived from cholesterol and are essential for fetal development.
There have been rare reports of congenital anomalies following intrauterine exposure to HMG-CoA reductase inhibitors. Severe congenital bone deformities, tracheo-esophageal fistula, and anal atresia (VATER association) were reported in a baby born to a woman who took the HMG-CoA reductase inhibitor lovastatin with dextroamphetamine sulfate during the first trimester of pregnancy. Atorvastatin should not be administered to women of childbearing potential when they are highly likely to conceive. If a woman becomes pregnant during atorvastatin therapy, the medication should be discontinued and the patient advised of the potential hazards to the fetus.
In rats, atorvastatin crosses the placenta and reaches a concentration in fetal liver tissue equal to that in maternal plasma. No evidence of teratogenicity was found in rats given doses of up to 300 mg/kg per day or in rabbits given doses of up to 100 mg/kg per day. These doses represent 30 and 20 times, respectively, the human exposure based on body surface area (mg/m$^2$).
Studies in rats given 20, 100, or 225 mg/kg per day, from gestation day 7 through lactation day 21 (weaning), have shown decreased pup survival at birth, neonate, weaning, and maturity in pups of mothers given doses of 225 mg/kg per day. On days 4 and 21, body weight was decreased in pups of mothers given doses of 100 mg/kg per day; body weight was decreased at birth and at days 4, 21, and 91 in pups of mothers given 225 mg/kg per day. Pup development was delayed, as determined by rotorod performance (mothers given 100 mg/kg per day) and acoustic startle (mothers given 225 mg/kg per day). Development was also delayed in pinnae detachment and eye opening (mothers given 225 mg/kg per day). These doses represent 6 times (100 mg/kg) and 22 times (225 mg/kg) the human exposure at 80 mg per day.

FDA Pregnancy Category X.

**Breast-feeding**
While it is not known whether atorvastatin is distributed into breast milk, atorvastatin is *contraindicated* in women who are breast-feeding because inhibition of cholesterol synthesis may cause serious adverse effects in the nursing infant. Atorvastatin is distributed into the milk of lactating rats. Plasma and liver atorvastatin concentrations in nursing rat pups have reached 50% and 40%, respectively, of that in the mother's milk.

**Pediatrics**
Appropriate studies on the relationship of age to the effects of atorvastatin have not been performed in the pediatric population. However, eight pediatric patients (none younger than 9 years of age) with homozygous familial hypercholesterolemia (FH) were treated with atorvastatin at doses of up to 80 mg per day for 1 year. No clinical or biochemical abnormalities were reported in these patients.

**Geriatrics**
Use of atorvastatin in patients 65 years of age and older has not demonstrated geriatrics-specific problems that would limit the usefulness of atorvastatin in the elderly. Safety and efficacy of atorvastatin in 221 patients $\geq 70$ years of age given doses of up to 80 mg per day were similar to those in younger patients. However, in healthy subjects $\geq 65$ years of age, atorvastatin plasma concentrations ($C_{max}$) are higher and the AUC is greater by approximately 40% and 30%, respectively, compared with those in younger adults. Reduction of low-density lipoprotein cholesterol (LDL-C) is comparable to that in younger patients given equal doses of atorvastatin.

### Pharmacogenetics
There is no clinically significant difference in LDL-C reduction with atorvastatin between men and women, although plasma concentrations of atorvastatin in women are approximately 20% higher for $C_{max}$ and 10% lower for AUC, compared with those in men.

### Surgical
Atorvastatin therapy should be temporarily withheld or discontinued in any patient having a risk factor, such as major surgery, predisposing to the development of renal failure secondary to rhabdomyolysis.

### Drug interactions and/or related problems
The following drug interactions and/or related problems have been selected on the basis of their potential clinical significance (possible mechanism in parentheses where appropriate)—not necessarily inclusive (» = major clinical significance):

Note: Combinations containing any of the following medications, depending on the amount present, may also interact with this medication.

Alcohol, substantial use of
(elevations in transaminase values may occur)

Antacids, aluminum and magnesium hydroxide–containing
(plasma concentrations decreased by approximately 35% when atorvastatin was administered concurrently with an aluminum and magnesium hydroxide–containing antacid; however, reduction of LDL-C was not altered)

» Azole antifungals or
» Erythromycin or
» Gemfibrozil or
» Immunosuppressants, especially cyclosporine or
» Niacin (nicotinic acid)
(increased risk of myopathy, such as rhabdomyolysis, with concurrent administration; inhibition of cytochrome P450 3A4 isozyme [the enzyme responsible for atorvastatin metabolism] by erythromycin may increase atorvastatin plasma concentrations by approximately 40% with concurrent administration)

Colestipol
(concurrent use may decrease plasma concentrations of atorvastatin by approximately 25%; however, LDL-C reduction may be greater with combination therapy than with either medication given alone)

Contraceptives, oral, such as:
Ethinyl estradiol
Norethindrone
(concurrent administration may increase AUC for ethinyl estradiol and norethindrone by approximately 20% and 30%, respectively)

Digoxin
(concurrent administration may increase steady-state digoxin plasma concentrations by approximately 20%)

Medications that may decrease the concentrations or activity of endogenous steroid hormones, such as:
Cimetidine
Ketoconazole
Spironolactone
(HMG-CoA reductase inhibitors interfere with cholesterol synthesis and could possibly blunt adrenal and/or gonadal steroid production; concurrent administration with these drugs may further decrease concentrations and/or inhibit the activity of endogenous steroid hormones)

### Laboratory value alterations
The following have been selected on the basis of their potential clinical significance (possible effect in parentheses where appropriate)—not necessarily inclusive (» = major clinical significance):

With physiology/laboratory test values
Creatine kinase (CK), serum
(increases of CK > 10 times the upper limit of normal [ULN], accompanied by muscle aches or weakness, are associated with myopathy, such as rhabdomyolysis; atorvastatin should be discontinued if marked elevations of creatine kinase occur)

Transaminases, serum
(elevations in liver enzyme values usually occur within the first 3 months of treatment; persistent increases [> three times ULN, occurring on two or more occasions] in transaminase values occurred in 0.7% of patients in clinical trials; elevations in transaminase values are not usually associated with clinical signs or symptoms, although one patient in clinical trials developed jaundice; if elevations in aspartate aminotransferase [AST (SGOT)] or alanine aminotransferase [ALT (SGPT)] are > three times the ULN and persist, atorvastatin dosage should be reduced or discontinued; patients should be monitored until the abnormal values are resolved)

### Medical considerations/Contraindications
The medical considerations/contraindications included have been selected on the basis of their potential clinical significance (reasons given in parentheses where appropriate)—not necessarily inclusive (» = major clinical significance).

*Except under special circumstances, this medication should not be used when the following medical problems exist:*

» Hepatic disease, active, including
»     Alcoholic liver disease, chronic
»     Childs-Pugh Index grade A disease
»     Childs-Pugh Index grade B disease or
» Elevations of transaminase values, unexplained, persistent
(the presence of hepatic disease may increase atorvastatin plasma concentrations. Plasma concentrations are significantly increased in patients with chronic alcoholic liver disease. In patients with Childs-Pugh Index grade A disease, $C_{max}$ and AUC are each fourfold greater. In patients with Childs-Pugh Index grade B disease, $C_{max}$ and AUC are approximately sixteen- and elevenfold greater, respectively)

» Hypersensitivity to atorvastatin

*Risk-benefit should be considered when the following medical problems exist:*

» Electrolyte, endocrine, or metabolic disorders, severe or
» Hypotension or
» Infection, severe acute or
» Seizures, uncontrolled or
» Surgery, major or
» Trauma
(these conditions may predispose a patient to the development of renal failure, secondary to rhabdomyolysis; atorvastatin should be discontinued or temporarily withheld)

Hepatic disease, history of
(elevations in transaminase values may occur)

### Patient monitoring
The following may be especially important in patient monitoring (other tests may be warranted in some patients, depending on condition; » = major clinical significance):

Creatine kinase (CK), serum
(periodic determinations recommended in patients who develop muscle pain, tenderness, or weakness during therapy or if concurrently receiving azole antifungals, erythromycin, gemfibrozil, immunosuppressive drugs such as cyclosporine, or niacin)

» Hepatic function determinations
(recommended prior to initiation of treatment and at 6 and 12 weeks of treatment or at a dosage increase, and periodically, such as every 6 months, thereafter)

» Lipid concentrations, serum, primarily:
Low-density lipoprotein cholesterol (LDL-C) and, if not available
Total cholesterol (total-C)
(determinations recommended within 2 to 4 weeks after initiation or at a dosage adjustment of atorvastatin)

## Side/Adverse Effects
Note: Brain hemorrhage was seen in a female dog given 120 mg per kg of body weight (mg/kg) per day of atorvastatin for 3 months. This dose represents approximately 16 times the human area under the plasma concentration–time curve ($AUC_{[0-24]}$) based on the maximum human dose of 80 mg per day. Brain hemorrhage and optic nerve vacuolation were seen after 11 weeks in another female dog given atorvastatin in escalating doses of up to 280 mg/kg per day.

In a 2-year study in male dogs, a single tonic convulsion was seen in two dogs; one had been given 10 mg/kg per day and the other had been given 120 mg/kg per day of atorvastatin.

Central nervous system vascular lesions, characterized by perivascular hemorrhages, edema, and mononuclear cell infiltration of perivascular spaces, have been observed in dogs treated with other HMG-CoA reductase inhibitors.

Optic nerve degeneration (Wallerian degeneration of retinogeniculate fibers) was reported in dogs given a chemically similar drug at plasma concentrations 30 times higher than mean plasma concentrations in humans administered the highest recommended human dose.

The following side/adverse effects have been selected on the basis of their potential clinical significance (possible signs and symptoms in parentheses where appropriate)—not necessarily inclusive:

### Those indicating need for medical attention
Incidence less frequent or rare
> *Muscle disorders, such as leg cramps; myalgia, uncomplicated* (muscle pain); *myopathy and/or rhabdomyolysis* (fever; muscle cramps, pain, stiffness, or weakness; unusual tiredness); *and myositis* (inflammation of muscle)

> Note: The degradation of muscle occurs in *rhabdomyolysis*, resulting in the release of myoglobin into the urine, which can lead to acute renal failure. *Myopathy* and/or rhabdomyolysis should be considered if symptoms occur in conjunction with creatine kinase (CK) value increases > 10 times the upper limit of normal. The risk of myopathy increases when HMG-CoA reductase inhibitors are administered with azole antifungals, erythromycin, gemfibrozil, immunosuppressants such as cyclosporine, or niacin. Patients should be monitored during the first months of therapy and during dosage increases of either drug, and should report immediately any unexplained symptoms of muscle pain, tenderness, or weakness, especially if accompanied by fever or malaise.

### Those indicating need for medical attention only if they continue or are bothersome
Incidence less frequent
> *Abdominal pain; constipation; diarrhea; dyspepsia* (heartburn; indigestion; stomach discomfort); *flatulence* (belching; excessive gas); *skin rash*

## Overdose
For more information on the management of overdose or unintentional ingestion, **contact a Poison Control Center** (see *Poison Control Center Listing*).

**Treatment of overdose**
Treatment is symptomatic and supportive.

Supportive care—Patients in whom intentional overdose is confirmed or suspected should be referred for psychiatric consultation.

## Patient Consultation
As an aid to patient consultation, refer to *Advice for the Patient, Atorvastatin (Systemic)—Introductory Version*.

In providing consultation, consider emphasizing the following selected information (» = major clinical significance):

### Before using this medication
» Conditions affecting use, especially:
  Hypersensitivity to atorvastatin
  Pregnancy—Contraindicated during pregnancy or in women planning to become pregnant in the near future
  Breast-feeding—Contraindicated in women who are breast-feeding
  Surgical—Increased risk of development of renal failure secondary to rhabdomyolysis with major surgery
  Other medications, especially azole antifungals; erythromycin; gemfibrozil; immunosuppressants, such as cyclosporine; or niacin
  Other medical problems, especially active hepatic disease, including chronic alcoholic liver disease, Childs-Pugh Index grade A disease and Childs-Pugh Index grade B disease; hypotension; major surgery; severe acute infection; severe electrolyte, endocrine, or metabolic disorders; trauma; uncontrolled seizures; or unexplained persistent elevations of transaminase values

### Proper use of this medication
Compliance with therapy; taking medication at the same time each day to maintain the antihyperlipidemic effect
Compliance with prescribed diet during treatment
» Proper dosing
  Missed dose: Taking as soon as possible; not taking if almost time for next dose; not doubling doses
» Proper storage

### Precautions while using this medication
Regular visits to physician to check progress
Notifying physician immediately if pregnancy is suspected because of possible harm to the fetus
Caution if any kind of surgery (including dental surgery) or emergency treatment is required
Not taking over-the-counter niacin preparations without consulting physician because of increased risk of rhabdomyolysis
Not using alcohol excessively because elevations of liver enzymes may occur
Notifying physician immediately if unexplained muscle pain, tenderness, or weakness occurs, especially if accompanied by unusual tiredness or fever

### Side/adverse effects
Signs of potential side effects, especially muscle disorders, such as leg cramps, uncomplicated myalgia, myopathy and/or rhabdomyolysis, and myositis

## General Dosing Information
Clinical response to atorvastatin is seen within 2 weeks, and maximum response is usually achieved within 4 weeks and maintained during long-term therapy.

Prior to starting atorvastatin therapy, secondary causes for hypercholesterolemia, such as poorly controlled diabetes mellitus, hypothyroidism, nephrotic syndrome, dysproteinemias, obstructive liver disease, other medication therapy, and alcoholism should be excluded and a lipid profile performed to measure total cholesterol (total-C), low-density lipoprotein cholesterol (LDL-C), high-density lipoprotein cholesterol (HDL-C), and triglycerides (TG).

Atorvastatin may be used with colestipol or cholestyramine for additive antihyperlipidemic effects.

### Diet/Nutrition
Prior to treatment with atorvastatin, control of hypercholesterolemia with diet, exercise, weight reduction in obese patients, and treatment of underlying medical problems should be attempted. The patient should be placed on a standard cholesterol-lowering diet before receiving atorvastatin and should continue on this diet during treatment with atorvastatin.

Atorvastatin may be taken with or without food.

For additional information on initial therapeutic guidelines related to the treatment of hyperlipidemia, see *Appendix III*.

## Oral Dosage Forms

### ATORVASTATIN CALCIUM TABLETS

**Usual adult dose**
Heterozygous familial and nonfamilial hypercholesterolemia and mixed dyslipidemia (Fredrickson Types IIa and IIb)—
  Oral, initially 10 mg once a day. The dosage range is 10 to 80 mg once a day, to be administered at any time of the day, with or without food. After initiation or titration of atorvastatin, lipid concentrations should be measured within 2 to 4 weeks and the dosage adjusted accordingly.

> Note: The goal of therapy is to lower LDL-C. The National Cholesterol Education Program (NCEP) recommends that LDL-C concentrations be used to initiate and assess treatment response. Only if LDL-C concentrations are not available should total-C be used to monitor therapy.

Homozygous familial hypercholesterolemia—
  Oral, 10 to 80 mg a day.

> Note: Atorvastatin should be used in these patients as an adjunct to other lipid-lowering treatments, such as LDL apheresis, or if such treatments are unavailable.

**Usual adult prescribing limits**
80 mg a day.

**Usual pediatric dose**
Homozygous familial hypercholesterolemia—
  Dosage has not been established.

**Strength(s) usually available**
U.S.—
  10 mg (Rx) [*Lipitor* (film-coated)].
  20 mg (Rx) [*Lipitor* (film-coated)].
  40 mg (Rx) [*Lipitor* (film-coated)].

**Packaging and storage**
Store at controlled room temperature between 20 and 25 °C (68 and 77 °F).

**Auxiliary labeling**
Do not take other medications without your doctor's advice

Developed: 10/29/97

# ATOVAQUONE Systemic

VA CLASSIFICATION (Primary): AP109.

Commonly used brand name(s): *Mepron*.

Note: For a listing of dosage forms and brand names by country availability, see *Dosage Forms* section(s).

## Category
Antiprotozoal.

## Indications

**Accepted**

Pneumonia, *Pneumocystis carinii* (PCP) (treatment)—Atovaquone is indicated in the treatment of mild to moderate *Pneumocystis carinii* pneumonia (A-a gradient $\leq$ 45 mmHg and pO$_2$ $\geq$ 60 mmHg on room air) in patients who are intolerant of sulfamethoxazole and trimethoprim combination.

Atovaquone has not been evaluated for the treatment of more severe episodes of PCP, in patients who are failing sulfamethoxazole and trimethoprim combination therapy, or as a chronic suppressive agent for PCP prophylaxis.

**Unaccepted**

Atovaquone is not effective therapy against bacterial, viral, or fungal pneumonias or mycobacterial disease.

## Pharmacology/Pharmacokinetics

**Physicochemical characteristics**
Chemical group—1,4-Hydroxynaphthoquinone.
Molecular weight—366.84.

**Mechanism of action/Effect**
Atovaquone has possible cidal activity against susceptible organisms. The action against *Pneumocystis carinii* is not fully understood. Atovaquone is structurally similar to ubiquinone, which inhibits the mitochondrial electron-transport chain at the site of the cytochrome $bc_1$ complex (complex III) in *Plasmodium* species. This may ultimately inhibit the synthesis of nucleic acid and ATP. Atovaquone also has been shown to have good *in vitro* activity against *Toxoplasma gondii*.

**Absorption**
The bioavailability of atovaquone is low and variable, and decreases significantly with single doses greater than 750 mg. A standard breakfast containing 23 grams of fat has been shown to enhance absorption significantly.
Oral suspension—The oral suspension provides a two-fold increase in bioavailability in fasting or fed conditions compared to the tablets. Bioavailability of the suspension increases two-fold when administered with meals; when administered with food, bioavailability is approximately 47%.
Tablets—Bioavailability increases three-fold when administered with meals; bioavailability of the tablets when administered with food is approximately 23%.

**Distribution**
Atovaquone is highly lipophilic, with low aqueous solubility. The cerebrospinal fluid (CSF) to plasma ratio is very low ($<$ 1%).
Vol$_D$ at steady state is approximately 0.6 liter per kg (L/kg).

**Protein binding**
Very high ($>$ 99.9%); primarily bound to albumin in serum.

**Biotransformation**
There is indirect evidence that atovaquone may undergo limited metabolism; however, a specific metabolite has not been identified.

**Half-life**
2.2 to 3.2 days in adult patients with acquired immunodeficiency syndrome (AIDS), adult healthy volunteers, and immunocompromised children (ages 5 months to 13 years).

**Time to peak concentration**
A double peak has been observed. The first peak was 1 to 8 hours after dosing; the second peak was 24 to 96 hours after dosing. This is suggestive of enterohepatic recycling.

**Peak plasma concentration**
Adults—
  Oral suspension:
    Approximately 24 mcg per mL (mcg/mL) in patients infected with human immunodeficiency virus (HIV) taking 750 mg two times a day with food.
  Tablets:
    Approximately 13 mcg/mL in AIDS patients taking 750 mg three times a day with food.
Children—
  Oral suspension:
    Ages 3 to 24 months (steady-state concentrations)—
      Approximately 5.7 mcg/mL in HIV-infected children after administration of 10 mg per kg of body weight (mg/kg).
      Approximately 8.9 mcg/mL in HIV-infected children after administration of 30 mg/kg.
    Ages 2 to 13 years—
      Approximately 16.8 mcg/mL in HIV-infected children after administration of 10 mg/kg.
      Approximately 37.1 mcg/mL in HIV-infected children after administration of 30 mg/kg.
  Tablets:
    Ages 5 months to 13 years—
      Steady-state average of 7.5 mcg/mL after administration of 10 mg per kg of body weight (mg/kg) once a day, and a steady-state average of 14 mcg/mL after administration of 40 mg/kg once a day.

There appears to be a correlation between plasma atovaquone concentrations and the likelihood of successful treatment and survival. Patients with atovaquone concentrations $<$ 5 mcg/mL were more likely to die than those with concentrations $\geq$ 5 mcg/mL. In one study, 0 of 6 (0%) patients with a plasma atovaquone concentration of $<$ 5 mcg/mL were successfully treated, compared to 30 of 38 (79%) patients with plasma concentrations of 10 to $<$ 15 mcg/mL and 18 of 19 (95%) patients with plasma concentrations of 15 to $<$ 20 mcg/mL.

Steady-state plasma concentrations in AIDS patients administered atovaquone tablets are about one-third to one-half of the levels achieved in asymptomatic HIV-infected patients; the reason for this is not yet known.

**Elimination**
Fecal; $>$ 94% of atovaquone was recovered in the feces over 21 days; $<$ 0.6% was excreted in the urine.

## Precautions to Consider

**Carcinogenicity**
Studies in rats and mice have not been completed.

**Mutagenicity**
Atovaquone was found to be negative with or without metabolic activation in the Ames *Salmonella* mutagenicity assay, the mouse lymphoma mutagenesis assay, and the cultured human lymphocyte cytogenic assay. No evidence of genotoxicity was seen in the *in vivo* mouse micronucleus assay.

**Pregnancy/Reproduction**
Pregnancy—Studies have not been done in pregnant women.
Atovaquone was not teratogenic and did not cause reproductive toxicity in rats with plasma concentrations up to 2 to 3 times the estimated human exposure. It did cause maternal toxicity in rabbits with plasma concentrations that were approximately equal to the estimated human exposure; mean fetal body lengths and weights were decreased and there were higher numbers of early resorption and post-implantation losses per dam. It is not clear whether these effects were caused by atovaquone or were secondary to maternal toxicity. Concentrations in rabbit fetuses averaged 30% of the concurrent maternal plasma concentrations. After a single $^{14}$C-radiolabeled dose, concentrations of radiocarbon in rat fetuses were 18% (middle gestation) and 60% (late gestation) of concurrent maternal plasma concentrations.

FDA Pregnancy Category C.

**Breast-feeding**
It is not known whether atovaquone is distributed into human breast milk. A study done in rats found that the concentration of atovaquone in the milk was 30% of the concurrent concentration in the maternal plasma.

**Pediatrics**
No information is available on the efficacy of atovaquone in pediatric patients. Clinical experience with atovaquone in children is limited to pharmacokinetic and safety data in immunocompromised children 1 month of age to 13 years of age. These data suggest that the pharmacokinetics of atovaquone are age dependent; also, no treatment-limiting adverse effects were seen.

**Geriatrics**
No information is available on the relationship of age to the effects of atovaquone in geriatric patients.

**Drug interactions and/or related problems**

The following drug interactions and/or related problems have been selected on the basis of their potential clinical significance (possible mechanism in parentheses where appropriate)—not necessarily inclusive (» = major clinical significance):

Note: Combinations containing any of the following medications, depending on the amount present, may also interact with this medication.

Highly plasma protein–bound medications
(because atovaquone is very highly plasma protein–bound, it could potentially displace other medications that are also very highly plasma protein–bound; this could increase the risk of toxicity from medications that have narrow therapeutic indexes; however, atovaquone protein binding has not been affected *in vitro* by therapeutic concentrations of phenytoin, and the binding of phenytoin has not been affected by atovaquone)

Rifabutin or
» Rifampin
(concurrent administration of oral rifampin with atovaquone suspension resulted in a 52% decrease in the average steady-state plasma concentration of atovaquone and a decrease in the elimination half-life of atovaquone from 82 hours to 50 hours; the average steady-state plasma concentration of rifampin increased by 37%; alternative agents to rifampin should be considered when treating patients with atovaquone. Although interaction trials have not been conducted with atovaquone and rifabutin, rifabutin is structurally similar to rifampin and it may have some of the same drug interactions as rifampin)

Sulfamethoxazole and trimethoprim combination
(concurrent administration of sulfamethoxazole and trimethoprim combination with atovaquone suspension resulted in an 8% and 17% decrease in the steady-state serum concentration of sulfamethoxazole and trimethoprim, respectively; this effect is thought to be minor and is not expected to produce clinically significant events)

Zidovudine
(concurrent administration of zidovudine with atovaquone tablets resulted in a decrease in zidovudine clearance by 24% and a 35% increase in the area under the plasma concentration-time curve [AUC] of zidovudine; the glucuronide metabolite:parent ratio of zidovudine decreased from a mean of 4.5 when zidovudine was administered alone to 3.1 when zidovudine was administered with atovaquone; this effect is thought to be minor and is not expected to produce clinically significant events; zidovudine has no effect on atovaquone pharmacokinetics)

**Laboratory value alterations**

The following have been selected on the basis of their potential clinical significance (possible effect in parentheses where appropriate)—not necessarily inclusive (» = major clinical significance):

With physiology/laboratory test values
Alanine aminotransferase (ALT [SGPT]) and
Alkaline phosphatase and
Amylase, serum, and
Aspartate aminotransferase (AST [SGOT])
(values may be increased)

Hemoglobin, serum, and
White blood cell count
(hemoglobin concentrations and neutrophil counts may be mildly and transiently decreased)

Sodium, serum
(concentrations may be decreased)

**Medical considerations/Contraindications**

The medical considerations/contraindications included have been selected on the basis of their potential clinical significance (reasons given in parentheses where appropriate)—not necessarily inclusive (» = major clinical significance):

*Except under special circumstances, this medication should not be used when the following medical problem exists:*
» Allergic reaction to atovaquone

*Risk-benefit should be considered when the following medical problems exist:*
» Gastrointestinal disorders that may inhibit absorption
(patients with gastrointestinal disorders that may inhibit the absorption of atovaquone may not achieve therapeutic plasma concentrations; this may increase the risk of treatment failure and, possibly, death)

**Patient monitoring**

The following may be especially important in patient monitoring (other tests may be warranted in some patients, depending on condition; » = major clinical significance):

Complete blood counts (CBCs)
(because atovaquone may cause anemia and neutropenia, hemoglobin concentrations and neutrophil counts should be monitored periodically)

Liver function tests
(liver function tests, including serum ALT [SGPT] and AST [SGOT] values, and serum amylase concentration, should be monitored periodically)

## Side/Adverse Effects

Note: Because many of the patients who participated in clinical trials with atovaquone had advanced HIV disease, it was often difficult to differentiate between the underlying medical condition and the adverse effects of atovaquone.

The following side/adverse effects have been selected on the basis of their potential clinical significance (possible signs and symptoms in parentheses where appropriate)—not necessarily inclusive:

**Those indicating need for medical attention**
Incidence more frequent
*Fever; skin rash*

**Those indicating need for medical attention only if they continue or are bothersome**
Incidence more frequent
*Cough; diarrhea; headache; insomnia* (trouble in sleeping); **nausea; vomiting**

## Patient Consultation

As an aid to patient consultation, refer to *Advice for the Patient, Atovaquone (Systemic)*.

In providing consultation, consider emphasizing the following selected information (» = major clinical significance):

**Before using this medication**
» Conditions affecting use, especially:
Hypersensitivity to atovaquone
Breast-feeding—Atovaquone is distributed into the milk of rats
Other medications, especially rifampin
Other medical problems, especially gastrointestinal disorders that may impair absorption

**Proper use of this medication**
» Taking with a meal
Crushing tablets if necessary to ease administration
» Atovaquone oral suspension and tablets are not bioequivalent and cannot be interchanged or substituted for each other.
Proper administration technique for oral liquid; not using after expiration date
» Compliance with full course of therapy
» Importance of not missing doses and taking at evenly spaced times
» Proper dosing
Missed dose: Taking as soon as possible; not taking if almost time for next dose; not doubling doses
» Proper storage

**Precautions while using this medication**
Checking with physician if no improvement within a few days

**Side/adverse effects**
Signs of potential side effects, especially fever and skin rash

## General Dosing Information

Atovaquone tablets are uncoated and may be crushed if necessary to ease administration.

**Diet/Nutrition**
Atovaquone should be taken with a meal to enhance absorption. Failure to take with a meal may result in lower plasma concentrations of atovaquone, which may limit the response to therapy.

**Bioequivalence information**
Atovaquone oral suspension and tablets are not bioequivalent and cannot be interchanged or substituted for each other.

## Oral Dosage Forms

### ATOVAQUONE ORAL SUSPENSION

**Usual adult and adolescent dose**
Pneumonia, *Pneumocystis carinii*—
　Oral, 750 mg taken with a meal two times a day for twenty-one days.

**Usual pediatric dose**
Dosage has not been established; however, doses of 40 mg per kg of body weight per day have been used in children.

**Strength(s) usually available**
U.S.—
　750 mg per 5 mL (Rx) [*Mepron*].
Canada—
　Not commercially available.

**Packaging and storage**
Store between 15 and 25 °C (59 and 77 °F). Dispense in a tight container. Do not freeze.

**Auxiliary labeling**
• Take with food.
• Continue medicine for full time of treatment.
• Shake well.
• Beyond-use date.

**Note**
When dispensing, include a calibrated liquid-measuring device.

### ATOVAQUONE TABLETS

**Usual adult and adolescent dose**
Pneumonia, *Pneumocystis carinii*—
　Oral, 750 mg taken with a meal three times a day for twenty-one days.

**Usual pediatric dose**
Dose has not been established; however, doses of 40 mg per kg of body weight per day have been used in children.

**Strength(s) usually available**
U.S.—
　Not commercially available.
Canada—
　250 mg (Rx) [*Mepron*].

**Packaging and storage**
Store between 15 and 25 °C (59 and 77 °F). Dispense in a well-closed container.

**Auxiliary labeling**
• Take with food.
• Continue medicine for full time of treatment.

Revised: 08/14/95

---

**ATRACURIUM**—See *Neuromuscular Blocking Agents (Systemic)*

---

**ATROPINE**—See *Anticholinergics/Antispasmodics (Systemic)*; *Atropine (Ophthalmic)*

---

# ATROPINE Ophthalmic

VA CLASSIFICATION (Primary): OP600

Commonly used brand name(s): *Atropair; Atropine Care; Atropine Sulfate S.O.P.; Atropisol; Atrosulf; I-Tropine; Isopto Atropine; Minims Atropine; Ocu-Tropine.*

Note: For a listing of dosage forms and brand names by country availability, see *Dosage Forms* section(s).

## Category
Cycloplegic; mydriatic.

## Indications
Note: Bracketed information in the *Indications* section refers to uses that are not included in U.S. product labeling.

**Accepted**

Refraction, cycloplegic—Atropine is indicated for measurement of refractive errors. Atropine is a commonly used cycloplegic for refraction in children up to 6 years of age and in children with convergent strabismus. It is not useful for refraction in adults, because of its long duration of action.

Uveitis (treatment)—Atropine is indicated for pupil dilation and ciliary muscle relaxation, which are desirable in acute inflammatory conditions of the iris and uveal tract.

[Synechiae, posterior (prophylaxis and treatment)]—Atropine may be used for pupil dilation to break posterior synechiae and decrease the possibility of serious complications resulting from synechiae. However, a more rapidly acting medication is usually used. Atropine may also be used to prevent formation of posterior synechiae.

[Mydriasis, preoperative and postoperative]—Atropine may be used for preoperative and postoperative mydriasis.

[Glaucoma, malignant (treatment)][1]—Atropine is used in the treatment of malignant (ciliary block) glaucoma, which may occur after inflammation, surgery, trauma, or use of miotics.

[1]Not included in Canadian product labeling.

## Pharmacology/Pharmacokinetics

**Mechanism of action/Effect**
Atropine (a belladonna alkaloid) is an anticholinergic agent that blocks the responses of the sphincter muscle of the iris and the accommodative muscle of the ciliary body to stimulation by acetylcholine. Dilation of the pupil (mydriasis) and paralysis of accommodation (cycloplegia) result.

**Duration of action**
Long-acting; effects on accommodation may last 6 days; mydriasis may persist for 12 days.

## Precautions to Consider

**Cross-sensitivity and/or related problems**
Patients sensitive to any of the other belladonna alkaloids may be sensitive to atropine also.

**Carcinogenicity/Mutagenicity**
Studies have not been done in either animals or humans to evaluate the carcinogenic or mutagenic potential of atropine.

**Pregnancy/Reproduction**
Fertility—Studies have not been done in either animals or humans to evaluate the potential of atropine impairing fertility.

Pregnancy—Studies have not been done in humans; however, ophthalmic atropine may be systemically absorbed.
Studies have not been done in animals.
FDA Pregnancy Category C.

**Breast-feeding**
Systemic atropine is distributed into breast milk in very small amounts. Ophthalmic atropine may be systemically absorbed and may possibly cause adverse effects, such as fast pulse, fever, or dry skin, in nursing infants of mothers using ophthalmic atropine.

**Pediatrics**
Atropine should not be used in children who have previously had a severe systemic reaction to atropine.

An increased susceptibility to atropine has been reported in infants and young children and in children with blond hair, blue eyes, Down's syndrome, spastic paralysis, or brain damage; therefore, atropine should be used with great caution in these patients.

The ointment dosage form is generally preferred for use in children, since use of the solution presents a greater chance of systemic absorption.

## Atropine (Ophthalmic)

**Geriatrics**
Geriatric patients are more susceptible to the effects of atropine, thus increasing the potential for systemic side effects.

**Drug interactions and/or related problems**
The following drug interactions and/or related problems have been selected on the basis of their potential clinical significance (possible mechanism in parentheses where appropriate)—not necessarily inclusive (» = major clinical significance):

Note: Combinations containing any of the following medications, depending on the amount present, may also interact with this medication.

Anticholinergics or medications with anticholinergic activity, other (See *Appendix II*)
(if significant systemic absorption of ophthalmic atropine occurs, concurrent use of other anticholinergics or medications with anticholinergic activity may result in potentiated anticholinergic effects)

Antiglaucoma agents, cholinergic, long-acting, ophthalmic
(concurrent use with atropine may antagonize the antiglaucoma and miotic actions of ophthalmic long-acting cholinergic antiglaucoma agents, such as demecarium, echothiophate, and isoflurophate; concurrent use with atropine may also antagonize the antiaccommodative convergence effects of these medications when they are used for the treatment of strabismus)

Antimyasthenics or
Potassium citrate or
Potassium supplements
(if significant systemic absorption of ophthalmic atropine occurs, concurrent use may increase the chance of toxicity and/or side effects of these systemic medications because of the anticholinergic-induced slowing of gastrointestinal motility)

Carbachol or
Physostigmine or
Pilocarpine
(concurrent use with atropine may interfere with the antiglaucoma action of carbachol, physostigmine, or pilocarpine. Also, concurrent use may counteract the mydriatic effect of atropine; this counteraction may be used to therapeutic advantage)

CNS depression–producing medications (See *Appendix II*)
(if significant systemic absorption of ophthalmic atropine occurs, concurrent use of medications having CNS effects, such as antiemetic agents, phenothiazines, or barbiturates, may result in opisthotonos, convulsions, coma, and extrapyramidal symptoms)

**Medical considerations/Contraindications**
The medical considerations/contraindications included have been selected on the basis of their potential clinical significance (reasons given in parentheses where appropriate)—not necessarily inclusive (» = major clinical significance).

*Except under special circumstances, this medication should not be used when the following medical problem exists:*
» Severe systemic reaction to atropine, especially in children, history of

*Risk-benefit should be considered when the following medical problems exist:*
Brain damage, in children
Down's syndrome (mongolism), in children and adults
» Glaucoma, primary, or predisposition to angle closure
Keratoconus
(atropine may produce fixed dilated pupil)
Sensitivity to atropine
Spastic paralysis, in children
Synechiae between the iris and lens

## Side/Adverse Effects

Note: An increased susceptibility to atropine has been reported in infants, young children, children with blond hair or blue eyes, adults and children with Down's syndrome, children with brain damage or spastic paralysis, and the elderly. This susceptibility increases the potential for systemic side effects.

Prolonged use of atropine may produce local irritation, resulting in follicular conjunctivitis, vascular congestion, edema, exudate, contact dermatitis, or an eczematoid dermatitis.

Severe reactions to atropine may occur and are evidenced by hypotension with progressive respiratory depression. Coma and death have been reported in the very young.

The following side/adverse effects have been selected on the basis of their potential clinical significance (possible signs and symptoms in parentheses where appropriate)—not necessarily inclusive:

**Those indicating need for medical attention**
Symptoms of systemic absorption
*Clumsiness or unsteadiness; confusion or unusual behavior; dizziness; dryness of skin; fever; flushing or redness of face; hallucinations; skin rash; slurred speech; swollen stomach in infants; tachycardia* (fast or irregular heartbeat); *unusual drowsiness; tiredness or weakness; xerostomia* (thirst or dryness of mouth)

**Those indicating need for medical attention only if they continue or are bothersome**
*Blurred vision; eye irritation not present before therapy; increased sensitivity of eyes to light; swelling of the eyelids*

## Overdose

For specific information on the agents used in the management of ophthalmic atropine overdose, see:
- Atropine in *Anticholinergics/Antispasmodics (Systemic)* monograph;
- Diazepam in *Benzodiazepines (Systemic)* monograph; and/or
- *Physostigmine (Systemic)* monograph.

For more information on the management of overdose or unintentional ingestion, **contact a Poison Control Center** (see *Poison Control Center Listing*).

**Treatment of overdose**
For accidental ingestion, emesis or gastric lavage with 4% tannic acid solution is recommended.

For systemic effects, 0.2 to 1 mg (0.2 mg in children) physostigmine should be administered intravenously, as a dilution containing 1 mg in 5 mL of normal saline. The solution should be injected over a period of not less than 2 minutes. Dosage may be repeated every 5 minutes up to a total dose of 2 mg in children and 6 mg in adults in each 30-minute period.

Physostigmine is contraindicated in hypertensive reactions.

ECG monitoring is recommended during physostigmine administration.

Excitement may be controlled by diazepam or a short-acting barbiturate.

It is recommended that 1 mg of atropine be available for immediate injection if the physostigmine causes bradycardia, convulsion, or bronchoconstriction.

Supportive therapy may require oxygen and assisted respiration; cool water baths for fever, especially in children; and catheterization for urinary retention. In infants and small children, the body surface should be kept moist.

## Patient Consultation

As an aid to patient consultation, refer to *Advice for the Patient, Atropine/Homatropine/Scopolamine (Ophthalmic)*.

In providing consultation, consider emphasizing the following selected information (» = major clinical significance):

**Before using this medication**
» Conditions affecting use, especially:
Sensitivity to atropine, homatropine, or scopolamine
Breast-feeding—Medication passes into the breast milk in very small amounts and may cause side effects, such as fast pulse, fever, or dry skin, in babies of nursing mothers using ophthalmic atropine
Use in children—Infants and young children and children with blond hair or blue eyes may be especially sensitive to the effects of atropine; this may increase the chance of side effects during treatment
Use in the elderly—Geriatric patients are more susceptible to the effects of atropine, thus increasing the potential for systemic side effects
Other medical problems, especially primary glaucoma or predisposition to angle closure

**Proper use of this medication**
Proper administration technique
Washing hands immediately after application to remove any medication that may be on them; if applying medication to infants or children, washing their hands immediately afterwards also, and not letting any medication get into their mouths; wiping off any medication that may have accidentally gotten on the infant or child, including his or her face and eyelids
Preventing contamination: Not touching applicator tip to any surface; keeping container tightly closed

» Importance of not using more medication than the amount prescribed
» Proper dosing
  Missed dose
    If dosing schedule is—
      Once a day: Applying as soon as possible if remembered same day; if remembered later, skipping missed dose and going back to regular dosing schedule; not doubling doses
      More than once a day: Applying as soon as possible; if almost time for next dose, skipping missed dose and going back to regular dosing schedule; not doubling doses
» Proper storage

**Precautions while using this medication**
» Medication causes blurred vision and increased sensitivity of the eyes to light; checking with physician if these effects continue for longer than 14 days after discontinuation of atropine

**Side/adverse effects**
Signs of potential side effects, especially symptoms of systemic absorption

## General Dosing Information

A stronger concentration may be required to produce adequate cycloplegia in eyes with hazel or brown irides than in eyes with blue or light-colored irides.

The ointment dosage form is generally preferred for use in children, since use of the solution presents a greater chance of systemic absorption.

**For ointment dosage form only**
If the ointment is used for refraction, it should be applied several hours prior to the examination; otherwise it may impair the transparency of the cornea and alter the regularity of its refraction.

**For solution dosage form only**
Although some manufacturers recommend a dose of 2 drops of an ophthalmic solution at appropriate intervals, the conjunctival sac will usually hold only 1 drop.

To avoid excessive systemic absorption, patient should press finger to the lacrimal sac during, and for 2 or 3 minutes following, instillation of the solution.

## Ophthalmic Dosage Forms

Note: Bracketed uses in the *Dosage Forms* section refer to categories of use and/or indications that are not included in U.S. product labeling.

### ATROPINE SULFATE OPHTHALMIC OINTMENT USP

**Usual adult and adolescent dose**
Uveitis—
  Topical, to the conjunctiva, 0.3 to 0.5 cm of a 1% ointment one or two times a day.

**Usual pediatric dose**
Cycloplegic refraction—
  Topical, to the conjunctiva, 0.3 cm of the following concentrations three times a day for one to three days prior to refraction:
    Children up to 2 years of age with blue irides:
      0.5%.
    Children up to 2 years of age with dark irides:
      1%.
    Children 2 years of age and over:
      1%.
Uveitis
[Postoperative mydriasis]—
  Topical, to the conjunctiva, 0.3 to 0.5 cm of a 0.5 or 1% ointment one to three times a day.

**Strength(s) usually available**
U.S.—
  0.5% (Rx) [*Atropine Sulfate S.O.P.* (chlorobutanol 0.5%)].
  1% (Rx) [*Atropair; Atropine Sulfate S.O.P.* (chlorobutanol 0.5%); *Ocu-Tropine* [GENERIC (may contain chlorobutanol)].
Canada—
  1% (Rx) [GENERIC (may contain methylparaben, propylparaben)].

**Packaging and storage**
Store below 40 °C (104 °F), preferably between 15 and 30 °C (59 and 86 °F), in a tight container, unless otherwise specified by manufacturer. Protect from freezing.

**Auxiliary labeling**
• For the eye.
• Keep container tightly closed.

### ATROPINE SULFATE OPHTHALMIC SOLUTION USP

**Usual adult and adolescent dose**
Uveitis—
  Topical, to the conjunctiva, 1 drop of a 1% solution one or two times a day. In some cases, up to four doses a day may be required.
[To break posterior synechiae]—
  Topical, to the conjunctiva, 1 drop of a 1 to 3% solution alternated with 1 drop of a 2.5 or 10% phenylephrine solution every ten minutes for three applications of each. Extreme caution should be used if 10% phenylephrine is administered.
[Mydriasis]—
  Preoperative: Topical, to the conjunctiva, 1 drop of a 1% solution supplemented with 1 drop of a 2.5 or 10% phenylephrine solution, prior to surgery. Extreme caution should be used if 10% phenylephrine is administered.
  Postoperative: Topical, to the conjunctiva, 1 drop of a 1 to 3% solution one to three times a day.
[Malignant (ciliary block) glaucoma][1]—
  Initial: Topical, to the conjunctiva, 1 drop of a 1 to 3% solution administered concurrently with 1 drop of a 2.5 or 10% phenylephrine solution, three or four times a day. Extreme caution should be used if 10% phenylephrine is administered.
  Maintenance: Topical, to the conjunctiva, 1 drop of a 1 to 3% solution once every other day or once a day.

**Usual pediatric dose**
Cycloplegic refraction—
  Topical, to the conjunctiva, 1 drop of the following concentrations two times a day for one to three days prior to refraction:
    Infants up to 1 year of age:
      0.125%.
    Children 1 to 5 years of age:
      0.25%.
    Children 5 years of age and over with blue irides:
      0.25%.
    Children 5 years of age and over with dark irides:
      0.5 or 1%.
Uveitis—
  Topical, to the conjunctiva, 1 drop of a 0.125 to 1% solution one to three times a day.
[Postoperative mydriasis]—
  Topical, to the conjunctiva, 1 drop of a 0.5% solution one to three times a day or as determined by physician.

**Strength(s) usually available**
U.S.—
  0.5% (Rx) [*Atropisol; Isopto Atropine* (benzalkonium chloride 0.01%)].
  1% (Rx) [*Atropair; Atropine Care; Atropisol; Atrosulf; Isopto Atropine* (benzalkonium chloride 0.01%); *I-Tropine; Ocu-Tropine* [GENERIC (may contain chlorobutanol)].
  2% (Rx) [*Atropisol* [GENERIC]].
Canada—
  1% (Rx) [*Atropisol* (benzalkonium chloride); *Isopto Atropine* (benzalkonium chloride); *Minims Atropine* [GENERIC (may contain benzalkonium chloride)].
Note: The 0.125 and 0.25% strengths are no longer commercially available; compounding required for prescriptions.

**Packaging and storage**
Store below 40 °C (104 °F), preferably between 15 and 30 °C (59 and 86 °F), unless otherwise specified by manufacturer. Store in a tight container. Protect from freezing.

**Auxiliary labeling**
• For the eye.
• Keep container tightly closed.

---

[1]Not included in Canadian product labeling.

Revised: 06/21/94
Interim revision: 05/01/95

# ATROPINE, HYOSCYAMINE, METHENAMINE, METHYLENE BLUE, PHENYL SALICYLATE, AND BENZOIC ACID  Systemic†

VA CLASSIFICATION (Primary): GU200
Commonly used brand name(s): *Atrosept; Dolsed; Hexalol; Prosed/DS; Trac Tabs 2X; UAA; Uridon Modified; Urimed; Urinary Antiseptic No. 2; Urised; Uriseptic; Uritab; Uritin; Uro-Ves.*

Note: For a listing of dosage forms and brand names by country availability, see *Dosage Forms* section(s).

†Not commercially available in Canada.

## Category
Anticholinergic-antibacterial-analgesic (urinary tract).

## Indications

**Accepted**

Irritative voiding, symptoms of (treatment)—Indicated for the relief of local symptoms, such as inflammation, hypermotility, and pain, which accompany lower urinary tract infections.

Diagnostic procedure–induced symptoms, urinary (treatment)—Indicated for the relief of urinary tract symptoms caused by diagnostic procedures.

**Unaccepted**

This combination has a labeled indication for the treatment of cystitis, urethritis, and trigonitis caused by organisms that maintain or produce an acid urine and are susceptible to formaldehyde. In addition, it has a labeled indication for the prevention of recurring urinary tract infections. However, the main value of this medication consists in the management of the symptomatology of lower urinary tract infections and it is best used when the acute infection has been destroyed by other antibacterial agents. It is not intended as the primary drug for treatment or as prophylactic therapy in these conditions.

## Pharmacology/Pharmacokinetics

**Mechanism of action/Effect**

Anticholinergic—
  Atropine; hyoscyamine: Relax smooth muscle spasm by inhibiting the muscarinic actions of acetylcholine on autonomic effectors innervated by postganglionic cholinergic nerves as well as on smooth muscle, which responds to endogenous acetylcholine but is not so innervated.

Antibacterial—
  Methenamine: Hydrolyzation of methenamine, in acidic urine, releases formaldehyde, which provides bactericidal or bacteriostatic action, depending on urine pH, volume, and flow rate.
  Methylene blue: Mild antiseptic activity may inhibit bacterial proliferation; relatively ineffective in the treatment of urinary tract infections.
  Benzoic acid: Mild antibacterial and antifungal action. It also helps maintain an acid pH in the urine necessary for the degradation of methenamine.

Analgesic—
  Phenyl salicylate: Produces analgesia through a peripheral action by blocking pain impulse generation and via a central action, possibly in the hypothalamus.

**Other actions/effects**

Phenyl salicylate—May produce antipyresis by acting centrally on the hypothalamic heat-regulating center to produce peripheral vasodilation, resulting in increased cutaneous blood flow, sweating, and heat loss.

**Absorption**

Well absorbed from gastrointestinal tract.

**Distribution**

Methenamine—Freely distributed to body tissues and fluids, but not clinically significant because methenamine does not hydrolyze at pH greater than 6.8.

**Protein binding**

Atropine; hyoscyamine—Moderate.
Methenamine—Some formaldehyde is bound to substances in the urine and the surrounding tissues.

**Biotransformation**

Atropine; hyoscyamine—Hepatic.
Methenamine—Urine (70 to 90% of methenamine reaches the urine unchanged where it is hydrolyzed if the urine is acidic).

**Elimination**

Renal.
Atropine—30 to 50% excreted unchanged.
Hyoscyamine—Majority excreted unchanged.
Methenamine—Almost completely (90%) excreted within 24 hours; of this amount at pH 5, approximately 20% is formaldehyde.
Methylene blue—75% excreted unchanged.

## Precautions to Consider

**Cross-sensitivity and/or related problems**

Patients sensitive to other belladonna alkaloids or other salicylates may be sensitive to this medication also.

**Pregnancy/Reproduction**

Pregnancy—Atropine, hyoscyamine, and methenamine cross the placenta. Studies have not been done in humans.
Studies have not been done in animals.
FDA Pregnancy Category C.

**Breast-feeding**

Methenamine and traces of atropine and hyoscyamine are distributed into breast milk. However problems in humans have not been documented.

**Pediatrics**

No information is available on the relationship of age to the effects of this combination in pediatric patients. However, it is known that infants and young children are especially susceptible to the toxic effects of the belladonna alkaloids.

Close supervision is recommended for infants and children with spastic paralysis or brain damage since an increased response to anticholinergics has been reported in these patients and dosage adjustments are often required.

When anticholinergics are given to children where the environmental temperature is high, there is risk of a rapid increase in body temperature because of these medications' suppression of sweat gland activity.

A paradoxical reaction characterized by hyperexcitability may occur in children taking large doses of anticholinergics.

**Geriatrics**

No information is available on the relationship of age to the effects of this combination in geriatric patients. However, it is known that geriatric patients may respond to the usual doses of the belladonna alkaloids with excitement, agitation, drowsiness, or confusion. Also, geriatric patients are especially susceptible to anticholinergic side effects, such as constipation, dryness of mouth, and urinary retention (especially in males).

In addition, caution is recommended when anticholinergics are given to geriatric patients, because of the danger of precipitating undiagnosed glaucoma.

Memory may become severely impaired in geriatric patients, especially those who already have memory problems, with the continued use of atropine and hyoscyamine since these medications block the action of acetylcholine, which is responsible for many functions of the brain, including memory functions.

**Dental**

Prolonged use of belladonna alkaloids may decrease or inhibit salivary flow, thus contributing to the development of caries, periodontal disease, oral candidiasis, and discomfort.

**Drug interactions and/or related problems**

The following drug interactions and/or related problems have been selected on the basis of their potential clinical significance (possible mechanism in parentheses where appropriate)—not necessarily inclusive (» = major clinical significance):

Note: Combinations containing any of the following medications, depending on the amount present, may also interact with this medication.

Only specific interactions between this combination medication and other oral medications have been identified in this monograph. However, because of atropine's and hyoscyamine's effects on gastrointestinal motility and gastric emptying, absorption of other oral medications may be decreased during concurrent use with this combination medication.

» Alkalizers, urinary, such as:
Antacids, calcium- and/or magnesium-containing
Carbonic anhydrase inhibitors
Citrates
Sodium bicarbonate or
» Diuretics, thiazide
(may cause the urine to become alkaline, thereby reducing the effectiveness of methenamine by inhibiting its conversion to formaldehyde; concurrent use is not recommended)
» Anticholinergics, other, or other medications with anticholinergic action
(See *Appendix II*)
(concurrent use of these medications may intensify anticholinergic effects of atropine and hyoscyamine; patients should be advised to report occurrence of gastrointestinal problems promptly since paralytic ileus may occur with concurrent therapy)
» Antacids or
» Antidiarrheals, adsorbent
(simultaneous use of these medications with this combination medication may reduce absorption of atropine and hyoscyamine, resulting in decreased therapeutic effectiveness; doses of these medications should be spaced 2 to 3 hours apart from doses of atropine and hyoscyamine)

(concurrent use of this combination medication with antacids, especially calcium carbonate–, magnesium-, or sodium bicarbonate–containing, may cause the urine to become alkaline, thereby reducing the effectiveness of methenamine by inhibiting its conversion to formaldehyde; simultaneous use may reduce absorption of atropine and hyoscyamine, resulting in decreased therapeutic effectiveness)
» Ketoconazole
(atropine and hyoscyamine may cause increased gastrointestinal pH; concurrent administration of ketoconazole with atropine and hyoscyamine may result in a marked reduction in absorption of ketoconazole; patients should be advised to take this combination at least 2 hours after ketoconazole)
Metoclopramide
(concurrent use of metoclopramide with atropine and hyoscyamine may antagonize the effects of metoclopramide on gastrointestinal motility)
Monoamine oxidase (MAO) inhibitors, including furazolidone, procarbazine, and selegiline
(concurrent use may result in intensified anticholinergic side effects because of these medications' secondary anticholinergic activities; also, concurrent use of MAO inhibitors may block detoxification of anticholinergics, thus potentiating their action)
Opioid (narcotic) analgesics
(concurrent use of opioids with atropine and hyoscyamine may result in increased risk of severe constipation, which may lead to paralytic ileus, and/or urinary retention)
» Potassium chloride, especially wax matrix preparations
(concurrent use with atropine and hyoscyamine may increase severity of potassium chloride–induced gastrointestinal lesions)
» Sulfonamides
(in acid urine, methenamine breaks down into formaldehyde, which may form an insoluble precipitate with certain sulfonamides and may also increase the danger of crystalluria; concurrent use is not recommended)

**Laboratory value alterations**
The following have been selected on the basis of their potential clinical significance (possible effect in parentheses where appropriate)—not necessarily inclusive (» = major clinical significance):
With diagnostic test results
Catecholamine determinations, urinary and
17-hydroxycorticosteroid (17-OHCS) determinations, urinary and
Vanillylmandelic acid (VMA), urinary
(methenamine may cause a false increase)
Estriol determinations, urinary and
5-Hydroxy indoleacetic acid (5-HIAA) determinations, urinary
(methenamine may cause a false decrease)
» Gastric acid secretion test
(atropine and hyoscyamine may antagonize the effect of pentagastrin and histamine in the evaluation of gastric acid secretory function; administration of this combination is not recommended during the 24 hours preceding the test)
» Phenolsulfonphthalein (PSP) excretion test
(methylene blue may cause a false positive)

Radionuclide gastric emptying studies
(atropine and hyoscyamine may result in delayed gastric emptying)
Urinary free formaldehyde and
Urine pH
(methylene blue may interfere with analysis)

**Medical considerations/Contraindications**
The medical considerations/contraindications included have been selected on the basis of their potential clinical significance (reasons given in parentheses where appropriate)—not necessarily inclusive (» = major clinical significance).

*Risk-benefit should be considered when the following medical problems exist:*
Brain damage, in children
(CNS effects may be exacerbated by atropine and hyoscyamine)
» Cardiac disease, especially cardiac arrhythmias, congestive heart failure, coronary heart disease, mitral stenosisor
Hemorrhage, acute, with tachycardia or
Hyperthyroidism or
Tachycardia
(increase in heart rate caused by atropine and hyoscyamine may be undesirable)
Dehydration, severe or
Renal function impairment
(inadequate concentrations of this combination medicine may be achieved in urine; salts of methenamine may precipitate, causing crystalluria in patients with low urine output)
» Esophagitis, reflux
(decrease in esophageal and gastric motility and relaxation of lower esophageal sphincter caused by atropine and hyoscyamine may promote gastric retention by delaying gastric emptying and may increase gastroesophageal reflux through an incompetent sphincter)
Fever
(may be increased through suppression of sweat gland activity caused by atropine and hyoscyamine)
» Gastrointestinal tract obstructive disease
(decrease in motility and tone caused by atropine and hyoscyamine may result in obstruction and gastric retention)
» Glaucoma, angle-closure, or predisposition to
(mydriatic effect caused by atropine and hyoscyamine may result in increased intraocular pressure and may precipitate an acute attack of angle-closure glaucoma)
» Glaucoma, open-angle
(mydriatic effect of atropine and hyoscyamine may cause a slight increase in intraocular pressure; glaucoma therapy may need to be adjusted)
Glucose-6-phosphate dehydrogenase (G6PD) deficiency
(use of methylene blue may induce hemolysis)
Hepatic function impairment
(decreased metabolism of atropine and hyoscyamine; methenamine may facilitate ammonia production in the intestinal tract)
» Hernia, hiatal, associated with reflux esophagitis
(atropine and hyoscyamine may aggravate condition)
Hypertension
(atropine and hyoscyamine may aggravate condition)
» Intestinal atony in the elderly or debilitated patient or
» Paralytic ileus
(atropine and hyoscyamine may result in obstruction)
Lung disease, chronic, especially in infants, small children, and debilitated patients
(reduction in bronchial secretion caused by atropine and hyoscyamine can lead to inspissation and formation of bronchial plugs)
» Myasthenia gravis
(condition may be aggravated because of inhibition of acetylcholine action)
Neuropathy, autonomic
(urinary retention and cycloplegia may be aggravated by atropine and hyoscyamine)
» Prostatic hypertrophy, nonobstructive or
» Urinary retention or
» Uropathy, obstructive, such as bladder neck obstruction due to prostatic hypertrophy
(urinary retention may be precipitated or aggravated by atropine and hyoscyamine)

Sensitivity to any of the medications in this combination
Spastic paralysis, in children
(response to atropine and hyoscyamine may be increased)
Toxemia of pregnancy
(hypertension may be aggravated by atropine and hyoscyamine)
Ulcerative colitis
(large doses of atropine and hyoscyamine may suppress intestinal motility, possibly causing paralytic ileus; also, use may precipitate or aggravate toxic megacolon)
Xerostomia
(prolonged use of atropine and hyoscyamine may further reduce limited salivary flow)
Caution in use is also recommended in patients over 40 years of age because of the danger of precipitating undiagnosed glaucoma.

**Patient monitoring**
The following may be especially important in patient monitoring (other tests may be warranted in some patients, depending on condition; » = major clinical significance):
Intraocular pressure determinations
(recommended at periodic intervals because atropine and hyoscyamine may increase the intraocular pressure by producing mydriasis)
Urine pH
(monitoring recommended before start of treatment and throughout therapy since the effectiveness of methenamine is increased if a pH of 5.5 or below is maintained. To check urine pH, phenaphthazine paper, which has a pH range of 4.5 to 7.5, may be used. However, the presence of methylene blue may interfere with urinary pH determination)

## Side/Adverse Effects

Note: This medication should be discontinued immediately if dizziness, increased pulse, or blurring of vision occurs.
Geriatric or debilitated patients may respond to usual doses of atropine and hyoscyamine with excitement, agitation, drowsiness, or confusion.

The following side/adverse effects have been selected on the basis of their potential clinical significance (possible signs and symptoms in parentheses where appropriate)—not necessarily inclusive:

**Those indicating need for medical attention**
Incidence less frequent or rare
*Allergic reaction* (skin rash or hives); *difficulty in eye accommodation* (blurred vision); *increased intraocular pressure* (eye pain)

**Those indicating need for medical attention only if they continue or are bothersome**
Incidence less frequent
*Difficult urination*—more frequent with large doses over a prolonged period of time; *dryness of mouth, nose, or throat; nausea or vomiting; stomach upset or pain*—more frequent with large doses over a prolonged period of time

**Those not indicating need for medical attention**
Incidence more frequent
*Blue or blue-green urine and/or stools*—due to excretion of methylene blue

## Overdose

For specific information on the agents used in the management of this combination product overdose, see:
• *Physostigmine* in *Systemic* monograph; and/or
• *Diazepam* in *Benzodiazepines (Systemic)* monograph.

For more information on the management of overdose or unintentional ingestion, **contact a Poison Control Center** (see *Poison Control Center Listing*).

**Clinical effects of overdose**
The following effects have been selected on the basis of their potential clinical significance (possible signs and symptoms in parentheses where appropriate)—not necessarily inclusive:

*Anticholinergic effects* (severe drowsiness; dizziness; fast heartbeat; flushing or redness of face; shortness of breath or troubled breathing); *hematuria; crystalluria* (blood in urine; lower back pain; pain or burning while urinating)—due to methenamine; *salicylate effects* (bloody stools; diarrhea; severe or continuing headache; dizziness; ringing or buzzing in ears; sweating; unusual tiredness or weakness)

**Treatment of overdose**
Recommended treatment for overdose includes:
To decrease absorption—
Emesis or gastric lavage.
Specific treatment—
Slow intravenous administration of physostigmine in doses of 1 to 4 mg (0.5 to 1 mg in children), repeated as needed in one to two hours, to reverse severe anticholinergic symptoms; use of physostigmine with caution and only with cardiac monitoring. Administration of small doses of diazepam to control excitement and seizures.
Supportive care—
Artificial respiration with oxygen if needed for respiratory depression. Adequate hydration. Symptomatic treatment as necessary. Patients in whom intentional overdose is known or suspected should be referred for psychiatric consultation.

## Patient Consultation

As an aid to patient consultation, refer to *Advice for the Patient, Atropine, Hyoscyamine, Methenamine, Methylene Blue, Phenyl Salicylate, and Benzoic Acid (Systemic)*.
In providing consultation, consider emphasizing the following selected information (» = major clinical significance):

**Before using this medication**
» Conditions affecting use, especially:
Sensitivity to any of the belladonna alkaloids or salicylates
Pregnancy—Crosses the placenta
Breast-feeding—Atropine, hyoscyamine, and methenamine distributed into breast milk
Use in children—Increased susceptibility to toxic effects of belladonna alkaloids; increased response to anticholinergics in children with spastic paralysis or brain damage; suppression of sweat gland activity in children; possibility of paradoxical reaction characterized by hyperexcitability
Use in the elderly—Increased susceptibility to CNS and anticholinergic effects of belladonna alkaloids; danger of precipitating undiagnosed glaucoma; possible impairment of memory
Dental—Possible development of dental problems because of decreased salivary flow
Other medications, especially antacids, other anticholinergics, antidiarrheals, ketoconazole, potassium chloride, sulfonamides, thiazide diuretics, or urinary alkalizers
Other medical problems, especially cardiac disease, fever, glaucoma, hemorrhage, hiatal hernia, intestinal atony or paralytic ileus, lung disease, myasthenia gravis, obstruction in gastrointestinal or urinary tract, prostatic hypertrophy, reflux esophagitis, ulcerative colitis, or xerostomia

**Proper use of this medication**
» Importance of not taking more medication than the amount prescribed
Maintaining fluid intake for adequate urinary output
» Compliance with full course of therapy
» Importance of maintaining acidic urine (pH 5.5 or below)
Measuring urine pH with phenaphthazine paper; adjusting urine pH with appropriate diet
» Proper dosing
Missed dose: Taking as soon as possible; if almost time for next dose, not taking at all; not doubling doses
» Proper storage

**Precautions while using this medication**
Checking with physician if no improvement within a few days
Caution during exercise or hot weather; overheating may result in heat stroke
» Caution if blurred vision occurs
Possible dryness of mouth, nose, or throat; using sugarless gum or candy, ice, or saliva substitute for relief; checking with dentist if dry mouth continues for more than 2 weeks
Avoid use of antacids and antidiarrheal medications within 2 or 3 hours of taking this medication

**Side/adverse effects**
Signs of potential side effects, especially allergic reaction, blurred vision, or eye pain
Blue or blue-green discoloration of urine and/or stools may be alarming to patient although medically insignificant

## General Dosing Information

An increase in the patient's fluid intake is not necessary; however, it is recommended that the patient drink enough liquids to satisfy normal fluid requirements and to maintain an adequate urine output.

In order to maintain a urine pH of 5.5 or below, most fruits (especially citrus fruits and juices), milk and other dairy products, and other alkalinizing foods should be avoided. A protein-rich diet with liberal amounts of cranberries (especially ascorbic acid–enriched cranberry juice), plums, or prunes may be helpful. If these measures do not produce a sufficiently acid urine, they may be supplemented with large doses of ascorbic acid (4 grams or more per day), arginine hydrochloride, or methionine. However, some brands of ascorbic acid may contain varying amounts of sodium ascorbate and may actually alkalinize the urine. Alternatively, ammonium chloride or sodium biphosphate may be given (caution—large doses of ammonium chloride may cause metabolic acidosis in patients with impaired renal function and may be contraindicated in patients with hepatic insufficiency).

Urea-splitting organisms (e.g., *Proteus mirabilis* and some strains of *Pseudomonas* and *Aerobacter*) may cause an increase in urine pH and thereby decrease the effectiveness of methenamine. Care should be taken to ensure urine acidification.

## Oral Dosage Forms

### ATROPINE SULFATE, HYOSCYAMINE, METHENAMINE, METHYLENE BLUE, PHENYL SALICYLATE, AND BENZOIC ACID TABLETS

**Usual adult and adolescent dose**
Oral, 1 or 2 tablets (depending on strength of product) four times a day.

**Usual pediatric dose**
Children up to 6 years of age—
  Use is not recommended.
Children 6 years of age and over—
  Dosage must be individualized by physician.

**Usual geriatric dose**
See *Usual adult and adolescent dose*.

Note: Geriatric patients may be more sensitive to the effects of the usual adult dose.

**Strength(s) usually available**
U.S.—
  30 mcg (0.03 mg) of atropine sulfate, 30 mcg (0.03 mg) of hyoscyamine, 40.8 mg of methenamine, 5.4 mg of methylene blue, 18.1 mg of phenyl salicylate, and 4.5 mg of benzoic acid, per tablet (Rx) [*Atrosept; Dolsed; Hexalol; UAA; Uridon Modified; Urimed; Urinary Antiseptic No. 2; Urised* (sugar-coated); *Uriseptic; Uritab; Uritin; Uro-Ves*].
  60 mcg (0.06 mg) of atropine sulfate, 30 mcg (0.03 mg) of hyoscyamine, 120 mg of methenamine, 6 mg of methylene blue, 30 mg of phenyl salicylate, and 7.5 mg of benzoic acid, per tablet (Rx) [*Trac Tabs 2X*].
  60 mcg (0.06 mg) of atropine sulfate, 60 mcg (0.06 mg) of hyoscyamine, 81.6 mg of methenamine, 10.8 mg of methylene blue, 36.2 mg of phenyl salicylate, and 9 mg of benzoic acid, per tablet (Rx) [*Prosed/DS*].

Note: Exact strengths of specific products may vary slightly, depending on manufacturer.

Canada—
  Not commercially available.

**Packaging and storage**
Store below 40 °C (104 °F), preferably between 15 and 30 °C (59 and 86 °F), unless otherwise specified by manufacturer.

**Auxiliary labeling**
• Take with a full glass of water.
• May discolor urine and/or stools.

**Note**
Instruct patient on taking adequate amounts of fluids with each dose and during therapy.

Revised: 05/11/93

---

**ATTAPULGITE**—The *Attapulgite (Oral-Local)* monograph is not included in this published version of the USP DI database. Copies of the monograph are available on request from Micromedex, Inc. - Reprint Requests, 6200 S. Syracuse Way, Suite 300, Englewood, CO 80111; telephone (303) 486-6400; telefax (303) 486-6464; Email: USPDI@MDX.COM.

---

**AURANOFIN**—See *Gold Compounds (Systemic)*

---

**AUROTHIOGLUCOSE**—See *Gold Compounds (Systemic)*

---

**AZATADINE**—See *Antihistamines (Systemic)*

---

# AZATHIOPRINE  Systemic

VA CLASSIFICATION (Primary/Secondary): IM600/MS109; GA400

Commonly used brand name(s): *Imuran*.

Note: For a listing of dosage forms and brand names by country availability, see *Dosage Forms* section(s).

## Category
Immunosuppressant; antirheumatic (disease-modifying); bowel disease (inflammatory) suppressant; lupus erythematosus suppressant.

## Indications
Note: Bracketed information in the *Indications* section refers to uses that are not included in U.S. product labeling.

**Accepted**
Transplant rejection, organ (prophylaxis)—Azathioprine is indicated as an adjunct for prevention of rejection in renal homotransplantation. [It is also used in the prevention of rejection in cardiac, hepatic, and pancreatic transplantation.]
Arthritis, rheumatoid (treatment)—Azathioprine is indicated for the management of severe, active, and erosive rheumatoid arthritis unresponsive to rest or conventional medications.
[Bowel disease, inflammatory (treatment)][1]
[Hepatitis, chronic active (treatment)][1]
[Cirrhosis, biliary (treatment)][1]
[Lupus erythematosus, systemic (treatment)][1]
[Glomerulonephritis (treatment)][1]
[Nephrotic syndrome (treatment)][1]
[Myopathy, inflammatory (treatment)][1]
[Myasthenia gravis (treatment)][1]
[Dermatomyositis, systemic (treatment)][1]
[Pemphigoid (treatment)][1] or
[Pemphigus (treatment)][1]—Azathioprine is also used in the treatment of other immunologic diseases including regional and ulcerative colitis, chronic active hepatitis and biliary cirrhosis, systemic lupus erythematosus (SLE), glomerulonephritis, nephrotic syndrome, inflammatory myopathy, myasthenia gravis, systemic dermatomyositis (polymyositis), pemphigus, and pemphigoid.

[1]Not included in Canadian product labeling.

## Pharmacology/Pharmacokinetics

**Physicochemical characteristics**
Molecular weight—277.26.

**Mechanism of action/Effect**
The exact mechanism of immunosuppressive action is unknown since the exact mechanism of the immune response itself is complex and not completely understood. The immunosuppressive effects of azathioprine involve a greater suppression of delayed hypersensitivity and cellular cytotoxicity tests than of antibody responses. Azathioprine antagonizes purine metabolism and may inhibit synthesis of DNA, RNA, and proteins; it may also interfere with cellular metabolism and inhibit mitosis.
The mechanism of action of azathioprine in rheumatoid arthritis and other immunologic diseases is unknown but may be related to immunosuppression. Azathioprine has a steroid-sparing effect, which allows a reduction in steroid dose when the two are combined in chronic inflammatory diseases.

**Absorption**
Well absorbed from the gastrointestinal tract.

**Protein binding**
Low (30%).

**Biotransformation**
Largely converted to 6-mercaptopurine and 6-thioinosinic acid (active metabolites). Further metabolism—Hepatic, largely by xanthine oxidase, and in erythrocytes. Proportions of metabolites vary among individual patients.

**Half-life**
Approximately 5 hours (unchanged drug and metabolites).

**Onset of action**
In rheumatoid arthritis—6 to 8 weeks.
In other inflammatory disorders—4 to 8 weeks.

**Time to peak concentration**
Serum—1 to 2 hours.

**Duration of action**
Immunosuppressant—Clinical effects may persist for long periods after the medication is eliminated.

**Elimination**
Hepatic (biliary).
Renal (1 to 2% unchanged).
In dialysis—Partially (minimally) removable by hemodialysis.

## Precautions to Consider

**Carcinogenicity**
Azathioprine has been shown to be carcinogenic in animals, and may be associated with an increased risk of development of carcinomas in humans, especially skin cancer and reticulum cell tumors or lymphomas in renal transplant patients and acute myelocytic leukemia and some solid tumors in rheumatoid arthritis patients. The risk of neoplastic toxicity appears to be lower in rheumatoid arthritis patients than in renal transplant patients; however, there is evidence that the risk is increased with prior use of alkylating agents.

**Mutagenicity**
Mutagenic effects have been reported in animals, and chromosomal abnormalities (reversible when azathioprine is discontinued) have been noted in humans.

**Pregnancy/Reproduction**
Fertility—Azathioprine has been reported to cause temporary depression in spermatogenesis and reduction in sperm viability and sperm count in mice at doses 10 times the human therapeutic dose; a reduced percentage of fertile matings occurred when animals received 5 mg per kg of body weight (mg/kg).

Pregnancy—Adequate and well-controlled studies in humans have not been done.

Azathioprine crosses the placenta.

Risk-benefit must be considered, especially during the first trimester, since azathioprine affects cell kinetics and can theoretically cause mutagenicity or teratogenicity.

There have been reports of limited immunologic abnormalities (lymphopenia, diminished IgG and IgM levels, cytomegalovirus [CMV] infection, and decreased thymic shadow; pancytopenia and severe immune deficiency) and other abnormalities (preaxial polydactyly in an infant whose mother received azathioprine and prednisone; meningomyelocele, bilateral dislocated hips, and bilateral *talipes equinovarus* in an infant whose father received azathioprine) in infants of renal homograft recipients treated with azathioprine.

Azathioprine is not recommended for use in pregnant women with rheumatoid arthritis.

Teratogenic effects (including skeletal malformations and visceral abnormalities) have been reported in rabbits and mice given doses equivalent to the human dose (5 mg/kg per day).

FDA Pregnancy Category D.

**Breast-feeding**
Azathioprine is distributed, at low concentrations, into breast milk. Nursing mothers should be advised to contact physician, since use by nursing mothers is not recommended because of possible adverse effects (especially tumorigenicity) on the infant.

**Pediatrics**
Appropriate studies performed to date have not demonstrated pediatrics-specific problems that would limit the usefulness of azathioprine in children.

**Geriatrics**
Although appropriate studies on the relationship of age to the effects of azathioprine have not been performed in the geriatric population, geriatrics-specific problems are not expected to limit the usefulness of this medication in the elderly. However, elderly patients are more likely to have age-related renal function impairment, which may require reduced dosage in patients receiving azathioprine.

**Dental**
The bone marrow depressant effects of azathioprine may result in an increased incidence of microbial infection, delayed healing, and gingival bleeding. Dental work, whenever possible, should be completed prior to initiation of therapy or deferred until blood counts have returned to normal. Patients should be instructed in proper oral hygiene during treatment, including caution in use of regular toothbrushes, dental floss, and toothpicks.

In addition, azathioprine rarely causes sores in the mouth and on the lips.

**Drug interactions and/or related problems**
The following drug interactions and/or related problems have been selected on the basis of their potential clinical significance (possible mechanism in parentheses where appropriate)—not necessarily inclusive (» = major clinical significance):

Note: Combinations containing any of the following medications, depending on the amount present, may also interact with this medication.

» Allopurinol
(allopurinol-induced inhibition of xanthine oxidase–mediated metabolism may result in greatly increased azathioprine activity and toxicity; concurrent use should be avoided if possible, especially in renal transplant patients, because of the high risk of 6-mercaptopurine [azathioprine metabolite] accumulation and consequent azathioprine toxicity if the transplanted kidney is rejected; if concurrent use is essential, it is recommended that azathioprine dosage be reduced to one quarter to one third of the usual dosage, the patient be carefully monitored, and subsequent dosage adjustments be based on patient response and evidence of toxicity)

Blood dyscrasia–causing medications (see *Appendix II*)
(leukopenic and/or thrombocytopenic effects of azathioprine may be increased with concurrent or recent therapy if these medications cause the same effects; dosage adjustment of azathioprine, if necessary, should be based on blood counts)

Bone marrow depressants, other (see *Appendix II*) or
Radiation therapy
(concurrent use with azathioprine may increase the bone marrow depressant effects of these medications and radiation therapy; dosage reduction may be required; use prior to azathioprine therapy may be associated with an increased risk of development of neoplasms)

» Immunosuppressants, other, such as:
Chlorambucil
Corticosteroids, glucocorticoid
Cyclophosphamide
Cyclosporine
Mercaptopurine
Muromonab-CD3
(concurrent use with azathioprine may increase the risk of infection and development of neoplasms)

Vaccines, killed virus
(because normal defense mechanisms may be suppressed by azathioprine therapy, the patient's antibody response to the vaccine may be decreased. The interval between discontinuation of medications that cause immunosuppression and restoration of the patient's ability to respond to the vaccine depends on the intensity and type of immunosuppression-causing medication used, the underlying disease, and other factors; estimates vary from 3 months to 1 year)

» Vaccines, live virus
(because normal defense mechanisms may be suppressed by azathioprine therapy, concurrent use with a live virus vaccine may potentiate the replication of the vaccine virus, may increase the side/adverse effects of the vaccine virus, and/or may decrease the patient's antibody response to the vaccine; immunization of these patients should be undertaken only with extreme caution after careful review of the patient's hematologic status and only with the knowledge and consent of the physician managing the azathioprine therapy. The interval between discontinuation of medications that cause immunosuppression and restoration of the patient's ability to respond to the vaccine depends on the intensity and type of immunosuppression-causing medication used, the underlying disease, and other factors; estimates vary from 3 months to 1 year. Patients with leukemia in remission should not receive live virus vaccine until at least 3 months after their last chemotherapy. In addition, immuni-

zation with oral poliovirus vaccine should be postponed in persons in close contact with the patient, especially family members)

**Laboratory value alterations**
The following have been selected on the basis of their potential clinical significance (possible effect in parentheses where appropriate)—not necessarily inclusive (» = major clinical significance):

With physiology/laboratory test values
Alanine aminotransferase (ALT [SGPT]) and
Alkaline phosphatase and
Amylase and
Aspartate aminotransferase (AST [SGOT]) and
Bilirubin
(serum values may be increased in association with toxic hepatitis and biliary stasis, primarily in allograft recipients; may also be increased as part of a gastrointestinal hypersensitivity reaction; uncommon in rheumatoid arthritis patients)
Albumin, plasma and
Hemoglobin and
Uric acid in blood and urine
(concentrations may be decreased)
Mean corpuscular volume (MCV)
(may be increased; occurs commonly, as a sign of macrocytosis)

**Medical considerations/Contraindications**
The medical considerations/contraindications included have been selected on the basis of their potential clinical significance (reasons given in parentheses where appropriate)—not necessarily inclusive (» = major clinical significance).

*Risk-benefit should be considered when the following medical problems exist:*
- » Chickenpox, existing or recent (including recent exposure) or
- » Herpes zoster
  (risk of severe generalized disease)
- » Gout
  (because of interaction with allopurinol)
- » Hepatic function impairment
- » Infection
- Pancreatitis
- » Renal function impairment
  (increased risk of hematologic toxicity; a lower dosage of azathioprine is recommended for patients with impaired renal function)
- » Sensitivity to azathioprine
- » Xanthine oxidase deficiency, severe
  (reduced metabolism may result in increased azathioprine activity and toxicity)
- » Caution should be used also in patients who have had previous cytotoxic drug therapy and radiation therapy.

**Patient monitoring**
The following may be especially important in patient monitoring (other tests may be warranted in some patients, depending on condition; » = major clinical significance):
- » Complete blood counts
  (recommended at least weekly during the first 2 months of therapy; frequency may be reduced to monthly once the patient is stabilized)

## Side/Adverse Effects

Note: The risk of hematologic and neoplastic toxicity appears to be lower in rheumatoid arthritis patients because of the lower doses used. Bone marrow depression may be more severe in renal transplant patients whose homografts are undergoing rejection.

The following side/adverse effects have been selected on the basis of their potential clinical significance (possible signs and symptoms in parentheses where appropriate)—not necessarily inclusive:

**Those indicating need for medical attention**
Incidence more frequent
**Leukopenia or infection** (leukopenia is usually asymptomatic; less frequently, fever or chills; cough or hoarseness; lower back or side pain; painful or difficult urination); **megaloblastic anemia** (unusual tiredness or weakness)
Note: *Leukopenia* may be severe or delayed and is dose-related. Not correlated with therapeutic effect.
The incidence of *infection* in renal transplant patients is 30 to 60 times that in patients taking azathioprine for rheumatoid arthritis.
*Infections* may be fatal.

Incidence less frequent—dose-related
**Hepatitis or biliary stasis** (asymptomatic); **thrombocytopenia** (usually asymptomatic; rarely, unusual bleeding or bruising; black, tarry stools; blood in urine or stools; pinpoint red spots on skin)
Note: *Hepatotoxicity* usually occurs within 6 months of transplantation and is reversible on withdrawal of azathioprine. It is uncommon (incidence less than 1%) in rheumatoid arthritis patients. Hepatotoxicity occurs more frequently at dosages above 2.5 mg per kg of body weight (mg/kg) per day.
*Thrombocytopenia* may be severe or delayed and is dose-related.

Incidence rare
**Gastrointestinal hypersensitivity reaction** (severe nausea and vomiting with diarrhea; sudden fever; joint pain; sudden unusual feeling of discomfort or illness); **hepatic veno-occlusive disease, potentially fatal** (stomach pain; swelling of feet or lower legs); **hypersensitivity** (fast heartbeat; sudden fever; muscle or joint pain; redness or blisters on skin); **pancreatitis, hypersensitivity** (severe stomach pain with nausea and vomiting); **pneumonitis** (cough; shortness of breath); **sores in mouth and on lips**
Note: Symptoms of the *gastrointestinal hypersensitivity reaction* usually develop within the first several weeks of therapy and are reversible on withdrawal of azathioprine, although they will recur within hours after the first dose on rechallenge. Hypotension may occasionally occur. Hepatic enzymes may also be elevated.
*Hypersensitivity* reactions usually occur after at least 1 week of therapy, and are reversible on withdrawal. The reaction may be more severe on rechallenge and can be fatal.

**Those indicating need for medical attention only if they continue or are bothersome**
Incidence more frequent
*Loss of appetite; nausea or vomiting*
Incidence less frequent
*Skin rash*

**Those indicating the need for medical attention if they occur after medication is discontinued**
*Bone marrow depression, delayed* (black, tarry stools; blood in urine; cough or hoarseness; fever or chills; lower back or side pain; painful or difficult urination; pinpoint red spots on skin; unusual bleeding or bruising)

## Patient Consultation

As an aid to patient consultation, refer to *Advice for the Patient, Azathioprine (Systemic)*.
In providing consultation, consider emphasizing the following selected information (» = major clinical significance):

**Before using this medication**
- » Conditions affecting use, especially:
  Sensitivity to azathioprine
    Pregnancy—Use not recommended because of mutagenic or teratogenic potential
    Breast-feeding—Not recommended because of risk of serious side effects
  Other medications, especially allopurinol, other immunosuppressants, or previous cytotoxic drug therapy or radiation therapy
  Other medical problems, especially chickenpox, herpes zoster, gout, hepatic function impairment, infection, or renal function impairment

**Proper use of this medication**
- » Importance of not taking more or less medication than the amount prescribed
- Caution with combination therapy; taking each medication at the right time
- » Checking with physician before discontinuing medication
- Possible nausea or vomiting; taking after meals or at bedtime to reduce stomach upset
- Checking with physician if vomiting occurs shortly after dose is taken
- » Proper dosing
  Missed dose—
    If dosing schedule is once a day—Not taking missed dose and not doubling next one
    If dosing schedule is several times a day—Taking as soon as possible or doubling next dose; checking with physician if more than one dose is missed
- » Proper storage

### Precautions while using this medication
» Importance of close monitoring by physician
» Avoiding immunizations unless approved by physician; other persons in patient's household should avoid immunizations with oral poliovirus vaccine; avoiding other persons who have taken oral poliovirus vaccine or wearing a protective mask that covers nose and mouth

*Caution if bone marrow depression occurs*
» Avoiding exposure to persons with bacterial or viral infections, especially during periods of low blood counts; checking with physician immediately if fever or chills, cough or hoarseness, lower back or side pain, or painful or difficult urination occurs
» Checking with physician immediately if unusual bleeding or bruising; black, tarry stools; blood in urine or stools; or pinpoint red spots on skin occur

Caution in use of regular toothbrush, dental floss, or toothpick; physician, dentist, or nurse may suggest alternatives; checking with physician before having dental work done

Not touching eyes or inside of nose unless hands washed immediately before

Using caution to avoid accidental cuts with use of sharp objects such as safety razor or fingernail or toenail cutters

Avoiding contact sports or other situations where bruising or injury could occur

### Side/adverse effects
Importance of discussing possible effects, including cancer, with physician

Signs of potential side effects, especially leukopenia, infection, megaloblastic anemia, hepatitis, biliary stasis, thrombocytopenia, gastrointestinal hypersensitivity reaction, hepatic veno-occlusive disease, hypersensitivity, pancreatitis, pneumonitis, and sores in mouth and on lips

Asymptomatic side effects, including hepatotoxicity

## General Dosing Information

Patients receiving azathioprine should be under supervision of a physician experienced in immunosuppressive therapy.

A variety of dosage schedules and regimens of azathioprine, alone or in combination with other immunosuppressive agents, are used. The prescriber may consult the medical literature as well as the manufacturers' literature in choosing a specific dosage.

Dosage must be adjusted to meet the individual requirements of each patient, on the basis of clinical response and appearance or severity of toxicity.

Cadaveric kidneys frequently develop a tubular necrosis with delayed onset of adequate function, necessitating a reduction in azathioprine dosage. If persistent negative nitrogen balance occurs, dosage should be reduced.

Because of the delayed action of azathioprine, dosage should be reduced or the medication withdrawn at the first sign of an abnormally large or persistent decrease in leukocyte count (to less than 3000 per cubic millimeter) or platelet count (to less than 100,000 per cubic millimeter) or other evidence of bone marrow depression. Therapy may be reinstituted at a lower dosage when leukocyte and platelet counts return to acceptable levels, usually after 7 to 10 days.

Special precautions are recommended in patients who develop thrombocytopenia as a result of administration of azathioprine. These may include extreme care in performing invasive procedures; regular inspection of intravenous sites, skin (including perirectal area), and mucous membrane surfaces for signs of bleeding or bruising; limiting frequency of venipuncture and avoiding intramuscular injections; testing urine, emesis, stool, and secretions for occult blood; care in use of regular toothbrushes, dental floss, toothpicks, safety razors, and fingernail and toenail cutters; avoiding constipation; and using caution to prevent falls and other injuries. Such patients should avoid alcohol and aspirin intake because of the risk of gastrointestinal bleeding. Platelet transfusions may be required.

Patients who develop leukopenia should be observed carefully for signs of infection. Antibiotic support may be required. In neutropenic patients who develop fever, broad-spectrum antibiotic coverage should be initiated empirically, pending bacterial cultures and appropriate diagnostic tests.

If an infection develops, it must be treated promptly; reduction of azathioprine dosage and/or use of other drugs may be necessary.

If symptoms of toxic hepatitis or biliary stasis appear, azathioprine therapy may have to be withdrawn. Patients with existing hepatic function impairment should be monitored carefully and treated with conservative doses (some clinicians recommend an initial dose of two thirds the usual dose). If hepatic veno-occlusive disease is clinically suspected, it is recommended that azathioprine be permanently withdrawn.

If signs of homograft rejection occur, a larger dose may be necessary. Other therapy should be considered if signs persist.

### For parenteral dosage forms
Azathioprine may be administered by intravenous push or infusion. Time for infusion is usually 30 to 60 minutes, but may range from 5 minutes to 8 hours.

### Diet/Nutrition
Gastrointestinal upset may be reduced by giving oral azathioprine in divided doses or after meals.

### Safety considerations for handling this medication
There is limited but increasing evidence and concern that personnel involved in preparation and administration of parenteral antineoplastics and immunosuppressants may be at some risk because of the potential mutagenicity, teratogenicity, and/or carcinogenicity of these agents, although the actual risk is unknown. USP advisory panels recommend cautious handling both in preparation and disposal of antineoplastic and immunosuppressant agents. Precautions that have been suggested include:

• Use of a biological containment cabinet during reconstitution and dilution of parenteral medications and wearing of disposable surgical gloves and masks.

• Use of proper technique to prevent contamination of the medication, work area, and operator during transfer between containers (including proper training of personnel in this technique).

• Cautious and proper disposal of needles, syringes, vials, ampuls, and unused medication.

A number of medical centers have developed detailed guidelines for handling of antineoplastic and immunosuppressant agents.

## Oral Dosage Forms

Note: Bracketed uses in the *Dosage Forms* section refer to categories of use and/or indications that are not included in U.S. product labeling.

### AZATHIOPRINE TABLETS USP

**Usual adult and adolescent dose**
Transplant rejection, organ (prophylaxis)—
  Initial: Oral, 3 to 5 mg per kg of body weight or 120 mg per square meter of body surface a day, one to three days before or at the time of surgery, the dosage being adjusted to maintain the homograft without causing toxicity.
  Maintenance: Oral, 1 to 2 mg per kg of body weight or 45 mg per square meter of body surface a day.
[Bowel disease, inflammatory][1] or
[Hepatitis, chronic active][1] or
[Cirrhosis, biliary][1] or
[Glomerulonephritis][1] or
[Nephrotic syndrome][1] or
[Myopathy, inflammatory][1] or
[Myasthenia gravis][1] or
[Dermatomyositis, systemic][1] or
[Pemphigoid][1] or
[Pemphigus][1]—
  Initial: Oral, 1 mg per kg of body weight per day, the dosage being increased in increments of 500 mcg (0.5 mg) per kg of body weight per day after six to eight weeks, then every four weeks as necessary up to a maximum dose of 2.5 mg per kg of body weight per day.
  Maintenance: Oral, the dosage being reduced to the minimum effective dose in decrements of 500 mcg (0.5 mg) per kg of body weight per day every four to eight weeks.
Rheumatoid arthritis or
[Lupus erythematosus, systemic][1]—
  Initial: Oral, 1 mg per kg of body weight per day, the dosage being increased in increments of 500 mcg (0.5 mg) per kg of body weight per day after six to eight weeks, then every four weeks as necessary up to a maximum dose of 2.5 mg per kg of body weight per day.
  Maintenance: Oral, the dosage being reduced to the minimum effective dose in decrements of 500 mcg (0.5 mg) per kg of body weight per day every four to eight weeks.

**Usual pediatric dose**
See *Usual adult and adolescent dose.*

**Strength(s) usually available**
U.S.—
  50 mg (Rx) [*Imuran* (scored; lactose) [GENERIC (scored)].
Canada—
  50 mg (Rx) [*Imuran* (scored)].

**Packaging and storage**
Store below 40 °C (104 °F), preferably between 15 and 30 °C (59 and 86 °F), in a well-closed container, unless otherwise specified by manufacturer. Protect from light.

## Parenteral Dosage Forms

Note: The dosing and strengths of the dosage form available are expressed in terms of azathioprine base.

### AZATHIOPRINE SODIUM FOR INJECTION USP

**Usual adult and adolescent dose**
Transplant rejection, organ (prophylaxis)—
  Initial: Intravenous 3 to 5 mg (base) per kg of body weight a day prior to, during, or soon after surgery, the dosage being adjusted to maintain the homograft without causing toxicity.
  Maintenance: Intravenous, 1 to 2 mg (base) per kg of body weight a day.

**Usual pediatric dose**
See *Usual adult and adolescent dose.*

**Size(s) usually available**
U.S.—
  100 mg (base) (Rx) [*Imuran;* GENERIC].
Canada—
  100 mg (base) (Rx) [*Imuran*].

**Packaging and storage**
Store below 40 °C (104 °F), preferably between 15 and 30 °C (59 and 86 °F). Protect from light, unless otherwise specified by manufacturer.

**Preparation of dosage form**
Azathioprine Sodium for Injection USP is reconstituted for intravenous use by adding 10 mL of sterile water for injection to the vial and swirling to dissolve.
Reconstituted solutions may be further diluted for administration by intravenous infusion with 0.9% sodium chloride injection or 5% dextrose and 0.9% sodium chloride injection.

**Stability**
Reconstituted solutions of azathioprine are stable for 24 hours at room temperature. Although solutions may be stable for longer periods, because there is no preservative, use within 24 hours is recommended for reasons of sterility.

**Incompatibilities**
Mixing with alkaline solutions, especially on warming, may result in conversion to 6-mercaptopurine. Conversion to mercaptopurine also occurs in the presence of sulfhydryl compounds such as cysteine, glutathione, and hydrogen sulfide.

---
[1]Not included in Canadian product labeling.

## Selected Bibliography
Korman N. Pemphigus. J Am Acad Dermatol 1988 Jun; 18: 1219-38.
Pugh MC, Pugh CB. Current concepts in clinical therapeutics: disease-modifying drugs for rheumatoid arthritis. Clin Pharm 1987 Jun; 6: 475-91.

---
Revised: 05/06/93
Interim revision: 07/22/97

---

# AZELAIC ACID   Topical†

VA CLASSIFICATION (Primary/Secondary): DE752/DE900
Commonly used brand name(s): *Azelex.*

Note: For a listing of dosage forms and brand names by country availability, see *Dosage Forms* section(s).

---
†Not commercially available in Canada.

---

## Category
Antiacne agent (topical); hypopigmentation agent (topical).

## Indications
Note: Bracketed information in the *Indications* section refers to uses that are not included in U.S. product labeling.

**Accepted**
Acne vulgaris(treatment)—Azelaic acid is indicated in the treatment of mild to moderate acne vulgaris.
[Melasma (treatment)]—Azelaic acid has been used to treat melasma, caused by hyperfunctioning melanocytes. Azelaic acid will not similarly affect the function of normal melanocytes; thus, it will not lighten freckles.

## Pharmacology/Pharmacokinetics

**Physicochemical characteristics**
Source—Dietary component (whole grain cereals and animal products).
Molecular weight—188.22.

**Mechanism of action/Effect**
Antiacne agent—
  The mechanism of action is not fully known but it is thought that azelaic acid causes antibacterial effects by inhibiting the synthesis of cellular protein in aerobic and anaerobic microorganisms, especially *Propionibacterium acnes* and *Staphylococcus epidermidis.* Within aerobic microorganisms, azelaic acid reversibly inhibits a variety of oxidoreductive enzymes including tyrosinase, mitochondrial enzymes of the respiratory chain, thioredoxin reductase, 5-alpha-reductase, and DNA polymerases. In anaerobic microorganisms, glycolysis is disrupted.
  Also, azelaic acid improves acne vulgaris by decreasing microcomedo formation and normalizing the keratin process. Azelaic acid may be effective against both inflamed and noninflamed lesions. Specifically, azelaic acid reduces the thickness of the stratum corneum, shrinks keratohyalin granules by reducing the amount and distribution of filaggrin (a component of keratohyalin) in epidermal layers, and lowers the number of keratohyalin granules.
Hypopigmentation agent—
  Azelaic acid's antityrosinase and antimitochondrial enzymatic activities may interrupt the hyperactivity of normal melanocytes and their resulting growth in melasma, a localized macular hyperpigmentation of facial or nuchal skin. Use of azelaic acid to treat hyperpigmentation disorders due to hyperactivity of abnormal melanocytes has not been consistently successful. The hypopigmentation action of azelaic acid may result, to a lesser extent, from its ability to scavenge free radicals that can cause hyperactivity of melanocytes. Free radicals are a metabolic product of peroxidation of cell membrane lipids, produced when cells are irradiated with ultraviolet light, including sunlight. There is no depigmenting effect on normal melanocytes.

**Other actions/effects**
Azelaic acid is being studied for potential antimycotic and antiviral properties.
In time- and dose-dependent *in vitro* studies, azelaic acid has been shown to selectively penetrate rapidly growing human and murine tumor cells that are undifferentiated and possess chromosomal abnormalities while not affecting normal cells. The antiproliferative and cytotoxic effects are attributed to the antityrosinase and antimitochondrial activity of azelaic acid. Further *in vivo* studies are needed to fully characterize the clinical course of azelaic acid within these cell lines.

**Absorption**
One study found the following levels of penetration after a single application to human skin *in vitro*—
  Stratum corneum: Approximately 3 to 5%.
  Dermis and epidermis: Up to 10%.
  Plasma: Approximately 4%.

**Elimination**
Renal, mainly unchanged.

## Precautions to Consider

**Carcinogenicity**
Carcinogenic animal studies were deemed unnecessary because azelaic acid is normally found in the human diet and is not considered to be a carcinogenic substance.

## Azelaic Acid (Topical)

**Mutagenicity**
The Ames test, hypoxanthine-guanine phosphoribosyltransferase (HGPRT) test in Chinese hamster ovary cells, human lymphocyte test, and dominant lethal assay in mice suggest that azelaic acid is nonmutagenic.

**Pregnancy/Reproduction**
Fertility—Adequate and well-controlled studies have not been done in humans.
Animal studies have shown no adverse effects.
Pregnancy—Systemically absorbed azelaic acid crosses the placenta; however, little systemic absorption of topical azelaic acid occurs. Adequate and well-controlled studies have not been done; problems in humans have not been documented.
In animal studies using toxic oral doses, embryotoxic effects occurred in Segment I and II studies of rats given doses of 2500 mg per kg of body weight (mg/kg) a day; similar effects were reported for Segment II studies in rabbits given doses of 150 to 500 mg/kg a day and monkeys given doses of 500 mg/kg a day. No teratogenic effects occurred. Animal studies using topical administration have not been done.
FDA Pregnancy Category B.

**Breast-feeding**
Azelaic acid may pass into breast milk, according to *in vitro* studies; however, the amount that is absorbed systemically from topical administration is insignificant and should not affect physiologic levels of azelaic acid. Problems in humans have not been documented.

**Pediatrics**
No information is available on the relationship of age to the effects of azelaic acid in pediatric patients. Safety and efficacy have not been established.

**Geriatrics**
No information is available on the relationship of age to the effects of azelaic acid in geriatric patients.

**Medical considerations/Contraindications**
The medical considerations/contraindications included have been selected on the basis of their potential clinical significance (reasons given in parentheses where appropriate)—not necessarily inclusive (» = major clinical significance).

*Risk-benefit should be considered when the following medical problem exists:*
Hypersensitivity to azelaic acid

## Side/Adverse Effects

The following side/adverse effects have been selected on the basis of their potential clinical significance (possible signs and symptoms in parentheses where appropriate)—not necessarily inclusive:

**Those indicating need for medical attention**
Incidence rare
*Hypopigmentation* (white spots or lightening of treated areas of dark skin)—in patients with dark complexions
Note: Azelaic acid will consistently lighten hyperpigmented skin (skin that is darker than normal for a given individual) but will not typically lighten skin beyond its normal color. Rarely, patients with dark complexions may notice *hypopigmentation* of skin.

**Those indicating need for medical attention only if they continue or are bothersome**
Incidence more frequent
*Desquamation* (peeling of skin); *dryness of skin; erythema* (redness of skin); *inflammatory reaction, mild* (burning, stinging, or tingling of skin, mild)—1 to 5% with continued use; *pruritus, mild* (itching of skin)—1 to 5% with continued use
Note: Mild burning, stinging, or tingling of skin and pruritus may occur at the start of each treatment and may last 5 to 20 minutes, especially if skin is inflamed or broken, but lessens with continued use. Dosage may be reduced until skin irritation lessens.

## Patient Consultation

As an aid to patient consultation, refer to *Advice for the Patient, Azelaic Acid (Topical)*.
In providing consultation, consider emphasizing the following selected information (» = major clinical significance):

**Before using this medication**
» Conditions affecting use, especially:
Hypersensitivity to azelaic acid

**Proper use of this medication**
Applying a small amount of medication as a thin film to clean, dry skin; gently and thoroughly rubbing into the affected area
Washing hands well after applying
» Not applying to mucous membranes and, if accidental contact occurs, washing affected area well with water immediately
» Compliance with full course of treatment
» Proper dosing
Missed dose: Applying as soon as possible; not applying if almost time for next dose; not doubling doses
» Proper storage

**Precautions while using this medication**
Contacting health care professional if acne worsens or does not improve in the first 4 weeks or if medication causes too much redness, dryness, or peeling of skin
May take longer than 4 weeks before full improvement is noticed
Other topical medications may be used but recommend applying them at different times during the day
Conservative use of water-base cosmetics is permissible with use of azelaic acid

## General Dosing Information

Some skin irritation may be expected with first use of topical azelaic acid; however, if skin irritation persists, dosage may be reduced to one time a day until irritation lessens. If skin irritation continues, azelaic acid treatment should be discontinued.

Patient should apply azelaic acid as a thin film to clean dry skin and rub into skin thoroughly. Improvement of acne or hyperpigmentation condition may take 4 weeks or longer.

**Safety considerations for handling this medication**
Wash hands thoroughly after handling topical azelaic acid.
Keep topical azelaic acid away from mouth, eyes, and other mucous membranes. If accidental contact occurs, large amounts of water should be used to wash affected area. If the eyes are involved and eye irritation persists after a thorough washing, contact a physician.

## Topical Dosage Form

Note: Bracketed uses in the *Dosage Forms* section refer to categories of use and/or indications that are not included in U.S. product labeling.

### AZELAIC ACID CREAM

**Usual adult and adolescent dose**
Antiacne agent or
[Hypopigmentation agent]—
Topical, to the affected area, two times a day (morning and evening).
Note: Initially, application once a day for a few days has been used for some patients sensitive to azelaic acid.

**Usual pediatric dose**
Safety and efficacy have not been established.

**Strength(s) usually available**
U.S.—
20% (Rx) [*Azelex*].
Canada—
Not commercially available.

**Packaging and storage**
Store below 40 °C (104 °F), preferably between 15 and 30 °C (59 and 86 °F), unless otherwise specified by manufacturer. Protect from freezing.

**Auxiliary labeling**
• External use only.

**Note**
Dermatologic use only; not for ophthalmic use.

## Selected Bibliography

Breathnach AS. Pharmacological properties of azelaic acid. Clin Drug Invest 1995; 10(Suppl 2): 27-33.

Developed: 06/27/96

# AZELASTINE Nasal—INTRODUCTORY VERSION†

VA CLASSIFICATION (Primary): NT400
Commonly used brand name(s): *Astelin*.
Note: For a listing of dosage forms and brand names by country availability, see *Dosage Forms* section(s).

†Not commercially available in Canada.

## Category
Antihistaminic ($H_1$-receptor), nasal.

## Indications
**Accepted**
Rhinitis, seasonal allergic (treatment)—Azelastine is indicated for symptomatic treatment of seasonal allergic rhinitis, including rhinorrhea, sneezing, and nasal pruritus, in adults and children 12 years of age and older.

## Pharmacology/Pharmacokinetics
**Physicochemical characteristics**
Chemical group—Phthalazinone derivative.
Molecular weight—418.37.
pH—Saturated solution: 5 to 5.4.
Commercial product: $6.8 \pm 0.3$.
Solubility—Sparingly soluble in water, methanol, and propylene glycol and slightly soluble in ethanol, octanol, and glycerine.

**Mechanism of action/Effect**
Azelastine acts by competing with histamine for $H_1$-receptor sites on effector cells.

**Absorption**
Systemic bioavailability is approximately 40% after nasal administration.

**Distribution**
$Vol_D$—14.5 liters per kg of body weight.

**Protein binding**
Azelastine—High (88%).
Desmethylazelastine—Very high (97%).

**Biotransformation**
Hepatic, by oxidation via the cytochrome P450 enzyme system. The exact cytochrome P450 isoenzyme involved has not been determined, but a nonspecific P450 inhibitor (cimetidine) was found to raise mean concentrations of azelastine significantly; no pharmacokinetic interaction could be demonstrated with a known CYP3A4 inhibitor (erythromycin).
The major metabolite, desmethylazelastine, also has $H_1$-receptor antagonist activity. Desmethylazelastine is undetectable in plasma following single intranasal doses of azelastine but concentrations range from 20 to 50% of azelastine concentrations at the steady-state.

**Half-life**
Elimination—
Azelastine (after intravenous or oral administration)—22 hours.
Desmethylazelastine (after oral administration of azelastine)—54 hours.
Note: According to limited data, the metabolite profile is similar for oral and intranasal administration of azelastine.

**Onset of action**
In dose-ranging trials, nasal azelastine was found to produce a statistically significant decrease in allergic symptoms within 3 hours after the initial dose.

**Time to peak concentration**
Plasma—2 to 3 hours.

**Peak plasma concentration**
Oral administration of azelastine produces linear responses in the maximum plasma concentration ($C_{max}$) and area under the plasma concentration–time curve (AUC). However, administration of intranasal doses of more than 2 sprays per nostril for 29 days has been found to produce greater than proportional increases in the $C_{max}$ and AUC.
In oral, single-dose studies, renal insufficiency (creatinine clearance less than 50 mL per minute) resulted in a 70 to 75% increase in the $C_{max}$ and AUC compared with those in normal subjects, although the time to peak plasma concentration was unchanged.

**Duration of action**
12 hours.

**Elimination**
Fecal—75% (less than 10% unchanged) after oral administration.

## Precautions to Consider
**Carcinogenicity**
Studies in rats and mice given oral doses of up to 30 and 25 mg per kg of body weight (mg/kg) per day, respectively (240 and 100 times the maximum recommended human daily intranasal dose on a mg per square meter of body surface area [mg/m$^2$] basis, respectively), found no evidence of carcinogenicity.

**Mutagenicity**
No evidence of mutagenicity caused by azelastine was found in the Ames test, DNA repair test, mouse lymphoma forward mutation assay, mouse micronucleus test, or chromosomal aberration test in rat bone marrow.

**Pregnancy/Reproduction**
Fertility—Studies in rats given oral doses of azelastine of up to 30 mg/kg per day (240 times the maximum recommended human daily intranasal dose on a mg/m$^2$ basis) found no effects on male or female fertility. However, at doses of 68.6 mg/kg per day (550 times the maximum recommended human daily intranasal dose on a mg/m$^2$ basis), duration of estrous cycles was prolonged and copulatory activity and the number of pregnancies were decreased. The numbers of corpora lutea and implantations were decreased, but the implantation ratio was not affected.
Pregnancy—Adequate and well-controlled studies in humans have not been done.
Studies in mice given an oral dose of 68.6 mg/kg per day (280 times the maximum recommended human daily intranasal dose on a mg/m$^2$ basis) found azelastine to be embryotoxic, fetotoxic, and teratogenic (external and skeletal abnormalities). Studies in rats given an oral dose of 30 mg/kg per day (240 times the maximum recommended human daily intranasal dose on a mg/m$^2$ basis) found delayed ossification (undeveloped metacarpus) and an increased incidence of 14th rib. At 68.6 mg/kg per day (550 times the maximum recommended human daily intranasal dose on a mg/m$^2$ basis), azelastine caused abortion and fetotoxic effects in rats.
It is recommended that risk-benefit be considered before using azelastine during pregnancy.
FDA Pregnancy Category C.

**Breast-feeding**
It is not known whether azelastine is distributed into breast milk.

**Pediatrics**
Safety and efficacy of azelastine in children up to 12 years of age have not been established.

**Geriatrics**
Although studies on the relationship of age to the effects of azelastine have not been performed in the geriatric population, placebo-controlled clinical trials included a small number of patients over 60 years of age, and adverse effects in this group were similar to those in younger individuals.

**Drug interactions and/or related problems**
The following drug interactions and/or related problems have been selected on the basis of their potential clinical significance (possible mechanism in parentheses where appropriate)—not necessarily inclusive (» = major clinical significance):

Note: Combinations containing any of the following medications, depending on the amount present, may also interact with this medication.

» Alcohol or
» CNS depression–producing medications, other (see *Appendix II*)
  (concurrent use may potentiate the CNS depressant effects of either these medications or azelastine)

» Cimetidine
  (concurrent use with azelastine results in significantly increased plasma concentrations of azelastine, as a result of inhibition of cytochrome P450 by cimetidine)

Ketoconazole
  (interferes with measurement of plasma azelastine concentrations)

**Laboratory value alterations**
The following have been selected on the basis of their potential clinical significance (possible effect in parentheses where appropriate)—not necessarily inclusive (» = major clinical significance):

Alanine aminotransferase (ALT [SGPT])
  (serum values may rarely be increased)

### Medical considerations/Contraindications

The medical considerations/contraindications included have been selected on the basis of their potential clinical significance (reasons given in parentheses where appropriate)—not necessarily inclusive (» = major clinical significance).

*Risk-benefit should be considered when the following medical problems exist:*

Renal function impairment
   (plasma concentrations may be increased)
Sensitivity to azelastine

## Side/Adverse Effects

Note: No significant effect on QT interval has been found in studies of orally or nasally administered azelastine at therapeutic doses.

The following side/adverse effects have been selected on the basis of their potential clinical significance (possible signs and symptoms in parentheses where appropriate)—not necessarily inclusive:

**Those indicating need for medical attention**
Incidence rare
   *Allergic reaction* (skin rash, hives, or itching); *bronchospasm* (shortness of breath, tightness in chest, troubled breathing, or wheezing); *cough; eye problems or pain* (eye pain or redness or blurred vision or other change in vision); *hematuria* (blood in urine); *stomatitis* (sores in mouth or on lips); *tachycardia* (rapid heartbeat)

**Those indicating need for medical attention only if they continue or are bothersome**
Incidence more frequent
   *Bitter taste*—incidence 19.7%; *somnolence* (drowsiness or sleepiness)
Incidence less frequent
   *Burning inside the nose; dizziness; dryness of mouth; epistaxis* (bloody mucus or unexplained nosebleeds); *fatigue* (unusual tiredness or weakness); *headache; myalgia* (muscle aches or pain); *nausea; pharyngitis* (sore throat); *sneezing, paroxysmal* (sudden outbursts of sneezing); *weight gain*

## Overdose

For more information on the management of overdose or unintentional ingestion, **contact a Poison Control Center** (see *Poison Control Center Listing*).

**Clinical effects of overdose**
There have been no reported incidents of azelastine overdose in humans; however, acute overdose would not be expected to result in clinically significant adverse effects other than increased somnolence, since one bottle contains 17 mg of azelastine hydrochloride and single oral doses of up to 16 mg have not produced serious adverse effects.
In mice, oral doses of greater than 120 mg per kg of body weight (mg/kg) (480 times the maximum recommended human daily intranasal dose on a mg per square meter of body surface area [mg/m$^2$] basis) produced significant mortality, preceded by tremor, convulsions, decreased muscle tone, and salivation. In dogs, single doses as high as 10 mg/kg (270 times the maximum recommended human daily intranasal dose on a mg/m$^2$ basis) were well tolerated, but single doses of 20 mg/kg were lethal.

**Treatment of overdose**
General supportive measures.

## Patient Consultation

As an aid to patient consultation, refer to *Advice for the Patient, Azelastine (Nasal)—Introductory Version*.
In providing consultation, consider emphasizing the following selected information (» = major clinical significance):

**Before using this medication**
» Conditions affecting use, especially:
   Sensitivity to azelastine
   Pregnancy—Risk-benefit should be considered; teratogenic in animals
   Use in children—Safety and efficacy not established in children up to 12 years of age
   Other medications, especially alcohol or other CNS depressants or cimetidine

**Proper use of this medication**
   Reading patient instructions carefully before using
   Clearing nasal passages by blowing nose before use
   Proper administration technique; reading patient directions carefully before use; before initial use, priming the pump with four sprays or until a fine mist appears; if not used for 3 or more days, priming the pump with two sprays or until a fine mist appears
   Preventing contamination: Wiping tip of applicator with clean, damp tissue; replacing cap right after use
» Importance of not using more medication than the amount prescribed
» Proper dosing
   Missed dose: Using as soon as possible; if almost time for next dose, skipping missed dose and going back to regular dosing schedule; not doubling doses
» Proper storage; storing upright at room temperature with pump tightly closed

**Precautions while using this medication**
» Avoiding use of alcohol or other CNS depressants
» Caution if dizziness or drowsiness occurs
» Avoiding spraying in the eyes

**Side/adverse effects**
   Signs of potential side effects, especially allergic reaction, bronchospasm, cough, eye problems or pain, hematuria, stomatitis, or tachycardia

## General Dosing Information

Before initial use, the pump should be primed with four sprays or until a fine mist appears. If not used for 3 or more days, the pump should be primed with two sprays or until a fine mist appears.
Prior to administration of azelastine, the nasal passages should be cleared.
Azelastine is dispensed in a package consisting of two bottles of medication (for a total of 200 metered sprays) and one pump assembly.

## Nasal Dosage Forms

### AZELASTINE HYDROCHLORIDE NASAL SOLUTION

**Usual adult and adolescent dose**
Rhinitis, seasonal allergic—
   Intranasal, 2 sprays in each nostril two times a day.

**Usual pediatric dose**
Rhinitis, seasonal allergic—
   Children 12 years of age and older: See *Usual adult and adolescent dose*.
   Children up to 12 years of age: Safety and efficacy have not been established.

**Strength(s) usually available**
U.S.—
   137 mcg per metered spray (1 mg per mL; 100 metered sprays per bottle) (Rx) [*Astelin* (benzalkonium chloride 125 mcg per mL; edetate disodium; hydroxypropyl methylcellulose; citric acid; dibasic sodium phosphate; sodium chloride; purified water)].

Note: Azelastine is dispensed in a package consisting of two bottles of medication (for a total of 200 metered sprays) and one pump assembly.

**Packaging and storage**
Store between 20 and 25 °C (68 and 77 °F). Protect from freezing.

**Stability**
The expiration date on the bottles applies to the unopened bottles.
Once the pump assembly has been inserted into the first bottle of the dispensing package, the pump assembly (and any unused portion of either bottle) should be discarded after 3 months, but not to exceed the original expiration date.

**Auxiliary labeling**
• Avoid spraying in eyes.
• For the nose.

---

Developed: 11/11/97
Interim revision: 07/15/98

# AZITHROMYCIN Systemic

VA CLASSIFICATION (Primary): AM200

Commonly used brand name(s): *Zithromax*.

Note: For a listing of dosage forms and brand names by country availability, see *Dosage Forms* section(s).

## Category
Antibacterial (systemic).

## Indications
Note: Bracketed information in the *Indications* section refers to uses that are not included in U.S. product labeling.

**General considerations**

Azithromycin is an azalide antibiotic, part of the macrolide family of antibacterials. It has *in vitro* activity against many gram-positive and gram-negative aerobic and anaerobic bacteria. It also has greater stability than erythromycin in the presence of acid.

Azithromycin is active against staphylococci, including *Staphylococcus aureus* and *Staphylococcus epidermidis*, as well as streptococci, such as *Streptococcus pyogenes* and *Streptococcus pneumoniae*. The minimum inhibitory concentration (MIC) of azithromycin is two to four times greater than that of erythromycin against staphylococcus and streptococcus. Most erythromycin-resistant strains of staphylococcus, enterococcus, and streptococcus, including methicillin-resistant *S. aureus*, are also resistant to azithromycin. Also, azithromycin is less potent than erythromycin and clarithromycin against erythromycin-sensitive enterococci.

Azithromycin has excellent activity against *Haemophilus influenzae*, being two to eight times more active than erythromycin and four to eight times more active than clarithromycin *in vitro*. MICs of 4 to 16 mcg per mL inhibit most *Escherichia coli*, *Salmonella*, *Shigella*, and *Aeromonas* species. *Pseudomonas aeruginosa*, *Klebsiella*, *Enterobacter*, *Citrobacter*, *Proteus*, *Providencia*, *Morganella*, and *Serratia* species are resistant to azithromycin.

Azithromycin is two- to fourfold more active than erythromycin against *Moraxella (Branhamella) catarrhalis*. Inhibition of anaerobes, such as *Clostridium perfringens*, is slightly better with azithromycin than with erythromycin, and azithromycin's inhibition of *Bacteroides fragilis* and other *Bacteroides* species is comparable to that of erythromycin. Azithromycin also has good *in vitro* activity against *Chlamydia trachomatis*, *Chlamydia pneumoniae*, *Mycoplasma pneumoniae*, *Legionella* species, *Borrelia burgdorferi*, *Ureaplasma urealyticum*, and *Gardnerella vaginalis*. Azithromycin has eightfold more activity than erythromycin against *Neisseria gonorrhoeae* and tenfold more activity against *Haemophilus ducreyi*. It has also been shown to inhibit *Toxoplasma gondii* *in vitro* and in animal models. However, no potentiation against *T. gondii* could be demonstrated when azithromycin was combined with pyrimethamine. Also, when azithromycin was administered as a single agent in the treatment of cerebral toxoplasmosis in two patients, it failed, although the patients responded to conventional treatment.

**Accepted**

Bronchitis, bacterial exacerbations (treatment) or

Otitis media, acute (treatment)—Azithromycin is indicated in the treatment of bacterial exacerbations of chronic bronchitis or acute otitis media due to *Haemophilus influenzae*, *Moraxella catarrhalis*, or *Streptococcus pneumoniae*. However, azithromycin is not recommended as the first line of therapy for otitis media.

Cervicitis, gonococcal (treatment) or

Cervicitis, nongonococcal (treatment) or

Urethritis, gonococcal (treatment) or

Urethritis, nongonococcal (treatment)—Azithromycin is indicated in the treatment of cervicitis or urethritis due to *Chlamydia trachomatis* or *Neisseria gonorrhoeae*.

Chancroid (treatment)—Azithromycin is indicated in the treatment of genital ulcer disease in men due to *Haemophilus ducreyi*.

*Mycobacterium avium* complex (MAC) disease, disseminated (prophylaxis)[1]—Azithromycin is indicated in the prevention of disseminated MAC disease in patients with advanced human immunodeficiency virus (HIV) infection.

Pelvic inflammatory disease (treatment)[1]—Azithromycin is indicated in the treatment of pelvic inflammatory disease due to *Chlamydia trachomatis*, *Mycoplasma hominis*, or *Neisseria gonorrhoeae*.

Pharyngitis (treatment) or

Tonsillitis (treatment)—Azithromycin is indicated in the treatment of pharyngitis or tonsillitis due to *Streptococcus pyogenes*.

Pneumonia, community-acquired (treatment)—Azithromycin is indicated in the treatment of community-acquired pneumonia due to *Chlamydia pneumoniae*[1], *Haemophilus influenzae*, *Legionella pneumophila*[1], *Moraxella catarrhalis*[1], *Mycoplasma pneumoniae*[1], *Staphylococcus aureus*[1], or *Streptococcus pneumoniae*.

Skin and soft tissue infections (treatment)—Azithromycin is indicated in the treatment of uncomplicated skin and soft tissue infections due to *Staphylococcus aureus*, *Streptococcus agalactiae*, or *Streptococcus pyogenes*.

[1]Not included in Canadian product labeling.

## Pharmacology/Pharmacokinetics

**Physicochemical characteristics**

Molecular weight—Azithromycin: 785.03.

**Mechanism of action/Effect**

Azithromycin binds to the 50S ribosomal subunit of the 70S ribosome of susceptible organisms, thereby inhibiting RNA-dependent protein synthesis.

Azithromycin is bactericidal for *Streptococcus pyogenes*, *Streptococcus pneumoniae*, and *Haemophilus influenzae*; it is bacteriostatic for staphylococci and most aerobic gram-negative species.

**Absorption**

For oral dosage forms—

Rapidly absorbed; bioavailability is approximately 37%.

Capsule form: Food decreases peak serum concentration ($C_{max}$) values by approximately 52% and area under the plasma concentration–time curve (AUC) values by approximately 43%.

Tablet form: Food increases $C_{max}$ values by approximately 23% and 34% for the 250- and 600-mg tablets, respectively, and has no effect on AUC values.

Oral suspension form (for adults): Food increases $C_{max}$ values by approximately 56% and has no effect on AUC values.

**Distribution**

Rapidly and widely distributed throughout the body. Concentrates intracellularly, resulting in tissue concentrations 10 to 100 times higher than those found in plasma or serum. Azithromycin is highly concentrated in phagocytes and fibroblasts. Phagocytes transport the drug to the site of infection and inflammation. Release of azithromycin from phagocytes is gradual, but it is enhanced by exposure to the cell membrane of bacteria. Release of azithromycin from fibroblasts is not enhanced by bacteria, but fibroblasts may act as reservoirs of the antibiotic, releasing azithromycin to phagocytes. Very low concentrations (< 0.01 mcg per mL [mcg/mL]) have been detected in the cerebrospinal fluid of human subjects with noninflamed meninges; however, higher concentrations were found in brain tissue in animal studies.

$Vol_D$—For oral dosage forms, approximately 31 L per kg (steady-state). For parenteral dosage forms, approximately 33 L per kg (following 1000- to 4000-mg doses at a concentration of 1 mg/mL infused over a 2-hour period).

**Protein binding**

Varies with concentration—Very low to moderate; approximately 7% at 1 mcg/mL, to 50% at 0.02 to 0.05 mcg/mL.

**Biotransformation**

Hepatic; approximately 35% metabolized by demethylation. Up to 10 metabolites, which are thought to have no significant antimicrobial activity, may be found in the bile.

**Half-life**

Peripheral leukocytes—34 to 57 hours (mean) after a single dose of 1200 mg (two 600-mg tablets).

Serum—11 to 14 hours when measured between 8 and 24 hours after a single, oral dose of 500 mg; however, after several doses, the half-life is approximately the same as the half-life in tissues.

Tissue—2 to 4 days.

**Time to peak concentration**

Adult subjects—For oral dosage forms: 2.1 to 3.2 hours.

For parenteral dosage forms: 1 to 2 hours.

Elderly subjects—3.8 to 4.4 hours.

**Peak plasma concentration**
For oral dosage forms, after a 500-mg loading dose on day 1, then 250 mg once a day on days 2 through 5—
  Day 1: Approximately 0.41 and 0.38 mcg/mL for healthy young and elderly adults, respectively.
  Day 5: Approximately 0.24 and 0.26 mcg/mL for healthy young and elderly adults, respectively.
For parenteral dosage forms—
  Approximately 1.1 mcg/mL after a 3-hour intravenous infusion of 500 mg at a concentration of 1 mg/mL.
  Approximately 3.6 mcg/mL after a 1-hour intravenous infusion of 500 mg at a concentration of 2 mg/mL.

**Elimination**
Over 50% of the dose is eliminated through biliary excretion as unchanged drug.
For oral dosage forms, approximately 4.5% of the dose is eliminated in the urine as unchanged drug within 72 hours.
For parenteral dosage forms, approximately 11 to 14% of the dose is eliminated in the urine as unchanged drug within 24 hours.

## Precautions to Consider

**Cross-sensitivity and/or related problems**
Patients who are hypersensitive to erythromycin or other macrolides may also be hypersensitive to azithromycin.

**Carcinogenicity**
Long-term studies have not been done in animals to evaluate the carcinogenic potential of azithromycin.

**Mutagenicity**
Azithromycin was not found to be mutagenic in the mouse lymphoma assay, the human lymphoctye clastogenic assay, or the mouse bone marrow clastogenic assay.

**Pregnancy/Reproduction**
Fertility—Adequate and well-controlled studies in humans have not been done.
Reproduction studies done in rats and mice given azithromycin at doses of up to moderately maternally toxic levels (i.e., 200 mg per kg of body weight [mg/kg] per day) have found no evidence of impaired fertility. On a mg per square meter of body surface area ($mg/m^2$) basis, these doses are estimated to be four and two times the human daily dose of 500 mg in rats and mice, respectively.
Pregnancy—Adequate and well-controlled studies in humans have not been done.
Reproduction studies done in rats and mice given azithromycin at doses of up to moderately maternally toxic levels (i.e., 200 mg/kg per day) have found no evidence of harm to the fetus. On a $mg/m^2$ basis, these doses are estimated to be four and two times the human daily dose of 500 mg in rats and mice, respectively.
FDA Pregnancy Category B.

**Breast-feeding**
It is not known if azithromycin is distributed into breast milk.

**Pediatrics**
Appropriate studies on the relationship of age to the effects of parenteral azithromycin or of the capsule or tablet dosage form of oral azithromycin have not been performed in children up to 16 years of age. Safety and efficacy have not been established. However, the oral suspension dosage form of azithromycin is approved for use in infants and children 6 months of age and older.

**Geriatrics**
Pharmacokinetic data in healthy elderly subjects (65 to 85 years old) were similar to those for younger volunteers (18 to 40 years old). A higher peak concentration (by 30 to 50%) was found in elderly women; however, no significant accumulation occurred. Dosage adjustment does not appear to be necessary in older patients with normal renal and hepatic function.

**Drug interactions and/or related problems**
The following drug interactions and/or related problems have been selected on the basis of their potential clinical significance (possible mechanism in parentheses where appropriate)—not necessarily inclusive (» = major clinical significance):
Note: Combinations containing any of the following medications, depending on the amount present, may also interact with this medication.

» Antacids, aluminum- and magnesium-containing
  (concurrent use with antacids decreases the peak serum concentration [$C_{max}$] of azithromycin by approximately 24%, but has no effect on the area under the plasma concentration–time curve [AUC]; oral azithromycin should be administered at least 1 hour before or 2 hours after aluminum- and magnesium-containing antacids)

Carbamazepine or
Cyclosporine or
Digoxin or
Hexobarbital or
Phenytoin or
Terfenadine
  (concurrent use with macrolide antibiotics has been associated with increased serum concentrations of carbamazepine, cyclosporine, digoxin, hexobarbital, phenytoin, and terfenadine; patients concurrently receiving azithromycin and any of these medications should be monitored carefully)

Dihydroergotamine or
Ergotamine
  (concurrent use with macrolide antibiotics has been associated with acute ergot toxicity characterized by severe peripheral vasospasm and dysesthesia; patients concurrently receiving azithromycin and either of these medications should be monitored carefully)

Theophylline
  (concurrent use with macrolide antibiotics has been associated with increased serum concentrations of theophylline; pending further investigation, plasma concentrations of theophylline should be monitored in patients concurrently receiving azithromycin and theophylline)

Triazolam
  (concurrent use with macrolide antibiotics has been associated with a decrease in the clearance of triazolam, which may increase its effects; patients concurrently receiving azithromycin and triazolam should be monitored carefully)

Warfarin
  (concurrent use with macrolide antibiotics has been associated with increased anticoagulant effects; prothrombin time should be monitored carefully in patients concurrently receiving azithromycin and warfarin)

**Laboratory value alterations**
The following have been selected on the basis of their potential clinical significance (possible effect in parentheses where appropriate)—not necessarily inclusive (» = major clinical significance):

With physiology/laboratory test values
  Alanine aminotransferase (ALT [SGPT]) and
  Aspartate aminotransferase (AST [SGOT]) and
  Creatine kinase and
  Gamma-glutamyltransferase and
  Lactate dehydrogenase
    (serum values may be increased)
  Bilirubin and
  Potassium, serum
    (concentrations may be increased)

**Medical considerations/Contraindications**
The medical considerations/contraindications included have been selected on the basis of their potential clinical significance (reasons given in parentheses where appropriate)—not necessarily inclusive (» = major clinical significance).

*Except under special circumstances, this medication should not be used when the following medical problem exists:*
» Hypersensitivity to azithromycin, erythromycins, or other macrolides

*Risk-benefit should be considered when the following medical problem exists:*
» Hepatic function impairment
  (because biliary excretion is the major route of elimination, caution should be used in patients with hepatic function impairment)

## Side/Adverse Effects

Note: Rarely, serious allergic reactions, such as anaphylaxis and angioedema, have been reported in patients taking azithromycin. Despite discontinuation of azithromycin and successful symptomatic treatment of the allergic reactions, allergic symptoms soon recurred in some patients when the symptomatic therapy was discontinued. These patients require prolonged periods of observation and symptomatic treatment.

The following side/adverse effects have been selected on the basis of their potential clinical significance (possible signs and symptoms in parentheses where appropriate)—not necessarily inclusive:

**Those indicating need for medical attention**
Incidence more frequent—for injection form only
   *Thrombophlebitis* (pain, redness, and swelling at site of injection)
Incidence rare
   *Acute interstitial nephritis* (fever; joint pain; skin rash); *allergic reactions* (difficulty in breathing; swelling of face, mouth, neck, hands, and feet; skin rash); *pseudomembranous colitis* (abdominal or stomach cramps or pain, severe; abdominal tenderness; diarrhea, watery and severe, which may also be bloody; fever)

**Those indicating need for medical attention only if they continue or are bothersome**
Incidence less frequent
   *Gastrointestinal disturbances* (abdominal pain; diarrhea, mild; nausea; vomiting)
Incidence rare
   *Dizziness; headache*

## Patient Consultation

As an aid to patient consultation, refer to *Advice for the Patient, Azithromycin (Systemic)*.
In providing consultation, consider emphasizing the following selected information (» = major clinical significance):

**Before using this medication**
» Conditions affecting use, especially:
   Hypersensitivity to azithromycin, erythromycins, or other macrolides
   Other medications, especially aluminum- and magnesium-containing antacids
   Other medical problems, especially hepatic function impairment

**Proper use of this medication**
   Azithromycin capsules and pediatric oral suspension should be given at least 1 hour before or 2 hours after meals
   Azithromycin tablets and adult single dose oral suspension may be taken with or without food
   Compliance with full course of therapy
» Importance of not taking more medication than prescribed; importance of not discontinuing medication without checking with physician
» Proper dosing
   Missed dose: Taking as soon as possible; not taking if almost time for next dose; not doubling doses
» Proper storage

**Precautions while using this medication**
   Checking with physician if no improvement within a few days or if condition becomes worse

**Side/adverse effects**
   Signs of potential side effects, especially thrombophlebitis, acute interstitial nephritis, allergic reactions, and pseudomembranous colitis

## General Dosing Information

No adjustment in dose is required in patients with mild renal function impairment (creatinine clearance ≥ 40 mL per minute [0.67 mL per second]). No data are available on the use of azithromycin in patients with more severe renal function impairment.

**Diet/Nutrition**
Azithromycin capsules and oral suspension in dropper bottles (for children) should be given at least 1 hour before or 2 hours after meals.
Azithromycin tablets and oral suspension in 1-gram packets (for adults) may be taken with or without food.

## Oral Dosage Forms

### AZITHROMYCIN CAPSULES USP

**Usual adult and adolescent dose**
Bronchitis, bacterial exacerbations or
Pharyngitis, streptococcal or
Pneumonia, due to *Streptococcus pneumoniae* or *Haemophilus influenzae*, or
Skin and soft tissue infections, uncomplicated, due to *Staphylococcus aureus*, *Streptococcus agalactiae*, or *Streptococcus pyogenes* or
Tonsillitis, streptococcal—
   Adults and adolescents 16 years of age and older: Oral, 500 mg as a single dose on the first day, then 250 mg once a day on days two through five.
   Adolescents up to 16 years of age: Safety and efficacy have not been established.

Cervicitis, nongonococcal or
Urethritis, nongonococcal—
   Adults and adolescents 16 years of age and older: Oral, 1000 mg as a single dose.
   Adolescents up to 16 years of age: Safety and efficacy have not been established.

**Usual pediatric dose**
Children up to 16 years of age—Safety and efficacy have not been established.

**Strength(s) usually available**
U.S.—
   250 mg (Rx) [*Zithromax* (lactose)].
Canada—
   250 mg (Rx) [*Zithromax* (lactose)].

**Packaging and storage**
Store below 40 °C (104 °F), preferably between 15 and 30 °C (59 and 86 °F) in a well-closed container.

**Auxiliary labeling**
• Do not take with food.
• Continue medicine for full time of treatment.

### AZITHROMYCIN FOR ORAL SUSPENSION USP

**Usual adult and adolescent dose**
Cervicitis, nongonococcal or
Chancroid, in men or
Urethritis, nongonococcal—
   Oral, 1 gram as a single dose.
Cervicitis, gonococcal or
Urethritis, gonococcal—
   Oral, 2 grams as a single dose.

**Usual pediatric dose**
Otitis media, acute or
Pneumonia, due to *Chlamydia pneumoniae*[1], *Haemophilus influenzae*, *Mycoplasma pneumoniae*[1], or *Streptococcus pneumoniae*—
   Infants and children 6 months to 12 years of age: Oral, 10 mg per kg of body weight, up to 500 mg, on the first day, then 5 mg per kg of body weight, up to 250 mg, on days two through five.
   Infants up to 6 months of age: Safety and efficacy have not been established.
Pharyngitis, streptococcal or
Tonsillitis, streptococcal—
   Children 2 to 12 years of age: Oral, 12 mg per kg of body weight, up to 500 mg, once a day for five days.
   Infants and children up to 2 years of age: Safety and efficacy have not been established.

**Usual pediatric prescribing limits**
500 mg per day for pharyngitis, tonsillitis, and the first day of dosing for otitis media and pneumonia.
250 mg per day for days two through five for otitis media and pneumonia.
U.S.—
   100 mg per 5 mL (when reconstituted according to manufacturer's instructions) (available in 300-mg bottles) (Rx) [*Zithromax* (sucrose)].
   200 mg per 5 mL (when reconstituted according to manufacturer's instructions) (available in 600-, 900-, and 1200-mg bottles) (Rx) [*Zithromax* (sucrose)].
   1 gram (single dose packet) (Rx) [*Zithromax* (sucrose)].
Canada—
   100 mg per 5 mL (when reconstituted according to manufacturer's instructions) (available in 300-mg bottles) (Rx) [*Zithromax* (sucrose)].
   200 mg per 5 mL (when reconstituted according to manufacturer's instructions) (available in 600- and 900-mg bottles) (Rx) [*Zithromax* (sucrose)].
   1 gram (single dose packet) (Rx) [*Zithromax* (sucrose)].

**Packaging and storage**
Prior to reconstitution, store between 5 and 30 °C (41 and 86 °F) in a tight container.
After reconstitution, the pediatric oral suspension should be stored between 5 and 30 °C (41 and 86 °F).

**Preparation of dosage form**
For the pediatric suspension—Add the indicated volume of water to the bottle and shake well.

| Azithromycin content | Final concentration | Total volume of water to be added |
|---|---|---|
| 300 mg | 100 mg/5 mL | 9 mL |
| 600 mg | 200 mg/5 mL | 9 mL |
| 900 mg | 200 mg/5 mL | 12 mL |
| 1200 mg | 200 mg/5 mL | 15 mL |

**502  Azithromycin (Systemic)**

For the adult single dose packets—Empty the entire contents of the packet into a glass containing 2 ounces (approximately 60 mL) of water and mix thoroughly. The suspension should be consumed immediately. Add an additional 2 ounces of water to the glass, mix, and drink to assure complete consumption of the dose. This packet should not be used to administer doses other than 1000 mg of azithromycin.

**Auxiliary labeling**
For the pediatric suspension—
- Refrigerate.
- Shake well.
- Do not take with food.
- Continue medicine for full time of treatment.

For the adult single dose packets—
- Reconstitute before taking.

## AZITHROMYCIN TABLETS

**Usual adult and adolescent dose**
Bronchitis, bacterial exacerbations or
Pharyngitis, streptococcal or
Pneumonia, due to *Chlamydia pneumoniae*[1], *Haemophilus influenzae*, *Mycoplasma pneumoniae*[1], or *Streptococcus pneumoniae* or
Skin and soft tissue infections or
Tonsillitis, streptococcal—
 Adults and adolescents 16 years of age and older: Oral, 500 mg as a single dose on the first day, then 250 mg once a day on days two through five.
 Adolescents up to 16 years of age: Safety and efficacy have not been established.
Cervicitis, nongonococcal or
Urethritis, nongonococcal—
 Adults and adolescents 16 years of age and older: Oral, 1000 mg as a single dose.
 Adolescents up to 16 years of age: Safety and efficacy have not been established.
*Mycobacterium avium* complex (MAC) disease, disseminated, prophylaxis[1]—
 Adults and adolescents 16 years of age and older: Oral, 1200 mg once a week, alone or in combination with an approved dosing regimen of rifabutin.
 Adolescents up to 16 years of age: Safety and efficacy have not been established.

**Usual pediatric dose**
Children up to 16 years of age—Safety and efficacy have not been established.

**Strength(s) usually available**
U.S.—
 250 mg (Rx) [*Zithromax* (scored; lactose)].
 600 mg (Rx) [*Zithromax* (lactose)].
Canada—
 250 mg (Rx) [*Zithromax* (scored; lactose)].

**Packaging and storage**
Store between 5 and 30 °C (41 and 86 °F).

**Auxiliary labeling**
- Continue medicine for full time of treatment.

## Parenteral Dosage Form
### AZITHROMYCIN FOR INJECTION

Note: Azithromycin for injection should be infused at a concentration of 1 mg per mL over a 3-hour period, or 2 mg per mL over a 1-hour period. Azithromycin should not be administered by bolus or intramuscular injection.

**Usual adult and adolescent dose**
Pelvic inflammatory disease[1]—
 Adults and adolescents 16 years of age and older: Intravenous infusion, 500 mg as a single dose once a day for the first one or two days of a seven-day course of therapy.
 Adolescents up to 16 years of age: Safety and efficacy have not been established.
Note: After the one- or two-day infusion therapy is complete, an oral dose of 250 mg should be administered once a day to complete the seven-day course of therapy.
Pneumonia[1], due to *Chlamydia pneumoniae*, *Haemophilus influenzae*, *Legionella pneumophila*, *Moraxella catarrhalis*, *Mycoplasma pneumoniae*, *Staphylococcus aureus*, or *Streptococcus pneumoniae*—
 Adults and adolescents 16 years of age and older: Intravenous infusion, 500 mg as a single dose once a day for at least the first two days of a seven- to ten-day course of therapy.
 Adolescents up to 16 years of age: Safety and efficacy have not been established.
Note: After the infusion therapy is complete, an oral dose of 500 mg should be administered once a day to complete the seven- to ten-day course of therapy.

**Usual pediatric dose**
Children up to 16 years of age—Safety and efficacy have not been established.

U.S.—
 500 mg (Rx) [*Zithromax* (sodium hydroxide)].
Canada—
 Not commercially available.

**Preparation of dosage form**
To prepare the initial solution for intravenous infusion, add 4.8 mL of sterile water for injection to each 500-mg vial and shake until all of the medication is dissolved. Further dilute this solution by transferring it into 250 or 500 mL of a suitable diluent (see manufacturer's package insert) to provide a final concentration of 2 or 1 mg per mL, respectively.

**Stability**
After reconstitution with sterile water for injection, the solution is stable for 24 hours when stored below 30 °C (86 °F). After dilution to 1 or 2 mg per mL in suitable diluent, solutions are stable for 24 hours at or below room temperature (30 °C [86 °F]), or for 7 days if stored at 5 °C (41 °F).

[1]Not included in Canadian product labeling.

## Selected Bibliography
Drew RH, Gallis HA. Azithromycin—spectrum of activity, pharmacokinetics, and clinical applications. Pharmacotherapy 1992; 12(3): 161-73.

Revised: 05/27/94
Interim revision: 06/28/94; 04/06/98

---

# AZTREONAM  Systemic†

VA CLASSIFICATION (Primary): AM130
Commonly used brand name(s): *Azactam*.
Note: For a listing of dosage forms and brand names by country availability, see *Dosage Forms* section(s).

†Not commercially available in Canada.

## Category
Antibacterial (systemic).
Note: Aztreonam is a narrow-spectrum antibacterial that is only active against aerobic, gram-negative organisms.

## Indications
Note: Bracketed information in the *Indications* section refers to uses that are not included in U.S. product labeling.

**Accepted**
Bronchitis (treatment) or
Pneumonia, gram-negative, bacterial (treatment)—Aztreonam is indicated as a secondary agent in the treatment of aerobic gram-negative bacterial bronchitis and pneumonia caused by *Enterobacter* species, *Escherichia coli*, *Haemophilus influenzae*, *Klebsiella pneumoniae*, *Proteus mirabilis*, *Pseudomonas aeruginosa*, and *Serratia marcescens*.

Skin and soft tissue infections (treatment)—Aztreonam is indicated as a secondary agent in the treatment of skin and soft tissue infections (including ulcers, burn wound infections, and postoperative wounds) caused by *Citrobacter* species, *Enterobacter* species, *E. coli*, *K. pneumoniae*, *P. mirabilis*, *Ps. aeruginosa*, and *S. marcescens*.

Cystitis (treatment) or
Urinary tract infections, bacterial (treatment)—Aztreonam is indicated as a secondary agent in the treatment of cystitis and complicated and uncomplicated urinary tract infections (including initial and recurrent pyelonephritis) caused by *Citrobacter* species, *E. cloacae*, *E. coli*, *K. oxytoca*, *K. pneumoniae*, *P. mirabilis*, *Ps. aeruginosa*, and *S. marcescens*.

Gynecologic infections (treatment)—Aztreonam is indicated as a secondary agent in the treatment of gynecologic infections (including endometritis and pelvic cellulitis) caused by *Enterobacter* species (including *E. cloacae*), *E. coli*, *K. pneumoniae*, and *P. mirabilis*.

Intra-abdominal infections (treatment)—Aztreonam is indicated as a secondary agent in the treatment of intra-abdominal infections (including peritonitis) caused by *Citrobacter* species (including *C. freundii*), *Enterobacter* species (including *E. cloacae*), *E. coli*, *Klebsiella* species (including *K. pneumoniae*), *Ps. aeruginosa*, and *Serratia* species (including *S. marcescens*).

Septicemia, bacterial (treatment)—Aztreonam is indicated as a secondary agent in the treatment of septicemia caused by *Enterobacter* species, *E. coli*, *K. pneumoniae*, *P. mirabilis*, *Ps. aeruginosa*, and *S. marcescens*.

[Bone and joint infections (treatment)]—Aztreonam is used as a secondary agent in the treatment of bone and joint infections caused by susceptible aerobic, gram-negative bacteria.

Aztreonam and aminoglycosides are synergistic *in vitro* against most strains of *Ps. aeruginosa*, many strains of Enterobacteriaceae, and other aerobic gram-negative bacilli.

Not all species or strains of a particular organism may be susceptible to aztreonam.

### Unaccepted
Aztreonam is not effective against gram-positive organisms (e.g., *Staphylococcus aureus*, enterococci, *Streptococcus pneumoniae*) and anaerobes (e.g., *Bacteroides* species and *Clostridium* species).

## Pharmacology/Pharmacokinetics

### Physicochemical characteristics
Molecular weight—435.43.

### Mechanism of action/Effect
Bactericidal; binds to penicillin-binding protein-3(PBP-3), which results in inhibition of bacterial cell wall synthesis, and often results ultimately in cell lysis and death; filamentation also occurs in Enterobacteriaceae and *Ps. aeruginosa*; does not induce beta-lactamase activity, but has a high degree of stability in the presence of bacterial beta-lactamases; does not bind appreciably to any essential PBPs in gram-positive or anaerobic organisms.

### Absorption
Oral—Less than 1% absorbed from the gastrointestinal tract following oral administration.
Intramuscular—Completely absorbed following intramuscular administration.

### Distribution
Rapidly and widely distributed to body fluids and tissues; distributed to bile; breast milk; bronchial secretions; and blister, pericardial, pleural, synovial, amniotic, peritoneal, and cerebrospinal fluids (inflamed meninges); also distributed to atrial appendages, endometrium, fallopian tubes, fat, femurs, gallbladder, kidneys, large intestine, liver, lungs, myometrium, ovaries, prostate, skeletal muscles, skin, and sternum; also crosses the placenta and enters fetal circulation.

$Vol_D$ (steady state)—
  Adults:
    0.11 to 0.21 L per kg.
  Burn patients:
    Approximately 0.31 L per kg.
  Pediatric patients:
    Premature neonates—0.29 to 0.36 L per kg.
    Neonates (up to 1 month old)—0.26 to 0.30 L per kg.
    Infants and children (1 month to 12 years)—0.20 to 0.29 L per kg.
    Cystic fibrosis patients—Approximately 0.25 L per kg.

### Protein binding
Normal renal function—Moderate (56 to 60%).
Impaired renal function (creatinine clearance <30 mL per min [0.50 mL per sec])—36 to 43%.

### Biotransformation
Approximately 6 to 16% metabolized to inactive metabolites by hydrolysis of the beta-lactam bond, resulting in an open-ring compound.

### Half-life
Adults—
  Normal renal function:
    1.4 to 2.2 hours.
  Impaired renal function:
    4.7 to 6.0 hours.
  Impaired hepatic function:
    Primary biliary cirrhosis—Approximately 2.2 hours.
    Alcoholic cirrhosis—Approximately 3.4 hours.
  In elderly males (65 to 75 years of age):
    Slightly prolonged (2.1 hours).
Pediatric patients—
  Premature neonates:
    3.1 to 5.7 hours.
  Neonates (up to 1 month old):
    2.4 to 2.6 hours.
  Infants and children (1 month to 12 years):
    1.5 to 1.7 hours.
  Cystic fibrosis patients:
    1.0 to 1.3 hours.

### Time to peak serum concentration
Intramuscular—Approximately 0.6 to 1.3 hours.

### Time to peak bile concentration
Intravenous—Approximately 2.4 hours.

### Peak serum concentration
Linear kinetics—
  Adults:
    Intramuscular—1 gram: 40 to 46.5 mcg per mL.
    Intravenous injection—1 gram: Approximately 125 mcg per mL.
    Intravenous infusion—1 gram: 90 to 164 mcg per mL.
  Pediatric patients:
    Intravenous injection (over 3 to 5 minutes)—30 mg per kg of body weight (mg/kg).
    Premature neonates—Approximately 80 mcg per mL.
    Neonates and children up to 12 years of age—90 to 120 mcg per mL.

### Peak bile concentration
Approximately 43 mcg per mL following a 1-gram intravenous dose.

### Urine concentration
Intramuscular—Approximately 500 and 1200 mcg per mL 2 hours following intramuscular doses of 500 mg and 1 gram, respectively.
Intravenous—Approximately 1100, 3500, and 6600 mcg per mL 2 hours following 30-minute intravenous infusions of 500 mg, 1 gram, and 2 grams, respectively.

### Elimination
Renal—
  Approximately 60 to 75% excreted unchanged in urine within 8 hours by active tubular secretion and glomerular filtration (in approximately equal amounts); excretion essentially complete within 12 hours; inactive metabolites also excreted in urine.
Biliary/fecal—
  Excreted unchanged in feces following oral administration.
  Approximately 1.5 to 3.5% (up to 12%) excreted unchanged in feces following parenteral administration; inactive metabolites also excreted in feces.
In dialysis—
  Hemodialysis: A 4-hour period of hemodialysis reduces plasma aztreonam concentrations by 27 to 58%.
  Peritoneal dialysis: Reduces plasma aztreonam concentrations by approximately 10%.

## Precautions to Consider

### Cross-sensitivity and/or related problems
Studies in rabbits have shown negligible cross-reactivity between antiaztreonam, antibenzylpenicillin, and anticephalothin antibodies.

In studies in normal volunteers, aztreonam was shown to be only weakly immunogenic in humans. Of 41 patients with immunoglobulin E (IgE) antibodies to one or more penicillin moieties, none reacted to aztreonam. In a study of 36 patients receiving multiple doses of aztreonam over a 7-day period, there were no IgE antibody responses. Only one patient had an IgG response. In a study of 22 patients with positive skin tests to penicillin reagents, three had positive skin tests to aztreonam. Of those three, one was negative on rechallenge and one was confirmed as positive. Of the 20 patients with negative aztreonam skin tests who received aztreonam, none showed immediate hypersensitivity reactions.

Since cross-reactivity only rarely occurs between aztreonam and beta-lactam antibacterials, aztreonam may usually be given without incident to patients with "rash-type" beta-lactam allergy. However, patients who have had immediate hypersensitivity (e.g., anaphylactic or urticarial) reactions to beta-lactams should be closely monitored while receiving aztreonam.

### Carcinogenicity
Studies in animals have not been done.

### Mutagenicity
Studies with aztreonam in several standard *in vivo* and *in vitro* laboratory models have shown no evidence of mutagenic potential at the chromosome or gene level.

## Pregnancy/Reproduction
Fertility—Two-generation reproduction studies in rats given doses up to 20 times the maximum recommended human dose (MRHD) prior to and during gestation and lactation have not shown any evidence of impaired fertility.

Pregnancy—Aztreonam crosses the placenta and enters the fetal circulation. Adequate and well-controlled studies in humans have not been done.

Studies in rats and rabbits given daily doses up to 15 and 5 times the MRHD, respectively, have not shown that aztreonam is embryotoxic, fetotoxic, or teratogenic. Studies in rats given 15 times the MRHD during late gestation and lactation have not shown any aztreonam-induced changes.

FDA Pregnancy Category B.

## Breast-feeding
Aztreonam is excreted in breast milk in concentrations that are less than 1% of maternal serum concentrations. However, aztreonam is not absorbed from the gastrointestinal tract.

## Pediatrics
There is little information currently available on the use of aztreonam in children, especially those up to the age of 12. However, studies to date have shown aztreonam to be clinically effective in pediatric patients, and the side effects seen in children appear to be similar to those seen in adults.

## Geriatrics
Studies performed to date have not demonstrated geriatrics-specific problems that would limit the usefulness of aztreonam in the elderly. However, elderly patients are more likely to have an age-related decrease in renal function, which may require a decrease in dosage in patients receiving aztreonam.

## Laboratory value alterations
The following have been selected on the basis of their potential clinical significance (possible effect in parentheses where appropriate)—not necessarily inclusive (» = major clinical significance):

With diagnostic test results
Coombs' (antiglobulin) tests
(may become positive during therapy)

With physiology/laboratory test values
Alanine aminotransferase (ALT [SGPT]), serum and
Alkaline phosphatase, serum and
Aspartate aminotransferase (AST [SGOT]), serum and
Lactate dehydrogenase (LDH), serum
(values may be transiently increased during therapy)

Creatinine, serum
(concentration may be transiently increased during therapy)

Partial thromboplastin time (PTT) and
Prothrombin time (PT)
(may be prolonged during therapy)

## Medical considerations/Contraindications
The medical considerations/contraindications included have been selected on the basis of their potential clinical significance (reasons given in parentheses where appropriate)—not necessarily inclusive (» = major clinical significance).

*Except under special circumstances, this medication should not be used when the following medical problem exists:*

» Previous allergic reaction to aztreonam

*Risk-benefit should be considered when the following medical problems exist:*

» Cirrhosis
(prolonged half-life; patients with cirrhosis may require a modest reduction in dose [20-25%] when receiving high-dose, long-term therapy with aztreonam)

» Renal function impairment
(it is recommended that aztreonam be administered in a reduced dosage to patients with impaired renal function)

## Side/Adverse Effects
The following side/adverse effects have been selected on the basis of their potential clinical significance (possible signs and symptoms in parentheses where appropriate)—not necessarily inclusive:

**Those indicating need for medical attention**
Incidence less frequent
*Hypersensitivity* (anaphylaxis; skin rash, redness, or itching); *thrombophlebitis* (inflammation or phlebitis at the injection site)

**Those indicating need for medical attention only if they continue or are bothersome**
Incidence less frequent or rare
*Gastrointestinal upset* (abdominal or stomach cramps; diarrhea; nausea; vomiting)

## Overdose
For more information on the management of overdose or unintentional ingestion, contact a **Poison Control Center** (see *Poison Control Center Listing*).

**Treatment of overdose**
Recommended treatment consists of the following:

Specific treatment—If necessary, hemodialysis to clear aztreonam from the serum.

Supportive care—Patients in whom intentional overdose is known or suspected should be referred for psychiatric consultation.

## Patient Consultation
As an aid to patient consultation, refer to *Advice for the Patient, Aztreonam (Systemic)*.

In providing consultation, consider emphasizing the following selected information (» = major clinical significance):

**Before receiving this medication**
» Conditions affecting use, especially:
Allergy to aztreonam or anaphylaxis to beta-lactam antibiotics
Pregnancy—Aztreonam crosses the placenta and enters the fetal circulation
Breast-feeding—Aztreonam is excreted in breast milk
Other medical problems, especially cirrhosis or renal function impairment

**Proper use of this medication**
» Importance of receiving medication for full course of therapy and on regular schedule
» Proper dosing

**Side/adverse effects**
Signs of potential side effects, especially hypersensitivity or thrombophlebitis

## General Dosing Information
Aztreonam may be administered intramuscularly or intravenously. In patients requiring single doses greater than 1 gram or in patients with bacterial septicemia, localized parenchymal abscesses, peritonitis, or other severe or life-threatening infections, the intravenous route is recommended.

Aztreonam may be administered slowly over a 3- to 5-minute period either by direct injection into a vein or by injection into the tubing of a suitable intravenous administration set.

Aztreonam may also be administered by intermittent intravenous infusion in 50 to 100 mL of a suitable fluid over a 20- to 60-minute period.

If aztreonam is administered via a volume-control administration set, the final dilution should not exceed 2% (20 mg per mL).

Because of the serious nature of infections caused by *Pseudomonas aeruginosa*, the recommended dose in the treatment of such infections is 2 grams every 6 to 8 hours.

Patients with renal function impairment may need an adjustment in dosage, based on creatinine clearance. Creatinine clearance (in mL per minute) may be calculated as follows:

Adult males: Creatinine clearance = $[(140 - \text{age}) \times (\text{ideal body weight in kg})]/[72 \times \text{serum creatinine (mg per dL)}]$

Adult females: Creatinine clearance = $[(140 - \text{age}) \times (\text{ideal body weight in kg})]/[72 \times \text{serum creatinine (mg per dL)}] \times 0.85$

Creatinine clearance may also be calculated in SI units (as mL per second) as follows:

Adult males: Creatinine clearance = $[(140 - \text{age}) \times (\text{ideal body weight in kg})]/[50 \times \text{serum creatinine (micromoles per L)}]$

Adult females: Creatinine clearance = $[(140 - \text{age}) \times (\text{ideal body weight in kg})]/[50 \times \text{serum creatinine (micromoles per L)}] \times 0.85$

**For treatment of adverse effects**
Recommended treatment consists of the following:
- Discontinuation of aztreonam and institution of supportive treatment (e.g., maintenance of ventilation and administration of epinephrine, pressor amines, antihistamines, corticosteroids) if serious hypersensitivity reactions or allergic reactions occur.

## Parenteral Dosage Forms

### AZTREONAM INJECTION

**Usual adult and adolescent dose**
Intravenous infusion over twenty to sixty minutes—
Moderately severe systemic infections: 1 to 2 grams every eight to twelve hours.
Severe systemic or life-threatening infections: 2 grams every six to eight hours.
Note: Urinary tract infections—Intravenous infusion over twenty to sixty minutes, 500 mg to 1 gram every eight to twelve hours.
Adults with impaired renal function require a reduction in dose as follows:

| Creatinine Clearance (mL/min)/(mL/sec) | Dose Loading Dose | Maintenance dose (every 6–12 hours) |
|---|---|---|
| >30/0.50 | | See *Usual adult and adolescent dose* |
| 10–30/0.17–0.50 | 1–2 grams | ½ of the loading dose |
| <10/0.17 | 500 mg–2 grams | ¼ of the loading dose; in serious or life-threatening infections, an additional ⅛ of the loading dose should be given after each hemodialysis period |

**Usual adult prescribing limits**
Up to a maximum of 8 grams daily.

**Usual pediatric dose**
Dosage has not been established.

**Strength(s) usually available**
U.S.—
 1 gram in 50 mL (Rx) [*Azactam*].
 2 grams in 50 mL (Rx) [*Azactam*].
Canada—
 Not commercially available.

**Packaging and storage**
Do not store above −20 °C (−4 °F), unless otherwise specified by manufacturer.

**Preparation of dosage form**
Thaw container at room temperature or in a refrigerator before administration, making sure that all ice crystals have melted.
Do not use minibags in series connections. This may result in air embolism because of residual air being drawn from the primary container before administration of intravenous solution from the secondary container is complete.

**Stability**
After thawing, solutions retain their potency for 48 hours at room temperature or for 14 days if refrigerated.
Once thawed, solutions should not be refrozen.
Do not use if the solution is cloudy or contains a precipitate.

**Incompatibilities**
Additives or other medication should not be added to, or infused simultaneously through the same intravenous line.

### AZTREONAM FOR INJECTION USP

**Usual adult and adolescent dose**
Intramuscular or intravenous
Moderately severe systemic infections: 1 to 2 grams every eight to twelve hours.
Severe systemic or life-threatening infections: 2 grams every six to eight hours.
Note: Urinary tract infections—Intramuscular or intravenous, 500 mg to 1 gram every eight to twelve hours.
Adults with impaired renal function require a reduction in dose as follows:

| Creatinine Clearance (mL/min)/(mL/sec) | Dose Loading Dose | Maintenance dose (every 6–12 hours) |
|---|---|---|
| >30/0.50 | | See *Usual adult and adolescent dose* |
| 10–30/0.17–0.50 | 1–2 grams | ½ of the loading dose |
| <10/0.17 | 500 mg–2 grams | ¼ of the loading dose; in serious or life-threatening infections, an additional ⅛ of the loading dose should be given after each hemodialysis period |

**Usual adult prescribing limits**
Up to a maximum of 8 grams daily.

**Usual pediatric dose**
Antibacterial—
 Dosage has not been established; however, the following doses have been reported in the literature:
 Infants up to 7 days of age—30 mg per kg of body weight every twelve hours.
 Infants 1 to 4 weeks of age—30 mg per kg of body weight every eight hours.
 Infants over 4 weeks of age—30 mg per kg of body weight every six to eight hours.
 Children with cystic fibrosis—50 mg per kg of body weight every six hours.

**Size(s) usually available**
U.S.—
 500 mg (Rx) [*Azactam* (L-arginine, 780 mg per gram)].
 1 gram (Rx) [*Azactam* (L-arginine, 780 mg per gram)].
 2 grams (Rx) [*Azactam* (L-arginine, 780 mg per gram)].
Canada—
 Not commercially available.

**Packaging and storage**
Prior to reconstitution, store below 40 °C (104 °F), preferably between 15 and 30 °C (59 and 86 °F), unless otherwise specified by manufacturer.

**Preparation of dosage form**
To prepare initial dilution for intramuscular use (15-mL vial), for each gram of aztreonam add at least 3 mL of sterile water for injection, bacteriostatic water for injection (preserved with benzyl alcohol or methyl- and propylparabens), 0.9% sodium chloride injection, or bacteriostatic sodium chloride injection (preserved with benzyl alcohol or methyl- and propylparabens).
To prepare initial dilution for direct intravenous use, add 6 to 10 mL of sterile water for injection to each 15-mL vial.
To prepare initial dilution for intravenous infusion (15-mL vial), for each gram of aztreonam add at least 3 mL of sterile water for injection. The resulting solution may be further diluted in 0.9% sodium chloride injection, Ringer's injection, lactated Ringer's injection, dextrose injection (5 or 10%), dextrose and sodium chloride injection, sodium lactate injection (M/6), dextrose and lactated Ringer's injection, or other electrolyte-containing solutions (see manufacturer's package insert).
For reconstitution of piggyback infusion bottles (100-mL), add at least 50 mL of suitable diluent (see manufacturer's package insert) for each gram of aztreonam. The final concentration should not exceed 2% (20 mg per mL).
After addition of the diluent, contents of the vial should be shaken immediately and vigorously.

**Stability**
Aztreonam vials are not intended for multiple-dose use. Unused solutions should be discarded.
Solutions range in color from colorless to light straw yellow, depending on the concentration and diluent.
Solutions may develop a slight pink tint on standing. This does not affect their potency.
After reconstitution for intramuscular use, solutions retain their potency for 48 hours at room temperature or for 7 days if refrigerated.
After reconstitution for intravenous use, solutions at concentrations not exceeding 2% (20 mg per mL) retain their potency for 48 hours at controlled room temperature (15 to 30 °C [59 to 86 °F]) or for 7 days if refrigerated at 2 to 8 °C (36 to 46 °F).

After reconstitution for intravenous use, solutions (except those reconstituted with sterile water for injection and sodium chloride injection) at concentrations exceeding 2% should be used promptly after reconstitution. Solutions reconstituted with sterile water for injection or sodium chloride injection retain their potency for 48 hours at controlled room temperature or for 7 days if refrigerated.

Frozen solutions (except those reconstituted with two untested diluents, 10% mannitol injection or dextrose and lactated Ringer's injection) retain their potency for up to 3 months at −20 °C (−4 °F). Frozen solutions may be thawed at controlled room temperature or by storage in a refrigerator overnight. Solutions that have been thawed and maintained at controlled room temperature or under refrigeration should be used within 24 or 72 hours, respectively. Once thawed, solutions should not be refrozen.

Admixtures of aztreonam and clindamycin phosphate, gentamicin sulfate, tobramycin sulfate, or cefazolin sodium in 0.9% sodium chloride injection or 5% dextrose injection retain their potency for 48 hours at room temperature or for 7 days if refrigerated.

Admixtures of aztreonam and ampicillin sodium in 0.9% sodium chloride injection retain their potency for 24 hours at room temperature (25 °C [77 °F]) or for 48 hours if refrigerated at 4 °C (39 °F). Admixtures containing aztreonam and ampicillin sodium in 5% dextrose injection retain their potency for 2 hours at room temperature (25 °C [77 °F]) or for 8 hours if refrigerated at 4 °C (39 °F).

Admixtures of aztreonam and cloxacillin sodium or aztreonam and vancomycin hydrochloride in peritoneal dialysis solution containing 4.25% dextrose retain their potency for 24 hours at room temperature.

**Incompatibilities**

Admixtures of aztreonam and nafcillin sodium, cephradine, vancomycin, or metronidazole are incompatible.

In general, admixtures of aztreonam and other medications are not recommended. However, certain admixtures have been shown to be compatible (see *Stability*).

Revised: 02/23/93

**BACAMPICILLIN**—See *Penicillins (Systemic)*

# BACILLUS CALMETTE-GUÉRIN (BCG) LIVE  Mucosal-Local

VA CLASSIFICATION (Primary): AN900
Commonly used brand name(s): *ImmuCyst; PACIS; TICE BCG; TheraCys.*
Note: For a listing of dosage forms and brand names by country availability, see *Dosage Forms* section(s).

## Category
Antineoplastic.

## Indications
Note: Bracketed information in the *Indications* section refers to uses that are not included in U.S. product labeling.

### Accepted
Carcinoma, bladder (prophylaxis and treatment)—BCG is used intravesically for prophylaxis and treatment of primary (multifocal, high grade) and relapsed superficial transitional cell bladder carcinoma. It is used to reduce frequency of tumor recurrence after transurethral resection and to eliminate existing tumors, including [Ta and T1 tumors] and carcinoma in situ (CIS tumors) with or without associated papillary tumors. It is not indicated for treatment of papillary tumors occurring alone.

### Unaccepted
The product labeled for use only in treatment of bladder carcinoma is not intended to be used as an immunizing agent for the prevention of tuberculosis; the product labeled for both uses can be used for both. BCG is not a vaccine for the prevention of cancer.

## Pharmacology/Pharmacokinetics

### Physicochemical characteristics
Source—It is a live culture of the attenuated bacillus Calmette-Guérin strain of *Mycobacterium bovis*. Commercially available strains (which are substrains of the Pasteur Institute strain) include the Armand-Frappier, Connaught, Glaxo/Evans, and Tice substrains; of these, only the Connaught and Tice strains are approved for bladder carcinoma.

### Mechanism of action/Effect
The effect of BCG against carcinoma is not completely understood. It may be related to an inflammatory response and possibly also to an immune response.
Intravesical BCG suspension produces a granulomatous response locally and in regional lymph nodes; the inflammatory response stimulates production of macrophages that have tumoricidal effects. The presence of interleukin-2, which is a substance produced by activated helper T lymphocytes and which activates natural killer cells, has also been noted in the urine of patients who responded to BCG treatment. However, the relationship of these effects to the antineoplastic effect of BCG is unknown.

### Other actions/effects
Induces active immunity against tuberculosis by unknown mechanism; may involve stimulating the reticuloendothelial system (RES) to produce macrophages and other activated cells that prevent multiplication of virulent *Mycobacterium tuberculosis*.
Viability and immunogenicity may vary between strains and viability varies between lots of any one strain. With intracavitary BCG, positive conversion of tuberculin (purified protein derivative [PPD]) skin test occurs in a majority of patients, usually after 3 to 12 weeks. Positive conversion of PPD skin test, when it occurs, is usually not permanent, although duration is variable and sometimes long.

## Precautions to Consider

### Tumorigenicity
Two cases of nephrogenic adenoma (adenomatous metaplasia of the bladder), which is usually benign and believed to result from chronic irritation or trauma, have been reported.

### Pregnancy/Reproduction
Pregnancy—Studies have not been done in humans.
Studies have not been done in animals.
FDA Pregnancy Category C.

### Breast-feeding
It is not known whether intravesical BCG is distributed into breast milk. However, problems in humans have not been documented.

### Pediatrics
No information is available on the relationship of age to the effects of BCG in pediatric patients. Safety and efficacy have not been established.

### Geriatrics
Studies performed to date have not demonstrated geriatrics-specific problems that would limit the usefulness of BCG as an antineoplastic in the elderly.

### Drug interactions and/or related problems
The following drug interactions and/or related problems have been selected on the basis of their potential clinical significance (possible mechanism in parentheses where appropriate)—not necessarily inclusive (» = major clinical significance):

Note: Combinations containing any of the following medications, depending on the amount present, may also interact with this medication.

Antimicrobial therapy
(potential negative effect on actions of BCG)
» Bone marrow depressants(see *Appendix II*) or
» Immunosuppressantsor
» Radiation
(may impair immune response to BCG. The interval between discontinuation of medications that cause immunosuppression and restoration of the patient's ability to respond to BCG depends on the intensity and type of immunosuppression-causing therapy used, the underlying disease, and other factors; estimates vary from 3 months to 1 year. Also, may increase the risk of osteomyelitis or disseminated BCG infection)

» Vaccines, killed or live virus
(concurrent administration with BCG is not recommended; it is recommended that live virus vaccines be given 6 to 8 weeks after BCG; it is recommended that killed virus vaccines be given 7 days before or 10 days after BCG)

### Laboratory value alterations
The following have been selected on the basis of their potential clinical significance (possible effect in parentheses where appropriate)—not necessarily inclusive (» = major clinical significance):

With physiology/laboratory test values
Hepatic function tests
(abnormalities have been reported rarely)
Tuberculin (purified protein derivative [PPD]) skin test
(positive conversion is produced in a majority of patients, usually after 3 to 12 weeks of intravesical BCG therapy; may complicate future interpretations of tuberculin skin test reactions in the diagnosis of suspected mycobacterial infections)
Microscopic examination of urine
(microscopic pyuria commonly seen; however, bacterial growth in urine is uncommon; returns to normal after completion of a course of BCG therapy)

### Medical considerations/Contraindications
The medical considerations/contraindications included have been selected on the basis of their potential clinical significance (reasons given in parentheses where appropriate)—not necessarily inclusive (» = major clinical significance).

*Except under special circumstances, this medication should not be used when the following medical problems exist:*
» Fever
(BCG should not be administered until the cause has been determined; if fever is caused by infection, BCG should be withheld until the patient is afebrile and off all therapy)
» Urinary tract infection
(risk of disseminated BCG infection; increased severity of bladder irritation)

*Risk-benefit should be considered when the following medical problems exist:*
» Hematuria, gross, existing
(risk of disseminated BCG infection; caution is necessary especially if the hematuria is induced by recent biopsy or resection, and it is recommended that intravesical BCG not be given until gross hematuria has cleared; if hematuria is from the tumor itself, BCG can

still be given, but with caution because irritable bladder symptoms may be increased)
» Impaired immune response
(decreased response to treatment; risk of osteomyelitis or disseminated BCG infection)
» Sensitivity to BCG live
Small bladder capacity
(increased incidence and severity of local irritation; in addition, therapy with BCG may rarely cause bladder contracture, which further decreases capacity)

**Patient monitoring**
The following may be especially important in patient monitoring (other tests may be warranted in some patients, depending on condition; » = major clinical significance):
» Bladder biopsy, cold cup
(recommended at regular intervals to assess response; also recommended for any suspicious area found by cystoscopy or cytology studies)
» Cystoscopy and
» Urine cytology studies
(recommended at regular intervals during and after treatment to assess response and confirm that the tumor is not progressing)
Hepatic function determinations
(recommended if persistent [e.g., 101 °F for longer than 2 days] or severe [e.g., greater than 103 °F] fever or continuing malaise occurs)
Needle biopsy of prostate in males
(recommended as indicated by presence of clinical signs of granulomatous prostatitis)
Tuberculin (PPD) skin test
(recommended before treatment and at periodic intervals during treatment. However, although it may predict responsiveness to BCG treatment in general, this is controversial and it is unlikely to provide a prognosis for a specific individual patient, especially since positive conversion does not occur in all patients who respond to BCG therapy)
Urine cultures
(recommended before and at periodic intervals during treatment; recommended if urinalysis or clinical symptoms suggest presence of urinary tract infection)

## Side/Adverse Effects

Note: Side/adverse effects are usually mild to moderate and transient, but may be cumulative.

The following side/adverse effects have been selected on the basis of their potential clinical significance (possible signs and symptoms in parentheses where appropriate)—not necessarily inclusive:

**Those indicating need for medical attention**
Incidence more frequent
*Bladder infection, secondary to bladder irritation*—usually asymptomatic; *bladder irritation* (blood in urine; frequent urge to urinate; increased frequency of urination; painful urination, severe or continuing); *flu-like syndrome* (fever and chills; joint pain; nausea and vomiting; in a few patients, has progressed to a severe systemic reaction with high fever, malaise, and anorexia); *granulomatous prostatitis* (appears as nodularity, enlargement, induration, and distortion of the prostate, which is clinically indistinguishable from prostatic carcinoma)—usually asymptomatic

Note: *Bladder infection* responds rapidly to antibiotic treatment.
*Bladder irritation* occurs in most patients, but is usually transient; may be severe in some patients. May predict antitumor response. Symptoms usually begin within 2 to 4 hours after a dose and last 24 to 72 hours. Granulomatous inflammation is seen on the histological examination; lesions that may be confused with tumors appear commonly within 4 weeks after BCG treatment; inflammation usually disappears within about 4 to 6 months after treatment.
Symptoms of the *flu-like syndrome* usually begin within 4 hours after a dose and last 24 to 72 hours.

Incidence rare
*Allergic reaction or erythema nodosum* (skin rash); *BCG infection, disseminated, with lung or liver involvement* (fever; cough); *bladder contracture; hepatic function impairment*—asymptomatic; *hypotension; leukopenia*—asymptomatic

Note: Symptoms of *disseminated BCG infection* may be difficult to distinguish from those of gram-negative sepsis or severe hypersensitivity reactions, or of progressing malignancy. Disseminated infection, with associated fever, may occur as late as 6 months or more after BCG therapy and may persist for 1 to 3 weeks after antituberculosis therapy is begun. It is usually diagnosed clinically based on the presence of fever (over 39 °C [103 °F] or persistently over 38 °C [101 °F] over 2 days) and chills, especially when associated with malaise and other systemic symptoms, negative blood and urine cultures, chest x-ray or computed tomography (CT) to exclude other pulmonary diseases, and hepatic function tests. Deaths have been reported.
*Hepatic function impairment* is usually mild and transient; abnormalities peak by 20 days and may persist months after BCG administration.

**Those indicating need for medical attention only if they continue or are bothersome**
Incidence more frequent
*Burning, slight, during first void after treatment*

**Those indicating the need for medical attention if they occur after medication is discontinued**
*BCG infection, disseminated, with lung or liver involvement* (fever; cough)

## Patient Consultation

As an aid to patient consultation, refer to *Advice for the Patient, Bacillus Calmette-Guérin (BCG) Live (Mucosal-Local).*
In providing consultation, consider emphasizing the following selected information (» = major clinical significance):

**Before using this medication**
» Conditions affecting use, especially:
Sensitivity to BCG
Other medications, especially bone marrow depressants or immunosuppressants or radiation therapy
Other medical problems, especially fever, gross hematuria, impaired immune response, or urinary tract infection

**Proper use of this medication**
Emptying bladder before instillation of each dose
» Following physician's instructions for holding solution in bladder; holding in bladder for 2 hours; telling physician if unable to retain solution for prescribed time; physician may recommend lying down for 15 minutes each in prone and supine positions, and on each side, during first hour; sitting down while voiding
» Importance of ample fluid intake for several hours after instillation
Bacteria will be present in urine; treating all urine voided within 6 hours after each instillation with an equal volume of 5% hypochlorite solution (undiluted household bleach; usually 6 to 8 ounces) and allowing to stand for 15 minutes before flushing
» Proper dosing

**Precautions while using this medication**
Avoiding persons with active tuberculosis for 6 to 12 weeks after treatment; telling physician about any exposure to active tuberculosis
Avoiding immunizations unless approved by physician

**Side/adverse effects**
Signs of potential side effects, especially bladder infection, bladder irritation, flu-like syndrome, allergic reaction, erythema nodosum, disseminated BCG infection, bladder contracture, and hypotension

## General Dosing Information

Patients receiving intravesical BCG should be under the supervision of a physician experienced in immunotherapy.

Prior to BCG administration, the bladder is emptied either by voiding or drainage through a urethral catheter inserted into the bladder under aseptic conditions. BCG is then instilled into the bladder by gravity flow via the catheter; the plunger should not be depressed to force the flow.

It is recommended that BCG instillation and equipment and materials used in preparation of the instillation be treated as biohazardous waste.

BCG should not be injected intravenously, subcutaneously, or intramuscularly.

Care and aseptic technique are necessary during administration of intravesical BCG therapy so as not to introduce contaminants into the urinary tract or to unduly traumatize the urinary mucosa.

If the physician believes that the bladder catheterization has been traumatic (e.g., associated with bleeding or possible false passage), instillation of BCG should be delayed by at least 1 week. However, beginning with the delayed dose, subsequent doses should be administered according to the original schedule (i.e., no doses should be omitted).

It is recommended that BCG therapy not be started until 7 to 14 days after bladder tumor resection or biopsy because fatalities from disseminated

BCG infection have been reported with use of BCG after traumatic catheterization.

If development of systemic BCG infection is suspected, it is recommended that BCG be withheld and fast-acting antituberculosis therapy initiated.

Patients who do not respond after two 6-week courses of BCG therapy are not likely to respond, and consideration of alternative therapy is recommended.

Most severe adverse effects can be prevented or reduced in severity with prophylactic isoniazid treatment given for 3 days beginning the morning of BCG treatment. Some clinicians also recommend use of antihistamines and nonsteroidal anti-inflammatory agents.

### Safety considerations for handling this medication
There is concern that personnel involved in preparation and administration of intravesical BCG may be at some risk because of the infectious potential of this agent, although the actual risk is unknown. USP advisory panels recommend cautious handling both in preparation and disposal of BCG for intravesical use. Precautions that have been suggested include:
- Use of a biological containment cabinet during reconstitution and dilution of parenteral medications and wearing of disposable surgical gloves and masks.
- Use of proper technique to prevent contamination of the medication, work area, and operator during transfer between containers (including proper training of personnel in this technique).
- Cautious and proper disposal of needles, syringes, vials, ampuls, and unused medication.

A number of medical centers have developed detailed guidelines for handling of antineoplastic and similar agents.

### For treatment of adverse effects
Most adverse effects respond to a reduction in BCG dose or temporary interruption of therapy; however, in some patients withdrawal of BCG therapy may be necessary.

Mild bladder irritation can usually be treated symptomatically with phenazopyridine hydrochloride and antispasmodics such as propantheline bromide or oxybutynin.

Recommended treatment of moderate to severe bladder irritation and flu-like syndrome may consist of the following:
- Isoniazid.
- Antihistamines, such as diphenhydramine hydrochloride.
- Nonsteroidal anti-inflammatory agents; parenteral narcotic analgesics may be necessary for severe bladder irritation.

Recommended treatment of disseminated BCG infection with liver and lung involvement consists of the following:
- Triple-drug antituberculosis therapy or
- A fast-acting antituberculosis medication such as cycloserine.

No specific treatment of granulomatous prostatitis secondary to BCG therapy is required.

## Topical Dosage Forms
### BCG LIVE (CONNAUGHT STRAIN)
**Usual adult dose**
Bladder carcinoma—
    Intracavitary, 1 vial (81 mg), reconstituted and then diluted with 50 mL of sterile, preservative-free 0.9% sodium chloride injection, to a final volume of 53 mL (less in patients with reduced bladder capacity), instilled into the empty bladder and retained for one to two hours (depending on irritative symptoms and the patient's ability to retain the solution). The procedure is repeated once a week for six weeks, followed by one treatment given at three, six, twelve, eighteen, and twenty-four months following the initial treatment or according to response.

Note: During the first hour after instillation, the patient may lie down for 15 minutes in the prone position, followed by the supine position, and on each side, then may be up for the second hour while the suspension is retained.
    The patient voids in a seated position.

**Usual pediatric dose**
Safety and efficacy have not been established.

**Size(s) usually available**
U.S.—
    81 mg (dry weight) or $10.5 \pm 8.7 \times 10^8$ colony-forming units (CFU) per vial (1 vial per package) (Rx) [*TheraCys* (monosodium glutamate 5% w/v plus diluent)].

Canada—
    Approximately $3 \times 10^8$ colony-forming units (CFU) per vial (3 vials per package) (Rx) [*ImmuCyst* (monosodium glutamate 5% w/v plus diluent)].

**Packaging and storage**
Store between 2 and 8 °C (36 and 46 °F). Protect from light.

**Preparation of dosage form**
BCG live (Connaught strain) is reconstituted by adding to the vial 1 mL of diluent provided by manufacturer. The vial is then shaken gently until a fine, even suspension results. The suspension is then diluted in a suitable quantity of sterile, preservative-free 0.9% sodium chloride injection for administration.

Note: Aseptic technique must be used for reconstitution and dilution.
    The product should not be handled by persons with a known immunologic deficiency.

**Stability**
Reconstituted suspension should be used immediately; otherwise, it should be refrigerated until use and should be discarded after 2 hours.

**Note**
Commercially available BCG strains are not interchangeable. *One product should not be substituted for another.* If patients are to be transferred from one to another, appropriate changes in dosage may be necessary.

**Additional information**
After usage, all equipment and materials used for instillation of BCG into the bladder should be placed immediately into plastic bags labeled as infectious waste and disposed of properly as biohazardous waste.

Any unused portion of reconstituted BCG, and urine voided for 6 hours after instillation, should be disinfected with an equal volume of 5% hypochlorite solution (undiluted household bleach) and allowed to stand for 15 minutes before being flushed.

### BCG LIVE (MONTREAL STRAIN)
**Usual adult dose**
Bladder carcinoma—
    Intracavitary, a single dose of 120 mg, reconstituted and then diluted with 50 mL of sterile, preservative-free 0.9% sodium chloride injection instilled into the bladder once a week for six weeks. The bladder should be drained via a urethral catheter under aseptic conditions prior to administration of the recommended dose. The induction therapy may be followed by a single instillation given at three, six, twelve, and twenty-four months following the initial treatment.

Note: During the first hour following instillation, the patient should lie down for 15 minutes in the prone position, supine position, and on each side. After this procedure, the patient should be allowed to be up; however, the suspension should be retained for another 60 minutes for a total of 2 hours. Some patients may not be able to retain the suspension for 2 hours and should be instructed to void in less time if necessary. At the end of treatment all patients should void in a seated position for safety reasons. Patients should be instructed to drink enough liquid after treatment to maintain adequate hydration.

**Usual pediatric dose**
Safety and efficacy have not been established.

**Size(s) usually available**
U.S.—
    Not commercially available.
Canada—
    2 to $10 \times 10^6$ colony-forming units (CFU) per vial (Rx) [*PACIS* (lactose 15% w/v plus diluent)].

**Packaging and storage**
Store between 2 and 8 °C (36 and 46 °F). Protect from light.

Note: Freezing will not harm the BCG; however, the sterile diluent should not be used if it has been frozen. At no time should the lyophilized preparation be exposed to sunlight, direct or indirect.

**Preparation of dosage form**
BCG live (Montreal strain) is reconstituted by adding to the vial 1 mL of diluent provided by manufacturer. The diluent should be left in contact with BCG live for about 1 minute. Then the suspension should be mixed by withdrawing it into the syringe and expelling it gently back to into the vial two or three times. To prevent the formation of foam, the suspension should not be shaken. The suspension is then diluted in a suitable quantity of sterile, preservative-free 0.9% sodium chloride injection for administration.

Note: BCG live (Montreal strain) should be handled as infectious material. Persons handling this product should wear masks and gloves. The product should not be handled by persons with a known immunologic deficiency.

### Stability
BCG live (Montreal strain) may be used for up to 6 hours after preparation if stored under artificial light at a temperature between 4 and 25 °C (39 and 77 °F) while still in the lyophilized state.

### Additional information
After usage, all equipment and materials used for instillation of BCG into the bladder should be placed immediately into plastic bags labeled as infectious waste and disposed of properly as biohazardous waste.

## BCG VACCINE (TICE STRAIN) USP

### Usual adult dose
Bladder carcinoma—
Intracavitary, 1 vial ( 1 to $8 \times 10^8$ colony-forming units [CFU]), reconstituted and then diluted to a total volume of 50 mL with sterile, preservative-free 0.9% sodium chloride injection (less in patients with reduced bladder capacity), instilled into the empty bladder and retained for one to two hours (depending on irritative symptoms and the patient's ability to retain the solution). The procedure is repeated once a week for six weeks; the schedule may be repeated once if circumstances warrant. This is followed by treatment at approximately monthly intervals for at least six to twelve months or according to response.

Note: During the first hour after instillation, the patient may lie for 15 minutes in the prone position, followed by the supine position, and on each side, then may be up for the second hour while the suspension is retained.

The patient voids in a seated position.

### Usual pediatric dose
Safety and efficacy have not been established.

### Size(s) usually available
U.S.—
1 to $8 \times 10^8$ CFU or approximately 50 mg (wet weight) per vial, (Rx) [*TICE BCG* (lactose)].

Canada—
Not commercially available.

### Packaging and storage
Store between 2 and 8 °C (36 and 46 °F). Protect from light.

### Preparation of dosage form
BCG Vaccine USP (Tice Strain) is reconstituted by adding 1 mL of sterile, preservative-free 0.9% sodium chloride injection to ampul, drawing the mixture back into the syringe and expelling it into the ampul three times to mix it thoroughly (minimizes clumping of mycobacteria). The suspension is then diluted in a suitable quantity of sterile, preservative-free 0.9% sodium chloride injection for administration.

Note: Aseptic technique must be used for reconstitution and dilution.
The product should not be handled by persons with a known immunologic deficiency.

### Stability
Reconstituted suspension should be used immediately and any unused portion discarded after 2 hours.

### Additional information
After usage, all equipment and materials used for instillation of BCG into the bladder should be placed immediately into plastic bags labeled as infectious waste and disposed of properly as biohazardous waste.

Any unused portion of reconstituted BCG, and urine voided for 6 hours after instillation, should be disinfected with an equal volume of 5% hypochlorite solution (undiluted household bleach) and allowed to stand for 15 minutes before being flushed.

Revised: 09/30/97
Interim revision: 08/14/98

---

# BACILLUS CALMETTE-GUÉRIN (BCG) LIVE    Systemic

Note: This monograph is specific for the Bacillus Calmette-Guérin (BCG) live vaccine, intended for immunization of uninfected (tuberculin negative) persons to induce tuberculin sensitivity as a protection against tuberculosis infection. Only BCG live vaccine labeled for use against tuberculosis infection should be used for immunization, or where labeled for use both against tuberculosis infection and bladder cancer (for bladder cancer see *Bacillus Calmette-Guérin (BCG) Live, Mucosal-Local*). The efficacy of the BCG vaccines currently available has not been demonstrated directly and can only be inferred.

VA CLASSIFICATION (Primary): IM100
Commonly used brand name(s): *TICE BCG*.

Note: For a listing of dosage forms and brand names by country availability, see *Dosage Forms* section(s).

## Category
Immunizing agent (active).

## Indications

### Accepted
Tuberculosis (prophylaxis)—BCG live vaccine is recommended for protection against tuberculosis in the following persons if tuberculin skin test (purified protein derivative [PPD]) result is negative.
- Infants and children who
 —Are at high risk of intimate and prolonged exposure to persistently untreated or ineffectively treated patients with infectious pulmonary tuberculosis and who cannot be removed from the source of exposure, and cannot be placed on long-term preventive therapy;
 —Are continuously exposed to persons with tuberculosis who have bacilli resistant to isoniazid and rifampin;
 —Are in groups in which the rate of new infections exceeds 1% per year and for whom the usual surveillance and treatment programs have been attempted but are not operatively feasible.
- Household contacts of untreated or insufficiently treated tuberculosis patients, especially patients with a positive sputum culture, when the contacts cannot be effectively shielded from prolonged exposure to the patients.

Selective vaccination is indicated for international travelers with a negative or weakly positive PPD who may be in a high-risk environment for prolonged periods without access to tuberculin testing surveillance.

Health care workers who are likely to be exposed continuously to multidrug-resistant tuberculosis may benefit from vaccination with BCG live.

### Unaccepted
Routine BCG vaccination is no longer recommended in the U.S. since the risk of infection is very low. Also, routine vaccination of health care workers repeatedly exposed to tuberculosis infection is not recommended; tuberculin testing surveillance and prophylactic isoniazid are preferable.

BCG live vaccine labeled for use only as an immunizing agent for the prevention of tuberculosis is not intended for use in the treatment of bladder carcinoma. BCG live vaccine labeled for use against tuberculosis infection and bladder cancer can be used for both. BCG vaccine has no value in the treatment of tuberculosis disease.

## Pharmacology/Pharmacokinetics

### Physicochemical characteristics
Source—A live culture of attenuated organisms of bacillus Calmette-Guérin (BCG) strain of *Mycobacterium bovis*. The original attenuated strain was distributed by Calmette and Guérin widely throughout the world for preparation of BCG vaccine. Until the development of lyophilization techniques, by which the seed culture is preserved currently, the strain was continued by repeated subculturing. This has resulted in the appearance of a number of seed strains with differing characteristics in various countries.

In the U.S., approved BCG live vaccine is prepared from an acceptable seed lot shown to produce vaccines that meet all the prescribed requirements for the product and that have been evaluated in clinical trials for their ability to induce tuberculin sensitivity. No data are available concerning the clinical efficacy of this strain.

The efficacy of any of the currently available BCG vaccines has not been demonstrated directly and can only be inferred.

### Mechanism of action/Effect
BCG live vaccine induces cell-mediated immunity against tuberculosis. However, its mechanism of action is unknown, and it is unclear whether BCG induces antitubercular antibodies.

### Other actions/effects
BCG live vaccine induces antibodies that bind to *Mycobacterium leprae* and may be effective in providing protection against leprosy.

### Protective effect
BCG live vaccination induces tuberculin sensitivity in more than 90% of vaccinated individuals. The protection afforded by BCG live vaccination has been reported from different field trials ranging from 0 to 80%, 50% in meta-analysis. However, there is poor correlation between tuberculin skin test conversion rates or size of induration and protective immunity. Protection, while prolonged, has not been judged to be permanent. In some clinical trials, protection has been negligible. The level of protection against meningitis or miliary tuberculosis in children has been found to be 64 to 86% in clinical trials and 75 to 83% in case control studies.

## Precautions to Consider

### Pregnancy/Reproduction
Fertility—Studies have not been done.

Pregnancy—Studies have not been done in humans. It is not known whether BCG vaccine can cause harm to the fetus when administered to a pregnant woman. BCG vaccine should be given to a pregnant woman or a woman of childbearing age only if the potential benefits outweigh the possible risks.

Studies have not been done in animals.

FDA Pregnancy Category C.

### Breast-feeding
It is not known whether BCG vaccine is distributed into breast milk. However, problems in humans have not been documented.

### Pediatrics
Infants less than 1 month of age should be given one-half of the usual dose. If a vaccinated infant remains tuberculin negative and the vaccine is still indicated, the vaccination should be repeated at full dose after the infant reaches 1 year of age. The World Health Organization (WHO) does not recommend tuberculin skin testing prior to BCG vaccination for infants and children, who are the largest group of individuals receiving BCG in the world. The WHO has recommended that, in populations where the risk of tuberculosis is high, human immunodeficiency virus (HIV)-infected children who are asymptomatic should receive BCG vaccine at birth or as soon as possible thereafter. However, in populations where the incidence of tuberculosis is low, the risk of disseminated BCG infection outweighs the potential benefit from BCG live vaccination. For unvaccinated infants, the Expanded Programme on Immunization (EPI) at WHO recommends simultaneous administration of BCG, measles, DTP, and polio vaccines. EPI, however, does not recommend mixing different vaccines in one syringe, and if vaccines cannot be given on the same day, then live vaccines should be separated by at least 4 weeks. These recommendations of the WHO are based on the fact that the separate administration of live vaccines is not practical or feasible in many developing countries where BCG usage is greatest.

### Geriatrics
Appropriate studies on the relationship of age to the effects of BCG vaccine have not been performed in the geriatric population. However, no geriatrics-specific problems have been documented to date.

### Drug interactions and/or related problems
The following drug interactions and/or related problems have been selected on the basis of their potential clinical significance (possible mechanism in parentheses where appropriate)—not necessarily inclusive (» = major clinical significance):

Note: Combinations containing any of the following medications, depending on the amount present, may also interact with this medication.

» Antitubercular agents
(antitubercular agents, such as isoniazid, rifampin, and streptomycin, inhibit multiplication of BCG; therefore, BCG vaccine may not be effective if administered during treatment with these medications)

» Corticosteroids
(possibility of the vaccine establishing a systemic infection)

» Immunosuppressant agents
(immunosuppressant agents may interfere with the development of the immune response and should be used only under medical supervision)

» Vaccines, killed or live virus
(concurrent administration with BCG is not recommended; it is recommended that live virus vaccines be given 6 to 8 weeks after BCG; and that killed virus vaccines be given 7 days before or 10 days after BCG)

### Laboratory value alterations
The following have been selected on the basis of their potential clinical significance (possible effect in parentheses where appropriate)—not necessarily inclusive (» = major clinical significance):

With diagnostic test results

Tuberculin, purified protein derivative (PPD)
(a positive reaction is produced in most patients, usually 6 to 12 weeks after BCG vaccination; however, administration of a tuberculin test a few years after BCG vaccination may result in either positive or negative reaction)

### Medical considerations/Contraindications
The medical considerations/contraindications included have been selected on the basis of their potential clinical significance (reasons given in parentheses where appropriate)—not necessarily inclusive (» = major clinical significance).

*Except under special circumstances, this medication should not be used when the following medical problems exist:*

» Fever
(BCG should not be administered until the cause of the fever has been determined; if the fever is caused by infection, BCG should be withheld until the patient is afebrile and off all therapy)

» Impaired immune response, including that associated with HIV infection
(BCG vaccine is less effective in patients with decreased natural immunity; in addition, the risk of disseminated BCG infection may be increased)

*Risk-benefit should be considered when the following medical problems exist:*

Extensive skin infections

Sensitivity to BCG live or any of its component substances

### Patient monitoring
The following may be especially important in patient monitoring (other tests may be warranted in some patients, depending on condition; » = major clinical significance):

Tuberculin, PPD skin test
(it is usually impossible to distinguish between tuberculin sensitivity caused by *M. tuberculosis* infection and tuberculin sensitivity resulting from the vaccine; therefore, caution should be exercised in interpreting tuberculin skin test reactions)

## Side/Adverse Effects

Note: The initial skin lesions, which are small red papules, appear in 10 to 14 days and reach a maximum diameter of 3 mm each after 4 to 6 weeks, which may scale and slowly subside. If not an abscess forms, which usually softens and tends to open spontaneously. The abscess heals within a few weeks, and, in such instances, a scar may form. The intensity and duration of the local reaction depend on the depth of penetration achieved in administration and the individual variation in tissue reaction.

The following side/adverse effects have been selected on the basis of their potential clinical significance (possible signs and symptoms in parentheses where appropriate)—not necessarily inclusive:

### Those indicating need for medical attention
Incidence more frequent
**Abscesses** (accumulation of pus); **dermatologic reactions** (peeling or scaling of the skin); **granulomas** (aggregation of inflammatory cells); **lymphadenitis** (inflammation of 1 or more lymph nodes); **ulceration at site of injection** (sores at place of injection)

Incidence rare
**Allergic reaction or erythema nodosum** (skin rash); **BCG infection, disseminated** (fever; cough); **osteomyelitis** (increase in bone pain)

Note: Symptoms of disseminated BCG infection may be difficult to distinguish from those of gram-negative sepsis or severe hypersensitivity reactions. Disseminated BCG infection is usually diagnosed based on the presence of fever and chills. Disseminated infection following BCG administration has occurred in individuals with impaired immune responses, especially children. It has also occurred following administration of BCG vaccine in patients with acquired immune deficiency syndrome (AIDS) and symptomatic HIV infection, and, rarely, in patients with asymptomatic HIV infection. If disseminated BCG infection is suspected in an individual who has received BCG live, appropriate antitubercular therapy should be initiated.

## Patient Consultation

As an aid to patient consultation, refer to *Advice for the Patient, Bacillus Calmette-Guérin (BCG) Live (Systemic)*.

In providing consultation, consider emphasizing the following selected information (» = major clinical significance):

### Before receiving this vaccine
» Conditions affecting use, especially:
  Sensitivity to BCG live
  Other medications, especially antitubercular agents, corticosteroids, immunosuppressant agents, or killed or live virus vaccines
  Other medical problems, especially fever, or impaired immune response, including symptomatic HIV infection

### Proper use of this vaccine
» Importance of telling the patient that the vaccine contains live organisms
» Proper dosing

### Side/adverse effects
Signs of potential side effects, especially abscesses, allergic reaction or erythema nodosum, dermatologic reactions, disseminated BCG infection, granulomas, lymphadenitis, oseteomyelitis, and ulceration at site of injection.

## General Dosing Information

The potency of BCG vaccines varies markedly and is related to several factors. These factors include the intrinsic immunogenicity of the particular strain, as well as other properties conferred by the method of preparation of the vaccine. In each country, the use of a particular vaccine depends on what is permitted by the national control authority and is based on the results of controlled field trials, which may not have included the particular national vaccine. The results have shown considerable variations, depending on the particular vaccines included, and may also be related to the immunity status of the subject population.

BCG live vaccine for immunization against tuberculosis should be administered according to the manufacturer's instructions.

Before the vaccine is administered, the risks and benefits of the vaccination should be fully explained to the patient, parent, or guardian.

The patient should be advised that the vaccine contains live organisms.

BCG live vaccine should be used with caution in individuals with asymptomatic HIV infection and in individuals known to be at high risk for HIV infection.

BCG live vaccine should be administered only to individuals with a negative tuberculin skin test. The tuberculin skin test (preferably done by Mantoux method) should be performed within 6 weeks prior to administration of BCG live vaccine. In persons highly sensitive to tuberculosis antigens, severe reactions may occur. However, the WHO does not recommend tuberculin skin testing prior to BCG vaccination for infants and children, who are the largest group of individuals receiving BCG in the world.

### For BCG vaccine (Tice strain)
BCG vaccine (Tice strain) is administered percutaneously, using a sterile multiple-puncture disk. The multiple-puncture disk is a thin wafer-like stainless steel plate from which 36 points protrude. The disk is held by magnet type holder. In this method of administration a drop of vaccine is placed on the patient's arm and spread with the wide edge of the disk. The disk is placed gently over the vaccine and the magnet is centered. The arm is grasped firmly from underneath, tensing the skin appreciably. Downward pressure is applied on the magnet so the points of the disk are well buried in the skin. With pressure still exerted, the disk is rocked forward and backward and from side to side several times. Pressure underneath the arm is then released and the magnet is slid off the disk. In a successful procedure, the points of the disk remain in the skin. If the points are on top of the skin, the procedure must be repeated. After a successful puncture, the disk is removed and the vaccine is spread evenly over the puncture area with the wide edge of the disk. Each disk should be used only once and discarded after autoclaving. The magnet should be sterilized after each individual vaccination.

### For BCG vaccine (Connaught strain)
BCG vaccine (Connaught strain) is administered intracutaneously into the outer surface of the upper arm. Repeat vaccination is advisable for individuals remaining tuberculin negative to the Mantoux test more than 3 months after the initial vaccination.

### For BCG vaccine (Montreal strain)
BCG vaccine (Montreal strain) is administered intradermally into the deltoid region of the arm or the upper external part of the thigh. Any unused portion of BCG vaccine and all material used for reconstituting the vaccine must be sterilized prior to disposal.

### For treatment of adverse effects
Recommended treatment consists of the following:
- Triple-drug antituberculosis therapy or
- Appropriate 3- or 4-drug antitubercular therapy.

## Parenteral Dosage Forms

### BCG VACCINE (TICE STRAIN) USP

**Usual adult and adolescent dose**
Tuberculosis (prophylaxis)—
  Percutaneous, 0.02 to 0.03 mL of the reconstituted vaccine.

**Usual pediatric dose**
See *Usual adult and adolescent dose*.

Note: If BCG live is indicated in neonates younger than 1 month of age, the dosage should be decreased by 50%. If indications persist and the tuberculin skin test is negative, a full dose of BCG live should be given after 1 year of age.

**Size(s) usually available**
U.S.—
  1 to $8 \times 10^8$ CFU, or approximately 50 mg (wet weight) per vial (Rx) [TICE BCG].
Canada—
  Not commercially available.

**Packaging and storage**
Store between 2 and 8 °C (35.6 and 46.4 °F). Protect from light.

**Preparation of dosage form**
Reconstituted by adding 1 mL (2 mL for neonates younger than 1 month of age) of sterile water for injection should be added to the vial using a sterile syringe. The mixture should then be drawn back into the syringe, and expelled again into the vial 3 times to mix it thoroughly.

### BCG VACCINE (CONNAUGHT STRAIN)

**Usual adult and adolescent dose**
Tuberculosis (prophylaxis)—
  Intracutaneous, 0.1 mL of the reconstituted vaccine.

**Usual pediatric dose**
Tuberculosis (prophylaxis)—
  Children 1 year of age and over: See *Usual adult and adolescent dose*.
  Children up to 1 year of age: Intracutaneous, 0.05 mL of the reconstituted vaccine.

**Size(s) usually available**
U.S.—
  Not commercially available.
Canada—
  Multi-dose vial (Rx) [GENERIC].

**Packaging and storage**
Store between 2 and 8 °C (35.6 and 46.4 °F). Protect from light.

**Stability**
Reconstituted vaccine should be used immediately and any that is unused by the end of the day should be destroyed. The reconstituted vaccine should be stored at 4 °C during the day of reconstitution.

### BCG VACCINE (MONTREAL STRAIN)

**Usual adult and adolescent dose**
Tuberculosis (prophylaxis)—
  Intradermal, 0.1 mL (0.075 mg of BCG) of the reconstituted vaccine.

**Usual pediatric dose**
Tuberculosis (prophylaxis)—
  Children 2 years of age and over: See *Usual adult and adolescent dose*.
  Children up to 2 years of age: Intradermal, 0.1 mL (0.0375 mg of BCG) of the reconstituted vaccine.

**Size(s) usually available**
U.S.—
  Not commercially available.
Canada—
  0.75 mg of freeze-dried vaccine per ampule (Rx) [GENERIC].

**Packaging and storage**
Store between 2 and 8 °C (35.6 and 46.4 °F). Protect from light.

**Preparation of dosage form**
1 mL (2 mL for children under 2 years of age) of the diluent supplied with the vaccine is added to the ampule via a sterile syringe. The suspension is then drawn into the syringe, and expelled again into the ampule, 2 times to ensure homogenicity. The ampule should not be shaken, to avoid frothing of the solution. The reconstituted solution should be allowed to stand for one minute before use.

## Selected Bibliography

Colditz GA, Brewer TF, Berkey CS, Wilson ME, Burdick E, Fineberg HV, et al. Efficacy of BCG vaccine in the prevention of tuberculosis. Meta-analysis of the published literature. JAMA 1994; 271(9): 698-702.

Centers for Disease Control. Use of BCG vaccines in the control of tuberculosis: a joint statement by the ACIP and the Advisory Committee for Elimination of Tuberculosis. MMWR. Morb Mortal Wkly Rep 1988; 37(43): 663-75.

Developed: 07/20/95

---

# BACLOFEN  Intrathecal-Systemic

VA CLASSIFICATION (Primary): MS200

Commonly used brand name(s): *Lioresal Intrathecal.*

Note: For a listing of dosage forms and brand names by country availability, see *Dosage Forms* section(s).

## Category
Antispastic.

## Indications

### General considerations
Although the manufacturer does not recommend that long-term intrathecal baclofen therapy be initiated in patients with spasticity due to traumatic injury until at least 1 year after the injury, some USP Advisory panelists recommend use sooner than 1 year in these patients.

Intrathecal baclofen may be used as an alternative to destructive neurosurgical procedures such as rhizotomies or phenol injections.

### Accepted
Spasticity, severe (treatment)—Intrathecal baclofen is indicated for the management of severe spasticity. It is used for the treatment of spasticity of spinal origin, including spinal cord trauma and multiple sclerosis, in patients who do not respond to or tolerate oral therapy. It is also used in patients with spasticity of cerebral origin, including traumatic brain injury and cerebral palsy.

## Pharmacology/Pharmacokinetics

### Physicochemical characteristics
Source—Analog of the inhibitory neurotransmitter gamma-aminobutyric acid (GABA).
Molecular weight—213.66.
pH—5 to 7.

### Mechanism of action/Effect
The precise mechanism of action of baclofen has not been fully determined. Baclofen exerts its effects as an agonist at presynaptic GABA-B (bicuculline-insensitive) receptors. It acts mainly at the spinal cord level to inhibit the transmission of both monosynaptic and polysynaptic reflexes, possibly by hyperpolarization of primary afferent fiber terminals, resulting in antagonism of the release of putative excitatory transmitters (i.e., glutamic and aspartic acids). Postsynaptic effects of baclofen have been demonstrated at concentrations above the therapeutic range. In addition, actions at the supraspinal sites may be involved.

### Other actions/effects
Baclofen has general central nervous system (CNS)–depressant actions. Animal studies demonstrated that baclofen also may have antinociceptive effects, possibly by acting at spinal and supraspinal sites to decrease the responsiveness of nociceptive neurons, thereby resulting in analgesia.

### Absorption
Following intrathecal administration of baclofen, concurrent plasma concentrations are expected to be low (0 to 5 nanograms per mL [nanograms/mL]).

### Distribution
Limited pharmacokinetic data suggest that baclofen injected into the lumbar cerebrospinal fluid (CSF) migrates upward. The concentration declines progressively upward along the neuroaxis during continuous infusion of therapeutic doses, thereby resulting in a lumbar-cisternal baclofen concentration gradient of approximately 4:1.

### Half-life
Elimination (CSF)—Following an intrathecal loading dose of 50 or 100 mcg over the first 4 hours: Approximately 1.5 hours.

### Onset of action
Following intrathecal loading dose of 50 or 100 mcg over the first 4 hours—Approximately 0.5 to 1 hour.
Following intrathecal continuous infusion—Approximately 6 to 8 hours.

### Time to peak concentration
Following intrathecal continuous infusion of 50 to 1200 mcg a day (time to CSF steady-state concentration)—Within 1 to 2 days.

### Peak serum concentration
Following intrathecal continuous infusion of 50 to 1200 mcg a day (peak CSF steady-state concentration)—Approximately 130 to 1240 nanograms/mL.

### Time to peak effect
Following intrathecal loading dose—Approximately 4 hours.
Following continuous infusion—Approximately 24 to 48 hours.

### Duration of action
Following intrathecal loading dose—Approximately 4 to 8 hours.

### Elimination
Following a loading dose of 50 or 100 mcg, the CSF clearance of intrathecal baclofen was 30 mL per minute (mL/min). CSF clearance of baclofen following intrathecal administration of a loading dose or continuous infusion approximates CSF turnover, which suggests that the elimination occurs by bulk flow removal of CSF.

## Precautions to Consider

### Tumorigenicity
Studies in animals to evaluate the tumorigenic potential of intrathecal baclofen have not been done. However, a 2-year study found no increase in tumors in rats receiving oral baclofen at 30 to 60 times the oral maximum recommended human dose (MRHD) on a mg per kg of body weight (mg/kg) basis (10 to 20 times the MRHD on a mg per square meter of body surface area [mg/m$^2$] basis).

### Mutagenicity
No mutagenicity assays have been done to evaluate the mutagenic potential of intrathecal baclofen.

### Pregnancy/Reproduction
Pregnancy—Adequate and well-controlled studies in humans have not been done.

Studies done in rats have found that oral doses of baclofen 13 times higher than the MRHD on a mg/kg basis (3 times the MRHD on a mg/m$^2$ basis) resulted in an increase in the incidence of omphaloceles (ventral hernias) in fetuses of rats. In addition, a reduction in weight gain and food intake occurred in the dams. However, an increased incidence of omphaloceles did not occur in fetuses of rabbits or mice.

FDA Pregnancy Category C.

### Breast-feeding
Although orally administered baclofen is distributed into breast milk, it is not known whether intrathecal baclofen is distributed into breast milk. However, problems in humans have not been documented.

### Pediatrics
Children 4 years of age and older: Appropriate studies performed to date have not demonstrated pediatrics-specific problems that would limit the usefulness of intrathecal baclofen in children. Children should be of sufficient body mass to accommodate the implantable pump for long-term infusion.

### Geriatrics
No information is available on the relationship of age to the effects of intrathecal baclofen in elderly patients. However, elderly patients are more likely to have age-related renal function impairment, which may require adjustment of dose or dosing interval in patients receiving intrathecal baclofen. In addition, caution should be used in those elderly patients who may be especially susceptible to baclofen-induced central nervous system (CNS) toxicity.

### Dental
Prolonged use of intrathecal baclofen may decrease or inhibit salivary flow, contributing to the develoment of caries, periodontal disease, oral candidiasis, and oral discomfort.

### Drug interactions and/or related problems
» Alcohol or
» CNS depression–producing medications, other (see *Appendix II*)
(concurrent use with intrathecal baclofen may enhance CNS depressant effects)
Opioid (narcotic) analgesics
(concurrent use of epidural morphine has been reported to result in hypotension and dyspnea)

### Medical considerations/Contraindications
The medical considerations/contraindications included have been selected on the basis of their potential clinical significance (reasons given in parentheses where appropriate)—not necessarily inclusive (» = major clinical significance).

*Risk-benefit should be considered when the following medical problems exist:*
» Autonomic dysreflexia
(abrupt withdrawal of intrathecal baclofen may precipitate an episode of dysreflexia)
Epilepsy
(baclofen may cause deterioration of seizure control)
» Psychiatric disorders, pre-existing
(increased risk of baclofen-induced psychiatric disorders; careful monitoring is recommended)
» Renal function impairment
(may result in increased concentrations of intrathecal baclofen in patients with renal function impairment; reduction in dosage may be required)
Sensitivity to baclofen

Note: Caution is also required in patients who depend on spasticity to maintain upright posture and balance or to obtain and/or maintain increased body function for optimal function and care.

## Side/Adverse Effects
The following side/adverse effects have been selected on the basis of their potential clinical significance (possible signs and symptoms in parentheses where appropriate)—not necessarily inclusive:

**Those indicating need for medical attention**
Incidence more frequent
*Seizures*

Incidence less frequent or rare
*Asthenia* (muscle weakness); *central nervous system (CNS) effects* (mental depression; ringing or buzzing in ears); *hallucinations* (seeing, hearing, or feeling things that are not there); *respiratory depression* (shortness of breath or troubled breathing); *syncope* (fainting); *visual disturbances* (blurred vision; double vision)

Note: Ovarian cysts have been found in female patients treated with oral baclofen for up to one year. However, there have been no reports to date of ovarian cysts in female patients using intrathecal baclofen.

**Those indicating need for medical attention only if they continue or are bothersome**
Incidence more frequent
*Constipation; difficult urination; dizziness; headache*—may be due to pump or catheter dislodgement or kinking; *hypotonia* (muscle weakness); *nausea and/or vomiting; paresthesia* (numbness or tingling in hands or feet); *somnolence* (sleepiness)

Incidence less frequent
*Ataxia* (clumsiness, unsteadiness, trembling, or other problems with muscle control); *diarrhea; dry mouth; edema* (swelling of ankles, feet, or lower legs); *frequent urge to urinate; hypotension* (dizziness or lightheadedness, especially when getting up from a lying or sitting position); *infection at the implantation site* (irritation of the skin at the site where the pump is located); *insomnia* (difficulty sleeping); *pruritus* (itching of the skin); *sexual dysfunction; slurred speech or other speech problems; tremor* (trembling or shaking)

**Those indicating the need for medical attention if they occur after medication is discontinued**
*Dysreflexia* (facial flushing; headache; increased sweating; slow heartbeat); *hallucinations* (seeing, hearing, or feeling things that are not there); *rebound spasticity* (increase in muscle spasms); *seizures*

## Overdose
For specific information on the agents used in the management of intrathecal baclofen overdose, see *Physostigmine (Systemic)* monograph.
For more information on the management of overdose, **contact a Poison Control Center** (see *Poison Control Center Listing*).

### Clinical effects of overdose
The following effects have been selected on the basis of their potential clinical significance (possible signs and symptoms in parentheses where appropriate)—not necessarily inclusive:

Acute and/or chronic
*Asthenia* (muscle weakness); *dizziness, drowsiness, or lightheadedness; excessive salivation* (increased watering of the mouth); *mental confusion; nausea and/or vomiting; respiratory depression* (shortness of breath or troubled breathing); *seizures*

Note: Special attention should be given to recognizing the signs and symptoms of overdose during the screening and dose titration phase of treatment. Extreme caution should be used when filling the implantable pump. These pumps should only be refilled through the reservoir refill septum. Some pumps are also equipped with a catheter access port that allows direct access to the intrathecal catheter. However, direct injection into the catheter access port may cause a life-threatening overdose.

### Treatment of overdose
Turn the pump off and remove residual baclofen intrathecal solution from the pump. If lumbar puncture is not contraindicated, withdrawal of 30 to 40 mL of cerebrospinal fluid (CSF) is recommended to reduce CSF baclofen concentration. However, according to some USP Advisory panelists, this method is not effective in all cases of overdose.

Specific treatment—Use of physostigmine to reverse the drowsiness and respiratory depression. Physostigmine has been associated with the induction of bradycardia, cardiac conduction disturbances, and seizures; therefore, it should be administered with caution. See the package insert or the *Physostigmine (Systemic)* monograph for specific guidelines for use of this product.

Supportive care—May include maintaining an open airway, supporting ventilation, maintaining proper fluid and electrolyte balance, correcting hypotension, and controlling seizures.

## Patient Consultation
As an aid to patient consultation, refer to *Advice for the Patient, Baclofen (Intrathecal-Systemic)*.
In providing consultation, consider emphasizing the following selected information (» = major clinical significance):

**Before using this medication**
» Conditions affecting use, especially:
Sensitivity to baclofen
Use in children—Safe use in children up to 4 years of age has not been established
Use in the elderly—Caution should be used in those elderly patients who may be especially susceptible to baclofen-induced central nervous system (CNS) toxicity
Other medications, especially alcohol or CNS depression–producing medications
Other medical problems, especially autonomic dysreflexia, pre-existing psychiatric disorders, or renal function impairment

**Precautions while using this medication**
Regular visits to physician to check progress during therapy
» Avoiding alcohol or other CNS depressants during therapy unless approved by physician
» Caution when driving or doing anything else requiring alertness because of possible dizziness, drowsiness, lightheadedness, impairment of physical or mental abilities, false sense of well-being, or visual disturbances
Possible dryness of mouth; using sugarless gum or candy, ice, or saliva substitute for relief; checking with physician or dentist if dry mouth continues for more than 2 weeks
Caution when getting up from a lying or sitting position

**Side/adverse effects**
Signs of potential side effects, especially asthenia, CNS effects, hallucinations, respiratory depression, seizures, syncope, and visual disturbances

## General Dosing Information
Intrathecal administration of baclofen requires the use of implantable pumps approved by the FDA. Refer to the manufacturer's manual for the implantable pump approved for intrathecal infusion and for more specific instructions and precautions for programming the pump and/or refilling the reservoir.

The pump may be programmed to administer higher doses at night to reduce spasms and lower doses during the day for patients who need some rigidity for ambulation. Infusion rates may range from as low as 0.1 mL per hour (mL/hr) to as high as 1 mL/hr. However, changes in flow rate should be programmed to start two hours before the time of the desired clinical effect.

Guidelines for pump implantation:
- Prescribing physicians should be trained and educated in long-term intrathecal infusion therapy.
- Prior to pump implantation and initiation of long-term infusion, patients must demonstrate a positive clinical response to a baclofen dose administered intrathecally during a screening period.
- Patients should be infection-free prior to the screening period.
- During the screening phase and dose-titration period immediately following implantation, patients must be monitored closely in a fully equipped and staffed environment.
- Strict aseptic technique in filling the implantable pump is required to avoid bacterial contamination and serious infection.
- Extreme caution should be used when filling an implantable pump. These pumps should only be refilled through the reservoir refill septum. Some pumps are also equipped with a catheter access port that allows direct access to the intrathecal catheter. However, direct injection into the catheter access port may cause a life-threatening overdose.
- The maintenance dose may need to be adjusted during the first few months of therapy while patients adjust to changes in lifestyle due to the alleviation of spasticity. A sudden large requirement for dose escalation may indicate a catheter complication. Most patients will require gradual increases in dose over time to maintain optimal response during long-term therapy. However, most patients obtain the optimal response within a year.
- For patients with programmable pumps who have achieved relatively satisfactory control of spasticity on continuous infusion, further benefit may be attained by using more complex dosing schedules for delivery of intrathecal baclofen.

During long-term treatment with intrathecal baclofen, approximately 5% of patients became refractory to increasing doses. Although there is insufficient experience of treatment for tolerance, tolerance has been treated in hospitalized patients with a drug holiday consisting of gradually reducing the dose of intrathecal baclofen over a 2- to 4-week period and switching to alternative methods of spasticity management. After a few days sensitivity to baclofen may return, then intrathecal baclofen should be restarted at the initial continuous infusion dose.

## Parenteral Dosage Forms

### Baclofen Injection

#### Usual adult and adolescent dose
Antispastic—
Screening phase: Intrathecal, 50 mcg in a volume of 1 mL, administered into the intrathecal space by barbotage over a period of not less than one minute.

Note: The patient should be monitored for four to eight hours for a positive response consisting of a significant decrease in muscle tone, frequency of spasms, and/or severity of spasms. If the initial response is less than desired, a second dose of 75 mcg of baclofen in a volume of 1.5 mL may be administered intrathecally twenty-four hours after the first dose, and the patient should be monitored for an interval of four to eight hours. If a response is still inadequate, a final screening dose of 100 mcg in 2 mL may be administered twenty-four hours later.

Patients who do not respond to a 100-mcg intrathecal screening dose should not be considered for implantation of a pump for long-term infusions.

Post-implantation dose titration period: To determine the initial total daily dose of intrathecal baclofen following implantation, the screening dose that gave a positive effect should be doubled and administered over a twenty-four-hour period. However, if the efficacy of the loading dose was maintained for more than eight hours, the starting daily dose should be the screening dose delivered over a twenty-four-hour period.

Spasticity of spinal cord origin—After the first twenty-four hours, the daily dose should be increased slowly by ten to thirty percent increments only once every twenty-four hours, until the desired clinical effect is achieved.

Spasticity of cerebral origin—After the first twenty-four hours, the daily dose should be increased slowly by five to fifteen percent only once every twenty-four hours, until the desired clinical effect is achieved.

Note: No dose increase should be given in the first twenty-four hours, until the steady state is achieved.

Maintenance:
Spasticity of spinal cord origin—Intrathecal, 12 to 2003 mcg per day for long-term continuous infusion.

Note: Most patients are adequately maintained on 300 to 800 mcg per day. During periodic refills of the pump, the daily dose may be increased by ten to forty percent, but no more than forty percent, to maintain adequate symptom control. However, there is limited experience with daily doses greater than 1000 mcg per day.

Spasticity of cerebral origin—Intrathecal, 22 to 1400 mcg per day for long-term continuous infusion.

Note: Most patients are adequately maintained on 90 to 703 mcg per day. During periodic refills of the pump, the daily dose may be increased by five to twenty percent, but no more than twenty percent, to maintain adequate symptom control.

The daily dose may be reduced by ten to twenty percent if patients experience intolerable side effects.

#### Usual pediatric dose
Antispastic—
Children 4 years of age and older: See *Usual adult and adolescent dose* for cerebral spasticity.

Note: In clinical trials, pediatric patients under 12 years of age required a lower daily dose than adults (average daily dose of 274 mcg per day). However, patients over 12 years of age had the same dosage requirements as adults.

#### Usual geriatric dose
See *Usual adult and adolescent dose*.

#### Strength(s) usually available
U.S.—
50 mcg per mL (Rx) [*Lioresal Intrathecal*].
500 mcg per mL (Rx) [*Lioresal Intrathecal*].
2000 mcg per mL (Rx) [*Lioresal Intrathecal*].
Canada—
50 mcg per mL (Rx) [*Lioresal Intrathecal*].
500 mcg per mL (Rx) [*Lioresal Intrathecal*].
2000 mcg per mL (Rx) [*Lioresal Intrathecal*].

#### Packaging and storage
Store below 30 °C (86 °F), preferably between 15 and 30 °C (59 and 86 °F). Protect from freezing.

#### Preparation of dosage form
Intrathecal baclofen may be prepared with sterile, preservative-free sodium chloride for injection.

Note: For screening—A 50-mcg-per-mL concentration should be used for injection into the subarachnoid space.

For maintenance—The solution must be diluted for patients who require concentrations other than 500 mcg per mL or 2000 mcg per mL.

## Selected Bibliography
Lewis KS, Mueller WM. Intrathecal baclofen for severe spasticity secondary to spinal cord injury. Ann Pharmacother 1993; 27: 767-73.
Albright AL. Baclofen in the treatment of cerebral palsy. J Child Neurol 1996; 11: 77-83.

Developed: 07/08/98

# BACLOFEN Systemic

VA CLASSIFICATION (Primary/Secondary): MS200/CN103
Commonly used brand name(s): *Alpha-Baclofen*; *Lioresal*; *PMS-Baclofen*.
Note: For a listing of dosage forms and brand names by country availability, see *Dosage Forms* section(s).

## Category
Antispastic analgesic (in trigeminal neuralgia).

## Indications
Note: Bracketed information in the *Indications* section refers to uses that are not included in U.S. product labeling.

## Accepted

**Spasticity (treatment)**—Baclofen is indicated to relieve the signs and symptoms of spasticity caused by multiple sclerosis, spinal cord diseases, or spinal cord injury. It is especially useful in relieving flexor spasms and concomitant pain, clonus, and muscular rigidity. Baclofen may also improve bowel and bladder function in some patients with spinal lesions; however, it may not improve spastic stiff gait or manual dexterity.

[**Neuralgia, trigeminal (treatment)**][1]—Baclofen is used to reduce the number and severity of attacks of trigeminal neuralgia in patients who are not able to tolerate, or who have become refractory to the effects of, carbamazepine. In some patients, baclofen may provide additional benefit when used concurrently with carbamazepine.

## Unaccepted

Baclofen should not be used in patients who require spasticity to sustain upright posture or balance in locomotion, or to obtain increased function.

Baclofen may not be effective, and is not recommended, in the treatment of patients with cerebrovascular accident, parkinsonism, cerebral palsy, or trauma-induced cerebral lesions.

Baclofen is not indicated in the treatment of skeletal muscle spasm caused by rheumatic disorders.

---

[1]Not included in Canadian product labeling.

## Pharmacology/Pharmacokinetics

**Physicochemical characteristics**
Molecular weight—213.66.

**Mechanism of action/Effect**
The precise mechanism of action of baclofen has not been fully determined. It acts mainly at the spinal cord level to inhibit the transmission of both monosynaptic and polysynaptic reflexes, possibly by hyperpolarization of primary afferent fiber terminals resulting in antagonism of the release of putative excitatory transmitters (i.e., glutamic and aspartic acids). Actions at supraspinal sites may also be involved.

**Other actions/effects:**
Baclofen has general central nervous system (CNS)–depressant actions.

**Absorption**
Rapid and extensive but subject to interpatient variation. Also, the rate and extent of absorption may decrease with increasing doses.

**Protein binding**
Low.

**Biotransformation**
Hepatic; only about 15% of a dose is metabolized.

**Half-life**
2.5 to 4 hours.

**Onset of action**
Highly variable; may range from hours to weeks.

**Time to peak concentration**
2 to 3 hours.

**Peak serum concentration**
500 to 600 nanograms per mL (ng/mL)(2.34 to 2.81 micromoles/L) following a 40-mg single dose; concentration remains above 200 ng/mL (0.94 micromoles/L) for 8 hours.

**Therapeutic serum concentration**
80 to 400 ng/mL (0.37 to 1.87 micromoles/L).

**Elimination**
Renal; 70 to 85% of a dose is excreted unchanged within 24 hours. Small amounts may also be excreted via the feces. About 40% of a dose is usually excreted within 6 hours, and excretion is usually complete within 3 days; however, with chronic use the rate of excretion is subject to interpatient variation.

## Precautions to Consider

**Pregnancy/Reproduction**
Pregnancy—Studies have not been done in humans.
Some studies in rats have shown that baclofen increases the incidence of omphaloceles (ventral hernias) and incomplete sternebral ossification in the fetus when given in doses approximately 13 times the maximum recommended human dose (MRHD). However, these abnormalities did not occur in studies using mice or rabbits. Also, studies in rabbits have shown that baclofen causes an increased incidence of unossified phalangeal nuclei of forelimbs and hindlimbs in the fetus when given in doses approximately 7 times the MRHD. In addition, some studies in mice have shown that baclofen causes a reduction in fetal birth weight with consequent delays in skeletal ossification when given in doses 17 times or 34 times the MHRD.

**Breast-feeding**
Baclofen is distributed into breast milk. However, problems in humans have not been documented.

**Pediatrics**
No information is available on the relationship of age to the effects of baclofen in pediatric patients. Safety and efficacy in children up to 12 years of age have not been established.

**Geriatrics**
Geriatric patients may be especially at risk for the development of CNS toxicity, leading to hallucinations, confusion or mental depression, other psychiatric disturbances, or incapacitating sedation, during baclofen therapy. Also, elderly patients are more likely to have age-related renal function impairment, which may require a reduction of dosage in patients receiving baclofen.

**Drug interactions and/or related problems**
The following drug interactions and/or related problems have been selected on the basis of their potential clinical significance (possible mechanism in parentheses where appropriate)—not necessarily inclusive (» = major clinical significance):

Note: Combinations containing any of the following medications, depending on the amount present, may also interact with this medication.

Antidepressants, tricyclic
(concurrent use with baclofen may result in pronounced muscle hypotonia; caution is recommended)

Antidiabetic agents, oral or
Insulin
(baclofen may increase blood glucose concentrations; dosage adjustments of these medications and/or of baclofen may be necessary during and after concurrent therapy)

Antihypertensives or
Other hypotension-producing medications
(concurrent use with baclofen may increase the risk of hypotension; dosage adjustment of the antihypertensive agent may be needed)

» CNS depression–producing medications, other (See *Appendix II*) or
Monoamine oxidase (MAO) inhibitors, including furazolidone, procarbazine, and selegiline
(concurrent use may result in increased CNS-depressant and hypotensive effects; caution is recommended and dosage of one or both agents should be reduced)

**Laboratory value alterations**
The following have been selected on the basis of their potential clinical significance (possible effect in parentheses where appropriate)—not necessarily inclusive (» = major clinical significance):

With physiology/laboratory test values
Alanine aminotransferase (ALT [SGPT]) and
Alkaline phosphatase and
Aspartate aminotransferase (AST [SGOT])
(values may be increased)

Glucose, blood
(concentration may be increased)

**Medical considerations/Contraindications**
The medical considerations/contraindications included have been selected on the basis of their potential clinical significance (reasons given in parentheses where appropriate)—not necessarily inclusive (» = major clinical significance).

*Risk-benefit should be considered when the following medical problems exist:*

Cerebral lesions or
Cerebrovascular accident
(increased risk of CNS, respiratory, or cardiovascular depression; ataxia; and psychiatric disturbances such as hallucinations, euphoria, and mental excitation, confusion, or depression)

Diabetes mellitus
(baclofen may increase blood glucose concentrations)

Epilepsy
(baclofen may cause deterioration of seizure control, electroencephalographic [EEG] changes)

Psychiatric disorders, pre-existing
(increased risk of baclofen-induced psychiatric disturbances)

Renal function impairment
(baclofen may accumulate; reduction in dosage may be required)

Sensitivity to baclofen

Caution is also required in geriatric patients, who may be especially susceptible to baclofen-induced CNS toxicity and who are more likely than younger adults to have renal function impairment.

**Patient monitoring**
The following may be especially important in patient monitoring (other tests may be warranted in some patients, depending on condition; » = major clinical significance):

Electroencephalogram (EEG) and clinical state determinations (increased or periodic monitoring recommended for epileptic patients because baclofen may cause deterioration of seizure control and EEG changes in these patients)

## Side/Adverse Effects

Note: Chronic administration of baclofen to female rats has caused a dose-related increase in the incidence of ovarian cysts and in enlarged and/or hemorrhagic adrenal glands. The clinical relevance of these findings to humans is not known.

Many of the CNS, visual, and genitourinary side effects listed below may be symptoms associated with the underlying spastic disease rather than baclofen-induced.

The following side/adverse effects have been selected on the basis of their potential clinical significance (possible signs and symptoms in parentheses where appropriate)—not necessarily inclusive:

**Those indicating need for medical attention**
Incidence rare
*Bloody or dark urine; chest pain; CNS toxicity* (visual and auditory hallucinations; mental depression or other mood changes; ringing or buzzing in ears); *dermatitis, allergic* (skin rash or itching); *syncope* (fainting)

**Those indicating need for medical attention only if they continue or are bothersome**
Incidence more frequent
*CNS effects* (drowsiness [up to 63%]; dizziness or lightheadedness [up to 15%]; weakness [up to 15%]; confusion [up to 11%]); *muscle weakness*—may be caused by CNS effect or become apparent if baclofen-induced reduction of muscle tone unmasks existing paresis; *nausea*—4 to 12%

Incidence less frequent or rare
*CNS effects* (clumsiness, unsteadiness, trembling, or other problems with muscle control; false sense of well-being; headache [up to 8%]; muscle pain; numbness or tingling in hands or feet; slurred speech or other speech problems; trouble in sleeping [up to 7%]; unexplained muscle stiffness; unusual excitement; unusual tiredness [up to 4%]); *constipation*—2 to 6%; *difficult or painful urination or decrease in amount of urine; fluid retention* (swelling of ankles; weight gain); *frequent urge to urinate; or uncontrolled urination*—2 to 6%; *gastrointestinal irritation* (abdominal or stomach pain or discomfort; diarrhea); *loss of appetite; low blood pressure*—up to 9%; *pounding heartbeat; sexual problems in males; stuffy nose*

**Those indicating need for medical attention and/or reinstitution of therapy if they occur after medication is abruptly discontinued**
*Convulsions; hallucinations, visual and auditory; increased spasticity; mood or mental changes such as paranoid ideation or manic psychosis; unusual nervousness or restlessness*

## Overdose

For specific information on the agents used in the management of baclofen overdose, see *Atropine* in *Anticholinergic/Antispasmodics (Systemic)* monograph.

For more information on the management of overdose or unintentional ingestion, **contact a Poison Control Center** (see *Poison Control Center Listing*).

**Clinical effects of overdose**
The following effects have been selected on the basis of their potential clinical significance (possible signs and symptoms in parentheses where appropriate)—not necessarily inclusive:

Acute and chronic
*CNS toxicity* (blurred or double vision; convulsions; myosis; mydriasis; severe muscle weakness; strabismus); *respiratory depression* (shortness of breath or unusually slow or troubled breathing); *vomiting*

**Treatment of overdose**
To decrease absorption—May include emptying the stomach by induction of emesis and/or gastric lavage.
Specific treatment—Administration of atropine has been recommended to increase ventilation, heart rate, blood pressure, and core body temperature. See the package insert or *Atropine* in *Anticholinergic/Antispasmodics (Systemic)* monograph.

Supportive care—May include maintaining adequate respiratory exchange. Respiratory stimulants should *not* be used. Patients in whom intentional overdose is known or suspected should be referred for psychiatric consultation.

## Patient Consultation

As an aid to patient consultation, refer to *Advice for the Patient, Baclofen (Systemic)*.

In providing consultation, consider emphasizing the following selected information (» = major clinical significance):

**Before using this medication**
» Conditions affecting use, especially:
Sensitivity to baclofen
Use in the elderly—Increased risk of adverse CNS effects
Other medications, especially other CNS depression-producing medications

**Proper use of this medication**
» Proper dosing
Missed dose: Taking if remembered within an hour or so; not taking if not remembered within an hour; not doubling doses
» Proper storage

**Precautions while using this medication**
» Checking with physician before discontinuing medication; gradual dosage reduction is necessary
» Avoiding alcohol or other CNS depressants
» Caution if drowsiness, dizziness, visual disturbances, or impaired coordination occur
Diabetics: May increase blood sugar concentrations

**Side/adverse effects**
» Convulsions, hallucinations, mood or mental changes, increased spasticity, or unusual nervousness or restlessness may occur following abrupt withdrawal
Signs and symptoms of potential side effects, especially bloody or dark urine, chest pain, CNS toxicity, allergic dermatitis, and syncope

## General Dosing Information

Side effects may be minimized by initiating therapy with low doses, which should be increased gradually until the desired response is obtained.

If the desired response is not achieved after a reasonable trial period, the medication should be slowly withdrawn.

Lower doses may be required in patients with renal function impairment.

Convulsions, hallucinations, other psychiatric disturbances, and exacerbation of spasticity have occurred following abrupt withdrawal of baclofen; gradual reduction of dosage over a period of 2 weeks or more is recommended before the medication is discontinued.

## Oral Dosage Forms

Note: Bracketed uses in the *Dosage Forms* section refer to categories of use and/or indications that are not included in U.S. product labeling.

### BACLOFEN TABLETS USP

**Usual adult and adolescent dose**
Antispastic and
[Analgesic (in trigeminal neuralgia)][1]—
Oral, 5 mg three times a day initially, then increased by increments of 5 mg per dose every three days until the desired response is achieved.

Note: A smoother response may be achieved in some patients if the total daily dose is given in four divided doses.

**Usual adult prescribing limits**
Up to 80 mg daily.

Note: Higher doses may be required in some patients.

**Usual pediatric dose**
Safety and efficacy have not been established.

**Strength(s) usually available**
U.S.—
10 mg (Rx) [*Lioresal* (scored); GENERIC].
20 mg (Rx) [*Lioresal* (scored); GENERIC].
Canada—
10 mg (Rx) [*Alpha-Baclofen; Lioresal* (scored); *PMS-Baclofen*].
20 mg (Rx) [*Alpha-Baclofen; Lioresal* (scored); *PMS-Baclofen*].

**Packaging and storage**
Store below 40 °C (104 °F), preferably between 15 and 30 °C (59 and 86 °F). Store in a well-closed container.

518  Baclofen (Systemic)

**Auxiliary labeling**
- May cause drowsiness.
- Avoid alcoholic beverages.

[1]Not included in Canadian product labeling.

Revised: 07/09/91
Interim revision: 06/13/95

# BARBITURATES  Systemic

This monograph includes information on the following: 1) Amobarbital; 2) Aprobarbital[†]; 3) Butabarbital; 4) Mephobarbital; 5) Metharbital*[†]; 6) Pentobarbital; 7) Phenobarbital; 8) Secobarbital; 9) Secobarbital and Amobarbital.

VA CLASSIFICATION (Primary/Secondary):
  Amobarbital
    Oral—CN301
    Parenteral—CN301/CN400
  Aprobarbital
    Oral—CN301
  Butabarbital
    Oral—CN301
  Mephobarbital
    Oral—CN400
  Metharbital
    Oral—CN400
  Pentobarbital
    Oral—CN301
    Parenteral—CN301/CN400
  Phenobarbital
    Oral—CN301/CN400; GA900
    Parenteral—CN301/CN400; GA900
  Secobarbital
    Oral—CN301
    Parenteral—CN301/CN400

Note:  Controlled substances in the U.S. and Canada as follows:

| Drug | U.S. | Canada |
| --- | --- | --- |
| Amobarbital | II | C |
| Aprobarbital | III | |
| Butabarbital | III | C |
| Mephobarbital | IV | C |
| Pentobarbital | | |
|   Oral | II | C |
|   Parenteral | II | C |
|   Rectal | III | C |
| Phenobarbital | IV | C |
| Secobarbital | | |
|   Oral | II | C |
|   Parenteral | II | C |
| Secobarbital and Amobarbital | II | C |

Commonly used brand name(s): *Alurate*[2]; *Amytal*[1]; *Ancalixir*[7]; *Barbita*[7]; *Busodium*[3]; *Butalan*[3]; *Butisol*[3]; *Gemonil*[5]; *Luminal*[7]; *Mebaral*[4]; *Nembutal*[6]; *Nova Rectal*[6]; *Novopentobarb*[6]; *Novosecobarb*[8]; *Sarisol No. 2*[3]; *Seconal*[8]; *Solfoton*[7]; *Tuinal*[9].

Note:  For a listing of dosage forms and brand names by country availability, see *Dosage Forms* section(s).

*Not commercially available in the U.S.
[†]Not commercially available in Canada.

## Category

Sedative-hypnotic—Amobarbital; Aprobarbital; Butabarbital; Pentobarbital; Phenobarbital (parenteral only); Secobarbital.
Anticonvulsant—Amobarbital (parenteral only); Mephobarbital; Metharbital; Pentobarbital (parenteral only); Phenobarbital; Secobarbital (parenteral only).
Antihyperbilirubinemic—Phenobarbital.

## Indications

Note:  Bracketed information in the *Indications* section refers to uses that are not included in U.S. product labeling.

**Accepted**

Anesthesia, adjunct—Amobarbital, butabarbital, pentobarbital, phenobarbital (parenteral), and secobarbital are indicated for use as preoperative medication to help reduce anxiety and facilitate induction of anesthesia.

Narcoanalysis—Amobarbital (parenteral) may be indicated in narcoanalysis.

Epilepsy, tonic-clonic seizure pattern (treatment) or
Epilepsy, simple partial seizure pattern (treatment)—Phenobarbital, a long-acting barbiturate, is indicated as long-term anticonvulsant therapy for the treatment of generalized tonic-clonic and simple partial (cortical focal) seizures; mephobarbital and metharbital, also long-acting barbiturates, may be indicated as alternatives to phenobarbital.

Convulsions (treatment)
Seizures (prophylaxis and treatment)
Status epilepticus (treatment) or
Tetanus (treatment adjunct)—Parenteral barbiturates, especially phenobarbital, are indicated in the emergency treatment of certain acute convulsive episodes such as those associated with status epilepticus, eclampsia, meningitis, and toxic reactions to strychnine. They are also indicated as adjunctive treatment for acute convulsive episodes associated with tetanus.

Phenobarbital is used in the prophylaxis and treatment of febrile seizures.[1]

[Hyperbilirubinemia (prophylaxis and treatment)][1]—Phenobarbital (oral and parenteral) is used in the prevention and treatment of hyperbilirubinemia in neonates. It is used also to lower bilirubin concentrations in patients with congenital nonhemolytic unconjugated hyperbilirubinemia or chronic intrahepatic cholestasis.

[Ischemia, cerebral (treatment)][1] or
[Hypertension, cerebral (treatment)][1]—Pentobarbital (parenteral) is used for induction of coma to protect the brain from various states, including ischemia and increased intracranial pressure that follow stroke and head trauma; however, this use is controversial and further studies are needed.

Amobarbital, aprobarbital, butabarbital, pentobarbital, phenobarbital, secobarbital, and secobarbital and amobarbital have been used for the short-term treatment of insomnia; however, they generally *have been replaced* by benzodiazepines. If barbiturates are used, they are not recommended for long-term use since they appear to lose their effectiveness in sleep induction and maintenance after 2 weeks or less.

Amobarbital, aprobarbital, butabarbital, mephobarbital, pentobarbital, phenobarbital, and secobarbital have also been used for routine sedation to relieve anxiety, tension, and apprehension; however, barbiturates generally *have been replaced* by benzodiazepines for daytime sedation.

**Unaccepted**

Amobarbital (parenteral) has been used as a diagnostic aid in schizophrenia but it generally has been replaced by other agents.

Amobarbital (parenteral) has also been used in the management of catatonic and negativistic reactions; however, phenothiazines generally are more appropriate therapy for catatonic reactions. It has also been used in the management of manic reactions, although benzodiazepines and lithium are usually preferred.

[Phenobarbital (oral and parenteral) has been used in the treatment of familial, senile, or essential action tremors; however, it generally has been replaced by other agents, such as benzodiazepines and beta-adrenergic blockers.]

[1]Not included in Canadian product labeling.

## Pharmacology/Pharmacokinetics

See *Table 1*, page 531.

**Physicochemical characteristics**
Molecular weight—
  Amobarbital: 226.27.
  Amobarbital sodium: 248.26.

Aprobarbital: 210.23.
Butabarbital sodium: 234.23.
Mephobarbital: 246.27.
Metharbital: 198.22.
Pentobarbital: 226.27.
Pentobarbital sodium: 248.26.
Phenobarbital: 232.24.
Phenobarbital sodium: 254.22.
Secobarbital sodium: 260.27.

### Mechanism of action/Effect
Barbiturates act as nonselective depressants of the central nervous system (CNS), capable of producing all levels of CNS mood alteration from excitation to mild sedation, hypnosis, and deep coma. In sufficiently high therapeutic doses, barbiturates induce anesthesia. Recent studies have suggested that the sedative-hypnotic and anticonvulsant effects of barbiturates may be related to their ability to enhance and/or mimic the inhibitory synaptic action of gamma-aminobutyric acid (GABA).

Sedative-hypnotic—
Barbiturates depress the sensory cortex, decrease motor activity, alter cerebral function, and produce drowsiness, sedation, and hypnosis. Although the mechanism of action has not been completely established, the barbiturates appear to have a particular effect at the level of the thalamus where they inhibit ascending conduction in the reticular formation, thus interfering with the transmission of impulses to the cortex.

The mechanism of action of pentobarbital in protecting the brain from ischemia and intracranial pressure is not completely understood; however, it is related to pentobarbital's anesthetic action (produced by sufficiently high dosage) and possibly to the depression of neuronal activity and metabolism.

Anticonvulsant—
Barbiturates are believed to act by depressing monosynaptic and polysynaptic transmission in the CNS. They also increase the threshold for electrical stimulation of the motor cortex.

Antihyperbilirubinemic—
Phenobarbital lowers serum bilirubin concentrations probably by induction of glucuronyl transferase, the enzyme which conjugates bilirubin.

### Other actions/effects
Barbiturates have little analgesic action at subanesthetic doses and may increase reaction to painful stimuli.

Although phenobarbital, mephobarbital, and metharbital are the only barbiturates effective as anticonvulsants in subhypnotic doses, all of the barbiturates exhibit anticonvulsant activity in anesthetic doses.

Barbiturates are respiratory depressants; the degree of respiratory depression is dose-dependent.

Barbiturates have been shown to reduce the rapid eye movement (REM) phase of sleep or dreaming stage. Also, Stages III and IV sleep (slow-wave sleep, SWS) are decreased.

Animal studies have shown that barbiturates cause reduction in the tone and contractility of the uterus, ureters, and urinary bladder; however, concentrations required to produce this effect in humans are not attained with sedative-hypnotic doses.

Barbiturates have been shown to induce liver microsomal enzymes, thereby increasing and altering the metabolism of other medications or compounds.

### Absorption
Absorbed in varying degrees following oral, parenteral, or rectal administration.

Barbiturate sodium salts are absorbed more rapidly than the free acids because of rapid dissolution.

The rate of absorption is increased if barbiturates are taken well diluted or on an empty stomach.

### Distribution
Rapidly distributed to all tissues and fluids with high concentrations in the brain, liver, and kidneys.

Lipid solubility is the primary factor in distribution within the body. The more lipid soluble the barbiturate, the more rapidly it penetrates all tissues of the body; phenobarbital has the lowest lipid solubility and secobarbital the highest.

### Biotransformation
Hepatic, primarily by the hepatic microsomal enzyme system.

About 75% of a single oral dose of mephobarbital is metabolized to phenobarbital in 24 hours.

Metharbital is metabolized to barbital.

### Onset of action
Oral or rectal—Varies from 20 to 60 minutes.
Intramuscular—Slightly faster than for oral or rectal.
Intravenous—Ranges from almost immediately for pentobarbital sodium to 5 minutes for phenobarbital sodium.

### Therapeutic serum concentration
Anticonvulsant—Phenobarbital: 10 to 40 mcg per mL (43 to 172 micromoles/L).

Note: The optimal blood phenobarbital concentration should be determined by response in seizure control and the appearance of toxic effects.

To achieve blood concentrations considered therapeutic in children, higher-per-kg dosages of phenobarbital and most other anticonvulsants generally are required.

### Time to peak effect
Phenobarbital—Maximal CNS depression may not occur for 15 minutes or more after intravenous administration of phenobarbital sodium.

## Precautions to Consider

### Cross-sensitivity and/or related problems
Patients sensitive to one of the barbiturates may be sensitive to other barbiturates also.

### Carcinogenicity/Tumorigenicity/Mutagenicity
For butabarbital and secobarbital—No long-term studies in animals have been done to determine the carcinogenic and mutagenic potential of butabarbital or secobarbital.

For pentobarbital—Adequate studies have not been done in humans or animals to determine the carcinogenic potential of pentobarbital.

For phenobarbital—Studies in animals have shown that phenobarbital is carcinogenic in mice and rats following lifetime administration. It produced benign and malignant liver cell tumors in mice and benign liver cell tumors very late in life in rats. A study in humans did not provide sufficient evidence that phenobarbital is carcinogenic in humans.

### Pregnancy/Reproduction
Fertility—For butabarbital: No long-term studies in animals have been done to determine the effects of butabarbital on fertility.

Pregnancy—Barbiturates readily cross the placenta following oral or parenteral administration. They are distributed throughout fetal tissues, the highest concentrations being found in the placenta, fetal liver, and brain. Following parenteral administration, fetal blood concentration approaches maternal blood concentration. Barbiturates have been shown to cause an increased incidence of fetal abnormalities. Risk-benefit must be carefully considered when the medication is required in life-threatening situations or in serious diseases for which other medications cannot be used or are ineffective.

Third trimester: Use of barbiturates throughout the last trimester of pregnancy may cause physical dependence with resulting withdrawal symptoms in the neonate. In infants suffering from long-term exposure in utero, the acute withdrawal syndrome of seizures and hyperirritability has been reported to occur from birth to a delayed onset of up to 14 days.

Use of long-acting barbiturates, especially phenobarbital, as anticonvulsants during pregnancy is reportedly associated with a neonatal coagulation defect that may cause bleeding during the early neonatal period (usually within 24 hours of birth). This coagulation defect is characterized by decreased concentrations of vitamin K–dependent clotting factors and prolongation of the prothrombin time and/or the partial thromboplastin time. Vitamin K should be given to the mother during delivery and to the infant (intramuscularly or subcutaneously) immediately after birth.

Also, one study in humans has suggested that prenatal exposure to barbiturates may be associated with an increased incidence of brain tumors.

FDA Pregnancy Category D.

Labor and delivery—Barbiturates in hypnotic doses do not appear to inhibit uterine activity; however, full anesthetic doses of barbiturates decrease the force and frequency of uterine contractions.

Use of barbiturates during labor may cause respiratory depression in the neonate, especially the premature neonate, because of immature hepatic function.

If barbiturates are used during labor and delivery, it is recommended that resuscitation equipment be readily available.

### Breast-feeding
Barbiturates are distributed into breast milk; use by nursing mothers may cause CNS depression in the infant.

### Pediatrics
Some children may react to barbiturates with paradoxical excitement.

### Geriatrics
Geriatric patients may react to usual doses of barbiturates with excitement, confusion, or mental depression.

## Barbiturates (Systemic)

The risk of barbiturate-induced hypothermia may be increased in elderly patients, especially with high doses or in acute overdose of barbiturates.

In addition, elderly patients are more likely to have age-related hepatic or renal function impairment, which may require a reduction of dosage in patients receiving a barbiturate.

### Drug interactions and/or related problems

The following drug interactions and/or related problems have been selected on the basis of their potential clinical significance (possible mechanism in parentheses where appropriate)—not necessarily inclusive (» = major clinical significance):

Note: Combinations containing any of the following medications, depending on the amount present, may also interact with this medication.

Acetaminophen
  (therapeutic effects of acetaminophen may be decreased when the medication is used concurrently in patients receiving chronic barbiturate therapy because of increased metabolism resulting from induction of hepatic microsomal enzymes; also, risk of hepatotoxicity with single toxic doses or prolonged use of high doses of acetaminophen may be increased in alcoholics or in patients regularly using hepatic enzyme inducers such as barbiturates)

Addictive medications, other, especially CNS depressants with habituating potential
  (prolonged concurrent use may increase the risk of habituation; caution is recommended)

» Adrenocorticoids, glucocorticoid and mineralocorticoid or
  Chloramphenicol or
» Corticotropin or
  Cyclosporine or
  Dacarbazine or
  Digitalis glycosides or
  Metronidazole or
  Quinidine
  (effects may be decreased when these medications are used concurrently with barbiturates, especially phenobarbital, because of enhanced metabolism resulting from induction of hepatic microsomal enzymes; dosage adjustment of these medications, with the exception of digoxin, may be necessary)

» Alcohol or
» CNS depression–producing medications, other (See *Appendix II*)
  (concurrent use may increase the CNS depressant effects of either these medications or barbiturates; caution is recommended and dosage of one or both agents should be reduced)

Amphetamines
  (concurrent use may cause a delay in the intestinal absorption of phenobarbital)

Anesthetics, halogenated hydrocarbon
  (chronic use of barbiturates prior to enflurane, halothane, or methoxyflurane anesthesia may increase anesthetic metabolism leading to increased risk of hepatotoxicity)

  (chronic use of barbiturates prior to methoxyflurane anesthesia may increase formation of nephrotoxic metabolites leading to increased risk of nephrotoxicity)

» Anticoagulants, coumarin- or indandione-derivative
  (effects may be decreased when these medications are used concurrently with barbiturates because of increased metabolism resulting from induction of hepatic microsomal enzymes; also, bleeding may result when the barbiturate is discontinued; periodic prothrombin-time determinations may be required to determine if dosage adjustments of anticoagulants are necessary)

Anticonvulsants, hydantoin
  (concurrent use with barbiturates appears to produce variable and unpredictable effects on the metabolism of hydantoin anticonvulsants; blood concentrations of hydantoin anticonvulsants should be closely monitored when these medications are used concurrently)

Anticonvulsants, succinimide or
» Carbamazepine
  (concurrent use with barbiturates may result in increased metabolism, leading to decreased serum concentrations and reduced elimination half-lives of carbamazepine or succinimide anticonvulsants because of induction of hepatic microsomal enzyme activity; monitoring of serum concentrations as a guide to dosage is recommended, especially when carbamazepine or a succinimide anticonvulsant is added to or withdrawn from an existing regimen)

Antidepressants, tricyclic
  (effects of tricyclic antidepressants may be decreased when these medications are used concurrently with barbiturates, especially phenobarbital, because of increased metabolism resulting from induction of hepatic microsomal enzymes)

Calcium channel blocking agents
  (caution is advised during titration of calcium channel blocker dosage for those patients taking medication known to promote hypotension, such as barbiturate preanesthetics, since the combination may result in excessive hypotension)

Carbonic anhydrase inhibitors
  (osteopenia induced by barbiturates, especially phenobarbital, may be enhanced when carbonic anhydrase inhibitors are used concurrently; it is recommended that patients receiving concurrent therapy be monitored for early signs of osteopenia and that the carbonic anhydrase inhibitor be discontinued and appropriate treatment initiated if necessary)

» Contraceptives, estrogen-containing, oral
  (concurrent use with barbiturates, especially phenobarbital, may result in reduced contraceptive reliability because of accelerated estrogen metabolism caused by induction of hepatic microsomal enzymes; use of a nonhormonal method of birth control or a progestin-only oral contraceptive may be necessary)

Cyclophosphamide
  (concurrent use with barbiturates, especially phenobarbital, may induce microsomal metabolism to increase formation of alkylating metabolites of cyclophosphamide, thereby reducing the half-life and increasing the leukopenic activity of cyclophosphamide)

Disopyramide
  (concurrent use with barbiturates, especially phenobarbital, may reduce serum disopyramide to ineffective concentrations; therefore, monitoring of its serum concentrations is necessary during concurrent therapy)

» Divalproex sodium or
» Valproic acid
  (concurrent use may decrease the metabolism of barbiturates, resulting in increased serum concentrations, which may lead to increased CNS depression and neurological toxicity; barbiturate serum concentrations should be monitored to determine if dosage adjustment is necessary when these medications are used concurrently; also, the half-life of valproic acid may be decreased and dosage adjustment may be necessary)

  (in addition, phenobarbital may enhance valproic acid hepatotoxicity, presumably through the formation of hepatotoxic valproate metabolites)

Doxycycline
  (half-life of doxycycline may be shortened when this medication is used concurrently with barbiturates, especially phenobarbital, probably because of increased metabolism resulting from induction of hepatic microsomal enzymes; this effect may continue for up to 2 weeks after barbiturate therapy is discontinued; adjustment of doxycycline dosage during and after therapy or substitution of another tetracycline may be necessary)

Fenoprofen
  (concurrent use with phenobarbital may decrease the elimination half-life of fenoprofen, possibly because of increased metabolism resulting from induction of hepatic microsomal enzyme activity; fenoprofen dosage adjustment may be required)

Griseofulvin
  (absorption may be decreased when this medication is used concurrently with barbiturates, especially phenobarbital, resulting in decreased serum concentrations; although the effect of decreased serum concentrations on therapeutic response has not been established, concurrent use preferably should be avoided)

Guanadrel or
Guanethidine
  (concurrent use with barbiturates may aggravate orthostatic hypotension)

Haloperidol
  (concurrent use with barbiturate anticonvulsants may cause a change in the pattern and/or frequency of epileptiform seizures; dosage adjustments of anticonvulsants may be necessary; serum concentrations of haloperidol may be significantly reduced)

Hypothermia-producing medications, other (See *Appendix II*)
  (concurrent use with barbiturates in high doses or acute overdose may increase the risk of hypothermia)

Ketamine
  (concurrent use of ketamine, especially in high doses or when rapidly administered, with barbiturate preanesthetics may increase the risk of hypotension and/or respiratory depression)

Leucovorin
: (large doses may counteract the anticonvulsant effects of barbiturate anticonvulsants)

Levothyroxine
: (concurrent use of barbiturates may increase hepatic degradation of levothyroxine, which may result in increased requirements; dosage adjustment may be necessary)

Loxapine or
Phenothiazines or
Thioxanthenes
: (may lower the seizure threshold; dosage adjustment of barbiturate anticonvulsants may be necessary)
: (concurrent use of chlorpromazine with phenobarbital has been shown to increase the metabolism of chlorpromazine; therefore, phenobarbital may decrease serum concentrations of phenothiazines when used concurrently)

Maprotiline
: (in addition to possibly enhancing CNS depressant effects, concurrent use of maprotiline may lower the convulsive threshold, at high doses, and decrease the effects of barbiturate anticonvulsants)

Methylphenidate
: (concurrent use may increase serum concentrations of barbiturate anticonvulsants, especially phenobarbital, because of metabolism inhibition, possibly resulting in toxicity; dosage adjustment of the barbiturate anticonvulsant may be necessary)

Mexiletine
: (concurrent use with barbiturates may accelerate metabolism and result in decreased plasma concentrations of mexiletine; plasma concentrations of mexiletine should be monitored during concurrent use to ensure efficacy is maintained)

Monoamine oxidase (MAO) inhibitors, including furazolidone, pargyline, and procarbazine
: (concurrent use may prolong the CNS depressant effects of barbiturates, probably because metabolism of the barbiturate is inhibited)
: (concurrent use with barbiturate anticonvulsants may cause a change in the pattern of epileptiform seizures; dosage adjustment of the barbiturate anticonvulsant may be necessary)

Phenylbutazone
: (concurrent use may decrease the efficacy of barbiturates by inducing hepatic microsomal enzymes and increasing their metabolism; also, hepatic enzyme inducers such as barbiturates may increase phenylbutazone metabolism and decrease its half-life)

Posterior pituitary
: (concurrent use with barbiturates may increase the risk of cardiac arrhythmias and coronary insufficiency)

Primidone
: (although concurrent use with barbiturate anticonvulsants is rarely indicated, since primidone is metabolized to phenobarbital, it may cause a change in the pattern of epileptiform seizures because of altered medication metabolism and also increase the sedative effect of either primidone or the barbiturate anticonvulsant; decreases in primidone dosage may be necessary)

Rifampin
: (concurrent use with rifampin may enhance the metabolism of hexobarbital by induction of hepatic microsomal enzymes, resulting in lower serum concentrations; there are conflicting data on rifampin's effect on phenobarbital; dosage adjustment may be required)

Vitamin D
: (effects may be reduced by barbiturates, especially phenobarbital, because of accelerated metabolism by hepatic microsomal enzyme induction; vitamin D supplementation may be required in patients on long-term barbiturate anticonvulsant therapy to prevent osteomalacia, although rickets is rare)

Xanthines, such as:
Aminophylline
Caffeine
Oxtriphylline
Theophylline
: (concurrent use with barbiturates, especially phenobarbital, may increase metabolism of the xanthines [except dyphylline] by induction of hepatic microsomal enzymes, resulting in increased theophylline clearance; also, concurrent use may antagonize hypnotic effects of barbiturates)

**Laboratory value alterations**
The following have been selected on the basis of their potential clinical significance (possible effect in parentheses where appropriate)—not necessarily inclusive (» = major clinical significance):

With diagnostic test results
Cyanocobalamin Co 57
: (absorption of radioactive cyanocobalamin may be impaired by concurrent use of barbiturate anticonvulsants, especially phenobarbital)

Metyrapone test
: (increased metabolism of metyrapone by an hepatic enzyme inducer such as a barbiturate may decrease the response to metyrapone)

Phentolamine test
: (barbiturates may cause a false-positive phentolamine test; it is recommended that all medications be withdrawn at least 24 hours, preferably 48 to 72 hours, prior to a phentolamine test)

With physiology/laboratory test values
Bilirubin, serum
: (concentrations may be decreased in neonates, in patients with congenital nonhemolytic unconjugated hyperbilirubinemia, and in epileptics; this effect is presumably due to induction of glucuronyl transferase, the enzyme responsible for the conjugation of bilirubin)

**Medical considerations/Contraindications**
The medical considerations/contraindications included have been selected on the basis of their potential clinical significance (reasons given in parentheses where appropriate)—not necessarily inclusive (» = major clinical significance).

*Except under special circumstances, this medication should not be used when the following medical problem exists:*

» Porphyria, acute intermittent or variegata, or history of
: (barbiturates may aggravate symptoms by inducing enzymes responsible for porphyrin synthesis)

*Risk-benefit should be considered when the following medical problems exist:*

Anemia, severe
: (may be complicated by barbiturate-induced respiratory depression, especially with phenobarbital)

Asthma, history of
: (hypersensitivity reactions such as bronchospasm more likely to occur in these patients)

Diabetes mellitus, especially with phenobarbital

» Drug abuse or dependence, history of
: (predisposition of patient to habituation and dependence)

» Hepatic coma, premonitory signs of, or
Hepatic function impairment
: (barbiturates metabolized in liver; medication should be administered with caution and, initially, in reduced dosage)

Hyperkinesis
: (condition may be exacerbated)

Hyperthyroidism
: (symptoms may be exacerbated because barbiturates displace thyroxine from plasma proteins)

Hypoadrenalism, borderline
: (systemic effects of exogenous hydrocortisone and endogenous cortisol may be diminished by barbiturates)

Mental depression and/or
Suicidal tendencies
: (condition may be exacerbated, especially in elderly patients)

» Pain, acute or chronic
: (paradoxical excitement may be induced or important symptoms may be masked)

Renal function impairment, especially with intermediate- and long-acting barbiturates
: (barbiturates excreted primarily by kidneys; dosage reduction may be necessary)

» Respiratory disease involving dyspnea or obstruction, particularly status asthmaticus
: (serious ventilatory depression may occur)

» Sensitivity to barbiturate prescribed
: (in patients sensitive to barbiturates, severe hepatic damage can occur from ordinary doses and is usually associated with dermatitis and involvement of parenchymatous organs)

Caution should be used also in debilitated patients because they may react to usual doses with marked excitement, mental depression, and confusion

*For parenteral dosage forms only*
Cardiac disease
: (adverse circulatory reactions may occur with intravenous administration, especially with too-rapid administration)

Hypertension
 (hypotension may occur with intravenous administration, especially in these patients; slow administration usually prevents this occurrence)

**Patient monitoring**
The following may be especially important in patient monitoring (other tests may be warranted in some patients, depending on condition; » = major clinical significance):

Folate concentrations, serum
 (determinations recommended periodically because of increased folate requirements of patients on long-term anticonvulsant therapy with phenobarbital and possibly mephobarbital)

Hematopoietic function and
Hepatic function and
Renal function
 (determinations recommended at periodic intervals during prolonged barbiturate therapy)

Barbital concentrations, serum
 (determinations recommended when clinically indicated during metharbital therapy)

Phenobarbital concentrations, serum
 (determinations recommended as clinically indicated when phenobarbital or mephobarbital is used as an anticonvulsant)

## Side/Adverse Effects

Note: Exfoliative dermatitis and Stevens-Johnson syndrome, possibly fatal, may occur rarely as hypersensitivity reactions to barbiturates. If dermatologic reactions occur, the barbiturate should be discontinued.

Severe respiratory depression, apnea, laryngospasm, bronchospasm, or hypertension may occur with intravenous administration of barbiturates, especially if administered too rapidly.

Prolonged barbiturate therapy may result in osteopenia or rickets.

Barbiturate dependence may occur, especially following prolonged use of high doses. The characteristics of dependence include: a strong desire or need to continue taking the barbiturate; a tendency to increase the dose; a psychological dependence on the effects of the medication; and a physical dependence on the effects of the medication requiring its presence for maintenance of homeostasis and resulting in an abstinence syndrome when the barbiturate is discontinued. Symptoms of withdrawal are related to the pharmacokinetics of the specific barbiturate and can be severe and may even cause death.

The following side/adverse effects have been selected on the basis of their potential clinical significance (possible signs and symptoms in parentheses where appropriate)—not necessarily inclusive:

**Those indicating need for medical attention**
Incidence less frequent
 *Sensitivity to barbiturates* (confusion)—especially in geriatric or debilitated patients; *mental depression*—especially in geriatric or debilitated patients; *paradoxical reaction* (unusual excitement)—especially in children or geriatric or debilitated patients

Incidence rare
 *Agranulocytosis* (sore throat and/or fever); *allergic reaction* (skin rash or hives; swelling of eyelids, face, or lips; wheezing or tightness in chest)—especially in patients who have asthma, urticaria, angioedema, and similar conditions; *exfoliative dermatitis* (fever; red, thickened, or scaly skin); *hallucinations; hypotension or megaloblastic anemia* (unusual tiredness or weakness)—with chronic barbiturate use; *Stevens-Johnson syndrome* (bleeding sores on lips; chest pain; muscle or joint pain; painful sores, ulcers, or white spots in mouth; skin rash or hives; sore throat or fever); *thrombocytopenia* (unusual bleeding or bruising); *thrombophlebitis* (soreness, redness, swelling, or pain at injection site)—for parenteral dosage forms only

With prolonged or chronic use
 *Hepatic damage* (yellow eyes or skin); *osteopenia or rickets* (bone pain, tenderness, or aching; loss of appetite; muscle weakness; unusual weight loss)

**Those indicating need for medical attention only if they continue or are bothersome**
Incidence more frequent
 *Clumsiness or unsteadiness; dizziness or lightheadedness; drowsiness; "hangover" effect*

Incidence less frequent
 *Anxiety or nervousness; constipation; feeling faint; headache; irritability; nausea or vomiting; nightmares or trouble in sleeping*

**Those indicating possible barbiturate withdrawal and need for medical attention if they occur after medication is discontinued**
Minor symptoms—may occur within 8 to 12 hours and usually occur in the following sequence:
 *Anxiety or restlessness; muscle twitching; trembling of hands; weakness; dizziness; vision problems; nausea; vomiting; trouble in sleeping, increased dreaming, or nightmares; orthostatic hypotension* (feeling faint; lightheadedness)

Major symptoms—may occur within 16 hours and last up to 5 days
 *Convulsions; hallucinations*

Note: Intensity of withdrawal symptoms gradually declines over a period of approximately 15 days.

## Overdose

For specific information on the agents used in the management of barbiturate overdose, see:
 • *Charcoal, Activated (Oral-Local)* monograph; and/or
 • *Ipecac (Oral-Local)* monograph.

For more information on the management of overdose or unintentional ingestion, **contact a Poison Control Center** (see *Poison Control Center Listing*).

**Clinical effects of overdose**
The following effects have been selected on the basis of their potential clinical significance (possible signs and symptoms in parentheses where appropriate)—not necessarily inclusive:

Acute
 *Confusion, severe; decrease in or loss of reflexes; drowsiness, severe; fever; hypothermia* (low body temperature); *shortness of breath or slow or troubled breathing; slow heartbeat; slurred speech; staggering; unusual movements of the eyes; weakness, severe*

Note: In acute barbiturate overdosage, CNS and respiratory depression may progress to Cheyne-Stokes respiration, areflexia, slight constriction of the pupils (in severe toxicity, pupils may be dilated), oliguria, tachycardia, lowered body temperature, and coma. Typical shock syndrome (apnea, circulatory collapse, respiratory arrest, and death) may occur.

In extreme barbiturate overdosage, all electrical activity in the brain may cease. In this case an electroencephalogram (EEG) may be "flat," but this does not necessarily indicate clinical death since, unless hypoxic damage occurs, this effect is fully reversible.

Complications in barbiturate overdosage such as pneumonia, pulmonary edema, cardiac arrhythmias, congestive heart failure, and renal failure may occur.

In acute overdosage, the blood barbiturate concentration for some of the barbiturates relative to the degree of CNS depression in nontolerant persons is as follows:
See *Table 2*, page 531.

Chronic
 *Confusion, severe; irritability, continuing; poor judgment; trouble in sleeping*

**Treatment of overdose**
Treatment of barbiturate overdose is primarily supportive and consists of the following

To decrease absorption—
 If the patient is conscious and has not lost the gag reflex, emesis may be induced with ipecac syrup; care should be taken to prevent pulmonary aspiration of vomitus. After vomiting is completed, 30 to 60 grams of activated charcoal in a glass of water or sorbitol may be administered to prevent absorption and increase excretion of the barbiturate.
 If emesis is contraindicated, gastric lavage may be performed with a cuffed endotracheal tube in place with the patient face down. Activated charcoal should be left in the stomach and a saline cathartic may be administered.

To enhance elimination—
 If renal function is normal, forced diuresis may help to eliminate the barbiturate.
 Alkalinization of the urine increases renal excretion of some barbiturates, especially phenobarbital, also aprobarbital, and mephobarbital (which is metabolized to phenobarbital).
 Although hemodialysis or hemoperfusion is not recommended as a routine procedure, it may be used in severe barbiturate poisoning or if the patient is anuric or in shock.

Monitoring—
 Vital signs and fluid balance should be monitored.

Supportive care—
  An adequate airway should be maintained, with assisted respiration and administration of oxygen as needed.
  Blood pressure and body temperature should be maintained.
  Fluid therapy and other standard treatment for shock should be administered, if necessary.
  A vasopressor may be required if hypotension occurs.
  Fluid or sodium overload should be avoided, especially if cardiovascular status is decreased.
  Chest physiotherapy should be administered.
  If pneumonia is suspected, appropriate cultures should be taken and antibiotics should be administered.
  Also, appropriate care should be taken to prevent hypostatic pneumonia, decubiti, aspiration, and other complications that may occur with altered states of consciousness.
  Patients in whom intentional overdose is known or suspected should be referred for psychiatric consultation.

## Patient Consultation

As an aid to patient consultation, refer to *Advice for the Patient, Barbiturates (Systemic)*.

In providing consultation, consider emphasizing the following selected information (» = major clinical significance):

### Before using this medication
» Conditions affecting use, especially:
  Sensitivity to barbiturates
  Pregnancy—Barbiturates readily cross placenta; increase in incidence of fetal abnormalities (FDA Pregnancy Category D); use during third trimester of pregnancy may cause physical dependence with resulting withdrawal symptoms in neonate; long-acting barbiturates associated with neonatal coagulation defect that may cause bleeding during early neonatal period; use during labor may cause respiratory depression in neonate
  Breast-feeding—Barbiturates distributed into breast milk; use by nursing mothers may cause CNS depression in infant
  Use in children—Children may react to barbiturates with paradoxical excitement
  Use in the elderly—Elderly patients may react to usual doses of barbiturates with excitement, confusion, or mental depression; risk of barbiturate-induced hypothermia may be increased in elderly patients; elderly patients more likely to have age-related hepatic or renal function impairment, which may require a dosage reduction of barbiturates
  Other medications, especially alcohol, adrenocorticoids, corticotropin, other CNS depression–producing medications, coumarin- or indandione-derivative anticoagulants, carbamazepine, divalproex sodium, estrogen-containing contraceptives, or valproic acid
  Other medical problems, especially history of drug abuse or dependence, premonitory signs of hepatic coma, acute or chronic pain, or respiratory disease involving dyspnea or obstruction (particularly status asthmaticus)
  Caution if any laboratory tests required; possible interference with results of metyrapone test.

### Proper use of this medication
» Importance of not using more medication than the amount prescribed because of habit-forming potential
» Not increasing dose if medication appears less effective after a few weeks; checking with physician
» For anticonvulsant use: Compliance with therapy; not missing any doses
» Proper dosing
  Missed dose: If on scheduled dosing regimen—Taking as soon as possible; not taking if almost time for next dose; not doubling doses
*Proper administration*
  *For extended-release dosage form*
    Swallowing capsule or tablet whole
    Not breaking, crushing, or chewing
  *For suppository dosage form*
    Proper administration technique
» Proper storage

### Precautions while using this medication
Regular visits to physician to check progress during prolonged therapy
Checking with physician before discontinuing medication after prolonged use; gradual dosage reduction may be necessary to avoid the possibility of withdrawal symptoms
» Avoiding use of alcohol or other CNS depressants
» Suspected psychological or physical dependence: Checking with physician
» Suspected overdose: Getting emergency help at once

» Caution if dizziness, lightheadedness, or drowsiness occurs
» Use of another or additional method of contraception if taking estrogen-containing oral contraceptives concurrently

### Side/adverse effects
Signs of potential side effects, especially allergic reaction or intolerance to barbiturate, blood dyscrasias, exfoliative dermatitis, hallucinations, hepatic damage (with prolonged or chronic use), mental depression, paradoxical reaction, osteopenia or rickets (with prolonged or chronic use), or Stevens-Johnson syndrome
Unusual excitement may be more likely to occur in children and in elderly or very ill patients
Confusion and mental depression may be more likely to occur in elderly or very ill patients

## General Dosing Information

See *Table 2*, page 531.

Dosage of the barbiturates must be individualized, based on the patient's age, weight, and condition.

In patients with impaired hepatic function, lower doses should be used initially. Lower doses may be required also in patients with impaired renal function.

Patients on dialysis may require an increase in dosage.

Tolerance may occur with repeated administration of the barbiturates, especially of the long-acting ones and with large doses of the shorter-acting ones.

Prolonged administration of barbiturates as hypnotics generally is not recommended because they have not been shown to be effective for a period of more than 2 weeks.

Prolonged uninterrupted use of barbiturates, particularly the short-acting ones, may result in psychic or physical dependence.

Chronic use of barbiturates at doses 3 to 4 times the therapeutic concentration will usually produce physical dependence in about 75% of patients.

Daily administration in excess of 400 mg of pentobarbital or secobarbital for approximately 90 days is likely to produce some degree of physical dependence; a dosage of 600 to 800 mg taken for at least 35 days is sufficient to produce withdrawal seizures. The average daily dose for the barbiturate addict generally is about 1.5 grams.

Barbiturates should be withdrawn gradually in order to avoid the possibility of precipitating withdrawal symptoms.

To minimize the possibility of acute or chronic overdosage, the least possible quantity of a barbiturate should be prescribed and dispensed at any one time.

The toxic dose of barbiturates varies but generally an oral dose of 1 gram of most barbiturates produces serious poisoning in an adult. Death commonly occurs after 2 to 10 grams of ingested barbiturate.

### Diet/Nutrition
Patients on long-term anticonvulsant therapy with phenobarbital and possibly mephobarbital may have increased folic acid requirements. In addition, patients on long-term therapy may require supplements of vitamin D to prevent osteomalacia.

### For parenteral dosage forms only
Prior to administration, parenteral solutions should be inspected visually for particulate matter and discoloration, if possible.

For intravenous injections, it is preferable to use the larger veins to minimize the risk of irritation and the possibility of resulting thrombosis. Administration into varicose veins is not recommended because of poor circulation in these veins.

Intravenous injections should be administered slowly and patients should be carefully monitored during administration. This requires maintenance of blood pressure, respiration, and cardiac function and recording of vital signs. Equipment for resuscitation and artificial ventilation should be readily available.

Intramuscular injections should be administered deeply into large muscles, such as the gluteus maximus or vastus lateralis because superficial intramuscular injection may be painful and may produce sterile abscesses or sloughs.

No more than 5 mL, regardless of drug concentration, should be injected intramuscularly at any one site because of possible tissue irritation.

Parenteral solutions of barbiturate salts are highly alkaline; therefore, caution should be used to avoid perivascular extravasation or intra-arterial injection, since extravasation may cause local tissue damage with subsequent necrosis and intra-arterial injection may cause spasm, severe pain, and possibly gangrene.

### For rectal dosage forms only
Barbiturates may be administered rectally when oral or parenteral administration may be undesirable. If the rectal dosage form is not available,

the soluble sodium salt of the barbiturate may be incorporated in a retention enema.

To assure accuracy in dosage, suppositories should not be divided.

Rectal administration of barbiturates is not recommended for status epilepticus; intravenous injection is the preferred route of administration for this condition.

### For treatment of dependence
Treatment of dependence consists of the following
- Gradual withdrawal of the barbiturate.
- An example of the different withdrawal regimens used (all of which require an extended period of time) involves substituting a 30-mg dose of phenobarbital for each 100- to 200-mg dose of the barbiturate that the patient has been taking. The total daily amount of phenobarbital then is administered as a single dose or in 3 or 4 divided doses, not to exceed 600 mg per day. If signs of withdrawal occur on the first day of treatment, a loading dose of 100 to 200 mg of phenobarbital may be administered intramuscularly in addition to the oral dose. After stabilization on phenobarbital, the total daily dose is decreased by 30 mg a day as long as withdrawal is proceeding smoothly. This regimen may be modified by initiating treatment at the patient's regular dosage level and decreasing the daily dosage by 10% if tolerated by the patient.
- For infants physically dependent on barbiturates, initially a dose of 3 to 10 mg of phenobarbital per kg of body weight per day may be given. After withdrawal symptoms (hyperactivity, disturbed sleep, tremors, hyperreflexia) are relieved, the dosage of phenobarbital should be gradually decreased and completely withdrawn over a 2-week period.
- Also, barbiturate withdrawal may be accomplished with benzodiazepines, such as diazepam.

### For treatment of adverse effects
For extravasation into subcutaneous tissues—Recommended treatment includes
- Application of moist heat to affected area.
- Injection of a 0.5% procaine solution into the affected area.

For accidental intra-arterial injection—Recommended treatment includes
- Release of tourniquet or restrictive garments to permit dilution of injected medication.
- Injection of 10 mL of a 1% procaine solution into the artery and, if necessary, brachial plexus block to relieve spasm.
- Anticoagulant therapy may prevent thrombosis.
- Supportive treatment.

---

## AMOBARBITAL

## Summary of Differences
Category:
　Parenteral amobarbital also may be indicated as an anticonvulsant.
Indications:
　Parenteral amobarbital also may be indicated in narcoanalysis; and has been used in diagnosis of schizophrenia and for catatonic, negativistic, and manic reactions, but generally has been replaced by other agents.
Pharmacology/pharmacokinetics:
　Long-acting barbiturate—
　　Onset of action: 60 minutes or longer.
　　Duration of action: 10 to 12 hours.
　Protein binding—
　　Moderate.

## Additional Dosing Information
See also *General Dosing Information*.

### For parenteral dosage forms only
The rate of intravenous injection should not exceed 100 mg per minute for adults or 60 mg per square meter of body surface per minute for children. Faster rates of administration may cause serious respiratory depression.

Superficial intramuscular or subcutaneous injections may be painful and may produce sterile abscesses or sloughs.

## Oral Dosage Forms
### AMOBARBITAL TABLETS USP
**Usual adult dose**
Sedative-hypnotic—
　Hypnotic:
　　Oral, 65 to 200 mg at bedtime.
　Sedative:
　　Daytime—Oral, 50 to 300 mg a day in divided doses.
Note: Geriatric and debilitated patients may react to usual doses with excitement, confusion, or mental depression. Lower doses may be required in these patients.

**Usual pediatric dose**
Sedative-hypnotic—
　Hypnotic:
　　Dosage has not been established.
　Sedative:
　　Daytime—Oral, 2 mg per kg of body weight or 60 mg per square meter of body surface three times a day.
　　Preoperative—Oral, 2 to 6 mg per kg of body weight, up to a maximum of 100 mg per dose.

**Strength(s) usually available**
U.S.—
　Not commercially available.
Canada—
　30 mg (Rx) [*Amytal*].
　100 mg (Rx) [*Amytal*].

**Packaging and storage**
Store below 40 °C (104 °F), preferably between 15 and 30 °C (59 and 86 °F), unless otherwise specified by manufacturer. Store in a well-closed container.

**Auxiliary labeling**
- Avoid alcoholic beverages.
- May cause drowsiness.

**Note**
Controlled substance in the U.S. and Canada.

### AMOBARBITAL SODIUM CAPSULES USP
**Usual adult dose**
Sedative-hypnotic—
　Hypnotic:
　　Oral, 65 to 200 mg at bedtime.
　Sedative:
　　Daytime—Oral, 50 to 300 mg a day in divided doses.
　　During labor—Oral, 200 to 400 mg, repeated every one to three hours, if necessary, up to a total dose of 1 gram.
　　Preoperative—Oral, 200 mg one to two hours before surgery.
Note: Geriatric and debilitated patients may react to usual doses with excitement, confusion, or mental depression. Lower doses may be required in these patients.

**Usual pediatric dose**
Sedative-hypnotic—
　Hypnotic:
　　Dosage has not been established.
　Sedative:
　　Daytime—Oral, 2 mg per kg of body weight or 60 mg per square meter of body surface three times a day.
　　Preoperative—Oral, 2 to 6 mg per kg of body weight, up to a maximum of 100 mg per dose.

**Strength(s) usually available**
U.S.—
　200 mg (Rx) [*Amytal*; GENERIC].
Canada—
　200 mg (Rx) [*Amytal*].

**Packaging and storage**
Store below 40 °C (104 °F), preferably between 15 and 30 °C (59 and 86 °F), unless otherwise specified by manufacturer. Store in a tight container.

**Auxiliary labeling**
- Avoid alcoholic beverages.
- May cause drowsiness.

**Note**
Controlled substance in the U.S. and Canada.

## Parenteral Dosage Forms
### AMOBARBITAL SODIUM STERILE USP
**Usual adult dose**
Sedative-hypnotic—
　Hypnotic:
　　Intramuscular or intravenous, 65 to 200 mg.
　Sedative:
　　Intramuscular or intravenous, 30 to 50 mg two or three times a day.

Anticonvulsant—
  Intravenous, 65 to 500 mg.
Note: Geriatric and debilitated patients may react to usual doses with excitement, confusion, or mental depression. Lower doses may be required in these patients.

**Usual adult prescribing limits**
Intramuscular, up to 500 mg per dose.
Intravenous, up to 1 gram per dose.

**Usual pediatric dose**
Sedative-hypnotic—
  Hypnotic:
    Children up to 6 years of age—
      Intramuscular, 2 to 3 mg per kg of body weight per dose.
    Children 6 years of age and over—
      Intramuscular, 2 to 3 mg per kg of body weight per dose.
      Intravenous, 65 to 500 mg per dose.
  Sedative:
    Preoperative—
      Intravenous, 65 to 500 mg or 3 to 5 mg per kg of body weight per dose.
Anticonvulsant—
  Children up to 6 years of age:
    Intramuscular or intravenous, 3 to 5 mg per kg of body weight or 125 mg per square meter of body surface per dose.
  Children 6 years of age and over:
    Intravenous, 65 to 500 mg per dose.

**Size(s) usually available**
U.S.—
  500 mg (Rx) [*Amytal*].
Canada—
  500 mg (Rx) [*Amytal*].

**Packaging and storage**
Prior to reconstitution, store below 40 °C (104 °F), preferably between 15 and 30 °C (59 and 86 °F), unless otherwise specified by manufacturer.

**Preparation of dosage form**
Solutions of amobarbital sodium should be prepared aseptically with sterile water for injection. For preparation of various concentrations of solutions for injection, see the manufacturer's package insert.

**Stability**
After reconstitution, solution should be used within 30 minutes since amobarbital sodium hydrolyzes in solution or upon exposure to air. Solution should not be used if it does not become absolutely clear within 5 minutes after reconstitution or if a precipitate forms after the solution clears.

**Note**
Controlled substance in the U.S. and Canada.

---

### APROBARBITAL

## Summary of Differences
Pharmacology/pharmacokinetics:
  Intermediate-acting barbiturate—
    Onset of action: 45 to 60 minutes.
    Duration of action: 6 to 8 hours.
  Protein binding—
    Low.

## Oral Dosage Forms
### APROBARBITAL ELIXIR
**Usual adult dose**
Sedative-hypnotic—
  Hypnotic: Oral, 40 to 160 mg at bedtime.
  Sedative: Daytime—Oral, 40 mg three times a day.
Note: Geriatric and debilitated patients may react to usual doses with excitement, confusion, or mental depression. Lower doses may be required in these patients.

**Usual pediatric dose**
Dosage has not been established.

**Strength(s) usually available**
U.S.—
  40 mg per 5 mL (Rx) [*Alurate* (alcohol 20%; dextrose; saccharin; sorbitol; sucrose; FD&C Yellow No. 6; FD&C Red No. 40)].
Canada—
  Not commercially available.

**Packaging and storage**
Store below 40 °C (104 °F), preferably between 15 and 30 °C (59 and 86 °F), in a tight, light-resistant container, unless otherwise specified by manufacturer. Protect from freezing.

**Auxiliary labeling**
- Avoid alcoholic beverages.
- May cause drowsiness.
- Keep container tightly closed.

**Note**
Controlled substance in the U.S.

---

### BUTABARBITAL

## Summary of Differences
Pharmacology/pharmacokinetics:
  Intermediate-acting barbiturate—
    Onset of action: 45 to 60 minutes.
    Duration of action: 6 to 8 hours.
  Protein binding—
    Low.

## Oral Dosage Forms
### BUTABARBITAL SODIUM ELIXIR USP
**Usual adult dose**
Sedative-hypnotic—
  Hypnotic:
    Oral, 50 to 100 mg at bedtime.
  Sedative:
    Daytime—Oral, 15 to 30 mg three or four times a day.
    Preoperative—Oral, 50 to 100 mg sixty to ninety minutes before surgery.
Note: Geriatric and debilitated patients may react to usual doses with excitement, confusion, or mental depression. Lower doses may be required in these patients.

**Usual pediatric dose**
Sedative-hypnotic—
  Hypnotic:
    Dosage must be individualized by physician.
  Sedative:
    Daytime—Oral, 2 mg per kg of body weight or 60 mg per square meter of body surface three times a day.
    Preoperative—Oral, 2 to 6 mg per kg of body weight, up to a maximum of 100 mg per dose.

**Strength(s) usually available**
U.S.—
  30 mg per 5 mL (Rx) [*Busodium; Butalan; Butisol* (alcohol [by volume] 7%; tartrazine); GENERIC].
Canada—
  Not commercially available.

**Packaging and storage**
Store below 40 °C (104 °F), preferably between 15 and 30 °C (59 and 86 °F), unless otherwise specified by manufacturer. Store in a tight container. Protect from freezing.

**Auxiliary labeling**
- Avoid alcoholic beverages.
- May cause drowsiness.
- Keep container tightly closed.

**Note**
Controlled substance in the U.S.

### BUTABARBITAL SODIUM TABLETS USP
**Usual adult dose**
See *Butabarbital Sodium Elixir USP*.

**Usual pediatric dose**
See *Butabarbital Sodium Elixir USP*.

**Strength(s) usually available**
U.S.—
  15 mg (Rx) [*Busodium; Butisol* (scored); GENERIC].
  30 mg (Rx) [*Busodium; Butisol* (scored; tartrazine); *Sarisol No. 2;* GENERIC].
  50 mg (Rx) [*Butisol* (scored; tartrazine)].
  100 mg (Rx) [*Busodium; Butisol* (scored); GENERIC].
Canada—
  15 mg (Rx) [*Butisol* (scored; sodium 2 mg)].

**526  Barbiturates (Systemic)**

30 mg (Rx) [*Butisol* (scored; sodium 3 mg; tartrazine)].
100 mg (Rx) [*Butisol* (scored; sodium 10 mg)].

### Packaging and storage
Store below 40 °C (104 °F), preferably between 15 and 30 °C (59 and 86 °F), unless otherwise specified by manufacturer. Store in a well-closed container.

### Auxiliary labeling
- Avoid alcoholic beverages.
- May cause drowsiness.

### Note
Controlled substance in the U.S. and Canada.

---

## MEPHOBARBITAL

## Summary of Differences
Category:
  Indicated only as an anticonvulsant.
Pharmacology/pharmacokinetics:
  Biotransformation—
    About 75% of a single dose metabolized to phenobarbital in 24 hours.
  Long-acting barbiturate—
    Onset of action: 60 minutes or longer.
    Duration of action: 10 to 12 hours.
Patient consultation:
  Compliance with therapy when used as an anticonvulsant.

## Additional Dosing Information
See also *General Dosing Information*.
In epilepsy
- Therapy with mephobarbital should begin with small doses, the dosage being gradually increased over a period of 4 to 5 days until the optimum dosage is determined.
- When used to replace another anticonvulsant, the dosage of mephobarbital should be gradually increased while the dosage of the other medication is maintained initially and then gradually decreased in order to maintain seizure control.
- Mephobarbital may be alternated with phenobarbital therapy.
- When used in conjunction with phenytoin, the dose of phenytoin may need to be reduced, but the full dose of mephobarbital may be given.
- Mephobarbital should be withdrawn slowly in order to avoid precipitating seizures or status epilepticus. When the dosage is to be reduced to a maintenance level or discontinued, the amount should be reduced over a period of 4 to 5 days or possibly longer.

## Oral Dosage Forms
### MEPHOBARBITAL TABLETS USP

**Usual adult dose**
Anticonvulsant—
  Oral, 200 mg at bedtime to 600 mg a day in divided doses.
Sedative-hypnotic—
  Sedative: Daytime—Oral, 32 to 100 mg three or four times a day.
Note: Geriatric and debilitated patients may react to usual doses with excitement, confusion, or mental depression. Lower doses may be required in these patients.

**Usual pediatric dose**
Anticonvulsant—
  Children up to 5 years of age: Oral, 16 to 32 mg three or four times a day.
  Children 5 years of age and over: Oral, 32 to 64 mg three or four times a day.
Sedative-hypnotic—
  Sedative: Daytime—Oral, 16 to 32 mg three or four times a day.

**Strength(s) usually available**
U.S.—
  32 mg (Rx) [*Mebaral* (scored; lactose; starch; stearic acid; talc)].
  50 mg (Rx) [*Mebaral* (lactose; starch; stearic acid; talc)].
  100 mg (Rx) [*Mebaral* (lactose; starch; stearic acid; talc)].
Canada—
  30 mg (Rx) [*Mebaral* (lactose 65 mg)].
  100 mg (Rx) [*Mebaral* (lactose 59 mg)].

### Packaging and storage
Store below 40 °C (104 °F), preferably between 15 and 30 °C (59 and 86 °F), unless otherwise specified by manufacturer. Store in a well-closed container.

### Auxiliary labeling
- Avoid alcoholic beverages.
- May cause drowsiness.

### Note
Controlled substance in the U.S. and Canada.

---

## METHARBITAL

## Summary of Differences
Category:
  Indicated only as an anticonvulsant.
Pharmacology/pharmacokinetics:
  Biotransformation—
    Metabolized to barbital.
  Long-acting barbiturate—
    Onset of action: 60 minutes or longer.
    Duration of action: 10 to 12 hours.
Patient consultation:
  Compliance with therapy.

## Additional Dosing Information
See also *General Dosing Information*.

Metharbital should be withdrawn gradually in order to avoid the possibility of precipitating seizures or status epilepticus.

When used to replace or supplement other anticonvulsant therapy, the dosage of metharbital should be gradually increased while the dosage of the other medication is maintained initially and then gradually decreased in order to maintain seizure control.

## Oral Dosage Forms
### METHARBITAL TABLETS

**Usual adult dose**
Anticonvulsant—
  Oral, initially 100 mg one to three times a day, the dosage being increased up to 800 mg per day, if necessary.
Note: Geriatric and debilitated patients may react to usual doses with excitement, confusion, or mental depression. Lower doses may be required in these patients.

**Usual pediatric dose**
Anticonvulsant—
  Oral, 50 mg one to three times a day; or 5 to 15 mg per kg of body weight per day in divided doses.

**Strength(s) usually available**
U.S.—
  Not commercially available.
Canada—
  Not commercially available.
In other countries—
  100 mg [*Gemonil* (scored; lactose)].

### Packaging and storage
Store below 40 °C (104 °F), preferably between 15 and 30 °C (59 and 86 °F), unless otherwise specified by manufacturer. Store in a tight container.

### Auxiliary labeling
- Avoid alcoholic beverages.
- May cause drowsiness.

---

## PENTOBARBITAL

## Summary of Differences
Category:
  Parenteral pentobarbital also may be indicated as an anticonvulsant.
Indications:
  Parenteral pentobarbital also used to protect brain from ischemia and increased intracranial pressure that follow stroke and head trauma.
Pharmacology/pharmacokinetics:
  Short-acting barbiturate—
    Onset of action: 10 to 15 minutes.
    Duration of action: 3 to 4 hours.
  Protein binding—
    Moderate to high.

## Additional Dosing Information
See also *General Dosing Information*.

When administered during labor, doses greater than 200 mg may cause respiratory depression in the newborn.

**For parenteral dosage forms only**

The injection is for intramuscular or intravenous use only; it is not recommended for subcutaneous administration.

Intravenous injections should be made slowly, not to exceed 50 mg per minute, to avoid adverse respiratory and circulatory reactions.

## Oral Dosage Forms
### PENTOBARBITAL ELIXIR USP
**Usual adult dose**
Sedative-hypnotic—
　Hypnotic:
　　Oral, 100 mg (pentobarbital sodium) at bedtime.
　Sedative:
　　Daytime—Oral, 20 mg (pentobarbital sodium) three or four times a day.
Note: Geriatric and debilitated patients may react to usual doses with excitement, confusion, or mental depression. Lower doses may be required in these patients.

**Usual pediatric dose**
Sedative-hypnotic—
　Hypnotic:
　　Dosage must be individualized by physician.
　Sedative:
　　Daytime—Oral, 2 to 6 mg (pentobarbital sodium) per kg of body weight per day.
　　Preoperative—Oral, 2 to 6 mg (pentobarbital sodium) per kg of body weight, up to a maximum of 100 mg per dose.

**Strength(s) usually available**
U.S.—
　20 mg of pentobarbital sodium (18.2 mg of pentobarbital) per 5 mL (Rx) [*Nembutal* (alcohol 18%)].
Canada—
　Not commercially available.

**Packaging and storage**
Store below 40 °C (104 °F), preferably between 15 and 30 °C (59 and 86 °F), unless otherwise specified by manufacturer. Store in a tight container. Protect from freezing.

**Auxiliary labeling**
- Avoid alcoholic beverages.
- May cause drowsiness.
- Keep container tightly closed.

**Note**
Controlled substance in the U.S.

### PENTOBARBITAL SODIUM CAPSULES USP
**Usual adult dose**
Sedative-hypnotic—
　Hypnotic: Oral, 100 mg at bedtime.
　Sedative: Preoperative—Oral, 100 mg.
Note: Geriatric and debilitated patients may react to usual doses with excitement, confusion, or mental depression. Lower doses may be required in these patients.

**Usual pediatric dose**
Sedative-hypnotic—
　Hypnotic: Dosage must be individualized by physician.
　Sedative: Preoperative—Oral, 2 to 6 mg per kg of body weight, up to a maximum of 100 mg per dose.

**Strength(s) usually available**
U.S.—
　50 mg (Rx) [*Nembutal;* GENERIC].
　100 mg (Rx) [*Nembutal* (tartrazine); GENERIC].
Canada—
　100 mg (Rx) [*Nembutal* (tartrazine); *Novopentobarb*].

**Packaging and storage**
Store below 40 °C (104 °F), preferably between 15 and 30 °C (59 and 86 °F), unless otherwise specified by manufacturer. Store in a tight container.

**Auxiliary labeling**
- Avoid alcoholic beverages.
- May cause drowsiness.

**Note**
Controlled substance in the U.S. and Canada.

## Parenteral Dosage Forms
### PENTOBARBITAL SODIUM INJECTION USP
**Usual adult dose**
Sedative-hypnotic—
　Hypnotic:
　　Intramuscular, 150 to 200 mg.
　　Intravenous, 100 mg initially; after one minute, additional small doses may be administered at one-minute intervals, if necessary, up to a total of 500 mg.
　Sedative:
　　Preoperative—Intramuscular, 150 to 200 mg.
Anticonvulsant—
　Intravenous, 100 mg initially; after one minute, additional small doses may be administered at one-minute intervals, if necessary, up to a total of 500 mg.
Note: Geriatric and debilitated patients may react to usual doses with excitement, confusion, or mental depression. Lower doses may be required in these patients.

**Usual pediatric dose**
Sedative-hypnotic—
　Hypnotic:
　　Intramuscular, 2 to 6 mg per kg of body weight, up to a maximum of 100 mg per dose.
　　Intravenous, 50 mg initially; after one minute, additional small doses may be administered at one-minute intervals, if necessary, until desired effect is obtained.
　Sedative:
　　Preoperative—Intramuscular, 2 to 6 mg per kg of body weight, up to a maximum of 100 mg per dose.
Anticonvulsant—
　Intramuscular or intravenous, 50 mg initially; after one minute, additional small doses may be administered at one-minute intervals, if necessary, until desired effect is obtained.

**Strength(s) usually available**
U.S.—
　50 mg per mL (Rx) [*Nembutal* (alcohol 10%; propylene glycol 40% v/v); GENERIC].
Canada—
　50 mg per mL (Rx) [*Nembutal* (alcohol 10%; propylene glycol 40%)].

**Packaging and storage**
Store below 40 °C (104 °F), preferably between 15 and 30 °C (59 and 86 °F), unless otherwise specified by manufacturer. Protect from freezing.

**Stability**
Do not use if solution is discolored or contains a precipitate.

**Note**
Controlled substance in the U.S. and Canada.

## Rectal Dosage Forms
### PENTOBARBITAL SODIUM SUPPOSITORIES
**Usual adult dose**
Sedative-hypnotic—
　Hypnotic:
　　Rectal, 120 to 200 mg at bedtime.
　Sedative:
　　Daytime—Rectal, 30 mg two to four times a day.
Note: Geriatric and debilitated patients may react to usual doses with excitement, confusion, or mental depression. Lower doses may be required in these patients.

**Usual pediatric dose**
Sedative-hypnotic—
　Hypnotic:
　　Children up to 2 months of age: Dosage has not been established.
　　Children 2 months to 1 year of age (4.5 to 9 kg): Rectal, 30 mg.
　　Children 1 to 4 years of age (9 to 18 kg): Rectal, 30 or 60 mg.
　　Children 5 to 12 years of age (18 to 36 kg): Rectal, 60 mg.
　　Children 12 to 14 years of age (36 to 50 kg): Rectal, 60 or 120 mg.
　Sedative:
　　Daytime—
　　　Rectal, 2 mg per kg of body weight or 60 mg per square meter of body surface three times a day.
　　Preoperative—
　　　Children up to 2 months of age: Dosage has not been established.

Children 2 months to 1 year of age: Rectal, 30 mg.
Children 1 to 4 years of age: Rectal, 30 or 60 mg.
Children 5 to 12 years of age: Rectal, 60 mg.
Children 12 to 14 years of age: Rectal, 60 or 120 mg.

**Strength(s) usually available**
U.S.—
- 30 mg (Rx) [*Nembutal* (semisynthetic glycerides)].
- 60 mg (Rx) [*Nembutal* (semisynthetic glycerides)].
- 120 mg (Rx) [*Nembutal* (semisynthetic glycerides)].
- 200 mg (Rx) [*Nembutal* (semisynthetic glycerides)].

Canada—
- 25 mg (Rx) [*Nova Rectal* (in a polyethylene glycol base)].
- 50 mg (Rx) [*Nova Rectal* (in a polyethylene glycol base)].

**Packaging and storage**
Store between 2 and 15 °C (36 and 59 °F), in a well-closed container, unless otherwise specified by manufacturer.

**Auxiliary labeling**
- For rectal use only.
- Avoid alcoholic beverages.
- May cause drowsiness.
- Refrigerate.

**Note**
Controlled substance in the U.S. and Canada.

---

## PHENOBARBITAL

## Summary of Differences
Category:
Also indicated as an anticonvulsant.
Oral and parenteral phenobarbital also used as an antihyperbilirubinemic; and has been used as an antitremor agent, although generally has been replaced by benzodiazepines and beta-adrenergic blockers.
Pharmacology/pharmacokinetics:
Distribution—
Distributed less rapidly than other barbiturates because it has lowest lipid solubility.
Time to peak effect—
Maximal CNS depression may not occur for 15 minutes or more after intravenous administration.
Long-acting barbiturate—
Onset of action: 60 minutes or longer.
Duration of action: 10 to 12 hours.
Protein binding—
Low to moderate.
Patient consultation:
Compliance with therapy when used as an anticonvulsant.

## Additional Dosing Information
See also *General Dosing Information*.
In epilepsy
- In children, higher-per-kg dosage of phenobarbital and most other anticonvulsants generally are required to achieve blood concentrations considered therapeutic.
- Several weeks of phenobarbital therapy may be required to achieve maximum antiepilepsy effects.
- Phenobarbital should be withdrawn slowly in order to avoid precipitating seizures or status epilepticus.
- When phenobarbital is replaced by another anticonvulsant, the dosage of phenobarbital should be maintained initially and then reduced gradually while, at the same time, the dosage of the replacement medication is increased gradually in order to maintain seizure control.
- When administered intravenously, phenobarbital sodium may require 15 minutes or more to attain peak concentrations in the brain; therefore, it is important to use the minimal dosage required and to wait for the anticonvulsant effect to develop before administering a second dose, in order to avoid the possibility of severe barbiturate-induced depression.

For parenteral dosage forms only
Sterile phenobarbital sodium may be administered subcutaneously after reconstitution, but phenobarbital sodium injection is not recommended for subcutaneous use.
The rate of the intravenous injection should not exceed 60 mg per minute. Faster rates of administration may cause serious respiratory depression.
Following intravenous administration, up to 30 minutes may be required for maximum effect.

**Bioequivalence information**
For phenobarbital tablets—
Bioavailability differences between generic products from different manufacturers have been reported in the past. However, no controlled studies systematically comparing the large number of tablets commercially available from different manufacturers have been conducted. In two studies published in 1979 and 1984 comparing phenobarbital tablets from different manufacturers in male volunteers, there were no significant differences in mean peak plasma concentrations ($C_{max}$) or relative area under the plasma concentration-time curve (AUC); however, statistically significant delays in reaching time of peak concentration ($t_{max}$) were demonstrated among products. In response to the potential problem of bio-inequivalence, official dissolution standards were changed, and problems have not been documented in the years following establishment of these standards. The current standard excludes slow-dissolving tablets.

## Oral Dosage Forms
Note: Bracketed uses in the *Dosage Forms* section refer to categories of use and/or indications that are not included in U.S. product labeling.

### PHENOBARBITAL CAPSULES
**Usual adult dose**
Anticonvulsant—
Oral, 60 to 250 mg (base) per day, as a single dose or in divided doses.
Sedative-hypnotic—
Hypnotic: Oral, 100 to 320 mg (base) at bedtime.
Sedative: Daytime—Oral, 30 to 120 mg (base) in two or three divided doses a day.
[Antihyperbilirubinemic][1]—
Oral, 30 to 60 mg (base) three times a day.

Note: Geriatric and debilitated patients may react to usual doses with excitement, confusion, or mental depression. Lower doses may be required in these patients.

**Usual pediatric dose**
Anticonvulsant—
Oral, 1 to 6 mg (base) per kg of body weight per day, as a single dose or in divided doses.
Sedative-hypnotic—
Hypnotic:
Dosage must be individualized by physician.
Sedative:
Daytime—Oral, 2 mg (base) per kg of body weight or 60 mg per square meter of body surface three times a day.
Preoperative—Oral, 1 to 3 mg (base) per kg of body weight.
[Antihyperbilirubinemic][1]—
Neonates: Oral, 5 to 10 mg (base) per kg of body weight per day for the first few days after birth.
Children up to 12 years of age: Oral, 1 to 4 mg (base) per kg of body weight three times a day.

**Strength(s) usually available**
U.S.—
- 15 mg (Rx) [*Solfoton*].

Canada—
Not commercially available.

**Packaging and storage**
Store below 40 °C (104 °F), preferably between 15 and 30 °C (59 and 86 °F), in a well-closed container, unless otherwise specified by manufacturer.

**Auxiliary labeling**
- Avoid alcoholic beverages.
- May cause drowsiness.

**Note**
Controlled substance in the U.S.

### PHENOBARBITAL ELIXIR USP
**Usual adult dose**
See *Phenobarbital Capsules*.

**Usual pediatric dose**
See *Phenobarbital Capsules*.

**Strength(s) usually available**
U.S.—
- 20 mg per 5 mL (Rx) [GENERIC].

Canada—
- 20 mg per 5 mL (Rx) [*Ancalixir*].

## Packaging and storage
Store below 40 °C (104 °F), preferably between 15 and 30 °C (59 and 86 °F), unless otherwise specified by manufacturer. Store in a tight, light-resistant container. Protect from freezing.

## Auxiliary labeling
- Avoid alcoholic beverages.
- May cause drowsiness.
- Keep container tightly closed.

## Note
Controlled substance in the U.S. and Canada.

## PHENOBARBITAL TABLETS USP
Note: Bioavailability differences between products from different manufacturers have been reported in the past. However, no controlled studies systematically comparing the large number of tablets commercially available from different manufacturers have been conducted. In two studies published in 1979 and 1984 comparing phenobarbital tablets from different manufacturers in male volunteers, there were no significant differences in mean peak plasma concentrations ($C_{max}$) or relative area under the plasma concentration-time curve (AUC); however, statistically significant delays in reaching time of peak concentration ($T_{max}$) were demonstrated among products. In response to the potential problem of bio-inequivalence, official dissolution standards were changed, and problems have not been documented in the years following establishment of these standards. The current standard excludes slow-dissolving tablets.

### Usual adult dose
See *Phenobarbital Capsules.*

### Usual pediatric dose
See *Phenobarbital Capsules.*

### Strength(s) usually available
U.S.—
   8 mg (Rx) [GENERIC].
   15 mg (Rx) [*Barbita; Solfoton;* GENERIC].
   30 mg (Rx) [GENERIC].
   60 mg (Rx) [GENERIC].
   100 mg (Rx) [GENERIC].
Canada—
   15 mg (Rx) [GENERIC].
   30 mg (Rx) [GENERIC].
   60 mg (Rx) [GENERIC].
   100 mg (Rx) [GENERIC].

### Packaging and storage
Store below 40 °C (104 °F), preferably between 15 and 30 °C (59 and 86 °F), unless otherwise specified by manufacturer. Store in a well-closed container.

### Auxiliary labeling
- Avoid alcoholic beverages.
- May cause drowsiness.

### Note
Controlled substance in the U.S. and Canada.

## Parenteral Dosage Forms
Note: Bracketed uses in the *Dosage Forms* section refer to categories of use and/or indications that are not included in U.S. product labeling.

## PHENOBARBITAL SODIUM INJECTION USP

### Usual adult dose
Anticonvulsant—
   Intravenous, 100 to 320 mg, repeated if necessary up to a total dose of 600 mg during a twenty-four-hour period.
   Status epilepticus: Intravenous (slow), 10 to 20 mg per kg of body weight, repeated if necessary.
Sedative-hypnotic—
   Hypnotic:
      Intramuscular or intravenous, 100 to 325 mg.
   Sedative:
      Daytime—Intramuscular or intravenous, 30 to 120 mg a day in two or three divided doses.
      Preoperative—Intramuscular, 130 to 200 mg sixty to ninety minutes before surgery.
Note: Geriatric and debilitated patients may react to usual doses with excitement, confusion, or mental depression. Lower doses may be required in these patients.

### Usual pediatric dose
Anticonvulsant—
   Initial: Intravenous, 10 to 20 mg per kg of body weight as a single loading dose.
   Maintenance: Intravenous, 1 to 6 mg per kg of body weight per day.
   Status epilepticus: Intravenous, 15 to 20 mg per kg of body weight, administered over a period of ten to fifteen minutes.
Sedative-hypnotic—
   Hypnotic: Dosage must be individualized.
   Sedative: Preoperative—Intramuscular or intravenous, 1 to 3 mg per kg of body weight, sixty to ninety minutes prior to surgery.
[Antihyperbilirubinemic][1]—
   Intramuscular, 5 to 10 mg per kg of body weight per day for the first few days after birth.

### Strength(s) usually available
U.S.—
   30 mg per mL (Rx) [GENERIC].
   60 mg per mL (Rx) [GENERIC].
   65 mg per mL (Rx) [GENERIC].
   130 mg per mL (Rx) [*Luminal* (alcohol 10%; propylene glycol 67.8% by volume); GENERIC].
Canada—
   30 mg per mL (Rx) [GENERIC].
   120 mg per mL (Rx) [GENERIC].

### Packaging and storage
Store below 40 °C (104 °F), preferably between 15 and 30 °C (59 and 86 °F), unless otherwise specified by manufacturer. Protect from freezing.

### Stability
Do not use if solution is discolored or contains a precipitate.

### Note
Controlled substance in the U.S. and Canada.

## PHENOBARBITAL SODIUM STERILE USP

### Usual adult dose
Anticonvulsant—
   Intravenous, 100 to 320 mg, repeated if necessary up to a total dose of 600 mg during a twenty-four-hour period.
   Status epilepticus: Intravenous (slow), 10 to 20 mg per kg of body weight, repeated if necessary.
Sedative-hypnotic—
   Hypnotic:
      Intramuscular, intravenous, or subcutaneous, 100 to 325 mg.
   Sedative:
      Daytime—Intramuscular, intravenous, or subcutaneous, 30 to 120 mg a day in two or three divided doses.
      Preoperative—Intramuscular, 130 to 200 mg sixty to ninety minutes before surgery.
Note: Geriatric and debilitated patients may react to usual doses of barbiturates with excitement, confusion, or mental depression. Lower doses may be required in these patients.

### Usual pediatric dose
Anticonvulsant—
   Initial: Intravenous, 10 to 20 mg per kg of body weight as a single loading dose.
   Maintenance: Intravenous, 1 to 6 mg per kg of body weight per day.
   Status epilepticus: Intravenous, 15 to 20 mg per kg of body weight, administered over a period of ten to fifteen minutes.
Sedative-hypnotic—
   Hypnotic: Dosage must be individualized.
   Sedative: Preoperative—Intramuscular, 1 to 3 mg per kg of body weight.
[Antihyperbilirubinemic][1]—
   Intramuscular, 5 to 10 mg per kg of body weight per day for the first few days after birth.

### Size(s) usually available
U.S.—
   120 mg (Rx) [GENERIC].
Canada—
   Not commercially available.

### Packaging and storage
Prior to reconstitution, store below 40 °C (104 °F), preferably between 15 and 30 °C (59 and 86 °F), unless otherwise specified by manufacturer.

### Preparation of dosage form
Solutions of phenobarbital sodium for subcutaneous or intramuscular injection may be prepared by dissolving 120 mg of anhydrous phenobarbital sodium powder in 1 mL of sterile water for injection. For intravenous use, 120 mg of anhydrous phenobarbital sodium powder should be dissolved in 3 mL of sterile water for injection. When solutions are

prepared, the sterile water for injection should be introduced slowly into the vial by means of a sterile syringe. Several minutes may be required for the medication to dissolve completely; solution should not be injected if it has not become clear after 5 minutes.

**Stability**
After reconstitution, solution should be used within thirty minutes since phenobarbital hydrolyzes in solution or upon exposure to air. Solution should not be used if it does not become absolutely clear within 5 minutes after reconstitution or if a precipitate forms after the solution clears.

**Note**
Controlled substance in the U.S.

[1]Not included in Canadian product labeling.

---

## SECOBARBITAL

## Summary of Differences
Category:
  Parenteral secobarbital also may be indicated as an anticonvulsant (in tetanus).
Pharmacology/pharmacokinetics:
  Distribution—
    Distributed more rapidly than other barbiturates because it has highest lipid solubility.
  Short-acting barbiturate—
    Onset of action: 10 to 15 minutes.
    Duration of action: 3 to 4 hours.
  Protein binding—
    Moderate to high.

## Additional Dosing Information
See also *General Dosing Information*.

**For parenteral dosage forms only**
The rate of the intravenous injection should not exceed 50 mg per 15-second period. Faster rates of administration may cause respiratory depression or apnea, laryngospasm, or vasodilation with fall in blood pressure.

**For rectal dosage forms only**
To prepare a solution for rectal administration, dilute the commercially available 5% secobarbital sodium injection with lukewarm tap water to a concentration of 10 to 15 mg per mL (1 to 1.5%).

## Oral Dosage Forms
### SECOBARBITAL SODIUM CAPSULES USP
**Usual adult dose**
Sedative-hypnotic—
  Hypnotic:
    Oral, 100 mg at bedtime.
  Sedative:
    Daytime—Oral, 30 to 50 mg three or four times a day.
    Preoperative—Oral, 200 to 300 mg one to two hours before surgery.
Note: Geriatric and debilitated patients may react to usual doses with excitement, confusion, or mental depression. Lower doses may be required in these patients.

**Usual pediatric dose**
Sedative-hypnotic—
  Sedative:
    Daytime—Oral, 2 mg per kg of body weight or 60 mg per square meter of body surface three times a day.
    Preoperative—Oral, 2 to 6 mg per kg of body weight, up to a maximum of 100 mg per dose, one to two hours before surgery.

**Strength(s) usually available**
U.S.—
  100 mg (Rx) [*Seconal*; GENERIC].
Canada—
  50 mg (Rx) [*Seconal*].
  100 mg (Rx) [*Novosecobarb; Seconal*].

**Packaging and storage**
Store below 40 °C (104 °F), preferably between 15 and 30 °C (59 and 86 °F), unless otherwise specified by manufacturer. Store in a tight container.

**Auxiliary labeling**
• Avoid alcoholic beverages.
• May cause drowsiness.

**Note**
Controlled substance in the U.S. and Canada.

## Parenteral Dosage Forms
### SECOBARBITAL SODIUM INJECTION USP
**Usual adult dose**
Sedative-hypnotic—
  Hypnotic:
    Intramuscular, 100 to 200 mg.
    Intravenous, 50 to 250 mg.
  Sedative:
    Dentistry—Intramuscular, 1.1 to 2.2 mg per kg of body weight ten to fifteen minutes before procedure.
    Nerve block—Intravenous, 100 to 150 mg.
Anticonvulsant (in tetanus)—
  Intramuscular or intravenous, 5.5 mg per kg of body weight, repeated every three to four hours as needed.
Note: Geriatric and debilitated patients may react to usual doses of barbiturates with excitement, confusion, or mental depression. Lower doses may be required in these patients.

**Usual pediatric dose**
Sedative-hypnotic—
  Hypnotic:
    Intramuscular—
      3 to 5 mg per kg of body weight or 125 mg per square meter of body surface, up to a maximum of 100 mg per dose.
    Rectal, the following doses as a 1 to 1.5% solution—
      Children weighing up to 40 kg: 5 mg per kg of body weight.
      Children weighing 40 kg and over: 4 mg per kg of body weight.
  Sedative:
    Preoperative—
      Intramuscular, 4 to 5 mg per kg of body weight.
Anticonvulsant (in tetanus)—
  Intramuscular or intravenous, 3 to 5 mg per kg of body weight or 125 mg per square meter of body surface per dose.

**Strength(s) usually available**
U.S.—
  50 mg per mL (Rx) [GENERIC].
Canada—
  Not commercially available.

**Packaging and storage**
Store between 2 and 8 °C (36 and 46 °F). Protect from light.

**Preparation of dosage form**
Secobarbital sodium injection may be administered in a concentration of 50 mg per mL or it may be diluted with sterile water for injection, 0.9% sodium chloride injection, or Ringer's injection.

**Stability**
Do not use if solution is discolored or contains a precipitate.

**Note**
Controlled substance in the U.S.

---

## SECOBARBITAL AND AMOBARBITAL

## Oral Dosage Forms
### SECOBARBITAL SODIUM AND AMOBARBITAL SODIUM CAPSULES USP
**Usual adult dose**
Sedative-hypnotic—
  Oral, 1 capsule at bedtime or one hour preoperatively.
Note: Geriatric and debilitated patients may react to usual doses with excitement, confusion, or mental depression. Lower doses may be required in these patients.

**Usual pediatric dose**
Dosage has not been established.

**Strength(s) usually available**
U.S.—
  50 mg of secobarbital and 50 mg of amobarbital (Rx) [*Tuinal*].
  100 mg of secobarbital and 100 mg of amobarbital (Rx) [*Tuinal*].
Canada—
  50 mg of secobarbital and 50 mg of amobarbital (Rx) [*Tuinal*].
  100 mg of secobarbital and 100 mg of amobarbital (Rx) [*Tuinal*].

**Packaging and storage**
Store below 40 °C (104 °F), preferably between 15 and 30 °C (59 and 86 °F), unless otherwise specified by manufacturer. Store in a well-closed container.

**Auxiliary labeling**
- Avoid alcoholic beverages.
- May cause drowsiness.

**Note**
Controlled substance in the U.S. and Canada.

Revised: 01/27/92
Interim revision: 08/29/94; 08/15/95

## Table 1. Pharmacology/Pharmacokinetics

| Drug | Protein Binding* (%) | Half-life (hr) Range | Half-life (hr) Mean | Onset of Action† (min) | Duration of Action‡ (hr) | Elimination/ % Excreted Unchanged§ |
|---|---|---|---|---|---|---|
| Long-acting | | | | 60 or longer | 10–12 | |
| Mephobarbital# | | 11–67 | 34 | | | Renal |
| Metharbital | | | | | | Renal/2%; 20% excreted as barbital |
| Phenobarbital | Low to Moderate (20–45) | 53–118** | 79 | | | Renal/25–50% |
| Intermediate-acting | | | | 45–60 | 6–8 | |
| Amobarbital | Moderate (61) | 16–40 | 25 | | | Renal/<1% |
| Aprobarbital | Low (20) | 14–34 | 24 | | | Renal/25–50% |
| Butabarbital | Low (26) | 34–42 | †† | | | Renal/<1% |
| Short-acting | | | | 10–15 | 3–4 | |
| Pentobarbital | Moderate to High (60–70) | 15–50 | ‡‡ | | | Renal/<1% |
| Secobarbital | Moderate to High (46–70) | 15–40 | 28 | | | Renal/5% |

*Bound to plasma and tissue proteins to a varying degree; binding increases proportionate to lipid solubility
†Following oral administration. Phenobarbital has the slowest, and secobarbital the fastest, onset of action
‡Following oral administration. Duration of action is related to the rate at which the barbiturates are redistributed throughout the body and is variable among individuals and in the same individual from time to time. Phenobarbital has the longest, and secobarbital the shortest, duration of action
§Metabolic products are excreted in the urine and, less commonly, in the feces. Inactive metabolites are excreted as conjugates of glucuronic acid. Peritoneal dialysis and hemodialysis remove phenobarbital from the body; serum phenobarbital concentrations should be determined during and after peritoneal dialysis and hemodialysis
#Activity due mostly to accumulation of phenobarbital
**Half-life is 60 to 180 hours in children (half-life 48 hours or less for newborns)
††One manufacturer states that the half-life of butabarbital is 100 hours
‡‡Dose-dependent; the mean half-life of elimination is 50 and 22 hours following a 50- and 100-mg dose, respectively

## Table 2. General Dosing Information

| Drug | Onset/Duration of Action | (1) | (2) | (3) | (4) | (5) |
|---|---|---|---|---|---|---|
| Pentobarbital | Fast/short | ≤2 | 0.5–3 | 10–15 | 12–25 | 15–40 |
| Secobarbital | Fast/short | ≤2 | 0.5–5 | 10–15 | 15–25 | 15–40 |
| Amobarbital | Intermediate/intermediate | ≤3 | 2–10 | 30–40 | 30–60 | 40–80 |
| Butabarbital | Intermediate/intermediate | ≤5 | 3–25 | 40–60 | 50–80 | 60–100 |
| Phenobarbital | Slow/long | ≤10 | 5–40 | 50–80 | 70–120 | 100–200 |

Barbiturate Blood Concentrations (mcg/mL) Categories of Degree of CNS Depression*

*Categories of degree of CNS depression in nontolerant persons:
(1) Under the influence and appreciably impaired for purposes of driving a motor vehicle or performing tasks requiring alertness and unimpaired judgment and reaction time.
(2) Sedated, therapeutic range, calm, relaxed, and easily aroused.
(3) Comatose, difficult to arouse, and significant respiratory depression.
(4) Comparable with death in aged or ill persons or in presence of obstructed airway, other toxic agents, or exposure to cold.
(5) Usual lethal concentration, the upper end of the range includes those who received some supportive treatment

# BARBITURATES AND ANALGESICS Systemic

This monograph includes information on the following: 1) Butalbital and Acetaminophen†; 2) Butalbital, Acetaminophen, Caffeine, and Codeine†; 3) Butalbital and Aspirin; 4) Butalbital, Aspirin‡, Caffeine, and Codeine; 5) Phenobarbital, ASA‡, and Codeine*

Pharmacy Equivalent Name (PEN):
Butalbital, Acetaminophen, and Caffeine—Co-bucafAPAP

INN: Acetaminophen—Paracetamol

VA CLASSIFICATION (Primary):
Butalbital and Acetaminophen—CN103
Butalbital, Acetaminophen, Caffeine, and Codeine—CN101
Butalbital and Aspirin—CN103
Butalbital, Aspirin, Caffeine, and Codeine—CN101
Phenobarbital, ASA‡, and Codeine—CN101

Note: Controlled substance classification—
Controlled substances in the U.S. and Canada, as follows—
Butalbital, Acetaminophen, Caffeine and Codeine:
U.S.—III.
Canada—Not available.
Butalbital and Aspirin:
U.S.—III.
Canada—C.
Butalbital, Aspirin, Caffeine, and Codeine:
U.S.—III.
Canada—N.
Phenobarbital, ASA‡, and Codeine:
U.S.—Not available.
Canada—N.

Commonly used brand name(s): *Amaphen*[1]; *Anolor-300*[1]; *Anoquan*[1]; *Arcet*[1]; *Ascomp with Codeine No.3*[4]; *Axotal*[3]; *Bancap*[1]; *Bucet*[1]; *Butace*[1]; *Butalbital Compound with Codeine*[4]; *Butalgen*[3]; *Butinal with Codeine No.3*[4]; *Conten*[1]; *Dolmar*[1]; *Endolor*[1]; *Esgic*[1]; *Esgic-Plus*[1]; *Ezol*[1]; *Femcet*[1]; *Fiorgen*[3]; *Fioricet*[1]; *Fioricet with Codeine*; *Fiorinal*[3]; *Fiorinal with Codeine No.3*[4]; *Fiorinal-C 1/2*[4]; *Fiorinal-C 1/4*[4]; *Fiormor*[3]; *Fortabs*[3]; *Idenal with Codeine*[4]; *Isobutal*[3]; *Isobutyl*[1]; *Isocet*[1]; *Isolin*[3]; *Isollyl*[3]; *Isollyl with Codeine*[4]; *Isopap*[1]; *Laniroif*[3]; *Lanorinal*[3]; *Marnal*[3]; *Medigesic*[1]; *Pacaps*[1]; *Pharmagesic*[1]; *Phenaphen with Codeine No.2*[5]; *Phenaphen with Codeine No.3*[5]; *Phenaphen with Codeine No.4*[5]; *Phrenilin*[1]; *Phrenilin Forte*[1]; *Repan*[1]; *Sedapap*[1]; *Tecnal*[3]; *Tecnal-C 1/2*[4]; *Tecnal-C 1/4*[4]; *Tencet*[1]; *Tencon*[1]; *Triad*[1]; *Triaprin*[1]; *Two-Dyne*[1]; *Vibutal*[3].

Note: For a listing of dosage forms and brand names by country availability, see *Dosage Forms* section(s).

*Not commercially available in U.S.
†Not commercially available in Canada.
‡In Canada, *Aspirin* is a brand name; acetylsalicylic acid is the generic name. ASA, a commonly used designation for aspirin (or acetylsalicylic acid) in both the U.S. and Canada, is the term used in Canadian product labeling.

## Category
Analgesic.

## Indications

Note: Bracketed information in the *Indications* section refers to uses that are not included in U.S. product labeling.

**Accepted**

Headache, tension-type (treatment)—Barbiturate and analgesic combinations are indicated for relief of the symptoms of occasional tension-type (muscle contraction) headache.

[Headache, migraine (treatment)]—Barbiturate and analgesic combinations are indicated to relieve occasional migraine[1] and coexisting migraine and tension-type headaches ("mixed" headache syndrome).

Note: Because of the risk of habituation, barbiturate and analgesic combinations are not recommended for treatment of frequent, especially daily, headaches.

To reduce analgesic use, underlying problems that may contribute to tension-type headaches, such as inflammation or structural abnormalities in the cervical or temporomandibular areas, should be identified and treated. In some patients, application of heat, muscle relaxants, and/or physical therapy may be helpful. Other medications having the potential to cause habituation (e.g., benzodiazepines) should be used as infrequently as possible.

Chronic tension-type headaches and severe migraines that occur more frequently than twice a month may require additional prophylactic treatment to reduce the frequency, severity, and/or duration of the headaches. The prophylactic agents most commonly used for tension-type headaches are tricyclic antidepressants, especially amitriptyline, and/or beta-adrenergic blocking agents, especially propranolol. For migraines, beta-adrenergic blocking agents, calcium channel blocking agents, tricyclic antidepressants, monoamine oxidase inhibitors, methysergide, pizotyline (not commercially available in the U.S.), and sometimes cyproheptadine (especially in children) are used for prophylaxis. The combination of amitriptyline plus propranolol has been found superior to either agent used alone in preventing "mixed" headaches.

Identification and avoidance of precipitating factors is also important in the overall management of the patient with migraine headaches. Relaxation and/or biofeedback techniques may also be helpful in controlling migraine headaches, and may reduce the need for medication.

[Pain (treatment)]—Barbiturate and analgesic combinations are also indicated for relief of pain other than headache, especially when an antianxiety or relaxant effect is desired.

[1]Not included in Canadian product labeling.

## Pharmacology/Pharmacokinetics

**Physicochemical characteristics**
Molecular weight—
Butalbital: 224.26.
Phenobarbital: 232.24.
Acetaminophen: 151.16.
Aspirin: 180.16.
Codeine phosphate: 406.37.
Caffeine (anhydrous): 194.19.
pKa—
Aspirin: 3.5.

**Mechanism of action/Effect**
Butalbital or
Phenobarbital—
Butalbital is a short- to intermediate-acting barbiturate; phenobarbital is a long-acting barbiturate. Barbiturates are nonselective depressants of the central nervous system (CNS). They are used in analgesic combinations for their antianxiety and relaxant effects.

Acetaminophen or
Aspirin—
The mechanism of analgesic action has not been fully determined. Acetaminophen and aspirin may act by inhibiting prostaglandin synthesis in the CNS and through a peripheral action by blocking pain-impulse generation. The peripheral action may also be due to inhibition of the synthesis of prostaglandins or to inhibition of the synthesis or actions of other substances that sensitize pain receptors to mechanical or chemical stimulation. Acetaminophen may act predominantly in the CNS, whereas aspirin may produce analgesia predominantly via peripheral actions.

Codeine—
Opioid analgesics bind with stereospecific receptors at many sites within the CNS to alter processes affecting both the perception of pain and the emotional response to pain. Precise sites and mechanisms of action have not been fully determined. It has been proposed that there are multiple subtypes of opioid receptors, each mediating various therapeutic and/or side effects of opioids. The actions of an opioid analgesic may therefore depend upon its binding affinity for each type of receptor and whether it acts as a full agonist or a partial agonist or is inactive at each type of receptor. At least two of these types of receptors (mu and kappa) mediate analgesia. Codeine probably produces its effects via agonist actions at the mu receptor.

Caffeine—
Caffeine-induced constriction of cerebral blood vessels, which leads to a decrease in cerebral blood flow and in the oxygen tension of the brain, may contribute to relief of some types of headache. Also, it has been suggested that the addition of caffeine to acetaminophen and/or aspirin may provide a more rapid onset of action and/or enhanced pain relief with lower doses of analgesics. However, the FDA has not accepted caffeine as an effective analgesic adjuvant.

**Other actions/effects**
Butalbital—
  Phenobarbital:
    Barbiturates have dose-dependent respiratory depressant effects. Phenobarbital is a potent inducer of the activity of the hepatic p-450 microsomal enzyme system and may alter the metabolism and efficacy of many other medications that are metabolized via this enzyme system. Butalbital may also have some enzyme-inducing activity.
    Phenobarbital also has anticonvulsant activity.
Acetaminophen—
  Has antipyretic activity.
Aspirin—
  Has antipyretic, anti-inflammatory, and platelet aggregation–inhibiting actions.
Codeine—
  Has CNS depressant, respiratory depressant, antidiarrheal, and antitussive actions.
Caffeine—
  Has CNS stimulating activity and may therefore inhibit sleep. Because sleep contributes to relief of migraine headaches, this action may be detrimental to the patient.

**Absorption**
Butalbital—
  Well absorbed from the gastrointestinal tract.
Acetaminophen—
  Rapid and almost complete; may be decreased if the medication is taken following a high-carbohydrate meal.
Aspirin—
  Generally rapid and complete but may vary according to factors such as tablet dissolution rate and gastric or intraluminal pH. Concurrent administration with food decreases the rate, but not the extent, of absorption.
Caffeine—
  Well absorbed from the gastrointestinal tract.
Note:  Gastric stasis that accompanies migraine headaches tends to inhibit absorption of orally administered medications, which may result in alteration of some of the pharmacokinetic values reported below. Consequently, the onset of action of these medications may be delayed and/or their efficacy decreased, especially if they are taken after a migraine is well established.

**Distribution**
In breast milk
  Acetaminophen—
    Peak concentrations of 10 to 15 mcg per mL (mcg/mL) (66.2 to 99.3 micromoles/L) have been measured 1 to 2 hours following maternal ingestion of a single 650-mg dose.
  Aspirin (as salicylate)—
    Peak salicylate concentrations of 173 to 483 mcg/mL (17.3 to 48.3 mg per 100 mL; 1.25 to 3.5 mmol/L) have been measured 5 to 8 hours after maternal ingestion of a single 650-mg dose.
  Codeine—
    Small quantities of codeine are distributed into breast milk.
  Caffeine—
    Small quantities of caffeine are distributed into breast milk.

**Protein binding**
Phenobarbital—
  Low to moderate (20 to 45%).
Acetaminophen—
  Not significant with usual analgesic doses.
Salicylate (from aspirin)—
  High (to albumin); decreases as plasma salicylate concentration increases, with reduced plasma albumin concentration or renal dysfunction, and during pregnancy.
Codeine—
  Very low.
Caffeine—
  Low.

**Biotransformation**
Phenobarbital and probably butalbital—
  Hepatic, primarily by the hepatic microsomal enzyme system.
Acetaminophen—
  Approximately 90 to 95% of a dose is metabolized in the liver, primarily by conjugation with glucuronic acid, sulfuric acid, and cysteine. An intermediate metabolite is hepatotoxic and possibly nephrotoxic.
Aspirin—
  Largely hydrolyzed in the gastrointestinal tract, liver, and blood to salicylate, which also has analgesic activity. Salicylate is further metabolized, primarily in the liver.
Codeine—
  Hepatic; about 10% of a dose is demethylated to morphine, which may contribute to the therapeutic actions.
Caffeine—
  Hepatic.

**Half-life**
Butalbital—
  About 35 hours.
Phenobarbital—
  May range between 53 and 118 hours (mean, 79 hours).
Acetaminophen—
  1 to 4 hours; does not change with renal failure but may be prolonged in some forms of hepatic disease, in overdose, in the elderly, and in the neonate; may be somewhat shortened in children.
  In breast milk: 1.35 to 3.5 hours.
Aspirin—
  15 to 20 minutes (for intact molecule); rapidly hydrolyzed to salicylate.
  In breast milk (as salicylate): 3.8 to 12.5 hours (average, 7.1 hours) following a single 650-mg dose.
Salicylate (from aspirin)—
  Dependent on dose and urinary pH; about 2 to 3 hours with usual analgesic doses.
Codeine—
  2.5 to 4 hours.
Caffeine—
  3 to 4 hours.

**Onset of action**
Phenobarbital—
  1 hour or longer.
Codeine—
  30 to 45 minutes.

**Time to peak concentration**
Butalbital—
  About 1.5 hours following a 100-mg dose.
Acetaminophen—
  0.5 to 2 hours.
Aspirin—
  Generally 1 to 2 hours with single doses.

**Peak serum concentration**
Butalbital—
  About 2 mcg/mL (8.9 micromoles/L), following a 100-mg dose.
Acetaminophen—
  5 to 20 mcg/mL (33.1 to 132.4 micromoles/L), with doses up to 650 mg.

**Therapeutic plasma concentration**
Aspirin (as salicylate)—
  25 to 50 mcg/mL (2.5 to 5 mg per 100 mL [0.18 to 0.36 mmol/L]); these concentrations are generally reached with doses of 325 to 650 mg.

**Time to peak effect**
Acetaminophen—
  1 to 3 hours.
Codeine—
  1 to 2 hours.

**Duration of action**
Phenobarbital—
  10 to 12 hours.
Acetaminophen—
  3 to 4 hours.
Codeine—
  4 to 6 hours.

**Elimination**
Butalbital—
  Primarily via hepatic metabolism, followed by renal excretion of metabolites; 50 to 88% of a dose is excreted in the urine, about 3.6% of a dose being excreted as unchanged butalbital and the remainder as metabolites.
Phenobarbital—
  Renal; 25 to 50% of a dose is eliminated as unchanged phenobarbital.
Acetaminophen—
  Renal, as metabolites, primarily conjugates; 3% of a dose may be excreted unchanged.
  In dialysis:
    Hemodialysis—120 mL per minute (for unmetabolized drug); metabolites also cleared rapidly.
    Hemoperfusion—200 mL per minute.
    Peritoneal dialysis—< 10 mL per minute.

Aspirin—
: Renal, primarily as free salicylic acid and conjugated metabolites. There are large interindividual variations in elimination kinetics. Also, the rate of excretion of total salicylate and the quantity of free salicylic acid eliminated are increased in alkaline urine and decreased in acidic urine.
  In dialysis: As salicylate:
    Hemodialysis: Clearances of 35 to 100 mL per minute have been reported.
    Peritoneal dialysis: Removed more slowly than with hemodialysis; clearances of 45 to 90 mL per hour have been reported in infants.

Codeine—
: Renal, primarily as metabolites (10% as unchanged or conjugated morphine); 5 to 15% of a dose may be excreted as unchanged codeine.

Caffeine—
: Renal, primarily as metabolites. About 10% of a dose is excreted unchanged.

## Precautions to Consider

Note: Information regarding precautions applying to the use of the individual ingredients in these combination medications is limited to brief summaries of the major precautions that may apply to occasional use of recommended doses. For more complete information that may apply, especially if these agents are ingested frequently or in higher-than-recommended doses, see—Butalbital: *Barbiturates (Systemic)*. Although butalbital is not specifically mentioned in that monograph, general precautions applying to all barbiturates may apply to butalbital also.

Phenobarbital: *Barbiturates (Systemic)*.
Acetaminophen: *Acetaminophen (Systemic)*.
Aspirin: *Salicylates (Systemic)*.
Codeine: *Opioid (Narcotic) Analgesics (Systemic)*.
Caffeine: *Caffeine (Systemic)*.

### Cross-sensitivity and/or related problems

*Butalbital and*
*Phenobarbital*—
: Patients sensitive to other barbiturates may be sensitive to butalbital and phenobarbital also.

*Acetaminophen*—
: Patients sensitive to aspirin are usually not sensitive to acetaminophen; however, mild bronchospastic reactions with acetaminophen have been reported in some aspirin-sensitive patients (fewer than 5% of those tested).

*Aspirin*—
: Patients sensitive to one salicylate, including methyl salicylate (oil of wintergreen), may be sensitive to aspirin also. However, patients sensitive to aspirin may not necessarily be sensitive to salicylamide.
  Patients sensitive to other nonsteroidal anti-inflammatory drugs (NSAIDs) may be sensitive to aspirin also.

### Pregnancy/Reproduction

Fertility—
  *Acetaminophen*—
    Chronic toxicity studies in animals have shown that high doses of acetaminophen cause testicular atrophy and inhibition of spermatogenesis; the relevance of this finding to use in humans is not known.

Pregnancy—Reproduction studies have not been done in humans or in animals with any of the butalbital and analgesic combinations. There is no information about the use of phenobarbital, aspirin, and codeine combination during pregnancy. However, the following information is available for individual ingredients in these formulations.

  *First trimester*
    Butalbital and
    Phenobarbital:
      Barbiturates readily cross the placenta and are distributed throughout fetal tissues. The highest concentrations are found in the placenta and in the fetal liver and brain. Prenatal exposure to barbiturates has been reported to increase the risk of fetal abnormalities and of brain tumors.
    Acetaminophen:
      Problems in humans have not been documented. Although controlled studies have not been done, it is known that acetaminophen crosses the placenta.
    Aspirin:
      Salicylate readily crosses the placenta. It has been reported that aspirin use during pregnancy may increase the risk of birth defects in humans. However, controlled studies using usual therapeutic doses of aspirin have not shown proof of teratogenicity.
      Studies in animals have shown that aspirin causes increased fetal resorptions and birth defects, including fissure of the spine and skull; facial clefts; eye defects; and malformations of the CNS, viscera, and skeleton (especially the vertebrae and ribs).
    Codeine:
      Codeine crosses the placenta. Although teratogenic effects in humans have not been documented, controlled studies have not been done.
      Studies in animals have not shown that codeine causes teratogenic effects in doses up to 150 times the human dose. However, a single dose of 100 mg per kg of body weight (mg/kg) caused delayed ossification in mice, and doses of 120 mg/kg caused increased resorptions in rats.
    Caffeine:
      Caffeine crosses the placenta and achieves fetal blood and tissue concentrations similar to maternal concentrations. Studies in humans have not shown that caffeine causes birth defects. However, excessive intake of caffeine by pregnant women has resulted in fetal arrhythmias.
      Studies in animals have shown that caffeine causes skeletal abnormalities in the digits and phalanges (when given in doses equivalent to the caffeine content of 12 to 24 cups of coffee daily throughout pregnancy or in very large single doses, i.e., 50 to 100 mg/kg) and retarded skeletal development (when given in lower doses).

  *Third trimester*
    Butalbital and
    Phenobarbital:
      Ingestion of a barbiturate shortly prior to delivery may cause respiratory depression in the neonate.
    Aspirin:
      Problems attributed to use of aspirin during the third trimester include prolonged gestation, increased risk of postmaturity syndrome, reduced birthweight, increased risk of stillbirth or neonatal death (possibly resulting from prepartum maternal or fetal hemorrhage or from premature closure of the fetal ductus arteriosus), and prolonged labor and complicated deliveries when the medication is used during the last few weeks of pregnancy. Although these problems have occurred with chronic, high-dose use or abuse of aspirin, it is recommended that pregnant women not take aspirin during the last trimester unless aspirin therapy is prescribed and monitored by a physician.
      Ingestion of aspirin during the last 2 weeks of pregnancy may increase the risk of maternal, fetal, or neonatal hemorrhage.
    Codeine:
      Ingestion of codeine shortly prior to delivery may cause respiratory depression in the neonate, especially the premature neonate.
      FDA Pregnancy Category C (butalbital, aspirin, and codeine combination).

### Breast-feeding

*Butalbital and*
*Phenobarbital*—
: Barbiturates are distributed into breast milk and may cause CNS depression in the infant.

*Acetaminophen*—
: Problems in humans have not been documented. Although peak concentrations of 10 to 15 mcg/mL (66.2 to 99.3 micromoles/L) have been measured in breast milk 1 to 2 hours following maternal ingestion of one 650-mg dose, neither acetaminophen nor its metabolites were detected in the urine of the nursing infants. The half-life in breast milk is 1.35 to 3.5 hours.

*Aspirin*—
: Problems in humans with usual analgesic doses have not been documented; however, salicylate is distributed into breast milk. In one study, peak salicylate concentrations of 173 to 483 mcg/mL (17.3 to 48.3 mg per 100 mL [1.25 to 3.5 mmol/L]) were measured in breast milk 5 to 8 hours after maternal ingestion of one 650-mg dose of aspirin. The half-life in breast milk was 3.8 to 12.5 hours (average 7.1 hours).

*Codeine*—
: Problems in humans have not been documented; however, codeine is distributed into breast milk in low concentrations.

*Caffeine*—
: Caffeine is distributed into breast milk in very small amounts; at recommended doses of caffeine-containing analgesic combinations,

concentration in the infant is considered insignificant. However, it is recommended that breast-feeding mothers limit their total daily intake of caffeine to 360 mg. Accumulation of caffeine in the infant, leading to signs of caffeine stimulation such as hyperactivity and wakefulness, may occur when a breast-feeding mother ingests large quantities of caffeine.

## Pediatrics
*Butalbital and*
*Phenobarbital*:
Some children react to barbiturates with paradoxical excitement.
*Acetaminophen—*
Studies performed to date have not demonstrated pediatrics-specific problems that would limit the usefulness of acetaminophen in children.
*Aspirin—*
Aspirin usage may be associated with the development of Reye's syndrome in children with acute febrile illnesses, especially influenza and varicella. It is recommended that aspirin not be administered to febrile pediatric patients until after the presence of such an illness has been ruled out. Other pediatric patients, especially those with fever and dehydration, may also be more susceptible to the toxic effects of salicylates.
*Codeine—*
Some children react to opioids with paradoxical excitement.
*Caffeine—*
Appropriate studies on the relationship of age to the effects of caffeine have not been performed in children up to 12 years of age. However, no pediatrics-specific problems have been documented to date.

## Adolescents
*Aspirin—*
Aspirin usage may be associated with the development of Reye's syndrome in adolescents with acute febrile illnesses, especially influenza and varicella. It is recommended that aspirin not be administered to febrile adolescent patients until after the presence of such an illness has been ruled out.

## Geriatrics
*Butalbital and*
*Phenobarbital—*
Geriatric patients may react to usual doses of barbiturates with excitement, confusion, or depression. Also, elderly patients are more likely to have age-related renal function impairment, which may require caution in patients receiving barbiturates.
*Acetaminophen—*
Studies performed to date have not demonstrated geriatrics-specific problems that would limit the usefulness of acetaminophen in the elderly.
*Aspirin—*
Geriatric patients may be more susceptible to the toxic effects of salicylates. Also, elderly patients may be more likely to have age-related renal function impairment, which may require caution in patients receiving aspirin.
*Codeine—*
Geriatric patients may be more susceptible to the effects, especially the respiratory depressant effects, of opioid analgesics such as codeine. Elderly patients tend to eliminate opioid analgesics more slowly than younger adults. Lower doses and/or longer intervals between doses may be required, and are usually effective, for these patients. Also, elderly patients are more likely to have age-related renal function impairment and/or prostatic hypertrophy or obstruction; opioid-induced urinary retention may be detrimental to these patients.
*Caffeine—*
No information is available on the relationship of age to the effects of caffeine in geriatric patients.

## Drug interactions and/or related problems
The following drug interactions and/or related problems have been selected on the basis of their potential clinical significance (possible mechanism in parentheses where appropriate)—not necessarily inclusive (» = major clinical significance):

Note: Combinations containing any of the following medications, depending on the amount present, may also interact with this medication.

*For barbiturates*
Addictive medications, other, especially CNS depressants with habituating potential
(caution in concurrent use is recommended because of the increased risk of habituation)

» Alcohol or
» CNS depression-producing medications, other (see *Appendix II*)
(concurrent use with a barbiturate may cause additive CNS depression; caution is recommended and dosage reduction of either or both medications may be needed)

Any medication that may be rendered less effective, because of accelerated metabolism, by hepatic enzyme induction, especially:
» Anticoagulants, coumarin- or indandione-derivative
» Carbamazepine
» Contraceptives, estrogen-containing, oral
» Corticosteroids, glucocorticoid and mineralocorticoid
» Corticotropin
(caution in concurrent use is recommended, especially with phenobarbital)

» Divalproex sodium or
» Valproic acid
(these agents may decrease barbiturate metabolism, possibly leading to increased barbiturate serum concentrations and risk of toxicity)
(concurrent use with a barbiturate may also increase the half-life and risk of hepatotoxicity of valproic acid)

*For acetaminophen*
» Alcohol, especially chronic abuse of or
Hepatic enzyme inducers (see *Appendix II*) or
Hepatotoxic medications, other (see *Appendix II*)
(risk of hepatotoxicity with single toxic doses of acetaminophen may be increased in alcoholics or in patients regularly taking other hepatotoxic medications or hepatic enzyme inducers)
(chronic use of barbiturates or primidone has been reported to decrease the therapeutic effects of acetaminophen, probably because of increased metabolism resulting from induction of hepatic microsomal enzyme activity; the possibility should be considered that similar effects may occur with other hepatic enzyme inducers; however, such problems have not been reported with occasional use of combination formulations containing butalbital and acetaminophen)

*For aspirin*
Acidifiers, urinary, such as:
Ammonium chloride
Ascorbic acid
Potassium or sodium phosphates
(acidification of the urine by these medications decreases salicylate [from aspirin] excretion, leading to increased salicylate plasma concentrations)

» Alkalizers, urinary, such as:
Carbonic anhydrase inhibitors
Citrates or
Antacids, chronic high-dose use, especially calcium- or magnesium-containing or sodium bicarbonate
(alkalinization of the urine by these agents increases salicylate [from aspirin] excretion, leading to decreased salicylate plasma concentrations, reduced effectiveness, and shortened duration of analgesic action)
(carbonic anhydrase inhibitors may also increase the risk of salicylate intoxication in patients receiving large doses of aspirin because metabolic acidosis induced by carbonic anhydrase inhibitors may increase penetration of salicylate into the brain; the increased risk of severe metabolic acidosis and salicylate toxicity must be considered if acetazolamide is used to produce forced alkaline diuresis in the treatment of aspirin overdose)

» Anticoagulants, coumarin- or indandione-derivative or
» Heparin or
» Thrombolytic agents, such as:
Alteplase
Anistreplase
Streptokinase
Urokinase
(because aspirin inhibits platelet aggregation and may induce gastrointestinal ulceration and/or bleeding, which may be hazardous to patients receiving anticoagulant or thrombolytic therapy, it is recommended that aspirin not be administered to patients receiving these agents except as part of a prescribed and monitored antithrombotic regimen)

Furosemide
(in addition to an increased risk of ototoxicity, concurrent use of furosemide with high doses of aspirin may lead to salicylate toxicity because of competition for renal excretory sites)

Laxatives, cellulose-containing
(concurrent use may reduce the salicylate effect because of physical binding or other absorptive hindrance; medications should be administered 2 hours apart)

» Methotrexate
(aspirin may displace methotrexate from its binding sites and decrease its renal clearance, leading to toxic plasma concentrations of methotrexate; if used concurrently, methotrexate dosage should be decreased, the patient observed for signs of toxicity, and/or methotrexate plasma concentration monitored; also, it is recommended that aspirin not be administered for 24 to 48 hours prior to administration of a high-dose methotrexate infusion, or until plasma methotrexate concentrations have decreased to a nontoxic level following the infusion [usually at least 12 hours])

Ototoxic medications, other (see *Appendix II*), especially
» Vancomycin
(concurrent or sequential administration of these medications with aspirin should be avoided because the potential for ototoxicity may be increased; hearing loss may occur and may progress to deafness even after discontinuation of the medication; these effects may be reversible, but usually are permanent)

» Probenecid or
» Sulfinpyrazone
(uricosuric effects of probenecid or sulfinpyrazone may be decreased by doses of aspirin that produce serum salicylate concentrations above 50 mcg/mL [5 mg per 100 mL; 0.36 mmol/L]; also, probenecid may decrease renal clearance and increase plasma concentrations of salicylate, thereby increasing the risk of toxicity)
(sulfinpyrazone may decrease salicylate [from aspirin] excretion and/or displace salicylate from its protein binding sites, possibly leading to increased salicylate concentrations and toxicity)

*For codeine*
Addictive medications, other, especially CNS depressants with habituating potential
(increased risk of habituation)

» Alcohol or
» CNS depression-producing medications, other (see *Appendix II*), including other opioid analgesics
(concurrent use with codeine may lead to additive CNS depression; caution is recommended and dosage reduction of either or both medications may be needed)

Anticholinergics, especially atropine and related compounds
(concurrent use with codeine may result in increased risk of severe constipation, possibly leading to paralytic ileus, and/or urinary retention)

Antidiarrheals, antiperistaltic
(risk of constipation, which may lead to paralytic ileus, as well as the risk of CNS and/or respiratory depression, may be increased)

Antihypertensives, especially ganglionic blocking agents such as guanadrel, guanethidine, and mecamylamine or
Diuretics or
Hypotension-producing medications, other (see *Appendix II*)
(codeine may potentiate the hypotensive effects of these medications, leading to an increased risk of orthostatic hypotension)

Metoclopramide
(codeine may antagonize the effects of metoclopramide on gastrointestinal motility)

Monoamine oxidase inhibitors, including furazolidone, procarbazine, and selegiline
(concurrent use with codeine should be undertaken with caution because concurrent use with meperidine has resulted in unpredictable, severe, and sometimes fatal reactions, including immediate excitation, sweating, rigidity, and severe hypertension or, in some patients, hypotension, severe respiratory depression, coma, seizures, hyperpyrexia, and cardiovascular collapse; it is recommended that codeine be administered in reduced dosage to patients receiving an MAO inhibitor)

Naloxone
(antagonizes the analgesic, CNS, and respiratory depressant effects of codeine and may precipitate withdrawal symptoms in physically dependent patients; dosage of the antagonist should be carefully titrated when used to treat codeine overdose in dependent patients)

» Naltrexone
(codeine should not be administered as an analgesic to patients receiving naltrexone, which blocks the therapeutic effects of opioids; also, naltrexone therapy should not be initiated in patients receiving codeine for therapeutic purposes)
(administration of naltrexone to a patient physically dependent on codeine will precipitate withdrawal symptoms; symptoms may appear within 5 minutes of naltrexone administration, persist for up to 48 hours, and be difficult to reverse)

Opioid analgesics, other
(concurrent use with codeine may result in additive CNS depressant, respiratory depressant, and hypotensive effects)
(opioid agonist/antagonist analgesics [butorphanol, nalbuphine, or pentazocine] may partially antagonize the therapeutic and CNS depressant effects of codeine; also, nalbuphine and pentazocine may precipitate withdrawal symptoms in patients who are physically dependent on codeine)

*For caffeine*
CNS stimulation-producing medications, other (see *Appendix II*)
(concurrent use with caffeine may result in excessive CNS stimulation, leading to unwanted effects such as nervousness, irritability, insomnia, or possibly convulsions or cardiac arrhythmias; close observation is recommended)

Lithium
(caffeine increases urinary excretion of lithium, and may thereby reduce its therapeutic effect)

Monoamine oxidase (MAO) inhibitors, including furazolidone, procarbazine, and selegiline
(the sympathomimetic side effects of caffeine may lead to cardiac arrhythmias or severe hypertension when large amounts of caffeine are used concurrently with MAO inhibitors; even small doses may cause tachycardia and a slight increase in blood pressure)

**Laboratory value alterations**
The following have been selected on the basis of their potential clinical significance (possible effect in parentheses where appropriate)—not necessarily inclusive (» = major clinical significance):

With diagnostic test results
*For barbiturates*
Cyanocobalamin Co 57 test for pernicious anemia or vitamin $B_{12}$ deficiency
(absorption of radioactive cyanocobalamin may be impaired by phenobarbital)

Metyrapone test for pituitary function
(induction of hepatic microsomal enzymes may increase metabolism of metyrapone, leading to a decreased response to the diagnostic agent)

Phentolamine test for pheochromocytoma
(barbiturates may cause false-positive test results; it is recommended that barbiturates not be administered for at least 24 hours, and preferably 48 to 72 hours, prior to the test)

*For acetaminophen*
Glucose, blood, determinations
(values may be falsely decreased by acetaminophen when measured by the glucose oxidase/peroxidase method but probably not when measured by the hexokinase/glucose-6-phosphate dehydrogenase [G6PD] method)
(values may be falsely increased when certain instruments are used in glucose analysis if high acetaminophen concentrations are present; consult manufacturer's instruction manual)

5-Hydroxyindoleacetic acid (5-HIAA), serum, determinations
(acetaminophen may cause false-positive results in qualitative screening tests using nitrosonaphthol reagent; the quantitative test is unaffected)

Pancreatic function determinations using bentiromide
(administration of acetaminophen prior to the bentiromide test will invalidate test results because acetaminophen is also metabolized to an arylamine and will thus increase the apparent quantity of para-aminobenzoic acid [PABA] recovered; it is recommended that acetaminophen be discontinued at least 3 days prior to administration of bentiromide)

Uric acid, serum, determinations
(falsely increased values may occur when the phosphotungstate uric acid test method is used)

*For aspirin*
Aceto-acetic acid, urine, via Gerhard test
(interference may occur because reaction with ferric chloride produces a reddish color that persists after boiling)

Glucose, urine, determinations using copper sulfate
(false-positive test results may occur with chronic use of 2.4 grams or more a day)

Glucose, urine, enzymatic determinations
  (false-negative test results may occur with chronic use of 2.4 grams or more a day)
5-Hydroxyindoleacetic acid (5-HIAA), urine, determinations
  (aspirin may alter results when fluorescent method is used)
Renal function test using phenolsulfonphthalein (PSP)
  (salicylate [from aspirin] may competitively inhibit renal tubular secretion of PSP, thereby decreasing urinary PSP concentration and invalidating test results)
Thyroid imaging, radionuclide
  (chronic aspirin administration may depress thyroid function; aspirin therapy should be discontinued at least 1 week prior to administration of the radiopharmaceutical; however, a rebound effect may occur following discontinuation of salicylate therapy, resulting in a period of 3 to 10 days of increased thyroidal uptake)
Thyroid-stimulating hormone (TSH) release, determined via protirelin stimulation
  (TSH response to protirelin may be decreased by 2 to 3.6 grams of aspirin daily; peak TSH concentrations occur at the same time after administration, but are reduced)
Vanillylmandelic acid (VMA), urine, determinations
  (values may be falsely increased or decreased, depending on method used)

*For codeine*
Gastric emptying studies
  (codeine may delay gastric emptying, thereby invalidating test results)
Hepatobiliary imaging using technetium Tc 99m disofenin
  (delivery of technetium Tc 99m disofenin may be prevented because of codeine-induced constriction of the sphincter of Oddi and increased biliary tract pressure; these actions result in delayed visualization and thus resemble obstruction of the common bile duct)

*For caffeine*
Myocardial perfusion studies, dipyridamole-assisted
  (caffeine may inhibit the effects of dipyridamole on myocardial blood flow, thereby interfering with test results; patients should be advised to avoid caffeine for at least 12 hours prior to the test)

With physiology/laboratory test values
*For barbiturates*
Bilirubin, serum
  (concentrations may be decreased in patients with congenital nonhemolytic unconjugated hyperbilirubinemia and in epileptics; this effect is presumably due to induction of glucuronyl transferase, the enzyme responsible for bilirubin conjugation)

*For acetaminophen*
Bilirubin, serum and
Lactate dehydrogenase, serum and
Prothrombin time and
Transaminase, serum
  (values may be increased indicating acetaminophen-induced hepatotoxicity, especially in alcoholics, patients taking hepatic enzyme–inducing agents, or those with pre-existing hepatic disease, when single toxic doses [>8–10 grams] are taken or with prolonged use of lower doses [>3–5 grams a day])

*For aspirin*
Bleeding time
  (may be prolonged by aspirin for 4 to 7 days because of suppressed platelet aggregation; as little as 40 mg of aspirin affects platelet function for at least 96 hours following administration; however, clinical bleeding problems have not been reported with small doses [150 mg or less])
Potassium, serum
  (concentrations may be decreased because of increased potassium excretion caused by direct effect on renal tubules)
Uric acid, serum
  (concentrations may be increased with doses producing plasma salicylate concentrations below 100 to 150 mcg/mL [10 to 15 mg per 100 mL; 0.724 to 1.09 mmol/L] or decreased with doses producing plasma salicylate concentrations higher than 100 to 150 mcg/mL [10 to 15 mg per 100 mL; 0.724 to 1.09 mmol/L])

*For codeine*
Amylase, plasma and
Lipase, plasma
  (values may be increased because codeine can cause contractions of the sphincter of Oddi and increased biliary tract pressure; the diagnostic utility of determinations of these enzymes may be compromised for up to 24 hours after medication has been given)

## Medical considerations/Contraindications
The medical considerations/contraindications included have been selected on the basis of their potential clinical significance (reasons given in parentheses where appropriate)—not necessarily inclusive (» = major clinical significance).

*Except under special circumstances, this medication should not be used when the following medical conditions exist:*

*For barbiturates*
» Porphyria, acute intermittent or variegata or history of
  (barbiturates may aggravate symptoms by inducing enzymes responsible for porphyrin synthesis)

*For aspirin*
» Angioedema, anaphylaxis or other severe allergic reaction induced by aspirin or other NSAIDs, history of
  (high risk of recurrence)
» Bleeding ulcers or
» Hemorrhagic states, other active
  (may be exacerbated)
» Hemophilia or other bleeding problems, including coagulation or platelet function disorders
  (increased risk of hemorrhage)
» Nasal polyps associated with aspirin-induced asthma or other allergies
  (high risk of severe allergic reactions)

*For codeine*
» Diarrhea caused by poisoning or antibiotic therapy, until toxic material has been eliminated from the gastrointestinal tract
  (codeine may slow elimination of toxic material)
» Respiratory depression, acute
  (may be exacerbated)

*Risk-benefit should be considered when the following medical problems exist:*

*For barbiturates*
» Allergic reaction to a barbiturate, history of
Asthma, history of
  (increased risk of bronchospastic allergic reactions)
Diabetes mellitus, especially with phenobarbital
» Drug abuse or dependence, history of
  (patient predisposed to habituation and dependence)
» Hepatic coma, premonitory signs of or
Hepatic function impairment
  (barbiturates metabolized in liver; caution and a reduction in barbiturate dosage is recommended)
Hyperkinesis
  (increased risk of barbiturate-induced paradoxical excitement)
Hyperthyroidism
  (symptoms may be exacerbated because barbiturates displace thyroxine from plasma proteins)
Mental depression or
Suicidal tendencies
  (condition may be exacerbated, especially in elderly patients)
Renal function impairment
  (barbiturates excreted via kidneys; reduction in barbiturate dosage may be necessary)
» Respiratory disease involving dyspnea or obstruction, particularly status asthmaticus
  (serious ventilatory depression may occur)
Caution is also recommended in geriatric or debilitated patients, who may be more sensitive to the effects of barbiturates and may react to usual doses of a barbiturate with excitement, depression, and confusion and in pediatric patients, who are especially susceptible to paradoxical excitement during barbiturate therapy.

*For acetaminophen*
» Alcohol abuse, current or
» Hepatic disease or
» Viral hepatitis
  (increased risk of hepatotoxicity)
Renal function impairment, severe
  (risk of adverse renal effects may be increased with prolonged use of high doses; occasional use is acceptable)
Sensitivity to acetaminophen, history of
  (increased risk of allergic reaction)

*For aspirin*
» Asthma
  (increased risk of bronchospastic allergic reactions)

» Gastritis, erosive or
» Peptic ulcer
(may be exacerbated because of ulcerogenic effects; risk of gastrointestinal bleeding is increased)

Gout
(aspirin may increase serum uric acid concentrations; also, may interfere with efficacy of uricosuric agents)

Hepatic function impairment
(salicylates metabolized in liver; also, in severe hepatic impairment, inhibition of platelet function by aspirin may increase risk of hemorrhage)

Hypoprothrombinemia or
Vitamin K deficiency
(increased risk of bleeding because of antiplatelet action of aspirin)

Mild sensitivity reaction to aspirin, history of
(increased risk of severe allergic reactions)

Renal function impairment
(salicylates excreted via kidneys)

*For codeine*
Allergic reaction to codeine, history of
» Asthma, acute attack or
» Respiratory impairment or disease, chronic
(codeine may decrease respiratory drive and increase airway resistance)

Cardiac arrhythmias or
Convulsions, history of
(may be induced or exacerbated)

Drug abuse or dependence, history of or
Emotional instability or
Suicidal ideation or attempts
(increased risk of abuse)

Gallbladder disease or gallstones
(codeine may cause biliary tract spasm)

Head injury or
Increased intracranial pressure, pre-existing or
Intracranial lesions
(risk of respiratory depression and further elevation of cerebrospinal fluid is increased; also, codeine may cause sedation and pupillary changes which may obscure clinical course of head injury)

Hepatic function impairment
(codeine metabolized in liver; may accumulate)

Hypothyroidism
(increased risk of respiratory depression and prolonged CNS depression)

» Inflammatory bowel disease, severe
(risk of toxic megacolon may be increased, especially with repeated dosing)

Prostatic hypertrophy or obstruction or
Urethral stricture
(codeine may cause urinary retention)

Renal function impairment
(codeine excreted primarily via kidneys; also, may cause urinary retention)

Caution is also advised in administration to very young, elderly, or very ill or debilitated patients, who may be more sensitive to the effects, especially the respiratory depressant effects, of codeine.

*For caffeine*
Cardiac disease, severe
(high doses of caffeine may increase risk of tachycardia or extrasystoles, which may lead to heart failure)

Sensitivity to caffeine, history of
(risk of allergic reaction)

## Side/Adverse Effects

Note: Barbiturates and codeine may cause dependence, especially following prolonged use of high doses, in any patient. The characteristics of dependence include: a strong desire or need to continue taking the medication; a tendency to increase the dose; a psychological dependence on the effects of the medication; and a physical dependence on the effects of the medication requiring its presence for maintenance of homeostasis and resulting in an abstinence syndrome when the medication is discontinued. With codeine, the severity of withdrawal symptoms depends upon the abruptness of withdrawal and the extent to which dependence has developed. However, codeine has lower dependence liability and potential for abuse than most other opioid agonists because of its relatively weak agonist activity with usual analgesic doses.

Frequent use of any analgesic for treatment of headaches (including analgesics that do not contain a barbiturate or an opioid) may lead to tolerance, an increased dosage requirement, dependence, withdrawal (rebound) headaches, and further use of the medication. Eventually, chronic (daily or near-daily) headaches may occur. This type of dependence may occur only in headache-prone patients; withdrawal headaches have not been reported in patients who take analgesics frequently for other types of pain. Chronic daily use of caffeine may also result in the development of physical dependence, leading to withdrawal headaches and medication abuse.

Aspirin-induced bronchospasm is most likely to occur in patients with the triad of aspirin-induced asthma, allergies, and nasal polyps. Aspirin-induced angioedema or urticaria may be more likely to occur in patients with a history of recurrent idiopathic angioedema or urticaria.

The side/adverse effects listed below are those that may occur with occasional use of recommended doses of these combination medications (including those that may result from an allergic or idiosyncratic response to individual ingredients in the formulations) or with an acute overdose. For additional information on side/adverse effects that may occur with individual ingredients in these medications, especially if these agents are ingested frequently or in higher-than-recommended doses, see—For butalbital: *Barbiturates (Systemic)*. Although butalbital is not specifically mentioned in that monograph, side effects that are likely to occur with other barbiturates may occur with butalbital also.

For phenobarbital: *Barbiturates (Systemic)*.

For acetaminophen: *Acetaminophen (Systemic)*.

For aspirin: *Salicylates (Systemic)*.

For codeine: *Opioid (Narcotic) Analgesics (Systemic)*.

For caffeine: *Caffeine (Systemic)*.

The following side/adverse effects have been selected on the basis of their potential clinical significance (possible signs and symptoms in parentheses where appropriate)—not necessarily inclusive:

### Those indicating need for medical attention
Incidence less frequent or rare

*For barbiturates*
**Agranulocytosis** (fever with or without chills; sores, ulcers, or white spots on lips or in mouth; sore throat); **angioedema** (large, hive-like swellings on eyelids, face, lips, and/or tongue); **bronchospastic allergic reaction** (shortness of breath; troubled breathing; tightness in chest; wheezing); **CNS (Central Nervous System) effects** (confusion; hallucinations; mental depression; unusual tiredness or weakness)—confusion or mental depression especially likely to occur in geriatric or debilitated patients; **CNS stimulation, paradoxical** (unusual excitement)—especially likely to occur in pediatric, geriatric, or debilitated patients; **dermatitis, allergic** (skin rash or hives); **dermatitis, exfoliative** (fever with or without chills; red, thickened, or scaly skin; swollen and/or painful glands; unusual bruising); **erythema multiforme** (fever with or without chills; muscle cramps or pain; skin rash; sores, ulcers, or white spots on lips or in mouth); **hypotension** (decreased blood pressure)—usually asymptomatic, but may lead to tiredness or weakness if severe; **Stevens-Johnson syndrome** (bleeding or crusting sores on lips; chest pain; fever with or without chills; muscle cramps or pain; skin rash; sores, ulcers, or white spots in mouth; sore throat); **thrombocytopenia** (usually asymptomatic; rarely, unusual bleeding or bruising; black, tarry stools; blood in urine or stools; pinpoint red spots on skin)

*For acetaminophen*
**Agranulocytosis** (fever with or without chills; sores, ulcers, or white spots on lips or in mouth; sore throat); **dermatitis, allergic** (skin rash, hives, or itching); **thrombocytopenia** (usually asymptomatic; rarely, unusual bleeding or bruising; black, tarry stools; blood in urine or stools; pinpoint red spots on skin)

*For aspirin*
**Anaphylaxis** (bluish discoloration or flushing or redness of skin; coughing; difficulty in swallowing; dizziness or feeling faint, severe; skin rash, hives [may include giant urticaria], and/or itching; stuffy nose; large, hive-like swellings on eyelids, face, lips, and/or tongue; tightness in chest, troubled breathing, and/or wheezing, especially in asthmatic patients); **bronchospastic allergic reaction** (shortness of breath, troubled breathing, tightness in chest, and/or wheezing); **dermatitis, allergic** (skin rash, hives, or itching); **necrolysis, toxic epidermal** (redness, tenderness, itching, burning, or peeling of skin; sore throat; fever with or without chills)

*For codeine*
**Angioedema** (large, hive-like swellings on face, eyelids, mouth, lips, and/or tongue); ***bronchoconstriction, laryngeal edema, or laryngospasm, allergic*** (shortness of breath, troubled breathing, tightness in chest, or wheezing); **CNS toxicity** (convulsions, hallucinations, trembling, and/or uncontrolled muscle movements; mental depression); ***dermatitis, allergic*** (skin rash, itching, or hives)

**Those indicating need for medical attention only if they continue or are bothersome**
Incidence more frequent
*For all barbiturate and analgesic combinations*
**CNS effects** (dizziness, drowsiness, or lightheadedness, mild); **gastrointestinal irritation** (bloated or "gassy" feeling, mild stomach pain, heartburn or indigestion, nausea with or without vomiting)—especially likely with formulations containing aspirin.

## Overdose
For specific information on the agents used in the management of barbiturates and analgesics overdose, see:
For acetaminophen
- *Acetylcysteine (Systemic)* monograph; and/or
- *Vitamin K— Phytonadione₁ (Systemic)* in *Vitamin K (Systemic)* monograph.

For aspirin
- *Vitamin K— Phytonadione₁ (Systemic)* in *Vitamin K (Systemic)* monograph.

For codeine
- *Naloxone (Systemic)* monograph.

For more information on the management of overdose or unintentional ingestion **contact a Poison Control Center** (see *Poison Control Center Listing*).

**Clinical effects of overdose**
The following effects have been selected on the basis of their potential clinical significance (possible signs and symptoms in parentheses where appropriate)—not necessarily inclusive:

*For barbiturates*
Acute
***Confusion; severe drowsiness or weakness; shortness of breath or unusually slow or troubled breathing; slow heartbeat; slurred speech; staggering; unusual movements of the eyes***

Note: In acute barbiturate overdosage, *CNS and respiratory depression* may lead to *Cheyne-Stokes respiration, areflexia,* slight *pupillary constriction* (in severe toxicity, pupils may be dilated), *oliguria, tachycardia, lowered body temperature,* and *coma.* Typical *shock syndrome* (apnea, circulatory collapse, respiratory arrest, and death) may occur.

In extreme barbiturate overdosage, all electrical activity in the brain may cease. In this case an electroencephalogram (EEG) may be "flat," but this does not necessarily indicate clinical death since, unless hypoxic damage occurs, this effect is fully reversible.

Complications in barbiturate overdosage such as *pneumonia, pulmonary edema, cardiac arrhythmias, congestive heart failure,* and *renal failure* may occur.

*For acetaminophen*
Acute
***Diarrhea; increased sweating; loss of appetite; nausea or vomiting; stomach cramps or pain***—may occur within 6 to 14 hours after ingestion of the overdose and persist for about 24 hours

Note: Early signs and symptoms often do not occur.

Chronic
***Hepatotoxicity*** (pain, tenderness, and/or swelling in upper abdominal area)—may occur 2 to 4 days after the overdose is ingested

Note: The first indications of overdosage may be signs and symptoms of possible *liver damage* and abnormalities in liver function tests, which may not occur until 2 to 4 days after ingestion of the overdose. Maximal changes in liver function tests usually occur 3 to 5 days after ingestion of the overdose.

Overt *hepatic disease or failure* may occur 4 to 6 days after ingestion of the overdose. *Hepatic encephalopathy* (with mental changes, confusion, agitation, or stupor), *convulsions, respiratory depression, coma, cerebral edema, coagulation defects, gastrointestinal bleeding, disseminated intravascular coagulation, hypoglycemia, metabolic acidosis, renal tubular necrosis leading to renal failure* (signs include bloody or cloudy urine and sudden decrease in amount of urine), *cardiac arrhythmias,* and *cardiovascular collapse* may occur.

*For aspirin*
Acute and chronic
[Mild overdose] Salicylism
***Continuing ringing or buzzing in ears, or hearing loss; confusion; severe or continuing diarrhea, stomach pain, and/or headache; dizziness or lightheadedness; severe drowsiness; fast or deep breathing; continuing nausea and/or vomiting; uncontrollable flapping movements of the hands, especially in elderly patients; increased thirst; vision problems***

Severe overdose
***Bloody urine; convulsions; hallucinations; severe nervousness, excitement, or confusion; shortness of breath or troubled breathing; unexplained fever***

Note: In young children, the only signs of an overdose may be *changes in behavior, severe drowsiness or tiredness,* and/or *fast or deep breathing.*

Laboratory findings in overdose may indicate encephalographic abnormalities; alterations in acid-base balance, especially *respiratory alkalosis* and *metabolic acidosis; hyperglycemia or hypoglycemia,* especially in children; *ketonuria; hyponatremia; hypokalemia;* and *proteinuria.*

*For codeine*
Acute / chronic
**CNS toxicity** (confusion, convulsions, severe dizziness, severe drowsiness, severe nervousness or restlessness, unconsciousness, severe weakness); ***cold, clammy skin; low blood pressure; pinpoint pupils of eyes; respiratory depression*** (shortness of breath or unusually slow or troubled breathing); ***slow heartbeat***

*For caffeine*
Acute and chronic
**CNS toxicity** (agitation, anxiety, excitement, or restlessness; confusion or delirium; increased sensitivity to touch or pain; irritability; ringing or other sounds in ears; seeing flashes of zig-zag" lights; seizures, usually tonic-clonic; trouble in sleeping); ***dehydration; fast or irregular heartbeat; fever; frequent urination; gastrointestinal effects*** ((abdominal or stomach pain; nausea and vomiting, sometimes with blood)); ***headache; muscle trembling or twitching***

**Treatment of overdose**
For all barbiturate and analgesic combinations—
To decrease absorption—Inducing emesis with ipecac syrup if the patient is conscious and has not lost the gag reflex. Care should be taken to prevent pulmonary aspiration of vomitus. If emesis is contraindicated, performing gastric lavage with a cuffed endotracheal tube in place with the patient face down.

After emesis is completed, administering activated charcoal in a glass of water or sorbitol to prevent absorption and increase excretion of the barbiturate. It is usually recommended that activated charcoal be left in the stomach. Also, a saline cathartic may be administered.

To enhance elimination—If renal function is normal, inducing forced diuresis, which may help to eliminate the barbiturate. Alkalinization of the urine increases renal excretion of some barbiturates.

Instituting hemodialysis or hemoperfusion in severe barbiturate poisoning or if the patient is anuric or in shock. However, hemodialysis or hemoperfusion is not recommended as a routine procedure.

Specific treatment—Administering fluid therapy and other standard treatment for shock, if necessary. A vasopressor may be required if hypotension occurs. Fluid or sodium overload should be avoided, especially if cardiovascular status is decreased.

Administering chest physiotherapy. If pneumonia is suspected, appropriate cultures should be taken and antibiotics should be administered. Also, appropriate care should be taken to prevent hypostatic pneumonia, decubiti, aspiration, and other complications that may occur with altered states of consciousness.

Supportive care—Maintaining an adequate airway, with assisted respiration and administration of oxygen as needed.

Monitoring vital signs and fluid balance.

For acetaminophen—
To enhance elimination—Instituting hemodialysis or hemoperfusion to remove acetaminophen from the circulation may be beneficial if acetylcysteine administration cannot be instituted within 24 hours following ingestion of a massive acetaminophen overdose. However, the efficacy of this treatment in preventing acetaminophen-induced hepatotoxicity is not known.

**Specific treatment**—Because activated charcoal may interfere with absorption of oral acetylcysteine (antidote used to protect against acetaminophen-induced hepatotoxicity), removal of activated charcoal via gastric lavage may be advisable prior to acetylcysteine administration. See the package insert or *Acetylcysteine (Systemic)* for specific dosing guidelines for use of this product.

**Administering acetylcysteine.** *It is recommended that acetylcysteine administration be instituted as soon as possible after ingestion of an overdose has been reported,* without waiting for the results of plasma acetaminophen determinations or other laboratory tests. Acetylcysteine is most effective if treatment is started within 10 to 12 hours after ingestion of the overdose; however, it may be of some benefit if treatment is started within 24 hours.

**Administering vitamin K₁** (if prothrombin time ratio exceeds 1.5) and fresh frozen plasma or clotting factor concentrate (if prothrombin time ratio exceeds 3.0). See the package insert or *Phytonadione* in *Vitamin K (Systemic)* for specific dosing guidelines for use of this product.

**Monitoring**—Determining plasma acetaminophen concentration at least 4 hours following ingestion of the overdose. Determinations performed prior to this time are not reliable for assessing potential hepatotoxicity. Initial plasma concentrations above 150 mcg per mL (mcg/mL) (993 micromoles/L) at 4 hours, 100 mcg/mL (662 micromoles/L) at 6 hours, 70 mcg/mL (463.4 micromoles/L) at 8 hours, 50 mcg/mL (331 micromoles/L) at 10 hours, 20 mcg/mL (132.4 micromoles/L) at 15 hours, 8 mcg/mL (53 micromoles/L) at 20 hours, or 3.5 mcg/mL (23.2 micromoles/L) at 24 hours postingestion indicate possible hepatotoxicity and the need for completing the full course of acetylcysteine treatment. If the initial determination indicates a plasma concentration below those listed at the times indicated, cessation of acetylcysteine therapy can be considered. However, some clinicians advise that more than one determination should be performed to ascertain peak absorption and half-life of acetaminophen prior to considering discontinuation of acetylcysteine.

Performing liver function tests (serum aspartate aminotransferase [AST; SGOT], serum alanine aminotransferase [ALT; SGPT], prothrombin time, and bilirubin) at 24-hour intervals for at least 96 hours postingestion if the plasma acetaminophen concentration indicates potential hepatotoxicity. If no abnormalities are detected within 96 hours, further determinations are not needed.

Monitoring renal and cardiac function and administering appropriate therapy as required.

**Supportive care**—Instituting supportive treatment, including maintaining fluid and electrolyte balance, and correcting hypoglycemia.

For aspirin—
**To enhance elimination**—Inducing forced alkaline diuresis to increase salicylate excretion. However, bicarbonate should not be administered orally for this purpose because salicylate absorption may be increased. Also, if acetazolamide is used, the increased risk of severe metabolic acidosis and salicylate toxicity (caused by increased penetration of salicylate into the brain because of metabolic acidosis) must be considered. Some emergency care practitioners recommend that acetazolamide not be used at all in the treatment of salicylate overdose. Others state that acetazolamide may be used, provided that precautions are taken to prevent systemic metabolic acidosis, such as concurrent administration of an alkaline intravenous solution, e.g., one that contains sodium bicarbonate or sodium lactate.

Institution of exchange transfusion, hemodialysis, peritoneal dialysis, or hemoperfusion as needed in severe overdose.

Administering blood or vitamin K₁ if necessary to treat hemorrhaging. See the package insert or *Phytonadione (Systemic)* in *Vitamin K (Systemic)* for specific dosing guidelines for use of this product.

**Monitoring**—Monitoring serum salicylate concentration until it is apparent that the concentration is decreasing to the nontoxic range. Salicylate concentrations of 500 mcg/mL (50 mg per 100 mL; 3.62 mmol/L) 2 hours after ingestion indicate serious toxicity; salicylate concentrations above 800 mcg/mL (80 mg per 100 mL; 5.79 mmol/ L) 2 hours after ingestion indicate possible fatality. In addition, prolonged monitoring may be necessary in massive overdosage because absorption may be delayed; if a determination performed prior to 6 hours after ingestion fails to show a toxic salicylate concentration, the determination should be repeated. Salicylate concentrations indicative of varying degrees of toxicity are as follows:

| Time After Ingestion | Salicylate Concentration | | |
|---|---|---|---|
| | mcg/mL | mg/100 mL | mmol/L |
| Mild toxicity | | | |
| 6 hr | 450–650 | 45–65 | 3.26–4.71 |
| 12 hr | 350–550 | 35–55 | 2.53–3.98 |
| Moderate toxicity | | | |
| 6 hr | 650–900 | 65–90 | 4.71–6.52 |
| 12 hr | 550–750 | 55–75 | 3.98–5.43 |
| Severe toxicity | | | |
| 6 hr | > 900 | > 90 | > 6.52 |
| 12 hr | > 750 | > 75 | > 5.43 |

Monitoring for pulmonary edema and instituting appropriate therapy if required.

**Supportive care**—Correcting hyperthermia; fluid, electrolyte, and acid-base imbalances; ketosis; and plasma glucose concentration as needed.

For codeine—
**Specific treatment**—Administering the opioid antagonist naloxone. See the package insert or *Naloxone (Systemic)* for specific dosing guidelines for use of this product.

**Monitoring**—Continuing to monitor the patient (mandatory because the duration of action of the opioid analgesic may exceed that of naloxone) so that additional antagonist may be administered as needed. Alternatively, initial treatment may be followed by continuous intravenous infusion of naloxone, with the rate of infusion being adjusted according to patient response. The fact that naloxone may also antagonize the analgesic actions of opioid analgesics and may precipitate withdrawal symptoms in physically dependent patients must be kept in mind.

**Supportive care**—Establishing adequate respiratory exchange through provision of a patent airway and institution of assisted or controlled respiration.

Administration of intravenous fluids, vasopressors, and other supportive measures as needed.

Note: Patients in whom intentional overdose is known or suspected should be referred for psychiatric consultation.

## Patient Consultation
See *Table 1,* page 545.

## General Dosing Information

When used for relief of headache, especially a migraine headache, a barbiturate and analgesic combination will be most effective if administered when the first symptoms appear (during the prodrome, for migraine with aura).

After the first dose has been administered, it is recommended that the patient lie down and relax in a quiet, darkened room, because this contributes to relief of headaches.

A reduction in dosage may be required for elderly or debilitated patients, who may react to usual doses of barbiturates with excitement, confusion, or depression. This is particularly important for the codeine-containing combinations, because these patients are also more sensitive to the respiratory depressant effects of codeine.

Tolerance may occur with repeated administration of large doses of barbiturates or codeine. Also, patients who are tolerant to the effects of other opioids may be at least partially cross-tolerant to the effects of codeine, and vice versa.

Prolonged uninterrupted use of codeine or barbiturates may result in psychic or physical dependence; in patients taking these medications for relief of pain other than headache pain, gradual withdrawal may be required to reduce the risk of precipitating withdrawal symptoms.

In headache-prone individuals, frequent use of analgesics may cause physical dependence, leading to both analgesic abuse and chronic (daily or near-daily) headaches. Chronic daily use of caffeine may also result in the development of physical dependence, leading to withdrawal (rebound) headaches when the medication is stopped and to further ingestion of caffeine-containing analgesics. Patients who experience frequent headaches may be dependent on a variety of medications, including opioid analgesics, nonopioid analgesics such as acetaminophen or aspirin, ergotamine-containing headache suppressants, and antianxiety agents or sedatives, as well as barbiturate and analgesic combinations.

Chronic headaches resulting from overmedication may be difficult to relieve, especially if the patient continues to take ergotamine-containing headache suppressants and/or analgesics. If such headaches occur, it is recommended that these medications be discontinued. In-patient treatment may be necessary during detoxification. Naproxen, alone or together with amitriptyline, may reduce the severity of the headaches. Repetitive intravenous administration of dihydroergotamine (in conjunction with metoclopramide [to control dihydroergotamine-induced nausea and vomiting]) is recommended by some headache specialists to relieve this type of headache. Appropriate treatment for symptoms of withdrawal from other substances frequently used or abused by chronic headache patients may also be needed. In addition, appropriate prophylactic treatment should be initiated or adjusted to reduce the frequency and severity of future headaches.

## BUTALBITAL AND ACETAMINOPHEN

## Summary of Differences
Pharmacology/pharmacokinetics:
  Mechanism of action/effect—Butalbital: A short- to intermediate-acting barbiturate.
  Biotransformation—Acetaminophen: An intermediate metabolite is hepatotoxic and possibly nephrotoxic.
Precautions:
  Cross-sensitivity and/or related problems—Acetaminophen: Low risk of cross-sensitivity with aspirin.
  Drug interactions and/or related problems—
  Butalbital: May be less likely than phenobarbital to cause significant interference with medications adversely affected by hepatic enzyme induction.
  Acetaminophen: Caution required with hepatic enzyme inducers and with other hepatotoxic medications.
  Laboratory value alterations—Acetaminophen: Interferes with blood glucose determinations, blood 5-hydroxyindoleacetic acid determinations, pancreatic function determinations using bentiromide, serum uric acid determinations. Hepatic function studies may indicate hepatotoxicity.
  Medical considerations/contraindications—Acetaminophen: Increased risk of hepatotoxicity in alcoholics and patients with hepatic disease or viral hepatitis.

## Oral Dosage Forms

### BUTALBITAL AND ACETAMINOPHEN CAPSULES

**Usual adult and adolescent dose**
Analgesic—
  Oral, 1 or 2 capsules containing 50 mg of butalbital and 325 mg of acetaminophen every four hours as needed, not to exceed 6 capsules a day; or
  Oral, 1 capsule containing 50 mg of butalbital and 650 mg of acetaminophen every four hours as needed, not to exceed 4 capsules a day.

**Usual pediatric dose**
Dosage has not been established.

**Strength(s) usually available**
U.S.—
  50 mg of butalbital and 325 mg of acetaminophen (Rx) [*Bancap; Triaprin*].
  50 mg of butalbital and 650 mg of acetaminophen (Rx) [*Bucet; Conten; Phrenilin Forte; Tencon*].
Canada—
  Not commercially available.

**Packaging and storage**
Store below 40 °C (104 °F), preferably between 15 and 30 °C (59 and 86 °F). Store in a tight container, unless otherwise specified by manufacturer.

**Auxiliary labeling**
• May cause drowsiness.
• Avoid alcoholic beverages.
• May be habit-forming.

### BUTALBITAL AND ACETAMINOPHEN TABLETS

**Usual adult and adolescent dose**
Analgesic—
  Oral, 1 or 2 tablets containing 50 mg of butalbital and 325 mg of acetaminophen every four hours as needed, not to exceed 6 tablets a day; or
  Oral, 1 tablet containing 50 mg of butalbital and 650 mg of acetaminophen every four hours as needed, not to exceed 4 tablets a day.

**Usual pediatric dose**
Dosage has not been established.

**Strength(s) usually available**
U.S.—
  50 mg of butalbital and 325 mg of acetaminophen (Rx) [*Phrenilin* (scored); GENERIC].
  50 mg of butalbital and 650 mg of acetaminophen (Rx) [*Sedapap* (scored)].
Canada—
  Not commercially available.

**Packaging and storage**
Store below 40 °C (104 °F), preferably between 15 and 30 °C (59 and 86 °F). Store in a tight container, unless otherwise specified by manufacturer.

**Auxiliary labeling**
• May cause drowsiness.
• Avoid alcoholic beverages.
• May be habit-forming.

### BUTALBITAL, ACETAMINOPHEN, AND CAFFEINE CAPSULES USP

**Usual adult and adolescent dose**
Analgesic—Oral, 1 or 2 capsules every four hours as needed, not to exceed 6 capsules a day.

**Usual pediatric dose**
Dosage has not been established.

**Strength(s) usually available**
U.S.—
  50 mg of butalbital, 325 mg of acetaminophen, and 40 mg of caffeine (Rx) [*Amaphen; Anolor-300; Anoquan; Butace; Dolmar; Endolor; Esgic; Ezol; Femcet; Isopap; Medigesic; Pacaps; Repan; Tencet; Triad; Two-Dyne*].
Canada—
  Not commercially available.

**Packaging and storage**
Store below 40 °C (104 °F), preferably between 15 and 30 °C (59 and 86 °F). Store in a tight container, unless otherwise specified by manufacturer.

**Auxiliary labeling**
• May cause drowsiness.
• Avoid alcoholic beverages.
• May be habit-forming.

### BUTALBITAL, ACETAMINOPHEN, AND CAFFEINE TABLETS USP

**Usual adult and adolescent dose**
Analgesic—
  Oral, 1 or 2 tablets containing 50 mg of butalbital and 325 mg of acetaminophen every four hours as needed, not to exceed 6 tablets a day; or
  Oral, 1 tablet containing 50 mg of butalbital and 500 mg of acetaminophen every four hours as needed, not to exceed 6 tablets a day.

**Usual pediatric dose**
Dosage has not been established.

**Strength(s) usually available**
U.S.—
  50 mg of butalbital, 325 mg of acetaminophen, and 40 mg of caffeine (Rx) [*Arcet; Dolmar; Esgic* (scored); *Fioricet; Isocet; Medigesic; Pharmagesic; Repan*; GENERIC].
  50 mg of butalbital, 500 mg of acetaminophen, and 40 mg of caffeine (Rx) [*Esgic-Plus* (scored)].
Canada—
  Not commercially available.

**Packaging and storage**
Store below 40 °C (104 °F), preferably between 15 and 30 °C (59 and 86 °F). Store in a tight container.

**Auxiliary labeling**
• May cause drowsiness.
• Avoid alcoholic beverages.
• May be habit-forming.

## BUTALBITAL, ACETAMINOPHEN, CAFFEINE, AND CODEINE

## Summary of Differences
Pharmacology/pharmacokinetics:
  Mechanism of action/effect—Butalbital: A short- to intermediate-acting barbiturate.

Other actions/effects—Codeine: Also has antidiarrheal and antitussive actions.

Biotransformation—Acetaminophen: An intermediate metabolite is hepatotoxic and possibly nephrotoxic.

Precautions:
Cross-sensitivity and/or related problems—Acetaminophen: Low risk of cross-sensitivity with aspirin.
Pregnancy—Codeine: Ingestion shortly prior to delivery may cause neonatal respiratory depression, especially in premature neonates.
Geriatrics—Codeine: Increased susceptibility to respiratory depressant effects.
Drug interactions and/or related problems—
Butalbital: May be less likely than phenobarbital to cause significant interference with medications adversely affected by hepatic enzyme induction.
Acetaminophen: Caution is required with hepatic enzyme inducers and with other hepatotoxic medications.
Codeine: Caution is also required with anticholinergics, antiperistaltic antidiarrheals, agents that may reduce blood pressure, metoclopramide, monoamine oxidase inhibitors, naloxone, naltrexone, and other opioid analgesics.
Laboratory value alterations—
Acetaminophen: Interferes with blood glucose determinations, blood 5-hydroxyindoleacetic acid determinations, pancreatic function determinations using bentiromide, serum uric acid determinations. Hepatic function studies may indicate hepatotoxicity.
Codeine: Interferes with gastric emptying studies and hepatobiliary imaging (radionuclide). Also, may increase plasma amylase and/or lipase concentrations.
Medical considerations/contraindications—
Acetaminophen: Increased risk of hepatotoxicity in alcoholics and patients with hepatic disease or viral hepatitis.
Codeine: Should not be used if the patient has diarrhea caused by poisoning or by antibiotic therapy, or in the presence of acute respiratory depression. Caution is also required in patients with asthma, chronic respiratory disease, and severe inflammatory bowel disease.
Side/adverse effects:
Codeine: May also cause laryngospasm or laryngeal edema.

## Oral Dosage Forms
### BUTALBITAL, ACETAMINOPHEN, CAFFEINE AND CODEINE PHOSPHATE CAPSULES

**Usual adult and adolescent dose**
Analgesic—
Oral, 1 or 2 capsules every four hours as needed, not to exceed 6 capsules a day.

**Usual pediatric dose**
Dosage has not been established.

**Strength(s) usually available**
U.S.—
50 mg of butalbital, 325 mg of acetaminophen, 40 mg of caffeine, and 30 mg of codeine phosphate (Rx) [*Fioricet with Codeine* ( propylparaben; carboxymethylcellulose; silicone dioxide and/or sodium propionate)].
Canada—
Not commercially available.

**Packaging and storage**
Store below 40 °C (86 °F). Store in a tight container, unless otherwise specified by manufacturer.

**Auxiliary labeling**
• May cause drowsiness.
• Avoid alcoholic beverages.
• May be habit-forming.

---

## BUTALBITAL AND ASPIRIN

## Summary of Differences
Pharmacology/pharmacokinetics:
Mechanism of action/effect—Butalbital: A short- to intermediate-acting barbiturate.
Other actions/effects—Aspirin: Also has platelet aggregation–inhibiting actions.
Precautions:
Cross-sensitivity and/or related problems—Aspirin: Risk of cross-sensitivity with other nonsteroidal anti-inflammatory drugs (NSAIDs); slight risk of cross-sensitivity with acetaminophen.
Pregnancy/reproduction—Aspirin:
First trimester—Reports of possible birth defects in humans, but teratogenicity not found in controlled studies with usual therapeutic doses.
Third trimester—Use not recommended; chronic, high-dose use has caused complications (including stillbirth or neonatal death) associated with prolonged gestation, premature closure of the fetal ductus arteriosus, prolonged labor, complicated deliveries, and maternal, fetal or neonatal bleeding.
Pediatrics—Aspirin: Risk of Reye's syndrome in children with acute febrile illness, especially influenza and varicella; febrile, dehydrated patients also more susceptible to other forms of salicylate toxicity.
Adolescents—Aspirin: Risk of Reye's syndrome in adolescents with acute febrile illness, especially influenza and varicella.
Geriatrics—Aspirin: Increased susceptibility to salicylate toxicity.
Drug interactions and/or related problems—
Butalbital: May be less likely than phenobarbital to cause significant interference with medications adversely affected by hepatic enzyme induction.
Aspirin: Caution also required with urinary acidifiers or alkalizers; anticoagulants; methotrexate; ototoxic medications; probenecid; sulfinpyrazone; and thrombolytic agents.
Laboratory value alterations—Aspirin: Interferes with determinations of urine aceto-acetic acid (Gerhard test), urine glucose (copper sulfate or enzymatic tests), urine 5-hydroxyindoleacetic acid, renal function test (phenolsulfonphthalein), thyroid imaging (radionuclide), thyroid-stimulating hormone release (protirelin-stimulated), vanillylmandelic acid. May also prolong bleeding time, decrease serum potassium concentrations, and cause dose-dependent increase or decrease in serum uric acid concentration.
Medical considerations/contraindications—Aspirin: Should not be used in patients with severe allergic or asthmatic reaction to aspirin or other NSAIDs (history of), bleeding ulcers or other active bleeding states, or hemophilia or other coagulation or platelet function defects. Caution also required in patients with gastrointestinal ulceration, gout, hypoprothrombinemia, and vitamin K deficiency.
Side/adverse effects: Aspirin—May also cause anaphylaxis and toxic epidermal necrolysis.

## Additional Dosing Information
See also *General Dosing Information*.

Medications containing aspirin should be administered with food or a full glass (240 mL) of water to lessen gastric irritation.

Dosage of aspirin should be reduced if fever or illness causes fluid depletion, especially in children.

In general, it is recommended that aspirin therapy be discontinued 5 days before surgery to reduce the risk of bleeding problems.

## Oral Dosage Forms
### BUTALBITAL AND ASPIRIN TABLETS USP

**Usual adult and adolescent dose**
Analgesic—
Oral, 1 tablet every four hours as needed, not to exceed 6 tablets a day.

**Usual pediatric dose**
Dosage has not been established.

**Strength(s) usually available**
U.S.—
50 mg of butalbital and 650 mg of aspirin (Rx) [*Axotal*].
Canada—
Not commercially available.

**Packaging and storage**
Store below 30 °C (86 °F), protected from moisture, unless otherwise specified by manufacturer. Store in a tight container.

**Auxiliary labeling**
• Avoid alcoholic beverages.
• May cause drowsiness.
• Take with food or with a full glass of water.

**Note**
Not a federally controlled substance in the U.S.; however, state regulations may apply.

### BUTALBITAL, ASPIRIN, AND CAFFEINE CAPSULES USP

**Usual adult and adolescent dose**
Analgesic—
Oral, 1 or 2 capsules every four hours as needed, not to exceed 6 capsules a day.

**Usual pediatric dose**
Dosage has not been established.

**Strength(s) usually available**
U.S.—
  50 mg of butalbital, 325 mg of aspirin, and 40 mg of caffeine (Rx) [*Butalgen; Fiorinal* (sodium bisulfite); *Isobutal; Isollyl; Laniroif; Lanorinal; Marnal;* GENERIC].
Canada—
  50 mg of butalbital, 330 mg of ASA, and 40 mg of caffeine (Rx) [*Fiorinal; Tecnal*].
Note: Because *Aspirin* is a brand name in Canada, ASA is the term used in Canadian product labeling.

**Packaging and storage**
Store below 25 °C (77 °F), in a well-closed container, unless otherwise specified by manufacturer.

**Auxiliary labeling**
• Avoid alcoholic beverages.
• May cause drowsiness.
• Take with food or with a full glass of water.

**Note**
Controlled substance in both the U.S. and Canada.

## BUTALBITAL, ASPIRIN, AND CAFFEINE TABLETS USP

**Usual adult and adolescent dose**
Analgesic—
  Oral, 1 or 2 tablets containing 50 mg of butalbital, 325 mg of aspirin, and 40 mg of caffeine every four hours as needed, not to exceed 6 tablets a day.

**Usual pediatric dose**
Dosage has not been established.

**Strength(s) usually available**
U.S.—
  50 mg of butalbital, 325 mg of aspirin, and 40 mg of caffeine (Rx) [*Butalgen; Fiorgen; Fiorinal* (lactose); *Fiormor; Fortabs; Isobutal; Isobutyl; Isolin; Isollyl; Laniroif; Lanorinal; Marnal; Vibutal;* GENERIC].
Canada—
  50 mg of butalbital, 330 mg of ASA, and 40 mg of caffeine (Rx) [*Fiorinal; Tecnal*].
Note: Because *Aspirin* is a brand name in Canada, ASA is the term used in Canadian product labeling.

**Packaging and storage**
Store below 30 °C (86 °F), preferably between 15 and 30 °C (59 and 86 °F), unless otherwise specified by manufacturer. Store in a tight container.

**Auxiliary labeling**
• Avoid alcoholic beverages.
• May cause drowsiness.
• Take with food or with a full glass of water.

**Note**
Products containing 325 mg of aspirin and 50 mg of butalbital per tablet are controlled substances in both the U.S. and Canada.

---

### BUTALBITAL, ASPIRIN, CAFFEINE, AND CODEINE

## Summary of Differences

Pharmacology/pharmacokinetics:
  Mechanism of action/effect—Butalbital: A short- to intermediate-acting barbiturate.
  Other actions/effects—
    Aspirin: Also has platelet aggregation–inhibiting actions.
    Codeine: Also has antidiarrheal and antitussive actions.
Precautions:
  Cross-sensitivity and/or related problems—Aspirin: Risk of cross-sensitivity with other nonsteroidal anti-inflammatory drugs (NSAIDs); slight risk of cross-sensitivity with acetaminophen.
  Pregnancy/reproduction—
    First trimester: Aspirin—Reports of possible birth defects in humans, but teratogenicity not found in controlled studies with usual therapeutic doses.
    Third trimester:
      Aspirin—Use not recommended; chronic, high-dose use has caused complications (including stillbirth or neonatal death) associated with prolonged gestation, premature closure of the fetal ductus arteriosus, prolonged labor, complicated deliveries, and maternal, fetal or neonatal bleeding.
    Codeine—Ingestion shortly prior to delivery may cause neonatal respiratory depression, especially in premature neonates.
  Pediatrics—Aspirin: Risk of Reye's syndrome in children with acute febrile illness, especially influenza and varicella; febrile, dehydrated patients also more susceptible to other forms of salicylate toxicity.
  Adolescents—Aspirin: Risk of Reye's syndrome in adolescents with acute febrile illness, especially influenza and varicella.
  Geriatrics—
    Aspirin: Increased susceptiblity to salicylate toxicity.
    Codeine: Increased susceptibility to respiratory depressant effects.
  Drug interactions and/or related problems—
    Butalbital: May be less likely than phenobarbital to cause significant interference with medications adversely affected by hepatic enzyme induction.
    Aspirin: Caution also required with urinary acidifiers or alkalizers; anticoagulants; methotrexate; ototoxic medications; probenecid; sulfinpyrazone; and thrombolytic agents.
    Codeine: Caution also required with anticholinergics, antiperistaltic antidiarrheals, agents that may reduce blood pressure, metoclopramide, monoamine oxidase inhibitors, naloxone, naltrexone, and other opioid analgesics.
  Laboratory value alterations—
    Aspirin: Interferes with determinations of urine aceto-acetic acid (Gerhard test), urine glucose (copper sulfate or enzymatic tests), urine 5-hydroxyindoleacetic acid, renal function test (phenolsulfonphthalein), thyroid imaging (radionuclide), thyroid-stimulating hormone release (protirelin-stimulated), vanillylmandelic acid. May also prolong bleeding time, decrease serum potassium concentrations, and cause dose-dependent increase or decrease in serum uric acid concentration.
    Codeine: Interferes with gastric emptying studies and hepatobiliary imaging (radionuclide). Also, may increase plasma amylase and/or lipase concentrations.
  Medical considerations/contraindications
    Aspirin: Should not be used in patients with severe allergic or asthmatic reaction to aspirin or other NSAIDs (history of), bleeding ulcers or other active bleeding states (current), or hemophilia or other coagulation or platelet function defects. Caution also required in patients with gastrointestinal ulceration, gout, hypoprothrombinemia, and vitamin K deficiency.
    Codeine: Should not be used if the patient has diarrhea caused by poisoning or by antibiotic therapy, or in the presence of acute respiratory depression. Caution also required in patients with asthma, chronic respiratory disease, and severe inflammatory bowel disease.
  Side/adverse effects:
    Aspirin: May also cause anaphylaxis and toxic epidermal necrolysis.
    Codeine: May also cause laryngospasm or laryngeal edema.

## Additional Dosing Information

See also *General Dosing Information*.

Medications containing aspirin should be administered with food or a full glass (240 mL) of water to lessen gastric irritation.

Dosage of aspirin should be reduced if fever or illness causes fluid depletion, especially in children.

In general, it is recommended that aspirin therapy be discontinued 5 days before surgery to reduce the risk of bleeding problems.

## Oral Dosage Forms

### BUTALBITAL, ASPIRIN, CAFFEINE, AND CODEINE PHOSPHATE CAPSULES USP

**Usual adult and adolescent dose**
Analgesic—
  Oral, 1 or 2 capsules every four hours as needed, not to exceed 6 capsules a day.

**Usual pediatric dose**
Dosage has not been established.

**Strength(s) usually available**
U.S.—
  50 mg of butalbital, 325 mg of aspirin, 40 mg of caffeine, and 30 mg of codeine phosphate (Rx) [*Ascomp with Codeine No.3; Butalbital Compound with Codeine; Butinal with Codeine No.3; Fiorinal with Codeine No.3; Idenal with Codeine; Isollyl with Codeine;* GENERIC].
Canada—
  50 mg of butalbital, 330 mg of ASA, 40 mg of caffeine, and 15 mg of codeine phosphate (Rx) [*Fiorinal-C ¼* (lactose); *Tecnal-C ¼*].

50 mg of butalbital, 330 mg of ASA, 40 mg of caffeine, and 30 mg of codeine phosphate (Rx) [*Fiorinal-C ½* (lactose); *Tecnal-C ½*].

Note: Because *Aspirin* is a brand name in Canada, ASA is the term used in Canadian product labeling.

**Packaging and storage**
Store below 25 °C (77 °F), in a well-closed container, unless otherwise specified by manufacturer.

**Auxiliary labeling**
• Avoid alcoholic beverages.
• May cause drowsiness.
• Take with food or with a full glass of water.
• May be habit-forming.

**Note**
Controlled substance in both the U.S. and Canada.

### BUTALBITAL, ASPIRIN, CAFFEINE, AND CODEINE PHOSPHATE TABLETS

**Usual adult and adolescent dose**
See *Butalbital, Aspirin, Caffeine, and Codeine Phosphate Capsules USP*.

**Usual pediatric dose**
Dosage has not been established.

**Strength(s) usually available**
U.S.—
    50 mg of butalbital, 325 mg of aspirin, 30 mg of codeine phosphate, and 40 mg of caffeine (Rx) [*Idenal with Codeine;* GENERIC].
Canada—
    Not commercially available.

**Packaging and storage**
Store below 25 °C (77 °F), in a well-closed container, unless otherwise specified by manufacturer.

**Auxiliary labeling**
• Avoid alcoholic beverages.
• May cause drowsiness.
• Take with food or with a full glass of water.
• May be habit-forming.

**Note**
Controlled substance in the U.S.

---

### PHENOBARBITAL, ASA, AND CODEINE

## Summary of Differences

Pharmacology/pharmacokinetics:
    Mechanism of action/effect—Phenobarbital: A long-acting barbiturate.
    Other actions/effects—
    Phenobarbital: Also has anticonvulsant activity.
    Aspirin: Also has platelet aggregation–inhibiting actions.
    Codeine: Also has antidiarrheal and antitussive actions.
Precautions:
    Cross-sensitivity and/or related problems—Aspirin: Risk of cross-sensitivity with other nonsteroidal anti-inflammatory drugs (NSAIDs); slight risk of cross-sensitivity with acetaminophen.
    Pregnancy/reproduction—
    First trimester: Aspirin—Reports of possible birth defects in humans, but teratogenicity not found in controlled studies with usual therapeutic doses.
    Third trimester: Aspirin—Use not recommended; chronic, high-dose use has caused complications (including stillbirth or neonatal death) associated with prolonged gestation, premature closure of the fetal ductus arteriosus, prolonged labor, complicated deliveries, and maternal, fetal or neonatal bleeding.
    Pediatrics—Aspirin: Risk of Reye's syndrome in children with acute febrile illness, especially influenza and varicella; febrile, dehydrated patients also more susceptible to other forms of salicylate toxicity.
    Adolescents—Aspirin: Risk of Reye's syndrome in adolescents with acute febrile illness, especially influenza and varicella.
    Geriatrics—
    Aspirin: Increased susceptiblity to salicylate toxicity.
    Codeine: Increased susceptibility to respiratory depressant effects.
    Drug interactions and/or related problems—
    Phenobarbital: More likely than butalbital to cause significant interference with medications adversely affected by hepatic enzyme induction.
    Aspirin: Caution also required with urinary acidifiers or alkalizers; anticoagulants; methotrexate; ototoxic medications; probenecid; sulfinpyrazone; and thrombolytic agents.
    Codeine: Caution also required with anticholinergics, antiperistaltic antidiarrheals, agents that may reduce blood pressure, metoclopramide, monoamine oxidase inhibitors, naloxone, naltrexone, and other opioid analgesics.
Laboratory value alterations—
Aspirin: Interferes with determinations of urine aceto-acetic acid (Gerhard test), urine glucose (copper sulfate or enzymatic tests), urine 5-hydroxyindoleacetic acid, renal function test (phenolsulfonphthalein), thyroid imaging (radionuclide), thyroid-stimulating hormone release (protirelin-stimulated), vanillylmandelic acid. May also prolong bleeding time, decrease serum potassium concentrations, and cause dose-dependent increase or decrease in serum uric acid concentration.
Codeine: Interferes with gastric emptying studies and hepatobiliary imaging (radionuclide). Also, may increase plasma amylase and/or lipase concentrations.
Medical considerations/contraindications
Aspirin: Should not be used in patients with severe allergic or asthmatic reaction to aspirin or other NSAIDs (history of), bleeding ulcers or other active bleeding states (current), or hemophilia or other coagulation or platelet function defects. Caution also required in patients with gastrointestinal ulceration, gout, hypoprothrombinemia, and vitamin K deficiency.
Codeine: Should not be used if the patient has diarrhea caused by poisoning or by antibiotic therapy, or in the presence of acute respiratory depression. Caution also required in patients with asthma, chronic respiratory disease, and severe inflammatory bowel disease.
Side/adverse effects:
    Aspirin—May also cause anaphylaxis and toxic epidermal necrolysis.
    Codeine—May also cause laryngospasm or laryngeal edema.

## Additional Dosing Information

See also *General Dosing Information*.

Medications containing aspirin should be administered with food or a full glass (240 mL) of water to lessen gastric irritation.

Dosage of aspirin should be reduced if fever or illness causes fluid depletion, especially in children.

In general, it is recommended that aspirin therapy be discontinued 5 days before surgery to reduce the risk of bleeding problems.

## Oral Dosage Forms

### PHENOBARBITAL, ASA, AND CODEINE PHOSPHATE CAPSULES

**Usual adult and adolescent dose**
Analgesic—
    Oral, 1 or 2 capsules containing 16.2 mg of phenobarbital, 325 mg of ASA, and 16.2 or 32.4 mg of codeine phosphate every three or four hours; or
    Oral, 1 capsule containing 16.2 mg of phenobarbital, 325 mg of ASA, and 64.8 mg of codeine phosphate every three or four hours.

**Usual pediatric dose**
Dosage has not been established.

**Strength(s) usually available**
U.S.—
    Not commercially available.
Canada—
    16.2 mg of phenobarbital, 325 mg of ASA, and 16.2 mg of codeine phosphate (Rx) [*Phenaphen with Codeine No.2*].
    16.2 mg of phenobarbital, 325 mg of ASA, and 32.4 mg of codeine phosphate (Rx) [*Phenaphen with Codeine No.3*].
    16.2 mg of phenobarbital, 325 mg of ASA, and 64.8 mg of codeine phosphate (Rx) [*Phenaphen with Codeine No.4*].

Note: Because *Aspirin* is a brand name in Canada, ASA is the term used in Canadian product labeling.

**Packaging and storage**
Store below 30 °C (86 °F), preferably between 15 and 30 °C (59 and 86 °F), unless otherwise specified by manufacturer.

**Auxiliary labeling**
• Avoid alcoholic beverages.
• May cause drowsiness.
• Take with food or with a full glass of water.

**Note**
Controlled substance in Canada.

## Selected Bibliography

Kunkel RS. Diagnosis and treatment of muscle contraction (tension-type) headaches. Med Clin N Amer 1991; 75: 595-603.

Elkind AH. Drug abuse and headache. Med Clin N Amer 1991; 75: 717-32.

Sands GH. A protocol for butalbital, aspirin, and caffeine (BAC) detoxification in headache patients. Headache 1990; 30: 491-6.

Revised: 07/13/92
Interim revision: 05/13/98

## Table 1. Patient Consultation

As an aid to patient consultation, refer to *Advice for the Patient, Butalbital and Acetaminophen (Systemic); Butalbital and Aspirin (Systemic); Butalbital, Acetaminophen, Caffeine, and Codeine (Systemic)* or *Barbiturates, Aspirin, and Codeine (Systemic)*.

In providing consultation, consider emphasizing the following selected information (» = major clinical significance):

Legend:
I = Butalbital and Acetaminophen
II = Butalbital, Acetaminophen, and Caffeine
III = Butalbital and Aspirin
IV = Butalbital, Aspirin, and Caffeine
V = Butalbital, Aspirin, Caffeine, and Codeine
VI = Phenobarbital, Aspirin, and Codeine
VII = Butalbital, Acetaminophen, Caffeine and Codeine

| | I | II | III | IV | V | VI | VII |
|---|---|---|---|---|---|---|---|
| **Before using this medication** | | | | | | | |
| » Conditions affecting use, especially: | | | | | | | |
|   Sensitivity to— | | | | | | | |
|     Butalbital, phenobarbital, or other barbiturates | ✓ | ✓ | ✓ | ✓ | ✓ | ✓ | ✓ |
|     Acetaminophen | ✓ | ✓ | | | | | ✓ |
|     Aspirin or other nonsteroidal anti-inflammatory drugs (NSAIDs) | | | ✓ | ✓ | ✓ | ✓ | |
|     Codeine | | | | | ✓ | ✓ | ✓ |
|     Caffeine | | ✓ | | ✓ | ✓ | | ✓ |
|   Pregnancy— | | | | | | | |
|     Barbiturates cross the placenta; may cause fetal abnormalities and/or an increased risk of brain tumors in the neonate; may also cause breathing problems in the neonate if taken shortly before delivery | ✓ | ✓ | ✓ | ✓ | ✓ | ✓ | ✓ |
|     Aspirin crosses the placenta; should not be taken during third trimester unless prescribed by physician; chronic, high-dose use may cause adverse effects on the circulation in fetus or neonate, bleeding in fetus and/or mother, prolonged gestation, and complicated deliveries | | | ✓ | ✓ | ✓ | ✓ | |
|     Codeine crosses the placenta; may cause breathing problems in the neonate if taken just before delivery | | | | | ✓ | ✓ | ✓ |
|     Caffeine crosses the placenta; total daily intake should be limited because of risk of fetal arrhythmias | | ✓ | | ✓ | ✓ | | ✓ |
|   Breast-feeding— | | | | | | | |
|     Barbiturates distributed into breast milk; may cause CNS depression in the infant | ✓ | ✓ | ✓ | ✓ | ✓ | ✓ | ✓ |
|     Caffeine distributed into breast milk; total daily intake should be limited because of risk of CNS stimulation in the infant | | ✓ | | ✓ | ✓ | | ✓ |
|   Use in children— | | | | | | | |
|     Possibility of barbiturate-induced paradoxical excitement | ✓ | ✓ | ✓ | ✓ | ✓ | ✓ | ✓ |
|     Not giving aspirin to children with symptoms of viral illness (especially influenza or varicella) without physician's permission because of risk of Reye's syndrome; children without a viral illness are also more susceptible to aspirin-induced toxicity | | | ✓ | ✓ | ✓ | ✓ | |
|     Possibility of codeine-induced paradoxical excitement | | | | | ✓ | ✓ | ✓ |
|   Use in teenagers—Checking with physician before giving to teenagers with symptoms of acute febrile illness, especially influenza or varicella, because of the risk of Reye's syndrome | | | | ✓ | ✓ | ✓ | |
|   Use in the elderly— | | | | | | | |
|     Increased sensitivity to barbiturates; may react to usual doses with confusion, depression, or excitement | ✓ | ✓ | ✓ | ✓ | ✓ | ✓ | ✓ |
|     Increased susceptibility to toxic effects of aspirin | | | ✓ | ✓ | ✓ | ✓ | |
|     Increased susceptibility to respiratory depressant and other adverse effects of opioid analgesics | | | | | ✓ | ✓ | ✓ |
|   Other medications, especially: | | | | | | | |
|     Alcohol | ✓ | ✓ | ✓ | ✓ | ✓ | ✓ | ✓ |
|     Alkalizers, urinary | | | ✓ | ✓ | ✓ | ✓ | |
|     Anticoagulants, coumarin- or indandione-derivative | ✓ | ✓ | ✓ | ✓ | ✓ | ✓ | ✓ |
|     Carbamazepine | ✓ | ✓ | ✓ | ✓ | ✓ | ✓ | ✓ |
|     Contraceptives, estrogen-containing, oral | ✓ | ✓ | ✓ | ✓ | ✓ | ✓ | ✓ |
|     Corticosteroids, glucocorticoid and mineralocorticoid | ✓ | ✓ | ✓ | ✓ | ✓ | ✓ | ✓ |
|     Corticotropin | ✓ | ✓ | ✓ | ✓ | ✓ | ✓ | ✓ |
|     CNS depressants | ✓ | ✓ | ✓ | ✓ | ✓ | ✓ | ✓ |
|     Divalproex sodium | ✓ | ✓ | ✓ | ✓ | ✓ | ✓ | ✓ |
|     Heparin | | | ✓ | ✓ | ✓ | ✓ | |

## Table 1. Patient Consultation (continued)

As an aid to patient consultation, refer to *Advice for the Patient, Butalbital and Acetaminophen (Systemic); Butalbital and Aspirin (Systemic); Butalbital, Acetaminophen, Caffeine, and Codeine (Systemic)* or *Barbiturates, Aspirin, and Codeine (Systemic)*.

In providing consultation, consider emphasizing the following selected information (» = major clinical significance):

Legend:
I = Butalbital and Acetaminophen
II = Butalbital, Acetaminophen, and Caffeine
III = Butalbital and Aspirin
IV = Butalbital, Aspirin, and Caffeine
V = Butalbital, Aspirin, Caffeine, and Codeine
VI = Phenobarbital, Aspirin, and Codeine
VII = Butalbital, Acetaminophen, Caffeine and Codeine

| | I | II | III | IV | V | VI | VII |
|---|---|---|---|---|---|---|---|
| Methotrexate | | | ✔ | ✔ | ✔ | ✔ | |
| Naltrexone | | | | | ✔ | ✔ | ✔ |
| Probenecid | | | ✔ | ✔ | ✔ | ✔ | |
| Sulfinpyrazone | | | ✔ | ✔ | ✔ | ✔ | |
| Valproic acid | ✔ | ✔ | ✔ | ✔ | ✔ | ✔ | ✔ |
| Vancomycin | | | ✔ | ✔ | ✔ | ✔ | |
| **Other medical problems, especially:** | | | | | | | |
| Alcohol abuse | ✔ | ✔ | | | | | ✔ |
| Asthma | ✔ | ✔ | | | | | |
| Bleeding ulcers, or other bleeding problems or coagulation defects | | | ✔ | ✔ | ✔ | ✔ | |
| Diarrhea caused by antibiotics or poisoning | | | | | | | |
| Drug abuse or history of | ✔ | ✔ | ✔ | ✔ | ✔ | ✔ | ✔ |
| Gastritis (erosive) or peptic ulcer, history of | | | ✔ | ✔ | ✔ | ✔ | |
| Inflammatory bowel disease, severe | | | | | ✔ | ✔ | ✔ |
| Liver disease | ✔ | ✔ | ✔ | ✔ | ✔ | ✔ | ✔ |
| Porphyria | ✔ | ✔ | ✔ | ✔ | ✔ | ✔ | ✔ |
| Porphyria | ✔ | ✔ | ✔ | ✔ | ✔ | ✔ | ✔ |
| Respiratory disease | ✔ | ✔ | ✔ | ✔ | ✔ | ✔ | ✔ |
| Viral hepatitis | ✔ | ✔ | | | | | ✔ |

**Proper use of this medication**

| | I | II | III | IV | V | VI | VII |
|---|---|---|---|---|---|---|---|
| » Taking with food or a full glass (240 mL) of water to minimize stomach irritation | | | ✔ | ✔ | ✔ | ✔ | |
| » Not taking medication if it has a strong vinegar-like odor | | | ✔ | ✔ | ✔ | ✔ | |
| » Importance of not taking more medication than the amount prescribed because of danger of: | | | | | | | |
| Habituation | ✔ | ✔ | ✔ | ✔ | ✔ | ✔ | ✔ |
| Hepatotoxicity | ✔ | ✔ | | | | | ✔ |
| Overdose | ✔ | ✔ | ✔ | ✔ | ✔ | ✔ | ✔ |
| » For relief of headache: | | | | | | | |
| Most effective when taken as soon as headache appears or at first sign of migraine attack (prodromal stage) | ✔ | ✔ | ✔ | ✔ | ✔ | ✔ | ✔ |
| Lying down in a quiet, dark room for a while after taking | ✔ | ✔ | ✔ | ✔ | ✔ | ✔ | ✔ |
| Compliance with prophylactic therapy, if prescribed | ✔ | ✔ | ✔ | ✔ | ✔ | ✔ | ✔ |
| » Proper dosing | ✔ | ✔ | ✔ | ✔ | ✔ | ✔ | ✔ |
| Missed dose (if on scheduled dosing regimen): Taking as soon as possible; not taking if almost time for next dose; not doubling doses | ✔ | ✔ | ✔ | ✔ | ✔ | ✔ | ✔ |
| » Proper storage | ✔ | ✔ | ✔ | ✔ | ✔ | ✔ | ✔ |

**Precautions while using this medication**

| | I | II | III | IV | V | VI | VII |
|---|---|---|---|---|---|---|---|
| » Checking with physician if effectiveness of medication decreases and/or frequency of headaches increases; possibility that tolerance to or physical dependence on the medication, leading to withdrawal headaches, has developed | ✔ | ✔ | ✔ | ✔ | ✔ | ✔ | ✔ |
| » Risk of overdose if taking other medications containing: | | | | | | | |
| Barbiturates | ✔ | ✔ | ✔ | ✔ | ✔ | ✔ | ✔ |
| Acetaminophen | ✔ | ✔ | | | | | ✔ |
| Aspirin or other salicylates | | | ✔ | ✔ | ✔ | ✔ | |
| Codeine or other opioids | | | | | ✔ | ✔ | ✔ |
| » Avoiding alcohol or other CNS depressants unless prescribed or otherwise approved by physician | ✔ | ✔ | ✔ | ✔ | ✔ | ✔ | ✔ |
| Alcohol consumption may increase probability of stomach problems | | | | ✔ | ✔ | ✔ | ✔ |
| Alcohol consumption may increase risk of hepatotoxicity, with high doses or prolonged use | ✔ | ✔ | | | | | ✔ |
| » Caution if dizziness, lightheadedness, drowsiness, or a false sense of well-being occurs | ✔ | ✔ | ✔ | ✔ | ✔ | ✔ | ✔ |
| Caution when getting up suddenly from a lying or sitting position | | | | | | ✔ | ✔ |
| Lying down if nausea or vomiting, or dizziness or lightheadedness occurs | | | | | ✔ | ✔ | ✔ |

### Table 1. Patient Consultation (continued)

| | | | | | | | |
|---|:-:|:-:|:-:|:-:|:-:|:-:|:-:|
| As an aid to patient consultation, refer to *Advice for the Patient, Butalbital and Acetaminophen (Systemic); Butalbital and Aspirin (Systemic); Butalbital, Acetaminophen, Caffeine, and Codeine (Systemic)* or *Barbiturates, Aspirin, and Codeine (Systemic)*.<br>In providing consultation, consider emphasizing the following selected information (» = major clinical significance): | | Legend:<br>I = Butalbital and Acetaminophen<br>II = Butalbital, Acetaminophen, and Caffeine<br>III = Butalbital and Aspirin<br>IV = Butalbital, Aspirin, and Caffeine<br>V = Butalbital, Aspirin, Caffeine, and Codeine<br>VI = Phenobarbital, Aspirin, and Codeine<br>VII = Butalbital, Acetaminophen, Caffeine and Codeine | | | | | |
| | I | II | III | IV | V | VI | VII |
| Need to inform physician or dentist of use of medication if any kind of surgery (including dental surgery) or emergency treatment is required | ✔ | ✔ | ✔ | ✔ | ✔ | ✔ | ✔ |
| Caution if any kind of surgery is required; aspirin should be discontinued 5 days prior to surgery unless otherwise directed by physician | | | ✔ | ✔ | ✔ | ✔ | |
| Diabetics: May cause false urine sugar test results with prolonged use of 8 or more capsules or tablets per day | | | ✔ | ✔ | ✔ | ✔ | |
| Caution if any laboratory tests required<br>  Possible interference with laboratory test results<br>  Not taking caffeine for 8 to 12 hours prior to dipyridamole-assisted myocardial perfusion studies | ✔ | ✔<br>✔ | ✔ | ✔<br>✔ | ✔<br>✔ | ✔ | ✔<br>✔ |
| » Checking with physician before discontinuing medication following prolonged use; gradual reduction in dosage may be required to reduce risk of withdrawal symptoms | ✔ | ✔ | ✔ | ✔ | ✔ | ✔ | ✔ |
| » Suspected overdose: Getting emergency help at once | ✔ | ✔ | ✔ | ✔ | ✔ | ✔ | ✔ |
| **Side/adverse effects**<br>Signs and symptoms of potential side effects, especially:<br>  Agranulocytosis<br>  Anaphylaxis<br>  Angioedema<br>  Bronchospastic allergic reaction<br>  CNS adverse effects<br>  CNS stimulation (paradoxical)<br>  Dermatitis, allergic<br>  Dermatitis, exfoliative<br>  Erythema multiforme<br>  Laryngeal edema, allergic<br>  Laryngospasm, allergic<br>  Stevens-Johnson syndrome<br>  Thrombocytopenia<br>  Toxic epidermal necrolysis | ✔<br><br>✔<br>✔<br>✔<br>✔<br>✔<br>✔<br><br><br>✔<br>✔<br> | ✔<br><br>✔<br>✔<br>✔<br>✔<br>✔<br>✔<br><br><br>✔<br>✔<br> | ✔<br>✔<br>✔<br>✔<br>✔<br>✔<br>✔<br>✔<br>✔<br><br><br>✔<br>✔<br>✔ | ✔<br>✔<br>✔<br>✔<br>✔<br>✔<br>✔<br>✔<br>✔<br><br><br>✔<br>✔<br>✔ | ✔<br>✔<br>✔<br>✔<br>✔<br>✔<br>✔<br>✔<br>✔<br>✔<br>✔<br>✔<br>✔<br>✔ | ✔<br>✔<br>✔<br>✔<br>✔<br>✔<br>✔<br>✔<br>✔<br>✔<br>✔<br>✔<br>✔<br>✔ | ✔<br>✔<br>✔<br>✔<br>✔<br>✔<br>✔<br>✔<br>✔<br>✔<br>✔<br>✔<br>✔<br>✔ |

---

**BARIUM SULFATE**—The *Barium Sulfate (Local)* monograph is not included in this published version of the USP DI database. Copies of the monograph are available on request from Micromedex, Inc. - Reprint Requests, 6200 S. Syracuse Way, Suite 300, Englewood, CO 80111; telephone (303) 486-6400; telefax (303) 486-6464; Email: USPDI@MDX.COM.

---

# BASILIXIMAB  Systemic—INTRODUCTORY VERSION

VA CLASSIFICATION (Primary): IM600
Commonly used brand name(s): *Simulect*.
Note: For a listing of dosage forms and brand names by country availability, see *Dosage Forms* section(s).

## Category

Immunosuppressant; monoclonal antibody.

## Indications

### General considerations

The efficacy of basiliximab was demonstrated in two placebo-controlled, multicenter trials in which basiliximab was administered in conjunction with cyclosporine and corticosteroids. The primary endpoint in the trials was the incidence of death, loss of the graft, or acute rejection within the first 6 months following transplantation. The incidence of the primary endpoint was lower in the basiliximab-treated group than it was in the placebo-treated group in both the U.S. study and the European and Canadian study ($P = 0.002$ and $0.003$, respectively).

Note: The finding of significance in this combined primary endpoint is attributed to the significant difference observed in the incidence of acute rejection in the basiliximab-treated group. The incidences of death and loss of graft were not significantly different between the control group and the basiliximab-treated group (see below).

A secondary endpoint in the trials was the incidence of death, loss of the graft, or acute rejection within the first 12 months following transplantation. The incidence of this secondary endpoint was lower in the basiliximab-treated group than it was in the placebo-treated group in both studies ($P = 0.001$ and $0.007$, respectively). The finding of significance in this combined endpoint is attributed to the significant difference in acute rejection between the placebo-treated group and the basiliximab-treated group.

Additional secondary endpoints in the trials were the incidences of biopsy-confirmed rejection at 6 and at 12 months. There was significantly less biopsy-confirmed rejection at 6 months and at 12 months in the basiliximab-treated group than in the placebo-treated group in both studies.

The trials also compared patient survival at 1 year following transplantation. Patient survival was not significantly different between the placebo-treated groups and the basiliximab-treated groups ($P = 0.56$ and $0.29$, respectively). There was no significant difference in the percentage of patients with a functioning graft at 12 months between the placebo-treated groups and the basiliximab-treated groups ($P = 0.5$ and $0.7$, respectively).

The incidences of lymphoproliferative disorders and opportunistic infections were not increased in the basiliximab-treated patients in the trials. However, only 363 patients were treated with basiliximab in these trials, and the follow-up period was short. Additional experience with basiliximab is needed to evaluate its potential for causing lymphoproliferative disorders and opportunistic infections.

The long-term ability of the immune system to respond to antigens first encountered while being treated with basiliximab is not known.

### Accepted

Transplant rejection, kidney (prophylaxis)—Basiliximab is indicated, in combination with cyclosporine and corticosteroids, for the prevention of acute rejection of transplanted kidneys.

## Pharmacology/Pharmacokinetics

### Physicochemical characteristics
Source—Composite of human and murine antibody sequences obtained through recombinant DNA technology.
Molecular weight—Approximately 144,000 daltons.
Solubility—Soluble in water.

### Mechanism of action/Effect
Basiliximab is an interleukin-2 (IL-2) receptor antagonist that binds to the alpha subunit of the IL-2 receptor complex and inhibits IL-2 binding. By inhibiting IL-2 binding, IL-2–mediated activation of lymphocytes is prevented, and the response of the immune system to antigens is impaired.

### Distribution
Volume of distribution ($Vol_D$)—
 Adults: 8.6 ± 4.1 liters (L).
 Children: 5.2 ± 2.8 L.
 Adolescents: 10.1 ± 7.6 L.

### Half-life
Elimination—
 Adults: 7.2 ± 3.2 days.
 Children: 11.5 ± 6.3 days.
 Adolescents: 7.2 ± 3.6 days.

### Duration of action
The mean duration of complete binding to the alpha subunit of the IL-2 receptor complex is 36 ± 14 days.

### Therapeutic serum concentration
Complete binding to the alpha subunit of the IL-2 receptor complex occurs when the serum concentration of basiliximab exceeds 0.2 microgram per milliliter (mcg/mL).

## Precautions to Consider

### Carcinogenicity
Studies have not been done to evaluate the carcinogenic potential of basiliximab. In the preapproval trials of basiliximab, there was not an increased incidence of lymphoproliferative disorders in the basiliximab-treated patients during the short follow-up period. Long-term follow-up studies are not available in these patients. However, it is known that patients receiving immunosuppressive therapy are at increased risk for developing malignancies.

### Mutagenicity
Basiliximab was not mutagenic in the Ames test or the V79 chromosomal aberration assay.

### Pregnancy/Reproduction
Fertility—Adequate and well-controlled studies have not been done.

Pregnancy—Basiliximab crosses the placenta. Adequate and well-controlled studies have not been done in humans. The manufacturer recommends that women of childbearing potential use effective contraception before beginning therapy with basiliximab and continuing for 2 months after completion of therapy with basiliximab.

FDA Pregnancy Category B.

### Breast-feeding
It is not known whether basiliximab is distributed into breast milk. The manufacturer recommends that patients receiving basiliximab discontinue breast-feeding.

### Pediatrics
Appropriate studies on the relationship of age to the effects of basiliximab have not been performed in pediatric patients. Preliminary data from the use of basiliximab in 12 pediatric patients 2 to 15 years of age suggest that pediatric patients receiving basiliximab experience similar incidences of graft rejection and adverse effects as those experienced by adult patients.

### Geriatrics
Geriatric patients were included in preapproval clinical trials of basiliximab in kidney transplantation. The adverse effect profile in geriatric patients was similar to that in younger adults.

### Dental
The immunosuppressive effects of basiliximab may result in an increased incidence of certain microbial infections and delayed healing. Dental work, whenever possible, should be completed prior to initiation of therapy and undertaken with caution during therapy. Patients should be instructed in proper oral hygiene.

### Drug interactions and/or related problems
Note: In clinical trials, basiliximab was administered to patients receiving other immunosuppressants (antilymphocyte globulin, antithymocyte globulin, azathioprine, corticosteroids, cyclosporine, muromonab-CD3, and mycophenolate mofetil). No drug interactions have been evaluated or reported with basiliximab.

### Laboratory value alterations
The following have been selected on the basis of their potential clinical significance (possible effect in parentheses where appropriate)—not necessarily inclusive (» = major clinical significance):

With physiology/laboratory test values
 Calcium, serum and
 Glucose, blood
 Potassium, serum
  (concentrations may be decreased or increased)

 Cholesterol, serum
  (values may be increased)

 Blood urea nitrogen (BUN) and
 Serum creatinine and
 Uric acid, serum
  (concentrations may be increased)

 Hematocrit value and
 Hemoglobin concentration
  (may be decreased or increased)

 Magnesium and
 Phosphate, serum
  (concentrations may be decreased)

 Platelets, blood
  (counts may be decreased)

### Medical considerations/Contraindications
The medical considerations/contraindications included have been selected on the basis of their potential clinical significance (reasons given in parentheses where appropriate)—not necessarily inclusive (» = major clinical significance).

*Except under special circumstances, this medication should not be used when the following medical problem exists:*

» Allergy to basiliximab, history of
  Note: Anaphylactoid reactions have not been reported following administration of basiliximab. However, anaphylactoid reactions are possible following administration of proteins.

*Risk-benefit should be considered when the following medical problems exist:*

Infection
 (immunosuppression may exacerbate infection)

Malignancy, current or history of
 (immunosuppression is associated with an increased incidence of some malignancies)

### Patient monitoring
The following may be especially important in patient monitoring (other tests may be warranted in some patients, depending on condition; » = major clinical significance):

Blood pressure and
Heart rate and
Respiratory rate
 (routine monitoring of vital signs is recommended while basiliximab is administered and for a short period of time following the infusion to monitor for anaphylactoid reaction)

Wound infection
 (basiliximab may cause an increased risk of wound infection)

Note: Although the incidences of malignancies and systemic infection were not increased in the basiliximab-treated group in preapproval clinical trials, patients receiving basiliximab should be monitored routinely for malignancy and systemic infection.

## Side/Adverse Effects

Note: The product labeling for basiliximab contains an extensive list of adverse effects observed in patients during clinical trials. Because all the patients were receiving other immunosuppressant drugs, some of the adverse effects may have resulted from the use of the other immunosuppressant drugs. Basiliximab did not seem to add additional side effects to those which would have been expected in transplant patients receiving standard immunosuppressant drug regimens. The incidence of adverse effects, including serious adverse effects, was similar between the basiliximab-treated group and the placebo-treated group. The side effect profile of basiliximab may become better known as additional experience is gained with its use.

The following side/adverse effects have been selected on the basis of their potential clinical significance (possible signs and symptoms in parentheses where appropriate)—not necessarily inclusive:

**Those indicating need for medical attention**
Incidence more frequent
*Abdominal pain; asthenia* (loss of energy or weakness); *back pain; candidiasis* (white patches in the mouth or throat or on the tongue); *cough; dizziness; dyspnea* (shortness of breath); *dysuria* (painful urination); *edema* (swelling of ankles, body, face, feet, or lower legs); *fever; hypertension*—asymptomatic; *infection* (fever or chills); *pharyngitis* (sore throat); *tremor* (trembling or shaking of hands or feet); *vomiting*

Incidence less frequent
*Abnormal vision; agitation; anxiety; arrhythmia* (dizziness)—may be asymptomatic; *chest pain; depression; fatigue; gastrointestinal bleeding* (blood in the stool)—usually asymptomatic; *gingival hyperplasia* (bleeding, tender, or enlarged gums); *hematoma* (bruising); *hypoesthesia* ("stocking and gloves" sensation of the hands or feet); *hypotension* (dizziness); *neuropathy* (numbness or pain in the legs); *paresthesia* (tingling); *pruritus* (itching); *pulmonary edema* (coughing; shortness of breath); *skin rash; stomatitis* (sores in the mouth); *urinary retention* (difficulty in urinating)

**Those indicating need for medical attention only if they continue or are bothersome**
Incidence more frequent
*Acne; constipation; diarrhea; dyspepsia* (heartburn); *headache; insomnia* (trouble in sleeping); *nausea; weight gain*

Incidence less frequent
*Arthralgia* (joint pain); *hypertrichosis* (excessive hair growth); *myalgia* (muscle pain)

## Overdose

There is no clinical experience with overdose of basiliximab, and a maximum tolerated dose has not been established. Some patients have received doses of up to 60 mg without any adverse effects.

## Patient Consultation

As an aid to patient consultation, refer to *Advice for the Patient, Basiliximab (Systemic)—Introductory Version*.

In providing consultation, consider emphasizing the following selected information (» = major clinical significance):

**Before using this medication**
» Conditions affecting use, especially:
 Allergy to basiliximab
 Carcinogenicity—Use of basiliximab may be associated with an increased risk of malignancy
 Pregnancy—Basiliximab crosses the placenta
 Breast-feeding—Use is not recommended
 Dental—Dental work should be completed prior to initiation of therapy whenever possible

**Proper use of this medication**
 Advisability of women of childbearing age using effective contraception before, during, and for 2 months after receiving basiliximab
» Proper dosing

**Precautions while receiving this medication**
» Importance of close monitoring by a physician

**Side/adverse effects**
 Signs of potential side effects, especially abdominal pain, asthenia, back pain, candidiasis, cough, dizziness, dyspnea, dysuria, edema, fever, hypertension, infection, pharyngitis, tremor, vomiting, abnormal vision, agitation, anxiety, arrhythmia, chest pain, depression, fatigue, gastrointestinal bleeding, gingival hyperplasia, hematoma, hypoesthesia, hypotension, neuropathy, paresthesia, pruritus, pulmonary edema, skin rash, stomatitis, and urinary retention

## General Dosing Information

Basiliximab should be used only by physicians experienced in the management of organ transplant patients. Medications for the treatment of severe hypersensitivity reactions should be immediately available when basiliximab is administered.

Shaking of the vial of prepared solution of basiliximab may cause foaming and should be avoided.

## Parenteral Dosage Forms

### BASILIXIMAB FOR INJECTION

**Usual adult dose**
Transplant rejection, kidney (prophylaxis)—
 Intravenous infusion over twenty to thirty minutes, 20 mg within two hours prior to transplantation surgery. The dose should be repeated four days after transplantation.

**Usual pediatric dose**
Transplant rejection, kidney (prophylaxis)—
 Intravenous infusion over twenty to thirty minutes, 12 mg per square meter of body surface area within two hours prior to transplantation surgery. The dose should be repeated four days after transplantation.

**Usual pediatric prescribing limits**
20 mg for each infusion

**Usual geriatric dose**
See *Usual adult dose*.

**Strength(s) usually available**
U.S.—
 20 mg (Rx) [*Simulect* (lyophilized powder; potassium phosphate monobasic 7.21 mg; disodium hydrogen phosphate [anhydrous] 0.99 mg; sodium chloride 1.61 mg; sucrose 20 mg; mannitol 80 mg; glycine 40 mg)].

**Packaging and storage**
Store between 2 and 8 °C (36 and 46 °F).

**Preparation of dosage form**
Reconstitute vial with 5 mL of Sterile Water for Injection USP. The reconstituted solution should be diluted to a volume of 50 mL with 0.9% sodium chloride injection or 5% dextrose injection.

**Stability**
Basiliximab does not contain preservatives. Prepared solutions of basiliximab should be used within 4 hours. If refrigerated at 4 °C (39 °F), solutions should be used within 24 hours. The prepared solution should be inspected for particulate matter and clarity before administration to the patient, and should be discarded if particulate matter is present.

**Incompatibilities**
There are no data on the compatibility or incompatibility of other drugs or solutions with basiliximab. Until more data are available, other drugs should not be infused simultaneously through the same intravenous line.

Developed: 07/09/98

# BECAPLERMIN Topical—INTRODUCTORY VERSION

VA CLASSIFICATION (Primary): DE900
Commonly used brand name(s): *Regranex*.
Note: For a listing of dosage forms and brand names by country availability, see *Dosage Forms* section(s).

## Category
Biological response modifier (topical); platelet-derived growth factor (topical).

## Indications

### Accepted
Ulcers, dermal (treatment)—Becaplermin is indicated in the treatment of neuropathic diabetic ulcers of the lower extremities that extend into the subcutaneous tissue or beyond when the ulcer has an adequate blood supply. It is used adjunctively with optimal wound care procedures that include initial sharp debridement, infection control, and pressure relief.

Use of becaplermin in the treatment of ulcers unrelated to diabetes mellitus or in ischemic or dermal ulcers that do not extend into the subcutaneous tissue (Stage I or II, International Association of Enterostomal Therapy [IAET] staging classification) has not been evaluated.

## Pharmacology/Pharmacokinetics

### Physicochemical characteristics
Source—Becaplermin is a recombinant human platelet-derived growth factor (rhPDGF-BB) produced by recombinant DNA technology by insertion of the gene for the B chain of platelet-derived growth factor into the yeast, *Saccharomyces cerevisiae*.
Chemical group—Becaplermin is a homodimer composed of two identical polypeptide chains bound together by disulfide bonds.
Molecular weight—Approximately 30,000.

### Mechanism of action/Effect
Similar in action to endogenous platelet-derived growth factor, becaplermin forms granulation tissue in diabetic ulcers, healing them by promoting the chemotatic recruitment and proliferation of cells involved in wound repair.

### Absorption
Apparent minimal systemic absorption.

## Precautions to Consider

### Cross-sensitivity and/or related problems
Allergy to product components, including parabens and metacresol.

### Carcinogenicity/Tumorigenicity
Carcinogenesis studies have not been done in humans or animals.

### Mutagenicity
Becaplermin is not mutagenic according to the following *in vitro* tests: bacterial or mammalian cell point mutation, chromosomal aberration for bacterial and mammalian cell point mutation, and chromosomal aberration and DNA damage/repair. Becaplermin is not mutagenic according to an *in vivo* assay for the induction of micronuclei in mouse bone marrow cells.

### Pregnancy/Reproduction
Pregnancy—No adequate or well-controlled studies have been done in pregnant women.
Reproductive studies have not been done in animals.
FDA Pregnancy Category C.

### Breast-feeding
It is not known if becaplermin is distributed into breast milk. Problems in humans have not been documented.

### Pediatrics
No information is available on the relationship of age to the effects of becaplermin in pediatrics patients 16 years of age or over. Safety and efficacy have not been established in children up to 16 years of age.

### Geriatrics
No information is available on the relationship of age to the effects of becaplermin in geriatric patients.

### Medical considerations/Contraindications
The medical considerations/contraindications included have been selected on the basis of their potential clinical significance (reasons given in parentheses where appropriate)—not necessarily inclusive (» = major clinical significance).

*Except under special circumstances, this medication should not be used when the following medical problems exist:*
» Skin neoplasms
  (use of becaplermin is not recommended with skin neoplasms at the site of application)
» Wounds closed by primary intention
  (becaplermin is a preserved, nonsterile product and is not recommended for wounds requiring a sterile product, such as wounds intentionally closed)

*Risk-benefit should be considered when the following medical problems exist:*
Wounds showing exposed joints, tendons, ligaments, or bone
  (effects of becaplermin in these types of wounds in humans have not been clinically assessed; however, animal studies show histologic changes indicative of stimulated connective tissue growth and accelerated bone remodeling as shown by periosteal hyperplasia, subperiosteal bone resorption, and exostosis)
Sensitivity to becaplermin or allergy to parabens or metacresol

### Patient monitoring
The following may be especially important in patient monitoring (other tests may be warranted in some patients, depending on condition; » = major clinical significance):
Regular visits to health care provider
  (becaplermin requires that the dose be recalculated weekly or biweekly according to the rate of change in the width and length of the diabetic ulcer)

## Side/Adverse Effects

The following side/adverse effects have been selected on the basis of their potential clinical significance (possible signs and symptoms in parentheses where appropriate)—not necessarily inclusive:

### Those indicating need for medical attention
Incidence less frequent
  *Erythematous rash, local* (reddened skin near ulcer; skin rash near ulcer)—incidence of 2%
  Note: *Local erythematous rashes* occurred at the same rate in patients using either becaplermin or placebo gel, but this effect did not occur for patients using only good ulcer care.

## Patient Consultation

As an aid to patient consultation, refer to *Advice for the Patient, Becaplermin (Topical)—Introductory Version*.
In providing consultation, consider emphasizing the following selected information (» = major clinical significance):

### Before using this medication
» Conditions affecting use, especially:
    Sensitivity to becaplermin or allergy to parabens or metacresol
    Other medical problems, especially skin neoplasms or wounds closed by primary intention

### Proper use of this medication
» Reading patient directions that come with medication carefully before using
» Importance of not contaminating medication; not placing the tube's tip onto the ulcer or on any other object
» Proper administration:
    Washing hands before administering
    Measuring proper amount as indicated by health care professional, according to ulcer size and tube size; expecting a change in dose weekly or biweekly
    Measuring dose carefully and accurately on a nonabsorbent surface, such as wax paper, and transferring to ulcer using an applicator aid, such as a cotton swab or tongue depressor
    Applying dose to ulcer in a leveled, thin, and continuous layer
    Applying a gauze pad moistened with 0.9% Sodium Chloride Irrigation USP to protect ulcer after applying becaplermin
    Removing remaining medication in ulcer by washing with water or 0.9% Sodium Chloride Irrigation USP after 12 hours
    Keeping the ulcer from becoming too dry. At the time of dressing changes, the bandage may need to be moistened with 0.9% Sodium Chloride Irrigation USP to prevent injury to healing tissues
    Placing a new gauze pad moistened with 0.9% Sodium Chloride Irrigation USP or moisture dressing on ulcer to protect it for 12 hours until the time of the next dose of becaplermin

» Proper dosing
  Missed dose: Use the missed dose as soon as possible. However, if you do not remember the missed dose until the next day, skip the missed dose and go back to your regular dosing schedule. Do not double doses.
» Proper storage

**Precautions while using this medication**
» Regular visits to physician
» Importance of using becaplermin with a good ulcer care program, including avoiding bearing weight on affected extremity
  Discussing continuing use of becaplermin with physician if ulcer is not improved by 30% in 10 weeks or there is no apparent improvement in ulcer healing beyond 20 weeks
  Understanding importance of using proper amounts, not using more than prescribed
  Not using medication beyond the expiration date that is imprinted on the crimped portion of the bottom of the tube

**Side/adverse effects**
Signs of potential side effects, especially erythematous rash, local

## General Dosing Information

Continuing becaplermin treatment should be reconsidered if the ulcer is not reduced in size by 30% within 10 weeks of treatment or complete healing has not occurred in 20 weeks. When expected reduction in ulcer size occurs successfully, the treatment is continued until the ulcer is completely healed.

Becaplermin should be used within a good ulcer care regimen that includes educating the patient not to bear weight on the affected extremity. This frequently requires the use of crutches or a wheelchair.

The gel is measured on a clean, nonabsorbent surface (for example, wax paper) and transferred to the ulcer using an applicator aid (for example, cotton swab or tongue depressor). The gel is spread as a thin, continuous film of one-sixteenth inch thickness onto the ulcer, covered with a gauze pad moistened with 0.9% Sodium Chloride Irrigation USP for 12 hours, then removed by washing any residual gel from ulcer with water or 0.9% Sodium Chloride Irrigation USP. Until time of next application of becaplermin in 24 hours, the ulcer is covered for 12 hours with a new gauze pad moistened with 0.9% Sodium Chloride Irrigation USP or with a moisture dressing.

Each square inch of ulcer surface area requires that 1.3 inches of gel be taken from a 2-gram tube or that a 0.6-inch length of gel be taken from a 7.5-gram tube or 15-gram tube. The formulas for dose calculations when measuring in inches include:
• For a 2-gram tube: (ulcer length in inches)(ulcer width in inches)(1.3)
• For 7.5-gram and 15-gram tubes: (ulcer length in inches)(ulcer width in inches)(0.6)

Alternatively, each square centimeter of ulcer surface area requires that 0.5 centimeter length of gel be taken from a 2-gram tube or that 0.25 centimeter length of gel be taken from a 7.5-gram tube or 15-gram tube. The formulas for dose calculations when measuring in centimeters include:
• For a 2-gram tube: (ulcer length in centimeters)(ulcer width in centimeters)/2.
• For 7.5-gram and 15-gram tubes: (ulcer length in centimeters)(ulcer width in centimeters)/4.

It is not known if use of other topical medications during the day will interfere with the use of becaplermin.

## Topical Dosage Forms

### BECAPLERMIN GEL

**Usual adult dose**
Ulcers, dermal—
  Topical, an amount of gel to be applied once a day for twelve hours is calculated weekly or biweekly, depending on the rate at which the ulcer changes, as measured in length and width.

**Usual pediatric dose**
Children up to 16 years of age: Safety and efficacy have not been established.
Children 16 years of age and over: See *Usual adult dose*.

**Usual geriatric dose**
See *Usual adult dose*.

**Strength(s) usually available**
U.S.—
  0.01% (Rx) [*Regranex* (glacial acetic acid; l-lysine hydrochloride; metacresol; methylparaben; propylparaben; sodium acetate trihydrate; sodium chloride; Water for Injection USP)].

**Packaging and storage**
Store between 2 and 8 °C (36 and 46 °F), unless otherwise specified by manufacturer. Protect from freezing.

**Auxiliary labeling**
• For external use only.
• Refrigerate. Do not freeze.

Developed: 03/30/98

---

**BECLOMETHASONE** — See *Corticosteroids (Inhalation-Local)*; *Corticosteroids (Nasal)*; *Corticosteroids (Topical)*

---

**BELLADONNA** — See *Anticholinergics/Antispasmodics (Systemic)*

---

# BELLADONNA ALKALOIDS AND BARBITURATES  Systemic

This monograph includes information on the following: 1) Atropine, Hyoscyamine, Scopolamine, and Phenobarbital; 2) Atropine and Phenobarbital; 3) Belladonna and Butabarbital; 4) Belladonna and Phenobarbital; 5) Hyoscyamine and Phenobarbital.

VA CLASSIFICATION (Primary): GA802

**NOTE:** The *Belladonna Alkaloids and Barbiturates (Systemic)* monograph is maintained on the USP DI electronic data base. For a printed copy of the most recent revision of the complete monograph, contact Micromedex, Inc. - Reprint Requests, 6200 S. Syracuse Way, Suite 300, Englewood, CO 80111; telephone (303) 486-6400; telefax (303) 486-6464; Email: USPDI@MDX.COM.

For information on the specific components of this combination, see the *USP DI* monographs for *Anticholinergics/Antispasmodics (Systemic)* and *Barbiturates (Systemic)*.

The information that follows is selectively abstracted from the complete monograph and is provided to facilitate drug use review and patient counseling.

Note: For a listing of dosage forms and brand names by country availability, see *Dosage Forms* section(s).

## Category

Anticholinergic-sedative.

## Indications

**Accepted**
Ulcer, peptic (treatment adjunct) or
Bowel syndrome, irritable (treatment adjunct)—FDA has classified these medications as possibly effective for use as adjunctive therapy in the treatment of peptic ulcer and irritable bowel syndrome (irritable colon, spastic colon, mucous colitis).

Note: Less than effective classification requires the submission of adequate and well-controlled studies in order to provide substantial evidence of effectiveness. In the past, FDA has notified manufacturers of the possible withdrawal from the market of products containing a combination of an anticholinergic and a sedative because their efficacy as fixed combinations had not been proven in adequately designed clinical trials. To date, no final action has been taken.

**Unaccepted**
Anticholinergic and sedative combinations have been used as adjuncts in the treatment of acute enterocolitis; however, their use for this condition is controversial since they cause a reduction in gastrointestinal motility resulting in retention of the causative organism or toxin and the consequent prolongation of symptoms.

## Patient Consultation

As an aid to patient consultation, refer to *Advice for the Patient, Belladonna Alkaloids and Barbiturates (Systemic)*.

In providing consultation, consider emphasizing the following selected information (» = major clinical significance):

### Before using this medication
» Conditions affecting use, especially:
  Sensitivity to any of the belladonna alkaloids or barbiturates
  Pregnancy—Use not recommended because belladonna alkaloids and barbiturates cross placenta; barbiturates may cause fetal abnormalities; phenobarbital may cause neonatal hemorrhage
  Breast-feeding—Distributed into breast milk; possible inhibition of lactation
  Use in children—Increased susceptibility to toxic effects of anticholinergics; increased response in infants and children with spastic paralysis or brain damage; risk of increased body temperature in hot weather; hyperexcitability (paradoxical reaction); hyperkinesis may be induced in hypersensitive children
  Use in the elderly—Increased susceptibility to mental and other toxic effects of anticholinergics and barbiturates; danger of precipitating undiagnosed glaucoma; possible impairment of memory
  Dental—Possible development of dental problems because of decreased salivary flow
  Other medications, especially adrenocorticoids or corticotropin, other anticholinergics, antacids, anticoagulants, antidiarrheals, ketoconazole, CNS depressants, MAO inhibitors, or potassium chloride
  Other medical problems, especially gastrointestinal obstructive disease, glaucoma, hepatic function impairment, renal function impairment, or urinary retention

### Proper use of this medication
Taking dose 30 to 60 minutes before meals unless otherwise directed by physician
» Importance of not taking more medication than the amount prescribed
» Proper dosing
  Missed dose: Taking as soon as possible; not taking if almost time for next dose; not doubling doses
» Proper storage

### Precautions while using this medication
» Avoiding use of alcohol or other CNS depressants
  Not taking antacids and antidiarrheal medications within 1 hour of taking this medication
» Caution during exercise and hot weather; overheating may result in heat stroke
  Possible increased sensitivity of eyes to light
» Caution if drowsiness or blurred vision occurs
  Possible dryness of mouth, nose, and throat; using sugarless candy or gum, ice, or saliva substitute for relief; checking with physician or dentist if dry mouth continues for more than 2 weeks

### Side/adverse effects
Signs of potential side effects, especially agranulocytosis, allergic reaction, hepatitis, increased intraocular pressure, and thrombocytopenia

---
## ATROPINE, HYOSCYAMINE, SCOPOLAMINE, AND PHENOBARBITAL
---

## Oral Dosage Forms

### ATROPINE SULFATE, HYOSCYAMINE SULFATE (or HYOSCYAMINE HYDROBROMIDE), SCOPOLAMINE HYDROBROMIDE, AND PHENOBARBITAL CAPSULES

**Usual adult and adolescent dose**
Anticholinergic-sedative—
  Oral, 1 or 2 capsules two to four times a day, the dosage being adjusted as needed and tolerated.

**Usual pediatric dose**
Dosage must be individualized by physician.

**Usual geriatric dose**
See *Usual adult and adolescent dose*.

Note: Geriatric patients may be more sensitive to the effects of the usual adult dose.

**Strength(s) usually available**
U.S.—
  19.4 mcg (0.0194 mg) of atropine sulfate, 104 mcg (0.104 mg) of hyoscyamine sulfate (or hydrobromide), 6.5 mcg (0.0065 mg) of scopolamine hydrobromide, and 16 mg of phenobarbital (Rx) [*Donnatal* (lactose); *Hyosophen*].

Note: Strengths of individual components may vary slightly among products of different manufacturers.

Canada—
  Not commercially available.

**Auxiliary labeling**
• May cause drowsiness.
• Avoid alcoholic beverages.

### ATROPINE SULFATE, HYOSCYAMINE SULFATE (or HYOSCYAMINE HYDROBROMIDE), SCOPOLAMINE HYDROBROMIDE, AND PHENOBARBITAL ELIXIR

**Usual adult and adolescent dose**
Anticholinergic-sedative—
  Oral, 5 to 10 mL three or four times a day, the dosage being adjusted as needed and tolerated.

**Usual pediatric dose**
Anticholinergic-sedative—
  Children 4.5 to 9 kg of body weight: Oral, 0.5 to 0.75 mL every four to six hours.
  Children 9 to 13.5 kg of body weight: Oral, 1.0 to 1.5 mL every four to six hours.
  Children 13.5 to 22.5 kg of body weight: Oral, 1.5 to 2 mL every four to six hours.
  Children 22.5 to 36.5 kg of body weight: Oral, 2.5 to 3.75 mL every four to six hours.
  Children 36.5 to 45.4 kg of body weight: Oral, 3.75 to 5 mL every four to six hours.
  Children 45.4 kg of body weight and over: Oral, 5 to 7.5 mL every four to six hours.

Note: Dosage must be adjusted for each patient as needed and tolerated.

**Usual geriatric dose**
See *Usual adult and adolescent dose*.

Note: Geriatric patients may be more sensitive to the effects of the usual adult dose.

**Strength(s) usually available**
U.S.—
  19.4 mcg (0.0194 mg) of atropine sulfate, 103.7 mcg (0.1037 mg) of hyoscyamine sulfate (or hydrobromide), 6.5 mcg (0.0065 mg) of scopolamine hydrobromide, and 16 mg of phenobarbital, per 5 ml (Rx) [*Barophen; Donnamor; Donnapine; Donnatal; Hyosophen; Spasmophen; Spasquid; Susano*].

Note: Contain 23% alcohol.

  34 mcg (0.034 mg) of atropine sulfate, 174 mcg (0.174 mg) of hyoscyamine sulfate (or hydrobromide), 10 mcg (0.01 mg) of scopolamine hydrobromide, and 21.6 mg of phenobarbital, per 5 mL (Rx) [*Barbidonna* (alcohol 15%)].

Canada—
  19 mcg (0.019 mg) of atropine sulfate, 104 mcg (0.104 mg) of hyoscyamine sulfate, 7 mcg (0.007 mg) of scopolamine hydrobromide, and 16.2 mg of phenobarbital, per 5 ml (Rx) [*Donnatal* (alcohol 23%)].

Note: Strengths of individual components may vary slightly among products of different manufacturers.

**Auxiliary labeling**
• May cause drowsiness.
• Avoid alcoholic beverages.
• Keep container tightly closed.

### ATROPINE SULFATE, HYOSCYAMINE SULFATE (or HYOSCYAMINE HYDROBROMIDE), SCOPOLAMINE HYDROBROMIDE, AND PHENOBARBITAL TABLETS

**Usual adult and adolescent dose**
Anticholinergic-sedative—
  Oral, 1 or 2 tablets two to four times a day, the dosage being adjusted as needed and tolerated.

**Usual pediatric dose**
Dosage must be individualized by physician.

**Usual geriatric dose**
See *Usual adult and adolescent dose*.

Note: Geriatric patients may be more sensitive to the effects of the usual adult dose.

**Strength(s) usually available**
U.S.—
  19.4 mcg (0.0194 mg) of atropine sulfate, 104 mcg (0.104 mg) of hyoscyamine sulfate (or hydrobromide), 6.5 mcg (0.0065 mg) of scopolamine hydrobromide, and 16 mg of phenobarbital (Rx) [*Bellalphen; Donnapine; Donnatal; Malatal; Relaxadon; Spaslin; Spasmolin; Susano;* GENERIC].
  19.4 mcg (0.0194) of atropine sulfate, 104 mcg (0.104 mg) of hyoscyamine sulfate, 6.5 mcg (0.0065 mg) of scopolamine hydrobromide, and 32 mg of phenobarbital (Rx) [*Donnatal No. 2*].
  20 mcg (0.02 mg) of atropine sulfate, 100 mcg (0.1 mg) of hyoscyamine sulfate (or hydrobromide), 6.0 mcg (0.006 mg) of scopolamine hydrobromide, and 15 mg of phenobarbital (Rx) [*Donphen; Spasmophen*].
  25 mcg (0.025 mg) of atropine sulfate, 128.6 mcg (0.1286 mg) of hyoscyamine sulfate (or hydrobromide), 7.4 mcg (0.0074 mg) of scopolamine hydrobromide, and 16 mg of phenobarbital (Rx) [*Barbidonna*].
  25 mcg (0.025 mg) of atropine sulfate, 128.6 mcg (0.1286 mg) of hyoscyamine sulfate (or hydrobromide), 7.4 mcg (0.0074 mg) of scopolamine hydrobromide, and 32 mg of phenobarbital (Rx) [*Barbidonna No. 2*].
Canada—
  19 mcg (0.019 mg) of atropine sulfate, 104 mcg (0.104 mg) of hyoscyamine sulfate, 7 mcg (0.007 mg) of scopolamine hydrobromide, and 16.2 mg of phenobarbital (Rx) [*Donnatal*].
Note: Strengths of individual components may vary slightly among products of different manufacturers.

**Auxiliary labeling**
- May cause drowsiness.
- Avoid alcoholic beverages.

### ATROPINE SULFATE, HYOSCYAMINE SULFATE, SCOPOLAMINE HYDROBROMIDE, AND PHENOBARBITAL CHEWABLE TABLETS

**Usual adult and adolescent dose**
Anticholinergic-sedative—
  Oral, 1 or 2 tablets three or four times a day, the dosage being adjusted as needed and tolerated.

**Usual pediatric dose**
Anticholinergic-sedative—
  Children up to 2 years of age: Use is not recommended.
  Children 2 to 12 years of age: Oral, ½ to 1 tablet three or four times a day, the dosage being adjusted as needed and tolerated.

**Usual geriatric dose**
See *Usual adult and adolescent dose*.
Note: Geriatric patients may be more sensitive to the effects of the usual adult dose.

**Strength(s) usually available**
U.S.—
  120 mcg (0.12 mg) of atropine sulfate, 120 mcg (0.12 mg) of hyoscyamine sulfate, 7 mcg (0.007 mg) of scopolamine hydrobromide, and 16 mg of phenobarbital (Rx) [*Kinesed*].
Canada—
  Not commercially available.

**Auxiliary labeling**
- May be chewed or swallowed with liquids.
- May cause drowsiness.
- Avoid alcoholic beverages.

### ATROPINE SULFATE, HYOSCYAMINE SULFATE, SCOPOLAMINE HYDROBROMIDE, AND PHENOBARBITAL EXTENDED-RELEASE TABLETS

**Usual adult and adolescent dose**
Anticholinergic-sedative—
  Oral, 1 tablet every eight to twelve hours, the dosage being adjusted as needed and tolerated.

**Usual pediatric dose**
Use is not recommended.

**Usual geriatric dose**
See *Usual adult and adolescent dose*.
Note: Geriatric patients may be more sensitive to the effects of the usual adult dose.

**Strength(s) usually available**
U.S.—
  58.2 mcg (0.0582 mg) of atropine sulfate, 311.1 mcg (0.3111 mg) of hyoscyamine sulfate, 19.5 mcg (0.0195 mg) of scopolamine hydrobromide, and 48.6 mg of phenobarbital (Rx) [*Donnatal Extentabs*].
Canada—
  58.2 mcg (0.0582 mg) of atropine sulfate, 311.1 mcg (0.3111 mg) of hyoscyamine sulfate, 19.5 mcg (0.0195 mg) of scopolamine hydrobromide, and 48.6 mg of phenobarbital (Rx) [*Donnatal Extentabs*].

**Auxiliary labeling**
- Swallow tablets whole.
- May cause drowsiness.
- Avoid alcoholic beverages.

---

## ATROPINE AND PHENOBARBITAL

## Oral Dosage Forms

### ATROPINE SULFATE AND PHENOBARBITAL CAPSULES

**Usual adult and adolescent dose**
Anticholinergic-sedative—
  Oral, 1 or 2 capsules two to four times a day, the dosage being adjusted as needed and tolerated.

**Usual pediatric dose**
Dosage must be individualized by physician.

**Usual geriatric dose**
See *Usual adult and adolescent dose*.
Note: Geriatric patients may be more sensitive to the effects of the usual adult dose.

**Strength(s) usually available**
U.S.—
  195 mcg (0.195 mg) of atropine sulfate and 16 mg of phenobarbital (Rx) [*Antrocol*].
Canada—
  Not commercially available.

**Auxiliary labeling**
- May cause drowsiness.
- Avoid alcoholic beverages.

### ATROPINE SULFATE AND PHENOBARBITAL ELIXIR

**Usual adult and adolescent dose**
Anticholinergic-sedative—
  Oral, 5 to 10 mL three or four times a day, the dosage being adjusted as needed and tolerated.

**Usual pediatric dose**
Anticholinergic-sedative—
  Children 7 to 14 kg of body weight: Oral, 0.5 to 1 mL every four to six hours.
  Children 14 to 21 kg of body weight: Oral, 1 to 1.5 mL every four to six hours.
  Children 21 to 28 kg of body weight: Oral, 1.5 to 2 mL every four to six hours.
  Children 28 to 35 kg of body weight: Oral, 2 to 2.5 mL every four to six hours.
  Children 41 kg of body weight and over: Oral, 3 mL every four to six hours.
Note: Dosage must be adjusted for each patient as needed and tolerated.

**Usual geriatric dose**
See *Usual adult and adolescent dose*.
Note: Geriatric patients may be more sensitive to the effects of the usual adult dose.

**Strength(s) usually available**
U.S.—
  195 mcg (0.195 mg) of atropine sulfate and 16 mg of phenobarbital, per 5 mL (Rx) [*Antrocol* (alcohol 20%)].
Canada—
  Not commercially available.

**Auxiliary labeling**
- May cause drowsiness.
- Avoid alcoholic beverages.
- Keep container tightly closed.

### ATROPINE SULFATE AND PHENOBARBITAL TABLETS

**Usual adult and adolescent dose**
Anticholinergic-sedative—
  Oral, 1 or 2 tablets three or four times a day, the dosage being adjusted as needed and tolerated.

**Usual pediatric dose**
Dosage must be individualized by physician.

**Usual geriatric dose**
See *Usual adult and adolescent dose*.

Note: Geriatric patients may be more sensitive to the effects of the usual adult dose.

**Strength(s) usually available**
U.S.—
    195 mcg (0.195 mg) of atropine sulfate and 16 mg of phenobarbital (Rx) [*Antrocol*].
Canada—
    Not commercially available.

**Auxiliary labeling**
• May cause drowsiness.
• Avoid alcoholic beverages.

---
### BELLADONNA AND BUTABARBITAL
---

## Oral Dosage Forms

### BELLADONNA EXTRACT AND BUTABARBITAL SODIUM ELIXIR

**Usual adult and adolescent dose**
Anticholinergic-sedative—
    Oral, 5 to 10 mL three or four times a day, the dosage being adjusted as needed and tolerated.

**Usual pediatric dose**
Anticholinergic-sedative—
    Children up to 6 years of age: Oral, 1.25 to 2.5 mL three or four times a day, the dosage being adjusted as needed and tolerated.
    Children 6 to 12 years of age: Oral, 2.5 to 5 mL three or four times a day, the dosage being adjusted as needed and tolerated.

**Usual geriatric dose**
See *Usual adult and adolescent dose*.

Note: Geriatric patients may be more sensitive to the effects of the usual adult dose.

**Strength(s) usually available**
U.S.—
    15 mg of belladonna extract and 15 mg of butabarbital sodium, per 5 mL (Rx) [*Butibel* (alcohol 7%)].
Canada—
    Not commercially available.

**Auxiliary labeling**
• May cause drowsiness.
• Avoid alcoholic beverages.
• Keep container tightly closed.

### BELLADONNA EXTRACT AND BUTABARBITAL SODIUM TABLETS

**Usual adult and adolescent dose**
Anticholinergic-sedative—
    Oral, 1 or 2 tablets three or four times a day, the dosage being adjusted as needed and tolerated.

**Usual pediatric dose**
Dosage must be individualized by physician.

**Usual geriatric dose**
See *Usual adult and adolescent dose*.

Note: Geriatric patients may be more sensitive to the effects of the usual adult dose.

**Strength(s) usually available**
U.S.—
    15 mg of belladonna extract and 15 mg of butabarbital sodium (Rx) [*Butibel*].
Canada—
    Not commercially available.

**Auxiliary labeling**
• May cause drowsiness.
• Avoid alcoholic beverages.

---
### BELLADONNA AND PHENOBARBITAL
---

## Oral Dosage Forms

### BELLADONNA EXTRACT AND PHENOBARBITAL TABLETS

**Usual adult and adolescent dose**
Anticholinergic-sedative—
    Oral, 1 or 2 tablets two to four times a day, the dosage being adjusted as needed and tolerated.

**Usual pediatric dose**
Dosage must be individualized by physician.

**Usual geriatric dose**
See *Usual adult and adolescent dose*.

Note: Geriatric patients may be more sensitive to the effects of the usual adult dose.

**Strength(s) usually available**
U.S.—
    15 mg of belladonna extract and 15 mg of phenobarbital (Rx) [*Chardonna-2*].
Canada—
    Not commercially available.

Note: Strengths of individual components may vary slightly among products of different manufacturers.

**Auxiliary labeling**
• May cause drowsiness.
• Avoid alcoholic beverages.

---
### HYOSCYAMINE AND PHENOBARBITAL
---

## Oral Dosage Forms

### HYOSCYAMINE SULFATE AND PHENOBARBITAL ELIXIR

**Usual adult and adolescent dose**
Anticholinergic-sedative—
    Oral, 5 to 10 mL every four hours, the dosage being adjusted as needed and tolerated.

**Usual pediatric dose**
Anticholinergic-sedative—
    Children up to 2 years of age: Oral, 1.25 to 2.5 mL every four hours.
    Children 2 to 10 years of age: Oral, 2.5 to 5 mL every four hours.
    Children 10 years of age and over: See *Usual adult and adolescent dose*.

Note: Dosage must be adjusted for each patient as needed and tolerated.

**Usual geriatric dose**
See *Usual adult and adolescent dose*.

Note: Geriatric patients may be more sensitive to the effects of the usual adult dose.

**Strength(s) usually available**
U.S.—
    125 mcg (0.125 mg) of hyoscyamine sulfate and 15 mg of phenobarbital, per 5 mL (Rx) [*Levsin with Phenobarbital* (alcohol 20%)].
Canada—
    Not commercially available.

**Auxiliary labeling**
• May cause drowsiness.
• Avoid alcoholic beverages.

### HYOSCYAMINE SULFATE AND PHENOBARBITAL ORAL SOLUTION

**Usual adult and adolescent dose**
Anticholinergic-sedative—
    Oral, 1 to 2 mL every four hours, the dosage being adjusted as needed and tolerated.

**Usual pediatric dose**
Anticholinergic-sedative—
    Children up to 1 year of age: Oral, 0.1 to 0.5 mL every four hours.
    Children 1 to 10 years of age: Oral, 0.5 to 1 mL every four hours.
    Children 10 years of age and over: See *Usual adult and adolescent dose*.

Note: Dosage must be adjusted for each patient as needed and tolerated.

**Usual geriatric dose**
See *Usual adult and adolescent dose*.

Note: Geriatric patients may be more sensitive to the effects of the usual adult dose.

**Strength(s) usually available**
U.S.—
   125 mcg (0.125 mg) of hyoscyamine sulfate and 15 mg of phenobarbital, per mL (Rx) [*Levsin-PB* (alcohol 5%)].
Canada—
   Not commercially available.

**Auxiliary labeling**
- May cause drowsiness.
- Avoid alcoholic beverages.

## HYOSCYAMINE SULFATE AND PHENOBARBITAL TABLETS

**Usual adult and adolescent dose**
Anticholinergic-sedative—
   Oral, 1 to 2 tablets three or four times a day, the dosage being adjusted as needed and tolerated.

**Usual pediatric dose**
Dosage must be individualized by physician.

**Usual geriatric dose**
See *Usual adult and adolescent dose*.

Note: Geriatric patients may be more sensitive to the effects of the usual adult dose.

**Strength(s) usually available**
U.S.—
   125 mcg (0.125 mg) of hyoscyamine sulfate and 15 mg of phenobarbital (Rx) [*Levsin with Phenobarbital*].

Canada—
   Not commercially available.

**Auxiliary labeling**
- May cause drowsiness.
- Avoid alcoholic beverages.

Revised: 01/13/92
Interim revision: 08/29/94

---

**BENAZEPRIL**—See *Angiotensin-converting Enzyme (ACE) Inhibitors (Systemic)*.

---

**BENDROFLUMETHIAZIDE**—See *Diuretics, Thiazide (Systemic)*.

---

**BENTIROMIDE**—The *Bentiromide (Systemic)* monograph is not included in this published version of the USP DI database. Copies of the monograph are available on request from Micromedex, Inc. - Reprint Requests, 6200 S. Syracuse Way, Suite 300, Englewood, CO 80111; telephone (303) 486-6400; telefax (303) 486-6464; Email: USPDI@MDX.COM.

---

# BENTOQUATAM Topical †

VA CLASSIFICATION (Primary): DE900
Commonly used brand name(s): *IvyBlock*.
Note: For a listing of dosage forms and brand names by country availability, see *Dosage Forms* section(s).

†Not commercially available in Canada.

## Category
Skin protectant, barrier (topical).

## Indications
**Accepted**
Dermatitis, allergic contact (prophylaxis)—Bentoquatam is indicated to prevent or reduce the severity of allergic contact dermatitis due to urushiol, the allergenic resin of poison ivy, poison oak, and poison sumac.

## Pharmacology/Pharmacokinetics
**Physicochemical characteristics**
Chemical group—Organoclay containing an ammonium compound, quaternium-18-bentonite.

**Mechanism of action/Effect**
The mechanism of action is unknown. It is thought topically applied bentoquatam acts as a physical barrier that interferes with the adsorption of antigens onto the skin and reduces absorption of antigens into the skin. It probably does not work by modifying the systemic allergic response.

## Precautions to Consider
**Cross-sensitivity and/or related problems**
Sensitivity to components of the formulation, such as methylparaben.

**Pregnancy/Reproduction**
Pregnancy—Problems in humans have not been documented.

**Breast-feeding**
Problems in humans have not been documented.

**Pediatrics**
Appropriate studies on the relationship of age to the effects of bentoquatam have not been performed in the pediatric population. However, no pediatrics-specific problems have been documented to date. Safety and efficacy have not been established in children up to 6 years of age. Use is not recommended unless instructed to do so by a physician.

**Geriatrics**
No information is available on the relationship of age to the effects of bentoquatam in geriatric patients.

**Medical considerations/Contraindications**
The medical considerations/contraindications included have been selected on the basis of their potential clinical significance (reasons given in parentheses where appropriate)—not necessarily inclusive (» = major clinical significance).

*Except under special circumstances, this medication should not be used when the following medical problem exists:*
» Dermatitis, allergic contact, due to poison ivy, poison oak, or poison sumac
   (bentoquatam should not be applied to the rash of poison ivy, poison oak, or poison sumac, and should be discontinued if such rash develops)

*Risk-benefit should be considered when the following medical problem exists:*
Sensitivity to components of formulation
   (in general, the Cosmetic Ingredient Review classified organoclays as nonirritating and nonsensitizing agents without toxic allergenic potential; however, other inactive ingredients of the formulation, such as methylparabens, have sensitivity potential for some individuals and should be considered)

## Side/Adverse Effects
The following side/adverse effects have been selected on the basis of their potential clinical significance (possible signs and symptoms in parentheses where appropriate)—not necessarily inclusive:

**Those indicating need for medical attention**
Incidence rare
   *Erythema, mild* (mild redness of skin)

## Patient Consultation
As an aid to patient consultation, refer to *Advice for the Patient, Bentoquatam (Topical)*.

In providing consultation, consider emphasizing the following selected information (» = major clinical significance):

## Bentoquatam (Topical)

**Before using this medication**
» Conditions affecting use, especially:
Sensitivity to components in formulation
Use in children—Use in children up to 6 of years of age is not recommended
Other medical problems, especially allergic contact dermatitis

**Proper use of this medication**
Avoiding allergen provides maximum protection against allergic contact dermatitis; understanding that use of this medication provides some protection, but not always complete protection
For external use only; keeping away from eyes; washing eyes for 20 minutes if accidental contact occurs
To apply the lotion: shaking lotion vigorously before use; rubbing sufficient amount on exposed skin to leave a smooth wet film; allowing film to dry for at least 15 minutes before potential exposure
Maximum protection lasts for 4 hours or as long as a dry film can be seen on the skin
Removing with soap and water when medication is no longer needed
» Proper dosing
» Proper storage

**Precautions while using this medication**
Discontinuing use and checking with health care professional if rash, irritation, or sensitivity develops

**Side/adverse effects**
Signs of potential side effects, especially mild erythema

## General Dosing Information

Bentoquatam is for external use only. Contact with eye area should be avoided, and eyes flushed for 20 minutes with water if contact does occur.

Bentoquatam should be applied in a sufficient quantity to provide a smooth film on exposed skin and allowed to dry at least 15 minutes before exposure to allergens. A visible coating indicates protection. Avoiding poison ivy, poison oak, and poison sumac provides maximum protection. Patient should be counseled that bentoquatam helps protect the skin from allergens when used properly but that incomplete protection can occur, especially when the film coating is compromised or solution is not reapplied after 4 hours.

Using soap and water is sufficient for removal when medication is no longer needed.

Treatment should be discontinued and a health care professional consulted if sensitivity develops or rash or irritation occurs, especially if incomplete protection occurs that results in the development of allergic contact dermatitis due to poison ivy, poison oak, or poison sumac.

## Topical Dosage Forms

### BENTOQUATAM LOTION

**Usual adult and adolescent dose**
Dermatitis, allergic contact (prophylaxis)—
Topical, to potentially involved or exposed area(s) of skin, applied at least fifteen minutes before allergen exposure as smooth wet film, drying to a visible coating. Reapply every four hours or sooner if needed to maintain the shield of dried coating.

**Usual pediatric dose**
Dermatitis, allergic contact (prophylaxis)—
For children 6 years of age and older: See *Usual adult and adolescent dose*.
For children up to 6 years of age: Safety and efficacy have not been established.

**Usual geriatric dose**
Dermatitis, allergic contact (prophylaxis)—
See *Usual adult and adolescent dose*.

**Strength(s) usually available**
U.S.—
5% (OTC) [*IvyBlock* (25% denatured alcohol; diisopropyl adipate bentonite; benzyl alcohol; methylparaben; purified water)].
Canada—
Not commercially available.

**Packaging and storage**
Store below 40 °C (104 °F), preferably between 15 and 30 °C (59 and 86 °F), unless otherwise specified by manufacturer. Store in a tight container.

**Auxiliary labeling**
• For external use only.
• Shake well.

## Selected Bibliography

Marks James G Jr, Fowler Joseph F Jr, Sherertz Elizabeth F, et al. Prevention of poison ivy and poison oak allergic contact dermatitis by quaternium-18 bentonite. J Am Acad Dermatol 1995; 33: 212-6.

Developed: 05/07/97

---

**BENZNIDAZOLE**—The *Benznidazole (Systemic)* monograph is not included in this published version of the USP DI database. Copies of the monograph are available on request from Micromedex, Inc. - Reprint Requests, 6200 S. Syracuse Way, Suite 300, Englewood, CO 80111; telephone (303) 486-6400; telefax (303) 486-6464; Email: USPDI@MDX.COM.

---

**BENZOCAINE**—See *Anesthetics (Mucosal-Local)*; *Anesthetics (Topical)*

---

**BENZOCAINE AND MENTHOL**—See *Anesthetics (Topical)*

---

# BENZODIAZEPINES  Systemic

This monograph includes information on the following: 1) Alprazolam; 2) Bromazepam*; 3) Chlordiazepoxide; 4) Clobazam*; 5) Clonazepam; 6) Clorazepate; 7) Diazepam; 8) Estazolam†; 9) Flurazepam; 10) Halazepam†; 11) Ketazolam*†; 12) Lorazepam; 13) Nitrazepam*; 14) Oxazepam; 15) Prazepam*†; 16) Quazepam†; 17) Temazepam; 18) Triazolam.

VA CLASSIFICATION (Primary/Secondary):
Alprazolam
Oral—CN302
Bromazepam
Oral—CN302
Chlordiazepoxide
Oral—CN302
Parenteral—CN302
Clobazam
Oral—CN400
Clonazepam
Oral—CN302/CN400
Clorazepate
Oral—CN302/CN400
Diazepam
Oral—CN302/CN400; MS200
Parenteral—CN302/CN400; MS200
Rectal—CN400
Estazolam
Oral—CN302
Flurazepam
Oral—CN302
Halazepam
Oral—CN302
Ketazolam
Oral—CN302
Lorazepam
Oral—CN302/MS200
Parenteral—CN302/CN400; MS200; GA605
Nitrazepam
Oral—CN302/CN400
Oxazepam
Oral—CN302
Prazepam
Oral—CN302

Quazepam
Oral—CN302
Temazepam
Oral—CN302
Triazolam
Oral—CN302

Note: All of the benzodiazepines in this monograph are controlled substances in the U.S.—Schedule IV

Commonly used brand name(s): *Alprazolam Intensol*[1]; *Alti-Alprazolam*[1]; *Alti-Bromazepam*[2]; *Alti-Clonazepam*[5]; *Alti-Triazolam*[18]; *Apo-Alpraz*[1]; *Apo-Chlordiazepoxide*[3]; *Apo-Clonazepam*[5]; *Apo-Clorazepate*[6]; *Apo-Diazepam*[7]; *Apo-Flurazepam*[9]; *Apo-Lorazepam*[12]; *Apo-Oxazepam*[14]; *Apo-Temazepam*[17]; *Apo-Triazo*[18]; *Ativan*[12]; *Clonapam*[5]; *Dalmane*[9]; *Diastat*[7]; *Diazemuls*; *Diazepam Intensol*[7]; *Dizac*[7]; *Doral*[16]; *Frisium*[4]; *Gen-Alprazolam*[1]; *Gen-Bromazepam*[2]; *Gen-Clonazepam*[5]; *Gen-Triazolam*[18]; *Halcion*[18]; *Klonopin*[5]; *Lectopam*[2]; *Librium*[3]; *Lorazepam Intensol*[12]; *Mogadon*[13]; *Novo-Alprazol*[1]; *Novo-Clopate*[6]; *Novo-Dipam*[7]; *Novo-Flupam*[9]; *Novo-Lorazem*[12]; *Novo-Poxide*[3]; *Novo-Temazepam*[17]; *Novo-Triolam*[18]; *Novoxapam*[14]; *Nu-Alpraz*[1]; *Nu-Loraz*[12]; *PMS-Clonazepam*[5]; *PMS-Diazepam*[7]; *Paxipam*[10]; *ProSom*[8]; *Restoril*[17]; *Rivotril*[5]; *Serax*[14]; *Somnol*[9]; *Tranxene*[6]; *Tranxene T-Tab*[6]; *Tranxene-SD*[6]; *Tranxene-SD Half Strength*[6]; *Valium*[7]; *Vivol*[7]; *Xanax*[1]; *Xanax TS*[1].

Note: For a listing of dosage forms and brand names by country availability, see *Dosage Forms* section(s).

*Not commercially available in the U.S.
†Not commercially available in Canada.

## Category

Note: **All of the benzodiazepines have similar pharmacologic actions; however, clinical uses among specific agents may vary because of actual pharmacokinetic differences, availability of specific testing, and/or availability of clinical-use data.**

Antianxiety agent—Alprazolam; Bromazepam; Chlordiazepoxide; Clorazepate; Diazepam; Halazepam; Ketazolam; Lorazepam; Oxazepam; Prazepam.
Sedative-hypnotic—Alprazolam; Bromazepam; Chlordiazepoxide; Clonazepam; Clorazepate; Diazepam; Estazolam; Flurazepam; Halazepam; Ketazolam; Lorazepam; Nitrazepam; Oxazepam; Prazepam; Quazepam; Temazepam; Triazolam.
Amnestic—Diazepam (parenteral only); Lorazepam (parenteral only).
Anticonvulsant—Clobazam; Clonazepam; Clorazepate; Diazepam; Lorazepam (parenteral only); Nitrazepam.
Antipanic agent—Alprazolam; Chlordiazepoxide (parenteral only); Clonazepam; Diazepam; Lorazepam.
Skeletal muscle relaxant adjunct—Diazepam; Lorazepam.
Antitremor agent—Alprazolam; Chlordiazepoxide (oral only); Diazepam (oral only); Lorazepam (oral only).
Antiemetic, in cancer chemotherapy—Lorazepam (parenteral only).

## Indications

Note: Because ketazolam and prazepam are not commercially available in the U.S. or Canada, the bracketed information and the use of the superscript 1 in this monograph reflect the lack of labeled (approved) indications for these medications.

Bracketed information in the *Indications* section refers to uses that are not included in U.S. product labeling.

### Accepted

Anxiety (treatment)—Alprazolam, bromazepam, chlordiazepoxide, clorazepate, diazepam, halazepam, [ketazolam][1], lorazepam, oxazepam, and [prazepam][1] are indicated for the management of anxiety disorders or for the short-term relief of the symptoms of anxiety. Chlordiazepoxide, [oral diazepam][1], and sublingual or intramuscular lorazepam are indicated for treatment of preoperative apprehension and anxiety.

Benzodiazepines are not indicated for the treatment of anxiety or tension associated with the stress of everyday life. Effectiveness of these medications for long-term management of anxiety has not been assessed in systematic clinical studies. The medication's efficacy in an individual patient should be reassessed at periodic intervals.

Anxiety associated with mental depression (treatment adjunct)[1]—Alprazolam, lorazepam (oral), and oxazepam are also indicated for the adjunctive management of anxiety associated with mental depression. Effectiveness of these medications for long-term use has not been assessed in systematic clinical studies. The medication's efficacy in an individual patient should be reassessed at periodic intervals.

Alcohol withdrawal (treatment)—Chlordiazepoxide, clorazepate, diazepam, [lorazepam][1], and oxazepam are indicated for the relief of acute alcohol withdrawal symptoms such as acute agitation, tremor, impending or acute delirium tremens, and hallucinosis.

Anesthesia, adjunct—Parenteral chlordiazepoxide and parenteral diazepam are indicated as premedication to relieve anxiety and tension in patients who are to undergo surgical procedures. Also, parenteral lorazepam is indicated in adults as preanesthetic medication to produce sedation, relief of anxiety, and anterograde amnesia.

Amnesia, in cardioversion or
Anxiety, in cardioversion (treatment)—Parenteral diazepam is indicated for intravenous administration prior to cardioversion to relieve anxiety and tension and to produce anterograde amnesia.

Amnesia, in endoscopic procedures or
Anxiety, in endoscopic procedures (treatment adjunct)—Parenteral diazepamand [parenteral lorazepam][1] are indicated as adjuncts prior to endoscopic procedures if apprehension, anxiety, or acute stress reactions are present and to diminish patient's recall of the procedure. Safety and efficacy have not been established for the use of diazepam prior to bronchoscopy or laryngoscopy.

[Sedation, conscious][1]—Parenteral diazepam is used in dentistry to relieve anxiety and produce amnesia in prolonged or difficult dental procedures. It is used frequently with a local anesthetic.

Insomnia (treatment)—Estazolam, flurazepam, nitrazepam, quazepam, temazepam, and triazolam are indicated for the short-term treatment of insomnia characterized by difficulty in falling asleep, frequent nocturnal awakenings, and/or early morning awakenings. Lorazepam[1] is indicated for insomnia due to anxiety or transient situational stress. Other benzodiazepines, such as [alprazolam][1], bromazepam[1], [diazepam][1], [ketazolam][1], [halazepam], and [prazepam][1], are also used in the treatment of insomnia. Failure of insomnia to remit after 7 to 10 days of treatment may indicate the presence of a primary psychiatric or medical illness. Worsening of insomnia or the emergence of new abnormalities of thinking or behavior may be the consequence of an unrecognized psychiatric or physical disorder.

[Short- and intermediate-acting benzodiazepine hypnotics may be useful in the prevention or treatment (short-term) of transient insomnia associated with a sudden sleep schedule change, such as occurs in transmeridian travel and shift-work rotation.][1]

Convulsions (treatment adjunct) or
Status epilepticus (treatment adjunct)—Diazepam injection, sterile emulsion[1], and [diazepam for rectal solution][1] are indicated as adjuncts in status epilepticus and severe recurrent convulsive seizures. They are not recommended for maintenance anticonvulsant therapy; therefore, once seizures are controlled, appropriate maintenance anticonvulsant therapy should be instituted. [Parenteral lorazepam also is used for the treatment of status epilepticus.]

Convulsive disorders (treatment adjunct)—Oral diazepam[1] is indicated as short-term (7 to 14 days) adjunctive therapy in convulsive disorders. It is not useful as sole therapy in convulsive disorders. [Clonazepam may be effective as an adjunct in convulsive disorders such as eclamptic convulsions, infantile spasms, reading epilepsy, and startle-induced seizures.][1]

Epilepsy (treatment adjunct)—Clobazam is indicated as an adjunct in the treatment of patients with epilepsy who are not adequately stabilized by their current anticonvulsant therapy.

Diazepam rectal gel is indicated to control bouts of increased seizure activity in patients with refractory epilepsy who are on stable regimens of antiepileptic medications. Diazepam rectal gel may be administered in the home by a competent caregiver who has been instructed in its proper use and who can distinguish the characteristic seizure clusters that may be treated with diazepam rectal gel from the patient's usual seizure activity.

Epilepsy, Lennox-Gastaut syndrome (treatment) or
Epilepsy, akinetic seizure pattern (treatment) or
Epilepsy, myoclonic seizure pattern (treatment)—Clonazepam is indicated for use alone or, more frequently, as an adjunct in the treatment of the Lennox-Gastaut syndrome (petit mal variant), akinetic, and myoclonic seizures.

Nitrazepam also is indicated for the treatment of myoclonic seizures.

[Epilepsy, myoclonic seizure pattern (treatment adjunct)][1]—Oral diazepam is used as adjunctive therapy in myoclonus. It is not useful as sole therapy in this condition.

Epilepsy, absence seizure pattern (treatment)—Clonazepam may be useful in the treatment of absence (petit mal) seizures refractory to the succinimide anticonvulsants or valproic acid.

Epilepsy, simple partial seizure pattern (treatment adjunct)[1] or
Epilepsy, complex partial seizure pattern (treatment adjunct)[1]—Clorazepate is indicated as adjunctive therapy in the management of partial seizures.

[Epilepsy, simple partial seizure pattern (treatment)][1] or
[Epilepsy, complex partial seizure pattern (treatment)][1]—Clonazepam may be effective in refractory seizures such as complex partial (psychomotor, temporal lobe) or elementary partial (focal) seizures.

[Epilepsy, tonic-clonic seizure pattern (treatment)][1]—Clonazepam may be effective in tonic-clonic (grand mal) seizures. However, when clonazepam is used in patients in whom several types of seizure disorders coexist, it may increase the incidence or rarely precipitate the onset of generalized tonic-clonic (grand mal) seizures; addition of another anticonvulsant and/or an increase in dosage may be required.

Panic disorders (treatment)—Alprazolam, [chlordiazepoxide (parenteral)], clonazepam[1], [diazepam][1], and [lorazepam][1] are used in the treatment of panic disorders.

Spasm, skeletal muscle (treatment adjunct)—Diazepam and [lorazepam][1] are indicated as adjunctive therapy for the relief of skeletal muscle spasm due to reflex spasm of local pathology (such as inflammation of the muscles or joints, or secondary to trauma); spasticity caused by upper motor neuron disorders (such as cerebral palsy and paraplegia); athetosis; stiff-man syndrome; and tetanus. [Diazepam also is used to relieve spasms of facial muscles associated with problems of occlusion and temporomandibular joint disorders.][1]

[Nausea and vomiting, cancer chemotherapy-induced (prophylaxis)][1]—Lorazepam injection, alone or in combination with other agents, reduces the severity and duration of nausea and vomiting associated with emetogenic cancer chemotherapy. In addition, lorazepam-induced amnesia can reduce anticipatory anxiety, nausea, and vomiting.

[Headache, tension (treatment)]—Chlordiazepoxide, diazepam[1], lorazepam[1], and possibly other benzodiazepines[1] are used in the treatment of tension headache.

[Tremors (treatment)][1]—Oral alprazolam, chlordiazepoxide, diazepam, and lorazepam are also used in the treatment of familial, senile, or essential action tremors.

[1]Not included in Canadian product labeling.

## Pharmacology/Pharmacokinetics

See *Table 1*, page 578.

**Physicochemical characteristics**
Molecular weight—
  Alprazolam: 308.77.
  Bromazepam: 316.16.
  Chlordiazepoxide: 299.76.
  Chlordiazepoxide hydrochloride: 336.22.
  Clonazepam: 315.72.
  Clorazepate dipotassium: 408.93.
  Diazepam: 284.75.
  Estazolam: 294.74.
  Flurazepam hydrochloride: 460.81.
  Halazepam: 352.74.
  Ketazolam: 368.82.
  Lorazepam: 321.16.
  Nitrazepam: 281.27.
  Oxazepam: 286.72.
  Prazepam: 324.81.
  Quazepam: 386.8.
  Temazepam: 300.75.
  Triazolam: 343.22.

**Mechanism of action/Effect**

In general, benzodiazepines act as depressants of the central nervous system (CNS), producing all levels of CNS depression from mild sedation to hypnosis to coma, depending on dose.

Although the precise mechanisms of action have not been completely established, it is believed that benzodiazepines enhance or facilitate the action of gamma-aminobutyric acid (GABA), the major inhibitory neurotransmitter in the CNS, by causing it to bind more tightly to the GABA type A (GABA$_A$) receptor.

Benzodiazepines reportedly act as agonists at the benzodiazepine receptors, which have been shown to form a component of a functional supramolecular unit known as the benzodiazepine-GABA receptor-chloride ionophore complex. This receptor complex, which resides on neuronal membranes, functions mainly in the gating of the chloride channel. Activation of the GABA receptor results in the opening of the chloride channel, allowing the flow of chloride ions into the neuron. This results in hyperpolarization, which inhibits firing of the neuron and translates into decreased neuronal excitability, thus attenuating the effects of subsequent depolarizing excitatory transmitters. Benzodiazepines reportedly increase the frequency of chloride channel opening. There is also evidence that benzodiazepines may act at GABA-independent receptors.

Antianxiety agent; sedative-hypnotic—Believed to stimulate GABA receptors in the ascending reticular activating system. Since GABA is inhibitory, receptor stimulation increases inhibition and blocks both cortical and limbic arousal following stimulation of the brain stem reticular formation.

Amnestic—Mechanism of action has not been determined. However, as may occur with all sedative-hypnotic medications, preanesthetic doses of diazepam and lorazepam impair recent memory and interfere with the establishment of the memory trace, thus producing anterograde amnesia for events occurring while therapeutic concentrations of the benzodiazepine are present.

Anticonvulsant—Hyperpolarization, which is enhanced by benzodiazepines, reduces the ability of the neuron to depolarize to the threshold required to produce an action potential. Thus, the seizure threshold is raised. Benzodiazepines suppress the spread of seizure activity produced by epileptogenic foci in the cortex, thalamus, and limbic structures but do not abolish the abnormal discharge of the focus.

Skeletal muscle relaxant adjunct—The exact mechanism of action of benzodiazepines has not been completely established but these medications appear to produce skeletal muscle relaxation primarily by inhibiting spinal polysynaptic afferent pathways; however, monosynaptic afferent pathways may also be inhibited. Benzodiazepines may also directly depress motor nerve and muscle function.

**Absorption**

Following oral administration—Benzodiazepines are well absorbed from the gastrointestinal tract, usually within 1 to 2 hours. Diazepam and clorazepate are among the most rapidly absorbed, and prazepam and oxazepam are the least rapidly absorbed.

Following intramuscular administration—Lorazepam absorption is rapid and complete, whereas chlordiazepoxide and diazepam absorption may be slow and erratic, depending upon the site of administration. When diazepam is injected into the deltoid muscle, absorption is usually rapid and complete.

Following rectal administration—Absorption of diazepam rectal solution and rectal gel is rapid.

**Biotransformation**
Hepatic.
Long half-life benzodiazepines—
  Chlordiazepoxide, flurazepam, halazepam, ketazolam, and quazepam are metabolized by oxidation to active, as well as inactive, metabolites before final inactivation as glucuronide conjugates.
  Diazepam undergoes hepatic demethylation and hydroxylation, involving the cytochrome P450 2C19 (CYP2C19) and CYP3A4 isoenzymes, followed by glucuronidation. Only one active metabolite, desmethyldiazepam, is present in clinically significant concentrations.
  Clorazepate and prazepam are metabolized in the stomach and liver, respectively, to desmethyldiazepam as a result of first-pass biotransformation prior to entering systemic circulation.

Short to intermediate half-life benzodiazepines—
  Alprazolam undergoes hydroxylation, which is catalyzed by the CYP3A isoenzymes, and is eliminated as glucuronide conjugates. One of alprazolam's metabolites has one half of the biological activity of alprazolam, but is present in very low plasma concentrations.
  Bromazepam undergoes hepatic microsomal oxidation and is eliminated primarily as glucuronide conjugates.
  Clobazam undergoes hepatic demethylation and hydroxylation to active and inactive metabolites before inactivation by conjugation.
  Clonazepam and nitrazepam undergo hepatic nitro-reduction to inactive metabolites. Clonazepam also undergoes oxidative hydroxylation and CYP3A isoenzymes may play an important role in clonazepam's metabolism.
  Estazolam undergoes oxidative metabolism and hydroxylation to metabolites with little activity and low plasma concentrations in comparison with the parent compound.
  Lorazepam, oxazepam, and temazepam are metabolized by direct conjugation with glucuronic acid.
  Triazolam undergoes hepatic microsomal oxidation to inactive hydroxylated metabolites that are eliminated primarily as glucuronide conjugates.

**Accumulation**

During repeated dosing with long half-life benzodiazepines, there is accumulation of the parent compound and/or any pharmacologically active metabolites. Accumulation continues until a steady-state plasma concentration is reached, which usually takes 5 days to 2 weeks after initiation of therapy. Following termination of treatment, drug elimination is slow since active metabolites may remain in the blood for several days or even weeks, possibly resulting in persistent effects.

During repeated dosing with short to intermediate half-life benzodiazepines, accumulation is minimal, and a steady-state plasma concentration is usually attained within a few days after initiation of therapy. Following termination of treatment, blood concentrations are subclinical in 24 hours and return rapidly to zero (in about 4 days or less).

**Onset of action**
After single oral doses, onset of action depends largely upon absorption rate. After multiple doses, effects depend partly upon rate and extent of drug accumulation, which in turn relate to elimination half-life and clearance.

**Duration of action**
After single oral doses, duration of action depends upon rate and extent of drug distribution, as well as rate of elimination once distribution is complete. After multiple doses, effects depend partly upon rate and extent of drug accumulation, which in turn relate to elimination half-life and clearance. The duration of clinical effects of the benzodiazepines is not always predictable from the elimination half-life.

## Precautions to Consider

### Cross-sensitivity and/or related problems
Patients sensitive to one of the benzodiazepines may be sensitive to the other benzodiazepines also.

### Carcinogenicity/Tumorigenicity
*Alprazolam*—In a 24-month study in rats, alprazolam at doses of up to 150 times the maximum recommended human dose (MRHD) showed no evidence of carcinogenic potential.
*Clobazam*—Hepatomas, thyroid adenomas, and malignancies of the liver and thyroid gland were seen in rodent studies; the significance of this finding to humans is unknown.
*Clonazepam*—Studies on carcinogenic potential have not been done.
*Diazepam*—An increased incidence of liver tumors was seen in male mice and rats following oral administration of diazepam to mice and rats of both sexes at doses that were approximately 6 and 12 times, respectively, the MRHD (1 mg per kg of body weight [mg/kg] per day) on a mg per square meter of body surface area (mg/m$^2$) basis for 80 and 104 weeks, respectively.
*Estazolam*—Studies of 24-months duration in mice and rats showed no evidence of tumorigenicity. However, the female mice given 3 and 10 mg/kg per day of estazolam over the 2-year period showed an increase in hyperplastic liver nodules; the significance of this finding is unknown.
*Halazepam*—In oral oncogenicity studies in rats and mice, halazepam at doses 5 to 50 times the usual daily human dose of 120 mg showed no evidence of carcinogenicity.
*Lorazepam*—In an 18-month study in rats, lorazepam showed no evidence of carcinogenic potential.
*Oxazepam*—A 24-month study in rats given oxazepam at doses 30 times the MRHD showed an increase in benign thyroid follicular cell tumors, testicular interstitial cell adenomas, and prostatic adenomas. In a 9-month study in mice, oxazepam in doses 35 to 100 times the usual daily human dose caused dose-related increases in liver adenomas, some of which were classified as carcinomas after microscopic examination.
*Quazepam*—Oral oncogenicity studies in mice and hamsters showed no evidence of carcinogenicity.
*Temazepam*—Long-term studies in mice and rats showed no evidence of carcinogenicity. However, hyperplastic liver nodules occurred in female mice at the highest dose used (160 mg/kg per day); the clinical significance of this finding is unknown.
*Triazolam*—In a 24-month study in mice, triazolam in doses up to 4000 times the human dose showed no evidence of carcinogenic potential.

### Mutagenicity
*Alprazolam*—Mutagenicity was not demonstrated in appropriate tests on mice or bacteria.
*Estazolam*—Mutagenicity was not demonstrated in appropriate tests on mice, rats, and bacteria.
*Diazepam*—Data are insufficient to determine mutagenic potential.
*Halazepam*—Halazepam demonstrated no mutagenic activity in the Ames test.
*Lorazepam, oxazepam, and temazepam*—Studies on mutagenic potential have not been done.
*Quazepam*—Mutagenicity was not demonstrated in tests on mice or bacteria.

### Pregnancy/Reproduction
Pregnancy—
  All benzodiazepines—
    Chlordiazepoxide, clonazepam, diazepam, estazolam, flurazepam, lorazepam, nitrazepam, temazepam, and triazolam cross the placenta. Alprazolam, bromazepam, clorazepate, halazepam, ketazolam, oxazepam, prazepam, and quazepam are assumed to cross the placenta because of their similarity to the other benzodiazepines.
    First trimester—Chlordiazepoxide and diazepam have been reported to increase the risk of congenital malformations when used during the first trimester of pregnancy. Because of the similarity of the benzodiazepines, the other benzodiazepines are assumed to be associated with this increased risk also. Risk-benefit must be considered carefully. However, since the use of benzodiazepines (with the possible exception of anticonvulsant use) is rarely a matter of urgency, it should be avoided during pregnancy, especially during the first trimester. The possibility that a woman of childbearing potential may already be pregnant should be considered when initiating benzodiazepine treatment.
    When benzodiazepines are used as anticonvulsants, risk-benefit must be considered. Reports suggest an increased incidence of congenital abnormalities in children whose mothers used anticonvulsants during pregnancy, although anticonvulsant medications have not been definitively shown to have a causative role and other factors, such as the epileptic condition itself, may be involved. The severity of the seizure disorder and the potential harm to the mother or fetus in the event of a seizure must be considered when deciding whether to continue anticonvulsant treatment during pregnancy.
    Regular use of benzodiazepines during pregnancy may cause physical dependence with resulting withdrawal symptoms in the neonate.
    Use of benzodiazepine hypnotics during the last weeks of pregnancy has resulted in neonatal CNS depression, neonatal flaccidity, feeding difficulties, hypothermia, and respiratory problems.
  *Chlordiazepoxide*—
    Reproduction studies in rats showed that chlordiazepoxide, at doses of 10, 20, and 80 mg per kg of body weight (mg/kg) per day, caused no congenital anomalies or adverse effects on the growth of the newborn animal. However, another study with chlordiazepoxide at doses of 100 mg/kg per day showed a significant decrease in the fertilization rate and a decrease in the viability and body weight of offspring, which may have been due to the sedative effect; also, one neonate in each of the first and second matings in this study showed skeletal deformities.
    FDA pregnancy category not presently included in product labeling.
  *Clonazepam*—
    Studies in rabbits have shown that clonazepam in oral doses of 0.2 to 10 mg/kg per day (low dose approximately 0.2 times the maximum recommended human dose [MRHD] for seizure disorders and approximately equivalent to the MRHD for panic disorder, on a mg/m$^2$ basis), given during organogenesis, caused a non–dose-related increased incidence of cleft palates, open eyelids, fused sternebrae, and limb defects.
    Withdrawal of clonazepam anticonvulsant prior to or during pregnancy should be considered only when seizures are mild and infrequent in the absence of the medication and where the possibility of status epilepticus and withdrawal symptoms is considered low.
    FDA Pregnancy Category D.
  *Diazepam*—
    Rodent studies have shown that single oral doses ≥ eight times the MRHD of 1 mg/kg per day on a mg/m$^2$ basis, administered during organogenesis, are teratogenic. Cleft palate and exencephaly were the most commonly and consistently reported malformations. Also, long-term changes in cellular immune response, brain neurochemistry, and behavior were seen in offspring of rodents given diazepam during pregnancy in doses similar to human clinical doses.
    FDA Pregnancy Category D.
  *Lorazepam*—
    Studies in rabbits have shown that lorazepam causes fetal resorption and increased fetal loss at oral doses of 40 mg/kg and intravenous doses of 4 mg/kg and higher; lorazepam was also shown to cause anomalies in rabbits without relationship to dosage.
    FDA Pregnancy Category D (parenteral).
  *Quazepam*—
    Reproduction studies in mice given 66 to 400 times the human dose of quazepam showed minor developmental variations including delayed ossification of the sternum, vertebrae, distal phalanges, and supraoccipital bones. Studies in mice given 60 to 180 times the human dose showed slight reductions in the pregnancy rate.
    FDA Pregnancy Category X.

*Temazepam*—
Studies in rats have shown that temazepam causes an increased incidence of fetal resorption at doses of 30 and 120 mg/kg, and an increased occurrence of rudimentary ribs (considered skeletal variants) at doses of 240 mg/kg or higher. Increased nursing mortality was seen in rats when oral doses of 60 mg/kg per day were given to the dam during the perinatal-postnatal period. Also, studies in rabbits have shown that temazepam causes an increased incidence of the 13th rib variant at doses of 40 mg/kg or higher, and occasional abnormalities such as exencephaly and fusion or asymmetry of ribs without relationship to dosage.

FDA Pregnancy Category X.

*Alprazolam; Halazepam*—FDA Pregnancy Category D.
*Estazolam; Triazolam*—FDA Pregnancy Category X.
*Clorazepate, flurazepam, and oxazepam*—FDA pregnancy categories not presently included in product labeling.

Labor—*All benzodiazepines*: Use of benzodiazepines just prior to or during labor may cause neonatal flaccidity.

Delivery—*Diazepam*: When diazepam is administered in doses of more than 30 mg (especially intramuscularly or intravenously) to women within 15 hours before delivery, the neonate may develop apnea, hypotonia, hypothermia, a reluctance to feed, and impaired metabolic response to cold stress.

### Breast-feeding
Chlordiazepoxide, diazepam, halazepam, quazepam, and their metabolites, including desmethyldiazepam (which is also the metabolite of clorazepate and prazepam) are distributed into breast milk; clobazam and nitrazepam are distributed into breast milk also; alprazolam, clonazepam, flurazepam, lorazepam, oxazepam, temazepam, and/or their metabolites are assumed to be distributed into breast milk because of their similarity to the other benzodiazepines. Although studies in humans have not been done, studies in rats have shown that bromazepam, estazolam, ketazolam, triazolam, and their metabolites are distributed into the milk of rats.

Chronic use of diazepam by nursing mothers has been reported to cause lethargy and weight loss in the infants. Since neonates metabolize benzodiazepines more slowly than adults and accumulation of the benzodiazepine and/or its metabolites may occur, use by nursing mothers may cause sedation, feeding difficulties, and/or weight loss in the infant.

### Pediatrics
*All benzodiazepines*—Children, especially the very young, are usually more sensitive to the CNS effects of benzodiazepines. Prolonged CNS depression may be produced in the neonate because of inability to biotransform the benzodiazepine into inactive metabolites.

*Clonazepam*—Risk-benefit must be considered in the long-term use of clonazepam to treat seizure disorders in pediatric patients because of the possibility that adverse effects on physical or mental development may occur and may not become apparent for many years.

### Geriatrics
Geriatric patients are usually more sensitive to the CNS effects of benzodiazepines. It is recommended that dosage be limited to the smallest effective dose and increased gradually, if necessary, to decrease the possibility of development of ataxia, dizziness, and oversedation, which may lead to falls and other accidents. A retrospective case-control study has shown that elderly patients receiving long-acting benzodiazepines are more likely than those receiving short-acting benzodiazepines to suffer falls and fall-related fractures. However, both groups had an increased risk of these sequelae as compared to older patients who did not receive benzodiazepines or who received other short-acting sedative-hypnotics.

The half-lives of benzodiazepines may be longer in elderly than in younger patients.

Parenteral administration of benzodiazepines may be more likely to cause apnea, hypotension, bradycardia, or cardiac arrest in geriatric patients.

### Pharmacogenetics
*Diazepam*—3 to 5% of white patients have little or no cytochrome P450 2C19 (CYP2C19) activity and are poor metabolizers of diazepam.

### Drug interactions and/or related problems
The following drug interactions and/or related problems have been selected on the basis of their potential clinical significance (possible mechanism in parentheses where appropriate)—not necessarily inclusive (» = major clinical significance):

Note: The cytochrome P450 2C19 (CYP2C19) isoenzyme is known to be involved in diazepam's metabolism. Medications that inhibit CYP2C19, such as cimetidine, quinidine, and tranylcypromine, may decrease the rate of elimination of diazepam. Likewise, medications that induce CYP2C19, such as rifampin, may increase the rate of diazepam's elimination.

The CYP3A isoenzymes are known to be involved in the metabolism of alprazolam, clonazepam, diazepam, and triazolam. Concurrent use with medications that inhibit CYP3A isoenzymes, other than those listed below, should be undertaken with caution, and reduction in benzodiazepine dosage should be considered.

Combinations containing any of the following medications, depending on the amount present, may also interact with this medication.

Addictive medications, other, especially CNS depressants with habituating potential
(prolonged concurrent use may increase the risk of habituation; caution is recommended)

» Alcohol or
» CNS depression–producing medications, other (see *Appendix II*)
(CNS depressant effects may be potentiated and the risk of apnea may be increased; use of alcohol during treatment with a benzodiazepine is not recommended; caution is recommended when another CNS depression–producing medication is used with a benzodiazepine, and dosage of one or both agents should be reduced)
(when a benzodiazepine is used with an opioid analgesic, the dosage of the opioid analgesic should be reduced by at least one third and administered in small increments)

Antacids
(concurrent use may delay, but not reduce, the absorption of chlordiazepoxide and diazepam; whether this effect applies to other benzodiazepines has not been determined)
(concurrent use with clorazepate may decrease the rate of conversion of clorazepate to desmethyldiazepam, but does not affect the degree of absorption)

Antidepressants, tricyclic
(in addition to possibly increasing CNS depressant effects, concurrent use with alprazolam in doses of up to 4 mg per day has been reported to increase steady-state plasma concentrations of imipramine and desipramine by an average of 31% and 20%, respectively; however, the clinical significance of these changes is unknown)

Carbamazepine
(induction of hepatic microsomal enzyme activity by carbamazepine may result in increased metabolism, decreased serum concentrations, and reduced elimination half-lives of benzodiazepines metabolized via the hepatic enzyme system, such as clonazepam; carbamazepine concentrations may be increased during concurrent use with a benzodiazepine; monitoring of carbamazepine blood concentrations as a guide to dosage is recommended, especially when carbamazepine is added to or withdrawn from existing benzodiazepine therapy)

Cimetidine or
Contraceptives, estrogen-containing, oral or
Diltiazem or
Disulfiram or
Erythromycin or
Fluoxetine or
» Fluvoxamine or
Grapefruit juice or
» Itraconazole or
» Ketoconazole or
» Nefazodone or
Propoxyphene or
Ranitidine or
Verapamil
(concurrent use may inhibit the hepatic metabolism of benzodiazepines that are metabolized by oxidation, resulting in delayed elimination and increased plasma concentrations; however, the hepatic metabolism of benzodiazepines that undergo direct glucuronide conjugation, such as lorazepam, oxazepam, and temazepam, is probably not affected)

(concurrent use of cimetidine or oral, estrogen-containing contraceptives may inhibit the hepatic metabolism of benzodiazepines that are metabolized primarily by nitro-reduction, such as nitrazepam, possibly resulting in delayed elimination, prolonged elimination half-life, and, during long-term use, increased serum concentrations)

(alprazolam's peak plasma concentration [$C_{max}$] has been almost doubled during concurrent use of cimetidine, fluvoxamine, or nefazodone; also, decreased psychomotor performance has been demonstrated during concurrent use of fluvoxamine; dosage reductions of alprazolam may be required [initial reductions of 50% are recommended in patients receiving fluvoxamine or nefazodone]; alprazolam's $C_{max}$ has been increased by approximately 50% during concurrent use of fluoxetine or propoxyphene; also, psychomotor performance has been decreased during concurrent use of fluoxetine)

(diazepam and desmethyldiazepam clearances have been reduced and patient psychomotor performance has been impaired during concurrent use of fluvoxamine; concurrent use is not recommended due to the potential for accumulation of diazepam and desmethyldiazepam)

(triazolam's area under the plasma concentration–time curve [AUC] has been increased 22 and 27 times during concurrent use of ketoconazole and itraconazole, respectively; concurrent use is not recommended; triazolam's AUC was increased fourfold and patient psychomotor performance was impaired during concurrent use of nefazodone; reductions in initial triazolam dosage of 75% are recommended in patients receiving nefazodone; triazolam's $C_{max}$ and half-life [$t_{1/2}$] have been doubled during concurrent use of cimetidine or erythromycin; dosage reductions may be necessary; triazolam's $C_{max}$, $t_{1/2}$, and AUC have been increased during concurrent use of ranitidine; caution is recommended; plasma concentration, AUC, and $t_{1/2}$ of triazolam have been increased by coadministration with grapefruit juice)

Clozapine
(collapse, sometimes accompanied by respiratory depression or arrest, has been reported in a few patients receiving clozapine concurrently with benzodiazepines. Caution is advised when clozapine is administered concomitantly with any agent that may depress respiration, and the dosage of clozapine should be titrated upward slowly. Some clinicians have recommended that benzodiazepines be discontinued at least 1 week prior to initiation of therapy with clozapine)

Fentanyl derivatives
(premedication with diazepam or lorazepam may decrease the dose of a fentanyl derivative required for induction of anesthesia and decrease the time to loss of consciousness with induction doses; also, administration of diazepam or lorazepam prior to or during surgery may decrease risk of patient recall of surgical events postoperatively; however, these potential benefits must be weighed against the potential risks of concurrent use, such as an increased risk of severe hypotension associated with decreases in systemic vascular resistance, increased risk of respiratory depression, and delayed recovery time, especially when the benzodiazepine is administered intravenously)

Hypotension-producing medications, other (see *Appendix II*)
(concurrent use may potentiate the hypotensive effects of benzodiazepine preanesthetics used in surgery; dosage adjustments may be necessary)

(concurrent use of mecamylamine or trimethaphan with benzodiazepine preanesthetics used in surgery may potentiate the hypotensive response, with increased risk of severe hypotension, shock, and cardiovascular collapse during surgery)

(caution is advised during titration of calcium channel blocker dosage for those patients taking medication known to promote hypotension, such as benzodiazepine preanesthetics, since the combination may result in excessive hypotension)

Isoniazid
(concurrent use may inhibit the elimination of diazepam and triazolam, resulting in increased plasma concentrations; whether this effect applies to other benzodiazepines has not been determined; dosage adjustment may be necessary)

Levodopa
(concurrent use with benzodiazepines may decrease the therapeutic effects of levodopa)

Omeprazole
(concurrent use of omeprazole may prolong the elimination of diazepam)

Probenecid
(concurrent use may impair glucuronide conjugation of lorazepam, oxazepam, or temazepam, resulting in increased effects and possibly excessive sedation)

Rifampin
(concurrent use may enhance the elimination of diazepam, resulting in decreased plasma concentrations; whether this effect applies to other benzodiazepines has not been determined; dosage adjustment may be necessary)

Scopolamine, systemic
(concurrent use of scopolamine with parenteral lorazepam is reported to have no added beneficial effect and their combined effect may increase the incidence of sedation, hallucination, and irrational behavior)

» Tubing, infusion, plastic
(diazepam adheres to plastic infusion tubing; if parenteral diazepam must be administered through tubing, it should be injected as closely as possible to the insertion point)

Zidovudine
(concurrent use with benzodiazepines may, in theory, competitively inhibit hepatic glucuronidation and decrease the clearance of zidovudine; the toxicity of zidovudine potentially could be increased)

**Laboratory value alterations**
The following have been selected on the basis of their potential clinical significance (possible effect in parentheses where appropriate)—not necessarily inclusive (» = major clinical significance):

With diagnostic test results
Metyrapone test
(chlordiazepoxide may interfere with the assay for urine 17-ketosteroids or 17-ketogenic steroids; in addition, the response to metyrapone may be decreased)

Sodium iodide I 123 and
Sodium iodide I 131
(benzodiazepines may decrease thyroidal uptake of I 123 and I 131)

**Medical considerations/Contraindications**
The medical considerations/contraindications included have been selected on the basis of their potential clinical significance (reasons given in parentheses where appropriate)—not necessarily inclusive (» = major clinical significance).

*Risk-benefit should be considered when the following medical problems exist:*

» Alcohol intoxication, acute, with depressed vital signs
(additive CNS depression)
» Coma or
» Shock
(hypnotic or hypotensive effects may be prolonged or intensified by benzodiazepines administered parenterally)

Drug abuse or dependence, history of
(patients predisposed to habituation and dependence)

Epilepsy or
Seizures, history of
(initiation or abrupt withdrawal of clonazepam or diazepam therapy may increase frequency and/or severity of tonic-clonic [grand mal] seizures; use of intravenous diazepam for absence [petit mal] status or Lennox-Gastaut syndrome [petit mal variant] status may precipitate tonic status epilepticus)

(abrupt withdrawal of clonazepam or diazepam used to treat these disorders may precipitate seizures or status epilepticus)

» Glaucoma, angle-closure, acute or predisposition to
(benzodiazepines may have anticholinergic effect)

Hepatic function impairment
(elimination half-life may be prolonged; minimal effect with oxazepam, lorazepam, and temazepam)

Hyperkinesis
(paradoxical reactions may occur)

Hypoalbuminemia
(may predispose patient to higher incidence of sedative side effects, especially with chlordiazepoxide and diazepam)

Mental depression, severe
(suicidal tendencies may be present; protective measures may be necessary; also benzodiazepines, when used alone, may increase depression; episodes of hypomania and mania reported with use of alprazolam in patients with mental depression)

» Myasthenia gravis
(condition may be exacerbated)

Organic brain disorders
(patients may be more prone to disinhibition and CNS depressant effects of benzodiazepines)

Porphyria
(condition may be exacerbated with the use of chlordiazepoxide)

Psychoses
(benzodiazepines are rarely effective as primary treatment for psychosis; also, paradoxical reactions may be more likely to occur in psychotic patients)

» Pulmonary disease, severe chronic obstructive
(compromised respiratory function may be exacerbated and increased salivation and bronchial secretions occurring with benzo-

diazepine use may cause problems in these patients; deaths occurring shortly after beginning treatment with alprazolam have been reported rarely in patients with severe pulmonary disease)

Renal function impairment
  (accumulation of renally excreted metabolites may occur)

Sensitivity to benzodiazepines

Sleep apnea, established or suspected
  (condition may be exacerbated)

Swallowing abnormality, in children
  (condition may be exacerbated because drooling and aspiration induced by benzodiazepines, such as nitrazepam, may delay cricopharyngeal relaxation; patient should be closely monitored)

Caution should also be used in surgical or nonambulatory patients because of the cough-suppressant effects of clonazepam.

## Patient monitoring

The following may be especially important in patient monitoring (other tests may be warranted in some patients, depending on condition; » = major clinical significance):

Assessment of amount and frequency of medication use
  (recommended at periodic intervals during long-term therapy to detect signs of dependence or abuse)

Reassessment of medication's efficacy as an antianxiety agent or a sedative-hypnotic
  (recommended at periodic intervals during therapy; see *Indications*)

## Side/Adverse Effects

Note: Although not all of these side effects have been attributed specifically to each benzodiazepine, a potential exists for their occurrence during the use of any benzodiazepine.

Psychological or physical dependence and tolerance may occur with benzodiazepine use, especially with high-dose or prolonged use.

Geriatric and debilitated patients, children (especially the very young), and patients with liver disease or low serum albumin are usually more sensitive to the CNS effects of benzodiazepines.

Parenteral administration of benzodiazepines may cause apnea, hypotension, bradycardia, or cardiac arrest, especially in geriatric or severely ill patients and in patients with limited pulmonary reserve or unstable cardiovascular status or if intravenous administration of medication is too rapid.

Parenteral benzodiazepines have produced hypotension or muscular weakness in some patients, especially when used concurrently with narcotics, barbiturates, or alcohol.

Coughing, depressed respiration, dyspnea, hyperventilation, laryngospasm, and pain in throat and chest have been reported when parenteral diazepam was administered in peroral endoscopic procedures.

The following side/adverse effects have been selected on the basis of their potential clinical significance (possible signs and symptoms in parentheses where appropriate)—not necessarily inclusive:

### Those indicating need for medical attention

Incidence less frequent
  *Anterograde amnesia* (lack of memory of events taking place after benzodiazepine is taken); *anxiety; confusion*—especially in the elderly and in patients with cerebral impairment; *mental depression; tachycardia/palpitation* (fast, pounding, or irregular heartbeat)

Note: *Anterograde amnesia* may be dose-related and may occur at a higher rate with triazolam than with other benzodiazepines. "Traveler's amnesia," which occurs in people taking benzodiazepines to avoid jet lag, may be associated with allowing insufficient time for sleep and/or concommitant use of alcohol.

Daytime *anxiety*, as well as wakefulness during the last third of the night, may develop over several weeks of nightly dosing with short to intermediate half-life benzodiazepines. These effects are thought to be due to the development of tolerance or adaptation, which leads to a relative deficiency of benzodiazepine receptor binding between nightly doses.

Incidence rare
  *Abnormal thinking; including delusions* (false beliefs that cannot be changed by facts); *depersonalization* (loss of sense of reality); *or disorientation; allergic reaction* (skin rash or itching); *behavior changes; including bizarre behavior; or decreased inhibition; blood dyscrasias, including agranulocytosis* (chills, fever, sore throat; unusual tiredness or weakness); *anemia* (unusual tiredness or weakness); *leukopenia* (chills, fever, sore throat); *neutropenia* (chills, fever, and/or sore throat; ulcers or sores in mouth or throat, continuing; unusual tiredness or weakness); *thrombocytopenia* (unusual bleeding or bruising); *extrapyramidal effects, dystonic* (uncontrolled movements of body, including the eyes); *hepatic dysfunction* (yellow eyes or skin); *hypotension* (low blood pressure); *muscle weakness; paradoxical reactions; including agitation; aggressive behavior; hallucinations* (seeing, hearing, or feeling things that are not there); *hostility or rage* (outbursts of anger); *insomnia* (trouble in sleeping); *unusual excitement, irritability, or nervousness; phlebitis or venous thrombosis* (redness, swelling, or pain at injection site)—for parenteral dosage forms only; *seizures*

Note: *Behavioral disturbances* associated with clonazepam are more likely to occur in children or in patients with pre-existing brain damage and/or mental retardation or a history of behavioral or psychiatric disturbances; if these effects occur, the medication should be discontinued.

*Paradoxical reactions* have occurred most often in patients who were receiving additional CNS-active medications, or who had underlying psychiatric conditions, a history of violent or aggressive behavior, a history of alcohol or substance abuse, or a history of unusual reactions to sedatives or alcohol. Benzodiazepine treatment should be discontinued if a paradoxical reaction occurs.

Incidence of *phlebitis* or *venous thrombosis* is more common with diazepam, less common with lorazepam, and rare with chlordiazepoxide.

There may be an increased incidence and severity of *seizures*, especially on initiation or abrupt withdrawal of clonazepam and diazepam, in patients with epilepsy or history of seizures.

### Those indicating need for medical attention only if they continue or are bothersome

Incidence more frequent
  *Ataxia* (clumsiness or unsteadiness)—especially in elderly or debilitated patients; *dizziness or lightheadedness; drowsiness, including residual daytime drowsiness when used as a hypnotic*—especially in elderly or debilitated patients; *slurred speech*

Note: *Ataxia* and *drowsiness* are dose-related and are most severe during initial therapy. They may decrease in severity or disappear with continued or long-term therapy.

*Residual daytime drowsiness* is dose-related.

Incidence less frequent or rare
  *Abdominal or stomach cramps or pain; blurred vision or other changes in vision; changes in libido* (changes in sexual desire or ability); *constipation; diarrhea; dryness of mouth or increased thirst; euphoria* (false sense of well-being); *headache; increased bronchial secretions or excessive salivation* (watering of mouth); *muscle spasm; nausea or vomiting; problems with urination; tremor* (trembling or shaking); *unusual tiredness or weakness*

Note: *Increased bronchial secretions* and *excessive salivation* may pose a risk of aspiration in infants and young children, and in elderly or bedridden patients as well as in patients with chronic respiratory disease.

### Those indicating possible withdrawal and the need for medical attention if they occur (usually within 2 to 3 days with short to intermediate half-life benzodiazepines and 10 to 20 days with long half-life benzodiazepines) after medication is discontinued

Incidence more frequent
  *Insomnia* (trouble in sleeping); *irritability; nervousness*

Note: When a benzodiazepine has been used as a hypnotic, withdrawal of the medication may cause a transient recurrence of symptoms known as rebound *insomnia*. Rebound insomnia may be more severe than the insomnia that originally led to treatment.

Incidence less frequent
  *Abdominal or stomach cramps; confusion; depersonalization* (loss of sense of reality); *increased sweating; mental depression; muscle cramps; nausea or vomiting; perceptual disturbances, including hyperacusis* (increased sense of hearing); *hypersensitivity to touch and pain; parasthesias* (tingling, burning, or prickly sensations); *or photophobia* (sensitivity of eyes to light); *tachycardia* (fast or pounding heartbeat); *tremor* (trembling or shaking)

Incidence rare
  *Convulsions; delirium* (confusion as to time, place, or person); *hallucinations; paranoid symptoms* (feelings of suspicion and distrust)

Note: *Withdrawal symptoms* are more common and often more severe in patients who have received high doses of a benzodiazepine over a prolonged period of time. However, symptoms have occurred following abrupt discontinuation of benzodiazepines that have been taken continuously, at therapeutic doses, for as few as 1 to 2 weeks. Abrupt discontinuation increases the chance of developing withdrawal symptoms, including life-threatening seizures. In some patients, withdrawal symptoms have occurred during gradual discontinuation or tapering of benzodiazepines. Withdrawal symptoms may be more likely to occur following the use of short-acting benzodiazepines than long-acting benzodiazepines.

## Overdose

For specific information on the agents used in the management of benzodiazepine overdose, see:
- *Charcoal, Activated (Oral-Local)* monograph;
- *Dopamine* and/or *Metaraminol* and/or *Norepinephrine* in *Sympathomimetic Agents—Cardiovascular Use (Parenteral-Systemic)* monograph; and/or
- *Flumazenil (Systemic)* monograph.

For more information on the management of overdose or unintentional ingestion, **contact a Poison Control Center** (see *Poison Control Center Listing*).

### Clinical effects of overdose
Note: Serious sequelae are rare unless other drugs or alcohol have been coingested. However, deaths have occurred after overdoses of benzodiazepines alone. Also, when benzodiazepines have been coingested with alcohol, deaths have occurred at benzodiazepine and alcohol plasma concentrations that were less than those usually associated with death by overdose with either agent alone.

The following effects have been selected on the basis of their potential clinical significance (possible signs and symptoms in parentheses where appropriate)—not necessarily inclusive:

***Confusion, continuing; decreased reflexes; drowsiness, severe, or coma; seizures; shakiness; slow heartbeat; slurred speech, continuing; staggering; troubled breathing; weakness, severe***

### Treatment of overdose
To decrease absorption—
If the patient is conscious (and not at risk of becoming obtunded, comatose, or convulsing based on ingestion), emesis should be induced mechanically or with emetics; also, activated charcoal may be administered orally to increase clearance as well as decrease absorption of the benzodiazepine.
If the patient is unconscious, gastric lavage may be performed with a cuffed endotracheal tube in place to prevent aspiration of vomitus.
To enhance elimination—
Intravenous fluids may be administered to promote diuresis.
Specific treatment—
After airway, ventilation, and intravenous access have been secured, flumazenil, a specific benzodiazepine receptor antagonist, may be administered to reverse sedative effects. Patients must be monitored for the return of sedation after the administration of flumazenil. Flumazenil may precipitate seizures, especially in patients who have been using benzodiazepines long-term or who have coingested a cyclic antidepressant. Because of the risk of seizure induction, flumazenil use is not recommended in epileptic patients who have been treated with benzodiazepines.
Oxygen should be administered if respiration is depressed.
Hypotension may be controlled, if necessary, by intravenous administration of vasopressors such as dopamine, norepinephrine, or metaraminol.
Monitoring—
Respiration, pulse, and blood pressure should be monitored.
Supportive care—
Maintenance of adequate pulmonary ventilation is essential.
Intravenous fluids should be administered to maintain blood pressure.
Patients in whom intentional overdose is confirmed or suspected should be referred for psychiatric consultation.
Note: If excitation occurs, barbiturates should *not* be used since they may exacerbate excitation and/or prolong CNS depression.
Dialysis is of no known value in the treatment of benzodiazepine overdose.

## Patient Consultation

As an aid to patient consultation, refer to *Advice for the Patient, Benzodiazepines (Systemic)*.
In providing consultation, consider emphasizing the following selected information (» = major clinical significance):

### Before using this medication
» Conditions affecting use, especially:
Sensitivity to benzodiazepines
Pregnancy—Benzodiazepines reported to increase risk of congenital malformations when used during first trimester of pregnancy; chronic use may cause physical dependence in the neonate with resulting withdrawal symptoms; use during last weeks of pregnancy may cause neonatal CNS depression; use just prior to or during labor may cause neonatal flaccidity
Breast-feeding—Some benzodiazepines and their metabolites distributed into breast milk and others may be distributed into breast milk; use by nursing mothers may cause sedation, and possibly feeding difficulties and weight loss in the infant
Use in children—Children, especially the very young, usually more sensitive to CNS effects of benzodiazepines
Use in the elderly—Elderly patients usually more sensitive to CNS effects of benzodiazepines
Other medications, especially other CNS depression–producing medications, fluvoxamine, itraconazole, ketoconazole, or nefazodone
Other medical problems, especially acute angle-closure glaucoma, myasthenia gravis, or severe chronic obstructive pulmonary disease

### Proper use of this medication
*For caregiver administering diazepam rectal gel*
Discussing with patient's physician when to use and proper administration
Discussing with patient's physician when to summon emergency help
Carefully reading instructions supplied with medication before use is needed
Monitoring patient after administration as instructed by physician
*Proper administration*
For extended-release dosage form of clorazepate
Swallowing tablets whole
Not crushing, breaking, or chewing
For concentrated oral solution dosage form of alprazolam, diazepam, or lorazepam
Measuring each dose with dropper provided with medication
Diluting dose with liquid or semisolid food such as water, soda or soda-like beverages, applesauce, or pudding is recommended
Consuming entire mixture immediately; not saving for later use
For sublingual tablet dosage form of lorazepam
Not chewing or swallowing tablet whole
Dissolving slowly under tongue; not swallowing for at least 2 minutes to allow sufficient absorption
» Importance of not taking more medication than the amount prescribed because of habit-forming potential
» Not increasing dose if medication is less effective after a few weeks; checking with physician
*For anticonvulsant use when on a regular dosing regimen*
» Compliance with therapy; not missing any doses
*For hypnotic use*
» Taking only when schedule will allow a full night's sleep to avoid amnesia and residual daytime sedation
*For flurazepam only*
» Maximum effectiveness of medication may not occur until 2 or 3 nights after initiation of therapy
» Proper dosing
Missed dose: If on scheduled dosing regimen (e.g., for epilepsy)—Taking right away if remembered within an hour or so; if remembered later, not taking at all; not doubling doses
» Proper storage

### Precautions while using this medication
Regular visits to physician to check progress during prolonged therapy (and during initial therapy for anticonvulsant use) and to evaluate need to continue benzodiazepine use
*For anticonvulsant use*
Carrying medical identification card or bracelet during therapy
*For sedative-hypnotic use*
Checking with physician if feel need to use medication for more than 7 to 10 days
Possibility of rebound insomnia after discontinuing medication
» Checking with physician if physical or psychological dependence is suspected
» Checking with physician before discontinuing medication after high-dose or prolonged use; gradual dosage reduction may be necessary to avoid the possibility of withdrawal symptoms and, in patients with epilepsy or history of seizures, the possibility of precipitating seizures
» Avoiding use of alcohol or other CNS depressants during therapy
» Suspected overdose: Getting emergency help at once
Caution if any laboratory tests required; possible interference with results of metyrapone test
» Not driving, riding a bicycle, or operating machinery until effects of medication are known or until effects of acute use have worn off, including residual daytime effects after use to treat insomnia, be-

cause of possible drowsiness, dizziness, lightheadedness, clumsiness, or unsteadiness; may be especially important for elderly patients

### Side/adverse effects
Signs of potential side effects, especially anterograde amnesia, anxiety, confusion, mental depression, abnormal thinking, allergic reaction, behavior changes, blood dyscrasias, extrapyramidal symptoms, hepatic dysfunction, hypotension, muscle weakness, paradoxical reactions, or seizures

Most side/adverse effects are more likely to occur in children, especially the very young, and in elderly patients; these patients are usually more sensitive to effects of benzodiazepines

For patients receiving chlordiazepoxide, diazepam, or lorazepam injection: Checking with physician if redness, swelling, or pain at injection site occurs

Possibility of withdrawal symptoms

## General Dosing Information

The possibility that a woman of childbearing potential may already be pregnant should be considered when initiating benzodiazepine treatment.

Geriatric or debilitated patients, children, or patients with hepatic or renal function impairment or low serum albumin should receive decreased initial dosage since elimination of benzodiazepines, especially those with long half-lives, may be decreased in these patients, resulting in increased CNS side effects such as oversedation, dizziness, or impaired coordination.

Benzodiazepines may suppress respiration, especially in the elderly, the very ill, the very young, and patients with limited pulmonary reserve. Lower doses may be required for these patients. Deaths occurring shortly after beginning treatment with alprazolam have been reported rarely in patients with severe pulmonary disease.

Optimal dosage of benzodiazepines varies with diagnosis and patient response. Individual dosage adjustments are important. The minimum effective dose should be used for the shortest period, with the need for continuing therapy with benzodiazepines reviewed regularly.

If daytime anxiety appears in a patient being treated for insomnia, discontinuation of the benzodiazepine should be considered.

Prolonged use and/or use of large doses of benzodiazepines increases the risk of developing psychological or physical dependence. However, withdrawal symptoms, including seizures, have occurred after short-term use at recommended doses of alprazolam. The risk of dependence among patients taking > 4 mg per day of alprazolam may be greater than among patients taking lower doses.

When a benzodiazepine is discontinued after treatment with a dose higher than the lowest dose for more than a few weeks, the medication should be withdrawn gradually to lessen the possibility of precipitating withdrawal symptoms, especially in patients with a history of seizures.

Depressed patients with suicidal tendencies, particularly those who use alcohol excessively, should not have access to large quantities of benzodiazepines.

### For parenteral dosage forms only
Following administration of parenteral dosage forms, patients should be kept under observation for a period of 3 to 8 hours or longer, based on the patient's clinical response and rate of recovery.

Too rapid intravenous administration may result in apnea, hypotension, bradycardia, or cardiac or respiratory arrest.

Inadvertent intra-arterial injection of benzodiazepines may produce arteriospasm, resulting in gangrene.

**When parenteral benzodiazepines are to be administered intravenously, equipment necessary to support respiration should be immediately available and a patent airway should be maintained.** This may be especially important in the elderly and in children.

### For treatment of dependence
Some clinicians substitute a long-acting benzodiazepine for short-acting agents before withdrawal is attempted.

Benzodiazepines should be tapered gradually, since there is some evidence that some withdrawal symptoms may be lessened in severity or avoided by gradual dosage reduction. Withdrawal schedules ranging from 4 to 16 weeks are usually suggested; however, some practitioners believe withdrawal should be completed within 2 weeks, thus exposing patients to withdrawal symptoms for a shorter length of time.

When necessary, the benzodiazepine may be reinstituted or another benzodiazepine may be substituted, at doses sufficient to suppress withdrawal symptoms, until restabilization allows continuance of the dosage taper, possibly at a slower rate.

---

# ALPRAZOLAM

## Summary of Differences
Category:
- In addition to being indicated as an antianxiety agent, indicated as an antipanic agent and used as an antitremor agent.

Indications:
- Also indicated for adjunctive management of anxiety associated with mental depression.

Pharmacology/pharmacokinetics:
- Short to intermediate half-life benzodiazepine.
- Accumulation is minimal during repeated dosing.
- Steady-state plasma concentration usually attained within a few (2 to 3) days.
- Elimination rapid following discontinuation of therapy.

Precautions:
- Drug interactions and/or related problems—Elevation of steady-state plasma concentrations of imipramine and desipramine reported with concurrent use of alprazolam.
- Medical considerations/contraindications—Episodes of hypomania and mania reported with use of alprazolam in patients with mental depression; deaths shortly after alprazolam therapy initiation reported rarely in patients with severe pulmonary disease.

## Additional Dosing Information
See also *General Dosing Information*.

Dosage should be reduced gradually when therapy is discontinued or the daily dosage is decreased. It is suggested that the daily dosage be decreased by no more than 500 mcg (0.5 mg) every 3 days. However, some patients may need a slower reduction in dosage.

The occurrence of early morning anxiety or the emergence of anxiety symptoms between doses of alprazolam in panic disorder patients may reflect the development of tolerance, or a time interval between doses that exceeds the duration of clinical action of the administered dose. The manufacturer states that when these effects occur, the prescribed dose is presumed to be insufficient to maintain plasma levels above those needed to prevent relapse, rebound, or withdrawal symptoms over the course of the interdosing interval; they recommend that the same total daily dose be administered in more frequently divided doses.

## Oral Dosage Forms

### ALPRAZOLAM ORAL SOLUTION

#### Usual adult dose
Antianxiety agent—
Oral, initially 250 to 500 mcg (0.25 to 0.5 mg) three times a day, the dosage being titrated to the needs of the patient up to a maximum total dose of 4 mg per day.

Note: Debilitated patients—Oral, initially 250 mcg (0.25 mg) two or three times a day, the dosage being increased as needed and tolerated.

The starting dosage may be decreased if adverse effects occur.

Antipanic agent—
Oral, initially 500 mcg (0.5 mg) three times a day, the dosage being increased as needed and tolerated up to a maximum of 10 mg per day.

#### Usual pediatric dose
Antianxiety or antipanic agent—
Children younger than 18 years of age: Safety and efficacy have not been established.

#### Usual geriatric dose
Antianxiety agent—
Oral, initially 250 mcg (0.25 mg) two or three times a day, the dosage being increased as needed and tolerated.

#### Strength(s) usually available
U.S.—
0.1 mg per mL (Rx) [GENERIC].
1 mg per mL (Rx) [*Alprazolam Intensol*].

Canada—
Not commercially available.

#### Packaging and storage
Store between 15 and 30 °C (59 and 86 °F), unless otherwise specified by manufacturer. Store in a tight, light-resistant container.

#### Preparation of dosage form
For concentrated oral solution (1 mg per mL)—Measure dose with calibrated dropper provided with product. It is recommended that each dose be gently stirred into liquid or semi-solid food, such as water, soda or

soda-like beverage, applesauce, or pudding, immediately before taking. Entire mixture should be consumed; no mixture should be stored for later use.

**Auxiliary labeling**
- Avoid alcoholic beverages.
- May cause drowsiness.

**Note**
Patient or caregiver should be instructed in proper measurement and, for concentrated oral solution (1 mg per mL), preparation of dose.
Controlled substance in the U.S.

### ALPRAZOLAM TABLETS USP

**Usual adult dose**
See *Alprazolam Oral Solution*.

**Usual pediatric dose**
See *Alprazolam Oral Solution*.

**Usual geriatric dose**
See *Alprazolam Oral Solution*.

**Strength(s) usually available**
U.S.—
- 0.25 mg (Rx) [*Xanax* (scored; lactose; sodium benzoate); GENERIC (may be scored)].
- 0.5 mg (Rx) [*Xanax* (scored; docusate sodium; lactose; sodium benzoate); GENERIC (may be scored)].
- 1 mg (Rx) [*Xanax* (scored; docusate sodium; lactose; sodium benzoate); GENERIC (may be scored)].
- 2 mg (Rx) [*Xanax* (multi-scored; docusate sodium; lactose; sodium benzoate); GENERIC].

Note: The multi-scored 2-mg tablet can be broken to provide doses of 0.5 or 1 mg.

Canada—
- 0.25 mg (Rx) [*Alti-Alprazolam* (scored; lactose); *Apo-Alpraz* (scored; sodium < 0.14 mg); *Gen-Alprazolam* (lactose); *Novo-Alprazol*; *Nu-Alpraz* (scored; sodium < 0.14 mg); *Xanax* (scored; lactose)].
- 0.5 mg (Rx) [*Alti-Alprazolam* (scored; lactose); *Apo-Alpraz* (scored; sodium < 0.14 mg); *Gen-Alprazolam* (lactose); *Novo-Alprazol*; *Nu-Alpraz* (scored; sodium < 0.14 mg); *Xanax* (scored; lactose)].
- 1 mg (Rx) [*Gen-Alprazolam* (lactose); *Xanax* (scored; lactose)].
- 2 mg (Rx) [*Gen-Alprazolam* (lactose); *Xanax TS* (triscored; lactose)].

Note: The triscored 2-mg tablet can be broken into four equal parts of 0.5 mg each.

**Packaging and storage**
Store between 15 and 30 °C (59 and 86 °F), unless otherwise specified by manufacturer. Store in a tight, light-resistant container.

**Auxiliary labeling**
- Avoid alcoholic beverages.
- May cause drowsiness.

**Note**
Controlled substance in the U.S.

---

### BROMAZEPAM

## Summary of Differences
Category:
  Indicated only as an antianxiety agent.
Pharmacology/pharmacokinetics:
  Short to intermediate half-life benzodiazepine.
  Accumulation is minimal during repeated dosing.
  Steady-state plasma concentration usually attained within a few (2 to 3) days.
  Elimination rapid following discontinuation of therapy.

## Oral Dosage Forms

### BROMAZEPAM TABLETS

**Usual adult dose**
Antianxiety agent—
  Oral, 6 to 30 mg per day in divided doses.
Note: Dosages of up to 60 mg may be used in severe cases.
  Debilitated patients—Initial daily dosage should not exceed 3 mg in divided doses, the dosage being carefully adjusted as needed and tolerated.

**Usual pediatric dose**
Antianxiety agent—
  Children younger than 18 years of age: Safety and efficacy have not been established.

**Usual geriatric dose**
Antianxiety agent—
  Oral, initially up to 3 mg, the dosage being carefully adjusted as needed and tolerated.

**Strength(s) usually available**
U.S.—
  Not commercially available.
Canada—
- 1.5 mg (Rx) [*Alti-Bromazepam* (scored; lactose); *Gen-Bromazepam* (scored; lactose); *Lectopam* (scored; lactose 96 mg)].
- 3 mg (Rx) [*Alti-Bromazepam* (scored; lactose); *Gen-Bromazepam* (scored; lactose); *Lectopam* (scored; lactose 94 mg)].
- 6 mg (Rx) [*Alti-Bromazepam* (scored; lactose); *Gen-Bromazepam* (scored; lactose); *Lectopam* (scored; lactose 91 mg)].

**Packaging and storage**
Store below 40 °C (104 °F), preferably between 15 and 30 °C (59 and 86 °F), in a well-closed container, unless otherwise specified by manufacturer.

**Auxiliary labeling**
- Avoid alcoholic beverages.
- May cause drowsiness.

---

### CHLORDIAZEPOXIDE

## Summary of Differences
Category:
  In addition to being indicated as an antianxiety agent and a sedative-hypnotic, oral chlordiazepoxide is used as an antitremor agent and parenteral chlordiazepoxide is used as an antipanic agent.
Indications:
  Also indicated for relief of acute alcohol withdrawal symptoms and as a preoperative medication.
  Also used in treatment of tension headache.
Pharmacology/pharmacokinetics:
  Absorption of intramuscular chlordiazepoxide may be slow and erratic.
  Long half-life benzodiazepine.
  Accumulation of chlordiazepoxide and its active metabolites is significant during repeated dosing.
  Steady-state plasma concentration usually attained in 5 days to 2 weeks.
  Elimination slow since metabolites remain in blood for several days or even weeks.
Precautions:
  Drug interactions and/or related problems—
    Antacids may delay the rate of but not reduce the extent of absorption of chlordiazepoxide.
  Medical considerations/contraindications—
    Hypoalbuminemia may predispose patient to an increased incidence of sedative side effects.
    Porphyria may be exacerbated by use of chlordiazepoxide.
Side/adverse effects:
  Intravenous chlordiazepoxide less likely to cause phlebitis or venous thrombosis than diazepam or lorazepam.

## Additional Dosing Information
See also *General Dosing Information*.

**For parenteral dosage forms only**
Intramuscular injections should be administered deeply into the muscle; absorption may be slow and erratic, but effects are usually seen in 15 to 30 minutes.
When more rapid effect is mandatory, chlordiazepoxide hydrochloride solution prepared with sterile physiological saline (0.9% sodium chloride injection) or sterile water for injection may be administered intravenously.
Intravenous administration of the intramuscular preparation is not recommended by the manufacturer because of the air bubbles that may form when the intramuscular diluent is added to the chlordiazepoxide hydrochloride powder.
Intravenous injections should be administered slowly over a 1-minute period.
The chlordiazepoxide hydrochloride solution prepared with sterile physiological saline (0.9% sodium chloride injection) or sterile water for injection should not be administered intramuscularly because of pain on injection.

## Oral Dosage Forms

### CHLORDIAZEPOXIDE HYDROCHLORIDE CAPSULES USP

**Usual adult dose**
Antianxiety agent—
  Oral, 5 to 25 mg three or four times a day.
  Note: Debilitated patients—Oral, 5 mg two to four times a day, the dosage being increased gradually as needed and tolerated.
Sedative-hypnotic—
  Alcohol withdrawal: Oral, initially 50 to 100 mg, repeated as needed, up to 400 mg per day, the dosage then reduced to maintenance levels.

**Usual pediatric dose**
Antianxiety agent—
  Children younger than 6 years of age: Safety and efficacy have not been established.
  Children 6 years of age and older: Oral, 5 mg two to four times a day, the dosage being increased, if necessary, to 10 mg two or three times a day.

**Usual geriatric dose**
Antianxiety agent—
  Oral, 5 mg two to four times a day, the dosage being increased gradually as needed and tolerated.

**Strength(s) usually available**
U.S.—
  5 mg (Rx) [*Librium* (lactose; Gelatin capsule shells may contain methyl and propyl parabens and potassium sorbate); GENERIC].
  10 mg (Rx) [*Librium* (lactose; Gelatin capsule shells may contain methyl and propyl parabens and potassium sorbate); GENERIC].
  25 mg (Rx) [*Librium* (lactose; Gelatin capsule shells may contain methyl and propyl parabens and potassium sorbate); GENERIC].
Canada—
  5 mg (Rx) [*Apo-Chlordiazepoxide; Novo-Poxide* (lactose)].
  10 mg (Rx) [*Apo-Chlordiazepoxide; Novo-Poxide* (lactose)].
  25 mg (Rx) [*Apo-Chlordiazepoxide; Novo-Poxide* (lactose)].

**Packaging and storage**
Store below 40 °C (104 °F), preferably between 15 and 30 °C (59 and 86 °F), unless otherwise specified by manufacturer. Store in a tight, light-resistant container.

**Auxiliary labeling**
- Avoid alcoholic beverages.
- May cause drowsiness.

**Note**
Controlled substance in the U.S.

## Parenteral Dosage Forms

Note: Bracketed uses in the *Dosage Forms* section refer to categories of use and/or indications that are not included in U.S. product labeling.

### CHLORDIAZEPOXIDE HYDROCHLORIDE FOR INJECTION USP

**Usual adult dose**
Antianxiety agent—
  Intramuscular or intravenous, initially 50 to 100 mg, then 25 to 50 mg three or four times a day, if necessary.
  Preoperative: Intramuscular, 50 to 100 mg one hour prior to surgery.
Sedative-hypnotic—
  Alcohol withdrawal: Intramuscular or intravenous, initially 50 to 100 mg, repeated in two to four hours, if necessary.
[Antipanic agent]—
  Intramuscular or intravenous, initially 50 to 100 mg, repeated in four to six hours if necessary.
  Note: Debilitated patients—Intramuscular or intravenous, 25 to 50 mg per dose.

**Usual adult prescribing limits**
300 mg per day.

**Usual pediatric dose**
Antianxiety agent or
Sedative-hypnotic—
  Children younger than 12 years of age: Safety and efficacy have not been established.
  Children 12 years of age and older: Intramuscular or intravenous, 25 to 50 mg per dose.

**Usual geriatric dose**
Antianxiety agent or
Sedative-hypnotic—
  Intramuscular or intravenous, 25 to 50 mg per dose.

**Size(s) usually available**
U.S.—
  100 mg, with 2 mL of special intramuscular diluent (Rx) [*Librium* (benzyl alcohol 1.5%; polysorbate 80 4%; propylene glycol 20%; maleic acid 1.6%; sodium hydroxide)].
Canada—
  Not commercially available.

**Packaging and storage**
Prior to reconstitution, store below 40 °C (104 °F), preferably between 15 and 30 °C (59 and 86 °F), unless otherwise specified by manufacturer. Protect from light.
Note: Chlordiazepoxide injectable diluent should be stored between 2 and 8 °C (36 and 46 °F).

**Preparation of dosage form**
Solutions of chlordiazepoxide hydrochloride for intramuscular or intravenous use should be prepared immediately before administration.
To prepare solution for intramuscular use, add 2 mL of the special intramuscular diluent (supplied by manufacturer) to the ampul containing 100 mg of chlordiazepoxide hydrochloride. The diluent solution should not be used if it is opalescent or hazy. The diluent should be added carefully to the ampul of powder to avoid bubble formation. Agitate the ampul gently until the powder is completely dissolved.
  Caution—Use of diluents containing benzyl alcohol is not recommended for preparation of medications for use in neonates (first 30 days of postnatal life). A fatal toxic syndrome consisting of metabolic acidosis, CNS depression, respiratory problems, renal failure, hypotension, and possibly seizures and intracranial hemorrhages has been associated with this use.
To prepare solution for intravenous use, add 5 mL of 0.9% sodium chloride injection or sterile water for injection to the ampul containing 100 mg of chlordiazepoxide hydrochloride. Agitate the ampul gently until the powder is completely dissolved.

**Stability**
If the diluent is stored at room temperature, it will remain stable for 18 to 20 months rather than until the expiration date, which reflects a stability period of 36 months. As the diluent alters, it develops slight opalescence; do not use if opalescent. Stability of diluent will not be affected by 2 to 4 weeks at room temperature.
After reconstitution, solution should be used immediately.
Any unused portion of the solution should be discarded.
Sterilization by heating should not be done.

**Note**
Controlled substance in the U.S.

---

### CLOBAZAM

## Summary of Differences

Category:
  Indicated as an anticonvulsant only.
Pharmacology/pharmacokinetics:
  Intermediate half-life benzodiazepine.

## Additional Dosing Information

See also *General Dosing Information*.

Daily dosages of up to 30 mg may be taken as a single dose at bedtime. If the daily dosage is divided, the larger portion should be taken at bedtime.

There have been reports of development of tolerance to the anticonvulsant effects of clobazam with continuous, long-term use. There are insufficient data to predict which patients will develop tolerance or when this might occur. Some studies in catamenial epilepsy have indicated that efficacy may be maintained with intermittent use. However, long-term results from intermittent-use studies are not available.

## Oral Dosage Forms

### CLOBAZAM TABLETS

**Usual adult dose**
Anticonvulsant—
  Oral, initially 5 to 15 mg per day. Dosage may be increased gradually as needed.
Note: Dosage should be reduced in patients with impaired hepatic or renal function.

**Usual adult prescribing limits**
80 mg per day.

**Usual pediatric dose**
Anticonvulsant—
  Children younger than 2 years of age: Oral, initially 0.5 to 1 mg per kg of body weight per day.
  Children 2 to 16 years of age: Oral, initially 5 mg per day. Dosage may be increased at five-day intervals.

**Usual pediatric prescribing limits**
Children 2 to 16 years of age—40 mg per day.

**Strength(s) usually available**
U.S.—
  Not commercially available.
Canada—
  10 mg (Rx) [*Frisium* (scored; lactose)].

**Packaging and storage**
Store in original container at room temperature, below 25 °C (77 °F), unless otherwise specified by manufacturer.

**Auxiliary labeling**
• May cause drowsiness or dizziness.
• Avoid alcoholic beverages.

---

## CLONAZEPAM

## Summary of Differences
Category:
  In addition to being indicated as an anticonvulsant, indicated as an antipanic agent.
Pharmacology/pharmacokinetics:
  Intermediate half-life benzodiazepine.
Precautions:
  Pregnancy—
    Increased incidence of congenital abnormalities in children whose mothers used anticonvulsants during pregnancy; studies in animals have shown that clonazepam causes a non–dose-related increased incidence of cleft palates, open eyelids, fused sternebrae, and limb defects; withdrawal of clonazepam prior to or during pregnancy should be considered only when seizures are mild and infrequent in absence of medication and the possibility of status epilepticus and withdrawal symptoms is considered low.
  Pediatrics—
    It is possible that long-term use of clonazepam may result in adverse effects on physical or mental development that may not become apparent for many years.
  Medical considerations/contraindications—
    Initiation or abrupt withdrawal of clonazepam in patients with epilepsy or a history of seizures may precipitate seizures or status epilepticus.
    Caution should be used in surgical or non-ambulatory patients because of cough suppressant effects of clonazepam.

## Additional Dosing Information
See also *General Dosing Information*.

In some studies, up to 30% of patients have shown loss of anticonvulsant activity after a few (often within 3) months of therapy; dosage adjustment may restore efficacy of clonazepam.

In order to maintain seizure control when clonazepam is used to replace other anticonvulsant therapy, the dosage of clonazepam should be increased gradually while the dosage of the other medication is decreased gradually; when clonazepam is used to supplement other anticonvulsant therapy, the dosage of clonazepam should be increased gradually until seizure activity is controlled adequately and then the dosage of the other medication may be decreased gradually if necessary.

Also, clonazepam should be withdrawn gradually, especially in patients being treated for epilepsy and in patients who have received long-term, high-dose therapy, since abrupt withdrawal may precipitate seizures or status epilepticus. During withdrawal of clonazepam, the simultaneous administration of another anticonvulsant may be indicated in patients with epilepsy. The manufacturer recommends clonazepam dosage be decreased by 0.125 mg two times a day every 3 days.

## Oral Dosage Forms
### CLONAZEPAM TABLETS USP
**Usual adult dose**
Anticonvulsant—
  Oral, initially up to 500 mcg (0.5 mg) three times a day; the dosage may be increased in increments of 500 to 1000 mcg (0.5 to 1 mg) every three days until seizures are controlled or until side effects prevent any further increase.
Note: Maintenance dose must be individualized, depending on patient's response.
Antipanic agent[1]—
  Oral, initially 250 mcg (0.25 mg) two times a day, the dosage being increased to 1000 mcg (1 mg) per day after three days in most patients. The dosage may be increased in increments of 125 to 250 mcg (0.125 to 0.25 mg) two times a day every three days until panic disorder is controlled or until side effects prevent further dosage increases. One dose may be taken at bedtime to minimize daytime somnolence.
Note: A fixed dose study comparing dosages of 1, 2, 3, and 4 mg per day in the treatment of panic disorder found that a dosage of 1000 mcg (1 mg) per day was the most effective and best tolerated dosage for most patients.

**Usual adult prescribing limits**
Anticonvulsant—
  20 mg per day.
Antipanic agent[1]—
  4 mg per day.

**Usual pediatric dose**
Anticonvulsant—
  Infants and children younger than 10 years of age or less than 30 kg of body weight: Oral, initially 10 to 30 mcg (0.01 to 0.03 mg), not to exceed 50 mcg (0.05 mg), per kg of body weight per day in two or three divided doses, the dosage being increased by no more than 250 to 500 mcg (0.25 to 0.5 mg) every third day until a maintenance dose of 100 to 200 mcg (0.1 to 0.2 mg) per kg of body weight per day is reached or until seizures are controlled or side effects prevent a further increase.
Note: The daily dose should be divided into three equal doses, if possible. If doses are not divided equally, the largest dose should be given at bedtime.
Antipanic agent[1]—
  Safety and efficacy have not been established in children up to 18 years of age.

**Strength(s) usually available**
U.S.—
  0.5 mg (Rx) [*Klonopin* (scored; lactose); GENERIC (may be scored)].
  1 mg (Rx) [*Klonopin* (lactose); GENERIC (may be scored)].
  2 mg (Rx) [*Klonopin* (lactose); GENERIC (may be scored)].
Canada—
  0.25 mg (Rx) [*PMS-Clonazepam* (lactose)].
  0.5 mg (Rx) [*Alti-Clonazepam* (scored; lactose); *Apo-Clonazepam* (scored); *Clonapam* (scored; lactose); *Gen-Clonazepam*; *PMS-Clonazepam* (scored; lactose); *Rivotril* (scored; lactose 122 mg)].
  1 mg (Rx) [*Clonapam* (scored; lactose); *PMS-Clonazepam* (lactose)].
  2 mg (Rx) [*Alti-Clonazepam* (cross-scored; lactose); *Apo-Clonazepam* (scored); *Clonapam* (scored; lactose); *Gen-Clonazepam*; *PMS-Clonazepam* (lactose); *Rivotril* (scored; lactose 122 mg)].

**Packaging and storage**
Store between 15 and 30 °C (59 and 86 °F). Store in a tight, light-resistant container.

**Auxiliary labeling**
• Avoid alcoholic beverages.
• May cause drowsiness.

**Note**
Controlled substance in the U.S.

---
[1]Not included in Canadian product labeling.

---

## CLORAZEPATE

## Summary of Differences
Category:
  In addition to being indicated as an antianxiety agent and a sedative-hypnotic, indicated as an anticonvulsant.

## Benzodiazepines (Systemic)

Indications:
  Also indicated for relief of acute alcohol withdrawal symptoms.
Pharmacology/pharmacokinetics:
  Drug precursor; metabolized to desmethyldiazepam before absorption.
  Orally, one of most rapidly absorbed benzodiazepines.
  Long half-life benzodiazepine.
  Accumulation of active metabolites is significant during repeated dosing.
  Steady-state plasma concentration usually attained in 5 days to 2 weeks.
  Elimination slow since metabolites remain in blood for several days or even weeks.
Precautions:
  Drug interactions and/or related problems—
    Antacids may decrease rate of conversion to desmethyldiazepam but do not affect degree of absorption.

## Additional Dosing Information

See also *General Dosing Information*.

When used for alcohol withdrawal, excessive reductions in the total amount of medication administered on successive days should be avoided.

## Oral Dosage Forms

### CLORAZEPATE DIPOTASSIUM CAPSULES

**Usual adult and adolescent dose**
Antianxiety agent—
  Oral, 7.5 to 15 mg two to four times a day; or 15 mg initially, as a single dose at bedtime, the dosage being adjusted as needed and tolerated.
  Note: Debilitated patients—Oral, initially, 3.75 to 15 mg per day, the dosage being increased gradually as needed and tolerated.
Sedative-hypnotic—
  Alcohol withdrawal: Oral, 30 mg initially, followed by 15 mg two to four times a day the first day; 15 mg three to six times a day the second day; 7.5 to 15 mg three times a day the third day; 7.5 mg two to four times a day the fourth day; and thereafter, 3.75 mg two to four times a day. Discontinue when patient's condition is stable.
Anticonvulsant[1]—
  Oral, initially up to 7.5 mg three times a day, the dosage being increased by no more than 7.5 mg per week, not to exceed 90 mg per day.

**Usual adult prescribing limits**
90 mg per day.

**Usual pediatric dose**
Children younger than 9 years of age: Safety and efficacy have not been established.
Anticonvulsant[1]—
  Children 9 to 12 years of age: Oral, initially up to 7.5 mg two times a day, the dosage being increased by no more than 7.5 mg per week, not to exceed 60 mg per day.
  Children 12 years of age and older: See *Usual adult and adolescent dose*.

**Usual geriatric dose**
Antianxiety agent—
  Oral, initially, 3.75 to 15 mg per day, the dosage being increased gradually as needed and tolerated.

**Strength(s) usually available**
U.S.—
  Not commercially available.
Canada—
  3.75 mg (Rx) [*Apo-Clorazepate; Novo-Clopate; Tranxene*].
  7.5 mg (Rx) [*Apo-Clorazepate; Novo-Clopate; Tranxene*].
  15 mg (Rx) [*Apo-Clorazepate; Novo-Clopate*].

**Packaging and storage**
Store below 40 °C (104 °F), preferably between 15 and 30 °C (59 and 86 °F), in a tight, light-resistant container, unless otherwise specified by manufacturer.

**Auxiliary labeling**
• Avoid alcoholic beverages.
• May cause drowsiness.

### CLORAZEPATE DIPOTASSIUM TABLETS USP

**Usual adult and adolescent dose**
See *Clorazepate Dipotassium Capsules*.

**Usual adult prescribing limits**
See *Clorazepate Dipotassium Capsules*.

**Usual pediatric dose**
See *Clorazepate Dipotassium Capsules*.

**Usual geriatric dose**
See *Clorazepate Dipotassium Capsules*.

**Strength(s) usually available**
U.S.—
  3.75 mg (Rx) [*Tranxene T-Tab* (scored); GENERIC (may be scored)].
  7.5 mg (Rx) [*Tranxene T-Tab* (scored); GENERIC (may be scored)].
  15 mg (Rx) [*Tranxene T-Tab* (scored); GENERIC (may be scored)].
Canada—
  Not commercially available.

**Packaging and storage**
Store between 15 and 30 °C (59 and 86 °F), in a tight, light-resistant container, unless otherwise specified by manufacturer.

**Stability**
Clorazepate dipotassium degrades in the presence of moisture. One of the degradation products is carbon dioxide gas, which tends to cause the tablets to "blow apart" and disintegrate very rapidly. The drug is also sensitive to heat and light. Pharmacists are advised to retain the desiccant when opening a new stock bottle of the product. If it is necessary to repackage the drug into unit doses, it is recommended that pharmacists be certain that the packaging materials used for unit-dose containers will produce a Class A package as defined in the USP. Multiple-dose containers should meet USP "tight" and "light-resistant" specifications. Pharmacists should consider using desiccant packets when dispensing a large number of tablets in a multiple-dose container. If shipping or mailing prescriptions, pharmacists should take into account these instability problems. Patients should be warned not to expose the product to moisture, light, or heat, and, when possible, to keep the tablets in the original containers.

**Auxiliary labeling**
• Avoid alcoholic beverages.
• May cause drowsiness.

**Note**
Controlled substance in the U.S.

### CLORAZEPATE DIPOTASSIUM EXTENDED-RELEASE TABLETS

**Usual adult and adolescent dose**
Not intended for initiation of therapy. Single daily dose of 11.25 mg may be substituted for prompt-release dosage forms in patients already stabilized on a dosage of 3.75 mg three times a day. Single daily dose of 22.5 mg may be substituted for prompt-release dosage forms in patients already stabilized on a dosage of 7.5 mg three times a day.

**Usual pediatric dose**
Children younger than 9 years of age—Safety and efficacy have not been established.
Children 9 to 12 years of age—See *Usual adult and adolescent dose*.

**Usual geriatric dose**
See *Usual adult and adolescent dose*.

**Strength(s) usually available**
U.S.—
  11.25 mg (Rx) [*Tranxene-SD Half Strength* (lactose; potassium carbonate; potassium chloride; castor oil wax; magnesium stearate; magnesium oxide; talc; FD&C Blue #2)].
  22.5 mg (Rx) [*Tranxene-SD* (iron oxide; lactose; potassium carbonate; potassium chloride; castor oil wax; magnesium stearate; magnesium oxide; talc)].
Canada—
  Not commercially available.

**Packaging and storage**
Store between 15 and 30 °C (59 and 86 °F), in a tight, light-resistant container, unless otherwise specified by manufacturer.

**Stability**
Clorazepate dipotassium degrades in the presence of moisture. One of the degradation products is carbon dioxide gas, which tends to cause the tablets to "blow apart" and disintegrate very rapidly. The drug is also sensitive to heat and light. Pharmacists are advised to retain the desiccant when opening a new stock bottle of the product. If it is necessary to repackage the drug into unit doses, it is recommended that pharmacists be certain that the packaging materials used for unit-dose containers will produce a Class A package as defined in the USP. Multiple-dose containers should meet USP "tight" and "light-resistant" specifications. Pharmacists should consider using desiccant packets when dispensing a large number of tablets in a multiple-dose container. If shipping or mailing prescriptions, pharmacists should take into account these instability problems. Patients should be warned not to expose the product to moisture, light, or heat, and, when possible, to keep the tablets in the original containers.

**Auxiliary labeling**
- Avoid alcoholic beverages.
- May cause drowsiness.
- Swallow tablets whole.

**Note**

Clorazepate dipotassium extended-release tablets are not intended to be used to initiate therapy, but to provide ease of dosing in patients who are already stabilized on clorazepate dipotassium at a dosage that allows direct substitution of the extended-release tablet for the prompt-release dosage forms.

Controlled substance in the U.S.

[1]Not included in Canadian product labeling.

---

## DIAZEPAM

## Summary of Differences

Category:
  In addition to being indicated as an antianxiety agent and a sedative-hypnotic, indicated as an anticonvulsant and a skeletal muscle relaxant adjunct and used as an antipanic agent.
  Parenteral diazepam also indicated as an amnestic.
  Oral diazepam also used as an antitremor agent.
Indications:
  Also indicated for relief of acute alcohol withdrawal symptoms, for the treatment of status epilepticus, and as a preoperative medication.
  Parenteral diazepam also indicated as an adjunct prior to endoscopic procedures; indicated prior to cardioversion; and used in dentistry to produce conscious sedation.
  Also used to relieve spasms of facial muscles associated with problems of occlusion and temporomandibular joint disorders, and for the treatment of tension headache.
Pharmacology/pharmacokinetics:
  Orally, the most rapidly absorbed benzodiazepine.
  Absorption of intramuscular diazepam may be slow and erratic, depending upon administration site; usually rapid and complete when injected into the deltoid muscle.
  Absorption of rectal diazepam gel or solution is rapid.
  Long half-life benzodiazepine.
  Accumulation of diazepam and its active metabolites is significant during repeated dosing.
  Steady-state plasma concentration usually attained in 5 days to 2 weeks.
  Elimination slow since metabolites remain in blood for several days or even weeks.
Precautions:
  Sensitivity—
    Sterile emulsion dosage form contains soybean oil.
  Pregnancy—
    Administration (especially intramuscular or intravenous) in doses of more than 30 mg within 15 hours before delivery may cause apnea, hypotonia, hypothermia, a reluctance to feed, and impaired metabolic response to cold stress in the neonate.
  Drug interactions and/or related problems—
    Antacids may delay but not reduce the absorption of diazepam.
    Premedication with diazepam may decrease dose of a fentanyl derivative required for induction of anesthesia and decrease time to loss of consciousness with induction doses.
    Diazepam in parenteral dosage forms adheres to plastic infusion tubing.
    Isoniazid may inhibit elimination of diazepam, resulting in increased plasma concentrations.
    Rifampin may enhance elimination of diazepam, resulting in decreased plasma concentrations.
  Medical considerations/contraindications—
    Initiation or abrupt withdrawal of diazepam in patients with epilepsy or a history of seizures may precipitate seizures or status epilepticus. Use of intravenous diazepam for absence status or Lennox-Gastaut syndrome status may precipitate tonic status epilepticus.
    Hypoalbuminemia may predispose patient to increased incidence of sedative side effects.
Side/adverse effects:
  Intravenous diazepam more likely to cause phlebitis or venous thrombosis than chlordiazepoxide or lorazepam.

## Additional Dosing Information

See also *General Dosing Information*.

**For oral dosage forms only**
When diazepam is used as an adjunct in treating convulsive disorders, the possibility of an increase in the frequency and/or severity of generalized tonic-clonic (grand mal) seizures may require an increase in dosage of standard anticonvulsant medication. Also, abrupt withdrawal of diazepam may result in a temporary increase in the frequency and/or severity of seizures.

**For parenteral dosage forms only**
Intravenous administration of diazepam is usually preferred, since absorption may be slow and erratic following intramuscular administration depending upon site of injection.
If intramuscular injections of diazepam are used, they should be administered deeply into the deltoid muscle.
For intravenous injections of diazepam, small veins such as those on the back of the hand or wrist should not be used and care should be taken to avoid intra-arterial administration or extravasation in order to reduce the possibility of venous thrombosis, phlebitis, local irritation, swelling, and, rarely, vascular impairment.
For intravenous injections, the medication should be injected slowly into a large vein, taking at least 1 minute for each 5 mg (1 mL) of medication given, due to the risk of thrombophlebitis.
When subsequent doses are administered within 1 to 4 hours, consideration should be given to the possibility that active metabolites may still be present from the initial dose.
Continuous intravenous infusion of diazepam is not recommended because of the possibility of precipitation of diazepam in intravenous fluids and adsorption of the medication to the plastic of infusion bags and tubing.
If diazepam cannot be administered by direct intravenous injection, it may be injected slowly through an infusion tubing as close as possible to the insertion point to minimize adsorption of the medication to the plastic tubing.
When intravenous diazepam is used to control seizures, a significant proportion of patients will return to seizure activity and will require additional doses.
When parenteral diazepam is used for peroral endoscopic procedures, the use of a topical anesthetic and availability of necessary countermeasures are recommended since these procedures may cause an increase in cough reflex and laryngospasm.

**For rectal gel dosage form only**
Diazepam rectal gel should be administered only by caregivers who are able to distinguish the distinct cluster of seizures to be treated, or the events accompanying their onset, from the patient's usual seizure activity, and who understand which seizure manifestations may or may not be treated with diazepam rectal gel. The caregiver also must be competent in the proper administration of the rectal gel and in monitoring the patient's response, including recognizing when professional medical attention is required.
Caregivers should be instructed to notify the physician immediately of any signs that are not typical of the patient's characteristic seizure episode.

## Oral Dosage Forms

### DIAZEPAM ORAL SOLUTION

**Usual adult dose**
Antianxiety agent—
  Oral, 2 to 10 mg two to four times a day.
Sedative-hypnotic—
  Alcohol withdrawal: Oral, 10 mg three or four times during the first twenty-four hours, the dosage being decreased to 5 mg three or four times a day as needed.
Anticonvulsant—
  Oral, 2 to 10 mg two to four times a day.
Skeletal muscle relaxant adjunct—
  Oral, 2 to 10 mg three or four times a day.
Note: Debilitated patients—Oral, 2 to 2.5 mg one or two times a day, the dosage being increased gradually as needed and tolerated.

**Usual pediatric dose**
Antianxiety agent or
Anticonvulsant or
Skeletal muscle relaxant adjunct—
  Children younger than 6 months of age: Use is not recommended.
  Children 6 months of age and older: Oral, 1 to 2.5 mg, 40 to 200 mcg (0.04 to 0.2 mg) per kg of body weight, or 1.17 to 6 mg per square meter of body surface, three or four times a day, the dosage being increased gradually as needed and tolerated.

**Usual geriatric dose**
Antianxiety agent or
Sedative-hypnotic or
Anticonvulsant or
Skeletal muscle relaxant adjunct—
  Oral, 2 to 2.5 mg one or two times a day, the dosage being increased gradually as needed and tolerated.

**Strength(s) usually available**
U.S.—
  5 mg per mL (Rx) [*Diazepam Intensol*].
  5 mg per 5 mL (Rx) [GENERIC].
Canada—
  1 mg per mL (Rx) [*PMS-Diazepam*].

**Packaging and storage**
Store below 40 °C (104 °F), preferably between 15 and 30 °C (59 and 86 °F), in a well-closed container, unless otherwise specified by manufacturer. Protect from freezing.

**Preparation of dosage form**
For concentrated oral solution (5 mg per mL)—Measure dose with calibrated dropper provided with product. It is recommended that each dose be mixed with liquid or soft food, such as water, juice, soda, pudding, or applesauce, immediately before taking. The entire mixture should be consumed; none of the mixture should be stored for later use.

**Auxiliary labeling**
- Avoid alcoholic beverages.
- May cause drowsiness.

**Note**
Patient or caregiver should be instructed in proper measurement of the dose and, for concentrated oral solution (5 mg per mL), preparation of the dose.

Controlled substance in the U.S.

## DIAZEPAM TABLETS USP

**Usual adult dose**
See *Diazepam Oral Solution*.

**Usual pediatric dose**
See *Diazepam Oral Solution*.

**Usual geriatric dose**
See *Diazepam Oral Solution*.

**Strength(s) usually available**
U.S.—
  2 mg (Rx) [*Valium* (scored); GENERIC].
  5 mg (Rx) [*Valium* (scored); GENERIC].
  10 mg (Rx) [*Valium* (scored); GENERIC].
Canada—
  2 mg (Rx) [*Apo-Diazepam* (scored); *Novo-Dipam* (scored); *Vivol* (double-scored; lactose; sodium < 1 mmol [trace])].
  5 mg (Rx) [*Apo-Diazepam* (scored); *Novo-Dipam* (scored); *Valium* (scored; lactose); *Vivol* (double-scored; lactose; sodium < 1 mmol [trace])].
  10 mg (Rx) [*Apo-Diazepam* (scored); *Novo-Dipam* (scored); *Valium* (scored; lactose 100 mg); *Vivol* (double-scored; lactose; sodium < 1 mmol [trace])].

**Packaging and storage**
Store below 40 °C (104 °F), preferably between 15 and 30 °C (59 and 86 °F), unless otherwise specified by manufacturer. Store in a tight, light-resistant container.

**Auxiliary labeling**
- Avoid alcoholic beverages.
- May cause drowsiness.

**Note**
Controlled substance in the U.S.

## Parenteral Dosage Forms

### DIAZEPAM INJECTION USP

**Usual adult dose**
Antianxiety agent—
  Preoperative medication: Dosage must be individualized; however, as a general guideline—Intramuscular or intravenous, 5 to 10 mg prior to surgery.
  Anxiety disorders or symptoms of anxiety: Intramuscular or intravenous, 2 to 10 mg (2 to 5 mg for moderate symptoms; 5 to 10 mg for severe symptoms), the dose being repeated in three or four hours, if necessary.

Sedative-hypnotic—
  Alcohol withdrawal: Intramuscular or intravenous, initially 10 mg, followed by 5 to 10 mg in three or four hours, if necessary.
Amnestic—
  Cardioversion:
    Intravenous, 5 to 15 mg five to ten minutes prior to the procedure.
  Endoscopic procedures:
    Intravenous (preferred route), up to 20 mg, the dosage being titrated to give the desired sedative response and administered immediately prior to the procedure.
    Intramuscular, 5 to 10 mg approximately thirty minutes prior to the procedure.
Anticonvulsant—
  Status epilepticus and severe recurrent convulsive seizures: Intravenous, initially 5 to 10 mg, the dose being repeated, if necessary, at ten- to fifteen-minute intervals up to a cumulative dose of 30 mg. If necessary, regimen may be repeated in two to four hours.
  Note: The intravenous route of administration is preferred; however, if intravenous administration is impossible, the intramuscular route of administration may be used.

  Some clinicians have used continuous intravenous infusions of diazepam in the treatment of selected patients with status epilepticus refractory to initial treatment. However, this method of administration is problematic due to inherent adsorption problems with plastic infusion bags and tubing.
Skeletal muscle relaxant adjunct—
  Muscle spasm: Intramuscular or intravenous, initially 5 to 10 mg, the dose being repeated in three or four hours, if necessary. For tetanus, larger doses may be required.
Note: Debilitated patients—Intramuscular or intravenous, initially 2 to 5 mg per dose, the dosage being increased gradually as needed and tolerated.

**Usual pediatric dose**
Neonates 30 days of age and younger: Safety and efficacy have not been established.
Anticonvulsant—
  Status epilepticus and severe recurrent convulsive seizures:
    Infants older than 30 days of age and children younger than 5 years of age—Intravenous (slow), 200 to 500 mcg (0.2 to 0.5 mg) every two to five minutes up to a cumulative dose of 5 mg. If necessary, regimen may be repeated in two to four hours.
    Children 5 years of age and older—Intravenous (slow), 1 mg every two to five minutes up to a cumulative dose of 10 mg. If necessary, regimen may be repeated in two to four hours.
  Note: The intravenous route of administration is preferred; however, if intravenous administration is impossible, the intramuscular route of administration may be used.
Skeletal muscle relaxant adjunct—
  Tetanus:
    Infants older than 30 days of age and children younger than 5 years of age—Intramuscular or intravenous, 1 to 2 mg, the dose being repeated every three or four hours as needed.
    Children 5 years of age and older—Intramuscular or intravenous, 5 to 10 mg, the dose being repeated every three or four hours as needed.
Note: In general, when the intravenous route is used in infants and children, it is recommended that the medication be administered slowly over a three-minute period in a dose not to exceed 250 mcg (0.25 mg) per kg of body weight. After an interval of fifteen to thirty minutes, the dose may be repeated. After an additional interval of fifteen to thirty minutes, the dose may be repeated a third time. If the third administration does not provide relief of symptoms, adjunctive treatment appropriate to the condition being treated should be considered.

  Caution—Medications containing benzyl alcohol are not recommended for use in neonates (first 30 days of postnatal life). A fatal toxic syndrome consisting of metabolic acidosis, CNS depression, respiratory problems, renal failure, hypotension, and possibly seizures and intracranial hemorrhages has been associated with this use.

**Usual geriatric dose**
Antianxiety agent or
Sedative-hypnotic or
Amnestic or
Anticonvulsant or
Skeletal muscle relaxant adjunct—
  Intramuscular or intravenous, initially 2 to 5 mg per dose, the dosage being increased gradually as needed and tolerated.

### Strength(s) usually available
U.S.—
  5 mg per mL (Rx) [*Valium* (benzoic acid; benzyl alcohol 1.5%; ethyl alcohol 10%; propylene glycol 40%; sodium benzoate 5%); GENERIC].
Canada—
  5 mg per mL (Rx) [*Valium* (benzyl alcohol 16 mg; ethyl alcohol 80 mg; propylene glycol 414 mg; sodium < 1 mmol; sodium benzoate; benzoic acid)].

### Packaging and storage
Store below 40 °C (104 °F), preferably between 15 and 30 °C (59 and 86 °F), unless otherwise specified by manufacturer. Protect from light. Protect from freezing.

### Stability
Do not mix or dilute this medication with other solutions, intravenous fluids, or medications, because the resulting admixtures are unstable.
Diazepam is adsorbed to the plastic of intravenous infusion bags and tubing.

### Incompatibilities
Diazepam injection is physically incompatible with aqueous solutions.

### Note
Controlled substance in the U.S.

## DIAZEPAM EMULSION STERILE

### Usual adult dose
Antianxiety agent—
  Preoperative medication: Dosage must be individualized; however, as a general guideline—Intramuscular or intravenous, 10 mg one to two hours prior to surgery.
  Anxiety disorders or symptoms of anxiety: Intramuscular or intravenous, 2 to 10 mg (2 to 5 mg for moderate symptoms; 5 to 10 mg for severe symptoms), the dose being repeated in three or four hours, if necessary.
Anticonvulsant[1]—
  Status epilepticus and severe recurrent convulsive seizures[1]: Intravenous, 5 to 10 mg, the dose being repeated at ten- to fifteen-minute intervals, if needed, up to a cumulative dose of 30 mg. Regimen may be repeated in two to four hours, if needed, keeping in mind the persistence of active metabolites in the circulation.
Sedative-hypnotic—
  Alcohol withdrawal: Intramuscular or intravenous, initially 10 mg, followed by 5 to 10 mg in three or four hours, if necessary.
Amnestic—
  Cardioversion: Intravenous, 5 to 15 mg ten to twenty minutes prior to the procedure.
  Endoscopic procedures: Intramuscular or intravenous, 5 to 10 mg about thirty minutes prior to procedure. Intravenous dose may be titrated to desired sedative response with slow administration immediately prior to the procedure; although ≤ 10 mg is generally adequate, up to 20 mg may be given, particularly when no concomitant narcotics are administered.
Skeletal muscle relaxant adjunct—
  Muscle spasm: Intramuscular or intravenous, initially 5 to 10 mg, the dose being repeated in three or four hours, if necessary. Larger doses may be required in tetanus.
Note: Debilitated patients and patients receiving other sedative medications—Intramuscular or intravenous, initially 2 to 5 mg per dose, the dosage being increased gradually as needed and tolerated.

### Usual pediatric dose
Antianxiety agent or
Amnestic—
  Neonates 30 days of age and younger: Safety and efficacy have not been established.
  Infants and children older than 30 days of age: Dosage must be individualized.
Anticonvulsant[1]—
  For status epilepticus and severe recurrent convulsive seizures[1]:
    Neonates 30 days of age and younger—Safety and efficacy have not been established.
    Infants older than 30 days of age and children younger than 5 years of age—Intravenous, 0.2 to 0.5 mg, administered slowly. May be repeated every two to five minutes, if needed, up to a cumulative dose of 5 mg. Regimen may be repeated in two to four hours, if needed, keeping in mind the persistence of active metabolites in the circulation.
    Children 5 years of age and older—Intravenous, 1 mg, administered slowly. May be repeated every two to five minutes, if needed, up to a cumulative dose of 10 mg. Regimen may be repeated in two to four hours, if needed, keeping in mind the persistence of active metabolites in the circulation.

Skeletal muscle relaxant adjunct—
  For tetanus[1]:
    Neonates 30 days of age and younger—Safety and efficacy have not been established.
    Infants older than 30 days of age and children younger than 5 years of age—Intravenous, 1 to 2 mg, administered slowly. May be repeated every three to four hours, if needed.
    Children 5 years of age and older—Intravenous, 5 to 10 mg, administered slowly. May be repeated every three to four hours, if needed.
Note: In general, when the intravenous route is used in infants and children, it is recommended that the medication be administered slowly over a three-minute period in a dose not to exceed 250 mcg (0.25 mg) per kg of body weight. After an interval of fifteen to thirty minutes, the dose may be repeated. After an additional interval of fifteen to thirty minutes, the dose may be repeated a third time. If the third administration does not provide relief of symptoms, adjunctive treatment appropriate to the condition being treated should be considered.

### Usual geriatric dose
Antianxiety agent or
Anticonvulsant[1] or
Sedative-hypnotic or
Amnestic or
Skeletal muscle relaxant adjunct—
  Intramuscular or intravenous, initially 2 to 5 mg per dose, the dosage being increased gradually as needed and tolerated.

### Strength(s) usually available
U.S.—
  5 mg per mL (Rx) [*Dizac* (fractionated soybean oil 150 mg/mL; deacetylated monoglycerides 50 mg/mL; fractionated egg yolk phospholipids 12 mg/mL; glycerin 22 mg/mL; water for injection; sodium hydroxide)].
Canada—
  5 mg per mL (Rx) [*Diazemuls* (acetylated monoglycerides 50 mg/mL; purified egg phospholipids 12 mg/mL; purified soybean oil 150 mg/mL; glycerol 22 mg/mL; sodium hydroxide)].
Note: Sterile diazepam emulsion is an oil/water emulsion with a pH of approximately 8.

### Packaging and storage
Store below 25 °C (77 °F), unless otherwise specified by manufacturer. Protect from freezing. Protect from light.

### Preparation of dosage form
When administered intravenously, sterile diazepam emulsion should be administered without prior dilution or mixing with other products or solutions. However, it may be mixed or diluted with its emulsion base (*Intralipid* or *Nutralipid*) but the admixture should be used within 6 hours.

### Stability
Sterile diazepam emulsion contains no preservatives and can support rapid microbial growth. Administration should be completed within 6 hours after the ampul has been opened.
Mixing or diluting sterile diazepam emulsion with products or solutions other than its own emulsion base (*Intralipid* or *Nutralipid*) may destabilize the emulsion. Although such an effect may not be recognized on visual inspection, it may result in potentially serious adverse reactions.

### Incompatibilities
Sterile diazepam emulsion is incompatible with morphine and glycopyrrolate.
Infusion sets containing polyvinyl chloride should not be used for administration of sterile diazepam emulsion.

### Note
For administration of sterile diazepam emulsion, polyethylene-lined or glass infusion sets and polyethylene/polypropylene plastic syringes are recommended.
Sterile diazepam emulsion should not be administered through a filter with a pore size of less than 5 microns, because the emulsion may be broken down.
Strict aseptic technique is required in the handling of sterile diazepam emulsion.
Controlled substance in the U.S.

## Rectal Dosage Forms
### DIAZEPAM FOR RECTAL SOLUTION

#### Usual adult and adolescent dose
Anticonvulsant—
  Status epilepticus and severe recurrent convulsive seizures: Rectal, 150 to 500 mcg (0.15 to 0.5 mg) of diazepam per kg of body weight, up to a maximum of 20 mg per dose.

### Usual pediatric dose
Anticonvulsant—
  Status epilepticus and severe recurrent convulsive seizures: Rectal, 200 to 500 mcg (0.2 to 0.5 mg) of diazepam per kg of body weight.

### Usual geriatric dose
Rectal, 200 to 300 mcg (0.2 to 0.3 mg) of diazepam per kg of body weight.

### Strength(s) usually available
U.S.—
  Not commercially available.
Canada—
  Not commercially available.

### Packaging and storage
Store below 40 °C (104 °F), preferably between 15 and 30 °C (59 and 86 °F), unless otherwise specified by manufacturer. Protect from light. Protect from freezing.

### Preparation of dosage form
For rectal administration, Diazepam Injection USP has been used. The parenteral preparation may be instilled via a cannula or catheter fitted to the syringe or directly from a needleless 1-mL syringe inserted 4 to 5 centimeters into the rectum to allow for optimum absorption. Alternatively, a dilution of Diazepam Injection USP with propylene glycol to make a solution containing 1 mg of diazepam per mL has been used.

### Stability
Do not mix or dilute this medication with other solutions, intravenous fluids, or medications, because the resulting admixtures are unstable.
Diazepam is adsorbed to the plastic of intravenous infusion bags and tubing.

### Incompatibilities
Diazepam injection is physically incompatible with aqueous solutions.

## DIAZEPAM RECTAL GEL

### Usual adult and adolescent dose
Anticonvulsant—
  Rectal, 200 mcg (0.2 mg) per kg of body weight rounded up to the next available unit dose. Dose may be repeated, if needed, in four to twelve hours.
Note: Geriatric or debilitated patients—Rounding down to the next available unit dose is recommended to avoid ataxia and oversedation.

### Usual pediatric dose
Anticonvulsant—
  Children younger than 2 years of age: Safety and efficacy have not been established.
  Children 2 to 6 years of age: Rectal, 500 mcg (0.5 mg) per kg of body weight rounded up to the next available unit dose. Dose may be repeated, if needed, in four to twelve hours.
  Children 6 to 12 years of age: Rectal, 300 mcg (0.3 mg) per kg of body weight rounded up to the next available unit dose. Dose may be repeated, if needed, in four to twelve hours.
  Children 12 years of age and older: See *Usual adult and adolescent dose*.

### Strength(s) usually available
U.S.—
  2.5 mg with pediatric (4.4 cm) rectal tip size (Rx) [*Diastat* (propylene glycol; ethyl alcohol 10%; hydroxypropyl methylcellulose; sodium benzoate; benzyl alcohol 1.5%; benzoic acid; water)].
  5 mg with pediatric (4.4 cm) rectal tip size (Rx) [*Diastat* (propylene glycol; ethyl alcohol 10%; hydroxypropyl methylcellulose; sodium benzoate; benzyl alcohol 1.5%; benzoic acid; water)].
  10 mg with pediatric (4.4 cm) rectal tip size (Rx) [*Diastat* (propylene glycol; ethyl alcohol 10%; hydroxypropyl methylcellulose; sodium benzoate; benzyl alcohol 1.5%; benzoic acid; water)].
  10 mg with adult (6 cm) rectal tip size (Rx) [*Diastat* (propylene glycol; ethyl alcohol 10%; hydroxypropyl methylcellulose; sodium benzoate; benzyl alcohol 1.5%; benzoic acid; water)].
  15 mg with adult (6 cm) rectal tip size (Rx) [*Diastat* (propylene glycol; ethyl alcohol 10%; hydroxypropyl methylcellulose; sodium benzoate; benzyl alcohol 1.5%; benzoic acid; water)].
  20 mg with adult (6 cm) rectal tip size (Rx) [*Diastat* (propylene glycol; ethyl alcohol 10%; hydroxypropyl methylcellulose; sodium benzoate; benzyl alcohol 1.5%; benzoic acid; water)].
Canada—
  Not commercially available.

### Packaging and storage
Store between 15 and 30 °C (59 and 86 °F), unless otherwise specified by manufacturer.

### Auxiliary labeling
- May cause drowsiness.
- For rectal use only.

### Caution
Medications containing benzyl alcohol are not recommended for use in neonates (first 30 days of postnatal life). A fatal toxic syndrome consisting of metabolic acidosis, CNS depression, respiratory problems, renal failure, hypotension, and possibly seizures and intracranial hemorrhages has been associated with this use.

It is recommended that diazepam rectal gel be used no more frequently than every 5 days, and no more than five times a month.

### Note
Caregiver must be instructed in the proper use of diazepam rectal gel, including when use is appropriate, how to administer, how to monitor the patient after administration, and when immediate medical attention is required.

Administration instructions for caregiver should be included with each prescription dispensed.

If a child requires a dose of 15 mg and the pediatric rectal tip size is desired, unit doses of 5 and 10 mg must be dispensed since the 15 mg unit dose is available only in the adult rectal tip size.

Controlled substance in the U.S.

### Additional information
The 2.5 mg unit dose size is intended for more precise dose titration or for the partial replacement of a dose that is expelled by the patient.

---

[1]Not included in Canadian product labeling.

---

## ESTAZOLAM

## Summary of Differences
Category:
  Indicated only as a sedative-hypnotic.
Indications:
  May be useful in prevention or treatment of transient insomnia associated with sudden sleep schedule changes.
Pharmacology/pharmacokinetics:
  Intermediate half-life benzodiazepine.
  Small degree of accumulation during repeated dosing.
  Steady-state plasma concentration usually attained within a few days.
  Intermediate rate of elimination following discontinuation of therapy.

## Oral Dosage Forms

### ESTAZOLAM TABLETS

#### Usual adult dose
Sedative-hypnotic—
  Oral, initially 1 mg at bedtime. A dose of 2 mg may be necessary in some patients.

#### Usual pediatric dose
Sedative-hypnotic—
  Children younger than 18 years of age: Safety and efficacy have not been established.

#### Usual geriatric dose
Sedative-hypnotic—
  Oral, initially 1 mg at bedtime. Dosage increases should be made cautiously.
Note: Small or debilitated older patients may be started at 0.5 mg.

#### Strength(s) usually available
U.S.—
  1 mg (Rx) [*ProSom* (scored; lactose); GENERIC (may be scored)].
  2 mg (Rx) [*ProSom* (scored; lactose); GENERIC (may be scored)].
Canada—
  Not commercially available.

#### Packaging and storage
Store below 30 °C (86 °F), in a well-closed container, unless otherwise specified by manufacturer.

#### Auxiliary labeling
- Avoid alcoholic beverages.
- May cause daytime drowsiness.

#### Note
Controlled substance in the U.S.

## FLURAZEPAM

### Summary of Differences
Category:
  Indicated only as a sedative-hypnotic.
Pharmacology/pharmacokinetics:
  Drug precursor; parent drug does not reach systemic circulation in significant amounts.
  Long half-life benzodiazepine.
  Accumulation of active metabolites is significant during repeated dosing.
  Steady-state plasma concentration usually attained in 7 to 10 days.
  Elimination slow since metabolites remain in blood for several days.

### Additional Dosing Information
See also *General Dosing Information*.

Flurazepam is increasingly effective on the second or third night of consecutive use, and for one or two nights after medication is discontinued both sleep latency and total wake time may still be decreased.

## Oral Dosage Forms

### FLURAZEPAM HYDROCHLORIDE CAPSULES USP
**Usual adult dose**
Sedative-hypnotic—
  Oral, 15 or 30 mg at bedtime.
Note: The usual adult dose is 30 mg, but 15 mg may be sufficient for some patients.
  Debilitated patients—Oral, initially 15 mg at bedtime, the dosage being increased as needed and tolerated.

**Usual pediatric dose**
Sedative-hypnotic—
  Children younger than 15 years of age: Safety and efficacy have not been established.

**Usual geriatric dose**
Sedative-hypnotic—
  Oral, initially 15 mg at bedtime, the dosage being increased as needed and tolerated.

**Strength(s) usually available**
U.S.—
  15 mg (Rx) [*Dalmane* (lactose; gelatin capsules may contain methyl and propyl parabens); GENERIC].
  30 mg (Rx) [*Dalmane* (lactose; gelatin capsules may contain methyl and propyl parabens); GENERIC].
Canada—
  15 mg (Rx) [*Apo-Flurazepam; Dalmane* (lactose 276 mg; methylparaben; propylparaben); *Novo-Flupam*].
  30 mg (Rx) [*Apo-Flurazepam; Dalmane* (lactose 263 mg; methylparaben; propylparaben); *Novo-Flupam*].

**Packaging and storage**
Store below 40 °C (104 °F), preferably between 15 and 30 °C (59 and 86 °F), unless otherwise specified by manufacturer. Store in a tight, light-resistant container.

**Auxiliary labeling**
- Avoid alcoholic beverages.
- May cause daytime drowsiness.

**Note**
Controlled substance in the U.S.

### FLURAZEPAM HYDROCHLORIDE TABLETS
**Usual adult dose**
See *Flurazepam Hydrochloride Capsules USP*.

**Usual pediatric dose**
See *Flurazepam Hydrochloride Capsules USP*.

**Usual geriatric dose**
See *Flurazepam Hydrochloride Capsules USP*.

**Strength(s) usually available**
U.S.—
  Not commercially available.
Canada—
  15 mg (Rx) [*Somnol* (scored; lactose)].
  30 mg (Rx) [*Somnol* (scored; lactose)].

**Packaging and storage**
Store between 8 and 15 °C (46 and 59 °F), in a well-closed container, unless otherwise specified by manufacturer.

**Auxiliary labeling**
- Avoid alcoholic beverages.
- May cause daytime drowsiness.

## HALAZEPAM

### Summary of Differences
Category:
  Indicated only as an antianxiety agent.
Pharmacology/pharmacokinetics:
  Long half-life benzodiazepine.
  Accumulation of active metabolite is significant during repeated dosing.
  Steady-state plasma concentration usually attained in 5 days to 2 weeks.
  Elimination slow since metabolite remains in blood for several days or even weeks.

## Oral Dosage Forms

### HALAZEPAM TABLETS
**Usual adult dose**
Antianxiety agent—
  Oral, 20 to 40 mg three or four times a day. Dosage may be adjusted upward or downward after several days if needed. The optimal dosage is usually 80 to 160 mg per day.
Note: Debilitated patients—Oral, 20 mg one or two times a day, the dosage being adjusted as needed and tolerated.

**Usual pediatric dose**
Antianxiety agent—
  Children younger than 18 years of age: Safety and efficacy have not been established.

**Usual geriatric dose**
Antianxiety agent—
  Oral, 20 mg one or two times a day, the dosage being adjusted as needed and tolerated.

**Strength(s) usually available**
U.S.—
  20 mg (Rx) [*Paxipam* (scored; lactose)].
  40 mg (Rx) [*Paxipam* (scored; lactose)].
Canada—
  Not commercially available.

**Packaging and storage**
Store between 2 and 30 °C (36 and 86 °F), in a well-closed container, unless otherwise specified by manufacturer.

**Auxiliary labeling**
- Avoid alcoholic beverages.
- May cause drowsiness.

**Note**
Controlled substance in the U.S.

## KETAZOLAM

### Summary of Differences
Category:
  Formerly indicated in Canada as an antianxiety agent only.
Pharmacology/pharmacokinetics:
  Long half-life benzodiazepine.
  Accumulation of active metabolites is significant during repeated dosing.
  Steady-state plasma concentration usually attained in 7 to 10 days.
  Elimination slow since metabolites remain in blood for several days.

## Oral Dosage Forms

### KETAZOLAM CAPSULES
**Usual adult dose**
[Antianxiety agent][1]—
  Oral, 15 mg one or two times a day, the dosage being increased in 15-mg increments as needed and tolerated.
Note: Debilitated patients—The recommended initial dosage is one half the lowest recommended initial adult dosage.

**Usual pediatric dose**
[Antianxiety agent][1]—
  Children younger than 18 years of age: Safety and efficacy have not been established.
Note: Use in infants is not recommended.

## Benzodiazepines (Systemic)

**Usual geriatric dose**
[Antianxiety agent][1]—
  Oral, 15 mg once a day, the dosage being increased in 15-mg increments as needed and tolerated.

**Strength(s) usually available**
U.S.—
  Not commercially available.
Canada—
  Not commercially available.

**Packaging and storage**
Store below 40 °C (104 °F), preferably between 15 and 30 °C (59 and 86 °F), in a well-closed container, unless otherwise specified by manufacturer.

**Auxiliary labeling**
- Avoid alcoholic beverages.
- May cause drowsiness.

---

[1]Not included in Canadian product labeling.

---

## LORAZEPAM

## Summary of Differences

Category:
  In addition to being indicated as an antianxiety agent and a sedative-hypnotic, lorazepam is indicated as an amnestic and used as an anticonvulsant (parenteral only), an antiemetic in cancer chemotherapy (parenteral only), an antipanic agent, an antitremor agent (oral only), and a skeletal muscle relaxant adjunct.

Indications:
  Oral lorazepam also indicated for adjunctive management of anxiety associated with mental depression.
  Parenteral lorazepam also indicated as a preanesthetic medication; and used as an adjunct prior to endoscopic procedures, as prophylaxis of cancer chemotherapy–induced nausea and vomiting, and for the treatment of status epilepticus.
  Oral and parenteral lorazepam also used for relief of acute alcohol withdrawal symptoms and for treatment of tension headache.

Pharmacology/pharmacokinetics:
  Absorption of intramuscular lorazepam is rapid and complete.
  Short to intermediate half-life benzodiazepine.
  Accumulation is minimal during repeated dosing.
  Steady-state plasma concentration usually attained within a few (2 to 3) days.
  Elimination rapid following discontinuation of therapy.

Precautions:
  Drug interactions and/or related problems—
    Cimetidine, oral estrogen-containing contraceptives, diltiazem, disulfiram, erythromycin, fluoxetine, fluvoxamine, grapefruit juice, itraconazole, ketoconazole, nefazodone, propoxyphene, ranitidine, or verapamil, which inhibit the oxidative metabolism of benzodiazepines, are less likely to affect lorazepam, which undergoes glucuronide conjugation.
    Premedication with lorazepam may decrease dose of a fentanyl derivative required for induction of anesthesia and reduce time to loss of consciousness with induction doses.
    Probenecid may impair glucuronide conjugation of lorazepam, resulting in increased effects and possibly excessive sedation.
  Medical considerations/contraindications—
    Prolongation of elimination half-life due to hepatic function impairment may be minimal with lorazepam.

Side/adverse effects:
  Intravenous lorazepam more likely than chlordiazepoxide but less likely than diazepam to cause phlebitis or venous thrombosis.

## Additional Dosing Information

See also *General Dosing Information*.

**For sublingual tablets only**
Do not swallow for at least 2 minutes to allow sufficient time for absorption.

**For parenteral dosage forms only**
Immediately prior to intravenous use, lorazepam injection must be diluted with an equal amount of a compatible diluent such as sterile water for injection, 0.9% sodium chloride injection, or 5% dextrose injection.
Following proper dilution, the medication may be injected directly into the vein or into the tubing of an intravenous infusion.
Intravenous injection should be made slowly and with repeated aspiration.
The rate of the intravenous injection should not exceed 2 mg per minute.
Intra-arterial injection and perivascular extravasation should be avoided. Intra-arterial injection may produce arteriospasm, possibly resulting in gangrene.
When administered intramuscularly, the injection (undiluted) should be injected deeply into the muscle mass.
When parenteral lorazepam is used for peroral endoscopic procedures, the use of topical or regional anesthesia is recommended to minimize the reflex activity associated with such procedures.
When lorazepam is administered intravenously as premedication prior to regional or local anesthesia, potential excessive sleepiness or drowsiness may interfere with patient cooperation in determining levels of anesthesia. This is more likely to occur when doses greater than 0.05 mg per kg of body weight (mg/kg) are given and narcotic analgesics are used concomitantly with recommended doses.

## Oral Dosage Forms

### LORAZEPAM ORAL CONCENTRATE USP

**Usual adult and adolescent dose**
Antianxiety agent—
  Oral, 1 to 3 mg two or three times a day.
Sedative-hypnotic—
  Oral, 2 to 4 mg as a single dose at bedtime.
Note: Debilitated patients—Oral, initially 1 to 2 mg per day in divided doses, the dosage being increased gradually as needed and tolerated.

**Usual adult prescribing limits**
10 mg per day.

**Usual pediatric dose**
Antianxiety agent or
Sedative-hypnotic[1]—
  Children younger than 12 years of age: Safety and efficacy have not been established.

**Strength(s) usually available**
U.S.—
  2 mg per mL (Rx) [*Lorazepam Intensol*].
Canada—
  Not commercially available.

**Packaging and storage**
Store between 2 and 8 °C (36 and 46 °F), unless otherwise specified by manufacturer. Store in a well-closed container. Protect from light.

**Preparation of dosage form**
The manufacturer recommends that each dose be mixed with water, juice, soda or soda-like beverages, or semisolid food, such as applesauce or pudding. The entire amount of the mixture should be consumed immediately after mixing; no part of the mixture should be saved for later use.

**Auxiliary labeling**
- Refrigerate.
- Avoid alcoholic beverages.
- May cause drowsiness.

**Note**
The patient or caregiver should be instructed in proper measurement of the dose using the calibrated dropper provided with the medication, and in preparation of the dose.

Controlled substance in the U.S.

### LORAZEPAM TABLETS USP

**Usual adult and adolescent dose**
Antianxiety agent—
  Oral, 1 to 3 mg two or three times a day.
Note: Debilitated patients—Oral, initially 0.5 to 2 mg per day in divided doses, the dosage being increased gradually as needed and tolerated.
Sedative-hypnotic[1]—
  Oral, 2 to 4 mg as a single dose at bedtime.
Note: Elderly and debilitated patients may require a lower dose.

**Usual pediatric dose**
Antianxiety agent or
Sedative-hypnotic[1]—
  Children younger than 12 years of age: Safety and efficacy have not been established.

**Usual geriatric dose**
Antianxiety agent—
  Oral, initially 0.5 to 2 mg per day in divided doses, the dosage being increased gradually as needed and tolerated.

### Strength(s) usually available
U.S.—
- 0.5 mg (Rx) [ *Ativan* (lactose); GENERIC (may be scored)].
- 1 mg (Rx) [*Ativan* (scored; lactose); GENERIC (may be scored)].
- 2 mg (Rx) [*Ativan* (scored; lactose); GENERIC (may be scored)].

Canada—
- 0.5 mg (Rx) [*Apo-Lorazepam* (sodium < 1 mmol [0.06 mg]); *Ativan* (lactose); *Novo-Lorazem*; *Nu-Loraz* (sodium < 1 mmol [0.06 mg])].
- 1 mg (Rx) [*Apo-Lorazepam* (scored; sodium < 1 mmol [0.13 mg]); *Ativan* (scored; lactose); *Novo-Lorazem* (scored); *Nu-Loraz* (scored; sodium < 1 mmol [0.13 mg])].
- 2 mg (Rx) [*Apo-Lorazepam* (scored; sodium < 1 mmol [0.16 mg]); *Ativan* (scored; lactose); *Novo-Lorazem* (scored); *Nu-Loraz* (scored; sodium < 1 mmol [0.16 mg]))].

### Packaging and storage
Store between 15 and 30 °C (59 and 86 °F), unless otherwise specified by manufacturer. Store in a tight, light-resistant container.

### Auxiliary labeling
- Avoid alcoholic beverages.
- May cause drowsiness.

### Note
Controlled substance in the U.S.

## LORAZEPAM SUBLINGUAL TABLETS

### Usual adult dose
Antianxiety agent—
  Sublingual, 2 to 3 mg per day in divided doses, the dosage being adjusted as needed, usually not exceeding 6 mg per day.

  Note: Debilitated patients—Sublingual, initially 500 mcg (0.5 mg) per day, the dosage being gradually adjusted as necessary.

  Preoperative: Sublingual, 50 mcg (0.05 mg) per kg of body weight, up to a maximum of 4 mg, one to two hours before surgery.

### Usual pediatric dose
Antianxiety agent—
  Children younger than 18 years of age: Safety and efficacy have not been established.

### Usual geriatric dose
Antianxiety agent—
  Sublingual, initially 500 mcg (0.5 mg) per day, the dosage being gradually adjusted as necessary.

### Strength(s) usually available
U.S.—
  Not commercially available.

Canada—
- 0.5 mg (Rx) [*Ativan* (lactose)].
- 1 mg (Rx) [*Ativan* (lactose)].
- 2 mg (Rx) [*Ativan* (lactose)].

### Packaging and storage
Store below 40 °C (104 °F), preferably between 15 and 30 °C (59 and 86 °F), in a well-closed container, unless otherwise specified by manufacturer.

### Auxiliary labeling
- Dissolve tablets under tongue.
- Avoid alcoholic beverages.
- May cause drowsiness.

## Parenteral Dosage Forms

Note: Bracketed uses in the *Dosage Forms* section refer to categories of use and/or indications that are not included in U.S. product labeling.

## LORAZEPAM INJECTION USP

### Usual adult dose
Antianxiety agent or
Sedative-hypnotic or
Amnestic—
  Intramuscular, 50 mcg (0.05 mg) per kg of body weight, up to a maximum of 4 mg. Dose should be administered at least two hours prior to surgery for optimum amnestic effect.

  Intravenous, initially 44 mcg (0.044 mg) per kg of body weight or a total dose of 2 mg, whichever is less. For greater amnestic effect, up to 50 mcg (0.05 mg) per kg of body weight, not to exceed a maximum of 4 mg, may be administered. Dose should be administered fifteen to twenty minutes prior to surgery for optimum amnestic effect.

[Antiemetic, in cancer chemotherapy][1]—
  Intravenous, initially 2 mg thirty minutes before initiation of chemotherapy, followed by 2 mg every four hours as needed.

[Anticonvulsant]—
  Status epilepticus: Intravenous, initially 50 mcg (0.05 mg) per kg of body weight up to a maximum of 4 mg, administered slowly. If seizures continue or recur after a ten- to fifteen-minute observation period, an additional dose of 50 mcg (0.05 mg) per kg may be administered. If seizure control is not evident after another ten to fifteen minutes, other measures to control status epilepticus should be used. The total cummulative dose should not exceed 8 mg of lorazepam in a twelve-hour period.

### Usual pediatric dose
Antianxiety agent or
Sedative-hypnotic or
Amnestic—
  Children younger than 18 years of age: Safety and efficacy have not been established.

Caution—
  Use of medications containing benzyl alcohol is not recommended for use in neonates (first 30 days of postnatal life). A fatal toxic syndrome consisting of metabolic acidosis, CNS depression, respiratory problems, renal failure, hypotension, and possibly seizures and intracranial hemorrhages has been associated with this use.

### Strength(s) usually available
U.S.—
- 2 mg per mL (Rx) [*Ativan* (benzyl alcohol 2%; polyethylene glycol 400 0.18 mL in propylene glycol); GENERIC].
- 4 mg per mL (Rx) [*Ativan* (benzyl alcohol 2%; polyethylene glycol 400 0.18 mL in propylene glycol); GENERIC].

Canada—
- 4 mg per mL (Rx) [*Ativan* (benzyl alcohol 2%; polyethylene glycol 18%; propylene glycol 80%)].

### Packaging and storage
Store between 2 and 8 °C (36 and 46 °F), unless otherwise specified by manufacturer. Protect from light. Protect from freezing.

### Preparation of dosage form
For intravenous administration—Immediately prior to use, lorazepam injection must be diluted with an equal volume of a compatible diluent, such as sterile water for injection, 0.9% sodium chloride injection, or 5% dextrose injection.

### Stability
Do not use if solution is discolored or contains a precipitate.

### Incompatibilities
Lorazepam injection is physically incompatible with buprenorphine injection.

### Note
Controlled substance in the U.S.

---

[1]Not included in Canadian product labeling.

---

# NITRAZEPAM

## Summary of Differences
Category:
  In addition to being indicated as a sedative-hypnotic, indicated as an anticonvulsant.

Pharmacology/pharmacokinetics:
  Absorption of nitrazepam is rapid.
  Short to intermediate half-life benzodiazepine.
  Accumulation is minimal during repeated dosing.
  Steady-state plasma concentration usually attained within a few (2 to 3) days.
  Elimination rapid following discontinuation of therapy.

Precautions:
  Drug interactions and/or related problems—Cimetidine or oral estrogen-containing contraceptives may inhibit the nitro-reduction of nitrazepam, resulting in delayed elimination and prolonged elimination half-life; serum concentrations may also be increased during long-term use.
  Medical considerations/contraindications—Nitrazepam may delay cricopharyngeal relaxation, exacerbating swallowing abnormalities in children.

## Oral Dosage Forms

### NITRAZEPAM TABLETS

#### Usual adult dose
Sedative-hypnotic—
  Oral, 5 or 10 mg at bedtime.

Note: Debilitated patients—Oral, initially 2.5 mg, the dosage being increased as needed and tolerated up to 5 mg.

**Usual pediatric dose**
Sedative-hypnotic—
  Dosage has not been established.
Anticonvulsant—
  Children up to 30 kg: Oral, initially the dosage should be below the usual recommended dosage range of 300 mcg (0.3 mg) to 1 mg per kg of body weight per day given in three divided doses, to determine response and tolerance. The dosage may be increased above the recommended range gradually, as needed and tolerated.
  Note: If doses are not equally divided, the larger dose should be given at bedtime.

**Usual geriatric dose**
Sedative-hypnotic—
  Oral, initially 2.5 mg, the dosage being increased as needed and tolerated up to 5 mg.

**Strength(s) usually available**
U.S.—
  Not commercially available.
Canada—
  5 mg (Rx) [*Mogadon* (scored; lactose)].
  10 mg (Rx) [*Mogadon* (scored; lactose)].

**Packaging and storage**
Store below 40 °C (104 °F), preferably between 15 and 30 °C (59 and 86 °F), in a well-closed container, unless otherwise specified by manufacturer. Protect from light.

**Auxiliary labeling**
• Avoid alcoholic beverages.
• May cause drowsiness.

---

### OXAZEPAM

## Summary of Differences
Indications:
  Also indicated for adjunctive management of anxiety associated with mental depression and relief of acute alcohol withdrawal symptoms.
Pharmacology/pharmacokinetics:
  Orally, one of least rapidly absorbed benzodiazepines.
  Short to intermediate half-life benzodiazepine.
  Accumulation is minimal during repeated dosing.
  Steady-state plasma concentration usually attained within a few days.
  Elimination rapid following discontinuation of therapy.
Precautions:
  Drug interactions and/or related problems—
    Cimetidine, oral estrogen-containing contraceptives, diltiazem, disulfiram, erythromycin, fluoxetine, fluvoxamine, grapefruit juice, itraconazole, ketoconazole, nefazodone, propoxyphene, ranitidine, and verapamil, which inhibit the oxidative metabolism of benzodiazepines, are less likely to affect oxazepam, which undergoes glucuronide conjugation.
    Probenecid may impair glucuronide conjugation of oxazepam, resulting in increased effects and possibly excessive sedation.
  Medical considerations/contraindications—
    Prolongation of elimination half-life due to hepatic function impairment may be minimal with oxazepam.

## Oral Dosage Forms

### OXAZEPAM CAPSULES USP

**Usual adult dose**
Antianxiety agent—
  Oral, 10 to 30 mg three or four times a day.
Sedative-hypnotic—
  Alcohol withdrawal: Oral, 15 or 30 mg three or four times a day.

**Usual pediatric dose**
Antianxiety agent or
Sedative-hypnotic—
  Children younger than 6 years of age: Safety and efficacy have not been established.
  Children 6 to 12 years of age: Dosage has not been established.

**Usual geriatric dose**
Antianxiety agent—
  Oral, initially 10 mg three times a day, the dosage being increased as needed and tolerated to 15 mg three or four times a day.

**Strength(s) usually available**
U.S.—
  10 mg (Rx) [*Serax* (lactose); GENERIC].
  15 mg (Rx) [*Serax* (lactose); GENERIC].
  30 mg (Rx) [*Serax* (lactose); GENERIC].
Canada—
  Not commercially available.

**Packaging and storage**
Store below 40 °C (104 °F), preferably between 15 and 30 °C (59 and 86 °F), in a well-closed container, unless otherwise specified by manufacturer.

**Auxiliary labeling**
• Avoid alcoholic beverages.
• May cause drowsiness.

**Note**
Controlled substance in the U.S.

### OXAZEPAM TABLETS USP

**Usual adult dose**
See *Oxazepam Capsules USP*.

**Usual pediatric dose**
See *Oxazepam Capsules USP*.

**Usual geriatric dose**
Antianxiety agent—
  Oral, initially 10 mg three times a day, the dosage being increased as needed and tolerated to 15 mg three or four times a day. Alternatively, an initial dosage of 5 mg one or two times a day has been recommended.

**Strength(s) usually available**
U.S.—
  15 mg (Rx) [*Serax* (tartrazine; lactose); GENERIC].
Canada—
  10 mg (Rx) [*Apo-Oxazepam* (scored); *Novoxapam* (scored); *Serax* (scored; lactose)].
  15 mg (Rx) [*Apo-Oxazepam* (scored); *Novoxapam* (scored); *Serax* (scored; lactose)].
  30 mg (Rx) [*Apo-Oxazepam* (scored; sodium < 1 mmol [0.49 mg]); *Novoxapam* (scored); *Serax* (scored; lactose)].

**Packaging and storage**
Store below 40 °C (104 °F), preferably between 15 and 30 °C (59 and 86 °F), in a well-closed container, unless otherwise specified by manufacturer.

**Auxiliary labeling**
• Avoid alcoholic beverages.
• May cause drowsiness.

**Note**
Controlled substance in the U.S.

---

### PRAZEPAM

## Summary of Differences
Category:
  Formerly indicated in the U.S. as an antianxiety agent only.
Pharmacology/pharmacokinetics:
  Drug precursor; metabolized to desmethyldiazepam before reaching systemic circulation.
  Orally, one of least rapidly absorbed benzodiazepines.
  Long half-life benzodiazepine.
  Accumulation of active metabolites is significant during repeated dosing.
  Steady-state plasma concentration usually attained in 5 days to 2 weeks.
  Elimination slow since metabolites remain in blood for several days.

## Oral Dosage Forms

### PRAZEPAM CAPSULES USP

**Usual adult dose**
[Antianxiety agent][1]—
  Oral, 10 mg three times a day (range, 20 to 60 mg per day); or 20 to 40 mg at bedtime.
Note: Debilitated patients—Oral, initially 10 to 15 mg per day in divided doses, the dosage being increased gradually as needed and tolerated.

**Usual pediatric dose**
[Antianxiety agent][1]—
Children younger than 18 years of age: Safety and efficacy have not been established.

**Usual geriatric dose**
[Antianxiety agent][1]—
Oral, initially 10 to 15 mg per day in divided doses, the dosage being increased gradually as needed and tolerated.

**Strength(s) usually available**
U.S.—
Not commercially available.
Canada—
Not commercially available.

**Packaging and storage**
Store between 15 and 30 °C (59 and 86 °F), unless otherwise specified by manufacturer. Store in a tight, light-resistant container.

**Auxiliary labeling**
- Avoid alcoholic beverages.
- May cause drowsiness.

[1]Not included in Canadian product labeling.

---

## QUAZEPAM

## Summary of Differences
Category:
Indicated only as a sedative-hypnotic.
Pharmacology/pharmacokinetics:
Long half-life benzodiazepine.
Accumulation of active metabolites may occur during repeated dosing.
Steady-state plasma concentrations usually attained within 7 to 13 days.
Elimination slow since metabolites remain in blood for several days.

## Oral Dosage Forms
### QUAZEPAM TABLETS
**Usual adult dose**
Sedative-hypnotic—
Oral, initially 15 mg, the dose being reduced to 7.5 mg as needed.
Note: Debilitated patients—Because of increased sensitivity to benzodiazepines, it is suggested that the nightly dose be reduced after one or two nights of treatment.

**Usual pediatric dose**
Sedative-hypnotic—
Children younger than 18 years of age: Safety and efficacy have not been established.

**Usual geriatric dose**
Sedative-hypnotic—
Oral, initially 15 mg, the dose being reduced to 7.5 mg after one or two nights.

**Strength(s) usually available**
U.S.—
7.5 mg (Rx) [*Doral* (lactose)].
15 mg (Rx) [*Doral* (lactose)].
Canada—
Not commercially available.

**Packaging and storage**
Store between 15 and 30 °C (59 and 86 °F), in a tight container, unless otherwise specified by manufacturer.

**Auxiliary labeling**
- Avoid alcoholic beverages.
- May cause daytime drowsiness.

**Note**
Controlled substance in the U.S.

---

## TEMAZEPAM

## Summary of Differences
Category:
Indicated only as a sedative-hypnotic.
Indications:
May be useful in prevention or treatment of transient insomnia associated with sudden sleep schedule changes.
Pharmacology/pharmacokinetics:
Short to intermediate half-life benzodiazepine.
Accumulation is minimal during repeated dosing.
Steady-state plasma concentration usually attained within a few (about 3) days.
Elimination rapid following discontinuation of therapy.
Precautions:
Drug interactions and/or related problems—
Cimetidine, oral estrogen-containing contraceptives, diltiazem, disulfiram, erythromycin, fluoxetine, fluvoxamine, grapefruit juice, itraconazole, ketoconazole, nefazodone, propoxyphene, ranitidine, and verapamil, which inhibit the oxidative metabolism of the benzodiazepines, are less likely to affect temazepam, which undergoes glucuronide conjugation.
Probenecid may impair glucuronide conjugation of temazepam, resulting in increased effects and possibly excessive sedation.
Medical considerations/contraindications—
Prolongation of elimination half-life due to hepatic function impairment may be minimal with temazepam.

## Oral Dosage Forms
### TEMAZEPAM CAPSULES USP
**Usual adult dose**
Sedative-hypnotic—
Oral, usually 15 mg at bedtime, although 7.5 mg may be sufficient for some patients and others may need 30 mg.
Note: In transient insomnia, 7.5 mg may be sufficient to improve sleep latency.
Debilitated patients—Oral, initially 7.5 mg, the dosage being adjusted as needed and tolerated.

**Usual pediatric dose**
Sedative-hypnotic—
Children younger than 18 years of age: Safety and efficacy have not been established.

**Usual geriatric dose**
Sedative-hypnotic—
Oral, initially 7.5 mg, the dosage being adjusted as needed and tolerated.

**Strength(s) usually available**
U.S.—
7.5 mg (Rx) [*Restoril* (lactose); GENERIC].
15 mg (Rx) [*Restoril* (lactose); GENERIC].
30 mg (Rx) [*Restoril* (lactose); GENERIC].
Canada—
15 mg (Rx) [*Apo-Temazepam; Novo-Temazepam; Restoril* (lactose)].
30 mg (Rx) [*Apo-Temazepam; Novo-Temazepam; Restoril* (lactose)].

**Packaging and storage**
Store between 15 and 30 °C (59 and 86 °F), in a tight, light-resistant container, unless otherwise specified by manufacturer.

**Auxiliary labeling**
- Avoid alcoholic beverages.
- May cause daytime drowsiness.

**Note**
Controlled substance in the U.S.

---

## TRIAZOLAM

## Summary of Differences
Category:
Indicated only as a sedative-hypnotic.
Indications:
May be useful in prevention or treatment of transient insomnia associated with sudden sleep schedule change.
Pharmacology/pharmacokinetics:
Short half-life benzodiazepine.
Accumulation is minimal during repeated dosing.
Elimination rapid following discontinuation of therapy.
Precautions:
Drug interactions and/or related problems—
Itraconazole and ketoconazole greatly increase the area under the plasma concentration–time curve (AUC) of triazolam; concurrent use is not recommended.
Nefazodone increases the AUC of triazolam fourfold, resulting in impairment of psychomotor function; a 75% reduction in triazolam dosage is recommended during concurrent use.
Cimetidine and erythromycin may inhibit the hepatic metabolism of triazolam, resulting in increased plasma concentrations and delayed clearance of triazolam; dosage reductions may be necessary.

Isoniazid may inhibit the elimination of triazolam, resulting in increased plasma concentrations.

Side/adverse effects:
Anterograde amnesia may be more likely to occur with triazolam than with most other benzodiazepines.
Because of the potency of triazolam, symptoms of overdose may occur at doses as low as 2 mg.

## Oral Dosage Forms
### TRIAZOLAM TABLETS USP
**Usual adult dose**
Sedative-hypnotic—
   Oral, 125 to 250 mcg (0.125 to 0.25 mg) at bedtime.

Note: A dose of 500 mcg (0.5 mg) may be necessary in some patients. However, this dose should be reserved for patients who do not respond adequately to lower doses, since the risk of side effects increases with dosage increases.
   Debilitated patients—Oral, initially 125 mcg (0.125 mg) at bedtime, the dosage being increased as needed and tolerated.

**Usual pediatric dose**
Sedative-hypnotic—
   Children younger than 18 years of age: Safety and efficacy have not been established.

**Usual geriatric dose**
Sedative-hypnotic—
   Oral, initially 125 mcg (0.125 mg) at bedtime, the dosage being increased as needed and tolerated.

**Strength(s) usually available**
U.S.—
   125 mcg (0.125 mg) (Rx) [*Halcion* (docusate sodium; lactose; sodium benzoate); GENERIC (may contain docusate sodium, lactose, and/or sodium benzoate)].
   250 mcg (0.25 mg) (Rx) [*Halcion* (scored; docusate sodium; lactose; sodium benzoate); GENERIC (may be scored; may contain docusate sodium, lactose, and/or sodium benzoate)].
Canada—
   125 mcg (0.125 mg) (Rx) [*Alti-Triazolam* (scored; docusate sodium; erythrosine sodium; lactose); *Apo-Triazo* (scored; sodium < 1 mmol [0.32 mg]); *Gen-Triazolam* (scored); *Halcion* (scored; docusate sodium; lactose); *Novo-Triolam* (scored) [GENERIC].
   250 mcg (0.25 mg) (Rx) [*Alti-Triazolam* (scored; docusate sodium; lactose); *Apo-Triazo* (scored; sodium < 1 mmol [0.32 mg]); *Gen-Triazolam* (scored); *Halcion* (scored; docusate sodium; lactose); *Novo-Triolam* (scored) [GENERIC].

**Packaging and storage**
Store between 15 and 30° C (59 and 86° F), unless otherwise specified by manufacturer. Store in a tight, light-resistant container.

**Auxiliary labeling**
• Avoid alcoholic beverages.
• May cause daytime drowsiness.

**Note**
Controlled substance in the U.S.

Revised: 08/07/98

## Table 1. Pharmacology/Pharmacokinetics
Note: Whether the half-life of a benzodiazepine is considered to be long, intermediate, or short is determined by the half-lives of any active metabolites, as well as the half-life of the parent compound.

| Drug | Protein binding (%) | Half-life* (hr) | Major active metabolites (half-life in hr) | Time to peak plasma concentration† (oral dose) (hr) | Elimination‡ (% excreted unchanged) |
|---|---|---|---|---|---|
| *Long half-life* | | | | | |
| Chlordiazepoxide | Very high (96) | 5–30 | Desmethylchlordiazepoxide (18) Demoxepam (14–95) Desmethyldiazepam (40–120) Oxazepam (5–15) | 0.5–4 | Renal (1–2); 3–6% as conjugate |
| Clorazepate§ | Desmethyldiazepam: Very high (95–98) | — | Desmethyldiazepam (40–120) Oxazepam (5–15) | 0.5–2 | Renal; fecal |
| Diazepam | Very high (98) | 20–80# | Desmethyldiazepam (40–120) Temazepam (8–15) Oxazepam (5–15) | 1–2 (injection: IM, 0.5–1.5; IV, within 0.25) (sterile emulsion: IM, > 2; IV, 0.13–0.25) (rectal gel: 1.5) | Renal |
| Flurazepam§** | Desalkylflurazepam: Very high (97) | 2.3 | Desalkylflurazepam (47–100) N-1-hydroxyethylflurazepam (2–4) | 0.5–1 | Renal |
| Halazepam | Very high (97) | 14 | Desmethyldiazepam (40–120) | 1–3 | Renal (< 1) |
| Ketazolam | Very high (93) | 2 | Desmethyldiazepam (40–120) N-methylketazolam (34–52) Diazepam (20–80)# | 3 | Renal; fecal ≤ 1% |
| Prazepam§ | Desmethyldiazepam: Very high (95–98) | — | Desmethyldiazepam (40–120) Oxazepam (5–15) | Desmethyldiazepam (single dose): 2.5–6 | Renal |
| Quazepam | Very high (> 95) | 39 | Desalkylflurazepam (47–100) 2-oxoquazepam (39) | 2 | Renal (trace); fecal |
| *Short to intermediate half-life* | | | | | |
| Alprazolam | High (80) | 11 (6.3–26.9) | None | 1–2 | Renal |
| Bromazepam | High (70) | 12 (8–19) | None | 1–4 | Renal |
| Clobazam | High (85) | 18 (10–30) | N-desmethylclobazam 42 (36–46) | 1–4 | Renal |
| Clonazepam | High (85) | 18–50 | None | 1–2†† | Renal (< 2) |

## Table 1. Pharmacology/Pharmacokinetics *(continued)*

Note: Whether the half-life of a benzodiazepine is considered to be long, intermediate, or short is determined by the half-lives of any active metabolites, as well as the half-life of the parent compound.

| Drug | Protein binding (%) | Half-life* (hr) | Major active metabolites (half-life in hr) | Time to peak plasma concentration† (oral dose) (hr) | Elimination‡ (% excreted unchanged) |
|---|---|---|---|---|---|
| Estazolam | Very high (93) | 10–24 | None | 2 (0.5–6) | Renal (< 5) |
| Lorazepam‡‡ | High (85) | 10–20 | None | 1–6 (IM, 1–1.5; sublingual, 1) | Renal |
| Nitrazepam | High (87) | 30 (18–57) | None | 2–3 | Renal (about 1); fecal |
| Oxazepam | Very high (97) | 5–15 | None | 1–4 | Renal; fecal |
| Temazepam | Very high (96) | 8–15 | None | 1–2 | Renal (< 1)§§ |
| Triazolam | High (89) | 1.5–5.5 | None | ≤ 2 | Renal (small amount)§§ |

*Elimination half-lives may be prolonged in children, especially premature and newborn infants, geriatric patients, and patients with hepatic disease; however, metabolic clearance of short to intermediate half-life benzodiazepines, especially lorazepam, oxazepam, temazepam, and triazolam, is affected less by age and hepatic disease than that of the long half-life benzodiazepines. The elimination half-life does not always predict the duration of clinical effects.
†With multiple dosing, steady-state plasma concentrations of long half-life benzodiazepines usually are achieved within 5 days to 2 weeks and those of short to intermediate half-life benzodiazepines within a few days.
‡Benzodiazepines are not significantly removed from the body by hemodialysis.
§Prodrugs or drug precursors; do not reach circulation in clinically significant amounts.
#Increases with age from approximately 20 hours in a 20-year-old patient to approximately 80 hours in an 80-year-old patient.
**Maximum effectiveness as a hypnotic may not be achieved for 2 to 3 days.
††Following a single dose; in some patients peak concentrations may not be achieved for 4 to 8 hours.
‡‡Peak amnestic effect: IM, within 2 hours; IV, 15 to 20 minutes.
§§Appears to be biphasic in its time course.

**BENZONATATE**—The *Benzonatate (Systemic)* monograph is not included in this published version of the USP DI database. Copies of the monograph are available on request from Micromedex, Inc. - Reprint Requests, 6200 S. Syracuse Way, Suite 300, Englewood, CO 80111; telephone (303) 486-6400; telefax (303) 486-6464; Email: USPDI@MDX.COM.

# BENZOYL PEROXIDE   Topical

VA CLASSIFICATION (Primary/Secondary): DE752/DE500

Commonly used brand name(s): *10 Benzagel; 10 Benzagel Acne Gel; 2.5 Benzagel Acne Gel; 2.5 Benzagel Acne Lotion; 5 Benzagel; 5 Benzagel Acne Gel; 5 Benzagel Acne Lotion; 5 Benzagel Acne Wash; 5 Benzagel Liquid Acne Soap; Acetoxyl 10 Gel; Acetoxyl 2.5 Gel; Acetoxyl 20 Gel; Acetoxyl 5 Gel; Acne-Aid Aqua Gel; Acne-Aid Vanishing Cream; Acnomel B.P. 5 Lotion; Ambi 10 Acne Medication; Benoxyl 10 Lotion; Benoxyl 20 Lotion; Benoxyl 5 Lotion; BenzaShave 10 Cream; BenzaShave 5 Cream; Benzac 10 Gel; Benzac 5 Gel; Benzac AC 10 Gel; Benzac AC 2½ Gel; Benzac AC 5 Gel; Benzac AC Wash 10; Benzac AC Wash 2½; Benzac AC Wash 5; Benzac W 10 Gel; Benzac W 10 Gel; Benzac W 2½ Gel; Benzac W 5 Gel; Benzac W 5 Gel; Benzac W Wash 10; Benzac W Wash 5; Brevoxyl-4 Cleansing Lotion; Brevoxyl-4 Gel; Brevoxyl-8 Cleansing Lotion; Brevoxyl-8 Gel; Clean & Clear Persagel 10; Clean & Clear Persagel 5; Clear By Design 2.5 Gel; Clearasil BP Plus 5 Lotion; Clearasil BP Plus Skin Tone Cream; Clearasil Maximum Strength Medicated Anti-Acne 10 Tinted Cream; Clearasil Maximum Strength Medicated Anti-Acne 10 Vanishing Cream; Clearasil Maximum Strength Medicated Anti-Acne 10 Vanishing Lotion; Clearplex 10; Clearplex 5; Cuticura Acne 5 Cream; Del-Aqua-10 Gel; Del-Aqua-5 Gel; Dermacne; Dermoxyl 10 Gel; Dermoxyl 20 Gel; Dermoxyl 5 Gel; Dermoxyl Aqua 5 Gel; Desquam-E 10 Gel; Desquam-E 2.5 Gel; Desquam-E 5 Gel; Desquam-X 10 Bar; Desquam-X 10 Gel; Desquam-X 10 Wash; Desquam-X 2.5 Gel; Desquam-X 5 Gel; Desquam-X 5 Wash; Exact 5 Tinted Cream; Exact 5 Vanishing Cream; Fostex 10 BPO Gel; Fostex 10 Bar; Fostex 10 Cream; Fostex 10 Wash; Fostex 5 Gel; H2Oxyl 10 Gel; H2Oxyl 2.5 Gel; H2Oxyl 20 Gel; H2Oxyl 5 Gel; Loroxide 5 Lotion; Loroxide 5.5 Lotion; Neutrogena Acne Mask 5; Noxzema Clear-ups Maximum Strength 10 Lotion; Noxzema Clear-ups On-The-Spot 10 Lotion; Oxy 10 Balance Emergency Spot Treatment Cover-Up Formula Gel; Oxy 10 Balance Emergency Spot Treatment Invisible Formula Gel; Oxy 10 Balance Maximum Medicated Face Wash; Oxy 5 Regular Strength Cover-Up Cream; Oxy 5 Regular Strength Vanishing Lotion; Oxy 5 Sensitive Skin Vanishing Lotion; Oxy Balance Deep Action Night Formula Lotion; Oxy Balance Emergency Spot Treatment Invisible Formula; Oxyderm 10 Lotion; Oxyderm 20 Lotion; Oxyderm 5 Lotion; PanOxyl 10 Bar; PanOxyl 10 Gel; PanOxyl 10 Wash; PanOxyl 15 Gel; PanOxyl 20 Gel; PanOxyl 5 Bar; PanOxyl 5 Gel; PanOxyl 5 Wash; PanOxyl AQ 10 Gel; PanOxyl AQ 2½ Gel; PanOxyl AQ 5 Gel; PanOxyl Aquagel 10; PanOxyl Aquagel 2.5; PanOxyl Aquagel 20; PanOxyl Aquagel 5; Solugel 4; Solugel 8; Student's Choice Acne Medication; Triaz; Triaz Cleanser; Xerac BP 5.*

Note: For a listing of dosage forms and brand names by country availability, see *Dosage Forms* section(s).

## Category

Antiacne agent (topical); keratolytic (topical).

## Indications

Note: Bracketed information in the *Indications* section refers to uses that are not included in U.S. product labeling.

### Accepted

Acne vulgaris(treatment)—Indicated for the topical treatment of mild to moderate acne vulgaris. In more severe acne, benzoyl peroxide may be indicated as an adjunct in therapeutic regimens including oral and topical antibiotics, retinoic acid preparations, and sulfur/salicylic acid–containing preparations.

[Ulcer, decubital (treatment)] or
[Ulcer, stasis (treatment)]—Benzoyl peroxide, usually in a 20% strength, is used as an oxidizing agent in the treatment of decubital or stasis ulcers.

## Pharmacology/Pharmacokinetics

### Physicochemical characteristics
Molecular weight—242.23 (hydrous).

### Mechanism of action/Effect
Benzoyl peroxide slowly releases active oxygen.

Acne vulgaris—Benzoyl peroxide has antibacterial action against *Propionibacterium acnes* in treatment of acne vulgaris. Benzoyl peroxide improves both inflammatory and noninflammatory lesions of acne. The medication also has some keratolytic effect, which produces comedo lysis, as well as drying and desquamative actions that contribute to its efficacy.

Decubital or statis ulcers—Benzoyl peroxide stimulates epithelial cell proliferation and the production of granulation tissue in treatment of decubital or stasis ulcers.

**Absorption**
Absorbed by the skin.

**Biotransformation**
Metabolized in skin to benzoic acid. About 5% of the metabolized medication is systemically absorbed and eliminated unchanged in the urine.

**Onset of action**
Improvement in condition is usually noticeable within 4 to 6 weeks.

**Elimination**
Renal; excreted as benzoic acid in urine.

## Precautions to Consider

### Carcinogenicity/Tumorigenicity
Benzoyl peroxide is not considered to be a carcinogen and does not show tumor-initiating ability; however, data from a study using mice known to be highly susceptible to cancer suggest that benzoyl peroxide acts as a tumor promoter.

### Pregnancy/Reproduction
Pregnancy—This medicine may be systemically absorbed. Studies have not been done in humans or animals.
FDA Pregnancy Category C.

### Breast-feeding
It is not known whether benzoyl peroxide is distributed into breast milk. Problems in humans have not been documented; however, benzoyl peroxide may be systemically absorbed.

### Pediatrics
Children up to 12 years of age—Appropriate studies on the relationship of age to the effects of benzoyl peroxide have not been performed in this age group. Safety and efficacy have not been established.

Children 12 years of age and over—Pediatrics-specific problems that would limit the usefulness of this medication in this age group are not expected.

### Geriatrics
Appropriate studies on the relationship of age to the effects of benzoyl peroxide have not been performed in the geriatric population. However, geriatrics-specific problems that would limit the usefulness of this medication in the elderly are not expected.

### Drug interactions and/or related problems
The following drug interactions and/or related problems have been selected on the basis of their potential clinical significance (possible mechanism in parentheses where appropriate)—not necessarily inclusive (» = major clinical significance):

Note: Combinations containing any of the following medications, depending on the amount present, may also interact with this medication.

Acne products, topical, or products containing a peeling agent, such as
  Resorcinol
  Salicylic acid
  Sulfur
Alcohol-containing products, topical, such as
  After-shave lotions
  Astringents
  Cosmetics or soaps with a strong drying effect
  Shaving creams or lotions or
Hair products, skin-irritating, such as hair permanents or hair removal products or
Isotretinoin or
Products containing lime or spices, topical or
Soaps or cleansers, abrasive
  (concurrent use with benzoyl peroxide on the same area of the skin may cause a cumulative irritant or drying effect, especially with the application of peeling, desquamating, or abrasive agents, resulting in excessive irritation of the skin. If irritation occurs, the strength or dose of benzoyl peroxide may need to be reduced or application temporarily discontinued until the skin is less sensitive)
Antibiotics, topical, such as clindamycin or erythromycin or
Retinoids, topical, such as adapalene or tretinoin
  (although these medications are used in a treatment regimen with benzoyl peroxide for therapeutic effect, their use on the same area of the skin at the same time is not recommended. The oxidizing action of benzoyl peroxide degrades antibiotics over time. A physical incompatibility between the use of the medications and benzoyl peroxide or a change in pH may reduce their efficacy if used simultaneously. When used together for clinical effect, it is recommended that these medications and benzoyl peroxide be used at different times of the day, such as morning and night, to minimize possible skin irritation, unless otherwise directed. If irritation occurs, changes in dose or frequency may be needed until the skin is less sensitive)

### Medical considerations/Contraindications
The medical considerations/contraindications included have been selected on the basis of their potential clinical significance (reasons given in parentheses where appropriate)—not necessarily inclusive (» = major clinical significance).

*Risk-benefit should be considered when the following medical problems exist:*

Dermatitis, seborrheic or
Eczema or
» Inflammation of skin, acute, or denuded skin, including sunburn
  (irritation may be increased; benzoyl peroxide should be discontinued until the skin is less sensitive)
Sensitivity to benzoyl peroxide or parabens

## Side/Adverse Effects
The following side/adverse effects have been selected on the basis of their potential clinical significance (possible signs and symptoms in parentheses where appropriate)—not necessarily inclusive:

### Those indicating need for medical attention
Incidence less frequent or rare
  *Allergic contact dermatitis* (burning, blistering, crusting, itching, severe redness, or swelling of skin); *irritant effect* (painful irritation of skin); *skin rash*

### Those indicating need for medical attention only if they continue or are bothersome
Incidence less frequent
  *Dryness or peeling of skin*—may occur after a few days; *feeling of warmth, mild stinging, or redness of skin*

## Overdose
For specific information on the agents used in the management of benzoyl peroxide overdose, see:
• *Corticosteroids (Topical)* monograph.

For more information on the management of overdose or unintentional ingestion, **contact a Poison Control Center** (see *Poison Control Center Listing*).

### Clinical effects of overdose
The following effects have been selected on the basis of their potential clinical significance (possible signs and symptoms in parentheses where appropriate)—not necessarily inclusive:

  *Burning, itching, scaling, redness, or swelling of skin, severe*

### Treatment of overdose
Medication should be discontinued. After symptoms and signs of overdosage subside, a reduced dosage schedule may be cautiously reinstated.

Specific treatment—Emollients, cool compresses, and/or topical corticosteroid preparations may be used to hasten resolution of overdosage.

## Patient Consultation
As an aid to patient consultation, refer to *Advice for the Patient, Benzoyl Peroxide (Topical)*.
In providing consultation, consider emphasizing the following selected information (» = major clinical significance):

### Before using this medication
» Conditions affecting use, especially:
  Sensitivity to benzoyl peroxide or to parabens
  Other medical problems, especially acute inflammation of skin or denuded skin, including sunburn

### Proper use of this medication
» Importance of not using more medication than the amount recommended
» Avoiding contact with the eyes, mucous membranes, and sensitive areas of the neck
» Not applying medication to raw or irritated skin, including windburned or sunburned skin, or, unless told otherwise, to open wounds
  Reading patient directions carefully before use

*Proper administration*
  For cream, gel, lotion, or stick dosage form
    Before applying—Washing affected area with nonmedicated soap and water or with a mild cleanser; gently patting dry

Applying enough medication to cover affected area and rubbing in gently
*For shave cream dosage form*
  Wetting area to be shaved; applying a small amount and gently rubbing over entire area; shaving; rinsing area and patting dry; not using after-shave lotions or other drying face products without checking with physician
*For cleansing bar or lotion or soap dosage form*
  Using to wash affected areas
*For facial mask dosage form*
  Before applying—Washing affected area with nonmedicated cleanser; rinsing and patting skin dry
  Using circular motion, applying thin layer of mask evenly over affected area
  Allowing mask to dry for 15 to 25 minutes
  Rinsing thoroughly with warm water and patting dry
  Washing hands afterwards to remove any lingering medication

» Proper dosing
  Missed dose: Applying as soon as possible
» Proper storage

## Precautions while using this medication
Possibility that skin will become irritated or that acne may appear to worsen during the first 3 weeks of therapy; checking with health care professional if skin problem has not improved within 4 to 6 weeks
Not washing the areas of the skin treated with benzoyl peroxide for at least 1 hour after application
» Avoiding use of any other topical product on the same area within 1 hour before or after application of benzoyl peroxide to avoid physical incompatibilities or excessive skin irritation
Either checking with health care professional before using or avoiding use of other topical acne or skin products containing a peeling agent (resorcinol, salicylic acid, sulfur, or tretinoin), irritating hair products (permanents or hair removal products), sun-sensitizing skin products (could contain lime or spices), alcohol-containing skin products, or drying or abrasive skin products (some cosmetics or soaps or skin cleansers); sometimes benzoyl peroxide is used with topical antibiotics or topical tretinoin but medication is applied at different times of the day to lessen skin irritation
» Medication may bleach hair or colored fabrics
Checking with doctor any time skin becomes too dry or too irritated; choosing proper skin products to reduce skin dryness or irritation

## Side/adverse effects
Signs of potential side effects, especially allergic contact dermatitis, irritant effect, or skin rash

# General Dosing Information
This medication contains an oxidizing agent that may bleach hair and colored fabrics.

## For treatment of acne
• Benzoyl peroxide should not be applied to acutely inflamed, denuded, or highly sensitive skin, unless otherwise directed by physician as in treating an ulceration.
• Therapy may be initiated with the 2.5 or 5% cream, gel, or lotion, then changed to the 10% strength after 3 to 4 weeks, if needed, or sooner if tolerance to the lower strengths has been determined.
• After treatment with benzoyl peroxide for approximately 8 to 12 weeks, maximum lesion reduction may be expected. Continued prophylactic use of benzoyl peroxide is usually required to maintain optimal therapeutic response.
• In fair-skinned patients or under excessively dry atmospheric conditions, it is recommended that therapy be initiated with one application daily and gradually increased up to 2 to 4 times a day (depending on the dosage form) as tolerated.

## For treatment of decubital or stasis ulcers
• A protective ointment should be applied to a wide area bordering the ulcer to decrease the possibility of irritant dermatosis of the surrounding skin.
• Ulcers should be treated by applying a sterile dressing of terry cloth moistened with normal saline and saturated with 20% lotion to the clean and surgically debrided ulcer. Occlude the dressed area with a plastic film and apply an abdominal dressing pad overall and tape firmly in place. Change the dressing every 8 hours in large ulcers and every 12 hours in small ulcers.
• For maximal therapeutic efficacy, the lotion dressing should be kept moist and as close to 37 °C (98.6 °F) as possible: the plastic film is used to retain moisture and the abdominal dressing pad is used to increase the local temperature through its insulating effect.
• Exuberant granulation tissue may be kept below the epidermal level with cauterization by a silver nitrate stick to facilitate ingrowth of epithelium.
• Severe ulcers may be treated by packing with surgical gauze saturated with 20% lotion to facilitate good contact with the walls of the cavity and then occluding.
• Large amounts of serous exudate appearing on the ulcer surface is a normal response to benzoyl peroxide therapy.
• Two weeks may pass before progress is visible in large chronic ulcers.

# Topical Dosage Forms
Note: Bracketed uses in the *Dosage Forms* section refer to categories of use and/or indications that are not included in U.S. product labeling.

## BENZOYL PEROXIDE CLEANSING BAR
### Usual adult and adolescent dose
Acne vulgaris—
  Topical, to the skin, as a 5 or 10% cleansing bar two or three times a day or as directed.
### Usual pediatric dose
Acne vulgaris—
  Children up to 12 years of age: Safety and efficacy have not been established.
  Children 12 years of age and over: See *Usual adult and adolescent dose*.
### Strength(s) usually available
U.S.—
  5% (OTC) [*PanOxyl 5 Bar*].
  10% (OTC) [*Desquam-X 10 Bar; Fostex 10 Bar; PanOxyl 10 Bar*].
Canada—
  5% (OTC) [*PanOxyl 5 Bar*].
  10% (Rx) [*PanOxyl 10 Bar*].
### Packaging and storage
Store below 40 °C (104 °F), preferably between 15 and 30 °C (59 and 86 °F), in a well-closed container, unless otherwise specified by manufacturer.
### Auxiliary labeling
• For external use only.

## BENZOYL PEROXIDE CLEANSING LOTION
### Usual adult and adolescent dose
Acne vulgaris—
  Topical, to the skin, as a 5 to 10% cleansing lotion one or two times a day.
### Usual pediatric dose
Acne vulgaris—
  Children up to 12 years of age: Safety and efficacy have not been established.
  Children 12 years of age and over: See *Usual adult and adolescent dose*.
### Strength(s) usually available
U.S.—
  2½% (Rx) [*Benzac AC Wash 2½*; GENERIC].
  4% (Rx) [*Brevoxyl-4 Cleansing Lotion* (cetyl alcohol)].
  5% (Rx) [*Benzac AC Wash 5 (Rx); Benzac W Wash 5 (Rx); Desquam-X 5 Wash (Rx)*; GENERIC].
  8% (Rx) [*Brevoxyl-8 Cleansing Lotion* (cetyl alcohol)].
  10% [*Benzac AC Wash 10 (Rx); Benzac W Wash 10 (Rx); Desquam-X 10 Wash (Rx); Fostex 10 Wash (OTC); Oxy 10 Balance Maximum Medicated Face Wash (OTC); Triaz Cleanser (Rx)*; GENERIC].
Canada—
  5% [*Benzac W Wash 5 (OTC); 5 Benzagel Acne Wash (OTC)* (cetyl alcohol; methylparaben; paraben); *5 Benzagel Liquid Acne Soap (OTC); Desquam-X 5 Wash (Rx); PanOxyl 5 Wash (Rx)* (parabens)].
  10% (Rx) [*Benzac W Wash 10; Desquam-X 10 Wash; PanOxyl 10 Wash* (parabens)].
### Packaging and storage
Store between 15 and 30 °C (59 and 86 °F), in a well-closed container, unless otherwise specified by manufacturer. Protect from freezing.
### Auxiliary labeling
• Shake well.
• For external use only.
Note: *Benzac W* does not require shaking.

## BENZOYL PEROXIDE CREAM
### Usual adult and adolescent dose
Acne vulgaris—
  Topical, to the skin, as a 5 to 10% cream one or two times a day.

**Usual pediatric dose**
Acne vulgaris—
  Children up to 12 years of age: Safety and efficacy have not been established.
  Children 12 years of age and over: See *Usual adult and adolescent dose*.

**Strength(s) usually available**
U.S.—
  5% [*BenzaShave 5 Cream (Rx)* (methylparaben; propylparaben); *Cuticura Acne 5 Cream (OTC)*; *Exact 5 Tinted Cream (OTC)* (parabens); *Exact 5 Vanishing Cream (OTC)* (parabens)].
  10% [*Ambi 10 Acne Medication (OTC)* (parabens); *Acne-Aid Vanishing Cream (OTC)* (methylparaben; propylparaben); *BenzaShave 10 Cream (Rx)* (methylparaben; propylparaben); *Clearasil Maximum Strength Medicated Anti-Acne 10 Tinted Cream (OTC)* (methylparaben; propylparaben); *Clearasil Maximum Strength Medicated Anti-Acne 10 Vanishing Cream (OTC)*; *Fostex 10 Cream (OTC)* (methylparaben; propylparaben)].
Canada—
  5% (OTC) [*Clearasil BP Plus Skin Tone Cream*; *Oxy 5 Regular Strength Cover-Up Cream*].

**Packaging and storage**
Store between 15 and 30 °C (59 and 86 °F), in a well-closed container, unless otherwise specified by manufacturer. Protect from freezing.

**Auxiliary labeling**
• For external use only.

## BENZOYL PEROXIDE FACIAL MASK

**Usual adult and adolescent dose**
Acne vulgaris—
  Topical, to the skin, as a 5% facial mask once a week to once a day, or as directed.

**Usual pediatric dose**
Acne vulgaris—
  Children up to 12 years of age: Safety and efficacy have not been established.
  Children 12 years of age and over: See *Usual adult and adolescent dose*.

**Strength(s) usually available**
U.S.—
  5% (OTC) [*Neutrogena Acne Mask 5*].
Canada—
  Not commercially available.

**Packaging and storage**
Store below 40 °C (104 °F), preferably between 15 and 30 °C (59 and 86 °F), in a well-closed container, unless otherwise specified by manufacturer. Protect from freezing.

**Auxiliary labeling**
• For external use only.

## BENZOYL PEROXIDE GEL USP

**Usual adult and adolescent dose**
Acne vulgaris—
  Topical, to the skin, as a 2.5 to 20% gel one or two times a day.

**Usual pediatric dose**
Acne vulgaris—
  Children up to 12 years of age: Safety and efficacy have not been established.
  Children 12 years of age and over: See *Usual adult and adolescent dose*.

**Strength(s) usually available**
U.S.—
  2.5% [*Acne-Aid Aqua Gel (OTC)*; *Benzac AC 2½ Gel (Rx)*; *Benzac W 2½ Gel (Rx)*; *Clear By Design 2.5 Gel (Rx)*; *Desquam-E 2.5 Gel (Rx)*; *Desquam-X 2.5 Gel (Rx)*; *PanOxyl AQ 2½ Gel (Rx)* (methylparaben); GENERIC].
  4% (Rx) [*Brevoxyl-4 Gel* (cetyl alcohol; stearyl alcohol)].
  5% [*5 Benzagel (Rx)*; *Benzac AC 5 Gel (Rx)*; *Benzac 5 Gel (Rx)* (alcohol 12%); *Benzac W 5 Gel (Rx)*; *Clean & Clear Persagel 5 (OTC)*; *Clearplex 5*; *Del-Aqua-5 Gel*; *Desquam-E 5 Gel (Rx)*; *Desquam-X 5 Gel (Rx)*; *Fostex 5 Gel (OTC)*; *Oxy Balance Emergency Spot Treatment Invisible Formula (OTC)*; *PanOxyl AQ 5 Gel (Rx)* (methylparaben); *PanOxyl 5 Gel (Rx)* (alcohol 20%); GENERIC].
  6% (Rx) [*Triaz*].
  8% (Rx) [*Brevoxyl-8 Gel* (cetyl alcohol; stearyl alcohol)].
  10% [*Benzac AC 10 Gel (Rx)*; *Benzac 10 Gel (Rx)* (alcohol 12%); *Benzac W 10 Gel (Rx)*; *10 Benzagel (Rx)*; *Clean & Clear Persagel 10 (OTC)*; *Clearplex 10 (OTC)*; *Del-Aqua-10 Gel (OTC)*; *Desquam-E 10 Gel (Rx)*; *Desquam-X 10 Gel (Rx)*; *Fostex 10 BPO Gel (OTC)*; *Oxy 10 Balance Emergency Spot Treatment Cover-Up Formula Gel (OTC)*; *Oxy 10 Balance Emergency Spot Treatment Invisible Formula Gel (OTC)*; *PanOxyl AQ 10 Gel (Rx)* (methylparaben); *PanOxyl 10 Gel (Rx)* (alcohol 20%); *Triaz (Rx)*; GENERIC].
Canada—
  2.5% [*Acetoxyl 2.5 Gel (Rx)* (acetone); *2.5 Benzagel Acne Gel (OTC)* (alcohol 15%); *H₂Oxyl 2.5 Gel (Rx)*; *PanOxyl Aquagel 2.5 (Rx)*].
  4% (Rx) [*Solugel 4*].
  5% [*Acetoxyl 5 Gel (Rx)* (acetone); *Benzac AC 5 Gel (Rx)*; *Benzac W 5 Gel (OTC)*; *5 Benzagel Acne Gel (OTC)* (alcohol 15%); *Dermoxyl Aqua 5 Gel (OTC)*; *Dermoxyl 5 Gel (OTC)* (acetone); *Desquam-X 5 Gel (Rx)*; *H₂Oxyl 5 Gel (Rx)*; *PanOxyl Aquagel 5 (Rx)*; *PanOxyl 5 Gel (Rx)* (alcohol); *Xerac BP 5 (Rx)*].
  8% (Rx) [*Solugel 8*].
  10% (Rx) [*Acetoxyl 10 Gel* (acetone); *Benzac AC 10 Gel*; *Benzac W 10 Gel*; *10 Benzagel Acne Gel* (alcohol 15%); *Dermoxyl 10 Gel* (acetone); *Desquam-X 10 Gel*; *H₂Oxyl 10 Gel*; *PanOxyl Aquagel 10*; *PanOxyl 10 Gel* (alcohol)].
  15% (Rx) [*PanOxyl 15 Gel* (alcohol)].
  20% (Rx) [*Acetoxyl 20 Gel* (acetone); *Dermoxyl 20 Gel* (acetone); *H₂Oxyl 20 Gel*; *PanOxyl Aquagel 20*; *PanOxyl 20 Gel* (alcohol)].

**Packaging and storage**
Store below 40 °C (104 °F), preferably between 15 and 30 °C (59 and 86 °F), unless otherwise specified by manufacturer. Store in a tight container. Protect from freezing.

**Auxiliary labeling**
• For external use only.

## BENZOYL PEROXIDE LOTION USP

**Usual adult and adolescent dose**
Acne vulgaris—
  Topical, to the skin, as a 5 to 10% lotion one to four times a day.
[Decubital ulcer] or
[Stasis ulcer]—
  Topical, to the ulcer, as a 20% lotion every 8 hours for large ulcers and every 12 hours for small ulcers.

**Usual pediatric dose**
Acne vulgaris—
  Children up to 12 years of age: Safety and efficacy have not been established.
  Children 12 years of age and over: See *Usual adult and adolescent dose*.

**Strength(s) usually available**
U.S.—
  5% (OTC) [*Benoxyl 5 Lotion*; GENERIC].
  5.5% (OTC) [*Loroxide 5.5 Lotion*].
  10% (OTC) [*Benoxyl 10 Lotion* (methylparaben; propylparaben); *Clearasil Maximum Strength Medicated Anti-Acne 10 Vanishing Lotion*; *Noxzema Clear-ups Maximum Strength 10 Lotion* (methylparaben; propylparaben); *Noxzema Clear-ups On-The-Spot 10 Lotion* (methylparaben; propylparaben); *Oxy Balance Deep Action Night Formula Lotion*; *Student's Choice Acne Medication*; GENERIC].
Canada—
  2.5% (OTC) [*2.5 Benzagel Acne Lotion*; *Oxy 5 Sensitive Skin Vanishing Lotion*].
  5% [*Acnomel B.P. 5 Lotion (OTC)*; *Benoxyl 5 Lotion (Rx)*; *5 Benzagel Acne Lotion (OTC)*; *Clearasil BP Plus 5 Lotion (OTC)*; *Dermacne (OTC)*; *Loroxide 5 Lotion (Rx)*; *Oxyderm 5 Lotion (Rx)*; *Oxy 5 Regular Strength Vanishing Lotion (OTC)*].
  10% (Rx) [*Benoxyl 10 Lotion*; *Oxyderm 10 Lotion*].
  20% (Rx) [*Benoxyl 20 Lotion*; *Oxyderm 20 Lotion*].

**Packaging and storage**
Store below 40 °C (104 °F), preferably between 15 and 30 °C (59 and 86 °F), unless otherwise specified by manufacturer. Store in a tight container. Protect from freezing.

**Preparation of dosage form**
In some products, benzoyl peroxide powder is packaged separately and must be added to the lotion before dispensing.

**Auxiliary labeling**
• Shake well.
• For external use only.

## BENZOYL PEROXIDE STICK

**Usual adult and adolescent dose**
Acne vulgaris—
  Topical, to the skin, as a 10% stick one to three times a day.

**Usual pediatric dose**
Acne vulgaris—
  Children up to 12 years of age: Safety and efficacy have not been established.
  Children 12 years of age and over: See *Usual adult and adolescent dose*.

**Strength(s) usually available**
U.S.—
  Not commercially available.
Canada—
  Not commercially available.

**Packaging and storage**
Store below 40 °C (104 °F), preferably between 15 and 30 °C (59 and 86 °F), in a well-closed container, unless otherwise specified by manufacturer.

**Auxiliary labeling**
• For external use only.

## Selected Bibliography
Berson DS, Shalita A. The treatment of acne: the role of combination therapies. J Am Acad Dermatol 1995; 32(5 Pt 3): S113-S115.
Leyden JJ, Shalita AR. Rational therapy for acne vulgaris: an update on topical treatment. J Am Acad Dermatol 1986 Oct; (4 Pt 2): 907-14.
Leyden JJ. New understandings of the pathogenesis of acne. J Am Acad Dermatol 1995; 32(5 Pt 3): S15-S25.

Revised: 07/29/98

---

**BENZPHETAMINE**—See *Appetite Suppressants (Systemic)*

**BENZTHIAZIDE**—See *Diuretics, Thiazide (Systemic)*

**BENZTROPINE**—See *Antidyskinetics (Systemic)*

**BENZYL BENZOATE**—The *Benzyl Benzoate (Topical)* monograph is not included in this published version of the USP DI database. Copies of the monograph are available on request from Micromedex, Inc. - Reprint Requests, 6200 S. Syracuse Way, Suite 300, Englewood, CO 80111; telephone (303) 486-6400; telefax (303) 486-6464; Email: USPDI@MDX.COM.

**BEPRIDIL**—See *Calcium Channel Blocking Agents (Systemic)*

---

# BERACTANT  Intratracheal-Local

VA CLASSIFICATION (Primary): RE700
Commonly used brand name(s): *Survanta*.
Another commonly used name is modified bovine surfactant extract.
Note: For a listing of dosage forms and brand names by country availability, see *Dosage Forms* section(s).

## Category
Pulmonary surfactant.

## Indications
**Accepted**
Respiratory distress syndrome, neonatal (prophylaxis and treatment)—Beractant intratracheal suspension is indicated for the prophylaxis (prevention strategy) and treatment (rescue strategy) of respiratory distress syndrome (RDS), also known as hyaline membrane disease, in premature infants.
  Beractant is used to prevent RDS in infants with birth weights of less than 1250 grams who are at risk of developing RDS or who show evidence of surfactant deficiency. For prevention of RDS, beractant should be given as soon as possible after the infant's birth, preferably within 15 minutes after birth.
  Beractant is used in the rescue treatment of RDS in infants who have developed RDS, confirmed by chest radiography, and who require mechanical ventilation. For rescue treatment, beractant should be given as soon as possible after diagnosis of RDS is confirmed and the infant is placed on a respirator, preferably within 8 hours after the infant's birth.

## Pharmacology/Pharmacokinetics
**Mechanism of action/Effect**
Beractant is a natural bovine lung extract containing phospholipids, neutral lipids, fatty acids, and the two hydrophobic, low-molecular-weight surfactant-associated proteins, SP-B and SP-C (beractant does not contain the hydrophilic, large-molecular-weight protein, SP-A). Colfosceril palmitate, palmitic acid, and tripalmitin are added to standardize the composition of beractant and make it similar to natural lung surfactant by optimizing surface tension-lowering properties. When beractant is used as a replacement for deficient endogenous lung surfactant, it is effective in lowering surface tension on alveolar surfaces during respiration and stabilizing the alveoli against collapse at resting transpulmonary pressures. Therefore, beractant reduces the incidence of RDS, mortality due to RDS, and air-leak complications.
Neonatal RDS develops primarily in premature infants because of pulmonary immaturity, including a deficiency of endogenous lung surfactant that results in higher alveolar surface tension and lower compliance properties. Without sufficient endogenous lung surfactant, progressive alveolar collapse occurs and both oxygen and carbon dioxide exchange are impaired. Also, RDS appears to be characterized by high pulmonary vascular permeability and increased lung tissue water. Fluid and protein that leak into alveoli inactivate both endogenous and exogenous surfactant, worsening lung function.
Natural lung surfactant is a mixture of lipids and apoproteins secreted by the alveolar cells into the alveoli and respiratory air passages. Surfactant reduces the surface tension of pulmonary fluids and thereby increases lung compliance. It exhibits not only surface tension-reducing properties (contributed by the lipids) but also rapid spreading and adsorption (contributed by the apoproteins). The major fraction of the lipid component of natural lung surfactant is dipalmitoylphosphatidylcholine (DPPC, colfosceril palmitate); this comprises up to 70% of the natural surfactant by weight.

**Absorption**
Biophysical activity occurs locally at alveolar surface with no systemic absorption.

**Onset of action**
Marked improvements in oxygenation may occur within minutes of administration.

**Duration of action**
Significant improvements in arterial-alveolar oxygen ratio ($PaO_2/PAO_2$), inspired oxygen fraction ($FIO_2$), and mean airway pressure (MAP) were sustained for 48 to 72 hours in several studies of beractant-treated infants who had RDS.

## Precautions to Consider
**Cross-sensitivity and/or related problems**
Circulating antibodies to bovine surfactant proteins, SP-B and SP-C, as analyzed by Western blot immunoassay, were not detected in blood specimens taken from infants 7 and 28 days of age who had been treated previously with beractant after development of severe respiratory distress syndrome. Also, serum samples taken from infants 6 and 12 months of age who had been previously treated with beractant were negative for circulating antibodies to surfactant-associated proteins. However, the potential for an allergic response to foreign protein still exists with beractant.

**Carcinogenicity**
Long-term studies have not been performed in animals to evaluate the carcinogenic potential of beractant.

**Mutagenicity**
Ames mutagenicity studies with beractant were negative.

# Beractant (Intratracheal-Local)

**Pregnancy/Reproduction**
Fertility—No adverse effect on fertility was observed in rats given beractant.
Pregnancy—No information is available on the use of beractant during pregnancy.

**Breast-feeding**
No information is available on the use of beractant during breast-feeding.

**Pediatrics**
Appropriate studies on the relationship of age to the effects of beractant have not been performed in the pediatric population. No information is available on administration more than 48 hours after birth.

**Geriatrics**
No information is available on the relationship of age to the effects of beractant.

**Patient monitoring**
The following may be especially important in patient monitoring (other tests may be warranted in some patients, depending on condition; » = major clinical significance):

» Arterial blood gases
(after both prophylactic and rescue dosing, frequent arterial and transcutaneous measurements of systemic oxygen and carbon dioxide are recommended to prevent hyperoxia and hypercarbia, which may occur within minutes of administration of beractant; if hyperoxia develops and transcutaneous oxygen saturation is in excess of 95%, $FIO_2$ should be reduced until saturation is 90 to 95%; failure to reduce inspiratory ventilator pressures rapidly can result in lung overdistention and pulmonary air leaks)

Heart rate and
Oxygen saturation
(continuous monitoring is recommended during dosing procedure; if transient episodes of bradycardia and decreased oxygen saturation occur, procedure must be stopped and appropriate measures taken to relieve condition; dosing procedure may be resumed after stabilization of the infant)

## Side/Adverse Effects

Note: In controlled clinical studies, infants treated with beractant were at no greater risk than control infants for developing patent ductus arteriosus, intracranial hemorrhage, necrotizing enterocolitis, apnea, post-treatment infections, and pulmonary hemorrhage. Infants treated with beractant were at less risk for developing pulmonary air leaks and pulmonary interstitial emphysema. No particular surfactant or method of surfactant delivery was related to an increased incidence of intracranial hemorrhage. Surfactant therapy, in itself, may initiate hemodynamic changes that could predispose an infant to intracranial hemorrhage in certain circumstances. Such changes can probably be compensated for by careful management of oxygenation and ventilation.

Beractant-treated infants were at significantly greater risk for post-treatment nosocomial sepsis than were premature infants in control groups. However, the increased risk of sepsis was not associated with increased mortality.

The most commonly reported adverse effects in clinical trials were associated with particular dosing procedures or methods of administration. These effects include endotracheal tube reflux (noted in single-dose studies) and transient bradycardia and decreased oxygenation (noted in multidose studies).

The following side/adverse effects have been selected on the basis of their potential clinical significance (possible signs and symptoms in parentheses where appropriate)—not necessarily inclusive:

**Those indicating need for medical attention**
Incidence more frequent
*Bradycardia, transient (<60 beats per minute); carbon dioxide tension, increased; oxygen desaturation; reflux, endotracheal tube*

Incidence less frequent (<1%)
*Apnea; blockage, endotracheal tube; hypercarbia or hypocarbia; hypertension or hypotension; pallor; vasoconstriction*

## General Dosing Information

Beractant should be used only by neonatologists and other clinicians who are experienced in neonatal intubation and ventilatory management. Also, instillation of this medication should be performed only by trained medical personnel experienced in airway and clinical management of unstable premature infants. Adequate personnel, facilities, equipment, and medications are required to optimize the perinatal outcome in these premature infants. In addition, continuous clinical attention should be given to all infants prior to, during, and after administration of this medication.

Review of audiovisual materials provided by the manufacturer is recommended before using beractant to obtain a description of its dosing and administration procedures.

Prior to administration of beractant, proper placement of the endotracheal tube tip in the trachea (not in the esophagus or the right or left mainstream bronchus) should be confirmed. The endotracheal tube may be suctioned at the discretion of the clinician to ensure patency before administration of beractant.

Beractant intratracheal suspension is administered only by instillation into the trachea through a No. 5 end-hole French catheter. The length of the catheter should be shortened so that the tip of the catheter protrudes just beyond the endotracheal tube above the infant's carina. The catheter can be inserted into the endotracheal tube without interrupting ventilation by passing the catheter through a neonatal suction valve attached to the endotracheal tube. The neonatal suction valve maintains a closed airway circuit system by sealing the valve around the catheter. The catheter must be rigid enough to pass through the endotracheal tube without twisting or curling within the suction valve. Alternatively, beractant can be instilled through the catheter by briefly disconnecting the endotracheal tube from the ventilator. The infant should be allowed to stabilize before the dosing proceeds.

Prior to administration, the suspension should be warmed by allowing the vial to stand at room temperature for at least 20 minutes or by warming it in the hand for at least 8 minutes. No artificial warming methods should be used. For prophylactic doses, warming must begin before the infant's birth.

Four doses of four aliquots each can be administered in the infant's first 48 hours of life; doses should be given at least 6 hours apart, as follows:

### FIRST DOSE

The total dose for both prevention and rescue strategies is determined from the dosing chart provided by the manufacturer and is dependent on the infant's birth weight.

To ensure homogeneous distribution of beractant throughout the lungs, the total dose (100 mg of phospholipids [4 mL of suspension] per kg of birth weight) is divided into 4 aliquots (25 mg [1 mL] per kg of birth weight). The infant is supine during the dosing procedure. The respective aliquots are administered with the infant held in the following positions: infant's head and body inclined slightly downward with head turned to the right; infant's head and body inclined downward with head turned to the left; infant's head and body inclined upward with head turned to the right; infant's head and body inclined upward with head turned to the left.

The entire contents of the vial are slowly drawn into a plastic syringe through a 20-gauge or larger needle without filtering or shaking. The catheter is attached to the syringe and filled with beractant suspension. Any excess suspension beyond the total dose is discarded through the catheter so that only the total dose remains in the syringe. With the infant positioned appropriately, the first aliquot is injected gently through the catheter into the endotracheal tube over 2 to 3 seconds.

Prevention strategy—The catheter is removed from the endotracheal tube after the first quarter-dose, and the infant is ventilated manually, by means of a hand-bag with sufficient oxygen to prevent cyanosis at a ventilation rate of 60 breaths per minute and with enough positive pressure to provide adequate air exchange and chest wall excursion.

Rescue strategy—The catheter is removed from the endotracheal tube after the first quarter-dose and the infant is placed on the mechanical ventilator.

Both strategies—The infant is then repositioned for administration of each of the next quarter-doses. Between aliquots, the catheter is removed and the infant is ventilated for at least 30 seconds or until the infant is stabilized. Immediately after the ventilation period, the next aliquot is instilled and the same procedure is followed until the entire dose is administered. After the final instillation, the catheter is removed without being flushed with air or liquid. The infant is not suctioned for at least 1 hour after dosing unless signs of significant airway obstruction appear.

After completion of the dosing procedure, usual ventilator management and clinical care are resumed.

### ADDITIONAL DOSES

The need for subsequent doses is determined based on evidence of continuing respiratory distress in the infant. The following criteria for redosing are used
- Dose no sooner than 6 hours after the preceding dose if the infant remains intubated and requires at least 30% inspired oxygen to maintain a $PaO_2$ not less than 80 torr.

- For infants who received beractant as a prevention dose initially, radiographic confirmation of RDS is required before any additional doses are administered.
- Repeat doses are also 100 mg of phospholipids (or 4 mL suspension) per kg of birth weight, administered in four aliquots. The infant should not be reweighed.

Manual hand-bag ventilation should not be used for repeat doses. The infant is ventilated mechanically with ventilator settings adjusted to maintain appropriate oxygenation and ventilation.

## Intratracheal Dosage Forms

### BERACTANT INTRATRACHEAL SUSPENSION

**Usual pediatric dose**
Pulmonary surfactant (prophylaxis)—
  Intratracheal, the equivalent of 100 mg of phospholipids (4 mL of suspension) per kg of birth weight for the first dose (administered as four quarter-doses) as soon as possible within 15 minutes after infant's birth; additional doses should be administered no sooner than 6 hours later to infants who remain intubated and require at least 30% inspired oxygen.

Pulmonary surfactant (treatment)—
  Intratracheal, the equivalent of 100 mg of phospholipids (4 mL of suspension) per kg of birth weight for the first dose (administered as four quarter-doses) as soon as possible after diagnosis of respiratory distress syndrome (RDS) is confirmed and infant is placed on a respirator, preferably within 8 hours after birth; additional doses should be administered no sooner than 6 hours later to infants who remain intubated and require at least 30% inspired oxygen.

Note: Each dose is administered in four quarter-doses, with each quarter-dose being equivalent to 25 mg of beractant (1 mL of suspension) per kg of birth weight. Each quarter-dose is instilled slowly over 2 to 3 seconds through the catheter.

**Strength(s) usually available**
U.S.—
  25 mg of phospholipids per mL (200 mg per 8-mL vial) (Rx) [*Survanta* (sodium chloride, 0.09%)].

Canada—
  25 mg of phospholipids per mL (200 mg per 8-mL vial) (Rx) [*Survanta* (sodium chloride, 0.09%)].

**Packaging and storage**
Store unopened vials between 2 and 8 °C (35 and 46 °F). Protect from light.

**Preparation of dosage form**
The suspension should be warmed by allowing the vial to stand at room temperature for at least 20 minutes or by warming it in the hand for at least 8 minutes. No artificial warming methods should be used. For prevention doses, warming must begin before the infant's birth.

**Stability**
The optimum color of the suspension is off-white to light brown. Visual inspection before use is necessary to detect any discoloration of the product.
If the suspension appears to have separated, the vial should be swirled gently (not shaken) to resuspend any particles that may have settled during storage.

**Additional information**
Unopened, unused vials of the suspension that have been warmed to room temperature may be returned to the refrigerator within 8 hours of warming and stored for future use. However, warmed, unopened vials should not be returned to the refrigerator more than once.
Each single-use vial should be entered with a needle only once. Any unused suspension must be discarded.

## Selected Bibliography

Liechty EA, Donovan E, Purohit D, et al. Reduction of neonatal mortality after multiple doses of bovine surfactant in low birth weight neonates with respiratory distress syndrome. Pediatrics 1991 July; 88(1): 19-28.

Reynolds MS, Wallander KA. Surfactant for neonatal respiratory distress syndrome. J Pediatr Health Care 1990 Jul-Aug; 4(4): 209-15.

Yee WFH, Scarpelli EM. Surfactant replacement therapy. Pediatr Pulmonol 1991; 11: 65-80.

Developed: 8/15/95

---

# BETA-ADRENERGIC BLOCKING AGENTS    Ophthalmic

This monograph includes information on the following: 1) Betaxolol; 2) Carteolol†; 3) Levobunolol; 4) Metipranolol†; 5) Timolol.

VA CLASSIFICATION (Primary): OP110

Commonly used brand name(s): *Apo-Timop*[5]; *Betagan C Cap B.I.D.*[3]; *Betagan C Cap Q.D.*[3]; *Betagan Standard Cap*[3]; *Betoptic*[1]; *Betoptic S*[1]; *Gen-Timolol*[5]; *Ocupress*[2]; *OptiPranolol*[4]; *Timoptic*[5]; *Timoptic in Ocudose*[5].

Note: For a listing of dosage forms and brand names by country availability, see *Dosage Forms* section(s).

†Not commercially available in Canada.

## Category

Antiglaucoma agent (ophthalmic).

## Indications

Note: Bracketed information in the *Indications* section refers to uses that are not included in U.S. product labeling.

**Accepted**

Glaucoma, open-angle (treatment) or
Hypertension, ocular (treatment)—Ophthalmic beta-adrenergic blocking agents are indicated in the treatment of chronic open-angle glaucoma. They also may be used in the treatment of ocular hypertension. They may be used alone or in combination with other antiglaucoma agents.

Glaucoma, in aphakic eyes (treatment) or
Glaucoma, secondary (treatment)—[Betaxolol][1], [carteolol][1], [levobunolol][1], [metipranolol][1], and timolol are indicated in the treatment of glaucoma in aphakic eyes and in some cases of secondary glaucoma.

[Glaucoma, angle-closure (treatment adjunct)]—Betaxolol[1], carteolol[1], levobunolol[1], metipranolol[1], and timolol may be used in conjunction with miotics to reduce intraocular pressure in acute and chronic angle-closure glaucoma. However, the ophthalmic beta-adrenergic blocking agent's action alone is unlikely to terminate an acute attack of angle-closure glaucoma, because the agent produces little or no constriction of the pupil. Constriction of the pupil is necessary to pull the iris away from the trabeculum to relieve blockage of the trabecular meshwork.

[Glaucoma, angle-closure, *during* or *after* iridectomy (treatment)][1] or
[Glaucoma, malignant (treatment)][1]—Ophthalmic beta-adrenergic blocking agents may be used to lower intraocular pressure in the treatment of angle-closure glaucoma *during* or *after* iridectomy and in the treatment of malignant glaucoma.

Ophthalmic betaxolol may be especially useful in the treatment of glaucoma in patients with pulmonary disease because it is a relatively selective beta-1-adrenergic antagonist. Although ophthalmic betaxolol can have significant effects on pulmonary function in persons with pulmonary disease, it appears to do so much less frequently than non-selective beta-antagonists.

[1]Not included in Canadian product labeling.

## Pharmacology/Pharmacokinetics

**Physicochemical characteristics**
Molecular weight—
  Betaxolol: 343.89.
  Carteolol: 328.84.
  Levobunolol: 327.85.
  Metipranolol: 309.40.
  Timolol: 432.49.

**Mechanism of action/Effect**
Betaxolol is a cardioselective (beta-1-adrenergic) receptor blocking agent. Carteolol, levobunolol, metipranolol, and timolol are beta-1 and beta-2 (nonselective) adrenergic blocking agents. The exact mechanism of the ocular hypotensive action of ophthalmic beta-adrenergic blocking agents has not been established. However, it appears that the ophthalmic beta-adrenergic blocking agents reduce aqueous humor production, as demonstrated by tonography and fluorophotometry. A slight increase in aqueous humor outflow may be an additional mechanism.

**Other actions/effects**
Ophthalmic beta-adrenergic blocking agents, if systemically absorbed, are capable of producing beta-adrenergic receptor blockade in the bronchi and bronchioles. (This is less likely to occur with ophthalmic betaxolol

because it is a relatively selective beta-1-adrenergic blocking agent.) This action results in an increase in airway resistance because of unopposed parasympathetic activity. This effect is in keeping with the beta-2-adrenergic blocking action of these medications. It is possible that carteolol, because of its partial beta-agonist activity, may have less of a beta-blockade effect than the other ophthalmic beta-2-adrenergic blocking agents; however, the possible protection conferred by the beta-agonist effect has not been clinically evaluated. Betaxolol 1% solution, when compared to a placebo, was not shown to have a significant effect on pulmonary function as measured by forced expiratory volume in 1 second ($FEV_1$), forced vital capacity (FVC), and $FEV_1$/VC. However, in clinical use, ophthalmic betaxolol has caused a worsening of respiratory symptoms in some patients with pulmonary disease.

Ophthalmic beta-adrenergic blocking agents, if systemically absorbed, are also capable of reducing heart rate, myocardial contractility, and cardiac output, resulting in bradycardia and hypotension, in both healthy individuals and patients with heart disease. This is in keeping with the beta-1-adrenergic blocking action of these medications.

The ophthalmic beta-adrenergic blocking agents do not have significant membrane-stabilizing (local anesthetic) activity.

Ophthalmic beta-adrenergic blocking agents reduce normal as well as elevated intraocular pressure (IOP), whether or not it is accompanied by glaucoma.

Ophthalmic beta-adrenergic blocking agents have little or no effect on pupil size or accommodation compared with miosis produced by cholinergic agents.

### Absorption
Ophthalmic beta-adrenergic blocking agents may be systemically absorbed.

### Onset of action
Betaxolol, metipranolol, and timolol—Within 30 minutes following a single dose.
Levobunolol—Within 1 hour following a single dose.

### Time to peak effect
Betaxolol, carteolol, and metipranolol—Approximately 2 hours following a single dose. This applies to both betaxolol ophthalmic solution and suspension.
Levobunolol—Between 2 and 6 hours following a single dose.
Timolol—Within 1 to 2 hours following a single dose.

### Duration of action
Betaxolol—12 hours, following a single dose of either the ophthalmic solution or suspension.
Carteolol—More than 6 to 8 hours.
Levobunolol and timolol—A significant lowering of intraocular pressure may be maintained for up to 24 hours following a single dose.
Metipranolol—A reduction in intraocular pressure can be demonstrated 24 hours following a single dose.

## Precautions to Consider

### Cross-sensitivity and/or related problems
Patients sensitive to any of the ophthalmic or systemic beta-adrenergic blocking agents, such as acebutolol, atenolol, betaxolol, bisoprolol, carteolol, labetalol, levobunolol, metipranolol, metoprolol, nadolol, oxprenolol, penbutolol, pindolol, propranolol, sotalol, or timolol, may be sensitive to any other beta-adrenergic blocking agent also.

### Carcinogenicity
*Betaxolol*—In lifetime studies in mice and rats, betaxolol has not been shown to be carcinogenic when administered orally at doses of 6, 20, or 60 mg per kg of body weight (mg/kg) per day (mice) and at doses of 3, 12, or 48 mg/kg per day (rats).
*Carteolol*—In 2-year studies in mice and rats, carteolol has not been shown to be carcinogenic when administered orally at doses of up to 40 mg/kg per day.
*Metipranolol*—In lifetime studies, metipranolol has not been shown to be carcinogenic when administered orally to mice at doses of 5, 50, and 100 mg/kg per day and to rats at doses of up to 70 mg/kg per day.
*Timolol*—In a lifetime study in mice, timolol increased the incidence of malignant pulmonary tumors and mammary adenocarcinomas in female mice when administered orally at doses of 500 mg/kg per day, but not at 5 or 50 mg/kg per day.

### Tumorigenicity
*Betaxolol and carteolol*—Unknown.
*Levobunolol*—In a lifetime study, levobunolol increased the incidence of benign leiomyomas in female mice when administered orally at doses of 200 mg/kg per day (14,000 times the recommended human dose for glaucoma), but did not produce this effect at doses of 12 or 50 mg/kg per day (850 and 3500 times the human dose). In a 2-year study in rats, levobunolol increased the incidence of benign hepatomas in male rats when administered orally at doses 12,800 times the recommended human dose for glaucoma. Similar differences were not observed in rats when levobunolol was administered at oral doses equivalent to 350 to 2000 times the recommended human dose for glaucoma.
*Metipranolol*—In lifetime studies, female mice had an increased number of pulmonary adenomas when they were given metipranolol at an oral dose of 5 mg/kg per day. However, doses of 50 and 100 mg/kg per day did not produce this effect.
*Timolol*—In a 2-year study in rats, timolol increased the incidence of adrenal pheochromocytomas in male rats when administered orally at doses of 300 mg/kg per day (which are 250 times the maximum recommended human oral dose of 30 mg [1 drop of ophthalmic timolol contains about 1/150th of this dose or about 0.2 mg of timolol]). However, similar effects were not observed in rats when timolol was administered at oral doses equivalent to 20 or 80 times the maximum recommended human oral dose. In a lifetime study in mice, timolol increased the incidence of benign pulmonary tumors and benign uterine polyps in female mice when administered orally at doses of 500 mg/kg per day. However, doses of 5 and 50 mg/kg per day did not produce this effect. In addition, timolol increased the overall incidence of neoplasms in female mice at oral doses of 500 mg/kg per day.

### Mutagenicity
*Betaxolol*—*In vitro* and *in vivo* bacterial and mammalian cell assays have not shown betaxolol to be mutagenic.
*Carteolol*—Carteolol was not shown to be mutagenic in the Ames test and recombinant (rec)-assay and in the *in vivo* cytogenetic and dominant lethal assays.
*Levobunolol*—In microbiological and mammalian *in vitro* and *in vivo* assays, levobunolol was not shown to be mutagenic.
*Metipranolol*—Metipranolol was nonmutagenic in *in vivo* and *in vitro* bacterial and mammalian cell assays.
*Timolol*—Timolol was not shown to be mutagenic when tested *in vivo* (mouse) in the micronucleus test and cytogenetic assay (at doses up to 800 mg/kg) and *in vitro* in a neoplastic cell transformation assay (up to 0.1 mg per mL).

### Pregnancy/Reproduction
Fertility—*Betaxolol*: Studies in rabbits and rats have shown that betaxolol, administered at oral doses above 12 mg/kg and 128 mg/kg, respectively, causes drug-related postimplantation loss.
*Carteolol*: Studies in rats and mice have not shown that carteolol causes any adverse effects on male and female fertility when administered at doses of up to 150 mg/kg per day.
*Levobunolol*: Reproduction and fertility studies in rats showed no adverse effects on male or female fertility when levobunolol was administered at doses of up to 1800 times the recommended human dose for glaucoma.
*Metipranolol*: Reproduction and fertility studies on metipranolol in rats and mice showed no adverse effect on female or male fertility at oral doses of up to 25 mg/kg per day and 50 mg/kg per day, respectively.
*Timolol*: Reproduction and fertility studies in rats have not shown that timolol causes any adverse effects on male and female fertility when administered at doses of up to 125 times the maximum recommended human oral dose.

Pregnancy—
*Betaxolol*—
    Adequate and well-controlled studies in humans have not been done.
    In animal studies, betaxolol was not shown to cause teratogenic effects or other adverse effects on reproduction at subtoxic doses.
    FDA Pregnancy Category C.
*Carteolol*—
    Although adequate and well-controlled studies in humans have not been done, carteolol may be absorbed systemically.
    In rabbits and rats, carteolol, administered in doses approximately 1052 and 5264 times the maximum recommended human oral dose of 10 mg per 70 kg of body weight per day, respectively, resulted in maternotoxicity, increased incidence of fetal resorptions, and decreased fetal weights. In rats, carteolol, administered in doses approximately 212 times the maximum recommended human oral dose, resulted in a dose-related increase in wavy ribs in the developing rat fetus. However, in mice, carteolol, administered in doses up to approximately 1052 times the maximum recommended human oral dose, did not result in wavy ribs.
    FDA Pregnancy Category C.
*Levobunolol*—
    Adequate and well-controlled studies in humans have not been done.
    Although levobunolol has been shown to cause fetotoxicity in rabbits when administered at doses equivalent to 200 and 700 times

the recommended dose for the treatment of glaucoma, similar studies in rats have not shown levobunolol to cause fetotoxic effects when administered at doses of up to 1800 times the human dose for glaucoma. Moreover, in teratogenicity studies in rats, levobunolol was not shown to cause fetal malformations when administered at doses of up to 25 mg/kg per day (1800 times the recommended human dose for glaucoma). Also, levobunolol was not shown to have adverse effects on the postnatal development of animal offspring.

FDA Pregnancy Category C.

*Metipranolol—*
Adequate and well-controlled studies in humans have not been done.

No metipranolol-related effects were reported for the segment II teratology study in fetal rats when metipranolol was administered orally to pregnant rats in doses of up to 50 mg/kg per day during organogenesis. However, metipranolol has been shown to increase fetal resorption, fetal death, and delayed development when administered orally to pregnant rabbits at 50 mg/kg during organogenesis.

FDA Pregnancy Category C.

*Timolol—*
Although adequate and well-controlled studies in humans have not been done, timolol may be absorbed systemically.

Studies in rats have shown that timolol at doses of up to 50 mg/kg per day (50 times the maximum recommended human oral dose) causes delayed fetal ossification; however, there were no adverse effects on postnatal development of offspring. Teratogenic studies in mice and rabbits have not shown that timolol at doses of up to 50 mg/kg per day causes fetal malformations. In mice, timolol at doses of 1 gram per kg per day (1000 times the maximum recommended human oral dose) was maternotoxic and resulted in increased incidence of fetal resorptions. In rabbits, timolol at doses 100 times the maximum recommended human oral dose caused increased incidence of fetal resorptions but not maternotoxicity.

FDA Pregnancy Category C.

**Breast-feeding**

*Betaxolol—*Systemic betaxolol is distributed into breast milk in large enough quantities to have pharmacological effects. However, it is not known whether ophthalmic betaxolol is distributed into breast milk and problems in humans have not been documented.

*Carteolol—*It is not known whether systemic or ophthalmic carteolol is distributed into human breast milk; however, carteolol has been shown to be distributed into animal milk.

*Levobunolol—*It is not known whether ophthalmic levobunolol is distributed into breast milk. However, problems in humans have not been documented.

*Metipranolol—*It is not known whether ophthalmic metipranolol is distributed into breast milk. However, problems in humans have not been documented.

*Timolol—*Systemic timolol is distributed into breast milk. Problems in humans have not been documented for ophthalmic timolol; however, ophthalmic timolol may be systemically absorbed and distributed into the breast milk, possibly causing serious adverse reactions in the infants of nursing mothers.

**Pediatrics**

Although appropriate studies on the relationship of age to the effects of beta-adrenergic blocking agents, including the ophthalmic blocking agents, have not been performed in the pediatric population, infants should be treated cautiously and monitored for signs of dyspnea. In addition, the use of nasolacrimal occlusion should be emphasized for both infants and children.

**Geriatrics**

Although appropriate studies on the relationship of age to the effects of ophthalmic beta-adrenergic blocking agents have not been performed in the geriatric population, no geriatrics-specific problems have been documented to date. However, if significant systemic absorption of ophthalmic beta-adrenergic blocking agents occurs, the same geriatrics-related problems may occur that are possible with the systemic beta-adrenergic blocking agents. These include bradycardia, increased myocardial depression because of reduced metabolic and excretory capabilities in many elderly patients, and the increased risk of beta-adrenergic blocking agent–induced hypothermia in elderly patients.

In addition, elderly patients are more likely to have age-related peripheral vascular disease, which may require caution in patients receiving beta-adrenergic blocking agents.

**Drug interactions and/or related problems**

The following drug interactions and/or related problems have been selected on the basis of their potential clinical significance (possible mechanism in parentheses where appropriate)—not necessarily inclusive (» = major clinical significance):

Note: Combinations containing any of the following medications, depending on the amount present, may also interact with this medication.

Information concerning interactions between ophthalmic beta-adrenergic blocking agents and other medications is still limited. Some of the following potential interactions apply to beta-adrenergic blocking agents in general and are stated for cautionary reference until additional information specific to the ophthalmic beta-adrenergic blocking agents is available.

Allergen immunotherapy or
Allergenic extracts for skin testing
(if significant systemic absorption of ophthalmic beta-adrenergic blocking agents occurs, concurrent use of these agents in patients using ophthalmic beta-adrenergic blocking agents may increase the potential for serious systemic reaction or anaphylaxis)

Amiodarone
(if significant systemic absorption of ophthalmic beta-adrenergic blocking agents occurs, concurrent use may potentiate bradycardia, sinus arrest, and atrioventricular [AV] block, especially in patients with underlying sinus function impairment)

Anesthetics, hydrocarbon inhalation, such as:
Chloroform
Cyclopropane
Enflurane
Halothane
Isoflurane
Methoxyflurane
Trichloroethylene
(if significant systemic absorption of ophthalmic beta-adrenergic blocking agents occurs, concurrent use of hydrocarbon inhalation anesthetics may increase the risk of myocardial depression and hypotension because the beta-adrenergic blockade reduces the ability of the heart to respond to beta-adrenergically mediated sympathetic reflex stimuli; if it is necessary to reverse the effects of beta-adrenergic blocking agents during surgery, agonists, such as dobutamine, dopamine, isoproterenol, or norepinephrine, may be used but should be administered with caution, especially in patients receiving halothane. Some clinicians recommend gradual withdrawal of beta-adrenergic blocking agents 48 hours prior to elective surgery; however, this recommendation is controversial)

Antidiabetic agents, oral or
Insulin
(systemic beta-adrenergic blocking agents may affect diabetes mellitus therapy. This may also occur with ophthalmic beta-adrenergic blocking agents if there is significant systemic absorption. Nonselective beta-adrenergic blocking agents impair glycogenolysis and the hyperglycemic response to endogenous epinephrine, leading to persistence of hypoglycemia. Also, beta-adrenergic blocking agents, especially nonselective agents, decrease the release of insulin in response to hyperglycemia. Dosage adjustment of the antidiabetic agent may be required to avoid a severe hypoglycemic reaction. In addition, beta-adrenergic blocking agents may complicate patient monitoring by masking symptoms of hypoglycemia caused by epinephrine, such as increased heart rate and increased blood pressure, but not dizziness and sweating. Although selective or relatively selective beta-adrenergic blocking agents usually cause fewer problems with blood glucose levels, they may still mask symptoms of hypoglycemia)

Beta-adrenergic blocking agents, systemic
(if significant systemic absorption of ophthalmic beta-adrenergic blocking agents occurs, concurrent use of these medications may result in an additive effect on intraocular pressure or in additive systemic effects of beta-adrenergic blockade)

Calcium channel blocking agents
(if significant systemic absorption of ophthalmic beta-adrenergic blocking agents occurs, concurrent use of calcium channel blocking agents, such as bepridil, diltiazem, flunarizine, isradipine, nicardipine, nifedipine, nimodipine, and verapamil, may result in atrioventricular conduction disturbances, left ventricular failure, and hypotension; in some patients, if a calcium antagonist is necessary, nicardipine or nifedipine may be preferred because they have less effect on heart rate and conduction, although they may also cause greater hypotension; concurrent use of calcium channel blockers

and ophthalmic beta-adrenergic blocking agents should be used with care in patients with impaired cardiac function)

Catecholamine-depleting medications, such as the rauwolfia alkaloids:
Alseroxylon
Deserpidine
Rauwolfia serpentina
Reserpine
(if significant systemic absorption of ophthalmic beta-adrenergic blocking agents occurs, concurrent use of catecholamine-depleting medications may result in additive and possibly excessive beta-adrenergic blockade; although this effect is largely theoretical, close observation is recommended, since bradycardia and marked hypotension may occur)

Cimetidine
(if significant systemic absorption of ophthalmic beta-adrenergic blocking agents occurs, concurrent use with cimetidine may reduce the clearance of hepatically metabolized beta-adrenergic blocking agents, resulting in elevations of plasma concentrations)

Clonidine
(if significant systemic absorption of ophthalmic beta-adrenergic blocking agents occurs during concurrent use, discontinuation of clonidine therapy may increase the risk of clonidine-withdrawal hypertensive crisis; ideally, beta-adrenergic blocking agents should be discontinued several days before clonidine is discontinued; blood pressure control may also be impaired when the 2 are combined)

Cocaine
(cocaine may inhibit the therapeutic effects of systemic beta-adrenergic blocking agents, and may also have this effect on ophthalmic beta-adrenergic blocking agents)
(concurrent use of cocaine with systemic beta-adrenergic blocking agents may increase the risk of hypertension, excessive bradycardia, and possibly heart block because beta-adrenergic blockade may leave cocaine's alpha-adrenergic activity unopposed. This may also occur with ophthalmic beta-adrenergic blocking agents if significant systemic absorption of the ophthalmic beta-adrenergic blocking agent occurs)

Contrast media, iodinated
(if significant systemic absorption of ophthalmic beta-adrenergic blocking agents occurs, concurrent use with intravenous contrast media may increase the risk of moderate to severe anaphylaxis; these reactions may be refractory to treatment. There was no consensus among USP experts as to whether or not this interaction was clinically significant)

Fentanyl and derivatives
(preoperative chronic use of ophthalmic beta-adrenergic blocking agents [with the possible exception of betaxolol] may increase the risk of initial bradycardia following induction doses of fentanyl or any of its derivatives)

Flecainide
(if significant systemic absorption of ophthalmic beta-adrenergic blocking agents occurs, concurrent use may result in additive negative cardiac inotropic effects, especially, or perhaps only, in patients with cardiac problems)

Hypotension-producing medications, other (See *Appendix II*)
(if significant systemic absorption of ophthalmic beta-adrenergic blocking agents [with the possible exception of betaxolol] occurs, concurrent use may potentiate the hypotensive effects of these medications)

Methacholine
(if significant systemic absorption of ophthalmic beta-adrenergic blocking agents occurs, methacholine inhalation challenge should not be performed, since the reaction to methacholine may be exaggerated or prolonged and may not respond as rapidly to treatment with bronchodilators)

Nicotine
(nicotine increases the metabolism of beta-adrenergic blocking agents; if significant systemic absorption of ophthalmic beta-adrenergic blocking agents occurs, patients undergoing smoking cessation may experience an increase in the frequency of side/adverse effects caused by the blocking agents because of the subsequent decrease in the blocking agents' metabolism. There was no consensus among USP experts as to whether or not this interaction was clinically significant)

Phenothiazines
(if significant systemic absorption of ophthalmic beta-adrenergic blocking agents occurs, concurrent use may result in an increased plasma concentration of either the phenothiazine or the ophthalmic beta-adrenergic blocking agent because of inhibition of metabolism. This may result in additive hypotensive effects, irreversible retinopathy, cardiac arrhythmias, or tardive dyskinesia. There was no consensus among USP experts as to whether or not this interaction was clinically significant)

Phenytoin, intravenous
(if significant systemic absorption of ophthalmic beta-adrenergic blocking agents occurs, concurrent use may cause additive cardiac depressant effects. There was no consensus among USP experts as to whether or not this interaction was clinically significant)

Sympathomimetics, systemic
(if significant systemic absorption of ophthalmic beta-adrenergic blocking agents occurs, concurrent use may result in inhibition of the beta-adrenergic effects of sympathomimetics; depending on the type of sympathomimetic, this inhibition will occur with the beta-1-adrenergic cardiac effects and/or the beta-2-adrenergic bronchodilating effect; betaxolol will block primarily the beta-1-adrenergic effects)
(concurrent use of norepinephrine may result in mutual inhibition of therapeutic effects)

Xanthines, such as:
Aminophylline
Caffeine
Dyphylline
Oxtriphylline
Theophylline
(if significant systemic absorption of ophthalmic beta-adrenergic blocking agents [with the possible exception of betaxolol] occurs, concurrent use may result in inhibition of therapeutic effects of xanthines; in addition, concurrent use of xanthines [except dyphylline] with the ophthalmic beta-adrenergic blocking agents [with the possible exception of betaxolol] may decrease theophylline clearance, especially in patients with increased theophylline clearance induced by smoking; concurrent use requires careful monitoring)
(concurrent use with caffeine may result in inhibition of caffeine's therapeutic effect)

## Medical considerations/Contraindications

The medical considerations/contraindications included have been selected on the basis of their potential clinical significance (reasons given in parentheses where appropriate)—not necessarily inclusive (» = major clinical significance).

*Except under special circumstances, this medication should not be used when the following medical problems exist:*

» Asthma, bronchial (or history of) or
» Pulmonary disease, obstructive, severe chronic
(severe respiratory reactions, including death due to bronchospasm, have been reported in patients with asthma, following administration of the ophthalmic beta-adrenergic blocking agents. Although betaxolol appears to have a minimal effect on pulmonary function, caution should be used in patients with severe restriction of pulmonary function)

» Cardiac failure, overt or
» Cardiogenic shock or
» Heart block, 2nd- or 3rd-degree atrioventricular (AV) or
» Sinus bradycardia
(risk of further myocardial depression may occur with the use of the ophthalmic beta-adrenergic blocking agents)

» Previous allergic reaction to the ophthalmic beta-adrenergic blocking agent prescribed

*Risk-benefit should be considered when the following medical problems exist:*

» Bronchitis, nonallergenic or chronic or
» Emphysema or
» Pulmonary function impairment, other
(use of the ophthalmic beta-adrenergic blocking agents may promote bronchospasm and block bronchodilation produced by endogenous and exogenous catecholamine stimulation of beta-2-receptors. Although the effects of betaxolol on pulmonary function have been shown in some studies to be minimal in patients with reactive airway disease, there have been reports of asthmatic attacks and pulmonary distress during betaxolol treatment)

Cerebrovascular insufficiency
(potential effects on blood pressure and pulse; if signs of reduced cerebral blood flow occur following initiation of therapy, alternative therapy should be considered)

» Congestive heart failure
(risk of further depression of myocardial contractility)

» Cardiac failure, history of or
Heart block, history of
(possible risk of myocardial depression; treatment should be discontinued at first signs of cardiac failure)
» Diabetes mellitus, especially labile diabetes or
» Hypoglycemia
(ophthalmic beta-adrenergic blocking agents may mask some signs and symptoms of hypoglycemia, such as tachycardia and tremor, although they do not mask dizziness and sweating)
» Hyperthyroidism
(ophthalmic beta-adrenergic blocking agents may mask certain signs and symptoms of hyperthyroidism; abrupt withdrawal may precipitate a thyroid storm)
Myasthenia gravis
(beta-adrenergic blockade may potentiate muscle weakness related to certain myasthenic symptoms, such as diplopia, ptosis, and generalized weakness)

**Patient monitoring**
The following may be especially important in patient monitoring (other tests may be warranted in some patients, depending on condition; » = major clinical significance):
Intraocular pressure determination
(recommended during, and following, the first month of therapy during which stabilization of the pressure-lowering response to the ophthalmic beta-adrenergic blocking agent usually occurs; thereafter, intraocular pressure should be determined as necessary)

## Side/Adverse Effects

Note: Even in patients *without* a history of cardiac failure, continued depression of the myocardium with beta-blockers, including ophthalmic beta-adrenergic blocking agents, over a period of time can lead to cardiac failure, if significant systemic absorption occurs. However, betaxolol and metipranolol may be less likely to cause myocardial depression. At the first sign or symptom of cardiac failure, the ophthalmic beta-adrenergic blocking agent should be discontinued.

Although ophthalmic beta-adrenergic blocking agents have minimal membrane-stabilizing (local anesthetic) action, decreased corneal sensitivity may occur following prolonged use, and has been reported rarely with the use of betaxolol, levobunolol, and timolol, but not with the use of metipranolol. In contrast, carteolol has been reported to occasionally cause increased corneal sensitivity.

Because of betaxolol's relatively selective beta-1-adrenergic receptor inhibition, betaxolol may have less potential for systemic side/adverse effects than have the other ophthalmic beta-adrenergic blocking agents, which are nonselective beta-1 and beta-2 adrenergic receptor inhibitors. This may be especially important for patients for whom beta-2 adrenergic blockade could be harmful.

The ophthalmic suspension dosage form of betaxolol appears to be less irritating to the eye than the ophthalmic solution dosage form, although eye irritation occurs more frequently than other side effects with both dosage forms.

The side effects listed below have been reported for one or more of the ophthalmic beta-adrenergic blocking agents. However, all of these side effects are possible with any of the ophthalmic beta-adrenergic blocking agents. In addition, since the ophthalmic beta-adrenergic blocking agents may be systemically absorbed, any of the side effects that are possible for the systemic beta-adrenergic blocking agents are also theoretically possible for the ophthalmic beta-adrenergic blocking agents.

The following side/adverse effects have been selected on the basis of their potential clinical significance (possible signs and symptoms in parentheses where appropriate)—not necessarily inclusive:

### Those indicating need for medical attention
Incidence more frequent
*Conjunctival hyperemia* (redness of eyes or inside of eyelids)—reported for carteolol, frequency 25%
Incidence less frequent or rare
*Anisocoria* (different size pupils of the eyes)—reported for betaxolol; *blepharitis*—reported for metipranolol and timolol; *blepharoconjunctivitis*—reported for carteolol and levobunolol; *conjunctivitis*—reported for metipranolol and timolol; *corneal punctate keratitis*—reported for betaxolol; *dermatitis of eyelid*—reported for metipranolol; *edema*—reported for carteolol and metipranolol; *iridocyclitis*—reported for levobunolol; *keratitis*—reported for betaxolol and timolol (severe swelling, irritation, or inflammation of eye or eyelid); *blepharoptosis* (droopy upper eyelid)—reported for carteolol and timolol; *corneal staining* (discoloration of the eyeball)—reported for betaxolol and carteolol; *decreased corneal sensitivity*—reported for betaxolol, levobunolol, and timolol; *diplopia* (seeing double)—reported for timolol; *eye pain*—reported for betaxolol suspension; *glossitis* (redness or irritation of the tongue)—reported for betaxolol; *vision disturbances* (blurred vision or other change in vision)—reported for betaxolol suspension, carteolol, metipranolol, and timolol

Symptoms of systemic absorption
*Allergic reaction* (skin rash, hives, or itching)—reported for all except levobunolol; *alopecia* (hair loss)—reported for betaxolol and timolol; *anxiety or nervousness*—reported for metipranolol only; *arthritis or myalgia* (muscle or joint aches or pain)—reported for metipranolol only; *ataxia* (clumsiness or unsteadiness)—reported for levobunolol only; *change in taste*—reported for carteolol only; *chest pain*—reported for timolol only; *confusion or mental depression*—reported for betaxolol, metipranolol, and timolol; *congestive heart failure* (swelling of feet, ankles, or lower legs)—reported for betaxolol and timolol; *coughing, wheezing, or troubled breathing, especially in patients with predisposition to bronchoconstriction*—reported for all; *diarrhea*—reported for timolol only; *dizziness or feeling faint*—reported for all; *drowsiness*—reported for metipranolol and timolol; *epistaxis* (bleeding nose)—reported for metipranolol and timolol; *hallucinations*—reported for timolol only; *headache*—reported for all; *heartblock*—reported for betaxolol and timolol; *hypertension*—reported for metipranolol and timolol; *impotence* (decreased sexual ability)—reported for timolol only; *insomnia* (trouble in sleeping)—reported for betaxolol and carteolol; *irregular, slow, or pounding heartbeat*—reported for all; *nasal congestion* (stuffy nose)—reported for timolol only; *nausea or vomiting*—reported for metipranolol and timolol; *paresthesia* (burning or prickling feeling on body)—reported for timolol only; *rhinitis or sinusitis* (runny nose)—reported for carteolol, metipranolol, and timolol; *systemic lupus erythematosus*—reported for timolol only; *toxic epidermal necrolysis* (raw or red areas of the skin)—reported for betaxolol; *unusual tiredness or weakness*—reported for all

### Those indicating need for medical attention only if they continue or are bothersome
Incidence more frequent
*Decreased night vision*—reported for carteolol; *stinging of eye or other eye irritation, transient upon administration of medication*—reported for betaxolol, levobunolol, and metipranolol
Incidence less frequent or rare
*Browache*—reported with carteolol and metipranolol; *corneal sensitivity*—reported for carteolol ; *crusting of eyelashes*—reported with betaxolol suspension; *dryness of eye*—reported with betaxolol suspension; *increased sensitivity of eye to light*—reported for betaxolol, carteolol, and metipranolol; *redness, itching, stinging, burning, or watering of eye or other eye irritation*—reported for all; more frequent for carteolol and levobunolol

## Overdose

For specific information on the agents used in the management of ophthalmic beta-adrenergic blocking agents overdose, see:
• *Aminophylline* in *Bronchodilators, Theophylline-derivative (Systemic)* monograph;
• *Atropine* in *Anticholinergics/Antispasmodics (Systemic)* monograph;
• *Charcoal, Activated (Oral-Local)* monograph;
• *Digitalis Glycosides (Systemic)* monograph;
• *Dobutamine* in *Sympathomimetic Agents-Cardiovascular Use (Parenteral-Systemic)* monograph;
• *Dopamine* in *Sympathomimetic Agents-Cardiovascular Use (Parenteral-Systemic)* monograph;
• *Glucagon (Systemic)* monograph;
• *Isoproterenol* in *Sympathomimetic Agents-Cardiovascular Use (Parenteral-Systemic)* monograph;
• *Norepinephrine* in *Sympathomimetic Agents-Cardiovascular Use (Parenteral-Systemic)* monograph; and/or
• *Theophylline* in *Bronchodilators, Theophylline-derivative (Systemic)* monograph.

For more information on the management of overdose or unintentional ingestion, **contact a Poison Control Center** (see *Poison Control Center Listing*).

### Treatment of overdose
If an ophthalmic overdose occurs, immediately flush the eyes with warm tap water.

If an ophthalmic beta-adrenergic blocking agent is accidentally ingested, activated charcoal or gastric lavage may be appropriate to decrease further absorption.

For symptoms of systemic toxicity, the medication should be discontinued. Depending on severity of toxicity, the following supportive and symptomatic treatments should be utilized if necessary:

For bradycardia: Atropine (0.25 to 2 mg) should be administered intravenously to induce vagal blockade. If bradycardia persists, intravenous isoproterenol hydrochloride may be administered with caution. A transvenous cardiac pacemaker may be used, if necessary.

For hypotension: Glucagon and sympathomimetic pressor agents, such as dobutamine, dopamine, or norepinephrine, may be used. (See *Drug interactions and/or related problems* for precautions in use of sympathomimetic vasopressors.)

For bronchospasm: Isoproterenol hydrochloride should be administered. Additional therapy with a beta-2-agonist or a theophylline derivative may be used, if necessary.

For cardiac failure, acute: Digitalis, diuretics, and oxygen should be administered immediately. Intravenous aminophylline may be used in refractory cases. Also, glucagon hydrochloride may be used, if necessary.

For heart block, second or third degree: Isoproterenol hydrochloride or a transvenous cardiac pacemaker should be used.

## Patient Consultation

As an aid to patient consultation, refer to *Advice for the Patient, Beta-adrenergic Blocking Agents (Ophthalmic)*.

In providing consultation, consider emphasizing the following selected information (» = major clinical significance):

### Before using this medication
» Conditions affecting use, especially:
  Allergy to any of the beta-adrenergic blocking agents, either ophthalmic or systemic, such as acebutolol, atenolol, betaxolol, bisoprolol, carteolol, labetalol, levobunolol, metipranolol, metoprolol, nadolol, oxprenolol, penbutolol, pindolol, propranolol, sotalol, or timolol
  Pregnancy—Ophthalmic beta-adrenergic blocking agents may be absorbed into the body. Studies in animals have not shown that betaxolol, levobunolol, metipranolol, or timolol causes birth defects. However, very large doses of carteolol given by mouth to pregnant rats have been shown to cause wavy ribs in rat babies. In addition, some studies in animals have shown that beta-adrenergic blocking agents increase the chance of death in the animal fetus
  Use in children—Infants may be especially sensitive to the effects of ophthalmic beta-adrenergic blocking agents, thus increasing the risk of side effects
  Use in the elderly—If significant systemic absorption of ophthalmic beta-adrenergic blocking agents occurs, the chance of side effects during treatment may be increased, since elderly people are especially sensitive to the effects of these medications
  Other medical problems, especially bronchial asthma, or history of, severe chronic obstructive pulmonary disease, overt cardiac failure, 2nd- or 3rd-degree atrioventricular (AV) heart block, cardiogenic shock, sinus bradycardia, nonallergenic or chronic bronchitis, emphysema or other pulmonary function impairment, congestive heart failure, history of cardiac failure, diabetes mellitus, spontaneous hypoglycemia, or hyperthyroidism

### Proper use of this medication
» Proper administration technique; using nasolacrimal occlusion is especially important in infants and children
  Preventing contamination: Not touching applicator tip to any surface; keeping container tightly closed
  Proper use of medication having compliance cap
» Importance of not using more medication than the amount prescribed
» Proper dosing
  Missed dose: If dosing schedule is—
    Once a day: Applying as soon as possible; not applying if not remembered until next day; applying regularly scheduled dose
    More than once a day: Applying as soon as possible; not applying if almost time for next dose; applying next dose at regularly scheduled time
» Proper storage

### Precautions while using this medication
  Regular visits to physician to check eye pressure during therapy
» Caution if any kind of surgery (including dental surgery) or emergency treatment is required
» Diabetics: May mask some signs of hypoglycemia, such as increased pulse rate and trembling, but not dizziness and sweating; also, may cause decreased or sometimes increased blood glucose concentrations

  Possible photophobia: Wearing sunglasses and avoiding too much exposure to bright light

### Side/adverse effects
  Signs of potential side effects, especially conjunctival hyperemia, anisocoria, blepharitis, blepharoconjunctivitis, conjunctivitis, corneal punctate keratitis, dermatitis of eyelid, edema, iridocyclitis, keratitis, blepharoptosis, corneal staining, decreased corneal sensitivity, diplopia, eye pain, glossitis, vision disturbances, or symptoms of systemic absorption

## General Dosing Information

Although some manufacturers recommend a dose of 2 drops of an ophthalmic solution at appropriate intervals, the conjunctival sac will usually hold 1 drop or less.

When one ophthalmic beta-adrenergic blocking agent is used to replace another, the original beta-blocker maybe discontinued simultaneously with initiation of therapy with the new one.

When an ophthalmic beta-adrenergic blocking agent is used to replace a single antiglaucoma agent other than another beta-blocker, the other antiglaucoma agent may be continued on the first day that the new beta-blocker is used but can be discontinued on the second day.

When an ophthalmic beta-adrenergic blocking agent is used to replace several concomitantly administered antiglaucoma agents, the patient's dosage should be individualized as required. If any of the other antiglaucoma agents used is a beta-blocker, it can be discontinued before the new ophthalmic beta-adrenergic blocking agent is added to the regimen. The other antiglaucoma agents being used may be continued on the first day that the new beta-blocker is used but one of the agents should be discontinued on the second day. Then the remaining antiglaucoma agents may be decreased or discontinued according to the patient's response. Additional adjustments usually should involve only one agent at a time and should be made at intervals of not less than one week.

Ophthalmic beta-adrenergic blocking agents may be used concurrently with direct and indirect cholinergic agonists (e.g., pilocarpine, echothiophate, carbachol), beta-agonists (e.g., ophthalmic epinephrine or dipivefrin), or systemic carbonic anhydrase inhibitors (such as acetazolamide), if necessary to control intraocular pressure.

In patients scheduled for major surgery, some practitioners recommend that beta-adrenergic blocking agents be gradually withdrawn 48 hours prior to surgery because beta-adrenergic receptor blockade impairs the ability of the heart to respond to beta-adrenergically mediated reflex stimuli. This recommendation is controversial. However, since ophthalmic beta-adrenergic blocking agents may be absorbed systemically, gradual withdrawal of the medication should be considered for patients undergoing elective surgery because prolonged severe hypotension during anesthesia has occurred in some patients receiving systemic beta-adrenergic blocking agents. If necessary during surgery, the effects of beta-adrenergic blocking agents may be reversed by sufficient doses of agonists, such as isoproterenol, dopamine, dobutamine, or norepinephrine.

To help reduce systemic side effects, the patient can be instructed to close the eyes gently and apply pressure to the inner canthus of each eye in order to block lacrimal drainage through the tear ducts after instillation of the ophthalmic drops.

---

### BETAXOLOL

## Summary of Differences

Indications:
  Betaxolol may be especially useful in the treatment of glaucoma in patients with pulmonary disease.
Pharmacology/pharmacokinetics:
  Mechanism of action/effect—Betaxolol is a cardioselective (beta-1-adrenergic) receptor blocking agent.
  Other actions/effects—Betaxolol is less likely to produce significant beta-adrenergic receptor blockade in the bronchi and bronchioles.
  Duration of action—12 hours.
Fertility:
  Studies in rabbits and rats have shown that betaxolol, at oral doses above 12 mg/kg and 128 mg/kg, respectively, causes drug-related postimplantation loss.
Breast-feeding:
  Systemic betaxolol is distributed into breast milk in large enough quantities to have pharmacological effects. However, it is not known whether ophthalmic betaxolol is distributed into breast milk and problems in humans have not been documented.

## Ophthalmic Dosage Forms

### BETAXOLOL HYDROCHLORIDE OPHTHALMIC SOLUTION USP

Note: The dosing and strength usually available are expressed in terms of betaxolol base.

**Usual adult and adolescent dose**
Ophthalmic antiglaucoma agent—
 Topical, to the conjunctiva, 1 drop of a 0.5% solution of betaxolol (base) two times a day.

**Usual pediatric dose**
Safety and efficacy have not been established.

**Strength(s) usually available**
U.S.—
 0.5% (5 mg base; 5.6 mg as hydrochloride) (Rx) [*Betoptic* (benzalkonium chloride 0.01%; edetate disodium; sodium chloride; hydrochloric acid; sodium hydroxide)].
Canada—
 0.5% (5 mg base; 5.6 mg as hydrochloride) (Rx) [*Betoptic* (benzalkonium chloride 0.01%; edetate disodium; sodium chloride; hydrochloric acid; sodium hydroxide)].

**Packaging and storage**
Store below 40 °C (104 °F), preferably between 15 and 30 °C (59 and 86 °F), in a tight container, unless otherwise specified by manufacturer. Protect from freezing.

**Auxiliary labeling**
• For the eye.
• Keep container tightly closed.

### BETAXOLOL HYDROCHLORIDE OPHTHALMIC SUSPENSION

**Usual adult and adolescent dose**
Ophthalmic antiglaucoma agent—
 Topical, to the conjunctiva, 1 drop of a 0.25% suspension of betaxolol (base) two times a day.

**Usual pediatric dose**
Safety and efficacy have not been established.

**Strength(s) usually available**
U.S.—
 0.25% (2.5 mg base; 2.8 mg as hydrochloride) (Rx) [*Betoptic S* (benzalkonium chloride 0.01%; mannitol; poly(styrene-divinyl benzene) sulfonic acid; Carbomer 934P; edetate disodium; hydrochloric acid; sodium hydroxide)].
Canada—
 Not commercially available.

**Packaging and storage**
Store below 40 °C (104 °F), preferably between 15 and 30 °C (59 and 86 °F), in a well-closed container, unless otherwise specified by manufacturer. Protect from freezing.

**Auxiliary labeling**
• Shake well.
• For the eye.
• Keep container tightly closed.

---

## CARTEOLOL

### Summary of Differences

Pharmacology/pharmacokinetics:
 Other actions/effects—Carteolol has intrinsic sympathomimetic activity.
 Duration of action—More than 6 to 8 hours.
Pregnancy:
 In rabbits and rats, carteolol, administered in doses approximately 1052 and 5264 times the maximum recommended human oral dose of 10 mg per 70 kg of body weight per day, respectively, resulted in maternotoxicity, increased incidence of fetal resorptions, and decreased fetal weights. In rats, carteolol, administered in doses approximately 212 times the maximum recommended human oral dose, resulted in a dose-related increase in wavy ribs in the developing rat fetus. However, in mice, carteolol, administered in doses up to approximately 1052 times the maximum recommended human oral dose, did not result in wavy ribs.
Breast-feeding:
 It is not known whether systemic or ophthalmic carteolol is distributed into human breast milk; however, carteolol has been shown to be distributed into animal milk.

## Ophthalmic Dosage Forms

### CARTEOLOL HYDROCHLORIDE OPHTHALMIC SOLUTION

**Usual adult and adolescent dose**
Ophthalmic antiglaucoma agent—
 Topical, to the conjunctiva, 1 drop two times a day.

**Usual pediatric dose**
Safety and efficacy have not been established.

**Strength(s) usually available**
U.S.—
 1% (10 mg carteolol hydrochloride per mL) (Rx) [*Ocupress* (benzalkonium chloride 0.005%; sodium chloride; monobasic sodium phosphate; dibasic sodium phosphate)].
Canada—
 Not commercially available.

**Packaging and storage**
Store between 15 and 25 °C (59 and 77 °F), in a well-closed container, unless otherwise specified by manufacturer. Protect from light. Protect from freezing.

**Auxiliary labeling**
• For the eye.
• Keep container tightly closed.

---

## LEVOBUNOLOL

### Summary of Differences

Pharmacology/pharmacokinetics:
 Onset of action—Within 1 hour.
 Time to peak effect—Between 2 and 6 hours.
 Duration of action—Up to 24 hours.
Pregnancy:
 Although levobunolol has been shown to cause fetotoxicity in rabbits when administered at doses equivalent to 200 and 700 times the recommended dose for the treatment of glaucoma, similar studies in rats have not shown levobunolol to cause fetotoxic effects when administered at doses of up to 1800 times the human dose for glaucoma. Moreover, in teratogenicity studies in rats, levobunolol was not shown to cause fetal malformations when administered at doses of up to 25 mg/kg per day (1800 times the recommended human dose for glaucoma). Also, levobunolol was not shown to have adverse effects on the postnatal development of animal offspring.

## Ophthalmic Dosage Forms

### LEVOBUNOLOL HYDROCHLORIDE OPHTHALMIC SOLUTION USP

**Usual adult and adolescent dose**
Ophthalmic antiglaucoma agent—
 Topical, to the conjunctiva, 1 drop of a 0.25% solution one or two times a day or 1 drop of a 0.5% solution once a day.

**Usual adult prescribing limits**
Dosages above 1 drop of a 0.5% solution two times a day are generally not more effective.

**Usual pediatric dose**
Safety and efficacy have not been established.

**Strength(s) usually available**
U.S.—
 0.25% (Rx) [*Betagan C Cap B.I.D.* (polyvinyl alcohol 1.4%; benzalkonium chloride 0.004%; sodium metabisulfite; edetate disodium; dibasic sodium phosphate; monobasic potassium phosphate; sodium chloride; hydrochloric acid; sodium hydroxide)].
 0.5% (Rx) [*Betagan C Cap B.I.D.* (polyvinyl alcohol 1.4%; benzalkonium chloride 0.004%; sodium metabisulfite; edetate disodium; dibasic sodium phosphate; monobasic potassium phosphate; sodium chloride; hydrochloric acid; sodium hydroxide); *Betagan C Cap Q.D.* (polyvinyl alcohol 1.4%; benzalkonium chloride 0.004%; sodium metabisulfite; edetate disodium; dibasic sodium phosphate; monobasic potassium phosphate; sodium chloride; hydrochloric acid; sodium hydroxide); *Betagan Standard Cap* (polyvinyl alcohol 1.4%; benzalkonium chloride 0.004%; sodium metabisulfite; edetate disodium; dibasic sodium phosphate; monobasic potassium phosphate; sodium chloride; hydrochloric acid; sodium hydroxide)].
Canada—
 0.25% (Rx) [*Betagan C Cap B.I.D.* (polyvinyl alcohol 1.4%; benzalkonium chloride 0.004%; sodium metabisulfite; edetate disodium;

dibasic sodium phosphate; monobasic potassium phosphate; sodium chloride; hydrochloric acid; sodium hydroxide)].

0.5% (Rx) [*Betagan C Cap B.I.D.* (polyvinyl alcohol 1.4%; benzalkonium chloride 0.004%; sodium metabisulfite; edetate disodium; dibasic sodium phosphate; monobasic potassium phosphate; sodium chloride; hydrochloric acid; sodium hydroxide); *Betagan Standard Cap* (polyvinyl alcohol 1.4%; benzalkonium chloride 0.004%; sodium metabisulfite; edetate disodium; dibasic sodium phosphate; monobasic potassium phosphate; sodium chloride; hydrochloric acid; sodium hydroxide)].

**Packaging and storage**
Store below 40 °C (104 °F), preferably between 15 and 30 °C (59 and 86 °F), in a tight container, unless otherwise specified by manufacturer. Protect from light. Protect from freezing.

**Auxiliary labeling**
- For the eye.
- Keep container tightly closed.

## METIPRANOLOL

## Summary of Differences
Pharmacology/pharmacokinetics: Duration of action—More than 24 hours.
Pregnancy: No metipranolol-related effects were reported for the segment II teratology study in fetal rats when metipranolol was administered orally to pregnant rats in doses of up to 50 mg/kg per day during organogenesis. However, metipranolol has been shown to increase fetal resorption, fetal death, and delayed development when administered orally to pregnant rabbits at 50 mg/kg during organogenesis.

## Ophthalmic Dosage Forms
### METIPRANOLOL HYDROCHLORIDE OPHTHALMIC SOLUTION
Note: The dosing and strengths usually available are expressed in terms of metipranolol base.

**Usual adult and adolescent dose**
Ophthalmic antiglaucoma agent—
  Topical, to the conjunctiva, 1 drop of a 0.3% solution of metipranolol (base) two times a day.

**Usual adult prescribing limits**
Dosages above 1 drop of a 0.3% solution two times a day are not known to be of benefit.

**Usual pediatric dose**
Safety and efficacy have not been established.

**Strength(s) usually available**
U.S.—
  0.3% (3 mg base per mL) (Rx) [*OptiPranolol* (benzalkonium chloride 0.004%; glycerol; sodium chloride; edetate disodium; povidone; hydrochloric acid; sodium hydroxide)].
Canada—
  Not commercially available.

**Packaging and storage**
Store below 40 °C (104 °F), preferably between 15 and 30 °C (59 and 86 °F), in a well-closed container, unless otherwise specified by manufacturer. Protect from freezing.

**Auxiliary labeling**
- For the eye.
- Keep container tightly closed.

## TIMOLOL

## Summary of Differences
Pharmacology/pharmacokinetics: Duration of action—Up to 24 hours.
Carcinogenicity: In a lifetime study in mice, timolol increased the incidence of malignant pulmonary tumors and mammary adenocarcinomas in female mice when administered orally at doses of 500 mg/kg per day, but not at 5 or 50 mg/kg per day.
Pregnancy: Studies in rats have shown that timolol at doses of up to 50 mg/kg per day (50 times the maximum recommended human oral dose) causes delayed fetal ossification; however, there were no adverse effects on postnatal development of offspring. Teratogenic studies in mice and rabbits have not shown that timolol at doses of up to 50 mg/kg per day causes fetal malformations. In mice, timolol at doses of 1 gram per kg per day (1000 times the maximum recommended human oral dose) was maternotoxic and resulted in increased incidence of fetal resorptions.
In rabbits, timolol at doses 100 times the maximum recommended human oral dose caused increased incidence of fetal resorptions but not maternotoxicity.
Breast-feeding: Systemic timolol is distributed into breast milk. Problems in humans have not been documented for ophthalmic timolol; however, ophthalmic timolol may be systemically absorbed and distributed into the breast milk, possibly causing serious adverse reactions in the infants of nursing mothers.

## Ophthalmic Dosage Forms
### TIMOLOL MALEATE OPHTHALMIC SOLUTION USP
Note: The dosing and strengths usually available are expressed in terms of timolol base.

**Usual adult and adolescent dose**
Ophthalmic antiglaucoma agent—
  Topical, to the conjunctiva, 1 drop of a 0.25 or 0.5% solution of timolol (base) one or two times a day.

**Usual pediatric dose**
Ophthalmic antiglaucoma agent—
  Infants and children up to 10 years of age: Topical, to the conjunctiva, 1 drop of a 0.25% solution of timolol (base) one or two times a day.
  Children 10 years of age and older: See *Usual adult and adolescent dose*.

Note: Nasolacrimal occlusion should be emphasized to patient.

**Strength(s) usually available**
U.S.—
  0.25% (2.5 mg base; 3.4 mg as maleate) (Rx) [*Timoptic* (benzalkonium chloride 0.01%; monobasic sodium phosphate; dibasic sodium phosphate; sodium hydroxide); *Timoptic in Ocudose* (monobasic sodium phosphate; dibasic sodium phosphate; sodium hydroxide)].
  0.5% (5 mg base; 6.8 mg as maleate) (Rx) [*Timoptic* (benzalkonium chloride 0.01%; monobasic sodium phosphate; dibasic sodium phosphate; sodium hydroxide); *Timoptic in Ocudose* (monobasic sodium phosphate; dibasic sodium phosphate; sodium hydroxide)].
Canada—
  0.25% (2.5 mg base; 3.4 mg as maleate) (Rx) [*Apo-Timop* (benzalkonium chloride 0.1%; monobasic sodium phosphate; dibasic sodium phosphate; sodium hydroxide); *Gen-Timolol* (benzalkonium chloride 0.01%; monobasic sodium phosphate; dibasic sodium phosphate); *Timoptic* (benzalkonium chloride 0.01%; monobasic sodium phosphate; dibasic sodium phosphate; sodium hydroxide)].
  0.5% (5 mg base; 6.8 mg as maleate) (Rx) [*Apo-Timop* (benzalkonium chloride 0.1%; monobasic sodium phosphate; dibasic sodium phosphate; sodium hydroxide); *Gen-Timolol* (benzalkonium chloride 0.01%; monobasic sodium phosphate; dibasic sodium phosphate); *Timoptic* (benzalkonium chloride 0.01%; monobasic sodium phosphate; dibasic sodium phosphate; sodium hydroxide)].

**Packaging and storage**
Store between 15 and 30 °C (59 and 86 °F), in a tight container, unless otherwise specified by manufacturer. Protect from freezing. Protect from light.

**Auxiliary labeling**
- For the eye.
- Keep container tightly closed.

## Selected Bibliography
**For levobunolol**
Gonzalez JP, Clissold SP. Ocular levobunolol. A review of its pharmacodynamic and pharmacokinetic properties, and therapeutic efficacy. Drugs 1987 Dec; 34(60): 648-61.

**For timolol**
Novack GD. Ophthalmic beta-blockers since timolol. Surv Ophthalmol 1987 Mar-Apr; 31(5): 307-27.

**For betaxolol**
Buckley MMT, et al. Ocular betaxolol. A review of its pharmacological properties, and therapeutic efficacy in glaucoma and ocular hypertension. Drugs 40. Auckland, New Zealand: ADIS Drug Information Services, 1990.

**For metipranolol**
Battershill PE, Sorkin EM. Ocular metipranolol. A preliminary review of its pharmacodynamic and pharmacokinetic properties, and therapeutic efficacy in glaucoma and ocular hypertension. Drugs 1988 Nov; 36(5): 601-15.

**General**
Bauer K, et al. Assessment of systemic effects of different ophthalmic beta-blockers in healthy volunteers. Clin Pharmacol Ther 1991 Jun; 49(6): 658-64.

Brooks AM, Gillies WE. Ocular beta-blockers in glaucoma management. Clinical pharmacological aspects. Drugs Aging 1992 May-Jun; 2(3): 208-21.

**For carteolol**
Chrisp P, Sorkin EM. Ocular carteolol. A review of its pharmacological properties, and therapeutic use in glaucoma and ocular hypertension. Drugs Aging 1992 Jan-Feb; 2(1): 58-77.

Revised: 05/12/93

# BETA-ADRENERGIC BLOCKING AGENTS  Systemic

This monograph includes information on the following: 1) Acebutolol; 2) Atenolol; 3) Betaxolol†; 4) Bisoprolol†; 5) Carteolol†; 6) Labetalol; 7) Metoprolol; 8) Nadolol; 9) Oxprenolol*; 10) Penbutolol†; 11) Pindolol; 12) Propranolol; 13) Sotalol; 14) Timolol.

VA CLASSIFICATION (Primary/Secondary):
 Acebutolol—CV100/CV250; CV300; CV409; CV900; CN900
 Atenolol—CV100/CV250; CV300; CV409; CV900; CN105; CN900
 Betaxolol—CV100/CV409
 Bisoprolol—CV100/CV409
 Carteolol—CV100/CV409
 Labetalol—CV100/CV250; CV409
 Metoprolol—CV100/CV250; CV300; CV409; CV900; CN105; CN900
 Nadolol—CV100/CV250; CV300; CV409; CV900; CN105; CN900
 Oxprenolol—CV100/CV250; CV300; CV409; CV900; CN900
 Penbutolol—CV100/CV409
 Pindolol—CV100/CV250; CV409; CN900
 Propranolol—CV100/CV250; CV300; CV409; CV900; CN105; CN900
 Sotalol—CV100/CV250; CV300; CV409; CV900; CN900
 Timolol—CV100/CV250; CV300; CV409; CV900; CN105; CN900; OP111

Commonly used brand name(s): *Apo-Atenolol*[2]; *Apo-Metoprolol*[7]; *Apo-Metoprolol (Type L)*[7]; *Apo-Propranolol*[12]; *Apo-Timol*[14]; *Betaloc*[7]; *Betaloc Durules*[7]; *Betapace*[13]; *Blocadren*[14]; *Cartrol*[5]; *Corgard*[8]; *Detensol*[12]; *Inderal*[12]; *Inderal LA*[12]; *Kerlone*[3]; *Levatol*[10]; *Lopresor*[7]; *Lopresor SR*[7]; *Lopressor*[7]; *Monitan*[1]; *Normodyne*[6]; *Novo-Atenol*[2]; *Novo-Pindol*[11]; *Novo-Timol*[14]; *Novometoprol*[7]; *Novopranol*[12]; *Nu-Metop*[7]; *Sectral*[1]; *Slow-Trasicor*[9]; *Sotacor*[13]; *Syn-Nadolol*[8]; *Syn-Pindolol*[11]; *Tenormin*[2]; *Toprol-XL*[7]; *Trandate*[6]; *Trasicor*[9]; *Visken*[11]; *Zebeta*[4]; *pms Propranolol*[12].

Note: For a listing of dosage forms and brand names by country availability, see *Dosage Forms* section(s).

*Not commercially available in U.S.
†Not commercially available in Canada.

## Category

Note: All of the beta-adrenergic blocking agents have similar pharmacologic actions; however, clinical uses among specific agents may vary because of pharmacologic or pharmacokinetic differences, availability of specific testing, and/or availability of clinical-use data.

Antiadrenergic—Acebutolol; Atenolol; Betaxolol; Carteolol; Labetalol; Metoprolol; Nadolol; Oxprenolol; Penbutolol; Pindolol; Propranolol; Sotalol; Timolol.
Antianginal—Acebutolol; Atenolol; Carteolol; Labetalol; Metoprolol; Nadolol; Oxprenolol; Penbutolol; Pindolol; Propranolol; Sotalol; Timolol.
Antiarrhythmic—Acebutolol; Atenolol; Metoprolol; Nadolol; Oxprenolol; Propranolol; Sotalol; Timolol.
Antihypertensive—Acebutolol; Atenolol; Betaxolol; Bisoprolol; Carteolol; Labetalol; Metoprolol; Nadolol; Oxprenolol; Penbutolol; Pindolol; Propranolol; Sotalol; Timolol.
Hypertrophic cardiomyopathy therapy adjunct—Acebutolol; Atenolol; Metoprolol; Nadolol; Oxprenolol; Pindolol; Propranolol; Sotalol; Timolol.
Myocardial infarction prophylactic and therapy—Acebutolol; Atenolol; Metoprolol; Nadolol; Oxprenolol; Propranolol; Sotalol; Timolol.
Neuroleptic–induced akathisia therapy—Betaxolol; Metoprolol; Nadolol; Propranolol.
Pheochromocytoma therapy adjunct—Acebutolol; Atenolol; Labetalol; Metoprolol; Nadolol; Oxprenolol; Propranolol; Sotalol; Timolol.
Vascular headache prophylactic—Atenolol; Metoprolol; Nadolol; Propranolol; Timolol.
Antitremor agent—Acebutolol; Atenolol; Metoprolol; Nadolol; Oxprenolol; Pindolol; Propranolol; Sotalol; Timolol.
Antianxiety therapy adjunct—Acebutolol; Metoprolol; Oxprenolol; Propranolol; Sotalol; Timolol.
Thyrotoxicosis therapy adjunct—Acebutolol; Atenolol; Metoprolol; Nadolol; Oxprenolol; Propranolol; Sotalol; Timolol.
Antiglaucoma agent—Timolol.

## Indications

Note: Bracketed information in the *Indications* section refers to uses that are not included in U.S. product labeling.

**Accepted**

Angina pectoris, chronic (treatment)—[Acebutolol], atenolol, [carteolol], [labetalol][1], metoprolol, nadolol, oxprenolol[1], [penbutolol], [pindolol], propranolol, [sotalol], and [timolol] are indicated in the treatment of classic angina pectoris, also referred to as "effort-associated angina."

Arrhythmias, cardiac (prophylaxis and treatment)—Propranolol is indicated in the control and correction of supraventricular arrhythmias, ventricular tachycardias, digitalis-induced tachyarrhythmias, and catecholamine-induced tachyarrhythmias during anesthesia (with extreme caution because of possible additive myocardial depression with general anesthesia). Propranolol by intravenous injection is recommended only in the treatment of cardiac arrhythmias that occur while the patient is unable to receive oral medication, or when a rapid and observable effect is desired. [Acebutolol][1], [atenolol][1], [metoprolol][1], [nadolol][1], oxprenolol[1], sotalol[1], and [timolol][1] are also used for their antiarrhythmic effects, especially in supraventricular arrhythmias and ventricular tachycardias. Acebutolol[1] is indicated in the control and correction of premature ventricular contractions.

Hypertension (treatment)—Acebutolol, atenolol, betaxolol, bisoprolol, carteolol, labetalol, metoprolol, nadolol, oxprenolol, penbutolol, pindolol, propranolol, [sotalol], and timolol are indicated in the treatment of hypertension when used alone or in combination with other antihypertensive medication.

Parenteral labetalol is indicated for treatment of severe hypertension. Intravenous metoprolol and propranolol are not recommended for the management of hypertensive emergencies. However, intravenous propranolol has proven useful in controlling hypertension during anesthesia and surgery.

Cardiomyopathy, hypertrophic (treatment)—[Acebutolol][1], [atenolol][1], [metoprolol][1], [nadolol][1], oxprenolol[1], [pindolol][1], propranolol, [sotalol][1], and [timolol][1] are indicated in the management of angina, palpitations, and syncope associated with hypertrophic subaortic stenosis.

Myocardial infarction (treatment and prophylaxis)—[Acebutolol][1], atenolol[1], metoprolol, [nadolol][1], oxprenolol[1], propranolol, [sotalol][1], and timolol are indicated in clinically stable patients recovering from an initial definite or suspected acute myocardial infarction in order to reduce cardiovascular mortality and to decrease the risk of reinfarction.

Pheochromocytoma (treatment adjunct)—Propranolol is indicated in the management of symptoms of tachycardia due to excessive beta-receptor stimulation in pheochromocytoma. However, it should be used only after primary treatment with an alpha-adrenergic blocking agent (since use without concomitant alpha-blockade could lead to serious blood pressure elevation). [Acebutolol][1], [atenolol][1], [labetalol (with caution)][1], [metoprolol][1], [nadolol][1], oxprenolol[1], [sotalol][1], and [timolol][1] also may be used.

Headache, vascular (prophylaxis)—Propranolol and timolol are indicated for reducing frequency and severity of migraine headaches but are not recommended for treatment of acute attacks. [Atenolol][1], [metoprolol][1], and [nadolol][1] are also useful for prophylaxis of migraine. A beta-adrenergic blocking agent is the drug of choice for vascular headache prophylaxis.

Tremors (treatment)—Propranolol is indicated in the treatment of essential, familial, and senile tremors. Propranolol also has been used to reduce the agitation and tremors of alcohol withdrawal. [Acebutolol][1], [atenolol][1], [metoprolol][1], [nadolol][1], oxprenolol[1], [pindolol][1], [sotalol][1], and [timolol][1] also may be used to treat tremors. Propranolol is the drug of choice for treatment of essential tremor.

Anxiety (treatment adjunct)—[Propranolol][1] is used to control the physical manifestations of anxiety such as tachycardia and tremor. It is not particularly useful for chronic anxiety or panic attacks but is most useful for reducing anxiety and improving performance in specific stressful situations. [Acebutolol][1], [metoprolol][1], oxprenolol[1], [sotalol][1], and [timolol][1] also have been used for this purpose.

Thyrotoxicosis (treatment adjunct)—[Propranolol][1] has been effective in the short-term preoperative management of thyrotoxic crises (until thioamide therapy is effective) by reducing symptoms such as fever, tachycardia, and hyperkinesia. There is no effect on the hormone production of the thyroid. Abrupt withdrawal of beta-blocker treatment may provoke "thyroid storm." [Acebutolol][1], [atenolol][1], [metoprolol][1], [nadolol][1], oxprenolol[1], [sotalol][1], and [timolol][1] are also used for thyrotoxicosis.

Mitral valve prolapse syndrome (treatment)—[Acebutolol][1], [atenolol][1], [metoprolol][1], [nadolol][1], oxprenolol[1], [pindolol][1], [propranolol][1], [sotalol][1], and [timolol][1] are used in the treatment of mitral valve prolapse syndrome.

[Hypotension, controlled (induction and maintenance)][1]—Parenteral labetalol is used to produce controlled hypotension during surgery to reduce bleeding into the surgical field.

[Glaucoma, open-angle (treatment)][1]—Timolol is used to lower intraocular pressure in the treatment of open-angle glaucoma.

[Neuroleptic-induced akathisia (treatment)][1]—Propranolol may be used to relieve the somatic and subjective symptoms associated with neuroleptic-induced akathisia (NIA). Betaxolol, metoprolol, and nadolol have also been used for NIA.

---

[1]Not included in Canadian product labeling.

## Pharmacology/Pharmacokinetics

See *Table 1*, page 608.

**Physicochemical characteristics**

Molecular weight—
  Acebutolol: 336.43.
  Atenolol: 266.34.
  Betaxolol hydrochloride: 343.89.
  Bisoprolol fumarate: 766.97.
  Carteolol hydrochloride: 328.84.
  Labetalol hydrochloride: 364.87.
  Metoprolol succinate: 652.83.
  Metoprolol tartrate: 684.82.
  Nadolol: 309.40.
  Oxprenolol hydrochloride: 301.81.
  Penbutolol sulfate: 680.94.
  Pindolol: 248.32.
  Propranolol hydrochloride: 295.81.
  Sotalol hydrochloride: 308.82.
  Timolol maleate: 432.49.

pKa—
  Acebutolol: 9.20.
  Carteolol: 9.74.
  Labetalol: 9.45.
  Metoprolol: 9.68.
  Nadolol: 9.67.
  Penbutolol: 9.3.
  Timolol: Approximately 9 in water at 25 °C.

Lipid solubility
  Acebutolol: Low.
  Atenolol: Very low (log partition coefficient for octanol/water=0.23).
  Bisoprolol: Moderate (equally hydrophilic and lipophilic).
  Carteolol: Low.
  Labetalol: Low.
  Metoprolol: Moderate.
  Nadolol: Low.
  Oxprenolol: Moderate.
  Penbutolol: Moderate.
  Pindolol: Moderate.
  Propranolol: High.
  Sotalol: Low.
  Timolol: Moderate.

### Mechanism of action/Effect

Beta-adrenergic blocking agents block the agonistic effect of the sympathetic neurotransmitters by competing for receptor binding sites. When they predominantly block the beta-1 receptors in cardiac tissue, they are said to be cardioselective. When they block both beta-1 receptors and beta-2 receptors (primarily located in tissues other than cardiac), they are said to be nonselective. In general, so-called cardioselective beta-adrenergic blocking agents are relatively cardioselective—at lower doses they block beta-1 receptors only but begin to block beta-2 receptors as the dose increases.

Some beta-adrenergic blocking agents also have intrinsic sympathomimetic activity (ISA or partial agonist activity), which is the ability to cause weak stimulation of beta-adrenergic receptors while simultaneously blocking the effect of endogenous catecholamines; however, the significance of this property has not been established. Possession of ISA theoretically may result in fewer adverse effects related to unopposed beta blockade (e.g., bradycardia, heart block, bronchoconstriction, peripheral vascular constriction), but studies have not proven clinical benefit. Pindolol exhibits the most ISA of the beta-adrenergic blocking agents currently available; carteolol, oxprenolol, and penbutolol have moderate ISA; acebutolol has mild to moderate ISA; and the other members of the group have little, if any, such activity.

Propranolol possesses moderate membrane-stabilizing (quinidine-like) activity; acebutolol, betaxolol, metoprolol, and oxprenolol have slight activity. The other beta-adrenergic blocking agents of this group show little, if any, such activity. At one time membrane-stabilizing activity was thought to be related to the antiarrhythmic effect, but it is no longer considered to be significant because it occurs only at very high (much greater than therapeutic) doses.

Antianginal—
  Reduction in myocardial oxygen demand through negative chronotropic and inotropic effects.

Antiarrhythmic—
  May involve beta-blockade–induced reduction in the rate of spontaneous firing of sinus and ectopic pacemakers and slowing of atrioventricular (AV) nodal conduction. In the Vaughan Williams classification of antiarrhythmics, beta-adrenergic blocking agents are considered to be class II agents.

Antihypertensive—
  The precise mechanism of antihypertensive effect is not known. Possible mechanisms include reduced cardiac output, decreased sympathetic outflow to peripheral vasculature, and inhibition of renin release by the kidneys; with labetalol, may also be related to reduced peripheral vascular resistance as a result of alpha-adrenergic blockade.

Hypertrophic cardiomyopathy therapy adjunct—
  Reduction of elevated outflow pressure gradient, which is exacerbated by beta-receptor stimulation.

Myocardial infarction therapy and prophylactic—
  Possible reduction in severity of myocardial ischemia by decrease of myocardial oxygen requirements; postinfarction mortality may also be reduced through an antiarrhythmic action.

Vascular headache prophylactic—
  Involves several mechanisms, including prevention of arterial dilation through beta-blockade, blockade of catecholamine-induced platelet aggregation and lipolysis, reduction of platelet adhesiveness, prevention of coagulation factor elevation during epinephrine release, promotion of oxygen release to tissues, and inhibition of renin secretion.

Antitremor agent—
  Precise mechanism not known, but antitremor effect may be mediated predominantly by peripheral beta-2 receptor mechanisms.

Antianxiety therapy adjunct—
  Precise mechanism unknown; however, thought to involve improvement of somatic symptoms secondary to beta-blockade.

Thyrotoxicosis therapy adjunct—
  Unknown, but probably related to reduction of symptoms such as tremor, tachycardia, and elevated blood pressure caused by increased sensitivity to catecholamines.

### Other actions/effects

Labetalol also has selective alpha-1-adrenergic blocking effects, which lead to vasodilation, reduced peripheral vascular resistance, and postural hypotension.

## Precautions to Consider

Note: In general, because of the similarity of effect and because the cardioselectivity of beta-1 blockers is relative, the same precautions, especially drug interactions and medical problems, apply to all beta-adrenergic blocking agents.

### Carcinogenicity/Tumorigenicity

*Acebutolol*—Studies in rats and mice given up to 300 mg per kg of body weight (mg/kg) per day (equivalent to 15 times the maximum recommended human dose) found no evidence of carcinogenicity. Diacetolol, the major metabolite, also did not produce evidence of carcinogenicity in rats given up to 1800 mg/kg per day.

*Atenolol*—Two 18- to 24-month studies in rats and one study for up to 18 months in mice given up to 150 times the maximum recommended human antihypertensive dose found no evidence of carcinogenicity. However, a 24-month study in rats given up to 750 times the maximum recommended human antihypertensive dose revealed increased incidences of benign adrenal medullary tumors in males and females, mammary fibroadenomas in females, and anterior pituitary adenomas and thyroid parafollicular cell carcinomas in males.

*Betaxolol*—Studies in mice given up to 60 mg/kg per day orally (up to 90 times the maximum recommended human dose based on 60-kg body weight) and in rats given up to 48 mg/kg per day orally (up to 72 times the maximum recommended human dose) found no evidence of carcinogenicity.

*Bisoprolol*—Studies in mice and rats given 625 and 312 times, respectively, the maximum recommended human dose by weight found no evidence of carcinogenicity.

*Carteolol*—A 2-year study in rats and mice given 280 times the maximum recommended human dose (10 mg per 70 kg of body weight per day) found no evidence of carcinogenicity.

*Labetalol*—Studies for 18 months in mice and 2 years in rats found no evidence of carcinogenicity.

*Metoprolol*—A 1-year study in dogs given up to 105 mg/kg per day orally, a 2-year study in rats given up to 800 mg/kg per day orally, and a 21-month study in mice given up to 750 mg/kg per day orally found no evidence of carcinogenicity, although the incidence of small benign adenomas of the lung was higher in the treated female mice. A repeat of the 21-month study in mice found no increased incidence of any type of tumor.

*Nadolol*—A 2-year study in rats and mice found no evidence of carcinogenicity.

*Oxprenolol*—Long-term studies in mice and rats found no evidence of carcinogenicity.

*Penbutolol*—A 21-month study in mice and a 2-year study in rats at doses up to 500 times the maximum recommended human dose found no evidence of carcinogenicity.

*Pindolol*—Two-year studies in rats and mice found no evidence of carcinogenicity at doses as high as 50 and 100 times, respectively, the maximum recommended human dose.

*Propranolol*—Eighteen-month studies in rats and mice given up to 150 mg/kg per day found no evidence of carcinogenicity.

*Timolol*—A 2-year study found an increased incidence of adrenal pheochromocytomas in male rats given 300 times (but not 25 or 80 times) the maximum recommended human dose. Another study found an increased incidence of benign and malignant pulmonary tumors and benign uterine polyps in female mice given 500 (but not 5 or 50) mg/kg per day and an increase in mammary adenocarcinomas associated with elevations in serum prolactin at 500 mg/kg per day.

**Mutagenicity**

*Acebutolol*—Ames mutagenicity studies with acebutolol and diacetolol were negative.

*Atenolol*—Mutagenicity studies were negative.

*Betaxolol*—Betaxolol was not found to be mutagenic in a variety of *in vitro* and *in vivo* bacterial and mammalian cell assays.

*Bisoprolol*—Bisoprolol was not found to be mutagenic in a variety of *in vitro* and *in vivo* assays.

*Carteolol*—Carteolol was not found to be mutagenic in the Ames test, recombinant (rec)-assay, *in vivo* cytogenetics tests, and dominant lethal assay.

*Labetalol*—Labetalol was not found to be mutagenic in dominant lethal assays in rats and mice or in modified Ames tests.

*Metoprolol*—Metoprolol was not found to be mutagenic in several tests, including a dominant lethal study in mice, chromosome studies in somatic cells, a *Salmonella*/mammalian-microsome mutagenicity test, and a nucleus anomaly test in somatic interphase nuclei.

*Penbutolol*—Penbutolol was not found to be mutagenic in the *Salmonella* mutagenicity test (Ames test), the point mutation induction test (*Saccharomyces*), or the micronucleus test.

*Timolol*—*In vivo* (mouse) and *in vitro* mutagenicity studies were negative; in Ames tests, some changes were seen, but not enough to make the test positive.

**Pregnancy/Reproduction**

Fertility—*Acebutolol:* No adverse effect on fertility was observed in male or female rats given up to 240 mg/kg per day of acebutolol and 1000 mg/kg per day of diacetolol.

*Atenolol:* No adverse effect on fertility was observed in male or female rats given 100 times the maximum recommended human dose.

*Betaxolol:* No adverse effect on fertility or mating performance was observed in male or female rats given 380 times the maximum recommended human dose.

*Bisoprolol:* No adverse effect on fertility was observed in rats given 375 times the maximum recommended human dose by weight.

*Carteolol:* No adverse effect on fertility was observed in male or female rats and mice given 1052 times the maximum recommended human dose.

*Metoprolol:* No adverse effect on fertility was observed in rats given up to 55.5 times the maximum human daily dose of 450 mg.

*Nadolol:* No adverse effect on fertility was observed in rats given nadolol.

*Pindolol:* Mortality and decreased weight gain were observed in male rats given 100 mg/kg per day. Decreased mating was associated with atrophy and/or decreased spermatogenesis at 30 mg/kg per day. Mating behavior decreased and offspring mortality increased in females given 100 mg/kg per day and 30 mg/kg per day. In addition, there was an increase in prenatal mortality at a dose of 10 mg/kg per day, although there was not a clear dose-response relationship. In females necropsied on the 15th day of gestation, an increased resorption rate was observed at a dose of 100 mg/kg per day.

*Propranolol:* No adverse effect on fertility was observed in animal studies.

*Timolol:* No adverse effect on fertility was observed in male or female rats at doses up to 125 times the maximum recommended human dose.

Pregnancy—Beta-adrenergic blocking agents cross the placenta. The safety of these agents in pregnancy is not fully established. Fetal and neonatal bradycardia, hypotension, hypoglycemia, and respiratory depression have been reported with administration of a cardioselective or a noncardioselective beta-adrenergic blocking agent to pregnant women. In addition, intrauterine growth retardation has been reported rarely with atenolol and nadolol. However, other reports seem to indicate successful treatment of maternal hypertension during pregnancy with no apparent effects on the fetus or neonate.

*Acebutolol*—

Acebutolol was not teratogenic in rats or rabbits given up to 31.5 and 6.8 times, respectively, the maximum recommended therapeutic dose in a 60-kg human. However, slight fetal growth retardation occurred in rabbits given 135 mg/kg per day. An elevation in postimplantation loss was seen in rabbit dams given 450 mg/kg per day of diacetolol.

FDA Pregnancy Category B.

*Atenolol*—

Dose-related increases in embryo/fetal resorptions were observed in rats given atenolol in doses greater than or equal to 25 times the maximum recommended human antihypertensive dose. This effect was not seen in rabbits given 12.5 times the maximum recommended human antihypertensive dose.

FDA Pregnancy Category D.

*Betaxolol*—

Administration of betaxolol to pregnant rats in doses up to 600 times the maximum recommended human dose was associated with increased postimplantation loss, reduced litter size and weight, and increased incidence of skeletal and visceral abnormalities, which may or may not have resulted from maternal drug toxicity. In another study, betaxolol, given at doses of up to 300 times the maximum recommended human dose, was associated with an increase in resorptions, but no teratogenicity. Administration of 380 times the maximum recommended human dose caused a marked increase in total litter loss within 4 days postpartum. A marked increase in postimplantation loss, but no teratogenicity, was observed in pregnant rabbits given up to 54 times the maximum recommended human dose.

FDA Pregnancy Category C.

*Bisoprolol*—

Bisoprolol was not teratogenic in rats or rabbits given 375 and 31 times, respectively, the maximum recommended human dose by weight. However, there was an increase in late resorptions in rats given bisoprolol at doses 125 times the maximum recommended human dose by weight.

FDA Pregnancy Category C.

*Carteolol*—

Increased resorptions and decreased fetal weights occurred in rabbits and rats given maternally toxic doses 1052 and 5264 times, respectively, the maximum recommended human dose. A dose-related increase in fetal wavy ribs was seen in pregnant rats given 212 times the maximum recommended human dose. However, this was not observed in mice given up to 1052 times the maximum recommended human dose.

FDA Pregnancy Category C.

*Labetalol—*
Teratogenic effects were not seen in rats and rabbits given 6 and 4 times, respectively, the maximum recommended human dose. Administration of labetalol to rats during late gestation through weaning at doses up to 2 to 4 times the maximum recommended human dose resulted in decreased neonatal survival.

FDA Pregnancy Category C.

*Metoprolol—*
Increased postimplantation loss and decreased neonatal survival were observed in rats given up to 55.5 times the maximum human daily dose of 450 mg. No evidence of teratogenicity was seen in animal studies.

FDA Pregnancy Category C.

*Nadolol—*
Evidence of embryotoxicity and fetotoxicity was found in rabbits given up to 10 times the maximum indicated human dose. However, these effects were not seen in rats or hamsters. Teratogenic effects were not seen in any of these species.

FDA Pregnancy Category C.

*Pindolol—*
No evidence of embryotoxicity or teratogenicity was found in rats and rabbits given doses exceeding 100 times the maximum recommended human dose.

FDA Pregnancy Category B.

*Propranolol—*
Embryotoxicity occurred in animals given 10 times the maximum recommended human dose.

FDA Pregnancy Category C.

*Timolol—*
No evidence of fetal malformations was observed in mice and rabbits given up to 50 times the maximum recommended human dose. In rats, at similar doses, delayed fetal ossification was observed, but there were no adverse effects on postnatal development of offspring. Increased fetal resorptions were seen in mice and rabbits given 1000 and 100 times, respectively, the maximum recommended human dose.

FDA Pregnancy Category C.

### Breast-feeding
Acebutolol (and diacetolol), atenolol, betaxolol, labetalol, metoprolol, nadolol, oxprenolol, pindolol, propranolol, sotalol, and timolol are distributed into breast milk. It is not known whether bisoprolol, carteolol, and penbutolol are distributed into breast milk. Cyanosis and bradycardia resulted from maternal therapy with atenolol in one breast-fed neonate; hypotension, bradycardia, and transient tachypnea resulted from maternal acebutolol therapy in another. Adverse neonatal effects resulting from maternal ingestion of other beta-adrenergic blocking agents have not been reported. Although the risk appears to be small, breast-fed infants should be monitored for signs of beta-adrenergic blockade, especially bradycardia, hypotension, respiratory distress, and hypoglycemia.

### Pediatrics
Use of beta-adrenergic blocking agents in a limited number of neonates, infants, and children has not demonstrated pediatrics-specific problems that would limit the usefulness of these medications in children.

### Geriatrics
Beta-adrenergic blocking agents have been used safely and efficaciously in elderly patients. However, elderly patients may be more susceptible to some adverse effects of these agents. Beta-adrenergic blocking agents have been reported to cause or exacerbate mental impairment in the elderly. However, other evidence suggests that these agents do not produce significant lethargy or impairment in mental performance. It is possible that the likelihood of central nervous system (CNS) effects may be related to lipophilicity of the beta-adrenergic blocking agent. However, this relationship has not been conclusively established.

Elderly patients are more likely to have age-related peripheral vascular disease, which may require caution in patients receiving beta-adrenergic blocking agents. In addition, the risk of beta-blocker–induced hypothermia may be increased in elderly patients.

### Surgical
Recent evidence suggests that withdrawal of antihypertensive therapy prior to surgery may be undesirable. However, the anesthesiologist must be aware of such therapy.

### Drug interactions and/or related problems
The following drug interactions and/or related problems have been selected on the basis of their potential clinical significance (possible mechanism in parentheses where appropriate)—not necessarily inclusive (» = major clinical significance):

Note: Combinations containing any of the following medications, depending on the amount present, may also interact with this medication.

Information concerning interactions between beta-adrenergic blocking agents and other medications is still limited. Therefore, some of the following potential interactions are stated for cautionary reference until additional information is available.

» Allergen immunotherapy or
» Allergenic extracts for skin testing
  (use of these agents in patients taking beta-adrenergic blocking agents may increase the potential for serious systemic reaction or anaphylaxis; if possible, another medication should be substituted for a beta-adrenergic blocking agent in patients on allergen immunotherapy; allergen immunotherapy for conditions that are not life-threatening should be avoided in patients who cannot discontinue beta-adrenergic blocking agent therapy)

Amiodarone
  (concurrent administration with beta-adrenergic blocking agents may result in additive depressant effects on conduction and negative inotropic effects, especially in patients with underlying sinus node dysfunction or atrioventricular node dysfunction)

Anesthetics, hydrocarbon inhalation, such as:
  Chloroform
  Cyclopropane
  Enflurane
» Halothane
  Isoflurane
  Methoxyflurane
  Trichloroethylene
  (concurrent use with beta-adrenergic blocking agents may increase the risk of myocardial depression and hypotension because beta-blockade reduces the ability of the heart to respond to beta-adrenergically mediated sympathetic reflex stimuli; if necessary to reverse the effects of beta-adrenergic blocking agents during surgery, agonists such as dobutamine, dopamine, isoproterenol, or norepinephrine may be used but should be administered with caution. In patients scheduled for major surgery, most practitioners believe the risk of precipitating myocardial infarction following abrupt cessation of beta-adrenergic blocking agent therapy prior to surgery outweighs the risks of continuing therapy while compensating for medication effects by anesthetic techniques)

  (high concentrations of halothane [3% or above] or high concentrations of other halogenated hydrocarbon anesthetics should not be used when labetalol is used to produce controlled hypotension during anesthesia because of the risk of excessive hypotension, large reduction in cardiac output, and increase in central venous pressure)

» Antidiabetic agents, oral or
» Insulin
  (concurrent use with beta-adrenergic blocking agents may impair glycemic control; there may be an increased risk of hyperglycemia secondary to a slight deterioration in carbohydrate metabolism and peripheral insulin resistance; beta-adrenergic blocking agents may impair recovery from hypoglycemia in diabetics because they block the effects of catecholamines, which promote glycogenolysis and mobilize glucose in response to hypoglycemia; beta-adrenergic blocking agents also may mask certain symptoms of developing hypoglycemia such as increases in pulse rate and blood pressure, thus complicating patient monitoring; labetalol and selective or relatively selective beta-adrenergic blocking agents, such as acebutolol, atenolol, betaxolol, bisoprolol, or metoprolol, may cause fewer problems with blood glucose levels, especially at lower dosages, although they may still mask the symptoms of hypoglycemia)

Anti-inflammatory drugs, nonsteroidal (NSAIDs), especially indomethacin
  (NSAIDs may reduce the antihypertensive effects of beta-adrenergic blocking agents, possibly by inhibiting renal prostaglandin synthesis and/or causing sodium and fluid retention)

Beta-adrenergic blocking agents, ophthalmic
  (if significant systemic absorption of the ophthalmic beta-adrenergic blocking agent occurs, concurrent use may result in an additive effect either on intraocular pressure or on systemic effects of beta-blockade)

» Calcium channel blocking agents or
» Clonidine or
  Diazoxide or

» Guanabenz or
Reserpine or
Hypotension-producing medications, other, (See *Appendix II*) with the exception of monoamine oxidase (MAO) inhibitors
(blood pressure control may be impaired when clonidine or guanabenz is used concurrently with a beta-adrenergic blocking agent; potentiation of antihypertensive effect should be anticipated when other hypotension-producing medications are used concurrently; although combinations of antihypertensive agents and/or diuretics are often used for therapeutic advantage, dosage adjustment may be needed when any hypotension-producing medication is added to or withdrawn from a regimen including a beta-adrenergic blocking agent)

(symptomatic bradycardia, with or without serious hemodynamic effects, has been reported during concurrent use of diltiazem or verapamil with systemic beta-adrenergic blocking agents;though these effects may occur in the absence of overt pre-existing sinoatrial disease, older patients and patients with left ventricular dysfunction or sinoatrial or atrioventricular conduction abnormalities may be at increased risk; concurrent use of nifedipine with beta-adrenergic blocking agents, although usually well tolerated, may produce excessive hypotension and in rare cases may increase the possibility of congestive heart failure)

(calcium channel blocking agents may decrease the hepatic metabolism of propranolol, metoprolol, and possibly other beta-adrenergic blocking agents with substantial hepatic biotransformation; although the clinical significance of this effect appears to be minimal, caution is warranted given the potential for additive cardiodepressant effects during concurrent use)

(concurrent use of diazoxide with beta-adrenergic blocking agents prevents the tachycardia produced by diazoxide but may also increase the hypotensive effects)

(concurrent use of reserpine with beta-adrenergic blocking agents may result in additive and possibly excessive beta-adrenergic blockade; close observation is recommended since bradycardia and hypotension may occur)

Cimetidine
(cimetidine may reduce the clearance of hepatically metabolized beta-adrenergic blocking agents, resulting in elevations of plasma concentrations)

» Cocaine
(cocaine may inhibit the therapeutic effects of beta-adrenergic blocking agents)

(although beta-adrenergic blocking agents are recommended to reduce tachycardia, myocardial ischemia, and/or arrhythmias induced by cocaine, concurrent use of a beta-adrenergic blocking agent with cocaine may increase the risk of hypertension, excessive bradycardia, and possibly heart block, because beta-adrenergic blockade may leave cocaine's alpha-adrenergic activity unopposed; the risk of these adverse effects may be decreased with labetalol because labetalol also has some alpha-adrenergic blocking activity, although its beta-adrenergic blocking activity predominates)

Contrast media, iodinated
(concurrent use of beta-adrenergic blocking agents with intravenous contrast media may increase the risk of moderate to severe anaphylaxis; an anaphylactic event may be refractory to treatment)

Estrogens
(concurrent use may decrease the antihypertensive effect of beta-adrenergic blocking agents because estrogen-induced fluid retention may lead to increased blood pressure)

Fentanyl and derivatives
(preoperative chronic use of systemic beta-adrenergic blocking agents may decrease the frequency and/or severity of hypertensive responses to surgery, especially during sternotomy and sternal spread in cardiac or coronary artery surgery; however, chronic preoperative use of systemic beta-adrenergic blocking agents may also increase the risk of initial bradycardia following induction doses of fentanyl or any of its derivatives)

Flecainide
(although there have been no reports of adverse effects during concurrent administration of flecainide with the beta-adrenergic blocking agents, caution is recommended because of the potential for additive negative inotropic effects, especially in patients with compromised left ventricular function [ejection fraction < 30%])

Lidocaine
(concurrent use with beta-adrenergic blocking agents may reduce lidocaine elimination and increase the risk of lidocaine toxicity because of reduced hepatic blood flow; lidocaine dosage should be adjusted on the basis of serum lidocaine concentrations)

Monoamine oxidase (MAO) inhibitors, including furazolidone, procarbazine, and selegiline
(significant hypertension theoretically may occur up to 14 days following discontinuation of the MAO inhibitor; although sufficient clinical reports are lacking, concurrent use with beta-adrenergic blocking agents is not recommended)

Neuromuscular blocking agents, nondepolarizing
(beta-adrenergic blocking agents may potentiate and prolong the action of nondepolarizing neuromuscular blocking agents when used concurrently; careful postoperative monitoring of the patient may be necessary following concurrent or sequential use, especially if there is a possibility of incomplete reversal of neuromuscular blockade)

Nicotine chewing gum or
Smoking deterrents, other or
Smoking, tobacco, cessation of
(smoking cessation may increase therapeutic effects of propranolol by decreasing metabolism, thereby increasing serum concentrations; dosage adjustments may be necessary)

Nitroglycerin
(labetalol reduces the reflex tachycardia caused by nitroglycerin and may increase the antihypertensive effect)

Phenothiazines
(concurrent use with beta-adrenergic blocking agents results in an increased plasma concentration of each medication)

Phenytoin
(concurrent use of propranolol, and probably other beta-adrenergic blocking agents, with intravenous phenytoin may produce additive cardiac depressant effects)

Phenoxybenzamine or
Phentolamine
(concurrent use with labetalol may result in additive alpha-adrenergic blocking effects)

Propafenone
(concurrent use with metoprolol or propranolol may result in significant increases in plasma concentrations and half-life of propranolol and metoprolol, without affecting plasma propafenone concentrations; dosage reduction of the beta-adrenergic blocking agent may be necessary)

» Sympathomimetics
(concurrent use of beta-adrenergic blocking agents with sympathomimetic amines having beta-adrenergic stimulant activity may result in mutual inhibition of therapeutic effects; for sympathomimetic agents with beta-adrenergic effects, beta-blockade may antagonize beta-1-adrenergic cardiac effects [dobutamine, dopamine] or the beta-2-adrenergic bronchodilating effect [albuterol, ethylnorepinephrine, isoetharine, isoproterenol, metaproterenol, terbutaline] or both [isoproterenol]; use of a cardioselective beta-1-adrenergic blocker [atenolol, betaxolol, or metoprolol] or labetalol [because of its alpha-blocking activity] at low doses may prevent antagonism of the bronchodilating effect)

(sympathomimetic agents with both alpha- and beta-adrenergic effects [amphetamines, ephedrine, epinephrine, metaraminol, norepinephrine, phenylephrine, pseudoephedrine], beta-blockade may result in unopposed alpha-adrenergic activity with a risk of hypertension and excessive bradycardia and possible heart block; risk should be less with labetalol because of its alpha-blocking activity; beta-blockade also antagonizes the bronchodilating effect of ephedrine and epinephrine)

» Xanthines, especially aminophylline or theophylline
(concurrent use with beta-adrenergic blocking agents may result in mutual inhibition of therapeutic effects; in addition, concurrent use with the xanthines [except dyphylline] may decrease xanthine clearance, especially in patients with increased theophylline clearance induced by smoking; concurrent use requires careful monitoring)

## Laboratory value alterations
The following have been selected on the basis of their potential clinical significance (possible effect in parentheses where appropriate)—not necessarily inclusive (» = major clinical significance):

With diagnostic test results
Amphetamine determinations, urinary
(labetalol may produce false-positive results when commercially available assay methods [thin-layer chromatographic assay or radioenzymatic assay] are used; during labetalol therapy, positive results should be confirmed with more specific methods, such as a gas chromatographic-mass spectrometer technique)

Catecholamine determinations
(urinary concentrations of catecholamines and/or their metabolites [metanephrine, normetanephrine, vanillylmandelic acid] may be falsely increased by labetalol when measured by fluorimetric or photometric methods; a specific method, such as high performance liquid chromatography assay with solid phase extraction, should be used instead)

Glaucoma screening test
(may be interfered with by systemic beta-blockade, which reduces intraocular pressure)

Radionuclide ventriculography
(beta-adrenergic blocking agents may blunt the exercise-induced changes in cardiac function in the evaluation of coronary artery disease by decreasing heart rate)

With physiology/laboratory test values
Alkaline phosphatase, serum and
Lactate dehydrogenase (LDH), serum and
Transaminases, serum
(may be increased by acebutolol, labetalol, or metoprolol; it is recommended that labetalol be withdrawn if jaundice or laboratory signs of hepatic function impairment occur)

Antinuclear antibody (ANA) titers
(may be increased by beta-adrenergic blocking agents; dose-related)

Blood glucose concentrations
(nonselective beta-adrenergic blocking agents impair glycogenolysis and the hyperglycemic response to endogenous epinephrine, leading to persistence of hypoglycemia and delayed recovery of blood glucose to normal levels, especially in diabetics; studies have shown no such effect in resting nondiabetics with therapeutic doses; beta-adrenergic blocking agents, especially nonselective agents, decrease the release of insulin in response to hyperglycemia; effects on blood glucose may be less likely with labetalol or cardioselective agents such as acebutolol, betaxolol, atenolol, and metoprolol, especially at lower doses)

Blood urea nitrogen (BUN) (usually in patients with severe heart disease) and
Potassium concentrations, serum and
Uric acid concentrations, serum
(may be increased)

Lipoproteins, serum and
Triglycerides, serum
(concentrations may be increased)

**Medical considerations/Contraindications**
The medical considerations/contraindications included have been selected on the basis of their potential clinical significance (reasons given in parentheses where appropriate)—not necessarily inclusive (» = major clinical significance).

Note: In general, because of the similarity of effect and because the cardioselectivity of beta-1 blockers is relative, the same precautions apply to all beta-adrenergic blocking agents.

*Except under special circumstances, this medication should not be used when the following medical problems exist:*

*For all indications*
» Cardiac failure, overt or
» Cardiogenic shock or
» Heart block, 2nd- or 3rd-degree atrioventricular (AV) block or
» Sinus bradycardia (heart rate less than 45 beats per minute)
(risk of further myocardial depression; risk may be less with carteolol, labetalol, oxprenolol, penbutolol, and pindolol; beta-adrenergic blocking agents may be used with extreme caution in some patients with cardiac failure [e.g., high output failure associated with thyrotoxicosis])

*For use in myocardial infarction*
» Hypotension
(patients dependent on sympathetic stimulation to maintain adequate cardiac output and blood pressure, such as patients with hypotension in the setting of myocardial infarction, may not benefit from beta-adrenergic blockade; studies of beta-adrenergic blockade in the treatment of myocardial infarction excluded patients with systolic pressures less than 100 mm Hg)

*Risk-benefit should be considered when the following medical problems exist:*

*For all beta-adrenergic blocking agents*
» Allergy, history of or
» Asthma, bronchial or
» Emphysema or nonallergenic bronchitis
(beta-adrenergic blocking agents may promote bronchospasm and block the bronchodilating effect of epinephrine; cardioselective agents such as acebutolol, atenolol, betaxolol, bisoprolol, and metoprolol, or agents with ISA such as carteolol, oxprenolol, penbutolol, or pindolol are theoretically less likely to cause such effects when used at lower doses; labetalol may also pose less risk of bronchoconstriction; however, caution is necessary with all beta-adrenergic blocking agents)

(severity and duration of anaphylactic reactions to allergens and allergen immunotherapy may be increased in some patients being treated with beta-adrenergic blocking agents; if possible, another medication should be substituted for a beta-adrenergic blocking agent in patients receiving allergen immunotherapy, or, for conditions that are not life-threatening, allergen immunotherapy should be avoided in patients who cannot discontinue beta-adrenergic blocking agent therapy; caution is also recommended during skin testing in patients on beta-adrenergic blocking agents)

» Congestive heart failure
(risk of further depression of myocardial contractility; betaxolol and agents with ISA such as carteolol, oxprenolol, penbutolol, pindolol, and possibly acebutolol may theoretically be associated with less risk and may be used with caution in patients who are well-compensated)

» Diabetes mellitus
(beta-adrenergic blocking agents may mask tachycardia associated with hypoglycemia, but not dizziness and sweating; beta-adrenergic blocking agents may adversely affect recovery from hypoglycemia and impair peripheral circulation; these effects may theoretically be more likely with the noncardioselective agents and less likely with labetalol and cardioselective agents)

Hepatic function impairment
(metabolism of beta-adrenergic blocking agents that undergo hepatic metabolism may be decreased; patients with impaired hepatic function may require lower doses of beta-adrenergic blocking agents [exceptions are atenolol, betaxolol, carteolol, metoprolol (except in severe impairment), and nadolol, which require no dosage adjustment]; such reduction in dosage frequently applies to geriatric patients, many of whom have reduced hepatic function)

» Hyperthyroidism
(beta-adrenergic blocking agents may mask tachycardic symptoms; abrupt withdrawal may intensify symptoms)

» Mental depression, or history of
(although the association between beta-adrenergic blocking agents and depression is not fully established, these medications should be used cautiously in these patients)

Myasthenia gravis
(beta-adrenergic blocking agents may potentiate a myasthenic condition, including muscle weakness and double vision)

Pheochromocytoma
(although labetalol is used to lower blood pressure, higher-than-usual doses may be required; paradoxical hypertensive responses to labetalol have been reported in a few patients; with other beta-adrenergic blocking agents, there is a risk of hypertension if effective alpha-adrenergic blockade is not achieved first)

Psoriasis
(may be exacerbated)

Renal function impairment
(may impair beta-adrenergic blocking agent clearance; risk of reduced renal blood flow; patients with impaired renal function may require reduced doses of beta-adrenergic blocking agents [exceptions are labetalol, metoprolol, oxprenolol, penbutolol, pindolol (unless impairment is severe), propranolol, and timolol, which require no dosage adjustment]; such reduction in dosage frequently applies to geriatric patients, many of whom have reduced renal function; specific dosage recommendations, where available, are included in the *Dosage Forms* section for the particular agent)

Sensitivity to the beta-blocker prescribed

*For all beta-adrenergic blocking agents except labetalol*
Raynaud's syndrome and other peripheral vascular diseases
(beta-adrenergic blocking agents may reduce peripheral circulation and worsen these conditions; cardioselective agents such as acebutolol, atenolol, betaxolol, bisoprolol, metoprolol, or agents with ISA such as acebutolol, carteolol, oxprenolol, penbutolol, or pindolol are theoretically less likely to produce adverse effect)

**Patient monitoring**
The following may be especially important in patient monitoring (other tests may be warranted in some patients, depending on condition; » = major clinical significance):

Blood cell counts and

» Blood glucose concentrations (for diabetic patients) and
» Cardiac function monitoring and
  Hepatic function determinations and
» Pulse rate determinations and
  Renal function determinations
    (may be required at periodic intervals)
» Blood pressure and
» Electrocardiogram (ECG) and
» Heart rate
    (should be carefully monitored during intravenous administration)
» Blood pressure determinations
    (recommended at periodic intervals to monitor efficacy and safety of therapy in patients being treated for hypertension; selected patients may be trained to perform blood pressure measurements at home and report the results at regular physician visits)

## Side/Adverse Effects

The following side/adverse effects have been selected on the basis of their potential clinical significance (possible signs and symptoms in parentheses where appropriate)—not necessarily inclusive:

### Those indicating need for medical attention
Incidence less frequent
  *Bradycardia, symptomatic* (dizziness); *bronchospasm* (difficulty breathing and/or wheezing); *congestive heart failure* (swelling of ankles, feet, and/or lower legs; shortness of breath); *mental depression; reduced peripheral circulation* (cold hands and feet)—except labetalol
  Note: Risk of *bronchospasm or reduced peripheral circulation* is theoretically reduced with acebutolol, atenolol, betaxolol, bisoprolol, carteolol, metoprolol, oxprenolol, penbutolol, or pindolol.
    *Mental depression* is usually reversible and mild, but may progress to catatonia.

Incidence rare
  *Allergic reaction* (skin rash); *arrhythmias* (irregular heartbeat); *back pain or joint pain; chest pain; confusion*—especially in the elderly; *hallucinations; hepatotoxicity* (dark urine, yellow eyes or skin)—for acebutolol, bisoprolol, or labetalol; *leukopenia* (fever, sore throat); *orthostatic hypotension* (dizziness or lightheadedness when getting up from a lying or sitting position); *psoriasiform eruption* (red, scaling, or crusted skin); *thrombocytopenia* (unusual bleeding and bruising)
  Note: *Hepatotoxicity* is usually reversible; however, hepatic necrosis and death have been reported with labetalol.

### Those indicating need for medical attention only if they continue or are bothersome
Incidence more frequent
  *Decreased sexual ability; drowsiness*—especially with higher doses; *trouble in sleeping; unusual tiredness or weakness*

Incidence less frequent
  *Anxiety and/or nervousness; constipation; diarrhea; nasal congestion* (stuffy nose); *nausea or vomiting; stomach discomfort*

Incidence rare
  *Changes in taste; dry, sore eyes; frequent urination*—for acebutolol or carteolol; *itching of skin; nightmares and vivid dreams; numbness and/or tingling of fingers, toes, or skin, especially the scalp*—for labetolol

### Those indicating the need for medical attention if they occur after medication is discontinued
  *Arrhythmias* (fast or irregular heartbeat); *chest pain; general feeling of discomfort, illness, or weakness; headache; shortness of breath, sudden; sweating; trembling*

## Overdose

For more information on the management of overdose or unintentional ingestion, **contact a Poison Control Center** (see *Poison Control Center Listing*).

### Clinical effects of overdose
The following effects have been selected on the basis of their potential clinical significance (possible signs and symptoms in parentheses where appropriate)—not necessarily inclusive:
  *Bradycardia; dizziness, severe, or fainting; hypotension; irregular heartbeat; difficulty breathing; bluish-colored fingernails or palms of hands; or seizures.*

### Treatment of overdose
Decreased absorption—Gastric lavage and administration of activated charcoal.

Specific treatment—
  *Atropine:* May be administered for severe bradycardia in the presence of hypotension.
  *Diazepam or lorazepam:* May be used intravenously to treat associated seizures.
  *Dobutamine, dopamine, epinephrine, norepinephrine, or isoproterenol:* May be administered for chronotropic and inotropic support and treatment of severe hypotension. However, the effects of sympathomimetic agents may be inhibited by the presence of significant beta-blockade. Therefore, hypotension and ensuing pump failure may be refractory to treatment with catecholamines.
  *Glucagon:* Glucagon has been used effectively in the treatment of bradycardia and hypotension in beta-adrenergic blocking agent overdose. Glucagon demonstrates major inotropic and less dramatic chronotropic effects. These effects appear to be independent of the beta-adrenergic receptor. Therefore, glucagon may be an advantageous alternative treatment to reverse the hemodynamic depression of beta-adrenergic blocking agent overdose.
  *Transvenous pacing:* May be necessary for heart block.
  *Other therapy:* May include furosemide or digitalis glycoside for pulmonary edemaor cardiac failure; or a beta-2 agonist such as isoproterenol and/or a theophylline derivative for bronchospasm.
  There is limited evidence that calcium chloride may be effective in improving myocardial contractility and hemodynamic status. It is speculated that hypocalcemia resulting from beta-adrenergic blocking agent overdose may contribute to a decline in myocardial contractility.

## Patient Consultation

As an aid to patient consultation, refer to *Advice for the Patient, Beta-adrenergic Blocking Agents (Systemic)*.
In providing consultation, consider emphasizing the following selected information (» = major clinical significance):

### Before using this medication
» Conditions affecting use, especially:
  Sensitivity to the beta-blocker prescribed
  Pregnancy—Beta-adrenergic blocking agents cross the placenta; risk of hypoglycemia, respiratory depression, bradycardia, and hypotension in the fetus and neonate
  Breast-feeding—Beta-adrenergic blocking agents pass into breast milk; bradycardia, cyanosis, hypotension, and tachypnea have been reported in breast-fed infants whose mothers ingested atenolol or acebutolol
  Use in the elderly—Older patients may be more susceptible to some side/adverse effects; increased risk of beta-blocker–induced hypothermia
  Other medications, especially allergen immunotherapy and allergenic extracts used for skin testing, oral antidiabetic agents, insulin, calcium channel blocking agents, clonidine, guanabenz, cocaine, MAO inhibitors, sympathomimetics, or xanthines
  Other medical problems, especially overt cardiac failure, cardiogenic shock, 2nd- or 3rd- degree AV block, sinus bradycardia, hypotension (when used in myocardial infarction), history of allergy, bronchial asthma, emphysema or nonallergenic bronchitis, congestive heart failure, diabetes mellitus, hyperthyroidism, or mental depression

### Proper use of this medication
  Proper administration of extended-release dosage forms: Swallowing whole without crushing, breaking (except with metoprolol succinate), or chewing
  *Proper use of concentrated oral propranolol solution*
  Measuring with calibrated dropper
  Mixing with liquid or semi-solid food such as water, juices, soda or soda-like beverages, applesauce, and puddings; making sure entire dose is taken
  Not storing after mixing
  Checking pulse, if directed to do so by physician, and notifying physician if pulse falls below the rate designated by physician
  Taking medication at the same time(s) each day to maintain the therapeutic effect
» Importance of not missing doses, especially with schedules of one dose per day
» Proper dosing
  Missed dose: Taking as soon as possible; not taking at all if within 4 hours of next scheduled dose (8 hours for atenolol, betaxolol, carteolol, labetalol, nadolol, penbutolol, sotalol, or extended-release oxprenolol or propranolol); not doubling doses

## Beta-adrenergic Blocking Agents (Systemic)

» Proper storage

*For use as an antihypertensive*
  Possible need for control of weight and diet, especially sodium intake
» Compliance with therapy; patient may not experience symptoms of hypertension; importance of taking medication only as directed and keeping appointments with physician, even if feeling well
» Does not cure, but helps control hypertension; possible need for lifelong therapy; checking with physician before discontinuing medication; serious consequences of untreated hypertension

**Precautions while using this medication**
  Making regular visits to physician to check progress
» Checking with physician before discontinuing medication; gradual dosage reduction may be necessary
  Having enough medication on hand to get through weekends, holidays, and vacations; possibly carrying second written prescription for emergency use
  Carrying medical identification card during therapy
» Caution if any kind of surgery (including dental surgery) or emergency treatment is required
» Diabetics: May mask signs and symptoms of hypoglycemia or may cause increased blood glucose concentrations or prolong hypoglycemia
» Caution when driving or doing things requiring alertness, because of possible drowsiness, dizziness, or lightheadedness
  Caution during exposure to cold weather because of possible increased sensitivity to cold
» Caution against overexertion in response to decreased chest pain
  Caution if any laboratory tests required; possible interference with test results
  Patients with allergies to foods, medications, or stinging insect venom: Possible increase in severity of allergic reactions; checking with physician immediately if severe allergic reaction occurs

*For use as an antihypertensive*
» Not taking other medications, especially nonprescription sympathomimetics, unless discussed with physician

*For oral labetalol only*
» Caution when getting up suddenly from a lying or sitting position, especially during initiation of therapy or when dosage is increased
» Caution in using alcohol, while standing for long periods or exercising, and during hot weather because of enhanced orthostatic hypotensive effects

*For parenteral labetalol only*
» Lying down during injection and for up to 3 hours after getting injection, then getting up gradually

**Side/adverse effects**
  Signs of potential side effects, especially bradycardia, breathing difficulty and/or wheezing, congestive heart failure, mental depression, reduced peripheral circulation, allergic reaction, arrhythmias, back pain or joint pain, chest pain, confusion, hallucinations, hepatotoxicity, leukopenia, psoriasiform eruption, thrombocytopenia, and withdrawal reaction
  For labetalol: Transient scalp tingling may occur, usually at beginning of treatment

## General Dosing Information

Although plasma concentrations of beta-adrenergic blocking agents can be ascertained, there is not always a predictable relationship between plasma concentration and pharmacological effects. Pharmacological effects have been observed when plasma concentrations were not discernible. Therefore, titration of dosage with measurement of heart rate and blood pressure is used to guide therapy.

In some patients, once-daily dosing is effective.

When beta-adrenergic blocking agent therapy is discontinued in patients concurrently receiving clonidine or guanabenz, the beta-adrenergic blocking agent should be gradually discontinued several days before the clonidine or guanabenz is gradually discontinued in order to avoid clonidine- or guanabenz-withdrawal hypertensive crisis.

**For oral dosage forms only**
When a beta-adrenergic blocking agent must be withdrawn from established therapy *(especially in patients with ischemic heart disease)*, it is recommended that the dosage be reduced gradually to minimize risk of exacerbation of angina or development of myocardial infarction. Dosage reduction should occur over a period of approximately 2 weeks. During this time the patient should avoid vigorous physical activity in order to minimize the danger of infarction or arrhythmias. If signs of withdrawal (e.g., angina) occur, beta-adrenergic blocking agent therapy should be reinstated temporarily and then carefully withdrawn after the patient has stabilized.

It is recommended that beta-adrenergic blocking agent therapy be withdrawn if drug-induced mental depression occurs.

**Diet/Nutrition**
Oral beta-adrenergic blocking agents may be taken either with food or on an empty stomach. Studies indicate that bioavailability of labetalol, propranolol, and possibly metoprolol may be enhanced by administration with food, which may slow the hepatic metabolism of the medication. Bioavailability of acebutolol, atenolol, nadolol, oxprenolol, penbutolol, and pindolol are not affected by food intake. Concurrent food intake may slow carteolol absorption, but does not affect bioavailability. Sotalol does not undergo significant first-pass metabolism. Food, especially milk and milk products, may reduce the bioavailability of sotalol.

---

### ACEBUTOLOL

## Summary of Differences

Pharmacology/pharmacokinetics:
  Mechanism of action/Effect—Mild to moderate intrinsic sympathomimetic activity (ISA); relatively cardioselective; low lipid solubility.
  Absorption—Bioavailability significantly reduced by first-pass metabolism but effect not reduced because of active metabolite.
  Protein binding—Low.
  Elimination—Removable by hemodialysis.
Precautions:
  Medical considerations/contraindications—Dosage reduction necessary in hepatic function and renal function impairment.
Side/adverse effects:
  Theoretical reduced risk of bronchospasm, hypoglycemia, and peripheral vasoconstriction because of cardioselectivity.

## Oral Dosage Forms

### ACEBUTOLOL HYDROCHLORIDE CAPSULES

**Usual adult dose**
Antiarrhythmic—
  Oral, 200 mg two times a day, the dosage being adjusted according to response, generally in the range of 600 to 1200 mg per day.
Antihypertensive—
  Oral, initially 400 mg per day as a single dose or in two divided daily doses, the dosage being adjusted according to response, with maintenance doses usually in the range of 400 to 800 mg per day.
Note: Geriatric patients may have increased or decreased sensitivity to the effects of the usual adult dose.

It is recommended that the dosage of acebutolol be reduced in patients with renal function impairment as follows:

| Creatinine clearance (mL/min/1.73m) | % of normal dose to be given |
|---|---|
| <50 | 50 |
| <25 | 25 |

**Usual geriatric prescribing limits**
In geriatric patients, daily doses should not exceed a total of 800 mg.

**Usual pediatric dose**
Dosage has not been established.

**Strength(s) usually available**
U.S.—
  200 mg (Rx) [*Sectral;* GENERIC].
  400 mg (Rx) [*Sectral;* GENERIC].
Canada—
  Not commercially available.

**Packaging and storage**
Store below 40 °C (104 °F), preferably between 15 and 30 °C (59 and 86 °F), in a well-closed container, unless otherwise specified by manufacturer.

**Auxiliary labeling**
• Do not take other medicine without your doctor's advice.

**Note**
Check refill frequency to determine compliance in hypertensive patients.

### ACEBUTOLOL HYDROCHLORIDE TABLETS

**Usual adult dose**
Antianginal—
  Oral, initially 200 mg two times a day, the dosage being adjusted according to response, generally in the range of 600 to 1200 mg per day.

Antihypertensive—
    Oral, initially 100 mg two times a day, the dosage being adjusted weekly according to response, up to a maximum of 400 mg two times a day.
Antiarrhythmic[1]—
    Oral, 200 mg two times a day, the dosage being adjusted according to response.

**Usual pediatric dose**
Dosage has not been established.

**Strength(s) usually available**
U.S.—
    Not commercially available.
Canada—
    100 mg (Rx) [*Monitan; Sectral* (scored)].
    200 mg (Rx) [*Monitan* (scored); *Sectral* (scored)].
    400 mg (Rx) [*Monitan* (scored); *Sectral* (scored)].

**Packaging and storage**
Store below 40 °C (104 °F), preferably between 15 and 30 °C (59 and 86 °F), in a well-closed container, unless otherwise specified by manufacturer.

**Auxiliary labeling**
• Do not take other medicines without your doctor's advice.

**Note**
Check refill frequency to determine compliance in hypertensive patients.

[1]Not included in Canadian product labeling.

---

### *ATENOLOL*

## Summary of Differences
Pharmacology/pharmacokinetics:
    Mechanism of action/Effect—Relatively cardioselective (beta-1); very low lipid solubility.
    Biotransformation—Minimal hepatic metabolism.
    Protein binding—Very low to low.
    Elimination—Removable by hemodialysis.
Precautions:
    Medical considerations/contraindications—Dosage reduction necessary in renal function impairment but not necessary in hepatic function impairment.
Side/adverse effects:
    Theoretical reduced risk of bronchospasm, hypoglycemia, and peripheral vasoconstriction when daily dosage is in the lower range, because of cardioselectivity.

## Oral Dosage Forms
### ATENOLOL TABLETS
**Usual adult dose**
Antianginal—
    Oral, initially 50 mg once a day, the dosage being increased gradually to 100 mg a day after one week if necessary and tolerated. Some patients may require up to 200 mg a day.
Antihypertensive—
    Oral, initially 25 to 50 mg once a day, the dosage being increased to 50 to 100 mg a day after two weeks if necessary and tolerated.
Myocardial infarction—
    In patients who tolerate the full intravenous dose: Oral, initially 50 mg ten minutes after the last intravenous dose, followed by another 50 mg twelve hours later. A dose of 100 mg once a day or 50 mg two times a day may then be given for six to nine days or until discharge from the hospital.
Note: Geriatric patients may have increased or decreased sensitivity to the effects of the usual adult dose.

    For patients with severe renal function impairment, the following maximum doses are recommended:

| Creatinine clearance (mL/min/1.73m) | Maximum dose |
|---|---|
| 15–35 | 50 mg per day |
| <15 | 50 mg every second day |

**Usual pediatric dose**
Dosage has not been established.

**Strength(s) usually available**
U.S.—
    25 mg (Rx) [*Tenormin;* GENERIC].
    50 mg (Rx) [*Tenormin* (scored); GENERIC].
    100 mg (Rx) [*Tenormin;* GENERIC].
Canada—
    50 mg (Rx) [*Apo-Atenolol; Novo-Atenol; Tenormin* (scored) [GENERIC].
    100 mg (Rx) [*Apo-Atenolol; Novo-Atenol; Tenormin* (scored) [GENERIC].

**Packaging and storage**
Store below 40 °C (104 °F), preferably between 15 and 30 °C (59 and 86 °F), in a well-closed container, unless otherwise specified by manufacturer. Protect from light.

**Auxiliary labeling**
• Do not take other medicine without your doctor's advice.

**Note**
Check refill frequency to determine compliance in hypertensive patients.

## Parenteral Dosage Forms
### ATENOLOL INJECTION
**Usual adult dose**
Myocardial infarction—
    Early treatment: Intravenous, 5 mg (over five minutes), the dose being repeated ten minutes later.
Note: Geriatric patients may have increased or decreased sensitivity to the effects of the usual adult dose.

    In patients who tolerate the full intravenous dose (10 mg), oral atenolol treatment should be initiated ten minutes after the last intravenous dose.

    For patients with severe renal function impairment, the following maximum doses are recommended:

| Creatinine clearance (mL/min/1.73m) | Maximum dose |
|---|---|
| 15–35 | 50 mg per day |
| <15 | 50 mg every second day |

**Usual pediatric dose**
Dosage has not been established.

**Strength(s) usually available**
U.S.—
    500 mcg (0.5 mg) per mL (Rx) [*Tenormin*].
Canada—
    Not commercially available.

**Packaging and storage**
Store between 2 and 30 °C (36 and 86 °F), unless otherwise specified by manufacturer. Protect from light. Protect from freezing.

---

### *BETAXOLOL*

## Summary of Differences
Pharmacology/pharmacokinetics:
    Mechanism of action/Effect—Relatively cardioselective; moderate lipid solubility.
    Protein binding—Moderate.
    Elimination—Not removable by hemodialysis.
Precautions:
    Medical considerations/contraindications—Dosage reduction may be recommended in renal function impairment; dosage reduction not necessary in hepatic function impairment.

## Oral Dosage Forms
### BETAXOLOL TABLETS
**Usual adult dose**
Antihypertensive—
    Oral, 10 mg once a day initially, the dosage being doubled, if necessary, after seven to fourteen days.
Note: Geriatric patients may have increased or decreased sensitivity to the effects of the usual adult dose. An initial dose of 5 mg should be considered for elderly patients.

    For patients with renal function impairment who are undergoing hemodialysis, an initial dose of 5 mg once a day is recommended, increased by 5 mg a day every fourteen days, as necessary, up to a maximum daily dose of 20 mg.

**Usual pediatric dose**
Dosage has not been established.

**Strength(s) usually available**
U.S.—
  10 mg (Rx) [*Kerlone* (scored)].
  20 mg (Rx) [*Kerlone*].
Canada—
  Not commercially available.

**Packaging and storage**
Store below 40 °C (104 °F), preferably between 15 and 30 °C (59 and 86 °F), unless otherwise specified by manufacturer.

**Auxiliary labeling**
• Do not take other medicine without your doctor's advice.

**Note**
Check refill frequency to determine compliance in hypertensive patients.

---

## BISOPROLOL

## Summary of Differences
Pharmacology/pharmacokinetics:
  Mechanism of action/Effect—Relatively cardioselective (beta-1).
  Protein binding—Low.
Precautions:
  Breast-feeding—Not known if distributed into breast milk.

## Oral Dosage Forms
### BISOPROLOL FUMARATE TABLETS

**Usual adult dose**
Antihypertensive—
  Oral, initially 5 mg once a day, the dosage being increased to 10 mg once a day if hypertension is not adequately controlled.
Note: An initial dose of 2.5 mg once a day may be appropriate for some patients, especially patients with bronchospastic disease.

**Usual adult prescribing limits**
20 mg once a day.

**Usual pediatric dose**
Dosage has not been established.

**Strength(s) usually available**
U.S.—
  5 mg (Rx) [*Zebeta* (scored)].
  10 mg (Rx) [*Zebeta*].
Canada—
  Not commercially available.

**Packaging and storage**
Store below 40 °C (104 °F), preferably between 15 and 30 °C (59 and 86 °F), in a tight container, unless otherwise specified by manufacturer.

**Auxiliary labeling**
• Do not take other medicine without your doctor's advice.

**Note**
Check refill frequency to determine compliance in hypertensive patients.

---

## CARTEOLOL

## Summary of Differences
Pharmacology/pharmacokinetics:
  Mechanism of action/Effect—Moderate intrinsic sympathomimetic activity (ISA); nonselective; low lipid solubility.
  Biotransformation—Minimal hepatic metabolism (one active metabolite).
  Protein binding—Low.
Precautions:
  Breast-feeding—Not known if distributed into breast milk.
  Medical considerations/contraindications—Dosage reduction necessary in renal function impairment but not necessary in hepatic function impairment.
Side/adverse effects:
  Theoretical reduced risk of bronchospasm, heart failure, and peripheral vasoconstriction because of ISA.

## Oral Dosage Forms
### CARTEOLOL HYDROCHLORIDE TABLETS

**Usual adult dose**
Antihypertensive—
  Oral, initially 2.5 mg once a day, the dosage being adjusted according to response, up to a maximum of 10 mg once a day.
Note: Geriatric patients may have increased or decreased sensitivity to the effects of the usual adult dose.
  It is recommended that the dosage interval be increased in patients with renal function impairment as follows:

| Creatinine clearance (mL/min) | Dosage interval (hrs) |
|---|---|
| >60 | 24 |
| 20–60 | 48 |
| <20 | 72 |

**Usual adult prescribing limits**
10 mg per day.

**Usual pediatric dose**
Dosage has not been established.

**Strength(s) usually available**
U.S.—
  2.5 mg (Rx) [*Cartrol* (lactose)].
  5 mg (Rx) [*Cartrol* (lactose)].
Canada—
  Not commercially available.

**Packaging and storage**
Store below 40 °C (104 °F), preferably between 15 and 30 °C (59 and 86 °F), in a well-closed container, unless otherwise specified by manufacturer.

**Auxiliary labeling**
• Do not take other medicine without your doctor's advice.

**Note**
Check refill frequency to determine compliance in hypertensive patients.

---

## LABETALOL

## Summary of Differences
Pharmacology/pharmacokinetics:
  Mechanism of action/Effect—Also has selective alpha-1-adrenergic blocking effects; nonselective beta-blocker; low lipid solubility.
  Absorption—Bioavailability significantly reduced by first-pass metabolism and enhanced by concurrent administration with food.
  Protein binding—Moderate.
  Elimination—Not removable by hemodialysis.
Precautions:
  Medical considerations/contraindications—May not exacerbate Raynaud's phenomenon or other peripheral vascular diseases; dosage reduction necessary in hepatic function impairment but not necessary in renal function impairment.
Side/adverse effects:
  Possible reduced risk of bradycardia, bronchoconstriction, cardiac failure, hypoglycemia, and peripheral vasoconstriction, and increased incidence of postural hypotension.

## Additional Dosing Information
See also *General Dosing Information*.

The hypotensive effect of labetalol may be especially pronounced when the patient is standing. If feasible, blood pressure should be taken in the supine position, after standing for 10 minutes, and immediately after exercise. Dosage increases should be made only if there has been no decrease in the standing blood pressure from previous levels.

Hospitalized patients should not be discharged until the effect of labetalol on their standing blood pressure has been determined.

Dosage reduction is indicated if the patient has excessive orthostatic fall in pressure and/or normal supine pressure.

Appropriate laboratory testing is recommended at the first sign and/or symptom of hepatotoxicity; if there is laboratory evidence of hepatotoxicity, it is recommended that labetalol be permanently withdrawn.

*For parenteral dosage form*

Labetalol hydrochloride injection may be administered as a direct intravenous injection (over a 2-minute period) or by continuous intravenous infusion.

When labetalol is administered by continuous intravenous infusion, it is recommended that it be administered by means of an infusion pump, a micro-drip regulator, or a similar device to allow precise adjustment of the flow rate.

To reduce the chance of postural hypotension, patients should remain supine for up to 3 hours after receiving parenteral labetalol. Ambulation should not be permitted until the ability of the patient to tolerate the upright position has been determined.

## Oral Dosage Forms

### LABETALOL HYDROCHLORIDE TABLETS USP

**Usual adult dose**
Antihypertensive—
  Initial: Oral, 100 mg two times a day, the dosage being adjusted in increments of 100 mg two times a day every two or three days until the desired response is achieved.
  Maintenance: Oral, 200 to 400 mg two times a day.
Note: Labetalol may be administered in three divided daily doses if necessary because of side effects such as nausea or dizziness.
  In severe hypertension, doses of 1.2 to 2.4 grams per day, in two or three divided doses, may be needed.
  Geriatric patients may have increased or decreased sensitivity to the effects of the usual adult dose.

**Usual pediatric dose**
Dosage has not been established.

**Strength(s) usually available**
U.S.—
  100 mg (Rx) [*Normodyne* (scored); *Trandate* (scored)].
  200 mg (Rx) [*Normodyne* (scored); *Trandate* (scored)].
  300 mg (Rx) [*Normodyne*; *Trandate* (scored)].
Canada—
  100 mg (Rx) [*Trandate* (scored)].
  200 mg (Rx) [*Trandate* (scored)].

**Packaging and storage**
Store between 2 and 30 °C (36 and 86 °F), unless otherwise specified by manufacturer. Store in a tight, light-resistant container.

**Auxiliary labeling**
• Do not take other medicines without your doctor's advice.

**Note**
Check refill frequency to determine compliance in hypertensive patients.

## Parenteral Dosage Forms

### LABETALOL HYDROCHLORIDE INJECTION USP

**Usual adult dose**
Antihypertensive—
  Intravenous, 20 mg (0.25 mg per kg of body weight for an 80-kg patient) injected slowly over a two-minute period; additional injections of 40 mg and 80 mg may be given at ten-minute intervals until the desired blood pressure is achieved or a total of 300 mg has been given; or
  Intravenous infusion, administered at a rate of 2 mg per minute, the dosage being adjusted according to response; the total dose necessary may range from 50 to 300 mg.
Note: Geriatric patients may have increased or decreased sensitivity to the effects of the usual adult dose.

**Usual pediatric dose**
Dosage has not been established.

**Strength(s) usually available**
U.S.—
  5 mg per mL (Rx) [*Normodyne*; *Trandate*].
Canada—
  5 mg per mL (Rx) [*Trandate*].

**Packaging and storage**
Store between 2 and 30 °C (36 and 86 °F), unless otherwise specified by manufacturer. Protect from light. Protect from freezing.

**Preparation of dosage form**
Labetalol hydrochloride may be prepared for administration by continuous intravenous infusion by either of the following methods—
Adding 200 mg to 160 mL of a commonly used intravenous fluid to produce 200 mL of solution containing 1 mg of labetalol hydrochloride per mL; or
Adding 200 mg to 250 mL of intravenous fluid to produce about 300 mL of solution containing approximately 2 mg of labetalol hydrochloride per 3 mL.

---

## METOPROLOL

## Summary of Differences

Pharmacology/pharmacokinetics:
  Mechanism of action/Effect—Relatively cardioselective (beta-1); moderate lipid solubility.
  Absorption—Bioavailability significantly reduced by first-pass metabolism.
  Protein binding—Low.
  Elimination—Not removable by hemodialysis.
Precautions:
  Medical considerations/contraindications—No dosage reduction necessary in hepatic function impairment (unless severe) or renal function impairment.
Side/adverse effects:
  Theoretical reduced risk of bronchospasm, hypoglycemia, and peripheral vasoconstriction when daily dosage does not exceed 200 mg, because of cardioselectivity; increased risk of central nervous system (CNS) side effects because of lipid solubility and relative ease of penetration into CNS.

## Oral Dosage Forms

Note: Bracketed uses in the *Dosage Forms* section refer to categories of use and/or indications that are not included in U.S. product labeling.

### METOPROLOL SUCCINATE EXTENDED-RELEASE TABLETS

**Usual adult dose**
Antihypertensive—
  Oral, 50 to 100 mg once a day, the dosage being increased at weekly (or longer) intervals as needed and tolerated up to a total of 400 mg a day.
Antianginal—
  Oral, 100 mg once a day, the dosage being increased gradually at weekly intervals as needed and tolerated up to a maximum of 400 mg a day.
[Vascular headache prophylactic][1]—
  Oral, 200 mg once a day.
Note: Geriatric patients may have increased or decreased sensitivity to the effects of the usual adult dose.

**Usual pediatric dose**
Dosage has not been established.

**Strength(s) usually available**
U.S.—
  50 mg (Rx) [*Toprol-XL* (scored)].
  100 mg (Rx) [*Toprol-XL* (scored)].
  200 mg (Rx) [*Toprol-XL* (scored)].
Canada—
  Not commercially available.

**Packaging and storage**
Store between 15 and 30 °C (59 and 86 °F), unless otherwise specified by manufacturer. Store in a tight container.

**Auxiliary labeling**
• Do not take other medicine without your doctor's advice.

**Note**
Check refill frequency to determine compliance in hypertensive patients.

### METOPROLOL TARTRATE TABLETS USP

**Usual adult dose**
Antianginal
Antihypertensive—
  Oral, initially 100 mg a day in single (hypertension) or divided (angina or hypertension) doses, the dosage being increased at one-week intervals as needed and tolerated up to a total of 450 mg a day if necessary.
Note: To maintain satisfactory blood pressure control, some patients may require division of the total daily dose into three separate doses.
Myocardial infarction—
  Early treatment: Oral, 50 mg (for patients who tolerate the full intravenous dose) or 25 to 50 mg (for patients who do not tolerate the full intravenous dose) every six hours starting fifteen minutes after the last intravenous dose or as soon as clinical condition allows. This dosage is continued for forty-eight hours, followed by
  Late treatment: Oral, 100 mg two times a day for at least three months and possibly for as long as one to three years.

[Vascular headache prophylactic][1]—
 Oral, 50 to 100 mg two to four times a day.

Note: Geriatric patients may have increased or decreased sensitivity to the effects of the usual adult dose.

### Usual pediatric dose
Dosage has not been established.

### Strength(s) usually available
U.S.—
 50 mg (Rx) [*Lopressor* (scored); GENERIC].
 100 mg (Rx) [*Lopressor* (scored); GENERIC].
Canada—
 50 mg (Rx) [*Apo-Metoprolol* (scored); *Apo-Metoprolol (Type L)*; *Betaloc* (scored); *Lopresor* (scored); *Novometoprol* (scored); *Nu-Metop* [GENERIC].
 100 mg (Rx) [*Apo-Metoprolol* (scored); *Apo-Metoprolol (Type L)*; *Betaloc* (scored); *Lopresor* (scored); *Novometoprol* (scored); *Nu-Metop* [GENERIC].

### Packaging and storage
Store between 15 and 30 °C (59 and 86 °F), unless otherwise specified by manufacturer. Store in a tight, light-resistant container.

### Auxiliary labeling
• Do not take other medicine without your doctor's advice.

### Note
Check refill frequency to determine compliance in hypertensive patients.

### METOPROLOL TARTRATE EXTENDED-RELEASE TABLETS

#### Usual adult dose
Antianginal
Antihypertensive—
 Oral, 100 to 400 mg administered once a day for maintenance of established dosage requirements.

Note: Geriatric patients may have increased or decreased sensitivity to the effects of the usual adult dose.

#### Usual pediatric dose
Dosage has not been established.

#### Strength(s) usually available
U.S.—
 Not commercially available.
Canada—
 100 mg (Rx) [*Lopresor SR*].
 200 mg (Rx) [*Betaloc Durules*; *Lopresor SR*].

#### Packaging and storage
Store below 40 °C (104 °F), preferably between 15 and 30 °C (59 and 86 °F), unless otherwise specified by manufacturer. Store in a light-resistant container.

#### Auxiliary labeling
• Do not take other medicine without your doctor's advice.

#### Note
Check refill frequency to determine compliance in hypertensive patients.

## Parenteral Dosage Forms

### METOPROLOL TARTRATE INJECTION USP

#### Usual adult dose
Myocardial infarction—
 Early treatment: Intravenous (rapid), 5 mg every two minutes for three doses.

Note: Geriatric patients may have increased or decreased sensitivity to the effects of the usual adult dose.

#### Usual pediatric dose
Dosage has not been established.

#### Strength(s) usually available
U.S.—
 1 mg per mL (Rx) [*Lopressor*; GENERIC].
Canada—
 1 mg per mL (Rx) [*Betaloc* (sodium chloride 45 mg per mL); *Lopresor* (sodium chloride 45 mg per mL)].

#### Packaging and storage
Store below 40 °C (104 °F), preferably between 15 and 30 °C (59 and 86 °F), unless otherwise specified by manufacturer. Protect from light. Protect from freezing.

[1]Not included in Canadian product labeling.

---

## NADOLOL

### Summary of Differences
Pharmacology/pharmacokinetics:
 Mechanism of action/Effect—Nonselective; low lipid solubility.
 Biotransformation—Not hepatically metabolized.
 Protein binding—Very low to low.
 Elimination—Removable by hemodialysis.
Precautions:
 Medical considerations/contraindications—Dosage reduction or increased dosing intervals recommended in renal function impairment; dosage reduction not necessary in hepatic function impairment.

## Oral Dosage Forms

Note: Bracketed uses in the *Dosage Forms* section refer to categories of use and/or indications that are not included in U.S. product labeling.

### NADOLOL TABLETS USP

#### Usual adult dose
Antianginal—
 Oral, 40 mg once a day initially, the dosage being increased by 40 to 80 mg at three- to seven-day intervals as needed and tolerated up to a total of 240 mg a day if necessary.
Antihypertensive—
 Oral, initially 40 mg once a day, the dosage being increased in increments of 40 to 80 mg at one-week intervals as needed and tolerated up to a total of 320 mg a day if necessary.
[Vascular headache prophylactic][1]—
 Oral, 20 to 40 mg once a day initially, the dosage being gradually increased as tolerated up to 120 mg per day if necessary.

Note: Geriatric patients may have increased or decreased sensitivity to the effects of the usual adult dose.

Because of the long half-life, once-a-day dosage is sufficient to provide stable plasma concentrations; however, such steady-state concentrations may not be achieved for up to 5 days following initiation of therapy or change of dose.

For patients with renal function impairment, the following dosage adjustments are recommended:

| Creatinine clearance (mL/min/1.73m) | Dosage interval (hours) |
|---|---|
| >50 | 24 |
| 31–50 | 24–36 |
| 10–30 | 24–48 |
| <10 | 40–60 |

#### Usual pediatric dose
Dosage has not been established.

#### Strength(s) usually available
U.S.—
 20 mg (Rx) [*Corgard* (scored); GENERIC].
 40 mg (Rx) [*Corgard* (scored); GENERIC].
 80 mg (Rx) [*Corgard* (scored); GENERIC].
 120 mg (Rx) [*Corgard* (scored); GENERIC].
 160 mg (Rx) [*Corgard* (scored); GENERIC].
Canada—
 40 mg (Rx) [*Corgard* (scored); *Syn-Nadolol* (scored) [GENERIC].
 80 mg (Rx) [*Corgard* (partially scored); *Syn-Nadolol* (partially scored) [GENERIC].
 160 mg (Rx) [*Corgard* (scored); *Syn-Nadolol* (scored) [GENERIC].

#### Packaging and storage
Store between 15 and 30 °C (59 and 86 °F), unless otherwise specified by manufacturer. Store in a tight, light-resistant container.

#### Auxiliary labeling
• Do not take other medicine without your doctor's advice.

#### Note
Check refill frequency to determine compliance in hypertensive patients.

[1]Not included in Canadian product labeling.

## OXPRENOLOL

### Summary of Differences
Pharmacology/pharmacokinetics:
  Mechanism of action/Effect—Moderate intrinsic sympathomimetic activity (ISA); nonselective; moderate lipid solubility.
  Absorption—Bioavailability significantly reduced by first-pass metabolism.
  Protein binding—High.
Precautions:
  Medical considerations/contraindications—Dosage reduction necessary in hepatic function impairment but not necessary in renal function impairment.
Side/adverse effects:
  Theoretical reduced risk of bronchospasm, heart failure, and peripheral vasoconstriction because of ISA.

### Oral Dosage Forms
Note: Dosage and strengths of the dosage forms available are expressed in terms of the hydrochloride salt.

### OXPRENOLOL TABLETS USP
**Usual adult dose**
Antihypertensive—
  Oral, 20 mg three times a day initially, the dosage being increased in increments of 60 mg per day every one to two weeks until the desired response is achieved, usually in the range of 120 to 320 mg a day.
Note: Once the optimal daily dose has been reached, twice-daily dosing may be used.
  Geriatric patients may have increased or decreased sensitivity to the effects of the usual adult dose.

**Usual adult prescribing limits**
480 mg per day.

**Usual pediatric dose**
Dosage has not been established.

**Strength(s) usually available**
U.S.—
  Not commercially available.
Canada—
  20 mg (hydrochloride) (Rx) [*Trasicor*].
  40 mg (hydrochloride) (Rx) [*Trasicor* (scored)].
  80 mg (hydrochloride) (Rx) [*Trasicor* (scored)].

**Packaging and storage**
Store below 40 °C (104 °F), preferably between 15 and 30 °C (59 and 86 °F), in a well-closed container, unless otherwise specified by manufacturer. Protect from light.

**Auxiliary labeling**
• Do not take other medicine without your doctor's advice.

**Note**
Check refill frequency to determine compliance in hypertensive patients.

### OXPRENOLOL EXTENDED-RELEASE TABLETS USP
**Usual adult dose**
Antihypertensive—
  Oral, usually 120 to 320 mg a day administered once a day in the morning for maintenance of established dosage requirements.
Note: Geriatric patients may have increased or decreased sensitivity to the effects of the usual adult dose.

**Usual pediatric dose**
Dosage has not been established.

**Strength(s) usually available**
U.S.—
  Not commercially available.
Canada—
  80 mg (hydrochloride) (Rx) [*Slow-Trasicor* (lactose)].
  160 mg (hydrochloride) (Rx) [*Slow-Trasicor* (lactose)].

**Packaging and storage**
Store below 40 °C (104 °F), preferably between 15 and 30 °C (59 and 86 °F), in a well-closed container, unless otherwise specified by manufacturer. Protect from light.

**Auxiliary labeling**
• Do not take other medicine without your doctor's advice.

**Note**
Check refill frequency to determine compliance in hypertensive patients.

## PENBUTOLOL

### Summary of Differences
Pharmacology/pharmacokinetics:
  Mechanism of action/Effect—Moderate intrinsic sympathomimetic activity (ISA); high lipid solubility; nonselective.
  Biotransformation—Although hepatically metabolized, penbutolol undergoes no significant first-pass effect.
  Protein binding—High to very high.
  Elimination—Not removable by hemodialysis.
Precautions:
  Breast-feeding—Not known whether distributed into breast milk.
  Medical considerations/contraindications—Dosage reduction necessary in hepatic function impairment but not necessary in renal function impairment.
Side/adverse effects:
  Theoretical reduced risk of bronchospasm, heart failure, and peripheral vasoconstriction because of ISA.

### Oral Dosage Forms
### PENBUTOLOL SULFATE TABLETS
**Usual adult dose**
Antihypertensive—
  Oral, 20 mg once a day.
Note: Geriatric patients may have increased or decreased sensitivity to the effects of the usual adult dose.

**Usual pediatric dose**
Dosage has not been established.

**Strength(s) usually available**
U.S.—
  20 mg (Rx) [*Levatol* (scored; lactose)].
Canada—
  Not commercially available.

**Packaging and storage**
Store below 40 °C (104 °F), preferably between 15 and 30 °C (59 and 86 °F), in a well-closed container, unless otherwise specified by manufacturer. Protect from light.

**Auxiliary labeling**
• Do not take other medicine without your doctor's advice.

**Note**
Check refill frequency to determine compliance in hypertensive patients.

## PINDOLOL

### Summary of Differences
Pharmacology/pharmacokinetics:
  Mechanism of action/Effect—Exhibits the most intrinsic sympathomimetic activity (ISA) of beta-blockers currently available; moderate lipid solubility; nonselective.
  Biotransformation—Although hepatically metabolized, pindolol undergoes no significant first-pass effect.
  Protein binding—Moderate.
Precautions:
  Medical considerations/contraindications—Dosage reduction necessary in hepatic function and severe renal function impairment.
Side/adverse effects:
  Theoretical reduced risk of bronchospasm, heart failure, and peripheral vasoconstriction because of ISA; overdose may produce tachycardia and hypertension.

### Oral Dosage Forms
Note: Bracketed uses in the *Dosage Forms* section refer to categories of use and/or indications that are not included in U.S. product labeling.

### PINDOLOL TABLETS USP
**Usual adult dose**
Antihypertensive—
  Oral, initially 5 mg two times a day, the dosage being increased in increments of 10 mg per day at two- or three-week intervals as needed and tolerated up to a maximum of 45 mg a day (Canada) or 60 mg a day (U.S.).
Note: Many hypertensive patients require a maintenance dose of only 5 mg of pindolol two times a day to provide an adequate reduction in blood pressure.

Once the optimal daily dose has been reached, once-daily dosing may be used.

Geriatric patients may have increased or decreased sensitivity to the effects of the usual adult dose.

[Antianginal]—
Oral, 5 mg three times a day, the dosage being increased at one to two week intervals up to a maximum of 40 mg per day.

### Usual adult prescribing limits
45 mg a day (Canada) or 60 mg a day (U.S.).

### Usual pediatric dose
Dosage has not been established.

### Strength(s) usually available
U.S.—
5 mg (Rx) [*Visken* (scored); GENERIC].
10 mg (Rx) [*Visken* (scored); GENERIC].
Canada—
5 mg (Rx) [*Novo-Pindol; Syn-Pindol; Visken* (scored) [GENERIC].
10 mg (Rx) [*Novo-Pindol; Syn-Pindol; Visken* (scored) [GENERIC].
15 mg (Rx) [*Novo-Pindol; Syn-Pindol; Visken* (scored) [GENERIC].

### Packaging and storage
Store below 40 °C (104 °F), preferably between 15 and 30 °C (59 and 86 °F), in a well-closed container, unless otherwise specified by manufacturer. Protect from light.

### Auxiliary labeling
• Do not take other medicine without your doctor's advice.

### Note
Check refill frequency to determine compliance in hypertensive patients.

---

## PROPRANOLOL

## Summary of Differences
Pharmacology/pharmacokinetics:
  Mechanism of action/Effect—Nonselective; high lipid solubility.
  Absorption—Bioavailability significantly reduced by first-pass metabolism.
  Protein binding—Very high.
  Elimination—Not removable by hemodialysis.
Precautions:
  Medical considerations/contraindications—Dosage reduction necessary in hepatic function impairment but not necessary in renal function impairment.
Side/adverse effects:
  Increased risk of CNS side effects because of high lipid solubility and ease of penetration into CNS.

## Oral Dosage Forms
Note: Bracketed uses in the *Dosage Forms* section refer to categories of use and/or indications that are not included in U.S. product labeling.

### PROPRANOLOL HYDROCHLORIDE EXTENDED-RELEASE CAPSULES USP
#### Usual adult dose
Antihypertensive—
Oral, 80 mg once a day, the dosage being increased gradually up to 160 mg once a day. Doses up to 640 mg per day may be needed in some patients.
Antianginal—
Oral, 80 mg once a day, the dosage being increased gradually at three- to seven-day intervals as needed up to 320 mg per day.
Vascular headache prophylaxis—
Oral, 80 mg once a day, the dosage being increased gradually as needed up to 240 mg once a day.
Note: Geriatric patients may have increased or decreased sensitivity to the effects of the usual adult dose.

#### Usual pediatric dose
Dosage has not been established.

#### Strength(s) usually available
U.S.—
60 mg (Rx) [*Inderal LA;* GENERIC].
80 mg (Rx) [*Inderal LA;* GENERIC].
120 mg (Rx) [*Inderal LA;* GENERIC].
160 mg (Rx) [*Inderal LA;* GENERIC].
Canada—
60 mg (Rx) [*Inderal LA* (sulfites)].
80 mg (Rx) [*Inderal LA* (sulfites)].
120 mg (Rx) [*Inderal LA* (sulfites)].
160 mg (Rx) [*Inderal LA* (sulfites)].

#### Packaging and storage
Store below 40 °C (104 °F), preferably between 15 and 30 °C (59 and 86 °F), unless otherwise specified by manufacturer. Protect from light.

#### Auxiliary labeling
• Do not take other medicine without your doctor's advice.

#### Note
Check refill frequency to determine compliance in hypertensive patients.

### PROPRANOLOL HYDROCHLORIDE ORAL SOLUTION
#### Usual adult dose
Antianginal—
Oral, 80 to 320 mg per day given in two, three, or four divided doses.
Antiarrhythmic—
Oral, 10 to 30 mg three or four times a day, the dosage being adjusted as needed and tolerated.
Antihypertensive—
Oral, 40 mg two times a day, the dosage being increased gradually as needed and tolerated, usually 120 to 240 mg a day; doses up to a total of 640 mg a day may be necessary (a total daily dose of 1 gram has been used by some clinicians).
Hypertrophic cardiomyopathy therapy adjunct—
Oral, 20 to 40 mg three or four times a day, the dosage being adjusted as needed and tolerated.
Myocardial infarction—
Oral, 180 to 240 mg a day in divided doses.
Pheochromocytoma therapy adjunct—
Oral, 20 mg three times a day to 40 mg three or four times a day (as necessary for sufficient beta-blockade) for three days prior to surgery, concomitantly with alpha-adrenergic blocking medication (should *never* be started until alpha-adrenergic blockade is at least partially established). Doses of 30 to 160 mg per day in divided doses have been used for management of inoperable tumor.
Vascular headache prophylactic—
Oral, 20 mg four times a day initially, the dosage being increased gradually as needed and tolerated up to a total of 240 mg a day if necessary.
Antitremor agent—
Oral, 40 mg two times a day, the dosage being adjusted as needed and tolerated, up to 120 mg a day; occasionally, doses up to 320 mg a day may be needed.
[Antianxiety therapy adjunct][1]—
Oral, 10 to 80 mg thirty to ninety minutes prior to the anxiety-provoking activity.
[Thyrotoxicosis therapy adjunct][1]—
Oral, 10 to 40 mg three or four times a day, the dosage being adjusted as needed and tolerated.
Note: Twice-daily or, in some patients, once-daily dosing may be effective for use as an antianginal, antihypertensive, or for myocardial infarction.
Geriatric patients may have increased or decreased sensitivity to the effects of the usual adult dose.

#### Usual pediatric dose
Antiarrhythmic
Antihypertensive—
Initial: Oral, 500 mcg (0.5 mg) to 1 mg per kg of body weight per day in two to four divided doses has been used as an initial dose, the dosage being adjusted as necessary to treat hypertension and prevent supraventricular tachycardia.
Maintenance: Oral, 2 to 4 mg per kg per day in two divided doses.

#### Strength(s) usually available
U.S.—
4 mg per mL (Rx) [GENERIC].
8 mg per mL (Rx) [GENERIC].
80 mg per mL (concentrated; must be diluted) (Rx) [GENERIC].
Canada—
Not commercially available.

#### Packaging and storage
Store below 40 °C (104 °F), preferably between 15 and 30 °C (59 and 86 °F), in a well-closed container, unless otherwise specified by manufacturer. Protect from light. Protect from freezing.

#### Preparation of dosage form
Propranolol concentrated oral solution is prepared for administration by mixing it with a liquid such as water, juice, or soda or soda-like beverage. After the patient drinks the mixture, the glass should be rinsed with more liquid to make sure all the medication is taken. Propranolol

concentrated oral solution may also be mixed with semi-solid food such as applesauce or pudding.

**Auxiliary labeling**
- Do not take other medicine without your doctor's advice.

**Note**
Check refill frequency to determine compliance in hypertensive patients.

### PROPRANOLOL HYDROCHLORIDE TABLETS USP

**Usual adult dose**
See *Propranolol Hydrochloride Oral Solution*.

**Usual pediatric dose**
See *Propranolol Hydrochloride Oral Solution*.

**Strength(s) usually available**
U.S.—
- 10 mg (Rx) [*Inderal* (scored); GENERIC].
- 20 mg (Rx) [*Inderal* (scored); GENERIC (may be scored)].
- 40 mg (Rx) [*Inderal* (scored); GENERIC (may be scored)].
- 60 mg (Rx) [*Inderal* (scored); GENERIC (may be scored)].
- 80 mg (Rx) [*Inderal* (scored); GENERIC (may be scored)].
- 90 mg (Rx) [*Inderal* (scored); GENERIC (may be scored)].

Canada—
- 10 mg (Rx) [*Apo-Propranolol* (scored); *Detensol* (scored); *Inderal* (scored); *Novopranol* (scored); *pms Propranolol* (scored) [GENERIC].
- 20 mg (Rx) [*Apo-Propranolol* (scored); *Novopranol* (scored); *Inderal* (scored) [GENERIC].
- 40 mg (Rx) [*Apo-Propranolol* (scored); *Detensol* (scored); *Inderal* (scored); *Novopranol* (scored); *pms Propranolol* (scored) [GENERIC].
- 80 mg (Rx) [*Apo-Propranolol* (scored); *Detensol* (scored); *Inderal* (scored); *Novopranol* (scored); *pms Propranolol* (scored) [GENERIC].
- 120 mg (Rx) [*Apo-Propranolol* (scored); *Inderal* (scored); *Novopranol* (scored); *pms Propranolol* (scored) [GENERIC].

**Packaging and storage**
Store below 40 °C (104 °F), preferably between 15 and 30 °C (59 and 86 °F), unless otherwise specified by manufacturer. Store in a well-closed, light-resistant container.

**Auxiliary labeling**
- Do not take other medicine without your doctor's advice.

**Note**
Check refill frequency to determine compliance in hypertensive patients.

## Parenteral Dosage Forms

### PROPRANOLOL HYDROCHLORIDE INJECTION USP

**Usual adult dose**
Antiarrhythmic—
Intravenous, 1 to 3 mg administered at a rate not to exceed 1 mg per minute, repeated after two minutes and again after four hours if necessary.

Note: An intravenous dose of one-tenth the oral dose may be used to temporarily replace oral dosing in patients undergoing surgery.
Geriatric patients may have increased or decreased sensitivity to the effects of the usual adult dose.

**Usual pediatric dose**
Antiarrhythmic—
Slow intravenous, 10 to 100 mcg (0.01 to 0.1 mg) per kg of body weight (up to a maximum of 1 mg per dose), repeated every six to eight hours if necessary.

**Strength(s) usually available**
U.S.—
- 1 mg per mL (Rx) [*Inderal*; GENERIC].

Canada—
- 1 mg per mL (Rx) [*Inderal*].

**Packaging and storage**
Store below 40 °C (104 °F), preferably between 15 and 30 °C (59 and 86 °F), unless otherwise specified by manufacturer. Store in a light-resistant container. Protect from freezing.

[1]Not included in Canadian product labeling.

---

## SOTALOL

## Summary of Differences
Pharmacology/pharmacokinetics:
Mechanism of action/Effect—Nonselective; no intrinsic sympathomimetic activity (ISA) or membrane-stabilizing activity; low lipid solubility.
Protein binding—Not protein bound.
Elimination—Removable by hemodialysis.

## Oral Dosage Forms
Note: Bracketed uses in the *Dosage Forms* section refer to categories of use and/or indications that are not included in U.S. product labeling.

### SOTALOL HYDROCHLORIDE TABLETS

**Usual adult dose**
[Antianginal]
[Antihypertensive]—
Initial: Oral, 80 mg two times a day, the dosage being increased in increments of 80 mg two times a day at weekly intervals as needed and tolerated.
Maintenance: Oral, 160 mg two times a day.

Note: Once-daily dosing may be effective in patients taking a total daily maintenance dose of 320 mg or less.
Geriatric patients may have increased or decreased sensitivity to the effects of the usual adult dose.

Antiarrhythmic[1]—
Initial: Oral, 80 mg two times a day, the dosage being increased gradually.
Maintenance: Oral, 160 to 320 mg per day, given in two or three divided doses.

Note: It is recommended that the dosage interval be increased in patients with renal function impairment as follows:

| Creatinine clearance (mL/min) | Dosage interval (hrs) |
|---|---|
| >60 | 12 |
| 30–60 | 24 |
| 10–30 | 36–48 |
| <10 | Dosage and dosing interval must be individualized |

**Usual adult prescribing limits**
For life-threatening arrhythmias—640 mg per day.
For other indications—480 mg per day.

**Usual pediatric dose**
Dosage has not been established.

**Strength(s) usually available**
U.S.—
- 80 mg (Rx) [*Betapace* (scored)].
- 120 mg (Rx) [*Betapace*].
- 160 mg (Rx) [*Betapace* (scored)].
- 240 mg (Rx) [*Betapace* (scored)].

Canada—
- 160 mg (Rx) [*Sotacor* (scored)].

**Packaging and storage**
Store below 40 °C (104 °F), preferably between 15 and 30 °C (59 and 86 °F), in a well-closed container, unless otherwise specified by manufacturer.

**Auxiliary labeling**
- Do not take other medicines without your doctor's advice.

**Note**
Check refill frequency to determine compliance in hypertensive patients.

[1]Not included in Canadian product labeling.

---

## TIMOLOL

## Summary of Differences
Pharmacology/pharmacokinetics:
Mechanism of action/Effect—Nonselective; no significant intrinsic sympathomimetic activity (ISA); moderate lipid solubility.
Absorption—Bioavailability significantly reduced by first-pass metabolism.
Protein binding—Very low.
Elimination—Not removable by hemodialysis.

## Oral Dosage Forms

Note: Bracketed uses in the *Dosage Forms* section refer to categories of use and/or indications that are not included in U.S. product labeling.

### TIMOLOL MALEATE TABLETS USP

**Usual adult dose**
Antihypertensive
[Antianginal]—
  Initial: Oral, 10 mg two times a day initially, the dosage being increased at one-week intervals as needed and tolerated.
  Maintenance: Oral, usually 20 to 40 mg per day; doses up to 60 mg per day divided into two doses may be necessary.
Myocardial infarction[1]—
  Oral, 10 mg two times a day prophylactically against reinfarction in clinically stable patients. Treatment is initiated one to four weeks following initial infarction.
Vascular headache prophylactic—
  Oral, 10 mg two times a day initially; maintenance, 20 mg a day (may be given as a single daily dose); maximum dose is 30 mg per day (10 mg in the morning and 20 mg at night).

Note: Geriatric patients may have increased or decreased sensitivity to the effects of the usual adult dose.

**Usual pediatric dose**
Dosage has not been established.

**Strength(s) usually available**
U.S.—
  5 mg (Rx) [*Blocadren;* GENERIC].
  10 mg (Rx) [*Blocadren* (scored); GENERIC].
  20 mg (Rx) [*Blocadren* (scored); GENERIC].
Canada—
  5 mg (Rx) [*Apo-Timol* (scored); *Blocadren* (scored); *Novo-Timol* [GENERIC].
  10 mg (Rx) [*Apo-Timol* (scored); *Blocadren* (scored); *Novo-Timol* [GENERIC].
  20 mg (Rx) [*Apo-Timol; Blocadren* (scored); *Novo-Timol* [GENERIC].

**Packaging and storage**
Store below 40 °C (104 °F), preferably between 15 and 30 °C (59 and 86 °F), unless otherwise specified by manufacturer. Store in a well-closed, light-resistant container.

**Auxiliary labeling**
• Do not take other medicine without your doctor's advice.

**Note**
Check refill frequency to determine compliance in hypertensive patients.

[1] Not included in Canadian product labeling.

## Selected Bibliography

**General**
Drayer DE. Lipophilicity, hydrophilicity, and the central nervous system side effects of beta blockers. Pharmacother 1987; 7(4): 87-91.
Gerber JG, Nies AS. Beta-adrenergic blocking drugs. Ann Rev Med 1985; 36: 145-64.
Prichard BN, Tomlinson B. The additional properties of beta adrenoreceptor blocking drugs. J Cardiovasc Pharmacol 1986; 8(Suppl 4): S1-S15.

**For acebutolol**
De Bono G, Kaye CM, Roland E, Summers AJH. Acebutolol: ten years of experience. Am Heart J 1985 May; 109: 1211-23.
Singh BN, Thoden WR, Wahl J. Acebutolol: a review of its pharmacology, pharmacokinetics, clinical uses, and adverse effects. Pharmacother 1986 Mar/Apr; 6: 45-63.
Anonymous. Acebutolol. Med Lett Drugs Ther 1985 Jul 5; 27: 58-9.

**For betaxolol**
Beresford R, Heel RC. Betaxolol. A review of its pharmacodynamic and pharmacokinetic properties, and therapeutic efficacy in hypertension. Drugs 1986; 31: 6-28.

**For bisoprolol**
Lancaster SG, Sorkin EM. Bisoprolol. A preliminary review of its pharmacodynamic and pharmacokinetic properties, and therapeutic efficacy in hypertension and angina pectoris. Drugs 1988; 36: 256-85.

**For carteolol**
Luther RR, Maurath CJ, Klepper MJ, et al. Carteolol treatment of essential hypertension. J Int Med Res 1986; 14: 175-84.
Luther RR, Glassman HN, Jordan DC, et al. Long-term treatment of angina pectoris with carteolol. J Int Med Res 1986; 14: 167-74.

**For labetalol**
Blakey B, Williams LL, Lopez LM, Stein GH. Labetalol HCl: alpha- and beta-blocking properties may offer advantages over pure beta-blockers. Hosp Form 1987 Oct; 22: 864-9.
Weintraub M, Evans P. Labetalol: an alpha-blocker for treatment of hypertension. Hosp Form 1984 Apr; 19: 295-305.
MacCarthy EP, Bloomfield SS. Labetalol: a review of its pharmacology, pharmacokinetics, clinical uses, and adverse effects. Pharmacother 1983 Jul/Aug; 3: 193-219.

**For oxprenolol**
Weintraub M, Standish R. Oxprenolol: a nonselective beta blocking agent with intrinsic sympathomimetic activity. Hosp Form 1984 May; 19: 359-65.

**For penbutolol**
Marone C, Perisic M, Borer M. Antihypertensive efficacy and tolerance of penbutolol. Results of a cooperative study in 227 patients. Curr Med Res Opin 1985; 9: 417-25.

**For sotalol**
Singh BN, Deedwania P, Nademanee K, Ward A, Sorkin EM. Sotalol. A review of its pharmacodynamic and pharmacokinetic properties, and therapeutic use. Drugs 1987; 34: 311-49.

Revised: 05/13/93
Interim revision: 08/20/97; 08/13/98

## Precautions:
Medical considerations/contraindications—Dosage reduction necessary in hepatic function impairment but not necessary in renal function impairment.

## Table 1. Pharmacology/Pharmacokinetics

| Drug | Site of Effect | Oral Absorption (%) | Protein Binding | Biotransformation | Half-life (hr) | Time to Peak Effect— Single dose (hr) | Elimination (% unchanged) | Removable by Hemodialysis |
|---|---|---|---|---|---|---|---|---|
| Acebutolol | Beta-1* | 70† | Low (26%) | Hepatic‡ | 3–4‡ | 2.5‡ | 30–40% Renal; 50–60% Biliary/fecal | Yes |
| Atenolol | Beta-1* | 50–60 | Very low to low (6–16%) | Hepatic (minimal) | 6–7§ | 2–4 | 85–100% Renal | Yes** |
| Betaxolol | Beta-1* | 80–89† | Moderate (50–55%) | Hepatic | 14–22§ | 3–4 | >80% (15) Renal | No |
| Bisoprolol | Beta-1 | 80–90 | Low (26–33%) | Hepatic | 9–12 | | Renal (50) <2% Fecal | No |
| Carteolol | Beta-1; Beta-2 | 85 | Low (23–30%) | Hepatic (minimal) | 6§ | 1–3 | Renal (50–70) | ? |

Table 1. Pharmacology/Pharmacokinetics (continued)

| Drug | Site of Effect | Oral Absorption (%) | Protein Binding | Biotransformation | Half-life (hr) | Time to Peak Effect— Single dose (hr) | Elimination (% unchanged) | Removable by Hemodialysis |
|---|---|---|---|---|---|---|---|---|
| Labetalol | Beta-1; Beta-2 | 100† | Moderate (50%) | Hepatic | 6–8 (oral); ~5.5 (IV) | 2–4 (oral); 5 min (IV) | 55–60% (<5) Renal; Biliary/fecal | No |
| Metoprolol | Beta-1* | 95† | Low (12%) | Hepatic | 3–7§ | 1–2 (oral—regular); 6–12 (oral—long-acting); 20 min (IV) | Renal (3–10) | No |
| Nadolol | Beta-1; Beta-2 | 30 | Very low to low (4 to 30%) | None | 20–24§ | 4 | Renal (70) | Yes |
| Oxprenolol | Beta-1; Beta-2 | 90† | High (80%) | Hepatic | 1.3–1.5 | ? | Renal (<5) | ? |
| Penbutolol | Beta-1; Beta-2 | 100 | High to very high (80–98%) | Hepatic | 5§ | 1.5–3 | 90% (0) Renal | No |
| Pindolol | Beta-1; Beta-2 | 90–100 | Moderate (40%) | Hepatic | 3–4§ | 1–2 | Renal (40) | ? |
| Propranolol | Beta-1; Beta-2 | 90† | Very high (93%) | Hepatic | 3–5 | 1–1.5 | Renal (<1) | No |
| Sotalol | Beta-1; Beta-2 | >80 | None | Hepatic | 7–18§ | 2–3 | Renal (75) | Yes |
| Timolol | Beta-1; Beta-2 | 90† | Very low (<10%) | Hepatic | 4 | 1–2 | Renal (20); Fecal | No |

\*Cardioselectivity tends to diminish with increased dosage.
†First-pass metabolism results in a decrease (usually significant) in bioavailability.
    Acebutolol—The effect is not reduced because of the active metabolite. Bioavailability of acebutolol may be increased 2-fold in the elderly because of reduced first-pass metabolism and renal function.
    Betaxolol—First-pass effect is small.
‡Acebutolol—Major metabolite (diacetolol) is pharmacologically active and even more cardioselective than acebutolol; time to peak effect is 3.5 hours; the half-life of diacetolol is 8 to 13 hours.
§Atenolol—Increased to 16–27 hours or more in patients with renal function impairment (up to 144 hours when severe).
  Betaxolol—Increased by approximately 33% in hepatic function impairment, but clearance unchanged.
    —Approximately doubled in renal function impairment; dosage reduction necessary.
  Carteolol—Prolonged in renal failure.
  Metoprolol—No change in renal failure.
  Nadolol—Increased in renal failure.
  Penbutolol—Increased in renal failure.
  Pindolol—Varies from 2.5 to more than 30 hours in patients with hepatic function impairment.
    —Increased to 3 to 11.5 hours in patients with renal function impairment.
    —Increased to an average of 7 hours (and as high as 15 hours) in the elderly.
  Sotalol—Increased in renal failure.
\*\*Atenolol—Patients should receive 50 mg of atenolol after each dialysis and remain under supervision since marked hypotension may occur.

# BETA-ADRENERGIC BLOCKING AGENTS AND THIAZIDE DIURETICS   Systemic

This monograph includes information on the following: 1) Atenolol and Chlorthalidone; 2) Bisoprolol and Hydrochlorothiazide; 3) Metoprolol and Hydrochlorothiazide; 4) Nadolol and Bendroflumethiazide; 5) Pindolol and Hydrochlorothiazide; 6) Propranolol and Hydrochlorothiazide; 7) Timolol and Hydrochlorothiazide.

VA CLASSIFICATION (Primary): CV401

NOTE:   The *Beta-adrenergic Blocking Agents and Thiazide Diuretics (Systemic)* monograph is maintained on the USP DI electronic data base. For a printed copy of the most recent revision of the complete monograph, contact Micromedex, Inc. - Reprint Requests, 6200 S. Syracuse Way, Suite 300, Englewood, CO 80111; telephone (303) 486-6400; telefax (303) 486-6464; Email: USPDI@MDX.COM.

For information on the specific components of this combination, see the *USP DI* monographs for *Beta-adrenergic Blocking Agents (Systemic)* and *Diuretics, Thiazide (Systemic)*.

The information that follows is selectively abstracted from the complete monograph and is provided to facilitate drug use review and patient counseling.

Note:   For a listing of dosage forms and brand names by country availability, see *Dosage Forms* section(s).

## Category
Antihypertensive.

## Indications

### Accepted
Hypertension (treatment)—Beta-adrenergic blocking agent (beta-blocker) and thiazide diuretic combinations are indicated in the management of hypertension.

Fixed-dosage combinations generally are not recommended for initial therapy, but are utilized in maintenance therapy after the required dose is established, in order to increase convenience, economy, and patient compliance.

## Patient Consultation

As an aid to patient consultation, refer to *Advice for the Patient, Beta-adrenergic Blocking Agents and Thiazide Diuretics (Systemic)*.
In providing consultation, consider emphasizing the following selected information (» = major clinical significance):

### Before using this medication
» Conditions affecting use, especially:
   Sensitivity to the beta-adrenergic blocking agent prescribed, or to any thiazide diuretic or other sulfonamide-type medications
   Pregnancy—Risk of hypoglycemia, respiratory depression, bradycardia, and hypotension with beta-adrenergic blocking agents; thiazide diuretics may cause jaundice, thrombocytopenia, hypokalemia in infant
   Breast-feeding—Distributed into breast milk; not known for bisoprolol
   Use in the elderly—Increased sensitivity to effects; increased risk of beta-blocker–induced hypothermia
   Other medications, especially allergen immunotherapy or skin testing, oral antidiabetic agents, calcium channel blocking agents, clonidine, cocaine, digitalis glycosides, guanabenz, insulin, lithium, MAO inhibitors, sympathomimetics, or xanthines
   Other medical problems, especially anuria or severe renal function impairment, bronchial asthma, cardiogenic shock, congestive heart failure, diabetes mellitus, emphysema or nonallergic bronchitis, history of allergy, hyperthyroidism, hypotension, mental depression, overt cardiac failure, second or third degree AV block, or sinus bradycardia

### Proper use of this medication
Possible need for control of weight and diet, especially sodium intake
» Compliance with therapy; patient may not experience symptoms of hypertension; importance of taking medication only as directed and keeping appointments with physician, even if feeling well
» Does not cure, but helps control hypertension; possible need for lifelong therapy; serious consequences of untreated hypertension
   Proper administration of extended-release dosage forms: Swallowing whole without crushing, breaking, or chewing
   Getting into habit of taking at same time each day to help increase compliance
   Checking pulse as directed (checking with physician if less than 50 beats per minute)
   Diuretic effects of the medication and timing of doses to minimize inconvenience of diuresis
» Importance of not missing doses, especially with schedules of one dose per day
» Proper dosing
   Missed dose: Taking as soon as possible; not taking at all if within 4 hours of next scheduled dose (8 hours for atenolol and chlorthalidone, nadolol and bendroflumethiazide, or extended-release propranolol and hydrochlorothiazide); not doubling doses
» Proper storage

### Precautions while using this medication
Regular visits to physician to check progress
» Checking with physician before discontinuing medication; gradual dosage reduction may be necessary
   Having enough medication on hand to get through weekends, holidays, and vacations; possibly carrying second written prescription for emergency use
   Carrying medical identification during therapy
» Not taking other medications, especially nonprescription sympathomimetics, unless discussed with physician
» Caution if any kind of surgery (including dental surgery) or emergency treatment is required
» Diabetics: May mask signs and symptoms of hypoglycemia or cause increased blood glucose concentrations
» Possibility of hypokalemia; possible need for additional potassium in diet; not changing diet without first checking with physician
   To prevent dehydration, checking with physician if severe nausea, vomiting, or diarrhea occurs and continues
» Caution when driving or doing things requiring alertness, because of possible drowsiness, dizziness, or lightheadedness
   Caution during exposure to cold weather because of possible increased sensitivity to cold
   Possible skin photosensitivity; avoiding unprotected exposure to sun; using protective clothing and sun block product; avoiding use of sunlamp, tanning bed, or tanning booth
   Caution if any laboratory tests required; possible interference with test results
   Patients with allergies to foods, medications, or stinging insect venom: Possible increase in severity of allergic reactions; checking with physician immediately if severe allergic reaction occurs

### Side/adverse effects
Signs of potential side effects, especially electrolyte imbalance, bradycardia, bronchospasm, congestive heart failure, mental depression, reduced peripheral circulation, allergic reaction, arrhythmias, agranulocytosis, back pain, joint pain, chest pain, cholecystitis, pancreatitis, confusion (especially in elderly), hallucinations, hepatotoxicity, hyperuricemia, gout, leukopenia, psoriasiform eruption, and thrombocytopenia

---
### ATENOLOL AND CHLORTHALIDONE
---

## Oral Dosage Forms

### ATENOLOL AND CHLORTHALIDONE TABLETS

**Usual adult dose**
Antihypertensive—
   Oral, 1 or 2 tablets once a day, as determined by individual titration with the component agents.

Note: Geriatric patients may have increased or decreased sensitivity to the effects of the usual adult dose.

**Usual pediatric dose**
Dosage has not been established.

**Strength(s) usually available**
U.S.—
   50 mg of atenolol and 25 mg of chlorthalidone (Rx) [*Tenoretic 50* (scored); GENERIC].
   100 mg of atenolol and 25 mg of chlorthalidone (Rx) [*Tenoretic 100*; GENERIC].
Canada—
   50 mg of atenolol and 25 mg of chlorthalidone (Rx) [*Tenoretic* (scored)].
   100 mg of atenolol and 25 mg of chlorthalidone (Rx) [*Tenoretic* (scored)].

**Auxiliary labeling**
• Do not take other medicines without your doctor's advice.

---
### BISOPROLOL AND HYDROCHLOROTHIAZIDE
---

## Oral Dosage Forms

### BISOPROLOL FUMARATE AND HYDROCHLOROTHIAZIDE TABLETS

**Usual adult dose**
Antihypertensive—
   Oral, 1 or 2 tablets once a day, as determined by individual titration with the component agents.

Note: Geriatric patients may have increased or decreased sensitivity to the effects of the usual adult dose.

**Usual pediatric dose**
Dosage has not been established.

**Strength(s) usually available**
U.S.—
   2.5 mg of bisoprolol and 6.25 mg of hydrochlorothiazide (Rx) [*Ziac*].
   5 mg of bisoprolol and 6.25 mg of hydrochlorothiazide (Rx) [*Ziac*].
   10 mg of bisoprolol and 6.25 mg of hydrochlorothiazide (Rx) [*Ziac*].
Canada—
   Not commercially available.

**Auxiliary labeling**
• Do not take other medicine without your doctor's advice.

---
### METOPROLOL AND HYDROCHLOROTHIAZIDE
---

## Oral Dosage Forms

### METOPROLOL TARTRATE AND HYDROCHLOROTHIAZIDE TABLETS USP

**Usual adult dose**
Antihypertensive—
   Oral, 1 or 2 tablets a day, as a single dose or in divided doses, as determined by individual titration with the component agents.

Note: Geriatric patients may have increased or decreased sensitivity to the effects of the usual adult dose.

**Usual pediatric dose**
Dosage has not been established.

**Strength(s) usually available**
U.S.—
  50 mg of metoprolol tartrate and 25 mg of hydrochlorothiazide (Rx) [*Lopressor HCT* (scored; lactose)].
  100 mg of metoprolol tartrate and 25 mg of hydrochlorothiazide (Rx) [*Lopressor HCT* (scored; lactose)].
  100 mg of metoprolol tartrate and 50 mg of hydrochlorothiazide (Rx) [*Lopressor HCT* (scored; lactose)].
Canada—
  Not commercially available.

**Auxiliary labeling**
• Do not take other medicines without your doctor's advice.

---

## NADOLOL AND BENDROFLUMETHIAZIDE

# Oral Dosage Forms

### NADOLOL AND BENDROFLUMETHIAZIDE TABLETS USP

**Usual adult dose**
Antihypertensive—
  Oral, 1 tablet once a day, as determined by individual titration with the component agents.

Note: Geriatric patients may have increased or decreased sensitivity to the effects of the usual adult dose.

**Usual pediatric dose**
Dosage has not been established.

**Strength(s) usually available**
U.S.—
  40 mg of nadolol and 5 mg of bendroflumethiazide (Rx) [*Corzide 40/5* (scored; lactose)].
  80 mg of nadolol and 5 mg of bendroflumethiazide (Rx) [*Corzide 80/5* (scored; lactose)].
Canada—
  40 mg of nadolol and 5 mg of bendroflumethiazide (Rx) [*Corzide* (scored)].
  80 mg of nadolol and 5 mg of bendroflumethiazide (Rx) [*Corzide* (scored)].

**Auxiliary labeling**
• Do not take other medicines without your doctor's advice.

---

## PINDOLOL AND HYDROCHLOROTHIAZIDE

# Oral Dosage Forms

### PINDOLOL AND HYDROCHLOROTHIAZIDE TABLETS

**Usual adult dose**
Antihypertensive—
  Oral, 1 or 2 tablets once a day, as determined by individual titration with the component agents.

Note: Geriatric patients may have increased or decreased sensitivity to the effects of the usual adult dose.

**Usual pediatric dose**
Dosage has not been established.

**Strength(s) usually available**
U.S.—
  Not commercially available.
Canada—
  10 mg of pindolol and 25 mg of hydrochlorothiazide (Rx) [*Viskazide*].
  10 mg of pindolol and 50 mg of hydrochlorothiazide (Rx) [*Viskazide*].

**Auxiliary labeling**
• Do not take other medicines without your doctor's advice.

---

## PROPRANOLOL AND HYDROCHLOROTHIAZIDE

# Oral Dosage Forms

### PROPRANOLOL HYDROCHLORIDE AND HYDROCHLOROTHIAZIDE EXTENDED-RELEASE CAPSULES USP

**Usual adult dose**
Antihypertensive—
  Oral, 1 capsule a day, as determined by individual titration with the component agents.

Note: Geriatric patients may have increased or decreased sensitivity to the effects of the usual adult dose.

**Usual pediatric dose**
Dosage has not been established.

**Strength(s) usually available**
U.S.—
  80 mg of propranolol hydrochloride and 50 mg of hydrochlorothiazide (Rx) [*Inderide LA* (lactose)].
  120 mg of propranolol hydrochloride and 50 mg of hydrochlorothiazide (Rx) [*Inderide LA* (lactose)].
  160 mg of propranolol hydrochloride and 50 mg of hydrochlorothiazide (Rx) [*Inderide LA* (lactose)].
Canada—
  Not commercially available.

**Auxiliary labeling**
• Do not take other medicines without your doctor's advice.

### PROPRANOLOL HYDROCHLORIDE AND HYDROCHLOROTHIAZIDE TABLETS USP

**Usual adult dose**
Antihypertensive—
  Oral, 1 or 2 tablets two times a day, as determined by individual titration with the component agents.

Note: Geriatric patients may have increased or decreased sensitivity to the effects of the usual adult dose.

**Usual pediatric dose**
Dosage has not been established.

**Strength(s) usually available**
U.S.—
  40 mg of propranolol hydrochloride and 25 mg of hydrochlorothiazide (Rx) [*Inderide* (scored); GENERIC (may be scored)].
  80 mg of propranolol hydrochloride and 25 mg of hydrochlorothiazide (Rx) [*Inderide* (scored); GENERIC (may be scored)].
Canada—
  40 mg of propranolol hydrochloride and 25 mg of hydrochlorothiazide (Rx) [*Inderide* (scored)].
  80 mg of propranolol hydrochloride and 25 mg of hydrochlorothiazide (Rx) [*Inderide* (scored)].

**Auxiliary labeling**
• Do not take other medicines without your doctor's advice.

---

## TIMOLOL AND HYDROCHLOROTHIAZIDE

# Oral Dosage Forms

### TIMOLOL MALEATE AND HYDROCHLOROTHIAZIDE TABLETS USP

**Usual adult dose**
Antihypertensive—
  Oral, 1 tablet two times a day or 2 tablets once a day, as determined by individual titration with the component agents.

Note: Geriatric patients may have increased or decreased sensitivity to the effects of the usual adult dose.

**Usual pediatric dose**
Dosage has not been established.

**Strength(s) usually available**
U.S.—
  10 mg of timolol maleate and 25 mg of hydrochlorothiazide (Rx) [*Timolide 10-25*].
Canada—
  10 mg of timolol maleate and 25 mg of hydrochlorothiazide (Rx) [*Timolide*].

**Auxiliary labeling**
• Do not take other medicine without your doctor's advice.

---

Revised: 08/23/94
Interim revision: 08/12/98

# BETA-CAROTENE Systemic

VA CLASSIFICATION (Primary/Secondary): VT050/DE890
Commonly used brand name(s): *Lumitene; Max-Caro.*
Note: For a listing of dosage forms and brand names by country availability, see *Dosage Forms* section(s).

## Category
Nutritional supplement (vitamin precursor); photosensitivity reaction suppressant in erythropoietic protoporphyria; polymorphous light eruption suppressant.

Note: Beta-carotene is a precursor to vitamin A (a fat-soluble vitamin).

## Indications
Note: Bracketed information in the *Indications* section refers to uses that are not included in U.S. product labeling.

**Accepted**

Vitamin A deficiency (prophylaxis)—Beta-carotene may be used for prevention of vitamin A deficiency states in most individuals. Vitamin A deficiency may occur as a result of inadequate nutrition or intestinal malabsorption but does not occur in healthy individuals receiving an adequate balanced diet. For prophylaxis of vitamin A deficiency, dietary improvement, rather than supplementation, is advisable. For treatment of vitamin A deficiency, supplementation with vitamin A is preferred.

Deficiency of vitamin A may lead to keratomalacia, xerophthalmia, and nyctalopia (night blindness).

Recommended intakes may be increased and/or supplementation may be necessary in the following conditions (based on documented vitamin A deficiency):
Fat malabsorption (steatorrhea)
Fever, chronic
Hepatic-biliary tract disease—hepatic function impairment, cirrhosis, obstructive jaundice
Infection, prolonged
Malabsorption syndromes associated with pancreatic insufficiency—pancreatic disease, cystic fibrosis
Protein deficiency, severe

Some unusual diets (e.g., reducing diets that drastically restrict food selection) may not supply minimum daily requirements of vitamin A. Supplementation is necessary in patients receiving total parenteral nutrition (TPN) or undergoing rapid weight loss or in those with malnutrition, because of inadequate dietary intake.

Recommended intakes for most vitamins and minerals are increased during pregnancy. Many physicians recommend that pregnant women receive multivitamin and mineral supplements, especially those pregnant women who do not consume an adequate diet and those in high-risk categories (i.e., women carrying more than one fetus, heavy cigarette smokers, and alcohol and drug abusers). Taking excessive amounts of a multivitamin and mineral supplement may be harmful to the mother and/or fetus and should be avoided.

Recommended intakes for most vitamins and minerals are increased during breast-feeding.

Recommended intakes of vitamin A may be increased by the following medications: Cholestyramine, colestipol, mineral oil, and neomycin.

[Photosensitivity reactions in erythropoietic protoporphyria (prophylaxis and treatment)][1]—Beta-carotene is indicated to reduce the severity of photosensitivity reactions in patients with erythropoietic protoporphyria (EPP).

[Polymorphous light eruption (prophylaxis and treatment)][1]—Beta-carotene is used in the prophylaxis and treatment of severe cases of polymorphous light eruption.

**Acceptance not established**

Although it has been documented that individuals who consume foods containing high levels of beta-carotene have a reduced risk of certain types of *cancer* and possibly *cardiovascular disease*, there are insufficient data to show the same relationship using beta-carotene supplements. Use cannot be recommended in individuals with a history of smoking and/or asbestos exposure, since two large trials have found an increased incidence of lung cancer when beta-carotene supplements were given to these populations. However, another large trial using beta-carotene supplements found no increased risk of lung cancer. Research is underway to determine whether beta-carotene may have raised cancer risks only in subpopulations (e.g., smokers, drinkers of alcohol). It is also possible that some formulations of beta-carotene may not raise beta-carotene concentrations as much as the preparations used in these two studies.

**Unaccepted**

Beta-carotene has not been proven effective as a sunscreen.

[1]Not included in Canadian product labeling.

## Pharmacology/Pharmacokinetics

**Mechanism of action/Effect**

Nutritional supplement—Beta-carotene is a precursor to vitamin A, which is essential for normal function of the retina; in the form of retinal, it combines with opsin (red pigment in the retina) to form rhodopsin (visual purple), which is necessary for visual adaptation to darkness. It is also necessary for growth of bone, testicular and ovarian function, and embryonic development, and for regulation of growth and differentiation of epithelial tissues.

Photosensitivity reaction—Beta-carotene quenches singlet oxygen and free radicals that are generated when porphyrin is exposed to light and air.

**Absorption**

Absorption of beta-carotene depends on the presence of dietary fat and bile in the intestinal tract.

**Storage**

Unchanged beta-carotene is found in various tissues, primarily fat tissues, adrenal glands, and ovaries. Small concentrations are found in the liver.

**Biotransformation**

Approximately 20 to 60% of beta-carotene is metabolized to retinaldehyde and then converted to retinol, primarily in the intestinal wall. A small amount of beta-carotene is converted to vitamin A in the liver. The proportion of beta-carotene converted to vitamin A diminishes inversely to the intake of beta-carotene, as long as the dosages are higher than one to two times the daily requirements. High doses of beta-carotene do not lead to abnormally high serum concentrations of vitamin A.

**Elimination**

Primarily fecal.

## Precautions to Consider

**Carcinogenicity**

Two large studies have found an increased incidence in lung cancers when beta-carotene supplements were given to individuals with a history of smoking and/or asbestos exposure. One study of 29,000 males with a history of smoking found an 18% increase in the incidence of lung cancer in the group receiving 20 mg of beta-carotene a day for 5 to 8 years as compared with those receiving placebo. Another study of 18,000 individuals found 28% more lung cancers in individuals with a history of smoking and/or asbestos exposure who took 30 mg of beta-carotene in addition to 25,000 Units of retinol a day for 4 years as compared with those receiving placebo. However, one study of 22,000 male physicians, some of them smokers and former smokers, found no increased risk of lung cancer at doses of 50 mg of beta-carotene every other day for 12 years.

**Mutagenicity**

*In vitro* and *in vivo* mutagenicity studies were negative.

**Pregnancy/Reproduction**

Fertility—No problems with fertility have been documented in women taking up to 30 mg (5000 retinol equivalents [RE]) of beta-carotene a day. The effects of doses greater than 30 mg a day are not known.

Beta-carotene did not affect fertility in male rats at doses of up to 100 times the recommended human dose.

Pregnancy—Beta-carotene crosses the placenta. Adequate and well-controlled studies in humans have not been done. However, no problems with pregnancy have been documented in women taking up to 30 mg (5000 RE) of beta-carotene a day. The effects of doses greater than 30 mg (5000 RE) a day are not known.

Studies in rats at doses 300 to 400 times the recommended human dose have shown that beta-carotene causes an increase in resorption rate. No increase in resorption rate was noted in rats receiving 75 times the recommended human dose or less.

FDA Pregnancy Category C.

**Breast-feeding**

Problems in humans have not been documented with intake of normal daily recommended amounts.

### Pediatrics
Problems in pediatrics have not been documented with intake of normal daily recommended amounts.

### Geriatrics
Problems in geriatrics have not been documented with intake of normal daily recommended amounts.

### Drug interactions and/or related problems
The following drug interactions and/or related problems have been selected on the basis of their potential clinical significance (possible mechanism in parentheses where appropriate)—not necessarily inclusive (» = major clinical significance):

Note: Combinations containing any of the following, depending on the amount present, may also interact with beta-carotene.

Asbestos exposure, or history of or
Smoking tobacco, or history of
(data from two large studies indicate an increased incidence of lung cancers when beta-carotene supplements were given to individuals with a history of smoking and/or asbestos exposure; use of beta-carotene supplements in these subgroups is not recommended)

Cholestyramine or
Colestipol or
Mineral oil or
Neomycin
(concurrent use may interfere with the absorption of beta-carotene or vitamin A; requirements for vitamin A may be increased in patients receiving these medications)

Vitamin A
(for treatment of vitamin A deficiency, vitamin A should fulfill normal vitamin A requirements; additional beta-carotene supplementation may not be necessary)

Vitamin E
(concurrent use of vitamin E may facilitate absorption and utilization of beta-carotene and may reduce toxicity of vitamin A)

### Medical considerations/Contraindications
The medical considerations/contraindications included have been selected on the basis of their potential clinical significance (reasons given in parentheses where appropriate)—not necessarily inclusive (» = major clinical significance).

*Risk-benefit should be considered when the following medical problems exist:*

Anorexia or
Hepatic function impairment or
Renal impairment
(may lead to an increase of serum beta-carotene concentrations)

Hypervitaminosis A
Sensitivity to beta-carotene

### Patient monitoring
The following may be especially important in patient monitoring (other tests may be warranted in some patients, depending on condition; » = major clinical significance):

Beta-carotene concentrations, plasma and
Vitamin A concentrations, plasma
(determinations recommended to confirm deficiency; plasma vitamin A concentrations are not necessarily indicative of vitamin A nutritional status because of significant hepatic storage, although low concentrations correlate with deficiency)

## Side/Adverse Effects

The following side/adverse effects have been selected on the basis of their potential clinical significance (possible signs and symptoms in parentheses where appropriate)—not necessarily inclusive:

**Those indicating need for medical attention only if they continue or are bothersome**
Incidence more frequent
*Carotenodermia* (yellowing of palms, hands, or soles of feet, and to a lesser extent the face)—develops after 2 to 6 weeks of therapy

Incidence rare
*Arthralgia* (joint pain); *diarrhea; dizziness; ecchymoses* (unusual bleeding or bruising)

## Patient Consultation

As an aid to patient consultation, refer to *Advice for the Patient, Beta-carotene—For Dietary Supplement (Vitamin) (Systemic)* and *Beta-carotene—For Photosensitivity (Systemic).*

In providing consultation, consider emphasizing the following selected information (» = major clinical significance):

### Description of use
Description should include function in the body; indications for use; signs of vitamin A deficiency; conditions that may cause deficiency of vitamin A; and unproven uses

### Importance of diet
For use as a dietary supplement
Importance of proper nutrition; supplement may be desired because of inadequate dietary intake
Importance of relationship between diet and decreased risk of heart disease and certain cancers
Food sources of beta-carotene; effects of processing
Not using vitamins as substitute for balanced diet

### Before using this medication
» Conditions affecting use, especially:
Sensitivity to beta-carotene

### Proper use of this medication
*For use as a dietary supplement*
» Proper dosing
Function of beta-carotene in body
Missed dose: No cause for concern because of length of time necessary for depletion; remembering to take as directed

*For use in photosensitivity*
» Proper dosing
Missed dose: Taking as soon as possible; not taking if almost time for next dose; not doubling doses
» Proper storage

### Precautions while using this medicine
Not taking beta-carotene supplements if history of smoking or asbestos exposure

### Side/adverse effects
Yellow discoloration of skin is to be expected; if taking as nutritional supplement, may be a sign that the dose is too high

## General Dosing Information

Because of the infrequency of vitamin A deficiency alone, combinations of several vitamins are commonly administered. Many commercial vitamin complexes are available.

Therapy as a nutritional supplement may be discontinued when liver storage of vitamin A is determined to be adequate.

### Diet/Nutrition
Although most manufacturers still label their beta-carotene products in terms of Units (U) of vitamin A activity, the preferred way of designating activity is in retinol equivalents (RE). Six micrograms of beta-carotene is equivalent to 1 RE and 10 Units of vitamin A activity.

It has been documented that individuals who consume diets containing high levels of dietary beta-carotene have a reduced risk of cardiovascular disease and certain types of cancer.

The best dietary sources of beta-carotene include carrots; dark green leafy vegetables, such as spinach; green leafy lettuce; sweet potatoes; broccoli; cantaloupe; and winter squash. Ordinary cooking does not destroy beta-carotene.

## Oral Dosage Forms

Note: Bracketed uses in the *Dosage Forms* section refer to categories of use and/or indications that are not included in U.S. product labeling.

### BETA-CAROTENE CAPSULES USP

**Usual adult and adolescent dose**
Vitamin A deficiency (prophylaxis)—
Oral, 1000 to 2500 RE (the equivalent of 10,000 to 25,000 Units of vitamin A activity or 6 to 15 mg of beta-carotene) per day.
[Photosensitivity reaction suppressant][1]—
Oral, 5000 to 50,000 RE (the equivalent of 50,000 to 500,000 Units of vitamin A activity or 30 to 300 mg of beta-carotene) per day.
[Polymorphous light eruption suppressant][1]—
Oral, 12,500 to 30,000 RE (the equivalent of 125,000 to 300,000 Units of vitamin A activity or 75 to 180 mg of beta-carotene) per day.

**Usual pediatric dose**
Vitamin A deficiency (prophylaxis)—
Oral, 500 to 1000 RE (the equivalent of 5000 to 10,000 Units vitamin A activity or 3 to 6 mg of beta-carotene) per day.
[Photosensitivity reaction suppressant][1] or
[Polymorphous light eruption suppressant][1]—
Oral, 5000 to 25,000 RE (the equivalent of 50,000 to 250,000 Units of vitamin A activity or 30 to 150 mg of beta-carotene) per day.

# Beta-carotene (Systemic)

**Strength(s) usually available**
U.S.—
- 10,000 Units of vitamin A activity (6 mg of beta-carotene) (OTC) [GENERIC].
- 25,000 Units of vitamin A activity (15 mg of beta-carotene) (OTC) [*Max-Caro;* GENERIC].
- 50,000 Units of vitamin A activity (30 mg of beta-carotene) (OTC) [*Lumitene*].

Canada—
- 10,000 Units of vitamin A activity (6 mg of beta-carotene) (OTC) [GENERIC].
- 25,000 Units of vitamin A activity (15 mg of beta-carotene) (OTC) [GENERIC].

Note: Some strengths of these beta-carotene preparations may exceed the dosage range recommended by USP DI Advisory Panels based on the amount necessary to meet normal nutritional needs.

**Packaging and storage**
Store below 40 °C (104 °F), preferably between 15 and 30 °C (59 and 86 °F), unless otherwise specified by manufacturer.

## BETA-CAROTENE TABLETS

**Usual adult and adolescent dose**
See *Beta-carotene Capsules USP*.

**Usual pediatric dose**
See *Beta-carotene Capsules USP*.

**Strength(s) usually available**
U.S.—
- 10,000 Units of vitamin A activity (6 mg of beta-carotene) (OTC) [GENERIC].
- 25,000 Units of vitamin A activity (15 mg of beta-carotene) (OTC) [GENERIC].

Canada—
- 25,000 Units of vitamin A activity (15 mg of beta-carotene) (OTC) [GENERIC].

Note: Some strengths of these beta-carotene preparations may exceed the dosage range recommended by USP DI Advisory Panels based on the amount necessary to meet normal nutritional needs.

**Packaging and storage**
Store below 40 °C (104 °F), preferably between 15 and 30 °C (59 and 86 °F), unless otherwise specified by manufacturer.

## BETA-CAROTENE CHEWABLE TABLETS

**Usual adult and adolescent dose**
See *Beta-carotene Capsules USP*.

**Usual pediatric dose**
See *Beta-carotene Capsules USP*.

**Strength(s) usually available**
U.S.—
Not commercially available.
Canada—
- 5000 Units of vitamin A activity (3 mg of beta-carotene) (OTC) [GENERIC].

**Packaging and storage**
Store below 40 °C (104 °F), preferably between 15 and 30 °C (59 and 86 °F), unless otherwise specified by manufacturer.

[1]Not included in Canadian product labeling.

Revised: 07/09/97

---

**BETAINE**—The *Betaine (Systemic)* monograph is not included in this published version of the USP DI database. Copies of the monograph are available on request from Micromedex, Inc. - Reprint Requests, 6200 S. Syracuse Way, Suite 300, Englewood, CO 80111; telephone (303) 486-6400; telefax (303) 486-6464; Email: USPDI@MDX.COM.

---

**BETAMETHASONE**—See *Corticosteroid—Glucocorticoid Effects (Systemic); Corticosteroids—Glucocorticoid Effects (Systemic); Corticosteroids (Ophthalmic); Corticosteroids (Otic); Corticosteroids (Topical)*

---

**BETAXOLOL**—See *Beta-adrenergic Blocking Agents (Ophthalmic); Beta-adrenergic Blocking Agents (Systemic)*

---

# BETHANECHOL  Systemic

VA CLASSIFICATION (Primary): AU300.
Commonly used brand name(s): *Duvoid; Urabeth; Urecholine*.

Note: For a listing of dosage forms and brand names by country availability, see *Dosage Forms* section(s).

## Category
Cholinergic.

## Indications

Note: Bracketed information in the *Indications* section refers to uses that are not included in U.S. product labeling.

**Accepted**

Urinary retention (treatment)—Although it generally has been replaced by more effective agents, bethanechol is indicated for the treatment of acute postoperative nonobstructive urinary retention and for neurogenic atony of the urinary bladder with retention.

[Atony, postoperative, gastric (treatment)][1] or
[Megacolon, congenital (treatment)][1]—Bethanechol is used in certain cases of gastric atony or stasis, and is also used in selected cases of congenital megacolon.

[Reflux, gastroesophageal (treatment)]—Oral bethanechol is used for treatment of gastroesophageal reflux associated with decreased pressure of the lower esophageal sphincter.

[1]Not included in Canadian product labeling.

## Pharmacology/Pharmacokinetics

**Physicochemical characteristics**
Molecular weight—196.68.

**Mechanism of action/Effect**
Bethanechol is a muscarinic cholinomimetic, which acts at cholinergic receptors in the smooth muscle of the urinary bladder and gastrointestinal tract. It increases the tone of the detrusor urinae muscle, producing an increase in the intravesical pressure. It may initiate micturition and empty the bladder; however, its clinical effectiveness in such conditions as voiding dysfunction has not been fully established. It also stimulates gastric and intestinal motility, and increases lower esophageal sphincter pressure.

**Other actions/effects**
Following oral or subcutaneous administration, cardiovascular effects and nicotinic activity are minimal.

**Onset of action**
Oral–Within 30 to 90 minutes.
Subcutaneous–Within 5 to 15 minutes.

**Time to peak effect**
Oral–About 1 hour.
Subcutaneous–Within 15 to 30 minutes.

**Duration of action**
Oral—Up to 6 hours, depending on dose.
Subcutaneous—About 2 hours.

## Precautions to Consider

**Pregnancy/Reproduction**
Pregnancy—Adequate and well-controlled studies in humans have not been done.
Studies have not been done in animals.
FDA Pregnancy Category C.

**Breast-feeding**
It is not known whether bethanechol is distributed into breast milk.

### Pediatrics
Appropriate studies on the relationship of age to the effects of bethanechol have not been performed in the pediatric population. However, no pediatrics-specific problems have been documented to date.

### Geriatrics
Appropriate studies on the relationship of age to the effects of bethanechol have not been performed in the geriatric population. However, geriatric-specific problems that would limit the usefulness of this medication in the elderly are not expected.

### Drug interactions and/or related problems
The following drug interactions and/or related problems have been selected on the basis of their potential clinical significance (possible mechanism in parentheses where appropriate)—not necessarily inclusive (» = major clinical significance):

Note: Combinations containing any of the following medications, depending on the amount present, may also interact with this medication.

Cholinergics, other, especially cholinesterase inhibitors
(concurrent use may increase the effects of either these medications or bethanechol and increase the potential for toxicity)

Ganglionic blocking agents, such as mecamylamine, pentolinium, and trimethaphan
(concurrent use with bethanechol may produce a critical fall in blood pressure, which is usually preceded by severe abdominal symptoms)

Procainamide or
Quinidine
(concurrent use may antagonize the cholinergic effects of bethanechol)

### Laboratory value alterations
The following have been selected on the basis of their potential clinical significance (possible effect in parentheses where appropriate)—not necessarily inclusive (» = major clinical significance):

With physiology/laboratory test values
Amylase, serum, and
Lipase, serum
(concentrations may be increased because bethanechol stimulates pancreatic secretion and constricts the sphincter of Oddi)

Aspartate aminotransferase, serum (AST [SGOT])
(concentrations may be increased because bethanechol impairs excretion by causing contractions in the sphincter of Oddi)

### Medical considerations/Contraindications
The medical considerations/contraindications included have been selected on the basis of their potential clinical significance (reasons given in parentheses where appropriate)—not necessarily inclusive (» = major clinical significance).

*Risk-benefit should be considered when the following medical problems exist:*
» Asthma, bronchial, active or latent
(bethanechol may cause bronchospasm and may precipitate asthmatic attack)

Atrioventricular conduction defects
(bethanechol may aggravate this condition by decreasing the rate of conduction)

» Bradycardia, pronounced
(bethanechol slows heart rate and may exacerbate the condition)

» Hypotension
(bethanechol may reduce blood pressure)

» Conditions in which increased muscular activity of the gastrointestinal tract or urinary bladder might be harmful, such as:
Anastomosis
Bladder surgery, recent
Gastrointestinal resection

» Conditions in which strength or integrity of gastrointestinal or bladder wall is questionable or
» Gastrointestinal obstruction or
Urinary tract obstruction
(increased muscular activity of the gastrointestinal tract or urinary bladder may be harmful)

» Coronary artery disease, especially occlusion
(bethanechol may decrease coronary blood flow)

Epilepsy
(although no causal relationship has been established, seizures have been reported in patients receiving bethanechol)

Hypertension
(bethanechol may cause sudden fall in blood pressure)

» Hyperthyroidism
(risk of atrial fibrillation may be increased)

» Peptic ulcer
(bethanechol may aggravate symptoms probably by increasing acid secretion and/or by increasing gastric motility)

Parkinsonism or
Vagotonia, marked
(bethanechol may exacerbate these conditions)

» Peritonitis
(bethanechol may increase cramping and exacerbate the condition and increase patient discomfort)

Sensitivity to bethanechol

## Side/Adverse Effects
Note: In addition to those side/adverse effects needing medical attention listed below, other severe symptoms of cholinergic overstimulation such as circulatory collapse, hypotension, bloody diarrhea, shock, or sudden cardiac arrest are likely to occur in cases of hypersensitivity or overdosage, and may occur rarely after subcutaneous administration.

The following side/adverse effects have been selected on the basis of their potential clinical significance (possible signs and symptoms in parentheses where appropriate)—not necessarily inclusive:

**Those indicating need for medical attention**
Incidence rare—more frequent with subcutaneous injection
*Shortness of breath, wheezing, or tightness in chest, especially in patients with predisposition to bronchoconstriction*

**Those indicating need for medical attention only if they continue or are bothersome**
Incidence less frequent or rare—more frequent with subcutaneous injection
*Belching; blurred vision or change in near or distance vision; diarrhea; frequent urge to urinate*
With high doses
*CNS stimulation* (sleeplessness, nervousness, or jitters); *orthostatic hypotension* (dizziness or lightheadedness; feeling faint); *parasympathetic stimulation* (headache; increased salivation or sweating; nausea or vomiting; redness or flushing of skin or feeling of warmth; stomach discomfort or pain); *seizures*

## Overdose
For specific information on the agents used in the management of bethanechol overdose, see:
• Atropine in *Anticholinergics/Antispasmodics* monograph.

For more information on the management of overdose or unintentional ingestion, **contact a Poison Control Center** (see *Poison Contol Center Listing*).

### Treatment of overdose
Specific treatment—
Treatment consists of subcutaneous administration of atropine in doses of 500 mcg (0.5 mg) to 1 mg for adults and 10 mcg (0.01 mg) per kg of body weight for infants and children, repeated as needed every 2 hours. In emergencies, intravenous injection of atropine may be used to counteract severe toxic cardiovascular or bronchoconstrictor effects of bethanechol.

## Patient Consultation
As an aid to patient consultation, refer to *Advice for the Patient, Bethanechol (Systemic)*.

In providing consultation, consider emphasizing the following selected information (» = major clinical significance):

**Before using this medication**
» Conditions affecting use, especially:
Sensitivity to bethanechol
Other medical problems, especially anastomosis, recent bladder surgery or gastrointestinal resection; asthma; pronounced bradycardia or hypotension; coronary artery disease; hyperthyroidism; peptic ulcer; peritonitis; or conditions in which the strength or integrity of the gastrointestinal or bladder wall is in question or in the presence of mechanical obstruction; or marked vagotonia

**Proper use of this medication**
» Taking medication on an empty stomach to minimize the possibility of nausea and vomiting, unless otherwise directed by physician
» Importance of not taking more medication than the amount prescribed

## Bethanechol (Systemic)

» Proper dosing
  Missed dose: Taking if remembered within an hour or so; not taking if remembered after 2 or more hours; not doubling doses
» Proper storage

**Precautions while using this medication**
Caution when getting up suddenly from a lying or sitting position

**Side/adverse effects**
Signs of potential side effects, especially shortness of breath, wheezing, or tightness in chest

## General Dosing Information

**For oral dosage forms only**
Preferably, bethanechol should be taken on an empty stomach to minimize the possibility of nausea and vomiting.

**For parenteral dosage forms only**
Bethanechol injection is for subcutaneous use *only*. It should *not* be given intravenously or intramuscularly because severe symptoms of cholinergic overstimulation may occur, and the selectivity of bethanechol's action may be decreased.

After administration of bethanechol, the patient should be observed for 30 minutes to 1 hour for possible severe reactions, and a syringe containing a dose of atropine should be immediately available during this period.

## Oral Dosage Forms

Note: Bracketed uses in the *Dosage Forms* section refer to categories of use and/or indications that are not included in U.S. product labeling.

### BETHANECHOL CHLORIDE TABLETS USP

**Usual adult and adolescent dose**
Cholinergic—
  Oral, 25 to 50 mg three or four times a day.
Note: The minimum effective dose may be determined by administering 5 or 10 mg initially and repeating the same dose at one- to two-hour intervals until a satisfactory response is obtained or up to a maximum of 50 mg; or by administering 10 mg initially, and repeating with 25 mg and then 50 mg at six-hour intervals until the desired response is obtained.
[Treatment of gastroesophageal reflux]—
  Oral, 10 to 25 mg four times a day, after meals and at bedtime.

**Usual pediatric dose**
Cholinergic—
  Oral, 0.6 mg per kg of body weight a day in 3 or 4 divided doses.
[Treatment of gastroesophageal reflux]—
  Oral, 0.4 mg per kg of body weight a day in 4 divided doses or 3 mg per square meter of body surface every eight hours.

**Usual geriatric dose**
See *Usual adult and adolescent dose*.

**Strength(s) usually available**
U.S.—
  5 mg (Rx) [*Urabeth*; *Urecholine* [GENERIC (may be scored)].
  10 mg (Rx) [*Duvoid* (scored); *Urabeth*; *Urecholine* (scored) [GENERIC (may be scored)].
  25 mg (Rx) [*Duvoid* (scored); *Urabeth*; *Urecholine* (scored) [GENERIC (may be scored)].
  50 mg (Rx) [*Duvoid* (scored); *Urabeth*; *Urecholine* (scored) [GENERIC (may be scored)].
Canada—
  10 mg (Rx) [*Duvoid* (scored); *Urecholine* (scored)].
  25 mg (Rx) [*Duvoid* (scored); *Urecholine* (scored)].
  50 mg (Rx) [*Duvoid* (scored)].

**Packaging and storage**
Store below 40 °C (104 °F), preferably between 15 and 30 °C (59 and 86 °F), unless otherwise specified by manufacturer. Store in a tight container.

## Parenteral Dosage Forms

### BETHANECHOL CHLORIDE INJECTION USP

**Usual adult and adolescent dose**
Cholinergic—
  Subcutaneous, 5 mg three or four times a day as needed.
Note: The minimum effective dose may be determined by administering 2.5 mg initially and repeating the same dose at 15- to 30-minute intervals up to a maximum of four doses until a satisfactory response is obtained.
  Single doses of 10 mg may be required. However, such a large dose may cause severe side effects and should be used only after single doses of 2.5 to 5 mg have proven to be ineffective.

**Usual pediatric dose**
Cholinergic—
  Subcutaneous, 0.2 mg per kg of body weight a day in 3 or 4 divided doses.

**Usual geriatric dose**
See *Usual adult and adolescent dose*.

**Strength(s) usually available**
U.S.—
  5 mg per mL (Rx) [*Urecholine*].
Canada—
  5 mg per mL (Rx) [*Urecholine*].

**Packaging and storage**
Store below 40 °C (104 °F), preferably between 15 and 30 °C (59 and 86 °F), unless otherwise specified by manufacturer. Protect from freezing.

**Note**
For subcutaneous use only. Discard unused portion.

Revised: 05/12/93
Interim revision: 06/27/94

---

**BICALUTAMIDE**— See *Antiandrogens, Nonsteroidal (Systemic)*

---

**BIOTIN**— The *Biotin (Systemic)* monograph is not included in this published version of the USP DI database. Copies of the monograph are available on request from Micromedex, Inc. - Reprint Requests, 6200 S. Syracuse Way, Suite 300, Englewood, CO 80111; telephone (303) 486-6400; telefax (303) 486-6464; Email: USPDI@MDX.COM.

---

**BIPERIDEN**— See *Antidyskinetics (Systemic)*

---

**BISACODYL**— See *Laxatives (Local)*

---

# BISMUTH SUBSALICYLATE   Oral-Local

VA CLASSIFICATION (Primary): GA208
Commonly used brand name(s): *Bismatrol*; *Bismatrol Extra Strength*; *Bismed*; *PMS-Bismuth Subsalicylate*; *Pepto-Bismol*; *Pepto-Bismol Easy-to-Swallow Caplets*; *Pepto-Bismol Maximum Strength*.
Note: For a listing of dosage forms and brand names by country availability, see *Dosage Forms* section(s).

## Category
Antidiarrheal (antisecretory); antacid; antiulcer agent.

## Indications
Note: Bracketed information in the *Indications* section refers to uses that are not included in U.S. product labeling.

**Accepted**
Diarrhea (treatment)—Bismuth subsalicylate is indicated for the symptomatic treatment of nonspecific diarrhea.

Gastric distress (treatment)—Bismuth subsalicylate is indicated for the symptomatic relief of upset stomach, including heartburn, acid indigestion, and nausea.

[Traveler's diarrhea (prophylaxis)][1]—Bismuth subsalicylate is used for the prevention of secretory diarrhea produced by enterotoxigenic *Escherichia coli* (traveler's diarrhea) and viral infections.

[Ulcer, duodenal, *Helicobacter pylori*-associated (treatment adjunct)][1] or

[Gastritis, *Helicobacter pylori*-associated (treatment adjunct)][1]—Bismuth subsalicylate is used, in combination with oral antibiotic therapy, in the treatment of *Helicobacter pylori*-associated gastritis and duodenal ulcer.

[1]Not included in Canadian product labeling.

## Pharmacology/Pharmacokinetics

**Physicochemical characteristics**
Molecular weight—362.09.

**Mechanism of action/Effect**
Antidiarrheal—Exact mechanism has not been determined. Bismuth subsalicylate may exert its antidiarrheal action not only by stimulating absorption of fluid and electrolytes across the intestinal wall (antisecretory action) but also, when hydrolyzed to salicylic acid, by inhibiting synthesis of a prostaglandin responsible for intestinal inflammation and hypermotility. In addition, bismuth subsalicylate binds toxins produced by *Escherichia coli*. Both bismuth subsalicylate and the intestinal reaction products, bismuth oxychloride and bismuth hydroxide, are believed to have bactericidal action.

Antacid—Bismuth has weak antacid properties.

**Absorption**
Following oral administration, absorption of the salicylate component from the small intestine is generally rapid and complete (>90%). In contrast to the salicylate, the amount of bismuth absorbed is negligible (<0.005%).

**Protein binding**
Salicylate—High (to albumin).

**Biotransformation**
Based on *in vitro* dissociation data and *in vivo* animal data, bismuth subsalicylate is believed to be largely hydrolyzed in the stomach to bismuth oxychloride and salicylic acid. In the small intestine, nondissociated bismuth subsalicylate reacts with other anions (bicarbonate and phosphate) to form insoluble bismuth salts. In the colon, nondissociated bismuth subsalicylate and other bismuth salts react with hydrogen sulfide to produce bismuth sulfide, a highly insoluble black salt responsible for the darkening of the stools.

**Elimination**
Bismuth—Fecal (>99% of the bismuth present in an oral dose); renal.
Salicylate—Renal (primarily excreted as free salicylic acid and conjugated metabolites).

## Precautions to Consider

**Cross-sensitivity and/or related problems**
Patients sensitive to salicylates including methyl salicylate(oil of wintergreen), or to other nonsteroidal anti-inflammatory drugs (NSAIDs), may be sensitive to bismuth subsalicylate also.

**Pregnancy/Reproduction**
The occasional use of bismuth subsalicylate during pregnancy is not likely to result in adverse effects on the fetus or newborn; however, based on what is known about salicylates, the following information should be considered with higher doses and longer therapy.

Fertility—Salicylates have caused increased numbers of fetal resorptions in animal studies.

Pregnancy—First trimester: Salicylates readily cross the placenta. Studies in animals have shown that salicylates cause birth defects including fissure of the spine and skull; facial clefts; eye defects; and malformations of the central nervous system (CNS), viscera, and skeleton (especially the vertebrae and ribs). It has been reported that salicylate use during pregnancy may increase the risk of birth defects in humans.

Third trimester: Chronic, high-dose salicylate therapy may result in prolonged gestation, increased risk of postmaturity syndrome (fetal damage or death due to decreased placental function if pregnancy is greatly prolonged), and increased risk of maternal antenatal hemorrhage. Also, ingestion of salicylates during the last 2 weeks of pregnancy may increase the risk of fetal or neonatal hemorrhage. The possibility that regular use late in pregnancy may result in constriction or premature closure of the fetal ductus arteriosus, possibly leading to persistent pulmonary hypertension and heart failure in the neonate, must also be considered.

Labor and delivery—Chronic, high-dose salicylate therapy late in pregnancy may result in prolonged labor, complicated deliveries, and increased risk of maternal or fetal hemorrhage.

**Breast-feeding**
Problems in humans have not been documented. However, salicylate is distributed into breast milk; with chronic, high-dose use, intake by the infant may be high enough to cause adverse effects.

**Pediatrics**
In infants and children up to 3 years of age with diarrhea, caution is recommended because of the risk of fluid and electrolyte loss; these patients should be referred to a physician.

Pediatric patients, especially those with fever and dehydration, may be more susceptible to the toxic effects of salicylates.

Although no cases have been documented with the use of bismuth subsalicylate, recent studies indicate that use of aspirin, a salicylate, may be associated with the development of Reye's syndrome in children with acute febrile illnesses, especially influenza and varicella. There is insufficient data to establish an association between the use of nonaspirin salicylates, such as bismuth subsalicylate, and the occurrence of Reye's syndrome. However, it is recommended that children and adolescents who have or are recovering from influenza or varicella not be given bismuth subsalicylate to treat nausea or vomiting. Since nausea or vomiting could be an early sign of Reye's syndrome, these patients should be referred to a physician.

Bismuth is more likely to cause impaction in children.

**Geriatrics**
In geriatric patients with diarrhea, caution is recommended because of the risk of fluid and electrolyte loss; these patients should be referred to a physician.

Also, elderly patients are more likely to have age-related renal function impairment, which may increase the risk of salicylate toxicity. Dosage reduction may be required to prevent accumulation of the medication.

Bismuth is more likely to cause impaction in elderly patients.

**Drug interactions and/or related problems**
The following drug interactions and/or related problems have been selected on the basis of their potential clinical significance (possible mechanism in parentheses where appropriate)—not necessarily inclusive (» = major clinical significance):

Note: Although significant interactions are unlikely with usual doses of bismuth subsalicylate in the treatment of diarrhea and for occasional relief of gastric distress, the higher doses and the longer therapy used in the prophylaxis of traveler's diarrhea increase the potential for significant drug interactions.

Combinations containing any of the following medications, depending on the amount present, may also interact with this medication.

» Anticoagulants, coumarin- or indandione-derivative or
» Heparin or
» Thrombolytic agents, such as:
  Alteplase (tissue-type plasminogen activator, recombinant)
  Anistreplase
  Streptokinase
  Urokinase
  (increased risk of bleeding may occur when these medications are used concurrently with salicylates)

» Antidiabetic agents, oral or
  Insulin
  (large doses of salicylate may enhance the hypoglycemic effect of these medications; dosage adjustment may be necessary)

» Probenecid or
» Sulfinpyrazone
  (concurrent use of salicylates is not recommended when these medications are used to treat hyperuricemia or gout because uricosuric effects of these medications may be decreased by doses of salicylates that produce serum salicylate concentrations above 50 mcg per mL)
  (probenecid may decrease renal clearance and increase plasma concentrations and toxicity of salicylates)

» Salicylates, other
  (ingestion of large repeated doses of bismuth subsalicylate, as for traveler's diarrhea, may produce substantial plasma salicylate concentrations thus increasing the risk of salicylate toxicity during concurrent use with other salicylates)

» Tetracyclines, oral
  (calcium carbonate contained in the tablet dosage form may decrease gastrointestinal absorption and bioavailability of tetracyclines; patients should be advised not to take bismuth subsalicylate tablets within 1 to 3 hours of oral tetracyclines)

**Laboratory value alterations**
The following have been selected on the basis of their potential clinical significance (possible effect in parentheses where appropriate)—not necessarily inclusive (» = major clinical significance):
With diagnostic test results
Copper sulfate urine sugar tests
(false-positive results may occur with chronic use of high doses of salicylate)
Gerhardt test for urine aceto-acetic acid
(may be interfered with because reaction of salicylate with ferric chloride produces a reddish color that persists after boiling)
Glucose enzymatic urine sugar tests
(false-negative results may occur with chronic use of high doses of salicylate)
Radiological examination of gastrointestinal tract
(radiopacity of bismuth may interfere with radiologic examination of the gastrointestinal tract)
Serum uric acid determinations
(falsely increased values may occur with colorimetric assay methods when plasma salicylate concentrations exceed 130 mcg per mL; the uricase assay method is not affected)
Thyroid imaging, radionuclide
(chronic salicylate administration may decrease thyroidal uptake of iodide I 131 or of pertechnetate ion because of depressed thyroid function; salicylate therapy should be discontinued at least 1 week prior to administration of the radiopharmaceutical; however, a rebound effect may occur following discontinuation of salicylate therapy, resulting in a period of 3 to 10 days of increased thyroidal uptake)
Urine vanillylmandelic acid (VMA) concentrations
(salicylate may falsely increase or decrease VMA concentrations, depending on method used)
With physiology/laboratory test values
Liver function tests, including:
Serum alanine aminotransferase(ALT [SGPT]) and
Serum alkaline phosphatase and
Serum aspartate aminotransferase (AST [SGOT])
(abnormalities may occur, especially in patients with juvenile rheumatoid arthritis, systemic lupus erythematosus, or history of liver disease, or when plasma salicylate concentrations exceed 250 mcg per mL)
Prothrombin time
(may be prolonged with large doses of salicylates, especially if plasma concentrations exceed 300 mcg per mL)
Serum potassium concentrations
(may be decreased because of increased potassium excretion caused by direct effect of salicylate on renal tubules)
Serum thyroxine ($T_4$) concentrations and
Serum triiodothyronine ($T_3$) concentrations
(large doses of salicylate may decrease serum $T_4$ and $T_3$ concentrations when determined by radioimmunoassay)
Serum uric acid concentrations
(may be increased or decreased, depending on salicylate dosage; plasma salicylate concentrations below 100 to 150 mcg per mL increase serum uric acid concentrations; salicylate concentrations above 100 to 150 mcg per mL decrease uric acid concentrations)
$T_3$ resin uptake
(may be increased with large doses of salicylate)
Urine phenolsulfonphthalein (PSP) concentrations
(may be decreased because of competition of salicylate with PSP for renal tubular secretion)

**Medical considerations/Contraindications**
The medical considerations/contraindications included have been selected on the basis of their potential clinical significance (reasons given in parentheses where appropriate)—not necessarily inclusive (» = major clinical significance):

*Risk-benefit should be considered when the following medical problems exist:*
» Bleeding ulcers or
» Hemorrhagic states, other active
(may be exacerbated by the salicylate)
» Dehydration
(rehydration therapy is essential if signs of dehydration, such as dry mouth, excessive thirst, wrinkled skin, decreased urination, dizziness or lightheadedness, are present with the diarrhea; fluid loss may have serious consequences, such as circulatory collapse and renal failure, especially in young children)
» Dysentery, acute, characterized by bloody stools and elevated temperature
(sole treatment with bismuth subsalicylate may be inadequate; antibiotic therapy may be required)
Gout
(salicylates may have variable dose-dependent effects on serum uric acid concentrations; also, salicylates may interfere with efficacy of uricosuric antigout agents)
» Hemophilia
(salicylate may increase risk of hemorrhage)
Renal function impairment
(increased risk of bismuth and salicylate toxicity because of decreased excretion)
Sensitivity to bismuth subsalicylate

## Side/Adverse Effects

The following side/adverse effects have been selected on the basis of their potential clinical significance (possible signs and symptoms in parentheses where appropriate)—not necessarily inclusive:

**Those indicating need for medical attention**
Incidence rare—reported with higher-than-recommended doses and/or chronic dosing; may also be signs of overdose
*Bismuth encephalopathy* (anxiety; confusion; difficulty in speaking or slurred speech; severe and/or continuing headache; mental depression; muscle spasms, especially of face, neck, and back; muscle weakness; trembling; uncontrolled body movements); *constipation, severe; salicylism, symptoms of* (any loss of hearing; confusion; severe or continuing diarrhea; dizziness or lightheadedness; severe drowsiness; fast or deep breathing; severe or continuing headache; increased sweating; increased thirst; severe or continuing nausea or vomiting; continuing ringing or buzzing in ears; severe or continuing stomach pain; uncontrollable flapping movements of the hands, especially in elderly patients; vision problems)

**Those not indicating need for medical attention**
Incidence more frequent
*Discoloration produced by bismuth* (darkening of tongue or grayish black stools)

## Overdose

For specific information on the agents used in the management of bismuth subsalicylate overdose, see:
• *Charcoal, Activated (Oral-Local)* monograph;
• *Acetazolamide* in *Carbonic Anhydrase Inhibitors (Systemic)* monograph; and/or
• *Vitamin K (Systemic)* monograph.

For more information on the management of overdose or unintentional ingestion, **contact a Poison Control Center** (see *Poison Control Center Listing*).

**Clinical effects of overdose**
The following effects have been selected on the basis of their potential clinical significance (possible signs and symptoms in parentheses where appropriate)—not necessarily inclusive:

*Bismuth encephalopathy* (anxiety; confusion; difficulty in speaking or slurred speech; severe and/or continuing headache; mental depression; muscle spasms, especially of face, neck, and back; muscle weakness; trembling; uncontrolled body movements); *symptoms of salicylism* (any loss of hearing; confusion; severe or continuing diarrhea; dizziness or lightheadedness; severe drowsiness; fast or deep breathing; severe or continuing headache; increased sweating; increased thirst; severe or continuing nausea or vomiting; continuing ringing or buzzing in ears; severe or continuing stomach pain; uncontrollable flapping movements of the hands, especially in elderly patients; vision problems)

**Treatment of overdose**
Recommended treatment of overdose may include:
To decrease absorption—Emptying the stomach via induction of emesis or gastric lavage; administering activated charcoal.
To enhance elimination—Institution of exchange transfusion, hemodialysis, peritoneal dialysis, or hemoperfusion as needed in severe overdose.
Specific treatment—Monitoring serum salicylate concentration until it is apparent that the concentration is decreasing to the nontoxic range. Salicylate concentrations of 500 mcg per mL 2 hours after ingestion indicate serious toxicity; salicylate concentrations above 800 mcg per mL 2 hours after ingestion indicate possible fatality.

In addition, prolonged monitoring may be necessary in massive overdosage because absorption may be delayed.

Inducing forced alkaline diuresis to increase salicylate excretion. However, bicarbonate should not be administered orally for this purpose because salicylate absorption may be increased. Also, if acetazolamide is used, the increased risk of severe metabolic acidosis and salicylate toxicity (caused by increased penetration of salicylate into the brain because of metabolic acidosis) must be considered. It is recommended that acetazolamide be given concurrently with an alkaline intravenous solution, e.g., one that contains sodium bicarbonate or sodium lactate.

Administering blood or vitamin K$_1$ if necessary to treat hemorrhaging.

Monitoring—Monitoring and supporting vital functions; monitoring for pulmonary edema and convulsions and instituting appropriate therapy if required.

Supportive care—Correcting hyperthermia; fluid, electrolyte, and acid-base imbalances; ketosis; and plasma glucose concentration as needed. Patients in whom intentional overdose is confirmed or suspected should be referred for psychiatric consultation.

## Patient Consultation

As an aid to patient consultation, refer to *Advice for the Patient, Bismuth Subsalicylate (Oral)*.

In providing consultation, consider emphasizing the following selected information (» = major clinical significance):

### Before using this medication
» Conditions affecting use, especially:
    Allergies to salicylates or other nonsteroidal anti-inflammatory drugs
    Pregnancy—Salicylates cross the placenta; concern only with high doses and long-term therapy because of salicylate effects
    Breast-feeding—Concern only with high doses and chronic use because of salicylate intake by infant
    Use in children—Risk of fluid and electrolyte loss due to diarrhea; increased susceptibility to toxic effects of salicylates if fever and dehydration present; risk of impaction due to bismuth
    Use in the elderly—Risk of fluid and electrolyte loss due to diarrhea; increased susceptibility to toxic effects of salicylates possibly due to decreased renal function; risk of impaction due to bismuth
    Other medications, especially anticoagulants, heparin, or thrombolytic agents; antidiabetic agents; probenecid or sulfinpyrazone; other salicylates; or oral tetracyclines (for tablet dosage form)
    Other medical problems, especially bleeding ulcers or other active hemorrhagic states, acute dysentery, dehydration, or hemophilia

### Proper use of this medication
Following physician's or manufacturer's instructions
» Not giving to children with symptoms of influenza or varicella without first checking with physician
Missed dose: If on a regular schedule—Taking as soon as possible; not taking if almost time for next dose; not doubling doses
» For use in treatment of diarrhea—Importance of maintaining adequate hydration and proper diet
» Proper dosing
» Proper storage

### Precautions while using this medication
» Caution if other medications containing aspirin or other salicylates are used
Diabetics:
Possibility of false urine sugar test results with prolonged use
Checking with health care professional, if changes in urine sugar test results occur, or if any other questions, especially if diabetes is not well-controlled
» Suspected overdose: Getting emergency help immediately
For antidiarrheal use
Checking with physician if—
Symptoms do not improve within 2 days or become worse
Diarrhea is accompanied by high fever

### Side/adverse effects
May cause encephalopathy, severe constipation, and/or salicylism with higher-than-recommended doses and/or chronic use
Dark tongue or grayish black stools may be alarming to patient although medically insignificant

## Oral Dosage Forms

Note: Bracketed uses in the *Dosage Forms* section refer to categories of use and/or indications that are not included in U.S. product labeling.

## BISMUTH SUBSALICYLATE ORAL SUSPENSION

### Usual adult and adolescent dose
Diarrhea (treatment); or
Gastric distress (treatment)—
    Oral, 524 or 528 mg every half-hour to one hour or 1048 or 1056 mg every hour if needed.
[Traveler's diarrhea (prophylaxis)][1]—
    Oral, 524 or 528 mg four times a day, starting one day prior to departure and continuing for two days after returning, but not to exceed three weeks of continued use.
[Ulcer, duodenal, *Helicobacter pylori*–associated (treatment adjunct)][1]; or
[Gastritis, *Helicobacter pylori*–associated (treatment adjunct)][1]—
    Dosage has not been established. However, in one study, 525 mg was administered orally three times a day one hour before meals, in conjunction with 500 mg of amoxicillin and 500 mg of metronidazole administered three times a day after meals, for one to two weeks.

### Usual adult prescribing limits
4.2 grams in twenty-four hours.

### Usual pediatric dose
Diarrhea (treatment); or
Gastric distress (treatment)—
    Children up to 3 years of age:
        According to weight as follows (may be repeated every four hours if needed, but not to exceed six doses in a day)—:
        Children weighing 6.4 to 8 13 kg: Oral, 44 mg.
        Children weighing over 13 kg: Oral, 88 mg.
    Children 3 to 6 years of age:
        Oral, 88 mg every half-hour to one hour but not to exceed 704 mg in a day.
    Children 6 to 9 years of age:
        Oral, 174.6 or 176 mg every half-hour to one hour but not to exceed 1.4 grams in a day.
    Children 9 to 12 years of age:
        Oral, 262 or 264 mg every half-hour to one hour but not to exceed 2.1 grams in a day.

### Usual geriatric dose
See *Usual adult and adolescent dose*.

Note: Geriatric patients with reduced renal function may be more sensitive to the effects of the usual adult dose and may require lower doses.

### Strength(s) usually available
U.S.—
    262 mg per 15 mL (OTC) [*Pepto-Bismol* (salicylate 130 mg; sodium <3 mg); GENERIC].
    525 mg per 15 mL (OTC) [*Bismatrol Extra Strength*; *Pepto-Bismol Maximum Strength* (salicylate 236 mg; sodium <5 mg)].
Canada—
    264 mg per 15 mL (OTC) [*Bismed* (alcohol 2%; sodium <18 mg); *Pepto-Bismol* (sodium <1.3 mg)].
    525 mg per 15 mL (OTC) [*PMS-Bismuth Subsalicylate*].

### Packaging and storage
Store below 40 °C (104 °F), preferably between 15 and 30 °C (59 and 86 °F), unless otherwise specified by manufacturer. Protect from freezing.

### Auxiliary labeling
• Shake well.
• May cause darkening of tongue and/or stools.

## BISMUTH SUBSALICYLATE TABLETS

### Usual adult and adolescent dose
Diarrhea (treatment); or
Gastric distress (treatment)—
    Oral, 524 or 600 mg every half-hour to one hour or 1050 or 1200 mg every hour if needed.
[Traveler's diarrhea (prophylaxis)][1]—
    Oral, 524 or 600 mg four times a day, starting one day prior to departure and continuing for two days after returning, but not to exceed three weeks of continued use.
[Ulcer, duodenal, *Helicobacter pylori*–associated (treatment adjunct)][1]
[Gastritis, *Helicobacter pylori*–associated (treatment adjunct)][1]—
    Dosage has not been established. However, in one study, 525 mg was administered orally three times a day one hour before meals, in conjunction with 500 mg of amoxicillin and 500 mg of metronidazole administered three times a day after meals, for one to two weeks.

### Usual adult prescribing limits
4.8 grams in twenty-four hours.

# Bismuth Subsalicylate (Oral-Local)

### Usual pediatric dose
Diarrhea (treatment); or
Gastric distress (treatment)—
  Children up to 9 years of age: The available strength of the tablet may not conform to the recommended dose for children up to 9 years of age; the bismuth subsalicylate oral suspension is the preferred dosage form for this age group.
  Children 9 to 12 years of age: Oral, 262 or 300 mg every half-hour to one hour but not to exceed 2.4 grams in a day.

### Usual geriatric dose
See *Usual adult and adolescent dose*.

Note: Geriatric patients with reduced renal function may be more sensitive to the effects of the usual adult dose and may require lower doses.

### Strength(s) usually available
U.S.—
  262 mg (OTC) [*Pepto-Bismol Easy-to-Swallow Caplets* (salicylate 99 mg)].
Canada—
  Not commercially available.

### Packaging and storage
Store below 40 °C (104 °F), preferably between 15 and 30 °C (59 and 86 °F), unless otherwise specified by manufacturer.

### Auxiliary labeling
- Swallow with water. Do not chew.
- May cause darkening of tongue and/or stools.

## BISMUTH SUBSALICYLATE CHEWABLE TABLETS

### Usual adult and adolescent dose
See *Bismuth Subsalicylate Tablets*.

### Usual pediatric dose
See *Bismuth Subsalicylate Tablets*.

### Usual geriatric dose
See *Bismuth Subsalicylate Tablets*.

### Strength(s) usually available
U.S.—
  262 mg (OTC) [*Bismatrol; Pepto-Bismol* (salicylate 102 mg; sodium <2 mg; calcium carbonate 350 mg); GENERIC].
Canada—
  262 mg (OTC) [*Pepto-Bismol* (sodium <2 mg; calcium carbonate 350 mg)].
  300 mg (OTC) [*Bismed* (calcium carbonate 350 mg); *PMS-Bismuth Subsalicylate* (calcium carbonate 350 mg)].

### Packaging and storage
Store below 40 °C (104 °F), preferably between 15 and 30 °C (59 and 86 °F), unless otherwise specified by manufacturer.

### Auxiliary labeling
- Chew or allow to disintegrate in mouth before swallowing.
- May cause darkening of tongue and/or stools.

[1] Not included in Canadian product labeling.

## Selected Bibliography
Bierer DW. Bismuth subsalicylate: History, chemistry, and safety. Rev Infect Dis 1990; 12(S1): S3-S7.
DuPont HL, Ericsson CD, Johnson PC, et al. Use of bismuth subsalicylate for the prevention of traveler's diarrhea. Rev Infect Dis 1990; 12: S64-S67.
Soriano-Brücher HE, Avendaño P, O'Ryan M, et al. Use of bismuth subsalicylate in acute diarrhea in children. Rev Infect Dis 1990; 12: S51-S55.

Revised: 02/03/92
Interim revision: 09/01/94

---

# BISMUTH SUBSALICYLATE, METRONIDAZOLE, AND TETRACYCLINE—FOR *H. PYLORI* Systemic—INTRODUCTORY VERSION

VA CLASSIFICATION (Primary): GA303
Commonly used brand name(s): *Helidac*.
Note: For a listing of dosage forms and brand names by country availability, see *Dosage Forms* section(s).

## Category
Antiulcer agents.

## Indications

### General considerations
The information in this monograph is specific only to the use of these products as indicated in this combination package. These products are intended only for use as described. The individual medications contained in this package should not be used alone or in combination for other purposes. For information on use of the individual components when dispensed as individual medications outside this combined use for treating *Helicobacter pylori*–associated duodenal ulcer, refer to the monographs for each individual agent.

### Accepted
Duodenal ulcer, active (treatment)—Bismuth subsalicylate, metronidazole, and tetracycline, administered in combination with a histamine H$_2$-receptor antagonist, are indicated for the treatment of patients with an active duodenal ulcer associated with *Helicobacter pylori* infection. Eradication of *H. pylori* has been shown to reduce the risk of ulcer recurrence.

Patients who are still infected with *H. pylori* following treatment with this combination plus a histamine H$_2$-receptor antagonist should be considered to have *H. pylori* resistant to metronidazole, and should not be re-treated with a regimen containing metronidazole.

## Pharmacology/Pharmacokinetics
Note: Pharmacokinetic parameters for bismuth subsalicylate, metronidazole, and tetracycline when coadministered have not been studied. There is no information about the gastric mucosal concentrations of these agents after concomitant administration or in combination with an acid-suppressive agent. Pharmacokinetic information provided below is based on studies of each medication when administered alone.

### Physicochemical characteristics
Molecular weight—Bismuth subsalicylate: 362.11.
Metronidazole: 171.16.
Tetracycline hydrochloride: 480.9.

### Mechanism of action/Effect
Bismuth subsalicylate, metronidazole, and tetracycline individually have demonstrated *in vitro* activity against most susceptible strains of *Helicobacter pylori* isolated from patients with duodenal ulcers. The relative contribution of systemic versus local antimicrobial activity against *H. pylori* for agents used in eradication therapy has not been established.
For further information regarding the mechanism of action of each agent in this combination therapy, refer to the individual monographs.

### Absorption
Bismuth subsalicylate—Following oral administration, bismuth subsalicylate is almost completely hydrolyzed in the gastrointestinal tract to bismuth and salicylic acid.
  Bismuth: Less than 1% of bismuth from oral doses of bismuth subsalicylate is absorbed into the systemic circulation.
  Salicylic acid: More than 80% of salicylic acid is absorbed from oral doses of bismuth subsalicylate chewable tablets.
Metronidazole—Well absorbed.
Tetracycline—Readily absorbed.

### Distribution
Bismuth—Absorbed bismuth is distributed throughout the body.
Salicylic acid—Volume of distribution (Vol$_D$): Approximately 170 mL per kg of body weight.
Metronidazole—Distributed into cerebrospinal fluid, saliva, and breast milk in concentrations similar to those found in plasma.
Tetracycline—Distributed into breast milk.

### Protein binding
Bismuth—Very high (90%).
Salicylic acid—High (about 90%).
Metronidazole—Low (<20%).
Tetracycline—Variable.

### Biotransformation

Bismuth subsalicylate—Almost completely hydrolyzed in the gastrointestinal tract to bismuth and salicylic acid. Salicylic acid is, in turn, extensively metabolized.

   Note: The metabolic clearance of salicylic acid is saturable; nonlinear pharmacokinetics are observed at bismuth subsalicylate doses greater than 525 mg. Metabolic clearance of salicylic acid is lower in females than in males.

Metronidazole—Metabolized primarily by side-chain oxidation to [1-(beta-hydroxyethyl)-2-hydroxymethyl-5-nitroimidazole and 2-methyl-5-nitroimidazole-1-yl-acetic acid], and by glucuronide conjugation.

### Half-life

Bismuth has multiple disposition half-lives, with an intermediate half-life of 5 to 11 days, and a terminal half-life of 21 to 72 days.

Salicylic acid has a terminal half-life of 2 to 5 hours after administration of a single oral dose of 525 mg of bismuth subsalicylate.

Metronidazole has an average elimination half-life of 8 hours in normal volunteers.

### Time to peak concentration

Metronidazole—Peak plasma concentrations occur 1 to 2 hours after administration.

### Peak plasma concentration

Salicylic acid—Mean peak plasma salicylic acid concentration was 13.1 ± 3.4 mcg per mL following administration of a single oral dose of 525 mg of bismuth subsalicylate under fasting conditions.

Metronidazole—Peak plasma concentrations following oral administration of 250 mg were 6 mcg per mL.

   Note: There are no significant bioavailability differences between males and females; however, because of weight differences, the resulting metronidazole plasma concentrations in males are generally lower.

### Steady-state serum concentration

Salicylic acid—Mean steady-state serum total salicylate concentration was 24 mcg per mL following 2 weeks of oral administration of 525-mg bismuth subsalicylate liquid suspension four times a day.

### Trough concentration

Bismuth—Mean trough blood bismuth concentration after 2 weeks of oral administration of 787-mg bismuth subsalicylate chewable tablets four times a day under fasting conditions was 5.1 ± 3.1 nanograms per mL.

### Elimination

Bismuth—Primarily eliminated in the urine and bile; renal clearance is 50 ± 18 mL per minute.

Salicylic acid—About 10% excreted unchanged in the urine.

Metronidazole—60 to 80% excreted in the urine and 6 to 15% in the feces; unchanged metronidazole accounts for approximately 20% of the total. Renal clearance of metronidazole is approximately 10 mL per minute per 1.73 square meter of body surface area.

Tetracycline—Concentrated by the liver in the bile; excreted in the urine and feces at high concentrations in a biologically active form.

## Precautions to Consider

### Cross-sensitivity and/or related problems

Patients sensitive to bismuth subsalicylate, metronidazole or other nitroimidazole derivatives, or any of the tetracyclines may be sensitive to this medication. In addition, although this product does not contain aspirin, it should not be administered to patients with a known allergy to aspirin or other salicylates.

### Carcinogenicity

Metronidazole has been shown to be carcinogenic in mice and rats.

No evidence of carcinogenicity has been shown in studies of tetracycline in mice and rats. However, some related antibiotics (oxytetracycline, minocycline) have shown evidence of oncogenic activity in rats.

No long-term studies have been performed to evaluate the effect of the combined use of bismuth subsalicylate, metronidazole, and tetracycline on carcinogenesis.

### Mutagenicity

Bismuth has not shown mutagenic potential in the NTP *salmonella* plate assay.

Metronidazole has shown mutagenic activity in a number of *in vitro* assay systems; however, *in vivo* studies in mammals have failed to demonstrate a potential for genetic damage.

In two *in vitro* mammalian cell assay systems (L51784y mouse lymphoma and Chinese hamster lung cells), there was evidence of mutagenicity by tetracycline at concentrations of 60 and 10 micrograms per mL, respectively.

No long-term studies have been performed to evaluate the effect of the combined use of bismuth subsalicylate, metronidazole, and tetracycline on mutagenesis.

### Pregnancy/Reproduction

This therapy is not recommended in pregnant women.

Fertility—No long-term studies have been performed to evaluate the effect of the combined use of bismuth subsalicylate, metronidazole, and tetracycline on fertility.

Pregnancy—Tetracycline should not be used in pregnant women. Animal studies have indicated that this medication crosses the placenta and may have toxic effects on the fetus, often related to retardation of skeletal development. Embryotoxicity has been reported in animals treated early in pregnancy.

In addition, use of tetracycline in the last half of pregnancy may affect tooth development, causing permanent discoloration (yellow-gray-brown) of the teeth of the child. This effect is more common during long-term use of tetracycline, but has been observed following repeated short-term courses. Enamel hypoplasia has also been reported.

Pregnant women with renal disease may be more prone to developing tetracycline-associated hepatic failure.

FDA Pregnancy Category D.

Labor and delivery—The effect of this combination therapy on labor and delivery is unknown.

### Breast-feeding

Metronidazole and tetracycline are both distributed into human milk. Because of the potential carcinogenicity from metronidazole and the potential for serious adverse reactions in nursing infants from tetracyclines, breast-feeding during this combination therapy is not recommended.

### Pediatrics

Infants and children up to 8 years of age should not take this combination therapy. Use of tetracycline during tooth development may cause permanent discoloration (yellow-gray-brown) of the teeth. This effect is more common during long-term use of tetracycline, but has been observed following repeated short-term courses. Enamel hypoplasia has also been reported.

Children or teenagers who have or who are recovering from chickenpox or influenza should not use this medication. Patients are advised to consult a physician if nausea or vomiting occurs after they have taken this combination therapy, because either could be an early sign of Reye's syndrome, a rare but serious illness.

In addition, the safety and efficacy of this therapy in pediatric patients infected with *H. pylori* have not been established.

### Geriatrics

Elderly patients are more likely to suffer from asymptomatic hepatic or renal function impairment. This therapy should not be given to patients with impairment of hepatic or renal function.

### Dental

Use of systemic tetracycline during pregnancy or in infants and children up to 8 years of age may cause permanent tooth discoloration and enamel hypoplasia.

### Surgical

Use of tetracycline concurrently with the inhalation anesthetic methoxyflurane may result in fatal renal toxicity (see *Drug interactions and/or related problems*).

### Drug interactions and/or related problems

The following drug interactions and/or related problems have been selected on the basis of their potential clinical significance (possible mechanism in parentheses where appropriate)—not necessarily inclusive (» = major clinical significance):

Note: Bismuth and/or the calcium carbonate excipient of bismuth subsalicylate tablets reduce(s) the systemic absorption of tetracycline. However, since the relative contribution of systemic versus local antimicrobial activity against *H. pylori* has not been established, the clinical significance of this interaction is unknown.

Combinations containing any of the following medications, depending on the amount present, may also interact with the medications in this combination therapy.

» Alcohol
   (it is recommended that alcohol not be consumed during metronidazole therapy and for at least 1 day afterward, to avoid potential abdominal cramps, nausea, vomiting, headaches, and flushing)

- Antacids, aluminum-, calcium-, or magnesium-containing or
- Iron or
- Milk or other dairy products or
- Sodium bicarbonate or
- Zinc
    (absorption of tetracycline may be impaired; antacids, milk or other dairy products, or sodium bicarbonate should not be taken within 1 to 2 hours of this medication; preparations containing iron or zinc, including vitamins, should not be taken within 2 to 3 hours of this medication)
- Anticoagulants, coumarin- or indandione-derivative
    (metronidazole may potentiate anticoagulant effects and prolong prothrombin time; salicylates may cause an increased risk of bleeding; tetracycline may depress plasma prothrombin activity; anticoagulant activity should be monitored while the patient is receiving this therapy concurrently)
- Antidiabetic agents, oral or
- Insulin
    (salicylates may enhance the hypoglycemic effects of these medications)
- Aspirin or
- Salicylates, other
    (risk of salicylate toxicity may be increased)
- Disulfiram
    (metronidazole should not be taken if less than 2 weeks have elapsed since ingestion of disulfiram; psychotic reactions have been reported in alcoholic patients taking these agents concurrently)
- Hepatic enzyme inducers, such as phenytoin or phenobarbital (see *Appendix II*)
    (elimination of metronidazole may be increased, resulting in reduced plasma concentrations; impaired clearance of phenytoin also has been reported)
- Hepatic enzyme inhibitors, such as cimetidine (see *Appendix II*)
    (half-life of metronidazole may be prolonged, resulting in decreased plasma clearance of metronidazole)
- Lithium
    (in patients taking relatively high doses of lithium, short-term metronidazole therapy has been associated with elevated serum lithium concentrations and a few cases of lithium toxicity; to detect any increase that may precede clinical symptoms of lithium intoxication, serum lithium and serum creatinine concentrations should be monitored for several days after beginning metronidazole)
- Methoxyflurane
    (concurrent use with tetracycline may result in fatal renal toxicity)
- Oral contraceptives
    (concurrent use with tetracycline may reduce the effectiveness of oral contraceptives; different or additional forms of contraception should be used while taking this combination therapy; breakthrough bleeding may occur)
- Penicillin
    (tetracycline may interfere with the bactericidal action of penicillin)
- Probenecid or
- Sulfinpyrazone
    (salicylates may decrease the effects of these medications)

**Laboratory value alterations**
The following have been selected on the basis of their potential clinical significance (possible effect in parentheses where appropriate)—not necessarily inclusive (» = major clinical significance):

With diagnostic test results
    Gastrointestinal radiographic procedures, diagnostic
        (bismuth absorbs x-rays)
    Note: Although bismuth subsalicylate may cause a temporary and harmless darkening of the stool, it does not interfere with standard tests for occult blood.

With physiology/laboratory test values
    Blood urea nitrogen (BUN)
        (concentrations may be increased)
    Alanine aminotransferase (ALT [SGPT]) and
    Aspartate aminotransferase (AST [SGOT]) and
    Hexokinase glucose and
    Lactate dehydrogenase (LDH) and
    Triglycerides
        (serum values of zero may be observed due to interference of metronidazole with assay methods that involve enzymatic coupling of the assay to oxidation-reduction of nicotine adenine dinucleotide)

**Medical considerations/Contraindications**
The medical considerations/contraindications included have been selected on the basis of their potential clinical significance (reasons given in parentheses where appropriate)—not necessarily inclusive (» = major clinical significance).

*Risk-benefit should be considered when the following medical problems exist:*
    Blood dyscrasias, or history of
        (metronidazole may cause leukopenia)
    Central nervous system (CNS) diseases
        (metronidazole may cause seizures and peripheral neuropathy; rarely, bismuth subsalicylate has been associated with neurotoxicity)
- Hepatic function impairment or
- Renal function impairment
    (metabolism of metronidazole and/or elimination of tetracycline may be decreased, leading to increased toxicity; use of tetracycline is not recommended in patients with renal function impairment)
    Sensitivity to bismuth subsalicylate, or known allergy to aspirin or other salicylates; sensitivity to metronidazole or other nitroimidazole derivatives; or sensitivity to any of the tetracyclines

## Side/Adverse Effects
Note: For additional adverse effects that may be due to any one agent of this combination, please refer to the individual monographs.

The following side/adverse effects have been selected on the basis of their potential clinical significance (possible signs and symptoms in parentheses where appropriate)—not necessarily inclusive:

### Those indicating need for medical attention
Incidence more frequent
    *Abdominal pain; diarrhea; melena* (bloody or black, tarry stools); *nausea*
Incidence less frequent
    *Dizziness; paresthesia* (burning, prickling, or tingling sensations); *vomiting*
Incidence rare
    *Dysphagia* (trouble in swallowing); *gastrointestinal hemorrhage* (black, tarry stools; bloody vomit); *glossitis* (irritation of tongue); *hypertension* (high blood pressure); *myocardial infarction* (heart attack); *pain; photosensitivity reaction* (sensitivity of skin to sunlight); *rheumatoid arthritis* (joint pain and swelling); *seizures; skin rash; stomatitis* (irritation of mouth); *syncope* (fainting)

### Those indicating need for medical attention only if they continue or are bothersome
Incidence less frequent or rare
    *Anal discomfort* (burning or itching around anus); *anorexia* (loss of appetite); *asthenia* (unusual tiredness or weakness); *constipation; insomnia* (trouble in sleeping); *malaise* (general feeling of discomfort or illness); *nervousness*

### Those not indicating need for medical attention
    *Discoloration produced by bismuth* (darkening of tongue; grayish-black stools)

## Overdose
For specific information on the agent used in the management of bismuth subsalicylate overdose, see *Charcoal, Activated (Oral-Local)* monograph.

For information on the management of overdose or unintentional ingestion of bismuth subsalicylate, metronidazole, and tetracycline, **contact a Poison Control Center** (see *Poison Control Center Listing*). If all three components of this therapy are involved in overdose, acute treatment should focus on the salicylate intoxication. There are no data suggesting an increased toxicity of the combination as compared with that of the individual components.

### Clinical effects of overdose
The following effects have been selected on the basis of their potential clinical significance (possible signs and symptoms in parentheses where appropriate)—not necessarily inclusive:

Bismuth subsalicylate
Since less than 1% of the bismuth is normally absorbed, treatment should focus on the salicylate overdose. Initial symptoms include:
    *Confusion; hyperpnea* (fast or deep breathing); *hyperpyrexia* (fever); *lethargy* (unusual tiredness); *nausea; tachycardia* (fast heartbeat); *tinnitus* (continuing ringing or buzzing in ears); *vomiting*

Metronidazole
*Ataxia* (clumsiness or unsteadiness); *nausea; peripheral neuropathy* (pain, numbness, or tingling in arms, legs, hands, or feet); *seizures; vomiting*

Tetracycline
*Diarrhea; nausea; vomiting*

### Treatment of overdose
Recommended treatment of overdose is symptomatic and supportive, and is based mainly on treatment of salicylate intoxication.

To decrease absorption—Induction of emesis or gastric lavage; administering activated charcoal.

To enhance elimination—Alkalinization of urine; institution of hemodialysis or hemoperfusion as needed in severe overdose. Hemodialysis may be preferred over hemoperfusion, since it aids in correcting acid-base disturbances.

Note:   Metronidazole is dialyzable. Tetracycline is not dialyzable.

Monitoring—Monitoring plasma salicylate concentrations may be useful.

Supportive care—Correcting fluid, electrolyte, and acid-base imbalances, and plasma glucose concentration as needed. Patients in whom intentional overdose is confirmed or suspected should be referred for psychiatric consultation.

## Patient Consultation
As an aid to patient consultation, refer to *Advice for the Patient, Bismuth Subsalicylate, Metronidazole, and Tetracycline—For H. Pylori (Systemic)—Introductory Version.*

In providing consultation, consider emphasizing the following selected information (» = major clinical significance):

### Before using this medication
» Conditions affecting use, especially:
  Sensitivity to bismuth subsalicylate, aspirin, or other salicylates; metronidazole or other nitroimidazole derivatives; or any of the tetracyclines
  Pregnancy—Use is not recommended during pregnancy since tetracycline may cause permanent discoloration of the teeth and enamel hypoplasia in the fetus; animal studies have shown tetracycline to be embryotoxic
  Breast-feeding—Metronidazole and tetracycline are distributed into breast milk
  Use in children—Tetracycline should not be used in children younger than 8 years of age because of risk of permanent tooth discoloration or enamel hypoplasia; bismuth subsalicylate should not be used in children and adolescents who have or are recovering from chickenpox or influenza, as it may mask early signs of Reye's syndrome
  Dental—Tetracycline should not be used during pregnancy or in children younger than 8 years of age because of risk of permanent tooth discoloration or enamel hypoplasia
  Surgical—Tetracycline used concurrently with methoxyflurane may result in fatal renal toxicity
  Other medications, especially alcohol; antacids; anticoagulants; antidiabetic agents; aspirin or other salicylates; disulfiram; hepatic enzyme inducers; hepatic enzyme inhibitors; insulin; methoxyflurane; milk or other dairy products; oral contraceptives; other medicines containing calcium, iron, magnesium, or zinc; penicillin; or sodium bicarbonate
  Other medical problems, especially hepatic function impairment or renal function impairment

### Proper use of this medication
Understanding patient instructions in package
Compliance with full course of therapy
» Proper dosing
  Missed dose: Continuing on regular dosing schedule until the medication is finished; not doubling doses; checking with physician if more than four doses are missed
» Proper storage

### Precautions while using this medication
» Avoiding use of aspirin and other salicylates
» Avoiding milk, milk formulas, and other dairy products within 1 to 2 hours of tetracycline
» Avoiding antacids or sodium bicarbonate within 1 to 2 hours of tetracycline; avoiding iron preparations withing 2 to 3 hours of tetracycline
» Avoiding use of alcohol
» Caution if dizziness or lightheadedness occurs
» Using an alternative or additional means of contraception if currently taking oral contraceptives
» Possible photosensitivity reactions

### Side/adverse effects
Signs of potential side effects, especially abdominal pain, diarrhea, melena, nausea, dizziness, paresthesia, vomiting, dysphagia, gastrointestinal hemorrhage, glossitis, hypertension, myocardial infarction, pain, photosensitivity reaction, rheumatoid arthritis, seizures, skin rash, stomatitis, and syncope

Darkening of tongue and grayish-black stools caused by bismuth subsalicylate may be alarming to patient although medically insignificant

## General Dosing Information
Each dose of this combination therapy consists of 3 tablets and 1 capsule (2 bismuth subsalicylate tablets, 1 metronidazole tablet, and 1 tetracycline capsule); these are packaged on a blister card containing a full day's dosage (a total of 12 tablets and 4 capsules). Patient information is included in the product packaging.

Administration of adequate amounts of fluid, particularly with the bedtime dose of tetracycline, will reduce the risk of esophageal irritation and ulceration.

### Diet/Nutrition
Milk and other dairy products may interfere with the absorption of tetracycline. Dairy products should not be taken within 1 to 2 hours of taking this medication. In addition, preparations containing iron or zinc, including vitamin preparations, should not be taken within 2 to 3 hours of taking this medication.

## Oral Dosage Forms

### BISMUTH SUBSALICYLATE CHEWABLE TABLETS, METRONIDAZOLE TABLETS, AND TETRACYCLINE CAPSULES

Note:   Each day's therapy is contained on a blister card and contains eight bismuth subsalicylate 262.4-mg chewable tablets, four metronidazole 250-mg tablets, and four tetracycline 500-mg capsules. They must be taken in combination with a histamine $H_2$-receptor antagonist.

### Usual adult dose
Duodenal ulcer associated with *H. pylori*.
  Oral, 525 mg bismuth subsalicylate, 250 mg metronidazole, and 500 mg tetracycline, taken four times a day (with meals and at bedtime) for fourteen days, in combination with the appropriate dose of a histamine $H_2$-receptor antagonist.

Note:   Each bismuth subsalicylate tablet should be chewed and swallowed. The metronidazole tablet and the tetracycline capsule should be swallowed with a full glass (eight ounces) of water.

### Usual pediatric dose
Safety and efficacy of this therapy in pediatric patients infected with *H. pylori* have not been established.

### Usual geriatric dose
See *Usual adult dose*.

### Strength(s) usually available
U.S.—
  Eight bismuth subsalicylate 262.4-mg chewable tablets, four metronidazole 250-mg tablets, and four tetracycline 500-mg capsules per card (Rx) [*Helidac* (each blister card contains one day's dosage, fourteen days' therapy [fourteen cards] per carton)].

### Packaging and storage
Store at controlled room temperature, between 20 and 25 °C (68 and 77 °F).

### Auxiliary labeling
• Follow patient instructions included with the product.

Revised: 07/28/98
Developed: 10/30/97

---

**BISOPROLOL**—See *Beta-adrenergic Blocking Agents (Systemic)*

---

**BITOLTEROL**—See *Bronchodilators, Adrenergic (Inhalation-Local)*

# BLEOMYCIN Systemic

VA CLASSIFICATION (Primary/Secondary): AN200/DE600
Commonly used brand name(s): *Blenoxane*.
Note: For a listing of dosage forms and brand names by country availability, see *Dosage Forms* section(s).

## Category
Antineoplastic.

## Indications
Note: Bracketed information in the *Indications* section refers to uses that are not included in U.S. product labeling.

**Accepted**
Carcinoma, head and neck (treatment)
Carcinoma, laryngeal (treatment)
[Carcinoma, paralaryngeal (treatment)]
[Carcinoma, esophageal (treatment)][1]
[Carcinoma, thyroid (treatment)][1]
Carcinoma, cervical (treatment)
Carcinoma, penile (treatment)
[Carcinoma, skin (treatment)]
Carcinoma, vulvar (treatment) or
Carcinoma, testicular (treatment)—Bleomycin is indicated for treatment of squamous cell carcinomas of the head and neck (including the mouth, tongue, tonsil, nasopharynx, oropharynx, sinus, palate, lip, buccal mucosa, gingiva, epiglottis, and larynx and paralarynx), cervix, penis, skin, and vulva. It is also indicated for treatment of testicular carcinoma (including embryonal cell carcinoma, choriocarcinoma, and teratocarcinoma), esophageal, and thyroid carcinomas.

Lymphomas, Hodgkin's (treatment) or
Lymphomas, non-Hodgkin's (treatment)—Bleomycin is indicated for treatment of Hodgkin's and non-Hodgkin's lymphomas.

[Kaposi's sarcoma, acquired immunodeficiency syndrome (AIDS)—associated (treatment)][1]—Bleomycin is indicated in the treatment of AIDS-associated Kaposi's sarcoma.

[Osteosarcoma (treatment)][1]—Bleomycin is indicated in the treatment of osteosarcoma.

[Malignant effusions, peritoneal (treatment)][1]
[Malignant effusions, pericardial (treatment)][1] or
Malignant effusions, pleural (treatment)—Bleomycin is indicated, by intracavitary administration, for treatment of peritoneal, pericardial, and pleural effusions.

[Melanoma, malignant (treatment)][1]—Bleomycin is indicated as reasonable medical therapy for the treatment of malignant melanoma (Evidence rating: IA).

[Tumors, germ cell, ovarian (treatment)][1]—Bleomycin is indicated for treatment of germ cell ovarian tumors.

[Tumors, trophoblastic, gestational (treatment)][1]—Bleomycin is indicated for treatment of gestational trophoblastic tumors.

[Mycosis fungoides (treatment)][1]—Bleomycin is indicated, in combination with other agents, for treatment of advanced stage mycosis fungoides.

[Verruca vulgaris (treatment)][1]—Bleomycin is indicated, by intralesional injection, for treatment of severe, recalcitrant common warts (verrucae vulgaris) not responding to conventional treatment.

Extreme caution is recommended in use of bleomycin for nonneoplastic conditions because of potential carcinogenicity with long-term use of this agent.

[1]Not included in Canadian product labeling.

## Pharmacology/Pharmacokinetics

**Physicochemical characteristics**
Hygroscopic; inactivated *in vitro* by agents containing sulfhydryl groups, hydrogen peroxide, and ascorbic acid.

**Mechanism of action/Effect**
Bleomycin is classed as an antibiotic but is not used as an antimicrobial agent. Although bleomycin is effective against both cycling and non-cycling cells, it seems to be most effective in the $G_2$ phase of cell division. Its exact mechanism of antineoplastic action is unknown but may involve binding to DNA, inducing lability of the DNA structure, and reduced synthesis of DNA, and, to a lesser extent, RNA and proteins.

**Absorption**
Approximately 45% of a dose is absorbed into the systemic circulation following intrapleural or intraperitoneal administration.

**Protein binding**
Very low (1%).

**Biotransformation**
Unknown; probably by enzyme degradation in tissues (based on animal studies). Tissue enzyme activity varies, which may determine toxicity and antitumor effect of bleomycin; enzyme activity is high in the liver and kidneys, as well as in bone marrow and lymph nodes, but is low in the skin and lungs. It is not known if any metabolites are active.

**Half-life**
Creatinine clearance greater than 35 mL per minute—115 minutes.
Creatinine clearance less than 35 mL per minute—Increases exponentially as creatinine clearance decreases.

**Elimination**
Renal, 60 to 70%, largely as unchanged drug; markedly reduced in renal failure.
In dialysis—Probably not dialyzable.

## Precautions to Consider

**Carcinogenicity/Mutagenicity**
Secondary malignancies are potential delayed effects of many antineoplastic agents, although it is not clear whether the effect is related to their mutagenic or immunosuppressive action. The effects of dose and duration of therapy are also unknown, although risk seems to increase with long-term use.
Carcinostatic antibiotics have been shown to be carcinogenic in animals, and have been associated with an increased risk of development of secondary carcinomas in humans.
Bleomycin has not been found to be mutagenic according to the Ames test. However, chromosomal aberrations were reported in bone marrow cells and spermatogonia of mice given very high doses.

**Pregnancy/Reproduction**
Fertility—Gonadal suppression, resulting in amenorrhea or azoospermia, may occur in patients taking antineoplastic therapy, especially with the alkylating agents. In general, these effects appear to be related to dose and length of therapy and may be irreversible. Prediction of the degree of testicular or ovarian function impairment is complicated by the common use of combinations of several antineoplastics, which makes it difficult to assess the effects of individual agents.

Pregnancy—First trimester: It is usually recommended that use of antineoplastics, especially combination chemotherapy, be avoided whenever possible, especially during the first trimester. Although information is limited because of the relatively few instances of antineoplastic administration during pregnancy, the mutagenic, teratogenic, and carcinogenic potential of these medications must be considered.
Other hazards to the fetus include adverse reactions seen in adults.
In general, use of a contraceptive is recommended during cytotoxic drug therapy.
Bleomycin has been found to be teratogenic in mice given intraperitoneal doses of 0.6 to 5 Units per kg of body weight on days 7 to 12 of gestation; increased fetal resorptions occurred at doses of 3 and 5 Units per kg of body weight.

**Breast-feeding**
Although very little information is available regarding distribution of antineoplastic agents into breast milk, breast-feeding is not recommended while bleomycin is being administered because of the risks to the infant (adverse effects, mutagenicity, carcinogenicity).

**Pediatrics**
Appropriate studies on the relationship of age to the effects of bleomycin have not been performed in the pediatric population. However, no pediatrics-specific problems have been documented to date.

**Geriatrics**
Although appropriate studies on the relationship of age to the effects of bleomycin have not been performed in the geriatric population, there may be an increased risk of pulmonary toxicity in the elderly (over 70 years of age). In addition, elderly patients are more likely to have age-related renal function impairment, which may require reduction of dosage in patients receiving bleomycin.

**Dental**
Bleomycin may cause mild stomatitis.

### Drug interactions and/or related problems

The following drug interactions and/or related problems have been selected on the basis of their potential clinical significance (possible mechanism in parentheses where appropriate)—not necessarily inclusive (» = major clinical significance):

» Anesthetics, general
(use in patients previously treated with bleomycin may result in rapid pulmonary deterioration because bleomycin causes sensitization of lung tissue to oxygen; even with concentrations of inspired oxygen considered to be safe, pulmonary fibrosis may develop postoperatively)

Antineoplastics, other or
Radiation therapy
(concurrent use may result in increased bleomycin toxicity, including bone marrow depression, which is rarely caused by bleomycin alone, and mucosal and pulmonary toxicity; dosage adjustment may be necessary)

Cisplatin
(cisplatin-induced renal function impairment may result in delayed clearance and bleomycin toxicity even at low doses; caution is recommended because of the frequent combined use of these two agents)

Vincristine
(sequential administration prior to bleomycin arrests cells in mitosis so that they are more susceptible to bleomycin; frequently used to therapeutic advantage)

### Medical considerations/Contraindications

The medical considerations/contraindications included have been selected on the basis of their potential clinical significance (reasons given in parentheses where appropriate)—not necessarily inclusive (» = major clinical significance).

*Risk-benefit should be considered when the following medical problems exist:*

Hepatic function impairment
(potential hepatotoxicity)

» Pulmonary function impairment

Raynaud's phenomenon or
Vascular disease, peripheral
(for intralesional use in treatment of warts; local Raynaud's phenomenon reported in fingers injected with bleomycin)

» Renal function impairment, severe—creatinine clearance less than 25 to 35 mL per minute
(toxicity of bleomycin may be increased; it is recommended that dosage of bleomycin be reduced in patients with renal function impairment)

Sensitivity to bleomycin

» Caution should be used also in patients who have had previous cytotoxic drug therapy or radiation therapy (especially chest irradiation), as well as in patients who smoke, because of the increased risk of pulmonary toxicity.

### Patient monitoring

» Auscultation of the lungs and
» Chest x-ray
(recommended prior to initiation of therapy and at periodic intervals during therapy)

Blood urea nitrogen (BUN) concentrations and
Creatinine concentrations, serum
(determinations recommended prior to initiation of therapy and at periodic intervals during therapy; frequency varies according to clinical state, agent, dose, and other agents being used concurrently)

» Pulmonary function studies, including single-breath carbon monoxide diffusion capacity (DLco) and forced vital capacity
(recommended at frequent intervals during therapy to detect early asymptomatic interstitial damage; however, DLco results are sometimes difficult to interpret because of the effects of weakness and anemia or the presence of an extensive lung tumor or effusion. Therapy with bleomycin should be discontinued at the first sign of pulmonary changes [for example, if forced vital capacity is reduced to 75% or less or DLco to 40% or less of pretreatment level]; if the changes are determined to be drug-related, bleomycin therapy should not be resumed)

## Side/Adverse Effects

Note: There is some evidence that administration of bleomycin by continuous intravenous infusion over 24 hours rather than intermittently may be associated with less pulmonary and idiosyncratic toxicity, although mucocutaneous toxicity may be increased.

The main reported side effect with intralesional use is local burning or pain within 24 to 48 hours after injection. Blackening and eschar occur at the site of the lesion within 1 or 2 weeks and healing usually occurs within 2 to 3 weeks without scarring. Cases of urticaria, nail loss, and Raynaud's phenomenon have also been reported.

When bleomycin is used in combination with vinblastine for testicular carcinoma, vasospasm is a common vascular toxicity.

The following side/adverse effects have been selected on the basis of their potential clinical significance (possible signs and symptoms in parentheses where appropriate)—not necessarily inclusive:

### Those indicating need for medical attention
Incidence more frequent
*Fever and chills; pneumonitis, progressing to pulmonary fibrosis* (cough; shortness of breath); *stomatitis, mild* (sores in mouth and on lips)—due to mucocutaneous toxicity

Note: *Fever and chills* occur in approximately 20 to 60% of patients, usually 3 to 6 hours after administration, last 4 to 12 hours, and become less frequent with continued use.

*Pulmonary toxicity* occurs in 10 to 40% of treated patients, usually 4 to 10 weeks after initiation of treatment; approximately 1% of treated patients have died of pulmonary fibrosis. Pulmonary toxicity is age- and dose-related, occurring most frequently in patients over 70 years of age and/or receiving a total dose greater than 400 Units (although it has been reported with doses as low as 20 to 60 Units). It may be irreversible and fatal; however, there is some evidence that in patients who survive, symptoms and pulmonary function parameters return to normal in approximately 2 years. It occurs at lower doses in patients who have received other antineoplastics or thoracic irradiation; mortality may be as high as 10% in patients who have received pulmonary irradiation. A low-dose allergic pneumonitis has also been reported.

The earliest signs of *pulmonary toxicity* are a decrease in diffusion capacity and fine rales. On chest x-ray, pneumonitis is seen as nonspecific patchy opacities, usually of the lower lung fields. Pulmonary function tests show a decrease in total lung volume and a decrease in vital capacity.

Incidence less frequent
*Idiosyncratic reaction* (confusion; faintness; fever and chills; wheezing)

Note: The *idiosyncratic reaction* occurs in approximately 1% of treated patients (1 to 6% of lymphoma patients). If not promptly treated, it may progress to sweating, dehydration, hypotension, and renal failure or cardiorespiratory collapse. It usually occurs at doses of 25 Units per square meter of body surface area or greater, although it has occurred with a dose of 7.5 Units. May be immediate or delayed by several hours, and occurs after the first or second dose.

Incidence rare
*Hepatic toxicity*—seen as changes in hepatic function tests; *pleuropericarditis* (sudden severe chest pain); *renal toxicity*—seen as changes in renal function tests; *vascular toxicity, including cerebral arteritis, cerebrovascular accident, myocardial infarction, and/or thrombotic microangiopathy* (sudden weakness in arms or legs; sudden, severe chest pain)

### Those indicating need for medical attention only if they continue or are bothersome
Incidence more frequent
*Mucocutaneous toxicity* (darkening or thickening of skin; itching of skin; skin rash or colored bumps on fingertips, elbows, or palms; skin redness or tenderness; dark stripes on skin; swelling of fingers; less frequently, changes in fingernails or toenails); *vomiting and loss of appetite*

Note: *Skin toxicity* occurs in 25 to 50% of treated patients, usually 2 to 4 weeks after initiation of therapy; it appears to be related to cumulative dose and usually develops after 150 to 200 Units have been given.

*Vomiting and loss of appetite* occur in 15 to 30% of treated patients.

Incidence less frequent
*Weight loss*

### Those not indicating need for medical attention
Incidence less frequent
*Loss of hair*

Note: *Loss of hair* begins after several weeks, with regrowth occurring several months later.

**Bleomycin (Systemic)**

Those indicating the need for medical attention if they occur after medication is discontinued
   *Pulmonary toxicity* (cough; shortness of breath)
   Note: *Pulmonary toxicity* may occur up to 1 month after bleomycin is discontinued.

## Patient Consultation
As an aid to patient consultation, refer to *Advice for the Patient, Bleomycin (Systemic)*.
In providing consultation, consider emphasizing the following selected information (» = major clinical significance):

### Before using this medication
» Conditions affecting use, especially:
   Sensitivity to bleomycin
   Pregnancy—Use not recommended because of mutagenic, teratogenic, and carcinogenic potential; advisability of using contraception; telling physician immediately if pregnancy is suspected
   Breast-feeding—Not recommended because of risk of serious side effects
   Use in the elderly—Increased risk of pulmonary toxicity
   Other medications, especially previous cytotoxic drug or radiation therapy
   Other medical problems, especially pulmonary function impairment, severe renal function impairment, or history of smoking

### Proper use of this medication
Caution in taking combination therapy; taking each medication at the proper time
Frequency of nausea, vomiting, and loss of appetite; importance of continuing medication despite stomach upset
» Proper dosing

### Precautions while using this medication
» Importance of close monitoring by physician
» Caution if any kind of surgery (including dental surgery) or emergency treatment is required

### Side/adverse effects
Signs of potential side effects, especially fever and chills, pneumonitis, pulmonary fibrosis, mild stomatitis due to mucocutaneous toxicity, idiosyncratic reaction, hepatic toxicity, pleuropericarditis, renal toxicity, or vascular toxicity, including cerebral arteritis, cerebrovascular accident, myocardial infarction, and/or thrombotic microangiopathy
Physician or nurse can help in dealing with side effects
Possibility of hair loss; normal hair growth should return after treatment has ended (may take several months)
Pulmonary toxicity more likely in smokers

## General Dosing Information
See also *Patient monitoring*.

It is recommended that bleomycin be administered to patients under supervision of a physician experienced in cancer chemotherapy. It is also recommended that equipment and medications (including epinephrine, oxygen, diphenhydramine, and intravenous corticosteroids) necessary for treatment of a possible anaphylactic reaction be readily available at each administration of bleomycin.

A variety of dosage schedules, routes, and regimens of bleomycin, alone or in combination with other antitumor agents, are used. The prescriber may consult the medical literature in choosing a specific dosage or route.

Because of the risk of an idiosyncratic reaction in lymphoma patients, one test dose of 1 or 2 Units or less of bleomycin (base) given 2 to 4 hours prior to initiation of therapy at regular dosage may be used, although the test dose does not always detect reactors.

Some clinicians recommend premedication of patients receiving bleomycin with acetaminophen, steroids, and diphenhydramine hydrochloride to reduce drug fever and the risk of anaphylaxis.

Bleomycin may be administered intravenously or intra-arterially slowly over a period of 10 minutes, or may be further diluted with 50 to 100 mL of the initial diluent for administration by regional infusion.

It is recommended that the dosage of bleomycin be reduced in patients with renal function impairment (creatinine clearance less than 25 to 35 mL per minute). For example, dosage may be adjusted as follows:

| Serum creatinine (mg/dL) | (micromoles per liter) | Fraction of normal dose to be given |
|---|---|---|
| 1.5–2 | 130–180 | 1/2 |
| 2.5–4 | 180–350 | 1/4 |
| 4–6 | 350–530 | 1/5 |
| 6–10 | 530–900 | 1/10–1/20 |

### Safety considerations for handling this medication
There is limited but increasing evidence and concern that personnel involved in preparation and administration of parenteral antineoplastics may be at some risk because of the potential mutagenicity, teratogenicity, and/or carcinogenicity of these agents, although the actual risk is unknown. USP advisory panels recommend cautious handling both in preparation and disposal of antineoplastic agents. Precautions that have been suggested include:
• Use of a biological containment cabinet during reconstitution and dilution of parenteral medications and wearing of disposable surgical gloves and masks.
• Use of proper technique to prevent contamination of the medication, work area, and operator during transfer between containers (including proper training of personnel in this technique).
• Cautious and proper disposal of needles, syringes, vials, ampuls, and unused medication.

A number of medical centers have developed detailed guidelines for handling of antineoplastic agents.

### Combination chemotherapy
Bleomycin is usually used in combination with other agents in various regimens. As a result, incidence and/or severity of side effects may be altered and different dosages (usually reduced) may be used. For example, bleomycin is part of the following chemotherapeutic combination (a commonly used acronym is in parentheses):
   —doxorubicin, bleomycin, vinblastine, and dacarbazine (ABVD).

For specific dosages and schedules, consult the literature. For information regarding each agent, consult the individual monographs.

### For treatment of adverse effects
Treatment of the idiosyncratic reaction is symptomatic and may consist of volume expansion, pressor agents, antihistamines, and corticosteroids.

## Parenteral Dosage Forms

Note: Bracketed uses in the *Dosage Forms* section refer to categories of use and/or indications that are not included in U.S. product labeling.
   A Unit of bleomycin is equal to the formerly used milligram activity. The term milligram activity is a misnomer and was changed to Units to be more precise.

### BLEOMYCIN FOR INJECTION USP
Note: The doses and strength of the available dosage form are expressed in terms of bleomycin base (not the sulfate salt).

#### Usual adult and adolescent dose
Squamous cell carcinoma
Non-Hodgkin's lymphomas
Testicular carcinoma—
   Intramuscular, intravenous, or subcutaneous, 0.25 to 0.5 Units (base) per kg of body weight or 10 to 20 Units per square meter of body surface area one or two times a week or
   Intravenous infusion, continuous, 0.25 Units (base) per kg of body weight or 15 Units per square meter of body surface area per day (over twenty-four hours) for four to five days.
Hodgkin's lymphomas—
   Initially, intramuscular, intravenous, or subcutaneous, 0.25 to 0.5 Units (base) per kg of body weight or 10 to 20 Units per square meter of body surface area one or two times a week.
   Maintenance: Intramuscular or intravenous, after a 50% response occurs, 1 Unit (base) a day or 5 Units a week.
Squamous cell carcinoma of the head, neck, or uterine cervix—
   Regional arterial infusion, 30 to 60 Units (base) a day over a period of one to twenty-four hours.

[Esophageal carcinoma][1] or
[Germ cell ovarian tumors][1] or
[Gestational trophoblastic tumors][1] or
[Kaposi's sarcoma, AIDS-associated][1] or
[Malignant melanoma][1] or
[Mycosis fungoides][1] or
[Osteosarcoma][1] or
[Paralaryngeal carcinoma][1] or
[Skin carcinoma][1] or
[Thyroid carcinoma][1]—
    Consult medical literature and manufacturer's literature for information on appropriate dosage.
[Malignant effusions][1]—
    Intrapleural, 15 to 120 Units (base) in 100 mL of sodium chloride injection, instilled, and after twenty-four hours, removed.
    Intraperitoneal, 60 to 120 Units (base) in 100 mL of sodium chloride injection, instilled, and after twenty-four hours, removed.
[Verruca vulgaris][1]—
    Intralesional, 0.2 to 0.8 Units (base) (according to size) one or more times at intervals of two to four weeks, up to a maximum total dose of 2 Units, using a solution of 15 Units of Sterile Bleomycin Sulfate USP in 15 mL of 0.9% sodium chloride injection or water for injection.

### Usual adult prescribing limits
Because of the risk of pulmonary toxicity, total doses exceeding 225 to 400 Units (base) (less in patients with renal or pulmonary function impairment) should be given with great caution. If bleomycin is administered intrapleurally or intraperitoneally, one half of the administered dose should be counted towards this total.

### Usual pediatric dose
See *Usual adult and adolescent dose*.

### Size(s) usually available
U.S.—
    15 Units (base) (Rx) [*Blenoxane*].
Canada—
    15 Units (base) (Rx) [*Blenoxane*].

### Packaging and storage
Store between 2 and 8 °C (36 and 46 °F).

### Preparation of dosage form
Sterile bleomycin sulfate may be prepared for intramuscular or subcutaneous use by dissolving the contents of the vial (15 Units [base]) in 1 to 5 mL of sterile water for injection, 0.9% sodium chloride for injection, or bacteriostatic water for injection.

U.S.—Sterile Bleomycin Sulfate USP may be prepared for intravenous use by dissolving the contents of the vial (15 Units [base]) in 5 mL or more of 0.9% sodium chloride injection.

Canada—Sterile bleomycin sulfate may be prepared for intravenous or intra-arterial use by dissolving the contents of the vial (15 Units [base]) in 5 to 20 mL of 0.9% sodium chloride for injection.

Use of diluents containing benzyl alcohol is not recommended for preparation of medications for use in neonates. A fatal toxic syndrome consisting of metabolic acidosis, central nervous system (CNS) depression, respiratory problems, renal failure, hypotension, and possibly seizures and intracranial hemorrhages has been associated with this use.

### Stability
U.S.—Reconstituted solutions of Sterile Bleomycin Sulfate USP in 0.9% sodium chloride injection are stable for 24 hours at room temperature, or for at least 14 days if refrigerated.

Canada—Reconstituted solutions are stable for 8 hours at room temperature and at least 48 hours when refrigerated.

[1]Not included in Canadian product labeling.

### Selected Bibliography
DeVita VT, Hellman S, Rosenberg SA, editors. Cancer: principles and practice of oncology. 5th ed. Philadelphia: Lippincott-Raven; 1997.

Revised: 06/24/98
Interim revision: 07/08/98

# BOTULINUM TOXIN TYPE A  Parenteral-Local

VA CLASSIFICATION (Primary): OP900
Commonly used brand name(s): *Botox*.
Note: For a listing of dosage forms and brand names by country availability, see *Dosage Forms* section(s).

## Category
Neuromuscular blocking agent (ophthalmic).

## Indications
Note: Bracketed information in the *Indications* section refers to uses that are not included in U.S. product labeling.

### Accepted
Blepharospasm (treatment) or
Strabismus (treatment)—Botulinum toxin type A is indicated for the treatment of strabismus, including horizontal strabismus up to 50 prism diopters, vertical strabismus, and persistent VI nerve palsy of 1 month or longer duration, and for blepharospasm associated with dystonia, including benign essential blepharospasm or VII nerve disorders.
[Hemifacial spasm (treatment)]
[Facial spasm (treatment)]
[Spasmodic dysphonia (treatment)] or
[Spasmodic torticollis (treatment)]—Botulinum toxin type A is also used to treat the above listed dystonias or dysphonias.

Botulinum toxin type A is of doubtful efficacy for the following indications, or multiple injections over time may be required: deviations over 50 prism diopters, restrictive strabismus, Duane's syndrome with lateral rectus weakness, and secondary strabismus caused by prior surgical over-recession of the antagonist.

### Unaccepted
Botulinum toxin type A is ineffective in chronic paralytic strabismus except to reduce antagonist contracture in conjunction with surgical repair.

## Pharmacology/Pharmacokinetics

### Physicochemical characteristics
Botulinum toxin type A is a sterile, lyophilized form of purified botulinum toxin type A that is produced from a culture of the Hall strain of *Clostridium botulinum*.

### Mechanism of action/Effect
Botulinum toxin type A blocks neuromuscular conduction by binding to receptor sites on motor nerve terminals, entering the nerve terminals, and inhibiting the release of acetylcholine. When injected intramuscularly in therapeutic doses, botulinum toxin type A produces a localized chemical denervation muscle paralysis. When the muscle is chemically denervated, it atrophies and may develop extrajunctional acetylcholine receptors. There is evidence that the nerve can sprout and reinnervate the muscle, thereby reversing the weakness. The paralytic effect on muscles injected with botulinum toxin type A reduces the excessive, abnormal contractions associated with blepharospasm. In the treatment of strabismus, it is postulated that the administration of botulinum toxin type A affects muscle pairs by inducing an atrophic lengthening of the injected muscle and a corresponding shortening of the muscle's antagonist. Following peri-ocular injection of botulinum toxin type A, distant muscles show electrophysiologic changes, but no clinical weakness or other clinical change, for a period of several weeks or months, corresponding to the duration of local clinical paralysis.

### Onset of action
In the treatment of blepharospasm, the initial effect of the injections is seen within 3 days and the effect reaches a peak 1 to 2 weeks after treatment.
In the treatment of strabismus, the initial doses typically create paralysis of injected muscles beginning 1 or 2 days after injection and increasing in intensity during the first week.

### Duration of action
In the treatment of blepharospasm, each treatment lasts approximately 3 months.
In the treatment of strabismus, the paralysis lasts for 2 to 6 weeks and gradually resolves over an additional 2 to 6 weeks.
In the treatment of hemifacial spasm, treatment may last 6 months.

## Precautions to Consider

**Carcinogenicity**
Long term studies in animals have not been done to evaulate the carcinogenic potential of botulinum toxin type A.

**Pregnancy/Reproduction**
Pregnancy—Studies have not been done in either animals or humans.
FDA Pregnancy Category C.

**Breast-feeding**
It is not known whether botulinum toxin type A is excreted in breast milk. However, problems in humans have not been documented.

**Pediatrics**
Appropriate studies on the relationship of age to the effect of botulinum toxin type A have not been performed in children up to 12 years of age. Safety and efficacy have not been established.

**Geriatrics**
Appropriate studies on the relationship of age to the effects of botulinum toxin type A have not been performed in the geriatric population. However, no geriatrics-specific problems have been documented to date.

**Drug interactions and/or related problems**
The following drug interactions and/or related problems have been selected on the basis of their potential clinical significance (possible mechanism in parentheses where appropriate)—not necessarily inclusive (» = major clinical significance):

Note: Combinations containing any of the following medications, depending on the amount present, may also interact with this medication.

Aminoglycoside antibiotics
(may potentiate the effects of botulinum toxin type A)

**Medical considerations/Contraindications**
The medical considerations/contraindications included have been selected on the basis of their potential clinical significance (reasons given in parentheses where appropriate)—not necessarily inclusive (» = major clinical significance).

*Risk-benefit should be considered when the following medical problems exist:*

Cardiac or other medical conditions that may worsen with rapidly increasing activity
(patients with blepharospasm may have been sedentary for a long time; sedentary patients should be cautioned to resume activity slowly and carefully following the administration of botulinum toxin type A)

Infection with *Clostridium botulinum* toxin, history of
(persons with a previous episode of botulism poisoning may have produced antibodies that may interfere with botulinum toxin type A therapy)

Sensitivity to botulinum toxin type A injection

## Side/Adverse Effects

Note: Treatment with botulinum toxin type A may cause the body to produce antibodies against the toxin. This may reduce the effectiveness of continued therapy. To forestall this, the dose of botulinum toxin type A should be kept as low as possible, and in any case below 200 units given in a one-month period.

Two persons previously incapacitated by blepharospasm experienced cardiac collapse within 3 weeks following treatment with botulinum toxin type A. The collapse was attributed to physical overexertion. Sedentary patients should be cautioned to resume activity slowly and carefully following treatment with botulinum toxin type A.

During the treatment of strabismus, retrobulbar hemorrhages sufficient to compromise retinal circulation have occurred from needle penetrations into the orbit. It is recommended that appropriate instruments to decompress the orbit be accessible.

Ocular (globe) penetrations by needles have also occurred. An ophthalmoscope should be available to diagnose this condition.

The injection procedure for the treatment of strabismus has also caused scleral perforations, vitreous hemorrhage, and pupillary change consistent with ciliary ganglion damage (Adies pupil).

During the treatment of blepharospasm, reduced blinking as a result of injection of botulinum toxin type A into the orbicularis muscle can lead to corneal exposure, persistent epithelial defect, and corneal ulceration, especially in patients with VII nerve disorders. In one case, in an aphakic eye, reduced blinking resulted in corneal perforation that subsequently required corneal grafting. Careful testing of corneal sensation in eyes previously operated upon, avoidance of injection into the lower lid area in order to avoid ectropion, and vigorous treatment of any epithelial defect should be employed. Treatment for the above problems may include protective drops, ointment, therapeutic soft contact lenses, or closure of the eye by patching or other means.

The following side/adverse effects have been selected on the basis of their potential clinical significance (possible signs and symptoms in parentheses where appropriate)—not necessarily inclusive:

**Those indicating need for medical attention**
Incidence more frequent
*After treatment for blepharospasm*
**Keratoconjunctivitis sicca** (dryness of the eye); ***lagophthalmos*** (inability to close the eyelid completely)

Incidence less frequent or rare
*After treatment for blepharospasm*
**Decreased blinking; ectropion** (turning outward of the edge of the eyelid); **entropion** (turning inward of the edge of the eyelid); **keratitis** (irritation of the cornea [colored portion] of the eye)

**Those indicating need for medical attention only if they continue or are bothersome**
Incidence more frequent
*After treatment for blepharospasm*
**Ecchymosis** (blue or purplish bruise on eyelid); ***irritation or watering of the eye; photophobia*** (sensitivity of the eye to light); **ptosis** (drooping of the upper eyelid)

*After treatment for horizontal strabismus*
**Ptosis** (drooping of the upper eyelid)—In trials, the average incidence was 10 to 20%; the incidence of ptosis was much less after inferior rectus injection (less than 1%) and much greater after superior rectus injection (30 to 40%); less than 1% of patients had ptosis lasting more than 180 days; **vertical deviation** (eye pointing upward or downward instead of straight ahead)—In trials, the incidence was 10 to 20%; 2% of patients had vertical deviation greater than 2 prism diopters lasting more than 180 days

Incidence less frequent
*After treatment for blepharospasm or strabismus*
**Skin rash, diffuse; swelling of the eyelid skin following injection into the eyelid**—may last several days

*After treatment for horizontal strabismus*
**Diplopia** (double vision); ***past-pointing or spatial disorientation*** (difficulty finding the location of objects)

Incidence rare (less than 1%)
*After treatment for blepharospasm*
**Diplopia** (double vision)

## Patient Consultation

As an aid to patient consultation, refer to *Advice for the Patient, Botulinum Toxin Type A (Parenteral-Local)*.

In providing consultation, consider emphasizing the following selected information (» = major clinical significance):

**Before using this medication**
» Conditions affecting use, especially:
Sensitivity to botulinum toxin type A
Use in children—No specific information about its use in children up to 12 years of age.

**Proper use of this medication**
» Proper dosing

**Precautions while using this medication**
Increasing activities slowly and carefully to allow the heart and body time to strengthen

**Side/adverse effects**
Signs of potential side effects, especially keratoconjunctivitis sicca, lagophthalmos, decreased blinking, ectropion, entropion, and keratitis

## General Dosing Information

The cumulative dose of botulinum toxin type A in the treatment of either strabismus or blepharospasm should not exceed 200 units (U) in a one-month period.

Physicians administering botulinum toxin type A should understand the standard electromyographic techniques as well as the relevant neuromuscular and orbital anatomy and any alterations to the anatomy because of prior surgical procedures.

**For treatment of blepharospasm**
For blepharospasm, the diluted medication is injected using a sterile, 27 to 30 gauge needle without electromyographic guidance.

### For treatment of strabismus
For strabismus, botulinum toxin type A is intended for injection into extraocular muscles utilizing the electrical activity recorded from the tip of the injection needle as a guide to placement within the target muscle. Injection without surgical exposure or electromyographic guidance should not be attempted.

The injection should be prepared by drawing an amount of the properly diluted toxin that is slightly greater than the intended dose into a sterile 1.0 mL tuberculin syringe. Any air bubbles should be expelled from the syringe barrel and the syringe should be attached to the electromyographic injection needle, which is preferably a 1½ inch, 27 gauge needle. The injection volume that is in excess of the intended dose should be expelled through the needle; this assures patency of the needle and confirms that there is no syringe-needle leakage. A new, sterile needle and syringe should be used to enter the vial on each occasion for dilution or removal of the medication.

To prepare the eye for the injection, it is recommended that several drops of a local anesthetic and an ocular decongestant be administered several minutes prior to injection.

### For treatment of adverse effects
Recommended treatment consists of the following:
- Should accidental injection or oral ingestion occur, the person should be medically supervised for several days on an office or outpatient basis for signs or symptoms of systemic weakness or muscle paralysis.

A vial containing 100 U of lyophilized *Clostridium botulinum* toxin type A is considered to be below the estimated dose for systemic toxicity in humans weighing 6 kg (13.2 lb) or greater.

## Parenteral Dosage Forms
Note: Bracketed uses in the Dosage Forms section refer to categories of use and/or indications that are not included in U.S. product labeling.

### BOTULINUM TOXIN TYPE A FOR INJECTION
#### Usual adult and adolescent dose
Strabismus—
  Vertical muscles; or horizontal strabismus of less than 20 prism diopters:
    Intramuscularly, initially, 1.25 to 2.5 units (U) into any one muscle.
  Horizontal strabismus of 20 to 50 prism diopters:
    Intramuscularly, initially, 2.5 to 5 U into any one muscle.
  Persistent VI nerve palsy of one month duration or longer:
    Intramuscularly, initially, 1.25 to 2.5 U into the medial rectus muscle.
  Note: The volume of botulinum toxin type A injected for treatment of strabismus should be between 0.05 to 0.15 mL per muscle.
    For initial treatment of strabismus—
    Use the lower of the initial doses for treatment of small deviations. Use the larger doses only for large deviations.

    The initial doses typically create paralysis of injected muscles beginning one or two days after injection and increasing in intensity during the first week. The paralysis usually lasts for two to six weeks and gradually resolves over an additional two to six weeks. Overcorrections lasting more than six months have been rare. About one half of patients will require subsequent doses because of inadequate paralytic response of the muscle to the initial dose, or because of mechanical factors, such as large deviations or restrictions, or because of the lack of binocular motor fusion to stabilize the alignment.

    For subsequent treatment of residual or recurrent strabismus—
    It is recommended that patients be reexamined seven to fourteen days after each injection to assess the effect of that dose.
    Patients who experience adequate paralysis of the target muscle and who require subsequent injections should receive a dose comparable to the initial dose.
    Subsequent doses for patients experiencing incomplete paralysis of the target muscle may be increased up to twice the previously administered dose.
    Subsequent injections should not be administered until the effects of the previous dose have dissipated, as evidenced by substantial function in the injected and adjacent muscles.
    The maximum recommended dose as a single injection into any one muscle is 25 U.

Blepharospasm—
  Intramuscularly, initially, 1.25 to 2.5 U (using 0.05 to 0.1 mL volume at each site), injected into the medial and lateral pre-tarsal orbicularis oculi of the upper lid and into the lateral pre-septal orbicularis oculi of the lower lid. An additional 2.5 to 5 U may be injected into the orbital portion of the orbicularis oculi at the zygomatic arch.

Note: In general, the initial effect of the injections is seen within three days and the effect reaches a peak one to two weeks after treatment.

Each treatment lasts approximately three months, following which the procedure can be repeated indefinitely.

At subsequent treatment sessions, the dose may be increased up to twofold if the response from the initial treatment is considered insufficient, which is usually defined as an effect that does not last longer than two months. There appears to be little benefit from injecting more than 5 U per site. In addition, some tolerance may occur when the medication is used in treating blepharospasm if the treatments are administered more frequently than every three months. Also, it is rare to have the effect be permanent.

[Spasmodic torticollis (cervical dystonia)]—
  Intramuscularly, the dosage should be individualized based on the patient's head and neck position, localization of pain and muscle hypertrophy, the patient's body weight, and individual patient response.
  The dosages used in clinical trials ranged between 140 and 280 U, however, in clinical practice dosages in the range of 200 to 360 U have been used effectively. It is not recommended that a total dose of 6 U per kg every 2 months be exceeded.
  Note: For injections into superficial muscles, a 25, 27, or 30 gauge needle may be used, and a 22 gauge needle may be used for deeper musculature. Localization of the involved muscles with electromyographic guidance may be useful.

    The use of multiple injection sites allows botulinum toxin type A to have more uniform contact with the innervation areas of the dystonic muscle, and are especially useful in larger muscles. The optimal number of injection sites is dependent upon the size of the muscle to be chemically denervated.

    Clinical improvement generally occurs within the first 2 weeks following the injection. The clinical benefit typically peaks approximately 6 weeks following the injection. Subsequent doses should be administered when the clinical effect of the previous injection diminishes, and no more frequently than every 2 months. The interval between injections reported in the clinical trials showed substantial variation (from 2 to 32 weeks), with a typical duration of approximately 12 to 16 weeks, depending on the patient's individual symptoms and responses.

Dosage Guide
Note: This dosing table is intended to provide guidelines for the injection of botulinum toxin type A in the treatment of cervical dystonia. This information is provided as guidance for the initial injection since the extent of muscle hypertrophy and the muscle groups involved in the dystonic posture may change over time, necessitating alterations in the dose of botulinum toxin type A and the muscles to be injected. The exact dosage and the sites to be injected should be individualized for each patient.

| Dosage Guide | | | |
|---|---|---|---|
| Classification of Cervical Dystonia | Muscle Groupings | Total Dosage | Number of Sites |
| Type I—Head rotated toward side of shoulder elevations | Sternocleidomastoid | 50–100 U | at least 2 sites |
| | Levator scapulae | 50 U | 1 or 2 sites |
| | Scalene | 25–50 U | 1 or 2 sites |
| | Splenius capitis | 25–75 U | 1 to 3 sites |
| | Trapezius | 25–100 U | 1 to 8 sites |
| Type II—Head rotation only | Sternocleidomastoid | 25–100 U | at least 2 sites if > 25 U given |
| Type III—Head tilted toward side of shoulder elevation | Sternocleidomastoid | 25–100 U | at posterior border; at least 2 sites if > 25 U given |
| | Levator scapulae | 25–100 U | at least 2 sites |
| | Scalene | 25–75 U | at least 2 sites |
| | Trapezius | 25–100 U | 1 to 8 sites |

## Dosage Guide (continued)

| Classification of Cervical Dystonia | Muscle Groupings | Total Dosage | Number of Sites |
|---|---|---|---|
| Type IV— Bilateral posterior cervical muscle spasm with elevation of the face | Splenius capitis and cervicis | 50–200 U | 2 to 8 sites; treat bilaterally |

**Usual pediatric dose**
Infants and children up to 12 years of age—Safety and efficacy have not been established.
Children 12 years of age and older—See *Usual adult and adolescent dose*.

**Size(s) usually available**
U.S.—
  100 units of lyophilized *Clostridium botulinum* toxin type A (Rx) [Botox (0.5 mg human albumin)].
Canada—
  100 units of lyophilized *Clostridium botulinum* toxin type A (Rx) [Botox (0.5 mg human albumin)].
Note: One unit corresponds to the calculated median lethal intraperitoneal dose (LD/50) in mice.

**Packaging and storage**
Lyophilized product—Store in a freezer at or below −5 °C (23 °F), unless otherwise specified by manufacturer.
Reconstituted product—Store in a refrigerator between 2 and 8 °C (36 and 46 °F), unless otherwise specified by manufacturer.

**Preparation of dosage form**
Botulinum toxin type A for injection should be reconstituted with sterile non–preserved normal saline, such as 0.9% sodium chloride injection.
Dilution Table

Note: The dilutions and doses listed below are calculated for an injection volume of 0.1 mL. A decrease or increase in the dose is also possible by administering a smaller or larger injection volume; from 0.05 mL (50% decrease in dose) to 0.15 mL (50% increase in dose).

| Amount of Diluent Added | Resulting dose in Units per 0.1 mL |
|---|---|
| 1 mL | 10 U |
| 2 mL | 5 U |
| 4 mL | 2.5 U |
| 8 mL | 1.25 U |

**Stability**
Botulinum toxin type A is denatured by bubbling or similar violent agitation; the diluent should be injected into the vial gently.
Discard the vial if its vacuum does not pull the diluent into the vial.
The lyophilized medication and the diluent to be used contain no preservatives.
The medication should be administered within 4 hours after reconstitution and should be stored in a refrigerator during those 4 hours. The date and time of reconstitution should be recorded on the vial.
Reconstituted botulinum toxin type A is clear, colorless, and free of particulate matter. The solution should be discarded if it is discolored or contains particulate matter.

## Selected Bibliography

Biglan AW, et al. Management of strabismus with botulinum A toxin. Ophthalmology 1989 Jul; 96(7): 935-43.

Biglan, AW, et al. Management of facial spasm with Clostridium botulinum toxin, type A (Oculinum). Arch Otolaryngol Head Neck Surg 1988 Dec; 114(12): 1407-12.

Kalra, HK, et al. Side effects of the use of botulinum toxin for treatment of benign essential blepharospasm and hemifacial spasm. Ophthalmic Surg 1990 May; 21(5): 335-8.

Revised: 08/14/98

---

# BRETYLIUM  Systemic

INN: Bretylium tosilate
VA CLASSIFICATION (Primary): CV300
Commonly used brand name(s): *Bretylate*; *Bretylol*.
Note: For a listing of dosage forms and brand names by country availability, see *Dosage Forms* section(s).

## Category
Antiarrhythmic.

## Indications

**Accepted**
Arrhythmias, ventricular (prophylaxis and treatment)—Bretylium is indicated in the prophylaxis and management of ventricular fibrillation.
  Bretylium is also indicated in the treatment of life-threatening ventricular arrhythmias (e.g., ventricular tachycardias) refractory to first-line treatment (lidocaine and cardioversion).

## Pharmacology/Pharmacokinetics

**Physicochemical characteristics**
Molecular weight—Bretylium tosylate: 414.37.

**Mechanism of action/Effect**
The exact mechanism of antiarrhythmic effects has not been fully determined. Bretylium is a quaternary ammonium compound that possesses both adrenergic and direct myocardial effects. Bretylium is selectively taken up into peripheral adrenergic nerve terminals where it produces an initial release of norepinephrine resulting in a sympathomimetic effect. After this initial release phase, bretylium inhibits norepinephrine release, producing adrenergic blockade. Finally, bretylium blocks the uptake of norepinephrine and epinephrine into adrenergic nerve endings. The importance of these effects in mediating bretylium's antiarrhythmic action is not clear.
Bretylium's direct myocardial effect includes prolongation of action potential duration and effective refractory period by inhibition of potassium conductance. However, it does not directly depress conduction velocity or automaticity. Bretylium elevates the ventricular fibrillation threshold. In infarcted canine hearts, bretylium reduces the disparity in action potential duration and refractory period between normal and infarcted regions and transiently improves conduction velocity in infarcted areas. In the Vaughan Williams classification of antiarrhythmics, bretylium is considered to be a class III agent.

**Other actions/effects**
Bretylium produces a positive inotropic effect, which may or may not be related to the norepinephrine release.

**Biotransformation**
Insignificant. No metabolites have been identified.

**Half-life**
Mean, 10 hours (range 4 to 17 hours); this variability may result partially from differences in renal function or administration procedures; increased to 16 to 31.5 hours in renal function impairment.

**Onset of action**

| | Onset of Effect after Administration | |
|---|---|---|
| | Ventricular Fibrillation (min) | Ventricular Tachycardia (min) |
| Intravenous | 5–10 | 20–120 |
| Intramuscular | 20–60 | 20–120 |

**Time to peak serum concentration**
Intramuscular, 1 hour.

**Duration of action**
6 to 24 hours.

**Elimination**
Renal, 90% (unchanged).
In dialysis—Removable by hemodialysis.

## Precautions to Consider

**Carcinogenicity/Mutagenicity**
No information is available on the carcinogenic or mutagenic potential of bretylium.

### Pregnancy/Reproduction
Pregnancy—Studies have not been done in humans.
Studies have not been done in animals.
FDA Pregnancy Category C.

### Breast-feeding
It is not known whether bretylium is distributed into breast milk.

### Pediatrics
Appropriate studies on the relationship of age to the effects of bretylium have not been performed in the pediatric population. Safety and efficacy have not been established.

### Geriatrics
No information is available on the relationship of age to the effects of bretylium in the geriatric population. However, elderly patients are more likely to have age-related renal function impairment, which may require reduction of dosage or increase of dosage intervals in patients receiving bretylium.

### Drug interactions and/or related problems
The following drug interactions and/or related problems have been selected on the basis of their potential clinical significance (possible mechanism in parentheses where appropriate)—not necessarily inclusive (» = major clinical significance):

» Digitalis glycosides
   (initial norepinephrine release caused by bretylium may aggravate digitalis toxicity; concurrent use is not recommended)

Procainamide or
Quinidine
   (concurrent administration may counteract inotropic effect of bretylium and potentiate hypotension)

Sympathomimetics, such as dopamine or norepinephrine
   (the pressor effects of these agents may be enhanced during concurrent administration with bretylium; blood pressure should be monitored closely during concurrent use and dilute solutions should be used)

### Medical considerations/Contraindications
The medical considerations/contraindications included have been selected on the basis of their potential clinical significance (reasons given in parentheses where appropriate)—not necessarily inclusive (» = major clinical significance).

*Risk-benefit should be considered when the following medical problems exist:*

Conditions with fixed cardiac output, such as:
  Aortic stenosis or
  Pulmonary hypertension, severe
   (severe hypotension may occur as a result of reduced peripheral resistance without a compensatory increase in cardiac output; bretylium may be used if necessary for survival, but vasoconstrictive catecholamines may be necessary if severe hypotension occurs)
Renal function impairment
   (elimination reduced; dosage intervals should be increased)
Sensitivity to bretylium

### Patient monitoring
The following may be especially important in patient monitoring (other tests may be warranted in some patients, depending on condition; » = major clinical significance):

Blood pressure determinations and
Electrocardiogram (ECG)
   (should be monitored continuously during administration)

## Side/Adverse Effects
Note: Hypotension (both postural and supine) occurs routinely, with an incidence of about 50% in supine patients, but is rarely symptomatic. Hypotension may occur at doses lower than those necessary to treat arrhythmias.

An initial increase in frequency of arrhythmias and a transient hypertension may occur as a result of the initial release of norepinephrine, and may last a few minutes to an hour. This effect may be reduced by slowing the rate of administration of bretylium.

The following side/adverse effects have been selected on the basis of their potential clinical significance (possible signs and symptoms in parentheses where appropriate)—not necessarily inclusive:

**Those indicating need for medical attention**
Incidence rare (less than 0.1%)
  *Hyperthermia; renal function impairment; respiratory depression from possible neuromuscular block*

Note: *Hyperthermia* has been reported in a small number of patients. Temperatures in excess of 106 °F have been observed. Temperature rise may begin within 1 hour or later after bretylium administration and may reach a peak within 1 to 3 days. If hyperthermia is suspected or diagnosed, bretylium should be discontinued and appropriate treatment instituted immediately.

**Those indicating need for medical attention only if they continue or are bothersome**
Incidence less frequent (3%)
  *Nausea and vomiting*—especially following rapid (less than 8 minutes) intravenous administration
Incidence rare
  *Angina* (chest pain); *bradycardia* (slow heartbeat); *feeling of pressure in the chest; postural hypotension* (dizziness or lightheadedness when getting up from a lying or sitting position; sudden fainting)

## Overdose
For more information on the management of overdose or unintentional ingestion, **contact a poison control center** (see *Poison Control Center Listing*).

### Clinical effects of overdose
The following effects have been selected on the basis of their potential clinical significance (possible signs and symptoms in parentheses where appropriate)—not necessarily inclusive:
*Hypertension, hypotension*

Note: Marked *hypertension* may be followed by marked refractory *hypotension*. This exaggerated hemodynamic response may be due to rapid injection of a very large dose of bretylium while some effective circulation is still present.

### Treatment of overdose
For hypertensive response—Administration of nitroprusside or other short-acting intravenous antihypertensive agent.

For hypotensive response—Appropriate fluid therapy and pressor agents such as dopamine or norepinephrine.

## General Dosing Information
Dosage must be adjusted to meet the individual requirements of each patient, on the basis of clinical response.

Bretylium injection is always diluted before intravenous administration, *except when used in life-threatening ventricular fibrillation* when it is administered undiluted and as rapidly as possible. Consult package insert for dilution information.

When administering bretylium by continuous intravenous infusion, an infusion pump or other suitable metering device should be used to control the rate of infusion.

Intramuscular administration should be limited to 5 mL, undiluted, at each injection site. The injection site should be rotated to avoid tissue destruction.

Bretylium is used clinically for short-term therapy only. It should be discontinued after 3 to 5 days by gradual dosage reduction and replaced with oral antiarrhythmic therapy if necessary.

Tolerance to the hypotensive effect of bretylium usually occurs within several days. Until that occurs, the patient should remain supine or be observed carefully for hypotension. No treatment is needed as long as the supine systolic blood pressure remains above 75 mm Hg, unless there are associated symptoms. If it falls to less than 75 mm Hg, treatment should consist of intravenous infusion of dobutamine, dopamine, or norepinephrine and volume replacement with blood or plasma and intravenous fluids if necessary. Hemodynamic monitoring is recommended in these unstable situations to help guide medication therapy.

## Parenteral Dosage Forms
### BRETYLIUM TOSYLATE INJECTION
**Usual adult and adolescent dose**
Ventricular fibrillation or
Ventricular tachycardia, hemodynamically unstable—
  Immediate suppression: Intravenous (rapid), 5 mg per kg of body weight administered *undiluted*. If the arrhythmia persists, the dosage may be increased to 10 mg per kg of body weight and repeated as necessary.
  Continuous suppression: Intravenous infusion, 1 to 2 mg per minute of the *diluted* solution. Alternatively, infuse the *diluted* solution at a dosage of 5 to 10 mg per kg of body weight over a period greater than eight minutes every six hours.

Note: For specific dilution information, see *Preparation of Dosage Form*.

**Ventricular arrhythmias, other—**
- Intravenous infusion, 5 to 10 mg per kg of body weight of the *diluted*-solution infused over a period greater than eight minutes. If the arrhythmia persists, additional doses may be given at one- to two-hour intervals. This same dosage may be administered every six hours, or a constant infusion of 1 to 2 mg per minute may be used for maintenance therapy; or
- Intramuscular, 5 to 10 mg per kg of body weight administered *undiluted*. If the arrhythmia persists, subsequent doses may be given at one- to two-hour intervals and thereafter maintaining the same dosage every six to eight hours.
- Note: The site of intramuscular injection should be rotated. No more than 5 mL should be injected intramuscularly into one site.

**Usual pediatric dose**
Safety and efficacy have not been established.

**Strength(s) usually available**
U.S.—
50 mg per mL (Rx) [*Bretylol* (preservative-free); GENERIC].
100 mg per mL (Rx) [GENERIC].
Canada—
50 mg per mL (Rx) [*Bretylate*].

**Packaging and storage**
Store between 15 and 30 °C (59 and 86 °F), unless otherwise specified by manufacturer. Protect from freezing.

**Preparation of dosage form**
For intravenous infusion—Using sterile environment and technique, dilute each 500 mg bretylium tosylate in at least 50 mL of 5% dextrose injection or 0.9% sodium chloride injection.

## BRETYLIUM TOSYLATE IN 5% DEXTROSE INJECTION

**Usual adult and adolescent dose**
Ventricular fibrillation or
Ventricular tachycardia, hemodynamically unstable—
Intravenous infusion, 1 to 2 mg per minute; or 5 to 10 mg per kg of body weight infused over a period greater than eight minutes every six hours.

**Usual pediatric dose**
Safety and efficacy have not been established.

**Strength(s) usually available**
U.S.—
1 mg per mL (Rx) [GENERIC].
2 mg per mL (Rx) [GENERIC].
4 mg per mL (Rx) [GENERIC].
Canada—
2 mg per mL (Rx) [GENERIC].
4 mg per mL (Rx) [GENERIC].

**Packaging and storage**
Store below 40 °C (104 °F), preferably between 15 and 30 °C (59 and 86 °F), unless otherwise specified by manufacturer. Protect from freezing.

## Selected Bibliography
Anderson JL. Bretylium tosylate: profile of the only available class III antiarrhythmic agent. Clin Ther 1985; 7(2): 205-24.

Revised: 06/28/96

---

# BRIMONIDINE    Ophthalmic—INTRODUCTORY VERSION

VA CLASSIFICATION (Primary): OP114
Commonly used brand name(s): *Alphagan*.
Note: For a listing of dosage forms and brand names by country availability, see *Dosage Forms* section(s).

## Category
Antiglaucoma agent (ophthalmic); antihypertensive, ocular.

## Indications
**Accepted**
Glaucoma, open-angle (treatment) or
Hypertension, ocular (treatment)—Brimonidine is used in the treatment of open-angle glaucoma or ocular hypertension.

## Pharmacology/Pharmacokinetics
**Physicochemical characteristics**
Molecular weight—442.24.
Other characteristics—The pH of brimonidine tartrate ophthalmic solution is 6.3 to 6.5.

**Mechanism of action/Effect**
Brimonidine is a relatively selective alpha$_2$-adrenergic agonist. It appears to act by decreasing aqueous humor production and increasing aqueous outflow.

**Other actions/effects**
Brimonidine has minimal cardiovascular or pulmonary effects after application to the conjunctiva.

**Absorption**
Some systemic absorption occurs after ocular instillation.

**Half-life**
For systemically absorbed brimonidine—Approximately 3 hours.

**Time to peak plasma concentration**
Approximately 1 to 4 hours after ocular instillation.

**Time to peak effect**
Approximately 2 hours.

**Elimination**
For systemically absorbed brimonidine—Primarily renal, as unchanged brimonidine and metabolites.

## Precautions to Consider
**Carcinogenicity**
Brimonidine was not carcinogenic in a 21-month study in mice given oral doses of 2.5 mg per kg of body weight (mg/kg) per day or in a 2-year study in rats given oral doses of 1 mg/kg per day. These doses provided plasma concentrations equivalent to 77 and 118 times, respectively, the human plasma concentration occurring after ocular instillation of a recommended dose.

**Mutagenicity**
Brimonidine was not mutagenic in several *in vitro* and *in vivo* studies including the Ames test, host-mediated assay, chromosomal aberration test in Chinese hamster ovary (CHO) cells, dominant lethal assay, and cytogenetic studies in mice.

**Pregnancy/Reproduction**
Fertility—Brimonidine did not impair fertility in rats given oral doses of 0.66 mg/kg, which produced plasma concentrations equivalent to 100 times the human plasma concentration occurring after ocular instillation of multiple doses.

Pregnancy—Studies in humans have not been done.
Animal studies have shown that limited quantities of brimonidine cross the placenta and enter the fetal circulation. However, no harm to the fetus occurred in rats given oral doses of 0.66 mg/kg of brimonidine, which produced plasma concentrations equivalent to 100 times the human plasma concentration occurring after ocular instillation of multiple doses.
FDA Pregnancy Category B.

**Breast-feeding**
It is not known whether brimonidine is distributed into human breast milk. However, brimonidine was detected in breast milk in animal studies.

**Pediatrics**
No information is available on the relationship of age to the effects of brimonidine in pediatric patients. Safety and efficacy have not been established.

**Geriatrics**
No information is available on the relationship of age to the effects of brimonidine in geriatric patients.

**Drug interactions and/or related problems**
The following drug interactions and/or related problems have been selected on the basis of their potential clinical significance (possible mechanism in parentheses where appropriate)—not necessarily inclusive (» = major clinical significance):

Note: Combinations containing any of the following medications, depending on the amount present, may also interact with this medication.

Antihypertensives or
Beta-adrenergic blocking agents or
Other cardiovascular agents
(although ophthalmic brimonidine had little effect on pulse or blood pressure in clinical studies, caution in concurrent use with these medications is recommended because alpha-adrenergic agonists such as brimonidine may decrease pulse rate and blood pressure)

Central nervous system (CNS) depressants
(caution in concurrent use is recommended because of the possibility of additive CNS depression)

» Monoamine oxidase (MAO) inhibitors
(brimonidine should not be administered during, or within 14 days following, the administration of an MAO inhibitor)

Tricyclic antidepressants
(whether tricyclic antidepressants may interfere with the ocular antihypertensive effect of ophthalmic brimonidine has not been determined, but they have been reported to decrease the antihypertensive effect of systemic clonidine)

(although the effect of ophthalmic brimonidine on systemic catecholamine concentrations has not been determined, caution is recommended in its concurrent use with tricyclic antidepressants because the antidepressants may alter the metabolism and uptake of circulating catecholamines)

**Medical considerations/Contraindications**
The medical considerations/contraindications included have been selected on the basis of their potential clinical significance (reasons given in parentheses where appropriate)—not necessarily inclusive (» = major clinical significance).

*Except under special circumstances, this medication should not be used when the following medical problem exists:*
» Sensitivity to brimonidine or other ingredients in the formulation

*Risk-benefit should be considered when the following medical problems exist:*
» Cardiovascular disease, severe or
Cerebral insufficiency or
Coronary insufficiency or
Hypotension, orthostatic or
Raynaud's disease or
Thromboangiitis obliterans
(caution is advised, although ocular instillation of brimonidine had minimal effect on blood pressure in clinical trials)

Hepatic function impairment or
Renal function impairment
(caution is recommended because studies have not been done in patients with these conditions)

Mental depression
(caution is recommended; some patients experienced mental depression during clinical trials with brimonidine)

**Patient monitoring**
The following may be especially important in patient monitoring (other tests may be warranted in some patients, depending on condition; » = major clinical significance):

» Intraocular pressure
(should be monitored regularly to determine that an adequate response to treatment is achieved and maintained; in clinical trials the efficacy of brimonidine decreased over time in some patients)

## Side/Adverse Effects

The following side/adverse effects have been selected on the basis of their potential clinical significance (possible signs and symptoms in parentheses where appropriate)–not necessarily inclusive:

**Those indicating need for medical attention**
Incidence more frequent (10 to 30%)
*Allergic reaction* (redness of eye or inner lining of eyelid; swelling of eyelid; itching; tearing; *conjunctival follicles; headache; ocular hyperemia* (redness of eye)

Incidence less frequent (9% or lower)
*Ache or pain in eye; blepharitis* (redness, swelling, and/or itching of eyelid); *blurred vision or other change in vision; conjunctival discharge* (oozing in eye); *conjunctival hemorrhage* (bloody eye); *corneal erosion; dizziness; edema of conjunctiva or eyelid* (swelling of eye or eyelid); *foreign body sensation* (feeling of something in the eye); *gastrointestinal symptoms* (nausea or vomiting); *increased blood pressure; mental depression; muscle pain; syncope* (fainting); *upper respiratory symptoms* (runny or stuffy nose; sneezing)

**Those indicating need for medical attention only if they continue or are bothersome**
Incidence more frequent (10 to 30%)
*Burning, stinging, or tearing; drowsiness or tiredness; dryness of mouth*

Incidence less frequent (9% or lower)
*Anxiety; conjunctival blanching* (paleness of eye or inner lining of eyelid); *corneal staining* (discoloration of white part of eye); *crusting on eyelid or corner of eye; dryness of eye; muscle weakness; photophobia* (increased sensitivity of eye to light); *pounding heartbeat; taste changes; trouble in sleeping*

## Overdose

There is no experience with brimonidine overdose. For information on the management of overdose or unintentional ingestion, **contact a Poison Control Center** (see *Poison Control Center Listing*).

**Treatment of overdose**
Treatment may consist of maintaining a patent airway and other supportive measures required to relieve observed symptoms.

## Patient Consultation

As an aid to patient consultation, refer to *Advice for the Patient, Brimonidine (Ophthalmic)—Introductory Version.*

In providing consultation, consider emphasizing the following selected information (» = major clinical significance)

**Before using this medication**
» Conditions affecting use, especially:
Sensitivity to brimonidine
Other medications, especially monoamine oxidase inhibitors
Other medical problems, especially severe cardiovascular disease

**Proper use of this medication**
Waiting at least 10 minutes between instillation of two different ophthalmic solutions
Proper administration technique; using a second drop if necessary; not touching applicator tip to any surface; keeping container tightly closed
» Importance of not using more medication than the amount prescribed
» Proper dosing
Missed dose: Using as soon as possible; not using if almost time for next dose; using next dose at regularly scheduled time; not doubling doses
» Proper storage

**Precautions while using this medication**
» Regular visits to physician to check eye pressure during therapy
» Medication may cause dizziness, drowsiness, or tiredness; using caution when driving, using machines, or doing anything else requiring alertness
» Contacting physician immediately if syncope occurs
» Soft contact lens users: Preservative in product may be absorbed by soft contact lenses; waiting at least 15 minutes after instilling medication before inserting lenses
Possible photophobia; wearing sunglasses or avoiding bright light

**Side/adverse effects**
Signs of potential side effects, especially allergic reaction, conjunctival follicles, headache, ocular hyperemia, ache or pain in eye, blepharitis, blurred vision or other change in vision, conjunctival discharge, conjunctival hemorrhage, corneal erosion, dizziness, edema of conjunctiva or eyelid, foreign body sensation, gastrointestinal symptoms, increased blood pressure, mental depression, muscle pain, syncope, or upper respiratory symptoms

## General Dosing Information

The intraocular pressure (IOP) lowering effect of brimonidine decreases over time. Although the onset of loss of effect is variable, in clinical studies some patients experienced inadequate control of IOP during the first month of treatment.

## Ophthalmic Dosage Forms

### BRIMONIDINE TARTRATE OPHTHALMIC SOLUTION

**Usual adult dose**
Open-angle glaucoma or
Ocular hypertension—
Topical, to the conjunctiva, 1 drop in the affected eye(s) three times a day.

**Usual pediatric dose**
Safety and efficacy have not been established.

**Strength(s) usually available**
U.S.—
- 0.2% (2 mg of brimonidine tartrate, equivalent to 1.32 mg of brimonidine base, per mL) (Rx) [*Alphagan* (benzalkonium chloride 0.05 mg per mL; polyvinyl alcohol; sodium chloride; citric acid; hydrochloric acid and/or sodium hydroxide to adjust pH)].

**Packaging and storage**
Store at or below 25 °C (77 °F).

**Auxiliary labeling**
- For the eye.

Developed: 04/01/97
Interim revision: 07/15/98

# BRINZOLAMIDE  Ophthalmic—INTRODUCTORY VERSION

VA CLASSIFICATION (Primary): OP112
Commonly used brand name(s): *Azopt*.

Note: For a listing of dosage forms and brand names by country availability, see *Dosage Forms* section(s).

## Category
Antiglaucoma agent (ophthalmic).

## Indications

**Accepted**
Glaucoma, open-angle (treatment) or
Hypertension, ocular (treatment)—Brinzolamide is indicated in the treatment of elevated intraocular pressure in patients with ocular hypertension or open-angle glaucoma.

**Acceptance not established**
Ophthalmic brinzolamide has not been studied in patients with acute angle-closure glaucoma.

## Pharmacology/Pharmacokinetics

**Physicochemical characteristics**
Chemical group—Sulfonamide.
Molecular weight—383.5.
pH—Brinzolamide ophthalmic suspension: 7.5.
Solubility—Insoluble in water, very soluble in methanol, and soluble in ethanol.

**Mechanism of action/Effect**
Brinzolamide is a sulfonamide and a carbonic anhydrase inhibitor. Carbonic anhydrase is an enzyme found in many tissues of the body, including the eye. Carbonic anhydrase catalyzes the reversible reaction involving the hydration of carbon dioxide and the dehydration of carbonic acid. In humans, carbonic anhydrase exists as a number of isoenzymes, the most active of which is carbonic anhydrase II. Carbonic anhydrase II is found primarily in red blood cells, but it also appears in other tissues.
Antiglaucoma agent—Brinzolamide inhibits human carbonic anhydrase II. Inhibition of carbonic anhydrase in the ciliary processes of the eye decreases aqueous humor secretion, presumably by slowing the formation of bicarbonate ions, with subsequent reduction in sodium and fluid transport. The result is a reduction in intraocular pressure, and thereby a reduction in the risk of optic nerve damage and glaucomatous visual field loss. In clinical studies of up to 3 months in duration in patients with glaucoma or ocular hypertension, brinzolamide had an intraocular pressure (IOP)-lowering effect of approximately 4 or 5 mm of mercury (mm Hg).

**Other actions/effects**
When brinzolamide was administered orally in doses of 1 mg twice a day for up to 32 weeks to healthy volunteers, inhibition of carbonic anhydrase II activity at steady state was approximately 70 to 75%, which was less than the degree of inhibition considered to be necessary for a pharmacological effect on renal function and respiration in healthy persons. (The oral dose of 1 mg twice daily approximates the amount of medication delivered systemically by ophthalmic administration of 1% brinzolamide to both eyes three times per day, and simulates systemic drug and metabolite concentrations similar to those achieved with long-term ophthalmic dosing.)

**Absorption**
Brinzolamide is systemically absorbed when applied to the eye. In a study designed to simulate systemic absorption during long-term ophthalmic administration, healthy subjects were given 1 mg of oral brinzolamide twice a day for up to 32 weeks. (The oral dose of 1 mg twice daily closely approximates the amount of medication delivered systemically by ophthalmic administration of 1% brinzolamide in both eyes three times a day). Saturation of red blood cell carbonic anhydrase II by brinzolamide (concentrations of approximately 20 micromolar) was reached within 4 weeks, and steady-state accumulation of the metabolite *N*-desethyl brinzolamide in red blood cells (6 to 30 micromolar) was reached within 20 to 28 weeks.

**Distribution**
During chronic dosing, brinzolamide accumulates in red blood cells by binding to carbonic anhydrase II. The *N*-desethyl metabolite also accumulates in red blood cells by binding primarily to carbonic anhydrase I in the presence of brinzolamide. Plasma concentrations of brinzolamide and the *N*-desethyl metabolite are generally below the minimum assay limit of 10 nanograms per mL.

**Protein binding**
Moderate (approximately 60%).

**Biotransformation**
To an *N*-desethyl metabolite that binds mainly to carbonic anhydrase I in the presence of brinzolamide.

**Half-life**
Following ophthalmic administration—In whole blood, approximately 111 days.

**Elimination**
Renal, primarily as unchanged drug. Metabolites *N*-desethyl brinzolamide and, in lower concentrations, the *N*-desmethoxypropyl and *O*-desmethyl metabolites also appear in the urine.

## Precautions to Consider

**Cross-sensitivity and/or related problems**
Patients sensitive to sulfonamides may also be sensitive to brinzolamide.

**Carcinogenicity**
Studies have not been done.

**Mutagenicity**
No evidence of mutagenicity was found in the *in vivo* mouse micronucleus assay, the *in vivo* sister chromatid exchange assay, or the Ames *Escherichia coli* test. The *in vitro* mouse lymphoma forward mutation assay was negative in the absence of microsomal activation, but positive in the presence of activation.

**Pregnancy/Reproduction**
Fertility—Studies in male and female rats at doses of up to 18 mg per kg of body weight (mg/kg) per day (375 times the recommended human ophthalmic dose) found no adverse effects on fertility.
Pregnancy—Adequate and well-controlled studies in humans have not been done.
Radiolabeled brinzolamide has been found to cross the placenta and appear in the fetal tissues and blood in pregnant rats. Studies in rabbits at oral brinzolamide doses of 1, 3, and 6 mg/kg per day (20, 62, and 125 times the recommended human ophthalmic dose, respectively) found maternal toxicity at the 6 mg/kg per day dose and a significant increase in the number of fetal variations (such as accessory skull bones) that was only slightly higher than the historic value at 1 and 6 mg/kg. Studies in female rats at oral doses of 18 mg/kg per day (375 times the recommended human ophthalmic dose) during gestation found statistically decreased body weights of fetuses that were proportional to the reduced maternal weight gain, with no statistically significant effects on organ or tissue development. Increases in unossified sternebrae, reduced ossification of the skull, and unossified hyoid that occurred at 6 and 18 mg/kg were not statistically significant. No treatment-related malformations have been seen.
It is recommended that risk-benefit be considered before using ophthalmic brinzolamide during pregnancy.
FDA Pregnancy Category C.

**Breast-feeding**
It is not known whether ophthalmic brinzolamide passes into human breast milk. A study in lactating rats at an oral dose of 15 mg/kg per day (312 times the recommended human ophthalmic dose) found decreases in body weight gain in offspring during lactation. When radiolabeled oral

brinzolamide was administered to lactating rats, radioactivity was found in milk at concentrations below those in the blood and plasma.

It is recommended that risk-benefit be considered before patients breast-feed during treatment with ophthalmic brinzolamide.

### Pediatrics
Safety and efficacy have not been established.

### Geriatrics
No information is available on the relationship of age to the effects of brinzolamide in geriatric patients.

### Drug interactions and/or related problems
The following drug interactions and/or related problems have been selected on the basis of their potential clinical significance (possible mechanism in parentheses where appropriate)—not necessarily inclusive (» = major clinical significance):

Note: Combinations containing any of the following medications, depending on the amount present, may also interact with this medication.

» Carbonic anhydrase inhibitors, oral
(potential additive systemic effect; concurrent use is not recommended)

Salicylates, high doses
(acid-base and electrolyte alterations have not been reported with the use of ophthalmic brinzolamide; however, in patients treated with oral carbonic anhydrase inhibitors, rare cases of adverse effects have occurred with concurrent high-dose salicylate therapy)

### Medical considerations/Contraindications
The medical considerations/contraindications included have been selected on the basis of their potential clinical significance (reasons given in parentheses where appropriate)—not necessarily inclusive (» = major clinical significance).

*Risk-benefit should be considered when the following medical problems exist:*

Hepatic function impairment
(although studies with brinzolamide have not been done in patients with hepatic function impairment, caution is advised when brinzolamide is administered to these patients)

» Renal function impairment, severe (creatinine clearance less than 30 mL per minute)
(although studies with brinzolamide have not been done in patients with renal function impairment, brinzolamide is eliminated renally, and the risk of side effects may be increased because of decreased elimination; use is not recommended)

» Sensitivity to brinzolamide

## Side/Adverse Effects
Note: Because it is absorbed systemically, there is a possibility that ophthalmic brinzolamide could cause serious side effects associated with other sulfonamides, including Stevens-Johnson syndrome, toxic epidermal necrolysis, fulminant hepatic necrosis, agranulocytosis, aplastic anemia, and other blood dyscrasias.

Carbonic anhydrase activity has been observed in both the cytoplasm and around the plasma membranes of the corneal endothelium. The effect of continued administration of ophthalmic brinzolamide on the corneal endothelium has not been fully evaluated.

The following side/adverse effects have been selected on the basis of their potential clinical significance (possible signs and symptoms in parentheses where appropriate)—not necessarily inclusive:

### Those indicating need for medical attention
Incidence less frequent
*Blepharitis* (redness or soreness of eyelid); *dermatitis* (skin rash); *feeling of something in the eye; headache; hyperemia* (redness of the eye); *keratitis* (eye redness, irritation, or pain); *ocular discharge* (discharge from the eye); *ocular pain* (eye pain)

Incidence rare
*Allergic reaction, ocular* (itching, redness, swelling, or other sign of eye or eyelid irritation); *alopecia* (hair loss); *chest pain; conjunctivitis* (redness of inner lining of eyelid); *diplopia* (seeing double); *dizziness; dyspnea* (shortness of breath); *hypertonia* (excessive muscle tone); *keratoconjunctivitis* (eye redness, irritation, or pain); *keratopathy* (eye redness, irritation, or pain); *kidney pain; pharyngitis* (sore throat); *urticaria* (hives)

### Those indicating need for medical attention only if they continue or are bothersome
Incidence more frequent
*Bitter, sour, or other unusual taste; blurred vision, transient, after application*

Incidence less frequent
*Burning, stinging, or discomfort when medicine is applied; dry eye; rhinitis* (runny nose)

## Overdose
For more information on the management of overdose or unintentional ingestion, **contact a Poison Control Center** (see *Poison Control Center Listing*).

**Clinical effects of overdose**
No human data are available. However, electrolyte imbalance, acidosis, and possible nervous system effects may occur with oral overdose.

**Treatment of overdose**
Monitoring of serum electrolyte concentrations (especially potassium) and blood pH is recommended.

## Patient Consultation
As an aid to patient consultation, refer to *Advice for the Patient, Brinzolamide (Ophthalmic)—Introductory Version*.

In providing consultation, consider emphasizing the following selected information (» = major clinical significance):

### Before using this medication
» Conditions affecting use, especially:
Sensitivity to brinzolamide or other sulfonamides
Pregnancy—Crosses the placenta in animals; maternal and fetal toxicity occurs in animals administered large doses of medication
Breast-feeding—Risk-benefit should be considered
Other medicines, especially oral carbonic anhydrase inhibitors
Other medical problems, especially renal function impairment

### Proper use of this medication
Shaking medication before each use
Proper administration technique; preventing contamination of medication in bottle
» Importance of using medication only as directed
Waiting 10 minutes between use of two different ophthalmic preparations to prevent "washing out" of the first one
» Proper dosing
Missed dose: Using as soon as possible; not using if almost time for next dose; not doubling doses
» Proper storage

### Precautions while using this medication
Regular visits to physician to check progress during therapy
» Checking with physician if signs of ocular allergic reaction occur
Removing soft contact lenses before instillation of suspension; may be reinserted 15 minutes after instillation
» Checking with physician about possible need for a fresh bottle of medication to use in case of surgery, injury, or infection
» Temporary blurring of vision may occur following administration; caution in driving or operating machinery

### Side/adverse effects
Signs of potential side effects, especially blepharitis, dermatitis, feeling of something in the eye, headache, hyperemia, keratitis, ocular discharge, ocular pain, ocular allergic reaction, alopecia, chest pain, conjunctivitis, diplopia, dizziness, dyspnea, hypertonia, keratoconjunctivitis, keratopathy, kidney pain, pharyngitis, or urticaria

## General Dosing Information
Because of the preservative benzalkonium chloride, the manufacturer recommends that patients remove soft contact lenses before instillation of brinzolamide. Lenses may be reinserted 15 minutes after instillation.

Brinzolamide may be used concurrently with other medications instilled in the eye to lower intraocular pressure. However, the medications should be administered at least 10 minutes apart.

It is recommended that brinzolamide be discontinued if signs of hypersensitivity or other serious reactions occur.

## Ophthalmic Dosage Forms

### BRINZOLAMIDE OPHTHALMIC SUSPENSION

**Usual adult dose**
Antiglaucoma agent (ophthalmic)—
Topical, to the conjunctiva, 1 drop in the affected eye(s) three times a day.

**Usual pediatric dose**
Antiglaucoma agent (ophthalmic)—
Safety and efficacy have not been established.

**Strength(s) usually available**
U.S.—
  1% (Rx) [*Azopt* (benzalkonium chloride 0.01%; mannitol; carbomer 974P; tyloxapol; edetate disodium; sodium chloride; hydrochloric acid and/or sodium hydroxide)].

**Packaging and storage**
Store between 4 and 30 °C (39 and 86 °F).

**Auxiliary labeling**
- For the eye.
- Shake well before using.

Developed: 08/06/98

---

**BROMAZEPAM**—See *Benzodiazepines (Systemic)*

---

# BROMOCRIPTINE  Systemic

VA CLASSIFICATION (Primary/Secondary): AU900/HS900
Commonly used brand name(s): *Alti-Bromocriptine; Apo-Bromocriptine; Parlodel; Parlodel SnapTabs.*
Note: For a listing of dosage forms and brand names by country availability, see *Dosage Forms* section(s).

## Category
Dopamine agonist; antihyperprolactinemic; infertility therapy adjunct; lactation inhibitor; antidyskinetic; growth hormone suppressant (acromegaly); neuroleptic malignant syndrome therapy.

## Indications
Note: Bracketed information in the *Indications* section refers to uses that are not included in U.S. product labeling.

**Accepted**

Prolactinomas, pituitary (treatment)—Bromocriptine is indicated in the treatment of prolactin-secreting pituitary tumors in men and women. Bromocriptine is usually considered to be the treatment of choice for microadenomas and for macroadenomas including those with visual defects. However, surgery may be required to treat macroadenomas in those patients who either cannot take bromocriptine or who exhibit a poor therapeutic response to bromocriptine. Bromocriptine may also be used as an adjunct to radiotherapy when the tumor is inoperable.

[Bromocriptine is used by some clinicians in the treatment of visual field defects that develop during pregnancy. Visual field defects that respond to bromocriptine are secondary to pituitary adenoma enlargement. ][1]

Amenorrhea, secondary, due to hyperprolactinemia (treatment) or
Galactorrhea due to hyperprolactinemia (treatment) or
Hypogonadism, male, due to hyperprolactinemia (treatment) or
Infertility due to hyperprolactinemia (treatment)—Bromocriptine is indicated in the short-term symptomatic treatment of amenorrhea and/or galactorrhea or male or female infertility associated with hyperprolactinemia. Its usefulness in normoprolactinemic amenorrhea or anovulation is controversial.

[Lactation, after second- or third-trimester pregnancy loss (prophylaxis)][1]—Bromocriptine can be used in selected individuals for the prevention of physiological lactation and breast engorgement after stillbirth, neonatal death, or abortion. However, in many patients, breast engorgement is a benign, self-limited condition, which may respond to breast support and mild analgesics, such as acetaminophen and ibuprofen. Once bromocriptine has been discontinued, 18 to 40% of patients experience rebound symptoms of breast secretion, congestion, or engorgement. Also, the relative risk of all of bromocriptine's rare, severe, or life-threatening side effects, which have included strokes, seizures, and myocardial infarction, has yet to be determined.

Parkinsonism (treatment)—Bromocriptine is indicated, usually as an adjunct to levodopa/carbidopa therapy, in the treatment of the signs and symptoms of idiopathic or postencephalic parkinsonism.

Acromegaly (treatment)—Bromocriptine is indicated in the treatment of some cases of acromegaly, usually as an adjunct to surgery or radiotherapy. There are some reports that patients who respond may have elevated prolactin as well as elevated growth hormone concentrations.

[Neuroleptic malignant syndrome (treatment)][1]—Although controlled clinical trials have not been conducted, bromocriptine is sometimes used as adjunctive therapy in the treatment of neuroleptic malignant syndrome. Individual case reports and the known pharmacological activity of bromocriptine indicate that it may have some utility in the treatment of this disorder, as well as a lower incidence of side effects, as compared with other modes of therapy for this condition.

**Unaccepted**

The routine use of bromocriptine for suppression of postpartum lactation is not recommended.

[1]Not included in Canadian product labeling.

## Pharmacology/Pharmacokinetics

**Physicochemical characteristics**
Chemical group—Bromocriptine is an ergot alkaloid derivative.
Molecular weight—750.70.

**Mechanism of action/Effect**
Dopamine agonist
Antihyperprolactinemic
Infertility therapy adjunct and
Lactation inhibitor—Reduction of serum prolactin concentrations by direct inhibition of release of prolactin from the anterior pituitary gland through binding to dopamine type 2 ($D_2$) receptors, resulting in restoration of testicular or ovarian function and suppression of lactation.
Antidyskinetic—In high doses, stimulation of post-synaptic dopamine type 2 ($D_2$) receptors in the neostriatum of the central nervous system (CNS); may also decrease dopamine turnover. At low doses, bromocriptine may worsen dyskinesia by stimulating presynaptic dopamine receptors. Is most effective when used concurrently with levodopa, as stimulation of $D_1$ receptors by levodopa enhances the antidyskinetic effects of post-synaptic $D_2$ receptor stimulation by bromocriptine.
Growth hormone suppressant (acromegaly)—Suppression of secretion and reduction of elevated growth hormone serum concentrations.
Neuroleptic malignant syndrome therapy—Some evidence exists that neuroleptic malignant syndrome may result from depletion of dopamine or blockade of dopamine receptors in the nigrostriatal, hypothalamic, and mesolimbic cortical pathways. Bromocriptine stimulates these dopamine receptors.

**Absorption**
Approximately 28% of an oral dose is absorbed from the gastrointestinal tract, but because of first-pass metabolism, only 6% reaches the systemic circulation unchanged.

**Protein binding**
Very high (90 to 96% to serum albumin).

**Biotransformation**
Hepatic.

**Half-life**
Biphasic—
  4 to 4.5 hours (alpha phase).
  15 hours (terminal).

**Onset of action**
Single dose:
  Serum prolactin-lowering effect: 2 hours.
  Antiparkinsonism effect: 30 to 90 minutes.
  Growth hormone-lowering effect: 1 to 2 hours.

**Time to peak concentration**
1 to 3 hours.

**Time to peak effect**
Serum prolactin-lowering effect—8 hours (after a single dose).
Note: The maximum obtainable reduction in serum prolactin occurs after approximately 4 weeks of continuous therapy. The average duration of therapy required to reinitiate menses is 6 to 8 weeks. In the

treatment of galactorrhea, a significant reduction in lactation usually occurs within 6 to 7 weeks, with cessation of lactation occurring by 12 to 13 weeks. Suppression of postpartum lactation requires 2 to 3 weeks of therapy; some clinicians believe that 3 weeks of therapy is necessary to prevent rebound lactation.

Antiparkinsonism effect—2 hours (after a single dose).

Growth hormone–lowering effect—A clinical response occurs within 4 to 8 weeks with continuous therapy.

**Duration of action**

Serum prolactin–lowering effect—Approximately 24 hours (after a single dose).

Note: Serum prolactin concentrations usually return to pretreatment levels within 2 months after bromocriptine is discontinued.

Growth hormone–lowering effect—4 to 8 hours.

**Elimination**

As metabolites—
  Biliary: Approximately 95%.
  Renal: 2.5 to 5.5%.

## Precautions to Consider

### Cross-sensitivity and/or related problems

Patients sensitive to other ergot derivatives may be sensitive to this medication also.

### Pregnancy/Reproduction

Fertility—Restoration of fertility may result in pregnancy with possible enlargement of a pituitary adenoma, leading to visual field defects, headaches, and excessive nausea and vomiting in the mother.

In general, use of a nonhormonal contraceptive is recommended in patients being treated for hyperprolactinemia until normal ovulatory menstrual cycles are established. At that time, contraception can be discontinued in patients desiring pregnancy, with careful monitoring to avoid inadvertent administration of bromocriptine after pregnancy is diagnosed.

Pregnancy—Bromocriptine is not generally recommended for use during pregnancy; however, it has been used in the treatment of acromegaly, Parkinson's disease, or prolactinoma in pregnant patients when deemed medically necessary. For patients who develop pregnancy-related hypertension or have recently developed hypertensive disorders of pregnancy, withdrawal of bromocriptine is recommended, unless discontinuation is considered medically contraindicated.

Large and long-term studies performed in humans have found no increased incidence of birth defects. In clinical use, successful pregnancies have occurred in humans taking bromocriptine both before conception and for periods ranging from the first 2 to 3 weeks to the full length of the pregnancy.

FDA Pregnancy Category B.

Postpartum—Bromocriptine should not be used during the postpartum period in women with a history of coronary artery disease or other severe cardiovascular conditions, unless withdrawal of bromocriptine is considered medically contraindicated. If bromocriptine is used during the postpartum period, the patient should be monitored for adverse events. Although causal relationship between bromocriptine and these adverse events has not been established, serious events that have occurred during bromocriptine treatment are seizures with or without hypertension, stroke, and myocardial infarction. Many postpartum patients who had seizures or strokes during bromocriptine therapy experienced severe headaches with possible visual disturbances for hours or days before the event occurred.

### Breast-feeding

This medication should not be administered to mothers who intend to breast-feed, since bromocriptine interferes with lactation.

### Pediatrics

Appropriate studies on the relationship of age to the effects of bromocriptine have not been performed in the pediatric population. Safety and efficacy have not been established.

### Adolescents

Appropriate studies performed to date have not demonstrated adolescent-specific problems that would limit the use of bromocriptine in adolescents 15 years of age and older. However, appropriate studies to establish safety and efficacy in adolescents younger than 15 years of age have not been performed.

### Geriatrics

Appropriate studies on the relationship of age to the effects of bromocriptine have not been performed in the geriatric population. However, clinical experience with the use of bromocriptine has shown that CNS effects may occur more frequently in the elderly.

### Dental

Use of large doses of bromocriptine (for example, in the treatment of acromegaly or parkinsonism) may decrease or inhibit salivary flow, thus contributing to the development of caries, periodontal disease, oral candidiasis, and discomfort.

### Drug interactions and/or related problems

The following drug interactions and/or related problems have been selected on the basis of their potential clinical significance (possible mechanism in parentheses where appropriate)—not necessarily inclusive (» = major clinical significance):

Note: Combinations containing any of the following medications, depending on the amount present, may also interact with this medication.

» Alcohol
  (disulfiram-like reaction may occur, including chest pain, confusion, fast or pounding heartbeat, flushing or redness of face, sweating, nausea, vomiting, throbbing headache, blurred vision, and severe weakness)

Clarithromycin or
» Erythromycin or
  Troleandomycin
  (concurrent use of erythromycin caused a 268% increase in bromocriptine's area under the plasma concentration–time curve (AUC) when standardized to body weight and a 4.7-fold increase in the peak bromocriptine plasma concentration ($C_{max}$). Patients should be monitored for bromocriptine toxicity if erythromycin is used concurrently. Although not reported, similar increases may be expected for clarithromycin or troleandomycin)

» Ergot alkaloids, other, or derivatives, including
  Dihydroergotamine
  Ergonovine
  Methylergonovine
  Methysergide
  (although there is no conclusive evidence of a drug interaction, rarely occurring cases of hypertension associated with the use of bromocriptine may be aggravated with use of ergot alkaloids or its derivatives)

Haloperidol or
Loxapine or
Methyldopa or
Metoclopramide or
Molindone or
Monoamine oxidase (MAO) inhibitors, including furazolidone, procarbazine, and selegiline or
Phenothiazines or
Pimozide or
Reserpine or
» Risperidone or
  Thioxanthenes
  (may increase serum prolactin concentrations and interfere with effects of bromocriptine; dosage adjustment of bromocriptine may be necessary)

Hypotension-producing medications, other (See *Appendix II*)
  (concurrent use may result in additive hypotensive effects; antihypertensive dosage adjustment may be necessary)

Levodopa
  (bromocriptine may produce additive effects, allowing reduction in levodopa dosage)

» Ritonavir
  (bromocriptine serum concentrations can increase threefold when given with ritonavir; 50% reduction of bromocriptine dose is recommended if the combination is necessary)

### Laboratory value alterations

The following have been selected on the basis of their potential clinical significance (possible effect in parentheses where appropriate)—not necessarily inclusive (» = major clinical significance):

With physiology/laboratory test values
  Growth hormone
    (plasma concentrations may be transiently increased in individuals with normal concentrations, paradoxically reduced in patients with acromegaly)

### Medical considerations/Contraindications

The medical considerations/contraindications included have been selected on the basis of their potential clinical significance (reasons given in parentheses where appropriate)—not necessarily inclusive (» = major clinical significance):

*Risk-benefit should be considered when the following medical problems exist:*

Hepatic function impairment
(metabolism may be reduced; dosage reduction may be required)

Hypertension, or history of or

Hypertension, pregnancy-induced, history of
(may be aggravated; cautious use and monitoring of blood pressure are indicated with these conditions)

Psychiatric disorders
(may be exacerbated)

Sensitivity to bromocriptine or other ergot alkaloids

**Patient monitoring**

The following may be especially important in patient monitoring (other tests may be warranted in some patients, depending on condition; » = major clinical significance):

» Blood pressure measurements
(recommended especially when used for suppression of postpartum lactation; commonly decreases or rarely increases)

» Imaging studies of sella turcica
(recommended prior to initiation of therapy for all patients with hyperprolactinemia, to rule out possible pituitary tumor, and once a year during therapy to detect enlargement of a tumor; after one or two years of therapy, this examination may be performed less frequently in asymptomatic patients)

» Pregnancy test
(recommended in patients being treated for amenorrhea once menses resumes, whenever a menstrual period is missed)

» Prolactin, serum
(measurement of serum concentrations is recommended monthly during initial treatment and twice yearly during maintenance treatment of hyperprolactinemia to assess effectiveness of bromocriptine)

Visual field assessment
(recommended if clinically indicated during pregnancy after treatment with bromocriptine in case of enlargement of a previously detected macroadenoma)

*For treatment of female infertility*

Anterior pituitary function
(complete evaluation may be warranted prior to initiation of treatment for infertility)

» Evaluation of ovulation, including:
  Daily basal body temperature and/or
  Progesterone, serum and/or
  Use of ovulation prediction test kits and

» Prolactin, serum
(measurement of baseline serum prolactin concentration is recommended, with subsequent measurements as needed, along with other tests as may be appropriate for the evaluation and treatment of female infertility)

*For treatment of male infertility*

FSH, serum and
LH, serum and
Prolactin, serum and
Testosterone, serum
(baseline serum concentration measurements recommended to rule out other causes of infertility and at 3- to 6-month intervals thereafter)

Prolactin, serum
(measurement of serum concentrations is recommended at 4- to 6-week intervals until normal levels are established, then at 3- to 6-month intervals)

Sperm counts
(recommended at periodic intervals beginning 3 months after initiation of treatment)

*For treatment of acromegaly*

» Growth hormone or
Insulin-like growth factor I concentrations (IGF-I), serum
(measurement of serum concentrations is recommended at periodic intervals to assess efficacy and aid in dosage adjustment)

Physical examination
(periodic examination, especially assessing changes in ring size, heel pad thickness, or soft-tissue volume)

## Side/Adverse Effects

Note: The most common side effects occur on initiation of therapy. Most side effects occurring with continuous therapy are dose-related.

Long-term treatment (6 to 36 months) with bromocriptine mesylate has rarely been associated with pulmonary infiltrates, pleural effusion, and thickening of the pleura. These occurred in a few patients taking doses ranging from 20 to 100 mg per day. When bromocriptine was discontinued, the changes slowly reversed toward normal.

The following side/adverse effects have been selected on the basis of their potential clinical significance (possible signs and symptoms in parentheses where appropriate)—not necessarily inclusive:

**Those indicating need for medical attention**
Incidence less frequent
*Confusion; dyskinesia* (uncontrolled movements of the body, such as the face, tongue, arms, hands, head, and upper body); *hallucinations*

Note: *Confusion*, *dyskinesia*, or *hallucinations* are usually associated with use of high doses but may occur in 20 to 25% of patients being treated for parkinsonism, even at low doses, and may persist for a week or more after bromocriptine is withdrawn.

Incidence rare
*Myocardial infarction* (severe chest pain; fainting; fast heartbeat; increased sweating; continuing or severe nausea and vomiting; nervousness; unexplained shortness of breath; weakness); *seizures or strokes* (atypical headache; vision changes, such as blurred vision or temporary blindness; sudden weakness)

Note: There have been a few reports of *myocardial infarction* occurring in patients treated with bromocriptine, including patients that were treated with bromocriptine to suppress lactation, although a direct causal relationship has not been established.

There have been a number of reports of postpartum hypertension, *seizures*, and *strokes* as well as reports of fatalities occurring in patients treated with bromocriptine to suppress lactation; however, further studies are being conducted to determine if a causal relationship exists between the incidence of hypertension, strokes, and seizures and the use of bromocriptine for suppression of lactation. Mean onset of the reactions was 9 days postpartum. The cases of cerebrovascular accident were all associated with hypertension. Use of bromocriptine should be re-evaluated in those patients who experience unexplained headaches and therapy discontinued if headache is severe and atypical.

*With high doses*
*Cerebrospinal fluid rhinorrhea* (continuing runny nose)—in patients treated for pituitary macroadenomas; *fainting*—has also occurred with low doses used in postpartum patients; *gastrointestinal hemorrhage or peptic ulcer* (black, tarry stools; blood in vomit; severe or continuing stomach pain); *retroperitoneal fibrosis* (continuing or severe abdominal or stomach pain; increased frequency of urination; continuing loss of appetite; lower back pain; continuing or severe nausea and vomiting; weakness)—with long-term use

**Those indicating need for medical attention only if they continue or are bothersome**
Incidence more frequent
*Hypotension, especially orthostatic hypotension* (dizziness or lightheadedness, especially when getting up from a lying or sitting position); *nausea*

Note: *Hypotension* occurs frequently, but is symptomatic only in 1 to 5% of patients (8% of postpartum patients). Rarely, hypotension may be severe. A "first-dose phenomenon" has been reported.

Incidence less frequent—more frequent with high doses (for example, when used for acromegaly or parkinsonism)
*Constipation; diarrhea; drowsiness or tiredness; dry mouth; leg cramps at night; loss of appetite; mental depression; Raynaud's phenomenon* (tingling or pain in fingers or toes when exposed to cold); *stomach pain; stuffy nose; vomiting*

## Patient Consultation

As an aid to patient consultation, refer to *Advice for the Patient, Bromocriptine (Systemic)*.

In providing consultation, consider emphasizing the following selected information (» = major clinical significance):

**Before using this medication**
» Conditions affecting use, especially:
  Sensitivity to bromocriptine or other ergot alkaloids
  Pregnancy—Use is not generally recommended
  Breast-feeding—Will prevent lactation in mothers who intend to breast-feed
  Use in the elderly—CNS effects may occur more frequently
  Dental—Reduced salivary flow caused by large doses may contribute to dental disorders
  Other medications, especially alcohol, ergot alkaloids or derivatives, erythromycin, risperidone, or ritonavir

### Proper use of this medication
Taking with meals or milk to reduce gastrointestinal irritation; taking dose at bedtime or the first doses vaginally to better tolerate nausea
» Proper dosing
Missed dose: Taking if remembered within 4 hours; otherwise not taking at all; not doubling doses
» Proper storage

### Precautions while using this medication
Regular visits to physician to check progress
» Caution when driving or doing jobs requiring alertness because of possible drowsiness or dizziness
Dizziness may be more likely to occur after initial dose; taking first dose at bedtime or lying down; getting up slowly from sitting or lying position; taking first dose vaginally, if necessary
» Possible dryness of mouth; using sugarless gum or candy, ice, or saliva substitute for relief; checking with physician or dentist if dry mouth continues for more than 2 weeks
Checking with physician before reducing dosage or discontinuing medication
» Possibility of disulfiram-like reaction with alcohol
*For treatment of acromegaly, amenorrhea, infertility, galactorrhea, or pituitary prolactinomas in females of child-bearing potential*
Advisability of using nonhormonal contraception during therapy or, when using bromocriptine for female infertility, until normal menstrual cycle is established; patients desiring pregnancy should discuss with physician proper time to discontinue use of contraception; telling physician immediately if pregnancy is suspected
» Telling physician right away if symptoms of enlargement of pituitary tumor (blurred vision, sudden headache, severe nausea and vomiting) occur

### Side/adverse effects
Signs of potential side effects, especially CNS effects, fainting, myocardial infarction, seizures, gastrointestinal hemorrhage, peptic ulcer, retroperitoneal fibrosis, rhinorrhea, and strokes

## General Dosing Information
Incidence and severity of side effects (especially nausea) may be reduced by initiating therapy at a low dose (for example, 1.25 mg at bedtime) and increasing gradually (increments of 2.5 mg every 14 to 28 days for parkinsonism and 3 to 7 days for other indications) to the minimum effective dose, and by administering bromocriptine with food. Also, dizziness and nausea may be better tolerated by administering some or all of the dose at bedtime or by administering one or more of the initial doses intravaginally. Since no first-pass effect occurs with a vaginal dose, a reduced first dose may be warranted in some cases and certainly with subsequent doses because higher serum concentrations may result.

Bromocriptine is used rarely to prevent postpartum lactation because of the risk of significant hypotension and other adverse effects. If it is used, the medication should be given only after the patient's vital signs are stable and no sooner than 4 hours after delivery.

Treatment of hyperprolactinemia with bromocriptine may be symptomatic rather than curative. Following withdrawal, rebound amenorrhea usually occurs within 4 to 24 weeks and galactorrhea within 2 to 12 weeks. Pituitary adenoma regrowth and increase in serum prolactin concentrations may occur after withdrawal of bromocriptine. Elevated growth hormone concentrations will also return when the medication is withdrawn if the cause of acromegaly is not eliminated.

## Oral Dosage Forms
Note: Bracketed uses in the *Dosage Forms* section refer to categories of use and/or indications that are not included in U.S. product labeling.

### BROMOCRIPTINE MESYLATE CAPSULES USP
Note: For doses less than 5 mg, use *Bromocriptine Mesylate Tablets USP*.

#### Usual adult dose
Amenorrhea, secondary, due to hyperprolactinemia or
Galactorrhea due to hyperprolactinemia or
Hypogonadism, male, due to hyperprolactinemia or
Infertility due to hyperprolactinemia—
Initial: Oral, 1.25 to 2.5 mg at bedtime with a snack. Dosage may be increased by 2.5 mg every three to seven days as needed to a total of 5 to 7.5 mg a day taken in divided doses with meals.
Maintenance: Oral, 2.5 mg two or three times a day with meals. Doses of up to 15 mg have been used.
Prolactinomas, pituitary—
Initial: Oral, 1.25 mg two or three times a day with meals. Dosage adjustment is gradual over several weeks to 10 to 20 mg a day taken in divided doses with meals. Occasionally, higher doses may be required.
Maintenance: Oral, 2.5 to 20 mg a day taken in divided doses with meals.
Parkinsonism—
Initial: Oral, 1.25 mg one or two times a day with meals; for single doses, at bedtime with a snack is preferred. Dosage may be increased by 2.5 mg increments every fourteen to twenty-eight days.
Maintenance: Oral, 2.5 to 40 mg a day, taken in divided doses with meals. Although higher doses have been used, safety and efficacy have not been established with doses greater than 100 mg a day.
Acromegaly—
Initial: Oral, 1.25 to 2.5 mg at bedtime with a snack for 3 days; dosage may be increased by 1.25 or 2.5 mg every three to seven days up to 30 mg a day taken in divided doses with meals or at bedtime with a snack.
Maintenance: Oral, 10 to 30 mg a day taken in divided doses with meals or at bedtime with a snack. Up to 100 mg per day has been used.
[Lactation suppression][1]—
Initial: Oral, 2.5 mg twice a day taken with meals. Patient may begin medication only after vital signs stabilize and no sooner than four hours after delivery.
Maintenance: Oral, 2.5 to 7.5 mg a day taken in divided doses with meals or at bedtime with a snack for fourteen days. Has been used for up to twenty-one days if needed.
[Neuroleptic malignant syndrome][1]—
Initial: Oral, 5 mg once a day taken at bedtime with a snack; dosage adjustment titrated according to patient response by 2.5 mg increments a day as needed, taken in divided doses with meals or at bedtime with a snack.
Maintenance: Oral, up to 20 mg a day taken in divided doses with meals or at bedtime with a snack.

#### Usual adult prescribing limits
Parkinsonism—40 mg a day.
Other indications—20 mg a day.
Note: Although higher doses have been used, safety and efficacy have not been established with doses greater than 100 mg a day.

#### Usual pediatric dose
Children up to 15 years of age: Dosage has not been established.
Children 15 years of age and older: See *Usual adult dose*.

#### Strength(s) usually available
U.S.—
  5 mg (Rx) [*Parlodel* (lactose; sodium bisulfite)].
Canada—
  5 mg (Rx) [*Parlodel* (lactose)].

#### Packaging and storage
Store below 25 °C (77 °F), unless otherwise specified by manufacturer. Store in a tight, light-resistant container.

#### Auxiliary labeling
• Avoid alcoholic beverages.
• Take with meals or milk.
• May cause drowsiness.

#### Note
Unit-dose repackaging by any process involving heat is not recommended.

### BROMOCRIPTINE MESYLATE TABLETS USP
Note: For doses 5 mg or greater, consider using *Bromocriptine Mesylate Capsules USP*.

#### Usual adult dose
See *Bromocriptine Mesylate Capsules USP*.

#### Usual pediatric dose
See *Bromocriptine Mesylate Capsules USP*.

#### Strength(s) usually available
U.S.—
  2.5 mg (Rx) [*Parlodel SnapTabs* (scored; lactose); GENERIC].
Canada—
  2.5 mg (Rx) [*Alti-Bromocriptine; Apo-Bromocriptine; Parlodel* (scored; lactose); GENERIC].

#### Packaging and storage
Store below 25 °C (77 °F), unless otherwise specified by manufacturer. Store in a tight, light-resistant container.

#### Auxiliary labeling
• Avoid alcoholic beverages.
• Take with meals or milk.
• May cause drowsiness.

#### Note
Unit-dose repackaging by any process involving heat is not recommended.

---
[1]Not included in Canadian product labeling.

## Selected Bibliography

Ho Ky, Thorner Mo. Therapeutic applications of bromocriptine in endocrine and neurological diseases. Drugs 1988; 36: 67-82.

The American Fertility Society. Guideline for practice: The use of bromocriptine. Birmingham: American Fertility Society, 1991.

Revised: 08/09/95
Interim revision: 08/20/97

**BROMODIPHENHYDRAMINE**—See *Antihistamines (Systemic)*

**BROMPHENIRAMINE**—See *Antihistamines (Systemic)*

# BRONCHODILATORS, ADRENERGIC  Inhalation-Local

This monograph includes information on the following: 1) Albuterol; 2) Bitolterol†; 3) Epinephrine; 4) Fenoterol*; 5) Isoetharine†; 6) Isoproterenol; 7) Metaproterenol; 8) Pirbuterol; 9) Procaterol*; 10) Salmeterol; 11) Terbutaline.

INN:
  Albuterol—Salbutamol
BAN:
  Albuterol—Salbutamol
  Epinephrine—Adrenaline
JAN:
  Albuterol—Salbutamol
  Metaproterenol—Orciprenaline
VA CLASSIFICATION (Primary/Secondary):
  Albuterol—RE102
  Bitolterol—RE102
  Epinephrine—RE102/RE900
  Fenoterol—RE102
  Isoetharine—RE102
  Isoproterenol—RE102
  Metaproterenol—RE102
  Pirbuterol—RE102
  Procaterol—RE102
  Salmeterol—RE102
  Terbutaline—RE102

Commonly used brand name(s): *Adrenalin Chloride*[3]; *Airet*[1]; *Alupent*[7]; *Apo-Salvent*[1]; *Arm-a-Med Isoetharine*[5]; *Arm-a-Med Metaproterenol*[7]; *AsthmaNefrin*[3]; *Asthmahaler Mist*[3]; *Berotec*[4]; *Beta-2*[5]; *Brethaire*[11]; *Bricanyl Turbuhaler*[11]; *Bronkaid Mist*[3]; *Bronkaid Mistometer*[3]; *Bronkaid Suspension Mist*[3]; *Bronkometer*[5]; *Bronkosol*[5]; *Dey-Lute Isoetharine*[5]; *Dey-Lute Metaproterenol*[7]; *Gen-Salbutamol Sterinebs P.F.*[1]; *Isuprel*[6]; *Isuprel Mistometer*[6]; *Maxair*[8]; *Maxair Autohaler*[8]; *Medihaler-Iso*[6]; *Nephron*[3]; *Novo-Salmol*[1]; *Primatene Mist*[3]; *Pro-Air*[9]; *Proventil*[1]; *Proventil HFA*[1]; *S-2*[3]; *Serevent*[10]; *Tornalate*[2]; *Vaponefrin*[3]; *Ventodisk*[1]; *Ventolin*[1]; *Ventolin Nebules*[1]; *Ventolin Nebules P.F.*[1]; *Ventolin Rotacaps*[1]; *microNefrin*[3].

Other commonly used names are:
  Adrenaline [Epinephrine]
  Orciprenaline [Metaproterenol]
  Salbutamol [Albuterol]

Note: For a listing of dosage forms and brand names by country availability, see *Dosage Forms* section(s).

*Not commercially available in U.S.
†Not commercially available in Canada.

## Category

Bronchodilator—Albuterol; Bitolterol; Epinephrine; Fenoterol; Isoetharine; Isoproterenol; Metaproterenol; Pirbuterol; Procaterol; Salmeterol; Terbutaline.
Croup therapy agent—Epinephrine.

## Indications

Note: Bracketed information in the *Indications* section refers to uses that are not included in U.S. product labeling.

**Accepted**

Bronchospasm, asthma-associated (treatment)—Albuterol, bitolterol, fenoterol, metaproterenol, pirbuterol, procaterol, and terbutaline are indicated as bronchodilators for the treatment of bronchospasm associated with asthma.

Adrenergic bronchodilators that are more selective for the beta$_2$-receptor and have a longer duration of action are preferred; therefore, epinephrine, isoetharine, and isoproterenol are generally not recommended for this indication.

Bronchospasm, asthma-associated (prophylaxis)—Salmeterol is indicated to prevent bronchospasm and reduce the frequency of acute asthma exacerbations in patients with chronic asthma who are receiving treatment with anti-inflammatory medication and still require regular treatment with an inhaled shorter-acting beta-adrenergic bronchodilator. During therapy with salmeterol, it is important for patients to have a fast-acting inhaled beta-adrenergic bronchodilator available for relief of acute attacks.

Generally, regularly scheduled, daily use of short-acting beta$_2$-agonists is not recommended.

Bronchospasm, exercise-induced (prophylaxis)—Albuterol, [bitolterol], [pirbuterol], procaterol, salmeterol[1], and [terbutaline][1] are indicated for the prevention of exercise-induced bronchospasm. With use of salmeterol, it is important for patients to also have a fast-acting inhaled beta-adrenergic bronchodilator available for relief of acute attacks. Adrenergic bronchodilators that are more selective for the beta$_2$-receptor and have a longer duration of action are preferred; therefore, epinephrine, isoetharine, and isoproterenol are generally not recommended for this indication.

Bronchospasm, chronic bronchitis–associated (prophylaxis and treatment)
Bronchospasm, pulmonary emphysema–associated (prophylaxis and treatment)
Bronchospasm, chronic obstructive pulmonary disease–associated (prophylaxis and treatment)—Albuterol, bitolterol, fenoterol, metaproterenol, pirbuterol, procaterol, and terbutaline are indicated as bronchodilators for the treatment of bronchospasm associated with chronic obstructive airway disease, including bronchitis and pulmonary emphysema. Patients may benefit from the addition of regularly scheduled doses of a beta$_2$-agonist to ipratropium. Adrenergic bronchodilators that are more selective for the beta$_2$-receptor and have a longer duration of action are preferred; therefore, epinephrine, isoetharine, and isoproterenol are generally not recommended for these indications.

Croup (treatment)—Racepinephrine and nebulized [epinephrine][1] are indicated in the treatment of postintubation and viral croup to temporarily reduce mucosal edema, thereby relieving acute respiratory distress.

**Acceptance not established**

Although albuterol, epinephrine, and racepinephrine have been used for treatment of *acute bronchiolitis in infants*, data are insufficient to prove that these medications are effective for this indication. Some studies indicate modest, short-term benefit; however, other results are conflicting.

**Unaccepted**

Salmeterol is not indicated for the treatment of acute or breakthrough asthma symptoms when rapid bronchodilation is needed because of its slower onset of action compared to shorter-acting adrenergic bronchodilators.

Salmeterol therapy should not be initiated in patients with significantly worsening or acutely deteriorating asthma (rapid worsening over hours to days).

[1]Not included in Canadian product labeling.

## Pharmacology/Pharmacokinetics

**Physicochemical characteristics**
Molecular weight—
  Albuterol: 239.32.
  Albuterol sulfate: 576.71.
  Bitolterol mesylate: 557.67.
  Epinephrine: 183.21.
  Epinephrine bitartrate: 333.30.
  Fenoterol hydrobromide: 303.36.
  Isoetharine hydrochloride: 275.78.
  Isoetharine mesylate: 335.42.
  Isoproterenol sulfate: 556.64.

Metaproterenol sulfate: 520.60.
Pirbuterol acetate: 300.36.
Procaterol hydrochloride: 326.82.
Salmeterol xinafoate: 603.76.
Terbutaline sulfate: 548.66.

### Mechanism of action/Effect
Bronchodilator—Adrenergic bronchodilators act by stimulating beta$_2$-adrenergic receptors in the lungs to relax bronchial smooth muscle, thereby relieving bronchospasm. This action is believed to result from increased production of cyclic adenosine 3,5-monophosphate (cyclic 3,5-AMP; cAMP) and ensuing reduction in intracellular calcium concentration caused by activation of the enzyme adenylate cyclase that catalyzes the conversion of adenosine triphosphate (ATP) to cAMP. Increased cAMP concentrations, in addition to relaxing bronchial smooth muscle, inhibit release of mediators of immediate hypersensitivity from cells, especially from mast cells.

Croup therapy agent—Epinephrine has alpha-adrenergic stimulating effects that produce constriction of arteries and veins. The resulting decreased mucosal edema is thought to be the mechanism by which epinephrine and racepinephrine are beneficial in the treatment of croup. The L-isomer of racepinephrine is the primary active isomer.

### Other actions/effects
Albuterol, bitolterol, fenoterol, isoetharine, pirbuterol, procaterol, salmeterol, and terbutaline have a relatively high degree of selectivity for beta$_2$-adrenergic receptors. Data indicate that there is a population of beta$_2$-receptors in the human heart existing in a concentration between 10 and 50% of the cardiac beta-adrenergic receptors; stimulation of these receptors produces tachycardia. Stimulation of beta$_2$-receptors located in skeletal muscle causes muscle tremor.

Epinephrine, isoproterenol, and metaproterenol have significant beta$_1$-adrenergic activity in the heart, resulting in an increased rate and force of cardiac contractions.

Other effects of epinephrine include alpha- and beta$_2$-receptor–mediated stimulation of glycogenolysis and gluconeogenesis.

Limited *in vitro* and *in vivo* animal studies and allergen challenge studies in asthmatics demonstrate that some adrenergic bronchodilators have inhibitory effects on several inflammatory response mediators. However, these medications are not considered to have clinically relevant anti-inflammatory effects.

### Absorption
Systemic absorption is rapid following aerosol administration; however, serum concentrations at recommended doses are very low or unmeasurable.

### Biotransformation
Bitolterol—A prodrug hydrolyzed by esterases in tissue and blood to the active compound colterol.

### Onset of action
Albuterol, bitolterol, epinephrine, fenoterol, isoetharine, isoproterenol, metaproterenol, pirbuterol, procaterol, and terbutaline—Rapid, within 5 minutes.
Salmeterol—Approximately 10 to 20 minutes.

### Time to peak effect
Epinephrine, isoetharine, and isoproterenol—Within 5 to 15 minutes.
Albuterol, bitolterol, fenoterol, metaproterenol, pirbuterol, procaterol, and terbutaline—Within 30 to 90 minutes; however, for albuterol, fenoterol, pirbuterol, and terbutaline, 75% of maximal effect is achieved within 5 minutes.
Salmeterol—3 to 4 hours; however, approximately 80% of the maximal increase in forced expiratory volume in 1 second (FEV$_1$) occurs within 1 hour after administration.

### Duration of action
Short-acting (less than 3 hours)—Epinephrine, isoetharine, and isoproterenol.
Intermediate-acting (3 to 6 hours)—Albuterol, bitolterol, fenoterol, metaproterenol, pirbuterol, procaterol, and terbutaline.
Long-acting—Salmeterol: Approximately 12 hours.

Note: It is believed that the sustained pharmacological action of salmeterol is due to its lipophilicity and long N-substituted side chain. The side chain has been shown to bind to the exo-site, an area in the beta$_2$-receptor adjacent to the active site. The phenylethanolamine portion of the salmeterol molecule is then in position to associate with and dissociate from the receptor's active site. This theory is supported by the fact that the pharmacologic effect of salmeterol *in vitro* is rapidly and completely reversed by beta-receptor antagonism and resumes once the antagonist is removed.

## Precautions to Consider

### Carcinogenicity/Tumorigenicity/Mutagenicity
*Albuterol*—A 2-year study in rats showed that albuterol, administered orally in doses that provided 93, 463, and 2315 times the maximum inhalational dose for a human weighing 50 kilograms (kg), caused a dose-related increase in the incidences of benign leiomyomas of the mesovarium. An 18-month study in mice and a lifetime study in hamsters showed no evidence of tumorigenicity. Studies with albuterol showed no evidence of mutagenesis.

*Bitolterol*—No tumorigenicity was observed in a 2-year study in rats given oral doses that provided 12 or 62 times the maximal daily human inhalational dose for the inhalation solution, or 23 or 114 times the maximal daily human dose for the metered-dose inhaler, or in an 18-month study in mice given oral doses that provided up to 312 times the maximal daily human inhalational dose for the inhalation solution, or 568 times the maximal daily human dose for the metered-dose inhaler. Bitolterol was not mutagenic in Ames Salmonella and mouse lymphoma mutation assays *in vitro*.

*Epinephrine and fenoterol*—Studies to evaluate the carcinogenic, tumorigenic, or mutagenic potential of epinephrine and fenoterol have not been done. There is no evidence from human data that use of these medications may cause problems.

*Isoetharine*—No evidence of carcinogenicity was observed in chronic toxicity studies in dogs given doses up to the equivalent of approximately 200 times the dose for a 70 kg human for 12 months or in rats given doses of up to the equivalent of approximately 450 times the dose for a 70 kg human.

*Isoproterenol*—Isoproterenol has not been evaluated for carcinogenicity or mutagenicity.

*Metaproterenol*—An 18-month study in mice given doses equivalent to 320 and 640 times the maximum recommended dose for a 50 kg human showed an increase in benign ovarian tumors. In a 2-year study in rats given 640 times the maximum recommended human dose, a nonsignificant incidence of benign mesovarian leiomyomas was noted. Mutagenic studies have not been conducted.

*Pirbuterol*—When administered orally to rats for 24 months and to mice for 18 months in doses equivalent to 200 times the maximum human inhalation dose, no evidence of carcinogenicity was observed. In a 12-month study in rats, direct intragastric administration of pirbuterol in doses equivalent to 6250 times the maximum recommended daily inhalation dose for humans resulted in no increased incidence of tumorigenicity. Studies with pirbuterol showed no evidence of mutagenicity.

*Procaterol*—A 23-month study in mice given procaterol orally showed no increased incidence of tumorigenicity. When administered orally to rats at doses of 5, 50, and 500 mg per kg per day, a dose-related incidence of mesovarian leiomyomas was observed. Procaterol has not been shown to be mutagenic.

*Salmeterol*—An 18-month study in mice showed that salmeterol, administered orally in doses that provided 9 and 63 times the human exposure (based on comparison of area under the plasma concentration–time curves [AUCs]), caused a dose-related increase in the incidences of smooth muscle hyperplasia, cystic glandular hyperplasia, leiomyomas of the uterus, and ovarian cysts. A 24-month study in rats given salmeterol orally and by inhalation in doses approximately 55 and 215 times, respectively, the recommended human clinical dose based on mg per square meter of body surface area (mg/m$^2$) showed dose-related increases in the incidences of mesovarian leiomyomas and ovarian cysts. Similar results have been reported with other beta-adrenergic bronchodilators. Salmeterol produced no significant carcinogenic effects in mice receiving doses that provided 1.3 times the human exposure based on AUC comparison, or in rats given 15 times the recommended human clinical dose based on mg/m$^2$. Salmeterol was not mutagenic in *in vitro* tests in microbial or mammalian genes or in human lymphocytes or in an *in vivo* rat micronucleus test.

*Terbutaline*—A 2-year study in rats given oral doses equivalent to 1042, 10,417, 20,833, and 41,667 times the recommended daily human adult dose showed dose-related increases in leiomyomas of the mesovarium. The incidence of ovarian cysts was significantly increased at all doses except the highest dose, and mesovarium hyperplasia was increased significantly at 10,417 and 41,667 times the recommended daily human adult dose. A 21-month study in mice given oral doses equivalent to 104, 1042, and 4167 times the recommended daily human adult dose showed no evidence of carcinogenicity. Studies to evaluate mutagenicity have not been done.

### Pregnancy/Reproduction
*Fertility—Albuterol, bitolterol, pirbuterol, procaterol, salmeterol, and terbutaline:* Reproduction studies in rats showed no significant effects on fertility after administration of these agents.

*Isoetharine, isoproterenol, and metaproterenol:* Studies with isoetharine, isoproterenol, and metaproterenol have not been done.

Pregnancy—
*All adrenergic bronchodilators—*
Although adequate and well-controlled studies in pregnant women have not been done with inhaled adrenergic bronchodilators, albuterol, bitolterol, fenoterol, isoetharine, isoproterenol, metaproterenol, pirbuterol, procaterol, salmeterol, and terbutaline (but not epinephrine) are used in pregnancy when any potential risk that may be associated with treatment is preferable to the risk of placental hypoxemia from uncontrolled pulmonary disease. Extensive use of adrenergic bronchodilators during pregnancy has provided no evidence that the sympathomimetic class effects seen in animal studies are relevant to human use.

*Albuterol—*
Adequate and well-controlled studies in humans have not been done.
Albuterol has been shown to be teratogenic in mice given doses equivalent to 14 times the human dose. Studies in mice given albuterol subcutaneously at doses comparable to 1.15, 11.5, and 115 times the maximum inhalation dose for a 50-kg human showed cleft palate formation in 0%, 4.5%, and 9.3% of fetuses, respectively. When rabbits were given oral albuterol at doses corresponding to 2315 times the maximum inhalation dose for a 50-kg human, cranioschisis occurred in 37% of their fetuses.
FDA Pregnancy Category C.

*Bitolterol—*
Adequate and well-controlled studies in humans have not been done.
No teratogenic effects were seen in rats and rabbits after administration of oral doses of bitolterol of up to 361 and 557 times the maximal daily human inhalation dose, or in mice after administration of oral doses of bitolterol of up to 188 and 284 times the maximal daily human inhalation doses, for the inhalation solution and the metered-dose inhaler, respectively. When bitolterol was injected subcutaneously into mice at doses of 2, 10, and 20 mg per kg of body weight, the incidence of cleft palate was 5.7%, 3.8%, and 3.3%, respectively.
FDA Pregnancy Category C.

*Epinephrine—*
Adequate and well-controlled studies in humans have not been done. Epinephrine crosses the placenta and, although systemic concentrations are generally low following inhalation therapy, epinephrine usually should be avoided during pregnancy due to its alpha-adrenergic effects; safer and more effective beta$_2$-adrenergic bronchodilators are preferred. The Collaborative Perinatal Project monitored 189 mother-child pairs exposed to subcutaneous epinephrine during the first trimester as well as anytime during pregnancy. An association was found between first trimester use and the incidence of fetal malformations. An association was also found between use anytime during pregnancy and the incidence of inguinal hernia. Interpretation of these data is complicated in that the severity of the mother's asthma may contribute to the effects on the fetus.
Epinephrine has been shown to be teratogenic in rats when given systemically in doses of about 25 times the human dose.
FDA Pregnancy Category C.

*Fenoterol—*
Adequate and well-controlled studies in humans have not been done. Direct blood and tissue studies in humans showed that the levels of fenoterol and its conjugates were 10 to 20 times lower in the fetus than in maternal tissues.
Autoradiographic studies in pregnant rats showed no detectable amounts of fenoterol in the fetus. Direct blood and tissue studies in several animal species showed that levels of fenoterol and its conjugates were 10 to 20 times lower in the fetus than in maternal tissues.
FDA Pregnancy Category B.

*Isoetharine—*
Studies have not been done in humans.
Studies have not been done in animals.
FDA Pregnancy Category C.

*Isoproterenol—*
Adequate and well-controlled studies have not been done in humans.
Studies performed in rats and rabbits at inhaled doses comparable to 15 times the human dose have not shown harm to the fetus.
FDA Pregnancy Category B.

*Metaproterenol—*
Adequate and well-controlled studies in humans have not been done.
Metaproterenol has been shown to be teratogenic and embryocidal in rabbits when given orally in doses comparable to 620 times the human inhalation dose. Effects included skeletal abnormalities and hydrocephalus with bone separation. Studies in mice, rats, and rabbits showed no teratogenic or embryocidal effects at doses corresponding to 310 times the recommended human inhalation dose.
FDA Pregnancy Category C.

*Pirbuterol—*
Adequate and well-controlled studies in humans have not been done.
Studies performed in rats and rabbits given inhaled pirbuterol at doses of up to 12 and 16 times the maximum human inhalation dose, respectively, showed no teratogenic effects.
FDA Pregnancy Category C.

*Procaterol—*
Adequate and well-controlled studies have not been done in humans.
Studies in rabbits and rats given large doses of inhaled procaterol showed no teratogenic or embryocidal effects.

*Salmeterol—*
Adequate and well-controlled studies have not been done in humans.
In rats, maternal exposure to salmeterol at doses of up to approximately 160 times the recommended human clinical dose based on mg per square meter of body surface (mg/m$^2$) produced no significant effects. However, Dutch rabbit fetuses exposed to high concentrations of salmeterol *in utero* developed effects considered to be characteristic of beta-adrenergic stimulation (i.e., precocious eyelid openings, cleft palate, sternebral fusion, limb and paw flexures, and delayed ossification of the frontal cranial bones). No significant effects occurred at 12 times the recommended human clinical dose based on AUC comparisons. In New Zealand rabbits, exposure to oral doses approximately 1600 times the recommended human clinical dose based on mg/m$^2$ produced only delayed ossification of frontal bones.
FDA Pregnancy Category C.

*Terbutaline—*
Adequate and well-controlled studies in humans have not been done.
Studies in rats and mice at doses of up to 1042 times the human dose showed no teratogenic effects.
FDA Pregnancy Category B.

Labor and delivery—Beta-adrenergic agonists have been shown to decrease uterine contractions when administered systemically. This effect is unlikely with inhaled beta-adrenergic bronchodilators.

**Breast-feeding**

It is not known whether albuterol, bitolterol, epinephrine, fenoterol, isoetharine, isoproterenol, metaproterenol, pirbuterol, procaterol, salmeterol, or terbutaline is distributed into the breast milk of humans.
Salmeterol is distributed into the milk of lactating rats in concentrations similar to those in plasma.

**Pediatrics**

Some children up to 5 years old may have difficulty using a metered dose or powder inhaler device correctly; therefore, use of an inhalation solution may be more appropriate. A spacer device is recommended for use with metered dose inhalers.

*Albuterol, bitolterol, epinephrine, isoproterenol, metaproterenol, pirbuterol, procaterol, salmeterol, and terbutaline*—Use of these medications in children has not demonstrated pediatrics-specific problems that would limit their usefulness.

*Fenoterol*—Appropriate studies on the relationship of age to the effects of fenoterol have not been performed in the pediatric population.

*Isoetharine*—Use of isoetharine in children is not recommended.

**Geriatrics**

Although not clearly proven, airway responsiveness to these medications may change with age. Additionally, older patients may also be more sensitive to the side effects of beta$_2$-agonists, including tremor and tachycardia, especially those with preexisting ischemic heart disease.

*Albuterol, bitolterol, epinephrine, fenoterol, isoetharine, isoproterenol, metaproterenol, pirbuterol, procaterol, and terbutaline*—Appropriate studies on the relationship of age to the effects of these agents have not been performed in the geriatric population. However, no geriatric-specific problems have been documented to date.

*Salmeterol*—Clinical studies have been conducted in 241 patients 65 years of age and older. No apparent differences in the efficacy and safety of salmeterol were observed in these patients compared with younger patients.

### Drug interactions and/or related problems
The following drug interactions and/or related problems have been selected on the basis of their potential clinical significance (possible mechanism in parentheses where appropriate)—not necessarily inclusive (» = major clinical significance):

Note: Because adrenergic bronchodilators produce low systemic concentrations following aerosol administration when compared to serum concentrations following systemic administration, drug interactions known to occur with sympathomimetics as a class, especially with those possessing alpha-adrenoceptor activity, are unlikely to occur with use of albuterol, bitolterol, epinephrine, fenoterol, isoetharine, isoproterenol, metaproterenol, pirbuterol, procaterol, salmeterol, or terbutaline at recommended doses.

Combinations containing any of the following medications, depending on the amount present, may also interact with this medication.

» Beta-adrenergic blocking agents, ophthalmic
(ophthalmic beta-adrenergic blocking agents are absorbed systemically via the nasolacrimal duct. Respiratory complications associated with the use of timolol have been reported and include bronchospasm, dyspnea, wheezing, decreased pulmonary function, and respiratory failure; therefore, concurrent use may result in inhibition of the beta-adrenergic effects of the adrenergic bronchodilators and worsening of bronchospasm)

» Beta-adrenergic blocking agents, systemic
(concurrent use with adrenergic bronchodilators may result in mutual inhibition of therapeutic effects; beta-blockade may antagonize the bronchodilating effect of these bronchodilators; although antagonists with beta$_1$-selectivity may be less antagonistic, extreme caution is recommended if these agents are used in patients with bronchospasm because beta-adrenergic blocking agents may induce bronchospasm; use of a nonselective beta-blocking agent also allows for alpha-adrenergic receptor stimulation when epinephrine is administered, which may result in increased vascular resistance when epinephrine aerosol is used in higher-than-recommended doses)

### Laboratory value alterations
The following have been selected on the basis of their potential clinical significance (possible effect in parentheses where appropriate)—not necessarily inclusive (» = major clinical significance):

With physiology/laboratory test values
Electrocardiogram
(transient ventricular premature contractions, atrial arrhythmia, inverted T waves, junctional rhythm, and prolongation of the QTc interval are reported rarely with adrenergic bronchodilators; effects may be more pronounced following nebulization, frequent use of higher doses or an overdose, or with use of fenoterol; arrhythmias may also result from hypoxia or hypokalemia)

Glucose, blood
(concentrations may be increased, possibly due to glycogenolysis; clinically significant changes may be more pronounced following nebulization or with frequent use of higher doses or an overdose)

Potassium, serum
(concentrations may be decreased, possibly through intracellular shunting; the decrease is dose-related, is usually transient, and may not require supplementation; effects may be more pronounced following nebulization, frequent use of higher doses or an overdose, or use of fenoterol)

### Medical considerations/Contraindications
The medical considerations/contraindications included have been selected on the basis of their potential clinical significance (reasons given in parentheses where appropriate)—not necessarily inclusive (» = major clinical significance).

*Risk-benefit should be considered when the following medical problems exist:*

Cardiac arrhythmias or
» Coronary insufficiency
(rarely, inhaled adrenergic bronchodilators, especially epinephrine, may make these conditions worse)

Hypertension, not optimally controlled
(rarely, inhaled epinephrine may make this condition worse)

Hyperthyroidism, not optimally controlled, or
Pheochromocytoma, diagnosed or suspected
(signs or symptoms of excessive beta-adrenergic stimulation are more likely to occur)

» Sensitivity to an adrenergic bronchodilator

» Sensitivity to sulfites contained in some isoetharine, isoproterenol, and racepinephrine solutions for inhalation

### Patient monitoring
The following may be especially important in patient monitoring (other tests may be warranted in some patients, depending on condition; » = major clinical significance):

Pulmonary function monitoring
(objective measures of lung function are essential for diagnosis and for guiding therapeutic decision-making in the treatment of asthma; measurement of forced expiratory airflow, using a spirometer or a peak expiratory flowmeter, is recommended at periodic intervals)

## Side/Adverse Effects
Note: The side effects of aerosolized adrenergic bronchodilators are due primarily to systemic absorption of the medication, which is limited with usual doses. Higher doses or administration via nebulization is more likely to be associated with side effects than are lower doses.

Fatalities have been reported in association with excessive use of inhaled sympathomimetics. The exact cause of death is unknown. Whether the fatalities are associated with disease severity, substandard quality of care, and/or patient noncompliance has not been established.

For side effects more commonly seen with an overdose, see the *Overdose* section of this monograph.

The following side/adverse effects have been selected on the basis of their potential clinical significance (possible signs and symptoms in parentheses where appropriate)—not necessarily inclusive:

### Those indicating need for medical attention
Incidence rare
*Bronchospasm, paradoxical or hypersensitivity-induced* (shortness of breath; troubled breathing; tightness in chest; wheezing); *dermatitis, hypersensitivity-induced* (angioedema [swelling of face, lips, or eyelids]; skin rash; urticaria [hives]); *laryngeal spasm, irritation, or swelling* (feeling of choking)—with salmeterol; *sensitivity reaction to sulfites* (chest pain; dizziness, severe, or feeling faint; flushing or redness of skin, continuing; skin rash, hives, or itching; swelling of face, lips, or eyelids; wheezing or difficulty in breathing)—for isoetharine, isoproterenol, and racepinephrine inhalation solutions containing sulfites

### Those indicating need for medical attention only if they continue or are bothersome
Incidence more frequent
*Fast heartbeat; headache; nervousness; trembling*

Incidence less frequent
*Coughing or other bronchial irritation; dizziness or lightheadedness; dryness or irritation of mouth or throat*

Incidence rare
*Chest discomfort or pain; drowsiness or fatigue* (weakness); *hypokalemia; increase in blood pressure*—with epinephrine; *irregular heartbeat; muscle cramps or twitching; nausea and/or vomiting; restlessness; trouble in sleeping*

### Those not indicating need for medical attention
Incidence more frequent
*Pinkish to red coloration of saliva*—with isoproterenol

Incidence less frequent
*Taste changes*

## Overdose
Although uncommon, fatalities have been reported in association with excessive use of inhaled sympathomimetics. The exact cause of death is unknown. Whether the fatalities are associated with disease severity, substandard quality of care, and/or patient noncompliance has not been established.

For specific information on the agents used in the management of adrenergic bronchodilator overdose, see:
• *Beta-adrenergic Blocking Agents (Systemic)* monograph.

For more information on the management of overdose, **contact a Poison Control Center** (see *Poison Control Center Listing*).

### Clinical effects of overdose
Note: The following effects are more likely to occur following oral or parenteral overdose with an adrenergic bronchodilator; however, they may occur following overdose via inhalation, if sufficient systemic concentrations of medication are achieved.

The following effects have been selected on the basis of their potential clinical significance (possible signs and symptoms in parentheses where appropriate)—not necessarily inclusive:

Acute overdose
More common
*Hyperglycemia; hypokalemia; hypotension* (dizziness or lightheadedness); *lactic acidosis; tachycardia* (fast heartbeat, continuing); *trembling, continuing; vomiting*
Less common
*Agitation; chest pain*—with epinephrine; *headache*—with epinephrine; *hypercalcemia; hypertension*—with epinephrine; *hypophosphatemia; leukocytosis; peripheral vasoconstriction*—with epinephrine; *respiratory alkalosis*
Rare
*Hallucinations*—with nebulized albuterol; *paranoia*—with nebulized albuterol; *seizures; tachyarrhythmias* (fast and irregular heartbeat, continuing)

Chronic overdose
More common
*Hypotension* (dizziness or lightheadedness); *tachycardia* (fast heartbeat, continuing); *trembling, continuing; vomiting*
Less common
*Agitation; chest pain*—with epinephrine; *headache*—with epinephrine; *hypertension*—with epinephrine; *peripheral vasoconstriction*—with epinephrine
Rare
*Seizures; tachyarrhythmias* (fast and irregular heartbeat, continuing)

**Treatment of overdose**
Specific treatment—
Therapy with any adrenergic bronchodilator should be stopped.
For tachyarrhythmias—Administering a cardioselective beta-adrenergic blocking agent, if necessary; however, caution is needed because beta-adrenergic blocking agents can induce bronchospasm.
Monitoring—
Monitoring the patient carefully, especially for cardiovascular status.
Supportive care—
Patients in whom intentional overdose is confirmed or suspected should be referred for psychiatric evaluation.

## Patient Consultation

As an aid to patient consultation, refer to *Advice for the Patient, Bronchodilators, Adrenergic (Inhalation)*.
In providing consultation, consider emphasizing the following selected information (» = major clinical significance):

**Before using this medication**
» Conditions affecting use, especially:
Sensitivity to sympathomimetics or sulfites contained in some isoetharine, isoproterenol, and racepinephrine solutions for inhalation
Pregnancy—Use of epinephrine is generally avoided
Other medications, especially beta-adrenergic blocking agents
Other medical problems, especially cardiovascular disease

**Proper use of this medication**
*For all adrenergic bronchodilators*
» Reading patient instructions carefully before using
» Importance of not using more medication than prescribed
» Proper dosing
Missed dose: If used regularly, using as soon as possible; resuming regular schedule; not doubling doses
» Proper storage
*For salmeterol*
» Importance of not using this medication to treat acute symptoms
» Having a rapid-acting inhaled beta-adrenergic bronchodilator available for symptomatic relief of acute asthma attacks
» Not using more than two times a day or less than 12 hours apart
» Missed dose: If used regularly, using as soon as possible; resuming regular schedule; not doubling doses; using rapid-acting inhaled bronchodilator if symptoms occur before next dose is due
*For epinephrine*
Not self-medicating without a diagnosis of asthma and follow-up by a physician, or unless directed by a physician if previously hospitalized for asthma; if taking a prescription drug for asthma, not using unless told to do so by physician
*For inhalation aerosol dosage form*
Avoiding contact with the eyes
Testing or priming inhaler before using first time if required
Proper administration technique
Technique for using spacer with inhaler
Proper cleaning procedure for inhaler
Saving inhaler, refill canister may be available
*For powder for inhalation dosage form*
Knowing correct administration technique for using inhaler
*For inhalation solution dosage form*
Knowing correct administration technique for using in a nebulizer
Not using if solution is discolored or cloudy
Not mixing with another inhalation solution in nebulizer unless directed

**Precautions while using this medication**
*For all adrenergic bronchodilators*
Regular visits to physician to check progress during therapy
» Checking with physician immediately if difficulty in breathing persists after use of this medication or if condition becomes worse
» For patients also using anti-inflammatory medication, checking with physician before stopping or reducing anti-inflammatory therapy
*For salmeterol*
» Checking with physician if using four or more inhalations per day of a rapid-acting beta-adrenergic bronchodilator for two or more consecutive days or more than one canister (200 inhalations per canister) in an eight-week period
*For albuterol, bitolterol, epinephrine, fenoterol, isoetharine, isoproterenol, metaproterenol, pirbuterol, procaterol, and terbutaline*
» Checking with physician immediately if more inhalations than usual of a rapid-acting beta-adrenergic bronchodilator are needed to relieve an acute attack
» If not using anti-inflammatory medication: checking with physician if using a rapid-acting beta-adrenergic bronchodilator to relieve symptoms more than two times per week
» If using anti-inflammatory medication: checking with physician if using more than one canister per month of a rapid-acting beta-adrenergic bronchodilator to relieve symptoms

**Side/adverse effects**
Signs of potential side effects, especially laryngeal spasm, irritation, or swelling, paradoxical bronchospasm or hypersensitivity

## General Dosing Information

For emergency department and hospital treatment of acute, severe bronchospasm associated with asthma, inhaled short-acting beta$_2$-agonist therapy using the higher dose and administered either as three treatments within the first hour or by continuous nebulization is recommended. Studies have shown that administration of high doses (6 to 12 puffs) of a short-acting beta$_2$-agonist via metered-dose inhaler with a spacer can produce equivalent bronchodilation when compared with nebulizer therapy. For outpatient management of an asthma exacerbation, two to four puffs of a short-acting beta$_2$-adrenergic bronchodilator via metered-dose inhaler every 20 minutes, for up to 1 hour if needed, or a single dose via nebulization is recommended as initial treatment.

The use of a spacer device with many adrenergic bronchodilators may be beneficial, especially for young children and older adults. By reducing the need for proper coordination of timing of inhalation with activation of the inhaler and reducing the velocity and mean diameter of the aerosol particles, a spacer reduces the amount of medication deposited in the upper airways and increases the amount deposited in the lower respiratory tract in patients with poor technique.

For dilution of adrenergic bronchodilator solutions for inhalation, only products that do not contain benzyl alcohol, preferably preservative-free products, should be used.

A metered-dose inhaler (MDI) should be primed before it is used for the first time or if it has not recently been used. The amount of medication in a dose from a MDI product may depend on how much time has elapsed since the preceding dose and the position in which the inhaler has been stored. One study found that the medication content of single sprays of albuterol MDI ranged between 23 and 208% of the label claim. Additionally, this study suggests that initial sprays from a new canister contain higher albuterol content than the final sprays from the same canister. Single, unprimed doses (doses taken 4 hours or more after the last spray) from canisters stored in the upright position and activated after 4 or 16 hours averaged a higher medication content than single, unprimed doses from canisters stored with the valve down. Primed sprays (those sprays that were taken within minutes of a previous spray), whether stored with the valve up or valve down, contained a mean of 92% of labeled medication content of single sprays of albuterol MDI. Specific information about when to prime an inhaler, other than the first time it is used, as well as the number of sprays that should be performed, remains to be defined. For salmeterol, the recommendation is to prime the inhaler if it has not been used for 4 weeks or longer, and that two priming sprays should be performed.

The contents of metered dose inhalers should generally not be floated in water to assess the contents since this method may not reliably predict the amount of medication remaining in the canister. A record should be kept of the number of inhalations used.

It is not clear whether clinically significant tachyphylaxis or tolerance to the bronchodilator effects of rapid-acting beta-adrenergic bronchodilators develops with repeated use. For longer-acting salmeterol, a 12-month study demonstrated that regular use does not lead to a loss of bronchodilatory effect. Decreased bronchoprotection was reported in one 8-week study in which the effects of salmeterol on bronchodilation and on airway hyperresponsiveness to methacholine were studied in a small number of asthmatics. In another study, duration of salmeterol's protective effect against exercise-induced bronchospasm, another potential marker of tolerance, decreased over a 4-week period in some patients. Systemic administration of corticosteroids has been shown to alter beta$_2$-receptor function on lymphocytes to prevent and reverse tolerance; however, the effect of inhaled or systemic corticosteroids on changes in bronchodilator responses in asthmatics is less clear. There is some evidence that inhaled corticosteroids are unable to prevent tolerance to long-acting beta$_2$-agonists.

As a way to protect the stratospheric ozone layer, the manufacture of chlorofluorocarbons (CFCs) is being phased out. The 1987 Montreal Protocol, an international treaty that is enforced in the U.S. by the Clean Air Act, banned CFC use as of January 1, 1996. CFC-containing inhalers have been granted a temporary exemption so that alternative propellants can be developed.

## ALBUTEROL

## Additional Dosing Information
See also *General Dosing Information*.

### Bioequivalenence information
Unless a generic albuterol metered-dose inhaler has proven bioequivalence, one product should not be substituted for another without the concurrence of the prescribing physician. Generic albuterol metered-dose inhalers distributed by Zenith Goldline and Dey Laboratories may be substituted for *Ventolin*. The generic product distributed by Warrick Pharmaceuticals may only be substituted for *Proventil*.

## Inhalation Dosage Forms
Note: The doses and strengths of the available dosage forms are expressed in terms of albuterol (not the sulfate salt).

### ALBUTEROL INHALATION AEROSOL
Note: Unless a generic albuterol metered-dose inhaler has proven bioequivalence, one product should not be substituted for another without the concurrence of the prescribing physician. Generic albuterol metered-dose inhalers distributed by Zenith Goldline and Dey Laboratories may be substituted for *Ventolin*. The generic product distributed by Warrick Pharmaceuticals may only be substituted for *Proventil*.

**Usual adult and adolescent dose**
Bronchodilator—
  Oral inhalation, 2 inhalations (180 or 200 mcg albuterol) every four to six hours. For some patients, 1 inhalation (90 or 100 mcg) every four to six hours may be sufficient.
Bronchospasm, exercise-induced (prophylaxis)—
  Oral inhalation, 2 inhalations (180 or 200 mcg) fifteen minutes prior to exercise.

**Usual pediatric dose**
Bronchodilator—
  Children up to 4 years of age: Dosage has not been established.
  Children 4 years of age and over: See *Usual adult and adolescent dose*.

**Strength(s) usually available**
U.S.—
  90 mcg albuterol per metered spray (Rx) [*Proventil* (dichlorodifluoromethane; trichloromonofluoromethane; oleic acid); *Ventolin* (dichlorodifluoromethane; trichloromonofluoromethane; oleic acid); GENERIC].
Canada—
  100 mcg albuterol per metered spray (Rx) [*Apo-Salvent; Novo-Salmol; Ventolin;* GENERIC].
Note: In Canada, metered dose inhalers are labeled according to the amount of medication delivered from the valve; in the U.S., metered dose inhalers are labeled according to the amount of medication delivered at the mouthpiece or actuator.

**Packaging and storage**
Store below 40 °C (104 °F), preferably between 15 and 30 °C (59 and 86 °F), unless otherwise specified by manufacturer.

**Auxiliary labeling**
• For oral inhalation only.
• Shake well before using.

**Note**
Include patient instructions when dispensing.

### ALBUTEROL SULFATE INHALATION AEROSOL
**Usual adult and adolescent dose**
Bronchodilator—
  Oral inhalation, 2 inhalations (180 mcg albuterol) every four to six hours. For some patients, 1 inhalation (90 mcg) every four hours may be sufficient.

**Usual pediatric dose**
Bronchodilator—
  Children up to 12 years of age: Dosage has not been established.
  Children 12 years of age and over: See *Usual adult and adolescent dose*.

**Strength(s) usually available**
U.S.—
  90 mcg (albuterol) per metered spray [*Proventil HFA* (CFC-free; hydrofluoroalkane-134a [1,1,1,2 tetrafluoroethane]; oleic acid; ethanol)].
Canada—
  Not commercially available.

**Packaging and storage**
Store between 15 and 25 °C (59 and 77 °F).

**Auxiliary labeling**
• For oral inhalation only.
• Shake well before using.

**Note**
Include patient instructions when dispensing.

### ALBUTEROL SULFATE INHALATION SOLUTION
**Usual adult and adolescent dose**
Bronchodilator—
  Oral inhalation, administered by nebulization, 2.5 mg (albuterol), delivered over approximately five to fifteen minutes, repeated every four to six hours.

**Usual pediatric dose**
Bronchodilator—
  Neonates and infants: Oral inhalation, administered by nebulization, 0.05 to 0.15 mg (albuterol) per kg of body weight delivered over approximately five to fifteen minutes, repeated every four to six hours.
  Children up to 12 years of age: Oral inhalation, administered by nebulization, 1.25 to 2.5 mg delivered over approximately five to fifteen minutes, repeated every four to six hours if necessary.
  Children 12 years of age and over: See *Usual adult and adolescent dose*.

**Strength(s) usually available**
U.S.—
  0.83 mg (albuterol) per mL (Rx) [*Airet; Proventil* (benzalkonium chloride); *Ventolin Nebules*; GENERIC].
  5 mg (albuterol) per mL (Rx) [*Proventil* (benzalkonium chloride); *Ventolin* (benzalkonium chloride); GENERIC].
Canada—
  0.5 mg (albuterol) per mL (Rx) [*Ventolin Nebules P.F.*].
  1 mg (albuterol) per mL (Rx) [*Gen-Salbutamol Sterinebs P.F.; Ventolin Nebules P.F.*].
  2 mg (albuterol) per mL (Rx) [*Gen-Salbutamol Sterinebs P.F.; Ventolin Nebules P.F.*].
  5 mg (albuterol) per mL (Rx) [*Apo-Salvent* (benzalkonium chloride); *Ventolin* (benzalkonium chloride); GENERIC].

**Packaging and storage**
Store below 40 °C (104 °F), preferably between 15 and 30 °C (59 and 86 °F), unless otherwise specified by manufacturer.

**Preparation of dosage form**
For preparation of the inhalation solution, diluents containing benzyl alcohol or preservatives other than benzalkonium chloride are not recommended since the safety of these preservatives has not been established for inhalation therapy.
The 0.5-, 0.83-, 1-, and 2-mg-per-mL solutions do not require dilution prior to administration. The 5-mg-per-mL solution is concentrated and must be diluted in 2.5 mL of sterile 0.9% sodium chloride solution prior to administration.

**Stability**
Albuterol inhalation solution is compatible with cromolyn and ipratropium inhalation solutions for up to 1 hour.

**Auxiliary labeling**
For oral inhalation only.

## Note
Include patient instructions when dispensing.

### ALBUTEROL SULFATE POWDER FOR INHALATION

**Usual adult and adolescent dose**
Bronchodilator—
  Oral inhalation, 200 or 400 mcg every four to six hours.
Bronchospasm, exercise-induced (prophylaxis) —
  Oral inhalation, 200 mcg, fifteen minutes before exercise.

**Usual pediatric dose**
Bronchodilator—
  Children up to 4 years of age: Dosage has not been established.
  Children 4 years of age and over: See *Usual adult and adolescent dose*.

**Strength(s) usually available**
U.S.—
  200 mcg per capsule (Rx) [*Ventolin Rotacaps* (lactose)].
Canada—
  200 mcg per blister or capsule (Rx) [*Ventodisk; Ventolin Rotacaps* (lactose)].
  400 mcg per blister or capsule (Rx) [*Ventodisk; Ventolin Rotacaps* (lactose)].

**Packaging and storage**
Store below 40 °C (104 °F), preferably between 15 and 30 °C (59 and 86 °F), in a well-closed container, unless otherwise specified by manufacturer.

**Auxiliary labeling**
• For oral inhalation only.

**Note**
Include patient instructions when dispensing.

Use of albuterol powder for inhalation requires a special device that separates the capsule into halves or pierces the blister and releases the medication.

---

## BITOLTEROL

## Summary of Differences
Pharmacology/pharmacokinetics: Biotransformation—A prodrug hydrolyzed by esterases in tissue and blood to the active compound colterol.

## Inhalation Dosage Forms
Note: Bracketed uses refer to categories of use and/or indications that are not included in U.S. product labeling.

### BITOLTEROL MESYLATE INHALATION AEROSOL

**Usual adult and adolescent dose**
Bronchodilator—
  Oral inhalation, 2 inhalations (740 mcg) every eight hours, or 2 inhalations (740 mcg) administered at least one to three minutes apart, followed by 1 additional inhalation (370 mcg) if needed. Dosage per day should not exceed 2 inhalations (740 mcg) every four hours or 3 inhalations (1.11 mg) every six hours.
[Bronchospasm, exercise-induced (prophylaxis)]—
  Oral inhalation, 2 inhalations (740 mcg) five minutes prior to exercise.

**Usual pediatric dose**
Bronchodilator—
  See *Usual adult and adolescent dose*.
[Bronchospasm, exercise-induced (prophylaxis)]—
  Oral inhalation, 1 or 2 inhalations (370 or 740 mcg) five minutes prior to exercise.

**Strength(s) usually available**
U.S.—
  370 mcg per metered spray (Rx) [*Tornalate* (alcohol 38%; dichlorodifluoromethane; dichlorotetrafluoroethane; saccharin)].
Canada—
  Not commercially available.

**Packaging and storage**
Store between 15 and 30 °C (59 and 86 °F).

**Auxiliary labeling**
• For oral inhalation only.

**Note**
Include patient instructions when dispensing.

### BITOLTEROL MESYLATE INHALATION SOLUTION

**Usual adult and adolescent dose**
Bronchodilator—
  Oral inhalation:
    Continuous flow nebulization—2.5 milligrams (mg) (range, 1.5 to 3.5 mg), diluted and delivered over ten to fifteen minutes, three to four times per day, not less than four hours apart.
    Intermittent flow nebulization—1 milligram (mg) (range, 0.5 to 1.5 mg), diluted and delivered over ten to fifteen minutes, three to four times per day, not less than four hours apart.

**Usual adult and adolescent prescribing limits**
The maximum daily dose should not exceed 8 mg with intermittent flow nebulization or 14 mg with continuous flow nebulization.

**Usual pediatric dose**
  Children up to 12 years of age: Dosage has not been established.
  Children 12 years of age and over: See *Usual adult and adolescent dose*.

**Strength(s) usually available**
U.S.—
  2 mg per mL (Rx) [*Tornalate* (alcohol 25%)].
Canada—
  Not commercially available.

**Packaging and storage**
Store between 15 and 30 °C (59 and 86 °F).

**Preparation of dosage form**
Bitolterol inhalation solution should be diluted to 2 to 4 mL with sterile 0.9% sodium chloride solution.

**Stability**
Bitolterol inhalation solution should not be mixed with other medications, such as cromolyn sodium or acetylcysteine, at clinically recommended doses due to chemical and/or physical incompatibilities.

---

## EPINEPHRINE

## Summary of Differences
Indications:
  Epinephrine and racepinephrine inhalation also indicated in treatment of postintubation and infectious croup.
Pharmacology/pharmacokinetics:
  Epinephrine also has alpha- and beta$_1$-adrenergic receptor action.
  Duration of action: Short-acting.
Pregnancy:
  Not recommended during pregnancy because of alpha-adrenergic agonist activity.
Medical considerations/contraindications:
  May worsen heart conditions or hypertension.

## Inhalation Dosage Forms
Note: The doses and strengths of the available dosage forms are expressed in terms of epinephrine (not the bitartrate or chloride salt).

Effective June 19, 1996, the Food and Drug Administration amended the final monograph for over-the-counter bronchodilator products by removing *pressurized metered-dose aerosol inhaler* dosage forms containing epinephrine and epinephrine bitartrate. Initial introduction of such a product now requires an application for approval of safety and efficacy. Products that are currently marketed contain a chlorofluorocarbon (CFC) propellant and will be phased out when the temporary exemption for CFCs expires.

### EPINEPHRINE INHALATION AEROSOL USP

**Usual adult and adolescent dose**
Bronchodilator—
  Oral inhalation, 1 inhalation (200 to 275 mcg), repeated after at least one minute, if necessary; subsequent dose(s) should not be administered for at least three hours.

**Usual pediatric dose**
Bronchodilator—
  Children up to 4 years of age: Dosage must be individualized by physician.
  Children 4 years of age and over: See *Usual adult and adolescent dose*.

**Strength(s) usually available**
U.S.—
  0.125% (OTC) [GENERIC].
  0.5% (200 mcg per metered spray) (OTC) [GENERIC].
  0.5% (220 mcg per metered spray) (OTC) [*Primatene Mist* (alcohol 34%; fluorocarbons)].

0.5% (250 mcg per metered spray) (OTC) [*Bronkaid Mist* (alcohol 33%; dichlorodifluoromethane; dichlorotetrafluoroethane)].

Canada—
0.5% (275 mcg per metered spray) (OTC) [*Bronkaid Mistometer* (alcohol 33%)].

**Packaging and storage**
Store below 40 °C (104 °F), preferably between 15 and 30 °C (59 and 86 °F), unless otherwise specified by manufacturer.

## EPINEPHRINE INHALATION SOLUTION USP

**Usual adult and adolescent dose**
Bronchodilator—
Oral inhalation, 10 drops administered by hand-bulb nebulizer, 1 to 3 inhalations. Doses should not be repeated more often than every three hours.

**Usual pediatric dose**
Bronchodilator—
Children up to 4 years of age: Dosage must be individualized by physician.
Children 4 years of age and over: See *Usual adult and adolescent dose.*

**Strength(s) usually available**
U.S.—
1% (epinephrine) (OTC) [*Adrenalin Chloride* (benzethonium chloride; sodium bisulfite)].

Canada—
Not commercially available.

Note: The solution intended for oral inhalation is more concentrated than those intended for injection and is not to be given parenterally.

**Packaging and storage**
Store below 40 °C (104 °F), preferably between 15 and 30 °C (59 and 86 °F), unless otherwise specified by manufacturer, in a tight, light-resistant container.

**Stability**
When exposed to air, the solution will turn pinkish to brownish in color because of oxidation. Also, light, heat, alkalies, and certain metals (for example, copper, iron, zinc) may promote deterioration. Do not use if solution is pinkish to brownish in color or contains a precipitate.

**Auxiliary labeling**
• For oral inhalation only.

## EPINEPHRINE BITARTRATE INHALATION AEROSOL USP

**Usual adult and adolescent dose**
Bronchodilator—
Oral inhalation, 1 inhalation (160 mcg epinephrine) repeated after one minute, if necessary; subsequent dose(s) should not be administered for at least three hours.

**Usual pediatric dose**
Bronchodilator—
Children up to 4 years of age: Dosage must be individualized by physician.
Children 4 years of age and over: See *Usual adult and adolescent dose.*

**Strength(s) usually available**
U.S.—
300 mcg (160 mcg [epinephrine]) per metered spray (OTC) [*Asthmahaler Mist* (dichlorodifluoromethane; dichlorotetrafluoroethane; trichloromonofluoromethane); *Bronkaid Suspension Mist*].

Canada—
Not commercially available.

**Packaging and storage**
Store below 40 °C (104 °F), preferably between 15 and 30 °C (59 and 86 °F), unless otherwise specified by manufacturer.

## RACEPINEPHRINE INHALATION SOLUTION USP

**Usual adult and adolescent dose**
Bronchodilator—
Oral inhalation, administered by hand-bulb nebulization, 0.5 mL (approximately 10 drops) to provide 1 to 3 inhalations, repeated after three hours if necessary.
Oral inhalation, administered by jet nebulization, 0.2 to 0.5 mL (approximately 4 to 10 drops) of diluted solution, delivered over approximately fifteen minutes, repeated every three or four hours.

**Usual pediatric dose**
Bronchodilator—
Children up to 4 years of age: Dosage must be individualized by physician.
Children 4 years of age and over: See *Usual adult and adolescent dose.*

Croup—
Oral inhalation, administered by nebulization, 0.05 mL per kg of body weight, diluted to 3 mL with 0.9% sodium chloride solution, delivered over approximately fifteen minutes, repeated not more frequently than every two hours, if needed.

**Usual pediatric prescribing limits**
Croup—
0.5 mL per dose.

**Strength(s) usually available**
U.S.—
2% (OTC) [*Vaponefrin* (sodium metabisulfite; chlorobutanol; benzoic acid; glycerin)].
2.25% (epinephrine) (OTC) [*AsthmaNefrin* (sodium bisulfite; benzoic acid; chlorobutanol); *microNefrin* (sodium bisulfite; potassium metabisulfite; chlorobutanol; benzoic acid; propylene glycol); *Nephron; S-2* (sodium bisulfite; potassium metabisulfite; chlorobutanol; benzoic acid; propylene glycol)].

Canada—
2.25% (epinephrine) (OTC) [*Vaponefrin* (sodium metabisulfite)].

**Packaging and storage**
Store below 40 °C (104 °F), preferably between 15 and 30 °C (59 and 86 °F), unless otherwise specified by manufacturer, in a tight, light-resistant container.

**Preparation of dosage form**
If administered via hand-bulb nebulizer, racepinephrine inhalation solution does not require dilution; however, if administered via jet nebulizer, it should be diluted to a volume of 3 to 5 mL with sterile 0.9% sodium chloride solution.

**Stability**
When exposed to air, the solution will turn pinkish to brownish in color because of oxidation. Also, light, heat, alkalies, and certain metals (for example, copper, iron, zinc) may promote deterioration. Do not use if solution is pinkish to brownish in color or contains a precipitate.

---

*FENOTEROL*

## Inhalation Dosage Forms

### FENOTEROL HYDROBROMIDE INHALATION AEROSOL

**Usual adult and adolescent dose**
Bronchodilator—
Oral inhalation, 2 inhalations (100 or 200 mcg), three to four times a day, if necessary, but not to be administered more often than every four hours. Dosage should not exceed 8 inhalations *of the 100 mcg per metered spray formulation* or 6 inhalations *of the 200 mcg per metered spray* formulation per day.

**Usual pediatric dose**
Bronchodilator—
Children up to 12 years of age: Dosage has not been established.
Children 12 years of age and over: See *Usual adult and adolescent dose.*

**Strength(s) usually available**
U.S.—
Not commercially available.

Canada—
100 mcg per metered spray (Rx) [*Berotec* (monofluorotrichloromethane; dichlorotetrafluoroethane; dichlorodifluoromethane)].
200 mcg per metered spray (Rx) [*Berotec* (monofluorotrichloromethane; dichlorotetrafluoroethane; dichlorodifluoromethane)].

**Packaging and storage**
Store below 40 °C (104 °F), preferably between 15 and 30 °C (59 and 86 °F), unless otherwise specified by manufacturer.

**Auxiliary labeling**
• For oral inhalation only.
• Shake well before using.

**Note**
Include patient instructions when dispensing.

### FENOTEROL HYDROBROMIDE INHALATION SOLUTION

**Usual adult and adolescent dose**
Bronchodilator—
Oral inhalation, administered via nebulization, 0.5 mg to 1 mg (up to 2.5 mg in some cases) of diluted solution, delivered over ten to

fifteen minutes. Dosage may be repeated every six hours, if necessary.

**Usual pediatric dose**
Bronchodilator—
Children up to 12 years of age: Dosage has not been established.
Children 12 years of age and over: See *Usual adult and adolescent dose*.

**Strength(s) usually available**
U.S.—
Not commercially available.
Canada—
1 mg per mL (Rx) [*Berotec* (benzalkonium chloride)].

**Packaging and storage**
Store below 40 °C (104 °F), preferably between 15 and 30 °C (59 and 86 °F), in a well-closed container, unless otherwise specified by manufacturer.

**Preparation of dosage form**
Fenoterol inhalation solution should be diluted to 5 mL with sterile 0.9% sodium chloride solution.

**Auxiliary labeling**
• For oral inhalation only.

## ISOETHARINE

## Summary of Differences
Pharmacology/pharmacokinetics: Duration of action—short-acting.
Precautions: Pediatrics—Use in children not recommended.

## Inhalation Dosage Forms
### ISOETHARINE INHALATION SOLUTION USP

**Usual adult dose**
Bronchodilator—
Oral inhalation, administered via nebulization, 2.5 to 10 mg, delivered over approximately fifteen to twenty minutes, repeated every four hours, if needed.

**Usual pediatric dose**
Use is not recommended.

**Strength(s) usually available**
U.S.—
0.062% (HCl) (Rx) [*Arm-a-Med Isoetharine*].
0.08% (Rx) [*Dey-Lute Isoetharine*].
0.1% (Rx) [*Dey-Lute Isoetharine;* GENERIC].
0.125% (Rx) [*Arm-a-Med Isoetharine;* GENERIC].
0.167% (Rx) [*Arm-a-Med Isoetharine;* GENERIC].
0.17% (Rx) [*Dey-Lute Isoetharine*].
0.2% (Rx) [*Arm-a-Med Isoetharine;* GENERIC].
0.25% (Rx) [*Arm-a-Med Isoetharine; Dey-Lute Isoetharine;* GENERIC].
1% (Rx) [*Beta-2* (sodium bisulfite); *Bronkosol* (acetone sodium bisulfite; glycerin; parabens; sodium chloride; sodium citrate); GENERIC].
Canada—
Not commercially available.

**Packaging and storage**
Store below 40 °C (104 °F), preferably between 15 and 30 °C (59 and 86 °F), unless otherwise specified by manufacturer, in a tight, light-resistant container.

**Preparation of dosage form**
For preparation of the inhalation solution, diluents containing benzyl alcohol or preservatives other than benzalkonium chloride are not recommended since the safety of these preservatives has not been established for inhalation therapy.
The 0.062 to 0.25% solutions do not require dilution prior to administration. The 1% solution is concentrated and must be diluted with 1 to 4 mL of sterile 0.9% sodium chloride solution prior to administration.

**Stability**
Do not use if solution is pinkish or darker than slightly yellow in color or if it contains a precipitate.

**Auxiliary labeling**
• For oral inhalation only.

### ISOETHARINE MESYLATE INHALATION AEROSOL USP

**Usual adult and adolescent dose**
Bronchodilator—
Oral inhalation, 1 or 2 inhalations (340 or 680 mcg) repeated every four hours as needed.

**Usual pediatric dose**
Use is not recommended.

**Strength(s) usually available**
U.S.—
0.61% (340 mcg per metered spray) (Rx) [*Bronkometer;* GENERIC].
Canada—
Not commercially available.

**Packaging and storage**
Store below 40 °C (104 °F), preferably between 15 and 30 °C (59 and 86 °F), unless otherwise specified by manufacturer.

**Auxiliary labeling**
• For oral inhalation only.
**Note:** Include patient instructions when dispensing.

## ISOPROTERENOL

## Summary of Differences
Pharmacology/pharmacokinetics:
Isoproterenol also has beta$_1$-adrenergic receptor activity.
Duration of action: Short-acting.
Side/adverse effects:
Pinkish to red coloration of saliva.

## Inhalation Dosage Forms
### ISOPROTERENOL INHALATION SOLUTION USP

**Usual adult and adolescent dose**
Bronchodilator—
Oral inhalation, administered via nebulization, 2.5 mg diluted, and delivered over approximately ten to twenty minutes, repeated every four hours if needed.

**Usual pediatric dose**
Bronchodilator—
Oral inhalation, administered via nebulization, 0.05 to 0.1 mg per kg up to 1.25 mg diluted, and delivered over approximately ten to twenty minutes, repeated every four hours if needed.

**Strength(s) usually available**
U.S.—
0.25% (2.5 mg per mL) (Rx) [GENERIC].
0.5% (5 mg per mL) (Rx) [*Isuprel* (sodium metabisulfite; chlorobutanol; citric acid; glycerin; sodium chloride); GENERIC (may contain sodium bisulfite)].
1% (10 mg per mL) (Rx) [*Isuprel* (sodium metabisulfite; chlorobutanol; saccharin; sodium chloride; sodium citrate; citric acid)].
Canada—
0.5% (5 mg per mL) (Rx) [*Isuprel* (chlorobutanol)].

**Packaging and storage**
Store below 40 °C (104 °F), preferably between 15 and 30 °C (59 and 86 °F), unless otherwise specified by manfacturer, in a tight, light-resistant container.

**Preparation of dosage form**
Isoproterenol inhalation solution should be diluted with 1.5 to 2 mL of sterile 0.9% sodium chloride solution.

**Stability**
When exposed to air, alkalies, or metals, isoproterenol solutions turn pinkish to brownish in color because of oxidation. Do not use if solution is pinkish to brownish in color or contains a precipitate.

**Auxiliary labeling**
• For oral inhalation only.

### ISOPROTERENOL HYDROCHLORIDE INHALATION AEROSOL USP

**Usual adult and adolescent dose**
Bronchodilator—
Oral inhalation, 1 inhalation (120 to 131 mcg) repeated after two to five minutes if necessary, every three to four hours.

**Usual pediatric dose**
Bronchodilator—
　Children up to 12 years of age: Use is not recommended.
　Children 12 years of age and over: See *Usual adult and adolescent dose*.

**Strength(s) usually available**
U.S.—
　120 mcg per metered spray (Rx) [GENERIC].
　131 mcg per metered spray (Rx) [*Isuprel Mistometer* (alcohol 33%; ascorbic acid; dichlorodifluoromethane; dichlorotetrafluoroethane)].
Canada—
　125 mcg per metered spray (Rx) [*Isuprel Mistometer* (ethyl alcohol; ascorbic acid; inert propellants)].

**Packaging and storage**
Store below 40 °C (104 °F), preferably between 15 and 30 °C (59 and 86 °F), unless otherwise specified by manufacturer.

**Auxiliary labeling**
• For oral inhalation only.
• Shake well before using.

**Note**
Include patient instructions when dispensing.

### ISOPROTERENOL SULFATE INHALATION AEROSOL USP

**Usual adult and adolescent dose**
Bronchodilator—
　Oral inhalation, 1 inhalation (80 mcg) repeated after two to five minutes if necessary, every four to six hours.

**Usual pediatric dose**
Bronchodilator—
　Children up to 12 years of age: Dosage has not been established.
　Children 12 years of age and over: See *Usual adult and adolescent dose*.

**Strength(s) usually available**
U.S.—
　80 mcg per metered spray (Rx) [*Medihaler-Iso* (dichlorodifluoromethane; dichlorotetrafluoroethane; trichloromonofluoromethane; sorbitan trioleate)].
Canada—
　Not commercially available.

**Packaging and storage**
Store below 40 °C (104 °F), preferably between 15 and 30 °C (59 and 86 °F), unless otherwise specified by manufacturer.

**Auxiliary labeling**
• For oral inhalation only.
• Shake well before using.

**Note**
Include patient instructions when dispensing.

---

### METAPROTERENOL

## Summary of Differences
Pharmacology/pharmacokinetics: Has significant beta$_1$-adrenergic activity.

## Inhalation Dosage Forms

### METAPROTERENOL SULFATE INHALATION AEROSOL USP

**Usual adult and adolescent dose**
Bronchodilator—
　Oral inhalation, 2 or 3 inhalations (1.3 to 1.95 mg) every three to four hours, not to exceed 12 inhalations per day.

**Usual pediatric dose**
Bronchodilator—
　Children up to 12 years of age: Oral inhalation, 1 to 3 inhalations (0.65 to 1.95 mg) every three to four hours, not to exceed 12 inhalations per day.
　Children 12 years of age and over: See *Usual adult and adolescent dose*.

**Strength(s) usually available**
U.S.—
　650 mcg per metered spray (Rx) [*Alupent* (dichlorodifluoromethane; dichlorotetrafluoroethane; trichloromonofluoromethane; sorbitan trioleate)].
Canada—
　750 mcg per metered spray (Rx) [*Alupent* (dichlorodifluoromethane; dichlorotetrafluoroethane; trichloromonofluoromethane; sorbitan trioleate)].
Note: In Canada, metered dose inhalers are labeled according to the amount of medication delivered from the valve; in the U.S., metered dose inhalers are labeled according to the amount of medication delivered at the mouthpiece or actuator.

**Packaging and storage**
Store below 40 °C (104 °F), preferably between 15 and 25 °C (59 and 77 °F), unless otherwise specified by manufacturer.

**Auxiliary labeling**
• For oral inhalation only.
• Shake well before using.

**Note**
Include patient instructions when dispensing.

### METAPROTERENOL SULFATE INHALATION SOLUTION USP

**Usual adult and adolescent dose**
Bronchodilator—
　Oral inhalation, administered via nebulization, 15 mg (range 10 to 15 mg), repeated three or four times a day, not more often than every four hours.

**Usual pediatric dose**
Bronchodilator—
　Children up to 6 years of age: Oral inhalation, administered via nebulization, 5 to 15 mg, repeated three or four times a day, not more often than every four hours.
　Children 6 years of age and over: See *Usual adult and adolescent dose*.

**Strength(s) usually available**
U.S.—
　0.4% (Rx) [*Alupent; Arm-a-Med Metaproterenol; Dey-Lute Metaproterenol;* GENERIC].
　0.6% (Rx) [*Alupent; Arm-a-Med Metaproterenol; Dey-Lute Metaproterenol;* GENERIC].
　5% (Rx) [*Alupent* (benzalkonium chloride); GENERIC].
Canada—
　5% (Rx) [*Alupent*].

**Packaging and storage**
Store below 40 °C (104 °F), preferably between 15 and 30 °C (59 and 86 °F), unless otherwise specified by manufacturer, in a tight, light-resistant container.

**Preparation of dosage form**
For preparation of the inhalation solution, diluents containing benzyl alcohol or preservatives other than benzalkonium chloride are not recommended since the safety of these preservatives has not been established for inhalation therapy.
The 0.4% and 0.6% solutions require no dilution prior to administration. The 5% solution is concentrated and must be diluted in approximately 2.5 mL of sterile 0.9% sodium chloride solution prior to administration.

**Stability**
Do not use solution if its color is pinkish or darker than slightly yellow or if it contains a precipitate.
Metaproterenol inhalation solution is compatible with cromolyn inhalation solution for up to 1 hour.

**Auxiliary labeling**
• For oral inhalation only.

---

### PIRBUTEROL

## Inhalation Dosage Forms
Note: Bracketed uses refer to categories of use and/or indications that are not included in U.S. product labeling.
　The doses and strengths of the available dosage forms are expressed in terms of pirbuterol (not the acetate salt).

### PIRBUTEROL ACETATE INHALATION AEROSOL

**Usual adult and adolescent dose**
Bronchodilator—
　Oral inhalation, 1 or 2 inhalations (200 or 400 mcg pirbuterol) every four to six hours, not to exceed a total dose of 12 inhalations (2.4 mg) per day.
[Bronchospasm, exercise-induced (prophylaxis)]—
　Oral inhalation, 2 inhalations (400 mcg pirbuterol) five minutes prior to exercise.

# Bronchodilators, Adrenergic (Inhalation-Local)

**Usual pediatric dose**
Bronchodilator—
   See *Usual adult and adolescent dose*.

**Strength(s) usually available**
U.S.—
   200 mcg (pirbuterol) per metered spray (Rx) [*Maxair* (dichlorodifluoromethane; trichloromonofluoromethane; sorbitan trioleate); *Maxair Autohaler* (dichlorodifluoromethane; trichloromonofluoromethane; sorbitan trioleate)].
Canada—
   250 mcg (pirbuterol) per metered spray (Rx) [*Maxair*].
Note: *Maxair Autohaler* is a breath-activated inhaler, which automatically releases a spray of medicine when the patient inhales.

**Packaging and storage**
Store below 40 °C (104 °F), preferably between 15 and 30 °C (59 and 86 °F), unless otherwise specified by manufacturer.

**Auxiliary labeling**
- For oral inhalation only.
- Shake well before using.

**Note**
Include patient instructions when dispensing.

---

## PROCATEROL

## Inhalation Dosage Forms

### PROCATEROL HYDROCHLORIDE HEMIHYDRATE INHALATION AEROSOL

**Usual adult and adolescent dose**
Bronchodilator—
   Oral inhalation, 1 or 2 inhalations (10 or 20 mcg) three times a day.
Bronchospasm, exercise-induced (prophylaxis)—
   Oral inhalation, 1 or 2 inhalations (10 or 20 mcg) at least fifteen minutes before exertion.

**Usual pediatric dose**
Bronchodilator—
   See *Usual adult and adolescent dose*.

**Strength(s) usually available**
U.S.—
   Not commercially available.
Canada—
   10 mcg per metered spray (Rx) [*Pro-Air* (monofluorotrichloromethane; tetrafluorodichloroethane; difluorodichloromethane)].
Note: Each canister provides at least 200 inhalations.

**Packaging and storage**
Store below 40 °C (104 °F), preferably between 15 and 30 °C (59 and 86 °F), unless otherwise specified by manufacturer.

**Auxiliary labeling**
- For oral inhalation only.
- Shake well before using.

**Note**
Include patient instructions when dispensing.

---

## SALMETEROL

## Summary of Differences

Indications:
   Salmeterol is *not indicated* for the treatment of acute or breakthrough asthma symptoms when rapid bronchodilation is needed because of its slower onset of action compared to shorter-acting adrenergic bronchodilators.
   Salmeterol therapy *should not be initiated* in patients with significantly worsening or acutely deteriorating asthma (rapid worsening over hours to days).
Pharmacology/pharmacokinetics:
   Onset of action—Approximately 10 to 20 minutes.
   Time to peak effect—3 to 4 hours; however, approximately 80% of the maximal increase in forced expiratory volume in 1 second ($FEV_1$) occurs within 1 hour after administration.
   Duration of action—Approximately 12 hours.

## Inhalation Dosage Forms

Note: The doses and strengths of the available dosage forms are expressed in terms of salmeterol (not the xinafoate salt).

### SALMETEROL XINAFOATE INHALATION AEROSOL

**Usual adult and adolescent dose**
Bronchospasm, asthma-associated (prophylaxis)—
   Oral inhalation, 2 inhalations (42 or 50 mcg salmeterol) two times a day, morning and evening, approximately twelve hours apart.
Bronchospasm, exercise-induced (prophylaxis)[1]—
   Oral inhalation, 2 inhalations (42 mcg salmeterol) at least thirty to sixty minutes before exercise.
Note: Patients receiving chronic therapy should not use additional salmeterol for prevention of exercise-induced bronchospasm. Patients using salmeterol for exercise-induced bronchospasm should not use additional doses for twelve hours after each prophylactic administration.

**Usual pediatric dose**
Bronchospasm, asthma-associated (prophylaxis)—
Bronchospasm, exercise-induced (prophylaxis)—
   Children up to 12 years of age: Dosage has not been established.
   Children 12 years of age and over: See *Usual adult and adolescent dose*.

**Strength(s) usually available**
U.S.—
   21 mcg (salmeterol) per metered spray (Rx) [*Serevent* (dichlorodifluoromethane; trichlorofluoromethane)].
Canada—
   25 mcg (salmeterol) per metered spray (Rx) [*Serevent* (dichlorodifluoromethane; trichlorofluoromethane)].
Note: In Canada, metered dose inhalers are labeled according to the amount of salmeterol delivered at the valve; in the U.S., metered dose inhalers are labeled according to the amount of salmeterol delivered at the mouthpiece or actuator.

**Packaging and storage**
Store below 40 °C (104 °F), preferably between 2 and 30 °C (36 and 86 °F).

**Auxiliary labeling**
- For oral inhalation only.
- Shake well before using.

**Note**
Include patient instructions when dispensing.

### SALMETEROL XINAFOATE POWDER FOR INHALATION

**Usual adult and adolescent dose**
Bronchospasm, asthma-associated (prophylaxis)—
   Oral inhalation, the contents of one blister (50 mcg salmeterol) two times a day.

**Usual pediatric dose**
Bronchospasm, asthma-associated (prophylaxis)—
   Children up to 12 years of age: Dosage has not been established.
   Children 12 years of age and over: See *Usual adult and adolescent dose*.

**Strength(s) usually available**
U.S.—
   Not commercially available.
Canada—
   50 mcg (salmeterol) per blister (Rx) [*Serevent*].

**Packaging and storage**
Store below 40 °C (104 °F), preferably between 15 and 30 °C (59 and 86 °F), unless otherwise specified by manufacturer.

**Auxiliary labeling**
- For oral inhalation only.

**Note**
Use of salmeterol powder for inhalation requires a special device that pierces the blister and releases the medication. Include patient instructions when dispensing.

[1]Not included in Canadian product labeling.

---

## TERBUTALINE

## Inhalation Dosage Forms

Note: Bracketed uses refer to categories of use and/or indications that are not included in U.S. product labeling.

## TERBUTALINE SULFATE INHALATION AEROSOL USP

**Usual adult and adolescent dose**
Bronchodilator—
  Oral inhalation, 2 inhalations (400 mcg) every four to six hours.
  Note: In Canada, the recommended dose from the *breath-actuated dry powder inhaler* is 1 inhalation (500 mcg), repeated after five minutes if needed. Doses should not exceed 6 inhalations per day.
[Bronchospasm, exercise-induced (prophylaxis)][1]—
  Oral inhalation, 2 inhalations (400 mcg) five to fifteen minutes prior to exercise.

**Usual pediatric dose**
Bronchodilator—
  See *Usual adult and adolescent dose*.

**Strength(s) usually available**
U.S.—
  200 mcg per metered spray (Rx) [*Brethaire* (dichlorodifluoromethane; dichlorotetrafluoroethane; trichloromonofluoromethane)].
Canada—
  500 mcg per metered spray (Rx) [*Bricanyl Turbuhaler*].
  Note: *Bricanyl Turbuhaler* is a *breath-actuated dry powder inhaler*, which automatically releases a dose of terbutaline, without carrier powders or propellants, when the patient inhales.

**Packaging and storage**
Store below 40 °C (104 °F), preferably between 15 and 30 °C (59 and 86 °F), unless otherwise specified by manufacturer.

**Auxiliary labeling**
- For oral inhalation only.
- Shake well before using.

**Note**
Include patient instructions when dispensing.

[1]Not included in Canadian product labeling.

### Selected Bibliography
Nelson H. Beta-adrenergic bronchodilators. N Engl J Med 1995; 333: 499-506.
Jenne JW, Tashkin DP. Beta-adrenergic agonists. In: Weiss EB, Stein M, editors. Bronchial asthma—mechanisms and therapeutics. Boston: Little, Brown and Co; 1993. p. 746-83.
National Asthma Education and Prevention Program. Expert panel report II. Guidelines for the diagnosis and management of asthma. National Heart, Lung, and Blood Institute, Feb 1997. Available from: http://www.nhlbi.nih.gov/nhlbi/lung/asthma/prof/asthgdln.htm.

Revised: 08/01/97

# BRONCHODILATORS, ADRENERGIC   Systemic

This monograph includes information on the following: 1) Albuterol; 2) Ephedrine; 3) Epinephrine; 4) Ethylnorepinephrine†; 5) Fenoterol*; 6) Isoproterenol; 7) Metaproterenol; 8) Terbutaline.

INN: Albuterol—Salbutamol

VA CLASSIFICATION (Primary/Secondary):
  Albuterol
    Oral— RE103
    Parenteral—RE900
  Ephedrine
    Oral—RE103/ RE200; CN809; DE890
    Parenteral—AU100/RE900; DE890
  Epinephrine
    Parenteral—AU100/RE900; CN205; OP900; DE900; RE900
  Ethylnorepinephrine
    Parenteral—RE900
  Fenoterol
    Oral—RE103
  Isoproterenol
    Oral—AU100/RE103
    Parenteral—AU100/RE900
  Metaproterenol
    Oral—RE103
  Terbutaline
    Oral—RE103/GU900
    Parenteral—AU100/RE900; GU900

Commonly used brand name(s): *Adrenalin*[3]; *Adrenalin Chloride Solution*[3]; *Alupent*[7]; *Ana-Guard*[3]; *Berotec*[5]; *Brethine*[8]; *Bricanyl*[8]; *Bronkephrine*[4]; *EpiPen Auto-Injector*[3]; *EpiPen Jr. Auto-Injector*[3]; *Isuprel*[6]; *Isuprel Glossets*[6]; *Metaprel*[7]; *Metaprel*[7]; *Novo-Salmol*[1]; *Prometa*[7]; *Proventil*[1]; *Proventil Repetabs*[1]; *Sus-Phrine*[3]; *Ventolin*[1]; *Volmax*[1].

Other commonly used names are:
  Orciprenaline [Metaproterenol]
  Salbutamol [Albuterol]
  Note: For a listing of dosage forms and brand names by country availability, see *Dosage Forms* section(s).

*Not commercially available in U.S.
†Not commercially available in Canada.

## Category
Bronchodilator—Albuterol; Ephedrine; Epinephrine; Ethylnorepinephrine; Fenoterol; Isoproterenol; Metaproterenol; Terbutaline.
Anesthetic (local) adjunct—Epinephrine Injection.
Antiallergic (systemic)—Epinephrine Injection.
Surgical aid (antihemorrhagic; decongestant; mydriatic)—Epinephrine Injection.
Antihemorrhagic (topical)—Epinephrine Injection.
Decongestant, nasal (systemic)—Ephedrine (Oral).
Central nervous system (CNS) stimulant—Ephedrine (Oral).
Labor (premature) inhibitor—Terbutaline (Oral and Parenteral).
Urticaria therapy adjunct—Ephedrine.
Priapism reversal agent—Epinephrine Injection.

## Indications
Note: Bracketed information in the *Indications* section refers to uses that are not included in U.S. product labeling.

**Accepted**
Asthma, bronchial (treatment);
Bronchitis (treatment);
Bronchospasm (treatment);
Emphysema, pulmonary (treatment);
Bronchiectasis (treatment); or
Pulmonary disease, obstructive, other (treatment)—Albuterol, epinephrine, ethylnorepinephrine, fenoterol, metaproterenol, and terbutaline are indicated for the symptomatic treatment of bronchial asthma. These medications are also indicated for the treatment of reversible bronchospasm associated with bronchitis, pulmonary emphysema, bronchiectasis, and other obstructive pulmonary diseases.

Also, ephedrine may be indicated for the symptomatic treatment of bronchial asthma and reversible bronchospasm associated with other obstructive pulmonary diseases; however, agents with less beta-1-adrenergic effects and more selective beta-2-adrenergic effects are generally preferred. In the treatment of acute bronchospasm, parenteral ephedrine is usually less effective than epinephrine.

Isoproterenol sublingual tablets may be used for the treatment of bronchial asthma and in the management of obstructive pulmonary disease, but isoproterenol inhalation is preferred because absorption after sublingual administration may be erratic and unpredictable.

Bronchospasm, during anesthesia (treatment)—Parenteral isoproterenol may be indicated in the management of bronchospasm during anesthesia. [Parenteral epinephrine and terbutaline may also be useful in the management of bronchospasm during anesthesia.]

Allergic reactions, drug-induced (treatment);
Anaphylactic reactions (treatment);
Angioedema (treatment);
Bites or stings, insect (treatment);
Laryngeal edema, acute noninfectious (treatment); or
Transfusion reactions, urticarial (treatment)—Epinephrine injection is indicated in the emergency treatment of severe allergic reactions to drugs, foods, sera, insect stings, or other allergens. It relieves symptoms such as bronchospasm, urticaria, pruritus, hives, angioedema, and swelling of lips, eyelids, tongue, and nasal mucosa. Epinephrine injection is also used in the treatment of acute noninfectious laryngeal edema.

Anesthesia, local, adjunct—Epinephrine injection is indicated for concurrent use with some local anesthetics to decrease the rate of vascular absorption and thereby localize anesthesia, prolong the duration of action, and decrease the risk of toxicity due to the local anesthetic. Epinephrine injection should be used cautiously and in carefully circumscribed quantities, if at all, with local anesthetics for anesthetizing areas with end arteries (such as the fingers, toes, or penis) or otherwise compromised blood supply because ischemia leading to gangrene may result.

Hemorrhage, superficial, in ocular surgery (treatment);
Congestion, conjunctival, during surgery (treatment);
Mydriasis, during surgery; or
Hypertension, ocular, during surgery (treatment)—Epinephrine may be injected intracamerally or subconjunctivally to control hemorrhage, produce conjunctival decongestion and mydriasis, and reduce intraocular pressure during ocular surgery.

Hemorrhage, superficial (treatment)—Epinephrine injection may be applied topically to control superficial bleeding from arterioles and capillaries in the skin, mucous membranes, or other tissues. However, only small doses should be used because topically applied epinephrine can be systemically absorbed.

Congestion, nasal (treatment); or
Congestion, sinus (treatment)—Oral ephedrine may be indicated for the local treatment of nasal congestion in acute coryza, vasomotor rhinitis, acute sinusitis, and hay fever. It may also be used in the treatment of sinus congestion.

Narcolepsy (treatment); or
Depression, mental (treatment)—Oral ephedrine may be indicated as a CNS stimulant in the treatment of narcolepsy and depressive states.

Status asthmaticus (treatment)—Parenteral albuterol is used for the treatment of status asthmaticus.

[Labor, premature (prophylaxis and treatment)][1]—Terbutaline (oral and parenteral) is used for prophylaxis and treatment of preterm labor.

[Urticaria (treatment adjunct)][1]—Ephedrine may be useful as an adjunct in the treatment of acute and chronic urticaria.

[Hemorrhage, gingival (treatment adjunct)][1]; or
[Hemorrhage, pulpal (treatment)][1]—Epinephrine injection is used topically as an adjunct in the treatment of gingival hemorrhage. It is also used in the treatment of pulpal hemorrhage.

[Priapism (treatment)][1]—Epinephrine injection, administered intracavernosally, has been reported to be effective in the treatment of priapism resulting from use of intracavernosal papaverine or phentolamine or from other causes. However, epinephrine should be used with caution because hypertension and ischemic electrocardiographic changes can occur.

**Unaccepted**
Oral ephedrine has been used in the treatment of enuresis and myasthenia gravis but it has been replaced by more effective agents.

[1]Not included in Canadian product labeling.

## Pharmacology/Pharmacokinetics

See *Table 1*, page 660.

**Physicochemical characteristics**
Molecular weight—
  Albuterol: 239.31.
  Albuterol sulfate: 576.70.
  Ephedrine sulfate: 428.54.
  Epinephrine: 183.21.
  Ethylnorepinephrine hydrochloride: 233.69.
  Fenoterol hydrobromide: 384.3.
  Isoproterenol hydrochloride: 247.72.
  Metaproterenol sulfate: 520.59.
  Terbutaline sulfate: 548.65.

**Mechanism of action/Effect**
Bronchodilator—
  Adrenergic bronchodilators act by stimulating beta-2-adrenergic receptors in the lungs to relax bronchial smooth muscle, thereby relieving bronchospasm, increasing vital capacity, decreasing residual volume, and reducing airway resistance. This action is believed to result from increased production of cyclic adenosine 3′,5′-monophosphate (cyclic 3′,5′-AMP or c-AMP) caused by activation of the enzyme adenyl cyclase, the enzyme that catalyzes the conversion of adenosine triphosphate (ATP) to c-AMP. Increased c-AMP concentrations, in addition to relaxing bronchial smooth muscle, inhibit release of mediators of immediate hypersensitivity from cells, especially from mast cells. Also, epinephrine acts by stimulating alpha-adrenergic receptors to constrict bronchial arterioles.
  Epinephrine also inhibits antigen-induced release of histamine and the slow-reacting substance of anaphylaxis and directly antagonizes histamine-induced bronchiolar constriction, vasodilation, and edema. Ephedrine and metaproterenol may also inhibit antigen-induced release of histamine, and isoproterenol may inhibit antigen-induced release of histamine and the slow-reacting substance of anaphylaxis.

Anesthetic (local) adjunct—
  Epinephrine acts on alpha-adrenergic receptors in the skin, mucous membranes, and viscera to produce vasoconstriction. This action decreases the rate of vascular absorption of the local anesthetic used with epinephrine, thereby localizing anesthesia, prolonging the duration of action, and decreasing the risk of toxicity due to the anesthetic.

Surgical aid (antihemorrhagic; decongestant; mydriatic)—
  Epinephrine acts on alpha-adrenergic receptors in the conjunctiva to produce vasoconstriction and hemostasis in bleeding from small vessels; also, conjunctival congestion is decreased. Epinephrine contracts the dilator muscle of the pupil by acting on alpha-adrenergic receptors, resulting in dilation of the pupil (mydriasis).

Antihemorrhagic (topical)—
  Epinephrine acts on alpha-adrenergic receptors in the skin, mucous membranes, and viscera to produce vasoconstriction and hemostasis in bleeding from small vessels.

Decongestant, nasal (systemic)—
  Ephedrine acts on alpha-adrenergic receptors of blood vessels in the nasal mucosa, producing vasoconstriction, which may result in nasal decongestion.

CNS stimulant—
  Ephedrine stimulates the cerebral cortex and subcortical centers to produce its effects in narcolepsy and depressive states.

Labor (premature) inhibitor—
  Terbutaline acts primarily as a beta-adrenergic stimulant to relax the uterine muscle, thereby inhibiting uterine contractions.

Urticaria therapy adjunct—
  Ephedrine acts on alpha-adrenergic receptors of blood vessels in the skin to produce vasoconstriction, which may help to reverse cutaneous vasodilation and thereby reduce the increased vascular permeability that results in localized edema in urticaria.

**Other actions/effects**
Other adrenergic effects include alpha-receptor–mediated contraction of gastrointestinal and urinary sphincters; beta-1-receptor–mediated lipolysis; and beta-2-receptor–mediated decrease in gastrointestinal tone, and increases in uterine relaxation, renin secretion, hepatic glycogenolysis/gluconeogenesis, and pancreatic beta cell secretion.

**Absorption**
Albuterol—
  Oral: Rapidly and well absorbed from the gastrointestinal tract.
Ephedrine—
  Rapidly absorbed after oral, intramuscular, or subcutaneous administration.
Epinephrine—
  Intramuscular or subcutaneous: Well absorbed. Both rapid and prolonged following administration of the aqueous suspension.
Isoproterenol—
  Parenteral: Rapidly absorbed.
  Sublingual: Variable and may be unreliable.
Metaproterenol—
  Oral: About 40% of an oral metaproterenol dose absorbed from gastrointestinal tract.
Terbutaline—
  Oral: About 30 to 70% of an oral dose absorbed from gastrointestinal tract. Food reduces the bioavailability of terbutaline by one-third.
  Subcutaneous: Well absorbed.

## Precautions to Consider

**Carcinogenicity/Tumorigenicity**
*Albuterol*—In one 2-year study in rats, albuterol given orally in doses corresponding to 3, 16, and 78 times the maximum human oral dose caused a significant dose-related increase in the incidence of benign leiomyomas of the mesovarium. In another study, this effect was blocked by the coadministration of propranolol. Studies have shown that other beta agonists also induce mesovarium tumors in rats. An 18-month study with albuterol in mice and a lifetime study in hamsters showed no evidence of tumorigenicity. The relevance of these findings to humans is not known.

*Epinephrine, ethylnorepinephrine, isoproterenol, and metaproterenol*—Long-term studies to evaluate carcinogenic potential in animals have not been done. There is no evidence from human data that epinephrine, ethylnorepinephrine, isoproterenol, or metaproterenol may be carcinogenic.

*Terbutaline*—An 18-month carcinogenicity study in NMRI strain mice showed that terbutaline administered orally in doses of 5, 50, and 200 mg per kg (500, 5000, and 20,000 times the clinical subcutaneous dose, respectively) caused no drug-related tumorigenicity. A 2-year carcinogenesis bioassay of terbutaline at oral doses of 50, 500, 1000, and 2000 mg per kg (corresponding to 167, 1667, 3333, and 6667 times the recommended daily adult oral dose, respectively) in Sprague-Dawley rats showed drug-related changes in the female genital system; female rats showed drug-related increases in leiomyomas of the mesovarium, which were significant at doses of 500, 1000, and 2000 mg per kg; the incidence of ovarian cysts was increased significantly at all dose levels except at 2000 mg per kg; and hyperplasia of the mesovarium was increased significantly at 500 and 2000 mg per kg. However, in a 21-month study in mice, terbutaline at oral doses of 5, 50, and 200 mg per kg (corresponding to 17, 167, and 667 times the recommended daily adult oral dose, respectively) showed no evidence of carcinogenicity.

**Mutagenicity**

*Albuterol*—Studies with albuterol have not shown any evidence of mutagenesis.

*Epinephrine, ethylnorepinephrine, isoproterenol, metaproterenol, and terbutaline*—Long-term mutagenicity studies in animals have not been done. There is no evidence from human data that epinephrine, ethylnorepinephrine, isoproterenol, metaproterenol, or terbutaline may be mutagenic.

**Pregnancy/Reproduction**

Fertility—*Albuterol*: Animal (rat) reproduction studies with albuterol have shown no evidence of impaired fertility.

*Terbutaline*: A reproduction study in rats with oral terbutaline at doses up to 50 mg per kg of body weight (mg/kg) (corresponding to 167 times the human oral dose) showed no adverse effects on fertility.

Pregnancy—
  *Albuterol*—
    Adequate and well-controlled studies in humans have not been done.
    Some studies in CD-1 mice have shown that albuterol causes cleft palate formation when given subcutaneously in doses of 0.25 mg per kg (corresponding to 0.4 times the maximum human oral dose) and 2.5 mg per kg. Another study in CD-1 mice has shown that albuterol causes malformations when given orally in doses of 25 and 50 mg per kg (corresponding to at least 32 times the maximum human oral daily dose). Also, a reproduction study in Stride Dutch rabbits has shown that albuterol causes cranioschisis when given in doses of 50 mg per kg (corresponding to 78 times the maximum human oral dose).
    FDA Pregnancy Category C.
  *Ephedrine*—
    Studies have not been done in humans.
    Studies have not been done in animals.
    FDA Pregnancy Category C.
  *Epinephrine*—
    Epinephrine crosses the placenta. Adequate and well-controlled studies in humans have not been done. Use of epinephrine during pregnancy may cause anoxia in the fetus.
    Studies in animals have shown that epinephrine causes teratogenic effects in rats when given in doses about 25 times the human dose.
    FDA Pregnancy Category C.
  *Ethylnorepinephrine and isoproterenol*—
    Studies have not been done in humans.
    Studies have not been done in animals.
    FDA Pregnancy Category C.
  *Fenoterol*—
    Problems in humans have not been documented.
  *Metaproterenol*—
    Adequate and well-controlled studies in humans have not been done.
    Studies in rabbits have shown that metaproterenol was teratogenic (effects included skeletal abnormalities and hydrocephalus with bone separation) and embryocidal when given orally in doses 62 times the human oral dose. Reproduction studies in mice, rats, and rabbits did not show metaproterenol to be teratogenic or embryocidal when given orally in doses up to 50 mg per kg (31 times the human oral dose). Studies in rabbits have shown metaproterenol to cause fetal loss and teratogenic effects when administered at and above oral doses of 50 and 100 mg/kg, respectively.
    FDA Pregnancy Category C.
  *Terbutaline*—
    Terbutaline crosses the placenta. Studies in humans have not been done. Parenteral administration of terbutaline during pregnancy has been reported to cause fetal tachycardia.
    Studies in animals (mice and rats) have not shown that terbutaline, at doses up to 1000 times the human dose, causes adverse effects on the fetus. Also, reproduction studies in mice with terbutaline at doses up to 1.1 mg/kg, administered subcutaneously (corresponding to 4 times the human oral dose and 110 times the human subcutaneous dose) and in rats and rabbits with terbutaline at doses up to 50 mg/kg orally (corresponding to 167 times the human oral dose and 5000 times the human subcutaneous dose) have shown no adverse effects on the fetus.
    FDA Pregnancy Category B.

Labor—*Albuterol*: Albuterol administered intravenously or orally reportedly inhibits uterine contractions. Although albuterol administered orally has been reported to delay preterm labor, there are no well-controlled studies that show it will stop preterm labor or prevent labor at term.

*Ephedrine*: When ephedrine is administered just prior to or during labor, its effect on the neonate or on the child's later growth and development is not known.

*Epinephrine*: Epinephrine is not recommended for use during labor since its action in relaxing the muscles of the uterus may delay the second stage. Also, when administered in high dosage sufficient to reduce uterine contractions, epinephrine may cause prolonged uterine atony with hemorrhage.

*Terbutaline*: Terbutaline inhibits uterine activity during the second and third trimesters of pregnancy and may inhibit labor. When administered during labor, terbutaline has been reported to cause serious adverse reactions such as transient hypokalemia, pulmonary edema, and hypoglycemia in the mother and hypoglycemia in neonates of mothers treated with parenteral terbutaline.

Delivery—*Ephedrine and epinephrine*: Parenteral administration of ephedrine or epinephrine to maintain blood pressure during spinal anesthesia for delivery can cause acceleration of the fetal heart rate and should not be used when maternal blood pressure exceeds 130/80.

**Breast-feeding**

*Albuterol*—Although it is not known whether albuterol is distributed into breast milk, problems in humans have not been documented. However, some animal studies have shown albuterol to be potentially tumorigenic.

*Ethylnorepinephrine, isoproterenol, and metaproterenol*—Although it is not known whether ethylnorepinephrine, isoproterenol, or metaproterenol is distributed into breast milk, problems in humans have not been documented.

*Ephedrine*—Ephedrine is distributed into breast milk. Use by nursing mothers is not recommended because of the higher than usual risks for infants.

*Epinephrine*—Epinephrine is distributed into breast milk; use by nursing mothers may cause serious adverse reactions in the infant.

*Fenoterol*—Problems in humans have not been documented.

*Terbutaline*—Problems in humans have not been documented. However, terbutaline is distributed into breast milk and some animal studies have shown this medication to be potentially tumorigenic.

**Pediatrics**

*Albuterol, ethylnorepinephrine, fenoterol, isoproterenol, metaproterenol, and terbutaline*—Appropriate studies on the relationship of age to the effects of adrenergic bronchodilators have not been performed in the pediatric population. However, no pediatrics-specific problems have been documented to date.

*Ephedrine*—Caution should be used in infants because of the higher than usual risks with the use of ephedrine in these patients.

*Epinephrine*—Epinephrine should be used with caution in infants and children since syncope has occurred following administration of epinephrine to asthmatic children.

**Geriatrics**

*Albuterol, epinephrine, ethylnorepinephrine, fenoterol, isoproterenol, metaproterenol, and terbutaline*—No information is available on the relationship of age to the effects of these medicines in geriatric patients.

*Ephedrine*—Although appropriate studies on the relationship of age to the effects of ephedrine have not been performed in the geriatric population, no geriatrics-specific problems have been documented to date. However, elderly patients are more likely to have age-related prostatic hypertrophy and caution should be used in patients receiving ephedrine.

**Dental**

*Epinephrine*—Epinephrine is used in gingival retraction cords. Systemic absorption of epinephrine can occur from application of retraction cords, especially to abraded surfaces. Epinephrine retraction cords should be used with caution in patients with cardiovascular problems, since the amount of epinephrine absorbed systemically cannot be predicted.

**Drug interactions and/or related problems**

The following drug interactions and/or related problems have been selected on the basis of their potential clinical significance (possible mechanism

in parentheses where appropriate)—not necessarily inclusive (» = major clinical significance):
See *Table 2*, page 661.

**Laboratory value alterations**
The following have been selected on the basis of their potential clinical significance (possible effect in parentheses where appropriate)—not necessarily inclusive (» = major clinical significance):

With physiology/laboratory test values
*For all adrenergic bronchodilators*
   Potassium concentrations, serum
      (may be decreased, possibly through intracellular shunting, when beta-agonists are given intravenously or in higher-than-recommended doses; decrease is usually transient, not requiring supplementation)
*For epinephrine*
   Blood glucose concentrations and
   Lactic acid concentrations, serum
      (may be increased)

**Medical considerations/Contraindications**
The medical considerations/contraindications included have been selected on the basis of their potential clinical significance (reasons given in parentheses where appropriate)—not necessarily inclusive (» = major clinical significance).

Note: A blank space usually signifies lack of information; it is not necessarily an indication that a given medical problem is of no concern. However, the pharmacologic similarity of these agents may suggest that if caution is required in particular medical problems for one agent, then it may be required for the others as well.
See *Table 3*, page 665.

## Side/Adverse Effects
Note: Hypokalemia may be induced by higher-than-recommended doses of beta-agonists, especially in those patients receiving digitalis glycosides or diuretics or who are prone to cardiac dysrhythmias.

Parenteral albuterol may induce reversible metabolic changes, including hyperglycemia and hypokalemia, which are more pronounced during intravenous infusion.

If high arterial blood pressure is inadvertently induced by parenteral epinephrine, it may result in angina pectoris, aortic rupture, or cerebral hemorrhage.
See *Table 4*, page 666.

## Overdose
**Treatment of overdose**
Recommended treatment consists of the following:
*For all adrenergic bronchodilators*
   • Reducing dosage or discontinuing medication.
   • Supportive therapy.
*For albuterol, ethylnorepinephrine, fenoterol, and metaproterenol*
   • For oral overdose, performing gastric lavage.
   • Administering a cardioselective beta-adrenergic blocker (e.g., acebutolol, atenolol, metoprolol), if necessary for cardiac arrhythmias; however, the beta-adrenergic blocker should be used with caution because it could induce severe bronchospasm or an asthmatic attack.
*For ephedrine*
   • Protecting patient's airway and supporting ventilation and perfusion.
   • Monitoring and maintaining, within acceptable limits, patient's vital signs, blood gases, and serum electrolytes. Also, monitoring electrocardiogram continuously.
   • In alert patients, removing ephedrine from the stomach by inducing emesis with ipecac, followed by activated charcoal (as long as ileus is not present); in depressed or hyperactive patients, removing ephedrine by airway-protected gastric lavage.
   • For supraventricular or ventricular tachycardias, administering a beta-adrenergic blocker, such as propranolol, by slow intravenous administration if necessary to control cardiac arrhythmias; however, in asthmatic patients, a cardioselective beta-adrenergic blocker (e.g., acebutolol, atenolol, metoprolol) may be more appropriate. The beta-blocker should be used with caution in asthmatic patients because it could induce severe bronchospasm or an asthmatic attack.
   • For marked hypertension, administering nitroprusside or phentolamine infusion, if necessary.
   • For "true" hypotension, administration of intravenous fluids, elevation of legs, or administration of inotropic vasopressors, such as norepinephrine, should be considered.
   • To control convulsions, administering diazepam. For refractory seizures, general anesthesia with thiopental or halothane and paralysis with a neuromuscular blocking agent may be necessary.
   • Controlling pyrexia by cool applications and by slow intravenous administration of 1 mg of dexamethasone per kg of body weight.
*For epinephrine*
   • Treatment primarily supportive since epinephrine is rapidly inactivated in the body.
   • For anxiety, administering sedatives.
   • To counteract pressor effects, administering rapidly acting vasodilators or alpha-adrenergic blockers, if necessary; however, if prolonged hypotension follows such measures, it may be necessary to administer another pressor agent such as norepinephrine.
   • For epinephrine-induced pulmonary edema that interferes with respiration, administering a rapidly acting alpha-adrenergic blocker, such as phentolamine, and/or intermittent positive-pressure respiration.
   • For arrhythmias, administering a beta-adrenergic blocker, such as propranolol; however, in asthmatic patients, a cardioselective beta-adrenergic blocker (e.g., acebutolol, atenolol, metoprolol) may be more appropriate. The beta-blocker should be used with caution in asthmatic patients because it could induce severe bronchospasm or an asthmatic attack.
*For isoproterenol*
   • For CNS stimulation, administering sedatives, such as barbiturates.
   • For tachycardia and arrhythmias induced by isoproterenol, administering a beta-adrenergic blocker, such as propranolol; however, in asthmatic patients, a cardioselective beta-adrenergic blocker (e.g., acebutolol, atenolol, metoprolol) may be more appropriate. The beta-blocker should be used with caution in asthmatic patients because it could induce severe bronchospasm or an asthmatic attack.
*For terbutaline*
   • In the alert patient who has taken excessive oral terbutaline, inducing emesis followed by gastric lavage.
   • In the unconscious patient, performing gastric lavage after the airway is secured with a cuffed endotracheal tube; not inducing emesis.
   • Instilling activated charcoal slurry to help reduce absorption of terbutaline.
   • Maintaining an adequate respiratory exchange.
   • Providing cardiac and respiratory support as needed.
   • Monitoring patient until symptom-free.

## Patient Consultation
See *Table 5*, page 667.

## General Dosing Information
Patients taking this medication for bronchial asthma, bronchitis, emphysema, or other obstructive pulmonary disease should be advised to contact their physician if they do not respond to the usual dose of this medication, since this may be a sign of seriously worsening asthma or bronchospasm that requires reassessment of therapy.

Following administration of an adrenergic bronchodilator, a sufficient interval of time should elapse before administration of another sympathomimetic agent.

---

## ALBUTEROL

## Summary of Differences
Indications:
   Parenteral albuterol also used in treatment of status asthmaticus.
Pharmacology/pharmacokinetics
Half-life—
   Elimination: 3.8 hours.
   Plasma: 2.7 to 5 hours.
Onset of action—
   Oral: 15 to 30 minutes.
Time to peak effect—
   Oral: 2 to 3 hours.
Duration of action—
   Oral: 8 hours or more (12 hours for extended-release tablets).
Elimination—
   Secondary route of elimination is fecal.
Precautions:
Pregnancy/reproduction:
   Labor—
      Albuterol administered intravenously or orally reportedly inhibits uterine contractions.

Medical considerations/contraindications—
Caution also needed in ketoacidosis when large parenteral doses of albuterol are administered.

Side/adverse effects:
Difficult or painful urination, drowsiness, flushing or redness of face or skin, heartburn, loss of appetite, muscle cramps or twitching, or unusual paleness may occur.

## Additional Dosing Information

See also *General Dosing Information*.

**For parenteral dosage forms only**
Parenteral albuterol is preferably administered by continuous intravenous infusion. However, if a rapid response is required, it may be administered by direct intravenous injection, followed by a continuous intravenous infusion. Albuterol injection may also be administered by intramuscular injection, if necessary.

## Oral Dosage Forms

### ALBUTEROL SULFATE ORAL SOLUTION

**Usual adult dose**
Bronchodilator—
Oral, 2 to 4 mg (base) three or four times a day.

**Usual pediatric dose**
Bronchodilator—
Children up to 2 years of age: Dosage has not been established.
Children 2 to 6 years of age: Oral, 100 mcg (0.1 mg) (base) per kg of body weight three or four times a day.
Children 6 to 12 years of age: Oral, 2 mg (base) three or four times a day.

**Strength(s) usually available**
U.S.—
Not commercially available.
Canada—
2 mg (base) per 5 mL (Rx) [*Ventolin*].

**Packaging and storage**
Store below 40 °C (104 °F), preferably between 15 and 30 °C (59 and 86 °F), unless otherwise specified by manufacturer. Protect from freezing.

### ALBUTEROL SULFATE SYRUP

**Usual adult and adolescent dose**
Bronchodilator—
Oral, 2 to 6 mg (base) three or four times a day initially, the dosage being increased as needed and tolerated up to a maximum of 8 mg four times a day.

Note: Patients sensitive to beta-adrenergic stimulants—Oral, 2 mg (base) three or four times a day initially, the dosage being increased as needed and tolerated up to a maximum of 8 mg three or four times a day.

**Usual pediatric dose**
Bronchodilator—
Children up to 2 years of age: Dosage has not been established.
Children 2 to 6 years of age: Oral, 100 mcg (0.1 mg) (base) per kg of body weight three times a day initially, the dosage being increased as needed and tolerated up to 200 mcg (0.2 mg) per kg of body weight, not to exceed 4 mg, three times a day.
Children 6 to 14 years of age: Oral, 2 mg (base) three or four times a day initially, the dosage being increased as needed and tolerated up to a maximum of 24 mg per day in divided doses.
Children 14 years of age and over: See *Usual adult and adolescent dose*.

**Usual geriatric dose**
Bronchodilator—
Oral, 2 mg (base) three or four times a day initially, the dosage being increased as needed and tolerated up to a maximum of 8 mg three or four times a day.

**Strength(s) usually available**
U.S.—
2 mg (base) per 5 mL (Rx) [*Proventil; Ventolin;* GENERIC].
Canada—
Not commercially available.

**Packaging and storage**
Store between 2 and 30 °C (36 and 86 °F), in a well-closed container, unless otherwise specified by manufacturer. Protect from light. Protect from freezing.

### ALBUTEROL TABLETS USP

**Usual adult and adolescent dose**
Bronchodilator—
Oral, 2 to 6 mg (base) three or four times a day initially, the dosage being increased as needed and tolerated up to a maximum of 8 mg four times a day.

Note: Patients sensitive to beta-adrenergic stimulants—Oral, 2 mg (base) three or four times a day initially, the dosage being increased as needed and tolerated up to a maximum of 8 mg three or four times a day.

**Usual pediatric dose**
Bronchodilator—
Children up to 6 years of age: Dosage has not been established.
Children 6 to 12 years of age: Oral, 2 mg (base) three or four times a day initially, the dosage being increased as needed and tolerated up to a maximum of 24 mg per day in divided doses.
Children 12 years of age and over: See *Usual adult and adolescent dose*.

**Usual geriatric dose**
Bronchodilator—
Oral, 2 mg (base) three or four times a day initially, the dosage being increased as needed and tolerated up to a maximum of 8 mg three or four times a day.

**Strength(s) usually available**
U.S.—
2 mg (base) (Rx) [*Proventil* ( scored); *Ventolin* (scored); GENERIC].
4 mg (base) (Rx) [*Proventil* (scored); *Ventolin* (scored); GENERIC].
5 mg (base) (Rx) [GENERIC].
Canada—
2 mg (base) (Rx) [*Novo-Salmol* (scored); *Ventolin* (scored)].
4 mg (base) (Rx) [*Novo-Salmol* (scored); *Ventolin* (scored)].

**Packaging and storage**
Store between 2 and 30 °C (36 and 86 °F), in a tight container, unless otherwise specified by manufacturer.

### ALBUTEROL SULFATE EXTENDED-RELEASE TABLETS

**Usual adult and adolescent dose**
Bronchodilator—
Oral, 4 or 8 mg (base) every twelve hours.

**Usual adult prescribing limits**
Up to 32 mg (base) per day.

**Usual pediatric dose**
Bronchodilator—
Children up to 12 years of age: Dosage has not been established.
Children 12 years of age and over: See *Usual adult and adolescent dose*.

**Strength(s) usually available**
U.S.—
4 mg (base) (Rx) [*Proventil Repetabs; Volmax*].
8 mg (base) (Rx) [*Volmax*].
Canada—
4 mg (base) (Rx) [*Volmax*].
8 mg (base) (Rx) [*Volmax*].

**Packaging and storage**
Store between 2 and 30 °C (36 and 86 °F), in a tight container, unless otherwise specified by manufacturer.

**Auxiliary labeling**
• Swallow tablets whole.

## Parenteral Dosage Forms

### ALBUTEROL SULFATE INJECTION

**Usual adult dose**
Bronchodilator—
Intramuscular, 500 mcg (0.5 mg) (base), or 8 mcg (0.008 mg) per kg of body weight, repeated every four hours as required up to a maximum dose of 2 mg per day.
Intravenous, 250 mcg (0.25 mg) (base), or 4 mcg (0.004 mg) per kg of body weight, administered over a period of two to five minutes, the dosage being repeated after fifteen minutes, if necessary, up to a maximum dose of 1 mg per day.
Intravenous infusion, administered at a rate of 5 mcg (0.005 mg) (base) per minute, the dosage being increased to 10 mcg (0.01 mg) per minute and then 20 mcg (0.02 mg) per minute at fifteen-to-thirty minute intervals, if necessary.

## Bronchodilators, Adrenergic (Systemic)

**Usual pediatric dose**
Dosage has not been established.

**Strength(s) usually available**
U.S.—
 Not commercially available.
Canada—
 50 mcg (0.05 mg) (base) per mL (Rx) [*Ventolin* (sodium 3.5 mg per mL)].
 500 mcg (0.5 mg) (base) per mL (Rx) [*Ventolin* (sodium 3.5 mg per mL)].

**Packaging and storage**
Store below 30 °C (86 °F), unless otherwise specified by manufacturer. Protect from light. Protect from freezing.

**Preparation of dosage form**
For an intravenous infusion, albuterol injection may be diluted in 0.9% sodium chloride injection, dextrose injection, or sodium chloride and dextrose injection.
An intravenous infusion may be prepared by diluting 10 mL of albuterol injection, 500 mcg (0.5 mg) (base) per mL, in 500 mL of an appropriate intravenous solution to provide an albuterol concentration of 10 mcg (0.01 mg) per mL.

**Stability**
Unused admixtures should be discarded 24 hours after preparation.

---

## EPHEDRINE

### Summary of Differences
Category:
 Oral ephedrine also indicated as a nasal decongestant and CNS stimulant.
 Oral and parenteral ephedrine also used as an urticaria therapy adjunct.
Indications:
 Oral ephedrine has been used in treatment of enuresis and myasthenia gravis, but has been replaced by more effective agents.
Pharmacology/pharmacokinetics:
 Ephedrine also has alpha- and beta-1-adrenergic receptor action.
 Half-life:
  Elimination—
   At urine pH 5—About 3 hours.
   At urine pH 6.3—About 6 hours.
 Onset of action—
  Oral: 15 to 60 minutes.
  Intramuscular: 10 to 20 minutes.
 Duration of action—
  Oral: 3 to 5 hours.
  Intramuscular or subcutaneous: 0.5 to 1 hour after 25 to 50 mg dose.
 Elimination—
  Mostly excreted unchanged; dependent on urinary pH; increased in acidic urine.
Precautions:
 Pregnancy/reproduction:
  Delivery—
   Parenteral administration of ephedrine to maintain blood pressure during spinal anesthesia for delivery can cause acceleration of fetal heart rate and should not be used when maternal blood pressure exceeds 130/80.
 Breast-feeding—
  Ephedrine excreted in breast milk; use by nursing mothers not recommended because of higher than usual risks for infants.
 Drug interactions and/or related problems—
  Caution also needed with glucocorticoid adrenocorticoids, corticotropin, urinary alkalizers, alpha-adrenergic blocking agents, diatrizoates, iothalamate, ioxaglate, ergot alkaloids, methysergide, oxytocin, doxapram, guanadrel, guanethidine, mazindol, mecamylamine, methyldopa, trimethaphan, methylphenidate, and rauwolfia alkaloids.
 Medical considerations/contraindications—
  Caution also needed in angle-closure glaucoma (or predisposition to) and prostatic hypertrophy.
Side/adverse effects:
 Hallucinations or mood or mental changes may occur rarely with high doses of ephedrine; also, difficult or painful urination, loss of appetite, or unusual paleness may occur.

### Additional Dosing Information
See also *General Dosing Information*.
Tolerance to ephedrine may develop with prolonged or excessive use. Discontinuation of the medication for a few days and subsequent readministration may restore its effectiveness.

**Bioequivalenence information**
For oral dosage forms only—
 Bioavailability or bioequivalence problems among different brands of Ephedrine Sulfate Capsules have not been documented.

**For oral dosage forms only**
To minimize the possibility of insomnia, the last dose of ephedrine for each day should be administered a few hours before bedtime.

**For parenteral dosage forms only**
When ephedrine is administered intravenously, the injection should be given slowly.

### Oral Dosage Forms
**EPHEDRINE SULFATE CAPSULES USP**

Note: Bioavailability or bioequivalence problems among different brands of Ephedrine Sulfate Capsules have not been documented.

**Usual adult dose**
Bronchodilator
decongestant, nasal (systemic) or
CNS stimulant—
 Oral, 25 to 50 mg every three or four hours, if necessary.

Note: Ephedrine has been used in the treatment of enuresis and myasthenia gravis. For enuresis, 25 to 50 mg once a day at bedtime; for myasthenia gravis, 25 mg three or four times a day.

**Usual pediatric dose**
Bronchodilator
decongestant, nasal (systemic) or
CNS stimulant—
 Oral, 3 mg per kg of body weight or 100 mg per square meter of body surface per day, in four to six divided doses.

**Strength(s) usually available**
U.S.—
 25 mg (OTC) [GENERIC].
 50 mg (OTC) [GENERIC].
Canada—
 Not commercially available.

**Packaging and storage**
Store below 40 °C (104 °F), preferably between 15 and 30 °C (59 and 86 °F), unless otherwise specified by manufacturer. Store in a tight, light-resistant container.

### Parenteral Dosage Forms
**EPHEDRINE SULFATE INJECTION USP**

**Usual adult dose**
Bronchodilator—
 Intramuscular, intravenous, or subcutaneous, 12.5 to 25 mg; subsequent dosage to be determined by patient response.

**Usual adult prescribing limits**
Up to 150 mg per twenty-four hours.

**Usual pediatric dose**
Bronchodilator—
 Intravenous or subcutaneous, 3 mg per kg of body weight or 100 mg per square meter of body surface per day, in four to six divided doses.

**Strength(s) usually available**
U.S.—
 25 mg per mL (Rx) [GENERIC].
 50 mg per mL (Rx) [GENERIC].
Canada—
 50 mg per mL (Rx) [GENERIC].

**Packaging and storage**
Store below 40 °C (104 °F), preferably between 15 and 30 °C (59 and 86 °F), unless otherwise specified by manufacturer. Store in a light-resistant container. Protect from freezing.

**Stability**
Ephedrine sulfate injection should not be used unless solution is clear. Unused portion should be discarded.

# EPINEPHRINE

## Summary of Differences
Category:
  Epinephrine injection also indicated as a local anesthetic adjunct, surgical aid (antihemorrhagic; decongestant; mydriatic), and topical antihemorrhagic.
Indications—
  Epinephrine injection also indicated in treatment of anaphylactic reactions; and may be used in management of bronchospasm during anesthesia.
Pharmacology/pharmacokinetics:
  Epinephrine also has alpha- and beta-1-adrenergic receptor action.
  Biotransformation—
    Also metabolized in sympathetic nerve endings and other tissues.
  Onset of action—
    Intramuscular: Variable.
    Subcutaneous: 6 to 15 minutes.
  Time to peak effect:
    Subcutaneous—
      0.3 hours.
  Duration of action—
    Intramuscular or subcutaneous: <1 to 4 hours.
  Elimination—
    Very small amount excreted unchanged.
Precautions:
  Pregnancy/reproduction—
    Epinephrine crosses placenta; use during pregnancy may cause anoxia in fetus; not recommended for use during labor since it may delay second stage; high doses, sufficient to reduce uterine contraction, may cause prolonged uterine atony with hemorrhage; parenteral administration of epinephrine to maintain blood pressure during spinal anesthesia for delivery can cause acceleration of fetal heart rate and should not be used when maternal blood pressure exceeds 130/80.
  Breast-feeding—
    Epinephrine excreted in breast milk; use by nursing mothers may cause serious adverse reactions in infant.
  Pediatrics—
    Syncope has occurred following administration of epinephrine to asthmatic children.
  Drug interactions and/or related problems—
    Caution also needed with alpha-adrenergic blocking agents, parenteral-local anesthetics, oral antidiabetic agents, insulin, diatrizoates, iothalamate, ioxaglate, ergot alkaloids, methysergide, oxytocin, doxapram, guanadrel, guanethidine, mazindol, mecamylamine, methyldopa, trimethaphan, methylphenidate, and rauwolfia alkaloids.
  Medical considerations/contraindications—
    Caution also needed in phenothiazine-induced circulatory collapse or hypotension; angle-closure glaucoma (or predisposition to); Parkinson's disease; prostatic hypertrophy; and cardiogenic, traumatic, or hemorrhagic shock.
Side/adverse effects:
  Hallucinations may occur with high doses of epinephrine; also, flushing or redness of face or skin may occur.

## Additional Dosing Information
See also *General Dosing Information*.
Tolerance to epinephrine may develop with prolonged or excessive use. Discontinuation of the medication for a few days and subsequent readministration may restore its effectiveness.

### For parenteral dosage forms only
The 1:1000 (1 mg/mL) concentration of epinephrine injection must be diluted before administering intracardially or intravenously.
If epinephrine injection is to be administered by intracardiac injection, it should be administered only by personnel well trained in the technique.
If the patient has been intubated, epinephrine can be injected via the endotracheal tube directly into the bronchial tree at the same dosage as for intravenous injection.
Intra-arterial administration of epinephrine injection is not recommended since marked vasoconstriction may result in gangrene.
It is recommended that sterile epinephrine suspension be administered with a tuberculin syringe and a 26-gauge, ½-inch needle.
After withdrawing a dose of sterile epinephrine suspension into the syringe, prompt injection is recommended to avoid settling of the suspension.
A single dose of sterile epinephrine suspension may be effective for up to 10 hours.
Repeated local injections may result in necrosis at the site of injection because of vascular constriction. Sites of injection should be rotated.
Intramuscular injection of epinephrine injection into the buttocks should be avoided since the vasoconstriction produced by the epinephrine reduces the oxygen tension of the tissues, enabling any anaerobic *Clostridium welchii* that may be present on the buttocks to multiply and possibly cause gas gangrene.

## Parenteral Dosage Forms

### EPINEPHRINE INJECTION USP

**Usual adult and adolescent dose**
Bronchodilator—
  Subcutaneous, initially 200 to 500 mcg (0.2 to 0.5 mg) (base), repeated every twenty minutes to four hours as needed, the dosage being increased up to a maximum of 1 mg per dose, if necessary.
Anaphylactic reactions—
  Intramuscular or subcutaneous, initially 200 to 500 mcg (0.2 to 0.5 mg) (base), repeated every ten to fifteen minutes as needed, the dosage being increased up to a maximum of 1 mg per dose if necessary.
Anesthetic (local) adjunct—
  For use with local anesthetics, 100 to 200 mcg (0.1 to 0.2 mg) (base) in a 1:200,000 to 1:20,000 solution.
  For use with intraspinal anesthetics, 200 to 400 mcg (0.2 to 0.4 mg) (base) added to the anesthetic spinal fluid mixture.
Surgical aid (antihemorrhagic; decongestant; mydriatic)—
  Intracameral or subconjunctival, a 0.01 to 0.1% (1:10,000 to 1:1000) (base) solution.
Antihemorrhagic (topical)—
  Topical, a 0.002 to 0.1% (1:50,000 to 1:1000) (base) solution.

**Usual pediatric dose**
Bronchodilator or
Anaphylactic reactions—
  Subcutaneous, 10 mcg (0.01 mg) (base) per kg of body weight or 300 mcg (0.3 mg) per square meter of body surface up to a maximum of 500 mcg (0.5 mg) per dose, repeated every fifteen minutes for two doses, then every four hours as needed.
Anesthetic (local) adjunct—
  See *Usual adult and adolescent dose*.
Surgical aid (antihemorrhagic; decongestant; mydriatic)—
  See *Usual adult and adolescent dose*.
Antihemorrhagic (topical)—
  See *Usual adult and adolescent dose*.

**Strength(s) usually available**
U.S.—
  10 mcg (0.01 mg) (base) per mL (Rx) [GENERIC].
  100 mcg (0.1 mg) (base) per mL (Rx) [GENERIC].
  500 mcg (0.5 mg) (base) per mL (Rx) [*EpiPen Jr. Auto-Injector* (sodium chloride 6 mg per mL; sodium metabisulfite 1.67 mg per mL)].
  1 mg (base) per mL (Rx) [*Adrenalin Chloride Solution* (benzyl alcohol; chlorobutanol 0.5%; sodium bisulfite not more than 0.1% in ampuls and 0.15% in vials; sodium chloride); *Ana-Guard* (not more than 5 mg chlorobutanol; not more than 1.5 mg sodium bisulfite per mL); *EpiPen Auto-Injector* (sodium chloride 6 mg per mL; sodium metabisulfite 1.67 mg per mL); GENERIC].
Canada—
  100 mcg (0.1 mg) (base) per mL (Rx) [GENERIC].
  500 mcg (0.5 mg) (base) per mL (Rx) [*EpiPen Jr. Auto-Injector* (sodium chloride 6 mg per mL; sodium metabisulfite 1.67 mg per mL)].
  1 mg (base) per mL (Rx) [*Adrenalin* (sodium chloride; sulfites); *EpiPen Auto-Injector* (sodium chloride 6 mg per mL; sodium metabisulfite 1.67 mg per mL)].
Note: The auto-injector containing 500 mcg (0.5 mg) (base) per mL delivers a single dose of 150 mcg (0.15 mg); and the auto-injector containing 1 mg (base) per mL delivers a single dose of 300 mcg (0.3 mg).

**Packaging and storage**
Store below 40 °C (104 °F), preferably between 15 and 30 °C (59 and 86 °F), unless otherwise specified by manufacturer. Store in a tight, light-resistant container. Protect from freezing.

**Preparation of dosage form**
For intracardiac or intravenous administration of epinephrine injection, dilute 0.5 mL (0.5 mg) of a 1:1000 (1 mg/mL) solution to 10 mL with 0.9% sodium chloride injection.

**Stability**
Epinephrine is readily destroyed by alkalies and oxidizing agents (for example, oxygen, chlorine, bromine, iodine, permanganates, chromates, nitrites, and salts of easily reducible metals, especially iron). Do not use if solution is pinkish or brownish in color or contains a precipitate.
Discard unused portion.

**Note**
For epinephrine auto-injector—Include patient instructions when dispensing.

### STERILE EPINEPHRINE SUSPENSION

**Usual adult dose**
Bronchodilator—
  Subcutaneous, 500 mcg (0.5 mg) initially, then 500 mcg (0.5 mg) to 1.5 mg not more often than every six hours as needed.

**Usual pediatric dose**
Bronchodilator—
  Subcutaneous, 25 mcg (0.025 mg) per kg of body weight or 625 mcg (0.625 mg) per square meter of body surface; dose may be repeated, if necessary, but not more often then every six hours.
Note: For children weighing 30 kg or less, the maximum single dose is 750 mcg (0.75 mg).

**Strength(s) usually available**
U.S.—
  5 mg per mL (Rx) [*Sus-Phrine* (ascorbic acid 10 mg; thioglycolic acid 6.6 mg [as sodium salts]; glycerin 325 mg; phenol 5 mg; sodium hydroxide)].
Canada—
  Not commercially available.

**Packaging and storage**
Store below 30 °C (86 °F), preferably between 2 and 8 °C (36 and 46 °F), unless otherwise specified by manufacturer. Store in a light-resistant container. Protect from freezing.

**Stability**
On removal of doses from the multiple dose vial, air is introduced which slowly oxidizes the epinephrine causing discoloration of the suspension and possible loss of potency. Do not use if suspension is pinkish or brownish in color.

**Auxiliary labeling**
• Shake well.
• Refrigerate.

---

## ETHYLNOREPINEPHRINE

### Summary of Differences
Pharmacology/pharmacokinetics:
  Ethylnorepinephrine also has beta-1-adrenergic receptor action.
  Onset of action—Intramuscular or subcutaneous: 6 to 12 minutes.
  Duration of action—Intramuscular or subcutaneous: 1 to 2 hours.

### Additional Dosing Information
See also *General Dosing Information*.

Intraneural or intravascular injection of ethylnorepinephrine should be avoided.

### Parenteral Dosage Forms

#### ETHYLNOREPINEPHRINE HYDROCHLORIDE INJECTION USP

**Usual adult dose**
Bronchodilator—
  Intramuscular or subcutaneous, 1 to 2 mg.
Note: Smaller doses of 600 mcg (0.6 mg) to 1 mg may be sufficient, depending on the severity of the asthmatic attack.

**Usual pediatric dose**
Bronchodilator—
  Intramuscular or subcutaneous, 200 mcg (0.2 mg) to 1 mg.

**Strength(s) usually available**
U.S.—
  2 mg per mL (Rx) [*Bronkephrine* (acetone sodium bisulfite 0.2%; sodium chloride 0.7%)].
Canada—
  Not commercially available.

**Packaging and storage**
Store below 40 °C (104 °F), preferably between 15 and 30 °C (59 and 86 °F), unless otherwise specified by manufacturer. Store in a light-resistant container. Protect from freezing.

---

## FENOTEROL

### Summary of Differences
Pharmacology/pharmacokinetics:
  Onset of action—
    Oral: 30 to 60 minutes.
  Time to peak effect—
    Oral: 2 to 3 hours.
  Duration of action—
    Oral: 6 to 8 hours.
Precautions:
  Medical considerations/contraindications—
    Caution also needed in angle-closure glaucoma (or predisposition to).
Side/adverse effects:
  Heartburn, or muscle cramps or twitching may occur.

### Oral Dosage Forms

#### FENOTEROL HYDROBROMIDE TABLETS

**Usual adult and adolescent dose**
Bronchodilator—
  Oral, 2.5 mg two times a day initially, the dosage being increased up to a maximum of 5 mg three times a day, if necessary, but not to be administered more often than every six hours.

**Usual pediatric dose**
Bronchodilator—
  Children up to 12 years of age: Dosage has not been established.
  Children 12 years of age and over: See *Usual adult and adolescent dose*.

**Strength(s) usually available**
U.S.—
  Not commercially available.
Canada—
  2.5 mg (Rx) [*Berotec* (scored; lactose)].

**Packaging and storage**
Store below 40 °C (104 °F), preferably between 15 and 30 °C (59 and 86 °F), in a well-closed container, unless otherwise specified by manufacturer.

---

## ISOPROTERENOL

### Summary of Differences
Pharmacology/pharmacokinetics:
  Isoproterenol also has beta-1-adrenergic receptor action.
  Absorption of sublingual tablets may be erratic and unpredictable.
  Biotransformation—
    Also metabolized in the lungs and other tissues.
  Onset of action—
    Intravenous: Immediate.
    Rectal: Within 30 minutes.
    Sublingual: 15 to 30 minutes.
  Duration of action—
    Intravenous: <1 hour.
    Rectal: 2 to 4 hours.
    Sublingual: 1 to 2 hours.
  Elimination—
    Intravenous: About 40 to 50% excreted unchanged.
    Oral: About 5 to 15% excreted unchanged.
Side/adverse effects:
  Irregular heartbeat, pinkish to red coloration of saliva (for sublingual dosage form only), and flushing or redness of face or skin may occur.

### Additional Dosing Information
See also *General Dosing Information*.

### Oral Dosage Forms

#### ISOPROTERENOL HYDROCHLORIDE TABLETS USP

**Usual adult dose**
Bronchodilator—
  Sublingual, 10 to 15 mg three or four times a day.

**Usual pediatric dose**
Bronchodilator—
  Sublingual, 5 to 10 mg three times a day.

**Strength(s) usually available**
U.S.—
  10 mg (Rx) [*Isuprel Glossets* (lactose; saccharin sodium; sodium metabisulfite 2 mg)].
Canada—
  Not commercially available.

**Packaging and storage**
Store below 40 °C (104 °F), preferably between 15 and 30 °C (59 and 86 °F), unless otherwise specified by manufacturer. Store in a well-closed, light-resistant container.

**Auxiliary labeling**
- Dissolve tablets under tongue.
- Keep container tightly closed.

## Parenteral Dosage Forms
### ISOPROTERENOL HYDROCHLORIDE INJECTION USP
**Usual adult dose**
Bronchodilator (bronchospasm during anesthesia)—
  Intravenous, 10 to 20 mcg (0.01 to 0.02 mg), repeated as needed.

**Usual pediatric dose**
Dosage must be individualized by physician.

**Strength(s) usually available**
U.S.—
  20 mcg (0.02 mg) per mL (Rx) [GENERIC].
  200 mcg (0.2 mg) per mL (Rx) [*Isuprel* (sodium metabisulfite; sodium chloride 7 mg; sodium lactate 1.8 mg; lactic acid 0.2 mg); GENERIC].
Canada—
  200 mcg (0.2 mg) per mL (Rx) [*Isuprel* (sodium lactate; sodium metabisulfite)].

**Packaging and storage**
Store below 40 °C (104 °F), preferably between 15 and 30 °C (59 and 86 °F), unless otherwise specified by manufacurer. Protect from light. Protect from freezing.

**Preparation of dosage form**
For preparation of solutions for injection, see manufacturer's package insert.

**Stability**
When exposed to air, alkalies, or metals, isoproterenol may turn pinkish to brownish in color because of oxidation. Do not use if solution is pinkish to brownish in color or contains a precipitate.

---
## METAPROTERENOL
---

## Summary of Differences
Pharmacology/pharmacokinetics:
  Onset of action—
    Oral: Within 15 to 30 minutes.
  Time to peak effect—
    Oral: Within 1 hour.
  Duration of action—
    Oral: Up to 4 hours.
  Elimination—
    Primarily excreted as glucuronic acid conjugates.
Precautions:
  Medical considerations/contraindications—
    Caution also needed in convulsive disorders.
Side/adverse effects:
  Muscle cramps or twitching may occur.

## Oral Dosage Forms
### METAPROTERENOL SULFATE SYRUP USP
**Usual adult and adolescent dose**
Bronchodilator—
  Oral, 20 mg three or four times a day.

**Usual pediatric dose**
Bronchodilator—
  Children up to 6 years of age: Dosage has not been established.
  Children 6 to 9 years of age and over; or
  Children weighing up to 27 kg: Oral, 10 mg three or four times a day.
  Children 9 years of age and over; or
  Children weighing 27 kg and over: See *Usual adult and adolescent dose*.

Note: Experience in children up to 6 years of age is limited; however, studies have shown a dose of 325 to 650 mcg (0.325 to 0.65 mg) per kg of body weight four times a day for this age group to be well tolerated.

**Strength(s) usually available**
U.S.—
  10 mg per 5 mL (Rx) [*Alupent; Metaprel; Prometa;* GENERIC].
Canada—
  10 mg per 5 mL (Rx) [*Alupent* (parabens; sorbitol; sodium <10 mg per 5 mL)].

**Packaging and storage**
Store below 40 °C (104 °F), preferably between 15 and 30 °C (59 and 86 °F), unless otherwise specified by manufacturer. Store in a tight, light-resistant container. Protect from freezing.

### METAPROTERENOL SULFATE TABLETS USP
**Usual adult and adolescent dose**
Bronchodilator—
  Oral, 20 mg three or four times a day.

**Usual pediatric dose**
Bronchodilator—
  Children up to 6 years of age: Dosage has not been established.
  Children 6 to 9 years of age and over; or
  Children weighing up to 27 kg: Oral, 10 mg three or four times a day.
  Children 9 years of age and over; or
  Children weighing 27 kg and over: See *Usual adult and adolescent dose*.

Note: Experience in children up to 6 years of age is limited; however, studies have shown a dose of 325 to 650 mcg (0.325 to 0.65 mg) per kg of body weight four times a day for this age group to be well tolerated.

**Strength(s) usually available**
U.S.—
  10 mg (Rx) [*Alupent* (scored); *Metaprel* (scored); GENERIC].
  20 mg (Rx) [*Alupent* (scored); *Metaprel* (scored); GENERIC].
Canada—
  20 mg (Rx) [*Alupent* (lactose)].

**Packaging and storage**
Store below 40 °C (104 °F), preferably between 15 and 30 °C (59 and 86 °F), unless otherwise specified by manufacturer. Store in a well-closed, light-resistant container.

---
## TERBUTALINE
---

## Summary of Differences
Category:
  Oral and parenteral terbutaline also used as a labor (premature) inhibitor; and parenteral terbutaline may be used in management of bronchospasm during anesthesia.
Pharmacology/pharmacokinetics:
  Biotransformation—
    Metabolized primarily to inactive sulfate conjugate.
  Onset of action—
    Oral: Within 60 to 120 minutes.
    Parenteral: Within 15 minutes.
  Time to peak effect—
    Oral: Within 2 to 3 hours.
    Parenteral: Within 0.5 to 1 hour.
  Duration of action—
    Oral: 4 to 8 hours.
    Parenteral: 1.5 to 4 hours.
Precautions:
  Pregnancy/reproduction—
    Pregnancy: Parenteral administration during pregnancy reported to cause fetal tachycardia.
    Labor and delivery: Inhibits uterine activity during the second and third trimesters of pregnancy and may inhibit labor; when administered during labor, reported to cause serious adverse reactions such as transient hypokalemia, pulmonary edema, and hypoglycemia in the mother and hypoglycemia in neonates of mothers treated with parenteral terbutaline.
  Medical considerations/contraindications—
    Caution also needed in ketoacidosis when large parenteral doses of terbutaline are administered and in patients with history of seizures.
Side/adverse effects:
  Irregular heartbeat, drowsiness, or muscle cramps or twitching may occur.

## Additional Dosing Information
See also *General Dosing Information*.

**For parenteral dosage forms only**
The subcutaneous injection is usually injected into the lateral deltoid area.

## Oral Dosage Forms
Note: Bracketed uses in the *Dosage Forms* section refer to categories of use and/or indications that are not included in U.S. product labeling.

### TERBUTALINE SULFATE TABLETS USP
**Usual adult dose**
Bronchodilator—
    Oral, 2.5 to 5 mg three times a day, administered at approximately six-hour intervals.
[Labor (premature) inhibitor][1]—
    Maintenance: Oral, 2.5 mg every four to six hours until term.

**Usual adult prescribing limits**
Up to 15 mg per twenty-four hours.

**Usual pediatric dose**
Bronchodilator—
    Children up to 12 years of age: Dosage has not been established.
    Children 12 to 15 years of age: Oral, 2.5 mg three times a day, administered at approximately six-hour intervals.

**Strength(s) usually available**
U.S.—
    2.5 mg (Rx) [*Brethine* (scored); *Bricanyl*].
    5 mg (Rx) [*Brethine* (scored); *Bricanyl* (scored)].
Canada—
    2.5 mg (Rx) [*Bricanyl* (scored)].
    5 mg (Rx) [*Bricanyl* (scored)].

**Packaging and storage**
Store between 15 and 30 °C (59 to 86 °F), in a tight container.

## Parenteral Dosage Forms
Note: Bracketed uses in the *Dosage Forms* section refer to categories of use and/or indications that are not included in U.S. product labeling.

### TERBUTALINE SULFATE INJECTION USP
**Usual adult dose**
Bronchodilator—
    Subcutaneous, 250 mcg (0.25 mg), repeated after fifteen to thirty minutes if necessary; a total dose of 500 mcg (0.5 mg) should not be exceeded within a four-hour period.
[Labor (premature) inhibitor][1]—
    Intravenous infusion, administered at a rate of 10 mcg (0.01 mg) per minute initially, the rate being increased by 5 mcg (0.005 mg) per minute every ten minutes until contractions cease or up to a maximum dose of 80 mcg (0.08 mg) per minute. After contractions cease for thirty minutes to one hour, the rate of administration is decreased by 5 mcg (0.005 mg) per minute to the lowest effective dose. The minimum effective dosage should be continued for four to eight hours after contractions cease.
    Subcutaneous, 250 mcg (0.25 mg) every hour until contractions cease.

**Usual pediatric dose**
Bronchodilator—
    Children up to 12 years of age: Dosage has not been established.

**Strength(s) usually available**
U.S.—
    1 mg (820 mcg [0.82 mg] [base]) per mL (Rx) [*Brethine* (sodium chloride); *Bricanyl* (sodium chloride)].
Canada—
    Not commercially available.

**Packaging and storage**
Store between 15 and 30 °C (59 and 86 °F). Protect from light.

**Stability**
Do not use if solution is discolored.

[1] Not included in Canadian product labeling.

Revised: 7/90
Interim revision: 09/12/94; 08/09/95; 08/01/97

## Table 1. Pharmacology/Pharmacokinetics

| Drug | Adrenergic Receptor Action (Primary) | Biotransformation | Half-life (hr) | Onset of Action (min) | Time to Peak Effect (hr) | Duration of Action (hr) | Elimination Primary (% unchanged)/ Secondary |
|---|---|---|---|---|---|---|---|
| Albuterol* Oral | Beta-2 | Hepatic† | Plasma: 2.7–5 | 15–30 | 2–3 | 8 or more (12 for extended-release tablets) | Renal/Fecal‡ |
| Ephedrine | Alpha; Beta-1; Beta-2 | Hepatic | Elimination: At urine pH 5— About 3 At urine pH 6.3— About 6 | | | | Renal (mostly unchanged); dependent on urinary pH; increased in acidic urine |
| Oral | | | | 15–60 | — | 3–5 | |
| Intramuscular | | | | 10–20 | — | 0.5–1 after 25–50 mg dose | |
| Subcutaneous | | | | — | — | 0.5–1 after 25–50 mg dose | |
| Epinephrine | Alpha; Beta-1; Beta-2 | Hepatic; also in sympathetic nerve endings and other tissues | | | | | Renal (very small amount) |
| Intramuscular | | | — | Variable | — | <1–4 | |
| Subcutaneous | | | — | 6–15 | 0.3 | <1–4 | |
| Ethylnorepine-phrine§ | Beta-1; Beta-2 | — | | | | | — |
| Intramuscular | | | — | 6–12 | — | 1–2 | |
| Subcutaneous | | | — | 6–12 | — | 1–2 | |
| Fenoterol* Oral | Beta-2 | — | — | 30–60 | 2–3 | 6–8 | Renal/Biliary/Fecal |

## Table 1. Pharmacology/Pharmacokinetics *(continued)*

| Drug | Adrenergic Receptor Action (Primary) | Biotransformation | Half-life (hr) | Onset of Action (min) | Time to Peak Effect (hr) | Duration of Action (hr) | Elimination Primary (% unchanged)/ Secondary |
|---|---|---|---|---|---|---|---|
| Isoproterenol | Beta-1; Beta-2 | Hepatic; also in lungs and other tissues | | | | | Renal (IV, about 40–50; oral, about 5–15) |
|   Intravenous | | | — | Immediate | — | <1 | |
|   Rectal | | | — | Within 30 | — | 2–4 | |
|   Sublingual | | | — | 15–30 | — | 1–2 | |
| Metaproterenol* | Beta-2 | Hepatic | | | | | Renal, primarily as glucuronic acid conjugates |
|   Oral | | | — | Within 15–30 | Within 1 | Up to 4 | |
| Terbutaline* | Beta-2 | Hepatic, partially; primarily to inactive sulfate conjugate | | | | | Renal |
|   Oral | | | — | Within 60–120 | Within 2–3 | 4–8 | |
|   Parenteral | | | — | Within 15 | Within 0.5–1 | 1.5–4 | |

*Has minor beta-1 activity.
†Primarily to albuterol 4′-0-sulfate, which has little or no beta-adrenergic stimulating effect and no beta-adrenergic blocking effect.
‡Oral—
  Renal: Approximately 65 to 90% of oral dose excreted over 3 days in urine, the majority of dose being excreted within first 24 hours, consisting of 60% as metabolite.
  Fecal: About 4% of oral dose may be excreted in feces.
§Has minor alpha activity.

## Table 2. Drug interactions and/or related problems

The following drug interactions and/or related problems have been selected on the basis of their potential clinical significance (possible mechanism in parentheses where appropriate)—not necessarily inclusive (» = major clinical significance):

Note: Combinations containing any of the following medications, depending on the amount present, may also interact with this medication.

Legend:
**I** = Albuterol    **V** = Fenoterol
**II** = Ephedrine    **VI** = Isoproterenol
**III** = Epinephrine    **VII** = Metaproterenol
**IV** = Ethylnorepinephrine    **VIII** = Terbutaline

| | I | II | III | IV | V | VI | VII | VIII |
|---|---|---|---|---|---|---|---|---|
| Alkalizers, urinary, such as:<br>  Antacids, calcium- and/or magnesium-containing<br>  Carbonic anhydrase inhibitors<br>  Citrates<br>  Sodium bicarbonate<br>    (urine alkalinization induced by these medications reduces urinary excretion of ephedrine and therefore may increase the half-life of ephedrine and prolong its duration of action, especially if the urine remains alkaline for several days or longer; patient should be monitored for ephedrine toxicity [e.g., nervousness, insomnia, excitability]; dosage adjustment of ephedrine may be necessary) | | ✓ | | | | | | |
| Alpha-adrenergic blocking agents, such as:<br>  Labetalol<br>  Phenoxybenzamine<br>  Phentolamine<br>  Prazosin<br>  Tolazoline, or<br>Other medications with alpha-adrenergic blocking action, such as:<br>  Haloperidol<br>  Loxapine<br>  Phenothiazines<br>  Thioxanthenes, or<br>Vasodilators, rapidly acting, such as nitrites<br>    (concurrent use may block the alpha-adrenergic effects of epinephrine, possibly resulting in severe hypotension and tachycardia)<br>    (concurrent use of ephedrine or epinephrine may reduce the antianginal effect of amyl nitrite) | | ✓ | ✓ ✓ | | | | | |

## Table 2. Drug interactions and/or related problems *(continued)*

The following drug interactions and/or related problems have been selected on the basis of their potential clinical significance (possible mechanism in parentheses where appropriate)—not necessarily inclusive (» = major clinical significance):

Note: Combinations containing any of the following medications, depending on the amount present, may also interact with this medication.

Legend:
I = Albuterol
II = Ephedrine
III = Epinephrine
IV = Ethylnorepinephrine
V = Fenoterol
VI = Isoproterenol
VII = Metaproterenol
VIII = Terbutaline

| | I | II | III | IV | V | VI | VII | VIII |
|---|---|---|---|---|---|---|---|---|
| » Anesthetics, hydrocarbon inhalation, such as: Chloroform, Cyclopropane, Enflurane, Halothane, Isoflurane, Methoxyflurane, Trichloroethylene | | | | | | | | |
| (concurrent use of chloroform, cyclopropane, halothane, or trichloroethylene with ephedrine, epinephrine, ethylnorepinephrine, or isoproterenol may increase the risk of severe ventricular arrhythmias because these anesthetics greatly sensitize the myocardium to the effects of sympathomimetics; these medications should be used with caution and in substantially reduced dosage in patients receiving hydrocarbon inhalation anesthetics) | | ✓ | ✓ | ✓ | | ✓ | | |
| (administration of high doses of albuterol, fenoterol, metaproterenol, or terbutaline prior to or shortly after anesthesia with chloroform, cyclopropane, halothane, or trichloroethylene may increase the risk of severe ventricular arrhythmias, especially in patients with pre-existing heart disease, because these anesthetics greatly sensitize the myocardium to the effects of sympathomimetics) | ✓ | | | | ✓ | | ✓ | ✓ |
| (enflurane, isoflurane, or methoxyflurane may also cause some sensitization of the myocardium to the effects of sympathomimetics; caution is recommended during concurrent use with the sympathomimetic) | ✓ | ✓ | ✓ | ✓ | ✓ | ✓ | ✓ | ✓ |
| » Anesthetics, parenteral-local (epinephrine shoud be used cautiously and in carefully circumscribed quantities, if at all, with local anesthetics for anesthetizing areas with end arteries [such as the fingers, toes, or penis] or otherwise compromised blood supply; ischemia leading to gangrene may result) | | | ✓ | | | | | |
| » Antidepressants, tricyclic, or » Maprotiline | | | | | | | | |
| (concurrent use may potentiate the cardiovascular effects of epinephrine or isoproterenol, possibly resulting in arrhythmias, tachycardia, or severe hypertension or hyperpyrexia) | | | ✓ | | | ✓ | | |
| (concurrent use of tricyclic antidepressants may potentiate the action of albuterol, metaproterenol, or terbutaline on the vascular system) | ✓ | | | | | | ✓ | ✓ |
| Antidiabetic agents, oral, or Insulin (effects may be decreased when these medications are used concurrently with epinephrine, since epinephrine increases blood glucose by inhibiting glucose uptake by peripheral tissues and by promoting glycogenolysis; dosage adjustments of oral antidiabetic agents or insulin may be necessary) | | | ✓ | | | | | |
| Antihypertensives or Diuretics used as antihypertensives (antihypertensive effects may be reduced when these medications are used concurrently with adrenergic bronchodilators; the patient should be carefully monitored to confirm that the desired effect is being obtained) | ✓ | ✓ | ✓ | ✓ | ✓ | ✓ | ✓ | ✓ |
| » Beta-adrenergic blocking agents, including ophthalmic agents (concurrent use with adrenergic bronchodilators may result in mutual inhibition of therapeutic effects) | ✓ | ✓ | ✓ | ✓ | ✓ | ✓ | ✓ | ✓ |
| (for adrenergic bronchodilators with both alpha- and beta-adrenergic effects [ephedrine, epinephrine], beta-adrenergic blockade may result in unopposed alpha-adrenergic activity with a risk of hypertension and excessive bradycardia with possible heart block; beta-blockade also antagonizes the beta-2-adrenergic bronchodilating effect of ephedrine and epinephrine) | | ✓ | ✓ | | | | | |
| (for adrenergic bronchodilators with beta-adrenergic effects, beta-blockade may antagonize the beta-2-adrenergic bronchodilating effect of albuterol, ethylnorepinephrine, fenoterol, metaproterenol, or terbutaline and the beta-1-adrenergic cardiac effect and the beta-2-adrenergic bronchodilating effect of isoproterenol; use of a cardioselective beta-1-adrenergic blocker, such as atenolol or metoprolol, at low doses may reduce antagonism of the bronchodilating effect) | ✓ | | | | ✓ | ✓ | ✓ | ✓ |
| CNS stimulation–producing medications, other (See *Appendix II*) (concurrent use with adrenergic bronchodilators may result in additive CNS stimulation to excessive levels, which may cause unwanted effects such as nervousness, irritability, insomnia, or possibly convulsions or cardiac arrhythmias; close observation is recommended) | ✓ | ✓ | ✓ | ✓ | ✓ | ✓ | ✓ | ✓ |

## Table 2. Drug interactions and/or related problems (continued)

The following drug interactions and/or related problems have been selected on the basis of their potential clinical significance (possible mechanism in parentheses where appropriate)—not necessarily inclusive (» = major clinical significance):

Note: Combinations containing any of the following medications, depending on the amount present, may also interact with this medication.

Legend:
I = Albuterol
II = Ephedrine
III = Epinephrine
IV = Ethylnorepinephrine
V = Fenoterol
VI = Isoproterenol
VII = Metaproterenol
VIII = Terbutaline

| Drug | I | II | III | IV | V | VI | VII | VIII |
|---|---|---|---|---|---|---|---|---|
| » Cocaine, mucosal-local (in addition to increasing CNS stimulation, concurrent use of a sympathomimetic may increase the cardiovascular effects of either or both medications and the risk of adverse effects) | ✓ | ✓ | ✓ | ✓ | ✓ | ✓ | ✓ | ✓ |
| (concurrent use of epinephrine with cocaine [especially intranasal application of "cocaine mud," a potentially lethal substance obtained by moistening cocaine powder with an epinephrine solution] is not recommended because of the high risk of hypertensive episodes and cardiac arrhythmias; also, concurrent use of cocaine and epinephrine is unnecessary because epinephrine does not provide additional local vasoconstriction or slow absorption of cocaine from the mucosa) | | | ✓ | | | | | |
| Corticosteroids, glucocorticoid, or Corticotropin, chronic therapeutic use of (concurrent use of glucocorticoid corticosteroids or chronic therapeutic use of corticotropin with ephedrine may increase the metabolic clearance of corticosteroids or corticotropin; glucocorticoid dosage adjustment may be required) | | ✓ | | | | | | |
| Diatrizoates or Iothalamate or Ioxaglate (neurologic effects of these medications, including paraplegia, may be increased during aortography when the medications are administered after hypertensive agents, such as parenteral ephedrine or epinephrine, used to increase contrast; increase of neurologic effects is due to contraction of vessels in the splanchnic circulation, forcing more of the contrast material into the vessels leading to the spine and spinal cord) | | ✓ | ✓ | | | | | |
| » Digitalis glycosides (concurrent use with adrenergic bronchodilators may increase the risk of cardiac arrhythmias; caution and close electrocardiographic monitoring are very important if concurrent use is necessary) | ✓ | ✓ | ✓ | ✓ | ✓ | ✓ | ✓ | ✓ |
| Dihydroergotamine or » Ergoloid mesylates or Ergonovine or » Ergotamine or Methylergonovine or Methysergide or Oxytocin (concurrent use of dihydroergotamine, ergonovine, methylergonovine, or methysergide with ephedrine or epinephrine may result in enhanced vasoconstriction; dosage adjustments may be necessary) | | ✓ | ✓ | | | | | |
| (concurrent use of ergoloid mesylates or ergotamine with ephedrine or epinephrine may produce peripheral vascular ischemia and gangrene and is not recommended) | | ✓ | ✓ | | | | | |
| (concurrent use of ergonovine, ergotamine, methylergonovine, or oxytocin may potentiate the pressor effect of ephedrine or epinephrine and result in severe hypertension; rarely, rupture of a cerebral blood vessel has occurred postpartum) | | ✓ | ✓ | | | | | |
| Doxapram (in addition to possibly increasing CNS stimulation, concurrent use may increase the pressor effects of either doxapram or ephedrine or epinephrine) | | ✓ | ✓ | | | | | |
| Guanadrel or Guanethidine (in addition to possibly decreasing the hypotensive effect of guanadrel or guanethidine, concurrent use may potentiate the pressor effect of ephedrine or epinephrine, as a result of inhibition of sympathomimetic uptake by adrenergic neurons, possibly resulting in hypertension and cardiac arrhythmias) | | ✓ | ✓ | | | | | |
| Levodopa (concurrent use with adrenergic bronchodilators may increase the possibility of cardiac arrhythmias; dosage reduction of the sympathomimetic is recommended) | ✓ | ✓ | ✓ | ✓ | ✓ | ✓ | ✓ | ✓ |
| Mazindol (in addition to possibly increasing CNS stimulation, concurrent use may potentiate the pressor effect of ephedrine or epinephrine; if necessary to administer a pressor amine agent to a patient who has recently received mazindol, initiating pressor therapy in reduced dosage and monitoring of blood pressure at frequent intervals are recommended) | | ✓ | ✓ | | | | | |
| Mecamylamine or Methyldopa or Trimethaphan (in addition to possibly decreasing the hypotensive effects of these medications, concurrent use may enhance the pressor response to ephedrine or epinephrine) | | ✓ | ✓ | | | | | |

## Table 2. Drug interactions and/or related problems *(continued)*

The following drug interactions and/or related problems have been selected on the basis of their potential clinical significance (possible mechanism in parentheses where appropriate)—not necessarily inclusive (» = major clinical significance):

Note: Combinations containing any of the following medications, depending on the amount present, may also interact with this medication.

Legend:
I = Albuterol
II = Ephedrine
III = Epinephrine
IV = Ethylnorepinephrine
V = Fenoterol
VI = Isoproterenol
VII = Metaproterenol
VIII = Terbutaline

| | I | II | III | IV | V | VI | VII | VIII |
|---|---|---|---|---|---|---|---|---|
| Methylphenidate (in addition to possibly increasing CNS stimulation, concurrent use may potentiate the pressor effects of ephedrine or epinephrine) | | ✔ | ✔ | | | | | |
| » Monoamine oxidase (MAO) inhibitors, including furazolidone and procarbazine (concurrent use may potentiate the action of albuterol, fenoterol, metaproterenol, or terbutaline on the vascular system) | ✔ | | | | ✔ | | ✔ | ✔ |
| (concurrent use may prolong and intensify cardiac stimulant and vasopressor effects of ephedrine because of release of catecholamines, which accumulate in intraneuronal storage sites during MAO inhibitor therapy, resulting in headache, cardiac arrhythmias, vomiting, or sudden and severe hypertensive and/or hyperpyretic crises; ephedrine should not be administered during or within 14 days following the administration of an MAO inhibitor) | | ✔ | | | | | | |
| Nitrates (concurrent use with adrenergic bronchodilators may reduce the antianginal effects of nitrates) | ✔ | ✔ | ✔ | ✔ | ✔ | ✔ | ✔ | ✔ |
| Papaverine, intracavernosal, or Phentolamine, intracavernosal (vasodilating effect of papaverine or phentolamine is reversed by epinephrine; epinephrine may be used to treat priapism or overdose due to these medications) | | | ✔ | | | | | |
| Rauwolfia alkaloids (concurrent use with ephedrine may decrease the hypotensive effects of rauwolfia alkaloids) | | ✔ | | | | | | |
| (in addition to possibly decreasing the hypotensive effects of rauwolfia alkaloids, concurrent use may theoretically prolong the action of direct-acting sympathomimetics, such as epinephrine, by preventing uptake into storage granules; a "denervation supersensitivity" response is also possible; although concurrent use with epinephrine is not known to produce severe adverse effects, a significant increase in blood pressure has been documented when phenylephrine ophthalmic drops have been administered to patients taking reserpine, and caution and close observation are recommended) | | | ✔ | | | | | |
| Ritodrine (concurrent use may increase the effect of either these medications or ritodrine and the potential for side effects) | ✔ | ✔ | ✔ | ✔ | ✔ | ✔ | ✔ | ✔ |
| Sympathomimetics, other (in addition to possibly increasing CNS stimulation, concurrent use may increase the cardiovascular effects of either the other sympathomimetic or the adrenergic bronchodilator and the potential for side effects; however, an aerosol bronchodilator of the adrenergic stimulant type may be used to relieve acute bronchospasm in patients receiving chronic oral adrenergic bronchodilator therapy) | ✔ | ✔ | ✔ | ✔ | ✔ | ✔ | ✔ | ✔ |
| Thallous chloride Tl 201 (in animal studies, concurrent use of isoproterenol increased myocardial uptake of thallous chloride Tl 201; human data are not available) | | | | | | ✔ | | |
| Thyroid hormones (concurrent use may increase the effects of either these medications or adrenergic bronchodilators; thyroid hormones enhance risk of coronary insufficiency when sympathomimetic agents are administered to patients with coronary artery disease; dosage adjustment is recommended, although problem is reduced in euthyroid patients) | ✔ | ✔ | ✔ | ✔ | ✔ | ✔ | ✔ | ✔ |
| Xanthines, such as: Aminophylline Caffeine Dyphylline Oxtriphylline Theophylline (in addition to possibly increasing CNS stimulation, concurrent use with adrenergic bronchodilators may result in other additive toxic effects) | ✔ | ✔ | ✔ | ✔ | ✔ | ✔ | ✔ | ✔ |

## Table 3. Medical considerations/Contraindications

Note: A blank space usually signifies lack of information; it is not necessarily an indication that a given medical problem is of no concern. However, the pharmacologic similarity of these agents may suggest that if caution is required in particular medical problems for one agent, then it may be required for the others as well.

The medical considerations/contraindications included have been selected on the basis of their potential clinical significance (reasons given in parentheses were appropriate)—not necessarily inclusive (» = major clinical signficance).

**Risk-benefit should be considered when the following medical problems exist:**

Legend:
I = Albuterol
II = Ephedrine
III = Epinephrine
IV = Ethylnorepinephrine
V = Fenoterol
VI = Isoproterenol
VII = Metaproterenol
VIII = Terbutaline

| | I | II | III | IV | V | VI | VII | VIII |
|---|---|---|---|---|---|---|---|---|
| » Brain damage, organic | | | ✔ | | | | | |
| » Cardiovascular disease, including: Angina pectoris | | ✔ | ✔ | | | ✔ | | |
| Cardiac arrhythmias | ✔ | ✔ | ✔ | | | | ✔ | ✔ |
| Cardiac arrhythmias associated with tachycardia | | | | | ✔ | ✔ | ✔ | |
| Cardiac asthma | | | | | | | | |
| Cardiac dilatation | | | | ✔ | | | | |
| Cerebral arteriosclerosis | | | | ✔ | | | | |
| Congestive heart failure | | | | ✔ | | ✔ | | |
| Coronary artery disease | | | | ✔ | ✔ | ✔ | ✔ | |
| Coronary insufficiency | ✔ | ✔ | ✔ | | | ✔ | | ✔ |
| Degenerative heart disease | | | | ✔ | | ✔ | | |
| Hypertension | ✔ | ✔ | ✔ | ✔ | ✔ | ✔ | ✔ | ✔ |
| Idiopathic hypertrophic subvalvular aortic stenosis | | | | | | ✔ | | |
| Ischemic heart disease | ✔ | | ✔ | | | | | |
| Limited cardiac reserve | | | | | | | | |
| Organic heart disease | | | | ✔ | | ✔ | | |
| Stroke, history of | | | | ✔ | | | | |
| Tachycardia caused by digitalis intoxication (condition may be exacerbated due to drug-induced cardiovascular effects) | | | | | | ✔ | | |
| Circulatory collapse or hypotension, phenothiazine-induced (pressor effect of epinephrine may be reversed by the phenothiazine, resulting in further lowering of blood pressure) | | | | ✔ | | | | |
| Convulsive disorders | | | | | | | ✔ | |
| Diabetes mellitus (potential drug-induced hyperglycemia may result in loss of diabetic control; dosage of insulin or hypoglycemic agents may need to be increased, especially with epinephrine) | ✔ | ✔ | ✔ | | ✔ | ✔ | ✔ | ✔ |
| Glaucoma, angle-closure, or predisposition to | | ✔ | ✔ | ✔ | | | | |
| Hyperthyroidism (adverse reactions more likely to occur) | ✔ | ✔ | ✔ | ✔ | ✔ | ✔ | ✔ | ✔✔ |
| Ketoacidosis (large parenteral doses of albuterol or terbutaline may aggravate condition) | ✔ | | | | | | | ✔ |
| Parkinson's disease (rigidity and tremor may be increased temporarily) | | | | ✔ | | | | |
| Pheochromocytoma, diagnosed or suspected | ✔ | ✔ | ✔ | ✔ | ✔ | ✔ | ✔ | ✔ |
| Prostatic hypertrophy | | ✔ | | | | | | |
| Psychoneurotic disorders (worsening of symptoms) | | | | ✔ | | | | |
| Seizures, history of | | | | | | | | ✔ |
| Sensitivity to sympathomimetics | ✔ | ✔ | ✔ | ✔ | ✔ | ✔ | ✔ | ✔ |
| » Shock, cardiogenic, traumatic, or hemorrhagic (increases myocardial oxygen demand in cardiogenic shock) | | | ✔ | | | | | |

## Table 4. Side/Adverse Effects*

The following side/adverse effects have been selected on the basis of their potential clinical significance (possible signs and symptoms in parentheses where appropriate)—not necessarily inclusive:

Legend:
**I** = Albuterol
**II** = Ephedrine
**III** = Epinephrine
**IV** = Ethylnorepinephrine
**V** = Fenoterol
**VI** = Isoproterenol
**VII** = Metaproterenol
**VIII** = Terbutaline

| | I | II | III | IV | V | VI | VII | VIII |
|---|---|---|---|---|---|---|---|---|
| **Medical attention needed** | | | | | | | | |
| Chest discomfort or pain, continuing or severe, or | ✔ | ✔ | ✔ | ✔ | ✔ | ✔ | ✔ | ✔ |
| Chills or fever or | | ✔ | ✔ | | | | | |
| Convulsions or | | | ✔ | ✔ | | | | |
| Dizziness or lightheadedness, continuing or severe, or | ✔ | ✔ | ✔ | ✔ | ✔ | ✔ | ✔ | ✔ |
| Fast heartbeat, continuing, or | ✔ | ✔ | ✔ | ✔ | ✔ | ✔ | ✔ | ✔ |
| Hallucinations or | | | ✔ | | | | | |
| Headache, continuing or severe, or | ✔ | ✔ | ✔ | | ✔ | ✔ | ✔ | ✔ |
| Increase in blood pressure, severe, or | ✔ | ✔† | ✔† | ✔ | ✔ | ✔ | ✔ | ✔ |
| Irregular heartbeat, continuing or severe, or | | ✔ | ✔ | ✔ | ✔ | ✔ | ✔ | ✔ |
| Mood or mental changes or | | ✔ | | | | | | |
| Muscle cramps, severe, or | | | | | ✔ | | | ✔ |
| Nausea or vomiting, continuing or severe, or | ✔ | ✔ | ✔ | ✔ | ✔ | ✔ | ✔ | ✔ |
| Pounding heartbeat, continuing or severe, or | ✔ | | | | | | | |
| Shortness of breath or troubled breathing, severe, or | | | | ✔ | | | | |
| Slow heartbeat or | | | | ✔ | | | | |
| Trembling, severe, or | ✔ | ✔ | ✔ | ✔ | ✔ | ✔ | ✔ | ✔ |
| Unusual anxiety, nervousness, or restlessness or | ✔ | ✔ | ✔ | ✔ | ✔ | ✔ | ✔ | ✔ |
| Unusually large pupils or blurred vision or | ✔ | | | ✔ | | | | |
| Unusual paleness and coldness of skin or | | | ✔ | ✔ | | | | |
| Weakness, severe (signs of overdose) | | ✔ | ✔ | ✔ | ✔ | | ✔ | ✔ |
| Chest discomfort or pain | R | R | R‡ | U | U | R | U | R |
| Hallucinations | U | § | § | U | U | U | U | U |
| Irregular heartbeat | U | | R‡ | U | U | R | U | R |
| Mood or mental changes | U | § | U | U | U | U | U | U |
| Numbness in hands or feet | U | U | U | U | U | U | U | U |
| Paradoxical bronchospasm (increase in wheezing or difficulty in breathing) | R | | R | R | R | | R | R |
| Unusual bruising | U | U | U | U | U | U | U | U |
| **Medical attention needed only if continuing or bothersome** | | | | | | | | |
| Difficult or painful urination | L | L | U | U | U | U | U | U |
| Dizziness or lightheadedness | L | L | L# | L | L | L | L | L |
| Drowsiness | L | U | U | U | U | U | U | L |
| Dryness or irritation of mouth or throat# | L | L | R | — | L | M | U | L |
| Fast heartbeat | M | L | M†† | L | L | L | L | L |
| Flushing or redness of face or skin | L | U | L# | U | U | L | U | U |
| Headache | L | L | L# | L | L | L | L | L |
| Heartburn | L | U | U | — | L | U | L | U |
| Increased sweating | L | L | L# | U | L | L | L | L |
| Increase in blood pressure | L** | L | L | L** | U | L** | L | L |
| Loss of appetite | R | L | U | U | U | U | U | U |
| Muscle cramps or twitching | L | U | U | U | L | U | L | L |
| Nausea | M | L | L# | L | L | L | L | L |
| Nervousness or restlessness | M | M | M†† | U | M | M | M | M |
| Pain or stinging at intramuscular injection site | L | U | U | U | — | U | — | — |
| Pounding heartbeat | M | L | M†† | L | L | L | L | L |
| Trembling | M | L | L# | L | M | L | L | M |
| Trouble in sleeping | L | M | L# | U | L | M | U | L |
| Unusual paleness | R | L | L# | U | U | U | U | U |
| Vomiting | L | L | L# | U | L | L | L | L |
| Weakness | L | L | L# | L | L | L | L | L |

## Table 4. Side/Adverse Effects *(continued)**

| The following side/adverse effects have been selected on the basis of their potential clinical significance (possible signs and symptoms in parentheses where appropriate)—not necessarily inclusive: | Legend:<br>**I**=Albuterol<br>**II**=Ephedrine<br>**III**=Epinephrine<br>**IV**=Ethylnorepinephrine | | | | **V**=Fenoterol<br>**VI**=Isoproterenol<br>**VII**=Metaproterenol<br>**VIII**=Terbutaline | | | |
|---|---|---|---|---|---|---|---|---|
| | **I** | **II** | **III** | **IV** | **V** | **VI** | **VII** | **VIII** |
| **Medical attention *not* needed**<br>    *Pinkish to red coloration of saliva* | — | — | — | — | — | M‡‡ | — | — |

*Differences in frequency of occurrence may reflect either lack of clinical-use data or actual pharmacologic distinctions among agents (although the agents' pharmacologic similarity suggests that side effects occurring with one may occur with the others). M=more frequent; L=less frequent; R=rare; U=unknown.
　†Or possibly a severe decrease in blood pressure.
　‡More frequent with high doses.
　§With high doses.
　#Less frequent with injection.
　**Or possibly a decrease in blood pressure.
　††More frequent with injection.
　‡‡For sublingual dosage form of isoproterenol.

## Table 5. Patient Consultation

| As an aid to patient consultation, refer to *Advice for the Patient, Bronchodilators, Adrenergic (Oral/Injection)*.<br><br>In providing consultation, consider emphasizing the following selected information (» = major clinical signficance): | Legend:<br>**I**=Albuterol<br>**II**=Ephedrine<br>**III**=Epinephrine<br>**IV**=Ethylnorepinephrine | | | | **V**=Fenoterol<br>**VI**=Isoproterenol<br>**VII**=Metaproterenol<br>**VIII**=Terbutaline | | | |
|---|---|---|---|---|---|---|---|---|
| | **I** | **II** | **III** | **IV** | **V** | **VI** | **VII** | **VIII** |
| **Before using this medication**<br>» Conditions affecting use, especially: | | | | | | | | |
| 　　Sensitivity to sympathomimetics | ✓ | ✓ | ✓ | ✓ | ✓ | ✓ | ✓ | ✓ |
| 　　Pregnancy— | | | | | | | | |
| 　　　　Studies in animals have shown albuterol, epinephrine, and metaproterenol to cause teratogenic effects when medication given in doses many times human dose | ✓ | | ✓ | | | | ✓ | |
| 　　　　Use of epinephrine during pregnancy may cause anoxia in fetus | | | ✓ | | | | | |
| 　　　　Parenteral administration of terbutaline during pregnancy reported to cause fetal tachycardia | | | | | | | | ✓ |
| 　　Labor and/or delivery— | | | | | | | | |
| 　　　　Albuterol given intravenously or orally reportedly inhibits uterine contractions | ✓ | | | | | | | |
| 　　　　Epinephrine is not recommended for use during labor because it may delay second stage; also may cause prolonged uterine atony with hemorrhage when given in sufficient dosage to reduce uterine contractions | | | ✓ | | | | | |
| 　　　　Terbutaline inhibits uterine activity during second and third trimesters of pregnancy and may inhibit labor; when administered during labor; terbutaline reported to cause serious adverse reactions (e.g., transient hypokalemia, pulmonary edema, hypoglycemia) in mother and hypoglycemia in neonates of mothers treated with parenteral terbutaline | | | | | | | | ✓ |
| 　　Breast-feeding— | | | | | | | | |
| 　　　　Not known if albuterol is distributed into breast milk; however, some animal studies have shown albuterol to be potentially tumorigenic | ✓ | | | | | | | |
| 　　　　Epinephrine distributed into breast milk; use by nursing mothers may cause serious adverse reactions in infant | | | ✓ | | | | | |
| 　　　　Terbutaline distributed into breast milk; some animal studies have shown terbutaline to be potentially tumorigenic | | | | | | | | ✓ |
| 　　Use in children—Epinephrine should be used with caution in infants and children, since syncope has occurred following administration of epinephrine in asthmatic children | | | ✓ | | | | | |
| 　　Dental—Epinephrine present in gingival retraction cords; systemic absorption of epinephrine from retraction cords may occur; epinephrine retraction cords should be used with caution in patients with cardiovascular problems | | | ✓ | | | | | |
| 　　Other medications, especially— | | | | | | | | |
| 　　　　Beta-adrenergic blocking agents | ✓ | ✓ | ✓ | ✓ | ✓ | ✓ | ✓ | ✓ |
| 　　　　Cocaine, mucosal-local | ✓ | ✓ | ✓ | ✓ | ✓ | ✓ | ✓ | ✓ |
| 　　　　Digitalis glycosides | ✓ | ✓ | ✓ | ✓ | ✓ | ✓ | ✓ | ✓ |
| 　　　　Ergoloid mesylates | | | ✓ | ✓ | | | | |
| 　　　　Ergotamine | | ✓ | ✓ | | | | | |
| 　　　　Maprotiline | ✓ | ✓ | ✓ | | | | ✓ | |
| 　　　　Monoamine oxidase (MAO) inhibitors | ✓ | ✓ | ✓ | | ✓ | ✓ | ✓ | ✓ |
| 　　　　Tricyclic antidepressants | ✓ | ✓ | ✓ | | | | ✓ | ✓ |
| 　　Other medical problems, especially— | | | | | | | | |
| 　　　　Brain damage, organic | | | ✓ | | | | | |
| 　　　　Cardiovascular disease | ✓ | ✓ | ✓ | ✓ | ✓ | ✓ | ✓ | ✓ |
| **Proper use of this medication** | | | | | | | | |
| 　　Not using if solution or suspension is pinkish to brownish in color or if solution contains a precipitate | | | ✓ | ✓ | | ✓ | | |

**668**     Bronchodilators, Adrenergic (Systemic)                                                                                                 *USP DI*

## Table 5. Patient Consultation *(continued)*

As an aid to patient consultation, refer to *Advice for the Patient, Bronchodilators, Adrenergic (Oral/Injection).*

In providing consultation, consider emphasizing the following selected information (» = major clinical signficance):

Legend:
I = Albuterol
II = Ephedrine
III = Epinephrine
IV = Ethylnorepinephrine
V = Fenoterol
VI = Isoproterenol
VII = Metaproterenol
VIII = Terbutaline

|   | I | II | III | IV | V | VI | VII | VIII |
|---|---|----|-----|----|---|----|-----|------|
| » Importance of not using more medication than the amount recommended | ✔ | ✔ | ✔ | ✔ | ✔ | ✔ | ✔ | ✔ |
| » Taking the medication a few hours before bedtime to minimize the possibility of insomnia |  | ✔ |  |  |  |  |  |  |
| » Proper dosing | ✔ | ✔ | ✔ | ✔ | ✔ | ✔ | ✔ | ✔ |
| Missed dose: If on scheduled dosing regimen, using as soon as possible; using any remaining doses for the day at regularly spaced intervals; not doubling doses | ✔ | ✔ | ✔ |  | ✔ | ✔ | ✔ | ✔ |
| *For extended-release tablet dosage form* <br> Swallowing tablet whole; not crushing, breaking, or chewing | ✔ |  |  |  |  |  |  |  |
| *For sublingual tablet dosage form* <br> Not chewing or swallowing tablet whole, but dissolving slowly under tongue; not swallowing until tablet completely dissolved |  |  |  |  |  | ✔ |  |  |
| *For injection dosage forms* <br> » Using only for conditions as prescribed by physician <br> Keeping ready for use at all times; also keeping telephone numbers for physician and nearest hospital emergency room readily available <br> Checking expiration date routinely; replacing medication before it expires <br> Knowing correct administration technique for self-administration; checking with physician if necessary |  |  | ✔ <br> ✔ <br> ✔ <br> ✔ | ✔ <br> ✔ <br> ✔ <br> ✔ |  |  |  |  |
| For emergency use in allergic reaction— <br> » Using medication immediately <br> Notifying physician immediately or going to nearest hospital emergency room <br> If stung by an insect, removing insect's stinger; applying ice packs or sodium bicarbonate soaks, if available, to area stung <br> For auto-injector use: <br> Importance of not removing safety cap on auto-injector before ready to use <br> Reading patient instructions carefully before need to use medication <br> Procedures for using— <br> Removing gray safety cap <br> Placing black tip on thigh at right angle to leg <br> Pressing hard into thigh until auto-injector functions; holding in place several seconds; removing and properly discarding <br> Massaging injection area for 10 seconds |  |  | ✔ |  |  |  |  |  |
| » Proper storage | ✔ | ✔ | ✔ | ✔ | ✔ | ✔ | ✔ | ✔ |
| **Precautions while using this medication** <br> Diabetics: May increase blood glucose concentrations |  |  |  | ✔ |  |  |  |  |
| **Side/adverse effects** <br> Signs of potential side effects, especially: <br> Allergic reaction to sulfites present in some preparations <br> Chest discomfort or pain <br> Hallucinations, with high doses <br> Irregular heartbeat <br> Mood or mental changes <br> Numbness in feet or hands <br> Paradoxical bronchospasm <br> Unusual bruising | <br><br><br>✔<br><br><br><br>✔ | <br>✔<br>✔<br><br><br><br><br>✔ | <br>✔<br>✔<br>✔<br>✔<br>✔<br><br>✔ | <br>✔<br>✔<br>✔<br>✔<br><br><br>✔ | <br>✔<br><br><br><br><br><br>✔ | <br>✔<br><br>✔<br>✔<br><br><br>✔ | <br><br><br><br><br><br><br>✔ | <br>✔<br><br>✔<br><br><br><br>✔ |
| In some animal studies, albuterol caused increased incidence of benign leiomyomas of mesovarium when administered at doses many times the maximum human inhalation or oral dose | ✔ |  |  |  |  |  |  |  |
| Some studies in animals have shown that terbutaline caused increased incidence of leiomyomas of mesovarium, ovarian cysts, and hyperplasia of mesovarium when administered at oral doses many times the recommended daily adult dose |  |  |  |  |  |  |  | ✔ |

# BRONCHODILATORS, THEOPHYLLINE  Systemic

This monograph includes information on the following: 1) Aminophylline; 2) Oxtriphylline; 3) Theophylline.

**INN:**
Oxtriphylline—Choline theophyllinate

**BAN:**
Oxtriphylline—Choline theophyllinate

**JAN:**
Oxtriphylline—Choline theophylline

**VA CLASSIFICATION** (Primary/Secondary):
Aminophylline

Injection—RE104/RE900
Oral solution—RE104/RE109; RE900
Tablets—RE104/RE109
Extended-release tablets—RE104/RE109
Oxtriphylline—RE104/RE109
Theophylline
Capsules—RE104/RE109
Extended-release capsules—RE104/RE109
Elixir—RE104/RE109; RE900
Oral solution—RE104/RE109; RE900
Syrup—RE104/RE109; RE900

Tablets—RE104/RE109
Extended-release tablets—RE104/RE109
Theophylline in Dextrose—RE104/RE900

Commonly used brand name(s): *Aerolate Sr*[3]; *Apo-Oxtriphylline*[2]; *Apo-Theo LA*[3]; *Asmalix*[3]; *Choledyl*[2]; *Choledyl SA*[2]; *Elixophyllin*[3]; *Lanophyllin*[3]; *PMS Theophylline*[3]; *PMS-Oxtriphylline*[2]; *Phyllocontin*[1]; *Phyllocontin-350*[1]; *Pulmophylline*[3]; *Quibron-T Dividose*[3]; *Quibron-T/SR Dividose*[3]; *Respbid*[3]; *Slo-Bid Gyrocaps*[3]; *Slo-Phyllin*[3]; *T-Phyl*[3]; *Theo-24*[3]; *Theo-Dur*[3]; *Theo-SR*[3]; *Theo-Time*[3]; *Theo-X*[3]; *Theobid Duracaps*[3]; *Theochron*[3]; *Theoclear L.A.-260*[3]; *Theoclear-80*[3]; *Theolair*[3]; *Theolair SR*[3]; *Theolair-SR*[3]; *Theovent Long-Acting*[3]; *Truphylline*[1]; *Truxophyllin*[3]; *Uni-Dur*[3]; *Uniphyl*[3].

Note: For a listing of dosage forms and brand names by country availability, see *Dosage Forms* section(s).

## Category

Bronchodilator—Aminophylline; Oxtriphylline; Theophylline.
Asthma prophylactic—Aminophylline; Oxtriphylline; Theophylline.
Stimulant, respiratory—Aminophylline Injection USP; Aminophylline Oral Solution USP; Theophylline Elixir; Theophylline Oral Solution; Theophylline Syrup.
Antidote (to dipyridamole toxicity)—Aminophylline Injection USP.

## Indications

Note: Bracketed information in the *Indications* section refers to uses that are not included in U.S. product labeling.

### Accepted

Asthma, bronchial (prophylaxis and treatment)—Aminophylline, oxtriphylline, and theophylline are indicated for the prevention and treatment of bronchial asthma symptoms. They improve pulmonary function and reduce the frequency and severity of symptoms such as wheezing, cough, shortness of breath, or dyspnea.

Some studies have shown that theophylline does not provide additional benefit in the initial treatment of *acute* airway obstruction when optimal therapy is provided with inhaled or injected beta-2-adrenergic bronchodilators and systemic glucocorticoids in patients not already receiving a methylxanthine. Although patients hospitalized with asthma may benefit from administration of aminophylline or theophylline, these medications should not be relied upon to produce immediate bronchodilation, even if therapeutic theophylline concentrations are rapidly achieved.

Aminophylline, oxtriphylline, and theophylline may benefit those patients with an inadequate response to anti-inflammatory medications and beta-adrenergic bronchodilators; however, theophylline bronchodilators are not considered to be first-line therapy.

Bronchitis, chronic (treatment)
Emphysema, pulmonary (treatment) or
Pulmonary disease, chronic obstructive, other (treatment)—Aminophylline, oxtriphylline, and theophylline may be indicated in the treatment of reversible airway obstruction associated with chronic bronchitis, emphysema, or other chronic obstructive pulmonary disease.

[Apnea, neonatal (treatment adjunct)][1]—Aminophylline oral solution and injection and theophylline oral liquids are used in the treatment of idiopathic apnea in neonates, characterized by cessation of respiration that lasts 20 seconds or longer. Aminophylline or theophylline should be considered in addition to administration of oxygen, sensory stimulation, or low pressure nasal continuous positive airway pressure.

Toxicity, dipyridamole (treatment)[1]—Parenteral aminophylline is used to reverse the adenosine-mediated adverse effects of dipyridamole, such as angina pectoris, ventricular arrhythmias, bronchospasm, and severe hypotension.

### Unaccepted

Parenteral aminophylline and theophylline have been used in the treatment of Cheyne-Stokes respiration. However, there is insufficient evidence to establish the efficacy of these medications for this indication.

[1]Not included in Canadian product labeling.

## Pharmacology/Pharmacokinetics

### Physicochemical characteristics

Source—
Aminophylline: Theophylline compound with ethylenediamine.
Oxtriphylline: The choline salt of theophylline.
Molecular weight—
Aminophylline: 420.43.
Oxtriphylline: 283.33.
Theophylline: 198.18.

### Mechanism of action/Effect

The exact mechanism of action by which theophylline produces its pharmacologic effect is unknown; it is likely to involve multiple mechanisms.

Bronchodilator; asthma prophylactic—Theophylline directly relaxes smooth muscle in the bronchial airways and pulmonary blood vessels. This action is believed to be mediated by selective inhibition of specific phosphodiesterases (PDEs), which in turn produces an increase in intracellular cyclic 3′,5′-adenosine monophosphate (cyclic AMP). *In vitro* study results demonstrate that the PDE isoenzyme types III and IV may play a primary role. Inhibition of these isoenzymes may also mediate certain theophylline side effects such as emesis, hypotension, and tachycardia. Theophylline also demonstrates adenosine receptor antagonism, which may contribute to its effect on bronchial airways.

Respiratory stimulant—Theophylline is believed to stimulate the medullary respiratory center, presumably by increasing sensitivity to the stimulatory actions of carbon dioxide.

Antidote (to dipyridamole toxicity)—Involves antagonism of the coronary vasodilatory effects of the increased concentrations of adenosine produced by intravenous administration of dipyridamole during myocardial perfusion studies.

### Other actions/effects

Theophylline may attenuate airway hyperreactivity associated with the late phase response that is induced by inhaled allergens by an undefined mechanism which is not attributable to PDE inhibition or adenosine antagonism. Theophylline also has been reported to increase the number and activity of suppressor T-cells in the peripheral blood. Whether these actions are clinically relevant is not clear.

Theophylline may produce other physiologic effects such as transient diuresis, stimulation of cardiac muscle, improved contractility of the diaphragm, reduction of systemic and pulmonary vascular resistance, increased gastric acid secretion, central nervous system stimulation, and cerebral vasoconstriction.

### Absorption

Immediate-release capsule, liquid, or tablet dosage forms—Rapidly and completely absorbed. The rate of absorption may be slowed by concurrent ingestion of food or magnesium-containing antacids; however, the effect on the extent of absorption is generally not clinically significant.

Delayed-release tablets—Enteric coating provides delayed and possibly incomplete absorption compared with immediate-release dosage forms.

Extended-release capsules or tablets—The rate of absorption varies among different formulations and is slower than with immediate-release products; the extent of absorption may also vary. Significant intra- and interindividual differences in absorption have been reported. Serum concentration fluctuations are most apparent in patients demonstrating increased theophylline clearance. Co-administration of antacids or food may only slow the rate of absorption from some extended-release formulations, while significantly altering the extent of absorption from others. Some formulations designed for once-a-day administration may be substantially affected by food.

Intramuscular—Slow absorption; medication may precipitate at the injection site.

Suppository—Slow and unreliable absorption.

### Distribution

Theophylline distributes rapidly into peripheral non-adipose tissues and body water, including breast milk and cerebrospinal fluid. It freely crosses the placenta. The apparent volume of distribution (Vol$_D$) for theophylline averages 0.45 L per kg of body weight (L/kg) and ranges from 0.3 to 0.7 L/kg (30 to 70% of ideal body weight) in both adults and children. The Vol$_D$ may be increased, probably due to altered protein binding, in premature neonates, adults with cirrhosis, patients with uncorrected acidemia, elderly patients, pregnant women during the third trimester, critically ill patients, mechanically ventilated adults, and children with protein-calorie malnutrition.

### Protein binding

Moderate (40%). Primarily to albumin. Patients with reduced protein binding may have low total serum theophylline concentrations when unbound theophylline is in the therapeutic range.

### Biotransformation

Aminophylline and oxtriphylline—
    Release free theophylline at physiologic pH.
Theophylline—
    Hepatic; no first-pass effect. Believed to occur over multiple parallel pathways, mediated by cytochrome P-450 isoenzymes P-4501A2, P-4503A3, and P-4502E1. In neonates, several of these pathways are undeveloped but mature slowly over the first year of life. Caffeine is a minor active metabolite, except in premature neonates and children less than 6 months of age, in whom caffeine's extremely

long half-life results in significant accumulation. The half-life of caffeine shortens over the first 6 months of life because of maturation of its metabolic pathway. Thereafter, caffeine does not accumulate in older children and adults. Major inactive metabolites in adults and children older than 6 months of age are 1,3-dimethyluric acid, 3-methylxanthine, and 1-methyluric acid.

Theophylline approximates first-order elimination kinetics, where serum concentrations follow a log-linear decay. However, zero-order kinetics, where elimination becomes dependent on the serum concentration, can be observed in patients at therapeutic concentrations. This is probably due to capacity limitations of the hepatic enzymes that metabolize theophylline, and is clinically relevant for some patients in that a small change in theophylline dosage may result in a disproportionately large change in serum concentration.

### Half-life
Elimination half-life and total body clearance values for theophylline in various patients are as follows—

| Patient characteristics | Half-life Mean (Range)* (hr) | Total body clearance Mean (Range)* (mL/kg/min) |
|---|---|---|
| **Age** | | |
| Premature neonates | | |
| 3–15 days† | 30 (17–43) | 0.29 (0.09–0.49) |
| 25–57 days† | 20 (9.4–30.6) | 0.64 (0.04–1.2) |
| Term infants | | |
| 1–2 days† | (25–26.5) | |
| 3–26 weeks† | 11 (6–29) | |
| Children | | |
| 1–4 yrs | 3.4 (1.2–5.6) | 1.7 (0.5–2.9) |
| 4–12 yrs | | 1.57 (0.83–2.31) |
| 13–15 yrs | | 0.88 (0.38–1.38) |
| 6–17 yrs‡ | 3.7 (1.5–5.9) | 1.4 (0.2–2.6) |
| Adults§ | 8.2 (6.1–12.8) | 0.65 (0.27–1.03) |
| Elderly# | 9.8 (1.6–18) | 0.41 (0.21–0.61) |
| **Concurrent illness or altered physiologic state** | | |
| Acute pulmonary edema | 19 (3.1–82)** | 0.33 (0.07–2.35)** |
| COPD†† | 11 (9.4–12.6) | 0.54 (0.44–0.64) |
| COPD and cor pulmonale | | 0.48 (0.08–0.88) |
| Cystic fibrosis‡‡ | 6 (1.8–10.2) | 1.25 (0.31–2.19) |
| Fever§§ | 7 (1–13) | |
| Hepatic disease | | |
| Acute hepatitis | 19.2 (16.6–21.8) | 0.35 (0.25–0.45) |
| Cholestasis | 14.4 (5.7–31.8) | 0.65 (0.25–1.45) |
| Cirrhosis | 32 (10–56)** | 0.31 (0.1–0.7)** |
| Hyperthyroidism | 4.5 (3.7–5.6) | 0.8 (0.68–0.97) |
| Hypothyroidism | 11.6 (8.2–25) | 0.38 (0.13–0.57) |
| Pregnancy | | |
| First trimester | 8.5 (3.1–13.9) | |
| Second trimester | 8.8 (3.9–13.8) | |
| Third trimester | 13.3 (8.4–17.6) | |
| Sepsis## | 18.8 (6.3–24.1) | 0.46 (0.19–1.9) |

*Reported or estimated range (mean ±2 SD) where actual range not reported.
†Postnatal age.
‡Elimination half-life and total body clearance gradually become slower until adult values are reached.
§Otherwise healthy, nonsmoking asthmatics.
#Nonsmokers with normal cardiac, liver, and renal function; 70 to 85 years of age.
**Median.
††Stable; older than 60 years of age; at least 1 year since stopped smoking.
‡‡Patients 14 to 28 years of age.
§§Associated with acute viral respiratory illness in children 9 to 15 years of age.
##With multi-organ failure.

### Time to peak concentration
Theophylline—
  Immediate-release capsules, tablets, or oral solution: 1 to 2 hours.
  Delayed-release tablets: Approximately 4 hours.
  Extended-release capsules and tablets: 4 to 13 hours depending upon the specific product.

### Therapeutic serum concentration
Bronchodilator—
  For most patients, a conservative goal of therapy would be to target peak steady-state serum concentrations in the range of 5 to 15 mcg/mL (27.5 to 82.5 micromoles/L). Although improved pulmonary function is evident over the range of 5 to 20 mcg/mL (27.5 to 110 micromoles/L), concentrations at the upper end of the therapeutic range may be associated with an increased potential for toxicity. When serum concentrations exceed 20 mcg/mL (110 micromoles/L), the probability of toxicity increases.
Respiratory stimulant—
  Neonatal apnea: Steady-state peak serum concentrations of 5 to 12 mcg per mL (27.5 to 66 micromoles per L).

### Elimination
Theophylline—
  Renal; approximately 10% excreted unchanged in the urine in adults; amount excreted unchanged may reach 50% in neonates.
  In dialysis: Charcoal hemoperfusion increases theophylline clearance 2 to 4 times. Hemodialysis and peritoneal dialysis are estimated to increase theophylline clearance by approximately 50% and 30%, respectively.

## Precautions to Consider

### Carcinogenicity/Tumorigenicity
Long-term studies have not been done in humans. The results of long-term carcinogenicity studies performed in mice and rats are pending.

### Mutagenicity
Theophylline has not been shown to be mutagenic in Ames salmonella, *in vivo* and *in vitro* cytogenetics, micronucleus and Chinese hamster ovary test systems.

### Pregnancy/Reproduction
Fertility—Studies in rodents have shown that theophylline impairs fertility in mice given oral doses approximately 1 to 3 times the human dose on a mg per square meter of body surface area (mg/m$^2$), and in rats given oral doses approximately 2 times the human dose on a mg/m$^2$ basis.

Pregnancy—Although adequate and well-controlled studies in pregnant women have not been done, these medications are used in pregnancy when the risk of treatment is preferable to the risk of placental hypoxemia from uncontrolled pulmonary disease. The Collaborative Perinatal Project monitored 193 mother-child pairs exposed to theophylline during the first trimester and found no evidence of association with teratogenicity.

Theophylline crosses the placenta; cord blood concentrations are approximately equal to the maternal serum concentration. Because of this, higher-than-recommended serum concentrations during pregnancy may result in potentially dangerous serum theophylline and caffeine concentrations in the neonate. Tachycardia, irritability, jitteriness, and vomiting have been reported; therefore, neonates of mothers taking these medications during pregnancy should be monitored for signs of theophylline toxicity.

Theophylline clearance is reported to be lower in the third trimester, which may necessitate more frequent theophylline serum concentration determinations and possible dosage reductions.

Theophylline was not teratogenic in mice or rats given oral doses approximately 2 and 3 times the recommended human dose on a mg/m$^2$ basis, respectively. Embryotoxicity was observed in rats given 220 mg per kg of body weight, in the absence of maternal toxicity.

FDA Pregnancy Category C.

Labor—Theophylline has been shown to slightly inhibit uterine contractions.

### Breast-feeding
Less than 1% of a maternal theophylline dose distributes into breast milk; this may cause irritability in the infant.

### Pediatrics
Caution is recommended in neonates and children less than 1 year of age, especially in premature neonates and in infants less than 3 months of age with renal function impairment, because theophylline clearance is reduced, resulting in lower dosage requirements. Clearance progressively increases over the first year of life, remains constant during the subsequent 9 years, and gradually declines to mean adult values by 16 years of age.

### Geriatrics
Caution is recommended when aminophylline, oxtriphylline, or theophylline is used in patients older than 60 years of age. Theophylline clearance in healthy adults older than 60 years of age is 30% lower than in healthy younger adults. These patients may require adjustment in dosage or dosing interval. Severe signs or symptoms of toxicity resulting from chronic overdose are more common in elderly patients, occurring in 65% of patients 60 years of age or older with serum theophylline concentrations 30 mcg per mL (165 micromoles per L).

### Drug interactions and/or related problems
The following drug interactions and/or related problems have been selected on the basis of their potential clinical significance (possible mechanism in parentheses where appropriate)—not necessarily inclusive (» = major clinical significance):

Note: Combinations containing any of the following medications, depending on the amount present, may also interact with this medication.

*Pharmacokinetic interactions*
Medications that decrease theophylline clearance
(the medications listed in the table below probably decrease theophylline clearance by inhibition of one or more hepatic cytochrome P-450 isoenzyme; changes in clearance of approximately 25% or greater can have clinical significance; monitoring of serum theophylline concentrations and/or dosage adjustments are strongly recommended when concurrent use of these medications with aminophylline, oxtriphylline, or theophylline is initiated or discontinued)

| Medication | Decrease in Clearance (avg. %) | Increase in Serum Concentration (avg. %)* |
|---|---|---|
| Alcohol† | 25 | 33 |
| Allopurinol‡ | 20 | 25 |
| » Cimetidine | 33 | 33–50 |
| Contraceptives, estrogen-containing, oral | 25–34 | 33–50 |
| Disulfiram§ | 21–33 | 25–50 |
| Fluoroquinolone antibiotics# | | |
| » Ciprofloxacin | 20–40 | 25–66 |
| » Enoxacin | 40–70 | 66–300 |
| » Fluvoxamine | 100 | >300 |
| » Interferon alpha, recombinant | 10–50 | 11–100 |
| Macrolide antibiotics** | | |
| » Clarithromycin | 20 | 25 |
| » Erythromycin | 5–35 | 5–50 |
| » Troleandomycin | 25–50†† | 33–100 |
| Methotrexate‡‡ | 15–25 | 18–33 |
| » Mexiletine | 43 | 75 |
| Propafenone | | 40§§ |
| » Pentoxifylline | | 30 (0–95) |
| » Propranolol | 30–50 | 40–100 |
| » Tacrine | 50 | 100 |
| » Thiabendazole | 66 | >200 |
| » Ticlopidine | 37 | 60 |
| Verapamil | 14–23 | 16–30 |

*Calculation based on reported change in clearance if actual change not reported.
†3 mL of whiskey per kg of body weight as a single dose decreased clearance up to 24 hrs.
‡≥600 mg per day.
§Dose-dependent, 250 and 500 mg.
#Norfloxacin, lomefloxacin, and ofloxacin are not considered to significantly decrease theophylline clearance.
**Azithromycin does not appear to alter theophylline clearance.
††Once-daily dose decreases clearance by average of 25%.
‡‡Low-dose intramuscular regimen of 15 mg per week.
§§Beta-2-antagonist effect may decrease effect of theophylline.

Medications that increase theophylline clearance
(the medications listed in the table below probably increase theophylline clearance by induction of one or more hepatic cytochrome P-450 isoenzyme; changes in clearance of approximately 25% or greater can have clinical significance; monitoring of serum theophylline concentrations and/or dosage adjustments are strongly recommended when concurrent use of these medications with aminophylline, oxtriphylline, or theophylline is initiated or discontinued)

| Medication | Increase in Clearance (avg. %) | Decrease in Serum Concentration (avg. %)* |
|---|---|---|
| Aminoglutethimide | 18–43 | 15–30 |
| Carbamazepine | 33 | 25 |
| Isoproterenol, intravenous | 21 | 17 |
| » Moricizine | 44–66 | 30–40 |
| Phenobarbital | 33 | 25 |
| » Phenytoin | 35–75 | 25–43 |
| » Rifampin | 64–100 | 40–50 |

*Calculation based on reported change in clearance if actual change not reported.

*Pharmacodynamic or other drug interactions*
Adenosine
(concurrent use with theophylline may antagonize the cardiovascular effects of adenosine; larger doses of adenosine may be required or alternative therapy should be used)

Benzodiazepines
(theophylline may reverse benzodiazepine sedation; caution is recommended when starting or stopping either medication)

» Beta-adrenergic blocking agents, including ophthalmic agents
(concurrent use with theophylline may result in inhibition of its bronchodilator effect; although agents with beta-1-selectivity may be less antagonistic, extreme caution is recommended if beta-adrenergic blocking agents are used in patients with bronchospasm)

Ephedrine
(concurrent use with theophylline may result in increased frequency of nausea, nervousness, or insomnia)

» Halothane
(ventricular arrhythmias have been reported when halothane is used concurrently with theophylline)

» Ketamine
(concurrent use with theophylline may lower the seizure threshold)

Lithium
(concurrent use of lithium with theophylline may increase renal elimination of lithium, thus decreasing its therapeutic effect)

Neuromuscular blocking agents, nondepolarizing
(concurrent use with theophylline may antagonize neuromuscular blocking effects; a larger dose of neuromuscular blocking agent may be required)

» Smoking tobacco or marijuana
(induces the hepatic metabolism of theophylline, resulting in increased clearance and decreased serum concentrations. Passive smoking may also increase theophylline clearance. Induction is attributed to the polyaromatic hydrocarbons in smoke. Following cessation of cigarette smoking, theophylline clearance begins to decrease after 1 week; however, normalization may require 6 months to 2 years. Dosage adjustments and/or additional theophylline serum determinations may be necessary when smoking is started or stopped)

Sucralfate
(concurrent use with aminophylline, oxtriphylline, or theophylline may result in adsorption of the theophylline bronchodilator if medications are administered less than 2 hours apart)

### Laboratory value alterations
The following have been selected on the basis of their potential clinical significance (possible effect in parentheses where appropriate)—not necessarily inclusive (» = major clinical significance):

With diagnostic test results
» Dipyridamole-assisted myocardial perfusion studies
(the theophylline bronchodilators reverse the effects of dipyridamole on myocardial blood flow, thereby interfering with test results; dipyridamole-assisted myocardial perfusion studies should not be performed if therapy with aminophylline, oxtriphylline, or theophylline cannot be withheld for 36 hours prior to the test)

With physiology/laboratory test values
Cholesterol and
Free cortisol excretion, urinary and
Free fatty acids and
Glucose, plasma and
HDL and HDL/LDL ratio and
Uric acid, plasma
(concentrations may be increased by theophylline serum concentrations within the therapeutic range)

Triiodothyronine, serum
(concentration may be transiently decreased by theophylline serum concentrations within the therapeutic range)

**Medical considerations/Contraindications**

The medical considerations/contraindications included have been selected on the basis of their potential clinical significance (reasons given in parentheses where appropriate)—not necessarily inclusive (» = major clinical significance).

*Risk-benefit should be considered when the following medical problems exist:*

- » Acute pulmonary edema or
- » Congestive heart failure or
  Fever, sustained or
- » Hepatic disease or
- » Hypothyroidism, not optimally controlled or
- » Sepsis
    (theophylline clearance may be decreased, resulting in increased theophylline serum concentrations)
    (the extent to which fever, as opposed to other complicating factors such as acute viral illness, affects theophylline clearance is controversial; however, some practitioners recommend additional monitoring and/or dose reduction when the body temperature is 102 °F or greater for at least 24 hours, or when a lower temperature elevation persists for a longer period)

  Gastritis, active or
  Peptic ulcer disease, active
    (may be exacerbated because theophylline increases gastric acid secretion)

  Gastroesophageal reflux
    (theophylline may decrease lower esophageal sphincter pressure, resulting in increased gastroesophageal reflux)

- » Seizure disorder
    (aminophylline, oxtriphylline, or theophylline may lower the seizure threshold; caution is recommended unless the patient is receiving appropriate anticonvulsant therapy)

  Tachyarrhythmias
    (condition may be exacerbated at higher theophylline serum concentrations)

- » Sensitivity to a theophylline bronchodilator or ethylenediamine

**Patient monitoring**

The following may be especially important in patient monitoring (other tests may be warranted in some patients, depending on condition; » = major clinical significance):

Caffeine concentrations, serum
  (determinations may be required in neonates; usually necessary only if adverse effects occur when the serum theophylline concentration is within the therapeutic range)

Pulmonary function tests
  (objective measures of lung function are essential for diagnosis and for guiding therapeutic decision making in asthma; measurement of forced expiratory airflow, using a spirometer or a peak expiratory flowmeter, is recommended at periodic intervals)

» Theophylline concentrations
  (dosage requirements are usually guided by measurement of the peak serum concentration obtained at the expected time of the peak, depending upon the specific product characteristics; the frequency of determinations should relate to the specific clinical situation)

  (theophylline determinations are recommended when initiating therapy, before increasing the dose when a patient fails to exhibit the expected results, at the appearance of any adverse reaction, whenever any change in physiologic state or medication known to alter theophylline elimination occurs, and upon the addition of any new medication with an unknown effect on theophylline elimination; also recommended at least every 6 to 12 months in stable patients)

  (blood samples obtained for guidance of therapy should be collected during steady-state conditions, which are generally reached after 48 to 72 hours of treatment, provided that the medication is taken at regular intervals, with no missed or extra doses. Steady-state conditions may not be reached for up to 5 days in patients with factors known to decrease theophylline clearance. On each occasion, blood samples should be obtained during the same dosing interval, due to the diurnal variation in the absorption of these medications)

  (for intravenous therapy, concentrations may be determined 30 to 60 minutes after an intravenous loading dose, approximately 8 to 12 hours after initiating continuous intravenous therapy, and at approximately 24-hour intervals during continuous intravenous therapy)

  (trough concentration may be useful when evaluating serum concentration–time profiles; determinations may be performed just before the next dose or, for once-daily evening administration of an extended-release product, the morning following a dose)

  (caution is recommended in interpreting serum theophylline concentrations in patients with low albumin; total serum theophylline concentrations may be low when unbound theophylline is in the therapeutic range; measurement of unbound serum theophylline concentration provides a more reliable basis for dosage adjustment)

  (caution is recommended in interpreting the results of rapid theophylline immunoassays for uremic patients, because falsely high values may occur. Also, when theophylline concentration is determined via high pressure liquid chromatography, sulfamethoxazole may cause inaccurate test results and large doses of ampicillin, cephalothin, or acetazolamide may cause falsely high concentrations. Determinations via specific immunoassay or high pressure liquid chromatography are not affected by caffeine or dyphylline. However, when theophylline is measured via spectrophotometry, caffeine [including caffeine-containing substances such as chocolate, coffee, tea, colas, or medications] or acetaminophen may cause falsely high concentrations)

Note: Concentrations in saliva are approximately 60% of serum concentrations; however, the saliva-to-serum concentration ratio may not remain constant within the same patient; caution is recommended in use and interpretation of the data without the use of special techniques.

## Side/Adverse Effects

Note: The less severe signs or symptoms of toxicity, such as continuing or severe abdominal pain, agitation, confusion or change in behavior, diarrhea, hematemesis, hypotension, trembling, and continued vomiting, do not always precede the more serious ones such as sinus tachycardia, ventricular arrhythmias, or seizures. Patients with chronic overdosage have a greater risk for serious toxicity at lower serum concentrations than patients with acute single overdosage. Severe signs or symptoms of toxicity resulting from chronic overdose are more common in elderly patients, occurring in 65% of patients 60 years of age or older with serum theophylline concentrations > 30 mcg/mL (165 micromoles/L). For additional information about acute or chronic overdose, refer to the *Overdose* section of this monograph.

Although some studies do not support the suggestion that theophylline has an adverse effect on behavioral and cognitive function in children, differences in individual response have been reported; monitoring for these effects may be advisable.

The following side/adverse effects have been selected on the basis of their potential clinical significance (possible signs and symptoms in parentheses where appropriate)—not necessarily inclusive:

**Those indicating need for medical attention**

Incidence less frequent
  *Gastroesophageal reflux* (heartburn; vomiting)
  Note: Aminophylline, oxtriphylline, or theophylline may relax the gastroesophageal sphincter; however, if *vomiting* occurs, theophylline toxicity should be considered.

Incidence rare
  *For aminophylline only*
    *Dermatitis, ethylenediamine hypersensitivity–induced* (hives; skin rash; sloughing of skin)
    Note: *Ethylenediamine hypersensitivity–induced dermatitis* can appear up to 48 hours after administration of aminophylline.

**Those indicating need for medical attention only if they continue or are bothersome**

Incidence less frequent
  *Headache; increased urination; insomnia* (trouble in sleeping); *nausea; nervousness; tachycardia* (fast heartbeat); *trembling*
  Note: These caffeine-like side effects may occur at therapeutic theophylline serum concentrations, especially if the concentrations are rapidly attained. Tolerance generally develops within 1 or 2 weeks; however, the symptoms may persist in < 3% of children and < 10% of adults with chronic therapydespite therapeutic serum theophylline concentrations. Starting therapy at a low dose and slowly increasing the dose by no more than 25% at no less than 3-day intervals until the desired daily dose is reached may prevent the caffeine-like side effects.

*For parenteral aminophylline and theophylline—with too rapid intravenous administration*
  **Anxiety; headache; nausea; vomiting**
  Note: *Hypotension and cardiac arrest have been reported following rapid direct administration through a central venous catheter.*

## Overdose

For specific information on the agents used in the management of theophylline overdose, see:
- *Anesthetics, Inhalation (Systemic)* monograph;
- *Benzodiazepines (Systemic)* monograph;
- *Charcoal, Activated (Oral-Local)* monograph;
- *Metoclopramide (Systemic)* monograph;
- *Neuromuscular Blocking Agents (Systemic)* monograph;
- *Ondansetron (Systemic)* monograph;
- *Phenobarbital* in *Barbiturates (Systemic)* monograph;
- *Polyethylene Glycol and Electrolytes (Local)* monograph; and/or
- *Thiopental* in *Anesthetics, Barbiturate (Systemic)* monograph.

For more information on the management of overdose or unintentional ingestion, **contact a Poison Control Center** (see *Poison Control Center Listing*).

Theophylline is associated with a significant potential for toxicity because of its narrow therapeutic index. The upper limit of the therapeutic serum concentration range is considered to be 20 mcg per mL (mcg/mL) (110 micromoles per L [micromoles/L]). Clinical symptoms of toxicity become evident in some patients with serum concentrations above 15 mcg/mL (82.5 micromoles/L), and increase in frequency when 20 mcg/mL (110 micromoles/L) is exceeded. Less severe toxicities do not always precede major toxicities. Serum theophylline concentrations do not always predict who will experience life-threatening toxicity. Theophylline demonstrates concentration-dependent elimination kinetics as its metabolic pathways become saturated, resulting in prolonged elimination.

Theophylline overdose is associated with significant morbidity and mortality, primarily due to the development of arrhythmias or seizures. Patients who develop seizures are at the highest risk for further morbidity and mortality from associated hypoxia, acidosis, rhabdomyolysis, or myoglobinuric renal failure. The type of theophylline overdose has significant influence on clinical outcome. Chronic theophylline overdose appears to be associated with a greater frequency of seizures and arrhythmias at lower theophylline concentrations, when compared with acute overdose outcomes; this is especially true in patients older than 60 years of age. Although there is a lack of correlation between serum theophylline concentrations and clinical course of a chronic overdose, serum theophylline concentrations > 40 mcg/mL (220 micromoles/L) are considered potentially life-threatening. Following an acute overdose, serum theophylline concentrations of > 90 mcg/mL (495 micromoles/L) are associated with major toxicity, especially seizures. The onset and duration of theophylline toxicity vary and depend on the formulation used, the route of administration, the amount ingested, time since the ingestion, and the patient's theophylline elimination capacity.

### Clinical effects of overdose

The following effects have been selected on the basis of their potential clinical significance (possible signs and symptoms in parentheses where appropriate)—not necessarily inclusive:

Acute and chronic effects
  ***Abdominal pain, continuing or severe; agitation*** (nervousness or restlessness, continuing); ***confusion or change in behavior; diarrhea; hematemesis*** (dark or bloody vomit); ***hyperglycemia; hypokalemia; hypotension*** (dizziness; lightheadedness); ***metabolic acidosis; seizures*** (convulsions); ***tachyarrhythmias*** (fast and irregular heartbeat); ***tachycardia*** (fast heartbeat); ***trembling, continuing; vomiting***

### Treatment of overdose

There is no antidote for theophylline overdose. Treatment is symptomatic and supportive.
  To decrease absorption—
    Regardless of the route or mode of exposure resulting in toxicity, oral activated charcoal (OAC) should be administered. OAC binds medication remaining in the gastrointestinal tract and decreases serum concentrations by interrupting enteroenteric recirculation of theophylline. Use of an aqueous activated charcoal preparation is recommended. If the total dose of OAC is not tolerated, more frequent administration of smaller doses, slow instillation through a nasogastric tube, or concurrent use of an antiemetic may be tried.
    The initial dose of charcoal may be followed by a single dose of sorbitol if the charcoal is not pre-mixed with sorbitol. Caution is recommended when giving more than a single dose of sorbitol since frequent administration may result in dehydration and electrolyte imbalance secondary to diarrhea. Sorbitol is reported to be more effective than magnesium-containing cathartics and is not associated with hypermagnesemia; however, the role of cathartics is questionable.
  **Ipecac syrup should generally be avoided** in the management of theophylline overdoses.
  Gastric lavage is generally not necessary if the patient has vomited. Lavage may provide some benefit if performed via a large bore orogastric tube less than 1 hour after a large ingestion. This procedure may not be very effective for large, poorly soluble tablets.
  Whole bowel irrigation with polyethylene glycol and electrolyte combination may be of some value if performed early in the treatment of large ingestions of extended-release dosage forms. Whole bowel irrigation with polyethylene glycol and electrolytes may also be useful when theophylline serum concentrations rapidly increase or when high concentrations persist despite other methods of removal.
  To enhance elimination—
    Repeated doses of OAC will at least double theophylline clearance and should be continued throughout the course of toxicity, until the patient is asymptomatic and serum concentration is below 20 mcg/mL (110 micromoles/L).
    Extracorporeal elimination of theophylline by charcoal hemoperfusion is the most effective means of increasing theophylline clearance. Hemodialysis is less effective; however, it may be used if hemoperfusion is unavailable. Peritoneal dialysis is considered ineffective. Controversy exists about when to initiate extracorporeal elimination. It may be indicated when serum theophylline concentrations are approaching 90 mcg/mL (495 micromoles/L) in an acute overdose or when serum theophylline concentrations are greater than 40 mcg/mL (220 micromoles/L) in a chronic overdose or in certain patients with other significant risk factors, such as age greater than 60 years or presence of complicating illness. In addition, use of extracorporeal elimination is recommended in the presence of intractable seizures or life-threatening cardiovascular symptoms, regardless of serum concentration.
  Nausea or vomiting—
    The presence of nausea or vomiting should not cause postponement of OAC administration. Antiemetic therapy with metoclopramide or ondansetron, administered intravenously, may be useful. See the package insert or the *Metoclopramide (Systemic)* or *Ondansetron (Systemic)* monograph for specific dosing guidelines for use of these products. Phenothiazine antiemetics such as prochlorperazine or perphenazine should be avoided since they can lower the seizure threshold.
  Seizures—
    Seizures associated with serum concentrations > 30 mcg/mL (165 micromoles/L) are often resistant to anticonvulsant therapy and may produce a toxic encephalopathy and permanent brain damage if not rapidly controlled. An intravenous benzodiazepine is the drug of choice. See the package insert or the *Benzodiazepines (Systemic)* monograph for specific dosing guidelines for use of these products.
    If seizures are repetitive or seizure prophylaxis is indicated in selected patients at high risk for theophylline-induced seizures, intravenous phenobarbital may be administered. In animal studies, the prophylactic use of phenobarbital in therapeutic doses has delayed the onset of theophylline-induced seizures and reduced mortality. There are no controlled studies in humans. See the package insert or the *Barbiturates (Systemic)* monograph for specific dosing guidelines for use of this product. Phenytoin is considered ineffective.
    Should use of a benzodiazepine and phenobarbital fail to control seizure activity, the addition of the barbiturate anesthetic agent, thiopental, may be considered. Use of a neuromuscular blocking agent may also be considered to decrease the muscular manifestations of persistent seizures. General anesthesia should be used with caution because flourinated volatile anesthetics may sensitize the myocardium to endogenous catecholamines released by theophylline. Enflurane appears less likely to be associated with this effect than does halothane. See the package insert or the *Anesthetics, Inhalation (Systemic)*, *Anesthetics, Barbiturate (Systemic)*, and/or *Neuromuscular Blocking Agents (Systemic)* monographs for specific dosing guidelines for use of these products.
  Ventricular tachyarrhythmias—
    Ventricular tachyarrhythmias considered to be life-threatening require antiarrhythmic therapy specific for the type of arrhythmia.

Monitoring—
Serial theophylline serum concentrations should be obtained to guide and assess treatment decisions. Serial monitoring should continue at periodic intervals after treatment has been discontinued until it is clear that the serum concentration is no longer rising. Serious rebound theophylline toxicity has been reported, due to bezoar formation composed of undissolved extended-release tablets.

All monitoring interventions should be continued until the serum concentration remains below 20 mcg/mL (110 micromoles/L) and the patient is asymptomatic.

Abdominal physical examination should be performed to determine the presence of distention and/or the absence of bowel sounds when repeated doses of OAC are administered. Arterial blood gases, electrocardiograph, serum electrolytes and glucose, stool output, and vital signs should also be monitored as required.

Supportive care—
Respiration should be supported by airway management, oxygen administration, or mechanical ventilation as required, especially if higher doses of a benzodiazepine, phenobarbital, or a neuromuscular blocking agent are used.

Standard measures should be used to manage hypotension and metabolic complications.

Patients in whom intentional overdose is known or suspected should be referred for psychiatric consultation.

## Patient Consultation

As an aid to patient consultation, refer to *Advice for the Patient, Bronchodilators, Theophylline (Systemic)*.
In providing consultation, consider emphasizing the following selected information (» = major clinical significance):

### Before using this medication
» Conditions affecting use, especially:
Sensitivity to theophylline bronchodilators or to ethylenediamine in aminophylline
Pregnancy—Crosses placenta; decreased elimination during third trimester may require more frequent serum concentration determinations
Breast-feeding—Distributes into breast milk; may result in irritability in infants
Use in children—Decreased theophylline clearance in children less than 1 year of age, especially neonates and infants less than 3 months of age with renal function impairment, results in lower dosage requirements; initially, use in children less than 1 year of age may require more frequent serum concentration determinations
Use in the elderly—Possible decreased theophylline clearance in patients 60 years of age or older may result in lower dosage requirements; severe signs or symptoms of toxicity are more common in these patients following chronic overdose that results in serum concentrations > 30 mcg per mL (165 micromoles per L)
Other medications, especially beta-adrenergic blocking agents; cimetidine; ciprofloxacin; clarithromycin; enoxacin; erythromycin; fluvoxamine; mexiletine; moricizine; pentoxifylline; phenytoin; rifampin; tacrine; thiabendazole; ticlopidine; or troleandomycin
Other medical problems, especially congestive heart failure, convulsions (seizures), hepatic disease, or hypothyroidism

### Proper use of this medication
» Proper administration
For liquids and immediate-release capsules or tablets: Taking on an empty stomach with a glass of water for faster absorption or, if necessary, taking with meals or immediately after meals to lessen gastrointestinal irritation, unless otherwise directed
For once-a-day dosage forms: Taking the medication either in the morning at least 1 hour before eating or in the evening with or without food, depending on the specific product; taking consistently with or without food; taking at approximately the same time each day
For enteric-coated or delayed-release tablet dosage form: Swallowing tablets whole; not breaking (unless scored for breakage), crushing, or chewing
For extended-release dosage forms: Swallowing capsules whole or opening capsules and sprinkling contents on soft food, then swallowing without crushing or chewing; not breaking (unless scored for breakage), crushing, or chewing tablets; taking on an empty stomach with a glass of water for faster absorption or, if necessary, taking with meals or immediately after meals to lessen gastrointestinal irritation, unless otherwise directed

» Importance of not using more than amount prescribed
» Compliance with therapy; not missing doses
» Proper dosing
Missed dose: Taking as soon as possible; not taking if almost time for next dose; not doubling doses
» Proper storage

### Precautions while using this medication
» Regular visits to physician required to check progress, including blood levels
» Not changing brands or dosage forms without first checking with physician
» Notifying physician of factors that may alter theophylline concentrations, such as:
—fever (≥102 °F ≥ 24 hours or a lower temperature elevation for a longer period)
—other medicines started or stopped
—smoking started or stopped
—an extended change in diet
Caution in eating or drinking large amounts of caffeine-containing foods or beverages during therapy with this medication

### Side/adverse effects
Signs of potential side effects, especially heartburn and/or vomiting, hives, skin rash, and sloughing of skin
Signs of toxicity

## General Dosing Information

The bronchodilator action of aminophylline, oxtriphylline, and theophylline depends upon their theophylline content. The anhydrous theophylline content of various theophylline salts is as follows:
Aminophylline anhydrous—86%.
Aminophylline dihydrate—79%.
Oxtriphylline—64%.
Theophylline monohydrate—91%.

Theophylline does not distribute into fatty tissue; therefore, all dosages should be calculated on the basis of lean (ideal) body weight.

The recommended doses are given as a guideline for use in the average patient. Dosage of aminophylline, oxtriphylline, or theophylline must be adjusted to meet the individual requirements of each patient on the basis of product selected, patient characteristics, clinical response, and steady-state serum theophylline concentrations.

Administration of a single loading dose of theophylline is intended to produce a serum concentration in the therapeutic range as quickly as possible. A theophylline loading dose may be considered for all patient groups, including neonates. Although the intravenous route of administration provides the most rapid effect, immediate-release oral liquids, tablets, or capsules may also be used. Delayed- or extended-release dosage forms should not be used when rapid achievement of a therapeutic serum theophylline concentration is required.

Before a loading dose is administered, it is extremely important to determine the time, amount, dosage form, and route of administration of previous doses of aminophylline, oxytriphylline, or theophylline.

Once the desired theophylline serum concentration is obtained with a loading dose, it can be maintained with an oral or intravenous dosage form.

The goal of chronic therapy is to obtain maximum potential benefit with minimal risk of adverse effects. Transient caffeine-like side effects and excessively high serum concentrations can be avoided in most patients by starting with a lower dose and slowly increasing the dose by 25% at three-day intervals, approximately.

For final dosage adjustment in chronic therapy after serum theophylline measurement, the following dosage adjustments are recommended:

| Steady-state Peak Serum Theophylline Concentration (mcg/mL) | Recommended Dosage Adjustment |
|---|---|
| Below 9.9 | If *clinically indicated*, about 25% increase to nearest dose increment; recheck serum theophylline concentration after 3 days for further dosage adjustment |
| 10–14.9 | If *clinically indicated*, maintain dose and recheck serum theophylline concentration at 6- to 12-month intervals; if symptoms are not controlled, consider adding additional medication to treatment regimen |
| 15–19.9 | Consider 10% decrease in dose to increase margin of safety even if current dosage is tolerated |

| Steady-state Peak Serum Theophylline Concentration (mcg/mL) | Recommended Dosage Adjustment |
|---|---|
| 20–24.9 | Decrease dose by 25% even if no adverse effects are present; recheck serum theophylline concentration after 3 days |
| 25–30 | Omit next dose; 25% decrease in subsequent doses even if no adverse effects are present; recheck serum theophylline concentration after 3 days; if symptomatic, consider whether overdose treatment is indicated |
| > 30 | Treatment of overdose may be indicated; when theophylline is resumed, decrease subsequent dose by at least 50%; recheck serum theophylline concentration after 3 days |

Note: If asthma is well controlled and there are no side effects or intervening factors that would alter dose requirements, follow-up serum concentration measurements can be obtained at 6- to 12-month intervals. However, **whenever a patient develops nausea, vomiting, CNS stimulation or any other symptom of theophylline toxicity, even if another cause is suspected (e.g., viral gastroenteritis), the next dose should be withheld and a serum concentration measurement obtained.** In addition, various drug interactions and physiologic abnormalities can alter theophylline elimination and require serum concentration measurement and/or dose adjustment.

**For oral dosage forms only**
The dosing frequency should be individualized. When rapidly absorbed dosage forms such as liquids or immediate-release capsules or tablets are used, dosing to maintain therapeutic serum concentrations usually requires administration every 6 hours, especially in children and smoking adults. A dosing interval of up to 8 hours may be appropriate in some nonsmoking adults, elderly or debilitated patients, and neonates due to a slower clearance rate. In premature neonates and patients with hepatic disease, dosing every 12 hours or longer will usually provide relatively constant serum concentrations.

Patients requiring higher-than-usual doses (i.e., patients with rapid clearance rates) may be more effectively controlled during chronic therapy by being given extended-release dosage forms. These products have the potential to achieve relatively constant serum concentrations with 12-hour dosing intervals. Patients who metabolize theophylline rapidly may require an extended-release product every 8 hours. Patients who metabolize theophylline at a normal or slow rate (elimination half-life longer than 8 hours) are potential candidates for once-a-day formulations.

Alcohol-free liquid dosage forms are generally preferred.

For patients who have difficulty in swallowing, some extended-release capsules may be opened and the contents sprinkled on a spoonful of soft, cold food such as applesauce or pudding, then taken without chewing.

**For parenteral dosage forms only**
Therapy can be converted from an intravenous to an oral product by dividing the total daily dose that produced the desired steady-state peak serum concentration into equal parts, and giving in amounts and at intervals appropriate for the product. The intravenous infusion can usually be discontinued when the first oral dose of medication is administered. Extreme caution is recommended if intravenous and oral therapy are overlapped, since this practice may lead to inadvertent theophylline toxicity.

Use of intravenous aminophylline or theophylline should be reassessed after 24 to 72 hours. Oral therapy should be substituted for intravenous therapy as soon as the patient is able to take medication orally.

**Diet/Nutrition**
Dietary changes are of clinical importance only if a sustained and extreme change in the usual eating pattern occurs. High-carbohydrate, low-protein diets have been shown to decrease theophylline elimination. Low-carbohydrate, high-protein diets and daily ingestion of charcoal-broiled beef have been shown to increase theophylline elimination.

Large amounts of caffeine-containing foods or beverages should be avoided, since they may increase CNS stimulant effects of theophylline bronchodilators.

**Bioequivalenence information**
For oral dosage forms only—
The formulation selected for maintenance therapy can have an important effect on the serum concentration–time profile. Selection of a theophylline product must be based upon the specific clinical indication, the absorption characteristics of the formulation, and the rate of theophylline elimination in the individual patient. Immediate-release oral formulations can generally be used interchangeably since they are not considered to have clinically important differences in rates of absorption. However, many brands of extended-release theophylline products have clinically important differences in their extent and/or rate of absorption. Different extended-release products having the same strength of active ingredient may not be equivalent due to formulation differences. Even with reliably absorbed extended-release formulations, a minority of patients can have marked day-to-day variations in absorption. When this occurs, alternative therapy should be considered.

Due to the significant variability in extended-release product characteristics, pharmacists should not substitute one brand for another without consulting the prescribing physician unless the product has proven bioequivalence, so that theophylline serum concentrations can be appropriately monitored.

---

*AMINOPHYLLINE*

## Summary of Differences
Category:
   Aminophylline (injection, oral solution) is also used as a respiratory stimulant in neonatal apnea; aminophylline injection is used as an antidote to dipyridamole toxicity.
Pharmacology/pharmacokinetics:
   Aminophylline is a theophylline compound with ethylenediamine.
   Aminophylline releases free theophylline at physiologic pH.
Side/adverse effects:
   Ethylenediamine in aminophylline may cause hives, skin rash, or sloughing of skin.
General dosing information:
   Aminophylline anhydrous contains about 86% of anhydrous theophylline.
   Aminophylline dihydrate contains about 79% of anhydrous theophylline.

## Additional Dosing Information
See also *General Dosing Information*.

The recommended doses are given as a guideline for use in the average patient. Dosage of aminophylline must be adjusted to meet the individual requirements of each patient on the basis of product selected, patient characteristics, clinical response, and steady-state serum theophylline concentrations.

**For parenteral dosage forms only**
Intramuscular administration of aminophylline injection is not recommended since precipitation may occur at the site of injection, resulting in severe local pain and slow absorption.

Aminophylline may be administered by direct intravenous injection or by intravenous infusion; however, it is recommended that intravenous aminophylline be administered slowly, at a rate *not exceeding* 25 mg per minute.

**For rectal dosage forms only**
USP DI Advisory Panels do not recommend the use of aminophylline suppositories because of the potential for slow and unreliable absorption. The suppositories may also cause local irritation.

## Oral Dosage Forms
Note: Bracketed uses in the *Dosage Forms* section refer to categories of use and/or indications that are not included in U.S. product labeling.

### AMINOPHYLLINE ORAL SOLUTION USP
**Usual adult dose**
Bronchodilator—
   Loading dose:
      For patients *not* currently receiving theophylline preparations—Oral, the equivalent of 5 mg of anhydrous theophylline per kg of lean (ideal) body weight as a single dose to provide an average peak serum concentration of 10 mcg per mL (55 micromoles per L), range 5 to 15 mcg per mL (27.5 to 82.5 micromoles per L).
      For patients currently receiving theophylline preparations—Obtaining a serum theophylline concentration prior to administering a partial loading dose is recommended. Once the theophylline concentration is known, the loading dose for theophylline is based on the principle that each 0.5 mg of theophylline per kg of lean (ideal) body weight will result in a 1 mcg per mL increase in serum theophylline concentration.

Maintenance:
　Oral, the equivalent of anhydrous theophylline, initially, 300 mg per day. After three days, the dosage may be increased, if tolerated, to 400 mg per day. After three more days, the dosage may be increased, if tolerated, to 600 mg per day without measurement of serum concentration.
　The total daily adult dose is administered in three or four divided doses given about six to eight hours apart. Patients with risk factors for impaired theophylline clearance may require a dosing interval of every twelve hours. Young adult smokers and patients with more rapid metabolism may require a dosing interval of every six hours.

　Note: **If the 600-mg-per-day dose is to be maintained or exceeded, monitoring of serum theophylline concentration and patient response is recommended to achieve the optimal therapeutic aminophylline dosage and minimize the risk of toxicity.**

**Usual pediatric dose**
Bronchodilator—
　Loading dose:
　　For patients not currently receiving theophylline preparations—Infants and children up to 16 years of age: Oral, the equivalent of 5 mg of anhydrous theophylline per kg of lean (ideal) body weight as a single dose to provide an average peak serum concentration of 10 mcg per mL (55 micromoles per L), range 5 to 15 mcg per mL (27.5 to 82.5 micromoles per L).
　　For patients currently receiving theophylline preparations—Obtaining a serum theophylline concentration prior to administering a partial loading dose is recommended. Once the theophylline concentration is known, the loading dose for theophylline is based on the principle that each 0.5 mg of theophylline per kg of lean (ideal) body weight will result in a 1 mcg per mL increase in serum theophylline concentration.
　Maintenance:
　　Premature infants, postnatal age less than 24 days—Oral, the equivalent of 1 mg of anhydrous theophylline per kg of body weight every twelve hours.
　　Premature infants, postnatal age 24 days and older—Oral, the equivalent of 1.5 mg of anhydrous theophylline per kg of body weight every twelve hours.
　　Full-term infants, postnatal age up to 52 weeks—Oral, the equivalent of anhydrous theophylline: total daily dose in mg per kg of body weight = (0.2)(postnatal age in weeks) + 5.
　　Note: For full-term infants up to 26 weeks of age, divide the total daily dose into three equal amounts administered eight hours apart.
　　　For full-term infants 26 to 52 weeks of age, divide the total daily dose into four equal amounts administered six hours apart.
　　Children 1 year of age and older, weighing less than 45 kg—Oral, the equivalent of anhydrous theophylline, 12 to 14 mg per kg of body weight, *up to a maximum of 300 mg*, per day in divided doses. The dosage may be increased, if tolerated, after three days to 16 mg per kg of body weight, *up to a maximum of 400 mg*, per day. After three more days, if tolerated, the dosage may be increased to 20 mg per kg of body weight, *up to a maximum of 600 mg*, per day. The total daily dose is administered in four to six divided doses and given every four to six hours.
　　Children weighing more than 45 kg—See *Usual adult dose*.

　Note: **If the above maintenance dose is to be maintained or exceeded, monitoring of serum theophylline concentration and patient response is recommended to achieve the optimal therapeutic aminophylline dosage and minimize the risk of toxicity.**

[Respiratory stimulant (neonatal apnea)][1]—
　Loading dose:
　　For patients *not* currently receiving theophylline preparations—Oral, the equivalent of 5 mg of anhydrous theophylline per kg of lean (ideal) body weight as a single dose to provide an average peak serum concentration of 10 mcg per mL (55 micromoles per L), range 5 to 15 mcg per mL (27.5 to 82.5 micromoles per L).
　　For patients currently receiving theophylline preparations—Obtaining a serum theophylline concentration prior to administering a partial loading dose is recommended. Once the theophylline concentration is known, the loading dose for theophylline is based on the principle that each 0.5 mg of theophylline per kg of lean (ideal) body weight will result in a 1 mcg per mL increase in serum theophylline concentration.

　Maintenance:
　　Premature infants, postnatal age less than 24 days—Oral, the equivalent of 1 mg of anhydrous theophylline per kg of body weight every twelve hours.
　　Premature infants, postnatal age 24 days and older—Oral, the equivalent of 1.5 mg of anhydrous theophylline per kg of body weight every twelve hours.

　Note: **If the above maintenance dose is to be maintained or exceeded, monitoring of serum theophylline concentration and patient response is recommended to achieve the optimal therapeutic aminophylline dosage and minimize the risk of toxicity.**

**Strength(s) usually available**
U.S.—
　105 mg of anhydrous aminophylline (equivalent to 90 mg of anhydrous theophylline) per 5 mL (Rx) [GENERIC].
Canada—
　Not commercially available.

**Packaging and storage**
Store between 15 and 30 °C (59 and 86 °F), unless otherwise specified by manufacturer. Store in a tight container.

## AMINOPHYLLINE TABLETS USP

**Usual adult dose**
See *Aminophylline Oral Solution USP*.

**Usual pediatric dose**
Bronchodilator—
　Loading dose:
　　For patients not currently receiving theophylline preparations—Infants and children up to 16 years of age: Oral, the equivalent of 5 mg of anhydrous theophylline per kg of lean (ideal) body weight as a single dose to provide an average peak serum concentration of 10 mcg per mL (55 micromoles per L), range 5 to 15 mcg per mL (27.5 to 82.5 micromoles per L).
　　For patients currently receiving theophylline preparations—Obtaining a serum theophylline concentration prior to administering a partial loading dose is recommended. Once the theophylline concentration is known, the loading dose for theophylline is based on the principle that each 0.5 mg of theophylline per kg of lean (ideal) body weight will result in a 1 mcg per mL increase in serum theophylline concentration.
　Maintenance:
　　Premature infants, postnatal age less than 24 days—Oral, the equivalent of 1 mg of anhydrous theophylline per kg of body weight every twelve hours.
　　Premature infants, postnatal age 24 days and older—Oral, the equivalent of 1.5 mg of anhydrous theophylline per kg of body weight every twelve hours.
　　Full-term infants, postnatal age up to 52 weeks—Oral, the equivalent of anhydrous theophylline: total daily dose in mg per kg of body weight = (0.2)(postnatal age in weeks) + 5.
　　Note: For full-term infants up to 26 weeks of age, divide the total daily dose into three equal amounts administered eight hours apart.
　　　For full-term infants 26 to 52 weeks of age, divide the total daily dose into four equal amounts administered six hours apart.
　　Children 1 year of age and older, weighing less than 45 kg—Oral, the equivalent of anhydrous theophylline, 12 to 14 mg per kg of body weight, *up to a maximum of 300 mg*, per day in divided doses. The dosage may be increased, if tolerated, after three days to 16 mg per kg of body weight, *up to a maximum of 400 mg*, per day. After three more days, if tolerated, the dosage may be increased to 20 mg per kg of body weight, *up to a maximum of 600 mg*, per day. The total daily dose is administered in four to six divided doses and given every four to six hours.
　　Children weighing more than 45 kg—See *Usual adult dose*.

　Note: **If the above maintenance dose is to be maintained or exceeded, monitoring of serum theophylline concentration and patient response is recommended to achieve the optimal therapeutic aminophylline dosage and minimize the risk of toxicity.**

**Strength(s) usually available**
U.S.—
　100 mg of hydrous aminophylline (equivalent to 79 mg of anhydrous theophylline) (Rx) [GENERIC (may be scored)].
　200 mg of hydrous aminophylline (equivalent to 158 mg of anhydrous theophylline) (Rx) [GENERIC (may be scored)].

Canada—
- 100 mg of hydrous aminophylline (equivalent to 79 mg of anhydrous theophylline) (Rx) [GENERIC (may be scored)].
- 200 mg of hydrous aminophylline (equivalent to 158 mg of anhydrous theophylline) (Rx) [GENERIC (may be scored)].

**Packaging and storage**
Store below 40 °C (104 °F), preferably between 15 and 30 °C (59 and 86 °F), unless otherwise specified by manufacturer. Store in a tight container.

## AMINOPHYLLINE EXTENDED-RELEASE TABLETS

**Usual adult dose**
Bronchodilator—
Oral, the equivalent of anhydrous theophylline, initially, 300 mg per day. If tolerated, the dosage may be increased after three days, to 400 mg per day. After three more days, the dosage may be increased, if tolerated, to 600 mg per day without measurement of serum concentration. One-half of the daily dose may be given at twelve-hour intervals. However, certain patients metabolize theophylline more rapidly, especially the young and those who smoke, and may require dosing at eight-hour intervals.

Note: **If the 600-mg-per-day dose is to be maintained or exceeded, monitoring of serum theophylline concentration and patient response is recommended to achieve the optimal therapeutic aminophylline dosage and minimize the risk of toxicity.**

**Usual pediatric dose**
Bronchodilator—
Children up to 6 years of age: Use is not recommended.
Children 6 to 16 years of age: See *Usual adult dose*.

**Strength(s) usually available**
U.S.—
- 225 mg of hydrous aminophylline (equivalent to 178 mg of anhydrous theophylline) (Rx) [*Phyllocontin* (scored)].

Canada—
- 225 mg of hydrous aminophylline (equivalent to 182.25 mg of anhydrous theophylline) (Rx) [*Phyllocontin* (scored)].
- 350 mg of hydrous aminophylline (equivalent to 283.5 mg of anhydrous theophylline (Rx) [*Phyllocontin-350* (scored)].

**Packaging and storage**
Store below 40 °C (104 °F), preferably between 15 and 30 °C (59 and 86 °F), in a well-closed container, unless otherwise specified by manufacturer.

# Parenteral Dosage Forms

Note: Bracketed uses in the *Dosage Forms* section refer to categories of use and/or indications that are not included in U.S. product labeling.

## AMINOPHYLLINE INJECTION USP

**Usual adult dose**
Bronchodilator—
Loading dose:
For patients *not* currently receiving theophylline preparations—Intravenous, the equivalent of 5 mg of anhydrous theophylline per kg of lean (ideal) body weight as a single dose, infused over twenty to thirty minutes, to provide an average peak serum concentration of 10 mcg per mL (55 micromoles per L), range 5 to 15 mcg per ml (27.5 to 82.5 micromoles per L).

For patients currently receiving theophylline preparations—Obtaining a serum theophylline concentration prior to administering a partial loading dose is recommended. Once the theophylline concentration is known, the loading dose for theophylline is based on the principle that each 0.5 mg of theophylline per kg of lean (ideal) body weight will result in a 1 mcg per mL increase in serum theophylline concentration.

Maintenance:
Young adult smokers—Intravenous infusion, the equivalent of anhydrous theophylline, 700 mcg (0.7 mg) per kg of body weight per hour.

Otherwise healthy nonsmoking adults—Intravenous infusion, the equivalent of anhydrous theophylline, 400 mcg (0.4 mg) per kg of body weight per hour.

Older patients and patients with cardiac decompensation, cor pulmonale, or hepatic function impairment—Intravenous infusion, the equivalent of anhydrous theophylline, 200 mcg (0.2 mg) per kg of body weight per hour.

Note: **If the above maintenance dose is to be maintained or exceeded, monitoring of serum theophylline concentration and patient response is recommended to achieve the optimal therapeutic aminophylline dosage and minimize the risk of toxicity.**

Antidote (to dipyridamole toxicity)[1]—
Intravenous, the equivalent of 50 to 100 mg (range, 50 mg up to a maximum dose of 250 mg) administered over thirty to sixty seconds.

**Usual pediatric dose**
Bronchodilator—
Loading dose:
For patients not currently receiving theophylline preparations—Children up to 16 years of age: Intravenous, the equivalent of 5 mg of anhydrous theophylline per kg of lean (ideal) body weight as a single dose over twenty to thirty minutes to provide an average peak serum concentration of 10 mcg per mL (55 micromoles per L), range 5 to 15 mcg per mL (27.5 to 82.5 micromoles per L).

For patients currently receiving theophylline preparations—Obtaining a serum theophylline concentration prior to administering a partial loading dose is recommended. Once the theophylline concentration is known, the loading dose for theophylline is based on the principle that each 0.5 mg of theophylline per kg of lean (ideal) body weight will result in a 1 mcg per mL increase in serum theophylline concentration.

Maintenance:
Premature infants, postnatal age less than 24 days—Intravenous, the equivalent of 1 mg of anhydrous theophylline per kg of body weight every twelve hours.

Premature infants, postnatal age 24 days and older—Intravenous, the equivalent of 1.5 mg of anhydrous theophylline per kg of body weight every twelve hours.

Full-term infants, postnatal age up to 52 weeks—Intravenous, the equivalent of anhydrous theophylline, total daily dose in mg per kg of body weight = $(0.2)$(postnatal age in weeks) $+ 5$.

For full-term infants up to 26 weeks of age, divide the total daily dose into three equal amounts administered eight hours apart. For full-term infants 26 to 52 weeks of age, divide the total daily dose into four equal amounts administered six hours apart.

Note: May also be administered to infants less than 1 year as an intravenous infusion, the equivalent of anhydrous theophylline, dose in mg per kg of body weight per hour = $(0.008)$(age in weeks) $+ 0.21$.

Children 1 to 9 years of age—Intravenous infusion, the equivalent of anhydrous theophylline, 800 mcg (0.8 mg) per kg of body weight per hour.

Children 9 to 16 years—Intravenous infusion, the equivalent of anhydrous theophylline, 700 mcg (0.7 mg) per kg of body weight per hour.

Note: **If the above maintenance dose is to be maintained or exceeded, monitoring of serum theophylline concentration and patient response is recommended to achieve the optimal therapeutic aminophylline dosage and minimize the risk of toxicity.**

[Respiratory stimulant (neonatal apnea)][1]—
Loading dose:
For patients *not* currently receiving theophylline preparations—Intravenous, the equivalent of 5 mg of anhydrous theophylline per kg of lean (ideal) body weight as a single dose over twenty to thirty minutes to provide an average peak serum concentration of 10 mcg per mL (55 micromoles per L), range 5 to 15 mcg per mL (27.5 to 82.5 micromoles per L).

For patients currently receiving theophylline preparations: Obtaining a serum theophylline concentration prior to administering a partial loading dose is recommended. Once the theophylline concentration is known, the loading dose for theophylline is based on the principle that each 0.5 mg of theophylline per kg of lean (ideal) body weight will result in a 1 mcg per mL increase in serum theophylline concentration.

Maintenance:
Premature infants, postnatal age less than 24 days—Intravenous, the equivalent of 1 mg of anhydrous theophylline per kg of body weight every twelve hours.

Premature infants, postnatal age 24 days and older—Intravenous, the equivalent of 1.5 mg of anhydrous theophylline per kg of body weight every twelve hours.

Note: **If the above maintenance dose is to be maintained or exceeded, monitoring of serum theophylline concentration and patient response is recommended to achieve the optimal therapeutic aminophylline dosage and minimize the risk of toxicity.**

**Strength(s) usually available**
U.S.—
  25 mg of hydrous aminophylline (equivalent to 19.7 mg of anhydrous theophylline) per mL (Rx) [GENERIC].
Canada—
  25 mg of hydrous aminophylline (equivalent to 19.7 mg of anhydrous theophylline) per mL (Rx) [GENERIC].
  50 mg of hydrous aminophylline (equivalent to 39.4 mg of anhydrous theophylline) per mL (Rx) [GENERIC].

**Packaging and storage**
Store below 40 °C (104 °F), preferably between 15 and 30 °C (59 and 86 °F), unless otherwise specified by manufacturer. Protect from light. Protect from freezing.

**Preparation of dosage form**
To dilute the injection for intravenous administration, dextrose 5% in water, sodium chloride, or dextrose-sodium chloride combinations may be used.

**Stability**
A slight yellowing of the solution can occur when aminophylline is added to some dextrose-containing solutions. Because the aminophylline content remains constant, the discoloration is believed to result from the decomposition of dextrose.
Aminophylline solutions whose concentration does not exceed 40 mg/mL are reported to be stable for at least 48 hours at 77 °F (25 °C).

**Incompatibilities**
Although aminophylline has been reported to precipitate in acidic media, this generally does not apply to the dilute solutions for intravenous infusions.
No additives should be made directly to the same intravenous bag or bottle of aminophylline because dosages are titrated to response, and because admixture incompatibilities exist with a number of other medications.
Doxapram hydrochloride is reported to be incompatible with aminophylline when combined in the same syringe.
Medications that are incompatible when injected into Y-sites of administration sets with a continuous infusion of aminophylline include amiodarone hydrochloride, ciprofloxacin, diltiazem hydrochloride, dobutamine hydrochloride, hydralazine hydrochloride, and ondansetron hydrochloride.

## Rectal Dosage Forms
### AMINOPHYLLINE SUPPOSITORIES USP
Note: USP DI Advisory Panels do not recommend the use of Aminophylline Suppositories USP because of the potential for slow and unreliable absorption.

**Strength(s) usually available**
U.S.—
  250 mg of hydrous aminophylline (equivalent to 197.5 mg of anhydrous theophylline) (Rx) [*Truphylline;* GENERIC].
  500 mg of hydrous aminophylline (equivalent to 395 mg of anhydrous theophylline) (Rx) [*Truphylline;* GENERIC].
Canada—
  Not commercially available.

---
[1]Not included in Canadian product labeling.

---

### OXTRIPHYLLINE

## Summary of Differences
Pharmacology/pharmacokinetics:
  Oxtriphylline is the choline salt of theophylline.
  Oxtriphylline releases free theophylline at physiologic pH.
General dosing information:
  Oxtriphylline contains about 64% of anhydrous theophylline.

## Additional Dosing Information
See also *General Dosing Information*.
The recommended doses are given as a guideline for use in the average patient. Dosage of oxtriphylline must be adjusted to meet the individual requirements of each patient on the basis of product selected, patient characteristics, clinical response, and steady-state serum theophylline concentrations.

## Oral Dosage Forms
### OXTRIPHYLLINE ORAL SOLUTION USP
**Usual adult dose**
Bronchodilator—
  Loading dose:
    For patients *not* currently receiving theophylline preparations—Oral, the equivalent of 5 mg of anhydrous theophylline per kg of lean (ideal) body weight as a single dose to provide an average peak serum concentration of 10 mcg per mL (55 micromoles per L), range 5 to 15 mcg per mL (27.5 to 82.5 micromoles per L).
    For patients currently receiving theophylline preparations—Obtaining a serum theophylline concentration prior to administering a partial loading dose is recommended. Once the theophylline concentration is known, the loading dose for theophylline is based on the principle that each 0.5 mg of theophylline per kg of lean (ideal) body weight will result in a 1 mcg per mL increase in serum theophylline concentration.
  Maintenance:
    Oral, the equivalent of anhydrous theophylline, initially, 300 mg per day. After three days, the dosage may be increased, if tolerated, to 400 mg per day. After three more days, the dosage may be increased, if tolerated, to 600 mg per day without measurement of serum concentration.
    The total daily adult dose is administered in three or four divided doses given about six to eight hours apart. Patients with risk factors for impaired theophylline clearance may require a dosing interval of every twelve hours. Young adult smokers and patients with more rapid metabolism may require a dosing interval of every six hours.
  Note: **If the 600-mg-per-day dose is to be maintained or exceeded, monitoring of serum theophylline concentration and patient response is recommended to achieve the optimal therapeutic oxtriphylline dosage and minimize the risk of toxicity.**

**Usual pediatric dose**
Use is not recommended in children due to high alcohol content.

**Strength(s) usually available**
U.S.—
  Not commercially available.
Canada—
  100 mg (equivalent to 64 mg of anhydrous theophylline) per 5 mL (Rx) [*Choledyl* (alcohol 20%); *PMS-Oxtriphylline* (alcohol 20%)].

**Packaging and storage**
Store below 40 °C (104 °F), preferably between 15 and 30 °C (59 and 86 °F), unless otherwise specified by manufacturer. Store in a tight container. Protect from freezing.

### OXTRIPHYLLINE SYRUP
**Usual adult dose**
See *Oxtriphylline Oral Solution USP*.

**Usual pediatric dose**
Bronchodilator—
  Loading dose:
    For patients not currently receiving theophylline preparations—Infants and children up to 16 years of age: Oral, the equivalent of 5 mg of anhydrous theophylline per kg of lean (ideal) body weight as a single dose to provide an average peak serum concentration of 10 mcg/mL (55 micromoles per L), range 5 to 15 mcg per mL (27.5 to 82.5 micromoles per L).
    For patients currently receiving theophylline preparations—Obtaining a serum theophylline concentration prior to administering a partial loading dose is recommended. Once the theophylline concentration is known, the loading dose for theophylline is based on the principle that each 0.5 mg of theophylline per kg of lean (ideal) body weight will result in a 1 mcg per mL increase in serum theophylline concentration.
  Maintenance:
    Premature infants, postnatal age less than 24 days—Oral, the equivalent of 1 mg of anhydrous theophylline per kg of body weight every twelve hours.
    Premature infants, postnatal age 24 days and older—Oral, the equivalent of 1.5 mg of anhydrous theophylline per kg of body weight every twelve hours.
    Full-term infants, postnatal age up to 52 weeks—Oral, the equivalent of anhydrous theophylline: Total daily dose in mg per kg of body weight = (0.2)(postnatal age in weeks) + 5.
  Note: For full-term infants up to 26 weeks of age, divide the total daily dose into three dosing intervals, eight hours apart.

For full-term infants 26 to 52 weeks of age, divide the total daily dose into four dosing intervals six hours apart.

Children 1 year of age and older, but weighing less than 45 kg—Oral, the equivalent of anhydrous theophylline, 12 to 14 mg per kg of body weight, *up to a maximum of 300 mg*, per day in divided doses. The dosage may be increased, if tolerated, after three days to 16 mg per kg of body weight, *up to a maximum of 400 mg per day*. After three more days, if tolerated, the dosage may be increased to 20 mg per kg of body weight *up to a maximum of 600 mg per day*. The total daily dose is administered in four to six divided doses given every four to six hours.

Children weighing more than 45 kg—See *Usual adult dose*.

Note: **If the above maintenance dose is to be maintained or exceeded, monitoring of serum theophylline concentration and patient response is recommended to achieve the optimal therapeutic oxtriphylline dosage and minimize the risk of toxicity.**

### Strength(s) usually available
U.S.—
Not commercially available.
Canada—
50 mg (equivalent to 32 mg of anhydrous theophylline) per 5 mL (Rx) [*Choledyl; PMS-Oxtriphylline*].

### Packaging and storage
Store below 40 °C (104 °F), preferably between 15 and 30 °C (59 and 86 °F), in a tight container, unless otherwise specified by manufacturer. Protect from freezing.

## OXTRIPHYLLINE TABLETS

### Usual adult dose
See *Oxtriphylline Oral Solution USP*.

### Usual pediatric dose
See *Oxtriphylline Syrup*.

### Strength(s) usually available
U.S.—
Not commercially available.
Canada—
100 mg (equivalent to 64 mg of anhydrous theophylline) (Rx) [*Apo-Oxtriphylline*].
200 mg (equivalent to 128 mg of anhydrous theophylline) (Rx) [*Apo-Oxtriphylline; Choledyl*].
300 mg (equivalent to 192 mg of anhydrous theophylline) (Rx) [*Apo-Oxtriphylline*].

### Packaging and storage
Store below 40 °C (104 °F), preferably between 15 and 30 °C (59 and 86 °F), unless otherwise specified by manufacturer. Store in a tight container.

## OXTRIPHYLLINE DELAYED-RELEASE TABLETS USP

### Usual adult dose
Bronchodilator—
Oral, the equivalent of anhydrous theophylline, initially, 300 mg per day. If tolerated, the dosage may be increased after three days to 400 mg per day. After three more days, the dosage may be increased, if tolerated, to 600 mg per day without measurement of serum concentration. The total daily adult dose is administered in three or four divided doses given about six to eight hours apart. Patients with risk factors for impaired theophylline clearance may require a dosing interval of every twelve hours. Young adult smokers and patients with more rapid metabolism may require a dosing interval of every six hours.

### Usual pediatric dose
Bronchodilator—
Children up to 6 years of age: Use is not recommended in children up to 6 years of age since this age group may not be capable of swallowing the tablets whole.
Children 6 to 16 years of age: See *Usual adult dose*.

### Strength(s) usually available
U.S.—
100 mg (equivalent to 64 mg of anhydrous theophylline) (Rx) [*Choledyl* (enteric, sugar-coated)].
200 mg (equivalent to 127 mg of anhydrous theophylline) (Rx) [*Choledyl* (enteric, sugar-coated)].
Canada—
Not commercially available.

### Packaging and storage
Store below 40 °C (104 °F), preferably between 15 and 30 °C (59 and 86 °F), unless otherwise specified by manufacturer. Store in a tight container.

### Auxiliary labeling
- Swallow tablets whole.

## OXTRIPHYLLINE EXTENDED-RELEASE TABLETS USP

### Usual adult dose
Bronchodilator—
Oral, the equivalent of anhydrous theophylline, initially, 300 mg per day. If tolerated, the dosage may be increased after three days to 400 mg per day. After three more days, the dosage may be increased, if tolerated, to 600 mg per day without measurement of serum concentration. One-half of the daily dose may be given at twelve-hour intervals. However, certain patients metabolize theophylline more rapidly, especially the young and those that smoke, and may require dosing at eight-hour intervals.

Note: **If the 600-mg-per-day dose is to be maintained or exceeded, monitoring of serum theophylline concentration and patient response is recommended to achieve the optimal therapeutic oxtriphylline dosage and minimize the risk of toxicity.**

### Usual pediatric dose
Bronchodilator—
Children up to 6 years of age: Use is not recommended.
Children 6 to 16 years of age: See *Usual adult dose*.

### Strength(s) usually available
U.S.—
400 mg (equivalent to 254 mg of anhydrous theophylline) (Rx) [*Choledyl SA* (confectioner's sugar)].
600 mg (equivalent to 382 mg of anhydrous theophylline) (Rx) [*Choledyl SA* (confectioner's sugar)].
Canada—
400 mg (equivalent to 254 mg of anhydrous theophylline) (Rx) [*Choledyl SA* (scored)].
600 mg (equivalent to 382 mg of anhydrous theophylline) (Rx) [*Choledyl SA* (scored)].

### Packaging and storage
Store below 40 °C (104 °F), preferably between 15 and 30 °C (59 and 86 °F), unless otherwise specified by manufacturer. Store in a tight container.

---

# THEOPHYLLINE

## Summary of Differences
Category: Theophylline oral liquids are also used as a respiratory stimulant in neonatal apnea.

## Additional Dosing Information
See also *General Dosing Information*.

The recommended doses are given as a guideline for use in the average patient. Dosage of theophylline must be adjusted to meet the individual requirements of each patient on the basis of product selected, patient characteristics, clinical response, and steady-state serum theophylline concentrations.

### For parenteral dosage forms only
The rate of administration of theophylline and dextrose injection should *not exceed* 25 mg per minute.

## Oral Dosage Forms
Note: Bracketed uses in the *Dosage Forms* section refer to categories of use and/or indications that are not included in U.S. product labeling.

## THEOPHYLLINE CAPSULES USP

### Usual adult dose
Bronchodilator—
Loading dose:
For patients *not* currently receiving theophylline preparations—Oral, the equivalent of 5 mg of anhydrous theophylline per kg of lean (ideal) body weight as a single dose to provide an average peak serum concentration of 10 mcg per mL (55 micromoles per L), range 5 to 15 mcg per mL (27.5 to 82.5 micromoles per L).

For patients currently receiving theophylline preparations—Obtaining a serum theophylline concentration prior to administering a partial loading dose is recommended. Once the theophylline concentration is known, the loading dose for theophylline is based on the principle that each 0.5 mg of theophylline per kg of lean (ideal) body weight will result in a 1 mcg per mL increase in serum theophylline concentration.

Maintenance:
Oral, the equivalent of anhydrous theophylline, initially, 300 mg per day. After three days, the dosage may be increased, if tolerated, to 400 mg per day. After three more days, the dosage may be increased, if tolerated, to 600 mg per day without measurement of serum concentration.

The total daily adult dose is administered in three or four divided doses given about six to eight hours apart. Patients with risk factors for impaired theophylline clearance may require a dosing interval of every twelve hours. Young adult smokers and patients with more rapid metabolism may require a dosing interval of every six hours.

Note: **If the 600-mg-per-day dose is to be maintained or exceeded, monitoring of serum theophylline concentration and patient response is recommended to achieve the optimal therapeutic theophylline dosage and minimize the risk of toxicity.**

### Usual pediatric dose
Bronchodilator—
Loading dose:
For patients *not* currently receiving theophylline preparations—Infants and children up to 16 years of age: Oral, the equivalent of 5 mg of anhydrous theophylline per kg of lean (ideal) body weight as a single dose to provide an average peak serum concentration of 10 mcg per mL (55 micromoles per L), range 5 to 15 mcg per mL (27.5 to 82.5 micromoles per L).

For patients currently receiving theophylline preparations—Obtaining a serum theophylline concentration prior to administering a partial loading dose is recommended. Once the theophylline concentration is known, the loading dose for theophylline is based on the principle that each 0.5 mg of theophylline per kg of lean (ideal) body weight will result in a 1 mcg per mL increase in serum theophylline concentration.

Maintenance:
Children 1 year of age and older, weighing less than 45 kg—Oral, the equivalent of anhydrous theophylline, 12 to 14 mg per kg of body weight, *up to a maximum of 300 mg*, per day in divided doses. The dosage may be increased, if tolerated, after three days to 16 mg per kg of body weight, *up to a maximum of 400 mg*, per day. After three more days, if tolerated, the dosage may be increased to 20 mg per kg of body weight *up to a maximum of 600 mg*, per day. The total daily dose is administered in four to six divided doses given every four to six hours.

Children weighing more than 45 kg—See *Usual adult dose*.

Note: **If the 600-mg-per-day dose is to be maintained or exceeded, monitoring of serum theophylline concentration and patient response is recommended to achieve the optimal therapeutic theophylline dosage and minimize the risk of toxicity.**

### Strength(s) usually available
U.S.—
100 mg (equivalent of anhydrous theophylline) (Rx) [*Elixophyllin*; GENERIC].
200 mg (equivalent of anhydrous theophylline) (Rx) [*Elixophyllin*; GENERIC].
300 mg (equivalent of anhydrous theophylline) (Rx) [GENERIC].

Canada—
Not commercially available.

### Packaging and storage
Store below 40 °C (104 °F), preferably between 15 and 30 °C (59 and 86 °F), unless otherwise specified by manufacturer. Store in a well-closed container.

## THEOPHYLLINE EXTENDED-RELEASE CAPSULES USP

Note: Due to the significant variability in extended-release product characteristics, pharmacists should not substitute one brand for another without consulting the prescribing physician unless the product has proven bioequivalence, so that theophylline serum concentrations can be appropriately monitored.

### Usual adult dose
Bronchodilator—
Oral, the equivalent of anhydrous theophylline, initially, 300 mg per day. If tolerated, the dosage may be increased after three days to 400 mg per day. After three more days, the dosage may be increased, if tolerated, to 600 mg per day without measurement of serum concentration. One-half of the daily theophylline dose may be given at twelve-hour intervals. However, certain patients metabolize theophylline more rapidly, especially the young and those that smoke, and may require dosing at eight-hour intervals.

Note: **If the 600-mg-per-day dose is to be maintained or exceeded, monitoring of serum theophylline concentration and patient response is recommended to achieve the optimal therapeutic theophylline dosage and minimize the risk of toxicity.**

### Usual pediatric dose
Bronchodilator—
Children 1 year of age and older, weighing less than 45 kg: Oral, the equivalent of anhydrous theophylline, 12 to 14 mg per kg of body weight, *up to a maximum of 300 mg*, per day in divided doses. The dosage may be increased, if tolerated, after three days to 16 mg per kg of body weight, *up to a maximum of 400 mg*, per day. After three more days, if tolerated, the dosage may be increased to 20 mg per kg of body weight *up to a maximum of 600 mg*, per day. One-half of the daily theophylline dose may be given as aminophylline at twelve-hour intervals. However, younger patients may require dosing at eight-hour intervals.

Children weighing more than 45 kg: See *Usual adult dose*.

Note: **If the 600-mg-per-day dose is to be maintained or exceeded, monitoring of serum theophylline concentration and patient response is recommended to achieve the optimal therapeutic theophylline dosage and minimize the risk of toxicity.**

### Strength(s) usually available
U.S.—
50 mg (equivalent of anhydrous theophylline) (Rx) [*Slo-Bid Gyrocaps*].
75 mg (equivalent of anhydrous theophylline) (Rx) [*Slo-Bid Gyrocaps*].
100 mg (equivalent of anhydrous theophylline) (Rx) [*Slo-Bid Gyrocaps; Theo-24*].
125 mg (equivalent of anhydrous theophylline) (Rx) [*Slo-Bid Gyrocaps; Theovent Long-Acting*].
200 mg (equivalent of anhydrous theophylline) (Rx) [*Slo-Bid Gyrocaps; Theo-24*].
250 mg (equivalent of anhydrous theophylline) (Rx) [*Theovent Long-Acting*].
260 mg (equivalent of anhydrous theophylline) (Rx) [*Aerolate Sr; Theobid Duracaps; Theoclear L.A.-260*].
300 mg (equivalent of anhydrous theophylline) (Rx) [*Slo-Bid Gyrocaps; Theo-24*].
400 mg (equivalent of anhydrous theophylline) (Rx) [*Theo-24*].

Canada—
50 mg (equivalent of anhydrous theophylline) (Rx) [*Slo-Bid Gyrocaps*].
100 mg (equivalent of anhydrous theophylline) (Rx) [*Slo-Bid Gyrocaps*].
200 mg (equivalent of anhydrous theophylline) (Rx) [*Slo-Bid Gyrocaps*].
300 mg (equivalent of anhydrous theophylline) (Rx) [*Slo-Bid Gyrocaps*].

### Packaging and storage
Store below 40 °C (104 °F), preferably between 15 and 30 °C (59 and 86 °F), unless otherwise specified by manufacturer. Store in a well-closed container.

### Additional information
Certain extended-release capsules may be opened and the contents sprinkled on soft food immediately prior to ingestion, then swallowed without crushing or chewing. Capsule contents should not be subdivided.

## THEOPHYLLINE ELIXIR

### Usual adult dose
See *Theophylline Capsules USP*.

### Usual pediatric dose
Use is not recommended in children due to the high alcohol content.

### Strength(s) usually available
U.S.—
27 mg (equivalent of anhydrous theophylline) per 5 mL (Rx) [*Asmalix* (alcohol 20%); *Elixophyllin* (alcohol 20%); *Lanophyllin* (alcohol 20%); *Truxophyllin*; GENERIC].

Canada—
27 mg (equivalent of anhydrous theophylline) per 5 mL (Rx) [*PMS Theophylline* (alcohol 18%); *Pulmophylline* (alcohol 20% [v/v]) [GENERIC].

### Packaging and storage
Store below 40 °C (104 °F), preferably between 15 and 30 °C (59 and 86 °F), in a tight container, unless otherwise specified by manufacturer. Protect from freezing.

**Stability**

Exposure to cold temperatures may cause theophylline crystallization to occur. At room temperature the crystals redissolve and solution gradually clears.

**Auxiliary labeling**
- Do not refrigerate.

## THEOPHYLLINE ORAL SOLUTION

**Usual adult dose**
See *Theophylline Capsules USP.*

**Usual pediatric dose**
Bronchodilator—
  Loading dose:
    For patients not currently receiving theophylline preparations—Infants and children up to 16 years of age: Oral, the equivalent of 5 mg of anhydrous theophylline per kg of lean (ideal) body weight as a single dose to provide an average peak serum concentration of 10 mcg per mL (55 micromoles per L), range 5 to 15 mcg per mL (27.5 to 82.5 micromoles per L).
    For patients currently receiving theophylline preparations—Obtaining a serum theophylline concentration prior to administering a partial loading dose is recommended. Once the theophylline concentration is known, the loading dose for theophylline is based on the principle that each 0.5 mg of theophylline per kg of lean (ideal) body weight will result in a 1 mcg per mL increase in serum theophylline concentration.
  Maintenance:
    Premature infants, postnatal age less than 24 days—Oral, the equivalent of 1 mg of anhydrous theophylline per kg of body weight every twelve hours.
    Premature infants, postnatal age 24 days and older—Oral, the equivalent of 1.5 mg of anhydrous theophylline per kg of body weight every twelve hours.
    Full-term infants, postnatal age up to 52 weeks—Oral, the equivalent of anhydrous theophylline: total daily dose in mg per kg of body weight = (0.2)(postnatal age in weeks) + 5.
    Note: For full-term infants up to 26 weeks of age, divide the total daily dose into three equal amounts administered eight hours apart.
    For full-term infants 26 to 52 weeks of age, divide the total daily dose into four equal amounts administered six hours apart.
  Children 1 year of age and older, weighing less than 45 kg: Oral, the equivalent of anhydrous theophylline, 12 to 14 mg per kg of body weight, *up to a maximum of 300 mg,* per day in divided doses. The dosage may be increased, if tolerated, after three days to 16 mg per kg of body weight, *up to a maximum of 400 mg,* per day. After three more days, if tolerated, the dosage may be increased to 20 mg per kg of body weight *up to a maximum of 600 mg,* per day. The total daily dose is administered in four to six divided doses given every four to six hours.
  Children weighing more than 45 kg: See *Usual adult dose.*
  Note: **If the above maintenance dose is to be maintained or exceeded, monitoring of serum theophylline concentration and patient response is recommended to achieve the optimal therapeutic theophylline dosage and minimize the risk of toxicity.**

[Respiratory stimulant (neonatal apnea)][1]—
  Loading dose:
    For patients *not* currently receiving theophylline preparations—Infants and children up to 16 years of age: Oral, the equivalent of 5 mg of anhydrous theophylline per kg of lean (ideal) body weight as a single dose to provide an average peak serum concentration of 10 mcg per mL (55 micromoles per L), range 5 to 15 mcg per mL (27.5 to 82.5 micromoles per L).
    For patients currently receiving theophylline preparations—Obtaining a serum theophylline concentration prior to administering a partial loading dose is recommended. Once the theophylline concentration is known, the loading dose for theophylline is based on the principle that each 0.5 mg of theophylline per kg of lean (ideal) body weight will result in a 1 mcg per mL increase in serum theophylline concentration.
  Maintenance:
    Premature infants, postnatal age less than 24 days—Oral, the equivalent of 1 mg of anhydrous theophylline per kg of body weight every twelve hours.
    Premature infants, postnatal age 24 days and older—Oral, the equivalent of 1.5 mg of anhydrous theophylline per kg of body weight every twelve hours.

Note: **If the above maintenance dose is to be maintained or exceeded, monitoring of serum theophylline concentration and patient response is recommended to achieve the optimal therapeutic theophylline dosage and minimize the risk of toxicity.**

**Strength(s) usually available**
U.S.—
  27 mg (equivalent of anhydrous theophylline) per 5 mL (Rx) [*Theolair;* GENERIC].
Canada—
  27 mg (equivalent of anhydrous theophylline) per 5 mL (Rx) [*Theolair*].

**Packaging and storage**
Store below 40 °C (104 °F), preferably between 15 and 30 °C (59 and 86 °F), in a well-closed container, unless otherwise specified by manufacturer. Protect from freezing.

**Stability**
Exposure to cold temperatures may cause theophylline crystallization to occur. At room temperature the crystals redissolve and solution gradually clears.

**Auxiliary labeling**
- Do not refrigerate.

## THEOPHYLLINE SYRUP

**Usual adult dose**
See *Theophylline Capsules USP.*

**Usual pediatric dose**
See *Theophylline Oral Solution.*

**Strength(s) usually available**
U.S.—
  27 mg (equivalent of anhydrous theophylline) per 5 mL (Rx) [*Slo-Phyllin; Theoclear-80*].
Canada—
  Not commercially available.

**Packaging and storage**
Store below 40 °C (104 °F), preferably between 15 and 30 °C (59 and 86 °F), in a well-closed container, unless otherwise specified by manufacturer. Protect from freezing.

**Stability**
Exposure to cold temperatures may cause theophylline crystallization to occur. At room temperature the crystals redissolve and solution gradually clears.

**Auxiliary labeling**
- Do not refrigerate.

## THEOPHYLLINE TABLETS USP

**Usual adult dose**
See *Theophylline Capsules USP.*

**Usual pediatric dose**
See *Theophylline Capsules USP.*

**Strength(s) usually available**
U.S.—
  100 mg (equivalent of anhydrous theophylline) (Rx) [*Slo-Phyllin* (scored); GENERIC].
  125 mg (equivalent of anhydrous theophylline) (Rx) [*Theolair* (scored)].
  200 mg (equivalent of anhydrous theophylline) (Rx) [*Slo-Phyllin* (scored); GENERIC].
  250 mg (equivalent of anhydrous theophylline) (Rx) [*Theolair* (scored)].
  300 mg (equivalent of anhydrous theophylline) (Rx) [*Quibron-T Dividose* (scored); GENERIC].
Canada—
  125 mg (equivalent of anhydrous theophylline) (Rx) [*Theolair* (scored)].
  250 mg (equivalent of anhydrous theophylline) (Rx) [*Theolair* (scored)].

**Packaging and storage**
Store below 40 °C (104 °F), preferably between 15 and 30 °C (59 and 86 °F), unless otherwise specified by manufacturer. Store in a well-closed container.

## THEOPHYLLINE EXTENDED-RELEASE TABLETS

Note: Due to the significant variability in extended-release product characteristics, pharmacists should not substitute one brand for another without consulting the prescribing physician unless the product has proven bioequivalence, so that theophylline serum concentrations can be appropriately monitored.

**Usual adult dose**
Bronchodilator—Oral, the equivalent of anhydrous theophylline, initially, 300 mg per day. If tolerated, the dosage may be increased after three days, to 400 mg per day. After three more days, the dosage may be increased, if tolerated, to 600 mg per day without measurement of serum concentration. One-half the daily theophylline dose may be given at twelve hour intervals. However, certain patients metabolize theophylline more rapidly, especially the young and those that smoke, and may require dosing at eight hour intervals.

Note: **If the 600-mg-per-day dose is to be maintained or exceeded, monitoring of serum theophylline concentration and patient response is recommended to achieve the optimal therapeutic theophylline dosage and minimize the risk of toxicity.**

**Usual pediatric dose**
Bronchodilator—
  Children 1 year of age and older, weighing less than 45 kg: Oral, the equivalent of anhydrous theophylline, 12 to 14 mg per kg of body weight, *up to a maximum of 300 mg*, per day in divided doses. The dosage may be increased, if tolerated, after three days to 16 mg per kg of body weight, *up to a maximum of 400 mg*, per day. After three more days, if tolerated, the dosage may be increased to 20 mg per kg of body weight *up to a maximum of 600 mg*, per day. One-half of the daily theophylline dose may be given at twelve-hour intervals. However, younger patients may require dosing at eight-hour intervals.
  Children weighing more than 45 kg: See *Usual adult dose.*
  Children 6 to 16 years of age: See *Usual adult dose.*

**Strength(s) usually available**
U.S.—
  100 mg (equivalent of anhydrous theophylline) (Rx) [*Theochron* (scored); *Theo-Dur* (scored); *Theo-Time; Theo-X;* GENERIC].
  200 mg (equivalent of anhydrous theophylline) (Rx) [*Theochron* (scored); *Theo-Dur* (scored); *Theolair-SR* (scored); *Theo-Time; Theo-X; T-Phyl* (scored); GENERIC].
  250 mg (equivalent of anhydrous theophylline) (Rx) [*Respbid* (scored); *Theolair-SR* (scored)].
  300 mg (equivalent of anhydrous theophylline) (Rx) [*Quibron-T/SR Dividose* (scored); *Theochron* (scored); *Theo-Dur* (scored); *Theolair-SR* (scored); *Theo-Time; Theo-X;* GENERIC].
  400 mg (equivalent of anhydrous theophylline) (Rx) [*Uni-Dur* (scored); *Uniphyl* (scored)].
  450 mg (equivalent of anhydrous theophylline) (Rx) [*Theo-Dur* (scored); GENERIC (may be scored)].
  500 mg (equivalent of anhydrous theophylline) (Rx) [*Respbid* (scored); *Theolair-SR* (scored)].
  600 mg (equivalent of anhydrous theophylline) (Rx) [*Uni-Dur* (scored)].
Canada—
  100 mg (equivalent of anhydrous theophylline) (Rx) [*Apo-Theo LA* (scored); *Theochron* (scored); *Theo-Dur* (scored )].
  200 mg (equivalent of anhydrous theophylline) (Rx) [*Apo-Theo LA* (scored); *Theochron* (scored); *Theo-Dur* (scored ); *Theolair-SR* (scored); *Theo-SR* (scored)].
  250 mg (equivalent of anhydrous theophylline) (Rx) [*Theolair SR* (scored)].
  300 mg (equivalent of anhydrous theophylline) (Rx) [*Apo-Theo LA* (scored); *Quibron-T/SR Dividose* (scored); *Theochron* (scored); *Theo-Dur* (scored ); *Theolair-SR* (scored); *Theo-SR* (scored)].
  400 mg (equivalent of anhydrous theophylline) (Rx) [*Uniphyl* (scored)].
  450 mg (equivalent of anhydrous theophylline) (Rx) [*Theo-Dur* (scored)].
  500 mg (equivalent of anhydrous theophylline) (Rx) [*Theolair-SR* (scored)].
  600 mg (equivalent of anhydrous theophylline) (Rx) [*Uniphyl* (scored)].

**Packaging and storage**
Store below 40 °C (104 °F), preferably between 15 and 30 °C (59 and 86 °F), in a well-closed container, unless otherwise specified by manufacturer.

**Auxiliary labeling**
• Swallow tablets whole, unless otherwise directed.

# Parenteral Dosage Forms

Note: Bracketed uses in the *Dosage Forms* section refer to categories of use and/or indications that are not included in U.S. product labeling.

## THEOPHYLLINE IN DEXTROSE INJECTION USP

**Usual adult dose**
Bronchodilator—
  Loading dose:
    For patients *not* currently receiving theophylline preparations—Intravenous, the equivalent of 5 mg of anhydrous theophylline per kg of lean (ideal) body weight as a single dose, infused over 20 to 30 minutes, to provide an average peak serum concentration of 10 mcg per mL (55 micromoles per L), range 5 to 15 mcg per mL (range 27.5 to 82.5 micromoles per L).
    For patients currently receiving theophylline preparations—Obtaining a serum theophylline concentration prior to administering a partial loading dose is recommended. Once the theophylline concentration is known, the loading dose for theophylline is based on the principle that each 0.5 mg of theophylline per kg of lean (ideal) body weight will result in a 1 mcg per mL increase in serum theophylline concentration.
  Maintenance:
    Young adult smokers—Intravenous infusion, the equivalent of anhydrous theophylline: 700 mcg (0.7 mg) per kg of body weight per hour
    Otherwise healthy nonsmoking adults—Intravenous infusion, the equivalent of anhydrous theophylline: 400 mcg (0.4 mg) per kg of body weight per hour.
    Older patients and patients with cardiac decompensation, cor pulmonale, or hepatic function impairment—Intravenous infusion, the equivalent of anhydrous theophylline: 200 mcg (0.2 mg) per kg of body weight per hour.

Note: **If the above maintenance dose is to be maintained or exceeded, monitoring of serum theophylline concentration and patient response is recommended to achieve the optimal therapeutic theophylline dosage and minimize the risk of toxicity.**

**Usual pediatric dose**
Bronchodilator—
  Loading dose:
    For patients *not* currently receiving theophylline preparations—Children 1 to 16 years of age: Intravenous, the equivalent of 5 mg of anhydrous theophylline per kg of lean (ideal) body weight as a single dose over twenty to thirty minutes to provide an average peak serum concentration of 10 mcg per mL (55 micromoles per L), range 5 to 15 mcg per mL (27.5 to 82.5 micromoles per L).
    For patients currently receiving theophylline preparations—Obtaining a serum theophylline concentration prior to administering a partial loading dose is recommended. Once the theophylline concentration is known, the loading dose for theophylline is based on the principle that each 0.5 mg of theophylline per kg of lean (ideal) body weight will result in a 1 mcg per mL increase in serum theophylline concentration.
  Maintenance:
    Full-term infants, postnatal age up to 52 weeks—Intravenous infusion, the equivalent of anhydrous theophylline: Dose in mg per kg of body weight per hour = (0.008)(age in weeks) + 0.21.
    Children 1 to 9 years of age—Intravenous infusion, the equivalent of anhydrous theophylline: 800 mcg (0.8 mg) per kg of body weight per hour.
    Children 9 to 16 years—Intravenous infusion, the equivalent of anhydrous theophylline: 700 mcg (0.7 mg) per kg of body weight per hour.

Note: **If the above maintenance dose is to be maintained or exceeded, monitoring of serum theophylline concentration and patient response is recommended to achieve the optimal therapeutic theophylline dosage and minimize the risk of toxicity.**

**Strength(s) usually available**
U.S.—
  Theophylline in 5% dextrose injection (Rx) [GENERIC] contains the following amounts of anhydrous theophylline:

| Volume (approx.) mL | Theophylline Anhydrous Total mg | mg/mL |
|---|---|---|
| 50 | 200 | 4 |
| 100 | 200 | 2 |
| 100 | 400 | 4 |
| 250 | 400 | 1.6 |
| 250 | 800 | 3.2 |
| 500 | 400 | 0.8 |
| 500 | 800 | 1.6 |
| 1000 | 400 | 0.4 |
| 1000 | 800 | 0.8 |

Canada—
Theophylline in 5% dextrose injection (Rx) [GENERIC] contains the following amounts of anhydrous theophylline:

| Volume (approx.) mL | Theophylline Anhydrous Total mg | mg/mL |
|---|---|---|
| 50 | 200 | 4 |
| 100 | 200 | 2 |
| 100 | 400 | 4 |
| 250 | 400 | 1.6 |
| 500 | 400 | 0.8 |
| 500 | 800 | 1.6 |
| 1000 | 400 | 0.4 |
| 1000 | 800 | 0.8 |

**Packaging and storage**
Store below 40 °C (104 °F), preferably between 15 and 30 °C (59 and 86 °F), unless otherwise specified by manufacturer. Protect from freezing.

**Stability**
Theophylline and dextrose solutions contain no bacteriostatic, antimicrobial agent, or added buffer; they are intended only for single-dose administration. When smaller doses are required, the unused portion should be discarded.

**Incompatibilities**
No additives should be made to theophylline and dextrose injection because dosages are titrated to response.
Hetastarch has been shown to be incompatible with theophylline in dextrose solution when injected into Y-sites of administration sets.

[1]Not included in Canadian product labeling.

## Selected Bibliography
Edwards DJ, Zarowitz BJ, Slaughter RL. Theophylline. In: Evans WE, Schentag JJ, Jusko WJ, editors. Applied Pharmacokinetics: principles of therapeutic drug monitoring. Vancouver, WA: Applied Therapeutics, 1992: 13-1–13-38.

Weinberger MM. Methylxanthines. In: Weiss EB, Stein M, editors. Bronchial asthma—mechanisms and therapeutics. Boston: Little, Brown and Co, 1993: 746-83.

National Asthma Education Program. Expert Panel Report. Guidelines for the diagnosis and management of asthma. National Heart, Lung and Blood Institute, 1991.

Revised: 8/11/95

**BUCLIZINE**—The *Buclizine (Systemic)* monograph is not included in this published version of the USP DI database. Copies of the monograph are available on request from Micromedex, Inc. - Reprint Requests, 6200 S. Syracuse Way, Suite 300, Englewood, CO 80111; telephone (303) 486-6400; telefax (303) 486-6464; Email: USPDI@MDX.COM.

**BUDESONIDE**—See *Corticosteroids (Inhalation-Local)*; *Corticosteroids (Nasal)*

**BUMETANIDE**—See *Diuretics, Loop (Systemic)*

**BUPIVACAINE**—See *Anesthetics (Parenteral-Local)*

# BUPRENORPHINE  Systemic

VA CLASSIFICATION (Primary/Secondary): CN101/CN206
Note: Controlled substance classification—
U.S.—V.
Commonly used brand name(s): *Buprenex*.
Note: For a listing of dosage forms and brand names by country availability, see *Dosage Forms* section(s).

## Category
Analgesic; anesthesia adjunct.
Note: Buprenorphine is an opioid agonist/antagonist analgesic.

## Indications
Note: Bracketed information in the *Indications* section refers to uses that are not included in U.S. product labeling.

**Accepted**
Pain (treatment)—Indicated for the treatment of moderate to severe pain.
[Anesthesia, general, adjunct]; or
[Anesthesia, local, adjunct]—Buprenorphine is used as an opioid analgesic adjunct to general and local anesthesia.

Prior to administration of buprenorphine, its antagonist activity and its high affinity for, and slow rate of dissociation from, receptor binding sites must be considered. Buprenorphine may precipitate withdrawal symptoms if administered to a patient physically dependent on an opioid analgesic. Also, buprenorphine may temporarily reduce or block the effects of subsequently administered opioid analgesics. In addition, buprenorphine-induced respiratory depression or other adverse effects may be difficult to reverse.

Buprenorphine (unlike pentazocine, which has cardiovascular effects that tend to increase cardiac work) may be administered to patients with angina pectoris or compromised cardiac function, following cardiac or cardiovascular surgery, and to relieve pain due to acute myocardial infarction.

## Pharmacology/Pharmacokinetics

**Physicochemical characteristics**
Molecular weight—504.11.
pKa—8.42 and 9.92.
Other characteristics—Weakly acidic; highly lipophilic

**Mechanism of action/Effect**
Analgesic—
Opioid analgesics bind with stereospecific receptors at many sites within the central nervous system (CNS) to alter processes affecting both the perception of pain and the emotional response to pain. Precise sites and mechanisms of action have not been fully determined, but may partially involve alterations in release of various neurotransmitters from afferent nerves sensitive to painful stimuli.

It has been proposed that there are multiple subtypes of opioid receptors, each mediating various therapeutic and/or side effects of opioid drugs. The actions of an opioid analgesic may therefore depend upon its binding affinity for each type of receptor and whether it acts as a full agonist or a partial agonist or is inactive at each type of receptor. At least two of these types of receptors (mu and kappa) mediate analgesia. Mu receptors are widely distributed throughout the CNS, especially in the limbic system (frontal cortex, temporal cortex, amygdala, and hippocampus), thalamus, striatum, hypothalamus, and midbrain as well as laminae I, II, IV, and V of the dorsal horn in the spinal cord. Kappa receptors are localized primarily in the spinal cord and in the cerebral cortex. A third type of receptor (sigma) may not mediate analgesia; actions at this receptor may produce the subjective and psychotomimetic effects characteristic of most opioids having mixed agonist/antagonist activity. Buprenorphine may act primarily as a partial agonist at the mu receptor; it may also have some agonist activity at the kappa receptor. Buprenorphine has little if any activity at the sigma receptor.

Antagonist—
Buprenorphine may displace mu-receptor opioid agonists from their receptor binding sites and competitively inhibit their actions. Because buprenorphine has high affinity for the mu receptor, but less intrinsic activity at this receptor than morphine or other potent mu-receptor agonists, it may precipitate withdrawal symptoms in physically dependent patients who are chronically receiving these agonists. However, because of its partial agonist activity, buprenorphine may attenuate spontaneous withdrawal symptoms caused by abrupt discontinuation of opioid agonists. Also, buprenorphine dissociates from the mu receptor very slowly and may reduce or block the effects of subsequently administered mu-receptor agonists. In some animal studies, the antagonist activity of buprenorphine was com-

parable to that of naloxone. One study indicates that buprenorphine may also have some antagonist activity at the kappa receptor.

**Other actions/effects**
Buprenorphine shares the CNS depressant, respiratory depressant, and hypotensive effects of opioid analgesics.

Buprenorphine may have less potential for causing habituation or abuse than other strong opioid analgesics. Studies in animals have indicated that it has less reinforcing efficacy than other opioids. Also, its slow rate of dissociation from the mu receptor reduces the risk that a severe abstinence syndrome will occur following abrupt withdrawal. Studies in opioid addicts have shown that withdrawal effects may not reach maximum intensity for up to 15 days following abrupt discontinuation. Withdrawal effects are morphine-like, mild to moderate, and may persist for 1 to 2 weeks. Despite the relatively low risk of habituation, abuse has been reported; further experience with this medication is necessary before its true abuse potential can be assessed.

Although studies in humans have not been done, animal studies have indicated that buprenorphine has potent, prolonged antitussive activity.

**Absorption**
Intramuscular—Rapid; 5 to 10 minutes following intramuscular administration, plasma concentrations are equivalent to those measured 10 minutes following intravenous administration.

**Protein binding**
Very high, primarily to alpha and beta globulin fractions; binding to albumin is not significant.

**Biotransformation**
Hepatic; undergoes extensive enterohepatic circulation.

**Half-life**
Triphasic—Following a dose of 0.3 mg intravenously—
  Distribution—2 minutes
  Redistribution—18 minutes
  Elimination—1.2 to 7.2 hours; average 2 to 3 hours.

**Onset of action**
Analgesic:
  Intramuscular: About 15 minutes
  Intravenous: More rapid than with intramuscular administration.
Antagonist:
  When used to antagonize effects of fentanyl or sufentanil used in conjunction with nitrous oxide for anesthesia: 15 minutes.
Respiratory depressant:
  1 to 3 hours following intramuscular administration.
Note: Pharmacokinetic studies have demonstrated no apparent relationship between the onset of buprenorphine's activity and its plasma concentration.

**Time to peak concentration**
Intramuscular—2 to 5 minutes
Intravenous—2 minutes

**Peak plasma concentration**
Intravenous—18 nanograms per mL following a 0.3-mg dose.

**Time to peak effect**
Analgesic—
  Intramuscular: 1 hour
  Intravenous: Somewhat less than with intramuscular injection.
Antagonist—
  When used to antagonize effects of fentanyl or sufentanil used in conjunction with nitrous oxide for anesthesia: 1.5 to 2 hours.

**Duration of action**
Analgesia
  Adults:
    Intramuscular or intravenous—Up to 6 hours in most patients, but 10 hours or longer in some studies.
    Epidural—12 hours following a 0.3-mg dose; 6 hours following a 0.15-mg dose (when administered concurrently with a local anesthetic).
  Children 2 to 12 years of age:
    4 to 5 hours
Antagonist—
  When used to antagonize effects of fentanyl or sufentanil used in conjunction with nitrous oxide for anesthesia: 4 hours.
  Following chronic administration of large doses of buprenorphine: In one study in opioid addicts receiving chronic administration of 8 mg per day of buprenorphine subcutaneously, the effects of large doses (up to 120 mg) of subsequently administered morphine were blocked for more than 30 hours following the last dose of buprenorphine.

Respiratory depression—
  May persist significantly longer than morphine-induced respiratory depression.
Note: Pharmacokinetic studies have demonstrated no apparent relationship between the duration of buprenorphine's activity and its plasma concentration. The medication's prolonged duration of action is more likely related to its slow rate of dissociation from receptor binding sites.

**Elimination**
Primarily biliary/fecal; about 68% (range 50 to 71%) of an intramuscular dose is eliminated in the feces as unchanged buprenorphine within 7 days. Up to 27% of an intramuscular dose may be excreted in the urine as conjugated buprenorphine and as a dealkylated metabolite; little if any unchanged buprenorphine appears in the urine. It has been proposed that the medication undergoes extensive enterohepatic circulation and is excreted into the bile as inactive conjugates, which are subsequently hydrolyzed in the gastrointestinal tract.

Note: A study in a limited number of pediatric patients 3 to 5 years of age showed that clearance of buprenorphine in children, although subject to high interpatient variability, may be more rapid than in adults.

## Precautions to Consider

**Carcinogenicity**
Studies in animals have not shown that buprenorphine has carcinogenic potential.

**Mutagenicity**
Studies utilizing *in vitro* and *in vivo* test systems have shown some evidence of mutagenicity with very high concentrations or doses in some test systems but not in others using similar concentrations or doses.

**Pregnancy/Reproduction**
Fertility—Reproduction studies with rats have not shown evidence of impaired fertility with subcutaneous or intramuscular administration of 0.05, 0.5, or 5 mg per kg of body weight per day (up to 1000 times the human dose).

Pregnancy—Adequate and well-controlled studies in humans have not been done.
Studies in rats administered up to 1000 times the human dose intramuscularly or up to 160 times the human dose intravenously showed no evidence of teratogenicity. However, studies in rabbits showed a dose-related trend toward extra rib formation, which was statistically significant with intramuscular administration of 1000 times the human dose. Also, studies in rats showed an increased incidence of postimplantation losses and early fetal deaths with intramuscular administration of 10 or 100, but not 1000, times the human dose per day. A slight increase in postimplantation losses, possibly treatment-related, also occurred in rats receiving up to 160 times the human dose intravenously. In addition, intramuscular administration of 1000 times the human dose per day to rats throughout gestation caused dystocia, a high incidence of neonatal mortality, and a slow growth rate in surviving offspring.

FDA Pregnancy Category C.

Labor and delivery—Safe use of buprenorphine in labor and delivery has not been established. However, it has been recommended that the medication not be used during labor because of potential respiratory depressant effects in the neonate, which may be very difficult to reverse.

**Breast-feeding**
Although it is not known whether buprenorphine is distributed into human breast milk, problems in humans have not been documented. Concentrations in the milk of lactating animals have been shown to equal or exceed maternal plasma concentrations; it is reasonable to assume that this highly lipophilic medication would be distributed into human breast milk also. In addition, animal studies have shown that administration of buprenorphine throughout the periods of gestation and lactation inhibits milk production.

**Pediatrics**
Appropriate studies performed to date have not demonstrated pediatrics-specific problems that would limit the usefulness of buprenorphine in children 2 years of age and older.

**Geriatrics**
Geriatric patients may be more sensitive to the effects, especially the respiratory depressant effects, of opioid analgesics, including buprenorphine. Also, elderly patients are more likely to have age-related renal function impairment, which may require caution and dosage adjustment in patients receiving buprenorphine. It is recommended that initial dosage for these patients be reduced by one-half. However, geriatric patients may also be more sensitive to the analgesic effects of the medication so that lower doses and/or a longer interval between doses may provide sufficient analgesia.

### Drug interactions and/or related problems

The following drug interactions and/or related problems have been selected on the basis of their potential clinical significance (possible mechanism in parentheses where appropriate)—not necessarily inclusive (» = major clinical significance):

Note: Combinations containing any of the following medications, depending on the amount present, may also interact with this medication.

Other interactions applying to opioid analgesics may apply to buprenorphine also, although documentation is currently not available.

» CNS depression–producing medications, other (See *Appendix II*) or Monoamine oxidase (MAO) inhibitors, including furazolidone, procarbazine, and selegiline
(concurrent use may increase the CNS depressant, respiratory depressant, and hypotensive effects of these medications and/or buprenorphine; caution is recommended; it is recommended that dosage of buprenorphine be reduced by one-half; a reduction in dosage of the other agent may also be required)

Naltrexone
(although not documented, the possibility must be considered that usual doses of buprenorphine will be ineffective if administered to a patient receiving naltrexone therapy [because naltrexone blocks the therapeutic effects of other potent opioids] and that administration of increased doses of buprenorphine to override naltrexone-induced blockade of opioid receptors may increase the risk of adverse effects)

» Opioid analgesics, other
(if administered prior to another opioid analgesic, buprenorphine may reduce the therapeutic effects of the other opioid; in one study in opioid addicts receiving chronic administration of 8 mg per day of buprenorphine, the effects of large doses [up to 120 mg] of morphine were blocked during buprenorphine therapy and for at least 30 hours following the last dose of buprenorphine)

(buprenorphine antagonizes the respiratory depressant effects of large doses of previously administered opioids; however, additive respiratory depression may occur if buprenorphine is administered in conjunction with low doses of other opioids)

(when administered following fentanyl derivative–assisted anesthesia, buprenorphine may reverse the respiratory depressant effects of fentanyl or its derivatives [alfentanil and sufentanil] while providing adequate postoperative analgesia; however, in one study, administration of 0.3 or 0.45 mg of buprenorphine intramuscularly every 6 hours following opioid-assisted anesthesia with total doses of 0.2 or 0.3 mg of fentanyl or 1.75 or 4 mg of phenoperidine [not available in the U.S.] caused a higher incidence of hypotension, respiratory depression, and CNS depression than equianalgesic doses [10 or 15 mg] of morphine intramuscularly every 6 hours)

(buprenorphine may precipitate withdrawal symptoms in physically dependent patients who are chronically receiving potent mu-receptor agonists such as morphine; however, because of its partial agonist activity, buprenorphine may partially suppress spontaneous withdrawal symptoms caused by abrupt discontinuation of opioid agonists)

### Laboratory value alterations

The following have been selected on the basis of their potential clinical significance (possible effect in parentheses where appropriate)—not necessarily inclusive (» = major clinical significance):

With diagnostic test results
Gastric emptying studies
(buprenorphine may delay gastric emptying, thereby invalidating test results)

Hepatobiliary imaging using technetium Tc 99m disofenin
(delivery of technetium Tc 99m disofenin to the small bowel may be prevented because of buprenorphine-induced constriction of the sphincter of Oddi and increased biliary tract pressure; these actions result in delayed visualization and thus resemble obstruction of the common bile duct)

With physiology/laboratory test values
Amylase, plasma and
Lipase, plasma
(values may be increased because buprenorphine can cause contractions of the sphincter of Oddi and increased biliary tract pressure; the diagnostic utility of determinations of these enzymes may be compromised for up to 24 hours after medication has been given)

Cerebrospinal fluid (CSF) pressure
(may be increased; effect is secondary to respiratory depression–induced carbon dioxide retention)

### Medical considerations/Contraindications

The medical considerations/contraindications included have been selected on the basis of their potential clinical significance (reasons given in parentheses where appropriate)—not necessarily inclusive (» = major clinical significance).

*Except under special circumstances, this medication should not be used when the following medical problems exist:*

» Diarrhea caused by poisoning, until toxic material has been eliminated from gastrointestinal tract
(may slow elimination of toxic material)

» Respiratory depression, acute
(may be exacerbated)

*Risk-benefit should be considered when the following medical problems exist:*

Abdominal conditions, acute
(diagnosis or clinical course may be obscured)

» Asthma, acute attack or
» Respiratory impairment or disease, chronic
(opioids may decrease respiratory drive and increase airway resistance in these patients; it is recommended that dosage be reduced by one-half, unless the patient is being mechanically ventilated)

Cardiac arrhythmias or
Seizures, history of
(may be induced or exacerbated by opioids)

Dependence on opioid analgesics, current
(buprenorphine may precipitate withdrawal symptoms if patient is currently receiving other opioids)

Drug abuse or dependence, history of, including acute alcoholism or
Emotional instability or
Suicidal ideation or attempts
(increased risk of opioid abuse)

Gallbladder disease or gallstones
(opioids may cause biliary colic)

Gastrointestinal tract surgery, recent
(opioids may alter gastrointestinal motility)

Head injury or
Increased intracranial pressure, pre-existing or
Intracranial lesions
(risk of respiratory depression and further elevation of cerebrospinal fluid pressure is increased; also, opioids may cause sedation and pupillary changes that may obscure clinical course of head injury)

Hepatic function impairment
(opioids metabolized in liver)

Hypothyroidism
(risk of respiratory depression and prolonged CNS depression is greatly increased)

» Inflammatory bowel disease, severe
(risk of toxic megacolon may be increased, especially with repeated dosing)

Prostatic hypertrophy or obstruction or
Urethral stricture or
Urinary tract surgery, recent
(opioids may cause urinary retention)

Renal function impairment
(buprenorphine metabolites excreted via kidneys; also, may cause urinary retention)

Sensitivity to buprenorphine, history of

Caution is also advised in administration to geriatric or very ill or debilitated patients, who may be more sensitive to the effects, especially the respiratory depressant effects, of buprenorphine.

## Side/Adverse Effects

Note: Buprenorphine appears less likely than other opioid agonist/antagonist analgesics to cause the subjective and psychotomimetic effects characteristic of this class of drugs. These effects may include several or all of the following, occurring as a group: confusion, delusions, feelings of depersonalization or unreality, hallucinations (usually visual), dysphoria, nightmares, and nervousness or anxiety. However, several of these effects have been reported individually (incidence < 1%) in patients receiving buprenorphine.

Buprenorphine may have less dependence or abuse liability than other potent opioid analgesics. However, abuse has been reported.

In some studies, the incidence and/or severity of nausea and vomiting occurring with buprenorphine was greater than that induced by meperidine or morphine.

Epidural administration of buprenorphine may be associated with a lower incidence of adverse effects, such as late respiratory depression, pruritus, and urinary retention, than has been reported with epidural morphine. However, early respiratory depression resistant to naloxone therapy has been reported. Also, signs of shock (pallor, cold skin, low blood pressure, and tachycardia) have been reported in a few patients following epidural buprenorphine. Although these signs eventually abated spontaneously, naloxone and other treatments were not effective in reversing them.

The following side/adverse effects have been selected on the basis of their potential clinical significance (possible signs and symptoms in parentheses where appropriate)—not necessarily inclusive:

### Those indicating need for medical attention
Incidence 1 to 5%
*Decreased blood pressure; respiratory depression, mild* (unusually slow breathing)

Note: Whether buprenorphine's respiratory depressant activity is subject to the same ceiling effect (i.e., the depth of respiratory depression is not increased with higher doses) reported for other opioid agonist/antagonist drugs has not been established in humans. Studies in animals indicate that such a ceiling effect may occur, but at higher dosage levels than with other opioid agonist/antagonist drugs.

Incidence <1%
*CNS effects* (confusion, hallucinations, mental depression or other mood or mental changes; psychosis; ringing or buzzing in ears); *conjunctivitis* (red and/or irritated eyes); *dermatitis, allergic* (skin rash, hives, or itching); *increased blood presssure; increased or decreased heart rate; paresthesia* (pain, numbness, tingling, or burning feeling in hands or feet); *respiratory depression, severe* (blue color of face, lips, or fingernails; difficult or troubled breathing); *urinary retention* (decrease in amount of urine; swelling of face, fingers, hands, feet, or lower legs; weight gain); *Wenckebach block*

### Those indicating need for medical attention only if they continue or are bothersome
Incidence up to 66%
*Drowsiness*

Incidence 5 to 10%
*Dizziness or lightheadedness; nausea*—especially in ambulatory patients

Incidence 1 to 5%
*Headache; increased sweating; vomiting*—especially in ambulatory patients

Incidence <1%
*Blurred vision or any change in vision; false sense of well-being; general feeling of discomfort or illness; pain, redness, or swelling at place of injection; slurred speech; trembling; unusual nervousness; unusual tiredness; unusual weakness*

### Those indicating possible withdrawal and the need for medical attention if they occur within 15 days after medication is discontinued
*Body aches; diarrhea; fast heartbeat; gooseflesh; increased sweating; loss of appetite; nausea or vomiting; nervousness, restlessness, or irritability; runny nose; shivering or trembling; sneezing; stomach cramps; trouble in sleeping; unexplained fever; unusually large pupils of eyes; weakness; yawning*

## Overdose
For specific information on the agents used in the management of buprenorphine overdose, see:
- *Naloxone (Systemic)* monograph; and/or
- *Doxapram (Systemic)* monograph.

For more information on the management of overdose or unintentional ingestion, **contact a Poison Control Center** (see *Poison Control Center Listing*).

### Clinical effects of overdose
The following effects have been selected on the basis of their potential clinical significance (possible signs and symptoms in parentheses where appropriate)—not necessarily inclusive:

Acute and chronic
*Cold, clammy skin; confusion; convulsions; dizziness, severe; drowsiness, severe; low blood pressure; nervousness or restlessness, severe; pinpoint pupils of eyes; slow heartbeat; slow or troubled breathing; unconsciousness; weakness, severe*

### Treatment of overdose
Specific treatment—Use of the opioid antagonist naloxone for buprenorphine-induced respiratory depression. However, even in doses as high as 16 mg, naloxone may not completely antagonize buprenorphine-induced respiratory depression or other adverse effects.

The respiratory stimulant doxapram may be administered if naloxone fails to reverse respiratory depression.

Assisted or controlled ventilation may be necessary despite administration of naloxone and/or doxapram.

Monitoring—May include monitoring the respiratory and cardiac status of the patient.

May include continual monitoring of the patient so that additional naloxone and/or doxapram may be administered as needed. Administration of these medications by continuous intravenous infusion, with the rate of infusion being adjusted according to patient response, may be preferable to intermittent administration.

Supportive care—May include establishing adequate respiratory exchange through provision of a patent airway and institution of assisted or controlled respiration using 100% oxygen if respiratory depression is severe; if respiratory depression is mild, i.e., a conscious and responsive patient is breathing unusually slowly (but without difficulty) and/or coaching the patient to breathe produces improvement, these measures may not be required.

May include administering intravenous fluids, vasopressors, and other supportive measures as needed.

## Patient Consultation
As an aid to patient consultation, refer to *Advice for the Patient, Narcotic Analgesics (Systemic—For Pain Relief)* and *Narcotic Analgesics (Systemic—For Surgery and Obstetrics)*.

In providing consultation, consider emphasizing the following selected information (» = major clinical significance):

### Before using this medication
» Conditions affecting use, especially:
  Allergic reaction to buprenorphine, history of
  Breast-feeding—Buprenorphine has inhibited milk production in animal studies
  Use in the elderly—Lower doses recommended because of increased sensitivity to opioids
  Other medications, especially other CNS depression–producing medications and other opioids
  Medical problems, especially diarrhea caused by poisoning, respiratory depression or disease (including asthma), and severe inflammatory bowel disease

### Proper use of this medication
Proper administration technique (if dispensed for home use)
» Importance of not taking more medication than the amount prescribed because of danger of overdose and habit-forming potential
» Not increasing dose if medication is less effective after a few weeks; checking with physician
Missed dose (if on scheduled dosing): Using as soon as possible; not using if almost time for next dose; not doubling doses
» Proper dosing
» Proper storage

### Precautions while using this medication
Regular visits to physician to check progress during long-term therapy
» Avoiding alcohol or other CNS depressants during therapy
» Caution if dizziness, drowsiness, lightheadedness, or false sense of well-being occurs
Caution when getting up suddenly from a lying or sitting position
Lying down if nausea, vomiting, dizziness, or lightheadedness occurs
Caution if any kind of surgery (including dental surgery) or emergency treatment is required
» Checking with physician before discontinuing medication after prolonged use of high doses; gradual dosage reduction may be necessary to avoid withdrawal symptoms
» Suspected overdose: Getting emergency help at once

### Side/adverse effects
Signs and symptoms of potential side effects, especially respiratory and/or CNS depression, allergic dermatitis, hallucinations, and overdose

## General Dosing Information
Intramuscular administration of 300 mcg (0.3 mg) of buprenorphine provides analgesia equivalent to that produced by intramuscular administration of 10 mg of morphine.

Buprenorphine may suppress respiration, especially in geriatric, very ill, or debilitated patients and patients with respiratory problems. It is recommended that dosage for these patients be reduced by one-half initially, then adjusted as required and tolerated. However, geriatric patients may also be more sensitive to the analgesic effects of the medication so that lower doses and/or a longer interval between doses may be sufficient to provide effective analgesia.

Dosage and dosing intervals should be individualized on the basis of the severity of pain, the condition of the patient, other medications given concurrently, and patient response.

Some clinicians recommend that patients in chronic pain due to neoplastic disease receive opioid analgesics on a fixed dosage schedule in order that they remain free of pain rather than on an as needed basis after pain recurs.

Concurrent administration of a non-opioid analgesic (such as aspirin or other salicylates, other nonsteroidal anti-inflammatory analgesics, or acetaminophen) with opioid analgesics provides additive analgesia and may permit lower doses of the opioid analgesic to be utilized.

Although buprenorphine may have less potential for causing habituation or abuse than other opioid analgesics, psychological and physical dependence may occur with chronic administration. An abstinence syndrome may be precipitated when the medication is abruptly discontinued. Although withdrawal symptoms may not reach maximum intensity for up to 15 days following discontinuation, if they occur they may persist for 1 to 2 weeks. Also, abuse has been reported.

Rapid intravenous injection of most opioid analgesics has caused anaphylactoid reactions, severe respiratory depression, hypotension, peripheral circulatory collapse, and cardiac arrest. Although these effects have not been documented with buprenorphine, the same precautions applying to other opioid analgesics may apply, i.e., administering the medication slowly, with an opioid antagonist and equipment for artificial ventilation available. It is recommended that intravenous injections of buprenorphine be administered over at least 2 minutes.

Frequent monitoring of the patient's respiratory status is recommended during buprenorphine therapy because of the risk of respiratory depression.

When an opioid analgesic is administered parenterally, the patient usually should be lying down and should remain recumbent for a period of time to minimize side effects such as hypotension, dizziness, lightheadedness, nausea, and vomiting. If these side effects occur in an ambulatory patient, they may be relieved if the patient lies down.

In patients with shock, impaired perfusion may prevent complete absorption following intramuscular injection. Repeated administration may result in overdose due to an excessive amount suddenly being absorbed when circulation is restored.

Tolerance to buprenorphine requiring increased dosage to maintain adequate analgesia has not occurred in long-term studies in cancer patients. However, tolerance has been demonstrated in studies with opioid addicts.

## Parenteral Dosage Forms

Note: The dosing and strength of the available dosage form are expressed in terms of buprenorphine base (not the hydrochloride salt).

### BUPRENORPHINE HYDROCHLORIDE INJECTION

**Usual adult and adolescent dose**
Analgesic—
Intramuscular or slow intravenous, 300 mcg (0.3 mg) (base) every six or more hours as needed. An additional dose of up to 300 mcg (0.3 mg) may be administered thirty to sixty minutes following the initial dose, if necessary.

Note: Dosage may be increased to 600 mcg (0.6 mg), or the frequency of administration may be increased to every four hours if necessary, depending upon the severity of pain and patient response. This larger dose should be administered only via the intramuscular route and only to patients who are not at high risk for opioid toxicity. Although doses exceeding 600 mcg (0.6 mg) have been administered in some studies, long-term use of such doses is not recommended because of insufficient data.

**Usual pediatric dose**
Analgesic—
Children up to 2 years of age: Dosage has not been established.
Children 2 to 12 years of age: Intramuscular or slow intravenous, 2 to 6 mcg (0.002 to 0.006 mg) (base) per kg of body weight every four to six hours or as needed.

Note: Because of interpatient variability in buprenorphine clearance, it is recommended that the appropriate dosing interval for an individual pediatric patient be determined before a fixed-interval dosing regimen is scheduled.

**Strength(s) usually available**
U.S.—
Without preservative
300 mcg (0.3 mg) (base) per mL (Rx) [*Buprenex* (dextrose 5%)].

**Packaging and storage**
Store below 40 °C (104 °F), preferably between 15 and 30 °C (59 and 86 °F), unless otherwise specified by manufacturer. Protect from freezing. Avoid prolonged exposure to light.

**Incompatibilities**
Buprenorphine injection is chemically incompatible with diazepam and with lorazepam.

**Auxiliary labeling**
• May cause drowsiness.
• Avoid alcoholic beverages.
• May be habit-forming.

**Note**
Controlled substance in the U.S.

Revised: 07/29/94

# BUPROPION  Systemic

INN: Amfebutamone
VA CLASSIFICATION (Primary/Secondary): CN609/AD600
Commonly used brand name(s): *Wellbutrin; Wellbutrin; Wellbutrin SR; Zyban*.

Note: For a listing of dosage forms and brand names by country availability, see *Dosage Forms* section(s).

## Category

Antidepressant; smoking cessation adjunct.

## Indications

**Accepted**
Depressive disorder, major (treatment)—Bupropion is indicated for the treatment of major depression. Treatment of acute depressive episodes typically requires 6 to 12 months of antidepressant therapy. Patients with recurrent or chronic depression may require long-term treatment.

Nicotine dependence (treatment adjunct)—The extended-release formulation of bupropion is indicated as an aid to smoking cessation treatment. A smoking cessation program should include behavioral interventions, counseling, and/or other support services.

## Pharmacology/Pharmacokinetics

**Physicochemical characteristics**
Chemical group—Aminoketone. Bupropion is structurally related to phenylethylamines and closely resembles diethylpropion.
Molecular weight—Bupropion hydrochloride: 276.21.
Solubility—Highly soluble in water.

**Mechanism of action/Effect**
Antidepressant—
Although the exact mechanism of antidepressant action is unclear, it is thought to be mediated by bupropion's noradrenergic and/or dopaminergic effects. Bupropion is a weak inhibitor of neuronal uptake of norepinephrine and dopamine, although inhibition of uptake occurs at doses higher than those required for bupropion's antidepressant effects. Hydroxybupropion, an active metabolite of bupropion, has weak norepinephrine reuptake blocking activity but it reaches concentrations high enough to produce significant norepinephrine blockade and may have clinically significant antidepressant effects. Animal studies have suggested that bupropion's antidepressant activity may be mediated through noradrenergic pathways involving the locus ceruleus. Bupropion and hydroxybupropion reduce the firing rates of noradrenergic neurons in the locus ceruleus in a dose-dependent manner; this action is similar to that of the tricyclic antidepressants.

Bupropion shows little affinity for the serotonergic transport system, and it does not inhibit monoamine oxidase.

**Smoking cessation adjunct—**
Although the exact mechanism of smoking cessation action is unclear, it is thought to be mediated by bupropion's noradrenergic and/or dopaminergic effects. Bupropion increases extracellular dopamine concentrations in the nucleus accumbens, as do all known addictive substances including nicotine. The nucleus accumbens, a part of the mesolimbic dopamine system, may be an important component of the neural circuitry of reward. Also, as nicotine concentrations drop with abstinence, the firing rates of noradrenergic neurons in the locus ceruleus increase, which may be the basis of withdrawal symptoms. Bupropion and its active metabolite, hydroxybupropion, reduce the firing rates of noradrenergic neurons in the locus ceruleus in a dose-dependent manner.

**Other actions/effects**
Although animal studies indicate that bupropion may be an inducer of hepatic microsomal enzymes, a study in humans using a dosage of 150 mg three times a day for 14 days found no evidence of autoinduction.
May produce dose-related central nervous system (CNS) stimulation.

**Absorption**
Approximately 80%; rapidly absorbed from the gastrointestinal tract; however, extensive presystemic metabolism limits bioavailability. Food increases extent of absorption insignificantly.

**Distribution**
Readily crosses the blood-brain barrier and placenta; a study of one subject demonstrated that bupropion and its metabolites are distributed into breast milk.

**Protein binding**
Bupropion—High (84%), to human plasma proteins.
Hydroxybupropion—High (77%).

**Biotransformation**
Bupropion is extensively metabolized, including presystemic metabolism. Three metabolites have shown activity in animal studies. Hydroxybupropion, formed principally by the cytochrome P450 2B6 (CYP2B6) isoenzyme, is comparable in potency to bupropion. Threohydrobupropion and erythrohydrobupropion, amino-alcohol isomers formed by hydroxylation and/or reduction, are one tenth to one half as potent as bupropion.

**Half-life**
Distribution—
 3 to 4 hours.
Elimination—
 Bupropion: Single-dose mean, approximately 14 (range, 8 to 24) hours. Single-dose studies demonstrate a first-order elimination pattern with a mean total body clearance of approximately 2 liters per hour per kilogram of body weight.
 Bupropion: Steady-state mean, 21 ± 9 hours.
 Hydroxybupropion: Mean, approximately 20 hours.

**Onset of action**
Antidepressant—1 to 3 weeks; full effect may require 4 or more weeks to achieve.

**Time to peak concentration**
Prompt-release formulation:
 Bupropion: Approximately 1.5 hours, followed by biphasic decline.
 Hydroxybupropion: Approximately 3 hours.
Extended-release formulation:
 Bupropion: Approximately 3 hours.
 Hydroxybupropion: Approximately 6 hours.

**Time to steady-state concentration**
Bupropion—Within 5 days.
Hydroxybupropion—Within 8 days.

**Steady-state plasma concentration**
Mean maximum concentration of bupropion was 136 nanograms per mL (0.492 micromoles per L) in healthy volunteers following a 150-mg dose of the extended-release tablet every 12 hours. Peak plasma concentration of hydroxybupropion at steady-state is approximately 10 times that of bupropion.

**Elimination**
Renal—
 Less than 1% excreted in urine unchanged. Over 60% excreted as metabolites within 24 hours, over 80% within 96 hours.
Fecal—
 Less than 10% excreted in feces, primarily as metabolites.

## Precautions to Consider

**Carcinogenicity**
In a lifetime study of rats, there was an increase in nodular proliferative lesions of the liver at doses of 100 mg to 300 mg per kg of body weight (mg/kg; approximately 3 to 10 times the maximum recommended human dose [MRHD] on a mg per square meter of body surface area [mg/m$^2$] basis) a day. However, whether such lesions may be precursors of neoplasms of the liver has not been resolved. Similar lesions were not seen in studies with mice given doses of up to 150 mg/kg a day (approximately two times the MRHD on a mg/m$^2$ basis).

**Tumorigenicity**
Studies in rodents showed no increase in malignant tumors of the liver or other organs.

**Mutagenicity**
In two of five strains in the Ames bacterial mutagenicity test, bupropion produced a mutation rate of two to three times the control mutation rate. In one of three *in vivo* bone marrow cytogenetic studies in rats, bupropion produced chromosomal aberrations.

**Pregnancy/Reproduction**
Fertility—Studies in rats and rabbits given doses of up to 300 mg/kg a day have shown no evidence of impaired fertility.
Pregnancy—Adequate and well-controlled studies in humans have not been done. However, bupropion readily crosses the placenta.
Studies in rats and rabbits given doses of up to 15 to 45 times the human daily dose have not shown that bupropion causes adverse effects in the fetus. In rabbits, two studies showed a slightly increased incidence of fetal abnormalities; however, there was no increase in any specific abnormality.
FDA Pregnancy Category B.
Labor and delivery—The effect of bupropion on labor and delivery in humans is unknown.

**Breast-feeding**
Bupropion accumulates in breast milk, and the potential exists for serious adverse reactions (such as seizures) in the infant.
The milk-to-plasma ratio of bupropion in one nursing mother who was receiving 100 mg of the prompt-release formulation of bupropion three times a day ranged from 2.51 to 8.58 over 6 hours, with the peak breast-milk concentration occurring 2 hours after bupropion dosing. The bupropion metabolite threohydrobupropion also accumulated in breast milk, with a milk-to-plasma ratio ranging from 1.23 to 1.57 over the same 6 hours. Hydroxybupropion concentrations in milk did not exceed corresponding plasma concentrations at any of the measure times. Neither bupropion nor its metabolites were detectable in serum taken from the infant, a 14-month-old boy, 3.75 hours after nursing, which occurred 9.5 hours after the mother's last dose of bupropion. No adverse effects were observed in the infant.

**Pediatrics**
Studies that included a small number of patients 6 to 16 years of age have not demonstrated pediatrics-specific problems that would limit the usefulness of bupropion in children. However, there is not sufficient evidence to establish safety and efficacy of bupropion in children up to 18 years of age.

**Geriatrics**
Studies that included patients 60 years of age and older have not demonstrated geriatrics-specific problems that would limit the usefulness of bupropion in the elderly. However, older patients are known to be more sensitive to the anticholinergic, sedative, and cardiovascular side effects of antidepressants. In addition, elderly patients are more likely to have age-related renal or hepatic function impairment, which may require dosage adjustment in patients receiving bupropion.

**Drug interactions and/or related problems**
The following drug interactions and/or related problems have been selected on the basis of their potential clinical significance (possible mechanism in parentheses where appropriate)—not necessarily inclusive (» = major clinical significance):

Note:  The cytochrome P450 2B6 (CYP2B6) isoenzyme is involved in the metabolism of bupropion to its active metabolite hydroxybupropion. A potential exists for interactions between bupropion and medications that affect CYP2B6, such as orphenadrine and cyclophosphamide.

Combinations containing any of the following medications, depending on the amount present, may also interact with this medication.

» Alcohol
 (concurrent use of or the cessation of chronic use of alcohol during therapy may lower the seizure threshold and increase the risk of seizures; patients should be advised to minimize alcohol consumption or avoid the use of alcohol completely)

Hepatic enzyme inducers (see *Appendix II*)
 (concurrent use with bupropion may increase the metabolism of bupropion; a study in patients receiving chronic carbamazepine

therapy showed significant decreases in bupropion peak plasma concentration and area under the plasma concentration–time curve [AUC] and increases in hydroxybupropion peak plasma concentration and AUC; a study in cigarette smokers showed no effect of smoking on the pharmacokinetics of bupropion)

Hepatic enzyme inhibitors (see *Appendix II*)
(these medications may inhibit hepatic microsomal enzymes, thereby decreasing metabolism and increasing serum concentrations of bupropion, thus increasing the risk of seizures; a study in patients receiving chronic valproic acid therapy showed no change in bupropion concentrations but increases in hydroxybupropion peak concentration and AUC)

Levodopa
(concurrent use with bupropion may result in a greater incidence of adverse effects; small initial doses of bupropion and gradual dosage increases are recommended during concurrent therapy)

» Monoamine oxidase (MAO) inhibitors, including furazolidone, procarbazine, and selegiline
(concurrent use of bupropion with these medications may increase the risk of acute toxicity of bupropion and is **contraindicated**; a medication-free interval of at least 14 days should elapse between discontinuation of the MAO inhibitor and initiation of bupropion therapy)

Nicotine
(although a nicotine transdermal system may be used concurrently with bupropion in the treatment of nicotine dependence, the combination has been associated with hypertension; blood pressure should be monitored in patients receiving this combination)

» Ritonavir
(although there is no experience with the combination, ritonavir has a high affinity for several cytochrome P450 isoenzymes and may increase bupropion plasma concentrations, thus increasing the risk of seizures; concurrent use should be approached with caution until more information is available)

» Seizure-threshold–lowering medications, other, such as:
Antidepressants, tricyclic or
Clozapine or
Fluoxetine or
Haloperidol or
Lithium or
Loxapine or
Maprotiline or
Molindone or
Phenothiazines or
Thioxanthenes or
Trazodone
(concurrent use of these medications with bupropion may increase the risk of major motor seizures; in addition, changes in treatment regimen, such as abrupt discontinuation of a benzodiazepine, may precipitate a seizure)

**Laboratory value alterations**
The following have been selected on the basis of their potential clinical significance (possible effect in parentheses where appropriate)—not necessarily inclusive (» = major clinical significance):

With physiology/laboratory test values
White blood cell count
(decreased by 10 to 14% during the first 2 months of therapy in one study; unknown clinical significance)

**Medical considerations/Contraindications**
The medical considerations/contraindications included have been selected on the basis of their potential clinical significance (reasons given in parentheses where appropriate)—not necessarily inclusive (» = major clinical significance).

***Except under special circumstances, this medication should not be used when the following medical problems exist:***

» Anorexia nervosa, or history of or
» Bulimia, or history of
(increased risk of seizures in patients with current or prior diagnosis of these conditions)

» Seizure disorders
(increased risk of seizures)

***Risk-benefit should be considered when the following medical problems exist:***

Bipolar disorder
(mania may be precipitated during the depressed phase in patients with manic-depressive illness)

» CNS tumor or
» Head trauma or
» Neurologic impairment, including developmental delay, or
» Spontaneous seizures, history of
(increased risk of seizures)

Drug abuse
(patients with a history of amphetamine or stimulant abuse may be attracted to bupropion because of its mild amphetamine-like activity, especially at higher doses; however, risk of seizures has prevented adequate testing)
(risk of seizures may be increased in patients with addiction to opiates, cocaine, or stimulants)

» Heart disease
(higher plasma concentrations of the active metabolites of bupropion may occur in patients with left ventricular dysfunction; in a short-term study of 36 patients with left ventricular impairment, ventricular arrhythmias, and/or conduction disease, mean systolic supine blood pressure readings increased by 5 ± 10 mm Hg, mean diastolic supine blood pressure readings increased by 3 ± 5 mm Hg, and two patients with mild hypertension at baseline discontinued use due to exacerbation of hypertension)

» Hepatic function impairment or
» Renal function impairment
(metabolism or excretion may be altered; bupropion treatment should be initiated at a reduced dosage and patient should be monitored closely)

Hypertension
(may be exacerbated)

Psychosis, especially schizoaffective disorder, depressed
(latent psychosis or mania may be activated in susceptible patients)

Sensitivity to bupropion

**Patient monitoring**
The following may be especially important in patient monitoring (other tests may be warranted in some patients, depending on condition; » = major clinical significance):

Blood pressure
(recommended in patients who are using a nicotine transdermal system concurrently with bupropion and in patients with baseline hypertension)

Careful supervision of depressed patients with suicidal tendencies
(recommended especially during early weeks of treatment for depression; hospitalization may be required as a protective measure)

## Side/Adverse Effects

The following side/adverse effects have been selected on the basis of their potential clinical significance (possible signs and symptoms in parentheses where appropriate)—not necessarily inclusive:

**Those indicating need for medical attention**
Incidence more frequent
*Agitation; anxiety*

Incidence less frequent
*Headache, severe; skin rash, hives, or itching; tinnitus* (buzzing or ringing in ears)

Incidence rare
*Fainting; neuropsychiatric effects, including confusion; delusions* (false beliefs that are not changed by facts); *hallucinations* (seeing, hearing, or feeling things that are not there); *paranoia* (extreme distrust); *or trouble in concentrating; seizures*—especially with higher doses

Note: The risk of *seizures* with bupropion may be greater than with other antidepressants. Seizures occur more frequently at higher doses. The incidence with use of the extended-release formulation is approximately 0.1% (3/3100 patients) at doses of up to 300 mg a day, and 0.4% (4/1000 patients) at a dose of 400 mg a day. With the use of the prompt-release formulation, seizure frequencies of 0.4% (13/3200 patients) at doses of 300 to 450 mg a day and almost tenfold higher at doses between 450 mg and 600 mg a day have been reported.

**Those indicating need for medical attention only if they continue or are bothersome**
Incidence more frequent
*Abdominal pain; anorexia* (decrease in appetite); *constipation; dizziness; dryness of mouth; increased sweating; insomnia* (trouble in sleeping); *nausea or vomiting; tremor* (trembling or shaking); *weight loss, unusual*

Note: *Dryness of mouth* and *insomnia* may be dose-related. Avoiding taking bupropion at bedtime may help to relieve insomnia.

Incidence less frequent or rare
*Blurred vision; drowsiness; palpitation* (feeling of fast or irregular heartbeat); *taste perversion* (change in sense of taste); *unusual feeling of well-being; urinary frequency*

## Overdose

For specific information on the agents used in the management of bupropion overdose, see:
- *Benzodiazepines (Systemic)* monograph; and/or
- *Charcoal, Activated (Oral-Local)* monograph.

For more information on the management of overdose or unintentional ingestion, **contact a Poison Control Center** (see *Poison Control Center Listing*).

### Clinical effects of overdose

Note: Deaths have occurred following massive overdose with bupropion alone.

The following effects have been selected on the basis of their potential clinical significance (possible signs and symptoms in parentheses where appropriate)—not necessarily inclusive:

Acute
*Hallucinations* (seeing, hearing, or feeling things that are not there); *loss of consciousness; nausea; seizures; tachycardia* (fast heartbeat)—possibly progressing to bradycardia or asystole; *vomiting*

Note: *Seizures* occur in about one third of bupropion overdose cases.

### Treatment of overdose

To decrease absorption—In comatose or stuporous patients, initiation of airway intubation followed by gastric lavage within the first 12 hours of ingestion, when absorption is not yet complete. Administration of activated charcoal every 6 hours within the first 12 hours of ingestion. Ipecac syrup should not be used to induce vomiting because of the possibility of seizures.

Specific treatment—Treatment of seizures with an intravenous benzodiazepine, although seizures may be resistant to benzodiazepine treatment.

Monitoring—Monitoring ECG and EEG for at least 48 hours. Monitoring acid-base and electrolyte balance in patients presenting in status epilepticus.

Supportive care—Maintenance of patent airway and adequate ventilation. Maintenance of adequate fluid intake. Patients in whom intentional overdose is confirmed or suspected should be referred for psychiatric consultation.

Note: Diuresis, dialysis, and hemoperfusion are not likely to be of benefit due to the slow diffusion of bupropion and its metabolites from tissue to plasma.

## Patient Consultation

As an aid to patient consultation, refer to *Advice for the Patient, Bupropion (Systemic)*.

In providing consultation, consider emphasizing the following selected information (» = major clinical significance):

### Before using this medication
» Conditions affecting use, especially:
    Sensitivity to bupropion
    Pregnancy—Crosses placenta
    Breast-feeding—Accumulates in breast milk; because of potential for serious adverse effects in the infant, use is not recommended
    Contraindicated medications MAO inhibitors
    Other medications, especially alcohol, other seizure-threshold-lowering medications, or ritonavir
    Other medical problems, especially anorexia nervosa, bulimia, CNS tumor, head trauma, heart disease, hepatic or renal function impairment, history of spontaneous seizures, neurologic impairment, or seizure disorders

### Proper use of this medication
» Compliance with therapy; not taking more or less medication than prescribed
» Taking doses of prompt-release tablets at least 4 hours apart; taking doses of extended-release tablets at least 8 hours apart to avoid occurrence of seizures
» Swallowing extended-release tablets whole; not crushing, breaking, or chewing
   Taking with food if needed to lessen gastrointestinal irritation

*For smoking cessation*
   Taking bupropion for 7 or more days prior to the date on which smoking will be discontinued

   Participating in smoking cessation support program, including behavioral interventions, counseling, and/or other support

*For mental depression*
   May require 4 weeks or longer for optimal antidepressant effects
» Proper dosing
   Missed dose: For extended-release and prompt-release tablets—Skipping the missed dose and returning to regular dosing schedule; not doubling doses
» Proper storage

### Precautions while using this medication
   Regular visits to physician to check progress during therapy
» Not taking bupropion within 14 days of taking an MAO inhibitor
» Not taking bupropion under different brand names concurrently because of dose-dependent incidence of seizures
» Minimizing or avoiding consumption of alcoholic beverages to reduce the risk of seizures
» Possible dizziness, drowsiness, or euphoria; caution when driving, using machinery, or doing other things requiring alertness and judgment

### Side/adverse effects
Signs of potential side effects, especially agitation; anxiety; severe headache; skin rash, hives, or itching; tinnitus; fainting; neuropsychiatric effects; or seizures

## General Dosing Information

Bupropion is marketed under different brand names for different approved indications; patients should not receive bupropion under different brand names concurrently due to the dose-dependent incidence of seizures.

To reduce the risk of agitation, anxiety, and insomnia, which are more frequent at initiation of therapy, increases in dosage must be made gradually.

Seizures occur more frequently at higher doses; the incidence with use of the extended-release formulation is approximately 0.1% (3/3100 patients) at doses of up to 300 mg a day, and 0.4% (4/1000 patients) at a dose of 400 mg a day. With use of the prompt-release formulation, seizure frequencies of 0.4% (13/3200 patients) at doses of 300 to 450 mg a day and almost tenfold higher at doses between 450 mg and 600 mg a day have been reported.

Patients being treated for nicotine dependence should continue to smoke during the first week of treatment with bupropion to allow the medication to reach steady-state plasma concentrations. A target date for discontinuation of smoking should be set for the second week of treatment. Bupropion treatment should be continued for 7 to 12 weeks. Longer treatment may be considered in individual patients. Treatment with bupropion should be reconsidered if significant progress toward abstinence is not seen by the seventh week of therapy, as the patient is unlikely to quit smoking on that attempt.

Full antidepressant action may not be evident for 4 weeks or longer.

Potentially suicidal patients should not have access to large quantities of this medication since depressed patients, particularly those who use alcohol excessively, may continue to exhibit suicidal tendencies until significant improvement occurs.

### Diet/Nutrition
Bupropion may be taken with food to lessen gastrointestinal irritation.

### Bioequivalence information
At steady-state, the prompt-release and the extended-release formulations of bupropion hydrochloride are bioequivalent with respect to both rate and extent of absorption.

### For prevention of seizures
The risk of seizures may be reduced if:
- The total daily dose of the prompt-release formulation does not exceed 450 mg and the total daily dose of the extended-release formulation does not exceed 400 mg when used as an antidepressant and 300 mg when used as an aid to smoking cessation.
- Each single dose of the prompt-release formulation or the extended-release formulation, when used as an aid to smoking cessation, does not exceed 150 mg, and each single dose of the extended-release formulation does not exceed 200 mg when used as an antidepressant.
- Doses of the prompt-release formulation are taken at least 4 hours apart and doses of the extended-release formulation are taken at least 8 hours apart.
- The dosage is increased gradually.
- Caution is used in patients with a history of seizures, cranial trauma, or other predisposition to seizures, and during concurrent use with other medications or treatment regimens, such as the abrupt discontinuation of benzodiazepines, that may lower the seizure threshold.

### For treatment of adverse effects
Recommended treatment consists of the following:
- For agitation, anxiety, or insomnia—Lowering dosage, and then increasing it gradually as needed and tolerated. Temporary sedative-hypnotic medication may be necessary, but is usually not required beyond the first week of treatment. Avoiding a bedtime bupropion dose may minimize insomnia. If effects are severe, discontinuation of bupropion may be necessary.
- For nausea and vomiting—Taking with meals, or decreasing and then gradually increasing the dosage.

## Oral Dosage Forms

### BUPROPION HYDROCHLORIDE EXTENDED-RELEASE TABLETS

#### Usual adult dose
Antidepressant—
Oral, initially 150 mg once a day in the morning for three days, then 150 mg two times a day if well tolerated. If no improvement is seen after several weeks, dosage may be increased to 200 mg two times a day.

Note: Doses should be taken at least eight hours apart to reduce the risk of seizures.

Smoking cessation adjunct—
Oral, initially 150 mg once a day for three days, then 150 mg two times a day for seven to twelve weeks.

Note: Doses should be taken at least eight hours apart to reduce the risk of seizures.

#### Usual adult prescribing limits
Antidepressant—
400 mg per day, with no single dose exceeding 200 mg.
Smoking cessation adjunct—
300 mg per day, with no single dose exceeding 150 mg.

#### Usual pediatric dose
Safety and efficacy have not been established in children younger than 18 years of age.

#### Strength(s) usually available
U.S.—
100 mg (Rx) [*Wellbutrin SR* (carnauba wax; cysteine hydrochloride; FD&C Blue No. 1 Lake; hydroxypropyl methylcellulose; magnesium stearate; microcrystalline cellulose; polyethylene glycol; polysorbate 80; titanium dioxide)].
150 mg (Rx) [*Wellbutrin SR* (carnauba wax; cysteine hydrochloride; FD&C Blue No. 2 Lake; FD&C Red No. 40 Lake; hydroxypropyl methylcellulose; magnesium stearate; microcrystalline cellulose; polyethylene glycol; polysorbate 80; titanium dioxide)]; *Zyban* (carnauba wax; cysteine hydrochloride; FD&C Blue No. 2 Lake; FD&C Red No. 40 Lake; hydroxypropyl methylcellulose; magnesium stearate; microcrystalline cellulose; polyethylene glycol; polysorbate 80; titanium dioxide)].

Canada—
100 mg (Rx) [*Wellbutrin SR* (carnauba wax; cysteine hydrochloride; FD&C Blue No. 1 Lake; hydroxypropyl methylcellulose; magnesium stearate; microcrystalline cellulose; polyethylene glycol; polysorbate 80; titanium dioxide)].
150 mg (Rx) [*Wellbutrin SR* (carnauba wax; cysteine hydrochloride; FD&C Blue No. 2 Lake; FD&C Red No. 40 Lake; hydroxypropyl methylcellulose; magnesium stearate; microcrystalline cellulose; polyethylene glycol; polysorbate 80; titanium dioxide)].

#### Packaging and storage
Store at controlled room temperature, 20 to 25 °C (68 to 77 °F), in a tight, light-resistant container, unless otherwise specified by manufacturer.

#### Auxiliary labeling
- Avoid alcoholic beverages.
- Swallow tablet whole. Do not break or chew.

#### Additional information
Bupropion is marketed under different brand names for different approved indications; patients should not receive bupropion under different brand names concurrently due to the dose-dependent incidence of seizures.

Note: Bupropion hydrochloride may have a characteristic odor.

### BUPROPION HYDROCHLORIDE TABLETS

#### Usual adult dose
Antidepressant—
Oral, initially 100 mg two times a day, the dosage being increased gradually, no sooner than three days after beginning therapy, to 100 mg three times a day as needed and tolerated.

Note: Doses should be taken at least four hours apart to reduce the risk of seizures.

#### Usual adult prescribing limits
450 mg per day, with no single dose exceeding 150 mg.

#### Usual pediatric dose
Safety and efficacy have not been established in children younger than 18 years of age.

#### Strength(s) usually available
U.S.—
75 mg (Rx) [*Wellbutrin* (D&C Yellow No. 10 Lake; FD&C Yellow No. 6 Lake; hydroxypropyl cellulose; hydroxypropyl methylcellulose; light mineral oil; microcrystalline cellulose; talc; titanium dioxide)].
100 mg (Rx) [*Wellbutrin* (FD&C Red No. 40 Lake; FD&C Yellow No. 6 Lake; hydroxypropyl cellulose; hydroxypropyl methylcellulose; light mineral oil; microcrystalline cellulose; talc; titanium dioxide)].

Canada—
Not commercially available.

#### Packaging and storage
Store below 40 °C (104 °F), preferably between 15 and 30 °C (59 and 86 °F), unless otherwise specified by manufacturer.

#### Auxiliary labeling
- Avoid alcoholic beverages.

#### Additional information
Bupropion is marketed under different brand names for different approved indications; patients should not receive bupropion under different brand names concurrently due to the dose-dependent incidence of seizures.

Note: Bupropion hydrochloride may have a characteristic odor.

Revised: 02/17/98
Interim revision: 08/07/98

---

# BUSERELIN Systemic*

VA CLASSIFICATION (Primary): AN500
Commonly used brand name(s): *Suprefact*.
Note: For a listing of dosage forms and brand names by country availability, see *Dosage Forms* section(s).

*Not commercially available in U.S.

## Category
Antineoplastic.

## Indications

### Accepted
Carcinoma, prostatic (treatment)—Buserelin is indicated for the palliative treatment of advanced prostatic carcinoma (stage D), especially as an alternative to orchiectomy or estrogen administration.

## Pharmacology/Pharmacokinetics

### Physicochemical characteristics
Molecular weight—1299.49.

### Mechanism of action/Effect
Buserelin is a synthetic luteinizing hormone–releasing hormone (LHRH) analog. Like naturally occurring LHRH that is produced by the hypothalamus, initial or intermittent administration of buserelin stimulates release of luteinizing hormone (LH) and follicle-stimulating hormone (FSH) from the anterior pituitary, which in turn transiently increases testosterone concentrations in males. However, continuous daily administration of buserelin in the treatment of prostatic carcinoma suppresses secretion of LH and FSH, with a resultant fall in testosterone concentrations and a "medical castration".

### Onset of action
Testosterone concentrations—Transient increase occurs within first week of therapy, but decline to castrate levels occurs within 2 to 4 weeks.

## Precautions to Consider

### Carcinogenicity
Studies in rats for two years at daily subcutaneous doses of 0.2 to 1.8 mcg per kg of body weight found no evidence of carcinogenicity.

### Mutagenicity
Mutagenicity studies in bacterial systems (Ames test in *Salmonella typhimurium* and *Escherichia coli*) and mammalian systems (micronuclei test in mice) found no evidence of mutagenic effects.

### Pregnancy/Reproduction
Fertility—Suppression of testosterone secretion results in impairment of fertility. Although it is not known whether fertility is restored after buserelin is withdrawn, reversal of fertility suppression does occur after withdrawal of similar analogs.

### Geriatrics
Appropriate studies on the relationship of age to the effects of buserelin have not been performed in the geriatric population. However, clinical trials were conducted mainly in older patients and geriatrics-specific problems that would limit the usefulness of this medication in the elderly are not expected.

### Laboratory value alterations
The following have been selected on the basis of their potential clinical significance (possible effect in parentheses where appropriate)—not necessarily inclusive (» = major clinical significance):

With physiology/laboratory test values
  Acid phosphatase
    (transient increases in serum values may occur early in treatment, but usually decrease to or near baseline by the fourth week; may decrease to below baseline levels if elevated concentrations were present before treatment)
  Testosterone
    (serum concentrations usually increase during the first week of therapy but then decrease; castrate levels are reached within 2 to 4 weeks)

### Medical considerations/Contraindications
The medical considerations/contraindications included have been selected on the basis of their potential clinical significance (reasons given in parentheses where appropriate)—not necessarily inclusive (» = major clinical significance).

*Risk-benefit should be considered when the following medical problems exist:*
  Obstructive uropathy, history of
    (increased incidence of disease flare during initial buserelin treatment because of the initial increase in serum testosterone concentrations)
  Sensitivity to buserelin
  Vertebral metastases
    (risk of spinal cord compression as a result of disease flare during initial buserelin treatment)

### Patient monitoring
The following may be especially important in patient monitoring (other tests may be warranted in some patients, depending on condition; » = major clinical significance):

  Acid phosphatase concentrations, plasma prostaticor serum or
  Prostatic specific antigen concentrations, serumand
  Testosterone concentrations, serum
    (recommended at periodic intervals to monitor response)

## Side/Adverse Effects
The following side/adverse effects have been selected on the basis of their potential clinical significance (possible signs and symptoms in parentheses where appropriate)—not necessarily inclusive:

### Those indicating need for medical attention
Incidence less frequent—approximately 1%
  *Possible disease flare* (bone pain; numbness or tingling of hands or feet; trouble in urinating; weakness in legs)
  Note: *Possible disease flare* includes a transient (usually less than 10 days' duration), sometimes severe, increase in bone or tumor pain that may occur shortly after initiation of therapy, usually associated with the increase in serum testosterone, but that usually subsides with continued buserelin treatment. Analgesics may be required during this time. Other signs and symptoms of prostatic carcinoma, including difficult urination, may also worsen transiently. In addition, worsening of neurologic signs and symptoms in patients with vertebral metastases may result in temporary weakness and paresthesias of the lower extremities.

### Those indicating need for medical attention only if they continue or are bothersome
Incidence more frequent—incidence about 50%
  *Hot flashes* (sudden sweating and feelings of warmth)—incidence about 50%; *impotence or decrease in sexual desire*—incidence about 80 to 90%
Incidence less frequent
  *Burning, itching, redness, or swelling at site of injection; diarrhea; dry or sore nose*—with intranasal use only; *headache*—with intranasal use only; *increased sweating*—with intranasal use only; *loss of appetite; nausea or vomiting; swelling and increased tenderness of breasts; swelling of feet or lower legs*

## Patient Consultation
As an aid to patient consultation, refer to *Advice for the Patient, Buserelin (Systemic).*

In providing consultation, consider emphasizing the following selected information (» = major clinical significance):

### Before using this medication
» Conditions affecting use, especially:
    Sensitivity to buserelin
    Pregnancy—Pregnancy/reproduction—May cause sterility

### Proper use of this medication
» Carefully reading and following patient instruction sheet contained in package
  For patients using the injection:
    Using disposable syringes provided in kit
    Proper disposal of used syringes
  For patients using the nasal solution:
    Using nebulizer provided
» Importance of not using more or less medication than the amount prescribed
» Importance of continuing medication despite side effects
» Proper dosing
  Missed dose: Using as soon as remembered; not using if almost time for next dose; not doubling doses
» Proper storage

### Precautions while using this medication
» Importance of close monitoring by the physician

### Side/adverse effects
  Signs of potential side effects, especially transient disease flare

## General Dosing Information
Patients receiving buserelin should be under supervision of a physician experienced in cancer therapy.

Buserelin has approximately 20 to 170 times the activity of naturally occurring luteinizing hormone–releasing hormone (LHRH) and a longer duration of action.

## Nasal Dosage Forms

### BUSERELIN ACETATE NASAL SOLUTION

#### Usual adult dose
Prostatic carcinoma—
  Maintenance: Intranasal, 400 mcg (0.4 mg) (base) (200 mcg in each nostril) every eight hours.
  Note: Initial treatment is by subcutaneous injection.
    Each pump action delivers 100 mcg (0.1 mL) of medication.

#### Strength(s) usually available
U.S.—
  Not commercially available.
Canada—
  1 mg (base) per mL (Rx) [*Suprefact* (benzyl alcohol 10 mg per mL; no propellants)].

#### Packaging and storage
Store below 25 °C (77 °F), unless otherwise specified by manufacturer. Protect from freezing.

#### Auxiliary labeling
• Do not freeze.

## Parenteral Dosage Forms

### BUSERELIN ACETATE INJECTION

**Usual adult dose**
Prostatic carcinoma—
   Initial: Subcutaneous, 500 mcg (0.5 mg) (base) every eight hours for seven days.
   Maintenance: Subcutaneous, 200 mcg (0.2 mg) (base) once a day.
   Note: Alternatively, the nasal solution may be used for maintenance dosing.

**Strength(s) usually available**
U.S.—
   Not commercially available.
Canada—
   1 mg (base) per mL (Rx) [*Suprefact* (benzyl alcohol 10 mg per mL)].

**Packaging and storage**
Store below 25 °C (77 °F), unless otherwise specified by manufacturer. Protect from freezing.

**Auxiliary labeling**
• Do not freeze.

## Selected Bibliography

Schroder FH (ed.). New treatment modalities in prostatic cancer: LHRH superagonists. Symposium held during World Congress of Oncology, Budapest, Hungary, August 26, 1986. Am J Clin Oncol 1988; 11 (Suppl 1): S1-46.

The management of clinically localized prostate cancer. National Institutes of Health Consensus Development Conference Statement 1987 June 15–17; 6(10).

Korman LB. Treatment of prostate cancer. Clin Pharm 1989 Jun; 8: 412-24.

Furr BJA, Woodburn JR. Luteinizing hormone–releasing hormone and its analogues: a review of biological properties and clinical uses. J Endocrinol Invest 1988 Jul–Aug; 11: 535-57.

Revised: 07/11/94

---

# BUSPIRONE    Systemic

VA CLASSIFICATION (Primary): CN304
Commonly used brand name(s): *BuSpar; BuSpar DIVIDOSE; Bustab*.
Note: For a listing of dosage forms and brand names by country availability, see *Dosage Forms* section(s).

## Category
Antianxiety agent.

## Indications

**General considerations**
The efficacy of buspirone in the treatment of generalized anxiety of moderate severity has been shown to be comparable to that of benzodiazepines such as diazepam, clorazepate, alprazolam, and lorazepam. However, unlike the benzodiazepines, buspirone appears to lack potential for physical dependence or abuse.

Buspirone has been shown to cause less sedation than other antianxiety agents, especially at lower doses. Therefore, it may be a useful alternative to other antianxiety agents in the treatment of generalized anxiety, particularly in patients hypersensitive to the sedative effects of the other agents.

**Accepted**
Anxiety (treatment)—Buspirone is indicated for the management of anxiety disorders or the short-term relief of the symptoms of anxiety. However, buspirone usually is not indicated for the treatment of anxiety or tension associated with the stress of everyday life.

The effectiveness of buspirone in the management of anxiety for more than 3 to 4 weeks has not been shown in controlled studies. However, buspirone has not been shown to cause adverse effects different from those seen with short-term use when used for up to 1 year. If buspirone is used for extended periods of time, efficacy of the medication should be reassessed at periodic intervals.

**Acceptance not established**
Buspirone has shown some effectiveness in small uncontrolled studies as an adjunct to antidepressant medications in the treatment of mental depression (Evidence rating: C-3).

Small uncontrolled studies and case reports indicate buspirone may be effective as a treatment of aggressive behavior in patients with neurological disorders or damage (Evidence rating: C-3).

## Pharmacology/Pharmacokinetics

**Physicochemical characteristics**
Chemical group—Azaspirodecanedione (an azapirone). Buspirone is not chemically or pharmacologically related to benzodiazepines, barbiturates, or other sedative/antianxiety agents.
Molecular weight—Buspirone hydrochloride: 421.97.
—Buspirone hydrochloride is very water soluble.

**Mechanism of action/Effect**
The exact mechanism of action of buspirone has not been determined. The medication is believed to have a unique anxioselective action, since it has no anticonvulsant or muscle relaxant activity and does not appear to cause physical dependence or significant sedation. Buspirone has a high affinity for serotonin 5-HT$_{1A}$ receptors. Serotonin 5-HT$_{1A}$ receptors are found in high concentrations in the dorsal raphe nucleus of the brain, where they are considered to be presynaptic, and in the hippocampal and cortical regions of the brain, where they are considered to be postsynaptic. Buspirone acts as an agonist at presynaptic 5-HT$_{1A}$ receptors, causing decreased firing of serotonergic neurons in the dorsal raphe nucleus, and decreased serotonin synthesis and release. Buspirone acts as a partial agonist at postsynaptic 5-HT$_{1A}$ receptors. Buspirone also has been shown to have a moderate affinity for brain dopamine D$_2$ receptors, where it acts as a weak antagonist both pre- and postsynaptically. It has no significant affinity for benzodiazepine receptors and does not affect gamma-aminobutyric acid (GABA) binding. The neuronal reuptake of monoamines is not blocked by buspirone. Some studies have suggested that buspirone may have indirect effects on other neurotransmitter systems.

In contrast to the benzodiazepines, the spontaneous firing rate of noradrenergic cells in the locus ceruleus is increased rather than decreased by buspirone. Differences in dependence and tolerance between benzodiazepines and buspirone are due to these site-specific differences.

**Other actions/effects**
Although increases in plasma prolactin and growth hormone concentrations to more than two times the upper limit of normal were seen in healthy male volunteers given buspirone in single doses of 30 mg or higher, these increases did not occur in another study using a buspirone dosage of 10 mg three times a day for 28 days.

**Absorption**
Rapidly and completely absorbed from the gastrointestinal tract; however, extensive first-pass metabolism limits the bioavailability of buspirone to approximately 4%. Although concurrent administration of food slows the rate of absorption of buspirone, the presence of food increases the amount of unchanged buspirone reaching systemic circulation.

**Distribution**
Apparent Vol$_D$—Healthy adult males: 5.3 ± 2.6 L per kg (L/kg).

**Protein binding**
Plasma—Very high (95%); about 70% is bound to albumin, and 30% is bound to alpha$_1$-acid glycoprotein. Although buspirone is highly protein-bound, it does not displace tightly protein-bound medications, such as warfarin, phenytoin, and propranolol, *in vitro*. However, buspirone does displace digoxin *in vitro*.

**Biotransformation**
Hepatic. Buspirone is rapidly metabolized and undergoes extensive first-pass metabolism. It is metabolized primarily by oxidation, producing several hydroxylated derivatives, and dealkylation. The *N*-dealkylated metabolite, 1-pyrimidinylpiperazine (1-PP), is pharmacologically active. In animal studies, 1-PP has been shown to have about one fourth the anxiolytic activity of buspirone.

A study on the effects of pretreatment with erythromycin or itraconazole on buspirone pharmacokinetics indicated that the cytochrome P450 3A4 (CYP3A4) isoenzyme plays a significant role in buspirone metabolism.

**Half-life**
Elimination—
   Mean, about 2 to 3 hours following single oral doses of 10 to 40 mg or a single intravenous dose of 1 mg in healthy males. Mean elimination half-life has ranged from 2 to 11 hours in other studies.

### Onset of action
May require up to 4 weeks to reach maximal effect, although some improvement may be seen in 1 week. Since buspirone does not cause muscle relaxation or significant sedation, patient may not immediately notice effects of medication.

### Time to peak plasma concentration
40 to 90 minutes following single oral doses of 20 mg; less than 1 hour following single oral doses of 10 mg.

### Peak plasma concentration
1 to 6 nanograms per mL following single oral doses of 20 mg. Following oral administration, plasma concentrations of unchanged buspirone are very low and vary about tenfold among individuals. One study in 15 subjects suggests that buspirone may exhibit nonlinear pharmacokinetics. Therefore, blood concentrations after dosage increases or multiple dosing may be higher than predicted by single-dose studies.

### Elimination
Clearance of a single 1-mg dose of buspirone in eight healthy males was 28 mL per kg of body weight per minute (mL/kg/min).
Renal—
    29 to 63% of the dose was excreted in urine within 24 hours in a single-dose study; less than 1% as unchanged drug.
Fecal—
    18 to 38% of the dose was excreted in feces in a single-dose study.
In dialysis—
    In six anuric patients, hemodialysis either decreased or had no effect on buspirone clearance.

## Precautions to Consider

### Carcinogenicity
Buspirone was not shown to be carcinogenic when it was administered to rats during a 24-month study at doses approximately 133 times the maximum recommended human dose (MRHD) or to mice during an 18-month study at doses approximately 167 times the MRHD.

### Mutagenicity
Buspirone was not shown to induce point mutations, with or without metabolic activation, in five strains of *Salmonella typhimurium* (Ames test) or mouse lymphoma L5178YTK⁺ cell cultures, nor was DNA damage observed with buspirone in Wi-38 human cells. Also, chromosomal abnormalities did not occur in bone marrow cells of mice given one or five daily doses of buspirone.

### Pregnancy/Reproduction
Fertility—Reproduction studies in rats and rabbits showed no impairment of fertility when buspirone was administered at doses approximately 30 times the maximum recommended human dose (MRHD).

Pregnancy—Adequate and well-controlled studies in humans have not been done.

Reproduction studies in rats and rabbits did not show buspirone to cause fetal damage when the medication was administered at doses approximately 30 times the MRHD.

FDA Pregnancy Category B.

Labor and delivery—Reproduction studies in rats have not shown buspirone to cause any adverse effects during labor and delivery.

### Breast-feeding
Problems in humans have not been documented. However, buspirone and its metabolites are distributed into the milk of rats.

### Pediatrics
Appropriate studies on the relationship of age to the effects of buspirone have not been performed in children up to 18 years of age. Safety and efficacy have not been established.

### Geriatrics
Although buspirone has not been systematically evaluated in older patients, clinical studies performed in several hundred elderly patients have not demonstrated geriatrics-specific problems that would limit the usefulness of buspirone in the elderly.

### Drug interactions and/or related problems
The following drug interactions and/or related problems have been selected on the basis of their potential clinical significance (possible mechanism in parentheses where appropriate)—not necessarily inclusive (» = major clinical significance):

Note: In one pharmacokinetics study, eight healthy females received erythromycin or itraconazole, at therapeutic doses, or placebo for four days. On the fourth day, a single 10-mg dose of buspirone was given and a series of blood samples was drawn. Buspirone area under the plasma concentration–time curve (AUC) and mean maximum plasma concentration ($C_{max}$) were greatly increased in the erythromycin and itraconazole pretreated subjects, indicating that the cytochrome P450 3A4 (CYP3A4) isoenzyme, which these medications inhibit, plays a significant role in buspirone metabolism. Interactions with medications that inhibit CYP3A4, other than those listed below, should be considered.

Combinations containing any of the following medications, depending on the amount present, may also interact with this medication.

Digoxin
    (may be displaced from serum protein binding sites when used concurrently with buspirone; however, the clinical significance is unknown)

» Erythromycin or
» Itraconazole
    (after pretreatment with erythromycin and itraconazole, $C_{max}$ of buspirone was increased 5-fold and 13-fold, respectively, and AUC of buspirone was increased 6-fold and 19-fold, respectively, in eight healthy female volunteers, probably due to decreased first-pass metabolism; also, an increased incidence of adverse effects was observed; decreased buspirone dosage is recommended)

» Monoamine oxidase (MAO) inhibitors, including furazolidone, procarbazine, and more than 10 mg a day of selegiline
    (elevations in blood pressure have been reported when buspirone was added to regimens that included MAO inhibitors)

### Medical considerations/Contraindications
The medical considerations/contraindications included have been selected on the basis of their potential clinical significance (reasons given in parentheses where appropriate)—not necessarily inclusive (» = major clinical significance).

*Risk-benefit should be considered when the following medical problems exist:*

» Hepatic function impairment
    (buspirone clearance is decreased in patients with impaired hepatic function; careful monitoring is recommended, and dosage adjustments may be necessary)

Renal function impairment
    (clearance of buspirone or its active metabolite, 1-pyrimidinylpiperazine [1-PP], may be decreased in patients with impaired renal function)

Sensitivity to buspirone

## Side/Adverse Effects

Note: Buspirone appears to lack potential for physical dependence or abuse.

Studies have shown that buspirone causes less sedation than other antianxiety agents (about one third of that occurring with benzodiazepines) and does not produce significant functional impairment. However, the CNS effects of buspirone in any individual patient may not be predictable.

Withdrawal symptoms or rebound anxiety has not been reported when the medication was abruptly discontinued.

The following side/adverse effects have been selected on the basis of their potential clinical significance (possible signs and symptoms in parentheses where appropriate)—not necessarily inclusive:

### Those indicating need for medical attention
Incidence rare
    *Chest pain; confusion; fast or pounding heartbeat; fever; mental depression; neurologic effects* (incoordination; muscle weakness; numbness, tingling, pain, or weakness in hands or feet; stiffness of arms or legs; uncontrolled movements of the body); *skin rash or hives; sore throat*

### Those indicating need for medical attention only if they continue or are bothersome
Incidence more frequent
    *Dizziness or lightheadedness*—especially when getting up from a sitting or lying position; *headache; nausea; syndrome of restlessness* (restlessness, nervousness, or unusual excitement)

Note: *Syndrome of restlessness* may occur shortly after buspirone therapy is initiated, and may be due to increased central noradrenergic activity or to dopaminergic effects.

Incidence less frequent or rare
    *Blurred vision; clamminess or sweating; decreased concentration; diarrhea; drowsiness*—more frequent with doses > 20 mg per day; *dryness of mouth; insomnia* (trouble in sleeping); *nightmares; or vivid dreams; musculoskeletal effects* (muscle pain, spasms, cramps, or stiffness); *ringing in the ears; unusual tiredness or weakness*

## Overdose

For more information on the management of overdose or unintentional ingestion, **contact a Poison Control Center** (see *Poison Control Center Listing*).

**Clinical effects of overdose**

Note: Buspirone is minimally toxic in overdose.
The following effects have been selected on the basis of their potential clinical significance (possible signs and symptoms in parentheses where appropriate)—not necessarily inclusive:

Acute
*Dizziness or lightheadedness; drowsiness, severe, or loss of consciousness; stomach upset, including nausea or vomiting; unusually small pupils*

**Treatment of overdose**

There is no known specific antidote to buspirone. Treatment is generally symptomatic and supportive.

To decrease absorption—Immediate (within 1 to 1.5 hours of ingestion) gastric lavage may be used.

Monitoring—Monitoring of respiration, pulse, and blood pressure is recommended. Patient should be observed for the development of extrapyramidal symptoms or behavior disturbances such as panic or mania.

Supportive care—Patients in whom intentional overdose is confirmed or suspected should be referred for psychiatric consultation.

## Patient Consultation

As an aid to patient consultation, refer to *Advice for the Patient, Buspirone (Systemic)*.

In providing consultation, consider emphasizing the following selected information (» = major clinical significance):

**Before using this medication**
» Conditions affecting use, especially:
Sensitivity to buspirone
Other medications, especially erythromycin, itraconazole, and monoamine oxidase (MAO) inhibitors
Other medical problems, especially hepatic function impairment

**Proper use of this medication**
» Importance of not using more medication than the amount prescribed
One to two weeks of therapy may be required before antianxiety effect is noticeable
» Proper dosing
Missed dose: Taking as soon as possible; not taking if almost time for next dose; not doubling doses
» Proper storage

**Precautions while using this medication**
Regular visits to physician to check progress during prolonged therapy
» Caution in driving or operating machinery until effects of medication are known
» Suspected overdose: Getting emergency help at once

**Side/adverse effects**
Signs of potential side effects, especially chest pain, confusion, fast or pounding heartbeat, fever, mental depression, neurologic effects, skin rash or hives, and sore throat

## General Dosing Information

Since buspirone does not exhibit cross-tolerance with benzodiazepines and other common sedative/hypnotic agents, the medication will not block the withdrawal syndrome associated with discontinuation of therapy with these agents. Therefore, prior to initiating therapy with buspirone, these agents should be withdrawn gradually, especially in patients who have been chronically using these CNS depressants.

A study that evaluated 120 patients meeting *Diagnostic and Statistical Manual of Mental Disorders, Third edition, Revised* (DSM IIIR) criteria for generalized anxiety disorder who had received buspirone 10 mg three times a day or 15 mg two times a day found no significant difference in efficacy or safety between the two regimens.

One to two weeks of therapy may be required before the antianxiety effect of buspirone is noticeable, as compared to the immediate effect of benzodiazepines.

## Oral Dosage Forms

### BUSPIRONE HYDROCHLORIDE TABLETS USP

**Usual adult dose**
Antianxiety agent—
Oral, initially 5 mg two or three times a day, or 7.5 mg two times a day, the dosage being increased by 5 mg per day at two- to three-day intervals until the desired response is obtained.

Note: The usual therapeutic dosage is 20 to 30 mg a day.

**Usual adult prescribing limits**
60 mg per day.

**Usual pediatric dose**
Safety and efficacy have not been established in children under 18 years of age.

**Usual geriatric dose**
Antianxiety agent—
See *Usual adult dose*.

**Strength(s) usually available**
U.S.—
5 mg (Rx) [*BuSpar* (scored; colloidal silicon dioxide; lactose; magnesium stearate; microcrystalline cellulose; sodium starch glycolate)].
10 mg (Rx) [*BuSpar* (scored; colloidal silicon dioxide; lactose; magnesium stearate; microcrystalline cellulose; sodium starch glycolate)].
15 mg (Rx) [*BuSpar DIVIDOSE* (multi-scored; colloidal silicon dioxide; lactose; magnesium stearate; microcrystalline cellulose; sodium starch glycolate)].

Note: The 15-mg tablet may be divided to provide doses of 5, 7.5, 10, or 15 mg.

Canada—
5 mg (Rx) [*BuSpar* (scored; lactose anhydrous); *Bustab*].
10 mg (Rx) [*BuSpar* (scored; lactose anhydrous); *Bustab*].

**Packaging and storage**
Store between 15 and 30 °C (59 and 86 °F), in a tight, light-resistant container, unless otherwise specified by manufacturer.

**Auxiliary labeling**
• May cause dizziness or drowsiness.

## Selected Bibliography

Fulton B, Brogden RN. Buspirone: an updated review of its clinical pharmacology and therapeutic applications. CNS Drugs 1997 Jan; 7(1): 68-88.

Revised: 03/17/98

# BUSULFAN Systemic

VA CLASSIFICATION (Primary): AN100

Commonly used brand name(s): *Myleran*.

Note: For a listing of dosage forms and brand names by country availability, see *Dosage Forms* section(s).

## Category

Antineoplastic.

## Indications

Note: Bracketed information in the *Indications* section refers to uses that are not included in U.S. product labeling.

**Accepted**

Leukemia, chronic myelocytic (treatment)—Busulfan is indicated for palliative treatment of chronic myelocytic leukemia. It is not useful in the blastic crisis phase.

[Leukemia, acute nonlymphocytic (treatment)][1]—Busulfan is used for treatment of acute nonlymphocytic leukemia.

[1]Not included in Canadian product labeling.

## Pharmacology/Pharmacokinetics

**Physicochemical characteristics**
Molecular weight—246.29.

# Busulfan (Systemic)

### Mechanism of action/Effect
Busulfan is a bifunctional alkylating agent of the alkylsulfonate type and is cell cycle–phase nonspecific. Its mechanism of action is not clear but is thought to consist of alkylation and cross-linking of strands of DNA and myelosuppression.

### Absorption
Completely absorbed from the gastrointestinal tract. Radioactivity is detected in the blood ½ to 2 hours after oral administration of radiolabeled busulfan.

### Biotransformation
Hepatic; rapid.

### Half-life
About 2.5 hours.

### Onset of action
A clinical response usually begins within 1 to 2 weeks after initiation of therapy.

### Elimination
Renal, slow, almost entirely as metabolites.

In dialysis—No information available; however, likely to have minimal effect because of poor water solubility of busulfan and prolonged retention of metabolites.

## Precautions to Consider

### Carcinogenicity
Secondary malignancies are potential delayed effects of many antineoplastic agents, although it is not clear whether the effect is related to their mutagenic or immunosuppressive action. The effect of dose and duration of therapy is also unknown, although risk seems to increase with long-term use. Although information is limited, available data seem to indicate that the carcinogenic risk is greatest with the alkylating agents.

Busulfan has been associated with development of acute leukemia in humans.

### Mutagenicity
Busulfan is mutagenic in mice. It has been reported to cause chromosome aberrations in human cells.

### Pregnancy/Reproduction
Fertility—Gonadal suppression, resulting in amenorrhea or azoospermia, may occur in patients taking antineoplastic therapy, especially with the alkylating agents. In general, these effects appear to be related to dose and length of therapy and may be irreversible. Prediction of the degree of testicular or ovarian function impairment is complicated by the common use of combinations of several antineoplastics, which makes it difficult to assess the effects of individual agents.

Busulfan produces sterility in the male and female offspring of rats due to germinal cell aplasia in testes and ovaries. It has also been associated with impairment of gonadal function in humans (ovarian suppression and amenorrhea with menopausal symptoms in premenopausal patients; sterility, azoospermia, and testicular atrophy in males).

Pregnancy—Adequate and well-controlled studies in humans have not been done. Although several successful pregnancies have been reported, one case of neonatal abnormalities has been reported in which the mother received radiation and combination chemotherapy including busulfan. In addition, there have been reports of small infants, especially after use of busulfan during the third trimester, and there is one report of mild anemia and neutropenia at birth after maternal administration of busulfan from the eighth week of pregnancy to term.

First trimester: It is usually recommended that use of antineoplastics, especially combination chemotherapy, be avoided whenever possible, especially during the first trimester. Although information is limited because of the relatively few instances of antineoplastic administration during pregnancy, the mutagenic, teratogenic, and carcinogenic potential of these medications must be considered.

Other hazards to the fetus include adverse reactions seen in adults.

In general, use of a contraceptive is recommended during cytotoxic drug therapy.

FDA Pregnancy Category D.

### Breast-feeding
Although very little information is available regarding distribution of antineoplastic agents into breast milk, breast-feeding is not recommended during chemotherapy because of the risks to the infant (adverse effects, mutagenicity, carcinogenicity). It is not known whether busulfan is distributed into breast milk.

### Pediatrics
Appropriate studies performed to date have not demonstrated pediatrics-specific problems that would limit the usefulness of busulfan in children.

### Geriatrics
Appropriate studies on the relationship of age to the effects of busulfan have not been performed in the geriatric population. However, geriatrics-specific problems that would limit the usefulness of this medication in the elderly are not expected.

### Dental
The bone marrow depressant effects of busulfan may result in an increased incidence of microbial infection, delayed healing, and gingival bleeding. Dental work, whenever possible, should be completed prior to initiation of therapy or deferred until blood counts have returned to normal. Patients should be instructed in proper oral hygiene during treatment, including caution in use of regular toothbrushes, dental floss, and toothpicks.

Busulfan may also cause stomatitis associated with considerable discomfort.

### Drug interactions and/or related problems
The following drug interactions and/or related problems have been selected on the basis of their potential clinical significance (possible mechanism in parentheses where appropriate)—not necessarily inclusive (» = major clinical significance):

Note: Combinations containing any of the following medications, depending on the amount present, may also interact with this medication.

Allopurinol or
Colchicine or
» Probenecid or
» Sulfinpyrazone
(busulfan may raise the concentration of blood uric acid; dosage adjustment of antigout agents may be necessary to control hyperuricemia and gout; allopurinol may be preferred to prevent or reverse busulfan-induced hyperuricemia because of risk of uric acid nephropathy with uricosuric antigout agents)

Blood dyscrasia–causing medications (see *Appendix II*)
(leukopenic and/or thrombocytopenic effects of busulfan may be increased with concurrent or recent therapy if these medications cause the same effects; dosage adjustment of busulfan, if necessary, should be based on blood counts)

» Bone marrow depressants, other (see *Appendix II*) or
» Radiation therapy
(additive bone marrow depression may occur; dosage reduction may be required when two or more bone marrow depressants, including radiation, are used concurrently or consecutively)

Vaccines, killed virus
(because normal defense mechanisms may be suppressed by busulfan therapy, the patient's antibody response to the vaccine may be decreased. The interval between discontinuation of medications that cause immunosuppression and restoration of the patient's ability to respond to the vaccine depends on the intensity and type of immunosuppression-causing medication used, the underlying disease, and other factors; estimates vary from 3 months to 1 year)

» Vaccines, live virus
(because normal defense mechanisms may be suppressed by busulfan therapy, concurrent use with a live virus vaccine may potentiate the replication of the vaccine virus, may increase the side/adverse effects of the vaccine virus, and/or may decrease the patient's antibody response to the vaccine; immunization of these patients should be undertaken only with extreme caution after careful review of the patient's hematologic status and only with the knowledge and consent of the physician managing the busulfan therapy. The interval between discontinuation of medications that cause immunosuppression and restoration of the patient's ability to respond to the vaccine depends on the intensity and type of immunosuppression-causing medication used, the underlying disease, and other factors; estimates vary from 3 months to 1 year. Patients with leukemia in remission should not receive live virus vaccine until at least 3 months after their last chemotherapy. In addition, immunization with oral poliovirus vaccine should be postponed in persons in close contact with the patient, especially family members)

### Laboratory value alterations
The following have been selected on the basis of their potential clinical significance (possible effect in parentheses where appropriate)—not necessarily inclusive (» = major clinical significance):

With diagnostic test results
Cytology studies of lung, bladder, breast, or uterine cervix tissue
(cytologic dysplasia caused by busulfan may be severe enough to cause difficulty in interpretation)

With physiology/laboratory test values
  Uric acid in blood and urine
    (concentrations may be increased)

**Medical considerations/Contraindications**
The medical considerations/contraindications included have been selected on the basis of their potential clinical significance (reasons given in parentheses where appropriate)—not necessarily inclusive (» = major clinical significance).

*Risk-benefit should be considered when the following medical problems exist:*
» Bone marrow depression
» Chickenpox, existing or recent (including recent exposure) or
» Herpes zoster
    (risk of severe generalized disease)
  Gout, history of or
  Urate renal stones, history of
    (risk of hyperuricemia)
» Infection
  Sensitivity to busulfan
  Caution is necessary when using very high doses of busulfan in patients with head trauma or a history of seizure disorder; some clinicians use prophylactic anticonvulsant therapy.
» Caution should be used also in patients who have had previous cytotoxic drug therapy or radiation therapy or who have evidence of myelofibrosis.

**Patient monitoring**
The following may be especially important in patient monitoring (other tests may be warranted in some patients, depending on condition; » = major clinical significance):

  Alanine aminotransferase values, serum and
  Alkaline phosphatase values, serum and
  Bilirubin concentrations, serum
    (recommended at periodic intervals to detect possible hepatotoxicity, including hepatic veno-occlusive disease)
» Hematocrit or hemoglobin or
» Leukocyte count, total and, if appropriate, differential and
  Platelet count
    (determinations recommended prior to initiation of therapy and at periodic intervals during therapy; frequency varies according to clinical state, agent, dose, and other agents being used concurrently; because of severe and delayed myelosuppression caused by busulfan, frequent monitoring is necessary so that therapy can be withdrawn promptly when indicated)
  Uric acid concentrations, serum
    (recommended prior to initiation of therapy and at periodic intervals during therapy; frequency varies according to clinical state, agent, dose, and other agents being used concurrently)

## Side/Adverse Effects

Note: Many "side effects" of antineoplastic therapy are unavoidable and represent the medication's pharmacologic action. Some of these (for example, leukopenia and thrombocytopenia) are actually used as parameters to aid in individual dosage titration.

Busulfan can cause cellular dysplasia in many tissues, including lungs, lymph nodes, pancreas, thyroid, adrenal gland, liver, bone marrow, bladder, breast, and uterine cervix.

Seizures have been reported in 2 of 130 patients receiving very high investigational doses (1 mg per kg of body weight [mg/kg] four times a day for four days, total dose 16 mg/kg).

Hepatic veno-occlusive disease has been reported following investigational use of very high doses of busulfan in combination with other chemotherapy prior to bone marrow transplantation.

Continuous treatment with a combination of busulfan and thioguanine in approximately 330 patients was associated with esophageal varices along with abnormal hepatic function tests and evidence of nodular regenerative hyperplasia on liver biopsy in 12 patients after six to forty-five months of therapy. No hepatic toxicity was found in the busulfan alone arm of the study.

The following side/adverse effects have been selected on the basis of their potential clinical significance (possible signs and symptoms in parentheses where appropriate)—not necessarily inclusive:

**Those indicating need for medical attention**
Incidence more frequent
  *Anemia; leukopenia or infection* (fever or chills; cough or hoarseness; lower back or side pain; painful or difficult urination)—usually asymptomatic; *thrombocytopenia* (unusual bleeding or bruising; black, tarry stools; blood in urine or stools; pinpoint red spots on skin)
  Note: Onset of *leukopenia* is usually 10 to 15 days after initiation of therapy (leukocyte counts usually increase transiently before this), with nadir of white cell count at 11 to 30 days; white cell counts may continue to fall for more than 1 month after withdrawal but usually recover within 12 to 20 weeks.
    *Bone marrow depression* may be severe and progressive, leading to pancytopenia. Recovery from pancytopenia after withdrawal of busulfan may take 1 month to 2 years.
    Symptoms of *bone marrow depression* may also indicate transformation of chronic myelocytic leukemia into the acute blastic form.

Incidence less frequent—occurring with long-term use or high dosage
  *Bronchopulmonary dysplasia with pulmonary fibrosis* (fever; cough; shortness of breath); *hyperuricemia or uric acid nephropathy* (joint pain; lower back or side pain; swelling of feet or lower legs); *stomatitis* (sores in mouth and on lips)
  Note: *Bronchopulmonary dysplasia with pulmonary fibrosis* usually occurs 8 months to 10 years (average 4 years) after initiation of therapy and is usually fatal within 6 months after diagnosis. Associated with decreased diffusion capacity and pulmonary compliance. Histologically resembles changes following pulmonary irradiation. Lung biopsy may be necessary to establish the diagnosis.
    *Hyperuricemia or uric acid nephropathy* occurs most commonly during initial treatment of patients with leukemia, as a result of rapid cell breakdown which leads to elevated serum uric acid concentrations.

Incidence rare
  *Cataracts* (blurred vision)—occur after prolonged administration

**Those indicating need for medical attention only if they continue or are bothersome**
Incidence more frequent
  *Amenorrhea and ovarian suppression* (missed or irregular menstrual periods); *darkening of skin*—5 to 10%

Incidence less frequent—occurring with long-term use
  *Confusion; diarrhea; hypotension* (dizziness); *loss of appetite; nausea and vomiting; unusual tiredness or weakness; sudden weight loss*
  Note: All of the above, as well as darkening of skin, may occur after prolonged therapy and may resemble adrenocortical insufficiency, although adrenocortical function is not suppressed in most patients. Symptoms are sometimes reversible on withdrawal of busulfan. Adrenal responsiveness to exogenous adrenocorticotropic hormone (ACTH) is usually normal, but pituitary function testing with metyrapone has shown blunted urinary 17-hydroxycorticosteroid excretion in some patients that returned to normal when busulfan was discontinued.

**Those indicating the need for medical attention if they occur after medication is discontinued**
  *Bone marrow depression, thrombocytopenia, pancytopenia* (unusual bleeding or bruising; black, tarry stools; blood in urine or stools; pinpoint red spots on skin; fever or chills; cough or hoarseness; lower back or side pain; painful or difficult urination); *pulmonary fibrosis* (fever; cough; shortness of breath)

## Overdose

For more information on the management of overdose or unintentional ingestion, **contact a Poison Control Center** (see *Poison Control Center Listing*).

**Treatment of overdose**
Induction of vomiting or gastric lavage followed by administration of charcoal if ingestion is recent.
Monitoring of hematologic status and supportive measures if necessary.

## Patient Consultation

As an aid to patient consultation, refer to *Advice for the Patient, Busulfan (Systemic)*.
In providing consultation, consider emphasizing the following selected information (» = major clinical significance):

**Before using this medication**
» Conditions affecting use, especially:
    Sensitivity to busulfan
    Pregnancy—Use not recommended because of mutagenic, teratogenic, and carcinogenic potential; advisability of using contraception; telling physician immediately if pregnancy is suspected

Breast-feeding—Not recommended because of risk of serious side effects

Other medications, especially probenecid, sulfinpyrazone, other bone marrow depressants, or previous cytotoxic drug therapy or radiation therapy

Other medical problems, especially chickenpox, herpes zoster, or other infections

**Proper use of this medication**

» Importance of not taking more or less medication than the amount prescribed

Taking each dose at the same time each day to ensure uniform effect

Importance of ample fluid intake and subsequent increase in urine output to aid in excretion of uric acid

» Possible nausea and vomiting; importance of continuing medication despite stomach upset

Checking with physician if vomiting occurs shortly after dose is taken
» Proper dosing
Missed dose: Not taking at all; not doubling doses
» Proper storage

**Precautions while using this medication**

» Importance of close monitoring by the physician
» Avoiding immunizations unless approved by physician; other persons in patient's household should avoid immunizations with oral poliovirus vaccine; avoiding persons who have taken oral poliovirus vaccine or wearing a protective mask that covers nose and mouth

*Caution if bone marrow depression occurs*

» Avoiding exposure to persons with infections, especially during periods of low blood counts; checking with physician immediately if fever or chills, cough or hoarseness, lower back or side pain, or painful or difficult urination occurs

» Checking with physician immediately if unusual bleeding or bruising; black, tarry stools; blood in urine or stools; or pinpoint red spots on skin occur

Caution in use of regular toothbrush, dental floss, or toothpick; physician, dentist, or nurse may suggest alternatives; checking with physician before having dental work done

Not touching eyes or inside of nose unless hands washed immediately before

Using caution to avoid accidental cuts with use of sharp objects such as safety razor or fingernail or toenail cutters

Avoiding contact sports or other situations where bruising or injury might occur

Caution if any laboratory tests required; possible interference with tissue study results

**Side/adverse effects**

May cause adverse effects such as lung or blood problems; importance of discussing possible effects with physician

Signs of potential side effects, especially anemia, leukopenia, infection, thrombocytopenia, bronchopulmonary dysplasia with pulmonary fibrosis, hyperuricemia, uric acid nephropathy, stomatitis, and cataracts

Physician or nurse can help in dealing with side effects

## General Dosing Information

Patients receiving busulfan should be under supervision of a physician experienced in cancer chemotherapy.

Dosage must be adjusted to meet the individual requirements of each patient, based on clinical response and degree of bone marrow depression.

Development of uric acid nephropathy in patients with leukemia may be prevented by adequate oral hydration and, in some cases, administration of allopurinol. Alkalinization of urine may be necessary if serum uric acid concentrations are elevated.

Busulfan therapy should be discontinued at the first sign of interstitial pulmonary fibrosis.

Because of the delayed effect, it is recommended that busulfan therapy be discontinued or dosage reduced at the first sign of a sudden large decrease in leukocyte (particularly granulocyte) count to prevent irreversible bone marrow depression.

Special precautions are recommended in patients who develop thrombocytopenia as a result of administration of busulfan. These may include extreme care in performing invasive procedures; regular inspection of intravenous sites, skin (including perirectal area), and mucous membrane surfaces for signs of bleeding or bruising; limiting frequency of venipuncture and avoiding intramuscular injections; testing urine, emesis, stool, and secretions for occult blood; care in use of regular toothbrushes, dental floss, toothpicks, safety razors, and fingernail and toenail cutters; avoiding constipation; and using caution to prevent falls and other injuries. Such patients should avoid alcohol and aspirin intake because of the risk of gastrointestinal bleeding. Platelet transfusions may be required.

Patients who develop leukopenia should be observed carefully for signs of infection. Antibiotic support may be required. In neutropenic patients who develop fever, broad-spectrum antibiotic coverage should be initiated empirically, pending bacterial cultures and appropriate diagnostic tests.

## Oral Dosage Forms

**BUSULFAN TABLETS USP**

**Usual adult dose**
Chronic myelocytic leukemia—
Induction—
  Oral, 1.8 mg per square meter of body surface or 60 mcg (0.06 mg) per kg of body weight a day until the white cell count falls below 15,000 cells per cubic millimeter. Usual dosage range is 4 to 8 mg per day but may range from 1 to 12 mg per day. During remission, treatment is resumed when a monthly white cell count reaches 50,000 cells per cubic millimeter.

Note: Some patients may be unusually sensitive to busulfan and develop myelosuppression more rapidly than usual. Therefore, frequent and careful monitoring of blood counts is necessary. The total leukocyte count decreases exponentially at a constant busulfan dose, so a weekly plot of leukocyte count on semi-logarithmic graph paper can aid in predicting when leukocyte counts will reach 15,000 and busulfan should be discontinued.

Maintenance—
  Oral, 1 to 3 mg per day.

Note: Maintenance therapy with busulfan is recommended only when a remission is shorter than 3 months.

**Usual pediatric dose**
Chronic myelocytic leukemia—
  Induction: Oral, 60 to 120 mcg (0.06 to 0.12 mg) per kg of body weight or 1.8 to 4.6 mg per square meter of body surface per day.

Note: Dosage is titrated to reduce and maintain a leukocyte count of about 20,000 cells per cubic millimeter.

**Strength(s) usually available**
U.S.—
  2 mg (Rx) [*Myleran* (scored)].
Canada—
  2 mg (Rx) [*Myleran* (scored)].

**Packaging and storage**
Store below 40 °C (104 °F), preferably between 15 and 25 °C (59 and 77 °F), unless otherwise specified by manufacturer. Store in a well-closed container.

## Selected Bibliography

Rushing D et al. Hydroxyurea versus busulfan in the treatment of chronic myelogenous leukemia. Am J Clin Oncol 1982; 5: 307-13.

Revised: 06/12/92
Interim revision: 05/02/94; 09/23/97

---

# BUTABARBITAL—See *Barbiturates (Systemic)*

---

# BUTACAINE—See *Anesthetics (Mucosal-Local)*

---

# BUTAMBEN—See *Anesthetics (Topical)*

# BUTENAFINE Topical—INTRODUCTORY VERSION

VA CLASSIFICATION (Primary): DE102
Commonly used brand name(s): *Mentax*.
Note: For a listing of dosage forms and brand names by country availability, see *Dosage Forms* section(s).

## Category
Antifungal (topical).

## Indications

**Accepted**
Tinea pedis (treatment) or
Tinea corporis (treatment) or
Tinea cruris (treatment)—Butenafine is indicated in the treatment of interdigital tinea pedis (athlete's foot), tinea corporis (ringworm), or tinea cruris (jock itch) due to *Epidermophyton floccosum*, *Trichophyton mentagrophytes*, *T. rubrum*, or *T. tonsurans*.

## Pharmacology/Pharmacokinetics

**Physicochemical characteristics**
Chemical group—Butenafine is a member of the benzylamines, which are structurally related to allylamines.
Molecular weight—Butenafine hydrochloride: 353.93.

**Mechanism of action/Effect**
Fungicidal; inhibits the epoxidation of squalene; this action blocks the biosynthesis of ergosterol, an important component of fungal cell membranes.

**Absorption**
The total amount absorbed into the systemic circulation following topical application has not been determined.
In a pharmacokinetic study, 6 and 20 grams of 1% butenafine cream applied once a day to the dorsal skin (3000 square centimeters) of healthy subjects produced measurable plasma concentrations of butenafine hydrochloride, which remained 7 days after the last dose application.
In a 4-week study of daily application of 1% butenafine cream to the affected and immediately surrounding skin area in 11 patients with tinea pedis, measurements 10 to 20 hours after dosing at 1, 2, and 4 weeks showed that plasma concentrations of butenafine hydrochloride ranged from undetectable to 0.3 nanogram per mL.
In a 2-week study of daily application of 1% butenafine cream to the affected and immediately surrounding skin area in 24 patients with tinea cruris (mean average daily dose of 1.3 grams), plasma concentrations of butenafine hydrochloride measured 0.5 to 65 hours after the last dose ranged from undetectable to 2.52 nanograms per mL. Four weeks after treatment, the plasma concentrations ranged from undetectable to 0.28 nanogram per mL.

**Biotransformation**
By hydroxylation at the terminal *t*-butyl side-chain.

**Half-life**
Following topical application—
  Initial: 35 hours.
  Terminal: More than 150 hours.

**Time to peak concentration**
Plasma—
Following topical application of 6 grams: 15 ± 8 hours.
Following topical application of 20 grams: 6 ± 6 hours.

**Peak plasma concentration**
Following topical application of 6 grams once a day—1.4 ± 0.8 nanograms per mL.
  Note: The mean area under the plasma concentration–time curve ($AUC_{0-24\ hours}$) was 23.9 ± 11.3 nanogram-hours per mL.

Following topical application of 20 grams once a day—5 ± 2 nanograms per mL.
  Note: The mean $AUC_{0-24\ hours}$ was 87.8 ± 45.3 nanogram-hours per mL.

**Elimination**
Renal.

## Precautions to Consider

**Cross-sensitivity and/or related problems**
Patients sensitive to allylamine antifungal agents may also be sensitive to butenafine.

**Carcinogenicity**
Long-term studies to evaluate the carcinogenic potential of butenafine have not been conducted.

**Mutagenicity**
*In vitro* and *in vivo* animal studies found no mutagenic or clastogenic potential for butenafine.

**Pregnancy/Reproduction**
Fertility—Studies in animals using a dose of approximately 25 mg per kg of body weight per day administered subcutaneously revealed no adverse effect on male or female fertility. This dose is approximately five to six times higher than the maximum recommended human topical dose.
Pregnancy—Adequate and well-controlled studies in humans have not been done.
Butenafine was not teratogenic when it was administered subcutaneously or topically at daily doses that were 5 to 12 times the maximum recommended human topical dose during organogenesis in rats and rabbits.
FDA Pregnancy Category B.

**Breast-feeding**
It is not known whether butenafine is distributed into breast milk. Problems in humans have not been documented.

**Pediatrics**
Appropriate studies on the relationship of age to the effects of butenafine have not been performed in the pediatric population. Safety and efficacy in children younger than 12 years of age have not been established.

**Geriatrics**
No information is available on the relationship of age to the effects of butenafine in geriatric patients. Although there is no specific information comparing use of butenafine in the elderly with use in other age groups, clinical studies included older patients. No geriatrics-specific problems have been documented to date.

**Medical considerations/Contraindications**
The medical considerations/contraindications included have been selected on the basis of their potential clinical significance (reasons given in parentheses where appropriate)—not necessarily inclusive (» = major clinical significance).

*Risk-benefit should be considered when the following medical problem exists:*
  Sensitivity to butenafine or allylamines

## Side/Adverse Effects
The following side/adverse effects have been selected on the basis of their potential clinical significance (possible signs and symptoms in parentheses where appropriate)—not necessarily inclusive:

**Those indicating need for medical attention**
Incidence rare
  *Contact dermatitis* (rash); **hypersensitivity** (blistering, burning, itching, oozing, stinging, swelling or other signs of skin irritation not present before use of this medicine); *redness*

## Patient Consultation

As an aid to patient consultation, refer to *Advice for the Patient, Butenafine (Topical)—Introductory Version*.
In providing consultation, consider emphasizing the following selected information (» = major clinical significance):

**Before using this medication**
» Conditions affecting use, especially:
    Sensitivity to butenafine or allylamines

**Proper use of this medication**
   Applying sufficient medication to cover affected and surrounding areas, and rubbing in gently
   Washing hands after application to remove any residual medication
» Avoiding contact with the eyes and mucous membranes such as the inside of the nose, mouth, or vagina
» Not bandaging or applying an occlusive dressing on the area being treated unless otherwise directed by physician
» Compliance with full course of therapy; fungal infections may require prolonged therapy

## 700 Butenafine (Topical)—Introductory Version — USP DI

» Proper dosing
  Missed dose: Applying as soon as possible; not applying if almost time for next dose
» Proper storage

**Precautions while using this medication**
  Checking with physician if no improvement within 4 weeks or if symptoms become worse
» Using hygienic measures to help cure infection and prevent reinfection
*For tinea pedis*
  Carefully drying feet, especially between toes, after bathing
  Avoiding socks made from wool or synthetic materials; wearing clean, cotton socks and changing them daily or more often if feet perspire excessively
  Wearing sandals or well-ventilated shoes
  Using a bland, absorbent powder liberally between toes, on feet, and in socks and shoes once or twice daily; using the powder after butenafine has been applied and has disappeared into the skin; not using the powder as the only therapy for fungal infection
*For tinea cruris*
  Carefully drying inguinal area after bathing
  Not wearing underwear that is tight-fitting or made from synthetic materials; wearing loose-fitting cotton underwear instead
  Using a bland, absorbent powder liberally once or twice daily; using the powder after butenafine has been applied and has disappeared into the skin; not using the powder as the only therapy for fungal infection
*For tinea corporis*
  Carefully drying the body after bathing
  Avoiding excess heat and humidity if possible; keeping moisture from accumulating on affected areas of the body
  Wearing well-ventilated clothing
  Using a bland, absorbent powder liberally once or twice daily; using the powder after butenafine has been applied and has disappeared into the skin; not using the powder as the only therapy for fungal infection

**Side/adverse effects**
  Signs of potential side effects, especially contact dermatitis, hypersensitivity, or redness

## Topical Dosage Forms

### BUTENAFINE HYDROCHLORIDE CREAM
**Usual adult and adolescent dose**
Tinea pedis, interdigital —
  Topical, to the affected skin and surrounding areas, once a day for four weeks , or
  Topical, to the affected skin and surrounding areas, twice a day for seven days.
Note: Because there is some evidence that the seven-day dosing regimen is less effective than the four-week regimen, caution is recommended before selecting the seven-day regimen for patients at risk for development of bacterial cellulitis of the lower extremity associated with interdigital cracking or fissuring.
Tinea corporis or
Tinea cruris—
  Topical, to the affected skin and surrounding areas, once a day for two weeks.

**Usual pediatric dose**
Tinea pedis, interdigital or
Tinea corporis or
Tinea cruris—
  Safety and efficacy in children younger than 12 years of age have not been established.
  Children 12 to 16 years of age: See *Usual adult and adolescent dose*.

**Strength(s) usually available**
U.S.—
  1% (Rx) [*Mentax* (benzyl alcohol; cetyl alcohol; diethanolamine; glycerin; glyceryl monostearate; polyoxyethylene cetyl ether; propylene glycol dicaprylate; sodium benzoate; stearic acid; white petrolatum)].

**Packaging and storage**
Store between 5 and 30 ºC (41 and 86 ºF).

**Auxiliary labeling**
• For external use only.
• Continue medicine for full time of treatment.

Developed: 11/12/97
Revised: 08/07/98

---

**BUTOCONAZOLE** — See *Antifungals, Azole (Vaginal)*

---

**BUTORPHANOL** — See *Opioid (Narcotic) Analgesics (Systemic)*

---

# BUTORPHANOL   Nasal-Systemic

VA CLASSIFICATION (Primary): CN101
Note: Controlled substance classification—Schedule II
Note: For information on parenteral administration of butorphanol, see *Opioid (Narcotic) Analgesics (Systemic)*.
Note: For a listing of dosage forms and brand names by country availability, see *Dosage Forms* section(s).

## Category
Analgesic.

## Indications

**Accepted**
Pain (treatment)—Intranasal butorphanol is indicated for relief of pain requiring treatment with an opioid analgesic. Butorphanol has been used to relieve moderate to severe pain following cesarean section, arthroscopic or abdominal surgery, and episiotomy.

**Acceptance not established**
Intranasal butorphanol may be appropriate for use as alternative therapy for migraine headache pain that has not responded to other abortive agents. However, more comparative clinical studies with first-line agents in the treatment of acute migraine headaches need to be done to determine the role of intranasal butorphanol as an alternative therapy.

**Unaccepted**
Intranasal butorphanol has not been evaluated, and is therefore not recommended, for relief of labor pain or for use as an adjunct to anesthesia.

## Pharmacology/Pharmacokinetics

**Physicochemical characteristics**
Source—Synthetic.
Chemical group—An opioid analgesic of the phenanthrene series.
Molecular weight—477.56.

**Mechanism of action/Effect**
Butorphanol is a mixed agonist/antagonist opioid analgesic. It has agonist activity at the kappa opioid receptor and mixed agonist and antagonist activity at the mu opioid receptor. Because of its antagonist activity, withdrawal symptoms may occur if a patient dependent on another opioid is abruptly transferred to butorphanol.
A 2-mg dose of intranasal butorphanol produces analgesic and/or respiratory depressant effects equivalent to those produced by 2 mg of intravenous butorphanol, 10 mg of intramuscular morphine or methadone, or 75 mg of intramuscular meperidine.
Note: See *Opioid (Narcotic) Analgesics (Systemic)* for additional information on the mechanisms of action of opioid analgesics.

**Other actions/effects**
Butorphanol has cardiovascular effects that tend to increase cardiac work. It produces alterations in cardiovascular resistance and capacitance that may lead to increases in left ventricular pressure, diastolic pressure, systemic arterial pressure, pulmonary arterial pressure, and pulmonary wedge pressure.
Butorphanol shares the central nervous system (CNS) depressant and respiratory depressant effects of other opioid analgesics.
Butorphanol also alters bronchomotor tone, gastrointestinal secretory and motor activity, and bladder sphincter activity; suppresses the cough reflex; stimulates emesis; and produces miosis.

### Absorption
After intranasal administration, absolute bioavailability averages 60 to 70%, although mean values of 48% and 75% have been determined for elderly females and elderly males, respectively.

Nasal mucosal blood vessels are surrounded by adrenergic nerves, and stimulation of adrenergic receptor produces a decrease in blood content and blood flow by vasoconstriction. However, concurrent use of a nasal vasoconstrictor (e.g., oxymetazoline) decreases the rate, but not the extent, of absorption. A study evaluating patients with rhinitis found that inflammation of the nasal mucosa and secretions from the nasal gland did not effect the rate or extent of absorption of transnasal butorphanol.

### Distribution
Butorphanol crosses the blood-brain barrier and the placenta and is distributed into breast milk.

### Protein binding
High (approximately 80%), with plasma concentrations of up to 7 nanograms per mL (nanograms/mL).

### Biotransformation
Hepatic; extensive, primarily to hydroxybutorphanol and, to a lesser extent, to norbutorphanol. These metabolites have some analgesic activity in animal models; possible analgesic activity in humans has not been investigated.

### Half-life
Elimination—
 Normal renal function:
  Young adults (20 to 40 years of age)—4.74 ± 1.57 (range, 2.89 to 8.79) hours.
  Elderly adults (> 65 years of age)—6.56 ± 1.51 (range, 3.75 to 9.17) hours.
 Renal function impairment (creatinine clearance < 30 mL per minute): Approximately 10.5 hours.

### Onset of action
Within 15 minutes, but may be delayed if administered concurrently with or immediately following a nasal vasoconstrictor (e.g., oxymetazoline).

### Time to peak concentration
Approximately 30 to 60 minutes.

### Peak serum concentration
Following a 1-mg dose—1.04 ± 0.4 (range, 0.35 to 1.97) nanograms/mL, in young adults with normal renal function. Values in individuals older than 65 years of age are more variable, ranging from 0.1 to 2.68 nanograms/mL, but mean values are not significantly different than in young adults. Single-dose values in patients with renal function impairment (creatinine clearance < 30 mL per minute) are not significantly different than those in individuals with normal renal function.

### Time to steady-state serum concentration
Within 2 days, when administered at 6-hour intervals.

### Time to peak effect
1 to 2 hours.

### Duration of action
4 to 5 hours.

### Elimination
Renal—Approximately 70 to 80% of a dose; 5% of a dose as unchanged butorphanol, 49% of a dose as hydroxybutorphanol, and < 5% of a dose as norbutorphanol.
Biliary/fecal: Approximately 15% of a dose.

## Precautions to Consider

### Carcinogenicity
The carcinogenic potential of butorphanol has not been adequately studied.

### Mutagenicity
No genotoxicity was demonstrated in assays in *Salmonella typhimurium* or *Escherichia coli*, or in unscheduled DNA synthesis and repair assays in cultured human fibroblast cells.

### Pregnancy/Reproduction
Fertility—A reduced pregnancy rate occurred in rats given 160 mg per kg of body weight (mg/kg) per day (944 mg per square meter of body surface area [mg/m$^2$] per day) orally, but not in rats given 2.5 mg/kg per day (14.75 mg/m$^2$) per day subcutaneously.

Pregnancy—Adequate and well-controlled studies in humans have not been done.
No teratogenicity occurred in reproduction studies in mice, rats, and rabbits given butorphanol during organogenesis. However, the rate of stillbirths was increased in pregnant rats given 1 mg/kg (5.9 mg/m$^2$) subcutaneously. Also, postimplantation losses were increased in rabbits given 60 mg/kg (10.2 mg/m$^2$) orally.

FDA Pregnancy Category C.
Labor—Intranasally administered butorphanol has not been studied, and is therefore not recommended, for relief of labor pain.

### Breast-feeding
Butorphanol has been detected in breast milk after intramuscular administration of 2 mg 4 times a day, producing estimated concentrations of 4 micrograms per mL (mcg/mL). Although there is no experience with intranasal administration of butorphanol in nursing women, it should be assumed that similar quantities are distributed into breast milk. However, the amount of butorphanol that might be ingested by a nursing infant is probably clinically insignificant.

### Pediatrics
No information is available on the relationship of age to the effects of butorphanol in patients up to 18 years of age. Safety and efficacy have not been established.

### Geriatrics
Studies in patients 65 years of age and older indicate that absorption may be decreased in elderly females, but not in elderly males. Butorphanol clearance is decreased in geriatric patients, resulting in a prolonged elimination half-life. Results from a long-term clinical trial also indicate that older individuals may be more sensitive to butorphanol-induced side effects. In particular, these patients may be less able than younger adults to tolerate dizziness that occurs during treatment. Due to the increase in sensitivity to the butorphanol induced side effects, it is recommended that the dosage and dosing interval be adjusted in elderly patients.

### Drug interactions and/or related problems
The following drug interactions and/or related problems have been selected on the basis of their potential clinical significance (possible mechanism in parentheses where appropriate)—not necessarily inclusive (» = major clinical significance):

Note: Combinations containing any of the following medications, depending on the amount present, may also interact with this medication
 See *Opioid (Narcotic) Analgesics (Systemic)* for additional drug interactions that apply to use of butorphanol.

» Alcohol or
» CNS depression–producing medications, other (See *Appendix II*)
 (concurrent use with opioid analgesics may result in increased CNS and/or respiratory depressant effects; the lowest effective dosage regimen for intranasal butorphanol should be used)

Decongestants, sympathomimetic, nasal
 (vasoconstriction induced by these medications decreases the rate, but not the extent, of butorphanol absorption through the nasal mucosa; a slower onset of action should be anticipated if butorphanol is administered concurrently with or immediately following a decongestant)

Enzyme inducers, hepatic, cytochrome P450 (See *Appendix II*) or
Enzyme inhibitors, hepatic, various (See *Appendix II*)
 (effects of these medications on the pharmacokinetics of butorphanol have not been established; dose or frequency of administration of butorphanol may need to be adjusted during concurrent use)

» Opioid analgesics, other
 (patients who have been receiving long-term treatment with other opioid analgesics may experience withdrawal symptoms if abruptly transferred to butorphanol)

### Laboratory value alterations
The following have been selected on the basis of their potential clinical significance (possible effect in parentheses where appropriate)—not necessarily inclusive (» = major clinical significance):

With physiology/laboratory test values
 Cerebrospinal fluid pressure
  (may be increased secondary to carbon dioxide retention)

Note: See *Opioid (Narcotic) Analgesics (Systemic)* for additional laboratory value alterations that apply to use of butorphanol.

### Medical considerations/Contraindications
The medical considerations/contraindications included have been selected on the basis of their potential clinical significance (reasons given in parentheses where appropriate)—not necessarily inclusive (» = major clinical significance).

*Except under special circumstances, this medication should not be used when the following medical problems exist:*
» CNS disease affecting respiratory function or
» Pulmonary disease affecting respiratory function or control or
» Respiratory depression, pre-existing

(risk of precipitating, or exacerbating pre-existing, respiratory depression)
» Physical dependence on other opioid analgesics
(butorphanol may precipitate withdrawal symptoms)

*Risk-benefit should be considered when the following medical problems exist:*

» Cardiovascular disease, including:
Coronary insufficiency
Myocardial infarction, acute
Ventricular function abnormalities
(butorphanol may increase the work of the heart, especially the pulmonary circuit, and should be administered only if the potential benefit clearly outweighs the potential risks)

Drug abuse, history of or
Emotional instability
(patient predisposition to drug abuse)

Head injury or
Increased intracranial pressure
(caution is recommended because butorphanol may increase cerebrospinal fluid pressure and may also cause miosis and alterations in mental state that may interfere with assessment of the clinical course of the patient)

Hepatic function impairment or
Renal function impairment
(clearance of butorphanol may be altered; it is recommended that the medication be given at 6- to 8-hour intervals, initially, until the patient's response has been characterized. Also, subsequent doses should be determined by patient response rather than scheduled at fixed intervals)

Sensitivity to butorphanol

Tolerance to other opioid analgesics, possibility of
(caution is recommended when patients receiving these medications are transferred to butorphanol because of difficulty in assessing the degree to which tolerance may have developed)

Note: See *Opioid (Narcotic) Analgesics (Systemic)* for additional medical considerations/contraindications that apply to use of butorphanol.

## Side/Adverse Effects

Note: A 2-mg dose of butorphanol produces respiratory depression equivalent to that caused by 10 mg of intramuscular morphine. In contrast to a pure opioid agonist such as morphine, which produces dose-related respiratory depression, butorphanol produces limited depression that reaches a plateau or ceiling at doses two to three times the analgesic dose. The duration, but not the depth, of butorphanol-induced respiratory depression is increased when these higher doses are given.

In addition to the side/adverse effects listed below, apnea or shallow breathing, convulsions, delusions, edema, hypertension, and mental depression have been reported during butorphanol therapy (incidence of each < 1%). However, a causal relationship has not been established.

Intranasal butorphanol can produce drug dependence and may potentially be abused. Studies have found the abuse potential to be similar to intramuscular butorphanol.

The following side/adverse effects have been selected on the basis of their potential clinical significance (possible signs and symptoms in parentheses where appropriate)—not necessarily inclusive:

**Those indicating need for medical attention**
Incidence more frequent (3 to 9%)
*Difficulty in breathing; nosebleeds; runny nose; sinus congestion; sore throat; tinnitus* (ringing or buzzing in ears); *upper respiratory infection* (fever; sneezing)

Note: Several side/adverse effects that are listed individually according to their reported frequencies of occurrence (bronchitis, cough, nasal congestion, runny nose, sinus congestion, sinusitis, sore throat) may also occur in conjunction with an *upper respiratory infection*.

Incidence less frequent (1 to 3%)
*Blurred vision; bronchitis* (congestion in chest; cough; difficult or painful breathing); *cough; ear pain; itching; sinusitis* (sinus congestion with pain)

Incidence rare (< 1%)
*Decrease in blood pressure; difficulty in urinating; fainting; hallucinations; skin rash or hives*

**Those indicating need for medical attention only if they continue or are bothersome**
Incidence more frequent (3 to 9% or as indicated)
*Confusion; constipation; dizziness*—incidence 19%; *drowsiness*—incidence 43%; *dry mouth; headache; irritation inside nose; loss of appetite; nasal congestion*—incidence 13%; *nausea or vomiting; sweating or clammy feeling; trouble in sleeping; unpleasant taste; vasodilation* (flushing); *weakness, severe*

Incidence less frequent (1 to 3%) or rare (< 1%)
*Anxiety; behavior changes; burning, crawling, or prickling feeling on skin; false sense of well-being; feeling hot; floating feeling; nervousness, sometimes with restlessness; pounding heartbeat; stomach pain; strange dreams; trembling*

**Those indicating possible withdrawal and/or the need for medical attention if they occur after medication is discontinued**
*Anxiety; diarrhea; nervousness and restlessness*

Note: See *Opioid (Narcotic) Analgesics (Systemic)* for additional signs and symptoms typical of opioid withdrawal.

## Overdose

For specific information on the agents used in the management of butorphanol overdose, see *Naloxone (Systemic)* monograph.

For more information on the management of overdose or unintentional ingestion, **contact a Poison Control Center** (see *Poison Control Center Listing*).

**Clinical effects of overdose**
The following effects have been selected on the basis of their potential clinical significance (possible signs and symptoms in parentheses where appropriate)—not necessarily inclusive:

Acute and chronic
*Cold, clammy skin; confusion; convulsions; low blood pressure; pinpoint pupils of eyes; severe dizziness, drowsiness, nervousness, restlessness, or weakness; slow heartbeat; slow or troubled breathing; unconsciousness*

Note: Excessive administration of transnasal butorphanol may cause saturation of the nasal mucosa and limited absorption. However, overdose occurs when butorphanol is administered after desaturation of the nasal mucosa.

**Treatment of overdose**
Primary importance should be given to maintaining adequate ventilation. Assessing the patient's respiratory status and, if necessary, administering oxygen or otherwise assisting respiration are essential. Provision of an artificial airway may be necessary in the presence of coma.

Specific treatment—Administering naloxone if necessary. See the package insert or *Naloxone (Systemic)* for specific dosing guidelines for naloxone.

Monitoring—Continuous monitoring of mental status, responsiveness, and vital signs is recommended. Oxygenation may be monitored via pulse oximetry.

Supportive care—Supportive measures include establishing intravenous lines, maintaining peripheral perfusion and normal body temperature, and treating hypotension. Patients in whom intentional overdose is confirmed or suspected should be referred for psychiatric consultation.

## Patient Consultation

In providing consultation, consider emphasizing the following selected information (» = major clinical significance):

**Before using this medication**
» Conditions affecting use, especially:
Sensitivity to butorphanol
Pregnancy—Safe use in pregnancy has not been established
Breast-feeding—Probably distributed into breast milk
Use in the elderly—Lower dosage regimen recommended because of increased susceptibility to effects of opioids and prolonged butorphanol half-life in geriatric patients
Other medications, especially other CNS depressants, including alcohol and, other opioid analgesics
Other medical problems, especially cardiovascular disease, CNS or pulmonary disease affecting respiratory function, physical dependence on other opioid analgesics or pre-existing respiratory depression

**Proper use of this medication**
» Reading patient instructions carefully
» Importance of not using more medication than the amount prescribed
*Priming the unit*
» Removing protective cover and clip

- » Keeping sprayer pointed away from patient, other people, or pets while priming
- » Prior to first use, pumping the activator 7 or 8 times until a fine, wide spray appears
- » Repriming by pumping the activator 1 or 2 times if unit has not been used in 48 hours

*Proper administration*
- » Blowing nose gently
- » To obtain a 1-mg dose, inserting spray unit into a nostril, closing off the other nostril with index finger, tilting head slightly forward and spraying once, sniffing gently with mouth closed
- » Removing unit from nostril, tilting head back, then sniffing gently again
- » To obtain a 2-mg dose, repeating procedure for obtaining a 1-mg dose using the other nostril
- » Replacing protective cover and clip after use
- » Proper dosing
  (if on scheduled dosing)
  Using as soon as possible; not using if almost time for next dose
- » Proper storage

**Precautions while using this medication**
- » Avoiding use of alcoholic beverages or other CNS depressants during therapy, unless prescribed or otherwise approved by physician
- » Caution if dizziness, drowsiness, lightheadedness, impairment of physical or mental abilities, or false sense of well-being occurs
- » Possibility of hypotension and syncope, especially during the first hour after administration; avoiding activities in which these effects could be hazardous

  Caution if any kind of surgery (including dental surgery) or emergency treatment is required

  Possible dryness of mouth; using sugarless candy or gum, ice, or saliva substitute for relief; checking with physician or dentists if dry mouth continues for more than 2 weeks

  Checking with physician before discontinuing medication after prolonged use; gradual dosage reduction may be necessary to avoid withdrawal symptoms
- » Suspected overdose: Getting emergency help at once

**Side/adverse effects**
  Checking with physician if difficulty in breathing, nosebleeds, runny nose, sinus congestion, sore throat, tinnitus, upper respiratory infection, blurred vision, bronchitis, cough, ear pain, itching, sinusitis, decrease in blood pressure, difficulty in urinating, fainting, hallucinations, or skin rash or hives occurs

## General Dosing Information

Dosage of butorphanol should be based on the patient's age, body weight, physical status, underlying pathological condition, and other medications being used concurrently.

## Nasal Dosage Forms

### BUTORPHANOL TARTRATE NASAL SOLUTION

**Usual adult dose**
Analgesic—
  Nongeriatric adults with normal hepatic and renal function: Intranasal, 1 mg (one spray in one nostril). If adequate pain relief is not achieved within sixty to ninety minutes, another 1-mg dose may be administered. This two-dose sequence may be repeated in three to four hours as needed. Alternatively, if pain is severe and the patient will be able to remain recumbent if drowsiness or dizziness occurs, a 2-mg dose (one spray in each nostril) may be administered. This dose may be repeated every three or four hours. The increased risk of adverse effects must be kept in mind if this higher dose is used.

  Patients with impaired hepatic or renal function: Intranasal, 1 mg (one spray in one nostril). If adequate pain relief is not achieved within ninety minutes to two hours, another 1-mg dose may be given. Subsequent doses should be administered according to patient response rather than at fixed intervals, but generally at not less than six-hour intervals.

**Usual pediatric dose**
Safety and efficacy in patients up to 18 years of age have not been established.

**Usual geriatric dose**
Analgesic—Intranasal, 1 mg (one spray in one nostril). If adequate pain relief is not achieved within ninety minutes to two hours, another 1-mg dose may be given. Subsequent doses should be administered according to patient response rather than at fixed intervals, but generally at not less than six-hour intervals.

**Strength(s) usually available**
U.S.—
  1% (10 mg per mL; 1 mg per metered spray) (Rx) [*Stadol NS* (benzethonium chloride; sodium chloride; purified water; sodium hydroxide and/or hydrochloric acid to adjust pH)].

Canada—
  1% (10 mg per mL; 1 mg per metered spray) (Rx) [*Stadol NS* (benzethonium chloride; citric acid; sodium chloride; purified water; sodium hydroxide and/or hydrochloric acid to adjust pH)].

Note: Each container provides an average of 14 to 15 doses (1 mg each). If frequent repriming is necessary, only 8 to 10 doses may be obtained from the unit.

**Packaging and storage**
Store below 30 °C (86 °F), unless otherwise specified by manufacturer.

**Auxiliary labeling**
- May cause drowsiness.
- Avoid alcoholic beverages.

**Note**
Controlled substance in the U.S.

**Additional information**
At the time of dispensing, the pharmacist should replace the screw cap on the bottle of nasal solution with the spray pump included in the package without removing the clear cover from the pump. The unit should be returned to the child-resistant vial before being given to the patient.

Developed: 03/30/98

# CABERGOLINE  Systemic—INTRODUCTORY VERSION

VA CLASSIFICATION (Primary/Secondary): AU900/HS900
Commonly used brand name(s): *Dostinex*.
Note: For a listing of dosage forms and brand names by country availability, see *Dosage Forms* section(s).

## Category
Dopamine agonist; antihyperprolactinemic.

## Indications

### Accepted
Hyperprolactinemic disorders (treatment) or
Prolactinomas, pituitary (treatment)—Cabergoline is indicated in the treatment of hyperprolactinemic disorders due to pituitary adenomas or to idiopathic etiology.

## Pharmacology/Pharmacokinetics

### Physicochemical characteristics
Chemical group—Cabergoline is an ergoline (ergot alkaloid derivative).
Molecular weight—451.62.

### Mechanism of action/Effect
Cabergoline is a long-acting, selective dopamine receptor agonist, exhibiting high affinity for $D_2$ receptors and low affinity for $D_1$, $alpha_1$- and $alpha_2$-adrenergic, and serotonin (5-hydroxytryptamine$_1$ and 5-hydroxytryptamine$_2$) receptors. Cabergoline inhibits the synthesis and release of prolactin from the anterior pituitary by directly stimulating the $D_2$ receptors of the pituitary lactotrophs in a dose-related fashion. While cabergoline doses up to 2 mg inhibited prolactin in healthy volunteers, similar inhibition did not occur for the other anterior pituitary hormones, including growth hormone, follicle-stimulating hormone, luteinizing hormone, corticotropin, and thyroid-stimulating hormone. Cabergoline did not affect serum cortisol concentrations.

### Absorption
Exhibits first-pass effect; absolute bioavailability is unknown.

### Distribution
Extensive tissue distribution; cabergoline concentrations are at least 100 times greater in the pituitary than in the serum. Studies done in rats showed significant concentrations of cabergoline in the mammary glands and uterine wall, and that cabergoline crosses the placenta.

### Protein binding
Moderate (40 to 42%), in a concentration-independent manner. Cabergoline's protein binding is unlikely to be influenced by concomitant treatment with other protein-bound medications.

### Biotransformation
Hepatic—Cabergoline undergoes hydrolysis to inactive metabolites without causing hepatic enzyme induction or inhibition; cytochrome P450–mediated metabolism is minimal. Although mild to moderate hepatic function impairment does not alter pharmacokinetic values for cabergoline, severe hepatic function impairment (Child-Pugh score greater than 10) can substantially increase the values of $C_{max}$ and area under the plasma concentration–time curve (AUC).

### Half-life
Elimination—63 to 69 hours.

### Time to peak concentration
Within 3 hours.

### Peak serum concentration
30 to 70 picograms/mL (66.4 to 155 picomoles/L), reported in healthy volunteers taking single doses of 0.5 to 1.5 mg cabergoline. The steady-state serum concentration in patients using multiple weekly doses is expected to be 2 to 3 times higher than that reported for single doses.

### Time to peak effect
48 hours (single 0.6-mg dose of cabergoline in hyperprolactinemic patients).

### Duration of action
Up to 14 days (single 0.6-mg dose of cabergoline in hyperprolactinemic patients).

### Elimination
At 20 days for five healthy patients given single doses—
  Fecal: 60%.
  Renal: 22% (4% unchanged).

Nonrenal clearance was 3.2 L per minute in healthy adults. Renal clearance was 0.08 L per minute, similar to that of hyperprolactinemic patients. Moderate-to-severe renal insufficiency did not alter cabergoline's pharmacokinetics.

## Precautions to Consider

### Cross-sensitivity and/or related problems
Patients sensitive to other ergot derivatives may be sensitive to cabergoline also.

### Carcinogenicity/Tumorigenicity
In studies of mice, a slight increase in cervical and uterine leiomyomas and uterine leiomyosarcomas occurred when cabergoline was given in doses seven times the maximum recommended human dose (MRHD)—a dose based on the body surface area (BSA) of a 50-kg human. Cabergoline, when given to rats at doses four times greater than the MRHD, caused a slight increase in interstitial cell adenomas and malignant tumors of the uterus and cervix. The relevance of these findings to humans is not clear because of the hormonal differences between humans and animals.

### Mutagenicity
Cabergoline was not found to be mutagenic in a series of *in vitro* tests, including the Ames test, gene mutation assay, chromosomal aberration test in human lymphocytes, and a DNA damage and repair test in bacteria. Cabergoline also produced a negative mouse bone marrow micronucleus test.

### Pregnancy/Reproduction
Fertility—Cabergoline doses equal to one twenty-eighth of the MRHD inhibited conception in studies of female rats.
Pregnancy—Adequate and well-controlled studies in humans have not been done. Cabergoline is not recommended for use during pregnancy.
Cabergoline crosses the placenta in animals. Researchers studied cabergoline's effect on reproduction in mice, rats, and rabbits. Maternotoxicity, but not teratogenicity, occurred in studies of mice given doses of cabergoline 55 times greater than the MRHD (based on body surface area of a 50-kg human). When given doses of cabergoline equal to one seventh of the MRHD, rats experienced embryofetal loss after embryo implantation. Similar studies in rabbits given doses 19 times greater than the MRHD produced maternotoxicity, exhibited as reduced food intake and body weight loss. Doses 150 times greater than the MRHD produced fetal malformations in rabbits in one study, a result not reproduced in another study using doses 300 times greater than the MRHD. The relevance of these findings to humans is not clear since prolactin affects the reproductive cycles of animals and humans differently.
FDA Pregnancy Category B.

### Breast-feeding
It is not known if cabergoline is distributed into breast milk. Cabergoline should not be used in breast-feeding women or women planning to begin breast-feeding within a short period of time since it inhibits lactation by suppressing prolactin release.
In a study in rats, continued treatment of female rats with cabergoline beginning 6 days before parturition resulted in arrested pup growth and death of the litter due to the decreased amount of available maternal milk.

### Pediatrics
Appropriate studies on the relationship of age to the effects of cabergoline have not been performed in the pediatric population. Safety and efficacy have not been established.

### Geriatrics
No information is available on the relationship of age to the effects of cabergoline in geriatric patients. Safety and efficacy have not been established.

### Drug interactions and/or related problems
The following drug interactions and/or related problems have been selected on the basis of their potential clinical significance (possible mechanism in parentheses where appropriate)—not necessarily inclusive (» = major clinical significance):

Note: Combinations containing any of the following medications, depending on the amount present, may also interact with this medication.

  Antihypertensives, including
    Methyldopa
    Reserpine
      (concurrent use may result in additive hypotensive effects; dosage adjustment of the antihypertensive agent may be needed)

» Dopaminergic blocking agents, including metoclopramide or
» Neuroleptics, including
   Haloperidol
   Phenothiazines
   Thioxanthenes
       (cabergoline may interfere with the dopamine-blocking effects of these medications, reducing their effectiveness and exacerbating the patient's underlying condition; dosage adjustment of either medication may be necessary)

### Medical considerations/Contraindications
The medical considerations/contraindications included have been selected on the basis of their potential clinical significance (reasons given in parentheses where appropriate)—not necessarily inclusive (» = major clinical significance).

*Except under special circumstances, this medication should not be used when the following medical problems exist:*
» Eclampsia, or history of or
» Hypertension, uncontrolled or
» Preeclampsia, or history of
    (may aggravate these conditions; although cabergoline usually lowers blood pressure, rarely, blood pressure can increase)
» Hepatic function impairment, severe
    (metabolism may be reduced with severe hepatic function impairment; dosage reduction may be required if cabergoline is used)

*Risk-benefit should be considered when the following medical problems exist:*
Hepatic function impairment, mild to moderate
    (although mild to moderate hepatic function impairment does not decrease cabergoline metabolism, special hepatic function and serum prolactin monitoring as a precaution may be warranted; a lower dose of cabergoline may be needed if condition worsens)
Sensitivity to cabergoline or other ergot derivatives

### Patient monitoring
The following may be especially important in patient monitoring (other tests may be warranted in some patients, depending on condition; » = major clinical significance):

Blood pressure measurements
    (initial doses of cabergoline above 1 mg can cause orthostatic hypotension; monitoring for possible hypotensive effects may be needed)
Prolactin, serum
    (periodic monitoring of serum prolactin concentrations is needed during treatment, after each dosing interval, or when cabergoline is discontinued to assess efficacy of treatment. If serum prolactin levels are normal for 6 months, cabergoline can be discontinued. Patient monitoring should be continued to assess if or when to reinstate the antihyperprolactinemic treatment)

## Side/Adverse Effects
Note: Side effects for cabergoline are dose-related. Patients using cabergoline for Parkinson's disease, an unlabeled use, receive much higher doses than do those patients with a hyperprolactinemic condition. At doses up to 11.5 mg of cabergoline a day, patients with Parkinson's disease have experienced the following additional side effects: dyskinesia, hallucinations, heart failure, pleural effusion, pulmonary fibrosis, gastric or duodenal ulcer, and, in one case, constrictive pericarditis.

The following side/adverse effects have been selected on the basis of their potential clinical significance (possible signs and symptoms in parentheses where appropriate)—not necessarily inclusive:

### Those indicating need for medical attention
Incidence less frequent—4 or 5%
   *Abdominal pain; vertigo* (sensation of motion, usually whirling, either of oneself or of one's surroundings)
Incidence rare— ≤ 1%
   *Anorexia* (loss of appetite associated with weight loss or gain); *edema, periorbital* (vision changes); *edema, peripheral* (swelling of hands, ankles, or feet); *impaired concentration; syncope or hypotension* (fainting or lightheadedness when getting up from a lying or sitting position; unusually fast heartbeat)—especially orthostatic hypotension

### Those indicating need for medical attention only if they continue or are bothersome
Incidence more frequent
   *Asthenia* (weakness)—incidence 6%; *constipation*—incidence 7%; *dizziness*—incidence 17%; *dyspepsia* (stomach discomfort following meals)—incidence 4%; *headache*—incidence 26%; *nausea*—incidence 29%
Incidence less frequent— < 3%
   *Diarrhea; dryness of mouth; flatulence* (stomach or intestinal gas); *flu-like symptoms* (general feeling of discomfort or illness; runny nose; sore throat); *hot flashes; insomnia* (trouble in sleeping); *mental depression; muscle or joint pain; paresthesia* (unusual feeling of burning or stinging of skin); *pruritus* (itching of skin); *somnolence* (sleepiness); *toothache; vomiting*

### Those not indicating need for medical attention
Incidence less frequent— < 1%
   *Acne; increased libido* (increased sex drive)

## Overdose
For more information on the management of overdose or unintentional ingestion, **contact a Poison Control Center** (see *Poison Control Center Listing*).

### Clinical effects of overdose
The following effects have been selected on the basis of their potential clinical significance (possible signs and symptoms in parentheses where appropriate)—not necessarily inclusive:

   *Hallucinations; nasal congestion; syncope* (fainting; lightheadedness; palpitations)

### Treatment of overdose
Monitoring—Blood pressure measurements.

Patients in whom intentional overdose is known or suspected should be referred for psychiatric consultation.

## Patient Consultation
As an aid to patient consultation, refer to *Advice for the Patient, Cabergoline (Systemic)—Introductory Version*.

In providing consultation, consider emphasizing the following selected information (» = major clinical significance):

### Before using this medication
» Conditions affecting use, especially:
    Sensitivity to cabergoline or other ergot derivatives
    Carcinogenicity/tumorigenicity—Studies in mice showed slight increase in cervical and uterine leiomyomas and uterine leiomyosarcomas; studies in rats showed a slight increase in malignant tumors of the uterus and cervix and interstitial cell adenomas. Relevancy to humans is not known because prolactin affects animals and humans differently
    Pregnancy—Not recommended for use during pregnancy
    Breast-feeding—Not known if cabergoline is distributed into breast milk; will prevent lactation in mothers who breast-feed or are planning to begin breast-feeding soon
    Other medications, especially dopaminergic blocking agents and neuroleptics
    Other medical problems, especially eclampsia (or history of), severe hepatic function impairment, hypertension (uncontrolled), or preeclampsia (or history of)

### Proper use of this medication
Compliance with therapy: Importance of not taking more or less medication than the amount prescribed
» Proper dosing
    Missed dose: Taking as soon as possible within 1 or 2 days; if missed dose is not remembered until time of next dose, doubling the dose if medication is generally well-tolerated, without causing nausea. If not well-tolerated, discussing with health care professional before taking missed dose
» Proper storage

### Precautions while using this medication
Regular visits to physician to check progress
» Caution when driving or doing jobs requiring alertness because of possible drowsiness or dizziness
Checking with physician immediately if pregnancy is suspected
Getting up slowly from sitting or lying position to decrease the incidence of dizziness, lightheadedness, or vertigo

### Side/adverse effects
Signs of potential side effects, especially abdominal pain, vertigo, anorexia, periorbital or peripheral edema, impaired concentration, or syncope or hypotension

## General Dosing Information
The use of cabergoline for longer than 24 months has not been established. After the patient's serum prolactin level is normal for 6 months, cabergoline may be discontinued. Treatment of hyperprolactinemia may be

symptomatic rather than curative; reinitiation of an antihyperprolactinemic agent may be needed.

## Oral Dosage Forms

### CABERGOLINE TABLETS

**Usual adult dose**
Antihyperprolactinemic—
    Oral, 0.25 mg two times a week. In accordance with patient's serum prolactin level, dosage may be increased in increments of 0.25 mg, up to 1 mg two times a week, waiting at least four weeks between each dosage increase.

**Usual adult prescribing limits**
2 mg a week.

**Usual pediatric dose**
Antihyperprolactinemic—
    Safety and efficacy have not been established.

**Usual geriatric dose**
Antihyperprolactinemic—
    See *Usual adult dose*.

**Strength(s) usually available**
U.S.—
    0.5 mg (Rx) [*Dostinex* (scored; lactose)].

**Packaging and storage**
Store below 40 °C (104 °F), preferably between 15 and 30 °C (59 and 86 °F), unless otherwise specified by manufacturer.

Developed: 06/26/97
Interim revision: 06/30/98

---

# CAFFEINE   Systemic

This monograph includes information on the following: 1) Caffeine; 2) Citrated Caffeine; 3) Caffeine and Sodium Benzoate†.

VA CLASSIFICATION (Primary/Secondary):
    Caffeine—CN809/RE900
    Caffeine, Citrated—CN809/RE900
    Caffeine and Sodium Benzoate—CN809

Commonly used brand name(s): *Caffedrine*[1]; *Caffedrine Caplets*[1]; *Dexitac*[1]; *Enerjets*[1]; *Keep Alert*[1]; *NoDoz*[1]; *NoDoz Maximum Strength Caplets*[1]; *Pep-Back*[1]; *Quick Pep*[1]; *Ultra Pep-Back*[1]; *Vivarin*[1]; *Wake-Up*[1].

Note:   For a listing of dosage forms and brand names by country availability, see *Dosage Forms* section(s).

†Not commercially available in Canada.

## Category

Central nervous system stimulant—Caffeine; Citrated Caffeine; Caffeine and Sodium Benzoate.
Analgesia adjunct—Caffeine.
Respiratory stimulant adjunct—Caffeine; Citrated Caffeine.

## Indications

Note:   Bracketed information in the *Indications* section refers to uses that are not included in U.S. product labeling.

**Accepted**
Fatigue or
Drowsiness (treatment)—Caffeine is used as a mild central nervous system stimulant to help restore mental alertness or wakefulness when fatigue or drowsiness is experienced.

[Apnea, neonatal (treatment adjunct)]—Caffeine or citrated caffeine (but not caffeine and sodium benzoate combination) is used in the management of neonatal apnea, especially primary apnea of prematurity, which is characterized by periodic breathing and apneic episodes of more than 15 seconds accompanied by cyanosis and bradycardia. However, caffeine should be considered only as an adjunct to nondrug measures such as decreased ambient temperature, oxygen, sensory stimulation, and mechanical support of ventilation. Caffeine may be considered a desirable alternative to theophylline when initiating therapy for premature neonatal apnea because some infants are unable to convert theophylline to caffeine, a major metabolite of theophylline in neonates. Caffeine also has a wider therapeutic index than theophylline. Caffeine therapy in the management of apnea is usually required for only a few weeks and rarely for more than a few months, the apnea usually resolving by about 34 to 36 weeks' gestational age.

[Apnea, infant, postoperative (prophylaxis)]—Caffeine or citrated caffeine has been used for the prevention of postoperative apnea in former preterm infants.

[Electroconvulsive therapy (ECT) (treatment adjunct)]—Caffeine pretreatment is used to augment ECT by increasing seizure duration and reducing the need for increases in stimulus intensity.

Caffeine is used in combination with ergotamine to treat vascular headaches such as migraine and cluster headaches (histaminic cephalalgia, migrainous neuralgia, Horton's headache).

Caffeine is also used, and has been shown to be effective, as an analgesic adjunct in combination with aspirin or acetaminophen and aspirin to enhance pain relief, although it has no analgesic activity of its own. However, caffeine's efficacy as an analgesic adjunct in combination with acetaminophen alone has been questioned.

**Unaccepted**
Caffeine and sodium benzoate combination has been used in conjunction with other supportive measures to treat respiratory depression associated with overdose with central nervous system (CNS) depressants such as narcotic analgesics or alcohol; however, because of the availability of specific antagonists, such as flumazenil and naloxone, and caffeine's questionable benefit and transient effect, most authorities believe caffeine should not be used for these conditions and, therefore, recommend other supportive therapy.

Caffeine is used in combination with other agents such as analgesics and diuretics to relieve tension and fluid retention associated with menstruation; however, its usefulness for this purpose is in doubt because of its minimal diuretic action.

## Pharmacology/Pharmacokinetics

**Physicochemical characteristics**
Source—
    Coffee, tea, some soft drinks, and cocoa or chocolate. May also be synthesized from urea or dimethylurea.
Chemical group—
    Methylated xanthine.
Molecular weight—
    Caffeine (anhydrous): 194.19.
    Citric acid: 192.12.
    Sodium benzoate: 144.11.

**Mechanism of action/Effect**
Central nervous system stimulant—Caffeine stimulates all levels of the CNS, although its cortical effects are milder and of shorter duration than those of amphetamines. In larger doses, caffeine stimulates medullary, vagal, vasomotor, and respiratory centers, promoting bradycardia, vasoconstriction, and increased respiratory rate. This action was previously believed to be primarily due to increased intracellular cyclic 3′,5′-adenosine monophosphate (cyclic AMP) following inhibition of phosphodiesterase, the enzyme that degrades cyclic AMP. More recent studies indicate that caffeine exerts its physiological effects in large part through antagonism of central adenosine receptors.

Analgesia adjunct—Caffeine constricts cerebral vasculature with an accompanying decrease in cerebral blood flow and in the oxygen tension of the brain. It has been suggested that the addition of caffeine to aspirin or aspirin and acetaminophen combinations may help to relieve headache by providing a more rapid onset of action and/or enhanced pain relief with a lower dose of the analgesic. In some patients, caffeine may reduce headache pain by reversing caffeine withdrawal symptoms. Recent studies with ergotamine indicate that the enhancement of effect by the addition of caffeine may be due to improved gastrointestinal absorption of ergotamine when administered with caffeine.

Respiratory stimulant adjunct—Although the exact mechanism of action has not been completely established, caffeine, as other methylxanthines, is believed to act primarily through stimulation of the medullary respiratory center. This action is seen in certain pathophysiological states, such as in Cheyne-Stokes respiration and in apnea of preterm infants, and when respiration is depressed by certain drugs, such as barbiturates and opioids. Methylxanthines appear to increase the sensitivity of the respiratory center to the stimulatory actions of carbon dioxide, increasing alveolar ventilation, thereby reducing the severity and frequency of apneic episodes.

### Other actions/effects
Cardiac—Caffeine produces a positive inotropic effect on the myocardium and a positive chronotropic effect on the sinoatrial node, causing transient increases in heart rate, force of contraction, and cardiac output. Low concentrations of caffeine may produce small decreases in heart rate, possibly as a result of stimulation of the medullary vagal nuclei. At higher concentrations, caffeine produces definite tachycardia and sensitive persons may experience other arrhythmias, such as premature ventricular contractions.

Vascular—Caffeine causes constriction of cerebral vasculature with an accompanying decrease in cerebral blood flow and in the oxygen tension in the brain. Caffeine also causes an increase in systemic vascular resistance, resulting in an increase in blood pressure. These effects are believed to be mediated by blockade of adenosine-induced vasodilation and activation of the sympathetic nervous system.

Skeletal muscles—Caffeine stimulates voluntary skeletal muscle, possibly by inducing the release of acetylcholine, increasing the force of contraction and decreasing muscle fatigue. This stimulation of diaphragmatic muscles decreases the work of breathing.

Gastrointestinal secretions—Caffeine causes secretion of both pepsin and gastric acid from parietal cells.

Renal—Caffeine increases renal blood flow and glomerular filtration rate and decreases proximal tubular reabsorption of sodium and water, resulting in a mild diuresis.

Caffeine also inhibits uterine contractions, increases plasma and urinary catecholamine concentrations, and transiently increases plasma glucose by stimulating glycogenolysis and lipolysis.

### Absorption
Readily absorbed after oral or parenteral administration. Absorption of methylxanthines relates more to lipophilicity than to water solubility.

### Distribution
Rapidly distributed to all body compartments; readily crosses the placenta and blood-brain barrier. Volume of distribution (Vol$_D$) in adults ranges from 0.4 to 0.6 liter per kg of body weight (L/kg). Vol$_D$ in neonates averages between 0.78 and 0.92 L/kg.

### Protein binding
Low (25–36%).

### Biotransformation
Hepatic. In adults, about 80% of a dose of caffeine is metabolized to paraxanthine (1,7-dimethylxanthine), about 10% is metabolized to theobromine (3,7-dimethylxanthine), and about 4% is metabolized to theophylline (1,3-dimethylxanthine). These compounds are further demethylated to monomethylxanthines and then to methyl uric acids. In premature neonates, theophylline is converted to caffeine.

### Half-life
Adults—3 to 7 hours.
Neonates—65 to 130 hours. Decreases to adult values by 4 to 7 months post-term.
Note: Half-life is increased in pregnant women and in patients with cirrhosis.

### Time to peak plasma concentration
50 to 75 minutes following oral administration in adults.

### Therapeutic plasma concentration
5 to 25 mcg per mL (25.8 to 128.8 micromoles per L).

### Elimination
Adults—Renal; primarily as metabolites; about 1 to 2% excreted unchanged.
Neonates—Renal; about 85% excreted unchanged.

## Precautions to Consider

### Cross-sensitivity and/or related problems
Patients sensitive to other xanthines (aminophylline, dyphylline, oxtriphylline, theobromine, theophylline) may be sensitive to caffeine also.

### Pregnancy/Reproduction
Pregnancy—Caffeine crosses the placenta and achieves blood and tissue concentrations in the fetus that are similar to maternal concentrations. Studies in humans have shown that heavy caffeine consumption by pregnant women may increase the risk of spontaneous abortion and intrauterine growth retardation. Also, excessive intake of caffeine by pregnant women has resulted in fetal arrhythmias. It is therefore recommended that pregnant women limit their intake of caffeine to less than 300 mg (3 cups of coffee) per day.

Studies in animals have shown that caffeine causes skeletal abnormalities in the digits and phalanges when given in doses equivalent to the caffeine content of 12 to 24 cups of coffee daily throughout pregnancy or when given in very large single doses (i.e., 50 to 100 mg per kg of body weight), and causes retarded skeletal development when given in lower doses.

FDA Pregnancy Category C.

### Breast-feeding
Caffeine is distributed into breast milk in very small amounts. Although the concentration of caffeine in breast milk is 1% of the mother's plasma concentration, caffeine can accumulate in the infant. The infant may show signs of caffeine stimulation such as hyperactivity and wakefulness when a breast-feeding mother drinks as much as 6 to 8 cups of caffeine-containing beverages. It is recommended that nursing mothers limit their intake of caffeine-containing beverages to 1 to 2 cups per day and avoid taking over-the-counter caffeine capsules or tablets. At recommended doses of caffeine-containing analgesic combinations, concentration in the infant is considered to be insignificant.

### Pediatrics
With the exception of infants, appropriate studies on the relationship of age to the effects of caffeine have not been performed in children up to 12 years of age; however, no pediatrics-specific problems have been documented to date.

Caffeine and sodium benzoate injection is not recommended in neonatal apnea because the benzoate may interact competitively with bilirubin at the albumin binding site, which could cause or increase jaundice. In addition, elevated serum concentrations of benzyl alcohol and benzoate have been associated with neurological disturbances, hypotension, gasping respirations, and metabolic acidosis.

### Geriatrics
No information is available on the relationship of age to the effects of caffeine in geriatric patients.

### Drug interactions and/or related problems
The following drug interactions and/or related problems have been selected on the basis of their potential clinical significance (possible mechanism in parentheses where appropriate)—not necessarily inclusive (» = major clinical significance):

Note: Combinations containing any of the following medications, depending on the amount present, may also interact with this medication.

Adenosine
(effects of adenosine are antagonized by caffeine; larger doses of adenosine may be required, or adenosine may be ineffective)

Barbiturates or
Primidone
(concurrent use of barbiturates or primidone [because of the phenobarbital metabolite] with caffeine may increase the metabolism of caffeine by induction of hepatic microsomal enzymes, resulting in increased clearance of caffeine; in addition, concurrent use may antagonize the hypnotic or anticonvulsant effects of the barbiturates)

Beta-adrenergic blocking agents, systemic or
Beta-adrenergic blocking agents, ophthalmic
(concurrent use of beta-blocking agents, including ophthalmic agents [significant systemic absorption possible] with caffeine may result in mutual inhibition of therapeutic effects)

Bronchodilators, adrenergic
(concurrent use with caffeine may result in additive CNS stimulation and other additive toxic effects)

» Caffeine-containing beverages (coffee, tea, or soft drinks) or
» Caffeine-containing medications, other or
» CNS stimulation–producing medications, other (See Appendix II)
(excessive CNS stimulation causing nervousness, irritability, insomnia, or possibly convulsions or cardiac arrhythmias may occur; close observation is recommended)

Calcium supplements
(concurrent use with excessive amounts of caffeine may inhibit absorption of calcium)

Cimetidine
(decreased hepatic metabolism of caffeine results in delayed elimination and increased blood concentrations)

Ciprofloxacin or
Enoxacin or
Norfloxacin
(hepatic metabolism and clearance of caffeine may be reduced, increasing the risk of caffeine-related CNS stimulation)

Contraceptives, oral
(concurrent use may decrease caffeine metabolism)

Disulfiram
(concurrent use may reduce the elimination rate of caffeine by inhibiting its metabolism; recovering alcoholic patients on disulfiram therapy are best advised to avoid the use of caffeine to prevent the possibility of complicating alcohol withdrawal by caffeine-induced cardiovascular and cerebral excitation)

Erythromycin or
Troleandomycin
(concurrent use may reduce the hepatic clearance of caffeine)

Hydantoin anticonvulsants, especially phenytoin
(concurrent use of phenytoin may increase the clearance of caffeine)

Lithium
(concurrent use with caffeine increases urinary excretion of lithium, possibly reducing its therapeutic effect)

Mexiletine
(concurrent use with caffeine reduces the elimination of caffeine by up to 50% and may increase the potential for adverse effects)

» Monoamine oxidase (MAO) inhibitors, including furazolidone, procarbazine, and selegiline
(large amounts of caffeine may produce dangerous cardiac arrhythmias or severe hypertension because of the sympathomimetic side effects of caffeine; concurrent use with small amounts of caffeine may produce tachycardia and a mild increase in blood pressure)

Smoking, tobacco
(concurrent use of tobacco increases the elimination rate of caffeine)

Xanthines, other, such as:
Aminophylline
Dyphylline
Oxtriphylline
Theobromine
Theophylline
(caffeine may decrease the clearance of theophylline and possibly other xanthines, increasing the potential for additive pharmacodynamic and toxic effects)

**Laboratory value alterations**
The following have been selected on the basis of their potential clinical significance (possible effect in parentheses where appropriate)—not necessarily inclusive (» = major clinical significance):

With diagnostic test results
Dipyridamole- or adenosine-assisted cardiac diagnostic studies
(caffeine antagonizes the effects of dipyridamole and adenosine on myocardial blood flow, thereby interfering with test results; patients should be instructed to avoid ingesting caffeine [from a dietary or medicinal source] for 8 to 12 hours prior to the test)

Urate measurements, serum
(false-positive elevations when measured by the Bittner method)

Vanillylmandelic acid (VMA) and
Catecholamines, including norepinephrine and epinephrine and
5-hydroxyindoleacetic acid
(urine concentrations are slightly increased; high urinary concentrations of VMA or catecholamines may result in a false-positive diagnosis of pheochromocytoma or neuroblastoma; caffeine intake should be avoided during tests)

With physiology/laboratory test values
Glucose, blood
(concentrations may be increased; glucose tolerance may be impaired in diabetic patients)

**Medical considerations/Contraindications**
The medical considerations/contraindications included have been selected on the basis of their potential clinical significance (reasons given in parentheses where appropriate)—not necessarily inclusive (» = major clinical significance).

*Risk-benefit should be considered when the following medical problems exist:*

» Anxiety disorders, including agoraphobia and panic attacks
(increased risk of anxiety, nervousness, fear, nausea, palpitations, rapid heartbeat, restlessness, and trembling)

» Cardiac disease, severe
(high doses not recommended because of increased risk of tachycardia or extrasystoles, which may lead to heart failure)

» Hepatic function impairment
(half-life of caffeine may be prolonged leading to toxic accumulation)

» Hypertension or
» Insomnia
(may be potentiated)

Sensitivity to caffeine or other xanthines

**Patient monitoring**
The following may be especially important in patient monitoring (other tests may be warranted in some patients, depending on condition; » = major clinical significance):

*For neonatal apnea*
Caffeine concentrations, plasma or serum
(determinations recommended 24 hours after loading dose, then 1 to 2 times a week; alternatively, some clinicians recommend checking caffeine concentrations every 2 weeks once the infant has been stabilized)

Theophylline concentrations, serum
(determinations may be indicated in the presence of adverse effects possibly caused by conversion of caffeine to theophylline in the neonate)

## Side/Adverse Effects

The following side/adverse effects have been selected on the basis of their potential clinical significance (possible signs and symptoms in parentheses where appropriate)—not necessarily inclusive:

**Those indicating need for medical attention**
Incidence more frequent
*CNS stimulation, excessive* (dizziness; fast heartbeat; irritability, nervousness, or severe jitters in neonates; tremors; trouble in sleeping); *gastrointestinal irritation* (diarrhea; nausea; vomiting)

**Those indicating need for medical attention only if they continue or are bothersome**
Incidence more frequent
*CNS stimulation, mild* (nervousness or jitters); *gastrointestinal irritation, mild* (nausea)

**Those indicating possible withdrawal if they occur after medication is abruptly discontinued after prolonged use**
*Anxiety; dizziness; headache; irritability; muscle tension; nausea; nervousness; stuffy nose; unusual tiredness*

## Overdose

For specific information on the agents used in the management of caffeine overdose, see:
- *Antacids (Oral-Local)* monograph;
- *Charcoal, Activated (Oral-Local)* monograph;
- *Diazepam* in *Benzodiazepines (Systemic)* monograph;
- *Ipecac (Oral-Local)* monograph;
- *Magnesium sulfate* in *Laxatives (Local)* monograph;
- *Phenobarbital* in *Barbiturates (Systemic)* monograph; and/or
- *Phenytoin* in *Anticonvulsants, Hydantoin (Systemic)* monograph.

For more information on the management of overdose or unintentional ingestion, **contact a Poison Control Center** (see *Poison Control Center Listing*).

**Clinical effects of overdose**
The following effects have been selected on the basis of their potential clinical significance (possible signs and symptoms in parentheses where appropriate)—not necessarily inclusive:
*Abdominal or stomach pain; agitation, anxiety, excitement, or restlessness; confusion or delirium; dehydration; fast or irregular heartbeat; fever; frequent urination; headache; increased sensitivity to touch or pain; irritability; muscle trembling or twitching; nausea and vomiting, sometimes with blood; painful, swollen abdomen or vomiting in neonates; ringing or other sounds in ears; seeing flashes of "zig-zag" lights; seizures, usually tonic-clonic seizures*—in acute overdose; *trouble in sleeping; whole body tremors in neonates*

**Treatment of acute overdose**
Acute caffeine toxicity has been reported rarely. Treatment is primarily symptomatic and supportive.

To decrease absorption—
Induction of emesis with ipecac syrup and/or gastric lavage if caffeine has been ingested within 4 hours in amounts over 15 mg per kg of body weight (mg/kg) and emesis has not been induced by caffeine.

Administration of activated charcoal may be useful within the first 4 hours if precautions are taken to minimize the risk of aspiration; magnesium sulfate cathartic may also be useful.

To enhance elimination—
Hemoperfusion is usually more effective than dialysis. Use of exchange transfusion in neonates, if necessary.

Specific treatment—
    Control of CNS stimulation or seizures with intravenous diazepam, phenobarbital, or phenytoin.
    Administration of antacids and iced saline lavage for hemorrhagic gastritis.
Supportive care—
    Maintenance of fluid and electrolyte balance. Maintenance of ventilation and oxygenation. Patients in whom intentional overdose is confirmed or suspected should be referred for psychiatric consultation.

## Patient Consultation

As an aid to patient consultation, refer to *Advice for the Patient, Caffeine (Systemic)*.
In providing consultation, consider emphasizing the following selected information (» = major clinical significance):

### Before using this medication
» Conditions affecting use, especially:
    Sensitivity to caffeine or other xanthines (aminophylline, dyphylline, oxtriphylline, theobromine, theophylline)
    Pregnancy—Crosses placenta; excessive use during pregnancy may result in spontaneous abortion, intrauterine growth retardation, or fetal arrhythmias; animal studies have shown skeletal abnormalities with large doses and retarded skeletal development with lower doses
    Breast-feeding—Distributed into breast milk in small amounts but accumulates in infant and may cause hyperactivity and wakefulness; nursing mothers should limit intake of caffeine from all sources
    Use in children—Caffeine and sodium benzoate injection is not recommended in neonates because of the benzoate content. However, caffeine citrate may be used safely
    Other medications, especially caffeine-containing medications or beverages, other CNS stimulation–producing medications, or monoamine oxidase (MAO) inhibitors
    Other medical problems, especially anxiety disorders including agoraphobia and panic attacks, severe cardiac disease, hepatic function impairment, hypertension, or insomnia

### Proper use of this medication
» Importance of not taking more medication and not taking it more often than directed because of increased risk of side effects and habit-forming potential; should be used only occasionally
    Proper administration of extended-release capsule: Swallowing whole; not breaking, crushing, or chewing
» Caution if tolerance develops; not increasing dose
» Proper dosing
» Proper storage

### Precautions while using this medication
» Checking with physician if fatigue or drowsiness persists or recurs often
    Caution in concurrently drinking large amounts of coffee, tea, or colas or using other medications containing caffeine since amount of caffeine in medication is about the same as in a cup of coffee; importance of knowing amount of caffeine in common foods and beverages
» Discontinuing caffeine-containing medications or foods if fast pulse, dizziness, or pounding heartbeat occurs
    Not taking too close to bedtime

### Side/adverse effects
Signs of potential side effects, especially excessive CNS stimulation or gastrointestinal irritation

## General Dosing Information

With prolonged use, habituation or psychological dependence and tolerance to cardiovascular, diuretic, and stimulant effects may occur.

Citrated caffeine injection or oral solution for use in neonatal apnea is not available commercially but must be prepared extemporaneously from citrated caffeine powder. Caffeine tablets may also be crushed and made into an oral suspension. Caffeine citrate powder may be combined with lactose to add to feedings.

Citrated caffeine injection should not be administered intramuscularly because of its acidic nature (pH 3 to 4). It may be administered intravenously.

Caffeine and sodium benzoate injection is not recommended in neonatal apnea because of the benzoate content.

### Diet/Nutrition
The amount of caffeine from dietary sources is as follows
    Coffee, brewed—40 to 180 mg per cup.
    Coffee, instant—30 to 120 mg per cup.
    Coffee, decaffeinated—3 to 5 mg per cup.
    Tea, brewed American—20 to 90 mg per cup.
    Tea, brewed imported—25 to 110 mg per cup.
    Tea, instant—28 mg per cup.
    Tea, canned iced—22 to 36 mg per 12 ounces.
    Cola and other soft drinks, caffeine-containing—36 to 90 mg per 12 ounces.
    Cola and other soft drinks, decaffeinated—0 mg per 12 ounces.
    Cocoa—4 mg per cup.
    Chocolate, milk—3 to 6 mg per ounce.
    Chocolate, bittersweet—25 mg per ounce.

---

## CAFFEINE

## Oral Dosage Forms

Note: Bracketed uses in the *Dosage Forms* section refer to categories of use and/or indications that are not included in U.S. product labeling.

### CAFFEINE EXTENDED-RELEASE CAPSULES

**Usual adult and adolescent dose**
Fatigue; drowsiness—
    Oral, 200 to 250 mg (anhydrous caffeine), the dosage to be repeated no sooner than three or four hours, as needed.

**Usual adult prescribing limits**
Up to 1 gram a day.

**Usual pediatric dose**
Fatigue; drowsiness—
    Children up to 12 years of age: Use is not recommended.

**Strength(s) usually available**
U.S.—
    200 mg (anhydrous caffeine) (OTC) [*Caffedrine; Caffedrine Caplets;* GENERIC].
    250 mg (anhydrous caffeine) (OTC) [*Dexitac;* GENERIC].
Canada—
    Not commercially available.

**Packaging and storage**
Store below 40 °C (104 °F), preferably between 15 and 30 °C (59 and 86 °F), in a well-closed container, unless otherwise specified by manufacturer.

**Auxiliary labeling**
• Do not take at bedtime.

### CAFFEINE TABLETS

**Usual adult and adolescent dose**
Fatigue; drowsiness—
    Oral, 100 to 200 mg (anhydrous caffeine), the dosage to be repeated no sooner than three or four hours, as needed.

**Usual adult prescribing limits**
Up to 1 gram a day.

**Usual pediatric dose**
Fatigue; drowsiness—
    Children up to 12 years of age: Use is not recommended.
[Neonatal apnea]—
    Initial: Oral, 10 mg (anhydrous caffeine) per kg of body weight.
    Maintenance: Oral, 2.5 mg (anhydrous caffeine) per kg of body weight a day, starting twenty-four hours after the initial dose, to maintain a serum concentration of 5 to 25 mcg per mL (25.8 to 128.8 micromoles per L).
Note: Caffeine tablets may be crushed and made into an oral suspension for use in neonatal apnea.

**Strength(s) usually available**
U.S.—
    75 mg (anhydrous caffeine) (OTC) [*Enerjets*].
    100 mg (anhydrous caffeine) (OTC) [*NoDoz; Pep-Back;* GENERIC].
    150 mg (anhydrous caffeine) (OTC) [*Quick Pep*].
    200 mg (anhydrous caffeine) (OTC) [*Keep Alert; NoDoz Maximum Strength Caplets; Ultra Pep-Back; Vivarin*].
Canada—
    100 mg (anhydrous caffeine) (OTC) [*Caffedrine*].
    100 mg (caffeine alkaloid) (OTC) [*Wake-Up*].

**Packaging and storage**
Store below 40 °C (104 °F), preferably between 15 and 30 °C (59 and 86 °F), in a well-closed container, unless otherwise specified by manufacturer.

**Auxiliary labeling**
• Do not take at bedtime.

## CAFFEINE, CITRATED

## Oral Dosage Forms

Note: Bracketed uses in the *Dosage Forms* section refer to categories of use and/or indications that are not included in U.S. product labeling.

### CITRATED CAFFEINE SOLUTION

**Usual pediatric dose**
[Neonatal apnea]—
  Initial: Oral, 20 mg (10 mg of anhydrous caffeine and 10 mg of anhydrous citric acid) per kg of body weight.
  Maintenance: Oral, 5 mg (2.5 mg of anhydrous caffeine and 2.5 mg of anhydrous citric acid) per kg of body weight a day, starting twenty-four hours after the initial dose, to maintain a serum concentration of 5 to 25 mcg per mL (25.8 to 128.8 micromoles per L).

Note: Premature neonates may require a smaller dose.

**Strength(s) usually available**
U.S.—
  Dosage form not commercially available. Compounding required.
Canada—
  Dosage form not commercially available. Compounding required.

**Preparation of dosage form**
Ten grams of citrated caffeine powder should be dissolved in 250 mL of sterile water for irrigation, and stirred until completely clear; then flavoring should be added (simple syrup and cherry syrup 2:1) to make 500 mL. The final concentration is 20 mg (10 mg of anhydrous caffeine and 10 mg of anhydrous citric acid) per mL.

**Stability**
Compounded product as described above is stable for 3 months at room temperature.

**Note**
Citrated caffeine powder may also be combined with lactose and added to infant feedings.

### CITRATED CAFFEINE TABLETS

**Usual adult and adolescent dose**
Fatigue; drowsiness—
  Oral, initially, 65 to 325 mg (32 to 162 mg of anhydrous caffeine and 32 to 162 mg of anhydrous citric acid) three times a day, as needed.

**Usual adult prescribing limits**
Up to 1 gram of anhydrous caffeine a day.

**Usual pediatric dose**
Children up to 12 years of age—
  Use is not recommended.

**Strength(s) usually available**
U.S.—
  65 mg (32.5 mg of anhydrous caffeine and 32.5 mg of anhydrous citric acid) (OTC) [GENERIC].
Canada—
  Not commercially available.

**Packaging and storage**
Store below 40 °C (104 °F), preferably between 15 and 30 °C (59 and 86 °F), unless otherwise specified by manufacturer.

**Auxiliary labeling**
• Do not take at bedtime.

## Parenteral Dosage Forms

Note: Bracketed uses in the *Dosage Forms* section refer to categories of use and/or indications that are not included in U.S. product labeling.

### CITRATED CAFFEINE INJECTION

**Usual pediatric dose**
[Neonatal apnea]—
  Initial: Intravenous, 20 mg (10 mg of anhydrous caffeine and 10 mg of anhydrous citric acid) per kg of body weight.
  Maintenance: Intravenous, 5 mg (2.5 mg of anhydrous caffeine and 2.5 mg of anhydrous citric acid) per kg of body weight a day, starting twenty-four hours after the initial dose, to maintain a serum concentration of 5 to 25 mcg per mL (25.8 to 128.8 micromoles per L).

**Strength(s) usually available**
U.S.—
  Dosage form not commercially available. Compounding required.
Canada—
  Dosage form not commercially available. Compounding required.

**Preparation of dosage form**
Ten grams of citrated caffeine powder should be dissolved in 250 mL of sterile water for injection and transferred to a 500-mL empty evacuated container (EEC). The container should be filled with sterile water to the 500-mL mark and filtered through a 0.22-micron filter into another 500-mL EEC. Then the solution should be transferred to 10-mL vials and autoclaved at 121 °C for 15 minutes and allowed to cool. The resulting concentration is 20 mg (10 mg of anhydrous caffeine and 10 mg of anhydrous citric acid) per mL.

**Stability**
Compounded product as described above is stable for 3 months at room temperature.

## CAFFEINE AND SODIUM BENZOATE

## Parenteral Dosage Forms

### CAFFEINE AND SODIUM BENZOATE INJECTION USP

**Usual adult and adolescent dose**
CNS stimulant—
  Intramuscular or intravenous, up to a maximum of 500 mg (250 mg of anhydrous caffeine and 250 mg of sodium benzoate), as needed and tolerated.

**Usual adult prescribing limits**
2.5 grams (1.25 grams of anhydrous caffeine and 1.25 grams of sodium benzoate) a day.

**Usual pediatric dose**
Dosage has not been established.

Note: Use not recommended in neonatal apnea because of benzoate content.

**Strength(s) usually available**
U.S.—
  250 mg (125 mg of anhydrous caffeine and 125 mg of sodium benzoate) per mL (Rx) [GENERIC].
Canada—
  Not commercially available.

**Packaging and storage**
Store below 40 °C (104 °F), preferably between 15 and 30 °C (59 and 86 °F), unless otherwise specified by manufacturer.

## Selected Bibliography

Nehlig A, Daval J-L, Debry G. Caffeine and the central nervous system: mechanisms of action, biochemical, metabolic and psychostimulant effects. Brain Res Rev 1992; 17: 139-70.

Revised: 07/12/94

---

**CAFFEINE, CITRATED**—See *Caffeine (Systemic)*

---

**CALAMINE**—The *Calamine (Topical)* monograph is not included in this published version of the USP DI database. Copies of the monograph are available on request from Micromedex, Inc. - Reprint Requests, 6200 S. Syracuse Way, Suite 300, Englewood, CO 80111; telephone (303) 486-6400; telefax (303) 486-6464; Email: USPDI@MDX.COM.

---

**CALCIFEDIOL**—See *Vitamin D and Analogs (Systemic)*

# CALCIPOTRIENE Topical

INN: Calcipotriol
BAN: Calcipotriol
VA CLASSIFICATION (Primary): DE802
Commonly used brand name(s): *Dovonex*.
Another commonly used name is MC 903.
Note: For a listing of dosage forms and brand names by country availability, see *Dosage Forms* section(s).

## Category
Antipsoriatic (topical).

## Indications
Note: Bracketed information in the *Indications* section refers to uses that are not included in U.S. product labeling.

### Accepted
Psoriasis (treatment)—Calcipotriene cream and ointment are indicated for the treatment of [mild] to moderate plaque psoriasis. [Calcipotriene cream and ointment also may be used in the treatment of extensive or severe chronic plaque psoriasis. However, its use in this type of psoriasis is generally not recommended because of increased risk of hypercalcemia, secondary to excessive absorption of the medication when there is extensive skin involvement. If calcipotriene is to be used for severe extensive psoriasis, it is necessary to monitor the serum and urinary calcium levels at regular intervals.]

[Calcipotriene ointment is also used in combination with ultraviolet B light (UVB) phototherapy in the treatment of psoriasis.]

Psoriasis, of scalp (treatment)—Calcipotriene topical solution is indicated to treat chronic, moderately severe psoriasis of the scalp.

## Pharmacology/Pharmacokinetics

### Physicochemical characteristics
Source—Synthetic vitamin $D_3$ derivative.
Molecular weight—412.6.

### Mechanism of action/Effect
Unknown; however, calcipotriene inhibits keratinocyte proliferation (without any evidence of cytotoxic effect) and induces terminal differentiation of keratinocytes, thus reversing the abnormal keratinocyte change in psoriasis. Calcipotriene exhibits a vitamin D–like effect by competing for the cellular receptors for calcitriol $(1,25[OH]_2D_3)$, a biologically active metabolite of vitamin D. These calcitriol receptors have been identified on keratinocytes of both normal and psoriatic skin. *In vitro* data suggest that calcipotriene is equal to calcitriol in its ability to inhibit proliferation and induce differentiation of many cell types. Animal data show calcipotriene to be 100 to 200 times less potent in its effects on calcium metabolism as compared with those of calcitriol.

In open studies involving 400 patients treated with topical calcipotriene for up to 1 year, half of the studies excluded patients who had responded poorly to previous use of calcipotriene. Calcipotriene used for 8 weeks resulted in:
- Ointment—With use of calcipotriene once a day, 57% of patients studied showed marked improvement and 6% complete clearing of psoriasis. In another study of patients using ointment twice a day, 70% of patients showed marked improvement and 11% complete clearing of psoriasis. Since these patients were not compared in the same study, the difference, among other factors, may be due to the population studied, the vehicle, and the time of the year when treated. Using calcipotriene twice a day is not considered to be superior in efficacy to its use once a day.
- Cream (used twice a day)—50% of patients showed marked improvement and 4% showed complete clearing in patients studied.
- Solution (used twice a day)—17% of patients showed marked improvement and 14% showed complete clearing in 31% of patients studied.

### Other actions/effects
Calcipotriene seems to have an immunoregulatory role that involves the skin immune system, and is associated with variable decreases in keratinocyte expression of markers of activation. Calcipotriene may reduce the release of cytokines from different cell lineages; it may also govern a down-regulation of cell adhesion molecules (CAMs) that are known to mediate the passage of activated T-lymphocytes in the dermis and in the epidermis, thereby producing a reduction of cellular infiltrates in psoriasis.

### Absorption
For the cream—Systemic absorption of the cream has not been studied but is thought to be less than that of the ointment.
For the ointment—Approximately 6% (± 3%, SD) of the applied dose of radiolabeled calcipotriene ointment is absorbed systemically when the ointment is applied topically to psoriasis plaques; about 5% (± 2.6%, SD) is absorbed when applied to normal skin.
For the solution—Approximately 1% of the applied dose is systemically absorbed.

### Protein binding
*In vitro*, the affinity of calcipotriene for human serum vitamin D–binding protein is 30 times less than that of calcitriol.

### Biotransformation
Clinical studies using radiolabeled calcipotriene ointment have shown that much of the active substance absorbed is converted to inactive metabolites within 24 hours following topical application to psoriasis plaques and normal skin. In animal studies, calcipotriene is rapidly metabolized in the liver following systemic uptake and converted to inactive metabolites identified as MC 1046 and MC 1080.

### Elimination
Only small amounts (< 1%) of radiolabeled calcipotriene were recovered in the urine and feces following topical application of this medication in 4 patients with psoriasis.

## Precautions to Consider

### Carcinogenicity
Long-term animal studies have not been conducted to evaluate the carcinogenic potential of calcipotriene.

### Mutagenicity
Calcipotriene did not show any mutagenic effects in the Ames mutagenicity assay, the mouse lymphoma TK locus assay, the human lymphocyte chromosome aberration test, and the mouse micronucleus test.

### Pregnancy/Reproduction
Fertility—Studies in rats given calcipotriene in doses up to 54 mcg per kg of body weight (mcg/kg) per day (318 mcg per square meter of body surface area [mcg/m$^2$] per day) showed no impairment of fertility or of general reproductive performance.

Pregnancy—Adequate and well-controlled studies have not been done in humans. There is evidence that calcitriol crosses the placenta; similar distribution is expected for calcipotriene.
Maternal and fetal toxicity increased in pregnant rabbits given oral doses of 12 mcg/kg per day (132 mcg/m$^2$ per day). Incomplete ossification of the fetal pubic bones and forelimb phalanges occurred at doses of 36 mcg/kg per day (396 mcg/m$^2$ per day). Skeletal abnormalities, such as enlarged fontanelles and extra ribs, occurred in the fetuses of pregnant rats given oral doses of 54 mcg/kg per day (318 mcg/m$^2$ per day). The effect of skeletal enlargement is probably due to the alteration of calcium metabolism by the medication.
The amount of the dose expected to be absorbed systemically from a topical application of calcipotriene is approximately 18.5 mcg/m$^2$ per day for the ointment (corresponding to about 5 to 6% of the applied dose) and approximately 0.13 mcg/m$^2$ per day for the scalp solution (corresponding to 1% of the applied dose).
Following oral administration (absorbed dose corresponds to 40 to 60% of oral dose), adverse fetal development or skeletal teratogenic effects occurred in rats at absorbed doses of approximately 156 mcg/m$^2$ per day. These effects also occurred in rabbits at absorbed doses of approximately 61 mcg/m$^2$ and 198 mcg/m$^2$ per day. No adverse fetal effects were seen at absorbed doses of 43.2 mcg/m$^2$ per day in rats or 17.6 mcg/m$^2$ per day in rabbits.
FDA Pregnancy Category C.

### Breast-feeding
It is not known whether calcipotriene is distributed into breast milk. However, problems in humans have not been documented.

### Pediatrics
Appropriate studies on the relationship of age to the effects of calcipotriene have not been performed in the pediatric population. Safety and efficacy have not been established. Because of a higher ratio of skin surface area to body mass, children are at greater risk than adults of systemic adverse effects when they are treated with topical medication.
Although the severity of stable psoriasis did not improve in pediatric patients enrolled in one prospective, placebo-controlled, double-blind study, 43 children between 2 and 14 years of age showed less skin redness and scaliness after being treated for 8 weeks with topical cal-

cipotriene. Treatment of less than 30% of total body surface area did not produce any short-term, detectable alterations of bone and calcium metabolism in these children.

**Geriatrics**
According to the manufacturer, about 12% of the total number of patients in the clinical studies of calcipotriene ointment were 65 years of age or older, while about 4% were 75 years of age and older. Skin-related adverse effects with use of the ointment were more severe in patients over 65 years of age than in those under 65 years of age.

**Laboratory value alterations**
The following have been selected on the basis of their potential clinical significance (possible effect in parentheses where appropriate)—not necessarily inclusive (» = major clinical significance):

With physiology/laboratory test values
» Calcium concentrations, serum
   (rapid, transient, and reversible increase may occur, which may or may not be dose-related; if increase in serum calcium is outside the normal range, treatment should be discontinued until normal calcium levels are restored)
» Calcium concentrations, urine
   (transient, reversible increase may occur, usually with excessive doses; one study showed an increase in urine calcium level when calcipotriene was used within the recommended maximum dose of 100 grams per week; this increase was attributed to the following mechanisms: increased absorption of calcium by the gut, increased mobilization from bone, or altered renal handling; urine calcium levels may rise even in the absence of any apparent change in the serum calcium levels)

**Medical considerations/Contraindications**
The medical considerations/contraindications included have been selected on the basis of their potential clinical significance (reasons given in parentheses where appropriate)—not necessarily inclusive (» = major clinical significance).

*Except under special circumstances, this medication should not be used when the following medical problem exists:*
» Psoriasis, of scalp, acute eruptions
   (solution should not be applied to acute psoriatic eruptions; medication should be discontinued if skin irritation develops on involved or surrounding uninvolved skin)

*Risk-benefit should be considered when the following medical problems exist:*
» Hypercalcemia or
» Hypercalciuria, pre-existing or
» Hypervitaminosis D
   (may result in renal impairment due to increased renal calculi formation, secondary to precipitation of calcium salts in the renal parenchyma [nephrocalcinosis])
   Hypersensitivity to calcipotriene or to other components of the preparation, history of
» Nephrolithiasis, history of
   (may further aggravate condition due to increased renal calculi formation)

**Patient monitoring**
The following may be especially important in patient monitoring (other tests may be warranted in some patients, depending on condition; » = major clinical significance):

» Calcium concentrations, serum
   (transient, reversible increase may occur; generally, treatment with calcipotriene at recommended doses of up to 100 grams per week does not result in changes in laboratory values of serum calcium; however, it is recommended that baseline serum calcium levels be obtained prior to treatment and that monitoring be done at regular intervals, especially if calcipotriene is used at doses in excess of 100 grams per week or if it is used for severe psoriasis with extensive skin involvement; if serum calcium levels become elevated, treatment with calcipotriene should be discontinued and serum calcium levels should be measured once a week until the levels return to normal; patients with marginally elevated serum calcium may be treated with calcipotriene, provided that the serum calcium is monitored at suitable intervals)
» Calcium concentrations, urine
   (transient, reversible increase may occur; urine calcium is considered a more sensitive indicator of toxicity than is serum calcium; patients with extensive psoriasis who may require a dose approaching 100 grams per week should be screened for hypercalciuria by obtaining baseline urine calcium levels prior to treatment; urine calcium of these patients should be monitored if this dose is continued for more than a few weeks)

## Side/Adverse Effects
The following side/adverse effects have been selected on the basis of their potential clinical significance (possible signs and symptoms in parentheses where appropriate)—not necessarily inclusive:

**Those indicating need for medical attention**
Incidence more frequent
   *Dermatitis* (redness and swelling of skin with itching)—incidence of 10 to 15% for cream and ointment and 1 to 5% for solution; *skin rash*—incidence of 1 to 10% for cream and ointment and 11% for solution; *worsening of psoriasis, including development of psoriasis of the face and scalp*—incidence of 1 to 10% for cream and ointment and 1 to 5% for solution

Note: The incidence of side/adverse effects may be somewhat under-reported since half of the open studies involving 400 patients treated with topical calcipotriene ointment for up to 1 year excluded patients who had responded poorly to previous use of calcipotriene.

Incidence rare—1% or less for ointment, not reported for cream or solution
   *Atrophy of skin* (thinning, weakness, or wasting away of skin); *folliculitis* (burning, itching, and pain in hairy areas; pus in the hair follicles); *hypercalcemia, severe* (high blood levels of calcium; in severe cases, abdominal pain, constipation, depression, easy fatigability, high blood pressure, loss of appetite, loss of weight, muscle weakness, nausea, thirst, and vomiting)—usually asymptomatic in mild cases; *hypercalciuria* (high urine levels of calcium)—usually asymptomatic

Note: *Hypercalcemia* and *hypercalciuria* are usually reversible upon withdrawal of the medication.

**Those indicating need for medical attention only if they continue or are bothersome**
Incidence more frequent
   *Burning, irritation, or itching of skin, transient*—incidence of 20% for cream and ointment and 23% for solution upon application; *dryness or peeling of skin*—incidence of 1 to 10% for cream and ointment and 1 to 5% for solution; *erythema* (redness of skin)—incidence of 1 to 10% for ointment

Incidence rare
   *Hyperpigmentation* (darkening of treated skin)—incidence of less than 1% for cream and ointment, not reported with solution

## Overdose
For specific information on the agents used in the management of calcipotriene overdose, see:
• *Corticosteroids/Corticotropin—Glucocorticoid Effects (Systemic)* monograph;
• *Diuretics, Loop (Systemic)* monograph; and/or
• *Potassium Supplements (Systemic)* monograph.

For more information on the management of overdose or unintentional ingestion, **contact a Poison Control Center** (see *Poison Control Center Listing*).

**Clinical effects of overdose**
The following effects have been selected on the basis of their potential clinical significance (possible signs and symptoms in parentheses where appropriate)—not necessarily inclusive:

Acute effects
   *Hypercalcemia and/or hypercalciuria, severe* (abdominal pain, constipation, depression, easy fatigability, high blood pressure, loss of appetite, loss of weight, muscle weakness, nausea, thirst, and vomiting)—less severe cases are usually asymptomatic

**Treatment of overdose**
To decrease absorption—For both mild and severe cases of hypercalcemia and/or hypercalciuria, treatment with calcipotriene should be discontinued. For mild cases, withdrawal of the medication should be sufficient treatment.

To enhance elimination—For severe hypercalcemia, intensive hydration to increase calcium excretion is necessary. Fluids should be given both orally and parenterally (sodium chloride given intravenously is most effective).

Specific treatment—Diuretics such as furosemide may be given in conjunction with vigorous hydration. Prednisone may also be effective. Sufficient potassium chloride with continuous cardiac monitoring may be given to prevent hypokalemia. For patients with impaired renal function, hemodialysis may be useful.

Monitoring—Fluid intake and output and serum and urine electrolytes should be monitored carefully.

Supportive care—Patients in whom intentional overdose is known or suspected should be referred for psychiatric consultation.

## Patient Consultation
As an aid to patient consultation, refer to *Advice for the Patient, Calcipotriene (Topical)*.
In providing consultation, consider emphasizing the following selected information (» = major clinical significance):

**Before using this medication**
» Conditions affecting use, especially:
   Hypersensitivity to calcipotriene or to other components of the preparation
   Pregnancy—Calcipotriene probably crosses placenta. Human studies have not been done; in animal studies, high oral doses have caused incomplete skeletal development and skeletal abnormalities in fetuses
   Use in children—Safety and efficacy have not been established. Children are at greater risk of developing adverse systemic effects than adults when treated with topical medications; however, problems in bone and calcium metabolism did not occur in 43 children between 2 and 14 years of age treated for 8 weeks with topical calcipotriene applied to less than 30% of their body surface areas
   Use in the elderly—Skin-related side effects may be more severe when they occur in patients over 65 years of age
   Other medical problems, especially acute psoriatic eruptions on the scalp (for topical solution), hypercalcemia, hypercalciuria, hypervitaminosis D, or nephrolithiasis

**Proper use of this medication**
» For external use only and not for ophthalmic, oral, or intravaginal use; using this medication only as directed by physician
   Compliance with full course of therapy
» Not using more than 100 grams of cream or ointment or 60 mL of solution per week or a total dose of more than 5 mg of calcipotriene a week
» Avoiding contact of medication with face, eyes, mucous membranes, or uninvolved skin; washing medication off with water if it accidentally gets onto face, into eyes or mucous membranes, or onto normal skin surrounding the psoriatic area(s)
   Applying medication sparingly in folds of skin because of risk of irritation of skin where there is natural occlusion
   Washing hands after application to avoid inadvertently transferring medication onto face or uninvolved areas of the skin
   Not using medication for any skin disorder other than that for which it was prescribed
*For cream and ointment dosage forms*
» Applying enough medication to cover affected area(s) of skin and rubbing in gently and completely; avoiding use of occlusive dressing
» When ointment is used in combination with ultraviolet B light (UVB) phototherapy, applying medication after ultraviolet light exposure. This avoids the vehicle's UV-blocking action. Also, UV light can inactivate calcipotriene.
*For solution dosage form*
   Properly preparing scalp before application by combing and removing scaly debris, parting hair for easy access to scalp lesions; applying medication only to visible lesions; rubbing it in gently and completely; not applying on acute psoriatic eruptions
» Proper dosing
   Missed dose: Applying as soon as possible; not applying if almost time for next dose; not doubling doses
» Proper storage

**Precautions while using this medication**
   Medication may cause transient irritation of lesions and surrounding uninvolved skin after application; not scratching irritated skin
» Discontinuing use and checking with physician if irritation persists, or if facial rash or other problems develop
   While using this medication, visiting physician regularly for monitoring of serum and urine calcium levels
   Checking with physician if skin problem has not improved (usually within 2 to 8 weeks) or if skin condition becomes worse

**Side/adverse effects**
   Signs of potential side effects, especially dermatitis, skin rash, worsening of psoriasis, atrophy of skin, folliculitis, hypercalcemia, and hypercalciuria

## General Dosing Information
Calcipotriene is for external use only and not for ophthalmic, oral, or intravaginal use.

Calcipotriene should not be used on the face since it may cause itching and erythema of the facial skin. Patients should be instructed to wash their hands after using calcipotriene to avoid inadvertent transfer of this medication to the face or eyes. Should facial dermatitis develop, therapy should be discontinued.

Excessive use (more than 100 grams of cream or ointment, 60 mL of solution, or a total calcipotriene dose of 5 mg per week) may cause elevated serum or urinary calcium, which rapidly subsides when treatment is discontinued.

**For cream and ointment dosage forms**
The patient should apply the cream or ointment only to lesions and rub in well. Calcipotriene should be used cautiously in skin folds, such as the intertriginous areas, where natural occlusion may increase the medication's irritant effect.

Treatment with calcipotriene ointment may be combined with ultraviolet light phototherapy. With this form of treatment, patients are allowed to expose their skin to sunlight. Calcipotriene ointment should not be applied the morning of exposure to ultraviolet (UV) light because of the significant UV-blocking action of the vehicle.

**For solution dosage form**
To properly apply the topical solution to the scalp, the patient should comb dry hair and remove any scaly debris, then part the hair for easy access to scalp lesions. The medication is then applied and gently rubbed thoroughly into visible lesions. Avoid applying to unaffected areas of skin, including forehead.

## Topical Dosage Forms

### CALCIPOTRIENE CREAM
**Usual adult dose**
Psoriasis—
   Topical, to the affected area(s) of skin, two times a day. Efficacy of treatment beyond eight weeks has not been established.

**Usual adult prescribing limits**
100 grams of cream per week, or a total dose of 5 mg of calcipotriene per week when using more than one formulation.

**Usual pediatric dose**
Safety and efficacy have not been established.

**Usual geriatric dose**
See *Usual adult dose*.

**Strength(s) usually available**
U.S.—
   0.005% (Rx) [*Dovonex* (cetearyl alcohol; ceteth-20; diazolidinyl urea; dichlorobenzyl alcohol; dibasic sodium phosphate; edetate disodium; glycerin; mineral oil; petrolatum; water)].
Canada—
   0.005% (Rx) [*Dovonex* (cetomacrogol 1000; chlorallyhexaminium chloride [dowicil 200]; disodium edetate; disodium phosphate dihydrate; glycerol 85%; liquid paraffin; purified water; white soft paraffin)].

**Packaging and storage**
Store between 15 and 25 °C (59 and 77 °F), unless otherwise specified by manufacturer. Protect from freezing.

**Auxiliary labeling**
• For external use only.

### CALCIPOTRIENE OINTMENT
**Usual adult dose**
Psoriasis—
   Topical, to the affected area(s) of skin, one or two times a day. Efficacy of treatment beyond eight weeks has not been established.

**Usual adult prescribing limits**
100 grams of ointment per week or a total dose of 5 mg of calcipotriene per week when more than one formulation is used.

**Usual pediatric dose**
Safety and efficacy have not been established.

**Usual geriatric dose**
See *Usual adult dose*.

**Strength(s) usually available**
U.S.—
   0.005% (Rx) [*Dovonex* (dibasic sodium phosphate; edetate disodium; mineral oil; petrolatum; propylene glycol; tocopherol; steareth-2; water)].

Canada—
0.005% (Rx) [*Dovonex* (disodium edetate; disodium phosphate dihydrate; D, L-alpha-tocopherol; liquid paraffin; polyoxyethylene-(2)-stearyl ether; propylene glycol; purified water; white soft paraffin)].

**Packaging and storage**
Store between 15 and 25 °C (59 and 77 °F), unless otherwise specified by manufacturer. Protect from freezing.

**Auxiliary labeling**
• For external use only.

## CALCIPOTRIENE SOLUTION

**Usual adult dose**
Psoriasis, of scalp—
Topical, to the scalp lesions, two times a day. Efficacy of treatment beyond eight weeks has not been established.

**Usual adult prescribing limits**
60 mL of solution per week, or a total dose of 5 mg of calcipotriene per week when other formulations are used.

**Usual pediatric dose**
Safety and efficacy have not been established.

**Usual geriatric dose**
See *Usual adult dose*.

**Strength(s) usually available**
U.S.—
0.005% (Rx) [*Dovonex* (hydroxypropyl cellulose; isopropanol 51% v/v; menthol; propylene glycol; sodium citrate; water)].

Canada—
0.005% (Rx) [*Dovonex* (hydroxypropyl cellulose; isopropanol; levomenthol; propylene glycol; purified water; sodium citrate)].

**Packaging and storage**
Store between 15 and 25 °C (59 and 77 °F), unless otherwise specified by manufacturer. Protect from freezing. Protect from light.

**Auxiliary labeling**
• For external use only.

**Additional information**
This medication contains alcohol and is flammable; keep away from open flame.

## Selected Bibliography

Bruce S, Epinette WW, Funicella T, et al. Comparative study of calcipotriene (MC 903) ointment and fluocinonide ointment in the treatment of psoriasis. J Am Acad Dermatol 1994; 31(5 Pt 1): 755-9.

Highton A, Quell J, The Calcipotriene Study Group. Calcipotriene ointment 0.005% for psoriasis: a safety and efficacy study. J Am Acad Dermatol 1995; 32(1): 67-72.

Cunliffe WJ, Berth-Jones J, Claudy A, et al. Comparative study of calcipotriol (MC 903) ointment and betamethasone 17-valerate ointment in patients with psoriasis vulgaris. J Am Acad Dermatol 1992; 26(5 Pt 1): 736-43.

Revised: 08/20/97

---

# CALCITONIN   Nasal-Systemic—INTRODUCTORY VERSION

VA CLASSIFICATION (Primary): HS900

Commonly used brand name(s): *Miacalcin*.

Note: For a listing of dosage forms and brand names by country availability, see *Dosage Forms* section(s).

## Category
Bone resorption inhibitor; osteoporosis therapy.

## Indications

**Accepted**
Osteoporosis, postmenopausal (treatment adjunct)—Intranasal calcitonin-salmon is indicated for the treatment of osteoporosis in women who are more than 5 years postmenopause and have low bone mass relative to healthy premenopausal women. It is used in conjunction with an adequate intake of calcium (1000 mg of elemental calcium a day) and vitamin D (400 IU a day). Calcitonin should be reserved for patients who refuse or cannot tolerate estrogens or those in whom estrogens are contraindicated.

Intranasal calcitonin has been shown to increase spinal bone mass in postmenopausal women with established osteoporosis, but not in early postmenopausal women.

## Pharmacology/Pharmacokinetics

**Mechanism of action/Effect**
Osteoporosis—Studies using injectable calcitonin have found that it inhibits bone resorption by reducing the number and/or function of osteoclasts. With prolonged injectable calcitonin use, there is a persistent, smaller decrease in the rate of bone resorption. In vitro studies using injectable calcitonin-salmon have found an inhibition of osteoclast function with loss of the ruffled osteoclast border that is responsible for resorption of bone. *In vitro* studies indicate that calcitonin may augment bone formation by increasing osteoblastic activity. Long-term studies indicate that injectable calcitonin therapy results in the formation of bone that is of normal quality.

**Other actions/effects**
There is a slight decrease in serum calcium concentrations associated with intranasal calcitonin-salmon use; however, serum calcium remains within normal limits.

Injectable calcitonin increases the excretion of filtered phosphate, calcium, and sodium by inhibiting their tubular reabsorption.

Short-term administration of injectable calcitonin decreases the volume and acidity of gastric juice, the content of trypsin and amylase, and the volume of pancreatic juice. However, studies have not been conducted with intranasal calcitonin.

**Absorption**
Rapidly absorbed by the nasal mucosa.

**Half-life**
Elimination—43 minutes after intranasal administration.

**Time to peak concentration**
Approximately 31 to 39 minutes after intranasal administration.

## Precautions to Consider

**Cross-sensitivity and/or related problems**
Although not specifically reported for intranasal calcitonin-salmon, patients who are allergic to proteins may be allergic to calcitonin, because calcitonin is a protein. Its use in not recommended in patients with suspected sensitivity to calcitonin who show a positive response to skin testing prior to initiating therapy.

**Carcinogenicity**
A 1-year toxicity study in Sprague-Dawley and Fischer 344 rats given subcutaneous calcitonin-salmon at doses of 80 IU per kg of body weight a day (16 to 19 times the recommended human parenteral dose and approximately 130 to 160 times the recommended human intranasal dose based on body surface area) found an increased incidence of nonfunctioning pituitary adenomas. It was suggested that calcitonin-salmon reduced the latency period for development of pituitary adenomas that do not produce hormones, probably through the perturbation of physiologic processes involved in the evolution of this commonly occurring endocrine lesion in the rat. Although calcitonin-salmon reduced the latency period, it did not induce the hyperplastic or neoplastic process.

**Mutagenicity**
Calcitonin-salmon was found nonmutagenic in studies using *Salmonella typhimurium* (five strains) and *Escherichia coli* (two strains), both with and without rat liver metabolic activation. Calcitonin-salmon also was found nonmutagenic in an *in vitro* chromosome aberration test in mammalian V79 cells of the Chinese hamster.

**Pregnancy/Reproduction**
Pregnancy—Adequate and well-controlled studies in humans have not been done. Intranasal calcitonin-salmon is not indicated for use in pregnancy.

Reproduction studies in rabbits given injectable calcitonin-salmon in doses ranging from 8 to 33 times the recommended human parenteral dose and 70 to 278 times the recommended human intranasal dose based on body surface area showed a decrease in fetal birth weights. Since calcitonin does not cross the placenta, these effects may have been due to metabolic effects on the pregnant animal.

FDA Pregnancy Category C.

**Breast-feeding**
It is not known whether intranasal calcitonin-salmon is distributed into human breast milk. Calcitonin has been shown to inhibit lactation in animals.

**Pediatrics**
There are no data to support the use of intranasal calcitonin-salmon in children.

**Geriatrics**
Appropriate studies performed to date have not demonstrated geriatrics-specific problems that would limit the usefulness of intranasal calcitonin-salmon in the elderly.

**Drug interactions and/or related problems**
The following drug interactions and/or related problems have been selected on the basis of their potential clinical significance (possible mechanism in parentheses where appropriate)—not necessarily inclusive (» = major clinical significance):

Bisphosphonates, such as alendronate, etidronate, and pamidronate
(prior bisphosphonate use has been reported to reduce the antiresorptive response to intranasal calcitonin-salmon in patients with Paget's disease; however, this effect has not been assessed in postmenopausal women)

**Medical considerations/Contraindications**
The medical considerations/contraindications included have been selected on the basis of their potential clinical significance (reasons given in parentheses where appropriate)—not necessarily inclusive (» = major clinical significance).

*Risk-benefit should be considered when the following medical problems exist:*

» Allergy to proteins (or history of) or
» Sensitivity to calcitonin
(although not reported specifically for intranasal calcitonin-salmon, serious systemic allergic reactions [e.g., bronchospasm, swelling of the tongue or throat, anaphylactic shock, death due to anaphylaxis] have been reported with use of injectable calcitonin-salmon; skin testing should be considered prior to treatment of patients with suspected sensitivity to calcitonin-salmon)

**Patient monitoring**
The following may be especially important in patient monitoring (other tests may be warranted in some patients, depending on condition; » = major clinical significance):

Alkaline phosphatase, serum and
Hydroxyproline, urinary
(effects of intranasal calcitonin-salmon on these markers of bone turnover have not been consistently demonstrated in studies of women with postmenopausal osteoporosis; therefore, these parameters alone should not be used to determine clinical response to calcitonin-salmon; values should decrease with treatment)

Bone mass
(periodic measurements of vertebral bone mass are recommended during treatment to document stabilization of bone loss or increases in bone density; bone mass values should increase with treatment)

Nasal examinations
(nasal examinations should be performed before treatment begins, and at any time that nasal complaints occur; mucosal alterations or transient nasal conditions have been reported in up to 9% of patients receiving intranasal calcitonin-salmon; the examination should consist of visualization of the nasal mucosa, turbinates, and septum and assessment of mucosal blood vessel status; therapy should be discontinued temporarily to allow healing if small ulcers occur, and discontinued permanently if severe ulceration [e.g., ulcers greater than 1.5 mm in diameter, ulcers that penetrate below the mucosa, or ulcers associated with heavy bleeding] occurs)

Urinalysis
(periodic examinations of urine sediment should be considered, since coarse granular casts containing renal tubular epithelial cells were found in the urine of individuals receiving injectable calcitonin-salmon while at bedrest; no urine sediment abnormalities were found in ambulatory patients receiving injectable calcitonin-salmon)

## Side/Adverse Effects

The following side/adverse effects have been selected on the basis of their potential clinical significance (possible signs and symptoms in parentheses where appropriate)—not necessarily inclusive:

**Those indicating need for medical attention**
Incidence more frequent (3 to 12%)
*Nasal symptoms, specifically development of crusts; dryness; epistaxis* (nose bleeds); *inflammation; irritation; itching; redness; rhinitis* (runny nose); *sores or wounds on nasal mucosa; or tenderness*
Note: Patients who develop these nasal symptoms should be examined by their physicians. Development of ulcers on the nasal mucosa may require temporary or permanent discontinuation of intranasal calcitonin-salmon.

Incidence less frequent (1 to 3%)
*Angina* (chest pain); *bronchospasm* (wheezing or troubled breathing, severe); *cystitis* (bloody or cloudy urine; difficult, burning, or painful urination; frequent urge to urinate); *hypertension* (dizziness; headaches, severe or continuing); *lymphadenopathy* (swollen glands); *respiratory tract infection, upper* (chest pain; chills; cough; ear congestion or pain; fever; head congestion; hoarseness or other voice changes; nasal congestion; runny nose; sneezing; sore throat)

Incidence rare (< 1%)
*Allergic reactions, specifically hives, itching, or skin rash*

**Those indicating need for medical attention only if they continue or are bothersome**
Incidence more frequent (3 to 12%)
*Arthralgia* (joint pain); *back pain; headache*

Incidence less frequent (1 to 3%) or rare (< 1%)
*Abdominal pain; conjunctivitis* (burning, dry, or itching eyes); *constipation; diarrhea; dizziness; dyspepsia* (upset stomach); *fatigue* (unusual tiredness or weakness); *flu-like symptoms; flushing; lacrimation, unusual* (unusual tearing of eyes); *mental depression; myalgia* (muscle pain); *nausea; skin rash*

## Overdose

For specific information on the agents used in the management of intranasal calcitonin-salmon overdose, see the *Calcium Supplements (Systemic)* monograph.

For more information on the management of overdose or unintentional ingestion, **contact a Poison Control Center** (see *Poison Control Center Listing*).

**Treatment of overdose**
Specific treatment—Administering parenteral calcium if hypocalcemic tetany develops.

Supportive care—Patients in whom intentional overdose is confirmed or suspected should be referred for psychiatric consultation.

## Patient Consultation

As an aid to patient consultation, refer to *Advice for the Patient, Calcitonin (Nasal-Systemic)—Introductory Version.*

In providing consultation, consider emphasizing the following selected information (» = major clinical significance):

**Before using this medication**
» Conditions affecting use, especially:
Allergies (history of) or sensitivity to calcitonin or other proteins
Pregnancy—Not indicated for use during pregnancy
Breast-feeding—Lactation inhibited in animal studies
Use in children—No data to support use

**Proper use of this medication**
» Reading patient instructions carefully
» Importance of not using more medication than the amount prescribed
» Importance of not reactivating pump before daily dose

*Assembling the unit (Note: If unit has been assembled by health care professional, this step is not necessary)*
» Removing bottle from refrigerator and allowing it to reach room temperature
» Lifting up blue plastic tab and pulling metal safety seal off bottle
» Keeping bottle upright while removing rubber stopper from bottle
» Holding pump unit while removing opaque plastic protective cap from bottom of unit
» Holding bottle upright while inserting nasal spray pump unit into bottle
» Turning pump unit clockwise and tightening until securely fastened

*Priming the unit (for first-time use of unit only)*
» Holding bottle upright while removing clear protective cap from nozzle
» Depressing the two white side arms several times until a faint spray is emitted

*Proper administration*
» Blowing nose gently before using spray
» Keeping head in upright position and placing nozzle firmly into one nostril
» Depressing pump toward bottle one time
» Not inhaling while spraying

# Calcitonin (Nasal-Systemic)—Introductory Version

» Replacing plastic cap
» Proper dosing
  Missed dose: Using as soon as possible; not using if almost time for next dose
» Proper storage

**Side/adverse effects**
Signs of potential side effects, especially nasal symptoms; angina; bronchospasm; cystitis; hypertension; lymphadenopathy; respiratory tract infection, upper; and allergic reaction

## General Dosing Information

Skin testing should be considered prior to treatment of patients with suspected sensitivity to calcitonin-salmon. The manufacturer's recommendation for preparing the solution for skin testing is as follows:
• Prepare a dilution of 10 IU per mL by withdrawing 0.05 mL of calcitonin-salmon into a tuberculin syringe.
• Fill syringe to 1 mL with 0.9% sodium chloride injection. Mix well.
• Discard 0.9 mL and inject 0.1 mL intracutaneously on the inner forearm.
• Observe injection site 15 minutes after injection.
• A positive response is considered to be the appearance of erythema or a wheal that is more than mild.

## Nasal Dosage Form

### CALCITONIN-SALMON NASAL SOLUTION

**Usual adult and adolescent dose**
Postmenopausal osteoporosis—
  Intranasal, 200 IU (one metered spray in one nostril) a day, alternating nostrils daily.

**Strength(s) usually available**
U.S.—
  200 IU per metered spray (Rx) [*Miacalcin*].

**Packaging and storage**
The unopened container should be stored between 2 and 8 °C (36 and 46 °F). Protect from freezing.

**Stability**
Once the pump has been activated, the bottle may be kept at room temperature until the medication is finished (2 weeks). Opened or unopened bottles left at room temperature for more than 30 days must be discarded.

Developed: 07/02/97

---

# CALCITONIN   Systemic

This monograph includes information on the following: 1) Calcitonin-Human[†]; 2) Calcitonin-Salmon.
VA CLASSIFICATION (Primary): HS304
Commonly used brand name(s): *Calcimar*[2]; *Cibacalcin*[1]; *Miacalcin*[2].
Note: For a listing of dosage forms and brand names by country availability, see *Dosage Forms* section(s).

[†]Not commercially available in Canada.

## Category

Bone resorption inhibitor; osteoporosis therapy adjunct; antihypercalcemic therapy adjunct.

## Indications

Note: Bracketed information in the *Indications* section refers to uses that are not included in U.S. product labeling.

**Accepted**
Paget's disease of bone (treatment)—Calcitonin-salmon and calcitonin-human are indicated in the treatment of moderate to severe symptomatic Paget's disease (osteitis deformans), characterized by abnormal and accelerated bone metabolism in one or more bones. Signs and symptoms may include bone pain, deformity, and/or fractures; increased concentrations of serum alkaline phosphatase and/or urinary hydroxyproline; neurologic disorders associated with skull lesions and spinal deformities; and elevated cardiac output and other vascular disorders associated with increased vascularity of bones. Calcitonin-human may be effective for treatment of patients who have developed resistance to calcitonin-salmon.

Osteoporosis, postmenopausal (treatment adjunct)—Calcitonin-salmon[1] is indicated [and calcitonin-human is used] for the treatment of osteoporosis in postmenopausal women in conjunction with an adequate intake of calcium (1.5 grams of elemental calcium per day) and vitamin D (400 IU per day) to aid in the prevention of the progressive loss of bone mass. An adequate diet is also essential.

Although calcitonin may increase bone mass or help slow the loss of bone mass in some patients, questions still remain as to whether treatment with calcitonin will actually decrease the incidence of compression fractures in postmenopausal women with osteoporosis.

Hypercalcemia (treatment adjunct)—Calcitonin-salmon is indicated [and calcitonin-human is used] with intravenous saline and other appropriate hypocalcemic agents in the treatment of hypercalcemic emergencies. Calcitonin has been shown to effectively lower serum calcium concentrations in patients with carcinoma, multiple myeloma, or, to a lesser degree, primary hyperparathyroidism. Calcitonin-salmon may be added to existing therapeutic regimens for the treatment of hypercalcemia, such as intravenous fluids, furosemide, oral phosphates, or adrenocorticoids.

[Osteoporosis, secondary (treatment adjunct)][1]—Calcitonin-human and calcitonin-salmon are used in conjunction with an adequate intake of calcium and vitamin D for the treatment of osteoporosis secondary to hormonal disturbances, drug therapy, immobilization, and other causes. Calcitonin therapy is initiated when treatment of the underlying etiology is not feasible.

[1]Not included in Canadian product labeling.

## Pharmacology/Pharmacokinetics

**Physicochemical characteristics**
Molecular weight—
  Calcitonin-human: 3527.20.
  Calcitonin-salmon: 3431.88.

**Mechanism of action/Effect**
Paget's disease—Calcitonin reduces the rate of bone turnover, possibly by an initial blocking of bone resorption, resulting in decreases in serum alkaline phosphatase (reflecting decreased bone formation) and decreases in urinary hydroxyproline excretion (reflecting decreased bone resorption, i.e., breakdown of collagen).

Osteoporosis or
Hypercalcemia—Calcitonin lowers serum calcium concentration primarily by a direct inhibition of bone resorption. The number and/or function of osteoclasts is reduced and a decrease in osteocytic resorption may also be involved. These effects may be mediated in part by a drug-induced increase in cyclic adenosine monophosphate concentration in bone cells and subsequent alteration of calcium and/or phosphate transport across the plasma membrane of the osteoclast.

**Other actions/effects**
Calcitonin also has a direct effect on the kidneys, increasing the excretion of calcium, phosphate, and sodium by inhibiting their tubular reabsorption. These effects are also mediated in part by cyclic adenosine monophosphate. However, in some patients, calcitonin-induced inhibition of bone resorption has a greater effect on calcium excretion than does the drug's direct renal action, so that urinary calcium is decreased rather than increased.

Short-term administration of calcitonin results in decreases in the volume and acidity of gastric juice, and in trypsin and amylase content and volume of pancreatic juice.

**Duration of effect**
Calcitonin-salmon—Hypercalcemia: 6 to 8 hours.

**Biotransformation**
Calcitonin is rapidly metabolized, primarily in the kidneys but also in blood and peripheral tissues.

**Half-life**
Calcitonin-human—60 minutes, after a single dose.
Calcitonin-salmon—70 to 90 minutes, after a single dose.

**Onset of therapeutic action**
Calcitonin-human and calcitonin-salmon—Maximum reductions of serum alkaline phosphatase and urinary hydroxyproline excretion in Paget's disease may take 6 to 24 months of continuous treatment.

**Time to peak effect**
Cacitonin-salmon—Hypercalcemia: 2 hours.

### Elimination
Renal; very small amounts are excreted unchanged.

## Precautions to Consider

### Cross-sensitivity and/or related problems
Patients who are allergic to proteins may be allergic to calcitonin, since calcitonin is a protein. Its use is not recommended in patients with suspected sensitivity who show a positive response to skin testing prior to initiating therapy. Since calcitonin-salmon is a foreign protein, it may induce antibodies with continued use. In short-term treatment (2 years or less), antibody titers appear in 30 to 60% of treated patients, but only 5 to 15% become resistant to treatment as a result. Long-term treatment may be possible in patients who are not limited by antibody formation. Because synthetic human calcitonin is identical to naturally occurring human calcitonin, antibody formation is rare, allowing longer term treatment that is not limited by antibody-mediated resistance.

### Carcinogenicity
No long-term studies have been done to evaluate carcinogenic potential of calcitonin. The incidence of osteogenic sarcoma is increased in Paget's disease with or without treatment. Pagetic lesions, with or without therapy, should be carefully evaluated to distinguish them from osteogenic sarcoma, since such lesions may show marked progression on x-ray, with possible loss of periosteal margins. Calcitonin does not appear to slow the progression of such sarcomas.

### Pregnancy/Reproduction
Pregnancy—No adequate and well-controlled studies in humans have been done. However, calcitonin does not cross the placenta.

In animal studies, calcitonin has been shown to decrease fetal birth weight, when given in doses 14 to 56 times the dose recommended for human use, possibly due to metabolic effects on the pregnant animal.

FDA Pregnancy Category C.

### Breast-feeding
Calcitonin is distributed into breast milk. However, problems in humans have not been documented. In animal studies, calcitonin has been shown to inhibit lactation.

### Pediatrics
Appropriate studies on the relationship of age to the effects of calcitonin have not been performed in the pediatric population.

### Geriatrics
Appropriate studies on the relationship of age to the effects of calcitonin have not been performed in the geriatric population. However, no geriatrics-specific problems have been documented to date.

### Drug interactions and/or related problems
The following drug interactions and/or related problems have been selected on the basis of their potential clinical significance (possible mechanism in parentheses where appropriate)—not necessarily inclusive (» = major clinical significance):

Note: Combinations containing any of the following medications, depending on the amount present, may also interact with this medication.

Calcium-containing preparations or
Vitamin D, including calcifediol and calcitriol
(in the treatment of hypercalcemia, concurrent use may antagonize the effect of calcitonin; in the treatment of other conditions, calcium-containing preparations may be given 4 hours after calcitonin)

### Medical considerations/Contraindications
The medical considerations/contraindications included have been selected on the basis of their potential clinical significance (reasons given in parentheses where appropriate)—not necessarily inclusive (» = major clinical significance).

*Risk-benefit should be considered when the following medical problems exist:*
» Allergy to proteins (or history of) or
» Sensitivity to calcitonin
(possibility of systemic allergic reaction, especially in patients with a history of severe allergy, even with a negative skin test reaction to calcitonin, because of the protein nature of calcitonin; allergic reaction is more likely with calcitonin-salmon)

### Patient monitoring
The following may be especially important in patient monitoring (other tests may be warranted in some patients, depending on condition; » = major clinical significance):

Alkaline phosphatase concentrations, serum and
Urinary hydroxyproline concentrations (24-hour)
(determinations recommended at periodic intervals during therapy with calcitonin-salmon in Paget's disease of bone; during therapy with calcitonin-human, biochemical determinations are recommended prior to initiation, and once during the first three months, and at approximately 3- to 6-month intervals during chronic treatment of Paget's bone disease to determine effectiveness and dosage of calcitonin; most clinicians prefer to measure serum alkaline phosphatase for routine use because urinary hydroxyproline concentrations are cumbersome to measure and expensive)

Calcium concentrations, serum
(determinations required at periodic intervals during therapy for hypercalcemia)

Skin testing for allergic reaction
(recommended prior to treatment for patients with suspected hypersensitivity to calcitonin or patients with a history of florid allergy to foreign proteins)

## Side/Adverse Effects
The following side/adverse effects have been selected on the basis of their potential clinical significance (possible signs and symptoms in parentheses where appropriate)—not necessarily inclusive:

### Those indicating need for medical attention
Incidence rare
*Allergic reactions, specifically; skin rash; and urticaria* (hives)

### Those indicating need for medical attention only if they continue or are bothersome
Incidence more frequent
*Flushing, redness, or tingling of face, ears, hands, or feet; gastrointestinal effects, specifically; diarrhea; loss of appetite; nausea or vomiting; and stomach pain; redness, soreness, or swelling at injection site*

Incidence less frequent
*Increased frequency of urination*

Incidence rare
*Chills; dizziness; headache; pressure in chest; stuffy nose; tenderness or tingling of hands or feet; trouble in breathing; weakness*

## Patient Consultation
As an aid to patient consultation, refer to *Advice for the Patient, Calcitonin (Systemic)*.

In providing consultation, consider emphasizing the following selected information (» = major clinical significance):

### Before using this medication
» Conditions affecting use, especially:
Allergies (history of) or sensitivity to calcitonin or other proteins
Breast-feeding—Distributed into breast milk; lactation inhibited in animal studies

### Proper use of this medication
Proper administration: Using aseptic technique; subcutaneous injection preferred for self-administration
Importance of using reconstituted solution of calcitonin-human within 6 hours
Importance of inspecting solution for particles or discoloration before administering
» Proper dosing
Missed dose: If dosage schedule is:
Two doses a day—Taking missed dose, if remembered within 2 hours, and continuing on schedule; if remembered later, skipping missed dose, not doubling doses, and continuing on schedule
One dose a day—Taking as soon as possible unless remembered the next day; then skipping missed dose and continuing on schedule, but not doubling doses
One dose every other day—Taking as soon as possible if on scheduled day; taking if remembered on alternate day, but skipping the following day and restarting schedule
One dose three times a week (Monday-Wednesday-Friday)—Taking missed dose the next day; setting each injection back a day and resuming regular schedule the following week
» Proper storage

### Precautions while using this medication
Regular visits to physician to check progress during therapy
Possible need for calcium and vitamin D restriction, including calcifediol and calcitriol, in patients with hypercalcemia

### Side/adverse effects
Signs of potential side effects, especially allergic reaction

## General Dosing Information

**For use in Paget's disease of bone**

Clinical or biochemical improvement (decreased serum alkaline phosphatase) usually occurs within the first few months of therapy if calcitonin is effective. A longer period of therapy, often more than a year, may be required for maximum improvement.

Dosage adjustments depend on clinical and radiologic evidence, changes in serum alkaline phosphatase and urinary hydroxyproline excretion, and severity of nausea or flushing.

Bedtime administration may help to reduce the severity of nausea or flushing. Reduction in dosage may also be helpful.

After at least 6 months of treatment for Paget's disease, if symptoms have been relieved, therapy may be reduced for 6 months, monitoring biochemical and clinical responses, before being discontinued. Since biochemical indexes will relapse after cessation of treatment, they cannot be relied on to indicate a need for restarting therapy.

---

### CALCITONIN-HUMAN

## Summary of Differences

Cross-sensitivity and/or related problems: May be used for longer term-treatment with less antibody formation or protein hypersensitivity than calcitonin-salmon.

## Additional Dosing Information

See also *General Dosing Information*.

More severe cases of Paget's disease of bone (evidence of weak bones with osteolytic lesions) may require doses of up to 1 mg a day, given in divided doses.

## Parenteral Dosage Forms

### CALCITONIN-HUMAN FOR INJECTION

**Usual adult dose**
Paget's disease of bone—
   Subcutaneous, initially 500 mcg (0.5 mg) a day, the dosage being reduced for some patients to 500 mcg (0.5 mg) two or three times a week, or 250 mcg (0.25 mg) a day.
Note: To diminish side effects, some clinicians recommend starting with a low dose and gradually increasing dosage over 2 weeks.

**Usual pediatric dose**
Dosage has not been established.

**Size(s) usually available**
U.S.—
   500 mcg (0.5 mg) (Rx) [*Cibacalcin*].
Canada—
   Not commercially available.

**Packaging and storage**
Store at a temperature not exceeding 25 °C (77 °F), unless otherwise specified by manufacturer. Protect from light. Do not refrigerate.

**Preparation of dosage form**
To reconstitute, push the barrel of the double-chambered syringe into the vial as far as possible, and press upward on the plunger to release the water into the dry powder. Shake gently to mix. Withdraw the reconstituted medication back into the syringe and inject.

**Stability**
The reconstituted solution should be used within 6 hours.

**Additional information**
One chamber of the dual syringe contains 0.5 mg of calcitonin-human for injection and mannitol (20 mg) in sterile, lyophilized form. The other chamber contains mannitol (30 mg) in 1 mL of water for injection.

---

### CALCITONIN-SALMON

## Summary of Differences

Cross-sensitivity and/or related problems: Risk of protein hypersensitivity and antibody-mediated resistance greater than with calcitonin-human.

## Additional Dosing Information

See also *General Dosing Information*.

This medicine is for intramuscular or subcutaneous injection. The subcutaneous route of administration is usually preferred for patient self-administration.

If the volume to be injected exceeds 2 mL, the intramuscular route of administration is usually preferred and multiple sites of injection should be used to minimize local inflammatory reactions.

Skin testing should be considered prior to treatment of patients with suspected sensitivity to calcitonin-salmon. The manufacturer's recommendation for preparing the solution for skin testing is as follows:
• Prepare a dilution of 10 IU per mL by withdrawing 0.05 mL into a tuberculin syringe (an insulin syringe with no "dead space" may be preferred for a more accurate dilution).
• Fill to 1 mL with 0.9% sodium chloride injection. Mix well.
• Discard 0.9 mL and inject 0.1 mL intracutaneously on the inner forearm.
• Observe injection site 15 minutes after injection.
• A positive response is considered to be the appearance of a more than mild erythema or wheal.

In any patient who has an acceptable initial response but later relapses, either clinically or biochemically, there is the possibility of antibody formation. Testing the patient for high antibody titer by an appropriate specialized test or by critical clinical evaluation should be considered. Alternatively, a trial of therapy with calcitonin-human may be considered. Patient compliance should also be assessed in the event of relapse.

In patients who have relapsed, a dosage increase above 100 IU per day does not appear to improve patient response.

## Parenteral Dosage Forms

### CALCITONIN-SALMON INJECTION

**Usual adult dose**
Paget's disease of bone—
   Intramuscular or subcutaneous, initially 100 IU a day, the dosage being decreased to 50 IU once a day, once every other day, or three times a week, in patients without serious deformity or bone involvement.
Hypercalcemia—
   Intramuscular or subcutaneous, initially 4 IU per kg of body weight every twelve hours, the dosage being increased, if necessary for a more satisfactory response, to 8 IU per kg of body weight every twelve hours, up to a maximum of 8 IU per kg of body weight every six hours.
Postmenopausal osteoporosis[1]—
   Intramuscular or subcutaneous, 100 IU once a day, once every other day, or three times a week.
Note: To diminish side effects, some clinicians recommend starting with a low dose and gradually increasing dosage over 2 weeks.

**Usual pediatric dose**
Dosage has not been established.

**Strength(s) usually available**
U.S.—
   200 IU per mL (Rx) [*Calcimar; Miacalcin*].
Canada—
   200 IU per mL (Rx) [*Calcimar*].

**Packaging and storage**
Store between 2 and 8 °C (36 and 46 °F), unless otherwise specified by manufacturer. Do not freeze.

**Auxiliary labeling**
• Refrigerate.

**Additional information**
May also contain 5 mg of phenol per mL, as a preservative.
The activity of calcitonin-salmon is stated in terms of International Units (IU), which are equal to Medical Research Council Units (MRC).

[1]Not included in Canadian product labeling.

Revised: 05/13/92
Interim revision: 06/27/94

---

**CALCITONIN-HUMAN**—See *Calcitonin (Systemic)*

---

**CALCITONIN-SALMON**—See *Calcitonin (Systemic)*

---

**CALCITRIOL**—See *Vitamin D and Analogs (Systemic)*

**CALCIUM ACETATE**—See *Calcium Supplements (Systemic)*

# CALCIUM ACETATE  Systemic—INTRODUCTORY VERSION

VA CLASSIFICATION (Primary): TN402
Commonly used brand name(s): *PhosLo*.

Note: For a listing of dosage forms and brand names by country availability, see *Dosage Forms* section(s).

## Category
Antihyperphosphatemic.

## Indications

**Accepted**

Hyperphosphatemia (treatment)—Calcium acetate is indicated in patients with end-stage renal failure to lower serum phosphate concentrations. It does not promote aluminum absorption.

## Pharmacology/Pharmacokinetics

**Physicochemical characteristics**
Molecular weight—158.17.

**Mechanism of action/Effect**
Calcium acetate, when taken with meals, combines with dietary phosphate to form insoluble calcium phosphate, which is excreted in the feces.

**Absorption**
Data from healthy subjects and renal dialysis patients under various conditions indicate that after oral administration of calcium acetate, approximately 40% is absorbed in the fasting state and approximately 30% is absorbed in the nonfasting state.

**Elimination**
Fecal.

## Precautions to Consider

**Carcinogenicity**
Long-term studies to evaluate carcinogenic potential of calcium acetate have not been performed.

**Pregnancy/Reproduction**
Fertility—Studies have not been done in either humans or animals.
Pregnancy—Studies in humans have not been done.
Studies in animals have not been done.
FDA Pregnancy Category C.

**Breast-feeding**
It is not known whether calcium acetate is distributed into breast milk.

**Pediatrics**
No information is available on the relationship of age to the effects of calcium acetate in pediatric patients. Safety and efficacy have not been established.

**Geriatrics**
No information is available on the relationship of age to the effects of calcium acetate in geriatric patients.

**Drug interactions and/or related problems**
The following drug interactions and/or related problems have been selected on the basis of their potential clinical significance (possible mechanism in parentheses where appropriate)—not necessarily inclusive (» = major clinical significance):

Note: Combinations containing any of the following, depending on the amount present, may also interact with this medication.

» Calcium-containing foods or preparations, including dietary supplements or antacids
(concurrent use may cause hypercalcemia; dietary calcium should be estimated daily initially and intake adjusted as needed)

» Digitalis glycosides
(concurrent use is not recommended because calcium acetate may cause hypercalcemia, which could precipitate cardiac arrhythmias)

Tetracyclines, oral
(concurrent administration may decrease the bioavailability of tetracyclines)

**Medical considerations/Contraindications**
The medical considerations/contraindications included have been selected on the basis of their potential clinical significance (reasons given in parentheses where appropriate)—not necessarily inclusive (» = major clinical significance).

*Except under special circumstances, this medication should not be used when the following medical problem exists:*
» Hypercalcemia
(calcium acetate may exacerbate the condition)

*Risk-benefit should be considered when the following medical problem exists:*
Sensitivity to calcium acetate

**Patient monitoring**
The following may be especially important in patient monitoring (other tests may be warranted in some patients, depending on condition; » = major clinical significance):

Calcium concentrations, serum and
Phosphate concentrations, serum
(serum calcium concentrations should be monitored twice a week early in the treatment during the dosage adjustment period; serum calcium concentrations > 10.5 mg per dL (mg/dL) indicate mild hypercalcemia and serum concentrations > 12 mg/dL indicate severe hypercalcemia; the product of the serum calcium concentration and the serum phosphate concentration should not exceed 66; if hypercalcemia develops, calcium acetate should be discontinued or the dosage reduced, depending on the severity of hypercalcemia; serum phosphate concentrations should be monitored periodically and the dosage adjusted as needed to keep concentrations below 6 mg per dL)

## Side/Adverse Effects

The following side/adverse effects have been selected on the basis of their potential clinical significance (possible signs and symptoms in parentheses where appropriate)—not necessarily inclusive:

**Those indicating need for medical attention**
Incidence rare
*Hypercalcemia, mild* (constipation; loss of appetite; nausea or vomiting); *hypercalcemia, severe* (confusion; full or partial loss of consciousness; incoherent speech)
Note: *Mild hypercalcemia* may be asymptomatic.

**Those indicating need for medical attention only if they continue or are bothersome**
Incidence less frequent
*Nausea; pruritus* (itching)
Note: *Pruritus* may represent an allergic reaction.

## Overdose

For more information on the management of overdose or unintentional ingestion, **contact a Poison Control Center** (see *Poison Control Center Listing*).

**Clinical effects of overdose**
The following effects have been selected on the basis of their potential clinical significance (possible signs and symptoms in parentheses where appropriate)—not necessarily inclusive:

Acute and/or chronic
*Hypercalcemia, mild* (constipation; loss of appetite; nausea and vomiting); *hypercalcemia, severe* (confusion; full or partial loss of consciousness; incoherent speech)
Note: *Mild hypercalcemia* may be asymptomatic.
Chronic *hypercalcemia* may lead to vascular calcification or other soft-tissue calcification.

**Treatment of overdose**
Mild hypercalcemia may be controlled by reducing the dose of calcium acetate or temporarily discontinuing therapy. Calcium acetate therapy should be discontinued in severe hypercalcemia.

To enhance elimination—Severe hypercalcemia should be treated by hemodialysis.

Monitoring—If chronic hypercalcemia develops, radiographic evaluation of the suspected anatomical region may detect soft-tissue calcification.

Supportive care—Patients in whom intentional overdose is confirmed or suspected should be referred for psychiatric consultation.

## Patient Consultation

As an aid to patient consultation, refer to *Advice for the Patient, Calcium Acetate (Systemic)—Introductory Version*.
In providing consultation, consider emphasizing the following selected information (» = major clinical significance):

**Before using this medication**
» Conditions affecting use, especially:
    Other medications, especially calcium-containing foods or preparations or digitalis glycosides
    Other medical problems, especially hypercalcemia

**Proper use of this medication**
Taking with meals
» Proper dosing
    Missed dose: Taking as soon as possible; not taking if almost time for next dose; not doubling doses
» Proper storage

**Precautions while using this medication**
Importance of close monitoring by physician
» Avoiding concurrent use with calcium-containing preparations, including dietary supplements and antacids
» Estimating daily dietary calcium intake and adjusting if needed

**Side/adverse effects**
Signs of potential side effects, especially mild and severe hypercalcemia

## General Dosing Information

Most patients require 3 to 4 tablets with each meal.

**Diet/Nutrition**
Calcium acetate should be taken with meals.
Daily intake of dietary calcium should be estimated initially and adjusted if needed.

## Oral Dosage Forms

### CALCIUM ACETATE TABLETS

**Usual adult and adolescent dose**
Antihyperphosphatemic—
    Oral, 2 tablets three times a day with meals. The dosage may be increased gradually to keep serum phosphate concentrations below 6 mg per dL.

**Usual pediatric dose**
Safety and efficacy have not been established.

**Strength(s) usually available**
U.S.—
    169 mg elemental calcium (667 mg calcium acetate) (Rx) [*PhosLo*].

**Packaging and storage**
Store below 40 °C (104 °F), preferably between 15 and 30 °C (59 and 86 °F), unless otherwise specified by the manufacturer.

**Auxiliary labeling**
• Take with meals.

Developed: 10/20/97

---

**CALCIUM CARBONATE**—See *Antacids (Oral-Local)*; *Calcium Supplements (Systemic)*

---

# CALCIUM CHANNEL BLOCKING AGENTS    Systemic

This monograph includes information on the following: 1) Bepridil†; 2) Diltiazem; 3) Felodipine; 4) Flunarizine*; 5) Isradipine†; 6) Nicardipine; 7) Nifedipine; 8) Nimodipine; 9) Verapamil.

VA CLASSIFICATION (Primary/Secondary):
    Bepridil—CV200/CV250
    Diltiazem—CV200/CV250; CV300; CV409
    Felodipine—CV200/CV409
    Flunarizine—CV200/CN105
    Isradipine—CV200/CV409
    Nicardipine—CV200/CV250; CV409
    Nifedipine—CV200/CV250; CV409
    Nimodipine—CV200
    Verapamil—CV200/CN105; CV250; CV300; CV409; CV900

Commonly used brand name(s): *Adalat*[7]; *Adalat CC*[7]; *Adalat PA*[7]; *Adalat XL*[7]; *Apo-Diltiaz*[2]; *Apo-Nifed*[7]; *Apo-Verap*[9]; *Calan*[9]; *Calan SR*[9]; *Cardene*[6]; *Cardizem*[2]; *Cardizem CD*[2]; *Cardizem SR*[2]; *Dilacor-XR*[2]; *DynaCirc*[5]; *Isoptin*[9]; *Isoptin SR*[9]; *Nimotop*[8]; *Novo-Diltazem*[2]; *Novo-Nifedin*[7]; *Novo-Veramil*[9]; *Nu-Diltiaz*[2]; *Nu-Nifed*[7]; *Nu-Verap*[9]; *Plendil*[3]; *Procardia*[7]; *Procardia XL*[7]; *Renedil*[3]; *Sibelium*[4]; *Syn-Diltiazem*[2]; *Vascor*[1]; *Verelan*[9].

Note: For a listing of dosage forms and brand names by country availability, see *Dosage Forms* section(s).

*Not commercially available in U.S.
†Not commercially available in Canada.

## Category

Antianginal—Bepridil; Diltiazem; Felodipine; Isradipine; Nicardipine; Nifedipine; Verapamil.
Antiarrhythmic—Diltiazem; Verapamil.
Antihypertensive—Diltiazem; Felodipine; Isradipine; Nicardipine; Nifedipine; Verapamil.
Hypertrophic cardiomyopathy therapy adjunct—Verapamil.
Subarachnoid hemorrhage therapy—Flunarizine; Nicardipine; Nimodipine.
Vascular headache prophylactic—Flunarizine; Verapamil.

## Indications

Note: Bracketed information in the *Indications* section refers to uses that are not included in U.S. product labeling.

**Accepted**

Angina pectoris, chronic (treatment)—Bepridil, diltiazem, [felodipine], [isradipine], nicardipine, nifedipine, and verapamil are indicated in the management of classic angina (chronic stable angina or effort-associated angina) with no evidence of vasospasm. Nicardipine [and other calcium channel blocking agents] may be used alone or in combination, with caution, with beta-adrenergic blocking agents.

Diltiazem, [felodipine], [isradipine], [nicardipine], nifedipine, and verapamil are also indicated in the management of vasospastic angina (Prinzmetal's variant, or at-rest angina) or unstable angina in patients who are unable to tolerate or whose symptoms are not relieved by adequate doses of beta-adrenergic blocking agents or organic nitrates. They are generally indicated when vasospastic angina is confirmed by: (a) the classical pattern accompanied by elevation of ST segment; (b) ergonovine-induced angina or coronary artery spasm; or (c) coronary artery spasm demonstrated by angiography, although they may also be used when a vasospastic component is indicated but not confirmed (e.g., where pain has a variable threshold on exertion or in unstable angina where electrocardiographic findings are compatible with intermittent vasospasm).

Tachycardia, supraventricular (treatment and prophylaxis)—Verapamil and parenteral diltiazem are indicated in the treatment of supraventricular tachyarrhythmias. Diltiazem and verapamil produce rapid conversion to sinus rhythm of paroxysmal supraventricular tachycardia (including those associated with accessory bypass tracts, such as Wolff-Parkinson-White [W-P-W] or Lown-Ganong-Levine [L-G-L] syndrome) in patients who do not respond to vagal maneuvers when the atrioventricular (AV) node is required for reentry to sustain tachycardia. Parenteral diltiazem and verapamil also produce temporary control of rapid ventricular rate in atrial flutter or atrial fibrillation. Oral verapamil is indicated, alone or in association with digitalis, for control of ventricular rate at rest and during stress in patients with chronic atrial flutter and/or atrial fibrillation (not otherwise controllable with digitalis), and for prophylaxis of repetitive paroxysmal supraventricular tachycardia. Diltiazem and verapamil do not produce class I, II, or III antiarrhythmic effects.

Hypertension (treatment)—Diltiazem, felodipine, isradipine, nicardipine, nifedipine, and verapamil are indicated, alone or in combination with other agents, for treatment of hypertension.

[Cardiomyopathy, hypertrophic (treatment adjunct)]—Verapamil is used in the treatment of hypertrophic cardiomyopathy to relieve ventricular outflow obstruction. However, extreme caution is recommended when hypertrophic cardiomyopathy is complicated by left ventricular obstruction, high pulmonary wedge pressure, paroxysmal nocturnal dyspnea or orthopnea, sinoatrial (SA) nodal function impairment, or severe heart block.

Raynaud's phenomenon (treatment)—[Felodipine], [isradipine], [nicardipine], and [nifedipine][1] are used for symptomatic treatment of Raynaud's phenomenon.

Subarachnoid hemorrhage–associated neurologic deficits (treatment)—Nimodipine is indicated for improvement of neurological outcome by reducing the incidence and severity of ischemic deficits in patients with subarachnoid hemorrhage from ruptured congenital intracranial aneurysms who are in good neurological condition post-ictus (e.g., Hunt and Hess Grades I–III). [Flunarizine] and [nicardipine] are also used for this indication.

Headache, vascular (prophylaxis)—Flunarizine and [verapamil] are indicated for reducing frequency and severity of vascular headaches, but are not recommended for treatment of acute attacks.

### Unaccepted
Sublingual use of nifedipine capsules for hypertensive crisis is not recommended because it has been associated with severe hypotension, acute myocardial infarction, stroke, and death.

[1]Not included in Canadian product labeling.

## Pharmacology/Pharmacokinetics
### Physicochemical characteristics
Molecular weight—
Bepridil hydrochloride: 421.02.
Diltiazem hydrochloride: 450.98.
Felodipine: 384.26.
Flunarizine hydrochloride: 477.42.
Isradipine: 371.39.
Nicardipine hydrochloride: 515.99.
Nifedipine: 346.34.
Nimodipine: 418.45.
Verapamil hydrochloride: 491.07.

### Mechanism of action/Effect
These agents are calcium-ion influx inhibitors (slow-channel blocking agents). Although their mechanism is not completely understood, they are thought to inhibit calcium ion entry through select voltage-sensitive areas termed "slow channels" across cell membranes. By reducing intracellular calcium concentration in cardiac and vascular smooth muscle cells, they dilate coronary arteries and peripheral arteries and arterioles and may reduce heart rate, decrease myocardial contractility (negative inotropic effect), and slow atrioventricular (AV) nodal conduction. Serum calcium concentrations are unchanged, although there is some evidence that elevated serum calcium concentrations may alter the therapeutic effect of verapamil.

Calcium channel blocking agents may be classified into subgroups according to structure—
Bepridil.
Benzothiazepine (diltiazem).
Diphenylpiperazine (flunarizine).
Dihydropyridine (felodipine, isradipine, nicardipine, nifedipine, nimodipine).
Diphenylalkylamine (verapamil).

Effects within each subgroup are generally the same—
Bepridil is a nonselective calcium channel blocking agent that affects both cardiac and smooth muscle. It also inhibits the fast sodium inward current in myocardial and vascular smooth muscle.
Piperazine derivatives act on vascular smooth muscle, with few or no direct myocardial effects.
Dihydropyridines are selective for vascular smooth muscle compared with myocardium and therefore act primarily as vasodilators. Hypotensive effects are accompanied by reflex tachycardia.
Diltiazem (a benzothiazepine) and verapamil (a diphenylalkylamine) are less selective vasodilators that also have direct effects on the myocardium, including depression of sinoatrial (SA) and atrioventricular (AV) nodal conduction.

See *Table 1*, page 733.
Antianginal—
Dilation of the peripheral vasculature reduces systemic pressure or cardiac afterload, which results in lessened myocardial wall tension and reduced oxygen requirements of the myocardial tissues. In vasospastic angina, a relaxation of coronary arteries and arterioles and inhibition of coronary artery spasm improves blood flow and oxygen supply to myocardial tissues. May also be related to enhanced left ventricular diastolic relaxation and decreased wall stiffness (improved diastolic compliance).

Antiarrhythmic—
The inhibited influx of calcium ions in cardiac tissues prolongs the effective refractory period and results in slowed AV nodal conduction. Normal sinus rhythm is usually not affected, except in some elderly patients or patients with sick sinus syndrome, in whom calcium channel blockade may interfere with sinus-node impulse generation and may induce sinus or sinoatrial block. Normal atrial action potential or intraventricular conduction are not altered, but in depressed atrial fibers amplitude, velocity of depolarization, and conduction velocity are decreased. The antegrade effective refractory period of the accessory bypass tract may be shortened.

Antihypertensive—
Reduction of total peripheral vascular resistance as a result of vasodilation.

Hypertrophic cardiomyopathy therapy adjunct—
Improvement of left ventricular outflow. May also be related to enhanced left ventricular diastolic relaxation and decreased wall stiffness.

Subarachnoid hemorrhage therapy—
Theoretically, nimodipine may prevent cerebral arterial spasm following subarachnoid hemorrhage, but that has not been confirmed by arteriography. Its exact mechanism of action in treatment of neurologic deficits caused by subarachnoid hemorrhage is not known.

Vascular headache prophylactic—
By inhibiting the vasoconstriction that occurs in the prodromal phase, calcium channel blockade may relieve or prevent reactive vasodilation.

### Other actions/effects
Inhibition of platelet aggregation. Decrease in esophageal contraction amplitude. Diltiazem and verapamil may inhibit cytochrome P450 metabolism, thereby inhibiting the metabolism of other medications or compounds. Flunarizine has antihistaminic effects. Isradipine has diuretic effects. Verapamil decreases gastrointestinal transit time.

### Absorption
Bepridil—Rapid and complete; bioavailability 60 to 70% because of first-pass metabolism; rate, but not extent of absorption, is reduced in the presence of food.
Diltiazem—Well absorbed; bioavailability approximately 40% because of first-pass metabolism; bioavailability may increase with chronic use and increasing dose (i.e., bioavailability is nonlinear).
Felodipine—Almost completely absorbed; bioavailability approximately 20% because of first-pass metabolism. Bioavailability is not affected in the presence of food; however, bioavailability more than doubled when felodipine was taken with doubly concentrated grapefruit juice as compared to when it was taken with water or orange juice (a similar, but lesser, effect is also seen with other dihydropyridines).
Flunarizine—Well absorbed.
Isradipine—Absorption is 90 to 95%; bioavailability approximately 15 to 24% because of first-pass metabolism; rate, but not extent, of absorption is reduced in the presence of food.
Nicardipine—Completely absorbed; bioavailability approximately 35% because of first-pass metabolism.
Nifedipine—Rapidly and completely absorbed; bioavailability approximately 60 to 75% because of first-pass metabolism. Bioavailability of extended-release formulations may be 10 to 15% lower than that of immediate-release formulations, but plasma concentrations are more stable, with smaller fluctuations over the dosing interval. Bioavailability of both formulations is increased with hepatic function impairment. Rate, but not extent, of absorption of *Procardia XL* may be reduced in the presence of food.
Nimodipine—Rapidly absorbed. Because of extensive first-pass metabolism, bioavailability is only about 13% (significantly increased [up to double the peak serum concentration] in patients with hepatic function impairment). The effect of food on absorption is unknown.
Verapamil—More than 90% of an oral dose is absorbed; bioavailability approximately 20 to 35% because of first-pass metabolism; bioavailability of oral verapamil may increase with chronic use and increasing dose (i.e., bioavailability is nonlinear).

### Distribution
Bepridil—In breast milk: Concentration is approximately one-third serum concentration.

### Protein binding
Bepridil—Very high (more than 99%).
Diltiazem—High (70 to 80%, 35 to 40% to albumin).
Felodipine—Very high (more than 99%).
Flunarizine—Very high (99%).

Isradipine—Very high (95%).
Nicardipine—Very high (more than 95%).
Nifedipine—Very high (92 to 98%).
Nimodipine—Very high (over 95%); independent of concentration.
Verapamil—Very high (approximately 90%).

**Biotransformation**
Hepatic; extensive and rapid, with a prominent first-pass effect.
Bepridil—At least 17 metabolites, 1 or more of which may have cardiovascular activity.
Diltiazem—By cytochrome P450 mixed function oxidase. A major metabolite, detected following oral and continuous intravenous administration but not rapid intravenous administration, is desacetyl diltiazem, which has one quarter to one half the coronary dilatation activity of the parent compound.
Felodipine—Six metabolites, accounting for 23% of an oral dose, have been identified; none has significant vasodilating activity.
Isradipine—Completely metabolized; six metabolites identified.
Nifedipine—No known active metabolites.
Verapamil—Principal metabolite is norverapamil, which has approximately 20% of the hypotensive cardiovascular activity of verapamil; 11 other metabolites occur only in trace amounts.

**Half-life**
Bepridil (biphasic)—
    Distribution:
        Approximately 2 hours.
    Elimination:
        Terminal: Average, 42 hours (range, 26 to 64 hours).
        Dosing interval: Less than 24 hours.
Diltiazem—
    Oral (biphasic):
        Extended-release capsules—
            *Cardizem CD*: Apparent—5 to 8 hours.
            *Cardizem SR*: Apparent—5 to 7 hours.
        Tablets—
            Early: 20 to 30 minutes.
            Terminal: Approximately 3.5 hours (5 to 8 hours with high and repetitive dosage).
    Intravenous:
        Approximately 3.4 hours.
Felodipine (polyphasic)—
    Terminal:
        11 to 16 hours.
Flunarizine—
    19 days.
Isradipine (biphasic)—
    Early: 1.5 to 2 hours.
    Terminal: About 8 hours.
Nicardipine (biphasic)—
    Early: 2 to 4 hours.
    Terminal: 8.6 hours.
Nifedipine—
    Approximately 2 hours.
        Extended-release tablets:
            *Adalat CC*: Terminal—Approximately 7 hours
            *Adalat PA*: Terminal—6 to 12 hours
            *Adalat XL, Procardia XL*: Not available. The gastrointestinal therapeutic system (GITS) is designed to deliver nifedipine by zero-order systemic absorption over a period of approximately 18 hours.
Nimodipine—
    Terminal: 8 to 9 hours. Earlier, more rapid elimination rates (equivalent to a half-life of 1 to 2 hours) necessitate frequent dosing.
Verapamil—
    Oral:
        Single dose—Range, 2.8 to 7.4 hours.
        Repetitive dosage—Range, 4.5 to 12 hours (half-life is increased because of saturation of hepatic enzyme systems as plasma verapamil concentrations increase).
    Intravenous (biphasic):
        Early—About 4 minutes.
        Terminal—2 to 5 hours.

**Onset of action**
Diltiazem—
    Oral:
        Extended-release capsules—2 to 3 hours.
        Tablets—30 to 60 minutes.
    Parenteral:
        Rapid intravenous injection—
            Reduction in heart rate or conversion of paroxysmal supraventricular tachycardia to sinus rhythm: Within 3 minutes.
Felodipine—
    Within 2 to 5 hours.
Isradipine—
    2 to 3 hours.
Nifedipine—
    Oral:
        Capsules—20 minutes.
Verapamil—
    Oral:
        1 to 2 hours.
    Intravenous:
        Antiarrhythmic—Within 1 to 5 minutes and usually less than 2 minutes.
        Hemodynamic—Within 3 to 5 minutes.

**Time to peak concentration**
Bepridil—
    2 to 3 hours.
Diltiazem—
    Oral (wide individual variation in concentrations achieved):
        Extended-release capsules—
            *Cardizem CD*: 10 to 14 hours.
            *Cardizem SR*: 6 to 11 hours.
        Tablets—
            2 to 3 hours.
Felodipine—
    2.5 to 5 hours. Peak plasma concentrations at steady state are about 20% higher than after a single dose.
Flunarizine—
    2 to 4 hours.
Isradipine—
    About 1.5 hours.
Nicardipine—
    30 minutes to 2 hours (mean, 1 hour).
Nifedipine—
    Capsules:
        About 30 to 60 minutes.
    Extended-release tablets:
        *Adalat CC*—2.5 to 5 hours
        *Adalat PA*—4 hours.
        *Adalat XL, Procardia XL*—Approximately 6 hours.
Nimodipine—
    Within 1 hour.
Verapamil—
    Oral:
        Extended-release capsules—7 to 9 hours.
        Tablets—1 to 2 hours (wide individual variation in concentrations achieved).
        Extended-release tablets—5 to 7 hours.

**Time to peak effect**
Bepridil—
    Time to steady-state plasma concentration: 8 days.
Diltiazem—
    Antihypertensive: Multiple doses—Within 2 weeks.
    Antiarrhythmic: Rapid intravenous injection—Hypotension or reduction in heart rate: Within 2 to 7 minutes.
Flunarizine—
    Multiple doses: Several weeks.
Isradipine—
    Antihypertensive: Multiple doses—2 to 4 weeks.
Nicardipine—
    Single dose: 1 to 2 hours.
Verapamil—
    Oral: About 30 to 90 minutes. The maximum effects from oral dosage are usually evident sometime during the first 24 to 48 hours of therapy (for some patients the time may be slightly extended because the half-life of verapamil tends to increase during this period).
    Intravenous: Within 3 to 5 minutes after completion of injection.

**Elimination**
Bepridil—
    Renal: 70% (none unchanged).
    Biliary/fecal: 22% (none unchanged).
    In dialysis: Not removable by hemodialysis.
Diltiazem—
    Biliary and renal (2 to 4% unchanged).
    In dialysis: Does not appear to be removable by hemodialysis or peritoneal dialysis.

Felodipine—
    Renal: 70% (less than 0.5% unchanged).
    Biliary/fecal: 10% (less than 0.5% unchanged).
Flunarizine—
    Drug and metabolites: Very slow and prolonged.
    Biliary/fecal: Less than 6% in the first 48 hours.
    Renal: Less than 0.2% in the first 48 hours.
Isradipine—
    Renal: 60 to 65% (none unchanged).
    Biliary/fecal: 25 to 30% (none unchanged).
    In dialysis: No information, but not likely to be removable by hemodialysis because of plasma protein binding.
Nicardipine—
    Renal: 60% (less than 1% unchanged).
    Biliary/fecal: 35%.
Nifedipine—
    Renal: 80% (as metabolites), only traces unchanged.
    Biliary/fecal: 20% (as metabolites).
    In dialysis: Does not appear to be removed by hemodialysis or chronic ambulatory peritoneal dialysis; however, plasmapheresis may be beneficial.
Nimodipine—
    Renal (less than 1% unchanged).
    Biliary/fecal.
    In dialysis: Because of extensive protein binding, unlikely to be significantly removed by hemodialysis or peritoneal dialysis.
Verapamil—
    Renal:
        As conjugated metabolites—70% as metabolites and 3 to 4% unchanged within 5 days.
        Unmetabolized—3%.
    Biliary/fecal:
        9 to 16%.
    In dialysis:
        Not removable by hemodialysis.

## Precautions to Consider

### Carcinogenicity/Mutagenicity
*For bepridil*—
    A lifetime study in mice at doses up to 60 times the maximum recommended human dose (MRHD) (based on a 60-kg subject) found no evidence of carcinogenicity. A lifetime study in rats at doses 20 times the usual recommended human dose found unilateral follicular adenomas of the thyroid.
    Mutagenicity studies (micronucleus test for chromosomal effects, liver microsome activated bacterial assay for mutagenicity, Chinese hamster ovary cell assay for mutagenicity, sister chromatid exchange assay) were negative.
*For diltiazem*—
    A 24-month study with diltiazem in rats and a 21-month study in mice found no evidence of carcinogenicity.
    There was no mutagenic response in *in vitro* bacterial tests.
*For felodipine*—
    A 2-year study in rats at doses of 7.7, 23.1, or 69.3 mg per kg of body weight (mg/kg) per day (up to 28 times the MRHD [based on a 50-kg subject]) found an increased incidence of benign interstitial cell tumors of the testes (Leydig cell tumors) in males, probably secondary to a reduction in testicular testosterone and corresponding increase in serum luteinizing hormone (which have not been observed in humans). In addition, a dose-related increase in the incidence of focal squamous cell hyperplasia in the esophageal groove of both males and females at all doses (humans have no anatomical structure comparable to the esophageal groove). Felodipine was not carcinogenic and did not increase the incidence of Leydig cell tumors in mice at doses up to 138.6 mg/kg per day (28 times the MRHD [based on a 50-kg subject]) for periods up to 80 and 99 weeks in males and females, respectively; no effect on the esophageal groove occurred.
    Mutagenicity studies (Ames test, mouse lymphoma forward mutation assay, mouse micronucleus test, human lymphocyte chromosome aberration assay) were negative.
*For flunarizine*—
    A 24-month study in 4 groups of 50 male and 50 female Wistar rats at doses of 0, 5, 20, or 40 mg/kg per day (the 40-mg/kg group received 80 mg/kg for the first 2 months) did not produce an effect on tumor rate or type; however, the validity of the study is questionable because of an extremely high mortality rate (more than 90% in the males and 80% in the females).
    Mutagenicity studies (Ames test, sister chromatid exchange test in human lymphocytes, sex-linked recessive lethal test in *Drosophila melanogaster*, micronucleus test in male rats, dominant lethal test in male and female mice) were negative.
*For isradipine*—
    A 2-year study in male rats at doses of 2.5, 12.5, or 62.5 mg/kg per day (approximately 6, 31, and 156 times the MRHD, respectively, based on a 50-kg subject) found a dose-dependent increase in the incidence of benign Leydig cell tumors and testicular hyperplasia relative to untreated control animals; these findings were replicated in a subsequent study. A 2-year study in mice at doses of 6, 38, and 200 times the MRHD found no evidence of oncogenicity.
    Mutagenicity studies were negative.
*For nicardipine*—
    A 2-year study in rats with nicardipine at dosage levels of 5, 15, or 45 mg/kg per day found a dose-dependent increase in thyroid hyperplasia and neoplasia (follicular adenoma/carcinoma). One- and three-month studies in the rat suggest that the mechanism for this effect is a nicardipine-induced reduction in plasma thyroxine ($T_4$) concentrations with a resulting increase in thyroid-stimulating hormone (TSH) concentrations, which is known to cause hyperstimulation of the thyroid; in rats on an iodine-deficient diet, one month of nicardipine administration produced thyroid hyperplasia that was prevented by $T_4$ supplementation. Studies in mice for up to 18 months at doses up to 100 mg/kg per day and in dogs for 1 year at doses up 25 mg/kg per day found no evidence of neoplasia of any tissue and no evidence of thyroid changes. No effects of nicardipine on thyroid function (plasma $T_4$ and TSH) have been reported in humans.
    No evidence of mutagenicity was found in a battery of genotoxicity tests conducted on microbial indicator organisms, in micronucleus tests in mice and hamsters, or in a sister chromatid exchange study in hamsters.
*For nifedipine*—
    Nifedipine was not shown to be carcinogenic when administered orally to rats for 2 years.
    *In vivo* mutagenic tests were negative.
*For nimodipine*—
    A 2-year study in rats found an increased incidence of adenocarcinoma of the uterus and Leydig-cell adenoma of the testes, but the increases were not significant. A 91-week study in mice found no evidence of carcinogenicity, although the life expectancy was shortened.
    Mutagenicity studies, including the Ames, micronucleus, and dominant lethal tests, have been negative.
*For verapamil*—
    A 2-year study in rats with verapamil at doses up to 12 times the MRHD found no evidence of carcinogenicity.
    There was no mutagenic response in the Ames test in 5 test strains at 3 mg per plate with or without metabolic activation.

### Pregnancy/Reproduction
Fertility—
*For felodipine*—
    No significant effect on reproductive performance was found in male or female rats given doses of 3.8, 9.6, or 26.9 mg/kg per day.
*For flunarizine*—
    In studies in male and female Wistar rats at doses of 0 and approximately 10, 40, and 160 mg/kg given for 60 days pre-mating in the males or 14 days pre-mating and 21 days of gestation in the females, treated animals were mated with non-treated animals. In treated females at the highest dose, there were no pregnancies and a large number of deaths; at the 40-mg/kg dose, there was decreased weight gain during pregnancy, decreased rate of pregnancy, increase in the number of resorbed fetuses, decreased litter size, and decreased weight of pups at birth. In non-treated females mated with treated males, a slight increase in resorption was seen only at the highest dose.
*For nifedipine*—
    Reduced fertility occurred in rats given 30 times the maximum recommended human dose (MRHD) prior to mating.
Pregnancy—
*For bepridil*—
    Adequate and well-controlled studies in humans have not been done.
    Studies in rats at maternal doses of 37 times the MRHD found reduced litter size at birth and decreased pup survival during lactation. No teratogenicity was observed in rats or rabbits at the same dose.
    FDA Pregnancy Category C.
*For diltiazem*—
    Well-controlled studies in humans have not been done.

Studies in mice, rats, and rabbits, using doses of diltiazem 5 to 10 times greater than the recommended daily dose on a mg/kg basis, resulted in embryo and fetal deaths, reduced neonatal survival rates, and skeletal abnormalities. In addition, there was an increased incidence of stillbirths at doses of 20 or more times the recommended human dose.

FDA Pregnancy Category C.

*For felodipine—*

Adequate and well-controlled studies in humans have not been done.

Studies in rabbits at doses of 0.46, 1.2, 2.3, and 4.6 mg/kg per day (from 0.4 to 4 times the MRHD [based on a 50-kg subject] on a mg per square meter of body surface area basis) found digital anomalies consisting of reduction in size and degree of ossification of the terminal phalanges in the fetuses. Frequency and severity of the changes were dose-related and occurred even at the lowest dose. These changes are similar to those occurring with other dihydropyridines and may be the result of compromised uterine blood flow. The anomalies did not occur in rats; abnormal position of the distal phalanges (but not reduction in size of the terminal phalanges) occurred in about 40% of cynomolgus monkey fetuses.

Studies in rats at doses of 9.6 mg/kg per day (4 times the MRHD [based on a 50-kg subject] on a mg per square meter of body surface area basis) produced a prolongation of parturition with a difficult labor and an increased frequency of fetal and early postnatal deaths.

Studies in rabbits at doses greater than or equal to 1.2 mg/kg per day (equal to the MRHD on a mg per square meter of body surface area basis) found significant enlargement (in excess of normal) of the mammary glands during pregnancy, which regressed during lactation. These effects were not observed in rats or monkeys.

FDA Pregnancy Category C.

*For flunarizine—*

Studies in humans have not been done.

There was a slight increase in resorptions and decrease in number of live fetuses in female Wistar rats given 40 mg/kg, with no effects seen at doses of 0, 10, or 20 mg/kg; there was no evidence of teratogenicity. There was a dose-related increase in the number of resorptions in New Zealand rabbits given doses of 0, 2.5, or 10 mg/kg from day 6 to day 18 of pregnancy, with a corresponding decrease in number of live births; there was no evidence of teratogenicity.

*For isradipine—*

Studies in humans have not been done.

Studies in rats at doses of 6, 20, or 60 mg/kg per day produced a significant reduction in maternal weight gain at the highest dose (150 times the MRHD), but with no lasting effects on the mother or offspring. Studies in rabbits at doses of 1, 3, or 10 mg/kg per day (2.5, 7.5, and 25 times the MRHD, respectively) found decreased maternal weight gain and increased fetal resorptions at the two highest doses. There was no evidence of embryotoxicity at doses that were not maternotoxic and no evidence of teratogenicity at any dose. With peri- and postnatal administration of doses of 20 and 60 mg/kg per day, reduced maternal weight gain during late pregnancy was associated with reduced birth weights and decreased peri- and postnatal pup survival.

FDA Pregnancy Category C.

*For nicardipine—*

Adequate and well-controlled studies in humans have not been done.

Studies in Japanese White rabbits at doses of 150 mg/kg per day during organogenesis (but not at doses of 50 mg/kg per day [25 times the MRHD]) found nicardipine to be embryocidal and to cause marked body weight gain suppression in the treated doe. Studies in rats with nicardipine at doses 50 times the MRHD found no evidence of embryolethality or teratogenicity, but dystocia, reduced birth weights, reduced neonatal survival, and reduced neonatal weight gain occurred.

FDA Pregnancy Category C.

*For nifedipine—*

Adequate and well-controlled studies in humans have not been done.

Nifedipine has been shown to be teratogenic in rodents and embryotoxic (increased fetal resorptions, reduced fetal weight, increase in stunted forms, increased fetal deaths, and decreased fetal survival) in rodents and rabbits at doses 30 times and 3 to 10 times the MRHD, respectively. In pregnant monkeys, small placentas and underdeveloped chorionic villi occurred at two thirds and two times the MRHD. In rats, three times or more the MRHD caused prolongation of pregnancy.

FDA Pregnancy Category C.

*For nimodipine—*

Adequate and well-controlled studies in humans have not been done.

Two studies in Himalayan rabbits found an increased incidence of teratogenic malformations in the fetuses at doses of 1 and 10 (but not 3) mg/kg per day given on days 6 through 18 of pregnancy; in these same studies, stunted fetuses were found at doses of 1 and 10 (but not 3) mg/kg per day in one study, and only at 1 mg/kg per day in the other. Studies in Long Evans rats at doses of 100 mg/kg per day given on days 6 through 15 found embryotoxicity, including fetal resorption and stunted fetal growth. In other rat studies, doses of 30 mg/kg per day from days 16 to 20 or 21 produced an increased incidence of skeletal variation, stunted fetuses, and stillbirths, but no malformations.

FDA Pregnancy Category C.

*For verapamil—*

Adequate and well-controlled studies in humans have not been done.

Verapamil crosses the placenta and can be detected in umbilical vein blood at delivery. Occasionally, rapid intravenous injection of verapamil in humans may cause maternal hypotension resulting in fetal distress.

Studies in rats, using doses of verapamil up to 6 times the recommended daily dose for humans, resulted in embryo deaths and slowed growth.

FDA Pregnancy Category C.

**Breast-feeding**

*For all calcium channel blocking agents—*

Although problems in humans have not been documented, bepridil, diltiazem, nifedipine, and verapamil, and possibly other calcium channel blocking agents, are distributed into breast milk.

*For felodipine only—*

It is not known whether felodipine is distributed into breast milk in humans.

*For flunarizine only—*

It is not known whether flunarizine is distributed into breast milk in humans; however, it is distributed into the milk of dogs, at concentrations much higher than in plasma.

*For nimodipine only—*

It is not known whether nimodipine is distributed into breast milk in humans; however, nimodipine and/or its metabolites have been found in the milk of treated rats, at concentrations much higher than maternal plasma concentrations.

**Pediatrics**

Although appropriate studies on the relationship of age to the effects of calcium channel blocking agents have not been performed in the pediatric population, pediatrics-specific problems that would limit the usefulness of calcium channel blocking agents in children are not expected. However, in rare instances, severe adverse hemodynamic effects have occurred after intravenous administration of verapamil in neonates and infants.

**Geriatrics**

*For diltiazem, nimodipine, verapamil, and possibly other calcium channel blocking agents—*

Half-life of calcium channel blocking agents may be increased in the elderly as a result of decreased clearance.

*For felodipine only—*

Plasma concentrations increase with age. Mean clearance at mean age of 76 was found to be only 45% of that at mean age of 26.

*For isradipine only—*

Bioavailability may be increased in patients over 65 years of age.

*For nicardipine only—*

Studies in patients 65 years of age and older found no difference in half-life or protein binding from that in young normal volunteers.

*For nimodipine only—*

Risk of hypotension may be increased.

*For all calcium channel blocking agents—*

Elderly patients are more likely to have age-related renal function impairment, which may require caution in patients receiving calcium channel blocking agents.

**Dental**

Gingival enlargement is a rare side effect that has been reported with diltiazem, felodipine, nifedipine, and verapamil. It usually starts as gingivitis or gum inflammation in the first 1 to 9 months of treatment. A strictly enforced program of teeth cleaning by a professional combined with plaque control by the patient will minimize growth rate and severity of gingival enlargement. Periodontal surgery may be indicated in some cases, and should be followed by careful plaque control to inhibit recurrence of gum enlargement.

**Drug interactions and/or related problems**
The following drug interactions and/or related problems have been selected on the basis of their potential clinical significance (possible mechanism in parentheses where appropriate)—not necessarily inclusive (» = major clinical significance):

Note: Information concerning interactions between calcium channel blocking agents and other medications is still limited. Therefore, some of the following potential interactions are stated for cautionary reference until additional information is available.

Combinations containing any of the following medications, depending on the amount present, may also interact with these medications.

Anesthetics, hydrocarbon inhalation
(concurrent use with calcium channel blocking agents may produce additive hypotension; although calcium channel blocking agents may be useful to prevent supraventricular tachycardias, hypertension, or coronary spasm during surgery, caution is recommended during use)

Anti-inflammatory drugs, nonsteroidal (NSAIDs), especially indomethacin
(indomethacin, and possibly other NSAIDs, may antagonize the antihypertensive effect of calcium channel blocking agents by inhibiting renal prostaglandin synthesis and/or by causing sodium and fluid retention; the patient should be carefully monitored to confirm that the desired effect is being obtained)

» Beta-adrenergic blocking agents, systemic or ophthalmic
(concurrent use of oral dosage forms with oral bepridil, diltiazem, or verapamil or intravenous verapamil usually results in no serious negative inotropic, chronotropic, or dromotropic effects. However, caution and careful monitoring are necessary since the additive effect may prolong sinoatrial [SA] and atrioventricular [AV] conduction [which may lead to severe hypotension, bradycardia, and cardiac failure], especially in patients with impaired ventricular function or abnormal cardiac conduction or sinus node depression. When verapamil and beta-adrenergic blocking agents are to be given intravenously, they should be administered at least a few hours apart since they may have additive depressant effects on myocardial contractility or SA or AV conduction, and asystole has been reported with concurrent use)

(in a single small study, diltiazem was reported to significantly increase the bioavailability of propranolol; in other studies, verapamil was found to decrease clearance of both metoprolol and propranolol, with a variable effect on atenolol)

(concurrent use with dihydropyridines, although usually well tolerated, may produce excessive hypotension, and in rare cases may increase the possibility of congestive heart failure. Occasionally, angina has occurred upon initiation of nicardipine or nifedipine therapy, especially after recent abrupt discontinuation of beta-adrenergic blocking agent therapy. If possible, it is recommended that beta-adrenergic blocking agent dosage be discontinued gradually, but especially before nicardipine or nifedipine therapy is begun. However, if concurrent use is necessary, nicardipine or nifedipine may be preferred over other calcium channel blocking agents in some patients because both have less effect on heart rate and conduction)

(if significant systemic absorption of an ophthalmic beta-adrenergic blocking agent occurs, concurrent use of calcium channel blocking agents may result in atrioventricular conduction disturbances, left ventricular failure, and hypotension; in some patients, if a calcium antagonist is necessary, nicardipine or nifedipine may be preferred because both have less effect on heart rate and conduction, although they may also cause greater hypotension; concurrent use of calcium channel blocking agents and ophthalmic beta-adrenergic blocking agents should be avoided in patients with impaired cardiac function)

Calcium supplements
(concurrent use in quantities sufficient to elevate serum calcium concentrations above normal may reduce the response to verapamil and probably other calcium channel blocking agents)

» Carbamazepine or
» Cyclosporine or
» Quinidine or
  Theophylline or
  Valproate
(diltiazem or verapamil may inhibit cytochrome P450 metabolism, resulting in increased concentrations and toxicity of these medications)

(an idiosyncratic reaction has been reported in which concurrent use of nifedipine and quinidine resulted in significantly reduced serum quinidine concentrations; caution is recommended when nifedipine therapy is initiated or discontinued in a patient stabilized on quinidine)

Cimetidine
(concurrent use may result in accumulation of the calcium channel blocking agent as a result of inhibition of first-pass metabolism; caution and careful titration of the calcium channel blocking agent dose is recommended on initiation of therapy in patients receiving cimetidine; ranitidine and famotidine do not appear to significantly affect calcium channel blocking agent metabolism)

» Digitalis glycosides
(concurrent use of digoxin with some calcium channel blocking agents [especially verapamil and, to a lesser extent, bepridil, diltiazem, and nifedipine] has been reported to increase the serum concentration of digoxin; the effect of verapamil on digoxin kinetics is enhanced in patients with hepatic function impairment; felodipine significantly increased peak plasma concentrations of digoxin, although there was no significant change in the area under the plasma concentration–time curve [AUC]; isradipine and nicardipine do not appear to have a significant effect. Digoxin serum concentrations should be monitored and dosage may need to be altered when concurrent dosage of the calcium channel blocking agent is initiated, changed, or discontinued. Concurrent use of oral digitalis preparations with oral diltiazem or verapamil or intravenous verapamil has resulted in no serious adverse effects when patients were closely monitored; however, both groups of medications slow AV conduction. Patients receiving them concurrently should be monitored for AV block or excessive bradycardia, especially during the first week of concurrent dosage. To avoid toxicity, dosage reduction of digitalis glycoside may be necessary)

» Disopyramide or
  Flecainide
(disopyramide should not be administered within 48 hours before or 24 hours following verapamil administration since both medications possess negative inotropic properties; deaths have been reported; caution is also recommended when disopyramide is used concurrently with diltiazem, nicardipine, or nifedipine; caution is also recommended when flecainide is used concurrently with a calcium channel blocking agent)

Estrogens
(estrogen-induced fluid retention tends to increase blood pressure; the patient should be carefully monitored to confirm that the desired effect is being obtained)

» Grapefruit juice
(concurrent administration with 200 mL of grapefruit juice has been shown to increase felodipine plasma concentration more than twofold by inhibiting first-pass metabolism in the gastrointestinal wall and/or the liver; a lesser effect also has been seen with two other dihydropyridines, nifedipine and nisoldipine)

Highly protein-bound medications, such as:
  Anticoagulants, coumarin- and indandione-derivative
  Anticonvulsants, hydantoin
  Anti-inflammatory drugs, nonsteroidal
  Quinine
  Salicylates
  Sulfinpyrazone
(caution is advised when these medications are used concurrently with nifedipine or verapamil since changes in serum concentrations of the free, unbound medications may occur)

» Hypokalemia-producing medications, such as:
  Amphotericin B, parenteral
  Carbonic anhydrase inhibitors
  Corticosteroids, glucocorticoid, especially those with significant mineralocorticoid activity
  Corticosteroids, mineralocorticoid
  Corticotropin (ACTH)
  Diuretics, potassium-depleting (such as bumetanide, ethacrynic acid, furosemide, indapamide, mannitol, or thiazides)
  Sodium phosphates
(risk of bepridil-induced arrhythmias may be increased)

Hypotension-producing medications, other (see *Appendix II*)
(antihypertensive effects may be potentiated when these medications are used concurrently with hypotension-producing calcium channel blocking agents; although some antihypertensive and/or diuretic combinations are frequently used for therapeutic advantage, when any hypotension-producing medication is used concurrently dosage adjustments may be necessary)

Lithium
(concurrent use with calcium channel blocking agents may result in neurotoxicity in the form of nausea, vomiting, diarrhea, ataxia, tremors, and/or tinnitus; caution is recommended)

Neuromuscular blocking agents
(verapamil may potentiate the activity of curare-like and depolarizing neuromuscular blocking agents; dosage reduction of either or both medications may be necessary during concurrent use)

Phenobarbital
(may increase clearance of verapamil)

Prazosin, and possibly other alpha-adrenergic blocking agents
(concurrent use with calcium channel blocking agents may produce an increased hypotensive effect, possibly related to impairment of compensatory responses by alpha-blockade and/or inhibition of prazosin metabolism by calcium channel blocking agents; caution is recommended)

» Procainamide or
» Quinidine or
» Other medications causing Q-T interval prolongation
(risk of increased Q-T interval prolongation)
(caution is recommended when procainamide or quinidine is used with a calcium channel blocking agent since both groups of medications possess negative inotropic properties)

Rifampin, and possibly other hepatic enzyme inducers
(rifampin may reduce the bioavailability of oral verapamil by induction of first-pass metabolism; other calcium channel blocking agents may also be affected, depending on the extent of first-pass metabolism)

Sympathomimetics
(concurrent use may reduce antihypertensive effects of calcium channel blocking agents; the patient should be carefully monitored to confirm that the desired effect is being obtained)

**Laboratory value alterations**
The following have been selected on the basis of their potential clinical significance (possible effect in parentheses where appropriate)—not necessarily inclusive (» = major clinical significance):

With physiology/laboratory test values
Antinuclear antibody (ANA) titers and
Direct Coombs test, with or without hemolytic anemia
(positive results have been reported during nifedipine therapy)
Arterial blood pressure
(may be reduced by calcium channel blocking agents [except bepridil and flunarizine])

Electrocardiograph (ECG) effects
P-R interval
(may be increased by diltiazem and verapamil)
Note: Increase tends to be proportional to serum concentration.
Q-T interval
(may be increased by bepridil)
T-wave morphology
(may be altered by bepridil)

Hepatic enzymes
(may rarely be increased after several days of therapy; concentrations return to normal upon withdrawal of therapy)

Prolactin
(serum concentrations may be slightly increased by flunarizine)

Note: Total serum calcium concentrations are not affected by the calcium channel blocking agents.

**Medical considerations/Contraindications**
The medical considerations/contraindications included have been selected on the basis of their potential clinical significance (reasons given in parentheses where appropriate)—not necessarily inclusive (» = major clinical significance).
See Table 2, page 733.

**Patient monitoring**
The following may be especially important in patient monitoring (other tests may be warranted in some patients, depending on condition; » = major clinical significance):
» Blood pressure determinations and
» ECG readings and
» Heart rate determinations
(recommended primarily during dosage titration or when dosage is increased from established maintenance dosage level, or during addition of medications affecting cardiac conduction or blood pressure; also recommended during intravenous verapamil administration)
(blood pressure determinations are recommended at periodic intervals in patients being treated for hypertension; selected patients may be trained to perform blood pressure measurements at home and report the results at regular physician visits)

Hepatic function determinations or
Renal function determinations
(may be required at periodic intervals during long-term therapy)

For bepridil
Potassium concentrations, serum
(recommended at periodic intervals during therapy to watch for hypokalemia)

For nimodipine
Neurological examinations
(recommended at periodic intervals during treatment)

## Side/Adverse Effects
See Table 3, page 735.

## Patient Consultation
As an aid to patient consultation, refer to USP DI, Advice for the Patient, Calcium Channel Blocking Agents (Systemic).
In providing consultation, consider emphasizing the following selected information (» = major clinical significance):

**Before using this medication**
» Conditions affecting use, especially:
Sensitivity to the calcium channel blocking agent prescribed
Pregnancy—High doses in animals cause birth defects, prolonged pregnancy, poor bone development, and stillbirth
Use in the elderly—Elderly patients may be more sensitive to effects
Other medications, especially parenteral amphotericin B (for bepridil), beta-adrenergic blocking agents, carbamazepine, carbonic anhydrase inhibitors, corticosteroids (for bepridil), cyclosporine, digitalis glycosides, disopyramide, grapefruit juice, potassium-depleting diuretics (for bepridil), procainamide, or quinidine
Other medical problems, especially arrhythmias (for bepridil), other cardiovascular problems, or hypokalemia (for bepridil)

**Proper use of this medication**
» Compliance with therapy; importance of not taking more medication than amount prescribed
» Proper dosing
Missed dose: Taking as soon as possible; not taking if almost time for next scheduled dose; not doubling doses
» Proper storage

For bepridil
If nausea occurs, may be taken with meals or at bedtime

For extended-release diltiazem capsules
Swallowing capsules whole without crushing or chewing
» Caution if switching brands; one is for once-daily dosing and one is for twice-daily dosing

For extended-release verapamil capsules
Swallowing capsules whole without crushing or chewing

For extended-release felodipine or nifedipine tablets
Swallowing tablets whole, without breaking, crushing, or chewing
For Adalat XL and Procardia XL—Patient may notice empty shell in stool left over after medication is absorbed
Taking Adalat CC on an empty stomach

For extended-release verapamil tablets
Swallowing tablets whole, without crushing or chewing; 240-mg tablet may be broken in half on instructions from physician
Taking with food or milk

For felodipine
Importance of not taking felodipine with grapefruit juice

For use as an antihypertensive
Importance of diet; possible need for sodium restriction and/or weight reduction
» Patient may not experience symptoms of hypertension; importance of taking medication even if feeling well
» Does not cure, but helps control hypertension; possible need for lifelong therapy; serious consequences of untreated hypertension

**Precautions while using this medication**
Regular visits to physician to check progress during therapy
Checking with physician before discontinuing medication; gradual dosage reduction may be necessary

» Discussing exercise or physical exertion limits with physician; reduced occurrence of chest pain may tempt patient to be overactive
Possible headache; checking with physician if continuing or severe
» Maintaining good dental hygiene and seeing dentist frequently for teeth cleaning to prevent tenderness, bleeding, and gum enlargement

*For use as an antihypertensive*
» Not taking other medications, especially nonprescription sympathomimetics, unless discussed with physician

*For patients taking bepridil, diltiazem, or verapamil*
» Checking pulse as directed; checking with physician if less than 50 beats per minute

*For patients taking flunarizine*
Caution when driving or doing other things requiring alertness because of risk of drowsiness

### Side/adverse effects
Signs of potential side effects, especially angina, arrhythmias, congestive heart failure or pulmonary edema, extrapyramidal effects (for flunarizine), galactorrhea (for flunarizine), peripheral edema, tachycardia, bradycardia, excessive hypotension, gingival enlargement, allergic reaction, mental depression (for flunarizine), arthritis (for nifedipine), thrombocytopenia, and transient blindness (for nifedipine)

## General Dosing Information

The results of several meta-analyses of clinical trials in post-myocardial infarction patients and patients with angina and of observational studies in hypertensive patients have suggested that taking short-acting nifedipine may increase the risk of adverse cardiovascular events and/or mortality, especially when given in high doses. Consequently, the National Heart, Lung, and Blood Institute (NHLBI) recommends that short-acting nifedipine be used with extreme caution in the treatment of hypertension or angina, especially when given in higher doses. Other drugs, such as beta-adrenergic blocking agents and diuretics, have been found to reduce the risk of major cardiovascular events and mortality in the treatment of hypertension and are recommended as preferred treatment by *The Fifth Report of the Joint National Committee on Detection, Evaluation, and Treatment of High Blood Pressure.*

### For oral dosage forms only
Oral dosage must be titrated for each patient as needed and tolerated.

Concurrent administration of nitroglycerin sublingually or long-acting nitrates with calcium channel blocking agents may produce an additive antianginal effect. Nitroglycerin may be used sublingually as required to abort acute angina attacks during calcium channel blocking agent therapy. Nitrate medication may be used during calcium channel blocking agent therapy for angina prophylaxis.

Although no "rebound effect" has been reported upon discontinuation of calcium channel blocking agents, a gradual decrease of dosage with physician supervision is recommended.

### Diet/Nutrition
Concurrent administration of felodipine with 200 mL of grapefruit juice has been shown to increase felodipine plasma concentration more than twofold by inhibiting first-pass metabolism in the gastrointestinal wall and/or the liver; a lesser effect also has been seen with two other dihydropyridines, nifedipine and nisoldipine

### For treatment of overdose or acute adverse effects
The following treatments have been proven effective for the indicated adverse effect:
- Hypotension, symptomatic—Intravenous fluids. Intravenous dopamine or dobutamine, calcium chloride, isoproterenol, metaraminol, or norepinephrine. For parenteral verapamil, placement of patient in Trendelenburg position.
- Tachycardia, rapid ventricular rate in patients with antegrade conduction in atrial flutter fibrillation, and accessory pathway with Wolff-Parkinson-White or Lown-Ganong-Levine syndrome—Direct-current cardioversion or intravenous procainamide. Intravenous fluids given by slow-drip.
- Bradycardia, rarely second- or third-degree atrioventricular (AV) block, with a few patients progressing to asystole—Intravenous atropine, isoproterenol, norepinephrine, or calcium chloride or use of electronic cardiac pacemaker.

---
**BEPRIDIL**
---

## Summary of Differences
Pharmacology/pharmacokinetics:
Nonselective calcium channel blocking agent; also affects fast sodium inward current.
Depresses sinoatrial (SA) and atrioventricular (AV) nodes; negative inotropic effect; causes bradycardia.
Precautions:
Laboratory value alterations—Increases Q-T interval and alters T-wave morphology.
Medical considerations/contraindications—Contraindicated in patients with history of serious ventricular arrhythmias or Q-T interval prolongation. Also, contraindicated in patients with second- or third-degree atrioventricular (AV) block or sinoatrial (SA) nodal function impairment, except in patients with a functioning artificial ventricular pacemaker. Extreme caution necessary in patients with hypokalemia.
Side/adverse effects:
Differences in frequencies are due to differences in pharmacological effects. Also causes agranulocytosis (rare); arrhythmias, including torsades de pointes (less common).

## Oral Dosage Forms
### BEPRIDIL HYDROCHLORIDE TABLETS
**Usual adult dose**
Antianginal—
Oral, initially 200 mg once a day, the dosage being increased after ten days, if necessary, to 300 mg once a day.

**Usual adult prescribing limits**
400 mg daily.

**Usual pediatric dose**
Safety and efficacy have not been established.

**Usual geriatric dose**
See *Usual adult dose.*

**Strength(s) usually available**
U.S.—
200 mg (Rx) [*Vascor*].
300 mg (Rx) [*Vascor*].
400 mg (Rx) [*Vascor*].
Canada—
Not commercially available.

**Packaging and storage**
Store below 40 °C (104 °F), preferably between 15 and 30 °C (59 and 86 °F), in a well-closed container, unless otherwise specified by manufacturer. Protect from light.

---
**DILTIAZEM**
---

## Summary of Differences
Pharmacology/pharmacokinetics:
Benzothiazepine structure.
Depresses sinoatrial (SA) and atrioventricular (AV) nodes; little or no negative inotropic effect; usually does not significantly alter heart rate, but may cause slight bradycardia.
Precautions:
Laboratory value alterations—Increases P-R interval.
Medical considerations/contraindications—Contraindicated in patients with second- or third-degree atrioventricular (AV) block, sinoatrial (SA) nodal function impairment, or Wolff-Parkinson-White or Lown-Ganong-Levine syndrome accompanied by atrial flutter or fibrillation, except in patients with a functioning artificial ventricular pacemaker.
Side/adverse effects:
Differences in frequencies are due to differences in pharmacological effects.

## Additional Dosing Information
See also *General Dosing Information.*
Dermatologic side effects usually disappear even with continued use. However, if skin eruptions persist, it is recommended that diltiazem therapy be withdrawn, since progression to erythema multiforme and/or exfoliative dermatitis or Stevens-Johnson syndrome have been reported rarely.

## Oral Dosage Forms
Note: Bracketed uses in the *Dosage Forms* section refer to categories of use and/or indications that are not included in U.S. product labeling.

## DILTIAZEM HYDROCHLORIDE EXTENDED-RELEASE CAPSULES

### Usual adult and adolescent dose
Antihypertensive—
    *Cardizem CD* or *Dilacor-XR*: Oral, 180 to 240 mg once a day, the dosage being adjusted after fourteen days as needed and tolerated.

Note: The total daily dose usually ranges from 240 to 360 mg.

    *Cardizem SR*: Oral, initially 60 to 120 mg two times a day, the dosage being adjusted after fourteen days as needed and tolerated.

Note: Geriatric patients may be more sensitive to the effects of the usual adult dose.

### Usual adult prescribing limits
360 mg daily.

### Usual pediatric dose
Dosage has not been established.

### Strength(s) usually available
U.S.—
    60 mg (Rx) [*Cardizem SR* (sucrose); GENERIC].
    90 mg (Rx) [*Cardizem SR* (sucrose); GENERIC].
    120 mg (Rx) [*Cardizem CD*; *Cardizem SR* (sucrose); *Dilacor-XR*; GENERIC].
    180 mg (Rx) [*Cardizem CD* (sucrose); *Dilacor-XR*].
    240 mg (Rx) [*Cardizem CD* (sucrose); *Dilacor-XR*].
    300 mg (Rx) [*Cardizem CD* (sucrose)].
Canada—
    90 mg (Rx) [*Cardizem SR*].
    120 mg (Rx) [*Cardizem SR*].

### Packaging and storage
Store below 40 °C (104 °F), preferably between 15 and 30 °C (59 and 86 °F), in a well-closed container, unless otherwise specified by manufacturer.

### Auxiliary labeling
• Do not take other medicines without physician's advice.

### Note
Check refill frequency to determine compliance in hypertensive patients.
*Cardizem CD* and *Cardizem SR* can be used interchangeably on a total daily mg-per-mg dosing basis.

## DILTIAZEM HYDROCHLORIDE TABLETS USP

### Usual adult and adolescent dose
Antianginal or [Antihypertensive][1]—
    Oral, initially 30 mg three or four times a day, the dosage being increased gradually at one- or two-day intervals as needed and tolerated.

Note: Geriatric patients may be more sensitive to the effects of the usual adult dose.

### Usual adult prescribing limits
360 mg daily.

### Usual pediatric dose
Dosage has not been established.

### Strength(s) usually available
U.S.—
    30 mg (Rx) [*Cardizem*; GENERIC].
    60 mg (Rx) [*Cardizem* (scored); GENERIC].
    90 mg (Rx) [*Cardizem* (scored); GENERIC].
    120 mg (Rx) [*Cardizem* (scored); GENERIC].
Canada—
    30 mg (Rx) [*Apo-Diltiaz*; *Cardizem*; *Novo-Diltiazem*; *Nu-Diltiaz*; *Syn-Diltiazem*; GENERIC].
    60 mg (Rx) [*Apo-Diltiaz*; *Cardizem* (scored); *Novo-Diltiazem* (scored); *Nu-Diltiaz*; *Syn-Diltiazem* (scored); GENERIC].
    90 mg (Rx) [*Cardizem*].
    120 mg (Rx) [*Cardizem*].

### Packaging and storage
Store below 40 °C (104 °F), preferably between 15 and 30 °C (59 and 86 °F), unless otherwise specified by manufacturer. Store in a tight container. Protect from light.

### Auxiliary labeling
• Do not take other medicines without physician's advice.

### Note
Check refill frequency to determine compliance in hypertensive patients.

## Parenteral Dosage Forms

## DILTIAZEM HYDROCHLORIDE INJECTION

### Usual adult and adolescent dose
Antiarrhythmic—
    Intravenous (rapid), 250 mcg (0.25 mg) per kg of actual body weight administered slowly over a two-minute period with continuous ECG and blood pressure monitoring. If response is not adequate, 350 mcg (0.35 mg) per kg of actual body weight may be administered fifteen minutes after completion of initial dose. Subsequent doses should be individualized.

Note: Some patients may respond to an initial dose of 150 mcg (0.15 mg) per kg of actual body weight, although the duration of action may be shorter.

    Intravenous infusion, continuous (for continued reduction of heart rate [up to twenty-four hours] in patients with atrial fibrillation or atrial flutter), initially 10 mg per hour beginning immediately after the last rapid intravenous dose. The rate of infusion may be increased in increments of 5 mg per hour as needed, up to a maximum rate of 15 mg per hour.

Note: Some patients may respond to an initial rate of 5 mg per hour.

### Usual pediatric dose
Safety and efficacy have not been established.

### Strength(s) usually available
U.S.—
    5 mg per mL (Rx) [*Cardizem*; GENERIC].
Canada—
    5 mg per mL (Rx) [*Cardizem*; GENERIC].

### Packaging and storage
Store between 2 and 8 °C (36 and 46 °F), unless otherwise specified by manufacturer. May be stored at room temperature for 1 month; destroy after 1 month at room temperature. Protect from freezing.

### Preparation of dosage form
Diltiazem hydrochloride injection may be prepared for administration by continuous intravenous infusion by diluting the appropriate quantity in the desired volume of 0.9% sodium chloride injection, 5% dextrose injection, or 5% dextrose in 0.45% sodium chloride injection, and mixing thoroughly, as follows:

| Diluent volume | Quantity of cardizem injection | Final concentrations | Administration Dose* | Infusion rate |
|---|---|---|---|---|
| 100 mL | 125 mg (25 mL) | 1.0 mg/mL | 10 mg/hr 15 mg/hr | 10 mL/hr 15 mL/hr |
| 250 mL | 250 mg (50 mL) | 0.83 mg/mL | 10 mg/hr 15 mg/hr | 12 mL/hr 18 mL/hr |
| 500 mL | 250 mg (50 mL) | 0.45 mg/mL | 10 mg/hr 15 mg/hr | 22 mL/hr 33 mL/hr |

*5 mg/hr may be appropriate for some patients.

### Stability
After dilution for administration by intravenous infusion, diltiazem hydrochloride injection should be refrigerated until use and should be used within 24 hours.

### Incompatibilities
Diltiazem hydrochloride injection is physically incompatible with furosemide solution.

[1] Not included in Canadian product labeling.

---

## FELODIPINE

## Summary of Differences

Pharmacology/pharmacokinetics:
    Dihydropyridine structure.
    Potent peripheral vasodilator; does not depress sinoatrial (SA) or atrioventricular (AV) node; reflex increase in heart rate in response to vasodilation masks negative inotropic effect.
Precautions:
    Medical considerations/contraindications—No caution necessary in renal function impairment.
Side/adverse effects:
    Differences in frequencies are due to differences in pharmacological effects.

## Oral Dosage Forms
### FELODIPINE EXTENDED-RELEASE TABLETS
**Usual adult dose**
Antihypertensive—
   Initial: Oral, 5 mg once a day, the dosage being adjusted as needed, usually at intervals of not less than two weeks.
   Maintenance: Oral, 5 to 10 mg once a day.
Antianginal—
   Oral, 10 mg once a day.
Note: Geriatric patients may be more sensitive to the effects of the usual adult dose.

**Usual adult prescribing limits**
20 mg once a day.

**Usual pediatric dose**
Safety and efficacy have not been established.

**Strength(s) usually available**
U.S.—
   2.5 mg [*Plendil*].
   5 mg (Rx) [*Plendil*].
   10 mg (Rx) [*Plendil*].
Canada—
   2.5 mg [*Plendil; Renedil*].
   5 mg (Rx) [*Plendil; Renedil*].
   10 mg (Rx) [*Plendil; Renedil*].

**Packaging and storage**
Store below 30 °C (86 °F), unless otherwise specified by manufacturer. Store in a tight container. Protect from light.

**Auxiliary labeling**
- Do not take other medicines without physician's advice.

**Note**
Check refill frequency to determine compliance in hypertensive patients.

---
## FLUNARIZINE

## Summary of Differences
Indications:
   Indicated for prophylaxis of migraine.
Pharmacology/pharmacokinetics:
   Diphenylpiperazine structure.
   Does not depress sinoatrial (SA) or atrioventricular (AV) node; no negative inotropic effect; no reflex increase in heart rate; no antihypertensive effect.
   Cerebroselective.
Precautions:
   Medical considerations/contraindications—Caution required in patients with history of mental depression or with Parkinsonian syndrome or other extrapyramidal disorders.
Side/adverse effects:
   Differences in frequencies are due to differences in pharmacological effects. Also causes parkinsonian extrapyramidal effects (less common), galactorrhea (rare), mental depression (less common), drowsiness (more common), dryness of mouth (less common), increased appetite and/or weight gain (more common).

## Oral Dosage Forms
### FLUNARIZINE HYDROCHLORIDE CAPSULES
**Usual adult dose**
Vascular headache prophylactic—
   Oral, 10 mg once a day in the evening.
Note: Geriatric patients may be more sensitive to the effects of the usual adult dose.

**Usual pediatric dose**
Dosage has not been established.

**Strength(s) usually available**
U.S.—
   Not commercially available.
Canada—
   5 mg (Rx) [*Sibelium*].

**Packaging and storage**
Store below 40 °C (104 °F), preferably between 15 and 30 °C (59 and 86 °F), in a well-closed container, unless otherwise specified by manufacturer. Protect from light.

---
## ISRADIPINE

## Summary of Differences
Pharmacology/pharmacokinetics:
   Dihydropyridine structure.
   Potent peripheral vasodilator; does not depress sinoatrial (SA) or atrioventricular (AV) node; reflex increase in heart rate in response to vasodilation masks negative inotropic effect.
Side/adverse effects:
   Differences in frequencies are due to differences in pharmacological effects.

## Oral Dosage Forms
### ISRADIPINE CAPSULES
**Usual adult dose**
Antihypertensive—
   Oral, initially 2.5 mg two times a day, alone or in combination with a thiazide diuretic, the dosage being increased, if necessary, in increments of 5 mg per day at two- to four-week intervals.
Note: Geriatric patients may be more sensitive to the effects of the usual adult dose.

**Usual adult prescribing limits**
10 mg two times a day.

**Usual pediatric dose**
Safety and efficacy have not been established.

**Strength(s) usually available**
U.S.—
   2.5 mg (Rx) [*DynaCirc*].
   5 mg (Rx) [*DynaCirc*].
Canada—
   Not commercially available.

**Packaging and storage**
Store below 40 °C (104 °F) between 15 and 30 °C (59 and 86 °F), unless otherwise specified by manufacturer. Store in a tight container. Protect from light.

**Auxiliary labeling**
- Do not take other medicines without physician's advice.

**Note**
Check refill frequency to determine compliance in hypertensive patients.

---
## NICARDIPINE

## Summary of Differences
Pharmacology/pharmacokinetics:
   Dihydropyridine structure.
   Potent peripheral vasodilator; does not depress sinoatrial (SA) or atrioventricular (AV) node; reflex increase in heart rate in response to vasodilation masks negative inotropic effect.
Precautions:
   Geriatrics—No change in half-life or protein binding.
   Medical considerations/contraindications—Caution necessary in patients with acute cerebral infarction or hemorrhage.
Side/adverse effects:
   Differences in frequencies are due to differences in pharmacological effects.

## Oral Dosage Forms
### NICARDIPINE HYDROCHLORIDE CAPSULES
**Usual adult and adolescent dose**
Antianginal or
Antihypertensive—
   Oral, initially 20 mg three times a day, the dosage being adjusted as needed and tolerated.

**Usual pediatric dose**
Dosage has not been established.

**Strength(s) usually available**
U.S.—
   20 mg (Rx) [*Cardene*; GENERIC].
   30 mg (Rx) [*Cardene*; GENERIC].
Canada—
   20 mg (Rx) [*Cardene*].
   30 mg (Rx) [*Cardene*].

## Calcium Channel Blocking Agents (Systemic)

**Packaging and storage**
Store between 15 and 25 °C (59 and 77 °F), in a well-closed, light-resistant container, unless otherwise specified by manufacturer.

**Auxiliary labeling**
- Do not take other medicines without physician's advice.

**Note**
Check refill frequency to determine compliance in hypertensive patients.

### NIFEDIPINE

## Summary of Differences
Pharmacology/pharmacokinetics:
   Dihydropyridine structure.
   Potent peripheral vasodilator; does not depress sinoatrial (SA) or atrioventricular (AV) node; reflex increase in heart rate in response to vasodilation masks negative inotropic effect.
Precautions:
   The results of several meta-analyses of clinical trials in post-myocardial infarction patients and patients with angina and of observational studies in hypertensive patients have suggested that taking short-acting nifedipine may increase the risk of adverse cardiovascular events and/or mortality, especially when given in high doses. Consequently, the National Heart, Lung, and Blood Institute (NHLBI) recommends that short-acting nifedipine be used with extreme caution in the treatment of hypertension or angina, especially at higher doses. Other drugs, such as beta-adrenergic blocking agents and diuretics, have been found to reduce the risk of major cardiovascular events and mortality in the treatment of hypertension and are recommended as preferred treatment by *The Fifth Report of the Joint National Committee on Detection, Evaluation, and Treatment of High Blood Pressure.*
Side/adverse effects:
   Differences in frequencies are due to differences in pharmacological effects. Also causes arthritis associated with elevated antinuclear antibody (ANA) titers (rare), transient blindness at peak plasma concentrations (rare).

## Additional Dosing Information
See also *General Dosing Information*.

In solution, degradation of nifedipine occurs more rapidly at 25 °C (77 °F) than at 4 °C (39 °F). However, when nifedipine solutions are protected from light and refrigerated, concentrations of nifedipine decline to approximately 90% of the original concentrations within 6 hours of preparation. It is recommended that extemporaneous preparations be made immediately before use.

## Oral Dosage Forms
Note: Bracketed uses in the *Dosage Forms* section refer to categories of use and/or indications that are not included in U.S. product labeling.

### NIFEDIPINE CAPSULES USP
**Usual adult and adolescent dose**
Antianginal or
[Antihypertensive][1]—
   Essential hypertension: Oral, initially 10 mg three times a day, the dosage being increased over a seven- to fourteen-day period as needed and tolerated.
Note: For hospitalized patients under close supervision, dosage may be increased by 10-mg increments over four- to six-hour periods until symptoms are controlled.
   When justified by symptom frequency and/or severity, dosage titration may be accomplished over a three-day period (medication given three times a day and increased stepwise from 10 mg to 20 mg, then to 30 mg per dose as needed and tolerated), but only if the patient is monitored frequently.
   Geriatric patients may be more sensitive to the effects of the usual adult dose.

**Usual adult prescribing limits**
Single dose, up to 30 mg; total daily dose, up to 180 mg (a total daily dose greater than 120 mg is rarely required).

**Usual pediatric dose**
Dosage has not been established.

**Strength(s) usually available**
U.S.—
   10 mg (Rx) [*Adalat; Procardia;* GENERIC].
   20 mg (Rx) [*Adalat; Procardia;* GENERIC].
Canada—
   5 mg (Rx) [*Adalat*].
   10 mg (Rx) [*Adalat; Apo-Nifed; Novo-Nifedin; Nu-Nifed*].

**Packaging and storage**
Store between 15 and 25 °C (59 and 77 °F), unless otherwise specified by manufacturer. Store in a tight, light-resistant container.

**Auxiliary labeling**
- Do not take other medicines without physician's advice.

**Note**
Check refill frequency to determine compliance in hypertensive patients.

### NIFEDIPINE EXTENDED-RELEASE TABLETS
**Usual adult and adolescent dose**
Antianginal—
   *Adalat XL* or *Procardia XL*:
     Oral, 30 or 60 mg once a day, the dosage being adjusted over a seven- to fourteen-day period as needed and tolerated.
Antihypertensive—
   *Adalat CC*:
     Initial—Oral, 30 mg once a day.
     Maintenance—Oral, 30 to 60 mg once a day, the dosage being adjusted over a seven- to fourteen-day period as needed and tolerated.
     Note: *Adalat CC* should be taken on an empty stomach.
   *Adalat PA*:
     Initial—Oral, 10 or 20 mg two times a day. The full antihypertensive effect may not be apparent for three weeks; therefore, a dosage increase, if needed, should occur at three-week intervals.
     Maintenance—Oral, 20 mg two times a day.
     Note: Geriatric patients may be more sensitive to the effects of the usual adult dose.
   *Adalat XL*:
     Initial—Oral, 30 or 60 mg once a day, the dosage being adjusted over a seven- to fourteen-day period as needed and tolerated.
     Maintenance—Oral, 60 to 90 mg once daily.
   *Procardia XL*:
     Oral, 30 or 60 mg once a day, the dosage being adjusted over a seven- to fourteen-day period as needed and tolerated

**Usual adult prescribing limits**
Antianginal—
   90 mg a day (*Adalat XL*, *Procardia XL*).
Antihypertensive—
   90 mg a day (*Adalat CC*), or 80 mg a day (*Adalat PA*), or 120 mg a day (*Adalat XL*, *Procardia XL*)

**Usual pediatric dose**
Dosage has not been established.

**Strength(s) usually available**
U.S.—
   30 mg (Rx) [*Adalat CC; Procardia XL*].
   60 mg (Rx) [*Adalat CC; Procardia XL*].
   90 mg (Rx) [*Adalat CC; Procardia XL*].
Canada—
   10 mg [*Adalat PA*].
   20 mg [*Adalat PA*].
   30 mg [*Adalat XL*].
   60 mg [*Adalat XL*].
Note: Although similar in appearance to conventional tablets, *Adalat XL* and *Procardia XL* consist of an osmotically active drug core surrounded by a semipermeable membrane which is designed to release nifedipine at a constant rate over 24 hours; following the release of the drug, the insoluble tablet shell is eliminated in the feces.

**Packaging and storage**
Store below 40 °C (104 °F), preferably between 15 and 30 °C (59 and 86 °F), in a well-closed container, unless otherwise specified by manufacturer.

**Auxiliary labeling**
- Do not take other medicines without physician's advice.
*Adalat CC*:
- Do not take other medicines without physician's advice.
- Take on empty stomach.

**Note**
Check refill frequency to determine compliance in hypertensive patients.

---
[1]Not included in Canadian product labeling.

## NIMODIPINE

### Summary of Differences
Indications:
    Indicated for treatment of subarachnoid hemorrhage–associated neurologic deficits.
Pharmacology/pharmacokinetics:
    Dihydropyridine structure.
    Potent peripheral vasodilator; does not depress sinoatrial (SA) or atrioventricular (AV) node; no negative inotropic effect; reflex increase in heart rate in response to vasodilation occurs.
    Cerebroselective.
Side/adverse effects:
    Differences in frequencies are due to differences in pharmacological effects. Also causes thrombocytopenia (rare).

### Oral Dosage Forms
#### NIMODIPINE CAPSULES
**Usual adult dose**
Subarachnoid hemorrhage–associated neurologic deficits—
    Oral, 60 mg every four hours, beginning within ninety-six hours after the subarachnoid hemorrhage and continuing for twenty-one days.
Note: In patients with hepatic function impairment, dosage should be reduced to 30 mg every four hours, with close monitoring of blood pressure and heart rate.
    Geriatric patients may be more sensitive to the effects of the usual adult dose.

**Usual pediatric dose**
Dosage has not been established.

**Strength(s) usually available**
U.S.—
    30 mg (Rx) [*Nimotop*].
Canada—
    30 mg (Rx) [*Nimotop*].

**Packaging and storage**
Store between 15 and 30 °C (59 and 86 °F), in a well-closed container, unless otherwise specified by manufacturer. Protect from light. Protect from freezing.

**Preparation of dosage form**
For patients who cannot take oral solids:
    For patients who cannot swallow, a hole may be made in both ends of the capsule with an 18 gauge needle and the contents of the capsule withdrawn into a syringe, and then emptied into the patient's nasogastric tube and washed down the tube with 30 mL of 0.9% sodium chloride solution.

## VERAPAMIL

### Summary of Differences
Indications:
    Indicated for treatment of supraventricular tachyarrhythmias; oral dosage form indicated for prophylaxis.
    Also used to treat hypertrophic cardiomyopathy.
Pharmacology/pharmacokinetics:
    Diphenylalkylamine structure.
    Depresses sinoatrial (SA) and atrioventricular (AV) nodes; usually does not significantly alter heart rate but may cause bradycardia; negative inotropic effect countered by reduction in afterload.
Precautions:
    Pediatrics—In rare instances, severe adverse hemodynamic effects have occurred after intravenous administration of verapamil in neonates and infants.
    Laboratory value alterations—Prolongs P-R interval in serum concentrations greater than 30 nanograms per mL.
    Medical considerations/contraindications—Contraindicated in patients with second- or third-degree atrioventricular (AV) block, sinoatrial (SA) nodal function impairment, or Wolff-Parkinson-White or Lown-Ganong-Levine syndrome accompanied by atrial flutter or fibrillation, except in patients with a functioning artificial ventricular pacemaker. Caution necessary in patients with neuromuscular transmission deficiency, and wide-complex ventricular tachycardia (with intravenous use).
Side/adverse effects:
    Differences in frequencies are due to differences in pharmacological effects.

### Additional Dosing Information
See also *General Dosing Information*.
Dermatologic side effects usually disappear even with continued use. However, if skin eruptions persist, it is recommended that verapamil therapy be withdrawn, since progression to erythema multiforme has been reported rarely.

**For parenteral dosage forms only**
Parenteral dosage is indicated in the management of cardiac arrhythmias with close monitoring. Emergency equipment and medications should be readily available.

### Oral Dosage Forms
Note: Bracketed uses in the *Dosage Forms* section refer to categories of use and/or indications that are not included in U.S. product labeling.

#### VERAPAMIL TABLETS USP
Note: The dosing and strengths of verapamil are expressed in terms of hydrochloride salt.

**Usual adult and adolescent dose**
Antianginal
Antiarrhythmic
Antihypertensive or[1]
[Hypertrophic cardiomyopathy therapy adjunct]—
    Oral, initially 80 to 120 mg (HCl) three times a day, the dosage being increased at daily or weekly intervals as needed and tolerated.
Note: An initial dose of 40 mg (HCl) three times a day is recommended in patients who may have an increased response to verapamil (e.g., those with hepatic function impairment, elderly patients, patients with poor left ventricular function).
    The total daily dose usually ranges from 240 to 480 mg.
    Because of prolongation of the half-life with repeated dosing, decreased frequency of dosing may be possible; dosage should be individualized.
    Geriatric patients may be more sensitive to the effects of the usual adult dose.

**Usual adult prescribing limits**
480 mg (HCl) daily in divided doses; has been used in doses up to 720 mg per day in the treatment of hypertrophic cardiomyopathy.

**Usual pediatric dose**
For infants less than 1 year and children 1 to 15 years of age—Oral, 4 to 8 mg (HCl) per kg of body weight per day in divided doses.

**Usual geriatric dose**
Oral, initially 40 mg (HCl) three times a day, the dosage being adjusted as needed and tolerated.

**Strength(s) usually available**
U.S.—
    40 mg (HCl) (Rx) [*Calan*; *Isoptin* (scored); GENERIC].
    80 mg (HCl) (Rx) [*Calan* (scored); *Isoptin* (scored); GENERIC].
    120 mg (HCl) (Rx) [*Calan* (scored); *Isoptin* (scored); GENERIC].
Canada—
    80 mg (HCl) (Rx) [*Apo-Verap*; *Isoptin*; *Novo-Veramil*; *Nu-Verap*; GENERIC].
    120 mg (HCl) (Rx) [*Apo-Verap*; *Isoptin*; *Novo-Veramil*; *Nu-Verap*; GENERIC].

**Packaging and storage**
Store below 40 °C (104 °F), preferably between 15 and 30 °C (59 and 86 °F), unless otherwise specified by manufacturer. Store in a tight container. Protect from light.

**Auxiliary labeling**
- Do not take other medicines without physician's advice.

**Note**
Check refill frequency to determine compliance in hypertensive patients.

#### VERAPAMIL HYDROCHLORIDE EXTENDED-RELEASE CAPSULES

**Usual adult and adolescent dose**
Antihypertensive—
    Oral, initially 240 mg once a day, the dosage being increased in increments of 120 mg per day at daily or weekly intervals as needed and tolerated.
Note: An initial dose of 120 mg per day is recommended in patients who may have an increased response to verapamil (e.g., elderly, small people, etc.).
    The total daily dose usually ranges from 240 to 480 mg.

Geriatric patients may be more sensitive to the effects of the usual adult dose.

**Usual pediatric dose**
Dosage has not been established.

**Strength(s) usually available**
U.S.—
- 120 mg (Rx) [*Verelan*].
- 180 mg (Rx) [*Verelan*].
- 240 mg (Rx) [*Verelan*].
- 360 mg (Rx) [*Verelan*].

Canada—
- 120 mg (Rx) [*Verelan*].
- 180 mg (Rx) [*Verelan*].
- 240 mg (Rx) [*Verelan*].

**Packaging and storage**
Store below 40 °C (104 °F), preferably between 15 and 30 °C (59 and 86 °F), unless otherwise specified by manufacturer. Store in a tight container. Protect from light.

**Auxiliary labeling**
- Do not take other medicines without physician's advice.

**Note**
Check refill frequency to determine compliance in hypertensive patients.

### VERAPAMIL HYDROCHLORIDE EXTENDED-RELEASE TABLETS

**Usual adult and adolescent dose**
*Antihypertensive*—
Oral, initially 180 mg once a day in the morning with food, the dosage being increased at daily or weekly intervals as needed and tolerated in the following order: 240 mg once a day in the morning; 180 mg every twelve hours or 240 mg in the morning and 120 mg in the evening; 240 mg every twelve hours.

Note: Lower initial doses (e.g., 120 mg per day) may be necessary in patients with a potential increased response to verapamil.

*Calan SR* and *Isoptin SR* 240 mg tablets may be broken in half, but should not be crushed or chewed.

Geriatric patients may be more sensitive to the effects of the usual adult dose.

**Usual pediatric dose**
Dosage has not been established.

**Strength(s) usually available**
U.S.—
- 120 mg (Rx) [*Calan SR; Isoptin SR*].
- 180 mg (Rx) [*Calan SR; Isoptin SR*].
- 240 mg (Rx) [*Calan SR* (scored); *Isoptin SR* (scored)].

Canada—
- 120 mg (Rx) [*Isoptin SR*].
- 180 mg (Rx) [*Isoptin SR*].
- 240 mg (Rx) [*Isoptin SR* (scored)].

**Packaging and storage**
Store below 40 °C (104 °F), preferably between 15 and 30 °C (59 and 86 °F), unless otherwise specified by manufacturer. Store in a tight, light-resistant container.

**Auxiliary labeling**
- Take with meals or milk.
- Do not take other medicines without physician's advice.

**Note**
Check refill frequency to determine compliance in hypertensive patients.

## Parenteral Dosage Forms

### VERAPAMIL INJECTION USP

Note: The dosing and strengths of verapamil are expressed in terms of hydrochloride salt.

**Usual adult dose**
Intravenous, initially 5 to 10 mg (HCl) (or 75 to 150 mcg [0.075 to 0.15 mg] per kg of body weight) administered slowly over a two-minute period with continuous ECG and blood pressure monitoring. If response is not adequate, 10 mg (or 150 mcg [0.15 mg] per kg of body weight) may be administered thirty minutes after completion of initial dose.

Note: In geriatric patients, the intravenous dose should be administered slowly over a three-minute period to minimize undesired effects.

**Usual pediatric dose**
The following doses should be administered slowly over a two-minute period, with continuous ECG monitoring. If response is not adequate, a repeat dose may be administered thirty minutes after completion of initial dose.

Infants up to 1 year of age—Initially, 100 to 200 mcg (HCl) (0.1 to 0.2 mg) per kg of body weight (usual single dose range, 0.75 to 2 mg).

Children 1 to 15 years of age—Initially, 100 to 300 mcg (HCl) (0.1 to 0.3 mg) per kg of body weight (usual single dose range, 2 to 5 mg) not to exceed a total of 5 mg. For repeat dose, thirty minutes after initial dose, do not exceed 10 mg as a single dose.

**Strength(s) usually available**
U.S.—
- 2.5 mg (HCl) per mL (Rx) [*Isoptin;* GENERIC (sodium chloride 8.5 mg per mL)].

Canada—
- 2.5 mg (HCl) per mL (Rx) [*Isoptin;* GENERIC].

**Packaging and storage**
Store between 15 and 30 °C (59 and 86 °F), unless otherwise specified by manufacturer. Protect from light. Protect from freezing.

**Stability**
Verapamil hydrochloride injection is physically and chemically compatible with Ringer's injection or 5% dextrose or 0.9% sodium chloride injection.

**Incompatibilities**
Verapamil hydrochloride injection is physically incompatible with albumin, amphotericin B injection, hydralazine hydrochloride injection, and sulfamethoxazole and trimethoprim injection. Precipitation of verapamil hydrochloride will occur in any solution with a pH greater than 6.

[1]Not included in Canadian product labeling.

## Selected Bibliography

**General**
Tracy TS, Black CD. Calcium modulators: future agents, future uses. Drug Intell Clin Pharm 1987 Jul/Aug; 21: 575-83.
Lam YW. Calcium metabolism, calcium-channel blocking agents, and hypertension management. Drug Intell Clin Pharm 1988 Sep; 22: 659-71.
Freedman DD, Waters DD. 'Second generation' dihydropyridine calcium antagonists. Greater vascular selectivity and some unique applications. Drugs 1987; 34: 578-98.

**Bepridil**
Flaim SF, Cummings DM. Bepridil hydrochloride: a review of its pharmacologic properties. Curr Ther Res 1986 Apr; 39: 568-97.

**Bepridil and nicardipine**
Hasegawa GR. Nicardipine, nitrendipine, and bepridil: new calcium antagonists for cardiovascular disorders. Clin Pharm 1988 Feb; 7: 97-108.

**Diltiazem**
McAuley BJ, Schroeder JS. The use of diltiazem hydrochloride in cardiovascular disorders. Pharmacother 1982 May/Jun; 2: 121-33.
Chaffman M, Brogden RN. Diltiazem. A review of its pharmacological properties and therapeutic efficacy. Drugs 1985 May; 29: 387-454.

**Felodipine**
Yedinak KC, Lopez LM. Felodipine: a new dihydropyridine calcium-channel antagonist. DICP Ann Pharmacother 1991 Nov; 25: 1193-1206.

**Flunarizine**
Holmes B, Brogden RN, Heel RC, et al. Flunarizine: a review of its pharmacodynamic and pharmacokinetic properties and therapeutic use. Drugs 1984; 27: 6-44.

**Isradipine**
Fitton A, Benfield P. Isradipine. A review of its pharmacodynamic and pharmacokinetic properties, and therapeutic use in cardiovascular disease. Drugs 1990; 40(1): 31-74.

**Nicardipine**
Sorkin EM, Clissold SP. Nicardipine. A review of its pharmacodynamic and pharmacokinetic properties, and therapeutic efficacy, in the treatment of angina pectoris, hypertension and related cardiovascular disorders. Drugs 1987; 33: 296-345.

**Nifedipine**
Ferlinz J. Nifedipine in myocardial ischemia, systemic hypertension, and other cardiovascular disorders. Ann Intern Med 1986 Nov; 105: 714-29.

**Nimodipine**
Allen GS, et al. A controlled trial of nimodipine in acute ischemic stroke. N Engl J Med 1988 Jan 28; 318: 203-7.
Petruk K, et al. Nimodipine treatment in poor-grade aneurysm patients. Results of a multicenter, double-blind, placebo-controlled trial. J Neurosurg 1988; 68: 505-17.

Pickard JD, Murray GD, Illingworth R, et al. Effect of oral nimodipine on cerebral infarction and outcome after subarachnoid hemorrhage: British aneurysm nimodipine trial. Br Med J 1989 Mar 11; 298: 636-42.

**Verapamil**
Baky SH, Singh BN. Verapamil hydrochloride: Pharmacological properties and role in cardiovascular therapeutics. Pharmacother 1982 Nov/Dec; 2: 328-53.

Revised: 08/21/92
Interim revision: 09/07/94; 04/13/95; 12/02/97; 08/13/98

## Table 1. Pharmacology/Pharmacokinetics

| Hemodynamic effect | Legend*: I = Bepridil; II = Diltiazem; III = Felodipine; IV = Flunarizine; V = Isradipine | | | | | VI = Nicardipine; VII = Nifedipine; VIII = Nimodipine; IX = Verapamil | | | |
|---|---|---|---|---|---|---|---|---|---|
| | I | II | III | IV | V | VI | VII | VIII | IX |
| Peripheral vasodilation | + | + | ++ | + | ++ | ++ | ++ | ++ | + |
| Heart rate | D | D | I† | N | I† | I† | I† | I† | D |
| Depression of sinoatrial (SA) or atrioventricular (AV) nodal conduction | + | + | − | − | − | − | − | − | + |
| Negative inotropic effect | +‡ | +/− | +/−‡ | − | +/−‡ | +/−‡ | +/−‡ | +/−‡ | +‡ |
| Antihypertensive effect | − | + | + | − | + | + | + | + | + |
| Cerebrovascular selectivity | | | | + | | + | | + | |

*Legend: I = Increase; D = Decrease; N = No effect; + = Some effect; ++ = Significant effect; − = No effect.
†Reflex increase occurs in response to vasodilating action. Isradipine causes only a slight increase or no change.
‡Bepridil's negative inotropic effect is small and tends to occur at high doses. For felodipine, isradipine, nicardipine, nifedipine, and nimodipine, the effect is masked by the reflex increase in heart rate. The effect of verapamil is countered by a reduction in afterload.

## Table 2. Medical Considerations/Contraindications

| The medical considerations/contraindications included have been selected on the basis of their potential clinical significance (reasons given in parentheses where appropriate)—not necessarily inclusive (» = major clinical significance). | Legend: I = Bepridil; II = Diltiazem; III = Felodipine; IV = Flunarizine; V = Isradipine | | | | | VI = Nicardipine; VII = Nifedipine; VIII = Nimodipine; IX = Verapamil | | | |
|---|---|---|---|---|---|---|---|---|---|
| | I | II | III | IV | V | VI | VII | VIII | IX |
| ***Except under special circumstances, this medication should not be used when the following medical problems exist:*** | | | | | | | | | |
| » Arrhythmias, ventricular, serious, history of or<br>» Q-T interval prolongation, history of<br>   (increased risk of bepridil-induced arrhythmias) | ✓ | | | | | | | | |
| » Heart block—2nd- or 3rd- degree atrioventricular (AV) block, except in patients with a functioning artificial ventricular pacemaker<br>   (use of calcium channel blocking agent may lead to excessive bradycardia) | ✓ | ✓ | | | | | | | ✓ |
| » Hypotension, severe | ✓ | ✓ | ✓ | | ✓ | ✓ | ✓ | ✓ | ✓ |
| » Sinoatrial (SA) nodal function impairment (sick sinus syndrome) except in patients with functioning artificial ventricular pacemaker<br>   (use of calcium channel blocking agent may lead to severe hypotension, bradycardia, and asystole) | ✓ | ✓ | | | | | | | ✓ |
| » Wolff-Parkinson-White or Lown-Ganong-Levine syndrome accompanied by atrial flutter or fibrillation, except in patients with a functioning artificial ventricular pacemaker<br>   (use of a calcium channel blocking agent for treatment of atrial fibrillation or flutter may precipitate severe ventricular arrhythmias) | | ✓ | | | | | | | ✓ |
| ***Risk-benefit should be considered when the following medical problems exist:***<br>Aortic stenosis, severe<br>   (increased risk of heart failure when a calcium channel blocking agent is initiated, because of fixed impedance to flow across aortic valve) | | ✓ | | | | ✓ | ✓ | | ✓ |

## Table 2. Medical Considerations/Contraindications *(continued)*

The medical considerations/contraindications included have been selected on the basis of their potential clinical significance (reasons given in parentheses where appropriate)—not necessarily inclusive (» = major clinical significance).

Legend:
I = Bepridil
II = Diltiazem
III = Felodipine
IV = Flunarizine
V = Isradipine
VI = Nicardipine
VII = Nifedipine
VIII = Nimodipine
IX = Verapamil

| | I | II | III | IV | V | VI | VII | VIII | IX |
|---|---|---|---|---|---|---|---|---|---|
| » Bradycardia, extreme, or<br>» Heart failure<br>(reduced sinus node and AV node activity may be worsened)<br>Note: When not severe or rate-related, heart failure should be controlled with digitalization and diuretics before administration of a calcium channel blocking agent. Heart failure, severe or moderately severe (pulmonary wedge pressure above 20 mm of mercury, ejection fraction less than 30%), may be acutely worsened by administration of a calcium channel blocking agent. | ✓ | ✓ | | | | | | | ✓ |
| Bradycardia, extreme, or<br>Heart failure<br>(because these agents have a slight negative inotropic effect, caution is recommended) | | | | ✓ | | ✓ | ✓ | ✓ | |
| » Cardiogenic shock | ✓ | ✓ | ✓ | | ✓ | ✓ | ✓ | ✓ | ✓ |
| Cerebral infarction or hemorrhage, acute | | | | | | ✓ | | | |
| Hepatic function impairment<br>(clearance and duration of effect may be prolonged; clearance of felodipine is reduced to about 60%; half-life of nicardipine may be increased to 19 hours in patients with severe hepatic function impairment; half-life of verapamil may be increased to 14 to 16 hours and plasma clearance reduced to about 30% of normal; dosage reduction may be necessary) | ✓ | ✓ | ✓ | ✓ | ✓ | ✓ | ✓ | ✓ | ✓ |
| » Hypokalemia<br>(risk of bepridil-induced arrhythmias may be increased) | ✓ | | | | | | | | |
| Hypotension, mild to moderate<br>(tendency to hypotension is augmented by the peripheral vasodilating effect of the calcium channel blocking agent) | | ✓ | ✓ | | ✓ | ✓ | ✓ | | ✓ |
| Mental depression, history of<br>(flunarizine may precipitate mental depression) | | | | ✓ | | | | | |
| » Myocardial infarction, acute, with pulmonary congestion documented by x-ray on admission<br>(associated heart failure may be acutely worsened by administration of a calcium channel blocking agent) | ✓ | ✓ | | | | | | | ✓ |
| Myocardial infarction, acute, with pulmonary congestion documented by x-ray on admission<br>(because these agents have a slight negative inotropic effect, there is a possibility that associated heart failure may be acutely worsened) | | | ✓ | | ✓ | ✓ | ✓ | ✓ | |
| Narrowing of the gastrointestinal tract, pathologic or iatrogenic, severe<br>(passage of the nondeformable extended-release nifedipine system [Procardia XL] may be impaired; obstructive symptoms may occur) | | | | | | | ✓ | | |
| Neuromuscular transmission deficiency<br>(verapamil has been reported to decrease neuromuscular transmission in patients with Duchenne's muscular dystrophy, and to prolong recovery from the neuromuscular blocking agent vecuronium; dosage reduction may be required) | | | | | | | | | ✓ |
| Parkinsonian syndrome or<br>Extrapyramidal disorders, other<br>(flunarizine may produce parkinsonian extrapyramidal symptoms not responsive to antiparkinsonian medications) | | | | ✓ | | | | | |
| Renal function impairment<br>(possible reduced clearance of the calcium channel blocking agent or metabolites, although half-life is only slightly increased; dosage adjustment may be necessary) | ✓ | ✓ | | | | ✓ | ✓ | ✓ | ✓ |
| (plasma concentrations of felodipine are unchanged; although reduced excretion results in increased concentrations of metabolites, they are inactive) | | | | ✓ | | | | | |
| » Sensitivity to the calcium channel blocking agent prescribed | ✓ | ✓ | ✓ | ✓ | ✓ | ✓ | ✓ | ✓ | ✓ |
| Ventricular tachycardia, wide-complex<br>(risk of ventricular fibrillation if intravenous diltiazem or verapamil administered) | | ✓ | | | | | | | ✓ |

## Table 3. Side/Adverse Effects

Note: Side/adverse effects tend to be dose-related and occur most frequently during periods of dosage titration.

Although not reported to occur in humans, lenticular changes and cataracts have developed during chronic dosage with verapamil in beagles. These effects resulted from daily dosage of 30 mg and more per kg of body weight and are considered likely to be species-specific.

A possible hyperglycemic effect has been reported with nicardipine (at a daily dose of 40 mg) and nifedipine therapy (when the daily dosage exceeds 60 mg). No significant effect on fasting serum glucose has been seen with felodipine.

Depression of atrioventricular (AV) and sinoatrial (SA) nodal conduction by bepridil, diltiazem, and verapamil may result in asymptomatic first-degree block and transient sinus bradycardia, sometimes accompanied by nodal escape rhythms.

Use of verapamil for hypertrophic cardiomyopathy, especially in patients with pre-existing risk factors, has resulted in serious side effects (including pulmonary edema, sinus bradycardia, severe hypotension, second-degree AV block, and sudden death).

| The following side/adverse effects have been selected on the basis of their potential clinical significance (possible signs and symptoms in parentheses where appropriate)—not necessarily inclusive:* | Legend:<br>I = Bepridil<br>II = Diltiazem<br>III = Felodipine<br>IV = Flunarizine<br>V = Isradipine | | | | | VI = Nicardipine<br>VII = Nifedipine<br>VIII = Nimodipine<br>IX = Verapamil | | | |
|---|---|---|---|---|---|---|---|---|---|
| | I | II | III | IV | V | VI | VII | VIII | IX |
| **Medical attention needed** | | | | | | | | | |
| *Agranulocytosis*—not symptomatic | R | U | U | U | U | U | U | U | U |
| *Allergic reaction* (skin rash) | R | L | L | R | L | R | R | R | L |
| Note: May disappear, even with continued diltiazem use. Rarely, may progress to erythema multiforme (diltiazem, verapamil), exfoliative dermatitis (diltiazem), or Stevens-Johnson syndrome (diltiazem, verapamil). | | | | | | | | | |
| *Angina* (chest pain)—may occur about 30 minutes after administration | U | R | L | U | L | L | R | U | R |
| Note: Rarely, especially in patients with severe obstructive coronary artery disease, increased frequency, duration, and/or severity of angina or acute myocardial infarction have occurred when therapy is initiated or dosage increased. | | | | | | | | | |
| *Arrhythmias, including torsades de pointes*—usually asymptomatic | L | U | U | U | U | U | U | U | U |
| *Arthritis* (painful, swollen joints)—associated with elevated ANA titers | U | U | U | U | U | U | R | U | U |
| *Blindness,* transient, at peak plasma concentration | U | U | U | U | U | U | R | U | U |
| *Bradycardia* less than 50 beats per minute; rarely, 2nd- or 3rd- degree AV block, with a few patients progressing to asystole (slow heartbeat) | L | R | X | U | X | X | X | X | L |
| *Congestive heart failure or pulmonary edema,* possible (breathing difficulty, coughing, or wheezing) | L | L | L | U | R | R | L | R | L |
| *Extrapyramidal effects, parkinsonian* (loss of balance control, mask-like face, shuffling walk, stiffness of arms or legs, trembling and shaking of hands and fingers, trouble in speaking or swallowing) | U | R | U | L | U | U | U | U | U |
| Note: Symptoms are not responsive to antiparkinsonian medications, but are reversible on withdrawal of flunarizine. | | | | | | | | | |
| *Galactorrhea* (unusual secretion of milk) | U | U | U | R | U | U | U | U | R |
| *Gingival enlargement* (bleeding, tender, or swollen gums) | U | R | R | U | U | R | R | U | R |
| *Hypotension*—usually not symptomatic; not orthostatic | R | L | R | U | L | L | L | L | L |
| *Hypotension, excessive* (fainting) | R | R | R | U | R | R | R | R | R |
| *Mental depression* | U | R | R | L | U | U | U | U | U |
| *Peripheral edema* (swelling of ankles, feet, or lower legs) | R | L | M | U | L | L | L | M | L |
| *Tachycardia* (irregular or fast, pounding heartbeat) | X | R | L | U | L | L | L | L | R |
| Note: In patients receiving verapamil, rapid ventricular rate may occur in patients with atrial flutter/fibrillation and an accessory AV pathway as with Wolff-Parkinson-White, or Lown-Ganong-Levine syndrome; in patients receiving felodipine, isradipine, nicardipine, nifedipine, or nimodipine, reflex tachycardia may occur because of its hypotensive effect. | | | | | | | | | |
| *Thrombocytopenia*—not symptomatic | U | R | U | U | U | U | U | R | U |
| **Medical attention needed only if continuing or bothersome** | | | | | | | | | |
| *Constipation* | L | L | L | U | R | R | L | U | L |
| *Diarrhea* | M | L | L | U | L | R | U | L | U |
| *Dizziness or lightheadedness* | M | L | L | L | L | L | M | L | L |
| *Drowsiness* | U | R | U | M | U | R | U | U | U |

*Differences in frequency of occurrence may reflect either lack of clinical-use data or actual pharmacologic distinctions among agents (although their pharmacologic similarity suggests that side effects occurring with one may occur with the others). M = more frequent; L = less frequent; R = rare; U = unknown; X = does not occur.

Table 3. Side/Adverse Effects *(continued)*

Note: Side/adverse effects tend to be dose-related and occur most frequently during periods of dosage titration.

Although not reported to occur in humans, lenticular changes and cataracts have developed during chronic dosage with verapamil in beagles. These effects resulted from daily dosage of 30 mg and more per kg of body weight and are considered likely to be species-specific.

A possible hyperglycemic effect has been reported with nicardipine (at a daily dose of 40 mg) and nifedipine therapy (when the daily dosage exceeds 60 mg). No significant effect on fasting serum glucose has been seen with felodipine.

Depression of atrioventricular (AV) and sinoatrial (SA) nodal conduction by bepridil, diltiazem, and verapamil may result in asymptomatic first-degree block and transient sinus bradycardia, sometimes accompanied by nodal escape rhythms.

Use of verapamil for hypertrophic cardiomyopathy, especially in patients with pre-existing risk factors, has resulted in serious side effects (including pulmonary edema, sinus bradycardia, severe hypotension, second-degree AV block, and sudden death).

The following side/adverse effects have been selected on the basis of their potential clinical significance (possible signs and symptoms in parentheses where appropriate)—not necessarily inclusive:*

Legend:
I = Bepridil
II = Diltiazem
III = Felodipine
IV = Flunarizine
V = Isradipine
VI = Nicardipine
VII = Nifedipine
VIII = Nimodipine
IX = Verapamil

| | I | II | III | IV | V | VI | VII | VIII | IX |
|---|---|---|---|---|---|---|---|---|---|
| *Dryness of mouth* | U | R | R | L | U | R | U | U | U |
| *Flushing and feeling of warmth* | U | L | L | U | L | M | M | R | R |
| *Headache* | L | L | M | U | M | L | M | L | L |
| *Increased appetite and/or weight gain* | U | U | U | M | U | U | U | U | U |
| *Nausea* | M | L | L | L | L | L | M | L | L |
| *Unusual tiredness or weakness* | L | L | L | L | L | L | L | U | L |

*Differences in frequency of occurrence may reflect either lack of clinical-use data or actual pharmacologic distinctions among agents (although their pharmacologic similarity suggests that side effects occurring with one may occur with the others). M = more frequent; L = less frequent; R = rare; U = unknown; X = does not occur.

---

**CALCIUM CHLORIDE**—See *Calcium Supplements (Systemic)*

**CALCIUM CITRATE**—See *Calcium Supplements (Systemic)*

**CALCIUM GLUBIONATE**—See *Calcium Supplements (Systemic)*

**CALCIUM GLUCEPTATE**—See *Calcium Supplements (Systemic)*

**CALCIUM GLUCEPTATE AND CALCIUM GLUCONATE**—See *Calcium Supplements (Systemic)*

**CALCIUM GLUCONATE**—See *Calcium Supplements (Systemic)*

**CALCIUM GLYCEROPHOSPHATE AND CALCIUM LACTATE**—See *Calcium Supplements (Systemic)*

**CALCIUM LACTATE**—See *Calcium Supplements (Systemic)*

**CALCIUM LACTATE-GLUCONATE AND CALCIUM CARBONATE**—See *Calcium Supplements (Systemic)*

**CALCIUM PANTOTHENATE**—See *Pantothenic Acid (Systemic)*

**CALCIUM PHOSPHATE, DIBASIC**—See *Calcium Supplements (Systemic)*

**CALCIUM PHOSPHATE, TRIBASIC**—See *Calcium Supplements (Systemic)*

---

# CALCIUM SUPPLEMENTS Systemic

This monograph includes information on the following: 1) Calcium Acetate†; 2) Calcium Carbonate; 3) Calcium Chloride; 4) Calcium Citrate†; 5) Calcium Glubionate‡§; 6) Calcium Gluceptate†; 7) Calcium Gluceptate and Calcium Gluconate*; 8) Calcium Gluconate; 9) Calcium Glycerophosphate and Calcium Lactate†; 10) Calcium Lactate; 11) Calcium Lactate-Gluconate and Calcium Carbonate*; 12) Dibasic Calcium Phosphate†; 13) Tribasic Calcium Phosphate†.

INN: Calcium Gluceptate—Calcium Glucoheptonate

VA CLASSIFICATION (Primary/Secondary):
Calcium Acetate
  Parenteral—TN402
Calcium Carbonate
  Oral—TN402/GA105
Calcium Chloride
  Parenteral—TN402/CV900
Calcium Citrate
  Oral—TN402

Calcium Glubionate
    Oral—TN402
Calcium Gluceptate
    Parenteral—TN402
Calcium Gluceptate and Calcium Gluconate
    Oral—TN402
Calcium Gluconate
    Oral—TN402
    Parenteral—TN402/CV900
Calcium Glycerophosphate and Calcium Lactate
    Parenteral—TN402
Calcium Lactate
    Oral—TN402
Calcium Lactate-Gluconate and Calcium Carbonate
    Oral—TN402
Dibasic Calcium Phosphate
    Oral—TN402
Tribasic Calcium Phosphate
    Oral—TN402

Commonly used brand name(s): *Alka-Mints*[2]; *Amitone*[2]; *Apo-Cal*[2]; *BioCal*[2]; *Cal-Plus*[2]; *Calcarb 600*[2]; *Calci-Chew*[2]; *Calci-Mix*[2]; *Calciday 667*[2]; *Calciject*[3]; *Calcilac*[2]; *Calcionate*[5]; *Calcite 500*[2]; *Calcium 600*[2]; *Calcium Stanley*[7]; *Calcium-Sandoz*[5]; *Calcium-Sandoz Forte*[11]; *Calglycine*[2]; *Calphosan*[9]; *Calsan*[2]; *Caltrate 600*[2]; *Caltrate Jr*[2]; *Chooz*[2]; *Citracal*[4]; *Citracal Liquitabs*[4]; *Dicarbosil*[2]; *Gencalc 600*[2]; *Gramcal*[11]; *Liqui-Cal*[2]; *Liquid Cal-600*[2]; *Maalox Antacid Caplets*[2]; *Mallamint*[2]; *Neo-Calglucon*[5]; *Nephro-Calci*[2]; *Nu-Cal*[2]; *Os-Cal*[2]; *Os-Cal 500*[2]; *Os-Cal Chewable*[2]; *OsCal 500 Chewable*[2]; *Oysco*[2]; *Oysco 500 Chewable*[2]; *Oyst-Cal 500*[2]; *Oystercal 500*[2]; *Posture*[13]; *Rolaids Calcium Rich*[2]; *Titralac*[2]; *Tums*[2]; *Tums 500*[2]; *Tums E-X*[2]; *Tums Extra Strength*[2]; *Tums Regular Strength*[2].

Note: For a listing of dosage forms and brand names by country availability, see *Dosage Forms* section(s).

*Not commercially available in U.S.
†Not commercially available in Canada.
‡Antacid product commonly recommended as calcium supplement.
§In Canada, calcium glubionate is known as calcium glucono-galacto gluconate.

## Category

Antihypocalcemic—Calcium Acetate; Calcium Carbonate; Calcium Chloride; Calcium Citrate; Calcium Glubionate; Calcium Gluceptate; Calcium Gluconate; Calcium Glycerophosphate and Calcium Lactate; Calcium Lactate; Calcium Lactate-Gluconate and Calcium Carbonate; Dibasic Calcium Phosphate; Tribasic Calcium Phosphate.
Electrolyte replenisher—Calcium Acetate; Calcium Chloride; Calcium Gluceptate; Calcium Gluconate Injection.
Cardiotonic—Calcium Chloride; Calcium Gluconate Injection.
Antihyperkalemic—Calcium Chloride; Calcium Gluconate Injection.
Antihypermagnesemic—Calcium Chloride; Calcium Gluceptate; Calcium Gluconate Injection.
Antacid—Calcium Carbonate.
Nutritional supplement (mineral)—Calcium Carbonate; Calcium Citrate; Calcium Glubionate, Oral; Calcium Gluceptate and Calcium Gluconate; Calcium Gluconate, Oral; Calcium Lactate; Calcium Lactate-Gluconate and Calcium Carbonate; Dibasic Calcium Phosphate; Tribasic Calcium Phosphate.
Antihyperphosphatemic—Calcium Carbonate; Calcium Citrate.

## Indications

Note: Bracketed information in the *Indications* section refers to uses that are not included in U.S. product labeling.

**Accepted**

Hypocalcemia, acute (treatment)—Parenteral calcium salts (i.e., acetate, chloride, gluceptate, and gluconate) are indicated in the treatment of hypocalcemia in conditions that require a rapid increase in serum calcium-ion concentration, such as in neonatal hypocalcemic tetany; tetany due to parathyroid deficiency; hypocalcemia due to "hungry bones" syndrome (remineralization hypocalcemia) following surgery for hyperparathyroidism; vitamin D deficiency; and alkalosis. Calcium salts have been used as adjunctive therapy for insect bites or stings, such as Black Widow Spider bites, and sensitivity reactions, especially when characterized by urticaria; and as an aid in the management of acute symptoms of lead colic. Parenteral calcium gluconate and calcium gluceptate are also used for the prevention of hypocalcemia during exchange transfusions.

Electrolyte depletion (treatment)—Calcium acetate, parenteral calcium chloride, calcium gluconate, and calcium gluceptate are used in conditions that require an increase in calcium ions for electrolyte adjustment.

Cardiac arrest (treatment adjunct)—Parenteral calcium chloride, [or calcium gluconate] may be used also as an adjunct in cardiac resuscitation, particularly after open heart surgery, to strengthen myocardial contractions, such as following defibrillation or when there is an inadequate response to catecholamines.

Hyperkalemia (treatment)—Calcium chloride and parenteral calcium gluconate, are used to decrease or reverse the cardiac depressant effects of hyperkalemia on electrocardiographic (ECG) function.

Hypermagnesemia (treatment adjunct)—Calcium chloride, [calcium gluceptate], and calcium gluconate injections have also been used as an aid in the treatment of central nervous system (CNS) depression due to overdosage of magnesium sulfate.

Hypocalcemia, chronic (treatment)—Oral calcium supplements provide a source of calcium ion for treating calcium depletion occurring in conditions such as chronic hypoparathyroidism, pseudohypoparathyroidism, osteomalacia, rickets, chronic renal failure, and hypocalcemia secondary to the administration of anticonvulsant medications. When chronic hypocalcemia is due to vitamin D deficiency, oral calcium salts may be administered concomitantly with vitamin D analogs. However, calcium phosphate should *not* be used in patients with hypoparathyroidism or renal failure, since phosphate levels may be too high and giving more phosphate would exacerbate the condition. Calcium supplements should not be used in hyperparathyroidism, unless the need for a calcium supplement is high and the patient is carefully monitored. For treatment of hypocalcemia, supplementation is preferred.

Calcium deficiency (prophylaxis)—Oral calcium salts are used as dietary supplemental therapy for persons who may not get enough calcium in their regular diet. However, for prophylaxis of calcium deficiency, dietary improvement, rather than supplementation, is preferred. Due to increased needs, children and pregnant women are at greatest risk. Pre- and postmenopausal women; adolescents, especially girls and the elderly may not receive adequate calcium in their diets. However, studies have shown that supplemental calcium in postmenopausal women without functioning ovaries does not lead to increases in bone density, even in the presence of supplemental vitamin D. Calcium supplements are used as part of the prevention and treatment of osteoporosis in patients with an inadequate calcium intake. The use of calcium citrate may reduce the risk of kidney stones in susceptible patients. The use of water-soluble salts of calcium (i.e., citrate, gluconate, and lactate) may be preferable to acid-soluble salts (i.e., carbonate and phosphate) for patients with reduced stomach acid or patients taking acid-inhibiting medication, such as the histamine $H_2$-receptor antagonists.

Some unusual diets (e.g., reducing diets that drastically restrict food selection) may not supply minimum daily requirements of calcium. Supplementation is necessary in patients receiving total parenteral nutrition (TPN) or undergoing rapid weight loss or in those with malnutrition, because of inadequate dietary intake.

Recommended intakes for all vitamins and most minerals are increased during pregnancy. Many physicians recommend that pregnant women receive multivitamin and mineral supplements, especially those pregnant women who do not consume an adequate diet and those in high-risk categories (i.e., women carrying more than one fetus, heavy cigarette smokers, and alcohol and drug abusers). Taking excessive amounts of a multivitamin and mineral supplement may be harmful to the mother and/or fetus and should be avoided.

Recommended intakes for all vitamins and most minerals are increased during breast-feeding.

Hyperacidity (treatment)—See *Calcium Carbonate, Antacids (Oral-Local)*.

[Hyperphosphatemia (treatment)]—Calcium carbonate is used in patients with end-stage renal failure (renal osteodystrophy) to lower serum phosphate concentrations. However, it should be used with caution in patients on chronic hemodialysis. See also *Patient monitoring*. Calcium citrate is also used in renal failure as a phosphate binder.

## Pharmacology/Pharmacokinetics

**Physicochemical characteristics**

Molecular weight—
    Calcium acetate: 158.17.
    Calcium carbonate, precipitated: 100.09.
    Calcium chloride: 147.01.
    Calcium citrate: 570.50.
    Calcium glubionate: 610.53.
    Calcium gluceptate: 490.43.
    Calcium gluconate: 430.38.
    Calcium lactate: 218.22 (anhydrous).

Calcium lactate-gluconate: 1551.5.
Calcium phosphate, dibasic: 136.06.
Calcium phosphate, tribasic: 503.31.

### Mechanism of action/Effect
Calcium is essential for the functional integrity of the nervous, muscular, and skeletal systems. It plays a role in normal cardiac function, renal function, respiration, blood coagulation, and cell membrane and capillary permeability. Also, calcium helps to regulate the release and storage of neurotransmitters and hormones, the uptake and binding of amino acids, absorption of vitamin $B_{12}$, and gastrin secretion. The major fraction (99%) of calcium is in the skeletal structure primarily as hydroxyapatite, $Ca_{10}(PO_4)_6(OH)_2$; small amounts of calcium carbonate and amorphous calcium phosphates are also present. The calcium of bone is in a constant exchange with the calcium of plasma. Since the metabolic functions of calcium are essential for life, when there is a disturbance in the calcium balance because of dietary deficiency or other causes, the stores of calcium in bone may be depleted to fill the body's more acute needs. Therefore, on a chronic basis, normal mineralization of bone depends on adequate amounts of total body calcium.

### Absorption
Approximately one-fifth to one-third of orally administered calcium is absorbed in the small intestine, depending on presence of vitamin D metabolites, pH in lumen, and on dietary factors, such as calcium binding to fiber or phytates. Calcium absorption is increased when a calcium deficiency is present or when a patient is on a low-calcium diet. In patients with achlorhydria or hypochlorhydria, calcium absorption, especially with the carbonate salt, may be reduced.

### Protein binding
Moderate, approximately 45% in plasma.

### Elimination
Renal (20%)—The amount excreted in the urine varies with degree of calcium absorption and whether there is excessive bone loss or failure of renal conservation.
Fecal (80%)—Consists mainly of nonabsorbed calcium, with only a small amount of endogenous fecal calcium excreted.

## Precautions to Consider

### Pregnancy/Reproduction
Pregnancy—Studies have not been done in humans. However, problems have not been documented with intake of normal daily recommended amounts.
Studies have not been done in animals.
Second and third trimesters: Some studies have shown that calcium supplementation begun in the second trimester may be effective in lowering blood pressure in pregnant women with pregnancy-induced hypertension or pre-eclampsia, both of which may possibly be associated with increased calcium demand of the fetus during the last trimester.
During pregnancy, there is an increased need for calcium to calcify fetal bones and to increase the maternal skeletal mass in preparation for lactation. This need is normally met by enhanced intestinal absorption of calcium, increased vitamin D production, and a concurrent increase in calcitonin secretion, which prevents unwanted bone resorption in the maternal skeleton. The maternal parathyroid glands undergo hyperplasia, producing greater amounts of parathyroid hormone, which acts indirectly to increase intestinal absorption of calcium, reabsorption at the distal renal tubules, and bone calcium mobilization. However, the prescribing of calcium supplements during pregnancy may be necessary since standard prenatal vitamins along with normal intake of dairy products may not provide sufficient elemental calcium for the average pregnant woman.
Calcium acetate, calcium chloride, calcium gluceptate, calcium gluconate injection—FDA Pregnancy Category C.
Other calcium salts—FDA pregnancy categories not currently included in product labeling.
Labor and delivery—The effect of calcium chloride, calcium gluceptate, and calcium gluconate on mother and fetus during labor and delivery is unknown.

### Breast-feeding
Problems in nursing babies have not been documented with intake of normal daily recommended amounts. Although some oral supplemental calcium may be distributed into breast milk, the concentration is not sufficient to produce an adverse effect in the neonate. It is not known whether calcium chloride or calcium gluconate is distributed into breast milk.

### Pediatrics
Problems in pediatrics have not been documented with intake of normal daily recommended amounts.

*Parenteral calcium preparations, especially calcium chloride—*
The extreme irritation and possibility of tissue necrosis and sloughing caused by intravenous injection of calcium preparations usually restricts its use in pediatric patients because of the small vasculature of this patient group.

*For calcium gluceptate injection only—*
It is not recommended that calcium gluceptate be administered intramuscularly to infants and children except in emergencies when the intravenous route is technically impossible, because of the possibility of severe tissue necrosis or sloughing.

### Geriatrics
Problems in geriatrics have not been documented with intake of normal daily recommended amounts. With advancing age, intestinal calcium absorption decreases. Therefore, calcium requirements are increased in the elderly, and dosages of oral supplements may need to be adjusted accordingly. Impaired absorption may be due to low levels of active vitamin D metabolites.

### Drug interactions and/or related problems
The following drug interactions and/or related problems have been selected on the basis of their potential clinical significance (possible mechanism in parentheses where appropriate)—not necessarily inclusive (» = major clinical significance):

Note: Combinations containing any of the following, depending on the amount present, may also interact with this medication.

Not all interactions between calcium supplements and other oral medications have been identified in this monograph. Because the rate and/or extent of absorption of other oral medications may vary when used concurrently with calcium supplements, especially calcium carbonate, patients should be advised not to take any other oral medications within 1 to 2 hours of calcium supplements.

Alcohol or
Caffeine, usually more than 8 cups of coffee a day or
Tobacco
(concurrent use of excessive amounts of these substances has been reported to decrease calcium absorption)

Antacids containing aluminum
(concurrent use with calcium citrate may enhance aluminum absorption)

Calcitonin
(concurrent use with calcium supplements may antagonize the effect of calcitonin in the treatment of hypercalcemia; however, when calcitonin is prescribed for osteoporosis or Paget's disease of the bone, calcium intake should be generous to prevent hypocalcemia which might generate secondary hyperparathyroidism; calcium-containing preparations may be given 4 hours after calcitonin)

Calcium-channel blocking agents
(concurrent use of these medications with calcium supplements in quantities sufficient to raise serum calcium concentrations above normal may reduce the response to verapamil and probably other calcium-channel blockers)

» Calcium-containing preparations, other or
Magnesium-containing preparations, oral
(concurrent use with calcium supplements may increase serum calcium or magnesium concentrations in susceptible patients, mainly patients with impaired renal function, leading to hypercalcemia or hypermagnesemia, respectively)

» Cellulose sodium phosphate
(concurrent use with calcium supplements may decrease effectiveness of cellulose sodium phosphate in preventing hypercalciuria)

Contraceptives, estrogen-containing, oral or
Estrogens
(concurrent use with calcium supplements may increase calcium absorption, which is used to therapeutic advantage when estrogens are prescribed for the treatment of postmenopausal osteoporosis)

» Digitalis glycosides
(concurrent use of parenteral calcium salts with digitalis glycosides may increase the risk of cardiac arrhythmias; therefore, when the parenteral administration of calcium salts to digitalized patients is deemed necessary, caution and close electrocardiographic [ECG] monitoring are recommended)

Diuretics, thiazide
(concurrent use with large doses of calcium supplements may result in hypercalcemia because of reduced calcium excretion)

» Etidronate
(concurrent use with calcium supplements may prevent absorption of etidronate; patients should be advised not to take etidronate within 2 hours of calcium supplements)

Fiber, found in bran, whole-grain breads and cereals or
Phytates, found in bran and whole-grain breads and cereals
(concurrent use of large amounts of fiber or phytates, especially in patients being treated for hypocalcemia, with calcium supplements may reduce calcium absorption by formation of nonabsorbable complexes)

Fluoroquinolones
(concurrent use with calcium carbonate may reduce absorption by chelation of fluoroquinolones, resulting in lower serum and urine concentrations of fluoroquinolones; therefore, concurrent use is not recommended)

» Gallium nitrate
(concurrent use with calcium supplements may antagonize the effect of gallium nitrate)

Iron supplements
(concurrent use with calcium carbonate and calcium phosphate will decrease the absorption of iron; iron supplements should not be taken within 1 or 2 hours of calcium carbonate or phosphate; however, when iron and calcium carbonate are present in multivitamin-with-minerals formulations, the absorption of iron is not significantly changed, possibly because the ascorbic acid in the formulation maintains the iron in the ferrous state, thus increasing its solubility and absorption)

» Magnesium sulfate, parenteral
(parenteral calcium salts may neutralize effects of parenteral magnesium sulfate and should be readily available to counteract the potentially serious risk of magnesium intoxication; also, calcium sulfate may precipitate when a calcium salt is admixed with magnesium sulfate in the same intravenous solution, although commercial nutritional solutions are formulated to avoid precipitation; calcium and magnesium should be administered through separate intravenous lines if required in post-parathyroidectomy "hungry bones" syndrome or tetany associated with hypocalcemia and hypomagnesemia)

Milk or milk products
(concurrent excessive and prolonged use with calcium supplements may result in the milk-alkali syndrome)

Neuromuscular blocking agents, except succinylcholine
(concurrent use with parenteral calcium salts usually reverses the effects of nondepolarizing neuromuscular blocking agents; also, concurrent use with calcium salts has been reported to enhance or prolong the neuromuscular blocking action of tubocurarine)

» Phenytoin
(concurrent use decreases the bioavailability of both phenytoin and calcium because of possible formation of a nonabsorbable complex; patients should be advised not to take calcium supplements within 1 to 3 hours of taking phenytoin; also, enteral feeding solutions containing calcium should not be administered through a nasogastric feeding tube together with phenytoin oral suspension; a 2-hour interval should elapse between the administration of the feeding solution and of the phenytoin)

Potassium phosphates or
Potassium and sodium phosphates
(concurrent use with calcium supplements may increase potential for deposition of calcium in soft tissues if serum ionized calcium is high)

Sodium bicarbonate
(concurrent and prolonged use with calcium supplements may result in milk-alkali syndrome)

Sodium fluoride
(concurrent use with calcium supplements may cause the calcium ions to complex with fluoride and inhibit absorption of both fluoride and calcium; however, if sodium fluoride is used with calcium supplements to treat osteoporosis, a one- to two-hour interval should elapse between doses)

» Tetracyclines, oral
(concurrent use with calcium supplements may decrease absorption of tetracyclines because of possible formation of nonabsorbable complexes and increase in intragastric pH; patients should be advised not to take calcium supplements within 1 to 3 hours of taking tetracyclines)

Vitamin A
(excessive intake, more than 7500 RE or 25,000 Units per day, of vitamin A may stimulate bone loss and counteract the effects of calcium supplementation and may cause hypercalcemia)

Vitamin D, especially calcifediol and calcitriol
(concurrent use of large doses of vitamin D with calcium supplements may excessively increase intestinal absorption of calcium, increasing risk of chronic hypercalcemia in susceptible patients; however, it may be therapeutically advantageous in elderly and high-risk groups when it is necessary to prescribe vitamin D or its derivatives with calcium; careful monitoring of serum calcium concentrations is essential during long-term therapy)

**Laboratory value alterations**
The following have been selected on the basis of their potential clinical significance (possible effect in parentheses where appropriate)—not necessarily inclusive (» = major clinical significance):

With physiology/laboratory test values
Phosphate, serum
(concentrations may be decreased by excessive and prolonged calcium use)

**Medical considerations/Contraindications**
The medical considerations/contraindications included have been selected on the basis of their potential clinical significance (reasons given in parentheses where appropriate)—not necessarily inclusive (» = major clinical significance).

*Except under special circumstances, these medications should not be used when the following medical problems exist:*

For all calcium supplements
» Hypercalcemia, primary or secondary or
» Hypercalciuria or
» Renal calculi, calcium
(risk of exacerbation)
» Sarcoidosis
(may potentiate hypercalcemia)

For calcium phosphate, dibasic or tribasic, only
» Hypoparathyroidism or
» Renal insufficiency
(may increase risk of hyperphosphatemia)

For parenteral calcium salts only
» Digitalis toxicity
(increased risk of arrhythmias)

*Risk-benefit should be considered when the following medical problems exist:*

For all calcium supplements
» Dehydration or
Electrolyte imbalance, other
(may increase risk of hypercalcemia)

Diarrhea or
Malabsorption, gastrointestinal, chronic
(fecal excretion of calcium may be increased, although patients with chronic diarrhea or malabsorption commonly need calcium supplements)

» Renal calculi, history of
(risk of recurrent stone formation)

» Renal function impairment, chronic
(may increase risk of hypercalcemia; however, calcium carbonate or calcium citrate may be used as a phosphate binder in renal failure; also, some patients with renal failure have symptomatic hypocalcemia and need cautious treatment with calcium salts)

For calcium carbonate and calcium phosphate only
Achlorhydria or hypochlorhydria
(calcium absorption may be decreased unless the calcium carbonate or phosphate is taken with meals)

For parenteral calcium salts only
» Cardiac function impairment
» Ventricular fibrillation during cardiac resuscitation
(increased risk of arrhythmias; however, calcium may increase strength of myocardial contraction, make fibrillation coarser, and help in electrical defibrillation, especially with concomitant hyperkalemia)

**Patient monitoring**
The following may be especially important in patient monitoring (other tests may be warranted in some patients, depending on condition; » = major clinical significance):

For hypocalcemia
Blood pressure determinations and
Electrocardiographic monitoring and
Magnesium, concentrations, serum and
Parathyroid hormone (PTH) concentrations, serum and
Phosphate concentrations, serum and
Potassium concentrations, serum and

Renal function determinations
(determinations recommended at initiation of therapy and at frequent intervals during treatment of hypocalcemia)
Note: In elderly patients or patients with hypertension, blood pressure should be monitored during intravenous administration, since a transient increase in blood pressure may occur.
» Calcium concentrations, serum or
» Ionized calcium concentrations, serum
(determinations recommended at frequent intervals during treatment of acute hypocalcemia to achieve normal serum calcium concentrations without exceeding them; at periodic intervals for patients on chronic hemodialysis to prevent hypercalcemia; for patients with chronic renal failure not yet on dialysis who are taking calcium as a phosphate binder; and during long-term therapy with oral calcium supplements. In patients with hypoparathyroidism, serum calcium concentrations should be kept in the low normal range, since significant hypercalciuria may occur intermittently or as a complication with higher concentrations, especially if vitamin D preparations are being used concurrently; serum ionized calcium concentrations are preferable to determine free and bound calcium, but may not be readily available from a reliable lab)

Calcium concentrations, urine
(urinary calcium excretion determinations are sometimes needed to avoid hypercalciuria)

## Side/Adverse Effects

Note: Side/adverse effects may be more likely to occur if oral calcium supplements are taken in much larger doses than recommended (greater than 2000 to 2500 mg a day), if they are taken for a longer period of time, or if they are taken by patients with renal function impairment or milk-alkali syndrome.

The following side/adverse effects have been selected on the basis of their potential clinical significance (possible signs and symptoms in parentheses where appropriate)—not necessarily inclusive:

### Those indicating need for medical attention
Incidence more frequent
*With parenteral dosage forms only*
**Hypotension** (dizziness); *flushing and/or sensation of warmth or heat; irregular heartbeat; nausea or vomiting; skin redness, rash, pain, or burning at injection site; sweating; tingling sensation; decrease in blood pressure, moderate*—with calcium chloride only
Note: *Tingling sensation* may result when intravenous injection is too rapid; *skin redness, rash, pain,* or *burning* may indicate extravasation and can precede sloughing or necrosis of skin.

Incidence rare
**Hypercalcemic syndrome, acute** (drowsiness; continuing nausea and vomiting; weakness); **renal calculi, calcific** (difficult or painful urination)—with oral dosage forms

Early symptoms of hypercalcemia
*Constipation, severe; dryness of mouth; headache, continuing; increased thirst; irritability; loss of appetite; mental depression; metallic taste; unusual tiredness or weakness*

Late symptoms of hypercalcemia
*Confusion; drowsiness; high blood pressure; increased sensitivity of eyes or skin to light, especially in hemodialysis patients; irregular, fast, or slow heartbeat; nausea and vomiting; unusually large amount of urine or increased frequency of urination*

Note: In severe *hypercalcemia*, ECG changes consisting of shortened Q-T intervals are also seen.

## Patient Consultation

As an aid to patient consultation, refer to *Advice for the Patient, Calcium Supplements (Systemic).*
In providing consultation, consider emphasizing the following selected information (» = major clinical significance):

### Description of use
Description should include function in the body, signs of deficiency, and conditions that may cause deficiency

### Importance of diet
Importance of proper nutrition, supplement may be needed because of inadequate dietary intake
Recommended daily intake for calcium
Importance of adequate weight-bearing exercise, especially during younger years, for building and maintaining dense bones to prevent osteoporosis in later life
Calcium content of selected foods

Importance of adequate amounts of vitamin D or exposure to sunlight for enhancement of calcium absorption; avoiding too much vitamin D
Importance of not using bonemeal or dolomite as a source of calcium because of potential lead contamination
Calcium content per tablet of supplements

### Before using this dietary supplement
» Conditions affecting use, especially:
Use in children—Use of injectable calcium preparations may cause extreme irritation and possible tissue necrosis and sloughing
Use in the elderly—Absorption is decreased; dosage adjustments may be necessary
Other medications, especially cellulose sodium phosphate, digitalis glycosides (for parenteral calcium salts only), etidronate, gallium nitrate, parenteral magnesium sulfate (for parenteral calcium salts only), phenytoin, oral tetracyclines, or other calcium-containing preparations
Other medical problems, especially hypercalcemia, hypercalciuria, calcium renal calculi, sarcoidosis, hypoparathyroidism (for calcium phosphate only), dehydration, diarrhea or malabsorption, renal function impairment, or achlorhydria or hypochlorhydria (for calcium carbonate and calcium phosphates only)

### Proper use of this dietary supplement
» Proper dosing
Drinking full glass (8 ounces) of water or juice with all oral dosage forms, except when taking calcium carbonate as a phosphate binder in renal dialysis
» Proper administration of calcium carbonate or phosphate: Taking tablets 1 to 1½ hours after meals, unless otherwise directed by physician
Proper administration of chewable tablet: Chewing tablets well before swallowing
Proper administration of syrup: Taking calcium glubionate syrup *before* meals; diluting syrup in water or fruit juice, if desired, for infants or children
Missed dose: If on scheduled dosing regimen—Taking as soon as possible; then going back to regular schedule
» Proper storage

### Precautions while using this dietary supplement
Regular visits to physician to check progress if taking dietary supplement in large doses or if taking regularly for long period of time
» Not taking within 1 or 2 hours of other oral medication, if possible
» Avoiding concurrent use with other preparations containing significant amounts of calcium, phosphates, magnesium, or vitamin D, unless otherwise directed or approved by health care professional
» Avoiding concomitant use with certain fiber-containing foods such as bran and whole-grain breads and cereals; not eating these foods within 1 or 2 hours of taking calcium supplements
» Avoiding excessive use of alcoholic beverages, tobacco, or caffeine-containing beverages
» Importance of using calcium carbonate products labeled "USP," to avoid differences in bioavailability

### Side/adverse effects
Signs of potential side effects, especially calcium renal calculi or hypercalcemia

## General Dosing Information

The action of calcium supplements depends upon their content of calcium ion. The various calcium salts contain the following amounts of elemental calcium:

| Calcium salt | Calcium (mg/gram) | Calcium (mEq/gram) | % Calcium |
|---|---|---|---|
| Calcium acetate | 253 | 12.2 | 25.3 |
| Calcium carbonate | 400 | 20 | 40 |
| Calcium chloride | 272 | 13.6 | 27.2 |
| Calcium citrate | 211 | 10.5 | 21.1 |
| Calcium glubionate | 65 | 3.2 | 6.5 |
| Calcium gluceptate | 82 | 4.1 | 8.2 |
| Calcium gluconate | 90 | 4.5 | 9 |
| Calcium lactate | 130 | 6.5 | 13 |
| Calcium phosphate | | | |
| Dibasic | 230 | 11.5 | 23 |
| Tribasic | 380 | 19 | 38 |

The following table includes the number of tablets of each calcium salt required to provide 1000 mg of elemental calcium:

| Calcium supplement | Amount of salt in tablet (in milligrams) | Amount of calcium per tablet (in milligrams) | Number of tablets to provide 1000 milligrams of calcium |
|---|---|---|---|
| Calcium carbonate | 625 | 250 | 4 |
|  | 650 | 260 | 4 |
|  | 750 | 300 | 4 |
|  | 835 | 334 | 3 |
|  | 1250 | 500 | 2 |
|  | 1500 | 600 | 2 |
| Calcium citrate | 950 | 200 | 5 |
| Calcium gluconate | 500 | 45 | 22 |
|  | 650 | 58 | 17 |
|  | 1000 | 90 | 11 |
| Calcium lactate | 325 | 42 | 24 |
|  | 650 | 84 | 12 |
| Calcium phosphate, dibasic | 500 | 115 | 9 |
| Calcium phosphate, tribasic | 800 | 304 | 4 |
|  | 1600 | 608 | 2 |

Administration of calcium supplements should not preclude the use of other measures intended to correct the underlying cause of calcium depletion.

In the prevention of osteoporosis, postmenopausal women are sometimes also given estrogens to prevent bone resorption and/or small doses of vitamin D (usually 400 IU per day) to enhance calcium absorption. If estrogens are prescribed, either cyclically or continuously for women who have not undergone a hysterectomy, it is recommended that a progestin such as medroxyprogesterone acetate also be given to reduce or prevent the possibility of adverse endometrial changes from occurring.

The Food and Drug Administration has issued warnings that bonemeal and dolomite (sometimes used as sources of calcium) may contain lead in sufficient quantities to be dangerous.

**For parenteral dosage forms only**
The injection should be warmed to body temperature prior to administration, unless precluded by an emergency situation. Following injection, the patient should remain recumbent for a short period of time to prevent dizziness.

Parenteral calcium salts are administered by *slow* intravenous injection (excepting calcium glycerophosphate and calcium lactate combination which is given by intramuscular injection) to prevent a high concentration of calcium from reaching the heart and causing cardiac syncope.

Side effects experienced by the conscious patient are often the result of too rapid a rate of intravenous administration of calcium salts. Administration should be temporarily discontinued with the appearance of abnormal electrocardiogram (ECG) readings or with patient complaints of discomfort; administration may be resumed when the abnormal reading or the discomfort has disappeared.

Severe necrosis, requiring skin grafting, and calcification can occur at the site of infiltration after intravenous injection, especially after push injection.

Transient increases in blood pressure, especially in the elderly or patients with hypertension, may occur during intravenous administration of calcium salts.

**Diet/Nutrition**
Oral calcium supplements are best taken 1 to 1½ hours after meals in 3 to 4 daily doses. However, calcium glubionate syrup should be administered before meals to enhance absorption.

In the elderly, who may be more prone than younger patients to impaired stomach acid production, calcium absorption may be increased by the use of a more soluble calcium salt, such as calcium citrate, gluconate, or lactate. The poor solubility of carbonate and phosphate salts makes them less desirable as antihypocalcemic agents in patients with known achlorhydria or hypochlorhydria.

Recommended dietary intakes for calcium are defined differently worldwide.

For U.S.—
The Recommended Dietary Allowances (RDAs) for vitamins and minerals are determined by the Food and Nutrition Board of the National Research Council and are intended to provide adequate nutrition in most healthy persons under usual environmental stresses.

In addition, a different designation may be used by the FDA for food and dietary supplement labeling purposes, as with Daily Value (DV). DVs replace the previous labeling terminology United States Recommended Daily Allowances (USRDAs).

For Canada—
Recommended Nutrient Intakes (RNIs) for vitamins, minerals, and protein are determined by Health and Welfare Canada and provide recommended amounts of a specific nutrient while minimizing the risk of chronic diseases.

Daily recommended intakes for calcium are generally defined as follows:

| Persons | U.S. (mg) | Canada (mg) |
|---|---|---|
| Infants and children |  |  |
| Birth to 3 years of age | 400–800 | 250–550 |
| 4 to 6 years of age | 800 | 600 |
| 7 to 10 years of age | 800 | 700–1100 |
| Adolescent and adult males | 800–1200 | 800–1100 |
| Adolescent and adult females | 800–1200 | 700–1100 |
| Pregnant females | 1200 | 1200–1500 |
| Breast-feeding females | 1200 | 1200–1500 |

The following table indicates the calcium content of selected foods:

| Food (amount) | Milligrams of calcium |
|---|---|
| Nonfat dry milk, reconstituted (1 cup) | 375 |
| Lowfat, skim, or whole milk (1 cup) | 290 to 300 |
| Yogurt (1 cup) | 275 to 400 |
| Sardines with bones (3 ounces) | 370 |
| Ricotta cheese, part skim (½ cup) | 340 |
| Salmon, canned, with bones (3 ounces) | 285 |
| Cheese, Swiss (1 ounce) | 272 |
| Cheese, cheddar (1 ounce) | 204 |
| Cheese, American (1 ounce) | 174 |
| Cottage cheese, lowfat (1 cup) | 154 |
| Tofu (4 ounces) | 154 |
| Shrimp (1 cup) | 147 |
| Ice milk (¾ cup) | 132 |

**For treatment of adverse effects**
Perivascular infiltration:Treatment may include the following—
- Immediate discontinuation of intravenous administration.
- Infusion of normal saline into the area by clysis.
- Local application of heat and elevation.

A serum calcium concentration exceeding 2.6 mmol per liter (10.5 mg per 100 mL) is considered a hypercalcemic condition. Withholding additional administration of calcium and any other medications that may cause hypercalcemia usually resolves mild hypercalcemia in asymptomatic patients, when patient renal function is adequate.

When serum calcium concentrations are greater than 2.9 mmol per liter (12 mg per 100 mL), immediate measures may be required with possible use of the following:
- Hydrating with intravenous 0.9% sodium chloride injection. Forcing diuresis with furosemide or ethacrynic acid may be used to rapidly increase calcium and sodium excretion when saline overload occurs.
- Monitoring of potassium and magnesium serum concentrations and starting replacement early to prevent complications of therapy.
- ECG monitoring and the possible use of beta-adrenergic blocking agents to protect the heart against serious arrhythmias.
- Possibly including hemodialysis, calcitonin, and corticosteroids in the treatment.
- Determining serum calcium concentrations at frequent intervals to guide therapy adjustments.

---

## *CALCIUM ACETATE*

## Summary of Differences
Category: Also used as an electrolyte replenisher.

## Additional Dosing Information
See also *General Dosing Information*.

For intravenous use only; subcutaneous or intramuscular injection may cause severe necrosis and sloughing.

Calcium acetate contains the equivalent of 253 mg of calcium ion per gram.

## Parenteral Dosage Forms

### CALCIUM ACETATE INJECTION

**Usual adult and adolescent dose**
Electrolyte replenisher or
Hypocalcemia (prophylaxis or treatment)—
  Intravenous infusion, as part of total parenteral nutrition solutions, the specific amount determined by individual patient need.

**Usual pediatric dose**
Electrolyte replenisher or
Hypocalcemia (prophylaxis or treatment)—
  Intravenous infusion, as part of total parenteral nutrition solutions, the specific amount determined by individual patient need.

**Strength(s) usually available**
U.S.—
  40 mg (10 mg [0.5 mEq] of calcium ion) per mL (Rx) [GENERIC].
Canada—
  Not commercially available.

**Packaging and storage**
Store below 40 °C (104 °F), preferably between 15 and 30 °C (59 and 86 °F), protected from light, unless otherwise specified by manufacturer. Protect from freezing.

**Incompatibilities**
Calcium acetate is precipitated by phosphates.

---

## CALCIUM CARBONATE

### Summary of Differences

Category:
  Also used as an antihyperphosphatemic and as an antacid (see *Calcium Carbonate, Antacids [Oral-Local]*).
Precautions:
  Drug interactions and/or related problems—Concurrent use with fluoroquinolones may decrease the absorption of fluoroquinolones, resulting in lower serum and urine concentrations of fluoroquinolones.
  Medical considerations/contraindications—Calcium absorption may be decreased in patients with achlorhydria or hypochlorhydria, unless the supplement is taken with meals.

### Additional Dosing Information

See also *General Dosing Information*.
Calcium carbonate contains the equivalent of 400 mg of calcium ion per gram.

### Oral Dosage Forms

Note: Bracketed uses in the *Dosage Forms* section refer to categories of use and/or indications that are not included in U.S. product labeling.

### CALCIUM CARBONATE CAPSULES

**Usual adult and adolescent dose**
Hypocalcemia (prophylaxis)—
  Oral, amount based on normal daily recommended intakes:

| Persons | U.S. (mg) | Canada (mg) |
|---|---|---|
| Adolescent and adult males | 800–1200 | 800–1100 |
| Adolescent and adult females | 800–1200 | 700–1100 |
| Pregnant females | 1200 | 1200–1500 |
| Breast-feeding females | 1200 | 1200–1500 |

Hypocalcemia (treatment)—
  Treatment dose is individualized by prescriber based on severity of deficiency.
Antacid—
  See *Calcium Carbonate, Antacids (Oral-Local)*.
[Antihyperphosphatemic]—
  Oral, 5 to 13 grams (2 to 5.2 grams of calcium ion) a day, in divided doses with meals.
  Note: Careful titration is recommended to prevent hypercalcemia, which has been reported with doses above 2 grams of calcium ion a day.

**Usual pediatric dose**
Dosage form not appropriate for use in children.

**Strength(s) usually available**
U.S.—
  1.25 grams (500 mg of calcium ion) (OTC) [*Calci-Mix*].
  1.5 grams (600 mg of calcium ion) (OTC) [*Liqui-Cal; Liquid Cal-600*].
Canada—
  1.25 grams (500 mg of calcium ion) (OTC) [*Calsan*].
Note: Some strengths of these calcium preparations may exceed the dosage range recommended by USP DI Advisory Panels based on the amount necessary to meet normal nutritional needs.

**Packaging and storage**
Store below 40 °C (104 °F), preferably between 15 and 30 °C (59 and 86 °F), in a well-closed container, unless otherwise specified by manufacturer.

**Auxiliary labeling**
• Drink a full glass of water.

Note: When taking as a phosphate binder in renal dialysis, patients should *not* be advised to take capsules with a glass of water.

### CALCIUM CARBONATE ORAL SUSPENSION USP

**Usual adult and adolescent dose**
Hypocalcemia (prophylaxis or treatment)—
  See *Calcium Carbonate Capsules*.
Antacid—
  See *Calcium Carbonate, Antacids (Oral-Local)*.
[Antihyperphosphatemic]—
  Oral, 5 to 13 grams (2 to 5.2 grams of calcium ion) a day, in divided doses with meals.
  Note: Careful titration is recommended to prevent hypercalcemia, which has been reported with doses above 2 grams of calcium ion a day.

**Usual pediatric dose**
Hypocalcemia (prophylaxis)—
  Oral, amount based on normal daily recommended intakes:

| Persons | U.S. (mg) | Canada (mg) |
|---|---|---|
| Infants and children | | |
| Birth to 3 years of age | 400–800 | 250–550 |
| 4 to 6 years of age | 800 | 600 |
| 7 to 10 years of age | 800 | 700–1100 |

Hypocalcemia (treatment)—
  Treatment dose is individualized by prescriber based on severity of deficiency.

**Strength(s) usually available**
U.S.—
  1 gram (400 mg of calcium ion) per 5 mL (OTC) [*Titralac*].
  1.25 grams (500 mg of calcium ion) per 5 mL (OTC) [GENERIC].
Canada—
  Not commercially available.
Note: Some strengths of these calcium preparations may exceed the dosage range recommended by USP DI Advisory Panels based on the amount necessary to meet normal nutritional needs.

**Packaging and storage**
Store below 40 °C (104 °F), preferably between 15 and 30 °C (59 and 86 °F), in a well-closed container, unless otherwise specified by manufacturer.

**Auxiliary labeling**
• Shake well before using.
• Drink a full glass of water.

Note: When taking as a phosphate binder in renal dialysis, patients should *not* be advised to take suspension with a glass of water.

### CALCIUM CARBONATE TABLETS USP

**Usual adult and adolescent dose**
Hypocalcemia (prophylaxis or treatment)—
  See *Calcium Carbonate Capsules*.
Antacid—
  See *Calcium Carbonate, Antacids (Oral-Local)*.
[Antihyperphosphatemic]—
  Oral, 5 to 13 grams (2 to 5.2 grams of calcium ion) a day, in divided doses with meals.
  Note: Careful titration is recommended to prevent hypercalcemia, which has been reported with doses above 2 grams of calcium ion a day.

**Usual pediatric dose**
See *Calcium Carbonate Oral Suspension USP*.

**Strength(s) usually available**
U.S.—
    650 mg (260 mg of calcium ion) (OTC) [GENERIC].
    667 mg (266.8 mg of calcium ion) (OTC) [*Calciday 667*].
    1 gram (OTC) [*Maalox Antacid Caplets*].
    1.25 grams (500 mg of calcium ion) (OTC) [*BioCal;* GENERIC].
    1.5 grams (600 mg of calcium ion) (OTC) [*Calcarb 600; Calcium 600; Cal-Plus; Caltrate 600; Gencalc 600; Nephro-Calci;* GENERIC].
Canada—
    625 mg (250 mg of calcium ion) (OTC) [*Apo-Cal*].
    1.25 grams (500 mg of calcium ion) (OTC) [*Apo-Cal*].
    1.5 grams (600 mg of calcium ion) (OTC) [*Caltrate 600;* GENERIC].
Note: Some strengths of these calcium preparations may exceed the dosage range recommended by USP DI Advisory Panels based on the amount necessary to meet normal nutritional needs.

**Packaging and storage**
Store below 40 °C (104 °F), preferably between 15 and 30 °C (59 and 86 °F), unless otherwise specified by manufacturer. Store in a well-closed container.

**Auxiliary labeling**
- Drink a full glass of water.

Note: When taking as a phosphate binder in renal dialysis, patients should *not* be advised to take tablets with a glass of water.

## CALCIUM CARBONATE TABLETS (CHEWABLE) USP

**Usual adult and adolescent dose**
Hypocalcemia (prophylaxis or treatment)—
    See *Calcium Carbonate Capsules*.
Antacid—
    See *Calcium Carbonate, Antacids (Oral-Local)*.
[Antihyperphosphatemic]—
    Oral, 5 to 13 grams (2 to 5.2 grams of calcium ion) a day, in divided doses with meals.
Note: Careful titration is recommended to prevent hypercalcemia, which has been reported with doses above 2 grams of calcium ion a day.

**Usual pediatric dose**
See *Calcium Carbonate Oral Suspension USP*.

**Strength(s) usually available**
U.S.—
    350 mg (140 mg calcium ion) (OTC) [*Amitone*].
    420 mg (168 mg of calcium ion) (OTC) [*Calcilac; Calglycine; Mallamint; Titralac*].
    500 mg (200 mg of calcium ion) (OTC) [*Chooz; Dicarbosil; Tums*].
    550 mg (220 mg of calcium ion) (OTC) [*Rolaids Calcium Rich*].
    750 mg (300 mg of calcium ion) (OTC) [*Caltrate Jr; Tums E-X*].
    850 mg (340 mg calcium ion) (OTC) [*Alka-Mints*].
    1.25 grams (500 mg of calcium ion) (OTC) [*Calci-Chew; OsCal 500 Chewable; Tums 500*].
    1.5 grams (600 mg of calcium ion) (OTC) [*Calcium 600*].
Canada—
    500 mg (200 mg of calcium ion) (OTC) [*Tums Regular Strength*].
    750 mg (300 mg of calcium ion) (OTC) [*Tums Extra Strength*].
    1250 mg (500 mg of calcium ion) (OTC) [*Calsan*].
Note: Some strengths of these calcium preparations may exceed the dosage range recommended by USP DI Advisory Panels based on the amount necessary to meet normal nutritional needs.

**Packaging and storage**
Store below 40 °C (104 °F), preferably between 15 and 30 °C (59 and 86 °F), unless otherwise specified by manufacturer. Store in a well-closed container.

**Auxiliary labeling**
- Chew tablets before swallowing.
- Drink a full glass of water.

Note: When taking as a phosphate binder in renal dialysis, patients should *not* be advised to take tablets with a glass of water.

## CALCIUM CARBONATE (OYSTER-SHELL DERIVED) TABLETS

**Usual adult and adolescent dose**
Hypocalcemia (prophylaxis or treatment)—
    See *Calcium Carbonate Capsules*.
Antacid—
    See *Calcium Carbonate, Antacids (Oral-Local)*.
[Antihyperphosphatemic]—
    Oral, 5 to 13 grams (2 to 5.2 grams of calcium ion) a day, in divided doses with meals.
Note: Careful titration is recommended to prevent hypercalcemia, which has been reported with doses above 2 grams of calcium ion a day.

**Usual pediatric dose**
Hypocalcemia (prophylaxis or treatment)—
    See *Calcium Carbonate Oral Suspension USP*.

**Strength(s) usually available**
U.S.—
    1.25 grams (500 mg of calcium ion) (OTC) [*Os-Cal 500; Oysco; Oyst-Cal 500; Oystercal 500;* GENERIC].
    1.562 grams (625 mg of calcium ion) (OTC) [GENERIC].
Canada—
    625 mg (250 mg of calcium ion) (OTC) [*Os-Cal*].
    1.25 grams (500 mg of calcium ion) (OTC) [*Calcite 500; Nu-Cal; Os-Cal*].
Note: Some strengths of these calcium preparations may exceed the dosage range recommended by USP DI Advisory Panels based on the amount necessary to meet normal nutritional needs.

**Packaging and storage**
Store below 40 °C (104 °F), preferably between 15 and 30 °C (59 and 86 °F), unless otherwise specified by manufacturer. Store in a well-closed container.

**Auxiliary labeling**
- Drink a full glass of water.

Note: When taking as a phosphate binder in renal dialysis, patients should *not* be advised to take tablets with a glass of water.

## CALCIUM CARBONATE (OYSTER-SHELL DERIVED) TABLETS (CHEWABLE)

**Usual adult and adolescent dose**
Antacid—
    See *Calcium Carbonate, Antacids (Oral-Local)*.
Hypocalcemia (prophylaxis or treatment)—
    See *Calcium Carbonate Capsules*.
[Antihyperphosphatemic]—
    Oral, 5 to 13 grams (2 to 5.2 grams of calcium ion) a day, in divided doses with meals.
Note: Careful titration is recommended to prevent hypercalcemia, which has been reported with doses above 2 grams of calcium ion a day.

**Usual pediatric dose**
See *Calcium Carbonate Oral Suspension USP*.

**Strength(s) usually available**
U.S.—
    1.25 grams (500 mg of calcium ion) (OTC) [*Oysco 500 Chewable;* GENERIC].
Canada—
    1.25 grams (500 mg of calcium ion) (OTC) [*Os-Cal Chewable*].
    1.875 grams (750 mg of calcium ion) (OTC) [*Os-Cal Chewable*].
Note: Some strengths of these calcium preparations may exceed the dosage range recommended by USP DI Advisory Panels based on the amount necessary to meet normal nutritional needs.

**Packaging and storage**
Store below 40 °C (104 °F), preferably between 15 and 30 °C (59 and 86 °F), unless otherwise specified by manufacturer. Store in a well-closed container.

**Auxiliary labeling**
- Chew tablets before swallowing.
- Drink a full glass of water.

Note: When taking as a phosphate binder in renal dialysis, patients should *not* be advised to take tablets with a glass of water.

---

### *CALCIUM CHLORIDE*

## Summary of Differences

Category: Also used as an electrolyte replenisher, a cardiotonic, an antihyperkalemic, and an antihypermagnesemic.

Precautions: Pediatrics—Parenteral calcium chloride use is usually restricted in pediatric patients due to possibility of irritation in small vasculature.

Side/adverse effects: Causes peripheral vasodilation with moderate decrease in blood pressure.

General dosing information: Has three times as much calcium per mL as calcium gluconate injection.

## Additional Dosing Information
See also *General Dosing Information*.

For intravenous use only; not to be administered intramuscularly, intramyocardially, subcutaneously, or permitted to extravasate into any body tissue; may cause severe tissue necrosis and/or sloughing and abscess formation.

Injected through a small-bore needle inserted into a large vein to minimize irritation.

Calcium chloride contains 272 mg of calcium ion per gram.

## Parenteral Dosage Forms
### CALCIUM CHLORIDE INJECTION USP
**Usual adult dose**
Hypocalcemia (prophylaxis)—
  Intravenous infusion, as part of total parenteral nutrition solutions, the specific amount determined by individual patient need.
Hypocalcemia (treatment) or
Electrolyte replenisher—
  Intravenous, 500 mg to 1 gram (136 to 272 mg of calcium ion) administered slowly at a rate not to exceed 0.5 mL (13.6 mg of calcium ion) to 1 mL (27.2 mg of calcium ion) a minute, the dosage being repeated at intervals of one to three days as indicated by patient response and serum calcium concentrations.
  Note: For use in cases such as hungry bones syndrome, some clinicians recommend that calcium chloride be diluted in saline or dextrose and given by continuous intravenous infusion at a dosage of 0.5 to 1 mg per minute (up to 2 or more mg per minute). The rate and/or concentration can be adjusted until oral calcium supplements can be given.
Cardiotonic—
  Intravenous, 500 mg to 1 gram (136 to 272 mg of calcium ion) administered at a rate not to exceed 1 mL (27.2 mg of calcium ion) a minute.
  Intraventricular, 200 to 800 mg (54.4 to 217.6 mg of calcium ion) administered directly into cavity as a single dose.
Note: Injection into the cardiac muscle must be avoided.
Antihyperkalemic—
  Dosage must be titrated by constant monitoring of ECG changes during administration.
Antihypermagnesemic—
  Intravenous, initially 500 mg (136 mg of calcium ion) repeated as indicated by patient response.

**Usual pediatric dose**
Hypocalcemia (treatment) or
Electrolyte replenisher—
  Intravenous, 25 mg (6.8 mg of calcium ion) per kg of body weight administered slowly.
Note: Calcium chloride injection is rarely used in pediatric patients, since a less irritating salt is preferred for use in the small vasculature.

**Strength(s) usually available**
U.S.—
  100 mg (27.2 mg [1.36 mEq] of calcium ion) per mL (Rx) [GENERIC].
Canada—
  100 mg (27.2 mg [1.36 mEq] of calcium ion) per mL (Rx) [*Calciject*; GENERIC].

**Packaging and storage**
Store below 40 °C (104 °F), preferably between 15 and 30 °C (59 and 86 °F), unless otherwise specified by manufacturer. Protect from freezing.

**Incompatibilities**
Calcium chloride is precipitated by carbonates or bicarbonates, phosphates, sulfates, and tartrates.

---
## CALCIUM CITRATE

## Summary of Differences
Indications:
  May reduce risk of kidney stones in susceptible patients.
  Also used to treat hyperphosphatenia in renal osteodystrophy.

## Additional Dosing Information
See also *General Dosing Information*.
Calcium citrate contains 211 mg of calcium ion per gram.

## Oral Dosage Forms
### CALCIUM CITRATE TABLETS
**Usual adult and adolescent dose**
Hypocalcemia (prophylaxis)—
  Oral, amount based on normal daily recommended intakes:

| Persons | U.S. (mg) | Canada (mg) |
|---|---|---|
| Adolescent and adult males | 800–1200 | 800–1100 |
| Adolescent and adult females | 800–1200 | 700–1100 |
| Pregnant females | 1200 | 1200–1500 |
| Breast-feeding females | 1200 | 1200–1500 |

Hypocalcemia (treatment)—
  Treatment dose is individualized by prescriber based on severity of deficiency.

**Usual pediatric dose**
Dosage form not appropriate for use in children.

**Strength(s) usually available**
U.S.—
  950 mg (200 mg of calcium ion) (OTC) [*Citracal*].
Canada—
  Not commercially available.
Note: The strength of this calcium preparation may exceed the dosage range recommended by USP DI Advisory Panels based on the amount necessary to meet normal nutritional needs.

**Packaging and storage**
Store below 40 °C (104 °F), preferably between 15 and 30 °C (59 and 86 °F), in a well-closed container, unless otherwise specified by manufacturer.

**Auxiliary labeling**
• Drink a full glass of water.

### CALCIUM CITRATE EFFERVESCENT TABLETS
**Usual adult and adolescent dose**
See *Calcium Citrate Tablets*.

**Usual pediatric dose**
Hypocalcemia (prophylaxis)—
  Oral, amount based on normal daily recommended intakes:

| Persons | U.S. (mg) | Canada (mg) |
|---|---|---|
| Infants and children | | |
| Birth to 3 years of age | 400–800 | 250–550 |
| 4 to 6 years of age | 800 | 600 |
| 7 to 10 years | 800 | 700–1100 |

Hypocalcemia (treatment)—
  Treatment dose is individualized by prescriber based on severity of deficiency.

**Strength(s) usually available**
U.S.—
  2.38 grams (500 mg calcium ion) (OTC) [*Citracal Liquitabs*].
Canada—
  Not commercially available.

**Packaging and storage**
Store below 40°C (104°F), preferably between 15 and 30 °C (59 and 86 °F), unless otherwise specified by manufacturer. Store in a tight container or original foil packaging.

**Auxiliary labeling**
• Take dissolved in glass of water.

---
## CALCIUM GLUBIONATE

## Oral Dosage Forms
### CALCIUM GLUBIONATE SYRUP USP
**Usual adult and adolescent dose**
Hypocalcemia (prophylaxis)—
  Oral, amount based on normal daily recommended intakes:

| Persons | U.S. (mg) | Canada (mg) |
|---|---|---|
| Adolescent and adult males | 800–1200 | 800–1100 |
| Adolescent and adult females | 800–1200 | 700–1100 |
| Pregnant females | 1200 | 1200–1500 |
| Breast-feeding females | 1200 | 1200–1500 |

Hypocalcemia (treatment)—
  Treatment dose is individualized by prescriber based on severity of deficiency

**Usual pediatric dose**
Hypocalcemia (prophylaxis)—
  Oral, amount based on normal daily recommended intakes:

| Persons | U.S. (mg) | Canada (mg) |
|---|---|---|
| Infants and children |  |  |
| Birth to 3 years of age | 400–800 | 250–550 |
| 4 to 6 years of age | 800 | 600 |
| 7 to 10 years | 800 | 700–1100 |

Hypocalcemia (treatment)—
  Treatment dose is individualized by prescriber based on severity of deficiency.

**Strength(s) usually available**
U.S.—
  1.8 grams (115 mg of calcium ion) per 5 mL (OTC) [*Calcionate; Neo-Calglucon*].
Canada—
  1.2 grams calcium lactobionate, 530 mg calcium gluconate (110 mg of calcium ion) per 5 mL (OTC) [*Calcium-Sandoz*].
Note: Some strengths of these calcium preparations may exceed the dosage range recommended by USP DI Advisory Panels based on the amount necessary to meet normal nutritional needs.

**Packaging and storage**
Store below 30 °C (86 °F) preferably between 15 and 30 °C (59 and 86 °F), unless otherwise specified by manufacturer. Store in a tight container. Protect from freezing.

## CALCIUM GLUCEPTATE

## Summary of Differences
Category: Also used as an electrolyte replenisher and as an antihypermagnesemic.
Precautions: Pediatrics—Administered intramuscularly to infants and children only in emergencies when intravenous route is technically impossible.

## Additional Dosing Information
See also *General Dosing Information*.
Calcium gluceptate contains 82 mg of calcium ion per gram.
May also be administered intramuscularly to adults.

## Parenteral Dosage Forms
Note: Bracketed uses in the *Dosage Forms* section refer to categories of use and/or indications that are not included in U.S. product labeling.

### CALCIUM GLUCEPTATE INJECTION USP
**Usual adult and adolescent dose**
Hypocalcemia (prophylaxis)—
  Intravenous infusion, as part of total parenteral nutrition solutions, the specific amount determined by individual patient need.
Hypocalcemia (treatment) or
Electrolyte replenisher—
  Intramuscular, 440 mg to 1.1 gram (36 to 90 mg of calcium ion).
  Note: When a dose of 5 mL (90 mg of calcium ion) or more is administered, injection should be in the gluteal region.
  Intravenous, 1.1 to 4.4 grams (90 to 360 mg of calcium ion) administered slowly at a rate not to exceed 2 mL (36 mg of calcium ion) a minute.
[Antihypermagnesemic]—
  Intravenous, initially 1.2 to 2.4 grams (98 to 196 mg of calcium ion) administered slowly at a rate not to exceed 2 mL (36 mg of calcium ion) a minute.

**Usual pediatric dose**
Hypocalcemia (prophylaxis)—
  Intravenous infusion, part of total parenteral nutrition solutions, the specific amount determined by individual patient need.
Hypocalcemia (treatment)—
  Intramuscular, 440 mg to 1.1 gram (36 to 90 mg of calcium ion).
  Note: Calcium gluceptate may be administered intramuscularly to infants and children only in emergencies when intravenous administration is impossible.

When a dose of 5 mL (90 mg of calcium ion) or more is administered to infants, injection should be administered in the lateral thigh.
  Intravenous, 440 mg to 1.1 gram (36 to 90 mg of calcium ion) as a single dose, administered at a rate not to exceed 2 mL (36 mg of calcium ion) a minute.
Exchange transfusions in newborns—
  Intravenous, 110 mg (9 mg of calcium ion) after every 100 mL of blood exchanged.

**Strength(s) usually available**
U.S.—
  220 mg (18 mg [0.9 mEq] of calcium ion) per mL (Rx) [GENERIC].
Canada—
  Not commercially available.

**Packaging and storage**
Store below 38 °C (100 °F), preferably between 15 and 30 °C (59 and 86 °F), unless otherwise specified by manufacturer. Store in a tight container. Protect from freezing.

**Stability**
Do not use if crystals are present.
Discard unused portion.

**Incompatibilities**
Calcium gluceptate is precipitated by carbonates or bicarbonates, phosphates, sulfates, and tartrates.

## CALCIUM GLUCEPTATE AND CALCIUM GLUCONATE

## Oral Dosage Forms

### CALCIUM GLUCEPTATE AND CALCIUM GLUCONATE ORAL SOLUTION
**Usual adult and adolescent dose**
Hypocalcemia (prophylaxis)—
  Oral, amount based on normal daily recommended intakes:

| Persons | U.S. (mg) | Canada (mg) |
|---|---|---|
| Adolescent and adult males | 800–1200 | 800–1100 |
| Adolescent and adult females | 800–1200 | 700–1100 |
| Pregnant females | 1200 | 1200–1500 |
| Breast-feeding females | 1200 | 1200–1500 |

Hypocalcemia (treatment)—
  Treatment dose is individualized by prescriber based on severity of deficiency.

**Usual pediatric dose**
Hypocalcemia (prophylaxis)—
  Oral, amount based on normal daily recommended intakes:

| Persons | U.S. (mg) | Canada (mg) |
|---|---|---|
| Infants and children |  |  |
| Birth to 3 years of age | 400–800 | 250–550 |
| 4 to 6 years of age | 800 | 600 |
| 7 to 10 years | 800 | 700–1100 |

Hypocalcemia (treatment)—
  Treatment dose is individualized by prescriber based on severity of deficiency.

**Strength(s) usually available**
U.S.—
  Not commercially available.
Canada—
  660 mg calcium gluceptate, and 560 mg calcium gluconate (total of 100 mg of calcium ion) per 5 mL (OTC) [*Calcium Stanley*].
Note: The strength of this calcium preparation may exceed the dosage range recommended by USP DI Advisory Panels based on the amount necessary to meet normal nutritional needs.

**Packaging and storage**
Store below 40 °C (104 °F), preferably between 15 and 30 °C (59 and 86 °F), unless otherwise specified by manufacturer.

## CALCIUM GLUCONATE

## Summary of Differences
Category: Injection may also be used as an electrolyte replenisher, a cardiotonic, an antihyperkalemic, and an antihypermagnesemic.

## Additional Dosing Information
See also *General Dosing Information*.

Calcium gluconate injection is for intravenous use only; it is not to be administered intramuscularly, intramyocardially, subcutaneously, or permitted to extravasate into any body tissue; may cause severe tissue necrosis and/or sloughing, and abscess formation.

Calcium gluconate contains 90 mg of calcium ion per gram.

## Oral Dosage Forms

### CALCIUM GLUCONATE TABLETS USP

**Usual adult and adolescent dose**
Hypocalcemia (prophylaxis)—
    Oral, amount based on normal daily recommended intakes:

| Persons | U.S. (mg) | Canada (mg) |
|---|---|---|
| Adolescent and adult males | 800–1200 | 800–1100 |
| Adolescent and adult females | 800–1200 | 700–1100 |
| Pregnant females | 1200 | 1200–1500 |
| Breast-feeding females | 1200 | 1200–1500 |

Hypocalcemia (treatment)—
    Treatment dose is individualized by prescriber based on severity of deficiency.

**Usual pediatric dose**
Dosage form not appropriate for use in children.

**Strength(s) usually available**
U.S.—
    325 mg (OTC) [GENERIC].
    500 mg (45 mg of calcium ion) (OTC) [GENERIC].
    650 mg (58.5 mg of calcium ion) (OTC) [GENERIC].
    975 mg (87.75 mg of calcium ion) (OTC) [GENERIC].
    1 gram (90 mg of calcium ion) (OTC) [GENERIC].
Canada—
    650 mg (60 mg of calcium ion) (OTC) [GENERIC].

Note: Some strengths of these calcium preparations may exceed the dosage range recommended by USP DI Advisory Panels based on the amount necessary to meet normal nutritional needs.

### CALCIUM GLUCONATE TABLETS (CHEWABLE) USP

**Usual adult and adolescent dose**
Hypocalcemia (prophylaxis)—
    Oral, amount based on normal daily recommended intakes:

| Persons | U.S. (mg) | Canada (mg) |
|---|---|---|
| Adolescent and adult males | 800–1200 | 800–1100 |
| Adolescent and adult females | 800–1200 | 700–1100 |
| Pregnant females | 1200 | 1200–1500 |
| Breast-feeding females | 1200 | 1200–1500 |

Hypocalcemia (treatment)—
    Treatment dose is individualized by prescriber based on severity of deficiency.

**Usual pediatric dose**
Hypocalcemia (prophylaxis)—
    Oral, amount based on normal daily recommended intakes:

| Persons | U.S. (mg) | Canada (mg) |
|---|---|---|
| Infants and children | | |
|   Birth to 3 years of age | 400–800 | 250–550 |
|   4 to 6 years of age | 800 | 600 |
|   7 to 10 years | 800 | 700–1100 |

Hypocalcemia (treatment)—
    Treatment dose is individualized by prescriber based on severity of deficiency.

**Strength(s) usually available**
U.S.—
    650 mg (58.5 mg of calcium ion) (OTC) [GENERIC].
    1 gram (90 mg of calcium ion) (OTC) [GENERIC].
Canada—
    Not commercially available.

Note: Some strengths of these calcium preparations may exceed the dosage range recommended by USP DI Advisory Panels based on the amount necessary to meet normal nutritional needs.

**Packaging and storage**
Store below 40 °C (104 °F), preferably between 15 and 30 °C (59 and 86 °F), unless otherwise specified by manufacturer. Store in a well-closed container.

**Auxiliary labeling**
- Chew tablets before swallowing.
- Drink a full glass of water.

## Parenteral Dosage Forms
Note: Bracketed uses in the *Dosage Forms* section refer to categories of use and/or indications that are not included in U.S. product labeling.

### CALCIUM GLUCONATE INJECTION USP

**Usual adult dose**
Hypocalcemia (prophylaxis)—
    Intravenous infusion, as part of total parenteral nutrition solutions, the specific amount determined by individual patient need.
Hypocalcemia (treatment) or
Electrolyte replenisher—
    Intravenous, 970 mg (94.7 mg of calcium ion), administered slowly at a rate not to exceed 5 mL (47.5 mg of calcium ion) a minute. The dosage may be repeated, if necessary, until tetany is controlled.
Note: For use in cases such as hungry bones syndrome, some clinicians recommend that calcium gluconate be diluted in isotonic solution and given by continuous intravenous infusion at a dosage of 0.5 to 1 mg per minute (up to 2 or more mg per minute). The rate and/or concentration can be adjusted until oral calcium supplements can be given.
Antihyperkalemic—
    Intravenous, 1 to 2 grams (94.7 to 189 mg of calcium ion), administered slowly at a rate not to exceed 5 mL (47.5 mg of calcium ion) a minute, the dosage being titrated and adjusted by constant monitoring of ECG changes during administration.
[Antihypermagnesemic]—
    Intravenous, 1 to 2 grams (94.7 to 189 mg of calcium ion), administered at a rate not to exceed 5 mL (47.5 mg of calcium ion) a minute.

**Usual adult prescribing limits**
15 grams (1.42 gram of calcium ion) a day.

**Usual pediatric dose**
Hypocalcemia (prophylaxis)—
    Intravenous infusion, as part of total parenteral nutrition solutions, the specific amount determined by individual patient need.
Hypocalcemia (treatment)—
    Intravenous, 200 to 500 mg (19.5 to 48.8 mg of calcium ion) as a single dose, administered slowly at a rate not to exceed 5 mL (47.5 mg of calcium ion) a minute, repeated if necessary until tetany is controlled.
Exchange transfusions in newborns—
    Intravenous, 97 mg (9.5 mg of calcium ion) administered after every 100 mL of citrated blood exchanged.

**Strength(s) usually available**
U.S.—
    100 mg (9.3 mg [0.465 mEq] of calcium ion) per mL (Rx) [GENERIC].
Canada—
    100 mg (9.3 mg [0.465 mEq] of calcium ion) per mL (Rx) [GENERIC].

**Packaging and storage**
Store below 40 °C (104 °F), preferably between 15 and 30 °C (59 and 86 °F), unless otherwise specified by manufacturer. Protect from freezing.

**Stability**
Only clear solutions should be administered. If any crystals form, they may be redissolved by warming to 30 to 40 °C (86 to 104 °F).

**Incompatibilities**
Calcium gluconate is precipitated by carbonates or bicarbonates, phosphates, sulfates, and tartrates.

**Additional information**
Injection also contains 3.5 mg of calcium d-saccharate tetrahydrate per mL for stabilization.

## CALCIUM GLYCEROPHOSPHATE AND CALCIUM LACTATE

### Additional Dosing Information
See also *General Dosing Information*.

Intramuscular administration does not produce inflammation or sloughing at site of injection.

### Parenteral Dosage Forms

#### CALCIUM GLYCEROPHOSPHATE AND CALCIUM LACTATE INJECTION

**Usual adult and adolescent dose**
Hypocalcemia (prophylaxis)—
  Intravenous infusion, as part of total parenteral nutrition solutions, the specific amount determined by individual patient need.
Hypocalcemia (treatment)—
  Intramuscular, initially 10 mL one or two times a week for four to five weeks, the dosage being repeated as needed to raise serum calcium concentrations.

**Usual pediatric dose**
Dosage has not been established.

**Strength(s) usually available**
U.S.—
  5 mg of calcium glycerophosphate and 5 mg of calcium lactate (0.08 mEq of calcium ion) per mL (Rx) [*Calphosan* (in sodium chloride solution; 0.25% phenol)].
Canada—
  Not commercially available.

**Packaging and storage**
Store below 40 °C (104 °F), preferably between 15 and 30 °C (59 and 86 °F), unless otherwise specified by manufacturer. Protect from light. Protect from freezing.

**Note**
May also be administered intravenously or subcutaneously because of neutral pH (approximately 7).

**Additional information**
Contains phenol 0.25% as a preservative.

## CALCIUM LACTATE

### Additional Dosing Information
See also *General Dosing Information*.

Calcium lactate contains 130 mg of calcium ion per gram.

### Oral Dosage Forms

#### CALCIUM LACTATE TABLETS USP

**Usual adult and adolescent dose**
Hypocalcemia (prophylaxis)—
  Oral, amount based on normal daily recommended intakes:

| Persons | U.S. (mg) | Canada (mg) |
|---|---|---|
| Adolescent and adult males | 800–1200 | 800–1100 |
| Adolescent and adult females | 800–1200 | 700–1100 |
| Pregnant females | 1200 | 1200–1500 |
| Breast-feeding females | 1200 | 1200–1500 |

Hypocalcemia (treatment)—
  Treatment dose is individualized by prescriber based on severity of deficiency.

**Usual pediatric dose**
Hypocalcemia (prophylaxis)—
  Oral, amount based on normal daily recommended intakes:

| Persons | U.S. (mg) | Canada (mg) |
|---|---|---|
| Infants and children | | |
|   Birth to 3 years of age | 400–800 | 250–550 |
|   4 to 6 years of age | 800 | 600 |
|   7 to 10 years | 800 | 700–1100 |

Hypocalcemia (treatment)—
  Treatment dose is individualized by prescriber based on severity of deficiency.

**Strength(s) usually available**
U.S.—
  325 mg (42.25 mg of calcium ion) (OTC) [GENERIC].
  650 mg (84.5 mg of calcium ion) (OTC) [GENERIC].
Canada—
  650 mg (84.5 mg of calcium ion) (OTC) [GENERIC].

Note: Some strengths of these calcium preparations may exceed the dosage range recommended by USP DI Advisory Panels based on the amount necessary to meet normal nutritional needs.

**Packaging and storage**
Store below 40 °C (104 °F), preferably between 15 and 30 °C (59 and 86 °F), unless otherwise specified by manufacturer. Store in a tight container.

**Auxiliary labeling**
• Drink a full glass of water.

## CALCIUM LACTATE-GLUCONATE AND CALCIUM CARBONATE

### Oral Dosage Forms

#### CALCIUM LACTATE-GLUCONATE AND CALCIUM CARBONATE EFFERVESCENT TABLETS

**Usual adult and adolescent dose**
Hypocalcemia (prophylaxis)—
  Oral, amount based on normal daily recommended intakes:

| Persons | U.S. (mg) | Canada (mg) |
|---|---|---|
| Adolescent and adult males | 800–1200 | 800–1100 |
| Adolescent and adult females | 800–1200 | 700–1100 |
| Pregnant females | 1200 | 1200–1500 |
| Breast-feeding females | 1200 | 1200–1500 |

Hypocalcemia (treatment)—
  Treatment dose is individualized by prescriber based on severity of deficiency.

**Usual pediatric dose**
Hypocalcemia (prophylaxis)—
  Oral, amount based on normal daily recommended intakes:

| Persons | U.S. (mg) | Canada (mg) |
|---|---|---|
| Infants and children | | |
|   Birth to 3 years of age | 400–800 | 250–550 |
|   4 to 6 years of age | 800 | 600 |
|   7 to 10 years | 800 | 700–1100 |

Hypocalcemia (treatment)—
  Treatment dose is individualized by prescriber based on severity of deficiency.

**Strength(s) usually available**
U.S.—
  Not commercially available.
Canada—
  2.37 grams calcium lactate-gluconate, and 1.75 grams calcium carbonate (total of 1000 mg of calcium ion) (OTC) [*Gramcal*].
  2.94 grams calcium lactate-gluconate, and 300 mg calcium carbonate (total of 500 mg of calcium ion) (OTC) [*Calcium-Sandoz Forte*].

Note: Some strengths of these calcium preparations may exceed the dosage range recommended by USP DI Advisory Panels based on the amount necessary to meet normal nutritional needs.

**Packaging and storage**
Store below 40 °C (104 °F), preferably between 15 and 30 °C (59 and 86 °F), in a well-closed container, unless otherwise specified by manufacturer.

## DIBASIC CALCIUM PHOSPHATE

### Summary of Differences
Medical considerations/contraindications:
  Calcium absorption may be decreased in patients with achlorhydria or hypochlorhydria, unless the supplement is taken with meals.
  Risk of hyperphosphatemia may be increased in patients with hypoparathyroidism or renal insufficiency.

## Additional Dosing Information
See also *General Dosing Information*.
Dibasic calcium phosphate contains 230 mg of calcium ion per gram.

## Oral Dosage Forms
### DIBASIC CALCIUM PHOSPHATE TABLETS USP
**Usual adult and adolescent dose**
Hypocalcemia (prophylaxis)—
　Oral, amount based on normal daily recommended intakes:

| Persons | U.S. (mg) | Canada (mg) |
|---|---|---|
| Adolescent and adult males | 800–1200 | 800–1100 |
| Adolescent and adult females | 800–1200 | 700–1100 |
| Pregnant females | 1200 | 1200–1500 |
| Breast-feeding females | 1200 | 1200–1500 |

Hypocalcemia (treatment)—
　Treatment dose is individualized by prescriber based on severity of deficiency.

**Usual pediatric dose**
Hypocalcemia (prophylaxis)—
　Oral, amount based on normal daily recommended intakes:

| Persons | U.S. (mg) | Canada (mg) |
|---|---|---|
| Infants and children | | |
| 　Birth to 3 years of age | 400–800 | 250–550 |
| 　4 to 6 years of age | 800 | 600 |
| 　7 to 10 years | 800 | 700–1100 |

Hypocalcemia (treatment)—
　Treatment dose is individualized by prescriber based on severity of deficiency.

**Strength(s) usually available**
U.S.—
　500 mg (115 mg of calcium ion) (OTC) [GENERIC].
Canada—
　Not commercially available.

Note: The strength of this calcium preparation may exceed the dosage range recommended by USP DI Advisory Panels based on the amount necessary to meet normal nutritional needs.

**Packaging and storage**
Store below 40 °C (104 °F), preferably between 15 and 30 °C (59 and 86 °F), unless otherwise specified by manufacturer. Store in a well-closed container.

**Auxiliary labeling**
• Drink a full glass of water.

---

### TRIBASIC CALCIUM PHOSPHATE

## Summary of Differences
Medical considerations/contraindications:
　Calcium absorption may be decreased in patients with achlorhydria or hypochlorhydria, unless the supplement is taken with meals.

Risk of hyperphosphatemia may be increased in patients with hypoparathyroidism or renal insufficiency.

## Additional Dosing Information
See also *General Dosing Information*.
Tribasic calcium phosphate contains 380 mg of calcium ion per gram.

## Oral Dosage Forms
### TRIBASIC CALCIUM PHOSPHATE TABLETS
**Usual adult dose**
Hypocalcemia (prophylaxis)—
　Oral, amount based on normal daily recommended intakes:

| Persons | U.S. (mg) | Canada (mg) |
|---|---|---|
| Adolescent and adult males | 800–1200 | 800–1100 |
| Adolescent and adult females | 800–1200 | 700–1100 |
| Pregnant females | 1200 | 1200–1500 |
| Breast-feeding females | 1200 | 1200–1500 |

Hypocalcemia (treatment)—
　Treatment dose is individualized by prescriber based on severity of deficiency.

**Usual pediatric dose**
Hypocalcemia (prophylaxis)—
　Oral, amount based on normal daily recommended intakes:

| Persons | U.S. (mg) | Canada (mg) |
|---|---|---|
| Infants and children | | |
| 　Birth to 3 years of age | 400–800 | 250–550 |
| 　4 to 6 years of age | 800 | 600 |
| 　7 to 10 years | 800 | 700–1100 |

Hypocalcemia (treatment)—
　Treatment dose is individualized by prescriber based on severity of deficiency.

**Strength(s) usually available**
U.S.—
　1.6 grams (600 mg of calcium ion) (OTC) [*Posture*].
Canada—
　Not commercially available.

Note: The strength of this calcium preparation may exceed the dosage range recommended by USP DI Advisory Panels based on the amount necessary to meet normal nutritional needs.

**Packaging and storage**
Store below 40 °C (104 °F), preferably between 15 and 30 °C (59 and 86 °F), in a well-closed container, unless otherwise specified by manufacturer.

**Auxiliary labeling**
• Drink a full glass of water.

Revised: 06/10/92
Interim revision: 08/22/94; 07/18/95

---

# CAPECITABINE   Systemic—INTRODUCTORY VERSION

VA CLASSIFICATION (Primary): AN300
Commonly used brand name(s): *Xeloda*.
Note: For a listing of dosage forms and brand names by country availability, see *Dosage Forms* section(s).

## Category
Antineoplastic.

## Indications
**Accepted**
Carcinoma, breast (treatment)—Capecitabine is indicated for treatment of metastatic breast carcinoma that is resistant to both paclitaxel and an anthracycline-containing chemotherapy regimen (i.e., has progressed during, or relapsed within 6 months following completion of, treatment). It is also indicated for treating patients whose disease is resistant to paclitaxel and who should not receive further anthracycline therapy (for example, patients who have received cumulative doses of 400 mg per square meter of body surface area of doxorubicin or doxorubicin equivalents).

## Pharmacology/Pharmacokinetics
**Physicochemical characteristics**
Chemical group—A fluoropyrimidine carbamate.
Molecular weight—359.35.
Solubility—In water: 26 mg per mL at 20 °C.

**Mechanism of action/Effect**
Capecitabine is relatively noncytotoxic *in vitro*; its activity occurs after *in vivo* conversion to 5-fluorouracil (5-FU; fluorouracil), which in turn is converted to two active metabolites, 5-fluoro-2-deoxyuridine monophosphate (FdUMP) and 5-fluorouridine triphosphate (FUTP). The cytotoxic effect is produced by two different mechanisms. First, FdUMP

and the folate cofactor $N^{5\text{-}10}$-methylenetetrahydrofolate bind to thymidylate synthase to form a ternary complex, thereby inhibiting thymidylate formation. Thymidylate is the precursor of thymidine triphosphate, which is essential for DNA synthesis; deficiency of this precursor leads to inhibition of cell division. Second, nuclear transcriptional enzymes can incorporate FUTP instead of uridine triphosphate during RNA synthesis, resulting in a metabolic error that interferes with RNA processing and protein synthesis.

**Absorption**
Readily absorbed. Both the rate and extent of absorption are decreased by concurrent administration with food.

**Protein binding**
Moderate (less than 60%), primarily to albumin (approximately 35%). Binding is not concentration-dependent.

**Biotransformation**
Capecitabine—
  Initially hepatic, hydrolyzed via a carboxyesterase to 5'-deoxy-5-fluorocytidine (5'-DFCR), which in turn is first converted to 5'-deoxy-5-fluorouridine (5'-DFUR) and then hydrolyzed to the active substance, fluorouracil, by cytidine deaminase and thymidine phosphorylase, respectively. These enzymes are found in most tissues, including tumors. Thymidine phosphorylase is expressed in higher concentrations by some human carcinomas than by surrounding normal tissues.
Fluorouracil—
  Metabolized in normal and tumor cells to the active metabolites FdUMP and FUTP. Also, metabolized by dihydropyrimidine dehydrogenase to 5-fluoro-5,6-dihydro-fluorouracil ($FUH_2$), which is much less toxic. This compound is further metabolized by cleavage of the pyrimidine ring to yield 5-fluoro-ureido-propionic acid (FUPA), which undergoes further cleavage to produce alpha-fluoro-beta-alanine (FBAL).

**Half-life**
Elimination—
  For both capecitabine and fluorouracil: Approximately 45 minutes.

**Time to peak concentration**
In blood—Approximately 1.5 hours for capecitabine and 2 hours for fluorouracil. Peak concentrations of both substances are delayed by 1.5 hours when capecitabine is administered concurrently with food.

**Peak blood concentration**
There is wide interpatient variability (> 85%) in the maximum concentration ($C_{max}$) and area under the plasma concentration–time curve (AUC) for fluorouracil.
In studies with doses ranging between 500 and 3500 mg per square meter of body surface area (mg/m²) per day, the pharmacokinetics of capecitabine and 5'-DFCR were dose-proportional and did not change over time. However, the increases in the AUCs of fluorouracil and 5'-DFUR were greater than proportional to the increase in dose, and the AUC of fluorouracil was 34% higher on day 14 than on day 1. In 13 patients with mild to moderate hepatic function impairment given single doses of 1255 mg/m² of capecitabine, $C_{max}$ and AUC values for the parent compound were 60% higher than in patients with normal hepatic function, but values for fluorouracil were not affected.
When capecitabine is administered concurrently with food, $C_{max}$ values for capecitabine and fluorouracil are decreased by 60% and 35%, respectively, and AUC values are reduced by 43% and 21%, respectively.

**Elimination**
Renal, more than 70% of a capecitabine dose as drug-related species (approximately 50% as FBAL).
In dialysis—
  Although there is no clinical experience, it is possible that 5'-DFUR (the low–molecular weight capecitabine metabolite that is the immediate precursor of fluorouracil) may be removable by dialysis.

## Precautions to Consider

**Cross-sensitivity and/or related problems**
Patients sensitive to fluorouracil may also be sensitive to capecitabine.

**Carcinogenicity**
Long-term studies in animals have not been done.

**Mutagenicity**
Capecitabine was not found to be mutagenic in in vitro bacterial tests (Ames test) or in mammalian cells (Chinese hamster V79/HPRT gene mutation assay). It was clastogenic to human peripheral blood lymphocytes in vitro but not to mouse bone marrow (micronucleus test) in vivo.
Fluorouracil causes mutations in bacteria and yeast and causes chromosomal abnormalities in the mouse micronucleus test in vivo.

**Pregnancy/Reproduction**
Fertility—Studies in female mice given oral doses of 760 mg per kg of body weight (mg/kg) per day found a reversible disturbance of estrus and a subsequent decrease in fertility; in mice that did become pregnant, no fetuses survived. The same dose in male mice produced degenerative changes in the testes, including decreases in the number of spermatocytes and spermatids. In mice, this dose produces area under the plasma concentration–time curve (AUC) values for the immediate precursor of fluorouracil (5'-deoxy-5-fluorouridine [5'-DFUR]) that are approximately 0.7 times the corresponding values in humans taking the recommended daily dose.
Pregnancy—Adequate and well-controlled studies in women have not been done. It is recommended that women of childbearing potential be advised to avoid becoming pregnant during treatment because of the potential risks to the fetus. Also, if the medication is used during pregnancy, or the patient becomes pregnant during treatment, the patient should be informed of the potential risks.
Capecitabine caused teratogenicity (cleft palate, anophthalmia, microphthalmia, oligodactyly, polydactyly, syndactyly, kinky tail, dilation of cerebral ventricles) and embryolethality in mice given doses of 198 mg/kg per day (producing AUC values for 5'-DFUR approximately 0.2 times the corresponding value in humans taking the recommended daily dose) during the period of organogenesis. It also caused fetal deaths in monkeys given 90 mg/kg per day (producing AUC values for 5'-DFUR approximately 0.6 times the corresponding value in humans taking the recommended daily dose) during organogenesis.
FDA Pregnancy Category D.

**Breast-feeding**
It is not known whether capecitabine is distributed into breast milk. However, breast-feeding is not recommended during treatment because of the potential risks to the infant.

**Pediatrics**
Studies on the relationship of age to the effects of capecitabine have not been performed in the pediatric population. Safety and efficacy in patients younger than 18 years of age have not been established.

**Geriatrics**
Geriatric patients may be pharmacodynamically more sensitive to the toxic effects of fluorouracil than younger adults. In particular, the risk of severe (National Cancer Institute [NCI] grade 3 or 4) gastrointestinal adverse effects (diarrhea, nausea, vomiting) may be increased in patients 80 years of age and older. Careful monitoring is recommended. Pharmacokinetic studies have not been performed in the geriatric population.

**Dental**
Capecitabine may cause stomatitis. In clinical trials, stomatitis occurred in up to 24%, and was severe enough to decrease food intake substantially (NCI grade 3) in 4 to 7%, of the patients.

**Drug interactions and/or related problems**
The following drug interactions and/or related problems have been selected on the basis of their potential clinical significance (possible mechanism in parentheses where appropriate)—not necessarily inclusive (» = major clinical significance):

Note: Combinations containing any of the following medications, depending on the amount present, may also interact with this medication.

Antacids, aluminum and magnesium–containing
  (administration of an aluminum and magnesium–containing antacid immediately after capecitabine in 12 patients produced small increases in blood concentrations of capecitabine and the metabolite 5'-deoxy-5-fluorocytidine [5'-DFCR], but did not affect the concentrations of other major metabolites)

Leucovorin
  (concurrent use may increase the therapeutic and toxic effects of fluorouracil as a result of increased concentrations; fatalities as a result of severe enterocolitis, diarrhea, and dehydration have been reported in elderly patients who received the two medications concurrently)

**Laboratory value alterations**
The following have been selected on the basis of their potential clinical significance (possible effect in parentheses where appropriate)—not necessarily inclusive (» = major clinical significance):

With physiology/laboratory test values
  Alkaline phosphatase and
  Alanine aminotransferase (ALT [SGPT]) and
  Aspartate aminotransferase (AST [SGOT]) and

Bilirubin
(elevations of serum bilirubin and concurrent increases in alkaline phosphatase and/or transaminase concentrations may occur, especially in patients with hepatic metastases)

### Medical considerations/Contraindications
The medical considerations/contraindications included have been selected on the basis of their potential clinical significance (reasons given in parentheses where appropriate)—not necessarily inclusive (» = major clinical significance).

*Risk-benefit should be considered when the following medical problems exist:*

Coronary artery disease, history of
(fluorinated pyrimidine therapy has been associated with cardiotoxicity, which may be more common in patients with a prior history of coronary artery disease)

» Hepatic function impairment
(caution is recommended because blood concentrations and AUC values for capecitabine may be increased, and the risk of grade 3 or 4 hyperbilirubinemia with concurrent increases in alkaline phosphatase and/or transaminases is higher, in patients with mild to moderate hepatic function impairment due to hepatic metastases; no information is available for patients with severe hepatic function impairment)

Sensitivity to capecitabine or fluorouracil

### Patient monitoring
The following may be especially important in patient monitoring (other tests may be warranted in some patients, depending on condition; » = major clinical significance):

Hepatic function
(monitoring recommended in patients with pre-existing hepatic function impairment because of the increased risk of hyperbilirubinemia and associated increases in alkaline phosphatase and/or transaminase values; temporary withdrawal of treatment is recommended if hyperbilirubinemia of NCI grade 2 [serum bilirubin 1.5 times normal values] or higher occurs. If treatment is reinstated after hyperbilirubinemia has resolved, a reduction in dosage may be needed)

## Side/Adverse Effects

The following side/adverse effects have been selected on the basis of their potential clinical significance (possible signs and symptoms in parentheses where appropriate)—not necessarily inclusive:

### Those indicating need for medical attention
Incidence more frequent

*Abdominal or stomach pain; anemia* (unusual tiredness or weakness)—usually asymptomatic; *diarrhea, moderate or severe; hand-and-foot syndrome* (blistering, peeling, redness, and/or swelling of palms of hands or bottoms of feet; numbness, pain, tingling, or unusual sensations in palms of hands or bottoms of feet); *neutropenia*—usually asymptomatic; *stomatitis* (pain, redness, and/or swelling in mouth and on lips; sores or ulcers in mouth and on lips); *thrombocytopenia*—usually asymptomatic

Note: *Diarrhea* is one of the dose-limiting toxicities of capecitabine. It may be severe and lead to dehydration. In clinical trials, diarrhea of any grade occurred in at least 50% of the patients, but was severe in relatively few, with National Cancer Institute (NCI) grades 3 and 4 diarrhea occurring in fewer than 12% and 3% of the patients, respectively. The median time to first occurrence of NCI grade 2 or higher diarrhea was 31 (range, 1 to 322) days.

*Hand-and-foot syndrome* (also known as palmar-plantar erythrodysesthesia or chemotherapy-induced acral erythema) may result in severe discomfort that interferes with the patient's ability to work or perform activities of daily living. A reaction of such severity requires immediate medical attention.

Bone marrow depression during treatment with capecitabine resulted in *anemia, neutropenia,* or *thrombocytopenia* in up to 74%, 26%, and 24%, respectively, of the patients in clinical trials. However, each of these hematologic toxicities reached a severity of NCI grade 3 or 4 in only 4% or fewer, and grade 3 or 4 coagulation disorders, pancytopenia, or thrombocytopenic purpura each occurred in only 0.2%, of the patients.

Incidence less frequent or rare

*Angina pectoris* (chest pain); *ataxia* (clumsiness or unsteadiness; problems with coordination); *bronchospasm; dyspnea; or respiratory distress* (shortness of breath, troubled breathing, tightness in chest, or wheezing); *cardiomyopathy* (fast or irregular heartbeat; shortness of breath or troubled breathing; tiredness or weakness, severe); *cholestatic hepatitis; hepatic fibrosis; or hepatitis* (dark urine; fever; itching; light-colored stools; pain, tenderness, and/or swelling in upper abdominal area; skin rash; swollen glands; yellow eyes or skin); *edema* (swelling of face, fingers, feet, or lower legs); *epistaxis* (unexplained nosebleeds); *fever; gastrointestinal tract toxicity* (abdominal or stomach cramping or pain, severe; bloody or black, tarry stools; constipation or diarrhea, severe; difficulty in swallowing or pain in back of throat or chest when swallowing; vomiting blood or material that looks like coffee grounds); *hypotension* (decreased blood pressure); *hypertension* (increased blood pressure); *infection* (cough or hoarseness; fever or chills; lower back or side pain; painful or difficult urination; sneezing; sore throat; stuffy nose; white spots in mouth or throat)—rarely, may be associated with neutropenia; *nausea*—severe enough to cause loss of appetite; *phlebitis; thrombophlebitis; or deep vein thrombosis* (hot, red skin on feet or legs; painful, swollen feet or legs); *pulmonary embolism* (shortness of breath or troubled breathing; pain in chest); *thrombocytopenic purpura* (unusual bleeding or bruising; black, tarry stools; blood in urine or stools; pinpoint red spots on skin); *vomiting*—two or more episodes in 24 hours

Note: *Gastrointestinal toxicity* may affect any area of the gastrointestinal tract and may result in colitis, duodenitis, esophagitis, gastritis, gastrointestinal or rectal bleeding, hematemesis, intestinal obstruction, or necrotizing enterocolitis.

Reported *infections* include oral, esophageal, or gastrointestinal candidiasis; upper respiratory tract infection; urinary tract infection; bronchitis, pneumonia, or bronchopneumonia; and sepsis. Each of these occurred in fewer than 5%, and was severe (NCI grade 3 or 4) in only 0.2% (0.4% for sepsis), of the patients in clinical trials.

Reported neurologic effects (in addition to *ataxia*) include decrease or loss of consciousness and encephalopathy.

### Those indicating need for medical attention only if they continue or are bothersome
Incidence more frequent

*Constipation, mild or moderate; dermatitis* (skin rash or itching); *diarrhea, mild; loss of appetite; nausea; unusual tiredness; vomiting*

Note: NCI grade 2 or greater *nausea* or *vomiting* requires immediate medical attention.

Incidence less frequent

*Changes in fingernails or toenails; dizziness; dyspepsia* (heartburn); *eye irritation* (red, sore eyes); *headache; insomnia* (trouble in sleeping); *myalgia* (muscle pain); *photosensitivity* (increased sensitivity of skin to sunlight); *radiation recall syndrome* (pain and redness of skin at place of earlier radiation treatment)

## Overdose

For more information on the management of overdose or unintentional ingestion, **contact a Poison Control Center** (see *Poison Control Center Listing*).

### Clinical effects of overdose
The following effects have been selected on the basis of their potential clinical significance (possible signs and symptoms in parentheses where appropriate)—not necessarily inclusive:

Acute and chronic

*Bone marrow depression* (black, tarry stools; blood in urine or stools; cough or hoarseness; fever or chills; lower back or side pain; painful or difficult urination; pinpoint red spots on skin; unusual bleeding or bruising); *gastrointestinal tract toxicity* (abdominal or stomach pain, severe; bloody or black, tarry stools; constipation or diarrhea, severe; difficulty in swallowing or pain in back of throat or chest when swallowing; nausea or vomiting, severe; vomiting blood or material that looks like coffee grounds)

### Treatment of overdose
Supportive care—Appropriate care to address the clinical manifestations.

Dialysis may be effective in removing circulating 5'-DFUR, the low-molecular weight metabolite that is the immediate precursor of fluorouracil.

## Patient Consultation

As an aid to patient consultation, refer to *Advice for the Patient, Capecitabine (Systemic—Introductory Version)*

In providing consultation, consider emphasizing the following selected information (» = major clinical significance):

### Before using this medication
» Conditions affecting use, especially:
Sensitivity to capecitabine or fluorouracil

Pregnancy—Avoiding pregnancy during treatment; telling physician immediately if pregnancy is suspected

Breast-feeding—Not recommended because of risk of serious side effects

Use in the elderly—Possible increased sensitivity to gastrointestinal adverse effects

Other medical problems, especially hepatic function impairment

**Proper use of this medication**
Taking within 30 minutes after a meal
Swallowing tablets with water
» Proper dosing
Missed dose: Not taking at all; not doubling doses; checking with physician
» Proper storage

**Precautions while using this medication**
» Importance of close monitoring by the physician
» Notifying physician immediately if fever of 100.5 °F or higher, or other evidence of an infection, occurs
» Stopping treatment and notifying physician immediately if symptoms indicative of NCI grade 2 (or higher) diarrhea, hand-and-foot syndrome, nausea, vomiting, or stomatitis occurs

**Side/adverse effects**
May cause adverse effects such as blood problems, hand-and-foot syndrome, and gastrointestinal tract toxicity; importance of discussing possible effects with physician

Signs of potential side effects, especially abdominal or stomach pain; anemia; diarrhea (moderate); hand-and-foot-syndrome; stomatitis; angina; ataxia; bronchospasm, dyspnea, or respiratory distress; cardiomyopathy; cholestatic hepatitis, hepatic fibrosis, or hepatitis; edema; epistaxis; fever; gastrointestinal toxicity; hypotension; hypertension; infection; phlebitis, thrombophlebitis, or deep venous thrombosis; pulmonary embolism; and thrombocytopenic purpura

Physician or nurse can help in dealing with side effects

## General Dosing Information

Patients receiving capecitabine should be under the supervision of a physician experienced in cancer chemotherapy.

Dosage must be adjusted to meet the individual requirements of each patient, based on appearance or severity of toxicity.

It is recommended that capecitabine be taken within 30 minutes after a meal and that the tablets be swallowed with water.

It is recommended that capecitabine be discontinued immediately if any of the following occur:
Diarrhea, grade 2 (an increase of 4 to 6 stools per day or nocturnal stools) or greater.
Hand-and-foot syndrome, grade 2 (painful erythema and swelling of the palms of the hands and/or the bottoms of the feet that results in discomfort affecting daily living activities) or greater.
Hyperbilirubinemia, grade 2 (bilirubin concentrations 1.5 times normal) or greater.
Nausea, grade 2 (sufficient to result in significantly decreased food intake, but the patient is able to eat intermittently) or greater.
Vomiting, grade 2 (2 to 5 episodes in a 24-hour period) or greater.
Stomatitis, grade 2 (painful erythema, edema, or ulcers of the mouth or tongue) or greater.

Once the effect has resolved or decreased to grade 1, capecitabine therapy may be reinstituted (depending on the number of times that the problem has occurred), but a reduction of dosage may be required.

**For treatment of adverse effects**
Withdrawal of capecitabine therapy is recommended for NCI grade 2 or higher adverse effects; dosage adjustment may be necessary if treatment is reinstituted.

For NCI grade 2 or higher diarrhea: Standard antidiarrheal treatment (e.g., loperamide). Severe diarrhea requires careful monitoring and possibly fluid and electrolyte replacement for dehydration.

For NCI grade 2 or higher nausea, vomiting, hand-and-foot syndrome, or stomatitis: Symptomatic treatment is recommended.

## Oral Dosage Forms

### CAPECITABINE TABLETS

**Usual adult dose**
Carcinoma, breast (treatment)—
Oral, 2500 mg per square meter of body surface per day, in two divided doses (approximately twelve hours apart) at the end of a meal. This dose is given for two weeks, followed by a one-week rest period, i.e., as three-week cycles.

Note: The development of adverse effects may require adjustment of capecitabine dosage, depending on severity (as graded according to NCI common toxicity criteria) as follows:

Grade 1 toxicity—No interruption or modification of therapy is needed.

Grade 2 toxicity—Therapy should be interrupted until the effect has resolved or improved to the grade 1 level, then reinstituted (or not) according to the following guidelines:
After a first occurrence—Treatment may be reinstituted using 100% of the starting dose.
After a second occurrence—Treatment may be reinstituted using 75% of the starting dose.
After a third occurrence—Treatment may be reinstituted using 50% of the starting dose.
After a fourth occurrence—Treatment should not be reinstituted.

Grade 3 toxicity—Therapy should be interrupted until the effect has resolved or improved to the grade 1 level, then reinstituted (or not) according to the following guidelines:
After a first occurrence—Treatment may be reinstituted using 75% of the starting dose.
After a second occurrence—Treatment may be reinstituted using 50% of the starting dose.
After a third occurrence—Treatment should not be reinstituted.

Grade 4 toxicity—Based on the clinician's judgement, treatment may be withdrawn permanently or, after the effect has resolved or improved to the grade 1 level, reinstituted using 50% of the starting dose.

**Usual pediatric dose**
Safety and efficacy in children younger than 18 years of age have not been established.

**Strength(s) usually available**
U.S.—
150 mg (Rx) [*Xeloda* (anhydrous lactose)].
500 mg (Rx) [*Xeloda* (anhydrous lactose)].

**Packaging and storage**
Store between 15 and 30 °C (59 and 86 °F), preferably at 25 °C (77 °F), in a tight container.

**Auxiliary labeling**
• Take with meals.

Developed: 06/25/98

---

# CAPREOMYCIN Systemic

VA CLASSIFICATION (Primary): AM500
Commonly used brand name(s): *Capastat*.
Note: For a listing of dosage forms and brand names by country availability, see *Dosage Forms* section(s).

## Category
Antibacterial (antimycobacterial).

## Indications

**Accepted**

Tuberculosis (treatment)—Capreomycin is indicated in combination with other antituberculosis medications in the treatment of pulmonary tuberculosis caused by *Mycobacterium tuberculosis* after failure with the primary medications (streptomycin, isoniazid, rifampin, pyrazinamide, and ethambutol) or when these cannot be used because of toxicity or development of resistant tubercle bacilli.

Since bacterial resistance may develop rapidly when capreomycin is administered alone, it should only be administered concurrently with other antituberculosis medications in the treatment of tuberculosis. Cross-

# Capreomycin (Systemic)

resistance has been documented with kanamycin; however, no cross-resistance has been found between capreomycin and other available antimycobacterial agents.

Not all species or strains of a particular organism may be susceptible to capreomycin.

## Pharmacology/Pharmacokinetics

**Mechanism of action/Effect**
Unknown; polypeptide complex with toxicities similar to those of the aminoglycosides.

**Absorption**
Not absorbed from the gastrointestinal tract in sufficient quantities; must be given intramuscularly.

**Distribution**
Does not penetrate into the cerebrospinal fluid (CSF); high concentrations are achieved in the urine. Crosses the placenta.

**Half-life**
Normal renal function—
  3 to 6 hours.
Impaired renal function—
  Prolonged.

**Time to peak serum concentration**
1 to 2 hours following intramuscular administration.

**Peak serum concentration**
Mean, 28 to 32 mcg/mL (range, 20 to 47 mcg/mL) after a 1-gram dose.

**Urine concentration**
Mean, 1680 mcg/mL after a 1-gram dose.

**Elimination**
Renal—
  50 to 60% excreted unchanged within 12 hours by glomerular filtration; capreomycin accumulates in the serum of patients with renal function impairment.
Biliary—
  Small amounts may also be excreted in the bile.

## Precautions to Consider

**Carcinogenicity/Mutagenicity**
Studies have not been performed with capreomycin to determine its potential for carcinogenicity or mutagenicity.

**Pregnancy/Reproduction**
Pregnancy—Capreomycin crosses the placenta. Studies in pregnant women have not been done.
Studies in rats have shown that capreomycin is teratogenic, causing a low incidence of "wavy ribs" when it is given in daily doses of 50 mg per kg of body weight (mg/kg) (3½ times the human dose) or more.
FDA Pregnancy Category C.

**Breast-feeding**
It is not known whether capreomycin is distributed into breast milk. However, problems in humans have not been documented.

**Pediatrics**
No information is available on the relationship of age to the effects of capreomycin in pediatric patients. Safety and efficacy have not been established.

**Geriatrics**
No information is available on the relationship of age to the effects of capreomycin in geriatric patients. However, elderly patients are more likely to have an age-related decrease in renal function, which may require a decrease in dosage or an increased dosing interval in patients receiving capreomycin.

**Drug interactions and/or related problems**
The following drug interactions and/or related problems have been selected on the basis of their potential clinical significance (possible mechanism in parentheses where appropriate)—not necessarily inclusive (» = major clinical significance):

Note: Combinations containing any of the following medications, depending on the amount present, may also interact with this medication.

» Aminoglycosides, parenteral
  (concurrent use of these medications with capreomycin should be avoided since the potential for ototoxicity, nephrotoxicity, and neuromuscular blockade may be increased; hearing loss may occur and may progress to deafness even after discontinuation of the drug and may be reversible, but usually is permanent; neuromuscular blockade may result in skeletal muscle weakness and respiratory depression or paralysis [apnea]; treatment with anticholinesterase agents or calcium salts may help reverse the blockade)

» Methoxyflurane or
» Polymyxins, parenteral
  (concurrent and/or sequential use of these medications with capreomycin should be avoided since the potential for nephrotoxicity and/or neuromuscular blockade may be increased; neuromuscular blockade may result in skeletal muscle weakness and respiratory depression or paralysis [apnea]; caution is also recommended when these medications are used concurrently during surgery or in the postoperative period; treatment with anticholinesterase agents or calcium salts to help reverse the blockade)

» Nephrotoxic medications (See *Appendix II*) or
» Ototoxic medications (See *Appendix II*)
  (concurrent and/or sequential use of these medications with capreomycin may increase the potential for ototoxicity and/or nephrotoxicity; hearing loss may occur and may progress to deafness even after discontinuation of the drug; hearing loss may be reversible, but usually is permanent; serial audiometric function determinations may be required with concurrent or sequential use of other ototoxic antibacterials; renal function determinations may be required)

» Neuromuscular blocking agents or other medications with neuromuscular blocking activity
  (concurrent use of medications with neuromuscular blocking activity, including halogenated hydrocarbon inhalation anesthetics and massive transfusions with citrate anticoagulated blood, with capreomycin should be carefully monitored since neuromuscular blockade may be enhanced, resulting in skeletal muscle weakness and respiratory depression or paralysis [apnea]; caution is recommended when these medications and capreomycin are used concurrently during surgery or in the postoperative period, especially if there is a possibility of incomplete reversal of neuromuscular blockade postoperatively; treatment with anticholinesterase agents or calcium salts may help reverse the blockade)

**Laboratory value alterations**
The following have been selected on the basis of their potential clinical significance (possible effect in parentheses where appropriate)—not necessarily inclusive (» = major clinical significance):

With physiology/laboratory test values
» Blood urea nitrogen (BUN) and
» Creatinine, serum
  (concentrations may be increased)

**Medical considerations/Contraindications**
The medical considerations/contraindications included have been selected on the basis of their potential clinical significance (reasons given in parentheses where appropriate)—not necessarily inclusive (» = major clinical significance).

*Risk-benefit should be considered when the following medical problems exist:*

Dehydration
  (possible increased risk of toxicity because of elevated serum concentrations)

» Eighth-cranial-nerve impairment
  (capreomycin may cause auditory and vestibular toxicity)

» Hypersensitivity to capreomycin

» Myasthenia gravis or
» Parkinsonism
  (capreomycin has produced a partial neuromuscular blockade after being administered in large intravenous doses; use of capreomycin may result in further skeletal muscle weakness)

» Renal function impairment
  (capreomycin may cause nephrotoxicity; it is recommended that capreomycin be administered in a reduced dosage at fixed intervals, or in normal doses at prolonged intervals to patients with impaired renal function)

**Patient monitoring**
The following may be especially important in patient monitoring (other tests may be warranted in some patients, depending on condition; » = major clinical significance):

» Audiograms and
» Vestibular function determinations
  (may be required prior to treatment, especially in patients with pre-existing renal or eighth-cranial-nerve impairment; twice-weekly or weekly audiometric testing to detect high-frequency hearing loss and periodic vestibular function determinations are recommended)

Potassium, serum
(concentrations may be required prior to and monthly during therapy since hypokalemia may occur; however, hypokalemia is less likely to occur when capreomycin is given 2 or 3 times weekly)

» Renal function determinations
(weekly renal function determinations may be required during therapy; patients with impaired renal function require a reduction in dose or withdrawal of the medication)

## Side/Adverse Effects

The following side/adverse effects have been selected on the basis of their potential clinical significance (possible signs and symptoms in parentheses where appropriate)—not necessarily inclusive:

**Those indicating need for medical attention**
Incidence more frequent
*Nephrotoxicity* (greatly increased or decreased frequency of urination or amount of urine; increased thirst; loss of appetite; nausea; vomiting)

Incidence less frequent
*Hypersensitivity* (skin rash; itching; redness; swelling; or fever); *hypokalemia* (irregular heartbeat; loss of appetite; nausea; muscle cramps or pain; unusual tiredness or weakness; vomiting); *neuromuscular blockade* (difficulty in breathing; drowsiness; unusual tiredness or weakness); *ototoxicity, auditory* (any loss of hearing; ringing or buzzing or a feeling of fullness in the ears); *ototoxicity, vestibular* (clumsiness or unsteadiness; dizziness; nausea or vomiting); *pain, hardness, unusual bleeding, or a sore at the place of injection*

## Patient Consultation

As an aid to patient consultation, refer to *Advice for the Patient, Capreomycin (Systemic)*.

In providing consultation, consider emphasizing the following selected information (» = major clinical significance):

**Before using this medication**
» Conditions affecting use, especially:
Hypersensitivity to capreomycin
Pregnancy—Capreomycin crosses the placenta; studies in rats have found capreomycin to be teratogenic
Use in the elderly—Geriatric patients may be at increased risk of renal toxicity because of an age-related decrease in renal function
Other medications, especially parenteral aminoglycosides, other nephrotoxic or ototoxic medications, methoxyflurane, parenteral polymyxins, or other agents with neuromuscular blocking activity
Other medical problems, especially eighth-cranial-nerve impairment, myasthenia gravis, parkinsonism, or renal function impairment

**Proper use of this medicine**
» Compliance with full course of therapy; for tuberculosis, therapy may take months or years
» Proper dosing
Missed dose: Using as soon as possible; not using if almost time for next dose; not doubling doses

**Side/adverse effects**
Signs of potential side effects, especially nephrotoxicity; hypersensitivity; hypokalemia; neuromuscular blockade; auditory and vestibular ototoxicity; and pain, hardness, unusual bleeding, or a sore at the place of injection

## General Dosing Information

Sterile capreomycin sulfate should be administered only by deep intramuscular injection into a large muscle mass since superficial injections may be associated with increased pain and development of sterile abscesses.

Patients with renal function impairment may need an adjustment in dosage, based on creatinine clearance.

## Parenteral Dosage Forms

Note: The dosing and dosage forms available are expressed in terms of capreomycin base.

### CAPREOMYCIN SULFATE STERILE USP

**Usual adult and adolescent dose**
Tuberculosis—
In combination with other antituberculosis medications: Intramuscular, 1 gram (base) once a day for sixty to one hundred and twenty days, followed by 1 gram two or three times a week.

Note: Adults with impaired renal function require a reduction in dose as follows:

| Creatinine Clearance (mL/min)/(mL/sec) | Dose (base) |
|---|---|
| >110/1.84 | See *Usual adult and adolescent dose* |
| 110/1.84 | 13.9 mg per kg every 24 hours |
| 100/1.67 | 12.7 mg per kg every 24 hours |
| 80/1.33 | 10.4 mg per kg every 24 hours |
| 60/1.00 | 8.2 mg per kg every 24 hours |
| 50/0.83 | 7 mg per kg every 24 hours; or 14 mg per kg every 48 hours |
| 40/0.67 | 5.9 mg per kg every 24 hours; or 11.7 mg per kg every 48 hours |
| 30/0.50 | 4.7 mg per kg every 24 hours; 9.5 mg per kg every 48 hours; or 14.2 mg per kg every 72 hours |
| 20/0.33 | 3.6 mg per kg every 24 hours; 7.2 mg per kg every 48 hours; or 10.7 mg per kg every 72 hours |
| 10/0.17 | 2.4 mg per kg every 24 hours; 4.9 mg per kg every 48 hours; or 7.3 mg per kg every 72 hours |
| 0/0 | 1.3 mg per kg every 24 hours; 2.6 mg per kg every 48 hours; or 3.9 mg per kg every 72 hours |

**Usual adult prescribing limits**
Up to a maximum of 20 mg (base) per kg of body weight daily.

**Usual pediatric dose**
Dosage has not been established.

**Size(s) usually available**
U.S.—
1 gram (base) (Rx) [*Capastat*].
Canada—
Sterile capreomycin sulfate (*Capastat*) is available in Canada on a restricted basis from the manufacturer. For information on how to obtain this product, contact Eli Lilly and Company in Canada.

**Packaging and storage**
Prior to reconstitution, store below 40 °C (104 °F), preferably between 15 and 30 °C (59 and 86 °F), unless otherwise specified by manufacturer.

**Preparation of dosage form**
To prepare initial dilution for intramuscular use, add 2 mL of 0.9% sodium chloride injection or sterile water for injection to each 1-gram vial. Two to three minutes may be required for complete dissolution.

**Stability**
After reconstitution, solutions retain their potency for 48 hours at room temperature or for up to 14 days if refrigerated.
Reconstituted solutions may vary in color from almost colorless to pale straw-colored and may darken in time. This variation does not affect their potency.

Revised: 06/27/94

---

# CAPSAICIN Topical

VA CLASSIFICATION (Primary): DE900
Commonly used brand name(s): *Zostrix; Zostrix–HP*.
Note: For a listing of dosage forms and brand names by country availability, see *Dosage Forms* section(s).

## Category

Analgesic, specific pain syndromes (topical); antineuralgic, specific pain syndromes (topical); antipruritic (topical).

## Indications

Note: Bracketed information in the *Indications* section refers to uses that are not included in U.S. product labeling.

## Accepted

Neuralgia (treatment)—Capsaicin is indicated for the treatment of neuralgias, such as the pain following herpes zoster (shingles) and painful diabetic neuropathy.

Osteoarthritis (treatment); or

Rheumatoid arthritis (treatment)—Capsaicin is indicated for the treatment of pain from osteoarthritis and rheumatoid arthritis.

[Pain, neurogenic, other (treatment)]—Capsaicin is used to treat the pain associated with postmastectomy pain syndrome (PMPS) and reflex sympathetic dystrophy syndrome (RSDS, causalgia).

[Pruritus, aquagenic (treatment) or,]

[Pruritus, hemodialysis-induced (treatment),]—Capsaicin is used in the treatment of pruritus associated with hemodialysis and exposure to water (aquagenic).

## Acceptance not established

Preliminary studies suggest capsaicin may be used to treat *pruritus associated with psoriasis*. However, there are currently insufficient data to establish the safety and efficacy of capsaicin for this indication.

## Pharmacology/Pharmacokinetics

### Physicochemical characteristics

Source—Capsaicin is a naturally occurring substance in plants of the Solanaceae family.

Molecular weight—305.4.

### Mechanism of action/Effect

The precise mechanism of action has not been fully elucidated. Capsaicin is a neuropeptide-active agent that affects the synthesis, storage, transport, and release of substance P. Substance P is thought to be the principal chemical mediator of pain impulses from the periphery to the central nervous system. In addition, substance P has been shown to be released into joint tissues where it activates inflammatory intermediates that are involved with the development of rheumatoid arthritis. Capsaicin renders skin and joints insensitive to pain by depleting and preventing reaccumulation of substance P in peripheral sensory neurons. With the depletion of substance P in the nerve endings, local pain impulses cannot be transmitted to the brain.

Note: Capsaicin is not a local anesthetic, since it only blocks the conduction of painful impulses carried by the type-C fibers, whereas local anesthetics block the conduction of impulses in all afferent neurons, which impairs all sensations including touch, pressure, heat, and vibration.

Capsaicin is not a traditional counterirritant, since it does not produce vasodilation.

## Precautions to Consider

### Pregnancy/Reproduction

Pregnancy—Problems in humans have not been documented.

### Breast-feeding

It is not known whether capsaicin, applied topically, is distributed into breast milk. However, problems in humans have not been documented.

### Pediatrics

Appropriate studies on the relationship of age to the effects of capsaicin have not been performed in infants and children up to 2 years of age. However, use in infants and children up to 2 years of age is not recommended.

### Geriatrics

Appropriate studies on the relationship of age to the effects of capsaicin have not been performed in the geriatric population. However, geriatrics-specific problems that would limit the usefulness of this medication in the elderly are not expected.

### Medical considerations/Contraindications

The medical considerations/contraindications included have been selected on the basis of their potential clinical significance (reasons given in parentheses where appropriate)—not necessarily inclusive (» = major clinical significance).

*Except under special circumstances, this medication should not be used when the following medical problem exists:*

» Broken or irritated skin on area to be treated
 (will cause pain and further irritation of skin)

*Risk-benefit should be considered when the following medical problem exists:*

Sensitivity to capsaicin or to the fruits of *Capsicum* plants (e.g., hot peppers)

## Side/Adverse Effects

Note: Capsaicin has no known systemic side effects.

Patients may experience a warm, stinging, or burning sensation at the site of application, especially during the initial few days of use. Although this sensation frequently disappears after the first several days of treatment, it may persist for 2 to 4 weeks or longer. This effect is related to the initial excitatory effect of capsaicin on type-C fibers and their release of substance P. The burning usually decreases in frequency and intensity with continued administration of capsaicin. However, application schedules of capsaicin of less than 3 or 4 times daily may prolong the burning sensation while not providing optimum pain relief. Environmental factors, such as heat or humidity; wrappings, such as clothing or bandages; bathing in warm water; or sweating may intensify the sensation. The incidence of the burning sensation has been variable in different studies. This may be related to the etiology and pathogenesis of the pain syndrome in different persons. For example, patients with arthritis generally experience less intense burning than do patients with peripheral neuropathies.

Removal of clothing or bedsheets that have covered the area of topical capsaicin application has been associated rarely with respiratory irritation, such as coughing, in the patient and bystanders who were present at the time. This has been attributed to the inhalation of the residue of the dried cream.

There is some concern that capsaicin may be potentially neurotoxic, although animal and clinical studies with topical capsaicin have not shown this to occur. Capsaicin is thought to be capable of elevating the heat-pain threshold in the treated skin areas, especially in patients with diabetic neuropathy; these patients often already have an elevated threshold for heat and pain.

The following side/adverse effects have been selected on the basis of their potential clinical significance (possible signs and symptoms in parentheses where appropriate)—not necessarily inclusive:

**Those indicating need for medical attention only if they continue or are bothersome**

Incidence more frequent
  *Warm, stinging, or burning sensation at the site of application*

## Patient Consultation

As an aid to patient consultation, refer to *Advice for the Patient, Capsaicin (Topical)*.

In providing consultation, consider emphasizing the following selected information (» = major clinical significance):

### Before using this medication

» Conditions affecting use, especially:
  Sensitivity to capsaicin or to the fruits of *Capsicum* plants (e.g., hot peppers)
  Use in children—Not recommended in infants and children up to 2 years of age, except under the direction of a physician
  Other medical problems, especially broken or irritated skin on area to be treated

### Proper use of this medication

If using capsaicin for treatment of neuralgia due to herpes zoster, not applying medicine until after zoster sores have healed

Washing areas to be treated will not cause harm, but is not necessary

Rubbing cream into the affected area well so that little or no cream is left on surface of skin

Washing hands with soap and water after applying capsaicin to avoid getting medicine in eyes or on other sensitive areas of body; however, if medication used on arthritic hands, not washing hands for at least 30 minutes after application

If bandage is being used, not applying tightly

Warm, stinging, or burning sensation may occur and is related to the action of capsaicin on the skin; usually disappears after first several days of treatment, however, may last 2 to 4 weeks or longer; heat, humidity, clothing, bathing in warm water, or sweating may increase sensation; sensation usually lessens in frequency and intensity the longer medication is used; reducing number of daily doses of capsaicin will not lessen sensation, and may prolong period of time that sensation occurs; reducing number of doses also will reduce amount of pain relief obtained

Relief from pain may not occur right away; also, time it takes for capsaicin to work differs depending on type of pain; with arthritis, pain relief usually begins within 1 or 2 weeks; with neuralgia, pain relief usually begins within 2 to 4 weeks; with head and neck neuralgias, pain relief may take 4 to 6 weeks

Using capsaicin 3 or 4 times a day or as directed by doctor; pain relief will last only as long as capsaicin is used regularly; if medicine is discontinued and pain recurs, capsaicin treatment may be restarted
» Proper dosage
Missed dose: Using as soon as possible; if almost time for next dose, skipping missed dose and returning to regular dosing schedule; not doubling doses
» Proper storage

**Precautions while using this medication**
If capsaicin gets into eyes, flushing with water; if capsaicin gets on other sensitive areas of body, washing with warm (not hot) soapy water
If condition worsens, or does not improve after 1 month, discontinuing use and checking with physician

## General Dosing Information

The cream should be applied sparingly and rubbed well into the affected area so that little or no cream is left on the surface of the skin.

During the first 1 or 2 weeks of treatment, application of a topical lidocaine product before capsaicin application may reduce initial discomfort.

A therapeutic pain response is usually achieved within 2 to 4 weeks. Most patients with arthritis notice an initial response within 1 or 2 weeks. Most patients with neuralgia pain begin to respond within 2 to 4 weeks, although patients with pain from head and neck neuralgias may take 4 to 6 weeks to respond.

Continued application of capsaicin 3 or 4 times daily is necessary to sustain pain relief. If the medicine is discontinued and pain recurs, capsaicin treatment may be restarted.

Persons using capsaicin to treat arthritis in their hands should avoid washing their hands for at least 30 minutes after application.

When capsaicin is used for the treatment of neuralgia due to herpes zoster, it should not be applied to the skin until after the zoster lesions have healed.

If a bandage is being used on the treated area, it should not be applied tightly.

## Topical Dosage Forms

### CAPSAICIN CREAM

**Usual adult and adolescent dose**
Topical, to the affected area, three or four times a day.

**Usual pediatric dose**
Infants and children up to 2 years of age—Use is not recommended.
Children 2 years of age and older—See *Usual adult and adolescent dose.*

**Strength(s) usually available**
U.S.—
  0.025% (OTC) [*Zostrix* (benzyl alcohol; cetyl alcohol)].
  0.075% (OTC) [*Zostrix-HP* (benzyl alcohol; cetyl alcohol)].
Canada—
  0.025% (OTC) [*Zostrix*].
  0.075% (OTC) [*Zostrix-HP*].

**Packaging and storage**
Store below 40 °C (104 °F), preferably between 15 and 30 °C (59 and 86 °F), unless otherwise specified by manufacturer. Protect from freezing.

**Auxiliary labeling**
• For external use only.
• Avoid contact with eyes.

## Selected Bibliography

Rumsfield JA, West DP. Topical capsaicin in dermatologic and peripheral pain disorders. DICP 1991 Apr; 25: 381-7.
Watson CP, et al. Post-herpetic neuralgia: 208 cases [abstract]. Pain 1988 Dec; 35(3): 289-97.

Revised: 07/14/92
Interim revision: 05/13/98

---

**CAPTOPRIL**—See *Angiotensin-converting Enzyme (ACE) Inhibitors (Systemic)*

---

# CARBACHOL  Ophthalmic

VA CLASSIFICATION (Primary/Secondary): OP118/OP900
Commonly used brand name(s): *Carboptic; Isopto Carbachol; Miostat.*
Another commonly used name is carbamylcholine.
Note: For a listing of dosage forms and brand names by country availability, see *Dosage Forms* section(s).

## Category

Antiglaucoma agent (ophthalmic)—Carbachol Ophthalmic Solution USP;
Miotic—Carbachol Intraocular Solution USP; Carbachol Ophthalmic Solution USP.

## Indications

Note: Bracketed information in the *Indications* section refers to uses that are not included in U.S. product labeling.

**Accepted**

Miosis induction, during surgery—Carbachol intraocular solution is indicated to produce pupillary miosis during surgery.

Glaucoma, open-angle (treatment)—Carbachol ophthalmic solution is indicated for lowering intraocular pressure in the treatment of chronic open-angle glaucoma. It is especially useful as a replacement drug, particularly in eyes that have become intolerant of, or resistant to, pilocarpine.

[Glaucoma, angle-closure (treatment)][1]—Carbachol ophthalmic solution is used for emergency treatment of angle-closure glaucoma; however, pilocarpine is usually preferred.

[Glaucoma, angle-closure, *during* or *after* iridectomy (treatment)][1]—Carbachol ophthalmic solution is used in the treatment of angle-closure glaucoma during or after iridectomy.

[Glaucoma, secondary (treatment)][1]—Carbachol ophthalmic solution is used in the treatment of secondary glaucoma if there is no active intraocular inflammation present.

---
[1]Not included in Canadian product labeling.

## Pharmacology/Pharmacokinetics

**Physicochemical characteristics**
Molecular weight—182.65.

**Mechanism of action/Effect**
Carbachol is a parasympathomimetic that directly stimulates cholinergic receptors. It may also act indirectly by promoting release of acetylcholine and by a weak anticholinesterase action. Carbachol produces contraction of the iris sphincter muscle resulting in pupillary constriction (miosis), constriction of the ciliary muscle resulting in increased accommodation, and a reduction in intraocular pressure associated with decreased resistance to aqueous humor outflow.

In chronic open-angle glaucoma, the exact mechanism by which carbachol lowers intraocular pressure is not precisely known; however, contraction of the ciliary muscle apparently opens the intertrabecular spaces and facilitates aqueous humor outflow.

In angle-closure glaucoma, constriction of the pupil apparently pulls the iris away from the trabeculum, thereby relieving blockage of the trabecular meshwork.

**Onset of action**
Ophthalmic solution—Miosis: Within 10 to 20 minutes.

**Time to peak effect**
Intraocular solution—Miosis: Within 2 to 5 minutes.
Ophthalmic solution—Reduction in intraocular pressure: Within 4 hours.

**Duration of action**
Intraocular solution—
  Miosis: About 24 hours.
Ophthalmic solution—
  Miosis: About 4 to 8 hours.
  Reduction in intraocular pressure: About 8 hours.

## Precautions to Consider

**Carcinogenicity**
Long-term animal studies have not been done.

## Carbachol (Ophthalmic)

**Pregnancy/Reproduction**
Pregnancy—Studies have not been done in humans. However, carbachol may be systemically absorbed.
Studies have not been done in animals.
FDA Pregnancy Category C.

**Breast-feeding**
Carbachol may be systemically absorbed. It is not known whether carbachol is distributed into breast milk. However, problems in humans have not been documented.

**Pediatrics**
Appropriate studies on the relationship of age to the effects of carbachol have not been performed in the pediatric population. However, no pediatrics-specific problems have been documented to date.

**Geriatrics**
Appropriate studies on the relationship of age to the effects of carbachol have not been performed in the geriatric population. However, no geriatrics-specific problems have been documented to date.

**Drug interactions and/or related problems**
The following drug interactions and/or related problems have been selected on the basis of their potential clinical significance (possible mechanism in parentheses where appropriate)—not necessarily inclusive (» = major clinical significance):

Note: Combinations containing any of the following medications, depending on the amount present, may also interact with this medication.

Belladonna alkaloids, ophthalmic or
Cyclopentolate
(concurrent use of these medications may interfere with the antiglaucoma action of carbachol. Also, concurrent use with carbachol counteracts the mydriatic effects of these medications; this counteraction may be used to therapeutic advantage)

Flurbiprofen, ophthalmic
(ophthalmic carbachol may be ineffective when administered following ophthalmic flurbiprofen; the pharmacologic basis for this interference is not known)

**Medical considerations/Contraindications**
The medical considerations/contraindications included have been selected on the basis of their potential clinical significance (reasons given in parentheses where appropriate)—not necessarily inclusive (» = major clinical significance).

*Risk-benefit should be considered when the following medical problems exist:*

Asthma, bronchial
Cardiac failure, acute
Corneal abrasion or injury
(possible excessive absorption of medication, which can produce systemic toxicity)
Gastrointestinal spasm
Hyperthyroidism
» Iritis, acute, or other conditions in which pupillary constriction is undesirable
Parkinson's disease
Peptic ulcer, active
Sensitivity to carbachol
Urinary tract obstruction

**Patient monitoring**
The following may be especially important in patient monitoring (other tests may be warranted in some patients, depending on condition; » = major clinical significance):

Intraocular pressure determinations
(recommended at periodic intervals during therapy when carbachol is used in the treatment of glaucoma)

## Side/Adverse Effects

Note: Corneal clouding, persistent bullous keratopathy, and post-operative iritis following cataract extraction have been reported occasionally when carbachol intraocular solution was used during cataract surgery.
With the exception of retinal detachment, the following side effects have not been reported following the use of carbachol intraocular solution.

The following side/adverse effects have been selected on the basis of their potential clinical significance (possible signs and symptoms in parentheses where appropriate)—not necessarily inclusive:

**Those indicating need for medical attention**
Incidence rare
*Retinal detachment* (veil or curtain appearing across part of vision)
Symptoms of systemic absorption
*Asthma* (shortness of breath, wheezing, or tightness in chest); *cardiac arrhythmia* (irregular heartbeat); *diarrhea, stomach cramps or pain, or vomiting; flushing or redness of face; frequent urge to urinate; hypotension* (unusual tiredness or weakness); *increased sweating; syncope* (fainting); *watering of mouth*

**Those indicating need for medical attention only if they continue or are bothersome**
Incidence more frequent
*Blurred vision or change in near or distance vision; eye pain; stinging or burning of the eye*
Incidence less frequent
*Headache; irritation or redness of eyes; twitching of eyelids*

## Overdose

For specific information on the agents used in the management of ophthalmic carbachol overdose, see:
• Atropine in *Anticholinergics/Antispasmodics (Systemic)* monograph.

For more information on the management of overdose or unintentional ingestion, **contact a Poison Control Center** (see *Poison Control Center Listing*).

**Treatment of overdose**
Atropine sulfate injection is used as an antidote to the systemic effects of carbachol.

## Patient Consultation

As an aid to patient consultation, refer to *Advice for the Patient, Carbachol (Ophthalmic)*.

In providing consultation, consider emphasizing the following selected information (» = major clinical significance):

**Before using this medication**
» Conditions affecting use, especially:
Sensitivity to carbachol
Other medical problems, especially acute iritis or other conditions in which pupillary constriction is undesirable

**Proper use of this medication**
*For the ophthalmic solution*
» Importance of not using more medication than the amount prescribed
Proper administration technique
Washing hands immediately after applying eye drops
Preventing contamination: Not touching applicator tip to any surface; keeping container tightly closed
» Proper dosing
Missed dose: Applying as soon as possible; not applying if almost time for next dose; applying next dose at regularly scheduled time
» Proper storage

**Precautions while using this medication**
*For the ophthalmic solution*
Regular visits to physician to check eye pressure during therapy
» Caution if driving or doing anything else at night or in dim light
» Caution if blurred vision or change in near or distance vision occurs

**Side/adverse effects**
Signs of potential side effects, especially retinal detachment or symptoms of systemic absorption

## General Dosing Information

**For ophthalmic solution**
Although some manufacturers recommend a dose of 2 drops of an ophthalmic solution at appropriate intervals, the conjunctival sac will usually hold only 1 drop.

More frequent instillation or use of a stronger solution may be required to produce an adequate reduction in intraocular pressure in eyes with hazel or brown irides than is needed in eyes with blue or light-colored irides.

To avoid excessive systemic absorption, patient should press finger to the lacrimal sac during and for 1 or 2 minutes following instillation of medication.

Tolerance to carbachol may develop with prolonged use. Effectiveness may be restored by changing to another miotic for a short time and then resuming the original medication.

## Ophthalmic Dosage Forms

### CARBACHOL INTRAOCULAR SOLUTION USP

**Usual adult and adolescent dose**
Miotic—
  Intraocular irrigation, no more than 0.5 mL of a 0.01% solution instilled into the anterior chamber.

**Usual pediatric dose**
See *Usual adult and adolescent dose*.

**Usual geriatric dose**
See *Usual adult and adolescent dose*.

**Strength(s) usually available**
U.S.—
  0.01% (Rx) [*Miostat*].
Canada—
  0.01% (Rx) [*Miostat*].

**Packaging and storage**
Store between 15 and 30 °C (59 and 86 °F), in a tight container. Protect from freezing.

**Auxiliary labeling**
• For single-dose intraocular use only.
• Discard unused portion.

### CARBACHOL OPHTHALMIC SOLUTION USP

**Usual adult and adolescent dose**
Antiglaucoma agent (ophthalmic)—
  Topical, to the conjunctiva, 1 drop of a 0.75 to 3% solution one to three times a day.

**Usual pediatric dose**
See *Usual adult and adolescent dose*.

**Usual geriatric dose**
See *Usual adult and adolescent dose*.

**Strength(s) usually available**
U.S.—
  0.75% (Rx) [*Isopto Carbachol* (benzalkonium chloride 0.005%)].
  1.5% (Rx) [*Isopto Carbachol* (benzalkonium chloride 0.005%)].
  2.25% (Rx) [*Isopto Carbachol* (benzalkonium chloride 0.005%)].
  3% (Rx) [*Carboptic; Isopto Carbachol* (benzalkonium chloride 0.005%)].
Canada—
  1.5% (Rx) [*Isopto Carbachol* (benzalkonium chloride)].
  3% (Rx) [*Isopto Carbachol* (benzalkonium chloride)].

**Packaging and storage**
Store below 40 °C (104 °F), preferably between 15 and 30 °C (59 and 86 °F), unless otherwise specified by manufacturer. Store in a tight container. Protect from freezing.

**Auxiliary labeling**
• For the eye.
• Keep container tightly closed.

Revised: 06/21/94
Interim revision: 05/01/95

---

# CARBAMAZEPINE Systemic

VA CLASSIFICATION (Primary/Secondary): CN400/CN103; CN900; HS900

Commonly used brand name(s): *Apo-Carbamazepine; Atretol; Carbatrol; Epitol; Novo-Carbamaz; Nu-Carbamazepine; Taro-Carbamazepine; Taro-Carbamazepine CR; Tegretol; Tegretol CR; Tegretol Chewtabs; Tegretol-XR*.

Note: For a listing of dosage forms and brand names by country availability, see *Dosage Forms* section(s).

## Category

Anticonvulsant; antineuralgic (specific pain syndromes); antimanic; antidiuretic; antipsychotic.

## Indications

Note: Bracketed information in the *Indications* section refers to uses that are not included in U.S. product labeling.

**Accepted**

Epilepsy (treatment)—Carbamazepine is indicated for the treatment of partial seizures with simple or complex symptomatology (psychomotor, temporal lobe); generalized tonic-clonic seizures (grand mal); mixed seizure patterns that include the above; or other partial or generalized seizures.

Carbamazepine is a first-choice anticonvulsant because of its relatively low behavioral and psychological toxicity and the rarity of serious adverse effects.

Neuralgia, trigeminal (treatment)—Carbamazepine is indicated for relief of pain due to true trigeminal neuralgia (tic douloureux) and glossopharyngeal neuralgia.

[Bipolar disorder (prophylaxis and treatment)]—Carbamazepine is used alone or in combination with lithium and/or antidepressants or antipsychotic agents to treat patients with manic-depressive illness who are unresponsive to, or cannot tolerate, lithium or neuroleptics alone.

[Pain, neurogenic, other (treatment)][1]—Carbamazepine may also be used in some patients to relieve the lightning pains of tabes dorsalis; neuralgic pain associated with multiple sclerosis, acute idiopathic neuritis (Guillain-Barré syndrome), peripheral diabetic neuropathy, phantom limb, restless leg syndrome (Ekbom's syndrome), and hemifacial spasm; post-traumatic neuropathy or neuralgia; and postherpetic neuralgia.

[Diabetes insipidus, central partial (treatment)][1]—Carbamazepine is used alone or with other agents such as clofibrate or chlorpropamide in the treatment of partial central diabetes insipidus.

[Alcohol withdrawal (treatment)][1]—Carbamazepine is used for the detoxification of alcoholics. It has been found to be effective in rapidly relieving anxiety and distress of acute alcohol withdrawal and for such symptoms as seizures, hyperexcitability, and sleep disturbances.

[Psychotic disorders (treatment)][1]—Carbamazepine has been shown to be effective in certain psychiatric disorders including schizoaffective illness, resistant schizophrenia, and dyscontrol syndrome, associated with limbic system dysfunction.

**Unaccepted**

*Carbamazepine is not a simple analgesic and should not be used to relieve general aches or pains.*

Carbamazepine is *not* indicated for atypical or generalized absence seizures (petit mal) or myoclonic or atonic seizures.

Although carbamazepine has also been reported to relieve dystonic attacks in children, reduce migraine attacks, and relieve intractable hiccups in some patients, its therapeutic efficacy in such cases has not been established.

Carbamazepine should not be used prophylactically during long periods of remission in trigeminal neuralgia.

---

[1]Not included in Canadian product labeling.

## Pharmacology/Pharmacokinetics

**Physicochemical characteristics**

Chemical group—Tricyclic iminostilbene derivative. Structurally resembles the psychoactive agents imipramine, chlorpromazine, and maprotiline; shares some structural features with the anticonvulsant agents phenytoin, clonazepam, and phenobarbital.
Molecular weight—236.27.
pKa—7.

**Mechanism of action/Effect**

Anticonvulsant—Exact mechanism unknown; may act postsynaptically by limiting the ability of neurons to sustain high frequency repetitive firing of action potentials through enhancement of sodium channel inactivation; in addition to altering neuronal excitability, may act presynaptically to block the release of neurotransmitter by blocking presynaptic sodium channels and the firing of action potentials, which in turn decreases synaptic transmission.

Antineuralgic—Exact mechanism unknown; may involve gamma-aminobutyric acid (GABA$_B$) receptors, which may be linked to calcium channels.

Antidiuretic—Exact mechanism unknown; may exert a hypothalamic effect on the osmoreceptors mediated via secretion of antidiuretic hormone (ADH), or may have a direct effect on the renal tubule.

Antimanic; antipsychotic—Exact mechanism unknown; may be related to either the anticonvulsant or the antineuralgic effects of carbamazepine, or to its effects on neurotransmitter modulator systems.

**Other actions/effects**
Anticholinergic, antidepressant, neuromuscular transmission-inhibiting, and antiarrhythmic actions have been reported.

**Absorption**
Slow and variable, but almost completely absorbed from gastrointestinal tract.

**Distribution**
Apparent volume of distribution ($vol_D$)—
    Carbamazepine: Ranges from 0.8 to 2 L per kg.
    Carbamazepine-10,11-epoxide: Ranges from 0.59 to 1.5 L per kg.
In breast milk—
    May reach 60% of the maternal plasma concentration.

**Protein binding**
Carbamazepine—Moderate (55 to 59% in children, 76% in adults).
Carbamazepine-10,11-epoxide—Moderate (50%).

**Biotransformation**
Hepatic (97%); may induce its own metabolism. One metabolite, carbamazepine-10,11-epoxide, has anticonvulsant, antidepressant, and antineuralgic activity.

**Half-life**
Carbamazepine—
    Initial single dose: May range from 25 to 65 hours.
    Chronic dosing: May decrease to 8 to 29 hours (average 12 to 17 hours) because of autoinduction of metabolism.
Carbamazepine-10,11-epoxide—
    5 to 8 hours.

**Onset of action**
Anticonvulsant effect—Varies from hours to days, depending on individual patient. A stable therapeutic concentration may require a month to achieve due to autoinduction of metabolism.
Relief of pain of trigeminal neuralgia—8 to 72 hours.
Antimanic response—Usually 7 to 10 days.

**Time to peak concentration**
Suspension—1.5 hours following chronic administration.
Tablets—4 to 5 hours following chronic administration.
Extended-release capsules—5.9 (range, 4.1 to 7.7) hours following chronic administration.
Extended-release tablets—3 to 12 hours following chronic administration.

**Therapeutic plasma concentrations**
4 to 12 mcg per mL (16.9 to 50.8 micromoles per L) (in adults); variations due to autoinduction of metabolism.

**Elimination**
Renal—72% (3% as unchanged drug).
Fecal—28%.
Clearance values ranged from 0.011 to 0.021 L per hour per kg following a single dose of carbamazepine in healthy volunteers, and from 0.025 to 0.540 L per hour per kg following multiple dosing in healthy volunteers and epilepsy patients.

Note: Large interindividual differences in apparent plasma half-life and total body clearance are related to the phenomenon of autoinduction, which reaches different levels in different individuals. Autoinduction may lead to time-dependent kinetics, in which clearance values increase with time and higher doses are required to maintain the same plasma concentrations. In healthy volunteers, it is estimated that a plateau for autoinduction is reached after 20 to 30 days; in epileptic patients, however, the time course may differ due to previous induction by other medications.

Although the pharmacokinetic parameters of carbamazepine disposition are similar in children and adults, there is a poor correlation between plasma concentrations and carbamazepine dose in children. Carbamazepine is more rapidly metabolized to the active 10,11-epoxide metabolite in younger age groups than in adults. In children younger than 15 years of age, there is an inverse relationship between the carbamazepine-10,11-epoxide to carbamazepine ratio (CBZ-E/CBZ) and increasing age.

# Precautions to Consider

### Cross-sensitivity and/or related problems
Patients who are sensitive to tricyclic antidepressants may be sensitive to carbamazepine also. Carbamazepine should be given with caution, if at all, to such patients.

**Carcinogenicity/Tumorigenicity**
Carbamazepine is considered carcinogenic in Sprague-Dawley rats because doses of 25, 75, and 250 mg per kg per day for 2 years caused a dose-related increase in the incidence of hepatocellular tumors in females and of benign interstitial cell adenomas in the testes of males. The significance of these findings for use of carbamazepine in humans is not known.

**Pregnancy/Reproduction**
Pregnancy—Carbamazepine crosses the placenta. Although adequate and well-controlled studies in humans have not been done, there have been reports of babies prenatally exposed to carbamazepine having small head circumferences, low birth weights, craniofacial defects, fingernail hypoplasia, developmental delays, and spina bifida. When it is essential to continue carbamazepine therapy during pregnancy, serum carbamazepine concentrations must be monitored closely, since adverse effects in the fetus have been associated with high blood concentrations.

Studies in animals have shown that carbamazepine caused kinked ribs in 1.5% of the offspring of rats receiving 250 mg per kg. Also, carbamazepine caused cleft palate, deformities of the foot, or anophthalmos in about 3% of the offspring of rats receiving 650 mg per kg. These doses are 10 to 25 times the human daily dose.

FDA Pregnancy Category C.

Also, it must be kept in mind that other anticonvulsants used during pregnancy have been implicated in birth defects in infants born to epileptic mothers. In addition, retrospective studies have suggested that there may be a higher incidence of teratogenic effects with the use of combinations of anticonvulsants than with monotherapy.

Delivery—To prevent neonatal bleeding disorders, administration of vitamin K to the mother during the last weeks of pregnancy has been recommended.

**Breast-feeding**
Carbamazepine is distributed into breast milk. Concentrations in breast milk and in the plasma of nursing infants have been reported to reach 60% of the maternal plasma concentration. Therefore, the possibility exists that carbamazepine may cause adverse effects in the nursing infant. In animal studies, nursing rats showed a lack of weight gain and an unkempt appearance with maternal doses of 200 mg per kg.

**Pediatrics**
Appropriate studies have not been performed in children up to 6 years of age. However, behavioral changes are more likely to occur in children.

**Geriatrics**
Geriatric patients may be more susceptible to carbamazepine-induced confusion or agitation, atrioventricular (AV) heart block, syndrome of inappropriate antidiuretic hormone (SIADH), and bradycardia than younger patients.

**Dental**
The leukopenic and thrombocytopenic effects of carbamazepine may result in an increased incidence of microbial infection, delayed healing, and gingival bleeding. If leukopenia or thrombocytopenia occurs, dental work should be deferred until blood counts have returned to normal. Patient instruction in proper oral hygiene should include caution in use of regular toothbrushes, dental floss, and toothpicks.

**Surgical**
Carbamazepine antagonizes the effects of nondepolarizing muscle relaxants, such as pancuronium. Patients should be monitored closely for more rapid recovery from neuromuscular blockade than expected.

### Drug interactions and/or related problems
The following drug interactions and/or related problems have been selected on the basis of their potential clinical significance (possible mechanism in parentheses where appropriate)—not necessarily inclusive (» = major clinical significance):

Note: Hepatic cytochrome P450 3A4 has been identified as the major isoform responsible for the metabolism of carbamazepine to carbamazepine-10,11-epoxide. Medications that inhibit or induce the CYP 3A4 isoenzymes may alter carbamazepine plasma concentrations. Similarly, carbamazepine may inhibit or induce the metabolism of other medications, thus altering their plasma concentrations.

Combinations containing any of the following medications, depending on the amount present, may also interact with this medication.

Acetaminophen
(risk of hepatotoxicity with single toxic doses or prolonged use of high doses of acetaminophen may be increased, and therapeutic effects of acetaminophen may be decreased, in patients taking hepatic enzyme-inducing agents such as carbamazepine)

Aminophylline or
Oxtriphylline or
Theophylline
(concurrent use with carbamazepine may stimulate hepatic metabolism of the xanthines [except dyphylline], resulting in increased theophylline clearance)

» Anticoagulants, coumarin- or indandione-derivative
(anticoagulant effects may be decreased because of induction of hepatic microsomal enzyme activity, resulting in increased anticoagulant metabolism leading to decreased anticoagulant plasma concentrations and elimination half-life; dosage adjustments based on monitoring of prothrombin time may be necessary during and after carbamazepine therapy)

» Anticonvulsants, hydantoin or
» Anticonvulsants, succinimide or
» Barbiturates or
» Benzodiazepines metabolized via hepatic microsomal enzymes, especially clonazepam or
» Primidone or
» Valproic acid
(concurrent use with carbamazepine may result in increased metabolism, leading to decreased serum concentrations and reduced elimination half-lives of these medications because of induction of hepatic microsomal enzyme activity; monitoring of serum concentrations as a guide to dosage is recommended, especially when any of these medications or carbamazepine is added to or withdrawn from an existing regimen)

(valproic acid may prolong the half-life and reduce the protein-binding of carbamazepine; the concentration of the active 10,11-epoxide metabolite may be increased)

(in addition, use of carbamazepine in combination with other anticonvulsants has been reported to be associated with an increased risk of congenital defects and with an alteration of thyroid function)

» Antidepressants, tricyclic or
Clozapine or
Haloperidol or
Loxapine or
Maprotiline or
Molindone or
Phenothiazines or
Pimozide or
Thioxanthenes
(concurrent use of these agents with carbamazepine may enhance the central nervous system [CNS] depressant effects of carbamazepine, lower the seizure threshold, and decrease the anticonvulsant effects of carbamazepine; dosage adjustments may be necessary to control seizures; anticholinergic effects may be potentiated, leading to confusion and delirium)

(also, concurrent use of haloperidol, and possibly other neuroleptics, with carbamazepine may decrease plasma concentrations of the neuroleptic by about 60% with or without adverse clinical effects; close observation of patient for clinical signs of ineffectiveness of the neuroleptic is recommended; dosage adjustment may be necessary)

Carbonic anhydrase inhibitors
(concurrent use may increase the risk of carbamazepine-induced osteopenia; it is recommended that patients receiving concurrent therapy be monitored for early signs of osteopenia and that the carbonic anhydrase inhibitor be discontinued and appropriate treatment initiated if necessary)

Chlorpropamide or
Desmopressin or
Lypressin or
Posterior pituitary or
Thiazide diuretics, when used for their paradoxical antidiuretic activity in the treatment of diabetes insipidus, or
Vasopressin
(concurrent use with carbamazepine may potentiate the antidiuretic effect, leading to a lower sodium concentration and causing adverse effects that include increased seizure activity; a reduction in dosage of either or both medications may be necessary for optimal therapeutic effect in the treatment of diabetes insipidus)

» Cimetidine
(concurrent use may result in increased plasma concentrations of carbamazepine by delaying its clearance, leading to carbamazepine toxicity)

Cisplatin or
Doxorubicin or
Rifampin
(concurrent use with carbamazepine may cause an increased rate of metabolism of carbamazepine, resulting in decreased plasma concentrations)

(rifampin also increases the plasma concentrations of the 10,11-epoxide metabolite)

» Clarithromycin
(administration of carbamazepine with clarithromycin has been shown to significantly increase the plasma concentration of carbamazepine; carbamazepine plasma concentrations should be monitored)

» Contraceptives, estrogen-containing, oral or
Cyclosporine or
Dacarbazine or
Digitalis glycosides, with the possible exception of digoxin or
Disopyramide or
» Estrogens, including estramustine or
Levothyroxine or
Methadone or
Mexiletine or
» Quinidine
(concurrent use may decrease the effects of these medications because of increased metabolism resulting from induction of hepatic microsomal enzyme activity; dosage adjustments may be necessary)

(in addition, concurrent use of oral, estrogen-containing contraceptives with carbamazepine may result in breakthrough bleeding and contraceptive failure due to the increased rate of hepatic enzyme metabolism of steroids induced by carbamazepine; the dose of the estrogenic substance in the oral contraceptive may be increased to diminish bleeding and decrease the risk of conception; parenteral medroxyprogesterone or nonhormonal methods of birth control may be considered as alternatives)

» Corticosteroids
(concurrent use may decrease the corticosteroid effect because of increased corticosteroid metabolism resulting from induction of hepatic microsomal enzymes)

Danazol or
» Diltiazem or
Felodipine or
Loratadine or
Niacinamide or
Terfenadine or
» Verapamil
(concurrent use of these agents with carbamazepine may inhibit carbamazepine metabolism, resulting in increased plasma concentrations and toxicity)

(carbamazepine toxicity may be delayed for several weeks after initiation of danazol therapy; carbamazepine dosage may need to be reduced)

(it is recommended that nifedipine be used as an alternative to verapamil or diltiazem)

Doxycycline
(concurrent use may decrease plasma concentration and elimination half-life of doxycycline because of induction of hepatic microsomal enzyme activity; if concurrent use cannot be avoided, doxycycline plasma concentrations or the therapeutic response to doxycycline should be closely monitored and dosage adjustments made as necessary)

Enflurane or
Halothane or
Methoxyflurane
(chronic use of a hepatic enzyme–inducing agent such as carbamazepine prior to anesthesia may increase the metabolism of these anesthetics, leading to an increased risk of hepatotoxicity)

(formation of nephrotoxic metabolites of methoxyflurane may be increased by chronic use of a hepatic enzyme–inducing agent such as carbamazepine prior to anesthesia, leading to increased risk of nephrotoxicity)

(in addition, cardiac arrhythmias may occur, possibly due to sensitization of the myocardium resulting from increased concentrations of norepinephrine)

» Erythromycin or
Troleandomycin
(concurrent use of these agents with carbamazepine may inhibit carbamazepine metabolism, resulting in increased plasma concen-

**Carbamazepine (Systemic)**

trations and toxicity; it is recommended that an alternate antibiotic to erythromycin or troleandomycin be used)

» Felbamate
(concurrent use may decrease carbamazepine plasma concentrations by about 20 to 30% and increase carbamazepine-10,11–epoxide plasma concentrations by about 60%, leading to an increase in adverse effects; enzyme induction by carbamazepine may lead to decreased felbamate plasma concentrations; carbamazepine dosage should be reduced by 20 to 33% when felbamate therapy is initiated, and plasma concentrations of carbamazepine should be monitored with further dosage adjustments made as clinically necessary)

Folic acid
(requirements for folic acid may be increased in patients receiving anticonvulsant therapy)

Fluoxetine or
» Fluvoxamine
(concurrent use with carbamazepine may inhibit the metabolism of carbamazepine, resulting in increased plasma concentrations and toxicity; carbamazepine plasma concentrations should be monitored)

Influenza virus vaccine
(concurrent use with carbamazepine may inhibit carbamazepine metabolism, resulting in increased plasma concentrations and toxicity; carbamazepine plasma concentrations may be increased on days 7 to 14 after influenza virus vaccination; dosage adjustments of carbamazepine based on the patient's clinical status and plasma carbamazepine concentrations may be necessary)

» Isoniazid
(carbamazepine may induce microsomal metabolism of isoniazid, increasing formation of a reactive intermediate and leading to hepatotoxicity; also, isoniazid administration may result in elevated plasma concentrations of carbamazepine and possible toxicity)

Isotretinoin
(concurrent use with carbamazepine alters the bioavailability and/or clearance of carbamazepine and its active 10,11–epoxide metabolite; plasma concentrations should be monitored)

» Itraconazole and
» Ketoconazole
(concurrent use with carbamazepine may inhibit the metabolism of carbamazepine, resulting in increased plasma concentrations and toxicity)
(concurrent use of carbamazepine with itraconazole may decrease itraconazole plasma concentrations, leading to treatment failure or relapse)

» Lamotrigine
(concurrent use with carbamazepine increases the clearance of lamotrigine; initial lamotrigine dosage and rate of lamotrigine dosage escalation should be based on concomitant anticonvulsant therapy; monitoring of plasma concentrations of lamotrigine and carbamazepine should be considered, especially during dosage adjustments)
(an increased incidence of CNS adverse effects, including ataxia, blurred vision, diplopia, dizziness, or increased excitation, may occur with concomitant use of lamotrigine; dose reduction of either lamotrigine or carbamazepine may decrease these effects)

Lithium
(concurrent use may decrease the antidiuretic effect of carbamazepine and increase the neurotoxic side effects even at nontoxic blood concentrations of both lithium and carbamazepine; however, the concurrent use of lithium with carbamazepine may be synergistic in the treatment of patients with manic-depressive illness who fail to respond to either drug alone)

Mebendazole
(in patients receiving high oral doses of mebendazole for treatment of tissue-dwelling organisms such as *Echinococcus multilocularis* or *granulosus* [Hydatid disease], carbamazepine has been shown to lower plasma mebendazole concentrations by induction of hepatic microsomal enzymes and to impair the therapeutic response; if carbamazepine is being used for seizures, replacement with another anticonvulsant is recommended; treatment of intestinal helminths such as whipworms or hookworms does not appear to be affected by the rate of hepatic metabolism of mebendazole)

Metoclopramide
(concurrent use with carbamazepine may increase the risk of neurotoxic side effects, even if plasma concentrations remain in the therapeutic range)

» Monoamine oxidase (MAO) inhibitors, including furazolidone and procarbazine
(concurrent use with carbamazepine has resulted in hyperpyretic crises, hypertensive crises, severe convulsions, and death; a medication-free interval of at least 14 days is recommended between discontinuation of MAO inhibitor therapy and initiation of carbamazepine therapy, or vice versa)
(MAO inhibitors may also cause a change in the pattern of epileptiform seizures in patients receiving carbamazepine as an anticonvulsant)

Pancuronium
(carbamazepine antagonizes the effects of nondepolarizing muscle relaxants; dosage of the muscle relaxant may need to be increased; patients should be monitored closely for more rapid recovery from neuromuscular blockade than expected)

Praziquantel
(one small, single-dose, controlled study found that epileptic patients taking carbamazepine had significantly lower plasma concentrations of praziquantel [7.9% of the control group]; this effect is thought to be due to induction of the cytochrome P450 microsomal enzyme system by carbamazepine; patients on carbamazepine may require a larger dose of praziquantel)

» Propoxyphene
(concurrent use with carbamazepine may inhibit carbamazepine metabolism, resulting in increased plasma concentrations and toxicity; an analgesic other than propoxyphene should be used)

» Risperidone
(chronic administration of carbamazepine may increase the clearance of risperidone)

Tiagabine
(tiagabine clearance is increased by 60% in patients taking carbamazepine)

Topiramate
(when these two medications were given concurrently, the mean carbamazepine area under the plasma concentration–time curve [AUC] was unchanged or changed by less than 10%, whereas the AUC of topiramate was decreased by 40%)

**Laboratory value alterations**
The following have been selected on the basis of their potential clinical significance (possible effect in parentheses where appropriate)—not necessarily inclusive (» = major clinical significance):

With diagnostic test results
» Metyrapone test
(increased metabolism of metyrapone by a hepatic enzyme inducer such as carbamazepine may decrease the response to metyrapone)

Pregnancy test
(false-negative results may occur with the use of tests that determine human chorionic gonadotropin [HCG])

With physiology/laboratory test values
Alanine aminotransferase (ALT [SGPT]), serum, and
Alkaline phosphatase, serum, and
Aspartate aminotransferase (AST [SGOT]), serum
(values may be increased)

Bilirubin, serum and
Blood urea nitrogen (BUN)
(concentrations may be increased)

Cholesterol, serum and
High-density lipoprotein cholesterol, serum and
Triglyceride, serum
(concentrations may occasionally be increased)

Free cortisol, urine
(may be increased)

Glucose, urine and
Protein (albumin), urine
(may be detected in the urine)

Ionized calcium, serum
(concentrations may be decreased)

Thyroid hormones
(serum concentrations of $T_3$, free $T_4$, and free $T_4$ index may be decreased due to increased hepatic metabolism of hormones during long-term therapy with carbamazepine; thyroid size may be increased as a compensatory mechanism)

**Medical considerations/Contraindications**
The medical considerations/contraindications included have been selected on the basis of their potential clinical significance (reasons given in

parentheses where appropriate)—not necessarily inclusive (» = major clinical significance).

***Except under special circumstances, this medication should not be used when the following medical problems exist:***

» Absence seizures, atypical or generalized or
» Atonic seizures or
» Myoclonic seizures
   (increased risk of generalized seizures)
» Atrioventricular (AV) heart block or
» Blood disorders characterized by serious abnormalities in blood count, platelets, or serum iron or
» Bone marrow depression, history of
   (increased risk of exacerbation)

***Risk-benefit should be considered when the following medical problems exist:***

Alcoholism, active
   (CNS depression may be potentiated; in addition, the metabolism of carbamazepine may be accelerated)
Behavioral disorders
   (latent psychosis may be activated, or agitation or confusion may be produced in elderly patients, especially when carbamazepine is used concurrently with other medications)
Cardiac damage, including organic heart disease and congestive heart disease or
Coronary artery disease
   (may be exacerbated)
Diabetes mellitus
   (elevated urine glucose concentrations may occur)
Glaucoma or
Increased intraocular pressure
   (may be exacerbated because of mild anticholinergic effects of carbamazepine)
Hematologic reactions, adverse, to other medications, history of
   (patients may be especially at risk for carbamazepine-induced bone marrow depression)
Hepatic function impairment
   (increased risk of liver damage)
Hyponatremia, dilutional, caused by syndrome of inappropriate antidiuretic hormone (SIADH) secretion or other conditions such as hypopituitarism, hypothyroidism, or adrenocortical insufficiency or
Urinary retention
   (may be exacerbated)
Renal function impairment
   (excretion of carbamazepine may be altered)
Sensitivity to carbamazepine or to tricyclic antidepressants
Caution is also advised in administration to patients who have had interrupted courses of therapy with carbamazepine.

## Patient monitoring

The following may be especially important in patient monitoring (other tests may be warranted in some patients, depending on condition; » = major clinical significance):

» Blood counts, complete (CBCs), including platelet and possibly reticulocyte counts and
» Iron concentrations, serum
   (determinations recommended prior to initiation of therapy as a baseline. Patients who develop low or decreased white blood cell or platelet counts during the course of treatment should be monitored closely and carbamazepine discontinued if there is any evidence of significant bone marrow depression)
BUN determinations and
Ophthalmologic examinations, including slit-lamp funduscopy and tonometry, where indicated, and
Urinalysis, complete
   (recommended prior to initiation of therapy and at periodic intervals during therapy)
» Carbamazepine concentrations, plasma
   (determinations recommended periodically as a guide to efficacy and safety; plasma concentrations of 6 to 12 mcg per mL [25 to 51 micromoles per L] are optimal for anticonvulsant activity and, in rare cases, concentrations may go up to 16 mcg per mL [68 micromoles per L]; when used to treat psychiatric disorders, carbamazepine plasma concentrations of 8 to 12 mcg per mL [34 to 51 micromoles per L] are optimal; taking sample prior to the morning dose to determine lowest daily concentration is suggested)

Electrocardiogram (ECG) readings and
Electrolyte concentrations, serum
   (determinations recommended prior to therapy and periodically during therapy because of possibility of hyponatremia)
» Ionized calcium concentrations, serum
   (recommended every 6 months or if seizure frequency increases after weeks or months of carbamazepine therapy, since hypocalcemia decreases seizure threshold)
Liver function tests
   (recommended prior to initiation of therapy and at periodic intervals during therapy; discontinuation of carbamazepine should be considered immediately upon evidence of aggravated liver function impairment or new disease)

## Side/Adverse Effects

Note: Carbamazepine-induced stimulation of antidiuretic hormone (ADH) release may cause water retention resulting in significant volume expansion and dilutional hyponatremia (syndrome of inappropriate secretion of antidiuretic hormone). Patients reporting lethargy, weakness, nausea, vomiting, confusion or hostility, neurological abnormalities, stupor, or increased seizure frequency should be suspected of being hyponatremic, although many of these symptoms may also be associated with other carbamazepine-induced side effects.

A case of aseptic meningitis accompanied by myoclonus and peripheral eosinophilia has been reported in a patient taking carbamazepine in conjunction with other medications; rechallenge with carbamazepine resulted in recurrence of meningitis.

The following side/adverse effects have been selected on the basis of their potential clinical significance (possible signs and symptoms in parentheses where appropriate)—not necessarily inclusive:

**Those indicating need for medical attention**
Incidence more frequent
   *CNS toxicity, including blurred or double vision; or nystagmus* (continuous back-and-forth eye movements)
Incidence less frequent
   *Allergic reaction; Stevens-Johnson syndrome; or toxic epidermal necrolysis* (skin rash, hives, or itching); *behavioral changes*—especially in children; *diarrhea, severe; hyponatremia, dilutional, or water intoxication (SIADH)* (confusion, agitation, or hostility, especially in the elderly; continuing headache; increase in seizure frequency; severe nausea and vomiting; unusual drowsiness; weakness); *systemic lupus erythematosus (SLE)-like syndrome* (skin rash, hives, or itching; fever; sore throat; bone or joint pain; unusual tiredness or weakness)
   Note: The risk of *hyponatremia* and *SIADH* appears to increase with patient age and serum concentration of carbamazepine; *hyponatremia* seemingly does not occur in children.
Incidence rare
   *Adenopathy or lymphadenopathy* (swollen glands); *blood dyscrasias, including aplastic anemia* (shortness of breath, troubled breathing, wheezing, or tightness in chest; sores, ulcers, or white spots on lips or in mouth; swollen or painful glands; unusual bleeding or bruising); *agranulocytosis* (chills; fever; sore throat; unusual tiredness or weakness); *eosinophilia* (fever); *leukopenia* (usually asymptomatic; rarely, fever or chills; cough or hoarseness; lower back or side pain; painful or difficult urination); *pancytopenia* (nosebleeds or other unusual bleeding or bruising); *and thrombocytopenia* (usually asymptomatic; rarely, unusual bleeding or bruising; black, tarry stools; blood in urine or stools; pinpoint red spots on skin); *bone marrow depression* (chills; fever; sore throat; unusual bleeding or bruising); *cardiovascular effects, including arrhythmias* (fast, slow, or irregular heartbeat); *atrioventricular (AV) heart block* (unusual weakness; pounding heartbeat; troubled breathing; fainting); *bradycardia* (slow heartbeat); *congestive heart failure* (chest pain; troubled breathing; swelling of feet or lower legs; rapid weight gain); *edema* (swelling of face, hands, feet, or lower legs); *hypertension, increased* (high blood pressure); *hypotension* (low blood pressure); *and syncope* (fainting); *CNS toxicity* (difficulty in speaking or slurred speech; mental depression with restlessness and nervousness; rigidity; ringing, buzzing, or other unexplained sounds in the ears; trembling; uncontrolled body movements; visual hallucinations; *hypersensitivity hepatitis* (darkening of urine; pale stools; yellow eyes or skin); *hypocalcemia* (increase in seizure frequency; muscle or abdominal cramps); *renal toxicity, renal failure, acute, or water intoxication (SIADH)* (frequent urination; sudden decrease in amount of urine; swelling of feet or lower legs); *paresthesias or peripheral neuritis* (numbness, tingling, pain, or weakness in hands and feet); *porphyria, acute intermittent* (darkening of urine); *pulmonary hypersensitivity* (fever; troubled breathing; cough; shortness of breath; tightness in

chest; wheezing); ***thrombophlebitis*** (pain, tenderness, bluish color, or swelling of leg or foot)

Note: Geriatric patients and those with a defective conduction system may be especially susceptible to *AV heart block* or *bradycardia* with carbamazepine.

*Hypocalcemia* may lead to osteopenia as a direct effect of carbamazepine on bone metabolism.

**Those indicating need for medical attention only if they continue or are bothersome**
Incidence more frequent, especially during initiation of therapy
***Clumsiness or unsteadiness; confusion; dizziness, mild, or lightheadedness; drowsiness, mild; nausea or vomiting, mild***

Incidence less frequent or rare
***Aching joints or muscles or leg cramps; alopecia*** (loss of hair); ***anorexia*** (loss of appetite); ***constipation; diaphoresis*** (increased sweating); ***diarrhea; dryness of mouth; glossitis or stomatitis*** (irritation or soreness of tongue or mouth); ***headache; increased sensitivity of skin to sunlight; sexual problems in males; stomach pain or discomfort; unusual tiredness or weakness***

## Overdose

Note: For specific information on the agents used in the management of carbamazepine overdose, see:
- *Barbiturates (Systemic)* monograph;
- *Benzodiazepines (Systemic)* monograph;
- *Charcoal, Activated (Oral-Local)* monograph; and/or
- *Laxatives (Local)* monograph.

For more information on the management of overdose or unintentional ingestion, **contact a Poison Control Center** (see *Poison Control Center Listing*).

**Clinical effects of overdose**
The following effects have been selected on the basis of their potential clinical significance (possible signs and symptoms in parentheses where appropriate)—not necessarily inclusive:

***Anuria, oliguria, or urinary retention*** (sudden decrease in amount of urine); ***cardiovascular effects, including conduction disorders or tachycardia*** (fast or irregular heartbeat); ***convulsions***—especially in small children; ***dizziness, severe; drowsiness, severe; dysmetria*** (poor control in body movements—for example, when reaching or stepping); ***hyperreflexia, followed by hyporeflexia*** (overactive reflexes, followed by underactive reflexes); ***hypertension or hypotension*** (high or low blood pressure); ***motor restlessness; muscular twitching; mydriasis*** (large pupils); ***nausea or vomiting, severe; neurological effects, including ataxia*** (clumsiness or unsteadiness); ***athetoid movements or ballism*** (abnormal body movements); ***opisthotonus*** (body spasm in which head and heels are bent backward and body bowed forward); ***respiratory depression*** (irregular, slow, or shallow breathing); ***shock*** (fainting); ***tremor***

Note: Signs and symptoms of acute toxicity may occur 1 to 3 hours following ingestion of an overdose. Neurological and neuromuscular symptoms predominate, followed by cardiovascular toxicity. Symptoms resemble those observed following overdose with tricyclic antidepressants. Cardiotoxic effects are more likely to occur in elderly and cardiopathic patients.

Laboratory findings in overdosage may indicate leukocytosis, reduced leukocyte count, glycosuria, acetonuria, and electroencephalogram (EEG) dysrhythmias.

**Treatment of overdose**
Recommended treatment consists of the following:
To decrease absorption—Induction of emesis or gastric lavage, followed by administration of activated charcoal or laxatives to reduce further absorption.

To enhance elimination—Forced diuresis may accelerate elimination. Dialysis is indicated only in severe poisoning associated with renal failure. In small children, severe poisoning may require replacement transfusion.

Specific treatment—For hypotension and shock, elevation of patient's legs and administration of a plasma volume expander. Use of a vasopressor may be considered if other measures are insufficient. Administration of a benzodiazepine or a barbiturate as required for seizures. The fact that these agents may aggravate respiratory depression (especially in children), hypotension, and coma must be considered. Also, barbiturates or benzodiazepines should not be used if the patient has taken a monoamine oxidase inhibitor within the previous 14 days.

Monitoring—Monitoring of respiration, cardiac function, blood pressure, body temperature, pupillary reflexes, and kidney and bladder function for several days.

Supportive care—Maintenance of a patent airway with tracheal intubation, artificial respiration, and/or administration of oxygen. Patients in whom intentional overdose is confirmed or suspected should be referred for psychiatric consultation.

## Patient Consultation

As an aid to patient consultation, refer to *Advice for the Patient, Carbamazepine (Systemic)*.

In providing consultation, consider emphasizing the following selected information (» = major clinical significance):

**Before using this medication**
» Conditions affecting use, especially:
  Sensitivity to tricyclic antidepressants or carbamazepine
  Pregnancy—Crosses placenta; babies reportedly born with small head circumference, low birth weight, craniofacial defects, fingernail hypoplasia, developmental delays, and spina bifida; animal studies have shown rib anomalies, cleft palate, foot deformities, or anophthalmos with doses 10 to 25 times the human dose
  Breast-feeding—Distributed into breast milk; animal studies have shown lack of weight gain and unkempt appearance of young at high doses
  Use in children—Appropriate studies have not been done in children up to 6 years of age; behavior changes more likely to occur in children
  Use in the elderly—Elderly more likely to have confusion or agitation, AV heart block, SIADH, or bradycardia than are younger people
  Dental—Increased incidence of blood dyscrasias that cause infection, delayed healing, or gingival bleeding; proper oral hygiene necessary
  Surgical—Recovery from neuromuscular blockade induced by nondepolarizing muscle relaxants such as pancuronium may be more rapid than expected due to antagonism by carbamazepine
  Other medications, especially anticoagulants, other anticonvulsants, tricyclic antidepressants, barbiturates, benzodiazepines metabolized via hepatic microsomal enzymes (especially clonazepam), cimetidine, clarithromycin, oral estrogen-containing contraceptives, corticosteroids, diltiazem, erythromycin, estrogens, isoniazid, fluvoxamine, itraconazole, ketoconazole, lamotrigine, MAO inhibitors, propoxyphene, quinidine, risperidone, or verapamil
  Other medical problems, especially absence, atonic, or myoclonic seizures; AV heart block; blood disorders; or bone marrow depression

**Proper use of this medication**
» Taking with food to lessen gastrointestinal irritation
» Compliance with therapy; not taking more or less medication than prescribed
» Not using medication for minor aches and pains
» Proper dosing
  Missed dose: Taking as soon as possible; not taking if almost time for next dose; not doubling doses; calling physician if more than one dose a day is missed
» Proper storage; not storing tablet dosage forms in bathroom or other high-moisture areas due to loss of potency and effectiveness

*For use in epilepsy*
» Checking with physician before discontinuing medication; gradual dosage reduction may be necessary to prevent seizures or status epilepticus

**Precautions while using this medication**
» Regular visits to physician to check progress of therapy
» Avoiding the use of alcoholic beverages and other CNS depressants while taking this medicine
» Possible drowsiness, dizziness, lightheadedness, blurred or double vision, weakness, or muscular incoordination; caution when driving or using machinery, or doing jobs requiring alertness and coordination
» Possible skin photosensitivity; avoiding unprotected exposure to sun; using protective clothing; using a sun block product that includes protection against both UVA-caused photosensitivity reactions and UVB-caused sunburn reactions; avoiding use of sunlamp, tanning bed, or tanning booth
» Using different or additional means of birth control than estrogen-containing oral contraceptives
  Diabetic patients: May increase urine sugar concentrations

Caution if any laboratory tests required; possible interference with results of metyrapone or pregnancy tests

» Caution if any kind of surgery, dental treatment, or emergency treatment is needed

Carrying medical identification card or bracelet during therapy

### Side/adverse effects

Signs of potential side effects, especially CNS toxicity, allergic reaction, Stevens-Johnson syndrome, toxic epidermal necrolysis, behavioral changes, severe diarrhea, dilutional hyponatremia or water intoxication (SIADH), SLE-like syndrome, adenopathy or lymphadenopathy, blood dyscrasias, bone marrow depression, cardiovascular effects, hypersensitivity hepatitis, hypocalcemia, renal toxicity or failure, paresthesias or peripheral neuritis, porphyria, pulmonary hypersensitivity, or thrombophlebitis

## General Dosing Information

Side effects may be minimized by initiating therapy with low doses, which should be increased gradually at weekly intervals until an adequate response is obtained; administering carbamazepine with meals, and giving the total daily dosage in 3 or 4 divided doses may also minimize side effects.

When carbamazepine is added to existing anticonvulsant therapy, it should be added gradually while the other anticonvulsants are maintained or gradually decreased, except for phenytoin, which may have to be increased.

The maintenance dosage of carbamazepine may need to be increased progressively over the first few weeks of treatment to avoid low plasma carbamazepine concentrations caused by autoinduction.

Abrupt discontinuation in a responsive epileptic patient may result in convulsions and possibly status epilepticus; gradual withdrawal is recommended.

Therapy should be discontinued if cardiovascular reactions or skin rashes occur.

When carbamazepine is used as an antineuralgic in specific pain syndromes, *an attempt should be made at least once every few months to reduce dosage or discontinue therapy* if the patient is totally free of pain.

Carbamazepine suspension should not be administered simultaneously with other liquid medications or diluents because of the possibility of precipitation of an orange rubbery mass. This phenomenon has been observed after mixing carbamazepine suspension with chlorpromazine solution or with liquid forms of thioridazine hydrochloride.

### Diet/Nutrition

Carbamazepine suspension and tablets should be taken with food to lessen gastrointestinal irritation. Carbamazepine extended-release capsules may be taken with or without food. The contents of carbamazepine extended-release capsules may also be sprinkled over food (such as a teaspoonful of applesauce or other similar food products); the capsule or its contents should not be crushed or chewed.

The requirements for folic acid may be increased in patients receiving anticonvulsant therapy.

### Bioequivalenence information

Administration of carbamazepine suspension results in higher peak serum concentrations than does the same dose administered as tablets. It is recommended that doses of the suspension be initially lower and be increased more slowly than doses of the tablets to avoid side effects.

### For treatment of adverse effects

Treatment of bone marrow depression includes the following:
- Discontinuing carbamazepine therapy.
- Daily CBC, platelet, and reticulocyte counts.
- Performing a bone marrow aspiration and trephine biopsy immediately and repeating with sufficient frequency to monitor recovery.
- Considering other studies that may be helpful, including white cell and platelet antibodies; $^{59}$Fe—ferrokinetic studies; peripheral blood cell typing; cytogenic studies on marrow and peripheral blood; bone marrow culture studies for colony-forming units; hemoglobin electrophoresis for A$^2$ and F hemoglobin; and serum folic acid and B$_{12}$ concentrations. If aplastic anemia develops, specialized consultation should be sought for appropriate monitoring and treatment.

## Oral Dosage Forms

Note: Bracketed uses in the *Dosage Forms* section refer to categories of use and/or indications that are not included in U.S. product labeling.

## CARBAMAZEPINE ORAL SUSPENSION USP

### Usual adult and adolescent dose

Anticonvulsant—
  Initial: Oral, 100 mg four times a day on the first day, the dosage being increased by up to 200 mg a day at weekly intervals. Some clinicians recommend initiating therapy at 100 mg a day and increasing to full therapeutic dosage slowly at weekly intervals to avoid side effects and potential noncompliance.
  Maintenance: Oral, usually 800 mg to 1.2 grams a day.

Antineuralgic—
  Initial: Oral, 50 mg four times a day on the first day, the dosage being increased by up to 200 mg a day, using increments of 50 mg four times a day only as needed until pain is relieved.
  Maintenance: Oral, 200 mg to 1.2 grams a day (average 400 to 800 mg a day) in divided doses.

[Antidiuretic][1]—
  Oral, 300 to 600 mg a day if used as sole therapy; or 200 to 400 mg a day if used concurrently with other antidiuretic agents.

[Antimanic][1] or
[Antipsychotic][1]—
  Oral, initially 200 to 400 mg a day in divided doses, the dosage being gradually increased at weekly intervals up to a maximum of 1.6 grams a day as needed and tolerated according to clinical response.

Note: Whenever possible, total daily dosage should be given in 3 or 4 divided doses.

### Usual adult and adolescent prescribing limits

Anticonvulsant—
  Patients 12 to 15 years of age:
    Dosage should generally not exceed 1 gram a day.
  Patients 15 years of age and over:
    Dosage should generally not exceed 1.2 grams a day. In rare instances, doses of up to 1.6 grams a day have been used in adults.

Antineuralgic—
  Dosage should not exceed 1.2 grams a day.

### Usual pediatric dose

Anticonvulsant—
  Children up to 6 years of age:
    Initial—Oral, 10 to 20 mg per kg of body weight a day in two or three divided doses, the dosage being increased by up to 100 mg a day at weekly intervals as needed and tolerated.
    Maintenance—Oral, adjusted to the minimum effective dosage, usually 250 to 350 mg a day, and generally not exceeding 400 mg or 35 mg per kg of body weight a day.
  Children 6 to 12 years of age:
    Initial—Oral, 50 mg four times a day on the first day, the dosage being increased by up to 100 mg a day at weekly intervals until the best response is obtained.
    Maintenance—Oral, adjusted to the minimum effective dosage, usually 400 to 800 mg a day.

Note: Dosage generally should not exceed 1 gram a day.
  Whenever possible, total daily dosage should be given in 3 or 4 divided doses.

### Strength(s) usually available

U.S.—
  100 mg per 5 mL (Rx) [*Tegretol* (citrus-vanilla flavor; sorbitol; sucrose)].

Canada—
  100 mg per 5 mL (Rx) [*Tegretol* (citrus-vanilla flavor; sorbitol; sucrose)].

### Packaging and storage

Store below 30 °C (86 °F), in a tight, light-resistant container, unless otherwise specified by manufacturer. Protect from freezing.

### Auxiliary labeling

- Shake well before using.
- May cause drowsiness.
- Take with meals.

## CARBAMAZEPINE TABLETS USP

### Usual adult and adolescent dose

Anticonvulsant—
  Initial: Oral, 200 mg two times a day on the first day, the dosage being increased by up to 200 mg a day at weekly intervals until the best response is obtained. Some clinicians recommend initiating therapy at 100 mg a day and increasing to full therapeutic dosage slowly at weekly intervals to avoid side effects and potential noncompliance.
  Maintenance: Oral, adjusted to the minimum effective dosage, usually 600 mg to 1.6 grams a day.

Antineuralgic—
: Initial: Oral, 100 mg two times a day on the first day, the dosage being increased by up to 200 mg a day, using increments of 100 mg every twelve hours only as needed until pain is relieved.
: Maintenance: Oral, 200 mg to 1.2 grams a day (average 400 to 800 mg a day) in divided doses.

[Antidiuretic][1]—
: Oral, 300 to 600 mg a day if used as sole therapy; or 200 to 400 mg a day if used concurrently with other antidiuretic agents.

[Antimanic][1] or
[Antipsychotic][1]—
: Oral, initially 200 to 400 mg a day in divided doses, the dosage being gradually increased at weekly intervals up to a maximum of 1.6 grams a day as needed and tolerated according to clinical response.

Note: Whenever possible, total daily dosage should be given in 3 or 4 divided doses.

### Usual adult and adolescent prescribing limits
Anticonvulsant—
: Patients 12 to 15 years of age:
: : Dosage should generally not exceed 1 gram a day.
: Patients 15 years of age and over:
: : Dosage should generally not exceed 1.2 grams a day. In rare instances, doses of up to 1.6 grams a day have been used in adults.

Antineuralgic—
: Dosage should not exceed 1.2 grams a day.

### Usual pediatric dose
Anticonvulsant—
: Children up to 6 years of age:
: : Initial—Oral, 10 to 20 mg per kg of body weight a day in two or three divided doses, the dosage being increased by up to 100 mg a day at weekly intervals as needed and tolerated.
: : Maintenance—Oral, adjusted to the minimum effective dosage, usually 250 to 350 mg a day, and generally not exceeding 400 mg or 35 mg per kg of body weight a day.
: Children 6 to 12 years of age:
: : Initial—Oral, 100 mg two times a day on the first day, the dosage being increased by 100 mg a day at weekly intervals until the best response is obtained.
: : Maintenance—Oral, adjusted to the minimum effective dosage, usually 400 to 800 mg a day.

Note: Dosage generally should not exceed 1 gram a day.
: Whenever possible, total daily dosage should be given in 3 or 4 divided doses.

### Strength(s) usually available
U.S.—
: 200 mg (Rx) [*Atretol* (scored); *Epitol* (scored); *Tegretol* (scored); GENERIC (scored)].

Canada—
: 200 mg (Rx) [*Apo-Carbamazepine* (double-scored); *Novo-Carbamaz* (scored); *Nu-Carbamazepine* (double-scored); *Taro-Carbamazepine* (double-scored); *Tegretol* (double-scored)].

### Packaging and storage
Store below 40 °C (104 °F), preferably between 15 and 30 °C (59 and 86 °F), unless otherwise specified by manufacturer. Store in a tight container.

### Auxiliary labeling
- May cause drowsiness.
- Take with meals.
- Store in a dry place.
- Protect from moisture.

## CARBAMAZEPINE TABLETS (CHEWABLE) USP

### Usual adult and adolescent dose
See *Carbamazepine Tablets USP*.

### Usual adult and adolescent prescribing limits
See *Carbamazepine Tablets USP*.

### Usual pediatric dose
See *Carbamazepine Tablets USP*.

### Strength(s) usually available
U.S.—
: 100 mg (Rx) [*Epitol* (scored); *Tegretol* (scored; sucrose) [GENERIC (scored)].

Canada—
: 100 mg (Rx) [*Tegretol Chewtabs* (scored)].
: 200 mg (Rx) [*Tegretol Chewtabs* (scored)].

### Packaging and storage
Store below 40 °C (104 °F), preferably between 15 and 30 °C (59 and 86 °F), unless otherwise specified by manufacturer. Store in a tight container.

### Auxiliary labeling
- May cause drowsiness.
- Take with meals.
- May be chewed.
- Store in a dry place.
- Protect from moisture.

## CARBAMAZEPINE EXTENDED-RELEASE CAPSULES

### Usual adult and adolescent dose
Anticonvulsant—
: Initial: Oral, 200 mg two times a day, the dosage being increased gradually as needed and tolerated. Some clinicians recommend increasing to full therapeutic dosage slowly at weekly intervals to avoid side effects and potential noncompliance.
: Maintenance: Oral, adjusted to the minimum effective dosage, usually 800 to 1200 mg a day.

Antineuralgic—
: Initial: Oral, 200 mg on the first day, the dosage being increased by up to 200 mg a day every twelve hours only as needed until pain is relieved.
: Maintenance: Oral, 200 mg to 1.2 grams a day (average 400 to 800 mg a day) in divided doses.

Note: As soon as pain relief is maintained, the dosage should be reduced to the minimum effective dose.
: Attempts should be made at intervals of not more than 3 months to reduce or discontinue use.

### Usual adult and adolescent prescribing limits
Anticonvulsant—
: Patients 12 to 15 years of age:
: : Dosage should generally not exceed 1 gram a day.
: Patients 15 years of age and over:
: : Dosage should generally not exceed 1.2 grams a day. In rare instances, doses of up to 1.6 grams a day have been used in adults.

Antineuralgic—
: Dosage should not exceed 1.2 grams a day.

### Usual pediatric dose
Anticonvulsant—
: Children up to 12 years of age:
: : Oral, doses of immediate-release carbamazepine of 400 mg or greater may be converted to the same total daily dose of extended-release carbamazepine capsules using the twice a day regimen. Ordinarily, optimal clinical response is achieved at daily doses below 35 mg per kg of body weight.

Note: When seizure relief is maintained, the dosage should be reduced gradually to the lowest effective dose.
: If satisfactory clinical response has not been achieved, plasma concentrations of carbamazepine should be measured to determine whether they are in the therapeutic range.
: Dosage generally should not exceed 1 gram a day.

### Strength(s) usually available
U.S.—
: 200 mg (Rx) [*Carbatrol*].
: 300 mg (Rx) [*Carbatrol*].

Canada—
: Not commercially available.

### Packaging and storage
Store at controlled room temperature, preferably between 15 and 25 °C (59 and 77 °F), in a tight container, unless otherwise specified by manufacturer. Protect from light.

### Auxiliary labeling
- May cause drowsiness.
- Do not chew.

## CARBAMAZEPINE EXTENDED-RELEASE TABLETS

### Usual adult and adolescent dose
Anticonvulsant—
: Initial: Oral, 100 to 200 mg one or two times a day with meals, the dosage being increased gradually as needed and tolerated. Some clinicians recommend initiating therapy at 100 mg a day and increasing to full therapeutic dosage slowly at weekly intervals to avoid side effects and potential noncompliance.
: Maintenance: Oral, adjusted to the minimum effective dosage, usually 800 to 1200 mg a day.

Antineuralgic—
: Oral, initially 100 mg two times a day on the first day, the dosage being increased by 200 mg a day (in increments of 100 mg every twelve hours) only as needed and tolerated until pain is relieved.

Note: As soon as pain relief is maintained, the dosage should be reduced to the minimum effective dose.

Attempts should be made at intervals of not more than 3 months to reduce or discontinue use.

**Usual adult and adolescent prescribing limits**
Anticonvulsant—
  Patients 12 to 15 years of age:
    Dosage should generally not exceed 1 gram a day.
  Patients 15 years of age and over:
    Dosage should generally not exceed 1.2 grams a day. In rare instances, doses of up to 1.6 grams a day have been used in adults.
Antineuralgic—
  Dosage should not exceed 1.2 grams a day.

**Usual pediatric dose**
Anticonvulsant—
  Children 6 to 12 years of age:
    Oral, initially 100 mg one to two times on the first day, the dosage being increased gradually by 100 mg a day as needed and tolerated until the best response is obtained.
  Note: When seizure relief is maintained, the dosage should be reduced gradually to the lowest effective dose.
    Dosage generally should not exceed 1 gram a day.

**Strength(s) usually available**
U.S.—
  100 mg (Rx) [*Tegretol-XR*].
  200 mg (Rx) [*Tegretol-XR*].
  400 mg (Rx) [*Tegretol-XR*].
Canada—
  200 mg (Rx) [*Taro-Carbamazepine CR; Tegretol CR* (scored)].
  400 mg (Rx) [*Taro-Carbamazepine CR; Tegretol CR* (scored)].

**Packaging and storage**
Store below 40 °C (104 °F), preferably between 15 and 30 °C (59 and 86 °F), in a tight container, unless otherwise specified by manufacturer.

**Auxiliary labeling**
• May cause drowsiness.
• Take with meals.
• Do not chew.

[1]Not included in Canadian product labeling.

Revised: 08/11/98

**CARBENICILLIN**—See *Penicillins (Systemic)*

# CARBIDOPA AND LEVODOPA   Systemic

Pharmacy Equivalent Name (PEN): Co-Careldopa
VA CLASSIFICATION (Primary): CN500
Commonly used brand name(s): *Sinemet; Sinemet CR 25-100; Sinemet CR 50-200*.
Note: For a listing of dosage forms and brand names by country availability, see *Dosage Forms* section(s).

## Category
Antidyskinetic.

## Indications
**Accepted**
Parkinsonism (treatment)—Carbidopa and levodopa combination is indicated in the treatment of idiopathic Parkinson's disease (paralysis agitans), postencephalitic parkinsonism, or symptomatic parkinsonism, which may follow injury to the nervous system by carbon monoxide intoxication or manganese intoxication, to permit achievement of symptomatic relief with a lower dosage of levodopa than with levodopa alone. Also, it permits a smoother and more rapid dosage titration, reduces nausea and vomiting, and allows concurrent administration of pyridoxine when necessary.

## Pharmacology/Pharmacokinetics
See also *Levodopa (Systemic)*.
**Physicochemical characteristics**
Molecular weight—Carbidopa: 244.25.
**Mechanism of action/Effect**
Carbidopa—Inhibits the peripheral decarboxylation of levodopa, thus slowing its conversion to dopamine in extracerebral tissues. This results in an increased availability of levodopa for transport to the brain where it undergoes decarboxylation to dopamine.
**Absorption**
Carbidopa and levodopa combination—
  Tablets: Absorption is rapid and virtually complete in 2 to 3 hours.
  Extended-release tablets: Absorption is gradual and continuous for 4 to 6 hours, although the majority of the dose is absorbed in 2 to 3 hours.
Bioavailability of carbidopa and levodopa extended-release tablets—
  Approximately 70 to 75% relative to the immediate-release tablets.
  Increased somewhat in the presence of food.
  Two half tablets approximately 20% more bioavailable than one intact tablet.
**Distribution**
Carbidopa—Widely distributed in body tissues other than the central nervous system (CNS).

**Protein binding**
Carbidopa—Moderate (approximately 36%).
**Biotransformation**
Carbidopa—Not extensive. Inhibits metabolism of levodopa in the gastrointestinal tract, thus increasing its absorption from the gastrointestinal tract and its concentration in plasma.
**Half-life**
Carbidopa—1 to 2 hours. When given in combination with levodopa, increases levodopa's plasma half-life from 1 hour to about 2 hours, and, in some cases to as long as 15 hours.
**Time to peak concentration**
Peak levodopa concentrations at steady state—
  Tablets:
    0.7 hours.
  Extended-release tablets:
    2.4 hours.
  Note: Peak plasma concentrations of levodopa are increased when the extended-release tablets are administered with food.
    Plasma concentrations of levodopa fluctuate less with the extended-release tablets than with the immediate release tablets.
**Elimination**
Carbidopa—Renal; 30% of dose of carbidopa excreted unchanged in urine within 24 hours. When given in combination with carbidopa, the amount of levodopa excreted unchanged in urine is increased by about 6%.

## Precautions to Consider
**Pregnancy/Reproduction**
Pregnancy—Studies in humans have not been done.
Reproduction studies in rodents have shown that levodopa, when given in doses in excess of 200 mg per kg of body weight (mg/kg) per day, depresses fetal and postnatal growth and viability. Also, studies in rabbits have shown that levodopa alone or in combination with carbidopa causes visceral and skeletal malformations.
FDA Pregnancy Category C.
**Breast-feeding**
Levodopa is distributed into breast milk. Although problems in humans have not been documented, breast-feeding is not recommended because of the potential for side effects in the infant.
Also, levodopa may inhibit lactation.
**Pediatrics**
Appropriate studies on the relationship of age to the effects of carbidopa and levodopa have not been performed in children up to 18 years of age. Safety and efficacy have not been established.

## Geriatrics
Smaller doses may be required in geriatric patients since they may have reduced tolerance to the effects of levodopa. Also, peripheral dopa decarboxylase, the enzyme responsible for decarboxylation, decreases with age, thus making large doses unnecessary.

Geriatric patients, especially those with osteoporosis, responsive to antiparkinsonian therapy should resume normal activity gradually and with caution because increased mobility may increase risk of fractures.

Psychic side effects, such as anxiety, confusion, or nervousness, are more common in geriatric patients receiving other antiparkinsonian medications, especially anticholinergics.

## Dental
Involuntary movements of jaws may result in poor retention of full dentures; dosage reduction may be required.

## Drug interactions and/or related problems
The following drug interactions and/or related problems have been selected on the basis of their potential clinical significance (possible mechanism in parentheses where appropriate)—not necessarily inclusive (» = major clinical significance):

Note: Combinations containing any of the following medications, depending on the amount present, may also interact with this medication.

Amantadine or
Benztropine or
Procyclidine or
Trihexyphenidyl
(concurrent use may result in increased efficacy of levodopa; however, concurrent use is not recommended if there is a history of psychosis)

» Anesthetics, hydrocarbon inhalation
(administration prior to anesthesia with these agents may result in cardiac arrhythmias because of increased endogenous dopamine concentration; carbidopa and levodopa combination should be discontinued 6 to 8 hours before the administration of these anesthetics, especially halothane)

» Anticonvulsants, hydantoin or
Benzodiazepines or
Droperidol or
» Haloperidol or
Loxapine or
Metyrosine or
Papaverine or
» Phenothiazines or
Rauwolfia alkaloids or
Thioxanthenes
(concurrent use may decrease the therapeutic effects of levodopa; hydantoin anticonvulsants increase the metabolism of levodopa, thus decreasing its therapeutic effects; since droperidol, haloperidol, loxapine, papaverine, phenothiazines, and the thioxanthenes block the dopamine receptors in the brain, they may induce extrapyramidal symptoms, thus aggravating parkinsonism and antagonizing the effects of levodopa; the rauwolfia alkaloids cause dopamine depletion in the brain, thus opposing the effects of levodopa)

Bromocriptine
(may produce additive effects, allowing reduction in levodopa dosage)

» Cocaine
(concurrent use with levodopa may increase the risk of cardiac arrhythmias; if use of cocaine is necessary in patients receiving levodopa, it is recommended that cocaine be administered with caution, in reduced dosage, and in conjunction with electrocardiographic monitoring)

Foods, especially high-protein
(concurrent or previous ingestion of food may decrease the absorption of levodopa from the gastrointestinal tract, consequently delaying its effect; in addition, proteins in food may be degraded into the amino acids that compete with levodopa for transport to the brain, thus decreasing and/or making erratic the response to levodopa; however, rather than cutting down on daily protein intake to avoid this effect on levodopa, it is recommended that the intake of proteins be distributed equally throughout the day)

Hypotension-producing medications, other (See *Appendix II*)
(concurrent use with levodopa may result in an increased hypotensive effect)

Methyldopa
(concurrent use with levodopa may alter the antiparkinsonian effects of levodopa and may also produce additive toxic CNS effects such as psychosis)

Metoclopramide
(gastric emptying of levodopa may be accelerated with concurrent use of metoclopramide, thus possibly increasing levodopa's rate and extent of absorption from the small intestine; the clinical significance of this interaction has not been determined)

Molindone
(concurrent use may inhibit antiparkinsonian effects of levodopa by blocking dopamine receptor in the brain; also, levodopa may counteract the antipsychotic effects of molindone)

» Monoamine oxidase (MAO) inhibitors, including furazolidone and procarbazine
(although high doses [300 to 400 mg a day] of carbidopa in combination with levodopa may help suppress the hypertensive reactions caused by concurrent use with MAO inhibitors, it is recommended that MAO inhibitors be discontinued for 2 to 4 weeks prior to initiation of carbidopa and levodopa combination therapy)

» Selegiline
(although sometimes used in conjunction with carbidopa and levodopa combination, selegiline may enhance levodopa-induced dyskinesias, nausea, orthostatic hypotension, confusion, and hallucinations; levodopa dosage should be reduced within 2 to 3 days after the initiation of selegiline therapy)

## Laboratory value alterations
The following have been selected on the basis of their potential clinical significance (possible effect in parentheses where appropriate)—not necessarily inclusive (» = major clinical significance):

With diagnostic test results
Coombs' (antiglobulin) test
(occasionally becomes positive after long-term levodopa therapy)

Gonadorelin test
(levodopa may elevate serum gonadotropin concentrations)

Glucose, urine
(tests using copper reduction methods may cause false-positive results; tests using glucose oxidase methods may cause false-negative results)

Ketones, urine
(tests using dipstick or test tape methods may cause false-positive results)

Norepinephrine, urine
(test shows false-positive results)

Protein, urine
(use of the Lowery test may cause false-positive results)

Thyroid function determinations
(chronic use of levodopa may inhibit the TSH response to protirelin)

Uric acid, serum and urine
(tests may show high concentrations with colorimetric measurements, but not with uricase)

With physiology/laboratory values
Alanine aminotransferase (ALT [SGPT]) and
Alkaline phosphatase and
Aspartate aminotransferase (AST [SGOT]) and
Bilirubin and
Lactate dehydrogenase (LDH) and
Protein-bound iodine (PBI)
(serum concentrations may be increased)

Blood urea nitrogen (BUN)
(concentrations may be increased)

Note: Concentrations of BUN, creatinine, and uric acid, although elevated during carbidopa and levodopa therapy, are elevated to a lesser degree than when levodopa is used alone.

## Medical considerations/Contraindications
The medical considerations/contraindications included have been selected on the basis of their potential clinical significance (reasons given in parentheses where appropriate)—not necessarily inclusive (» = major clinical significance).

### Risk-benefit should be considered when the following medical problems exist:
» Bronchial asthma, emphysema, and other severe pulmonary diseases
(respiratory effects of levodopa may aggravate condition)

» Cardiovascular disease, severe
(increased risk of cardiac arrhythmias)

Convulsive disorders, history of
(use of levodopa may precipitate seizures)

Diabetes mellitus
(use of levodopa may adversely affect control of glucose in blood)

Endocrine diseases
(use of levodopa may adversely affect hypothalamus or pituitary function)
» Glaucoma, angle-closure, or predisposition to
(mydriatic effect resulting in increased intraocular pressure may precipitate an acute attack of angle closure glaucoma)
Glaucoma, open-angle, chronic
(mydriatic effect may cause a slight increase in intraocular pressure; glaucoma therapy may need to be adjusted)
Hepatic function impairment
» Melanoma, history of or suspected
(use of levodopa may activate a malignant melanoma)
» Myocardial infarction, history of, with residual arrhythmias
(use of levodopa may precipitate or aggravate condition)
» Peptic ulcer, history of
(increased risk of upper gastrointestinal hemorrhage)
» Psychotic states
(increased risk of developing depression and suicidal tendencies)
» Renal function impairment
(use of levodopa may lead to urinary retention)
Sensitivity to carbidopa and/or levodopa
» Urinary retention
(use of levodopa may precipitate or aggravate condition)

**Patient monitoring**
The following may be especially important in patient monitoring (other tests may be warranted in some patients, depending on condition; » = major clinical significance):
Blood cell counts and
Hemoglobin determinations and
Hepatic function determinations and
Ophthalmologic examinations for glaucoma and monitoring of intraocular pressure in patients with open angle glaucoma and
Renal function determinations
(recommended at periodic intervals for patients on long-term levodopa therapy; also, blood cell counts and hepatic and renal function determinations are recommended after withdrawal of levodopa therapy as part of the evaluation of a patient with suspected neuroleptic malignant–like syndrome)
Cardiovascular monitoring for detection of arrhythmias or orthostatic hypotensive tendencies
(recommended during the period of initial dosage adjustment)
Serum creatine phosphokinase concentrations
(determinations recommended after discontinuation of levodopa therapy, especially if fever is present; an elevated serum creatine phosphokinase level may be an early indication of the presence of neuroleptic malignant–like syndrome)

## Side/Adverse Effects

Note: Carbidopa, in doses used to inhibit peripheral decarboxylation of levodopa, has no significant ability to produce side effects. However, it allows certain CNS side effects of levodopa, such as dyskinesias and mental effects, to develop sooner and at lower levodopa doses because of the resultant greater efficiency per dose of levodopa.

Patients receiving carbidopa and levodopa combination for one to several years may experience sudden, unexpected akinesia, tremor, and rigidity, such as the "on-off" phenomenon. Emotional stress may precipitate akinesia paradoxica or "start hesitation" in these patients.

A syndrome resembling neuroleptic malignant syndrome, which includes intermittent dystonia alternating with substantial agitation, hyperthermia and mental changes, has been reported after the abrupt discontinuation of levodopa therapy.

Convulsions have been reported but a causal relationship to the use of levodopa or carbidopa and levodopa combination has not been established.

The following side/adverse effects have been selected on the basis of their potential clinical significance (possible signs and symptoms in parentheses where appropriate)—not necessarily inclusive:

**Those indicating need for medical attention**
Incidence more frequent
**Mental depression; mood or mental changes, such as aggressive behavior; uncontrolled movements of the body, including the face, tongue, arms, hands, head, and upper body**—may indicate excessive concentration of dopamine in the corpus striatum

Note: *Mental depression, mood or mental changes, and uncontrolled movements of the body* tend to appear earlier during therapy with carbidopa and levodopa than with levodopa alone.
*Choreiform and other involuntary movements* occur in 50 to 80% of patients and are usually dose-related.

Incidence less frequent
**Difficult urination; irregular heartbeat; nausea or vomiting, severe or continuing; orthostatic hypotension** (dizziness or lightheadedness when getting up from a lying or sitting position); **spasm or closing of eyelids**—possible early sign of overdose

Note: *Nausea and vomiting* may occur frequently in early carbidopa and levodopa therapy with tolerance being gradually achieved during continued use. The concurrent use of carbidopa with levodopa often reduces the frequency and severity of nausea and vomiting, although approximately 15% of patients continue to experience these side effects.

Incidence rare
*Duodenal ulcer* (stomach pain); **hemolytic anemia** (unusual tiredness or weakness); **hypertension** (high blood pressure)

**Those indicating need for medical attention only if they continue or are bothersome**
Incidence more frequent
*Anxiety, confusion, or nervousness*—especially in elderly patients receiving other antiparkinsonian medication

Incidence less frequent
*Anorexia* (loss of appetite); **blurred vision; constipation; diarrhea; dryness of mouth; flushing of skin; headache; insomnia** (trouble in sleeping); **muscle twitching; nightmares; unusual tiredness or weakness**

**Those not indicating need for medical attention**
Incidence less frequent
*Darkening in color of urine or sweat*

## Overdose

For more information on the management of overdose or unintentional ingestion, **contact a Poison Control Center** (See *Poison Control Center Listing*).

**Clinical effects of overdose**
*Spasm or closing of eyelids*—possible early sign of overdose

**Treatment of overdose**
Since there is no specific antidote for acute overdose with carbidopa and levodopa, treatment is symptomatic and supportive, with possible utilization of the following
To decrease absorption—Immediate gastric lavage.
Specific treatment—
Antiarrhythmic medication, if necessary.
Pyridoxine is not effective in reversing the actions of carbidopa and levodopa combination.
The value of dialysis in the treatment of overdose is not known.
Supportive care—Patients in whom intentional overdose is confirmed or suspected should be referred for psychiatric consultation.

## Patient Consultation

As an aid to patient consultation, refer to *Advice for the Patient, Levodopa (Systemic)*.

In providing consultation, consider emphasizing the following selected information (» = major clinical significance):

**Before using this medication**
» Conditions affecting use, especially:
Sensitivity to carbidopa and/or levodopa
Pregnancy—No studies in humans; depressed growth and malformations in animal studies
Breast-feeding—Levodopa is distributed into breast milk; may inhibit lactation
Use in the elderly—Reduced tolerance to effects of levodopa; caution in resuming normal activity, especially in patients with osteoporosis; psychic effects more common with concurrent use of anticholinergics
Dental—Possible difficulty in retention of full dentures
Other medications, especially haloperidol, hydantoin anticonvulsants, hydrocarbon inhalation anesthetics, phenothiazines, cocaine, MAO inhibitors, and selegiline
Other medical problems, especially severe cardiovascular disease, severe pulmonary diseases, glaucoma, melanoma (history of or suspected), peptic ulcer (history of), psychosis, renal function impairment, or urinary retention

### Proper use of this medication
» Taking food shortly after taking medication to relieve gastric irritation; taking food before or concurrently may retard levodopa's effect
» Compliance with therapy; taking medication only as directed; not stopping medication unless ordered by physician
» Maximum effectiveness of medication may not occur for several weeks or months after therapy is initiated
   Missed dose: Taking as soon as possible; skipping dose if next scheduled dose is within 2 hours; not doubling doses
» Proper storage

### Precautions while using this medication
Caution if any kind of surgery (including dental surgery) or emergency treatment is required
For diabetic patients—May interfere with urine tests for sugar and ketones
» Caution if drowsiness occurs
» Caution when getting up suddenly from lying or sitting position; dizziness and fainting may occur
Possibility of "on-off" phenomenon

### Side/adverse effects
Occasional darkening of urine or sweat may be alarming to patient although medically insignificant
Signs of potential side effects, especially difficult urination, duodenal ulcer, hemolytic anemia, hypertension, irregular heartbeat, mental depression, mood or mental changes, severe nausea or vomiting, orthostatic hypotension, spasm or closing of eyelids, or uncontrolled movements of body

## General Dosing Information
Titrated dosage is necessary to achieve the individual therapeutic blood concentration requirements and to avoid side effects. This is especially important for geriatric patients and patients receiving other medications.

Postencephalitic and geriatric patients often require and tolerate lower dosage levels than other parkinsonism patients.

Levodopa must be discontinued at least 8 hours before the carbidopa and levodopa combination dosage is begun. Levodopa may be discontinued in the evening and the carbidopa and levodopa combination started the following morning.

The concurrent administration of carbidopa may permit the dose of levodopa to be reduced by up to 75% with no decrease in therapeutic results. Carbidopa also reduces the adverse effect of pyridoxine on levodopa.

Because carbidopa and levodopa extended-release tablets are 25 to 30% less systemically bioavailable than Carbidopa and Levodopa Tablets USP, increased daily doses of the extended-release tablets may be required to achieve the same level of symptomatic relief.

Amantadine or anticholinergic medications are often used concurrently with carbidopa and levodopa in the more advanced cases of parkinsonism or when response to carbidopa and levodopa decreases. However, gradual dosage reduction of these medications is recommended during initiation of therapy with carbidopa and levodopa and after optimum dosage is reached to maintain proper control of patient's condition.

When carbidopa and levodopa combination is to be discontinued, dosage should be reduced gradually to prevent the occurrence of a syndrome that resembles the neuroleptic malignant syndrome. Careful patient monitoring after withdrawal of carbidopa and levodopa will allow early diagnosis and treatment of neuroleptic malignant–like syndrome.

### Diet/Nutrition
Food should be eaten shortly after carbidopa and levodopa combination is taken to relieve gastric irritation; taking food before or concurrently may retard levodopa's effects.

High protein diets should be avoided, because amino acid degradation products compete with levodopa for transport to the brain, resulting in a decreased or erratic response to levodopa. It is recommended that intake of normal amounts of protein be distributed equally throughout the day.

### For treatment of adverse effects
Immediate relief of nausea and vomiting may sometimes be obtained by reducing the daily dose, giving smaller individual doses at more frequent intervals, or having patient take food shortly after each dose; however, high-protein foods should be avoided since they may decrease levodopa's effect as well (see *Drug interactions and/or related problems*). Since the nausea results primarily from the CNS effects of levodopa, non-phenothiazine antiemetics are sometimes successfully used. Phenothiazine antiemetics may be more effective but should not be used because of their tendency to negate levodopa's therapeutic effect.

The appearance of choreiform and other involuntary movements may require a reduction in dosage since tolerance usually does not develop.

Serious psychiatric disturbances, such as severe mental depression, with or without suicidal tendencies, may require reduction in dosage or complete withdrawal of levodopa.

After discontinuation of levodopa therapy, dantrolene and/or bromocriptine may be used in patients with evidence of neuroleptic malignant-like syndrome, to help reduce fever and thus avoid a potentially lethal complication.

## Oral Dosage Forms

### CARBIDOPA AND LEVODOPA TABLETS USP

**Usual adult dose**
Antidyskinetic—
   For patients not being converted from levodopa therapy:
      Oral, initially, 10 mg of carbidopa and 100 mg of levodopa three or four times a day or 25 mg of carbidopa and 100 mg of levodopa three times a day, the dosage per day being increased gradually at one- or two-day intervals as needed and tolerated.
   For patients being converted from levodopa therapy (levodopa must be discontinued for at least eight hours prior to conversion to carbidopa and levodopa therapy):
      Patients who require less than 1.5 grams of levodopa per day—
         Oral, 10 mg of carbidopa and 100 mg of levodopa or 25 mg of carbidopa and 100 mg of levodopa three or four times a day initially, the dosage per day being increased gradually at one- or two-day intervals as needed and tolerated.
      Patients who require more than 1.5 grams of levodopa per day—
         Oral, 25 mg of carbidopa and 250 mg of levodopa three or four times a day initially, the dosage per day being increased gradually at one- or two-day intervals as needed and tolerated.
   Note: Postencephalitic patients may be more sensitive to the effects of the usual adult dose.
      For patients being converted from levodopa therapy, the initial dose of carbidopa and levodopa per day should provide approximately 25% of the total dosage of levodopa per day previously required.

**Usual adult prescribing limits**
Up to 200 mg of carbidopa and 2 grams of levodopa in combination daily.
Note: Additional levodopa may be administered alone if it is required and tolerated.

**Usual pediatric dose**
Children up to 18 years of age—Safety and efficacy have not been established.

**Usual geriatric dose**
See *Usual adult dose*.
Note: Geriatric patients may be more sensitive to the effects of the usual adult dose.

**Strength(s) usually available**
U.S.—
   10 mg of carbidopa and 100 mg of levodopa (Rx) [*Sinemet* (scored); GENERIC].
   25 mg of carbidopa and 100 mg of levodopa (Rx) [*Sinemet* (scored); GENERIC].
   25 mg of carbidopa and 250 mg of levodopa (Rx) [*Sinemet* (scored); GENERIC].
Canada—
   10 mg of carbidopa and 100 mg of levodopa (Rx) [*Sinemet* (scored)].
   25 mg of carbidopa and 100 mg of levodopa (Rx) [*Sinemet* (scored)].
   25 mg of carbidopa and 250 mg of levodopa (Rx) [*Sinemet* (scored)].

**Packaging and storage**
Store below 40 °C (104 °F), preferably between 15 and 30 °C (59 and 86 °F), unless otherwise specified by manufacturer. Store in a well-closed, light-resistant container.

**Auxiliary labeling**
• May darken urine or sweat.

### CARBIDOPA AND LEVODOPA EXTENDED-RELEASE TABLETS

**Usual adult dose**
Antidyskinetic—
   Initial dosage
      For patients not receiving levodopa therapy
         Mild to moderate disease:
            Oral, initially, 50 mg of carbidopa and 200 mg of levodopa twice a day, at intervals of at least 6 hours.
      For patients currently treated with conventional carbidopa-levodopa preparations

Dosage with the extended-release tablets should be substituted at an amount that provides approximately 10% more levodopa per day, although this may need to be increased to 30% more levodopa per day based on clinical response. The interval between doses of the extended-release tablets should be 4 to 8 hours during the waking day, although a few patients may require more frequent dosing.

Guidelines for initial conversion from Carbidopa and Levodopa Tablets USP to carbidopa and levodopa extended-release tablets:

| Total daily dose of levodopa (mg) | Suggested dosage regimen of carbidopa and levodopa extended-release tablets (based on levodopa content) |
|---|---|
| 300–400 | 200 mg twice a day |
| 500–600 | 300 mg twice a day or 200 mg three times a day |
| 700–800 | A total of 800 mg in 3 or more divided doses (e.g., 300 mg a.m., 300 mg early p.m., and 200 mg later p.m.) |
| 900–1000 | A total of 1000 mg in 3 or more divided doses (e.g., 400 mg a.m., 400 mg early p.m., and 200 mg later p.m.) |

For patients currently treated with levodopa without a decarboxylase inhibitor:
  Levodopa must be discontinued at least 8 hours before initiating therapy with carbidopa and levodopa extended-release tablets. The extended-release tablets should be substituted at a dosage of approximately 25% of the previous levodopa dosage.
  Mild to moderate disease: Oral, initially, 50 mg of carbidopa and 200 mg of levodopa twice a day.

Maintenance dosing—
  Depending upon therapeutic response, doses and dosing intervals may be increased or decreased following initiation of therapy. An interval of at least 3 days between dosage adjustments is recommended. Most patients have been adequately treated with 400 to 1600 mg of levodopa per day, administered as divided doses at intervals ranging from 4 to 8 hours. A few patients may require higher doses (12 or more tablets per day) and shorter intervals (less than 4 hours).
  When the extended-release tablets are given at less than 4-hour intervals, and/or if the divided doses are not equal, the smaller doses should be given at the end of the day.
  Carbidopa and Levodopa Tablets USP may be added to the dosage regimen in selected patients with advanced disease who need additional levodopa for a brief time during daytime hours. Usually one-half or one tablet of carbidopa 10 mg and levodopa 100 mg or carbidopa 25 mg and levodopa 100 mg is added.

**Usual pediatric dose**
Children up to 18 years of age—Safety and efficacy have not been established.

**Usual geriatric dose**
See *Usual adult dose*.

**Strength(s) usually available**
U.S.—
  25 mg of carbidopa and 100 mg of levodopa (Rx) [*Sinemet CR 25-100*].
  50 mg of carbidopa and 200 mg of levodopa (Rx) [*Sinemet CR 50-200* (scored)].
Canada—
  25 mg of carbidopa and 100 mg of levodopa (Rx) [*Sinemet CR 25-100*].
  50 mg of carbidopa and 200 mg of levodopa (Rx) [*Sinemet CR 50-200* (scored)].

**Packaging and storage**
Store below 40 °C (104 °F), preferably between 15 and 30 °C (59 and 86 °F), unless otherwise specified by manufacturer. Store in a well-closed, light-resistant container.

**Auxiliary labeling**
• May darken urine or sweat.
• Do not chew or crush tablets.

Revised: 08/18/92
Interim revision: 05/23/94

---

**CARBINOXAMINE**—See *Antihistamines (Systemic)*

---

# CARBOHYDRATES AND ELECTROLYTES  Systemic

This monograph includes information on the following: 1) Dextrose and Electrolytes; 2) Oral Rehydration Salts§*; 3) Rice Syrup Solids and Electrolytes†.

VA CLASSIFICATION (Primary): TN490

Other commonly used names are oral rehydration salts, ORS-bicarbonate, and ORS-citrate.§

Note:  For a listing of dosage forms and brand names by country availability, see *Dosage Forms* section(s).

*Not commercially available in U.S.
†Not commercially available in Canada.
§Distributed by the World Health Organization (WHO).

## Category
Electrolyte replenisher.

## Indications
**Accepted**
Diarrhea (treatment) and
Electrolyte depletion (prophylaxis and treatment)—Carbohydrate and electrolytes solutions are indicated for oral replacement of fluids and electrolytes (especially sodium and potassium) in the treatment of clinically evident dehydration caused by diarrhea; to prevent severe dehydration by replacing losses early in the course of diarrhea; and to maintain hydration in the presence of continuing fluid loss. Oral rehydration therapy (ORT) consists of rehydration (the expansion of intravascular volume and deficit replacement); replacement of ongoing abnormal losses of fluids and electrolyte salts from continuing diarrhea and vomiting and normal water losses through skin and respiration; and the maintenance of fluids and electrolytes in the body until adequate nutrition can be restored. Acute diarrhea is not immediately terminated by oral rehydration therapy, but it is usually self-limiting. Some carbohydrate and electrolytes solutions are also used for maintenance of water and electrolytes when food and liquid intake has been discontinued after surgery, and some are indicated for maintenance of hydration only, rather than for rehydration.

ORT is recommended by the World Health Organization (WHO) Diarrheal Disease Control Program and United Nations Children's Fund (UNICEF) as a fundamental treatment for acute diarrheal disease in infants and children and provides the basis for all national programs of diarrhea control. The WHO formulations of ORS-bicarbonate or ORS-citrate rehydration salts, consisting of preweighed sodium chloride, potassium chloride, sodium citrate or sodium bicarbonate, and dextrose, are distributed in aluminum foil or polyethylene packets to be prepared at home and given at the onset of diarrhea. The solutions are simple to prepare (i.e., the contents of each packet are dissolved in one liter of potable water) and are very effective, inexpensive, and therapeutically appropriate for routine use in prevention and treatment of dehydration from diarrhea of any cause in all age groups. These powders are not widely used or commercially available in the U.S.

Some commercial carbohydrate and electrolytes solutions available in the U.S. and Canada have a lower sodium content than the recommended WHO formulas. This reflects the concern that the higher sodium content of the WHO solution may cause hypernatremia, especially in developed countries, due to the use of high solute diets and the lower incidence of malnutrition in young children. However, there is no evidence that the WHO solution causes hypernatremia when used as directed. Carbohydrate and electrolytes solutions with a lower sodium content have been found to be as effective as the WHO formulas.

Intravenous replacement of fluids and electrolytes is not used routinely in treatment of diarrhea, but it may be necessary to treat severe dehydration (fluid loss of 10% or more of body weight) or impending shock.

## Pharmacology/Pharmacokinetics

**Physicochemical characteristics**
Molecular weight—
    Calcium chloride: 147.02.
    Citric acid: 192.12.
    Dextrose (anhydrous): 180.16.
    Dextrose (monohydrate): 198.17.
    Dibasic sodium phosphate: 268.07.
    Magnesium chloride: 203.30.
    Potassium chloride: 74.55.
    Potassium citrate: 324.41.
    Sodium bicarbonate: 84.01.
    Sodium chloride: 58.44.
    Sodium citrate (anhydrous): 258.07.
    Sodium citrate (dihydrate): 294.1.

**Mechanism of action/Effect**
During normal digestion, about 9 liters of fluid a day in adults and about 3 to 6 liters a day in infants and children pass through the duodenum, where most of the dietary sugars, fats, and amino acids are absorbed. The fluid, containing ingested food and liquids and digestive secretions, reaches the ileum mainly as an isotonic salt solution that is similar to plasma in its ionic sodium and potassium content. The ileum absorbs most of this isotonic solution by various active transport mechanisms, but about 1 liter a day is emptied into the colon, where all but about 100 mL is absorbed. The rest is excreted into the feces to prevent desiccation. In addition, cells in the small intestine both absorb and secrete water and electrolytes, but less secretion occurs than absorption, so that the net effect of small-bowel transport is absorption. In acute diarrheal states, various infectious agents produce alterations in the intestinal mucosa, inhibiting absorption or stimulating secretion. The large volume of secretions thus produced cannot be fully absorbed by the colon and are expelled as watery diarrhea. Essential water and salts are lost in stools and vomitus, and dehydration results when blood volume is decreased because of fluid loss from the extracellular fluid compartment. Thirst is the first sign of dehydration when fluid loss is less than 5% of the body weight. Tachycardia, decreased skin elasticity, sunken eyes, hypotension, irritability, oliguria or anuria, severe thirst, and stupor or coma develop rapidly when fluid loss is greater than 5% of the body weight. Shock occurs when the deficit equals about 10% of body weight, and death is caused by greater losses of fluids.

  Preservation of the facilitated glucose-sodium cotransport system in the small-bowel mucosa is the rationale of oral rehydration therapy. Glucose is actively absorbed in the normal intestine and carries sodium with it in about an equimolar ratio. Therefore, there is a greater net absorption of an isotonic salt solution with glucose than of one without it. During acute diarrhea, the absorption of sodium is impaired and an isotonic salt solution without glucose can increase stool volume by passing through the intestine unabsorbed. Since the glucose absorption system usually remains intact during diarrheal illnesses, the net absorption of water and electrolytes from an isotonic dextrose-salt or a hypotonic rice-salt solution can equal or exceed diarrheal stool volume, even if the loss is rapid. Sucrose (ordinary sugar) may be substituted for dextrose in the dextrose-based oral rehydration solutions, but twice the amount of sugar is needed for near-equal efficacy. However, excessive use of dextrose or sucrose to increase palatability of the solution or to increase nutritive value for small children may exacerbate diarrhea, because of the osmotic effect of unabsorbed glucose. A solution with 2 to 2.5% dextrose in the dextrose-based oral rehydration solutions is optimal for promoting coupled absorption of sodium from the intestine.

  Rice-based oral rehydration solutions use starch rather than dextrose as a base. The ingested starch gradually releases glucose which along with sodium preserves the glucose-sodium transport system in the manner described above. The rice-based formula has the advantage of a lower osmotic effect and provides a few more calories than the dextrose-based electrolytes solution. This formula has also been found to be more effective in reducing stool output and shortening the duration of diarrhea.

  Potassium replacement during acute diarrhea prevents below-normal serum concentrations of potassium, especially in children, in whom stool potassium losses are higher than in adults.

  When added to oral rehydration solutions, bicarbonate and citrate are equally effective in correcting the metabolic acidosis caused by diarrhea and dehydration. However, citrate is used instead of the bicarbonate in the WHO formulation, to prevent the occurrence of bicarbonate-induced discoloration and decomposition of the dextrose in the packets.

  Treatment started early in the course of diarrhea minimizes vomiting, anorexia, lethargy, or coma, which interfere with continued feeding; allows the homeostatic mechanisms of thirst and renal function to remain intact; and avoids the risk of death from severe dehydration. Thirst determines the amount of rehydration required, and normal renal function allows the excretion of any excess water and salts.

**Time to peak effect**
8 to 12 hours.

## Precautions to Consider

**Pregnancy/Reproduction**
Pregnancy—Problems in humans have not been documented.

**Breast-feeding**
Problems in humans have not been documented. Continued breast-feeding during the treatment and maintenance phases of oral rehydration therapy is vital for the management of diarrhea.

**Pediatrics**
Although oral rehydration therapy appears to be safe and effective in neonates, it has not been evaluated in premature infants. The range of sodium concentrations recommended by the American Academy of Pediatrics Committee on Nutrition is 40 to 60 mEq per liter for maintenance solutions and 75 to 90 mEq per liter for rehydration solutions. To allow adequate intake of free water in the prevention of hypernatremia with the use of WHO ORS-bicarbonate or citrate solutions, feeding (including breast milk) may continue, and/or the infant may be given a separate feeding of plain water after every two doses of undiluted WHO solution.

**Geriatrics**
Carbohydrate and electrolytes solutions are well tolerated by elderly patients.

**Medical considerations/Contraindications**
The medical considerations/contraindications included have been selected on the basis of their potential clinical significance (reasons given in parentheses where appropriate)—not necessarily inclusive (» = major clinical significance).

*Except under special circumstances, this medication should not be used when the following medical problems exist:*

» Anuria or
» Oliguria
    (since normal renal function is required to allow the excretion of any excess water or salt, patients with prolonged anuria or oliguria usually require precise parenteral administration of water and electrolytes; however, transient oliguria is a feature of dehydration due to diarrhea and is not a contraindication for oral rehydration therapy)

» Dehydration, severe, with symptoms of shock
    (oral rehydration is too slow; rapid intravenous therapy is necessary; symptoms of severe dehydration include severe thirst, rapid heartbeat, decreased skin turgor, hypotension, oliguria or anuria, sunken eyes, loss of body weight, convulsions, stupor, and coma; if symptoms of severe dehydration appear after oral therapy has been attempted, rehydration must be achieved with parenteral therapy)

» Diarrhea, severe
    (when amounts of diarrhea exceed 30mL per kg of body weight per hour, patient may be unable to drink enough fluids to replace continuing loss)

» Glucose malabsorption
    (diarrhea is exacerbated and dehydration worsened when oral rehydration solutions are given to patients with this problem; volume of stool greatly increases and contains large amounts of glucose; rehydration therapy should be discontinued)

» Inability to drink or
» Vomiting, severe and sustained
    (parenteral therapy is required for patients unable to drink because of extreme fatigue, stupor, coma, or uncontrollable vomiting)

» Intestinal obstruction or
» Paralytic ileus or
» Perforated bowel
    (delayed passage of carbohydrate and electrolytes solutions through the gastrointestinal tract may increase risk of gastrointestinal irritation)

**Patient monitoring**
The following may be especially important in patient monitoring (other tests may be warranted in some patients, depending on condition; » = major clinical significance):

Blood pressure measurements
    (recommended to detect shock due to severe dehydration)

Body weight
    (recommended periodically to determine the degree of rehydration or the recurrence of dehydration)

Electrolytes, serum and
pH, serum
    (recommended to help determine status of individual ions and acid-base status)

Glucose malabsorption tests
(recommended when oral rehydration solution appears to exacerbate diarrhea; infant's feces should be monitored for reducing substances to detect transient monosaccharide malabsorption, which may occur during acute infectious diarrhea; sugar intake should be eliminated or decreased if glucose intolerance is present; intravenous fluid replacement may be required)

Observation for signs of rehydration
(observation of patients with frequent diarrhea is recommended every 3 to 6 hours for signs of rehydration, i.e., normal skin turgor, normal urine flow, normal pulse rate and volume, and a sense of well-being)

Stool volume measurements
(recommended periodically to determine the dose and continued need for maintenance therapy; the volume of ingested replacement solution should equal the volume of stool losses; if stool volume cannot be measured, an intake of 10 to 15 mL of rehydration solution per kilogram of body weight per hour is suggested)

## Side/Adverse Effects

The following side/adverse effects have been selected on the basis of their potential clinical significance (possible signs and symptoms in parentheses where appropriate)—not necessarily inclusive:

**Those indicating need for medical attention**
Incidence rare
*Hypernatremia* (dizziness; fast heartbeat; high blood pressure; irritability; muscle twitching; restlessness; seizures; swelling of feet or lower legs; weakness)

Symptoms of overhydration
*Puffy eyelids*
Note: Therapy may need to be discontinued temporarily.

**Those indicating need for medical attention only if they continue or are bothersome**
Incidence more frequent
*Vomiting, mild*
Note: *Mild vomiting* may occur when oral therapy is begun, but therapy should be continued with frequent, small amounts of solution administered slowly.

## Patient Consultation

As an aid to patient consultation, refer to *Advice for the Patient, Carbohydrates and Electrolytes (Systemic)*.
In providing consultation, consider emphasizing the following selected information (» = major clinical significance):

**Before using this medication**
» Conditions affecting use, especially:
Other medical problems, especially renal function impairment, severe dehydration, severe and continuing diarrhea, glucose malabsorption, inability to drink, severe and continuing vomiting, intestinal obstruction, paralytic ileus, or perforated bowel

**Proper use of this medication**
Importance of helping infants and small children to drink solution slowly and frequently in small amounts, given with a spoon
Importance of not taking for a longer time than recommended by physician
» Proper dosing
» Proper storage

*For patients using the commercial powder form*
Adding recommended amount of boiled, cooled drinking water to contents of packet; stirring or shaking container for 2 or 3 minutes to dissolve completely
Not adding more water to the solution after it is mixed
Not boiling solution
Making and using fresh solution each day

*For patients using the freezer pop form*
Removing from box and not separating before freezing
Freezing pop for best taste; cutting wrapper and pushing from bottom to eat frozen pop
Cutting wrapper and pouring unfrozen pop in glass or cup to drink

*For patients using the powder form distributed by the World Health Organization (WHO)*
Adding powder to recommended amount of drinking water; shaking container for 2 or 3 minutes to dissolve completely
Not adding more water to the solution after it is mixed
Not boiling solution
Making and using fresh solution each day

**Precautions while using this medication**
Eating soft foods, such as cereals, bananas, cooked peas and beans, and potatoes, to maintain nutrition
Giving breast milk to breast-fed infants between doses of solution
Checking with physician if diarrhea does not improve in a day or 2 or becomes worse during treatment with this medication
Checking with physician as soon as possible if signs of severe dehydration occur, including doughy skin (decreased skin turgor), sunken eyes, dizziness or lightheadedness, weakness or tiredness, irritability, and weight loss

*For patients taking ORS-citrate or ORS-bicarbonate*
Drinking water between doses of rehydration solution (except breast-fed infants)

*For patients taking the premixed liquid form*
Avoiding other electrolyte-containing foods or liquids, such as fruit juices or foods with added salt, until rehydration solutions are discontinued, to prevent excessive electrolyte ingestion or osmotic diarrhea

**Side/adverse effects**
Signs of potential side effects, especially hypernatremia

## General Dosing Information

Infants and young children should be given small, frequent, and slowly administered amounts of oral rehydration fluid. Infants who finish 150 mL of solution per kg of body weight in less than 24 hours should be encouraged to drink plain water to prevent hypernatremia and to quench thirst.

The commercially prepared solutions do not require additional water intake because of the generally lower sodium content.

Rehydration solutions must not be diluted with water, because dilution decreases the absorptive properties of the glucose-sodium cotransport system.

Acute watery diarrhea, dysentery, and persistent diarrhea in children can also result in tissue catabolism, which may in turn lead to malnutrition. This can be further aggravated by the common practice of withholding fluids and nutrition during diarrhea. Although early feeding may result in slightly increased stool volume, nutrient absorption is increased and weight loss is lessened. Therefore, continued feeding (including breast milk) of infants and children and supplementation with plain drinking water during the maintenance phase of oral rehydration therapy are important for maintaining hydration and nutrition in the management of diarrhea.

The oral rehydration solution should be taken alternately with soft foods, such as rice cereal, bananas, cooked legumes, potatoes, or other non–lactose-containing, carbohydrate-rich food. Older children and adults should resume their normal diets as soon as the appetite returns. Other electrolyte-containing foods or liquids such as fruit juices or foods with added salt should be withheld until oral rehydration solutions are discontinued, to prevent excessive electrolyte ingestion or osmotic diarrhea.

Cow's milk should be discontinued only if diarrhea worsens considerably after feeding and the stool becomes acidic and contains reducing substances. This reflects a depression of lactase activity, which may occur when the brush borders of jejunal mucosal cells are damaged. Soy formulas without lactose are given alternately with carbohydrate and electrolytes solutions for the first 24 to 48 hours.

If the initial dehydration is severe, rehydration must be achieved by intravenous administration of an appropriate isotonic electrolyte solution, after which the oral solution may be used for maintenance when tolerance to oral intake has been established.

Parenteral rehydration therapy should be started if symptoms of dehydration reappear after aggressive oral replacement of fluids and electrolytes has been attempted.

---

### DEXTROSE AND ELECTROLYTES

## Oral Dosage Forms
### DEXTROSE AND ELECTROLYTES SOLUTION
**Usual adult and adolescent dose**
*For oral solution dosage form—*
Rehydration:
Mild dehydration—Oral, initially 50 mL of solution per kg of body weight over four to six hours, the amounts and rates being adjusted as needed and tolerated, depending on thirst and response to therapy.

## Carbohydrates and Electrolytes (Systemic)

Moderate dehydration—Oral, initially 100 mL of solution per kg of body weight over six hours, the amounts and rates being adjusted as needed and tolerated, depending on thirst and response to therapy.

Note: Severe dehydration must be treated with intravenous electrolyte solutions.

Maintenance of hydration:
  Mild continuing diarrhea—Oral, 100 to 200 mL of solution per kg of body weight over twenty-four hours until diarrhea stops.
  Severe continuing diarrhea—Oral, 15 mL of solution per kg of body weight every hour until diarrhea stops.

*For freezer pop dosage form—*
  Rehydration: Oral, freezer pop may be given as frequently as desired.

**Usual adult prescribing limits**
1000 mL per hour.

**Usual pediatric dose**
*For oral solution dosage form—*
  Rehydration:
    Children up to 2 years of age—Oral, initially 150 mL of solution per kg of body weight over twenty-four hours (75 mL per kg of body weight during the first eight hours, and 75 mL per kg of body weight during the next sixteen hours), the amounts and rates being adjusted as needed and tolerated, depending on thirst and response to therapy.
    Children 2 to 10 years of age with moderate to severe dehydration—Oral, initially 50 mL of solution per kg of body weight over the first four to six hours, and 100 mL of solution per kg of body weight over the next eighteen to twenty-four hours, the amounts and rates being adjusted as needed and tolerated, depending on thirst and response to therapy.

Note: No more than 100 mL of fluid should be given during any 20-minute period.

    Children over 10 years of age—See *Usual adult and adolescent dose.*

*For freezer pop dosage form—*
  Rehydration:—
    Children older than 1 year of age—Oral, freezer pop may be given as frequently as desired.
    Children up to 1 year of age—Consult physician before use.

**Strength(s) usually available**

| Product | Na+ | K+ | Cl− | Citrate | Mg++ | Ca++ | Phosphate |
|---|---|---|---|---|---|---|---|
| U.S.— | | | | | | | |
| Kao Lectrolyte* (OTC) | 50 | 20 | | 30 | | | |
| Naturalyte† (OTC) | 45 | 20 | 35 | 48 | | | |
| Oralyte† (OTC) | 45 | 20 | 35 | 48 | | | |
| Pedialyte† (OTC) | 45 | 20 | 35 | 30 | | | |
| Pedialyte Freezer Pops† (OTC) | 45 | 20 | 35 | 30 | | | |
| Rehydralyte† (OTC) | 75 | 20 | 65 | 30 | | | |
| Resol* (OTC) | 50 | 20 | 50 | 34 | 4 | 4 | 5 |
| Canada— | | | | | | | |
| Lytren* (OTC) | 50 | 25 | 45 | 30 | | | |
| Pedialyte† (OTC) | 45 | 20 | 35 | 30 | | | |

*Dextrose content = 20 grams per liter.
†Dextrose content = 25 grams per liter.

Note: *Resol* is available to hospitals only.
  Generic name product is available in the U.S.

**Packaging and storage**
Store below 40 °C (104 °F), preferably between 15 and 30 °C (59 and 86 °F), unless otherwise specified by manufacturer.

---

## ORAL REHYDRATION SALTS

## Oral Dosage Forms

### ORAL REHYDRATION SALTS (FOR ORAL SOLUTION) USP

**Usual adult and adolescent dose**
Rehydration—
  Mild dehydration: Oral, initially 50 mL of solution per kg of body weight over four to six hours, the amounts and rates being adjusted as needed and tolerated, depending on thirst and response to therapy.
  Moderate dehydration: Oral, initially 100 mL of solution per kg of body weight over six hours, the amounts and rates being adjusted as needed and tolerated, depending on thirst and response to therapy.

Note: Severe dehydration must be treated with intravenous electrolyte solutions.

Maintenance of hydration—
  Mild continuing diarrhea: Oral, 100 to 200 mL of solution per kg of body weight over twenty-four hours until diarrhea stops.
  Severe continuing diarrhea: Oral, 15 mL of solution per kg of body weight every hour until diarrhea stops.

**Usual adult prescribing limits**
Up to 1000 mL per hour.

**Usual pediatric dose**
Rehydration—
  Mild or moderate dehydration: Oral, initially 50 to 100 mL per kg of body weight during the first four hours, the dosage being adjusted to 100 mL per kg of body weight per day until diarrhea stops, the amounts and rates being adjusted as needed and tolerated, depending on thirst and response to therapy.

**Strength(s) usually available**

| Product | Na+ | K+ | Cl− | Bicarbonate | Citrate |
|---|---|---|---|---|---|
| U.S.— | | | | | |
| Not commercially available. | | | | | |
| Canada— | | | | | |
| Gastrolyte* (OTC) | 60 | 20 | 60 | 10 | |
| Rapolyte† (OTC) | 90 | 20 | 80 | 30 | |
| Other— | | | | | |
| ORS-bicarbonate† | 90 | 20 | 80 | 30 | |
| ORS-citrate† | 90 | 20 | 80 | | 30 |

*Dextrose content = 17.8 grams per liter.
†Dextrose content = 20 grams per liter.

**Packaging and storage**
Store below 30 °C (86 °F), preferably between 15 and 30 °C (59 and 86 °F). Store in a tight container.

**Preparation of dosage form**
Packets distributed by WHO—To one quart or liter of drinking water, add contents of one packet containing sodium chloride, potassium chloride, sodium bicarbonate or citrate, and dextrose. Stir or shake well for 2 or 3 minutes to dissolve.
Packets available commercially—Add 200 mL (7 ounces) of boiled, cooled tap water to the contents of one packet containing sodium chloride, potassium chloride, sodium bicarbonate, and dextrose. Stir or shake well for 2 or 3 minutes to dissolve.
To prepare extemporaneous oral rehydration solution—Add 3.5 grams (0.5 teaspoonful) sodium chloride (table salt), 1.5 grams (1.2 teaspoonfuls) potassium chloride or potassium salt, 2.5 grams (0.5 teaspoonful) sodium bicarbonate (baking soda), and 40 grams (4 tablespoonfuls) sucrose (table sugar) to one liter of potable water.

**Stability**
The constituted solution may be stored in a refrigerator for up to a maximum of 24 hours after constitution, after which time the unused portion should be discarded.
ORS-bicarbonate can be stored up to 3 years if the product is dry, filled and sealed in a dry atmosphere in air-tight aluminum laminate, and stored at temperatures below 30 °C. In conditions other than these, the product may deteriorate (caramelize) and change color (yellow to brown).
ORS-citrate can be stored for at least 3 years. If moisture is absorbed, the product will lump or harden with no change in color and no effect on its dissolution in water.

### Additional information
The WHO oral rehydration solution contains sodium chloride 3.5 grams, potassium chloride 1.5 grams, sodium bicarbonate 2.5 grams or sodium citrate (dihydrate) 2.9 grams, and dextrose 20.0 grams, per liter of water.

---

### RICE SYRUP SOLIDS AND ELECTROLYTES

## Oral Dosage Forms

### RICE SYRUP SOLIDS AND ELECTROLYTES SOLUTION

**Usual adult and adolescent dose**
See *Dextrose and Electrolytes Solution*.

**Usual pediatric dose**
See *Dextrose and Electrolytes Solution*.

**Strength(s) usually available**

| Product | Na+ | K+ | Cl− | Citrate |
|---|---|---|---|---|
| U.S.— | | | | |
| Infalyte* (OTC) | 50 | 25 | 45 | 36 |
| Canada— | | | | |
| Not commercially available. | | | | |

*Rice syrup solids content = 30 grams per liter.

### Packaging and storage
Store below 40 °C (104 °F), preferably between 15 and 30 °C (59 and 86 °F), unless otherwise specified by manufacturer.

### Stability
The manufacturer of the rice-based oral electrolytes solution recommends that the product be refrigerated and used within 48 hours after opening.

Revised: 12/02/92
Interim revision: 08/09/94; 07/20/95; 08/11/97; 05/21/98

---

**CARBOL-FUCHSIN**—The *Carbol-Fuchsin (Topical)* monograph is not included in this published version of the USP DI database. Copies of the monograph are available on request from Micromedex, Inc. - Reprint Requests, 6200 S. Syracuse Way, Suite 300, Englewood, CO 80111; telephone (303) 486-6400; telefax (303) 486-6464; Email: USPDI@MDX.COM.

---

# CARBONIC ANHYDRASE INHIBITORS   Systemic

This monograph includes information on the following: 1) Acetazolamide; 2) Dichlorphenamide†; 3) Methazolamide.

INN: Dichlorphenamide—Diclofenamide

VA CLASSIFICATION (Primary/Secondary):
  Acetazolamide—CV703/OP113; CN400; MS900; GU900
  Dichlorphenamide—CV703/OP113
  Methazolamide—CV703/OP113

Commonly used brand name(s): *Acetazolam*[1]; *Ak-Zol*[1]; *Apo-Acetazolamide*[1]; *Daranide*[2]; *Dazamide*[1]; *Diamox*[1]; *Diamox Sequels*[1]; *MZM*[3]; *Neptazane*[1]; *Storzolamide*[1].

Note: For a listing of dosage forms and brand names by country availability, see *Dosage Forms* section(s).

†Not commercially available in Canada.

## Category
Antiglaucoma agent (systemic)—Acetazolamide; Dichlorphenamide; Methazolamide.
Anticonvulsant—Acetazolamide (tablets and injection).
Altitude sickness (acute) prophylactic and therapeutic agent—Acetazolamide.
Antiparalytic (familial periodic paralysis)—Acetazolamide.
Diuretic, urinary alkalinizing—Acetazolamide (parenteral).
Antiurolithic (uric acid calculi; cystine calculi)—Acetazolamide Tablets USP.

## Indications
Note: Bracketed information in the *Indications* section refers to uses that are not included in U.S. product labeling.

**Accepted**
Glaucoma, open-angle (treatment)
Glaucoma, secondary (treatment)
Glaucoma, angle-closure (treatment) or
[Glaucoma, malignant (treatment)]—Carbonic anhydrase inhibitors are indicated primarily as adjuncts to other agents in the treatment of open-angle (chronic simple) glaucoma and secondary glaucoma, and to lower intraocular pressure prior to surgery for some types of glaucoma.

These medications should not be used for long-term therapy in non-congestive angle-closure (closed-angle) glaucoma; organic closure of the angle may occur while the worsening condition is masked by the lowered intraocular pressure.

[Acetazolamide is used to lower intraocular pressure in the treatment of malignant (ciliary block) glaucoma, which may occur after inflammation, surgery, trauma, or use of miotics.]

Epilepsy, absence seizure pattern (treatment)
Epilepsy, tonic-clonic seizure pattern (treatment)
Epilepsy, mixed seizure pattern (treatment)
Epilepsy, simple partial seizure pattern (treatment) or
Epilepsy, myoclonic seizure pattern (treatment)—Acetazolamide is indicated as an adjunct to other anticonvulsants in the management of absence seizures (petit mal), generalized tonic-clonic seizures (grand mal), mixed seizure patterns, simple partial seizure patterns, and myoclonic seizure patterns. It may be especially useful for intermittent therapy in females who experience increased seizure activity at the time of menstruation.

Altitude sickness (prophylaxis)[1] or
Altitude sickness (treatment)[1]—Oral acetazolamide is indicated to decrease the incidence and/or severity of symptoms (such as headache, nausea, shortness of breath, dizziness, drowsiness, and fatigue) associated with acute altitude sickness in mountain climbers who are attempting rapid ascent and in those who are very susceptible to altitude sickness despite gradual ascent. Gradual ascent is desirable for prevention of acute altitude sickness even when acetazolamide is used. However, prompt descent may still be necessary if severe manifestations of acute altitude sickness, such as pulmonary edema or cerebral edema, occur.

[Paralysis, familial periodic (treatment)][1]—Acetazolamide is used to treat both the hypokalemic and hyperkalemic forms of familial periodic paralysis. It terminates the acute attacks and, with chronic use, prevents their recurrence. It may be the drug of choice in the hypokalemic form of the condition.

[Toxicity, weakly acidic medications (treatment)]—Parenteral acetazolamide is used to produce a forced alkaline diuresis as a method of increasing the elimination of certain weakly acidic medications.

[Renal calculi, uric acid (prophylaxis)][1] or
[Renal calculi, cystine (prophylaxis)][1]—Oral acetazolamide is used to alkalinize the urine as a means of preventing the occurrence or recurrence of uric acid renal stones, especially in patients receiving uricosuric antigout agents, or of cystine renal stones.

**Unaccepted**
Acetazolamide has also been used to prevent or counteract metabolic alkalosis, including that which may occur following open-heart surgery; however, it is no longer used for these indications.

Acetazolamide has also been used as a diuretic in the treatment of edema due to congestive heart disease and drug-induced edema. However, it has been replaced by newer diuretics for these indications.

[1]Not included in Canadian product labeling.

## Pharmacology/Pharmacokinetics

**Physicochemical characteristics**
Molecular weight—
  Acetazolamide—222.24.
  Acetazolamide sodium—244.22.
  Dichlorphenamide—305.15.
  Methazolamide—236.26.

## Mechanism of action/Effect
Nonbacteriostatic sulfonamide derivatives. Inhibition of the enzyme carbonic anhydrase decreases formation of hydrogen and bicarbonate ions from carbon dioxide and water and reduces the availability of these ions for active transport. These agents reduce plasma bicarbonate concentration and increase plasma chloride concentration, producing systemic metabolic acidosis. Although all of these medications may produce diuresis with acute or intermittent administration, loss of diuretic effect occurs with chronic administration. Therefore, dichlorphenamide and methazolamide are not used as diuretics, and acetazolamide is now being used only to produce alkaline diuresis in certain cases of drug overdose. Methazolamide has less diuretic effect and less influence on urinary bicarbonatethan do other carbonic anhydrase inhibitors with doses used in glaucoma.

Antiglaucoma agent—
  Lowers intraocular pressure by decreasing the production of aqueous humor by 50 to 60%. The mechanism is not completely understood but probably involves a decrease of the bicarbonate ion concentration in ocular fluids. These agents have no effect on the facility of aqueous outflow. The ocular action is independent of any diuretic action.

Acetazolamide
  Anticonvulsant:
    Mechanism of action has not been fully determined. Inhibition of carbonic anhydrase in the central nervous system (CNS) may increase carbon dioxide tension, resulting in a retardation of neuronal conduction. The production of systemic metabolic acidosis may also be involved. This action is independent of any diuretic action.
  Altitude sickness, acute, prophylactic and therapeutic agent:
    May act by producing metabolic acidosis resulting in increased respiratory drive and arterial oxygen tension and/or by causing diuresis.
    In clinical trials, pulmonary function, such as minute ventilation, expired vital capacity, and peak flow, was greater in climbers treated with acetazolamide, whether they had acute altitude sickness or were asymptomatic. Acetazolamide-treated climbers also had less difficulty sleeping.
  Antiparalytic (for familial periodic paralysis):
    May stabilize muscle membranes against abnormal fluxes of potassium ions. Alternatively, may produce metabolic acidosis resulting in prevention of the intracellular shift of potassium.
  Diuretic, urinary alkalinizing:
    Induces alkaline diuresis by lowering hydrogen ion concentration in the renal tubule and increasing excretion of bicarbonate, sodium, potassium, and water. This increases the solubility in urine of weakly acidic drugs and promotes their excretion.
  Antiurolithic:
    Alkalinization of the urine increases the solubility in urine of uric acid and cystine, thereby reducing the formation of uric acid- or cystine-containing renal stones.

## Absorption
Well absorbed; methazolamide absorbed more slowly than acetazolamide or dichlorphenamide.

## Protein binding
Acetazolamide—Very high (90%).
Methazolamide—Moderate.

## Half-life
Acetazolamide (tablets)—10 to 15 hours.
Methazolamide—14 hours.

## Time to peak concentration
Acetazolamide tablets—2 to 4 hours after a 500-mg dose.
Acetazolamide extended-release capsules—8 to 12 hours after a 500-mg dose.

## Peak serum concentration
Acetazolamide tablets—12 to 27 mcg per mL with a 500-mg dose.
Acetazolamide extended-release capsules—6 mcg per mL with a 500-mg dose.

## Elimination
Acetazolamide—Renal; as unchanged drug; 90 to 100% of a dose is excreted within 24 hours after administration of oral tablets or intravenous injection; 47% of a dose is excreted within 24 hours after administration of extended-release capsules.
Dichlorphenamide—Unknown.
Methazolamide—Renal; 15 to 30% excreted unchanged. Remainder unknown.

### Effects on intraocular pressure

| Drug | Onset of Action | Peak Effect | Duration of Action (hr) |
|---|---|---|---|
| Acetazolamide | | | |
| Extended-release capsules | 2 hr | 8–12 hr | 18–24 |
| Tablets | 1–1.5 hr | 2–4 hr | 8–12 |
| Intravenous | 2 min | 15 min | 4–5 |
| Dichlorphenamide | | | |
| Tablets | 0.5–1 hr | 2–4 hr | 6–12 |
| Methazolamide | | | |
| Tablets | 2–4 hr | 6–8 hr | 10–18 |

## Precautions to Consider

### Cross-sensitivity and/or related problems
Patients sensitive to antibacterial sulfonamides, thiazide diuretics, or other sulfonamide-derivative diuretics may be sensitive to carbonic anhydrase inhibitors also.

### Carcinogenicity
Long-term studies in animals have not been conducted using carbonic anhydrase inhibitors.

### Mutagenicity
*Acetazolamide*—In a bacterial mutagenicity assay, acetazolamide was not mutagenic when evaluated with and without metabolic activation.
*Methazolamide*—In the Ames bacterial test, methazolamide was not mutagenic.

### Pregnancy/Reproduction
Fertility—*Acetazolamide:* Acetazolamide had no effect on fertility of male and female rats administered oral daily doses of up to 4 times the recommended human dose of 1000 mg in a 50 kg individual.
*Dichlorphenamide* and *methazolamide:* Long-term studies in animals have not been conducted.

Pregnancy—Adequate and well-controlled studies have not been done using carbonic anhydrase inhibitors in humans.
  *Acetazolamide*—
    Acetazolamide has been shown to cause limb defects in mice, rats, hamsters, and rabbits.
    FDA Pregnancy Category C.
  *Dichlorphenamide and methazolamide* —
    Dichlorphenamide and methazolamide, when given in large doses, have been shown to cause skeletal anomalies in rats.
    FDA Pregnancy Category C.

### Breast-feeding
Because of the potential for serious adverse reactions, a decision should be made whether to discontinue nursing during therapy with carbonic anhydrase inhibitors.
*Acetazolamide*—Acetazolamide may be distributed into breast milk.
*Dichlorphenamide* and *methazolamide*—It is not known whether dichlorphenamide or methazolamide is distributed into breast milk.

### Pediatrics
Appropriate studies on the relationship of age to the effects of carbonic anhydrase inhibitors have not been performed in the pediatric population. However, no pediatrics-specific problems have been documented to date.

### Geriatrics
No information is available on the relationship of age to the effects of carbonic anhydrase inhibitors in geriatric patients. However, elderly patients are more likely to have age-related renal function impairment, which may require caution in patients receiving these medications.

### Dental
Acetazolamide may cause facial paresthesia, such as numbness, tingling, or burning feeling of the mouth, tongue, or lips. Other carbonic anhydrase inhibitors may cause similar side effects.

### Drug interactions and/or related problems
The following drug interactions and/or related problems have been selected on the basis of their potential clinical significance (possible mechanism in parentheses where appropriate)—not necessarily inclusive (» = major clinical significance):

Note: Combinations containing any of the following medications, depending on the amount present, may also interact with this medication.

Corticosteroids, glucocorticoid, especially with significant mineralocorticoid activity or
Corticosteroids, mineralocorticoid or
Amphotericin B, parenteral or
Corticotropin, especially prolonged therapeutic use
   (concurrent use with carbonic anhydrase inhibitors may result in severe hypokalemia and should be undertaken with caution; serum potassium concentrations and cardiac function should be monitored during concurrent use)
   (concurrent use of corticosteroids or corticotropin with acetazolamide sodium may increase the risk of hypernatremia and/or edema because these medications cause sodium and fluid retention; the risk with corticosteroids or corticotropin may depend on the patient's sodium requirement as determined by the condition being treated)
   (the possibility should be considered that concurrent chronic use of corticosteroids or corticotropin with carbonic anhydrase inhibitors may increase the risk of hypocalcemia and osteoporosis because these medications increase calcium excretion)

» Amphetamines or
Anticholinergics, especially atropine and related compounds or
» Mecamylamine or
» Quinidine
   (therapeutic and/or side effects may be enhanced or prolonged when these medications are used concurrently with carbonic anhydrase inhibitors, especially acetazolamide, as a result of decreased excretion caused by alkalinization of urine; concurrent use with mecamylamine is not recommended; dosage adjustments of the other medications may be needed when carbonic anhydrase inhibitor therapy is initiated or discontinued or if the dosage is changed)

Antidiabetic agents, oral or
Insulin
   (hypoglycemic response may be decreased during concurrent use because carbonic anhydrase inhibitors may cause hyperglycemia and glycosuria in diabetic patients; dosage adjustments may be required)

Barbiturates, especially phenobarbital or
Carbamazepine or
Phenytoin or other hydantoin anticonvulsants or
Primidone
   (osteopenia induced by these agents may be enhanced; it is recommended that patients receiving concurrent therapy be monitored for early signs of osteopenia and that the carbonic anhydrase inhibitor be discontinued and appropriate treatment initiated if necessary)

Ciprofloxacin
   (urinary alkalizers, such as carbonic anhydrase inhibitors, may reduce the solubility of ciprofloxacin in the urine; patients should be observed for signs of crystalluria and nephrotoxicity)

Digitalis glycosides
   (concurrent use with carbonic anhydrase inhibitors may enhance the possibility of digitalis toxicity associated with hypokalemia)

Diuretics, other
   (diuretic effects may be enhanced during concurrent therapy; however, the hypokalemic and hyperuricemic effects of many diuretics may also be enhanced during concurrent therapy)

Ephedrine
   (urine alkalinization induced by carbonic anhydrase inhibitors may increase the half-life of ephedrine and prolong its duration of action, especially if the urine remains alkaline for several days or longer; dosage adjustment of ephedrine may be necessary)

Mannitol or
Urea
   (concurrent use with carbonic anhydrase inhibitors may lead to increased reduction of intraocular pressure as well as increased diuresis)

» Methenamine
   (efficacy may be reduced because alkaline urine produced by carbonic anhydrase inhibitors inhibits methenamine conversion to formaldehyde, which is the active bacteriostatic derivative of methenamine; concurrent use is not recommended)

Mexiletine
   (marked alkalinization of urine by carbonic anhydrase inhibitors may retard renal excretion of mexiletine)

Neuromuscular blocking agents, nondepolarizing
   (hypokalemia induced by carbonic anhydrase inhibitors may enhance the blockade of nondepolarizing neuromuscular blocking agents, possibly leading to increased or prolonged respiratory depression or paralysis [apnea]; serum potassium concentration determinations may be necessary prior to administration of a nondepolarizing neuromuscular blocking agent)

Salicylates
   (the risk of salicylate intoxication in patients receiving large doses of salicylates may be increased during concurrent therapy because metabolic acidosis induced by carbonic anhydrase inhibitors may increase penetration of salicylate into the brain. Anorexia, tachypnea, lethargy, coma, and death have been reported with concurrent use of high-dose aspirin and carbonic anhydrase inhibitors. In addition, the increased risk of severe metabolic acidosis and salicylate toxicity should be considered if acetazolamide is used to produce forced alkaline diuresis in the treatment of salicylate overdose. With average doses of salicylates, alkalinization of the urine results in increased salicylate excretion and decreased salicylate plasma concentrations)

**Laboratory value alterations**
The following have been selected on the basis of their potential clinical significance (possible effect in parentheses where appropriate)—not necessarily inclusive (» = major clinical significance):

With diagnostic test results
   Urine 17-hydroxysteroid (17-OHCS) determinations
      (may produce false-positive results by interfering with absorbance in the modified Glenn-Nelson technique)
   Urine protein determinations
      (may produce false-positive results with bromophenol blue test reagent and with sulfosalicylic acid, heat and acetic acid, and nitric acid ring test methods because of alkalinization of urine)

With physiology/laboratory test values
   Ammonia concentrations, blood and
   Bilirubin concentrations, serum and
   Urobilinogen concentrations, urine
      (may be increased)
   Bicarbonate concentrations, plasma
      (usually are decreased)
   Calcium concentrations, urine
      (may be increased or unchanged)
   Chloride concentrations, plasma
      (may be increased, especially with acetazolamide)
   Citrate concentrations, urine
      (may be decreased; in combination with increased or unchanged urine calcium concentrations may result in renal calculi and ureteral colic)
   Glucose concentrations, blood and
   Glucose concentrations, urine
      (may be increased, especially in diabetic or prediabetic patients receiving acetazolamide; patients not predisposed to diabetes are not significantly affected)
   Iodine uptake by the thyroid gland
      (may be decreased in hyperthyroid patients or those with normal thyroid function but not in hypothyroid patients)
   Potassium concentrations, serum
      (may be decreased, especially when therapy is initiated or with intermittent dosage; with continuous therapy, serum potassium concentrations usually return to normal)
   Uric acid concentrations, serum
      (may be increased; rarely, gout may be exacerbated)

**Medical considerations/Contraindications**
The medical considerations/contraindications included have been selected on the basis of their potential clinical significance (reasons given in parentheses where appropriate)—not necessarily inclusive (» = major clinical significance).

***Risk-benefit should be considered when the following medical problems exist:***
» Adrenal gland failure or adrenocortical insufficiency (Addison's disease)
      (patients more susceptible to electrolyte imbalances)
   Diabetes mellitus
      (may increase blood and urine sugar concentrations)
   Gout, except when used to prevent uric acid calculi in patients receiving uricosuric antigout agents or
» Hyperchloremic acidosis or
» Hypokalemia, hyponatremia, or other electrolyte imbalance or
   Respiratory acidosis
      (may be exacerbated)

» Hepatic disease, including cirrhosis, or impairment
(patients more susceptible to electrolyte imbalances; increased risk of hepatic coma and hepatotoxicity)
Impaired alveolar ventilation due to pulmonary disease, edema, infection, or obstruction
(respiratory acidosis may be induced or increased)
» Renal failure, disease, or impairment
(excessively high plasma concentrations may result and the acidosis of renal failure may be aggravated)
» Renal calculi, calcium-containing, or history of
(may be exacerbated or induced during therapy)
Sensitivity to carbonic anhydrase inhibitors

**Patient monitoring**

The following may be especially important in patient monitoring (other tests may be warranted in some patients, depending on condition; » = major clinical significance):

Complete blood cell (CBC) count
Platelet count
(baseline CBC and platelet counts recommended prior to initiating therapy and at regular intervals during therapy. If significant changes occur, medication should be promptly discontinued and appropriate therapy instituted)

» Electrolyte concentrations, serum
(recommended prior to initiation of therapy and at periodic intervals during therapy, especially in patients for whom hypokalemia or other electrolyte imbalances would be detrimental, such as those with hepatic cirrhosis or those receiving potassium-wasting medications or digitalis)

Urologic examinations
(may be necessary to detect possible renal problems, especially crystalluria or renal calculi)

## Side/Adverse Effects

Note: Serious side/adverse effects occur infrequently; many of the serious adverse effects are those that are common to all sulfonamide derivatives, such as Stevens-Johnson syndrome, toxic epidermal necrolysis, fulminant hepatic necrosis, agranulocytosis, aplastic anemia, and other blood dyscrasias. Rarely, these serious adverse effects have caused fatalities. Many side effects are dose-related and may respond to a reduction of dosage.

Hypokalemia may occur if diuresis is brisk and may be especially likely to occur if hepatic cirrhosis is present, if potassium intake is inadequate, or if other potassium-wasting drugs are used concurrently. Potassium supplementation may be necessary in some patients.

Severe metabolic acidosis or acidotic coma may occur rarely during long-term carbonic anhydrase inhibitor therapy and may be corrected by administration of bicarbonate.

| The following side/adverse effects have been selected on the basis of their potential clinical significance (possible signs and symptoms in parentheses where appropriate)—not necessarily inclusive:* | Legend: I=Acetazolamide II=Dichlorphenamide III=Methazolamide | | |
|---|---|---|---|
| | I | II | III |
| Medical attention needed | | | |
| *Acidosis* (shortness of breath, troubled breathing)# | R | R | R |
| *Blood dyscrasias* (fever and sore throat, unusual bruising or bleeding)† | R | R | R |
| *Bloody or black, tarry stools* | R | R | R |
| *Cholestatic jaundice* (darkening of urine, pale stools, yellow eyes or skin) | R | U | U |
| *Clumsiness or unsteadiness* | R | R | R |
| *Confusion* | R | R | R |
| *Convulsions* | R | R | R |
| *Crystalluria, renal calculus, or sulfonamide-like nephrotoxicity* (blood in urine, difficult urination, pain in lower back, pain or burning while urinating, sudden decrease in amount of urine)† | L | L | L |
| *Hypersensitivity* (fever, hives, itching, skin rash or sores) | R | R | R |

| The following side/adverse effects have been selected on the basis of their potential clinical significance (possible signs and symptoms in parentheses where appropriate)—not necessarily inclusive:* | Legend: I=Acetazolamide II=Dichlorphenamide III=Methazolamide | | |
|---|---|---|---|
| | I | II | III |
| *Hypokalemia* (dryness of mouth, increased thirst, irregular heartbeats, mood or mental changes, muscle cramps or pain, nausea or vomiting, unusual tiredness or weakness, weak pulse)‡ | R | R | R |
| *Mental depression* | L | L | L |
| *Nearsightedness*§ | R | R | R |
| *Ringing or buzzing in ears* | R | R | R |
| *Severe muscle weakness or trembling* | R | R | R |
| *Unusual tiredness or weakness*** | M | M | M |
| Medical attention needed only if continuing or bothersome | | | |
| *Constipation* | U | R | U |
| *Diarrhea* | M | M | M |
| *Dizziness or lightheadedness* | U | L | L |
| *Drowsiness* | L | L | L |
| *Feeling of choking or lump in throat* | U | R | U |
| *General feeling of discomfort or illness* | M | M | M |
| *Headache* | R | R | R |
| *Increase in frequency of urination or amount of urine* | M | M | R |
| *Increased sensitivity of eyes to sunlight* | R | U | R |
| *Loss of appetite* | M | M | M |
| *Loss of taste and smell* | R | R | R |
| *Metallic taste in mouth* | M | M | M |
| *Nausea or vomiting* | M | M | M |
| *Nervousness or irritability* | U | R | U |
| *Numbness, tingling, or burning in hands, fingers, feet, toes, mouth, tongue, lips, or anus*† | M | M | M |
| *Weight loss* | M | M | M |

*Acetazolamide is the most widely used carbonic anhydrase inhibitor; most of the data concerning side effects have been reported for that medication. The comparatively infrequent reports of side effects with other agents of this group may reflect their less frequent usage rather than actual reduced incidence. The pharmacologic similarity of these medications suggests that side effects occurring with one may potentially occur with the others. However, many side effects may not occur with the same severity or frequency with all carbonic anhydrase inhibitors, and patients unable to tolerate one of these medications may be able to tolerate another. Frequency of side effects (generalized): M = more frequent; L = less frequent; R = rare; U = unknown.

†May be more likely to occur with acetazolamide and least likely to occur with methazolamide.

‡May be more likely to occur with dichlorphenamide.

§Transient myopia may occur when therapy is initiated and usually responds to a reduction in dosage or withdrawal of therapy. Transient myopia may not recur if therapy is restarted.

#May be less likely to occur with dichlorphenamide.

**Usually part of a general feeling of malaise induced by these agents but should be evaluated because rarely may indicate acidosis, blood dyscrasias, or hypokalemia.

## Patient Consultation

As an aid to patient consultation, refer to *Advice for the Patient, Carbonic Anhydrase Inhibitors (Systemic)*.

In providing consultation, consider emphasizing the following selected information (» = major clinical significance):

### Before using this medication

» Conditions affecting use, especially:
Sensitivity to carbonic anhydrase inhibitors, antibacterial sulfonamides, thiazide diuretics, or other sulfonamide-derivative diuretics
Pregnancy—Studies in animals have shown teratogenic (skeletal anomalies) and embryocidal effects

Breast-feeding—Use is not recommended, because these medicines may be distributed into breast milk and have the potential for serious adverse reactions

Other medications, especially amphetamines, mecamylamine, methenamine, or quinidine

Other medical problems, especially adrenal gland failure or adrenocortical insufficiency; hepatic disease, including cirrhosis or impairment; hyperchloremic acidosis; hypokalemia, hyponatremia, or other electrolyte imbalance; renal calculi, calcium-containing, or history of; or renal failure, disease, or impairment

**Proper use of this medication**
» Importance of not taking more medication than the amount prescribed
Taking medication with meals to lessen gastrointestinal upset
How to minimize inconvenience of unwanted diuresis
» Proper dosing
Missed dose: Taking as soon as possible; not taking if almost time for next dose; not doubling doses
» Proper storage

**Precautions while using this medication**
» Caution if drowsiness, dizziness, lightheadedness, or tiredness occurs
Regular visits to physician to check progress during therapy
» Possibility of hypokalemia
Diabetics: May increase blood and urine glucose concentrations
Importance of adequate fluid intake during therapy to help prevent kidney stones
Checking with physician before discontinuing acetazolamide (when used as anticonvulsant); gradual dosage reduction may be desirable

**Side/adverse effects**
Signs of potential side effects, especially acidosis; blood dyscrasias; bloody or black, tarry stools; cholestatic jaundice; clumsiness or unsteadiness; confusion; convulsions; crystalluria, renal calculus, sulfonamide-like nephrotoxicity; hypersensitivity; hypokalemia; mental depression; nearsightedness; ringing or buzzing in ears; severe muscle weakness or trembling; or unusual tiredness or weakness

## General Dosing Information

Carbonic anhydrase inhibitors are usually used concurrently with other antiglaucoma agents including miotics, mydriatics, and osmotic agents.

Dosage should be adjusted according to the requirements and response of the individual patient as indicated by measurement of ocular tension and symptomatology.

Carbonic anhydrase inhibitors may be given with meals to minimize gastrointestinal upset.

Maintenance of a high fluid intake may be advisable, especially in patients with hypercalciuria or gout, to reduce the risk of renal calculi.

Patients unable to tolerate one carbonic anhydrase inhibitor because of side effects may be able to tolerate another.

If a satisfactory lowering of intraocular pressure is not achieved or maintained with one carbonic anhydrase inhibitor, one of the other agents in this group may provide a beneficial effect.

It is recommended that various brands of acetazolamide marketed by different manufacturers not be used interchangeably unless data indicating therapeutic equivalence are available; bioequivalence problems have been reported.

It is recommended that carbonic anhydrase inhibitor therapy be discontinued if hematopoietic reactions, fever, skin rash, or renal problems occur.

If potassium supplementation is needed in a patient receiving a carbonic anhydrase inhibitor, the fact that plasma chloride concentration may be elevated should be kept in mind and a potassium preparation chosen that does not contain chloride.

---

### ACETAZOLAMIDE

## Summary of Differences

Indications: Also indicated as an anticonvulsant, to prevent or reduce severity of symptoms of acute altitude sickness, to treat toxicity caused by weakly acidic medications, to treat familial periodic paralysis, and to prevent uric acid or cystine renal calculi.

Side effects: See *Side/Adverse Effects*.

## Additional Dosing Information

See also *General Dosing Information*.

When acetazolamide is added to existing anticonvulsant therapy, an initial daily dose of 4 to 5 mg per kg of body weight per day in addition to existing medication is recommended. Dosage may be increased as necessary. Changes from other anticonvulsants to acetazolamide or withdrawal of acetazolamide therapy should be gradual to prevent increased seizure activity and possible status epilepticus.

Tolerance to the anticonvulsant effect of acetazolamide develops rapidly, over weeks or months in some patients.

For oral dosage forms only:
• Both the acetazolamide tablets and extended-release capsules are indicated for use in glaucoma and for prophylaxis and treatment of acute altitude sickness. Although the extended release capsules may be better tolerated than the acetazolamide tablets or the tablets of the other carbonic anhydrase inhibitors, they may be less effective in some patients.

For parenteral dosage forms only:
• Direct intravenous administration is preferred; intramuscular injection is not recommended, because it is painful due to the alkaline pH of the solution.
• Parenteral administration is usually used when the patient cannot take oral medication or when a rapid initial intraocular pressure-lowering action is necessary. Therapy is usually continued with oral acetazolamide, depending on the patient's condition and response.

## Oral Dosage Forms

Note: Bracketed uses in the *Dosage Forms* section refer to categories of use and/or indications that are not included in U.S. product labeling.

### ACETAZOLAMIDE EXTENDED-RELEASE CAPSULES

**Usual adult and adolescent dose**
Antiglaucoma agent—
Oral, 500 mg two times a day, in the morning and evening.
Note: In the treatment of glaucoma, dosage greater than 1 gram per day usually does not produce an increased effect.
Altitude sickness, acute, prophylactic and therapeutic agent[1]—
Oral, 500 mg one or two times a day.
Note: During rapid ascent, such as in rescue or military operations, 1,000 mg a day is recommended. Therapy should preferably be initiated 24 to 48 hours before ascent and, while at high altitude, continued for 48 hours or longer as necessary to control symptoms.
The use of acetazolamide for rapid ascent does not obviate the need for prompt descent if severe forms of high altitude sickness, such as high altitude pulmonary edema (HAPE) or high altitude cerebral edema, occur.

**Usual pediatric dose**
Safety and efficacy have not been established.

**Strength(s) usually available**
U.S.—
500 mg (Rx) [*Diamox Sequels*].
Canada—
500 mg (Rx) [*Diamox Sequels*].

**Packaging and storage**
Store between 15 and 30 °C (59 and 86 °F), in a well-closed container, unless otherwise specified by manufacturer.

**Auxiliary labeling**
• May cause drowsiness.

### ACETAZOLAMIDE TABLETS USP

**Usual adult and adolescent dose**
Antiglaucoma agent—
Open-angle glaucoma:
Initial—Oral, 250 mg one to four times a day.
Maintenance—To be titrated according to patient response; lower doses may be sufficient.
Secondary glaucoma and preoperative lowering of intraocular pressure:
Oral, 250 mg every four hours. Some patients may respond to 250 mg two times a day. In some acute cases, an initial dose of 500 mg followed by 125 or 250 mg every four hours may be preferable.
Malignant (ciliary block) glaucoma:
Oral, 250 mg four times a day to reduce intraocular pressure.
Anticonvulsant—
Oral, 4 to 30 mg (usually 10 mg initially) per kg of body weight a day in up to 4 divided doses; usually 375 mg to 1 gram a day.
Altitude sickness, acute, prophylactic and therapeutic agent[1]—
Oral, 250 mg two to four times a day.
Note: During rapid ascent, such as in rescue or military operations, 1,000 mg a day is recommended. Therapy should preferably be initiated 24 to 48 hours before ascent and, while at high altitude,

continued for 48 hours or longer as necessary to control symptoms.

The use of acetazolamide for rapid ascent does not obviate the need for prompt descent if severe forms of high altitude sickness, such as high altitude pulmonary edema (HAPE) or high altitude cerebral edema, occur.

[Antiparalytic][1]—
Oral, 250 mg to 1.5 grams a day in divided doses.

[Antiurolithic][1]—
Oral, 250 mg daily at bedtime.

Note: For use as an anticonvulsant or in open-angle glaucoma, dosage greater than 1 gram per day usually does not produce an increased effect.

**Usual pediatric dose**
Glaucoma—
Oral, 8 to 30 mg per kg of body weight, usually 10 to 15 mg per kg, or 300 to 900 mg per square meter of body surface area a day in divided doses.

Anticonvulsant—
See *Usual adult and adolescent dose*.

**Strength(s) usually available**
U.S.—
125 mg (Rx) [*Diamox* (scored); GENERIC].
250 mg (Rx) [*Ak-Zol; Dazamide; Diamox* (scored); *Storzolamide*; GENERIC].
Canada—
250 mg (Rx) [*Acetazolam; Apo-Acetazolamide; Diamox*].

**Packaging and storage**
Store between 15 and 30 °C (59 and 86 °F), in a well-closed container, unless otherwise specified by manufacturer.

**Preparation of dosage form**
For pediatric patients or adults unable to swallow tablets—An acetazolamide oral suspension may be prepared by crushing acetazolamide tablets and suspending the resultant powder in a highly flavored syrup (cherry, raspberry, chocolate, etc.). Up to 500 mg may be suspended in 5 mL of syrup, but a suspension containing 250 mg per 5 mL is more palatable. Such a suspension is stable for 1 week. Refrigeration may improve the taste but does not increase or lengthen stability. Elixirs or other vehicles containing alcohol or glycerin will not provide a palatable suspension.

**Auxiliary labeling**
• May cause drowsiness.

## Parenteral Dosage Forms

Note: Bracketed uses in the *Dosage Forms* section refer to categories of use and/or indications that are not included in U.S. product labeling.

### ACETAZOLAMIDE SODIUM STERILE USP

**Usual adult and adolescent dose**
Antiglaucoma agent—
For rapid initial lowering of intraocular pressure: Intravenous, the equivalent of acetazolamide—500 mg.

Note: Parenteral administration may be repeated in two to four hours in some acute cases, but therapy is usually continued with oral acetazolamide, depending on the patient's response.

[Diuretic (urinary alkalinizing)]—
Intravenous, 5 mg per kg of body weight or as required to achieve and maintain a forced alkaline diuresis.

Note: For other uses or when the patient is unable to take oral medication, acetazolamide may be given parenterally in dosages equivalent to those recommended for the oral tablets. (See *Acetazolamide Tablets USP*.)

**Usual pediatric dose**
Antiglaucoma agent—
Acute glaucoma: Intravenous, the equivalent of acetazolamide—5 to 10 mg per kg of body weight every six hours.

[Diuretic (urinary alkalinizing)]—
Intravenous, the equivalent of acetazolamide: 5 mg per kg of body weight or 150 mg per square meter of body surface area once a day in the morning for one or two days alternated with a drug-free day.

**Strength(s) usually available**
U.S.—
500 mg (Rx) [*Diamox*; GENERIC].
Canada—
500 mg (Rx) [*Diamox*].

**Packaging and storage**
Prior to reconstitution, store below 40 °C (104 °F), preferably between 15 and 30 °C (59 and 86 °F), unless otherwise specified by manufacturer.

**Preparation of dosage form**
Sterile Acetazolamide Sodium USP is reconstituted for parenteral use by adding at least 5 mL of Sterile Water for Injection USP to the vial and shaking to dissolve. A solution prepared using 5 mL of diluent contains the equivalent of 100 mg of acetazolamide per mL.

**Stability**
After reconstitution, solutions retain their potency for 1 week if refrigerated. However, because they contain no preservative, use within 24 hours is strongly recommended.

[1]Not included in Canadian product labeling.

---

## DICHLORPHENAMIDE

## Summary of Differences
Side effects: See *Side/Adverse Effects*.

## Oral Dosage Forms

### DICHLORPHENAMIDE TABLETS USP

**Usual adult and adolescent dose**
Antiglaucoma agent—
Initial: 100 to 200 mg for the first dose followed by 100 mg every twelve hours until the desired response is obtained.
Maintenance: 25 to 50 mg one to three times a day.

**Usual pediatric dose**
Safety and efficacy have not been established.

**Strength(s) usually available**
U.S.—
50 mg (Rx) [*Daranide* (scored)].
Canada—
Not commercially available.

**Packaging and storage**
Store below 40 °C (104 °F), preferably between 15 and 30 °C (59 and 86 °F), in a well-closed container, unless otherwise specified by manufacturer.

**Auxiliary labeling**
• May cause drowsiness.

---

## METHAZOLAMIDE

## Summary of Differences
Side effects: See *Side/Adverse Effects*.

## Oral Dosage Forms

### METHAZOLAMIDE TABLETS USP

**Usual adult and adolescent dose**
Antiglaucoma agent—
Oral, 50 to 100 mg two or three times a day.

**Usual pediatric dose**
Safety and efficacy have not been established.

**Strength(s) usually available**
U.S.—
25 mg (Rx) [*MZM; Neptazane*; GENERIC].
50 mg (Rx) [*MZM; Neptazane* (scored); GENERIC].
Canada—
50 mg (Rx) [*Neptazane*].

**Packaging and storage**
Store between 15 and 30 °C (59 and 86 °F), in a well-closed container, unless otherwise specified by manufacturer.

**Auxiliary labeling**
• May cause drowsiness.

Revised: 06/21/94
Interim revision: 01/24/95

# CARBOPLATIN Systemic

VA CLASSIFICATION (Primary): AN900
Commonly used brand name(s): *Paraplatin; Paraplatin-AQ*.
Note: For a listing of dosage forms and brand names by country availability, see *Dosage Forms* section(s).

## Category
Antineoplastic.

## Indications
Note: Bracketed information in the *Indications* section refers to uses that are not included in U.S. product labeling.

**Accepted**
Carcinoma, ovarian, epithelial (treatment)—Carboplatin is indicated for palliative treatment of epithelial ovarian carcinoma refractory to standard chemotherapy that did or did not include cisplatin. It is also indicated for initial treatment of advanced ovarian carcinoma in established combination with other approved chemotherapeutic agents.

[Carcinoma, endometrial (treatment)][1]—Carboplatin is indicated as reasonable medical therapy in the treatment of endometrial carcinoma. (Evidence rating: IIID)

[Carcinoma, lung, small cell (treatment)][1]
[Carcinoma, lung, non–small cell (treatment)][1]
[Carcinoma, head and neck (treatment)][1]
[Carcinoma, testicular (treatment)][1] or
[Seminoma (treatment)][1]—Carboplatin is indicated for treatment of small cell and non–small cell lung carcinoma, head and neck tumors, nonseminomatous testicular carcinoma, and seminoma.

[Retinoblastoma (treatment)][1]—Carboplatin is indicated as reasonable medical therapy in the treatment of retinoblastoma. (Evidence rating: IIID)

[Tumors, brain, primary (treatment)][1]—Carboplatin is indicated for treatment of primary brain tumors.

[Malignant melanoma (treatment)][1]—Carboplatin is indicated for treatment of malignant melanoma.

[1]Not included in Canadian product labeling.

## Pharmacology/Pharmacokinetics

**Physicochemical characteristics**
Molecular weight—371.26.

**Mechanism of action/Effect**
Carboplatin resembles an alkylating agent. Although the exact mechanism of action is unknown, action is thought to be similar to that of the bifunctional alkylating agents, that is, possible cross-linking and interference with the function of DNA. It is cell cycle–phase nonspecific.

**Protein binding**
Very low; however, platinum from carboplatin is irreversibly bound to plasma proteins and is slowly eliminated with a minimum half-life of 5 days.

**Biotransformation**
By hydrolysis in solution (aquation), at a rate slower than occurs with cisplatin, to the active species that reacts with DNA.

**Half-life**
Alpha phase—1.1 to 2 hours.
Beta phase—2.6 to 5.9 hours.

**Elimination**
Renal (71% within 24 hours at creatinine clearances of 60 mL per minute and greater).

## Precautions to Consider

**Cross-sensitivity and/or related problems**
Patients sensitive to cisplatin or other platinum-containing compounds may be sensitive to carboplatin also.

**Carcinogenicity**
Secondary malignancies are potential delayed effects of many antineoplastic agents, although it is not clear whether the effect is related to their mutagenic or immunosuppressive action. The effect of dose and duration of therapy is also unknown, although risk seems to increase with long-term use. Although information is limited, available data seem to indicate that the carcinogenic risk is greatest with the alkylating agents.

**Mutagenicity**
Both *in vivo* and *in vitro* studies have shown carboplatin to be mutagenic.

**Pregnancy/Reproduction**
Fertility—Gonadal suppression, resulting in amenorrhea or azoospermia, may occur in patients taking antineoplastic therapy, especially with the alkylating agents. In general, these effects appear to be related to dose and length of therapy and may be irreversible. Prediction of the degree of testicular or ovarian function impairment is complicated by the common use of combinations of several antineoplastics, which makes it difficult to assess the effects of individual agents.

Pregnancy—Carboplatin is embryotoxic and teratogenic in rats.
First trimester: It is usually recommended that use of antineoplastics, especially combination chemotherapy, be avoided whenever possible, especially during the first trimester. Although information is limited because of the relatively few instances of antineoplastic administration during pregnancy, the mutagenic, teratogenic, and carcinogenic potential of these medications must be considered.

Other hazards to the fetus include adverse reactions seen in adults.
In general, use of a contraceptive is recommended during cytotoxic drug therapy.

FDA Pregnancy Category D.

**Breast-feeding**
Although very little information is available regarding distribution of antineoplastic agents into breast milk, breast-feeding is not recommended while carboplatin is being administered because of the risks to the infant (adverse effects, mutagenicity, carcinogenicity). It is not known whether carboplatin is distributed into breast milk.

**Pediatrics**
No information is available on the relationship of age to the effects of carboplatin in pediatric patients.

**Geriatrics**
Incidence of peripheral neurotoxicity is increased and myelotoxicity may be more severe in patients older than 65 years of age. In addition, elderly patients are more likely to have age-related renal function impairment, which may require dosage reduction and careful monitoring of blood counts in patients receiving carboplatin.

**Dental**
The bone marrow depressant effects of carboplatin may result in an increased incidence of microbial infection, delayed healing, and gingival bleeding. Dental work, whenever possible, should be completed prior to initiation of therapy or deferred until blood counts have returned to normal. Patients should be instructed in proper oral hygiene during treatment, including caution in use of regular toothbrushes, dental floss, and toothpicks.

Carboplatin rarely may also cause mucositis or stomatitis associated with considerable discomfort.

**Drug interactions and/or related problems**
The following drug interactions and/or related problems have been selected on the basis of their potential clinical significance (possible mechanism in parentheses where appropriate)—not necessarily inclusive (» = major clinical significance):

Note: Combinations containing any of the following medications, depending on the amount present, may also interact with this medication.

Blood dyscrasia–causing medications (see *Appendix II*)
(leukopenic and/or thrombocytopenic effects of carboplatin may be increased with concurrent or recent therapy if these medications cause the same effects; dosage adjustment of carboplatin, if necessary, should be based on blood counts)

» Bone marrow depressants, other (see *Appendix II*) or
Radiation therapy
(concurrent use may increase the total effects of these medications and radiation therapy; dosage reduction is recommended)

Cisplatin
(incidence of carboplatin-induced neurotoxicity or ototoxicity is increased in patients previously treated with cisplatin; use of carboplatin worsens pre-existing cisplatin-induced neurotoxicity [in about 30% of those patients] or ototoxicity; additive nephrotoxicity has not been reported)

Nephrotoxic medications, other (see *Appendix II*) or
Ototoxic medications, other (see *Appendix II*)
(concurrent and/or sequential administration may increase the potential for ototoxicity and nephrotoxicity)

Vaccines, killed virus
(because normal defense mechanisms may be suppressed by carboplatin therapy, the patient's antibody response to the vaccine may be decreased. The interval between discontinuation of medications that cause immunosuppression and restoration of the patient's ability to respond to the vaccine depends on the intensity and type of immunosuppression-causing medication used, the underlying disease, and other factors; estimates vary from 3 months to 1 year)

» Vaccines, live virus
(because normal defense mechanisms may be suppressed by carboplatin therapy, concurrent use with a live virus vaccine may potentiate the replication of the vaccine virus, may increase the side/adverse effects of the vaccine virus, and/or may decrease the patient's antibody response to the vaccine; immunization of these patients should be undertaken only with extreme caution after careful review of the patient's hematologic status and only with the knowledge and consent of the physician managing the carboplatin therapy. The interval between discontinuation of medications that cause immunosuppression and restoration of the patient's ability to respond to the vaccine depends on the intensity and type of immunosuppression-causing medication used, the underlying disease, and other factors; estimates vary from 3 months to 1 year. In addition, immunization with oral poliovirus vaccine should be postponed in persons in close contact with the patient, especially family members)

**Laboratory value alterations**
The following have been selected on the basis of their potential clinical significance (possible effect in parentheses where appropriate)—not necessarily inclusive (» = major clinical significance):

With physiology/laboratory test values
Bilirubin concentrations, serum and
Alkaline phosphatase values, serum and
Aspartate aminotransferase (AST [SGOT]) values, serum
(may be increased; increases are usually mild and are reversible in 50% of cases; severe abnormalities occur at carboplatin doses of more than four times the recommended dose)

Blood urea nitrogen (BUN) concentrations and
Creatinine concentrations, serum
(may be increased, indicating nephrotoxicity; usually mild; reversible in about 50% of cases)

Calcium and
Magnesium and
Potassium and
Sodium
(serum concentrations may be decreased)

**Medical considerations/Contraindications**
The medical considerations/contraindications included have been selected on the basis of their potential clinical significance (reasons given in parentheses where appropriate)—not necessarily inclusive (» = major clinical significance).

*Risk-benefit should be considered when the following medical problems exist:*

Ascites or
Pleural effusion
(increased risk of toxicity)
Bleeding, significant
» Bone marrow depression
» Chickenpox, existing or recent (including recent exposure) or
» Herpes zoster
(risk of severe generalized disease)
Hearing impairment
» Infection
» Renal function impairment
(reduced elimination; increased bone marrow depression; incidence and severity of nephrotoxicity may be increased. A lower dosage of carboplatin is recommended in patients with impaired renal function and careful monitoring of blood counts between courses is recommended)
Sensitivity to carboplatin
» Caution should be used also in patients who have had previous cytotoxic drug therapy or radiation therapy.

**Patient monitoring**
The following may be especially important in patient monitoring (other tests may be warranted in some patients, depending on condition; » = major clinical significance):

Audiometric testing
(recommended prior to initiation of therapy and if ototoxicity is suspected during therapy)
Blood urea nitrogen (BUN) concentrations and
» Creatinine clearance and
Creatinine concentrations, serum
(recommended prior to initiation of therapy and before each course of carboplatin to adjust dosage and detect renal toxicity)
Calcium concentrations, serum and
Magnesium concentrations, serum and
Potassium concentrations, serum and
Sodium concentrations, serum
(recommended at periodic intervals during therapy)
» Hematocrit or hemoglobin and
» Leukocyte count, total and, if appropriate, differential, and
» Platelet count
(determinations recommended prior to initiation of therapy and at periodic intervals during therapy; frequency varies according to clinical state, agent, dose, and other agents being used concurrently)
Neurologic function studies
(recommended prior to initiation of therapy and at periodic intervals during therapy)

## Side/Adverse Effects

Note: Many "side effects" of antineoplastic therapy are unavoidable and represent the medication's pharmacologic action. Some of these (for example, leukopenia and thrombocytopenia) are actually used as parameters to aid in individual dosage titration.
Carboplatin infrequently causes mild renal toxicity, which may be detected initially only by means of renal function tests.

The following side/adverse effects have been selected on the basis of their potential clinical significance (possible signs and symptoms in parentheses where appropriate)—not necessarily inclusive:

**Those indicating need for medical attention**
Incidence more frequent—dose-related
*Anemia* (unusual tiredness or weakness)—usually asymptomatic; *leukopenia or neutropenia* (fever or chills; cough or hoarseness; lower back or side pain; painful or difficult urination)—usually asymptomatic; *pain at site of injection; thrombocytopenia* (unusual bleeding or bruising; black, tarry stools; blood in urine or stools; pinpoint red spots on skin)—usually asymptomatic

Note: *Anemia* may be cumulative; transfusions are frequently necessary.
With *leukopenia and thrombocytopenia*, nadir of leukocyte and platelet counts occurs after 21 days and counts usually recover by 30 days after a dose. Nadir of granulocyte counts usually occurs after 21 to 28 days and counts usually recover by day 35.
*Leukopenia and thrombocytopenia* are dose-dependent and cumulative; in a small percentage of patients (less than 10%) they are unpredictable.

Incidence less frequent
*Allergic reaction* (skin rash or itching; wheezing); *peripheral neurotoxicity* (numbness or tingling in fingers or toes); *ototoxicity* (ringing in ears)—usually asymptomatic

Note: An *allergic reaction* occurs within minutes of administration.
*Neurotoxicity* may be cumulative.
With *ototoxicity*, hearing loss usually occurs first with high frequencies (above speech tones) and may be unilateral or bilateral.

Incidence rare
*Blurred vision; mucositis or stomatitis* (sores in mouth and on lips)

**Those indicating need for medical attention only if they continue or are bothersome**
Incidence more frequent
*Asthenia* (unusual tiredness or weakness); *nausea and vomiting*

Note: Less frequently, *asthenia* may be related to anemia.
*Nausea and vomiting* occur in about 65% of patients; these are severe in about one third of those. Nausea alone occurs in about 10 to 15% of patients. Symptoms usually begin 6 to 12 hours after a dose, and vomiting may persist for 24 hours. May be treated or prevented by antiemetic medication.

Incidence less frequent
*Constipation or diarrhea; loss of appetite*

Those not indicating need for medical attention
Incidence less frequent
*Loss of hair*

## Patient Consultation

As an aid to patient consultation, refer to *Advice for the Patient, Carboplatin (Systemic)*.

In providing consultation, consider emphasizing the following selected information (» = major clinical significance):

### Before using this medication
» Conditions affecting use, especially:
    Sensitivity to cisplatin or other platinum-containing compounds, or to carboplatin
    Pregnancy—Use not recommended because of mutagenic, teratogenic, and carcinogenic potential; advisability of using contraception; telling physician immediately if pregnancy is suspected
    Breast-feeding—Not recommended because of risk of serious side effects
    Use in the elderly—Increased incidence of peripheral neurotoxicity and severity of myelotoxicity
    Other medications, especially other bone marrow depressants or previous cytotoxic drug or radiation therapy
    Other medical problems, especially chickenpox, herpes zoster, other infections, or renal function impairment

### Proper use of this medication
Caution if taking combination therapy; taking each medication at the right time
Frequency of nausea and vomiting; importance of continuing medication despite stomach upset
» Proper dosing

### Precautions while using this medication
» Importance of close monitoring by the physician
» Avoiding immunizations unless approved by physician; other persons in patient's household should avoid immunizations with oral poliovirus vaccine; avoiding persons who have taken oral poliovirus vaccine within the past several months or wearing a protective mask that covers nose and mouth

*Caution if bone marrow depression occurs*
» Avoiding exposure to persons with infections, especially during periods of low blood counts; checking with physician immediately if fever or chills, cough or hoarseness, lower back or side pain, or painful or difficult urination occurs
» Checking with physician immediately if unusual bleeding or bruising; black, tarry stools; blood in urine or stools; or pinpoint red spots on skin occur
Caution in use of regular toothbrush, dental floss, or toothpick; physician, dentist, or nurse may suggest alternatives; checking with physician before having dental work done
Not touching eyes or inside of nose unless hands washed immediately before
Using caution to avoid accidental cuts with use of sharp objects such as safety razor or fingernail or toenail cutters
Avoiding contact sports or other situations where bruising or injury might occur

### Side/adverse effects
May cause adverse effects such as ear and kidney problems, blood problems, and cancer; importance of discussing possible effects with physician
Signs of potential side effects, especially anemia, leukopenia or neutropenia, pain at site of injection, thrombocytopenia, allergic reaction, peripheral neurotoxicity, ototoxicity, blurred vision, and mucositis or stomatitis
Physician or nurse can help in dealing with side effects
Possibility of hair loss; normal hair growth should resume after treatment has ended

## General Dosing Information

It is recommended that carboplatin be administered to patients under supervision of a physician experienced in cancer chemotherapy. It is also recommended that equipment and medications (including epinephrine, oxygen, antihistamines, and intravenous corticosteroids) necessary for treatment of a possible anaphylactic reaction be readily available at each administration of carboplatin.

Dosage must be adjusted to meet the individual requirements of each patient, on the basis of clinical response and appearance or severity of toxicity.

Carboplatin may be used in combination with other agents in various regimens. As a result, incidence and/or severity of side effects may be altered and different dosages (usually reduced) may be used.

It is recommended that carboplatin be administered as an intravenous infusion, usually over 15 to 60 minutes. No pre- or post-treatment hydration or forced diuresis is required.

Carboplatin has also been administered as a continuous intravenous infusion over 24 hours or by dividing the total dose into five consecutive daily pulse doses; this method of administration appears to reduce nausea and vomiting but not nephrotoxicity or ototoxicity.

It is recommended that courses of carboplatin be administered no more frequently than every 4 weeks to allow recovery of bone marrow.

Administration of subsequent doses of carboplatin is not recommended before platelet levels return to at least 100,000 per cubic millimeter and leukocyte levels to at least 2000 per cubic millimeter.

Special precautions are recommended in patients who develop thrombocytopenia as a result of administration of carboplatin. These may include extreme care in performing invasive procedures; regular inspection of intravenous sites, skin (including perirectal area), and mucous membrane surfaces for signs of bleeding or bruising; limiting frequency of venipuncture and avoiding intramuscular injections; testing urine, emesis, stool, and secretions for occult blood; care in use of regular toothbrushes, dental floss, toothpicks, safety razors, and fingernail and toenail cutters; avoiding constipation; and using caution to prevent falls and other injuries. Such patients should avoid alcohol and aspirin intake because of the risk of gastrointestinal bleeding. Platelet transfusions may be required.

Patients who develop leukopenia should be observed carefully for signs of infection. Antibiotic support may be required. In neutropenic patients who develop fever, broad-spectrum antibiotic coverage should be initiated empirically, pending bacterial cultures and appropriate diagnostic tests.

### Safety considerations for handling this medication

There is limited but increasing evidence and concern that personnel involved in preparation and administration of parenteral antineoplastics may be at some risk because of the potential mutagenicity, teratogenicity, and/or carcinogenicity of these agents, although the actual risk is unknown. USP advisory panels recommend cautious handling both in preparation and disposal of antineoplastic agents. Precautions that have been suggested include:

- Use of a biological containment cabinet during reconstitution and dilution of parenteral medications and wearing of disposable surgical gloves and masks.
- Use of proper technique to prevent contamination of the medication, work area, and operator during transfer between containers (including proper training of personnel in this technique).
- Cautious and proper disposal of needles, syringes, vials, ampuls, and unused medication.

A number of medical centers have developed detailed guidelines for handling of antineoplastic agents.

## Parenteral Dosage Forms

Note: Bracketed uses in the *Dosage Forms* section refer to categories of use and/or indications that are not included in U.S. product labeling.

### CARBOPLATIN FOR INJECTION

**Usual adult dose**
Carcinoma, ovarian, epithelial—
Initial: Intravenous, according to the formula Total dose (mg) = (target AUC) × (GFR + 25) where AUC (area under the plasma concentration–time curve) is expressed in mg per mL·min and GFR (glomerular filtration rate) is expressed in mL per minute.

The target AUC of 4 to 6 mg per mL·min using carboplatin monotherapy appears to provide the most appropriate dose range in previously treated patients.

Additional dosing option: Advanced, initial treatment—Intravenous, 300 mg per square meter of body surface area once every four weeks (day 1) for six cycles, in combination with cyclophosphamide 600 mg per square meter of body surface area intravenously once every four weeks (day 1) for six cycles.

Refractory to other chemotherapy: Intravenous, 360 mg per square meter of body surface area once every four weeks (day 1).

Note: An initial dose of 250 mg per square meter of body surface area is recommended in patients with creatinine clearance of 41 to 59 mL per minute; an initial dose of 200 mg per square meter of body surface area is recommended in patients with creatinine clearance of 16 to 40 mL per minute.

**782  Carboplatin (Systemic)**

A suggested dosage adjustment schedule for subsequent doses is:

| Nadir after prior dose (cells per cubic millimeter) | | % of Prior dose to be given |
|---|---|---|
| Neutrophils | Platelets | |
| >2000 | >100,000 | 125 |
| 500–2000 | 50,000–100,000 | 100 |
| <500 | <50,000 | 75 |

Note: Only one dose escalation should be made.
Geriatric patients may require lower doses.

[Carcinoma, endometrial][1] or
[Carcinoma, head and neck][1] or
[Carcinoma, lung, non–small cell][1] or
[Carcinoma, lung, small cell][1] or
[Malignant melanoma][1] or
[Retinoblastoma][1] or
[Seminoma][1] or
[Tumors, brain, primary][1]—
  Consult medical literature or manufacturer's literature for information on dosage.

### Usual pediatric dose
Dosage has not been established.

### Size(s) usually available
U.S.—
  50 mg (Rx) [*Paraplatin* (mannitol, equal quantity by weight)].
  150 mg (Rx) [*Paraplatin* (mannitol, equal quantity by weight)].
  450 mg (Rx) [*Paraplatin* (mannitol, equal quantity by weight)].
Canada—
  50 mg (Rx) [*Paraplatin* (mannitol, equal quantity by weight)].
  150 mg (Rx) [*Paraplatin* (mannitol, equal quantity by weight)].
  450 mg (Rx) [*Paraplatin* (mannitol, equal quantity by weight)].

### Packaging and storage
Store between 15 and 30 °C (59 and 86 °F), unless otherwise specified by manufacturer. Protect from light.

### Preparation of dosage form
Carboplatin for injection is reconstituted for intravenous use by adding 5, 15, or 45 mL of sterile water for injection, 5% dextrose injection, or 0.9% sodium chloride injection to the 50-mg, 150-mg, or 450-mg vial, respectively, producing a solution containing 10 mg of carboplatin per mL. The resulting solution may be further diluted to a concentration as low as 500 mcg (0.5 mg) per mL with 5% dextrose injection or 0.9% sodium chloride injection if further dilution for administration by intravenous infusion is required.

### Stability
Reconstituted solutions of carboplatin are stable for 8 hours at 25 °C (77 °F).
Caution—A black platinum precipitate will form if carboplatin comes in contact with aluminum.

### Incompatibilities
Do not use needles, intravenous sets, or equipment containing aluminum for administration since carboplatin is incompatible with aluminum.

## CARBOPLATIN INJECTION

### Usual adult dose
See *Carboplatin for injection*.

### Usual pediatric dose
Dosage has not been established.

### Strength(s) usually available
U.S.—
  Not commercially available.
Canada—
  10 mg per mL (Rx) [*Paraplatin-AQ*].

### Packaging and storage
Store between 15 and 30 °C (59 and 86 °F), unless otherwise specified by manufacturer. Protect from light. Protect from freezing.

### Stability
Caution—A black platinum precipitate will form if carboplatin comes in contact with aluminum.

### Incompatibilities
Do not use needles, intravenous sets, or equipment containing aluminum for administration since carboplatin is incompatible with aluminum.

[1]Not included in Canadian product labeling.

Revised: 06/24/98

---

# CARBOPROST  Systemic

VA CLASSIFICATION (Primary/Secondary): HS200/GU600
Commonly used brand name(s): *Hemabate*; *Prostin/15M*.
Note: For a listing of dosage forms and brand names by country availability, see *Dosage Forms* section(s).

## Category
Oxytocic; abortifacient; antihemorrhagic (postpartum and postabortal uterine bleeding).

## Indications
Note: Bracketed information in the *Indications* section refers to uses that are not included in U.S. product labeling.

### Accepted
Abortion or
[Abortion, incomplete (treatment)][1]—Carboprost is used for aborting midtrimester pregnancy (between the thirteenth and twentieth weeks of gestation as calculated from the first day of the last normal menstrual period). Carboprost is also indicated for second trimester abortion when other methods lead to failure of expulsion of the fetus, premature rupture of membranes with insufficient or absent uterine activity, and requirement of a repeat intrauterine instillation of drug for expulsion of the fetus, or when rupture of membranes in the presence of a previable fetus occurs without adequate activity for expulsion. Carboprost can be used for abortion in the early weeks of pregnancy, but its use is associated with an increased incidence of side effects and failures. Carboprost is sometimes used in combination with hypertonic saline, urea, or oxytocin.

Carboprost is used for induction of labor in cases of intrauterine fetal death.

Postpartum hemorrhage (treatment)[1]—Carboprost is indicated to reduce blood loss and correct uterine atony during the postpartum period in patients unresponsive to conventional treatment such as oxytocin, ergonovine, or methylergonovine.

[Hydatidiform mole, benign (treatment)][1] or
[Induction of labor][1] or
[Cervical ripening][1]—Carboprost has been used in the treatment of benign hydatidiform mole, for medically indicated induction of labor at term, and to ripen the cervix prior to abortion procedures such as vacuum curettage. However, experience with the use of carboprost for these indications is limited.

[1]Not included in Canadian product labeling.

## Pharmacology/Pharmacokinetics

### Physicochemical characteristics
Chemical name—Prosta-5,13-dien-1-oic acid, 9,11,15-trihydroxy-15-methyl, (5Z,9 alpha,11 alpha,13E,15S)-, compound with 2-amino-2-(hydroxymethyl)-1,3-propanediol (1:1).
Chemical group—Carboprost tromethamine is the tromethamine salt of the (15S)-15 methyl analog of naturally occurring prostaglandin $F_{2\text{-alpha}}$.
Molecular weight—489.65.

### Mechanism of action/Effect
Carboprost appears to act directly on the myometrium, but this has not been completely established. Carboprost stimulates myometrial contractions in the gravid uterus similar to the contractions occurring in the term uterus during natural labor. These contractions are usually sufficient to cause abortion. Uterine response to prostaglandins increases gradually throughout pregnancy. Carboprost also facilitates cervical dilatation and softening.

### Other actions/effects
Carboprost stimulates the smooth muscle of the gastrointestinal tract, arterioles, and bronchioles.

### Biotransformation
Primarily hepatic oxidation and some enzymatic dehydrogenation in maternal lung tissues; occur more slowly than with prostaglandin $F_{2\text{alpha}}$, due to the presence of a 15-methyl group.

**Time to peak concentration**
15 to 60 minutes.

**Peak serum concentration**
2060 picograms of 15-methyl-prostaglandin $F_{2alpha}$ per mL at 30 minutes after a single intramuscular dose of 250 mcg, declining to 770 picograms per mL after 2 hours; slightly increased to 2663 picograms per mL at 30 minutes post-dosing with a second dose 2 hours later, declining to 1047 picograms per mL after 2 hours.

**Time to peak effect**
The mean abortion time with carboprost is about 16 hours.

**Elimination**
Primarily renal as metabolites; rapid and nearly complete at 24 hours after intravenous, subcutaneous, or intramuscular dosing.

## Precautions to Consider

**Carcinogenicity**
Studies have not been done in either animals or humans.

**Mutagenicity**
No evidence of mutagenicity was found in the micronucleus test or Ames assay.

**Pregnancy/Reproduction**
Pregnancy—Although studies have not been done in humans, any pregnancy termination with carboprost that fails should be completed by another method.
Proliferation of bone has been reported with clinical use of prostaglandin $E_1$ during prolonged therapy. However, there is no evidence to date that the short-term use of carboprost causes proliferation of bone in the fetus.
Studies in rats and rabbits found that carboprost causes embryotoxicity. Carboprost did not cause teratogenicity in animal studies. Prostaglandins of the E and F series have caused proliferation of bone with high doses in other animal studies.
FDA Pregnancy Category C.
Labor and delivery—Use of high doses may result in excessive uterine tone, causing decreased uterine blood flow and fetal distress. Carboprost is not feticidal and may result in delivery of a live fetus.

**Drug interactions and/or related problems**
The following drug interactions and/or related problems have been selected on the basis of their potential clinical significance (possible mechanism in parentheses where appropriate)—not necessarily inclusive (» = major clinical significance):

Oxytocin or other oxytocics
(concurrent use with carboprost may result in uterine hypertonus, possibly causing uterine rupture or cervical laceration, especially in the absence of adequate cervical dilatation; although combinations are sometimes used for therapeutic advantage, patient should be monitored closely when this combination is used)

**Laboratory value alterations**
The following have been selected on the basis of their potential clinical significance (possible effect in parentheses where appropriate)—not necessarily inclusive (» = major clinical significance):

With physiology/laboratory test values
Blood pressure, maternal or
Heart rate, maternal
(may be decreased or increased, especially with large doses)
Body temperature
(a temperature increase of greater than 1.1 °C [2 °F] usually occurs within 1 to 16 hours after the first injection, and the temperature returns to normal within several hours after the last injection)

**Medical considerations/Contraindications**
The medical considerations/contraindications included have been selected on the basis of their potential clinical significance (reasons given in parentheses where appropriate)—not necessarily inclusive (» = major clinical significance).

*Except under special circumstances, this medication should not be used when the following medical problems exist:*
» Allergy or intolerance to carboprost or other oxytocics
» Asthma, or history of
(increased risk of bronchospasm)
» Pulmonary disease, active
(use of carboprost may decrease pulmonary blood flow and increase pulmonary arterial pressure)

*Risk-benefit should be considered when the following medical problems exist:*
Adrenal disease, history of
(carboprost stimulates steroid production)
Anemia
(increased incidence of excessive uterine bleeding may occur with the use of prostaglandins in performance of abortion)
» Cardiac disease, active
(decrease in blood pressure and bradycardia may result in cardiovascular collapse and angina pectoris)
Cardiovascular disease, history of or
Hypertension, or history of or
Hypotension, or history of or
Preeclampsia
(may be aggravated by possible vasoconstriction or decreased blood pressure)
Cervical stenosis or
Uterine fibroids or
Uterine surgery, history of
(increased risk of uterine rupture)
Diabetes mellitus, history of
Epilepsy, or history of
(rarely, seizures have occurred during the use of prostaglandins)
Glaucoma
(increase in intraocular pressure and miosis have occurred rarely during the use of prostaglandins)
» Hepatic disease, active, or
Hepatic disease, history of
(metabolism of carboprost may be impaired, resulting in prolonged half-life)
Hypersensitivity to carboprost or
Multiparity
(excessive dosage or use with oxytocin may cause uterine hypertonicity with spasm and tetanic contraction, which can lead to posterior cervical perforations, cervical lacerations, uterine rupture, and hemorrhage)
Jaundice, history of
» Pelvic inflammatory disease, acute
(induction of uterine contractions is not generally recommended)
» Renal disease, active
Renal disease, history of

**Patient monitoring**
The following may be especially important in patient monitoring (other tests may be warranted in some patients, depending on condition; » = major clinical significance):

Contractions—frequency, duration and force of and
Temperature, pulse, and blood pressure, maternal and
Uterine tone, resting
(monitoring of these parameters is recommended at frequent intervals during abortion procedure or labor and delivery)
Vaginal examination
(recommended prior to each dose and postabortion or postdelivery to check for signs of cervical trauma)

## Side/Adverse Effects

The following side/adverse effects have been selected on the basis of their potential clinical significance (possible signs and symptoms in parentheses where appropriate)—not necessarily inclusive:

**Those indicating need for medical attention**
Incidence less frequent or rare
*Anaphylaxis, generalized* (swelling of face, inside the nose, and eyelids; hives; shortness of breath; trouble in breathing; tightness in chest; wheezing); *bradycardia* (slow heartbeat); *bronchoconstriction* (wheezing; trouble in breathing; tightness in chest)—most likely in asthmatic patients; *hypertension* (severe and continuing headache)—with very large doses; *ileus, adynamic* (constipation; tender or mildly bloated abdomen); *increased uterine pain accompanying abortion*—correlates with efficacy; *inflammation and pain at injection site; peripheral vasoconstriction, possibly severe* (pale, cool, or blotchy skin on arms or legs; weak or absent pulse in arms or legs); *substernal pressure or pain* (pressing or painful feeling in chest); *tachycardia* (fast heartbeat)

**Those indicating need for medical attention only if they continue or are bothersome**
Incidence more frequent
*Diarrhea*—about 67%; *nausea*—about 33%; *vomiting*—about 67%

Incidence less frequent
> *Chills or shivering; dizziness; fever, transient*—about 12%; *flushing or redness of face*—about 7%; *headache; stomach cramps or pain*

Those indicating possible postabortion complications and the need for medical attention if they occur after medication is discontinued
> *Endometritis* (continuing chills; shivering; continuing fever—usually on third day after abortion; foul-smelling vaginal discharge; pain in lower abdomen); *unusual increase in uterine bleeding*

## Overdose

For more information on the management of overdose or unintentional ingestion, **contact a Poison Control Center** (see *Poison Control Center Listing*).

**Treatment of overdose**
Supportive therapy—Emphasis on intravenous fluid replacement.

## Patient Consultation

As an aid to patient consultation, refer to *Advice for the Patient, Carboprost (Systemic)*.
In providing consultation, consider emphasizing the following selected information (» = major clinical significance):

**Before using this medication**
» Conditions affecting use, especially:
  Allergies or intolerance to carboprost or other oxytocics
  Pregnancy—Because some prostaglandins are teratogenic in animals, any pregnancy termination with carboprost that fails should be completed by another method
  Other medical problems, especially lung disease, cardiac disease, liver disease, pelvic inflammatory disease, or renal disease

**Proper use of this medication**
» Proper dosing

**Side/adverse effects**
Signs of potential side effects, especially adynamic ileus, anaphylaxis, bradycardia, bronchoconstriction, chest pain or pressure, endometritis, fever, hypertension, inflammation and pain at injection site, peripheral vasoconstriction, tachycardia, and uterine bleeding or pain

## General Dosing Information

Carboprost is sometimes used in combination with hypertonic saline or urea in the performance of abortion.

It is recommended that antiemetic and antidiarrheal medications be administered prior to or concurrently with carboprost to decrease the incidence and severity of gastrointestinal side effects. Narcotic analgesics may be given for uterine pain.

If carboprost is ineffective, it is recommended that alternative methods such as hypertonic saline not be used until the uterus has stopped contracting. Continuous administration of carboprost for more than two days is not recommended.

Caution should be taken to prevent exposure of skin to carboprost tromethamine. If carboprost injection is spilled on the skin, it should be washed off immediately with soap and water.

## Parenteral Dosage Forms

Note: Bracketed uses in the *Dosage Forms* section refer to indications and/or categories of use that are not included in U.S. product labeling.

### CARBOPROST TROMETHAMINE INJECTION USP

**Usual adult and adolescent dose**
Abortifacient—
  [Intra-amniotic, 2.5 mg (base) administered over five minutes. An additional dose of 2.5 mg may be administered twenty-four hours after the initial dose if abortion has not occurred, provided the membranes are intact] or
  Deep intramuscular, initially 250 mcg (0.25 mg) (base), the dosage being repeated every one and one-half to three and one-half hours, depending on uterine response. Dose may be increased to 500 mcg (0.5 mg) if uterine contractility is inadequate after several doses of 250 mcg (0.25 mg).

Note: An optional test dose of 100 mcg (0.1 mg) of carboprost (base) may be administered initially.
  Continuous administration for more than two days is not recommended.

Antihemorrhagic, postpartum and postabortal uterine bleeding[1]—
  Deep intramuscular, 250 mcg (0.25 mg) (base). If necessary, the dosage may be repeated at fifteen- to ninety-minute intervals on the basis of response.

**Usual adult prescribing limits**
Abortifacient—
  Intra-amniotic: 5 mg (base).
  Intramuscular: 6 to 12 mg (base), cumulative. Continuous administration for more than two days is not recommended.
Antihemorrhagic, postpartum and postabortal uterine bleeding[1]—
  2 mg (base), cumulative.

**Strength(s) usually available**
U.S.—
  250 mcg (0.25 mg) (base) per mL (Rx) [*Hemabate*].
Canada—
  250 mcg (0.25 mg) (base) per mL (Rx) [*Prostin/15M*].

**Packaging and storage**
Store between 2 and 8 °C (36 and 46 °F).

---
[1]Not included in Canadian product labeling.
---

Revised: 10/26/92
Interim revision: 06/08/94

---

**CARISOPRODOL**—See *Skeletal Muscle Relaxants (Systemic)*

---

# CARMUSTINE    Implantation-Local—INTRODUCTORY VERSION

VA CLASSIFICATION (Primary): AN100
Commonly used brand name(s): *Gliadel Wafer*.
Another commonly used name is BCNU.
Note: For a listing of dosage forms and brand names by country availability, see *Dosage Forms* section(s).

## Category
Antineoplastic.

## Indications

**Accepted**
Tumors, brain (treatment)—Carmustine implants are indicated, by insertion into the surgical resection cavity, to prolong survival of patients who require surgery for recurrent glioblastoma multiforme.

## Pharmacology/Pharmacokinetics

Note: Pharmacokinetic studies of carmustine and the biodegradable polyanhydride copolymer with which it is formulated into the implant dosage form have not been done in patients following implantation into brain tissue. However, in animal studies, carmustine was not detected in the plasma or cerebrospinal fluid of rabbits implanted with the medication.

**Mechanism of action/Effect**
Carmustine is an alkylating agent of the nitrosourea type. Carmustine's antineoplastic effect involves alkylation of DNA and RNA and cross-linking of DNA by carmustine and/or an active metabolite.

**Biotransformation**
Biotransformation of carmustine occurs spontaneously and/or metabolically. A metabolite, thought to be chloroethyl carbonium ion, is an active alkylating agent.

Note: The anhydride bonds of the copolymer with which carmustine is formulated into the implantable dosage form are hydrolyzed upon exposure to the aqueous environment of the tumor resection cavity, yielding carboxyphenoxypropane and sebacic acid and releasing carmustine. More than 70% of the copolymer is degraded within 3 weeks after implantation.

## Precautions to Consider

### Tumorigenicity
Carmustine caused an increase in the incidence of tumors, predominantly subcutaneous and lung tumors, in all treated animals (mice given 2.5 or 5 mg per kg of body weight [mg/kg] and rats given 1.5 mg/kg intraperitoneally three times a week for 6 months). These doses are equivalent to one fifth, one third, and one fourth, respectively, of the recommended human dose of eight 7.7-mg implants on a mg per square meter of body surface area (mg/m$^2$) basis.

### Mutagenicity
Carmustine is mutagenic *in vitro* (in the Ames test and the human lymphoblast HGPRT assay) and clastogenic both *in vitro* (in the micronucleus assay in V79 hamster cells) and *in vivo* (in the SCE assay in rodent brain tumors and the mouse bone marrow micronucleus assay).

### Pregnancy/Reproduction
Fertility—Intraperitoneal administration of 8 mg/kg of carmustine (equivalent to approximately 1.3 times the recommended human dose on a mg/m$^2$ basis) per week for 8 weeks caused testicular degeneration in male rats.

Pregnancy—Adequate and well-controlled studies have not been done in humans.

Reproductive studies with implanted carmustine have not been done in animals. However, carmustine was teratogenic in rats, causing anophthalmia, micrognathia, and omphalocele, when administered intraperitoneally on days 6 through 15 of gestation in doses of 1 mg/kg (equivalent to approximately one sixth of the recommended human dose on a mg/m$^2$ basis) or higher. Also, carmustine was embryotoxic in rabbits, causing increased embryo and fetal deaths, reduced numbers of litters, and reduced litter sizes, at a dose of 4 mg/kg per day intravenously (approximately 1.2 times the recommended human dose on a mg/m$^2$ basis).

FDA Pregnancy Category D.

### Breast-feeding
It is not known whether carmustine or the breakdown products of the copolymer with which it is formulated into the implant are distributed into breast milk. However, because of the potential for severe carmustine-induced adverse effects in nursing infants, it is recommended that breast-feeding be discontinued after insertion of the implants.

### Pediatrics
Appropriate studies on the relationship of age to the effects of carmustine implants have not been performed in pediatric patients. Safety and efficacy have not been established.

### Geriatrics
No information is available on the relationship of age to the effects of carmustine implants in geriatric patients.

### Diagnostic interference
The following have been selected on the basis of their potential clinical significance (possible effect in parentheses where appropriate)—not necessarily inclusive (» = major clinical significance):

*With diagnostic test results*
Tumor progression assessment
(implant-induced edema and inflammation in brain tissue surrounding the resection cavity may produce enhancement similar to that produced by tumor progression in computerized tomographic or magnetic resonance imaging studies)

### Medical considerations/Contraindications
The medical considerations/contraindications included have been selected on the basis of their potential clinical significance (reasons given in parentheses where appropriate)—not necessarily inclusive (» = major clinical significance).

*Except under special circumstances, this medication should not be used when the following medical problem exists:*
» Hypersensitivity to carmustine or other components of the implant, history of

### Patient monitoring
The following may be especially important in patient monitoring (other tests may be warranted in some patients, depending on condition; » = major clinical significance):
» Abnormal wound healing and
» Brain edema and
» Convulsions and
» Intracranial infections and
» Other complications of craniotomy
(patients should be monitored for the occurrence of such complications following implantation)

## Side/Adverse Effects

Note: In general, adverse effects reported following implantation of carmustine are typical of those occurring in patients undergoing craniotomy for resection of malignant gliomas. In clinical trials, most of the reported adverse effects did not occur significantly more often in treated patients than in controls (recipients of implants containing only the biodegradable copolymer).

Although a causal relationship has not been established, the following adverse effects were also reported in clinical trials (frequencies of occurrence varying from less than 1 to 3%): allergic reaction; asthenia; back, chest, eye, or neck pain; central nervous system (CNS) effects, including ataxia, cerebral hemorrhage, cerebral infarct, coma, diplopia, dizziness, hydrocephalus, and monoplegia; gastrointestinal tract effects, including constipation, diarrhea, dysphagia, fecal incontinence, and gastrointestinal hemorrhage; hematologic abnormalities, including leukocytosis and thrombocytopenia; hypertension or hypotension; metabolic abnormalities, including hyperglycemia, hypokalemia, and hyponatremia; musculoskeletal system infection; peripheral edema; psychological changes, including abnormal thinking, amnesia, insomnia, mental depression, and paranoid reaction; respiratory infection or aspiration pneumonia; sepsis; visual field defects; and urinary incontinence.

The following side/adverse effects have been selected on the basis of their potential clinical significance (possible signs and symptoms in parentheses where appropriate)—not necessarily inclusive:

### Those indicating need for medical attention
Incidence more frequent (> 10%)
**Convulsions; fever; hemiplegia** (inability to move legs or arms); **surgical site healing abnormalities; urinary tract infection** (blood in urine; burning, painful, or difficult urination; lower back or side pain)

Note: In clinical trials, new or worsened *convulsions*, usually mild to moderate in severity, occurred as frequently in control patients as in treated patients. The first new or worsened convulsion occurred within the first 5 days postoperatively in 54% of the treated patients and 9% of the controls who experienced this complication; the median time to onset in the two groups was 3.5 days and 61 days, respectively. The beneficial effect of the active treatment on survival was not affected.

Reported *surgical site healing abnormalities* included cerebrospinal fluid (CSF) leaks, subdural fluid accumulation, subgaleal effusions, wound breakdown, and wound effusions.

Incidence less frequent (4 to 10%)
*Aphasia* (problems in speaking); **brain edema; infection, including abscess or meningitis** (confusion; fever; headache; stiff neck); **intracranial hypertension** (headache; nausea and vomiting; papilledema); **pain; rash; stupor** (extremely severe sleepiness)

Note: *Brain edema* may result in a mass effect (characterized by bradycardia, hypertension, pupillary enlargement, slow breathing, and stupor) that is unresponsive to corticosteroid treatment. In some cases, reoperation and removal of the implant or its remnants may be necessary.

### Those indicating need for medical attention only if they continue or are bothersome
Incidence more frequent (≥ 10%)
*Confusion*—without other symptoms of infection; **drowsiness; headache**—without other symptoms of infection or intracranial hypertension; **nausea or vomiting**—without other symptoms of intracranial hypertension

## Overdose
There is no experience with overdose of the carmustine implants.

## Patient Consultation
As an aid to patient consultation, refer to *Advice for the Patient, Carmustine (Implantation-Local)—Introductory Version*.

In providing consultation, consider emphasizing the following selected information (» = major clinical significance):

### Before receiving this medication
» Conditions affecting use, especially:
Hypersensitivity to carmustine or other components of the implant, history of
Pregnancy—Potential risk because carmustine is tumorigenic, embryotoxic, and teratogenic in animals; informing physician immediately if pregnancy is suspected
Breast-feeding—Not recommended because of potential for carmustine-induced serious adverse effects in the infant

**Precautions after receiving this medication**
» Importance of close monitoring by the physician

**Side/adverse effects**
Signs of potential side effects, especially convulsions, fever, hemiplegia, urinary tract infection, aphasia, brain edema, infection, intracranial hypertension, pain, rash, or stupor

## General Dosing Information

Carmustine implants are inserted into the surgical resection cavity after the tumor has been resected, tumor pathology has been confirmed, and hemostasis has been achieved. Prior to implantation, communication between the surgical resection cavity and the ventricular system, if present, should be closed. This measure is needed to prevent the implants from migrating into the ventricular system and causing obstructive hydrocephalus.

After the implants are in place, a layer of oxidized regenerated cellulose may be placed over the implants to secure them against the surface of the surgical resection cavity. The resection cavity should be irrigated prior to closing the dura in a watertight fashion.

**Safety considerations for handling this medication**
The packets containing the implants should be handled carefully. They should be brought into the operating room unopened and remain sealed until the time of implantation.

The implants should be handled only by individuals wearing surgical gloves; contact with carmustine may cause severe burning and hyperpigmentation of the skin. It is recommended that two pairs of gloves be worn. The outer pair should be discarded into a biohazard container after use.

It is recommended that the implantation be performed using a surgical instrument dedicated to the handling of the implants.

If a repeat procedure is performed in an implanted area, any implant or remnant remaining in the surgical field should be treated as a potentially cytotoxic agent.

## Implantation Dosage Forms

### CARMUSTINE IMPLANTS

**Usual adult dose**
Tumors, brain—
Implantation, into the surgical resection cavity, up to 8 implants, depending on the capacity of the cavity. As much of the cavity as possible should be covered. Slight overlapping is acceptable.

Note: Implants that have been broken in half may be used, but any that have been broken into more than two pieces should be discarded into a biohazard container.

**Usual adult prescribing limits**
Up to 8 implants per procedure.

**Usual pediatric dose**
Safety and efficacy have not been established.

**Strength(s) usually available**
U.S.—
7.7 mg (Rx) [*Gliadel Wafer* (polifeprosan 20 [biodegradable polyanhydride copolymer] 192.3 mg)].

**Packaging and storage**
Store at or below −20 °C (−4 °F). However, unopened foil packets may be kept at room temperature for no longer than 6 hours at a time.

Note: Carmustine implants are packaged in two aluminum foil pouches. The sterile inner packet is designed to protect the implant from moisture as well as to maintain sterility. The outer surface of the overwrap is not sterile.

Developed: 04/01/97

---

# CARMUSTINE  Systemic

VA CLASSIFICATION (Primary/Secondary): AN100/DE600
Commonly used brand name(s): *BiCNU*.
Another commonly used name is BCNU.
Note: For a listing of dosage forms and brand names by country availability, see *Dosage Forms* section(s).

## Category
Antineoplastic.

## Indications
Note: Bracketed information in the *Indications* section refers to uses that are not included in U.S. product labeling.

**Accepted**
Tumors, brain, primary (treatment)
[Carcinoma, gastric (treatment)] or
[Carcinoma, colorectal (treatment)]—Carmustine is indicated as palliative therapy as a single agent or in combination therapy for treatment of primary brain tumors (glioblastoma, brain stem glioma, medulloblastoma, astrocytoma, ependymoma, and metastatic brain tumors) and for gastric and colorectal carcinoma.

Lymphomas, Hodgkin's (treatment) or
Lymphomas, non-Hodgkin's (treatment)—Carmustine is indicated for treatment of Hodgkin's disease and non-Hodgkin's lymphomas. Carmustine is indicated as secondary therapy in combination with other approved drugs in patients who relapse while being treated with primary therapy, or who fail to respond to primary therapy.

Multiple myeloma (treatment)—Carmustine is indicated for treatment of multiple myeloma, in combination with prednisone.

[Melanoma, malignant (treatment)]—Carmustine is used for treatment of disseminated malignant melanoma, in combination with vincristine sulfate.

[Mycosis fungoides (treatment)][1]—Carmustine is used topically for treatment of mycosis fungoides.

[Waldenström's macroglobulinemia (treatment)][1]—Carmustine is used for treatment of Waldenström's macroglobulinemia.

[1]Not included in Canadian product labeling.

## Pharmacology/Pharmacokinetics

**Physicochemical characteristics**
Molecular weight—214.05.

**Mechanism of action/Effect**
Carmustine is an alkylating agent of the nitrosourea type. Carmustine and/or its metabolites alkylate and interfere with the function of DNA and RNA and are also capable of cross-linking DNA. It is cell cycle–phase nonspecific. Carmustine may also act by protein modification.

**Distribution**
Crosses the blood-brain barrier (because of high lipid solubility and relative lack of ionization at physiological pH).

**Biotransformation**
Hepatic; rapid (active metabolites).

**Half-life**
Biologic—Approximately 15 to 30 minutes.
Chemical—Approximately 5 minutes.
Metabolites may persist in the plasma for several days, which may explain the delayed hematologic toxicity.

**Elimination**
Renal—60 to 70% (less than 1% unchanged); some enterohepatic circulation believed to occur.
Fecal—1%.
Respiratory—10% (as carbon dioxide).

## Precautions to Consider

**Carcinogenicity/Mutagenicity**
Secondary malignancies are potential delayed effects of many antineoplastic agents, although it is not clear whether the effect is related to their mutagenic or immunosuppressive action. The effect of dose and duration of therapy is also unknown, although risk seems to increase with long-term use. Although information is limited, available data seem to indicate that the carcinogenic risk is greatest with the alkylating agents.

Carmustine is carcinogenic in rats and mice at doses approximating the clinical dose and has been associated with development of secondary malignancies, including acute leukemia, in humans.

**Pregnancy/Reproduction**
Fertility—Gonadal suppression, resulting in amenorrhea or azoospermia, may occur in patients taking antineoplastic therapy, especially with the

alkylating agents. In general, these effects appear to be related to dose and length of therapy and may be irreversible. Prediction of the degree of testicular or ovarian function impairment is complicated by the common use of combinations of several antineoplastics, which makes it difficult to assess the effects of individual agents.

Carmustine affects fertility in male rats at doses somewhat higher than the human dose.

Pregnancy—Adequate and well-controlled studies in humans have not been done.

First trimester: It is usually recommended that use of antineoplastics, especially combination chemotherapy, be avoided whenever possible, especially during the first trimester. Although information is limited because of the relatively few instances of antineoplastic administration during pregnancy, the mutagenic, teratogenic, and carcinogenic potential of these medications must be considered.

Other hazards to the fetus include adverse reactions seen in adults.

In general, use of a contraceptive is recommended during cytotoxic drug therapy.

Carmustine is embryotoxic and teratogenic in rats and embryotoxic in rats and rabbits at doses equivalent to the human dose.

FDA Pregnancy Category D.

### Breast-feeding
It is not known whether carmustine is distributed into milk. Although very little information is available regarding distribution of antineoplastic agents into breast milk, breast-feeding is not recommended while carmustine is being administered because of the risks to the infant (adverse effects, mutagenicity, carcinogenicity).

### Pediatrics
Appropriate studies on the relationship of age to the effects of carmustine have not been performed in the pediatric population. However, pediatrics-specific problems that would limit the usefulness of this medication in children are not expected.

Delayed, sometimes fatal, pulmonary fibrosis has been reported to occur up to 15 years after treatment with carmustine in childhood and early adolescence in cumulative doses ranging from 770 to 1800 mg per square meter of body surface in combination with cranial radiotherapy for intracranial tumors.

### Geriatrics
No information is available on the relationship of age to the effects of carmustine in geriatric patients. However, geriatric patients are more likely to have age-related renal function impairment, which may require caution in patients receiving carmustine.

### Dental
The bone marrow depressant effects of carmustine may result in an increased incidence of microbial infection, delayed healing, and gingival bleeding. Dental work, whenever possible, should be completed prior to initiation of therapy or deferred until blood counts have returned to normal. Patients should be instructed in proper oral hygiene during treatment, including caution in use of regular toothbrushes, dental floss, and toothpicks.

Carmustine may also cause stomatitis associated with considerable discomfort.

### Drug interactions and/or related problems
The following drug interactions and/or related problems have been selected on the basis of their potential clinical significance (possible mechanism in parentheses where appropriate)—not necessarily inclusive (» = major clinical significance):

Note: Combinations containing any of the following medications, depending on the amount present, may also interact with this medication.

Blood dyscrasia–causing medications (see *Appendix II*)
(leukopenic and/or thrombocytopenic effects of carmustine may be increased with concurrent or recent therapy if these medications cause the same effects; dosage adjustment of carmustine, if necessary, should be based on blood counts)

» Bone marrow depressants, other (see *Appendix II*) or
Radiation therapy
(additive bone marrow depression may occur; dosage reduction may be required when two or more bone marrow depressants, including radiation, are used concurrently or consecutively)

Hepatotoxic medications, other (see *Appendix II*) or
Nephrotoxic medications, other (see *Appendix II*)
(concurrent use with carmustine may result in enhanced hepatotoxicity or nephrotoxicity; either or both medications should be discontinued at the first sign of impairment)

Vaccines, killed virus
(because normal defense mechanisms may be suppressed by carmustine therapy, the patient's antibody response to the vaccine may be decreased. The interval between discontinuation of medications that cause immunosuppression and restoration of the patient's ability to respond to the vaccine depends on the intensity and type of immunosuppression-causing medication used, the underlying disease, and other factors; estimates vary from 3 months to 1 year)

» Vaccines, live virus
(because normal defense mechanisms may be suppressed by carmustine therapy, concurrent use with a live virus vaccine may potentiate the replication of the vaccine virus, may increase the side/adverse effects of the vaccine virus, and/or may decrease the patient's antibody response to the vaccine; immunization of these patients should be undertaken only with extreme caution after careful review of the patient's hematologic status and only with the knowledge and consent of the physician managing the carmustine therapy. The interval between discontinuation of medications that cause immunosuppression and restoration of the patient's ability to respond to the vaccine depends on the intensity and type of immunosuppression-causing medication used, the underlying disease, and other factors; estimates vary from 3 months to 1 year. Immunization with oral poliovirus vaccine should also be postponed in persons in close contact with the patient, especially family members)

### Laboratory value alterations
The following have been selected on the basis of their potential clinical significance (possible effect in parentheses where appropriate)—not necessarily inclusive (» = major clinical significance):

With physiology/laboratory test values
Alkaline phosphatase values, serum and
Aspartate aminotransferase (AST [SGOT]) values, serum and
Bilirubin concentrations, serum
(may be increased, indicating hepatotoxicity)

Blood urea nitrogen (BUN)
(concentrations may be increased, indicating nephrotoxicity)

### Medical considerations/Contraindications
The medical considerations/contraindications included have been selected on the basis of their potential clinical significance (reasons given in parentheses where appropriate)—not necessarily inclusive (» = major clinical significance).

*Risk-benefit should be considered when the following medical problems exist:*

» Bone marrow depression
» Chickenpox, existing or recent (including recent exposure) or
» Herpes zoster
(risk of severe generalized disease)
Hepatic function impairment
(carmustine may cause mild hepatotoxicity)
» Infection
» Pulmonary function impairment, existing or history of
» Renal function impairment
» Sensitivity to carmustine
» Caution should be used also in patients who have had previous cytotoxic drug therapy or radiation therapy, especially to the mediastinum, and in patients who smoke, because of the possible increased risk of pulmonary toxicity.

### Patient monitoring
The following may be especially important in patient monitoring (other tests may be warranted in some patients, depending on condition; » = major clinical significance):

Alanine aminotransferase (ALT [SGPT]) values, serum and
Aspartate aminotransferase (AST [SGOT]) values, serum and
Bilirubin concentrations, serum and
Lactate dehydrogenase (LDH) values, serum
(recommended prior to initiation of therapy and at periodic intervals during therapy; frequency varies according to clinical state, agent, dose, and other agents being used concurrently)

Blood urea nitrogen (BUN) concentrations and
Creatinine concentrations, serum
(recommended prior to initiation of therapy and at periodic intervals during therapy; frequency varies according to clinical state, agent, dose, and other agents being used concurrently)

» Hematocrit or hemoglobin and
» Leukocyte count, total and, if appropriate, differential and
» Platelet count
(determinations recommended prior to initiation of therapy and at periodic intervals during therapy; frequency varies according to clinical state, agent, dose, and other agents being used concurrently)

## Carmustine (Systemic)

» Pulmonary function studies
  (recommended prior to initiation of therapy and at frequent intervals during systemic therapy)

Uric acid concentrations, serum
  (recommended prior to initiation of therapy and at periodic intervals during therapy; frequency varies according to clinical state, agent, dose, and other agents being used concurrently)

## Side/Adverse Effects

Note: Many "side effects" of antineoplastic therapy are unavoidable and represent the medication's pharmacologic action. Some of these (for example, leukopenia and thrombocytopenia) are actually used as parameters to aid in individual dosage titration.

Encephalomyelopathy has been reported in patients who have received high-dose carmustine therapy.

Ocular toxicity has been associated with intra-arterial use.

The following side/adverse effects have been selected on the basis of their potential clinical significance (possible signs and symptoms in parentheses where appropriate)—not necessarily inclusive:

### Those indicating need for medical attention
Incidence more frequent
  *Leukopenia or infection* (fever or chills; cough or hoarseness; lower back or side pain; painful or difficult urination)—usually asymptomatic; *phlebitis* (pain or redness at site of injection); *pneumonitis or pulmonary fibrosis* (cough; shortness of breath); *thrombocytopenia* (unusual bleeding or bruising; black, tarry stools; blood in urine or stools; pinpoint red spots on skin)—usually asymptomatic

  Note: Maximum *leukopenia* occurs about 5 to 6 weeks after a dose. Recovery usually occurs within 6 to 7 weeks but may take up to 10 to 12 weeks after prolonged therapy. Severity of bone marrow depression varies and determines subsequent dosage of carmustine.

  *Burning at the injection site* is associated with rapid intravenous infusion; true thrombosis is rare.

  *Pneumonitis or pulmonary fibrosis* was initially thought to occur after high cumulative doses (greater than 1200 to 1400 mg per square meter of body surface) or several courses (greater than 5) or months of therapy; however, there have been several reports of pulmonary toxicity after only 1 or 2 courses or low doses. Symptoms may be insidious or acute in onset, and damage may be reversible or irreversible. Fatalities have occurred. The relationship of pulmonary toxicity to dose is not yet clear and other factors (previous radiation to mediastinum, concurrent administration of cyclophosphamide or agents associated with pulmonary toxicity, history of lung disease or smoking) may be significant. Delayed pulmonary fibrosis has been reported to occur up to 15 years after treatment with carmustine in childhood and early adolescence in cumulative doses ranging from 770 to 1800 mg per square meter of body surface in combination with cranial radiotherapy for intracranial tumors. Chest x-rays demonstrated pulmonary hypoplasia with upper zone contraction, gallium scans were normal, and thoracic computed tomography (CT) scans demonstrated an unusual pattern of upper zone fibrosis. Late reduction of pulmonary function was noted in a substantial number of cases. This form of lung fibrosis may be slowly progressive and has been fatal in some cases.

  Maximum *thrombocytopenia* occurs about 4 to 5 weeks after a dose. Recovery usually occurs within 6 to 7 weeks but may take up to 10 to 12 weeks after prolonged therapy. Severity of bone marrow depression varies and determines subsequent dosage of carmustine.

Incidence less frequent
  *Anemia* (unusual tiredness or weakness); *flushing of face; stomatitis* (sores in mouth and on lips)

  Note: *Flushing of face* is caused by rapid intravenous infusion. Flushing occurs within 2 hours after a dose and persists approximately 4 hours.

Incidence rare
  *Hepatotoxicity*—asymptomatic; *renal toxicity and failure* (decrease in urination; swelling of feet or lower legs)

  Note: *Renal toxicity and failure* usually occur in patients who have received large cumulative doses after prolonged therapy, but has occasionally been reported with lower cumulative doses.

### Those indicating need for medical attention only if they continue or are bothersome
Incidence more frequent
  *Nausea and vomiting*

  Note: *Nausea and vomiting* occur within 2 hours after a dose and usually last 4 to 6 hours; dose-related.

Incidence less frequent
  *Central nervous system (CNS) toxicity* (dizziness; trouble in walking); *diarrhea; discoloration of skin along vein of injection; loss of appetite; skin rash and itching; trouble in swallowing*

### Those not indicating need for medical attention
Incidence less frequent
  *Loss of hair*

### Those indicating the need for medical attention if they occur after medication is discontinued
  *Bone marrow depression* (fever or chills; cough or hoarseness; lower back or side pain; painful or difficult urination; unusual bleeding or bruising; black, tarry stools; blood in urine or stools; pinpoint red spots on skin); *pneumonitis or pulmonary fibrosis* (cough or shortness of breath)

  Note: Cumulative *myelosuppression* may occur with repeated doses.

## Patient Consultation

As an aid to patient consultation, refer to *Advice for the Patient, Carmustine (Systemic)*.

In providing consultation, consider emphasizing the following selected information (» = major clinical significance):

### Before using this medication
» Conditions affecting use, especially:
    Sensitivity to carmustine
    Pregnancy—Use not recommended because of mutagenic, teratogenic, and carcinogenic potential; advisability of using contraception; telling physician immediately if pregnancy is suspected
    Breast-feeding—Not recommended because of risk of serious side effects
    Other medications, especially other bone marrow depressants, or previous cytotoxic drug therapy or radiation therapy
    Other medical problems, especially chickenpox, herpes zoster, infection, pulmonary function impairment, renal function impairment, or smoking

### Proper use of this medication
  Caution in taking combination therapy; taking each medication at the right time
  Frequency of nausea and vomiting; importance of continuing medication despite stomach upset
» Proper dosing

### Precautions while using this medication
» Importance of close monitoring by the physician
» Avoiding immunizations unless approved by physician; other persons in patient's household should avoid immunizations with oral poliovirus vaccine; avoiding persons who have taken oral poliovirus vaccine or wearing a protective mask that covers nose and mouth

*Caution if bone marrow depression occurs*
» Avoiding exposure to persons with infections, especially during periods of low blood counts; checking with physician immediately if fever or chills, cough or hoarseness, lower back or side pain, or painful or difficult urination occurs
» Checking with physician immediately if unusual bleeding or bruising; black, tarry stools; blood in urine or stools; or pinpoint red spots on skin occur
  Caution in use of regular toothbrush, dental floss, or toothpick; physician, dentist, or nurse may suggest alternatives; checking with physician before having dental work done
  Not touching eyes or inside of nose unless hands washed immediately before
  Using caution to avoid accidental cuts with use of sharp objects such as safety razor or fingernail or toenail cutters
  Avoiding contact sports or other situations where bruising or injury could occur
» Possibility of local tissue injury and scarring if infiltration of intravenous solution occurs; telling doctor or nurse right away about redness, pain, or swelling at injection site

### Side/adverse effects
  Importance of discussing possible adverse effects, including cancer, with physician
  Signs of potential side effects, especially leukopenia, infection, phlebitis, pneumonitis, pulmonary fibrosis, thrombocytopenia, anemia, flushing of face, stomatitis, and renal toxicity and failure

- Asymptomatic side effects, including leukopenia, thrombocytopenia, and hepatotoxicity
- Physician or nurse can help in dealing with side effects
- Possibility of hair loss; growth should return after treatment has ended
- Pulmonary toxicity more likely to occur in smokers

## General Dosing Information

Patients receiving carmustine should be under supervision of a physician experienced in cancer chemotherapy.

A variety of dosage schedules and regimens of carmustine, alone or in combination with other antitumor agents, are used. The prescriber may consult the medical literature as well as the manufacturer's literature in choosing a specific dosage.

Dosage of carmustine subsequent to the initial course should be adjusted to meet the individual requirements of each patient, based on hematologic response of the patient to the previous dose. An additional course of carmustine should be given only after circulating blood elements have returned to acceptable levels (leukocytes above 4000 per cubic millimeter and platelets above 100,000 per cubic millimeter).

Because of the delayed and cumulative bone marrow suppression caused by carmustine, the medication should be given no more frequently than every 6 weeks.

Some cross-resistance has been reported between carmustine and lomustine.

Frequency and duration of nausea and vomiting may be reduced in some patients by administration of antiemetics prior to dosing.

Intravenous infusion solutions should be administered over 1 to 2 hours to prevent irritation at the injection site. Some clinicians also recommend flushing the line with 5 to 10 mL of 0.9% sodium chloride injection or 5% dextrose injection both before and after administration of carmustine.

Special precautions are recommended in patients who develop thrombocytopenia as a result of administration of carmustine. These may include extreme care in performing invasive procedures; regular inspection of intravenous sites, skin (including perirectal area), and mucous membrane surfaces for signs of bleeding or bruising; limiting frequency of venipuncture and avoiding intramuscular injections; testing urine, emesis, stool, and secretions for occult blood; care in use of regular toothbrushes, dental floss, toothpicks, safety razors, and fingernail and toenail cutters; avoiding constipation; and using caution to prevent falls and other injuries. Such patients should avoid alcohol and aspirin intake because of the risk of gastrointestinal bleeding. Platelet transfusions may be required.

Patients who develop leukopenia should be observed carefully for signs of infection. Antibiotic support may be required. In neutropenic patients who develop fever, broad-spectrum antibiotic coverage should be initiated empirically, pending bacterial cultures and appropriate diagnostic tests.

Carmustine has been injected intra-arterially (hepatic artery) in the investigational treatment of hepatic tumors in a dose of 200 mg per square meter of body surface administered over 20 to 60 minutes.

### Safety considerations for handling this medication

There is limited but increasing evidence and concern that personnel involved in preparation and administration of parenteral antineoplastics may be at some risk because of the potential mutagenicity, teratogenicity, and/or carcinogenicity of these agents, although the actual risk is unknown. USP advisory panels recommend cautious handling both in preparation and disposal of antineoplastic agents. Precautions that have been suggested include:
- Use of a biological containment cabinet during reconstitution and dilution of parenteral medications and wearing of disposable surgical gloves and masks.
- Use of proper technique to prevent contamination of the medication, work area, and operator during transfer between containers (including proper training of personnel in this technique).
- Cautious and proper disposal of needles, syringes, vials, ampuls, and unused medication.

A number of medical centers have developed detailed guidelines for handling of antineoplastic agents.

### Combination chemotherapy

Carmustine may be used in combination with other agents in various regimens. As a result, incidence and/or severity of side effects may be altered and different dosages (usually reduced) may be used. For example, carmustine is part of the following chemotherapeutic combination:
—carmustine, cyclophosphamide, vinblastine, procarbazine, and prednisone (BCVPP).

For specific dosages and schedules, consult the literature. For information regarding each agent, consult the individual monographs.

## Parenteral Dosage Forms

Note: Bracketed uses in the *Dosage Forms* section refer to categories of use and/or indications that are not included in U.S. product labeling.

### CARMUSTINE FOR INJECTION

**Usual adult and adolescent dose**
Tumors, brain, primary or
[Carcinoma, colorectal or]
[Carcinoma, gastric] or
Lymphomas, Hodgkin's or
Lymphomas, non-Hodgkin's or
Multiple myeloma or
[Melanoma, malignant]—
   Intravenous, 150 to 200 mg per square meter of body surface as a single dose every six to eight weeks, or 75 to 100 mg per square meter of body surface on two successive days every six weeks, or 40 mg per square meter of body surface on five successive days every six weeks.

A suggested dosage adjustment schedule for subsequent doses is:

| Nadir after Prior Dose (cells per cubic millimeter) | | % of Prior Dose to Be Given |
|---|---|---|
| Leukocytes | Platelets | |
| >4000 | >100,000 | 100 |
| 3000–3999 | 75,000–99,999 | 100 |
| 2000–2999 | 25,000–74,999 | 70 |
| <2000 | <25,000 | 50 |

**Usual pediatric dose**
See *Usual adult and adolescent dose*.

**Size(s) usually available**
U.S.—
   100 mg (Rx) [*BiCNU*].
Canada—
   100 mg (Rx) [*BiCNU*].

**Packaging and storage**
Store between 2 and 8 °C (36 and 46 °F), unless otherwise specified by manufacturer. Exposure of the dry material to temperatures of 30.5 to 32 °C (86.9 to 89.6 °F) or above will cause the drug to decompose and liquefy, appearing as an oily film in the bottom of the vial; if this occurs, the vial must be discarded.

**Preparation of dosage form**
Carmustine for injection is reconstituted for intravenous use by adding 3 mL of sterile diluent (dehydrated alcohol injection) supplied by the manufacturer to dissolve it, then adding 27 mL of sterile water for injection, producing a clear, colorless solution containing 3.3 mg of carmustine per mL.

Reconstituted solutions may be further diluted with 0.9% sodium chloride injection or 5% dextrose injection for administration by intravenous infusion.

**Stability**
Reconstituted solutions are stable for 8 hours at 25 °C (77 °F) or 24 hours at 4 °C (39 °F). Reconstituted solutions diluted further for administration by infusion are stable for 48 hours when refrigerated and an additional 8 hours at 25 °C (77 °F) under normal room fluorescent light. Freezing does not alter the potency. Because the product contains no preservative, it should not be used as a multiple-dose vial.

**Note**
Avoid contact of the reconstituted solution with skin and eyes; it will cause burning and brown staining of skin. If accidental contact with skin or mucosa occurs, the area should be washed immediately and thoroughly with soap and water.

Revised: 07/15/94
Interim revision: 09/24/97

---

**CARTEOLOL**—See *Beta-adrenergic Blocking Agents (Ophthalmic)*; *Beta-adrenergic Blocking Agents (Systemic)*

# CARVEDILOL Systemic—INTRODUCTORY VERSION

VA CLASSIFICATION (Primary/Secondary): CV100/CV409
Commonly used brand name(s): *Coreg*.
Note: For a listing of dosage forms and brand names by country availability, see *Dosage Forms* section(s).

## Category
Antihypertensive; congestive heart failure treatment adjunct.

## Indications
**Accepted**
Congestive heart failure (treatment adjunct)—Carvedilol is indicated, in conjunction with digitalis, diuretics, and/or angiotensin-converting enzyme (ACE) inhibitors, for the treatment of mild or moderate (New York Heart Association [NYHA] class II or III) heart failure of ischemic or cardiomyopathic origin, to slow the progression of disease as evidenced by cardiovascular death, cardiovascular hospitalization, or the need to adjust other heart failure medications. Carvedilol may be used in patients unable to tolerate an ACE inhibitor or in patients who are or are not receiving digitalis, hydralazine, or nitrate therapy.

Hypertension (treatment)—Carvedilol is indicated, either alone or in combination with other antihypertensive agents, such as thiazide diuretics, in the treatment of essential hypertension.

## Pharmacology/Pharmacokinetics
**Physicochemical characteristics**
Molecular weight—406.5.

**Mechanism of action/Effect**
Carvedilol is a nonselective beta-adrenergic blocking agent with alpha$_1$-adrenergic blocking activity and no intrinsic sympathomimetic activity. The exact mechanism of the antihypertensive effect produced by beta-adrenergic blockade is not known, but may involve suppression of renin production. The beta-adrenergic blocking activity of carvedilol decreases cardiac output, exercise- and/or isoproterenol-induced tachycardia, and reflex orthostatic tachycardia. The alpha$_1$-adrenergic blocking activity of carvedilol blunts the pressor effect of phenylephrine, causes vasodilation, and reduces peripheral vascular resistance. The effect of alpha$_1$-adrenergic blockade is a reduction in standing blood pressure (more than supine), potentiating symptoms of postural hypotension and possibly syncope.

The mechanism by which carvedilol produces a beneficial effect in congestive heart failure is not known, but may be attributable to beta-adrenergic blockade and vasodilation.

**Absorption**
Carvedilol is rapidly and extensively absorbed. Absolute bioavailability of carvedilol is 25 to 35%, due to significant first-pass metabolism. Food slows the rate of absorption but does not appear to affect the extent of the bioavailability of carvedilol.

**Distribution**
Volume of distribution (Vol$_D$)—Steady-state: Approximately 115 L.

**Protein binding**
Very high (98%), primarily to albumin; concentration-independent.

**Biotransformation**
Hepatic; carvedilol is extensively metabolized, primarily by aromatic ring oxidation and glucuronidation by the cytochrome P450 2D6 enzyme. Other isozymes, such as P450 2C9 and P450 3A4, are involved to a lesser extent. Three active metabolites with beta-receptor blocking activity are produced by demethylation and hydroxylation at the phenol ring. The active metabolites show weak vasodilating (alpha$_1$-antagonist) activity when compared with carvedilol; however, in preclinical studies, the beta-blockade effect of the 4'-hydroxyphenyl metabolite was found to be approximately 13 times more potent than that of carvedilol.

**Half-life**
Elimination—
Apparent mean terminal: 7 to 10 hours; may be affected by induction or inhibition of cytochrome P450 enzymes.

**Elimination**
Fecal (biliary).
In dialysis—
Carvedilol does not appear to be cleared significantly by hemodialysis.

## Precautions to Consider
**Carcinogenicity**
No evidence of carcinogenicity was found in 2-year studies in rats and mice given doses of up to 75 mg per kg of body weight (mg/kg) per day (12 times the maximum recommended human dose [MRHD] on a mg per square meter of body surface area [mg/m$^2$] basis) and 200 mg/kg per day (16 times the MRHD on a mg/m$^2$ basis), respectively.

**Mutagenicity**
Mutagenicity was not detected in the Ames test or the CHO/HGPRT assay. Clastogenicity was not detected in the *in vitro* hamster micronucleus or the *in vivo* human lymphocyte cell tests.

**Pregnancy/Reproduction**
Fertility— Impaired fertility was observed in rats given doses ≥ 200 mg/kg per day (≥ 32 times the MRHD on a mg/m$^2$ basis). Administration of carvedilol at this dose was associated with a reduced number of successful matings, prolonged mating time, significantly fewer corpora lutea and implants per dam, and complete resorption of 18% of the litters.

Pregnancy—Adequate and well-controlled studies in humans have not been done.

Reproduction studies in rats and rabbits revealed increased postimplantation loss in rats at doses of 300 mg/kg per day (50 times the MRHD on a mg/m$^2$ basis) and in rabbits at doses of 75 mg/kg per day (25 times the MRHD on a mg/m$^2$ basis). In rats, a decrease in fetal body weight and an increase in the frequency of fetuses with delayed skeletal development (missing or stunted 13th rib) also occurred.

FDA Pregnancy Category C.

**Breast-feeding**
It is not known whether carvedilol is distributed into breast milk. Studies in lactating rats have shown that carvedilol and/or its metabolites were distributed into milk and caused an increased mortality in rat neonates. Because of the potential for a serious reaction in nursing infants from beta-adrenergic blockade (bradycardia), a decision should be made about whether to discontinue nursing or to discontinue carvedilol.

**Pediatrics**
No information is available on the relationship of age to the effects of carvedilol in pediatric patients. Safety and efficacy in pediatric patients have not been established.

**Geriatrics**
Use of carvedilol in patients 65 years of age and older has not demonstrated geriatric-specific problems that would limit the usefulness of carvedilol in the elderly. However, plasma levels of carvedilol in the elderly are about 50% higher on the average as compared with younger subjects, and the incidence of dizziness as a side effect is higher in the elderly than in younger patients.

**Pharmacogenetics**
In clinical trials, black patients with hypertension were less responsive to the antihypertensive beta-adrenergic blocking effects of carvedilol than nonblack patients.

Patients who are poor metabolizers of debrisoquin, a marker for the cytochrome P450 2D6 isozyme, may experience two- to threefold increases in carvedilol plasma concentrations, increasing the risk of adverse effects.

**Surgical**
Use of carvedilol perioperatively with anesthetic agents, such as cyclopropane, ether, and trichloroethylene, may further depress myocardial function.

**Drug interactions and/or related problems**
The following drug interactions and/or related problems have been selected on the basis of their potential clinical significance (possible mechanism in parentheses where appropriate)—not necessarily inclusive (» = major clinical significance):

Note: Combinations containing any of the following medications, depending on the amount present, may also interact with this medication.

Anesthetics, general, such as:
Cyclopropane
Ether
Trichloroethylene
(concurrent use with carvedilol may further depress myocardial function)

» Antidiabetic agents, sulfonylurea or
» Insulin
(concurrent use with carvedilol may increase the serum glucose–lowering effects of insulin and sulfonylurea antidiabetic agents; regular monitoring of blood glucose is recommended when using carvedilol and insulin or sulfonylurea antidiabetic agents concurrently)

» Calcium channel blocking agents, especially
Diltiazem or
Verapamil
(concurrent use of carvedilol with diltiazem has resulted in isolated cases of conduction disturbances; electrocardiogram and blood pressure measurements are recommended when carvedilol is used concurrently with calcium channel blocking agents)

Catecholamine-depleting agents, such as:
Monoamine oxidase inhibitors
Reserpine
(concurrent use of carvedilol with drugs that can deplete catecholamines may cause hypotension and bradycardia)

Clonidine
(concurrent use with carvedilol may have additive blood pressure– and heart rate–lowering effects)

Digoxin
(in hypertensive patients, concurrent use with carvedilol increased steady-state area under the plasma concentration–time curve [AUC] and trough concentrations of digoxin by 14% and 16%, respectively; slowing of atrioventricular [AV] conduction may be additive; monitoring of plasma digoxin concentrations is recommended when carvedilol is used concurrently)

Enzyme inducers, hepatic, cytochrome P450 (see *Appendix II*), such as
Rifampin or
Enzyme inhibitors, hepatic, cytochrome P450 (see *Appendix II*), such as:
Cimetidine
Fluoxetine
Paroxetine
Propafenone
Quinidine
(concurrent use may affect the metabolism and pharmacokinetics of carvedilol by inducing or inhibiting cytochrome P450 enzymes; in healthy male subjects, concurrent use of rifampin decreased the AUC and peak plasma concentration [$C_{max}$] of carvedilol by about 70%; in healthy male subjects, concurrent use of cimetidine increased the steady-state AUC of carvedilol by 30% with no change in $C_{max}$)

**Laboratory value alterations**
The following have been selected on the basis of their potential clinical significance (possible effect in parentheses where appropriate)—not necessarily inclusive (» = major clinical significance):

With physiology/laboratory test values
Bilirubin concentrations, serum or
Transaminase values, serum
(increases have occurred rarely; carvedilol should be withdrawn if laboratory signs of liver injury or jaundice occur)

Glucose, serum
(beta-adrenergic blocking agents, e.g., carvedilol, increase the serum glucose–lowering effects of insulin and sulfonylurea antidiabetic agents and delay the recovery of serum glucose levels; however, in patients with both diabetes and congestive heart failure, hyperglycemia may be worsened; in clinical trials with congestive heart failure patients, the incidence of hyperglycemia was 12.2%)

**Medical considerations/Contraindications**
The medical considerations/contraindications included have been selected on the basis of their potential clinical significance (reasons given in parentheses where appropriate)—not necessarily inclusive (» = major clinical significance).

*Except under special circumstances, this medication should not be used when the following medical problems exist:*
» Asthma, bronchial or
» Bronchospastic conditions, related
(carvedilol aggravates bronchial asthma and related bronchospastic conditions by blocking endogenous and exogenous beta agonists; two cases of death from status asthmaticus have been reported in patients receiving a single dose of carvedilol)
» Atrioventricular (AV) block, 2nd- or 3rd-degree or
» Bradycardia, severe or
» Cardiogenic shock or

» Sick sinus syndrome, without a pacemaker
(risk of further depression of myocardial contractility and conduction)
» Cardiac failure, decompensated, severe, requiring intravenous inotropic therapy, New York Heart Association (NYHA) class IV
(in clinical trials, area under the plasma concentration–time curve [AUC] and time to peak plasma concentration [$C_{max}$] increased by 50 to 100% in six patients with NYHA class IV heart failure; myocardial contractility may be further depressed in these patients)
» Hepatic function impairment, clinically manifested
(because carvedilol is hepatically metabolized, blood concentrations may be increased approximately four- to sevenfold following a single dose)
» Hypersensitivity to carvedilol

*Risk-benefit should be considered when the following medical problems exist:*
» Anaphylactic reaction to a variety of allergens, severe, history of
(administration of beta-adrenergic blocking agents may make these patients more reactive to allergen exposure and less responsive to the usual doses of epinephrine used to treat the allergic reaction)

Angina, Prinzmetal's variant
(nonselective beta-adrenergic blocking agents, such as carvedilol, may provoke chest pain in patients with this condition; caution should be used)

» Bronchospastic conditions, nonallergic, such as:
Chronic bronchitis and
Emphysema
(because carvedilol blocks the effect of endogenous and exogenous beta-adrenergic agonists, nonallergic bronchospastic conditions may be aggravated by carvedilol; only the smallest effective dose of carvedilol should be used, if it is used at all; in clinical trials, patients with congestive heart failure and bronchospastic disease received carvedilol only if treatment of their bronchospastic condition did not require oral or inhaled medication)

Congestive heart failure, if accompanied by:
Hypotension (systolic blood pressure < 100 mm Hg) or
Ischemic heart disease or
Renal insufficiency or
Vascular disease, diffuse
(patients with these conditions may be at risk for worsening of renal function if treated with carvedilol; renal function should be monitored and a dosage adjustment or discontinuation of carvedilol may be necessary if renal function deteriorates; heart failure may be worsened or fluid retention may occur when the dosage of carvedilol is increased; in such cases, dosages of diuretics should be increased, and carvedilol dosage increases should be postponed until the patient is clinically stable; carvedilol dosage may need to be reduced or temporarily discontinued in such cases. The AUC and $C_{max}$ may be increased in patients with congestive heart failure)

» Diabetes or
» Hypoglycemia
(beta-adrenergic blocking agents may mask symptoms of hypoglycemia, especially tachycardia; insulin-induced hypoglycemia may be potentiated and the recovery of serum glucose levels may be delayed; in patients with diabetes and congestive heart failure, hyperglycemia may be worsened with use of carvedilol; blood glucose concentrations should be monitored at each dosage adjustment)

» Hyperthyroidism
(beta-adrenergic blocking agents, such as carvedilol, may mask symptoms of hyperthyroidism, such as tachycardia; abrupt withdrawal of beta-adrenergic blocking agents may potentiate symptoms of hyperthyroidism or precipitate thyroid storm)

Peripheral vascular disease
(carvedilol may precipitate or aggravate symptoms of arterial insufficiency)

Pheochromocytoma
(in patients with this condition, therapy with alpha-adrenergic blocking agents should be initiated prior to beta-adrenergic blocking therapy; although carvedilol has both alpha- and beta-adrenergic blocking activity, there is no experience with use of carvedilol in this condition)

Renal function impairment
(increases in carvedilol plasma concentrations of approximately 40 to 50%, based on mean AUC data, were reported in patients with moderate to severe renal function impairment; peak plasma levels were approximately 12 to 26% higher in patients with renal function impairment)

## Carvedilol (Systemic)—Introductory Version

### Patient monitoring
The following may be especially important in patient monitoring (other tests may be warranted in some patients, depending on condition; » = major clinical significance):

» Blood pressure determinations, standing systolic
(measurements should be taken about 1 hour after dosing as a guide for tolerance and after 7 to 14 days to determine whether a dose increase is needed; monitoring is recommended when carvedilol is used concurrently with calcium channel blocking agents)

Blood glucose concentrations
(for diabetic patients)

Electrocardiogram (ECG) determinations
(monitoring is recommended when carvedilol is used concurrently with calcium channel blocking agents, such as diltiazem and verapamil, because of the possibility of cardiac conduction disturbances)

» Heart rate determinations
(in clinical trials in hypertensive patients, heart rate decreased by 7.5 beats per minute with a 50-mg per day dose of carvedilol; if heart rate drops below 55 beats per minute, the carvedilol dosage should be reduced)

Hepatic function determinations
(monitoring may be necessary)

Renal function determinations
(monitoring may be necessary, especially in patients with congestive heart failure, during dosage increases)

### Side/Adverse Effects

Use of carvedilol in patients with congestive heart failure has resulted in deterioration of renal function. Renal function returned to baseline when carvedilol was discontinued. Other rare side/adverse effects that have occurred with carvedilol therapy are complete atrioventricular (AV) block, bundle branch block, and myocardial ischemia.

The following side/adverse effects have been selected on the basis of their potential clinical significance (possible signs and symptoms in parentheses where appropriate)—not necessarily inclusive:

#### Those indicating need for medical attention
Incidence more frequent
*Allergy*—increased sensitivity to allergens; **bradycardia** (slow heartbeat)—incidence 2% in patients with hypertension and 9% in patients with congestive heart failure; **chest pain**—incidence 14.4% in patients with congestive heart failure; **dizziness**—incidence 6% in patients with hypertension and 32% in patients with congestive heart failure; **dyspnea** (shortness of breath); **edema, generalized** (generalized swelling); **edema, peripheral** (swelling of feet, ankles, or lower legs); **hypotension** (dizziness, lightheadedness, or fainting); **pain**—incidence 8.6% in patients with congestive heart failure; **syncope** (fainting); **weight increase**—incidence 9.7% in patients with congestive heart failure; may be a sign of fluid retention and worsening of heart failure

Note: *Hypotension* and postural hypotension were reported in 9.7% and *syncope* was reported in 3.4% of patients with congestive heart failure. In patients with hypertension, postural hypotension was reported in 1.8% and syncope in 0.1%. These problems may occur following the initial dose or at the time of a dosage increase.

Incidence less frequent
**Fever**—incidence 3.1% in patients with congestive heart failure; **hematuria** (blood in urine); **hepatic injury** (pruritus; dark urine; persistent anorexia; yellow eyes or skin; influenza (flu)-like symptoms; right upper quadrant tenderness); **depression, mental; thrombocytopenia** (unusual bleeding or bruising)

Note: Mild, reversible *hepatic injury* with minimal symptoms has been reported after short- and long-term therapy with carvedilol. Carvedilol should be discontinued if jaundice or laboratory evidence of hepatic injury occurs.

#### Those indicating need for medical attention only if they continue or are bothersome
Incidence more frequent
**Back pain; diarrhea; fatigue** (unusual tiredness or weakness); **paresthesia** (prickling or tingling sensation)

Incidence less frequent
**Abdominal pain; arthralgia** (joint pain); **blurred vision; headache; insomnia** (trouble in sleeping); **lacrimation, decreased** (decreased tearing)—in patients who wear contact lenses; **myalgia** (muscle pain); **nausea; pharyngitis** (sore throat); **rhinitis** (stuffy or runny nose); **sweating, increased; vomiting**

### Overdose
For specific information on the agents used in the management of carvedilol overdose, see:
- *Aminophylline* in *Bronchodilators, Theophylline (Systemic)* monograph;
- *Atropine* in *Anticholinergics/Antispasmodics (Systemic)* monograph;
- *Bronchodilators, Adrenergic (Inhalation-Local)* monograph;
- *Bronchodilators, Adrenergic (Systemic)* monograph;
- *Clonazepam* and *Diazepam* in *Benzodiazepines (Systemic)* monograph;
- *Dobutamine, Epinephrine, Isoproterenol,* and *Norepinephrine* in *Sympathomimetic Agents—Cardiovascular Use (Parenteral-Systemic)* monograph; and/or
- *Glucagon (Systemic)* monograph.

For more information on the management of overdose or unintentional ingestion, **contact a Poison Control Center** (see *Poison Control Center Listing*).

#### Clinical effects of overdose
The following effects have been selected on the basis of their potential clinical significance (possible signs and symptoms in parentheses where appropriate)—not necessarily inclusive:

Acute and chronic
***Bradycardia, severe; bronchospasm; cardiac arrest; cardiac insufficiency; cardiogenic shock; hypotension, severe; lapses of consciousness; respiratory problems; seizures, generalized; vomiting***

#### Treatment of overdose
For symptoms of shock (with severe intoxication), treatment with antidotes must be continued for an appropriate length of time consistent with the 7- to 10-hour half-life of carvedilol. Treatment is symptomatic and supportive and may include the following:

Monitoring—
The patient should be placed in a supine position and observed and treated under intensive care conditions.

To decrease absorption—
If overdose was recently ingested, gastric lavage or drug-induced emesis may be used.

Specific treatment—
For excessive bradycardia—Intravenous atropine may be used. If bradycardia is resistant to therapy, pacemaker therapy is recommended.
For bronchospasm—Intravenous or inhaled beta-adrenergic sympathomimetics or intravenous aminophylline is recommended.
For cardiovascular support—Intravenous glucagon or sympathomimetics such as dobutamine, isoproterenol, or epinephrine may be used.
For peripheral vasodilation—Epinephrine or norepinephrine with continuous monitoring is recommended.
For seizures—Intravenous diazepam or clonazepam is recommended.

Supportive care—
Patients in whom intentional overdose is confirmed or suspected should be referred for psychiatric consultation.

### Patient Consultation
As an aid to patient consultation, refer to *Advice for the Patient, Carvedilol (Systemic)—Introductory Version*.

In providing consultation, consider emphasizing the following selected information (» = major clinical significance):

#### Before using this medication
» Conditions affecting use, especially:
Hypersensitivity to carvedilol
Breast-feeding—Not recommended in mothers who are breast-feeding because of potential for serious reaction in nursing infant
Other medications, especially sulfonylurea antidiabetic agents; calcium channel blocking agents, especially diltiazem or verapamil; or insulin
Other medical problems, especially bronchial asthma or related bronchospastic conditions; atrioventricular block, 2nd- or 3rd-degree; bradycardia, severe; history of severe anaphylactic reaction to a variety of allergens; bronchospastic conditions, nonallergic; cardiac failure, decompensated, NYHA class IV; cardiogenic shock; diabetes or hypoglycemia; hepatic function impairment, clinically evident; hyperthyroidism; or sick sinus syndrome, without a pacemaker

#### Proper use of this medication
Taking medication at the same time each day to maintain the therapeutic effect
Taking medication with food

Not interrupting or discontinuing medication without consulting the physician

» Proper dosing

**Missed dose:**
Taking as soon as possible; not taking if almost time for next dose; not doubling doses

» Proper storage

**Precautions while using this medication**
Making regular visits to physician to check progress
Not taking other medications unless discussed with physician
Caution when driving or doing other tasks requiring alertness, because of the possible dizziness, lightheadedness, or fainting due to postural hypotension
Caution when standing quickly because of possible drop in blood pressure, which may result in dizziness or fainting; sitting or lying down may help alleviate these symptoms
Checking with physician if experiencing dizziness or faintness; a dosage adjustment may be necessary
Caution if any kind of surgery (including dental surgery) or emergency treatment is required
For diabetic patients—Checking with physician if any changes in blood sugar concentrations occur
For congestive heart failure patients—Checking with physician if experiencing weight gain or increasing shortness of breath, because of possible worsening of heart failure
For patients who wear contact lenses—Checking with physician if decreased lacrimation occurs

**Side/adverse effects**
Signs of potential side effects, especially allergy; bradycardia; chest pain; dizziness; dyspnea; edema, generalized; edema, peripheral; hypotension; pain; syncope; weight increase; fever; hematuria; hepatic injury; depression, mental; and thrombocytopenia

## General Dosing Information

Dosage must be adjusted to meet the individual requirements of each patient, on the basis of clinical response.

When concurrent carvedilol and clonidine treatment is to be discontinued, carvedilol should be discontinued before clonidine is discontinued. Clonidine should be withdrawn gradually; dosage should be decreased over several days.

When carvedilol is discontinued, its dosage should be tapered over a 1- to 2-week period, especially in patients with ischemic heart disease.

If the patient's pulse rate drops to below 55 beats per minute, the dosage of carvedilol should be reduced.

Hypotensive effects may be additive and orthostatic hypotension may be exaggerated when carvedilol therapy is added to diuretic therapy, or vice versa.

**Diet/Nutrition**
Taking carvedilol with food may slow the rate of absorption and minimize the risk of orthostatic hypotension.

## Oral Dosage Forms

### CARVEDILOL TABLETS

**Usual adult dose**
Congestive heart failure—
Initial: Oral, 3.125 mg two times a day for two weeks, taken with food. If tolerated, the dose may be increased to 6.25 mg two times a day. The dosage may then be doubled every two weeks to the highest dose tolerated by the patient.
At each dosage increase, the patient should be observed for one hour for signs of dizziness or lightheadedness.
In patients currently receiving digitalis, diuretics, and/or angiotensin-converting enzyme (ACE) inhibitors, the dosages of these medications should be stabilized prior to starting carvedilol therapy. Before each carvedilol dosage increase, tolerability of carvedilol should be determined by evaluation of the patient for symptoms of worsening heart failure, vasodilation (dizziness, lightheadedness, symptomatic hypotension), or bradycardia. Transient worsening of heart failure may be treated with increased doses of diuretics or it may be necessary to lower the carvedilol dose or temporarily discontinue it. Symptoms of vasodilation may respond to a reduction in the dose of diuretics or ACE inhibitors, and, if still not relieved, a reduction in the carvedilol dose. The dose of carvedilol should not be increased until symptoms of worsening heart failure or vasodilation have stabilized.
Hypertension—
Initial: Oral, 6.25 mg two times a day, taken with food. Dose should be maintained for seven to fourteen days and then increased to 12.5 mg two times a day, if tolerated, if blood pressure is not adequately controlled (based on trough blood pressure). If after the new dose is maintained for seven to fourteen days blood pressure is still not controlled, the dose may be increased to 25 mg two times a day, if tolerated. Standing systolic blood pressure taken one hour after dosing may be used as a guide for tolerance.
Maintenance: Oral, 6.25 to 25 mg two times a day. The full antihypertensive effect occurs within seven to fourteen days.

**Usual adult prescribing limits**
Congestive heart failure—
25 mg two times a day in patients weighing less than 85 kg (187 lbs) and 50 mg two times a day in patients weighing more than 85 kg.
Hypertension—
25 mg two times a day.

**Usual pediatric dose**
Children younger than 18 years of age—Safety and efficacy have not been established.

**Strength(s) usually available**
U.S.—
3.125 mg (Rx) [*Coreg*].
6.25 mg (Rx) [*Coreg*].
12.5 mg (Rx) [*Coreg*].
25 mg (Rx) [*Coreg*].

**Packaging and storage**
Store between 15 and 30 °C (59 and 86 °F) in a tight, light-resistant container. Protect from moisture.

**Auxiliary labeling**
• Do not take other medicines without your doctor's advice.
• Take with food.

Revised: 11/11/97
Developed: 04/07/97

---

**CASANTHRANOL** — See *Laxatives (Local)*

---

**CASCARA SAGRADA** — See *Laxatives (Local)*

---

**CASTOR OIL** — See *Laxatives (Local)*

---

**CEFACLOR** — See *Cephalosporins (Systemic)*

---

**CEFADROXIL** — See *Cephalosporins (Systemic)*

---

**CEFAMANDOLE** — See *Cephalosporins (Systemic)*

---

**CEFAZOLIN** — See *Cephalosporins (Systemic)*

---

**CEFEPIME** — See *Cephalosporins (Systemic)*

---

**CEFIXIME** — See *Cephalosporins (Systemic)*

**CEFONICID**—See *Cephalosporins (Systemic)*

**CEFOPERAZONE**—See *Cephalosporins (Systemic)*

**CEFOTAXIME**—See *Cephalosporins (Systemic)*

**CEFOTETAN**—See *Cephalosporins (Systemic)*

**CEFOXITIN**—See *Cephalosporins (Systemic)*

**CEFPODOXIME**—See *Cephalosporins (Systemic)*

**CEFPROZIL**—See *Cephalosporins (Systemic)*

**CEFTAZIDIME**—See *Cephalosporins (Systemic)*

**CEFTIBUTEN**—See *Cephalosporins (Systemic)*

**CEFTIZOXIME**—See *Cephalosporins (Systemic)*

**CEFTRIAXONE**—See *Cephalosporins (Systemic)*

**CEFUROXIME**—See *Cephalosporins (Systemic)*

**CELLULOSE SODIUM PHOSPHATE**—The *Cellulose Sodium Phosphate (Systemic)* monograph is not included in this published version of the USP DI database. Copies of the monograph are available on request from Micromedex, Inc. - Reprint Requests, 6200 S. Syracuse Way, Suite 300, Englewood, CO 80111; telephone (303) 486-6400; telefax (303) 486-6464; Email: USPDI@MDX.COM.

**CEPHALEXIN**—See *Cephalosporins (Systemic)*

# CEPHALOSPORINS   Systemic

This monograph includes information on the following: 1) Cefaclor; 2) Cefadroxil; 3) Cefamandole; 4) Cefazolin; 5) Cefepime; 6) Cefixime; 7) Cefonicid†; 8) Cefoperazone†; 9) Cefotaxime; 10) Cefotetan; 11) Cefoxitin; 12) Cefpodoxime†; 13) Cefprozil; 14) Ceftazidime; 15) Ceftibuten†; 16) Ceftizoxime; 17) Ceftriaxone; 18) Cefuroxime; 19) Cephalexin; 20) Cephalothin*; 21) Cephapirin†; 22) Cephradine†.

VA CLASSIFICATION (Primary):
Cefaclor—AM116
Cefadroxil—AM115
Cefamandole—AM116
Cefazolin—AM115
Cefepime—AM118
Cefixime—AM117
Cefonicid—AM116
Cefoperazone—AM117
Cefotaxime—AM117
Cefotetan—AM116
Cefoxitin—AM116
Cefpodoxime—AM117
Cefprozil—AM116
Ceftazidime—AM117
Ceftibuten—AM117
Ceftizoxime—AM117
Ceftriaxone—AM117
Cefuroxime—AM116
Cephalexin—AM115
Cephalothin—AM115
Cephapirin—AM115
Cephradine—AM115

Commonly used brand name(s): *Ancef*[4]; *Apo-Cefaclor*[1]; *Apo-Cephalex*[19]; *Ceclor*[1]; *Ceclor CD*[1]; *Cedax*[15]; *Cefadyl*[21]; *Cefizox*[16]; *Cefobid*[8]; *Cefotan*[10]; *Ceftin*[18]; *Cefzil*[13]; *Ceporacin*[20]; *Ceptaz*[14]; *Claforan*[9]; *Duricef*[2]; *Fortaz*[14]; *Keflex*[19]; *Keflin*[20]; *Keftab*[19]; *Kefurox*[18]; *Kefzol*[4]; *Mandol*[3]; *Maxipime*[5]; *Mefoxin*[11]; *Monocid*[7]; *Novo-Lexin*[19]; *Nu-Cephalex*[19]; *PMS-Cephalexin*[19]; *Rocephin*[17]; *Suprax*[6]; *Tazicef*[14]; *Tazidime*[14]; *Vantin*[12]; *Velosef*[22]; *Zinacef*[18].

Note: For a listing of dosage forms and brand names by country availability, see *Dosage Forms* section(s).

*Not commercially available in U.S.
†Not commercially available in Canada.

## Category
Antibacterial (systemic).

## Indications
Note: Bracketed information in the *Indications* section refers to uses that are not included in U.S. product labeling.

### General considerations
Cephalosporins have been classified by "generation" based on their spectrum of antibacterial activity, providing a useful, although somewhat arbitrary, means of grouping the many cephalosporins available. Several of the newer cephalosporins with an expanded spectrum of activity do not fit into any one generation but overlap into others. These medications have been placed into the generation that most closely describes their antibacterial spectrum.

First-generation cephalosporins include cefadroxil, cefazolin, cephalexin, cephalothin, cephapirin, and cephradine.

Second-generation cephalosporins include cefaclor, cefamandole, cefonicid, cefotetan, cefoxitin, cefprozil, and cefuroxime.

Third-generation cephalosporins include cefixime, cefoperazone, cefotaxime, cefpodoxime, ceftazidime, ceftibuten, ceftizoxime, and ceftriaxone.

The fourth-generation cephalosporin is cefepime.

Selection of any antimicrobial agent usually is based on the organism(s) that is present or most likely to be present, site(s) of infection, resistance patterns, and the side effects, cost, and pharmacokinetic properties of the cephalosporin. (See also *Table 1* and *Table 2*.)

First-generation cephalosporins have the highest degree of activity compared with other cephalosporins against most gram-positive bacteria, including beta-lactamase–producing *Staphylococcus aureus* and most streptococci; exceptions include methicillin-resistant staphylococci and penicillin-resistant *Streptococcus pneumoniae*. No cephalosporin is effective against *Enterococcus faecalis*, *Enterococcus faecium*, or *Listeria monocytogenes* infections. Gram-negative bacteria coverage is generally limited to *Escherichia coli*, *Klebsiella pneumoniae*, and *Proteus mirabilis*; cephalothin, cephapirin, and cephradine are also active, although poorly, against *Haemophilus influenzae*. Cephalothin and cefazolin have similar spectra of activity *in vitro*. Although cefazolin is more active against *E. coli* and *Klebsiella* species, it is more susceptible to staphylococcal penicillinases than is cephalothin. Cephalexin, cefadroxil, and cephradine all have very similar activities *in vitro* and are available only in an oral dosage form.

First-generation cephalosporins are used to treat bacterial endocarditis, bone and joint infections, otitis media, pneumonia, septicemia, skin and soft tissue infections, including burn wound infections, and urinary tract infections caused by susceptible bacterial organisms. They are not effective in treating meningitis. These medications are possible alternatives to the penicillins for staphylococcal and nonenterococcal streptococcal infections, including pneumonias, bone and joint infections, and bacterial endocarditis. Cefazolin is the preferred agent for use in perioperative prophylaxis because of its longer half-life. Because first-generation cephalosporins provide inconsistent coverage against gram-negative bacilli, their empiric use as therapy for nosocomial infections is not recommended.

Second-generation cephalosporins have enhanced activity, compared with the first-generation cephalosporins, against *E. coli*, *Klebsiella* species, and *P. mirabilis*; in addition, they have greater activity *in vitro* against a larger number of gram-negative bacteria, including *H. influenzae*, indole-positive *Proteus*, *Moraxella (Branhamella) catarrhalis*, *Neisseria meningitidis*, *Neisseria gonorrhoeae*, and some strains of *Serratia* and *Enterobacter* species. *Serratia* and *Enterobacter* species may induce beta-lactamases that inactivate the drug after a period of exposure to the cephalosporin, producing a resistance that may be expressed late; this resistance may not be detectable by disc sensitivity techniques. The second-generation cephalosporins have slightly less or variable activity against most gram-positive cocci, and none have activity against *Acinetobacter* species or *Pseudomonas aeruginosa*.

Cefaclor and cephalexin have comparable activity *in vitro* against most gram-positive cocci; however, cefaclor has better activity than cephalexin against *H. influenzae*, *E. coli*, *M. catarrhalis*, and *P. mirabilis*. Cefamandole, cefonicid, and cefuroxime all have similar activities *in vitro*. However, cefuroxime may be more stable against plasmid-encoded beta-lactamases (e.g., TEM-1) than is cefamandole, and cefonicid has less activity *in vitro* against *S. aureus*. Cefuroxime sodium is the only second-generation cephalosporin to penetrate into the cerebrospinal fluid (CSF). Cefprozil has *in vitro* activity that covers a broad range of organisms, including many gram-positive and gram-negative organisms that are typically covered by first-generation cephalosporins. It also has good activity against *H. influenzae*, *M. catarrhalis*, *Citrobacter diversus*, penicillinase-producing strains of *N. gonorrhoeae*, and *P. mirabilis*.

Second-generation cephalosporins are used in the treatment of bone and joint infections, pneumonia, septicemia, skin and soft tissue infections, including burn wound infections, and urinary tract infections caused by susceptible bacterial organisms. Cefuroxime is commonly used to treat community-acquired pneumonias because of its activity against *S. pneumoniae*, *S. aureus*, and *H. influenzae*. It has been used to treat meningitis caused by *S. pneumoniae*, *H. influenzae* (including ampicillin-resistant strains), and *N. meningitidis*, although third-generation cephalosporins have better penetration into the CSF. Also, delayed sterilization of the CSF has been reported in children being treated with cefuroxime for bacterial meningitis. Because cefaclor has good activity against many strains of *H. influenzae*, it is used in the treatment of amoxicillin-resistant otitis media and sinusitis. This is also true of cefuroxime axetil, an oral prodrug that is hydrolyzed to cefuroxime after absorption. It has been used to treat mild to moderate bronchitis, Lyme disease, otitis media, pharyngitis and tonsillitis, sinusitis, skin and soft tissue infections, uncomplicated gonococcal urethritis, and urinary tract infections. Cefprozil is also used to treat bronchitis, otitis media, pharyngitis and tonsillitis, sinusitis, and skin and soft tissue infections.

Cefoxitin and cefotetan have the greatest activity of all the cephalosporins against anaerobes, particularly the *Bacteroides fragilis* group. Cefoxitin has the greatest stability in the presence of beta-lactamases produced by the *B. fragilis* group. Cefotetan has activity similar to that of cefoxitin against *B. fragilis*, but cefotetan has greater activity than cefoxitin against aerobic gram-negative bacilli in general. Most strains of *Bacteroides distasonis*, *Bacteroides ovatus*, and *Bacteroides thetaiotaomicron* are resistant to cefotetan *in vitro*. Many of the second- and third-generation cephalosporins that are active against anaerobic organisms are not effective against resistant strains of the *B. fragilis* group.

Cefoxitin and cefotetan are used primarily in the treatment of mixed aerobic-anaerobic bacterial infections, including aspiration pneumonia, diabetic foot infections, intra-abdominal infections, and female pelvic infections. They are also used prophylactically to help prevent perioperative infections that may result from colorectal surgery and appendectomies, and in the treatment of penicillin-resistant strains of gonorrhea.

Most third-generation cephalosporins have a high degree of stability in the presence of beta-lactamases (penicillinases and cephalosporinases), and, therefore, have excellent activity against a wide spectrum of gram-negative bacteria, including penicillinase-producing strains of *N. gonorrhoeae* and most Enterobacteriaceae (*Citrobacter*, *E. coli*, *Enterobacter*, *Klebsiella*, *Morganella*, *Proteus*, *Providencia*, and *Serratia* species). However, third-generation cephalosporins in general are susceptible to hydrolysis by chromosomally encoded beta-lactamases. Cefoperazone tends to have slightly less activity against Enterobacteriaceae than the other third-generation cephalosporins because of its greater susceptibility to plasmid-encoded beta-lactamases (e.g., TEM-1, TEM-2). Strains of *P. aeruginosa*, *Serratia*, and *Enterobacter* species may develop resistance to the cephalosporin after a period of exposure due to induction of beta-lactamases. The third-generation cephalosporins are generally not as active against gram-positive cocci as are the first- and second-generation cephalosporins. Cefotaxime, ceftizoxime, and ceftriaxone all have similar activity *in vitro*. Cefixime, one of three oral third-generation cephalosporins, has the most activity of all oral cephalosporins against *Streptococcus pyogenes*, *S. pneumoniae*, and all gram-negative bacilli, including beta-lactamase–producing strains of *H. influenzae*, *M. catarrhalis*, and *N. gonorrhoeae*. Cefixime has little activity against staphylococci, and no activity against *P. aeruginosa*. Cefpodoxime is also an oral third-generation cephalosporin; its spectrum of activity is very similar to that of cefixime, except that cefpodoxime also has some activity against *S. aureus* and *Staphylococcus saprophyticus*. Most species of *Enterobacter*, *Enterococcus*, *Pseudomonas*, *Morganella*, and *Serratia* are resistant to cefpodoxime. Ceftibuten is the oral third-generation cephalosporin that is most resistant to beta-lactamases. It has a broad spectrum of activity *in vitro* against many gram-negative and selected gram-positive microorganisms, including *H. influenzae*, *M. catarrhalis*, *S. pneumoniae*, and *S. pyogenes*.

Ceftazidime has the greatest activity of the third-generation cephalosporins against *P. aeruginosa*. Cefoperazone is less effective than ceftazidime, but more effective than cefotaxime, against *P. aeruginosa*. The other third-generation cephalosporins tend to have variable activity against this pathogen. Cefoperazone achieves higher biliary concentrations than the other third-generation cephalosporins but has poor CSF penetration.

Third-generation cephalosporins and aminoglycosides (amikacin, gentamicin, netilmicin, or tobramycin) are synergistic *in vitro* against certain susceptible and resistant strains of *P. aeruginosa* as well as *Serratia marcescens* and other Enterobacteriaceae, including *Enterobacter cloacae*, *E. coli*, *K. pneumoniae*, and *P. mirabilis*.

Third-generation cephalosporins are used in the treatment of serious gram-negative bacterial infections, including bone and joint infections, female pelvic infections, intra-abdominal infections, gram-negative pneumonia, septicemia, skin and soft tissue infections, including burn wound infections, and complicated urinary tract infections caused by susceptible organisms. Cefotaxime, ceftazidime, ceftizoxime, and ceftriaxone are used to treat meningitis in both children and adults. Single-dose cefixime, cefotaxime, cefpodoxime, ceftizoxime, and ceftriaxone have been found to be effective in the treatment of uncomplicated gonorrhea; single-dose ceftriaxone is used to treat acute otitis media; and cefuroxime axetil, [ceftriaxone], and [cefotaxime] are also effective in the treatment of Lyme disease.

The fourth-generation cephalosporin cefepime generally is more resistant to hydrolysis by beta-lactamases than are the third-generation cephalosporins. However, some medical experts group cefepime with the third-generation cephalosporins. Cefepime is stable against plasmid-encoded beta-lactamases (e.g., TEM-1, TEM-2, SHV-1) and is also relatively resistant to the inducible chromosomally encoded beta-lactamases; in addition, it penetrates rapidly into gram-negative bacteria and targets multiple essential penicillin-binding proteins. These properties of cefepime make it a useful agent in treating infections caused by many Enterobacteriaceae, including *Citrobacter freundii* and *E. cloacae*, that are resistant to other cephalosporins. Although cefepime has similar activity to ceftazidime against *P. aeruginosa* and other gram-negative bacteria, cefepime is less active than ceftazidime against other *Pseudomonas* species and *Stenotrophomonas (Pseudomonas) maltophilia*. The activity against gram-positive microorganisms is similar for cefepime, cefotaxime, and ceftriaxone. Cefepime is inactive against *B. fragilis*, methicillin-resistant staphylococci, and penicillin-resistant pneumococci.

Cefepime is effective in the treatment of complicated intra-abdominal infections, pneumonia, uncomplicated skin and soft tissue infections, complicated and uncomplicated urinary tract infections, and in the empiric treatment of febrile neutropenia. [It is also used in the treatment of bronchitis and septicemia.]

## Accepted

Biliary tract infections (treatment)[1]—Cefazolin is indicated in the treatment of biliary tract infections caused by susceptible organisms.

Bone and joint infections (treatment)—[Cefaclor][1], [cefadroxil][1], cefamandole, cefazolin, [cefixime][1], cefonicid[1], [cefoperazone][1], cefotaxime[1], cefotetan, cefoxitin, [cefpodoxime][1], [cefprozil][1], ceftazidime, ceftizoxime, ceftriaxone, cefuroxime, cephalexin, [cephalothin][1], cephapirin[1], and [cephradine][1] are indicated in the treatment of bone and joint infections caused by susceptible organisms.

Bronchitis (treatment)—Cefaclor, cefixime, cefprozil[1], and cefuroxime axetil are indicated in the treatment of secondary bacterial infections of acute bronchitis caused by susceptible organisms.

Bronchitis, bacterial exacerbations (treatment)—Cefaclor[1], [cefepime], cefixime[1], cefpodoxime[1], cefprozil[1], ceftibuten[1], and cefuroxime axetil[1] are indicated in the treatment of bacterial exacerbations of chronic bronchitis caused by susceptible organisms.

Endocarditis, bacterial (treatment)—Cefazolin, [cephalothin][1], cephapirin[1], and [cephradine][1] are indicated in the treatment of bacterial endocarditis caused by susceptible organisms.

Genitourinary tract infections (treatment)—Cefazolin, cefoperazone[1], cefotaxime, cephalexin, [cephalothin], and cephradine[1] are indicated in the treatment of genitourinary tract infections, including epididymitis and prostatitis.

Gonorrhea, disseminated (treatment)[1]—Cefuroxime is indicated in the treatment of disseminated gonorrhea.

Gonorrhea, uncomplicated (treatment)—Cefixime, cefotaxime, cefpodoxime[1], ceftizoxime[1], ceftriaxone, cefuroxime, and cefuroxime axetil are indicated in the treatment of uncomplicated gonorrhea.

Impetigo (treatment)[1]—Cefadroxil, cefuroxime axetil, and [cephalexin] (Evidence rating: III), are indicated in the treatment of impetigo.

Intra-abdominal infections (treatment)—Cefamandole, cefepime, cefoperazone[1], cefotaxime, cefotetan, cefoxitin, ceftazidime, ceftizoxime, ceftriaxone, and [cephalothin] are indicated in the treatment of intra-abdominal infections caused by susceptible organisms.

Lyme disease (treatment)[1]—[Cefotaxime], [ceftriaxone], and cefuroxime axetil are indicated in the treatment of Lyme disease.

Meningitis (treatment)—Cefotaxime, ceftazidime, ceftizoxime[1], ceftriaxone, and cefuroxime are indicated in the treatment of meningitis caused by susceptible organisms.

Although indicated, cefuroxime is no longer considered a medication of choice in the treatment of bacterial meningitis due to its poor coverage of penicillin-resistant *S. pneumoniae* and subsequent therapeutic failures.

Neutropenia, febrile (treatment)—Cefepime and [ceftazidime][1] are indicated for empiric treatment of febrile neutropenia.

In patients at high risk for severe infection, including patients with a history of recent bone marrow transplantation, with hypotension at presentation, with an underlying hematologic malignancy, or with severe or prolonged neutropenia, antimicrobial therapy alone may not be appropriate.

Otitis media (treatment)—Cefaclor, [cefadroxil][1], [cefazolin][1], cefixime, cefpodoxime[1], cefprozil, ceftibuten[1], ceftriaxone[1], cefuroxime axetil, cephalexin, [cephalothin][1], [cephapirin][1], and cephradine[1] are indicated in the treatment of otitis media caused by susceptible organisms.

Pelvic infections, female (treatment)—Cefoperazone[1], cefotaxime, cefotetan, cefoxitin, cefpodoxime[1], ceftazidime[1], ceftizoxime[1], and ceftriaxone[1] are indicated in the treatment of female pelvic infections caused by susceptible organisms.

Perioperative infections (prophylaxis)—Cefamandole[1], cefazolin, cefonicid[1], cefotaxime, cefotetan, cefoxitin, ceftriaxone, cefuroxime, [cephalothin], and cephapirin[1] are indicated for the prophylaxis of perioperative infections caused by susceptible organisms.

Pharyngitis, bacterial (treatment) or
Tonsillitis (treatment)—Cefaclor, cefadroxil, cefixime, cefpodoxime[1], cefprozil, ceftibuten[1], cefuroxime axetil, cephalexin, and cephradine[1] are indicated in the treatment of bacterial pharyngitis and tonsillitis caused by susceptible organisms.

Penicillin is the usual medication of choice in the treatment of streptococcal infections, including the prophylaxis of rheumatic fever. These cephalosporins are generally effective in the eradication of streptococci from the nasopharynx; however, substantial data establishing the efficacy of cephalosporins in the prevention of subsequent rheumatic fever are not available at present.

Pneumonia, bacterial (treatment)—Cefaclor, [cefadroxil], cefamandole, cefazolin, cefepime, cefotaxime, cefoxitin, cefpodoxime[1], [cefprozil][1], ceftazidime, ceftriaxone[1], cefuroxime, [cefuroxime axetil], [cephalothin], and cephradine[1] are indicated in the treatment of bacterial pneumonia caused by susceptible organisms.

Pulmonary infections, in cystic fibrosis (treatment)—[Cefaclor], [cefamandole], and ceftazidime[1] are indicated in the treatment of pulmonary infections due to susceptible organisms in patients with cystic fibrosis.

Septicemia, bacterial (treatment)—Cefamandole, cefazolin, [cefepime], cefonicid[1], cefoperazone[1], cefotaxime, [cefotetan][1], cefoxitin, ceftazidime, ceftizoxime, ceftriaxone, cefuroxime[1], [cephalothin], cephapirin[1], and [cephradine][1] are indicated in the treatment of bacterial septicemia caused by susceptible organisms.

Sinusitis (treatment)—[Cefixime], cefprozil, and cefuroxime axetil are indicated in the treatment of sinusitis due to susceptible organisms.

Skin and soft tissue infections (treatment)—Cefaclor, cefadroxil, cefamandole, cefazolin, cefepime, [cefixime][1], cefonicid[1], cefoperazone[1], cefotaxime, cefotetan, cefoxitin, cefpodoxime[1], cefprozil[1], ceftazidime, ceftizoxime, ceftriaxone, cefuroxime, cefuroxime axetil, cephalexin, [cephalothin], cephapirin[1], and cephradine[1] are indicated in the treatment of skin and soft tissue infections caused by susceptible organisms.

Urinary tract infections, bacterial (treatment)—Cefaclor, cefadroxil, cefamandole, cefazolin, cefepime, cefixime, cefonicid[1], cefoperazone[1], cefotaxime, cefotetan, cefoxitin, cefpodoxime[1], [cefprozil], ceftazidime, ceftizoxime, ceftriaxone, cefuroxime, cefuroxime axetil[1], cephalexin, [cephalothin], cephapirin[1], and cephradine[1] are indicated in the treatment of bacterial urinary tract infections caused by susceptible organisms.

Ventriculitis (treatment)—Cefotaxime is indicated in the treatment of ventriculitis caused by susceptible organisms.

[Endocarditis, bacterial (prophylaxis)][1]—Cefadroxil, cefazolin, and cephalexin are indicated in the prevention of bacterial endocarditis caused by susceptible organisms. However, cefazolin and cephalexin are not recommended for genitourinary tract procedures.

[Sinusitis, amoxicillin-resistant (treatment)][1]—Cefaclor is used in the treatment of sinusitis resistant to amoxicillin.

## Unaccepted

None of the cephalosporins is considered to be effective against enterococci, *Listeria* species, chlamydia, *Clostridium difficile*, or methicillin-resistant *Staphylococcus epidermidis* or *S. aureus*.

---

[1]Not included in Canadian product labeling.

## Pharmacology/Pharmacokinetics

See *Table 1*, page 824, and *Table 2*, page 826.

### Physicochemical characteristics

Molecular weight—
- Cefaclor: 385.83.
- Cefadroxil: 381.41.
- Cefamandole nafate: 512.51.
- Cefazolin sodium: 476.5.
- Cefepime: 480.57.
- Cefepime hydrochloride: 571.51.
- Cefixime: 507.51.
- Cefonicid sodium: 586.54.
- Cefoperazone sodium: 667.66.
- Cefotaxime sodium: 477.46.
- Cefotetan disodium: 619.6.
- Cefoxitin sodium: 449.44.
- Cefpodoxime proxetil: 557.61.
- Cefprozil: 407.45.
- Ceftazidime: 636.67.
- Ceftibuten: 410.43.
- Ceftizoxime sodium: 405.39.
- Ceftriaxone sodium: 661.61.
- Cefuroxime axetil: 510.4.
- Cefuroxime sodium: 446.38.
- Cephalexin: 365.41.
- Cephalothin sodium: 418.43.
- Cephapirin sodium: 445.46.
- Cephradine: 349.41.

### Mechanism of action/Effect

Bactericidal; action depends on ability to reach and bind penicillin-binding proteins located in bacterial cytoplasmic membranes. Cephalosporins inhibit bacterial septum and cell wall synthesis, probably by acylation of membrane-bound transpeptidase enzymes. This prevents cross-linkage of peptidoglycan chains, which is necessary for bacterial cell wall strength and rigidity. Also, cell division and growth are inhibited, and elongation of susceptible bacteria and lysis frequently occur. Rapidly dividing bacteria are those most susceptible to the action of cephalosporins.

**Distribution**
Widely distributed throughout the body and reach therapeutic concentrations in most tissues and body fluids, including synovial, pericardial, pleural, and peritoneal fluids; bile; sputum; and urine. Also distributed into bone, the gallbladder, the myocardium, and skin and soft tissue. Most cephalosporins cross the placenta and are distributed into breast milk.

Cefoperazone and ceftriaxone reach the highest concentration in bile. Cefuroxime and ceftazidime reach the highest levels in the aqueous humor. Cefotaxime, ceftazidime, ceftizoxime, ceftriaxone, and cefuroxime are the only cephalosporins to achieve therapeutic concentrations in the cerebrospinal fluid (CSF).

**Time to peak bile concentration**
Cefoperazone— 1 to 3 hours.

**Bile concentration**
Cefixime—Approximately 56.9 mcg per mL following a single 200-mg oral dose.
Cefoperazone—Approximately 65, 1940, and 6000 mcg per mL 0.5, 1, and 3 hours, respectively, following a 2-gram intravenous bolus dose.

## Precautions to Consider

**Cross-sensitivity and/or related problems**
Patients allergic to one cephalosporin or cephamycin may be allergic to other cephalosporins or cephamycins also.
Patients allergic to penicillins, penicillin derivatives, or penicillamine may be allergic to cephalosporins or cephamycins also. Cephalosporin cross-reactivity is approximately 3 to 7% in patients with a documented history of penicillin allergy. Although cephalosporins have been administered without incident to some patients with rash-type penicillin allergy, caution is recommended when cephalosporins are administered to patients with a history of penicillin anaphylaxis since anaphylaxis may also occur after cephalosporin administration.

**Carcinogenicity**
*Cefaclor, cefadroxil, cefazolin, cefepime, cefixime, cefonicid, cefoperazone, cefotaxime, cefotetan, cefoxitin, cefpodoxime, cefprozil, ceftazidime, ceftibuten, ceftizoxime, ceftriaxone, cefuroxime, cefuroxime axetil, and cephradine*—Long-term studies in animals to evaluate the carcinogenic potential of these cephalosporins have not been done.

**Mutagenicity**
*Cefaclor, cefadroxil, cefazolin, cefoxitin, and cephradine*—Long-term studies in animals to evaluate the mutagenic potential of cefaclor, cefadroxil, cefazolin, cefoxitin, and cephradine have not been done.
*Cefepime, cefixime, cefonicid, cefoperazone, cefotaxime, cefotetan, cefpodoxime, cefprozil, ceftazidime, ceftibuten, ceftizoxime, ceftriaxone, cefuroxime, and cefuroxime axetil*—Studies have not shown that these cephalosporins are mutagenic.

**Pregnancy/Reproduction**
Fertility—
  *Cefamandole, cefoperazone, and cefotetan*—
    Adequate and well-controlled studies in humans have not been done.
    Beta-lactam antibacterials containing the N-methylthiotetrazole (NMTT) side chain have not been shown to cause adverse effects on fertility in rats exposed *in utero*, in neonatal rats (4 days of age or younger) that were treated prior to initiation of spermatogenesis, or in older rats (more than 40 days of age) after exposure for up to 6 months. Beta-lactam antibacterials containing the NMTT side chain have been shown to cause delayed maturation of the testicular germinal epithelium when given to neonatal rats during initial spermatogenic development (6 to 40 days of age), although the effect was slight in rats given 30 to 100 mg per kg of body weight (mg/kg) daily. However, in those neonatal rats given 1000 mg/kg per day (approximately 5 to 20 times the usual human dose), delayed maturation was pronounced and was associated with decreased testicular weight, arrested spermatogenesis, a reduced number of germinal cells, and vacuolation of Sertoli's cell cytoplasm. In addition, some neonatal rats given 1000 mg/kg per day from days 6 to 40 were infertile after reaching sexual maturity.
  *Other cephalosporins*—
    Adequate and well-controlled studies in humans have not been done.
    However, studies in animals have not shown that these cephalosporins cause impaired fertility.
Pregnancy—
  *Cefamandole, cefoperazone, and cefotetan*—
    Cefamandole, cefoperazone, and cefotetan cross the placenta. Adequate and well-controlled studies in humans have not been done.
    Studies in mice, rats, and monkeys given doses of up to 10 times the usual human dose have not shown that cefamandole, cefoperazone, or cefotetan causes adverse effects in the fetus.
    FDA Pregnancy Category B.
  *Cefotaxime*—
    Cefotaxime crosses the placenta. Adequate and well-controlled studies in humans have not been done.
    Studies in rats given parenteral cefotaxime have not shown that cefotaxime is teratogenic or fetotoxic. However, a slight decrease in fetal and neonatal weight was observed.
    FDA Pregnancy Category B.
  *Cefoxitin*—
    Cefoxitin crosses the placenta. Adequate and well-controlled studies in humans have not been done.
    Studies in rats and mice given parenteral doses of approximately 1 to 7.5 times the maximum recommended human dose have not shown that cefoxitin is teratogenic or fetotoxic. However, a slight decrease in fetal weight was observed. Studies in rabbits have shown that cefoxitin, although not teratogenic, causes a high incidence of abortion and maternal death.
    FDA Pregnancy Category B.
  *Other cephalosporins*—
    Cephalosporins cross the placenta. Adequate and well-controlled studies in humans have not been done.
    However, studies in animals have not shown that these cephalosporins cause adverse effects in the fetus.
    FDA Pregnancy Category B—Cefaclor, cefadroxil, cefazolin, cefepime, cefixime, cefonicid, cefpodoxime, cefprozil, ceftazidime, ceftibuten, ceftizoxime, ceftriaxone, cefuroxime, cefuroxime axetil, cephalexin, cephapirin, and cephradine.

**Breast-feeding**
*Cefadroxil, cefixime, and ceftibuten*—It is not known whether cefadroxil, cefixime, or ceftibuten is distributed into breast milk. However, problems in humans have not been documented to date.
*Other cephalosporins*—Other cephalosporins are distributed into breast milk, usually in low concentrations. However, problems in humans have not been documented to date.

**Pediatrics**
*All cephalosporins*—Lower metabolic and/or renal clearance of cephalosporins, with resulting prolonged half-life, has been reported in newborn infants. However, ceftriaxone has been found to have a shorter half-life in infants than it does in adults.
*Cefaclor and cefazolin*—Appropriate studies on the relationship of age to the effects of cefaclor or cefazolin have not been performed in premature infants and infants up to 1 month of age. However, no pediatrics-specific problems have been documented to date in children 1 month of age and older.
*Cefamandole*—Appropriate studies on the relationship of age to the effects of cefamandole have not been performed in premature infants and infants up to 6 months of age. However, no pediatrics-specific problems have been documented to date in children 6 months of age and older.
*Cefepime, cefoperazone, and cefotetan*—Appropriate studies on the relationship of age to the effects of cefepime, cefoperazone, or cefotetan have not been performed in the pediatric population.
*Cefixime, cefprozil, and ceftibuten*—Appropriate studies on the relationship of age to the effects of cefixime, cefprozil, or ceftibuten have not been performed in children up to 6 months of age.
*Cefonicid*—Cefonicid has been used in children 1 year of age and older, and no pediatrics-specific problems have been documented to date.
*Cefoxitin*—In children 3 months of age and older, higher doses of cefoxitin have been associated with an increased incidence of eosinophilia and elevated aspartate aminotransferase (AST [SGOT]).
*Cefpodoxime*—Appropriate studies on the relationship of age to the effects of cefpodoxime have not been performed in children up to 5 months of age.
*Ceftazidime L-arginine*—The safety of the arginine component of ceftazidime L-arginine has not been established in children. If treatment with ceftazidime is indicated for children younger than 12 years of age, the ceftazidime sodium product should be used.
*Ceftizoxime*—Although studies have been done in children up to 6 months of age, ceftizoxime is not indicated for use in this age group. In children 6 months of age and older, the use of ceftizoxime has been associated with transient elevated eosinophil counts and increased concentrations of alanine aminotransferase (ALT [SGPT]), aspartate aminotransferase (AST [SGOT]), and creatine kinase (CK).
*Ceftriaxone*—Because ceftriaxone is very highly bound to plasma proteins, it may be more likely than some other cephalosporins to displace bilirubin from serum albumin. Ceftriaxone should be used with caution in hyperbilirubinemic neonates, especially premature neonates.

*Cefuroxime, cefuroxime axetil, and cephapirin*—Appropriate studies on the relationship of age to the effects of cefuroxime, cefuroxime axetil, and cephapirin have not been performed in children up to 3 months of age. However, no pediatrics-specific problems have been documented to date in children 3 months of age and older.

*Cephradine*—Appropriate studies on the relationship of age to the effects of cephradine have not been performed in children up to 9 months of age. However, no pediatrics-specific problems have been documented to date in children 9 months of age and older.

*Other cephalosporins*—Appropriate studies on the relationship of age to the effects of these cephalosporins have not been performed in the pediatric population. However, no pediatrics-specific problems have been documented to date.

## Geriatrics
Cephalosporins have been used in the geriatric population, and no geriatrics-specific problems have been documented to date. However, elderly patients are more likely to have an age-related decrease in renal function, which may require an adjustment in dosage and/or dosing interval in patients receiving cephalosporins.

## Dental
Long-term therapy with cephalosporins may allow for the overgrowth of *Candida albicans*, resulting in oral candidiasis.

## Drug interactions and/or related problems
The following drug interactions and/or related problems have been selected on the basis of their potential clinical significance (possible mechanism in parentheses where appropriate)—not necessarily inclusive (» = major clinical significance):

Note: Combinations containing any of the following medications, depending on the amount present, may also interact with this medication.

» Alcohol
(concurrent use of alcohol with cefamandole, cefoperazone, or cefotetan is not recommended since these cephalosporins, because of their NMTT side chain, may inhibit the enzyme acetaldehyde dehydrogenase, resulting in accumulation of acetaldehyde in the blood)

(disulfiram-like effects such as abdominal or stomach cramps, facial flushing, headache, hypotension, nausea, palpitations, shortness of breath, sweating, tachycardia, or vomiting may occur following ingestion of alcohol or administration of intravenous alcohol-containing solutions; these effects usually occur within 15 to 30 minutes following ingestion of alcohol and usually subside spontaneously over several hours)

(patients should be advised not to drink alcoholic beverages, take alcohol-containing medications, or receive intravenous alcohol-containing solutions while receiving these cephalosporins and for several days after discontinuing them)

Antacids or
Ranitidine or
Histamine $H_2$-receptor antagonists, other
(concurrent use of high doses of antacids or $H_2$-receptor antagonists with cefpodoxime decreases absorption of cefpodoxime by 27 to 32%, and decreases peak plasma levels by 24 to 42%)

(concurrent use of ranitidine with ceftibuten increases the plasma concentration of ceftibuten by 23% and systemic exposure by 16%; the clinical relevance of these increases is not known)

(the extent of absorption of cefaclor is decreased with concurrent use of aluminum hydroxide– or magnesium-containing antacids; cefaclor should not be taken within 1 hour of taking these antacids)

» Anticoagulants, coumarin- or indandione-derivative, or
» Heparin or
» Thrombolytic agents
(concurrent use of these medications with cefamandole, cefoperazone, or cefotetan may increase the risk of bleeding because of the NMTT side chain on these medications; however, critical illness, poor nutritional status, and the presence of liver disease may be more important risk factors for hypoprothrombinemia and bleeding; because all cephalosporins can inhibit vitamin K synthesis by suppressing gut flora, prophylactic vitamin K therapy is recommended when any of these medications is used for prolonged periods in malnourished or seriously ill patients; dosage adjustments of anticoagulants may be necessary during and after therapy with cefamandole, cefoperazone, or cefotetan; concurrent use of any of these three cephalosporins with thrombolytic agents may increase the risk of severe hemorrhage and is not recommended)

(an increased anticoagulant effect has been reported with concurrent use of cefaclor and oral anticoagulants)

Nephrotoxic medications (see *Appendix II*)
(cephalothin has been associated with an increased incidence of nephrotoxicity when used concurrently with aminoglycosides; this effect has rarely been seen with other commercially available cephalosporins used at appropriate doses; the potential for increased nephrotoxicity exists when cephalosporins are used with other nephrotoxic medications, such as loop diuretics, especially in patients with pre-existing renal function impairment; renal function should be monitored carefully in patients receiving cephalosporins and aminoglycosides concurrently)

» Platelet aggregation inhibitors, other (see *Appendix II*)
(hypoprothrombinemia induced by large doses of salicylates and/or cephalosporins, and the gastrointestinal ulcerative or hemorrhagic potential of nonsteroidal anti-inflammatory drugs [NSAIDs], salicylates, or sulfinpyrazone may increase the risk of hemorrhage)

» Probenecid
(probenecid decreases renal tubular secretion of those cephalosporins excreted by this mechanism, resulting in increased and prolonged cephalosporin serum concentrations, prolonged elimination half-life, and increased risk of toxicity; probenecid has no effect on the excretion of cefoperazone, ceftazidime, or ceftriaxone; however, other cephalosporins and probenecid might be used concurrently in the treatment of infections, such as sexually transmitted diseases [STDs], or other infections in which high and/or prolonged antibiotic serum and tissue concentrations are required)

## Laboratory value alterations
The following have been selected on the basis of their potential clinical significance (possible effect in parentheses where appropriate)—not necessarily inclusive (» = major clinical significance):

With diagnostic test results
» Coombs' (antiglobulin) tests
(a positive Coombs' reaction appears frequently in patients who receive large doses of a cephalosporin; hemolysis rarely occurs, but has been reported; test may become positive in neonates whose mothers received cephalosporins before delivery)

Corticosteroids, urinary
(high concentrations of cefoxitin in the urine may produce false increases in the measurement of urinary 17-hydroxycorticosteroids by the Porter-Silber reaction)

Creatinine, serum and urine
(cefotetan, cefoxitin, or cephalothin may falsely elevate test values when Jaffe's reaction method is used; serum samples should not be obtained within 2 hours after administration)

Glucose, blood
(cefprozil, cefuroxime, or cefuroxime axetil may give false-negative test results with ferricyanide tests; glucose enzymatic or hexokinase tests are recommended to determine blood glucose concentrations)

» Glucose, urine
(most cephalosporins [cefaclor, cefamandole, cefazolin, cefepime, cefixime, cefoperazone, cefotetan, cefoxitin, cefprozil, ceftazidime, cefuroxime, cefuroxime axetil, cephalexin, cephalothin, cephapirin, cephradine] may produce false-positive or falsely elevated test results with copper-reduction tests [Benedict's, Fehling's, or *Clinitest*]; glucose enzymatic tests, such as *Clinistix* and *Tes-Tape*, are not affected)

Ketones, urine
(cefixime may produce a false-positive reaction for ketones in the urine with tests using nitroprusside; tests using nitroferricyanide are not affected)

Protein, urine
(cefamandole may produce false-positive test results for proteinuria with acid and denaturation-precipitation tests)

» Prothrombin time (PT)
(may be prolonged; cephalosporins may inhibit vitamin K synthesis by suppressing gut flora; also, ceftazidime and cephalosporins with the NMTT side chain [cefamandole, cefoperazone, cefotetan] have been associated with an increased incidence of hypoprothrombinemia; patients who are critically ill, malnourished, or have liver function impairment may be at the highest risk of bleeding)

With physiology/laboratory test values
Alanine aminotransferase (ALT [SGPT]) or
Alkaline phosphatase or
Aspartate aminotransferase (AST [SGOT]) or
Lactate dehydrogenase (LDH)
(serum values may be increased)

Bilirubin, serum or
Blood urea nitrogen (BUN) or
Creatinine, serum
   (concentrations may be increased)
Complete blood count (CBC) or
Platelet count
   (transient leukopenia, neutropenia, agranulocytosis, thrombocytopenia, eosinophilia, lymphocytosis, and thrombocytosis have been seen on rare occasions)

**Medical considerations/Contraindications**
The medical considerations/contraindications included have been selected on the basis of their potential clinical significance (reasons given in parentheses where appropriate)—not necessarily inclusive (» = major clinical significance).

*Except under special circumstances, this medication should not be used when the following medical problem exists:*
» Previous allergic reaction (anaphylaxis) to penicillins, penicillin derivatives, penicillamine, or cephalosporins

*Risk-benefit should be considered when the following medical problems exist:*
» Bleeding disorders, history of
   (cefamandole, cefoperazone, and cefotetan, which contain the NMTT side chain, have been associated with an increased risk of bleeding; however, all cephalosporins may cause hypoprothrombinemia and, potentially, bleeding)
» Gastrointestinal disease, history of, especially ulcerative colitis, regional enteritis, or antibiotic-associated colitis
   (cephalosporins may cause pseudomembranous colitis)
» Hepatic function impairment
   (cefoperazone is primarily excreted in bile; may also cause elevated AST [SGOT], ALT [SGPT], and alkaline phosphatase; it is recommended that patients with both severe liver disease and significant renal disease receive a reduced dosage of cefoperazone)
   Phenylketonuria
   (cefprozil for oral suspension contains 28 mg of phenylalanine per 5 mL)
» Renal function impairment
   (many cephalosporins are excreted renally; a reduced dosage is recommended in patients with renal function impairment receiving cefadroxil, cefamandole, cefazolin, cefepime, cefixime, cefonicid, cefotaxime, cefotetan, cefoxitin, cefpodoxime, cefprozil, ceftazidime, ceftibuten, ceftizoxime, cefuroxime, cephalothin, cephapirin, and cephradine)

**Patient monitoring**
The following may be especially important in patient monitoring (other tests may be warranted in some patients, depending on condition; » = major clinical significance):

*For all cephalosporins*
   Bleeding time and/or
» Prothrombin time (PT)
   (determinations may be required in selected patients prior to and during therapy since hypoprothrombinemia and decreased vitamin K–dependent clotting factors may occur on rare occasion, resulting in significant hemorrhage; administration of vitamin K promptly reverses the hypoprothrombinemia, which usually occurs in elderly, debilitated, malnourished, or other seriously ill patients with deficient vitamin K stores; prophylactic daily or periodic administration of vitamin K may be required, especially in such patients receiving cefamandole, cefoperazone, or cefotetan)

*For antibiotic-associated pseudomembranous colitis (AAPMC)*
   Stool examinations
   (cytotoxin assays of stool samples to document the presence of *Clostridium difficile* and/or its cytotoxin, which are neutralizable by *Clostridium sordellii* antitoxin, may be required prior to treatment in patients with AAPMC; however, *C. difficile* and its cytotoxin may persist following treatment with oral vancomycin, cholestyramine, bacitracin, or metronidazole, despite clinical improvement; follow-up cytotoxin assays are generally not recommended with complete clinical improvement)

## Side/Adverse Effects

The following side/adverse effects have been selected on the basis of their potential clinical significance (possible signs and symptoms in parentheses where appropriate)—not necessarily inclusive:

**Those indicating need for medical attention**
Incidence less frequent or rare
*For all cephalosporins*
   **Hypoprothrombinemia** (unusual bleeding or bruising)—more frequent for cefamandole, cefoperazone, and cefotetan; **pseudomembranous colitis** (abdominal or stomach cramps and pain, severe; abdominal tenderness; diarrhea, watery and severe, which may also be bloody; fever)
Incidence rare
*For all cephalosporins*
   **Allergic reactions, specifically anaphylaxis** (bronchospasm; hypotension); **erythema multiforme or Stevens-Johnson syndrome** (blistering, peeling, or loosening of skin and mucous membranes, which may involve the eyes or other organ systems); **hearing loss**—has occurred rarely in pediatric patients being treated for meningitis, but more frequently with cefuroxime; **hemolytic anemia, immune, drug-induced** (unusual tiredness or weakness; yellowing of the eyes or skin)—has occurred with many cephalosporins, but has been reported more commonly with cefotetan; **hypersensitivity reactions** (fever; skin itching, rash, or redness; swelling)—has occurred with many cephalosporins, but has been reported more commonly with cefazolin; **renal dysfunction** (decrease in urine output or decrease in urine-concentrating ability); **serum sickness–like reactions** (fever; joint pain; skin rash)—may be more frequent with cefaclor; **seizures**—especially with high doses and in patients with renal function impairment; **thrombophlebitis** (pain, redness, and swelling at site of injection)

   Note: Since the risk of serum sickness–like reaction to cefaclor may be as high as 0.5%, it is recommended that another cephalosporin or a similar medication, such as loracarbef, be substituted as appropriate.

*For ceftriaxone only*
   **Biliary "sludge" or pseudolithiasis** (anorexia; epigastric pain; nausea and vomiting)—more likely when administered by intravenous bolus over 3 to 5 minutes

**Those indicating need for medical attention only if they continue or are bothersome**
Incidence more frequent—less frequent with some cephalosporins
   **Gastrointestinal reactions** (abdominal cramps; diarrhea, mild; nausea or vomiting); **headache; oral candidiasis** (sore mouth or tongue); **vaginal candidiasis** (vaginal itching and discharge)

**Those indicating possible pseudomembranous colitis and the need for medical attention if they occur after medication is discontinued**
   *Abdominal or stomach cramps and pain, severe; abdominal tenderness; diarrhea, watery and severe, which may also be bloody; fever*

## Overdose

For more information on the management of overdose or unintentional ingestion, **contact a Poison Control Center** (see *Poison Control Center Listing*).

**Treatment of overdose**
To decrease absorption—Activated charcoal may aid in decreasing the absorption of cefaclor and cephalexin; gastric lavage may be used to decrease the absorption of cefixime.

To enhance elimination—Hemodialysis may be used to aid in the removal of cefamandole, cefepime, cefotetan, cefpodoxime, cefprozil, ceftibuten, cefuroxime axetil, and cephalothin; peritoneal dialysis may also be used for cefpodoxime and cefuroxime axetil.

Supportive care—Patients in whom intentional overdose is confirmed or suspected should be referred for psychiatric consultation.

## Patient Consultation

As an aid to patient consultation, refer to *Advice for the Patient, Cephalosporins (Systemic)*.

In providing consultation, consider emphasizing the following selected information (» = major clinical significance):

**Before using this medication**
» Conditions affecting use, especially:
   Allergies to penicillins, penicillin derivatives, penicillamine, or cephalosporins
   Pregnancy—Cephalosporins cross the placenta
   Breast-feeding—Most cephalosporins are distributed into breast milk; however, it is not known whether cefadroxil, cefixime, or ceftibuten is distributed into breast milk; no problems in humans have been documented
   Use in children—Accumulation of cephalosporins, with resulting prolonged half-life, has been reported in newborn infants. Ce-

foxitin and ceftizoxime have been associated with an increased incidence of eosinophilia and elevated aspartate aminotransferase (AST [SGOT]). Ceftizoxime also has been associated with elevated alanine aminotransferase (ALT [SGPT]) and creatine kinase (CK). Ceftriaxone should be used with caution in hyperbilirubinemic neonates since it may be more likely than other cephalosporins to displace bilirubin from serum albumin

Other medications, especially alcohol, anticoagulants, heparin, other platelet aggregation inhibitors, probenecid, or thrombolytic agents

Other medical problems, especially a history of bleeding disorders; a history of gastrointestinal disease, such as colitis; hepatic function impairment; or renal function impairment

**Proper use of this medication**
Taking on a full or empty stomach, or taking with food if gastrointestinal irritation occurs; cefaclor extended-release tablets, cefpodoxime proxetil, and cefuroxime axetil oral suspension should be taken with food; ceftibuten oral suspension should be taken on an empty stomach.

Proper administration technique for oral liquids; not using after expiration date

» Compliance with full course of therapy, especially in streptococcal infections
» Importance of not missing doses and of taking at evenly spaced times
» Proper dosing

Missed dose: Taking as soon as possible; not taking if almost time for next dose; not doubling doses

» Proper storage

**Precautions while using this medication**
Checking with physician if no improvement of symptoms within a few days
» Diabetics: False-positive reactions with copper-reduction tests for urine glucose may occur
» Patients with phenylketonuria (PKU): Cefprozil oral suspension contains phenylalanine
» For severe diarrhea, checking with physician before taking any antidiarrheals; for mild diarrhea, kaolin- or attapulgite-containing, but not other, antidiarrheals may be tried; checking with physician or pharmacist if mild diarrhea continues or worsens
» Avoiding alcoholic beverages or other alcohol-containing preparations while receiving, and for several days after discontinuing, cefamandole, cefoperazone, or cefotetan

Not taking antacids within 1 hour of taking cefaclor

**Side/adverse effects**
Signs of potential side effects, especially hypoprothrombinemia, pseudomembranous colitis, allergic reactions, erythema multiforme or Stevens-Johnson syndrome, hearing loss, hemolytic anemia, hypersensitivity reactions, renal dysfunction, serum sickness–like reactions, seizures, thrombophlebitis, or biliary "sludge" or pseudolithiasis

## General Dosing Information

Therapy should be continued for at least 10 days in group A beta-hemolytic streptococcal infections to help prevent the occurrence of acute rheumatic fever or glomerulonephritis.

### For oral dosage forms only
Most cephalosporins may be taken either on a full or empty stomach. Taking them with food may help if gastrointestinal irritation occurs. Cefaclor extended-release tablets, cefpodoxime proxetil, and cefuroxime axetil oral suspension should be taken with food. Ceftibuten oral suspension should be taken on an empty stomach, 2 hours before or 1 hour after a meal.

### For parenteral dosage forms only
Perioperative (preoperative, intraoperative, and postoperative) prophylactic administration of parenteral cephalosporins usually should be discontinued within 24 hours following surgery.

### For treatment of adverse effects
For antibiotic-associated pseudomembranous colitis (AAPMC)—
Some patients may develop AAPMC, caused by *Clostridium difficile* toxin, during or following administration of cephalosporins. Mild cases may respond to discontinuation of the drug alone. Moderate to severe cases may require fluid, electrolyte, and protein replacement.

In cases not responding to the above measures or in more severe cases, oral doses of metronidazole, bacitracin, cholestyramine, or vancomycin may be used. Oral vancomycin is effective in doses of 125 to 500 mg every 6 hours for 7 to 10 days. The dose of metronidazole is 250 to 500 mg every 8 hours; cholestyramine, 4 grams four times a day; and bacitracin, 25,000 units, orally, four times a day for 5 to 10 days. Recurrences are not uncommon and may be treated with a second course of these medications.

Cholestyramine and colestipol resins have been shown to bind *C. difficile* toxin *in vitro*. If cholestyramine or colestipol resin is administered in conjunction with oral vancomycin, the medications should be administered several hours apart since the resins have been shown to bind oral vancomycin also.

In addition, AAPMC may result in severe watery diarrhea, which may occur during therapy or up to several weeks after therapy is discontinued. If diarrhea occurs, administration of antiperistaltic antidiarrheals (e.g., atropine and dephenoxylate combination, loperamide, opiates) is not recommended since they may delay the removal of toxins from the colon, thereby prolonging and/or worsening damage to the colon because of toxin retention.

If hypersensitivity reactions occur, cephalosporins should be discontinued and the patient should be treated with the usual agents (antihistamines, corticosteroids, or epinephrine or other pressor amines), oxygen, and airway management, including intubation.

If seizures occur, cephalosporins should be discontinued. Anticonvulsants may be administered if clinically indicated.

---

### CEFACLOR

## Summary of Differences
Category: Second-generation cephalosporin.
Indications: Good activity against *Haemophilus influenzae*.
  Used for amoxicillin-resistant sinusitis.
Drug interactions: Increased anticoagulant effect with oral anticoagulants.
Side/adverse effects: Serum sickness–like reactions more common.

## Additional Dosing Information

Renal function impairment usually does not require a reduction in dose.

Cefaclor should not be taken within 1 hour of taking antacids.

Cefaclor extended-release tablets 500 mg two times a day are bioequivalent to the capsule formulation 250 mg three times a day, but are not bioequivalent to other cefaclor formulations 500 mg three times a day.

Extended-release tablets should be taken with food. They should not be cut, crushed, or chewed.

## Oral Dosage Forms
Note: Bracketed uses in the *Dosage Forms* section refer to categories of use and/or indications that are not included in U.S. product labeling.

### CEFACLOR CAPSULES USP

**Usual adult and adolescent dose**
[Bronchitis] or
Pharyngitis or
Pneumonia or
Skin and soft tissue infections, due to *Staphylococcus aureus* or *Streptococcus pyogenes* or
Tonsillitis or
Urinary tract infections—
  Oral, 250 to 500 mg every eight hours.

**Usual adult prescribing limits**
2 grams per day; however, 4 grams per day have been administered.

**Usual pediatric dose**
This dosage form is usually not used for children. See *Cefaclor for Oral Suspension USP*.

**Usual geriatric dose**
See *Usual adult and adolescent dose*.

**Strength(s) usually available**
U.S.—
  250 mg (Rx) [*Ceclor*; GENERIC].
  500 mg (Rx) [*Ceclor*; GENERIC].
Canada—
  250 mg (Rx) [*Apo-Cefaclor*; *Ceclor*].
  500 mg (Rx) [*Apo-Cefaclor*; *Ceclor*].

**Packaging and storage**
Store below 40 °C (104 °F), preferably between 15 and 30 °C (59 and 86 °F), unless otherwise specified by manufacturer. Store in a tight container.

**Auxiliary labeling**
• Continue medicine for full time of treatment.

### CEFACLOR FOR ORAL SUSPENSION USP

**Usual adult and adolescent dose**
See *Cefaclor Capsules USP*.

**Usual adult prescribing limits**
See *Cefaclor Capsules USP*.

**Usual pediatric dose**
[Bronchitis] or
Pneumonia or
Skin and soft tissue infections, due to *Staphylococcus aureus* or *Streptococcus pyogenes* or
Urinary tract infections—
  Infants and children 1 month of age and older: Oral, 6.7 to 13.4 mg per kg of body weight every eight hours.
  Infants up to 1 month of age: Safety and efficacy have not been established.
Otitis media or
Pharyngitis or
Tonsillitis—
  Infants and children 1 month of age and older: Oral, 6.7 to 13.4 mg per kg of body weight every eight hours; or 10 to 20 mg per kg of body weight every twelve hours.
  Infants up to 1 month of age: Safety and efficacy have not been established.

**Usual pediatric prescribing limits**
Doses of up to 60 mg per kg of body weight per day have been used. However, in older children, the maximum dose should not exceed 1.5 grams per day.

**Usual geriatric dose**
See *Cefaclor Capsules USP*.

**Strength(s) usually available**
U.S.—
  125 mg per 5 mL (when reconstituted according to manufacturer's instructions) (available in 75- and 150-mL bottles) (Rx) [*Ceclor* (sucrose); GENERIC (may contain sucrose)].
  187 mg per 5 mL (when reconstituted according to manufacturer's instructions) (available in 50- and 100-mL bottles) (Rx) [*Ceclor* (sucrose); GENERIC (may contain sucrose)].
  250 mg per 5 mL (when reconstituted according to manufacturer's instructions) (available in 75- and 150-mL bottles) (Rx) [*Ceclor* (sucrose); GENERIC (may contain sucrose)].
  375 mg per 5 mL (when reconstituted according to manufacturer's instructions) (available in 50- and 100-mL bottles) (Rx) [*Ceclor* (sucrose); GENERIC (may contain sucrose)].
Canada—
  125 mg per 5 mL (when reconstituted according to manufacturer's instructions) (available in 100- and 150-mL bottles) (Rx) [*Apo-Cefaclor*; *Ceclor* (sucrose)].
  250 mg per 5 mL (when reconstituted according to manufacturer's instructions) (available in 100- and 150-mL bottles) (Rx) [*Apo-Cefaclor*; *Ceclor* (sucrose)].
  375 mg per 5 mL (when reconstituted according to manufacturer's instructions) (available in 70- and 100-mL bottles) (Rx) [*Apo-Cefaclor*; *Ceclor* (sucrose)].

**Packaging and storage**
Prior to reconstitution, store below 40 °C (104 °F), preferably between 15 and 30 °C (59 and 86 °F), unless otherwise specified by manufacturer. Store in a tight container.

**Preparation of dosage form**
See manufacturer's labeling for instructions.

**Stability**
After reconstitution, suspensions retain their potency for 14 days if refrigerated.

**Auxiliary labeling**
- Refrigerate.
- Shake well.
- Continue medicine for full time of treatment.
- Beyond-use date.

**Note**
When dispensing, include a calibrated liquid-measuring device.

### CEFACLOR EXTENDED-RELEASE TABLETS

**Usual adult and adolescent dose**
Bronchitis or
Bronchitis, bacterial exacerbations—
  Adults and adolescents 16 years of age and older: Oral, 500 mg every twelve hours for seven days.
  Adolescents up to 16 years of age: Safety and efficacy have not been established.
Pharyngitis or
Tonsillitis—
  Adults and adolescents 16 years of age and older: Oral, 375 mg every twelve hours for ten days.
  Adolescents up to 16 years of age: Safety and efficacy have not been established.
Skin and soft tissue infections, uncomplicated, due to *Staphylococcus aureus*—
  Adults and adolescents 16 years of age and older: Oral, 375 mg every twelve hours for seven to ten days.
  Adolescents up to 16 years of age: Safety and efficacy have not been established.

**Usual pediatric dose**
Children up to 16 years of age—Safety and efficacy have not been established.

**Usual geriatric dose**
See *Usual adult and adolescent dose*.

**Strength(s) usually available**
U.S.—
  375 mg (Rx) [*Ceclor CD* (mannitol)].
  500 mg (Rx) [*Ceclor CD* (mannitol)].
Canada—
  Not commercially available.

**Packaging and storage**
Store at room temperature (15 to 30 °C [59 to 86 °F]).

**Auxiliary labeling**
- Take with food.
- Swallow whole.
- Continue medicine for full time of treatment.

---

## CEFADROXIL

## Summary of Differences
Category: First-generation cephalosporin.

## Additional Dosing Information
May be taken with food.

## Oral Dosage Forms
Note: Bracketed uses in the *Dosage Forms* section refer to categories of use and/or indications that are not included in U.S. product labeling.

### CEFADROXIL CAPSULES USP

**Usual adult and adolescent dose**
[Endocarditis, prophylaxis][1]—
  Oral, 2 grams one hour prior to the start of surgery.
Pharyngitis or
Tonsillitis—
  Oral, 500 mg every twelve hours, or 1 gram once a day, for ten days.
[Pneumonia]—
  Oral, 500 mg to 1 gram every twelve hours.
Skin and soft tissue infections—
  Oral, 500 mg every twelve hours; or 1 gram once a day.
Urinary tract infections, uncomplicated—
  Oral, 500 mg or 1 gram every twelve hours; or 1 or 2 grams once a day.

Note: After an initial loading dose of 1 gram, adults with impaired renal function may require a reduction in dose as follows:

| Creatinine clearance (mL/min)/(mL/sec) | Dose |
|---|---|
| > 50/0.83 | See *Usual adult and adolescent dose* |
| 25–50/0.42–0.83 | 500 mg every 12 hours |
| 10–25/0.17–0.42 | 500 mg every 24 hours |
| 0–10/0–0.17 | 500 mg every 36 hours |

**Usual adult prescribing limits**
4 grams per day.

**Usual pediatric dose**
This dosage form usually is not used for children. See *Cefadroxil for Oral Suspension USP*.

**Usual pediatric prescribing limits**
2 grams for prophylaxis of endocarditis.

**Usual geriatric dose**
See *Usual adult and adolescent dose*.

## 802  Cephalosporins (Systemic)

**Strength(s) usually available**
U.S.—
 500 mg (Rx) [*Duricef*; GENERIC].
Canada—
 500 mg (Rx) [*Duricef* (lactose)].

**Packaging and storage**
Store below 40 °C (104 °F), preferably between 15 and 30 °C (59 and 86 °F), unless otherwise specified by manufacturer. Store in a tight container.

**Auxiliary labeling**
• Continue medicine for full time of treatment.

### CEFADROXIL FOR ORAL SUSPENSION USP

**Usual adult and adolescent dose**
See *Cefadroxil Capsules USP*.

**Usual pediatric dose**
[Endocarditis, prophylaxis][1]—
 Oral, 50 mg per kg of body weight one hour prior to the start of surgery.
Impetigo[1] or
Pharyngitis or
Tonsillitis—
 Oral, 15 mg per kg of body weight every twelve hours, or 30 mg per kg of body weight once a day, for ten days.
Skin and soft tissue infections or
Urinary tract infections—
 Oral, 15 mg per kg of body weight every twelve hours.

**Usual pediatric prescribing limits**
See *Cefadroxil Capsules USP*.

**Usual geriatric dose**
See *Cefadroxil Capsules USP*.

**Strength(s) usually available**
U.S.—
 125 mg per 5 mL (when reconstituted according to manufacturer's instructions) (available in 50- and 100-mL bottles) (Rx) [*Duricef* (sodium benzoate; sucrose)].
 250 mg per 5 mL (when reconstituted according to manufacturer's instructions) (available in 50- and 100-mL bottles) (Rx) [*Duricef* (sodium benzoate; sucrose)].
 500 mg per 5 mL (when reconstituted according to manufacturer's instructions) (available in 50-, 75-, and 100-mL bottles) (Rx) [*Duricef* (sodium benzoate; sucrose)].
Canada—
 Not commercially available.

**Packaging and storage**
Prior to reconstitution, store below 40 °C (104 °F), preferably between 15 and 30 °C (59 and 86 °F), unless otherwise specified by manufacturer. Store in a tight container.

**Preparation of dosage form**
The bottle should be tapped to loosen the powder. The indicated volume of water should be added in two portions, shaking well after each addition.

| Bottle size | Total volume of water to be added |
|---|---|
| 50 mL | 34 mL |
| 75 mL | 51 mL |
| 100 mL | 67 mL |

**Stability**
After reconstitution, suspensions retain their potency for 14 days if refrigerated.

**Auxiliary labeling**
• Refrigerate.
• Shake well.
• Continue medicine for full time of treatment.
• Beyond-use date.

**Note**
When dispensing, include a calibrated liquid-measuring device.

### CEFADROXIL TABLETS USP

**Usual adult and adolescent dose**
See *Cefadroxil Capsules USP*.

**Usual adult prescribing limits**
See *Cefadroxil Capsules USP*.

**Usual pediatric dose**
This dosage form usually is not used for children. See *Cefadroxil for Oral Suspension USP*.

**Usual geriatric dose**
See *Cefadroxil Capsules USP*.

**Strength(s) usually available**
U.S.—
 1 gram (Rx) [*Duricef*].
Canada—
 Not commercially available.

**Packaging and storage**
Store below 40 °C (104 °F), preferably between 15 and 30 °C (59 and 86 °F), unless otherwise specified by manufacturer. Store in a tight container.

**Auxiliary labeling**
• Continue medicine for full time of treatment.

---

[1]Not included in Canadian product labeling.

---

## CEFAMANDOLE

## Summary of Differences

Category: Second-generation cephalosporin.
Pharmacology/pharmacokinetics: Contains *N*-methylthiotetrazole (NMTT) side chain.
Precautions:
 Drug interactions and/or related problems—Interacts with alcohol (disulfiram-like reaction), oral anticoagulants, and other medications that affect blood clotting.
 Laboratory value alterations—May produce false-positive test results for proteinuria with acid and denaturation-precipitation tests.
 Medical considerations/contraindications—Caution required in patients with history of bleeding problems.
 Patient monitoring—PT determinations may be required.
Side/adverse effects: May cause unusual bleeding or bruising.

## Parenteral Dosage Forms

Note: The dosing and strengths of the dosage forms available are expressed in terms of cefamandole base (not the nafate salt).

### CEFAMANDOLE NAFATE FOR INJECTION USP

**Usual adult and adolescent dose**
Perioperative prophylaxis[1]—
 Cesarean-section patients: Intramuscular or intravenous, 1 or 2 grams (base) as soon as the umbilical cord is clamped.
 Other surgery patients: Intramuscular or intravenous, 1 or 2 grams (base) one-half to one hour prior to the start of surgery; and 1 or 2 grams every six hours following surgery for twenty-four to forty-eight hours.
Pneumonia, uncomplicated or
Skin and soft tissue infections—
 Intramuscular or intravenous, 500 mg (base) every six hours.
Urinary tract infections—
 Intramuscular or intravenous, 500 mg to 1 gram (base) every eight hours.
For all other infections—
 Severe: Intramuscular or intravenous, 1 gram (base) every four to six hours.
 Life-threatening: Intramuscular or intravenous, up to 2 grams (base) every four hours.
Note: After an initial loading dose of 1 to 2 grams (base), adults with impaired renal function may require a reduction in dose as follows:

| Creatinine clearance (mL/min)/(mL/sec) | Dose (base) Severe infections | Life-threatening infections (maximum) |
|---|---|---|
| > 80/1.33 | 1–2 grams every 6 hours | 2 grams every 4 hours |
| 50–80/0.83–1.33 | 750 mg–1.5 grams every 6 hours | 1.5 grams every 4 hours; or 2 grams every 6 hours |
| 25–50/0.42–0.83 | 750 mg–1.5 grams every 8 hours | 1.5 grams every 6 hours; or 2 grams every 8 hours |
| 10–25/0.17–0.42 | 500 mg–1 gram every 8 hours | 1 gram every 6 hours; or 1.25 grams every 8 hours |
| 2–10/0.03–0.17 | 500–750 mg every 12 hours | 670 mg every 8 hours; or 1 gram every 12 hours |
| < 2/0.03 | 250–500 mg every 12 hours | 500 mg every 8 hours; or 750 mg every 12 hours |

**Usual adult prescribing limits**
12 grams (base) per day.

**Usual pediatric dose**
Perioperative prophylaxis[1]—
  Infants and children 3 months of age and older: Intramuscular or intravenous, 12.5 to 25 mg (base) per kg of body weight one-half to one hour prior to the start of surgery; and 12.5 to 25 mg per kg of body weight every six hours following surgery for twenty-four to forty-eight hours.
  Premature infants and infants up to 3 months of age: Dosage has not been established.
Mild to moderate infections—
  Infants and children 1 month of age and older: Intramuscular or intravenous, 8.3 to 33.3 mg (base) per kg of body weight every four to eight hours.
  Premature infants and infants up to 1 month of age: Dosage has not been established.
Severe infections—
  Infants and children 1 month of age and older: Intramuscular or intravenous, 25 to 50 mg (base) per kg of body weight every four to eight hours.
  Premature infants and infants up to 1 month of age: Dosage has not been established.

**Usual pediatric prescribing limits**
150 mg (base) per kg of body weight, or the maximum adult and adolescent dose, per day.

**Usual geriatric dose**
See *Usual adult and adolescent dose*.

**Usual geriatric prescribing limits**
1.5 grams (base) every six hours for patients older than seventy-five years of age, even if serum creatinine concentrations are normal.

**Strength(s) usually available**
U.S.—
  1 gram (base) (available in ADD-Vantage® vials) (Rx) [*Mandol* (sodium 3.3 mEq per gram)].
  2 grams (base) (available in ADD-Vantage® vials) (Rx) [*Mandol* (sodium 3.3 mEq per gram)].
  10 grams (base) (Rx) [*Mandol* (sodium 3.3 mEq per gram)].
Canada—
  1 gram (base) (also available in ADD-Vantage® vials) (Rx) [*Mandol* (sodium 3.3 mEq per gram)].
  2 grams (base) (Rx) [*Mandol* (sodium 3.3 mEq per gram)].

**Packaging and storage**
Prior to reconstitution, store below 40 °C (104 °F), preferably between 15 and 30 °C (59 and 86 °F), unless otherwise specified by manufacturer.

**Preparation of dosage form**
To prepare initial dilution for intramuscular use, 3 mL of sterile water for injection, bacteriostatic water for injection, 0.9% sodium chloride injection, or bacteriostatic sodium chloride injection should be added to each 1-gram vial, or 6 mL of diluent should be added to each 2-gram vial. Also, up to 10 mL of 0.5 to 2% lidocaine hydrochloride injection (without epinephrine) may be added to each 1-gram vial.
To prepare initial dilution for direct intermittent intravenous use, 10 mL of sterile water for injection, 5% dextrose injection, or 0.9% sodium chloride injection should be added to each 1-gram vial, or 20 mL of diluent should be added to each 2-gram vial. The resulting solution may be administered over a 3- to 5-minute period.
To prepare initial dilution for continuous intravenous infusion, 10 mL of sterile water for injection should be added to each 1-gram vial, or 20 mL of diluent should be added to each 2-gram vial. The resulting solution may be further diluted in suitable diluents (see manufacturer's package insert).
For reconstitution of piggyback infusion bottles or pharmacy bulk vials, see manufacturer's labeling for instructions.

**Stability**
After reconstitution, solutions retain their potency for 24 hours at room temperature (25 °C [77 °F]) or for 96 hours if refrigerated (5 °C [41 °F]).
If frozen immediately after reconstitution with sterile water for injection, 5% dextrose injection, or 0.9% sodium chloride injection, solutions retain their potency in the original container for 6 months at −20 °C (−4 °F). After being warmed to a maximum of 37 °C (98.6 °F), the solution should not be heated after thawing is complete. Once thawed, solutions should not be refrozen.
Solutions range in color from light yellow to amber depending on the concentration and diluent used. Solutions should not be used if they are of a different color or if they contain a precipitate.

Caution—During storage at room temperature, carbon dioxide develops inside the vial after reconstitution. This is of little or no consequence if the solution is added to sufficient quantities of intravenous fluids. However, if reconstituted cefamandole nafate is repackaged into certain types of syringes, continued production of carbon dioxide may cause leakage, or the rubber closure may be forced out of the barrel of the syringe. Therefore, syringes should be filled immediately prior to use.

**Incompatibilities**
The admixture of beta-lactam antibacterials (penicillins and cephalosporins) and aminoglycosides may result in substantial mutual inactivation. If they are administered concurrently, they should be administered in separate sites. Do not mix them in the same intravenous bag or bottle.
Since cefamandole nafate contains sodium carbonate, it may be incompatible with magnesium or calcium ions (including Ringer's injection and lactated Ringer's injection).

**Additional information**
Cefamandole nafate is rapidly hydrolyzed to cefamandole after initial dilution. Both compounds have microbiologic activity *in vivo*.
A solution containing 1 gram in 22 mL of sterile water for injection is isotonic.

[1]Not included in Canadian product labeling.

---

## *CEFAZOLIN*

## Summary of Differences
Category: First-generation cephalosporin.

## Parenteral Dosage Forms
Note: Bracketed uses in the *Dosage Forms* section refer to categories of uses and/or indications that are not included in U.S. product labeling.
  The dosing and strengths of the dosage forms available are expressed in terms of cefazolin base (not the sodium salt).

### CEFAZOLIN INJECTION USP
**Usual adult and adolescent dose**
[Endocarditis, prophylaxis][1]—
  Intravenous infusion, 1 gram (base) one-half hour prior to the start of surgery.
Perioperative prophylaxis—
  Intravenous infusion, 1 gram (base) one-half to one hour prior to the start of surgery; 500 mg to 1 gram during surgery; and 500 mg to 1 gram every six to eight hours following surgery for up to twenty-four hours.
Pneumonia, pneumococcal—
  Intravenous infusion, 500 mg (base) every twelve hours.
Urinary tract infections, acute, uncomplicated—
  Intravenous infusion, 1 gram (base) every twelve hours.
For all other infections—
  Mild: Intravenous infusion, 250 to 500 mg (base) every eight hours.
  Moderate to severe: Intravenous infusion, 500 mg to 1 gram (base) every six to eight hours.
  Severe to life-threatening: Intravenous infusion, 1 to 1.5 grams (base) every six hours.
Note: After an initial loading dose appropriate to the severity of the infection, adults with impaired renal function may require a reduction in dose as follows:

| Creatinine clearance (mL/min)/(mL/sec) | Dose (base) |
| --- | --- |
| ≥ 55/0.92 | See *Usual adult and adolescent dose* |
| 35–54/0.58–0.9 | Full dose every 8 hours or less frequently |
| 11–34/0.18–0.57 | ½ usual dose every 12 hours |
| ≤ 10/0.17 | ½ usual dose every 18–24 hours |

**Usual adult prescribing limits**
6 grams (base) per day; however, doses of up to 12 grams per day have been used in rare instances.

**Usual pediatric dose**
[Endocarditis, prophylaxis][1]—
  Intravenous infusion, 25 mg (base) per kg of body weight one-half hour prior to the start of surgery.

## 804 Cephalosporins (Systemic)

For all other infections—
Infants and children 1 month of age and older: Intravenous infusion, 6.25 to 25 mg (base) per kg of body weight every six hours; or 8.3 to 33.3 mg per kg of body weight every eight hours.
Neonates and infants up to 1 month of age: Intravenous infusion, 20 mg (base) per kg of body weight every eight to twelve hours.

Note: After an initial loading dose, children with impaired renal function may require a reduction in dose as follows:

| Creatinine clearance (mL/min)/(mL/sec) | Dose (base) |
|---|---|
| > 70/1.17 | See *Usual pediatric dose* |
| 40–70/0.67–1.17 | 7.5–30 mg per kg of body weight every 12 hours |
| 20–40/0.33–0.67 | 3.1–12.5 mg per kg of body weight every 12 hours |
| 5–20/0.08–0.33 | 2.5–10 mg per kg of body weight every 24 hours |

**Usual pediatric prescribing limits**
1 gram (base) for prophylaxis of bacterial endocarditis.

**Usual geriatric dose**
See *Usual adult and adolescent dose*.

**Usual geriatric prescribing limits**
500 mg (base) every eight hours for patients older than seventy-five years of age, even if serum creatinine concentrations are normal.

**Strength(s) usually available**
U.S.—
500 mg (base) per 50 mL (Rx) [*Ancef* (sodium 2 mEq per gram)].
1 gram (base) per 50 mL (Rx) [*Ancef* (sodium 2 mEq per gram)].
Canada—
Not commercially available.

**Packaging and storage**
Store between −25 and −10 °C (−13 and 14 °F), unless otherwise specified by manufacturer.

**Preparation of dosage form**
The container should be thawed at room temperature (25 °C [77 °F]) or under refrigeration (5 °C [41 °F]) before administration, making sure that all ice crystals have melted. Thawing should not be forced by immersion in water baths or by microwave irradiation.
Do not use minibags in series connections. This may result in air embolism because of residual air being drawn from the primary container before administration of intravenous solution from the secondary container is complete.

**Stability**
After thawing, solutions retain their potency for 48 hours at room temperature or for 30 days if refrigerated at 5 °C (41 °F). Once thawed, solutions should not be refrozen.
Do not use if the solution is cloudy or contains a precipitate.

**Incompatibilities**
The admixture of cefazolin sodium injection with other medications, including pentamidine isethionate, is not recommended.
The admixture of beta-lactam antibacterials (penicillins and cephalosporins) and aminoglycosides may result in substantial mutual inactivation. If they are administered concurrently, they should be administered at separate sites. Do not mix them in the same intravenous bag or bottle.

## CEFAZOLIN FOR INJECTION USP

**Usual adult and adolescent dose**
[Endocarditis, prophylaxis][1]—
Intramuscular or intravenous, 1 gram (base) one-half hour prior to the start of surgery.
Perioperative prophylaxis—
Intramuscular or intravenous, 1 gram (base) one-half to one hour prior to the start of surgery; 500 mg to 1 gram during surgery; and 500 mg to 1 gram every six to eight hours following surgery for up to twenty-four hours.
Pneumonia, pneumococcal—
Intramuscular or intravenous, 500 mg (base) every twelve hours.
Urinary tract infections, acute, uncomplicated—
Intramuscular or intravenous, 1 gram (base) every twelve hours.
For all other infections—
Mild: Intramuscular or intravenous, 250 to 500 mg (base) every eight hours.
Moderate to severe: Intramuscular or intravenous, 500 mg to 1 gram (base) every six to eight hours.
Severe to life-threatening: Intramuscular or intravenous, 1 to 1.5 grams (base) every six hours.

Note: Adults with renal function impairment may require a reduction in dose. See *Cefazolin Injection USP*.

**Usual adult prescribing limits**
See *Cefazolin Injection USP*.

**Usual pediatric dose**
[Endocarditis, prophylaxis][1]—
Intramuscular or intravenous, 25 mg (base) per kg of body weight one-half hour prior to the start of surgery.
For all other infections—
Infants and children 1 month of age and older: Intramuscular or intravenous, 6.25 to 25 mg (base) per kg of body weight every six hours; or 8.3 to 33.3 mg per kg of body weight every eight hours.
Neonates and infants up to 1 month of age: Intravenous infusion, 20 mg (base) per kg of body weight every eight to twelve hours.

Note: Children with renal function impairment may require a reduction in dose. See *Cefazolin Injection USP*.

**Usual pediatric prescribing limits**
See *Cefazolin Injection USP*.

**Usual geriatric dose**
See *Cefazolin Injection USP*.

**Usual geriatric prescribing limits**
See *Cefazolin Injection USP*.

**Strength(s) usually available**
U.S.—
500 mg (base) (may be available in ADD-Vantage® vials) (Rx) [*Ancef* (sodium 46 mg per gram); *Kefzol* (sodium 46 mg per gram); GENERIC].
1 gram (base) (may be available in ADD-Vantage® vials) (Rx) [*Ancef* (sodium 46 mg per gram); *Kefzol* (sodium 46 mg per gram); GENERIC].
5 grams (base) (Rx) [*Ancef* (sodium 46 mg per gram)].
10 grams (base) (Rx) [*Ancef* (sodium 46 mg per gram); *Kefzol* (sodium 46 mg per gram); GENERIC].
Canada—
50 mg (base) (may be available in Add-Vantage® vials) (Rx) [*Kefzol*].
500 mg (base) (may be available in ADD-Vantage® vials) (Rx) [*Ancef* (sodium 46 mg per gram); *Kefzol*; GENERIC].
1 gram (base) (also may be available in ADD-Vantage® vials) (Rx) [*Ancef* (sodium 46 mg per gram); *Kefzol*; GENERIC].
10 grams (base) (Rx) [*Ancef* (sodium 46 mg per gram); *Kefzol*; GENERIC].

**Packaging and storage**
Prior to reconstitution, store below 40 °C (104 °F), preferably between 15 and 30 °C (59 and 86 °F), unless otherwise specified by manufacturer.

**Preparation of dosage form**
To prepare initial dilution for intramuscular use, 2 mL of sterile water for injection should be added to each 500-mg vial, or 2.5 mL of diluent should be added to each 1-gram vial.
To prepare initial dilution for intravenous use, 2 mL of sterile water for injection should be added to each 500-mg vial, or 2.5 mL of diluent should be added to each 1-gram vial. For direct intravenous use further dilute with approximately 5 to 10 mL of sterile water for injection (see manufacturer's labeling instructions), and the resulting solution may be administered over a 3- to 5-minute period. For intermittent or continuous intravenous use, the solution may be further diluted in 50 to 100 mL of suitable diluent (see manufacturer's package insert).
For reconstitution of piggyback infusion bottles, pharmacy bulk vials, and dual-compartment vials, see manufacturer's labeling for instructions.

**Stability**
Prior to reconstitution, powders in their original containers are stable for up to 24 months.
After reconstitution, solutions retain their potency for 24 hours at room temperature or for 10 days if refrigerated (5 °C [41 °F]).
Reconstituted solutions may range in color from pale yellow to yellow without a change in potency.

**Incompatibilities**
The admixture of cefazolin with other medications, including pentamidine isethionate, is not recommended.
The admixture of beta-lactam antibacterials (penicillins and cephalosporins) and aminoglycosides may result in substantial mutual inactivation. If they are administered concurrently, they should be administered at separate sites. Do not mix them in the same intravenous bag or bottle.

---

[1]Not included in Canadian product labeling.

## CEFEPIME

### Summary of Differences
Category: Fourth-generation cephalosporin.

### Additional Dosing Information
Cefepime should be administered over a period of 30 minutes.

### Parenteral Dosage Forms
Note: Bracketed uses is the *Dosage Forms* section refer to categories of use and/or indications that are not included in U.S. product labeling. The dosing and strengths of the dosage form available are expressed in terms of cefepime base (not the hydrochloride salt).

#### CEFEPIME HYDROCHLORIDE FOR INJECTION
**Usual adult and adolescent dose**
Intra-abdominal infections, complicated—
   Intravenous, 2 grams (base), in combination with metronidazole, every twelve hours for seven to ten days.
[Septicemia] or
Skin and soft tissue infections, uncomplicated, moderate to severe or
Urinary tract infections, severe—
   Intravenous, 2 grams (base) every twelve hours for ten days.
Neutropenia, febrile—
   Intravenous, 2 grams (base) every eight hours for seven days or until resolution of neutropenia.
Note: In patients whose fever resolves but who remain neutropenic for more than seven days, the need for continued antimicrobial therapy should be re-evaluated frequently.
Pneumonia, moderate to severe—
   Intravenous, 1 to 2 grams (base) every twelve hours for ten days.
Urinary tract infections, mild to moderate—
   Intramuscular or intravenous, 500 mg to 1 gram (base) every twelve hours for seven to ten days.
Note: After an initial loading dose equal to that of patients with normal renal function, patients with renal function impairment may require a reduction in dose as follows:

| Creatinine clearance (mL/min)/(mL/sec) | Recommended dosing schedule for normal renal function, based on severity of infection ||||
|---|---|---|---|---|
| > 60/1 | 500 mg every 12 hours | 1 gram every 12 hours | 2 grams every 12 hours | 2 grams every 8 hours |
| | Recommended maintenance dosing schedule for renal function impairment, based on severity of infection ||||
| 30–60/0.5–1 | 500 mg every 24 hours | 1 gram every 24 hours | 2 grams every 24 hours | 2 grams every 12 hours |
| 11–29/0.18–0.49 | 500 mg every 24 hours | 500 mg every 24 hours | 1 gram every 24 hours | 2 grams every 24 hours |
| < 11/0.18 | 250 mg every 24 hours | 250 mg every 24 hours | 500 mg every 24 hours | 1 gram every 24 hours |
| Hemodialysis patients | Repeat the initial dose at the completion of each dialysis session. ||||
| Peritoneal dialysis patients | Administer normally recommended dose at 48-hour intervals. ||||

**Usual pediatric dose**
Children up to 12 years of age—Safety and efficacy have not been established.

**Usual geriatric dose**
See *Usual adult and adolescent dose.*

**Strength(s) usually available**
U.S.—
   500 mg (base) (Rx) [*Maxipime* (L-arginine 725 mg per gram)].
   1 gram (base) (also available in ADD-Vantage® vials) (Rx) [*Maxipime* (L-arginine 725 mg per gram)].
   2 grams (base) (also available in ADD-Vantage® vials) (Rx) [*Maxipime* (L-arginine 725 mg per gram)].

Canada—
   500 mg (base) (Rx) [*Maxipime* (L-arginine 725 mg per gram)].
   1 gram (base) (Rx) [*Maxipime* (L-arginine 725 mg per gram)].
   2 grams (base) (Rx) [*Maxipime* (L-arginine 725 mg per gram)].

**Packaging and storage**
Prior to reconstitution, store between 2 and 25 °C (36 and 77 °F). Protect from light.

**Preparation of dosage form**
To prepare initial dilution for intramuscular use, 1.3 mL of sterile water for injection, 0.9% sodium chloride injection, 5% dextrose injection, 0.5% or 1% lidocaine hydrochloride, or sterile bacteriostatic water for injection containing either parabens or benzyl alcohol should be added to each 500-mg vial, or 2.4 mL of diluent should be added to each 1-gram vial.

To prepare initial dilution for intravenous administration, 5 mL of suitable diluent (see manufacturer's labeling instructions) should be added to each 500-mg vial, or 10 mL of diluent should be added to each 1- or 2-gram vial. The resulting solution should be further diluted in 50 to 100 mL of a suitable diluent and administered over a period of 30 minutes.

For reconstitution of piggyback infusion bottles and ADD-Vantage® vials, dilute in 50 or 100 mL of suitable diluent (see manufacturer's labeling instructions), and administer over a period of 30 minutes.

**Stability**
After reconstitution, intramuscular solutions, intravenous solutions at concentrations from 1 to 40 mg per mL, and ADD-Vantage® vials at concentrations from 10 to 20 mg per mL retain their potency for up to 24 hours at room temperature (20 to 25 °C [68 to 77 °F]) or for 7 days if refrigerated (2 to 8 °C [36 to 46 °F]).
Solutions range in color from colorless to amber.

**Incompatibilities**
Cefepime should not be added to ampicillin solutions of a strength greater than 40 mg per mL, or to aminophylline, gentamicin, metronidazole, netilmicin, tobramycin, or vancomycin solutions. If these medications are administered concurrently with cefepime, they should be administered at separate sites.

## CEFIXIME

### Summary of Differences
Category: Third-generation cephalosporin. One of three oral third-generation cephalosporins.
Laboratory values: May produce false-positive reaction for ketones in urine with tests using nitroprusside.

### Additional Dosing Information
The oral suspension form of cefixime results in higher peak blood concentrations than the tablet when administered at the same dose. Therefore, the tablet should not be substituted for the oral suspension in the treatment of otitis media.

### Oral Dosage Forms
#### CEFIXIME FOR ORAL SUSPENSION USP
**Usual adult and adolescent dose**
Bronchitis or
Bronchitis, bacterial exacerbations[1] or
Pharyngitis or
Tonsillitis or
Urinary tract infections, uncomplicated—
   Oral, 200 mg every twelve hours; or 400 mg once a day.
Gonorrhea, cervical or urethral, uncomplicated—
   Oral, 400 mg as a single dose.
Note: Patients with renal function impairment may require a reduction in dose as follows:

| Creatinine clearance (mL/min)/(mL/sec) | Dose |
|---|---|
| > 60/1 | See *Usual adult and adolescent dose* |
| 21–60/0.35–1 or hemodialysis patients | 75% of standard dosage at standard dosing interval |
| < 20/0.33 or CAPD patients | 50% of standard dosage at standard dosing interval |

**806    Cephalosporins (Systemic)**

**Usual pediatric dose**
Bronchitis or
Bronchitis, bacterial exacerbations[1] or
Otitis media or
Pharyngitis or
Tonsillitis or
Urinary tract infections, uncomplicated—
   Children 50 kg of body weight and over: See *Usual adult and adolescent dose*.
   Infants and children 6 months to 12 years of age and up to 50 kg of body weight: Oral, 4 mg per kg of body weight every twelve hours; or 8 mg per kg of body weight once a day.
   Infants up to 6 months of age: Dosage has not been established.

**Usual geriatric dose**
See *Usual adult and adolescent dose*.

**Strength(s) usually available**
U.S.—
   100 mg per 5 mL (when reconstituted according to manufacturer's instructions) (available in 50-, 75-, and 100-mL bottles) (Rx) [*Suprax* (sodium benzoate; sucrose)].
Canada—
   100 mg per 5 mL (when reconstituted according to manufacturer's instructions) (available in 50-, 75-, and 100-mL bottles) (Rx) [*Suprax* (sodium benzoate; sucrose)].

**Packaging and storage**
Prior to reconstitution, store below 40 °C (104 °F), preferably between 15 and 30 °C (59 and 86 °F), unless otherwise specified by manufacturer. Store in a tight container.

**Preparation of dosage form**
The bottle should be tapped to loosen the powder. The indicated volume of water should be added in two portions, shaking well after each addition.

| Bottle size | Total volume of water to be added |
|---|---|
| 50 mL | 36 mL |
| 75 mL | 52 mL |
| 100 mL | 69 mL |

**Stability**
After reconstitution, suspension retains its potency for 14 days at room temperature or if refrigerated.

**Auxiliary labeling**
• Does not require refrigeration.
• Shake well.
• Continue medicine for full time of treatment.
• Beyond-use date.

**Note**
When dispensing, include a calibrated liquid-measuring device.

**CEFIXIME TABLETS USP**

**Usual adult and adolescent dose**
See *Cefixime for Oral Suspension USP*.

**Usual pediatric dose**
See *Cefixime for Oral Suspension USP*.
Note: Otitis media should be treated with cefixime for oral suspension since the suspension results in higher peak blood levels than the tablet when administered at the same dose.

**Usual geriatric dose**
See *Cefixime for Oral Suspension USP*.

**Strength(s) usually available**
U.S.—
   200 mg (Rx) [*Suprax* (scored)].
   400 mg (Rx) [*Suprax* (scored)].
Canada—
   200 mg (Rx) [*Suprax* (scored)].
   400 mg (Rx) [*Suprax* (scored)].

**Packaging and storage**
Store below 40 °C (104 °F), preferably between 15 and 30 °C (59 and 86 °F), unless otherwise specified by manufacturer. Store in a tight container.

**Auxiliary labeling**
• Continue medicine for full time of treatment.

[1]Not included in Canadian product labeling.

---

## CEFONICID

## Summary of Differences
Category: Second-generation cephalosporin.

## Additional Dosing Information
Intramuscular doses of 2 grams should be administered as divided doses in different sites.

## Parenteral Dosage Forms
Note: The dosing and strengths of the dosage forms available are expressed in terms of cefonicid base (not the sodium salt).

### CEFONICID INJECTION USP

**Usual adult and adolescent dose**
Perioperative prophylaxis[1]—
   Cesarean-section patients: Intramuscular or intravenous, 1 gram (base) as soon as the umbilical cord is clamped.
   Other surgical patients: Intramuscular or intravenous, 1 gram (base) one hour prior to the start of surgery.
Urinary tract infections, uncomplicated[1]—
   Intramuscular or intravenous, 500 mg (base) every twenty-four hours.
For all other infections[1]—
   Mild to moderate: Intramuscular or intravenous, 1 gram (base) every twenty-four hours.
   Severe to life-threatening: Intramuscular or intravenous, 2 grams (base) every twenty-four hours.

Note: After an initial loading dose of 7.5 mg (base) per kg of body weight, adults with impaired renal function may require a reduction in dose as follows:

| Creatinine clearance (mL/min)/(mL/sec) | Dose (base) Mild to moderate infections | Dose (base) Severe infections |
|---|---|---|
| ≥ 80/1.33 | See *Usual adult and adolescent dose* | See *Usual adult and adolescent dose* |
| 60–79/1–1.31 | 10 mg/kg every 24 hours | 25 mg/kg every 24 hours |
| 40–59/0.67–0.98 | 8 mg/kg every 24 hours | 20 mg/kg every 24 hours |
| 20–39/0.33–0.65 | 4 mg/kg every 24 hours | 15 mg/kg every 24 hours |
| 10–19/0.17–0.32 | 4 mg/kg every 48 hours | 15 mg/kg every 48 hours |
| 5–9/0.08–0.15 | 4 mg/kg every 3 to 5 days | 15 mg/kg every 3 to 5 days |
| < 5/0.08 | 3 mg/kg every 3 to 5 days | 4 mg/kg every 3 to 5 days |

**Usual pediatric dose**
Antibacterial—
   Safety and efficacy have not been established; however, cefonicid has been used in children 1 year of age and older, and no pediatrics-specific problems have been reported.

**Usual geriatric dose**
See *Usual adult and adolescent dose*.

**Usual geriatric prescribing limits**
25 mg (base) every twenty-four hours for patients older than seventy-five years of age, even if serum creatinine concentrations are normal.

**Strength(s) usually available**
U.S.—
   500 mg (base) (Rx) [*Monocid* (sodium 3.7 mEq per gram)].
   1 gram (base) (Rx) [*Monocid* (sodium 3.7 mEq per gram)].
   10 grams (base) (Rx) [*Monocid* (sodium 3.7 mEq per gram)].
Canada—
   Not commercially available.

**Packaging and storage**
Prior to reconstitution, store in the refrigerator (2 to 8 °C [36 to 46 °F]). Protect from light.

**Preparation of dosage form**
To prepare initial dilution for intramuscular or intravenous use, 2 mL of sterile water for injection should be added to each 500-mg vial, or 2.5 mL of diluent should be added to each 1-gram vial. For direct intravenous use, the resulting solution may be administered over a 3- to 5-minute period. For intravenous infusions, the resulting solution may be

further diluted in 50 to 100 mL of suitable fluids (see manufacturer's package insert).

For reconstitution of piggyback infusion bottles or pharmacy bulk vials, see manufacturer's labeling for instructions.

**Stability**

After reconstitution for intramuscular or intravenous use, solutions retain their potency for 24 hours at room temperature or for 72 hours if refrigerated at 5 °C (41 °F).

Slight yellowing of cefonicid solutions does not affect their potency.

**Incompatibilities**

The admixture of beta-lactam antibacterials (penicillins and cephalosporins) and aminoglycosides may result in substantial mutual inactivation. If they are administered concurrently, they should be administered in separate sites. Do not mix them in the same intravenous bag or bottle.

**Additional information**

A solution containing 1 gram in 18 mL of sterile water for injection is isotonic.

[1]Not included in Canadian product labeling.

---

## CEFOPERAZONE

## Summary of Differences

Category: Third-generation cephalosporin.
Pharmacology/pharmacokinetics:
  Achieves high biliary concentrations.
  Contains *N*-methylthiotetrazole (NMTT) side chain.
Precautions:
  Drug interactions and/or related problems—Interacts with alcohol (disulfiram-like reaction), oral anticoagulants, and other medications that affect blood clotting.
  Does not interact with probenecid.
  Medical considerations/contraindications—Caution required in patients with history of bleeding problems, and in patients with both severe hepatic function impairment and renal dysfunction.
  Patient monitoring—PT determinations may be required.
  Side/adverse effects—May cause unusual bleeding or bruising.

## Additional Dosing Information

Cefoperazone should be administered intramuscularly, by intermittent intravenous infusion over a 15- to 30-minute period, or by continuous intravenous infusion. Rapid bolus injection is not recommended.

Patients with impaired renal function generally do not require a reduction in dose since cefoperazone is excreted primarily in the bile. Also, patients with impaired hepatic function or biliary obstruction who are not receiving maximum doses generally do not require a reduction in dose since a corresponding increase in renal excretion (up to 90% or more) usually compensates, to a large degree, for reduced biliary excretion.

Patients with combined renal and hepatic function impairment require a reduction in dose since cefoperazone is not significantly metabolized and toxic serum concentrations may occur.

## Parenteral Dosage Forms

Note: The dosing and strengths of the dosage forms available are expressed in terms of cefoperazone base (not the sodium salt).

### CEFOPERAZONE INJECTION USP

**Usual adult dose**

Mild to moderate infections[1]—
  Intravenous infusion, 1 to 2 grams (base) every twelve hours.
Severe infections[1]—
  Intravenous infusion, 2 to 4 grams (base) every eight hours; or 3 to 6 grams every twelve hours.
Note: Adults with impaired hepatic function and/or biliary obstruction should not receive more than 4 grams (base) per day.
  Adults with combined hepatic and renal function impairment should not receive more than 1 to 2 grams (base) per day.
  In patients who are receiving hemodialysis treatments, a dose should be administered following hemodialysis.

**Usual adult prescribing limits**

12 grams (base) per day. However, up to 16 grams per day have been given by continuous infusion in severely immunocompromised patients without adverse effect.

**Usual pediatric dose**

Safety and efficacy have not been established.

**Usual geriatric dose**

See *Usual adult and adolescent dose*.

**Strength(s) usually available**

U.S.—
  1 gram in 50 mL (base) (Rx) [*Cefobid* (sodium 1.5 mEq per gram)].
  2 grams in 50 mL (base) (Rx) [*Cefobid* (sodium 1.5 mEq per gram)].
Canada—
  Not commercially available.

**Packaging and storage**

Store between −25 and −10 °C (−13 and 14 °F), unless otherwise specified by manufacturer.

**Preparation of dosage form**

The container should be thawed at room temperature (25 °C [77 °F]) or under refrigeration (5 °C [41 °F]) before administration, making sure that all ice crystals have melted. Thawing should not be forced by immersion in water baths or by microwave irradiation.

Do not use minibags in series connections. This may result in air embolism because of residual air being drawn from the primary container before administration of intravenous solution from the secondary container is complete.

**Stability**

After thawing, solutions retain their potency for 48 hours at room temperature or for 14 days if refrigerated at 5 °C (41 °F). Once thawed, solutions should not be refrozen.

Do not use if the solution is cloudy or contains a precipitate.

**Incompatibilities**

The admixture of cefoperazone with other medications, including pentamidine isethionate, is not recommended.

The admixture of beta-lactam antibacterials (penicillins and cephalosporins) and aminoglycosides may result in substantial mutual inactivation. If they are administered concurrently, they should be administered in separate sites. Do not mix them in the same intravenous bag or bottle.

### CEFOPERAZONE FOR INJECTION USP

**Usual adult dose**

Mild to moderate infections[1]—
  Intramuscular or intravenous, 1 to 2 grams (base) every twelve hours.
Severe infections[1]—
  Intramuscular or intravenous, 2 to 4 grams (base) every eight hours; or 3 to 6 grams every twelve hours.
Note: Adults with impaired hepatic function and/or biliary obstruction should not receive more than 4 grams (base) per day.
  Adults with combined hepatic and renal function impairment should not receive more than 1 to 2 grams (base) per day.
  In patients who are receiving hemodialysis treatments, a dose should be administered following hemodialysis.

**Usual adult prescribing limits**

See *Cefoperazone Injection USP*.

**Usual pediatric dose**

See *Cefoperazone Injection USP*.

**Usual geriatric dose**

See *Usual adult and adolescent dose*.

**Strength(s) usually available**

U.S.—
  1 gram (base) (Rx) [*Cefobid* (sodium 1.5 mEq per gram)].
  2 grams (base) (Rx) [*Cefobid* (sodium 1.5 mEq per gram)].
  10 grams (base) (Rx) [*Cefobid* (sodium 1.5 mEq per gram)].
Canada—
  Not commercially available.

**Packaging and storage**

Prior to reconstitution, store below 40 °C (104 °F), preferably between 15 and 30 °C (59 and 86 °F), unless otherwise specified by manufacturer. Protect from light.

**Preparation of dosage form**

To prepare initial dilution for intramuscular use resulting in final concentrations of less than 250 mg per mL, any suitable diluent (see manufacturer's package insert) may be used.

To prepare initial dilution for intramuscular use resulting in final concentrations of 250 mg per mL, 2.8 mL of sterile water for injection should be added to each 1-gram vial and shaken well until dissolution is complete. Then 1 mL of 2% lidocaine hydrochloride injection (without epinephrine) should be added and mixed well. Add 5.4 mL of sterile water for injection and 1.8 mL of 2% lidocaine hydrochloride injection to each 2-gram vial in the above manner. When a diluent other than lidocaine hydrochloride injection is used, follow the manufacturer's labeling instructions.

To prepare initial dilution for intramuscular use resulting in final concentrations of 333 mg per mL, 2 mL of sterile water for injection should be added to each 1-gram vial and shaken well until dissolution is complete. Then 0.6 mL of 2% lidocaine hydrochloride injection (without epinephrine) should be added and mixed well. Add 3.8 mL of sterile water for injection and 1.2 mL of 2% lidocaine hydrochloride injection to each 2-gram vial in the above manner. When a diluent other than lidocaine hydrochloride injection is used, follow the manufacturer's labeling instructions.

To prepare initial dilution for intravenous use, a minimum of 2.8 mL (5 mL preferred) of a suitable diluent (see manufacturer's package insert) should be added for each gram of cefoperazone. For intermittent infusion, the resulting solution should be further diluted in a suitable diluent (see manufacturer's package insert) and administered over a 15- to 30-minute period. For continuous infusion, the resulting solution should be further diluted to a final concentration of 2 to 25 mg per mL.

The solution should be allowed to stand following reconstitution. This allows the foam to dissipate, thus permitting visual inspection for complete dissolution. Vigorous and prolonged shaking may be required for complete dissolution, especially at higher concentrations (> 333 mg per mL). The maximum solubility of cefoperazone is approximately 475 mg per mL of compatible diluent.

For reconstitution of piggyback infusion bottles, see manufacturer's labeling for instructions.

### Stability
After reconstitution, solutions stored in bacteriostatic water for injection containing benzyl alcohol or parabens, most dextrose-containing injections, dextrose and sodium chloride injection, lactated Ringer's injection, 0.5% lidocaine hydrochloride injection, 0.9% sodium chloride injection, or other electrolyte-containing injections (see manufacturer's package insert) at concentrations of 2 to 300 mg per mL retain their potency for 24 hours at room temperature (15 to 25 °C [59 to 77 °F]) or for 5 days if refrigerated at 2 to 8 °C (36 to 46 °F).

Solutions stored in 5% dextrose injection, or 5% dextrose and 0.2 or 0.9% sodium chloride injection at concentrations of 2 or 50 mg per mL, respectively, retain their potency for 3 weeks if frozen at −20 to −10 °C (−4 to 14 °F).

Solutions stored in 0.9% sodium chloride injection or sterile water for injection at concentrations of 300 mg per mL retain their potency for 5 weeks if frozen at −20 to −10 °C (−4 to 14 °F).

Frozen solutions should be thawed at room temperature prior to use. Once thawed, solutions should not be refrozen.

Solutions may vary in color from colorless to straw yellow, depending on concentration.

### Incompatibilities
The admixture of cefoperazone with other medications, including pentamidine isethionate, is not recommended.

The admixture of beta-lactam antibacterials (penicillins and cephalosporins) and aminoglycosides may result in substantial mutual inactivation. If they are administered concurrently, they should be administered in separate sites. Do not mix them in the same intravenous bag or bottle.

---

[1]Not included in Canadian product labeling.

---

## CEFOTAXIME

## Summary of Differences
Category: Third-generation cephalosporin.

## Additional Dosing Information
Intramuscular doses of 2 grams should be administered as divided doses in different sites.

## Parenteral Dosage Forms
Note: The dosing and strengths of the dosage forms available are expressed in terms of cefotaxime free acid.

### CEFOTAXIME INJECTION USP
**Usual adult and adolescent dose**
Perioperative prophylaxis—
  Cesarean section patients: Intravenous infusion, 1 gram (free acid) as soon as the umbilical cord is clamped; then 1 gram every six hours for a maximum of two doses.
  Other surgery patients: Intravenous infusion, 1 gram (free acid) one-half to one and one-half hours prior to the start of surgery.
Septicemia—
  Intravenous infusion, 2 grams (free acid) every six to eight hours.
For all other infections—
  Uncomplicated: Intravenous infusion, 1 gram (free acid) every twelve hours.
  Moderate to severe: Intravenous infusion, 1 to 2 grams (free acid) every eight hours.
  Life-threatening: Intravenous infusion, 2 grams (free acid) every four hours.
Note: For patients with renal function impairment (< 20 mL per minute), one half the *Usual adult and adolescent dose* should be used at the same dosing intervals given above.

**Usual adult prescribing limits**
12 grams (free acid) per day.

**Usual pediatric dose**
Antibacterial—
  Neonates up to 1 week of age: Intravenous infusion, 50 mg (free acid) per kg of body weight every twelve hours.
  Neonates 1 to 4 weeks of age: Intravenous infusion, 50 mg (free acid) per kg of body weight every eight hours.
  Infants and children 1 month of age and older up to 50 kg of body weight: Intravenous infusion, 8.3 to 30 mg (free acid) per kg of body weight every four hours; or 12.5 to 45 mg per kg of body weight every six hours.
  Children 50 kg of body weight and over: See *Usual adult and adolescent dose*.

**Usual pediatric prescribing limits**
Infants and children up to 50 kg of body weight should not exceed 180 mg (free acid) per kg of body weight per day.
Children 50 kg of body weight and over should not exceed 12 grams (free acid) per day.

**Usual geriatric dose**
See *Usual adult and adolescent dose*.

**Strength(s) usually available**
U.S.—
  1 gram (free acid) in 50 mL (Rx) [*Claforan* (sodium 2.2 mEq per gram)].
  2 grams (free acid) in 50 mL (Rx) [*Claforan* (sodium 2.2 mEq per gram)].
Canada—
  Not commercially available.

**Packaging and storage**
Store between −25 and −10 °C (−13 and 14 °F), unless otherwise specified by manufacturer.

**Preparation of dosage form**
The container should be thawed at room temperature or under refrigeration (at or below 5 °C [41 °F]) before administration, making sure that all ice crystals have melted. Thawing should not be forced by immersion in water baths or by microwave irradiation.
Do not use minibags in series connections. This may result in air embolism because of residual air being drawn from the primary container before administration of intravenous solution from the secondary container is complete.

**Stability**
After thawing, solutions retain their potency for 24 hours at room temperature (22 °C [72 °F]) or for 10 days if refrigerated at 5 °C (41 °F). Once thawed, solutions should not be refrozen.
Do not use if the solution is cloudy or contains a precipitate.

**Incompatibilities**
The admixture of cefotaxime with other medications, including pentamidine isethionate, is not recommended.
The admixture of beta-lactam antibacterials (penicillins and cephalosporins) and aminoglycosides may result in substantial mutual inactivation. If they are administered concurrently, they should be administered in separate sites. Do not mix them in the same intravenous bag or bottle.

### CEFOTAXIME FOR INJECTION USP
**Usual adult and adolescent dose**
Gonorrhea, cervical or urethral or
Gonorrhea, rectal, in females—
  Intramuscular, 500 mg (free acid) as a single dose.
Gonorrhea, rectal, in males—
  Intramuscular, 1 gram (free acid) as a single dose.
Perioperative prophylaxis—
  Cesarean section patients: Intravenous, 1 gram (free acid) as soon as the umbilical cord is clamped; then 1 gram, intramuscularly or intravenously, every six hours for a maximum of two doses.
  Other surgery patients: Intramuscular or intravenous, 1 gram (free acid) one-half to one and one-half hours prior to the start of surgery.

Septicemia—
    Intravenous, 2 grams (free acid) every six to eight hours.
For all other infections—
    Uncomplicated: Intramuscular or intravenous, 1 gram (free acid) every twelve hours.
    Moderate to severe: Intramuscular or intravenous, 1 to 2 grams (free acid) every eight hours.
    Life-threatening: Intravenous, 2 grams (free acid) every four hours.
Note: For patients with renal function impairment (< 20 mL per minute), one half the *Usual adult and adolescent dose* should be used at the same dosing interval given above.

### Usual adult prescribing limits
See *Cefotaxime Injection USP*.

### Usual pediatric dose
For bacterial infections—
    Neonates up to 1 week of age: Intravenous, 50 mg (free acid) per kg of body weight every twelve hours.
    Neonates 1 to 4 weeks of age: Intravenous, 50 mg (free acid) per kg of body weight every eight hours.
    Infants and children 1 month of age and older up to 50 kg of body weight: Intramuscular or intravenous, 8.3 to 30 mg (free acid) per kg of body weight every four hours; or 12.5 to 45 mg per kg of body weight every six hours.
    Children 50 kg of body weight and over: See *Usual adult and adolescent dose*.

### Usual pediatric prescribing limits
See *Cefotaxime Injection USP*.

### Usual geriatric dose
See *Usual adult and adolescent dose*.

### Strength(s) usually available
U.S.—
    500 mg (free acid) (Rx) [*Claforan* (sodium 2.2 mEq per gram)].
    1 gram (free acid) (available in ADD-Vantage® vials) (Rx) [*Claforan* (sodium 2.2 mEq per gram)].
    2 grams (free acid) (available in ADD-Vantage® vials) (Rx) [*Claforan* (sodium 2.2 mEq per gram)].
    10 grams (free acid) (Rx) [*Claforan* (sodium 2.2 mEq per gram)].
Canada—
    500 mg (free acid) (Rx) [*Claforan*].
    1 gram (free acid) (also available in ADD-Vantage® vials) (Rx) [*Claforan*].
    2 grams (free acid) (Rx) [*Claforan*].

### Packaging and storage
Prior to reconstitution, store below 30 °C (86 °F), preferably between 15 and 30 °C (59 and 86 °F). Protect from excessive light.

### Preparation of dosage form
To prepare initial dilution for intramuscular use, 2, 3, or 5 mL of sterile water for injection or bacteriostatic water for injection should be added to each 500-mg, 1-gram, or 2-gram vial, respectively.
To prepare initial dilution for intravenous use, 10 mL of sterile water for injection should be added to each 500-mg, 1-gram, or 2-gram vial. For direct intravenous use, the resulting solution should be administered over a 3- to 5-minute period.
For reconstitution of piggyback infusion bottles or pharmacy bulk vials, see manufacturer's labeling for instructions.
Caution—Use of diluents containing benzyl alcohol is not recommended for preparation of medications for use in neonates. A fatal toxic syndrome consisting of metabolic acidosis, central nervous system (CNS) depression, respiratory problems, renal failure, hypotension, and possibly seizures and intracranial hemorrhages has been associated with this use.

### Stability
After reconstitution for intramuscular use, solutions retain at least 90% of their potency for 12 hours at room temperature (22 °C [72 °F]), for at least 5 days in plastic syringes or 7 days in the original container if refrigerated (5 °C [41 °F]), or for 13 weeks if frozen.
After reconstitution for intravenous use, solutions retain at least 90% of their potency for 12 hours (2-gram vial) or for 24 hours (500-mg and 1-gram vials) at room temperature, for at least 5 days in plastic syringes or 7 days in the original container if refrigerated, or for 13 weeks in plastic syringes or the original container if frozen. Reconstituted solutions further diluted up to 1000 mL in suitable diluents (see manufacturer's package insert) retain their potency for 24 hours at room temperature or for at least 5 days if refrigerated.
Frozen solutions should be thawed at room temperature before use. Once thawed, solutions should not be refrozen.
Reconstituted solutions exhibit maximum stability at pH 5 to 7. Therefore, sterile cefotaxime sodium should not be reconstituted with diluents having a pH above 7.5 (e.g., sodium bicarbonate injection).
Solutions range in color from pale yellow to light amber, depending on the concentration and diluent used. However, solutions tend to darken during storage. This does not affect their potency when stored per manufacturer's recommendations.

### Incompatibilities
The admixture of cefotaxime with other medications, including pentamidine isethionate, is not recommended.
The admixture of beta-lactam antibacterials (penicillins and cephalosporins) and aminoglycosides may result in substantial mutual inactivation. If they are administered concurrently, they should be administered in separate sites. Do not mix them in the same intravenous bag or bottle.

### Additional information
A solution containing 1 gram in 14 mL of sterile water for injection is isotonic.

---

## CEFOTETAN

### Summary of Differences
Category: Cephamycin; second-generation cephalosporin.
Indications: Good activity against anaerobic organisms.
Pharmacology/pharmacokinetics: Contains *N*-methylthiotetrazole (NMTT) side chain.
Precautions:
    Drug interactions and/or related problems—Interacts with alcohol (disulfiram-like reaction), oral anticoagulants, and other medications that affect blood clotting.
    Laboratory value alterations—May falsely elevate serum and urine creatinine concentrations when Jaffe's reaction method is used.
    Medical considerations/contraindications—Caution required in patients with history of bleeding problems.
    Patient monitoring—PT determinations may be required.
Side/adverse effects: May cause unusual bleeding or bruising.

### Parenteral Dosage Forms
Note: The dosing and strengths of the dosage forms available are expressed in terms of cefotetan base (not the disodium salt).

### CEFOTETAN INJECTION
Note: Cefotetan injection should be administered over a period of 20 to 60 minutes.

### Usual adult and adolescent dose
Perioperative prophylaxis—
    Cesarean section patients: Intravenous infusion, 1 or 2 grams (base) as soon as the umbilical cord is clamped.
    Other surgical patients: Intravenous infusion, 1 or 2 grams (base) one-half to one hour prior to the start of surgery.
Skin and soft tissue infections—
    Mild to moderate, due to *Klebsiella pneumoniae*: Intravenous infusion, 1 or 2 grams (base) every twelve hours for five to ten days.
    Mild to moderate, due to other organisms: Intravenous infusion, 1 gram (base) every twelve hours for five to ten days; or 2 grams every twenty-four hours for five to ten days.
    Severe: Intravenous infusion, 2 grams (base) every twelve hours for five to ten days.
Urinary tract infections—
    Intravenous infusion, 500 mg (base) every twelve hours for five to ten days; or 1 or 2 grams every twelve or twenty-four hours for five to ten days.
For all other infections—
    Mild to moderate: Intravenous infusion, 1 or 2 grams (base) every twelve hours for five to ten days.
    Severe: Intravenous infusion, 2 grams (base) every twelve hours for five to ten days.
    Life-threatening: Intravenous infusion, 3 grams (base) every twelve hours for five to ten days.

Note: Adults with renal function impairment may require a reduction in dose as follows:

| Creatinine clearance (mL/min)/(mL/sec) | Dose (base) determined by type and severity of infection |
|---|---|
| > 30/0.5 | See *Usual adult and adolescent dose* |
| 10–30/0.17–0.5 | Usual adult dose every 24 hours; or one half the usual adult dose every 12 hours |
| < 10/0.17 | Usual adult dose every 48 hours; or one fourth the usual adult dose every 12 hours |
| Hemodialysis patients | One fourth the usual adult dose every 24 hours on the days between hemodialysis sessions; and one half the usual adult dose on the day of hemodialysis |

**Usual adult prescribing limits**
6 grams (base) per day.

**Usual pediatric dose**
Safety and efficacy have not been established.

**Usual geriatric dose**
See *Usual adult and adolescent dose*.

**Strength(s) usually available**
U.S.—
   1 gram (base) in 50 mL [*Cefotan* (sodium 3.5 mEq per gram)].
   2 grams (base) in 50 mL [*Cefotan* (sodium 3.5 mEq per gram)].
Canada—
   Not commercially available.

**Packaging and storage**
Store at −20 °C (−4 °F).

**Preparation of dosage form**
The container should be thawed at room temperature (25 °C [77 °F]) or under refrigeration (5 °C [41 °F]) before administration. Thawing should not be forced by immersion in water baths or microwave irradiation.

Do not use minibags in series connections. This may result in air embolism because of residual air being drawn from the primary container before administration of intravenous solution from the secondary container is complete.

**Stability**
After thawing, solutions retain their potency for 48 hours at room temperature, or for 21 days if refrigerated. Once thawed, solutions should not be refrozen.

Do not use if the solution is cloudy or contains a precipitate.

**Incompatibilities**
The admixture of beta-lactam antibacterials (penicillins and cephalosporins) and aminoglycosides may result in substantial mutual inactivation. If they are administered concurrently, they should be administered in separate sites. Do not mix them in the same intravenous bag or bottle.

## CEFOTETAN FOR INJECTION USP

**Usual adult and adolescent dose**
Perioperative prophylaxis—
   Cesarean section patients: Intravenous, 1 or 2 grams (base) as soon as the umbilical cord is clamped.
   Other surgical patients: Intravenous, 1 or 2 grams (base) one-half to one hour prior to the start of surgery.
Skin and soft tissue infections—
   Mild to moderate, due to *Klebsiella pneumoniae*: Intramuscular or intravenous, 1 or 2 grams (base) every twelve hours for five to ten days.
   Mild to moderate, due to other organisms: Intramuscular or intravenous, 1 gram (base) every twelve hours for five to ten days; or 2 grams, intravenously, every twenty-four hours for five to ten days.
   Severe: Intravenous, 2 grams (base) every twelve hours for five to ten days.
Urinary tract infections—
   Intramuscular or intravenous, 500 mg (base) every twelve hours, or 1 or 2 grams every twelve or twenty-four hours, for five to ten days.
For all other infections—
   Mild to moderate: Intramuscular or intravenous, 1 or 2 grams (base) every twelve hours for five to ten days.
   Severe: Intravenous, 2 grams (base) every twelve hours for five to ten days.
   Life-threatening: Intravenous, 3 grams (base) every twelve hours for five to ten days.

Note: Adults with renal function impairment may require a reduction in dose. See *Cefotetan Injection*.

**Usual adult prescribing limits**
See *Cefotetan Injection*.

**Usual pediatric dose**
Safety and efficacy have not been established.

**Usual geriatric dose**
See *Usual adult and adolescent dose*.

**Strength(s) usually available**
U.S.—
   1 gram (base) (available in ADD-Vantage® vials) (Rx) [*Cefotan* (sodium 3.5 mEq per gram)].
   2 grams (base) (available in ADD-Vantage® vials) (Rx) [*Cefotan* (sodium 3.5 mEq per gram)].
   10 grams (base) (Rx) [*Cefotan* (sodium 3.5 mEq per gram)].
Canada—
   1 gram (base) (Rx) [*Cefotan* (sodium 3.4 mEq per gram)].
   2 grams (base) (Rx) [*Cefotan* (sodium 3.4 mEq per gram)].

**Packaging and storage**
Prior to reconstitution, do not store above 22 °C (72 °F), unless otherwise specified by manufacturer. Protect from light.

**Preparation of dosage form**
To prepare initial dilution for intramuscular use, 2 mL of sterile water for injection, bacteriostatic water for injection, 0.9% sodium chloride injection, or 0.5 or 1% lidocaine hydrochloride injection (without epinephrine) should be added to each 1-gram vial, or 3 mL of diluent should be added to each 2-gram vial.

To prepare initial dilution for intravenous use, 10 mL of sterile water for injection should be added to each 1-gram vial, or 10 to 20 mL of diluent should be added to each 2-gram vial. For direct intermittent intravenous use, the resulting solution should be administered over a 3- to 5-minute period.

For reconstitution of piggyback infusion bottles, add 50 to 100 mL of 5% dextrose injection or 0.9% sodium chloride injection to each bottle. If the Y-type method of administration is used, the primary infusion should be temporarily discontinued during infusion of cefotetan.

For reconstitution of ADD-Vantage® vials, see manufacturer's package labeling for instructions.

**Stability**
After reconstitution for intramuscular or intravenous use, solutions retain their potency for 24 hours at room temperature (25 °C [77 °F]), for 96 hours if refrigerated at 5 °C (41 °F), or for at least 1 week if frozen at −20 °C (−4 °F). Solutions stored in disposable glass or plastic syringes retain their potency for 24 hours at room temperature or for 96 hours if refrigerated.

Frozen solutions should be thawed at room temperature prior to use. Thawed solutions retain their potency for the time periods indicated above. Once thawed, solutions should not be refrozen.

After reconstitution of ADD-Vantage® vials, solutions retain their potency for 24 hours at room temperature. Solutions in ADD-Vantage® vials should not be refrigerated or frozen.

Solutions range from colorless to yellow in color, depending on the concentration.

**Incompatibilities**
The admixture of beta-lactam antibacterials (penicillins and cephalosporins) and aminoglycosides may result in substantial mutual inactivation. If they are administered concurrently, they should be administered in separate sites. Do not mix them in the same intravenous bag or bottle.

## CEFOXITIN

## Summary of Differences
Category: Cephamycin; second-generation cephalosporin.
Indications: Good activity against anaerobic organisms.
Precautions:
   Pediatrics—Higher doses associated with increased incidence of eosinophilia and elevated AST (SGOT).
   Laboratory value alterations—May falsely elevate serum and urine creatinine concentrations when Jaffe's reaction method is used.

## Parenteral Dosage Forms
Note: The dose and strengths of the dosage forms available are expressed in terms of cefoxitin base (not the sodium salt).

## CEFOXITIN INJECTION USP

### Usual adult and adolescent dose
Mild or uncomplicated infections—
  Intravenous, 1 gram (base) every six to eight hours.
Moderately severe or severe infections—
  Intravenous, 1 gram (base) every four hours; or 2 grams every six to eight hours.
Life-threatening infections—
  Intravenous, 2 grams (base) every four hours; or 3 grams every six hours.
Perioperative prophylaxis—
  Cesarean section patients: Intravenous, 2 grams (base) as soon as the umbilical cord is clamped; or 2 grams as soon as the umbilical cord is clamped, and 2 grams four and eight hours after the first dose.
  Other surgical patients: Intravenous, 2 grams (base) one-half to one hour prior to the start of surgery, and 2 grams every six hours after the first dose for up to twenty-four hours.
Note: After an initial loading dose of 1 to 2 grams (base), adults with impaired renal function may require a reduction in dose as follows:

| Creatinine clearance (mL/min)/(mL/sec) | Dose (base) |
| --- | --- |
| > 50/0.83 | See *Usual adult and adolescent dose* |
| 30–50/0.5–0.83 | 1–2 grams every 8–12 hours |
| 10–29/0.17–0.48 | 1–2 grams every 12–24 hours |
| 5–9/0.08–0.15 | 500 mg–1 gram every 12–24 hours |
| < 5/0.08 | 500 mg–1 gram every 24–48 hours |

### Usual pediatric dose
Perioperative prophylaxis—
  Intravenous infusion, 30 to 40 mg (base) per kg of body weight one-half to one hour prior to the start of surgery; and 30 to 40 mg per kg of body weight every six hours after the first dose for up to twenty-four hours.
For all other infections—
  Infants and children 3 months of age and older: Intravenous infusion, 13.3 to 26.7 mg (base) per kg of body weight every four hours; or 20 to 40 mg per kg of body weight every six hours.
  Infants 1 to 3 months of age: Intravenous infusion, 20 to 40 mg (base) per kg of body weight every six to eight hours.
  Infants 1 to 4 weeks of age: Intravenous infusion, 20 to 40 mg (base) per kg of body weight every eight hours.
  Premature infants weighing 1500 grams or over to neonates up to 1 week of age: Intravenous infusion, 20 to 40 mg (base) per kg of body weight every twelve hours.
Note: Pediatric patients with renal function impairment should receive a modified dose and a modified frequency of dosing consistent with the recommendations for adults. See *Usual adult and adolescent dose*.

### Usual pediatric prescribing limits
12 grams (base) per day.

### Usual geriatric dose
See *Usual adult and adolescent dose*.

### Usual geriatric prescribing limits
2 grams (base) every eight hours for patients older than seventy-five years of age, even if serum creatinine concentrations are normal.

### Strength(s) usually available
U.S.—
  1 gram in 50 mL (Rx) [*Mefoxin* (sodium 2.3 mEq per gram)].
  2 grams in 50 mL (Rx) [*Mefoxin* (sodium 2.3 mEq per gram)].
Canada—
  Not commercially available.

### Packaging and storage
Store between −25 and −10 °C (−13 and 14 °F), unless otherwise specified by manufacturer.

### Preparation of dosage form
The container should be thawed at room temperature (25 °C [77 °F]) or under refrigeration (2 to 8 °C [36 to 46 °F]) before administration, making sure that all ice crystals have melted. Thawing should not be forced by immersion in water baths or by microwave irradiation.
Do not use minibags in series connections. This may result in air embolism because of residual air being drawn from the primary container before administration of intravenous solution from the secondary container is complete.

### Stability
After thawing, solutions retain their potency for 24 hours at room temperature or for 21 days if refrigerated at 2 to 8 °C (36 to 46 °F). Once thawed, solutions should not be refrozen.
Do not use if the solution is cloudy or contains a precipitate.

### Incompatibilities
The admixture of cefoxitin with other medications, including pentamidine isethionate, is not recommended.
The admixture of beta-lactam antibacterials (penicillins and cephalosporins) and aminoglycosides may result in substantial mutual inactivation. If they are administered concurrently, they should be administered in separate sites. Do not mix them in the same intravenous bag or bottle.

## CEFOXITIN FOR INJECTION USP

### Usual adult and adolescent dose
See *Cefoxitin Injection USP*.

### Usual pediatric dose
See *Cefoxitin Injection USP*.

### Usual pediatric prescribing limits
See *Cefoxitin Injection USP*.

### Usual geriatric dose
See *Cefoxitin Injection USP*.

### Usual geriatric prescribing limits
See *Cefoxitin Injection USP*.

### Strength(s) usually available
U.S.—
  1 gram (available in ADD-Vantage® vials) (Rx) [*Mefoxin* (sodium 2.3 mEq per gram)].
  2 grams (available in ADD-Vantage® vials) (Rx) [*Mefoxin* (sodium 2.3 mEq per gram)].
  10 grams (Rx) [*Mefoxin* (sodium 2.3 mEq per gram)].
Canada—
  1 gram (also may be available in ADD-Vantage® vials) (Rx) [*Mefoxin* (sodium 2.3 mEq per gram); GENERIC].
  2 grams (also may be available in ADD-Vantage® vials) (Rx) [*Mefoxin* (sodium 2.3 mEq per gram); GENERIC].
  10 grams (Rx) [*Mefoxin* (sodium 2.3 mEq per gram)].

### Packaging and storage
Prior to reconstitution, store below 40 °C (104 °F), preferably between 15 and 30 °C (59 and 86 °F), unless otherwise specified by manufacturer.

### Preparation of dosage form
To prepare initial dilution for intravenous use, at least 10 mL of sterile water for injection, bacteriostatic water for injection, 0.9% sodium chloride injection, or 5% dextrose injection should be added to each 1-gram vial, or 10 or 20 mL of diluent should be added to each 2-gram vial. For continuous intravenous infusion, the resulting solution may be further diluted in 50 to 1000 mL of suitable diluent (see manufacturer's package insert).
To prepare initial dilution for direct intermittent intravenous use, 10 mL of sterile water for injection should be added to each 1- or 2-gram vial. The resulting solution should be administered over a 3- to 5-minute period.
For reconstitution of piggyback infusion bottles or pharmacy bulk vials, see manufacturer's labeling for instructions.
Caution—Use of diluents containing benzyl alcohol is not recommended for preparation of medications for use in neonates. A fatal toxic syndrome consisting of metabolic acidosis, CNS depression, respiratory problems, renal failure, hypotension, and possibly seizures and intracranial hemorrhages has been associated with this use.

### Stability
After reconstitution for intravenous use to a concentration of 1 gram per 10 mL with sterile water for injection, bacteriostatic water for injection, 0.9% sodium chloride injection, or 5% dextrose injection, solutions retain their potency for 6 hours at room temperature, or for 7 days if refrigerated (below 5 °C). Initial dilutions retain their potency for an additional 18 hours at room temperature or for an additional 48 hours if refrigerated when diluted in 50 to 1000 mL of suitable diluents (see manufacturer's package insert).
Solutions range from clear to light amber in color but tend to darken depending on storage conditions. This does not affect their potency.

### Incompatibilities
The admixture of cefoxitin with other medications, including pentamidine isethionate, is not recommended.
The admixture of beta-lactam antibacterials (penicillins and cephalosporins) and aminoglycosides may result in substantial mutual inactivation. If they are administered concurrently, they should be administered in separate sites. Do not mix them in the same intravenous bag or bottle.

## CEFPODOXIME

### Summary of Differences
Category: Third-generation cephalosporin, with broad *in vitro* activity. One of three oral third-generation cephalosporins.
Precautions:
  Drug interactions and/or related problems—Interacts with antacids and histamine $H_2$-receptor antagonists.

### Additional Dosing Information
The tablet dosage form should be taken with food.

The oral suspension dosage form may be taken with or without food.

### Oral Dosage Forms
Note: The dosing and strengths of the dosage forms available are expressed in terms of cefpodoxime base (not the proxetil salt).

#### CEFPODOXIME PROXETIL FOR ORAL SUSPENSION
**Usual adult and adolescent dose**
Gonorrhea, cervical[1] or urethral[1] or
Gonorrhea, rectal, in women[1]—
  Oral, 200 mg (base) as a single dose.
Pharyngitis[1] or
Tonsillitis[1]—
  Oral, 100 mg (base) every twelve hours for five to ten days.
Pneumonia, community-acquired[1]—
  Oral, 200 mg (base) every twelve hours for fourteen days.
Skin and soft tissue infections[1]—
  Oral, 400 mg (base) every twelve hours for seven to fourteen days.
Urinary tract infections, uncomplicated[1]—
  Oral, 100 mg (base) every twelve hours for seven days.
Note: Adults with renal function impairment may require a reduction in dose as follows:

| Creatinine clearance (mL/min)/(mL/sec) | Dosing interval |
|---|---|
| ≥ 30/0.5 | Every 12 hours |
| <30/0.5 | Every 24 hours |
| Hemodialysis patients | 3 times a week after hemodialysis |

**Usual pediatric dose**
Otitis media[1]—
  Infants and children 5 months to 12 years of age: Oral, 10 mg (base) per kg of body weight, up to 400 mg, every twenty-four hours for ten days; or 5 mg per kg of body weight, up to 200 mg, every twelve hours for ten days.
  Infants up to 5 months of age: Safety and efficacy have not been established.
Pharyngitis[1] or
Tonsillitis[1]—
  Infants and children 5 months to 12 years of age: Oral, 5 mg (base) per kg of body weight, up to 100 mg, every twelve hours for five to ten days.
  Infants up to 5 months of age: Safety and efficacy have not been established.

**Usual pediatric prescribing limits**
For otitis media, 400 mg per day. For pharyngitis or tonsillitis, 200 mg per day.

**Usual geriatric dose**
See *Usual adult and adolescent dose*.

**Strength(s) usually available**
U.S.—
  50 mg (base) per 5 mL (when reconstituted according to manufacturer's instructions) (available in 50-, 75-, and 100-mL bottles) (Rx) [*Vantin* (lactose; sodium benzoate; sucrose)].
  100 mg (base) per 5 mL (when reconstituted according to manufacturer's instructions) (available in 50-, 75-, and 100-mL bottles) (Rx) [*Vantin* (lactose; sodium benzoate; sucrose)].
Canada—
  Not commercially available.

**Packaging and storage**
Prior to reconstitution, store between 15 and 30 °C (59 and 86 °F), unless otherwise specified by manufacturer. Store in a tight container.

**Preparation of dosage form**
The bottle should be tapped to loosen the granules. The total volume of water should be added in two portions, shaking well after each addition.

| Final concentration | Bottle size | Total volume of water to be added |
|---|---|---|
| 50 mg/5 mL | 100 mL | 58 mL |
|  | 75 mL | 44 mL |
|  | 50 mL | 29 mL |
| 100 mg/5 mL | 100 mL | 57 mL |
|  | 75 mL | 43 mL |
|  | 50 mL | 29 mL |

**Stability**
After reconstitution, suspension retains its potency for 14 days if refrigerated at 2 to 8 °C (36 to 46 °F).

**Auxiliary labeling**
• Refrigerate.
• Shake well.
• May be taken with or without food.
• Continue medicine for full time of treatment.
• Beyond-use date.

**Note**
When dispensing, include a calibrated liquid-measuring device.

#### CEFPODOXIME PROXETIL TABLETS
**Usual adult and adolescent dose**
Bronchitis, bacterial exacerbations[1]—
  Oral, 200 mg (base) every twelve hours for ten days.
Gonorrhea, cervical[1] or urethral[1] or
Gonorrhea, rectal, in women[1]—
  Oral, 200 mg (base) as a single dose.
Pharyngitis[1] or
Tonsillitis[1]—
  Oral, 100 mg (base) every twelve hours for five to ten days.
Pneumonia, community-acquired[1]—
  Oral, 200 mg (base) every twelve hours for fourteen days.
Skin and soft tissue infections[1]—
  Oral, 400 mg (base) every twelve hours for seven to fourteen days.
Urinary tract infections, uncomplicated[1]—
  Oral, 100 mg (base) every twelve hours for seven days.

**Usual pediatric dose**
This dosage form usually is not used for children. See *Cefpodoxime Proxetil for Oral Suspension*.

**Usual geriatric dose**
See *Usual adult and adolescent dose*.

**Strength(s) usually available**
U.S.—
  100 mg (base) (Rx) [*Vantin* (lactose)].
  200 mg (base) (Rx) [*Vantin* (lactose)].
Canada—
  Not commercially available.

**Packaging and storage**
Store between 15 and 30 °C (59 and 86 °F), unless otherwise specified by manufacturer. Store in a tight container.

**Auxiliary labeling**
• Continue medicine for full time of treatment.
• Take with food.

[1]Not included in Canadian product labeling.

## CEFPROZIL

### Summary of Differences
Category: Second-generation cephalosporin, with broad *in vitro* activity.
Precautions:
  Medical considerations/contraindications—Cefprozil for oral solution contains 28 mg of phenylalanine per 5 mL.

### Oral Dosage Forms
Note: Bracketed uses in the *Dosage Forms* section refer to categories of use and/or indications that are not included in U.S. product labeling.

#### CEFPROZIL FOR ORAL SUSPENSION USP
**Usual adult and adolescent dose**
Bronchitis[1] or
Bronchitis, bacterial exacerbations[1]—
  Oral, 500 mg every twelve hours for ten days.
Pharyngitis or
Tonsillitis—
  Oral, 500 mg every twenty-four hours for ten days.

Sinusitis, acute—
  Oral, 250 or 500 mg every twelve hours for ten days.
Skin and soft tissue infections—
  Oral, 250 or 500 mg every twelve hours for ten days; or 500 mg every twenty-four hours for ten days.
[Urinary tract infections, uncomplicated]—
  Oral, 500 mg every twenty-four hours.
Note: Adults with renal function impairment may require a reduction in dose as follows:

| Creatinine clearance (mL/min)/(mL/sec) | Usual dose (%) |
|---|---|
| ≥ 30/0.5 | 100 |
| 0–30/0–0.5 | 50 |
| Hemodialysis patients | 100, after hemodialysis |

**Usual pediatric dose**
Otitis media—
  Infants and children 6 months to 12 years of age: Oral, 15 mg per kg of body weight every twelve hours for ten days.
  Infants up to 6 months of age: Safety and efficacy have not been established.
Pharyngitis or
Tonsillitis—
  Children 2 to 12 years of age: Oral, 7.5 mg per kg of body weight every twelve hours for ten days.
  Infants and children up to 2 years of age: Safety and efficacy have not been established.
Sinusitis, acute—
  Infants and children 6 months to 12 years of age: Oral, 7.5 or 15 mg per kg of body weight every twelve hours for ten days.
  Infants up to 6 months of age: Safety and efficacy have not been established.
Skin and soft tissue infections—
  Children 2 to 12 years of age: Oral, 20 mg per kg of body weight every twenty-four hours for ten days.
  Infants and children up to 2 years of age: Safety and efficacy have not been established.

**Usual pediatric prescribing limits**
1 gram per day.

**Usual geriatric dose**
See *Usual adult and adolescent dose*.

**Strength(s) usually available**
U.S.—
  125 mg per 5 mL (when reconstituted according to manufacturer's instructions) (available in 50-, 75-, and 100-mL bottles) (Rx) [*Cefzil* (phenylalanine 28 mg per 5 mL; sodium benzoate; sodium chloride; sucrose)].
  250 mg per 5 mL (when reconstituted according to manufacturer's instructions) (available in 50-, 75-, and 100-mL bottles) (Rx) [*Cefzil* (phenylalanine 28 mg per 5 mL; sodium benzoate; sodium chloride; sucrose)].
Canada—
  125 mg per 5 mL (when reconstituted according to manufacturer's instructions) (available in 75- and 100-mL bottles) (Rx) [*Cefzil* (phenylalanine 28 mg per 5 mL; sodium benzoate; sodium chloride; sucrose)].
  250 mg per 5 mL (when reconstituted according to manufacturer's instructions) (available in 75- and 100-mL bottles) (Rx) [*Cefzil* (phenylalanine 28 mg per 5 mL; sodium benzoate; sodium chloride; sucrose)].

**Packaging and storage**
Prior to reconstitution, store between 15 and 30 °C (59 and 86 °F), unless otherwise specified by manufacturer. Store in a tight container.

**Preparation of dosage form**
The bottle should be tapped to loosen the granules. The total volume of water indicated below should be added in two portions, shaking well after each addition.

| Bottle size | Total volume of water to be added |
|---|---|
| 50 mL | 36 mL |
| 75 mL | 54 mL |
| 100 mL | 72 mL |

**Stability**
After reconstitution, suspension retains its potency for 14 days if refrigerated.

**Auxiliary labeling**
• Refrigerate.
• Shake well.
• Continue medicine for full time of treatment.
• Beyond-use date.

**Note**
When dispensing, include a calibrated liquid-measuring device.

## CEFPROZIL TABLETS USP

**Usual adult and adolescent dose**
See *Cefprozil for Oral Suspension USP*.

**Usual pediatric dose**
See *Cefprozil for Oral Suspension USP*.

**Usual pediatric prescribing limits**
See *Cefprozil for Oral Suspension USP*.

**Usual geriatric dose**
See *Cefprozil for Oral Suspension USP*

**Strength(s) usually available**
U.S.—
  250 mg (Rx) [*Cefzil*].
  500 mg (Rx) [*Cefzil*].
Canada—
  250 mg (Rx) [*Cefzil*].
  500 mg (Rx) [*Cefzil*].

**Packaging and storage**
Store between 15 and 30 °C (59 and 86 °F), unless otherwise specified by manufacturer. Store in a tight container.

**Auxiliary labeling**
• Continue medicine for full time of treatment.

---

[1]Not included in Canadian product labeling.

---

## CEFTAZIDIME

## Summary of Differences
Category: Third-generation cephalosporin.
Indications: Good activity against *Pseudomonas aeruginosa*.
Precautions:
  Drug interactions and/or related problems—Does not interact with probenecid.

## Additional Dosing Information
Patients with impaired hepatic function do not require a reduction in dose.

## Parenteral Dosage Forms
Note: The dosing and strengths of the dosage form available are expressed in terms of ceftazidime base (not the sodium salt).

## CEFTAZIDIME INJECTION USP

**Usual adult and adolescent dose**
Bone and joint infections—
  Intravenous infusion, 2 grams (base) every twelve hours.
Intra-abdominal infections or
Meningitis or
Pelvic infections, female[1] or
Septicemia—
  Intravenous infusion, 2 grams (base) every eight hours.
Pneumonia, uncomplicated or
Skin and soft tissue infections—
  Intravenous infusion, 500 mg to 1 gram (base) every eight hours.
Pulmonary infections in cystic fibrosis, due to *Pseudomonas*[1]—
  Intravenous infusion, 30 to 50 mg (base) per kg of body weight every eight hours, up to 6 grams per day.
Urinary tract infections, complicated—
  Intravenous infusion, 500 mg (base) every eight to twelve hours.
Urinary tract infections, uncomplicated—
  Intravenous infusion, 250 mg (base) every twelve hours.
For all other infections, severe to life-threatening, especially in immunocompromised patients—
  Intravenous infusion, 2 grams (base) every eight hours.

## 814  Cephalosporins (Systemic)

Note: After an initial loading dose of 1 gram, adults with impaired renal function (including dialysis patients) may require a reduction in dose as follows:

| Creatinine clearance (mL/min)/(mL/sec) | Dose (base) |
|---|---|
| > 50/0.83 | See *Usual adult and adolescent dose* |
| 31–50/0.52–0.83 | 1 gram every 12 hours |
| 16–30/0.27–0.5 | 1 gram every 24 hours |
| 6–15/0.1–0.25 | 500 mg every 24 hours |
| < 5/0.08 | 500 mg every 48 hours |
| Hemodialysis patients | 1 gram after each hemodialysis period |
| Peritoneal dialysis patients | 500 mg every 24 hours |

**Usual pediatric dose**
For bacterial infections—
  Neonates up to 4 weeks of age: Intravenous infusion, 30 mg (base) per kg of body weight every twelve hours.
  Infants and children 1 month to 12 years of age: Intravenous infusion, 30 to 50 mg (base) per kg of body weight every eight hours.

**Usual pediatric prescribing limits**
6 grams (base) per day.

**Usual geriatric dose**
See *Usual adult and adolescent dose*.

**Usual geriatric prescribing limits**
1 gram (base) every twenty-four hours for patients older than seventy-five years of age, even if serum creatinine concentrations are normal.

**Strength(s) usually available**
U.S.—
  1 gram in 50 mL (Rx) [*Fortaz* (sodium 2.3 mEq per gram)].
  2 grams in 50 mL (Rx) [*Fortaz* (sodium 2.3 mEq per gram)].
Canada—
  Not commercially available.

**Packaging and storage**
Store between −25 and −10 °C (−13 and 14 °F), unless otherwise specified by manufacturer.

**Preparation of dosage form**
The container should be thawed at room temperature (25 °C [77 °F]) or under refrigeration (5 °C [41 °F]) before administration, making sure that all ice crystals have melted. Thawing should not be forced by immersion in water bath or by microwave irradiation.

Do not use minibags in series connections. This may result in air embolism because of residual air being drawn from the primary container before administration of intravenous solution from the secondary container is complete.

**Stability**
After thawing, solutions retain their potency for 24 hours at room temperature or for 7 days if refrigerated. Once thawed, solutions should not be refrozen.

Do not use if the solution is cloudy or contains a precipitate.

**Incompatibilities**
The admixture of ceftazidime with other medications, including aminophylline, amsacrine, fluconazole, idarubicin hydrochloride, pentamidine isethionate, sargramostim, and vancomycin, is not recommended.

The admixture of beta-lactam antibacterials (penicillins and cephalosporins) and aminoglycosides may result in substantial mutual inactivation. If they are administered concurrently, they should be administered in separate sites. Do not mix them in the same intravenous bag or bottle.

Vancomycin is physically incompatible with ceftazidime and a precipitate may form, depending on the concentration. Therefore, the intravenous lines should be flushed between the administration of these two medications if they are to be given through the same tubing.

## CEFTAZIDIME FOR INJECTION USP

**Usual adult and adolescent dose**
Bone and joint infections—
  Intravenous, 2 grams (base) every twelve hours.
Intra-abdominal infections or
Meningitis or
Pelvic infections, female[1] or
Septicemia—
  Intravenous, 2 grams (base) every eight hours.
Pneumonia, uncomplicated or
Skin and soft tissue infections—
  Intramuscular or intravenous, 500 mg to 1 gram (base) every eight hours.

Pulmonary infections in cystic fibrosis, due to *Pseudomonas*[1]—
  Intravenous, 30 to 50 mg (base) per kg of body weight every eight hours, up to 6 grams per day.
Urinary tract infections, complicated—
  Intramuscular or intravenous, 500 mg (base) every eight to twelve hours.
Urinary tract infections, uncomplicated—
  Intramuscular or intravenous, 250 mg (base) every twelve hours.
For all other infections, severe to life-threatening, especially in immunocompromised patients—
  Intravenous, 2 grams (base) every eight hours.

Note: Adults with renal function impairment may require a reduction in dose. See *Ceftazidime Injection USP*.

**Usual pediatric dose**
Meningitis—
  Infants and children 1 month to 12 years of age: Intravenous, 50 mg (base) per kg of body weight every eight hours.
  Neonates up to 1 month of age: Intravenous, 25 to 50 mg (base) per kg of body weight every twelve hours.
For all other infections—
  Infants and children 1 month to 12 years of age: Intravenous, 30 to 50 mg (base) per kg of body weight every eight hours.
  Neonates up to 4 weeks of age: Intravenous, 30 mg (base) per kg of body weight every twelve hours.

Note: The safety of the arginine component in the ceftazidime L-arginine formulation has not been established for neonates, infants, or children up to 12 years of age. If treatment with ceftazidime is indicated, the sodium formulation should be used.

**Usual pediatric prescribing limits**
See *Ceftazidime Injection USP*.

**Usual geriatric dose**
See *Usual adult and adolescent dose*.

**Usual geriatric prescribing limits**
See *Ceftazidime Injection USP*.

**Strength(s) usually available**
U.S.—
  500 mg (Rx) [*Fortaz* (sodium 2.3 mEq per gram); *Tazidime* (sodium 2.3 mEq per gram)].
  1 gram (may be available in ADD-Vantage® vials) (Rx) [*Ceptaz* (L-arginine 349 mg per gram); *Fortaz* (sodium 2.3 mEq per gram); *Tazicef* (sodium 2.3 mEq per gram); *Tazidime* (sodium 2.3 mEq per gram)].
  2 grams (may be available in ADD-Vantage® vials) (Rx) [*Ceptaz* (L-arginine 349 mg per gram); *Fortaz* (sodium 2.3 mEq per gram); *Tazicef* (sodium 2.3 mEq per gram); *Tazidime* (sodium 2.3 mEq per gram)].
  6 grams (Rx) [*Fortaz* (sodium 2.3 mEq per gram); *Tazicef* (sodium 2.3 mEq per gram); *Tazidime* (sodium 2.3 mEq per gram)].
  10 grams (Rx) [*Ceptaz* (L-arginine 349 mg per gram)].
Canada—
  500 mg (Rx) [*Fortaz; Tazidime* (sodium 2.3 mEq per gram)].
  1 gram (also may be available in ADD-Vantage® vials) (Rx) [*Ceptaz* (L-arginine); *Fortaz; Tazidime* (sodium 2.3 mEq per gram)].
  2 grams (also may be available in ADD-Vantage® vials) (Rx) [*Ceptaz* (L-arginine); *Fortaz; Tazidime* (sodium 2.3 mEq per gram)].
  6 grams (Rx) [*Fortaz; Tazidime* (sodium 2.3 mEq per gram)].
  10 grams (Rx) [*Ceptaz* (L-arginine)].

**Packaging and storage**
Prior to reconstitution, store between 15 and 30 °C (59 and 86 °F), unless otherwise specified by manufacturer. Protect from light.

**Preparation of dosage form**
To prepare solution for intramuscular use, 1.5 mL of suitable diluent (see manufacturer's package insert) should be added to each 500-mg vial, or 3 mL of diluent should be added to each 1-gram vial.

To prepare initial dilution for intravenous use, 3 or 5 mL of suitable diluent (see manufacturer's package insert) should be added to each 500-mg vial, or 10 mL of diluent should be added to each 1- or 2-gram vial, according to manufacturer's labeling instructions. For direct intermittent intravenous use, the resulting solution should be administered slowly over a 3- to 5-minute period. For intravenous infusion, the resulting solution may be further diluted in suitable fluids according to the manufacturer's labeling instructions.

For reconstitution of piggyback infusion bottles and pharmacy bulk vials, see manufacturer's labeling for instructions. If the Y-type method of administration is used, the primary infusion should be temporarily discontinued during infusion of ceftazidime.

After reconstitution of the sodium carbonate formulation, carbon dioxide is formed, causing positive pressure inside the vial. This may require venting.

Do not use minibags in series connections. This may result in air embolism because of residual air being drawn from the primary container before administration of intravenous solution from the secondary container is complete.

Caution—Use of diluents containing benzyl alcohol is not recommended for preparation of medications for use in neonates. A fatal toxic syndrome consisting of metabolic acidosis, CNS depression, respiratory problems, renal failure, hypotension, and possibly seizures and intracranial hemorrhages has been associated with this use.

**Stability**
After reconstitution for intramuscular use with sterile water for injection, bacteriostatic water for injection, or lidocaine hydrochloride injection, solutions retain their potency for at least 18 hours at room temperature or for 7 days if refrigerated. Solutions that are frozen immediately after reconstitution in the original container retain their potency for at least 3 months at −20 °C (−4 °F).

After reconstitution for intravenous use, solutions retain their potency for at least 18 hours at room temperature or for 7 days if refrigerated. Solutions that are frozen immediately after reconstitution with sterile water for injection in the original container retain their potency for at least 3 months at −20 °C (−4 °F).

Once thawed, solutions should not be refrozen. Thawed solutions retain their potency for at least 8 hours at room temperature or for at least 4 days if refrigerated.

Intravenous infusions at concentrations from 1 to 40 mg per mL retain their potency for at least 18 hours at room temperature or for 7 days if refrigerated, when stored in suitable fluids (see manufacturer's package insert). However, storage in sodium bicarbonate injection is not recommended since ceftazidime is less stable in sodium bicarbonate than in other fluids.

Solutions range in color from light yellow to amber, depending on the diluent and volume. Ceftazidime powder and solutions tend to darken, depending on storage conditions. This does not affect their potency.

**Incompatibilities**
The admixture of ceftazidime with other medications, including pentamidine isethionate, is not recommended.

The admixture of beta-lactam antibacterials (penicillins and cephalosporins) and aminoglycosides may result in substantial mutual inactivation. If they are administered concurrently, they should be administered in separate sites. Do not mix them in the same intravenous bag or bottle.

Vancomycin is physically incompatible with ceftazidime and a precipitate may form, depending on the concentration. Therefore, the intravenous lines should be flushed between the administration of these two medications if they are to be given through the same tubing.

[1]Not included in Canadian product labeling.

---

### CEFTIBUTEN

## Summary of Differences
Category: Third-generation. One of three oral third-generation cephalosporins.

## Additional Dosing Information
The capsule and oral suspension dosage forms are bioequivalent.

The oral suspension should be taken at least 2 hours before or 1 hour after a meal.

## Oral Dosage Forms

### CEFTIBUTEN CAPSULES

**Usual adult and adolescent dose**
Bronchitis, bacterial exacerbations[1] or
Otitis media[1] or
Pharyngitis[1] or
Tonsillitis[1]—
  Oral, 400 mg once a day for ten days.

Note: Adults with renal function impairment may require a reduction in dose as follows:

| Creatinine clearance (mL/min)/(mL/sec) | Dosing Capsules | Oral suspension |
|---|---|---|
| > 50/0.83 | See *Usual adult and adolescent dose* | 9 mg/kg once every 24 hours |
| 30–49/0.5–0.82 | 200 mg once every 24 hours | 4.5 mg/kg once every 24 hours |
| 5–29/0.1–0.49 | 100 mg once every 24 hours | 2.25 mg/kg once every 24 hours |

For patients undergoing hemodialysis two or three times a week, a single dose of 400 mg (capsules) or 9 mg/kg, up to 400 mg (oral suspension), may be administered at the end of each hemodialysis session.

**Usual adult and adolescent prescribing limits**
400 mg per day.

**Usual pediatric dose**
This dosage form usually is not used for children. See *Ceftibuten for Oral Suspension*.

**Usual geriatric dose**
See *Usual adult and adolescent dose*.

**Strength(s) usually available**
U.S.—
  400 mg (Rx) [*Cedax* (benzyl alcohol; butylparaben; methylparaben; propylparaben)].
Canada—
  Not commercially available.

**Packaging and storage**
Store between 2 and 25 °C (36 and 77 °F) in a tight container.

**Auxiliary labeling**
• Continue medicine for full time of treatment.

### CEFTIBUTEN FOR ORAL SUSPENSION

**Usual adult and adolescent dose**
See *Ceftibuten Capsules*.

**Usual adult and adolescent prescribing limits**
See *Ceftibuten Capsules*.

**Usual pediatric dose**
Otitis media[1] or
Pharyngitis[1] or
Tonsillitis[1]—
  Infants and children 6 months to 12 years of age: Oral, 9 mg per kg of body weight once a day for ten days.
  Infants up to 6 months of age: Safety and efficacy have not been established.

**Usual pediatric prescribing limits**
400 mg per day.

**Usual geriatric dose**
See *Ceftibuten Capsules*.

**Strength(s) usually available**
U.S.—
  90 mg per 5 mL (when reconstituted according to manufacturer's instructions) (available in 30-, 60-, 90-, and 120-mL bottles) (Rx) [*Cedax* (sodium benzoate; sucrose 1 gram per 5 mL)].
  180 mg per 5 mL (when reconstituted according to manufacturer's instructions) (available in 30-, 60-, and 120-mL bottles) (Rx) [*Cedax* (sodium benzoate; sucrose 1 gram per 5 mL)].
Canada—
  Not commercially available.

**Packaging and storage**
Store between 2 and 25 °C (36 and 77 °F).

**Preparation of dosage form**
The bottle should be tapped to loosen the powder. The total volume of water indicated below should be added in two portions, shaking well after each addition.

| Final concentration | Bottle size | Total amount of water |
|---|---|---|
| 90 mg/5 mL | 30 mL | 28 mL |
|  | 60 mL | 53 mL |
|  | 90 mL | 78 mL |
|  | 120 mL | 103 mL |
| 180 mg/5 mL | 30 mL | 28 mL |
|  | 60 mL | 53 mL |
|  | 120 mL | 103 mL |

## Stability
After reconstitution, the suspension may be stored for up to 14 days between 2 and 8 °C (36 and 46 °F).

## Auxiliary labeling
- Refrigerate.
- Shake well.
- Take on an empty stomach, at least 2 hours before or 1 hour after meals.
- Continue medicine for full time of treatment.
- Beyond-use date.

---

[1]Not included in Canadian product labeling.

---

# CEFTIZOXIME

## Summary of Differences
Category: Third-generation cephalosporin.
Precautions:
  Pediatrics—Associated with transient elevation in eosinophils, ALT (SGPT), AST (SGOT), and CK.

## Additional Dosing Information
Intramuscular doses of 2 grams should be administered as divided doses in different sites.

## Parenteral Dosage Forms
Note: The dosing and strengths of the dosage forms available are expressed in terms of ceftizoxime base (not the sodium salt).

### CEFTIZOXIME INJECTION USP
**Usual adult and adolescent dose**
Pelvic inflammatory disease[1]—
  Intravenous infusion, 2 grams (base) every eight hours.
Urinary tract infections, uncomplicated—
  Intravenous infusion, 500 mg (base) every twelve hours.
For all other infections—
  Mild to moderate: Intravenous infusion, 1 gram (base) every eight to twelve hours.
  Severe or refractory: Intravenous infusion, 1 gram (base) every eight hours; or 2 grams every eight to twelve hours.
  Life-threatening: Intravenous infusion, 3 to 4 grams (base) every eight hours.
Note: Dosages of up to 2 grams every four hours have been given for life-threatening infections.

After an initial loading dose of 500 mg to 1 gram (base), adults with impaired renal function may require a reduction in dose as follows:

| Creatinine clearance (mL/min)/(mL/sec) | Dose (base) Less severe infections | Life-threatening infections |
|---|---|---|
| ≥80/1.33 | See *Usual adult and adolescent dose* | See *Usual adult and adolescent dose* |
| 50–79/0.83–1.32 | 500 mg every 8 hours | 750 mg to 1.5 grams every 8 hours |
| 5–49/0.08–0.82 | 250 to 500 mg every 12 hours | 500 mg to 1 gram every 12 hours |
| 0–4/0–0.07 | 500 mg every 48 hours; or 250 mg every 24 hours | 500 mg to 1 gram every 48 hours; or 500 mg every 24 hours |

**Usual pediatric dose**
For bacterial infections—
  Children 6 months of age and older: Intravenous infusion, 50 mg (base) per kg of body weight every six to eight hours.
  Infants up to 6 months of age: Safety and efficacy have not been established.

**Usual pediatric prescribing limits**
200 mg (base) per kg of body weight (not to exceed the maximum adult dose for serious infection).

**Usual geriatric dose**
See *Usual adult and adolescent dose*.

**Usual geriatric prescribing limits**
1.5 grams (base) for patients older than seventy-five years of age, even if serum creatinine concentrations are normal.

**Strength(s) usually available**
U.S.—
  1 gram (base) per 50 mL (Rx) [*Cefizox* (sodium 2.6 mEq per gram)].
  2 grams (base) per 50 mL (Rx) [*Cefizox* (sodium 2.6 mEq per gram)].
Canada—
  Not commercially available.

**Packaging and storage**
Store between −25 and −10 °C (−13 and 14 °F), unless otherwise specified by manufacturer.

**Preparation of dosage form**
The container should be thawed at room temperature (25 °C [77 °F]) or under refrigeration (5 °C [41 °F]) before administration, making sure that all ice crystals have melted. Thawing should not be forced by immersion in water baths or by microwave irradiation.
Do not use minibags in series connections. This may result in air embolism because of residual air being drawn from the primary container before administration of intravenous solution from the secondary container is complete.

**Stability**
After thawing, solutions retain their potency for 48 hours at room temperature or for 28 days if refrigerated at 5 °C (41 °F). Once thawed, solutions should not be refrozen.
Do not use if the solution is cloudy or contains a precipitate.

**Incompatibilities**
The admixture of beta-lactam antibacterials (penicillins and cephalosporins) and aminoglycosides may result in substantial mutual inactivation. If they are administered concurrently, they should be administered in separate sites. Do not mix them in the same intravenous bag or bottle.

### CEFTIZOXIME FOR INJECTION USP
**Usual adult and adolescent dose**
Gonorrhea, uncomplicated[1]—
  Intramuscular, 1 gram (base) as a single dose.
Pelvic inflammatory disease[1]—
  Intravenous, 2 grams (base) every eight hours.
Urinary tract infections, uncomplicated—
  Intramuscular or intravenous, 500 mg (base) every twelve hours.
For all other infections—
  Mild to moderate: Intramuscular or intravenous, 1 gram (base) every eight to twelve hours.
  Severe or refractory: Intramuscular or intravenous, 1 gram (base) every eight hours; or 2 grams every eight to twelve hours.
  Life-threatening: Intravenous, 3 to 4 grams (base) every eight hours.
Note: Dosages of up to 2 grams (base) every four hours have been given for life-threatening infections.

Adults with renal function impairment may require a reduction in dose. See *Ceftizoxime Injection USP*.

**Usual pediatric dose**
For bacterial infections—
  Children 6 months to 12 years of age: Intramuscular or intravenous, 50 mg (base) per kg of body weight every six to eight hours.
  Infants and children up to 6 months of age: Safety and efficacy have not been established.

**Usual pediatric prescribing limits**
See *Ceftizoxime Injection USP*.

**Usual geriatric dose**
See *Usual adult and adolescent dose*.

**Usual geriatric prescribing limits**
See *Ceftizoxime Injection USP*.

**Strength(s) usually available**
U.S.—
  500 mg (base) (Rx) [*Cefizox* (sodium 2.6 mEq per gram)].
  1 gram (base) (Rx) [*Cefizox* (sodium 2.6 mEq per gram)].
  2 grams (base) (Rx) [*Cefizox* (sodium 2.6 mEq per gram)].
  10 grams (base) (Rx) [*Cefizox* (sodium 2.6 mEq per gram)].
Canada—
  1 gram (base) (Rx) [*Cefizox* (sodium 2.6 mEq per gram)].
  2 grams (base) (Rx) [*Cefizox* (sodium 2.6 mEq per gram)].

**Packaging and storage**
Prior to reconstitution, store below 40 °C (104 °F), preferably between 15 and 30 °C (59 and 86 °F), unless otherwise specified by manufacturer. Protect from excess light.

**Preparation of dosage form**
To prepare initial dilution for intramuscular use, 1.5, 3, or 6 mL of sterile water for injection should be added to each 500-mg, 1-gram, or 2-gram vial, respectively.

To prepare initial dilution for intravenous use, 5, 10, or 20 mL of sterile water for injection should be added to each 500-mg, 1-gram, or 2-gram vial, respectively. For direct intravenous use, the resulting solution should be administered slowly over a 3- to 5-minute period. For continuous or intermittent infusions, the resulting solution should be further diluted in 50 to 100 mL of suitable fluids (see manufacturer's package insert).

For reconstitution of piggyback infusion bottles and pharmacy bulk vials, see manufacturer's labeling for instructions.

### Stability
After reconstitution for intramuscular or intravenous use with suitable diluents (see manufacturer's package insert), solutions retain their potency for 24 hours at room temperature or for 48 to 96 hours (see manufacturer's package insert) if refrigerated at 5 °C (41 °F).

Solutions may vary in color from yellow to amber. This does not affect their potency.

### Incompatibilities
The admixture of beta-lactam antibacterials (penicillins and cephalosporins) and aminoglycosides may result in substantial mutual inactivation. If they are administered concurrently, they should be administered in separate sites. Do not mix them in the same intravenous bag or bottle.

### Additional information
A solution containing 1 gram in 13 mL of sterile water for injection is isotonic.

[1]Not included in Canadian product labeling.

## CEFTRIAXONE

## Summary of Differences
Category: Third-generation cephalosporin.
Pharmacology/pharmacokinetics: Long half-life; may be dosed once a day.
Precautions:
  Pediatrics—Should be used with caution when administered to hyperbilirubinemic neonates, especially premature neonates.
  Drug interactions and/or related problems—Does not interact with probenecid.
Side/adverse effects: Associated with "biliary sludge" or pseudolithiasis.

## Additional Dosing Information
Patients with impaired hepatic function do not generally require a reduction in dose. However, in patients with both impaired hepatic and renal function, the daily dose should not exceed 2 grams.

Intravenous infusion should be administered over a period of 30 minutes.

## Parenteral Dosage Forms
Note: The dosing and strengths of the dosage forms available are expressed in terms of ceftriaxone base (not the sodium salt).

### CEFTRIAXONE INJECTION USP
#### Usual adult and adolescent dose
Perioperative prophylaxis—
  Intravenous infusion, 1 gram (base) one-half to two hours prior to the start of surgery.
For all other infections—
  Intravenous infusion, 1 to 2 grams (base) every twenty-four hours; or 500 mg to 1 gram every twelve hours.

#### Usual adult and adolescent prescribing limits
4 grams (base) per day.

#### Usual pediatric dose
Meningitis—
  Intravenous infusion, 100 mg (base) per kg of body weight, up to 4 grams, on the first day; then 100 mg per kg of body weight every twenty-four hours, or 50 mg per kg of body weight every twelve hours, up to 4 grams per day, for seven to fourteen days.
Skin and soft tissue infections—
  Intravenous infusion, 50 to 75 mg (base) per kg of body weight every twenty-four hours, or 25 to 37.5 mg per kg of body weight every twelve hours, up to 2 grams per day.
For all other infections, serious—
  Intravenous infusion, 25 to 37.5 mg (base) per kg of body weight every twelve hours, up to 2 grams per day.

#### Usual pediatric prescribing limits
4 grams (base) per day for meningitis, and 2 grams per day for all other infections.

#### Usual geriatric dose
See Usual adult and adolescent dose.

#### Strength(s) usually available
U.S.—
  1 gram (base) in 50 mL (Rx) [*Rocephin* (sodium 3.6 mEq per gram)].
  2 grams (base) in 50 mL (Rx) [*Rocephin* (sodium 3.6 mEq per gram)].
Canada—
  Not commercially available.

#### Packaging and storage
Store between −25 and −10 °C (−13 and 14 °F), unless otherwise specified by manufacturer.

#### Preparation of dosage form
The container should be thawed at room temperature before administration, making sure that all ice crystals have melted.

Do not use minibags in series connections. This may result in air embolism because of residual air being drawn from the primary container before administration of intravenous solution from the secondary container is complete.

#### Stability
Once thawed, solutions should not be refrozen.
Do not use if the solution is cloudy or contains a precipitate.

#### Incompatibilities
The admixture of ceftriaxone with other medications, including pentamidine isethionate, or with labetalol hydrochloride is not recommended.

The admixture of beta-lactam antibacterials (penicillins and cephalosporins) and aminoglycosides may result in substantial mutual inactivation. If they are administered concurrently, they should be administered in separate sites. Do not mix them in the same intravenous bag or bottle.

### CEFTRIAXONE FOR INJECTION USP
#### Usual adult and adolescent dose
Gonorrhea, uncomplicated—
  Intramuscular, 250 mg (base) as a single dose.
Perioperative prophylaxis—
  Intravenous, 1 gram (base) one-half to two hours prior to the start of surgery.
For all other infections—
  Intramuscular or intravenous, 1 to 2 grams (base) every twenty-four hours; or 500 mg to 1 gram every twelve hours.

#### Usual adult prescribing limits
See *Ceftriaxone Injection USP*.

#### Usual pediatric dose
Meningitis—
  Intramuscular or intravenous, 100 mg (base) per kg of body weight, up to 4 grams, on the first day; then 100 mg per kg of body weight every twenty-four hours, or 50 mg per kg of body weight every twelve hours, up to 4 grams per day, for seven to fourteen days.
Otitis media[1]—
  Intramuscular, 50 mg (base) per kg of body weight, up to 1 gram, as a single dose.
Skin and soft tissue infections—
  Intramuscular or intravenous, 50 to 75 mg (base) per kg of body weight every twenty-four hours, or 25 to 37.5 mg per kg of body weight every twelve hours, up to 2 grams per day.
For all other serious infections—
  Intramuscular or intravenous, 25 to 37.5 mg (base) per kg of body weight every twelve hours, up to 2 grams per day.

#### Usual pediatric prescribing limits
See *Ceftriaxone Injection USP*.

#### Usual geriatric dose
See *Usual adult and adolescent dose*.

#### Strength(s) usually available
U.S.—
  250 mg (base) (Rx) [*Rocephin* (sodium 3.6 mEq per gram)].
  500 mg (base) (Rx) [*Rocephin* (sodium 3.6 mEq per gram)].
  1 gram (base) (also available in ADD-Vantage® vials) (Rx) [*Rocephin* (sodium 3.6 mEq per gram)].
  2 grams (base) (also available in ADD-Vantage® vials) (Rx) [*Rocephin* (sodium 3.6 mEq per gram)].
  10 grams (base) (Rx) [*Rocephin* (sodium 3.6 mEq per gram)].
Canada—
  250 mg (base) (Rx) [*Rocephin* (sodium 3.6 mEq per gram)].
  1 gram (base) (also available in ADD-Vantage® vials) (Rx) [*Rocephin* (sodium 3.6 mEq per gram)].
  2 grams (base) (Rx) [*Rocephin* (sodium 3.6 mEq per gram)].
  10 grams (base) (Rx) [*Rocephin* (sodium 3.6 mEq per gram)].

#### Packaging and storage
Prior to reconstitution, store below 25 °C (77 °F), preferably between 15 and 30 °C (59 and 86 °F), unless otherwise specified by manufacturer. Protect from light.

## Preparation of dosage form

To prepare initial dilution for intramuscular use, 0.9 mL of sterile water for injection, 0.9% sodium chloride injection, 5% dextrose injection, bacteriostatic water for injection (with 0.9% benzyl alcohol), or 1% lidocaine hydrochloride injection (without epinephrine) should be added to each 250-mg vial, 1.8 mL of diluent should be added to each 500-mg vial, 3.6 mL of diluent should be added to each 1-gram vial, or 7.2 mL of diluent should be added to each 2-gram vial to provide a concentration of approximately 250 mg per mL. Alternatively, to reduce the volume of intramuscular injection, a solution of 350 mg per mL may be prepared by adding 1 mL of diluent to each 500-mg vial, 2.1 mL of diluent to each 1-gram vial, or 4.2 mL of diluent to each 2-gram vial. The 350-mg-per-mL solution is bioequivalent to a 250-mg-per-mL solution.

To prepare initial dilution for intravenous use, 2.4 mL of appropriate diluent (see manufacturer's package insert) should be added to each 250-mg vial, 4.8 mL of diluent should be added to each 500-mg vial, 9.6 mL of diluent should be added to each 1-gram vial, or 19.2 mL of diluent should be added to each 2-gram vial to provide a concentration of approximately 100 mg per mL. The reconstituted solution may be further diluted to 50 or 100 mL with an appropriate diluent for intravenous infusion.

For reconstitution of piggyback infusion bottles and pharmacy bulk vials, see manufacturer's labeling for instructions.

Caution—Use of diluents containing benzyl alcohol is not recommended for preparation of medications for use in neonates. A fatal toxic syndrome consisting of metabolic acidosis, CNS depression, respiratory problems, renal failure, hypotension, and possibly seizures and intracranial hemorrhages has been associated with this use.

## Stability

After reconstitution for intramuscular use, solutions retain at least 90% of their potency for 1 to 3 days at room temperature (25 °C [77 °F]) or for 3 to 10 days if refrigerated at 4 °C (39 °F), depending on concentration and diluent.

After reconstitution for intravenous use, solutions retain at least 90% of their potency for 3 days at room temperature (25 °C [77 °F]) or for 10 days if refrigerated at 4 °C (39 °F), when stored in glass or polyvinyl chloride (PVC) containers in suitable diluents (see manufacturer's package insert).

After reconstitution for intravenous use with 5% dextrose injection or 0.9% sodium chloride injection, solutions at concentrations of 10 to 40 mg per mL retain their potency for 26 weeks at −20 °C (−4 °F) when stored in PVC or polyolefin containers. Frozen solutions should be thawed at room temperature. Once thawed, solutions should not be refrozen.

Solutions may vary in color from light yellow to amber, depending on length of time in storage, concentration, and diluent.

## Incompatibilities

The admixture of ceftriaxone with other medications, including pentamidine isethionate, or with labetalol hydrochloride is not recommended.

The admixture of beta-lactam antibacterials (penicillins and cephalosporins) and aminoglycosides may result in substantial mutual inactivation. If they are administered concurrently, they should be administered in separate sites. Do not mix them in the same intravenous bag or bottle.

[1]Not included in Canadian product labeling.

---

# CEFUROXIME

## Summary of Differences

Category: Second-generation cephalosporin.
Pharmacology/pharmacokinetics:
  Cefuroxime oral suspension reaches only 91% of the area under the plasma concentration–time curve (AUC) and 71% of the peak serum concentration that cefuroxime tablets reach.
  Parenteral cefuroxime is the only second-generation cephalosporin to adequately penetrate into the CSF; however, sterilization is delayed compared with third-generation cephalosporins.
Precautions:
  Laboratory value alteration—May give false-negative test result with ferricyanide blood glucose test.

## Additional Dosing Information

For oral dosage forms only:
- Cefuroxime axetil tablets may be given without regard to meals; however, absorption is enhanced when they are given with food.
- Cefuroxime axetil oral suspension should be taken with food.
- Cefuroxime axetil tablets and oral suspension are not bioequivalent and are not substitutable on a mg-per-mg basis.

## Oral Dosage Forms

Note: Bracketed uses in the *Dosage Forms* section refer to categories of use and/or indications that are not included in U.S. product labeling. The dosing and strengths of the dosage forms available are expressed in terms of cefuroxime base (not the axetil salt).

### CEFUROXIME AXETIL FOR ORAL SUSPENSION

**Usual adult and adolescent dose**
The oral suspension usually is used only for children. See *Cefuroxime Axetil Tablets USP*.

**Usual pediatric dose**
Impetigo[1] or
Otitis media, acute—
  Infants and children 3 months to 12 years of age: Oral, 15 mg (base) per kg of body weight every twelve hours, up to 1000 mg per day, for ten days.
  Infants up to 3 months of age: Safety and efficacy have not been established.
Pharyngitis or
Tonsillitis—
  Infants and children 3 months to 12 years of age: Oral, 10 mg (base) per kg of body weight every twelve hours, up to 500 mg per day, for ten days.
  Infants up to 3 months of age: Safety and efficacy have not been established.

**Usual pediatric prescribing limits**
500 mg per day for pharyngitis and tonsillitis, and 1000 mg per day for impetigo and otitis media.

**Strength(s) usually available**
U.S.—
  125 mg per 5 mL (when reconstituted according to manufacturer's instructions) (available in 50- and 100-mL bottles) (Rx) [*Ceftin* (sucrose)].
  250 mg per 5 mL (when reconstituted according to manufacturer's instructions) (available in 50- and 100-mL bottles) (Rx) [*Ceftin* (sucrose)].
Canada—
  125 mg per 5 mL (when reconstituted according to manufacturer's instructions) (available in 70- and 100-mL bottles) (Rx) [*Ceftin* (sucrose)].
  250 mg single dose packets (Rx) [*Ceftin* (sucrose)].

**Packaging and storage**
Prior to reconstitution, store between 2 and 30 °C (36 and 86 °F), in a well-closed container, unless otherwise specified by manufacturer.

**Preparation of dosage form**
Cefuroxime axetil should not be reconstituted with milk, hot water, or other hot fluids.
For the oral suspension—The bottle should be shaken to loosen the powder. The total amount of water for reconstitution should be added as indicated below. The solution should be shaken vigorously to reconstitute.

| Final concentration | Labeled volume after reconstitution | Total volume of water to be added |
|---|---|---|
| 125 mg/5 mL | 50 mL | 20 mL |
|  | 70 mL | 27 mL |
|  | 100 mL | 37 mL |
| 250 mg/5 mL | 50 mL | 19 mL |
|  | 100 mL | 35 mL |

For the single dose packets—Empty the contents of the packet into a glass. Add 10 mL or more of cold water; apple, grape, or orange juice; or lemonade. Stir well and consume the entire volume immediately.

**Stability**
After reconstitution, suspension retains its potency for 10 days if refrigerated or stored at room temperature (between 2 and 25 °C [36 and 77 °F]).

**Auxiliary labeling**
- Take with food.
- Does not require refrigeration.
- Continue medicine for full time of treatment.
- Shake well.
- Beyond-use date.

**Note**
When dispensing, include a calibrated liquid-measuring device.

## CEFUROXIME AXETIL TABLETS USP

**Usual adult and adolescent dose**
Bronchitis, bacterial exacerbations[1] or
Skin and soft tissue infections—
    Oral, 250 or 500 mg (base) two times a day for ten days.
Bronchitis—
    Oral, 250 or 500 mg (base) two times a day for five to ten days.
Gonorrhea, uncomplicated—
    Oral, 1000 mg (base) as a single dose.
Lyme disease, early[1]—
    Oral, 500 mg (base) two times a day for twenty days.
Pharyngitis or
Sinusitis, acute maxillary or
Tonsillitis—
    Oral, 250 mg (base) two times a day for ten days.
[Pneumonia]—
    Oral, 500 mg (base) two times a day.
Urinary tract infections, uncomplicated[1]—
    Oral, 125 or 250 mg (base) two times a day for seven to ten days.

**Usual pediatric dose**
Otitis media, acute—
    Children who can swallow tablets whole: Oral, 250 mg (base) two times a day for ten days.
    Children who cannot swallow tablets whole: See *Cefuroxime Axetil for Oral Suspension*.
Pharyngitis or
Tonsillitis—
    Children who can swallow tablets whole: Oral, 125 mg (base) two times a day for ten days.
    Children who cannot swallow tablets whole: See *Cefuroxime Axetil for Oral Suspension*.

**Usual geriatric dose**
See *Usual adult and adolescent dose*.

**Strength(s) usually available**
U.S.—
    125 mg (base) (Rx) [*Ceftin* (methylparaben; propylparaben; sodium benzoate)].
    250 mg (base) (Rx) [*Ceftin* (methylparaben; propylparaben)].
    500 mg (base) (Rx) [*Ceftin* (methylparaben; propylparaben)].
Canada—
    250 mg (base) (Rx) [*Ceftin* (methylparaben; propylparaben)].
    500 mg (base) (Rx) [*Ceftin* (methylparaben; propylparaben)].

**Packaging and storage**
Store between 15 and 30 °C (59 and 86 °F), unless otherwise specified by manufacturer. Store in a tight container.

**Auxiliary labeling**
- Continue medicine for full time of treatment.

# Parenteral Dosage Forms

Note: The dosing and strengths of the dosage forms available are expressed in terms of cefuroxime base (not the sodium salt).

## CEFUROXIME INJECTION USP

**Usual adult and adolescent dose**
Bone and joint infections—
    Intravenous infusion, 1.5 grams (base) every eight hours.
Gonococcal infections, disseminated[1] or
Pneumonia, uncomplicated or
Skin and soft tissue infections or
Urinary tract infections, uncomplicated—
    Intravenous infusion, 750 mg (base) every eight hours.
Meningitis, bacterial—
    Intravenous infusion, up to 3 grams (base) every eight hours.
Perioperative prophylaxis—
    Open heart surgery patients: Intravenous infusion, 1.5 grams (base) at the induction of anesthesia, then 1.5 grams every twelve hours, for a total of 6 grams.
    Other surgery patients: Intravenous infusion, 1.5 grams (base) one-half to one hour prior to the start of surgery, then 750 mg every eight hours thereafter.
For all other infections—
    Severe or complicated: Intravenous infusion, 1.5 grams (base) every eight hours.
    Life-threatening: Intravenous infusion, 1.5 grams (base) every six hours.

Note: Adults with impaired renal function may require a reduction in dose as follows:

| Creatinine clearance (mL/min)/(mL/sec) | Dose (base) |
|---|---|
| > 20/0.33 | 750 mg to 1.5 grams every 8 hours |
| 10–20/0.17–0.33 | 750 mg every 12 hours |
| < 10/0.17 | 750 mg every 24 hours |
| Hemodialysis patients | 750 mg at the end of each dialysis period |

**Usual pediatric dose**
Bone and joint infections—
    Intravenous infusion, 50 mg (base) per kg of body weight, up to 1.5 grams, every eight hours.
Meningitis, bacterial—
    Infants and children 1 month of age and older: Intravenous infusion, 50 to 80 mg (base) per kg of body weight every six to eight hours.
    Neonates up to 4 weeks of age: Intravenous infusion, 33.3 to 50 mg (base) per kg of body weight every eight to twelve hours.
For all other infections—
    Infants and children 1 month of age and older: Intravenous infusion, 12.5 to 33.3 mg (base) per kg of body weight every six to eight hours.
    Neonates up to 4 weeks of age: Intravenous infusion, 10 to 50 mg (base) per kg of body weight every eight to twelve hours.
Note: Pediatric patients with impaired renal function may require a reduction in the frequency of dosing consistent with adult dosing recommendations in renal impairment. See *Usual adult and adolescent dose*.

**Usual pediatric prescribing limits**
Up to the maximal adult dosage for the indication.

**Usual geriatric dose**
See *Usual adult and adolescent dose*

**Strength(s) usually available**
U.S.—
    750 mg in 50 mL (Rx) [*Zinacef* (sodium 4.8 mEq)].
    1.5 grams in 50 mL (Rx) [*Zinacef* (sodium 4.8 mEq)].
Canada—
    Not commercially available.

**Packaging and storage**
Store between −25 and −10 °C (−13 and 14 °F), unless otherwise specified by manufacturer.

**Preparation of dosage form**
The container should be thawed at room temperature (25 °C [77 °F]) or under refrigeration (5 °C [41 °F]) before administration, making sure that all ice crystals have melted. Thawing should not be forced by immersion in water baths or by microwave irradiation.
Do not use minibags in series connections. This may result in air embolism because of residual air being drawn from the primary container before administration of intravenous solution from the secondary container is complete.

**Stability**
After thawing, solutions retain their potency for 24 hours at room temperature or for 28 days if refrigerated at 5 °C (41 °F). Once thawed, solutions should not be refrozen.
Do not use if the solution is cloudy or contains a precipitate.
Solution ranges in color from light yellow to amber.

**Incompatibilities**
The admixture of cefuroxime with other antibacterials is not recommended.
The admixture of beta-lactam antibacterials (penicillins and cephalosporins) and aminoglycosides may result in substantial mutual inactivation. If they are administered concurrently, they should be administered in separate sites. Do not mix them in the same intravenous bag or bottle.

## CEFUROXIME FOR INJECTION USP

**Usual adult and adolescent dose**
Bone and joint infections—
    Intramuscular or intravenous, 1.5 grams (base) every eight hours.
Gonococcal infections, disseminated[1] or
Pneumonia, uncomplicated or
Skin and soft tissue infections or
Urinary tract infections, uncomplicated—
    Intramuscular or intravenous, 750 mg (base) every eight hours.
Gonorrhea, uncomplicated—
    Intramuscular, 1.5 grams (base) as a single dose at two different sites, in combination with 1 gram of oral probenecid.

**820    Cephalosporins (Systemic)**                                                     USP DI

Meningitis, bacterial—
  Intravenous, up to 3 grams (base) every eight hours.
Perioperative prophylaxis—
  Open heart surgery patients: Intravenous, 1.5 grams (base) at the induction of anesthesia, then 1.5 grams every twelve hours, for a total of 6 grams.
  Other surgery patients: Intravenous, 1.5 grams (base) one-half to one hour prior to the start of surgery, then 750 mg (intramuscularly or intravenously) every eight hours thereafter.
For all other infections—
  Severe or complicated: Intramuscular or intravenous, 1.5 grams (base) every eight hours.
  Life-threatening: Intramuscular or intravenous, 1.5 grams (base) every six hours.
Note: Adults with renal function impairment may require a reduction in dose. See *Cefuroxime Sodium Injection USP*.

**Usual pediatric dose**
Bone and joint infections—
  Intramuscular or intravenous, 50 mg (base) per kg of body weight, up to 1.5 grams, every eight hours.
Meningitis, bacterial—
  Infants and children 1 month of age and older: Intravenous, 50 to 80 mg (base) per kg of body weight every six to eight hours.
  Neonates up to 4 weeks of age: Intravenous, 33.3 to 50 mg (base) per kg of body weight every eight to twelve hours.
For all other infections—
  Infants and children 1 month of age and older: Intramuscular or intravenous, 12.5 to 33.3 mg (base) per kg of body weight every six to eight hours.
  Neonates up to 4 weeks of age: Intravenous, 10 to 50 mg (base) per kg of body weight every eight to twelve hours.
Note: Pediatric patients with renal function impairment may require a reduction in the frequency of dosing consistent with adult dosing recommendations in renal impairment. See *Cefuroxime Sodium Injection USP*.

**Usual pediatric prescribing limits**
See *Cefuroxime Injection USP*.

**Usual geriatric dose**
See *Usual adult and adolescent dose*.

**Strength(s) usually available**
U.S.—
  750 mg (also may be available in ADD-Vantage® vials) (Rx) [*Kefurox* (sodium 2.4 mEq per gram); *Zinacef* (sodium 2.4 mEq per gram); GENERIC].
  1.5 grams (also may be available in ADD-Vantage® vials) (Rx) [*Kefurox* (sodium 2.4 mEq per gram); *Zinacef* (sodium 2.4 mEq per gram); GENERIC].
  7.5 grams (Rx) [*Kefurox* (sodium 2.4 mEq per gram); *Zinacef* (sodium 2.4 mEq per gram); GENERIC].
Canada—
  750 mg (also may be available in ADD-Vantage® vials) (Rx) [*Kefurox* (sodium 2.4 mEq per gram); *Zinacef*].
  1.5 grams (also may be available in ADD-Vantage® vials) (Rx) [*Kefurox* (sodium 2.4 mEq per gram); *Zinacef*].
  7.5 grams (Rx) [*Kefurox* (sodium 2.4 mEq per gram); *Zinacef*].

**Packaging and storage**
Prior to reconstitution, store below 40 °C (104 °F), preferably between 15 and 30 °C (59 and 86 °F), unless otherwise specified by manufacturer. Protect from light.

**Preparation of dosage form**
To prepare initial dilution for intramuscular use, 3 or 3.6 mL of sterile water for injection (see manufacturer's labeling instructions) should be added to each 750-mg vial and the entire volume withdrawn to provide a concentration of approximately 220 mg per mL.
To prepare initial dilution for intravenous use, see manufacturer's labeling instructions. For direct intermittent intravenous use, the resulting solution should be administered slowly over a 3- to 5-minute period. For infusion, each 750-mg or 1.5-gram dose may be diluted with 50 to 100 mL of appropriate diluent (see manufacturer's package insert).
For reconstitution of piggyback infusion bottles and pharmacy bulk vials, see manufacturer's labeling for instructions. If the Y-type method of administration is used, the primary infusion should be temporarily discontinued during infusion of cefuroxime.

**Stability**
After reconstitution for intramuscular use, suspensions retain their potency for 24 hours at room temperature or for 48 hours if refrigerated at 5 °C (41 °F).
After reconstitution for intravenous use, solutions retain their potency for 24 hours at room temperature or for 48 hours if refrigerated at 5 °C (41 °F). Solutions stored in polyvinyl chloride (PVC) minibags in 50 or 100 mL of 5% dextrose injection or 0.9% sodium chloride injection retain their potency for 6 months at −20 °C (−4 °F).
Frozen solutions should be thawed at room temperature. Thawing should not be forced by immersion in water baths or by microwave irradiation. Thawed solutions retain their potency for up to 24 hours at room temperature or for 7 days if refrigerated.
Intravenous infusions at concentrations of 7.5 and 15 mg per mL in sterile water for injection, 5% dextrose injection, or 0.9% sodium chloride injection retain their potency for 24 hours at room temperature or for 7 days if refrigerated. Use of sodium bicarbonate is not recommended for dilution.
Solutions may vary in color from light yellow to amber, depending on concentration and diluent. In addition, cefuroxime powder, suspensions, and solutions tend to darken, depending on storage conditions. This does not affect their potency.

**Incompatibilities**
The admixture of beta-lactam antibacterials (penicillins and cephalosporins) and aminoglycosides may result in substantial mutual inactivation. If they are administered concurrently, they should be administered in separate sites. Do not mix them in the same intravenous bag or bottle.

[1]Not included in Canadian product labeling.

---

## CEPHALEXIN

## Summary of Differences
Category: First-generation cephalosporin.

## Additional Dosing Information
When daily doses greater than 4 grams are required, parenteral cephalosporins should be considered.
No dosage adjustment is necessary for renal function impairment.

## Oral Dosage Forms
Note: Bracketed uses in the *Dosage Forms* section refer to categories of use and/or indications that are not included in U.S. product labeling.

### CEPHALEXIN CAPSULES USP
**Usual adult and adolescent dose**
Cystitis, uncomplicated or
Pharyngitis or
Skin and soft tissue infections or
Tonsillitis—
  Oral, 500 mg every twelve hours.
  Note: Treatment of cystitis should be administered only to adults and adolescents 15 years of age and older, and should continue for seven to fourteen days.
[Endocarditis, prophylaxis][1]—
  Oral, 2 grams as a single dose one hour prior to the start of surgery.
For all other infections—
  Mild to moderate: Oral, 250 mg every six hours.
  Severe: Oral, up to 1 gram every six hours.

**Usual adult prescribing limits**
4 grams per day.

**Usual pediatric dose**
This dosage form usually is not used for children. See *Cephalexin for Oral Suspension USP*.

**Usual geriatric dose**
See *Usual adult and adolescent dose*.

**Strength(s) usually available**
U.S.—
  250 mg (Rx) [*Keflex*; GENERIC].
  500 mg (Rx) [*Keflex*; GENERIC].
Canada—
  250 mg (Rx) [*Novo-Lexin*].
  500 mg (Rx) [*Novo-Lexin*].

**Packaging and storage**
Store below 40 °C (104 °F), preferably between 15 and 30 °C (59 and 86 °F), unless otherwise specified by manufacturer. Store in a tight container. Protect from light.

**Auxiliary labeling**
• Continue medicine for full time of treatment.

## CEPHALEXIN FOR ORAL SUSPENSION USP

**Usual adult and adolescent dose**
See *Cephalexin Capsules USP*.

**Usual adult prescribing limits**
See *Cephalexin Capsules USP*.

**Usual pediatric dose**
[Endocarditis, prophylaxis][1]—
    Children over 40 kg of body weight: See *Usual adult and adolescent dose*.
    Children 1 year of age and older, and up to 40 kg of body weight: Oral, 50 mg per kg of body weight one hour prior to the start of surgery.
[Impetigo][1]—
    Oral, 15 mg per kg of body weight three times per day for ten days.
Otitis media—
    Children over 40 kg of body weight: See *Usual adult and adolescent dose*.
    Children 1 year of age and older, and up to 40 kg of body weight: Oral, 18.75 to 25 mg per kg of body weight every six hours.
Pharyngitis or
Skin and soft tissue infections or
Tonsillitis—
    Children over 40 kg of body weight: See *Usual adult and adolescent dose*.
    Children 1 year of age and older, and up to 40 kg of body weight: Oral, 12.5 to 25 mg per kg of body weight every twelve hours.
For all other infections—
    Children over 40 kg of body weight: See *Usual adult and adolescent dose*.
    Children 1 year of age and older, and up to 40 kg of body weight:
        Mild to moderate—Oral, 12.5 to 25 mg per kg of body weight every twelve hours; or 6.25 to 12.5 mg per kg of body weight every six hours.
        Severe—Oral, 25 to 50 mg per kg of body weight every twelve hours; or 12.5 to 25 mg per kg of body weight every six hours.
    Infants and children 1 month to 1 year of age: Oral, 6.25 to 12.5 mg per kg of body weight every six hours.

**Usual pediatric prescribing limits**
2 grams for prophylaxis of bacterial endocarditis.

**Usual geriatric dose**
See *Cephalexin Capsules USP*.

**Strength(s) usually available**
U.S.—
    125 mg per 5 mL (when reconstituted according to manufacturer's instructions) (may be available in 100- and 200-mL bottles) (Rx) [*Keflex* (sucrose); GENERIC (may contain sucrose)].
    250 mg per 5 mL (when reconstituted according to manufacturer's instructions) (may be available in 100- and 200-mL bottles) (Rx) [*Keflex* (sucrose); GENERIC (may contain sucrose)].
Canada—
    125 mg per 5 mL (when reconstituted according to manufacturer's instructions) (may be available in 100-, 150-, and 200-mL bottles) (Rx) [*Keflex* (sodium); *Novo-Lexin* (sodium); *PMS-Cephalexin* (sodium)].
    250 mg per 5 mL (when reconstituted according to manufacturer's instructions) (may be available in 100-, 150-, and 200-mL bottles) (Rx) [*Keflex* (sodium); *Novo-Lexin* (sodium); *PMS-Cephalexin* (sodium)].

**Packaging and storage**
Prior to reconstitution, store below 40 °C (104 °F), preferably between 15 and 30 °C (59 and 86 °F), unless otherwise specified by manufacturer. Store in a tight container.

**Preparation of dosage form**
See manufacturer's labeling for instructions.

**Stability**
After reconstitution, suspensions retain their potency for 14 days if refrigerated.

**Auxiliary labeling**
- Refrigerate.
- Shake well.
- Continue medicine for full time of treatment.
- Beyond-use date.

**Note**
When dispensing, include a calibrated liquid-measuring device.

## CEPHALEXIN TABLETS USP

**Usual adult and adolescent dose**
See *Cephalexin Capsules USP*.

**Usual adult prescribing limits**
See *Cephalexin Capsules USP*.

**Usual pediatric dose**
This dosage form usually is not used for children. See *Cephalexin for Oral Suspension USP*.

**Usual geriatric dose**
See *Cephalexin Capsules USP*.

**Strength(s) usually available**
U.S.—
    250 mg (Rx) [GENERIC (may be scored)].
    500 mg (Rx) [GENERIC (may be scored)].
Canada—
    250 mg (Rx) [*Apo-Cephalex* (scored); *Keflex; Novo-Lexin; Nu-Cephalex; PMS-Cephalexin*].
    500 mg (Rx) [*Apo-Cephalex* (scored); *Keflex; Novo-Lexin; Nu-Cephalex; PMS-Cephalexin*].

**Packaging and storage**
Store below 40 °C (104 °F), preferably between 15 and 30 °C (59 and 86 °F), unless otherwise specified by manufacturer. Store in a tight container.

**Auxiliary labeling**
- Continue medicine for full time of treatment.

## CEPHALEXIN HYDROCHLORIDE TABLETS USP

**Usual adult dose**
See *Cephalexin Capsules USP*.

**Usual adult prescribing limits**
See *Cephalexin Capsules USP*.

**Usual pediatric dose**
Safety and efficacy have not been established.

**Usual geriatric dose**
See *Cephalexin Capsules USP*.

**Strength(s) usually available**
U.S.—
    500 mg (Rx) [*Keftab* (sucrose)].
Canada—
    Not commercially available.

**Packaging and storage**
Store between 15 and 30 °C (59 and 86 °F), unless otherwise specified by manufacturer. Store in a tight container.

**Auxiliary labeling**
- Continue medicine for full time of treatment.

---

[1] Not included in Canadian product labeling.

---

## CEPHALOTHIN

### Summary of Differences
Category: First-generation cephalosporin.
Precautions:
    Drug interactions and/or related problems—May be more likely to interact with nephrotoxic medications.
    Laboratory value alterations—May falsely elevate serum and urine creatinine concentrations when Jaffe's reaction method is used.

### Additional Dosing Information
Since pain, induration, tenderness, and elevated temperature may occur on intramuscular administration, cephalothin should be administered by deep intramuscular injection or by intravenous injection.

When intravenous doses greater than 6 grams daily are given for more than 3 days, thrombophlebitis may occur. To help minimize the incidence of thrombophlebitis, larger veins may be used.

### Parenteral Dosage Forms
Note: Bracketed uses in the *Dosage Forms* section refer to categories of use and/or indications that are not included in U.S. product labeling. The dosing and strengths of the dosage forms available are expressed in terms of cephalothin base (not the sodium salt).

## CEPHALOTHIN FOR INJECTION USP

**Usual adult and adolescent dose**
[Furunculosis, with cellulitis] or
[Pneumonia, uncomplicated] or
[Urinary tract infections]—
    Intramuscular or intravenous, 500 mg (base) every six hours.

[Perioperative prophylaxis]—
  Intravenous, 2 grams (base) one-half to one hour prior to the start of surgery; 2 grams during surgery; and 2 grams every six hours following surgery for up to forty-eight hours.
[For all other infections]—
  Intramuscular or intravenous, 500 mg to 2 grams (base) every four to six hours.

Note: After an initial loading dose of 1 to 2 grams (base), adults with renal function impairment may require a reduction in dose as follows:

| Creatinine clearance (mL/min)/(mL/sec) | Dose (base) |
|---|---|
| > 80/1.33 | See *Usual adult and adolescent dose* |
| 50–80/0.83–1.33 | Up to 2 grams every 6 hours |
| 25–50/0.42–0.83 | Up to 1.5 grams every 6 hours |
| 10–25/0.17–0.42 | Up to 1 gram every 6 hours |
| 2–10/0.03–0.17 | Up to 500 mg every 6 hours |
| <2/0.03 | Up to 500 mg every 8 hours |

**Usual adult prescribing limits**
12 grams (base) per day.

**Usual pediatric dose**
[For bacterial infections]—
  Intramuscular or intravenous, 13.3 to 26.6 mg (base) per kg of body weight every four hours; or 20 to 40 mg per kg of body weight every six hours.

**Usual geriatric dose**
See *Usual adult and adolescent dose*.

**Strength(s) usually available**
U.S.—
  Not commercially available.
Canada—
  1 gram (base) (may be available in ADD-Vantage® vials) (Rx) [*Ceporacin; Keflin* (sodium 2.8 mEq per gram)].

**Packaging and storage**
Prior to reconstitution, store below 40 °C (104 °F), preferably between 15 and 30 °C (59 and 86 °F), unless otherwise specified by manufacturer.

**Preparation of dosage form**
To prepare initial dilution for intramuscular use, 4.5 mL of sterile water for injection should be added to each 1-gram vial.
To prepare initial dilution for intravenous use, 10 mL of sterile water for injection, 5% dextrose injection, or 0.9% sodium chloride injection should be added to each 1-gram vial. For direct or intermittent use, the resulting solution should be administered over a 3- to 5-minute period. For continuous infusion, the resulting solution should be further diluted in suitable fluids (see manufacturer's package insert).

**Stability**
After reconstitution, solutions retain their potency for 8 hours at room temperature or for 72 hours if refrigerated. Solutions reconstituted with bacteriostatic diluent and used for intramuscular administration retain their potency for up to 7 days when refrigerated.
Concentrated solutions will darken in color, especially at room temperature. However, slight discoloration does not affect potency.

**Incompatibilities**
The admixture of beta-lactam antibacterials (penicillins and cephalosporins) and aminoglycosides may result in substantial mutual inactivation. If they are administered concurrently, they should be administered in separate sites. Do not mix them in the same intravenous bag or bottle.

---

## CEPHAPIRIN

## Summary of Differences
Category: First-generation cephalosporin.

## Additional Dosing Information
Cephapirin should be administered by deep intramuscular injection or by intravenous injection only.

## Parenteral Dosage Forms

Note: The dosing and strengths of the dosage forms available are expressed in terms of cephapirin base (not the sodium salt).

### CEPHAPIRIN FOR INJECTION USP

**Usual adult and adolescent dose**
Perioperative prophylaxis[1]—
  Intramuscular or intravenous, 1 to 2 grams (base) one-half to one hour prior to the start of surgery; 1 to 2 grams during surgery; and 1 to 2 grams every six hours following surgery for up to twenty-four hours.
Skin and soft tissue infections[1] or
Urinary tract infections[1]—
  Intramuscular or intravenous, 500 mg (base) every four to six hours.
For all other infections[1]—
  Serious: Intramuscular or intravenous, 1 gram (base) every four to six hours.
  Very serious or life-threatening: Intravenous, up to 12 grams (base) per day.

Note: Patients with impaired renal function (moderately severe oliguria or serum creatinine above 5 mg per 100 mL) may receive 7.5 to 15 mg (base) per kg of body weight every twelve hours.
  Patients with severely reduced renal function and who are to be dialyzed should receive 7.5 to 15 mg (base) per kg of body weight just prior to dialysis and every twelve hours thereafter.

**Usual adult prescribing limits**
12 grams (base) per day.

**Usual pediatric dose**
For bacterial infections[1]—
  Infants up to 3 months of age: Dosage has not been established.
  Infants and children 3 months of age and older: Intramuscular or intravenous, 10 to 20 mg (base) per kg of body weight every six hours.

**Usual geriatric dose**
See *Usual adult and adolescent dose*.

**Strength(s) usually available**
U.S.—
  500 mg (base) (Rx) [*Cefadyl* (sodium 2.36 mEq per gram)].
  1 gram (base) (Rx) [*Cefadyl* (sodium 2.36 mEq per gram)].
  2 grams (base) (Rx) [*Cefadyl* (sodium 2.36 mEq per gram)].
  4 grams (base) (Rx) [*Cefadyl* (sodium 2.36 mEq per gram)].
  20 grams (base) (Rx) [*Cefadyl* (sodium 2.36 mEq per gram)].
Canada—
  Not commercially available.

**Packaging and storage**
Prior to reconstitution, store below 40 °C (104 °F), preferably between 15 and 30 °C (59 and 86 °F), unless otherwise specified by manufacturer.

**Preparation of dosage form**
To prepare initial dilution for intramuscular use, 1 mL of sterile water for injection or bacteriostatic water for injection should be added to each 500-mg vial, or 2 mL of diluent should be added to each 1-gram vial.
To prepare initial dilution for intravenous use, 10 mL or more of bacteriostatic water for injection, dextrose injection, or 0.9% sodium chloride injection should be added to each 500-mg, 1-gram, or 2-gram vial. For direct injection, the resulting solution should be administered slowly over a 3- to 5-minute period. For intermittent infusion, the resulting solution should be diluted with suitable fluids (see manufacturer's package insert).
For reconstitution of pharmacy bulk vials or piggyback infusion bottles, see manufacturer's labeling for instructions.

**Stability**
After reconstitution, solutions retain their potency for 12 to 48 hours at room temperature (25 °C [77 °F]), depending on the diluent, or for 10 days if refrigerated at 4 °C (39 °F). Color changes during the indicated storage times do not affect potency.
If frozen immediately after reconstitution with sterile water for injection, bacteriostatic water for injection containing either benzyl alcohol or parabens, 0.9% sodium chloride injection, or 5% dextrose injection, solutions retain their potency for up to 60 days at −15 °C (5 °F). After thawing at room temperature, solutions retain their potency for at least 12 hours at room temperature or for 10 days if refrigerated at 4 °C (39 °F).
At concentrations of 2 to 30 mg per mL in suitable fluids (see manufacturer's package insert), intravenous infusions retain their potency for 24 hours at room temperature. At a concentration of 4 mg per mL in suitable fluids (see manufacturer's package insert), intravenous infusions retain their potency for 10 days if refrigerated or for 14 days if frozen at −15 °C (5 °F). After thawing at room temperature, these infusions retain their potency for 24 hours at room temperature.

**Incompatibilities**
The admixture of beta-lactam antibacterials (penicillins and cephalosporins) and aminoglycosides may result in substantial mutual inactivation. If they are administered concurrently, they should be administered in separate sites. Do not mix them in the same intravenous bag or bottle.

---

[1]Not included in Canadian product labeling.

## CEPHRADINE

### Summary of Differences
Category: First-generation cephalosporin.

### Additional Dosing Information
May be taken with or without food.

## Oral Dosage Forms

### CEPHRADINE CAPSULES USP

**Usual adult and adolescent dose**
Pneumonia, lobar[1] or
Prostatitis[1] or
Urinary tract infections, serious[1]—
  Oral, 500 mg every six hours; or 1 gram every twelve hours.
Respiratory tract infections, other than lobar pneumonia[1] or
Skin and soft tissue infections[1]—
  Oral, 250 mg every six hours; or 500 mg every twelve hours.
Urinary tract infections, uncomplicated[1]—
  Oral, 500 mg every twelve hours.
For all other infections, severe or chronic[1]—
  Oral, up to 1 gram every six hours.

Note: Adults with impaired renal function may require a reduction in dose as follows:

| Creatinine clearance (mL/min)/(mL/sec) | Dose |
| --- | --- |
| > 20/0.33 | 500 mg every 6 hours |
| 5–20/0.08–0.33 | 250 mg every 6 hours |
| < 5/0.08 | 250 mg every 12 hours |
| Chronic intermittent hemodialysis patients | 250 mg at the start of hemodialysis; 250 mg after 12 hours; and 250 mg 36–48 hours after start |

**Usual adult prescribing limits**
4 grams per day.

**Usual pediatric dose**
This dosage form usually is not used for children. See *Cephradine for Oral Suspension USP*.

**Usual geriatric dose**
See *Usual adult and adolescent dose*.

**Strength(s) usually available**
U.S.—
  250 mg (Rx) [*Velosef* (lactose); GENERIC].
  500 mg (Rx) [*Velosef* (lactose); GENERIC].
Canada—
  Not commercially available.

**Packaging and storage**
Store below 30 °C (86 °F), preferably between 15 and 30 °C (59 and 86 °F), unless otherwise specified by manufacturer. Store in a tight container.

**Auxiliary labeling**
• Continue medicine for full time of treatment.

### CEPHRADINE FOR ORAL SUSPENSION USP

**Usual adult and adolescent dose**
See *Cephradine Capsules USP*.

**Usual adult prescribing limits**
See *Cephradine Capsules USP*.

**Usual pediatric dose**
Otitis media, due to *Haemophilus influenzae*[1]—
  Infants and children 9 months of age and older: Oral, 18.75 to 25 mg per kg of body weight every six hours; or 37.5 to 50 mg per kg of body weight every twelve hours.
  Infants up to 9 months of age: Oral, 18.75 to 25 mg per kg of body weight every six hours.
For all other infections[1]—
  Infants and children 9 months of age and older:
    Mild or moderate—Oral, 6.25 to 12.5 mg per kg of body weight every six hours; or 12.5 to 25 mg per kg of body weight every twelve hours.
    Severe or chronic—Oral, up to 1 gram every six hours.
  Infants up to 9 months of age:
    Mild or moderate—Oral, 6.25 to 12.5 mg per kg of body weight every six hours.
    Severe—Oral, up to 1 gram every six hours.

Note: Pediatric patients with renal function impairment may require a reduction in dose proportional to their weight and severity of infection.

**Usual pediatric prescribing limits**
4 grams per day.

**Usual geriatric dose**
See *Cephradine Capsules USP*.

**Strength(s) usually available**
U.S.—
  125 mg per 5 mL (when reconstituted according to manufacturer's instructions) (available in 100- and 200-mL bottles) (Rx) [*Velosef* (sucrose); GENERIC (may contain sucrose)].
  250 mg per 5 mL (when reconstituted according to manufacturer's instructions) (available in 100- and 200-mL bottles) (Rx) [*Velosef* (sucrose); GENERIC (may contain sucrose)].
Canada—
  Not commercially available.

**Packaging and storage**
Prior to reconstitution, store below 40 °C (104 °F), preferably between 15 and 30 °C (59 and 86 °F), unless otherwise specified by manufacturer. Store in a tight container.

**Preparation of dosage form**
See manufacturer's labeling instructions.

**Stability**
After reconstitution, suspensions retain their potency for 7 days at room temperature or for 14 days if refrigerated.

**Auxiliary labeling**
• Refrigerate.
• Shake well.
• Continue medicine for full time of treatment.
• Beyond-use date.

**Note**
When dispensing, include a calibrated liquid-measuring device.

---

[1]Not included in Canadian product labeling.

Revised: 08/03/98

## Table 1. Pharmacology/Pharmacokinetics

| Drug | Bioavailability (%) | Half-life (hr) Normal renal function | Half-life (hr) Impaired renal function | Time to peak serum concentration (hr) | Peak serum concentration after dose mcg/mL | Peak serum concentration after dose Dose | Peak urine concentration after dose mcg/mL | Peak urine concentration after dose Dose |
|---|---|---|---|---|---|---|---|---|
| **First generation** | | | | | | | | |
| Cefadroxil Oral | 95 | 1.5 | 20–25 | 1.5–2 | 16 | 500 mg | 1800 | 500 mg |
| | | | | | 28 | 1 gram | | |
| Cefazolin IM | | 1.4–2* | 40–70 | | 17 | 250 mg | 2400 | 500 mg |
| | | | | | 38 | 500 mg | 4000 | 1 gram |
| | | | | | 64 | 1 gram | | |
| IV | | | | End of infusion | 188 | 1 gram | | |
| Cephalexin Oral | 95 | 0.9–1.5 | 20–40 | 1–2 | 9 | 250 mg | 1000 | 250 mg |
| | | | | | 18 | 500 mg | 2200 | 500 mg |
| | | | | | 32 | 1 gram | 5000 | 1 gram |
| Cephalothin IM | | 0.5–1† | 3–18 | 0.5 | 10 | 500 mg | 800 | 500 mg |
| | | | | | 20 | 1 gram | 2500 | 1 gram |
| IV | | | | 0.25–0.5 | 30 | 1 gram | | |
| | | | | | 80–100 | 2 grams | | |
| Cephapirin IM | | 0.5–0.8 | 1.5–2.7 | 0.5–1 | 9 | 500 mg | 900 | 500 mg |
| | | | | | 16 | 1 gram | | |
| IV | | | | End of infusion | 35 | 500 mg | | |
| | | | | | 67 | 1 gram | | |
| | | | | | 129 | 2 grams | | |
| Cephradine Oral | 95 | 1.3 | 6–15 | 1‡ | 9 | 250 mg | 1600 | 250 mg |
| | | | | | 17 | 500 mg | 3200 | 500 mg |
| | | | | | 24 | 1 gram | 4000 | 1 gram |
| **Second generation** | | | | | | | | |
| Cefaclor Capsules, oral suspension | 95 | 0.6–0.9 | 2.3–2.8 | 0.5–1‡ | 7 | 250 mg | 600 | 250 mg |
| | | | | | 13 | 500 mg | 900 | 500 mg |
| | | | | | 23 | 1 gram | 1900 | 1 gram |
| Extended-release tablets | | | | 2.5–2.7 | 3.7§ | 375 mg | | |
| | | | | | 8.2§ | 500 mg | | |
| Cefamandole IM | | 0.5–1.2 | 3–11 | 0.5–2 | 13 | 500 mg | 254 | 500 mg |
| | | | | | 25 | 1 gram | 1357 | 1 gram |
| IV | | | | End of infusion | 139 | 1 gram | 750 | 1 gram |
| | | | | | 240 | 2 grams | 1380 | 2 grams |
| | | | | | 533 | 3 grams | | |
| | | | | | 666 | 4 grams | | |
| Cefonicid IM | | 3.5–4.5 | 17–56 | 1 | 99 | 1 gram | 385 | 500 mg |
| IV | | | | End of infusion | 220 | 1 gram | | |
| Cefotetan IM | | 3–4.6 | Prolonged | 1–3 | 71 | 1 gram | | |
| | | | | | 91 | 2 grams | | |
| IV | | | | End of infusion | 158 | 1 gram | 1700 | 1 gram |
| | | | | | 237 | 2 grams | 3500 | 2 grams |
| Cefoxitin IV | | 0.7–1.1# | 13–20 | End of infusion | 110 | 1 gram | | |
| | | | | | 244 | 2 grams | | |
| Cefprozil Oral | 90–95 | 1.3** | 5–6 | 1.5–1.7 | 6.1 | 250 mg | 700 | 250 mg |
| | | | | | 10.5 | 500 mg | 1000 | 500 mg |
| | | | | | 18.3 | 1 gram | 2900 | 1 gram |

## Table 1. Pharmacology/Pharmacokinetics (continued)

| Drug | Bioavailability (%) | Half-life (hr) Normal renal function | Half-life (hr) Impaired renal function | Time to peak serum concentration (hr) | Peak serum concentration after dose mcg/mL | Peak serum concentration after dose Dose | Peak urine concentration after dose mcg/mL | Peak urine concentration after dose Dose |
|---|---|---|---|---|---|---|---|---|
| Ceftibuten Oral | | 2–2.6†† | 7–22 | 1.7–3†† | 10††<br>15<br>23 | 200 mg††<br>400 mg<br>800 mg | | |
| Cefuroxime Oral suspension | | 1.2–1.9‡‡ | 3–17 | 2.7–3.6 | 3.3<br>5.1<br>7 | 10 mg/kg<br>15 mg/kg<br>20 mg/kg | | |
| Tablet | After food§§ (52–68)<br>Fasting (37) | | | 2.2–3 | 2<br>4<br>7<br>13.6 | 125 mg<br>250 mg<br>500 mg<br>1 gram | | |
| IM | | | | 0.75 | 27 | 750 mg | 1300 | 750 mg |
| IV | | | | End of infusion | 50<br>100 | 750 mg<br>1.5 grams | 1150<br>2500 | 750 mg<br>1.5 grams |
| **Third generation** | | | | | | | | |
| Cefixime Oral | 40–50 | 3–4 | 6.4–11.5 | 2–6 | 1–1.3<br>2–3<br>3.5–4.4 | 100 mg<br>200 mg<br>400 mg | 73<br>107<br>164 | 100 mg<br>200 mg<br>400 mg |
| Cefoperazone IM | | 1.6–2.4## | 2.1## | 1–2 | 65–75<br>97 | 1 gram<br>2 grams | 1000 | 2 grams |
| IV | | | | End of infusion | 153<br>252<br>340<br>506 | 1 gram<br>2 grams<br>3 grams<br>4 grams | > 2200 | 2 grams |
| Cefotaxime IM | 90–95 | 1 | 2.6–3 | 0.5 | 12<br>21 | 500 mg<br>1 gram | | |
| IV | | | | | 39<br>102<br>214 | 500 mg<br>1 gram<br>2 grams | | |
| Cefpodoxime Oral | 50§§ | 2.1–2.8 | 3.5–9.8 | 2–3 | 1.4<br>2.3<br>3.9 | 100 mg<br>200 mg<br>400 mg | | |
| Ceftazidime IM | | 1.4–2 | 13 | 1 | 17<br>39 | 500 mg<br>1 gram | 2100 | 500 mg |
| IV | | | | End of infusion | 42<br>69<br>170 | 500 mg<br>1 gram<br>2 grams | 12,100 | 2 grams |
| Ceftizoxime IM | | 1.4–1.7 | 30 | 1 | 14<br>39 | 500 mg<br>1 gram | | |
| IV | | | | End of infusion | 60<br>132<br>220 | 1 gram<br>2 grams<br>3 grams | > 6000 | 1 gram |

*The half-life of cefazolin in neonates less than 1 week old is 4.5 to 5 hours.
†The half-life of cephalothin in neonates less than 1 week old is 1.5 to 2 hours.
‡Delayed in presence of food.
§With food. Peak serum concentration is decreased when administered under fasting conditions.
#The half-life of cefoxitin is 5.6 hours in neonates 0 to 7 days of age; 2.5 hours in neonates 7 days to 1 month of age; and 1.7 hours in infants 1 to 3 months of age.
**In children, the half-life of cefprozil is 1.8 to 2.1 hours.
††In children, the half-life of ceftibuten is 1.4 to 2.6 hours; the time to peak serum concentration is 2 hours; and the peak serum concentration is 13 mcg/mL after a dose of 9 mg/kg. In geriatric patients, the peak serum concentration is 17 mcg/mL after a dose of 200 mg.
‡‡In neonates, the half-life of cefuroxime can be three to five times longer than it is in adults.
§§Bioavailability is increased when this medication is administered with food.
##In adults, not significantly different from normal values during hemodialysis; 2.8 to 4.2 hours between hemodialysis periods; 3 to 7 hours with impaired hepatic function and/or biliary obstruction. In pediatric patients, 6 to 10 hours in low-birth-weight neonates; 4 to 6 hours in infants approximately 1 month of age; 2.2 hours in infants and children 2 months to 11 years of age.
***The half-life of ceftriaxone in pediatric patients with meningitis after a 50- or 75-mg-per-kg dose.

## Table 1. Pharmacology/Pharmacokinetics (continued)

| Drug | Bioavailability (%) | Half-life (hr) Normal renal function | Half-life (hr) Impaired renal function | Time to peak serum concentration (hr) | Peak serum concentration after dose mcg/mL | Peak serum concentration after dose Dose | Peak urine concentration after dose mcg/mL | Peak urine concentration after dose Dose |
|---|---|---|---|---|---|---|---|---|
| Ceftriaxone | | | | | | | | |
| IM | | 5.8–8.7 | 12–24 | 2–3 | 38 | 500 mg | 425 | 500 mg |
| | | | | | 76 | 1 gram | 628 | 1 gram |
| IV | | 4.3–4.6*** | | End of infusion | 82 | 500 mg | 526 | 500 mg |
| | | | | | 151 | 1 gram | 995 | 1 gram |
| | | | | | 257 | 2 grams | 2692 | 2 grams |
| **Fourth generation** | | | | | | | | |
| Cefepime | 100 | 2 | 14 | | | | | |
| IM | | | | 1–2 | 14 | 500 mg | | |
| | | | | | 30 | 1 gram | | |
| | | | | | 57 | 2 grams | | |
| IV | | | | End of infusion | 18 | 250 mg | | |
| | | | | | 39 | 500 mg | | |
| | | | | | 82 | 1 gram | | |
| | | | | | 164 | 2 grams | | |

*The half-life of cefazolin in neonates less than 1 week old is 4.5 to 5 hours.
†The half-life of cephalothin in neonates less than 1 week old is 1.5 to 2 hours.
‡Delayed in presence of food.
§With food. Peak serum concentration is decreased when administered under fasting conditions.
#The half-life of cefoxitin is 5.6 hours in neonates 0 to 7 days of age; 2.5 hours in neonates 7 days to 1 month of age; and 1.7 hours in infants 1 to 3 months of age.
**In children, the half-life of cefprozil is 1.8 to 2.1 hours.
††In children, the half-life of ceftibuten is 1.4 to 2.6 hours; the time to peak serum concentration is 2 hours; and the peak serum concentration is 13 mcg/mL after a dose of 9 mg/kg. In geriatric patients, the peak serum concentration is 17 mcg/mL after a dose of 200 mg.
‡‡In neonates, the half-life of cefuroxime can be three to five times longer than it is in adults.
§§Bioavailability is increased when this medication is administered with food.
##In adults, not significantly different from normal values during hemodialysis; 2.8 to 4.2 hours between hemodialysis periods; 3 to 7 hours with impaired hepatic function and/or biliary obstruction. In pediatric patients, 6 to 10 hours in low-birth-weight neonates; 4 to 6 hours in infants approximately 1 month of age; 2.2 hours in infants and children 2 months to 11 years of age.
***The half-life of ceftriaxone in pediatric patients with meningitis after a 50- or 75-mg-per-kg dose.

## Table 2. Pharmacology/Pharmacokinetics*

| Drug | Protein binding (%) | Hepatic and renal biotransformation (%) | Renal excretion (% unchanged/hr) | Vol$_D$ (L/kg) | Removal by dialysis HD | Removal by dialysis PD |
|---|---|---|---|---|---|---|
| **First generation** | | | | | | |
| Cefadroxil | Low (15–20) | No | 93/24 (GF; TS) | 0.31 | Yes | |
| Cefazolin | High (85) | No | 60–89/6; 70–86/24 (GF; TS) | 0.12 | Moderate | No |
| Cephalexin | Low (10–15) | No | 80/6; 90/8 (TS; GF) | 0.26 | Moderate | Yes |
| Cephalothin | Moderate (70) | Yes; 20–30 | 60–70/6 (30 as metabolite/6) (TS) | 0.26 | Moderate | |
| Cephapirin | Moderate (44–50) | Yes; 40 | 70/6 (TS; GF; TR) | 0.13 | Slight | |
| Cephradine | Very low to low (8–17) | No | 60–90/6 (TS) | 0.25 | Signif | Yes |
| **Second generation** | | | | | | |
| Cefaclor | Low (25) | No | 60–85/8 | 0.35 | Moderate | Yes |
| Cefamandole | High (70–80) | No | 65–85/8 (GF; TS) | 0.16 | Moderate | Slight |
| Cefonicid | Very high (> 90) | No | 99/24 | 0.11 | Slight | |
| Cefotetan | High to very high (78–91) | No | 50–80/24 | 0.19 | Slight | NS |
| Cefoxitin | High (70–80) | Slight; 0.2–5 (inactive metabolite) | 85/6 (GF; TS) | 0.16 | Moderate | NS |

## Table 2. Pharmacology/Pharmacokinetics *(continued)**

| Drug | Protein binding (%) | Hepatic and renal biotransformation (%) | Renal excretion (% unchanged/hr) | Vol$_D$ (L/kg) | Removal by dialysis HD | PD |
|---|---|---|---|---|---|---|
| Cefprozil | Moderate (36–45) | No | 60–70/8 | 0.17–0.23 | Moderate | |
| Ceftibuten | High (65–77) | | 95/24 | 0.21† | Yes | |
| Cefuroxime | Low to moderate (33–50) | | | 0.82 | Moderate | |
| Oral | | No; prodrug rapidly hydrolyzed to cefuroxime | 50/12 (GF; TS) | | | |
| IM, IV | | | 90/6; 96/24 | | | |
| **Third generation** | | | | | | |
| Cefixime | High (65–70) | No | 50/24 | 0.11 | NS | No |
| Cefoperazone | High to very high (82–93) | No | 20–30/12‡ (GF) | 0.14–2 | Slight | |
| Cefotaxime | Low to moderate (30–50) | Yes; 30–50 (active and inactive metabolites) | 50–60/6 (15–25 as active metabolite) (GF) | 0.25–0.39 | Moderate | NS |
| Cefpodoxime | Low to moderate (21–40) | No; prodrug de-esterified to cefpodoxime | 29–33/12 40/24 | 0.7–1.15 | Moderate | |
| Ceftazidime | Very low to low (5–17) | No | 80–90/24 (GF) | 0.21–0.28 | Yes | Yes |
| Ceftizoxime | Low (30) | No | 70–100/24 | 0.35–0.4 | Moderate | |
| Ceftriaxone | High to very high (83–96) | | 33–67/24 | 0.12–0.14§ | No | No |
| **Fourth generation** | | | | | | |
| Cefepime | Low (20) | Yes; 15 | 80–85/12 (G/F) | 0.25# | Yes | Slight |

*Abbreviations: GF = glomerular filtration; HD = hemodialysis; PD = peritoneal dialysis; TR = tubular reabsorption; TS = tubular secretion; NS = not significant; Signif = significant.
†In pediatric patients 6 months to 12 years of age, the Vol$_D$ = 0.5 L/kg.
‡75% excreted unchanged in bile; 15 to 30% (range: 10 to 36%) excreted unchanged in urine within 6 to 12 hours, primarily by glomerular filtration; up to 90% or more excreted in urine in patients with severe hepatic function impairment or biliary obstruction.
§In pediatric patients, the Vol$_D$ = 0.3 L/kg.
#In pediatric patients 2 months to 16 years of age, the Vol$_D$ = 0.33 L/kg.

---

**CEPHALOTHIN**—See *Cephalosporins (Systemic)*

**CEPHRADINE**—See *Cephalosporins (Systemic)*

**CEPHAPIRIN**—See *Cephalosporins (Systemic)*

---

# CERIVASTATIN Systemic—INTRODUCTORY VERSION

VA CLASSIFICATION (Primary): CV601
Commonly used brand name(s): *Baycol*.
Note: For a listing of dosage forms and brand names by country availability, see *Dosage Forms* section(s).

## Category
Antihyperlipidemic; HMG-CoA reductase inhibitor.

## Indications
**Accepted**
Hyperlipidemia (treatment)—Cerivastatin is indicated as an adjunct to diet to reduce elevated total cholesterol (total-C) and low-density lipoprotein cholesterol (LDL-C) concentrations in patients with primary hypercholesterolemia (heterozygous familial and nonfamilial) and mixed dyslipidemia (Fredrickson Types IIa and IIb) when response to dietary restriction of saturated fat and cholesterol and other nonpharmacological measures alone has been inadequate.

## Pharmacology/Pharmacokinetics
**Physicochemical characteristics**
Molecular weight—481.5.

**Mechanism of action/Effect**
3-Hydroxy-3-methylglutaryl coenzyme A (HMG-CoA) reductase inhibitors competitively inhibit the enzyme that catalyzes the conversion of HMG-CoA to mevalonate, a precursor to cholesterol. The primary site of action of HMG-CoA reductase inhibitors is the liver, which is the principal site of cholesterol synthesis and low-density lipoprotein clearance. Cholesterol and triglycerides circulate in the bloodstream as part of lipoprotein complexes. These complexes are composed of high-density lipoprotein (HDL), intermediate-density lipoprotein (IDL), low-density lipoprotein (LDL), and very low-density lipoprotein (VLDL). Triglycerides (TG) and cholesterol are synthesized in the liver and incorporated into VLDL for release into the plasma and delivery to the peripheral tissues. LDL is formed from VLDL and is catabolized primarily through the LDL receptor. Elevated plasma concentrations of total cholesterol (total-C), LDL-cholesterol (LDL-C), and apolipoprotein B (apo B) pro-

mote human atherosclerosis and are risk factors for developing cardiovascular disease. Increased plasma concentrations of HDL-cholesterol (HDL-C) are associated with decreased cardiovascular risk. The reduction of cholesterol synthesis in the liver by cerivastatin reduces the level of cholesterol in hepatic cells, stimulating the synthesis of hepatic LDL receptors on the cell-surface and enhancing the uptake of LDL particles. The end result is a reduction in total-C, LDL-C, and apo B. Cerivastatin also reduces plasma triglycerides and increases plasma HDL-C.

**Other actions/effects**
Because HMG-CoA reductase inhibitors interfere with cholesterol synthesis, thereby lowering cholesterol levels, theoretically they may blunt adrenal or gonadal steroid hormone production.

**Absorption**
The mean absolute bioavailability of a 0.2-mg dose is 60%; range, 39 to 101%.

**Distribution**
Volume of distribution ($Vol_D$)—0.3 liter per kg (L/kg).

**Protein binding**
Very high (> 99%; 80% to albumin), concentration-independent up to 100 mg per liter (mg/L).

**Biotransformation**
The parent compound, cerivastatin, is primarily responsible for the cholesterol-lowering effects. Two metabolites, M1 and M23, are pharmacologically active and circulate in the blood with cerivastatin. Metabolite M1 is formed by demethylation of the benzylic methyl ether and metabolite M23 is formed by hydroxylation of the methyl group in the 6-isopropyl moiety. The combination of both reactions leads to formation of metabolite M24. Metabolites M1 and M23 are approximately 50% and 80% as potent as the parent compound, respectively. Mean $C_{max}$ values for cerivastatin, M1, and M23 were 3, 0.2, and 0.5 micrograms per liter (mcg/L), respectively, following a 0.3-mg dose of cerivastatin to six healthy volunteers.

**Half-life**
Elimination—
  2 to 3 hours.

**Time to peak concentration**
Approximately 2.5 hours.

**Peak serum concentration**
The mean value of the maximum serum concentrations ($C_{max}$) following an evening dose of 0.3 mg of cerivastatin is 3.8 mcg/L.

**Elimination**
Cerivastatin is not found in either urine or feces; M1 and M23 are the major metabolites excreted by the following routes:
Renal—Approximately 24%.
Fecal—Approximately 70%.
In dialysis—
  Because cerivastatin is highly protein bound, it is not expected to be cleared significantly by hemodialysis.

## Precautions to Consider

**Carcinogenicity**
Tumor incidences in treated rats were comparable to those in controls in all treatment groups in a 2-year study in which rats were given average daily doses of 0.007, 0.034, or 0.158 mg per kg of body weight (mg/kg) of cerivastatin. The high dosage level corresponded to area under the plasma concentration–time curve (AUC) values of approximately one to two times the mean human plasma drug concentrations after a 0.3-mg oral dose. A significant increase in hepatocellular adenomas occurred in both male and female mice at doses ≥ 9.1 mg/kg of cerivastatin in a 2-year study in which mice were given average daily doses of 0.4, 1.8, 9.1, or 55 mg/kg of cerivastatin. The incidence of hepatocellular carcinomas was increased significantly in male mice given ≥ 1.8 mg/kg of cerivastatin. These doses were comparable to a 0.3 mg per day human dose.

**Mutagenicity**
Genotoxicity was not observed *in vitro*, with or without metabolic activation, in the following assays: microbial mutagen tests using mutant strains of *Salmonella typhimurium* or *Escherichia coli*, Chinese hamster ovary forward mutation assay, unscheduled DNA synthesis in rat primary hepatocytes, chromosome aberrations in Chinese hamster ovary cells, or spindle inhibition in human lymphocytes. Genotoxicity was not observed *in vivo* in a mouse micronucleus test; however, there was equivocal evidence of mutagenicity in a mouse dominant lethal test.

**Pregnancy/Reproduction**
Fertility—No adverse effects on fertility or reproductive performance were seen in male and female rats given daily doses of up to 0.1 mg/kg of cerivastatin. This dose produced peak plasma drug concentrations ($C_{max}$) about one to two times higher than mean plasma drug concentrations for humans receiving 0.3 mg of cerivastatin per day. The length of gestation was marginally prolonged, the number of stillbirths was increased, and the rate of pup survival up to postpartum day 4 was decreased in rats given a daily dose of 0.3 mg/kg ($C_{max}$ four to five times the human concentration). A marginal reduction in fetal weight and delay in bone development was observed in the F1 generation of fetuses. In the mating of the F1 generation, there was a reduced number of female rats that littered.

A study in dogs given long-term daily doses of 0.008 mg/kg of cerivastatin (approximately two times the human exposure at doses of 0.3 mg, based on $C_{max}$) resulted in testicular atrophy, vacuolization of the germinal epithelium, spermatidic giant cells, and focal oligospermia. Another 1-year study in dogs given daily doses of 0.1 mg/kg of cerivastatin (approximately 23 times the human exposure at doses of 0.3 mg, based on $C_{max}$) resulted in a reduction in ejaculate volume and decreased libido. Semen analysis revealed an increased number of morphologically altered spermatozoa, indicating disturbances of epididymal sperm maturation that were reversible when drug administration was discontinued.

Pregnancy—Cerivastatin therapy is *contraindicated* in pregnant women because it decreases cholesterol synthesis and possibly the synthesis of other biologically active substances, such as steroids and cell membranes, that are derived from cholesterol and are essential for fetal development.

There have been rare reports of congenital anomalies following intrauterine exposure to HMG-CoA reductase inhibitors. Incidences of congenital anomalies, spontaneous abortions and fetal deaths and/or stillbirths did not exceed what would be expected in the general population in the review of approximately 100 pregnancies that were prospectively followed in women exposed to simvastatin or lovastatin. The number of cases that were reviewed is adequate only to exclude a three- to fourfold increase in congenital anomalies over the background incidence. In 89% of the prospectively followed pregnancies, pharmacologic treatment was initiated prior to pregnancy and was discontinued at some point during the first trimester when pregnancy was detected. Cerivastatin should not be administered to women of childbearing potential when they are highly likely to conceive. If a woman becomes pregnant during cerivastatin therapy, the medication should be discontinued and the patient advised of the potential hazards to the fetus.

A significant increase in the incidence of incomplete ossification of the lumbar center of the vertebrae occurred in rats given an oral dose of 0.72 mg/kg of cerivastatin. Anomalies or malformations did not occur in rabbits given oral doses of up to 0.75 mg/kg of cerivastatin. These doses resulted in a $C_{max}$ six to seven times the human exposure for rats and three to four times the human exposure for rabbits (based upon a human dose of 0.3 mg). In pregnant rats given a single oral 2-mg/kg dose, cerivastatin crossed the placenta and was found in fetal liver, gastrointestinal tract, and kidneys.

FDA Pregnancy Category X.

**Breast-feeding**
Cerivastatin is distributed into breast milk at a milk to plasma concentration ratio of 1.3 to 1. Cerivastatin is *contraindicated* in women who are breast-feeding because of the potential for serious adverse effects in the nursing infant resulting from the inhibition of cholesterol synthesis.

**Pediatrics**
No information is available on the relationship of age to the effects of cerivastatin in pediatric patients. Safety and efficacy have not been established.

**Geriatrics**
Cerivastatin plasma concentrations in healthy male subjects > 65 years of age are similar to those of males < 40 years of age.

**Pharmacogenetics**
$C_{max}$ is approximately 12% higher and AUC is approximately 16% greater in females than in males.

**Surgical**
Cerivastatin therapy should be withheld temporarily or discontinued in any patient having a risk factor, such as major surgery, predisposing to the development of renal failure secondary to rhabdomyolysis.

**Drug interactions and/or related problems**
The following drug interactions and/or related problems have been selected on the basis of their potential clinical significance (possible mechanism in parentheses where appropriate)—not necessarily inclusive (» = major clinical significance):

Note: Combinations containing any of the following medications, depending on the amount present, may also interact with this medication.

Alcohol, substantial use of
(elevations in transaminase values may occur; caution should be used)
» Antifungals, azole or
» Erythromycin or
» Gemfibrozil or
» Immunosuppressants, especially cyclosporine or
» Niacin (nicotinic acid)
(concurrent administration with these medications may increase the risk of myopathy, such as rhabdomyolysis; 10 days of concurrent erythromycin administration in hypercholesterolemic patients resulted in increases in cerivastatin AUC and $C_{max}$ of approximately 50% and 24%, respectively; use of gemfibrozil alone has been associated with myopathy and concurrent use with cerivastatin is not recommended)

Cholestyramine
(concurrent administration of 0.2 mg of cerivastatin and 12 grams of cholestyramine in 12 healthy volunteers resulted in a decrease of more than 22% and 40% for AUC and $C_{max}$ of cerivastatin, respectively; however, administration of 12 grams of cholestyramine 1 hour before the evening meal and 0.3 mg of cerivastatin approximately 4 hours after the same evening meal resulted in a decrease in the AUC of less than 8% and a decrease in $C_{max}$ of approximately 30%; it is recommended that cholestyramine be dosed before the evening meal and cerivastatin be dosed at bedtime in order to avoid a significant decrease in the bioavailability and clinical effect of cerivastatin)

Medications that may decrease the concentrations or activity of endogenous steroid hormones, such as:
Cimetidine or
Ketoconazole or
Spironolactone
(HMG-CoA reductase inhibitors interfere with cholesterol synthesis and could possibly blunt adrenal and/or gonadal steroid production; concurrent administration with these medications may further decrease concentrations and/or inhibit the activity of endogenous steroid hormones)

### Laboratory value alterations
The following have been selected on the basis of their potential clinical significance (possible effect in parentheses where appropriate)—not necessarily inclusive (» = major clinical significance):

With physiology/laboratory test values
Creatine kinase (CK), serum
(increases in CK values to > 10 times the upper limit of normal [ULN] occurred in < 0.2% of patients in cerivastatin clinical trials in the U.S.; cerivastatin should be discontinued if marked elevations of creatine kinase occur; if these elevations are accompanied by diffuse muscle aches, tenderness, or weakness, myopathy should be considered)

Transaminases, serum
(elevations in liver enzyme values usually occur within the first 3 months of treatment; if elevations in aspartate aminotransferase [AST (SGOT)] or alanine aminotransferase [ALT (SGPT)] are > three times the ULN and persist, it is recommended that cerivastatin be discontinued; persistent increases in transaminase values [> three times ULN, occurring on two or more occasions] have been reported in < 1% of patients treated with cerivastatin over an average period of 11 months; most elevations in transaminase values occurred during the first 6 weeks of treatment, resolved after discontinuation of cerivastatin, and were not associated with cholestasis)

### Medical considerations/Contraindications
The medical considerations/contraindications included have been selected on the basis of their potential clinical significance (reasons given in parentheses where appropriate)—not necessarily inclusive (» = major clinical significance).

***Except under special circumstances, this medication should not be used when the following medical problems exist:***
» Elevations of transaminase values, unexplained, persistent or
» Hepatic disease, active
(cerivastatin has not been studied in patients with active liver disease; the presence of hepatic disease may increase cerivastatin plasma concentrations and/or potentiate further deterioration of liver function)
» Hypersensitivity to cerivastatin

***Risk-benefit should be considered when the following medical problems exist:***
» Electrolyte, endocrine, or metabolic disorders, severe or
» Hypotension or
» Infection, severe acute or
» Seizures, uncontrolled or
» Surgery, major or
» Trauma
(these conditions may predispose a patient to the development of renal failure, secondary to rhabdomyolysis; cerivastatin should be discontinued or temporarily withheld)

Hepatic disease, history of
(elevations in transaminase values may occur; caution is recommended in the use of cerivastatin in these patients)

Renal function impairment
(AUC and $C_{max}$ may be increased by up to 60% and 23%, respectively, in patients with significant renal function impairment [creatinine clearance ≤ 60 mL per minute]; cerivastatin half-life may be prolonged by a period of up to 47% when compared with subjects with normal renal function; caution should be used)

### Patient monitoring
The following may be especially important in patient monitoring (other tests may be warranted in some patients, depending on condition; » = major clinical significance):

Creatine kinase (CK), serum
(periodic determinations recommended in patients who develop muscle pain, tenderness, or weakness during therapy or who concurrently are receiving azole antifungals, erythromycin, gemfibrozil, immunosuppressive agents such as cyclosporine, or niacin)

» Hepatic function determinations
(recommended prior to initiation of treatment and at 6 and 12 weeks of treatment or at a dosage increase, and periodically, such as every 6 months, thereafter; increased transaminase concentrations should be monitored with a second liver function evaluation followed by frequent liver function tests until the abnormalities are resolved)

» Lipid concentrations, serum, primarily:
High-density lipoprotein cholesterol (HDL-C) and
Low-density lipoprotein cholesterol (LDL-C) and
Total cholesterol (total-C) and
Triglycerides (TG)
(the goal of treatment is to lower LDL-C concentrations; if laboratory testing of LDL-C concentrations is not available, total-C concentrations may be used to monitor therapy; determinations recommended at 4 weeks after initiation of cerivastatin therapy)

## Side/Adverse Effects

Note: Long-term administration of cerivastatin to a variety of species has resulted in the following abnormalities: hemorrhage and edema in multiple organs and tissues including the central nervous system (CNS) in dogs; cataracts in dogs; degeneration of muscle fibers in dogs, rats, and mice; hyperkeratosis in the nonglandular stomach (no human equivalent) in rats and mice; and liver lesions in dogs, rats, and mice.

CNS lesions, characterized by multifocal bleeding with fibrinoid degeneration of vessel walls in the plexus choroideus of the brain stem and in the ciliary body of the eye, occurred in dogs given daily doses of 0.1 mg per kg of body weight (mg/kg) of cerivastatin. This dose resulted in maximum plasma concentrations ($C_{max}$) of cerivastatin that were about 23 times higher than the mean values in humans, based on a daily 0.3-mg dose of cerivastatin. CNS lesions were not observed in mice and rats after long-term treatment with cerivastatin for up to 2 years. In mice, the $C_{max}$ was up to seven times higher than that in humans, based on a daily 0.3-mg dose, and in rats, the $C_{max}$ was up to two times higher than that in humans.

Because HMG-CoA reductase inhibitors interfere with cholesterol synthesis, theoretically they may blunt adrenal or gonadal steroid hormone production. Patients who develop clinical evidence of endocrine dysfunction should be evaluated appropriately.

The following side/adverse effects have been selected on the basis of their potential clinical significance (possible signs and symptoms in parentheses where appropriate)—not necessarily inclusive:

### Those indicating need for medical attention
Incidence less frequent or rare
***Abdominal pain; chest pain; edema, peripheral*** (ankle, feet, and leg swelling); ***muscle disorders, such as leg cramps; myalgia, uncomplicated*** (muscle pain); ***myopathy and/or rhabdomyolysis*** (fever; muscle cramps, pain, stiffness, or weakness; unusual tiredness); ***and myositis*** (inflammation of muscle); ***skin rash***

Note: Degradation of muscle occurs in *rhabdomyolysis*, resulting in the release of myoglobin into the urine, which can lead to acute renal failure. *Myopathy* and/or rhabdomyolysis should be considered if symptoms occur in conjunction with creatine kinase (CK) value increases that are > 10 times the upper limit of normal. The risk of myopathy increases when HMG-CoA reductase inhibitors are administered with azole antifungals, erythromycin, gemfibrozil, immunosuppressants such as cyclosporine, or niacin. Patients should be monitored during the first months of therapy and during dosage increases of either drug, and should report immediately any unexplained symptoms of muscle pain, tenderness, or weakness, especially if accompanied by fever or malaise.

**Those indicating need for medical attention only if they continue or are bothersome**
Incidence more frequent
*Constipation; diarrhea; dizziness; dyspepsia* (heartburn; indigestion; stomach discomfort); *flatulence* (belching; excessive gas); *insomnia* (trouble in sleeping); *nausea*

## Overdose

For more information on the management of overdose or unintentional ingestion, **contact a Poison Control Center** (see *Poison Control Center Listing*).

**Treatment of overdose**
No information is available concerning the treatment of cerivastatin overdose.
Treatment should be symptomatic and supportive.
Supportive care—Patients in whom intentional overdose is confirmed or suspected should be referred for psychiatric consultation.

## Patient Consultation

As an aid to patient consultation, refer to *Advice for the Patient, Cerivastatin (Systemic)—Introductory Version*.
In providing consultation, consider emphasizing the following selected information (» = major clinical significance):

**Before using this medication**
» Conditions affecting use, especially:
  Hypersensitivity to cerivastatin
  Carcinogenicity—Hepatocellular adenomas and carcinomas have occurred in mice
  Pregnancy—Contraindicated during pregnancy or in women planning to become pregnant in the near future
  Breast-feeding—Contraindicated in women who are breast-feeding
  Surgical—Increased risk of development of myopathy with major surgery
  Other medications, especially azole antifungals; erythromycin; gemfibrozil; immunosuppressants, such as cyclosporine; or niacin (nicotinic acid)
  Other medical problems, especially active hepatic disease; hypotension; major surgery; severe acute infection; severe electrolyte, endocrine, or metabolic disorders; trauma; uncontrolled seizures; or unexplained persistent elevations of transaminase values

**Proper use of this medication**
Compliance with therapy; taking medication at the same time each day to maintain the antihyperlipidemic effect
Compliance with prescribed diet during treatment
» Proper dosing
Missed dose: Taking as soon as possible; not taking if almost time for next dose; not doubling doses
» Proper storage

**Precautions while using this medication**
Regular visits to physician to check progress
Notifying physician immediately if pregnancy is suspected because of possible harm to the fetus
Caution if any kind of surgery (including dental surgery) or emergency treatment is required
Not taking over-the-counter niacin preparations without consulting physician because of increased risk of rhabdomyolysis
Not using alcohol excessively because elevations of liver enzymes may occur
Notifying physician immediately if unexplained muscle pain, tenderness, or weakness occurs, especially if accompanied by unusual tiredness or fever because of risk of rhabdomyolysis

**Side/adverse effects**
Signs of potential side effects, especially abdominal pain; chest pain; peripheral edema; muscle disorders, such as leg cramps, uncomplicated myalgia, myopathy and/or rhabdomyolysis, and myositis; and skin rash

## General Dosing Information

Prior to starting cerivastatin therapy, secondary causes for hypercholesterolemia, such as poorly controlled diabetes mellitus, hypothyroidism, nephrotic syndrome, dysproteinemias, obstructive liver disease, other medication therapy, and alcoholism should be excluded and a lipid profile performed to measure total cholesterol (total-C), high-density lipoprotein cholesterol (HDL-C), and triglycerides (TG).

For patients with TG concentrations > 400 mg per dL (mg/dL), low-density lipoprotein cholesterol (LDL-C) concentrations should be measured directly. Cerivastatin is not indicated in hypertriglyceridemic patients in whom total-C is elevated and LDL-C is low or normal.

Cerivastatin may be given with cholestyramine for additional lipid-lowering effects on LDL-C and total-C. Cerivastatin should be given at least 2 hours after cholestyramine.

Maximum response is usually achieved within 4 weeks and maintained during long-term therapy, at which time lipid determinations should be performed.

**Diet/Nutrition**
Prior to treatment with cerivastatin, control of hypercholesterolemia with diet, exercise, weight reduction in obese patients, and treatment of underlying medical problems should be attempted. The patient should be placed on a standard cholesterol-lowering diet before receiving cerivastatin and should continue on this diet during treatment with cerivastatin.

For additional information on initial therapeutic guidelines related to the treatment of hyperlipidemia, see *Appendix III*.

## Oral Dosage Forms

### CERIVASTATIN SODIUM TABLETS

**Usual adult dose**
Heterozygous familial and nonfamilial and mixed dyslipidemia (Fredrickson Types IIa and IIb)—
  Oral, 0.3 mg once daily in the evening, taken with or without food.
  The recommended starting dose in patients with significant renal impairment (creatinine clearance ≤ 60 mL/min) is 0.2 mg once daily in the evening.

**Usual adult prescribing limits**
0.3 mg per day.

**Usual pediatric dose**
Safety and efficacy have not been established.

**Strength(s) usually available**
U.S.—
  0.2 mg (Rx) [*Baycol*].
  0.3 mg (Rx) [*Baycol*].

**Packaging and storage**
Store below 25 °C (77 °F). Protect from moisture. Dispense in a tight container.

**Auxiliary labeling**
• Do not take other medications without your doctor's advice.

Developed: 11/12/97

---

**CETIRIZINE**—See *Antihistamines (Systemic)*

# CHARCOAL, ACTIVATED Oral-Local

This monograph includes information on the following: 1) Activated Charcoal; 2) Activated Charcoal and Sorbitol.

**VA CLASSIFICATION (Primary):** AD900

Commonly used brand name(s): *Actidose with Sorbitol*[2]; *Actidose-Aqua*[1]; *Aqueous Charcodote*[1]; *Charac-50*[1]; *Charac-tol 50*[2]; *CharcoAid 2000*[1]; *Charcoaid*[2]; *Charcocaps*[1]; *Charcodote*[2]; *Charcodote TFS-25*[2]; *Charcodote TFS-50*[2]; *Insta-Char Aqueous*[1]; *Insta-Char with Sorbitol*[2]; *Liqui-Char*[1]; *Liqui-Char with Sorbitol*[2]; *Pediatric Aqueous Charcodote*[1]; *Pediatric Aqueous Insta-Char*[1]; *Pediatric Charcodote*[2].

Note: For a listing of dosage forms and brand names by country availability, see *Dosage Forms* section(s).

## Category

Antidote (adsorbent)—Activated Charcoal USP; Activated Charcoal Oral Suspension.
Antidote (adsorbent)-laxative—Activated Charcoal and Sorbitol Oral Suspension.
Antidiarrheal (adsorbent)—Activated Charcoal Capsules.
Antiflatulent—Activated Charcoal Capsules; Activated Charcoal Tablets.

## Indications

**Accepted**

Toxicity, nonspecific (treatment)—Activated charcoal powder (prepared as an aqueous slurry) and oral suspension and activated charcoal and sorbitol oral suspension are indicated for use as an emergency antidote in the treatment of poisoning by most drugs and chemicals. However, activated charcoal is relatively ineffective in adsorbing caustic alkalis, boric acid, lithium, petroleum distillates (e.g., kerosene, gasoline, coal oil, fuel oil, paint thinner, cleaning fluid), ethanol, methanol, iron salts, and mineral acids.

Diarrhea (treatment) or
Gas, intestinal (treatment)—Activated charcoal capsules and tablets are indicated in the treatment of diarrhea and as a temporary aid in the adsorption of intestinal gas causing flatulence; however, enough studies have not been done to confirm its efficacy for these uses.

## Pharmacology/Pharmacokinetics

**Mechanism of action/Effect**

Activated charcoal—
  Antidote (adsorbent): Adsorbs the toxic substance ingested, thus inhibiting gastrointestinal absorption.
  Antidiarrheal (adsorbent): Adsorbs many toxic irritants that cause diarrhea and gastrointestinal discomfort.
  Antiflatulent: Adsorbs intestinal gas to relieve discomfort.
Sorbitol—
  Laxative, hyperosmotic: Hygroscopic action results in increased water in the large intestine and increased intraluminal pressure, thus stimulating catharsis.
  Flavoring agent: Provides a sweet vehicle to enhance palatability.

**Absorption**

Activated charcoal—Not absorbed from the gastrointestinal tract.
Sorbitol—Poorly absorbed from the gastrointestinal tract.

**Biotransformation**

Activated charcoal—Not metabolized.
Sorbitol—Hepatic; slowly converted to fructose.

**Elimination**

Activated charcoal—Intestinal.

## Precautions to Consider

**Pregnancy/Reproduction**

Pregnancy—Problems in humans have not been documented.

**Breast-feeding**

Problems in humans have not been documented.

**Pediatrics**

*For use as an antidote—*
  Preparations of activated charcoal with sorbitol are usually not recommended for use in children under 1 year of age because of the risk of excessive catharsis. In older children, the weight of the child must be taken into account to determine a safe dosage of sorbitol, which should not exceed 3 grams per kg of body weight.

Children should not receive preparations of activated charcoal with sorbitol unless they are under the direct supervision of a physician, so proper attention may be given to the patients' fluid and electrolyte needs.

*For antidiarrheal or antiflatulent use (preparations without sorbitol only)—*
  When used as an antidiarrheal or antiflatulent, prolonged use of activated charcoal in infants and children under 3 years of age is not recommended since it may possibly interfere with nutrition.
  In pediatric patients with diarrhea, caution is recommended because of the risk of fluid and electrolyte loss; these patients should be referred to a physician.

**Geriatrics**

*For use as an antidote—*
  Although adequate and well-controlled studies have not been done in the geriatric population, caution is recommended when using preparations of activated charcoal with sorbitol because of the increased risk of catharsis, which may result in fluid and electrolyte loss in geriatric patients.

*For antidiarrheal use (preparations without sorbitol only)—*
  In geriatric patients with diarrhea, caution is recommended because of the risk of fluid and electrolyte loss; these patients should be referred to a physician.

**Drug interactions and/or related problems**

The following drug interactions and/or related problems have been selected on the basis of their potential clinical significance (possible mechanism in parentheses where appropriate)—not necessarily inclusive (» = major clinical significance):

» Acetylcysteine, oral
  (effectiveness of orally administered acetylcysteine as antidote in acetaminophen overdose may be decreased because of adsorption by activated charcoal; activated charcoal is recommended if ingestion of other substances [in addition to acetaminophen] is confirmed or suspected, but its removal by gastric lavage may be advisable prior to acetylcysteine administration)

Chocolate syrup or
Ice cream or sherbet
  (should not be used as vehicles for the administration of activated charcoal since they will decrease the adsorptive capacity of the activated charcoal)

Ipecac
  (if both ipecac and activated charcoal are to be used in the treatment for oral poisoning, it is generally recommended that the charcoal be administered only after vomiting has been induced and completed; however, in some clinical trials in which activated charcoal was administered pre-emesis 10 minutes after high doses of ipecac, the emetic properties of ipecac were not inhibited)

Oral medications, other
  (the effectiveness of other concurrently used medications may be decreased because of adsorption and increased elimination by the activated charcoal; patients should be advised not to take any other medication within 2 hours of the activated charcoal)

**Medical considerations/Contraindications**

The medical considerations/contraindications included have been selected on the basis of their potential clinical significance (reasons given in parentheses where appropriate)—not necessarily inclusive (» = major clinical significance).

*Risk-benefit should be considered when the following medical problems exist:*

» Bowel sounds, absence of
  (increased risk of gastrointestinal complications, such as gastrointestinal obstruction)

*For antidiarrheal use only (preparations without sorbitol only)*
» Dehydration
  (rehydration therapy is essential if signs of dehydration, such as dry mouth, excessive thirst, wrinkled skin, decreased urination, dizziness or lightheadedness, are present; fluid loss may have serious consequences, such as circulatory collapse and renal failure, especially in young children and the elderly)

Diarrhea, parasite-associated, suspected
  (use of adsorbent antidiarrheals may make recognition of parasitic causes of diarrhea more difficult; if parasitic agents are suspected pathogens, appropriate stool analyses should be performed prior to therapy with adsorbents)

» Dysentery, acute, characterized by bloody stools and elevated temperature
   (sole treatment with adsorbent antidiarrheals may be inadequate; antibiotic therapy may be required)

## Side/Adverse Effects

The following side/adverse effects have been selected on the basis of their potential clinical significance (possible signs and symptoms in parentheses where appropriate)—not necessarily inclusive:

Note: Dehydration, cardiac arrest, and brain damage occurred as a result of sorbitol overdose in a 3-year-old child who was being treated with activated charcoal and sorbitol combination for an overdose of a drug used to treat asthma.

**Those indicating need for medical attention**
Incidence less frequent or rare
*Swelling of abdomen or pain*

**Those indicating need for medical attention only if they continue**
Incidence more frequent—with sorbitol-containing preparations
*Diarrhea or vomiting*

Note: *Diarrhea or vomiting* may persist for several hours; precautions should be taken against possible fluid and electrolyte loss.

**Those not indicating need for medical attention**
Incidence more frequent
*Black stools*

## Patient Consultation

As an aid to patient consultation, refer to *Advice for the Patient, Charcoal, Activated (Oral)*.
In providing consultation, consider emphasizing the following selected information (» = major clinical significance):

**Before using this medication**
» Conditions affecting use, especially:
   Use in children—Preparations with sorbitol are not recommended for children up to 1 year of age and should be used only under a physician's supervision in older children because of risk of excessive catharsis; prolonged use of activated charcoal as an antidiarrheal/antiflatulent in children under 3 years of age may interfere with nutrition; risk of dehydration associated with diarrhea (for antidiarrheal use)
   Use in the elderly—Risk of fluid and electrolyte loss with preparations containing sorbitol; risk of dehydration associated with diarrhea (for antidiarrheal use)
   Other medical problems, especially absence of bowel sounds (for antidote use); dehydration and acute dysentery (for antidiarrheal/antiflatulent use)

**Proper use of this medication**
» Importance of not taking medication mixed with chocolate syrup, ice cream, or sherbet
» Proper dosing
» Proper storage
*When used as an antidote only*
» Calling poison control center, physician, or emergency room before taking medication
» Importance of shaking the oral liquid dosage form well; taking full dose
» Taking medication only after vomiting has been induced and completed if ipecac syrup is used also
*When used as an antidiarrheal/antiflatulent only*
   Taking doses of other oral medications at least 2 hours before or after doses of activated charcoal
*When used as an antidiarrheal only*
» Importance of maintaining adequate hydration and proper diet

**Precautions while using this medication**
*When used as an antidiarrheal/antiflatulent only*
   Checking with physician if condition has not improved after 7 days (when used as an antiflatulent only)
   Checking with physician if diarrhea continues after medication has been used for 2 days or if fever is present with diarrhea

**Side/adverse effects**
   Signs of potential side effects, especially continuing diarrhea or vomiting (for sorbitol-containing preparations)
   Medication will color stools black, which may be alarming to patient although medically insignificant

## General Dosing Information

**For use as an antidote only**

Activated charcoal is most effective when it is administered early in acute poisoning, preferably within 30 minutes following ingestion of the poison.

When the amount of toxic substance ingested is known, the dose of activated charcoal recommended is usually 5 to 10 times the amount of toxic substance ingested; however, a dose of 50 grams is considered the minimum adult dose by many clinicians.

Tablets or granules of activated charcoal are less effective than the powder form of the medication and should not be used in the treatment of poisoning.

The administration of activated charcoal as an aqueous slurry is generally preferred. However, to improve the palatability of activated charcoal, it has been administered in combination with suspending agents such as bentonite or carboxymethylcellulose. Also, a flavoring agent such as chocolate syrup has been added to the combination at the time of administration. However, some studies have shown that these agents, especially the flavoring agents, decrease the adsorptive capacity of activated charcoal and should not be used.

Following administration of activated charcoal, it is recommended that a cathartic be administered to enhance removal of the drug/charcoal complex since failure to excrete the drug/charcoal complex promptly may result in enhanced toxicity. However, administration of a cathartic may not be necessary when an activated charcoal product containing sorbitol is used.

Multiple-dose activated charcoal therapy may be useful in severe poisonings to prevent desorption from the charcoal; to hasten elimination of chronically used medications by the gastrointestinal tract (gastrointestinal dialysis); also, to increase clearance of certain drugs or substances that undergo enterohepatic circulation, to prevent their reabsorption. Some substances for which multiple-dose activated charcoal therapy has been demonstrated to be effective are amitriptyline, carbamazepine, diazepam, digoxin, doxepin, meprobamate, methotrexate, nortriptyline, phenobarbital, piroxicam, salicylates, and theophylline.

When multiple doses of activated charcoal are required, preparations that contain sorbitol should not be used in each dose of the multiple-dose regimen since they may produce excessive catharsis, which may result in dehydration and hypotension. Instead, doses of activated charcoal preparations without sorbitol should be alternated with the sorbitol-containing products.

The presence of normal bowel sounds is necessary to determine whether to continue multiple-dose activated charcoal therapy. If bowel sounds are absent or hypoactive, continuing multiple dosing of activated charcoal with or without sorbitol is not recommended because of the possibility of constipation (or aggravation of) and the possibility of pooling of fluids in the colon if sorbitol continues to be administered with the activated charcoal.

If catharsis does not occur within four to eight hours after use of an activated charcoal preparation containing sorbitol, an additional dose of sorbitol (1.5 grams per kg of body weight) or a saline laxative, such as magnesium citrate, may be administered.

---
### ACTIVATED CHARCOAL
---

## Oral-Local Dosage Forms

### ACTIVATED CHARCOAL USP

**Usual adult and adolescent dose**
Antidote (adsorbent)—
   Oral, 25 to 100 grams, as a slurry in water.

**Usual pediatric dose**
Antidote (adsorbent)—
   Oral, 1 gram per kg of body weight, or 25 to 50 grams, as a slurry in water.

**Usual geriatric dose**
See *Usual adult and adolescent dose*.

**Size(s) usually available**
U.S.—
   15 grams (OTC) [GENERIC].
   30 grams (OTC) [GENERIC].
   40 grams (OTC) [GENERIC].
   120 grams (OTC) [GENERIC].
   125 grams (OTC) [GENERIC].
   240 grams (OTC) [GENERIC].
   500 grams (OTC) [GENERIC].

Canada—
25 grams (OTC) [GENERIC].

**Packaging and storage**
Store below 40 °C (104 °F), preferably between 15 and 30 °C (59 and 86 °F), unless otherwise specified by manufacturer. Store in a well-closed container.

**Note**
If this medication is to be used as an antidote for emergency use in poisoning, consider providing on the label the telephone number for physician, poison control center, or emergency room.

### ACTIVATED CHARCOAL CAPSULES

Note: Activated charcoal capsules should not be used as an antidote for emergency use in poisoning.

**Usual adult and adolescent dose**
Antidiarrheal (adsorbent)—
  Oral, 520 mg, repeated every thirty minutes to one hour as needed up to 4.16 grams per day.
Antiflatulent—
  Oral, 1.04 to 3.9 grams three times a day after meals.

**Usual pediatric dose**
Antidiarrheal (adsorbent)—
  Infants and children up to 3 years of age: Dosage must be individualized by physician.
  Children 3 years of age and over: See *Usual adult and adolescent dose*.
Antiflatulent—
  Dosage must be individualized by physician.

**Usual geriatric dose**
See *Usual adult and adolescent dose*.

**Strength(s) usually available**
U.S.—
  250 mg (OTC) [*Charcocaps*].
  260 mg (OTC) [*Charcocaps;* GENERIC].
Canada—
  Content information not available (OTC) [GENERIC].

**Packaging and storage**
Store below 40 °C (104 °F), preferably between 15 and 30 °C (59 and 86 °F), in a well-closed container, unless otherwise specified by manufacturer.

### ACTIVATED CHARCOAL ORAL SUSPENSION

**Usual adult and adolescent dose**
Antidote (adsorbent)—
  Oral, 25 to 100 grams as a single dose.
Note: For multiple-dose therapy—Oral, 25 to 50 grams every four to six hours.

**Usual pediatric dose**
Antidote (adsorbent)—
  Children up to 1 year of age: Oral, 1 gram per kg of body weight as a single dose.
  Children 1 to 12 years of age: Oral, 25 to 50 grams as a single dose.
Note: For multiple-dose therapy, dose may be repeated every four to six hours.

**Usual geriatric dose**
See *Usual adult and adolescent dose*.

**Strength(s) usually available**
U.S.—
  12.5 grams per 60 mL (OTC) [*Liqui-Char;* GENERIC].
  15 grams per 72 mL (OTC) [*Actidose-Aqua;* GENERIC].
  15 grams per 75 mL (OTC) [*Liqui-Char*].
  15 grams per 120 mL (OTC) [*Pediatric Aqueous Insta-Char*].
  25 grams per 120 mL (OTC) [*Actidose-Aqua; Liqui-Char; Pediatric Aqueous Insta-Char;* GENERIC].
  30 grams per 120 mL (OTC) [*Liqui-Char*].
  50 grams per 240 mL (OTC) [*Actidose-Aqua; CharcoAid 2000; Insta-Char Aqueous; Liqui-Char;* GENERIC].
Canada—
  15 grams per 120 mL [*Insta-Char Aqueous*].
  25 grams per 125 mL [*Pediatric Aqueous Charcodote*].
  50 grams per 225 mL [*Charac-50*].
  50 grams per 240 mL [*Insta-Char Aqueous*].
  50 grams per 250 mL [*Aqueous Charcodote*].
Note: In Canada, this medication has not been assigned either Rx or OTC status. However, it may not be sold or dispensed directly to the patient.

**Packaging and storage**
Store below 40 °C (104 °F), preferably between 15 and 30 °C (59 and 86 °F), in a well-closed container, unless otherwise specified by manufacturer. Protect from freezing.

**Auxiliary labeling**
• Shake well.

**Note**
If this medication is to be used as an antidote for emergency use in poisoning, consider providing on the label the telephone number for poison control center, physician, or emergency room.

### ACTIVATED CHARCOAL TABLETS

Note: Activated charcoal tablets should not be used as an antidote for emergency use in poisoning.

**Usual adult and adolescent dose**
Antiflatulent—
  Oral, 975 mg to 3.9 grams three times a day after meals.

**Usual pediatric dose**
Antiflatulent—
  Dosage must be individualized by physician.

**Usual geriatric dose**
See *Usual adult and adolescent dose*.

**Strength(s) usually available**
U.S.—
  260 mg (OTC) [*Charcocaps*].
  325 mg (OTC) [GENERIC].
  650 mg (OTC) [GENERIC].
Canada—
  Not commercially available.

**Packaging and storage**
Store below 40 °C (104 °F), preferably between 15 and 30 °C (59 and 86 °F), in a well-closed container, unless otherwise specified by manufacturer.

---

## ACTIVATED CHARCOAL AND SORBITOL

## Oral-Local Dosage Forms

### ACTIVATED CHARCOAL AND SORBITOL ORAL SUSPENSION

**Usual adult and adolescent dose**
Antidote (adsorbent)—
  Oral, 50 grams of activated charcoal as a single dose.
Note: For multiple-dose therapy—Use is not recommended because of excessive catharsis, unless repeat doses are alternated with activated charcoal preparations that contain no sorbitol.

  Sorbitol content is different among the different preparations available. Product label should be consulted to determine the amount of sorbitol. For adults, the usual dose of sorbitol 70% (70 grams per 100 mL) is 50 to 150 mL.

**Usual pediatric dose**
Antidote (adsorbent)—
  Children up to 1 year of age: Use is not recommended.
  Children 1 to 12 years of age: Oral, 25 to 50 grams of activated charcoal as a single dose.
Note: For multiple-dose therapy—Use is not recommended because of excessive catharsis, unless repeat doses are alternated with activated charcoal preparations that contain no sorbitol.

  Sorbitol content is different among the different preparations available. Product label should be consulted to determine the amount of sorbitol. For children, the usual dose of sorbitol 70% (70 grams per 100 mL) is 2 mL per kg of body weight, or a dose not to exceed 3 grams of sorbitol per kg of body weight.

**Usual geriatric dose**
See *Usual adult and adolescent dose*.

**Strength(s) usually available**
U.S.—
  25 grams of activated charcoal and 25 grams of sorbitol per 120 mL (OTC) [*Insta-Char with Sorbitol*].
  25 grams of activated charcoal and 27 grams of sorbitol per 120 mL (OTC) [*Liqui-Char with Sorbitol*].
  25 grams of activated charcoal and 48 grams of sorbitol per 120 mL (OTC) [*Actidose with Sorbitol*].
  30 grams of activated charcoal and 62 grams of sorbitol per 150 mL (OTC) [*Charcoaid*].

50 grams of activated charcoal and 50 grams of sorbitol per 240 mL (OTC) [*Insta-Char with Sorbitol*].

50 grams of activated charcoal and 54 grams of sorbitol per 240 mL (OTC) [*Liqui-Char with Sorbitol*].

50 grams of activated charcoal and 96 grams of sorbitol per 240 mL (OTC) [*Actidose with Sorbitol*].

Canada—

25 grams of activated charcoal and 25 grams of sorbitol per 125 mL [*Charcodote TFS-25*].

25 grams of activated charcoal and 90 grams (approximately) of sorbitol per 125 mL [*Pediatric Charcodote*].

50 grams of activated charcoal and 50 grams of sorbitol per 250 mL [*Charac-tol 50; Charcodote TFS-50*].

50 grams of activated charcoal and 180 grams (approximately) of sorbitol per 250 mL [*Charcodote*].

Note: In Canada, this medication has not been assigned either Rx or OTC status. However, it may not be sold or dispensed directly to the patient.

**Packaging and storage**
Store below 40 °C (104 °F), preferably between 15 and 30 °C (59 and 86 °F), in a well-closed container, unless otherwise specified by manufacturer. Protect from freezing.

**Auxiliary labeling**
• Shake well.

**Note**
If this medication is to be used as an antidote for emergency use in poisoning, consider providing on the label the telephone number for physician, poison control center, or emergency room.

## Selected Bibliography
Pond S. Role of repeated oral doses of activated charcoal in clinical toxicology. Med Toxicol 1986; 1: 3-11.

Albertson TE, et al. Superiority of activated charcoal alone compared with ipecac and activated charcoal in the treatment of acute toxic ingestions. Ann Emerg Med 1989; 18: 56-59.

Revised: 08/16/91
Interim revision: 06/14/95

---

**CHENODIOL**—The *Chenodiol (Systemic)* monograph is not included in this published version of the USP DI database. Copies of the monograph are available on request from Micromedex, Inc. - Reprint Requests, 6200 S. Syracuse Way, Suite 300, Englewood, CO 80111; telephone (303) 486-6400; telefax (303) 486-6464; Email: USPDI@MDX.COM.

---

**CHLOPHEDIANOL**—The *Chlophedianol (Systemic)* monograph is not included in this published version of the USP DI database. Copies of the monograph are available on request from Micromedex, Inc. - Reprint Requests, 6200 S. Syracuse Way, Suite 300, Englewood, CO 80111; telephone (303) 486-6400; telefax (303) 486-6464; Email: USPDI@MDX.COM.

---

# CHLORAL HYDRATE  Systemic

VA CLASSIFICATION (Primary): CN309

Note: Controlled substance in the U.S.

Commonly used brand name(s): *Aquachloral Supprettes; Novo-Chlorhydrate; PMS-Chloral Hydrate*.

Note: For a listing of dosage forms and brand names by country availability, see *Dosage Forms* section(s).

## Category
Sedative-hypnotic.

## Indications
Note: Bracketed information in the *Indications* section refers to uses that are not included in U.S. product labeling.

**Accepted**
Anesthesia, adjunct—Chloral hydrate is indicated preoperatively to relieve anxiety and produce sedation and/or sleep.

[Sedation for procedures in pediatric patients]—Chloral hydrate is used to produce sedation in pediatric patients for certain dental and medical procedures.

Chloral hydrate has been used for the treatment of insomnia. However, this medication is effective as a hypnotic only for short-term use; it has been shown to lose its effectiveness for both inducing and maintaining sleep after 2 weeks of administration. In addition, chloral hydrate generally *has been replaced* by agents with better pharmacokinetic and pharmacodynamic profiles.

Chloral hydrate has been used as a routine sedative. However, it generally *has been replaced* by safer and more effective agents.

Chloral hydrate also has been used as an adjunct to opiates and analgesics in postoperative care and control of pain. However, it generally *has been replaced* by agents with better pharmacokinetic and pharmacodynamic profiles.

**Unaccepted**
Chloral hydrate is not recommended for use in infants and children when repetitive dosing would be necessary. With repeated dosing, accumulation of the trichloroethanol and trichloroacetic acid metabolites may increase the potential for excessive CNS depression, predispose neonates to conjugated and nonconjugated hyperbilirubinemia, decrease albumin binding of bilirubin, and contribute to metabolic acidosis.

## Pharmacology/Pharmacokinetics
**Physicochemical characteristics**
Molecular weight—165.40.

**Mechanism of action/Effect**
The central nervous system (CNS) depressant effects of chloral hydrate are believed to be due to its active metabolite trichloroethanol. The mechanism of action is not known.

**Absorption**
Readily absorbed from the gastrointestinal tract, following oral administration.

**Protein binding**
Trichloroethanol (the active metabolite)—35 to 41%.

**Biotransformation**
Chloral hydrate is metabolized in the liver and erythrocytes to the active metabolite trichloroethanol, which may be further metabolized to inactive metabolites. It is also metabolized directly to inactive metabolites by the liver and kidneys.

**Half-life**
The plasma half-life of trichloroethanol, the active metabolite, is about 7 to 10 hours.

**Onset of action**
Oral—Within 30 minutes.

**Duration of action**
About 4 to 8 hours.

**Elimination**
Renal; approximately 40% of dose excreted in 24 hours.

## Precautions to Consider
**Carcinogenicity/Mutagenicity**
Long-term studies in animals have not been done.

**Pregnancy/Reproduction**
Pregnancy—Chloral hydrate crosses the placenta. Studies on teratogenicity have not been done in humans. Chronic use of chloral hydrate during pregnancy may cause withdrawal symptoms in the neonate.

Studies on teratogenicity have not been done in animals.

FDA Pregnancy Category C.

**Breast-feeding**
Chloral hydrate is distributed into breast milk; use by nursing mothers may cause sedation in the infant.

**Pediatrics**
Appropriate studies on the relationship of age to the effects of chloral hydrate have not been performed in the pediatric population. *Deaths have occurred prior to or following diagnostic or therapeutic procedures, particularly in pediatric patients, after chloral hydrate was administered to induce sedation before the procedure. The current Guidelines*

for Monitoring and Management of Pediatric Patients During and After Sedation For Diagnostic and Therapeutic Procedures established by the American Academy of Pediatrics recommend that *sedatives be administered only at the health care facility*, where appropriate monitoring can be instituted. Monitoring must continue until the child's level of consciousness has returned to a state that meets appropriate approved discharge criteria. In addition, particular care must be taken in calculating and administering the proper dose appropriate to the age and weight of pediatric patients. Also, children with sleep apnea, especially obstructive sleep apnea with tonsillar hypertrophy, are particularly prone to respiratory compromise.

Chloral hydrate is not recommended for use in infants and children when repetitive dosing would be necessary. With repeated dosing, accumulation of the trichloroethanol and trichloroacetic acid metabolites may increase the potential for excessive CNS depression, predispose neonates to conjugated and nonconjugated hyperbilirubinemia, decrease albumin binding of bilirubin, and contribute to metabolic acidosis.

### Geriatrics
No information is available on the relationship of age to the effects of chloral hydrate in geriatric patients. However, elderly patients are more likely to have age-related hepatic function impairment and renal function impairment, which may require reduction of dosage in patients receiving chloral hydrate.

### Drug interactions and/or related problems
The following drug interactions and/or related problems have been selected on the basis of their potential clinical significance (possible mechanism in parentheses where appropriate)—not necessarily inclusive (» = major clinical significance):

Note: Combinations containing any of the following medications, depending on the amount present, may also interact with this medication.

  Addictive medications, other, especially CNS depressants with habituating potential
  (prolonged concurrent use may increase the risk of habituation; caution is recommended)

» Alcohol or
» CNS depression–producing medications, other (See *Appendix II*)
  (concurrent use may increase the CNS depressant effects of either these medications or chloral hydrate; caution is recommended and dosage of one or both agents should be reduced)

» Anticoagulants, coumarin- or indandione-derivative
  (hypoprothrombinemic effects may be increased when these medications are used concurrently with chloral hydrate, particularly during the first 2 weeks of concurrent therapy, because of displacement of the anticoagulant from its plasma protein binding sites; with continued concurrent use, anticoagulant activity may return to baseline level or be decreased; frequent prothrombin-time determinations may be required, especially during initiation of chloral hydrate therapy, to determine if dosage adjustment of the anticoagulant is necessary)

  Furosemide, intravenous
  (administration of chloral hydrate followed by intravenous furosemide within 24 hours may result in diaphoresis, hot flashes, and variable blood pressure, including hypertension, due to a hypermetabolic state caused by displacement of thyroxine from its bound state)

### Laboratory value alterations
The following have been selected on the basis of their potential clinical significance (possible effect in parentheses where appropriate)—not necessarily inclusive (» = major clinical significance):

With diagnostic test results
  Fluorometric tests for urine catecholamines
  (it is recommended that chloral hydrate not be administered for 48 hours preceding the test)

  Glucose, urine
  (determinations may give false-positive test results with Benedict's solution, and possibly with cupric sulfate tablets, but not with glucose enzymatic tests)

  Phentolamine test
  (chloral hydrate may cause false-positive phentolamine test; it is recommended that all medications be withdrawn at least 24 hours, preferably 48 to 72 hours, prior to a phentolamine test)

  Urinary 17-hydroxycorticosteroid determinations
  (when using the Reddy, Jenkins, and Thorn procedure)

### Medical considerations/Contraindications
The medical considerations/contraindications included have been selected on the basis of their potential clinical significance (reasons given in parentheses where appropriate)—not necessarily inclusive (» = major clinical significance).

*Risk-benefit should be considered when the following medical problems exist:*
  Cardiac disease, severe
  (condition may be exacerbated by large doses of chloral hydrate)
  Alcohol abuse or dependence, history of or
  Drug abuse or dependence, history of
  (dependence on chloral hydrate may develop)
» Esophagitis or
» Gastritis or
» Ulcers, gastric or duodenal
  (condition may be exacerbated—for oral dosage forms only)
» Hepatic function impairment, severe
  (chloral hydrate metabolized in liver)
  Porphyria, intermittent
  (acute attacks may be precipitated by chloral hydrate)
  Proctitis or colitis
  (condition may be exacerbated—for rectal dosage forms only)
» Renal function impairment, severe
  (chloral hydrate excreted via kidneys)
» Sleep apnea in pediatric patients (especially with tonsillar hypertrophy)
  (increased risk of respiratory compromise)
  Sensitivity to chloral hydrate

## Side/Adverse Effects
The following side/adverse effects have been selected on the basis of their potential clinical significance (possible signs and symptoms in parentheses where appropriate)—not necessarily inclusive:

**Those indicating need for medical attention**
Incidence less frequent
  *Allergic reaction* (skin rash or hives)
Incidence rare
  *Confusion; paradoxical reaction* (hallucinations; unusual excitement)

**Those indicating need for medical attention only if they continue or are bothersome**
Incidence more frequent
  *Nausea; stomach pain; vomiting*
Incidence less frequent
  *Clumsiness or unsteadiness; diarrhea; dizziness or lightheadedness; drowsiness; "hangover" effect*

**Those indicating possible withdrawal and the need for medical attention if they occur after medication is discontinued**
  *Confusion; hallucinations; nausea or vomiting; nervousness; restlessness; stomach pain; trembling; unusual excitement*

## Overdose
For more information on the management of overdose or unintentional ingestion, **contact a Poison Control Center** (see *Poison Control Center Listing*).

### Clinical effects of overdose
The following have been selected on the basis of their potential clinical significance (possible signs and symptoms in parentheses where appropriate)—not necessarily inclusive:

  *Confusion, continuing; convulsions; difficulty in swallowing; drowsiness, severe; low body temperature; nausea, vomiting, or stomach pain, severe; shortness of breath or troubled breathing; slow or irregular heartbeat; slurred speech; staggering; weakness, severe*

Note: Hepatic and renal function may be impaired, resulting in transient jaundice and albuminuria during recovery from chloral hydrate overdose.

### Treatment of overdose
Treatment of chloral hydrate overdose consists of the following:
To decrease absorption—
  Gastric lavage following oral overdose (endotracheal tube with inflated cuff should be in place to prevent aspiration of vomitus).
To enhance elimination—
  Hemodialysis may be effective in promoting the clearance of trichloroethanol.
Monitoring—
  Continuous cardiac monitoring is important, especially in patients with predisposing cardiac disease.

**Supportive care—**
Support of respiration and circulation.
Maintenance of normal body temperature.
Artificial respiration with oxygen may be required.
Appropriate fluid and electrolyte therapy should be administered and an adequate urinary output maintained.
Patients in whom intentional overdose is known or suspected should be referred for psychiatric consultation.

## Patient Consultation

As an aid to patient consultation, refer to *Advice for the Patient, Chloral Hydrate (Systemic)*.

In providing consultation, consider emphasizing the following selected information (» = major clinical significance):

**Before using this medication**
» Conditions affecting use, especially:
Sensitivity to chloral hydrate
Pregnancy—Chloral hydrate crosses placenta; chronic use during pregnancy may cause withdrawal symptoms in neonate
Breast-feeding—Chloral hydrate is distributed into breast milk; use by nursing mothers may cause sedation in the infant
Other medications, especially alcohol or other CNS depression–producing medications or coumarin- or indandione-derivative anticoagulants
Other medical problems, especially esophagitis, gastritis, gastric or duodenal ulcers, hepatic function impairment, renal function impairment, or sleep apnea in children, especially with tonsillar hypertrophy

**Proper use of this medication**
» Importance of not using more medication than the amount prescribed because of habit-forming potential

*Proper administration*
For capsule dosage form
Swallowing capsule whole; not chewing because of unpleasant taste
Taking with a full glass (240 mL) of water, fruit juice, or ginger ale to reduce gastric irritation
For syrup dosage form
Taking each dose mixed with clear liquid (e.g., water, apple juice, ginger ale) to improve flavor and reduce gastric irritation
For suppository dosage form
Proper administration technique
Chilling in refrigerator for 30 minutes or running cold water over suppository before removing foil wrapper if too soft for insertion
» Proper dosing
Missed dose: Not taking missed dose; not doubling doses
» Proper storage

**Precautions while using this medication**
Regular visits to physician to check progress during prolonged therapy
Checking with physician before discontinuing medication after prolonged use; gradual dosage reduction may be necessary to avoid the possibility of withdrawal symptoms
» Avoiding use of alcohol or other CNS depressants
» Suspected overdose: Getting emergency help at once
» Caution if dizziness, lightheadedness, or drowsiness occurs

**Side/adverse effects**
Signs of potential side effects, especially allergic reaction, confusion, and paradoxical reaction

## General Dosing Information

*Deaths have occurred prior to or following diagnostic or therapeutic procedures, particularly in pediatric patients, after chloral hydrate was administered to induce sedation before the procedure.* The current Guidelines for Monitoring and Management of Pediatric Patients During and After Sedation For Diagnostic and Therapeutic Procedures established by the American Academy of Pediatrics recommend that *sedatives be administered only at the health care facility*, where appropriate monitoring can be instituted. Monitoring must continue until the child's level of consciousness has returned to a state that meets appropriate approved discharge criteria. In addition, particular care must be taken in calculating and administering the proper dose appropriate to the age and weight of pediatric patients.

Use of chloral hydrate in infants and children is not recommended when repetitive dosing would be necessary.

Children with sleep apnea, especially obstructive sleep apnea with tonsillar hypertrophy, are particularly prone to respiratory compromise.

Tolerance may develop by the second week of continual administration.

Prolonged use of larger than usual therapeutic doses may result in psychic or physical dependence.

Following prolonged administration, chloral hydrate should be withdrawn gradually in order to avoid the possibility of precipitating withdrawal symptoms.

**For oral dosage forms only**
Chloral hydrate capsules should be administered with a full glass (240 mL) of water, fruit juice, or ginger ale to reduce gastric irritation.

Each dose of chloral hydrate syrup should be diluted in clear liquid (e.g., water, apple juice, ginger ale) to improve flavor and reduce gastric irritation.

In patients with gastritis, oral chloral hydrate preparations may be dissolved in olive oil or cottonseed oil and administered rectally.

## Oral Dosage Forms

### CHLORAL HYDRATE CAPSULES USP

**Usual adult dose**
Sedative-hypnotic—
Hypnotic:
Oral, 500 mg to 1 gram fifteen to thirty minutes before bedtime.
Sedative:
Daytime—Oral, 250 mg three times a day after meals.
Preoperative—Oral, 500 mg to 1 gram thirty minutes before surgery.

**Usual adult prescribing limits**
Up to 2 grams daily.

**Usual pediatric dose**
Sedative-hypnotic—
Premedication prior to dental or medical procedures: Oral, 50 mg per kg of body weight, up to a maximum of 1 gram per single dose. Doses of 25 to 100 mg per kg of body weight may be used in individual patients. The total dose should not exceed 100 mg per kg of body weight or 2 grams.
Premedication prior to electroencephalographic evaluation: Oral, 25 mg per kg of body weight.

Note: *Deaths have occurred prior to or following diagnostic or therapeutic procedures, particularly in pediatric patients, after chloral hydrate was administered to induce sedation before the procedure.* The current Guidelines for Monitoring and Management of Pediatric Patients During and After Sedation For Diagnostic and Therapeutic Procedures established by the American Academy of Pediatrics recommend that *sedatives be administered only at the health care facility*, where appropriate monitoring can be instituted. Monitoring must continue until the child has returned to the presedation level of consciousness or meets appropriate approved discharge criteria. In addition, particular care must be taken in calculating and administering the proper dose appropriate to the age and weight of pediatric patients.

**Strength(s) usually available**
U.S.—
250 mg (Rx) [GENERIC].
500 mg (Rx) [GENERIC].
Canada—
500 mg (Rx) [*Novo-Chlorhydrate*].

**Packaging and storage**
Store between 15 and 30 °C (59 and 86 °F), in a tight container.

**Stability**
Clarity of the capsules may vary without affecting the potency.

**Auxiliary labeling**
• Swallow capsules whole.
• Avoid alcoholic beverages.
• May cause drowsiness.
• Keep container tightly closed.

**Note**
Controlled substance in the U.S.

### CHLORAL HYDRATE SYRUP USP

**Usual adult dose**
See *Chloral Hydrate Capsules USP*.

**Usual adult prescribing limits**
See *Chloral Hydrate Capsules USP*.

**Usual pediatric dose**
See *Chloral Hydrate Capsules USP*.

**Strength(s) usually available**
U.S.—
  250 mg per 5 mL (Rx) [GENERIC].
  500 mg per 5 mL (Rx) [GENERIC].
Canada—
  500 mg per 5 mL (Rx) [*PMS-Chloral Hydrate;* GENERIC].

**Packaging and storage**
Store below 40 °C (104 °F), preferably between 15 and 30 °C (59 and 86 °F), unless otherwise specified by manufacturer. Store in a tight, light-resistant container. Protect from freezing.

**Auxiliary labeling**
• Avoid alcoholic beverages.
• May cause drowsiness.

**Note**
Controlled substance in the U.S.

## Rectal Dosage Forms

### CHLORAL HYDRATE SUPPOSITORIES

**Usual adult dose**
Sedative-hypnotic—
  Hypnotic: Rectal, 500 mg to 1 gram as a single dose at bedtime.
  Sedative: Rectal, 325 mg three times a day.

**Usual adult prescribing limits**
Up to 2 grams daily.

**Usual pediatric dose**
Sedative-hypnotic—
  Premedication prior to dental or medical procedures: Rectal, 50 mg per kg of body weight, up to a maximum of 1 gram per single dose. Doses of 25 to 100 mg per kg of body weight may be used in individual patients. The total dose should not exceed 100 mg per kg of body weight or 2 grams.
  Premedication prior to electroencephalographic evaluation: Rectal, 25 mg per kg of body weight.

Note: *Deaths have occurred prior to or following diagnostic or therapeutic procedures, particularly in pediatric patients, after chloral hydrate was administered to induce sedation before the procedure.* The current Guidelines for Monitoring and Management of Pediatric Patients During and After Sedation For Diagnostic and Therapeutic Procedures established by the American Academy of Pediatrics recommend that *sedatives be administered only at the health care facility,* where appropriate monitoring can be instituted. Monitoring must continue until the child has returned to the presedation level of consciousness or meets appropriate approved discharge criteria. In addition, particular care must be taken in calculating and administering the proper dose appropriate to the age and weight of pediatric patients.

**Strength(s) usually available**
U.S.—
  325 mg (Rx) [*Aquachloral Supprettes* (tartrazine)].
  500 mg (Rx) [GENERIC].
  650 mg (Rx) [*Aquachloral Supprettes* (tartrazine)].
Canada—
  Not commercially available.

**Packaging and storage**
Store below 40 °C (104 °F), preferably between 15 and 30 °C (59 and 86 °F), in a well-closed container, unless otherwise specified by manufacturer.

**Auxiliary labeling**
• For rectal use only.
• Avoid alcoholic beverages.
• May cause drowsiness.

**Note**
Controlled substance in the U.S.

Revised: 08/02/94
Interim revision: 03/31/95

# CHLORAMBUCIL  Systemic

VA CLASSIFICATION (Primary/Secondary): AN100/IM600
Commonly used brand name(s): *Leukeran.*
Note: For a listing of dosage forms and brand names by country availability, see *Dosage Forms* section(s).

## Category
Antineoplastic; immunosuppressant.

## Indications
Note: Bracketed information in the *Indications* section refers to uses that are not included in U.S. product labeling.

**Accepted**
Leukemia, chronic lymphocytic (treatment)—Chlorambucil is indicated for palliative treatment of chronic lymphocytic leukemia.

Lymphomas, Hodgkin's (treatment) or
Lymphomas, non-Hodgkin's (treatment)—Chlorambucil is indicated for palliative treatment of Hodgkin's disease and other malignant lymphomas including lymphosarcoma and giant follicular lymphoma.

[Carcinoma, ovarian, epithelial (treatment)][1]—Chlorambucil is indicated for the treatment of epithelial ovarian carcinoma.

[Lymphomas, cutaneous T-cell (treatment)][1]—Chlorambucil is indicated for the treatment of cutaneous T-cell lymphomas.

[Tumors, trophoblastic, gestational (treatment)][1]—Chlorambucil is indicated for the treatment of trophoblastic gestational tumors.

[Waldenström's macroglobulinemia (treatment)][1]—Chlorambucil is indicated for the treatment of Waldenström's macroglobulinemia.

[Leukemia, hairy cell (treatment)][1]—Chlorambucil is indicated for the treatment of hairy cell leukemia.

[Nephrotic syndrome (treatment)][1]—Chlorambucil has been used as an immunosuppressant, in combination with prednisone, in the treatment of steroid-resistant or frequently relapsing steroid-sensitive minimal-change nephrotic syndrome in children and adults, although there are significant risks associated with its use. The most common dose-limiting short-term toxicity is bone marrow depression. Because of potential long-term toxicity (male sterility, leukemia), use of chlorambucil is recommended only for patients unresponsive to or seriously intolerant of steroid treatment.

**Extreme caution is recommended in use of chlorambucil for non-neoplastic conditions because of potential carcinogenicity with long-term use of this agent.**

[1]Not included in Canadian product labeling.

## Pharmacology/Pharmacokinetics

**Physicochemical characteristics**
Molecular weight—304.22.
pKa—5.8.

**Mechanism of action/Effect**
Chlorambucil is a bifunctional alkylating agent of the nitrogen mustard type. Chlorambucil is cell cycle–phase nonspecific, although it is also cytotoxic to nonproliferating cells. Activity occurs as a result of formation of an unstable ethylenimmonium ion, which alkylates or binds with many intracellular molecular structures, including nucleic acids. Its cytotoxic action is primarily due to cross-linking of strands of DNA, which inhibits nucleic acid synthesis.

**Other actions/effects**
Also has immunosuppressant activity.

**Absorption**
Rapidly and completely absorbed from the gastrointestinal tract.

**Protein binding**
Very high (99%), specifically to albumin.

**Biotransformation**
Hepatic, extensive and rapid. The primary metabolite, phenylacetic acid mustard (an aminophenyl acetic acid derivative), is active. Also undergoes spontaneous degradation, forming monohydroxy and dihydroxy derivatives.

**Half-life**
Chlorambucil—Approximately 1.5 hours.
Aminophenyl acetic acid derivative metabolite—2.4 hours.

**Time to peak plasma concentration**
1 hour.

### Elimination
Renal, less than 1% as chlorambucil or phenylacetic acid mustard.
In dialysis—Not dialyzable.

## Precautions to Consider

### Cross-sensitivity and/or related problems
Patients sensitive to other alkylating agents (i.e., those who experience skin rash) may also be sensitive to chlorambucil.

### Carcinogenicity
Secondary malignancies are potential delayed effects of many antineoplastic agents, although it is not clear whether the effect is related to their mutagenic or immunosuppressive action. The effect of dose and duration of therapy is also unknown, although risk seems to increase with long-term use. Although information is limited, available data seem to indicate that the carcinogenic risk is greatest with the alkylating agents.

Chlorambucil has been shown to be carcinogenic in mice. There are many reports of acute leukemia occurring in patients treated with chlorambucil for both malignant and nonmalignant diseases, often in combination with radiation or other chemotherapy. Risk appears to be related to cumulative dose and duration of therapy, but a threshold cumulative dose has not been defined.

### Mutagenicity
Chlorambucil has been shown to cause chromatid or chromosome damage in humans.

### Pregnancy/Reproduction
Fertility—Gonadal suppression, resulting in amenorrhea or azoospermia, may occur in patients taking antineoplastic therapy, especially with the alkylating agents. In general, these effects appear to be related to dose and length of therapy and may be irreversible. Prediction of the degree of testicular or ovarian function impairment is complicated by the common use of combinations of several antineoplastics, which makes it difficult to assess the effects of individual agents.

However, there have been numerous reports of prolonged or permanent azoospermia and permanent sterility with long-term use of chlorambucil, especially in prepubertal and pubertal males. Amenorrhea has been reported in pubertal and adult females; autopsy studies of ovaries from women treated with combination therapy including chlorambucil have shown varying degrees of fibrosis, vasculitis, and depletion of primordial follicles.

Pregnancy—Adequate and well-controlled studies in humans have not been done. Although several successful pregnancies have been reported with chlorambucil use, two cases of an infant with an absent kidney and ureter have also been reported.

First trimester: It is usually recommended that use of antineoplastics, especially combination chemotherapy, be avoided whenever possible, especially during the first trimester. Although information is limited because of the relatively few instances of antineoplastic administration during pregnancy, the mutagenic, teratogenic, and carcinogenic potential of these medications must be considered.

Other hazards to the fetus include adverse reactions seen in adults.

In general, use of a contraceptive is recommended during cytotoxic drug therapy.

In rats, urogenital malformations including absence of a kidney have been reported.

FDA Pregnancy Category D.

### Breast-feeding
Although very little information is available regarding distribution of antineoplastic agents into breast milk, breast-feeding is not recommended during chemotherapy because of the risks to the infant (adverse effects, mutagenicity, carcinogenicity). It is not known whether chlorambucil is distributed into breast milk.

### Pediatrics
Appropriate studies performed to date generally have not demonstrated pediatrics-specific problems that would limit the usefulness of chlorambucil in children. However, children taking chlorambucil for nephrotic syndrome are reported to have an increased risk of seizures.

### Geriatrics
No information is available on the relationship of age to the effects of chlorambucil in geriatric patients.

### Dental
The bone marrow depressant effects of chlorambucil may result in an increased incidence of microbial infection, delayed healing, and gingival bleeding. Dental work, whenever possible, should be completed prior to initiation of therapy or deferred until blood counts have returned to normal. Patients should be instructed in proper oral hygiene during treatment, including caution in use of regular toothbrushes, dental floss, and toothpicks.

Chlorambucil may also infrequently cause stomatitis, which is associated with considerable discomfort.

### Drug interactions and/or related problems
The following drug interactions and/or related problems have been selected on the basis of their potential clinical significance (possible mechanism in parentheses where appropriate)—not necessarily inclusive (» = major clinical significance):

Note: Combinations containing any of the following medications, depending on the amount present, may also interact with this medication.

Allopurinol or
Colchicine or
» Probenecid or
» Sulfinpyrazone
(chlorambucil may raise the concentration of blood uric acid; dosage adjustment of antigout agents may be necessary to control hyperuricemia and gout; allopurinol may be preferred to prevent or reverse chlorambucil-induced hyperuricemia because of risk of uric acid nephropathy with uricosuric antigout agents)

Antidepressants, tricyclic or
Bupropion or
Clozapine or
Haloperidol or
Loxapine or
Maprotiline or
Molindone or
Monoamine oxidase (MAO) inhibitors, including furazolidone and procarbazine or
Phenothiazines or
Pimozide or
Thioxanthenes
(these medications may lower the seizure threshold and increase the risk of chlorambucil-induced seizures)

Blood dyscrasia–causing medications (see *Appendix II*)
(leukopenic and/or thrombocytopenic effects of chlorambucil may be increased with concurrent or recent therapy if these medications cause the same effects; dosage adjustment of chlorambucil, if necessary, should be based on blood counts)

» Bone marrow depressants, other (see *Appendix II*) or
» Radiation therapy
(additive bone marrow depression may occur; dosage reduction may be required when two or more bone marrow depressants, including radiation, are used concurrently or consecutively)

» Immunosuppressants, other, such as:
Azathioprine
Corticosteroids, glucocorticoid
Corticotropin (ACTH)
Cyclophosphamide
Cyclosporine
Cytarabine
Mercaptopurine
Muromonab-CD3
Tacrolimus
(concurrent use with chlorambucil may increase the risk of infection and development of neoplasms)

Vaccines, killed virus
(because normal defense mechanisms may be suppressed by chlorambucil therapy, the patient's antibody response to the vaccine may be decreased. The interval between discontinuation of medications that cause immunosuppression and restoration of the patient's ability to respond to the vaccine depends on the intensity and type of immunosuppression-causing medication used, the underlying disease, and other factors; estimates vary from 3 months to 1 year)

» Vaccines, live virus
(because normal defense mechanisms may be suppressed by chlorambucil therapy, concurrent use with a live virus vaccine may potentiate the replication of the vaccine virus, may increase the side/adverse effects of the vaccine virus, and/or may decrease the patient's antibody response to the vaccine; immunization of these patients should be undertaken only with extreme caution after careful review of the patient's hematologic status and only with the knowledge and consent of the physician managing the chlorambucil therapy. The interval between discontinuation of medications that cause immunosuppression and restoration of the patient's ability to respond to the vaccine depends on the intensity and type of immunosuppression-causing medication used, the underlying disease, and other factors; estimates vary from 3 months to 1 year. Patients with leukemia in remission should not receive live virus vaccine until at least 3 months after their last chemotherapy. In addition, immuni-

zation with oral poliovirus vaccine should be postponed in persons in close contact with the patient, especially family members)

**Laboratory value alterations**
The following have been selected on the basis of their potential clinical significance (possible effect in parentheses where appropriate)—not necessarily inclusive (» = major clinical significance):

With physiology/laboratory test values
    Alkaline phosphatase and
    Aspartate aminotransferase (AST [SGOT])
        (values may rarely be increased, indicating hepatotoxicity)
    Uric acid
        (concentrations in blood and urine may be increased)

**Medical considerations/Contraindications**
The medical considerations/contraindications included have been selected on the basis of their potential clinical significance (reasons given in parentheses where appropriate)—not necessarily inclusive (» = major clinical significance).

*Risk-benefit should be considered when the following medical problems exist:*
» Bone marrow depression
» Chickenpox, existing or recent (including recent exposure) or
» Herpes zoster
    (risk of severe generalized disease)
  Gout, history of or
  Urate renal stones, history of
    (risk of hyperuricemia)
  Head trauma or
  Seizure disorder, history of
    (increased risk of seizures)
» Infection
  Sensitivity to chlorambucil
» Tumor cell infiltration of bone marrow
» Caution should be used also in patients who have had previous cytotoxic drug therapy or radiation therapy.

**Patient monitoring**
The following are especially important in patient monitoring (other tests may be warranted in some patients, depending on condition; » = major clinical significance):

  Alanine aminotransferase (ALT [SGPT]) values and
  Alkaline phosphatase values and
  Aspartate aminotransferase (AST [SGOT]) values and
  Lactate dehydrogenase (LDH) values
    (recommended prior to initiation of therapy and at frequent intervals during therapy; frequency varies according to clinical state, agent, dose, and other agents being used concurrently)
» Hematocrit or hemoglobin and
» Leukocyte count, total and, if appropriate, differential and
» Platelet count
    (determinations recommended prior to initiation of therapy and at periodic intervals during therapy; frequency varies according to clinical state, agent, dose, and other agents being used concurrently)
  Uric acid concentrations, serum
    (recommended prior to initiation of therapy and at periodic intervals during therapy; frequency varies according to clinical state, agent, dose, and other agents being used concurrently)

## Side/Adverse Effects

Note: Many "side effects" of antineoplastic therapy are unavoidable and represent the medication's pharmacologic action. Some of these (for example, leukopenia and thrombocytopenia) are actually used as parameters to aid in individual dosage titration.

The following side/adverse effects have been selected on the basis of their potential clinical significance (possible signs and symptoms in parentheses where appropriate)—not necessarily inclusive:

**Those indicating need for medical attention**
Incidence more frequent—dose-related
  **Lymphopenia, leukopenia, neutropenia, immunosuppression, or infection** (fever or chills; cough or hoarseness; lower back or side pain; painful or difficult urination)—usually asymptomatic; **thrombocytopenia** (unusual bleeding or bruising; black, tarry stools; blood in urine or stools; pinpoint red spots on skin)—usually asymptomatic

Note: With a short course of therapy, *leukopenia* and *thrombocytopenia* may not occur until the third week of treatment and usually persist for 1 to 2 weeks (or sometimes up to 3 to 4 weeks) after withdrawal of chlorambucil. The neutrophil count may continue to decrease for up to 10 days after the last dose. After a single high dose of chlorambucil, the nadir of the leukocyte and platelet counts occurs after 7 to 14 days, with recovery in 2 to 3 weeks.

In general, short intermittent courses are thought to cause less risk of serious bone marrow depression than continuous therapy, by allowing bone marrow regeneration between courses. Excessive doses or prolonged therapy (a total dose of 6.5 mg per kg of body weight [mg/kg] in a single course) may result in pancytopenia and irreversible bone marrow damage.

Incidence less frequent
  *Allergic reaction* (skin rash); **hyperuricemia or uric acid nephropathy** (joint pain; lower back or side pain; swelling of feet or lower legs); **stomatitis** (sores in mouth and on lips)

Note: *Skin rash* has been reported to progress rarely to erythema multiforme, toxic epidermal necrolysis, and Stevens-Johnson syndrome.

*Hyperuricemia or uric acid nephropathy* occurs most commonly during initial treatment of patients with leukemia or lymphoma, as a result of rapid cell breakdown that leads to elevated serum uric acid concentrations.

*Stomatitis* may be associated with neutropenia.

Incidence rare
  **Drug fever; hepatotoxicity, hepatic necrosis, or cirrhosis** (yellow eyes or skin); **neurotoxicity** (agitation; confusion; hallucinations; muscle twitching; seizures; severe weakness or paralysis; tremors; trouble in walking); **pulmonary fibrosis** (cough; shortness of breath)—occurs after long-term use; **skin reactions, severe, including erythema multiforme, epidermal necrolysis, and Stevens-Johnson syndrome** (blisters on skin; severe skin rash; sores in mouth; fever may also be associated with Stevens-Johnson syndrome)

Note: Rare, focal and/or generalized seizures have been reported in both children and adults at therapeutic daily doses, and in pulse dosing regimens and acute overdose. However, the risk may be increased in children with nephrotic syndrome (seizures may occur 6 to 90 days after initiation of treatment) and in patients receiving high pulse doses. *Neurotoxicity* is usually reversible on withdrawal of chlorambucil.

*Pulmonary fibrosis* is usually reversible after chlorambucil is withdrawn, but fatalities have been reported.

**Those indicating need for medical attention only if they continue or are bothersome**
Incidence less frequent or rare
  *Changes in menstrual period; dermatitis* (itching of skin); **nausea and vomiting**

Note: *Nausea and vomiting* are associated with single oral doses of 20 mg or more, usually last less than 24 hours, and become less frequent with continued therapy; may persist up to 7 days after a single high dose.

**Those indicating need for medical attention if they occur after medication is discontinued**
  *Bone marrow damage, possibly irreversible* (fever or chills; cough or hoarseness; lower back or side pain; painful or difficult urination; unusual bleeding or bruising; black, tarry stools; blood in urine or stools; pinpoint red spots on skin); **pulmonary toxicity** (cough; shortness of breath)

## Overdose

For more information on the management of overdose or unintentional ingestion, **contact a Poison Control Center** (see *Poison Control Center Listing*).

**Clinical effects of overdose**
The following effects have been selected on the basis of their potential clinical significance (possible signs and symptoms in parentheses where appropriate)—not necessarily inclusive:

Symptoms of overdose, in order of frequency
  **Pancytopenia, reversible** (fever or chills; cough or hoarseness; lower back or side pain; painful or difficult urination; unusual bleeding or bruising; black, tarry stools; blood in urine or stools; pinpoint red spots on skin); **neurotoxicity, including ataxia** (trouble in walking); **agitation and seizures**

**Treatment of overdose**
To enhance elimination—Immediate evacuation of the stomach.
Monitoring—Monitoring of blood counts at least three times a week for at least 3 weeks or until bone marrow function has recovered.

Supportive care—Supportive, symptomatic treatment. Patients in whom intentional overdose is confirmed or suspected should be referred for psychiatric consultation.

## Patient Consultation

As an aid to patient consultation, refer to *Advice for the Patient, Chlorambucil (Systemic)*.
In providing consultation, consider emphasizing the following selected information (》 = major clinical significance):

### Before using this medication
》 Conditions affecting use, especially:
Sensitivity to chlorambucil or other alkylating agents
Pregnancy—Use not recommended because of mutagenic, teratogenic, and carcinogenic potential; advisability of using contraception; telling physician immediately if pregnancy is suspected
Breast-feeding—Not recommended because of risk of serious side effects
Other medications, especially probenecid, sulfinpyrazone, other bone marrow depressants, other immunosuppressants, or previous cytotoxic drug or radiation therapy
Other medical problems, especially chickenpox, herpes zoster, or infection

### Proper use of this medication
》 Importance of not taking more or less medication than the amount prescribed
Caution in taking combination therapy; taking each medication at the right time
Importance of ample fluid intake and subsequent increase in urine output to aid in excretion of uric acid
》 Possible nausea and vomiting; importance of continuing medication despite stomach upset
Checking with physician if vomiting occurs shortly after dose is taken
》 Proper dosing
Missed dose: If dosing schedule is—
Once a day: Taking as soon as possible if remembered same day; if not remembered until next day, skipping missed dose and taking next regularly scheduled dose
Several times a day: Taking as soon as possible; however, if almost time for next dose, not taking missed dose; not doubling doses
》 Proper storage

### Precautions while using this medication
》 Importance of close monitoring by the physician
》 Avoiding immunizations unless approved by physician; other persons in patient's household should avoid immunizations with oral poliovirus vaccine; avoiding persons who have taken oral poliovirus vaccine or wearing a protective mask that covers nose and mouth
*Caution if bone marrow depression occurs*
》 Avoiding exposure to persons with infections, especially during periods of low blood counts; checking with physician immediately if fever or chills, cough or hoarseness, lower back or side pain, or painful or difficult urination occurs
》 Checking with physician immediately if unusual bleeding or bruising; black, tarry stools; blood in urine or stools; or pinpoint red spots on skin occur
Caution in use of regular toothbrush, dental floss, or toothpick; physician, dentist, or nurse may suggest alternatives; checking with physician before having dental work done
Not touching eyes or inside of nose unless hands washed immediately before
Using caution to avoid accidental cuts with use of sharp objects such as safety razor or fingernail or toenail cutters
Avoiding contact sports or other situations where bruising or injury might occur

### Side/adverse effects
May cause adverse effects such as blood problems and cancer
Signs of potential side effects, especially lymphopenia, leukopenia, neutropenia, immunosuppression, infection, thrombocytopenia, allergic reaction, hyperuricemia, uric acid nephropathy, stomatitis, drug fever, hepatotoxicity, hepatic necrosis, cirrhosis, neurotoxicity, pulmonary fibrosis, and severe skin reactions
Physician or nurse can help in dealing with side effects

## General Dosing Information

Patients receiving chlorambucil should be under supervision of a physician experienced in use of alkylating agents.

A variety of dosage schedules and regimens of chlorambucil, alone or in combination with other antitumor agents, are used. The prescriber may consult the medical literature as well as the manufacturer's literature in choosing a specific dosage.

Dosage must be adjusted to meet the individual requirements of each patient, based on clinical response and degree of bone marrow depression.

Development of uric acid nephropathy in patients with leukemia or lymphoma may be prevented by adequate oral hydration and, in some cases, administration of allopurinol. Alkalinization of urine may be necessary if serum uric acid concentrations are elevated.

It is recommended that chlorambucil be withdrawn if signs of pulmonary toxicity or a severe skin reaction occurs.

Because of the risk of enhanced bone marrow toxicity, use of chlorambucil is not recommended within 4 to 6 weeks of radiation therapy or chemotherapy with drugs that depress bone marrow function.

Because the decrease in neutrophil count may continue for 10 days after the last dose of chlorambucil, caution is necessary as the total dose approaches 6.5 mg per kg of body weight (mg/kg) because of the risk of pancytopenia.

If the white blood cell count (particularly granulocyte count) falls suddenly, a reduction in dosage or withdrawal of therapy plus continued monitoring is required until leukocyte and platelet levels become adequate. Persistence of low neutrophil and platelet counts or presence of peripheral lymphocytosis may indicate bone marrow infiltration; if that is confirmed by bone marrow examination, the daily dosage of chlorambucil should not exceed 100 mcg (0.1 mg) per kg of body weight.

Special precautions are recommended in patients who develop thrombocytopenia as a result of administration of chlorambucil. These may include extreme care in performing invasive procedures; regular inspection of intravenous sites, skin (including perirectal area), and mucous membrane surfaces for signs of bleeding or bruising; limiting frequency of venipuncture and avoiding intramuscular injections; testing urine, emesis, stool, and secretions for occult blood; care in use of regular toothbrushes, dental floss, toothpicks, safety razors, and fingernail and toenail cutters; avoiding constipation; and using caution to prevent falls and other injuries. Such patients should avoid alcohol and aspirin intake because of the risk of gastrointestinal bleeding. Platelet transfusions may be required.

Patients who develop leukopenia should be observed carefully for signs of infection. Antibiotic support may be required. In neutropenic patients who develop fever, broad-spectrum antibiotic coverage should be initiated empirically, pending bacterial cultures and appropriate diagnostic tests.

### Combination chemotherapy

Although chlorambucil is usually used alone, it may be used in combination with other agents in various regimens. As a result, incidence and/or severity of side effects may be altered and different dosages (usually reduced) may be used. For example, chlorambucil is part of the following chemotherapeutic combination (a commonly used acronym is in parentheses):
—chlorambucil and prednisone (CHL + PRED).

For specific dosages and schedules, consult the literature. For information regarding each agent, consult the individual monographs.

## Oral Dosage Forms

Note: Bracketed uses in the *Dosage Forms* section refer to categories of use and/or indications that are not included in U.S. product labeling.

### CHLORAMBUCIL TABLETS USP

**Usual adult dose**
Leukemia, chronic lymphocytic or
Lymphomas, Hodgkin's or
Lymphomas, non-Hodgkin's—
Initiation or short course: Oral, 100 to 200 mcg (0.1 to 0.2 mg) per kg of body weight a day or 3 to 6 mg per square meter of body surface area, usually 4 to 10 mg, a day, as a single dose or in divided doses, for three to six weeks.

Note: An intermittent, biweekly, or once-monthly pulse course of therapy may produce less hematologic toxicity; an initial dose of 400 mcg (0.4 mg) per kg of body weight or 12 mg per square meter of body surface area is increased by 100 mcg (0.1 mg) per kg of body weight or 3 mg per square meter of body surface area until an effective or toxic dose is reached, then adjusted as necessary.

[Nephrotic syndrome][1]—
Oral, 100 to 200 mcg (0.1 to 0.2 mg) per kg of body weight per day, in a single dose, for eight to twelve weeks.

Note: The maximum recommended cumulative dose is 14 mg per kg of body weight or a maximum duration of treatment of 12 weeks; some clinicians recommend a maximum cumulative dose of 8.2 mg per kg of body weight or a maximum of 6 weeks of treatment.

**Usual adult prescribing limits**
Presence of lymphocytic infiltration of bone marrow or hypoplastic bone marrow—Up to 100 mcg (0.1 mg) per kg of body weight per day.

**Usual pediatric dose**
Leukemia, chronic lymphocytic or
Lymphomas, Hodgkin's or
Lymphomas, non-Hodgkin's—
 Oral, 100 to 200 mcg (0.1 to 0.2 mg) per kg of body weight or 4.5 mg per square meter of body surface area a day, as a single dose or in divided daily doses.
[Nephrotic syndrome][1]—
 See *Usual adult dose*.

**Strength(s) usually available**
U.S.—
 2 mg (Rx) [*Leukeran* (lactose; sucrose)].
Canada—
 2 mg (Rx) [*Leukeran*].

**Packaging and storage**
Store below 40 °C (104 °F), preferably between 15 and 30 °C (59 and 86 °F), unless otherwise specified by manufacturer. Store in a well-closed, light-resistant container.

[1]Not included in Canadian product labeling.

Revised: 09/22/97

**CHLORAMPHENICOL**—The *Chloramphenicol (Ophthalmic)* monograph is not included in this published version of the USP DI database. Copies of the monograph are available on request from Micromedex, Inc. - Reprint Requests, 6200 S. Syracuse Way, Suite 300, Englewood, CO 80111; telephone (303) 486-6400; telefax (303) 486-6464; Email: USPDI@MDX.COM.

**CHLORAMPHENICOL**—The *Chloramphenicol (Otic)* monograph is not included in this published version of the USP DI database. Copies of the monograph are available on request from Micromedex, Inc. - Reprint Requests, 6200 S. Syracuse Way, Suite 300, Englewood, CO 80111; telephone (303) 486-6400; telefax (303) 486-6464; Email: USPDI@MDX.COM.

# CHLORAMPHENICOL Systemic

VA CLASSIFICATION (Primary): AM900
Commonly used brand name(s): *Chloromycetin; Novochlorocap*.
Note: For a listing of dosage forms and brand names by country availability, see *Dosage Forms* section(s).

## Category
Antibacterial (systemic).

## Indications

**General considerations**
Chloramphenicol has *in vitro* activity against a large number of organisms, including various aerobic gram-positive and gram-negative bacteria, anaerobic bacteria, rickettsiae, spirochetes, and chlamydia. *Haemophilus influenzae, Streptococcus pneumoniae,* and *Neisseria meningitidis* are highly susceptible to chloramphenicol, which is considered to be bactericidal against these organisms. Chloramphenicol has bacteriostatic activity against *Staphylococcus aureus, Streptococcus pyogenes, S. viridans,* group B streptococcus, *Escherichia coli, Klebsiella pneumoniae, Proteus mirabilis, Salmonella typhi, S. paratyphi A, Shigella* species, *Pseudomonas pseudomallei,* and nearly all anaerobes, including *Bacteroides fragilis.* Bacteria that are generally considered to be resistant to chloramphenicol include *Pseudomonas aeruginosa, Acinetobacter* species, *Enterobacter* species, *Serratia marcescens,* indole positive *Proteus* species, methicillin-resistant staphylococcus, and *Enterococcus faecalis.*

Because of this drug's serious toxicities, chloramphenicol is indicated only for the treatment of serious infections in which less toxic antibacterials are ineffective or contraindicated. Other medications, such as the third-generation cephalosporins for the treatment of meningitis, and clindamycin or metronidazole for the treatment of anaerobic infections, have generally replaced chloramphenicol; however, under certain circumstances, chloramphenicol may still be the most appropriate drug to use.

Chloramphenicol is also used in the treatment of rickettsial infections that require parenteral treatment when other antibiotics are contraindicated.

**Chloramphenicol should be reserved for serious infections in which less toxic antibacterials are ineffective or contraindicated.**

**Accepted**
Brain abscess (treatment)—Chloramphenicol is indicated in the treatment of brain abscess caused by *B. fragilis* or other susceptible organisms.
Ehrlichiosis (treatment)—Chloramphenicol is indicated in the treatment of ehrlichiosis caused by *Ehrlichia canis.*
Meningitis (treatment)—Chloramphenicol is indicated in the treatment of meningitis caused by *H. influenzae, S. pneumoniae,* and *N. meningitidis.*
Paratyphoid fever (treatment)—Chloramphenicol is indicated in the treatment of paratyphoid fever caused by *S. paratyphi A.*
Q fever (treatment)—Chloramphenicol is indicated in the treatment of Q fever caused by *Coxiella burnetii.*
Rocky Mountain spotted fever (treatment)—Chloramphenicol is indicated in the treatment of Rocky Mountain spotted fever caused by *Rickettsia* species.
Typhoid fever (treatment)—Chloramphenicol is indicated in the acute treatment of typhoid fever only, caused by *S. typhi.*
Typhus infections (treatment)—Chloramphenicol is indicated in the treatment of typhus infections caused by *Rickettsia* species.

Not all species or strains of a particular organism may be susceptible to chloramphenicol.

**Unaccepted**
Chloramphenicol is not indicated in the routine treatment of typhoid carrier states; in the treatment of trivial infections, colds, influenza, or throat infections; or in the prophylaxis of infections.

## Pharmacology/Pharmacokinetics

**Physicochemical characteristics**
Molecular weight—Chloramphenicol: 323.13.
Chloramphenicol palmitate: 561.54.
Chloramphenicol sodium succinate: 445.19.

**Mechanism of action/Effect**
Chloramphenicol, a broad-spectrum antibiotic, is bacteriostatic. However, it may be bactericidal in high concentrations or when used against highly susceptible organisms.
Chloramphenicol, which is lipid soluble, diffuses through the bacterial cell membrane and reversibly binds to the 50 S subunit of bacterial ribosomes where transfer of amino acids to growing peptide chains is prevented (perhaps by suppression of peptidyl transferase activity), thus inhibiting peptide bond formation and subsequent protein synthesis.
The mechanism for the irreversible aplastic anemia following use of chloramphenicol has not been established.
The mechanism for the dose-related reversible bone-marrow depression during and following use of chloramphenicol is thought to be by inhibition of mitochondrial protein synthesis in bone-marrow cells.

**Absorption**
Rapidly and completely absorbed from gastrointestinal tract.
Well absorbed after intramuscular administration; achieves serum concentrations comparable to intravenous administration.
Intravenous bioavailability—70%.
Oral bioavailability—80%.

**Distribution**
Chloramphenicol diffuses rapidly and is widely, but not uniformly, distributed throughout the body to—
 Liver and kidneys: Highest concentrations.
 Urine: High concentrations.
 Placenta: Fetal serum concentrations may be 30 to 80% of maternal serum concentrations.
 Eye: Therapeutic concentrations in aqueous and vitreous humor.
 Cerebrospinal fluid (CSF): Concentrations may be 21 to 50% of serum concentrations through uninflamed meninges and may be 45 to 89% of serum concentrations through inflamed meninges.

Other: Pleural fluid, ascitic fluid, synovial fluid, breast milk, and saliva (bitter aftertaste).
Vol$_D$ = 0.6–1.0 L/kg.

### Protein binding
Adults—Moderate (50–60%).
Premature neonates—Low (32%).

### Biotransformation
Hepatic (free drug); 90% conjugated to inactive glucuronide.
Chloramphenicol palmitate is hydrolyzed to free drug in the gastrointestinal tract prior to absorption.
Chloramphenicol sodium succinate is hydrolyzed to free drug in the plasma, liver, lungs, and kidneys.
In the fetus and neonates, the immature liver cannot conjugate chloramphenicol, and toxic concentrations of active drug accumulate. In neonates and infants this may result in the "gray syndrome."

### Half-life
Adults—
  Normal renal and hepatic function: 1.5 to 3.5 hours.
  Impaired renal function: 3 to 4 hours.
  Severely impaired hepatic function: Prolonged (4.6 to 11.6 hours).
Children (1 month to 16 years old)—
  3 to 6.5 hours.
Infants:
  1 to 2 days old: 24 hours or longer; highly variable, especially in low-birth-weight infants.
  10 to 16 days old: 10 hours.

### Time to peak serum concentration:
Intravenous—1 to 1.5 hours.
Oral—1 to 3 hours.

### Peak serum concentration
Adults—Oral, 12.5 mg per kg of body weight (mg/kg): 11.2 to 18.4 mcg/mL.
Children—Oral and intravenous: 25 mg/kg—19 to 28 mcg/mL.

### Elimination
Renal, by glomerular filtration; 5 to 10% excreted unchanged within 24 hours; 80% rapidly excreted by tubular secretion as inactive metabolites. Inactive metabolites can accumulate in premature and newborn infants because of immaturity of renal tubular secretion mechanisms.
Fecal/biliary; small amounts excreted unchanged following oral administration.
Dialysis—Dialysis does not remove significant amounts of chloramphenicol from the blood. Charcoal hemoperfusion has been reported to lower blood concentrations in an infant.

## Precautions to Consider

### Pregnancy/Reproduction
Chloramphenicol readily crosses the placenta; fetal serum concentrations may be 30 to 80% of maternal serum concentrations. Although birth defects in humans have not been documented, use is not recommended in pregnancy at term or during labor because of potential toxicity ("gray syndrome" or bone marrow depression) in premature or full-term infants.

### Breast-feeding
Chloramphenicol is excreted in breast milk in concentrations up to 25 mcg per mL. Use is not recommended in nursing mothers because of the possibility of adverse effects, especially bone marrow depression, in the infant.

### Pediatrics
In the fetus and neonates, the immature liver cannot conjugate chloramphenicol, and toxic concentrations of active drug accumulate. In neonates and infants this may result in the "gray syndrome."
In infants 1 to 2 days old, the half-life is 24 hours or longer and may be highly variable, especially in low-birth-weight infants. In infants 10 to 16 days old, the half-life is 10 hours.
Inactive metabolites can accumulate in premature and newborn infants because of immaturity of renal tubular secretion mechanisms.
Serum concentrations must be performed in pediatric patients with impaired or immature metabolic functions or in patients who are receiving medications that are also metabolized by the liver (e.g., phenytoin, phenobarbital, acetaminophen, theophylline).

### Geriatrics
No information is available on the relationship of age to the effects of chloramphenicol in geriatric patients.

### Dental
The bone marrow–depressant effects of chloramphenicol may result in an increased incidence of microbial infection, delayed healing, and gingival bleeding. Dental work, whenever possible, should be completed prior to initiation of therapy or deferred until blood counts have returned to normal. Patients should be instructed in proper oral hygiene during treatment, including caution in use of regular toothbrushes, dental floss, and toothpicks.

### Drug interactions and/or related problems
The following drug interactions and/or related problems have been selected on the basis of their potential clinical significance (possible mechanism in parentheses where appropriate)—not necessarily inclusive (» = major clinical significance):

Note: Combinations containing any of the following medications, depending on the amount present, may also interact with this medication.

» Alfentanil
  (chronic preoperative or perioperative use of chloramphenicol, an hepatic enzyme inhibitor, may decrease the plasma clearance and prolong the duration of action of alfentanil)

» Anticonvulsants, hydantoin or
  Blood dyscrasia–causing medications (See *Appendix II*) or
» Bone marrow depressants, other (See *Appendix II* ) or
» Radiation therapy
  (concurrent use with chloramphenicol may increase the bone marrow–depressant effects of these medications and radiation therapy; dosage reduction may be required)

» Antidiabetic agents, oral
  (concurrent use of chloramphenicol with tolbutamide and chlorpropamide may enhance their hypoglycemic effect by inhibiting the hepatic metabolism of these medications and increasing their serum levels; dosage adjustments may be necessary; glipizide and glyburide, due to their non-ionic binding characteristics, may not be affected as much as the other oral antidiabetic agents; however, caution with concurrent use is recommended)

Contraceptives, estrogen-containing, oral
  (concurrent long-term use of chloramphenicol may result in reduced contraceptive reliability and increased incidence of breakthrough bleeding)

» Clindamycin or
» Erythromycins or
» Lincomycin
  (may be displaced from or prevented from binding to 50 S subunits of bacterial ribosomes by chloramphenicol, thus antagonizing the effects of erythromycins and lincomycins; concurrent use is not recommended)

Hepatic enzyme inducers
  (concurrent use of chloramphenicol with hepatic microsomal enzyme inducing drugs, including phenobarbital and rifampin, can increase the metabolism of chloramphenicol, decreasing chloramphenicol serum concentrations)

Penicillins
  (since bacteriostatic drugs may interfere with the bactericidal effects of penicillins in the treatment of meningitis or in other situations in which a rapid bactericidal effect is necessary, it is best to avoid concurrent therapy; however, chloramphenicol and ampicillin are sometimes administered concurrently in pediatric patients)

» Phenobarbital or
» Phenytoin or
» Warfarin or
» Other medications metabolized by mixed-function oxidase system
  (inhibition of the cytochrome P-450 enzyme system by chloramphenicol may cause a decrease in the hepatic metabolism of these medications, resulting in delayed elimination and increased blood concentrations)

Vitamin B$_{12}$
  (concurrent use may antagonize hematopoietic response to vitamin B$_{12}$; monitoring of hematologic status or use of an alternate antibiotic is recommended)

### Laboratory value alterations
The following have been selected on the basis of their potential clinical significance (possible effect in parentheses where appropriate)—not necessarily inclusive (» = major clinical significance):

With diagnostic test results
  Bentiromide
    (concurrent administration of chloramphenicol during a bentiromide test period will invalidate test results since chloramphenicol is also metabolized to arylamines and will thus increase the percent of PABA recovered; discontinuation of chloramphenicol at least 3 days prior to the administration of bentiromide is recommended)

Urine glucose determinations
(chloramphenicol may give false-positive test results with copper sulfate urine glucose tests)

### Medical considerations/Contraindications
The medical considerations/contraindications included have been selected on the basis of their potential clinical significance (reasons given in parentheses where appropriate)—not necessarily inclusive (» = major clinical significance).

*Except under special circumstances, this medication should not be used when the following medical problems exist:*
» Previous allergy or toxic reaction to chloramphenicol

*Risk-benefit should be considered when the following medical problems exist:*
» Bone marrow depression
(chloramphenicol may cause a dose-related bone marrow depression, an idiosyncratic aplastic anemia, and other blood dyscrasias)
» Hepatic function impairment
(chloramphenicol is metabolized in the liver; patients with impaired or immature hepatic or renal function, especially neonates and infants, or adults with both impaired hepatic and renal function, may require a reduction in dose; serum concentrations should be monitored)
» Risk-benefit should be considered in patients who have had previous cytotoxic drug therapy or radiation therapy also.

### Patient monitoring
The following may be especially important in patient monitoring (other tests may be warranted in some patients, depending on condition; » = major clinical significance):
» Chloramphenicol levels, serum
(serum concentrations must be performed in low-birth-weight infants because the pharmacokinetics of chloramphenicol are so variable in this age group; serum concentrations should also be monitored in patients with impaired or immature metabolic functions or in patients who are receiving medications that are also metabolized by the liver; the desired serum concentration should fall within the range of 10 to 25 mcg/mL, the concentration to which most susceptible organisms respond; concentrations in excess of these increase the risk of reversible bone marrow depression and "gray syndrome")
» Complete blood counts (CBCs)
(may be required frequently during therapy to detect dose-related reversible bone marrow depression; chloramphenicol should be discontinued if reticulocytopenia, leukopenia, thrombocytopenia, anemia, or other blood dyscrasias occur; however, CBCs are not useful in predicting aplastic anemia, which usually appears after treatment has been completed)
(patients should be informed of the importance of having blood counts followed closely during therapy)

## Side/Adverse Effects
Note: The hematologic toxicity of chloramphenicol can manifest itself in 1 of 2 ways—either as a reversible bone marrow depression or an idiosyncratic aplastic anemia. Bone marrow depression is dose-related and most commonly seen when serum concentrations exceed 25 mcg/mL. Bone marrow changes are usually reversible when chloramphenicol is discontinued. Aplastic anemia is an idiosyncratic reaction that occurs in 1 of every 25,000 to 40,000 courses of treatment. It is not related to dose or duration of therapy. Most cases have been associated with oral chloramphenicol, and the onset of aplasia may not occur until weeks or months after treatment with chloramphenicol has been discontinued.

Gray syndrome (or "gray baby syndrome") almost always occurs in newborn infants treated with inappropriately high doses of chloramphenicol. Typically, the infant has been started on chloramphenicol within the first 48 hours of life; symptoms first appear after 3 to 4 days of continued treatment with high doses of chloramphenicol; and serum levels are high, often between 40 and 200 mcg/mL. If caught early and chloramphenicol is discontinued, the infant may have a complete recovery. On rare occasion, older patients, including adults with severe liver disease, have also had a gray syndrome–type reaction.

The following side/adverse effects have been selected on the basis of their potential clinical significance (possible signs and symptoms in parentheses where appropriate)—not necessarily inclusive:

*Those indicating need for medical attention*
Incidence less frequent
*Blood dyscrasias* (pale skin; sore throat and fever; unusual bleeding or bruising; unusual tiredness or weakness)
Incidence rare
*Gray syndrome* (abdominal distension; blue-gray skin color; low body temperature; uneven breathing; unresponsiveness; cardiovascular collapse)—in neonates only; *hypersensitivity reactions* (skin rash; fever; shortness of breath); *neurotoxic reactions* (confusion; delirium; headache); *optic neuritis* (eye pain, blurred vision, or loss of vision); *peripheral neuritis* (numbness, tingling, burning pain, or weakness in the hands or feet)

*Those indicating need for medical attention only if they continue or are bothersome*
Incidence less frequent
*Gastrointestinal reaction* (diarrhea; nausea; vomiting)

*Those indicating possible fatal, irreversible bone marrow depression, leading to aplastic anemia, and the need for immediate medical attention if they occur weeks or months after medication is discontinued*
*Pale skin; sore throat and fever; unusual bleeding or bruising; unusual tiredness or weakness*

## Patient Consultation
As an aid to patient consultation, refer to *Advice for the Patient, Chloramphenicol (Systemic)*.
In providing consultation, consider emphasizing the following selected information (» = major clinical significance):

### Before using this medication
» Conditions affecting use, especially:
Allergies or toxic reactions to chloramphenicol
Pregnancy—Chloramphenicol crosses the placenta; use at term or during labor may cause "gray syndrome" in infants
Breast-feeding—Chloramphenicol is excreted in breast milk; may cause bone marrow depression in the infant
Use in children—Because of possible accumulation and toxic reactions, serum concentrations must be measured in premature and newborn infants
Dental—May result in an increased incidence of infection, delayed healing, and gingival bleeding
Other medications, especially alfentanil, hydantoin anticonvulsants, bone marrow depressants, radiation therapy, oral antidiabetic agents, erythromycins, lincomycins, phenobarbital, phenytoin, warfarin, or other medicines metabolized by mixed-function oxidase system
Other medical problems, especially bone marrow depression, liver dysfunction, previous cytotoxic drug therapy, or radiation therapy

### Proper use of this medication
Taking on an empty stomach
Proper administration technique for oral liquids
» Compliance with full course of therapy
» Proper dosing
Missed dose: Taking as soon as possible; not taking if almost time for next dose; not doubling doses
» Proper storage

### Precautions while using this medication
Checking with physician if no improvement within a few days
» Regular visits to physician to check for blood problems
Using caution in use of regular toothbrushes, dental floss, and toothpicks; completing dental work prior to initiation of therapy or deferring dental work until blood counts have returned to normal; checking with physician or dentist concerning proper oral hygiene
» Diabetics: False-positive reactions with copper sulfate urine glucose tests may occur

### Side/adverse effects
May also cause bone marrow aplasia and "gray syndrome"
Signs of potential side effects, especially blood dyscrasias, gray syndrome, optic neuritis, peripheral neuritis, neurotoxic reactions, or hypersensitivity reactions

## General Dosing Information
Treatment should be continued no longer than required to produce a cure, yet long enough to provide little or no risk of relapse.
Repeated courses of the drug should be avoided if at all possible since reversible bone marrow depression may occur.

# Chloramphenicol (Systemic)

The serum chloramphenicol concentration should fall within the range of 10 to 25 mcg/mL, the concentration to which most susceptible organisms respond; concentrations higher than 30 mcg/mL increase the risk of bone marrow depression and "gray syndrome."

**For oral dosage forms only**
Chloramphenicol should preferably be taken with a full glass (240 mL) of water on an empty stomach (either 1 hour before or 2 hours after meals) to optimize absorption.

Chloramphenicol palmitate must be hydrolyzed in the gastrointestinal tract to chloramphenicol before being absorbed. The rate of absorption may be decreased in neonates or increased in older children, depending on the individual rate of hydrolysis. Serum concentrations are usually similar to those resulting from oral base administration of chloramphenicol.

## Oral Dosage Forms

### CHLORAMPHENICOL CAPSULES USP

**Usual adult and adolescent dose**
Antibacterial—
   Oral, 12.5 mg (base) per kg of body weight every six hours.

**Usual adult prescribing limits**
Up to a maximum of 4 grams (base) daily.

**Usual pediatric dose**
Antibacterial—
   Premature and full-term infants up to 2 weeks of age: Oral, 6.25 mg (base) per kg of body weight every six hours.
   Infants 2 weeks of age and over: Oral, 12.5 mg (base) per kg of body weight every six hours; or 25 mg per kg of body weight every twelve hours.
Note:   In severe infections, such as bacteremia or meningitis, doses up to 75 to 100 mg (base) per kg of body weight daily may be used.
   Serum determinations are recommended in patients with impaired or immature metabolic functions.

**Strength(s) usually available**
U.S.—
   250 mg (base) (Rx) [*Chloromycetin;* GENERIC].
Canada—
   250 mg (base) (Rx) [*Novochlorocap*].

**Packaging and storage**
Store below 30 °C (86 °F), preferably between 15 and 30 °C (59 and 86 °F), unless otherwise specified by manufacturer. Store in a tight container.

**Auxiliary labeling**
• Continue medicine for full time of treatment.
• Take on empty stomach.

### CHLORAMPHENICOL PALMITATE ORAL SUSPENSION USP

**Usual adult and adolescent dose**
See *Chloramphenicol Capsules USP*.

**Usual adult prescribing limits**
See *Chloramphenicol Capsules USP*.

**Usual pediatric dose**
See *Chloramphenicol Capsules USP*.

**Strength(s) usually available**
U.S.—
   150 mg (base) per 5 mL (Rx) [*Chloromycetin* (sodium benzoate 2.5 mg per 5 mL)].
Canada—
   Not commercially available.

**Packaging and storage**
Store below 40 °C (104 °F), preferably between 15 and 30 °C (59 and 86 °F), unless otherwise specified by manufacturer. Store in a tight, light-resistant container. Protect from freezing.

**Auxiliary labeling**
• Shake well.
• Continue medicine for full time of treatment.
• Take on empty stomach.

**Note**
When dispensing, include a calibrated liquid-measuring device.

**Additional information**
The oral suspension is tasteless.

## Parenteral Dosage Forms

Note:   The dosing and strengths of the dosage forms available are expressed in terms of chloramphenicol base.

### STERILE CHLORAMPHENICOL SODIUM SUCCINATE USP

**Usual adult and adolescent dose**
Antibacterial—
   Intravenous, 12.5 mg (base) per kg of body weight every six hours.

**Usual adult prescribing limits**
Up to a maximum of 4 grams (base) daily.

**Usual pediatric dose**
Antibacterial—
   Premature and full-term infants up to 2 weeks of age: Intravenous, 6.25 mg (base) per kg of body weight every six hours.
   Infants 2 weeks of age and over: Intravenous, 12.5 mg (base) per kg of body weight every six hours; or 25 mg per kg of body weight every twelve hours.
Note:   In severe infections, such as bacteremia or meningitis, doses up to 75 to 100 mg (base) per kg of body weight daily may be used.
   Serum determinations are recommended in patients with impaired or immature metabolic functions.

**Size(s) usually available**
U.S.—
   1 gram (base) (Rx) [*Chloromycetin* (sodium 2.25 mEq per gram); GENERIC].
Canada—
   1 gram (base) (Rx) [*Chloromycetin*].

**Packaging and storage**
Prior to reconstitution, store below 40 °C (104 °F), preferably between 15 and 30 °C (59 and 86 °F), unless otherwise specified by manufacturer.

**Preparation of dosage form**
To prepare a 10% (100-mg-per-mL) solution, add 10 mL of an aqueous diluent such as sterile water for injection or 5% dextrose injection to each 1-gram vial.

**Stability**
After reconstitution, solutions (100-mg-per-mL) retain their potency for 2 to 30 days if stored at room temperature or if refrigerated, depending on the manufacturer.
Diluted solutions are stable for 24 to 48 hours if stored at room temperature or if refrigerated, depending on the manufacturer.
If frozen, solutions retain their potency for up to 6 months, depending on the manufacturer.
Do not use if solution is cloudy.

**Additional information**
Chloramphenicol sodium succinate must be hydrolyzed in the body to chloramphenicol; therefore, there may be a delay in achieving adequate serum concentrations of active drug.
May be given intravenously over at least a 1-minute period.
Chloramphenicol may also be given intramuscularly, achieving serum concentrations comparable to intravenous administration.

---

Revised: 05/13/92
Interim revision: 03/17/94; 06/20/95

---

# CHLORDIAZEPOXIDE—See *Benzodiazepines (Systemic)*

# CHLORDIAZEPOXIDE AND AMITRIPTYLINE  Systemic

VA CLASSIFICATION (Primary): CN900

NOTE: The *Chlordiazepoxide and Amitriptyline (Systemic)* monograph is maintained on the USP DI electronic data base. For a printed copy of the most recent revision of the complete monograph, contact Micromedex, Inc. - Reprint Requests, 6200 S. Syracuse Way, Suite 300, Englewood, CO 80111; telephone (303) 486-6400; telefax (303) 486-6464; Email: USPDI@MDX.COM.

For information on the specific components of this combination, see the *USP DI* monographs for *Antidepressants, Tricyclic (Systemic)* and *Benzodiazepines (Systemic)*.

The information that follows is selectively abstracted from the complete monograph and is provided to facilitate drug use review and patient counseling.

Note: For a listing of dosage forms and brand names by country availability, see *Dosage Forms* section(s).

## Category
Antianxiety agent–antidepressant.

## Indications

### Accepted
Anxiety associated with mental depression (treatment)—The combination of chlordiazepoxide and amitriptyline is indicated in the treatment of moderate to severe anxiety associated with moderate to severe depression.

The therapeutic response to chlordiazepoxide and amitriptyline combination may occur earlier than when either agent is used alone. Symptoms most likely to respond to therapy in the first week are feelings of guilt or worthlessness, insomnia, agitation, anxiety, suicidal thoughts, and anorexia.

## Patient Consultation
As an aid to patient consultation, refer to *Advice for the Patient, Chlordiazepoxide and Amitriptyline (Systemic)*.

In providing consultation, consider emphasizing the following selected information (» = major clinical significance):

### Before using this medication
» Conditions affecting use, especially:
Sensitivity to other benzodiazepines or tricyclic antidepressants
Pregnancy—Chlordiazepoxide: Crosses placenta; chronic use may cause physical dependence in mother and withdrawal symptoms in neonate; reported to increase risk of congenital malformations when used during first trimester; during delivery, may cause neonatal flaccidity when used just prior to or during labor
Amitriptyline: Animal studies have shown teratogenic effects when given in doses many times larger than the human dose; reports of cardiac problems, muscle spasms, respiratory distress, or urinary retention in neonates of mothers taking amitriptyline just prior to delivery
Breast-feeding—Chlordiazepoxide excreted in breast milk; may cause sedation, feeding difficulties, or weight loss in infant
Use in children—Adolescents are more likely to exhibit dose sensitivity to chlordiazepoxide and amitriptyline combination, requiring a lower initial dose
Use in the elderly—Elderly tend to develop CNS and anticholinergic effects at lower doses; close supervision necessary for patients with cardiac problems, glaucoma, urinary retention, and/or gastrointestinal problems; elderly may better tolerate divided doses
Dental—Dryness of mouth may contribute to development of caries, periodontal disease, oral candidiasis, and discomfort; possible dyscrasias caused by amitriptyline may increase incidence of microbial infection, delayed healing, and gingival bleeding
Other medications, especially other addictive medications, antacids, antithyroid agents, cimetidine, clonidine, guanadrel, guanethidine, alcohol or other CNS depression-producing medications, monoamine oxidase (MAO) inhibitors, metrizamide, or sympathomimetics
Other medical problems, especially alcoholism, active or in remission; seizure disorders; glaucoma; hepatic function impairment; latent psychosis; bipolar disorder; blood, cardiovascular, or gastrointestinal disorders; hyperthyroidism; prostatic hypertrophy; or urinary retention

### Proper use of this medication
Taking after meals or with food to reduce gastric irritation
» Several weeks of therapy may be required to produce optimal therapeutic effects.
» Importance of not taking more medication than the amount prescribed because of habit-forming potential
» Not increasing dose if medication is less effective after a few weeks; checking with physician
» Proper dosing
Missed dose: Not taking dose at all; continuing on schedule; not doubling doses
» Proper storage

### Precautions while using this medication
Regular visits to physician to check progress of therapy
» Checking with physician before discontinuing medication; gradual dosage reduction may be needed to avoid the possibility of withdrawal symptoms
» Avoiding use of alcoholic beverages or other CNS depressants during therapy; not taking other medication unless discussed with physician
Diabetics: May affect blood sugar determinations
Caution if any laboratory tests required; possible interference with results of metyrapone test
» Caution if any kind of surgery, dental treatment, or emergency treatment is required
» Possible drowsiness; caution when driving or doing things requiring alertness
» Possible dizziness; caution when getting up suddenly from a lying or sitting position
Possible dryness of mouth; using sugarless candy or gum, ice, or saliva substitute for relief; checking with dentist or physician if dry mouth continues for more than 2 weeks
Possible skin photosensitivity; avoiding unprotected exposure to sun; using protective clothing; using a sun block product that includes protection against both UVA-caused photosensitivity reactions and UVB-caused sunburn reactions; avoiding use of sunlamp, tanning bed, or tanning booth

### Side/adverse effects
Signs of potential side effects, especially aggravation of glaucoma, agranulocytosis, allergic reactions, anticholinergic effects, convulsions, hallucinations, hypotension, irregular heartbeat, jaundice, mood or mental changes, muscle tremors, or paradoxical CNS stimulation

## Oral Dosage Forms

### CHLORDIAZEPOXIDE AND AMITRIPTYLINE HYDROCHLORIDE TABLETS USP

**Usual adult and adolescent dose**
Antianxiety agent–antidepressant—
Oral, 5 mg of chlordiazepoxide and 12.5 mg of amitriptyline hydrochloride or 10 mg of chlordiazepoxide and 25 mg of amitriptyline hydrochloride three or four times a day initially, the dosage being adjusted as needed and tolerated.

Note: The larger portion of the daily dose may be taken at bedtime. A single bedtime dose may be adequate for some patients.

**Usual adult prescribing limits**
10 mg of chlordiazepoxide and 25 mg of amitriptyline hydrochloride up to six times a day.

**Usual pediatric dose**
Antianxiety agent–antidepressant—
Children up to 12 years of age: Dosage has not been established.
Children 12 years of age and over: See *Usual adult and adolescent dose*.

**Strength(s) usually available**
U.S.—
  5 mg of chlordiazepoxide and 12.5 mg of amitriptyline hydrochloride (Rx) [*Limbitrol;* GENERIC].
  10 mg of chlordiazepoxide and 25 mg of amitriptyline hydrochloride (Rx) [*Limbitrol DS;* GENERIC].
Canada—
  Not commercially available.

**Auxiliary labeling**
• May cause drowsiness.
• Avoid alcoholic beverages.

Revised: 03/19/93

# CHLORDIAZEPOXIDE AND CLIDINIUM    Systemic

VA CLASSIFICATION (Primary): GA802

NOTE: The *Chlordiazepoxide and Clidinium (Systemic)* monograph is maintained on the USP DI electronic data base. For a printed copy of the most recent revision of the complete monograph, contact Micromedex, Inc. - Reprint Requests, 6200 S. Syracuse Way, Suite 300, Englewood, CO 80111; telephone (303) 486-6400; telefax (303) 486-6464; Email: USPDI@MDX.COM.

For information on the specific components of this combination, see the *USP DI* monographs for *Anticholinergics/Antispasmodics (Systemic)* and *Benzodiazepines (Systemic)*.

The information that follows is selectively abstracted from the complete monograph and is provided to facilitate drug use review and patient counseling.

Note: For a listing of dosage forms and brand names by country availability, see *Dosage Forms* section(s).

## Category
Anticholinergic-sedative.

## Indications
**Accepted**
Ulcer, peptic (treatment adjunct) or
Bowel syndrome, irritable (treatment)—FDA has classified chlordiazepoxide and clidinium combination as possibly effective as adjunctive therapy in the treatment of peptic ulcer and irritable bowel syndrome.

Note: The less-than-effective classifications require submission of adequate and well-controlled studies to provide substantial evidence of effectiveness. FDA has notified manufacturers of the possible withdrawal from the market of products containing a combination of an anticholinergic and a sedative because their efficacy as fixed combinations has not been proven in adequately designed clinical trials. To date, no final action has been taken.

**Unaccepted**
Anticholinergic and sedative combinations have been used as adjuncts in the treatment of acute enterocolitis; however, their use for this condition is controversial since they cause a reduction in gastrointestinal motility, resulting in retention of the causative organism or toxin and the consequent prolongation of symptoms.

## Patient Consultation
As an aid to patient consultation, refer to *Advice for the Patient, Chlordiazepoxide and Clidinium (Systemic)*.
In providing consultation, consider emphasizing the following selected information (» = major clinical significance):

**Before using this medication**
» Conditions affecting use, especially:
  Sensitivity to clidinium and chlordiazepoxide or to other benzodiazepines or any of the belladonna alkaloids
  Pregnancy—Use is not recommended; chronic use of chlordiazepoxide may cause physical dependence and withdrawal symptoms in the neonate; chlordiazepoxide increases risk of congenital malformations in first trimester
  Breast-feeding—Chlordiazepoxide distributed into breast milk; clidinium may cause inhibition of lactation
  Use in children—Increased susceptibility to anticholinergic effects of clidinium and to CNS effects of chlordiazepoxide
  Use in the elderly—Increased susceptibility to mental and other anticholinergic effects of clidinium and to CNS effects of chlordiazepoxide; danger of precipitating undiagnosed glaucoma; possible impairment of memory
  Dental—Possible development of dental problems because of decreased salivary flow
  Other medications, especially other anticholinergics, antacids, antidiarrheals, CNS depressants, ketoconazole, or potassium chloride
  Other medical problems, especially cardiac disease, glaucoma, hepatic disease, hiatal hernia with reflux esophagitis, intestinal atony, myasthenia gravis, obstruction in gastrointestinal or urinary tract, ulcerative colitis, or urinary retention

**Proper use of this medication**
Taking dose 30 to 60 minutes before meals unless told otherwise by physician
» Taking medication only as directed
» Proper dosing
  Missed dose: Taking as soon as possible; not taking if almost time for next dose; not doubling doses
» Proper storage

**Precautions while using this medication**
Regular visits to physician to check progress of therapy if used for extended period of time
Avoiding medicine for diarrhea within 1 to 2 hours of taking this medication
» Caution if dizziness, lightheadedness, drowsiness, or blurred vision occurs
» Avoiding use of alcohol or other CNS depressants during and for a few days following therapy
» Caution during exercise and hot weather; overheating may result in heat stroke
  Possible dryness of mouth, nose, and throat; using sugarless gum or candy, ice, or saliva substitute for relief; checking with dentist if mouth continues to feel dry for more than 2 weeks
» Checking with physician if constipation occurs
  Checking with physician before discontinuing medication after prolonged use; gradual dosage reduction may be necessary to avoid the possibility of withdrawal symptoms

**Side/adverse effects**
Signs of potential side effects, especially agranulocytosis, granulocytopenia, or leukopenia; allergic reaction; CNS depression; increased intraocular pressure; jaundice; and paradoxical reaction

## Oral Dosage Forms

### CHLORDIAZEPOXIDE HYDROCHLORIDE AND CLIDINIUM BROMIDE CAPSULES USP

**Usual adult dose**
Oral, 1 or 2 capsules one to four times a day, thirty to sixty minutes before meals or food, the dosage then being adjusted as needed and tolerated.

Note: Debilitated patients—See *Usual geriatric dose*.

**Usual adult prescribing limits**
Up to a total of 8 capsules daily (40 mg of chlordiazepoxide hydrochloride and 20 mg of clidinium bromide).

**Usual pediatric dose**
Dosage has not been established.

**Usual geriatric dose**
Oral, initially no more than 1 capsule two times a day, the dosage then being adjusted as needed and tolerated.

**Strength(s) usually available**
U.S.—
  5 mg of chlordiazepoxide hydrochloride and 2.5 mg of clidinium bromide per capsule (Rx) [*Clindex; Clinoxide; Clipoxide; Librax; Lidox; Lidoxide; Zebrax;* GENERIC].
Canada—
  5 mg of chlordiazepoxide hydrochloride and 2.5 mg of clidinium bromide per capsule (Rx) [*Apo-Chlorax; Corium; Librax*].

**Auxiliary labeling**
• Take before meals.
• Avoid alcoholic beverages.
• May cause drowsiness.

Revised: 01/29/92
Interim revision: 08/10/94

# CHLORHEXIDINE Mucosal-Local

VA CLASSIFICATION (Primary/Secondary): OR500/DE101
Commonly used brand name(s): *Oro-Clense; Peridex; PerioGard.*
Note: For a listing of dosage forms and brand names by country availability, see *Dosage Forms* section(s).

## Category
Antibacterial (dental).

## Indications
Note: Bracketed information in the *Indications* section refers to uses that are not included in U.S. product labeling.

**Accepted**

Gingivitis (treatment)—Chlorhexidine is indicated for use between dental visits for the treatment of gingivitis that is characterized by redness and swelling of the gingivae or gingival bleeding upon probing.

[Gingivitis, necrotizing ulcerative, acute (treatment)]—Chlorhexidine is used along with other measures in the treatment of acute necrotizing ulcerative gingivitis (ANUG).

[Mouth infections (prophylaxis)] or
[Mouth infections (treatment)]—Chlorhexidine is used in the treatment of mouth infections in cancer patients who are being prepared for bone marrow transplants. Chlorhexidine is also used in the management of the oral complications that occur in leukemia patients.

Chlorhexidine is also used following periodontal surgery to promote healing by minimizing mouth infections and plaque that may lead to increased inflammation and infection during the healing process.

[Stomatitis, denture (treatment)]—Chlorhexidine is used in the treatment of inflammation of the oral mucosa caused by bacterial or fungal actions associated with the wearing of dentures but should not be used when inflammation is caused by poor fit or other mechanical factors associated with dentures.

[Stomatitis, aphthous (treatment)]—Chlorhexidine is used in the management of minor aphthous ulcers.

[Plaque, dental (prophylaxis)]—Chlorhexidine is used for reduction of dental plaque.

Microorganisms with high susceptibility to chlorhexidine include some staphylococci, *Streptococcus mutans*, *Streptococcus salivarius*, *Candida albicans*, *Escherichia coli*, *Selenomonas*, and anaerobic propionic bacteria. *Streptococcus sanguis* has moderate susceptibility. Microorganisms with low susceptibility to chlorhexidine include *Proteus* strains, *Pseudomonas*, *Klebsiella*, and gram-negative cocci resembling *Veillonella*.

Samples of plaque taken during a 6-month period of use with chlorhexidine oral rinse showed a 54 to 97% reduction in certain aerobic and anaerobic bacteria. However, 3 months after chlorhexidine was discontinued, the number of bacteria in the plaque had returned to baseline levels.

A 6-month clinical study did not show any significant changes in bacterial resistance, overgrowth of potentially opportunistic organisms, or other adverse changes in the oral microbial ecosystem during the use of chlorhexidine. In addition, 3 months after chlorhexidine was discontinued, the resistance of plaque bacteria to the medication was found to be the same as before therapy was initiated.

## Pharmacology/Pharmacokinetics

**Physicochemical characteristics**
Molecular weight—Chlorhexidine gluconate: 897.77.

**Mechanism of action/Effect**
Because of its positive charge, chlorhexidine gluconate is adsorbed during oral rinsing onto the surfaces of teeth, plaque, and oral mucosa, which have a net negative charge. Subsequently, the adsorbed medication is gradually released from these sites by diffusion for up to 24 hours as the concentration of chlorhexidine gluconate in the saliva decreases. This release provides a continuing bacteriostatic effect.

Chlorhexidine gluconate is adsorbed onto the cell walls of microorganisms, which causes leakage of intracellular components. At low concentrations, chlorhexidine gluconate is bacteriostatic; at higher concentrations, chlorhexidine gluconate is bactericidal.

**Absorption**
Pharmacokinetic studies indicate that approximately 30% of chlorhexidine gluconate is retained in the oral cavity following rinsing and subsequently is slowly released into the oral fluids.

Studies using humans and animals have shown that chlorhexidine gluconate is poorly absorbed from the gastrointestinal tract. In humans, the mean plasma level of chlorhexidine gluconate reached a peak of 0.206 mcg per gram 30 minutes following an oral dose of 300 mg.

**Elimination**
Following oral doses of 300 mg of chlorhexidine gluconate, excretion of chlorhexidine gluconate was primarily through the feces (approximately 90%); less than 1% of chlorhexidine gluconate was excreted in the urine. In addition, 12 hours after chlorhexidine gluconate was administered, it was not detectable in the plasma.

## Precautions to Consider

**Cross-sensitivity and/or related problems**
Patients sensitive to disinfectant skin cleansers containing chlorhexidine may be sensitive to chlorhexidine oral rinse also.

**Carcinogenicity**
Carcinogenesis was not observed in a drinking water study in rats where the highest dose of chlorhexidine used was 38 mg per kg of body weight (mg/kg) per day. This dose is at least 500 times the amount that would be ingested from the recommended human daily dose of chlorhexidine oral rinse.

**Mutagenicity**
Mutagenicity was not observed in 2 mammalian *in vivo* mutagenic studies with chlorhexidine.

**Pregnancy/Reproduction**
Fertility—Fertility studies have shown no evidence of impaired fertility in rats given chlorhexidine in doses of up to 100 mg/kg per day. This dose is approximately 100 times greater than the dose a person would receive if he/she ingested 30 mL (2 capfuls) of chlorhexidine oral rinse per day.

Pregnancy—Well-controlled studies in humans have not been done.
In animal studies, no evidence of harm to the fetus was observed in rats and rabbits given doses of chlorhexidine of up to 300 mg/kg per day and up to 40 mg/kg per day, respectively. These doses are approximately 300 and 40 times, respectively, greater than the dose a person would receive if she ingested 30 mL (2 capfuls) of chlorhexidine oral rinse per day.

FDA Pregnancy Category B.

**Breast-feeding**
Although it is not known whether chlorhexidine is distributed into breast milk, problems in humans have not been documented. In addition, studies in rats have shown no evidence of impaired parturition and no evidence of toxic effects to suckling pups when chlorhexidine was administered to dams at doses over 100 times greater than the dose a person would receive if she ingested 30 mL (2 capfuls) of chlorhexidine oral rinse per day.

**Pediatrics**
Appropriate studies on the relationship of age to the effects of this medicine have not been performed in the pediatric population. Safety and efficacy have not been established.

**Geriatrics**
Appropriate studies on the relationship of age to the effects of this medicine have not been performed in the geriatric population. However, no geriatrics-specific problems have been documented to date.

**Medical considerations/Contraindications**
The medical considerations/contraindications included have been selected on the basis of their potential clinical significance (reasons given in parentheses where appropriate)—not necessarily inclusive (» = major clinical significance).

*Risk-benefit should be considered when the following medical problems exist:*

Anterior tooth restorations (front-tooth fillings)
(anterior tooth restorations having rough surfaces or margins may develop permanent discoloration from chlorhexidine, necessitating replacement for cosmetic reasons)

Periodontitis
(during clinical tests, an increase in supragingival calculus was noted in patients using chlorhexidine; it is not known whether use of chlorhexidine results in an increase in subgingival calculus)
(since gingival inflammation and bleeding may occur with both periodontitis and gingivitis and chlorhexidine oral rinse may reduce these signs, the presence or absence of these signs should not be

# Chlorhexidine (Mucosal-Local)

used as indicators of periodontitis after the patient has been treated with chlorhexidine)

Sensitivity to chlorhexidine

**Patient monitoring**

The following may be especially important in patient monitoring (other tests may be warranted in some patients, depending on condition; » = major clinical significance):

Dental examination and prophylaxis
(tartar [calculus] deposits should be removed before therapy is initiated and during therapy at intervals of 6 months or less; the patient's condition should be reevaluated at intervals of 6 months or less, including monitoring of gingival pockets, because of the possible masking of coexisting periodontitis by chlorhexidine)

## Side/Adverse Effects

Note: Chlorhexidine causes staining of oral surfaces. Staining may be visible as early as 1 week after therapy; after 6 months of use, approximately 50% of patients may have a measurable increase in tooth stain and approximately 10% may have heavy staining. Staining is more pronounced in patients who have heavier accumulations of plaque. Tooth restorations having rough surfaces or margins may develop permanent staining. If this occurs on anterior surfaces, it may be necessary to replace the tooth restoration for cosmetic reasons.

Some patients develop an alteration in taste perception during treatment with chlorhexidine. This effect usually becomes less noticeable with continued treatment. No cases of permanent taste alteration have been reported.

No serious systemic side/adverse effects associated with the use of chlorhexidine oral rinse were reported during the clinical trials.

The following side/adverse effects have been selected on the basis of their potential clinical significance (possible signs and symptoms in parentheses where appropriate)—not necessarily inclusive:

**Those indicating need for medical attention**
Incidence rare
*Allergic reaction* (nasal congestion; shortness of breath or troubled breathing; skin rash, hives, or itching; swelling of face)

**Those indicating need for medical attention only if they continue or are bothersome**
Incidence more frequent
*Change in taste; increase in tartar (calculus) on teeth; staining of teeth, mouth, tooth restorations (fillings), and dentures or other mouth appliances*
Incidence less frequent or rare
*Parotid duct obstruction or parotitis* (swollen glands on side of face or neck); *superficial desquamative lesions* (mouth irritation)—reported mainly in children ages 10 to 18 years; the lesions are transient and may be painless; *tongue tip irritation*

## Overdose

For more information on the management of overdose or unintentional ingestion, **contact a Poison Control Center** (see *Poison Control Center Listing*).

**Treatment of overdose**
Medical attention and symptomatic treatment are recommended if signs of alcohol intoxication develop or if more than 4 ounces of chlorhexidine oral rinse is ingested by a child weighing approximately 10 kg (22 pounds) or less.

## Patient Consultation

As an aid to patient consultation, refer to *Advice for the Patient, Chlorhexidine (Dental)*.

In providing consultation, consider emphasizing the following selected information (» = major clinical significance):

**Before using this medication**
» Conditions affecting use, especially:
Allergy to chlorhexidine or to disinfectant skin cleansers containing chlorhexidine

**Proper use of this medication**
Using medication after brushing and flossing; rinsing toothpaste completely from mouth with water before using oral rinse; not eating or drinking for several hours after using oral rinse
Using the cap of the original container to measure the dose or acquiring another measuring device to use; asking your pharmacist for help
» Swishing medication around in mouth for 30 seconds and spitting out; using full strength; not swallowing

» Proper dosing
Missed dose: Using as soon as possible; not using if almost time for next dose; not doubling doses
» Proper storage

**Precautions while using this medication**
Not rinsing mouth with water immediately after using medication, since doing so will increase medication's bitter aftertaste and may decrease medication's effect
Medication causes change in taste; change may last up to 4 hours after dose; change in taste should be less noticeable as medication is continued; after medication is discontinued, taste should return to normal
Staining and increase in tartar (calculus) may occur; brushing with tartar-control toothpaste and flossing teeth daily to help reduce tartar build-up; visiting dentist at least every 6 months for teeth cleaning and gum examination
» Getting emergency help at once if a child weighing 22 pounds (10 kg) or less drinks more than 4 ounces of dental rinse or if any child experiences symptoms of alcohol intoxication, such as slurred speech, sleepiness, or staggering or stumbling walk, after drinking the dental rinse

**Side/adverse effects**
Signs of potential side effects, especially allergic reaction

## Dental Dosage Forms

Note: Bracketed uses in the *Dosage Forms* section refer to categories of use and/or indications that are not included in U.S. product labeling.

### CHLORHEXIDINE GLUCONATE ORAL RINSE

**Usual adult dose**
Gingivitis—
Topical, to the gingival membranes, 15 mL of a 0.12% oral rinse for 30 seconds two times a day after brushing and flossing teeth.
Note: Therapy with chlorhexidine oral rinse should start immediately following a dental prophylaxis.
[Denture stomatitis]—
Soak the dentures in chlorhexidine oral rinse 0.12% for 1 to 2 minutes two times a day. Rinsing the mouth for 30 seconds two times a day or brushing the gums or dentures two times a day with chlorhexidine oral rinse 0.12% may also be required.

**Usual pediatric dose**
Children up to 18 years of age—Safety and efficacy have not been established.

**Strength(s) usually available**
U.S.—
0.12% (Rx) [*Peridex* (alcohol 11.6%); *PerioGard* (alcohol 11.6%); GENERIC].
Canada—
0.12% (Rx) [*Oro-Clense* (alcohol); *Peridex* (alcohol)].

**Packaging and storage**
Store above freezing at a temperature not exceeding 25 °C (77 °F), unless otherwise specified by manufacturer. Protect from light.

**Preparation of dosage form**
If the medication is not commercially available, it may be compounded as follows—3 mL chlorhexidine gluconate 20% should be added to approximately 200 mL distilled water. Separately, 5 mL essence of peppermint should be combined with 5 mL ethanol 95% and then 15 mL glycerin should be added. This mixture should be combined with the chlorhexidine and water solution and enough distilled water added to make 500 mL.

**Auxiliary labeling**
• Do not swallow.
• Do not dilute.

**Note**
Dispense with patient package insert.
Dispense in original container, which includes a measuring cap, or in an amber glass container and include a device for measuring 15 mL (½ fluid ounce).

---

Revised: 05/16/94
Interim revision: 08/22/94; 08/14/98

---

**CHLOROPROCAINE**—See *Anesthetics (Parenteral-Local)*

# CHLOROQUINE Systemic

VA CLASSIFICATION (Primary/Secondary): AP101/MS109; TN900

Commonly used brand name(s): *Aralen; Aralen HCl.*

Note: For a listing of dosage forms and brand names by country availability, see *Dosage Forms* section(s).

## Category

Antiprotozoal—Chloroquine.
Antihypercalcemic—Chloroquine (Oral).
Antirheumatic (disease-modifying)—Chloroquine (Oral).
Lupus erythematosus suppressant—Chloroquine (Oral).
Polymorphous light eruption suppressant—Chloroquine (Oral).
Porphyria cutanea tarda suppressant—Chloroquine (Oral).

## Indications

Note: Bracketed information in the *Indications* section refers to uses that are not included in U.S. product labeling.

### General considerations

Chloroquine-resistant strains of *Plasmodium falciparum*, originally seen only in Southeast Asia and South America, are now documented in all malarious areas except Central America west of the Canal Zone, the Middle East, and the Caribbean. Chloroquine is still the drug of choice for the treatment of susceptible strains of *P. falciparum* and the other 3 malarial species; however, chloroquine-resistant *P. vivax* has recently been reported.

### Accepted

Malaria (prophylaxis and treatment)—Chloroquine is indicated in the suppressive treatment and the treatment of acute attacks of malaria caused by *P. vivax, P. malariae, P. ovale*, and chloroquine-susceptible strains of *P. falciparum*. The radical cure for *P. vivax* and *P. ovale* malaria requires the concurrent or subsequent administration of primaquine. However, there have been reports of chloroquine-resistant *P. vivax* in patients who have traveled to Papua New Guinea and Indonesia.

Liver abscess, amebic (treatment)—Chloroquine is indicated in the treatment of amebic liver abscess, usually in combination with an effective intestinal amebicide. However, it is not considered a primary drug.

[Hypercalcemia, sarcoid-associated (treatment)][1]—Chloroquine (oral) is used to reduce urinary calcium excretion and the levels of 1,25-dihydroxy vitamin D in the serum of sarcoid patients who are unable to take corticosteroids.

[Arthritis, juvenile (treatment)][1]—Chloroquine (oral) is used in the treatment of juvenile arthritis.

[Arthritis, rheumatoid (treatment)][1]—Chloroquine (oral) is indicated in the treatment of acute and chronic rheumatoid arthritis in patients who do not respond adequately to other less toxic antirheumatics. Chloroquine may be used in addition to nonsteroidal anti-inflammatory agents.

[Lupus erythematosus, discoid (treatment)][1] or
[Lupus erythematosus, systemic (treatment)][1]—Chloroquine (oral) is used as a suppressant for chronic discoid and systemic lupus erythematosus.

[Polymorphous light eruption (treatment)][1]—Chloroquine (oral) is used as a suppressant for polymorphous light eruption.

[Porphyria cutanea tarda (treatment)][1]—Chloroquine (oral) is used in the treatment of porphyria cutanea tarda.

[Urticaria, solar (treatment)][1] or
[Vasculitis, chronic cutaneous (treatment)][1]—Chloroquine is also used in the treatment of solar urticaria and chronic cutaneous vasculitis unresponsive to other therapy.

### Unaccepted

Chloroquine does not prevent relapses in patients with *P. vivax* or *P. ovale* malaria since it is not effective against exo-erythrocytic forms of the parasite. In these species, "hypnozoites," which remain dormant in the liver, are responsible for relapses.

Chloroquine is not indicated in the treatment of acute amebic dysentery or asymptomatic carriers.

[1] Not included in Canadian product labeling.

## Pharmacology/Pharmacokinetics

Note: Because chloroquine concentrates in the cellular fraction of blood, chloroquine concentrations measured in the blood are higher than those measured in the plasma, with concentration ratios between blood and plasma ranging from 1 to 25.

### Physicochemical characteristics

Molecular weight—Chloroquine: 319.88.
Chloroquine hydrochloride: 392.80.
Chloroquine phosphate: 515.87.

### Mechanism of action/Effect

Antiprotozoal—Malaria: Unknown, but may be based on ability of chloroquine to bind to and alter the properties of DNA. Chloroquine is also taken up into the acidic food vacuoles of the parasite in the erythrocyte. It increases the pH of the acid vesicles, interfering with vesicle functions and possibly inhibiting phospholipid metabolism. In suppressive treatment, chloroquine inhibits the erythrocytic stage of development of plasmodia. In acute attacks of malaria, chloroquine interrupts erythrocytic schizogony of the parasite. Its ability to concentrate in parasitized erythrocytes may account for its selective toxicity against the erythrocytic stages of plasmodial infection.

Antirheumatic—Chloroquine is thought to act as a mild immunosuppressant, inhibiting the production of rheumatoid factor and acute phase reactants. It also accumulates in white blood cells, stabilizing lysosomal membranes and inhibiting the activity of many enzymes, including collagenase and the proteases that cause cartilage breakdown.

### Absorption

Rate of absorption is variable; chloroquine is almost completely absorbed from the gastrointestinal tract. Bioavailability of tablets is approximately 89%.

### Distribution

Widely distributed in body tissues such as the eyes, heart, kidneys, liver, and lungs where retention is prolonged. Concentrations are 2 to 5 times higher in erythrocytes than in plasma. Very low concentrations are found in intestinal wall. Chloroquine crosses the placenta and is distributed into breast milk.

Apparent $Vol_D$ (in plasma)=204 L per kg (range, 116 to 285 L per kg); may be as large as 800 L per kg.

### Protein binding

Moderate (50 to 65%).

### Biotransformation

Hepatic (partially), to active de-ethylated metabolites. Principal metabolite is desethylchloroquine.

### Half-life

Terminal elimination half-life—1 to 2 months.

### Time to peak concentration

Adults (healthy, in plasma):
Oral: Approximately 3.5 hours.
Parenteral (IV, IM, SQ): 30 minutes.
Children (with malaria, via nasogastric tube, in whole blood):
7.5 hours (range, 1 to 12 hours) after an initial dose of 10 mg [base] per kg of body weight and 5 mg [base] per kg of body weight six hours later.

### Peak concentrations

Adults (in plasma)—
Oral:
300 mg (base) in healthy patients—73 to 76 mcg per L.
Parenteral:
Intravenous infusion, 300 mg (base) over 24 minutes in healthy patients—Approximately 837 mcg per L.
Intramuscular, 3 mg (base) per kg of body weight in malaria patients—236 to 256 mcg per L.
Subcutaneous, 3 mg (base) per kg of body weight in malaria patients—Approximately 265 mcg per L.
Children (with malaria, in whole blood)—
Oral (after an initial dose of 10 mg [base] per kg of body weight and 5 mg [base] per kg of body weight six hours later) via nasogastric tube: 897 mcg per L (491 to 1589 mcg per L).
Parenteral (after first dose):
Intravenous infusion, 5 mg (base) per kg of body weight over 4 hours—790 mcg per L (538 to 1249 mcg per L).
Intramuscular, 3.5 mg (base) per kg of body weight—Approximately 718 mcg per L.
Subcutaneous, 3.5 mg (base) per kg of body weight—Approximately 946 mcg per L.

### Elimination

Renal; 42 to 47% of chloroquine is excreted unchanged in the urine; 7 to 12% desethylchloroquine is excreted in urine. Chloroquine is excreted very slowly and may persist in urine for months or years after medication is discontinued. Urine acidification increases renal excretion by 20 to 90%.

**Hemodialysis**—Hemodialysis increases the clearance of chloroquine; however, due to chloroquine's large volume of distribution, hemodialysis may not remove appreciable amounts in an overdose.

## Precautions to Consider

### Cross-sensitivity and/or related problems
Patients hypersensitive to hydroxychloroquine may also be hypersensitive to chloroquine, a structurally similar 4-aminoquinoline compound.

### Pregnancy/Reproduction
Chloroquine crosses the placenta. Use is not recommended during pregnancy except in the suppression or treatment of malaria or hepatic amebiasis since malaria poses greater potential danger to the mother and fetus (i.e., abortion and death) than prophylactic administration of chloroquine. Chloroquine, given in weekly chemoprophylactic doses, has not been shown to cause adverse effects on the fetus. However, risk-benefit must be considered since chloroquine, given in therapeutic doses, has been shown to cause central nervous system (CNS) damage, including ototoxicity (auditory and vestibular); congenital deafness; retinal hemorrhages; and abnormal retinal pigmentation.

Chloroquine has been shown to accumulate selectively in melanin structures of fetal eyes of mice. It may be retained in ocular tissues for up to 5 months after elimination from the blood.

### Breast-feeding
Chloroquine is distributed into breast milk. Although problems in humans have not been documented, risk-benefit must be considered since infants and children are especially sensitive to the effects of chloroquine.

### Pediatrics
Infants and children are especially sensitive to the effects of chloroquine. Fatalities have been reported following the ingestion of as little as 300 mg of chloroquine base in a 12-month-old child. In addition, severe reactions and sudden death have been reported following parenteral administration of chloroquine in children. If chloroquine hydrochloride injection is given intravenously in pediatric patients, it should be diluted and administered very slowly.

### Geriatrics
No information is available on the relationship of age to the effects of chloroquine in geriatric patients.

### Drug interactions and/or related problems
The following drug interactions and/or related problems have been selected on the basis of their potential clinical significance (possible mechanism in parentheses where appropriate)—not necessarily inclusive (» = major clinical significance):

Note: Combinations containing any of the following medications, depending on the amount present, may also interact with this medication.

Penicillamine
(concurrent use of penicillamine with chloroquine may increase penicillamine plasma concentrations, increasing the potential for serious hematologic and/or renal adverse reactions, as well as the possibility of severe skin reactions)

### Medical considerations/Contraindications
The medical considerations/contraindications included have been selected on the basis of their potential clinical significance (reasons given in parentheses where appropriate)—not necessarily inclusive (» = major clinical significance).

*Risk-benefit should be considered when the following medical problems exist:*

» Blood disorders, severe
(chloroquine may cause blood dyscrasias, including agranulocytosis, aplastic anemia, neutropenia, or thrombocytopenia)

Gastrointestinal disorders, severe
(chloroquine may cause gastrointestinal irritation)

Glucose-6-phosphate dehydrogenase (G6PD) deficiency
(chloroquine may cause hemolytic anemia in G6PD-deficient patients, although this is unlikely when chloroquine is given in therapeutic doses)

» Hepatic function impairment
(because chloroquine is metabolized in the liver, hepatic function impairment may increase blood concentrations of chloroquine, increasing the risk of side effects)

Hypersensitivity to chloroquine or hydroxychloroquine

» Neurological disorders, severe
(chloroquine may cause polyneuritis, ototoxicity, seizures, or neuromyopathy)

Porphyria
(chloroquine may cause exacerbation of porphyria)

Psoriasis
(chloroquine may precipitate severe attacks of psoriasis)

» Retinal or visual field changes, presence of
(chloroquine may cause corneal opacities, keratopathy, or retinopathy)

### Patient monitoring
The following may be especially important in patient monitoring (other tests may be warranted in some patients, depending on condition; » = major clinical significance):

» Complete blood counts (CBCs)
(recommended periodically during prolonged daily therapy with chloroquine; if severe blood dyscrasias occur that are not attributable to the disease being treated, discontinuation of chloroquine should be considered)

» Neuromuscular examinations, including knee and ankle reflexes
(recommended periodically during long-term therapy with chloroquine to detect muscle weakness; if muscle weakness occurs, chloroquine should be discontinued)

» Ophthalmologic examinations, including visual acuity, expert slit-lamp, funduscopic, and visual field tests
(recommended before and at least every 3 to 6 months during prolonged daily therapy since irreversible retinal damage has been reported with long-term or high-dosage therapy; serious ocular injury has been thought to be correlated with a total cumulative dose of greater than 100 grams [base] of chloroquine; however, a daily dose of greater than 150 mg [base], or 2.4 mg [base] per kg daily, of chloroquine may be a more important determinant; any retinal or visual abnormality that is not fully explainable by difficulties of accommodation or corneal opacities should be monitored following discontinuation of therapy, since retinal changes and visual disturbances may progress even after cessation of therapy)

## Side/Adverse Effects

Note: Side/adverse effects of chloroquine are usually dose-related. When chloroquine is used for the short-term treatment of malaria or other parasitic diseases, side/adverse effects are usually mild and reversible. However, following prolonged use and/or high-dose therapy such as in the treatment of rheumatoid arthritis, lupus erythematosus, or polymorphous light eruption, side/adverse effects may be serious and sometimes irreversible.

Irreversible retinal damage may be more likely to occur when the daily dosage equals or exceeds the equivalent of 150 mg (base), or 2.4 mg (base) per kg per day of chloroquine.

The following side/adverse effects have been selected on the basis of their potential clinical significance (possible signs and symptoms in parentheses where appropriate)—not necessarily inclusive:

### Those indicating need for medical attention
Incidence less frequent
*Ocular toxicity such as corneal opacities* (blurred vision or any other change in vision); *keratopathy* (blurred vision or any other change in vision); *or retinopathy* (blurred vision or any other change in vision)

Incidence rare
*Blood dyscrasias such as agranulocytosis* (sore throat and fever); *aplastic anemia* (weakness; fatigue); *neutropenia* (sore throat and fever); *or thrombocytopenia* (bleeding; bruising); *cardiovascular toxicity such as hypotension* (feeling faint or lightheaded); *or prolonged QRS interval; emotional changes or psychosis* (mood or other mental changes); *neuromyopathy* (increased muscle weakness); *ototoxicity* (any loss of hearing, ringing or buzzing in ears)—usually in patients with pre-existing auditory damage; *seizures*

### Those indicating need for medical attention only if they continue or are bothersome
Incidence more frequent
*Ciliary muscle dysfunction* (difficulty in reading); *gastrointestinal irritation* (diarrhea; loss of appetite; nausea; stomach cramps or pain; vomiting); *headache; itching*—especially in black patients, but not an indication for discontinuing their therapy

Incidence less frequent
*Bleaching of hair or increased hair loss; blue-black discoloration of skin, fingernails, or inside of mouth*—with prolonged oral therapy; *skin rash or itching*

### Those indicating possible retinal changes or visual disturbances and the need for medical attention if they occur or progress after medication is discontinued
*Blurred vision or any other change in vision*

## Overdose

For specific information on the agents used in the management of chloroquine overdose, see:
- *Charcoal, Activated (Oral-Local)* monograph;
- *Diazepam* in *Benzodiazepines (Systemic)* monograph; and/or
- *Sympathomimetic Agents—Cardiovascular Use (Parenteral-Systemic)* monograph.

For more information on the management of overdose or unintentional ingestion, **contact a Poison Control Center** (see *Poison Control Center Listing*).

After ingestion of an overdose of chloroquine, toxic symptoms may occur within 30 minutes, and death may occur as soon as 3 hours post-ingestion. Doses of chloroquine phosphate as small as 300 mg in children, and 2.25 to 3 grams in adults, may be fatal.

### Clinical effects of overdose

The following effects have been selected on the basis of their potential clinical significance (possible signs and symptoms in parentheses where appropriate)—not necessarily inclusive:

Acute
*Cardiovascular toxicities* (conduction disturbances; hypotension); *neurotoxicity* (drowsiness; headache; hyperexcitability; seizures; coma); *respiratory and cardiac arrest; visual disturbances* (blurred vision)

### Treatment of overdose

Since there is no specific antidote, treatment of chloroquine overdose should be symptomatic and supportive.

To decrease absorption—
Gastric lavage may be performed to empty the stomach. Activated charcoal should be administered with a cathartic. The dose of activated charcoal should be 5 to 10 times the estimated dose of chloroquine ingested.

To enhance elimination—
Forcing diuresis and acidifying the urine, with ammonium chloride, for example, can help promote urinary excretion of chloroquine. The dose of the acidifying agent should be adjusted to maintain a urinary pH of 5.5 to 6.5. Monitoring of plasma potassium is recommended. Use with caution in patients with renal function impairment and/or metabolic acidosis.

Specific treatment—
For repetitive seizures or status epilepticus: Treat with intravenous diazepam (in 2.5 to 5.0 mg increments).

For life-threatening ventricular arrhythmias or cardiac arrest: Manage appropriately, as per Advanced Cardiac Life Support guidelines.

For hypotension and circulatory shock: Fluids should be administered at a sufficient rate to maintain urine output. Intravenous pressors and/or inotropic drugs, such as norepinephrine, dopamine, isoproterenol, or dobutamine, may be administered if required. High-dose diazepam infusion has been reported to improve hemodynamic function. Epinephrine has been shown to decrease the myocardial depressant and vasodilatory effects of chloroquine.

Supportive care—
Supportive measures such as securing and maintaining a patent airway, administering oxygen, and instituting assisted or controlled respiration may be required. In severe overdoses, early mechanical ventilation has been suggested to prevent hypoxemia. Patients in whom intentional overdose is confirmed or suspected should be referred for psychiatric consultation.

## Patient Consultation

As an aid to patient consultation, refer to *Advice for the Patient, Chloroquine (Systemic)*.

In providing consultation, consider emphasizing the following selected information (» = major clinical significance):

### Before using this medication
» Conditions affecting use, especially:
Hypersensitivity to chloroquine or hydroxychloroquine
Pregnancy—May cause toxicity to the fetus when given to mother in therapeutic doses; however, chloroquine has not been shown to cause adverse effects in the fetus when used as a prophylactic agent against malaria or hepatic amebiasis
Use in children—Infants and children are especially sensitive to effects of chloroquine
Other medical problems, especially impaired hepatic function, severe blood disorders, severe neurologic disorders, or presence of retinal or visual field changes

### Proper use of this medication
» Taking with meals or milk to minimize possible gastrointestinal irritation
» Keeping medication out of reach of children; fatalities reported with as little as 300 mg of chloroquine base (1 tablet) in a 12-month-old child
» Importance of not taking more medication than the amount prescribed
» Compliance with full course of therapy
» Importance of not missing doses and taking medication on regular schedule
» Proper dosing
Missed dose: If dosing schedule is—
Every 7 days: Taking as soon as possible
Once a day: Taking as soon as possible; not taking if not remembered until next day; not doubling doses
More than once a day: Taking right away if remembered within an hour or so; not taking if not remembered until later; not doubling doses
» Proper storage

*For prevention of malaria*
Starting medication 1 to 2 weeks before entering malarious area to ascertain patient response and allow time to substitute another medication if reactions occur
» Continuing medication while staying in area and for 4 weeks after leaving area; checking with physician immediately if fever develops while traveling or within 2 months after departure from endemic area

### Precautions while using this medication
» Regular visits to physician to check for blood problems, muscle weakness, and ophthalmologic examinations during or after long-term therapy
Checking with physician if no improvement within a few days (or a few weeks or months for arthritis)
» Caution if blurred vision, difficulty in reading, or other change in vision occurs

*Mosquito-control measures to reduce the chance of getting malaria:*
Avoiding exposure to mosquitoes, especially at peak feeding times (between dusk and dawn)
Sleeping in screened or air-conditioned room or under mosquito netting sprayed with insecticide
Wearing long-sleeved shirts or blouses and long trousers to protect arms and legs between dusk and dawn
Applying mosquito repellent to uncovered areas of skin between dusk and dawn
Using mosquito coils or spray

### Side/adverse effects
Signs of potential side effects, especially ocular toxicity such as corneal opacities, keratopathy, or retinopathy; blood dyscrasias such as agranulocytosis, aplastic anemia, or thrombocytopenia; cardiovascular toxicity such as hypotension or prolonged QRS interval; emotional changes or psychosis; neuromyopathy; ototoxicity; and seizures

## General Dosing Information

Long-term and/or high-dosage therapy may cause irreversible retinal damage and/or neurosensorial deafness.

Chloroquine should be discontinued if any of the following problems occur: any abnormality in visual acuity, visual fields, retinal macular changes, or any visual symptoms; muscle weakness; or severe blood disorders.

Malaria-suppressive therapy should be started 1 to 2 weeks before the patient enters a malarious area and should be continued for 4 weeks after patient leaves the area. Starting the medication in advance will help to determine the patient's tolerance to the medication and allow time to substitute other antimalarials if the patient develops allergies to the medication or other adverse effects.

### For oral dosage form only

Chloroquine should be taken with meals or milk to minimize the possibility of gastrointestinal irritation.

When chloroquine is used in the treatment of rheumatoid arthritis, up to 6 months of therapy may be required for it to reach its maximum effectiveness.

### For parenteral dosage forms only

If chloroquine hydrochloride injection is given intravenously in pediatric patients, it should be diluted and administered very slowly.

## Oral Dosage Forms

Note: Bracketed uses in the *Dosage Forms* section refer to categories of use and/or indications that are not included in U.S. product labeling.

## CHLOROQUINE PHOSPHATE TABLETS USP

**Usual adult and adolescent dose**
Malaria—
  Suppressive: Oral, 500 mg (300 mg base) once every seven days.
  Therapeutic: Oral, 1 gram (600 mg base) initially, followed by 500 mg (300 mg base) in six to eight hours, and 500 mg (300 mg base) once a day on the second and third days.
Liver abscess, amebic—
  In combination with other "tissue-acting" antiprotozoals: Oral, 250 mg (150 mg base) four times a day for two days, followed by 250 mg (150 mg base) two times a day for at least two to three weeks.
  Note: The dosage schedule may be revised up or down, if necessary, or the course of therapy may be repeated.
[Antirheumatic (disease-modifying)][1]—
  Oral, up to 4 mg (2.4 mg base) per kg of lean body weight daily.
[Lupus erythematosus suppressant][1]—
  Oral, up to 4 mg (2.4 mg base) per kg of lean body weight daily.
[Polymorphous light eruption suppressant][1]—
  Oral, 250 mg (150 mg base) two times a day for two weeks; then 250 mg (150 mg base) once a day.

**Usual pediatric dose**
Malaria—
  Suppressive: Oral, 8.3 mg (5 mg base) per kg of body weight, not to exceed the adult dose, once every seven days.
  Therapeutic: Oral, 41.7 mg (25 mg base) per kg of body weight administered over a period of three days as follows: 16.7 mg (10 mg base) per kg of body weight, not to exceed a single dose of 1 gram (600 mg base); then 8.3 mg (5 mg base) per kg of body weight, not to exceed a single dose of 500 mg (300 mg base), six, twenty-four, and forty-eight hours after the first dose.
Liver abscess, amebic—
  Oral, 10 mg (6 mg base) per kg of body weight (up to a maximum of 500 mg [300 mg base]) per day for three weeks.
Note: Children are especially sensitive to the effects of chloroquine.

**Strength(s) usually available**
U.S.—
  250 mg (equivalent to 150 mg base) (Rx) [GENERIC].
  500 mg (equivalent to 300 mg base) (Rx) [Aralen; GENERIC].
Canada—
  250 mg (equivalent to 150 mg base) (Rx) [Aralen].

**Packaging and storage**
Store below 40 °C (104 °F), preferably between 15 and 30 °C (59 and 86 °F), unless otherwise specified by manufacturer. Store in a well-closed container.

**Auxiliary labeling**
• Continue medication for full time of treatment.
• Keep out of reach of children.
• Take with food or milk.

**Note**
Explain potential danger of accidental overdose in children.
Consider dispensing in unit-dose packaging in child-resistant containers ("double-barrier" packaging).

## Parenteral Dosage Forms

### CHLOROQUINE HYDROCHLORIDE INJECTION USP

**Usual adult and adolescent dose**
Malaria—
  Intramuscular, initially 200 to 250 mg (160 to 200 mg base), repeated in six hours if necessary, not to exceed 1 gram (800 mg base) in the first twenty-four hours.
Liver abscess, amebic—
  Intramuscular, 200 to 250 mg (160 to 200 mg base) per day for ten to twelve days.
Note: Slow intravenous infusion, over at least four hours, has not been associated with any increase in side effects compared with oral administration.

**Usual pediatric dose**
Malaria—
  Intramuscular or subcutaneous, 4.4 mg (3.5 mg base) per kg of body weight, repeated in six hours if necessary, not to exceed a total dose of 12.5 mg (10 mg base) per kg of body weight per twenty-four hours.
  Intravenous infusion, initially 16.6 mg (13.3 mg base) per kg of body weight over eight hours, followed by 8.3 mg (6.6 mg base) per kg of body weight every six to eight hours over at least four hours.
Liver abscess, amebic—
  Intramuscular, 7.5 mg (6 mg base) per kg of body weight per day for ten to twelve days.
Note: In no instance should a single intramuscular or subcutaneous dose exceed 6.25 mg (5 mg base) per kg of body weight, since children are especially sensitive to the effects of the 4-aminoquinolines. Severe reactions and sudden death have been reported following parenteral administration in children.

**Strength(s) usually available**
U.S.—
  50 mg (equivalent to 40 mg base) per mL (Rx) [Aralen HCl].
Canada—
  Not commercially available.

**Packaging and storage**
Store below 40 °C (104 °F), preferably between 15 and 30 °C (59 and 86 °F), unless otherwise specified by manufacturer. Protect from freezing.

[1] Not included in Canadian product labeling.

Revised: 8/11/95

---

**CHLOROTHIAZIDE**—See *Diuretics, Thiazide (Systemic)*

---

**CHLOROTRIANISENE**—See *Estrogens (Systemic)*

---

**CHLOROXINE**—The *Chloroxine (Topical)* monograph is not included in this published version of the USP DI database. Copies of the monograph are available on request from Micromedex, Inc. - Reprint Requests, 6200 S. Syracuse Way, Suite 300, Englewood, CO 80111; telephone (303) 486-6400; telefax (303) 486-6464; Email: USPDI@MDX.COM.

---

**CHLORPHENESIN**—See *Skeletal Muscle Relaxants (Systemic)*

---

**CHLORPHENIRAMINE**—See *Antihistamines (Systemic)*

---

**CHLORPROMAZINE**—See *Phenothiazines (Systemic)*

---

**CHLORPROPAMIDE**—See *Antidiabetic Agents, Sulfonylurea (Systemic)*

---

**CHLORPROTHIXENE**—See *Thioxanthenes (Systemic)*

---

**CHLORTETRACYCLINE**—See *Tetracyclines (Ophthalmic); Tetracyclines (Topical)*

---

**CHLORTHALIDONE**—See *Diuretics, Thiazide (Systemic)*

---

**CHLORZOXAZONE**—See *Skeletal Muscle Relaxants (Systemic)*

# CHLORZOXAZONE AND ACETAMINOPHEN Systemic

**INN:** Acetaminophen—Paracetamol
**VA CLASSIFICATION (Primary):** MS200
**NOTE:** The *Chlorzoxazone and Acetaminophen (Systemic)* monograph is maintained on the USP DI electronic data base. For a printed copy of the most recent revision of the complete monograph, contact Micromedex, Inc. - Reprint Requests, 6200 S. Syracuse Way, Suite 300, Englewood, CO 80111; telephone (303) 486-6400; telefax (303) 486-6464; Email: USPDI@MDX.COM.

For information on the specific components of this combination, see the *USP DI* monographs for *Acetaminophen (Systemic)* and *Skeletal Muscle Relaxants (Systemic)*.

The information that follows is selectively abstracted from the complete monograph and is provided to facilitate drug use review and patient counseling.

Note: For a listing of dosage forms and brand names by country availability, see *Dosage Forms* section(s).

## Category
Analgesic–skeletal muscle relaxant.

## Indications
**Accepted**
Spasm, skeletal muscle, accompanied by pain (treatment)—Chlorzoxazone and acetaminophen combination is indicated as an adjunct to other measures, such as rest and physical therapy, for relief of pain and muscle spasm associated with acute, painful musculoskeletal conditions.

## Patient Consultation
As an aid to patient consultation, refer to *Advice for the Patient, Chlorzoxazone and Acetaminophen (Systemic)*.
In providing consultation, consider emphasizing the following selected information (» = major clinical significance):

**Before using this medication**
» Conditions affecting use, especially:
  Sensitivity to acetaminophen, aspirin, or chlorzoxazone
  Pregnancy—Acetaminophen crosses the placenta
  Breast-feeding—Acetaminophen is distributed into breast milk
  Other medications, especially alcohol or other CNS depression–producing medications
  Other medical problems, especially alcoholism (active), hepatic function impairment or other hepatic disease, and viral hepatitis

**Proper use of this medication**
» Importance of not taking more medication than the amount prescribed; acetaminophen may cause liver damage with long-term use or greater-than-recommended doses
» Proper dosing
  Missed dose: Taking as soon as possible; not taking if almost time for next dose; not doubling doses
» Proper storage

**Precautions while using this medication**
Regular visits to physician if long-term therapy is prescribed
» Risk of overdose if other medications containing acetaminophen are used
» Avoiding alcohol or other CNS depressants during therapy unless prescribed or otherwise approved by physician
» Risk of hepatotoxicity may be increased if acetaminophen used with alcohol
Not taking aspirin or other anti-inflammatory analgesics concurrently for more than a few days, unless directed by physician
» Caution if drowsiness, dizziness, or lightheadedness occurs
Possible interference with some laboratory tests; preferably discussing use of the medication with physician in charge 3 to 4 days ahead of time; if this is not possible, informing physician in charge if acetaminophen taken within the past 3 or 4 days
Diabetics: Possible false results with blood glucose tests; checking with physician, nurse, or pharmacist if changes in test results noted

» Suspected overdose: Getting emergency help at once even if no symptoms apparent; symptoms of severe acetaminophen overdosage may be delayed, but treatment must be begun as soon as possible; treatment started 24 hours or more after the overdose may be ineffective in preventing liver damage or fatality

**Side/adverse effects**
Medication may color the urine orange or reddish purple
Signs of potential side effects, especially agranulocytosis, anemia, angioedema, allergic dermatitis, gastrointestinal bleeding, hepatitis, renal colic, renal failure, sterile pyuria, and thrombocytopenia

## Oral Dosage Forms
### CHLORZOXAZONE AND ACETAMINOPHEN TABLETS
**Usual adult and adolescent dose**
Analgesic–skeletal muscle relaxant—
  Oral, 500 mg of chlorzoxazone and 600 mg of acetaminophen four times a day.

**Usual pediatric dose**
Administration of this combination medication to a child depends upon whether the appropriate dose of each ingredient, which must be individualized according to the child's age and weight, can be provided. Dosage of chlorzoxazone ranges between 125 and 500 mg, administered three or four times a day. The quantity of acetaminophen in one tablet of the chlorzoxazone and acetaminophen combination (300 mg) may be administered to children six years of age or older, but the quantity present in two tablets (600 mg) is higher than the maximum dose recommended for children younger than twelve years of age.

**Strength(s) usually available**
U.S.—
  Not commercially available.
Canada—
  250 mg of chlorzoxazone and 300 mg of acetaminophen (OTC) [*Parafon Forte* (scored; sodium bisulfite; tartrazine)].

**Auxiliary labeling**
• May cause drowsiness.
• Avoid alcoholic beverages.

Revised: 08/29/94

---

**CHOLECYSTOGRAPHIC AGENTS, ORAL**—The *Cholecystographic Agents, Oral (Systemic)* monograph is not included in this published version of the USP DI database. Copies of the monograph are available on request from Micromedex, Inc. - Reprint Requests, 6200 S. Syracuse Way, Suite 300, Englewood, CO 80111; telephone (303) 486-6400; telefax (303) 486-6464; Email: USPDI@MDX.COM.

---

**CHOLECYSTOKININ**—The *Cholecystokinin (Systemic)* monograph is not included in this published version of the USP DI database. Copies of the monograph are available on request from Micromedex, Inc. - Reprint Requests, 6200 S. Syracuse Way, Suite 300, Englewood, CO 80111; telephone (303) 486-6400; telefax (303) 486-6464; Email: USPDI@MDX.COM.

---

**CHOLERA VACCINE**—The *Cholera Vaccine (Systemic)* monograph is not included in this published version of the USP DI database. Copies of the monograph are available on request from Micromedex, Inc. - Reprint Requests, 6200 S. Syracuse Way, Suite 300, Englewood, CO 80111; telephone (303) 486-6400; telefax (303) 486-6464; Email: USPDI@MDX.COM.

---

# CHOLESTYRAMINE Oral-Local

VA CLASSIFICATION (Primary/Secondary): CV352/AD400; DE890; GA400; GU900
Commonly used brand name(s): *Questran; Questran Light*.

Note: For a listing of dosage forms and brand names by country availability, see *Dosage Forms* section(s).

# Cholestyramine (Oral-Local)

## Category
Antihyperlipidemic; antipruritic (cholestasis); antidiarrheal (postoperative colonic bile acids); antidote (anion-exchange resin); antihyperoxaluric.

## Indications
Note: Bracketed information in the *Indications* section refers to uses that are not included in U.S. product labeling.

### Accepted
Hyperlipidemia (treatment)—Cholestyramine is indicated for use in patients with primary hypercholesterolemia (type IIa hyperlipidemia) and a significant risk of coronary artery disease who have not responded to diet or other measures alone. Cholestyramine reduces plasma total cholesterol and low density lipoprotein (LDL) concentrations, but causes no change or a slight increase in serum triglyceride concentrations, and so is not useful in patients with elevated triglyceride concentrations alone. Its use is limited in other types of hyperlipidemia (including type IIb) because it may cause further elevation of triglycerides.

Studies have suggested that control of elevated cholesterol and triglycerides may not lessen the danger of cardiovascular disease and mortality, although incidence of nonfatal myocardial infarctions may be decreased.

For additional information on initial therapeutic guidelines related to the treatment of hyperlipidemia, see *Appendix III*.

Cholestyramine is indicated to reduce the risks of atherosclerotic heart disease and myocardial infarctions.

Pruritus, associated with partial biliary obstruction (treatment)—Cholestyramine is indicated for the relief of pruritus associated with partial biliary obstruction (including primary biliary cirrhosis and various other forms of bile stasis). It is not useful in patients with complete biliary obstruction or with pruritus due to other causes.

[Diarrhea, due to bile acids (treatment)]—Cholestyramine has also been used to treat diarrhea caused by increased bile acids in the colon after surgery, although the risk of steatorrhea is increased.

[Hyperoxaluria (treatment)][1]—Cholestyramine is also being used in the treatment of hyperoxaluria.

[Cholestyramine has been used in the treatment of digitalis glycoside overdose; however, it generally has been replaced by other agents such as digoxin immune fab.]

[1] Not included in Canadian product labeling.

## Pharmacology/Pharmacokinetics

### Physicochemical characteristics
Cholestyramine is an anion-exchange resin

### Mechanism of action/Effect
Cholestyramine binds with bile acids in the intestine, preventing their reabsorption and producing an insoluble complex, which is excreted in the feces.

Antihyperlipidemic—
Cholestyramine binds with bile acids in the intestine, causing an increase in hepatic synthesis of bile acids from cholesterol. This depletion of hepatic cholesterol increases hepatic low-density lipoprotein (LDL) receptor activity, which removes LDL cholesterol from the plasma. Cholestyramine may also increase hepatic very-density lipoprotein (VLDL) production, thereby increasing the plasma concentration of triglycerides, especially in patients with hypertriglyceridemia.

Antipruritic (cholestasis)—
Reduction of serum bile acids and subsequent reduction of excess bile acids, which are deposited in dermal tissue, may lead to reduced pruritus.

Antidiarrheal (postoperative colonic bile acids)—
Cholestyramine binds with and removes bile acids.

Antidote (anion-exchange resin)—
Because it is an anion-exchange resin, cholestyramine is capable of binding negatively charged medications as well as some others, causing a decreased effect or shortened half-life.

### Absorption
Not absorbed from the gastrointestinal tract.

### Onset of action
Reduction of plasma cholesterol concentrations—Generally reduced within 1 to 2 weeks after initiation of cholestyramine therapy, but may continue to fall for up to 1 year. In some patients, after the initial decrease, serum cholesterol concentrations return to or exceed baseline levels with continued therapy.

Relief of pruritus associated with biliary stasis—Usually occurs within 1 to 3 weeks after initiation of therapy.

Relief of diarrhea associated with bile acids—Within 24 hours.

### Duration of action
Reduction of plasma cholesterol concentrations—After withdrawal of cholestyramine, cholesterol concentrations return to baseline in about 2 to 4 weeks.

Relief of pruritus associated with biliary stasis—Pruritus returns within 1 to 2 weeks when the medication is withdrawn.

## Precautions to Consider

### Tumorigenicity
Cholestyramine was found to increase the incidence of intestinal tumors in rats receiving potent carcinogens.

### Pregnancy/Reproduction
Pregnancy—Problems in humans have not been documented. Cholestyramine is almost totally unabsorbed after oral administration; however, adverse effects on the fetus may potentially occur because of impaired maternal absorption of vitamins and nutrients.

### Breast-feeding
Problems in humans have not been documented. Cholestyramine is almost totally unabsorbed after oral administration. However, the possible impaired maternal vitamin and nutrient absorption may have an effect on nursing infants.

### Pediatrics
Several studies performed to date have not demonstrated pediatrics-specific problems that would limit the usefulness of cholestyramine in children. However, experience with cholestyramine in children younger than 10 years of age is limited. Therefore, caution is recommended since cholesterol is required for normal development.

### Geriatrics
Appropriate studies on the relationship of age to the effects of cholestyramine have not been performed in the geriatric population. However, patients over 60 years of age may be more likely to experience gastrointestinal side effects, as well as adverse nutritional effects.

### Drug interactions and/or related problems
The following drug interactions and/or related problems have been selected on the basis of their potential clinical significance (possible mechanism in parentheses where appropriate)—not necessarily inclusive (» = major clinical significance):

Note: Combinations containing any of the following medications, depending on the amount present, may also interact with this medication.

» Anticoagulants, coumarin- or indandione-derivative
(concurrent use may significantly increase the anticoagulant effect as a result of depletion of vitamin K, but cholestyramine may also bind with oral anticoagulants in the gastrointestinal tract and reduce their effects; administration at least 6 hours before cholestyramine and adjustment of anticoagulant dosage based on frequent prothrombin-time determinations are recommended)

Chenodiol or
Ursodiol
(effect may be decreased when chenodiol or ursodiol is used concurrently with cholestyramine, which binds these medications and decreases their absorption and also tends to increase cholesterol saturation of bile)

» Digitalis glycosides, especially digitoxin
(cholestyramine may reduce the half-life of these medications by decreasing intestinal reabsorption and enterohepatic circulation; caution is recommended, especially when cholestyramine is withdrawn from a patient who was stabilized on the digitalis glycoside while receiving cholestyramine, because of the potential for serious toxicity; some clinicians recommend administration of cholestyramine approximately 8 hours after the digitalis glycoside)

» Diuretics, thiazide, oral or
» Penicillin G, oral or
» Phenylbutazone or
» Propranolol, oral or
» Tetracyclines, oral
(concurrent use with cholestyramine may result in binding of these medications, thus decreasing their absorption; an interval of several hours between administration of cholestyramine and any of these medications is recommended)

Folic acid
(concurrent use with cholestyramine may interfere with absorption of folic acid; folic acid supplementation recommended in patients receiving cholestyramine for prolonged periods)

» Thyroid hormones, including dextrothyroxine
(concurrent use with cholestyramine may decrease the effects of thyroid hormones by binding and delaying or preventing absorption; an interval of 4 to 5 hours between administration of the two medications and regular monitoring of thyroid function tests are recommended)

» Vancomycin, oral
(cholestyramine has been shown to bind oral vancomycin significantly when used concurrently, resulting in decreased stool concentrations and marked reduction in antibacterial activity of vancomycin; concurrent use is not recommended; patients should be advised to take oral vancomycin and cholestyramine several hours apart)

Vitamins, fat-soluble
(cholestyramine may interfere with absorption of fat-soluble vitamins as a result of its interference with fat absorption; supplemental vitamins A and D in water-miscible or parenteral form are recommended in patients receiving cholestyramine for prolonged periods; supplemental vitamin K may be required in some patients who develop bleeding tendencies)

Medications, other
(cholestyramine may delay or reduce absorption of other medications administered concurrently because of its anion-binding activity; administration of other medications 1 to 2 hours before or 4 to 6 hours after cholestyramine is recommended, although absorption of some medications is impaired even then; caution is recommended when cholestyramine is withdrawn because of the risk of toxicity when suddenly increased absorption of the other medication leads to higher serum concentrations)

**Laboratory value alterations**

The following have been selected on the basis of their potential clinical significance (possible effect in parentheses where appropriate)—not necessarily inclusive (» = major clinical significance):

With physiology/laboratory test values
Alkaline phosphatase values and
Aspartate aminotransferase (AST [SGOT]) values and
Chloride concentrations, serum and
Phosphorus concentrations, serum
(may be increased)

Calcium
(serum concentrations may be decreased due to impaired absorption; may lead to osteoporosis, especially in patients with biliary cirrhosis who already have impaired calcium absorption)

Potassium and
Sodium
(serum concentrations may be decreased)

Prothrombin time (PT)
(may be prolonged)

Schilling test for absorption of vitamin $B_{12}$
(test may be falsely abnormal due to drug binding with intrinsic factor, which prevents the formation of an intrinsic factor-vitamin $B_{12}$ complex needed for absorption)

**Medical considerations/Contraindications**

The medical considerations/contraindications included have been selected on the basis of their potential clinical significance (reasons given in parentheses where appropriate)—not necessarily inclusive (» = major clinical significance).

*Risk-benefit should be considered when the following medical problems exist:*

Bleeding disorders or
Gallstones or
Gastrointestinal function impairment or
Hypothyroidism or
Malabsorption states, especially steatorrhea or
Peptic ulcer
(these conditions may be exacerbated)

» Complete biliary obstruction or complete atresia
(no bile acids in gastrointestinal tract for cholestyramine to bind)

» Constipation
(risk of fecal impaction)

Coronary artery disease and
Hemorrhoids
(exacerbation of these conditions may occur because of the risks associated with severe constipation)

» Phenylketonuria
(sensitivity to phenylalanine in aspartame, which is included in sugar-free preparation)

Renal function impairment
(increased risk of development of hyperchloremic acidosis)

Sensitivity to cholestyramine

**Patient monitoring**

The following may be especially important in patient monitoring (other tests may be warranted in some patients, depending on condition; » = major clinical significance):

Calcium concentrations, serum
(recommended periodically because of decreased absorption of calcium associated with chronic use of cholestyramine)

Cholesterol concentrations, serum and
Triglyceride concentrations, serum
(determinations recommended prior to initiation of therapy of hyperlipidemia and at periodic intervals during therapy to confirm efficacy and determine that a positive response is maintained)

Prothrombin-time (PT) determinations
(recommended periodically because vitamin K deficiency associated with chronic use of cholestyramine may increase bleeding tendency)

## Side/Adverse Effects

Note: Side effects are more likely to occur with high doses and in patients over 60 years of age.

Less frequently, osteoporosis has been reported as a result of chronic long-term cholestyramine use.

The following side/adverse effects have been selected on the basis of their potential clinical significance (possible signs and symptoms in parentheses where appropriate)—not necessarily inclusive:

### Those indicating need for medical attention
Incidence more frequent
*Constipation*—usually mild and transient, but may be severe and lead to fecal impaction

Incidence rare
*Gallstones or pancreatitis* (severe stomach pain with nausea and vomiting); *gastrointestinal bleeding or peptic ulcer* (black, tarry stools); *steatorrhea or malabsorption syndrome* (sudden loss of weight)

### Those indicating need for medical attention only if they continue or are bothersome
Incidence more frequent
*Heartburn or indigestion; nausea or vomiting; stomach pain*

Incidence less frequent
*Belching; bloating; diarrhea; dizziness; headache*

## Patient Consultation

As an aid to patient consultation, refer to *Advice for the Patient, Cholestyramine (Oral)*.

In providing consultation, consider emphasizing the following selected information (» = major clinical significance):

### Before using this medication
» Conditions affecting use, especially:
Sensitivity to cholestyramine
Use in children—Caution with use in children less than 10 years of age since cholesterol is required for normal development
Use in the elderly—Increased incidence of gastrointestinal side effects and potentially adverse nutritional effects in patients over 60 years of age
Other oral medications, especially anticoagulants, digitalis glycosides, thiazide diuretics, penicillin G, phenylbutazone, propranolol, tetracyclines, thyroid hormones, or vancomycin
Other medical problems, especially complete biliary obstruction or complete atresia, constipation, or phenylketonuria

### Proper use of this medication
» Importance of not taking more or less medication than the amount prescribed
» Proper dosing
Missed dose: Taking as soon as possible; not taking if almost time for next dose; not doubling doses
» Proper storage
» Importance of mixing with fluids before taking; instructions for measuring and mixing—Placing in 2 ounces of any beverage and stirring vigorously, then adding 2 to 4 ounces of beverage and shaking vigorously (does not dissolve); rinsing glass and drinking to make sure all medication is taken; may also be mixed with milk in cereals, thin soups, or pulpy fruits

## 856 Cholestyramine (Oral-Local)

*For use as an antihyperlipidemic*
- » Diet as preferred therapy; importance of following prescribed diet
   This medication does not cure the condition but rather helps control it

**Precautions while using this medication**
- » Importance of close monitoring by the physician
- » Not taking any other medication unless discussed with physician

*For use as an antihyperlipidemic*
- » Checking with physician before discontinuing medication; blood lipid concentrations may increase significantly

**Side/adverse effects**
Signs of potential side effects, especially constipation, gallstones, pancreatitis, gastrointestinal bleeding, peptic ulcer, and steatorrhea or malabsorption syndrome

## General Dosing Information

To prevent accidental inhalation or esophageal distress with the dry form, it is recommended that cholestyramine for suspension be mixed with at least 120 to 180 mL of water or other fluids before being ingested. It may also be taken in soups or with cereals or pulpy fruits.

Reduction in cholestyramine dosage or withdrawal of the medication may be necessary in some patients if constipation occurs or worsens, to prevent impaction. Administration of a laxative or stool softener or increased fluid intake may be helpful.

**For use as an antihyperlipidemic**
If a paradoxical increase in plasma cholesterol concentrations occurs, it is recommended that cholestyramine therapy be withdrawn.

If response is inadequate after 1 to 3 months of treatment, cholestyramine therapy should be withdrawn, except in the case of xanthoma tuberosum, which may require up to 1 year of treatment as long as reduction in size and/or number of xanthomata occurs.

**For use as an antipruritic**
Dosage may be reduced when relief of pruritus occurs.

## Oral Dosage Forms

Note: Bracketed uses in the *Dosage Forms* section refer to categories of use and/or indications that are not included in U.S. product labeling.

### CHOLESTYRAMINE FOR ORAL SUSPENSION USP

**Usual adult and adolescent dose**
Antihyperlipidemic; or
Antipruritic (cholestasis); or
[Antidiarrheal, postoperative colonic bile acids]—
   Initial: Oral, 4 grams (anhydrous cholestyramine) one or two times a day before meals, adjusted according to response.
   Maintenance: Oral, 8 to 24 grams (anhydrous cholestyramine) a day, in two to six divided doses.

Note: A single daily dose or two divided daily doses are equally effective, but up to six divided daily doses may be administered and may be more convenient for the patient, especially with the larger doses.

**Usual adult prescribing limits**
Antihyperlipidemic—24 grams (anhydrous cholestyramine) a day.
Antipruritic (cholestasis)—Up to 16 grams (anhydrous cholestyramine) a day.

**Usual pediatric dose**
Antihyperlipidemic—
   Initial: Oral, 4 grams (anhydrous cholestyramine) a day, in two divided doses.
   Maintenance: Oral, 8 to 24 grams (anhydrous cholestyramine) a day, in two or more divided doses.

**Size(s) usually available**
U.S.—
   5 grams (4 grams of anhydrous cholestyramine) per packet or level scoop (Rx) [*Questran Light* (aspartame; phenylalanine 16.8 mg per 5-gram dose)].
   9 grams (4 grams of anhydrous cholestyramine) per packet or level scoop (Rx) [*Questran* (sucrose)].
Canada—
   5 grams (4 grams of anhydrous cholestyramine) per packet or level scoop (Rx) [*Questran Light* (aspartame; phenylalanine 16.8 mg per 5-gram dose)].
   9 grams (4 grams of anhydrous cholestyramine) per packet or level scoop (Rx) [*Questran*].

**Packaging and storage**
Store below 40 °C (104 °F), preferably between 15 and 30 °C (59 and 86 °F), unless otherwise specified by manufacturer. Store in a tight container.

**Preparation of dosage form**
Cholestyramine is prepared for administration by placing the measured powder in 2 ounces of any beverage and stirring vigorously. An additional 2 to 4 ounces of beverage should then be added, again shaking vigorously (does not dissolve). After the patient drinks the suspension, the glass should be rinsed with more liquid to make sure all the medication is taken. Cholestyramine may also be mixed with milk in hot or regular breakfast cereals, in thin soups (tomato or chicken noodle), or in pulpy fruits such as pineapple, pears, peaches, or fruit cocktail.

**Stability**
Variations in color do not reflect changes in potency of the product.

**Auxiliary labeling**
• Take mixed in cold water or juice.

## Selected Bibliography

The Expert Panel. Report of the National Cholesterol Education Program Expert Panel on Detection, Evaluation, and Treatment of High Blood Cholesterol in Adults. Arch Intern Med 1988; 148: 36-69.

NIH Consensus Conference. Lowering blood cholesterol to prevent heart disease. JAMA 1985; 253: 2080-6.

Knodel LC, Talbert RL. Adverse effects of hypolipidaemic drugs. Med Toxicol 1987; 2: 10-32.

Revised: 08/02/94
Interim revision: 08/13/98

---

**CHOLINE SALICYLATE**—See *Salicylates (Systemic)*

---

# CHONDROCYTES, AUTOLOGOUS CULTURED Implantation-Local—INTRODUCTORY VERSION

VA CLASSIFICATION (Primary): MS900
Commonly used brand name(s): *Carticel*.
Note: For a listing of dosage forms and brand names by country availability, see *Dosage Forms* section(s).

## Category
Cartilage repair adjunct.

## Indications

**Accepted**
Cartilaginous defects, femoral (treatment)—Autologous cultured chondrocytes are indicated, in conjunction with arthrotomy (during which debridement and placement of a periosteal flap are first performed) and a post-implantation rehabilitation program, for repair of clinically significant, symptomatic, cartilaginous defects of the medial, lateral, or trochlear femoral condyle caused by acute or repetitive trauma.

Chondrocyte transplantation is **not** recommended for repairing femoral cartilage damage associated with osteoarthritis.

Note: The extent to which each treatment component (debridement, chondrocyte transplantation, and rehabilitation) contributes to the outcome is unknown.

Data regarding long-term functional improvement (beyond 3 years) is limited. Also, the long-term effect on knee function of cartilage harvesting and the long-term safety of cartilage implantation are unknown.

## Pharmacology/Pharmacokinetics

**Physicochemical characteristics**
Source—Harvested from the patient's normal, femoral cartilage and expanded via cell culture techniques.

### Mechanism of action/Effect

Implantation of autologous cultured chondrocytes beneath an autologous periosteal flap induces the formation of hyaline cartilage consisting of ≤ 5% chondrocytes and an extracellular matrix containing a variety of macromolecules, including type II collagen and proteoglycan. The structure of this extracellular matrix helps the cartilage absorb shock and withstand shearing and compression forces.

Note: Other cartilage repair procedures tend to promote growth of fibrocartilage, which has lesser ability than hyaline cartilage to withstand shock and shearing forces.

## Precautions to Consider

### Pregnancy/Reproduction
Whether the harvesting and implantation procedures should be done during pregnancy should be determined on an individual basis by the patient and her physician.

### Breast-feeding
Whether the harvesting and implantation procedures should be done in a breast-feeding woman should be determined on an individual basis by the patient and her physician.

### Pediatrics
No information is available on the relationship of age to the effects of chondrocyte implantation in pediatric patients. Safety and efficacy have not been established.

### Geriatrics
No information is available on the relationship of age to the effects of chondrocyte implantation in geriatric patients.

### Medical considerations/Contraindications
The medical considerations/contraindications included have been selected on the basis of their potential clinical significance (reasons given in parentheses where appropriate)—not necessarily inclusive (» = major clinical significance).

*Except under special circumstances, this medication should not be used when the following medical problems exist:*

» Anaphylactic reaction to gentamicin, history of
(product may contain trace quantities of gentamicin, which is present in the media used to transport the cartilage biopsies and early in cell culturing)

» Sensitivity to bovine-derived materials, history of
(product may contain trace quantities of bovine serum, which is present in the medium used during cell culturing)

*Risk-benefit should be considered when the following medical problem exists:*

Malignancy in area of cartilage harvesting or implantation
(potential for *in vitro* expansion and subsequent implantation of any malignant or dysplastic cells present in the harvested tissue; also, although there have been no reported instances in humans, the possibility exists that implantation might stimulate growth of nearby malignant cells)

### Patient monitoring
The following may be especially important in patient monitoring (other tests may be warranted in some patients, depending on condition; » = major clinical significance):

Arthroscopy
(recommended if the patient shows signs of tissue hypertrophy after implantation)

## Side/Adverse Effects

Note: Any intra- or postoperative complication associated with arthrotomy of the knee may occur in conjunction with the chondrocyte implantation procedure.

In addition to the side/adverse effects reported below, joint swelling not related to hypertrophic synovitis and formation of a keloid-like scar each occurred in fewer than 1% of the patients in clinical studies.

The following side/adverse effects have been selected on the basis of their potential clinical significance (possible signs and symptoms in parentheses where appropriate)—not necessarily inclusive:

### Those indicating need for medical attention
Incidence more frequent
*Tissue hypertrophy* ("crackling" sound when moving joint; joint "catching" or stiffness; pain when moving joint)

Note: In clinical trials, *tissue hypertrophy* at the site of transplantation was present at follow-up arthroscopy in 43% of the patients who were monitored for at least 18 months after surgery. The extent of overgrowth ranged from a small quantity of diffuse excess tissue at the implantation site to a distinct ridge of tissue at the implant margin to widespread hypertrophy throughout the entire joint. Symptoms generally resolved after arthroscopic resection, but the problem recurred and required additional treatment in 10% of the affected patients.

Incidence less frequent
*Adhesions* (joint stiffness); *hematoma formation* (bruising, severe); *synovitis, hypertrophic* (joint pain and swelling); *wound infection, superficial* (heat, redness, swelling, and/or oozing at the place of surgery)

Note: In clinical studies, *adhesions* within the joint and of the *bursa suprapatellaris* occurred in 8% and 2%, respectively, of the patients. Severe adhesions leading to "frozen knee" and requiring lysis occurred in approximately 1% of the patients.

Incidence rare
*Fever and pain, postoperative; pannus formation* (inability to move joint)

## Patient Consultation

As an aid to patient consultation, refer to *Advice for the Patient, Chondrocytes, Autologous Cultured (Implantation-Local—Introductory Version).*

In providing consultation, consider emphasizing the following selected information (» = major clinical significance):

### Before receiving this product
» Conditions affecting use, especially:
Sensitivity to gentamicin or material of bovine origin

### Proper use of this medication
» Proper dosing

### Precautions after receiving this product
» Using crutches for first 6 to 7 weeks, using a normal gait; placing no more than 25% of body weight on the treated knee for the first 3 weeks, then gradually increasing the amount of weight
» Checking with physician immediately if sharp pain with locking or swelling occurs
» Adherence to prescribed rehabilitation protocol; starting slowly with leg-supported exercises and gradually increasing number of repetitions; if pain and/or swelling develops, reducing activity to previous level until pain resolves and using ice packs to reduce swelling

### Side/adverse effects
Signs of adverse effects that may occur relatively shortly after surgery, including hematoma, superficial wound infection, and postoperative pain and fever
Signs of adverse effects that may appear after initial healing, including tissue hypertrophy, adhesions, hypertrophic synovitis, and pannus formation

## General Dosing Information

The biopsy harvesting and autologous cultured chondrocyte implantation procedures should be performed only by physicians who have completed the manufacturer's surgical training program. The harvested tissue is to be shipped for culturing only in the transport kit provided by the manufacturer.

The implantation is performed during arthrotomy. The procedure requires preparation of the defect bed and creation of a periosteal flap. Periosteal fixation and cell implantation should be performed only after complete hemostasis has been achieved. Complete instructions for the surgical procedure are available from the manufacturer.

The success of the procedure may be adversely affected by instability of the knee or abnormal weight distribution within the affected joint; these conditions should be corrected prior to implantation. Also, abnormal patellar tracking should be corrected, if possible, when treating trochlear defects. In addition, it should be kept in mind that the implant may be jeopardized by abnormal varus loading of the medial compartment.

After the procedure the patient should resume physical activity according to a predetermined rehabilitation plan. Too-vigorous activity may compromise the long-term success of the procedure.

### Safety considerations for handling this medication
Autologous cultured chondrocytes have not been tested for biohazards. Therefore, the product should be handled as if infectious materials are present.

**For treatment of adverse effects**
Recommended treatment consists of the following:
- For postoperative swelling—Application of ice packs is recommended.
- For symptomatic tissue hypertrophy—Arthroscopic resection of hypertrophic tissue may be needed.
- For adhesions resulting in "frozen knee"—Lysis may be necessary.

## Implantation Dosage Forms

### AUTOLOGOUS CULTURED CHONDROCYTES FOR IMPLANTATION

**Usual adult dose**
Cartilaginous defects, femoral—
   Surgical implantation, 0.64 million to 3.3 million (median number in clinical trials 1.6 million) cells per square centimeter of defect.

Note: The cells are transplanted using a tuberculin syringe attached to an intraspinal catheter. The catheter tip should be inserted through the superior opening of the periosteal chamber at the site of the defect, then advanced to the most inferior aspect of the defect. To ensure even distribution of cells throughout the defect, the dose should be injected slowly while the catheter tip is being moved from side to side and withdrawn proximally.

**Usual pediatric dose**
Safety and efficacy have not been established.

**Size(s) usually available**
U.S.—
   12 million cells per vial (Rx) [*Carticel* (buffered Dulbecco's modified eagle's medium)].

Note: An assay is performed prior to final packaging to confirm that cell viability is at least 80%.

**Packaging and storage**
Store at room temperature, in the unopened shipping container (which is capable of maintaining the appropriate storage temperature for up to 72 hours), until the time of implantation. Do not refrigerate, freeze, or incubate the shipping container or its contents.

**Preparation of dosage form**
Resuspending and withdrawing the cells for implantation involves—
- Following strict sterile technique protocols at all times. The exterior of the vial is not sterile.
- After removing the lid from the vial, wiping the vial surface and lid with alcohol and inspecting the vial contents for particles, discoloration, or turbidity. A yellowish clump of cells should be present in the bottom of the vial. The product should not be used if turbidity is apparent prior to resuspension.
- While holding the vial in a vertical position, inserting an intraspinal catheter into the vial and positioning the needle just above the fluid level, then slowly removing the inner needle from the catheter (leaving the flexible tip behind) and attaching a tuberculin syringe to the catheter.
- Lowering the catheter tip into the medium, positioned just above the pellet of cells, then aspirating all of the medium from the vial.
- Slowly expelling the medium back into the vial, to break the cell pellet and resuspend the cells in the medium.
- Lowering the catheter tip to the base of the vial, aspirating the entire contents, then slowly reinjecting them back into the vial. This step may be repeated as needed to ensure that all of the cells have been resuspended. Complete resuspension is achieved when cell particles are no longer apparent and a consistent, cloudy mixture has been attained.
- Aspirating the entire contents of the vial into the syringe, which should be kept in a vertical position so that the air pocket remains at the proximal end.

If more than one vial of cells is required, the contents of one vial at a time should be resuspended, aspirated, and injected.

**Stability**
The cultured cells are shipped in a container capable of maintaining cell viability for up to 72 hours and must be used within the time limit specified on the individual package.

**Caution:**
The product is for autologous use only.
The tissue has not been tested for biohazards and should be handled as a potentially infectious material.

Developed: 08/14/98

---

# CHORIONIC GONADOTROPIN   Systemic

VA CLASSIFICATION (Primary/Secondary): HS106/DX900; HS900
Note:  Controlled substance classification—U.S.—Schedule IV
Commonly used brand name(s): *A.P.L; Pregnyl; Profasi; Profasi HP*.
Another commonly used name is human chorionic gonadotropin (hCG).
Note:  For a listing of dosage forms and brand names by country availability, see *Dosage Forms* section(s).

## Category

Gonadotropin; cryptorchidism therapy adjunct; infertility therapy adjunct; diagnostic aid (hypogonadism).

## Indications

Note:  Bracketed information in the *Indications* section refers to uses that are not included in U.S. product labeling.

**Accepted**
[Cryptorchidism (diagnosis)][1] or
Cryptorchidism (treatment)—Chorionic gonadotropin is indicated both as a diagnostic trial and for treatment of prepubertal cryptorchidism not due to anatomical obstruction. Treatment with chorionic gonadotropin usually begins at 4 to 9 years of age. If no signs of improvement occur during the initial course, surgery is indicated.

Infertility, male (treatment)—Chorionic gonadotropin is indicated, alone or in combination with menotropins or clomiphene, for treatment of male hypogonadism due to pituitary deficiency. Males who have been hypogonadotropic for prolonged periods may require treatment with testosterone instead.

Infertility, female (treatment)—Chorionic gonadotropin is indicated in conjunction with menotropins, urofollitropin, or in some cases, clomiphene, to stimulate ovulation. In general, use of chorionic gonadotropin with menotropins or urofollitropin is the treatment of choice for induction of ovulation in patients who do not respond to clomiphene.

Reproductive technologies, assisted—Chorionic gonadotropin is indicated, in conjunction with menotropins or urofollitropin, to stimulate the development and maturation of multiple oocytes in ovulatory patients who are attempting to conceive by means of assisted reproductive technologies, such as gamete intrafallopian transfer (GIFT) or *in vitro* fertilization (IVF).

[Hypogonadism, male (diagnosis)][1]—Chorionic gonadotropin is also used to test the ability of the testes to respond to gonadotropin stimulation in males with delayed puberty.

[Corpus luteum insufficiency (treatment)][1]—Chorionic gonadotropin is used to treat corpus luteum dysfunction. Treatment should begin in the cycle of conception and not after the first missed menses. It is continued until hormone production is taken over by the placenta after 7 to 10 weeks of gestation.

**Unaccepted**
Chorionic gonadotropin has not been found effective and is not indicated for weight reduction.

[1]Not included in Canadian product labeling.

## Pharmacology/Pharmacokinetics

**Physicochemical characteristics**
Source—Produced by the placenta; extracted from urine of pregnant women.

**Mechanism of action/Effect**
The action of chorionic gonadotropin is almost identical to that of pituitary luteinizing hormone (LH). It is generally used as a substitute for LH.
Prepubertal cryptorchidism—
   Stimulates androgen production by the testes, which may stimulate descent of the testes. The effect is usually permanent but may be temporary. In use as a diagnostic trial, chorionic gonadotropin administration should stimulate increased serum testosterone concentrations.
Hypogonadotropic hypogonadism—
   Stimulates androgen production by the testes, which leads to the development of male secondary sexual characteristics.

For induction of ovulation and assisted reproductive technologies (ART)—
Clomiphene, menotropins, or urofollitropin prepare the ovarian follicle for ovulation. The combination of follicle-stimulating hormone (FSH) and LH stimulates follicular growth and maturation. Chorionic gonadotropin, whose actions are nearly identical to those of LH, is administered following administration of clomiphene, menotropins, or urofollitropin to mimic the naturally occurring surge of LH that triggers ovulation.
Diagnostic aid (hypogonadism)—
Should stimulate increased production of testosterone.
Corpus luteum insufficiency—
Promotes maintenance of the corpus luteum; stimulates ovarian production of progesterone.

**Half-life**
Biphasic, 11 and 23 hours (serum).

**Time to peak effect**
Females—Ovulation usually occurs within 32 to 36 hours after administration of chorionic gonadotropin.

**Elimination**
Renal, unchanged; 10 to 12% within 24 hours.

## Precautions to Consider

**Carcinogenicity/Mutagenicity**
Studies have not been done in either animals or humans.

**Pregnancy/Reproduction**
Fertility—Use of chorionic gonadotropin in conjunction with menotropins or urofollitropin to induce ovulation is associated with a high incidence of multiple gestations and multiple births. As a result, this may increase the risk of neonatal prematurity, as well as other complications associated with multiple gestations.
Pregnancy—Appropriate studies have not been done in either animals or humans.
Ovarian hyperstimulation syndrome (OHS), which may occur during chorionic gonadotropin therapy, may be more common, more severe, and protracted in patients who conceive.
FDA Pregnancy Category C.

**Pediatrics**
Precocious puberty has been reported in males treated with chorionic gonadotropin for cryptorchidism. Generally, therapy is withdrawn and the use of chorionic gonadotropin re-evaluated if signs of precocious puberty appear. Also, prolonged or high doses of chorionic gonadotropin may cause abnormally rapid advancement of skeletal maturation and lead to premature epiphyseal fusion. This could result in reduced final adult height.

**Laboratory value alterations**
The following have been selected on the basis of their potential clinical significance (possible effect in parentheses where appropriate)—not necessarily inclusive (» = major clinical significance):

With diagnostic test results
Immunologic assay for endogenous chorionic gonadotropin
(pregnancy test should be performed at least 10 days or longer after administration of chorionic gonadotropin to avoid false-positive result)

With physiology/laboratory test values
17-Hydroxycorticosteroids and
17-Ketosteroids
(urine concentrations may be increased)

**Medical considerations/Contraindications**
The medical considerations/contraindications included have been selected on the basis of their potential clinical significance (reasons given in parentheses where appropriate)—not necessarily inclusive (» = major clinical significance).

***Except under special circumstances, this medication should not be used when the following medical problems exist:***

*For all indications*
» Pituitary hypertrophy or tumor
(pituitary enlargement may occur)

*For treatment of cryptorchidism*
» Precocious puberty

*For induction of ovulation*
» Abnormal vaginal bleeding, undiagnosed
(may indicate the presence of endometrial hyperplasia or carcinoma, which may be exacerbated by ovulation-induced increases in estrogen serum concentrations; other possible endocrinopathies should also be ruled out)
» Fibroid tumors of the uterus or
» Ovarian cyst or enlargement not associated with polycystic ovarian disease
(risk of further enlargement)
» Thrombophlebitis, active
(increased risk of arterial thromboembolism due to elevations in serum estrogen concentrations)

*For males only*
» Prostatic carcinoma or other androgen-dependent neoplasm
(may be exacerbated by hCG-induced increases in testosterone serum concentrations)

***Risk-benefit should be considered when the following medical problems exist:***
Sensitivity to chorionic gonadotropin or other gonadotropins

*For induction of ovulation*
» Polycystic ovarian disease
(an exaggerated response to hCG may occur; lower dosage may be required)

**Patient monitoring**
The following may be especially important in patient monitoring (other tests may be warranted in some patients, depending on condition; » = major clinical significance):

*For induction of ovulation*
» Estradiol
(measurement of serum concentrations is recommended as needed, continuing through the day of chorionic gonadotropin administration; recommended to determine optimal dose and to lessen the risk of ovarian hyperstimulation)
» Ultrasound examination
(recommended prior to chorionic gonadotropin therapy to provide information on the number and size of mature follicles, to follow follicular development, and to lessen the risk of ovarian hyperstimulation syndrome and multiple gestation)
Daily basal body temperature
(can be used in ovulation induction to determine if ovulation has occurred; if basal body temperature following a treatment cycle is biphasic and is not followed by menses, a pregnancy test is recommended)
Progesterone
(measurement of serum concentrations can be performed after therapy to detect luteinized ovarian follicles)

*For treatment of male infertility (hypogonadism)*
Testosterone
(measurement of baseline serum concentrations recommended before and after chorionic gonadotropin administration to rule out other causes and evaluate success of treatment; should increase after chorionic gonadotropin therapy)
Sperm count and determinations of sperm motility
(to evaluate success of treatment)

*For diagnosis of male hypogonadism (delayed puberty)*
Testosterone
(measurement of baseline and post-treatment serum concentrations recommended prior to and 1 day following the course; should double if testes are normal)

## Side/Adverse Effects

Note: Use of chorionic gonadotropin in conjunction with other ovulation-inducing agents is associated with an increased risk of thromboembolic events, possibly due to increased serum estrogen concentrations.

The following side/adverse effects have been selected on the basis of their potential clinical significance (possible signs and symptoms in parentheses where appropriate)—not necessarily inclusive:

**Those indicating need for medical attention**
Incidence more frequent
*For induction of ovulation only*
**Ovarian cysts or mild to moderate, uncomplicated ovarian enlargement** (mild bloating, stomach or pelvic pain)
Note: Symptoms of *ovarian cysts or enlargement* are usually mild to moderate and abate within 2 or 3 weeks.

Incidence less frequent or rare
  For induction of ovulation only
    **Severe ovarian hyperstimulation syndrome** (severe abdominal or stomach pain; feeling of indigestion; moderate to severe bloating; decreased amount of urine; continuing or severe nausea, vomiting, or diarrhea; severe pelvic pain; rapid weight gain; shortness of breath; swelling of lower legs); **peripheral edema** (swelling of feet or lower legs; rapid weight gain)
  Note: *Ovarian hyperstimulation syndrome (OHS)* may occur in patients treated with hCG for ovulation induction. OHS may often occur 7 to 10 days after ovulation or completion of therapy. OHS is usually avoided or short-lived in patients for whom chorionic gonadotropin is withheld. OHS differs from uncomplicated ovarian enlargement and can rapidly progress to cause serious medical problems. With OHS, a marked increase in vascular permeability results in rapid accumulation of fluid in the peritoneal, pleural, and pericardial cavities (third-spacing of fluids). Medical complications ultimately arising from this increased vascular permeability may include hypovolemia, hemoconcentration, electrolyte imbalance, ascites, hemoperitoneum, pleural effusions, hydrothorax, acute pulmonary distress, and thromboembolic events. OHS is more common, more severe, and protracted in patients who conceive.

Incidence less frequent
  *In treatment of cryptorchidism only*
    **Precocious puberty** (acne; enlargement of penis or testes; growth of pubic hair; rapid increase in height)—generally requires discontinuance of chorionic gonadotropin and re-evaluation

Those indicating need for medical attention only if they continue or are bothersome
Incidence less frequent
  **Enlargement of breasts; headache; irritability; mental depression; pain at injection site; tiredness**

## Patient Consultation
As an aid to patient consultation, refer to *Advice for the Patient, Chorionic Gonadotropin (Systemic)*.
In providing consultation, consider emphasizing the following selected information (» = major clinical significance):

**Before using this medication**
» Conditions affecting use, especially:
    Sensitivity to chorionic gonadotropin
    Use in children—Use of chorionic gonadotropin for treatment of cryptorchidism has resulted in precocious puberty
  Other medical problems, especially:
    For all indications—Pituitary hypertrophy or tumor
    For induction of ovulation—Abnormal vaginal bleeding, uterine fibroids, ovarian cyst or enlargement, polycystic ovarian disease, or thrombophlebitis
    For treatment of male hypogonadism—Prostatic carcinoma or other androgen-dependent neoplasm

**Proper use of this medication**
» Proper dosing

**Precautions while using this medication**
» Importance of close monitoring by physician
» May take a long time to work; importance of continuing treatment
*For induction of ovulation*
» Importance of following physician's instructions for recording of basal body temperature and timing of intercourse, when recommended by physician

**Side/adverse effects**
  Signs of potential side effects, especially peripheral edema, ovarian enlargement, cysts, or hyperstimulation syndrome (for ovulation induction), and precocious puberty (for treatment of cryptorchidism)

## General Dosing Information
Patients receiving chorionic gonadotropin should be under supervision of a physician experienced in the treatment of gynecologic or endocrine disorders.

**For induction of ovulation**
Dosage varies considerably and must be adjusted to meet the individual requirements of each patient, on the basis of clinical response.
Conception should be attempted within 48 hours of ovulation. It is recommended that the couple have intercourse or insemination performed daily or every other day beginning the day after chorionic gonadotropin is administered until ovulation is thought to have occurred.
If ovulation does not occur after any cycle of therapy, the therapeutic regimen employed should be re-evaluated. After 3 cycles of non-ovulatory menses, the appropriateness of continuing the use of chorionic gonadotropin for ovulation induction should be reconsidered.

**For corpus luteum insufficiency**
Treatment must begin in the cycle of conception and not after the first missed menses.
Administration of chorionic gonadotropin should continue until hormone production is taken over by the placenta after 7 to 10 weeks gestation.

**For treatment of adverse effects**
Ovarian enlargement or ovarian cyst formation
  • Discontinuing therapy until ovarian size has returned to baseline. Chorionic gonadotropin should also be withheld for that cycle.
  • Prohibiting intercourse until ovarian size has returned to baseline to prevent cyst rupture.
  • Reducing dosage in next course of therapy.
Ovarian hyperstimulation syndrome (OHS)
  Acute phase
    • Discontinuing therapy. Chorionic gonadotropin should also be withheld for that cycle.
    • Prohibiting intercourse until ovarian size has returned to baseline to prevent cyst rupture.
    • Most cases of OHS will spontaneously resolve when menses begins. In selected cases, hospitalization of the patient with bed rest may be necessary.
    • Utilizing therapy to prevent hemoconcentration and minimize risk of thromboembolism and renal injury.
    • Correcting (cautiously) electrolyte imbalance while maintaining acceptable intravascular volume; in the acute phase, intravascular volume deficit cannot be completely corrected without increasing third space fluid volume.
    • Monitoring fluid intake and output, body weight, hematocrit, serum and urine electrolytes, urine specific gravity, blood urea nitrogen (BUN), creatinine, and abdominal girth daily or as often as required.
    • Monitoring serum potassium concentrations for development of hyperkalemia.
    • Limiting performance of pelvic examinations since they may result in rupture of ovarian cysts and hemoperitoneum.
    • Administering intravenous fluids, electrolytes, and human serum albumin, as needed to maintain adequate urine output and to avoid hemoconcentration.
    • Administering analgesics as needed.
    • Avoiding diuretic use since it reduces intravascular volume further.
    • Removing ascitic, pleural, or pericardial fluid *only* if it is imperative for relief of symptoms such as respiratory distress or cardiac tamponade; to do so may increase risk of injury to the ovary.
    • In patients who require surgery to control bleeding from ovarian cyst rupture, employing surgical measures that also maximally conserve ovarian tissue.
  Intermediate phase
    • Once patient is stabilized, minimizing third spacing of fluids by cautiously replacing potassium, sodium, and fluids as required, based on monitoring of serum electrolyte concentrations.
    • Avoiding diuretic use.
  Resolution phase
    • The third space fluid shifts to intravascular compartment, resulting in decreased hematocrit value and increased urinary output.
    • Peripheral and/or pulmonary edema may result if third space fluid volume mobilized exceeds renal output.
    • Administering diuretics when required, to manage pulmonary edema.

## Parenteral Dosage Forms
Note: Bracketed uses in the *Dosage Forms* section refer to categories of use and/or indications that are not included in U.S. product labeling.

### CHORIONIC GONADOTROPIN FOR INJECTION USP
**Usual adult dose**
Hypogonadotropic hypogonadism in males—
  Intramuscular, 1000 to 4000 Units two to three times a week for several weeks to months; may be continued indefinitely as long as a response occurs.
  For induction of spermatogenesis in infertility, treatment is usually continued for 6 months or longer. If sperm counts are still not adequate (> 5 million per mL), menotropins or urofollitropin may be added to the regimen. It may be necessary to continue a combined regimen for up to 12 additional months.

USP DI

[Corpus luteum insufficiency][1]—
  Intramuscular, 1500 Units (average; dosage will vary depending upon patient) every other day from the day of ovulation until the time of expected menses or confirmed pregnancy. After pregnancy is confirmed, this dose may be continued for up to 10 weeks gestation.
Induction of ovulation or
Assisted reproductive technologies—
  Intramuscular, 5000 to 10,000 Units one day following the last dose of menotropins or urofollitropin or five to nine days following the last dose of clomiphene.
  Note: If the ovaries are abnormally enlarged or the serum estradiol concentration is excessively elevated on the last day of menotropins or urofollitropin therapy, chorionic gonadotropin should not be given for that cycle.
  Dosage varies considerably and must be adjusted to meet the individual requirements of each patient, on the basis of clinical response.

**Usual pediatric dose**
Prepubertal cryptorchidism—
  Intramuscular, 1000 to 5000 Units two to three times a week for a maximum of 10 doses, discontinuing when the desired response is achieved.
  Note: Treatment with more than 10 doses is not recommended if progressive descent does not occur.
  Several dosage schedules have been used; dosage will vary depending on the degree of sexual development already present.
[Diagnostic aid (hypogonadism) in males][1]—
  Intramuscular, 2000 Units once a day for three days.

**Size(s) usually available**
U.S.—
  5000 Units (Rx) [*A.P.L; Profasi;* GENERIC].
  10,000 Units (Rx) [*A.P.L; Pregnyl; Profasi;* GENERIC].
  20,000 Units (Rx) [*A.P.L;* GENERIC].
Canada—
  5000 Units (Rx) [GENERIC].
  10,000 Units (Rx) [*A.P.L; Profasi HP;* GENERIC].
  20,000 Units (Rx) [GENERIC].

**Packaging and storage**
Store below 40 °C (104 °F), preferably between 15 and 30 °C (59 and 86 °F), unless otherwise specified by manufacturer.

**Preparation of dosage form**
Using standard aseptic technique, add 1 to 10 mL of diluent provided to each vial, depending upon manufacturer labeling.

**Stability**
Reconstituted solution is stable in the refrigerator for 60 or 90 days, depending on manufacturer.

[1]Not included in Canadian product labeling.

Revised: 07/26/92
Interim revision: 06/03/94

---

**CHROMIC CHLORIDE**—See *Chromium Supplements (Systemic)*

---

**CHROMIC PHOSPHATE P 32**—The *Chromic Phosphate P 32 (Parenteral-Local)* monograph is not included in this published version of the USP DI database. Copies of the monograph are available on request from Micromedex, Inc. - Reprint Requests, 6200 S. Syracuse Way, Suite 300, Englewood, CO 80111; telephone (303) 486-6400; telefax (303) 486-6464; Email: USPDI@MDX.COM.

---

**CHROMIUM**—See *Chromium Supplements (Systemic)*

---

# CHROMIUM SUPPLEMENTS Systemic

This monograph includes information on the following: 1) Chromic Chloride†; 2) Chromium.
VA CLASSIFICATION (Primary): TN490
Commonly used brand name(s): *Chroma-Pak*[1].
Note: For a listing of dosage forms and brand names by country availability, see *Dosage Forms* section(s).

†Not commercially available in Canada.

## Category
Nutritional supplement (mineral).

## Indications
**Accepted**
Chromium deficiency (prophylaxis and treatment)—Chromium supplements are indicated in the prevention and treatment of chromium deficiency, which may result from inadequate nutrition, protein malnutrition, or intestinal malabsorption but does not occur in healthy individuals receiving an adequate balanced diet. For prophylaxis of chromium deficiency, dietary improvement, rather than supplementation, is advisable. For treatment of chromium deficiency, supplementation is preferred.
Deficiency of chromium may lead to glucose intolerance and peripheral or central neuropathy.
Some unusual diets (e.g., reducing diets that drastically restrict food selection) may not supply minimum daily requirements of chromium. Supplementation may be necessary in patients receiving total parenteral nutrition (TPN) or undergoing rapid weight loss or in those with malnutrition, because of inadequate dietary intake.

**Acceptance not established**
There are insufficient data to show that chromium supplementation is beneficial in improving *glucose tolerance*.

## Pharmacology/Pharmacokinetics
**Physicochemical characteristics**
Molecular weight—
  Chromic chloride: 266.45.
  Elemental chromium: 52.

**Mechanism of action/Effect**
Chromium is part of the glucose tolerance factor (GTF), which is believed to potentiate the action of insulin at the cellular level. Chromium may also play a role in lipoprotein metabolism.

**Absorption**
Oral chromium is poorly absorbed. Oral chromium products may be chelated to increase absorption. The absorption of inorganic chromic salts is 0.5 to 1%.

**Protein binding**
10 to 17% bound to transferrin.

**Elimination**
Primarily in urine, with small amounts excreted in bile.

## Precautions to Consider
**Pregnancy/Reproduction**
Pregnancy—Problems in humans have not been documented with intake of normal daily recommended amounts. However, adequate and well-controlled studies in humans have not been done.
Adequate and well-controlled studies in animals have not been done.
FDA Pregnancy Category C (parenteral chromium).

**Breast-feeding**
Problems in humans have not been documented with intake of normal daily recommended amounts.

**Pediatrics**
Problems in pediatrics have not been documented with intake of normal daily recommended amounts.

Chromic chloride injection that contains benzyl alcohol as a preservative should not be used in newborn and immature infants. The use of benzyl alcohol in neonates has been associated with a fatal toxic syndrome consisting of metabolic acidosis and CNS, respiratory, circulatory, and renal function impairment.

### Geriatrics
Problems in geriatrics have not been documented with intake of normal daily recommended amounts.

### Drug interactions and/or related problems
The following drug interactions and/or related problems have been selected on the basis of their potential clinical significance (possible mechanism in parentheses where appropriate)—not necessarily inclusive (» = major clinical significance):

Note: Combinations containing any of the following medications, depending on the amount present, may also interact with chromium supplements.

Insulin
(some studies have found that administration of chromium supplements to a chromium deficient patient may improve glucose tolerance; this could decrease insulin requirements; careful monitoring of blood glucose may be necessary with chromium therapy to avoid hypoglycemia)

### Laboratory value alterations
The following have been selected on the basis of their potential clinical significance (possible effect in parentheses where appropriate)—not necessarily inclusive (» = major clinical significance):

With physiology/laboratory test values
Glucose
(serum concentrations may be decreased, as chromium has been reported to improve glucose tolerance and potentiate the action of insulin)

### Medical considerations/Contraindications
The medical considerations/contraindications included have been selected on the basis of their potential clinical significance (reasons given in parentheses where appropriate)—not necessarily inclusive (» = major clinical significance).

*Risk-benefit should be considered when the following medical problem exists:*

Diabetes mellitus
(some studies have found that administration of chromium supplements to a chromium deficient patient may improve glucose tolerance; this could decrease insulin requirements; careful monitoring of blood glucose may be necessary with chromium therapy to avoid hypoglycemia)

### Patient monitoring
The following may be especially important in patient monitoring (other tests may be warranted in some patients, depending on condition; » = major clinical significance):

Glucose determinations, serum
(determinations may be recommended at periodic intervals, especially in diabetes mellitus, to avoid hypoglycemia)

Hemoglobin A$_1$
(some clinicians recommend that hemoglobin A$_1$ be monitored in patients receiving long-term TPN therapy because it is a more accurate method of assessing glucose tolerance)

Glucose tolerance
(response to glucose tolerance tests or a change in insulin requirements during chromium supplementation may be useful in determining chromium status)

## Side/Adverse Effects
No side effects or overdoses have been reported with chromium supplements.

## Patient Consultation
As an aid to patient consultation, refer to *Advice for the Patient, Chromium Supplements (Systemic)*.
In providing consultation, consider emphasizing the following selected information (» = major clinical significance):

**Description of use**
Description should include function in the body, signs of deficiency, conditions that may cause chromium deficiency

**Importance of diet**
Importance of proper nutrition; supplement may be needed because of inadequate dietary intake

Food sources of chromium
Recommended daily intake for chromium

**Proper use of this dietary supplement**
» Proper dosing
Missed dose: No cause for concern because of length of time necessary for depletion; remembering to take as directed.
» Proper storage

## General Dosing Information
Because of the infrequency of chromium deficiency alone, combinations of several vitamins and/or minerals are commonly administered. Many commercial vitamin-mineral complexes are available.

**For parenteral dosage forms only**
In most cases, parenteral administration is indicated only when oral administration is not acceptable (for example, in nausea, vomiting, preoperative and postoperative conditions) or possible (for example, in malabsorption syndromes or following gastric resection).

**Diet/Nutrition**
Recommended dietary intakes for chromium are defined differently worldwide.

For U.S.—The Recommended Dietary Allowances (RDAs) for vitamins and minerals are determined by the Food and Nutrition Board of the National Research Council and are intended to provide adequate nutrition in most healthy persons under usual environmental stresses. In addition, a different designation may be used by the FDA for food and dietary supplement labeling purposes, as with Daily Value (DV). DVs replace the previous labeling terminology United States Recommended Daily Allowances (USRDAs).

For Canada—Recommended Nutrient Intakes (RNIs) for vitamins, minerals, and protein are determined by Health and Welfare Canada and provide recommended amounts of a specific nutrient while minimizing the risk of chronic diseases.

There is no RDA or RNI established for chromium. Normal daily recommended intakes for chromium are generally defined as follows:
Infants and children:
Birth to 3 years of age: 10 to 80 mcg.
4 to 6 years of age: 30 to 120 mcg.
7 to 10 years of age: 50 to 200 mcg.
Adolescents and adults:
50 to 200 mcg.
The best dietary sources of chromium include brewer's yeast, calf liver, American cheese, and wheat germ.

---
### CHROMIC CHLORIDE
---

## Parenteral Dosage Forms
### CHROMIC CHLORIDE INJECTION USP

**Usual adult and adolescent dose**
Deficiency (prophylaxis)—
Intravenous, 10 to 15 mcg (.01 to .015 mg) a day, added to total parenteral nutrition (TPN).
Deficiency (treatment)—
Intravenous, 20 mcg (.02 mg) a day, added to total parenteral nutrition (TPN).

**Usual pediatric dose**
Deficiency (prophylaxis or treatment)—
Intravenous, 0.14 to 0.2 mcg per kilogram of body weight a day, added to total parenteral nutrition (TPN).

Note: Chromic chloride injection that contains benzyl alcohol as a preservative should not be used in newborn and immature infants. The use of benzyl alcohol in neonates has been associated with a fatal toxic syndrome consisting of metabolic acidosis and CNS, respiratory, circulatory, and renal function impairment.

**Strength(s) usually available**
U.S.—
20.5 mcg (.0205 mg) (4 mcg elemental chromium) per mL (Rx) [*Chroma-Pak* (0.9% benzyl alcohol); GENERIC].
102.5 mcg (.1025 mg) (20 mcg elemental chromium) per mL (Rx) [*Chroma-Pak;* GENERIC].
Canada—
Not commercially available.

**Packaging and storage**
Store below 40 °C (104 °F), preferably between 15 and 30 °C (59 and 86 °F), unless otherwise specified by manufacturer.

**Preparation of dosage form**
Chromic chloride is compatible with amino acids, dextrose, electrolytes, and vitamins usually used for total parenteral nutrition (TPN).

---

## CHROMIUM

### CHROMIUM CAPSULES

**Usual adult and adolescent dose**
Deficiency (prophylaxis)—
 Oral, amount based on normal daily recommended intakes: 50 to 200 mcg.
Deficiency (treatment)—
 Treatment dose is individualized by prescriber based on severity of deficiency.

**Usual pediatric dose**
Deficiency (prophylaxis)—Oral, amount based on normal daily recommended amounts—
 Birth to 3 years of age—10 to 80 mcg.
 4 to 6 years of age—30 to 120 mcg.
 7 to 10 years of age—50 to 200 mcg.
Deficiency (treatment)—
 Treatment dose is individualized by prescriber based on severity of deficiency.

**Strength(s) usually available**
U.S.—
 200 mcg (0.2 mg) elemental chromium (OTC) [GENERIC].
Canada—
 Not commercially available.
Note: This chromium preparation may exceed the dosage range recommended by USP DI Advisory Panels based on the amount necessary to meet normal nutritional needs.

**Packaging and storage**
Store below 40 °C (104 °F), preferably between 15 and 30 °C (59 and 86 °F), unless otherwise specified by manufacturer.

### CHROMIUM TABLETS

**Usual adult and adolescent dose**
See *Chromium Capsules*.

**Usual pediatric dose**
See *Chromium Capsules*.

**Strength(s) usually available**
U.S.—
 100 mcg (0.1 mg) elemental chromium (OTC) [GENERIC].
 200 mcg (0.2 mg) elemental chromium (OTC) [GENERIC (yeast)].
 1 mg elemental chromium (OTC) [GENERIC (amino acids)].
Canada—
 200 mcg (0.2 mg) elemental chromium (OTC) [GENERIC (yeast)].
Note: Some strengths of these chromium preparations may exceed the dosage range recommended by USP DI Advisory Panels based on the amount necessary to meet normal nutritional needs.

**Packaging and storage**
Store below 40 °C (104 °F), preferably between 15 and 30 °C (59 and 86 °F), unless otherwise specified by manufacturer.

### Selected Bibliography
Mooradian A, Morely J. Micronutrient status in diabetes mellitus. Am J Clin Nutr 1987; 45: 877-95.

Revised: 03/24/92
Interim revision: 08/01/94; 05/26/95

---

**CHYMOPAPAIN**—The *Chymopapin (Parenteral-Local)* monograph is not included in this published version of the USP DI database. Copies of the monograph are available on request from Micromedex, Inc. - Reprint Requests, 6200 S. Syracuse Way, Suite 300, Englewood, CO 80111; telephone (303) 486-6400; telefax (303) 486-6464; Email: USPDI@MDX.COM.

---

# CICLOPIROX Topical

VA CLASSIFICATION (Primary): DE102
Commonly used brand name(s): *Loprox*.
Note: For a listing of dosage forms and brand names by country availability, see *Dosage Forms* section(s).

## Category
Antifungal (topical).
Note: Ciclopirox is a broad-spectrum antifungal, which has an antifungal spectrum similar to that of the imidazoles.

## Indications
Note: Bracketed information in the *Indications* section refers to uses that are not included in U.S. product labeling.

**Accepted**
Candidiasis, cutaneous (treatment)—Ciclopirox is indicated as a primary agent in the topical treatment of cutaneous candidiasis (moniliasis) caused by *Candida albicans (Monilia albicans)*.
Tinea corporis (treatment)
Tinea cruris (treatment) or
Tinea pedis (treatment)—Ciclopirox is indicated as a primary agent in the topical treatment of tinea corporis (ringworm of the body), tinea cruris (ringworm of the groin; jock itch), or tinea pedis (ringworm of the foot; athlete's foot) caused by *Trichophyton rubrum, T. mentagrophytes, Epidermophyton floccosum (Acrothesium floccosum)*, and *Microsporum canis*.
Tinea versicolor (treatment)—Ciclopirox is indicated as a primary agent in the topical treatment of tinea versicolor (pityriasis versicolor; "sun fungus") caused by *Pityrosporon orbiculare (Malassezia furfur)*.
[Onychomycosis (treatment)]—Ciclopirox is used as a secondary agent in the topical adjunctive treatment of onychomycosis (tinea unguium; ringworm of the nails).
Not all species or strains of a particular organism may be susceptible to ciclopirox.

## Pharmacology/Pharmacokinetics

**Physicochemical characteristics**
Molecular weight—268.36.
pH—The 1% cream and 1% lotion have a pH of 7.

**Mechanism of action/Effect**
Exact mechanism unknown; fungicidal *in vitro* against *Trichophyton rubrum, T. mentagrophytes, Epidermophyton floccosum (Acrothesium floccosum), Microsporum canis*, and *Candida albicans (Monilia albicans)*; may inhibit transport of certain essential substrates into fungal cells; may also interfere with the synthesis of proteins, RNA, and DNA in growing fungal cells; alterations in cell permeability, osmotic fragility, and endogenous respiration are affected only at high concentrations of ciclopirox.

**Other actions/effects**
Also has some activity against a wide variety of gram-positive and gram-negative bacteria.

**Absorption**
1% Solution in polyethylene glycol 400—Rapid, but minimal; 1.3% of dose absorbed following topical application to 750 cm$^2$ of skin on the back, followed by occlusion for 6 hours.
1% Cream—In penetration studies of human cadaveric skin from the back, 0.8 to 1.6% of the dose was present in the stratum corneum 1.5 to 6 hours following application. In addition, the levels in the dermis were still 10 to 15 times the minimum inhibitory concentrations (MICs).
1% Lotion—Penetration studies have indicated that the penetration of the 1% cream and the 1% lotion are equivalent.
Ciclopirox olamine also penetrates into hair and through the epidermis and hair follicles into sebaceous glands and dermis.

**Protein binding**
Very high (94-97%).

**Half-life**
1% Solution in polyethylene glycol 400—1.7 hours.

## Elimination
1% Solution in polyethylene glycol 400—
  Renal: Absorbed portion rapidly and almost completely excreted in urine; only 0.01% of dose remains in urine 2 days following topical application.
  Fecal: Negligible.

## Precautions to Consider

### Carcinogenicity/Tumorigenicity
A study in female mice given cutaneous doses of ciclopirox twice a week for 50 weeks, followed by a six-month drug-free period, has shown that ciclopirox is not carcinogenic or tumorigenic at the application site.

### Mutagenicity
Several studies have shown that ciclopirox is not mutagenic.

### Pregnancy/Reproduction
Fertility—Studies in mice, rats, rabbits, and monkeys given ciclopirox by various routes at doses of 10 or more times the topical human dose have not shown that ciclopirox causes impaired fertility.

Pregnancy—Adequate and well-controlled studies in humans have not been done.
Studies in rats have shown that ciclopirox crosses the placenta in very small amounts. Studies in mice, rats, rabbits, and monkeys given ciclopirox by various routes at doses of 10 or more times the topical human dose have not shown that ciclopirox causes adverse effects in the fetus.

FDA Pregnancy Category B.

### Breast-feeding
It is not known whether ciclopirox is distributed into breast milk. However, problems in humans have not been documented.

### Pediatrics
Appropriate studies on the relationship of age to the effects of ciclopirox have not been performed in infants and children up to 10 years of age. Safety and efficacy have not been established.

### Geriatrics
Appropriate studies on the relationship of age to the effects of ciclopirox have not been performed in the geriatric population. However, no geriatrics-specific problems have been documented to date.

### Medical considerations/Contraindications
The medical considerations/contraindications included have been selected on the basis of their potential clinical significance (reasons given in parentheses where appropriate)—not necessarily inclusive (» = major clinical significance).

*Risk-benefit should be considered when the following medical problem exists:*
  Sensitivity to ciclopirox

## Side/Adverse Effects
The following side/adverse effects have been selected on the basis of their potential clinical significance (possible signs and symptoms in parentheses where appropriate)—not necessarily inclusive:

### Those indicating need for medical attention
Incidence rare
  *Local irritation* (burning, itching, redness, swelling, or other signs of irritation not present before therapy)

## Patient Consultation
As an aid to patient consultation, refer to *Advice for the Patient, Ciclopirox (Topical)*.
In providing consultation, consider emphasizing the following selected information (» = major clinical significance):

### Before using this medication
» Conditions affecting use, especially:
    Sensitivity to ciclopirox

### Proper use of this medication
  Applying sufficient medication to cover affected and surrounding areas, and rubbing in gently
» Avoiding contact with the eyes
» Not applying occlusive dressing over this medication unless directed to do so by physician
» Compliance with full course of therapy; fungal infections may require prolonged therapy
» Proper dosing
    Missed dose: Applying as soon as possible; not applying if almost time for next dose
» Proper storage

### Precautions while using this medication
  Checking with physician if no improvement within 2 to 4 weeks
» Using hygienic measures to cure infection and prevent reinfection:
*For tinea cruris*
  Avoiding underwear that is tight-fitting or made from synthetic materials; wearing loose-fitting cotton underwear instead
  Using a bland, absorbent powder or an antifungal powder on the skin; using the powder between administration times for ciclopirox
*For tinea pedis*
  Carefully drying feet, especially between toes, after bathing
  Avoiding socks made from wool or synthetic materials; wearing clean, cotton socks and changing them daily or more often if feet perspire excessively
  Wearing sandals or well-ventilated shoes
  Using a bland, absorbent powder or an antifungal powder between toes, on feet, and in socks and shoes liberally once or twice daily; using the powder between administration times for ciclopirox

### Side/adverse effects
  Signs of potential side effects, especially local irritation

## General Dosing Information
Use of topical antifungals may lead to skin sensitization, resulting in hypersensitivity reactions with subsequent topical use of the medication.

To reduce the possibility of recurrence, *Candida* infections, tinea cruris, tinea corporis, and tinea versicolor should be treated for at least 2 weeks to 1 month; tinea pedis should be treated for at least 1 month or longer.

When this medication is used in the treatment of candidiasis, occlusive dressings should be avoided, since they provide conditions that favor growth of yeast and release of its irritating endotoxin.

## Topical Dosage Forms

### CICLOPIROX OLAMINE CREAM USP

**Usual adult and adolescent dose**
Antifungal—
  Topical, to the skin and surrounding areas, two times a day, morning and evening.

**Usual pediatric dose**
Antifungal—
  Infants and children up to 10 years of age: Safety and efficacy have not been established.
  Children 10 years of age and over: See *Usual adult and adolescent dose*.

**Strength(s) usually available**
U.S.—
  1% (Rx) [*Loprox*].
Canada—
  1% (Rx) [*Loprox*].

**Packaging and storage**
Store between 15 and 30 °C (59 and 86 °F). Store in a collapsible tube.

**Auxiliary labeling**
• For external use only.
• Continue medicine for full time of treatment.

### CICLOPIROX OLAMINE LOTION

**Usual adult and adolescent dose**
See *Ciclopirox Olamine Cream USP*.

**Usual pediatric dose**
See *Ciclopirox Olamine Cream USP*.

**Strength(s) usually available**
U.S.—
  1% (Rx) [*Loprox*].
Canada—
  1% (Rx) [*Loprox*].

**Packaging and storage**
Store between 15 and 30 °C (59 and 86 °F). Protect from freezing.

**Auxiliary labeling**
• Shake well.
• For external use only.
• Continue medicine for full time of treatment.

Revised: 05/26/94

# CIDOFOVIR    Systemic—INTRODUCTORY VERSION†

VA CLASSIFICATION (Primary): AM802

Commonly used brand name(s): *Vistide*.

Note: For a listing of dosage forms and brand names by country availability, see *Dosage Forms* section(s).

†Not commercially available in Canada.

## Category
Antiviral (systemic).

## Indications

### General considerations
All cidofovir-resistant cytomegalovirus (CMV) isolates have been found to be resistant to ganciclovir, but remained susceptible to foscarnet.

### Accepted
Cytomegalovirus retinitis (treatment)—Cidofovir is indicated, in combination with probenecid, for the treatment of cytomegalovirus (CMV) retinitis in patients with acquired immunodeficiency syndrome. Safety and efficacy have not been established for the treatment of CMV disease in non–HIV infected people, other CMV infections, or congenital or neonatal CMV disease.

## Pharmacology/Pharmacokinetics

### Physicochemical characteristics
Molecular weight—Cidofovir: 315.22.
Cidofovir anhydrous: 279.19.

### Mechanism of action/Effect
Cidofovir diphosphate, the active intracellular metabolite of cidofovir, suppresses cytomegalovirus (CMV) replication by selectively inhibiting viral DNA polymerase. Cidofovir diphosphate inhibits herpesvirus polymerases at concentrations that are 8- to 600-fold lower than those needed to inhibit the human cellular polymerases alpha, beta, and gamma. Reduction in the rate of viral DNA synthesis is due to incorporation of cidofovir into the growing viral DNA chain.

### Distribution
Volume of distribution is 537 mL per kg (mL/kg) without concurrent probenecid administration and 410 mL/kg with concurrent probenecid administration.

Concentrations of cidofovir were undetectable 15 minutes after the end of a 1-hour infusion in one patient who had a corresponding serum concentration of 8.7 mcg per mL (mcg/mL).

### Protein binding
Low (less than 6%).

### Time to peak concentration
End of infusion.

### Peak serum concentration
With concurrent probenecid administration—
3 mg per kg of body weight (mg/kg): 9.8 mcg/mL.
5 mg/kg: 19.6 mcg/mL.

Without concurrent probenecid administration—
3 mg/kg: 7.3 mcg/mL.
5 mg/kg: 11.5 mcg/mL.

### Elimination
Renal (without concurrent probenecid administration)—Approximately 80 to 100% of an administered cidofovir dose was recovered unchanged in the urine within 24 hours.

Renal (with concurrent probenecid administration)—Approximately 70 to 85% of an administered cidofovir dose was recovered unchanged in the urine within 24 hours. The renal clearance of cidofovir was reduced to that of creatinine clearance, suggesting that probenecid blocks active renal tubular secretion of cidofovir.

In dialysis—The effect of hemodialysis on the pharmacokinetics of cidofovir is not known.

## Precautions to Consider

### Carcinogenicity
Cidofovir should be considered a carcinogen in rats and a potential carcinogen in humans.

Chronic, two-year carcinogenicity studies in rats and mice have not been done. However, a 26-week toxicology study was done in rats evaluating once weekly subscapular subcutaneous injections of cidofovir. The study was terminated at 19 weeks because palpable mammary adenocarcinomas were detected in females after only six doses. These masses developed at doses as low as 0.6 mg per kg (mg/kg) per week, which is equivalent to 0.04 times the human systemic exposure at the recommended cidofovir dose based on area under the plasma concentration–time curve (AUC) comparisons.

There was also a significant increase in mammary adenocarcinomas in female rats and a significant incidence of Zymbal's gland carcinomas in male and female rats administered 15 mg/kg of cidofovir once weekly; this was not seen at the 0.6 or 3 mg/kg doses. The 15 mg/kg dose is equivalent to 1.1 times the human systemic exposure at the recommended dose of cidofovir, based on AUC.

### Tumorigenicity
No tumors were detected in cynomologus monkeys who received intravenous cidofovir, alone and in conjunction with concomitant oral probenecid, once a week for 52 weeks. This dose is equivalent to approximately 0.7 times the human systemic exposure. However, due to the small number of animals and the short duration of treatment, this study was not designed as a carcinogenicity study.

### Mutagenicity
There was no mutagenic response observed in microbial mutagenicity assays involving *Salmonella typhimurium* (Ames) and *Escherichia coli* in the presence and absence of metabolic activation. There was an increase in micronucleated polychromatic erythrocytes *in vivo* seen in mice receiving $\geq$ 2000 mg/kg, a dose approximately 65-times higher than the maximum recommended clincial dose of cidofovir, based on body surface area estimations. Cidofovir induced chromosomal aberrations in human peripheral blood lymphocytes *in vitro* without metabolic activation. At the four doses tested, the percentage of damaged metaphases and the number of aberrations per cell increased in a concentration-dependent manner.

### Pregnancy/Reproduction
Fertility—Cidofovir was shown to cause inhibition of spermatogenesis in rats and monkeys. However, there were no reported adverse effects on fertility or reproduction in male rats administered once-weekly intravenous injections for thirteen consecutive weeks at doses up to 15 mg/kg per week; this is equivalent to 1.1 times the recommended human dose based on AUC comparisons. Female rats dosed intravenously at 1.2 mg/kg per week (equivalent to 0.09 times the recommended human dose based on AUC) or higher for up to six weeks prior to mating, and for two weeks after mating, had decreased litter size and live births per litter, as well as an increased incidence of early resorptions per litter. Peri- and postnatal development studies in which female rats were administered subcutaneous cidofovir at doses up to 1 mg/kg per day from day 7 of gestation through day 21 postpartum (approximately five weeks) resulted in no adverse effects on viability, growth, behavior, sexual maturation, or reproductive capacity in the offspring.

Pregnancy—Adequate and well-controlled studies in humans have not been done. Cidofovir should be administered only if the potential benefit justifies the potential risk to the fetus.

Cidofovir was found to be embryotoxic (reduced fetal body weight) in rats administered 1.5 mg/kg per day and in rabbits given 1 mg/kg per day during the period of organogenesis; these doses were also maternotoxic. There was also an increased incidence of fetal external soft tissue and skeletal anomalies, such as meningocele, short snout, and short maxillary bones, seen in rabbits administered 1 mg/kg per day, which was also maternally toxic. The no-observable-effect levels for embryotoxicity in rats (0.5 mg/kg per day) and in rabbits (0.25 mg/kg per day) were approximately 0.04 and 0.05 times the human maintenance dose, respectively, based on AUC.

FDA Pregnancy Category C.

### Breast-feeding
It is not known whether cidofovir is distributed into breast milk. However, it is recommended that HIV-infected women not breast-feed their infants to avoid postnatal transmission of HIV to a child who may not be infected.

### Pediatrics
No information is available on the relationship of age to the effects of cidofovir in pediatric patients. Safety and efficacy have not been established. However, cidofovir should be used with caution in children with HIV infection because of the potential risk of long-term carcinogenicity and reproductive toxicity.

### Geriatrics
No studies have been done assessing the safety and efficacy of cidofovir in patients over the age of 60. However, elderly patients are more likely

to have age-related renal function impairment, which may require adjustment of dosage in patients receiving cidofovir.

**Drug interactions and/or related problems**
The following drug interactions and/or related problems have been selected on the basis of their potential clinical significance (possible mechanism in parentheses where appropriate)—not necessarily inclusive (» = major clinical significance):

Note: Combinations containing any of the following medications, depending on the amount present, may also interact with this medication.

» Nephrotoxic medications (see *Appendix II*)
(because cidofovir has been reported to be associated with severe renal function impairment, concurrent use with other nephrotoxic medications, such as aminoglycosides, amphotericin B, foscarnet, nonsteroidal anti-inflammatory drugs, and pentamidine, may increase the risk of nephrotoxicity and is contraindicated; it is recommended that patients undergo at least a 7-day washout period before receiving cidofovir)

» Probenecid
(probenecid must be administered concurrently with cidofovir; probenecid is known to interact with the metabolism or renal tubular excretion of many medications, such as acetaminophen, acyclovir, aminosalicylic acid, angiotensin-converting enzyme inhibitors, barbiturates, benzodiazepines, bumetanide, clofibrate, famotidine, furosemide, methotrexate, nonsteroidal anti-inflammatory agents, theophylline, and zidovudine; these medications should be used with caution when used concurrently with probenecid)

Zidovudine
(concurrent use with cidofovir, without probenecid, showed no evidence of an effect on the pharmacokinetics of zidovudine)

**Laboratory value alterations**
The following have been selected on the basis of their potential clinical significance (possible effect in parentheses where appropriate)—not necessarily inclusive (» = major clinical significance):

With physiology/laboratory test values
Creatinine, serum and
Protein, urine
(may be increased)
Bicarbonate, serum and
Neutrophils
(may be decreased)

**Medical considerations/Contraindications**
The medical considerations/contraindications included have been selected on the basis of their potential clinical significance (reasons given in parentheses where appropriate)—not necessarily inclusive (» = major clinical significance):

*Except under special circumstances, this medication should not be used when the following medical problem exists:*
» Hypersensitivity to cidofovir or probenecid

*Risk-benefit should be considered when the following medical problem exists:*
» Renal function impairment
(because cidofovir has been reported to be associated with severe renal function impairment, cidofovir is contraindicated in patients with a serum creatinine 1.5 mL per dL, a creatinine clearance ≤ 55 mL per minute [0.92 mL per second], or a urine protein ≥ 100 mg per dL [equivalent to ≥ 2+ proteinuria])

**Patient monitoring**
The following may be especially important in patient monitoring (other tests may be warranted in some patients, depending on condition; » = major clinical significance):

» Creatinine, serum and
» Protein, urine and
» White blood cell count with differential
(because cidofovir has been reported to cause severe renal function impairment and cause neutropenia, these laboratory parameters should be monitored prior to each dose of cidofovir)

» Intraocular pressure
» Visual acuity
(because cidofovir can cause ocular hypotony, especially in patients with preexisting diabetes, intraocular pressure and visual acuity should be monitored periodically)

## Side/Adverse Effects

Note: Nephrotoxicity, the major dose-limiting toxicity of cidofovir therapy, was manifested as > 1+ proteinuria, serum creatinine concentration ≥ 0.4 mg per dL, or a decrease in creatinine clearance to ≤ 55 mL per min (0.92 mL per second) in 53% of patients receiving a maintenance dose of 5 mg per kg of body weight every other week. Proteinuria may be an early indicator of cidofovir-related nephrotoxicity and continued administration may lead to additional proximal tubular cell injury, resulting in glycosuria, decreases in serum phosphate, uric acid, and bicarbonate, and elevations in serum creatinine. Patients with these side effects and meeting a criteria of Fanconi's syndrome have been reported. There have also been reports of severe renal function impairment associated with cidofovir use. To help reduce the risk of nephrotoxicity, patients must be prehydrated with at least 1 liter of 0.9% sodium chloride solution and probenecid must be administered at proper times. Dosage adjustment or discontinuation is necessary when changes in renal function occur during therapy.

Neutropenia (≤ 500 cells/mm$^3$) occurred in 20% of patients receiving the 5 mg per kg of body weight maintenance dose in clinical trials. Granulocyte colony stimulating factor was used in 34% of patients.

Ocular hypotony (≥ 50% change from baseline) was reported in 5 of 42 patients receiving the 5 mg per kg of body weight maintenance dose in clinical studies. Hypotony was reported in one patient with concomitant diabetes mellitus; the risk of ocular hypotony may be increased in patients with pre-existing diabetes.

Two percent of study patients were diagnosed with Fanconi's syndrome, manifested by multiple abnormalities of proximal tubule function. Decreases in serum bicarbonate to ≤ 16 milliequivalents per liter associated with evidence of renal tubular damage occurred in approximately 9% of patients.

The following side/adverse effects have been selected on the basis of their potential clinical significance (possible signs and symptoms in parentheses where appropriate)—not necessarily inclusive:

**Those indicating need for medical attention**
Incidence more frequent
*Nephrotoxicity* (decreased urination; increased thirst and urination); *neutropenia* (fever, chills, or sore throat)
Incidence less frequent
*Fever*
Incidence rare
*Ocular hypotony* (decreased vision or any change in vision)

**Those indicating need for medical attention only if they continue or are bothersome**
Incidence more frequent
*Gastrointestinal effects* (diarrhea; loss of appetite; nausea; vomiting); *headache*
Incidence less frequent
*Asthenia* (generalized weakness; loss of strength)

## Overdose

Overdosage with cidofovir has not been reported. However, probenecid may reduce potential nephrotoxicity through reduction of active tubular secretion. Hemodialysis and hydration may reduce plasma cidofovir concentrations.

For more information on the management of overdose or unintentional ingestion, **contact a Poison Control Center** (see *Poison Control Center Listing*).

## Patient Consultation

As an aid to patient consultation, refer to *Advice for the Patient, Cidofovir (Systemic)—Introductory Version*.

In providing consultation, consider emphasizing the following selected information (» = major clinical significance):

**Before using this medication**
» Conditions affecting use, especially:
Hypersensitivity to cidofovir or probenecid

Carcinogenicity—Cidofovir is a carcinogen in animals and should be considered a potential carcinogen in humans
Pregnancy—Cidofovir was embryotoxic and maternotoxic in animals; cidofovir should be administered only if the potential benefit justifies the potential risk to the fetus
Breast-feeding—It is not known whether cidofovir is distributed into breast milk; however, it is recommended that HIV-infected women not breast-feed their infants to avoid postnatal transmission of HIV to a child who may not be infected
Use in children—Safety and efficacy have not been established; however, cidofovir should be used with caution in HIV-infected

children because of the potential risk of long-term carcinogenicity and reproductive toxicity
- Other medications, especially nephrotoxic medications and probenecid
- Other medical problems, especially renal function impairment

**Proper use of this medication**
» Importance of receiving medication for full course of therapy and on a regular schedule
» Proper dosing

**Precautions while using this medication**
» Regular visits to physician to check blood counts
» Regular visits to ophthalmologist to examine eyes since progression of retinitis and visual loss may occur during cidofovir therapy

**Side/adverse effects**
Signs of potential side effects, especially, nephrotoxicity, neutropenia, fever, and ocular hypotony

## General Dosing Information

Cidofovir must not be administered by intraocular injection. Direct injection may result in significant decreases in intraocular pressure and vision impairment.

Because cidofovir has been reported to be associated with severe renal function impairment, the recommended dosage, frequency, or infusion rate must not be exceeded. Cidofovir must be diluted in 100 mL of 0.9% sodium chloride injection prior to administration. Probenecid and intravenous sodium chloride prehydration must be administered with each cidofovir infusion to minimize potential nephrotoxicity. The dose of cidofovir must be reduced or discontinued if changes in renal function occur during therapy. Serum creatinine and urine protein must be monitored within 48 hours prior to each dose of cidofovir.

The dose of cidofovir must be reduced or discontinued if changes in renal function occur during therapy. For increases in serum creatinine of 0.3 to 0.4 mg per dL (mg/dL) above baseline, the dose of cidofovir must be reduced from 5 mg per kg (mg/kg) to 3 mg/kg. Cidofovir must be discontinued for an increase in serum creatinine of 0.5 mg/dL above baseline or development of 3+ proteinuria. Patients with 2+ proteinuria should be observed carefully; dose reduction or temporary discontinuation of treatment should be considered.

Two grams of probenecid should be administered 3 hours prior to each dose of cidofovir and 1 gram should be administered 2 and 8 hours after the completion of the 1-hour infusion (total 4 grams).

Each dose of cidofovir should be administered with 1 liter of 0.9% sodium chloride injection, infused over 1 to 2 hours immediately before the cidofovir infusion. If the patient can tolerate the fluid load, a second liter of 0.9% sodium chloride injection should be started either at the beginning of the cidofovir infusion or immediately afterwards, over a 1- to 3-hour period.

Ingestion of food before each dose of probenecid may reduce nausea and vomiting associated with probenecid administration. Administration of an antiemetic may also reduce the potential for nausea.

**Safety considerations for handling this medication**
Due to the mutagenic potential of cidofovir, use of appropriate safety equipment is recommended for the preparation, administration, and disposal of cidofovir. The National Institutes of Health recommends that cidofovir be prepared in a Class II laminar flow biological safety cabinet and that personnel preparing this medication wear surgical gloves and a closed-front surgical-type gown with knit cuffs. If cidofovir contacts the skin, membranes should be washed and flushed thoroughly with water. Excess cidofovir and materials used in the admixture and administration procedures should be placed in a leak-proof, puncture-proof container. High temperature incineration is the recommended method of disposal.

## Parenteral Dosage Forms

### CIDOFOVIR INJECTION

**Usual adult dose**
Antiviral—
   Induction: Intravenous infusion, 5 mg per kg of body weight, administered continuously over one hour, once a week for two consecutive weeks. Probenecid must be administered with each dose of cidofovir. Two grams of probenecid should be administered three hours prior to each dose of cidofovir and 1 gram should be administered two and eight hours after the completion of the one-hour infusion (total 4 grams).
   Maintenance: Intravenous infusion, 5 mg per kg of body weight, administered continuously over one hour, once every two weeks. Probenecid must be administered with each dose of cidofovir. Two grams of probenecid should be administered three hours prior to each dose of cidofovir and 1 gram should be administered two and eight hours after the completion of the one-hour infusion (total 4 grams).

Note: Cidofovir has not been studied in patients with pre-existing renal function impairment. The most appropriate dose of cidofovir for patients with a serum creatinine 1.5 mg per mL or a creatinine clearance ≤ 55 mL per min (mL/min) is not known. However, the following doses (in mg per kg of body weight) are recommended when the benefits of cidofovir exceed the potential risks:

| Creatinine clearance (mL/min) | Induction (once weekly for 2 weeks) | Maintenance (once every 2 weeks) |
|---|---|---|
| 41–55 | 2 mg per kg | 2 mg per kg |
| 30–40 | 1.5 mg per kg | 1.5 mg per kg |
| 20–29 | 1 mg per kg | 1 mg per kg |
| ≤ 19 | 0.5 mg per kg | 0.5 mg per kg |

**Usual pediatric dose**
Safety and efficacy have not been established.

**Strength(s) usually available**
U.S.—
   375 mg per 5 mL (Rx) [*Vistide*].

**Packaging and storage**
Store at room temperature between 20 and 25 ºC (68 and 77 ºF).

**Preparation of dosage form**
The vial should be visually inspected for particulate matter and discoloration prior to administration and discarded if particulate matter or discoloration is observed.

The appropriate volume of cidofovir should be extracted from the vial and the dose transferred to an infusion bag containing 100 mL of 0.9% sodium chloride solution. The entire volume should be infused into the patient at a constant rate over a 1-hour period. It is recommended that a standard infusion pump be used for administration.

**Stability**
It is recommended that cidofovir admixtures be administered within 24 hours of preparation and that refrigeration or freezer storage not be used to extend this 24-hour limit.

If admixtures are not intended for immediate use, they may be refrigerated (between 2 and 8 ºC [36 and 46 ºF]) for no more than 24 hours. Refrigerated admixtures should be allowed to equilibrate to room temperature prior to use.

**Incompatibilities**
Compatibility with Ringer's solution, Lactated Ringer's solution, or bacteriostatic infusion fluids has not been evaluated.

The chemical stability of cidofovir admixtures was determined in polyvinyl chloride composition and ethylene/propylene copolymer composition commercial infusion bags, and in glass bottles.

**Note**
Great care should be taken to prevent exposure of the skin to cidofovir. The use of gloves is recommended. Any cidofovir that comes in contact with the skin should be washed off thoroughly with soap and water.

Developed: 02/27/97

---

**CIMETIDINE**—See *Histamine H₂-receptor Antagonists (Systemic)*

---

**CINOXACIN**—The *Cinoxacin (Systemic)* monograph is not included in this published version of the USP DI database. Copies of the monograph are available on request from Micromedex, Inc. - Reprint Requests, 6200 S. Syracuse Way, Suite 300, Englewood, CO 80111; telephone (303) 486-6400; telefax (303) 486-6464; Email: USPDI@MDX.COM.

---

**CIPROFLOXACIN**—See *Fluoroquinolones (Systemic)*

# CIPROFLOXACIN Ophthalmic

VA CLASSIFICATION (Primary): OP201
Commonly used brand name(s): *Ciloxan.*
Note: For a listing of dosage forms and brand names by country availability, see *Dosage Forms* section(s).

## Category
Antibacterial (ophthalmic).

## Indications

**Accepted**

*Corneal ulcers, bacterial* (treatment)—Ophthalmic ciprofloxacin is indicated in the treatment of corneal ulcers caused by susceptible strains of bacteria, including *Pseudomonas aeruginosa, Serratia marcescens, Staphylococcus aureus, Staphylococcus epidermidis, Streptococcus pneumoniae,* and *Streptococcus (Viridans Group).*

*Conjunctivitis, bacterial* (treatment)—Ophthalmic ciprofloxacin is indicated in the treatment of conjunctivitis caused by susceptible strains of *Staphylococcus aureus, Staphylococcus epidermidis,* and *Streptococcus pneumoniae.*

Note: Not all species or strains of a particular organism may be susceptible to ciprofloxacin. Streptococcal species are often less susceptible.

## Pharmacology/Pharmacokinetics

**Physicochemical characteristics**
Chemical group—Fluoroquinolone.
Molecular weight—385.82.

**Mechanism of action/Effect**
Ciprofloxacin's bactericidal action results from interference with the enzyme DNA gyrase, which is needed for the synthesis of bacterial DNA.

**Absorption**
During the patient's waking hours, ciprofloxacin was administered in each eye every 2 hours for 2 days followed by every 4 hours for an additional 5 days. The maximum reported plasma concentration of ciprofloxacin was less than 5 nanograms per mL. The mean concentration was usually less than 2.5 nanograms per mL.

## Precautions to Consider

**Cross-sensitivity and/or related problems**
Patients sensitive to other quinolones, such as cinoxacin, nalidixic acid, norfloxacin, or ofloxacin, may be sensitive to this medication also.

**Carcinogenicity**
Rats and mice administered ciprofloxacin orally for up to 2 years did not show carcinogenic effects.

**Mutagenicity**
Ciprofloxacin was not found to be mutagenic in the following *in vitro* tests: *Salmonella*/Microsome test, *E. coli* DNA Repair assay, Chinese Hamster V$_{79}$ Cell HGPRT test, Syrian Hamster Embryo Cell Transformation assay, *Saccharomyces cerevisiae* Point Mutation assay, and *Saccharomyces cerevisiae* Mitotic Crossover and Gene Conversion assay. In addition, ciprofloxacin was not found to be mutagenic in the following *in vivo* tests: Rat Hepatocyte DNA Repair assay, Micronucleus test (mice), and Dominant Lethal test (mice). However, ciprofloxacin was found to be mutagenic in the *in vitro* Mouse Lymphoma Cell Forward Mutation assay and the *in vitro* Rat Hepatocyte DNA Repair assay.

**Pregnancy/Reproduction**
*Fertility*—Studies performed in rats and mice administered ciprofloxacin in oral doses up to 6 times the usual daily human oral dose revealed no evidence of impaired fertility.

*Pregnancy*—Adequate and well-controlled studies in humans have not been done. However, problems in humans have not been documented.
Reproduction studies performed in rats and mice administered ciprofloxacin in oral doses up to 6 times the usual daily human oral dose revealed no evidence of harm to the fetus. In rabbits, ciprofloxacin, like most antimicrobial agents, when administered in oral doses of 30 and 100 mg per kg of body weight (mg/kg) per day produced gastrointestinal disturbances resulting in maternal weight loss and an increased incidence of abortion. However, no teratogenicity was observed at either dose. Ciprofloxacin administered intravenously in doses of up to 20 mg/kg, produced no embryotoxicity or teratogenicity.

FDA Pregnancy Category C.

**Breast-feeding**
It is not known whether ophthalmic ciprofloxacin is distributed into breast milk. However, oral ciprofloxacin was shown to be distributed into breast milk after a single 500 mg dose.

**Pediatrics**
Appropriate studies on the relationship of age to the effects of ciprofloxacin have not been performed in children up to 12 years of age. Safety and efficacy have not been established.
Although ciprofloxacin and other quinolones cause arthropathy in immature animals after oral administration, ophthalmic ciprofloxacin administered to immature animals did not cause any arthropathy. In addition, there is no evidence that the ophthalmic dosage form has any effect on the weight bearing joints.

**Geriatrics**
No information is available on the relationship of age to the effects of ciprofloxacin in geriatric patients.

**Medical considerations/Contraindications**
The medical considerations/contraindications included have been selected on the basis of their potential clinical significance (reasons given in parentheses where appropriate)—not necessarily inclusive (» = major clinical significance).

*Risk-benefit should be considered when the following medical problem exists:*
Sensitivity to ciprofloxacin

## Side/Adverse Effects

Note: In corneal ulcer studies, frequent administration of ophthalmic ciprofloxacin resulted in white crystalline precipitates in the eyes of 17% of patients. This precipitate did not prevent the continued use of the medication and did not adversely affect treatment outcome.

The following side/adverse effects have been selected on the basis of their potential clinical significance (possible signs and symptoms in parentheses where appropriate)—not necessarily inclusive:

**Those indicating need for medical attention**
Incidence rare
*Corneal infiltrates; corneal staining; decreased vision; keratopathy* (blurred vision or other change in vision); *keratitis* (severe irritation or redness of eye); *nausea; skin rash*

**Those indicating need for medical attention only if they continue or are bothersome**
Incidence more frequent
*Burning or other discomfort of the eye; crusting or crystals in corner of eye*

Incidence less frequent
*Bad taste following instillation; foreign body sensation* (feeling of something in eye); *hyperemia, conjunctival* (redness of the lining of the eyelids); *itching of eye*

Rare
*Lid edema* (swelling of eyelid); *photophobia* (increased sensitivity of eyes to light); *tearing of eye*

## Patient Consultation

As an aid to patient consultation, refer to *Advice for the Patient, Ciprofloxacin (Ophthalmic).*
In providing consultation, consider emphasizing the following selected information (» = major clinical significance):

**Before using this medication**
» Conditions affecting use, especially:
  Sensitivity to ciprofloxacin or other quinolones
  Breast-feeding—Oral ciprofloxacin is distributed into breast milk; it is not known whether ophthalmic ciprofloxacin is distributed into breast milk
  Use in children—Safety and efficacy have not been established in children up to 12 years of age

**Proper use of this medication**
Proper administration technique
» Compliance with full course of therapy
» Proper dosing
Missed dose: Applying as soon as possible; not applying if almost time for next dose
» Proper storage

### Precautions while using this medication
Checking with physician if no improvement within a few days
Possible photophobic reactions; wearing sunglasses and avoiding prolonged exposure to bright light

### Side/adverse effects
Signs of potential side effects, especially corneal infiltrates, corneal staining, decreased vision, keratopathy, keratitis, nausea, or skin rash

## General Dosing Information
Ciprofloxacin ophthalmic solution is not for injection into the eye.

Although some manufacturers recommend doses of 2 drops of ophthalmic solutions at appropriate intervals, the conjunctival sac usually holds less than 1 drop.

If hypersensitivity develops, therapy with ophthalmic ciprofloxacin should be discontinued.

### For treatment of adverse effects
Recommended treatment includes
- For mild hypersensitivity reaction—Administering antihistamines and, if necessary, glucocorticoids.
- For severe hypersensitivity or anaphylactic reaction—Administering epinephrine. Antihistamines and/or glucocorticoids may also be administered as required.

## Ophthalmic Dosage Forms
Note: The dosing and strengths of the dosage forms available are expressed in terms of ciprofloxacin base.

### CIPROFLOXACIN HYDROCHLORIDE OPHTHALMIC SOLUTION USP

**Usual adult and adolescent dose**
Bacterial conjunctivitis—
Topical, to the conjunctiva, 1 drop in each eye every two hours, while patient is awake, for two days, then 1 drop every four hours, while patient is awake, for the next five days.

Corneal ulcers—
Topical, to the conjunctiva, 1 drop into the affected eye every fifteen minutes for six hours, then 1 drop every thirty minutes, while patient is awake, for the rest of day one; 1 drop every hour, while patient is awake, on day two; and 1 drop every four hours, while patient is awake, on days three through fourteen. If corneal re-epithelialization has not occurred after fourteen days of treatment, treatment may be continued.

Note: During the initial 24 to 48 hours, additional doses may be necessary during the night in some cases.

**Usual pediatric dose**
Bacterial conjunctivitis or
Corneal ulcers—
Infants and children up to 12 years of age: Safety and efficacy have not been established.
Children over 12 years of age: See *Usual adult and adolescent dose*.

**Strength(s) usually available**
U.S.—
3.5 mg (3 mg base) (Rx) [*Ciloxan* (benzalkonium chloride 0.006%)].
Canada—
3.5 mg (3 mg base) (Rx) [*Ciloxan*].

**Packaging and storage**
Store below 40 °C (104 °F), preferably between 15 and 30 °C (59 and 86 °F), unless otherwise specified by manufacturer. Store in a tight container. Protect from light.

**Auxiliary labeling**
- For the eye.
- Continue medicine for full time of treatment.

## Selected Bibliography
Yolton DP. New antibacterial drugs for topical ophthalmic use. Optom Clin 1992; 2(4): 59-72.

Revised: 07/29/93

---

# CISAPRIDE Systemic

VA CLASSIFICATION (Primary): GA900
Commonly used brand name(s): *Prepulsid; Propulsid*.

Note: For a listing of dosage forms and brand names by country availability, see *Dosage Forms* section(s).

## Category
Cholinergic enhancer; gastrointestinal emptying (delayed) adjunct.

## Indications
Note: Bracketed information in the *Indications* section refers to uses that are not included in U.S. product labeling.

**Accepted**
Reflux, gastroesophageal (prophylaxis and treatment)—Cisapride is indicated for the symptomatic treatment of nocturnal [and daytime] heartburn, and of esophagitis due to reflux and delayed gastric emptying. Treatment may continue for up to 8 weeks; however, tolerance to cisapride may develop at some point in therapy. Because of the risk of serious and sometimes fatal cardiac arrythmias, cisapride generally should be reserved for patients who have not responded adequately to lifestyle modifications, and who are not concomitantly taking any contraindicated medications (*see Drug interactions and/or related problems*).

Note: In current Canadian labeling, cisapride is contraindicated for use in premature infants (i.e., born at gestational age < 36 weeks) during the first 3 months after delivery.

[Gastroparesis (treatment)]—Cisapride is indicated in the treatment of gastroparesis, including idiopathic, diabetic, and intestinal pseudo-obstruction. Treatment may continue for up to 8 weeks; however, tolerance to cisapride may develop at some point in therapy.

## Pharmacology/Pharmacokinetics
**Physicochemical characteristics**
Molecular weight—465.95.

**Mechanism of action/Effect**
Cisapride exerts its effect by increasing the release of acetylcholine from the postganglionic nerve endings of the myenteric plexus. This release of acetylcholine increases esophageal activity and increases esophageal sphincter tone, thereby improving esophageal clearance and decreasing reflux of gastric contents into the esophagus. Cisapride enhances gastric and duodenal emptying as a result of increased gastric and duodenal contractivity and antroduodenal coordination. Duodenogastric reflux is also decreased. Cisapride improves transit in both small and large bowel.

**Absorption**
Rapid and complete.

**Protein binding**
97.5% bound to plasma proteins, primarily albumin.

**Biotransformation**
Hepatic.

**Half-life**
Elimination—7 to 10 hours after both single and multiple oral dosing regimens.

**Onset of action**
30 to 60 minutes.

**Time to peak concentration**
1 to 2 hours.

**Elimination**
Renal and fecal.

## Precautions to Consider
**Carcinogenicity/Tumorigenicity**
No tumorigenicity was demonstrated in rats receiving up to 80 mg of cisapride per kilogram of body weight (mg/kg) (50 times the maximum recommended human dose for a 50 kg person) a day for 25 months or in mice receiving up to 80 mg/kg (50 times the maximum recommended human dose) of cisapride a day for 19 months.

## Mutagenicity
No mutagenicity was demonstrated in the following *in vitro* and *in vivo* models: Ames test, chromosomal aberration assay on human lymphocytes, sex-linked recessive lethal test in *Drosophila melanogaster*, dominant lethal test in male and female mice germ cells, and micronucleus test in rats.

## Pregnancy/Reproduction
Fertility—At oral doses of up to 160 mg/kg a day (100 times the maximum recommended human dose), cisapride was found to have no effect on fertility in male rats. In female rats at oral doses of 40 mg/kg a day and higher, cisapride prolonged the breeding interval required for impregnation. These effects were also observed at maturity in the female offspring of female rats treated with oral doses of cisapride at 10 mg/kg a day or higher. At doses of 160 mg/kg a day, cisapride exerted contragestational/pregnancy disrupting effects in female rats.

Pregnancy—Adequate and well-controlled studies in humans have not been done.

Studies in rats (at doses of up to 160 mg/kg) and rabbits (at doses of up to 40 mg/kg) found no evidence of a teratogenic potential of cisapride. Studies in rats at doses of up to 160 mg/kg a day (100 times the maximum recommended human dose) and in rabbits at doses of 20 mg/kg (approximately 12 times the maximum recommended human dose) a day or higher found cisapride to be embryotoxic and fetotoxic. Doses of cisapride at 40 and 160 mg/kg a day reduced birth weights of pups in rats and adversely affected pup survival.

FDA Pregnancy Category C.

## Breast-feeding
Problems in humans have not been documented; however, risk-benefit must be considered since cisapride is distributed into breast milk at concentrations approximately one twentieth of those in plasma.

## Pediatrics
Serious adverse effects including death have been reported in infants and children treated with cisapride (see *Side/Adverse Effects*). Cisapride should be used with caution, and recommended doses should not be exceeded.

## Geriatrics
Appropriate studies performed to date have not demonstrated geriatrics-specific problems that would limit the usefulness of cisapride in the elderly. However, the elimination half-life of cisapride has been found to be longer in some elderly patients, which may require adjustment of dosage in patients receiving cisapride.

## Drug interactions and/or related problems
The following drug interactions and/or related problems have been selected on the basis of their potential clinical significance (possible mechanism in parentheses where appropriate)—not necessarily inclusive (» = major clinical significance):

Note: Only specific interactions between cisapride and other oral medications have been identified in this monograph. However, because of increased gastrointestinal motility and decreased gastric emptying time caused by cisapride, absorption of medications from the stomach may be decreased, while absorption from the small intestine may be enhanced.

Medications that inhibit the hepatic cytochrome P450 3A4 isoenzyme can lead to elevated cisapride levels. Rare cases of serious cardiac arrhythmias, including ventricular tachycardia, ventricular fibrillation, torsades de pointes, and QT prolongation, have been reported both in patients with a positive cardiac history and in patients with no known cardiac history. Fatalities have occurred.

Combinations containing any of the following medications, depending on the amount present, may also interact with this medication.

Alcohol or
Benzodiazepines
(cisapride has been reported to increase the rate of absorption of these agents)

» Anticholinergics or other medications with anticholinergic activity (see *Appendix II*)
(concurrent use may antagonize the effects of cisapride on gastrointestinal motility)

Cimetidine or
Ranitidine
(cisapride accelerates the absorption of cimetidine and ranitidine)
(cimetidine coadministration causes increased peak plasma concentration and area under the plasma concentration–time curve [AUC] of cisapride)

» Clarithromycin or
» Erythromycin or
» Troleandomycin
(concurrent use of clarithromycin, erythromycin, or troleandomycin with cisapride is contraindicated; concurrent use may result in elevated plasma concentrations of cisapride through inhibition of the cytochrome P450 3A4 enzyme; this has led to serious cardiac arrhythmias including ventricular tachycardia, ventricular fibrillation, torsades de pointes, and QT prolongation; some of these events have been fatal)

» Fluconazole or
» Itraconazole or
» Ketoconazole or
» Miconazole
(concurrent use of fluconazole, itraconazole, ketoconazole, or intravenous miconazole with cisapride is contraindicated; concurrent use may result in elevated plasma concentrations of cisapride through inhibition of the cytochrome P450 3A4 enzyme; this has led to serious cardiac arrhythmias including ventricular tachycardia, ventricular fibrillation, torsades de pointes, and QT prolongation; some of these events have been fatal)

» Human immunodeficiency virus (HIV) protease inhibitors including:
Indinavir or
Nelfinivir or
Ritonavir or
(concurrent use of indinavir, nelfinivir, or ritonavir with cisapride is contraindicated; concurrent use may result in elevated plasma concentrations of cisapride through inhibition of the cytochrome P450 3A4 isoenzyme; serious cardiac arrhythmias including ventricular tachycardia, ventricular fibrillation, torsades de pointes, and QT prolongation have occurred; some of these events have been fatal)

» Medications that prolong the QT interval and increase the risk of arrhythmias, including:
Antidepressants, tricyclic
Astemizole
Calcium channel blocking agents, especially bepridil
Class IA antiarrhythmics, especially procainamide or quinidine
Class III antiarrhythmics, especially sotalol
Maprotiline
Phenothiazines
Sertindole
Sparfloxacin
Terodiline
(concurrent use of these medications with cisapride is contraindicated; serious cardiac arrhythmias including ventricular tachycardia, ventricular fibrillation, torsades de pointes, and QT prolongation have occurred; some of these events have been fatal)

» Nefazodone
(concurrent use of nefazodone with cisapride is contraindicated; serious cardiac arrhythmias including ventricular tachycardia, ventricular fibrillation, torsades de pointes, and QT prolongation have occurred; some of these events have been fatal)

» Potassium-wasting diuretics, including:
Bumetanide
Ethacrynic acid
Furosemide and
Thiazide diuretics
(concurrent use of these medications with cisapride is contraindicated in patients who might experience a rapid reduction in plasma potassium levels; serious, possibly fatal, cardiac arrhythmias may result)

» Terfenadine
(concurrent use of cisapride with terfenadine may increase risk of cardiac arrhythmias, which are seen on electrocardiogram [ECG] as prolongation of the QT interval)

## Medical considerations/Contraindications
The medical considerations/contraindications included have been selected on the basis of their potential clinical significance (reasons given in parentheses where appropriate)—not necessarily inclusive (» = major clinical significance).

*Except under special circumstances, this medication should not be used when the following medical problems exist:*

» Cardiac disease, including:
Congestive heart failure
History of long QT syndrome
History of prolonged electrocardiogram (ECG) QT intervals
History of second or third degree atrioventricular block

History of sinus node dysfunction
History of ventricular arrhythmias, including torsades de pointes
Ischemic heart disease
(increased risk of serious, possibly fatal, cardiac arrhythmias)
» Gastrointestinal hemorrhage, mechanical obstruction or perforation
(stimulation of gastrointestinal motility may aggravate these conditions)
» Intake of medications known to prolong the QT interval or
» Renal failure or
» Respiratory failure or
» Uncorrected electrolyte disorders, including:
Hypokalemia
Hypomagnesemia
(increased risk of serious, possibly fatal, cardiac arrhythmias)

*Risk-benefit should be considered when the following medical problems exist:*
Conditions predisposing the patient to development of electrolyte imbalances, including:
Dehydration, severe
Emergent insulin use to treat hypoglycemia with ketoacidosis
Malnutrition
Vomiting, severe
(increased risk of serious, possibly fatal, cardiac arrhythmias)
Conditions predisposing the patient to development of serious cardiac arrhythmias, including:
Advanced cancer
Apnea
Chronic obstructive pulmonary disease
Multiple organ failure
(increased risk of serious, possibly fatal, cardiac arrhythmias)
Hepatic function impairment or
Renal function impairment
(clearance of cisapride may be decreased; dosage reductions may be recommended)
Sensitivity to cisapride

## Side/Adverse Effects

Serious cardiac arrhythmias, including ventricular tachycardia, ventricular fibrillation, torsades de pointes (sometimes with syncope), and QT prolongation leading to cardiac arrest and sudden death have been reported in patients taking cisapride. Some, but not all, of these patients had pre-existing cardiac disease or risk factors for arrhythmias. Fatalities have occurred.

Serious adverse effects including death have been reported in infants and children treated with cisapride. Several pediatric deaths were due to cardiovascular events including third degree heart block and ventricular tachycardia; pediatric deaths have been associated with seizures, and there has been at least one case of sudden unexplained death in a 3-month-old infant. Other potentially serious events reported in pediatric patients include presence of antinuclear antibodies (ANA), anemia, hemolytic anemia, methemoglobinemia, hyperglycemia, hypoglycemia with acidosis, unexplained apneic episodes, confusion, impaired concentration, depression, apathy, visual changes accompanied by amnesia, and severe photosensitivity reaction.

The following side/adverse effects have been selected on the basis of their potential clinical significance (possible signs and symptoms in parentheses where appropriate)—not necessarily inclusive:

**Those indicating need for medical attention**
Incidence rare
*Cardiac arrhythmias* (dizziness; fainting or feeling faint; fast or racing heartbeat; pounding or irregular heartbeat); *edema* (swelling of face, hands, lower legs, and/or feet; unusual weight gain); *seizures; vision abnormalities* (blurred vision or other changes in vision)

**Those indicating need for medical attention only if they continue or are bothersome**
Incidence less frequent or rare
*Abdominal pain or cramping; constipation; diarrhea; dryness of mouth; dyspepsia* (heartburn or indigestion); *fatigue* (unusual tiredness or weakness); *flatulence* (gas); *migraine or other headache; nausea; rhinitis* (runny nose); *somnolence* (drowsiness); *tremor*
Note: Abdominal pain, constipation, diarrhea, flatulence, and rhinitis may be dose-related.

## Overdose

For specific information on the agents used in the management of cisapride overdose, see *Charcoal, Activated (Oral-Local)* monograph.

For more information on the management of overdose or unintentional ingestion, **contact a Poison Control Center** (see *Poison Control Center Listing*).

**Treatment of overdose**
Recommended treatment consists of the following:
Stopping administration of medication.
To decrease absorption—Use of gastric lavage and/or administration of activated charcoal.
Monitoring—Patients should be evaluated for possible QT prolongation and for factors that may predispose the patient to ventricular arrhythmias, including torsades de pointes.
Supportive care—Patients in whom intentional overdose is confirmed or suspected should be referred for psychiatric consultation.

## Patient Consultation

As an aid to patient consultation, refer to *Advice for the Patient, Cisapride (Systemic)*.
In providing consultation, consider emphasizing the following selected information (» = major clinical significance):

**Before using this medication**
» Conditions affecting use, especially:
Sensitivity to cisapride
Pregnancy—High doses in animals shown to be embryotoxic and fetotoxic
Breast-feeding—Distributed into breast milk in small amounts
Other medications, especially anticholinergics, clarithromycin, erythromycin, fluconazole, HIV protease inhibitors, itraconazole, ketoconazole, medications that prolong the QT interval, miconazole, nefazodone, potassium-wasting diuretics, terfenadine, and troleandomycin
Other medical problems, especially cardiac disease; gastrointestinal bleeding, mechanical obstruction, or perforation; intake of medications that prolong the QT interval; renal failure; respiratory failure; and uncorrected electrolyte disorders

**Proper use of this medication**
» Taking 15 minutes before meals and at bedtime with a beverage
» Proper dosing
Missed dose: Taking as soon as possible; not taking if almost time for next dose
» Proper storage

**Precautions while using this medication**
» Checking with physician before using alcohol
» Caution if drowsiness occurs
» Obtaining medical attention if fainting, dizziness, irregular heartbeat or pulse, or other unusual symptoms occur

**Side/adverse effects**
Cardiac arrhythmias, edema, seizures, vision abnormalities

## General Dosing Information

Cisapride should be taken 15 minutes before meals and bedtime.

In patients with hepatic or renal function impairment, the initial daily dose should be reduced and adjusted depending on the therapeutic effect or possible side effects. In patients with hepatic insufficiency, the dosage should be reduced by half.

Cisapride should be discontinued if relief of nocturnal heartburn does not occur. If relief is obtained, the minimum effective dose should be used. The recommended dose should not be exceeded.

## Oral Dosage Forms

Note: Bracketed uses in the *Dosage Forms* section refer to categories of use and/or indications that are not included in U.S. product labeling.

### CISAPRIDE ORAL SUSPENSION

**Usual adult and adolescent dose**
Gastroesophageal reflux—
Prophylaxis:
Oral, 10 mg two times a day, before breakfast and at bedtime or 20 mg a day at bedtime.
Note: Dose used in prophylaxis may be increased to a maximum of 20 mg two times a day with severe disease.
Treatment:
Oral, 5 to 10 mg three to four times a day, fifteen minutes before meals and at bedtime.
Note: Some patients may require a dose of 20 mg four times a day, taken fifteen minutes before meals and at bedtime.

# Cisapride (Systemic)

[Gastroparesis]—
Treatment:
Oral, 10 mg three to four times a day, fifteen minutes before meals and at bedtime.
Note: Dose may be increased to a maximum of 20 mg three times a day, fifteen minutes before meals.

**Usual pediatric dose**
Gastroesophageal reflux or
[Gastroparesis]—
Treatment: Oral, 0.15 to 0.3 mg per kg of body weight three or four times a day, before meals.

**Strength(s) usually available**
U.S.—
1 mg per mL (Rx) [*Propulsid*].
Canada—
1 mg per mL (Rx) [*Prepulsid*].

**Packaging and storage**
Store between 15 and 25 °C (59 and 77 °F), unless otherwise specified by manufacturer. Protect from light.

**Auxiliary labeling**
• Shake well.

## CISAPRIDE TABLETS

**Usual adult and adolescent dose**
See *Cisapride Oral Suspension*.

**Usual pediatric dose**
See *Cisapride Oral Suspension*.

**Strength(s) usually available**
U.S.—
10 mg (Rx) [*Propulsid* (scored)].
20 mg (Rx) [*Propulsid*].
Canada—
5 mg (Rx) [*Prepulsid*].
10 mg (Rx) [*Prepulsid*].
20 mg (Rx) [*Prepulsid*].

**Packaging and storage**
Store between 15 and 25 °C (59 and 77 °F), unless otherwise specified by manufacturer. Protect the 20 mg tablets from light.

### Selected Bibliography
McCallum R, Prakash C, Campoli-Richards D, Goa K. Cisapride: a preliminary review of its pharmacodynamic and pharmacokinetic properties, and therapeutic use as a prokinetic agent in gastrointestinal motility disorders. Drugs 1988; 36: 652-81.

Revised: 7/29/96
Interim revision: 01/07/98; 8/10/98

---

# CISATRACURIUM Systemic

INN: Cisatracurium Besilate
VA CLASSIFICATION (Primary): MS300
Commonly used brand name(s): *Nimbex*.
Note: For a listing of dosage forms and brand names by country availability, see *Dosage Forms* section(s).

## Category
Neuromuscular blocking agent.

## Indications

**Accepted**
Muscle (skeletal) relaxation, for surgery—Cisatracurium is indicated as an adjunct to general anesthesia to facilitate endotracheal intubation and to induce skeletal muscle relaxation in surgical patients. It is also indicated to facilitate endotracheal intubation and to induce skeletal muscle relaxation in patients who require mechanical ventilation in the intensive care unit[1]. However, cisatracurium has an intermediate onset of action and is therefore not recommended for rapid-sequence endotracheal intubation.

[1]Not included in Canadian product labeling.

## Pharmacology/Pharmacokinetics

**Physicochemical characteristics**
Source—Synthetic; one of the 10 isomers of atracurium besylate.
Molecular weight—Cisatracurium: 929.2.
Cisatracurium besylate: 1243.51.
pH—Cisatracurium injection: 3.25 to 3.65.

**Mechanism of action/Effect**
Cisatracurium is a nondepolarizing neuromuscular blocking agent. Nondepolarizing neuromuscular blocking agents inhibit neuromuscular transmission by competing with acetylcholine for the cholinergic receptors at the motor end plate, thereby antagonizing the action of acetylcholine. This type of competitive neuromuscular blockade is usually antagonized by anticholinesterase agents.
Neuromuscular blocking agents have no effect on consciousness or pain threshold.

**Distribution**
Volume of distribution (Vol$_D$)—Steady-state: 0.145 liter per kg of body weight (L/kg) in patients receiving opioid anesthesia; approximately 21% greater in patients receiving inhalation anesthesia and slightly greater in geriatric patients than in younger adults.
Note: A value of 0.28 ± 0.103 L/kg was calculated during the terminal elimination phase in intensive care patients receiving cisatracurium infusions for 24 to 48 hours. However, this value is an underestimate because elimination from the peripheral compartment was not included in the calculation.

**Biotransformation**
Eighty percent of a dose is metabolized via Hofmann elimination, a pH- and temperature-dependent process that is independent of renal or hepatic function. Some hepatic biotransformation also occurs. The primary metabolites are a monoquaternary acrylate derivative, which is further metabolized via Hofmann elimination (but more slowly than the parent compound) and via hydrolysis by nonspecific plasma esterases, and laudanosine, which is further metabolized to desmethyl metabolites that are subsequently conjugated with glucuronic acid. Neither metabolite has neuromuscular blocking activity, although laudanosine causes transient hypotension and, in higher doses, cerebral excitatory effects in animals. Whether laudanosine may contribute to the development of seizures during long-term cisatracurium administration has not been established.

**Half-life**
Elimination—
Cisatracurium:
Approximately 22 to 29 minutes, following administration of a single intravenous dose to surgical patients. The half-life is not substantially affected by the duration of administration (approximately 26 ± 11 minutes in intensive care patients receiving cisatracurium via intravenous infusion for 24 to 48 hours), type of anesthesia, or hepatic or renal function impairment, but is slightly longer in geriatric patients than in younger adults.
In individuals undergoing coronary artery bypass surgery with induced hypothermia (body temperature of 25 to 28 °C [77 to 82.4 °F]), the half-life during hypothermia is prolonged as compared with the half-life during normothermia.
Laudanosine:
6.6 ± 4.1 hours, in intensive care patients receiving long-term therapy via intravenous infusion; increased in patients with hepatic or renal function impairment.

**Onset of action**
Time to achieve intubating conditions in adults—Dose-dependent; 2 minutes following administration of 0.15 mg per kg of body weight (mg/kg) and 1.5 minutes following administration of 0.2 mg/kg. The dose of 0.2 mg/kg is four times the ED$_{95}$ (the dose required to produce 95% suppression of the twitch response to peripheral nerve stimulation).

**Peak serum concentration**
For laudanosine, in intensive care patients receiving cisatracurium via intravenous infusion for 24 to 48 hours—707 ± 360 nanograms per mL (1.98 ± 1 micromoles per L [micromoles/L]); higher in patients with renal or hepatic function impairment.

**Time to peak effect**
Time to maximum blockade—
  Adults:
    Dose-dependent; 3.5 (range, 1.6 to 6.8) minutes following administration of 0.15 mg/kg and 2.9 (range, 1.9 to 5.2) minutes following administration of 0.2 mg/kg in young adults with normal renal and hepatic function receiving opioid anesthesia.
  Note: After administration of 0.1 mg/kg, mean times to achieve maximum blockade are approximately 1 minute longer in geriatric patients and in patients with end-stage renal function impairment, and approximately 1 minute shorter in patients with end-stage hepatic function impairment than in young adults with normal renal and hepatic function.
  Children 2 to 12 years of age:
    2.8 (range, 1.8 to 6.7) minutes following administration of 0.1 mg/kg.

**Duration of action**
Note: Values reported below for adults undergoing surgery were determined in young adults with normal renal and hepatic function receiving opioid-nitrous oxide-oxygen anesthesia. No clinically significant differences in recovery parameters were found in geriatric patients or in patients with hepatic or renal function impairment. However, greater variability in duration of effect was observed in patients with renal function impairment. Values reported below for children 2 to 12 years of age were determined in surgical patients receiving stable halothane or opioid anesthesia.

The duration of action of cisatracurium may be prolonged in patients receiving a potent inhalation anesthetic (e.g., enflurane, isoflurane).

The duration of action may be prolonged in patients with acidosis or hypothermia.

Administration of an anticholinesterase agent such as edrophonium or neostigmine after some spontaneous recovery has occurred will decrease the recovery times reported below.

Duration of clinical effect (time for spontaneous recovery of the twitch response to peripheral nerve stimulation to 25% of the control value [$T_{25}$])—
  Adults undergoing surgery:
    Dose-dependent; 55 (range, 44 to 74) minutes following administration of 0.15 mg/kg and 65 (range, 43 to 103) minutes following administration of 0.2 mg/kg.
  Children 2 to 12 years of age undergoing surgery:
    28 (range, 21 to 38) minutes following administration of 0.1 mg/kg.
Time for spontaneous recovery of the twitch response to peripheral nerve stimulation to 95% of the control value ($T_{95}$)—
  Adults undergoing surgery:
    Dose-dependent; 76 (range, 60 to 103) minutes following administration of 0.15 mg/kg and 81 (range, 53 to 114) minutes following administration of 0.2 mg/kg.
  Children 2 to 12 years of age undergoing surgery:
    46 (range, 37 to 58) minutes following administration of 0.1 mg/kg.
Recovery index (time for the twitch response to nerve stimulation to increase spontaneously from 25% to 75% of the control value [$T_{25-75}$])—
  Adults undergoing surgery:
    Dose-dependent; 13 (range, 11 to 16) minutes following administration of 0.15 mg/kg and 12 (range, 2 to 30) minutes following administration of 0.2 mg/kg.
  Children 2 to 12 years of age undergoing surgery:
    10 (range, 7 to 12) minutes following administration of 0.1 mg/kg.
Time to spontaneous recovery of the $T_4:T_1$ ratio (train-of-four stimulation) to ≥ 70%—
  Adults undergoing surgery:
    Dose-dependent; 75 (range, 63 to 98) minutes following administration of 0.15 mg/kg and 85 (range, 55 to 114) minutes following administration of 0.2 mg/kg.
  Adults receiving long-term intravenous infusion (up to 6 days) in intensive care situations:
    55 (range, 20 to 270) minutes in one study; 50 (range, 20 to 175) minutes in another.
  Children 2 to 12 years of age undergoing surgery:
    44 (range, 36 to 58) minutes following administration of 0.1 mg/kg.

**Elimination**
Renal, 95%, mostly as metabolites. Less than 10% of a dose is eliminated as unchanged cisatracurium. About 4% of a dose is eliminated in the feces.

## Precautions to Consider

**Cross-sensitivity and/or related problems**
Patients allergic to benzylisoquinolinium compounds, such as atracurium, doxacurium, and mivacurium, may be allergic to cisatracurium also.

**Carcinogenicity**
Studies have not been done.

**Mutagenicity**
Positive results occurred in the mouse lymphoma assay, both in the presence and absence of exogenous metabolic activation (rat liver S-9). In the absence of metabolic activation, cisatracurium was positive at *in vitro* concentrations of 40 micrograms per mL (mcg/mL) or higher. In the presence of S-9, cisatracurium was mutagenic at a concentration of 300 mcg/mL, but not at lower or higher concentrations. No mutagenicity was found in the Ames *Salmonella* mutation test, a rat bone marrow cytogenic assay, or an *in vitro* human lymphocyte cytogenic assay.

**Pregnancy/Reproduction**
Pregnancy—Adequate and well-controlled studies have not been done in humans.
No maternal or fetal toxicity or teratogenicity was found in studies in nonventilated rats receiving maximum subparalyzing doses of 4 mg/kg subcutaneously (equivalent to eight times the intravenous human $ED_{95}$ [dose required to produce 95% suppression of the twitch response to peripheral nerve stimulation]) or in ventilated rats receiving paralyzing doses of 0.5 or 1 mg/kg intravenously (equivalent to 10 or 20 times the intravenous human $ED_{95}$, respectively).
FDA Pregnancy Category B.
Labor and delivery—Use of cisatracurium during labor, vaginal delivery, or cesarean section has not been studied in humans. Whether administration to the mother may affect the fetus has not been determined. However, potentiation of neuromuscular blockade may occur if magnesium salts are used for management of toxemia of pregnancy.
Administration of 0.2 or 0.4 mg/kg of cisatracurium to female beagles undergoing cesarean section produced negligible quantities of the medication in umbilical vessel blood and no adverse effects on the offspring.

**Breast-feeding**
It is not known whether cisatracurium is distributed into breast milk.

**Pediatrics**
Neonates—Multiple-dose vials of cisatracurium injection contain benzyl alcohol. Administration of excessive doses of benzyl alcohol to neonates has been associated with neurologic and other complications.
Infants and children up to 2 years of age—Appropriate studies on the relationship of age to the effects of cisatracurium have not been performed in infants and children up to 2 years of age.
Children 2 to 12 years of age—Appropriate studies on the relationship of age to the effects of cisatracurium have shown that the $ED_{95}$ of cisatracurium is lower, the onset of action is faster, the duration of action is shorter, and recovery time after administration of a reversal agent is more rapid than in adults. However, pediatrics-specific adverse effects or other problems that would limit the use of cisatracurium in children have not been documented.

**Geriatrics**
Clinical trials that included 145 patients 65 years of age or older, some of whom had cardiovascular disease, did not demonstrate geriatrics-specific problems that would limit the usefulness of cisatracurium in the elderly. These studies showed the time to achieve maximum neuromuscular blockade to be approximately 1 minute longer in elderly patients than in younger adults. However, despite some minor differences in pharmacokinetic parameters between elderly patients and younger adults, there were no clinically significant differences in recovery following a single dose of 0.1 mg/kg.

**Drug interactions and/or related problems**
The following drug interactions and/or related problems have been selected on the basis of their potential clinical significance (possible mechanism in parentheses where appropriate)—not necessarily inclusive (» = major clinical significance):
Note: Combinations containing any of the following medications, depending on the amount present, may also interact with this medication.

» Aminoglycosides or
» Anesthetics, parenteral-local or
  Bacitracin or
» Clindamycin or
  Colistimethate sodium or
  Colistin or
» Lincomycin or
  Lithium or

» Magnesium salts, large doses (e.g., for management of toxemia of pregnancy) or
» Polymyxins or
» Procainamide or
» Quinidine or
   Tetracyclines
      (these agents may enhance the effects of nondepolarizing neuromuscular blocking agents)

Aminophylline or
Theophylline
    (resistance to neuromuscular blockade may occur; higher doses of cisatracurium may be needed)

Anesthetics, hydrocarbon inhalation, especially:
   Enflurane
   Isoflurane
     (these agents may prolong the clinically effective duration of initial and maintenance doses of cisatracurium; although adjustment of the initial dose of cisatracurium should not be necessary when it is administered shortly after the start of inhalation anesthesia, during long surgical procedures, less frequent maintenance dosing and/or lower maintenance doses may be necessary; average infusion rate requirements during enflurane or isoflurane administration may be decreased by 30 to 40% or more)

Carbamazepine or
Phenytoin
    (resistance to the effects of other nondepolarizing neuromuscular blocking agents has been reported in patients receiving long-term anticonvulsant therapy; although the effects of such treatment on the efficacy of cisatracurium have not been established, a slightly shorter duration of neuromuscular blockade and increased infusion rate requirements should be anticipated)

Corticosteroids
    (a syndrome of prolonged paralysis and/or skeletal muscle weakness has occurred in intensive care patients receiving neuromuscular blocking agents to assist mechanical ventilation; the use of corticosteroids has been associated with the development of this syndrome)

Succinylcholine
    (the time to onset of maximum neuromuscular blockade is decreased by approximately 2 minutes when cisatracurium is administered following either 10% recovery or 95% recovery from a 1 mg/kg intubating dose of succinylcholine, but the duration of action of initial or maintenance doses of cisatracurium is not altered)

    (cisatracurium infusion requirements following prior administration of succinylcholine are similar to or slightly higher than are needed without initial use of succinylcholine)

    (administration of cisatracurium prior to succinylcholine, to attenuate some of succinylcholine's adverse effects, has not been studied)

Note: No interactions occurred when atracurium, pancuronium, or vecuronium was administered after varying degrees of recovery from single doses or infusions of cisatracurium.

### Medical considerations/Contraindications
The medical considerations/contraindications included have been selected on the basis of their potential clinical significance (reasons given in parentheses where appropriate)—not necessarily inclusive (» = major clinical significance).

*Risk-benefit should be considered when the following medical problems exist:*

Acid-base or electrolyte imbalance
    (action of nondepolarizing neuromuscular blocking agents may be antagonized or potentiated)

Burns
    (resistance to neuromuscular blockade may occur, resulting in an increase in the dosage requirement and a shorter duration of action of cisatracurium; the extent to which the response is altered may depend on the size of the burn and the time elapsed since the burn injury)

Carcinomatosis or
Neuromuscular disease, such as myasthenia gravis or myasthenic syndrome or
Other conditions in which prolonged neuromuscular blockade is a possibility
    (effect of neuromuscular blocking agents may be enhanced and/or prolonged; it is recommended that the patient be carefully monitored with a peripheral nerve stimulator, and that the initial cisatracurium dose be limited to 0.02 mg/kg)

Hemiparesis or
Paraparesis
    (affected limb or limbs may be resistant to neuromuscular blockade; a nonparetic limb should be used to monitor effect and recovery)

Sensitivity to cisatracurium or related compounds

### Patient monitoring
The following may be especially important in patient monitoring (other tests may be warranted in some patients, depending on condition; » = major clinical significance):

Muscle function
    (onset, degree, and recovery from neuromuscular blockade should be assessed periodically using a peripheral nerve stimulator; grip strength and/or ability to maintain a 5-second head lift may also be used to assess recovery)

## Side/Adverse Effects

Note: Cisatracurium does not increase plasma histamine concentrations in doses up to eight times the $ED_{95}$ (dose required to produce 95% suppression of the twitch response to peripheral nerve stimulation). Also, cisatracurium has no clinically significant effect on blood pressure or heart rate in children 2 to 12 years of age receiving doses of up to two times the pediatric $ED_{95}$; healthy adult surgical patients receiving doses as high as eight times the adult $ED_{95}$, administered over 5 to 10 seconds; or adult patients with cardiovascular disease undergoing coronary artery bypass surgery receiving doses as high as six times the adult $ED_{95}$, administered over 5 to 10 seconds. However, anaphylactic and anaphylactoid reactions have been reported with the use of cisatracurium.

The following side/adverse effects have been selected on the basis of their potential clinical significance (possible signs and symptoms in parentheses where appropriate)—not necessarily inclusive:

**Those indicating need for medical attention**
Incidence rare—less than 0.5%

*Bradycardia; bronchospasm; flushing, cutaneous; hypotension; skin rash*

Note: The above side/adverse effects were reported in surgical patients. *Bronchospasm* was also reported in one intensive care patient receiving a long-term cisatracurium infusion. Also, in clinical trials in intensive care patients, prolonged recovery following discontinuation of long-term infusion therapy occurred in 2 of 28 patients receiving cisatracurium (in comparison, prolonged recovery occurred in 13 of 30 patients receiving vecuronium).

## Overdose
For specific information on the agents used in the management of cisatracurium overdose, see:
- *Atropine* in *Anticholinergics/Antispasmodics (Systemic)* monograph;
- *Edrophonium (Systemic)* monograph;
- *Glycopyrrolate* in *Anticholinergics/Antispasmodics (Systemic)* monograph; and/or
- *Neostigmine* in *Antimyasthenics (Systemic)* monograph.

For more information on the management of an overdose **contact a Poison Control Center** (see *Poison Control Center Listing*).

**Clinical effects of overdose**
The following effect has been selected on the basis of its potential clinical significance (possible signs and symptoms in parentheses where appropriate)—not necessarily inclusive:

Acute
*Paralysis, prolonged*

**Treatment of overdose**
Recommended treatment includes maintaining a patent airway and assisting ventilation until adequate recovery has occurred.

Specific treatment—With the onset of spontaneous recovery, further recovery may be facilitated by administering an anticholinesterase agent (e.g., edrophonium or neostigmine). The reversal agent should be given in conjunction with a suitable anticholinergic agent (e.g., atropine or glycopyrrolate).

Monitoring—Recovery may be assessed by monitoring functions such as grip strength and/or ability to maintain a 5-second head lift, as well as by peripheral nerve stimulation.

## General Dosing Information
Neuromuscular blocking agents have no clinically significant effect on consciousness or pain threshold and should therefore always be used in conjunction with adequate anesthesia (surgical patients) or sedation and, if necessary, analgesia (intensive care patients).

Neuromuscular blocking agents should be administered only by personnel experienced in the techniques of resuscitation and life support (e.g., tracheal intubation, artificial respiration, oxygen administration). Facilities for these procedures and an antagonist (e.g., edrophonium, neostigmine) should be immediately available.

Cisatracurium is given intravenously; there are no data to support administration by intramuscular injection.

The $ED_{95}$ of cisatracurium (dose required to produce 95% suppression of the twitch response to peripheral nerve stimulation) is approximately 0.05 (range, 0.048 to 0.053) mg per kg of body weight (mg/kg) in adults and approximately 0.04 mg/kg in children 2 to 12 years of age. However, higher doses are used clinically to reduce the time to achieve adequate intubating conditions and maximum blockade and to prolong the duration of effective muscle relaxation. The stated initial doses for adults and children are equivalent to three and four times the adult $ED_{95}$ and 1.5 times the pediatric $ED_{95}$, respectively.

The stated doses are given only as guidelines. Actual dosage must be individualized. It is recommended that a peripheral nerve stimulator be used to monitor response, need for additional doses, and recovery.

**For use in surgical patients**

It has been established that the duration of action of initial and subsequent doses of cisatracurium may be prolonged when the medication is given after anesthesia with a potent inhalation anesthetic (e.g., enflurane, isoflurane). Less frequent maintenance dosing and/or lower maintenance doses of cisatracurium may be required; infusion rate requirements may be decreased by 30 to 40% or more. However, alteration of initial dosage should not be necessary if cisatracurium is administered shortly after the start of anesthesia.

Repeated administration of maintenance doses of cisatracurium, or administration by continuous intravenous infusion for up to 3 hours, does not result in cumulative effects or tachyphylaxis.

The time needed for recovery from a maintenance dose is not affected by the number of doses given, if partial recovery is allowed to occur between doses. Maintenance doses therefore may be given at regular intervals.

**For use in intensive care patients**

Use of cisatracurium for longer than 6 days has not been studied.

Dosage requirements may increase or decrease with time. It is recommended that cisatracurium use be monitored via peripheral nerve stimulation. Cisatracurium infusion therapy should be discontinued temporarily if there is no response to stimulation, and treatment resumed, if necessary, only after a definite response is obtained.

The effects of procedures such as hemodialysis, hemoperfusion, or hemofiltration on the plasma concentrations of cisatracurium or its metabolites have not been determined.

Multiple-dose vials of cisatracurium for injection contain benzyl alcohol. Administration of excessive doses of benzyl alcohol to neonates has been associated with a fatal toxic syndrome consisting of metabolic acidosis, CNS depression, respiratory problems, renal failure, hypotension, and possibly seizures and intracranial hemorrhage. Administration of excessive doses of benzyl alcohol is more likely during prolonged use of cisatracurium, which may occur in intensive care patients.

**For reversal of neuromuscular blockade**

The effect of cisatracurium may be reversed by an anticholinesterase agent (e.g., 1 mg per kg of body weight [mg/kg] of edrophonium or 0.04 to 0.07 mg/kg of neostigmine), which should be administered concurrently with a suitable anticholinergic agent (e.g., atropine or glycopyrrolate). However, the antagonist should not be given until some spontaneous recovery has begun. The time required for recovery increases with the depth of neuromuscular blockade at the time the reversal agent is administered. Also, recovery may be delayed if certain medical conditions (e.g., carcinomatosis, debilitation, cachexia) are present, or if medications that enhance neuromuscular blockade (e.g., anesthetic agents, various antibiotics) and/or independently cause respiratory depression have been given.

Even after administration of a reversal agent, ventilatory assistance should be continued until the patient is able to maintain an adequate respiratory exchange unassisted.

Evidence of adequate recovery, such as grip strength and/or ability to maintain a 5-second head lift, should be evaluated after administration of a reversal agent.

## Parenteral Dosage Forms

Note: Cisatracurium injection contains cisatracurium besylate. However, the dosage and strengths of the injection are stated in terms of cisatracurium base (not the besylate salt).

### CISATRACURIUM INJECTION

**Usual adult and adolescent dose**
Skeletal muscle relaxation—
  Initial (intubating dose), for surgical or intensive care patients:
    Intravenous, 150 mcg (0.15 mg) (base) per kg of body weight, to produce intubating conditions in approximately two minutes and approximately fifty-five minutes of relaxation, or
    Intravenous, 200 mcg (0.2 mg) (base) per kg of body weight, to produce intubating conditions in approximately one and one-half minutes and approximately sixty-one minutes of relaxation.
  Maintenance:
    Surgical patients—
      Intravenous, 30 mcg (0.03 mg) (base) per kg of body weight, administered after the effects of the intubating dose begin to subside and at approximately twenty-minute intervals thereafter, although dosage may be adjusted as necessary to provide shorter or longer durations of action, or
      Intravenous infusion, 3 mcg (0.003 mg) (base) per kg of body weight per minute, initially, then decreased to 1 to 2 mcg (0.001 to 0.002 mg) per kg of body weight per minute.
    Note: In individuals undergoing coronary artery bypass surgery with induced hypothermia (body temperature of 25 to 28 °C [77 to 82.4 °F]), maintenance infusion rate requirements during hypothermia may be reduced to approximately 50% of those needed during normothermia.
      Less frequent maintenance dosing or lower maintenance doses may be required in patients who have been exposed to potent inhalation anesthetics (e.g., enflurane, isoflurane). Infusion rate requirements may be decreased by 30 to 40% or more.
    Intensive care patients—
      Intravenous infusion, 3 mcg (0.003 mg) (base) per kg of body weight per minute, initially, then adjusted as needed.[1] Dosage requirements are subject to wide interpatient variability; doses ranging from 0.5 to 10.2 mcg (0.0005 to 0.0102 mg) per kg of body weight per minute have been used. Also, dosage requirements may increase or decrease over time.
    Note: If significant recovery from neuromuscular blockade occurs when an infusion is stopped temporarily, administration of an intubating dose may be needed to re-establish neuromuscular blockade quickly before the infusion is resumed.

**Usual pediatric dose**
Skeletal muscle relaxation—
  Infants and children up to 2 years of age:
    Dosage has not been established.
  Children 2 years of age and older:
    Initial—
      Intravenous, 100 mcg (0.1 mg) (base) per kg of body weight, administered over five to ten seconds, to produce maximum blockade in approximately two minutes, forty-eight seconds and approximately twenty-eight minutes of relaxation.
    Maintenance—
      Surgical patients:
        Intravenous infusion, 3 mcg (0.003 mg) (base) per kg of body weight per minute, initially, then decreased to 1 to 2 mcg (0.001 to 0.002 mg) per kg of body weight per minute.
  Note: In individuals undergoing coronary artery bypass surgery with induced hypothermia (body temperature of 25 to 28 °C [77 to 82.4 °F]), maintenance infusion rate requirements during hypothermia may be reduced to approximately 50% of those needed during normothermia.
    Less frequent maintenance dosing or lower maintenance doses may be required in patients who have been exposed to potent inhalation anesthetics (e.g., enflurane, isoflurane). Infusion rate requirements may be decreased by 30 to 40% or more.
      Intensive care patients:
        Intravenous infusion, 3 mcg (0.003 mg) (base) per kg of body weight per minute, initially, then adjusted as needed.[1] Dosage requirements are subject to wide interpatient variability; doses ranging from 0.5 to 10.2 mcg (0.0005 to 0.0102 mg) per kg of body weight per minute have been used in adults. Also, dosage requirements may increase or decrease with time.
  Note: If significant recovery from neuromuscular blockade occurs when an infusion is stopped temporarily, administration of an intubating dose may be needed to re-establish neuromuscular blockade quickly before the infusion is resumed.

**Strength(s) usually available**
U.S.—
  2 mg (base) per mL (Rx) [*Nimbex* (benzenesulfonic acid; benzyl alcohol 0.9% [10-mL multiple-dose vial only])].
  10 mg (base) per mL (Rx) [*Nimbex* (benzenesulfonic acid)].
Canada—
  2 mg (base) per mL (Rx) [*Nimbex* (benzenesulfonic acid; benzyl alcohol 0.9% [10-mL multiple-dose vial only])].
  10 mg (base) per mL (Rx) [*Nimbex* (benzenesulfonic acid)].
Note: The 10-mg-per-mL strength is intended only for preparing intravenous infusions for adults to be used in the intensive care unit. The 10-mg-per-mL vials contain benzyl alcohol and should not be used to prepare infusions for neonates.

**Packaging and storage**
Store between 2 and 8 °C (36 and 46 °F) in the original carton. Protect from light and freezing.

**Preparation of dosage form**
For preparation of intravenous infusions, cisatracurium injection may be diluted with a suitable quantity of 5% dextrose injection, 0.9% sodium chloride injection, or 5% dextrose and 0.9% sodium chloride injection. The quantity of infusion required will depend on the concentration of cisatracurium, desired dose, and patient's body weight. The patient's fluid requirement also should be considered when determining an appropriate infusion volume. Cisatracurium injection may be infused through intravenous lines (i.e., by Y-site) administering solutions of droperidol, fentanyl citrate, midazolam hydrochloride, or sufentanil citrate, prepared according to the manufacturers' specifications.

**Stability**
Undiluted cisatracurium injection, when kept under refrigeration at 5 °C (41 °F), loses potency at a rate of approximately 5% per year. The rate of potency loss increases to 5% per month at room temperature (25 °C [77 °F]). The injection should be used within 21 days after it is brought to room temperature, even if it is subsequently re-refrigerated.
Cisatracurium infusions prepared by dilution to a concentration of 0.1 mg per mL with 5% dextrose injection, 0.9% sodium chloride injection, or 5% dextrose and 0.9% sodium chloride injection may be stored under refrigeration or at room temperature for up to 24 hours without significant loss of potency. Cisatracurium infusions prepared by dilution to a concentration of 0.1 or 0.2 mg per mL with 5% dextrose and lactated Ringer's injection are stable for up to 24 hours at 5 °C (41 °F).

**Incompatibilities**
Cisatracurium injection is incompatible with lactated Ringer's injection.
Cisatracurium injection is acidic and may not be compatible with injections having a pH greater than 8.5 (e.g., barbiturate injections).
Cisatracurium injection is incompatible with propofol injection or ketorolac injection for Y-site administration.

[1]Not included in Canadian product labeling.

Revised: 04/27/98

# CISPLATIN  Systemic

VA CLASSIFICATION (Primary): AN900
Commonly used brand name(s): *Platinol*; *Platinol-AQ*.
Note: For a listing of dosage forms and brand names by country availability, see *Dosage Forms* section(s).

## Category
Antineoplastic.

## Indications
Note: Bracketed information in the *Indications* section refers to uses that are not included in U.S. product labeling.

**Accepted**
Carcinoma, bladder (treatment)—Cisplatin is indicated as a single agent for treatment of transitional cell cancer of the bladder that is no longer amenable to local treatments such as surgery and/or radiotherapy.
Carcinoma, ovarian (treatment)—Cisplatin is indicated in combination with other chemotherapeutic agents for treatment of metastatic ovarian tumors in patients who have already received appropriate surgical and/or radiotherapeutic procedures. It is indicated, as a single agent, as secondary therapy of metastatic ovarian tumors refractory to standard chemotherapy that did not include cisplatin.
Carcinoma, testicular (treatment)—Cisplatin is indicated in combination with other chemotherapeutic agents for treatment of metastatic testicular tumors in patients who have already received appropriate surgical and/or radiotherapeutic procedures.
[Carcinoma, adrenocortical (treatment)][1]
[Carcinoma, breast (treatment)][1]
[Carcinoma, cervical (treatment)][1]
[Carcinoma, endometrial (treatment)][1]
[Carcinoma, esophageal (treatment)][1]
[Carcinoma, gastric (treatment)][1]
[Carcinoma, lung, non–small cell (treatment)][1]
[Carcinoma, lung, small cell (treatment)][1]
[Neuroblastoma (treatment)][1]
[Carcinoma, pancreatic (treatment)][1]
[Carcinoma, prostatic (treatment)][1]
[Carcinoma, head and neck (treatment)][1]
[Carcinoma, hepatocellular, primary (treatment)][1]
[Carcinoma, thyroid (treatment)][1] or
[Thymoma (treatment)][1]—Cisplatin is indicated for treatment of adrenocortical carcinoma, breast carcinoma, cervical carcinoma, endometrial carcinoma, esophageal carcinoma, gastric carcinoma, non–small cell lung carcinoma, small cell lung carcinoma, neuroblastoma in children, pancreatic carcinoma, prostatic carcinoma, squamous cell carcinoma of the head and neck, primary hepatocellular carcinoma, thyroid carcinoma, and thymoma.
[Carcinoma, anal (treatment)][1]—Cisplatin is indicated for treatment of anal carcinoma (Evidence rating: IIID).
[Melanoma, malignant (treatment)][1]—Cisplatin is indicated for treatment of malignant melanoma.
[Lymphoma, Hodgkin's (treatment)][1] or
[Lymphoma, non-Hodgkin's (treatment)][1]—Cisplatin is indicated for treatment of Hodgkin's and non-Hodgkin's lymphomas.
[Hepatoblastoma (treatment)][1]
[Tumors, germ cell, ovarian (treatment)][1]
[Tumors, germ cell (treatment)][1]
[Tumors, trophoblastic, gestational (treatment)][1] or
[Wilms' tumor (treatment)][1]—Cisplatin is indicated for treatment of hepatoblastoma in children, ovarian germ cell tumors, germ cell tumors in children, gestational trophoblastic tumors, and Wilms' tumors in children.
[Osteosarcoma (treatment)][1]—Cisplatin is indicated for treatment of osteosarcoma in children.
[Sarcoma, soft tissue (treatment)][1]—Cisplatin is indicated, in combination with other chemotherapeutic agents, for treatment of soft tissue sarcomas (Evidence rating: IA).
[Kaposi's sarcoma, acquired immunodeficiency syndrome (AIDS)–associated (treatment)][1]—Cisplatin is indicated for treatment of AIDS-associated Kaposi's sarcoma.

[1]Not included in Canadian product labeling.

## Pharmacology/Pharmacokinetics

**Physicochemical characteristics**
Molecular weight—300.06.

**Mechanism of action/Effect**
Cisplatin resembles an alkylating agent. Although the exact mechanism of action is unknown, action is thought to be similar to that of the bifunctional alkylating agents, that is, possible cross-linking and interference with the function of DNA and a small effect on RNA. It is cell cycle phase–nonspecific. Stimulation of the host immune system is also possible.

**Distribution**
Does not readily cross the blood-brain barrier.

**Protein binding**
Metabolites—Very high (more than 90%) during excretory (beta) phase.

**Biotransformation**
By rapid nonenzymatic conversion to inactive metabolites.

**Half-life**
Alpha phase—
  25 to 49 minutes.

Beta phase (in hours)—
  Normal: 58 to 73.
  Anuric: Up to 240.

**Duration of action**
Inhibition of DNA persists for several days following administration.

**Elimination**
Renal (27 to 43% after 5 days); platinum may be detected in tissues for 4 months or more after administration.

In dialysis—Cisplatin is removable by dialysis, but only within 3 hours after administration.

## Precautions to Consider

### Carcinogenicity
Secondary malignancies are potential delayed effects of many antineoplastic agents, although it is not clear whether the effect is related to their mutagenic or immunosuppressive action. The effect of dose and duration of therapy is also unknown, although risk seems to increase with long-term use. Although information is limited, available data seem to indicate that the carcinogenic risk is greatest with the alkylating agents.

Development of acute leukemia has been reported to occur rarely in patients treated with cisplatin, usually in combination with other leukemogenic agents.

In studies of 50 BD IX rats administered intraperitoneal doses of cisplatin at 1 mg per kg of body weight (mg/kg) three times per week for 3 weeks, 33 animals died within 455 days after the first application. Thirteen of the deaths were related to malignancies (12 cases of leukemias and 1 of fibrosarcoma).

### Mutagenicity
Cisplatin is mutagenic in bacteria and has been shown to cause chromosome aberrations in animal cells in tissue culture.

### Pregnancy/Reproduction
Fertility—Gonadal suppression, resulting in amenorrhea or azoospermia, may occur in patients taking antineoplastic therapy, especially with the alkylating agents. In general, these effects appear to be related to the dose and length of therapy and may be irreversible. Prediction of the degree of testicular or ovarian function impairment is complicated by the common use of combinations of several antineoplastics, which makes it difficult to assess the effects of individual agents.

Pregnancy—Cisplatin may be toxic to the fetal urogenital tract.

First trimester: It is usually recommended that use of antineoplastics, especially combination chemotherapy, be avoided whenever possible, especially during the first trimester. Although information is limited because of the relatively few instances of antineoplastic administration during pregnancy, the mutagenic, teratogenic, and carcinogenic potential of these medications must be considered.

Other hazards to the fetus include adverse reactions seen in adults.

In general, use of a contraceptive is recommended during cytotoxic drug therapy.

Cisplatin is embryotoxic and teratogenic in mice.

FDA Pregnancy Category D.

### Breast-feeding
Although very little information is available regarding distribution of antineoplastic agents into breast milk, breast-feeding is not recommended during chemotherapy because of the risks to the infant (adverse effects, mutagenicity, carcinogenicity).

### Pediatrics
Ototoxic effects of cisplatin may be more severe in children.

### Geriatrics
No information is available on the relationship of age to the effects of cisplatin in geriatric patients. However, elderly patients are more likely to have age-related renal function impairment, which may require reduction of dosage in patients receiving cisplatin.

### Dental
The bone marrow depressant effects of cisplatin may result in an increased incidence of microbial infection, delayed healing, and gingival bleeding. Dental work, whenever possible, should be completed prior to initiation of therapy or deferred until blood counts have returned to normal. Patients should be instructed in proper oral hygiene during treatment, including caution in use of regular toothbrushes, dental floss, and toothpicks.

Cisplatin may also rarely cause stomatitis associated with considerable discomfort.

### Drug interactions and/or related problems
The following drug interactions and/or related problems have been selected on the basis of their potential clinical significance (possible mechanism in parentheses where appropriate)—not necessarily inclusive (» = major clinical significance):

Note: Combinations containing any of the following medications, depending on the amount present, may also interact with this medication.

Allopurinol or
Colchicine or
» Probenecid or
» Sulfinpyrazone
  (cisplatin may raise the concentration of blood uric acid; dosage adjustment of antigout agents may be necessary to control hyperuricemia and gout; allopurinol may be preferred to prevent or reverse cisplatin-induced hyperuricemia because of risk of uric acid nephropathy with uricosuric antigout agents)

Antihistamines or
Buclizine or
Cyclizine or
Loxapine or
Meclizine or
Phenothiazines or
Thioxanthenes or
Trimethobenzamide
  (concurrent use with cisplatin may mask the symptoms of ototoxicity, such as tinnitus, dizziness, or vertigo)

Bleomycin
  (cisplatin-induced renal function impairment may result in bleomycin toxicity even at low doses; caution is recommended because of the frequent combination of these two agents)

Blood dyscrasia–causing medications (see *Appendix II*)
  (leukopenic and/or thrombocytopenic effects of cisplatin may be increased with concurrent or recent therapy if these medications cause the same effects; dosage adjustment of cisplatin, if necessary, should be based on blood counts)

» Bone marrow depressants, other (see *Appendix II*) or
Radiation therapy
  (concurrent use may increase the total effects of these medications and radiation therapy; dosage reduction is recommended)

» Nephrotoxic medications, other (see *Appendix II*) or
» Ototoxic medications, other (see *Appendix II*)
  (concurrent and/or sequential administration should be avoided since the potential for ototoxicity and nephrotoxicity may be increased, especially in the presence of renal function impairment)

Vaccines, killed virus
  (because normal defense mechanisms may be suppressed by cisplatin therapy, the patient's antibody response to the vaccine may be decreased. The interval between discontinuation of medications that cause immunosuppression and restoration of the patient's ability to respond to the vaccine depends on the intensity and type of immunosuppression-causing medication used, the underlying disease, and other factors; estimates vary from 3 months to 1 year)

» Vaccines, live virus
  (because normal defense mechanisms may be suppressed by cisplatin therapy, concurrent use with a live virus vaccine may potentiate the replication of the vaccine virus, may increase the side/adverse effects of the vaccine virus, and/or may decrease the patient's antibody response to the vaccine; immunization of these patients should be undertaken only with extreme caution after careful review of the patient's hematologic status and only with the knowledge and consent of the physician managing the cisplatin therapy. The interval between discontinuation of medications that cause immunosuppression and restoration of the patient's ability to respond to the vaccine depends on the intensity and type of immunosuppression-causing medication used, the underlying disease, and other factors; estimates vary from 3 months to 1 year. In addition, immunization with oral poliovirus vaccine should be postponed in persons in close contact with the patient, especially family members)

### Laboratory value alterations
The following have been selected on the basis of their potential clinical significance (possible effect in parentheses where appropriate)—not necessarily inclusive (» = major clinical significance):

With physiology/laboratory test values
  Aspartate aminotransferase (AST [SGOT]), serum
    (values may be increased transiently)
  Bilirubin, serum
    (concentrations may be increased transiently)
  Blood urea nitrogen (BUN) and
  Creatinine, serum and
  Uric acid, serum
    (concentrations may be increased, indicating nephrotoxicity)

Calcium, serum and
Creatinine clearance and
Magnesium, serum and
Phosphate, serum and
Potassium, serum and
Sodium, serum
  (may be decreased, probably as a result of renal toxicity; rarely, tetany associated with hypocalcemia and hypomagnesemia has occurred)
Coombs' test
  (positive results, associated with hemolytic anemia, have been reported)

### Medical considerations/Contraindications
The medical considerations/contraindications included have been selected on the basis of their potential clinical significance (reasons given in parentheses where appropriate)—not necessarily inclusive (» = major clinical significance).

*Risk-benefit should be considered when the following medical problems exist:*
» Bone marrow depression
» Chickenpox, existing or recent (including recent exposure) or
» Herpes zoster
  (risk of severe generalized disease)
  Gout, history of or
  Urate renal stones, history of
  (risk of hyperuricemia)
» Hearing impairment
» Infection
» Renal function impairment
  (reduced excretion; a lower dosage of cisplatin is recommended)
  Sensitivity to cisplatin
» Caution should be used also in patients who have had previous cytotoxic drug therapy or radiation therapy.

### Patient monitoring
The following are especially important in patient monitoring (other tests may be warranted in some patients, depending on condition; » = major clinical significance):
» Audiometric testing and
» Neurologic function studies
  (determinations recommended prior to initiation of therapy and at periodic intervals during therapy)
  Blood urea nitrogen (BUN) and
» Creatinine clearance and
  Creatinine, serum
  (determinations recommended prior to initiation of therapy and before each course of cisplatin to detect renal toxicity)
  Calcium, serum and
  Magnesium, serum and
  Phosphate, serum and
  Potassium, serum
  (determinations recommended at periodic intervals during therapy)
» Hematocrit or hemoglobin and
» Leukocyte count, total and, if appropriate, differential and
» Platelet count
  (determinations recommended prior to initiation of therapy and at periodic intervals during therapy; frequency varies according to clinical state, agent, dose, and other agents being used concurrently)
  Uric acid, serum
  (determinations recommended prior to initiation of therapy and at periodic intervals during therapy; frequency varies according to clinical state, agent, dose, and other agents being used concurrently)

## Side/Adverse Effects
Note: Many "side effects" of antineoplastic therapy are unavoidable and represent the medication's pharmacologic action. Some of these (for example, leukopenia and thrombocytopenia) are actually used as parameters to aid in individual dosage titration.

Side effects are more pronounced at doses of cisplatin greater than 50 mg per square meter of body surface area.

Vascular toxicities have been reported rarely when cisplatin is given in combination with other antineoplastic agents, although it is unknown whether the toxicity is related to cisplatin administration or to other factors. Vascular toxicities reported include myocardial infarction, cerebrovascular accident, thrombotic microangiopathy, cerebral arteritis, and Raynaud's phenomenon.

The following side/adverse effects have been selected on the basis of their potential clinical significance (possible signs and symptoms in parentheses where appropriate)—not necessarily inclusive:

### Those indicating need for medical attention
*Incidence more frequent*—severity increases with repeated doses
**Anemia secondary to myelosuppression** (unusual tiredness or weakness)—usually asymptomatic; **leukopenia** (fever or chills; cough or hoarseness; lower back or side pain; painful or difficult urination)—usually asymptomatic; **nephrotoxicity, hyperuricemia, or uric acid nephropathy** (joint pain; lower back or side pain; swelling of feet or lower legs); **neurotoxicity** (loss of reflexes; loss of taste; numbness or tingling in fingers or toes; seizures; trouble in walking; rarely, muscle cramps); **ototoxicity** (loss of balance; ringing in ears; trouble in hearing); **thrombocytopenia** (unusual bleeding or bruising; black, tarry stools; blood in urine or stools; pinpoint red spots on skin)—usually asymptomatic

Note: *Myelosuppression (leukopenia, thrombocytopenia, anemia)* is more pronounced at higher doses. Nadir of leukocyte and platelet counts occurs after 18 to 23 days and counts usually recover by 39 days after a dose.

Cisplatin frequently causes *nephrotoxicity* in the form of acute renal dysfunction, which may be detected initially only by means of renal function tests. Laboratory abnormalities occur during the second week after a dose. Nephrotoxicity is dose-related and cumulative; it is usually reversible, but may become irreversible at high doses or with repeated treatments, and is occasionally fatal.

Hypocalcemia and hypomagnesemia may occur due to *nephrotoxicity*. Rarely, tetany associated with hypocalcemia may occur, and tremors or seizures may occur as a result of hypomagnesemia.

With *hyperuricemia*, peak uric acid concentrations occur 3 to 5 days after a dose.

*Neurotoxicity*, usually characterized by peripheral neuropathies, may occur after a single dose or prolonged therapy (4 to 7 months) and may be severe and irreversible. Signs and symptoms of neuropathy usually develop during treatment, but may rarely begin 3 to 8 weeks after the last dose, and may progress even after withdrawal of cisplatin. Muscle cramps (localized, painful, involuntary skeletal contractions of sudden onset and short duration) have been reported, usually in patients receiving a relatively high cumulative dose of cisplatin and in a relatively advanced symptomatic stage of peripheral neuropathy. Lhermitte's sign, dorsal column myelopathy, and autonomic neuropathy have also been reported.

*Ototoxicity* may be more severe in children and may not be reversible. Ototoxicity may also occur more frequently and may be more severe in patients of any age who have received prior cranial radiotherapy. Ototoxicity is cumulative; hearing loss usually occurs first with high frequencies (above speech tones) and may be unilateral or bilateral.

*Incidence less frequent*
**Anaphylactic reaction, occurring within a few minutes after administration** (dizziness or fainting; fast heartbeat; swelling of face; wheezing); **extravasation** (pain or redness at site of injection)

Note: *Extravasation* may rarely produce local soft tissue toxicity, the severity of which is related to the concentration of the solution. Infusion of solutions containing cisplatin in a concentration greater than 500 mcg (0.5 mg) per mL may result in tissue cellulitis, fibrosis, and necrosis.

*Incidence rare*
**Hemolytic anemia** (unusual tiredness or weakness)—usually asymptomatic; **optic neuritis, papilledema, or cerebral blindness** (blurred vision; change in ability to see colors, especially blue or yellow); **stomatitis** (sores in mouth and on lips); **syndrome of inappropriate antidiuretic hormone (SIADH) secretion** (dizziness, confusion, or agitation; unusual tiredness or weakness)

Note: A Coombs'-positive *hemolytic anemia* has also been reported.
*Optic neuritis, papilledema, or cerebral blindness* is usually reversible after withdrawal of cisplatin. Fundoscopic examination usually finds only irregular retinal pigmentation of the macular area.

### Those indicating need for medical attention only if they continue or are bothersome
*Incidence more frequent*—occurs in most patients
**Nausea and vomiting, severe**

Note: *Nausea and vomiting* usually begin 1 to 4 hours after a dose, and vomiting may persist for 24 hours. Nausea and anorexia may persist for up to 1 week. Serotonin antagonists (e.g., ondansetron), high-dose intravenous metoclopramide, or corticosteroids have been found to be useful in preventing severe nausea and vomiting; however, severe nausea and vomiting may require discontinuation of cisplatin.

Incidence less frequent
*Loss of appetite*

**Those indicating need for medical attention if they occur after medication is discontinued**
*Myelosuppression* (black, tarry stools; blood in urine or stools; cough or hoarseness; fever or chills; lower back or side pain; painful or difficult urination; pinpoint red spots on skin; unusual bleeding or bruising); *nephrotoxicity* (decrease in urination; swelling of feet or lower legs); *neurotoxicity* (loss of reflexes; loss of taste; numbness or tingling in fingers or toes; seizures; trouble in walking); *ototoxicity* (loss of balance; ringing in ears; trouble in hearing)

## Patient Consultation
As an aid to patient consultation, refer to *Advice for the Patient, Cisplatin (Systemic)*.

In providing consultation, consider emphasizing the following selected information (» = major clinical significance):

**Before using this medication**
» Conditions affecting use, especially:
Sensitivity to cisplatin
Pregnancy—Use not recommended because of mutagenic, teratogenic, and carcinogenic potential; advisability of using a contraceptive; telling physician immediately if pregnancy is suspected
Breast-feeding—Not recommended because of serious side effects
Use in children—Ototoxicity may be more severe
Other medications, especially probenecid, sulfinpyrazone, other bone marrow depressants, other nephrotoxic medications, other ototoxic medications, live virus vaccines, or previous cytotoxic drug therapy or radiation therapy
Other medical problems, especially chickenpox, herpes zoster, hearing impairment, infection, or renal function impairment

**Proper use of this medication**
Caution if taking combination therapy; taking each medication at the right time
Importance of ample fluid intake and subsequent increase in urine output to aid in excretion of uric acid
Frequency of severe nausea and vomiting; importance of continuing medication despite stomach upset
» Proper dosing

**Precautions while using this medication**
» Importance of close monitoring by the physician
» Avoiding immunizations unless approved by physician; other persons in patient's household should avoid immunizations with oral poliovirus vaccine; avoiding persons who have taken oral poliovirus vaccine or wearing a protective mask that covers nose and mouth
*Caution if bone marrow depression occurs*
» Avoiding exposure to persons with infections, especially during periods of low blood counts; checking with physician immediately if fever or chills, cough or hoarseness, lower back or side pain, or painful or difficult urination occurs
» Checking with physician immediately if unusual bleeding or bruising; black, tarry stools; blood in urine or stools; or pinpoint red spots on skin occur
Caution in use of regular toothbrush, dental floss, or toothpick; physician, dentist, or nurse may suggest alternatives; checking with physician before having dental work done
Not touching eyes or inside of nose unless hands washed immediately before
Using caution to avoid accidental cuts with use of sharp objects such as safety razor or fingernail or toenail cutters
Avoiding contact sports or other situations where bruising or injury could occur
» Possibility of local tissue injury and scarring if infiltration of intravenous solution occurs; telling doctor or nurse right away about redness, pain, or swelling at injection site

**Side/adverse effects**
Importance of discussing possible effects, including cancer, with physician
Signs of potential side effects, especially anemia, leukopenia, nephrotoxicity, hyperuricemia, uric acid nephropathy, neurotoxicity, ototoxicity, thrombocytopenia, anaphylactic reaction, extravasation, hemolytic anemia, optic neuritis, papilledema, cerebral blindness, stomatitis, and SIADH secretion
Physician or nurse can help in dealing with side effects

## General Dosing Information
It is recommended that cisplatin be administered to patients in an appropriate setting under supervision of a physician or nurse experienced in cancer chemotherapy. It is also recommended that equipment and medications (including epinephrine, oxygen, antihistamines, and intravenous corticosteroids) necessary for treatment of a possible anaphylactic reaction be readily available at each administration of cisplatin.

A variety of dosage schedules and regimens of cisplatin, alone or in combination with other antitumor agents, are used. The prescriber may consult the medical literature as well as the manufacturer's literature in choosing a specific dosage.

It is recommended that cisplatin be administered with vigorous parenteral infusion to increase hydration; this is intended to maintain urine output and reduce nephrotoxicity and ototoxicity, although it will not prevent them.

Vigorous pretreatment intravenous hydration, followed by adequate hydration and urinary output for 24 hours, are recommended. Mannitol or furosemide may also be used to produce acute diuresis, provided that salt and water depletion are avoided.

Cisplatin has also been administered as a continuous intravenous infusion over periods ranging from 24 hours to 5 days; this method of administration appears to reduce nausea and vomiting but not nephrotoxicity or ototoxicity. It is very important that orders for the total dose to be given over the entire course of the infusion *not* be misinterpreted as a daily dose, because of the risk of fatal overdose.

Development of uric acid nephropathy may be prevented by adequate oral hydration and, in some cases, administration of allopurinol. Alkalinization of urine may be necessary if serum uric acid concentrations are elevated.

It is recommended that courses of cisplatin be administered no more frequently than every 3 to 4 weeks, to reduce the risk of cumulative nephrotoxicity.

Subsequent doses of cisplatin must not be given before renal function approaches normal (measured by BUN, creatinine clearance, and serum creatinine). Administration of subsequent doses of cisplatin also is not recommended before platelet levels return to at least 100,000 per cubic millimeter and leukocyte levels to at least 4000 per cubic millimeter, or before auditory acuity is confirmed to be within normal limits.

Therapy with cisplatin should be discontinued at the first sign of significant neurotoxicity, which may be irreversible.

Special precautions are recommended in patients who develop thrombocytopenia as a result of administration of cisplatin. These may include extreme care in performing invasive procedures; regular inspection of intravenous sites, skin (including perirectal area), and mucous membrane surfaces for signs of bleeding or bruising; limiting frequency of venipuncture and avoiding intramuscular injections; testing urine, emesis, stool, and secretions for occult blood; care in use of regular toothbrushes, dental floss, toothpicks, safety razors, and fingernail and toenail cutters; avoiding constipation; and using caution to prevent falls and other injuries. Such patients should avoid alcohol and aspirin intake because of the risk of gastrointestinal bleeding. Platelet transfusions may be required.

Patients who develop leukopenia should be observed carefully for signs of infection. Antibiotic support may be required. In neutropenic patients who develop fever, broad-spectrum antibiotic coverage should be initiated empirically, pending bacterial cultures and appropriate diagnostic tests.

## Safety considerations for handling this medication
There is limited but increasing evidence and concern that personnel involved in preparation and administration of parenteral antineoplastics may be at some risk because of the potential mutagenicity, teratogenicity, and/or carcinogenicity of these agents, although the actual risk is unknown. USP advisory panels recommend cautious handling both in preparation and disposal of antineoplastic agents. Precautions that have been suggested include:
- Use of a biological containment cabinet during reconstitution and dilution of parenteral medications and wearing of disposable surgical gloves and masks.
- Use of proper technique to prevent contamination of the medication, work area, and operator during transfer between containers (including proper training of personnel in this technique).
- Cautious and proper disposal of needles, syringes, vials, ampuls, and unused medication.

A number of medical centers have developed detailed guidelines for handling of antineoplastic agents.

## Cisplatin (Systemic)

**Combination chemotherapy**
Cisplatin may be used in combination with other agents in various regimens. As a result, incidence and/or severity of side effects may be altered and different dosages (usually reduced) may be used. For example, cisplatin is part of the following chemotherapeutic combination (some commonly used acronyms are in parentheses):
—cyclophosphamide, doxorubicin, and cisplatin (CISCA or CAP).

For specific dosages and schedules, consult the literature. For information regarding each agent, consult the individual monographs.

## Parenteral Dosage Forms

Note: Bracketed uses in the *Dosage Forms* section refer to categories of use and/or indications that are not included in U.S. product labeling.

### CISPLATIN INJECTION

**Usual adult and adolescent dose**
Metastatic testicular tumors—
   Intravenous, 20 mg per square meter of body surface area a day for five days per twenty-one–day cycle.
Metastatic ovarian tumors—
   Intravenous, 75 to 100 mg per square meter of body surface area once every four weeks (day 1), in combination with 600 mg of cyclophosphamide per square meter of body surface area intravenously every four weeks on day 1 (administered sequentially), or
   Intravenous, 100 mg per square meter of body surface area once every four weeks (as a single agent), or
   Intravenous, 75 mg per square meter of body surface area once every three weeks, given in combination with 135 mg of paclitaxel (given over twenty-four hours) per square meter of body surface area every three weeks, for six courses.
Advanced bladder cancer—
   Intravenous, 50 to 70 mg per square meter of body surface area every three to four weeks (as a single agent). The lower end of the dosage range is recommended in patients heavily pretreated with radiation or chemotherapy.
[Carcinoma, adrenocortical (treatment)][1] or
[Carcinoma, breast (treatment)][1] or
[Carcinoma, cervical (treatment)][1] or
[Carcinoma, endometrial (treatment)][1] or
[Carcinoma, esophageal (treatment)][1] or
[Carcinoma, gastric (treatment)][1] or
[Carcinoma, lung, non–small cell (treatment)][1] or
[Carcinoma, lung, small cell (treatment)][1] or
[Neuroblastoma (treatment)][1] or
[Carcinoma, pancreatic (treatment)][1] or
[Carcinoma, prostatic (treatment)][1] or
[Carcinoma, head and neck (treatment)][1] or
[Carcinoma, hepatocellular, primary (treatment)][1] or
[Carcinoma, thyroid (treatment)][1] or
[Thymoma (treatment)][1] or
[Carcinoma, anal (treatment)][1] or
[Melanoma, malignant (treatment)][1] or
[Lymphoma, Hodgkin's (treatment)][1] or
[Lymphoma, non-Hodgkin's (treatment)][1] or
[Hepatoblastoma (treatment)][1] or
[Tumors, germ cell, ovarian (treatment)][1] or
[Tumors, germ cell (treatment)][1] or
[Tumors, trophoblastic, gestational (treatment)][1] or
[Wilms' tumor (treatment)][1] or
[Osteosarcoma (treatment)][1] or
[Sarcoma, soft tissue (treatment)][1] or
[Kaposi's sarcoma, acquired immunodeficiency syndrome (AIDS)–associated (treatment)][1]—
   Consult medical literature and manufacturer's literature for specific dosage.

**Usual adult prescribing limits**
Total dose for a single *course* of cisplatin (whether given as a single daily infusion or as a continuous infusion over several days, to be repeated every three to four weeks) should not exceed 120 mg per square meter of body surface area. Administration of higher doses in a single course may lead to potentially fatal overdose. Exceptions should be made, and care of these patients should be handled, only by medical professionals who fully understand and are prepared to deal with the potential toxicities of such dosing.

**Usual pediatric dose**
See *Usual adult and adolescent dose*.

**Strength(s) usually available**
U.S.—
   1 mg per mL (50-, and 100-mL vials) (Rx) [*Platinol-AQ* (sodium chloride 9 mg per mL)].
Canada—
   500 mcg (0.5 mg) per mL (20-, 50-, and 100-mL vials) (Rx) [*Platinol-AQ* (sodium chloride 9 mg per mL); GENERIC].
   1 mg per mL (10-, 50-, and 100-mL vials) [*Platinol-AQ* (sodium chloride 9 mg per mL)].

**Packaging and storage**
Store between 15 and 25 °C (59 and 77 °F), unless otherwise specified by manufacturer. Do not refrigerate.

**Stability**
Caution—A black platinum precipitate will form if cisplatin comes in contact with aluminum.
Solution remaining in amber vial following initial entry is stable for 28 days protected from light or for 7 days under fluorescent room light.

**Incompatibilities**
Do not use needles, intravenous sets, or equipment containing aluminum for administration since cisplatin is incompatible with aluminum.

**Note**
No more than 120 mg per square meter of body surface area per course (with each course separated by three to four weeks) should be dispensed without verbal or written confirmation by the prescribing physician. To reduce the risk of fatal overdose, no more than the amount for one course should be dispensed at one time.

### CISPLATIN FOR INJECTION USP

**Usual adult and adolescent dose**
See *Cisplatin Injection*.

**Usual adult prescribing limits**
See *Cisplatin Injection*.

**Usual pediatric dose**
See *Cisplatin Injection*.

**Size(s) usually available**
U.S.—
   Not commercially available.
Canada—
   10 mg (Rx) [*Platinol*].
   50 mg (Rx) [*Platinol*].

**Packaging and storage**
Store below 40 °C (104 °F), preferably between 15 and 30 °C (59 and 86 °F), unless otherwise specified by manufacturer. Protect from light.

**Preparation of dosage form**
Cisplatin for injection is reconstituted for intravenous use by adding 10 or 50 mL of sterile water for injection to the 10-mg or 50-mg vial, respectively, producing a clear, colorless solution containing 1 mg of cisplatin per mL. It is recommended that 5% dextrose injection in 0.3 or 0.45% sodium chloride injection be used if further dilution for administration by intravenous solution is required, in order to ensure stability.

**Stability**
Reconstituted solutions of cisplatin are stable for 20 hours at 27 °C (80 °F). Solution removed from the amber vial should be protected from light if it is not to be used within 6 hours.

**Incompatibilities**
Do not use needles, intravenous sets, or equipment containing aluminum for administration since cisplatin is incompatible with aluminum.

**Caution**
A precipitate will form if reconstituted solutions are refrigerated.
A black platinum precipitate will form if cisplatin comes in contact with aluminum.

**Note**
No more than 120 mg per square meter of body surface area per course (with each course separated by three to four weeks) should be dispensed without verbal or written confirmation by the prescribing physician. To reduce the risk of fatal overdose, no more than the amount for one course should be dispensed at one time.

[1]Not included in Canadian product labeling.

Revised: 06/24/98

# CITRATES Systemic

This monograph includes information on the following: 1) Potassium Citrate; 2) Potassium Citrate and Citric Acid; 3) Potassium Citrate and Sodium Citrate; 4) Sodium Citrate and Citric Acid; 5) Tricitrates.

VA CLASSIFICATION (Primary/Secondary):
Potassium Citrate—TN410/GU900
Potassium Citrate and Citric Acid—TN410/GU900; TN900
Potassium Citrate and Sodium Citrate—TN410/GU900
Sodium Citrate and Citric Acid—TN410/GU900; TN900
Tricitrates—TN410/GU900; TN900

Commonly used brand name(s): *Bicitra*[4]; *Citrolith*[3]; *Oracit*[4]; *Polycitra Syrup*[5]; *Polycitra-K*[2]; *Polycitra-K Crystals*[2]; *Polycitra-LC*[5]; *Urocit-K*[1].

Other commonly used names for sodium citrate and citric acid are Albright's solution and modified Shohl's solution.

Note: For a listing of dosage forms and brand names by country availability, see *Dosage Forms* section(s).

## Category

Antiurolithic, uric acid calculi—Potassium Citrate; Potassium Citrate and Citric Acid; Potassium Citrate and Sodium Citrate; Sodium Citrate and Citric Acid; Tricitrates.

Antiurolithic, cystine calculi—Potassium Citrate; Potassium Citrate and Citric Acid; Potassium Citrate and Sodium Citrate; Sodium Citrate and Citric Acid; Tricitrates.

Antiurolithic, calcium oxalate calculi—Potassium Citrate; Potassium Citrate and Citric Acid.

Antiurolithic, calcium phosphate calculi—Potassium Citrate; Potassium Citrate and Citric Acid.

Alkalizer, systemic—Potassium Citrate and Citric Acid; Sodium Citrate and Citric Acid; Tricitrates.

Alkalizer, urinary—Potassium Citrate; Potassium Citrate and Citric Acid; Potassium Citrate and Sodium Citrate; Sodium Citrate and Citric Acid; Tricitrates.

Buffer, neutralizing—Sodium Citrate and Citric Acid; Tricitrates.

## Indications

### Accepted

Renal calculi, cystine (prophylaxis and treatment) or
Renal calculi, uric acid (prophylaxis and treatment)—Citrates are indicated as urinary alkalizers in the prevention and treatment of uric acid or cystine lithiasis. They are often used in gout therapy as urinary alkalizers to prevent crystallization of urates.

Renal calculi, calcium (prophylaxis and treatment) or
Hypocitraturia (prophylaxis and treatment)—Potassium citrate and potassium citrate and citric acid are also indicated to increase urinary citrate in the prevention and treatment of calcium phosphate, calcium oxalate, or uric acid kidney stones in such conditions as renal tubular acidosis with calcium stones, hypocitraturic calcium oxalate nephrolithiasis of any etiology, and uric acid or cystine lithiasis with or without calcium stones.

Acidosis, in renal tubular disorders (treatment)—Potassium citrate and citric acid, sodium citrate and citric acid, and tricitrates are also used in the treatment of chronic metabolic acidosis resulting from chronic renal insufficiency or the syndrome of renal tubular acidosis. Sodium citrate is especially useful when the administration of potassium salts is undesirable or contraindicated.

Pneumonitis, aspiration (prophylaxis)—Sodium citrate and citric acid and tricitrates are used in preanesthesia medication as nonparticulate acid-neutralizing buffers of gastric acid to lessen the danger from acid-aspiration pneumonitis in patients at risk. Citrates have generally been replaced by the equally or more effective $H_2$-receptor antagonists in the prevention of acid aspiration in elective surgery. However, citrates and other antacids have a more rapid onset of action than $H_2$-receptor antagonists and may be more useful in emergency situations.

## Pharmacology/Pharmacokinetics

### Physicochemical characteristics

Molecular weight—
Potassium citrate: 324.41.
Sodium citrate: 258.07 (anhydrous).
Citric acid: 192.12.

### Mechanism of action/Effect

Alkalizer, urinary or
Antiurolithic, uric acid calculi or
Antiurolithic, cystine calculi—Sodium citrate and potassium citrate are metabolized to bicarbonates, which increase urinary pH by increasing the excretion of free bicarbonate ions, without producing systemic alkalosis when administered in recommended doses. A rise in urinary pH increases the solubility of cystine in the urine and the ionization of uric acid to more soluble urate ion. By maintaining an alkaline urine, the actual dissolution of uric acid stones may be accomplished.

Antiurolithic, calcium calculi—Metabolism of absorbed potassium citrate produces an alkaline load, raising urinary pH and increasing urinary citrate by augmenting citrate clearance. Thus, potassium citrate therapy appears to increase urinary citrate mainly by changing the renal handling of citrate, and, to a smaller extent, by increasing the filterable load of citrate. Increased urinary citrate and pH decreases calcium ion activity by increasing calcium complexation to dissociated anions and thus decreasing the saturation of calcium oxalate.

Potassium citrate also inhibits the crystallization and spontaneous nucleation of calcium oxalate and calcium phosphate in hypocitraturic calcium nephrolithiasis. However, potassium citrate does not alter the urinary saturation of calcium phosphate, because the effect of increased citrate complexation of calcium is antagonized by the rise in pH-dependent dissociation of phosphate. Calcium phosphate stones are more stable in alkaline urine.

Alkalizer, systemic—Increases the plasma bicarbonate, buffers excess hydrogen ion concentration, and raises blood pH, thereby reversing the clinical manifestations of acidosis.

Neutralizing buffer—Reacts chemically to neutralize or buffer existing quantities of gastric hydrochloric acid but has no direct effect on its output.

### Biotransformation

Oxidized in the body to form potassium bicarbonate or sodium bicarbonate. Effects are essentially those of chlorides before absorption and those of bicarbonates after absorption.

### Onset of action

Potassium citrate—Single dose: Within 1 hour.

### Duration of action

Potassium citrate tablets—
Single dose: Up to 12 hours.
Multiple doses: 3 days.

Potassium citrate and citric acid oral solution—Up to 24 hours at dosage of—
10 to 15 mL four times a day: Maintains a urine pH of 6.5 to 7.4.
15 to 20 mL four times a day: Maintains a urine pH of 7.0 to 7.6.

Tricitrates oral solution—Up to 24 hours at dosage of—
10 to 15 mL four times a day—Maintains a urine pH of 6.5 to 7.4.
15 to 20 mL four times a day—Maintains a urine pH of 7.0 to 7.6.

### Elimination

Urinary; less than 5% unchanged.

## Precautions to Consider

### Carcinogenicity

Long-term carcinogenicity studies in animals have not been performed.

### Pregnancy/Reproduction

Pregnancy—Studies have not been done in humans.
Studies have not been done in animals.

*Potassium citrate;* and *potassium citrate* and *sodium citrate*—FDA Pregnancy Category C.

### Breast-feeding

It is not known whether citrates are distributed into breast milk. However, problems in humans have not been documented.

### Pediatrics

Appropriate studies on the relationship of age to the effects of citrates have not been performed in the pediatric population. However, no pediatrics-specific problems have been documented to date.

### Geriatrics

No information is available on the relationship of age to the effects of citrates in geriatric patients.

### Drug interactions and/or related problems

The following drug interactions and/or related problems have been selected on the basis of their potential clinical significance (possible mechanism in parentheses where appropriate)—not necessarily inclusive (» = major clinical significance):

Note: Combinations containing any of the following medications, depending on the amount present, may also interact with this medication.

Amphetamines or
Ephedrine or
Pseudoephedrine or
» Quinidine
(concurrent use with citrates may inhibit urinary excretion and prolong the duration of action of these medications)

» Antacids, especially those containing aluminum or sodium bicarbonate
(concurrent use with citrates may result in systemic alkalosis)
(concurrent use of sodium citrate with sodium bicarbonate may promote the development of calcium stones in patients with uric acid stones, due to sodium ion opposition to the hypocalciuric effect of the alkaline load; may also cause hypernatremia)
(concurrent use of aluminum-containing antacids with citrate salts can increase aluminum absorption, possibly resulting in acute aluminum toxicity, especially in patients with renal insufficiency)

Anticholinergics or other medications with anticholinergic activity (See *Appendix II*)
(concurrent use with potassium citrate may increase risk of gastrointestinal irritation because of slowed gastrointestinal transit time; patients should be carefully monitored endoscopically for evidence of lesions)

» Angiotensin-converting enzyme (ACE) inhibitors or
» Anti-inflammatory drugs, nonsteroidal (NSAIDs) or
Cyclosporine or
» Diuretics, potassium-sparing or
» Heparin or
» Low-salt milk or
» Potassium-containing medications, other or
» Salt substitutes
(concurrent use with potassium citrate may increase serum potassium concentrations, which may cause severe hyperkalemia and lead to cardiac arrest, especially in renal insufficiency; low-salt milk may contain up to 60 mEq of potassium per liter and most salt substitutes contain substantial amounts of potassium)

Ciprofloxacin or
Norfloxacin or
Ofloxacin
(citrates may reduce the solubility of ciprofloxacin, norfloxacin, or ofloxacin in the urine; patients should be observed for signs of crystalluria and nephrotoxicity)

» Digitalis glycosides
(concurrent use with potassium citrate may increase risk of hyperkalemia in digitalized patients; careful monitoring of serum potassium concentrations during concurrent use is recommended)

Laxatives
(concurrent administration with citrates may have an additive effect since sodium or potassium citrate may act as a saline laxative; however, these medications may be used concurrently as a preoperative for therapeutic advantage)

Lithium
(concurrent use with sodium citrate may increase the urinary excretion of lithium and reduce its therapeutic effects, possibly due to the sodium content of the citrate and/or the effect of urinary alkalinization)

» Methenamine
(concurrent use with citrates is not recommended because alkalinizing the urine may inhibit the effects of methenamine)

Salicylates
(concurrent use with citrates may increase the urinary excretion and decrease the therapeutic effects of salicylates due to alkalinization of the urine)

Sodium-containing medications
(concurrent use with sodium citrate may increase the risk of hypernatremia, especially in patients with renal disease)

**Medical considerations/Contraindications**

The medical considerations/contraindications included have been selected on the basis of their potential clinical significance (reasons given in parentheses where appropriate)—not necessarily inclusive (» = major clinical significance).

*Except under special circumstances, this medication should not be used when the following medical problems exist:*

*For potassium citrate– and/or sodium citrate–containing*
» Aluminum toxicity
(citrate salts have been found to increase aluminum absorption and may exacerbate the condition, especially in renal insufficiency)

» Heart failure or
» Myocardial damage, severe
(because of impaired mechanisms for excreting potassium, potentially fatal asymptomatic hyperkalemia can develop, rapidly leading to cardiovascular failure and cardiac arrest)
(sodium retention may result when patients with congestive heart failure are administered sodium citrate)

» Renal impairment, severe, with azotemia or oliguria or
» Renal insufficiency, when glomerular filtration rate (GFR) is less than 0.7 mL per kg per minute
(danger of soft tissue calcification; increased risk of hyperkalemia or alkalosis)
(sodium retention may occur with use of sodium citrate)

» Urinary tract infection, active, with urea-splitting or other organisms, in association with calcium or struvite stones
(bacterial enzymatic degradation of citrate may occur, preventing it from increasing urinary citrate; also, the rise in urinary pH may promote further bacterial growth)

*For potassium citrate–containing only (in addition to those listed above)*
» Hyperkalemia, or conditions predisposing to hyperkalemia such as:
Adrenal insufficiency
Dehydration, acute
Diabetes mellitus, uncontrolled
Physical exercise, strenuous, in unconditioned persons
Renal failure, chronic
Tissue breakdown, extensive
(increased serum potassium concentrations leading to cardiac arrest may occur; exercise-induced hyperkalemia is transient and is a problem only in patients with renal insufficiency from dehydration or those taking medications that increase serum potassium)

» Peptic ulcer
(increased risk of gastrointestinal lesions with potassium citrate, especially with tablets)

*For potassium citrate tablets only (in addition to those listed above)*
» Gastric emptying, delayed or
» Esophageal compression or
» Intestinal obstruction or stricture
(delayed passage of tablets through gastrointestinal tract may increase risk of gastrointestinal irritation)

*Risk-benefit should be considered when the following medical problems exist:*

*For potassium citrate– and sodium citrate–containing*
» Acidosis, renal tubular, severe or
Diarrheal syndromes, chronic, such as ulcerative colitis, regional enteritis, or jejuno-ileal bypass surgery
(when urinary citrate in these conditions is very low [below 100 mg per day], citrates may be relatively ineffective in raising urinary citrate; higher doses may be required to produce the desired citraturic response; when urinary pH is high in renal tubular acidosis, citrates may produce only a small rise in pH; rapid transit time associated with diarrheal syndromes may prevent proper breakdown of tablets [especially wax matrix], liquid preparations should be used in diarrheal syndromes)

*For sodium citrate–containing only (in addition to those listed above)*
Edema, peripheral or pulmonary or
Hypertension or
Toxemia of pregnancy
(sodium salts should be used cautiously in patients with these conditions to prevent exacerbation; also, patients on sodium restricted diets should not take sodium citrate)

**Patient monitoring**

The following may be especially important in patient monitoring (other tests may be warranted in some patients, depending on condition; » = major clinical significance):

Acid-base balance, serum, including pH and carbon dioxide and
Complete blood counts, including hematocrit and hemoglobin and
Creatinine concentrations, serum and
Electrolyte concentrations, serum, including sodium, potassium, chloride, and bicarbonate
(determinations recommended every 4 months during therapy, especially for patients with renal disease; treatment should be discontinued if there is a significant rise in serum potassium or in serum creatinine, or a significant fall in hematocrit or hemoglobin values)

Citrate, urinary, 24-hour, determinations and/or
pH determinations, urinary
(recommended at start of therapy, to determine adequacy of initial dosage, and every 4 months thereafter; patients taking citrate solu-

tions should frequently check urinary pH to maintain alkalinity at all times)

Electrocardiogram (ECG)
(recommended periodically, especially in patients with cardiac disease; characteristic changes such as peaking of T-wave, loss of P-wave, depression of ST-segment, and prolongation of the QT-interval may indicate asymptomatic hyperkalemia)

## Side/Adverse Effects

The following side/adverse effects have been selected on the basis of their potential clinical significance (possible signs and symptoms in parentheses where appropriate)—not necessarily inclusive:

**Those indicating need for medical attention**
Incidence rare

*For potassium citrate– and sodium citrate–containing*
**Metabolic alkalosis** (mood or mental changes; muscle pain or twitching; nervousness or restlessness; slow breathing; unpleasant taste; unusual tiredness or weakness)

*For potassium citrate–containing only (in addition to those listed above)*
**Bowel obstruction or bowel perforation** (abdominal or stomach cramps or pain; black, tarry stools; severe vomiting, sometimes with blood)—for tablet dosage form only; *hyperkalemia* (confusion; irregular heartbeat; numbness or tingling in hands, feet, or lips; shortness of breath or difficult breathing; unexplained anxiety; unusual tiredness or weakness; weakness or heaviness of legs)

Note: *Bowel obstruction* or *bowel perforation* caused by high concentration of potassium ions in region of dissolving tablets. Because the wax matrix is not an enteric coating, improper release of some of the potassium ions from the wax matrix into the stomach may cause upper gastrointestinal bleeding with the same frequency as other wax-matrix potassium products; if these adverse effects occur, potassium citrate should be discontinued immediately.

*Hyperkalemia* may often be asymptomatic or manifested only by characteristic ECG changes. Late signs may include muscle paralysis and cardiac arrest. When citrates are used at recommended doses, hyperkalemia is rare in patients without predisposing conditions.

*For sodium citrate–containing only (in addition to those listed for potassium citrate– or sodium citrate–containing)*
**Hypernatremia** (dizziness; fast heartbeat; high blood pressure; irritability; muscle twitching; restlessness; seizures; swelling of feet or lower legs; weakness)—occurs very rarely

**Those indicating need for medical attention only if they continue or are bothersome**
Incidence less frequent

*For potassium citrate– and sodium citrate–containing*
**Laxative effect** (diarrhea or loose bowel movements)

*For potassium citrate only (in addition to those listed above)*
**Irritation, contact** (mild abdominal or stomach soreness or pain; nausea or vomiting)—for tablet dosage form only

Note: *Contact irritation* may be due to possible contact with ulcerous areas or high concentration of potassium ions in one area resulting from improper release of potassium ions from wax-matrix dosage form or delayed passage of dosage form through alimentary tract.

## Patient Consultation

As an aid to patient consultation, refer to *Advice for the Patient, Citrates (Systemic)*.

In providing consultation, consider emphasizing the following selected information (» = major clinical significance):

**Before using this medication**
» Conditions affecting use, especially:
   Other medications, especially—
      *For all citrates*: Quinidine, calcium-containing medications, methenamine, antacids
      *For potassium citrate–containing only*: Angiotensin-converting enzyme (ACE) inhibitors, digitalis glycosides, heparin, non-steroidal anti-inflammatory drugs (NSAIDs), potassium-sparing diuretics, other potassium-containing medications
   Other medical problems, especially—
      *For potassium citrate– and/or sodium citrate–containing*: Aluminum toxicity, heart failure, severe myocardial damage, severe renal function impairment with azotemia or oliguria, renal insufficiency, or urinary tract infection
      *For potassium citrate–containing only*: Hyperkalemia or conditions predisposing to hyperkalemia, peptic ulcer, or severe renal tubular acidosis
      *For potassium citrate tablets only*: Delayed gastric emptying, esophageal compression, or intestinal obstruction or stricture

**Proper use of this medication**
Proper administration:

*For tablet dosage form*
Swallowing tablet whole; not crushing, chewing, or sucking
Taking with a full glass (240 mL) of water or juice
» Checking with physician at once if trouble in swallowing tablets or if tablets seem to stick in the throat

*For oral liquid dosage form*
Diluting with 6 ounces of water or juice before swallowing; after swallowing, following with additional water, if desired
Chilling, but *not* freezing, before swallowing to enhance palatability

*For crystals dosage form*
Adding contents of one packet to at least 6 ounces of cool water or juice; stirring well to dissolve completely
Following with additional water after swallowing mixture, if desired

» Taking each dose immediately after a meal or within 30 minutes after a meal or bedtime snack to lessen gastrointestinal pain or saline laxative effect
» Importance of high fluid intake (at least 3 liters per day) to prevent supersaturation of urine and to assure a minimum urine volume of 2.5 liters per day
Compliance with therapy, especially when taking with diuretics and digitalis
» Proper dosing
Missed dose: Taking as soon as possible if remembered within 2 hours; not taking if almost time for next dose; not doubling doses
» Proper storage

**Precautions while using this medication**
Regular visits to physician to check progress of therapy
Checking with physician before starting strenuous physical exercise if out of condition, to prevent possible hyperkalemia

*For potassium citrate–containing only*
Not taking salt substitutes or drinking low-salt milk unless prescribed by physician

*For sodium citrate–containing only*
Avoiding salty foods and use of extra table salt

» Checking with physician at once if black, tarry stools or other signs of gastrointestinal bleeding are observed
Not being alarmed at appearance of "whole" tablet in stools; checking with physician

**Side/adverse effects**
Signs of potential side effects, especially:
*For potassium citrate– or sodium citrate–containing*—Metabolic alkalosis or diarrhea or loose bowel movements
*For potassium citrate–containing only*—Hyperkalemia
*For potassium citrate tablets only*—Bowel perforation or obstruction, or contact irritation resulting from improper release from wax matrix of tablets
*For sodium citrate–containing only*—Hypernatremia

## General Dosing Information

For patients on sodium-restricted diets, potassium citrate preparations may be preferable as urinary alkalizers; conversely, sodium citrate may be used when potassium citrate is contraindicated.

The goal of therapy with potassium citrate tablets or potassium citrate and citric acid solution is to increase the urinary citrate to normal (greater than 320 mg a day) and as close to the normal mean (640 mg a day) as possible, and to increase urinary pH to 6.0 to 7.0.

The rise in urinary citrate is directly dependent on the dosage of potassium citrate tablets or potassium citrate and citric acid oral solution. After long-term treatment, a dosage of 6.5 grams of potassium citrate (60 mEq of potassium ion) a day raises urinary citrate by approximately 400 mg a day and increases urinary pH by approximately 0.7 units. When treatment is withdrawn, urinary citrate begins to fall toward the pretreatment level of the first day.

Potassium citrate tablets and potassium citrate and citric acid oral solution are equally efficacious in raising urinary pH and citrate excretion.

**Diet/Nutrition**
Each dose should be taken immediately after a meal or within 30 minutes after a meal or bedtime snack, to lessen gastrointestinal pain or the saline laxative effect.

High fluid intake (at least 3 liters a day) is important to prevent supersaturation of urine and to assure a minimum urine volume of 2.5 liters a day.

Low-salt milk may contain up to 60 mEq of potassium per liter, and salt substitutes may contain substantial amounts of potassium. Both should be avoided if a patient is taking a potassium citrate–containing product, to prevent hyperkalemia.

### For treatment of adverse effects
*For hyperkalemia*
Treatment includes:
- Discontinuing foods and medications containing potassium, including salt substitutes, ACE inhibitors, nonsteroidal anti-inflammatory drugs (NSAIDs), heparin, cyclosporine, and potassium-sparing diuretics.
- Administering 10% dextrose injection containing 10 to 20 units of insulin per liter at a rate of 300 to 500 mL of solution per hour. Monitoring for serial EKG and serum potassium concentration is recommended.
- Correcting acidosis with intravenous sodium bicarbonate.
- Using exchange resins, hemodialysis, or peritoneal dialysis.
- Observing caution when treating hyperkalemia in digitalized patients, since rapid reduction of serum potassium concentrations may induce digitalis toxicity.

*For hypernatremia*
Treatment includes:
- Discontinuing foods and medications containing sodium.
- If acute hypernatremia, administering hypotonic or isotonic saline solution intravenously to maintain fluid volume. In infants, to avoid a too rapid fall in serum sodium concentrations, use of a saline solution containing less than 70 mEq per liter is not recommended. Serum osmolality should be corrected over a 24- to 48-hour period.

*For metabolic alkalosis*
Treatment includes:
- Controlling symptoms by having patient rebreathe expired air into a paper bag or mask.
- Administering calcium gluconate injection if alkalosis is severe, to control tetany.

---

## POTASSIUM CITRATE

## Summary of Differences
Indications: Also used to prevent or treat hypocitraturia in patients with calcium renal calculi.
Precautions: Medical considerations/contraindications—May increase risk of gastrointestinal lesions in peptic ulcer disease; may increase risk of gastrointestinal irritation in delayed gastric emptying, esophageal compression, or intestinal obstruction.
Side/adverse effects: Tablets may cause severe abdominal or stomach pain; black, tarry stools; or severe vomiting, sometimes with blood.

## Additional Dosing Information
May be used as a urinary alkalizer when sodium citrate is contraindicated.

## Oral Dosage Forms
### POTASSIUM CITRATE TABLETS
**Usual adult dose**
Antiurolithic or
Alkalizer, urinary—
Mild to moderate hypocitraturia (more than 150 mg of urinary citrate a day): Oral, initially 1.08 grams (10 mEq of potassium ion) three times a day with meals.
Severe hypocitraturia (less than 150 mg of urinary citrate a day): Oral, initially, 2.16 grams (20 mEq of potassium ion) three times a day, with meals or within thirty minutes after a meal or bedtime snack; or 1.62 grams (15 mEq of potassium ion) four times a day, with meals or within thirty minutes after a meal or bedtime snack.
Note: Dosage should be adjusted as determined by 24-hour fasting urinary citrate and/or urinary pH measurements.

**Usual adult prescribing limits**
10.8 grams of potassium citrate (100 mEq of potassium ion) a day.

**Usual pediatric dose**
Dosage has not been established.

**Strength(s) usually available**
U.S.—
540 mg (5 mEq of potassium ion) (Rx) [*Urocit-K*].
1080 mg (10 mEq of potassium ion) (Rx) [*Urocit-K*].

**Packaging and storage**
Store below 40 °C (104 °F), preferably between 15 and 30 °C (59 and 86 °F), in a tight container, unless otherwise specified by manufacturer.

**Auxiliary labeling**
- Swallow tablets whole
- Take with a full glass of water.
- Take with meals or snack.

**Note**
Dispense in original container.

**Additional information**
Intact wax matrix may appear in the feces.

---

## POTASSIUM CITRATE AND CITRIC ACID

## Summary of Differences
Indications: Also used to prevent or treat hypocitraturia in patients with calcium renal calculi.

## Additional Dosing Information
May be used as a urinary alkalizer when sodium citrate is contraindicated.

## Oral Dosage Forms
### POTASSIUM CITRATE AND CITRIC ACID ORAL SOLUTION USP
**Usual adult dose**
Antiurolithic or
Alkalizer, systemic or
Alkalizer, urinary—
Oral, initially 10 to 15 mL (2.2 to 3.3 grams of potassium citrate [20 to 30 mEq of potassium ion]) four times a day, after meals and at bedtime, the dosage being adjusted as needed and tolerated.
Note: Dosage should be adjusted as determined by 24-hour fasting urinary citrate and/or urinary pH measurements.

**Usual pediatric dose**
Alkalizer, urinary—Oral, initially 5 to 15 mL (1.1 to 3.3 grams of potassium citrate [10 to 30 mEq of potassium ion]) four times a day, after meals and at bedtime, the dosage being adjusted as needed and tolerated.

**Strength(s) usually available**
U.S.—
1.1 grams of potassium citrate (10 mEq of potassium ion) and 334 mg of citric acid per 5 mL (Rx) [*Polycitra-K*].

**Packaging and storage**
Store below 40 °C (104 °F), preferably between 15 and 30 °C (59 and 86 °F), unless otherwise specified by manufacturer. Store in a tight container. Protect from freezing and excessive heat.

**Auxiliary labeling**
- Dilute with water or juice.
- Take with meals or snack.

**Additional information**
Citric acid is present as a temporary buffer with only a transient effect on the systemic acid-base balance.

### POTASSIUM CITRATE AND CITRIC ACID FOR ORAL SOLUTION
**Usual adult dose**
Antiurolithic or
Alkalizer, systemic or
Alkalizer, urinary—
Oral, initially 3.3 grams of potassium citrate (30 mEq of potassium ion) four times a day, after meals and at bedtime, the dosage being adjusted as needed and tolerated.
Note: Dosage should be adjusted as determined by 24-hour fasting urinary citrate and/or urinary pH measurements.

**Usual pediatric dose**
Use is not recommended.
Note: Because of the difficulty of regulating dosage with this dosage form, the oral solution is not recommended for pediatric patients.

**Size(s) usually available**
U.S.—
3.3 grams of potassium citrate (30 mEq of potassium ion) and 1 gram of citric acid (Rx) [*Polycitra-K Crystals*].

*USP DI*                                                                                             **Citrates (Systemic)**

**Packaging and storage**
Store below 40 °C (104 °F), preferably between 15 and 30 °C (59 and 86 °F), in a tight container, unless otherwise specified by manufacturer.

**Preparation of dosage form**
Add contents of one packet to at least 6 ounces of cool water or juice. Stir well to dissolve.

**Auxiliary labeling**
- Dilute with water or juice.
- Take with meals or snack.

**Additional information**
Each packet provides the same amounts of potassium citrate and citric acid as 15 mL of potassium citrate and citric acid oral solution.
Citric acid is present as a temporary buffer with only a transient effect on the systemic acid-base balance.

---

### POTASSIUM CITRATE AND SODIUM CITRATE

## Summary of Differences
Indications: Used as a urinary alkalizing agent only, in patients with uric acid or cystine calculi.

## Oral Dosage Forms
### POTASSIUM CITRATE AND SODIUM CITRATE TABLETS

**Usual adult dose**
Antiurolithic or
Alkalizer, urinary—
    Oral, initially, 1 to 4 tablets (50 to 200 mg of potassium citrate [0.45 to 1.8 mEq of potassium ion] and 950 mg to 3.8 grams of sodium citrate [9.5 to 38 mEq of sodium ion]) after meals and at bedtime.

**Usual pediatric dose**
Dosage has not been established.

**Strength(s) usually available**
U.S.—
    50 mg of potassium citrate (0.45 mEq of potassium ion) and 950 mg of sodium citrate (9.5 mEq of sodium ion) (Rx) [*Citrolith*].

**Packaging and storage**
Store below 40 °C (104 °F), preferably between 15 and 30 °C (59 and 86 °F), in a well-closed container, unless otherwise specified by manufacturer.

**Auxiliary labeling**
- Swallow tablets whole.
- Take with a full glass of water.
- Take with meals or snack.

---

### SODIUM CITRATE AND CITRIC ACID

## Summary of Differences
Indications: Also used to prevent acid-aspiration pneumonitis.

## Additional Dosing Information
May be used when potassium citrate is contraindicated.

## Oral Dosage Forms
### SODIUM CITRATE AND CITRIC ACID ORAL SOLUTION USP

**Usual adult dose**
Antiurolithic or
Alkalizer, systemic or
Alkalizer, urinary—
    Oral, initially 10 to 30 mL (1 to 3 grams of sodium citrate [10 to 30 mEq of sodium ion]) four times a day, after meals and at bedtime, diluted in 30 to 90 mL of water, the dosage being adjusted as needed.
Note: Dosage should be adjusted as determined by urinary pH measurements.
Neutralizing buffer—
    Oral, 15 to 30 mL (1.5 to 3 grams of sodium citrate [15 to 30 mEq of sodium ion]), as a single dose, or diluted in 15 to 30 mL of water.

**Usual adult prescribing limits**
Up to 150 mL (15 grams of sodium citrate [150 mEq of sodium ion]) a day.

**Usual pediatric dose**
Alkalizer, systemic—Oral, initially 5 to 15 mL (500 mg to 1.5 grams of sodium citrate [5 to 15 mEq of sodium ion]) four times a day, after meals and at bedtime, diluted in 30 to 90 mL of water, the dosage being adjusted as needed.

**Strength(s) usually available**
U.S.—
    490 mg of sodium citrate (5 mEq of sodium ion) and 640 mg of citric acid per 5 mL (Rx) [*Oracit* (not USP)].
    500 mg of sodium citrate (5 mEq of sodium ion) and 334 mg of citric acid per 5 mL (Rx) [*Bicitra*].
Canada—
    490 mg of sodium citrate (5 mEq of sodium ion) and 640 mg of citric acid per 5 mL (OTC) [*Oracit*].

**Packaging and storage**
Store below 40 °C (104 °F), preferably between 15 and 30 °C (59 and 86 °F), unless otherwise specified by manufacturer. Store in a tight container. Protect from freezing.

**Auxiliary labeling**
- Dilute with water or juice.
- Take with meals or snack.

**Additional information**
Citric acid is a temporary buffer with only a transient effect on systemic acid-base balance.

---

### TRICITRATES

## Summary of Differences
Indications: Also used to treat chronic metabolic acidosis and to prevent acid-aspiration pneumonitis.

## Oral Dosage Forms
### TRICITRATES ORAL SOLUTION USP

**Usual adult dose**
Antiurolithic or
Alkalizer, systemic or
Alkalizer, urinary—
    Oral, initially 15 to 30 mL (1.6 to 3.3 grams of potassium citrate [15 to 30 mEq of potassium ion] and 1.5 to 3 grams of sodium citrate [15 to 30 mEq of sodium ion]) four times a day after meals and at bedtime, the dosage being adjusted as needed.
Note: Dosage should be adjusted as determined by urinary pH measurements.
Neutralizing buffer—
    Oral, 15 mL (1.65 grams of potassium citrate [15 mEq of potassium ion] and 1.5 grams of sodium citrate [15 mEq of sodium ion]), as a single dose, diluted in 15 mL of water.

**Usual pediatric dose**
Alkalizer, systemic or
Alkalizer, urinary—
    Oral, initially 5 to 10 mL (550 mg to 1.10 grams of potassium citrate [5 to 10 mEq of potassium ion] and 500 mg to 1 gram of sodium citrate [5 to 10 mEq of sodium ion]) four times a day after meals and at bedtime, the dosage being adjusted as needed.

**Strength(s) usually available**
U.S.—
    550 mg of potassium citrate (5 mEq of potassium ion), 500 mg of sodium citrate (5 mEq of sodium ion), and 334 mg of citric acid per 5 mL (Rx) [*Polycitra-LC; Polycitra Syrup* (sucrose)].

**Packaging and storage**
Store below 40 °C (104 °F), preferably between 15 and 30 °C (59 and 86 °F), unless otherwise specified by manufacturer. Store in a tight container. Protect from freezing.

**Auxiliary labeling**
- Dilute with water or juice.
- Take with meals or snack.

**Additional information**
Citric acid is a temporary buffer with only a transient effect on the systemic acid-base balance.

---

Revised: 01/18/93
Interim revision: 08/29/94

# CLADRIBINE Systemic

VA CLASSIFICATION (Primary): AN300
Commonly used brand name(s): *Leustatin*.
Other commonly used names are 2-chlorodeoxyadenosine and 2-CdA.

Note: For a listing of dosage forms and brand names by country availability, see *Dosage Forms* section(s).

## Category
Antineoplastic.

## Indications
Note: Bracketed information in the *Indications* section refers to uses that are not included in U.S. product labeling.

**Accepted**

Leukemia, hairy cell (treatment)—Cladribine is indicated for active treatment of hairy cell leukemia as defined by clinically significant anemia, neutropenia, thrombocytopenia, or disease-related symptoms.

[Leukemia, chronic lymphocytic (treatment)][1]—Cladribine is accepted for treatment of B-cell chronic lymphocytic leukemia (CLL) in both previously untreated patients and patients refractory to previous treatment, based upon reports of objective tumor responses, most of which were partial, in noncomparative studies.

[Lymphomas, non-Hodgkin's (treatment)][1]—Cladribine is accepted for treatment of low-grade non-Hodgkin's lymphomas in patients refractory to previous treatment, based upon reports of objective tumor responses, most of which were partial, in two noncomparative studies.

[Waldenstrom macroglobulinemia (treatment)][1]—Cladribine is accepted for treatment of Waldenstrom macroglobulinemia, based upon reports of objective tumor responses in one noncomparative study.

[1] Not included in Canadian product labeling.

## Pharmacology/Pharmacokinetics

**Physicochemical characteristics**
Source—Synthetic.
Chemical group—Cladribine is a halogenated purine nucleoside analog of deoxyadenosine.
Molecular weight—285.7.

**Mechanism of action/Effect**
Cladribine is an antimetabolite. The exact mechanism of action in hairy cell leukemia is unknown. Cladribine is resistant to the action of adenosine deaminase (ADA), which deaminates deoxyadenosine to deoxyinosine. The phosphorylated metabolites of cladribine accumulate in cells with a high ratio of deoxycytidine kinase activity to 5' nucleotidase activity (lymphocytes, monocytes) and are converted to the active triphosphate deoxynucleotide. Intracellular accumulation of toxic deoxynucleotides selectively kills these cells, which become unable to properly repair single-strand DNA breaks, leading to disruption of cell metabolism. In addition, there is some evidence that deoxynucleotides are incorporated into the DNA of dividing cells and impair DNA synthesis. Cladribine also induces apoptosis (a form of programmed cell death in sensitive cells).

Cladribine's action is cell cycle–phase nonspecific; cladribine equally affects dividing and resting lymphocytes.

**Other actions/effects**
Cladribine has immunosuppressant activity; restoration of lymphocyte subsets after treatment takes at least 6 to 12 months, although clinical immunocompetence is usually restored after about a month. Significant reductions in T and B lymphocytes occur during treatment (both CD4 and CD8 are affected) and CD4 counts recover more slowly after treatment.

**Distribution**
Cladribine crosses the blood-brain barrier.

**Protein binding**
Moderate (approximately 20%).

**Biotransformation**
Metabolized in all cells with deoxycytidine kinase activity to 2-chloro-2'-deoxyadenosine-5'-triphosphate.

**Half-life**
Distribution—With continuous intravenous infusion: Approximately 30 minutes.
Terminal—With continuous intravenous infusion: 7 hours.

**Onset of action**
Time to achieve response—Median 4 months. (Response is defined as absence of hairy cells in bone marrow and peripheral blood together with normalization of peripheral blood parameters.)
Pharmacologic—Toxicity to lymphocytes: 7 days.

**Duration of action**
Median duration of response—Greater than 8 months (range, up to and greater than 25 months).

**Elimination**
Unknown.
In dialysis or hemofiltration—Unknown.

## Precautions to Consider

**Carcinogenicity**
No studies have been done with cladribine in animals.
Secondary malignancies are potential delayed effects of many antineoplastic agents, although it is not clear whether the effect is related to their mutagenic or immunosuppressive action. The effect of dose and duration of therapy is also unknown, although risk seems to increase with long-term use. Although information is limited, available data seem to indicate that the carcinogenic risk is greatest with the alkylating agents.
Antimetabolites have been shown to be carcinogenic in animals and may be associated with an increased risk of development of secondary carcinomas in humans, although the risk appears to be less than with alkylating agents.

**Mutagenicity**
In mammalian cells in culture, cladribine has been shown to cause an imbalance of intracellular deoxyribonucleotide triphosphate pools. This imbalance resulted in the inhibition of DNA synthesis and DNA repair, yielding DNA strand breaks and subsequently cell death. Inhibition of thymidine incorporation into human lymphoblastic cells was 90% at concentrations of 0.3 micromolar. Cladribine was also incorporated into DNA of these cells. Cladribine was not mutagenic to bacteria and did not induce unscheduled DNA synthesis in primary rat hepatocyte cultures.

**Pregnancy/Reproduction**
Fertility—Gonadal suppression, resulting in amenorrhea or azoospermia, may occur in patients taking antineoplastic therapy, especially with the alkylating agents. In general, these effects appear to be related to dose and length of therapy and may be irreversible. Prediction of the degree of testicular or ovarian function impairment is complicated by the common use of combinations of several antineoplastics, which makes it difficult to assess the effects of individual agents.

Intravenous administration of cladribine to Cynomolgus monkeys has been shown to cause suppression of rapidly generating cells, including testicular cells.

Pregnancy—Adequate and well-controlled studies in women have not been done.

First trimester: It is usually recommended that use of antineoplastics, especially combination chemotherapy, be avoided whenever possible, especially during the first trimester. Although information is limited because of the relatively few instances of antineoplastic administration during pregnancy, the mutagenic, teratogenic, and carcinogenic potential of these medications must be considered.

Other hazards to the fetus include adverse reactions seen in adults.

In general, use of contraception is recommended during cytotoxic drug therapy.

Cladribine has been shown to cause a significant increase in fetal variations in mice at a dose of 1.5 mg per kg of body weight (mg/kg) (4.5 mg per square meter of body surface) per day, and to cause increased resorptions, reduced litter size, and increased fetal malformations in mice at a dose of 3 mg/kg (9 mg per square meter of body surface) per day. Cladribine was shown to cause fetal death and malformations in rabbits at a dose of 3 mg/kg (33 mg per square meter of body surface) per day. No fetal effects were produced in mice at a dose of 0.5 mg/kg (1.5 mg per square meter of body surface) per day or in rabbits at a dose of 1 mg/kg (11 mg per square meter of body surface) per day.

FDA Pregnancy Category D.

**Breast-feeding**
Although very little information is available regarding distribution of antineoplastic agents into breast milk, breast-feeding is not recommended during chemotherapy because of the potential risks to the infant (adverse effects, mutagenicity, carcinogenicity). It is not known whether cladribine is distributed into breast milk.

### Pediatrics
No information is available on the relationship of age to the effects of cladribine in pediatric patients. However, phase I and phase II studies in children have been reported and some studies of cladribine for acute myelocytic leukemia and acute lymphocytic leukemia have included children.

### Geriatrics
Although appropriate studies on the relationship of age to the effects of cladribine have not been performed in the geriatric population, clinical trials have included patients over 65 years of age and geriatrics-specific problems that would limit the usefulness of this medication in the elderly are not expected.

### Dental
The bone marrow depressant effects of cladribine may result in an increased incidence of microbial infection, delayed healing, and gingival bleeding. Dental work, whenever possible should be completed prior to initiation of therapy or deferred until blood counts have returned to normal. Patients should be instructed in proper oral hygiene during treatment, including caution in use of regular toothbrushes, dental floss, and toothpicks.

### Drug interactions and/or related problems
The following drug interactions and/or related problems have been selected on the basis of their potential clinical significance (possible mechanism in parentheses where appropriate)—not necessarily inclusive (» = major clinical significance):

Note: Combinations containing any of the following medications, depending on the amount present, may also interact with this medication.

Allopurinol or
Colchicine or
» Probenecid or
» Sulfinpyrazone
(cladribine may raise the concentration of blood uric acid; dosage adjustment of antigout agents may be necessary to control hyperuricemia and gout; allopurinol may be preferred to prevent or reverse cladribine-induced hyperuricemia because of risk of uric acid nephropathy with uricosuric antigout agents)

Blood dyscrasia–causing medications (See *Appendix II*)
(leukopenic and/or thrombocytopenic effects of cladribine may be increased with concurrent or recent therapy if these medications cause the same effects; dosage adjustment of cladribine, if necessary, should be based on blood counts)

» Bone marrow depressants, other (See *Appendix II*) or
Radiation therapy
(additive bone marrow depression may occur; dosage reduction may be required when two or more bone marrow depressants, including radiation, are used concurrently or consecutively)

Vaccines, killed virus
(because normal defense mechanisms may be suppressed by cladribine therapy, the patient's antibody response to the vaccine may be decreased. The interval between discontinuation of medications that cause immunosuppression and restoration of the patient's ability to respond to the vaccine depends on the intensity and type of immunosuppression-causing medication used, the underlying disease, and other factors)

» Vaccines, live virus
(because normal defense mechanisms may be suppressed by cladribine therapy, concurrent use with a live virus vaccine may potentiate the replication of the vaccine virus, may increase the side/adverse effects of the vaccine virus, and/or may decrease the patient's antibody response to the vaccine; immunization of these patients should be undertaken only with extreme caution after careful review of the patient's hematologic status and only with the knowledge and consent of the physician managing the cladribine therapy. The interval between discontinuation of medications that cause immunosuppression and restoration of the patient's ability to respond to the vaccine depends on the intensity and type of immunosuppression-causing medication used, the underlying disease, and other factors. In addition, immunization with oral poliovirus vaccine should be postponed in persons in close contact with the patient, especially family members)

### Laboratory value alterations
The following have been selected on the basis of their potential clinical significance (possible effect in parentheses where appropriate)—not necessarily inclusive (» = major clinical significance):

With physiology/laboratory test values
Uric acid concentrations in blood and urine
(may be increased as part of a tumor lysis syndrome, especially in patients with a large tumor burden)

### Medical considerations/Contraindications
The medical considerations/contraindications included have been selected on the basis of their potential clinical significance (reasons given in parentheses where appropriate)—not necessarily inclusive (» = major clinical significance).

*Risk-benefit should be considered when the following medical problems exist:*

» Bone marrow depression
» Chickenpox, existing or recent (including recent exposure) or
» Herpes zoster
(risk of severe generalized disease)
Gout, history of or
Urate renal stones, history of
(risk of hyperuricemia)
» Infection
» Sensitivity to cladribine
» Caution should be used also in patients who have had previous cytotoxic drug therapy or radiation therapy.

### Patient monitoring
The following are especially important in patient monitoring (other tests may be warranted in some patients, depending on condition; » = major clinical significance):

CD4 T lymphocyte count and
CD8 T lymphocyte count
(recommended prior to initiation of therapy and at periodic intervals during and after therapy)
» Hematocrit or hemoglobin and
» Leukocyte count, total and, if appropriate, differential and
» Platelet count
(determinations recommended prior to initiation of therapy and at periodic intervals during therapy; frequency varies according to clinical state, agent, dose, and other agents being used concurrently)

Uric acid concentrations, serum
(recommended prior to initiation of therapy and at periodic intervals during therapy; frequency varies according to clinical state, agent, dose, and other agents being used concurrently)

## Side/Adverse Effects
Note: Percentage figures for frequency of side/adverse effects listed below are based on a single study of patients with hairy cell leukemia and are included only as an indication of relative frequency of reported side/adverse effects.

Cladribine has considerable hematopoietic stem cell toxicity.

In patients with hairy cell leukemia, anemia, neutropenia, and thrombocytopenia may worsen during the first two weeks of cladribine therapy, before recovery begins.

Prolonged bone marrow hypocellularity has been observed after treatment with cladribine.

Administration of repeated courses for indications other than hairy cell leukemia has been associated with prolonged, dose-limiting thrombocytopenia, occasional pancytopenia, and prolonged erythroid macrocytosis.

Neurotoxicity (paraparesis/quadraparesis of upper and/or lower extremities consistent with a demyelinating disease) and acute renal failure (possibly necessitating hemodialysis) occurred frequently in patients who received cladribine for indications other than hairy cell leukemia in doses above 0.26 mg per kg of body weight (mg/kg) per day for 10 to 14 days (4 to 9 times the recommended dose for hairy cell leukemia) in conjunction with alkylating agents, total body irradiation, and allogeneic bone marrow transplantation.

The following side/adverse effects have been selected on the basis of their potential clinical significance (possible signs and symptoms in parentheses where appropriate)—not necessarily inclusive:

### Those indicating need for medical attention
Incidence more frequent
**Anemia, severe** (usually asymptomatic)—37%; **fever**—40–70%; **infection** (fever or chills; cough or hoarseness; lower back or side pain; painful or difficult urination)—28%; **neutropenia, severe** (usually asymptomatic)—up to 70%; **skin rash**—27%; **thrombocytopenia** (unusual bleeding or bruising; black, tarry stools; blood in urine or stools; pinpoint red spots on skin)—12%

Note: *Anemia* may increase transfusion requirements during the first month of therapy; median time to normalization of hemoglobin has been reported to be 8 weeks.

*Fever* (temperature above 100 °F [38 °C]) usually begins between the fifth and seventh day of therapy and lasts a few days. Severe fever (temperature of 104 °F [40 °C] or higher) occurs in about 10% of patients. In most patients, fever is associated with neutropenia, although non-neutropenic fever may also occur. Documented infections (including those related to central intravenous catheters) occur in fewer than one-third of patients who experience severe fever. Fever has generally not been reported when cladribine was used for indications other than hairy cell leukemia.

*Infections* may be bacterial, viral, protozoal (e.g., *Pneumocystis*), or fungal, may occur even in the absence of neutropenia, and may be life-threatening. Cladribine causes prolonged depression of CD4 and CD8 lymphocyte subset counts; recovery of counts takes at least 6 to 12 months.

The highest incidence of *severe neutropenia* is in patients with pre-existing neutropenia related to prior therapy. Median time to normalization of absolute neutrophil counts (ANC) has been reported to be 5 weeks.

With *thrombocytopenia* occurring during cladribine therapy of hairy cell leukemia, median time to normalization of platelet counts has been reported to be 12 days. However, thrombocytopenia may become prolonged and dose-limiting with repeated courses (i.e., when cladribine is used for indications other than hairy cell leukemia).

Incidence less frequent—less than 10%
   *Cough; edema* (swelling of feet or lower legs); *injection site reaction* (pain or redness at site of injection)—9%; *phlebitis* (pain or redness at site of injection)—2%; *shortness of breath; stomach pain; tachycardia* (unusually fast heartbeat)

**Those indicating need for medical attention only if they continue or are bothersome**
Incidence more frequent
   *Anorexia* (loss of appetite)—17%; *headache*—22%; *nausea*—28%; *unusual tiredness*—45%; *vomiting*—13%
   Note: *Nausea* is usually mild and does not usually require treatment with antiemetics.
   *Skin rashes* are usually mild.
Incidence less frequent—less than 10%
   *Constipation; diarrhea; dizziness; itching; malaise* (general feeling of discomfort or illness); *myalgia or arthralgia* (muscle or joint pain); *sweating; trouble in sleeping; weakness*
   Note: *Dizziness* may be a neurologic effect.

## Overdose
For more information on the management of overdose or unintentional ingestion, **contact a Poison Control Center** (see *Poison Control Center Listing*).

**Treatment of overdose**
Treatment consists of:
   Withdrawal of cladribine.
   Observation.
   Supportive therapy.

## Patient Consultation
As an aid to patient consultation, refer to *Advice for the Patient, Cladribine (Systemic)*.
In providing consultation, consider emphasizing the following selected information (» = major clinical significance):

**Before using this medication**
» Conditions affecting use, especially:
   Sensitivity to cladribine
   Pregnancy—Use not recommended because of mutagenic, teratogenic, and carcinogenic potential; advisability of using contraception; telling physician immediately if pregnancy is suspected
   Breast-feeding—Not recommended because of risk of serious side effects
   Other medications, especially probenecid, sulfinpyrazone, other bone marrow depressants, or other cytotoxic drug or radiation therapy
   Other medical problems, especially chickenpox, herpes zoster, or infection

**Proper use of this medication**
   Possibility of nausea and vomiting; importance of continuing medication despite stomach upset
» Proper dosing

**Precautions while using this medication**
» Importance of close monitoring by the physician
» Avoiding immunizations unless approved by physician; other persons in patient's household should avoid immunizations with oral poliovirus vaccine; avoiding other persons who have taken oral poliovirus vaccine or wearing a protective mask that covers nose and mouth

*Caution if bone marrow depression occurs*
» Avoiding exposure to persons with bacterial infections, especially during periods of low blood counts; checking with physician immediately if fever or chills, cough or hoarseness, lower back or side pain, or painful or difficult urination occur
» Checking with physician immediately if unusual bleeding or bruising; black, tarry stools; blood in urine or stools; or pinpoint red spots on skin occur
   Caution in use of regular toothbrush, dental floss, or toothpick; physician, dentist, or nurse may suggest alternatives; checking with physician before having dental work done
   Not touching eyes or inside of nose unless hands washed immediately before
   Using caution to avoid accidental cuts with use of sharp objects such as safety razor or fingernail or toenail cutters
   Avoiding contact sports or other situations where bruising or injury could occur

**Side/adverse effects**
   May cause adverse effects such as blood problems; importance of discussing possible effects with physician
   Signs of potential side effects, especially anemia, fever, infection, neutropenia, thrombocytopenia, cough, edema, injection site reaction or phlebitis, shortness of breath, stomach pain, and tachycardia
   Asymptomatic side effects including anemia and leukopenia
   Physician or nurse can help in dealing with side effects

## General Dosing Information
Patients receiving cladribine should be under supervision of a physician experienced in cancer chemotherapy.

Cladribine injection must be diluted prior to administration by intravenous infusion.

If fever occurs, it is recommended that the patient be evaluated for possible infection.

Development of uric acid nephropathy in patients with leukemia or lymphoma may be prevented by adequate oral hydration and, in some cases, administration of allopurinol. Alkalinization of urine may be necessary if serum uric acid concentrations are elevated.

Special precautions are recommended in patients who develop thrombocytopenia as a result of administration of cladribine. These may include extreme care in performing invasive procedures; regular inspection of intravenous sites, skin (including perirectal area), and mucous membrane surfaces for signs of bleeding or bruising; limiting frequency of venipuncture and avoiding intramuscular injections; testing urine, emesis, stool, and secretions for occult blood; care in use of regular toothbrushes, dental floss, toothpicks, safety razors, and fingernail and toenail cutters; avoiding constipation; and using caution to prevent falls and other injuries. Such patients should avoid alcohol and aspirin intake because of the risk of gastrointestinal bleeding. Platelet transfusions may be required.

Subsequent courses of cladribine should not be administered until hematological effects from the previous course have subsided and then only with great caution.

Patients who develop leukopenia should be observed carefully for signs of infection. Antibiotic support may be required. In neutropenic patients who develop fever, broad-spectrum antibiotic coverage should be initiated empirically, pending bacterial cultures and appropriate diagnostic tests.

Red blood cell transfusions may be required for anemia.

If neurotoxicity occurs, it is recommended that withholding or discontinuation of cladribine be considered.

**Safety considerations for handling this medication**
There is limited but increasing evidence and concern that personnel involved in preparation and administration of parenteral antineoplastics may be at some risk because of the potential mutagenicity, teratogenicity, and/or carcinogenicity of these agents, although the actual risk is unknown. USP advisory panels recommend cautious handling both in

preparation and disposal of antineoplastic agents. Precautions that have been suggested include:
- Use of a biological containment cabinet during reconstitution and dilution of parenteral medications and wearing of disposable surgical gloves and masks.
- Use of proper technique to prevent contamination of the medication, work area, and operator during transfer between containers (including proper training of personnel in this technique).
- Cautious and proper disposal of needles, syringes, vials, ampuls, and unused medication.

A number of medical centers have developed detailed guidelines for handling of antineoplastic agents.

## Parenteral Dosage Forms

### CLADRIBINE INJECTION

**Usual adult dose**
Hairy cell leukemia—
  Intravenous (by continuous infusion), 100 mcg (0.1 mg) per kg of body weight per day for seven days.

Note: Cladribine is usually given for only one course for treatment of hairy cell leukemia.

Early studies used an actual dose of 0.09 mg per kg of body weight per day as a result of a slight calculation error during formulation, but in most recent studies the patients received the 0.1 mg per kg dose.

**Usual adult prescribing limits**
A dose of 0.1 mg per kg of body weight per day by continuous infusion for seven days has been established as the maximum-tolerated dose (MTD) in phase I studies.

**Usual pediatric dose**
Dosage has not been established.

**Strength(s) usually available**
U.S.—
  1 mg per mL (Rx) [*Leustatin* (sodium chloride 9 mg [0.15 mEq] per mL)].
Canada—
  1 mg per mL (Rx) [*Leustatin* (sodium chloride 9 mg [0.15 mEq] per mL)].

**Packaging and storage**
Store between 2 and 8 °C (36 and 46 °F), unless otherwise specified by manufacturer. Protect from light. Not adversely affected by freezing; if freezing occurs, thawing naturally to room temperature is recommended (heat or microwave should not be used), and the solution should not be refrozen.

**Preparation of dosage form**
Cladribine injection must be diluted before administration. (Since the product contains no antimicrobial preservative or bacteriostatic agent, proper aseptic technique and environmental precautions are necessary.)

Cladribine injection is prepared for administration by a single 24-hour intravenous infusion (to be repeated daily for 7 days) by adding the calculated daily dose to an infusion bag containing 500 mL of 0.9% sodium chloride injection.

Cladribine injection is prepared for administration by a continuous 7-day intravenous infusion by adding the calculated 7-day dose to the infusion reservoir through a sterile 0.22 micron disposable hydrophilic syringe filter. Then bacteriostatic 0.9% sodium chloride injection (0.9% benzyl alcohol preserved) is added through the filter, in an amount sufficient to make a total of 100 mL.

Caution—Use of diluents containing benzyl alcohol is not recommended for preparation of medications for use in neonates. A fatal toxic syndrome consisting of metabolic acidosis, CNS depression, respiratory problems, renal failure, hypotension, and possibly seizures and intracranial hemorrhages has been associated with this use.

**Stability**
Reconstituted solutions contain no preservative and should be used immediately or stored between 2 and 8 °C (36 and 46 °F) and used within 8 hours of reconstitution.

**Incompatibilities**
Use of 5% dextrose injection is not recommended for dilution of cladribine injection because increased degradation of cladribine will occur.

## Selected Bibliography

Beutler E. Cladribine (2-chlorodeoxyadenosine). Lancet 1992 Oct 17; 340: 952-6.

Saven A, Piro LD. Treatment of hairy cell leukemia. Blood 1992 Mar 1; 79: 1111-20.

Bryson HM, Sorkin EM. Cladribine. A review of its pharmacodynamic and pharmacokinetic properties and therapeutic potential in haematological malignancies. Drugs 1993; 46(5): 872-94.

Developed: 07/26/94
Interim revision: 08/15/94

# CLARITHROMYCIN   Systemic

VA CLASSIFICATION (Primary/Secondary): AM200/AM900
Commonly used brand name(s): *Biaxin*.

Note: For a listing of dosage forms and brand names by country availability, see *Dosage Forms* section(s).

## Category
Antibacterial (systemic); antimycobacterial.

## Indications

Note: Bracketed information in the *Indications* section refers to uses that are not included in U.S. product labeling.

**General considerations**
Clarithromycin is a macrolide antibiotic with *in vitro* activity against many gram-positive and gram-negative aerobic and anaerobic organisms. The minimum inhibitory concentrations (MICs) of clarithromycin are generally two- to fourfold lower than those of erythromycin against gram-positive bacteria, such as methicillin-sensitive *Staphylococcus aureus* and most *Streptococcus* species. However, sensitivities vary and *S. aureus* strains that are resistant to erythromycin, methicillin, or oxacillin also have been found to be resistant to clarithromycin. Clarithromycin is bactericidal against *Streptococcus pyogenes* and *Streptococcus pneumoniae*; however, *Streptococcus* strains resistant to one macrolide antibiotic have demonstrated cross resistance to other macrolide antibiotics.

The activity of erythromycin is twice that of clarithromycin against *Haemophilus influenzae*; however, clarithromycin's active metabolite, 14-hydroxyclarithromycin, is as active as erythromycin. When clarithromycin and 14-hydroxyclarithromycin are combined, their MIC is two- to fourfold lower than that of erythromycin, suggesting additive or synergistic *in vitro* activity against *H. influenzae*.

Clarithromycin displays *in vitro* activity against *Mycobacterium avium* complex (MAC), being eight- to thirty-two–fold more active than erythromycin. High intracellular concentrations are achieved with clarithromycin, and it has been found to be effective against MAC in human macrophages. Clarithromycin may act synergistically with other agents used to treat MAC. It is also very active against many different species of mycobacteria. *In vitro* and *in vivo* activity against *Mycobacterium leprae* has been demonstrated, and there has been good clinical response to the treatment of cutaneous disease, including disseminated disease, caused by *Mycobacterium chelonae*. However, clarithromycin has not been found to have *in vitro* activity against *Mycobacterium tuberculosis*.

Clarithromycin has been found to have greater *in vitro* activity than erythromycin against *Legionella pneumophila*, *Moraxella (Branhamella) catarrhalis*, *Chlamydia trachomatis*, and *Ureaplasma urealyticum*. Its activity is variable and similar to that of erythromycin against *Neisseria gonorrhoeae*, anaerobic gram-positive cocci, and *Bacteroides* species. Clarithromycin also has good *in vitro* activity against *Helicobacter pylori* and has been clinically effective, when combined with amoxicillin and lansoprazole, omeprazole, or ranitidine bismuth citrate, in the treatment of duodenal ulcers.

**Accepted**
Bronchitis, bacterial exacerbations (treatment)
Otitis media (treatment) or
Sinusitis, acute maxillary (treatment)—Clarithromycin is indicated in the treatment of bacterial exacerbations of chronic bronchitis, otitis media, or acute maxillary sinusitis due to *H. influenzae*, *M. catarrhalis*, or *S. pneumoniae*.

*Mycobacterium avium* complex (MAC) disease, disseminated (prophylaxis)[1]—Clarithromycin is indicated for the prevention of disseminated

MAC disease in patients with advanced human immunodeficiency virus (HIV) infection.

*Mycobacterium avium* complex (MAC) disease, disseminated (treatment)—Clarithromycin is indicated, in combination with other antimycobacterials, in the treatment of disseminated MAC disease due to *M. avium* or *Mycobacterium intracellulare*.

Acquired resistance of *M. avium* complex to clarithromycin has been found to develop when clarithromycin is used as monotherapy. Clarithromycin should be used in combination with other antimycobacterials to prevent the development of resistance.

Pharyngitis (treatment) or
Tonsillitis (treatment)—Clarithromycin is indicated in the treatment of pharyngitis or tonsillitis due to *S. pyogenes*.

The usual drug of choice in the treatment of streptococcal infections and the prophylaxis of rheumatic fever is penicillin. Clarithromycin is generally effective in the eradication of *S. pyogenes* from the nasopharynx. However, data establishing the efficacy of clarithromycin in the subsequent prevention of rheumatic fever are not available at present.

Ulcer, duodenal, *Helicobacter pylori*–associated (treatment adjunct)—Clarithromycin is indicated in combination with amoxicillin and lansoprazole[1], omeprazole, or ranitidine bismuth citrate[1] for the treatment of duodenal ulcer associated with *H. pylori* infection.

Pneumonia, bacterial (treatment)—Clarithromycin is indicated in the treatment of pneumonia due to *Chlamydia pneumoniae*, *Mycoplasma pneumoniae*, or *S. pneumoniae*.

Skin and soft tissue infections (treatment)—Clarithromycin is indicated in the treatment of uncomplicated skin and soft tissue infections due to susceptible strains of *S. aureus* or *S. pyogenes*. However, clarithromycin should not be used as first-line treatment where resistance may occur.

[Legionnaires' disease (treatment)][1]—Clarithromycin is used in the treatment of Legionnaires' disease caused by *L. pneumophila*.

[1]Not included in Canadian product labeling.

## Pharmacology/Pharmacokinetics

**Physicochemical characteristics**
Molecular weight—747.96.

**Mechanism of action/Effect**
Clarithromycin binds to the 50S ribosomal subunit of the 70S ribosome of susceptible organisms, thereby inhibiting bacterial RNA-dependent protein synthesis.

**Absorption**
Well absorbed from the gastrointestinal tract; stable in gastric acid; food delays the rate, but not the extent, of absorption; bioavailability is approximately 55% in healthy volunteers. In adults, the bioavailability of the oral suspension was similar to that of the tablets.

**Distribution**
Widely distributed into tissues and fluids; high concentrations found in nasal mucosa, tonsils, and lungs; concentrations in tissues are higher than those in serum because of high intracellular concentrations; readily enters leukocytes and macrophages.
Vol$_D$—243 to 266 liters.

**Protein binding**
High (65 to 75%).

**Biotransformation**
Hepatically metabolized via three main pathways, demethylation, hydroxylation, and hydrolysis, to eight metabolites. One metabolite, 14-hydroxyclarithromycin, has *in vitro* antimicrobial activity comparable to that of clarithromycin and may act synergistically with clarithromycin against *Haemophilus influenzae*. Saturation of metabolism involves the demethylation and hydroxylation pathways, and accounts for an increase in serum half-life.

**Half-life**
Normal renal function
    Clarithromycin:
        250 mg every 12 hours—3 to 4 hours.
        500 mg every 12 hours—5 to 7 hours.
    14-Hydroxyclarithromycin:
        250 mg every 12 hours—5 to 6 hours.
        500 mg every 12 hours—Approximately 7 hours.

Renal function impairment (creatinine clearance of < 30 mL per minute [0.5 mL per second])—Clarithromycin: Approximately 22 hours.
    14-Hydroxyclarithromycin: Approximately 47 hours.

**Time to peak concentration**
2 to 3 hours.

**Peak serum concentration**
Adults—
    Clarithromycin (at steady state):
        250 mg (suspension) every 12 hours—Approximately 2 mcg/mL.
        250 mg (tablet) every 12 hours—Approximately 1 mcg/mL.
        500 mg (tablet) every 12 hours—2 to 3 mcg/mL.
    14-Hydroxyclarithromycin (at steady state):
        250 mg (suspension) every 12 hours—Approximately 0.7 mcg/mL.
        250 mg (tablet) every 12 hours—Approximately 0.6 mcg/mL.
        500 mg (tablet) every 12 hours—Up to 1 mcg/mL.

Children—
    Clarithromycin (at steady state):
        7.5 mg per kg of body weight (mg/kg) (suspension) every 12 hours—3 to 7 mcg/mL.
        15 mg/kg (suspension) every 12 hours—6 to 15 mcg/mL.
    14-Hydroxyclarithromycin (at steady state):
        7.5 mg/kg (suspension) every 12 hours—1 to 2 mcg/mL.

**Elimination**
Renal—Approximately 20 and 30% of the dose of 250- and 500-mg tablets, respectively, given twice a day, is excreted in the urine as unchanged drug. Approximately 40% of the dose of 250-mg suspension given twice a day is excreted in the urine as clarithromycin. 14-Hydroxyclarithromycin accounts for 10 and 15% of the dose excreted in the urine after doses of 250 and 500 mg, respectively, given twice a day.
Fecal—Approximately 4% of a 250-mg dose is excreted in the feces.

## Precautions to Consider

**Cross-sensitivity and/or related problems**
Patients who are hypersensitive to erythromycin or other macrolides may also be hypersensitive to clarithromycin.

**Carcinogenicity/Mutagenicity**
Clarithromycin was not found to be mutagenic in the *Salmonella*/mammalian microsome tests, the bacterial induced mutation frequency test, the rat hepatocyte DNA synthesis assay, the mouse lymphoma assay, the mouse dominant lethal assay, or the mouse micronucleus test. However, the *in vitro* chromosome aberration test was weakly positive in one test and negative in another. The Ames test was negative when performed on clarithromycin metabolites.

**Pregnancy/Reproduction**
Fertility—Adequate and well-controlled studies in humans have not been done.
Studies in male and female rats given 160 mg per kg of body weight (mg/kg) per day (plasma concentrations equivalent to approximately two times the human serum concentrations) showed no adverse effects on the estrous cycle, fertility, parturition, or the number and viability of offspring.

Pregnancy—Adequate and well-controlled studies in humans have not been done.
Monkeys administered oral doses of 150 mg/kg per day (plasma concentrations equivalent to three times the human serum concentrations) had embryonic loss, which was attributed to marked maternal toxicity at this dose. *In utero* fetal loss occurred in rabbits given intravenous doses of 33 mg per square meter of body surface area (mg/m$^2$), which is equivalent to 17 times less than the maximum recommended human daily dose.
Clarithromycin was not found to be teratogenic in four rat studies (three with oral doses and one with intravenous doses of up to 160 mg/kg per day administered during the period of major organogenesis) or in two rabbit studies (at oral doses of up to 125 mg/kg per day or intravenous doses of 30 mg/kg per day administered during gestation days 6 through 18). Two additional studies in a different rat strain demonstrated a low incidence of cardiovascular anomalies at oral doses of 150 mg/kg per day administered during gestation days 6 to 15. Cleft palate was seen at doses of 500 mg/kg per day. Fetal growth retardation was seen in monkeys given an oral dose of 70 mg/kg per day, which produced plasma concentrations that were equivalent to two times the human serum concentrations.

FDA Pregnancy Category C.

**Breast-feeding**
Clarithromycin and its active metabolite are distributed into breast milk.

**Pediatrics**
Appropriate studies on the relationship of age to the effects of clarithromycin have not been performed in children up to 6 months of age. Safety and efficacy have not been established.

**Geriatrics**
One study performed in healthy elderly subjects found increased peak steady-state concentrations of clarithromycin and 14-hydroxyclarith-

romycin; this was thought to be due to an age-related decrease in renal function. There was no increase in side effects in elderly patients compared with younger subjects. Elderly patients with severe renal function impairment may require a decrease in dose.

**Drug interactions and/or related problems**
The following drug interactions and/or related problems have been selected on the basis of their potential clinical significance (possible mechanism in parentheses where appropriate)—not necessarily inclusive (» = major clinical significance):

Note: Combinations containing any of the following medications, depending on the amount present, may also interact with this medication.

» Astemizole
(QTc-interval prolongation and torsades de pointes have been reported with concurrent use of astemizole and erythromycin; since clarithromycin is also metabolized by the cytochrome P450 enzyme system, concurrent use of clarithromycin and astemizole is not recommended)

Anticoagulants, coumarin- or indandione-derivative or
» Warfarin
(concurrent administration with clarithromycin has been shown to potentiate the effects of warfarin; prothrombin time should be monitored closely in patients receiving oral anticoagulants and clarithromycin concurrently)

» Carbamazepine or
Other medications metabolized by the cytochrome P450 enzyme system
(concurrent administration with clarithromycin has been shown to significantly increase the plasma concentrations of carbamazepine and other medications metabolized by the cytochrome P450 enzyme system; serum concentrations of carbamazepine and these other medications should be monitored)

» Cisapride or
» Pimozide or
» Terfenadine
(concurrent administration with clarithromycin has resulted in cardiac arrhythmias, including QTc-interval prolongation, ventricular tachycardia, ventricular fibrillation, and torsades de pointes; fatalities have also occurred; the most likely cause is the inhibition of hepatic metabolism of these medications by clarithromycin; concurrent use is **contraindicated**)

» Digoxin
(concurrent administration with clarithromycin has been shown to increase serum digoxin concentrations; monitoring of digoxin serum concentrations is recommended in patients receiving digoxin and clarithromycin concurrently)

» Rifabutin or
» Rifampin
(concurrent use with clarithromycin causes a decrease in the serum concentration of clarithromycin by > 50%)

» Theophylline
(concurrent administration with clarithromycin has been shown to increase the area under the plasma concentration–time curve [AUC] of theophylline by 17%; monitoring of theophylline serum concentrations is recommended in patients receiving high doses of theophylline or in patients with theophylline serum concentrations in the upper therapeutic range)

» Zidovudine
(concurrent administration with clarithromycin causes a decrease in the steady-state concentration of zidovudine; doses of clarithromycin and zidovudine should be taken at least 4 hours apart)

**Laboratory value alterations**
The following have been selected on the basis of their potential clinical significance (possible effect in parentheses where appropriate)—not necessarily inclusive (» = major clinical significance):

With physiology/laboratory test values
Alanine aminotransferase (ALT [SGPT]) or
Aspartate aminotransferase (AST [SGOT])
(rarely, serum values may be elevated)
Blood urea nitrogen (BUN)
(rarely, concentration may be elevated)

**Medical considerations/Contraindications**
The medical considerations/contraindications included have been selected on the basis of their potential clinical significance (reasons given in parentheses where appropriate)—not necessarily inclusive (» = major clinical significance).

*Risk-benefit should be considered when the following medical problems exist:*
Hypersensitivity to clarithromycin, erythromycins, or other macrolides
» Renal function impairment, severe
(the elimination of clarithromycin is reduced in patients with renal function impairment, especially those with a creatinine clearance of < 30 mL/min [0.5 mL/second] with or without coexisting hepatic function impairment; the dose of clarithromycin should be halved, or the dosing interval doubled, in patients with a creatinine clearance of < 30 mL/min [0.5 mL/second])

(liver function impairment alters the pharmacokinetics of clarithromycin by decreasing the amount of metabolites formed and increasing the renal clearance of the parent drug; however, steady-state concentrations in patients with mild to severe hepatic function impairment do not differ from those in patients with normal hepatic function, unless there is also concurrent severe renal function impairment; no dosage adjustment is necessary in patients with hepatic function impairment if renal function is normal)

## Side/Adverse Effects
The following side/adverse effects have been selected on the basis of their potential clinical significance (possible signs and symptoms in parentheses where appropriate)—not necessarily inclusive:

**Those indicating need for medical attention**
Incidence rare
*Hepatotoxicity* (fever; nausea and vomiting; yellow eyes or skin); *hypersensitivity reaction* (shortness of breath; skin rash and itching); *pseudomembranous colitis* (abdominal or stomach cramps and pain, severe; abdominal tenderness; diarrhea, watery and severe, which may also be bloody; fever); *thrombocytopenia* (unusual bleeding and bruising)

**Those indicating need for medical attention only if they continue or are bothersome**
Incidence less frequent
*Abnormal sensation of taste*—3%; *gastrointestinal disturbances* (abdominal discomfort or pain; diarrhea; nausea; vomiting)—2 to 3%; *headache*—2%

## Patient Consultation
As an aid to patient consultation, refer to *Advice for the Patient, Clarithromycin (Systemic)*.
In providing consultation, consider emphasizing the following selected information (» = major clinical significance):

**Before using this medication**
» Conditions affecting use, especially:
Hypersensitivity to clarithromycin, erythromycins, or other macrolides
Pregnancy—Clarithromycin has produced embryotoxicity and fetal toxicity in animals
Breast-feeding—Passes into breast milk
Contraindicated medications—Cisapride, pimozide, and terfenadine
Other medications, especially astemizole, carbamazepine, digoxin, rifabutin, rifampin, theophylline, warfarin, and zidovudine
Other medical problems, especially severe renal function impairment

**Proper use of this medication**
May be taken with food or milk or on an empty stomach
Taking at least 4 hours apart from taking zidovudine
» Compliance with full course of therapy
Proper administration technique for oral liquids
» Proper dosing
Missed dose: Taking as soon as possible; not taking if almost time for next dose; not doubling doses
» Proper storage

**Precautions while using this medication**
» Not taking with cisapride, pimozide, or terfenadine
Checking with physician if no improvement within a few days

**Side/adverse effects**
Signs of potential side effects, especially hepatotoxicity, hypersensitivity reaction, pseudomembranous colitis, and thrombocytopenia

## General Dosing Information
Clarithromycin tablets and suspension may be taken with meals or milk or on an empty stomach.

# Oral Dosage Forms

## CLARITHROMYCIN FOR ORAL SUSPENSION

**Usual adult and adolescent dose**

Bronchitis, bacterial exacerbations due to *Haemophilus influenzae*—
   Oral, 500 mg every twelve hours for seven to fourteen days.

Bronchitis, bacterial exacerbations due to other organisms or
Pneumonia, chlamydial, mycoplasmal, or streptococcal or
Skin and soft tissue infections, uncomplicated—
   Oral, 250 mg every twelve hours for seven to fourteen days.

*Mycobacterium avium* complex disease, disseminated, prophylaxis[1]—
   Oral, 500 mg two times a day.

*Mycobacterium avium* complex disease, disseminated, treatment—
   Oral, 500 mg two times a day in combination with other antimycobacterial agents; clarithromycin therapy should continue for life if clinical and mycobacterial improvements are observed.

Pharyngitis, streptococcal or
Tonsillitis—
   Oral, 250 mg every twelve hours for ten days.

Sinusitis, acute maxillary—
   Oral, 500 mg every twelve hours for fourteen days.

Note: The dose of clarithromycin should be adjusted in patients with severe renal function impairment (creatinine clearance [CrCl] < 30 mL/min [0.5 mL/sec]). The following dosing guidelines are suggested:

| Dose for CrCl of > 30 mL/min (0.5 mL/sec) | Adjusted dose for CrCl of < 30 mL/min (0.5 mL/sec) |
|---|---|
| 500 mg two times a day | 500 mg loading dose, then 250 mg two times a day |
| 250 mg two times a day | 250 mg once a day |

Dosage should not be continued beyond 14 days in patients with severe renal function impairment.

**Usual pediatric dose**

Otitis media, acute or
Pharyngitis, streptococcal or
Pneumonia, chlamydial, mycoplasmal, or streptococcal, or
Sinusitis, acute maxillary[1] or
Skin and soft tissue infections or
Tonsillitis[1]—
   Infants and children 6 months of age and older: Oral, 7.5 mg per kg of body weight every twelve hours for ten days.
   Infants up to 6 months of age: Safety and efficacy have not been established.

*Mycobacterium avium* complex disease, disseminated, prophylaxis[1]—
   Infants and children 6 months of age and older: Oral, 7.5 mg per kg of body weight, up to 500 mg, two times a day.
   Infants up to 6 months of age: Safety and efficacy have not been established.

*Mycobacterium avium* complex disease, disseminated, treatment—
   Infants and children 6 months of age and older: Oral, 7.5 mg per kg of body weight, up to 500 mg, two times a day in combination with other antimycobacterial agents; clarithromycin therapy should continue for life if clinical and mycobacterial improvements are observed.
   Infants up to 6 months of age: Safety and efficacy have not been established.

Note: The dose of clarithromycin should be halved, or the dosing interval doubled, in pediatric patients with severe renal function impairment (CrCl < 30 mL per minute [0.5 mL per second]), with or without co-existing hepatic function impairment.

**Usual pediatric prescribing limits**
1000 mg per day.

**Strength(s) usually available**

U.S.—
   125 mg per 5 mL (when reconstituted according to manufacturer's instructions) (available in 50- and 100-mL bottles) (Rx) [*Biaxin* (sucrose)].
   250 mg per 5 mL (when reconstituted according to manufacturer's instructions) (available in 50- and 100-mL bottles) (Rx) [*Biaxin* (sucrose)].

Canada—
   125 mg per 5 mL (when reconstituted according to manufacturer's instructions) (available in 60-, 105-, and 150-mL bottles) (Rx) [*Biaxin* (saccharine; sodium chloride; sucrose)].

**Packaging and storage**
Store between 15 and 30 °C (59 and 86 °F) in a well-closed container. Protect from light.

**Preparation of dosage form**
Add the total volume of water indicated below, in two portions, shaking well after each addition.

| Country available | Clarithromycin concentration after reconstitution | Total amount of water to be added | Total volume after reconstitution |
|---|---|---|---|
| U.S. | 125 mg/5 mL | 27 mL | 50 mL |
|  | 125 mg/5 mL | 55 mL | 100 mL |
|  | 250 mg/5 mL | 27 mL | 50 mL |
|  | 250 mg/5 mL | 55 mL | 100 mL |
| Canada | 125 mg/5 mL | 32 mL | 60 mL |
|  | 125 mg/5 mL | 56 mL | 105 mL |
|  | 125 mg/5 mL | 80 mL | 150 mL |

**Stability**
After reconstitution, suspension retains its potency for 14 days. Do not refrigerate.

**Auxiliary labeling**
- Shake well.
- Do not refrigerate.
- Continue for full time of treatment.
- Beyond-use date.

**Note**
When dispensing, include a calibrated liquid-measuring device.

## CLARITHROMYCIN TABLETS USP

**Usual adult and adolescent dose**

Bronchitis, bacterial exacerbations or
*Mycobacterium avium* complex disease, disseminated, prophylaxis[1] or treatment or
Pharyngitis, streptococcal or
Pneumonia, chlamydial, mycoplasmal, or streptococcal or
Sinusitis, acute maxillary or
Skin and soft tissue infections, uncomplicated or
Tonsillitis—
   See *Clarithromycin for Oral Suspension*.

Ulcer, duodenal, *Helicobacter pylori*–associated, treatment adjunct with amoxicillin and lansoprazole[1]—
   Oral, 500 mg in combination with amoxicillin 1000 mg and lansoprazole 30 mg every twelve hours for fourteen days.

Ulcer, duodenal, *H. pylori*–associated, treatment adjunct with omeprazole—
   Oral, 500 mg three times a day in combination with omeprazole 40 mg once a day for fourteen days, followed by omeprazole alone 20 mg once a day for fourteen days.

Ulcer, duodenal, *H. pylori*–associated, treatment adjunct with ranitidine bismuth citrate[1]—
   Oral, 500 mg three times a day in combination with ranitidine bismuth citrate 400 mg two times a day for fourteen days, followed by ranitidine bismuth citrate alone 400 mg two times a day for fourteen days.

Note: Combination therapy with clarithromycin and ranitidine bismuth citrate is not recommended for patients with creatinine clearance of less than 25 mL per minute (0.41 mL per second).

**Usual pediatric dose**
This product may not be suitable for young children. See *Clarithromycin for Oral Suspension*.

**Strength(s) usually available**

U.S.—
   250 mg (Rx) [*Biaxin*].
   500 mg (Rx) [*Biaxin*].

Canada—
   250 mg (Rx) [*Biaxin*].
   500 mg (Rx) [*Biaxin*].

**Packaging and storage**
Store below 40 °C (104 °F), preferably between 15 and 30 °C (59 and 86 °F), unless otherwise specified by manufacturer. Protect from light. Preserve in tight containers.

**Auxiliary labeling**
- Continue medicine for full time of treatment.

---

[1]Not included in Canadian product labeling.

**CLEMASTINE**—See *Antihistamines (Systemic)*

**CLIDINIUM**—See *Anticholinergics/Antispasmodics (Systemic)*

# CLINDAMYCIN  Systemic

VA CLASSIFICATION (Primary/Secondary): AM350/AP101

Commonly used brand name(s): *Cleocin; Cleocin Pediatric; Dalacin C; Dalacin C Flavored Granules; Dalacin C Phosphate.*

Note:  For a listing of dosage forms and brand names by country availability, see *Dosage Forms* section(s).

## Category

Antibacterial (systemic); antiprotozoal.

## Indications

Note:  Bracketed information in the *Indications* section refers to uses that are not included in U.S. product labeling.

**Accepted**

Bone and joint infections (treatment)—Parenteral clindamycin is indicated in the adjunctive surgical treatment of chronic bone and joint infections, and acute hematogenous osteomyelitis caused by staphylococci.

Pelvic infections, female (treatment)—Clindamycin is indicated in the treatment of female pelvic infections, including endometritis, nongonococcal tubo-ovarian abscess, pelvic cellulitis, and postsurgical vaginal cuff infections caused by anaerobes.

Intra-abdominal infections (treatment)—Clindamycin is indicated in the treatment of intra-abdominal infections (such as peritonitis and abscesses) caused by anaerobes.

Pneumonia, anaerobic (treatment)
Pneumonia, pneumococcal (treatment)
Pneumonia, staphylococcal (treatment) or
Pneumonia, streptococcal (treatment)—Clindamycin is indicated as a primary agent in the treatment of pneumonia, including serious respiratory tract infections (such as empyema, pneumonitis, and lung abscess) caused by anaerobes. Clindamycin is indicated as a secondary agent in the treatment of pneumonia caused by susceptible strains of pneumococci, staphylococci, and streptococci.

Septicemia, bacterial (treatment)—Oral and parenteral clindamycin are indicated in the treatment of septicemia caused by anaerobes. In addition, parenteral clindamycin is indicated in the treatment of septicemia caused by streptococci and staphylococci.

Skin and soft tissue infections (treatment)—Clindamycin is indicated in the treatment of serious skin and soft tissue infections caused by anaerobes, streptococci, and staphylococci.

[Actinomycosis (treatment)][1]—Clindamycin is used in the treatment of actinomycosis.

[Babesiosis (treatment)][1]—Clindamycin is used concurrently with quinine in the treatment of severe babesiosis caused by *Babesia microti*.

[Erysipelas (treatment)][1]—Clindamycin is used in the treatment of erysipelas.

[Malaria (treatment)][1]—Clindamycin is used in combination with quinine in the treatment of chloroquine-resistant malaria caused by *Plasmodium falciparum* in patients for whom standard therapy is contraindicated (e.g., children, pregnant women, sulfa allergy).

[Otitis media, chronic suppurative (treatment)][1]—Clindamycin is used in the treatment of chronic suppurative otitis media.

[Pneumonia, *Pneumocystis carinii* (treatment)][1]—Clindamycin is used in combination with primaquine in the treatment of *Pneumocystis carinii* pneumonia (PCP) in patients unresponsive or intolerant to standard therapy.

[Sinusitis (treatment)][1]—Clindamycin is used in the treatment of sinusitis.

[Toxoplasmosis, central nervous system (CNS) (treatment)][1]—Clindamycin is used in combination with pyrimethamine in the treatment of CNS toxoplasmosis in patients who are unresponsive or intolerant to standard therapy.

Not all species or strains of a particular organism may be susceptible to clindamycin.

**Unaccepted**

Clindamycin is not indicated in the treatment of meningitis since it penetrates poorly into cerebrospinal fluid (CSF), even in the presence of inflamed meninges.

[1]Not included in Canadian product labeling.

## Pharmacology/Pharmacokinetics

**Physicochemical characteristics**

Molecular weight—Clindamycin hydrochloride: 461.44.
Clindamycin palmitate hydrochloride: 699.86.
Clindamycin phosphate: 504.96.

**Mechanism of action/Effect**

Antibacterial (systemic)—The lincomycins inhibit protein synthesis in susceptible bacteria by binding to the 50 S subunits of bacterial ribosomes and preventing peptide bond formation. They are usually considered bacteriostatic, but may be bactericidal in high concentrations or when used against highly susceptible organisms.

**Absorption**

Rapidly absorbed from the gastrointestinal tract following oral administration; not inactivated by gastric acid. Approximately 90% absorbed orally in fasting state; absorption unaffected by food.

**Distribution**

Widely and rapidly distributed to most fluids and tissues, except cerebrospinal fluid (CSF); high concentrations in bone, bile, and urine. Readily crosses the placenta. Also excreted in breast milk.

$Vol_D$—
  Adults: Approximately 0.66 liter per kg.
  Children: Approximately 0.86 liter per kg.

**Protein binding**

Very high (92–94%).

**Biotransformation**

Hepatic; some metabolites may possess antibacterial activity. Clindamycin palmitate and clindamycin phosphate are inactive; they are rapidly hydrolyzed *in vivo* to active clindamycin.

**Half-life**

Normal renal function—
  Adults: 2.4 to 3.0 hours.
  Infants and children: 2.5 to 3.4 hours.
  Premature infants: 6.3 to 8.6 hours.
End-stage renal failure or severe hepatic impairment—
  Slightly increased (3 to 5 hours in adults).

**Time to peak serum concentration**

Oral—0.75 to 1 hour.
Intramuscular—1 hour (children); 3 hours (adults).
Intravenous—End of infusion.

**Peak serum concentration**

Adults (steady-state)—
  300 mg intravenously over 10 minutes every 8 hours: Approximately 7 mcg/mL.
  600 mg intravenously over 20 minutes every 8 hours: Approximately 10 mcg/mL.
  900 mg intravenously over 30 minutes every 12 hours: Approximately 11 mcg/mL.
  1200 mg intravenously over 45 minutes every 12 hours: Approximately 14 mcg/mL.
  300 mg intramuscularly every 8 hours: Approximately 6 mcg/mL.
  600 mg intramuscularly every 12 hours: Approximately 9 mcg/mL.
Children (first dose)—
  5 to 7 mg per kg of body weight (mg/kg) intravenously over 1 hour: Approximately 10 mcg/mL.
  3 to 5 mg/kg intramuscularly: Approximately 4 mcg/mL.
  5 to 7 mg/kg intramuscularly: Approximately 8 mcg/mL.

---

## Selected Bibliography

Piscitelli SC, Danziger LH, Rodvold KA. Clarithromycin and azithromycin: new macrolide antibiotics. Clin Pharm 1992; 11: 137-52.
Peters DH, Clissold SP. Clarithromycin. Drugs 1992; 44(1): 117-64.

Revised: 07/24/95
Interim revision: 03/26/98

## Elimination
Approximately 10% of a total dose is eliminated in the urine and 3.6% in the feces as active drug. The remainder is excreted as inactive metabolites.

Dialysis—Not removed from the blood by hemodialysis or peritoneal dialysis.

## Precautions to Consider

### Cross-sensitivity and/or related problems
Patients hypersensitive to lincomycin may be hypersensitive to clindamycin also. There is also a report of a possible cross-sensitivity between clindamycin and doxorubicin.

### Pregnancy/Reproduction
Pregnancy—Clindamycin crosses the placenta and may be concentrated in the fetal liver. However, problems in humans have not been documented.

### Breast-feeding
Clindamycin is excreted in breast milk. However, problems in humans have not been documented.

### Pediatrics
Clindamycin should be used with caution in infants up to 1 month of age. Clindamycin phosphate injection contains benzyl alcohol, which has been associated with a fatal gasping syndrome in infants.

### Geriatrics
No information is available on the relationship of age to the effects of clindamycin in geriatric patients.

### Drug interactions and/or related problems
The following drug interactions and/or related problems have been selected on the basis of their potential clinical significance (possible mechanism in parentheses where appropriate)—not necessarily inclusive (» = major clinical significance):

Note: Combinations containing any of the following medications, depending on the amount present, may also interact with this medication.

» Anesthetics, hydrocarbon inhalation or
» Neuromuscular blocking agents
(concurrent use of these medications with clindamycin, if necessary, should be carefully monitored since neuromuscular blockade may be enhanced, resulting in skeletal muscle weakness and respiratory depression or paralysis [apnea]; caution is also recommended when these medications are used concurrently with clindamycin during surgery or in the postoperative period; treatment with anticholinesterase agents or calcium salts may help reverse the blockade)

» Antidiarrheals, adsorbent
(concurrent use of kaolin- or attapulgite-containing antidiarrheals with oral clindamycin may significantly delay the absorption of oral clindamycin; concurrent use should be avoided or patients should be advised to take adsorbent antidiarrheals not less than 2 hours before or 3 to 4 hours after oral lincomycins)

Antimyasthenics
(concurrent use of medications with neuromuscular blocking action may antagonize the effect of antimyasthenics on skeletal muscle; temporary dosage adjustments of antimyasthenics may be necessary to control symptoms of myasthenia gravis during and following concurrent use)

» Chloramphenicol or
» Erythromycins
(may displace clindamycin from or prevent its binding to 50 S subunits of bacterial ribosomes, thus antagonizing clindamycin's effects; concurrent use is not recommended)

Opioid (narcotic) analgesics
(respiratory depressant effects of drugs with neuromuscular blocking activity may be additive to central respiratory depressant effects of opioid analgesics, possibly leading to increased or prolonged respiratory depression or paralysis [apnea]; caution and careful monitoring of the patient are recommended)

### Laboratory value alterations
The following have been selected on the basis of their potential clinical significance (possible effect in parentheses where appropriate)—not necessarily inclusive (» = major clinical significance):

With diagnostic test results
Alanine aminotransferase (ALT [SGPT]), serum and
Alkaline phosphatase, serum and
Aspartate aminotransferase (ALT [SGOT]), serum
(concentrations may be increased)

### Medical considerations/Contraindications
The medical considerations/contraindications included have been selected on the basis of their potential clinical significance (reasons given in parentheses where appropriate)—not necessarily inclusive (» = major clinical significance).

*Risk-benefit should be considered when the following medical problems exist:*

» Gastrointestinal disease, history of, especially ulcerative colitis, regional enteritis, or antibiotic-associated colitis
(clindamycin may cause pseudomembranous colitis)

» Hepatic function impairment, severe
(the half-life of clindamycin is prolonged in patients with severe hepatic function impairment; this may require an adjustment in dosage)

Hypersensitivity to lincomycins or doxorubicin

Renal function impairment, severe
(patients with impaired renal function do not generally require a reduction in dose unless the impairment is severe; however, patients receiving clindamycin with very severe renal impairment and/or very severe hepatic impairment accompanied by severe metabolic abnormalities may require a reduction in dosage)

### Patient monitoring
The following may be especially important in patient monitoring (other tests may be warranted in some patients, depending on condition; » = major clinical significance):

*For antibiotic-associated pseudomembranous colitis (AAPMC)*
Colonoscopy and/or
Proctosigmoidoscopy
(proctosigmoidoscopy and/or colonoscopy may be required in selected, severely ill patients with persistent symptoms of AAPMC to document the presence of pseudomembranes; it is no longer recommended as a routine monitoring parameter)

Stool examinations
(cytotoxin assays of stool samples for the presence of *Clostridium difficile* and its cytotoxin, neutralizable by *C. sordellii* antitoxin, may be required prior to treatment in patients with AAPMC to document the presence of *C. difficile* and/or its cytotoxin; however, *C. difficile* and its cytotoxin may persist following treatment with oral vancomycin despite clinical improvement; follow-up cytotoxin assays are generally not recommended with complete clinical improvement)

## Side/Adverse Effects
The following side/adverse effects have been selected on the basis of their potential clinical significance (possible signs and symptoms in parentheses where appropriate)—not necessarily inclusive:

### Those indicating need for medical attention
Incidence more frequent
*Pseudomembranous colitis* (severe abdominal or stomach cramps and pain; abdominal tenderness; diarrhea, watery and severe, which may also be bloody; fever)

Incidence less frequent
*Hypersensitivity* (skin rash, redness, and itching); *neutropenia* (sore throat and fever); *thrombocytopenia* (unusual bleeding or bruising)

### Those indicating need for medical attention only if they continue or are bothersome
Incidence more frequent
*Gastrointestinal disturbances* (abdominal pain; diarrhea; nausea and vomiting)

Incidence less frequent
*Fungal overgrowth* (itching of rectal or genital areas)

### Those indicating possible pseudomembranous colitis and the need for medical attention if they occur after medication is discontinued
Severe abdominal or stomach cramps and pain; abdominal tenderness; watery and severe diarrhea, which may also be bloody; fever

## Patient Consultation
As an aid to patient consultation, refer to *Advice for the Patient, Clindamycin (Systemic)*.

In providing consultation, consider emphasizing the following selected information (» = major clinical significance):

### Before using this medication
» Conditions affecting use, especially:
Hypersensitivity to clindamycin, lincomycin, or doxorubicin
Pregnancy—Clindamycin crosses the placenta
Breast-feeding—Clindamycin is excreted in breast milk

Use in children—Clindamycin should be used cautiously in infants up to 1 month of age; clindamycin injection contains benzyl alcohol, which has been associated with a fatal gasping syndrome in infants

Other medications, especially hydrocarbon inhalation anesthetics, neuromuscular blocking agents, adsorbent antidiarrheals, chloramphenicol, or erythromycins

Other medical problems, especially a history of gastrointestinal disease, particularly ulcerative colitis, or severe hepatic function impairment

**Proper use of this medication**
» Taking clindamycin capsules with a full glass of water or with meals to avoid esophageal ulceration

Proper administration technique for clindamycin oral solution; not using after expiration date
» Compliance with full course of therapy, especially in streptococcal infections
» Importance of not missing doses and taking at evenly spaced times
» Proper dosing
Missed dose: Taking as soon as possible; not taking if almost time for next dose; not doubling doses
» Proper storage

**Precautions while using this medication**
Regular visits to physician to check progress
Checking with physician if no improvement within a few days
» For severe diarrhea, checking with physician before taking any antidiarrheals; for mild diarrhea, taking attapulgite-containing antidiarrheals at least 2 hours before or 3 to 4 hours after taking oral clindamycin; other antidiarrheals may worsen or prolong the diarrhea; checking with physician or pharmacist if mild diarrhea continues or worsens
Caution if surgery with general anesthesia is required

**Side/adverse effects**
Signs of potential side effects, especially pseudomembranous colitis, hypersensitivity, neutropenia, and thrombocytopenia

## General Dosing Information

Therapy should be continued for at least 10 days in group A beta-hemolytic streptococcal infections to help prevent the occurrence of acute rheumatic fever.

For oral dosage forms only:
- The capsule dosage form should be taken with food or a full glass (240 mL) of water to avoid esophageal irritation.

**For treatment of adverse effects**
*For antibiotic-associated pseudomembranous colitis (AAPMC)*
- Some patients may develop antibiotic-associated pseudomembranous colitis (AAPMC), caused by *Clostridium difficile* toxin, during or following administration of lincomycins. Mild cases may respond to discontinuation of the drug alone. Moderate to severe cases may require fluid, electrolyte, and protein replacement.
- In cases not responding to the above measures or in more severe cases, oral doses of metronidazole, bacitracin, cholestyramine, or vancomycin may be used. Oral vancomycin is effective in doses of 125 to 500 mg every 6 hours for 5 to 10 days. The dose of metronidazole is 250 to 500 mg every 8 hours; cholestyramine, 4 grams four times a day; and bacitracin, 25,000 units, orally, four times a day. Recurrences may be treated with a second course of these medications.
- Cholestyramine and colestipol resins have been shown to bind *C. difficile* toxin *in vitro*. If cholestyramine or colestipol resin is administered in conjunction with oral vancomycin, the medications should be administered several hours apart since the resins have been shown to bind oral vancomycin also.
- In addition, antibiotic-associated pseudomembranous colitis may result in severe watery diarrhea, which may occur during therapy or up to several weeks after therapy is discontinued. If diarrhea occurs, administration of antiperistaltic antidiarrheals (e.g., opiates, diphenoxylate and atropine combination, loperamide) is not recommended since they may delay the removal of toxins from the colon, thereby prolonging and/or worsening the condition.

## Oral Dosage Forms

Note: Bracketed uses in the *Dosage Forms* section refer to categories of use and/or indications that are not included in U.S. product labeling.

### CLINDAMYCIN HYDROCHLORIDE CAPSULES USP
**Usual adult and adolescent dose**
Antibacterial—
Oral, 150 to 300 mg (base) every six hours.

[Malaria (treatment)][1]—
Oral, 900 mg (base) three times a day for three days.

[Pneumonia, *Pneumocystis carinii* (treatment)][1]—
Oral, 1200 to 1800 mg (base) per day in divided doses in combination with 15 to 30 mg of primaquine daily.

[Toxoplasmosis, central nervous system (CNS) (treatment)][1]—
Oral, 1200 to 2400 mg (base) per day in divided doses in combination with 50 to 100 mg of pyrimethamine daily.

**Usual pediatric dose**
Antibacterial—
Infants up to 1 month of age: Dosage must be individualized by physician. Use with caution.
Infants 1 month of age and over: Oral, 2 to 5 mg (base) per kg of body weight every six hours; or 2.7 to 6.7 mg per kg of body weight every eight hours.

Note: In children weighing 10 kg or less, the minimum recommended dose is 37.5 mg every eight hours.

[Malaria (treatment)][1]—
Oral, 6.7 to 13.3 mg per kg of body weight three times a day for three days.

**Strength(s) usually available**
U.S.—
75 mg (base) (Rx) [*Cleocin* (tartrazine); GENERIC].
150 mg (base) (Rx) [*Cleocin* (tartrazine); GENERIC].
300 mg (base) (Rx) [*Cleocin* (tartrazine)].
Canada—
150 mg (base) (Rx) [*Dalacin C*].
300 mg (base) (Rx) [*Dalacin C*].

**Packaging and storage**
Store below 40 °C (104 °F), preferably between 15 and 30 °C (59 and 86 °F), unless otherwise specified by manufacturer. Store in a tight container.

**Auxiliary labeling**
- Take with food or water.
- Continue medicine for full time of treatment.

### CLINDAMYCIN PALMITATE HYDROCHLORIDE FOR ORAL SOLUTION USP
**Usual adult and adolescent dose**
See *Clindamycin Hydrochloride Capsules USP*.

**Usual pediatric dose**
See *Clindamycin Hydrochloride Capsules USP*.

**Strength(s) usually available**
U.S.—
75 mg per 5 mL (base) (when reconstituted according to manufacturer's instructions) (Rx) [*Cleocin Pediatric* (sucrose)].
Canada—
75 mg per 5 mL (base) (when reconstituted according to manufacturer's instructions) (Rx) [*Dalacin C Flavored Granules*].

**Packaging and storage**
Prior to reconstitution, store below 40 °C (104 °F), preferably between 15 and 30 °C (59 and 86 °F), unless otherwise specified by manufacturer. Store in a tight container. Do not refrigerate the reconstituted solution since it may thicken and be difficult to pour when chilled.

**Stability**
After reconstitution, solutions retain their potency for 14 days at room temperature.

**Auxiliary labeling**
- Do not refrigerate.
- Shake well.
- Continue medicine for full time of treatment.
- Beyond-use date.

**Note**
When dispensing, include a calibrated liquid-measuring device.

## Parenteral Dosage Forms

Note: Bracketed uses in the *Dosage Forms* section refer to categories of use and/or indications that are not included in U.S. product labeling.

### CLINDAMYCIN PHOSPHATE INJECTION USP
**Usual adult and adolescent dose**
Antibacterial—
Intramuscular or intravenous, 300 to 600 mg (base) every six to eight hours; or 900 mg every eight hours.

**896    Clindamycin (Systemic)**

[Babesiosis (treatment)][1]—
  Intravenous, 300 to 600 mg clindamycin (base) four times a day with concurrent oral administration of 650 mg of quinine, three or four times a day for seven to ten days.
[Pneumonia, *Pneumocystis carinii* (treatment)][1]—
  Intravenous, 2400 to 2700 mg (base) per day in divided doses in combination with 15 to 30 mg of primaquine daily.
[Toxoplasmosis, central nervous system (CNS) (treatment)][1]—
  Intravenous, 1200 to 4800 mg (base) per day in divided doses in combination with 50 to 100 mg of pyrimethamine daily.

**Usual adult prescribing limits**
Up to 2.7 grams (base) daily.
Note: Doses up to 4.8 grams daily have been used. However, some medical experts recommend a maximum dose of 2.7 grams daily.

**Usual pediatric dose**
Antibacterial—
  Infants up to 1 month of age: Intramuscular or intravenous, 3.75 to 5 mg (base) per kg of body weight every six hours; or 5 to 6.7 mg per kg of body weight every eight hours.
  Infants 1 month of age and over: Intramuscular or intravenous, 3.75 to 10 mg (base) per kg of body weight or 87.5 to 112.5 mg per square meter of body surface every six hours; or 5 to 13.3 mg per kg of body weight or 116.7 to 150 mg per square meter of body surface every eight hours.
Note: In children, regardless of body weight, the minimum recommended dose is 300 mg (base) daily for severe infections.
  Bone infection—Intramuscular or intravenous, 7.5 mg per kg of body weight every six hours.
[Babesiosis (treatment)][1]—
  Dosage has not been established; however, based on one case report in an infant, the suggested dose is: Intravenous or intramuscular, 20 mg per kg of body weight per day of clindamycin with concurrent oral administration of 25 mg per kg of body weight per day of quinine for seven to ten days.

**Strength(s) usually available**
U.S.—
  300 mg (base) in 2 mL (Rx) [*Cleocin* (benzyl alcohol 9.45 mg); GENERIC].
  600 mg (base) in 4 mL (Rx) [*Cleocin* (benzyl alcohol 9.45 mg); GENERIC].
  900 mg (base) in 6 mL (Rx) [*Cleocin* (benzyl alcohol 9.45 mg); GENERIC].
  9000 mg (base) in 60 mL (Rx) [GENERIC].
Canada—
  300 mg (base) in 2 mL (Rx) [*Dalacin C Phosphate* (benzyl alcohol)].
  600 mg (base) in 4 mL (Rx) [*Dalacin C Phosphate* (benzyl alcohol)].
  900 mg (base) in 6 mL (Rx) [*Dalacin C Phosphate* (benzyl alcohol)].

**Packaging and storage**
Store below 40 °C (104 °F), preferably between 15 and 30 °C (59 and 86 °F), unless otherwise specified by manufacturer. Protect from freezing.

**Preparation of dosage form**
To prepare initial dilution for intravenous use, each dose must be diluted as follows (it must not be administered undiluted as a bolus):

| Dose (mg) | Diluent (mL) | Duration of Administration (min) |
|---|---|---|
| 300 | 50 | 10 |
| 600 | 100 | 20 |
| 900 | 100 | 30 |

Caution: Products containing benzyl alcohol are not recommended for use in neonates. A fatal toxic syndrome consisting of metabolic acidosis, CNS depression, respiratory problems, renal failure, hypotension, and possibly seizures and intracranial hemorrhages has been associated with this use.

**Stability**
Clindamycin phosphate retains its potency for 24 hours at room temperature in intravenous infusions containing sodium chloride, dextrose, potassium, vitamin B complex, cephalothin, kanamycin, gentamicin, penicillin, or carbenicillin.

**Incompatibilities**
Clindamycin phosphate is physically incompatible with ampicillin, phenytoin sodium, barbiturates, aminophylline, calcium gluconate, and magnesium sulfate.

**Additional information**
Clindamycin phosphate may also be administered as a single rapid infusion (initial dose) followed by continuous intravenous infusion as follows:

| Clindamycin Serum Concentrations (desired maintenance—mcg/mL) | Infusion Rate and Duration (initial) Rate (mg/min) | Duration (min) | Infusion Rate (continuous—mg/min) |
|---|---|---|---|
| >4 | 10 | 30 | 0.75 |
| >5 | 15 | 30 | 1.00 |
| >6 | 20 | 30 | 1.25 |

[1]Not included in Canadian product labeling.

Revised: 08/12/92
Interim revision: 03/18/94; 04/19/95; 08/14/98

# CLINDAMYCIN    Topical

VA CLASSIFICATION (Primary/Secondary): DE752/DE101
Commonly used brand name(s): *Cleocin T Gel; Cleocin T Lotion; Cleocin T Topical Solution; Clinda-Derm; Dalacin T Topical Solution.*
Note: For a listing of dosage forms and brand names by country availability, see *Dosage Forms* section(s).

## Category
Antiacne agent (topical); antibacterial (topical).

## Indications
Note: Bracketed information in the *Indications* section refers to uses that are not included in U.S. product labeling.

**Accepted**
Acne vulgaris (treatment)—Topical clindamycin is indicated in the treatment of acne vulgaris. It may be effective in grades II and III acne, which are characterized by inflammatory lesions such as papules and pustules. Topical antibacterials are not generally considered to be as effective as systemic antibacterials in the treatment of acne, especially more severe inflammatory acne. However, some studies have shown that clindamycin phosphate topical solution may be as effective as low-dose tetracycline for moderate cases of inflammatory acne.

[Skin infections, bacterial, minor (treatment)][1]—Topical clindamycin is used in the topical treatment of erythrasma caused by *Corynebacterium minutissimum*, rosacea, periorificial facial dermatitis, folliculitis, stasis, chronic lymphedema, and familial pemphigus.

[Ulcer, dermal (treatment)][1]—Clindamycin phosphate topical solution is used in the treatment of dermal ulcers.

Not all species or strains of a particular organism may be susceptible to clindamycin.

**Unaccepted**
Topical clindamycin is not effective in the treatment of deep cystic lesions or noninflammatory lesions.

[1]Not included in Canadian product labeling.

## Pharmacology/Pharmacokinetics
**Physicochemical characteristics**
Molecular weight—504.96.

**Mechanism of action/Effect**
Antiacne agent (topical)—Probably due to its antibacterial activity. Topical clindamycin is thought to reduce free fatty acid concentrations on the skin and to suppress the growth of *Propionibacterium acnes (Corynebacterium acnes)*, an anaerobe found in sebaceous glands and follicles. *P. acnes* produces proteases, hyaluronidases, lipases, and chemotactic factors, all of which can produce inflammatory components or inflammation directly.

**Absorption**
Approximately 1.7% absorbed through the skin following topical application of the solution every 12 hours for 4 days to approximately 300 cm$^2$ of skin surface.

**Mean comedonal extract concentration**
597 mcg per gram after 4 weeks of topical application.

**Biotransformation**
Clindamycin phosphate is inactive *in vitro*, but is rapidly hydrolyzed *in vivo* by tissue phosphatases to active clindamycin.

**Peak serum concentration**
<1 to 6 nanograms per mL following topical application of the solution every 12 hours for 4 days.

**Urine concentration**
<1 to 53 nanograms per mL following topical application of the solution every 12 hours for 4 days.

**Elimination**
Renal—0.15 to 0.25% of cumulative dose excreted in urine following topical application of the solution every 12 hours.

## Precautions to Consider

**Cross-sensitivity and/or related problems**
Patients sensitive to one lincomycin may be sensitive to other lincomycins also.

**Pregnancy/Reproduction**
Fertility—Studies in rats and mice receiving subcutaneous and oral doses of clindamycin ranging from 100 to 600 mg per kg per day have not shown that clindamycin causes impaired fertility.

Pregnancy—Adequate and well-controlled studies in humans have not been done.

Studies in rats and mice receiving subcutaneous and oral doses of clindamycin ranging from 100 to 600 mg per kg per day have not shown that clindamycin causes adverse effects on the fetus.

FDA Pregnancy Category B.

**Breast-feeding**
It is not known whether topical clindamycin is distributed into breast milk. Since systemically administered clindamycin is distributed into breast milk, topical clindamycin may be also. However, clindamycin is unlikely to be distributed into breast milk in significant amounts following topical administration, since the total daily dose is small and only approximately 1.7% of the dose is absorbed through the skin.

**Pediatrics**
Appropriate studies on the relationship of age to the effects of topical clindamycin have not been performed in children up to 12 years of age. Safety and efficacy have not been established.

**Geriatrics**
No information is available on the relationship of age to the effects of topical clindamycin in geriatric patients.

**Drug interactions and/or related problems**
The following drug interactions and/or related problems have been selected on the basis of their potential clinical significance (possible mechanism in parentheses where appropriate)—not necessarily inclusive (» = major clinical significance):

Note: Combinations containing any of the following medications, depending on the amount present, may also interact with this medication.

Abrasive or medicated soaps or cleansers or
Acne preparations or preparations containing a peeling agent, such as:
  Resorcinol
  Salicylic acid
  Sulfur, or
Alcohol-containing preparations, topical, such as:
  After-shave lotions
  Astringents
  Perfumed toiletries
  Shaving creams or lotions, or
Cosmetics or soaps with a strong drying effect or
Isotretinoin or
Medicated cosmetics or "cover-ups"
  (concurrent use with clindamycin phosphate topical solution may cause a cumulative irritant or drying effect, especially with the application of peeling, desquamating, or abrasive agents, resulting in excessive irritation of the skin)

**Medical considerations/Contraindications**
The medical considerations/contraindications included have been selected on the basis of their potential clinical significance (reasons given in parentheses where appropriate)—not necessarily inclusive (» = major clinical significance).

*Except under special circumstances, this medication should not be used when the following medical problem exists:*
» Sensitivity to clindamycin or lincomycin

*Risk-benefit should be considered when the following medical problems exist:*
Antibiotic-associated colitis, ulcerative colitis, or regional enteritis, history of
  (topical clindamycin may precipitate problems that may occur days, weeks, or months after start of therapy; also may occur up to several weeks after discontinuation of therapy)
Atopic reactions, history of

**Patient monitoring**
The following may be especially important in patient monitoring (other tests may be warranted in some patients, depending on condition; » = major clinical significance):

Endoscopy, large bowel
  (if severe diarrhea not controlled by administration of vancomycin occurs and persists during therapy, large bowel endoscopy may be required as an aid in the diagnosis of pseudomembranous colitis)

## Side/Adverse Effects

The following side/adverse effects have been selected on the basis of their potential clinical significance (possible signs and symptoms in parentheses where appropriate)—not necessarily inclusive:

**Those indicating need for medical attention**
Incidence less frequent
  *Contact dermatitis or hypersensitivity* (skin rash, itching, redness, swelling, or other sign of irritation not present before therapy)
Incidence rare
  *Pseudomembranous colitis* (abdominal or stomach cramps, pain, and bloating, severe; diarrhea, watery and severe, which may also be bloody; fever; increased thirst; nausea or vomiting; unusual tiredness or weakness; weight loss, unusual)

**Those indicating need for medical attention only if they continue or are bothersome**
Incidence more frequent
  *Dryness, scaliness, or peeling of skin*—for the topical solution
Incidence less frequent
  *Gastrointestinal disturbances* (abdominal pain; mild diarrhea); *irritation, sensitization or oiliness of skin; stinging or burning feeling of skin*—for the topical solution

**Those indicating possible pseudomembranous colitis and the need for medical attention if they occur after medication is discontinued**
*Abdominal or stomach cramps, pain, and bloating, severe; diarrhea, watery and severe, which may also be bloody; fever; increased thirst; nausea or vomiting; unusual tiredness or weakness; weight loss, unusual*

## Patient Consultation

As an aid to patient consultation, refer to *Advice for the Patient, Clindamycin (Topical)*.

In providing consultation, consider emphasizing the following selected information (» = major clinical significance):

**Before using this medication**
» Conditions affecting use, especially:
  Sensitivity to clindamycin or lincomycin
  Breast-feeding—May be distributed into breast milk in small quantities since systemic clindamycin is distributed into breast milk
  Other medical problems, especially a history of antibiotic-associated colitis, ulcerative colitis, or regional enteritis

**Proper use of this medication**
Before applying, washing affected areas with warm water and soap, rinsing, and patting dry
» Importance of applying medication to entire affected area
Avoiding too frequent washing of affected areas
» Compliance with full course of therapy, which may take months or longer
» Proper dosing
Missed dose: Applying as soon as possible; not applying if almost time for next dose
» Proper storage
*For topical solution only*
  Waiting 30 minutes after washing or shaving before applying
» Not using near heat, near open flame, or while smoking
  Proper administration technique for applicator-tip bottle:

» Avoiding contact with eyes, nose, mouth, or other mucous membranes
  Not using more often than prescribed
*For topical suspension only*
» Shaking well before using

**Precautions while using this medication**
Checking with physician or pharmacist if no improvement within about 6 weeks
Applying other medications at different times
Checking with physician if treated skin becomes excessively dry (for topical solution only)
» For severe diarrhea, checking with physician before taking any antidiarrheals; for mild diarrhea, taking attapulgite-containing, but not other, antidiarrheals; checking with physician or pharmacist if mild diarrhea continues or worsens
Using only "water-base" cosmetics; not applying too heavily or too often

**Side/adverse effects**
Signs of potential side effects, especially hypersensitivity reactions and pseudomembranous colitis

## General Dosing Information

Use of topical antibacterials may lead to skin sensitization, resulting in hypersensitivity reactions with subsequent topical or systemic use of the medication.

In the treatment of acne with topical clindamycin, noticeable improvement is usually seen after about 6 weeks in most patients. However, 8 to 12 weeks of treatment may be required before maximum benefit is seen.

**For treatment of adverse effects**
Some patients may develop antibiotic-associated pseudomembranous colitis (AAPMC), caused by *Clostridium difficile* toxin, during or following administration of topical clindamycin. Mild cases may respond to discontinuation of the drug alone. Moderate to severe cases may require fluid, electrolyte, and protein replacement.

In cases not responding to the above measures or in more severe cases, oral vancomycin, oral bacitracin, or oral metronidazole may be used. Oral vancomycin is effective in doses of 125 to 500 mg every 6 hours for 7 to 10 days. Recurrences may be treated with a second course of these medications.

Cholestyramine and colestipol resins have been shown to bind *C. difficile* toxin *in vitro*. If cholestyramine or colestipol resin is administered in conjunction with oral vancomycin, the medications should be administered several hours apart since the resins have been shown to bind oral vancomycin also.

In addition, AAPMC may result in severe watery diarrhea, which may occur during antibiotic therapy or up to several weeks after therapy is discontinued. If diarrhea occurs, administration of antiperistaltic antidiarrheals (e.g., opiates, diphenoxylate and atropine combination, loperamide) is *not* recommended since they may delay the removal of toxins from the colon, thereby prolonging and/or worsening the condition.

## Topical Dosage Forms

### CLINDAMYCIN PHOSPHATE GEL USP

**Usual adult and adolescent dose**
Antiacne agent (topical)—
  Topical, to the skin, a thin film applied two times a day to the affected areas.

**Usual pediatric dose**
Children up to 12 years of age—Safety and efficacy have not been established.

**Strength(s) usually available**
U.S.—
  1% (base) (Rx) [*Cleocin T Gel* (methylparaben; propylene glycol; sodium hydroxide)].

Canada—
  Not commercially available.

**Packaging and storage**
Store below 40 °C (104 °F), preferably between 15 and 30 °C (59 and 86 °F), unless otherwise specified by manufacturer. Store in a tight container. Protect from freezing.

**Auxiliary labeling**
• For external use only.
• Continue medicine for full time of treatment.

**Additional information**
Clindamycin phosphate gel is an aqueous, nonalcoholic, nondrying formulation.

### CLINDAMYCIN PHOSPHATE TOPICAL SOLUTION USP

**Usual adult and adolescent dose**
Antiacne agent (topical)—
  Topical, to the skin, two times a day to the affected areas.

Note:   Solutions have been used one to four times a day.

**Usual pediatric dose**
See *Clindamycin Phosphate Gel USP*.

**Strength(s) usually available**
U.S.—
  1% (base) (Rx) [*Cleocin T Topical Solution*; *Clinda-Derm* (isopropyl alcohol 50%; propylene glycol); GENERIC].
Canada—
  1% (base) (Rx) [*Dalacin T Topical Solution* (isopropyl alcohol 50%; propylene glycol)].

**Packaging and storage**
Store below 40 °C (104 °F), preferably between 15 and 30 °C (59 and 86 °F), unless otherwise specified by manufacturer. Store in a tight container. Protect from freezing.

**Auxiliary labeling**
• For external use only.
• Continue medicine for full time of treatment.
• Keep container tightly closed.
• Flammable—Keep away from heat and flame.

### CLINDAMYCIN PHOSPHATE TOPICAL SUSPENSION USP

**Usual adult and adolescent dose**
Antiacne agent (topical)—
  See *Clindamycin Phosphate Topical Solution USP*.

**Usual pediatric dose**
See *Clindamycin Phosphate Topical Solution USP*.

**Strength(s) usually available**
U.S.—
  1% (base) (Rx) [*Cleocin T Lotion* (cetostearyl alcohol 2.5%; isostearyl alcohol 2.5%)].
Canada—
  Not commercially available.

**Packaging and storage**
Store below 40 °C (104 °F), preferably between 15 and 30 °C (59 and 86 °F), unless otherwise specified by manufacturer. Store in a tight container. Protect from freezing.

**Auxiliary labeling**
• Shake well.
• For external use only.
• Continue medicine for full time of treatment.

Revised: 02/22/94

# CLINDAMYCIN   Vaginal

VA CLASSIFICATION (Primary): GU309
Commonly used brand name(s): *Cleocin*; *Dalacin*.
Note:   For a listing of dosage forms and brand names by country availability, see *Dosage Forms* section(s).

## Category
Anti-infective (vaginal).

## Indications

**Accepted**
Vaginosis, bacterial (treatment)—Vaginal clindamycin is indicated in the local treatment of bacterial vaginosis (previously known as *Haemophilus* vaginitis, *Gardnerella* vaginitis, nonspecific vaginitis, *Corynebacterium* vaginitis, or anaerobic vaginosis).

In addition to its use in nonpregnant patients, vaginal clindamycin is indicated for use during the second and third trimesters of pregnancy.

However, in a controlled clinical trial, no difference was found between vaginal clindamycin and placebo in reducing the risk of adverse pregnancy outcomes, such as premature rupture of the membranes, preterm labor, or preterm delivery. The best results are achieved when high-risk pregnant patients are screened early in the second trimester and asymptomatic high-risk and symptomatic low-risk patients are treated with oral metronidazole or oral clindamycin. Although some experts prefer the use of systemic therapy for low-risk pregnant patients to treat possible subclinical upper genital tract infections, vaginal metronidazole may be used in low-risk pregnant patients as an alternative therapy.

Not all species or strains of a particular organism may be susceptible to clindamycin.

### Unaccepted
Vaginal clindamycin is not effective in the treatment of vulvovaginitis caused by *Trichomonas vaginalis*, *Chlamydia trachomatis*, *Neisseria gonorrhoeae*, *Candida albicans*, or *Herpes simplex* virus.

## Pharmacology/Pharmacokinetics

### Physicochemical characteristics
Molecular weight—Clindamycin phosphate: 504.97.

### Mechanism of action/Effect
Clindamycin phosphate is hydrolyzed *in vivo* to clindamycin, which inhibits protein synthesis in susceptible bacteria by binding to the 50 S subunits of bacterial ribosomes and prevents peptide bond formation.

### Absorption
Approximately 2 to 8% of the administered dose (100 mg) is absorbed systemically; little or no systemic accumulation has been produced with multiple dosing.

### Biotransformation
Inactive clindamycin phosphate undergoes rapid hydrolysis *in vivo* to active clindamycin.

### Half-life
Systemic—1.5 to 2.6 hours.

### Time to peak concentration
Approximately 16 hours (range, 8 to 24 hours).

### Peak serum concentration
Steady state—Approximately 16 mcg/L (0.032 micromoles/L).

## Precautions to Consider

### Cross-sensitivity and/or related problems
Patients hypersensitive to lincomycin may be hypersensitive to clindamycin also.

### Carcinogenicity/Tumorigenicity
Long-term studies in animals have not been done.

### Mutagenicity
No evidence of mutagenicity was found in tests, including the Ames test and a rat micronucleus test.

### Pregnancy/Reproduction
Fertility—No evidence of adverse effects on fertility was found in rats when they were treated with oral doses of 300 mg per kg of body weight (mg/kg) a day (31 times the human exposure based on mg per square meter [mg/m$^2$] of body surface area).

Pregnancy—Systemic clindamycin crosses the placenta; up to 8% of vaginal clindamycin is systemically absorbed.

Well-controlled clinical trials using vaginal clindamycin during the second and third trimesters showed no adverse effects in the fetus; there is inadequate information on its use during the first trimester.

Although vaginal clindamycin is effective in treating bacterial vaginosis in pregnant and nonpregnant women, it frequently causes cervicitis or vaginitis with or without candidiasis, especially in pregnant patients. Pregnant patients were not re-treated in clinical trials even though bacterial vaginosis returned in about 50% of patients several weeks after initial treatment. In general, best results for treatment and pregnancy outcomes are associated with treatment early in the second trimester. The incidence of bacterial vaginosis appears to lessen by an unknown mechanism as pregnancy continues into the third trimester.

Reproduction studies in animals in which high systemic doses of clindamycin were used showed no evidence of fetal malformations, except one small study in which the fetuses of treated mice developed cleft palates. This result has not been duplicated in other animals or other mouse strains.

FDA Pregnancy Category B.

### Breast-feeding
Systemic clindamycin is distributed into breast milk. Problems in humans have not been documented. It is not known if vaginally administered clindamycin phosphate is distributed into breast milk.

### Pediatrics
No information is available on the relationship of age to the effects of vaginal clindamycin in pediatric patients. Safety and efficacy have not been established.

### Geriatrics
No information is available on the relationship of age to the effects of clindamycin in geriatric patients.

### Medical considerations/Contraindications
The medical considerations/contraindications included have been selected on the basis of their potential clinical significance (reasons given in parentheses where appropriate)—not necessarily inclusive (» = major clinical significance).

*Risk-benefit should be considered when the following medical problems exist:*

» Gastrointestinal disease, history of, especially ulcerative colitis, regional enteritis, or antibiotic-associated colitis
   (systemically and topically administered clindamycin may cause diarrhea and, rarely with topical administration, colitis—including pseudomembranous colitis; although only up to 8% of the vaginal dose may be systemically absorbed, vaginal use may potentially worsen these conditions)

» Hypersensitivity to lincomycin or clindamycin

## Side/Adverse Effects
Note: The side effects listed below are those reported in studies with vaginal clindamycin administration. Systemic side effects may occur since up to 8% of the vaginal dose is absorbed systemically. Pseudomembranous colitis has occurred rarely with topical use of clindamycin but has not been reported with vaginal administration.

The following side/adverse effects have been selected on the basis of their potential clinical significance (possible signs and symptoms in parentheses where appropriate)—not necessarily inclusive:

**Those indicating need for medical attention**
Incidence more frequent
  *Cervicitis, vaginitis, or vulvovaginal pruritus, primarily due to Candida albicans* (itching of the vagina or genital area; pain during sexual intercourse; thick, white vaginal discharge with no odor or with a mild odor)—incidence of 33% for pregnant patients and 16% for nonpregnant patients
Incidence less frequent
  *CNS effects* (dizziness; headache); *gastrointestinal disturbances* (diarrhea; nausea or vomiting; stomach pain or cramps)
Incidence rare
  *Hypersensitivity* (burning, itching, redness, skin rash, swelling, or other signs of skin irritation not present before therapy)

**Those indicating possible need for medical attention if they occur after medication is discontinued**
  *Cervicitis, vaginitis, or vulvovaginal pruritus, primarily due to Candida albicans* (itching of the vagina or genital area; pain during sexual intercourse; thick, white vaginal discharge with no odor or with a mild odor)

## Patient Consultation
As an aid to patient consultation, refer to *Advice for the Patient, Clindamycin (Vaginal)*.

In providing consultation, consider emphasizing the following selected information (» = major clinical significance):

**Before using this medication**
» Conditions affecting use, especially:
   Hypersensitivity to clindamycin or lincomycin
   Pregnancy—Systemic clindamycin crosses the placenta; up to 8% of vaginal clindamycin is systemically absorbed
   Breast-feeding—Systemically administered clindamycin is distributed into breast milk. It is not known if vaginal clindamycin also is distributed into breast milk
   Other medical problems, especially history of gastrointestinal disease (particularly ulcerative colitis, regional enteritis, or antibiotic-associated colitis)

### Proper use of this medication
Washing hands immediately before and after vaginal administration
Avoiding getting medication into the eyes; washing eyes out immediately with large amounts of cool tap water if medication does get into eyes; checking with physician if eyes continue to be painful
Reading patient directions carefully before use
Proper administration technique: Following directions regarding the filling of the applicator, insertion technique, and discarding the applicator after each use
» Compliance with full course of therapy, even during menstruation
» Not missing doses; using at evenly spaced times
» Proper dosing
Missed dose: Inserting as soon as possible; not inserting if almost time for next dose
» Proper storage

### Precautions while using this medication
Checking with physician if no improvement within a few days
Follow-up visit to physician after treatment for bacterial vaginosis to ensure that infection has been properly treated
Caution if dizziness occurs
Protecting clothing because of possible soiling with vaginal clindamycin; avoiding use of tampons
» Using hygienic measures to help cure infection and prevent reinfection, e.g., wearing freshly washed cotton panties instead of synthetic panties
» Sexual abstinence is recommended during treatment to prevent a dilution of the dose, which may result in reduced efficacy of the medication and a relapse of the infection
» Not using latex contraceptives for up to 72 hours after vaginal clindamycin treatment, as oils in the clindamycin weaken latex products and may affect their efficacy

### Side/adverse effects
Signs of potential side effects, especially cervicitis, vaginitis, or vulvovaginal pruritus, due to *Candida albicans*; CNS effects; gastrointestinal disturbances; and hypersensitivity

## General Dosing Information
Use of vaginal latex or rubber products, such as condoms, cervical caps, or diaphragms, is not recommended for up to 72 hours after completion of vaginal clindamycin treatment. Vaginal clindamycin cream contains mineral oil that can weaken or damage these products and reduce their efficacy.

Concurrent treatment of the male partner is generally unnecessary when treating bacterial vaginosis.

Vaginal applicators should be used with caution after the sixth month of pregnancy.

## Vaginal Dosage Form
### CLINDAMYCIN PHOSPHATE VAGINAL CREAM USP
#### Usual adult and adolescent dose
Anti-infective (vaginal)—
For nonpregnant females: Intravaginal, 100 mg (one applicatorful) into vagina once a day, preferably at bedtime, for three or seven consecutive days.
For pregnant females (second or third trimesters): Intravaginal, 100 mg (one applicatorful) into vagina once a day, preferably at bedtime, for seven consecutive days.

#### Usual pediatric dose
Safety and efficacy have not been established.

#### Strength(s) usually available
U.S.—
  2% (Rx) [*Cleocin* (benzyl alcohol; cetostearyl alcohol; mineral oil)].
Canada—
  2% (Rx) [*Dalacin* (benzyl alcohol; cetostearyl alcohol; mineral oil)].

### Packaging and storage
Store below 40 °C (104 °F), preferably between 15 and 30 °C (59 and 86 °F), unless otherwise specified by manufacturer. Store in well-closed containers.

### Auxiliary labeling
• May cause dizziness.
• Continue medicine for full time of treatment.
• For vaginal use only.

### Note
Include patient package insert (PPI) when dispensing.

### Selected Bibliography
Fischbach F, Petersen EE, Weissenbacher ER, et al. Efficacy of clindamycin vaginal cream versus oral metronidazole in the treatment of bacterial vaginosis. Obstet Gynecol 1993 Sep; 82(3): 405-10.
Livengood CH, Thomason JL, Hill GB. Bacterial vaginosis: diagnostic and pathogenetic findings during topical clindamycin therapy. Am J Obstet Gynecol 1990 Aug; 163(2): 515-20.

Revised: 08/11/98

---

**CLIOQUINOL** — The *Clioquinol (Topical)* monograph is not included in this published version of the USP DI database. Copies of the monograph are available on request from Micromedex, Inc. - Reprint Requests, 6200 S. Syracuse Way, Suite 300, Englewood, CO 80111; telephone (303) 486-6400; telefax (303) 486-6464; Email: USPDI@MDX.COM.

---

**CLIOQUINOL AND HYDROCORTISONE** — The *Clioquinol and Hydrocortisone (Topical)* monograph is not included in this published version of the USP DI database. Copies of the monograph are available on request from Micromedex, Inc. - Reprint Requests, 6200 S. Syracuse Way, Suite 300, Englewood, CO 80111; telephone (303) 486-6400; telefax (303) 486-6464; Email: USPDI@MDX.COM.

---

**CLOBAZAM** — See *Benzodiazepines (Systemic)*

---

**CLOBETASOL** — See *Corticosteroids (Topical)*

---

**CLOBETASONE** — See *Corticosteroids (Topical)*

---

**CLOCORTOLONE** — See *Corticosteroids (Topical)*

---

**CLOFAZIMINE** — The *Clofazimine (Systemic)* monograph is not included in this published version of the USP DI database. Copies of the monograph are available on request from Micromedex, Inc. - Reprint Requests, 6200 S. Syracuse Way, Suite 300, Englewood, CO 80111; telephone (303) 486-6400; telefax (303) 486-6464; Email: USPDI@MDX.COM.

---

# CLOFIBRATE  Systemic

VA CLASSIFICATION (Primary): CV603
Commonly used brand name(s): *Abitrate; Atromid-S; Claripex; Novofibrate.*
Note: For a listing of dosage forms and brand names by country availability, see *Dosage Forms* section(s).

## Category
Antihyperlipidemic; antidiuretic (central diabetes insipidus).

## Indications
Note: Bracketed information in the *Indications* section refers to uses that are not included in U.S. product labeling.

### Accepted
**Hyperlipidemia (treatment)**—Clofibrate is indicated in the treatment of hyperlipidemia. Because of risks associated with its use (see *Side/Adverse Effects*), clofibrate is recommended for use as an adjunct only in patients with severe primary hyperlipidemia (type III hyperlipidemia) and a significant risk of coronary artery disease who have not responded to diet or other measures alone. Clofibrate reduces plasma triglyceride concentrations to a greater extent than plasma cholesterol concentrations, and so is not useful in patients with elevated cholesterol concentrations alone. Its use is limited in type II hyperlipidemia because of its variable effect on cholesterol concentrations. Clofibrate is not recommended for community-wide prevention of ischemic heart disease.

Studies have suggested that control of elevated cholesterol and triglycerides may not lessen the danger of cardiovascular disease and mortality, although incidence of nonfatal myocardial infarctions may be decreased.

For additional information on initial therapeutic guidelines related to the treatment of hyperlipidemia, see *Appendix III*.

[Clofibrate has been used in the treatment of partial central diabetes insipidus in patients with some residual posterior pituitary function; however, it generally has been replaced by other agents.][1]

### Unaccepted
Although clofibrate alters platelet function (decreases platelet adhesiveness), it has not shown significant efficacy as an antiplatelet drug.

---

[1]Not included in Canadian product labeling.

## Pharmacology/Pharmacokinetics

### Physicochemical characteristics
Molecular weight—242.70.
pKa—2.95.

### Mechanism of action/Effect
*Antihyperlipidemic*—Not completely understood, but may involve inhibition of biosynthesis of cholesterol before mevalonate formation, increased secretion and fecal excretion of neutral sterols, enhanced catabolism of very low–density lipoproteins (VLDL) due to increased lipoprotein lipase activity in extrahepatic tissues, and/or increased clearance of triglycerides (VLDL) from the circulation.
*Antidiuretic*—May stimulate release of antidiuretic hormone (ADH) from the posterior pituitary.

### Absorption
Completely but slowly absorbed from the intestine.

### Protein binding
Very high (96%).

### Biotransformation
Hepatic and gastrointestinal; rapid de-esterification occurs in the gastrointestinal tract and/or on first-pass metabolism to produce the active form, clofibric acid (chlorophenoxy isobutyric acid [CPIB]).

### Half-life
Single dose—
  Normal: 6 to 25 hours.
  Anuria: 113 hours.
Steady state—
  Normal: 54 hours.

### Onset of action
Plasma VLDL concentrations are reduced within 2 to 5 days.

### Time to peak plasma concentration
2 to 6 hours after a dose.

### Time to peak effect
3 weeks (with continued use).

### Duration of action
Return to pretreatment VLDL concentrations occurs within 3 weeks after clofibrate is withdrawn.

### Elimination
Renal; 10 to 20% of clofibric acid excreted unchanged; also as glucuronide conjugate (60%).

## Precautions to Consider

### Carcinogenicity
Clofibrate, in doses 5 to 8 times the human dose, has been found to increase the incidence of malignant hepatic tumors in rodents.

### Pregnancy/Reproduction
*Pregnancy*—Studies have not been done in humans. However, clofibrate may cross the placenta, and the fetus may not have developed the enzyme system required to excrete it; use is not recommended during pregnancy. If a pregnancy is planned, clofibrate therapy should be withdrawn several months before conception.
Studies in rabbits indicate that fetal serum concentrations of clofibrate may be higher than maternal serum concentrations.
FDA Pregnancy Category C.

### Breast-feeding
Clofibrate is distributed into breast milk. Use of clofibrate during breast-feeding is not recommended because of potentially serious adverse effects on nursing infants.

### Pediatrics
Appropriate studies on the relationship of age to the effects of clofibrate have not been performed in the pediatric population. However, use in children under 2 years of age is not recommended since cholesterol is required for normal development.

### Geriatrics
Although appropriate studies on the relationship of age to the effects of clofibrate have not been performed in the geriatric population, geriatrics-specific problems that would limit the usefulness of this medication in the elderly are not expected. However, elderly patients are more likely to have age-related renal function impairment, which may require dosage adjustment in patients receiving clofibrate.

### Drug interactions and/or related problems
The following drug interactions and/or related problems have been selected on the basis of their potential clinical significance (possible mechanism in parentheses where appropriate)—not necessarily inclusive (» = major clinical significance):

Note: Combinations containing any of the following medications, depending on the amount present, may also interact with this medication.

» Anticoagulants, coumarin- or indandione-derivative
  (concurrent use with clofibrate may significantly increase the anticoagulant effect; adjustment of anticoagulant dosage based on frequent prothrombin-time determinations is recommended; some clinicians recommend reduction of the anticoagulant dosage by one-half)

Antidiabetic agents, oral, especially tolbutamide
  (concurrent use of clofibrate with oral antidiabetic agents may enhance the hypoglycemic effect through displacement from serum proteins; dosage adjustments may be necessary. Glipizide and glyburide, due to their non-ionic binding characteristics, may not be affected as much as the other oral agents; however, caution with concurrent use is recommended)

Chenodiol or
Ursodiol
  (effect may be decreased when chenodiol or ursodiol is used concurrently with clofibrate since clofibrate tends to increase cholesterol saturation of bile)

HMG-CoA reductase inhibitors
  (concurrent use with clofibrate may increase the risk of rhabdomyolysis; cases of rhabdomyolysis have not been reported with concurrent use of clofibrate and HMG-CoA reductase inhibitors; however, there have been reported cases of rhadomyolysis with concurrent use of another fibrate, gemfibrozil, and lovastatin)

Oral contraceptives
  (concurrent use may alter the effectiveness of clofibrate)

Probenecid
  (concurrent use of probenecid may decrease renal and metabolic clearances and alter the protein binding of clofibrate, increasing the therapeutic and toxic effects of clofibrate)

Rifampin
  (concurrent use with clofibrate may enhance the metabolism of clofibrate by induction of hepatic microsomal enzymes, resulting in significantly lower serum clofibrate concentrations)

### Laboratory value alterations
The following have been selected on the basis of their potential clinical significance (possible effect in parentheses where appropriate)—not necessarily inclusive (» = major clinical significance):

With physiology/laboratory test values
  Alanine aminotransferase (ALT [SGPT]) and
  Aspartate aminotransferase (AST [SGOT])
    (serum concentrations may be increased, indicating hepatotoxicity)
  Amylase
    (serum concentrations may be increased)

Beta-lipoprotein, plasma
(low-density lipoprotein [LDL] or cholesterol concentrations may be increased as a paradoxical response to a large decrease in very low–density lipoprotein [VLDL] concentrations)

Creatine kinase (CK)
(concentrations may be increased, especially in patients with renal failure or hypoalbuminemia)

Fibrinogen
(plasma concentrations may be decreased)

### Medical considerations/Contraindications
The medical considerations/contraindications included have been selected on the basis of their potential clinical significance (reasons given in parentheses where appropriate)—not necessarily inclusive (» = major clinical significance).

*Except under special circumstances, this medication should not be used when the following medical problem exists:*
» Primary biliary cirrhosis
  (use of clofibrate may further raise the cholesterol)

*Risk-benefit should be considered when the following medical problems exist:*
Cardiovascular disease
  (condition may be exacerbated)
Gallstones
  (increased risk of biliary complications)
» Hepatic function impairment
  (protein binding of clofibrate is reduced but half-life is not altered. It is recommended that patients with impaired hepatic function receive a reduced dose of clofibrate; some clinicians recommend reduction of dosage by one-half in patients with cirrhosis)
Hypothyroidism
  (may predispose to clofibrate-induced myopathy)
Peptic ulcer
  (reactivation has been reported)
» Renal function impairment
  (reduced protein binding and clearance of clofibrate leads to increased incidence of side effects, especially myopathy and rhabdomyolysis. It is recommended that clofibrate be administered in reduced dosage to patients with impaired renal function. However, dosage reduction is not necessary in nephrotic syndrome when renal function is not impaired, since steady-state concentration of unbound drug is unchanged in spite of markedly reduced protein binding and half-life)
Sensitivity to clofibrate

### Patient monitoring
The following may be especially important in patient monitoring (other tests may be warranted in some patients, depending on condition; » = major clinical significance):
» Cholesterol, serum concentrations and
» Triglyceride, serum concentrations
  (determinations recommended prior to initiation of therapy, at 2-week intervals during the first few months of therapy, at monthly intervals thereafter to detect a paradoxical rise in serum cholesterol or triglyceride concentrations as well as to confirm efficacy, then every few months when concentrations stabilize)
Complete blood counts
  (recommended prior to initiation of therapy and at periodic intervals during therapy if signs of anemia or leukopenia occur)
Creatine kinase (CK) concentrations
  (recommended at periodic intervals in uremic patients receiving clofibrate)
Liver function tests, including serum transaminase concentrations
  (determinations recommended prior to initiation of therapy, every month for the first 2 months, then every 2 months until an effect is observed, and every 4 months thereafter)

## Side/Adverse Effects
Note: The suggestion that long-term use of clofibrate may increase the risk of death from noncardiovascular causes (malignancy, postcholecystectomy complications, pancreatitis) was made after results first published in 1978 of a large prospective study (the WHO study). This suggestion has been controversial, in part because other studies (for example, the Coronary Drug Project report published in 1975) have not reached a similar conclusion, although both major studies agree that the risk of cholelithiasis and cholecystitis requiring surgery is greatly increased in clofibrate users. Clofibrate has been found to increase the risk of development of peripheral vascular disease, pulmonary embolism, thrombophlebitis, angina pectoris, arrhythmias, and intermittent claudication. Clofibrate, in doses 5 to 8 times the human dose, has been found to increase the incidence of malignant hepatic tumors in rodents.

Rhabdomyolysis and severe hyperkalemia have been reported in patients with pre-existing renal function impairment.

The following side/adverse effects have been selected on the basis of their potential clinical significance (possible signs and symptoms in parentheses where appropriate)—not necessarily inclusive:

**Those indicating need for medical attention**
Incidence rare
  *Anemia or leukopenia* (fever or chills; cough or hoarseness; lower back or side pain; painful or difficult urination); *angina* (chest pain; shortness of breath); *cardiac arrhythmias* (irregular heartbeat); *gallstones or pancreatitis* (severe stomach pain with nausea and vomiting); *renal toxicity* (blood in urine; decrease in urination; painful urination; swelling of feet and lower legs)
  Note: Increased creatine kinase (CK) and serum transaminase concentrations may be caused by clofibrate rather than myocardial infarction.

**Those indicating need for medical attention only if they continue or are bothersome**
Incidence more frequent
  *Diarrhea; nausea*
Incidence less frequent or rare
  *Decreased sexual ability; flu-like syndrome or myositis* (muscle aches or cramps; unusual tiredness or weakness); *headache; increased appetite or weight gain, slight; stomach pain, gas, or heartburn; stomatitis* (sores in mouth and on lips); *vomiting*
  Note: *Flu-like syndrome* or *myositis* occurs more frequently in patients with existing renal disease, and usually is accompanied by increased CK and serum transaminases.

## Patient Consultation
As an aid to patient consultation, refer to *Advice for the Patient, Clofibrate (Systemic)*.
In providing consultation, consider emphasizing the following selected information (» = major clinical significance):

**Before using this medication**
Potential serious toxicity; WHO study controversy
Diet as preferred therapy
» Conditions affecting use, especially:
  Sensitivity to clofibrate
  Pregnancy—May cross placenta; enzyme system required for excretion may not be developed in fetus; withdrawal of clofibrate therapy several months before conception is recommended if pregnancy is planned
  Breast-feeding—Use not recommended while nursing because of potentially serious adverse effects on nursing infants
  Use in children—Not recommended in children less than 2 years of age since cholesterol is required for normal development
  Other medications, especially anticoagulants
  Other medical problems, especially primary biliary cirrhosis, hepatic function impairment, or renal function impairment

**Proper use of this medication**
» Importance of not taking more or less medication than the amount prescribed
» Compliance with prescribed diet
  Taking with meals to prevent possible gastric irritation
» Proper dosing
  Missed dose: Taking as soon as possible; not taking if almost time for next dose; not doubling doses
» Proper storage

**Precautions while using this medication**
» Importance of close monitoring by the physician
» Checking with physician before discontinuing medication; blood lipid concentrations may increase significantly

**Side/adverse effects**
Signs of potential side effects, especially angina, cardiac arrhythmias, leukopenia, anemia, pancreatitis, gallstones, and renal toxicity

## General Dosing Information
If response is inadequate after 3 months of treatment, clofibrate therapy should be withdrawn, except in the case of xanthoma tuberosum, which may require up to 1 year of treatment as long as reduction in size and/or number of xanthomata occurs.

If results of hepatic function tests rise significantly or show significant abnormalities, it is recommended that clofibrate therapy be withdrawn and not resumed; laboratory abnormalities are usually reversible.

If an increase in serum amylase concentrations or a paradoxical increase in plasma cholesterol or plasma LDL concentrations occurs, it is recommended that clofibrate therapy be withdrawn.

When clofibrate is discontinued, an appropriate hypolipidemic diet and monitoring of serum lipids are recommended until the patient stabilizes, since a rise in serum cholesterol and triglyceride concentrations to or above the original base may occur.

**Diet/Nutrition**
It is recommended that clofibrate be taken with food to minimize gastrointestinal upset.

## Oral Dosage Forms

### CLOFIBRATE CAPSULES USP

**Usual adult dose**
Antihyperlipidemic—
 Oral, 1.5 to 2 grams per day in two to four divided doses.

Note: Clofibrate has been used in the treatment of diabetes insipidus at an oral dose of 6 to 8 grams per day in two or four divided doses.

**Usual adult prescribing limits**
Antihyperlipidemic—
 2 grams daily.

**Usual pediatric dose**
Dosage has not been established.

**Strength(s) usually available**
U.S.—
 500 mg (Rx) [*Abitrate; Atromid-S;* GENERIC].
Canada—
 500 mg (Rx) [*Atromid-S; Claripex; Novofibrate*].
 1 gram (Rx) [*Atromid-S*].

**Packaging and storage**
Store below 40 °C (104 °F), preferably between 15 and 30 °C (59 and 86 °F), unless otherwise specified by manufacturer. Store in a well-closed, light-resistant container.

**Auxiliary labeling**
• Take with meals.

## Selected Bibliography

The Expert Panel. Report of the National Cholesterol Education Program Expert Panel on Detection, Evaluation and Treatment of High Blood Cholesterol in Adults. Arch Intern Med 1988 Jan; 148: 36-69.
NIH Consensus Conference. Lowering blood cholesterol to prevent heart disease. JAMA 1985 Apr 12; 253: 2080-6.
Knodel LC, Talbert RL. Adverse effects of hypolipidaemic drugs. Med Toxicol 1987; 2: 10-32.

Revised: 11/24/92
Interim revision: 04/14/94; 08/12/98

# CLOMIPHENE Systemic

INN: Clomifene
JAN: Clomifene citrate
VA CLASSIFICATION (Primary/Secondary): HS106/DX900; HS900
Commonly used brand name(s): *Clomid; Milophene; Serophene*.
Note: For a listing of dosage forms and brand names by country availability, see *Dosage Forms* section(s).

## Category
Antiestrogen; infertility therapy adjunct; diagnostic aid (ovarian function; hypothalamic-pituitary-gonadal axis function).

## Indications
Note: Bracketed information in the *Indications* section refers to uses that are not included in U.S. product labeling.

**Accepted**
Infertility, female (treatment)—Clomiphene is indicated in the treatment of anovulation or oligo-ovulation in patients desiring pregnancy, whose sexual partners have adequate sperm, and who have potentially functional hypothalamic-hypophyseal-ovarian systems and adequate endogenous estrogen.

[Corpus luteum insufficiency (treatment)][1]—Clomiphene may be used to treat corpus luteum dysfunction.

[Hypothalamic-pituitary-gonadal axis function, in males (diagnosis)][1]—Clomiphene is used to detect abnormalities of the hypothalamic-pituitary-gonadal axis in males.

[Infertility, male (treatment)][1]—Clomiphene is used to treat infertility in males with oligospermia.

[Ovarian function studies][1]—Clomiphene is sometimes given as a test dose to aid in predicting whether an ovulatory response might occur.

[1]Not included in Canadian product labeling.

## Pharmacology/Pharmacokinetics

**Physicochemical characteristics**
Source—Synthetic; nonsteroidal geometric isomer (30 to 50% is cis-clomiphene zuclomiphene and the remainder is trans-enclomiphene).
Molecular weight—598.10.

**Mechanism of action/Effect**
Clomiphene has mainly antiestrogenic effects and some estrogenic effects. The mechanism in stimulating ovulation is unknown but is believed to be related to its antiestrogenic properties. By clomiphene competing with estrogen for binding sites at the hypothalamic level, the gonadotropins, follicle-stimulating hormone (FSH) and luteinizing hormone (LH), secretion is increased, which results in ovarian follicle maturation, followed by the preovulatory LH surge, ovulation, and the subsequent development of the corpus luteum. Usefulness in male infertility is also likely related to the increases in FSH and LH secretion.

**Absorption**
Readily absorbed from gastrointestinal tract; undergoes enterohepatic recycling, especially with cis-zuclomiphene.

**Biotransformation**
Hepatic.

**Half-life**
Plasma—5 to 7 days.

**Time to peak effect**
Ovulation usually occurs 4 to 10 days (average 7 days) after the last day of treatment; this period of time may vary by patient and by cycle. In rare cases, ovulation may occur as late as 14 days after the last day of treatment.

**Elimination**
Biliary/fecal—Up to 42% of the oral dose; can be detectable in feces for up to 6 weeks.
Renal—Up to 8% of the oral dose.

## Precautions to Consider

**Carcinogenicity/Tumorigenicity/Mutagenicity**
Long-term carcinogenicity or mutagenicity studies have not been done. Studies are ongoing to determine the additional risk, if any, of developing ovarian cancer in women taking fertility medication beyond that contributed by infertility. Although a causal relationship between hyperstimulation of the ovaries and ovarian cancer has not been established, a correlation does exist for certain risk factors, including ovarian cancer, nulliparity, and increasing age. In addition, prolonged use of clomiphene may contribute to the risk of a borderline or invasive ovarian tumor, which should be considered whenever ovarian cysts do not regress with clomiphene therapy. Two cases of bilateral female breast carcinoma and one case of testicular carcinoma have occurred during clomiphene therapy.

**Pregnancy/Reproduction**
Fertility—Clomiphene may cause a decrease in quantity or change in quality of cervical mucus, which may interfere with sperm function, fertilization, and, subsequently, the occurrence of pregnancy.

Pregnancy—Clomiphene is not recommended during pregnancy. Controlled studies in humans have not been done. However, there have been reports of congenital malformations and fetal death occurring with clomiphene administration in humans. In clinical use, the cumulative rate of congenital abnormalities associated with ovulation induction therapy does not appear to be greater than that reported in the general population for spontaneous pregnancy. However, because a direct causal relationship has not been established, careful monitoring of the patient is recommended to prevent inadvertent administration of clomiphene during pregnancy.

Use of clomiphene is associated with an increased incidence of multiple pregnancies and, therefore, possible premature deliveries, as well as ectopic and heterotopic pregnancy. The incidence of reported multiple pregnancies was 7.98% (6.9% twins, 0.5% triplets, 0.3% quadruplets, and 0.1% quintuplets) with about an 83.3% survival rate, or a lower rate (73%) when including stillbirths, spontaneous abortions, or neonatal deaths. The ratio of monozygotic twins to dizygotic twins is 1 to 5.

Studies in rats and rabbits have shown clomiphene to be teratogenic. The observed malformations were similar to those produced by *in utero* exposure to diethylstilbestrol and may include vaginal adenosis and other defects in the vaginal, uterine, and Fallopian tube structures.

FDA Pregnancy Category X.

### Breast-feeding
It is not known whether clomiphene is distributed into breast milk. However, clomiphene suppresses lactation.

### Laboratory value alterations
The following have been selected on the basis of their potential clinical significance (possible effect in parentheses where appropriate)—not necessarily inclusive (» = major clinical significance):

With physiology/laboratory test values
 Desmosterol (only with long-term use, possibly indicating interference with cholesterol synthesis) and
 Sex hormone–binding globulin and
 Transcortin
  (plasma concentrations may be increased)

### Medical considerations/Contraindications
The medical considerations/contraindications included have been selected on the basis of their potential clinical significance (reasons given in parentheses where appropriate)—not necessarily inclusive (» = major clinical significance).

*Except under special circumstances, this medication should not be used when the following medical problems exist:*
» Hepatic function impairment, active
  (potential for reduced clearance of clomiphene, leading to higher plasma concentrations or hepatotoxicity)
» Mental depression
  (may be exacerbated)
» Ovarian cyst, not associated with polycystic ovary syndrome or
» Ovarian enlargement, not associated with polycystic ovary syndrome
  (risk of further enlargement)
» Thrombophlebitis, active
  (increased risk of thrombophlebitis in susceptible individuals can be caused by elevated estradiol levels associated with ovulation induction by clomiphene)

*Risk-benefit should be considered when the following medical problems exist:*
» Abnormal vaginal bleeding, undiagnosed
  (careful evaluation recommended; neoplastic lesions should be ruled out)
» Endometriosis
  (implants may be aggravated by elevated estradiol levels associated with ovulation induction)
» Fibroid tumors of the uterus
  (risk of further enlargement)
» Hepatic function impairment, history of
  (potential for reduced clearance of clomiphene, leading to higher plasma concentrations or hepatotoxicity)
» Polycystic ovary syndrome or
 Sensitivity to pituitary gonadotropins
  (patient may have an exaggerated response to clomiphene; lower dose or shorter duration of therapy may be necessary)
 Sensitivity to clomiphene

### Patient monitoring
The following may be especially important in patient monitoring (other tests may be warranted in some patients, depending on condition; » = major clinical significance):

Immunologic assay for human chorionic gonadotropin (HCG)
 (recommended for detection of pregnancy if menses does not occur before start of next course of clomiphene; should be measured 10 days or later after exogenous HCG is administered)

Liver function tests
 (recommended in some patients prior to initiation of therapy with clomiphene, especially in patients with risk factors increasing their susceptibility to hepatic dysfunction)
Ophthalmologic, including slit-lamp, examination
 (recommended if treatment with clomiphene is continued for more than 1 year or if visual disturbances occur)
» Urinary luteinizing hormone surge testing
 (may be used as adjunctive therapy to predict ovulation)

## Side/Adverse Effects

Note: At the recommended dosage, adverse effects usually are rare. Incidence and severity of adverse effects tend to be related to dose and duration of treatment and are usually reversible after clomiphene therapy is discontinued. Doses over 100 mg a day for five days have been associated with a higher incidence of side effects; patients receiving these doses should be carefully monitored.

Rare reports of ovarian cancer have been associated with fertility medications but a causal relationship has not been determined partly because it is not possible to predict beyond the risk that infertility brings to developing ovarian cancer.

The following side/adverse effects have been selected on the basis of their potential clinical significance (possible signs and symptoms in parentheses where appropriate)—not necessarily inclusive:

### Those indicating need for medical attention
Incidence more frequent—> 5%
 *Ovarian cyst formation; ovarian enlargement; premenstrual syndrome; uterine fibroid enlargement* (abdominal bloating; stomach pain; pelvic pain)

Note: Maximum *ovarian enlargement* occurs several days after clomiphene therapy is discontinued.

A patient's report of *abdominal pain* during clomiphene therapy indicates the need for immediate pelvic examination. If ovarian enlargement or cyst formation has occurred, it is recommended that clomiphene therapy be withdrawn until the ovaries have returned to pretreatment size, usually within a few days or weeks. Dosage and duration of the next course of clomiphene should be reduced.

Incidence less frequent or rare
 *Hepatotoxicity* (yellow eyes or skin); *vision changes, especially afterimages* (persistence of visual images); *blurred vision*—especially with larger doses; *diplopia* (double vision); *floaters* (spots in visual field caused by protein deposits in the vitreous fluid of the eye); *phosphenes* (seeing flashes of light); *photophobia* (increased sensitivity of eyes to light); *scotoma* (area of decreased vision in visual field surrounded by normal or less-diminished vision)

Note: If the patient receiving clomiphene experiences any *visual disturbances*, it is recommended that clomiphene therapy be withdrawn and a complete ophthalmologic examination performed. Ocular side effects usually disappear within a few days or weeks after the last dose of clomiphene.

### Those indicating need for medical attention only if they continue or are bothersome
Incidence more frequent—10%
 *Hot flashes*

Incidence less frequent or rare—1 to 2%
 *Breast discomfort in women; gynecomastia in men* (enlargement of breasts); *dizziness or lightheadedness; headache; menorrhagia* (increased amount of menstrual bleeding at regular monthly periods); *mental depression; nausea or vomiting; nervousness; restlessness; spotting* (light uterine bleeding between regular menstrual periods); *tiredness; trouble in sleeping*

## Patient Consultation

As an aid to patient consultation, refer to *Advice for the Patient, Clomiphene (Systemic)*.

In providing consultation, consider emphasizing the following selected information (» = major clinical significance):

### Before using this medication
» Conditions affecting use, especially:
 Sensitivity to clomiphene
  Pregnancy—Use during pregnancy is not recommended since animal studies have shown teratogenicity
  Breast-feeding—Suppresses lactation
  Other medical problems, especially hepatic function impairment, mental depression, ovarian cyst, ovarian enlargement, throm-

bophlebitis, undiagnosed abnormal vaginal bleeding, endometriosis, uterine fibroids, and polycystic ovary syndrome

**Proper use of this medication**
» Compliance with therapy; clarification of schedule; taking at same time every day to aid in remembering each dose
» Proper dosing
Missed dose: Taking as soon as possible; doubling dose if not remembered until time of next dose; checking with physician if more than one dose missed
» Proper storage

**Precautions while using this medication**
» Importance of close monitoring by physician
» Importance of following physician's instructions for timing of intercourse
» Telling physician immediately if pregnancy is suspected; importance of not taking medication while pregnant
» Caution when driving or doing jobs requiring alertness because of visual disturbances, dizziness, or lightheadedness

**Side/adverse effects**
Signs of potential side effects, especially ovarian cyst formation, ovarian enlargement, uterine fibroid enlargement, premenstrual syndrome, hepatotoxicity, or vision changes

## General Dosing Information

Patients receiving clomiphene should be under supervision of a physician experienced in the treatment of gynecologic or endocrine disorders.

Patients who have been hypoestrogenic for prolonged periods may require pretreatment with estrogen to provide a more normal endometrium for ovum implantation. Estrogen therapy should be discontinued immediately before initiation of clomiphene therapy.

Properly timed coitus in relation to ovulation is important and may be predicted from ovulation test kits (the preferred method) or other appropriate tests for ovulation such as taking basal body temperature. Couples should be advised to have frequent intercourse at or around the time that ovulation is anticipated. Ovulation generally occurs 7 days (average) after the last dose of clomiphene (range is 5 to 10 days).

In some patients, a single injection of 5000 to 10,000 USP Units of human chorionic gonadotropin (HCG) given 5 to 9 days after the last dose of clomiphene to simulate the midcycle LH surge that results in ovulation may increase the efficacy of clomiphene.

If ovulation does not occur after 3 to 4 cycles of clomiphene therapy at the maximum dose, or if pregnancy does not result after a treatment interval of 3 to 6 months with documented ovulation, or if ovulatory menses does not occur, further treatment with clomiphene is not recommended and the diagnosis should be re-evaluated.

## Oral Dosage Forms

### CLOMIPHENE CITRATE TABLETS USP

**Usual adult dose**
Female infertility—
Oral, 50 mg a day for five days, starting on the fifth day of the menstrual cycle or at any time if the patient has had no recent uterine bleeding. If ovulation without conception occurs, this cycle is repeated until conception or for three or four cycles. A smaller dose or shorter duration may be necessary for individuals unusually sensitive to clomiphene, such as women with polycystic ovary sydrome. If ovulation does not occur, the dose is increased to 75 to 100 mg a day for five days (the next course beginning as early as thirty days after the previous course), repeated if ovulation without conception occurs. Rarely, patients require up to 250 mg a day to induce ovulation.

Note: A physical exam prior to the first and each subsequent treatment is needed to exclude pregnancy, ovarian enlargement, or ovarian cysts (not due to polycystic ovary syndrome) and to ensure normal liver function and no abnormal uterine bleeding before next course of clomiphene may be initiated.

**Strength(s) usually available**
U.S.—
50 mg (Rx) [*Clomid* (scored; lactose; sucrose); *Milophene* (scored; lactose; sucrose); *Serophene* (scored) [GENERIC].
Canada—
50 mg (Rx) [*Clomid* (scored; sucrose; lactose); *Serophene*].

**Packaging and storage**
Store below 40 °C (104 °F), preferably between 15 and 30 °C (59 and 86 °F), unless otherwise specified by manufacturer. Store in a well-closed container. Protect from light.

Revised: 08/08/95

---

**CLOMIPRAMINE**—See *Antidepressants, Tricyclic (Systemic)*

---

**CLONAZEPAM**—See *Benzodiazepines (Systemic)*

---

# CLONIDINE   Parenteral-Local—INTRODUCTORY VERSION

VA CLASSIFICATION (Primary): CN103
Commonly used brand name(s): *Duraclon*.
Note: For a listing of dosage forms and brand names by country availability, see *Dosage Forms* section(s).

## Category
Analgesic.

## Indications

**Accepted**
Pain, cancer (treatment adjunct)—Clonidine is indicated in combination with opiates for the treatment of severe pain in cancer patients that is not adequately relieved by opioid analgesics alone. Epidural clonidine is likely to be more effective in relieving neuropathic pain, characterized as electrical, burning, or shooting in nature, that is localized to a dermatomal or peripheral nerve distribution area, rather than in relieving pain that is diffuse, poorly localized, or visceral in origin.

## Pharmacology/Pharmacokinetics

**Physicochemical characteristics**
Chemical group—Imidazoline derivative.
Molecular weight—266.56.

**Mechanism of action/Effect**
Clonidine, administered epidurally, is thought to produce analgesia by preventing pain-signal transmission to the brain at presynaptic and postjunctional alpha$_2$-adrenoceptors in the spinal cord. Analgesia occurs in body regions innervated by the spinal segments where clonidine concentrates. Clonidine-associated analgesia is dose-dependent and is not antagonized by opiate antagonists.

**Other actions/effects**
Clonidine decreases sympathetic outflow to the heart, kidneys, and peripheral vasculature, resulting in decreased peripheral resistance, renal vascular resistance, heart rate, and blood pressure.

**Distribution**
Clonidine is highly lipid soluble and is distributed into extravascular sites, including the central nervous system (CNS).
Volume of distribution (Vol$_D$)—2.1 ± 0.4 liters per kg (L/kg).

**Protein binding**
Low (20 to 40%, *in vitro*), primarily to albumin.

**Biotransformation**
Clonidine is metabolized through minor pathways. The major metabolite, *p*-hydroxyclonidine, is present in concentrations less than 10% of those of unchanged clonidine in urine.

**Half-life**
Elimination from plasma—
22 ± 15 hours. Half-life may be prolonged by up to 41 hours in patients with renal function impairment.

**Time to peak plasma concentration**
19 ± 27 minutes.

### Elimination
Renal—72%, of which 40 to 50% is unchanged clonidine.
In dialysis—Only 5% of clonidine body stores was removed in subjects undergoing hemodialysis. Therefore, it is not necessary to administer supplemental clonidine to patients undergoing routine hemodialysis.

## Precautions to Consider

### Carcinogenicity
Clonidine was not found to be carcinogenic in a study in rats given a dietary admixture of clonidine at a dose representing five to eight times the 50 mcg per kg (mcg/kg) maximum recommended human daily dose (MRHDD) for [the treatment of] hypertension, based on body surface area.

### Mutagenicity
Clonidine was not found to be mutagenic in the Ames mutagenicity test.

### Pregnancy/Reproduction
Fertility—No effect on fertility was found in studies in male or female rats given oral doses of clonidine of up to 150 mcg/kg. This dose represents approximately 0.5 times the MRHDD. In a separate study, fertility appeared to be affected in female rats given oral doses of 500 to 2000 mcg/kg. These doses represent two to seven times the MRHDD.

Pregnancy—Clonidine crosses the placenta and reaches concentrations in umbilical cord plasma equal to those in maternal plasma. Concentrations in amniotic fluid may be four times those found in serum. Adequate and well-controlled studies have not been done in pregnant women during early gestation when organ formation occurs. Clonidine use during pregnancy is not recommended unless the potential benefits outweigh the potential risks to the fetus.

Teratogenic or embryotoxic potential was not found in reproduction studies in rabbits given clonidine in doses of up to approximately the MRHDD. A study in female rats given doses at one third the MRHDD for 2 months prior to mating resulted in an increase in resorptions. However, an increase in resorptions did not occur when female rats were given clonidine in the same doses or doses of up to 0.5 times the MRHDD on days 6 to 15 of gestation. An increase in resorptions was observed during a study in rats and mice given clonidine doses equivalent to seven times the MRHDD on days 1 to 14 of gestation.

FDA Pregnancy Category C.

Labor—Studies using epidural clonidine during labor have not shown any apparent adverse effects in the infant at the time of delivery, although hemodynamic effects in the infant on the days following delivery were not monitored. Adequate and well-controlled trials to evaluate dosing, safety, and effectiveness of epidural clonidine in obstetrics have not been done. The use of clonidine as an analgesic during labor and delivery is not recommended, essentially because maternal perfusion of the placenta is dependent on blood pressure.

### Breast-feeding
Clonidine is distributed into human breast milk, reaching concentrations that are approximately twice those found in maternal plasma. Clonidine is not recommended for use in nursing mothers because of the potential for severe adverse reactions in the infant.

### Pediatrics
No specific information is available on the relationship of age to the effects of epidurally administered clonidine in pediatric patients. Safety and efficacy have been established only in patients old enough to tolerate placement and management of an epidural catheter. Clonidine should be used in pediatric patients only for severe intractable pain associated with malignancy that is unresponsive to epidural or spinal opiates or other analgesic techniques.

### Geriatrics
No information is available on the relationship of age to the effects of clonidine in geriatric patients.

### Pharmacogenetics
Women have a lower mean plasma clearance rate, longer mean plasma half-life, and higher mean peak concentration of clonidine in both plasma and cerebro-spinal fluid (CSF) than do men.
Hypotension as a side effect of epidural clonidine was observed more frequently in women.

### Surgical
Epidural clonidine has been reported to cause a marked hypotensive response when used for intra- or postoperative analgesia.

### Drug interactions and/or related problems
The following drug interactions and/or related problems have been selected on the basis of their potential clinical significance (possible mechanism in parentheses where appropriate)—not necessarily inclusive (» = major clinical significance):

Note: Combinations containing any of the following medications, depending on the amount present, may also interact with this medication.

Alcohol or
Barbiturates or
Other CNS depression–producing medications (see *Appendix II*), including
  Analgesics, narcotic
    (concurrent use may cause CNS depressive effects and potentiation of hypotensive effects of clonidine)
Anesthetics, local, epidural
  (concurrent use with clonidine may prolong the duration of effects of these drugs, including both sensory and motor blockade effects)
Antidepressants, tricyclic
  (effects on clonidine's analgesic effects are unknown, but tricyclic antidepressants may antagonize the hypotensive effects of clonidine)
» Beta-adrenergic blocking agents
  (concurrent use may cause potentiation of the hypertensive response seen with clonidine withdrawal and may exacerbate bradycardia and atrioventricular [AV] block)
Fluphenazine
  (acute delirium was reported in one patient using oral clonidine concurrently; the symptoms resolved upon withdrawal of clonidine and recurred upon rechallenge)
Medications affecting sinus node function or AV nodal conduction, such as:
  Digitalis glycosides
  Calcium channel blocking agents
    (concurrent use may exacerbate bradycardia and atrioventricular [AV] block)

### Medical considerations/Contraindications
The medical considerations/contraindications included have been selected on the basis of their potential clinical significance (reasons given in parentheses where appropriate)—not necessarily inclusive (» = major clinical significance).

*Except under special circumstances, this medication should not be used when the following medical problems exist:*
» Allergic reaction to clonidine, history of or
» Sensitization to clonidine, history of
» Anticoagulant therapy or
» Hemorrhagic diathesis
  (because of the potential for hemorrhage into the spinal epidural space, epidural administration should not be used in these settings)
» Infection present at the injection site
  (increased risk of development of meningitis or epidural abscess)

*Risk-benefit should be considered when the following medical problems exist:*
Cardiovascular disease, severe or
Hemodynamic instability, such as:
  Bradycardia or
  Hypotension
    (increased risk of severe hypotension, further worsening these conditions; clonidine may also mask the increase in heart rate associated with hypovolemia)
Obstetrical pain or
Perioperative pain or
Postpartum pain
  (clonidine administration is associated with hypotension and/or bradycardia, which may not be tolerated by these patients)
Renal function impairment
  (elimination half-life may be prolonged; dosage adjustment may be necessary)

### Patient monitoring
The following may be especially important in patient monitoring (other tests may be warranted in some patients, depending on condition; » = major clinical significance):

» Blood pressure determinations
» Body temperature
» Heart rate determinations
» Respiratory rate
  (frequent monitoring recommended, especially during the first few days of therapy)

## Side/Adverse Effects

Note: Epidural clonidine may rarely cause atrioventricular (AV) block greater than first degree and may also mask the increase in heart rate associated with hypovolemia.

The following side/adverse effects may be related to administration of either clonidine or morphine and have been selected on the basis of their potential clinical significance (possible signs and symptoms in parentheses where appropriate)—not necessarily inclusive:

### Those indicating need for medical attention
Incidence more frequent
*Bradycardia* (slow heart rate); **hypotension** (dizziness, lightheadedness, or fainting)

  Note: In a study of cancer patients administered epidural clonidine at 30 mcg per hour (mcg/hr) in addition to epidural morphine, the incidence of *hypotension* was 45%. Hypotension occurred most often within the first 4 days after initiation of epidural clonidine, but also occurred throughout the duration of the study. Hypotension occurred more commonly in women, in patients with higher serum clonidine concentrations, and in patients with lower than average body weight. More pronounced hypotension may occur when clonidine is infused into the upper thoracic spinal segments. Severe hypotension may occur even with prior intravenous fluid treatment.

Incidence less frequent
*Chest pain; fever; hallucinations* (seeing, feeling, or hearing things that are not there); **hypoventilation** (extremely shallow or slow breathing); *mental depression; sedation; tachycardia* (fast heartbeat); **vomiting**

  Note: *Fever* occurring in a patient receiving clonidine therapy may be associated with catheter-related infection such as meningitis and/or epidural abscess. Catheter-related infections occur in 5 to 20% of patients, depending on the kind of catheter used, catheter placement technique, quality of catheter care, and duration of catheter placement.

  Clonidine activates alpha-adrenoreceptors in the brain stem and may cause *sedation*. High doses of clonidine may cause sedation and *hypoventilation*, although tolerance to these effects may develop with long-term administration. Bolus doses that are significantly larger than the infusion rate recommended for treating cancer pain have been associated with these effects.

  *Mental depression* has been associated with administration of oral or transdermal clonidine. Depression occurs commonly in cancer patients and may be potentiated by clonidine therapy. Patients should be monitored for signs and symptoms of depression, especially patients with a known history of affective disorders.

### Those indicating need for medical attention only if they continue or are bothersome
Incidence more frequent
*Anxiety and/or confusion; dizziness; dryness of mouth; nausea; somnolence* (sleepiness)

Incidence less frequent
*Asthenia* (weakness); **constipation; sweating, unusual; tinnitus** (ringing, noises, or buzzing in the ear)

### Those indicating possible rebound hypertension and/or the need for medical attention if they occur after medication is abruptly discontinued
*Agitation; headache; nervousness; and/or tremor, accompanied or followed by a rapid rise in blood pressure*

  Note: The *abrupt withdrawal* of clonidine in some patients has resulted in the above symptoms. These symptoms may be more likely to occur after administration of higher doses of clonidine or with concurrent use of beta-adrenergic blocking agents. Rarely, hypertensive encephalopathy, cerebrovascular accidents, and death have occurred after abrupt withdrawal of clonidine. Patients with a history of hypertension and/or other cardiovascular conditions may be particularly susceptible to the symptoms of abrupt clonidine withdrawal. In clinical trials, 4 of 38 patients receiving 720 mcg of epidural clonidine per day experienced rebound hypertension following abrupt withdrawal of clonidine; one of these 4 patients subsequently experienced a cerebrovascular accident.

## Overdose
For specific information on the agents used in the management of clonidine overdose, see:
- *Atropine* in *Anticholinergics/Antispasmodics (Systemic)* monograph; and/or
- *Diazoxide (Parenteral-Systemic)* monograph; and/or
- *Furosemide* in *Diuretics, Loop (Systemic)* monograph; and/or
- Vasopressor agents, including *Ephedrine* in *Sympathomimetic Agents—Cardiovascular Use (Parenteral-Systemic)* monograph; and/or
- *Naloxone (Systemic)* monograph; and/or
- *Phentolamine (Systemic)* monograph.

For more information on the management of overdose or unintentional ingestion, **contact a Poison Control Center** (see *Poison Control Center Listing*).

### Clinical effects of overdose
The following effects have been selected on the basis of their potential clinical significance (possible signs and symptoms in parentheses where appropriate)—not necessarily inclusive:

Acute and/or chronic
*Bradycardia* (slow heart rate); **decreased or absent reflexes; drowsiness; hallucinations; hypertension; hypotension; hypothermia; irritability; miosis** (blurred vision); **respiratory depression**

  Note: *Hypertension* may develop early and may be followed by *hypotension* and the above clinical effects.

Large oral overdoses
*Apnea* (cessation in breathing); **cardiac conduction defects or arrhythmias, reversible; coma; seizures**

### Treatment of overdose
Treatment is symptomatic and supportive.
  Specific treatment—
    For bradycardia—Atropine.
    For hypotension—Intravenous fluids and/or vasopressor agents, such as ephedrine.
    For hypertension—Intravenous furosemide, diazoxide, or alpha-adrenergic blocking agents, such as phentolamine. Use of tolazoline has shown inconsistent results and is not recommended as first-line therapy.
    For respiratory depression, hypotension, and/or coma—Naloxone.
  Monitoring—
    The administration of naloxone occasionally has resulted in paradoxical hypertension; blood pressure should be monitored.
  Supportive care—
    Patients in whom intentional overdose is confirmed or suspected should be referred for psychiatric consultation.

## Patient Consultation
As an aid to patient consultation, refer to *Advice for the Patient, Clonidine (Injection)—Introductory Version*.

In providing consultation, consider emphasizing the following selected information (» = major clinical significance):

### Before using this medication
» Conditions affecting use, especially:
    History of allergic reaction or sensitization to clonidine
    Pregnancy—Clonidine crosses the placenta; not recommended for use during pregnancy
    Breast-feeding—Clonidine is distributed into breast milk; not recommended for use in nursing mothers
    Use in children—Safety and efficacy have not been established; should be used only for severe intractable pain due to malignancy unresponsive to opiates or other analgesic techniques
    Pharmacogenetics—In women, plasma clearance rate may be lower and plasma half-life may be longer; peak concentration in plasma and cerebrospinal fluid (CSF) may be higher; hypotension may occur more frequently
    Surgical—Epidural clonidine has been reported to cause a marked hypotensive response when used for intra- or postoperative analgesia
  Other medications, especially beta-adrenergic blocking agents
  Other medical problems, especially anticoagulant therapy, hemorrhagic diathesis, infection present at the injection site

### Proper use of this medication
  Proper administration of epidural clonidine
» Proper dosing
    Missed dose: Notifying physician immediately if clonidine administration is interrupted for any reason
» Proper storage

### Precautions while using this medication
Not discontinuing therapy without consultation with and supervision by physician because of the possibility of serious adverse effects occurring with abrupt withdrawal

Caution when driving or doing other things requiring alertness because of possible sedation and hypotensive effects of clonidine

Getting up slowly from a lying or sitting position to prevent dizziness or faintness from hypotension

Caution in use of alcohol or other CNS depressants because of additional sedation or hypotensive effects

### Side/adverse effects
Signs of potential side effects, especially bradycardia, hypotension, chest pain, fever, hallucinations, hypoventilation, mental depression, sedation, tachycardia, and vomiting

## General Dosing Information
Abrupt withdrawal of clonidine has resulted in serious adverse effects in some patients. To discontinue epidural clonidine therapy, the dose should be reduced gradually over 2 to 4 days to avoid withdrawal symptoms. In patients concurrently receiving a beta-adrenergic blocking agent, the beta-blocking agent should be discontinued several days before the epidural clonidine is gradually discontinued.

The epidural administration of clonidine above the C4 dermatome is contraindicated because of the lack of adequate safety data supporting this use. Inadvertent administration of clonidine intrathecally has not been associated with a significant increase in adverse events, although there is a lack of adequate data supporting safety and efficacy.

Familiarization with the continuous epidural infusion device and monitoring or inspecting the device and catheter tubing for obstruction or dislodgment are necessary in order to reduce the risk of inadvertent abrupt withdrawal of epidural clonidine.

In patients with renal function impairment, the dosage should be adjusted according to the degree of impairment; careful monitoring is recommended.

### For treatment of adverse effects
Recommended treatment consists of the following:
- Symptomatic bradycardia may be treated with atropine.
- Hypotension may be treated with intravenous fluids and, if necessary, parenteral ephedrine.

For treatment of withdrawal symptoms—
Recommended treatment consists of the following:
- Hypertension following discontinuation of epidural clonidine may be treated by administration of clonidine or by intravenous phentolamine. For specific information on phentolamine, see *Phentolamine (Systemic)* monograph.

## Parenteral Dosage Forms

### CLONIDINE HYDROCHLORIDE INJECTION

**Usual adult dose**
Analgesic—
Initially, by continuous epidural infusion, 30 mcg per hour. The dosage is titrated to the degree of pain relief and occurrence of adverse effects; patients should be closely monitored for the first few days to assess their response.

**Usual adult prescribing limits**
Experience is limited with infusion rates above 40 mcg per hr.

**Usual pediatric dose**
Analgesic—
Initially, by continuous epidural infusion, 0.5 mcg per kg per hour, adjusted based on the clinical response.

Note: Safety and efficacy of epidural clonidine have been established only in pediatric patients who are old enough to tolerate placement and management of an epidural catheter.

**Strength(s) usually available**
U.S.—
100 mcg per mL (Rx) [*Duraclon* (individually packaged 10 mL vials, preservative-free)].

**Packaging and storage**
Store at controlled room temperature, between 15 and 30 °C (59 and 86 °F). Discard unused portion.

**Auxiliary labeling**
- Do not take other medicines without your doctor's advice.
- Avoid alcoholic beverages.

Developed: 11/04/97
Interim revision: 08/14/98

---

# CLONIDINE  Systemic

VA CLASSIFICATION (Primary/Secondary):
Oral—CV409/DX900; CN105; CN900
Transdermal—CV409

Commonly used brand name(s): *Catapres; Catapres-TTS; Dixarit*.

Note: For a listing of dosage forms and brand names by country availability, see *Dosage Forms* section(s).

## Category
Antihypertensive—Clonidine Hydrochloride Tablets; Clonidine Transdermal Systems.
Menopausal syndrome therapy adjunct—Clonidine Hydrochloride Tablets.
Vascular headache prophylactic—Clonidine Hydrochloride Tablets.
Antidysmenorrheal—Clonidine Hydrochloride Tablets.
Opioid withdrawal syndrome suppressant—Clonidine Hydrochloride Tablets.

## Indications
Note: Bracketed information in the *Indications* section refers to uses that are not included in U.S. product labeling.

**Accepted**
Hypertension (treatment)—Oral and transdermal dosage forms of clonidine are indicated in the treatment of hypertension. Because it causes only mild postural hypotension, clonidine may be useful as a substitute for guanethidine or other adrenergic blockers in patients who cannot tolerate these agents because of severe orthostatic hypotension.

[Oral clonidine is also used in the urgent treatment of hypertensive emergencies.][1]

[Pheochromocytoma (diagnosis)][1]—A clonidine suppression test is used in the diagnosis of pheochromocytoma.

[Headache, vascular (prophylaxis)][1]—Clonidine has been used orally in the prevention of migraine.

[Dysmenorrhea (treatment)][1] or
[Menopause, vasomotor symptoms of (treatment)][1]—Clonidine is used orally as an adjunct in the treatment of dysmenorrhea and menopausal flushing.

[Opioid (narcotic) abstinence syndrome (treatment)][1]—Clonidine is also used to control symptoms and aid in rapid detoxification in the treatment of opioid withdrawal.

[Nicotine dependence (treatment adjunct)][1]—Clonidine is used as an adjunct in the treatment of nicotine withdrawal.

[Gilles de la Tourette's syndrome (treatment)][1]—Clonidine is used in the treatment of Gilles de la Tourette's syndrome.

[1]Not included in Canadian product labeling.

## Pharmacology/Pharmacokinetics

**Physicochemical characteristics**
Molecular weight—Clonidine: 230.10.
Clonidine hydrochloride: 266.56.

**Mechanism of action/Effect**
Alpha-adrenergic agonist; also has some alpha-adrenergic antagonist effects.
Antihypertensive—
Thought to be due to central alpha$_2$-adrenergic stimulation, which results in a decreased sympathetic outflow to the heart, kidneys, and peripheral vasculature; this results in decreased peripheral vascular resistance, decreased systolic and diastolic blood pressure, and decreased heart rate.
Vascular headache prophylactic—
May block central vasomotor reflexes.
Dysmenorrhea therapy adjunct; or menopausal syndrome therapy adjunct—
Unknown, although may act as peripheral vascular stabilizer to reduce menopausal flushing.

Opioid withdrawal syndrome suppressant—
May be result of alpha-adrenergic inhibiting activity in areas of the brain such as the locus ceruleus.

**Other actions/effects**
Stimulates the release of growth hormone acutely, but not chronically.

**Absorption**
Oral—Well absorbed following oral administration. Bioavailability following chronic administration is approximately 65%.
Transdermal—Greatest from the chest and upper arm, and least from the thigh. Absorbed through the skin at a constant rate.

**Protein binding**
Low to moderate (20 to 40%).

**Biotransformation**
Hepatic (about 50% of the absorbed dose).

**Half-life**
Normal renal function—Range, 12 to 16 hours.
Renal function impairment—Up to 41 hours.

**Onset of effect**
Antihypertensive:
Oral: 30 to 60 minutes.
Transdermal: 2 to 3 days.

**Time to peak plasma concentration**
Oral—1.5 to 2.5 hours.
Transdermal—2 to 3 days.

**Time for peak effect**
Antihypertensive—Oral: 2 to 4 hours.

**Duration of action**
Antihypertensive—
Oral:
Up to 8 hours (24 to 36 hours in some patients).
Transdermal:
About 7 days with the system in place; about 8 hours after removal.

**Elimination**
Renal—40 to 60% (as unchanged drug) in 24 hours.
Biliary/fecal—20% (probably via enterohepatic circulation).
In dialysis—Very little (maximum 5%) removable by hemodialysis.

## Precautions to Consider

**Cross-sensitivity and/or related problems**
Patients sensitive to ophthalmic apraclonidine may be sensitive to clonidine.

**Carcinogenicity**
Studies in rats at doses 32 to 46 times the maximum recommended human dose for 132 weeks found no evidence of carcinogenicity.

**Pregnancy/Reproduction**
Fertility—Studies in male and female rats at doses up to 3 times the maximum recommended human dose found no impairment of fertility. However, fertility was affected in female rats given 10 to 40 times the maximum recommended human dose.

Pregnancy—Adequate and well-controlled studies in humans have not been done.

Studies in rats at doses as low as one-third the maximum recommended human dose given for 2 months prior to mating found an increased incidence of resorptions; this effect did not occur at doses of one-third to 3 times the maximum recommended human dose given on days 6 to 15 of gestation. Increased resorptions also occurred in rats and mice given doses up to 40 times the maximum recommended human dose on days 1 to 14 of gestation. No teratogenicity or embryotoxicity was observed in rabbits given up to 3 times the maximum recommended human dose.

FDA Pregnancy Category C.

**Breast-feeding**
Clonidine is distributed into breast milk. However, problems in humans have not been documented.

**Pediatrics**
Appropriate studies on the relationship of age to the effects of clonidine have not been performed in the pediatric population. However, there are numerous reports describing accidental clonidine overdose in the pediatric population. These reports seem to indicate that neonates, infants, and children are especially sensitive to the effects of clonidine. Caution is recommended.

**Geriatrics**
The elderly may be more sensitive than younger adults to clonidine's hypotensive effects. In addition, elderly patients are more likely to have age-related renal function impairment, which may require reduction of dosage in patients receiving clonidine.

**Dental**
Use of clonidine may decrease or inhibit salivary flow, thus contributing to the development of caries, periodontal disease, oral candidiasis, and discomfort.

**Drug interactions and/or related problems**
The following drug interactions and/or related problems have been selected on the basis of their potential clinical significance (possible mechanism in parentheses where appropriate)—not necessarily inclusive (» = major clinical significance):

Note: Combinations containing any of the following medications, depending on the amount present, may also interact with this medication.

Alcohol or
Central nervous system (CNS) depression–producing medications (See *Appendix II*)
(concurrent use may enhance the CNS depressant effects of either these medications or clonidine)

» Antidepressants, tricyclic, or
Appetite suppressants, with the exception of fenfluramine
(concurrent use may decrease the hypotensive effects of clonidine)

Anti-inflammatory drugs, nonsteroidal (NSAIDs), especially indomethacin
(NSAIDs may reduce the antihypertensive effects of clonidine, possibly by inhibiting renal prostaglandin synthesis and/or causing sodium and fluid retention; the patient should be carefully monitored to confirm that the desired effect is being obtained)

» Beta-adrenergic blocking agents (systemic)
(discontinuation of clonidine therapy during concurrent use of beta-adrenergic blocking agents may increase the risk of clonidine-withdrawal hypertensive crisis; ideally, beta-adrenergic blocking agents should be discontinued several days before clonidine is discontinued; blood pressure control may also be impaired when the 2 are combined)

Fenfluramine
(concurrent use may increase the hypotensive effects of clonidine)

Hypotension-producing medications, other, (See *Appendix II*) with the exception of systemic beta-adrenergic blocking agents and tricyclic antidepressants
(concurrent use may potentiate antihypertensive effects; although some antihypertensive and/or diuretic combinations are frequently used for therapeutic advantage, dosage adjustments may be necessary during concurrent use)

Sympathomimetics
(concurrent use may reduce the antihypertensive effects of clonidine; the patient should be carefully monitored to confirm that the desired effect is being obtained)

**Laboratory value alterations**
The following have been selected on the basis of their potential clinical significance (possible effect in parentheses where appropriate)—not necessarily inclusive (» = major clinical significance):

With physiology/laboratory test values
Catecholamine concentrations, urinary, and
Vanillylmandelic acid (VMA) excretion, urinary
(may be decreased but may increase on abrupt withdrawal)

Direct antiglobulin (Coombs') tests
(may produce weakly positive results)

Growth hormone concentrations, plasma
(may be increased transiently because of stimulation of growth hormone release, but are not elevated chronically with long-term use of clonidine)

**Medical considerations/Contraindications**
The medical considerations/contraindications included have been selected on the basis of their potential clinical significance (reasons given in parentheses where appropriate)—not necessarily inclusive (» = major clinical significance):

*Risk-benefit should be considered when the following medical problems exist:*

Atrioventricular (AV) node function impairment
(vagal effect of clonidine may exacerbate condition)

Cerebrovascular disease or
Coronary insufficiency or
Myocardial infarction, recent
(lowered blood pressure may decrease perfusion and worsen ischemia)

Mental depression, history of or
Raynaud's syndrome
(may be exacerbated by clonidine)
Renal function impairment, chronic
(reduces the elimination of clonidine and may increase the risk of toxicity; dosage reduction may be necessary)
Sensitivity to clonidine
Sinus node function impairment
(function may be further impaired)
Thromboangiitis obliterans

*For transdermal dosage form only (in addition to above)*
Polyarteritis nodosa or
Scleroderma or
Systemic lupus erythematosus (SLE)
(absorption may be decreased; placement of patches on affected areas should be avoided)
Skin irritation or abrasion
(absorption may be increased; placement of patches on irritated or abraded areas should be avoided)

### Patient monitoring
The following may be especially important in patient monitoring (other tests may be warranted in some patients, depending on condition; » = major clinical significance):
» Blood pressure measurements
(recommended at periodic intervals in patients being treated for hypertension; selected patients may be taught to monitor their blood pressure at home and report the results at regular physician visits)

## Side/Adverse Effects

Note: Incidence and severity of adverse systemic effects may be reduced with the transdermal dosage form, possibly because this form of administration maintains lower peak blood concentrations than occur with oral administration and decreases fluctuation in blood concentration.

Administration of clonidine for 6 months or longer to albino rats has resulted in a dose-related increase in the incidence and severity of spontaneously occurring retinal degeneration. These effects have not been observed in humans.

The following side/adverse effects have been selected on the basis of their potential clinical significance (possible signs and symptoms in parentheses where appropriate)—not necessarily inclusive:

### Those indicating need for medical attention
Incidence more frequent— about 15 to 20%, with transdermal systems only
*Itching or redness of skin*
Note: Patients who develop either a localized or an extended allergic reaction to the transdermal system may also experience a generalized allergic skin rash if oral clonidine is substituted.

Incidence less frequent
*Mental depression; sodium and water retention or edema* (swelling of feet and lower legs)

Incidence rare
*Raynaud's phenomenon* (paleness or cold feeling in fingertips and toes); *vivid dreams or nightmares*

### Those indicating need for medical attention only if they continue or are bothersome
Incidence more frequent
*Constipation*—about 10%; *dizziness*—about 16% with oral use; *drowsiness*—about 33% with oral use; *dryness of mouth*—about 40% with oral use; *unusual tiredness or weakness*—about 10%

Incidence less frequent—1 to 5%
*Anorexia* (loss of appetite); *darkening of skin*—with transdermal systems only; *decreased sexual ability; dry, itching, or burning eyes; orthostatic hypotension* (dizziness, lightheadedness, or fainting, especially when getting up from a lying or sitting position); *nausea or vomiting; nervousness*

### Those indicating possible rebound hypertension and need for medical attention if they occur after medication is abruptly discontinued
*Angina* (chest pain); *anxiety or tenseness; headache; increased salivation; nausea; nervousness; palpitations* (pounding heartbeat); *restlessness; shaking or trembling of hands and fingers; stomach cramps; sweating; tachycardia* (fast heartbeat); *trouble in sleeping; vomiting*

Note: *Rebound hypertension* may occur but is symptomatic in only 5 to 20% of patients. It is more likely to occur after abrupt withdrawal of clonidine in patients who had been receiving doses exceeding 1.2 mg per day or if clonidine therapy is discontinued before or at the same time as concurrent beta-adrenergic blocking agent therapy.

## Overdose
For more information on the management of overdose or unintentional ingestion, **contact a Poison Control Center** (see *Poison Control Center Listing*).

### Clinical effects of overdose
The following effects have been selected on the basis of their potential clinical significance (possible signs and symptoms in parentheses where appropriate)—not necessarily inclusive:
*Apnea or respiratory depression* (difficulty in breathing); *bradycardia* (slow heartbeat); *hypotension* (dizziness or faintness); *hypothermia* (feeling cold); *lethargy* (unusual tiredness or weakness, extreme); *miosis* (pinpoint pupils of eyes)

Note: Overdose may result in hypertension, especially in pediatric patients.
Toxicity may occur with ingestion of 100 mcg (0.1 mg) in children.

### Treatment of overdose
Specific treatment—
Recommended treatment for clonidine overdose is usually symptomatic and supportive and may include use of intravenous fluids.
For significant bradycardia: Atropine.
For hypotension: Dopamine infusion.
For hypertension: Intravenous furosemide, diazoxide, phentolamine, or nitroprusside.
Tolazoline infusion if necessary.

## Patient Consultation
As an aid to patient consultation, refer to *Advice for the Patient, Clonidine (Systemic)*.
In providing consultation, consider emphasizing the following selected information (» = major clinical significance):

### Before using this medication
» Conditions affecting use, especially:
Sensitivity to clonidine or to ophthalmic apraclonidine
Pregnancy—Increased resorptions in rats and mice
Breast-feeding—Distributed into breast milk
Use in children—Caution recommended in children because accidental overdoses have been reported
Use in the elderly—Hypotensive effects may be more likely
Other medications, especially tricyclic antidepressants or beta-adrenergic blocking agents

### Proper use of this medication
Proper administration of the transdermal dosage form:
» Compliance with therapy; reading patient instructions carefully
Not trimming or cutting patch
Applying to clean, dry skin area on upper arm or torso; area should be free of hair, scars, cuts, or irritation
Should remain in place even during showering, bathing, or swimming; applying adhesive overlay to loose systems; replacing systems that have loosened excessively or fallen off
Alternating application sites
Folding used patches in half with adhesive sides together; disposing of patch carefully, out of reach of children
Taking or applying medication at the same time(s) each day or week to maintain the therapeutic effect
» Proper dosing
Missed dose: Taking or using as soon as possible; checking with physician if miss two or more oral doses in a row or if are late in changing the transdermal system by 3 or more days; possible severe reaction if stopped abruptly
» Proper storage

*For use as an antihypertensive*
Possible need for control of weight and diet, especially sodium intake
» Patient may not experience symptoms of hypertension; importance of taking medication even if feeling well
» Does not cure, but helps control hypertension; possible need for lifelong therapy; serious consequences of untreated hypertension

### Precautions while using this medication
Regular visits to physician to check progress
» Checking with physician before discontinuing medication; gradual dosage reduction may be necessary to avoid serious rebound hypertension
» Having enough medication on hand to get through weekends, holidays, and vacations; possibly carrying second prescription for emergency use

- » Caution in taking alcohol or other CNS depressants
- » Caution when driving or doing things requiring alertness, because of possible drowsiness
- » Caution if any kind of surgery or emergency treatment is required
  Caution when getting up suddenly from a lying or sitting position
  Caution in using alcohol, while standing for long periods or exercising, and during hot weather, because of enhanced orthostatic hypotensive effects
  Possible dryness of mouth; using sugarless candy or gum, ice, or saliva substitute for relief; checking with physician or dentist if dry mouth continues for more than 2 weeks

*For use as an antihypertensive*
- » Not taking other medications, especially nonprescription sympathomimetics, unless discussed with physician

### Side/adverse effects
Signs of potential side effects, especially itching or redness of skin (transdermal), mental depression, sodium and water retention, edema, Raynaud's phenomenon, vivid dreams or nightmares, and withdrawal reaction

## General Dosing Information

With continued use, apparent tolerance to the antihypertensive effects of clonidine may develop as a result of fluid retention and expanded plasma volume. Concurrent administration of a diuretic may decrease this likelihood and will enhance the antihypertensive effects of clonidine. Other antihypertensives have also been used concurrently with clonidine. If combination therapy is indicated, individual titration is required to ensure the lowest possible therapeutic dose of each drug.

The abrupt interruption of clonidine therapy, including several consecutive missed doses, may result in rebound hypertension, which may be severe (acute post-treatment syndrome), or, in rare cases, overshoot hypertension, occurring within 12 to 48 hours of discontinuing therapy and lasting several days. Some patients may experience associated symptoms such as nervousness, agitation, and headache. At cessation of therapy, dosage should be gradually reduced (in the case of the transdermal system, by reducing patch strength and, if necessary, administering oral clonidine) over a 2- to 4-day period. Alternative therapy should be considered for unreliable or noncompliant patients. An excessive rise in blood pressure may be treated by resumption of oral clonidine therapy or by intravenous administration of diazoxide or an alpha-adrenergic blocking agent.

It is recommended that this medication be discontinued if mental depression occurs.

### For oral dosage form only
It is recommended that the last daily dose be taken at bedtime to ensure overnight control of blood pressure and reduce daytime drowsiness.

If clonidine therapy must be interrupted for surgery, it is recommended that the last dose be given no later than 4 to 6 hours prior to surgery, that parenteral hypotensive medication be administered throughout the procedure, and that clonidine therapy be reinstituted as soon as possible afterwards.

Clonidine has been used investigationally for rapid detoxification in the treatment of opioid withdrawal. One protocol used consists of a test dose of 5 to 6 mcg (0.005 to 0.006 mg) of clonidine hydrochloride per kg of body weight on the first day. Patients showing a positive response then receive 17 mcg (0.017 mg) of clonidine hydrochloride per kg of body weight in divided daily doses for 9 or 10 days (adjusted to avoid hypotension and oversedation), followed by a reduction to 50% of the dose on Days 11, 12, and 13, and no medication on Day 14. Dosage must be individualized according to each patient's tolerance.

### For transdermal dosage form only
Because the onset of action of transdermal clonidine is 2 to 3 days, when a patient is being switched from oral to transdermal therapy, the dose of oral clonidine should be gradually reduced over 2 to 3 days after transdermal therapy is begun, to avoid a withdrawal reaction.

Application should preferably be made at the same time of day each week to areas of clean, dry, hairless skin on the upper arm or torso. Skin areas with extensive scarring, calluses, or irritation should be avoided. Application sites should be alternated to avoid causing skin irritation.

The transdermal units *should not* be cut or trimmed in an attempt to adjust dosage.

If the transdermal system begins to loosen, the adhesive overlay provided by the manufacturer should be applied over the unit to hold it in place. A new dosage unit should be applied if the first becomes overly loosened or falls off.

If local skin irritation occurs before the system has been in place for 7 days, the system may be removed and a new one placed on a different site. If contact sensitization persists, withdrawal of transdermal therapy may be necessary.

## Oral Dosage Forms

Note: Bracketed uses in the *Dosage Forms* section refer to categories of use and/or indications that are not included in U.S. product labeling.

### CLONIDINE HYDROCHLORIDE TABLETS USP

**Usual adult dose**
Antihypertensive—
  Initial: Oral, 100 mcg (0.1 mg) two times a day, the dosage being increased by 100 or 200 mcg (0.1 or 0.2 mg, respectively) per day every two to four days if necessary for control of blood pressure.
  Maintenance: Oral, 200 to 600 mcg (0.2 to 0.6 mg) per day, in divided doses.
  Severe hypertension in the urgent but not emergency situation (loading dose): Oral, 200 mcg (0.2 mg), followed by 100 mcg (0.1 mg) every hour until diastolic blood pressure is controlled or a total of 800 mcg (0.8 mg) has been given; the patient is then controlled on a normal maintenance dose.
[Vascular headache prophylactic][1]—
  Oral, 25 mcg (0.025 mg) two to four times a day up to 50 mcg (0.05 mg) three times a day.
[Antidysmenorrheal][1]—
  Severe dysmenorrhea: Oral, 25 mcg (0.025 mg) two times a day for fourteen days before and during menses.
[Menopausal syndrome therapy adjunct]—
  Oral, 25 to 75 mcg (0.025 to 0.075 mg) two times a day.
Note: Geriatric patients may be more sensitive to the effects of the usual adult dose.

**Usual adult prescribing limits**
Antihypertensive—2.4 mg daily.

**Usual pediatric dose**
Safety and efficacy have not been established.

**Strength(s) usually available**
U.S.—
  100 mcg (0.1 mg) (Rx) [*Catapres* (scored; lactose) [GENERIC (may be scored; may contain lactose)].
  200 mcg (0.2 mg) (Rx) [*Catapres* (scored; lactose) [GENERIC (may be scored; may contain lactose)].
  300 mcg (0.3 mg) (Rx) [*Catapres* (scored; lactose) [GENERIC (may be scored; may contain lactose)].
Note: Not commercially available in 25-mcg (0.025-mg) strength used for indications other than hypertension; extemporaneous compounding required.
Canada—
  25 mcg (0.025 mg) (Rx) [*Dixarit* (lactose)].
  100 mcg (0.1 mg) (Rx) [*Catapres* (scored)].
  200 mcg (0.2 mg) (Rx) [*Catapres* (scored)].
Note: 100 mcg of the hydrochloride salt is equivalent to 87 mcg of the free base.

**Packaging and storage**
Store below 40 °C (104 °F), preferably between 15 and 30 °C (59 and 86 °F), unless otherwise specified by manufacturer. Store in a well-closed container.

**Auxiliary labeling**
- Avoid alcoholic beverages.
- Do not miss doses.
- Do not take other medicines without your doctor's advice.

**Note**
Check refill frequency to determine compliance in hypertensive patients.

## Topical Dosage Forms

### CLONIDINE TRANSDERMAL SYSTEM

**Usual adult dose**
Antihypertensive—
  Topical, to the intact skin, 1 transdermal dosage system, beginning with the system delivering 100 mcg (0.1 mg) per day, once a week. Dosage adjustments may be made every one or two weeks by changing to the next larger dosage system or a combination of systems.

**Usual pediatric dose**
Dosage has not been established.

**Strength(s) usually available**
U.S.—
  2.5 mg (delivering 100 mcg [0.1 mg] per day) (Rx) [*Catapres-TTS*].
  5.0 mg (delivering 200 mcg [0.2 mg] per day) (Rx) [*Catapres-TTS*].
  7.5 mg (delivering 300 mcg [0.3 mg] per day) (Rx) [*Catapres-TTS*].

Note: All systems are designed to release a constant, controlled dose of clonidine. The actual dose delivered will be as labeled and as intended, but less than the total content of each system.

Canada—
Not commercially available.

**Packaging and storage**
Store below 30 °C (86 °F), unless otherwise specified by manufacturer.

**Auxiliary labeling**
- Avoid alcoholic beverages.
- For external use only.
- Do not miss doses.
- Do not take other medicines without your doctor's advice.

**Note**
Include patient instructions when dispensing.
Check refill frequency to determine compliance in hypertensive patients.

[1]Not included in Canadian product labeling.

**Selected Bibliography**
Transdermal clonidine for hypertension. Med Lett Drugs Ther 1985 Nov 8; 27: 95-6.
The fifth report of the Joint National Committee on Detection, Evaluation, and Treatment of High Blood Pressure (JNC V). Arch Intern Med 1993; 153(2): 154-83.

Revised: 05/17/93
Interim revision: 08/13/98

# CLONIDINE AND CHLORTHALIDONE Systemic

VA CLASSIFICATION (Primary): CV401

**NOTE:** The *Clonidine and Chlorthalidone (Systemic)* monograph is maintained on the USP DI electronic data base. For a printed copy of the most recent revision of the complete monograph, contact Micromedex, Inc. - Reprint Requests, 6200 S. Syracuse Way, Suite 300, Englewood, CO 80111; telephone (303) 486-6400; telefax (303) 486-6464; Email: USPDI@MDX.COM.

For information on the specific components of this combination, see the *USP DI* monographs for *Clonidine (Systemic)* and *Diuretics, Thiazide (Systemic)*.

The information that follows is selectively abstracted from the complete monograph and is provided to facilitate drug use review and patient counseling.

Note: For a listing of dosage forms and brand names by country availability, see *Dosage Forms* section(s).

## Category
Antihypertensive.

## Indications

**Accepted**
Hypertension (treatment)—The combination of clonidine and chlorthalidone is indicated for treatment of hypertension.

Fixed-dosage combinations are generally not recommended for initial therapy and are useful for subsequent therapy only when the proportion of the component agents corresponds to the dose of the individual agents, as determined by titration.

## Patient Consultation
As an aid to patient consultation, refer to *Advice for the Patient, Clonidine and Chlorthalidone (Systemic)*.
In providing consultation, consider emphasizing the following selected information (» = major clinical significance):

**Before using this medication**
» Conditions affecting use, especially:
   Sensitivity to clonidine or to ophthalmic apraclonidine, or to sulfonamide-type medications
   Pregnancy—Chlorthalidone: Risk of jaundice, thrombocytopenia, hypokalemia in infant
   Breast-feeding—Distributed into breast milk; may suppress lactation
   Use in children—Caution recommended in children because accidental overdoses have been reported
   Use in the elderly—Hypotensive and hypokalemic effects may be more likely
   Other medications, especially tricyclic antidepressants, beta-adrenergic blocking agents, cholestyramine, colestipol, digitalis glycosides, or lithium
   Other medical problems, especially severe renal function impairment

**Proper use of this medication**
Diuretic effects of the medication and timing of doses to minimize inconvenience of diuresis
Possible need for control of weight and diet, especially sodium intake
» Patient may not experience symptoms of hypertension; importance of taking medication even if feeling well

» Does not cure, but helps control hypertension; possible need for lifelong therapy; serious consequences of untreated hypertension
Compliance with therapy; taking medication at the same time each day to maintain the therapeutic effect
» Proper dosing
Missed dose: Taking as soon as remembered; checking with physician if two or more doses in a row are missed
» Proper storage

**Precautions while using this medication**
Making regular visits to physician to check progress
» Checking with physician before discontinuing medication; gradual dosage reduction may be necessary to avoid serious rebound hypertension
» Having enough medication on hand to get through weekends, holidays, and vacations; possibly carrying second prescription for emergency use
» Caution if any kind of surgery or emergency treatment is required
» Not taking other medications, especially nonprescription sympathomimetics, unless discussed with physician
» Caution in taking alcohol or other central nervous system (CNS) depressants
» Caution when driving or doing things requiring alertness, because of possible drowsiness
Caution when getting up suddenly from a lying or sitting position
Caution in using alcohol, while standing for long periods or exercising, and during hot weather because of enhanced orthostatic hypotensive effects
» Possibility of hypokalemia; possible need for additional potassium in diet; not changing diet without first checking with physician
To prevent dehydration, checking with physician if severe nausea, vomiting, or diarrhea occurs and continues
Diabetics: May increase blood sugar levels
Possible photosensitivity; avoiding unprotected exposure to sun; using protective clothing and sun block product; avoiding use of sunlamp, tanning bed, or tanning booth
Possible dryness of mouth; using sugarless candy or gum, ice, or saliva substitute for relief; checking with physician or dentist if dry mouth continues for more than 2 weeks

**Side/adverse effects**
Signs of potential side effects, especially electrolyte imbalance, mental depression, sodium and water retention or edema, agranulocytosis, allergic reaction, cholecystitis or pancreatitis, hyperuricemia or gout, hepatic function impairment, Raynaud's phenomenon, thrombocytopenia, and vivid dreams or nightmares

## Oral Dosage Forms

### CLONIDINE HYDROCHLORIDE AND CHLORTHALIDONE TABLETS USP

**Usual adult dose**
Oral, 1 or 2 tablets two to four times a day, as determined by individual titration with the component agents.

Note: Geriatric patients may be more sensitive to the effects of the usual adult dose.

**Usual adult prescribing limits**
2.4 mg of clonidine hydrochloride daily.

**Usual pediatric dose**
Dosage has not been established.

**Strength(s) usually available**
U.S.—
 100 mcg (0.1 mg) clonidine hydrochloride and 15 mg chlorthalidone (Rx) [*Combipres* (scored; lactose); GENERIC].
 200 mcg (0.2 mg) clonidine hydrochloride and 15 mg chlorthalidone (Rx) [*Combipres* (scored; lactose); GENERIC].
 300 mcg (0.3 mg) clonidine hydrochloride and 15 mg chlorthalidone (Rx) [*Combipres* (scored; lactose); GENERIC].
Canada—
 100 mcg (0.1 mg) clonidine hydrochloride and 15 mg chlorthalidone (Rx) [*Combipres* (scored)].

Note: 100 mcg of clonidine hydrochloride is equivalent to 87 mcg of the free base.

**Auxiliary labeling**
• Avoid alcoholic beverages.
• Do not miss doses.
• Do not take other medicines without your doctor's advice.

Revised: 08/02/94
Interim revision: 08/13/98

# CLOPIDOGREL  Systemic—INTRODUCTORY VERSION

VA CLASSIFICATION (Primary): BL117
Commonly used brand name(s): *Plavix*.
Note: For a listing of dosage forms and brand names by country availability, see *Dosage Forms* section(s).

## Category
Antithrombotic; platelet aggregation inhibitor.

## Indications
**Accepted**
Myocardial infarction (prophylaxis) or
Stroke, thromboembolic (prophylaxis) or
Vascular death (prophylaxis)—Clopidogrel is indicated for reducing the risk of atherosclerotic events (myocardial infarction, stroke, and vascular death) in patients with atherosclerosis documented by recent myocardial infarction, recent stroke, or established peripheral arterial disease.

## Pharmacology/Pharmacokinetics
**Physicochemical characteristics**
Molecular weight—419.9.
Solubility—Practically insoluble in water at neutral pH, but freely soluble at pH 1; freely soluble in methanol, sparingly soluble in methylene chloride, and practically insoluble in ethyl ether.

**Mechanism of action/Effect**
Clopidogrel is an inhibitor of platelet aggregation; doses of 75 mg per day inhibit platelet aggregation by 40 to 60% at steady state, which occurs within 3 to 7 days.
Clopidogrel inhibits adenosine diphosphate (ADP) binding to its platelet receptor and subsequent ADP-mediated activation of the glycoprotein GPIIb/IIIa complex, thus inhibiting platelet aggregation. Because clopidogrel irreversibly modifies the ADP receptor, platelets are affected for the remainder of their lifespan. An active metabolite, not yet isolated, is responsible for the medication's activity. Platelet aggregation induced by agonists other than ADP is also inhibited by blocking the amplification of platelet activation by released ADP. Clopidogrel does not inhibit phosphodiesterase activity.

**Absorption**
Rapid, at least 50%. Bioavailability has not been found to be affected by food.

**Protein binding**
Very high, for clopidogrel and its main circulating metabolite (98% and 94%, respectively). Binding is nonsaturable *in vitro* up to a concentration of 100 micrograms per mL.

**Biotransformation**
Hepatic, extensive and rapid, by hydrolysis to the main circulating metabolite, a carboxylic acid derivative, which accounts for approximately 85% of the circulating drug-related compounds. A glucuronic acid derivative of the carboxylic acid derivative has also been found in plasma and urine. Neither the parent compound nor the carboxylic acid derivative has a platelet inhibiting effect.

**Half-life**
Elimination—
 Carboxylic acid derivative: 8 hours (after single and multiple doses).
Note: Covalent binding to platelets has accounted for 2% of radiolabeled clopidogrel with a half-life of 11 days.

**Onset of action**
Dose-dependent inhibition of platelet aggregation:
 After a single oral dose: 2 hours.
 After repeated doses of 75 mg: On the first day.

**Time to peak concentration**
Plasma—Approximately 1 hour for the carboxylic acid derivative.

**Peak plasma concentration**
Approximately 3 mg per liter (carboxylic acid derivative) after repeated doses of 75 mg. Pharmacokinetics of the main circulating metabolite are linear (increased in proportion to dose) in a dose range of 50 to 150 mg.

**Time to peak effect**
Steady-state inhibition of platelet aggregation with repeated doses of 75 mg per day usually occurs between day 3 and day 7.

**Duration of action**
Platelet aggregation and bleeding time gradually return to baseline levels within about 5 days after treatment is withdrawn.

**Elimination**
Renal, approximately 50%, five days after dosing with radiolabeled clopidogrel.
Fecal, approximately 46%, five days after dosing with radiolabeled clopidogrel

**Pharmacogenetics**
No significant differences in clopidogrel pharmacokinetics or pharmacodynamics were observed between male and female subjects.
Pharmacokinetic differences in different race populations have not been studied.

## Precautions to Consider
**Tumorigenicity**
Studies in mice and rats for 78 and 104 weeks, respectively, at doses of up to 77 mg per kg of body weight (mg/kg) per day (producing plasma exposures more than 25 times those in humans at the recommended daily dose of 75 mg) found no evidence of tumorigenicity.

**Mutagenicity**
Clopidogrel was not found to be genotoxic in four *in vitro* tests (Ames test, DNA-repair test in rat hepatocytes, gene mutation assay in Chinese hamster fibroblasts, and metaphase chromosome analysis of human lymphocytes) or in one *in vivo* test (micronucleus test by oral route in mice).

**Pregnancy/Reproduction**
Fertility—Studies in rats and rabbits at doses of up to 500 and 300 mg/kg per day (65 and 78 times the recommended daily human dose on a mg per square meter of body surface area [mg/m$^2$] basis), respectively, found no evidence of impaired fertility. Studies in male and female rats at oral doses of up to 400 mg/kg per day (52 times the recommended human dose on a mg/m$^2$ basis) also found no evidence of impaired fertility.

Pregnancy—Adequate and well-controlled studies in humans have not been done.
Studies in rats and rabbits at doses of up to 500 and 300 mg/kg per day (65 and 78 times the recommended daily human dose on a mg/m$^2$ basis), respectively, found no evidence of fetotoxicity.
Consideration of risk-benefit is recommended before using clopidogrel during pregnancy.

FDA Pregnancy Category B.

### Breast-feeding
It is not known whether clopidogrel is distributed into human breast milk. Clopidogrel and/or its metabolites are distributed into the milk of lactating rats. Consideration of risk-benefit is recommended in making decisions about using clopidogrel in breast-feeding women or continuing breast-feeding in women taking clopidogrel.

### Pediatrics
Appropriate studies on the relationship of age to the effects of clopidogrel have not been performed in the pediatric population. Safety and efficacy have not been established.

### Geriatrics
Plasma concentrations of the main circulating metabolite have been found to be significantly higher in elderly individuals ($\geq$ 75 years of age) than in young healthy volunteers, but these higher concentrations have not been found to be associated with differences in platelet aggregation and bleeding time. No dosage adjustment is recommended for elderly patients.

### Dental
Because of the risk of increased surgical blood loss, it is recommended that clopidogrel be discontinued 7 days prior to elective dental surgery if an antiplatelet effect is not desired.

### Surgical
Because of the risk of increased surgical blood loss, it is recommended that clopidogrel be discontinued 7 days prior to elective surgery if an antiplatelet effect is not desired.

### Drug interactions and/or related problems
The following drug interactions and/or related problems have been selected on the basis of their potential clinical significance (possible mechanism in parentheses where appropriate)—not necessarily inclusive ($\gg$ = major clinical significance):

$\gg$ Aspirin or
$\gg$ Nonsteroidal anti-inflammatory drugs (NSAIDs)
(concurrent use of clopidogrel with these agents may increase the risk of gastrointestinal bleeding)
(aspirin has not been found to modify the clopidogrel-mediated inhibiton of ADP-induced platelet aggregation, nor has it been found to increase the prolongation of bleeding time induced by clopidogrel; however, clopidogrel potentiated the effect of aspirin on collagen-induced platelet aggregation)

Fluvastatin or
Nonsteroidal anti-inflammatory drugs (NSAIDs) or
Phenytoin or
Tamoxifen or
Tolbutamide or
Torsemide or
Warfarin
(because clopidogrel inhibits hepatic cytochrome P450 enzyme activity at high concentrations *in vitro*, a possibility exists that it could interfere with the metabolism of these medications; caution is recommended)

Heparin or
Warfarin
(safety of concurrent use has not been established; caution is recommended)

### Laboratory value alterations
The following have been selected on the basis of their potential clinical significance (possible effect in parentheses where appropriate)—not necessarily inclusive ($\gg$ = major clinical significance):

With physiology/laboratory test values
Bilirubin, serum concentrations and
Hepatic enzymes, serum values
(may be increased)
Cholesterol, total
(serum concentrations may be increased)
Neutrophil count and
Platelet count
(may be decreased)
Nonprotein nitrogen (NPN)
(serum concentrations may be increased)
Uric acid
(serum concentrations may be increased)

### Medical considerations/Contraindications
The medical considerations/contraindications included have been selected on the basis of their potential clinical significance (reasons given in parentheses where appropriate)—not necessarily inclusive ($\gg$ = major clinical significance).

*Except under special circumstances, this medication should not be used when the following medical problems exist:*
$\gg$ Bleeding, active, such as:
  Intracranial hemorrhage
  Peptic ulcer
    (risk of severe bleeding)

*Risk-benefit should be considered when the following medical problems exist:*
$\gg$ Any condition in which there is a significant risk of bleeding, such as:
  Gastrointestinal ulceration
  Surgery
  Trauma
Hepatic function impairment
  (caution is recommended; experience is limited in patients with severe hepatic function impairment, who may have bleeding diatheses)
Sensitivity to clopidogrel

## Side/Adverse Effects
The following side/adverse effects have been selected on the basis of their potential clinical significance (possible signs and symptoms in parentheses where appropriate)—not necessarily inclusive:

### Those indicating need for medical attention
Incidence more frequent ($\geq$ 5%)
*Chest pain*—incidence 8.3%; *pain, generalized*—incidence 6.4%; *purpura* (red or purple spots on skin, varying in size from pinpoint to large bruises)—incidence 5.3%; *upper respiratory infection* (cough; runny nose; sneezing; sore throat)—incidence 8.7%

Incidence less frequent (1 to < 5%)
*Atrial fibrillation; or palpitations* (irregular heartbeat); *bronchitis* (cough; shortness of breath)—incidence 3.7%; *dyspnea* (shortness of breath)—incidence 4.5%; *edema* (swelling of feet or lower legs)—incidence 4.1%; *epistaxis* (nosebleed)—incidence 2.9%; *gastrointestinal hemorrhage* (vomiting of blood or material that looks like coffee grounds)—incidence 2%; *gout* (joint pain); *hypertension*—incidence 4.3%; *syncope* (fainting); *urinary tract infection* (frequent urination; painful or difficult urination)

Note: Incidence of *gastrointestinal hemorrhage* is increased in patients receiving aspirin. Approximately 0.7% of patients receiving clopidogrel have experienced gastrointestinal hemorrhage severe enough to require hospitalization.

Incidence rare (< 1%)
*Intracranial hemorrhage* (headache, sudden severe; weakness, sudden)—incidence 0.4%; *neutropenia, including agranulocytosis* (fever, chills, sore throat, other signs of infection; ulcers, sores, or white spots in mouth); *peptic, gastric, or duodenal ulcer* (stomach pain, severe)—incidence 0.7%; *skin reactions, severe* (blistering, flaking, or peeling of skin)—incidence 0.7%; *thrombocytopenia* (unusual bleeding or bruising; black, tarry stools; blood in urine or stools; pinpoint red spots on skin)—usually asymptomatic

### Those indicating need for medical attention only if they continue or are bothersome
Incidence more frequent ($\geq$ 5%)
*Abdominal or stomach pain*—incidence 5.6%; *arthralgia* (joint pain)—incidence 6.3%; *back pain*—incidence 5.8%; *dizziness*—incidence 6.2%; *dyspepsia* (heartburn)—incidence 5.2%; *flu-like symptoms* (aching muscles; fever and chills; general feeling of discomfort or illness; headache)—incidence 7.5%; *headache*—incidence 7.6%

Incidence less frequent (< 5%)
*Anxiety; asthenia* (weakness); *constipation; cough*—incidence 3.1%; *diarrhea*—incidence 4.5%; *fatigue* (unusual tiredness)—incidence 3.3%; *hypoesthesia or paresthesia* (numbness or tingling); *insomnia* (trouble in sleeping); *itching*—incidence 3.3%; *leg cramps; mental depression*—incidence 3.6%; *nausea*—incidence 3.4%; *rhinitis* (runny nose)—incidence 4.2%; *skin rash*—incidence 4.2%; *vomiting*

## Overdose
For more information on the management of overdose or unintentional ingestion, **contact a Poison Control Center** (see *Poison Control Center Listing*).

### Clinical effects of overdose
No adverse effects have been reported after ingestion of up to fourteen 75-mg tablets; bleeding time after six 75-mg tablets was prolonged by about the same amount as with the usual therapeutic dose of one 75-mg tablet.

The lethal single oral dose in mice and rats was 1500 or 2000 mg per kg of body weight (mg/kg) and in baboons was 3000 mg/kg. Symptoms of acute toxicity included vomiting (in baboons), prostration, difficult breathing, and gastrointestinal hemorrhage in all species.

**Treatment of overdose**
If quick reversal of pharmacologic effects is required, platelet transfusions may be useful.

## Patient Consultation
In providing consultation, consider emphasizing the following selected information (» = major clinical significance):

**Before using this medication**
» Conditions affecting use, especially:
   Sensitivity to clopidogrel
   Dental—Risk of increased blood loss during dental procedures
   Surgical—Risk of increased blood loss during surgical procedures
   Other medications, especially aspirin or nonsteroidal anti-inflammatory drugs (NSAIDs)
   Other medical problems, especially bleeding, including bleeding from a stomach ulcer

**Proper use of this medication**
Compliance with prescribed treatment regimen
» Proper dosing
   Missed dose: Taking as soon as possible; not taking if almost time for next dose; not doubling doses
» Proper storage

**Precautions while using this medication**
» Need to inform all health care providers of use of medicine
» Caution if any kind of surgery (including dental surgery) is required
» Notifying physician immediately if signs and symptoms of bleeding occur

**Side/adverse effects**
Signs of potential side effects, especially chest pain, generalized pain, purpura, upper respiratory infection, atrial fibrillation or palpitations, bronchitis, edema, epistaxis, gastrointestinal hemorrhage, gout, hypertension, syncope, urinary tract infection, intracranial hemorrhage, neutropenia, agranulocytosis, gastrointestinal ulcers, severe skin reactions, thrombocytopenia

## General Dosing Information
It is recommended that clopidogrel be discontinued 7 days prior to elective surgery because of the risk of increased blood loss.

**Diet/Nutrition**
Clopidogrel tablets may be taken with or without food.

## Oral Dosage Forms

### CLOPIDOGREL BISULFATE TABLETS
Note: Strength and dosage are expressed in terms of base.

**Usual adult dose**
Antithrombotic—
   Oral, 75 mg (base) once a day.

**Usual pediatric dose**
Safety and efficacy have not been established.

**Usual geriatric dose**
See *Usual adult dose.*

**Strength(s) usually available**
U.S.—
   75 mg (base) (Rx) [*Plavix* (lactose)].

**Packaging and storage**
Store between 15 and 30 °C (59 and 86 °F), preferably at 25 °C (77 °F).

Developed: 05/22/98

---

**CLORAZEPATE**—See *Benzodiazepines (Systemic)*

---

**CLOTRIMAZOLE**—See *Antifungals, Azole (Vaginal); Clotrimazole (Oral-Local); Clotrimazole (Topical)*

---

# CLOTRIMAZOLE   Oral-Local †

VA CLASSIFICATION (Primary): AM700
Commonly used brand name(s): *Mycelex Troches.*
Note: For a listing of dosage forms and brand names by country availability, see *Dosage Forms* section(s).

†Not commercially available in Canada.

## Category
Antifungal (oral-local).
Note: Clotrimazole is a broad-spectrum antifungal.

## Indications

**Accepted**
Candidiasis, oropharyngeal (treatment)—Oral clotrimazole is indicated as a primary agent in nonimmunosuppressed and immunosuppressed patients in the local treatment of oropharyngeal candidiasis (thrush) caused by *Candida* species.

Candidiasis, oropharyngeal (prophylaxis)—Oral clotrimazole is indicated as a primary agent in immunosuppressed patients in the local prophylaxis of oropharyngeal candidiasis caused by *Candida* species.

Not all species or strains of a particular organism may be susceptible to clotrimazole.

**Unaccepted**
Clotrimazole lozenges are not indicated in the treatment of systemic mycoses.

## Pharmacology/Pharmacokinetics

**Physicochemical characteristics**
Molecular weight—344.84.

**Mechanism of action/Effect**
Fungistatic; may be fungicidal, depending on concentration; inhibits biosynthesis of ergosterol or other sterols, damaging the fungal cell wall membrane and altering its permeability; as a result, loss of essential intracellular elements may occur; also inhibits biosynthesis of triglycerides and phospholipids by fungi; in addition, inhibits oxidative and peroxidative enzyme activity, resulting in intracellular buildup of toxic concentrations of hydrogen peroxide, which may contribute to deterioration of subcellular organelles and cellular necrosis. In *Candida albicans,* inhibits transformation of blastospores into invasive mycelial form.

**Other actions/effects**
Also has some antibacterial activity.

**Absorption**
Poorly and erratically absorbed, even when swallowed.

**Binding**
Apparently bound to oral mucosa from which it is slowly released.

**Biotransformation**
When swallowed, absorbed clotrimazole is metabolized in the liver to inactive compounds; induces hepatic microsomal enzyme activity, resulting in acceleration of its own catabolism.

**Saliva concentration**
Sufficient to inhibit most species of *Candida* present in saliva (5.2 to 15 mcg per mL after dissolution of troche).

**Duration of action**
Up to 3 hours.

**Elimination**
Fecal.

## Precautions to Consider

**Carcinogenicity**
An 18-month study in rats has not shown any carcinogenic effects.

**Pregnancy/Reproduction**
Pregnancy—Adequate and well-controlled studies in humans have not been done.
Studies in rats and mice, given doses 100 times the usual adult human dose (in mg per kg), have shown that clotrimazole is embryotoxic. In addition, clotrimazole, given orally to mice in doses 120 times the usual human dose, has been shown to cause impairment of mating, decreased number of viable young, and decreased survival to weaning. No effects were seen at doses 60 times the usual human dose. When given to rats at doses 50 times the usual human dose, clotrimazole caused a slight decrease in the number of pups per litter and decreased pup viability.

However, no teratogenic effects were seen in mice, rabbits, or rats given doses up to 200, 180, and 100 times the usual human dose, respectively.

FDA Pregnancy Category C.

**Breast-feeding**
It is not known whether clotrimazole is excreted in breast milk; however, clotrimazole is poorly and erratically absorbed, even when swallowed.

**Pediatrics**
Use of clotrimazole troches is not recommended in infants and children up to 5 years of age since this age group may not be capable of using the lozenge safely. No pediatrics-specific problems have been documented to date in children over 5 years old.

**Geriatrics**
Appropriate studies on the relationship of age to the effects of clotrimazole have not been performed in the geriatric population. However, no geriatrics-specific problems have been documented to date.

**Laboratory value alterations**
The following have been selected on the basis of their potential clinical significance (possible effect in parentheses where appropriate)—not necessarily inclusive (» = major clinical significance):

With physiology/laboratory test values
  Aspartate aminotransferase (AST [SGOT]), serum
    (concentration may be minimally increased in up to 15% of patients)

**Medical considerations/Contraindications**
The medical considerations/contraindications included have been selected on the basis of their potential clinical significance (reasons given in parentheses where appropriate)—not necessarily inclusive (» = major clinical significance).

*Risk-benefit should be considered when the following medical problem exists:*
  Hypersensitivity to clotrimazole

## Side/Adverse Effects
The following side/adverse effects have been selected on the basis of their potential clinical significance (possible signs and symptoms in parentheses where appropriate)—not necessarily inclusive:

**Those indicating need for medical attention only if they continue or are bothersome**
Incidence more frequent—when swallowed
  *Gastrointestinal disturbance* (abdominal or stomach cramping or pain; diarrhea; nausea or vomiting)

## Patient Consultation
As an aid to patient consultation, refer to *Advice for the Patient, Clotrimazole (Oral)*.
In providing consultation, consider emphasizing the following selected information (» = major clinical significance):

**Before using this medication**
» Conditions affecting use, especially:
  Hypersensitivity to clotrimazole
  Use in children—Use is not recommended in children up to 5 years of age

**Proper use of this medication**
  Proper administration technique:
    Holding lozenge in mouth and allowing it to dissolve slowly and completely
    Swallowing saliva during this time
» Not chewing or swallowing lozenge whole
» Not giving to infants or children under 4 to 5 years of age
» Compliance with full course of therapy; fungal infections may require prolonged therapy
» Proper dosing
  Missed dose: Using as soon as possible; not using if almost time for next dose
» Proper storage

**Precautions while using this medication**
  Checking with physician if no improvement within 1 week

## General Dosing Information
To provide prolonged oral contact with the medication and to achieve maximum effect, clotrimazole lozenges should be held in the mouth and allowed to dissolve slowly (and completely) over a 15- to 30-minute period. Saliva should be swallowed during this time. Clotrimazole lozenges should not be chewed or swallowed whole.

Since only limited data are available on the safety and efficacy of clotrimazole lozenges during prolonged administration, short-term administration is recommended whenever possible. However, clotrimazole lozenges have been used daily for approximately 3 months in renal transplant patients without apparent ill effects.

## Oral Dosage Forms

### CLOTRIMAZOLE LOZENGES

**Usual adult and adolescent dose**
Antifungal—
  Treatment: Oral, as a lozenge dissolved slowly and completely in the mouth, 10 mg five times a day for fourteen days or longer, especially in immunosuppressed patients.
  Prophylaxis: Oral, as a lozenge dissolved slowly and completely in the mouth, 10 mg three times a day in immunosuppressed patients.

**Usual pediatric dose**
Antifungal—
  Infants and children up to 5 years of age: Use is not recommended in infants and children up to 5 years of age since this age group may not be capable of using the lozenge safely.
  Children 5 years of age and over: See *Usual adult and adolescent dose*.

**Strength(s) usually available**
U.S.—
  10 mg (Rx) [*Mycelex Troches*].
Canada—
  Not commercially available.

**Packaging and storage**
Store below 30 °C (86 °F), in a tight container, unless otherwise specified by manufacturer.

**Auxiliary labeling**
• Dissolve slowly in mouth.
• Continue medicine for full time of treatment.

Revised: 02/23/93

---

# CLOTRIMAZOLE Topical

VA CLASSIFICATION (Primary): DE102

Commonly used brand name(s): *Canesten Cream; Canesten Solution; Canesten Solution with Atomizer; Clotrimaderm Cream; Lotrimin AF Cream; Lotrimin AF Lotion; Lotrimin AF Solution; Lotrimin Cream; Lotrimin Lotion; Lotrimin Solution; Mycelex Cream; Mycelex Solution; Myclo Cream; Myclo Solution; Myclo Spray Solution; Neo-Zol Cream.*

Note: For a listing of dosage forms and brand names by country availability, see *Dosage Forms* section(s).

## Category
Antifungal (topical).

## Indications
Note: Bracketed information in the *Indications* section refers to uses that are not included in U.S. product labeling.

**Accepted**
Candidiasis, cutaneous (treatment)—Topical clotrimazole is indicated in the treatment of cutaneous candidiasis (moniliasis) caused by *Candida albicans (Monilia albicans)*.

Tinea corporis (treatment)
Tinea cruris (treatment) or
Tinea pedis (treatment)—Topical clotrimazole is indicated in the treatment of tinea corporis (ringworm of the body), tinea cruris (ringworm of the groin; jock itch), and tinea pedis (ringworm of the foot; athlete's foot) caused by *Trichophyton rubrum, T. mentagrophytes, Epidermophyton floccosum (Acrothesium floccosum),* and *Microsporum canis*.

Tinea versicolor (treatment)—Topical clotrimazole is indicated in the treatment of tinea versicolor (pityriasis versicolor; "sun fungus") caused by *Pityrosporon orbiculare (Malassezia furfur)*.

[Paronychia (treatment)][1]
[Tinea barbae (treatment)][1] or
[Tinea capitis (treatment)][1]—Topical clotrimazole is used in the treatment of paronychia, tinea barbae, and tinea capitis.

Not all species or strains of a particular organism may be susceptible to clotrimazole.

[1] Not included in Canadian product labeling.

## Pharmacology/Pharmacokinetics

### Physicochemical characteristics
Molecular weight—344.84.

### Mechanism of action/Effect
Fungistatic; may be fungicidal, depending on concentration; inhibits biosynthesis of ergosterol or other sterols, damaging the fungal cell wall membrane and altering its permeability; as a result, loss of essential intracellular elements may occur; also inhibits biosynthesis of triglycerides and phospholipids by fungi; in addition, inhibits oxidative and peroxidative enzyme activity, resulting in intracellular buildup of toxic concentrations of hydrogen peroxide, which may contribute to deterioration of subcellular organelles and cellular necrosis. In *Candida albicans*, inhibits transformation of blastospores into invasive mycelial form.

### Absorption
Dermal penetration; minimal systemic absorption.

## Precautions to Consider

### Carcinogenicity
Studies in rats given oral doses of clotrimazole for 18 months have not shown that clotrimazole is carcinogenic.

### Mutagenicity
Studies in Chinese hamsters given clotrimazole in five oral doses of 100 mg per kg of body weight (mg/kg) prior to testing have shown no mutagenic effects in the spermatophore chromosomes.

### Pregnancy/Reproduction
Fertility—Clotrimazole caused impairment of mating in studies in mice and rats given oral doses of 50 to 120 mg per kg (mg/kg).

Pregnancy—Adequate and well-controlled studies in humans have not been done during the first trimester. Studies in humans given intravaginal clotrimazole during the second and third trimesters have not shown that clotrimazole causes adverse effects on the fetus.

Studies in rats given intravaginal doses of up to 100 mg/kg have not shown that clotrimazole causes adverse effects on the fetus. However, clotrimazole caused embryotoxicity, decreased litter size and number of viable young, and decreased pup survival to weaning in studies in mice and rats given oral doses of 50 to 120 mg/kg. Clotrimazole was not shown to be teratogenic in studies in mice, rabbits, and rats given oral doses of up to 200, 180, and 100 mg/kg, respectively.

FDA Pregnancy Category B.

### Breast-feeding
It is not known whether clotrimazole, applied topically, is distributed into breast milk. However, problems in humans have not been documented.

### Pediatrics
Appropriate studies performed to date have not demonstrated pediatrics-specific problems that would limit the usefulness of topical clotrimazole in children.

### Geriatrics
Appropriate studies on the relationship of age to the effects of topical clotrimazole have not been performed in the geriatric population. However, no geriatrics-specific problems have been documented to date.

### Medical considerations/Contraindications
The medical considerations/contraindications included have been selected on the basis of their potential clinical significance (reasons given in parentheses where appropriate)—not necessarily inclusive (» = major clinical significance).

*Risk-benefit should be considered when the following medical problem exists:*
Sensitivity to clotrimazole

## Side/Adverse Effects

The following side/adverse effects have been selected on the basis of their potential clinical significance (possible signs and symptoms in parentheses where appropriate)—not necessarily inclusive:

*Those indicating need for medical attention*
Hypersensitivity (skin rash, hives, blistering, burning, itching, peeling, redness, stinging, swelling, or other sign of skin irritation not present before therapy)

## Patient Consultation

As an aid to patient consultation, refer to *Advice for the Patient, Clotrimazole (Topical).*

In providing consultation, consider emphasizing the following selected information (» = major clinical significance):

**Before using this medication**
» Conditions affecting use, especially:
Sensitivity to clotrimazole

**Proper use of this medication**
Proper administration technique
» Avoiding contact with the eyes
» Not applying occlusive dressing over this medication unless directed to do so by physician
» Compliance with full course of therapy
» Proper dosing
Missed dose: Applying as soon as possible; not applying if almost time for next dose
» Proper storage

**Precautions while using this medication**
Checking with physician if no improvement within 4 weeks

**Side/adverse effects**
Signs of potential side effects, especially hypersensitivity reactions

## General Dosing Information

Use of topical antifungals may lead to skin sensitization, resulting in hypersensitivity reactions with subsequent topical use of the medication.

Improvement of condition, with relief of pruritus, usually occurs within the first week of therapy.

When this medication is used in the treatment of candidiasis, occlusive dressings should be avoided since they provide conditions that favor growth of yeast and release of its irritating endotoxin.

## Topical Dosage Forms

### CLOTRIMAZOLE CREAM USP

**Usual adult and adolescent dose**
Antifungal (topical)—
Topical, to the affected area of skin and surrounding areas, two times a day, morning and evening.

**Usual pediatric dose**
Antifungal (topical)—
See *Usual adult and adolescent dose.*

**Strength(s) usually available**
U.S.—
1% (10 mg per gram) (Rx/OTC) [*Lotrimin AF Cream (OTC)* (benzyl alcohol 1%); *Lotrimin Cream (Rx)* (benzyl alcohol 1%); *Mycelex Cream (OTC)* (benzyl alcohol 1%); GENERIC].
Canada—
1% (10 mg per gram) (Rx) [*Canesten Cream* (benzyl alcohol 1%); *Clotrimaderm Cream* (benzyl alcohol 1%); *Myclo Cream; Neo-Zol Cream*].

**Packaging and storage**
Store between 2 and 30 °C (36 and 86 °F). Store in a collapsible tube or in a tight container. Protect from freezing.

**Auxiliary labeling**
• For external use only.
• Continue medicine for full time of treatment.

### CLOTRIMAZOLE LOTION USP

**Usual adult and adolescent dose**
Antifungal (topical)—
See *Clotrimazole Cream USP.*

**Usual pediatric dose**
Antifungal (topical)—
See *Clotrimazole Cream USP.*

**Strength(s) usually available**
U.S.—
1% (10 mg per gram) (Rx/OTC) [*Lotrimin AF Lotion (OTC)* (benzyl alcohol; ceteryl alcohol); *Lotrimin Lotion (Rx)* (benzyl alcohol; ceteryl alcohol)].
Canada—
Not commercially available.

**Packaging and storage**
Store between 2 and 30 °C (36 and 86 °F). Store in a tight container. Protect from freezing.

**Auxiliary labeling**
- Shake well.
- For external use only.
- Continue medicine for full time of treatment.

## CLOTRIMAZOLE TOPICAL SOLUTION USP

**Usual adult and adolescent dose**
Antifungal (topical)—
    See *Clotrimazole Cream USP*.

**Usual pediatric dose**
Antifungal (topical)—
    See *Clotrimazole Cream USP*.

**Strength(s) usually available**
U.S.—
    1% (10 mg per mL) (Rx/OTC) [*Lotrimin AF Solution (OTC)* (polyethylene glycol); *Lotrimin Solution (Rx)* (polyethylene glycol); *Mycelex Solution (OTC)* (polyethylene glycol)].
Canada—
    1% (10 mg per mL) (Rx) [*Canesten Solution* (isopropyl alcohol); *Canesten Solution with Atomizer* (isopropyl alcohol); *Myclo Solution* (isopropyl alcohol); *Myclo Spray Solution* (isopropyl alcohol)].

**Packaging and storage**
Store between 2 and 30 °C (36 and 86 °F). Store in a tight container. Protect from freezing.

**Auxiliary labeling**
- For external use only.
- Keep container tightly closed.
- Continue medicine for full time of treatment.

Revised: 03/29/94

---

# CLOTRIMAZOLE AND BETAMETHASONE   Topical

VA CLASSIFICATION (Primary): DE250

**NOTE:** The *Clotrimazole and Betamethasone (Topical)* monograph is maintained on the USP DI electronic data base. For a printed copy of the most recent revision of the complete monograph, contact Micromedex, Inc. - Reprint Requests, 6200 S. Syracuse Way, Suite 300, Englewood, CO 80111; telephone (303) 486-6400; telefax (303) 486-6464; Email: USPDI@MDX.COM.

For information on the specific components of this combination, see the *USP DI* monographs for *Clotrimazole (Topical)* and *Corticosteroids (Topical)*.

The information that follows is selectively abstracted from the complete monograph and is provided to facilitate drug use review and patient counseling.

Note:   For a listing of dosage forms and brand names by country availability, see *Dosage Forms* section(s).

## Category
Antifungal-corticosteroid (topical).

Note:   Clotrimazole is a broad-spectrum antifungal agent.

## Indications
Note:   Bracketed information in the *Indications* section refers to uses that are not included in U.S. product labeling.

**Accepted**
Tinea corporis (treatment)
Tinea cruris (treatment) or
Tinea pedis (treatment)—Clotrimazole and betamethasone dipropionate combination is indicated [as a secondary agent] in the topical treatment of tinea corporis (ringworm of the body), tinea cruris (jock itch; ringworm of the groin), and tinea pedis (athlete's foot; ringworm of the foot), [accompanied by inflammation], caused by *Epidermophyton floccosum (Acrothesium floccosum)*, *Microsporum canis*, *Trichophyton rubrum*, and *T. mentagrophytes*.

The use of clotrimazole and betamethasone dipropionate combination has been shown to provide greater benefit than either clotrimazole or betamethasone dipropionate alone [during the first few days of treatment or for as long as inflammation persists, except on the palms of the hands and soles of the feet. After this time, USP medical experts recommend the use of plain clotrimazole or other topical antifungal agents].

[Candidiasis, cutaneous (treatment)][1]—Clotrimazole and betamethasone dipropionate combination is used as a secondary agent in the topical treatment of cutaneous candidiasis (moniliasis), accompanied by inflammation, caused by *Candida albicans (Monilia albicans)*.

Not all species or strains of a particular organism may be susceptible to clotrimazole.

**Unaccepted**
Since corticosteroids may cause thinning of the skin and telangiectasias when used on the face or in intertriginous areas (e.g., axilla, genitals, perineum, groin, between the toes), clotrimazole and betamethasone dipropionate combination is not recommended for use in these areas for longer than a few days.

Clotrimazole is not effective against bacteria, protozoa, or viruses.

[1]Not included in Canadian product labeling.

## Patient Consultation
As an aid to patient consultation, refer to *Advice for the Patient, Clotrimazole and Betamethasone (Topical)*.

In providing consultation, consider emphasizing the following selected information (» = major clinical significance):

**Before using this medication**
» Conditions affecting use, especially:
    Allergies to imidazoles or corticosteroids
    Pregnancy—Not recommended in pregnancy because of possibility of teratogenicity, especially when used on extensive surface areas, in large amounts, or for prolonged periods of time
    Breast-feeding—May cause systemic effects, such as growth suppression
    Use in children—May cause HPA axis suppression, Cushing's syndrome, intracranial hypertension, or growth suppression
    Other medical problems, especially eczema vaccinatum, herpes simplex, tubercular infections of the skin, vaccinia, varicella, or other viral infections of the skin

**Proper use of this medication**
    Before applying, washing affected area with soap and water, and drying thoroughly
» Not for ophthalmic use
*To use*
» Checking with physician before using medication on other skin problems
    Applying a thin layer of medication to affected area(s) and surrounding skin; rubbing in gently and thoroughly
» Not applying occlusive dressing over this medication unless directed to do so by physician; wearing loose-fitting clothing when using on inguinal area; avoiding tight-fitting diapers and plastic pants on diaper area of children
» Compliance with full course of therapy; not using more often or for longer than directed by physician; excessive use on thin skin areas may result in skin atrophy and stretch marks
» Proper dosing
    Missed dose: Applying as soon as possible; not applying if almost time for next dose
» Proper storage

**Precautions while using this medication**
    Checking with physician if no improvement within a few days
» Using hygienic measures to help cure infection and to help prevent reinfection:

*For tinea pedis*
  Carefully drying feet, especially between toes, after bathing
  Not wearing socks made from wool or synthetic materials; wearing clean, cotton socks and changing them daily or more often if feet perspire excessively
  Wearing well-ventilated shoes or sandals
  Using a bland, absorbent powder or an antifungal powder liberally between toes, on feet, and in socks and shoes once or twice daily; using the powder after cream has been applied and has disappeared into the skin; not using the powder as sole therapy for your fungal infection

*For tinea cruris*
  Carefully drying inguinal area after bathing
  Not wearing underwear that is tight-fitting or made from synthetic materials; wearing loose-fitting cotton underwear instead
  Using a bland, absorbent powder or an antifungal powder liberally once or twice daily; using the powder after cream has been applied and has disappeared into the skin; not using the powder as sole therapy for your fungal infection

*For tinea corporis*
  Carefully drying the body after bathing
  Avoiding excess heat and humidity if possible; keeping moisture from accumulating on affected areas of the body
  Wearing well-ventilated clothing
  Using a bland, absorbent powder or an antifungal powder liberally once or twice daily; using the powder after cream has been applied and has disappeared into the skin; not using the powder as sole therapy for your fungal infection

» Diabetics: May rarely cause hyperglycemia and glucosuria, especially with severe diabetes and use of large amounts; checking with physician before changing diet or dosage of antidiabetic medication

**Side/adverse effects**
Signs of potential side effects, especially hypersensitivity and long-term effects, including skin atrophy

## Topical Dosage Forms

### CLOTRIMAZOLE AND BETAMETHASONE DIPROPIONATE CREAM USP

**Usual adult and adolescent dose**
Tinea corporis; or
Tinea cruris; or
Tinea pedis—
  Topical, to the affected area(s) and surrounding skin, two times a day, morning and evening.

**Usual pediatric dose**
Infants and children up to 12 years of age—Safety and efficacy have not been established.
Children 12 years of age and over—See *Usual adult and adolescent dose*.

**Strength(s) usually available**
U.S.—
  1% of clotrimazole and 0.05% of betamethasone (base) (Rx) [*Lotrisone* (propylene glycol; benzyl alcohol)].
Canada—
  1% of clotrimazole and 0.05% of betamethasone (base) (Rx) [*Lotriderm* (propylene glycol; benzyl alcohol)].

**Auxiliary labeling**
• For external use only.
• Continue medication for full time of treatment.
• Do not use in the eyes.

Revised: 02/10/92
Interim revision: 07/01/94

---

**CLOXACILLIN**—See *Penicillins (Systemic)*

---

# CLOZAPINE  Systemic

VA CLASSIFICATION (Primary): CN709
Commonly used brand name(s): *Clozaril*.
Note: In the U.S. and Canada, clozapine is available only through pharmacies that agree to participate with physicians in a program to monitor patients' blood tests; a supply of medication sufficient to continue therapy until the next scheduled blood test may be dispensed if the results of the blood tests are within acceptable parameters.
Note: For a listing of dosage forms and brand names by country availability, see *Dosage Forms* section(s).

## Category
Antipsychotic.
Note: Clozapine is an atypical antipsychotic.

## Indications
**Accepted**
Schizophrenia (treatment)—Clozapine is indicated only in the management of severely ill schizophrenic patients who have failed to respond to other neuroleptic agents or who cannot tolerate the adverse effects produced by those agents. Clozapine may produce a significant improvement in both the positive and negative symptoms of schizophrenia.

Because of the significant risk of agranulocytosis and seizures associated with clozapine use, the patient should be given adequate trials with at least two different standard antipsychotic medications before clozapine therapy is initiated.

## Pharmacology/Pharmacokinetics

**Physicochemical characteristics**
Chemical group—Tricyclic dibenzodiazepine derivative.
Molecular weight—326.83.
Very slightly soluble in water.

**Mechanism of action/Effect**
The mechanism by which clozapine exerts its antipsychotic effect has not been defined. Clozapine shows more dopamine blocking activity in the limbic region of the brain than in the nigrostriatum. This may account for the low extrapyramidal side effect profile of clozapine. Clozapine interferes weakly with the binding of dopamine at $D_1$, $D_2$, $D_3$, and $D_5$ receptors, and potently at $D_4$ receptors. At alpha-adrenergic, cholinergic, histaminergic, and serotonergic receptors, clozapine acts as an antagonist. It is unclear whether a combination of these effects accounts for clozapine's efficacy. Clozapine has little or no effect on serum prolactin concentrations, because it does not bind to the tuberoinfundibular dopamine tract.

**Other actions/effects**
Clozapine may cause significant bone marrow suppression, which can lead to agranulocytosis. Deaths have occurred. The development of agranulocytosis has not been linked clearly to any patient characteristics and cannot be predicted reliably by either dose or duration of treatment. However, the greatest incidences have been seen during the first 6 months of clozapine use, in patients older than 50 years of age, and in patients of Jewish descent.
Electroencephalographic (EEG) studies show that clozapine increases delta and theta activity and slows dominant alpha frequencies. Sharp wave activity and spike and wave complexes may also develop. In some patients, the proportion of time spent in rapid eye movement (REM) sleep increases greatly and the REM sleep latency decreases greatly. Also, dose-related seizures are associated with clozapine use at a cumulative incidence at 1 year of approximately 5% in patients receiving 600 to 900 mg per day. Seizure incidence in patients receiving less than 300 mg per day of clozapine is about 1 to 2%.
Clozapine has potent anticholinergic effects.

**Absorption**
Rapid and nearly complete. However, first-pass metabolism results in an absolute bioavailability of 50 to 60%. Food does not affect the systemic bioavailability of clozapine.

**Distribution**
Rapid and extensive; crosses the blood-brain barrier.

**Protein binding**
Very high (95%).

**Biotransformation**
Extensive hepatic metabolism to metabolites with limited or no activity.
  The cytochrome P450 1A2 (CYP1A2) isoenzyme is the primary isoenzyme involved in clozapine metabolism. CYP2D6 is involved in clozapine metabolism to a lesser extent.

## Clozapine (Systemic)

**Half-life**
Elimination—
  8 hours (range, 4 to 12 hours) after a single 75-mg dose; 12 hours (range, 4 to 66 hours) after reaching steady-state dosing of 100 mg twice a day.

**Time to peak concentration**
Average, 2.5 hours (range, 1 to 6 hours). Steady-state concentrations are attained in 8 to 10 days.

**Peak serum concentration**
Steady-state peak and minimum plasma concentrations of clozapine average 319 nanograms per mL (range, 102 to 771 nanograms per mL) and 122 nanograms per mL (range, 41 to 343 nanograms per mL), respectively, at a dosage of 100 mg two times a day. At steady-state, administration of 37.5 mg, 75 mg, and 100 mg of clozapine two times a day produced linearly dose-proportional changes in the area under the plasma concentration–time curve and in the peak and minimum plasma concentrations of clozapine.

**Duration of action**
4 to 12 hours.

**Elimination**
Renal—
  Approximately 50% of an administered dose, only trace amounts as unchanged clozapine.
Fecal—
  Approximately 30% of an administered dose, only trace amounts as unchanged clozapine.

## Precautions to Consider

**Carcinogenicity**
Long-term studies in mice and rats given clozapine in doses approximately seven times the typical human dose on a mg per kg of body weight (mg/kg) basis demonstrated no potential carcinogenicity.

**Tumorigenicity**
Animal studies have shown no abnormalities.

**Mutagenicity**
Clozapine was not found to be genotoxic or mutagenic when assayed in appropriate bacterial and mammalian tests.

**Pregnancy/Reproduction**
Pregnancy—Clozapine crosses the placenta. Adequate and well-controlled studies in humans have not been done.
Studies in animals have not shown that clozapine causes adverse effects on the fetus.
FDA Pregnancy Category B.

**Breast-feeding**
Animal studies have suggested that clozapine may be distributed into breast milk. Clozapine may cause sedation, decreased suckling, restlessness or irritability, seizures, and cardiovascular instability in the nursing infant.

**Pediatrics**
Appropriate studies on the relationship of age to the effects of clozapine have not been performed in children up to 16 years of age. Safety and efficacy have not been established.

**Geriatrics**
No information is available on the relationship of age to the effects of clozapine in geriatric patients. However, the elderly may be at greater risk for orthostatic hypotension, and for anticholinergic side effects such as confusion and excitement. Also, elderly males are more likely to have age-related prostatic hypertrophy, which requires caution in the use of clozapine.

**Dental**
Although hypersalivation occurs as a frequent consequence of clozapine administration, peripheral anticholinergic effects of clozapine may decrease or inhibit salivary flow, thus contributing to the development of caries, periodontal disease, oral candidiasis, and discomfort.
The leukopenic and thrombocytopenic effects of clozapine may result in an increased incidence of microbial infection, delayed healing, and gingival bleeding. If leukopenia or thrombocytopenia occurs, dental work should be deferred until blood counts have returned to normal, and patients should be instructed in proper oral hygiene, including caution in the use of regular toothbrushes, dental floss, and toothpicks.

**Drug interactions and/or related problems**
The following drug interactions and/or related problems have been selected on the basis of their potential clinical significance (possible mechanism in parentheses where appropriate)—not necessarily inclusive (» = major clinical significance):

Note: Clozapine metabolism is mediated mainly by cytochrome P450 1A2 (CYP1A2) and to a lesser extent by CYP2D6. Interactions with other medications that are metabolized by these isoenzymes (e.g., encainide, flecainide, propafenone) or that induce or inhibit (e.g., quinidine) the cytochrome P450 enzymes, in addition to those listed below, should be considered. Dosage adjustments of either clozapine or the other medication may be required.
Combinations containing any of the following medications, depending on the amount present, may also interact with this medication.

» Alcohol or
» Central nervous system (CNS) depression–producing medications, other (see *Appendix II*)
  (concurrent use with clozapine may increase the severity and frequency of CNS depressant effects)

Anticholinergics, other (see *Appendix II*)
  (concurrent use with clozapine may potentiate the anticholinergic effects of these medications)

» Bone marrow depressants, other (see *Appendix II*)
  (concurrent use with clozapine may potentiate the myelosuppressive effects of these medications)

Carbamazepine or
Phenytoin or
Smoking tobacco
  (concurrent use may decrease the plasma concentrations of clozapine, reducing the effectiveness of a given clozapine dose; discontinuation may increase the plasma concentrations of clozapine)

Cimetidine or
Erythromycin
  (clozapine plasma concentrations may be increased, increasing the risk of developing adverse effects)

Highly protein-bound medications, other, such as:
  Digitoxin
  Warfarin
  (concurrent use with clozapine may result in increased serum concentrations of these medications; also, clozapine may be displaced from its binding sites by these medications)

» Hypotension-producing medications, other (see *Appendix II*), especially
Benzodiazepines or
Psychotropic medications, other
  (concurrent use with clozapine may cause additive hypotensive effects; epinephrine should not be used in the treatment of clozapine-induced hypotension because of a possible reverse epinephrine effect)
  (very rarely, circulatory collapse, respiratory arrest, and cardiac arrest have accompanied orthostatic hypotension in patients receiving clozapine alone or with benzodiazepines or other psychotropic medications; although drug interaction has not been established as the mechanism for these events, clozapine should be introduced with caution in patients receiving other psychotropic medications)

» Lithium
  (concurrent use with clozapine may increase the risk of seizures, confusional states, neuroleptic malignant syndrome, and dyskinesias)

» Selective serotonin reuptake inhibitors (SSRIs)
  (tenfold elevations in clozapine serum concentrations have been reported during concurrent use with fluvoxamine; lesser elevations have been reported during concurrent use with other SSRIs [fluoxetine, paroxetine, sertraline]; patients should be monitored closely, and a reduced clozapine dosage should be considered)

**Medical considerations/Contraindications**
The medical considerations/contraindications included have been selected on the basis of their potential clinical significance (reasons given in parentheses where appropriate)—not necessarily inclusive (» = major clinical significance).

*Except under special circumstances, this medication should not be used when the following medical problems exist:*

» CNS depression, severe
  (may be potentiated)

» Myeloproliferative disorders, specifically:
  Blood dyscrasias, or history of
  Bone marrow depression
    (may be potentiated)

***Risk-benefit should be considered when the following medical problems exist:***
- Cardiovascular disorders
  (increased risk of blood pressure alterations and arrhythmias)
- » Glaucoma, narrow-angle, predisposition to or
- » Intestinal motility impairment or
- » Prostatic hypertrophy
  (conditions may be exacerbated by the potent anticholinergic effects of clozapine)
- Hepatic function impairment
  (metabolism of clozapine may be altered; also, hepatitis has been reported with clozapine use in patients with normal hepatic function and in patients with impaired hepatic function)
- Renal function impairment
  (excretion of clozapine may be altered)
- » Seizure disorders, or history of
  (risk of seizures may be increased)

**Patient monitoring**

The following may be especially important in patient monitoring (other tests may be warranted in some patients, depending on condition; » = major clinical significance):

» White blood cell (WBC) and differential counts
  (WBC and differential counts are required prior to initiation of therapy. If the baseline WBC count is less than 3500 per mm³, clozapine therapy should not be initiated. WBC counts are required at specified intervals during therapy, and weekly for 4 weeks after clozapine is discontinued. Clozapine is supplied to the patient in quantities sufficient to continue treatment only until the next required blood test and only if the previous blood tests have been performed and the results are within an acceptable range. Repeat WBC and differential counts are recommended if, at any time during clozapine therapy, any of the following three events occurs: the WBC count drops below 3500 per mm³; the WBC count drops substantially [≥ 3000 per mm³ either as a single drop or as a cumulative drop over 3 weeks or less], even if total WBC count remains above 3500 per mm³; or immature forms are present)

(for the first 6 months of continuous clozapine therapy, WBC counts should be performed weekly. If during this 6-month period the patient has an interruption in clozapine therapy of ≤ 1 month, and there have been no abnormal blood events [WBC count < 3000 per mm³ or absolute neutrophil count (ANC) < 1500 per mm³], the 6-month period of weekly monitoring may be resumed from where it was left off. However, if the patient has an interruption in clozapine therapy of > 1 month, weekly monitoring is required for a 6-month period starting from the date of reinitiation of clozapine. If the patient has had no abnormal blood events through 6 months of weekly monitoring, and in the clinical judgment of the physician it is deemed appropriate, monitoring frequency may be decreased to once every other week)

(if a patient has met the criteria for every-other-week monitoring and subsequently has an interruption in clozapine therapy of ≤ 1 year, monitoring may be resumed at a frequency of once every other week with reinitiation of clozapine. However, if there is an interruption in clozapine therapy of > 1 year, a 6-month period of weekly monitoring with no abnormal blood events must again be completed before monitoring frequency may be decreased to once every other week)

(if any abnormal blood event that does not require permanent discontinuation of clozapine occurs [WBC count of 2000 to 3000 per mm³ or ANC of 1000 to 1500 per mm³], regardless of how long the patient has been taking clozapine or whether the patient is on a weekly or every-other-week monitoring schedule, monitoring should be performed every week for 6 months following the event)

(if WBC and differential counts reveal a WBC count of 3000 to 3500 per mm³ and an ANC > 1500 per mm³, WBC and differential counts should be performed twice weekly)

(if the WBC count falls below 3000 per mm³ or the ANC falls below 1500 per mm³, clozapine should be discontinued, WBC and differential counts performed daily, and the patient monitored for flu-like symptoms or other symptoms suggesting infection. If, subsequently, the WBC count exceeds 3000 per mm³, the ANC exceeds 1500 per mm³, and no signs of infection develop in these patients, clozapine may be resumed; however, WBC and differential counts should be performed at least twice weekly until the WBC count is greater than 3500 per mm³)

(if a differential count reveals an eosinophil count above 4000 per mm³, clozapine should be discontinued until the eosinophil count falls below 3000 per mm³)

(if the WBC count falls below 2000 per mm³ or the ANC falls below 1000 per mm³, clozapine should be *permanently discontinued* and WBC and differential counts should be performed daily; bone marrow aspiration should be considered to ascertain the patient's granulopoietic status; protective isolation and antibiotic therapy should be instituted if indicated. These patients should *not* be rechallenged with clozapine, because agranulocytosis may occur with a shorter latency period)

(after discontinuation of clozapine, WBC counts should be performed every week for 4 weeks even if no abnormal blood events occurred during treatment)

## Side/Adverse Effects

The following side/adverse effects have been selected on the basis of their potential clinical significance (possible signs and symptoms in parentheses where appropriate)—not necessarily inclusive:

**Those indicating need for medical attention**
Incidence more frequent
  ***Cardiovascular effects, specifically tachycardia*** (fast or irregular heartbeat); ***hypotension*** (low blood pressure); ***or orthostatic hypotension*** (dizziness or fainting)—especially when getting up from a lying or sitting position; ***fever***

Note: *Cardiovascular effects* can be minimized by increasing dosage gradually and tend to subside with continued use of clozapine.
  *Fever* usually occurs within the first 3 weeks of therapy and usually is benign and self-limiting. Occasionally, fever may be associated with an increase or decrease in white blood cell count. Any patient with fever should be evaluated to rule out underlying infectious processes or the development of agranulocytosis. If a high fever occurs in conjunction with severe muscle rigidity and autonomic changes, the possibility of neuroleptic malignant syndrome should be considered.

Incidence less frequent
  ***Agitation*** (unusual anxiety, nervousness, or irritability); ***akathisia*** (restlessness or need to keep moving); ***confusion; difficulty in accommodation*** (blurred vision); ***electrocardiogram (ECG) changes; hypertension*** (dizziness; severe or continuing headaches; increase in blood pressure); ***syncope*** (fainting)

Incidence rare
  ***Blood dyscrasias, specifically agranulocytosis*** (chills; fever; sore throat; unusual tiredness or weakness); ***eosinophilia*** (fever); ***granulocytopenia*** (chills; fever; sore throat; sores, ulcers, or white spots on lips or in mouth; unusual tiredness or weakness); ***leukopenia*** (chills; fever; sore throat); ***or thrombocytopenia*** (unusual bleeding or bruising); ***deep-vein thrombosis*** (swelling or pain in leg); ***or pulmonary embolism*** (chest pain; cough; fainting; fast heartbeat; sudden shortness of breath); ***extrapyramidal effects, specifically akinesia or hypokinesia*** (absence of or decrease in movement); ***rigidity*** (severe muscle stiffness); ***or tremor*** (trembling or shaking)—less frequent; ***hepatitis*** (dark urine; decreased appetite; nausea; vomiting; yellow eyes or skin); ***hyperglycemia*** (increased appetite; increased thirst; increased urination; weakness); ***impotence*** (decreased sexual ability); ***insomnia or disturbed sleep*** (trouble in sleeping); ***mental depression; neuroleptic malignant syndrome (NMS)*** (convulsions; difficult or fast breathing; fast heartbeat or irregular pulse; fever; high or low [irregular] blood pressure; increased sweating; loss of bladder control; severe muscle stiffness; unusually pale skin; unusual tiredness or weakness); ***seizures; tardive dyskinesia*** (lip smacking or puckering; puffing of cheeks; rapid or worm-like movements of tongue; uncontrolled chewing movements; uncontrolled movements of arms and legs); ***trouble in urinating***

Note: Liver function tests should be performed immediately in any patient who develops signs or symptoms of *hepatitis* during treatment with clozapine. If test values are significantly elevated or if the patient shows signs of jaundice, clozapine should be discontinued.

Several cases of *NMS* have occurred in patients receiving clozapine alone or concomitantly with lithium or other CNS-active agents.

For *seizures*, a dose-dependent relationship has been suggested, with *seizures* occurring in 1 to 2% of patients receiving low doses (< 300 mg per day), in 3 to 4% of patients receiving moderate doses (300 to 599 mg per day), and in 5% of patients receiving high doses (≥ 600 mg per day) of clozapine. Patients with a history of epilepsy or other predisposing factors may be at greater risk of developing seizures.

Although no confirmed cases of *tardive dyskinesia* have been attributed to clozapine, the possibility of occurrence cannot be ruled out. The smallest dose and shortest duration of treatment should be used, with periodic reassessment of need for clozapine treatment.

**Those indicating need for medical attention only if they continue or are bothersome**
Incidence more frequent
  *Constipation; dizziness or lightheadedness; drowsiness; headache; hypersalivation* (increased watering of mouth); *nausea or vomiting; unusual weight gain*
  Note: *Salivation* may be profuse, very fluid, and especially prevalent during sleep. It has been suggested by the manufacturer that this effect may be ameliorated in some cases by a reduction of clozapine dosage or by use of a peripherally acting anticholinergic medication; however, caution should be used since additive anticholinergic effects may lead to toxicity in some patients.

Incidence less frequent
  *Abdominal discomfort or heartburn; dryness of mouth; hyperhidrosis* (increased sweating)

## Overdose

For specific information on the agents used in the management of clozapine overdose, see:
  *Charcoal, Activated (Oral-Local)* monograph;
  *Dihydroergotamine* in *Vascular Headache Suppressants, Ergot Derivative–containing (Systemic)* monograph;
  *Norepinephrine* in *Sympathomimetic Agents—Cardiovascular Use (Parenteral-Systemic)* monograph; and/or
  *Physostigmine (Systemic)* monograph.

For more information on the management of overdose or unintentional ingestion, **contact a Poison Control Center** (see *Poison Control Center Listing*).

**Clinical effects of overdose**
The following effects have been selected on the basis of their potential clinical significance (possible signs and symptoms in parentheses where appropriate)—not necessarily inclusive:
  *Cardiac arrhythmias or tachycardia* (fast, slow, or irregular heartbeat); *delirium* (unusual excitement, nervousness, or restlessness; hallucinations); *drowsiness, severe or coma; hypersalivation* (increased watering of the mouth); *hypotension* (dizziness or fainting); *respiratory depression or failure* (slow, irregular, or troubled breathing); *seizures*
  Note: Aspiration pneumonia has also been reported.
    Deaths have occurred, generally at clozapine doses > 2500 mg. However, overdoses as low as 400 mg in adults and 50 to 200 mg in young children have resulted in coma. Patients have recovered from doses > 4000 mg.

**Treatment of overdose**
There is no specific antidote for clozapine. Treatment of overdose is symptomatic and supportive.

To decrease absorption—Initiation of gastric lavage or administration of activated charcoal within 6 hours of ingestion, if possible. Administration of activated charcoal, which may be used with sorbitol, may be as effective as or more effective than induction of emesis or gastric lavage.

Specific treatment—Considering use of physostigmine, dihydroergotamine, angiotensin, or norepinephrine to counteract anticholinergic symptoms. *Not* using epinephrine or derivatives in treatment of hypotension. *Not* using quinidine or procainamide in treatment of cardiac arrhythmias.

Monitoring—Monitoring of cardiac and vital signs; continued monitoring of patient for several days because of risk of delayed effects.

Supportive care—Establishment and maintenance of a patent airway, ensuring adequate oxygenation and ventilation. Patients in whom intentional overdose is confirmed or suspected should be referred for psychiatric consultation.

Note: Forced diuresis, dialysis, hemoperfusion, and exchange transfusions are not likely to be of benefit due to clozapine's high degree of protein binding.

## Patient Consultation

As an aid to patient consultation, refer to *Advice for the Patient, Clozapine (Systemic)*.
In providing consultation, consider emphasizing the following selected information (» = major clinical significance):

**Before using this medication**
» Conditions affecting use, especially:
    Pregnancy—Crosses the placenta
    Breast-feeding—May cause sedation, decreased suckling, and restlessness or irritability in nursing infant

  Use in the elderly—Greater risk of orthostatic hypotension and anticholinergic side effects in these patients
  Dental—Clozapine-induced blood dyscrasias may result in infections, delayed healing, and bleeding; dry mouth may cause caries and candidiasis; hypersalivation occurs frequently
  Other medications, especially alcohol, other CNS depression–producing medications, other bone marrow depressants, other hypotension-producing medications, lithium, or selective serotonin reuptake inhibitors
  Other medical problems, especially severe CNS depression, myeloproliferative disorders, predisposition to narrow-angle glaucoma, intestinal motility impairment, prostatic hypertrophy, and seizure disorders

**Proper use of this medication**
» Compliance with therapy; not taking more or less medication than prescribed
» Proper dosing
  Missed dose: Taking as soon as possible; not taking if almost time for next dose; not doubling doses; not taking if clozapine has not been taken in 2 or more days but contacting physician for instructions
» Proper storage

**Precautions while using this medication**
» Regular visits to physician to check progress of therapy and to laboratory for blood tests required to continue treatment
» Contacting physician for instruction before resuming clozapine use if clozapine has not been taken for ≥ 2 days
  Checking with physician before discontinuing medication; gradual dosage reduction may be needed
  Avoiding use of alcoholic beverages or other CNS depressants during therapy
» Immediately reporting to physician any lethargy, weakness, fever, sore throat, or other sign or symptom of infection that occurs during clozapine treatment because of the risk of blood dyscrasias
  Possible drowsiness, blurred vision, or seizures; not driving, swimming, climbing, operating machinery, or doing other things that require alertness or accurate vision
  Possible orthostatic hypotension; caution when getting up from a lying or sitting position
  Possible dryness of mouth; using sugarless gum or candy, ice, or saliva substitute for relief; checking with physician or dentist if dryness of mouth continues for more than 2 weeks

**Side/adverse effects**
Signs of potential side effects, especially cardiovascular effects, fever, agitation, akathisia, confusion, difficulty in accommodation, ECG changes, hypertension, syncope, blood dyscrasias, deep-vein thrombosis or pulmonary embolism, extrapyramidal effects, hepatitis, hyperglycemia, impotence, insomnia or disturbed sleep, mental depression, neuroleptic malignant syndrome, seizures, tardive dyskinesia, or trouble in urinating

## General Dosing Information

Clozapine dosage must be individualized by cautious titration from the lower dosage range. A divided dosing schedule should be used, the need for clozapine periodically reassessed, and the patient maintained at the lowest possible dosage level. Cautious titration and divided doses are necessary to minimize the risks of hypotension, seizure, and sedation.

Because of the risk of blood dyscrasias, the patient should be instructed to report immediately any lethargy, weakness, fever, sore throat, or other sign or symptom of infection that occurs during clozapine treatment.

Because of the continuing risks of seizure and agranulocytosis, a patient who does not show acceptable clinical benefit should not receive extended clozapine therapy.

If clozapine is to be discontinued, the dosage should be tapered gradually over 1 to 2 weeks if possible. However, if abrupt termination is necessary, the patient should be monitored for recurrence of psychotic symptoms, as rapid decompensation has occurred after sudden withdrawal.

Caution should be exercised in restarting clozapine. The mechanisms by which clozapine's adverse effects occur are unknown. The possibility exists that agranulocytosis will be more likely and more severe when clozapine is restarted in a patient who has previously received clozapine if, for example, an immune-mediated mechanism is involved. Any patient whose white blood cell (WBC) count falls below 2000 per mm$^3$ or whose absolute neutrophil count falls below 1000 per mm$^3$ should *not* be restarted on clozapine.

### For treatment of adverse effects
Neuroleptic malignant syndrome (NMS)—
Treatment is essentially symptomatic and supportive and may include the following:
- *Discontinuing clozapine immediately.*
- Hyperthermia—Administering antipyretics (aspirin or acetaminophen); using cooling blanket.
- Dehydration—Restoring fluids and electrolytes.
- Cardiovascular instability—Monitoring blood pressure and cardiac rhythm closely. Use of sodium nitroprusside may allow vasodilation with subsequent heat loss from the skin in patients with less dominant muscle rigidity.
- Hypoxia—Administering oxygen; considering airway insertion and assisted ventilation.
- Muscle rigidity—Administering dantrolene sodium (100 to 300 mg a day orally in divided doses; or 1.25 to 1.5 mg per kg of body weight [mg/kg], intravenously); or administering amantadine (100 mg twice daily) or bromocriptine (5 mg three times a day) to restore central balance of dopamine and acetylcholine at the receptor site.

Tardive dyskinesia—
No known effective treatment. Although no confirmed cases of tardive dyskinesia have been attributed to clozapine, the dosage of clozapine should be lowered or medication discontinued at earliest signs of tardive dyskinesia to prevent irreversible effects.

Agranulocytosis—
If the WBC count falls below 2000 per mm³ or the granulocyte count falls below 1000 per mm³:
- *Discontinuing clozapine immediately.*
- Considering bone marrow aspiration to determine granulopoietic status.
- Placing patient in protective isolation with close observation if granulopoiesis is deficient.
- Monitoring WBC and differential counts daily until normal levels return.
- Performing appropriate cultures and instituting appropriate antibiotic therapy if signs of infection occur.
- *Not* rechallenging patient with clozapine.

## Oral Dosage Forms

### CLOZAPINE TABLETS

**Usual adult dose**
Antipsychotic—
Oral, initially 12.5 mg (one half of a 25-mg tablet) one or two times a day, the dosage being increased in increments of 25 to 50 mg a day, if tolerated, to achieve a dose of 300 to 450 mg a day by the end of two weeks. Subsequent dosage increments should not exceed 100 mg one or two times a week.

If reinitiating clozapine treatment two or more days since the last dose was taken, an initial dosage of 12.5 mg (one half of a 25-mg tablet) one or two times a day is recommended. However, titration to an effective dosage may proceed more rapidly than initial titration if the medication is well-tolerated. In any patient who experienced respiratory or cardiac arrest during initial dosing but who was then successfully titrated to a therapeutic dosage, titration of clozapine following reinitiation should proceed with great caution after an interruption in therapy of ≥ 24 hours duration.

Note: For malnourished patients, or those with hepatic, renal, or cardiovascular disease, dosage should be titrated more slowly than for other patients.

**Usual adult prescribing limits**
900 mg per day.

**Usual pediatric dose**
Children younger than 16 years of age—
Safety and efficacy have not been established.

**Strength(s) usually available**
U.S.—
25 mg (Rx) [*Clozaril* (scored; lactose) [GENERIC (scored)].
100 mg (Rx) [*Clozaril* (scored; lactose) [GENERIC (scored)].
Canada—
25 mg (Rx) [*Clozaril* (scored; lactose)].
100 mg (Rx) [*Clozaril* (scored; lactose)].

**Packaging and storage**
Store below 30 °C (86 °F), in a tight container, unless otherwise specified by manufacturer.

**Auxiliary labeling**
- Avoid alcoholic beverages.

**Note**
Clozapine may be dispensed only upon presentation of acceptable white blood cell (WBC) count results and only in a quantity sufficient to cover the time until the next scheduled blood test.

Revised: 08/07/98

---

**COAL TAR**—The *Coal Tar (Topical)* monograph is not included in this published version of the USP DI database. Copies of the monograph are available on request from Micromedex, Inc. - Reprint Requests, 6200 S. Syracuse Way, Suite 300, Englewood, CO 80111; telephone (303) 486-6400; telefax (303) 486-6464; Email: USPDI@MDX.COM..

---

# COCAINE Mucosal-Local

VA CLASSIFICATION (Primary/Secondary): NT300/OR600
Note: Controlled substance classification—
U.S.—Schedule II
Canada—N
Note: For a listing of dosage forms and brand names by country availability, see *Dosage Forms* section(s).

## Category
Anesthetic-vasoconstrictor (mucosal-local).

## Indications

**Accepted**
Anesthesia, local[1]—Cocaine hydrochloride is indicated to provide local anesthesia and vasoconstriction of accessible mucous membranes, especially in the oral, laryngeal, and nasal cavities, prior to instrumentation (e.g., bronchoscopy) or surgical procedures. Cocaine's toxicity must be considered prior to its use, especially when it is being applied to the tracheobronchial tree.

Although cocaine is an acceptable topical anesthetic for dental procedures, it is no longer extensively used in dentistry because of its toxicity.

**Unaccepted**
Cocaine is not indicated for administration by injection and is not recommended for application to "closed" mucous surfaces, such as those of the urethra or bladder, because of the increased risk of severe toxic reactions.

[1]Not included in Canadian product labeling.

## Pharmacology/Pharmacokinetics

**Physicochemical characteristics**
Molecular weight—339.82.

**Mechanism of action/Effect**
Anesthetic, local—Acts primarily by blocking both the initiation and conduction of nerve impulses by decreasing the neuronal membrane's permeability to sodium ions. This reversibly stabilizes the membrane and inhibits depolarization, resulting in the failure of a propagated action potential and subsequent conduction blockade.

Vasoconstrictor—Cocaine is a potent indirect-acting sympathomimetic agent, i.e., it interferes with the uptake of norepinephrine by adrenergic nerve terminals and increases the concentration of this neurotransmitter at postsynaptic receptor sites. Norepinephrine acts on alpha-adrenergic receptors in blood vessels to produce vasoconstriction, which facilitates examination and surgery by reducing congestion, swelling, and bleeding at the site of application.

**Other actions/effects**
Cocaine's indirect sympathetic nervous system–stimulating activity results in potentiation of the effects of endogenous catecholamines, i.e., epinephrine and dopamine as well as norepinephrine. This leads to systemic, as well as local, vasoconstriction; increased heart rate, arterial blood pressure, and blood glucose concentrations; mydriasis; and a risk

of cardiac arrhythmias. Tachycardia and hypertension may increase myocardial work and oxygen demand; in some patients, especially those with predisposing cardiovascular disease, myocardial ischemia may result.

Cocaine is a potent central nervous system (CNS) stimulant.

Cocaine has pyrogenic activity that may result from CNS stimulation–induced increases in muscular activity (which increases heat production) as well as vasoconstriction (which decreases heat loss through the skin). There is some evidence that cocaine also produces pyresis via a direct effect on the heat-regulating centers in the CNS.

Cocaine has convulsant activity that may result from its pyrogenic activity as well as from its CNS effects.

Cocaine also blocks the uptake of dopamine, thereby increasing the concentration of dopamine at postsynaptic receptor sites and stimulating dopaminergic neurotransmission. However, repeated use of cocaine may cause dopamine depletion in the CNS. Studies have indicated that dopaminergic stimulation may be responsible for the development of cocaine-induced euphoria, whereas dopamine depletion may be responsible for the occurrence of dysphoria and/or mental depression following cessation of repeated cocaine use and may lead to psychological dependence on the drug. Cocaine abuse may also lead to physical dependence.

Topical application of cocaine to the oral or nasal mucosa decreases local sensory acuity; i.e., reduces or abolishes senses of taste and smell.

### Absorption
Cocaine is readily absorbed from all mucous membranes. Although cocaine's local vasoconstrictive effect may limit to some extent its rate of absorption (measurable quantities have been reported to remain in the nasal mucosa for 3 hours after application), the rate of absorption may exceed the rate of metabolism and/or excretion, leading to a significant risk of systemic toxicity. Entry of cocaine into the brain may be especially rapid following application to the nasal mucosa, particularly if the medication is applied as a fine-mist spray. Also, cocaine is more readily absorbed from inflamed or damaged tissue.

### Biotransformation
Cocaine is hydrolyzed by plasma and hepatic cholinesterases. The primary metabolites are benzoylecgonine and ecgonine methyl ester. Small quantities are also demethylated in the liver to an active metabolite, norcocaine, which has local anesthetic activity and, *in vitro*, inhibits norepinephrine uptake. Metabolism of cocaine is generally rapid, but may be significantly decreased or slowed in individuals with low levels of plasma or hepatic cholinesterase activity.

### Half-life
Elimination—1 to 1.5 hours; subject to wide inter- and intraindividual variability, but independent of the route of administration.

### Onset of action
Approximately 1 minute.

### Time to peak effect
Approximately 5 minutes.

### Duration of action
Approximately 30 minutes to 1 hour (average, 20 to 40 minutes), depending on the concentration.

### Elimination
Renal, primarily as metabolites. Approximately 10 to 20% of a dose may be excreted as unchanged cocaine, depending on the acidity of the urine (with larger quantities being excreted in acidic urine). The rate at which cocaine and its metabolites are cleared from the body is dose-dependent. Following intranasal administration of a single dose of about 100 mg, significant quantities of cocaine may appear in the urine for at least 10 hours, and significant quantities of its major metabolites may appear in the urine for 2 to 2.5 days.

In breast milk—Cocaine is excreted in breast milk.

## Precautions to Consider

### Carcinogenicity/Mutagenicity
Long-term studies have not been done.

### Pregnancy/Reproduction
Pregnancy—Cocaine has high water and lipid solubility and may therefore cross the placenta by simple diffusion. Although studies have not been done in pregnant women receiving cocaine clinically, the possibility should be considered that pregnant women may be especially sensitive to the effects of cocaine because of reduced plasma cholinesterase activity resulting in decreased or slower cocaine metabolism. Human fetuses and neonates also exhibit low cholinesterase activity. Use of cocaine by a pregnant woman 1 or 2 days prior to delivery may result in the appearance of measurable quantities of benzoylecgonine in the neonate's urine for up to 5 days after birth.

Studies in cocaine-abusing pregnant women have shown that cocaine may increase the risk of spontaneous abortion; premature labor and stillbirth associated with abruptio placentae, with onset of labor occurring shortly after use of cocaine during the third trimester; congenital malformations; decreased fetal growth (reduced neonatal birth weight, length, and head circumference); and neonatal neurobehavioral impairment. The congenital malformations reported in these studies include transposition of the great arteries, hypoplastic right heart syndrome, exencephaly, interparietal encephalocele, parietal bone defects, and, in one infant, major malformations of the urinary tract, with bilateral hydronephrosis and bilateral cryptorchidism. Also, one infant born to a mother who had used cocaine intranasally 15 hours prior to delivery displayed convulsions, right-sided muscle weakness, intermittent tachycardia, and hypertension at birth and was found to have had a cerebral infarction. It has been proposed that these effects result from cocaine-induced placental vasoconstriction as well as maternal hypertension, cardiac arrhythmias, and hyperpyrexia, which decrease the flow of blood and nutrients to the fetus and also increase the risk of spontaneous abortion or premature labor. Because of these adverse effects, and because less toxic local anesthetics are available, it is recommended that cocaine not be administered to pregnant women.

In animal studies, cocaine increased the fetal resorption rate in rats and mice, decreased fetal weight in rats, and caused edema in the rat fetus. In another study, administration of cocaine to CF-1 mice on one of Days 7 through 12 of gestation caused skeletal abnormalities (malformed sternebrae, fused sternebrae, and polysternebrae), exencephaly, cryptorchidism, hydronephrosis, butterfly xiphoid, ocular defects (including anophthalmia or malformed or missing lenses), and delayed ossification of the paws or skull. The occurrence of specific malformations or abnormalities was dependent on the day of administration and coincided with the period of ontogenesis for the structures involved. Also, in a study in pregnant ewes, cocaine increased maternal blood pressure and uterine vascular resistance, decreased uterine blood flow, and caused hypoxemia, hypertension, and tachycardia in the fetuses.

FDA Pregnancy Category C.

### Breast-feeding
Cocaine is distributed into human breast milk. Symptoms of cocaine intoxication, including tachycardia, tachypnea, hypertension, irritability, and tremulousness, occurred in a breast-fed infant whose mother used cocaine intranasally. The symptoms appeared within 3 hours after the mother first used cocaine and persisted for as long as significant quantities of the drug and/or its metabolites appeared in the infant's urine. Cocaine and benzoylecgonine were present in the breast milk for up to 36 hours, and in the infant's urine for up to 60 hours, after the mother's last dose of the drug. Another infant, whose mother applied cocaine to her nipples to relieve soreness prior to breast-feeding, developed convulsions. Neonates may be especially susceptible to cocaine-induced toxicity because of low levels of cholinesterase activity resulting in decreased and/or slowed inactivation of the drug. If clinical use of cocaine is unavoidable, temporary cessation of breast-feeding is recommended.

### Pediatrics
Because of cocaine's toxicity, it is recommended that the medication not be administered to children younger than 6 years of age. For children 6 years of age or older, it is recommended that cocaine be used with caution and in reduced dosage.

### Geriatrics
The risk of cocaine-induced adverse effects may be increased in geriatric patients, who are more likely to have cerebrovascular disease, and are therefore more likely to be adversely affected by sympathetic stimulation, than are younger adults. Also, elderly males may be especially sensitive to the effects of cocaine because of reduced plasma cholinesterase activity resulting in decreased or slower cocaine metabolism. A reduction in dosage is recommended.

### Drug interactions and/or related problems
The following drug interactions and/or related problems have been selected on the basis of their potential clinical significance (possible mechanism in parentheses where appropriate)—not necessarily inclusive (» = major clinical significance):

Note: Combinations containing any of the following medications, depending on the amount present, may also interact with this medication.

Anesthetics, hydrocarbon inhalation, such as:
»   Chloroform
»   Cyclopropane
    Enflurane
»   Halothane
    Isoflurane
    Methoxyflurane

» Trichloroethylene
(administration of cocaine prior to or shortly after anesthesia with chloroform, cyclopropane, halothane, or trichloroethylene may increase the risk of ventricular fibrillation or other severe ventricular arrhythmias, especially in patients with pre-existing heart disease, because these anesthetics greatly sensitize the myocardium to the effects of sympathomimetics; great caution and especially careful patient monitoring are recommended if concurrent use is necessary)
(isoflurane, and, to a lesser extent, enflurane or methoxyflurane, may also sensitize the myocardium to the effects of sympathomimetics; caution in concurrent use is recommended)

Antidepressants, tricyclic or
Digitalis glycosides or
» Levodopa or
» Methyldopa
(concurrent use with cocaine may increase the risk of cardiac arrhythmias; if use of cocaine is necessary in patients receiving these medications, it is recommended that cocaine be administered with caution, in reduced dosage, and in conjunction with electrocardiographic monitoring)

Antihypertensives, especially:
» Postganglionic blocking antihypertensive agents, i.e., guanadrel or guanethidine
(cocaine may decrease the antihypertensive effects of these medications; careful monitoring of the patient is recommended)
(postganglionic blocking agents such as guanadrel or guanethidine may potentiate cocaine-induced sympathetic stimulation; concurrent use may increase the risk of hypertension and cardiac arrhythmias)

» Beta-adrenergic blocking agents, possibly including ophthalmic betaxolol, levobunolol, metipranolol or timolol
(cocaine may inhibit the therapeutic effects of systemic beta-adrenergic blocking agents)
(although systemic beta-adrenergic blocking agents are recommended to reduce tachycardia, myocardial ischemia, and/or arrhythmias induced by cocaine [see *Treatment of overdose*], concurrent use of a systemic beta-adrenergic blocking agent with cocaine may increase the risk of hypertension, excessive bradycardia, and possibly heart block, because beta-blockade may leave cocaine's alpha-adrenergic activity unopposed; the risk of these adverse effects may be decreased with labetalol because labetalol also has some alpha-adrenergic blocking activity, although its beta-adrenergic blocking activity predominates; the possibility of adverse effects should also be considered if cocaine is administered to patients receiving ophthalmic beta-adrenergic blocking agents, which are extensively absorbed and cause significant systemic beta-adrenergic blockade)

» Cholinesterase inhibitors, such as:
Antimyasthenics
Cyclophosphamide
Demecarium
Echothiophate
Insecticides, neurotoxic, possibly including large quantities of topical malathion
Isoflurophate
Thiotepa
(inhibition of cholinesterase activity by these agents reduces or slows cocaine metabolism, thereby increasing and/or prolonging its effects and increasing the risk of toxicity; cholinesterase inhibition caused by echothiophate, demecarium, or isoflurophate may persist for weeks or months after the medication has been discontinued)

» CNS stimulation–producing medications, other (see *Appendix II*)
(concurrent use with cocaine may result in excessive CNS stimulation, leading to nervousness, irritability, insomnia, or possibly convulsions or cardiac arrhythmias; close observation is recommended)

» Monoamine oxidase (MAO) inhibitors, including furazolidone, procarbazine, and selegiline
(MAO inhibitors may prolong and intensify the cardiac stimulant and vasopressor effects of cocaine because of release of catecholamines that accumulate in intraneuronal storage sites during MAO inhibitor therapy, resulting in headache, cardiac arrhythmias, vomiting, or sudden and severe hypertensive and/or hyperpyretic crises; cocaine should not be administered during, or within 14 days following, administration of an MAO inhibitor)
(phenelzine also inhibits cholinesterase activity and may reduce or slow cocaine metabolism, thereby increasing and/or prolonging its effects and increasing the risk of toxicity)

Nitrates
(cocaine may reduce the antianginal effects of these medications)
» Sympathomimetics, other, especially:
Dobutamine or
Dopamine or
Epinephrine, topical
(in addition to increasing CNS stimulation, concurrent use may increase the cardiovascular effects of either or both medications and the risk of adverse effects)
(concurrent use of epinephrine with cocaine [especially intranasal application of "cocaine mud", a potentially lethal substance obtained by moistening cocaine crystals or flakes with an epinephrine solution] is not recommended because of the high risk of hypertensive episodes and cardiac arrhythmias; also, concurrent topical use of cocaine and epinephrine is unnecessary because epinephrine does not provide additional local vasoconstriction, slow absorption of cocaine from the mucosa, or prolong cocaine's duration of action)

Thyroid hormones
(concurrent use may increase the effects of either these medications or cocaine; thyroid hormones enhance the risk of coronary insufficiency when sympathomimetic agents are administered to patients with coronary artery disease; dosage adjustment is recommended, although the risk is reduced in euthyroid patients)

**Laboratory value alterations**
The following have been selected on the basis of their potential clinical significance (possible effect in parentheses where appropriate)—not necessarily inclusive (» = major clinical significance):

With physiology/laboratory test values
Blood pressure and
Body temperature and
Glucose, blood, concentrations and
Heart rate
(may be increased; even low doses of cocaine may increase blood pressure by 15 to 20% and heart rate by 30 to 50%, although transient bradycardia may occur initially; the extent to which these values are increased may depend on patient predisposition as well as dosage)

**Medical considerations/Contraindications**
The medical considerations/contraindications included have been selected on the basis of their potential clinical significance (reasons given in parentheses where appropriate)—not necessarily inclusive (» = major clinical significance).

*Risk-benefit should be considered when the following medical problems exist:*
» Cardiovascular disease, especially
» Angina pectoris or
» Myocardial infarction, history of
(risk of severe hypertension, myocardial ischemia, angina, and/or myocardial infarction in patients with these predisposing conditions)
» Cardiac arrhythmias or history of or
» Convulsions, history of
(may be induced or exacerbated by cocaine)
» Cerebrovascular disease
(risk of cerebrovascular accident and subarachnoid hemorrhage)
» Decreased cholinesterase activity, genetic or induced by disease, including carcinoma or hepatic disease; administration of or exposure to cholinesterase inhibitors; or, to a lesser extent, pregnancy
(metabolism of cocaine is decreased or slowed, leading to increased and/or prolonged effects and increased risk of toxicity)
» Hypertension, not optimally controlled or
» Thyrotoxicosis
(cocaine-induced potentiation of endogenous catecholamines is detrimental to patients with these conditions; extreme caution is warranted)
Infection, local, at area of application
(may alter pH at area of application, leading to decrease or loss of local anesthetic effect)
Sensitivity to cocaine, history of
» Tourette's syndrome
(may be exacerbated, probably because of cocaine's dopaminergic activity)
» Traumatized mucosa, severe
(increased risk of systemic toxicity because of enhanced cocaine absorption)

» Caution is also required in elderly, debilitated, or acutely ill patients, who may be especially sensitive to the effects of the medication.

**Patient monitoring**

The following may be especially important in patient monitoring (other tests may be warranted in some patients, depending on condition; » = major clinical significance):

» Blood pressure and
» Cardiac rhythm and
  Core body temperature and
» Heart rate
  (monitoring recommended because of the risk of hypertension, tachycardia, ventricular arrhythmias, and hyperpyrexia; when low doses are administered, tachycardia may initially be preceded by bradycardia caused by central vagal stimulation, although only tachycardia caused by central and peripheral sympathetic stimulation occurs following moderate or high doses)

## Side/Adverse Effects

Note: Many of cocaine's systemic adverse effects are due to excessive sympathetic activity and may be caused by rapid absorption, decreased patient tolerance, or, rarely, hypersensitivity. Toxic reactions are relatively uncommon with appropriate use of usual clinical doses.

The fatal dose of cocaine has been reported to be 1.2 grams. However, patient sensitivity to the effects of the medication is highly variable; adverse effects have been reported with as little as 20 mg.

Acute toxicity may occur very rapidly. Manifestations of systemic cocaine toxicity may occur in 3 stages (early stimulation, advanced stimulation, and depression). Although many of the signs and symptoms of early stimulation would not necessarily require medical intervention under other circumstances, their occurrence following use of cocaine indicates that prompt action is required, because progression from one stage of toxicity to the next may be very rapid.

The following side/adverse effects have been selected on the basis of their potential clinical significance (possible signs and symptoms in parentheses where appropriate)—not necessarily inclusive:

**Those indicating need for medical attention**

Signs and symptoms of systemic toxicity

*Early stimulation*

*Cardiac/cardiovascular effects, including increased blood pressure; increased heart rate; premature ventricular contractions* (irregular heartbeat); *vasoconstriction; chills and fever; CNS effects, including agitation; excitement; nervousness; restlessness; apprehension; irritability; confusion; dizziness or lightheadedness; hallucinations; sudden headache; inability to remain still; mood or mental changes, including elation or euphoria; dysphoria or dysphoric agitation; paranoid ideation or psychosis; preconvulsive movements; talkativeness; generalized tics or twitching of small muscles*—especially of the face, fingers, or feet; *gastrointestinal effects, including abdominal pain; nausea or vomiting; grinding of teeth; increased sweating; rapid breathing; unusually large pupils*—sometimes with bulging of eyes

Note: *Hallucinations* may be auditory, gustatory, olfactory, visual (e.g., "snow lights"), and/or tactile (e.g., formication ["cocaine bugs"], which may induce picking or stroking movements).

*Tachycardia* occurring after low doses of cocaine may initially be preceded by *bradycardia*.

*Advanced stimulation*

*Cardiac arrhythmias, including ventricular arrhythmias such as ventricular tachycardia and fibrillation* (blue discoloration of fingernails, lips, or skin; decreased blood pressure; rapid, irregular, or weak pulse); *CNS hemorrhage; congestive heart failure; convulsions, tonic-clonic*—may progress to status epilepticus; *decreased responsiveness to stimuli; delirium; hyperreflexia; loss of bladder or bowel control; malignant encephalopathy; myocardial ischemia; respiratory and/or cardiac weakness*

*Depression*

*Loss of reflexes; flaccid muscular paralysis; fixed, dilated pupils; loss of consciousness; ashen gray cyanosis; pulmonary edema; cardiac, circulatory, and/or respiratory failure*—may be fatal

**Those indicating need for medical attention only if continuing or bothersome**

Incidence more frequent—following application to oral or nasal mucosa
  *Loss of sense of smell and/or taste*

With repeated intranasal application
  *Rebound hyperemia* (stuffy nose); *rhinitis, chronic* (sneezing or sniffling, continuing)—may lead to chronic sinusitis and increased risk of upper respiratory infections

Note: With repeated or prolonged intranasal use, *ischemic damage to the mucosa* may occur and may lead to *atrophy of the nasal mucosa, necrosis of septal tissue*, and *septal perforation*.

## Overdose

For specific information on the agents used in the management of cocaine overdose, see:
  • *Benzodiazepines (Systemic)* monograph;
  • *Beta-adrenergic Blocking Agents (Systemic)* monograph;
  • *Calcium Channel Blocking Agents (Systemic)* monograph;
  • *Lidocaine (Systemic)* monograph;
  • *Nitrates (Systemic)* monograph;
  • *Nitroprusside (Systemic)* monograph;
  • *Phentolamine (Systemic)* monograph;
  • *Sodium Bicarbonate (Systemic)* monograph; and/or
  • *Thiopental* in *Anesthetics, Barbiturate (Systemic)* monograph.

For more information on the management of overdose or unintentional ingestion, **contact a Poison Control Center** (see *Poison Control Center Listing*).

**Clinical effects of overdose**

The following effects have been selected on the basis of their potential clinical significance (possible signs and symptoms in parentheses where appropriate)—not necessarily inclusive:

Acute
  *Cardiac arrhythmias; cardiovascular depression; convulsions; hypertension; hyperthermia; metabolic acidosis; myocardial ischemia*

**Treatment of overdose**

To decrease absorption—
  Measures to limit absorption in cases of overdosage (with recreational use of cocaine), such as administration of activated charcoal or gastric lavage (if the drug had been ingested orally) or application of a tourniquet (if the drug had been injected), may be of some value if they can be instituted rapidly. However, because severe cocaine toxicity may develop very quickly, *instituting the measures described below for treatment of cocaine-induced toxicity must always take precedence*.

Specific treatment—
  For cardiac arrhythmias—Administering propranolol (1 mg intravenously, repeated at 1-minute intervals as needed up to a total of 6 mg) or other beta-adrenergic blocking agents is recommended to treat tachycardia or other cardiac arrhythmias. However, pure beta-adrenergic blocking agents such as propranolol do not reduce cocaine-induced hypertension and may actually increase the risk of hypertension, bradycardia, and possibly heart block by leaving unopposed cocaine's alpha-adrenergic stimulating activity. Labetalol, which also has some alpha-adrenergic blocking activity (although its beta-adrenergic blocking activity predominates) has been recommended instead. Administration of a pure alpha-adrenergic blocking agent such as phentolamine (5 mg intravenously, repeated every 15 to 20 minutes as needed) may also be required. Lidocaine hydrochloride (50 to 100 mg as a single intravenous injection, followed by infusion at a rate of 2 to 4 mg per minute as needed) or other antiarrhythmics may also be administered. In addition, cardiac massage and/or electrical defibrillation may be required for ventricular fibrillation.

  For cardiovascular depression—Placing the patient in a 30-degree head down (Trendelenburg) position is recommended to increase venous return to the heart. Blood pressure should be maintained with intravenous fluids; administration of vasopressors is dangerous. For severe cardiovascular depression, cardiopulmonary resuscitation may be required, but inotropic agents should be given with great caution.

  For convulsions—If convulsions do not respond to respiratory support, administration of a benzodiazepine such as diazepam (5 to 10 mg intravenously, repeated as needed) or an ultrashort-acting barbiturate such as thiopental or thiamylal (in 50- to 100-mg increments every 2 to 3 minutes, intravenously) is recommended. The fact that these agents, especially the barbiturates, may cause circulatory depression when administered intravenously must be kept in mind. A neuromuscular blocking agent has also been recommended to decrease the muscular manifestations of persistent convulsions; artificial respiration is mandatory if such an agent is used. However, succinylcholine may cause fasciculations and/or malignant hyperthermia, which may cause further problems in these patients. Other neuromuscular blocking agents may be less hazardous.

For hypertension—Administering phentolamine, labetalol, or a vasodilator such as nitroprusside.

For hyperthermia—Applying external cooling measures, such as a cooling blanket, sponging with ice water, and/or using fans.

For metabolic acidosis—Administering bicarbonate.

For myocardial ischemia—Administering nitrates, cardioselective beta-adrenergic blocking agents, and/or calcium-channel blocking agents.

Monitoring—
Monitoring vital signs and core body temperature continuously.

Supportive care—
Securing and maintaining a patent airway, administering 100% oxygen, and instituting assisted or controlled respiration as required. In some patients, endotracheal intubation may be necessary.

Establishing intravenous lines using an isotonic or hypotonic intravenous solution; hypertonic or hyperosmolar solutions should be avoided. All medications must be administered intravenously because cocaine-induced vasoconstriction may prevent absorption following intramuscular administration.

Minimizing all forms of sensory stimulation may be advisable, since these hyperstimulated patients may be agitated and/or paranoid and may become aggressive.

Patients in whom intentional overdose is known or suspected should be referred for psychiatric consultation.

## Patient Consultation

As an aid to patient consultation, refer to *Advice for the Patient, Cocaine (Mucosal-Local)*.

In providing consultation, consider emphasizing the following selected information (» = major clinical significance):

### Before receiving this medication
» Conditions affecting use, especially:
   Sensitivity to cocaine
   Pregnancy—Cocaine crosses the placenta; spontaneous abortions, premature labor, and adverse effects on the fetus or neonate have resulted from cocaine abuse during pregnancy
   Breast-feeding—Cocaine is distributed into breast milk and has caused convulsions, high blood pressure, fast heartbeat, breathing problems, trembling, and unusual irritability in nursing infants
   Use in children—Caution required because of cocaine's toxicity
   Use in the elderly—Increased risk of adverse effects
   Other medications, especially beta-adrenergic blocking agents, guanadrel, guanethidine, levodopa, methyldopa, other CNS stimulants, cholinesterase inhibitors, monoamine oxidase inhibitors, and other sympathomimetics
   Other medical problems, especially cardiovascular, cardiac, or cerebrovascular disease, conditions predisposing to decreased pseudocholinesterase activity, convulsions (history of), hypertension, thyrotoxicosis, Tourette's syndrome, and severely traumatized mucosa

### Proper use of this medication
Proper dosing

### Precautions after receiving this medication
Caution if being tested for possible drug use because cocaine and/or its metabolites may be present in blood and/or urine for several days after administration

### Side/adverse effects
Signs and symptoms of potential side effects, especially abdominal pain; chills; confusion; dizziness or lightheadedness; excitement, nervousness, or restlessness; fast or irregular heartbeat; general feeling of discomfort or illness; hallucinations; headache, sudden; increased sweating; mood or mental changes; and nausea

## General Dosing Information

Safe and effective clinical use of cocaine depends upon careful patient selection, proper dosage, correct administration technique, adequate precautions, and readiness for emergencies. *Resuscitative equipment, trained personnel, oxygen, and other required medications should be immediately available.*

The dosage of cocaine depends on the technique of anesthesia, the area to be anesthetized, the vascularity of the tissues at the application site, and the patient's tolerance. Because of cocaine's toxicity, the lowest dosage that provides adequate anesthesia should be used.

The recommended adult doses are given as a guideline for use in the average adult. *The actual dosage and maximum dosage must be individualized,* based on the age, size, and physical status of the patient and the expected rate of systemic absorption from the administration site. Lower concentrations and/or lower total dosage are recommended for pediatric, geriatric, acutely ill, or debilitated patients.

A standard textbook should be consulted for specific techniques and procedures applicable to the use of mucosal-local anesthetics for individual diagnostic procedures.

Premedication with a benzodiazepine such as diazepam, which has anxiolytic, anticonvulsant, and muscle relaxant properties, may reduce the incidence and/or severity of some cocaine-induced adverse effects.

Tolerance to the effects of cocaine may develop with repeated application.

Repeated use of cocaine may lead to the development of psychological and physical dependence.

### For treatment of adverse effects
Recommended treatment consists of the following:
   • Minimizing all forms of sensory stimulation may be advisable, since these hyperstimulated patients may be agitated and/or paranoid and may become aggressive.
   • Treatment of CNS effects in patients who are not in immediate danger may include administering diazepam (2.5 to 5 mg) or a short-acting barbiturate (50 to 75 mg of amobarbital or secobarbital) for symptoms of CNS stimulation, such as hyperactivity or agitation; chlorpromazine or haloperidolfor paranoia or psychosis; or tricyclic antidepressants(with great caution, because of the risk of cardiac arrhythmias) for mental depression associated with heavy cocaine abuse or withdrawal.

## Mucosal-Local Dosage Forms

### COCAINE HYDROCHLORIDE (CRYSTALS/FLAKES) USP

**Usual adult dose**
Anesthetic-vasoconstrictor (mucosal-local)[1]—
   Topical, to the mucosa, a known (preweighed) quantity being applied via moistened cotton-tipped applicators.

**Usual adult prescribing limits**
400 mg, although the lowest effective dose should be used.

**Usual pediatric dose**
Dosage has not been established.

**Size(s) usually available**
U.S.—
   Available as bulk chemical.
Canada—
   Available as bulk chemical.

**Packaging and storage**
Store below 40 °C (104 °F), preferably between 15 and 30 °C (59 and 86 °F), unless otherwise specified by manufacturer. Store in a well-closed, light-resistant container.

**Note**
Controlled substance in both the U.S. and Canada.

### COCAINE HYDROCHLORIDE TABLETS FOR TOPICAL SOLUTION USP

**Usual adult dose**
Anesthetic-vasoconstrictor (mucosal-local)—
   Topical, to the mucosa, as a 1 to 4% solution. The medication may be applied by means of cotton applicators, packs, or spray, or by instillation.Concentrations greater than 4% are generally not recommended because of difficulty in controlling dosage and the increased risk of toxic reactions.

**Usual adult prescribing limits**
400 mg, although the lowest effective dose should be used.

**Usual pediatric dose**
Children up to 6 years of age—Use is not recommended.
Children 6 years of age and older—Dosage must be individualized by the physician.

**Strength(s) usually available**
U.S.—
   135 mg (Rx) [GENERIC (lactose)].
Canada—
   Not commercially available.

Note: This product is not to be dispensed directly to the patient.

**Packaging and storage**
Store below 40 °C (104 °F), preferably between 15 and 30 °C (59 and 86 °F), unless otherwise specified by manufacturer. Store in a well-closed, light-resistant container.

**Preparation of dosage form**
To prepare a 4% solution—Dissolve 1 tablet in 3.4 mL of distilled water.

**Incompatibilities**
Solutions of cocaine hydrochloride are incompatible with alkali and with alkaloidal precipitants.

**Note**
Controlled substance in the U.S.

### COCAINE HYDROCHLORIDE TOPICAL SOLUTION

**Usual adult dose**
Anesthetic-vasoconstrictor (mucosal-local)—
  Topical, to the mucosa, as a 1 to 4% solution. The medication may be applied by means of cotton applicators, packs, or spray, or by instillation. Concentrations greater than 4% are generally not recommended because of the difficulty in controlling dosage and the increased risk of toxic reactions.

**Usual adult prescribing limits**
400 mg, although the lowest effective dose should be used.

**Usual pediatric dose**
Children up to 6 years of age—Use is not recommended.
Children 6 years of age and older—Dosage must be individualized by the physician.

**Strength(s) usually available**
U.S.—
  4% (40 mg per mL) (Rx) [GENERIC].
  4% (40 mg per mL) (Rx) [GENERIC (sterile)].
  10% (100 mg per mL) (Rx) [GENERIC].
  10% (100 mg per mL) (Rx) [GENERIC (sterile)].
Canada—
  Not commercially available. Compounding (using cocaine hydrochloride crystals/flakes) is required for preparation of this dosage form.

Note: This product is not to be dispensed directly to the patient.

**Packaging and storage**
Store between 15 and 30 °C (59 and 86 °F), unless otherwise specified by manufacturer.

**Stability**
Ethylene oxide is recommended for sterilization of the external surface of glass bottles containing the solution. Do not steam autoclave.

**Incompatibilities**
Solutions of cocaine hydrochloride are incompatible with alkali and with alkaloidal precipitants.

**Note**
Controlled substance in the U.S.

### COCAINE HYDROCHLORIDE VISCOUS TOPICAL SOLUTION

**Usual adult dose**
Anesthetic-vasoconstrictor (mucosal-local)—
  Topical, to the mucosa, as a 1 to 4% solution. The medication may be applied by means of cotton applicators or packs, or by instillation. Concentrations greater than 4% are generally not recommended because of the difficulty in controlling dosage and the increased risk of toxic reactions.

**Usual adult prescribing limits**
400 mg, although the lowest effective dose should be used.

**Usual pediatric dose**
Children up to 6 years of age—Use is not recommended.
Children 6 years of age and older—Dosage must be individualized by the physician.

**Strength(s) usually available**
U.S.—
  4% (40 mg per mL) (Rx) [GENERIC].
  10% (100 mg per mL) (Rx) [GENERIC].
Canada—
  Not commercially available.

Note: This product is not to be dispensed directly to the patient.

**Packaging and storage**
Store between 15 and 30 °C (59 and 86 °F), unless otherwise specified by manufacturer.

**Stability**
Ethylene oxide is recommended for sterilization of the external surface of glass bottles containing the solution. Do not steam autoclave.

**Incompatibilities**
Solutions of cocaine hydrochloride are incompatible with alkali and with alkaloidal precipitants.

**Note**
Controlled substance in the U.S.

[1]Not included in Canadian product labeling.

Revised: 08/08/92
Interim revision: 08/12/97

---

**CODEINE**—See *Opioid (Narcotic) Analgesics (Systemic)*

---

# COLCHICINE Systemic

VA CLASSIFICATION (Primary): MS400
Note: For a listing of dosage forms and brand names by country availability, see *Dosage Forms* section(s).

## Category
Anti-inflammatory; antigout agent; familial Mediterranean fever suppressant; calcium pyrophosphate deposition disease suppressant; amyloidosis suppressant.

## Indications
Note: Bracketed information in the *Indications* section refers to uses that are not included in U.S. product labeling.

Note: The toxicity and narrow margin of safety of therapeutic doses of colchicine (e.g., doses required to relieve an acute attack of gout or calcium pyrophosphate deposition disease) must be carefully considered before treatment is initiated, especially when the medication is to be administered intravenously. However, long-term administration of prophylactic doses for chronic gout or other chronic conditions responsive to such treatment is relatively unlikely to cause serious toxicity in patients with normal renal and hepatic function.

### Accepted
Gouty arthritis, chronic (treatment) or
Gouty arthritis, acute (prophylaxis and treatment)—Colchicine is indicated to reduce the frequency and severity of acute attacks of gouty arthritis in patients with chronic gout. Complete remission of such attacks may occur in some patients. Prophylactic administration of colchicine may be especially important during the first several months of treatment with an antihyperuricemic agent (allopurinol, probenecid, or sulfinpyrazone) because the frequency of acute attacks may be increased when such therapy is initiated.

Although colchicine is also indicated to relieve the pain and inflammation of acute attacks of gouty arthritis, it has generally been replaced by less toxic medications for this purpose. Nonsteroidal anti-inflammatory drugs (NSAIDs) or corticosteroids (preferably via intrasynovial injection) are recommended for relief of an acute attack. Therapeutic doses of colchicine should be reserved for patients in whom these other agents are contraindicated or ineffective.

Intravenous administration of colchicine may be considered for treatment of acute attacks of gouty arthritis when oral administration is ineffective, gastrointestinal side effects limit administration of effective oral doses, or an especially rapid response is needed. Although the risk of gastrointestinal toxicity is considerably lower with intravenous administration than with oral administration, the risk of other forms of toxicity is very high, especially in patients with renal and/or hepatic function impairment; fatalities have been reported. It is recommended that the medication be administered intravenously with caution, in low doses, and only to carefully selected patients, if at all.

[Mediterranean fever, familial (prophylaxis and treatment)]—Colchicine is indicated to reduce the frequency and severity of acute attacks of familial Mediterranean fever (familial recurrent polyserositis). Complete remission of such attacks may occur in some patients.

Prophylactic use of colchicine prevents amyloidosis and amyloidosis-induced renal failure in patients with familial Mediterranean fever, including patients whose acute attacks are not suppressed by such treatment. Colchicine therapy must be started before nephrotic syndrome or uremia develops; initiation of treatment after either of these conditions is present will not prevent further deterioration of renal function. However, after renal transplantation, prophylactic colchicine prevents amyloid deposition and resultant tissue damage in the transplanted kidney. Prophylactic use of colchicine is therefore recommended for all patients with familial Mediterranean fever, even when frequent, severe attacks continue to occur despite colchicine administration.

Although colchicine may also be effective in aborting an acute attack of febrile polyserositis if taken at the earliest sign of an attack, it will not relieve or shorten a severe attack that is already in progress.

[Calcium pyrophosphate deposition disease, acute (prophylaxis and treatment)][1]—Colchicine is used for the symptomatic relief of acute attacks of calcium pyrophosphate deposition disease (chondrocalcinosis articularis; pseudogout; synovitis, crystal-induced). Intravenous administration of the medication is reported to be more consistently effective than oral administration for relief of an acute attack. However, the high risk of toxicity associated with intravenous administration of colchicine must be considered. Prophylactic use of oral colchicine may prevent repeat acute attacks.

[Arthritis, sarcoid (treatment)][1]—Colchicine is used to relieve acute arthritic symptoms associated with sarcoidosis.

[Amyloidosis (treatment)][1]—Colchicine is indicated to decrease amyloid deposition and resultant tissue damage in patients with primary amyloidosis or amyloidosis secondary to conditions such as psoriatic arthritis, ankylosing spondylitis, or familial Mediterranean fever. Colchicine has been used together with melphalan and prednisone for the treatment of primary amyloidosis.

[Behçet's syndrome (treatment)][1]—Colchicine is used in the treatment of patients with Behçet's syndrome. It relieves or prevents erythema nodosum and arthralgias and may also reduce the frequency or severity of oral and/or genital ulcerations in some patients. However, colchicine does not reduce the frequency or severity of ocular lesions associated with this disease or improve visual acuity in affected patients.

[Cirrhosis, biliary (treatment)][1]—Colchicine is used in the treatment of primary biliary cirrhosis. Biochemical indicators of disease activity (serum albumin, bilirubin, alkaline phosphatase, cholesterol, and aminotransferases) improve during treatment. Although colchicine may retard the development of fibrosis and hepatic failure in patients with biliary cirrhosis, it does not relieve symptoms, prevent or reverse histological changes characteristic of the disease, or decrease the need for hepatic transplantation. In a few studies colchicine-treated patients survived significantly longer than control patients. Colchicine may provide additional benefit when used concurrently with ursodiol for this indication. However, colchicine clearance is substantially reduced in patients with alcoholic cirrhosis. Caution and careful attention to dosage are recommended to prevent accumulation and toxicity if colchicine is administered to these patients.

[Pericarditis, recurrent (treatment)][1]—Limited data indicate that colchicine may be useful for preventing acute attacks of pericarditis that recur despite treatment with NSAIDs and/or corticosteroids. Colchicine has permitted withdrawal of corticosteroid therapy in some patients with this condition.

---

[1]Not included in Canadian product labeling.

## Pharmacology/Pharmacokinetics

### Physicochemical characteristics
Source—Colchicine is the active alkaloidal principle derived from various species of *Colchicum*.
Molecular weight—399.44.
pKa—1.7 and 12.4.

### Mechanism of action/Effect
Anti-inflammatory and—
Antigout agent:
The precise mechanism of action has not been completely established. In patients with gout, colchicine apparently interrupts the cycle of monosodium urate crystal deposition in joint tissues and the resultant inflammatory response that initiates and sustains an acute attack. Colchicine decreases leukocyte chemotaxis and phagocytosis and inhibits the formation and release of a chemotactic glycoprotein that is produced during phagocytosis of urate crystals. Colchicine also inhibits urate crystal deposition, which is enhanced by a low pH in the tissues, probably by inhibiting oxidation of glucose and subsequent lactic acid production in leukocytes. Colchicine has no analgesic or antihyperuricemic activity.

Note: Colchicine inhibits microtubule assembly in various cells, including leukocytes, probably by binding to and interfering with polymerization of the microtubule subunit tubulin. Although some studies have found that this action probably does not contribute significantly to colchicine's antigout action, a recent *in vitro* study has shown that it may be at least partially involved.

Colchicine's effect on microtubule assembly and/or leukocyte function may be involved in the medication's efficacy in conditions other than gout. In patients with biliary cirrhosis, interference with microtubule formation may inhibit collagen production, thereby retarding the development of hepatic fibrosis. Colchicine may also increase degradation of collagen by stimulating production of collagenase. Also, colchicine corrects some of the abnormalities of lymphocyte and monocyte function that have been identified in patients with active biliary cirrhosis. In addition, colchicine has been found to reverse abnormalities in neutrophil activity that are present in patients with Behçet's disease, i.e., increased migration and reduced superoxide scavenging activity.

Familial Mediterranean fever suppressant and—
Amyloidosis suppressant:
The mechanism by which colchicine suppresses acute attacks of febrile polyserositis in patients with familial Mediterranean fever has not been determined, but it may differ from the mechanism responsible for suppression of amyloidosis in patients with this disease. Colchicine inhibits secretion of serum amyloid A in patients with familial Mediterranean fever. It has also been suggested that colchicine may interfere with polymerization of amyloid subunits into mature amyloid fibrils.

### Other actions/effects
By inhibiting microtubule assembly, colchicine interferes with mitotic spindle formation, thereby arresting mitosis in metaphase.
Colchicine decreases body temperature, depresses the respiratory center, constricts blood vessels, and causes hypertension via central vasomotor stimulation.

### Absorption
Colchicine is rapidly absorbed after oral administration, probably from the jejunum and ileum. However, the rate and extent of absorption are variable, depending on the tablet dissolution rate; variability in gastric emptying, intestinal motility, and pH at the absorption site; and the extent to which colchicine is bound to microtubules in gastrointestinal mucosal cells.

### Distribution
Colchicine is rapidly distributed to peripheral leukocytes. Concentrations in these cells may exceed those in plasma. The medication can be detected in leukocytes for 9 to 10 days following administration of a single dose. Colchicine also concentrates in the kidneys, liver, and spleen. Accumulation in these tissues may lead to toxicity. Colchicine is distributed into breast milk; peak concentrations of 1.2 to 2.5 nanograms per mL (< 0.001 micromole per liter) have been measured 40 to 50 minutes after administration of a 0.6-mg dose to a patient receiving long-term therapy with 0.6 mg twice a day.

### Protein binding
In plasma—Low to moderate (30 to 50%).

### Biotransformation
Probably hepatic. Although colchicine metabolites have not been identified in humans, metabolism by mammalian hepatic microsomes has been demonstrated *in vitro*.

### Half-life
Distribution—3 to 5 minutes
Elimination—Approximately 1 hour in healthy subjects, although a study with an extended sampling time reported mean terminal elimination half-life values of approximately 9 to 10.5 hours. Other studies have reported half-life values of approximately 2 hours in patients with alcoholic cirrhosis and approximately 2.5 hours in patients with familial Mediterranean fever.

### Onset of action
Acute gouty arthritis (following first dose)—
Intravenous: Within 6 to 12 hours
Oral: Within 12 hours

### Time to peak concentration
Oral—0.5 to 2 hours

### Time to peak effect
Acute gouty arthritis—
  Relief of pain and inflammation: 24 to 48 hours following the first oral dose.
  Relief of swelling: May require several days.

### Elimination
Primarily biliary, with enterohepatic recirculation; 10 to 20% renal. Renal elimination may be increased in patients with hepatic disease. Because of the high degree of tissue uptake, only 10% of a single dose is eliminated within 24 hours; elimination of colchicine from the body may continue for 10 days or more after cessation of administration. Also, elimination is slower in patients with biliary disease; in one study mean clearance rates of 10.65 mL per minute per kg of body weight (mL/min/kg) and 4.22 mL/min/kg were measured in healthy control subjects and in patients with alcoholic cirrhosis, respectively.

In dialysis—Because of the high degree of tissue binding, colchicine is not dialyzable.

## Precautions to Consider

### Pregnancy/Reproduction
Fertility—Colchicine arrests cell division in animals and plants. Although colchicine has been reported to cause reversible azoospermia and fertility problems in male patients receiving long-term treatment with prophylactic doses, several studies in patients receiving such treatment have shown no significant reproductive difficulties, abnormalities in sperm counts, or alterations in testosterone, prolactin, luteinizing hormone, or follicle-stimulating hormone concentrations. Administration of colchicine does not increase, and may actually reduce, the risk of serious fertility problems in women with familial Mediterranean fever, who are subject to formation of fibrous adhesions, ovulatory disturbances, and, consequently, sterility.

Pregnancy—Controlled studies in pregnant women have not been done, but colchicine has been used prior to and throughout pregnancy by patients receiving long-term prophylaxis for familial Mediterranean fever. Although several miscarriages have been reported, the miscarriage rate in untreated women with this disease is high. A large majority of the pregnancies in female patients and wives of male patients receiving colchicine produced healthy, normal, full-term infants. However, a group of investigators reported 2 cases of trisomy 21 (in 91 pregnancies) and recommend that amniocentesis be performed when either parent is receiving colchicine.

Colchicine has been shown to be teratogenic in mice given doses of 0.5 mg per kg of body weight (mg/kg) or more, causing microtia, exencephaly, microphthalmia, anophthalmia, skeletal malformations, gastrochisis, abnormalities of the liver and stomach, dextrocardia, missing pulmonary lobe, and cleft palate. Colchicine has also produced fetotoxic and teratogenic effects in hamsters given 10 mg/kg. Administration to hamsters on Day 8 of pregnancy resulted in fatalities in 50% of the fetuses and congenital malformations including microphthalmia, anophthalmia, exencephaly, rib fusions and other skeletal anomalies, and umbilical hernias in a large number of the surviving fetuses. In other studies, colchicine was embryotoxic in rabbits and cattle, but not monkeys. Studies in rats produced contradictory results.

FDA Pregnancy Category D.

### Breast-feeding
Colchicine is distributed into breast milk; peak concentrations of 1.2 to 2.5 nanograms per mL (< 0.001 micromole per liter) have been measured 40 to 50 minutes after administration of a 0.6-mg dose to a patient receiving long-term therapy with 0.6 mg twice a day. No adverse effects were apparent in the breast-fed infant during the first 6 months of life.

### Pediatrics
For gouty arthritis—Appropriate studies on the relationship of age to the effects of colchicine have not been performed in the pediatric population (in whom gouty arthritis rarely if ever occurs). Safety and efficacy for this indication have not been established.

For familial Mediterranean fever—Studies in pediatric patients 3 years of age and older receiving long-term prophylactic treatment have not demonstrated pediatrics-specific problems that would limit the usefulness of colchicine for this indication in children.

### Geriatrics
Geriatric patients, even those with normal renal and hepatic function, may be more susceptible to cumulative toxicity with colchicine. Also, elderly patients are more likely to have age-related renal function impairment, which increases the risk of myopathy and other toxic effects in patients receiving colchicine. Caution and careful attention to dosage are recommended.

### Dental
The leukopenic and thrombocytopenic effects of colchicine may result in an increased incidence of microbial infection, delayed healing, and gingival bleeding. If leukopenia or thrombocytopenia occurs, dental work should be deferred until blood counts have returned to normal and patients should be instructed in proper oral hygiene, including caution in use of regular toothbrushes, dental floss, and toothpicks.

### Drug interactions and/or related problems
The following drug interactions and/or related problems have been selected on the basis of their potential clinical significance (possible mechanism in parentheses where appropriate)—not necessarily inclusive (» = major clinical significance):

Note: Combinations containing any of the following medications, depending on the amount present, may also interact with this medication.

In addition to the interactions listed below, the possibility should be considered that colchicine, because of its potential for causing gastrointestinal hemorrhage, thrombocytopenia (with chronic use), and coagulation defects including disseminated intravascular coagulation (with an overdose), may cause increased risk to patients receiving other medications that may impair blood clotting or cause hemorrhage. Such medications may include anticoagulants (coumarin- or indandione-derivative) or other hypoprothrombinemia-inducing medications; heparin; thrombolytic agents; platelet aggregation inhibitors; other thrombocytopenia-inducing medications; and other medications having significant potential for causing gastrointestinal ulceration or hemorrhage.

Alcohol
  (concurrent use with orally administered colchicine increases the risk of gastrointestinal toxicity, especially in alcoholics; also, alcohol increases blood uric acid concentrations and may decrease the efficacy of prophylactic gout therapy)

Anti-inflammatory drugs, nonsteroidal (NSAIDs), especially
» Phenylbutazone
  (concurrent use of phenylbutazone with colchicine may increase the risk of leukopenia, thrombocytopenia, or bone marrow depression)
  (concurrent use of any NSAID with colchicine may increase the risk of gastrointestinal ulceration or hemorrhage; also, NSAID-induced inhibition of platelet aggregation may increase the risk of bleeding in areas other than the gastrointestinal tract should colchicine-induced thrombocytopenia or clotting defects [with overdose] also occur)

Antineoplastic agents, rapidly cytolytic
  (these medications may increase serum uric acid concentrations and decrease the efficacy of prophylactic gout therapy)

Blood dyscrasia–causing medications (See *Appendix II*)
  (the leukopenic and/or thrombocytopenic effects of colchicine may be intensified with concurrent or recent therapy if these medications cause the same effects; blood counts should be monitored if concurrent or sequential use cannot be avoided)

» Bone marrow depressants, other (See *Appendix II*) or
Radiation therapy
  (additive bone marrow depression may occur; dosage reductions may be required when 2 or more bone marrow depressants, including radiation, are used concurrently or consecutively)

Vitamin $B_{12}$
  (absorption of this vitamin may be impaired by chronic administration or high doses of colchicine; requirement may be increased)

### Laboratory value alterations
The following have been selected on the basis of their potential clinical significance (possible effect in parentheses where appropriate)—not necessarily inclusive (» = major clinical significance):

With diagnostic test results
  Hemoglobin, in urine, or
  Red blood cells (RBC), in urine
    (colchicine may cause false-positive test results)

  17-Hydroxycorticosteroid determinations, in urine
    (interference may occur when the Reddy, Jenkins, and Thorn procedure is used)

With physiology/laboratory test values
  Alkaline phosphatase, serum and
  Aspartate aminotransferase (AST [SGOT]), serum
    (values may be increased)
  Platelet count
    (may be decreased)

**Medical considerations/Contraindications**
The medical considerations/contraindications included have been selected on the basis of their potential clinical significance (reasons given in parentheses where appropriate)—not necessarily inclusive (» = major clinical significance).

*Except under special circumstances, this medication should not be used when the following medical problems exist:*
» Hepatic and renal disease, concurrent
(risk of toxicity is very high, especially with intravenous administration)
» Renal function impairment, severe
(high risk of myopathy and other forms of toxicity; use in patients with severe renal function impairment [i.e., creatinine clearance 10 mL per minute (0.17 mL per second) or less] is not recommended)

*For intravenous administration only*
» Hepatic function impairment, severe
(intravenous administration is not recommended because of the high risk of impaired elimination and resultant toxicity)
» Leukopenia
(may be exacerbated; intravenous administration is not recommended)

*Risk-benefit should be considered when the following medical problems exist:*
Alcoholism, active
(increased risk of gastrointestinal toxicity with oral administration; parenteral administration is preferred; however, it is recommended that hepatic and renal function, which may be impaired in alcoholics, be assessed prior to initiation of therapy in these patients)
» Blood dyscrasias
(may be exacerbated)
» Cardiac disorders or
» Hepatic function impairment or
» Renal function impairment
(increased risk of cumulative toxicity, with the risk increasing as the severity of impairment increases; colchicine should be given with caution, with the dose being reduced and/or the intervals between doses being increased; it has been recommended that half of the usual dose be administered to patients with creatinine clearances of 50 mL per minute [0.83 mL per second] or less)
» Gastrointestinal disorders
(the risk of colchicine-induced damage to gastrointestinal tissues may be increased; also, colchicine's gastrointestinal toxicity may be particularly hazardous to patients with these conditions)
Sensitivity to colchicine, history of

Caution is also advised in administration to geriatric or debilitated patients, who may be more susceptible to cumulative toxicity.

**Patient monitoring**
The following may be especially important in patient monitoring (other tests may be warranted in some patients, depending on condition; » = major clinical significance):
Complete blood counts
(recommended at periodic intervals during long-term treatment because bone marrow depression with agranulocytosis, thrombocytopenia, or aplastic anemia may occur)

## Side/Adverse Effects

Note: There is no clear separation of nontoxic, toxic, and lethal doses of colchicine. Various sources report lethal doses ranging between 20 and 65 mg, although considerably lower doses may be fatal, especially in patients with renal and/or hepatic function impairment and with intravenous administration. Fatalities have occurred after ingestion of single doses as low as 7 mg or intravenous administration of cumulative doses of only 5 mg.

The following side/adverse effects have been selected on the basis of their potential clinical significance (possible signs and symptoms in parentheses where appropriate)—not necessarily inclusive:

**Those indicating need for medical attention**
Incidence rare
*Hypersensitivity reactions including dermatoses* (skin rash, hives); *and angioedema* (large, hive-like swellings on face, eyelids, mouth, lips, and/or tongue)
Note: Skin rash not associated with hypersensitivity may occur, especially with long-term treatment in patients with renal or hepatic function impairment.

*With intravenous administration*
*Cardiac arrhythmias*—with too-rapid administration; *localized reactions such as irritation, inflammation, or thrombophlebitis; median nerve neuritis in injected arm* (pain; tenderness; feeling of burning,"crawling," or tingling in the skin over the affected nerve); *or necrosis of the skin and soft tissues* (peeling of skin)—if extravasation occurs

*With prolonged or long-term use*
*Bone marrow depression with agranulocytosis* (fever with or without chills; sores, ulcers, or white spots on lips or in mouth; sore throat); *aplastic anemia* (unusual tiredness or weakness; headache; difficulty in breathing, exertional); *and thrombocytopenia* (usually asymptomatic; rarely, unusual bleeding or bruising; black, tarry stools; blood in urine or stools; pinpoint red spots on skin); *myopathy* (muscle weakness); *neuropathy* (mild numbness in fingers or toes)
Note: Myopathy is more likely to occur in patients with impaired renal or hepatic function who are receiving long-term treatment with prophylactic doses of colchicine. This condition is characterized by proximal muscle weakness, spontaneous activity in the electromyelogram, and elevated creatine kinase values. Because these findings are also present in patients with polymyositis, a muscle biopsy may be necessary to differentiate between the 2 conditions.

**Those indicating need for medical attention only if they continue or are bothersome**
Incidence more frequent (up to 80%) with therapeutic doses of oral colchicine; rare with intravenous administration
*Gastrointestinal toxicity* (diarrhea; nausea or vomiting; stomach pain)—early symptoms
Incidence less frequent
*Loss of appetite*
With long-term use or following recovery from severe toxicity
*Loss of hair*
Note: Hair loss may start to occur as soon as 2 to 3 weeks after initiation of long-term therapy; the risk is dose-dependent. Regrowth usually begins 3 to 12 weeks after discontinuation of the medication.

## Overdose

For specific information on the agents used in the management of colchicine overdose, see:
- Atropine in *Anticholinergics/Antispasmodics (Systemic)* monograph;
- *Benzodiazepines (Systemic)* monograph;
- *Charcoal, Activated (Oral-Local)* monograph;
- *Opioid (Narcotic) Analgesics (Systemic)* monograph; and/or
- *Vitamin K (Systemic)* monograph.

For more information on the management of overdose or unintentional ingestion, **contact a Poison Control Center** (see *Poison Control Center Listing*).

**Clinical effects of overdose**
The following effects have been selected on the basis of their potential clinical significance (possible signs and symptoms in parentheses where appropriate)—not necessarily inclusive:

Acute—usually begins within 24 to 72 hours after an acute overdose
*Fever*—may be the first sign of this stage and may be associated with septicemia; *cerebral edema; CNS toxicity*; (ascending paralysis of the CNS; convulsions; delirium) *multiple organ failure caused by tissue damage, including bone marrow hypoplasia*; (agranulocytosis or leukopenia; thrombocytopenia and disseminated intravascular coagulation or other coagulation abnormalities) *hepatocellular damage, possibly with necrosis muscle damage, including rhabdomyolysis*; (myoglobinuria; severe muscle weakness or paralysis) *or necrosis, possibly resulting in adult respiratory distress syndrome or other forms of respiratory distress*; (fast, shallow breathing) *pulmonary edema, and hypoxia, and/or myocardial injury*; (ST segment elevation in electrocardiogram; decreased cardiac contractility, creatine kinase elevation, hemorrhages and microinfarctions in the myocardium) *paralytic ileus renal damage*; (with hematuria; and oliguric renal failure)
Note: After a cumulative overdose has been administered intravenously, symptoms associated with *bone marrow depression* may be the first indications of toxicity. In some patients, *disseminated intravascular coagulation* may be the first hemato-

logic sign of toxicity, with the most severe coagulopathy occurring about 25 hours following administration of a large overdose.

*Fluid and electrolyte disturbances* often occur in colchicine toxicity. *Hypovolemia* may lead to *hypokalemia, hyponatremia*, and *metabolic acidosis*. Also, *hypocalcemia, hypokalemia, hypophosphatemia*, and/or *metabolic acidosis* may occur in association with *renal damage*.

Fatalities may result from *shock, respiratory or cardiac arrest*, or *rapidly progressive multiple organ failure*.

Chronic—may occur several hours after an acute overdose
**Burning feeling in the throat or skin; gastrointestinal toxicity** (burning feeling in the stomach; severe abdominal pain; diarrhea; nausea, and/or vomiting); ***sloughing of the gastrointestinal mucosa and/or hemorrhagic gastroenteritis*** (bloody diarrhea)—with oral ingestion only; ***vascular damage***

Note: Early *gastrointestinal symptoms* generally do not occur in overdosage caused by intravenous administration.

*Vascular damage* may lead to *fluid extravasation* which, together with fluid losses caused by severe *diarrhea* and *vomiting*, may cause profound dehydration, hypotension, and shock. Also, *septicemia* secondary to severe intestinal damage may result in *septic shock*.

Chronic—generally begins about 10 days after an acute overdose
**Alopecia** (hair loss)—reversible; ***rebound leukocytosis; stomatitis*** (sores, ulcers, or white spots on lips or in mouth)

**Treatment of overdose**
For early signs of overdose (gastrointestinal symptoms)—
Immediate discontinuation of colchicine administration (when used for short-term relief of an acute attack) or reducing the dose (when used prophylactically).
Specific treatment—Use of morphine or atropine for stomach pain.
Use of an opioid or other antidiarrheal agents for diarrhea.
For irritation caused by extravasation: Applying heat or cold to the affected area and administering analgesics.
For severe overdose—
To decrease absorption—May include removing unabsorbed medication (if taken orally) via gastric lavage and/or administration of activated charcoal. Because of colchicine's extensive biliary elimination and enterohepatic recirculation, repeated doses of activated charcoal are recommended to bind absorbed colchicine that re-enters the intestinal tract, which interrupts enterohepatic recirculation and hastens elimination.
To enhance elimination—Due to colchicine's high degree of uptake and binding in various tissues, forced diuresis, peritoneal dialysis, hemodialysis, charcoal hemoperfusion, or exchange transfusion cannot be expected to remove significant quantities of the medication from the body.
Specific treatment—
For treatment of convulsions caused by overdose:
Administering an anticonvulsant. A benzodiazepine, such as diazepam, may be administered. Since intravenously administered benzodiazepines may cause respiratory and circulatory depression, especially when administered rapidly, and respiratory distress and shock are also potential consequences of colchicine overdose, medications and equipment needed for support of respiration and for resuscitation must be immediately available.
For bone marrow suppression and resultant coagulation defects:
Vitamin $K_1$, fresh frozen plasma, platelets, and/or red blood cells may be administered as needed.
Note: One patient with colchicine induced aplastic anemia has been successfully treated with a single 300-mg subcutaneous dose of granulocyte colony-stimulating factor
For fever, leukopenia, and/or sepsis:
Use of broad-spectrum antibiotics.
Monitoring— May include monitoring hemodynamic, cardiac, and respiratory status and blood electrolytes. Prolonged observation is recommended because the most severe toxic effects generally do not appear until 24 hours or more after ingestion of an acute overdose.
Supportive care—
May include correcting dehydration via fluid replacement and instituting other measures to prevent or treat shock, including administration of a vasopressor, if necessary.
Correcting electrolyte imbalances and metabolic acidosis.
For respiratory distress, securing and maintaining a patent airway, administering oxygen, and instituting assisted or controlled respiration as needed. Endotracheal intubation may be required.

## Patient Consultation

As an aid to patient consultation, refer to *Advice for the Patient, Colchicine (Systemic)*.
In providing consultation, consider emphasizing the following selected information (» = major clinical significance):

**Before using this medication**
» Conditions affecting use, especially:
Sensitivity to colchicine
Use in the elderly—Increased susceptibility to cumulative toxicity
Other medications, especially other bone marrow depressants or radiation therapy
Other medical problems, especially blood dyscrasias, severe cardiac disorders, gastrointestinal disorders, renal function impairment, or hepatic function impairment

**Proper use of this medication**
» Importance of not taking more medication than prescribed
*For prophylactic use*
Compliance with therapy
Not using additional colchicine to relieve an acute gout attack that occurs during prophylactic therapy, unless otherwise directed by physician; using alternative treatment as prescribed
*For intermittent use to relieve acute attack*
Starting medication at earliest sign of attack
» Stopping medication when pain is relieved; at first sign of diarrhea, nausea or vomiting, or stomach pain; or when maximum dosage is reached (even if symptoms are not relieved)
Noting total quantity of colchicine taken before gastrointestinal symptoms occur and, in subsequent attacks, stopping treatment before this cumulative dose has been reached
» Not taking additional colchicine for 3 days after using therapeutic oral doses to relieve an acute attack or for 7 days after receiving intravenous colchicine
» Continuing other gout medication (if applicable) while taking colchicine
» Proper dosing
Missed dose: If on fixed-dosage chronic therapy—Taking as soon as possible; not taking if almost time for next dose; not doubling doses
» Proper storage

**Precautions while using this medication**
Regular visits to physician to check progress and possibly to be tested for adverse effects during long-term therapy
» Possibility that large quantities of alcohol may increase the risk of gastrointestinal toxicity; also, alcohol may increase uric acid concentrations and thereby decrease the effectiveness of medication when used for gout
Not discontinuing prophylactic treatment without first consulting physician if acute attacks continue to occur

**Side/adverse effects**
» Checking with physician if diarrhea, nausea, vomiting, or stomach pain occurs and continues for more than 3 hours after medication is discontinued
» Checking with physician immediately if symptoms of angioedema, bone marrow depression, or overdose occur
Signs and symptoms of other potential side effects, especially skin rash or hives, localized reactions to extravasation after intravenous administration, myopathy, and neuropathy

## General Dosing Information

Colchicine's toxicity and narrow margin of safety must be considered before therapeutic doses of the medication are administered, especially intravenously. Fatalities have occurred after ingestion of single doses as low as 7 mg or intravenous administration of cumulative doses of 5 mg.

If colchicine is used to relieve an acute attack of gout or to abort an acute attack of familial Mediterranean fever, therapy should be instituted at the first sign of the attack. Delay in starting treatment reduces the medication's effectiveness.

A reduction in the size of individual doses, an increase in the interval between doses, or a reduction in the total daily dosage may be necessary in patients with renal or hepatic function impairment. Specifically, it is recommended that dosage be reduced by half (for prophylactic use, limited to no more than 600 mcg [0.6 mg] per day, orally) if the patient's creatinine clearance is 50 mL per minute (0.83 mL per second) or less and that the medication not be used at all if the patient's creatinine clearance is 10 mL per minute (0.17 mL per second) or less.

Oral administration of colchicine is preferable for prophylactic treatment of recurrent or chronic gout; intravenous administration should be reserved for patients who are temporarily unable to take medications orally.

**The risk of colchicine-induced toxicity depends on the total dose given over a period of time, as well as on the size of single doses, especially with intravenous administration.** The following measures are recommended to reduce the risk of cumulative toxicity:

When therapeutic doses of colchicine are given for relief of an acute attack, **the oral and intravenous routes of administration should not be used concurrently or sequentially. Additional colchicine should not be administered for at least 3 days after a course of oral treatment or for at least 7 days (21 days for geriatric patients) after a course of intravenous treatment.**

Patients who are receiving prophylactic doses of colchicine should not increase the dose to therapeutic levels if an acute attack of gout occurs. An alternative agent (e.g., a nonsteroidal anti-inflammatory drug [NSAID] or a corticosteroid, preferably via intrasynovial injection) should be used instead of additional colchicine.

Maximum dosage should be reduced if intravenous administration of colchicine cannot be avoided in geriatric patients and/or patients who are receiving prophylactic doses of colchicine.

Desensitization has been successfully accomplished in several patients with familial Mediterranean fever who were unable to tolerate prophylactic doses of colchicine. The regimen used in a patient in whom adverse effects occurred with 1 mg per day of colchicine consisted of administering 1 mcg (0.001 mg) diluted in sodium chloride solution on the first day, doubling the dose each day until the tenth day, when 500 mcg (0.5 mg) was given, then increasing the dose to 750 mcg (0.75 mg) per day after 3 months and to 1 mg per day after another 3 months.

**For oral dosage forms only**
Treatment with therapeutic doses of colchicine should be discontinued immediately, even if symptoms of the acute attack have not been relieved, when gastrointestinal symptoms (abdominal pain, diarrhea, nausea, or vomiting) occur. The patient should be instructed to note the total dose taken prior to the appearance of these symptoms and, during subsequent attacks, to discontinue treatment before this cumulative dose has been reached.

A reduction in prophylactic dosage is recommended if weakness, loss of appetite, nausea, vomiting, or diarrhea occurs.

**For parenteral dosage forms only**
Colchicine must be given intravenously because severe local irritation occurs if it is administered subcutaneously or intramuscularly. Also, care must be taken to ensure that the needle is properly positioned in the vein and to avoid extravasation because local irritation, inflammation, thrombophlebitis, and sloughing of the skin and subcutaneous tissues may occur.

It is recommended that the injection be diluted with 10 to 20 mL of 0.9% sodium chloride injection prior to administration. Alternatively, the medication may be injected into a large vein via an established intravenous line through which 0.9% sodium chloride injection is being infused.

The intravenous injection should be administered slowly, over a period of at least 2 to 5 minutes. Some clinicians recommend administering an intravenous dose over a period of 10 minutes.

Gastrointestinal symptoms occur rarely with intravenous administration and therefore cannot be used as an indicator of impending toxicity or guide to dosage. **The total dose administered and the duration of treatment should be limited and the patient carefully monitored.**

**Nutrition**
Colchicine impairs absorption of vitamin $B_{12}$ from the terminal ileum. Patients receiving long-term treatment may require supplementation with this vitamin.

# Oral Dosage Forms

Note: Bracketed uses in the *Dosage Forms* section refer to categories of use and/or indications that are not included in U.S. product labeling.

## COLCHICINE TABLETS USP

### Usual adult dose
Antigout agent and
[Calcium pyrophosphate deposition disease suppressant][1]—
   Prophylactic:
      Oral, 500 or 600 mcg (0.5 or 0.6 mg) once a day, initially. If necessary, dosage may be increased to 500 or 600 mcg (0.5 or 0.6 mg) two or, rarely, three times a day. However, in mild cases, administration of a single dose one to four times a week may be sufficient.

In patients with gout who are undergoing surgery—Oral, 500 or 600 mcg (0.5 or 0.6 mg) three times a day for three days before and three days after surgery.

Therapeutic (relief of acute attack)—
   Oral, 1 or 2 tablets (500 or 600 mcg [0.5 or 0.6 mg] each), or a single 1-mg tablet, initially; then 500 or 600 mcg (0.5 or 0.6 mg) every one or two hours or 1 to 1.2 mg every two hours until pain is relieved; nausea, vomiting, or diarrhea occurs; or the maximum dose of 6 mg has been taken.

[Familial Mediterranean fever suppressant and]
[Amyloidosis suppressant][1]—
   Prophylactic—
      Oral, 500 or 600 mcg (0.5 or 0.6 mg) a day, initially. Dosage may be increased, if necessary and tolerated, up to a maximum of 2 mg a day in divided doses.

   Note: Patients with familial Mediterranean fever who continue to experience frequent, severe acute attacks at a prophylactic dose of 2 mg a day are not likely to obtain relief with higher doses. However, prophylactic colchicine has been shown to prevent amyloidosis in these patients and therefore should not be discontinued.

   Therapeutic (suppression of acute attack)—
      Oral, 600 mcg (0.6 mg) every hour for four doses, then every two hours for two additional doses on the first day; followed by 1.2 mg every twelve hours for two additional days. Administration may be discontinued at any time during this three-day regimen if it is apparent that the attack has been suppressed.

[Anti-inflammatory, in Behçet's disease][1]—
   Oral, 1 to 1.8 mg a day in two or three divided doses.
[Anti-inflammatory, in biliary cirrhosis][1]—
   Oral, 1 or 1.2 mg a day in two divided doses.
[Anti-inflammatory, in recurrent pericarditis][1]—
   Oral, 1 mg a day in two divided doses. After a beneficial response has been attained, some patients may be maintained on 500 mcg (0.5 mg) a day.

### Usual adult prescribing limits
Antigout agent—
   Prophylactic:
      Patients with renal function impairment (creatinine clearance between 10 and 50 mL per minute [0.17 and 0.83 mL per second])—600 mcg (0.6 mg) once a day.
   Therapeutic (relief of acute attacks):
      Patients with normal hepatic and renal function—6 mg.
      Patients with renal function impairment (creatinine clearance between 10 and 50 mL per minute [0.17 and 0.83 mL per second])—3 mg.

### Usual pediatric dose
[Familial Mediterranean fever suppressant]—
   Children younger than 5 years of age: Oral, 500 mcg (0.5 mg) once a day.
   Children 5 years of age and older: Oral, 500 mcg (0.5 mg) two times a day.
   Other indications—Safety and efficacy have not been established.

Note: Dosage adjustment may be required as the child grows. One study found that children who were younger than 5 years of age when treatment was initiated often required an increase in dosage (to two 500–mcg [0.5–mg] doses a day) at about 7 years of age, and that children who were older than 5 years of age when treatment was initiated often required an increase in dosage (to three 500–mcg [0.5–mg] doses a day) at about 12.5 years of age.

### Strength(s) usually available
U.S.—
   500 mcg (0.5 mg) (Rx) [GENERIC].
   600 mcg (0.6 mg) (Rx) [GENERIC].
Canada—
   600 mcg (0.6 mg) (Rx) [GENERIC].
   1 mg (Rx) [GENERIC].

### Packaging and storage
Store below 40 °C (104 °F), preferably between 15 and 30 °C (59 and 86 °F). Store in a well-closed, light-resistant container.

# Parenteral Dosage Forms

Note: Bracketed uses in the *Dosage Forms* section refer to categories of use and/or indications that are not included in U.S. product labeling.

## COLCHICINE INJECTION USP

### Usual adult dose
Antigout agent and
[Calcium pyrophosphate deposition disease suppressant][1]—
  Prophylactic:
    Intravenous, 500 mcg (0.5 mg) to 1 mg one or two times a day. Some clinicians recommend that single and total daily intravenous doses should be no larger than one-half of the doses recommended for oral administration if the intravenous route cannot be avoided.
  Therapeutic (relief of acute attack):
    Intravenous, 2 mg initially, then 500 mcg (0.5 mg) every six hours or 1 mg every six to twelve hours until the desired response is obtained or a maximum of 4 mg has been administered. However, some clinicians recommend administering an initial dose not higher than 1 mg, followed by 500 mcg (0.5 mg) one or two times a day. Other clinicians recommend that single and cumulative intravenous doses should be no larger than one-half of the doses recommended for oral administration

Note: Administration of one-half of the above prophylactic and therapeutic doses is recommended for patients with renal function impairment (creatinine clearance between 10 and 50 mL per minute [0.17 and 0.83 mL per second]).

### Usual adult prescribing limits
The cumulative dose administered over twenty-four hours or more is not to exceed—
For nongeriatric patients with normal renal and hepatic function: 4 mg. **After this quantity of colchicine has been administered, additional colchicine should not be administered by any route for at least seven days.**
For nongeriatric patients with renal function impairment (creatinine clearance between 10 and 50 mL per minute [0.17 and 0.83 mL per second]): 2 mg.
For geriatric patients: 2 mg. **After this quantity of colchicine has been administered, additional colchicine should not be administered by any route for at least twenty-one days.**

Note: It is recommended that patients who have been receiving oral prophylactic therapy receive total doses even lower than those recommended above. Specifically, a maximum dose of 1 or 2 mg is recommended for nongeriatric adults with normal hepatic and renal function.

### Usual pediatric dose
Safety and efficacy have not been established.

### Strength(s) usually available
U.S.—
  1 mg per 2-mL ampul (500 mcg [0.5 mg] per mL) (Rx) [GENERIC].
Canada—
  Not commercially available.

### Packaging and storage
Store below 40 °C (104 °F), preferably between 15 and 30 °C (59 and 86 °F), unless otherwise specified by manufacturer. Protect from freezing. Protect from light.

### Preparation of dosage form
To reduce the risk of sclerosis and other local reactions, it is recommended that the contents of 1 ampul (2 mL) be diluted to at least 10 to 20 mL with 0.9% sodium chloride injection. However, any solution that becomes turbid upon dilution should not be injected.

### Incompatibilities
It is recommended that colchicine injection **not** be diluted with or injected into intravenous tubing containing 5% dextrose injection, solutions containing a bacteriostatic agent, or any other fluid that might change the pH of the colchicine solution, because precipitation may occur.

[1]Not included in Canadian product labeling.

## Selected Bibliography
Levy M, Spino M, Read SE. Colchicine: a state-of-the-art review. Pharmacotherapy 1991; 11: 196-211.
Star VL, Hochberg MC. Prevention and management of gout. Drugs 1993; 45: 212-22.
Zemer D, Livneh A, Danon YL, Pras M, Sohar E. Long-term colchicine treatment in children with familial Mediterranean fever. Arthritis Rheum 1991; 34: 973-7.
Henderson A, Emmerson BT, Bailey NL, Pond SM. Colchicine overdose in 6 patients. Prospects for prevention and therapy. Drug Invest 1993; 6: 114-7.

Revised: 01/31/94

---

# COLESTIPOL   Oral-Local

VA CLASSIFICATION (Primary/Secondary): CV602/DE890; GA208
Commonly used brand name(s): *Colestid*.
Note: For a listing of dosage forms and brand names by country availability, see *Dosage Forms* section(s).

## Category
Antihyperlipidemic; antipruritic (cholestasis); antidiarrheal (postoperative colonic bile acids).

## Indications
Note: Bracketed information in the *Indications* section refers to uses that are not included in U.S. product labeling.

### Accepted
Hyperlipidemia (treatment)—Colestipol is indicated for use as an adjunct only in patients with primary hypercholesterolemia (type IIa hyperlipidemia) and a significant risk of coronary artery disease who have not responded to diet or other measures alone. Colestipol reduces plasma cholesterol concentrations but causes no change or a slight increase in serum triglyceride concentrations, and so is not useful in patients with elevated triglyceride concentrations alone. Its use is limited in other types of hyperlipidemia (including type IIb) because it may cause further elevation of triglycerides.

Studies have suggested that control of elevated cholesterol and triglycerides may not lessen the danger of cardiovascular disease and mortality, although incidence of nonfatal myocardial infarctions may be decreased.

For additional information on initial therapeutic guidelines related to the treatment of hyperlipidemia, see *Appendix III*.

[Pruritus, associated with partial biliary obstruction (treatment)][1]—Colestipol is also used for the relief of pruritus associated with partial biliary obstruction (including primary biliary cirrhosis and various other forms of bile stasis). It is not useful in patients with complete biliary obstruction or with pruritus due to other causes.

[Diarrhea, due to bile acids (treatment)][1]—Colestipol may also be used to treat diarrhea caused by increased bile acids in the colon after surgery, although the risk of steatorrhea is increased.

[Colestipol has been used in the treatment of digitalis glycoside overdose and hyperoxaluria; however, it generally has been replaced by more effective agents.][1]

[1]Not included in Canadian product labeling.

## Pharmacology/Pharmacokinetics

### Physicochemical characteristics
Colestipol is an anion-exchange resin.

### Mechanism of action/Effect
Colestipol binds with bile acids in the intestine, preventing their reabsorption and producing an insoluble complex, which is excreted in the feces.
Antihyperlipidemic—
  Colestipol binds with bile acids in the intestine, causing an increase in hepatic synthesis of bile acids from cholesterol. This depletion of hepatic cholesterol increases hepatic low-density lipoprotein (LDL) receptor activity, which removes LDL cholesterol from the plasma. Colestipol may also increase hepatic very low-density lipoprotein (VLDL) production, thereby increasing plasma concentration of triglycerides, especially in patients with hypertriglyceridemia.
Antipruritic (cholestasis)—
  Reduction of serum bile acids and subsequent reduction of excess bile acids, which are deposited in dermal tissue, may lead to reduced pruritus.
Antidiarrheal (postoperative colonic bile acids)—
  Colestipol binds with and removes bile acids.

**Other actions/effects**
Because it is an anion-exchange resin, colestipol is capable of binding negatively charged medications as well as some others, causing a decreased effect or shortened half-life.

**Absorption**
Not absorbed from the gastrointestinal tract.

**Onset of action**
Plasma cholesterol concentrations are generally reduced within 24 to 48 hours after initiation of colestipol therapy.

**Time to peak effect**
Within 1 month. In some patients, after the initial decrease, serum cholesterol concentrations return to or exceed baseline levels with continued therapy.

**Duration of action**
After withdrawal of colestipol, cholesterol concentrations return to baseline in about 1 month.

## Precautions to Consider

**Tumorigenicity**
Tumorigenicity/Mutagenicity—In rats given colestipol for 18 months, no evidence of drug-related intestinal tumor formation was found. Colestipol was not mutagenic in the Ames assay.

**Pregnancy/Reproduction**
Pregnancy—Studies have not been done in humans. Because colestipol is almost totally unabsorbed after oral administration, adverse effects on the fetus may potentially occur because of impaired maternal absorption of vitamins and nutrients.
Studies have not been done in animals.

**Breast-feeding**
Problems in humans have not been documented.

**Pediatrics**
Appropriate studies on the relationship of age to the effects of colestipol have not been performed in the pediatric population. However, use in children under 2 years of age is not recommended since cholesterol is required for normal development.

**Geriatrics**
Appropriate studies on the relationship of age to the effects of colestipol have not been performed in the geriatric population. However, patients over 60 years of age may be more likely to experience gastrointestinal side effects, as well as adverse nutritional effects.

**Drug interactions and/or related problems**
The following drug interactions and/or related problems have been selected on the basis of their potential clinical significance (possible mechanism in parentheses where appropriate)—not necessarily inclusive (» = major clinical significance):

Note: Combinations containing any of the following medications, depending on the amount present, may also interact with this medication.

» Anticoagulants, coumarin- or indandione-derivative
(concurrent use may significantly increase the anticoagulant effect as a result of depletion of vitamin K, but colestipol may also bind with oral anticoagulants in the gastrointestinal tract and reduce their effects; administration at least 6 hours before colestipol and adjustment of anticoagulant dosage based on frequent prothrombin-time determinations are recommended)

Chenodiol or
Ursodiol
(effect may be decreased when chenodiol or ursodiol is used concurrently with colestipol, which binds the medication and decreases its absorption and also tends to increase cholesterol saturation of bile)

» Digitalis glycosides
(colestipol may reduce the half-life of these medications by decreasing intestinal reabsorption and enterohepatic circulation; caution is recommended, especially when colestipol is withdrawn from a patient who was stabilized on the digitalis glycoside while receiving colestipol, because of the potential for serious toxicity; some clinicians recommend administration of colestipol approximately 8 hours after the digitalis glycoside)

» Diuretics, thiazide, oral or
» Penicillin G, oral or
» Propranolol, oral or
» Tetracyclines, oral
(concurrent administration with colestipol has been found to impair absorption of these medications; an interval of several hours between administration of colestipol and any of these medications is recommended; effects on absorption of other beta-blockers has not been determined)

» Thyroid hormones, including dextrothyroxine
(concurrent use with colestipol may decrease the effects of thyroid hormones by binding and delaying or preventing absorption; an interval of 4 to 5 hours between administration of the 2 medications and regular monitoring of thyroid function tests are recommended)

» Vancomycin, oral
(colestipol has been shown to bind oral vancomycin significantly when used concurrently, resulting in decreased stool concentrations and marked reduction in antibacterial activity of vancomycin; concurrent use is not recommended; patients should be advised to take oral vancomycin and colestipol several hours apart)

Vitamins, fat-soluble
(colestipol may interfere with absorption of fat-soluble vitamins as a result of its interference with fat absorption; supplemental vitamin A and D in water-miscible or parenteral form are recommended in patients receiving colestipol for prolonged periods; supplemental vitamin K may be required in some patients who develop bleeding tendencies)

Medications, other
(colestipol may delay or reduce absorption of other medications administered concurrently because of its anion-binding activity; administration of other medications 1 to 2 hours before or 4 hours after colestipol is recommended, although absorption of some medications is impaired even then; caution is recommended when colestipol is withdrawn because of the risk of toxicity when suddenly increased absorption of the other medication leads to higher serum concentrations)

**Laboratory value alterations**
The following have been selected on the basis of their potential clinical significance (possible effect in parentheses where appropriate)—not necessarily inclusive (» = major clinical significance):

With physiology/laboratory test values
Alkaline phosphatase and
Aspartate aminotransferase (AST [SGOT]), serum and
Chloride, serum and
Phosphorus, serum
(concentrations may be increased)

Potassium and
Sodium
(serum concentrations may be decreased)

Prothrombin time (PT)
(may be prolonged)

**Medical considerations/Contraindications**
The medical considerations/contraindications included have been selected on the basis of their potential clinical significance (reasons given in parentheses where appropriate)—not necessarily inclusive (» = major clinical significance).

*Except under special circumstances, this medication should not be used when the following medical problem exists:*

» Primary biliary cirrhosis
(may further raise the cholesterol concentration)

*Risk-benefit should be considered when the following medical problems exist:*

Bleeding disorders and
Gallstones and
Gastrointestinal dysfunction and
Hypothyroidism and
Malabsorption states, especially steatorrhea and
Peptic ulcer
(these conditions may be exacerbated)

» Complete biliary obstruction or complete atresia
(no bile acids in gastrointestinal tract for colestipol to bind)

» Constipation
(risk of fecal impaction)
Coronary artery disease and
Hemorrhoids
(because of the risks associated with severe constipation)

Renal function impairment
(increased risk of development of hyperchloremic acidosis)

Sensitivity to colestipol

### Patient monitoring

The following may be especially important in patient monitoring (other tests may be warranted in some patients, depending on condition; » = major clinical significance):

Cholesterol and
Triglyceride
   (serum concentration determinations recommended prior to initiation of therapy for hyperlipidemia and every 2 months after stabilization to confirm efficacy and determine that a positive response is maintained)

Prothrombin-time (PT) determinations
   (recommended periodically because vitamin K deficiency associated with chronic use of colestipol may increase bleeding tendency)

## Side/Adverse Effects

The following side/adverse effects have been selected on the basis of their potential clinical significance (possible signs and symptoms in parentheses where appropriate)—not necessarily inclusive:

### Those indicating need for medical attention
Incidence more frequent—about 10%
   *Constipation*—usually mild and transient, but may be severe and lead to fecal impaction
Incidence rare
   *Gallstones* (severe stomach pain with nausea and vomiting); *gastrointestinal bleeding or peptic ulcer* (black, tarry stools); *steatorrhea or malabsorption syndrome, especially with doses greater than 30 grams a day* (sudden loss of weight)

### Those indicating need for medical attention only if they continue or are bothersome
Incidence less frequent
   *Belching; bloating; diarrhea; dizziness; headache; nausea or vomiting; stomach pain*

## Patient Consultation

As an aid to patient consultation, refer to *Advice for the Patient, Colestipol (Oral)*.

In providing consultation, consider emphasizing the following selected information (» = major clinical significance):

### Before using this medication
Diet as preferred therapy; importance of following prescribed diet
This medication does not cure the condition but rather helps control it
» Conditions affecting use, especially:
   Sensitivity to colestipol
   Use in children—Not recommended in children under 2 years of age since cholesterol is required for normal development
   Use in the elderly—Increased incidence of gastrointestinal side effects and adverse nutritional effects in patients over 60 years of age
   Other medications, especially anticoagulants, digitalis glycosides, oral penicillin G, oral tetracyclines, oral propranolol, thyroid hormones, thiazide diuretics, or oral vancomycin
   Other medical problems, especially primary biliary cirrhosis, complete biliary obstruction or complete atresia, or constipation

### Proper use of this medication
» Importance of not taking more or less medication than the amount prescribed
» Compliance with prescribed diet
» Importance of mixing with fluids before taking; instructions for mixing: Stirring until completely mixed (does not dissolve); rinsing glass and drinking to make sure all medication is taken; may also be mixed with milk in cereals, thin soups, or pulpy fruits
» Proper dosing
   Missed dose: Taking as soon as possible; not taking if almost time for next dose; not doubling doses
» Proper storage

### Precautions while using this medication
» Importance of close monitoring by the physician
» Checking with physician before discontinuing medication; blood lipid concentrations may increase significantly
» Not taking any other medication unless discussed with physician

### Side/adverse effects
Signs of potential side effects, especially constipation, gallstones, gastrointestinal bleeding, peptic ulcer, and steatorrhea or malabsorption syndrome

## General Dosing Information

To prevent accidental inhalation or esophageal distress with the dry form, it is recommended that colestipol be mixed with at least 90 mL of water or other fluids (i.e., carbonated beverages, flavored drinks, juices, or milk) before being ingested. It may also be taken in soups or with cereals or pulpy fruits.

Reduction in colestipol dosage or withdrawal of the medication may be necessary in some patients if constipation occurs or worsens, to prevent impaction. Administration of a laxative or stool softener or increased fluid intake may be helpful.

### For use as an antihyperlipidemic
If a paradoxical increase in plasma cholesterol levels occurs, it is recommended that colestipol therapy be withdrawn.

If response is inadequate after 3 months of treatment, colestipol therapy should be withdrawn, except in the case of xanthoma tuberosum, which may require up to 1 year of treatment as long as reduction in size and/or number of xanthomata occurs.

## Oral Dosage Forms

### COLESTIPOL HYDROCHLORIDE FOR ORAL SUSPENSION USP

#### Usual adult dose
Antihyperlipidemic—
   Oral, 15 to 30 grams a day before meals in two to four divided doses.
Note:  Colestipol has been used to treat digitalis glycoside toxicity at an oral dose of 10 grams, followed by 5 grams every six to eight hours.

#### Usual pediatric dose
Safety and efficacy have not been established.

#### Size(s) usually available
U.S.—
   5 grams per packet or level scoop (Rx) [*Colestid*].
Canada—
   5 grams per packet or level scoop (Rx) [*Colestid*].

#### Packaging and storage
Store below 40 °C (104 °F), preferably between 15 and 30 °C (59 and 86 °F), unless otherwise specified by manufacturer. Store in a tight container.

#### Preparation of dosage form
Colestipol is prepared for administration by adding the measured powder to the liquid and stirring to mix thoroughly (does not dissolve). After the patient drinks the suspension, the glass should be rinsed with more liquid to make sure all the medication is taken. Colestipol may also be mixed with milk in hot or regular breakfast cereals, in thin soups (tomato or chicken noodle), or with pulpy fruits such as pineapples, pears, peaches, or fruit cocktail.

#### Auxiliary labeling
• Take mixed in cold water or juice.

## Selected Bibliography

The Expert Panel. Report of the national cholesterol education program expert panel on detection, evaluation and treatment of high blood cholesterol in adults. Arch Intern Med 1988; 148: 36-69.

NIH Consensus Conference. Lowering blood cholesterol to prevent heart disease. JAMA 1985 Apr 12; 253: 2080-6.

Knodel LC, Talbert RL. Adverse effects of hypolipidaemic drugs. Med Toxicol 1987; 2: 10-32.

Revised: 10/21/92
Interim revision: 04/14/94; 08/12/98

# COLFOSCERIL, CETYL ALCOHOL, AND TYLOXAPOL  Intratracheal-Local

VA CLASSIFICATION (Primary): RE700

Commonly used brand name(s): *Exosurf Neonatal*.

Other commonly used names for colfosceril are colfosceril palmitate, dipalmitoylphosphatidylcholine, DPPC, and synthetic lung surfactant.

Note: For a listing of dosage forms and brand names by country availability, see *Dosage Forms* section(s).

## Category

Pulmonary surfactant.

## Indications

### Accepted

Respiratory distress syndrome, neonatal (prophylaxis and treatment)—Colfosceril, cetyl alcohol, and tyloxapol combination is indicated for the prophylactic treatment of infants with birth weights of less than 1350 grams who are at risk of developing respiratory distress syndrome (RDS) and of infants with birth weights greater than 1350 grams who show evidence of pulmonary immaturity.

Colfosceril, cetyl alcohol, and tyloxapol combination is also indicated for rescue treatment of infants who have developed RDS. Infants considered for rescue treatment with this medication should be on mechanical ventilation, and have a diagnosis of RDS based on the presence of respiratory distress that is not due to causes other than RDS (as shown by clinical and laboratory assessments) and on chest radiographic findings consistent with the diagnosis of RDS.

## Pharmacology/Pharmacokinetics

### Mechanism of action/Effect

Neonatal respiratory distress syndrome (RDS) develops primarily in premature infants because of pulmonary immaturity, including a deficiency of endogenous lung surfactant that results in higher alveolar surface tension and lower compliance properties. Without sufficient endogenous lung surfactant, progressive alveolar collapse occurs and both oxygen and carbon dioxide exchange are impaired. Also, RDS appears to be characterized by high pulmonary vascular permeability and increased lung tissue water. Fluid and protein that leak into alveoli inactivate both endogenous and exogenous surfactant, worsening lung function.

Natural lung surfactant is a mixture of lipids and apoproteins secreted by the alveolar cells into the alveoli and respiratory air passages. It reduces the surface tension of pulmonary fluids and thereby increases lung compliance. Surfactant exhibits not only surface tension–reducing properties (contributed by the lipids), but also rapid spreading and adsorption (contributed by the apoproteins). The major fraction of the lipid component of natural lung surfactant is dipalmitoylphosphatidylcholine (DPPC); this comprises up to 70% of the natural surfactant by weight.

Although the colfosceril (also known as DPPC) contained in the synthetic protein-free lung surfactant reduces surface tension, it alone is ineffective in RDS because it spreads and adsorbs poorly due to slow dispersion at air-fluid interfaces. Cetyl alcohol acts as the spreading agent for the colfosceril at the air-fluid interface, resulting in surface-tension effects that are similar to those of endogenous lung surfactant. Tyloxapol, a polymeric long-chain repeating alcohol, is a nonionic surfactant that acts to disperse both colfosceril and cetyl alcohol. Therefore, colfosceril, cetyl alcohol, and tyloxapol combination, when used as a replacement for deficient endogenous lung surfactant, is effective in reducing the surface tension of pulmonary fluids, thereby increasing lung compliance properties in RDS to prevent alveolar collapse and decrease work in breathing. The possibility exists that it may also improve ventilation/perfusion matching, independent of its direct effect on lung compliance.

### Absorption

In nonclinical studies, it has been shown that DPPC can be absorbed from the alveolus into lung tissue where it can be catabolized extensively and reutilized for further phospholipid synthesis and secretion. However, human pharmacokinetic studies on the absorption, biotransformation, and excretion of the components of colfosceril, cetyl alcohol, and tyloxapol combination have not been performed.

### Distribution

The lung surfactant administered endotracheally is distributed to the lung lobes, distal airways, and alveolar spaces. As the lung surfactant is distributed to the bronchi, bronchioles, and alveoli after administration in the upper airway, its concentration is highest at the alveolar air-fluid interface where it remains as a monolayer.

The lung surfactant does not enter systemic circulation from normal, healthy lungs; however, when the integrity of the alveolar lining is disrupted, as occurs in infants with RDS, the surfactant may be distributed outside the lungs into systemic circulation.

## Precautions to Consider

### Carcinogenicity

Long-term studies have not been performed in animals to evaluate the carcinogenic potential of colfosceril, cetyl alcohol, and tyloxapol combination.

### Mutagenicity

Colfosceril, at concentrations up to 10,000 mcg per plate, was not mutagenic in the Ames Salmonella assay.

### Pregnancy/Reproduction

Fertility—The effects of colfosceril, cetyl alcohol, and tyloxapol combination on fertility have not been studied.

Pregnancy—No information is available on the use of colfosceril, cetyl alcohol, and tyloxapol combination during pregnancy.

### Breast-feeding

No information is available on the use of colfosceril, cetyl alcohol, and tyloxapol combination during breast-feeding.

### Pediatrics

Appropriate studies performed to date have not demonstrated pediatrics-specific problems that would limit the usefulness of colfosceril, cetyl alcohol, and tyloxapol combination in children.

### Geriatrics

No information is available on the relationship of age to the effects of colfosceril, cetyl alcohol, and tyloxapol combination.

### Patient monitoring

The following may be especially important in patient monitoring (other tests may be warranted in some patients, depending on condition; » = major clinical significance):

Arterial blood gases

(after both prophylactic and rescue dosing, frequent arterial blood gas monitoring is recommended to prevent post-dosing hyperoxia and hypocarbia)

(if arterial or transcutaneous carbon dioxide [$CO_2$] measurements are < 30 torr, ventilation should be reduced at once; failure to reduce ventilator pressure or rate in such cases may result in severe hypocarbia, which can cause barotrauma and reduce brain blood flow)

(if the infant becomes pink and transcutaneous oxygen saturation is in excess of 95%, the fraction of inspired oxygen [$FIO_2$] should be reduced in small but repeated increments, until saturation is 90 to 95%, without waiting for confirmation of elevated arterial oxygen partial pressure [$PaO_2$] by blood gas assessment; failure to reduce $FIO_2$ in such cases may result in hyperoxia)

Arterial blood pressure and
Electrocardiogram (ECG)

(continuous monitoring of ECG during dosing is recommended; in most infants treated prophylactically, monitoring of ECG should be initiated prior to administration of the first dose of colfosceril, cetyl alcohol, and tyloxapol combination; for subsequent doses, arterial blood pressure monitoring during dosing is also recommended)

Chest expansion and
Color and
Endotracheal tube patency and position and
Heart rate and
Oxygen saturation, transcutaneous

(prior to dosing, it should be verified that the endotracheal tube tip is correctly positioned in mid-trachea; also, brisk and symmetrical chest movement with each mechanical inspiration and equal breath sounds in the two axillae should be confirmed)

(monitoring of chest expansion, color, endotracheal tube patency and position, heart rate, and transcutaneous oxygen saturation during dosing is recommended; if heart rate slows, the infant becomes dusky or agitated, or the medication backs up in the endotracheal tube, dosing should be slowed or stopped and, if necessary, the peak inspiratory pressure, ventilator rate, or $FIO_2$ should be increased; if transcutaneous oxygen saturation decreases during dosing, administration of the medication should be stopped and, if necessary, peak inspiratory pressure on the ventilator should be increased by 4 to 5 cm water for up to 15 to 20 minutes, depending on the infant's degree of tolerance versus oxygenation/ventilation compromise; increases of FIO$_2$ may also be required for 15 to 20 minutes; however, rapid improvement in lung function may require immediate reduction in peak inspiratory pressure, ventilator rate, or FIO$_2$)

(at the end of dosing, the proper position of the endotracheal tube should be confirmed by listening for equal breath sounds in the axillae; chest expansion, color, and transcutaneous oxygen saturation should also be checked; continuous monitoring of the patient for at least 30 minutes after dosing is recommended, since rapid lung function changes require immediate changes in peak inspiratory pressure, ventilator rate, or FIO$_2$)

(if chest expansion improves substantially after dosing, peak ventilator inspiratory pressure should be reduced immediately, without waiting for confirmation of respiratory improvement by blood gas assessment; failure to reduce inspiratory ventilator pressure rapidly in such cases may result in lung overdistention and pulmonary air leak)

## Side/Adverse Effects

Note: In controlled clinical studies of infants receiving colfosceril, cetyl alcohol, and tyloxapol combination, there was an increased incidence in some of the conditions associated with prematurity and RDS, including apnea and pulmonary hemorrhage. Hypoxia and bradycardia can occur during treatment and are directly related to the dosing procedure.

Infants treated with synthetic surfactant may develop apnea because they are taken off the ventilator sooner due to their improved respiratory status. Thus, apnea is not considered a direct side effect of this medication and is, in fact, associated with a favorable rather than an untoward outcome. Apneic infants, whether or not they received colfosceril, cetyl alcohol, and tyloxapol combination, had fewer episodes of grade III intraventricular hemorrhage or periventricular echodensities or both, fewer air leaks, and better survival rates than did nonapneic infants.

Pulmonary hemorrhage occurred more frequently in infants who were younger, smaller ($<$ 700 grams at birth), or male, or in those who had a patent ductus arteriosus; it usually occurred in the first two days of life. Infants treated with colfosceril, cetyl alcohol, and tyloxapol combination who received steroids more than 24 hours prior to delivery or indomethacin postnatally had a lower rate of pulmonary hemorrhage than other infants treated with this medication.

Controlled clinical studies of infants receiving colfosceril, cetyl alcohol, and tyloxapol combination also showed a decreased incidence of pulmonary air leak and bronchopulmonary dysplasia, which are associated with mechanical ventilation in premature infants. Some studies have shown that, with rescue surfactant treatment, synthetic surfactant improved the chance of survival through 28 days without bronchopulmonary dysplasia.

During an open uncontrolled study, colfosceril, cetyl alcohol, and tyloxapol combination decreased oxygen (O$_2$) saturation ($\geq$ 20%) in 6% of infants on prophylactic treatment and in 22% of infants on rescue treatment; increased O$_2$ saturation ($\geq$ 10%) in 5% of infants on prophylactic treatment and in 6% of infants on rescue treatment; decreased transcutaneous oxygen partial pressure (PaO$_2$) ($\geq$ 20 mm Hg) in 1% of infants on prophylactic treatment and in 8% of infants on rescue treatment; increased transcutaneous PO$_2$ ($\geq$ 20 mm Hg) in 2% of infants on prophylactic treatment and in 5% of infants on rescue treatment; decreased transcutaneous carbon dioxide partial pressure (PaCO$_2$) ($\geq$ 20 mm Hg) in $<$ 1% of infants on prophylactic treatment and in 1% of infants on rescue treatment; and increased transcutaneous PCO$_2$ ($\geq$ 20 mm Hg) in 1% of infants on prophylactic treatment and in 3% of infants on rescue treatment.

The following side/adverse effects have been selected on the basis of their potential clinical significance (possible signs and symptoms in parentheses where appropriate)—not necessarily inclusive:

### Those indicating need for medical attention
Incidence rare
    *Apnea; bradycardia ($<$ 60 beats per minute); pulmonary air leak—due to excess ventilation caused by rapid improvement in lung; pulmonary hemorrhage; tachycardia ($>$ 200 beats per minute)*

### Those indicating need for medical attention only if they continue or are bothersome
Incidence less frequent or rare
    *Gagging*

## General Dosing Information

Colfosceril, cetyl alcohol, and tyloxapol combination should be used only by neonatologists and other clinicians who are experienced at neonatal intubation and ventilatory management. Also, instillation of this medication should be performed only by trained medical personnel experienced in airway and clinical management of unstable premature infants. Adequate personnel, facilities, equipment, and medications are required to optimize the perinatal outcome in these premature infants. In addition, continuous clinical attention should be given to all infants prior to, during, and after administration of this medication.

Colfosceril, cetyl alcohol, and tyloxapol combination should be administered only by instillation into the trachea.

To ensure accurate dosing, the current weight of the infant should be accurately determined.

Colfosceril, cetyl alcohol, and tyloxapol combination for intratracheal suspension is to be used with one of the 5 special endotracheal tube adapters with a special right-angle Luer-lock sideport, supplied by the manufacturer. The adapters are used as follows:
- An adapter size should be selected that corresponds to the inside diameter of the endotracheal tube.
- The adapter is inserted into the endotracheal tube with a firm push-twist motion.
- The breathing circuit "Y" is connected to the adapter.
- The cap is removed from the sideport on the adapter and the syringe containing the medication is attached to the sideport.
- After completion of dosing, the syringe is removed and the sideport is capped.

Colfosceril, cetyl alcohol, and tyloxapol for intratracheal suspension is administered through the sideport on the special endotracheal tube adapter without interrupting mechanical ventilation.

Prior to dosing with colfosceril, cetyl alcohol, and tyloxapol combination, proper placement of the endotracheal tube tip in the trachea and not in the esophagus or right or left mainstem bronchus should be confirmed. Brisk and symmetrical chest movement with each mechanical inspiration and equal breath sounds in the two axillae should also be confirmed prior to dosing. In prophylactic treatment, dosing with colfosceril, cetyl alcohol, and tyloxapol combination should not be delayed pending radiographic confirmation of the endotracheal tube tip position. In rescue treatment, bedside confirmation of the endotracheal tube tip position is usually sufficient if at least one chest radiograph subsequent to the last intubation confirms proper position of the endotracheal tube tip. If the endotracheal tube tip is too low, some lung areas could remain undosed.

Infants whose ventilation becomes severely impaired during or shortly after dosing may have mucous plugging of the endotracheal tube, especially if pulmonary secretions were prominent prior to administration of the medication. Therefore, prior to administration of colfosceril, cetyl alcohol, and tyloxapol combination, the infant should be suctioned to lessen the chance of mucous plugs obstructing the endotracheal tube. If endotracheal tube obstruction is suspected, and suctioning is ineffective in removing the obstruction, the blocked endotracheal tube should be replaced immediately. Following administration of colfosceril, cetyl alcohol, and tyloxapol combination, the infant should not be suctioned for 2 hours except when it is clinically necessary.

In infants weighing 500 to 700 grams, a single prophylactic dose of colfosceril, cetyl alcohol, and tyloxapol combination has been shown to significantly improve the fraction of inspired oxygen (FIO$_2$) and ventilator settings, reduce pneumothorax, and reduce the incidence of death from respiratory distress syndrome (RDS), but it has also been shown to increase pulmonary hemorrhage. The effects of multiple doses of colfosceril, cetyl alcohol, and tyloxapol combination in infants in this weight group are not known; therefore, clinicians should carefully consider the potential risks and benefits of this medication in these infants.

Each dose is administered in two half-doses, with each half-dose being equivalent to 33.75 mg of colfosceril palmitate (2.5 mL of reconstituted suspension) per kg of body weight. Each half-dose is instilled slowly over a minimum of 1 to 2 minutes (30 to 50 mechanical breaths) in small bursts timed with inspiration. After the first half-dose (the equivalent of 33.75 mg of colfosceril palmitate [2.5 mL of reconstituted suspension] per kg of body weight) is administered in the midline position, the infant's head and torso are turned 45° to the right for 30 seconds while mechanical ventilation is continued. Then the infant is returned to the midline position, and the second half-dose (the equivalent of 33.75 mg of colfosceril palmitate [2.5 mL of reconstituted suspension] per kg of body weight) is given in an identical manner. The infant's head and torso are then turned 45° to the left for 30 seconds while mechanical ventilation is continued, after which the infant is turned back to the midline position. Using these maneuvers allows gravity to assist in the lung distribution of the colfosceril, cetyl alcohol, and tyloxapol combination.

The dosage volume of the equivalent of 67.5 mg of colfosceril palmitate (5 mL reconstituted suspension) per kg of body weight may cause transient impairment of gas exchange by physical blockage of the airway, especially in infants on low ventilator setting. This may result in a drop in oxygen saturation during dosing, especially if these infants are on low ventilator settings prior to dosing. These transient effects may be overcome by increasing peak inspiratory pressure on the ventilator during dosing. $FIO_2$ may also be increased if necessary. In infants who are especially fragile or reactive to external stimuli, increasing peak inspiratory pressure just prior to dosing may minimize any transient decrease in oxygenation. However, the infant should be returned to pre-dose settings within a very short time after dosing is completed.

Rapid administration of colfosceril, cetyl alcohol, and tyloxapol combination may cause reflux of the medication into the endotracheal tube during dosing. If reflux occurs, administration of the medication should be stopped and, if necessary, the peak inspiratory pressure on the ventilator should be increased until the endotracheal tube clears.

In controlled clinical studies with infants receiving colfosceril, cetyl alcohol, and tyloxapol combination, infants who received steroids more than 24 hours prior to delivery or indomethacin postnatally had a lower rate of pulmonary hemorrhage than did other infants treated with this medication. Careful attention should be given to early treatment (unless contraindicated) of patent ductus arteriosus during the first 2 days of life (while the ductus arteriosus is often clinically silent).

## Intratracheal Dosage Forms

### COLFOSCERIL PALMITATE, CETYL ALCOHOL, AND TYLOXAPOL FOR INTRATRACHEAL SUSPENSION

**Usual pediatric dose**

Pulmonary surfactant (prophylaxis)—
Intratracheal, the equivalent of 67.5 mg of colfosceril palmitate (5 mL of reconstituted suspension) per kg of body weight for the first dose, administered (in two half-doses) as soon as possible after birth; second and third doses (each given in two half-doses) should be administered approximately twelve and twenty-four hours later to all infants remaining on mechanical ventilation at those times.

Pulmonary surfactant (rescue treatment)—
Intratracheal, initially the equivalent of 67.5 mg of colfosceril palmitate (5 mL of reconstituted suspension) per kg of body weight administered (in two half-doses) as soon as possible after diagnosis of respiratory distress syndrome (RDS) is confirmed; a second dose (given in two half-doses) should be administered approximately twelve hours after the first dose, provided that the infant remains on mechanical ventilation. Administration of a third or fourth dose when signs of RDS persist or recur was not shown to be of overall clinical benefit.

Note: Each dose is administered in two half-doses, with each half-dose being equivalent to 33.75 mg of colfosceril palmitate (2.5 mL of reconstituted suspension) per kg of body weight. Each half-dose is instilled slowly over a minimum of one to two minutes (thirty to fifty mechanical breaths) in small bursts timed with inspiration.

**Strength(s) usually available**

U.S.—
108 mg of colfosceril palmitate, 12 mg of cetyl alcohol, and 8 mg of tyloxapol per vial (13.5 mg of colfosceril palmitate, 1.5 mg of cetyl alcohol, and 1 mg of tyloxapol per mL, when reconstituted with 8 mL of Sterile Water for Injection supplied by manufacturer) (Rx) [*Exosurf Neonatal* (sodium chloride 47 mg per vial)].

Canada—
108 mg of colfosceril palmitate, 12 mg of cetyl alcohol, and 8 mg of tyloxapol per vial (13.5 mg of colfosceril palmitate, 1.5 mg of cetyl alcohol, and 1 mg of tyloxapol per mL, when reconstituted with 8 mL of Sterile Water for Injection supplied by manufacturer) (Rx) [*Exosurf Neonatal* (sodium chloride 47 mg per vial)].

**Packaging and storage**
Store below 40 °C (104 °F), preferably between 15 and 30 °C (59 and 86 °F), unless otherwise specified by manufacturer.

**Preparation of dosage form**
Colfosceril, cetyl alcohol, and tyloxapol combination should be reconstituted immediately before use because it does not contain antibacterial preservatives.

Solutions containing buffers or preservatives should not be used for reconstitution; Bacteriostatic Water for Injection USP should also not be used.

Each vial of colfosceril, cetyl alcohol, and tyloxapol combination should be reconstituted only with 8 mL of the preservative-free Sterile Water for Injection provided by the manufacturer, as follows:
A 10- or 12-mL syringe is filled with 8 mL of preservative-free Sterile Water for Injection, using an 18- or 19-gauge needle.
The vacuum in the vial should be allowed to draw the sterile water into the vial.
As much of the 8 mL as possible should be aspirated out of the vial into the syringe (while maintaining the vacuum), then the syringe plunger suddenly released; this step should be repeated three or four times to assure adequate mixing of the vial contents. If a vacuum is not present, the vial of colfosceril, cetyl alcohol, and tyloxapol combination should not be used.
The appropriate dosage volume for the entire dose (5 mL [equivalent of 67.5 mg of colfosceril palmitate] per kg of body weight) should then be drawn into the syringe from below the froth in the vial (while maintaining the vacuum).
Following reconstitution, the colfosceril, cetyl alcohol, and tyloxapol combination preparation is a milky white suspension with a total volume of 8 mL per vial.

**Stability**
The reconstituted suspension is chemically and physically stable and remains sterile for up to 24 hours following reconstitution (using aseptic technique) when stored at 2 to 30 °C (36 to 86 °F); however, the manufacturer's labeling states that it is best to reconstitute the colfosceril palmitate, cetyl alcohol, and tyloxapol combination immediately before use because the product does not contain antibacterial preservatives.
If the suspension appears to separate, the vial should be gently shaken or swirled to resuspend the preparation.
The reconstituted product should be inspected visually for homogeneity immediately before administration; if persistent large flakes or particulates are present, the vial should not be used.

## Selected Bibliography

Corbet A, Bucciarelli R, Goldman S, et al. Decreased mortality rate among small premature infants treated at birth with a single dose of synthetic surfactant: a multicenter controlled trial. J Pediatr 1991; 118: 277-84.

Jobe AH. Pulmonary surfactant therapy. N Engl J Med 1993; 32: 861-8.

Long W, Thompson T, Sundell H, et al. Effects of two rescue doses of a synthetic surfactant on mortality rate and survival without bronchopulmonary dysplasia in 700- to 1350-gram infants with respiratory distress syndrome. J Pediatr 1991; 118: 595-605.

Developed: 05/10/95

# COLISTIN, NEOMYCIN, AND HYDROCORTISONE Otic

VA CLASSIFICATION (Primary): OT250
Commonly used brand name(s): *Coly-Mycin Otic*; *Coly-Mycin S Otic*.
Note: For a listing of dosage forms and brand names by country availability, see *Dosage Forms* section(s).

## Category
Antibacterial-corticosteroid (otic).

## Indications
Note: Bracketed information in the *Indications* section refers to uses that are not included in U.S. product labeling.

**Accepted**
Ear canal infections, external (treatment) or
Mastoidectomy cavity infections (treatment)[1]—Colistin, neomycin, and hydrocortisone otic combination is indicated in the treatment of superficial external ear canal infections and superficial mastoidectomy and fenestration cavity infections caused by susceptible organisms, including *Pseudomonas aeruginosa*, *Staphylococcus aureus*, *Klebsiella* species, *Enterobacter (Aerobacter)* species, and *Escherichia coli*.

[Otitis media, chronic suppurative (treatment)][1]—Colistin, neomycin, and hydrocortisone otic combination is used in the treatment of chronic suppurative otitis media.

# Colistin, Neomycin, and Hydrocortisone (Otic)

Note: Not all species or strains of a particular organism may be susceptible to colistin and neomycin.

[1]Not included in Canadian product labeling.

## Pharmacology/Pharmacokinetics

**Physicochemical characteristics**
Molecular weight—Hydrocortisone acetate: 404.50.
Family—Colistin sulfate: Polymyxins; also known as polymyxin E.
Neomycin sulfate: Aminoglycosides.
Hydrocortisone acetate: Corticosteroids.

**Mechanism of action/Effect**
Colistin is bactericidal and active against *Pseudomonas aeruginosa* and other gram-negative bacteria. It is a surface-active basic polypeptide that binds to anionic phospholipid sites in bacterial cytoplasmic membranes, disrupts membrane structure, and alters membrane permeability to allow leakage of intracellular contents. Its action is antagonized by calcium and magnesium.

Neomycin is an aminoglycoside, bactericidal against most aerobic gram-negative bacilli and *Staphylococcus aureus*, but not effective against *Pseudomonas*. It is actively transported across the bacterial cell membrane, binds to a specific receptor protein on the 30 S subunit of bacterial ribosomes, and interferes with an initiation complex between mRNA (messenger RNA) and the 30 S subunit, thus inhibiting protein synthesis.

Hydrocortisone is a corticosteroid that diffuses across cell membranes and complexes with specific cytoplasmic receptors. These complexes then enter the cell nucleus, bind to DNA (chromatin), and stimulate transcription of mRNA and subsequent protein synthesis of various enzymes thought to be ultimately responsible for the anti-inflammatory effects of corticosteroids applied topically to the skin or ear.

**Absorption**
Colistin and hydrocortisone—Not absorbed when applied to the ear.
Neomycin—May possibly be absorbed if the eardrum is perforated or the skin of the ear canal is abraded.

## Precautions to Consider

**Cross-sensitivity and/or related problems**
Patients intolerant of one aminoglycoside or polymyxin may be intolerant of other aminoglycosides or polymyxins also.

**Pregnancy/Reproduction**
Problems in humans have not been documented.

**Breast-feeding**
Problems in humans have not been documented.

**Pediatrics**
Appropriate studies on the relationship of age to the effects of this medicine have not been performed in the pediatric population. However, no pediatrics-specific problems have been documented to date.

**Geriatrics**
Appropriate studies on the relationship of age to the effects of this medicine have not been performed in the geriatric population. However, no geriatrics-specific problems have been documented to date.

**Medical considerations/Contraindications**
The medical considerations/contraindications included have been selected on the basis of their potential clinical significance (reasons given in parentheses where appropriate)—not necessarily inclusive (» = major clinical significance).

*Risk-benefit should be considered when the following medical problems exist:*

Intolerance to colistin, neomycin, hydrocortisone, other aminoglycosides, polymyxins, or thimerosal

*For colistin and/or neomcyin*
Otitis media, chronic or
Perforated eardrum
(neomycin may cause ototoxicity)

*For hydrocortisone*
» Herpes simplex or
» Herpes zoster oticus or
» Tubercular or fungal infections of the ear or
» Vaccinia, varicella, or other viral disease of the ear
(may be exacerbated)

## Side/Adverse Effects

The following side/adverse effects have been selected on the basis of their potential clinical significance (possible signs and symptoms in parentheses where appropriate)—not necessarily inclusive:

**Those indicating need for medical attention**
Incidence more frequent
*Hypersensitivity* (itching, skin rash, redness, swelling, or other sign of irritation not present before therapy)

## Patient Consultation

As an aid to patient consultation, refer to *Advice for the Patient, Colistin, Neomycin, and Hydrocortisone (Otic)*.

In providing consultation, consider emphasizing the following selected information (» = major clinical significance):

**Before using this medication**
» Conditions affecting use, especially:
Intolerance to colistin, neomycin, hydrocortisone, other aminoglycosides, polymyxins, or thimerosal
Other medical problems, especially herpes simplex, herpes zoster oticus, tubercular or fungal infections of the ear, vaccinia, varicella, or other viral disease of the ear

**Proper use of this medication**
Thoroughly cleaning and drying external auditory canal with sterile cotton applicator before inserting medication
Warming otic suspension to body temperature before inserting
Proper administration technique for otic suspension
Not touching dropper to any surface; keeping container tightly closed
» Not using longer than 10 days unless otherwise directed by physician
» Compliance with full course of therapy
» Proper dosing
Missed dose: Inserting as soon as possible; not inserting if almost time for next dose
» Proper storage

**Precautions while using this medication**
Checking with physician if no improvement within 1 week or immediately if symptoms become worse

**Side/adverse effects**
Signs of potential side effects, especially hypersensitivity reactions

## General Dosing Information

Prior to administration, the external auditory canal should be thoroughly cleaned and dried with a sterile cotton applicator.

This medication may be warmed prior to administration, but not above body temperature in order to avoid loss of potency.

A cotton wick may be placed in the ear canal and then saturated with the suspension. The wick should be kept moist by adding suspension every four to eight hours and it should be replaced at least once daily.

Therapy should not be continued for more than 10 days unless directed by physician.

## Otic Dosage Forms

### COLISTIN AND NEOMYCIN SULFATES AND HYDROCORTISONE ACETATE OTIC SUSPENSION USP

**Usual adult and adolescent dose**
Topical, to the ear canal, 4 drops every six to eight hours.

**Usual pediatric dose**
Topical, to the ear canal, up to 3 drops every six to eight hours.

**Strength(s) usually available**
U.S.—
3 mg of colistin (base), 3.3 mg of neomycin (base), and 10 mg of hydrocortisone acetate per mL (Rx) [Coly-Mycin S Otic (thimerosal 0.002%)].
Canada—
3 mg of colistin (base), 3.3 mg of neomycin (base), and 10 mg of hydrocortisone acetate per mL (Rx) [Coly-Mycin Otic].

**Packaging and storage**
Store below 40 °C (104 °F), preferably between 15 and 30 °C (59 and 86 °F), unless otherwise specified by manufacturer. Store in a tight container. Protect from freezing.

**Stability**
Stable for 18 months at room temperature.

**Auxiliary labeling**
• Shake well.
• For the ear.
• Continue medicine for full time of treatment.

Revised: 05/25/95

# COLONY STIMULATING FACTORS  Systemic

This monograph includes information on the following: 1) Filgrastim; 2) Sargramostim†.

VA CLASSIFICATION (Primary): BL400

Commonly used brand name(s): *Leukine*[2]; *Neupogen*[1].

Other commonly used names for filgrastim are: Granulocyte colony stimulating factor, recombinant, rG-CSF, recombinant methionyl human granulocyte colony stimulating factor, and r-met HuG-CSF. Other commonly used names for sargramostim are: Granulocyte-macrophage colony stimulating factor, recombinant, recombinant human granulocyte-macrophage colony stimulating factor, rGM-CSF, and rHu GM-CSF.

Note: For a listing of dosage forms and brand names by country availability, see *Dosage Forms* section(s).

†Not commercially available in Canada.

## Category
Hematopoietic stimulant; antineutropenic.

## Indications
Note: Bracketed information in the *Indications* section refers to uses that are not included in U.S. product labeling.

**Accepted**

Neutropenia, chemotherapy-related (treatment)—Filgrastim (rG-CSF) and [sargramostim (rGM-CSF)] are indicated to decrease the incidence of infection, as manifested by febrile neutropenia, in patients with non-myeloid malignancies receiving myelosuppressive anticancer drugs associated with a significant incidence of severe neutropenia with fever.

Sargramostim is indicated for decreasing the duration of neutropenia after the completion of acute myelocytic leukemia (AML) induction chemotherapy in older adult patients (55 years of age and older).

Filgrastim[1] is indicated for decreasing the duration of neutropenia after the completion of AML induction or consolidation chemotherapy in adult patients.

Note: Caution is recommended in patients with myeloid malignancies such as AML because of the potential of colony stimulating factors to stimulate leukemic blasts. Filgrastim and sargramostim are not recommended for administration before or with chemotherapy in patients with AML. Criteria to define patients at increased risk (e.g., those with refractory anemia with excess blasts [RAEB] or refractory anemia with excess blasts in transformation [RAEBT], or cytogenetic abnormality) have been proposed but not established.

The theoretical risk that use of increased doses of chemotherapy permitted by administration of colony stimulating factors may result in an increase in other hematologic or nonhematologic toxicities not affected by colony stimulating factors has not been adequately studied, but caution is recommended.

Myeloid engraftment following bone marrow transplantation, promotion of (treatment adjunct)—Filgrastim is indicated for acceleration of myeloid recovery in patients undergoing autologous or allogeneic BMT following myeloablative chemotherapy for non-myeloid malignancies. [Filgrastim] and sargramostim are indicated for acceleration of myeloid recovery in patients with non-Hodgkin's lymphomas, acute lymphoblastic leukemia, and Hodgkin's disease undergoing autologous bone marrow transplantation (BMT). Sargramostim is indicated for acceleration of myeloid recovery in patients undergoing [autologous] or allogeneic BMT following myeloablative chemotherapy for non-myeloid malignancies. [Filgrastim] and sargramostim are indicated for acceleration of myeloid recovery in patients undergoing allogeneic BMT following myeloablative chemotherapy for myeloid malignancies.

Myeloid engraftment following bone marrow transplantation, failure or delay of (treatment)—[Filgrastim][1] and sargramostim are indicated for prolonging survival in patients who have undergone allogeneic or autologous BMT in whom engraftment is delayed or has failed, in the presence or absence of infection.

Note: Filgrastim and sargramostim are effective in patients receiving unpurged bone marrow or bone marrow purged with monoclonal (e.g., anti-B lymphocyte) antibodies; however, *in vitro* marrow purging with chemical agents may significantly reduce the number of responsive hematopoietic progenitors and prevent a response. The bone marrow purging process should preserve more than $1.2 \times 10^4$ progenitors per kg of body weight.

The effect may also be limited in patients who received extensive radiotherapy to hematopoietic sites for treatment of primary disease in the abdomen or chest or who have been exposed to multiple myelotoxic agents (alkylating agents, anthracycline antibiotics, and antimetabolites) before autologous BMT.

Peripheral progenitor cell yield, enhancement of (treatment adjunct)—Filgrastim and sargramostim are indicated as adjuncts to enhance peripheral progenitor cell yield in autologous hematopoietic stem cell transplantation. However, the yield (quantity and quality) of peripheral progenitor cells is dependent on the extent of prior chemotherapy.

Myeloid engraftment following hematopoietic stem cell transplantation, promotion of (treatment adjunct)—[Filgrastim] and sargramostim are indicated for acceleration of myeloid recovery in patients who have undergone hematopoietic stem cell transplantation following myeloablative chemotherapy.

[Myeloid engraftment following hematopoietic stem cell transplantation, failure or delay of (treatment)]—Sargramostim is indicated for prolonging survival in patients who have undergone autologous or allogeneic hematopoietic stem cell transplantation in whom engraftment is delayed or has failed, in the presence or absence of infection.

Neutropenia, AIDS-associated (treatment)—[Filgrastim][1] and [sargramostim] are indicated to treat acquired immunodeficiency syndrome (AIDS) patients with neutropenia caused by the disease itself or infection of opportunistic organisms (such as cytomegalovirus), or antiretroviral agents (zidovudine, ganciclovir).

The effects of colony stimulating factors on infections, hospitalization, or survival have not been established.

Because there is some evidence that sargramostim (but not filgrastim) may increase human immunodeficiency virus (HIV) replication, it is recommended that sargramostim only be given in combination with an antiretroviral agent.

Ganciclovir is toxic to stem cells. If neutrophil counts decrease despite use of colony stimulating factor, dose reduction or withdrawal of ganciclovir is recommended.

Myelodysplastic syndromes (treatment)—[Filgrastim][1] and [sargramostim] are indicated to enhance neutrophil function in patients with myelodysplastic syndromes and a history of infection.

Note: Caution is necessary because of the risk that colony stimulating factors may precipitate transformation of myelodysplastic syndromes into acute myelocytic leukemia. Assessment of risk is complicated by the fact that progression to acute leukemia may occur in the natural course of the disease.

Colony stimulating factors do not have a consistent effect on erythrocytes or platelets in these conditions.

Neutropenia, severe chronic (treatment)—Filgrastim and [sargramostim] are indicated for treatment of severe chronic neutropenia, including congenital neutropenia (Kostmann's syndrome), idiopathic neutropenia, and cyclic neutropenia.

Neutropenia, drug-induced (treatment)—[Filgrastim][1] and [sargramostim] are indicated for treatment of drug-induced neutropenia.

[1]Not included in Canadian product labeling.

## Pharmacology/Pharmacokinetics

**Physicochemical characteristics**

Source—

Filgrastim (rG-CSF): Synthetic. A protein chain of 175 amino acids produced by a recombinant DNA process involving genetically engineered *Escherichia coli* (the human granulocyte colony stimulating factor gene has been inserted into the bacteria). The protein has an amino acid sequence identical to the sequence in naturally occurring human granulocyte colony stimulating factor (G-CSF), predicted from human DNA sequence analysis, except for the addition of an N-terminal methionine necessary for expression in *E. coli*. In addition, unlike G-CSF isolated from a human cell, filgrastim is non-glycosylated. Purification is done by conventional means; prior to final purification, filgrastim is allowed to oxidize to its native state and final purity is achieved by sequential passage over a series of chromatography columns; the product is then formulated in an acetate buffer with mannitol and Tween 80.

Sargramostim (rGM-CSF): Synthetic. The commercially available form is a glycoprotein chain of 127 amino acids, characterized by 3 primary molecular species, produced by a recombinant DNA process involving a yeast (*S. cerevisiae*) expression system. The amino acid sequence differs from that of natural human granulocyte-macrophage colony stimulating factor (GM-CSF) by a substitution of leucine at position 23, and the carbohydrate moiety may be different.

Sargramostim produced in a yeast system is glycosylated; rGM-CSF produced in other systems may not be.

Chemical group—
Related to naturally occurring colony stimulating factors, which are hormone-like glycoprotein growth factors also known as cytokines.

Molecular weight—
Filgrastim: 18,800 daltons.
Sargramostim: Contains 3 primary molecular species with molecular masses of 19,500, 16,800, and 15,500 daltons.

**Mechanism of action/Effect**
In general, endogenous colony stimulating factors act on hematopoietic cells by binding to specific cell surface receptors and stimulating proliferation (clonal expansion), differentiation, and some end-cell functional activation. The recombinant colony stimulating factors have the same biological activity as the endogenous hormones. The actions of these growth factors promote differentiation of myeloid progenitor cells into granulocytes and monocytes; other pathways produce erythrocytes and platelets.

Filgrastim is a class II hematopoietic growth factor. It acts on progenitor cells capable of forming only one differentiated cell type—the neutrophil granulocyte; it is said to be lineage-specific. Sargramostim, a class I hematopoietic growth factor, stimulates formation of granulocytes (neutrophils, eosinophils) and macrophages and is therefore non–lineage specific.

Administration of colony stimulating factor to patients whose bone marrow has been depleted by myelotoxic agents or diseases such as acquired immunodeficiency syndrome (AIDS) results in an increased number of circulating hematopoietic progenitor cells. Filgrastim acts only on mature progenitor cells that are already committed to one pathway, the granulocyte pathway, and therefore increases only neutrophil concentrations. Sargramostim acts on progenitor cells at an earlier stage of development and can promote more than one lineage; it promotes formation of granulocyte, macrophage, and mixed granulocyte-macrophage colonies, resulting in increased concentrations of eosinophils and monocytes as well. Neither has a consistent effect on red cell or platelet counts.

**Other actions/effects**
Colony stimulating factors may have a proliferative effect on myeloid and erythroid leukemic cells. Sargramostim has been reported in some studies to increase replication of human immunodeficiency virus. Sargramostim has been reported to reduce low-density lipoprotein (LDL) concentrations in blood, with a variable effect on high-density lipoproteins (HDL); it has also been reported to transiently decrease cholesterol concentrations. Filgrastim has been reported to decrease serum cholesterol with variable changes in triglycerides; these changes return to normal or near baseline within 1 or 2 weeks after it is withdrawn.

**Absorption**
Filgrastim or sargramostim—Detected in serum within 5 minutes after subcutaneous administration.

**Half-life**
Distribution—
Sargramostim:
Intravenous (2-hour infusion)—
12 to 17 minutes.
Elimination—
Filgrastim:
Approximately 3.5 hours.
Sargramostim:
Intravenous (2-hour infusion)—Approximately 1 hour.
Subcutaneous—Approximately 3 hours.

**Onset of action**
Filgrastim—Decrease in circulating neutrophils occurs within the first 5 minutes of intravenous administration; after 4 hours, counts begin to rise, with an initial peak within 24 hours.
Sargramostim—Decrease in circulating neutrophils, eosinophils, and monocytes occurs, with a nadir at 30 minutes, and rebound to baseline or above by 2 hours. In addition, there is an apparent biphasic response over time; an initial plateau in leukocyte counts occurs after 3 to 7 days, which is followed by another increase and another plateau.

**Time to peak concentration**
Filgrastim—After subcutaneous administration: 2 to 8 hours.
Sargramostim—After subcutaneous administration: 2 hours.

**Time to peak effect**
Varies according to chemotherapy regimen, underlying disease and prior treatment history, and dose of colony stimulating factor.

## Precautions to Consider

**Cross-sensitivity and/or related problems**
Patients sensitive to *Escherichia coli*–derived proteins may also be sensitive to filgrastim (rG-CSF).
Patients sensitive to yeast-derived products may also be sensitive to sargramostim (rGM-CSF).

**Carcinogenicity**
Studies have not been done.

**Mutagenicity**
Filgrastim did not induce bacterial gene mutations in either the presence or absence of a drug-metabolizing enzyme system.

**Pregnancy/Reproduction**
Fertility—
*Filgrastim*—
No effect has been observed on the fertility of male or female rats or on gestation at doses up to 500 mcg per kg of body weight (mcg/kg).
*Sargramostim*—
Studies in animals have not been done due to species specificity of the human protein.

Pregnancy—Adequate and well-controlled studies in humans have not been done.
*Filgrastim*—
In pregnant rabbits, adverse effects have been observed at doses of 2 to 10 times the human dose. Studies in rabbits at doses of 80 mcg/kg per day found increased abortion and embryolethality. Studies in rabbits at doses of 100 mcg/kg per day during the period of organogenesis found increased fetal resorption, genitourinary bleeding, developmental abnormalities, and decreased body weight, live births, and food consumption; external abnormalities were not observed in the fetuses. Studies in rats at daily intravenous doses up to 575 mcg/kg per day during the period of organogenesis found no associated lethal, teratogenic, or behavioral effects on fetuses.

FDA Pregnancy Category C.

*Sargramostim*—
Studies in animals have not been donedue to species specificity of the human protein.

FDA Pregnancy Category C.

**Breast-feeding**
It is not known whether filgrastim or sargramostim is distributed into breast milk. However, problems in humans have not been documented.

**Pediatrics**
Appropriate studies on the relationship of age to the effects of colony stimulating factors have not been performed in the pediatric population. However, clinical trials have been conducted in infants and children; no differences in pharmacokinetics compared to studies in adults were found and no differences in type or incidence of adverse effects from those seen in adults have been documented to date. Subclinical increases in spleen size (seen during chronic use) detected by computed tomography (CT) or magnetic resonance imaging (MRI) studies were reported more often in children than in adults, but clinical significance of this is unknown.

Sargramostim liquid injection contains benzyl alcohol. Administration of benzyl alcohol to neonates has been associated with neurological and other complications.

**Geriatrics**
Appropriate studies on the relationship of age to the effects of colony stimulating factors have not been performed in the geriatric population. However, studies commonly include older patients, and geriatrics-specific problems that would limit the usefulness of these medications in the elderly are not expected.

**Laboratory value alterations**
The following have been selected on the basis of their potential clinical significance (possible effect in parentheses where appropriate)—not necessarily inclusive (» = major clinical significance):

With physiology/laboratory test values

*For filgrastim and sargramostim*
Blood pressure
(transient decreases occur uncommonly; hypotension has been associated with a rare "first-dose reaction" to sargramostim)

*For filgrastim only (in addition to the above)*
Alkaline phosphatase, leukocyte (LAP scores) and serum values and
Lactic dehydrogenase (LDH), serum values and

Uric acid, serum concentrations
(commonly increased in patients receiving filgrastim; the increases coincide with the rise in neutrophil counts. Concentrations return to normal within 1 or 2 weeks after withdrawal of filgrastim)

*For sargramostim only (in addition to the above)*
Albumin, serum
(decreases have been reported during sargramostim therapy; possibly related to capillary leak syndrome)
Bilirubin, serum values and
Creatinine, serum concentrations and
Hepatic enzymes, serum values
(reportedly increased by sargramostim in some patients with renal or hepatic function impairment)

**Medical considerations/Contraindications**
The medical considerations/contraindications included have been selected on the basis of their potential clinical significance (reasons given in parentheses where appropriate)—not necessarily inclusive (» = major clinical significance).

***Risk-benefit should be considered when the following medical problems exist:***

*For filgrastim and sargramostim*
Autoimmune disease, history of, e.g., autoimmune thrombocytopenia or
Inflammatory conditions, e.g., vasculitis
(may be exacerbated)
Cardiovascular disease, pre-existing
(supraventricular arrhythmia has been reported occasionally in patients receiving sargramostim, especially in patients with a history of cardiac arrhythmia; myocardial infarction and arrhythmias have been reported with filgrastim)
» Excessive leukemic myeloid blasts in the bone marrow or peripheral blood (10% or more)
(growth of leukemic blasts may be stimulated by colony stimulating factors, especially at high doses)
» Sensitivity to the colony stimulating factor prescribed
Sepsis
(theoretical potential of adult respiratory distress syndrome as a result of possible influx of neutrophils at the site of inflammation)
Caution should be used also in timing of colony stimulating factor administration to patients receiving chemotherapy or radiation therapy.

*For filgrastim only (in addition to the above)*
» Sensitivity to *E. coli*-derived proteins

*For sargramostim only (in addition to the above)*
Congestive heart failure or
Fluid retention, pre-existing (including peripheral edema, capillary leak syndrome, pleural and/or pericardial effusion) or
Pulmonary infiltrates
(sargramostim may aggravate fluid retention)
Hepatic function impairment or
Renal function impairment
(elevation of serum creatinine or bilirubin and hepatic enzymes by sargramostim has been reported; monitoring of function is recommended at least biweekly during treatment)
Pulmonary disease, including hypoxia
(caution is recommended because sargramostim causes sequestration of granulocytes in the pulmonary circulation; dyspnea has been reported)
» Sensitivity to yeast-derived proteins

**Patient monitoring**
The following may be especially important in patient monitoring (other tests may be warranted in some patients, depending on condition; » = major clinical significance):

*For filgrastim and sargramostim*
Cardiac monitoring
(recommended in patients with pre-existing cardiac conditions)
» Complete blood count (CBC) with differential (including examination for the presence of blast cells) and
Platelet counts
(recommended twice weekly during treatment to monitor the neutrophil count to assess the hematopoietic response and avoid excessive leukocytosis)
Hepatic function and/or
Renal function
(monitoring recommended at least biweekly in patients with hepatic and/or renal function impairment)

*For sargramostim only (in addition to the above)*
Body weight and
Hydration status
(recommended during treatment with sargramostim)

## Side/Adverse Effects

Note: There are relatively few side/adverse effects directly associated with colony stimulating factor administration alone. Most side/adverse effects reported are due to the underlying malignancy or cytotoxic therapy. Neutropenic effects caused by cytotoxic therapy (fever, infection, mucositis) are decreased in frequency when colony stimulating factor is used. Only those side/adverse effects specifically caused by colony stimulating factor are listed below.

Development of antibodies to filgrastim (rG-CSF) has not been detected during treatment in 500 patients for up to almost 2 years and no blunting or diminishing of response has occurred. Neutralizing antibodies have been detected in 5 of 165 patients (3%) treated with sargramostim (rGM-CSF); because all 5 had impaired hematopoiesis prior to treatment, assessment of the effect of antibody development on normal hematopoiesis was not possible.

The following side/adverse effects have been selected on the basis of their potential clinical significance (possible signs and symptoms in parentheses where appropriate)—not necessarily inclusive:

**Those indicating need for medical attention**
*For filgrastim*
Incidence less frequent
**Excessive leukocytosis**—usually asymptomatic; **redness or pain at site of subcutaneous injection**

Incidence rare
**Allergic or anaphylactic reaction** (wheezing); **splenomegaly**—usually asymptomatic; **supraventricular arrhythmia, transient** (rapid or irregular heartbeat); **Sweet's syndrome** (fever; sores on skin); **vasculitis** (sores on skin)

Note: *Splenomegaly* has been reported in patients receiving filgrastim for cyclic neutropenia. Subclinical splenomegaly occurs in approximately one-third of patients and clinical splenomegaly in about 3% of patients receiving chronic treatment with filgrastim.

*Sweet's syndrome* (also known as acute febrile neutrophilic dermatosis) appears to coincide with the increase in neutrophils.

*For sargramostim*
Incidence less frequent
**Capillary leak syndrome, including fluid retention, peripheral edema, or pleural and/or pericardial effusion** (swelling of feet or lower legs; sudden weight gain; shortness of breath); **fever; excessive leukocytosis**—usually asymptomatic; **redness or pain at site of subcutaneous injection; shortness of breath**

Note: *Capillary leak syndrome* is dose-related and dose-limiting; pleural and/or pericardial effusion usually occurs at doses above 32 mcg per kg of body weight per day. Fluid retention occurs at usual doses.

*Fever* is usually mild and dose-related. It occurs in about 50% of patients. It is not related to leukopenia, but may complicate assessment of fever associated with neutropenia. Fever resolves on withdrawal of sargramostim or administration of antipyretics such as acetaminophen.

*Shortness of breath* may be the result of sequestration of granulocytes in the pulmonary circulation. An adult respiratory distress syndrome has been reported.

Incidence rare
**Allergic or anaphylactic reaction** (wheezing); **pericarditis** (chest pain; shortness of breath); **supraventricular arrhythmia, transient** (rapid or irregular heartbeat); **thrombophlebitis**—may occur during continuous infusion into small veins; **thromboses around tip of venous catheter; vasculitis** (sores on skin)

Note: *Pericarditis* is a dose-limiting effect.
Development of *thromboses* is a dose-limiting effect.

**Those indicating need for medical attention only if they continue or are bothersome**
*For filgrastim and sargramostim*
Incidence more frequent
**Arthralgias or myalgias** (pain in joints or muscles); **medullary bone pain** (pain in lower back or pelvis; pain in arms or legs); **mild to moderate headache; skin rash or itching**

Note: *Arthralgias or myalgias* seem to occur when granulocyte counts are returning to normal. Pain usually occurs in the lower extremities.

*Bone pain* is usually mild to moderate and is alleviated by analgesics. It occurs in 20 to 50% of patients and is dose-related. It disappears within hours after withdrawal of colony stimulating factor, but usually resolves even with continued treatment. Bone pain is probably secondary to bone marrow expansion; it occurs over the 1- to 3-day period before myeloid recovery and the rise in peripheral blood neutrophils. It originates from sites containing bone marrow, including the sternum, spine, pelvis, and long bones.

*Skin rash* is usually generalized and mild.

*For sargramostim only (in addition to the above)*
Incidence less frequent or rare
    **First-dose reaction, with flushing, hypotension, and syncope** (flushing of face; dizziness or faintness); **weakness**
  Note: The *first-dose reaction* does not recur with the first dose of each course, although it may occur with the first dose of more than one course. The first-dose reaction has been described more consistently with bacterially-derived GM-CSF (molgramostim; not commercially available), and included tachycardia, musculoskeletal pain, and dyspnea.

## Overdose

There are no data on massive overdoses of filgrastim or sargramostim. However, sargramostim was administered to four patients at dosages sixteen times the recommended dose for 7 to 18 days in an uncontrolled study.

For more information on the management of overdose or unintentional ingestion, **contact a Poison Control Center** (see *Poison Control Center Listing*).

**Clinical effects of sargramostim overdose**
The following effects have been selected on the basis of their potential clinical significance (possible signs and symptoms in parentheses where appropriate)—not necessarily inclusive:

Acute and chronic
    **Chills; dyspnea** (shortness of breath); **excessive leukocytosis**—usually asymptomatic; **fever; headache; malaise** (general feeling of bodily discomfort); **nausea; skin rash; tachycardia** (rapid heartbeat)

**Treatment of overdose**
Treatment of sargramostim overdose—
    Specific treatment: Sargramostim should be discontinued.
    Monitoring: Respiratory status and white blood cell counts should be monitored.
    Patients in whom intentional overdose is confirmed or suspected should be referred for psychiatric consultation.

## Patient Consultation

As an aid to patient consultation, refer to *Advice for the Patient, Colony Stimulating Factors (Systemic)*.
In providing consultation, consider emphasizing the following selected information (» = major clinical significance):

**Before using this medication**
» Conditions affecting use, especially:
    Sensitivity to the colony stimulating factor prescribed
    Pregnancy—Adverse effects with filgrastim found in rabbits

**Proper use of this medication**
*For subcutaneous use*
» Compliance with therapy
» Reading patient directions carefully with regard to
    • Preparation of the injection
    • Use of disposable syringes
    • Proper administration technique
    • Stability of the injection
» Proper dosing
    Missed dose: Checking with physician
» Proper storage

**Precautions while using this medication**
» Importance of close monitoring by physician
» Telling physician right away if signs or symptoms of infection (fever, chills) occur
  Possibility of mild bone pain as bone marrow begins to recover; usually relieved by mild analgesics; checking with physician if severe

**Side/adverse effects**
*Signs of potential side effects, especially:*
  For filgrastim—Redness or pain at site of subcutaneous injection, allergic or anaphylactic reaction, arrhythmias, and Sweet's syndrome and other dermatoses
  For sargramostim—Fluid retention, peripheral edema, pleural and/or pericardial effusion, fever, redness or pain at site of subcutaneous injection, shortness of breath, allergic or anaphylactic reaction, arrhythmias, pericarditis, and Sweet's syndrome and other dermatoses

## General Dosing Information

Patients receiving colony stimulating factor should be under supervision of a physician experienced in cytokine and/or cancer chemotherapy.

It is recommended that appropriate precautions be taken in the event that an allergic reaction occurs. If a serious allergic or anaphylactic reaction occurs, colony stimulating factor should be immediately discontinued and appropriate therapy initiated.

It is recommended that colony stimulating factor be discontinued when the absolute neutrophil count (ANC) reaches or exceeds 10,000 per cubic millimeter after the ANC nadir has occurred, to avoid excessive leukocytosis.

Colony stimulating factor should not be administered within 24 hours before or after administration of the last dose of chemotherapy or within 12 hours before or after radiotherapy, because of potential sensitivity of rapidly dividing hematopoietic progenitor cells to cytotoxic chemotherapy or radiologic therapies.

---

### FILGRASTIM

## Summary of Differences

Pharmacology/pharmacokinetics: Mechanism of action—Lineage-specific; stimulates production of neutrophil granulocytes.
Side/adverse effects: Causes splenomegaly with chronic use, Sweet's syndrome; development of antibodies not reported.

## Additional Dosing Information

Filgrastim may be administered subcutaneously (by rapid injection or as a continuous 24-hour infusion) or intravenously (as a short 30-minute or continuous 24-hour infusion). *Intravenous administration should be by infusion over at least 30 minutes*, because there is a decrease in efficacy when filgrastim is administered by rapid intravenous injection; in addition, it is preferable not to flush the intravenous line after administration is complete.

A variety of dosage schedules are used, depending on the indication and the individual patient, for indications not included in the official labeling. The prescriber may consult the medical literature in choosing a specific dosage.

The chemotherapy-induced nadir usually occurs 2 or 3 days earlier during cycles in which filgrastim is administered.

Bone pain usually responds to treatment with non-narcotic analgesics; infrequently, it may be severe enough to require narcotic analgesics.

## Parenteral Dosage Forms

Note: Bracketed information in the *Dosage Forms* section refers to uses that are not included in U.S. product labeling.

### FILGRASTIM INJECTION

**Usual adult dose**
Neutropenia, chemotherapy-related—
  Intravenous or subcutaneous, 5 mcg (0.005 mg) per kg of body weight once a day, beginning no earlier than twenty-four hours after administration of the last dose of cytotoxic chemotherapy. This is continued for up to two weeks, until the absolute neutrophil count (ANC) reaches ten thousand per cubic millimeter following the nadir; in patients receiving dose intensified chemotherapy, filgrastim should be continued until two consecutive ANC's of at least ten thousand per cubic millimeter are documented. Dosage may be increased, if necessary, in increments of 5 mcg (0.005 mg) per kg of body weight for each chemotherapy cycle.

Myeloid engraftment following bone marrow transplantation, promotion of—
  Intravenous infusion (over four or twenty-four hours) or subcutaneous, 10 mcg (0.01 mg) per kg of body weight a day for twenty-one days beginning two to four hours after bone marrow infusion, and not less than twenty-four hours after the last dose of chemotherapy. When the ANC reaches one thousand per cubic millimeter, the dose of filgrastim may be lowered to 5 mcg (0.005 mg) per kg of body weight a day. If the ANC exceeds one thousand per cubic millimeter

for three additional days, filgrastim may be discontinued. If the ANC subsequently falls below one thousand per cubic millimeter, filgrastim may be resumed at 5 mcg (0.005 mg) per kg of body weight a day. If ANC decreases to less than one thousand per cubic millimeter at any time while the patient is receiving 5 mcg (0.005 mg) per kg of body weight a day, the dose may be increased to 10 mcg (0.01 mg) per kg of body weight a day.

[Myeloid engraftment following bone marrow transplantation, failure or delay (treatment)][1]—
  Intravenous or subcutaneous, 5 mcg (0.005 mg) per kg of body weight a day for fourteen days; course of therapy may be repeated after seven days if engraftment has not occurred. If engraftment has not occurred within seven days after the second fourteen-day course of therapy, a course of 10 mcg (0.01 mg) per kg of body weight a day for fourteen days may be tried.

[Myeloid engraftment following hematopoietic stem cell transplantation, promotion of]—
  Subcutaneous, continuous or intermittent injection, or intravenous infusion, 5 mcg (0.005 mg) per kg of body weight a day.

Peripheral progenitor cell yield, enhancement of—
  Subcutaneous, continuous or intermittent injection, 10 mcg (0.01 mg) per kg of body weight a day for at least four days prior to the first leukapheresis, and continuing until the last leukapheresis.

Note: The optimal schedule of filgrastim administration and leukapheresis has not been established. The administration of filgrastim for six or seven days, with leukapheresis on days five, six, and seven, was found to be effective in clinical trials.

Neutropenia, severe chronic—
  Congenital neutropenia:
    Subcutaneous, 6 mcg (0.006 mg) per kg of body weight two times a day.
  Idiopathic or cyclic neutropenia:
    Subcutaneous, 5 mcg (0.005 mg) per kg of body weight a day.

Note: The dose must be adjusted based on the clinical condition of the patient and the ANC. In some clinical trials, the target ANC was fifteen hundred per cubic millimeter.

Note: The calculated dose may be rounded off, within reason, to the nearest vial size (300 or 480 mcg) to reduce wastage.

**Usual adult prescribing limits**
Not defined. Patients have received doses as high as 115 mcg (0.115 mg) per kg of body weight a day without toxic effects.

**Usual pediatric dose**
Dosage has not been established.

**Strength(s) usually available**
U.S.—
  300 mcg (0.3 mg) per mL (300 mcg per 1-mL vial or 480 mcg per 1.6-mL vial) (Rx) [*Neupogen* (acetate 0.59 mg per mL; mannitol 50 mg per mL; 0.004% of Tween 80; sodium 0.035 mg per mL)].
Canada—
  300 mcg (0.3 mg) per mL (300 mcg per 1-mL vial or 480 mcg per 1.6-mL vial) (Rx) [*Neupogen* (acetate 0.59 mg per mL; 0.004% of Tween 80; sodium 0.035 mg per mL)].

Note: The specific activity is $1 \pm 0.6 \times 10^8$ Units per mg as measured by a cell mitogenesis assay.

**Packaging and storage**
Store between 2 and 8 °C (36 and 46 °F), unless otherwise specified by manufacturer. Protect from freezing. Avoid shaking.

**Preparation of dosage form**
Filgrastim injection may be diluted for administration by intravenous infusion in 5% dextrose injection to produce a concentration greater than or equal to 15 mcg of filgrastim per mL. If the final concentration is to be between 2 and 15 mcg per mL, addition of human albumin to the dextrose injection before addition of filgrastim injection is necessary to prevent adsorption to the components of the drug delivery system. The concentration of human albumin in the final solution should be 0.2% (2 mg per mL); this can be achieved with 2 mL of 5% human albumin in 50 mL of 5% dextrose injection.

**Stability**
Filgrastim injection contains no preservative. Before use, filgrastim injection may be allowed to reach room temperature for a maximum of 6 hours; after that period of time, the vial should be discarded.

**Auxiliary labeling**
• Do not shake.

---

[1]Not included in Canadian product labeling.

## SARGRAMOSTIM

### Summary of Differences
Pharmacology/pharmacokinetics: Mechanism of action—Non–lineage specific; stimulates production of granulocytes, macrophages, and eosinophils.
Precautions: Medical considerations/contraindications—Pulmonary disease.
Side/adverse effects: Causes capillary leak syndrome and fluid retention, fever, shortness of breath, pericarditis, thrombophlebitis, thromboses, first-dose reaction, and weakness.

### Additional Dosing Information
Sargramostim is administered as an intravenous infusion via a central venous line. An in-line membrane filter should not be used. Sargramostim may also be administered subcutaneously.

A variety of dosage schedules are used, depending on the indication and the individual patient, for indications not included in the official labeling. The prescriber may consult the medical literature in choosing a specific dosage.

Systemic adverse effects (bone pain, fever, asthenia, etc.) are usually prevented or reversed by administration of analgesics and antipyretics such as acetaminophen.

Fluid retention is reversible on withdrawal or dose reduction, with or without diuretic treatment.

If dyspnea occurs during sargramostim administration, the rate of administration should be reduced by half. The standard dosing schedule may be used, with careful monitoring, for subsequent infusions. If dyspnea persists following infusion rate reduction, the infusion should be discontinued.

If the absolute neutrophil count (ANC) exceeds 20,000 or the platelet count exceeds 500,000, sargramostim treatment should be discontinued or the dose reduced by half. Excessive blood counts usually return to normal or baseline levels within 3 to 7 days following withdrawal of sargramostim.

If progression of the underlying neoplastic disease (non-Hodgkin's lymphoma, acute lymphocytic leukemia, Hodgkin's disease) occurs during sargramostim therapy, it is recommended that sargramostim be discontinued.

If blast cells appear, it is recommended that sargramostim be discontinued.

### Parenteral Dosage Forms
Note: Bracketed information in the *Dosage Forms* section refers to uses that are not included in U.S. product labeling.

### SARGRAMOSTIM FOR INJECTION
**Usual adult dose**
Myeloid engraftment following bone marrow transplantation, promotion of—
  Intravenous infusion (over two hours) or subcutaneous, 250 mcg (0.25 mg) per square meter of body surface area a day for twenty-one days beginning two to four hours after allogeneic or autologous bone marrow infusion, and not less than twenty-four hours after the last dose of chemotherapy or radiotherapy and continued until an absolute neutrophil count (ANC) of fifteen hundred per cubic millimeter is achieved and maintained for three consecutive days.

Myeloid engraftment following hematopoietic stem cell transplantation, promotion of—
  Intravenous infusion (continuous) or subcutaneous, 250 mcg (0.25 mg) per square meter of body surface area a day through the period of peripheral blood progenitor cell (PBPC) collection, then immediately following infusion of progenitor cells and continued until an ANC of fifteen hundred per cubic millimeter is achieved and maintained for three consecutive days.

Myeloid engraftment following bone marrow transplantation, failure or delay—
  Intravenous infusion (over two hours) or subcutaneous, 250 mcg (0.25 mg) per square meter of body surface area a day for fourteen days; course of therapy may be repeated after seven days if engraftment has not occurred. If engraftment has not occurred within seven days after the second fourteen-day course of therapy, a course of 500 mcg (0.5 mg) per square meter of body surface area a day for fourteen days may be tried.

Neutropenia, chemotherapy-related, in older adult patients (55 years of age and older) with acute myelocytic leukemia (AML)—
  Intravenous infusion (over four hours) or subcutaneous, 250 mcg (0.25 mg) per square meter of body surface area a day beginning approximately day eleven (or four days after completion of induction

chemotherapy) if the bone marrow is hypoplastic with fewer than five percent blasts on day ten.

[Neutropenia, chemotherapy-related]—
Intravenous infusion (over two hours) or subcutaneous, 250 mcg (0.25 mg) per square meter of body surface area a day beginning no earlier than twenty-four hours after administration of the last dose of cytotoxic chemotherapy. This is continued for up to two weeks, until the ANC reaches ten thousand per cubic millimeter following the nadir; in patients receiving dose intensified chemotherapy, sargramostim should be continued until two consecutive ANC's of at least ten thousand per cubic millimeter are documented. Dosage may be increased, if necessary, in an increment of 250 mcg (0.25 mg) per square meter of body surface area, up to 500 mcg (0.5 mg) per square meter of body surface area.

Peripheral progenitor cell yield, enhancement of—
Intravenous infusion (continuous) or subcutaneous, 250 mcg (0.25 mg) per square meter of body surface area a day through the period of peripheral blood progenitor cell (PBPC) collection, then immediately following infusion of progenitor cells and continued until an ANC of fifteen hundred per cubic millimeter is achieved and maintained for three consecutive days.

Note: The calculated dose may be rounded off, within reason, to the nearest vial size (250 or 500 mcg) to reduce wastage.

**Usual pediatric dose**
Dosage has not been established.

**Size(s) usually available**
U.S.—
250 mcg (0.25 mg) (Rx) [*Leukine* (lyophilized; mannitol 40 mg; sucrose 10 mg; tromethamine 1.2 mg)].
500 mcg (0.5 mg) (Rx) [*Leukine* (lyophilized; mannitol 40 mg; sucrose 10 mg; tromethamine 1.2 mg)].
Canada—
Not commercially available.

Note: The specific activity is approximately $5 \times 10^7$ colony forming units per mg in a normal human bone marrow colony formation assay.

**Packaging and storage**
Store between 2 and 8 °C (36 and 46 °F), unless otherwise specified by manufacturer. Protect reconstituted solution from freezing. Avoid shaking solution.

**Preparation of dosage form**
Lyophilized sargramostim for injection is reconstituted by adding 1 mL of sterile water for injection (without preservative) to the vial containing 250 or 500 mcg, producing a clear, colorless solution containing 250 or 500 mcg of sargramostim per mL, respectively. To avoid foaming during dissolution, the diluent should be directed at the side of the vial and the contents swirled gently; excessive or vigorous agitation should be avoided; the vial should not be shaken.

The reconstituted solution is diluted further for administration by intravenous infusion with 0.9% sodium chloride injection. If the final concentration of sargramostim is to be less than 10 mcg per mL, addition of human albumin to the saline before addition of sargramostim solution is necessary to prevent adsorption to the components of the drug delivery system. The concentration of human albumin in the final solution should be 0.1% (1 mg per mL); this can be achieved with 1 mL of 5% human albumin in 50 mL of 0.9% sodium chloride injection.

**Stability**
Because lyophilized sargramostim contains no antibacterial preservative, solutions reconstituted with sterile water for injection (without preservative) should be used within 6 hours and any unused portion should be discarded. Lyophilized sargramostim reconstituted with bacteriostatic water for injection may be stored for 20 days between 2 and 8 °C (36 and 46 °F).

**Auxiliary labeling**
• Do not shake.

## SARGRAMOSTIM INJECTION

**Usual adult dose**
See *Sargramostim for Injection*.

**Usual pediatric dose**
Dosage has not been established.

**Strength(s) usually available**
U.S.—
500 mcg (0.5 mg) per mL (Rx) [*Leukine* (benzyl alcohol 1.1%; mannitol 40 mg; sucrose 10 mg; tromethamine 1.2 mg)].
Canada—
Not commercially available.

**Packaging and storage**
Store between 2 and 8 °C (36 and 46 °F), unless otherwise specified by manufacturer. Protect reconstituted solution from freezing.

**Preparation of dosage form**
Sargramostim injection for administration by intravenous infusion is diluted with 0.9% sodium chloride injection. The solution should not be shaken. If the final concentration of sargramostim is to be less than 10 mcg per mL, it is necessary to add human albumin to the saline before addition of sargramostim solution in order to prevent adsorption of sargramostim onto the components of the drug delivery system. The concentration of human albumin in the final solution should be 0.1% (1 mg per mL); this can be achieved with 1 mL of 5% human albumin in 50 mL of 0.9% sodium chloride injection.

**Stability**
After the vial has been entered, undiluted sargramostim injection may be stored for 20 days between 2 and 8 °C (36 and 46 °F). Unopened vials of sargramostim injection are stable for 14 days when stored at 30 °C (86 °F). After dilution with 0.9% sodium chloride injection in polyvinyl chloride bags to final concentrations of sargramostim of 2.5 mcg per mL (mcg/mL), 8 mcg/mL, or 12 mcg/mL, sargramostim injection may be stored for 48 hours between 2 and 8 °C (36 and 46 °F) or 25 °C (77 °F).

**Auxiliary labeling**
• Do not shake.

Revised: 10/01/97
Interim revision: 06/24/98

---

**CONDOMS**—The *Condoms* monograph is not included in this published version of the USP DI database. Copies of the monograph are available on request from Micromedex, Inc. - Reprint Requests, 6200 S. Syracuse Way, Suite 300, Englewood, CO 80111; telephone (303) 486-6400; telefax (303) 486-6464; Email: USPDI@MDX.COM.

---

# CONJUGATED ESTROGENS AND MEDROXYPROGESTERONE FOR OVARIAN HORMONE THERAPY (OHT) Systemic†

This monograph includes information on the following: 1) Conjugated Estrogens, and Conjugated Estrogens and Medroxyprogesterone†; 2) Conjugated Estrogens and Medroxyprogesterone†

Note: For information pertaining to the use of only estrogens or progestins, see *Estrogens (Systemic)* or *Progestins (Systemic)*.

VA CLASSIFICATION (Primary/Secondary):
Conjugated Estrogens—HS102/MS900
Conjugated Estrogens and Medroxyprogesterone Acetate—HS105/MS900

Commonly used brand name(s): *Premphase*[1]; *Prempro*[2].

Note: For a listing of dosage forms and brand names by country availability, see *Dosage Forms* section(s).

†Not commercially available in Canada.

## Category

Estrogen-progestin; osteoporosis prophylactic; ovarian hormone therapy agent.

## Indications

**General considerations**
Estrogen deficiency in women without a uterus is best treated with unopposed estrogen therapy; combined estrogen-progestin therapy is not needed.

**Accepted**
Menopause, vasomotor symptoms of (treatment) or
Vaginitis, atrophic (treatment) or
Vulvar atrophy (treatment)—Conjugated estrogens and medroxyprogesterone tablets are indicated to treat symptoms of estrogen deficiency,

including vasomotor symptoms of menopause, atrophic vaginitis, and vulvar atrophy. The progestin component, medroxyprogesterone acetate, is given only to modify estrogen's effect on the uterus, significantly reducing the incidence of endometrial hyperplasia.

Osteoporosis, postmenopausal (prophylaxis)—Conjugated estrogens and medroxyprogesterone are indicated to prevent osteoporosis due to estrogen deficiency in postmenopausal women who have a uterus. Proper diet, calcium supplementation, and physical activity also help lower the risk of osteoporosis. Although in one study estrogen reduced the rate of bone loss when it was given 6 years after the onset of menopause, the greatest benefit is achieved when treatment is initiated at menopause. Patient selection must be individualized according to the risks and benefits, and periodically re-evaluated for discontinuation when long-term treatment is prescribed. Although studies show that progestins positively influence bone density in postmenopausal women, a progestin is given mainly to oppose the effects of estrogen on the uterus; adding a progestin to increase bone mass is not warranted.

### Unaccepted
Although a few studies show that estrogens have some effect on neurotransmitters and may improve memory and cognitive function, estrogen and progestin therapy is not indicated or effective in the treatment of clinical depression.

## Pharmacology/Pharmacokinetics
### Physicochemical characteristics
Source—
Conjugated estrogens are a mixture of many estrogenic substances found in equine urine; the complete profile of the mixture is not known. The primary estrogens are considered to be sodium estrone sulfate and sodium equilin sulfate. Other estrogens defined as concomitant components are the sodium sulfated conjugates of 17-alpha-dihydroequilin, 17-alpha-estradiol, and 17-beta-dihydroequilin.

Chemical group—
Estrogen: Conjugated estrogens.
Progestin: Medroxyprogesterone acetate.

Molecular weight—
Medroxyprogesterone acetate: 386.53.

### Mechanism of action/Effect
Estrogen-progestin—
Both hormones diffuse into the nucleus of cells and bind to DNA via the receptor proteins; and, either a transcription process begins—messenger RNA (mRNA) increases, resulting in subsequent protein synthesis—or a transrepression process occurs. Transrepression occurs if transcription is not properly stimulated, resulting in no gene expression or protein synthesis. According to the cell's genetic makeup, the two hormones can affect different target tissues or dissimilarly affect the same responsive tissue. Depending on the target tissue, an increased concentration of a hormone can enhance, impede, or even negate its own effect (negative feedback mechanisms) or influence the effect of other hormones (either via receptor down-regulation or upregulation). The magnitude of estrogen's effect and its influence with different hormones depends on the endogenous estrogen concentration, product formulation, and type and dose of exogenous estrogen administered. For example, medroxyprogesterone reduces the number of estrogen receptors in the uterus and reduces estrogen's effect on DNA. In the absence of the estrogen effect, protein synthesis decreases and endometrial proliferation is decreased or stopped, depending on the estrogen and progestin doses.

Ovarian hormone therapy agent—
Tissues especially responsive to estrogens include female urogenital organs, breasts, hypothalamus, and pituitary; breast and uterine tissues are especially responsive to progestins. Estrogens maintain tone and elasticity of the urogenital structures, improving tissue function. Women taking physiologic doses of estrogen during menopause experience less urinary urgency or stress incontinence, burning on urination, irritation or inflammation of the vagina or vulva, and vaginal dryness. Use of continuous or cyclic progestin with estrogen lessens hyperplastic changes of the endometrium either by inducing menstrual-like periods to slough off endometrial lining or by producing endometrial atrophy. Amenorrhea occurs over time. In addition, estrogens in physiologic doses given to postmenopausal women restore their vasomotor stability with fewer hot flushes.

Osteoporosis prophylactic—
Although the exact mechanism of this action is not known, it is thought that use of estrogens slows down the rate of bone loss by nearly restoring equilibrium between bone loss and bone formation, potentially reducing the risk of fractures. Estrogen's effect on bone loss depends on the dose and the initial bone mass density, and is independent of patient age or the route of estrogen administration. In the short term, a new, lower rate of bone loss is established within 24 months with significant gain in the first 12 months, regardless of whether a patient is 1 or 10 years past menopause. Women of heavy and light body weights gain similar amounts of bone, more so in the spine than in the hip. With discontinuation of estrogen therapy, the rate of bone mass loss returns to the rate usually observed in the immediate postmenopausal period; the rate of loss is greater in women of lighter weight than in heavier women.

Beginning estrogen therapy early in menopause and continuing for at least 7 years imparts some long-term protection against accelerated bone loss, but investigators of the Framingham study suggest that 7 to 10 years of estrogen use may not be enough to protect women 75 years of age or older from fractures. When estrogen was used for 10 years or more in the Framingham study, women younger than 75 years of age had a 44% reduction in the risk of hip fracture at the femoral neck and 52% risk reduction at the trochanter.

### Other actions/effects
Estrogens help develop and maintain the female reproductive system and secondary sex characteristics. Estrogens may enhance mood and cognitive function by increasing serotonin and free tryptophan levels in the brain, and by modifying estrogen receptors in the pituitary, hypothalamus, limbic forebrain, and cerebral cortex. Estrogens, acting with other hormones and cytokines, stimulate the growth and development of breast tissue and skeleton formation, and are integral to the physiology of puberty, menstruation, ovulatory cycles, and pregnancy.

Estrogens prevent vessel constriction when challenged through a direct vessel wall effect and, to a lesser extent, improve the lipoprotein cholesterol profile; both effects are significant for cardioprotectionand reduction of arteriosclerosis. Concomitant progestin therapy can diminish the magnitude of improvement induced by estrogens in the lipoprotein cholesterol profile.

Locally, progestins relax the uterine smooth muscle, decrease the immune response, and cause sodium and water retention.

### Absorption
Conjugated estrogens and medroxyprogesterone—Well absorbed.
The following changes in absorption occur when conjugated estrogens and medroxyprogesterone are taken with a high-fat meal:
Continuous cycle (0.625 mg of conjugated estrogens and 2.5 mg of medroxyprogesterone):
Estrone—Peak plasma concentration ($C_{max}$) decreased by 34%;
Equilin—$C_{max}$ not affected; and
Medroxyprogesterone acetate—$C_{max}$ doubled, resulting in a 30% increase in the plasma concentration–time curve (AUC).
Phasic cycle (0.625 mg of conjugated estrogens continuously, and 14 days of 5 mg of medroxyprogesterone):
Estrone—$C_{max}$ decreased by 18%;
Equilin—$C_{max}$ increased by 38%; and
Medroxyprogesterone acetate—$C_{max}$ doubled, resulting in a 20% increase in AUC.

### Protein binding
Conjugated estrogens and medroxyprogesterone acetate—Moderate to high (50 to 80%). Conjugated estrogens bind mainly to albumin, and unconjugated estrogens bind to both albumin and sex hormone–binding globulin (SHBG). Medroxyprogesterone binds mainly to albumin or to other plasma proteins, but not to SHBG.

### Biotransformation
Primarily hepatic.

### Half-life
Apparent terminal-phase half-life—Conjugated estrogens: 10 to 24 hours. Medroxyprogesterone: 38 to 46 hours.

### Time to peak concentration
Conjugated or unconjugated estrogens—4 to 10 hours.
Medroxyprogesterone—Within 2 to 4 hours.

### Elimination
Conjugated estrogens—
Renal: Major route, as acidic ionized conjugates.
Fecal: Minimal; reabsorbed from intestines and returned through portal venous system.
Medroxyprogesterone—
Renal: Minor route; excreted mainly as glucuronide conjugates, with some sulfate metabolites.
Fecal: Major route; excreted as hydroxylated and conjugated metabolites.

## Precautions to Consider

### Carcinogenicity/Tumorigenicity
Estrogens may increase the incidence of breast cancer in some postmenopausal women. Long-term studies are still needed to fully characterize potential risk. The majority of data available does not seem to support a significant increase in risk for patients using physiologic doses. Patients using estrogens in either high doses or low doses for a prolonged period, especially longer than 10 years, potentially may have greater risk. Some studies suggest but do not prove that the risk doubles for patients with an individual risk factor (such as early menarche, late menopause, or nulliparity) or familial risk (such as patients whose mother or sister have had breast cancer). Short-term use of estrogens during menopause for treatment of menopausal symptoms does not appear to increase risk, and no additional risk has been attributed to adding a progestin to the therapy. Regular breast examinations or mammography will help detect any developing abnormality.

Studies show a lower incidence of endometrial hyperplasia and, potentially, endometrial cancer when patients take a progestin for a minimum of 10 to 14 days a month along with an estrogen cycle. One study reported an incidence of less than 1% for continuous or cyclic regimens of conjugated estrogens and medroxyprogesterone after 1 year of use. When nonusers were compared to users of an estrogen-only cycle, no risk of endometrial hyperplasia was shown for the first year of use. When unopposed estrogens were taken for a prolonged period or at higher than physiologic doses, risk increased 2- to 12-fold. Furthermore, the risk increased as high as 24-fold when estrogen alone was used for 5 years or longer. Although the magnitude of risk decreases substantially within 6 months after unopposed oral estrogen therapy is discontinued, some risk can continue for 8 to 15 years.

In certain animal species, long-term, continuous administration of estrogens increases the frequency of cancers of the breast, cervix, liver, pancreas, testes, uterus, and vagina. Results of animal studies may not apply to humans because of the general hormonal differences of sex steroids among species.

### Mutagenicity
There was no mutagenic response in the Ames and micronucleus tests for medroxyprogesterone.

### Pregnancy/Reproduction
Pregnancy—Use of a combination of conjugated estrogens and medroxyprogesterone is not recommended during pregnancy. Pregnancy occurs rarely in menopausal women because of the natural change in their hormone milieu; on the rare chance of occurrence, a fetus surviving to term is unlikely. Conjugated estrogens and medroxyprogesterone do not demonstrate teratogenic effects, although medroxyprogesterone can lessen intrauterine fetal growth. Although the association is questionable, a few cases of polysyndactyly in the infants occurred when the mother used parenteral medroxyprogesterone in the first trimester. Other progestins produced hypospadias in male infants, and virilized the external genitalia in female infants.

FDA Pregnancy Category X.

### Breast-feeding
Conjugated estrogens and medroxyprogesterone are distributed into breast milk. This combination is not recommended for use by nursing mothers.

### Drug interactions and/or related problems
The following drug interactions and/or related problems have been selected on the basis of their potential clinical significance (possible mechanism in parentheses where appropriate)—not necessarily inclusive (» = major clinical significance):

Note: Combinations containing any of the following medications, depending on the amount present, may also interact with this medication.

Antidiabetic or antihypertensive agents, antihyperlipidemics, or antifibrinolytics may need a dosage adjustment if adding or deleting estrogens or progestins causes slight changes in the patient's underlying condition.

» Aminoglutethimide
(may significantly lower the serum concentrations of oral medroxyprogesterone by an undetermined mechanism; it has been suggested that aminoglutethimide may decrease the intestinal absorption of medroxyprogesterone)

(although not considered clinically significant, aminoglutethimide inhibits estrogen production from androgens in peripheral tissues by blocking the aromatase enzyme; it may also enhance metabolism of estrone sulfate)

» Barbiturates, especially phenobarbital or
» Carbamazepine or
» Hydantoins, especially phenytoin or

Rifabutin or
» Rifampin
(hepatic enzyme–inducing properties of these drugs may reduce the activity of conjugated estrogens or medroxyprogesterone; rifabutin appears to be a less potent enzyme inducer of the hepatic cytochrome P450 system than rifampin)

(drug interaction data are not available for rifabutin, but because its structure is similar to that of rifampin, similar precautions may be warranted)

Calcium supplements
(concurrent use with estrogens may increase calcium absorption and exacerbate nephrolithiasis in susceptible individuals; this action can be used to therapeutic advantage to increase bone mass)

Corticosteroids, glucocorticoid
(concurrent use with estrogens may alter the metabolism and protein binding of the glucocorticoids, leading to decreased clearance, increased elimination half-life, and increased therapeutic and toxic effects of the glucocorticoids; glucocorticoid dosage adjustment may be required during and following concurrent use)

Corticotropin (long-term therapeutic use)
(concurrent use with estrogens may potentiate the anti-inflammatory effects of endogenous cortisol induced by corticotropin)

» Cyclosporine
(estrogens have been reported to inhibit cyclosporine metabolism and thereby increase plasma concentrations of cyclosporine, possibly increasing the risk of hepatotoxicity and nephrotoxicity; concurrent use is recommended only with great caution and frequent monitoring of blood cyclosporine concentrations and hepatic and renal function)

» Hepatotoxic medications, especially dantrolene and isoniazid (see Appendix II)
(concurrent use of these medications with estrogens may increase the risk of hepatotoxicity; fatal hepatitis has occurred)

Medications associated with pancreatitis, especially
Didanosine or
Lamivudine or
Zalcitabine
(estrogens should be used with caution with medications that cause pancreatitis, especially if patient has pre-existing risk factors, such as high triglyceride concentrations; however, physiologic doses of estrogen would not be expected to induce pancreatitis)

» Protease inhibitors, such as ritonavir
(ritonavir has decreased the area under the plasma concentration–time curve [AUC] of ethinyl estradiol by 40%; similar effects may occur with other estrogens or with other protease inhibitors)

Smoking, tobacco
(smoking increases the metabolism of estrogens and can result in a decreased estrogenic effect)

(smokers have an increased risk of coronary heart disease and are more likely to experience myocardial infarction and angina pectoris. Although data are unavailable for menopausal or postmenopausal patients who smoke tobacco, it is unlikely that the use of physiologic doses of estrogen in these patients increases risk. Smokers do have an increased risk of hip fractures, and estrogens provide some degree of protection)

Tamoxifen
(estrogens may interfere with tamoxifen's effect)

### Laboratory value alterations
The following have been selected on the basis of their potential clinical significance (possible effect in parentheses where appropriate)—not necessarily inclusive (» = major clinical significance):

*With diagnostic test results*
Biopsy
(pathologist should be notified of relevant specimens)

Metyrapone stimulation test
(response is lower than expected)

*With physiology/laboratory test values*
Antithrombin III, plasma and
Fibrinogen, plasma
(decreased levels are related to estrogen dose and duration of treatment. In one study, antithrombin III levels decreased by 5% from baseline in patients taking the continuous regimen of 0.625 mg conjugated estrogens and 2.5 mg medroxyprogesterone for 1 year. At the end of the year's treatment, patients taking the 0.625 mg conjugated estrogens and 5 mg medroxyprogesterone tablet showed a slight increase in antithrombin III activity. A 1% decrease occurred in the same 1-year study of patients taking the cyclical regimen)

Calcium, serum
  (concentrations may be increased, especially for immobilized patients or patients with breast cancer or bone metastases)
Cholesterol, total, serum and
Folic acid, serum and
Lipoprotein (a), plasma and
Lipoprotein cholesterol, low-density (LDLC), serum
  (concentrations may be decreased)
    (lower total cholesterol occurs because cyclic doses of 5 mg or continuous doses of 2.5 or 5 mg medroxyprogesterone attenuate most of the favorable increase in the HDLC component produced from a continuously administered dose of 0.625 mg conjugated estrogens)
Coagulation factors, plasma, such as Factors II, VII, VIII, IX, X, and XII and
Plasminogen, plasma and
Platelet count, whole blood
  (concentrations may be increased)
    (in one large clinical trial, patients taking either the continuous or phasic regimens of conjugated estrogen and medroxyprogesterone increased the plasminogen activity by 14% and the Factor X concentrations by 13% over their baseline values. In this same study, the magnitude of increase in the Factor VII concentration was 20% for the continuous regimen as compared with 8% for the cyclical regimen)
Insulin, serum or plasma and
Glucose, 2-hour postprandial, serum or plasma
  (minimal effect on glucose metabolism and unlikely to influence heart disease risk. While the fasting serum insulin and glucose show little or change, the 2-hour serum glucose may be slightly increased and the insulin concentration may be slightly decreased)
Lipoprotein cholesterol, high-density (HDLC), serum and
Triglycerides (TG), serum
  (concentrations are increased)
    (5-mg doses of the cyclic or continuous doses of 2.5 or 5 mg medroxyprogesterone attentuate much of the favorable increase of the HDLC component induced by 0.625 mg conjugated estrogens)
    (triglycerides are increased with the use of continuous doses of 2.5 or 5 mg medroxyprogesterone with 0.625 mg conjugated estrogens, but the increase is approximately half as great as that produced from use of 0.625 mg conjugated estrogens alone)
Liver profile test, serum
  (values may be increased; if abnormal, liver tests may be repeated 4 to 6 months after medication is discontinued)
Plasma binding globulins, such as
  Corticotropin-binding globulin (CBG), serum
  Sex hormone–binding globulin (SHBG), serum
  Thyroxine-binding globulin (TBG), serum
Plasma proteins, other than plasma binding globulins, such as
  Alpha$_1$-antitrypsin, serum
  Ceruloplasmin, serum
  Renin, plasma
    (concentrations may be increased from baseline; compensatory mechanisms keep the free serum concentrations of cortisol, sex steroids, and thyroid hormones unchanged)
Prothrombin time (PT), plasma and
Partial thromboplastin time (PTT), plasma and
Platelet aggregation time, plasma
  (time to coagulation may be shortened)
Triiodothyronine T$_3$, total, serum and
Triiodothyronine T$_3$ uptake test, serum
  (values for the T$_3$ uptake test may be decreased because of an increase in thyroid-binding globulin [TBG]; free T$_3$, thyroxine [T$_4$], and thyroid-stimulating hormone [TSH] concentrations remain unaltered and patient remains euthyroid even though the amount of total bound thyroid hormone may be increased)

**Medical considerations/Contraindications**
The medical considerations/contraindications included have been selected on the basis of their potential clinical significance (reasons given in parentheses where appropriate)—not necessarily inclusive (» = major clinical significance).

*Except under special circumstances, these medications should not be used when the following medical problems exist:*
» Genital or uterine bleeding, abnormal or undiagnosed
    (use of estrogens or progestins may delay diagnosis; on occurrence, estrogen should be discontinued until clinical evaluation is completed. Condition may worsen if cause of abnormal uterine bleeding is endometrial hyperplasia or uterine cancer)
» Hepatic function impairment, severe, including benign or malignant liver tumors
    (condition may worsen with use of oral estrogen or progestin. Hepatic function impairment may decrease estrogen or progestin metabolism and delay their elimination; medication should be discontinued)
» Hypercalcemia, associated with bone metastases or breast cancer or
» Neoplasia, estrogen-dependent, known or suspected
    (oral conjugated estrogens may promote tumor growth or interfere with the action of antiestrogen treatment regimens; when these conditions are present, estrogen medication should be discontinued)
    (estrogens can elevate calcium levels by altering calcium and phosphorus metabolism and can result in severe hypercalcemia or aggravate the hypercalcemia associated with breast cancer or bone metastases)
» Thrombophlebitis or thromboembolic disease, active
    (estrogens should be discontinued if thromboembolic events occur)

*Risk-benefit should be considered when the following medical problems exist:*
Asthma or
Cardiac insufficiency, significant or
Epilepsy or
Hypertension or
Migraine headaches or
Renal impairment, severe
    (rarely, the fluid retention caused by estrogens and progestins may aggravate these conditions; blood pressure, cardiovascular risk factors, and migraine headaches may improve with estrogen use)
Diabetes mellitus
    (minimal risk of altered carbohydrate metabolism; however, some postmenopausal patients, with or without diabetes mellitus, who are taking conjugated estrogens and medroxyprogesterone in physiologic doses may experience a slight decrease in the glucose tolerance by an unknown mechanism, as shown by an increased 2-hour postprandial blood glucose concentration test)
Endometriosis
    (endometrial implants may be aggravated by use of estrogens)
Gallbladder disease, or history of, especially gallstones
    (conflicting evidence exists as to whether an increased risk of recurrence or exacerbation of gallbladder disease occurs secondary to oral estrogen use at physiologic doses)
Hepatic function impairment, history of, including
Jaundice, or history of during pregnancy
  Porphyria, hepatic—acute, intermittent, or variegate or
    (impaired hepatic function may decrease the metabolism of conjugated estrogens and medroxyprogesterone and cause these conditions to worsen or recur)
Hyperlipoproteinemia, familial or
Pancreatitis
    (medroxyprogesterone, by lowering the beneficial effect of estrogens in decreasing LDLC and increasing HDLC levels, can rarely aggravate hyperlipidemia; estrogens at the premenopausal level can substantially increase serum triglycerides, which may lead to pancreatitis, especially in patients with familial defects in lipoprotein metabolism)
Leiomyomas, uterine
    (may increase in size during estrogen therapy)
Sensitivity to estrogens or progestins
Thromboembolic disorders, including cerebrovascular disease, pulmonary embolism, and retinal thrombosis, history of or
Thrombophlebitis, history of
    (may be exacerbated; hypercoagulability information for postmenopausal women with these conditions is not available. Estrogens and progestins have been used cautiously in women with predisposing risk factors but the medication should be discontinued if thromboembolic events occur)

**Patient monitoring**
The following may be especially important in patient monitoring (other tests may be warranted in some patients, depending on condition; » = major clinical significance):

Blood pressure determinations and
Physical examinations
    (annual monitoring; special attention given to abdomen, breasts, and pelvic organs, including counseling patient about periodic self-examination of breasts. During treatment of vasomotor symptoms of menopause and vulvar or vaginal atrophy, patient should be eval-

uated every 3 to 6 months to determine whether continued use of therapy is appropriate)

(generally, blood pressure remains the same or decreases with physiologic doses of estrogen and continuous 2.5- or cyclic 5-mg doses of medroxyprogesterone; idiosyncratic increases in blood pressure have occurred. A large clinical trial showed that 2 to 4% of postmenopausal women had transient increases in systolic blood pressure of 40 mm Hg and transient increases in diastolic blood pressure of 20 mm Hg)

Endometrial evaluation

(routine or baseline evaluation is not needed for women with an intact uterus who use combination estrogens and progestins unless unexpected uterine bleeding problems occur. An endometrial evaluation should be considered if unexpected withdrawal bleeding occurs during Days 5 to 15 when a progestin is given on Days 1 to 10 for cyclic estrogen-progestin therapy; or, for continuous estrogen-progestin therapy, if bleeding is heavier than a normal period, lasts longer than 10 days at a time, or occurs more often than monthly. Also, an endometrial evaluation should be considered if endometrial atrophy does not occur within 10 months after initiation of treatment with continuous estrogen-progestin therapy)

(transvaginal sonography is commonly used for endometrial monitoring. Endometrial biopsy may be needed instead, if irregular uterine bleeding persists after the first year of continuous therapy; if uterine bleeding is refractory to an increase in the progestin dose; if irregular bleeding occurs after a period of amenorrhea; or if transvaginal sonography shows an endometrial thickness of greater than 4 millimeters)

Hepatic function determinations and
Lipid profile determinations

(recommended annually or as determined by physician, especially if hepatic disease exists or is suspected)

Mammography or
Papanicolaou (Pap) test

(recommended annually or as determined by physician; especially important for those patients on long-term estrogen therapy)

(sensitivity or specificity of mammography is decreased during estrogen use due to detection problems caused by estrogen-induced breast tissue growth, especially if the postmenopausal breast is fibrous. Ordering mammography during the week of no hormone use or after cessation of therapy may help recognize false-positive or false-negative mammograms)

## Side/Adverse Effects

Note: The risk of any serious adverse effect is minimal for healthy women using low doses of estrogen and progestins. Even women who have special risk factors successfully use estrogens and progestins.

The following side/adverse effects have been selected on the basis of their potential clinical significance (possible signs and symptoms in parentheses where appropriate)—not necessarily inclusive:

Those indicating need for medical attention
  Incidence more frequent
    **Amenorrhea** (absence of menstrual periods)—usually occurring within 10 months; **changes in uterine bleeding pattern, including abnormal timing or amount of flow for withdrawal bleeding, breakthrough bleeding or spotting**—effects tapering off within 6 months; *vulvovaginal candidiasis* (vaginal itching or irritation; thick, white vaginal discharge)

    Note: *Withdrawal bleeding* or menstrual-like bleeding frequently will occur when patients who have a uterus are placed on cyclic estrogen-progestin therapy. Any unusual uterine bleeding persisting longer than 3 to 6 months should be investigated. With continuous estrogen-progestin therapy, withdrawal bleeding is eliminated, and endometrial atrophy and *amenorrhea* are produced in most patients after 2 to 3 months and, in the remaining patients, after 7 to 13 months. Amenorrhea is highly desired by many women and not considered to be an adverse effect.

  Incidence less frequent
    **Breast tumors** (breast lumps; discharge from breast); *skin rash*
  Incidence rare
    **Gallbladder obstruction, hepatitis, or pancreatitis** (yellow eyes or skin; pain or tenderness in stomach, side, or abdomen)

Those indicating need for medical attention only if they continue or are bothersome
  Incidence more frequent
    **Abdominal pain or cramping; arthralgia** (joint pain); **breast enlargement, pain, or tenderness; diarrhea; dizziness; dyspepsia** (stomach discomfort following meals); **dysmenorrhea** (painful menstrual periods); *flatulence* (passing of gas); *leukorrhea* (increase in amount of clear vaginal discharge); **mental depression; nausea; pruritus** (itching); **unusual tiredness**
  Incidence less frequent
    **Headaches including migraine headaches; hypertonia** (tense muscles); **increase in libido** (increase in sexual desire); **peripheral edema** (bloating or swelling of face, ankles, or feet; unusual weight gain or loss)
  Incidence rare
    *CNS disturbances, such as mood changes, or nervousness; trouble in sleeping; vomiting*

## Patient Consultation

As an aid to patient consultation, refer to *Advice for the Patient, Conjugated Estrogens and Medroxyprogesterone For Ovarian Hormone Therapy (OHT) (Systemic)*.

In providing consultation, consider emphasizing the following selected information (» = major clinical significance):

### Before using this medication
» Conditions affecting use, especially:
    Sensitivity to estrogens or progestins
    Carcinogenicity—The risk of breast cancer for patients taking estrogens or progestins is not fully understood or easily quantified; however, estrogen use in patients for 4 years or longer or at doses greater than physiologic doses shows a small but significantly increased risk. Also, significantly increased risk of endometrial hyperplasia and endometrial cancer exists for patients with an intact uterus who are placed on unopposed estrogen replacement therapy, but this risk decreases significantly with the use of a progestin in combination with the estrogen
    Pregnancy—Although not usually a concern for perimenopausal patients, conjugated estrogens and medroxyprogesterone are not recommended during pregnancy because of associated congenital abnormalities; physician should be informed immediately if pregnancy is suspected
    Breast-feeding—Although not usually a concern for perimenopausal patients, conjugated estrogens and medroxyprogesterone are not recommended because estrogens and progestins are distributed into breast milk
    Other medications, especially aminoglutethimide, barbiturates, carbamazepine, cyclosporine, hydantoins, hepatotoxic medications, protease inhibitors, or rifampin
    Other medical problems, especially abnormal or undiagnosed genital or uterine bleeding; estrogen-dependent neoplasia (known or suspected); hypercalcemia due to bone metatases or breast cancer; hepatic function impairment (severe); or thrombophlebitis or thromboembolic disease (active)

### Proper use of this medication
    Reading patient directions
» Importance of not taking more or less medication than the amount prescribed or for longer time than needed
» If taking combination therapy, taking each medication at the right time
» Taking with food if nausea occurs, especially for first few weeks after treatment initiation
» Proper dosing
    Missed dose: Taking as soon as possible; not taking if almost time for next dose; not doubling doses
» Proper storage

### Precautions while using this medication
» Regular visits to physician once every year, or more often, as determined by physician
» Checking breast by self-examination regularly and having clinical examination and mammography as required by physician; reporting unusual breast lumps or discharge
» Understanding that menstrual bleeding may begin again but, with continuous therapy, will stop by 10 months
» Understanding that intermenstrual vaginal bleeding will occur for the first 3 months; importance of not stopping medicine; checking with doctor immediately if uterine bleeding is unusual or continuous, missed period occurs, or pregnancy is suspected
    If scheduled for laboratory tests, telling physician about taking estrogens or progestins; certain blood tests and tissue biopsies are affected

### Side/adverse effects
Signs of potential side effects, especially amenorrhea; changes in uterine bleeding; vulvovaginal candidiasis; breast tumors; gallbladder obstruction, hepatitis, or pancreatitis; or skin rash

## General Dosing Information
It is recommended that the patient package insert (PPI) be given to patients.

Use of the continuous regimen for both conjugated estrogen and medroxyprogesterone is a good choice for women who do not want to resume menses. If spotting or uterine bleeding occurs during the first 6 months, a higher dose of progestin may be used for a short time until endometrial atrophy occurs.

Decisions to treat menopausal symptoms with hormones for a limited time (1 to 5 years) or to use hormones to prevent diseases in postmenopausal women for a longer period of time (10 to 20 years) or a lifetime should be made separately.

Counseling asymptomatic postmenopausal women about the benefits and risks of using long-term estrogen and progestin hormone replacement therapy to prevent osteoporosis and coronary heart disease and to increase life expectancy is complex. Risk estimates are based on observational studies; the true estimates for long-term risk and benefit await controlled clinical trials. Women should understand that the benefits and risks of preventive hormone therapy depend on their risk status, and that women at higher risk for developing osteoporosis or coronary heart disease can derive the greatest benefit.

For women with a uterus, adding a progestin to estrogen therapy may benefit postmenopausal women at risk for osteoporosis and slightly increase the risk of breast cancer over that of nonusers.

During treatment of vasomotor symptoms of menopause or vulvar and vaginal atrophy, patient should be evaluated every 3 to 6 months to determine whether continued use of estrogens is appropriate.

### Diet/Nutrition
Estrogen therapy may cause nausea, especially in the morning. Although this nausea is primarily of central origin, eating solid food often provides some relief.

---

### CONJUGATED ESTROGENS, AND CONJUGATED ESTROGENS AND MEDROXYPROGESTERONE

## Oral Dosage Forms

### CONJUGATED ESTROGENS TABLETS USP
### CONJUGATED ESTROGENS AND MEDROXYPROGESTERONE ACETATE TABLETS

**Usual adult dose**
Menopause, vasomotor symptoms of or
Osteoporosis, postmenopausal, prophylaxis or
Vaginitis, atrophic or
Vulvar atrophy—
  Oral, one tablet containing 0.625 mg conjugated estrogens a day on Days 1 through 14. Then one tablet containing 0.625 mg conjugated estrogens and 5 mg medroxyprogesterone a day is taken on Days 15 through 28. Repeat cycle.
Note: Other regimens may differ but also may be appropriate.

**Strength(s) usually available**
U.S.—
  0.625 mg of conjugated estrogens, and 0.625 mg of conjugated estrogens and 5 mg of medroxyprogesterone acetate (Rx) [*Premphase*].
  Note: *Premphase* contains twenty-eight tablets: fourteen tablets of Conjugated Estrogens Tablets USP 0.625 mg inscribed with the brand name *Premarin*, and fourteen tablets containing two hormones, conjugated estrogens 0.625 mg and medroxyprogesterone acetate 5 mg, inscribed with the brand name *Premphase*.

Canada—
  Not commercially available.

**Packaging and storage**
Store below 40 °C (104 °F), preferably between 15 and 30 °C (59 and 86 °F), unless otherwise specified by manufacturer.

**Note**
Include mandatory patient package insert (PPI) when dispensing.

---

### CONJUGATED ESTROGENS AND MEDROXYPROGESTERONE

## Oral Dosage Forms

### CONJUGATED ESTROGENS AND MEDROXYPROGESTERONE ACETATE TABLETS

**Usual adult dose**
Menopause, vasomotor symptoms of or
Osteoporosis, postmenopausal, prophylaxis or
Vaginitis, atrophic or
Vulvar atrophy—
  Oral, one tablet containing 0.625 mg conjugated estrogens and 2.5 mg medroxyprogesterone once a day for a continuous (nonphasic) regimen. Dose may be increased to one tablet containing 0.625 mg conjugated estrogens and 5 mg medroxyprogesterone once a day for a continuous (nonphasic) regimen in patients who continue to have undesired uterine bleeding or spotting.

**Strength(s) usually available**
U.S.—
  0.625 mg of conjugated estrogens and 2.5 mg of medroxyprogesterone acetate (Rx) [*Prempro*].
  0.625 mg of conjugated estrogens and 5 mg of medroxyprogesterone acetate (Rx) [*Prempro*].
  Note: Available as a twenty-eight-day cycle.

Canada—
  Not commercially available.

**Packaging and storage**
Store below 40 °C (104 °F), preferably between 15 and 30 °C (59 and 86 °F), unless otherwise specified by manufacturer.

**Note**
Include mandatory patient package insert (PPI) when dispensing.

## Selected Bibliography
American College of Physicians. Guidelines for counseling postmenopausal women about preventive hormone therapy. Ann Intern Med 1992; 117(12): 1038-41.

Hammond CB. Menopause and hormone replacement therapy: an overview. Obstet Gynecol 1996; 87 Suppl: 2-15.

Revised: 06/30/98

---

**COPPER GLUCONATE** — See *Copper Supplements (Systemic)*

---

**COPPER INTRAUTERINE DEVICES (IUDs)** — The *Copper Intrauterine Devices (IUDs)* monograph is not included in this published version of the USP DI database. Copies of the monograph are available on request from Micromedex, Inc. - Reprint Requests, 6200 S. Syracuse Way, Suite 300, Englewood, CO 80111; telephone (303) 486-6400; telefax (303) 486-6464; Email: USPDI@MDX.COM.

# COPPER SUPPLEMENTS Systemic†

This monograph includes information on the following: 1) Copper Gluconate†; 2) Cupric Sulfate†.

VA CLASSIFICATION (Primary): TN499

Commonly used brand name(s): *Cupri-Pak*².

Note: For a listing of dosage forms and brand names by country availability, see *Dosage Forms* section(s).

†Not commercially available in Canada.

## Category
Nutritional supplement (mineral).

## Indications

### Accepted
Copper deficiency (prophylaxis and treatment)—Copper supplements are indicated in the prevention and treatment of copper deficiency, which may result from inadequate nutrition or intestinal malabsorption, but does not occur in healthy individuals receiving an adequate balanced diet. For prophylaxis of copper deficiency, dietary improvement, rather than supplementation, is advisable. For treatment of copper deficiency, supplementation is preferred.

Deficiency of copper may lead to hypochromic and microcytic anemias, neutropenia, and bone demineralization.

Recommended intakes may be increased and/or supplementation may be necessary in the following persons or conditions (based on documented copper deficiency):
Burns
Gastrectomy
Infants—premature
Intestinal diseases—celiac, diarrhea, sprue
Malabsorption syndromes associated with pancreatic insufficiency—cystic fibrosis
Malnutrition, especially protein
Renal disease—nephrotic syndrome
Stress, prolonged

Some unusual diets (e.g., reducing diets that drastically restrict food selection) may not supply minimum daily requirements of copper. Supplementation may be necessary in patients receiving total parenteral nutrition (TPN) or undergoing rapid weight loss or in those with malnutrition, because of inadequate dietary intake.

Recommended intakes may be increased by the following: penicillamine, trientine, oral zinc supplements.

### Unaccepted
Copper supplements should not be used as emetics, as death has been reported.

A potential role for copper supplements in the treatment of rheumatoid arthritis and psoriasis has not been proven.

## Pharmacology/Pharmacokinetics

### Physicochemical characteristics
Molecular weight—
  Copper gluconate: 453.84.
  Copper sulfate: 249.7.
  Elemental copper: 63.54.

### Mechanism of action/Effect
Copper is necessary for the proper functioning of many metalloenzymes, including ceruloplasmin, monoamine oxidase, ferroxidase II, tyrosinase, dopamine beta-hydroxylase, and cytochrome-C-oxidase. Physiological functions that are copper dependent include oxidation of iron, erythro- and leukopoiesis, bone mineralization, elastin and collagen cross-linking, oxidative phosphorylation, catecholamine metabolism, melanin formation, myelin formation, glucose homeostasis, and antioxidant protection of the cell.

### Absorption
Approximately 40 to 60% of dietary copper is absorbed, primarily from the stomach and duodenum. Copper absorption increases in copper deficiency and decreases with adequate copper status. After absorption, copper is bound to the carrier protein, metallothionein.

### Protein binding
Copper is 90 to 95% bound to ceruloplasmin, 1 to 2% bound to amino acids or free, and the remaining is reversibly bound to albumin.

### Storage
Copper is stored primarily in the liver, with small amounts found in peripheral tissues.

### Biotransformation
Hepatic.

### Elimination
Primarily in bile, with small amounts eliminated in urine, sweat, and epidermal shedding.

## Precautions to Consider

### Pregnancy/Reproduction
Pregnancy—Problems in humans have not been documented with intake of normal daily recommended amounts. However, adequate and well-controlled studies in humans have not been done.

Studies have not been done in animals.

FDA Pregnancy Category C (parenteral copper).

### Breast-feeding
Problems in humans have not been documented with intake of normal daily recommended amounts.

### Pediatrics
Problems in pediatrics have not been documented with intake of normal daily recommended amounts.

Infusion of free amino acids of the total parenteral nutrition (TPN) solution has been reported to produce copper diuresis in infants.

Copper injection that contains benzyl alcohol as a preservative should not be used in newborn and immature infants. The use of benzyl alcohol in neonates has been associated with a fatal toxic syndrome consisting of metabolic acidosis and CNS, respiratory, circulatory, and renal function impairment.

### Geriatrics
Problems in geriatrics have not been documented with intake of normal daily recommended amounts.

### Drug interactions and/or related problems
The following drug interactions and/or related problems have been selected on the basis of their potential clinical significance (possible mechanism in parentheses where appropriate)—not necessarily inclusive (» = major clinical significance):

Note: Combinations containing any of the following, depending on the amount present, may also interact with copper supplements.

Copper-containing preparations, other
  (concurrent use with copper supplements may increase serum copper concentrations)

» Penicillamine or
» Trientine
  (copper chelation by penicillamine or trientine may lead to decreased serum copper concentrations; penicillamine or trientine should be given 2 hours before copper supplements)

» Zinc supplements, oral
  (large doses of zinc supplements may inhibit copper absorption in the intestine; copper supplements should be taken 2 hours after zinc supplements)

### Medical considerations/Contraindications
The medical considerations/contraindications included have been selected on the basis of their potential clinical significance (reasons given in parentheses where appropriate)—not necessarily inclusive (» = major clinical significance).

*Except under special circumstances, this medication should not be used when the following medical problem exists:*

» Wilson's disease
  (condition may be exacerbated)

*Risk-benefit should be considered when the following medical problems exist:*

» Biliary tract disease or
  Hepatic disease
  (may cause an accumulation of copper, since copper is normally eliminated in bile; a reduction in copper dosage may be necessary)

### Patient monitoring
The following may be especially important in patient monitoring (other tests may be warranted in some patients, depending on condition; » = major clinical significance):
- » Ceruloplasmin concentrations, serum or
- » Copper concentrations, serum, plasma, or urinary
  (determinations recommended monthly; however, these monitoring parameters are subject to many variables and may not be good indicators of copper overload)

## Overdose
For specific information on the agents used in the management of copper overdose, see:
- *Calcium Edetate Disodium (Systemic)* monograph;
- *Dimercaprol (Systemic)* monograph; and/or
- *Penicillamine (Systemic)*.

For more information on the management of overdose or unintentional ingestion, **contact a Poison Control Center** (see *Poison Control Center Listing*).

### Clinical effects of overdose
The following effects have been selected on the basis of their potential clinical significance (possible signs and symptoms in parentheses where appropriate)—not necessarily inclusive:
*Coma; diarrhea; epigastric pain and discomfort* (heartburn); *hematuria* (blood in urine; lower back pain; pain or burning while urinating); *hepatotoxicity* (black or bloody vomit; severe or continuing headache; loss of appetite; severe or continuing nausea; pain in abdomen; yellow eyes or skin); *hypotension* (dizziness or fainting); *jaundice* (yellow eyes or skin); *metallic taste; vomiting*

### Treatment of overdose
Dilution with milk or water
  To decrease absorption—
    Emptying stomach contents by emesis or gastric lavage if patient is not already vomiting
  Specific treatment—
    If patient is symptomatic, instituting chelation therapy with one of the following chelating agents:
      Calcium edetate disodium—
        Intravenous, 50 mg per kg of body weight (mg/kg) a day for 5 days; course may be repeated after a 2-day interval.
        Intramuscular, 12.5 mg/kg every 4 to 6 hours for 5 days; course may be repeated after a 2-day interval.
      Dimercaprol—Intramuscular, 3 to 5 mg/kg every 4 hours for 2 days, then 3 mg/kg every 6 hours for 2 days, then 3 mg/kg every 12 hours for up to 7 days or until recovery is complete.
      Penicillamine—Orally, 10 mg/kg in 4 divided doses a day (not to exceed 1 gram a day) for no longer than 1 week; if symptoms recur, allow 3 to 5 days before resuming therapy.

## Patient Consultation
As an aid to patient consultation, refer to *Advice for the Patient, Copper Supplements (Systemic)*.
In providing consultation, consider emphasizing the following selected information (» = major clinical significance):

### Description of use
  Description should include function in the body, signs of deficiency, conditions that may cause copper deficiency, unproven uses

### Importance of diet
  Importance of proper nutrition; supplement may be needed because of inadequate dietary intake
  Food sources of copper; effects of processing
  Recommended daily intake for copper

### Before using this dietary supplement
- » Conditions affecting use, especially:
    Other medications or dietary supplements, especially penicillamine, trientine, or oral zinc supplements
    Other medical problems, especially Wilson's disease and biliary tract disease

### Proper use of this dietary supplement
- » Proper dosing
    Missed dose: No cause for concern because of length of time necessary for depletion; remembering to take as directed
- » Proper storage

### Precautions while using this dietary supplement
  Not taking copper supplements within 2 hours of zinc supplements

## General Dosing Information
Because of the infrequency of copper deficiency alone, combinations of several vitamins and/or minerals are commonly administered. Many commercial vitamin/mineral complexes are available.

### For parenteral dosage forms only
In most cases, parenteral administration is indicated only when oral administration is not acceptable (for example, in nausea, vomiting, and preoperative and postoperative conditions) or possible (for example, in malabsorption syndromes or following gastric resection).

### Diet/Nutrition
Recommended dietary intakes for copper are defined differently worldwide.
For U.S.—
  The Recommended Dietary Allowances (RDAs) for vitamins and minerals are determined by the Food and Nutrition Board of the National Research Council and are intended to provide adequate nutrition in most healthy persons under usual environmental stresses. In addition, a different designation may be used by the FDA for food and dietary supplement labeling purposes, as with Daily Value (DV). DVs replace the previous labeling terminology United States Recommended Daily Allowances (USRDAs).
For Canada—
  Recommended Nutrient Intakes (RNIs) for vitamins, minerals, and protein are determined by Health and Welfare Canada and provide recommended amounts of a specific nutrient while minimizing the risk of chronic diseases.
There is no RDA or RNI established for copper. The following daily intakes are considered adequate for all individuals:
  Infants and children:
    Birth to 3 years of age: 0.4 to 1 mg.
    4 to 6 years of age: 1 to 1.5 mg.
    7 to 10 years of age: 1 to 2 mg.
  Adolescent and adult males:
    1.5 to 2.5 mg.
  Adolescent and adult females:
    1.5 to 3 mg.
The best sources of copper include organ meats (especially liver), seafoods, beans, nuts, and whole-grains. Additional copper can come from the interaction of drinking water with copper pipes, copper cookware, and copper-containing fungicides sprayed on agricultural products. The amount of copper in foods may be decreased as a result of prolonged storage in tin cans under acidic conditions.

---

### COPPER GLUCONATE

## Oral Dosage Forms
### COPPER GLUCONATE TABLETS
**Usual adult and adolescent dose**
Deficiency (prophylaxis)—Oral, amount based on normal daily recommended intakes:—
  Adolescent and adult males—1.5 to 2.5 mg.
  Adolescent and adult females—1.5 to 3 mg.
Deficiency (treatment)—
  Treatment dose is individualized by prescriber based on severity of deficiency.

**Usual pediatric dose**
Deficiency (prophylaxis)—Oral, amount based on normal daily recommended intakes:—
  Birth to 3 years of age—0.4 to 1 mg.
  4 to 6 years of age—1 to 1.5 mg.
  7 to 10 years of age—1 to 2 mg.
Deficiency (treatment)—
  Treatment dose is individualized by prescriber based on severity of deficiency.

**Strength(s) usually available**
U.S.—
  3 mg elemental copper (OTC) [GENERIC].
Canada—
  Not commercially available.
Note: The strength of this preparation may exceed the dosage range recommended by USP DI Advisory Panels based on the amount necessary to meet normal nutritional needs.

**Packaging and storage**
Store below 40 °C (104 °F), preferably between 15 and 30 °C (59 and 86 °F), unless otherwise specified by manufacturer. Store in a tight container.

# Copper Supplements (Systemic)

## CUPRIC SULFATE

### Parenteral Dosage Forms

Note: Injectable copper products must be diluted prior to intravenous administration.

### CUPRIC SULFATE INJECTION USP

**Usual adult and adolescent dose**
Deficiency (prophylaxis)—
  Intravenous infusion, 0.5 to 1.5 mg of elemental copper a day added to TPN.
Deficiency (treatment)—
  Intravenous infusion, 3 mg of elemental copper a day added to total parenteral nutrition (TPN).

**Usual pediatric dose**
Deficiency (prophylaxis)—
  For full-term infants and children:
    Intravenous infusion, 20 mcg elemental copper per kg of body weight per day added to TPN.
Deficiency (treatment)—
  For full-term infants and children:
    Intravenous infusion, 20 to 30 mcg elemental copper per kg of body weight per day added to TPN.
Note: Copper injection that contains benzyl alcohol as a preservative should not be used in newborn and immature infants. The use of benzyl alcohol in neonates has been associated with a fatal toxic syndrome consisting of metabolic acidosis and CNS, respiratory, circulatory, and renal function impairment.

**Strength(s) usually available**
U.S.—
  0.4 mg elemental copper per mL (1.57 mg cupric sulfate) (Rx) [*Cupri-Pak;* GENERIC].
  2 mg elemental copper per mL (7.85 mg cupric sulfate) (Rx) [GENERIC].
Canada—
  Not commercially available.

**Packaging and storage**
Store below 40 °C (104 °F), preferably between 15 and 30 °C (59 and 86 °F), unless otherwise specified by manufacturer. Protect from freezing.

**Preparation of dosage form**
The manufacturer states that copper sulfate can be added to TPN solutions, and is physically compatible with amino acid solutions, dextrose solutions, and most vitamins with the exception of ascorbic acid.

**Incompatibilities**
Large doses of ascorbic acid are physically incompatible with copper. The manufacturer recommends that copper sulfate and other trace metal additives be added to TPN solutions immediately prior to infusion to avoid potential incompatibilities.

Revised: 09/01/91
Interim revision: 06/25/92; 08/17/94; 05/26/95

---

# CORTICORELIN OVINE   Systemic-Diagnostic—INTRODUCTORY VERSION

VA CLASSIFICATION (Primary): DX900
Commonly used brand name(s): ACTHREL.
Note: For a listing of dosage forms and brand names by country availability, see *Dosage Forms* section(s).

## Category
Diagnostic aid (ACTH production).

## Indications

**Accepted**
Adrenocorticotropic hormone (ACTH) production, origin of (diagnosis)—
  Corticorelin ovine triflutate is indicated for differentiating pituitary and ectopic production of ACTH in patients with ACTH-dependent Cushing's syndrome in which hypercortisolism is caused by hypersecretion of ACTH by pituitary adenomas or nonadenomatous hyperplasia, possibly of hypothalamic origin (Cushing's disease), or by ectopic secretion of ACTH by nonpituitary tumors.

## Pharmacology/Pharmacokinetics

**Physicochemical characteristics**
Molecular weight—4670.35 daltons.

**Mechanism of action/Effect**
Corticorelin ovine triflutate is an analog of the naturally occurring human corticotropin-releasing hormone (hCRH) peptide. Both are potent stimulators of the release of adrenocorticotropic hormone (ACTH) from the anterior pituitary. ACTH in turn stimulates cortisol production in the adrenal cortex. In healthy subjects, administration of corticorelin ovine triflutate results in a rapid and sustained increase in plasma ACTH concentrations and a near parallel increase in plasma cortisol. In patients with pituitary hypersecretion of ACTH (Cushing's disease), the negative feedback mechanism that regulates the release of cortisol from the pituitary is impaired. Despite high basal concentrations, administration of corticorelin ovine triflutate stimulates additional release of ACTH and cortisol. Patients with Cushing's syndrome caused by ectopic ACTH production have very high basal concentrations of ACTH and cortisol that show little to no change in response to the corticorelin test.

**Distribution**
$Vol_D$—Mean: $6.2 \pm 0.5$ liters.

**Half-life**
Following a single intravenous injection of 1 mcg per kg of body weight (mcg/kg) in healthy males—
  Fast component: $11.6 \pm 1.5$ minutes.
  Slow component: $73 \pm 8$ minutes.

**Time to peak concentration**
Following doses $\geq 0.3$ mcg/kg in healthy volunteers:
  Plasma ACTH concentrations: 10 to 15 minutes.
  Plasma cortisol concentrations: 30 to 60 minutes.

**Peak serum concentration**
Following morning and evening administration of 1 mcg/kg or 100 mcg in healthy volunteers—
  ACTH:
    Morning—68 (range 39 to 114) picograms per mL (picograms/mL).
    Evening—30 (range 25 to 42) picograms/mL.
  Cortisol:
    Morning—21 (range 17 to 25) picograms/mL.
    Evening—16 (range 15 to 18) picograms/mL.

**Duration of action**
ACTH and cortisol responses remain elevated for 2 hours following a 1 mcg/kg dose.

## Precautions to Consider

**Carcinogenicity/Mutagenicity**
Studies to evaluate the carcinogenic and mutagenic potential of corticorelin ovine triflutate have not been done in animals.

**Pregnancy/Reproduction**
Pregnancy—Studies have not been done in humans.
Studies have not been done in animals.
FDA Pregnancy Category C.

**Breast-feeding**
It is not known whether corticorelin ovine triflutate is distributed into breast milk.

**Pediatrics**
Studies performed in healthy children and in children with multiple hypothalamic and/or pituitary deficiencies or tumors have not demonstrated pediatrics-specific problems that would limit the usefulness of corticorelin ovine triflutate in children.

**Geriatrics**
No information is available on the relationship of age to the effects of corticorelin ovine triflutate in geriatric patients.

**Drug interactions and/or related problems**
The following drug interactions and/or related problems have been selected on the basis of their potential clinical significance (possible mechanism in parentheses where appropriate)—not necessarily inclusive (» = major clinical significance):
Note: Combinations containing any of the following medications, depending on the amount present, may also interact with this medication.

Dexamethasone
(in healthy volunteers pretreated with dexamethasone, plasma ACTH responses to corticorelin ovine triflutate have been inhibited or blunted)
» Heparin
(concurrent use may cause severe hypotension; use of heparin to maintain intravenous cannula patency is not recommended during the corticorelin test)

## Side/Adverse Effects

The following side/adverse effects have been selected on the basis of their potential clinical significance (possible signs and symptoms in parentheses where appropriate)—not necessarily inclusive:

### Those indicating need for medical attention
Incidence less frequent
*Dyspnea* (shortness of breath); *flushing of face, neck, or upper chest, prolonged; hypotension; tachycardia* (fast heartbeat); *tightness in chest*

Note: *Dyspnea; prolonged flushing of face, neck, or upper chest; hypotension; tachycardia;* and *tightness in chest* were associated with doses > 3 mcg per kg of body weight (mcg/kg). Hypotension and tachycardia were significant at doses > 5 mcg/kg.
Cardiovascular effects began 2 to 3 minutes following injection and lasted for 30 to 60 minutes.
Flushing lasted for up to 4 hours in some patients.
All effects were milder when corticorelin ovine triflutate was administered as a 30-second infusion rather than as a bolus injection.

### Those indicating need for medical attention only if they continue or are bothersome
Incidence more frequent
*Flushing of face, neck, and upper chest, transient*—incidence 15%

Note: *Transient flushing of face, neck, and upper chest* began almost immediately following injection and lasted for 3 to 5 minutes.

Incidence less frequent
*Urge to take a deep breath*—incidence 5%

## Overdose

For more information on the management of overdose or unintentional ingestion, **contact a Poison Control Center** (see *Poison Control Center Listing*).

### Clinical effects of overdose
The following effects have been selected on the basis of their potential clinical significance (possible signs and symptoms in parentheses where appropriate)—not necessarily inclusive:

*Cardiovascular changes; dyspnea* (shortness of breath); *flushing of face, severe*

### Treatment of overdose
Clinical effects of overdose should be treated symptomatically.

## General Dosing Information

Basal adrenocorticotropic hormone (ACTH) and cortisol concentrations usually are higher in the morning than in the evening.

The physician administering the corticorelin test should be familiar with hypothalamic-pituitary-adrenal physiology, normal hormonal values, the clinical status of the patient, and the standards used by the laboratory performing the assays.

The corticorelin test requires a minimum of five blood samples. The procedure for determining ACTH and cortisol concentrations is as follows:
• Venous blood samples should be drawn 15 minutes and immediately prior to administration of corticorelin ovine triflutate. The two samples are averaged to determine the baseline concentration.
• Corticorelin ovine triflutate is administered over 30 to 60 seconds.
• Venous blood samples should then be drawn at 15, 30, and 60 minutes following administration of corticorelin.
• Blood samples should be handled as recommended by the particular laboratory performing the assay. Inter- and intra-assay variability may affect test results.

The corticorelin test results may be interpreted as follows:
• In patients with high basal plasma ACTH and cortisol concentrations—Administration of corticorelin ovine triflutate results in increased plasma ACTH and cortisol concentrations, indicating ACTH production of pituitary origin (Cushing's disease).
• In patients with high or very high basal ACTH concentrations and high basal plasma cortisol concentrations—Administration of corticorelin ovine triflutate results in little or no change in plasma ACTH and cortisol concentrations, indicating ectopic ACTH production.

False-negative results occur in approximately 5 to 10% of patients with Cushing's disease. In rare instances, patients with ectopic ACTH production also have responded to the corticorelin test.

## Parenteral Dosage Forms

### CORTICORELIN OVINE TRIFLUTATE FOR INJECTION

#### Usual adult dose
Diagnostic aid (ACTH production)—
Intravenous, 1 mcg per kg of body weight over thirty to sixty seconds.

Note: If a repeat evaluation is needed, it is recommended that the repeat dose be given at the same time of day as the original dose because there are differences in basal and peak response concentrations following morning or evening administration.

#### Usual adult prescribing limits
1 mcg per kg of body weight.

#### Usual pediatric dose
See *Usual adult dose*.

#### Size(s) usually available
U.S.—
100 mcg (Rx) [ACTHREL (ascorbic acid 0.88 mg; lactose 10 mg; cysteine hydrochloride monohydrate 26 mg)].

#### Packaging and storage
Store between 2 and 8 °C (36 and 46 °F). Protect from light.

#### Preparation of dosage form
Corticorelin ovine triflutate is reconstituted with 2 mL of 0.9% sodium chloride injection. The vial should be rolled, not shaken, to dissolve the drug. The resulting solution contains 50 mcg of corticorelin ovine triflutate per mL.

#### Stability
The reconstituted solution is stable for up to 8 hours when refrigerated.

#### Auxiliary labeling
• Refrigerate.

Developed: 11/10/97

---

# CORTICOSTEROIDS   Inhalation-Local

This monograph includes information on the following: 1) Beclomethasone; 2) Budesonide; 3) Dexamethasone†; 4) Flunisolide; 5) Triamcinolone.

INN:   Beclomethasone—Beclometasone
JAN:   Beclomethasone—Beclometasone dipropionate
VA CLASSIFICATION (Primary/Secondary): RE101/RE109

Commonly used brand name(s): *AeroBid*[4]; *AeroBid-M*[4]; *Azmacort*[5]; *Beclodisk*[1]; *Becloforte*[1]; *Becloyent*[1]; *Beclovent Rotacaps*[1]; *Bronalide*[4]; *Decadron Respihaler*[3]; *Pulmicort Nebuamp*[2]; *Pulmicort Turbuhaler*[2]; *Vanceril*[1]; *Vanceril 84 mcg Double Strength*[1].

Other commonly used names for beclomethasone are beclomethasone dipropionate, beclometasone, and beclometasone dipropionate.

Note: For a listing of dosage forms and brand names by country availability, see *Dosage Forms* section(s).

†Not commercially available in Canada.

## Category
Anti-inflammatory (inhalation); antiasthmatic.

## Indications

### Accepted
Asthma, bronchial, chronic (treatment)—Beclomethasone, budesonide, flunisolide, and triamcinolone are indicated as primary maintenance treatment in patients with persistent symptoms of chronic bronchial

asthma. Regular, continuous use controls chronic airway inflammation, decreases airway hyperresponsiveness, controls asthma symptoms, and reduces the frequency of asthma exacerbations. In clinical studies, inhaled corticosteroids appear to be effective in all types of asthma and in patients of all ages.

Initiation of therapy with daily doses of inhaled corticosteroids shortly after a diagnosis of chronic asthma (even if mild) may prevent irreversible structural changes in the airways resulting from uncontrolled inflammation, may decrease progression of severe disease, and may reduce the need for administration of systemic corticosteroids.

Information comparing dose-related systemic effects or the ratios of local to systemic activity of beclomethasone, budesonide, flunisolide, and triamcinolone is limited. However, since conclusive evidence is lacking and further studies are needed, the concept of using the lowest possible dose of an inhaled corticosteroid to achieve the desired clinical improvement in asthma seems prudent.

Because of the potent anti-inflammatory effects of inhaled corticosteroids and the potential morbidity and mortality associated with theophylline treatment, inhaled corticosteroids in conventional low doses are preferred to theophylline as first-line therapy for chronic asthma.

Guidelines for the treatment of children with asthma recommend that inhaled nonsteroidal anti-inflammatory medications, such as cromolyn and nedocromil, be considered as the first choice after beta-adrenergic bronchodilators. The use of beta-adrenergic bronchodilators more than three times a week suggests inadequate asthma control. An inhaled corticosteroid is then recommended to be substituted when asthma is not well controlled with cromolyn or nedocromil.

### Unaccepted

Corticosteroid inhalation therapy does not relieve acute bronchospasm and is not indicated for the primary treatment of status asthmaticus or other acute asthmatic episodes requiring more intensive or rapid treatment measures.

Corticosteroid inhalation therapy is not indicated in the treatment of non-asthmatic bronchitis.

Dexamethasone inhalation is not recommended for use in asthma because it has demonstrated a significantly higher incidence of systemic effects with no additional benefit over other inhaled corticosteroids. The high ratio of systemic glucocorticoid activity to local anti-inflammatory activity of inhaled dexamethasone may be due to its greater water solubility and longer metabolic half-life after absorption relative to the other inhaled corticosteroids.

## Pharmacology/Pharmacokinetics

### Physicochemical characteristics
Molecular weight—
 Beclomethasone dipropionate: 521.05.
 Budesonide: 430.54.
 Dexamethasone sodium phosphate: 516.41.
 Flunisolide: 443.51.
 Triamcinolone acetonide: 434.50.

### Mechanism of action/Effect
In the treatment of chronic bronchial asthma, orally inhaled corticosteroids have many probable sites of action. The net effect is to reduce the chronic inflammation in asthmatic airways.

The potent anti-inflammatory action may be due to an inhibition of the secretion of growth factors, endothelial activating and other cytokines from lymphocytes, eosinophils, macrophages, fibroblasts, and mast cells. The results are decreased influx of inflammatory cells into the bronchial walls, due in part to inhibition of expression of adhesion molecules on the endothelium and in the tissue. Decreased activation and survival of eosinophils in the lung tissue and a reduction in numbers of mast cells are further effects.

Corticosteroids may inhibit release of mediators from basophils and enzymes from macrophages. There is decreased permeability through vasoconstriction and direct inhibition of endothelial cell contraction.

Beta-adrenergic-receptor numbers may be increased, which results in an enhanced response to beta-adrenergic bronchodilators and reduced down-regulation of beta-receptors after prolonged beta-agonist exposure.

Inhaled corticosteroids also inhibit mucus secretion in airways, possibly by a direct action on submucosal gland cells and an indirect inhibitory effect caused by the reduction in inflammatory mediators that stimulate mucus secretion. The amount and viscosity of sputum are reduced.

The effect of inhaled corticosteroids on bronchial asthma is to block the late inflammatory response to inhaled allergens and reduce over time the response to nonspecific triggers such as exercise. Bronchial wall inflammation and edema are reduced, sputum production is diminished, and the airways become less hyperresponsive to direct and indirect challenges.

### Absorption
Beclomethasone, budesonide, and flunisolide are rapidly absorbed from the lungs and gastrointestinal tract. Triamcinolone is absorbed more slowly.

Without the use of a spacer, approximately 10 to 25% of an inhaled corticosteroid dose is deposited in the airways; the remainder is deposited in the mouth and throat, and swallowed. A greater percentage of the inhaled dose may reach the respiratory tract with the use of a spacer device.

### Biotransformation
For beclomethasone dipropionate—
 Rapidly transformed in the lungs to beclomethasone monopropionate, an active metabolite, which significantly increases the topical potency of beclomethasone.
For budesonide, flunisolide, and triamcinolone acetonide—
 Absorbed unchanged. Those portions of each drug absorbed through the lungs or absorbed after being swallowed are rapidly and extensively transformed to inactive metabolites in the liver.

### Half-life
For budesonide—120 minutes (plasma).
For flunisolide—90 to 120 minutes (plasma).

### Onset of action
Maximum improvement in pulmonary function and symptoms may take up to 4 weeks, while reduction in airway responsiveness occurs gradually over a period of weeks to months.

### Elimination
Fecal and renal.

## Precautions to Consider

### Pregnancy/Reproduction
Pregnancy—Chronic administration of systemic corticosteroids to pregnant women has shown decreased birth weight and a slight increase in the incidence of premature deliveries. In animal studies, decreases in fetal survival and weight have been demonstrated with systemic corticosteroids.

The use of conventional doses of inhaled corticosteroids by pregnant asthmatic women has not been reported to be associated with an increased incidence of congenital abnormalities in the newborn. Inhaled corticosteroids may be used during pregnancy when clinically necessary, since poorly controlled asthma and loss of pulmonary function and hypoxia present a greater risk to the mother and may cause fetal hypoxia. If inhaled corticosteroids are effective before pregnancy, it is advisable to continue regular maintenance dosing during pregnancy.

Beclomethasone is the preferred inhaled corticosteroid during pregnancy in the U.S. because of more extensive clinical experience with its use than with flunisolide or triamcinolone.

FDA Pregnancy Category C.

### Breast-feeding
It is not known whether inhaled corticosteroids are distributed into breast milk. However, problems in humans have not been documented. Although systemic corticosteroids are distributed into breast milk, it is unlikely that inhaled corticosteroids would reach significant quantities in maternal serum and the concentration in breast milk would probably be of minor clinical significance.

### Pediatrics
Inhaled corticosteroids in conventional low doses have been shown to be safe and effective in children with asthma. However, there have been reports that prolonged treatment and/or use of higher doses may, with great individual patient variation, result in systemic effects, such as decreased short-term growth rate and reduced cortisol secretion.

Studies have shown that high doses of inhaled corticosteroids may decrease short-term lower log linear growth but are not associated with long-term statural growth suppression. Minor degrees of growth suppression may be attributed to the transient drop in growth rate associated with delayed puberty in many asthmatic children, without the use of corticosteroids, suggesting that severity of asthma may influence growth. Monitoring of growth is advised in children who regularly require higher doses of inhaled corticosteroids.

Use of prolonged, high daily doses of inhaled corticosteroids may cause a reduction in secretion of endogenous cortisol, although there have been no reports of clinically significant adrenal insufficiency in children treated with inhaled corticosteroids only. However, monitoring for the possibility of some suppression of the hypothalamic-pituitary-adrenal axis may be advisable in children receiving prolonged treatment.

Using a spacer device, rinsing the mouth after inhalations, using the lowest possible doses, and reducing doses after favorable responses have been obtained appear to minimize the risk of adverse systemic and local side effects. A spacer device may enhance inhalation techniques and thus improve intrapulmonary delivery of inhaled corticosteroids and increase compliance in pediatric patients.

Children who are taking systemic corticosteroids in immunosuppressant doses may be more susceptible to infectious diseases, especially chickenpox and measles. Although it is highly unlikely that inhaled corticosteroids in usual doses would be associated with an increased risk of serious infection, some precautions are advisable for children who are taking larger than usual doses of inhaled corticosteroids and who have not had these diseases. Particular care should be taken to avoid exposure to chickenpox and measles and to immunize at an early age against infectious diseases for which there are vaccines, such as measles.

### Geriatrics
Appropriate studies on the relationship of age to the effects of inhaled corticosteroids have not been performed in the geriatric population. However, in studies that have included patients over 65 years of age, geriatrics-specific problems that would limit the usefulness of this medication in the elderly have not been documented.

### Drug interactions and/or related problems
Significant drug interactions are unlikely to occur with usual doses of inhaled corticosteroids. Although there are no defined drug interactions with inhaled corticosteroids, if these medications are used in high doses for a long time and systemic absorption occurs, some of the interactions seen with systemic corticosteroids have a potential to occur. (See *Corticosteroids—Glucocorticoid Effects [Systemic]*.)

### Laboratory value alterations
The following have been selected on the basis of their potential clinical significance (possible effect in parentheses where appropriate)—not necessarily inclusive (» = major clinical significance):

With physiology/laboratory test values
Note: The following values may be affected with chronic use of larger-than-recommended doses of inhalation corticosteroids.

Adrenal function and
Hypothalamic-pituitary-adrenal (HPA) axis function as assessed by 24-hour urinary free cortisol, morning serum cortisol concentration, or short tetracosactrin cortisol test
(may be decreased if significant absorption of inhaled corticosteroid occurs, especially in children)

Glucose, blood or urine
(high-dose therapy may be associated with an increase in fasting insulin, peak glucose, and insulin to glucose ratios after glucose tolerance tests)

Hematologic status
(neutrophils and total white blood cell count may be increased; eosinophils and lymphocytes may be decreased; clinical relevance of these systemic effects may be insignificant)

Osteocalcin, serum
(may be decreased in children and adults taking inhaled corticosteroids; however, decrease may also be seen in asthma patients not taking corticosteroids)

### Medical considerations/Contraindications
The medical considerations/contraindications included have been selected on the basis of their potential clinical significance (reasons given in parentheses where appropriate)—not necessarily inclusive (» = major clinical significance).

*Risk-benefit should be considered when the following medical problems exist:*

Osteoporosis
(may be exacerbated in postmenopausal women taking high doses over a prolonged time and not receiving an estrogen supplement)

Tuberculosis
(may be reactivated during prolonged inhaled corticosteroid therapy unless chemoprophylaxis is administered concurrently; asthmatic patients with a positive Mantoux test who are using inhaled corticosteroids should be carefully monitored for manifestation or reactivation, especially in countries with a high incidence of tuberculosis; inhaled corticosteroids should be avoided or used with great caution in patients with drug-resistant pulmonary tuberculosis or atypical tuberculosis)

### Patient monitoring
The following may be especially important in patient monitoring (other tests may be warranted in some patients, depending on condition; » = major clinical significance):

Adrenal function assessment
(may be advisable periodically during, and for several months following, transfer of a patient from systemic to inhalation corticosteroid therapy)

(may be advisable every year during treatment in both children and adults if dosing guidelines are exceeded, especially if systemic corticosteroids are used concurrently or prior to inhaled corticosteroids)

Growth and development in children
(careful observation may be advisable periodically during prolonged therapy with inhaled corticosteroids)

Inhalation technique
(frequent assessment of inhalation technique and patient education on the importance of continuous prophylactic treatment with inhaled corticosteroids is recommended to ensure compliance, enhance delivery of medication to lungs, and reduce local and systemic side effects)

Pulmonary function assessment
(periodic assessment is advisable during, and for several months following, transfer of a patient from systemic to inhalation corticosteroid therapy; frequent pulmonary function monitoring may be necessary in some patients for as long as 4 to 8 months after discontinuation of oral corticosteroids; daily outpatient peak expiratory flow rate [PEFR] measurements are useful in following the course of asthma and the patient's response to therapy)

## Side/Adverse Effects

Note: Significant systemic absorption of inhaled corticosteroids has been reported to cause hypothalamic-pituitary-adrenal (HPA) axis suppression, growth inhibition in children, and possibly osteoporosis, glaucoma, and cataracts. However, most studies to date have been unable to correlate measurable effects on laboratory values with clinically important complications.

Generally, systemic adverse effects do not often occur with the use of conventional inhalation corticosteroid doses. However, the potential for systemic side effects increases with factors that affect absorption, such as high doses, prolonged therapy, the inspiratory technique used and the delivery system employed, patient variations in absorption in relation to lung anatomy and steroid pharmacokinetics, presence of bronchitis, and/or combination therapy with oral corticosteroids.

Side effects from usual doses of inhaled corticosteroids are generally limited to local effects on the upper airways caused by deposition of the inhaled corticosteroid in the oropharynx. Some of these effects may be prevented or alleviated with the use of a spacer and/or mouth rinsing after each treatment.

The following side/adverse effects have been selected on the basis of their potential clinical significance (possible signs and symptoms in parentheses where appropriate)—not necessarily inclusive:

**Those indicating need for medical attention**
Incidence less frequent
*Oropharyngeal candidiasis or thrush* (creamy white, curd-like patches in mouth or throat; pain when eating or swallowing)

Incidence rare
*Bronchospasm, increased* (increased wheezing; tightness in chest; difficulty in breathing); *esophageal candidiasis* (pain or burning in chest); *psychic change* (nervousness; restlessness; mental depression; behavioral changes)—reported with budesonide only

**Those indicating need for medical attention only if they continue or are bothersome**
Incidence more frequent
*Cough; dry mouth; dysphonia* (hoarseness or other voice changes); *throat irritation*

Incidence less frequent
*Dry throat; headache; nausea; skin bruising or thinning; unpleasant taste*

## Patient Consultation

As an aid to patient consultation, refer to *Advice for the Patient, Corticosteroids (Inhalation)*.

In providing consultation, consider emphasizing the following selected information (» = major clinical significance):

**Before using this medication**
» Conditions affecting use, especially:
Sensitivity to corticosteroids
Use in children—Higher doses may result in retarded growth rate and reduced cortisol secretion; monitoring of growth and development and adrenal function is important with prolonged or high-dose therapy. The use of a spacer is necessary for better compliance and improved airway delivery. Exposure to chickenpox or measles should be avoided

**Proper use of this medication**
» Not using to relieve acute asthma attack; continuing use even if using other medication for asthma attack
» Importance of not using more medication than the amount prescribed
» Compliance with therapy by using every day in regularly spaced doses; patients who are not taking systemic corticosteroids when inhalation therapy started may require up to 4 weeks for initial improvement and several months for full benefits
  Gargling and rinsing mouth with water after each dose; not swallowing rinse water
» Reading patient instructions carefully; checking frequently with health care professional for proper use of inhaler
» Proper dosing
  Missed dose: Using as soon as possible; using any remaining doses for that day at regularly spaced intervals
  Checking with pharmacist to determine availability of refills for aerosol inhalers; saving inhaler if refills available
» Proper storage
  Proper dose may not be delivered if aerosol canister is cold

*For beclomethasone, flunisolide, or triamcinolone inhalation aerosol dosage form*
  Testing or priming the inhaler before using first time
  Proper administration technique
  Proper administration technique with use of spacer device
  Proper cleaning procedure for inhaler

*For beclomethasone capsule for inhalation dosage form*
» Not swallowing capsules; medication not effective if swallowed
  Proper loading technique for inhaler
  Proper administration technique
  Proper cleaning procedure for inhaler

*For beclomethasone powder for inhalation dosage form*
  Proper loading technique for inhaler
  Proper administration technique
  Proper cleaning procedure for inhaler

*For budesonide powder for inhalation dosage form*
  Proper loading technique for inhaler
  Proper administration technique

*For budesonide suspension for inhalation dosage form*
  Using in a power-operated nebulizer with an adequate flow rate and equipped with face mask or mouthpiece
  Preparation of medication for use in nebulizer
  Proper administration technique
  Proper cleaning procedure for nebulizer

**Precautions while using this medication**
» Checking with physician if
  Unusual physical stress occurs, such as surgery, injury, or infections
  Asthma attack is not responsive to bronchodilator
  Any sign indicating possible mouth, throat, or lung infection occurs
  Symptoms do not improve or condition becomes worse
  Carrying medical identification card stating that supplemental systemic corticosteroid therapy may be required in emergency situations, periods of unusual stress, or acute asthma attack
» Caution if any kind of surgery or emergency treatment is required; informing physician or dentist in charge that inhalation corticosteroid is being used

*For patients receiving systemic corticosteroid therapy*
» Importance of not discontinuing systemic corticosteroid therapy without physician's advice; carefully reducing dose or discontinuing treatment if so directed
» Importance of regular visits to physician during time that systemic corticosteroid therapy is being withdrawn; obtaining physician's instructions to follow if severe asthma attack occurs, medical or surgical treatment is needed, or symptoms of corticosteroid withdrawal occur

**Side/adverse effects**
  Signs of potential side effects, especially increased bronchospasm, oropharyngeal or esophageal candidiasis, and, with budesonide, psychic changes

## General Dosing Information

Pharmacologic doses of inhaled corticosteroids should be carefully titrated to minimum effective doses to control asthma symptoms and prevent systemic effects.

Gargling and rinsing the mouth with water after each dose are recommended to help prevent hoarseness, throat irritation, and oral candidiasis; the rinse water should not be swallowed. Rinsing the mouth without swallowing can also significantly reduce the amount of inhaled corticosteroid absorbed from the gastrointestinal tract.

The use of a spacer device with a metered dose inhaler may decrease the incidence of some adverse effects, especially oropharyngeal candidiasis and dysphonia. By reducing the need for proper coordination of timing of inhalation with activation of the inhaler and reducing the velocity and mean diameter of the aerosol particles, a spacer reduces the amount of medication deposited in the upper airways and increases the amount deposited in the lower respiratory tract. This enhances the local efficacy of the inhaled corticosteroid without significantly increasing systemic activity.

Some patients may require relatively high doses of inhaled corticosteroids to prevent severe asthma relapse. For this purpose, the highly concentrated beclomethasone aerosol inhalation product available outside the U.S. facilitates the clinical use of high doses. The risk of local side effects may be minimized by twice-daily dosing and the use of a spacer device. However, these measures do not eliminate the risk of systemic side effects associated with prolonged use of high doses.

Patients whose asthma is controlled by their usual dose of inhaled corticosteroids may require temporary emergency use of systemic corticosteroids, if their asthma control is rapidly deteriorating. The use of peak flow monitoring at home once or twice daily will provide objective information to the patient and the physician when this is necessary.

**For patients also receiving systemic corticosteroid therapy**

Caution is required when transferring patients from systemic corticosteroids to inhaled corticosteroids. Deaths due to severe asthma relapse or possibly adrenal insufficiency have occurred in asthmatic patients during and after the transfer.

Systemic corticosteroids should be continued initially when inhalation therapy is instituted. After 1 to 2 weeks of inhalation therapy, systemic corticosteroid dosage may be reduced gradually at 1- or 2-week intervals, depending on patient response. *Dosage reductions must be made very slowly and in small decrements* when patient has been receiving prolonged systemic therapy or when systemic corticosteroid dose (prednisone or equivalent) is less than 10 to 15 mg daily.

Some patients may not be able to discontinue use of systemic corticosteroids. A minimal oral maintenance dose may be required along with the inhaled corticosteroid.

Continued monitoring of the patient for signs of adrenal insufficiency is recommended following complete withdrawal of systemic corticosteroid therapy. Recovery of adrenal function may require up to 12 months in some patients, depending on the dosage and duration of systemic therapy.

Supplementation with systemic corticosteroids may be advisable during periods of pronounced physical stress, such as during surgery or severe infections. Supplementation is usually recommended in any patient who has had systemic corticosteroid therapy in the past year and who needs general anesthesia.

Severe asthma relapse may occur upon withdrawal of the systemic corticosteroid. Reinstitution of systemic therapy may be required if a severe asthma attack occurs. Frequent pulmonary function monitoring (peak expiratory flow rate measurements) may be needed for some patients for as long as four to eight months after discontinuation of the systemic corticosteroid.

A syndrome of pseudo-rheumatism (consisting of joint or muscle pain, joint swelling, peripheral edema, lethargy, anorexia, and nausea) may occur when systemic corticosteroid is withdrawn. This syndrome can be avoided or minimized if the dosage of systemic corticosteroids is reduced slowly, using an alternate-day regimen. If the syndrome occurs, the symptoms may be alleviated by treatment with acetaminophen or nonsteroidal anti-inflammatory drugs (NSAIDs) in asthmatic patients who are not sensitive to NSAIDs. Resumption of systemic corticosteroid therapy may not be required.

**For treatment of adverse effects**

For laryngeal or pharyngeal candidiasis—Recommended treatment includes
• Administration of an oral or systemic antifungal medication.
• Change in frequency of inhaled corticosteroid dosing from 4 to 2 times a day without decreasing the total daily dose. This may allow recovery and clearing of thrush or prevent its occurrence while maintaining therapeutic efficacy.
• Discontinuation of the inhaled corticosteroid is rarely necessary.

## BECLOMETHASONE

## Inhalation Dosage Forms

### BECLOMETHASONE DIPROPIONATE INHALATION AEROSOL

**Usual adult and adolescent dose**
Antiasthmatic—
  For the 42- or 50-mcg-per-metered-spray products:
    Oral inhalation, 2 inhalations (84 or 100 mcg) three or four times a day. Alternatively, a dosage of 4 inhalations two times a day has been shown to be effective for some patients.
  For severe asthma: Oral inhalation, initially, 12 to 16 inhalations a day. Dosage should then be decreased according to the patient's response.
  For the 84-mcg-per-metered-spray product:
    Oral inhalation, 2 inhalations (168 mcg) two times a day.
    For severe asthma, initially, 6 to 8 inhalations a day. Dosage should then be decreased according to the patient's response.

**Usual adult and adolescent prescribing limits**
For the 42- or 50-mcg-per-metered-spray products—20 inhalations (840 or 1000 mcg) per day.
For the 84-mcg-per-metered-spray product—10 inhalations (840 mcg) per day.

**Usual pediatric dose**
Antiasthmatic—
  Children up to 6 years of age:
    Dosage has not been established.
  Children 6 to 12 years of age:
    For the 42- or 50-mcg-per-metered-spray products—
      Oral inhalation, 1 or 2 inhalations three or four times a day. Alternatively, a dosage of 4 inhalations two times a day has been shown to be effective for some patients.
    For the 84-mcg-per-metered-spray product—
      Oral inhalation, 2 inhalations two times a day.
  Children older than 12 years of age:
    See *Usual adult and adolescent dose*.

**Usual pediatric prescribing limits**
For the 42- or 50-mcg-per-metered-spray products—
  10 inhalations (420 or 500 mcg) per day.
For the 84-mcg-per-metered-spray product—
  5 inhalations (420 mcg) per day.

**Strength(s) usually available**
U.S.—
  42 mcg (0.042 mg) per metered spray (Rx) [*Beclovent; Vanceril*].
  84 mcg (0.084 mg) per metered spray (Rx) [*Vanceril 84 mcg Double Strength* (chlorofluorocarbons)].
  Note: Each canister contains medication for about 200 inhalations.
Canada—
  50 mcg (0.05 mg) per metered spray (Rx) [*Beclovent; Vanceril*].
  Note: Each canister contains medication for about 200 inhalations.
  250 mcg (0.25 mg) per metered spray (Rx) [*Becloforte*].
  Note: The 250-mcg-per-metered-spray product is used only when the total daily dose equals or exceeds 500 mcg per day.
    Each canister contains medication for about 80 or 200 inhalations.

**Packaging and storage**
Store at temperature below 49 °C (120 °F) or between 2 and 30 °C (36 and 86 °F), depending on product, unless otherwise specified by manufacturer.

**Auxiliary labeling**
• Shake well before using.
• For oral inhalation only.
• Store away from heat and direct sunlight.

**Note**
Include patient instructions when dispensing.
Demonstrate administration technique.

**Additional information**
In Canada, metered dose inhalers are labeled according to the amount of beclomethasone delivered at the valve; in the U.S., metered dose inhalers are labeled according to the amount of beclomethasone delivered at the mouthpiece or actuator. Thus, 50 mcg of beclomethasone delivered at the valve is equivalent to 42 mcg delivered at the mouthpiece.
This product contains dichlorodifluoromethane and trichloromonofluoromethane, substances that harm public health and the environment by destroying ozone in the upper atmosphere.

### BECLOMETHASONE DIPROPIONATE FOR INHALATION (CAPSULES)

**Usual adult dose**
Antiasthmatic—
  Oral inhalation, 200 mcg (0.2 mg) three or four times a day. Dosage should then be decreased according to patient response; many patients may be maintained on 400 mcg (0.4 mg) a day.

**Usual pediatric dose**
Antiasthmatic—
  Children up to 6 years of age: Dosage has not been established.
  Children 6 to 14 years of age: Oral inhalation, 100 mcg (0.1 mg) two to four times a day. Dosage should then be decreased according to patient response.
  Children over 14 years of age: See *Usual adult dose*.

**Usual pediatric prescribing limits**
Up to 500 mcg (0.5 mg) per day.

**Strength(s) usually available**
U.S.—
  Not commercially available.
Canada—
  100 mcg (0.1 mg) per capsule (Rx) [*Beclovent Rotacaps* (lactose)].
  200 mcg (0.2 mg) per capsule (Rx) [*Beclovent Rotacaps* (lactose)].

**Packaging and storage**
Store below 40 °C (104 °F), preferably between 15 and 30 °C (59 and 86 °F), in a well-closed container, unless otherwise specified by manufacturer.

**Auxiliary labeling**
• Do not swallow capsule.

**Note**
Include patient instructions when dispensing.
Demonstrate administration technique.
Use of beclomethasone for oral inhalation (capsules) requires a special device that separates the capsule into halves and releases the medication.

### BECLOMETHASONE DIPROPIONATE FOR INHALATION (POWDER)

**Usual adult dose**
See *Beclomethasone Dipropionate for Inhalation (Capsules)*.

**Usual pediatric dose**
See *Beclomethasone Dipropionate for Inhalation (Capsules)*.

**Usual pediatric prescribing limits**
Up to 500 mcg (0.5 mg) per day.

**Strength(s) usually available**
U.S.—
  Not commercially available.
Canada—
  100 mcg (0.1 mg) per blister (Rx) [*Beclodisk*].
  200 mcg (0.2 mg) per blister (Rx) [*Beclodisk*].

**Packaging and storage**
Store below 30 °C (86 °F), in a well-closed container, unless otherwise specified by manufacturer.

**Note**
Include patient instructions when dispensing.
Demonstrate administration technique.
Use of beclomethasone for oral inhalation (powder) requires a special device that penetrates the blister and releases the medication.

## BUDESONIDE

## Inhalation Dosage Forms

### BUDESONIDE FOR INHALATION (POWDER)

**Usual adult dose**
Antiasthmatic—
  Previous asthma therapy consisting of bronchodilators alone:
    Oral inhalation, 1 to 2 inhalations (200 to 400 mcg) two times a day.
  Previous asthma therapy including inhaled corticosteroids:
    Oral inhalation, 1 to 2 inhalations (200 to 400 mcg) two times a day. Dosage may be increased as needed and as tolerated to a maximum of 4 inhalations (800 mcg) two times a day.

## Corticosteroids (Inhalation-Local)

Previous asthma therapy including systemic corticosteroids:
Oral inhalation, 2 to 4 inhalations (400 to 800 mcg) two times a day.

**Usual adult prescribing limits**
1600 mcg a day for patients previously treated with inhaled or systemic corticosteroids or 800 mcg a day for patients previously treated with bronchodilators alone.

**Usual pediatric dose**
Antiasthmatic—
  Children up to 6 years of age:
    Safety and efficacy have not been established.
  Children 6 years of age and older:
    Oral inhalation, 1 inhalation (200 mcg) two times a day. Dosage may be increased as needed and as tolerated to a maximum of 2 inhalations (400 mcg) two times a day.

**Usual pediatric prescribing limits**
800 mcg a day.

**Strength(s) usually available**
U.S.—
  200 mcg (0.2 mg) (Rx) [*Pulmicort Turbuhaler*].
Canada—
  100 mcg (0.1 mg) (Rx) [*Pulmicort Turbuhaler*].
  200 mcg (0.2 mg) (Rx) [*Pulmicort Turbuhaler*].
  400 mcg (0.4 mg) (Rx) [*Pulmicort Turbuhaler*].

**Packaging and storage**
Store between 15 and 30 °C (59 and 86 °F), unless otherwise specified by manufacturer. Protect from light.

**Auxiliary labeling**
• For oral inhalation only.

### BUDESONIDE SUSPENSION FOR INHALATION

**Usual adult and adolescent dose**
Antiasthmatic—
  Initial: Oral inhalation, 1 to 2 mg, diluted with sterile sodium chloride inhalation solution, if necessary, to a volume of two to four mL, and administered via nebulization over a period of ten to fifteen minutes two times a day.
  Note: For severe asthma, dosage may be increased according to patient response.
  Maintenance: After the desired clinical effect has been obtained, the maintenance dose should be reduced gradually to the smallest dose necessary for control of symptoms.

**Usual pediatric dose**
Antiasthmatic—
  Children up to 3 months of age: Dosage has not been established.
  Children 3 months to 12 years of age:
    Initial—Oral inhalation, 250 mcg (0.25 mg) to 1 mg, diluted with sterile sodium chloride inhalation solution, if necessary, to a volume of two to four mL, and administered via nebulization over a period of ten to fifteen minutes two times a day.
    Maintenance—After the desired clinical effect has been obtained, the maintenance dose should be reduced gradually to the smallest dose necessary for control of symptoms.

**Strength(s) usually available**
U.S.—
  Not commercially available.
Canada—
  125 mcg (0.125 mg) per mL (250 mcg per 2-mL ampul) (Rx) [*Pulmicort Nebuamp*].
  250 mcg (0.25 mg) per mL (500 mcg per 2-mL ampul) (Rx) [*Pulmicort Nebuamp*].
  500 mcg (0.5 mg) per mL (1000 mcg per 2-mL ampul) (Rx) [*Pulmicort Nebuamp*].

**Packaging and storage**
Store between 15 and 30 °C (59 and 86 °F), unless otherwise specified by manufacturer. Protect from freezing. Protect from light.

**Stability**
Any unused suspension remaining in an opened ampul may be stored for later use as long as it is protected from light and is used within 12 hours after the ampul was opened. The entire contents of an ampul must be used within 12 hours after it is first opened.
Ampuls in an opened envelope should be used within 3 months.

**Auxiliary labeling**
• For oral inhalation only.
• Shake gently before using.

**Note**
When dispensing, include patient instructions for preparation of solution.

**Additional information**
For nebulization of budesonide inhalation suspension, a gas flow (oxygen or compressed air) of 6 to 10 liters per minute should be used. Nebulizers with either a facemask or mouthpiece have been used. Ultrasonic nebulizers are not recommended.

---

## DEXAMETHASONE

### Inhalation Dosage Forms

#### DEXAMETHASONE SODIUM PHOSPHATE INHALATION AEROSOL USP

Note: USP DI Advisory Panels do not recommend the use of Dexamethasone Sodium Phosphate Inhalation Aerosol USP, because of the potential for extensive systemic absorption and the long metabolic half-life after absorption resulting in an increased risk of adverse effects with usual inhalation doses.

**Strength(s) usually available**
U.S.—
  100 mcg (0.1 mg) dexamethasone phosphate per metered spray (Rx) [*Decadron Respihaler* (alcohol 2%)].

---

## FLUNISOLIDE

### Inhalation Dosage Forms

#### FLUNISOLIDE INHALATION AEROSOL

**Usual adult and adolescent dose**
Antiasthmatic—
  Oral inhalation, 500 mcg (0.5 mg—2 metered sprays) two times a day, morning and evening.

**Usual adult prescribing limits**
Oral inhalation, 2 mg per day (4 metered sprays twice a day).

**Usual pediatric dose**
Antiasthmatic—
  Children up to 4 years of age: Dosage has not been established.
  Children 4 years of age and older: See *Usual adult and adolescent dose*.
  Note: Doses higher than 1 mg per day have not been studied in children 4 to 15 years of age. In the U.S., dosage has not been established for children under 6 years of age.

**Strength(s) usually available**
U.S.—
  250 mcg (0.25 mg) per metered spray (Rx) [*AeroBid; AeroBid-M* (menthol)].
Canada—
  250 mcg (0.25 mg) per metered spray (Rx) [*Bronalide*].
Note: Each canister delivers at least 100 inhalations.

**Packaging and storage**
Store below 49 °C (120 °F), preferably between 15 and 30 °C (59 and 86 °F), unless otherwise specified by manufacturer.

**Auxiliary labeling**
• Shake well before using.
• For oral inhalation only.

**Note**
Include patient instructions when dispensing.
Demonstrate administration technique.

**Additional information**
This product contains dichlorodifluoromethane, trichloromonomethane, and dichlorotetrafluoroethane, substances that harm public health and the environment by destroying ozone in the upper atmosphere.

---

## TRIAMCINOLONE

### Inhalation Dosage Forms

#### TRIAMCINOLONE ACETONIDE INHALATION AEROSOL

**Usual adult and adolescent dose**
Antiasthmatic—
  Initial: Oral inhalation, 200 mcg (0.2 mg—2 metered sprays) three or four times a day. For severe asthma—Oral inhalation, 1.2 to 1.6 mg (12 to 16 metered sprays) a day.

Maintenance: Dosage to be decreased according to patient response; maintenance may be achieved in some patients by administering the total daily dose in two divided doses.

**Usual pediatric dose**
Antiasthmatic—
  Children up to 6 years of age: Dosage has not been established.
  Children 6 to 12 years of age: Oral inhalation, 100 to 200 mcg (0.1 to 0.2 mg—1 or 2 metered sprays) three or four times a day. Dosage must be adjusted according to patient response.

**Usual pediatric prescribing limits**
Up to 1.2 mg (12 metered sprays) per day.

**Strength(s) usually available**
U.S.—
  100 mcg (0.1 mg) per metered spray (Rx) [*Azmacort* (alcohol 1%)].
Canada—
  100 mcg (0.1 mg) per metered spray (Rx) [*Azmacort* (alcohol 1%)].
Note: Each canister delivers at least 240 inhalations. Canister should not be used after 240 inhalations.

**Packaging and storage**
Store at temperatures below 49 °C (120 °F), preferably between 15 and 30 °C (59 and 86 °F), unless otherwise specified by manufacturer.

**Auxiliary labeling**
- Shake well before using.
- For oral inhalation only.

**Note**
Include patient instructions when dispensing.
Demonstrate administration technique.

**Additional information**
Each actuation releases approximately 200 mcg of triamcinolone acetonide, of which approximately 100 mcg are delivered from the unit.
This product contains dichlorodifluoromethane, a substance that harms public health and the environment by destroying ozone in the upper atmosphere.

Revised: 09/02/94
Interim revision: 10/13/94; 12/22/97

# CORTICOSTEROIDS   Nasal

This monograph includes information on the following: 1) Beclomethasone; 2) Budesonide*; 3) Dexamethasone†; 4) Flunisolide; 5) Triamcinolone.

INN: Beclomethasone—Beclometasone

VA CLASSIFICATION (Primary): NT201

Commonly used brand name(s): *Beconase*[1]; *Beconase AQ*[1]; *Decadron Turbinaire*[3]; *Nasacort*[5]; *Nasalide*[4]; *Rhinalar*[4]; *Rhinocort Aqua*[2]; *Rhinocort Turbuhaler*[2]; *Vancenase*[1]; *Vancenase AQ*[1].

Note: For a listing of dosage forms and brand names by country availability, see *Dosage Forms* section(s).

*Not commercially available in U.S.
†Not commercially available in Canada.

## Category
Anti-inflammatory (steroidal), nasal; corticosteroid (nasal).

## Indications
Note: Bracketed information in the *Indications* section refers to uses that are not included in U.S. product labeling.

**Accepted**
Rhinitis, perennial (treatment)
Rhinitis, seasonal (treatment) or
[Rhinitis, seasonal (prophylaxis)]—Nasal corticosteroids are indicated in the treatment of seasonal or perennial rhinitis in patients who have exhibited significant side effects from, or have exhibited poor response to, other therapies, such as antihistamines and decongestants. Antihistamines and decongestants are generally considered primary therapies for these disorders. However, some clinicians consider nasal corticosteroids primary therapy for perennial or seasonal rhinitis because they are more effective.

[Nasal corticosteroids are used in some patients for prophylaxis of seasonal rhinitis. This form of therapy is generally reserved for patients who have consistently demonstrated a need for nasal corticosteroids to control seasonal rhinitis symptoms. Antihistamines and decongestants are considered primary therapies for this disorder.]

Dexamethasone nasal aerosol is less frequently used because its use results in a significantly higher incidence of systemic adverse effects with no additional benefit over other nasal corticosteroids.

Allergic disorders, nasal (treatment)
Inflammatory conditions, noninfectious, nasal (treatment) or
Polyps, nasal (treatment)—Nasal corticosteroids are indicated in the treatment of allergic or inflammatory nasal conditions and nasal polyps.

Polyps, nasal, postsurgical recurrence of (prophylaxis)—Beclomethasone is indicated [and budesonide nasal solution, dexamethasone, flunisolide, and triamcinolone are used] to prevent recurrence of nasal polyps following their surgical removal and sufficient mucosal healing.

[Rhinitis, vasomotor (treatment)]—Budesonide is used in the treatment of vasomotor rhinitis in patients who are unresponsive to conventional therapy. Antihistamines are generally considered the primary therapy for this disorder.

## Pharmacology/Pharmacokinetics

**Physicochemical characteristics**
Molecular weight—
  Beclomethasone dipropionate: 521.05 (anhydrous).
  Beclomethasone dipropionate monohydrate: 539.07.
  Budesonide: 430.54.
  Dexamethasone sodium phosphate: 516.41.
  Flunisolide: 443.51.
  Triamcinolone acetonide: 434.5.

**Mechanism of action/Effect**
In the treatment of nasal symptoms, the primary action of nasally applied corticosteroids is anti-inflammatory. Nasal corticosteroids inhibit the IgE- and mast cell–mediated early-phase allergic reaction. They also inhibit the migration of inflammatory cells into the nasal tissue (the late-phase or late-onset allergic reaction), which may play a significant role in the pathology of chronic rhinitis.

During the late-phase allergic reaction, eosinophils, neutrophils, basophils, and mononuclear cells produce inflammatory mediators, which cause a reappearance of nasal symptoms.

**Absorption**
Beclomethasone dipropionate—Rapidly absorbed from the nasal mucosa; more slowly from the gastrointestinal tract.
Budesonide—Very little is absorbed from the nasal mucosa.
Flunisolide—50% of dose is absorbed from the nasal mucosa.
Dexamethasone sodium phosphate—Rapidly and extensively absorbed from the nasal mucosa; readily absorbed from the gastrointestinal mucosa.

**Distribution**
A portion of the drug administered nasally is swallowed.

**Protein binding**
Beclomethasone—87%, to albumin and transcortin.
Dexamethasone sodium phosphate—High (65–90%) to albumin and transcortin.
Flunisolide—Moderate, to albumin and transcortin.

**Biotransformation**
Beclomethasone—Hepatic to free beclomethasone and other inactive metabolites. The portion of the dose that is swallowed and absorbed from the gastrointestinal tract undergoes extensive first-pass metabolism to inactive compounds. Initially hydrolyzed to beclomethasone-17-propionate by fecal esterases.
Budesonide—Rapid; hepatic.
Flunisolide—Rapid; hepatic to less active 6-beta-hydroxy metabolites. The portion of the dose that is swallowed and absorbed from the gastrointestinal tract undergoes extensive first-pass metabolism to inactive compounds.
Triamcinolone acetonide—Hepatic to 3 less active metabolites, 6-beta-hydroxytriamcinolone acetonide, 21-carboxytriamcinolone acetonide, and 21-carboxy-6-beta-hydroxytriamcinolone acetonide.

**Half-life**
Beclomethasone dipropionate—
  15 hours (plasma).

Budesonide—
   Approximately 2 hours (plasma).
Dexamethasone sodium phosphate—
   190 minutes (plasma).
Flunisolide—
   1 to 2 hours (plasma).
Triamcinolone acetonide—
   Intravenous: Approximately 90 minutes (plasma).
   Intranasal: Apparent half-life is 4 hours (plasma) (range, 1 to 7 hours); however, this value probably reflects lingering absorption.

**Onset of action**
Beclomethasone and flunisolide—Usually 5 to 7 days; however, may rarely be as long as 2 to 3 weeks in some patients.
Triamcinolone acetonide—As early as 12 hours.

**Time to peak concentration**
Budesonide—
   Oral, approximately 3 hours.
   Inhalation, within 1 hour.
Flunisolide—
   10 to 30 minutes.
Triamcinolone acetonide—
   Average of 3.4 hours (range, 0.5 to 8 hours).

**Peak plasma concentration**
Flunisolide—0.4 to 1.0 nanogram per mL.
Triamcinolone acetonide—Less than 1 nanogram per mL.

**Time to maximum benefit**
Beclomethasone and flunisolide—Up to 3 weeks in some patients.
Budesonide—Usually 2 or 3 days, but up to 3 weeks in some patients.
Triamcinolone acetonide—Usually 3 to 4 days.

**Elimination**
Beclomethasone—Fecal; renal, 12 to 15%.
Dexamethasone sodium phosphate—Renal.
Flunisolide—Renal, 50%; fecal, 40%.
Triamcinolone acetonide—Primarily fecal.

## Precautions to Consider

### Cross-sensitivity and/or related problems
Patients intolerant of benzalkonium chloride, disodium edetate, or phenylethanol may be intolerant of some nasal corticosteroid preparations, since they may contain these substances as preservatives.
Beclomethasone, dexamethasone, and triamcinolone aerosols also contain fluorocarbon propellants; beclomethasone monohydrate and flunisolide dosage forms contain no fluorocarbon propellants.
Flunisolide solution contains propylene glycol and polyethylene glycols.

### Carcinogenicity
*Beclomethasone*—No evidence of carcinogenicity was demonstrated in rats receiving beclomethasone for 95 weeks (13 weeks by inhalation and 82 weeks orally).
*Flunisolide*—In long-term studies, flunisolide given orally caused an increase in the incidence of pulmonary adenomas in mice but not in rats. Also, as reported for other corticosteroids, flunisolide caused an increased incidence of mammary adenocarcinoma in female rats receiving the highest oral doses.
*Triamcinolone*—No evidence of carcinogenicity was demonstrated in a 2-year study on male and female rats administered oral doses of 1 mcg per kg of body weight (mcg/kg) a day and male and female mice administered oral doses of 3 mcg/kg a day.

### Mutagenicity
*Beclomethasone*—Studies on mutagenicity have not been done.
*Triamcinolone*—Studies on mutagenicity have not been done.

### Pregnancy/Reproduction
*Fertility*—*Beclomethasone:* Female dogs administered beclomethasone orally showed impaired fertility (inhibition of the estrous cycle). However, this effect was not observed following administration of the medication via inhalation.
*Dexamethasone:* Dexamethasone may increase or decrease spermatozoa count or motility in some patients.
*Flunisolide:* Studies in female rats showed some evidence of impaired fertility.
*Triamcinolone:* Male and female rats administered triamcinolone acetonide orally at doses of up to 15 mcg/kg per day (maternally toxic doses are 2.5 to 15 mcg/kg per day) exhibited no evidence of impaired fertility. However, a few female rats administered 8 or 15 mcg/kg per day exhibited dystocia and prolonged delivery.

*Pregnancy*—Corticosteroids cross the placenta. Studies in humans have not been done with budesonide, dexamethasone, flunisolide, or triamcinolone nasal formulations.

Studies in animals have shown that corticosteroids are embryotoxic, fetotoxic, and/or teratogenic. However, teratogenic effects have not been confirmed in humans receiving systemic corticosteroids.
Infants born to mothers who have received substantial doses of corticosteroids during pregnancy should be carefully observed for signs of hypoadrenalism.
*Beclomethasone*—
   In one study of orally inhaled beclomethasone in humans, beclomethasone did not cause teratogenic or other adverse effects.
   Studies in rats, mice, and rabbits have shown that subcutaneously administered beclomethasone causes increased fetal resorptions and birth defects, including cleft palate, agnathia, microstomia, absence of tongue, delayed ossification, and partial agenesis of the thymus.
   FDA Pregnancy Category C.
*Budesonide*—
   Studies in rats, mice, and rabbits have shown that subcutaneously administered budesonide causes fetal malformations, primarily skeletal defects.
*Dexamethasone*—
   Although studies in humans have not been done with dexamethasone nasal aerosol, risk-benefit must be considered, since studies in animals have shown systemically administered dexamethasone to be teratogenic.
*Flunisolide*—
   Adequate and well-controlled studies in humans have not been done.
   Studies in rabbits and rats have shown that systemically administered flunisolide causes teratogenic and fetotoxic effects.
   FDA Pregnancy Category C.
*Triamcinolone*—
   Adequate and well-controlled studies in humans have not been done.
   Developmental toxicity, which included increases in fetal resorptions and stillbirths and decreases in pup body weight and survival, occurred at oral maternal doses of 2.5 to 15 mcg/kg per day. Studies in rats and rabbits administered systemic doses of 20 to 80 mcg/kg per day have shown teratogenic effects, including a low incidence of cleft palate and/or internal hydrocephaly and axial skeletal defects. Studies in non-human primates administered systemic doses of 500 mcg/kg per day have shown teratogenic effects, including CNS and cranial malformations. Administration of triamcinolone nasal aerosol to pregnant rats and rabbits resulted in embryotoxic and fetotoxic effects that were comparable to those produced by administration by other routes.
   FDA Pregnancy Category C.

### Breast-feeding
Distribution of significant quantities of corticosteroids into breast milk may suppress growth, interfere with endogenous corticosteroid production, or cause other adverse effects in the nursing infant.
*Beclomethasone, budesonide, flunisolide, and triamcinolone*—It is not known whether beclomethasone, budesonide, flunisolide, or triamcinolone is distributed into breast milk. However, systemic corticosteroids are distributed into breast milk.
*Dexamethasone*—Dexamethasone is distributed into breast milk. Nursing while receiving pharmacologic doses of dexamethasone is not recommended.

### Pediatrics
Significant suppression of growth has not been well documented with the use of usual doses of nasal beclomethasone and flunisolide. If significant systemic absorption of nasal corticosteroids occurs in pediatric patients, adrenal suppression and growth suppression may result. Prolonged or high-dose therapy with these medications, especially dexamethasone, requires careful attention to dosage and close monitoring of growth and development.

### Geriatrics
Appropriate studies with nasal corticosteroids have not been performed in the geriatric population. However, geriatrics-specific problems that would limit the usefulness of this medication in the elderly are not expected.

### Laboratory value alterations
The following have been selected on the basis of their potential clinical significance (possible effect in parentheses where appropriate)—not necessarily inclusive (» = major clinical significance):

With diagnostic test results
For dexamethasone
   Nitroblue tetrazolium test for bacterial infection
      (dexamethasone may produce false-negative results)

With physiology/laboratory test values
Adrenal function as assessed by corticotropin (ACTH) stimulation or measurement of plasma cortisol and
Hypothalamic-pituitary-adrenal (HPA) axis function
(may be decreased if significant absorption occurs, especially in children; most likely with dexamethasone)
Glucose concentration, blood and urine
(may be increased if significant absorption occurs because of intrinsic hyperglycemic activity of glucocorticoids; most likely with dexamethasone)
Hematologic status
(should be monitored during long-term therapy)

### Medical considerations/Contraindications
The medical considerations/contraindications included have been selected on the basis of their potential clinical significance (reasons given in parentheses where appropriate)—not necessarily inclusive (» = major clinical significance).

*Risk-benefit should be considered when the following medical problems exist:*
Amebiasis, latent or active
(dexamethasone or other corticosteroids may activate latent amebiasis)
Glaucoma
(may increase intraocular pressure)
Hepatic function impairment
Hypothyroidism
» Infections, fungal, bacterial, or systemic viral or
» Ocular herpes simplex
(corticosteroids may mask infection)
Intolerance to corticosteroids
Nasal septal ulcers, recent or
Nasal surgery, recent or
Nasal trauma, recent
(corticosteroids inhibit wound healing)
» Tuberculosis, latent or active, of respiratory tract

### Patient monitoring
The following may be especially important in patient monitoring (other tests may be warranted in some patients, depending on condition; » = major clinical significance):
Adrenal function assessment
(assessment of HPA axis function may be advisable at periodic intervals in patients receiving long-term nasal corticosteroid therapy; especially important in patients receiving usual doses of dexamethasone or greater-than-recommended doses of beclomethasone, flunisolide, or triamcinolone)
» Otolaryngologic examination
(should be performed in patients on long-term therapy to monitor nasal mucosa and nasal passages for infection, nasal septal perforation, nasal membrane ulceration, or other histologic changes)

## Side/Adverse Effects
Note: The risk of systemic effects is minimal with usual doses of nasal beclomethasone and flunisolide. Side effects from usual doses of beclomethasone are generally limited to local effects.

Systemic effects including hypothalamic-pituitary-adrenal (HPA) axis suppression may occur with usual doses of nasal dexamethasone or greater-than-recommended doses of beclomethasone, flunisolide, or triamcinolone. (Doses of 440 mcg of triamcinolone acetonide administered daily for 42 days did not measurably affect adrenal response to a 6-hour cosyntropin test.) If the patient is particularly sensitive or has recently used systemic corticosteroids prior to using nasal corticosteroids, the patient may also be predisposed to hypercorticism.

The following side/adverse effects have been selected on the basis of their potential clinical significance (possible signs and symptoms in parentheses where appropriate)—not necessarily inclusive:

**Those indicating need for medical attention**
Incidence more frequent
*For triamcinolone*
**Headache**—incidence 18%
Incidence less frequent
*For all nasal corticosteroids*
**Crusting inside nose or epistaxis** (bloody mucus or unexplained nosebleeds)—especially if spray is improperly aimed toward nasal septum, rather than onto the turbinates; **sore throat; ulceration of nasal mucosa** (sores inside nose)
*For dexamethasone*
**Allergic reaction or bronchial asthma** (shortness of breath, troubled breathing, tightness in chest, hives, or wheezing)
*For beclomethasone (monohydrate), budesonide, dexamethasone, and flunisolide*
**Cough; dizziness or lightheadedness; headache; hoarseness**—not reported for budesonide; **lethargy** (unusual tiredness or weakness); **loss of sense of taste or smell**—reported for dexamethasone and flunisolide only; **nausea or vomiting; rhinorrhea, continuing** (runny nose); **stuffy nose, continuing; watery eyes, continuing**—not reported for budesonide; **stomach pains**—not reported for budesonide
Incidence rare
*For all nasal corticosteroids*
**Nasal candidiasis** (white patches inside nose); **nasal septal perforation** (bloody mucus or unexplained nosebleeds); **ocular hypertension** (eye pain; nausea; vomiting; gradual loss of vision); **pharyngeal candidiasis** (white patches in throat)
*For beclomethasone*
**Hypersensitivity reaction, delayed or immediate** (hives; rash; shortness of breath or troubled breathing; swelling of eyelids, face, or lips); **rhinitis, atrophic** (bad smell; dry or stuffy nose; headache behind eye sockets)
*For budesonide*
**Dermatitis** (rash); **urticaria** (hives)
*For triamcinolone*
**Burning or stinging, continuing, after use of spray; irritation inside nose**
Symptoms of chronic overdose
**Acneiform lesions** (acne); **Cushing's syndrome** (fullness or rounding of the face); **menstrual changes**

**Those indicating need for medical attention only if they continue or are bothersome**
Incidence more frequent
*For all nasal corticosteroids*
**Burning, dryness, or other irritation inside the nose, mild and transient**
*For beclomethasone and flunisolide*
**Irritation of throat**—possibly due to vehicle in nasal spray; **sneezing attacks**—may be more common in children using beclomethasone aerosol or flunisolide spray
Incidence less frequent
*For all nasal corticosteroids*
**Sneezing**
*For budesonide*
**Throat itching**
*For triamcinolone*
**Sinus congestion** (stuffy nose or headache); **stuffy nose; throat discomfort**

## Overdose
For more information on the management of overdose or unintentional ingestion, **contact a Poison Control Center** (see *Poison Control Center Listing*).

**Treatment of overdose**
For acute overdose—Adverse effects due to acute overdose are unlikely with the small quantities of corticosteroid contained in each canister.
For chronic overdose—If symptoms of chronic overdose occur, nasal corticosteroids should be discontinued slowly.

## Patient Consultation
As an aid to patient consultation, refer to *Advice for the Patient, Corticosteroids (Nasal)*.
In providing consultation, consider emphasizing the following selected information (» = major clinical significance):

**Before using this medication**
» Conditions affecting use, especially:
Intolerance to corticosteroids
Pregnancy—Risk-benefit must be considered, since systemic corticosteroids cross the placenta and have demonstrated embryotoxicity, fetotoxicity, and teratogenicity in animals; beclomethasone oral inhalation study in humans has shown no adverse effects on fetus; infants born to mothers who received substan-

## 964 Corticosteroids (Nasal)

tial doses of corticosteroids during pregnancy should be observed for hypoadrenalism

Breast-feeding—Use of dexamethasone is not recommended, since dexamethasone is distributed into breast milk

Use in children—Significant effect on growth by beclomethasone or flunisolide has not been documented; importance of monitoring growth and development with prolonged or high-dose therapy

Other medical problems, especially fungal, bacterial, or systemic viral infections, ocular herpes simplex, or latent or active tuberculosis of respiratory tract

### Proper use of this medication

» Proper administration technique; reading patient directions carefully before use

Blowing nose to clear nasal passages before administration; aiming spray away from nasal septum (aiming towards the inner corner of eye)

» Compliance with therapy; may require up to 3 weeks for full benefit

» Importance of not using more medication than the amount prescribed, because of potential enhanced absorption and increased severity of side effects

» Checking with physician before using medication for other nasal problems

Saving special inhaler used for beclomethasone or dexamethasone; refills may be available

» Proper dosing

Missed dose: Using as soon as possible if remembered within an hour or so; if remembered later, not using at all; not doubling doses

» Proper storage; not storing budesonide powder in damp places, especially if cap has not been tightly screwed on; decreased efficacy if aerosol canister is cold; not puncturing, breaking, or burning aerosol container; discarding unused portion of beclomethasone solution or flunisolide solution 3 months after opening package

### Precautions while using this medication

Regular visits to physician to check progress during prolonged therapy

» Checking with physician if:
—signs of infection of nose, throat, or sinuses occur
—no improvement within 7 days (for dexamethasone)
—no improvement within 3 weeks (for beclomethasone, budesonide, flunisolide, or triamcinolone)
—condition becomes worse

### Side/adverse effects

Signs of potential side effects, especially headache, crusting inside nose or epistaxis, sore throat, ulceration of nasal mucosa, allergic reaction or bronchial asthma, cough, dizziness or lightheadedness, hoarseness, lethargy, loss of sense of taste or smell, nausea or vomiting, continuing rhinorrhea, continuing stuffy nose, continuing watery eyes, stomach pains, nasal candidiasis, nasal septal perforation, ocular hypertension, pharyngeal candidiasis, delayed or immediate hypersensitivity reaction, atrophic rhinitis, dermatitis, urticaria, continuing burning or stinging after use of spray, or irritation inside nose

## General Dosing Information

In patients with blocked nasal passages, a topical decongestant may be used just prior to use of the nasal corticosteroid. However, because prolonged use of topical nasal decongestants may cause congestive rebound, they should preferably be used for a maximum of 3 to 5 days. An oral decongestant is recommended for chronic nasal congestion.

The smallest dose of a nasal corticosteroid required to control symptoms should be used as a maintenance dose after the desired clinical response is achieved.

The dosage of other corticosteroids being administered concurrently by other routes of administration, including oral inhalation, should be taken into account when determining the usual adult prescribing limits of nasal corticosteroids.

---

### BECLOMETHASONE

## Summary of Differences

Pharmacology/pharmacokinetics: See *Pharmacology/Pharmacokinetics*.

Precautions: Cross-sensitivity and/or related problems—Nasal spray dosage form contains no fluorocarbon propellants.

Side/adverse effects: See *Side/Adverse Effects*.

## Additional Dosing Information

Regular use is required to obtain full therapeutic benefit. Medication should be discontinued if improvement is not evident after 3 weeks.

See also *General Dosing Information*.

## Nasal Dosage Forms

### BECLOMETHASONE DIPROPIONATE NASAL AEROSOL

**Usual adult and adolescent dose**
Anti-inflammatory (steroidal), nasal—
Nasal, 42 or 50 mcg (0.042 or 0.05 mg) (1 metered spray) in each nostril two to four times a day (total daily dose, 168 to 400 mcg [0.168 to 0.4 mg]).

**Usual adult prescribing limits**
Nasal, 1 mg per day.

Note: If orally inhaled beclomethasone is used concurrently, the combined total daily dose should not exceed 1 mg.

**Usual pediatric dose**
Anti-inflammatory (steroidal), nasal—
Children up to 6 years of age: Safety and efficacy have not been established.
Children 6 to 12 years of age: Nasal, 42 or 50 mcg (0.042 or 0.05 mg) (1 metered spray) in each nostril three or four times a day (total daily dose, 252 mcg [0.252 mg] to 400 mcg [0.4 mg]).
Children 12 years of age and over: See *Usual adult and adolescent dose*.

**Usual pediatric prescribing limits**
Nasal, 500 mcg (0.5 mg) per day. If orally inhaled beclomethasone is used concurrently, the combined total daily dose should not exceed 500 mcg (0.5 mg).

**Strength(s) usually available**
U.S.—
42 mcg (0.042 mg) per metered spray (Rx) [*Beconase* (fluorocarbons); *Vancenase* (fluorocarbons)].
Canada—
50 mcg (0.05 mg) per metered spray (Rx) [*Beconase; Vancenase* (fluorocarbons) [GENERIC].

**Packaging and storage**
Store between 2 and 30 °C (36 and 86 °F), unless otherwise specified by manufacturer.

**Auxiliary labeling**
• For the nose.
• Shake well.

**Note**
When dispensing, include patient instructions.
Explain administration technique.

### BECLOMETHASONE DIPROPIONATE MONOHYDRATE NASAL SOLUTION

**Usual adult and adolescent dose**
Anti-inflammatory (steroidal), nasal—
Nasal, 42 to 100 mcg (0.042 to 0.1 mg) (1 or 2 metered sprays) in each nostril two times a day (total daily dose, 168 to 400 mcg [0.168 to 0.4 mg]).

**Usual adult prescribing limits**
Nasal, 600 mcg (0.6 mg) (12 metered sprays) per day.

Note: If orally inhaled beclomethasone is used concurrently, the combined total daily dose should not exceed 1 mg.

**Usual pediatric dose**
Anti-inflammatory (steroidal), nasal—
Children up to 6 years of age: Safety and efficacy have not been established.
Children 6 years of age and over: See *Usual adult and adolescent dose*.

**Usual pediatric prescribing limits**
Nasal, 400 mcg (0.4 mg) (8 metered sprays) per day. If orally inhaled beclomethasone is used concurrently, the combined total daily dose should not exceed 500 mcg (0.5 mg).

**Strength(s) usually available**
U.S.—
42 mcg (0.042 mg) per metered spray (Rx) [*Beconase AQ* (benzalkonium chloride; phenylethanol 0.25%); *Vancenase AQ* (benzalkonium chloride; phenylethanol 0.25%)].
Canada—
50 mcg (0.05 mg) per metered spray (Rx) [*Beconase AQ* [GENERIC].

**Packaging and storage**
Store between 15 and 30 °C (59 and 86 °F), unless otherwise specified by manufacturer.

**Auxiliary labeling**
- For the nose.
- Shake well.

**Note**
When dispensing, include patient instructions.
Explain administration technique.

---

### BUDESONIDE

## Summary of Differences
Pharmacology/pharmacokinetics: See *Pharmacology/Pharmacokinetics*.
Side/adverse effects: See *Side/Adverse Effects*.

## Additional Dosing Information
Regular use is required to obtain full therapeutic benefit. Treatment should not be continued beyond 3 weeks in the absence of significant symptomatic improvement.

See also *General Dosing Information*.

## Nasal Dosage Forms
### BUDESONIDE NASAL POWDER

**Usual adult and adolescent dose**
Anti-inflammatory (steroidal), nasal—
  Nasal inhalation, initially 200 mcg (0.2 mg) (2 metered inhalations) in each nostril once a day in the morning (total daily dose, 400 mcg [0.4 mg]), the dosage then being decreased to the lowest effective dose according to patient response.

**Usual adult prescribing limits**
Nasal inhalation, 800 mcg (0.8 mg) (8 metered inhalations) per day.

**Usual pediatric dose**
Anti-inflammatory (steroidal), nasal inhalation—
  Children up to 6 years of age: Safety and efficacy have not been established.
  Children 6 years of age and older: See *Usual adult and adolescent dose*.

**Usual pediatric prescribing limits**
Nasal inhalation, 400 mcg (0.4 mg) (4 metered inhalations) per day.

**Strength(s) usually available**
U.S.—
  Not commercially available.
Canada—
  100 mcg (0.1 mg) per metered inhalation (Rx) [*Rhinocort Turbuhaler*].

**Packaging and storage**
Store below 40 °C (104 °F), preferably between 15 and 30 °C (59 and 86 °F), unless otherwise specified by manufacturer.

**Auxiliary labeling**
- For the nose.

**Note**
When dispensing, include patient instructions.
Explain administration technique.

### BUDESONIDE NASAL SOLUTION

**Usual adult and adolescent dose**
Anti-inflammatory (steroidal), nasal—
  Initial: Nasal, 200 mcg (0.2 mg) (2 metered sprays) in each nostril once a day in the morning (total daily dose, 400 mcg [0.4 mg]).
  Maintenance: Nasal, 100 mcg (0.1 mg) (1 metered spray) in each nostril once a day in the morning (total daily dose, 200 mcg [0.2 mg]).

**Usual adult prescribing limits**
Nasal, 800 mcg (0.8 mg) per day.

**Usual pediatric dose**
Anti-inflammatory (steroidal), nasal—
  Children up to 6 years of age: Safety and efficacy have not been established.
  Children 6 years of age and older: See *Usual adult and adolescent dose*.

**Usual pediatric prescribing limits**
Nasal, 400 mcg (0.4 mg) per day.

**Strength(s) usually available**
U.S.—
  Not commercially available.
Canada—
  100 mcg (0.1 mg) per metered spray (Rx) [*Rhinocort Aqua*].

**Packaging and storage**
Store below 40 °C (104 °F), preferably between 15 and 30 °C (59 and 86 °F), unless otherwise specified by manufacturer. Protect from freezing.

**Auxiliary labeling**
- For the nose.
- Shake well.

**Note**
When dispensing, include patient instructions.
Explain administration technique.

---

### DEXAMETHASONE

## Summary of Differences
Indications:
  Less frequently used due to significantly increased incidence of adverse effects.
Pharmacology/pharmacokinetics:
  See *Pharmacology/Pharmacokinetics*.
Precautions:
  Laboratory value alterations—False-negative results may occur with nitroblue tetrazolium test for bacterial infections.
Side/adverse effects:
  HPA axis suppression or other systemic corticosteroid effects may occur with usual nasal inhalation doses.
  See also *Side/Adverse Effects*.

## Additional Dosing Information
When medication is to be discontinued, dosage usually should be reduced gradually according to the dose, frequency, and duration of therapy.

Patients whose conditions do not improve within 7 days should be re-evaluated. Use of dexamethasone should be limited to a maximum of 2 weeks.

See also *General Dosing Information*.

## Nasal Dosage Forms
### DEXAMETHASONE SODIUM PHOSPHATE NASAL AEROSOL

**Usual adult and adolescent dose**
Anti-inflammatory (steroidal), nasal—
  Nasal, initially 200 mcg (0.2 mg) (2 metered sprays) of dexamethasone phosphate in each nostril two or three times a day (total daily dose, 800 mcg [0.8 mg] to 1.2 mg of dexamethasone phosphate), the dosage then being decreased according to patient response.
Note: Some patients may be maintained on 100 mcg (0.1 mg) (1 metered spray) of dexamethasone phosphate in each nostril two times a day.
  Therapy should be discontinued as soon as possible. If symptoms recur, therapy may be reinstituted.

**Usual adult prescribing limits**
Nasal, 1.2 mg (12 metered sprays) of dexamethasone phosphate per day.

**Usual pediatric dose**
Anti-inflammatory (steroidal), nasal—
  Children up to 6 years of age: Use is not recommended.
  Children 6 to 12 years of age: Nasal, 100 or 200 mcg (0.1 or 0.2 mg) (1 or 2 metered sprays) of dexamethasone phosphate in each nostril two times a day (total daily dose, 400 or 800 mcg [0.4 or 0.8 mg] of dexamethasone phosphate).

**Usual pediatric prescribing limits**
Nasal, 800 mcg (0.8 mg) (8 metered sprays) of dexamethasone phosphate per day.

**Strength(s) usually available**
U.S.—
  100 mcg (0.1 mg) phosphate per metered spray (Rx) [*Decadron Turbinaire* (alcohol 2%; fluorocarbons)].
Canada—
  Not commercially available.

**Packaging and storage**
Store below 49 °C (120 °F), preferably between 15 and 30 °C (59 and 86 °F), unless otherwise specified by manufacturer. Protect from freezing.

**Auxiliary labeling**
- For the nose.
- Shake well.

## FLUNISOLIDE

### Summary of Differences
Pharmacology/pharmacokinetics: See *Pharmacology/Pharmacokinetics*.
Precautions: Cross-sensitivity and/or related problems—Dosage form contains no fluorocarbon propellants.
Side/adverse effects: See *Side/Adverse Effects*.

### Additional Dosing Information
Regular use is required to obtain full therapeutic benefits. Medication should be discontinued if improvement is not evident after 3 weeks.

See also *General Dosing Information*.

### Nasal Dosage Forms

**FLUNISOLIDE NASAL SOLUTION USP**

**Usual adult dose**
Anti-inflammatory (steroidal), nasal—
  Initial: Nasal, 50 mcg (0.05 mg) (2 metered sprays) in each nostril two times a day (total daily dose, 200 mcg [0.2 mg]); if necessary, dosing frequency may be increased to three times a day (total daily dose, 300 mcg [0.3 mg]).
  Maintenance: Nasal, as little as 25 mcg (0.025 mg) (1 metered spray) in each nostril once a day has been effective (total daily dose, 50 mcg [0.05 mg]).

**Usual adult prescribing limits**
Nasal, 400 mcg (0.4 mg) per day.

**Usual pediatric dose**
Anti-inflammatory (steroidal), nasal—
  Children up to 6 years of age:
    Safety and efficacy have not been established.
  Children 6 to 14 years of age:
    Initial—Nasal, 25 mcg (0.025 mg) (1 metered spray) in each nostril three times a day; or 50 mcg (0.05 mg) (2 metered sprays) in each nostril two times a day; (total daily dose, 150 or 200 mcg [0.15 or 0.2 mg]).
    Maintenance—Nasal, as little as 25 mcg (0.025 mg) (1 metered spray) in each nostril once a day has been effective (total daily dose, 50 mcg [0.05 mg]).
  Children 14 years of age and older:
    See *Usual adult dose*.

**Usual pediatric prescribing limits**
Nasal, 200 mcg (0.2 mg) per day.

**Strength(s) usually available**
U.S.—
  25 mcg (0.025 mg) per metered spray (Rx) [*Nasalide* (benzalkonium chloride; disodium edetate)].
Canada—
  25 mcg (0.025 mg) per metered spray (Rx) [*Rhinalar* (benzalkonium chloride)].

**Packaging and storage**
Store between 15 and 30 °C (59 and 86 °F). Store in a tight container. Protect from light.

**Stability**
Opened container should be discarded after 3 months.

**Auxiliary labeling**
• For the nose.

**Note**
When dispensing, include patient instructions.
Explain administration technique.

## TRIAMCINOLONE

### Summary of Differences
Pharmacology/pharmacokinetics: See *Pharmacology/Pharmacokinetics*.
Side/adverse effects: See *Side/Adverse Effects*.

### Additional Dosing Information
Regular use is required to obtain full therapeutic benefit. Medication should be discontinued if improvement is not evident after 3 weeks.

See also *General Dosing Information*.

### Nasal Dosage Forms

**TRIAMCINOLONE ACETONIDE NASAL AEROSOL**

**Usual adult and adolescent dose**
Anti-inflammatory (steroidal), nasal—
  Nasal, 110 mcg (0.11 mg) (2 metered sprays) in each nostril once a day (total daily dose, 220 mcg [0.22 mg]).

**Usual adult prescribing limits**
Nasal, 440 mcg (0.44 mg) (8 metered sprays) per day.

**Usual pediatric dose**
Anti-inflammatory (steroidal), nasal—
  Children up to 12 years of age: Safety and efficacy have not been established.
  Children 12 years of age and older: See *Usual adult and adolescent dose*.

**Strength(s) usually available**
U.S.—
  55 mcg (0.055 mg) per metered spray (Rx) [*Nasacort* (dehydrated alcohol 0.7% w/w; fluorocarbons)].
Canada—
  55 mcg (0.055 mg) per metered spray (Rx) [*Nasacort* (dehydrated alcohol 0.7% w/w; fluorocarbons)].

**Packaging and storage**
Store between 15 and 30 °C (59 and 86 °F), unless otherwise specified by manufacturer.

**Auxiliary labeling**
• For the nose.
• Shake well.

**Note**
When dispensing, include patient instructions.
Explain administration technique.

Revised: 05/16/94
Interim revision: 08/12/98

# CORTICOSTEROIDS   Ophthalmic

This monograph includes information on the following: 1) Betamethasone*; 2) Dexamethasone; 3) Fluorometholone; 4) Hydrocortisone*; 5) Medrysone; 6) Prednisolone.

VA CLASSIFICATION (Primary):
  Betamethasone—OP301
  Dexamethasone—OP301
  Fluorometholone—OP301
  Hydrocortisone—OP301
  Medrysone—OP301
  Prednisolone—OP301

Commonly used brand name(s): *AK-Dex*[2]; *AK-Pred*[6]; *AK-Tate*[6]; *Baldex*[2]; *Betnesol*[1]; *Cortamed*[4]; *Decadron*[2]; *Dexair*[2]; *Dexotic*[2]; *Diodex*[2]; *Econopred*[6]; *Econopred Plus*[6]; *Eflone*[3]; *FML Forte*[3]; *FML Liquifilm*[3]; *FML S.O.P*[3]; *Flarex*[3]; *Fluor-Op*[3]; *HMS Liquifilm*[5]; *I-Pred*[6]; *Inflamase Forte*[6]; *Inflamase Mild*[6]; *Lite Pred*[6]; *Maxidex*[2]; *Ocu-Dex*[2]; *Ocu-Pred*[6]; *Ocu-Pred Forte*[6]; *Ocu-Pred-A*[6]; *Ophtho-Tate*[6]; *PMS-Dexamethasone Sodium Phosphate*[2]; *Pred Forte*[6]; *Pred Mild*[6]; *Predair*[6]; *Predair A*[6]; *Predair Forte*[6]; *R.O.-Dexasone*[2]; *Spersadex*[2]; *Storz-Dexa*[2]; *Ultra Pred*[6].

Another commonly used name for hydrocortisone is cortisol.

Note: For a listing of dosage forms and brand names by country availability, see *Dosage Forms* section(s).

*Not commercially available in U.S.

### Category
Corticosteroid (ophthalmic); anti-inflammatory (steroidal), ophthalmic
Note: Ophthalmic dosage forms of betamethasone and hydrocortisone are not commercially available in the U.S.; therefore, there is no U.S. product labeling identifying approved indications.

## Indications
Note: Bracketed information in the *Indications* section refers to uses that are not included in U.S. product labeling.

### Accepted
Ophthalmic disorders (treatment)—Ophthalmic corticosteroids are indicated in the treatment of corticosteroid-responsive allergic and inflammatory conditions of the palpebral and bulbar conjunctiva, cornea, and anterior segment of the globe.

Fluorometholone (0.1%), medrysone, or prednisolone (0.12 or 0.125%) may be preferred for long-term treatment because they are least likely to increase intraocular pressure.

Very severe ocular disorders that do not respond to topical corticosteroid therapy may require treatment with systemic corticosteroids. In some cases, concurrent topical and systemic corticosteroid therapy may be utilized.

See *Table 1*, page 971.

### Unaccepted
Topical corticosteroids for ophthalmic use are not indicated in the treatment of degenerative ocular disorders. Also, if corticosteroid therapy is required for the treatment of disorders involving deep ocular structures, the medication should be administered systemically because topical application will not be effective.

## Pharmacology/Pharmacokinetics

### Physicochemical characteristics
Molecular weight—
  Betamethasone sodium phosphate: 516.41.
  Dexamethasone: 392.47.
  Dexamethasone sodium phosphate: 516.41.
  Fluorometholone: 376.47.
  Fluorometholone acetate: 418.51.
  Hydrocortisone acetate: 404.50.
  Medrysone: 344.49.
  Prednisolone acetate: 402.49.
  Prednisolone sodium phosphate: 484.39.

### Mechanism of action/Effect
Corticosteroids diffuse across cell membranes and complex with specific cytoplasmic receptors. These complexes then enter the cell nucleus, bind to DNA, and stimulate transcription of mRNA and subsequent protein synthesis of enzymes ultimately responsible for anti-inflammatory effects of topical application of corticosteroids to the eye. In high concentrations, which may be achieved after topical application, corticosteroids may exert direct membrane effects. Corticosteroids decrease cellular and fibrinous exudation and tissue infiltration, inhibit fibroblastic and collagen-forming activity, retard epithelial regeneration, diminish postinflammatory neovascularization, and reduce toward normal levels the excessive permeability of inflamed capillaries.

### Absorption
Absorbed into aqueous humor, cornea, iris, choroid, ciliary body, and retina. Systemic absorption occurs, but may be significant only at higher dosages or in extended pediatric therapy.

## Precautions to Consider

### Carcinogenicity/Mutagenicity
Dexamethasone—Long-term animal studies have not been conducted to evaluate the carcinogenicity of dexamethasone.

Fluorometholone, medrysone, and prednisolone—Studies in animals or humans have not been conducted to evaluate the carcinogenic or mutagenic potential of fluorometholone, medrysone, and prednisolone.

### Pregnancy/Reproduction
Pregnancy—Problems in humans have not been documented; however, adequate and well-controlled studies with these agents have not been done.

Infants born to mothers who have received substantial doses of corticosteroids during pregnancy should be carefully observed for signs of hypoadrenalism.

Studies in rabbits have shown that corticosteroids produce fetal resorptions and multiple abnormalities, including those of the head, ears, limbs, and palate.

*Dexamethasone, hydrocortisone, and prednisolone*—
  Studies in pregnant mice have shown that these medications, when applied to both eyes 5 times a day on Days 10–13 of gestation, caused a significant increase in fetal cleft palate.
  Dexamethasone and prednisolone—FDA Pregnancy Category C.

*Fluorometholone*—
  Studies in pregnant rabbits have shown that fluorometholone is teratogenic and embryocidal when applied to the eyes at various dosage levels on Days 6–18 of gestation.
  FDA Pregnancy Category C.

*Medrysone*—
  Studies in pregnant rabbits have indicated that medrysone (doses 10 and 30 times the human dose or higher) is embryocidal. Also, application to the eyes (2 drops 4 times a day on Days 6–18 of gestation) of pregnant rabbits caused an increase in early resorptions.
  FDA Pregnancy Category C.

### Breast-feeding
Problems in humans have not been documented.

### Pediatrics
Corticosteroids should be used with caution in children 2 years of age or younger because the different dose/weight ratio for children increases the risk of adrenal suppression. This risk increases with the length of therapy, which, therefore, should be limited to the shortest possible time (preferably less than 5 days).

### Geriatrics
Appropriate studies on the relationship of age to the effects of ophthalmic corticosteroids have not been performed in the geriatric population. However, no geriatrics-specific problems have been documented to date.

### Drug interactions and/or related problems
The following drug interactions and/or related problems have been selected on the basis of their potential clinical significance (possible mechanism in parentheses where appropriate)—not necessarily inclusive (» = major clinical significance):

Note: Combinations containing any of the following medications, depending on the amount present, may also interact with this medication.

Antiglaucoma agents
  (chronic or intensive use of ophthalmic corticosteroids may increase intraocular pressure and decrease the efficacy of antiglaucoma agents)

Anticholinergics, especially atropine and related compounds
  (risk of intraocular hypertension may be increased with prolonged corticosteroid therapy; may be more likely to occur during use of cycloplegic/mydriatic agents in patients predisposed to acute angle closure)

Contact lenses
  (risk of infection increased)

### Medical considerations/Contraindications
The medical considerations/contraindications included have been selected on the basis of their potential clinical significance (reasons given in parentheses where appropriate)—not necessarily inclusive (» = major clinical significance).

*Except under special circumstances, these medications should not be used when the following medical problems exist:*
» Fungal diseases, ocular, or
» Herpes simplex keratitis, acute superficial, or
» Tuberculosis, ocular, active or history of, or
» Viral disease, acute, infectious
  (corticosteroids decrease human resistance to bacterial, fungal, and viral infections; application may exacerbate existing infections and encourage the development of new or secondary infections)

*Risk-benefit should be considered when the following medical problems exist:*
» Cataracts
    (may be exacerbated)
  Diabetes mellitus
    (patient may be predisposed toward increases in intraocular pressure and/or cataract formation)
  Diseases causing thinning of the cornea or sclera
    (use may result in perforation)
» Glaucoma, chronic, open-angle, or family history of
    (may be precipitated or exacerbated)
» Infections of the cornea or conjunctiva, other
    (risk of exacerbation or development of secondary infections)
  Sensitivity to corticosteroids

## Patient monitoring

The following may be especially important in patient monitoring (other tests may be warranted in some patients, depending on condition; » = major clinical significance):

Ophthalmologic examinations, especially tonometry and slit-lamp examination

(initial ophthalmologic examinations should be performed 2 to 3 weeks following onset of chronic therapy; subsequent examinations are performed at intervals as determined by patient status or risk factors)

## Side/Adverse Effects

Note: Frequent or intensive use of ophthalmic corticosteroids may retard corneal healing.

Systemic absorption occurs, but may be significant only at higher dosages or in extended pediatric therapy. The different dose/weight ratio for children increases the risk of adrenal suppression.

The following side/adverse effects have been selected on the basis of their potential clinical significance (possible signs and symptoms in parentheses where appropriate)—not necessarily inclusive:

### Those indicating need for medical attention
Incidence less frequent or rare
*Corneal thinning and/or globe perforation* (decreased vision; watering of the eyes); *glaucoma; ocular hypertension; optic nerve damage; posterior subcapsular cataract; visual acuity and field defects* (gradual blurring or loss of vision; eye pain; nausea; vomiting); *secondary ocular infection*

### Those indicating need for medical attention only if they continue or are bothersome
Incidence more frequent
*Temporary mild blurred vision*—may be expected to occur after use of ointments

Incidence less frequent or rare
*Burning, stinging, redness, or watering of the eyes*

## Overdose

For more information on the management of overdose or unintentional ingestion, **contact a Poison Control Center** (see *Poison Control Center Listing*).

### Treatment of overdose
Generally, acute oral overdose of ophthalmic corticosteroids does not result in serious adverse effects. Dilution with fluids is the mainstay of therapy.

## Patient Consultation

As an aid to patient consultation, refer to *Advice for the Patient, Corticosteroids (Ophthalmic)*.

In providing consultation, consider emphasizing the following selected information (» = major clinical significance):

### Before using this medication
» Conditions affecting use, especially:
Sensitivity to corticosteroids
Use in children—Cautious and short-term use recommended
Other medical problems, especially eye infections (other), cataracts, or glaucoma

### Proper use of this medication
For contact lens wearers: Checking with ophthalmologist prior to use; contact lenses should not be worn during, and possibly for a time following, application of these medications because of an increased risk of infection
Shaking suspensions vigorously before applying
Proper administration technique
Preventing contamination: Not touching applicator tip to any surface and keeping container tightly closed
» Importance of not using more medication than the amount prescribed (especially in children)
» Checking with physician before using medication for future eye problems
» Proper dosing
Missed dose: Using as soon as possible; not using if almost time for next dose
» Proper storage

### Precautions while using this medication
Need for ophthalmologic examinations during long-term therapy
Checking with physician if there is no improvement after 5 to 7 days of therapy or if condition worsens

### Side/adverse effects
Signs of potential side effects, especially corneal thinning and/or globe perforation, glaucoma, ocular hypertension, optic nerve damage, posterior subcapsular cataract, visual acuity and field defects, or secondary ocular infection

## General Dosing Information

The severity and location of ocular inflammation often requires dosage to be higher and/or more frequent than the usual adult dose initially, then gradually reduced to as little as necessary to maintain the therapeutic effect. If infections do not respond promptly, the ophthalmic corticosteroid should be discontinued until the infection has been controlled.

Increasing the frequency of administration is usually as effective as, or more effective than, using higher concentrations of the medication.

The duration of treatment may vary from a few days to several weeks or months in some cases, depending on the condition being treated. Daily or alternate-day therapy may be indicated for extended periods in certain situations, such as following penetrating keratoplasty.

Although ophthalmic corticosteroids should not be used longer than is medically necessary, it is recommended that treatment be continued after apparent response, with the dosage gradually tapered to avoid relapse.

At night, the ophthalmic ointment, where available, may be used as an adjunct to the ophthalmic solution or suspension to provide prolonged contact with the eye.

---

### BETAMETHASONE

## Ophthalmic Dosage Forms

### BETAMETHASONE SODIUM PHOSPHATE OPHTHALMIC/OTIC SOLUTION

Note: The dosing and strengths of the dosage form available are expressed in terms of betamethasone base.

**Usual adult and adolescent dose**
Ophthalmic disorders (treatment)—
Topical, to the conjunctiva, 1 or 2 drops of a 0.1% (base) solution every one or two hours initially, with dosage gradually being decreased as inflammation subsides.

**Usual pediatric dose**
See *Usual adult and adolescent dose*.

**Usual geriatric dose**
See *Usual adult and adolescent dose*.

**Strength(s) usually available**
U.S.—
Not commercially available.
Canada—
0.1% (base) (Rx) [*Betnesol*].

**Packaging and storage**
Store below 40 °C (104 °F), preferably between 15 and 30 °C (59 and 86 °F), unless otherwise specified by manufacturer. Protect from freezing.

**Auxiliary labeling**
• For the eye.

**Note**
Dispense in original unopened container.

---

### DEXAMETHASONE

## Ophthalmic Dosage Forms

### DEXAMETHASONE OPHTHALMIC OINTMENT

**Usual adult and adolescent dose**
Ophthalmic disorders (treatment)—
Topical, to the conjunctiva, a thin strip (approximately 1 cm) of a 0.1% ointment three or four times a day initially. After a favorable response is obtained, the number of applications per day may be gradually reduced prior to discontinuation.

**Usual pediatric dose**
See *Usual adult and adolescent dose*.

**Usual geriatric dose**
See *Usual adult and adolescent dose*.

**Strength(s) usually available**
U.S.—
Not commercially available.

Canada—
    0.1% (Rx) [*Maxidex* (methylparaben; propylparaben)].

**Packaging and storage**
Store below 40 °C (104 °F), preferably between 15 and 30 °C (59 and 86 °F), unless otherwise specified by manufacturer. Store in a tight container. Protect from freezing.

**Auxiliary labeling**
• For the eye.

**Note**
Dispense in original unopened container.

### DEXAMETHASONE OPHTHALMIC SUSPENSION USP

**Usual adult and adolescent dose**
Ophthalmic disorders (treatment)—
    Topical, to the conjunctiva, 1 or 2 drops of a 0.1% suspension four to six times a day.

Note:  In severe conditions, treatment may be initiated with 1 or 2 drops every hour, with dosage gradually being decreased as inflammation subsides.

**Usual pediatric dose**
See *Usual adult and adolescent dose*.

**Usual geriatric dose**
See *Usual adult and adolescent dose*.

**Strength(s) usually available**
U.S.—
    0.1% (Rx) [*Maxidex;* GENERIC].
Canada—
    0.1% (Rx) [*Maxidex* (benzalkonium chloride)].

**Packaging and storage**
Store below 40 °C (104 °F), preferably between 15 and 30 °C (59 and 86 °F), unless otherwise specified by manufacturer. Store in a tight container. Protect from freezing.

**Auxiliary labeling**
• For the eye.
• Shake well.

**Note**
Dispense in original unopened container.

### DEXAMETHASONE SODIUM PHOSPHATE OPHTHALMIC OINTMENT USP

Note:  The dosing and strengths of the dosage form available are expressed in terms of dexamethasone phosphate not dexamethasone sodium phosphate.

**Usual adult and adolescent dose**
Ophthalmic disorders (treatment)—
    Topical, to the conjunctiva, a thin strip (approximately 1 cm) of a 0.05% (phosphate) ointment three or four times a day initially. After a favorable response is obtained, the number of applications per day may be gradually reduced prior to discontinuation.

**Usual pediatric dose**
See *Usual adult and adolescent dose*.

**Usual geriatric dose**
See *Usual adult and adolescent dose*.

**Strength(s) usually available**
U.S.—
    0.05% (phosphate) (Rx) [*AK-Dex* (methylparaben, propylparaben); *Baldex* (methylparaben; propylparaben); *Decadron; Dexair* (methylparaben; propylparaben); *Maxidex; Ocu-Dex;* GENERIC].
Canada—
    Not commercially available.

**Packaging and storage**
Store below 40 °C (104 °F), preferably between 15 and 30 °C (59 and 86 °F), unless otherwise specified by manufacturer. Protect from freezing.

**Auxiliary labeling**
• For the eye.

**Note**
Dispense in original unopened container.

### DEXAMETHASONE SODIUM PHOSPHATE OPHTHALMIC SOLUTION USP

Note:  The dosing and strengths of the dosage form available are expressed in terms of dexamethasone phosphate not dexamethasone sodium phosphate.

**Usual adult and adolescent dose**
Ophthalmic disorders (treatment)—
    Topical, to the conjunctiva, 1 or 2 drops of a 0.1% (phosphate) solution up to six times a day.

Note:  In severe conditions, treatment may be initiated with 1 or 2 drops every hour, with dosage gradually being decreased as inflammation subsides.

**Usual pediatric dose**
See *Usual adult and adolescent dose*.

**Usual geriatric dose**
See *Usual adult and adolescent dose*.

**Strength(s) usually available**
U.S.—
    0.1% (phosphate) (Rx) [*AK-Dex* (benzalkonium chloride); *Baldex* (sodium bisulfite; benzalkonium chloride); *Decadron* (sodium bisulfite 0.1%; benzalkonium chloride); *Dexair* (sodium bisulfite 0.1%; benzalkonium chloride); *Dexotic; Ocu-Dex; Storz-Dexa;* GENERIC].
Canada—
    0.1% (phosphate) (Rx) [*Decadron* (sodium bisulfite 0.1%; benzalkonium chloride); *Diodex* (disodium edetate; benzalkonium chloride); *PMS-Dexamethasone Sodium Phosphate; R.O.-Dexasone* (benzalkonium chloride); *Spersadex* (disodium edetate; benzalkonium chloride)].

**Packaging and storage**
Store below 40 °C (104 °F), preferably between 15 and 30 °C (59 and 86 °F), unless otherwise specified by manufacturer. Store in a tight, light-resistant container. Protect from freezing.

**Auxiliary labeling**
• For the eye.

**Note**
Dispense in original unopened container.

---

## *FLUOROMETHOLONE*

## Ophthalmic Dosage Forms

### FLUOROMETHOLONE OPHTHALMIC OINTMENT

**Usual adult and adolescent dose**
Ophthalmic disorders (treatment)—
    Topical, to the conjunctiva, a thin strip (approximately 1 cm) of a 0.1% ointment one to three times a day.

Note:  In severe conditions, treatment may be initiated with application every four hours, with dosage gradually being decreased as inflammation subsides.

**Usual pediatric dose**
See *Usual adult and adolescent dose*.

**Usual geriatric dose**
See *Usual adult and adolescent dose*.

**Strength(s) usually available**
U.S.—
    0.1% (Rx) [*FML S.O.P* (phenylmercuric acetate)].
Canada—
    Not commercially available.

**Packaging and storage**
Store below 40 °C (104 °F), preferably between 15 and 30 °C (59 and 86 °F), unless otherwise specified by manufacturer. Protect from freezing.

**Auxiliary labeling**
• For the eye.

**Note**
Dispense in original unopened container.

### FLUOROMETHOLONE OPHTHALMIC SUSPENSION USP

**Usual adult and adolescent dose**
Ophthalmic disorders (treatment)—
    Topical, to the conjunctiva, 1 or 2 drops of a 0.1% or 0.25% suspension two to four times a day.

Note:  In severe conditions, treatment may be initiated with 1 or 2 drops every hour, with dosage gradually being decreased as inflammation subsides.

**Usual pediatric dose**
See *Usual adult and adolescent dose*.

**Usual geriatric dose**
See *Usual adult and adolescent dose*.

**Strength(s) usually available**
U.S.—
   0.1% (Rx) [*Fluor-Op* (benzalkonium chloride); *FML Liquifilm* (benzalkonium chloride)].
   0.25% (Rx) [*FML Forte* (benzalkonium chloride)].
Canada—
   0.1% (Rx) [*FML Liquifilm* (benzalkonium chloride)].
   0.25% (Rx) [*FML Forte* (benzalkonium chloride)].

**Packaging and storage**
Store below 40 °C (104 °F), preferably between 15 and 30 °C (59 and 86 °F), unless otherwise specified by manufacturer. Store in a tight container. Protect from freezing.

**Auxiliary labeling**
- For the eye.
- Shake well.

**Note**
Dispense in original unopened container.

### FLUOROMETHOLONE ACETATE OPHTHALMIC SUSPENSION

**Usual adult and adolescent dose**
Ophthalmic disorders (treatment)—
   Topical, to the conjunctiva, 1 or 2 drops of a 0.1% suspension two to four times a day.

Note: In severe conditions, treatment may be initiated with 2 drops every two hours during the initial twenty-four to forty-eight hours. Dosage should be gradually decreased as inflammation subsides.

**Usual pediatric dose**
See *Usual adult and adolescent dose*.

**Usual geriatric dose**
See *Usual adult and adolescent dose*.

**Strength(s) usually available**
U.S.—
   0.1% (Rx) [*Eflone; Flarex* (benzalkonium chloride)].
Canada—
   0.1% (Rx) [*Flarex* (benzalkonium chloride)].

**Packaging and storage**
Store below 40 °C (104 °F), preferably between 15 and 30 °C (59 and 86 °F), unless otherwise specified by manufacturer. Protect from freezing.

**Auxiliary labeling**
- For the eye.
- Shake well.

---

## HYDROCORTISONE

## Ophthalmic Dosage Forms

### HYDROCORTISONE ACETATE OPHTHALMIC OINTMENT USP

**Usual adult and adolescent dose**
Ophthalmic disorders (treatment)—
   Topical, to the conjunctiva, a thin strip (approximately 1 cm) of a 2.5% ointment three or four times a day initially, with frequency of application gradually being decreased as inflammation subsides.

**Usual pediatric dose**
See *Usual adult and adolescent dose*.

**Usual geriatric dose**
See *Usual adult and adolescent dose*.

**Strength(s) usually available**
U.S.—
   Not commercially available.
Canada—
   2.5% (Rx) [*Cortamed*].

**Packaging and storage**
Store below 40 °C (104 °F), preferably between 15 and 30 °C (59 and 86 °F), unless otherwise specified by manufacturer. Protect from freezing.

**Auxiliary labeling**
- For the eye.

**Note**
Dispense in original unopened container.

---

## MEDRYSONE

## Ophthalmic Dosage Forms

### MEDRYSONE OPHTHALMIC SUSPENSION USP

**Usual adult and adolescent dose**
Ophthalmic disorders (treatment)—
   Topical, to the conjunctiva, 1 drop of a 1% suspension up to every four hours.

**Usual pediatric dose**
See *Usual adult and adolescent dose*.

**Usual geriatric dose**
See *Usual adult and adolescent dose*.

**Strength(s) usually available**
U.S.—
   1% (Rx) [*HMS Liquifilm* (benzalkonium chloride)].
Canada—
   1% (Rx) [*HMS Liquifilm* (benzalkonium chloride)].

**Packaging and storage**
Store below 40 °C (104 °F), preferably between 15 and 30 °C (59 and 86 °F), unless otherwise specified by manufacturer. Store in a tight, light-resistant container. Protect from freezing.

**Auxiliary labeling**
- For the eye.
- Shake well.

**Note**
Dispense in original unopened container.

---

## PREDNISOLONE

## Ophthalmic Dosage Forms

### PREDNISOLONE ACETATE OPHTHALMIC SUSPENSION USP

**Usual adult and adolescent dose**
Ophthalmic disorders (treatment)—
   Topical, to the conjunctiva, 1 or 2 drops of a 0.12 to 1% suspension two to four times a day.

Note: In severe conditions, treatment may be initiated with 1 or 2 drops every hour, with dosage gradually being decreased as inflammation subsides.

**Usual pediatric dose**
See *Usual adult and adolescent dose*.

**Usual geriatric dose**
See *Usual adult and adolescent dose*.

**Strength(s) usually available**
U.S.—
   0.12% (Rx) [*Pred Mild* (sodium bisulfite; benzalkonium chloride)].
   0.125% (Rx) [*Econopred* (benzalkonium chloride)].
   1% (Rx) [*AK-Tate* (benzalkonium chloride); *Econopred Plus* (benzalkonium chloride); *Ocu-Pred-A; Predair A* (sodium bisulfite; benzalkonium chloride); *Pred Forte* (sodium bisulfite; benzalkonium chloride); *Ultra Pred;* GENERIC].
Canada—
   0.12% (Rx) [*Pred Mild* (sodium bisulfite; benzalkonium chloride); GENERIC].
   1% (Rx) [*AK-Tate* (sodium bisulfite); *Ophtho-Tate; Pred Forte* (sodium bisulfite; benzalkonium chloride); GENERIC].

**Packaging and storage**
Store between 8 and 24 °C (46 and 75 °F), unless otherwise specified by manufacturer. Store in a tight container. Protect from light. Protect from freezing.

**Auxiliary labeling**
- For the eye.
- Shake well.

**Note**
Dispense in original unopened container.

## PREDNISOLONE SODIUM PHOSPHATE OPHTHALMIC SOLUTION USP

**Usual adult and adolescent dose**
Ophthalmic disorders (treatment)—
Topical, to the conjunctiva, 1 or 2 drops of a 0.125 or 1% solution up to six times a day.

Note: In severe conditions, treatment may be initiated with 1 or 2 drops every hour, with dosage gradually being decreased as inflammation subsides.

**Usual pediatric dose**
See *Usual adult and adolescent dose.*

**Usual geriatric dose**
See *Usual adult and adolescent dose.*

**Strength(s) usually available**
U.S.—
0.125% (Rx) [*AK-Pred* (sodium bisulfite; benzalkonium chloride); *Inflamase Mild* (benzalkonium chloride); *I-Pred* (sodium metabisulfite; benzalkonium chloride); *Lite Pred; Ocu-Pred; Predair* (sodium bisulfite; benzalkonium chloride); GENERIC].
1% (Rx) [*AK-Pred* (sodium bisulfite; benzalkonium chloride); *Inflamase Forte* (benzalkonium chloride); *I-Pred* (sodium metabisulfite; benzalkonium chloride); *Ocu-Pred Forte; Predair Forte* (sodium bisulfite; benzalkonium chloride); GENERIC].
Canada—
0.125% (Rx) [*Inflamase Mild* (benzalkonium chloride)].
1% (Rx) [*Inflamase Forte* (benzalkonium chloride)].

**Packaging and storage**
Store below 40 °C (104 °F), preferably between 15 and 30 °C (59 and 86 °F), unless otherwise specified by manufacturer. Store in a tight, light-resistant container. Protect from freezing.

**Auxiliary labeling**
• For the eye.

**Note**
Dispense in original unopened container.

Revised: 01/05/94
Interim revision: 05/16/94; 01/27/95; 08/12/98

---

### Table 1. Indications*

Note: Bracketed information refers to uses that are not included in U.S. product labeling.
Ophthalmic dosage forms of betamethasone and hydrocortisone are not commercially available in the U.S.; therefore, there is no U.S. product labeling identifying approved indications.

Legend:
I=Betamethasone  IV=Hydrocortisone
II=Dexamethasone  V=Medrysone
III=Fluorometholone  VI=Prednisolone

| | I | II | III | IV | V | VI |
|---|---|---|---|---|---|---|
| Indicated in the treatment of corticosteroid-responsive inflammatory conditions of the palpebral and bulbar conjunctiva, cornea, and anterior segment of the globe, such as: | | | | | | |
| Allergic disorders, ophthalmic (treatment) | ✔ | ✔ | ✔ | ✔ | | ✔ |
| Anterior segment disease, inflammatory (treatment) | | ✔ | ✔ | ✔ | | ✔ |
| Conjunctivitis, allergic (treatment) | ✔ | ✔ | ✔ | ✔ | ✔ | ✔ |
| Corneal injuries (treatment) | ✔ | ✔ | ✔ | ✔ | | ✔ |
| Cyclitis (treatment) | ✔ | ✔ | ✔ | ✔ | | ✔ |
| Episcleritis (treatment) | ✔ | ✔ | ✔ | ✔ | ✔ | ✔ |
| Iridocyclitis (treatment) | ✔ | ✔ | ✔ | ✔ | [✔]1 | ✔ |
| Keratitis, herpes zoster (treatment) | | ✔ | ✔ | ✔ | [✔]1 | ✔ |
| Keratitis not associated with herpes simplex or fungal infection (treatment) | ✔ | ✔ | ✔ | ✔ | [✔]1 | ✔ |
| Keratitis, punctate, superficial (treatment) | ✔ | ✔ | ✔ | ✔ | [✔]1 | ✔ |
| Keratitis, vernal (treatment) | | | | | [✔]1 | |
| Keratoconjunctivitis, allergic (treatment) | ✔ | ✔ | ✔ | ✔ | [✔]1 | ✔ |
| Keratoconjunctivitis, vernal (treatment) | ✔ | ✔ | ✔ | ✔ | ✔ | ✔ |
| Ocular infections, superficial (treatment adjunct)† | ✔ | ✔ | ✔ | ✔ | [✔]1 | ✔ |
| Ocular sensitivity to epinephrine (treatment) | ✔ | ✔ | ✔ | ✔ | ✔ | ✔ |
| Ophthalmia sympathetic (treatment) | ✔ | ✔ | ✔ | ✔ | [✔]1 | ✔ |
| Rosacea, ocular (treatment) | ✔ | ✔ | ✔ | ✔ | [✔]1 | ✔ |

*Indications for specific agents may vary because of lack of specific testing and/or clinical-use data. Although all of these medications are used for all of the listed indications, medrysone may be less effective than the other ophthalmic corticosteroids for any condition other than conjunctivitis.
†Use in the treatment of ocular infection requires that the risk of corticosteroid-induced exacerbation of existing infection or development of secondary infections be weighed against the need for reducing inflammation and edema. [Appropriate anti-infective therapy should also be administered as required.]
[1]Not included in Canadian product labeling.

---

# CORTICOSTEROIDS Otic

This monograph includes information on the following: 1) Betamethasone*; 2) Dexamethasone; 3) Hydrocortisone*.

VA CLASSIFICATION (Primary): OT200

Note: Otic corticosteroid formulations are identical to the corresponding ophthalmic formulations listed in *Corticosteroids (Ophthalmic)*. However, only the specific brand name products listed below are labeled for otic use.

Commonly used brand name(s): *AK-Dex*[2]; *Betnesol*[1]; *Cortamed*[3]; *Decadron*[2]; *I-Methasone*[2].

Another commonly used name for hydrocortisone is cortisol.

Note: For a listing of dosage forms and brand names by country availability, see *Dosage Forms* section(s).

*Not commercially available in U.S.

## Category
Corticosteroid (otic); Anti-inflammatory (steroidal), otic.

## Indications

Note: Bracketed information in the *Indications* section refers to uses that are not included in U.S. product labeling.

# Corticosteroids (Otic)

## Accepted

Otic corticosteroids are indicated in the treatment of corticosteroid-responsive inflammatory disorders of the external auditory meatus such as:
Otitis externa, allergic (treatment)
Otitis, infective (treatment adjunct)
[Lichen simplex chronicus, localized (treatment)]
[Otitis externa, eczematoid, chronic (treatment)] or
[Otitis externa, seborrheic (treatment)]—Dexamethasone, betamethasone, and hydrocortisone are used in the treatment of these and other corticosteroid-responsive disorders of the external auditory meatus.

Use in the treatment of infective otitis requires that the risk of corticosteroid-induced exacerbation of existing infection or development of secondary infections be weighed against the need for reducing inflammation and edema. Appropriate anti-infective therapy should also be administered as required.

Dexamethasone is indicated in the treatment of lichen simplex chronicus of the external auditory meatus.

## Pharmacology/Pharmacokinetics

### Physicochemical characteristics
Molecular weight—
Betamethasone sodium phosphate: 516.41.
Dexamethasone sodium phosphate: 516.41.
Hydrocortisone acetate: 404.50.

### Mechanism of action/Effect
Corticosteroids diffuse across cell membranes and complex with specific cytoplasmic receptors. These complexes then enter the cell nucleus, bind to DNA, and stimulate transcription of messenger RNA and subsequent protein synthesis of enzymes responsible for anti-inflammatory effects of otic corticosteroids. In the high concentrations that may be achieved after otic use, corticosteroids may exert direct membrane effects. Corticosteroids decrease cellular and fibrinous exudation and tissue infiltration, inhibit fibroblastic and collagen-forming activity, retard epithelial regeneration, diminish postinflammatory neovascularization, and reduce toward normal levels the excessive permeability of inflamed capillaries.

## Precautions to Consider

### Carcinogenicity/Mutagenicity
For dexamethasone—Long-term animal studies have not been conducted to evaluate the carcinogenicity of dexamethasone ophthalmic/otic solution.

### Pregnancy/Reproduction
Problems in humans have not been documented.

### Breast-feeding
Problems in humans have not been documented.

### Pediatrics
Appropriate studies on the relationship of age to the effects of otic corticosteroids have not been performed in the pediatric population. However, pediatrics-specific problems that would limit the usefulness of these medications in children are not expected.

### Geriatrics
Appropriate studies on the relationship of age to the effects of otic corticosteroids have not been performed in the geriatric population. However, geriatrics-specific problems that would limit the usefulness of these medications in the elderly are not expected.

### Medical considerations/Contraindications
The medical considerations/contraindications included have been selected on the basis of their potential clinical significance (reasons given in parentheses where appropriate)—not necessarily inclusive (» = major clinical significance).

*Except under special circumstances, these medications should not be used when the following medical problems exist:*
» Fungal diseases, aural or
» Tuberculosis, aural or
» Viral infection, acute, infectious
(corticosteroids decrease human resistance to bacterial, fungal, and viral infections; application may mask or exacerbate existing infections and encourage the development of new or secondary infections)
» Otitis media, chronic, history of or
» Perforation of ear drum membrane
(possibility of ototoxicity)
Sensitivity to corticosteroids

*Risk-benefit should be considered when the following medical problems exist:*
Infections, ear, acute or
Infections, ear, chronic or
Otitis media, especially in children
(risk of exacerbation or development of secondary infections)

## Side/Adverse Effects

The following side/adverse effects have been selected on the basis of their potential clinical significance (possible signs and symptoms in parentheses where appropriate)—not necessarily inclusive:

**Those indicating need for medical attention only if they continue or are bothersome**
Incidence less frequent or rare
*Burning or stinging of the ear*

## Patient Consultation

As an aid to patient consultation, refer to *Advice for the Patient, Corticosteroids (Otic)*.
In providing consultation, consider emphasizing the following selected information (» = major clinical significance):

### Before using this medication
» Conditions affecting use, especially:
Sensitivity to corticosteroids
Other medical problems, especially other ear infections, viral infections, or perforated ear drum

### Proper use of this medication
Proper administration technique
Preventing contamination: Not touching applicator tip to any surface and keeping container tightly closed
» Importance of not using more medication than the amount prescribed
» Checking with physician before using medication for future ear problems
» Proper dosing
Missed dose: Using as soon as possible; not using if almost time for next dose
» Proper storage

### Precautions while using this medication
Checking with physician if no improvement after 5 to 7 days of therapy or if condition worsens

## General Dosing Information

To allow optimum contact between the medication and affected surfaces of the ear canal, all cerumen and debris should be carefully removed by a physician or a trained assistant prior to initiation of therapy.

Otic solutions may be instilled directly into the ear canal or administered by use of a saturated gauze or cotton wick gently placed into the canal. The wick should be kept moist with additional solution and replaced every 12 to 24 hours.

The duration of treatment may vary from a few days to several weeks or months in some cases, depending on the condition being treated. Daily or alternate-day therapy may be indicated for extended periods in certain situations.

Treatment should be continued after apparent response, with the dosage being gradually tapered to avoid relapse.

---

## BETAMETHASONE

## Otic Dosage Forms

### BETAMETHASONE SODIUM PHOSPHATE OPHTHALMIC/OTIC SOLUTION

#### Usual adult and adolescent dose
Topical, to the ear canal, 2 or 3 drops of a 0.1% (base) solution every 2 or 3 hours initially, with dosage gradually being decreased as inflammation subsides.

#### Usual pediatric dose
See *Usual adult and adolescent dose*.

#### Usual geriatric dose
See *Usual adult and adolescent dose*.

#### Strength(s) usually available
U.S.—
Not commercially available.
Canada—
0.1% (base) (Rx) [*Betnesol*].

## DEXAMETHASONE

### Otic Dosage Forms

**DEXAMETHASONE SODIUM PHOSPHATE OPHTHALMIC SOLUTION (Otic use) USP**

**Usual adult and adolescent dose**
Topical, to the ear canal, 3 or 4 drops of a 0.1% (phosphate) solution two or three times a day. After a favorable response is obtained, dosage may be gradually reduced if required to provide continuing control of symptoms prior to discontinuation.

**Usual pediatric dose**
See *Usual adult and adolescent dose*.

**Usual geriatric dose**
See *Usual adult and adolescent dose*.

**Strength(s) usually available**
U.S.—
 0.1% (phosphate) (Rx) [*AK-Dex* (benzalkonium chloride 0.01%; sodium edetate); *Decadron* (sodium bisulfite 0.1%; benzalkonium chloride 0.02%; disodium edetate; phenylethanol 0.25%); *I-Methasone* (benzalkonium chloride 0.01%; disodium edetate)].
Canada—
 0.1% (phosphate) (Rx) [*AK-Dex* (benzalkonium chloride 0.1%; sodium edetate); *Decadron* (sodium bisulfite 0.1%; benzalkonium chloride 0.02%; disodium edetate 0.05%; phenylethanol 0.25%,)].

**Packaging and storage**
Store below 40 °C (104 °F), preferably between 15 and 30 °C (59 and 86 °F), unless otherwise specified by manufacturer. Store in a tight, light-resistant container. Protect from freezing.

**Auxiliary labeling**
• For the ear.

**Note**
Dispense in original unopened container.

## HYDROCORTISONE

### Otic Dosage Forms

**HYDROCORTISONE ACETATE OPHTHALMIC OINTMENT (Otic use) USP**

**Usual adult and adolescent dose**
Topical, to the external ear canal, a thin coating of a 2.5% ointment two or three times a day initially, with frequency of application gradually being decreased as inflammation subsides.

**Usual pediatric dose**
Children up to 2 years of age—Dosage has not been established.
Children 2 years of age and older—See *Usual adult and adolescent dose*.

**Usual geriatric dose**
See *Usual adult and adolescent dose*.

**Strength(s) usually available**
U.S.—
 Not commercially available.
Canada—
 2.5% (Rx) [*Cortamed*].

**Packaging and storage**
Store below 40 °C (104 °F), preferably between 15 and 30 °C (59 and 86 °F), unless otherwise specified by manufacturer. Protect from freezing.

**Auxiliary labeling**
• For the ear.

**Note**
Dispense in original unopened container.

Revised: 03/31/92
Interim revision: 02/17/94

---

# CORTICOSTEROIDS Rectal

This monograph includes information on the following: 1) Betamethasone*; 2) Budesonide*; 3) Hydrocortisone; 4) Tixocortol*.

INN: Hydrocortisone—Cortisol
BAN: Hydrocortisone—Cortisol
JAN: Hydrocortisone—Cortisol
VA CLASSIFICATION (Primary):
 Betamethasone—RS100
 Budesonide—RS100
 Hydrocortisone—RS100
 Tixocortol—RS100

Commonly used brand name(s): *Anu-Med HC*[3]; *Anucort-HC*[3]; *Anuprep HC*[3]; *Anusol-HC*[3]; *Anutone-HC*[3]; *Anuzone-HC*[3]; *Betnesol*[1]; *Cort-Dome*[3]; *Cortenema*[3]; *Cortifoam*[3]; *Cortiment-10*[3]; *Cortiment-40*[3]; *Entocort*[2]; *Hemorrhoidal HC*[3]; *Hemril-HC Uniserts*[3]; *Hycort*[3]; *Proctocort*[3]; *Proctosol-HC*[3]; *Rectocort*[3]; *Rectosol-HC*[3]; *Rectovalone*[4].

Note: For a listing of dosage forms and brand names by country availability, see *Dosage Forms* section(s).

*Not commercially available in U.S.

## Category

Corticosteroid (rectal); anti-inflammatory, steroidal (rectal).

## Indications

Note: Bracketed information in the *Indications* section refers to uses that are not included in U.S. product labeling.

**Accepted**
Colitis, ulcerative (treatment)—Rectal corticosteroids are indicated to induce remission in acute exacerbations of mild to moderate ulcerative colitis, especially the distal forms including ulcerative proctitis, ulcerative proctosigmoiditis, and left-sided ulcerative colitis. They also are used as adjuncts to systemic corticosteroids or other pharmacological therapies in severe disease and in mild to moderate disease extending proximal to the reach of topical therapy. Hydrocortisone enema has proven useful in some cases of ulcerative colitis involving the transverse and ascending colons. Systemic effects, such as adrenal suppression, preclude the use of corticosteroids for long-term or maintenance therapy.

Cryptitis (treatment)
Hemorrhoids (treatment) or
Proctitis, factitial (treatment)—Hydrocortisone suppositories are indicated in the treatment of inflammatory rectal disorders including cryptitis, inflamed hemorrhoids, and proctitis caused by radiation (factitial).

Pruritus, anogenital (treatment)—Hydrocortisone rectal dosage forms are indicated for treatment of anogenital pruritus.

[Crohn's disease (treatment)]—Hydrocortisone enema is indicated as an adjunct in the treatment of Crohn's disease (regional enteritis) with left-sided involvement.

## Pharmacology/Pharmacokinetics

**Physicochemical characteristics**
Molecular weight—
 Betamethasone sodium phosphate: 516.41.
 Budesonide: 430.54.
 Hydrocortisone: 362.47.
 Hydrocortisone acetate: 404.51.
 Tixocortol pivalate: 462.65.
Solubility
 Hydrocortisone acetate: 1 mg per 100 mL in water.
pH
 Hydrocortisone enema: Between 5.5 and 7.

**Mechanism of action/Effect**
Rectal corticosteroids appear to exert a local anti-inflammatory effect on the colonic mucosa. Corticosteroids decrease or prevent tissue re-

sponses to inflammatory processes, thereby reducing development of symptoms of inflammation without affecting the underlying cause. Corticosteroids inhibit accumulation of inflammatory cells including macrophages, monocytes, endothelial cells, fibroblasts, and lymphocytes at sites of inflammation, in part by induction of lipocortin, a protein that inhibits phospholipase $A_2$. As a result, there is a decrease in the production and release of cytokines, an inhibition of the synthesis of arachidonic acid–derived mediators of inflammation (leukotrienes and prostaglandins), and decreased extravasation of leukocytes to areas of injury. An immunosuppressant effect of corticosteroids also may contribute to the anti-inflammatory effect, possibly because both involve inhibition of specific functions of leukocytes.

### Absorption
Betamethasone—There is some systemic absorption following administration of the enema.
Budesonide—Rapid and essentially complete within 3 hours following a 2-mg low viscosity enema in healthy volunteers. Systemic availability is 15 ± 12%.
Hydrocortisone—Partially absorbed following rectal administration. In ulcerative colitis patients, up to 50% may be absorbed.
Hydrocortisone acetate—In normal healthy subjects, approximately 26% of the dose is absorbed following rectal administration of a suppository. However, absorption across abraded or inflamed surfaces may be increased. Systemic absorption may be greater from the foam dosage form than from the enema, because the foam is not expelled.
Tixocortol—Rapidly and well absorbed following rectal administration.

### Protein binding
Budesonide—High (88%); to plasma proteins.

### Biotransformation
Budesonide—Extensive (approximately 90%) first-pass metabolism via oxidative and reductive pathways to major metabolites, 6 beta-hydroxybudesonide and 16 alpha-hydroxyprednisolone. Glucocorticoid activity of metabolites is less than 1% that of budesonide.
Tixocortol—In the blood and liver; transformed into inactive metabolites.

### Half-life
Budesonide—Plasma: 2 to 3 hours.

### Time to peak concentration
Budesonide—1.5 hours.
Tixocortol—20 minutes.

### Peak plasma concentration
Budesonide—3 ± 2 nanomoles per L.

### Elimination
Tixocortol—Urinary and fecal excretion generally are completed within 72 to 96 hours.

## Precautions to Consider

### Carcinogenicity
Long-term animal studies have not been conducted to determine the carcinogenicity of rectal corticosteroids.

### Pregnancy/Reproduction
Fertility—
  *For betamethasone—*
    Motility and number of spermatozoa may be increased or decreased.
Pregnancy—
  *For corticosteroids—*
    Appropriate studies have not been done in humans. Corticosteroids should not be used extensively, in large amounts, or for prolonged periods in patients who are pregnant or planning to become pregnant.
  *For budesonide—*
    Budesonide crosses the placenta. High doses of budesonide administered subcutaneously produced fetal malformations (primarily skeletal defects) in rabbits, rats, and mice. However, the relevance of these findings to humans has not been established.
  *For hydrocortisone and hydrocortisone acetate—*
    In laboratory animals, low doses administered to gestating females have been associated with an increase in the incidence of fetal abnormalities.
    FDA Pregnancy Category C (hydrocortisone acetate).

### Breast-feeding
It is not known whether rectal corticosteroids are distributed into breast milk. Systemic corticosteroids are distributed into breast milk and may cause unwanted effects, such as growth suppression, in the infant. Rectal corticosteroids are not recommended for use by breast-feeding mothers.

### Pediatrics
*For corticosteroids—*
  Infants born to mothers who received corticosteroids during pregnancy should be monitored closely for signs of hypoadrenalism. Growth and development should be carefully observed in infants and children. Growth suppression may be a complication of corticosteroid therapy or of ulcerative colitis. Alternate-day therapy may minimize this effect.
*For budesonide and tixocortol—*
  Safety and efficacy have not been established.

### Geriatrics
Appropriate studies on the relationship of age to the effects of rectal corticosteroids have not been performed in the geriatric population. However, geriatrics-specific problems that would limit the usefulness of these medications in the elderly are not expected.

### Drug interactions and/or related problems
The following drug interactions and/or related problems have been selected on the basis of their potential clinical significance (possible mechanism in parentheses where appropriate)—not necessarily inclusive (» = major clinical significance):

Anti-inflammatory drugs, nonsteroidal (NSAIDs) or
Aspirin
  (potential for gastrointestinal ulceration or hemorrhage)
  (caution is recommended when aspirin is used concurrently with corticosteroids in patients with hypoprothrombinemia)

Phenytoin
  (therapeutic effect of the corticosteroid may be decreased because of increased metabolism and decreased plasma concentration, which may result from phenytoin's induction of hepatic microsomal enzymes; an increase in corticosteroid dosage may be necessary)

» Vaccines, live virus, or other immunizations
  (immunizations are not recommended because of the increased risk of neurological complications and the possibility of decreased or absent antibody response)

### Laboratory value alterations
The following have been selected on the basis of their potential clinical significance (possible effect in parentheses where appropriate)—not necessarily inclusive (» = major clinical significance):

With diagnostic test values
  Skin tests
    (reactions may be suppressed)

With physiology/laboratory test values
  Calcium, serum
    (concentrations may be decreased)
  Glucose
    (because of the intrinsic hyperglycemic activity of corticosteroids, blood and urine concentrations may be increased if significant absorption of the corticosteroid occurs)
» Hypothalamic-pituitary-adrenal (HPA) axis function as assessed by:
  Adrenocorticotropic hormone (ACTH, corticotropin) or
  Cortisol, blood or
  Cortisol, urine (24-hour) or
  17-hydroxycorticosteroids, urine (24-hour)
    (may be decreased)
    (because budesonide is almost completely eliminated during first-pass metabolism, it has minimal systemic effect on HPA axis function at a therapeutic dose)
  Osteocalcin, serum
    (may be decreased; serum osteocalcin concentrations are correlated with bone turnover; however, the clinical significance of the effect of rectal corticosteroids on these concentrations is not known)

### Medical considerations/Contraindications
The medical considerations/contraindications included have been selected on the basis of their potential clinical significance (reasons given in parentheses where appropriate)—not necessarily inclusive (» = major clinical significance).

*Except under special circumstances, this medication should not be used when the following medical problems exist:*

» Herpes simplex, ocular
  (corneal perforation or ulceration may be more likely to develop with use of corticosteroids)

» Psychosis, acute
  (may be aggravated)

» Tuberculosis, active, latent, or questionably healed
  (may be exacerbated or reactivated; appropriate antitubercular chemotherapy or prophylaxis should be administered concurrently)

*Risk-benefit should be considered when the following medical problems exist:*
- » Abscess, fecal or
- » Anastomoses, intestinal, fresh or
- » Diverticulitis or
- » Fistulas, intestinal, extensive or
- » Obstruction, intestinal or
- » Perforation, intestinal or
- » Peritonitis or
- » Sinus tracts
    (rectal corticosteroids should be used with caution to prevent local damage to the mucosa)
    (signs and symptoms of perforation and peritonitis may be masked)

Cirrhosis or
Hypothyroidism
    (effects of corticosteroids may be enhanced)

Coronary disease, acute or
Glomerulonephritis, acute or
Hypertension or
Hyperthyroidism or
Limited cardiac reserve or
Myasthenia gravis or
Renal function impairment or
Thrombophlebitis
    (corticosteroids should be used with caution)

Diabetes mellitus
    (loss of control of diabetes may occur due to possible elevations in blood glucose; manifestations of latent diabetes may be precipitated; an increase in the dose of insulin or oral antidiabetic medication may be needed)

Glaucoma
    (intraocular pressure may be increased)

Ileocolostomy, postoperative
    (corticosteroids may inhibit wound healing)

- » Infection, local or systemic or
- » Chickenpox or
- » Measles
    (signs of infection may be masked; new infection may develop; resistance and ability to localize infection may be decreased; if infection occurs during therapy, appropriate antimicrobial therapy should be instituted)
    (chickenpox and measles may be more serious or even fatal in non-immune children and adults using corticosteroids; prophylaxis with varicella zoster immune globulin may be indicated following exposure to chickenpox, and prophylaxis with immune globulin intravenous may be indicated following exposure to measles; if chickenpox develops, treatment with the appropriate antiviral agent should be considered)

Osteoporosis
    (may be exacerbated)

Peptic ulcer, active or latent
    (may cause hyperacidity)

Sensitivity to betamethasone, budesonide, hydrocortisone, or tixocortol
- » Ulcerative disease, severe
    (increased risk of perforation of the bowel wall; when surgery is imminent, it is hazardous to delay surgery while awaiting response to treatment)

**Patient monitoring**
The following may be especially important in patient monitoring (other tests may be warranted in some patients, depending on condition; » = major clinical significance):
- » Adrenal function assessment, may include adrenocorticotropic hormone (ACTH) stimulation test, blood or urine cortisol concentrations, or urine 17-hydroxycorticosteroids concentration
    (periodic monitoring may be advisable if therapy is prolonged)

Biopsy and
Endoscopy and
Sigmoidoscopy and
Stool examinations
    (recommended to confirm the presence of colitis and rule out infectious causes and to determine dosage adjustment, duration of therapy, and rate of improvement)
    (endoscopy is recommended to diagnose peptic ulcer when corticosteroid therapy is prolonged and accompanied by epigastric pain, hematemesis, melena, and/or nausea and vomiting)

Intraocular pressure
    (should be measured when rectal corticosteroids are used in the presence of glaucoma)

## Side/Adverse Effects

Note: The risk of systemic effects, including adrenal suppression, with the use of rectal corticosteroids, although less than with oral or systemic preparations, generally increases with increasing dosage and duration of therapy.

The risk of systemic effects following the use of conventional corticosteroids, such as betamethasone and hydrocortisone, is greater than the risk with budesonide or tixocortol. Although budesonide and tixocortol are well absorbed, tixocortol is rapidly transformed into an inactive metabolite and budesonide is almost completely eliminated during first-pass metabolism. As a result, the systemic effects of these two agents on adrenal and hypothalamic-pituitary-adrenal (HPA) axis function are minimal at therapeutic doses. However, a decrease in cortisol concentrations has been seen following rectal administration of a high dose (10 mg) of budesonide.

For several months to 1 year after discontinuation of prolonged corticosteroid therapy, acute adrenal insufficiency may be precipitated by periods of unusual stress. The risk of occurrence may be minimized by gradual dosage reduction, but if adrenal insufficiency occurs, it may require reinstatement of corticosteroid therapy or an increase in dosage.

The following side/adverse effects have been selected on the basis of their potential clinical significance (possible signs and symptoms in parentheses where appropriate)—not necessarily inclusive:

**Those indicating the need for medical attention**
Incidence less frequent or rare
    *Allergic contact dermatitis* (burning and itching of skin); *chills; decreased glucose tolerance; diarrhea; fever; folliculitis* (painful, red or itchy, pus-containing blisters in hair follicles); *infection, secondary; rectal irritation* (rectal bleeding, burning, dryness, itching, or pain not present before therapy); *neuropathy* (sensation of pins and needles; stabbing pain); *psychic disturbances* (depression; false sense of well-being; mood swings; personality changes); *tenesmus* (straining while passing stool)—with tixocortol only

**Those occurring principally during prolonged use indicating need for medical attention**
    *Acne; adrenal suppression; cataracts, posterior subcapsular* (gradual blurring or loss of vision); *Cushing's syndrome effects including backache; filling or rounding out of the face; hirsutism or hypertrichosis* (unusual increase in hair growth, especially on the face); *hunchback; hypertension; impotence* (unusual decrease in sexual desire or ability in men); *menstrual irregularities; muscle weakness; or striae* (reddish purple lines on arms, face, legs, trunk, or groin); *decreased resistance to infection; ecchymosis* (nonelevated blue or purplish patch on the skin); *fluid or sodium retention* (rapid weight gain; swelling of feet or lower legs); *glaucoma with possible damage to optic nerves* (blurred vision or other change in vision; eye pain); *growth suppression*—in children; *hypokalemia* (dryness of mouth; increased thirst; irregular heartbeat; mood or mental changes; muscle cramps or pain; nausea or vomiting; unusual tiredness or weakness; weak pulse); *impaired wound healing; increased intracranial pressure* (headache; insomnia; unusual tiredness or weakness); *necrotizing angiitis* (chills; coughing; coughing up blood; headache; loss of appetite; pain in joints or muscles; shortness of breath; skin rash; unusual tiredness; unusual weight loss); *ocular infection, secondary, fungal or viral* (blurred vision or other change in vision; eye pain; redness of eye; sensitivity of eye to light; tearing); *osteopenia, osteoporosis, or bone fractures; pancreatitis* (abdominal pain; chills; nausea or vomiting); *peptic ulcer* (stomach pain); *thrombophlebitis* (pain or discomfort over vein)

**Those indicating need for medical attention only if they continue or are bothersome**
Incidence less frequent or rare
    *Dry, scaly skin; flatulence* (passing of gas)—with budesonide only; *headache; hypopigmentation* (lightened skin color); *increased sweating; increase in appetite; insomnia* (trouble in sleeping); *nausea; skin rash; thin, fragile skin; thinning hair on scalp; unusual weight gain; vertigo* (dizziness; sensation of spinning)

Incidence rare—with tixocortol only
    *Anorexia* (loss of appetite); *unusual tiredness or weakness; unusual weight loss*

## Overdose

For more information on the management of overdose or unintentional ingestion, **contact a Poison Control Center** (see *Poison Control Center Listing*).

### Clinical effects of overdose
The following effects have been selected on the basis of their potential clinical significance (possible signs and symptoms in parentheses where appropriate)—not necessarily inclusive:

Chronic
*Adrenal suppression; cataracts, posterior subcapsular; Cushing's syndrome; glaucoma; growth suppression*—in children; *impaired wound healing; osteoporosis; pancreatitis; peptic ulcer; psychosis*

### Treatment of overdose
Since there is no specific antidote available, treatment is symptomatic and supportive, and consists of discontinuing corticosteroid therapy. Acute overdose usually does not require tapering of the dosage. However, corticosteroids should be withdrawn gradually following prolonged use.

## Patient Consultation

As an aid to patient consultation, refer to *Advice for the Patient, Corticosteroids (Rectal)*.

In providing consultation, consider emphasizing the following selected information (» = major clinical significance):

### Before using this medication
» Conditions affecting use, especially:
  Sensitivity to betamethasone, budesonide, hydrocortisone, or tixocortol
  Fertility—Motility and number of spermatozoa may be increased or decreased in men using betamethasone
  Pregnancy—High doses and long-term use are not recommended; budesonide crosses the placenta
  Breast-feeding—Not recommended for use by breast-feeding mothers
  Use in children—Infants born to mothers who received corticosteroids during pregnancy should be monitored for signs of hypoadrenalism; growth suppression also may occur
  Other medications, especially live virus vaccines or other immunizations
  Other medical problems, especially acute psychosis; chickenpox; diverticulitis; extensive intestinal fistulas; fecal abscess; fresh, intestinal anastamoses; intestinal obstruction or perforation; local or systemic infection; measles; ocular herpes simplex; peritonitis; severe ulcerative disease; sinus tracts; or tuberculosis

### Proper use of this medication
» Regular visits to physician to check progress
  Proper administration technique; reading patient directions carefully
» Importance of not using more medication than the amount prescribed
» Proper dosing
  Missed dose: Using as soon as possible; not using if almost time for next dose
» Proper storage

### Precautions while using this medication
» Checking with physician before discontinuing medication; gradual dosage reduction may be necessary
» Checking with physician if symptoms do not improve within 2 or 3 weeks or if condition becomes worse
» Checking with physician immediately if bleeding occurs
  Staining of fabric may occur following use of suppositories
» Caution in receiving skin tests
» Caution if any kind of surgery or emergency treatment is required
» Caution if serious infections or injuries occur
» Avoiding exposure to chickenpox or measles (especially for children); telling physician right away if exposure occurs
» Caution in receiving vaccinations or other immunizations
  For diabetic patients: May increase blood sugar concentrations

### Side/adverse effects
Signs of potential side effects, especially allergic contact dermatitis, chills, decreased glucose tolerance, diarrhea, fever, folliculitis, secondary infection, rectal irritation, neuropathy, psychic disturbances, and tenesmus

Signs of potential side effects occurring principally during prolonged therapy, especially acne; adrenal suppression; posterior subcapsular cataracts; Cushing's syndrome effects; decreased resistance to infection; ecchymosis; fluid or sodium retention; glaucoma with possible damage to optic nerves; growth suppression (in children); hypokalemia; impaired wound healing; increased intracranial pressure; necrotizing angiitis; secondary ocular infection (fungal or viral); osteopenia, osteoporosis, or bone fractures; pancreatitis; peptic ulcer; and thrombophlebitis

## General Dosing Information

A complete colorectal examination should be performed before rectal corticosteroid therapy commences to rule out serious pathology and to gauge the extent of the disease process.

If rectal corticosteroid therapy is to be successful in treating the disease, the medication must reach the diseased mucosa. Therefore, the choice of dosage form should be determined by the upper extent of the disease. The spread of the enema dosage form reaches the splenic flexure, whereas the spread of the foam and suppositories dosage forms is restricted to the rectum and sigmoid colon. Many patients prefer the foam to the enema because it allows ambulation immediately after application, interferes less with daily activities, and is easier to retain.

The enema should be retained for at least 1 to 3 hours, but it is preferable to retain it overnight. This may be facilitated by prior sedation and/or antidiarrheal medication, especially early in therapy when the urge to evacuate is the greatest.

Rectal corticosteroids for treatment of ulcerative colitis should be used in conjunction with rational dietary control, sedatives, antidiarrheal agents, antimicrobial therapy, and blood replacement, if necessary. However, anticholinergics, antidiarrheals, and antispasmodics should be used with caution because of the risk of inducing paralytic ileus or toxic megacolon.

The lowest possible dose of rectal corticosteroid should be used to control the condition under treatment. Also, corticosteroid therapy should be withdrawn gradually as soon as possible after a patient reaches remission. At that time, other agents may be used to maintain remission and/or to reduce the likelihood or frequency of relapse.

Satisfactory response to rectal corticosteroid therapy usually occurs within 1 or 2 weeks and is marked by a decrease in symptoms. However, symptomatic improvement (decreased diarrhea and bleeding, weight gain, improved appetite, reduced fever, and decreased leukocytosis) may be misleading and should not be the sole criterion for evaluating efficacy.

If there is no evidence of clinical or colorectal improvement within 2 or 3 weeks, or if the patient's condition worsens, rectal corticosteroid therapy should be discontinued.

In the presence of an infection, appropriate antimicrobial therapy should be instituted. If a favorable response does not occur promptly, the corticosteroid should be discontinued until the infection has been adequately controlled.

---

### BETAMETHASONE

## Summary of Differences

Pharmacology/pharmacokinetics: Some systemic absorption.
Precautions: Fertility—May increase or decrease motility and number of spermatozoa.
Side/adverse effects: Risk of systemic effects greater than with budesonide or tixocortol.

## Rectal Dosage Forms

### BETAMETHASONE SODIUM PHOSPHATE ENEMA

**Usual adult dose**
Colitis, ulcerative—
  Rectal, 5 mg as a retention enema every night for two to four weeks.

**Usual pediatric dose**
Dosage has not been established.

U.S.—
  Not commercially available.
Canada—
  5 mg per 100 mL (Rx) [*Betnesol*].

**Packaging and storage**
Store below 40 °C (104 °F), preferably between 15 and 30 °C (59 and 86 °F), unless otherwise specified by manufacturer. Protect from freezing.

**Auxiliary labeling**
• For rectal use only.

**Note**
When dispensing, explain administration technique.

## BUDESONIDE

### Summary of Differences
Pharmacology/pharmacokinetics:
  Biotransformation—Undergoes extensive first-pass metabolism.
  Potency ranking—High.
Precautions:
  Pregnancy—Crosses the placenta.
Side/adverse effects:
  Minimal systemic effect on hypothalamic-pituitary-adrenal axis function at a therapeutic dose.

## Rectal Dosage Forms
### BUDESONIDE ENEMA
**Usual adult dose**
Colitis, ulcerative—
  Rectal, 2 mg as a retention enema every night for four to eight weeks.

**Usual pediatric dose**
Safety and efficacy have not been established.

**Usual geriatric dose**
See *Usual adult dose*.

U.S.—
  Not commercially available.
Canada—
  2 mg per 100 mL (Rx) [*Entocort* (tablet 2.3 mg)].

**Packaging and storage**
Store between 15 and 30 °C (59 and 86 °F), unless otherwise specified by manufacturer.

**Preparation of dosage form**
For each dose, 1 tablet should be added to the enema bottle, then the bottle should be shaken vigorously for 10 seconds or until the tablet dissolves completely. The resulting 115-mL (15 mL is residual volume) suspension will be slightly yellowish in color, and should be used immediately.

**Auxiliary labeling**
• For rectal use only.

**Note**
When dispensing, explain administration technique.

## HYDROCORTISONE

### Summary of Differences
Indications: Also indicated in cryptitis, hemorrhoids, factitial proctitis, and anogenital pruritus; and used in left-sided Crohn's disease.
Pharmacology/pharmacokinetics: Potency ranking—Low (acetate and base).
Side/adverse effects: Risk of systemic effects is greater than with budesonide or tixocortol.

## Rectal Dosage Forms
Note:  Bracketed uses in the *Dosage Forms* section refer to categories of use and/or indications that are not included in U.S. product labeling.

### HYDROCORTISONE ENEMA USP
**Usual adult dose**
Colitis, ulcerative—
  Rectal, 100 mg as a retention enema at bedtime for two or three weeks or until there is clinical and proctologic remission. Refractory cases may require treatment for up to two to three months.
[Crohn's disease]—
  Rectal, 100 mg as a retention enema at bedtime for two or three weeks.
Note:  If it is necessary to continue therapy beyond three weeks, therapy should be discontinued gradually by reducing administration to every other night for two or three weeks.

**Usual pediatric dose**
Dosage has not been established.

U.S.—
  100 mg per 60 mL (Rx) [*Cortenema*; GENERIC].
Canada—
  100 mg per 60 mL (Rx) [*Cortenema*; *Hycort*].

**Packaging and storage**
Store between 15 and 30 °C (59 and 86 °F), unless otherwise specified by manufacturer. Store in a tight container. Protect from freezing and from light.

**Auxiliary labeling**
• For rectal use only.
• Shake well before use.

**Note**
When dispensing, explain administration technique.

### HYDROCORTISONE ACETATE FOAM
Note:  Each applicatorful delivers approximately 900 mg of foam containing approximately 90 mg of hydrocortisone acetate (80 mg of hydrocortisone base).

**Usual adult dose**
Colitis, ulcerative—
  Rectal, 1 applicatorful one or two times a day for two or three weeks, then 1 applicatorful every second day.

**Usual pediatric dose**
Dosage has not been established.

U.S.—
  10% (Rx) [*Cortifoam* (inert propellants isobutane and propane)].
Canada—
  10% (Rx) [*Cortifoam*].

**Packaging and storage**
Store between 15 and 30 °C (59 and 86 °F), unless otherwise specified by manufacturer.

**Auxiliary labeling**
• For rectal use only.
• Shake well before use.

**Note**
When dispensing, explain administration technique.

### HYDROCORTISONE ACETATE SUPPOSITORIES
**Usual adult dose**
Colitis, ulcerative—
  Rectal, 25 or 30 mg in the morning and at night for two weeks. In more severe cases, 25 or 30 mg three times a day or 50 or 60 mg two times a day.
Proctitis, factitial—
  Rectal, 25 or 30 mg in the morning and at night for six to eight weeks, according to response.
Cryptitis or
Hemorrhoids or
Pruritus, anogenital—
  Rectal, 20 to 30 mg a day for three days; or 40 to 80 mg a day, as needed.

**Usual pediatric dose**
Dosage has not been established.

**Strength(s) usually available**
U.S.—
  25 mg (Rx) [*Anucort-HC*; *Anu-Med HC*; *Anuprep HC*; *Anusol-HC*; *Anutone-HC*; *Anuzone-HC*; *Cort-Dome*; *Hemril-HC Uniserts*; *Hemorrhoidal HC*; *Proctosol-HC*; *Rectosol-HC*; GENERIC].
  30 mg (Rx) [*Proctocort*].
Canada—
  10 mg (Rx) [*Cortiment-10*].
  10 mg (base) (Rx) [*Rectocort*].
  40 mg (Rx) [*Cortiment-40*].

**Packaging and storage**
Store below 30 °C (86 °F), unless otherwise specified by manufacturer. Store in a well-closed container. Protect from freezing.

**Auxiliary labeling**
• For rectal use only.
• Store in a cool place.
• May be refrigerated.

**Note**
When dispensing, explain administration technique.

## TIXOCORTOL

## Rectal Dosage Forms
### TIXOCORTOL PIVALATE ENEMA
**Usual adult dose**
Colitis, ulcerative—
  Rectal, 250 mg as a retention enema at bedtime for twenty-one consecutive days. If there is no improvement after twenty-one days, an alternative method of treatment should be considered.

# Corticosteroids (Rectal)

**Usual pediatric dose**
Safety and efficacy have not been established.

U.S.—
Not commercially available.

Canada—
250 mg per 100 mL (Rx) [*Rectovalone* (benzyl alcohol)].

**Packaging and storage**
Store below 40 °C (104 °F), preferably between 15 and 30 °C (59 and 86 °F), unless otherwise specified by manufacturer. Protect from freezing.

**Auxiliary labeling**
- For rectal use only.
- Shake well before use.

**Note**
When dispensing, explain administration technique.

## Selected Bibliography
Kornbluth A, Sachar DB. Ulcerative colitis practice guidelines in adults. Am J Gastroenterol 1997; 92: 204-11.

Developed: 07/24/98

---

# CORTICOSTEROIDS  Topical

This monograph includes information on the following: 1) Alclometasone†; 2) Amcinonide; 3) Beclomethasone*; 4) Betamethasone; 5) Clobetasol; 6) Clobetasone*; 7) Clocortolone†; 8) Desonide; 9) Desoximetasone; 10) Dexamethasone†; 11) Diflorasone; 12) Diflucortolone*; 13) Flumethasone*; 14) Fluocinolone; 15) Fluocinonide; 16) Flurandrenolide; 17) Fluticasone†; 18) Halcinonide; 19) Halobetasol†; 20) Hydrocortisone; 21) Mometasone; 22) Triamcinolone.

INN:
Beclomethasone—Beclometasone
Flumethasone—Flumetasone
Flurandrenolide—Fludroxycortide
Halobetasol—Ulobetasol
Hydrocortisone—Cortisol

VA CLASSIFICATION (Primary):
Alclometasone
Topical—DE200
Amcinonide
Topical—DE200
Beclomethasone
Topical—DE200
Betamethasone
Topical—DE200
Clobetasol
Topical—DE200
Clobetasone
Topical—DE200
Clocortolone
Topical—DE200
Desonide
Topical—DE200
Desoximetasone
Topical—DE200
Dexamethasone
Topical—DE200
Diflorasone
Topical—DE200
Diflucortolone
Topical—DE200
Flumethasone
Topical—DE200
Fluocinolone
Topical—DE200
Fluocinonide
Topical—DE200
Flurandrenolide
Topical—DE200
Fluticasone
Topical—DE200
Halcinonide
Topical—DE200
Halobetasol
Topical—DE200
Hydrocortisone
Dental—OR900
Topical—DE200
Mometasone
Topical—DE200
Triamcinolone
Dental—OR900
Topical—DE200

Commonly used brand name(s): *9-1-1*[20]; *Aclovate*[1]; *Acticort 100*[20]; *Aeroseb-Dex*[10]; *Aeroseb-HC*[20]; *Ala-Cort*[20]; *Ala-Scalp HP*[20]; *Allercort*[20]; *Alphaderm*[20]; *Alphatrex*[4]; *Anusol-HC*[20]; *Aristocort*[22]; *Aristocort A*[22]; *Aristocort C*[22]; *Aristocort D*[22]; *Aristocort R*[22]; *Bactine*[20]; *Barriere-HC*[20]; *Beben*[4]; *Beta-HC*[20]; *Beta-Val*[4]; *Betacort Scalp Lotion*[4]; *Betaderm*[4]; *Betaderm Scalp Lotion*[4]; *Betatrex*[4]; *Betnovate*[4]; *Betnovate-1/2*[4]; *Bio-Syn*[14]; *CaldeCORT Anti-Itch*[20]; *CaldeCORT Light*[20]; *Carmol-HC*[20]; *Celestoderm-V*[4]; *Celestoderm-V/2*[4]; *Cetacort*[20]; *Cloderm*[7]; *Cordran*[16]; *Cordran SP*[16]; *Cort-Dome*[20]; *Cortacet*[20]; *Cortaid*[20]; *Cortate*[20]; *Cortate*[20]; *Cortef*[20]; *Cortef Feminine Itch*[20]; *Corticaine*[20]; *Corticreme*[20]; *Cortifair*[20]; *Cortoderm*[20]; *Cortril*[20]; *Cutivate*[17]; *Cyclocort*[2]; *Decaderm*[10]; *Decadron*[10]; *Decaspray*[10]; *Delacort*[20]; *Delta-Tritex*[22]; *Dermabet*[4]; *Dermacort*[20]; *Dermarest DriCort*[20]; *DermiCort*[20]; *Dermovate*[5]; *Dermovate Scalp Lotion*[5]; *Dermtex HC*[20]; *DesOwen*[8]; *Diprolene*[4]; *Diprolene AF*[4]; *Diprosone*[4]; *Drenison*[16]; *Drenison-1/4*[16]; *Ectosone Mild*[4]; *Ectosone Regular*[4]; *Ectosone Scalp Lotion*[4]; *Elocom*[21]; *Elocon*[21]; *Emo-Cort*[20]; *Emo-Cort Scalp Solution*[20]; *Epifoam*[20]; *Eumovate*[6]; *Florone*[11]; *Florone E*[11]; *Fluocet*[14]; *Fluocin*[15]; *Fluoderm*[14]; *Fluolar*[14]; *Fluonid*[14]; *Fluonide*[14]; *Flurosyn*[14]; *Flutex*[22]; *FoilleCort*[20]; *Gly-Cort*[20]; *Gynecort*[20]; *Gynecort 10*[20]; *Halog*[18]; *Halog-E*[18]; *Hi-Cor 1.0*[20]; *Hi-Cor 2.5*[20]; *Hyderm*[20]; *Hydro-Tex*[20]; *Hytone*[20]; *Kenac*[22]; *Kenalog*[22]; *Kenalog in Orabase*[22]; *Kenalog-H*[22]; *Kenonel*[22]; *LactiCare-HC*[20]; *Lanacort*[20]; *Lanacort 10*[20]; *Lemoderm*[20]; *Licon*[15]; *Lidemol*[15]; *Lidex*[15]; *Lidex-E*[15]; *Locacorten*[13]; *Locoid*[20]; *Lyderm*[15]; *Maxiflor*[11]; *Maximum Strength Cortaid*[20]; *Maxivate*[4]; *Metaderm Mild*[4]; *Metaderm Regular*[4]; *MyCort*[20]; *Nerisone*[12]; *Nerisone Oily*[12]; *Novobetamet*[4]; *Novohydrocort*[20]; *Nutracort*[20]; *Orabase-HCA*[20]; *Oracort*[22]; *Oralone*[22]; *Penecort*[20]; *Pentacort*[20]; *Pharma-Cort*[20]; *Prevex B*[4]; *Prevex HC*[20]; *Propaderm*[3]; *Psorcon*[11]; *Rederm*[20]; *Rhulicort*[20]; *S-T Cort*[20]; *Sarna HC 1.0%*[20]; *Sential*[20]; *Synacort*[20]; *Synalar*[14]; *Synalar-HP*[14]; *Synamol*[14]; *Synemol*[14]; *Teladar*[4]; *Temovate*[5]; *Temovate Scalp Application*[5]; *Texacort*[20]; *Topicort*[9]; *Topicort LP*[9]; *Topicort Mild*[9]; *Topilene*[4]; *Topisone*[4]; *Topsyn*[15]; *Triacet*[22]; *Triaderm*[22]; *Trianide Mild*[22]; *Trianide Regular*[22]; *Triderm*[22]; *Tridesilon*[8]; *Ultravate*[19]; *Unicort*[20]; *Uticort*[4]; *Valisone*[4]; *Valisone Reduced Strength*[4]; *Valisone Scalp Lotion*[4]; *Valnac*[4]; *Westcort*[20].

Other commonly used names are:
Beclometasone [Beclomethasone]
Cortisol [Hydrocortisone]
Fludroxycortide [Flurandrenolide]
Flumetasone [Flumethasone]
Ulobetasol [Halobetasol]

Note: For a listing of dosage forms and brand names by country availability, see *Dosage Forms* section(s).

*Not commercially available in U.S.
†Not commercially available in Canada.

## Category
Corticosteroid (topical); anti-inflammatory, steroidal (topical).

Note: Beclomethasone, Clobetasone, Diflucortolone, and Flumethasone are not commercially available in the U.S. Therefore, there is no U.S. product labeling identifying approved indications for these medications.

## Indications
Note: Bracketed information in the *Indications* section refers to uses that are not included in U.S. product labeling.

### Accepted
Skin disorders (treatment)
Topical corticosteroids are indicated to provide symptomatic relief of inflammation and/or pruritus associated with acute and chronic corticosteroid-responsive disorders.

The location of the skin lesion to be treated should be considered in selecting a formulation. In areas with thinner skin, such as facial, eye, and intertriginous areas, low-potency corticosteroid preparations are preferred for long-term therapy. Low- to medium-potency products may be used on the ears, trunk, arms, legs, and scalp. Medium- to very high–potency formulations may be required for treatment of dermatologic disorders in areas with thicker skin, such as the palms and soles. Lotion, aerosol, and gel formulations are cosmetically better suited for hairy areas.

The type of lesion to be treated should also be considered in product selection. For dry, scaly, cracked, thickened, or hardened skin, ointments of medium potency are often used. Medium-potency lotions, aerosols, or creams are preferred in treating moister, weeping lesions or areas or in treating conditions with intense inflammation. High- to very high–potency ointments may be required to treat hyperkeratotic or thick skin lesions.

Topical corticosteroids of low to medium potency (See *Table 1, Pharmacology/Pharmacokinetics*, page 995) are used in the treatment of the following dermatologic disorders. Occlusive dressings may also be required for chronic or severe cases of lichen simplex chronicus, psoriasis, eczema, atopic dermatitis, or chronic hand eczema. The more potent topical corticosteroids and/or occlusive dressings may be required for conditions such as discoid lupus erythematosus, lichen planus, granuloma annulare, psoriatic plaques, and psoriasis affecting the palms, soles, elbows, or knees.
Dermatitis, atopic, mild to moderate
Dermatitis, contact
Dermatitis, nummular, mild
Dermatitis, seborrheic, facial and intertriginous areas
Dermatoses, inflammatory, other, mild to moderate
Dermatitis, other forms of, mild to moderate
Intertrigo
Lichen planus, facial and intertriginous areas
Lupus erythematosus, discoid, facial and intertriginous areas
Polymorphous light eruption
Pruritus, anogenital
Pruritus senilis
Psoriasis, facial and intertriginous areas or
Xerosis, inflammatory phase

Topical corticosteroids of medium to very high potency (See *Table 1, Pharmacology/Pharmacokinetics*, page 995) are used in the treatment of the following dermatologic disorders. Systemic therapy with, or intralesional injection of, a corticosteroid may be required for some of the disorders, as determined by the type and severity of the condition or inadequate response to topical therapy. Occlusive dressings may also be required for conditions such as discoid lupus erythematosus; bullous disorders; lichen planus; granuloma annulare; psoriatic plaques; and psoriasis affecting the palms, soles, elbows, or knees.
Alopecia areata
Dermatitis, atopic, moderate to severe
Dermatitis, exfoliative, generalized
Dermatitis, nummular, moderate to severe
Dermatoses, inflammatory, other, moderate to severe
Dermatitis, other forms of, moderate to severe
Granuloma annulare
Keloids, reduction of associated itching
Lichen planus
Lichen simplex chronicus
Lichen striatus
Lupus erythematosus, discoid and subacute cutaneous
Myxedema, pretibial
Necrobiosis lipoidica diabeticorum
Pemphigoid
Pemphigus
Pityriasis rosea
Psoriasis
Sarcoidosis or
Sunburn

Oral lesions, inflammatory or ulcerative (treatment)
Hydrocortisone acetate and triamcinolone acetonide dental pastes are indicated for adjunctive treatment and temporary relief of symptoms associated with nonherpetic oral inflammatory and ulcerative lesions, including recurrent aphthous stomatitis. [Formulations of high potency gels and very high potency ointments are also used in the treatment of aphthous stomatitis.][1]

[These agents are also used to treat other gingival disorders, such as desquamative gingivitis and oral lichen planus when the diagnosis has been confirmed by biopsy testing. Gel formulations of high potency corticosteroids and dental triamcinolone are used in the treatment of lichen planus of the mucous membranes. ][1]

[Other topical corticosteroids are also used to treat gingival disorders.][1]

**Unaccepted**
Medium to very high potency topical corticosteroids should not be used in the treatment of rosacea and perioral dermatitis. Although topical corticosteroids may initially reduce the burning and pustulation associated with rosacea, a severe rebound flare-up may occur upon discontinuance of the steroid.

Topical corticosteroids should not be used in the treatment of acne.

Topical corticosteroids are not indicated for routine gingivitis, which should be treated by the removal of local causative factors and an improvement in oral hygiene.

[1]Not included in Canadian product labeling.

## Pharmacology/Pharmacokinetics
See *Table 1*, page 995.
### Physicochemical characteristics
Molecular weight—
  Alclometasone dipropionate: 521.05.
  Amcinonide: 502.58.
  Beclomethasone dipropionate: 521.05.
  Betamethasone: 392.47.
  Betamethasone benzoate: 496.57.
  Betamethasone dipropionate: 504.59.
  Betamethasone sodium phosphate: 516.41.
  Betamethasone valerate: 476.58.
  Clobetasol propionate: 466.99.
  Clobetasone butyrate: 479.
  Clocortolone pivalate: 495.03.
  Desonide: 416.51.
  Desoximetasone: 376.47.
  Dexamethasone: 392.47.
  Dexamethasone sodium phosphate: 516.41.
  Diflorasone diacetate: 494.53.
  Diflucortolone valerate: 478.6.
  Flumethasone pivalate: 494.57.
  Fluocinolone acetonide: 452.5.
  Fluocinolone acetonide, dihydrate: 488.53.
  Fluocinonide: 494.53.
  Flurandrenolide: 436.52.
  Fluticasone propionate: 500.57.
  Halcinonide: 454.97.
  Halobetasol propionate: 484.97.
  Hydrocortisone: 362.47.
  Hydrocortisone acetate: 404.5.
  Hydrocortisone butyrate: 432.56.
  Hydrocortisone valerate: 446.58.
  Mometasone furoate: 521.44.
  Triamcinolone acetonide: 434.5.

### Mechanism of action/Effect
Corticosteroids diffuse across cell membranes and complex with specific cytoplasmic receptors. These complexes then enter the cell nucleus, bind to DNA (chromatin), and stimulate transcription of messenger RNA (mRNA) and subsequent protein synthesis of various inhibitory enzymes responsible for anti-inflammatory effects of topical corticosteroids. These anti-inflammatory effects include inhibition of early processes such as edema, fibrin deposition, capillary dilatation, movement of phagocytes into the area, and phagocytic activities. Later processes, such as capillary production, collagen deposition, and keloid formation, are also inhibited by corticosteroids. The overall actions of topical corticosteroids are catabolic.

Factors that increase the clinical efficacy and potential for adverse effects of topical corticosteroids include enhancement of pharmacologic activity of the compound by altering molecular structure, increasing stratum corneum penetration of the compound, and increasing bioavailability of the compound from the vehicle.

The pharmacologic activity of topical corticosteroids is increased by several changes in molecular structure. Addition of a 9-alpha-fluorine atom increases the anti-inflammatory glucocorticoid activity, but simultaneously increases undesired mineralocorticoid activity. Mineralocorticoid activity is diminished by addition of a 16-hydroxy or 16-methyl group. Substitution or masking of 16- or 17-hydroxy groups with longer side chains such as acetonide, propionate, or valerate increases lipophilicity and subsequently stratum corneum penetration.

Dental paste in dental dosage forms acts as an adhesive vehicle for application of corticosteroids to oral mucosa. The vehicle also reduces pain by serving as a protective covering.

# Corticosteroids (Topical)

## Absorption
Absorbed systemically across the stratum corneum.

Stratum corneum penetration is primarily enhanced by increasing skin hydration and/or temperature, or by changes in molecular structure of the compound.

Hydrating the skin with occlusive dressings such as plastic wrap, a tight-fitting diaper or one covered with plastic pants, plastic tape, or dermatological patches can increase corticosteroid penetration by up to tenfold. Ointment bases inhibit evaporation of moisture from skin. Intertriginous areas (axillae and groin) are self-occluding. Intertriginous areas and the face also have inherently thinner skin, are more macerated and therefore, allow for increased absorption.

Absorption of topical corticosteroids has been greatly increased by altering the product vehicle or the drug substance itself. Vehicles containing substances that solubilize the corticosteroid enhance absorption. Increasing the concentration of the drug increases skin penetration but may also increase wastage of the drug. Decreasing drug particle size has been shown to increase topical bioavailability.

Increased percutaneous absorption of corticosteroids also occurs when the skin or mucosa is abraded or inflamed, when body temperature is elevated, with prolonged use, or with extensive use.

There is some systemic absorption of topical corticosteroids through the oral mucosa; absorption increases with increased potency and prolonged use.

## Biotransformation
Primarily in skin; once absorbed systemically, in the liver. Corticosteroids that contain substituted 17-hydroxyl groups or that are fluorinated are resistant to local metabolism in the skin. Repeated application results in a cumulative depot effect in the skin, which may lead to a prolonged duration of action, increased side effects, and increased systemic absorption.

The following topical corticosteroids contain substituted 17-hydroxyl groups (S) and/or are fluorinated (F) compounds:
- Alclometasone dipropionate—S
- Amcinonide—S, F
- Beclomethasone dipropionate—S
- Betamethasone—F
- Betamethasone benzoate—S, F
- Betamethasone dipropionate—S, F
- Betamethasone valerate—S, F
- Clobetasol propionate—S, F
- Clobetasone butyrate—S, F
- Clocortolone pivalate—S, F
- Desonide—S
- Desoximetasone—S (17-hydrogen), F
- Dexamethasone—F
- Dexamethasone sodium phosphate—F
- Diflorasone diacetate—S, F
- Diflucortolone valerate—F
- Flumethasone pivalate—F
- Fluocinolone acetonide—S, F
- Fluocinonide—S, F
- Flurandrenolide—S, F
- Fluticasone propionate—S, F
- Halcinonide—S, F
- Halobetasol propionate—S, F
- Hydrocortisone butyrate—S
- Hydrocortisone valerate—S
- Mometasone furoate—S
- Triamcinolone acetonide—S, F

## Precautions to Consider

### Carcinogenicity
Long-term animal studies have not been conducted on the carcinogenicity of topical corticosteroids.

### Mutagenicity
*Fluticasone*—No mutagenicity was shown with fluticasone propionate in the Ames test, *E. coli* fluctuation test, *S. cerevisiae* gene conversion test, or Chinese hamster ovarian cell assay. Fluticasone was not clastogenic in mouse micronucleus or cultured human lymphocyte tests.

*Halobetasol*—Halobetasol propionate was not found to be genotoxic in the Ames/*Salmonella* assay, sister chromatid exchange test in Chinese hamster somatic cells, chromosome aberration studies of germinal and somatic cells of rodents, and a mammalian spot test to determine point mutations. It was found to be mutagenic in a Chinese hamster micronucleus test, and in a mouse lymphoma gene mutation assay *in vitro*.

*Hydrocortisone* and *prednisolone*—Studies on mutagenicity with hydrocortisone and prednisolone yielded negative results.

*Mometasone*—No mutagenicity was shown with mometasone in the Ames test, mouse lymphoma assay, and a micronucleus test.

### Pregnancy/Reproduction
*Pregnancy*—Topical corticosteroids, especially the more potent ones, should not be used extensively, in large amounts, or for protracted periods in pregnant patients or in patients who are planning to become pregnant.

Appropriate studies in humans have not been done.

Studies in animals have shown that topical corticosteroids are systemically absorbed and may cause fetal abnormalities, especially when used in large amounts, with occlusive dressings, for prolonged periods of time, or if the more potent agents are used.

*Betamethasone*: A dose-related increase in fetal resorptions was observed in rabbits and mice given betamethasone dipropionate intramuscularly. This effect was not observed in rats. Teratogenic effects (umbilical hernia, cephalocele, cleft palate) were observed in rabbits when betamethasone dipropionate was administered intramuscularly.

*Desoximetasone*: In studies in mice, rats, and rabbits, desoximetasone has been shown to be teratogenic and embryotoxic with subcutaneous or dermal use.

*Fluticasone*: In studies in mice, fluticasone was found to be teratogenic (cleft palate) with subcutaneous usage of doses approximately 14 and 45 times the usual human topical dose.

*Halobetasol*: In studies in rats and rabbits, halobetasol propionate administered systemically was shown to be teratogenic at doses 3 to 33 times the usual human topical dose. Cleft palate was observed in both species. Omphalocele was seen in rats only. Halobetasol propionate was shown to be embryotoxic in rabbits but not in rats.

*Hydrocortisone dental dosage form*: Studies have not been done in animals.

FDA Pregnancy Category C.

### Breast-feeding
It is not known whether topical corticosteroids are distributed into breast milk. However, problems in humans have not been documented.

Systemic corticosteroids are distributed into breast milk and may cause unwanted effects in the infant such as growth suppression.

Topical corticosteroids should not be applied to the breasts prior to nursing.

### Pediatrics
Children and adolescents have a large skin surface area to body weight ratio and less developed, thinner skin, which may result in absorption of greater amounts of topical corticosteroids compared with older patients. Absorption is also greater in premature infants than in full term newborns, due to inadequate development of the stratum corneum.

Adrenal suppression, Cushing's syndrome, intracranial hypertension, and growth retardation due to the systemic absorption of topical corticosteroids have been documented in children. Therefore, special care must be exercised when these agents are used in children and growing adolescents, especially if factors that increase absorption are involved. It is recommended that only low-potency, unfluorinated topical corticosteroids that have a free 17-hydroxyl group be used in children or growing adolescents unless there is a demonstrated need for one of the other topical corticosteroids.

Generally, pediatric therapy continuing for longer than 2 weeks and consisting of doses in excess of one daily application (with medium- or high-potency corticosteroids) or two daily applications (with low-potency corticosteroids) should be evaluated carefully by the physician. This is especially important if medication is applied to more than 5 to 10% of the body surface or if an occlusive dressing is used. A tight-fitting diaper or one covered with plastic pants may constitute an occlusive dressing.

### Geriatrics
Although appropriate studies with topical corticosteroids have not been performed in the geriatric population, geriatrics-specific problems are not expected to limit the usefulness of topical corticosteroids in the elderly. However, elderly patients may be more likely to have preexisting skin atrophy secondary to aging. Purpura and skin lacerations that may raise the skin and subcutaneous tissue from deep fascia may be more likely to occur with the use of topical corticosteroids in geriatric patients. Therefore, topical corticosteroids should be used infrequently, for brief periods, or under close medical supervision in patients with evidence of pre-existing skin atrophy. Use of lower potency topical corticosteroids may also be necessary in some patients.

### Laboratory value alterations
The following have been selected on the basis of their potential clinical significance (possible effect in parentheses where appropriate)—not necessarily inclusive (» = major clinical significance):

With physiology/laboratory test values
  Adrenal function as assessed by corticotropin (ACTH) stimulation, measurement of 24-hour urine free cortisol or 17-hydroxycorticosteroids, or measurement of plasma cortisol and

Hypothalamic-pituitary-adrenal (HPA) axis function
(may be decreased if significant absorption of the corticosteroid occurs, especially in children)
Eosinophil count, total
(may be decreased as plasma cortisol concentration is decreased)
Glucose
(blood and urine concentrations may be increased if significant absorption of the corticosteroid occurs, because of intrinsic hyperglycemic activity of corticosteroids)

**Medical considerations/Contraindications**
The medical considerations/contraindications included have been selected on the basis of their potential clinical significance (reasons given in parentheses where appropriate)—not necessarily inclusive (» = major clinical significance).

*Risk-benefit should be considered when the following medical problems exist:*
Allergy to corticosteroids
Infection at treatment site
(may be exacerbated if no appropriate antimicrobial agent is used concurrently)
Skin atrophy, pre-existing
(may be exacerbated due to atrophigenic properties of corticosteroids)
For use in the oral cavity
Herpes simplex at treatment site
(may be transmitted to other sites, including the eye)
With long-term use of more potent formulations or if substantial absorption occurs
Cataracts
(corticosteroids may promote progression of cataracts, especially with the use of high- to very high–potency products in periorbital area)
Diabetes mellitus
(loss of control of diabetes may occur due to possible elevations in blood glucose)
Glaucoma
(intraocular pressure may be increased, especially with the use of high- to very high–potency products in periorbital area)
Tuberculosis
(may be exacerbated or reactivated; appropriate antitubercular chemotherapy or prophylaxis should be administered concurrently)

**Patient monitoring**
The following may be especially important in patient monitoring (other tests may be warranted in some patients, depending on condition; » = major clinical significance):
Adrenal function assessment, such as urine or plasma cortisol concentration or ACTH stimulation test
(may be advisable during and following use if factors that increase percutaneous absorption are involved and treatment is prolonged)

## Side/Adverse Effects

Note: Generally, local or systemic adverse effects do not often occur with the use of low-potency topical corticosteroids. However, as with all topical corticosteroids, the incidence and severity of local or systemic side effects increase with factors that increase percutaneous absorption.

Percutaneous absorption of topical corticosteroids has resulted in systemic side effects such as hyperglycemia, glycosuria, and hypothalamic-pituitary-adrenal (HPA) axis suppression. HPA axis suppression has resulted from use of low doses of very high–potency products. HPA axis suppression has also resulted from use of less potent topical steroid preparations when occlusive dressings or excessive quantities were used. In all cases of HPA axis suppression, the effect was reversible upon discontinuation of therapy.

The following side/adverse effects have been selected on the basis of their potential clinical significance (possible signs and symptoms in parentheses where appropriate)—not necessarily inclusive:

**Those indicating the need for medical attention**
Incidence less frequent or rare
*Allergic contact dermatitis* (burning and itching of skin; apparent chronic therapeutic failure)—may also be caused by vehicle ingredients; *folliculitis, furunculosis, pustules, pyoderma, or vesiculation* (painful, red or itchy, pus-containing blisters in hair follicles)—more frequent with occlusion or use of ointments in intertriginous areas; *hyperesthesia* (increased skin sensitivity); *numbness in fingers; purpura* (blood-containing blisters on skin); *skin atrophy* (thinning of skin with easy bruising, especially when used on facial or intertriginous areas); *skin infection, secondary*—more frequent with occlusion; *stripping of epidermal layer*—for tape dosage forms; *telangiectasia* (raised, dark red, wart-like spots on skin, especially when used on the face)
Incidence rare—with prolonged use or other factors that increase absorption
*Acneiform eruptions* (acne or oily skin, especially when used on the face); *cataracts, posterior subcapsular* (gradual blurring or loss of vision)—reported with use of systemic corticosteroids; caution advised with use of high- and very high–potency topical corticosteroids in periorbital area; *Cushing's syndrome* (filling or rounding out of the face; unusual tiredness or weakness; backache; irritability; mental depression; menstrual irregularities; in men—unusual decrease in sexual desire or ability); *dermatitis, perioral* (irritation of skin around mouth); *ecchymosis; edema* (increased blood pressure; swelling of feet or lower legs; rapid weight gain); *gastric ulcer* (loss of appetite; nausea; stomach bloating, pain, cramping, or burning; vomiting; weight loss); *glaucoma, secondary* (eye pain; gradual decrease in vision; nausea; vomiting)—with use of high- and very high–potency topical corticosteroids in periorbital area; *hirsutism or hypertrichosis* (unusual increase in hair growth, especially on the face); *hypertension; hypokalemic syndrome* (severe weakness of extremities and trunk; loss of appetite; nausea; vomiting; irregular heartbeat; muscle cramps or pain); *hypopigmentation* (lightened skin color); *or skin pigmentation changes, other; infection, aggravation of; miliaria rubra* (burning and itching of skin with pinhead-sized red blisters); *protein depletion* (muscle weakness); *skin laceration* (tearing of skin); *skin maceration* (softening of skin); *striae* (reddish purple lines on arms, face, legs, trunk, or groin); *subcutaneous tissue atrophy; unusual loss of hair*—especially on the scalp

**Those indicating need for medical attention only if they continue or are bothersome**
Incidence less frequent or rare
*Burning, dryness, irritation, itching, or redness of skin, mild and transient; increased redness or scaling of skin lesions, mild and transient; skin rash, minor and transient*

## Overdose

For more information on the management of overdose or unintentional ingestion, **contact a Poison Control Center** (see *Poison Control Center Listing*).

**Treatment of overdose**
For chronic topical overdose—Since there is no specific antidote available, treatment is symptomatic, supportive, and consists of discontinuance of topical corticosteroid therapy. Gradual withdrawal of the preparation may be necessary.

For acute oral overdose—Since there is no specific antidote available and serious adverse effects are unlikely, treatment consists of dilution with fluids.

## Patient Consultation

As an aid to patient consultation, refer to *Advice for the Patient, Corticosteroids (Dental)* or *Corticosteroids (Rectal)*. For alclometasone, clocortolone, desonide, flumethasone, flurandrenolide (*Drenison-¼* only), hydrocortisone, hydrocortisone acetate, and dexamethasone—*Corticosteroids—Low Potency (Topical)*. For amcinonide, betamethasone, clobetasol, clobetasone, desoximetasone, diflorasone, fluocinolone, fluocinonide, flurandrenolide (except *Drenison-¼*), fluticasone, halcinonide, halobetasol, hydrocortisone butyrate, hydrocortisone valerate, mometasone, and triamcinolone—*Corticosteroids—Medium to Very High Potency (Topical)*.

In providing consultation, consider emphasizing the following selected information (» = major clinical significance):

**Before using this medication**
» Conditions affecting use, especially:
Allergies to corticosteroids
Pregnancy—Use restricted because of possible fetal abnormalities
Breast-feeding—Should not be applied to the breasts prior to nursing
Use in children—Adrenal suppression, Cushing's syndrome, intracranial hypertension, growth retardation possible with improper use
Use in the elderly—Caution recommended because purpura, skin lacerations may be more likely

**Proper use of this medication**
Proper administration technique:

*For all topical corticosteroids*
    Keeping away from eyes
» Not bandaging or otherwise wrapping the treated skin area unless directed to do so by physician
    Proper use of occlusive dressing, if prescribed

*For dental paste dosage forms*
    Applying with cotton applicator; pressing, not rubbing, paste on lesion
    Applying at bedtime and after meals for maximum effect

*For aerosol dosage forms*
    Reading and following patient directions carefully
    Avoiding breathing vapors of spray
    Avoiding getting vapors of spray in eyes
    Not smoking while using aerosols
    Not using aerosols near open flame

*For flurandrenolide tape*
    Reading and following patient directions carefully

» Importance of not using more medication than the amount prescribed or recommended on package
» Checking with physician before using medication for other dental, skin, or rectal problems
    Missed dose: Using as soon as possible; not using if almost time for next dose
» Proper storage

**Precautions while using this medication**
» Checking with physician or dentist if symptoms do not improve within 1 week or condition becomes worse

*For topical dosage forms*
    Not using tight-fitting diapers or plastic pants on a child if the diaper area is being treated with this medication

**Side/adverse effects**
    Possible stinging when gel, lotion, solution, or aerosol form of medication is applied
    Signs of potential side effects, especially development of additional dermatologic problems

## General Dosing Information

**For topical dosage forms**
To minimize the possibility of significant systemic absorption of corticosteroids during long term therapy, treatment may be interrupted periodically, small amounts of the preparation may be applied, or one area of the body may be treated at a time.

Occlusion, whether by oleaginous ointment, a thin film of polyethylene, dermatological patch, or tape, promotes increased hydration of the stratum corneum and increased absorption. Rarely, body temperature may be elevated if large areas are covered with an occlusive dressing; occlusive dressings should not be used if body temperature is elevated. Use of intermittent, rather than continuous, occlusion may decrease the risk of side effects. Generally, occlusive dressings should be changed every 24 hours or more frequently. Very high–potency topical corticosteroid formulations should not be used with occlusive dressings.

Rarely, gradual withdrawal of therapy or supplemental systemic corticosteroid therapy may be required to avoid symptoms of steroid withdrawal. Gradual withdrawal of therapy by decreasing frequency of application or by using products of decreasing potency may be necessary also to avoid a rebound flare-up of certain conditions such as psoriasis. Tachyphylaxis may also result from continual usage.

Certain topical corticosteroids may be used as adjunctive therapy to antimicrobial agents for controlling inflammation, erythema, and pruritus associated with bacterial or fungal skin infections. If symptomatic relief is not noted within a few days to one week, the topical corticosteroid should be discontinued until the infection is controlled.

**For dental dosage forms only**
Applying the paste with a cotton applicator will help to eliminate any possible absorption from contact with the skin.

The paste should be pressed, not rubbed, on the lesion. Rubbing the paste on the lesion will result in a granular, gritty sensation and cause the medication to crumble. A smooth, slippery film forms after application.

If significant repair or regeneration of oral tissues has not occurred in 7 days, the etiology of the lesion should be reinvestigated.

**For treatment of adverse effects**
If a local infection develops at the site of application, discontinue occlusive dressings (if used) and institute appropriate antimicrobial therapy. Until the infection is controlled, discontinuance of the topical corticosteroid may be necessary.

If irritation or sensitization occurs at the site of application, discontinue use of the topical corticosteroid and institute appropriate symptomatic treatment.

---

## ALCLOMETASONE

### Summary of Differences
Pharmacology/pharmacokinetics:
    Substituted; non-fluorinated.
    Potency ranking—Low.

### Topical Dosage Forms

**ALCLOMETASONE DIPROPIONATE CREAM USP**

**Usual adult dose**
Topical, to the skin, as a 0.05% cream two or three times a day.

**Usual pediatric dose**
Children and adolescents—Dosage has not been established.

**Strength(s) usually available**
U.S.—
    0.05% (Rx) [*Aclovate* (chlorocresol)].
Canada—
    Not commercially available.

**Packaging and storage**
Store below 40 °C (104 °F), preferably between 15 and 30 °C (59 and 86 °F), unless otherwise specified by manufacturer. Store in a tight container.

**Auxiliary labeling**
• For external use only.
• Do not use in or around the eye.

**ALCLOMETASONE DIPROPIONATE OINTMENT USP**

**Usual adult dose**
Topical, to the skin, as a 0.05% ointment two or three times a day.

**Usual pediatric dose**
Children and adolescents—Dosage has not been established.

**Strength(s) usually available**
U.S.—
    0.05% (Rx) [*Aclovate*].
Canada—
    Not commercially available.

**Packaging and storage**
Store below 40 °C (104 °F), preferably between 15 and 30 °C (59 and 86 °F), unless otherwise specified by manufacturer. Store in a tight container.

**Auxiliary labeling**
• For external use only.
• Do not use in or around the eye.

---

## AMCINONIDE

### Summary of Differences
Pharmacology/pharmacokinetics:
    Substituted; fluorinated.
    Potency ranking—High.

### Topical Dosage Forms

**AMCINONIDE CREAM USP**

**Usual adult dose**
Topical, to the skin, as a 0.1% cream two or three times a day.

**Usual pediatric dose**
Topical, to the skin, as a 0.1% cream once a day.

**Strength(s) usually available**
U.S.—
    0.1% (Rx) [*Cyclocort* (benzyl alcohol 2%)].
Canada—
    0.1% (Rx) [*Cyclocort* (benzyl alcohol 2%)].

**Packaging and storage**
Store below 40 °C (104 °F), preferably between 15 and 30 °C (59 and 86 °F), unless otherwise specified by manufacturer. Store in a tight container. Protect from freezing.

**Auxiliary labeling**
• For external use only.
• Do not use in or around the eye.

## AMCINONIDE LOTION

**Usual adult dose**
Topical, to the skin, as a 0.1% lotion two or three times a day.

**Usual pediatric dose**
Topical, to the skin, as a 0.1% lotion once a day.

**Strength(s) usually available**
U.S.—
  0.1% (Rx) [*Cyclocort* (benzyl alcohol 1%)].
Canada—
  0.1% (Rx) [*Cyclocort* (benzyl alcohol 1%)].

**Packaging and storage**
Store below 40 °C (104 °F), preferably between 15 and 30 °C (59 and 86 °F), in a well-closed container, unless otherwise specified by manufacturer. Protect from freezing.

**Auxiliary labeling**
• For external use only.
• Do not use in or around the eye.

## AMCINONIDE OINTMENT USP

**Usual adult dose**
Topical, to the skin, as a 0.1% ointment two times a day.

**Usual pediatric dose**
Topical, to the skin, as a 0.1% ointment once a day.

**Strength(s) usually available**
U.S.—
  0.1% (Rx) [*Cyclocort* (benzyl alcohol)].
Canada—
  0.1% (Rx) [*Cyclocort* (benzyl alcohol 2%)].

**Packaging and storage**
Store below 40 °C (104 °F), preferably between 15 and 30 °C (59 and 86 °F), unless otherwise specified by manufacturer. Store in a tight container. Protect from freezing.

**Auxiliary labeling**
• For external use only.
• Do not use in or around the eye.

---

### BECLOMETHASONE

## Summary of Differences

Pharmacology/pharmacokinetics:
  Substituted; non-fluorinated.
  Potency ranking—Medium.

## Topical Dosage Forms

### BECLOMETHASONE DIPROPIONATE CREAM

**Usual adult dose**
Topical, to the skin, as a 0.025% cream one or two times a day.

**Usual pediatric dose**
Dosage has not been established.

**Strength(s) usually available**
U.S.—
  Not commercially available.
Canada—
  0.025% (Rx) [*Propaderm*].

**Packaging and storage**
Store below 40 °C (104 °F), preferably between 15 and 30 °C (59 and 86 °F), unless otherwise specified by manufacturer.

**Auxiliary labeling**
• For external use only.
• Do not use in or around the eye.

### BECLOMETHASONE DIPROPIONATE LOTION

**Usual adult dose**
Topical, to the skin, as a 0.025% lotion one or two times a day.

**Usual pediatric dose**
Dosage has not been established.

**Strength(s) usually available**
U.S.—
  Not commercially available.
Canada—
  0.025% (Rx) [*Propaderm*].

**Packaging and storage**
Store below 40 °C (104 °F), preferably between 15 and 30 °C (59 and 86 °F), unless otherwise specified by manufacturer.

**Auxiliary labeling**
• For external use only.
• Do not use in or around the eye.

### BECLOMETHASONE DIPROPIONATE OINTMENT

**Usual adult dose**
Topical, to the skin, as a 0.025% ointment one or two times a day.

**Usual pediatric dose**
Dosage has not been established.

**Strength(s) usually available**
U.S.—
  Not commercially available.
Canada—
  0.025% (Rx) [*Propaderm*].

**Packaging and storage**
Store below 40 °C (104 °F), preferably between 15 and 30 °C (59 and 86 °F), unless otherwise specified by manufacturer.

**Auxiliary labeling**
• For external use only.
• Do not use in or around the eye.

---

### BETAMETHASONE

## Summary of Differences

Pharmacology/pharmacokinetics:
  Substituted (benzoate, dipropionate, valerate); fluorinated (base, benzoate, dipropionate, valerate).
  Potency ranking—
    Betamethasone benzoate, Medium.
    Betamethasone dipropionate (except for *Diprolene* and *Diprolene AF* products), High.
    *Diprolene* and *Diprolene AF* products, Very high.
    Betamethasone valerate, Medium.

## Topical Dosage Forms

### BETAMETHASONE BENZOATE CREAM

**Usual adult dose**
Topical, to the skin, as a 0.025% cream two to four times a day.

**Usual pediatric dose**
Topical, to the skin, as a 0.025% cream once a day.

**Strength(s) usually available**
U.S.—
  0.025% (Rx) [*Uticort*].

**Packaging and storage**
Store between 15 and 30 °C (59 and 86 °F), in a well-closed container, unless otherwise specified by manufacturer. Protect from freezing.

**Auxiliary labeling**
• For external use only.
• Do not use in or around the eye.

### BETAMETHASONE BENZOATE GEL USP

**Usual adult dose**
Topical, to the skin, as a 0.025% gel two to four times a day.

**Usual pediatric dose**
Topical, to the skin, as a 0.025% gel once a day.

**Strength(s) usually available**
U.S.—
  0.025% (Rx) [*Uticort* (alcohol 13.8%)].
Canada—
  0.025% (base) (Rx) [*Beben* (alcohol)].

**Packaging and storage**
Store below 40 °C (104 °F), preferably between 15 and 30 °C (59 and 86 °F), unless otherwise specified by manufacturer. Store in a tight container. Protect from freezing.

**Auxiliary labeling**
• For external use only.
• Do not use in or around the eye.

### BETAMETHASONE BENZOATE LOTION

**Usual adult dose**
Topical, to the skin, as a 0.025% lotion two to four times a day.

**Usual pediatric dose**
Topical, to the skin, as a 0.025% lotion once a day.

**Strength(s) usually available**
U.S.—
    0.025% (Rx) [*Uticort* (butylparaben; propylparaben; methylparaben)].

**Packaging and storage**
Store below 40 °C (104 °F), preferably between 15 and 30 °C (59 and 86 °F), in a well-closed container, unless otherwise specified by manufacturer. Protect from freezing.

**Auxiliary labeling**
- For external use only.
- Do not use in or around the eye.
- Shake well.

### BETAMETHASONE DIPROPIONATE CREAM (AUGMENTED)

Note: The dosing and strengths of betamethasone dipropionate cream (augmented) are expressed in terms of betamethasone base.

**Usual adult dose**
Topical, to the skin, as a 0.05% (base) cream one or two times a day. Augmented betamethasone dipropionate cream may be used for only a short duration of therapy and on small surface areas. Occlusive dressings should not be used.

**Usual pediatric dose**
Children up to 12 years of age—Use is not recommended.

**Strength(s) usually available**
U.S.—
    0.05% (base) (Rx) [*Diprolene AF*].
Canada—
    0.05% (base) (Rx) [*Diprolene*].

**Packaging and storage**
Store below 40 °C (104 °F), preferably between 15 and 30 °C (59 and 86 °F), unless otherwise specified by manufacturer. Store in a tight container. Protect from freezing.

**Auxiliary labeling**
- For external use only.
- Do not use in or around the eye.

### BETAMETHASONE DIPROPIONATE CREAM USP

Note: The dosing and strengths of betamethasone dipropionate cream are expressed in terms of betamethasone base.

**Usual adult dose**
Topical, to the skin, as a 0.05% (base) cream one or two times a day.

**Usual pediatric dose**
Topical, to the skin, as a 0.05% (base) cream once a day.

**Strength(s) usually available**
U.S.—
    0.05% (base) (Rx) [*Alphatrex; Diprosone; Maxivate; Teladar;* GENERIC].
Canada—
    0.05% (base) (Rx) [*Diprosone; Topilene; Topisone*].

**Packaging and storage**
Store below 40 °C (104 °F), preferably between 15 and 30 °C (59 and 86 °F), unless otherwise specified by manufacturer. Store in a tight container. Protect from freezing.

**Auxiliary labeling**
- For external use only.
- Do not use in or around the eye.

### BETAMETHASONE DIPROPIONATE GEL

Note: The dosing and strengths of betamethasone dipropionate gel are expressed in terms of betamethasone base.

**Usual adult dose**
Topical, to the skin, as a 0.05% (base) gel one or two times a day. Betamethasone dipropionate gel may be used for only a short duration of therapy and on small surface areas. Occlusive dressings should not be used.

**Usual pediatric dose**
Children up to 12 years of age—Use is not recommended.

**Strength(s) usually available**
U.S.—
    0.05% (base) (Rx) [*Diprolene*].
Canada—
    Not commercially available.

**Packaging and storage**
Store below 40 °C (104 °F), preferably between 15 and 30 °C (59 and 86 °F), unless otherwise specified by manufacturer. Store in a tight container. Protect from freezing.

**Auxiliary labeling**
- For external use only.
- Do not use in or around the eye.

### BETAMETHASONE DIPROPIONATE LOTION (AUGMENTED)

Note: The dosing and strengths of betamethasone dipropionate lotion (augmented) are expressed in terms of betamethasone base.

**Usual adult dose**
Topical, to the skin, as a 0.05% (base) lotion two times a day. Augmented betamethasone dipropionate lotion may be used for only a short duration of therapy and on small surface areas. Occlusive dressings should not be used.

**Usual pediatric dose**
Children up to 12 years of age—Dosage has not been established.

**Strength(s) usually available**
U.S.—
    0.05% (base) (Rx) [*Diprolene*].
Canada—
    Not commercially available.

**Packaging and storage**
Store below 40 °C (104 °F), preferably between 15 and 30 °C (59 and 86 °F), unless otherwise specified by manufacturer. Store in a tight container. Protect from light. Protect from freezing.

**Auxiliary labeling**
- For external use only.
- Do not use in or around the eye.
- Shake well.

### BETAMETHASONE DIPROPIONATE LOTION USP

Note: The dosing and strengths of betamethasone dipropionate lotion are expressed in terms of betamethasone base.

**Usual adult dose**
Topical, to the skin, as a 0.05% (base) lotion two times a day.

**Usual pediatric dose**
Topical, to the skin, as a 0.05% (base) lotion once a day.

**Strength(s) usually available**
U.S.—
    0.05% (base) (Rx) [*Alphatrex; Diprosone; Maxivate;* GENERIC].
Canada—
    0.05% (base) (Rx) [*Diprosone; Topisone*].

**Packaging and storage**
Store below 40 °C (104 °F), preferably between 15 and 30 °C (59 and 86 °F), unless otherwise specified by manufacturer. Store in a tight container. Protect from light. Protect from freezing.

**Auxiliary labeling**
- For external use only.
- Do not use in or around the eye.
- Shake well.

### BETAMETHASONE DIPROPIONATE OINTMENT (AUGMENTED)

Note: The dosing and strengths of betamethasone dipropionate ointment (augmented) are expressed in terms of betamethasone base.

**Usual adult dose**
Topical, to the skin, as a 0.05% (base) ointment one or two times a day. Augmented betametasone dipropionate ointment may be used for only a short duration of therapy and on small surface areas. Occlusive dressings should not be used.

**Usual pediatric dose**
Children up to 12 years of age—Use is not recommended.

**Strength(s) usually available**
U.S.—
    0.05% (base) (Rx) [*Diprolene*].
Canada—
    0.05% (base) (Rx) [*Diprolene*].

**Packaging and storage**
Store below 40 °C (104 °F), preferably between 15 and 30 °C (59 and 86 °F), unless otherwise specified by manufacturer. Store in a well-closed container. Protect from freezing.

## BETAMETHASONE DIPROPIONATE OINTMENT USP

Note: The dosing and strengths of betamethasone dipropionate ointment are expressed in terms of betamethasone base.

**Usual adult dose**
Topical, to the skin, as a 0.05% (base) ointment one or two times a day.

**Usual pediatric dose**
Topical, to the skin, as a 0.05% (base) ointment once a day.

**Strength(s) usually available**
U.S.—
    0.05% (base) (Rx) [*Alphatrex; Diprosone; Maxivate;* GENERIC].
Canada—
    0.05% (base) (Rx) [*Diprosone; Topilene; Topisone*].

**Packaging and storage**
Store below 40 °C (104 °F), preferably between 15 and 30 °C (59 and 86 °F), unless otherwise specified by manufacturer. Store in a well-closed container. Protect from freezing.

**Auxiliary labeling**
- For external use only.
- Do not use in or around the eye.

## BETAMETHASONE DIPROPIONATE TOPICAL AEROSOL

Note: The dosing and strengths of betamethasone dipropionate topical aerosol are expressed in terms of betamethasone base.

**Usual adult dose**
Topical, to the skin, a three-second spray of a 0.1% (base) aerosol three times a day.

**Usual pediatric dose**
Topical, to the skin, as a 0.1% (base) aerosol once a day.

**Strength(s) usually available**
U.S.—
    0.1% (base) (Rx) [*Diprosone* (isobutane; isopropyl alcohol 10%; propane)].
Canada—
    Not commercially available.

Note: A three-second spray delivers the equivalent of 60 mcg (0.06 mg) of betamethasone.

**Packaging and storage**
Store below 40 °C (104 °F), preferably between 2 and 30 °C (36 and 86 °F), unless otherwise specified by manufacturer. Protect from freezing.

**Auxiliary labeling**
- For external use only.
- Do not use in or around the eye.

**Note**
Explain administration technique.
When dispensing, include patient instructions.

## BETAMETHASONE VALERATE CREAM USP

Note: The dosing and strengths of betamethasone valerate cream are expressed in terms of betamethasone base.

**Usual adult dose**
Topical, to the skin, as a 0.01 or 0.1% (base) cream one to three times a day.

**Usual pediatric dose**
Topical, to the skin, as a 0.01% (base) cream one or two times a day; or a 0.1% (base) cream once a day.

**Strength(s) usually available**
U.S.—
    0.01% (base) (Rx) [*Valisone Reduced Strength*].
    0.1% (base) (Rx) [*Betatrex; Beta-Val; Dermabet; Valisone; Valnac;* GENERIC].
Canada—
    0.05% (base) (Rx) [*Betaderm; Betnovate-½; Celestoderm-V/2; Ectosone Mild; Metaderm Mild; Novobetamet; Prevex B*].
    0.1% (base) (Rx) [*Betaderm; Betnovate; Celestoderm-V; Ectosone Regular; Metaderm Regular; Novobetamet*].

**Packaging and storage**
Store below 40 °C (104 °F), preferably between 15 and 30 °C (59 and 86 °F), unless otherwise specified by manufacturer. Store in a tight container. Protect from freezing.

**Auxiliary labeling**
- For external use only.
- Do not use in or around the eye.

## BETAMETHASONE VALERATE LOTION USP

Note: The dosing and strengths of betamethasone valerate lotion are expressed in terms of betamethasone base.

**Usual adult dose**
Topical, to the skin, as a 0.1% (base) lotion one or two times a day.

**Usual pediatric dose**
Topical, to the skin, as a 0.1% (base) lotion once a day.

**Strength(s) usually available**
U.S.—
    0.1% (base) (Rx) [*Betatrex; Beta-Val; Valisone;* GENERIC].
Canada—
    0.05% (base) (Rx) [*Betnovate-½; Ectosone Mild*].
    0.1% (base) (Rx) [*Betacort Scalp Lotion; Betaderm Scalp Lotion; Betnovate; Ectosone Regular; Ectosone Scalp Lotion; Valisone Scalp Lotion*].

**Packaging and storage**
Store between 15 and 30 °C (59 and 86 °F). Store in a tight, light-resistant container. Protect from freezing.

**Auxiliary labeling**
- For external use only.
- Do not use in or around the eye.
- Shake well.

## BETAMETHASONE VALERATE OINTMENT USP

Note: The dosing and strengths of betamethasone valerate ointment are expressed in terms of betamethasone base.

**Usual adult dose**
Topical, to the skin, as a 0.1% (base) ointment one to three times a day.

**Usual pediatric dose**
Topical, to the skin, as a 0.1% (base) ointment once a day.

**Strength(s) usually available**
U.S.—
    0.1% (base) (Rx) [*Betatrex; Beta-Val; Valisone; Valnac;* GENERIC].
Canada—
    0.05% (base) (Rx) [*Betaderm; Betnovate-½; Celestoderm-V/2; Metaderm Mild*].
    0.1% (base) (Rx) [*Betaderm; Betnovate; Celestoderm-V; Metaderm Regular*].

**Packaging and storage**
Store below 40 °C (104 °F), preferably between 15 and 30 °C (59 and 86 °F). Store in a tight container. Protect from freezing.

**Auxiliary labeling**
- For external use only.
- Do not use in or around the eye.

---

# CLOBETASOL

## Summary of Differences

Pharmacology/pharmacokinetics:
    Substituted; fluorinated.
    Potency rating: Very high.

## Topical Dosage Forms

### CLOBETASOL PROPIONATE CREAM

**Usual adult dose**
Topical, to the skin, as a 0.05% cream two or three times a day. Clobetasol propionate cream may be used for only a short duration of therapy and on small surface areas. Occlusive dressings should not be used.

**Usual pediatric dose**
Children up to 12 years of age—Use is not recommended.

**Strength(s) usually available**
U.S.—
    0.05% (Rx) [*Temovate*].
Canada—
    0.05% (Rx) [*Dermovate*].

**Packaging and storage**
Store below 40 °C (104 °F), preferably between 15 and 30 °C (59 and 86 °F), in a well-closed container, unless otherwise specified by manufacturer. Do not refrigerate. Protect from freezing.

**Auxiliary labeling**
- For external use only.
- Do not use in or around the eye.

### CLOBETASOL PROPIONATE SOLUTION

**Usual adult dose**
Topical, to the scalp, as a 0.05% solution two times a day. Clobetasol propionate solution may be used for only a short duration of therapy and on small surface areas. Occlusive dressings should not be used.

**Usual pediatric dose**
Children up to 12 years of age—Use is not recommended.

**Strength(s) usually available**
U.S.—
   0.05% (Rx) [*Temovate Scalp Application* (isopropyl alcohol)].
Canada—
   0.05% (Rx) [*Dermovate Scalp Lotion* (alcohol)].

**Packaging and storage**
Store below 40 °C (104 °F), preferably between 15 and 30 °C (59 and 86 °F), in a well-closed container, unless otherwise specified by manufacturer. Protect from freezing.

**Auxiliary labeling**
- For external use only.
- Do not use in or around the eye.

### CLOBETASOL PROPIONATE OINTMENT

**Usual adult dose**
Topical, to the skin, as a 0.05% ointment two or three times a day. Clobetasol propionate ointment may be used for only a short duration of therapy and on small surface areas. Occlusive dressings should not be used.

**Usual pediatric dose**
Children up to 12 years of age—Use is not recommended.

**Strength(s) usually available**
U.S.—
   0.05% (Rx) [*Temovate*].
Canada—
   0.05% (Rx) [*Dermovate*].

**Packaging and storage**
Store below 40 °C (104 °F), preferably between 15 and 30 °C (59 and 86 °F), in a well-closed container, unless otherwise specified by manufacturer. Protect from freezing.

**Auxiliary labeling**
- For external use only.
- Do not use in or around the eye.

---

## CLOBETASONE

## Summary of Differences
Pharmacology/pharmacokinetics:
   Substituted; fluorinated.
   Potency rating—Medium.

## Topical Dosage Forms

### CLOBETASONE BUTYRATE CREAM

**Usual adult dose**
Topical, to the skin, as a 0.05% cream two or three times a day.

**Usual adult prescribing limits**
Topical, to the skin, up to 100 grams per week.

**Usual pediatric dose**
Dosage has not been established.

**Strength(s) usually available**
U.S.—
   Not commercially available.
Canada—
   0.05% (Rx) [*Eumovate*].

**Packaging and storage**
Store below 40 °C (104 °F), preferably between 15 and 30 °C (59 and 86 °F), unless otherwise specified by manufacturer.

**Auxiliary labeling**
- For external use only.
- Do not use in or around the eye.

### CLOBETASONE BUTYRATE OINTMENT

**Usual adult dose**
Topical, to the skin, as a 0.05% ointment two or three times a day.

**Usual adult prescribing limits**
Topical, to the skin, up to 100 grams per week.

**Usual pediatric dose**
Dosage has not been established.

**Strength(s) usually available**
U.S.—
   Not commercially available.
Canada—
   0.05% (Rx) [*Eumovate*].

**Packaging and storage**
Store below 40 °C (104 °F), preferably between 15 and 30 °C (59 and 86 °F), unless otherwise specified by manufacturer.

**Auxiliary labeling**
- For external use only.
- Do not use in or around the eye.

---

## CLOCORTOLONE

## Summary of Differences
Pharmacology/pharmacokinetics:
   Substituted; fluorinated.
   Potency rating—Low.

## Topical Dosage Forms

### CLOCORTOLONE PIVALATE CREAM USP

**Usual adult dose**
Topical, to the skin, as a 0.1% cream three times a day.

**Usual pediatric dose**
Dosage has not been established.

**Strength(s) usually available**
U.S.—
   0.1% (Rx) [*Cloderm* (methylparaben; propylparaben)].
Canada—
   Not commercially available.

**Packaging and storage**
Store below 40 °C (104 °F), preferably between 15 and 30 °C (59 and 86 °F), unless otherwise specified by manufacturer. Store in a tight, light-resistant container. Protect from freezing.

**Auxiliary labeling**
- For external use only.
- Do not use in or around the eye.

---

## DESONIDE

## Summary of Differences
Pharmacology/pharmacokinetics:
   Substituted; non-fluorinated.
   Potency rating—Low.

## Topical Dosage Forms

### DESONIDE CREAM

**Usual adult dose**
Topical, to the skin, as a 0.05% cream two to four times a day.

**Usual pediatric dose**
Topical, to the skin, as a 0.05% cream once a day.

**Strength(s) usually available**
U.S.—
   0.05% (Rx) [*DesOwen; Tridesilon;* GENERIC].
Canada—
   0.05% (Rx) [*Tridesilon*].

**Packaging and storage**
Store between 15 and 30 °C (59 and 86 °F), in a tight container, unless otherwise specified by manufacturer. Protect from freezing.

**Auxiliary labeling**
- For external use only.
- Do not use in or around the eye.

### DESONIDE LOTION
**Usual adult dose**
Topical, to the skin, as a 0.05% lotion two to four times a day.

**Strength(s) usually available**
U.S.—
    0.05% (Rx) [*DesOwen*].
Canada—
    Not commercially available.

**Packaging and storage**
Store between 15 and 30 °C (59 and 86 °F), in a tight container, unless otherwise specified by manufacturer. Protect from freezing.

**Auxiliary labeling**
- For external use only.
- Shake well before using.
- Do not use in or around the eye.

### DESONIDE OINTMENT
**Usual adult dose**
Topical, to the skin, as a 0.05% ointment two to four times a day.

**Usual pediatric dose**
Topical, to the skin, as a 0.05% ointment once a day.

**Strength(s) usually available**
U.S.—
    0.05% (Rx) [*DesOwen; Tridesilon*].
Canada—
    0.05% (Rx) [*Tridesilon*].

**Packaging and storage**
Store between 15 and 30 °C (59 and 86 °F), in a tight container, unless otherwise specified by manufacturer. Protect from freezing.

**Auxiliary labeling**
- For external use only.
- Do not use in or around the eye.

---

## *DESOXIMETASONE*

## Summary of Differences
Pharmacology/pharmacokinetics:
    Substituted (17-H); fluorinated.
    Potency rating—
        High (except cream 0.05%).
        Cream 0.05%, Medium.

## Topical Dosage Forms

### DESOXIMETASONE CREAM USP
**Usual adult dose**
Topical, to the skin, as a 0.05 or 0.25% cream two times a day.

**Usual pediatric dose**
Topical, to the skin, as a 0.05 or 0.25% cream once a day.

**Strength(s) usually available**
U.S.—
    0.05% (Rx) [*Topicort LP;* GENERIC].
    0.25% (Rx) [*Topicort;* GENERIC].
Canada—
    0.05% (Rx) [*Topicort Mild*].
    0.25% (Rx) [*Topicort*].

**Packaging and storage**
Store between 15 and 30 °C (59 and 86 °F), in a well-closed container, unless otherwise specified by manufacturer. Protect from freezing.

**Auxiliary labeling**
- For external use only.
- Do not use in or around the eye.

### DESOXIMETASONE GEL USP
**Usual adult dose**
Topical, to the skin, as a 0.05% gel two times a day.

**Usual pediatric dose**
Topical, to the skin, as a 0.05% gel once a day.

**Strength(s) usually available**
U.S.—
    0.05% (Rx) [*Topicort* (alcohol 20%)].
Canada—
    0.05% (Rx) [*Topicort* (alcohol)].

**Packaging and storage**
Store between 15 and 30 °C (59 and 86 °F), in well-closed container, unless otherwise specified by manufacturer. Protect from freezing.

**Auxiliary labeling**
- For external use only.
- Do not use in or around the eye.

### DESOXIMETASONE OINTMENT USP
**Usual adult dose**
Topical, to the skin, as a 0.25% ointment two times a day.

**Usual pediatric dose**
Topical, to the skin, as a 0.25% ointment once a day.

**Strength(s) usually available**
U.S.—
    0.25% (Rx) [*Topicort*].
Canada—
    Not commercially available.

**Packaging and storage**
Store between 15 and 30 °C (59 and 86 °F), in well-closed container, unless otherwise specified by manufacturer. Protect from freezing.

**Auxiliary labeling**
- For external use only.
- Do not use in or around the eye.

---

## *DEXAMETHASONE*

## Summary of Differences
Pharmacology/pharmacokinetics:
    Unsubstituted; fluorinated.
    Potency rating—Low.

## Topical Dosage Forms

### DEXAMETHASONE GEL USP
**Usual adult dose**
Topical, to the skin, as a 0.1% gel three or four times a day.

**Usual pediatric dose**
Topical, to the skin, as a 0.1% gel one or two times a day.

**Strength(s) usually available**
U.S.—
    0.1% (Rx) [*Decaderm*].
Canada—
    Not commercially available.

**Packaging and storage**
Store below 30 °C (86 °F), in a tight container. Protect from freezing.

**Auxiliary labeling**
- For external use only.
- Do not use in or around the eye.

### DEXAMETHASONE TOPICAL AEROSOL (SOLUTION) USP
**Usual adult dose**
Topical, to the skin, as a 0.01 or 0.04% aerosol two to four times a day.

**Usual pediatric dose**
Topical, to the skin, as a 0.01 or 0.04% aerosol one or two times a day.

**Strength(s) usually available**
U.S.—
    0.01% (Rx) [*Aeroseb-Dex* (alcohol 59%)].
    0.04% (Rx) [*Decaspray*].
Note: Each one-second spray of 0.01% and 0.04% aerosols delivers 20 mcg (0.02 mg) and 75 mcg (0.075 mg) of dexamethasone, respectively.
Canada—
    Not commercially available.

**Packaging and storage**
Store below 40 °C (104 °F). Protect from freezing.

**Auxiliary labeling**
- For external use only.
- Do not use in or around the eye.
- Shake gently.

**Note**
Explain administration technique.

When dispensing, include patient instructions.

This medication comes with a special applicator tube for use on the scalp.

## DEXAMETHASONE SODIUM PHOSPHATE CREAM USP

**Usual adult dose**
Topical, to the skin, as a 0.1% (phosphate) cream three or four times a day.

**Usual pediatric dose**
Topical, to the skin, as a 0.1% (phosphate) cream once a day.

**Strength(s) usually available**
U.S.—
    0.1% (phosphate) (Rx) [*Decadron* (methylparaben)].
Canada—
    Not commercially available.

**Packaging and storage**
Store below 40 °C (104 °F), preferably between 15 and 30 °C (59 and 86 °F), unless otherwise specified by manufacturer. Store in a tight container. Protect from freezing.

**Auxiliary labeling**
- For external use only.
- Do not use in or around the eye.

---

## DIFLORASONE

### Summary of Differences
Pharmacology/pharmacokinetics:
    Substituted; fluorinated.
    Potency rating—
        High (except *Psorcon* ointment).
        *Psorcon* ointment, Very high.

### Topical Dosage Forms

#### DIFLORASONE DIACETATE CREAM USP

**Usual adult dose**
Topical, to the skin, as a 0.05% cream one to four times a day.

Note: Some patients may be maintained with once daily applications after the initial acute symptoms subside. Once daily dosage may also be used to taper therapy before discontinuance.

**Usual pediatric dose**
Topical, to the skin, as a 0.05% cream once a day.

**Strength(s) usually available**
U.S.—
    0.05% (Rx) [*Florone; Florone E; Maxiflor*].
Canada—
    0.05% (Rx) [*Florone*].

**Packaging and storage**
Store between 15 and 30 °C (59 and 86 °F), in a well-closed container, unless otherwise specified by manufacturer. Protect from freezing.

**Auxiliary labeling**
- For external use only.
- Do not use in or around the eye.

#### DIFLORASONE DIACETATE OINTMENT USP

**Usual adult dose**
Topical, to the skin, as a 0.05% ointment one to four times a day.

Note: Some patients may be maintained with once daily applications after the initial acute symptoms subside. Once daily dosage may also be used to taper therapy before discontinuance.
    *Psorcon* may be used for only a short duration of therapy and on small surface areas. Occlusive dressings should not be used with *Psorcon*.

**Usual pediatric dose**
Topical, to the skin, as a 0.05% ointment once a day.

Note: *Psorcon* should be used cautiously in patients up to 12 years of age.

**Strength(s) usually available**
U.S.—
    0.05% (Rx) [*Florone; Maxiflor; Psorcon*].
Canada—
    0.05% (Rx) [*Florone*].

**Packaging and storage**
Store between 15 and 30 °C (59 and 86 °F), in a well-closed container, unless otherwise specified by manufacturer. Protect from freezing.

**Auxiliary labeling**
- For external use only.
- Do not use in or around the eye.

---

## DIFLUCORTOLONE

### Summary of Differences
Pharmacology/pharmacokinetics:
    Unsubstituted; fluorinated.
    Potency rating—Medium.

### Topical Dosage Forms

#### DIFLUCORTOLONE VALERATE CREAM

**Usual adult dose**
Topical, to the skin, as a 0.1% cream one to three times a day.

Note: Some patients may be maintained with once daily applications after the initial acute symptoms subside. Once daily dosage may also be used to taper therapy before discontinuance.

**Usual adult prescribing limits**
Topical, to the skin, up to 100 grams per week.

**Usual pediatric dose**
Dosage has not been established.

**Strength(s) usually available**
U.S.—
    Not commercially available.
Canada—
    0.1% (Rx) [*Nerisone; Nerisone Oily*].

**Packaging and storage**
Store below 40 °C (104 °F), preferably between 15 and 30 °C (59 and 86 °F), unless otherwise specified by manufacturer.

**Auxiliary labeling**
- For external use only.
- Do not use in or around the eye.

#### DIFLUCORTOLONE VALERATE OINTMENT

**Usual adult dose**
Topical, to the skin, as a 0.1% ointment one to three times a day.

Note: Some patients may be maintained with once daily applications after the initial acute symptoms subside. Once daily dosage may also be used to taper therapy before discontinuance.

**Usual adult prescribing limits**
Topical, to the skin, up to 100 grams per week.

**Usual pediatric dose**
Dosage has not been established.

**Strength(s) usually available**
U.S.—
    Not commercially available.
Canada—
    0.1% (Rx) [*Nerisone*].

**Packaging and storage**
Store below 40 °C (104 °F), preferably between 15 and 30 °C (59 and 86 °F), unless otherwise specified by manufacturer.

**Auxiliary labeling**
- For external use only.
- Do not use in or around the eye.

---

## FLUMETHASONE

### Summary of Differences
Pharmacology/pharmacokinetics:
    Unsubstituted; fluorinated.
    Potency rating—Low.

### Topical Dosage Forms

#### FLUMETHASONE PIVALATE CREAM USP

**Usual adult dose**
Topical, to the skin, as a 0.03% cream one to three times a day.

**Usual pediatric dose**
Topical, to the skin, as a 0.03% cream once a day.

**Strength(s) usually available**
U.S.—
    Not commercially available.
Canada—
    0.03% (Rx) [*Locacorten* (methylparaben; propylparaben)].

### Packaging and storage
Store below 40 °C (104 °F), preferably between 15 and 30 °C (59 and 86 °F), in a well-closed container, unless otherwise specified by manufacturer. Protect from freezing.

### Auxiliary labeling
- For external use only.
- Do not use in or around the eye.

## FLUMETHASONE PIVALATE OINTMENT

### Usual adult dose
Topical, to the skin, as a 0.03% ointment one to three times a day.

### Usual pediatric dose
Topical, to the skin, as a 0.03% ointment once a day.

### Strength(s) usually available
U.S.—
  Not commercially available.
Canada—
  0.03% (Rx) [*Locacorten* (methylparaben; propylparaben)].

### Packaging and storage
Store below 40 °C (104 °F), preferably between 15 and 30 °C (59 and 86 °F), in a well-closed container, unless otherwise specified by manufacturer. Protect from freezing.

### Auxiliary labeling
- For external use only.
- Do not use in or around the eye.

---
## FLUOCINOLONE
---

## Summary of Differences
Pharmacology/pharmacokinetics:
  Substituted; fluorinated.
  Potency rating—
    Medium (except cream 0.2%).
    Cream 0.2%, High.

## Topical Dosage Forms

### FLUOCINOLONE ACETONIDE CREAM USP

#### Usual adult dose
Topical, to the skin, as a 0.01 to 0.2% cream two to four times a day.

#### Usual pediatric dose
Topical, to the skin, as a 0.01% cream one or two times a day; or as a 0.025 or 0.2% cream once a day.

Note: The 0.2% strength is not recommended for use in children up to 2 years of age, should not be used for long periods, and should not be used in quantities greater than 2 grams per day.

#### Strength(s) usually available
U.S.—
  0.01% (Rx) [*Bio-Syn; Fluocet; Flurosyn; Synalar;* GENERIC].
  0.025% (Rx) [*Bio-Syn; Fluocet; Flurosyn; Synalar; Synemol;* GENERIC].
  0.2% (Rx) [*Synalar-HP*].
Canada—
  0.01% (Rx) [*Fluoderm; Fluolar; Fluonide; Synalar; Synamol*].
  0.025% (Rx) [*Fluoderm; Fluolar; Fluonide; Synalar; Synamol*].

#### Packaging and storage
Store below 40 °C (104 °F), preferably between 15 and 30 °C (59 and 86 °F), unless otherwise specified by manufacturer. Store in a tight container. Protect from freezing.

#### Auxiliary labeling
- For external use only.
- Do not use in or around the eye.

### FLUOCINOLONE ACETONIDE OINTMENT USP

#### Usual adult dose
Topical, to the skin, as a 0.025% ointment two to four times a day.

#### Usual pediatric dose
Topical, to the skin, as a 0.025% ointment once a day.

#### Strength(s) usually available
U.S.—
  0.025% (Rx) [*Flurosyn; Synalar;* GENERIC].
Canada—
  0.01% (Rx) [*Fluoderm*].
  0.025% (Rx) [*Fluoderm; Synalar*].

#### Packaging and storage
Store below 40 °C (104 °F), preferably between 15 and 30 °C (59 and 86 °F), unless otherwise specified by manufacturer. Store in a tight container. Protect from freezing.

#### Auxiliary labeling
- For external use only.
- Do not use in or around the eye.

### FLUOCINOLONE ACETONIDE TOPICAL SOLUTION USP

#### Usual adult dose
Topical, to the skin, as a 0.01% solution two to four times a day.

#### Usual pediatric dose
Topical, to the skin, as a 0.01% solution one or two times a day.

#### Strength(s) usually available
U.S.—
  0.01% (Rx) [*Fluonid; Synalar;* GENERIC].
Canada—
  0.01% (Rx) [*Synalar*].

#### Packaging and storage
Store below 40 °C (104 °F), preferably between 15 and 30 °C (59 and 86 °F), unless otherwise specified by manufacturer. Store in a tight container. Protect from freezing.

#### Auxiliary labeling
- For external use only.
- Do not use in or around the eye.

---
## FLUOCINONIDE
---

## Summary of Differences
Pharmacology/pharmacokinetics:
  Substituted; fluorinated.
  Potency rating—High.

## Topical Dosage Forms

### FLUOCINONIDE CREAM USP

#### Usual adult dose
Topical, to the skin, as a 0.05% cream two to four times a day.

#### Usual pediatric dose
Topical, to the skin, as a 0.05% cream once a day.

#### Strength(s) usually available
U.S.—
  0.05% (Rx) [*Fluocin; Licon; Lidex; Lidex-E;* GENERIC].
Canada—
  0.01% (Rx) [*Lidex*].
  0.05% (Rx) [*Lidemol; Lidex; Lyderm*].

#### Packaging and storage
Store below 40 °C (104 °F), preferably between 15 and 30 °C (59 and 86 °F), unless otherwise specified by manufacturer. Store in a tight container. Protect from freezing.

#### Auxiliary labeling
- For external use only.
- Do not use in or around the eye.

### FLUOCINONIDE GEL USP

#### Usual adult dose
Topical, to the skin, as a 0.05% gel two to four times a day.

#### Usual pediatric dose
Topical, to the skin, as a 0.05% gel once a day.

#### Strength(s) usually available
U.S.—
  0.05% (Rx) [*Lidex;* GENERIC].
Canada—
  0.05% (Rx) [*Topsyn*].

#### Packaging and storage
Store below 40 °C (104 °F), preferably between 15 and 30 °C (59 and 86 °F), unless otherwise specified by manufacturer. Protect from freezing. Store in a tight container.

#### Auxiliary labeling
- For external use only.
- Do not use in or around the eye.

## FLUOCINONIDE OINTMENT USP

**Usual adult dose**
Topical, to the skin, as a 0.05% ointment two to four times a day.

**Usual pediatric dose**
Topical, to the skin, as a 0.05% ointment once a day.

**Strength(s) usually available**
U.S.—
 0.05% (Rx) [*Lidex*; GENERIC].
Canada—
 0.01% (Rx) [*Lidex*].
 0.05% (Rx) [*Lidex*].

**Packaging and storage**
Store below 40 °C (104 °F), preferably between 15 and 30 °C (59 and 86 °F), unless otherwise specified by manufacturer. Store in a tight container. Protect from freezing.

**Auxiliary labeling**
• For external use only.
• Do not use in or around the eye.

## FLUOCINONIDE TOPICAL SOLUTION USP

**Usual adult dose**
Topical, to the skin, as a 0.05% solution two to four times a day.

**Usual pediatric dose**
Topical, to the skin, as a 0.05% solution once a day.

**Strength(s) usually available**
U.S.—
 0.05% (Rx) [*Lidex* (alcohol 35%); GENERIC].
Canada—
 0.05% (Rx) [*Lidex* (alcohol 35%)].

**Packaging and storage**
Store below 40 °C (104 °F), preferably between 15 and 30 °C (59 and 86 °F), unless otherwise specified by manufacturer. Store in a tight container. Protect from freezing.

**Auxiliary labeling**
• For external use only.
• Do not use in or around the eye.

---

### *FLURANDRENOLIDE*

## Summary of Differences

Pharmacology/pharmacokinetics:
 Substituted; fluorinated.
 Potency ranking—
  Medium (except cream and ointment 0.0125%).
  Cream and ointment 0.0125%, Low.

## Topical Dosage Forms

### FLURANDRENOLIDE CREAM USP

**Usual adult dose**
Topical, to the skin, as a 0.025 or 0.05% cream two or three times a day.

**Usual pediatric dose**
Topical, to the skin, as a 0.025% cream one or two times a day; or as a 0.05% cream once a day.

**Strength(s) usually available**
U.S.—
 0.025% (Rx) [*Cordran SP*].
 0.05% (Rx) [*Cordran SP*].
Canada—
 0.0125% (Rx) [*Drenison-¼*].
 0.05% (Rx) [*Drenison*].

**Packaging and storage**
Store below 40 °C (104 °F), preferably between 15 and 30 °C (59 and 86 °F), unless otherwise specified by manufacturer. Store in a tight container. Protect from light. Protect from freezing.

**Auxiliary labeling**
• For external use only.
• Do not use in or around the eye.

### FLURANDRENOLIDE LOTION USP

**Usual adult dose**
Topical, to the skin, as a 0.05% lotion two or three times a day.

**Usual pediatric dose**
Topical, to the skin, as a 0.05% lotion once a day.

**Strength(s) usually available**
U.S.—
 0.05% (Rx) [*Cordran*; GENERIC].
Canada—
 Not commercially available.

**Packaging and storage**
Store below 40 °C (104 °F), preferably between 15 and 30 °C (59 and 86 °F). Store in a tight container. Protect from light. Protect from freezing.

**Auxiliary labeling**
• For external use only.
• Do not use in or around the eye.
• Shake well.

### FLURANDRENOLIDE OINTMENT USP

**Usual adult dose**
Topical, to the skin, as a 0.025 or 0.05% ointment two or three times a day.

**Usual pediatric dose**
Topical, to the skin, as a 0.025% ointment one or two times a day; or as a 0.05% ointment once a day.

**Strength(s) usually available**
U.S.—
 0.025% (Rx) [*Cordran*].
 0.05% (Rx) [*Cordran*].
Canada—
 0.0125% (Rx) [*Drenison-¼*].
 0.05% (Rx) [*Drenison*].

**Packaging and storage**
Store below 40 °C (104 °F), preferably between 15 and 30 °C (59 and 86 °F), unless otherwise specified by manufacturer. Store in a tight container. Protect from light. Protect from freezing.

**Auxiliary labeling**
• For external use only.
• Do not use in or around the eye.

### FLURANDRENOLIDE TAPE USP

**Usual adult dose**
Topical, to the skin, as a tape containing 4 mcg (0.004 mg) of flurandrenolide per square centimeter, to be replaced every twelve to twenty-four hours.

**Usual pediatric dose**
Topical, to the skin, as a tape containing 4 mcg (0.004 mg) of flurandrenolide per square centimeter; to be replaced once a day.

**Strength(s) usually available**
U.S.—
 4 mcg (0.004 mg) per square centimeter (Rx) [*Cordran*].
Canada—
 4 mcg (0.004 mg) per square centimeter (Rx) [*Drenison*].

**Packaging and storage**
Store between 15 and 30 °C (59 and 86 °F).

**Auxiliary labeling**
• For external use only.

**Note**
Explain administration technique.
When dispensing, include patient instructions.

**Additional information**
Tape of flexible polyethylene film impregnated with flurandrenolide in the acrylic adhesive serves as an occlusive dressing, and should not be used in intertriginous areas or applied to lesions exuding serum.

---

### *FLUTICASONE*

## Summary of Differences

Pharmacology/pharmacokinetics:
 Substituted; fluorinated.
 Potency ranking—Medium.

## Topical Dosage Forms

### FLUTICASONE PROPIONATE CREAM

**Usual adult dose**
Topical, to the skin, as a 0.05% cream two times a day.

**Usual pediatric dose**
Dosage has not been established.

**Strength(s) usually available**
U.S.—
0.05% (Rx) [*Cutivate*].
Canada—
Not commercially available.

**Packaging and storage**
Store below 40 °C (104 °F), preferably between 2 and 30 °C (36 and 86 °F), in a well-closed container, unless otherwise specified by manufacturer.

**Auxiliary labeling**
• For external use only.
• Do not use in or around the eye.

### FLUTICASONE PROPIONATE OINTMENT

**Usual adult dose**
Topical, to the skin, as a 0.005% ointment two times a day.

**Usual pediatric dose**
Dosage has not been established.

**Strength(s) usually available**
U.S.—
0.005% (Rx) [*Cutivate*].
Canada—
Not commercially available.

**Packaging and storage**
Store below 40 °C (104 °F), preferably between 2 and 30 °C (36 and 86 °F), in a well-closed container, unless otherwise specified by manufacturer.

**Auxiliary labeling**
• For external use only.
• Do not use in or around the eye.

## HALCINONIDE

## Summary of Differences
Pharmacology/pharmacokinetics:
    Substituted; fluorinated.
    Potency ranking—High.

## Topical Dosage Forms

### HALCINONIDE CREAM USP

**Usual adult dose**
Topical, to the skin, as a 0.025 or 0.1% cream one to three times a day.

**Usual pediatric dose**
Topical, to the skin, as a 0.025 or 0.1% cream once a day.

**Strength(s) usually available**
U.S.—
0.025% (Rx) [*Halog*].
0.1% (Rx) [*Halog; Halog-E*].
Canada—
0.1% (Rx) [*Halog*].

**Packaging and storage**
Store between 15 and 30 °C (59 and 86 °F), unless otherwise specified by manufacturer. Store in a well-closed container. Protect from freezing.

**Auxiliary labeling**
• For external use only.
• Do not use in or around the eye.

### HALCINONIDE OINTMENT USP

**Usual adult dose**
Topical, to the skin, as a 0.1% ointment two or three times a day.

**Usual pediatric dose**
Topical, to the skin, as a 0.1% ointment once a day.

**Strength(s) usually available**
U.S.—
0.1% (Rx) [*Halog*].
Canada—
0.1% (Rx) [*Halog*].

**Packaging and storage**
Store below 40 °C (104 °F), preferably between 15 and 30 °C (59 and 86 °F), unless otherwise specified by manufacturer. Store in a well-closed container. Protect from freezing.

**Auxiliary labeling**
• For external use only.
• Do not use in or around the eye.

### HALCINONIDE TOPICAL SOLUTION USP

**Usual adult dose**
Topical, to the skin, as a 0.1% solution two or three times a day.

**Usual pediatric dose**
Topical, to the skin, as a 0.1% solution once a day.

**Strength(s) usually available**
U.S.—
0.1% (Rx) [*Halog*].
Canada—
0.1% (Rx) [*Halog*].

**Packaging and storage**
Store below 40 °C (104 °F), preferably between 15 and 30 °C (59 and 86 °F), unless otherwise specified by manufacturer. Store in a well-closed container. Protect from freezing.

**Auxiliary labeling**
• For external use only.
• Do not use in or around the eye.

## HALOBETASOL

## Summary of Differences
Pharmacology/pharmacokinetics:
    Substituted; fluorinated.
    Potency ranking—Very high.

## Topical Dosage Forms

### HALOBETASOL PROPIONATE CREAM

**Usual adult dose**
Topical, to the skin, as a 0.05% cream one or two times a day. Halobetasol propionate cream may be used for only a short duration of therapy and on small surface areas. Occlusive dressings should not be used.

**Usual pediatric dose**
Dosage has not been established.

**Strength(s) usually available**
U.S.—
0.05% (Rx) [*Ultravate*].
Canada—
Not commercially available.

**Packaging and storage**
Store below 40 °C (104 °F), preferably between 2 and 30 °C (36 and 86 °F), in a well-closed container, unless otherwise specified by manufacturer.

**Auxiliary labeling**
• For external use only.
• Do not use in or around the eye.

### HALOBETASOL PROPIONATE OINTMENT

**Usual adult dose**
Topical, to the skin, as a 0.05% ointment one or two times a day. Halobetasol propionate ointment may be used for only a short duration of therapy and on small surface areas. Occlusive dressings should not be used.

**Usual pediatric dose**
Dosage has not been established.

**Strength(s) usually available**
U.S.—
0.05% (Rx) [*Ultravate*].
Canada—
Not commercially available.

**Packaging and storage**
Store below 40 °C (104 °F), preferably between 2 and 30 °C (36 and 86 °F), in a well-closed container, unless otherwise specified by manufacturer.

**Auxiliary labeling**
• For external use only.
• Do not use in or around the eye.

## HYDROCORTISONE

### Summary of Differences
Pharmacology/pharmacokinetics:
    Substituted (butyrate, valerate); non-fluorinated.
    Potency ranking—Low (acetate and base); Medium (butyrate and valerate).

## Dental Dosage Forms

### HYDROCORTISONE ACETATE DENTAL PASTE

**Usual adult dose**
Topical, to the oral mucous membranes, as a 0.5% paste two or three times a day after meals and at bedtime.

**Usual pediatric dose**
Dosage has not been established.

**Strength(s) usually available**
U.S.—
    0.5% (Rx) [*Orabase-HCA*].
Canada—
    Not commercially available.

**Packaging and storage**
Store between 4 and 30 °C (39 and 86 °F), unless otherwise specified by manufacturer. Protect from light. Protect from freezing.

**Auxiliary labeling**
- For use in the mouth only.

## Topical Dosage Forms

### HYDROCORTISONE CREAM USP

**Usual adult dose**
Topical, to the skin, as a 0.25 to 2.5% cream one to four times a day.

**Usual pediatric dose**
Children up to 2 years of age—Dosage has not been established.
Children 2 years of age and older—Topical, to the skin, as a 0.25 to 0.5% cream one to four times a day; or as a 1% cream one or two times a day.

**Strength(s) usually available**
U.S.—
    0.25% (OTC) [*Cort-Dome*].
    0.5% (OTC) [*Bactine; Cort-Dome; Cortifair; DermiCort; Dermtex HC; Hydro-Tex* (sodium bisulfite); *Hytone;* GENERIC].
    1% (Rx) [*Ala-Cort; Allercort; Alphaderm; Cort-Dome; Cortifair; Dermacort; Hi-Cor 1.0; Hydro-Tex* (sodium bisulfite); *Hytone; Lemoderm; Nutracort; Penecort; Synacort;* GENERIC].
    2.5% (Rx) [*Allercort; Anusol-HC; Hi-Cor 2.5; Hytone; Lemoderm; Penecort; Synacort;* GENERIC].
Canada—
    0.5% (OTC) [*Cortate; Unicort*].
    0.5% (Rx) [*Sential* (urea 4%)].
    1% (Rx) [*Barriere-HC; Emo-Cort; Prevex HC; Unicort*].
    2.5% (Rx) [*Emo-Cort*].

**Packaging and storage**
Store below 40 °C (104 °F), preferably between 15 and 30 °C (59 and 86 °F), unless otherwise specified by manufacturer. Store in a tight container. Protect from freezing.

**Auxiliary labeling**
- For external use only.
- Do not use in or around the eye.

### HYDROCORTISONE LOTION USP

**Usual adult dose**
Topical, to the skin, as a 0.25 to 2.5% lotion one to four times a day.

**Usual pediatric dose**
Children up to 2 years of age—Dosage has not been established.
Children 2 years of age and older—Topical, to the skin, as a 0.25 to 0.5% lotion one to four times a day; or as a 1% lotion one or two times a day; or as a 2.5% lotion once a day.

**Strength(s) usually available**
U.S.—
    0.25% (OTC) [*Cetacort; Cort-Dome*].
    0.5% (OTC) [*Cetacort; Delacort; MyCort; S-T Cort;* GENERIC].
    1% (Rx) [*Acticort 100; Ala-Cort; Allercort; Beta-HC; Cetacort; Dermacort; Gly-Cort; Hytone; LactiCare-HC; Lemoderm; Nutracort; Pentacort; Rederm;* GENERIC].
    2% (Rx) [*Ala-Scalp HP*].
    2.5% (Rx) [*Hytone; LactiCare-HC; Nutracort*].
Canada—
    0.5% (OTC) [*Cortate; Emo-Cort*].
    1% (Rx) [*Emo-Cort; Sarna HC 1.0%*].
    2.5% (Rx) [*Emo-Cort*].

**Packaging and storage**
Store below 40 °C (104 °F), preferably between 15 and 30 °C (59 and 86 °F), unless otherwise specified by manufacturer. Store in a tight container. Protect from freezing.

**Auxiliary labeling**
- For external use only.
- Do not use in or around the eye.
- Shake well.

### HYDROCORTISONE OINTMENT USP

**Usual adult dose**
Topical, to the skin, as a 0.5 to 2.5% ointment one to four times a day.

**Usual pediatric dose**
Children up to 2 years of age—Dosage has not been established.
Children 2 years of age and older—Topical, to the skin, as a 0.5% ointment one to four times a day; or as a 1% ointment one or two times a day; or as a 2.5% ointment once a day.

**Strength(s) usually available**
U.S.—
    0.5% (OTC) [GENERIC].
    1% [*Allercort; Cortril; Hytone; Lemoderm*].
    2.5% (Rx) [*Allercort; Hytone;* GENERIC].
Canada—
    0.5% (OTC) [*Cortate*].
    1% (Rx) [*Cortate; Cortef*].

**Packaging and storage**
Store below 40 °C (104 °F), preferably between 15 and 30 °C (59 and 86 °F), unless otherwise specified by manufacturer. Store in a well-closed container. Protect from freezing.

**Auxiliary labeling**
- For external use only.
- Do not use in or around the eye.

### HYDROCORTISONE TOPICAL SOLUTION

**Usual adult dose**
Topical, to the skin, as a 2.5% solution one to four times a day.

**Usual pediatric dose**
Topical, to the skin, as a 1% solution one or two times a day.

**Strength(s) usually available**
U.S.—
    0.5% (OTC) [*Aeroseb-HC* (alcohol 58%); *CaldeCORT Anti-Itch* (alcohol 89.5%); *Cortaid* (alcohol 46%; parabens); GENERIC].
    1% (OTC) [*Maximum Strength Cortaid* (alcohol 55%; parabens)].
    1% (Rx) [*Penecort* (alcohol 57%); *Texacort* (alcohol 33%)].
    2.5% (Rx) [*Texacort* (alcohol 49%)].
Canada—
    2.5% (Rx) [*Emo-Cort Scalp Solution* (alcohol)].

**Packaging and storage**
Store below 40 °C (104 °F), preferably between 15 and 30 °C (59 and 86 °F), in a well-closed container, unless otherwise specified by manufacturer. Protect from freezing.

**Auxiliary labeling**
- For external use only.
- Do not use in or around the eye.

### HYDROCORTISONE ACETATE CREAM USP

**Usual adult dose**
Topical, to the skin, as a 0.1 to 1% cream one to four times a day.

**Usual pediatric dose**
Children up to 2 years of age—Dosage has not been established.
Children 2 years of age and older—Topical, to the skin, as a 0.5 or 1% cream one to four times a day.

**Strength(s) usually available**
U.S.—
    0.5% (OTC) [*Corticaine; FoilleCort; Gynecort; Lanacort; 9-1-1; Pharma-Cort;* GENERIC].
    0.5% (base) (OTC) [*CaldeCORT Light; Cortaid; Cortef Feminine Itch;* GENERIC].
    1% (OTC) [*Anusol-HC; Gynecort 10; Lanacort 10*].
    1% (base) (OTC) [*Dermarest DriCort; Maximum Strength Cortaid*].
    1% (Rx) [*Carmol-HC* (sodium bisulfite); GENERIC].

Canada—
    0.1% (Rx) [*Corticreme*].
    0.5% (OTC) [*Cortacet; Hyderm; Novohydrocort*].
    1% (Rx) [*Corticreme; Hyderm; Novohydrocort*].

**Packaging and storage**
Store below 40 °C (104 °F), preferably between 15 and 30 °C (59 and 86 °F), unless otherwise specified by manufacturer. Store in a well-closed container. Protect from freezing.

**Auxiliary labeling**
• For external use only.
• Do not use in or around the eye.

### HYDROCORTISONE ACETATE TOPICAL AEROSOL FOAM

**Usual adult dose**
Topical, to the skin, as a 1% foam one to four times a day.

**Usual pediatric dose**
Topical, to the skin, as a 1% foam one or two times a day.

**Strength(s) usually available**
U.S.—
    1% (Rx) [*Epifoam* (butane; methylparaben; propane; propylparaben)].
Canada—
    Not commercially available.

**Packaging and storage**
Store below 49 °C (120 °F), unless otherwise specified by manufacturer.

**Auxiliary labeling**
• Shake well.
• For external use only.
• Do not use in or around the eye.

### HYDROCORTISONE ACETATE LOTION USP

**Usual adult dose**
Topical, to the skin, as a 0.5% lotion one to four times a day.

**Usual pediatric dose**
Children up to 2 years of age—Dosage has not been established.
Children 2 years of age and older—See *Usual adult dose*.

**Strength(s) usually available**
U.S.—
    0.5% (base) (OTC) [*Cortaid; Rhulicort*].
Canada—
    Not commercially available.

**Packaging and storage**
Store below 40 °C (104 °F), preferably between 15 and 30 °C (59 and 86 °F), unless otherwise specified by manufacturer. Store in a tight container. Protect from freezing.

**Auxiliary labeling**
• For external use only.
• Do not use in or around the eye.
• Shake well.

### HYDROCORTISONE ACETATE OINTMENT USP

**Usual adult dose**
Topical, to the skin, as a 0.5 to 2.5% ointment one to four times a day.

**Usual pediatric dose**
Children up to 2 years of age—Dosage has not been established.
Children 2 years of age and older—Topical, to the skin, as a 0.5% ointment one to four times a day; or as a 1% ointment one or two times a day; or as a 2.5% ointment once a day.

**Strength(s) usually available**
U.S.—
    0.5% (OTC) [*Lanacort*].
    0.5% (base) (OTC) [*Cortaid*].
    1% (Rx) [GENERIC].
    1% (base) (OTC) [*Maximum Strength Cortaid*].
Canada—
    0.5% (OTC) [*Cortoderm; Novohydrocort*].
    1% (Rx) [*Cortef; Cortoderm; Novohydrocort*].

**Packaging and storage**
Store below 40 °C (104 °F), preferably between 15 and 30 °C (59 and 86 °F), unless otherwise specified by manufacturer. Store in a well-closed container. Protect from freezing.

**Auxiliary labeling**
• For external use only.
• Do not use in or around the eye.

### HYDROCORTISONE BUTYRATE CREAM USP

**Usual adult dose**
Topical, to the skin, as a 0.1% cream two or three times a day.

**Usual pediatric dose**
Topical, to the skin, as a 0.1% cream one or two times a day.

**Strength(s) usually available**
U.S.—
    0.1% (Rx) [*Locoid* (methylparaben)].
Canada—
    Not commercially available.

**Packaging and storage**
Store below 40 °C (104 °F), preferably between 15 and 30 °C (59 and 86 °F), unless otherwise specified by manufacturer. Store in a well-closed container. Protect from freezing.

**Auxiliary labeling**
• For external use only.
• Do not use in or around the eye.

### HYDROCORTISONE BUTYRATE OINTMENT

**Usual adult dose**
Topical, to the skin, as a 0.1% ointment two or three times a day.

**Usual pediatric dose**
Topical, to the skin, as a 0.1% ointment one or two times a day.

**Strength(s) usually available**
U.S.—
    0.1% (Rx) [*Locoid*].
Canada—
    Not commercially available.

**Packaging and storage**
Store below 40 °C (104 °F), preferably between 15 and 30 °C (59 and 86 °F), unless otherwise specified by manufacturer. Protect from freezing.

**Auxiliary labeling**
• For external use only.
• Do not use in or around the eye.

### HYDROCORTISONE VALERATE CREAM USP

**Usual adult dose**
Topical, to the skin, as a 0.2% cream two or three times a day.

**Usual pediatric dose**
Topical, to the skin, as a 0.2% cream once a day.

**Strength(s) usually available**
U.S.—
    0.2% (Rx) [*Westcort*].
Canada—
    0.2% (Rx) [*Westcort*].

**Packaging and storage**
Store below 25 °C (77 °F), unless otherwise specified by manufacturer. Store in a well-closed container. Protect from freezing.

**Auxiliary labeling**
• For external use only.
• Do not use in or around the eye.

### HYDROCORTISONE VALERATE OINTMENT

**Usual adult dose**
Topical, to the skin, as a 0.2% ointment two or three times a day.

**Usual pediatric dose**
Topical, to the skin, as a 0.2% ointment once a day.

**Strength(s) usually available**
U.S.—
    0.2% (Rx) [*Westcort*].
Canada—
    0.2% (Rx) [*Westcort*].

**Packaging and storage**
Store below 26 °C (78 °F), in a well-closed container, unless otherwise specified by manufacturer. Protect from freezing.

**Auxiliary labeling**
• For external use only.
• Do not use in or around the eye.

## MOMETASONE

### Summary of Differences
Pharmacology/pharmacokinetics:
  Substituted; non-fluorinated.
  Potency ranking—Medium.

## Topical Dosage Forms
### MOMETASONE FUROATE CREAM

**Usual adult dose**
Topical, to the skin, as a 0.1% cream once a day.

**Usual pediatric dose**
Dosage has not been established.

**Strength(s) usually available**
U.S.—
  0.1% (Rx) [*Elocon*].
Canada—
  0.1% (Rx) [*Elocom*].

**Packaging and storage**
Store below 40 °C (104 °F), preferably between 2 and 30 °C (36 and 86 °F), in a well-closed container, unless otherwise specified by manufacturer.

**Auxiliary labeling**
- For external use only.
- Do not use in or around the eye.

### MOMETASONE FUROATE LOTION

**Usual adult dose**
Topical, to the skin, as a 0.1% lotion once a day.

**Usual pediatric dose**
Dosage has not been established.

**Strength(s) usually available**
U.S.—
  0.1% (Rx) [*Elocon* (isopropyl alcohol 40%)].
Canada—
  0.1% (Rx) [*Elocom*].

**Packaging and storage**
Store below 40 °C (104 °F), preferably between 2 and 30 °C (36 and 86 °F), in a well-closed container, unless otherwise specified by manufacturer.

**Auxiliary labeling**
- For external use only.
- Do not use in or around the eye.

### MOMETASONE FUROATE OINTMENT

**Usual adult dose**
Topical, to the skin, as a 0.1% ointment once a day.

**Usual pediatric dose**
Dosage has not been established.

**Strength(s) usually available**
U.S.—
  0.1% (Rx) [*Elocon*].
Canada—
  0.1% (Rx) [*Elocom*].

**Packaging and storage**
Store below 40 °C (104 °F), preferably between 2 and 30 °C (36 and 86 °F), in a well-closed container, unless otherwise specified by manufacturer.

**Auxiliary labeling**
- For external use only.
- Do not use in or around the eye.

## TRIAMCINOLONE

### Summary of Differences
Pharmacology/pharmacokinetics:
  Substituted; fluorinated.
  Potency ranking—
    Medium (except cream and ointment 0.5%).
    Cream and ointment 0.5%, High.

## Dental Dosage Forms
### TRIAMCINOLONE ACETONIDE DENTAL PASTE USP

**Usual adult dose**
Topical, to the oral mucous membranes, as a 0.1% paste two or three times a day after meals and at bedtime.

**Usual pediatric dose**
Dosage has not been established.

**Strength(s) usually available**
U.S.—
  0.1% (Rx) [*Kenalog in Orabase; Oracort; Oralone*].
Canada—
  0.1% (Rx) [*Kenalog in Orabase*].

**Packaging and storage**
Store below 40 °C (104 °F), preferably between 15 and 30 °C (59 and 86 °F), unless otherwise specified by manufacturer. Store in a tight container. Protect from freezing.

**Auxiliary labeling**
- For use in the mouth only.

## Topical Dosage Forms
### TRIAMCINOLONE ACETONIDE CREAM USP

**Usual adult dose**
Topical, to the skin, as a 0.025 to 0.5% cream two to four times a day.

**Usual pediatric dose**
Topical, to the skin, as a 0.025% cream one or two times a day; or as a 0.1 or 0.5% cream once a day.

**Strength(s) usually available**
U.S.—
  0.025% (Rx) [*Aristocort; Aristocort A; Flutex; Kenac; Kenalog; Kenonel; Triacet;* GENERIC].
  0.1% (Rx) [*Aristocort; Aristocort A; Delta-Tritex; Flutex; Kenac; Kenalog; Kenalog-H; Kenonel; Triacet; Triderm;* GENERIC].
  0.5% (Rx) [*Aristocort; Aristocort A; Flutex; Kenalog; Kenonel; Triacet;* GENERIC].
Canada—
  0.025% (Rx) [*Aristocort D; Triaderm; Trianide Mild*].
  0.1% (Rx) [*Aristocort R; Kenalog; Triaderm; Trianide Regular*].
  0.5% (Rx) [*Aristocort C*].

**Packaging and storage**
Store below 40 °C (104 °F), preferably between 15 and 30 °C (59 and 86 °F), unless otherwise specified by manufacturer. Store in a tight container. Protect from freezing.

**Auxiliary labeling**
- For external use only.
- Do not use in or around the eye.

### TRIAMCINOLONE ACETONIDE LOTION USP

**Usual adult dose**
Topical, to the skin, as a 0.025 or 0.1% lotion two to four times a day.

**Usual pediatric dose**
Topical, to the skin, as a 0.025% lotion one or two times a day; or as a 0.1% lotion once a day.

**Strength(s) usually available**
U.S.—
  0.025% (Rx) [*Kenalog;* GENERIC].
  0.1% (Rx) [*Kenalog; Kenonel;* GENERIC].
Canada—
  Not commercially available.

**Packaging and storage**
Store between 15 and 30 °C (59 and 86 °F), unless otherwise specified by manufacturer. Store in a tight container. Protect from freezing.

**Auxiliary labeling**
- For external use only.
- Do not use in or around the eye.
- Shake well.

### TRIAMCINOLONE ACETONIDE OINTMENT USP

**Usual adult dose**
Topical, to the skin, as a 0.025 to 0.5% ointment two to four times a day.

**Usual pediatric dose**
Topical, to the skin, as a 0.025% ointment one or two times a day; or as a 0.1 or 0.5% ointment once a day.

**Strength(s) usually available**
U.S.—
   0.025% (Rx) [*Flutex; Kenalog;* GENERIC].
   0.1% (Rx) [*Aristocort; Aristocort A; Flutex; Kenac; Kenalog; Kenonel;* GENERIC].
   0.5% (Rx) [*Aristocort; Flutex; Kenalog;* GENERIC].
Canada—
   0.025% (Rx) [*Aristocort D; Triaderm*].
   0.1% (Rx) [*Aristocort R; Kenalog; Triaderm*].

**Packaging and storage**
Store below 40 °C (104 °F), preferably between 15 and 30 °C (59 and 86 °F), unless otherwise specified by manufacturer. Store in a well-closed container. Protect from freezing.

**Auxiliary labeling**
- For external use only.
- Do not use in or around the eye.

## TRIAMCINOLONE ACETONIDE TOPICAL AEROSOL USP

**Usual adult dose**
Topical, to the skin, as a 0.015% aerosol spray three or four times a day.

**Usual pediatric dose**
Topical, to the skin, as a 0.015% aerosol spray one or two times a day.

**Strength(s) usually available**
U.S.—
   0.015% (Rx) [*Kenalog* (alcohol 10.3%)].
Note: A 2-second spray delivers 0.2 mg of triamcinolone acetonide. Product applied to skin contains approximately 0.2% triamcinolone acetonide.
Canada—
   Not commercially available.

**Packaging and storage**
Store below 40 °C (104 °F), preferably between 15 and 30 °C (59 and 86 °F). Protect from freezing.

**Auxiliary labeling**
- For external use only.
- Do not use in or around the eye.

**Note**
Explain administration technique.
When dispensing, include patient instructions.

Revised: 11/18/92
Interim revision: 09/29/98

## Table 1. Pharmacology/Pharmacokinetics

Note: The following table lists topical corticosteroid products available in the U.S. and/or Canada. A potency rank is also listed for each preparation: Low, Medium, High, or Very High.

Products with a Low potency ranking have a modest anti-inflammatory effect and are safest for chronic application. These products are also the safest products for use on the face and intertriginous areas, with occlusion, and in infants and young children.

Products with a Medium potency ranking are used in moderate inflammatory dermatoses. Examples of conditions for which these products are frequently used include chronic eczematous dermatoses such as hand eczema and atopic eczema. Medium potency preparations may be used on the face and intertriginous areas for a limited duration.

High potency preparations are used in more severe inflammatory dermatoses. Examples of conditions for which these products are frequently used include more severe eczematous dermatoses, lichen simplex chronicus, and psoriasis. They may be used for an intermediate duration, or for longer periods in areas with thickened skin due to chronic conditions. High potency preparations may also be used on the face and intertriginous areas but only for a short treatment duration.

Very High potency products are used primarily as an alternative to systemic corticosteroid therapy when local areas are involved. Examples of conditions for which Very High potency products are frequently used include thick, chronic lesions caused by psoriasis, lichen simplex chronicus, and discoid lupus erythematosus. There is a high likelihood of skin atrophy with the use of Very High potency preparations. They may be used for only a short duration of therapy and on small surface areas. Occlusive dressings should not be used with these products.

| Generic drug name | Dosage Form(s) | Strength (%) | Potency Ranking |
|---|---|---|---|
| Alclometasone dipropionate | | | |
| | Cream | 0.05 | Low |
| | Ointment | 0.05 | Low |
| Amcinonide | | | |
| | Cream | 0.1 | High |
| | Lotion | 0.1 | High |
| | Ointment | 0.1 | High |
| Beclomethasone dipropionate | | | |
| | Cream | 0.025 | Medium |
| | Lotion | 0.025 | Medium |
| | Ointment | 0.025 | Medium |
| Betamethasone benzoate | | | |
| | Cream | 0.025 | Medium |
| | Gel | 0.025 | Medium |
| | Lotion | 0.025 | Medium |
| Betamethasone dipropionate | | | |
| | Cream | | |
| | *Diprolene AF* | 0.05 | Very high |
| | Others | 0.05 | High |
| | Gel | | |
| | *Diprolene* | 0.05 | Very high |
| | Lotion | | |
| | *Diprolene* | 0.05 | Very high |
| | Others | 0.05 | High |
| | Ointment | | |
| | *Diprolene* | 0.05 | Very high |
| | Others | 0.05 | High |
| | Topical aerosol | 0.1 | High |

| Generic drug name | Dosage Form(s) | Strength (%) | Potency Ranking |
|---|---|---|---|
| Betamethasone valerate | | | |
| | Cream | 0.01 | Medium |
| | Cream | 0.05 | Medium |
| | Cream | 0.1 | Medium |
| | Lotion | 0.05 | Medium |
| | Lotion | 0.1 | Medium |
| | Ointment | 0.05 | Medium |
| | Ointment | 0.1 | Medium |
| Clobetasol propionate | | | |
| | Cream | 0.05 | Very high |
| | Ointment | 0.05 | Very high |
| | Solution | 0.05 | Very high |
| Clobetasone butyrate | | | |
| | Cream | 0.05 | Medium |
| | Ointment | 0.05 | Medium |
| Clocortolone pivalate | | | |
| | Cream | 0.1 | Low |
| Desonide | | | |
| | Cream | 0.05 | Low |
| | Lotion | 0.05 | Low |
| | Ointment | 0.05 | Low |
| Desoximetasone | | | |
| | Cream | 0.05 | Medium |
| | Cream | 0.25 | High |
| | Gel | 0.05 | High |
| | Ointment | 0.25 | High |

## Table 1. Pharmacology/Pharmacokinetics *(continued)*

| Generic drug name | Dosage Form(s) | Strength (%) | Potency Ranking |
|---|---|---|---|
| Dexamethasone | | | |
| | Gel | 0.1 | Low |
| | Topical aerosol | 0.01 | Low |
| | Topical aerosol | 0.04 | Low |
| Dexamethasone sodium phosphate | | | |
| | Cream | 0.1 (phosphate) | Low |
| Diflorasone diacetate | | | |
| | Cream | 0.05 | High |
| | Ointment | | |
| | *Psorcon* | 0.05 | Very high |
| | Others | 0.05 | High |
| Diflucortolone valerate | | | |
| | Cream | 0.1 | Medium |
| | Ointment | 0.1 | Medium |
| Flumethasone pivalate | | | |
| | Cream | 0.03 | Low |
| | Ointment | 0.03 | Low |
| Fluocinolone acetonide | | | |
| | Cream | 0.01 | Medium |
| | Cream | 0.025 | Medium |
| | Cream | 0.2 | High |
| | Ointment | 0.01 | Medium |
| | Ointment | 0.025 | Medium |
| | Topical solution | 0.01 | Medium |
| Fluocinonide | | | |
| | Cream | 0.01 | High |
| | Cream | 0.05 | High |
| | Gel | 0.05 | High |
| | Ointment | 0.01 | High |
| | Ointment | 0.05 | High |
| | Topical solution | 0.05 | High |
| Flurandrenolide | | | |
| | Cream | 0.0125 | Low |
| | Cream | 0.025 | Medium |
| | Cream | 0.05 | Medium |
| | Lotion | 0.05 | Medium |
| | Ointment | 0.0125 | Low |
| | Ointment | 0.025 | Medium |
| | Ointment | 0.05 | Medium |
| | Tape | 4 mcg/cm | Medium |
| Fluticasone propionate | | | |
| | Cream | 0.05 | Medium |
| | Ointment | 0.005 | Medium |
| Halcinonide | | | |
| | Cream | 0.025 | High |
| | Cream | 0.1 | High |
| | Ointment | 0.1 | High |
| | Topical solution | 0.1 | High |

| Generic drug name | Dosage Form(s) | Strength (%) | Potency Ranking |
|---|---|---|---|
| Halobetasol propionate | | | |
| | Cream | 0.05 | Very high |
| | Ointment | 0.05 | Very high |
| Hydrocortisone | | | |
| | Cream | 0.25 | Low |
| | Cream | 0.5 | Low |
| | Cream | 1 | Low |
| | Cream | 2.5 | Low |
| | Lotion | 0.25 | Low |
| | Lotion | 0.5 | Low |
| | Lotion | 1 | Low |
| | Lotion | 2 | Low |
| | Lotion | 2.5 | Low |
| | Ointment | 0.5 | Low |
| | Ointment | 1 | Low |
| | Ointment | 2.5 | Low |
| | Topical aerosol solution | 0.5 | Low |
| | Topical spray solution | 0.5 | Low |
| | Topical solution | 1 | Low |
| | Topical solution | 2.5 | Low |
| Hydrocortisone acetate | | | |
| | Cream | 0.1 | Low |
| | Cream | 0.5 | Low |
| | Cream | 1 | Low |
| | Lotion | 0.5 | Low |
| | Ointment | 0.5 | Low |
| | Ointment | 1 | Low |
| | Topical aerosol foam | 1 | Low |
| Hydrocortisone butyrate | | | |
| | Cream | 0.1 | Medium |
| | Ointment | 0.1 | Medium |
| Hydrocortisone valerate | | | |
| | Cream | 0.2 | Medium |
| | Ointment | 0.2 | Medium |
| Mometasone furoate | | | |
| | Cream | 0.1 | Medium |
| | Lotion | 0.1 | Medium |
| | Ointment | 0.1 | Medium |
| Triamcinolone acetonide | | | |
| | Cream | 0.025 | Medium |
| | Cream | 0.1 | Medium |
| | Cream | 0.5 | High |
| | Lotion | 0.025 | Medium |
| | Lotion | 0.1 | Medium |
| | Ointment | 0.025 | Medium |
| | Ointment | 0.1 | Medium |
| | Ointment | 0.5 | High |
| | Topical aerosol | 0.015 | Medium |

# CORTICOSTEROIDS AND ACETIC ACID  Otic

This monograph includes information on the following: 1) Desonide and Acetic Acid; 2) Hydrocortisone and Acetic Acid.

VA CLASSIFICATION (Primary): OT250

Commonly used brand name(s): *Otic Tridesilon Solution*[1]; *VoŠol HC*[2].

Another commonly used name for hydrocortisone is cortisol.

Note: For a listing of dosage forms and brand names by country availability, see *Dosage Forms* section(s).

## Category

Corticosteroid-antiseptic (otic); anti-inflammatory (steroidal), otic.

## Indications

Note: Bracketed information in the *Indications* section refers to uses that are not included in U.S. product labeling.

### Accepted

Ear canal infections, external (treatment)—Corticosteroid and acetic acid combinations are indicated in the treatment of superficial external ear canal infections that are accompanied by inflammation.

[Ear canal infections, external (prophylaxis)]—Hydrocortisone and acetic acid combination is indicated in the prophylaxis of external ear canal infections.

[Otitis externa, eczematoid, chronic (prophylaxis and treatment)]—Hydrocortisone and acetic acid combination is indicated in the prophylaxis and treatment of chronic eczematoid otitis externa.

[Otitis externa, seborrheic (prophylaxis and treatment)]—Hydrocortisone and acetic acid combination is indicated in the prophylaxis and treatment of seborrheic otitis externa.

## Pharmacology/Pharmacokinetics

**Physicochemical characteristics**
Molecular weight—
  Acetic acid: 60.05.
  Desonide: 416.51.
  Hydrocortisone: 362.47.

**Mechanism of action/Effect**
Corticosteroids—
  Otic corticosteroids possess anti-inflammatory, anti-allergic, and antipruritic actions.
  Corticosteroids diffuse across cell membranes and complex with specific cytoplasmic receptors. These complexes then enter the cell nucleus, bind to DNA, and stimulate transcription of messenger RNA (mRNA) and subsequent protein synthesis of enzymes ultimately responsible for anti-inflammatory effects of otic corticosteroids. In high concentrations, which may be achieved locally after topical application, corticosteroids may exert direct membrane effects. Corticosteroids decrease cellular and fibrinous exudation and tissue infiltration, inhibit fibroblastic and collagen-forming activity, retard epithelial regeneration, diminish post-inflammatory neovascularization, and reduce toward normal levels the excessive permeability of inflamed capillaries.
Acetic acid—
  Possesses antibacterial, astringent, and antifungal properties.

## Precautions to Consider

**Pregnancy/Reproduction**
Pregnancy—For desonide and acetic acid: Although problems in humans have not been documented, adequate and well-controlled studies have not been done.
FDA Pregnancy Category C.
For hydrocortisone and acetic acid: Problems in humans have not been documented.

**Breast-feeding**
Problems in humans have not been documented.

**Pediatrics**
Appropriate studies with these medications have not been performed in the pediatric population. However, pediatrics-specific problems that would limit the usefulness of these medications in children are not expected.

**Geriatrics**
Appropriate studies with these medications have not been performed in the geriatric population. However, geriatrics-specific problems that would limit the usefulness of these medications in the elderly are not expected.

**Medical considerations/Contraindications**
The medical considerations/contraindications included have been selected on the basis of their potential clinical significance (reasons given in parentheses where appropriate)—not necessarily inclusive (» = major clinical significance).

*Risk-benefit should be considered when the following medical problems exist:*
» Infection, aural, fungal or
» Infection, aural, acute untreated or
» Tuberculosis, auralor
  Viral infection, acute, infectious
    (infections may be exacerbated)
» Perforation of the ear drum membrane
    (possibility of ototoxicity)
  Sensitivity to acetic acid
  Sensitivity to corticosteroids

## Side/Adverse Effects

The following side/adverse effects have been selected on the basis of their potential clinical significance (possible signs and symptoms in parentheses where appropriate)—not necessarily inclusive:

**Those indicating need for medical attention only if they continue or are bothersome**
*Stinging, itching, irritation, or burning in the ear*

## Patient Consultation

As an aid to patient consultation, refer to *Advice for the Patient, Corticosteroids and Acetic Acid (Otic)*.

In providing consultation, consider emphasizing the following selected information (» = major clinical significance):

**Before using this medication**
» Conditions affecting use, especially:
    Sensitivity to acetic acid or corticosteroids
    Other medical problems, especially other untreated ear infections or perforated ear drum

**Proper use of this medication**
  Proper administration technique
  Preventing contamination: Avoid touching applicator tip to any surface; keeping container tightly closed
» Not washing dropper or applicator tip (to prevent dilution of medication with water)—applicable only to the hydrocortisone and acetic acid formulation; if necessary, wiping with clean tissue after use
  Importance of not using more medication than the amount prescribed
» Checking with physician before using medication for future ear problems
» Proper dosing
  Missed dose: Using as soon as possible; not using if almost time for next dose
» Proper storage

**Precautions while using this medication**
  Checking with physician if no improvement after 5 to 7 days of therapy or if ear condition becomes worse

## General Dosing Information

To allow optimum contact between the medication and infected surfaces of the ear canal, all cerumen and debris should be carefully removed by a physician or a trained assistant before initiation of therapy.

Otic solutions may be instilled directly into the ear canal or administered by use of a saturated gauze or cotton wick gently placed into the canal. The wick should be kept moist with additional solution and replaced every 12 to 24 hours.

The duration of treatment may vary from a few days to several weeks or months in some cases, depending on the condition being treated. Daily or alternate-day therapy may be indicated for extended periods in certain situations. In severe or persistent cases of external ear canal infections, more intensive anti-infective therapy may be required.

Treatment should be continued after apparent response, with the dosage being tapered gradually to avoid relapse.

---

### DESONIDE AND ACETIC ACID

## Otic Dosage Forms

### DESONIDE AND ACETIC ACID OTIC SOLUTION

**Usual adult and adolescent dose**
Topical, to the ear canal, 3 or 4 drops of the solution three or four times a day.

**Usual pediatric dose**
See *Usual adult and adolescent dose*.

**Usual geriatric dose**
See *Usual adult and adolescent dose*.

**Strength(s) usually available**
U.S.—
  0.05% desonide and 2% acetic acid (Rx) [*Otic Tridesilon Solution*].

**Packaging and storage**
Store below 30 °C (86 °F), unless otherwise specified by manufacturer. Protect from freezing.

**Auxiliary labeling**
• For the ear.
• Keep container tightly closed.

**Note**
Dispense in original unopened container.

---

### HYDROCORTISONE AND ACETIC ACID

## Otic Dosage Forms

Note: Bracketed uses in the *Dosage Forms* section refer to categories of use and/or indications that are not included in U.S. product labeling.

## HYDROCORTISONE AND ACETIC ACID OTIC SOLUTION USP

### Usual adult and adolescent dose
[Prophylaxis]—Topical, to each ear canal, 2 drops of solution in the morning and evening.

Treatment—Topical, to the ear canal, 2 to 5 drops of the solution three or four times a day.

Note: To promote continuous contact for initial 24 to 48 hours, a saturated wick may be inserted into the ear canal. The wick should be moistened with 3 to 5 drops of solution every 4 to 6 hours.

### Usual pediatric dose
See *Usual adult and adolescent dose*.

### Usual geriatric dose
See *Usual adult and adolescent dose*.

### Strength(s) usually available
U.S.—
1% hydrocortisone and 2% acetic acid (Rx) [*VoSol HC* (benzethonium chloride 0.02%; propylene glycol diacetate 3%)].

Canada—
1% hydrocortisone and 2% acetic acid (Rx) [*VoSol HC* (benzethonium chloride 0.02%; propylene glycol diacetate 3%)].

### Packaging and storage
Store below 40 °C (104 °F), preferably between 15 and 30 °C (59 and 86 °F), unless otherwise specified by manufacturer. Store in a tight, light-resistant container. Protect from freezing.

### Auxiliary labeling
- For the ear.
- Keep container tightly closed.

### Note
Dispense in original unopened container.

Revised: 03/31/92
Interim revision: 04/01/94

# CORTICOSTEROIDS—GLUCOCORTICOID EFFECTS   Systemic

This monograph includes information on the following: 1) Betamethasone; 2) Cortisone; 3) Dexamethasone; 4) Hydrocortisone; 5) Methylprednisolone; 6) Prednisolone; 7) Prednisone; 8) Triamcinolone.

VA CLASSIFICATION (Primary/Secondary):
Betamethasone—HS051/IM600
Cortisone—HS051/IM600
Dexamethasone—HS051/DX900; GA605; IM600
Hydrocortisone—HS051/GA605; IM600
Methylprednisolone—HS051/IM600
Prednisolone—HS051/IM600
Prednisone—HS051/GA605; IM600
Triamcinolone—HS051/IM600

Commonly used brand name(s): *A-hydroCort*[4]; *A-methaPred*[5]; *AK-Dex*[3]; *Amcort*[8]; *Apo-Prednisone*[7]; *Aristocort*[8]; *Aristocort Forte*[8]; *Aristocort Intralesional*[8]; *Aristospan Intra-articular*[8]; *Aristospan Intralesional*[8]; *Articulose-50*[6]; *Articulose-L.A*[8]; *Betnelan*[1]; *Betnesol*[1]; *Celestone*[1]; *Celestone Phosphate*[1]; *Celestone Soluspan*[1]; *Cenocort A-40*[8]; *Cenocort Forte*[8]; *Cinalone 40*[8]; *Cinonide 40*[8]; *Cortef*[4]; *Cortone*[2]; *Cortone Acetate*[2]; *Dalalone*[3]; *Dalalone D.P.*[3]; *Dalalone L.A*[3]; *Decadrol*[3]; *Decadron*[3]; *Decadron Phosphate*[3]; *Decadron-LA*[3]; *Decaject*[3]; *Decaject-L.A.*[3]; *Delta-Cortef*[6]; *Deltasone*[7]; *Depo-Medrol*[5]; *Depo-Predate 40*[5]; *Depo-Predate 80*[5]; *Depoject-40*[5]; *Depoject-80*[5]; *Depopred-40*[5]; *Depopred-80*[5]; *Deronil*[3]; *Dexacen LA-8*[3]; *Dexacen-4*[3]; *Dexamethasone Intensol*[3]; *Dexasone*[3]; *Dexasone-LA*[3]; *Dexone*[3]; *Dexone 0.5*[3]; *Dexone 0.75*[3]; *Dexone 1.5*[3]; *Dexone 4*[3]; *Dexone LA*[3]; *Duralone-40*[5]; *Duralone-80*[5]; *Hexadrol*[3]; *Hexadrol Phosphate*[3]; *Hydeltra T.B.A.*[6]; *Hydeltrasol*[6]; *Hydrocortone*[4]; *Hydrocortone Acetate*[4]; *Hydrocortone Phosphate*[4]; *Kenacort*[8]; *Kenacort Diacetate*[8]; *Kenaject-40*[8]; *Kenalog-10*[8]; *Kenalog-40*[8]; *Key-Pred 25*[6]; *Key-Pred 50*[6]; *Key-Pred SP*[6]; *Liquid Pred*[7]; *Medralone-40*[5]; *Medralone-80*[5]; *Medrol*[5]; *Meprolone*[5]; *Meticorten*[7]; *Mymethasone*[3]; *Nor-Pred T.B.A.*[6]; *Oradexon*[3]; *Orasone 1*[7]; *Orasone 10*[7]; *Orasone 20*[7]; *Orasone 5*[7]; *Orasone 50*[7]; *Pediapred*[6]; *Predaject-50*[6]; *Predalone 50*[6]; *Predalone T.B.A.*[6]; *Predate 50*[6]; *Predate S*[6]; *Predate TBA*[6]; *Predcor-25*[6]; *Predcor-50*[6]; *Predcor-TBA*[6]; *Predicort-50*[6]; *Predicort-RP*[6]; *Prednisone Intensol*[7]; *Prednicen-M*[7]; *Prelone*[6]; *Rep-Pred 40*[5]; *Rep-Pred 80*[5]; *Selestoject*[1]; *Solu-Cortef*[4]; *Solu-Medrol*[5]; *Solurex*[3]; *Solurex-LA*[3]; *Sterapred*[7]; *Sterapred DS*[7]; *Tac-3*[8]; *Tri-Kort*[8]; *Triam-A*[8]; *Triam-Forte*[8]; *Triamolone 40*[8]; *Triamonide 40*[8]; *Trilog*[8]; *Trilone*[8]; *Tristoject*[8]; *Winpred*[7]; *depMedalone 40*[5]; *depMedalone 80*[5].

Another commonly used name for hydrocortisone is cortisol.

Note: For a listing of dosage forms and brand names by country availability, see *Dosage Forms* section(s).

## Category

Corticosteroid—Betamethasone; Cortisone; Dexamethasone; Hydrocortisone; Methylprednisolone; Prednisolone; Prednisone; Triamcinolone.
Anti-inflammatory (steroidal)—Betamethasone; Cortisone; Dexamethasone; Hydrocortisone; Methylprednisolone; Prednisolone; Prednisone; Triamcinolone.
Diagnostic aid (Cushing's syndrome)—Dexamethasone Elixir USP; Dexamethasone Oral Solution; Dexamethasone Tablets USP; Dexamethasone Sodium Phosphate Injection USP.
Immunosuppressant—Betamethasone; Cortisone; Dexamethasone; Hydrocortisone; Methylprednisolone; Prednisolone; Prednisone; Triamcinolone.
Antiemetic, in cancer chemotherapy—Dexamethasone Elixir USP; Dexamethasone Tablets USP; Dexamethasone Sodium Phosphate Injection USP; Hydrocortisone (oral and parenteral); Prednisone.
Diagnostic aid (endogenous depression)—Dexamethasone (oral dosage forms).

## Indications

See *Table 1*, page 1015.

### Accepted

Corticosteroids are indicated (in physiologic doses) as replacement therapy in the treatment of adrenal insufficiency states.

In patients with known or suspected adrenal insufficiency, intravenous or intramuscular administration of a rapidly acting corticosteroid is indicated prior to surgery, including dental surgery, or if shock, severe trauma, illness, or other stress conditions occur. Patients already receiving replacement therapy require supplemental pharmacologic doses.

Glucocorticoids are indicated for their anti-inflammatory and immunosuppressant effects in the treatment of many disorders. Agents having minimal mineralocorticoid activity are preferred. For most indications, glucocorticoid administration provides symptomatic relief but has no effect on the underlying disease processes. Use of these medications does not eliminate the need for other therapies that may be required.

Corticosteroid therapy for conditions other than adrenocortical insufficiency, adrenogenital syndrome, or severe or life-threatening conditions is generally instituted only after less toxic therapies have proven ineffective.

## Pharmacology/Pharmacokinetics

See *Table 2*, page 1019 and *Table 3*, page 1020.

### Physicochemical characteristics

Molecular weight—
 Betamethasone—392.47
  Acetate: 434.50
  Sodium phosphate: 516.41
 Cortisone acetate—402.49
 Dexamethasone—392.47
  Acetate: 452.52
  Sodium phosphate: 516.41
 Hydrocortisone—362.47
  Acetate: 404.50

Cypionate: 486.65
Sodium phosphate: 486.41
Sodium succinate: 484.52
Methylprednisolone—374.48
Acetate: 416.51
Sodium succinate: 496.53
Prednisolone—360.45 (anhydrous); 387.47 (sesquihydrate)
Acetate: 402.49
Sodium phosphate: 484.39
Tebutate: 458.59
Prednisone—358.43
Triamcinolone—394.44
Acetonide: 434.50
Diacetate: 478.51
Hexacetonide: 532.65

**Mechanism of action/Effect**

Corticosteroids—Diffuse across cell membranes and complex with specific cytoplasmic receptors. These complexes then enter the cell nucleus, bind to DNA, and stimulate transcription of messenger RNA (mRNA) and subsequent protein synthesis of various enzymes thought to be ultimately responsible for two categories of effects of systemic corticosteroids. However, these agents may suppress transcription of mRNA in some cells (e.g., lymphocytes).

For glucocorticoid effects—
Anti-inflammatory (steroidal)—Glucocorticoids decrease or prevent tissue responses to inflammatory processes, thereby reducing development of symptoms of inflammation without affecting the underlying cause. Glucocorticoids inhibit accumulation of inflammatory cells, including macrophages and leukocytes, at sites of inflammation. They also inhibit phagocytosis, lysosomal enzyme release, and synthesis and/or release of several chemical mediators of inflammation. Although the exact mechanisms are not completely understood, actions that may contribute significantly to these effects include blockade of the action of macrophage inhibitory factor (MIF), leading to inhibition of macrophage localization; reduction of dilatation and permeability of inflamed capillaries and reduction of leukocyte adherence to the capillary endothelium, leading to inhibition of both leukocyte migration and edema formation; and increased synthesis of lipomodulin (macrocortin), an inhibitor of phospholipase $A_2$–mediated arachidonic acid release from membrane phospholipids, with subsequent inhibition of the synthesis of arachidonic acid–derived mediators of inflammation (prostaglandins, thromboxanes, and leukotrienes). Immunosuppressant actions may also contribute significantly to the anti-inflammatory effect.

Immunosuppressant—Mechanisms of immunosuppressant action are not completely understood but may involve prevention or suppression of cell-mediated (delayed hypersensitivity) immune reactions as well as more specific actions affecting the immune response. Glucocorticoids reduce the concentration of thymus-dependent lymphocytes (T-lymphocytes), monocytes, and eosinophils. They also decrease binding of immunoglobulin to cell surface receptors and inhibit the synthesis and/or release of interleukins, thereby decreasing T-lymphocyte blastogenesis and reducing expansion of the primary immune response. Glucocorticoids may also decrease passage of immune complexes through basement membranes and decrease concentrations of complement components and immunoglobulins.

For mineralocorticoid effects—
Water and electrolyte balance: Sodium reabsorption, and potassium and hydrogen excretion, along with subsequent water retention, are mediated through an action of mineralocorticoids on the renal distal tubule that facilitates sodium transport. Cation transport in other secretory cells is similarly affected; excretion of water and electrolytes by the large intestine and by salivary and sweat glands is also altered, but to a lesser extent. Only cortisone and hydrocortisone have clinically useful mineralocorticoid activity.

For specific indications—
Adrenogenital syndrome: Glucocorticoids inhibit corticotropin (adrenocorticotropin or ACTH) secretion, leading to suppression of adrenal hypersecretion of androgens responsible for the androgenism associated with various enzyme deficiencies.

Hypercalcemia: Glucocorticoids reduce plasma calcium concentration by decreasing gastrointestinal absorption of calcium, probably by interfering with intestinal calcium transport (by decreasing the effect of vitamin D), and increasing calcium excretion.

Respiratory distress syndrome prophylaxis: Glucocorticoids may induce enzymes which accelerate or increase production of lung surfactant by type 2 pneumonocytes.

**Other actions/effects**

Pharmacologic (supraphysiologic) doses of exogenous corticosteroids produce hypothalamic-pituitary-adrenal (HPA) axis suppression via a negative feedback mechanism, i.e., they inhibit pituitary ACTH secretion, thereby reducing ACTH-mediated production of corticosteroids and androgens in the adrenal cortex. The development of adrenocortical insufficiency and the time required for recovery of adrenal function depend primarily on the duration of corticosteroid therapy and, to a lesser extent, on dosage, timing, and frequency of administration, as well as on the potency and biologic (tissue) half-life of the specific agent. Adrenal insufficiency may occur in approximately 5 to 7 days with daily administration of doses equivalent to 20 to 30 mg of prednisone or in up to 30 days with lower doses. Following discontinuation of short-term (up to 5 days) high-dose use, adrenal recovery may occur within 1 week. Following prolonged high-dose use, complete recovery of adrenal function may require up to 1 year and, in some patients, may never occur.

Glucocorticoids stimulate protein catabolism and induce enzymes responsible for metabolism of amino acids. They decrease synthesis and increase degradation of protein in lymphoid tissue, connective tissue, muscle, and skin. With prolonged use, atrophy of these tissues may occur.

Glucocorticoids increase glucose availability by inducing hepatic enzymes involved in gluconeogenesis, stimulating protein catabolism (which increases hepatic concentrations of amino acids required for gluconeogenesis), and decreasing peripheral utilization of glucose. These actions lead to increased hepatic glycogen storage, increased blood glucose concentrations, and insulin resistance.

Glucocorticoids increase lipolysis and mobilize fatty acids from adipose tissues, leading to increased plasma fatty acid concentrations. With prolonged use, an abnormal redistribution of fat may occur.

Glucocorticoids decrease bone formation and increase bone resorption. They reduce plasma calcium concentration, leading to secondary hyperparathyroidism and subsequent stimulation of osteoclasts, and directly inhibit osteoblasts. These actions, together with a decrease in the protein matrix of bone secondary to increased protein catabolism, may lead to inhibition of bone growth in children and adolescents and the development of osteoporosis at any age.

**Absorption**

Oral—
Rapidly and almost completely absorbed.
Parenteral—
Intramuscular:
Freely soluble esters (sodium phosphate, sodium succinate)—Rapidly absorbed.
Poorly soluble derivatives (acetate, acetonide, diacetate, hexacetonide, tebutate)—Slowly but completely absorbed.
Local:
Freely soluble esters—Less rapidly absorbed than with intramuscular injection.
Poorly soluble derivatives—Slowly but completely absorbed.

**Biotransformation**

Primarily hepatic (rapid); also renal and tissue; mostly to inactive metabolites. Cortisone and prednisone are inactive until metabolized to the active metabolites hydrocortisone and prednisolone, respectively. Fluorinated corticosteroids are metabolized more slowly than other members of the group.

**Duration of action**

Duration of action depends upon the route/site of administration, solubility of the dosage form, dose administered, and the condition being treated. Following oral or intravenous administration, the duration of action depends upon the biological (tissue) half-life. Following intramuscular administration, the duration of action depends upon the solubility of the dosage form as well as the biological (tissue) half-life. Following local injections, the duration of action depends upon the solubility of the dosage form and the specific route/site of administration.

## Elimination
Primarily by renal excretion of inactive metabolites.

## Precautions to Consider

### Pregnancy/Reproduction
Fertility—Corticosteroids have been reported to increase or decrease the number or motility of spermatozoa. However, it is not known whether reproductive capacity in humans is adversely affected.

Pregnancy—
*For corticosteroids*—
Corticosteroids cross the placenta. Although adequate studies have not been done in humans, there is some evidence that pharmacologic doses of corticosteroids may increase the risk of placental insufficiency, decreased birthweight, or stillbirth. However, teratogenic effects in humans have not been confirmed.

Infants born to mothers who have received substantial doses of corticosteroids during pregnancy should be carefully observed for signs of hypoadrenalism and replacement therapy administered as required.

Prenatal administration of betamethasone or dexamethasone to the mother to prevent respiratory distress syndrome in the premature neonate has not been shown to affect the child's growth or development adversely. Physiologic replacement doses of corticosteroids administered for treatment of maternal adrenal insufficiency are also unlikely to adversely affect the fetus or neonate.

Studies in animals have shown that corticosteroids increase the incidence of cleft palate, placental insufficiency, spontaneous abortions, and intrauterine growth retardation.

FDA Pregnancy Category C.

### Breast-feeding
For corticosteroids—Problems in humans have not been documented. Administration of physiologic doses or low pharmacologic doses (the equivalent or less of 25 mg of cortisone or 5 mg of prednisone per day) is not considered likely to affect the infant adversely. Less than 1% of the administered dose of prednisolone is distributed into breast milk. However, breast-feeding during the use of higher pharmacologic doses is not recommended because corticosteroids are distributed into breast milk and may cause unwanted effects, such as growth suppression and inhibition of endogenous steroid production, in the infant.

### Pediatrics
Because infections such as chickenpox or measles may be more serious (or even fatal) in children receiving immunosuppressant doses of corticosteroids, extra care to avoid exposure to these infections is recommended. Prophylactic therapy with varicella zoster immune globulin (VZIG) or immune globulin intravenous (IGIV) or intramuscular (IGIM), as appropriate, may be indicated in exposed patients. Therapy with an antiviral agent may be indicated if chickenpox develops.

Chronic use of corticosteroids may suppress growth and development of the pediatric or adolescent patient and should be undertaken with caution. Use of long-acting glucocorticoids (betamethasone and dexamethasone) or daily doses of any corticosteroid that are larger than replacement therapy doses are especially likely to inhibit growth and are not recommended for any form of chronic therapy. For long-term therapy, a short-acting agent (cortisone or hydrocortisone) or an intermediate-acting agent (methylprednisolone, prednisolone, prednisone, or triamcinolone) is recommended. Alternate-day therapy with an oral intermediate-acting corticosteroid may decrease growth retardation effects. Some clinicians recommend that only cortisone, hydrocortisone, or prednisone be used for long-term replacement therapy. Also, pediatric patients may be at increased risk of developing osteoporosis, avascular necrosis of the femoral heads, glaucoma, or cataracts during prolonged therapy. Children and adolescents receiving prolonged therapy should be closely monitored.

Pediatric dosage is determined more by the severity of the condition and the response of the patient than by age or body weight. Also, for treatment of adrenocortical insufficiency, pediatric dosage is preferably determined in terms of mg per square meter of body surface area. Determination of pediatric dosage in terms of mg per kg of body weight (mg/kg) increases the possibility of overdosage, especially in very young, short, or heavy children.

### Geriatrics
Geriatric patients may be more likely to develop hypertension during corticosteroid therapy. Geriatric patients, especially postmenopausal women, may also be more likely to develop glucocorticoid-induced osteoporosis.

### Drug interactions and/or related problems
The following drug interactions and/or related problems have been selected on the basis of their potential clinical significance (possible mechanism in parentheses where appropriate)—not necessarily inclusive (» = major clinical significance):

See also *Laboratory value alterations*.

Note: Combinations containing any of the following medications, depending on the amount present, may also interact with this medication.

Interactions listed below involving alterations in serum potassium concentration and/or changes in sodium or fluid balance are especially likely to occur with corticosteroids having significant mineralocorticoid activity. However, these interactions may also occur with other corticosteroids, depending on dosage and patient predisposition.

Acetaminophen
(induction of hepatic enzymes by corticosteroids may increase the formation of a hepatotoxic acetaminophen metabolite, thereby increasing the risk of hepatotoxicity, when they are used concurrently with chronic or high-dose acetaminophen therapy)

Alcohol or
Anti-inflammatory drugs, nonsteroidal (NSAIDs)
(risk of gastrointestinal ulceration or hemorrhage may be increased when these substances are used concurrently with glucocorticoids; however, concurrent use of NSAIDs in the treatment of arthritis may provide additive therapeutic benefit and permit glucocorticoid dosage reduction)

» Aminoglutethimide
(aminoglutethimide suppresses adrenal function so that glucocorticoid supplementation may be required; however, aminoglutethimide accelerates the metabolism of dexamethasone so that dexamethasone half-life may be reduced two-fold; hydrocortisone is recommended instead because its metabolism is not known to be altered by aminoglutethimide and because its mineralocorticoid activity may also be required)

» Amphotericin B, parenteral or
Carbonic anhydrase inhibitors
(concurrent use with corticosteroids may result in severe hypokalemia and should be undertaken with caution; serum potassium concentrations and cardiac function should be monitored during concurrent use)

(the use of hydrocortisone to control adverse reactions to amphotericin B has resulted in cases of cardiac enlargement and congestive heart failure)

(concurrent use of corticosteroids with acetazolamide sodium may increase the risk of hypernatremia and/or edema because corticosteroids cause sodium and fluid retention; the risk with corticosteroids may depend on the patient's sodium requirement as determined by the condition being treated)

(the possibility should be considered that concurrent chronic use of both carbonic anhydrase inhibitors and corticosteroids may increase the risk of hypocalcemia and osteoporosis because carbonic anhydrase inhibitors also increase calcium excretion)

Anabolic steroids or
Androgens
(concurrent use with glucocorticoids may increase the risk of edema; also, concurrent use may promote the development of severe acne)

» Antacids
(concurrent chronic use with prednisone or dexamethasone may decrease absorption of these glucocorticoids; efficacy may be decreased sufficiently to require dosage adjustment in patients receiving small doses, but probably not in those receiving large doses, of the corticosteroid)

Anticholinergics, especially atropine and related compounds
(concurrent long-term use with glucocorticoids may increase intraocular pressure)

Anticoagulants, coumarin- or indandione-derivative or
Heparin or
Streptokinase or
Urokinase
(effects of coumarin or indandione derivatives are usually decreased [but may be increased in some patients] when these medications are used concurrently with glucocorticoids; dosage adjustments based on prothrombin time determinations may be necessary during and after glucocorticoid therapy)

(the potential occurrence of gastrointestinal ulceration or hemorrhage during glucocorticoid therapy, and the effects of glucocorticoids on vascular integrity, may cause increased risk to patients receiving anticoagulant or thrombolytic therapy)

Antidepressants, tricyclic
(these medications do not relieve, and may exacerbate, corticosteroid-induced mental disturbances; they should not be used for treatment of these adverse effects)
» Antidiabetic agents, sulfonylurea or
» Insulin
(glucocorticoids may increase blood glucose concentration; dosage adjustment of one or both agents may be necessary during concurrent use; dosage readjustment of the hypoglycemic agent may also be required when glucocorticoid therapy is discontinued)
Antithyroid agents or
Thyroid hormones
(changes in the thyroid status of the patient that may occur as a result of administration, changes in dosage, or discontinuation of thyroid hormones or antithyroid agents may necessitate adjustment of corticosteroid dosage because metabolic clearance of corticosteroids is decreased in hypothyroid patients and increased in hyperthyroid patients. Dosage adjustment should be based on results of thyroid function tests)
Asparaginase
(glucocorticoids, especially prednisone, may increase the hyperglycemic effect of asparaginase and the risk of neuropathy and disturbances in erythropoiesis; the toxicity appears to be less pronounced when asparaginase is administered following, rather than before or with, these medications)
Contraceptives, oral, estrogen-containing or
Estrogens
(estrogens may alter the metabolism and protein binding of glucocorticoids, leading to decreased clearance, increased elimination half-life, and increased therapeutic and toxic effects of the glucocorticoid; glucocorticoid dosage adjustment may be required during and following concurrent use)
» Digitalis glycosides
(concurrent use with glucocorticoids may increase the possibility of arrhythmias or digitalis toxicity associated with hypokalemia)
» Diuretics
(natriuretic and diuretic effects of these medications may be decreased by sodium- and fluid-retaining actions of corticosteroids, and vice versa)
(concurrent use of potassium-depleting diuretics with corticosteroids may result in severe hypokalemia; monitoring of serum potassium concentration and cardiac function is recommended)
(effects of potassium-sparing diuretics and/or corticosteroids on serum potassium concentration may be decreased during concurrent use; monitoring of serum potassium concentration is recommended)
Ephedrine
(ephedrine may increase the metabolic clearance of corticosteroids; corticosteroid dosage adjustment may be required during and following concurrent use)
Folic acid
(requirements may be increased in patients receiving long-term corticosteroid therapy)
» Hepatic enzyme–inducing agents (see *Appendix II*)
(concurrent use may decrease the corticosteroid effect because of increased corticosteroid metabolism resulting from induction of hepatic microsomal enzymes)
Immunosuppressant agents, other
(concurrent use with immunosuppressant doses of glucocorticoids may increase the risk of infection and possibly the development of lymphomas or other lymphoproliferative disorders; these neoplasms may be associated with Epstein-Barr virus infections; a few studies in organ transplant patients receiving immunosuppressant therapy indicate that progression of the neoplasm may be reversed after immunosuppressant dosage is decreased or therapy is discontinued)
Iophendylate or
Metrizamide
(concurrent intrathecal administration of metrizamide or iophendylate with intrathecal administration of glucocorticoids may increase the risk of arachnoiditis)
Isoniazid
(glucocorticoids, especially prednisolone, may increase hepatic metabolism and/or excretion of isoniazid, leading to decreased plasma concentration and effectiveness of isoniazid, especially in patients who are rapid acetylators; isoniazid dosage adjustment may be required during and following concurrent use)
Mexiletine
(concurrent use with glucocorticoids may accelerate mexiletine metabolism, leading to decreased mexiletine plasma concentration)

» Mitotane
(mitotane suppresses adrenocortical function; glucocorticoid supplementation is usually required during mitotane administration, but higher doses than those generally used for replacement therapy may be required because mitotane alters glucocorticoid metabolism)
Neuromuscular blocking agents, nondepolarizing
(hypokalemia induced by glucocorticoids may enhance the blockade of nondepolarizing neuromuscular blocking agents, possibly leading to increased or prolonged respiratory depression or paralysis [apnea]; serum potassium determinations may be necessary prior to administration of these agents)
(hydrocortisone and prednisone have also been reported to decrease the efficacy of pancuronium by an unknown mechanism; increased dosage of pancuronium or use of an alternate neuromuscular blocking agent may be necessary)
» Potassium supplements
(effects of these medications and/or corticosteroids on serum potassium concentration may be decreased when these medications are used concurrently; monitoring of serum potassium concentration is recommended)
» Ritodrine
(concurrent use may cause pulmonary edema in the mother; maternal death has been reported; both medications should be discontinued at the first sign of pulmonary edema)
Salicylates
(although concurrent use with glucocorticoids in the treatment of arthritis may provide additive therapeutic benefit and permit glucocorticoid dosage reduction, glucocorticoids may increase salicylate excretion and reduce salicylate plasma concentrations so that the salicylate dosage requirement may be increased; salicylism may occur when glucocorticoid dosage is subsequently decreased or discontinued, especially in patients receiving large [antirheumatic] doses of salicylates; also, the risk of gastrointestinal ulceration or hemorrhage may be increased during concurrent use)
» Sodium-containing medications or foods
(concurrent use with pharmacologic doses of glucocorticoids may result in edema and increased blood pressure, possibly to hypertensive levels)
(although patients receiving replacement doses of glucocorticoids may require sodium supplementation, adjustment of dietary sodium intake may be required when a medication having a high sodium content is also administered concurrently)
» Somatrem or
» Somatropin
(inhibition of the growth response to somatrem or somatropin may occur with chronic therapeutic use of daily doses [per square meter of body surface] in excess of:

|  | Oral | Parenteral |
| --- | --- | --- |
| Betamethasone | 300–450 mcg | 150–225 mcg |
| Cortisone | 12.5–18.8 mg | 6.25–9.4 mg |
| Dexamethasone | 375–563 mcg | 187.5–281.5 mcg |
| Hydrocortisone | 10–15 mg | 5–7.5 mg |
| Methylprednisolone | 2–3 mg | 1–1.5 mg |
| Prednisolone | 2.5–3.75 mg | 1.25–1.88 mg |
| Prednisone | 2.5–3.75 mg |  |
| Triamcinolone | 2–3 mg | 1–1.5 mg |

It is recommended that these doses not be exceeded during somatrem or somatropin therapy; if larger doses are required, administration of somatrem or somatropin should be postponed)
Streptozocin
(concurrent use with glucocorticoids may increase the risk of hyperglycemia)
Troleandomycin
(troleandomycin may decrease metabolism of methylprednisolone and possibly other glucocorticoids, leading to increased plasma concentration, elimination half-life, and therapeutic and toxic effects; glucocorticoid dosage adjustment may be required during and following concurrent use)
» Vaccines, live virus, or other immunizations
(administration of live virus vaccines to patients receiving pharmacologic [immunosuppressant] doses of glucocorticoids may potentiate replication of the vaccine virus, thereby increasing the risk of the patient's developing the viral disease, and/or decrease the patient's antibody response to the vaccine and is not recommended; the patient's immunologic status should be evaluated prior to administration of a live virus vaccine; also, immunization with oral poliovirus vaccine should be postponed in persons in close contact with the patient, especially family members)

(other immunizations are not recommended in patients receiving pharmacologic [immunosuppressant] doses of glucocorticoids because of the increased risk of neurological complications and the possibility of decreased or absent antibody response)

(immunizations may be administered to patients receiving glucocorticoids via routes or in quantities that are not likely to cause immunosuppression, for example, those receiving local injections, short-term [less than 2 weeks] therapy, or physiologic doses)

**Laboratory value alterations**
The following have been selected on the basis of their potential clinical significance (possible effect in parentheses where appropriate)—not necessarily inclusive (» = major clinical significance):
With results of dexamethasone suppression tests
*Due to other medications*
Alcohol (chronic abuse) or
Glutethimide or
Meprobamate or
Methaqualone or
Methyprylon
(may cause false-positive results in test for endogenous depression)

Benzodiazepines (high doses) or
Cyproheptadine (high doses) or
Glucocorticoid therapy, long-term or
Indomethacin
(may cause false-negative results in test for endogenous depression)

Ephedrine or
Estrogens (high doses) or
Hepatic enzyme–inducing agents (see *Appendix II*)
(may cause false-positive results in tests for Cushing's disease or endogenous depression)

*Due to medical problems or conditions*
Adrenal hyperfunction (Cushing's disease) or
Anorexia nervosa or malnutrition leading to extreme weight loss, recent or
Carcinoma, disseminated, with concurrent serious infection or
Cardiac failure or
Dehydration or
Diabetes mellitus, unstable or
Fever or
Hypertension or
Pregnancy or
Renal failure or
Temporal lobe disease
(may cause false-positive results in test for endogenous depression)

Adrenal insufficiency or
Hypopituitarism
(may cause false-negative results in test for endogenous depression)

Psychiatric disorders such as acute psychosis, mania, chronic schizophrenia, and primary degenerative dementia
(may interfere with results of test for endogenous depression)

With *other* diagnostic test results
Brain imaging using sodium pertechnetate Tc 99m, technetium Tc 99m gluceptate, or technetium Tc 99m pentetate
(uptake of these diagnostic aids into cerebral tumors may be decreased in patients receiving large doses of glucocorticoids because of glucocorticoid-induced reduction of peritumor edema)

Gonadorelin test for hypothalamic-pituitary-gonadal axis function
(glucocorticoids may alter the results of the gonadorelin test by affecting pituitary secretion of gonadotropins through a complicated feedback mechanism)

Nitroblue-tetrazolium test for bacterial infection
(false-negative test results may occur)

Protirelin test for thyroid function
(physiologic doses of corticosteroids have no effect, but pharmacologic doses may reduce the thyroid-stimulating hormone [TSH] response to protirelin; however, withdrawal of corticosteroids in patients with known hypopituitarism is generally not recommended)

Skeletal imaging using technetium Tc 99m medronate, technetium Tc 99m oxidronate, or technetium Tc 99m pyrophosphate
(long-term use of glucocorticoids may induce bone calcium depletion, thus causing decreased bone uptake of these diagnostic aids)

Skin tests, including tuberculin and histoplasmin skin tests and patch tests for allergy
(reactions may be suppressed, especially with daily administration of large doses of corticosteroids)

Thyroid $^{123}$I or $^{131}$I uptake
(may be decreased)

With physiology/laboratory test values
Adrenal function as assessed by ACTH stimulation or measurement of plasma or urinary free cortisol
(may be decreased with pharmacologic doses of glucocorticoids, especially in children)

Basophil count and
Eosinophil count and
Lymphocyte count and
Monocyte count
(may be decreased)

Calcium
(serum concentrations may be decreased)

Cholesterol and
Lipid (fatty acid)
(serum concentrations may be increased)

Glucose
(blood and urine concentrations may be increased because of intrinsic hyperglycemic activity)

17-Hydroxysteroid (17-OHCS) and
17-Ketosteroid (17-KS)
(urine concentrations may be decreased by potent corticosteroids)

Platelet count
(may be increased or decreased)

Polymorphonuclear leukocyte count
(may be increased)

Potassium
(serum concentrations may be decreased because of increased potassium excretion, especially with agents having significant mineralocorticoid activity)

Sodium
(serum concentrations may be increased because of sodium retention, especially with glucocorticoids having significant mineralocorticoid activity)

Uric acid
(serum concentrations may be increased in patients with acute leukemia; may be decreased in other patients because of weak uricosuric effect)

**Medical considerations/Contraindications**
The medical considerations/contraindications included have been selected on the basis of their potential clinical significance (reasons given in parentheses where appropriate)—not necessarily inclusive (» = major clinical significance).
See also *Laboratory value alterations*.
Note: The medical problems listed below apply only to pharmacologic (supraphysiologic) doses of glucocorticoids, unless otherwise stated.

***Except under special circumstances, these medications should not be used when the following medical problems exist:***
*For intra-articular injection*
» Arthroplasty of joint, prior
   (increased risk of infection)
» Blood clotting disorders
   (risk of intra- and extra-articular hemorrhage)
» Fracture, intra-articular
   (healing may be retarded)
» Infection, periarticular, current or history of
   (may be exacerbated or reactivated)
» Osteoporosis, juxta-articular, non-arthritic
   (may be exacerbated)
» Unstable joint

*For neonatal respiratory distress syndrome prophylaxis*
» Amnionitis
» Bleeding, uterine
» Febrile illness or infection, especially tuberculosis, maternal or
» Herpes type II infection, active, maternal or
» Keratitis, viral, maternal
   (may be exacerbated; if corticosteroid administration is essential, appropriate antimicrobial therapy must be administered concurrently)
» Placental insufficiency
» Premature membrane rupture
   (increased risk of maternal infection; the glucocorticoid should be administered immediately if this occurs, since the risk of infection increases with time)

*Risk-benefit should be considered when the following medical problems exist:*

*For all indications*
» Acquired immunodeficiency syndrome (AIDS) or
» Human immunodeficiency virus (HIV) infection
(although pharmacologic doses of corticosteroids can be effective in the treatment of certain HIV-related diseases, careful medical evaluation of the risks and benefits of this therapy must be done, due to the possible increased risk of severe uncontrollable infections and/or neoplasms; in one study in patients given tapering doses of intravenous methylprednisolone starting with 60 mg every 6 hours for 8 days as an adjunct to antipneumocystis therapy, an increase in frequency or severity of life-threatening opportunistic infections was observed; in a study of similar patients given tapering doses of prednisone starting at 40 mg two times a day for 21 days, no increase in the incidence of Kaposi's sarcoma or life-threatening opportunistic infections was observed, though the incidence of oral candidiasis and mucocutaneous herpes simplex infection did increase)

» Anastomoses, intestinal, recent
» Cardiac disease or
» Congestive heart failure or
Hypertension or
» Renal function impairment or disease, severe
(edema may be hazardous, especially with agents having significant mineralocorticoid activity)
(patients undergoing dialysis may have increased risk of avascular necrosis with long-term corticosteroid use)

» Chickenpox, existing or recent (including recent exposure) or
» Measles, existing or recent (including recent exposure)
(risk of severe, potentially fatal, generalized disease; extra care to avoid exposure to these infections is recommended; prophylactic therapy with varicella zoster immune globulin [VZIG] or immune globulin intravenous [IGIV] or intramuscular [IGIM], as appropriate, may be indicated in exposed patients; therapy with an antiviral agent may be indicated if chickenpox develops)

Colitis, ulcerative nonspecific, with possibility of impending perforation, abscess, or other infection or
Diverticulitis or
» Esophagitis, gastritis, or peptic ulcer, active or latent
(symptoms of progression or reactivation may be masked; hemorrhage and/or perforation may occur without warning)

» Diabetes mellitus or predisposition to
(may be exacerbated or activated)

» Fungal infections, systemic
(may be exacerbated; pharmacologic doses should not be given unless the patient is concurrently receiving an antifungal agent)

Glaucoma, open-angle
(intraocular pressure may be increased)

Hepatic function impairment or disease
(increased risk of glucocorticoid toxicity, especially if hypoalbuminemia present; possibility of impaired conversion of cortisone or prednisone to their active metabolites, although effect may be offset by decreased protein binding or clearance and/or conversion in other tissues)

» Herpes simplex, ocular
(possible corneal perforation)

Herpetic lesions, oral
Hyperlipidemia
(concentrations of fatty acids or cholesterol may be increased)

Hyperthyroidism
(glucocorticoid effect may be impaired because of accelerated metabolism; may be especially important with physiologic doses or low pharmacologic doses)

Hypoalbuminemia or conditions predisposing to, including hepatic cirrhosis or nephrotic syndrome
(increased risk of toxicity because reduced availability of albumin for glucocorticoid binding leads to increased serum concentration of unbound drug; reduction in initial dosage is recommended)

Hypothyroidism
(decreased metabolism of corticosteroid may result)

Infections, viral or bacterial, uncontrolled, systemic or at site of local injection
(may be exacerbated; concurrent antimicrobial therapy required)

Intolerance to corticosteroids

» Myasthenia gravis
(muscle weakness may be increased initially, possibly leading to respiratory distress; patient should be hospitalized, and respiratory support should be immediately available, when glucocorticoid therapy is initiated)

Osteoporosis
(may be exacerbated)

Renal function impairment, mild to moderate, or stones
(fluid retention may exacerbate these conditions; increased risk of edema, especially with agents having mineralocorticoid activity)
(patients receiving dialysis may have increased risk of avascular necrosis with long-term corticosteroid use)

Systemic lupus erythematosus (SLE)
(cautious use is recommended because of an increased risk of aseptic necrosis)

» Tuberculosis—active, positive skin test, latent, or history of
(may be exacerbated or reactivated; appropriate antitubercular chemotherapy or prophylaxis should be administered concurrently)

**Patient monitoring**

The following may be especially important in patient monitoring (other tests may be warranted in some patients, depending on condition; » = major clinical significance):

Glucose concentrations, blood or urine or
Glucose tolerance test
(may be required for patients with diabetes mellitus or a predisposition to diabetes mellitus)

Growth and development determinations
(recommended in children and adolescents receiving prolonged therapy)

Hypothalamic-pituitary-adrenal (HPA) axis function determination
(may be required during, and following withdrawal of, high-dose or long-term [more than 3 weeks] therapy to assess adrenal function; complete recovery of adrenal function may require up to 1 year following prolonged use, especially with high doses; in some patients receiving prolonged, high-dose therapy, complete recovery may never occur)

Ophthalmologic examinations
(may be required at periodic intervals for adults or children receiving therapy for more than 6 weeks to detect the presence of cataracts, increased intraocular pressure, glaucoma, or ocular infections)

Serum electrolyte determinations and
Stool tests for occult blood loss
(may be required during long-term therapy)

## Side/Adverse Effects

Note: The risk of adverse effects with pharmacologic doses of corticosteroids generally increases with the duration of therapy and frequency of administration and, to a lesser extent, with dosage.

Chronic administration of physiologic replacement doses of corticosteroids rarely causes adverse effects.

Administration of glucocorticoids via local injection reduces the risk of systemic effects. The risk of both systemic and local adverse effects is still present to a degree, however, and increases with the frequency of injections.

Pharmacologic doses of glucocorticoids lower resistance to infection; the patient may be predisposed to systemic infections during, and for a time following, therapy. Increased susceptibility to infection may occur with short-term high-dose use ("pulse" therapy) as well as with more prolonged use. Also, symptoms of onset or progression of infections may be masked.

The following side/adverse effects have been selected on the basis of their potential clinical significance (possible signs and symptoms in parentheses where appropriate)—not necessarily inclusive:

### Those indicating need for medical attention

Incidence less frequent
*Cataracts* (decreased or blurred vision); *diabetes mellitus* (decreased or blurred vision; frequent urination; increased thirst)

Incidence rare
*Generalized allergic reaction* (skin rash or hives); *local allergic reaction or infection at injection site* (redness, swelling, pain, or other signs of infection or allergic reaction); *sudden blindness; burning, numbness, pain, or tingling at or near place of injection; psychic disturbances such as delirium* (confusion; excitement; restlessness); *disorientation; euphoria* (false sense of well-being); *hallucinations* (seeing, hearing, or feeling things that are not there); *manic-depressive*

*episodes* (sudden, wide mood swings); *mental depression, or paranoia* (mistaken feelings of self-importance or being mistreated)

Note: *Sudden blindness* following injection into sites in the head or neck area, such as nasal turbinates or scalp, due to possible entry of drug crystals into ocular blood vessels.

*Psychic disturbances* are more likely in patients with chronic debilitating illnesses that predispose them to psychic disturbances and in patients receiving higher daily dosages. Psychic disturbances may be related to dose rather than duration of therapy; symptoms may appear within a few days to 2 weeks after initiation of therapy and are usually associated with doses equivalent to 40 mg or more of prednisone per day. Additionally, euphoria or fear of relapse may lead to psychological dependence or abuse of corticosteroids.

With rapid intravenous administration of high doses ("pulse" therapy)
*Generalized anaphylaxis* (swelling of face, nasal membranes, and eyelids; hives; shortness of breath; tightness in chest; troubled breathing; wheezing); *flushing of face or cheeks; irregular or pounding heartbeat; seizures*

Note: *Rapid intravenous administration of high doses* of corticosteroids has been reported to cause convulsions, angioedema and/or anaphylactic reactions, and sudden death associated with cardiac arrhythmias. Monitoring of the electrocardiogram (ECG) is recommended. Equipment, medications, and trained personnel necessary for treating these complications should be immediately available.

**Those occurring principally during long-term use indicating need for medical attention**

*Acne or other skin problems; avascular necrosis* (hip or shoulder pain); *Cushing's syndrome* (filling or rounding out of the face); *edema* (swelling of feet or lower legs; rapid weight gain); *endocrine imbalance* (menstrual irregularities); *gastrointestinal irritation* (nausea; vomiting); *hypokalemic syndrome* (irregular heartbeat; muscle cramps or pain; unusual tiredness or weakness); *osteoporosis or bone fractures* (pain in back, ribs, arms, or legs)—includes vertebral compression and long bone pathologic fractures; *pancreatitis* (continuing abdominal or stomach pain or burning; nausea; vomiting); *peptic ulceration or intestinal perforation* (continuing abdominal or stomach pain or burning; bloody or black, tarry stools); *scarring at injection site; steroid myopathy* (muscle weakness); *striae* (reddish purple lines on arms, face, legs, trunk, or groin); *tendon rupture*—with local injection; *cutaneous or subcutaneous tissue atrophy* (thin, shiny skin; pitting or depression of skin at place of injection)—with frequent repository injections; *unusual bruising; wounds that will not heal*

**Those indicating need for medical attention only if they continue or are bothersome**

Incidence more frequent
*Increased appetite; indigestion; nervousness or restlessness; trouble in sleeping*

For triamcinolone
*Loss of appetite*

Incidence less frequent or rare
*Changes in skin color or hypopigmentation* (darkening or lightening of skin color); *dizziness or lightheadedness; flushing of face or cheeks; headache*—following intranasal injection; *increased joint pain*—following intra-articular injection; *increased sweating; nosebleeds*—following intranasal injection; *unusual increase in hair growth on body or face*

Note: *Hypopigmentation* is more likely at the injection site.
*Flushing of face or cheeks* may persist for 24 to 48 hours.
*Increased joint pain* may occur within a few hours postinjection and persist for up to 48 hours.

**Those occurring principally after medication is discontinued, indicating a corticosteroid withdrawal syndrome and the need for medical attention**

*Withdrawal syndrome* (abdominal or back pain; dizziness; fainting; frequent or continuing unexplained headaches; low-grade fever; muscle or joint pain; nausea; prolonged loss of appetite; rapid weight loss; reappearance of disease symptoms; shortness of breath; unusual tiredness or weakness; vomiting)

Note: Too-rapid *withdrawal of therapy*, especially after prolonged use, may cause acute, possibly life-threatening, adrenal insufficiency and/or a withdrawal syndrome not related to HPA axis suppression.

## Patient Consultation

As an aid to patient consultation, refer to *Advice for the Patient, Corticosteroids—Glucocorticoid Effects (Systemic)*.

In providing consultation, consider emphasizing the following selected information (» = major clinical significance):

**Before using this medication**
» Conditions affecting use, especially:
  Allergies to corticosteroids
  Pregnancy—Pharmacologic doses in animals show some evidence of increased risk of placental insufficiency, decreased birthweight, or stillbirths; other animal studies show increased incidence of cleft palate, placental insufficiency, spontaneous abortions, or intrauterine growth retardation. Hypoadrenalism may occur in infants if mothers received substantial doses of corticosteroids prenatally
  Breast-feeding—Breast-feeding is not recommended during use of higher doses
  Use in children—Close monitoring required since chronic therapy may result in suppression of growth and development; possible increased severity of chickenpox or measles in children receiving immunosuppressant doses; discussing possible effects with physician
  Use in the elderly—Increased risk of osteoporosis (especially in postmenopausal females) or hypertension
  Other medications, especially aminoglutethimide, parenteral amphotericin B, antacids, sulfonylurea antidiabetic agents, insulin, digitalis glycosides, diuretics, hepatic enzyme–inducing agents, mitotane, potassium supplements, ritodrine, sodium-containing medications, human growth hormone, or immunizations
  Other medical problems, especially
    For all uses—AIDS, systemic or local infections, gastrointestinal disorders, cardiac disease, chickenpox, congestive heart failure, renal diseases, diabetes mellitus, measles, or myasthenia gravis
    For intra-articular injection only—Arthroplasty, clotting disorders, fracture, osteoporosis, or unstable joint
    For neonatal respiratory distress syndrome prophylaxis only—Amnionitis, uterine bleeding, febrile illness, placental insufficiency, or premature membrane rupture

**Proper use of this medication**
*For oral dosage forms*
» Taking with food to minimize gastrointestinal irritation
  Possibility that alcohol may enhance ulcerogenic effects of medication
» Importance of not using more medication than the amount prescribed
» Proper dosing
  Missed dose: If dosing schedule is—
    Every other day: Taking as soon as possible if remembered same morning; if remembered later, not taking until next morning, then skipping a day
    Once a day: Taking as soon as possible; not taking if almost time for next dose; not doubling doses
    Several times a day: Taking as soon as possible; doubling if time for next dose
» Proper storage

**Precautions while using this medication**
» Regular visits to physician to check progress during and following therapy
» Checking with physician before discontinuing medication; gradual dosage reduction may be necessary
  Checking with physician if symptoms recur or worsen when dose decreased or therapy discontinued
» Possible need for calorie and/or sodium restriction or potassium supplementation during long-term therapy
  Possible need for increased protein intake during long-term therapy
  Ophthalmologic examinations during long-term therapy
  Carrying medical identification card indicating use of medication during long-term therapy
» Caution in receiving skin tests
» Caution if any kind of surgery or emergency treatment is required
» Avoiding exposure to chickenpox or measles (especially for children); telling physician right away if exposure occurs
» Caution in receiving vaccinations or other immunizations or coming in contact with persons receiving oral poliovirus vaccine
» Caution if serious infections or injuries occur
  Diabetics: May increase blood sugar concentrations

*For parenteral dosage forms*
  Restricting use of joint following intra-articular injection
  Checking with physician if redness or swelling occurs, and continues or becomes worse, following local injection

### Side/adverse effects

Signs of potential side effects, especially visual disturbances, diabetes mellitus, local irritation, allergic reactions, local or systemic infection, psychic disturbances, seizures, hypertension, tachycardia, musculoskeletal disorders, Cushing's syndrome, edema, endocrine imbalance, hypokalemic syndrome, gastrointestinal effects, myopathy, striae, tissue atrophy, scarring at injection site, bruising, or delayed wound healing

## General Dosing Information

See *Table 4*, page 1020.

For replacement therapy in chronic adrenocortical insufficiency states, corticosteroid therapy must be continued for the life of the patient. It is recommended that dosage of cortisone or hydrocortisone be timed to simulate endogenous corticosteroid secretion, with two-thirds of the daily dose administered in the morning and one-third in the evening. Other corticosteroids are usually given once a day.

For treatment of adrenogenital syndrome, suppression of corticotropin secretion is required to decrease hypersecretion of adrenal androgens. This is usually achieved by administering one-third of the daily dose of cortisone or hydrocortisone in the morning and two-thirds in the evening or giving one-third of the daily dose three times a day at evenly spaced intervals. Other corticosteroids are usually given once a day.

Except in severe conditions or emergency situations, it is recommended that therapy be instituted with low doses that should be increased as necessary to provide the desired effect. For most conditions, administration in the lowest effective dose for the shortest time possible is recommended. Dosage requirements are variable and should be individualized according to the disease being treated and patient response rather than by age or body weight. Whenever possible, local administration is recommended in order to concentrate the medication at the affected site and reduce the risk of systemic effects. After a favorable response is obtained, the dosage should be decreased gradually to the lowest dose that will maintain an adequate clinical response.

Frequent monitoring of drug effect is required. Situations that may necessitate dosage adjustments include remissions or exacerbations of the disease process and the patient's response to the medication.

Clinically significant hypothalamic-pituitary-adrenal (HPA) axis suppression leading to adrenal insufficiency may occur more readily with multiple daily doses or evening administration than with single doses given every morning or every other morning. Administration of a single daily dose of a short- or intermediate-acting corticosteroid prior to 9 a.m. may reduce the risk of HPA axis suppression (because maximum endogenous corticosteroid secretion occurs in the morning) and is recommended for daily administration whenever possible. However, some disease conditions may require multiple daily doses.

Following discontinuation of short-term (up to 5 days) high-dose use, adrenal recovery may occur within 1 week; however, following prolonged high-dose administration, complete recovery of adrenal function may require up to 1 year. Following very prolonged suppression, complete recovery may never occur. During the recovery period, monitoring of adrenal function may be required to assess the patient's ability to respond to stress.

Patients with known or suspected adrenal insufficiency, including those already receiving replacement therapy, require an increase in dosage or reinstitution of therapy prior to, during, and for a time following, exposure to emotional stress or physical stress such as severe infection, surgery (including dental surgery), or injury. Administration of sodium and/or a mineralocorticoid may also be required. Dosage and duration of such therapy are dependent on the severity of the stress.

When medication is to be discontinued, dosage should be reduced gradually. The rate at which dosage can be decreased and the time required for complete withdrawal of therapy are variable, depending on the specific agent used; dose, frequency, and route of administration; duration of therapy; condition being treated; and patient response.

### For oral dosage forms only

If oral long-term use is required for disease therapy, an alternate-day regimen using an intermediate-acting corticosteroid is recommended to minimize HPA axis suppression and possibly other adverse effects. An intermediate-acting corticosteroid is one that suppresses HPA axis activity for 12 to 36 hours following a single dose. Administration of longer-acting corticosteroids on an alternate-day schedule does not reduce the risk of HPA axis suppression and is not recommended.

Alternate-day therapy utilizes a single dose administered every other morning, usually in a quantity equivalent to, or somewhat higher than, twice the usual or pre-established daily dose. The patient should have a normal or moderately responsive HPA axis.

If treatment has been initiated with daily administration, changes to alternate-day therapy should be made gradually, after the patient's condition has stabilized. However, for some diseases, such as childhood nephrosis, therapy may be initiated with alternate-day dosing.

Alternate-day therapy may not be effective in treating hematologic disorders, malignancies, ulcerative colitis, or severe conditions. Also, some patients, such as those with asthma or rheumatoid arthritis, may experience exacerbation of symptoms on the second day. Administration of (or increasing the dosage of) suitable supplemental therapy on the second day may provide sufficient symptomatic relief to permit alternate-day dosing in some patients.

### For parenteral dosage forms only

For acute adrenocortical insufficiency, initiation of corticosteroid therapy by intravenous injection followed by slow intravenous infusion or intramuscular administration is recommended. Certain other acute conditions may also require initiation of therapy with intravenous administration or intramuscular administration of a rapidly acting formulation.

In severe or life-threatening conditions, single-dose or short-term intravenous administration of a very high dose ("pulse" therapy) may produce the required therapeutic response with a minimum risk of prolonged HPA axis suppression or other adverse effects. Such therapy has been recommended for treating conditions such as organ transplant rejection reactions, acute nephritis associated with systemic lupus erythematosus, vasculitis, adult respiratory distress syndrome, and shock. However, rapid intravenous administration of high doses of corticosteroids has been reported to cause potentially life-threatening side effects and appropriate precautions should be observed.

When the suspension dosage forms are administered intramuscularly, they should be injected deeply into the gluteal muscle to prevent local tissue atrophy. It is recommended that the deltoid muscle not be used because of a higher incidence of local atrophy. In addition, do not inject repeatedly into the same site.

A standard textbook should be consulted for specific techniques and procedures applicable to local injection of corticosteroids for various indications.

It is recommended that intra-articular injections be repeated no more often than once every 3 weeks. Frequent repeated injections may cause joint damage.

Following intra-articular injection, the injected joint should not be overused, even if pain is relieved, because of the increased risk of joint damage or deterioration. It is recommended that weight-bearing joints be rested for 24 to 48 hours postinjection.

Administration of a local anesthetic concurrently with intra-articular or soft tissue injection of a corticosteroid may reduce the pain of injection and provide immediate relief of symptoms. However, a post-injection flare of pain may occur when the local anesthetic effect subsides.

Dosages for local injections (e.g., intra-articular, intrabursal, intradermal, intralesional) are given as ranges only. The actual dosage depends upon the size of the joint or lesion and the severity of the condition being treated.

### Diet/Nutrition

Administration of oral dosage forms with food may relieve indigestion or mild gastrointestinal irritation that may occur.

Patients receiving prolonged therapy with pharmacologic doses of corticosteroids, especially those with significant mineralocorticoid activity, may require sodium restriction and/or potassium supplementation during therapy.

Because corticosteroids promote protein catabolism, increased protein intake may be necessary during prolonged therapy.

Administration of calcium and vitamin D and, if the patient's condition permits, exercise or physical therapy may reduce the risk of corticosteroid-induced osteoporosis during prolonged therapy.

### For treatment of adverse effects

Recommended treatment consists of the following

- For gastrointestinal effects—Administration of antacids between meals may relieve indigestion or mild gastrointestinal irritation that may occur during parenteral, as well as oral, corticosteroid therapy. However, the efficacy of antacids or other antiulcer medications in preventing severe gastrointestinal problems, such as ulceration, hemorrhage, and/or bowel perforation, during corticosteroid therapy has not been established.

- For mental depression or psychoses—If possible, decrease corticosteroid dosage or discontinue therapy. A phenothiazine may be administered if necessary; lithium has also been recommended. Some patients may require electroconvulsive therapy if severe depression persists. Tricyclic antidepressants should not be used since they do not relieve, and may exacerbate, corticosteroid-induced mental disturbances. Prophylactic administration of an antipsychotic agent may be indicated if ad-

ditional courses of corticosteroid therapy are required by a patient with a history of corticosteroid-induced psychosis.
• For withdrawal effects (non-HPA axis suppression)—Administration of aspirin or another nonsteroidal anti-inflammatory drug may alleviate some of the symptoms of this condition.

## BETAMETHASONE

## Summary of Differences
Indications: See *Table 1*, 1015.
Pharmacology/pharmacokinetics: See *Table 2*, 1019 and *Table 3*, 1020.
Precautions: Pediatrics—Not recommended for chronic use; especially likely to inhibit growth.
General dosing information: See *Table 4*, 1020.

## Oral Dosage Forms

### BETAMETHASONE SYRUP USP
**Usual adult and adolescent dose**
Oral, 600 mcg (0.6 mg) to 7.2 mg a day as a single dose or in divided doses.

**Usual pediatric dose**
Adrenocortical insufficiency—
   Oral, 17.5 mcg (0.0175 mg) per kg of body weight or 500 mcg (0.5 mg) per square meter of body surface a day in three divided doses.
Other indications—
   Oral, 62.5 to 250 mcg (0.0625 to 0.25 mg) per kg of body weight or 1.875 to 7.5 mg per square meter of body surface a day in three or four divided doses.

**Strength(s) usually available**
U.S.—
   600 mcg (0.6 mg) per 5 mL (Rx) [*Celestone* (alcohol <1%)].

**Packaging and storage**
Store between 2 and 30 °C (36 and 86 °F), protected from light. Store in a well-closed container. Protect from freezing.

### BETAMETHASONE TABLETS USP
**Usual adult and adolescent dose**
Oral, 600 mcg (0.6 mg) to 7.2 mg a day as a single dose or in divided doses.

**Usual pediatric dose**
Adrenocortical insufficiency—
   Oral, 17.5 mcg (0.0175 mg) per kg of body weight or 500 mcg (0.5 mg) per square meter of body surface a day in three divided doses.
Other indications—
   Oral, 62.5 to 250 mcg (0.0625 to 0.25 mg) per kg of body weight or 1.875 to 7.5 mg per square meter of body surface a day in three or four divided doses.

**Strength(s) usually available**
U.S.—
   600 mcg (0.6 mg) (Rx) [*Celestone* (scored)].
Canada—
   500 mcg (0.5 mg) (Rx) [*Betnelan* (scored); *Celestone* (scored)].

**Packaging and storage**
Store between 2 and 30 °C (36 and 86 °F). Store in a well-closed container.
Note: Protect the 21-tablet pack from excessive moisture.

### BETAMETHASONE EFFERVESCENT TABLETS
**Usual adult and adolescent dose**
Oral, 600 mcg (0.6 mg) to 7.2 mg a day as a single dose or in divided doses.

**Usual pediatric dose**
Adrenocortical insufficiency—
   Oral, 17.5 mcg (0.0175 mg) per kg of body weight or 500 mcg (0.5 mg) per square meter of body surface a day in three divided doses.
Other indications—
   Oral, 62.5 to 250 mcg (0.0625 to 0.25 mg) per kg of body weight or 1.875 to 7.5 mg per square meter of body surface a day in three or four divided doses.

**Strength(s) usually available**
U.S.—
   Not commercially available.
Canada—
   500 mcg (0.5 mg) (Rx) [*Betnesol* (scored)].

**Packaging and storage**
Store below 40 °C (104 °F), preferably between 15 and 30 °C (59 and 86 °F), in a well-closed container, unless otherwise specified by manufacturer. Protect from moisture.

**Preparation of dosage form**
Dissolve in water immediately prior to ingestion.

**Note**
When dispensing, explain dissolution requirement to patient.

### BETAMETHASONE SODIUM PHOSPHATE EXTENDED-RELEASE TABLETS
**Usual adult and adolescent dose**
Oral, 2 to 6 mg per day initially, then adjusted according to patient response.

**Usual pediatric dose**
Adrenocortical insufficiency—
   Oral, 17.5 mcg (0.0175 mg) per kg of body weight or 500 mcg (0.5 mg) per square meter of body surface a day in three divided doses.
Other indications—
   Oral, 62.5 to 250 mcg (0.0625 to 0.25 mg) per kg of body weight or 1.875 to 7.5 mg per square meter of body surface a day in three or four divided doses.

**Strength(s) usually available**
U.S.—
   Not commercially available.
Canada—
   1 mg (Rx) [*Celestone*].

**Packaging and storage**
Store below 40 °C (104 °F), preferably between 15 and 30 °C (59 and 86 °F), in a well-closed container, unless otherwise specified by manufacturer.

## Parenteral Dosage Forms
Note: The dosing and strengths of the dosage forms available are expressed in terms of betamethasone base.

### BETAMETHASONE SODIUM PHOSPHATE INJECTION USP
**Usual adult and adolescent dose**
Intra-articular, intralesional, or soft-tissue injection, up to 9 mg (base), repeated as needed.
Intramuscular or intravenous, up to 9 mg (base) a day.

**Usual pediatric dose**
Adrenocortical insufficiency—
   Intramuscular, 17.5 mcg (0.0175 mg) (base) per kg of body weight or 500 mcg (0.5 mg) (base) per square meter of body surface a day (in three divided doses) every third day; or 5.8 to 8.75 mcg (0.0058 to 0.00875 mg) (base) per kg of body weight or 166 to 250 mcg (0.166 to 0.25 mg) (base) per square meter of body surface once a day.
Other indications—
   Intramuscular, 20.8 to 125 mcg (0.021 to 0.125 mg) (base) per kg of body weight or 625 mcg (0.625 mg) to 3.75 mg (base) per square meter of body surface every twelve to twenty-four hours.

**Strength(s) usually available**
U.S.—
   3 mg (base) (4 mg sodium phosphate) per mL (Rx) [*Celestone Phosphate* (sodium bisulfite 3.2 mg); *Selestoject* (sodium bisulfite); GENERIC].

**Packaging and storage**
Store below 40 °C (104 °F), preferably between 15 and 30 °C (59 and 86 °F), protected from light, unless otherwise specified by manufacturer. Protect from freezing.

### STERILE BETAMETHASONE SODIUM PHOSPHATE AND BETAMETHASONE ACETATE SUSPENSION USP
**Usual adult and adolescent dose**
Intra-articular, 1.5 to 12 mg, depending upon the size of the affected joint, repeated as needed.
Intrabursal, 6 mg, repeated as needed.
Intradermal or intralesional, 1.2 mg per square centimeter of affected skin up to a total amount of 6 mg, repeated at one-week intervals, if necessary.
Intramuscular, 500 mcg (0.5 mg) to 9 mg a day.

**Usual pediatric dose**
Dosage has not been established.

**Strength(s) usually available**
U.S.—
  6 mg (3 mg of betamethasone acetate and 3 mg of betamethasone base) per mL (Rx) [*Celestone Soluspan*].
Canada—
  6 mg (3 mg of betamethasone acetate and 3 mg of betamethasone base) per mL (Rx) [*Celestone Soluspan*].

**Packaging and storage**
Store between 2 and 25 °C (36 and 77 °F), protected from light, unless otherwise specified by manufacturer. Protect from freezing.

**Incompatibilities**
This medication should *not* be mixed with parenteral-local anesthetic formulations containing parabens, phenol, or other such preservatives, because flocculation of the corticosteroid may occur. Withdraw the required quantity of corticosteroid suspension into a syringe, then add the local anesthetic. *Do not introduce the local anesthetic directly into the multiple-dose vial.*

**Auxiliary labeling**
• Shake well.

**Additional dosing information**
For administration of injections, see manufacturer's labeling.
Do not administer this medication intravenously.

---

## CORTISONE

### Summary of Differences
Indications: See *Table 1*, 1015.
Pharmacology/pharmacokinetics: See *Table 2*, 1019 and *Table 3*, 1020.
General dosing information: See *Table 4*, 1020.

## Oral Dosage Forms
### CORTISONE ACETATE TABLETS USP

**Usual adult and adolescent dose**
Oral, 25 to 300 mg a day as a single dose or in divided doses.

**Usual pediatric dose**
Adrenocortical insufficiency—
  Oral, 700 mcg (0.7 mg) per kg of body weight or 20 to 25 mg per square meter of body surface a day in divided doses.
Other indications—
  Oral, 2.5 to 10 mg per kg of body weight or 75 to 300 mg per square meter of body surface a day as a single dose or in divided doses.

**Strength(s) usually available**
U.S.—
  5 mg (Rx) [GENERIC (scored; lactose)].
  10 mg (Rx) [GENERIC (scored)].
  25 mg (Rx) [*Cortone Acetate* (scored); GENERIC (scored; sucrose)].
Canada—
  5 mg (Rx) [*Cortone* (lactose)].
  25 mg (Rx) [*Cortone* (scored; lactose) [GENERIC].

**Packaging and storage**
Store below 40 °C (104 °F), preferably between 15 and 30 °C (59 and 86 °F). Store in a well-closed container.

## Parenteral Dosage Forms
### STERILE CORTISONE ACETATE SUSPENSION USP

**Usual adult and adolescent dose**
Intramuscular, 20 to 300 mg a day.

**Usual pediatric dose**
Adrenocortical insufficiency—
  Intramuscular, 700 mcg (0.7 mg) per kg of body weight or 37.5 mg per square meter of body surface a day every third day; or 233.33 to 350 mcg (0.23333 to 0.350 mg) per kg of body weight or 12.5 mg per square meter of body surface once a day.
Other indications—
  Intramuscular, 833 mcg (0.833 mg) to 5 mg per kg of body weight or 25 to 150 mg per square meter of body surface every twelve to twenty-four hours.

**Strength(s) usually available**
U.S.—
  25 mg per mL (Rx) [GENERIC].
  50 mg per mL (Rx) [*Cortone Acetate*; GENERIC].
Canada—
  50 mg per mL (Rx) [*Cortone*].

**Packaging and storage**
Store below 40 °C (104 °F), preferably between 15 and 30 °C (59 and 86 °F), unless otherwise specified by manufacturer. Protect from freezing.

**Stability**
Dilutions or admixtures of this medication with other products are not recommended because the state of suspension or the rate of absorption may be affected.
This medication is heat-sensitive and should not be autoclaved.

**Auxiliary labeling**
• Shake well.

**Additional information**
Do not administer this medication intravenously.

---

## DEXAMETHASONE

### Summary of Differences
Category: Also, diagnostic aid (Cushing's syndrome and endogenous depression) and antiemetic (in cancer chemotherapy).
Indications: See *Table 1*, 1015.
Pharmacology/pharmacokinetics: See *Table 2*, 1019 and *Table 3*, 1020.
Precautions: Pediatrics—Not recommended for chronic use; especially likely to inhibit growth.
General dosing information: See *Table 4*, 1020.

## Oral Dosage Forms
### DEXAMETHASONE ELIXIR USP

**Usual adult and adolescent dose**
Oral, 500 mcg (0.5 mg) to 9 mg a day as a single dose or in divided doses.
Dexamethasone suppression test—
  Test for Cushing's syndrome: Oral, 1 mg as a single dose at 11:00 p.m. or 500 mcg (0.5 mg) every six hours for forty-eight hours.
  Test to distinguish Cushing's syndrome due to pituitary ACTH excess from Cushing's syndrome due to other causes: Oral, 2 mg every six hours for forty-eight hours.
  Depression diagnosis: Oral, 1 mg as a single dose at 11:00 p.m.
In cerebral edema associated with recurrent or inoperable brain tumor—
  Oral, 2 mg two or three times a day, administered as maintenance therapy after cerebral edema has initially been controlled using parenteral dexamethasone sodium phosphate.

**Usual pediatric dose**
Adrenocortical insufficiency—
  Oral, 23.3 mcg (0.0233 mg) per kg of body weight or 670 mcg (0.67 mg) per square meter of body surface a day in three divided doses.
Other indications—
  Oral, 83.3 to 333.3 mcg (0.0833 to 0.3333 mg) per kg of body weight or 2.5 to 10 mg per square meter of body surface a day in three or four divided doses.

**Strength(s) usually available**
U.S.—
  500 mcg (0.5 mg) per 5 mL (Rx) [*Decadron* (alcohol 5%); *Hexadrol* (alcohol 5%); *Mymethasone* (alcohol 5%); GENERIC].

**Packaging and storage**
Store below 40 °C (104 °F), preferably between 15 and 30 °C (59 and 86 °F), unless otherwise specified by manufacturer. Store in a tight container. Protect from freezing.

**Auxiliary labeling**
• Keep container tightly closed.

### DEXAMETHASONE ORAL SOLUTION

**Usual adult and adolescent dose**
Oral, 500 mcg (0.5 mg) to 9 mg a day as a single dose or in divided doses.
Dexamethasone suppression test—
  Test for Cushing's syndrome: Oral, 1 mg as a single dose at 11:00 p.m. or 500 mcg (0.5 mg) every six hours for forty-eight hours.
  Test to distinguish Cushing's syndrome due to pituitary ACTH excess from Cushing's syndrome due to other causes: Oral, 2 mg every six hours for forty-eight hours.
  Depression diagnosis: Oral, 1 mg as a single dose at 11:00 p.m.
In cerebral edema associated with recurrent or inoperable brain tumor—
  Oral, 2 mg two or three times a day, administered as maintenance therapy after cerebral edema has initially been controlled using parenteral dexamethasone sodium phosphate.

**Usual pediatric dose**
Adrenocortical insufficiency—
  Oral, 23.3 mcg (0.0233 mg) per kg of body weight or 670 mcg (0.67 mg) per square meter of body surface a day in three divided doses.

Other indications—
  Oral, 83.3 to 333.3 mcg (0.0833 to 0.3333 mg) per kg of body weight or 2.5 to 10 mg per square meter of body surface a day in three or four divided doses.

**Strength(s) usually available**
U.S.—
  500 mcg (0.5 mg) per 5 mL (Rx) [GENERIC].
  1 mg per mL (Rx) [*Dexamethasone Intensol* (alcohol 30%)].

**Packaging and storage**
Store below 40 °C (104 °F), preferably between 15 and 30 °C (59 and 86 °F), in a well-closed container, unless otherwise specified by manufacturer. Protect from freezing.

## DEXAMETHASONE TABLETS USP

**Usual adult and adolescent dose**
Oral, 500 mcg (0.5 mg) to 9 mg a day as a single dose or in divided doses.
Dexamethasone suppression test—
  Test for Cushing's syndrome: Oral, 1 mg as a single dose at 11:00 p.m. or 500 mcg (0.5 mg) every six hours for forty-eight hours.
  Test to distinguish Cushing's syndrome due to pituitary ACTH excess from Cushing's syndrome due to other causes: Oral, 2 mg every six hours for forty-eight hours.
  Depression diagnosis: Oral, 1 mg as a single dose at 11:00 p.m.
In cerebral edema associated with recurrent or inoperable brain tumor—
  Oral, 2 mg two or three times a day, administered as maintenance therapy after cerebral edema has initially been controlled using parenteral dexamethasone sodium phosphate.

**Usual pediatric dose**
Adrenocortical insufficiency—
  Oral, 23.3 mcg (0.0233 mg) per kg of body weight or 670 mcg (0.67 mg) per square meter of body surface a day in three divided doses.
Other indications—
  Oral, 83.3 to 333.3 mcg (0.0833 to 0.3333 mg) per kg of body weight or 2.5 to 10 mg per square meter of body surface a day in three or four divided doses.

**Strength(s) usually available**
U.S.—
  250 mcg (0.25 mg) (Rx) [*Decadron* (scored); GENERIC].
  500 mcg (0.5 mg) (Rx) [*Decadron* (scored); *Dexone 0.5* (scored); *Hexadrol* (scored); GENERIC].
  750 mcg (0.75 mg) (Rx) [*Decadron* (scored); *Dexone 0.75* (scored); *Hexadrol* (scored); GENERIC].
  1 mg (Rx) [GENERIC (scored)].
  1.5 mg (Rx) [*Decadron* (scored); *Dexone 1.5* (scored); *Hexadrol* (scored); GENERIC].
  2 mg (Rx) [GENERIC (scored)].
  4 mg (Rx) [*Decadron* (scored); *Dexone 4* (scored); *Hexadrol* (scored); GENERIC].
  6 mg (Rx) [*Decadron* (scored); GENERIC].
Canada—
  500 mcg (0.5 mg) (Rx) [*Deronil* (scored); *Dexasone* (scored)].
  750 mcg (0.75 mg) (Rx) [*Deronil* (scored); *Dexasone* (scored)].
  4 mg (Rx) [*Deronil* (scored); *Dexasone* (scored); *Hexadrol* (scored); *Oradexon* (scored)].

**Packaging and storage**
Store below 40 °C (104 °F), preferably between 15 and 30 °C (59 and 86 °F). Store in a well-closed container.

# Parenteral Dosage Forms

Note: The dosing and strengths of the dosage forms available are expressed in terms of dexamethasone base.

## STERILE DEXAMETHASONE ACETATE SUSPENSION USP

**Usual adult and adolescent dose**
Intra-articular or soft-tissue injection, 4 to 16 mg of dexamethasone (base), repeated at one- to three-week intervals, if necessary.
Intralesional, 800 mcg (0.8 mg) to 1.6 mg of dexamethasone (base) per injection site, repeated as needed.
Intramuscular, 8 to 16 mg of dexamethasone (base), repeated at one- to three-week intervals, if necessary.

**Usual pediatric dose**
Dosage has not been established.

**Strength(s) usually available**
U.S.—
  8 mg (base) per mL (Rx) [*Dalalone L.A* (sodium bisulfite); *Decadron-LA* (sodium bisulfite 1 mg); *Decaject-L.A.* (sodium bisulfite); *Dexacen LA-8* (benzyl alcohol; sodium bisulfite); *Dexasone-LA*; *Dexone LA* (sodium bisulfite); *Solurex-LA* (sodium bisulfite); GENERIC].
  16 mg (base) per mL (Rx) [*Dalalone D.P.* (sodium bisulfite 1 mg)].

**Packaging and storage**
Store below 40 °C (104 °F), preferably between 15 and 30 °C (59 and 86 °F), unless otherwise specified by manufacturer. Protect from freezing.

**Stability**
This medication is heat-sensitive and should not be autoclaved.

**Auxiliary labeling**
• Shake well.

**Additional information**
For administration of injections, see manufacturer's labeling.
Do not administer this medication intravenously.
The suspension containing the equivalent of 16 mg of dexamethasone per mL is not for intralesional use.

## DEXAMETHASONE SODIUM PHOSPHATE INJECTION USP

**Usual adult and adolescent dose**
Intra-articular, intralesional, or soft-tissue injection, 200 mcg (0.2 mg) to 6 mg of dexamethasone (phosphate), repeated at three-day to three-week intervals, if necessary.
Intramuscular or intravenous, 500 mcg (0.5 mg) to 9 mg of dexamethasone (phosphate) a day.
For cerebral edema—
  Initial: Intravenous, 10 mg (phosphate), followed by 4 mg (phosphate) intramuscularly every six hours until symptoms subside. Dosage may be reduced after two to four days and gradually discontinued over a period of five to seven days, unless a brain tumor, which must be treated before dexamethasone can be discontinued, is present.
  Maintenance (for recurrent or inoperable brain tumors): Intramuscular, 2 mg (phosphate) two or three times a day initially, then adjusted according to patient response.
For shock—
  The following regimens have been utilized:
    Intravenous, 20 mg (phosphate) as a single dose initially, followed by 3 mg (phosphate) per kg of body weight per 24 hours via continuous intravenous infusion, or
    Intravenous, 2 to 6 mg (phosphate) per kg of body weight as a single injection, or
    Intravenous, 40 mg (phosphate) as a single dose, administered every two to six hours as needed, or
    Intravenous, 1 mg (phosphate) per kg of body weight as a single injection.
  Note: Administration of high-dose therapy for shock should be discontinued after the patient's condition has stabilized and is usually continued for no longer than two to three days.

**Usual adult prescribing limits**
80 mg daily.

**Usual pediatric dose**
Adrenocortical insufficiency—
  Intramuscular, 23.3 mcg (0.0233 mg) (phosphate) per kg of body weight or 670 mcg (0.67 mg) (phosphate) per square meter of body surface a day (in three divided doses) every third day; or 7.76 to 11.65 mcg (0.00776 to 0.01165 mg) (phosphate) per kg of body weight or 233 to 335 mcg (0.233 to 0.335 mg) (phosphate) per square meter of body surface once a day.
Other indications—
  Intramuscular, 27.76 to 166.65 mcg (0.02776 to 0.16665 mg) (phosphate) per kg of body weight or 0.833 to 5 mg (phosphate) per square meter of body surface every twelve to twenty-four hours.

**Strength(s) usually available**
U.S.—
  4 mg (phosphate) per mL (Rx) [*AK-Dex*; *Dalalone* (sodium bisulfite); *Decadrol*; *Decadron Phosphate* (sodium bisulfite 1 mg); *Decaject* (sodium bisulfite); *Dexacen-4* (sodium bisulfite); *Dexone* (sodium bisulfite); *Hexadrol Phosphate* (sodium sulfite 1 mg); *Solurex* (sodium bisulfite); GENERIC (sodium metabisulfite)].
  10 mg (phosphate) per mL (Rx) [*Hexadrol Phosphate* (sodium sulfite 1.5 mg); GENERIC (sodium metabisulfite)].
  20 mg (phosphate) per mL (Rx) [*Hexadrol Phosphate* (sodium sulfite 1.75 mg); GENERIC (sodium metabisulfite)].
  24 mg (phosphate) per mL (Rx) [*Decadron Phosphate* (sodium bisulfite 1 mg); GENERIC (sodium metabisulfite)].

Canada—
- 4 mg (phosphate) per mL (Rx) [*Decadron* (sodium bisulfite 1 mg) [GENERIC (sodium metabisulfite)].
- 10 mg (phosphate) per mL (Rx) [GENERIC (sodium metabisulfite)].

### Packaging and storage
Store below 40 °C (104 °F), preferably between 15 and 30 °C (59 and 86 °F), unless otherwise specified by manufacturer. Protect from light. Protect from freezing.

### Stability
This medication is heat-sensitive and should not be autoclaved.

### Additional information
For administration of injections, see manufacturer's labeling.
Dosage forms containing 24 mg (phosphate) per mL are for intravenous use only.

---

## HYDROCORTISONE

### Summary of Differences
Indications: See *Table 1*, 1015.
Pharmacology/pharmacokinetics: See *Table 2*, 1019 and *Table 3*, 1020.
General dosing information: See *Table 4*, 1020.

## Oral Dosage Forms

### HYDROCORTISONE TABLETS USP

**Usual adult and adolescent dose**
Oral, 20 to 240 mg a day as a single dose or in divided doses.

**Usual pediatric dose**
Adrenocortical insufficiency—
  Oral, 560 mcg (0.56 mg) per kg of body weight or 15 to 20 mg per square meter of body surface a day as a single dose or in divided doses.
Other indications—
  Oral, 2 to 8 mg per kg of body weight or 60 to 240 mg per square meter of body surface a day as a single dose or in divided doses.

**Strength(s) usually available**
U.S.—
- 5 mg (Rx) [*Cortef* (scored)].
- 10 mg (Rx) [*Cortef* (scored); *Hydrocortone* (scored); GENERIC].
- 20 mg (Rx) [*Cortef* (scored); *Hydrocortone* (scored); GENERIC (scored)].

Canada—
- 10 mg (Rx) [*Cortef* (scored)].
- 20 mg (Rx) [*Cortef* (scored)].

**Packaging and storage**
Store below 40 °C (104 °F), preferably between 15 and 30 °C (59 and 86 °F). Store in a well-closed container.

### HYDROCORTISONE CYPIONATE ORAL SUSPENSION USP

**Usual adult and adolescent dose**
Oral, 20 to 240 mg (base) a day as a single dose or in divided doses.

**Usual pediatric dose**
Adrenocortical insufficiency—
  Oral, 560 mcg (0.56 mg) (base) per kg of body weight or 15 to 20 mg per square meter of body surface a day as a single dose or in divided doses.
Other indications—
  Oral, 2 to 8 mg (base) per kg of body weight or 60 to 240 mg per square meter of body surface a day as a single dose or in divided doses.

**Strength(s) usually available**
U.S.—
- 10 mg (base) per 5 mL (Rx) [*Cortef*].

**Packaging and storage**
Store below 40 °C (104 °F), preferably between 15 and 30 °C (59 and 86 °F), unless otherwise specified by manufacturer. Store in a tight, light-resistant container. Protect from freezing.

**Auxiliary labeling**
- Shake well.

## Parenteral Dosage Forms

### STERILE HYDROCORTISONE SUSPENSION USP

**Usual adult and adolescent dose**
Intramuscular, 15 to 240 mg a day.

**Usual pediatric dose**
Adrenocortical insufficiency—
  Intramuscular, 560 mcg (0.56 mg) per kg of body weight or 30 to 37.5 mg per square meter of body surface a day every third day; or 186 to 280 mcg (0.186 to 0.28 mg) per kg of body weight or 10 to 12.5 mg per square meter of body surface once a day.
Other indications—
  Intramuscular, 666 mcg (0.666 mg) to 4 mg per kg of body weight or 20 to 120 mg per square meter of body surface every twelve to twenty-four hours.

**Strength(s) usually available**
U.S.—
- 25 mg per mL (Rx) [GENERIC].
- 50 mg per mL (Rx) [GENERIC].

**Packaging and storage**
Store below 40 °C (104 °F), preferably between 15 and 30 °C (59 and 86 °F), unless otherwise specified by manufacturer. Protect from freezing.

**Auxiliary labeling**
- Shake well.

**Additional information**
Do not administer this medication intravenously.

### STERILE HYDROCORTISONE ACETATE SUSPENSION USP

**Usual adult and adolescent dose**
Intra-articular, intralesional, or soft-tissue injection, 5 to 75 mg, repeated at two- to three-week intervals.

Note: Severe conditions may require doses at one-week intervals.

**Usual pediatric dose**
Dosage has not been established.

**Strength(s) usually available**
U.S.—
- 25 mg per mL (Rx) [*Hydrocortone Acetate*; GENERIC].
- 50 mg per mL (Rx) [*Hydrocortone Acetate*; GENERIC].

**Packaging and storage**
Store below 40 °C (104 °F), preferably between 15 and 30 °C (59 and 86 °F), unless otherwise specified by manufacturer. Protect from freezing.

**Stability**
For concurrent use of a parenteral-local anesthetic, withdraw the required quantity of corticosteroid suspension into a syringe, then add the local anesthetic. *Do not introduce the local anesthetic directly into the multiple-dose vial.* Also, inject the mixture immediately and discard any unused portion.
This medication is heat-sensitive and should not be autoclaved.

**Auxiliary labeling**
- Shake well.

**Additional information**
For administration of injections, see manufacturer's labeling.
Do not administer this medication intravenously.

### HYDROCORTISONE SODIUM PHOSPHATE INJECTION USP

**Usual adult and adolescent dose**
Intramuscular, intravenous, or subcutaneous, 100 to 500 mg (base); may be repeated every two to six hours, depending upon patient condition and response.

**Usual pediatric dose**
Adrenocortical insufficiency—
  Intramuscular or intravenous, 186 to 280 mcg (0.186 to 0.28 mg) (base) per kg of body weight or 10 to 12 mg (base) per square meter of body surface a day in three divided doses.
Other indications—
  Intramuscular, 666 mcg (0.666 mg) to 4 mg (base) per kg of body weight or 20 to 120 mg (base) per square meter of body surface every twelve to twenty-four hours.

**Strength(s) usually available**
U.S.—
- 50 mg (base) per mL (Rx) [*Hydrocortone Phosphate* (sodium bisulfite 3.2 mg); GENERIC (Quad—sodium metabisulfite 2 mg)].

**Packaging and storage**
Store below 40 °C (104 °F), preferably between 15 and 30 °C (59 and 86 °F), unless otherwise specified by manufacturer. Protect from freezing.

**Stability**
This medication is heat-sensitive and should not be autoclaved.

**Additional information**
For administration of injections, see manufacturer's labeling.

## HYDROCORTISONE SODIUM SUCCINATE FOR INJECTION USP

**Usual adult and adolescent dose**
Intramuscular or intravenous, 100 to 500 mg (base); may be repeated every two to six hours, depending upon patient condition and response.

Note: Initial intravenous dosage should be administered over a period of thirty seconds (100-mg dose) to ten minutes (doses 500 mg or higher).
Maintenance dosage (if required) should be no less than 25 mg per day.

**Usual pediatric dose**
Adrenocortical insufficiency—
Intramuscular or intravenous, 186 to 280 mcg (0.186 to 0.28 mg) (base) per kg of body weight or 10 to 12 mg (base) per square meter of body surface a day in three divided doses.
Other indications—
Intramuscular, 666 mcg (0.666 mg) to 4 mg (base) per kg of body weight or 20 to 120 mg (base) per square meter of body surface every twelve to twenty-four hours.

**Size(s) usually available**
U.S.—
    100 mg (base) (Rx) [*A-hydroCort; Solu-Cortef;* GENERIC].
    250 mg (base) (Rx) [*A-hydroCort; Solu-Cortef;* GENERIC].
    500 mg (base) (Rx) [*A-hydroCort; Solu-Cortef;* GENERIC].
    1 gram (base) (Rx) [*A-hydroCort; Solu-Cortef;* GENERIC].
Canada—
    100 mg (base) (Rx) [*Solu-Cortef*].
    250 mg (base) (Rx) [*Solu-Cortef*].
    500 mg (base) (Rx) [*Solu-Cortef*].
    1 gram (base) (Rx) [*Solu-Cortef*].

**Packaging and storage**
Store below 40 °C (104 °F), preferably between 15 and 30 °C (59 and 86 °F), unless otherwise specified by manufacturer.

**Stability**
Reconstituted solution should be used only if it is clear and should be discarded after 3 days.
After reconstitution, protect the solution from light.

**Additional information**
For preparation and administration of injections, see manufacturer's labeling.

---

## METHYLPREDNISOLONE

### Summary of Differences
Indications: See *Table 1*, 1015.
Pharmacology/pharmacokinetics: See *Table 2*, 1019 and *Table 3*, 1020.
General dosing information: See *Table 4*, 1020.

### Oral Dosage Forms

#### METHYLPREDNISOLONE TABLETS USP

**Usual adult and adolescent dose**
Oral, 4 to 48 mg a day as a single dose or in divided doses.
In multiple sclerosis—
Oral, 160 mg a day for one week, then 64 mg every other day for one month.

**Usual pediatric dose**
Adrenocortical insufficiency—
Oral, 117 mcg (0.117 mg) per kg of body weight or 3.33 mg per square meter of body surface a day in three divided doses.
Other indications—
Oral, 417 mcg (0.417 mg) to 1.67 mg per kg of body weight or 12.5 to 50 mg per square meter of body surface per day in three or four divided doses.

**Strength(s) usually available**
U.S.—
    2 mg (Rx) [*Medrol* (scored)].
    4 mg (Rx) [*Medrol* (scored); *Meprolone;* GENERIC].
    8 mg (Rx) [*Medrol* (scored)].
    16 mg (Rx) [*Medrol* (scored); GENERIC].
    24 mg (Rx) [*Medrol* (scored; tartrazine); GENERIC].
    32 mg (Rx) [*Medrol* (scored); GENERIC].
Canada—
    2 mg (Rx) [*Medrol* (scored)].
    4 mg (Rx) [*Medrol* (scored)].
    16 mg (Rx) [*Medrol* (scored)].

**Packaging and storage**
Store below 40 °C (104 °F), preferably between 15 and 30 °C (59 and 86 °F), unless otherwise specified by manufacturer. Store in a tight container.

### Parenteral Dosage Forms

Note: Bracketed uses in the *Dosage Forms* section refer to categories of use and/or indications that are not included in U.S. product labeling.

#### STERILE METHYLPREDNISOLONE ACETATE SUSPENSION USP

**Usual adult and adolescent dose**
Intra-articular, intralesional, or soft-tissue injection, 4 to 80 mg, repeated at one- to five-week intervals, if necessary.
Intramuscular, 40 to 120 mg, repeated at one-day to two-week intervals, if necessary.
For acute exacerbations of multiple sclerosis—
Intramuscular, 177.6 mg per day for one week, then 71 mg every other day for one month.

**Usual pediatric dose**
Adrenocortical insufficiency—
Intramuscular, 117 mcg (0.117 mg) per kg of body weight or 3.33 mg per square meter of body surface a day (in three divided doses) every third day; or 39 to 58.5 mcg (0.039 to 0.0585 mg) per kg of body weight or 1.11 to 1.66 mg per square meter of body surface once a day.
Other indications—
Intramuscular, 139 to 835 mcg (0.139 to 0.835 mg) per kg of body weight or 4.16 to 25 mg per square meter of body surface every twelve to twenty-four hours.

**Strength(s) usually available**
U.S.—
    20 mg per mL (Rx) [*Depo-Medrol;* GENERIC].
    40 mg per mL (Rx) [*depMedalone 40; Depoject-40; Depo-Medrol; Depopred-40; Depo-Predate 40; Duralone-40; Medralone-40; Rep-Pred 40;* GENERIC].
    80 mg per mL (Rx) [*depMedalone 80; Depoject-80; Depo-Medrol; Depopred-80; Depo-Predate 80; Duralone-80; Medralone-80; Rep-Pred 80;* GENERIC].
Canada—
    40 mg per mL (Rx) [*Depo-Medrol* (lidocaine 10 mg)].

**Packaging and storage**
Store below 40 °C (104 °F), preferably between 15 and 30 °C (59 and 86 °F), unless otherwise specified by manufacturer. Protect from freezing.

**Incompatibilities**
It is recommended that this medication not be diluted or mixed with other solutions because of possible physical incompatibility.

**Auxiliary labeling**
- Shake well.

**Additional information**
For preparation and administration of injections, see manufacturer's labeling.
Do not administer this medication intrathecally or intravenously.

#### METHYLPREDNISOLONE SODIUM SUCCINATE FOR INJECTION USP

**Usual adult and adolescent dose**
Intramuscular or intravenous, 10 to 40 mg (base), repeated as needed.
For high-dose ("pulse") therapy—
Intravenous, 30 mg (base) per kg of body weight administered over at least thirty minutes. This dose may be repeated every four to six hours as needed.
For acute exacerbations of multiple sclerosis—
Intramuscular or intravenous, 160 mg (base) per day for one week, followed by 64 mg every other day for one month.
[For treatment of acute spinal cord injury][1]—
Intravenous, 30 mg (base) per kg of body weight administered over fifteen minutes, followed in forty-five minutes by a continuous infusion of 5.4 mg per kg of body weight per hour, for twenty-three hours.
[For adjunctive treatment in AIDS-associated *Pneumocystis carinii* pneumonia][1]—
Intravenous, 30 mg (base) two times a day on days one through five, 30 mg once a day on days six through ten, and 15 mg once a day on days eleven through twenty-one.

**Usual pediatric dose**
Adrenocortical insufficiency—
Intramuscular, 117 mcg (0.117 mg) (base) per kg of body weight or

3.33 mg (base) per square meter of body surface a day (in three divided doses) every third day; or 39 to 58.5 mcg (0.039 to 0.0585 mg)(base) per kg of body weight or 1.11 to 1.66 mg (base) per square meter of body surface once a day.

[For treatment of acute spinal cord injury][1]—
    Intravenous, 30 mg (base) per kg of body weight administered over fifteen minutes, followed in forty-five minutes by a continuous infusion of 5.4 mg per kg of body weight per hour, for twenty-three hours.

Other indications—
    Intramuscular, 139 to 835 mcg (0.139 to 0.835 mg) (base) per kg of body weight or 4.16 to 25 mg (base) per square meter of body surface every twelve to twenty-four hours.

[For adjunctive treatment in AIDS-associated *Pneumocystis carinii* pneumonia][1]—
    Children 13 years of age and younger: Dosage has not been established.
    Children over 13 years of age: See *Usual adult and adolescent dose*.

### Size(s) usually available
U.S.—
- 40 mg (base) (Rx) [*A-methaPred; Solu-Medrol;* GENERIC].
- 125 mg (base) (Rx) [*A-methaPred; Solu-Medrol;* GENERIC].
- 500 mg (base) (Rx) [*A-methaPred; Solu-Medrol;* GENERIC].
- 1 gram (base) (Rx) [*A-methaPred; Solu-Medrol;* GENERIC].
- 2 grams (base) (Rx) [*Solu-Medrol*].

Canada:
- 40 mg (base) (Rx) [*Solu-Medrol*].
- 125 mg (base) (Rx) [*Solu-Medrol*].
- 500 mg (base) (Rx) [*Solu-Medrol*].
- 1 gram (base) (Rx) [*Solu-Medrol*].

### Packaging and storage
Store below 40 °C (104 °F), preferably between 15 and 30 °C (59 and 86 °F), unless otherwise specified by manufacturer.

### Stability
Use reconstituted solution within 48 hours. Do not use if solution is cloudy or contains a precipitate.

### Additional information
For preparation and administration of injections, see manufacturer's labeling.

When used intravenously, Methylprednisolone Sodium Succinate for Injection USP should be administered over a period of 1 to several minutes.

---

[1]Not included in Canadian product labeling.

---

## PREDNISOLONE

## Summary of Differences
Indications: See *Table 1*, 1015.
Pharmacology/pharmacokinetics: See *Table 2*, 1019 and *Table 3*, 1020.
General dosing information: See *Table 4*, 1020.

## Oral Dosage Forms

### PREDNISOLONE SYRUP USP

#### Usual adult and adolescent dose
Oral, 5 to 60 mg a day as a single dose or in divided doses.
For acute exacerbations of multiple sclerosis—
    Oral, 200 mg per day for one week, followed by 80 mg every other day for one month.

#### Usual adult prescribing limits
250 mg daily.

#### Usual pediatric dose
Adrenocortical insufficiency—
    Oral, 140 mcg (0.14 mg) per kg of body weight or 4 mg per square meter of body surface a day in three divided doses.
Other indications—
    Oral, 500 mcg (0.5 mg) to 2 mg per kg of body weight or 15 to 60 mg per square meter of body surface a day in three or four divided doses.

#### Strength(s) usually available
U.S.—
- 15 mg per 5 mL (Rx) [*Prelone* (alcohol 5%)].

#### Packaging and storage
Store below 40 °C (104 °F), preferably between 15 and 30 °C (59 and 86 °F), in a well-closed container, unless otherwise specified by manufacturer. Protect from freezing.

### PREDNISOLONE TABLETS USP

#### Usual adult and adolescent dose
Oral, 5 to 60 mg a day as a single dose or in divided doses.
For acute exacerbations of multiple sclerosis—
    Oral, 200 mg per day for one week, followed by 80 mg every other day for one month.

#### Usual adult prescribing limits
Oral, up to 250 mg a day.

#### Usual pediatric dose
Adrenocortical insufficiency—
    Oral, 140 mcg (0.14 mg) per kg of body weight or 4 mg per square meter of body surface a day in three divided doses.
Other indications—
    Oral, 500 mcg (0.5 mg) to 2 mg per kg of body weight or 15 to 60 mg per square meter of body surface a day in three or four divided doses.

#### Strength(s) usually available
U.S.—
- 5 mg (Rx) [*Delta-Cortef* (scored); GENERIC (scored)].

#### Packaging and storage
Store below 40 °C (104 °F), preferably between 15 and 30 °C (59 and 86 °F). Store in a well-closed container.

### PREDNISOLONE SODIUM PHOSPHATE ORAL SOLUTION

#### Usual adult and adolescent dose
Oral, 5 to 60 mg (base) a day as a single dose or in divided doses.
For acute exacerbations of multiple sclerosis—
    Oral, 200 mg (base) per day for one week, followed by 80 mg every other day for one month.

#### Usual adult prescribing limits
Oral, up to 250 mg (base) a day.

#### Usual pediatric dose
Adrenocortical insufficiency—
    Oral, 140 mcg (0.14 mg) (base) per kg of body weight or 4 mg per square meter of body surface a day in three divided doses.
Other indications—
    Oral, 500 mcg (0.5 mg) (base) to 2 mg per kg of body weight or 15 to 60 mg per square meter of body surface a day in three or four divided doses.

#### Strength(s) usually available
U.S.—
- 5 mg (base) per 5 mL (Rx) [*Pediapred*].

#### Packaging and storage
Store below 40 °C (104 °F), preferably between 15 and 30 °C (59 and 86 °F). Protect from freezing.

#### Auxiliary labeling
- Keep container tightly closed.

## Parenteral Dosage Forms

### STERILE PREDNISOLONE ACETATE SUSPENSION USP

#### Usual adult and adolescent dose
Intra-articular, intralesional, or soft-tissue injection, 4 to 100 mg, repeated as needed.
Intramuscular, 4 to 60 mg a day.

#### Usual pediatric dose
Adrenocortical insufficiency—
    Intramuscular, 140 mcg (0.14 mg) per kg of body weight or 4 mg per square meter of body surface a day (in three divided doses) every third day; or 46 to 70 mcg (0.046 to 0.07 mg) per kg of body weight or 1.33 to 2 mg per square meter of body surface once a day.
Other indications—
    Intramuscular, 166 mcg (0.166 mg) to 1 mg per kg of body weight or 5 to 30 mg per square meter of body surface every twelve to twenty-four hours.

#### Strength(s) usually available
U.S.—
- 25 mg per mL (Rx) [*Key-Pred 25; Predcor-25;* GENERIC].
- 50 mg per mL (Rx) [*Articulose-50; Key-Pred 50; Predaject-50; Predalone 50; Predate 50; Predcor-50; Predicort-50;* GENERIC].

#### Packaging and storage
Store below 40 °C (104 °F), preferably between 15 and 30 °C (59 and 86 °F), unless otherwise specified by manufacturer. Protect from freezing.

#### Auxiliary labeling
- Shake well.

### Additional information
Do not administer this medication intravenously.

### STERILE PREDNISOLONE ACETATE AND PREDNISOLONE SODIUM PHOSPHATE SUSPENSION

#### Usual adult and adolescent dose
Intra-articular, intramuscular, or intrasynovial, 20 to 80 mg of prednisolone acetate and 5 to 20 mg of prednisolone sodium phosphate, repeated at three-day to four-week intervals, if necessary.

#### Usual pediatric dose
Dosage has not been established.

#### Strength(s) usually available
U.S.—
    80 mg of prednisolone acetate and 20 mg of prednisolone sodium phosphate per mL (Rx) [GENERIC].

#### Packaging and storage
Store below 40 °C (104 °F), preferably between 15 and 30 °C (59 and 86 °F), unless otherwise specified by manufacturer. Protect from light. Protect from freezing.

#### Auxiliary labeling
- Shake well.

#### Additional information
Do not administer this medication intravenously.

### PREDNISOLONE SODIUM PHOSPHATE INJECTION USP

#### Usual adult and adolescent dose
Intra-articular, intralesional, or soft-tissue injection, 2 to 30 mg of prednisolone phosphate, repeated at three-day to three-week intervals, if necessary.
Intramuscular or intravenous, 4 to 60 mg of prednisolone phosphate a day.

#### Usual pediatric dose
Adrenocortical insufficiency—
    Intramuscular, 140 mcg (0.14 mg) (phosphate) per kg of body weight or 4 mg (phosphate) per square meter of body surface a day (in three divided doses) every third day; or 46 to 70 mcg (0.046 to 0.07 mg)(phosphate) per kg of body weight or 1.33 to 2 mg (phosphate) per square meter of body surface once a day.
Other indications—
    Intramuscular, 166 mcg (0.166 mg) to 1 mg (phosphate) per kg of body weight or 5 to 30 mg (phosphate) per square meter of body surface every twelve to twenty-four hours.

#### Strength(s) usually available
U.S.—
    20 mg (phosphate) per mL (Rx) [*Hydeltrasol* (sodium bisulfite 1 mg); *Key-Pred SP* (sodium bisulfite); *Predate S; Predicort-RP* (sodium bisulfite); GENERIC].

#### Packaging and storage
Store below 40 °C (104 °F), preferably between 15 and 30 °C (59 and 86 °F), unless otherwise specified by manufacturer. Protect from light. Protect from freezing.

#### Stability
This medication is heat-sensitive and should not be autoclaved.

#### Additional information
For preparation and administration of injections, see manufacturer's labeling.

### STERILE PREDNISOLONE TEBUTATE SUSPENSION USP

#### Usual adult and adolescent dose
Intra-articular, intralesional, or soft-tissue injection, 4 to 40 mg, repeated at two- to three-week intervals, if necessary.
Note: Severe conditions may require doses at one-week intervals.

#### Usual pediatric dose
Dosage has not been established.

#### Strength(s) usually available
U.S.—
    20 mg per mL (Rx) [*Hydelta T.B.A.; Nor-Pred T.B.A.; Predalone T.B.A.; Predate TBA.; Predcor-TBA.;* GENERIC].

#### Packaging and storage
Store below 40 °C (104 °F), preferably between 15 and 30 °C (59 and 86 °F), protected from light, unless otherwise specified by manufacturer. Protect from freezing.

#### Stability
For concurrent use of a parenteral-local anesthetic, withdraw the required quantity of corticosteroid suspension into a syringe, then add the local anesthetic. *Do not introduce the local anesthetic directly into the multiple-dose vial. Also, inject the mixture immediately and discard any unused portion.*
This medication is heat-sensitive and should not be autoclaved.

#### Auxiliary labeling
- Shake well.

#### Additional information
For preparation and administration of injections, see manufacturer's labeling.
Do not administer this medication intravenously.

---

## PREDNISONE

## Summary of Differences
Indications: See *Table 1*, 1015.
Pharmacology/pharmacokinetics: See *Table 2*, 1019 and *Table 3*, 1020.
General dosing information: See *Table 4*, 1020.

## Oral Dosage Forms
Note: Bracketed uses in the *Dosage Forms* section refer to categories of use and/or indications that are not included in U.S. product labeling.

### PREDNISONE ORAL SOLUTION USP

#### Usual adult and adolescent dose
    Oral, 5 to 60 mg a day as a single dose or in divided doses.
For acute exacerbations of multiple sclerosis—
    Oral, 200 mg a day for one week followed by 80 mg every other day for one month.
For adrenogenital syndrome—
    Oral, 5 to 10 mg a day as a single dose.
[For adjunctive treatment in AIDS-associated *Pneumocystis carinii* pneumonia][1]—
    Oral, 40 mg two times a day on days one through five, 40 mg once a day on days six through ten, and 20 mg once a day on days eleven through twenty-one.

#### Usual adult prescribing limits
250 mg daily.

#### Usual pediatric dose
For nephrosis—
    Children up to 18 months of age: Dosage has not been established.
    Children 18 months to 4 years of age: Oral, initially 7.5 to 10 mg four times a day.
    Children 4 to 10 years of age: Oral, initially 15 mg four times a day.
    Children 10 years of age and older: Oral, initially 20 mg four times a day.
For rheumatic carditis, leukemia, tumors—
    Oral, 500 mcg (0.5 mg) per kg of body weight or 15 mg per square meter of body surface four times a day for two to three weeks; then 375 mcg (0.375 mg) per kg of body weight or 11.25 mg per square meter of body surface four times a day for four to six weeks.
For tuberculosis (with concurrent antitubercular therapy)—
    Oral, 500 mcg (0.5 mg) per kg of body weight or 15 mg per square meter of body surface four times a day for two months.
    Note: Medication should be gradually discontinued.
For adrenogenital syndrome—
    Oral, 5 mg per square meter of body surface area a day in two divided doses.
[For adjunctive treatment in AIDS-associated *Pneumocystis carinii* pneumonia][1]—
    Children 13 years of age and younger: Dosage has not been established.
    Children over 13 years of age: See *Usual adult and adolescent dose*.

#### Strength(s) usually available
U.S.—
    5 mg per 5 mL (Rx) [GENERIC (alcohol 5%)].
    5 mg per mL (Rx) [*Predisone Intensol* (alcohol 30%)].

#### Packaging and storage
Store below 40 °C (104 °F), preferably between 15 and 30 °C (59 and 86 °F), in a light-resistant container, unless otherwise specified by manufacturer. Store in a tight container. Protect from freezing.

### PREDNISONE SYRUP USP

#### Usual adult and adolescent dose
    Oral, 5 to 60 mg a day as a single dose or in divided doses.

For acute exacerbations of multiple sclerosis—
    Oral, 200 mg a day for one week followed by 80 mg every other day for one month.
For adrenogenital syndrome—
    Oral, 5 to 10 mg a day as a single dose.
[For adjunctive treatment in AIDS-associated *Pneumocystis carinii* pneumonia][1]—
    Oral, 40 mg two times a day on days one through five, 40 mg once a day on days six through ten, and 20 mg once a day on days eleven through twenty-one.

**Usual adult prescribing limits**
250 mg daily.

**Usual pediatric dose**
For nephrosis—
    Children up to 18 months of age: Dosage has not been established.
    Children 18 months to 4 years of age: Oral, initially 7.5 to 10 mg four times a day.
    Children 4 to 10 years of age: Oral, initially 15 mg four times a day.
    Children 10 years of age and older: Oral, initially 20 mg four times a day.
For rheumatic carditis, leukemia, tumors—
    Oral, 500 mcg (0.5 mg) per kg of body weight or 15 mg per square meter of body surface four times a day for two to three weeks; then 375 mcg (0.375 mg) per kg of body weight or 11.25 mg per square meter of body surface four times a day for four to six weeks.
For tuberculosis (with concurrent antitubercular therapy)—
    Oral, 500 mcg (0.5 mg) per kg of body weight or 15 mg per square meter of body surface four times a day for two months.
    Note: Medication should be gradually discontinued.
For adrenogenital syndrome—
    Oral, 5 mg per square meter of body surface area a day in two divided doses.
[For adjunctive treatment in AIDS-associated *Pneumocystis carinii* pneumonia][1]—
    Children 13 years of age and younger: Dosage has not been established.
    Children over 13 years of age: See *Usual adult and adolescent dose*.

**Strength(s) usually available**
U.S.—
    5 mg per 5 mL (Rx) [*Liquid Pred* (alcohol 5%)].

**Packaging and storage**
Store below 40 °C (104 °F), preferably between 15 and 30 °C (59 and 86 °F), in a light-resistant container, unless otherwise specified by manufacturer. Store in a tight container. Protect from freezing.

### PREDNISONE TABLETS USP

**Usual adult and adolescent dose**
Oral, 5 to 60 mg a day as a single dose or in divided doses.
For acute exacerbations of multiple sclerosis—
    Oral, 200 mg per day for one week followed by 80 mg every other day for one month.
For adrenogenital syndrome—
    Oral, 5 to 10 mg a day as a single dose.
[For adjunctive treatment in AIDS-associated *Pneumocystis carinii* pneumonia][1]—
    Oral, 40 mg two times a day on days one through five, 40 mg once a day on days six through ten, and 20 mg once a day on days eleven through twenty-one.

**Usual adult prescribing limits**
250 mg daily.

**Usual pediatric dose**
For nephrosis—
    Children up to 18 months of age: Dosage has not been established.
    Children 18 months to 4 years of age: Oral, initially 7.5 to 10 mg four times a day.
    Children 4 to 10 years of age: Oral, initially 15 mg four times a day.
    Children 10 years of age and older: Oral, initially 20 mg four times a day.
For rheumatic carditis, leukemia, tumors—
    Oral, 500 mcg (0.5 mg) per kg of body weight or 15 mg per square meter of body surface four times a day for two to three weeks; then 375 mcg (0.375 mg) per kg of body weight or 11.25 mg per square meter of body surface four times a day for four to six weeks.
For tuberculosis (with concurrent antitubercular therapy)—
    Oral, 500 mcg (0.5 mg) per kg of body weight or 15 mg per square meter of body surface four times a day for two months.
    Note: Medication should be gradually discontinued.
For adrenogenital syndrome—
    Oral, 5 mg per square meter of body surface area a day in two divided doses.
[For adjunctive treatment in AIDS-associated *Pneumocystis carinii* pneumonia][1]—
    Children 13 years of age and younger: Dosage has not been established.
    Children over 13 years of age: See *Usual adult and adolescent dose*.

**Strength(s) usually available**
U.S.—
    1 mg (Rx) [*Meticorten; Orasone 1* (scored); GENERIC (scored)].
    2.5 mg (Rx) [*Deltasone* (scored); GENERIC (scored)].
    5 mg (Rx) [*Deltasone* (scored); *Orasone 5* (scored); *Prednicen-M* (scored); *Sterapred;* GENERIC (scored)].
    10 mg (Rx) [*Deltasone* (scored); *Orasone 10* (scored); *Sterapred DS* (scored); GENERIC (scored)].
    20 mg (Rx) [*Deltasone* (scored); *Orasone 20* (scored); GENERIC (scored)].
    25 mg (Rx) [GENERIC (scored)].
    50 mg (Rx) [*Deltasone* (scored); *Orasone 50* (scored); GENERIC (scored)].
Canada—
    1 mg (Rx) [*Apo-Prednisone* (scored); *Winpred*].
    5 mg (Rx) [*Apo-Prednisone* (scored); *Deltasone* (scored); *Winpred* (scored) [GENERIC (scored)].
    50 mg (Rx) [*Apo-Prednisone* (scored); *Deltasone* (scored)].

**Packaging and storage**
Store below 40 °C (104 °F), preferably between 15 and 30 °C (59 and 86 °F). Store in a well-closed container.

[1]Not included in Canadian product labeling.

---

### TRIAMCINOLONE

## Summary of Differences
Indications: See *Table 1*, 1015.
Pharmacology/pharmacokinetics: See *Table 2*, 1019 and *Table 3*, 1020.
General dosing information: See *Table 4*, 1020.

## Oral Dosage Forms
### TRIAMCINOLONE TABLETS USP

**Usual adult and adolescent dose**
Adrenocortical insufficiency—
    Oral, 4 to 12 mg a day as a single dose or in divided doses.
Other indications—
    Oral, 4 to 48 mg a day as a single dose or in divided doses.
    Note: In some patients (e.g., those with systemic lupus erythematosus, acute rheumatic carditis, or certain hematologic disorders), initial doses as high as 60 mg per day may be required.

**Usual pediatric dose**
Adrenocortical insufficiency—
    Oral, 117 mcg (0.117 mg) per kg of body weight or 3.3 mg per square meter of body surface a day as a single dose or in divided doses.
Other indications—
    Oral, 416 mcg (0.416 mg) to 1.7 mg per kg of body weight or 12.5 to 50 mg per square meter of body surface a day as a single dose or in divided doses.
    Note: Some pediatric patients with neoplastic disease (acute leukemia) may require initial doses as high as 2 mg per kg of body weight per day.

**Strength(s) usually available**
U.S.—
    1 mg (Rx) [*Aristocort* (scored)].
    2 mg (Rx) [*Aristocort* (scored)].
    4 mg (Rx) [*Aristocort* (scored); *Kenacort;* GENERIC].
    8 mg (Rx) [*Aristocort* (scored); *Kenacort* (scored; tartrazine)].
    16 mg (Rx) [*Aristocort* (scored)].
Canada—
    2 mg (Rx) [*Aristocort* (scored)].
    4 mg (Rx) [*Aristocort* (scored); *Kenacort* (scored)].

**Packaging and storage**
Store below 40 °C (104 °F), preferably between 15 and 30 °C (59 and 86 °F). Store in a well-closed container.

### TRIAMCINOLONE DIACETATE SYRUP USP

**Usual adult and adolescent dose**
Adrenocortical insufficiency—
    Oral, 4 to 12 mg (base) a day as a single dose or in divided doses.
Other indications—
    Oral, 4 to 48 mg (base) a day as a single dose or in divided doses.

**1014　Corticosteroids—Glucocorticoid Effects (Systemic)**　　*USP DI*

Note: After an initial response has been attained, this medication may be administered on an intermittent schedule. An example of this schedule is as follows: three or four days of medication followed by three medication-free days.

In some patients (e.g., those with systemic lupus erythematosus, acute rheumatic carditis, or certain hematologic disorders), initial doses as high as 60 mg (base) per day may be required.

### Usual pediatric dose
Adrenocortical insufficiency—
　Oral, 117 mcg (0.117 mg) (base) per kg of body weight or 3.3 mg per square meter of body surface a day as a single dose or in divided doses.
Other indications—
　Oral, 416 mcg (0.416 mg) to 1.7 mg (base) per kg of body weight or 12.5 to 50 mg per square meter of body surface a day as a single dose or in divided doses.

Note: Some pediatric patients with neoplastic disease (acute leukemia) may require initial doses as high as 2 mg (base) per kg of body weight per day.

### Strength(s) usually available
U.S.—
　2 mg (diacetate) per 5 mL (Rx) [*Aristocort*].
　4.85 mg anhydrous diacetate (4 mg base) per 5 mL (Rx) [*Kenacort Diacetate*].
Canada—
　2 mg (diacetate) per 5 mL (Rx) [*Aristocort*].

### Packaging and storage
Store below 40 °C (104 °F), preferably between 15 and 30 °C (59 and 86 °F), unless otherwise specified by manufacturer. Store in a tight, light-resistant container. Protect from freezing.

## Parenteral Dosage Forms
### STERILE TRIAMCINOLONE ACETONIDE SUSPENSION USP

#### Usual adult and adolescent dose
Intra-articular, intrabursal, or tendon-sheath injection, 2.5 to 15 mg.
Intradermal or intralesional, up to 1 mg per injection site, repeated at one-week or less frequent intervals, if necessary.
Intramuscular, 40 to 80 mg, repeated at four-week intervals, if necessary.

#### Usual pediatric dose
Children up to 6 years of age—
　Use is not recommended.
Children 6 to 12 years of age—
　Intra-articular, intrabursal, or tendon-sheath injection, 2.5 to 15 mg, repeated as needed.
　Intramuscular, 40 mg, repeated at four-week intervals if necessary; or 30 to 200 mcg (0.03 to 0.2 mg) per kg of body weight or 1 to 6.25 mg per square meter of body surface, repeated at one- to seven-day intervals.

#### Strength(s) usually available
U.S.—
　3 mg per mL (Rx) [*Tac-3*].
　10 mg per mL (Rx) [*Kenalog-10*].
　40 mg per mL (Rx) [*Cenocort A-40; Cinonide 40; Kenaject-40; Kenalog-40; Triam-A; Triamonide 40; Tri-Kort; Trilog;* GENERIC].
Canada—
　10 mg per mL (Rx) [*Kenalog-10*].
　40 mg per mL (Rx) [*Kenalog-40*].

#### Packaging and storage
Store below 40 °C (104 °F), preferably between 15 and 30 °C (59 and 86 °F), unless otherwise specified by manufacturer. Protect from light. Protect from freezing.

#### Auxiliary labeling
- Shake well.

#### Additional information
For preparation and administration of injections, see manufacturer's labeling.
Do not administer this medication intravenously.
Do not administer the 40-mg-per-mL strength intradermally or intralesionally.
Do not administer the 10-mg-per-mL strength intramuscularly.

### STERILE TRIAMCINOLONE DIACETATE SUSPENSION USP

#### Usual adult and adolescent dose
Intra-articular, intrasynovial, intralesional, sublesional, or soft-tissue injection, 3 to 48 mg, repeated at one- to eight-week intervals, if necessary.
Intramuscular, 40 mg once a week. Alternatively, a dose equal to four to seven times the predetermined oral daily dose may be administered as a single injection and repeated at four-day to four-week intervals as required.

#### Usual pediatric dose
Children up to 6 years of age—Use is not recommended.
Children 6 to 12 years of age—Intramuscular, 40 mg once a week.

#### Strength(s) usually available
U.S.—
　25 mg per mL (Rx) [*Aristocort Intralesional*].
　40 mg per mL (Rx) [*Amcort; Aristocort Forte; Articulose-L.A; Cenocort Forte; Cinalone 40; Triam-Forte; Triamolone 40 (benzyl alcohol); Trilone; Tristoject;* GENERIC].
Canada—
　25 mg per mL (Rx) [*Aristocort Intralesional*].
　40 mg per mL (Rx) [*Aristocort Forte* [GENERIC]].

#### Packaging and storage
Store below 40 °C (104 °F), preferably between 15 and 30 °C (59 and 86 °F), unless otherwise specified by manufacturer. Protect from freezing.

#### Stability
Admixtures containing local anesthetics will retain their potency for one full week.

#### Incompatibilities
This medication should *not* be mixed with parenteral-local anesthetic formulations containing preservatives such as parabens or phenol because flocculation of the corticosteroid may occur.

#### Auxiliary labeling
- Shake well.

#### Additional information
For preparation and administration of injections, see manufacturer's labeling.
Do not administer this medication intravenously.

### STERILE TRIAMCINOLONE HEXACETONIDE SUSPENSION USP

#### Usual adult and adolescent dose
Intra-articular, 2 to 20 mg, repeated at three- or four-week intervals, if necessary.
Intralesional or sublesional, up to 500 mcg (0.5 mg) per square inch of affected skin, repeated as needed.

#### Usual pediatric dose
Dosage has not been established.

#### Strength(s) usually available
U.S.—
　5 mg per mL (Rx) [*Aristospan Intralesional*].
　20 mg per mL (Rx) [*Aristospan Intra-articular*].
Canada—
　20 mg per mL (Rx) [*Aristospan Intra-articular*].

#### Packaging and storage
Store below 40 °C (104 °F), preferably between 15 and 30 °C (59 and 86 °F), unless otherwise specified by manufacturer. Protect from freezing.

#### Stability
Admixtures containing local anesthetics will retain their potency for one full week.

#### Incompatibilities
This medication should *not* be mixed with parenteral-local anesthetic formulations containing parabens, phenol, or other such preservatives because flocculation of the corticosteroid may occur.

#### Auxiliary labeling
- Shake well.

#### Additional information
For preparation and administration of injections, see manufacturer's labeling.
Do not administer this medication intravenously.
The 5-mg-per-mL strength is recommended for intralesional and sublesional injections only.
The 20-mg-per-mL strength is recommended for intra-articular injection only.

---

Revised: 04/14/92
Interim revision: 08/09/94; 04/01/96; 09/30/97

## Table 1. Indications

Note: Bracketed information refers to uses or routes that are not included in U.S. product labeling.

| Indication | Oral | IM; IV; SC† | Local‡ |
|---|---|---|---|
| **Adrenocortical function abnormalities** | | | |
| Adrenocortical insufficiency, acute (treatment)—Hydrocortisone and cortisone are preferred as replacement therapy because of their significant mineralocorticoid activity. Medication should be administered IV or by IM injection of a rapidly acting preparation initially. Replacement of sodium and fluids is also required. In some patients, additional mineralocorticoid replacement may also be necessary. | | ✓ | |
| Adrenocortical insufficiency, chronic primary (Addison's disease) (treatment)—Hydrocortisone and cortisone are preferred as replacement therapy for most patients because of their significant mineralocorticoid activity. Administration of sodium (as dietary salt) is recommended; however, additional mineralocorticoid supplementation may also be required in some patients. If a glucocorticoid other than hydrocortisone or cortisone is administered, mineralocorticoid supplementation is usually mandatory. Rarely, however, a patient will have only a glucocorticoid deficiency and will not require mineralocorticoid or sodium supplementation. | ✓ | ✓ | |
| Adrenocortical insufficiency, secondary (treatment)—Glucocorticoid replacement is usually sufficient; a mineralocorticoid is not always required. | ✓ | ✓ | |
| Adrenogenital syndrome (adrenal hyperplasia, congenital) (treatment)—Indicated to reduce virilization caused by enzyme deficiency–induced adrenal androgen hypersecretion. Corticosteroid and supplemental therapy depends upon the enzyme deficiency involved and form of disease present. In salt-losing forms, hydrocortisone or cortisone, plus increased sodium intake, may be preferred. However, additional mineralocorticoid supplementation may be required. In salt-retaining or hypertensive forms, a glucocorticoid having minimal mineralocorticoid activity is preferred. However, long-acting glucocorticoids are best avoided because of the increased risk of growth retardation and difficulty in dosage adjustment. | ✓ | ✓ | |
| Cushing's syndrome (diagnosis)—Dexamethasone is indicated in the diagnosis of Cushing's syndrome and to distinguish Cushing's syndrome caused by excessive corticotropin secretion from that due to other causes. | ✓ | ✓ | |
| **Allergic disorders**—Indicated for the treatment of severe or incapacitating allergic disorders intractable to adequate trials of conventional treatment, such as: | | | |
| Allergic reactions, drug-induced (treatment) | ✓ | ✓ | |
| Anaphylactic or anaphylactoid reactions (treatment adjunct)—Use of glucocorticoids is generally reserved for prolonged reactions (those not responding to other forms of treatment within 1 hour), reactions requiring cardiovascular or respiratory resuscitation, or situations in which there is a significant risk of relapse. Medication should be administered IV or by IM injection of a rapidly acting preparation initially. | ✓ | ✓ | |
| Angioedema (treatment adjunct)—Medication should be administered IV or by IM injection of a rapidly acting preparation initially. | ✓ | ✓ | |
| Laryngeal edema, acute noninfectious (treatment adjunct)—If a corticosteroid is used, it should be administered IV or by IM injection of a rapidly acting preparation initially. (Epinephrine is the drug of first choice) | ✓ | ✓ | |
| Rhinitis, allergic, perennial or seasonal, severe (treatment) | ✓ | ✓ | [✓][1] |
| Serum sickness (treatment) | ✓ | ✓ | |
| Transfusion reactions, urticarial (treatment)—Medication should be administered IV or by IM injection of a rapidly acting preparation initially. | | ✓ | |
| **Collagen disorders (treatment)**—Indicated during an acute exacerbation or as maintenance therapy in selected cases of: | | | |
| Carditis, rheumatic [or nonrheumatic][1], acute | ✓ | ✓ | |
| Dermatomyositis, systemic (polymyositis)—Glucocorticoids may be the treatment of choice in children with this condition. | ✓ | ✓ | |
| Lupus erythematosus, systemic | ✓ | ✓ | |
| [Arteritis, giant-cell (temporal)][1] | ✓ | ✓ | |
| [Connective tissue disease, mixed][1] | ✓ | ✓ | |
| [Polyarteritis nodosa][1] | ✓ | ✓ | |
| [Polychondritis, relapsing][1] | ✓ | ✓ | |
| [Polymyalgia rheumatica][1] | ✓ | ✓ | |
| [Vasculitis][1] | ✓ | ✓ | |

*Unless otherwise specified in text, any glucocorticoid may be administered, subject to availability of a dosage form suitable for the recommended route of administration.

†IM=intramuscular; IV=intravenous; SC=subcutaneous. See Table 4 for specific dosage forms.

‡Routes of local injection may include intra-articular, intrabursal, intralesional, intrasynovial, soft tissue, or [intranasal (intraturbinal)], depending on condition being treated. See Table 4 for specific dosage forms.

[1] Not included in Canadian product labeling.

# Table 1. Indications (continued)

Note: Bracketed information refers to uses or routes that are not included in U.S. product labeling.

| Indication | Oral | IM; IV; SC† | Local‡ |
|---|---|---|---|
| [Depression, mental, endogenous (diagnosis)][1]—Dexamethasone is used in diagnosing endogenous depression and in evaluating the efficacy of treatment. Dexamethasone reduces plasma cortisol to a greater extent in control subjects than in hospitalized patients with diagnosed depression; values return toward those of control subjects as the patient responds to therapy. However, the dexamethasone suppression test is less sensitive in patients with mild to moderate depression; also, many medications, medical problems, and other psychiatric disorders have been reported to interfere with the test results. The Health and Public Policy Committee of the American College of Physicians recommends that the dexamethasone suppression test not be used as a screening test for depression. | ✓ | | |
| **Dermatologic disorders (treatment)**—Indicated in the treatment of dermatologic disorders, such as: | | | |
|    Alopecia areata | | | ✓ |
|    Dermatitis, atopic | ✓ | ✓ | |
|    Dermatitis, contact | ✓ | ✓ | |
|    Dermatitis, exfoliative | ✓ | ✓ | |
|    Dermatitis herpetiformis, bullous | ✓ | ✓ | |
|    Dermatitis, seborrheic, severe | ✓ | ✓ | |
|    Dermatoses, inflammatory, severe | ✓ | ✓ | ✓ |
|    Erythema multiforme, severe (Stevens-Johnson syndrome) | ✓ | ✓ | |
|    Granuloma annulare | | | ✓ |
|    Keloids | | | ✓ |
|    Lichen planus | | | ✓ |
|    Lichen simplex chronicus | | | ✓ |
|    Lupus erythematosus, discoid | | | ✓ |
|    Mycosis fungoides | ✓ | ✓ | |
|    Necrobiosis lipoidica diabeticorum | | | ✓ |
|    Pemphigus | ✓ | ✓ | |
|    Psoriasis, severe | ✓ | ✓ | ✓ |
|    [Eczema, severe] | ✓ | | |
|    [Pemphigoid][1] | ✓ | ✓ | |
|    [Sarcoid, localized cutaneous][1] | | | ✓ |
| **Gastrointestinal disorders (treatment)**—Indicated in the treatment of inflammatory bowel disease as listed below. Oral or parenteral dosage forms are indicated when systemic therapy is required during a critical period of the disease; long-term use is not recommended. | | | |
|    Bowel disease, inflammatory, including colitis, ulcerative: | ✓ | ✓ | |
|    Enteritis, regional (Crohn's disease) | ✓ | ✓ | |
|    [Celiac disease, severe][1] | ✓ | ✓ | |
| **Hematologic disorders (treatment)**—Indicated in the treatment of: | | | |
|    Anemia, hemolytic, acquired (autoimmune) | ✓ | ✓ | |
|    Anemia, hypoplastic, congenital (erythroid) | ✓ | ✓ | |
|    Anemia, red blood cell (erythroblastopenia) | ✓ | ✓ | |
|    Thrombocytopenia, secondary, in adults | ✓ | ✓ | |
|    Thrombocytopenic purpura, idiopathic, in adults: Oral or IV only; IM injections are contraindicated. | ✓ | ✓ | |
|    [Hemolysis][1] | ✓ | ✓ | |
| **[Hepatic disease (treatment)][1]**—Although their use is controversial, methylprednisolone, prednisolone, and prednisone are used in the treatment of: | | | |
|    [Hepatitis, alcoholic, with encephalopathy][1] | ✓ | ✓ | |
|    [Hepatitis, chronic active][1] | ✓ | ✓ | |
|    [Hepatitis, nonalcoholic, in women][1] | ✓ | ✓ | |
|    [Necrosis, hepatic, subacute][1] | ✓ | ✓ | |
| **Hypercalcemia associated with neoplasms [or sarcoidosis][1] (treatment)** | ✓ | ✓ | |
| **Inflammation, nonrheumatic (treatment)**—Indicated during an acute episode or exacerbation of the disorders listed below. Local injections are preferred when only a few joints or areas are affected. | | | |
|    Bursitis, acute or subacute | ✓ | ✓ | ✓ |
|    Epicondylitis | ✓ | ✓ | ✓ |
|    Tenosynovitis, nonspecific acute | ✓ | ✓ | ✓ |

## Table 1. Indications (continued)

Note: Bracketed information refers to uses or routes that are not included in U.S. product labeling.

| Indication | Glucocorticoids* Oral | Glucocorticoids* IM; IV; SC† | Glucocorticoids* Local‡ |
|---|:---:|:---:|:---:|
| **[Nausea and vomiting, cancer chemotherapy–induced (prophylaxis)][1]**—Dexamethasone, hydrocortisone, and prednisone are used to prevent nausea and vomiting induced by antineoplastic agents. The medication is administered prior to and following each course of chemotherapy. However, the advisability of administering a potent glucocorticoid to a cancer patient, unless indicated for palliation of the disease, has been questioned. Although an increased incidence of infection has not been reported in patients receiving such therapy, the possibility must be considered. | ✓ | ✓ | |
| **Neoplastic disease**—Indicated in conjunction with appropriate specific antineoplastic disease therapy for the palliative management of the following neoplastic diseases and related problems: | | | |
| Leukemia, acute or chronic lymphocytic (treatment) | ✓ | ✓ | |
| Lymphomas, Hodgkin's or non-Hodgkin's (treatment) | ✓ | ✓ | |
| [Carcinoma, breast (treatment)][1] | ✓ | ✓ | |
| [Carcinoma, prostatic (treatment)][1] | ✓ | ✓ | |
| [Fever, due to malignancy (treatment adjunct)][1] | ✓ | ✓ | |
| [Multiple myeloma (treatment)][1] | ✓ | ✓ | |
| [Tumors, brain, primary (treatment adjunct)][1] | ✓ | ✓ | |
| Waldenström's macroglobulinemia (treatment) | ✓ | | |
| **Nephrotic syndrome (treatment)**—Indicated to induce diuresis or remission of proteinuria in idiopathic nephrotic syndrome (without uremia), and to improve renal function in patients with lupus erythematosus. In idiopathic nephrotic syndrome, long-term therapy may be required to prevent frequent relapses. | ✓ | ✓ | |
| **Neurologic disease** | | | |
| Meningitis, tuberculous (treatment adjunct)—Indicated for administration concurrently with appropriate antitubercular chemotherapy in patients with concurrent or impending subarachnoid block. | ✓ | ✓ | |
| Multiple sclerosis (treatment)[1]—Indicated for treatment of acute exacerbations of the disease. | ✓ | ✓ | |
| [Myasthenia gravis (treatment)][1]—Used for treatment of severe cases not controlled by antimyasthenic agents alone. Glucocorticoid therapy may be more effective following thymectomy and in patients having disease onset after age 40. Long-term therapy may be required. | ✓ | | |
| **Neurotrauma**— Note: Use in neurotrauma, except in conjunction with brain surgery and spinal cord injury, is controversial. Glucocorticoids are considered effective in preventing neurosurgery-associated cerebral edema and in treating edema caused by glioblastomas or metastatic brain tumors. They may be less effective in treating edema caused by astrocytomas or meningiomas. Beneficial effects in closed head injury or ischemic brain edema have not been established. Because very high doses are required, only those glucocorticoids having little or no mineralocorticoid activity should be used. | | | |
| Edema, cerebral, especially when associated with primary or metastatic brain tumor, craniotomy, or head injury ([prophylaxis and][1] treatment)—Dexamethasone (oral dosage forms and dexamethasone sodium phosphate injection) are indicated [and prednisone is used][1]. | ✓ | ✓ | |
| [Ischemia, cerebral (treatment)][1]—Dexamethasone is used. | ✓ | ✓ | |
| [Pseudotumor cerebri (treatment)][1]—Dexamethasone is used. | ✓ | ✓ | |
| [Spinal cord injury (treatment)][1]—Methylprednisolone is used. A large study concluded that patients receiving high-dose methylprednisolone therapy within 8 hours of acute spinal cord injury recover more motor and sensory function, as compared with those receiving placebo or naloxone. However, methylprednisolone did not improve patient prognosis when dosing was commenced more than 8 hours after spinal cord injury. | ✓ | ✓ | |
| **Ophthalmic disorders (treatment)**—Indicated in the treatment of severe acute or chronic allergic and inflammatory ophthalmic conditions, such as: | | | |
| Chorioretinitis | ✓ | ✓ | |
| Choroiditis, posterior, diffuse | ✓ | ✓ | |
| Conjunctivitis, allergic (not controlled topically) | ✓ | ✓ | |
| Herpes zoster | ✓ | ✓ | |
| Iridocyclitis | ✓ | ✓ | |
| Keratitis not associated with herpes simplex or fungal infection | ✓ | ✓ | |
| Neuritis, optic | ✓ | ✓ | |
| Ophthalmia sympathetic | ✓ | ✓ | |
| Uveitis, posterior, diffuse | ✓ | ✓ | |

*Unless otherwise specified in text, any glucocorticoid may be administered, subject to availability of a dosage form suitable for the recommended route of administration.

†IM=intramuscular; IV=intravenous; SC=subcutaneous. See Table 4 for specific dosage forms.

‡Routes of local injection may include intra-articular, intrabursal, intralesional, intrasynovial, soft tissue, or [intranasal (intraturbinal)], depending on condition being treated. See Table 4 for specific dosage forms.

[1] Not included in Canadian product labeling.

## Table 1. Indications *(continued)*

Note: Bracketed information refers to uses or routes that are not included in U.S. product labeling.

| Indication | Glucocorticoids* Oral | IM; IV; SC† | Local‡ |
|---|:---:|:---:|:---:|
| **[Oral disorders (treatment)][1]**—Systemic corticosteroids are indicated for treatment of oral lesions unresponsive to topical therapy. The presence of an oral herpetic lesion must be ruled out prior to initiation of glucocorticoid therapy. | | | |
| [Gingivitis, desquamative (when the diagnosis is confirmed via immunofluorescent biopsy assay)][1] | ✔ | | |
| [Lesions, oral, associated with corticosteroid-responsive disorders, such as systemic lupus erythematosus; discoid lupus erythematosus; pemphigus; pemphigoid; erythema multiforme, severe (Stevens-Johnson syndrome); and lichen planus][1] | ✔ | | |
| [Stomatitis, aphthous, recurrent (recurrent aphthous ulcers)][1] | ✔ | | |
| **[Pericarditis (treatment)][1]**—Used to relieve inflammation and fever | ✔ | ✔ | |
| **Polyps, nasal (treatment)**[1] | ✔ | ✔ | |
| **[Polyps, nasal, severe (treatment)][1]** | | | ✔ |
| **Respiratory disorders (treatment [and prophylaxis][1])**— | | | |
| [Prophylactic uses include administration prior to or during extracorporeal circulation in heart surgery if the patient has a pre-existing pulmonary disorder, and administration prior to, during, and following oral, facial, or neck surgery to prevent edema that may threaten the airway.][1] | | | |
| Indicated in the treatment of respiratory disorders, such as: | | | |
| Asthma, bronchial | ✔ | ✔ | |
| Berylliosis | ✔ | ✔ | |
| Loeffler syndrome (eosinophilic pneumonitis or hypereosinophilic syndrome) | ✔ | ✔ | |
| Pneumonitis, aspiration | ✔ | ✔ | |
| Sarcoidosis, symptomatic | ✔ | ✔ | |
| Tuberculosis, pulmonary, disseminated or fulminating (treatment adjunct): Administered concurrently with appropriate antituberculosis chemotherapy | ✔ | ✔ | |
| [Bronchitis, asthmatic, acute or chronic][1] | ✔ | ✔ | |
| [Edema, pulmonary, noncardiogenic (protamine sensitivity–induced)][1]—Medication should be administered IV or by IM injection of a rapidly acting preparation initially. | ✔ | ✔ | |
| [Hemangioma, airway-obstructing, in infants][1]—Medication should be administered IV or by IM injection of a rapidly acting preparation initially. | ✔ | ✔ | |
| [Pneumonia, *Pneumocystis carinii*, associated with immunodeficiency syndrome, acquired (treatment adjunct)][1]—In a small number of studies, early use of corticosteroids (e.g., corticosteroid therapy begun within 24 to 72 hours of initial antipneumocystis therapy) as an adjunct to specific antipneumocystis therapy was shown to significantly reduce the risk of oxygenation deterioration, respiratory failure, and death in patients being treated for moderate-to-severe AIDS-associated pneumocystis pneumonia. The specific corticosteroids used in these studies were prednisone and intravenous methylprednisolone. No improvement in clinical outcome was shown in another study when adjunctive corticosteroid therapy was begun after the onset of respiratory failure and after the initiation of primary antipneumocystis therapy. Therefore, if adjunctive corticosteroid therapy is used, it should be started at the initiation of primary therapy for pneumocystis pneumonia in adults and children over 13 years of age who have documented or suspected HIV infection and documented or suspected pneumocystis pneumonia, accompanied by moderate-to-severe pulmonary dysfunction (PaO$_2$ < 70 mm Hg on room air or A-a gradient > 35 mm Hg). The diagnosis of HIV infection and pneumocystis pneumonia should be confirmed as soon as possible. | ✔ | ✔ | |
| [Pulmonary disease, chronic obstructive (not controlled with theophylline and beta-adrenergic agonists)] | ✔ | ✔ | |
| [Status asthmaticus]—Medication should be administered IV or by IM injection of a rapidly acting preparation initially. | | ✔ | |
| **[Respiratory distress syndrome, neonatal (prophylaxis)][1]**—Betamethasone, dexamethasone, and hydrocortisone are used to reduce the incidence and severity of respiratory distress syndrome (hyaline membrane disease) in premature neonates. Long-acting agents (betamethasone or dexamethasone) are preferred. The medication is administered to the mother, preferably 24 to 48 hours prior to delivery to allow time for it to produce an effect. Corticosteroids will not be effective when delivery is imminent. If necessary, ritodrine may be administered to delay delivery. If delivery does not occur within several days to 1 week following corticosteroid administration, but the risk of premature delivery persists, administration of a second course of corticosteroid therapy may be necessary. Glucocorticoids are not effective in the treatment of respiratory distress syndrome in the premature neonate. | | ✔ | |
| **[Respiratory distress syndrome, adult (treatment)][1]**—Dexamethasone is used in the treatment of respiratory distress syndrome in adults, especially those with post-traumatic pulmonary insufficiency or burns, and during or following massive blood transfusions. However, the benefits of such treatment have not been established. | | ✔ | |
| **Rheumatic disorders (treatment)**— | | | |
| Note: Local injections are preferred when only a few joints or areas are involved. | | | |
| Indicated as adjunctive therapy during an acute episode or exacerbation of rheumatic disorders, such as: | | | |
| Ankylosing spondylitis | ✔ | ✔ | |
| Arthritis, psoriatic | ✔ | ✔ | ✔ |
| Arthritis, rheumatoid (including juvenile arthritis): [Long-term use in the treatment of rheumatoid arthritis is controversial. It is recommended that such treatment be reserved for patients not responsive to other measures, such as aspirin or other nonsteroidal anti-inflammatory drugs, rest, and physical therapy.][1] | ✔ | ✔ | ✔ |

## Table 1. Indications (continued)

Note: Bracketed information refers to uses or routes that are not included in U.S. product labeling.

| Indication | Oral | IM; IV; SC† | Local‡ |
|---|---|---|---|
| Gouty arthritis, acute | ✔ | ✔ | ✔ |
| Osteoarthritis, post-traumatic | ✔ | ✔ | ✔ |
| Synovitis of osteoarthritis | ✔ | ✔ | ✔ |
| [Calcium pyrophosphate deposition disease, acute (pseudogout; chondrocalcinosis articularis; synovitis, crystal-induced)][1] | ✔ | ✔ | ✔ |
| [Polymyalgia rheumatica][1] | ✔ | ✔ | |
| [Reiter's disease][1] | ✔ | ✔ | |
| [Rheumatic fever (especially if carditis is present)] | ✔ | ✔ | |
| **Shock (treatment)**—Glucocorticoids are indicated in the treatment of shock caused by adrenocortical insufficiency (Addisonian shock) and as adjuncts in treating shock associated with anaphylactic or anaphylactoid reactions. Medication should be administered IV or by IM injection of a rapidly acting preparation initially.<br>[Intravenous glucocorticoids are also being used as adjuncts in the treatment of septic shock. Such use is very controversial because efficacy has not been established and superimposition of new infections has been reported. Specifically, methylprednisolone has been shown to be ineffective, and hazardous, in the treatment of septic shock and is not recommended.] | ✔ | ✔<br><br>✔ | |
| **Thyroiditis, nonsuppurative (treatment)** | ✔ | ✔ | |
| [**Transplant rejection, organ (prophylaxis and treatment)**][1]—Indicated concurrently with other immunosuppressants such as azathioprine or cyclosporine to reduce the risk of rejection of transplanted organs.<br>[High doses of rapidly acting corticosteroids are also indicated in the treatment of rejection reactions.][1] | ✔ | ✔<br><br>✔ | |
| **Trichinosis (treatment)**—Indicated for the treatment of trichinosis with neurological or myocardial involvement. | ✔ | ✔ | |
| **Tumors, cystic, of a tendon or aponeurosis (treatment)** | | | ✔ |

*Unless otherwise specified in text, any glucocorticoid may be administered, subject to availability of a dosage form suitable for the recommended route of administration.
†IM=intramuscular; IV=intravenous; SC=subcutaneous. See Table 4 for specific dosage forms.
‡Routes of local injection may include intra-articular, intrabursal, intralesional, intrasynovial, soft tissue, or [intranasal (intraturbinal)], depending on condition being treated. See Table 4 for specific dosage forms.
[1] Not included in Canadian product labeling.

## Table 2. Pharmacology/Pharmacokinetics*

| Drug and Route | Onset of Action | Peak Effect | Duration of Action | Drug and Route | Onset of Action | Peak Effect | Duration of Action |
|---|---|---|---|---|---|---|---|
| Betamethasone | | | | Hydrocortisone | | | |
|   Oral | | 1–2 hr | 3.25 days |   Oral | | 1 hr | 1.25–1.5 days |
|   Sodium phosphate | | | |   IM | | 4–8 hr | |
|     IV | Rapid | | |   Acetate | | | |
|     IM | Rapid | | |     IA, IS, IB, IL, ST | | 24–48 hr | 3 days–4 wk |
|   Acetate/Sodium phosphate | | | |   Cypionate | | | |
|     IM | 1–3 hr | | 1 wk |     Oral | Slower than tablet | 1–2 hr | |
|     IA, IS | | | 1–2 wk |   Sodium phosphate | | | |
|     IL, ST | | | 1 wk |     IV | Rapid | | |
| Cortisone acetate | | | |     IM | Rapid | 1 hr | |
|   Oral | Rapid | 2 hr | 1.25–1.5 days |   Sodium succinate | | | |
|   IM | Slow | 20–48 hr | |     IV | Rapid | | |
| Dexamethasone | | | |     IM | Rapid | 1 hr | Variable |
|   Oral | | 1–2 hr | 2.75 days | | | | |
|   Acetate | | | | | | | |
|     IM | | 8 hr | 6 days | | | | |
|     IA, ST, IL | | | 1–3 wk | | | | |
|   Sodium phosphate | | | | | | | |
|     IV | Rapid | | | | | | |
|     IM | Rapid | | | | | | |
|     IA, IS, IL, ST | | | 3 days–3 wk | | | | |

*Abbreviations: IA=intra-articular; IB=intrabursal; IL=intralesional; IM=intramuscular; IS=intrasynovial; ST=soft tissue.

## Table 2. Pharmacology/Pharmacokinetics* (continued)

| Drug and Route | Onset of Action | Peak Effect | Duration of Action |
|---|---|---|---|
| Methylprednisolone | | | |
|   Oral | | 1–2 hr | 1.25–1.5 days |
|  Acetate | | | |
|   IM | Slow 6–48 hr | 4–8 days | 1–4 wk |
|   IA, IL, ST | Very slow | 7 days | 1–5 wk |
|  Sodium succinate | | | |
|   IV | Rapid | | |
|   IM | Rapid | | |
| Prednisolone | | | |
|   Oral | | 1–2 hr | 1.25–1.5 days |
|  Acetate | | | |
|   IM | Slow | | |
|  Acetate/Sodium phosphate | | | |
|   IM | | | Up to 4 wk |
|   IB, IS, IA, ST | | | 3 days–4 wk |
|  Sodium phosphate | | | |
|   IV | Rapid | 1 hr | |
|   IM | Rapid | 1 hr | |
|   IA, IL, ST | | | 3 days–3 wk |
|  Tebutate | | | |
|   IA, IL, ST | Slow 1–2 days | | 1–3 wk |

| Drug and Route | Onset of Action | Peak Effect | Duration of Action |
|---|---|---|---|
| Prednisone | | | |
|   Oral | | 1–2 hr | 1.25–1.5 days |
| Triamcinolone | | | |
|   Oral | | 1–2 hr | 2.25 days |
|  Acetonide | | | |
|   IM | Slow 24–48 hr | | 1–6 wk |
|   IB, IA, IS, IL, ST | | | Several wk |
|  Diacetate | | | |
|   Oral | | 1–2 hr | |
|   IM | Slow | | 4 days–4 wk |
|   IL | | | 1–2 wk |
|   IA, IS, ST | | | 1–8 wk |
|  Hexacetonide | | | |
|   IA, IL | | | 3–4 wk |

*Abbreviations: IA=intra-articular; IB=intrabursal; IL=intralesional; IM=intramuscular; IS=intrasynovial; ST=soft tissue.

## Table 3. Pharmacology/Pharmacokinetics

| | Relative Potency | | | Protein Binding§ | Half-life (hr) | |
|---|---|---|---|---|---|---|
| | Glucocorticoid Dose (mg)* | Glucocorticoid Activity† | Mineralocorticoid Activity‡ | | Plasma | Biological (Tissue) |
| **Corticosteroids** | | | | | | |
| *Short-acting* | | | | | | |
|  Cortisone | 25 | 0.8 | 2+ | Very high | 0.5 | 8–12 |
|  Hydrocortisone | 20 | 1 | 2+ | | 1.5–2 | 8–12 |
| *Intermediate-acting* | | | | | | |
|  Methylprednisolone | 4 | 5 | 0# | | >3.5 | 18–36 |
|  Prednisolone | 5 | 4 | 1+ | High | 2.1–3.5 | 18–36 |
|  Prednisone | 5 | 4 | 1+ | High to very high | 3.4–3.8 | 18–36 |
|  Triamcinolone | 4 | 5 | 0# | High | 2–>5 | 18–36 |
| *Long-acting* | | | | | | |
|  Betamethasone | 0.6 | 20–30 | 0# | High | 3–5 | 36–54 |
|  Dexamethasone | 0.5–0.75 | 20–30 | 0# | High | 3–4.5 | 36–54 |

*Approximate; applies to oral or intravenous administration only.
†Anti-inflammatory, immunosuppressant, metabolic effects.
‡Sodium and water retention, potassium depletion.
§Hydrocortisone binds to transcortin (corticosteroid binding globulin; CBG) and to albumin. Prednisone, but not betamethasone, dexamethasone, or triamcinolone, also binds to CBG.
#Although these glucocorticoids are considered not to have significant mineralocorticoid activity, hypokalemia and/or sodium and fluid retention may occur, depending on dosage and patient predisposition.

## Table 4. General Dosing Information*

| Drug | Parenteral Routes of Administration† | | | | | | | | |
|---|---|---|---|---|---|---|---|---|---|
| | Systemic | | | Local | | | | | |
| | IM | IV | SC | IA | IB | IL | IS | ST | [IT][1] |
| **Betamethasone** | | | | | | | | | |
|  Sodium phosphate | ✓ | ✓ | | ✓ | | ✓ | | ✓ | |
|  Acetate/Sodium phosphate | ✓ | | | ✓ | | ✓ | ✓ | ✓ | |
| **Cortisone Acetate** | ✓ | | | | | | | | |
| **Dexamethasone** | | | | | | | | | |
|  Acetate | ✓ | | | ✓ | | ✓ | | ✓ | |
|  Sodium phosphate | ✓ | ✓ | | ✓ | | ✓ | ✓ | ✓ | |
| **Hydrocortisone** | | | | | | | | | |
|  Sterile suspension | ✓ | | | | | | | | |
|  Acetate | | | | ✓ | ✓ | ✓ | ✓ | ✓ | |

## Table 4. General Dosing Information* *(continued)*

| Drug | Parenteral Routes of Administration† |||||||||
|---|---|---|---|---|---|---|---|---|---|
| | Systemic ||| Local ||||||
| | IM | IV | SC | IA | IB | IL | IS | ST | [IT][1] |
| Sodium phosphate | ✔ | ✔ | ✔ | | | | | | |
| Sodium succinate | ✔ | ✔ | | | | | | | |
| Methylprednisolone | | | | | | | | | |
|   Acetate | ✔ | | | ✔ | | | ✔ | ✔ | |
|   Sodium succinate | ✔ | ✔ | | | | | | | |
| Prednisolone | | | | | | | | | |
|   Acetate | ✔ | | | | | | | | |
|   Acetate/Sodium phosphate | | | | ✔ | ✔ | | ✔ | ✔ | |
|   Sodium phosphate | ✔ | ✔ | | ✔ | | ✔ | ✔ | | |
|   Tebutate | | | | ✔ | | | | ✔ | [✔][1] |
| Triamcinolone | | | | | | | | | |
|   Acetonide | ✔ | | | ✔ | ✔ | ✔ | | | [✔][1] |
|   Diacetate | ✔ | | | ✔ | | ✔ | ✔ | ✔ | [✔][1] |
|   Hexacetonide | | | | ✔ | ✔ | | | | [✔][1] |

*Bracketed information refers to routes of administration that are not included in U.S. product labeling.
†Abbreviations: Systemic—IM=intramuscular; IV=intravenous; SC=subcutaneous. Local—IA=intra-articular; IB=intrabursal; IL=intralesional; IS=intrasynovial; ST=soft tissue; IT=intraturbinal.
[1]Not included in Canadian product labeling.

# CORTICOTROPIN Systemic

VA CLASSIFICATION (Primary):
  Corticotropin for Injection—DX900
  Repository Corticotropin—CN400

Commonly used brand name(s): *ACTH; Acthar; Acthar Gel (H.P.); Acthar Powder; H.P. Acthar Gel.*

Another commonly used name is ACTH.

Note: For a listing of dosage forms and brand names by country availability, see *Dosage Forms* section(s).

## Category

Diagnostic aid (adrenocortical function)—Corticotropin for Injection USP.
Anticonvulsant (specific in infantile myoclonic seizures)—Repository Corticotropin Injection USP.

## Indications

Note: Bracketed information in the *Indications* section refers to uses that are not included in U.S. product labeling.

**Accepted**

Adrenocortical insufficiency (diagnosis)—Corticotropin for injection is indicated as an aid in diagnosing adrenocortical insufficiency; however, the synthetic fragment of corticotropin, cosyntropin, is the preferred diagnostic aid because it is less antigenic. Additionally, corticotropin is purified from animal pituitary glands and can contain significant amounts of vasopressin and other peptides, which are not found in cosyntropin.

[Seizures, myoclonic, infantile (treatment)][1]—Repository corticotropin is used in the treatment of infantile myoclonic seizures (infantile spasms), although there are only limited data suggesting that it has greater efficacy than do glucocorticoids.

**Unaccepted**

Corticotropin is no longer recommended for its anti-inflammatory and immunosuppressant properties. Although corticotropin is FDA-approved for the treatment of secondary adrenocortical insufficiency and many nonendocrine disorders that are responsive to glucocorticoid therapy, treatment with a corticosteroid is preferred.

[1]Not included in Canadian product labeling.

## Pharmacology/Pharmacokinetics

**Physicochemical characteristics**
Hormone; obtained from porcine pituitary glands.

**Mechanism of action/Effect**
Diagnostic aid (adrenocortical function)—Corticotropin combines with a specific receptor on the adrenal cell plasma membrane. In patients with normal adrenocortical function, it stimulates the initial reaction involved in the synthesis of adrenal steroids (including cortisol, cortisone, weak androgenic substances, and a limited quantity of aldosterone) from cholesterol by increasing the quantity of cholesterol within the mitochondria. Corticotropin does *not* significantly increase serum cortisol concentrations in patients with primary adrenocortical insufficiency (Addison's disease).

Anticonvulsant (specific in infantile myoclonic seizures)—The mechanism of action of corticotropin in the treatment of infantile myoclonic seizures is unknown.

**Other actions/effects**
Corticotropin is not a corticosteroid. However, it shares many actions of the corticosteroids due to its ability to increase endogenous corticosteroid synthesis.

**Absorption**
Corticotropin is rapidly absorbed following intramuscular administration; the repository dosage form is slowly absorbed over approximately 8 to 16 hours.

**Half-life**
About 15 minutes following intravenous administration.

**Time to peak effect**
Peak plasma cortisol concentrations are usually achieved within 1 hour after intramuscular or rapid intravenous administration of corticotropin for injection.

**Duration of action**
Following intramuscular or rapid intravenous administration of corticotropin, peak plasma cortisol concentrations begin to decrease after 2 to 4 hours.
The effects of repository corticotropin may last up to 3 days.

## Precautions to Consider

**Cross-sensitivity and/or related problems**
Patients allergic to proteins of porcine origin or cosyntropin may also be allergic to corticotropin.

**Carcinogenicity**
Adequate and well-controlled animal studies have not been done in animals; however, use in humans has not shown an increase in malignant disease.

**Pregnancy/Reproduction**
Fertility—Studies have not been done in humans or in animals.
Pregnancy—Adequate and well-controlled studies have not been done in humans.
Studies in animals have shown that corticotropin is embryocidal.
FDA Pregnancy Category C.

**Breast-feeding**
It is not known whether corticotropin is distributed into breast milk. However, problems in humans have not been documented.

## Corticotropin (Systemic)

**Pediatrics**
Appropriate studies performed to date using corticotropin have not demonstrated pediatrics-specific problems that would limit the usefulness of corticotropin in children. However, prolonged use of corticotropin in children will inhibit skeletal growth; therefore, close monitoring is recommended.

**Geriatrics**
Appropriate studies performed to date using corticotropin have not demonstrated geriatrics-specific problems that would limit the usefulness of corticotropin in the elderly.

**Drug interactions and/or related problems**
The following drug interactions and/or related problems have been selected on the basis of their potential clinical significance (possible mechanism in parentheses where appropriate)—not necessarily inclusive (» = major clinical significance):

Note: Combinations containing any of the following medications, depending on the amount present, may also interact with this medication.

Estrogens
(estrogen may cause abnormally high plasma cortisol concentrations before and after corticotropin administration; however, a normal incremental response to corticotropin still occurs)

» Immunizations
(during chronic therapy, patients should not be vaccinated against smallpox; extreme caution is recommended if other immunizations are to be given, because of the risk of neurological complications and lack of antibody response)

Verapamil
(limited data show that chronic administration of oral verapamil may blunt the effect of corticotropin, resulting in a false negative diagnostic test result)

**Laboratory value alterations**
The following have been selected on the basis of their potential clinical significance (possible effect in parentheses where appropriate)—not necessarily inclusive (» = major clinical significance):
With results of adrenocortical function testing
*Due to other medications*
» Corticosteroids, glucocorticoid
(if competitive protein binding assays or immunoassays showing cross-reactivity with prednisone or cortisone are used, a high baseline cortisol concentration with no response to corticotropin may be seen in patients taking these medications)

**Medical considerations/Contraindications**
The medical considerations/contraindications included have been selected on the basis of their potential clinical significance (reasons given in parentheses where appropriate)—not necessarily inclusive (» = major clinical significance).

*Except under special circumstances, this medication should not be used when the following medical problems exist:*
» Infections, serious bacterial or viral, especially varicella
(possible immunosupression may lead to infectious complications with chronic use)

*Risk-benefit should be considered when the following medical problems exist:*
» Allergy to corticotropin, cosyntropin, or porcine derivatives
(risk of allergic reaction)

**Patient monitoring**
The following may be especially important in patient monitoring (other tests may be warranted in some patients, depending on condition; » = major clinical significance):

*For treatment of infantile myoclonic seizures*
» Blood pressure and
» Calcium, serum and
» Electroencephalogram, waking and sleeping and
» Electrolytes, serum and
» Glucose, urine and
» Phosphorus, serum and
» Urinalysis and
» Weight
(recommended at periodic intervals during therapy to assess therapeutic and/or adverse effects)

» Calcium, serum and
» Complete blood count and
» Electrolytes, serum and
» Endocrine profile and
» Glucose, serum, fasting and 2-hour postprandial and
» Phosphorus, serum, and
» Renal function tests and
» Urinalysis
(recommended prior to initiation of therapy; caution in using corticotropin is recommended if any of these tests are abnormal)

## Side/Adverse Effects

Note: Except for rare allergic reactions, there are no side/adverse effects associated with the use of corticotropin as a diagnostic aid.

The following side/adverse effects have been selected on the basis of their potential clinical significance (possible signs and symptoms in parentheses where appropriate)—not necessarily inclusive:

**Those indicating need for medical attention**
Incidence less frequent—with chronic use only
*Cerebral ventriculomegaly; congestive heart failure; hyperglycemia; hypertension; hypothalamic-pituitary suppression; metabolic abnormalities, such as; hypernatremia; hypokalemia; hypocalcemia; hypophosphatemia; sepsis*
Incidence rare
*Allergic reaction* (dizziness; nausea and vomiting; shock; skin rash); *worsening of seizures*—with chronic use only

**Those indicating need for medical attention only if they continue or are bothersome**
Incidence more frequent—with chronic use only
*Irritability, extreme*

**Those not indicating need for medical attention**
Incidence more frequent—with chronic use only
*Cushingoid facies; cutaneous pigmentation; hirsutism; seborrheic dermatitis*

## General Dosing Information

Following administration of corticotropin as a diagnostic agent, adrenal insufficiency can be confirmed when a plasma, serum, or urinary free cortisol concentration does not increase above a baseline concentration.

During chronic therapy of infantile myoclonic seizures, patients should not be vaccinated against smallpox. Extreme caution is recommended if other immunizations are to be given, because of the risk of neurological complications and lack of antibody response.

**For treatment of adverse effects**
Recommended treatment for hypertension that may develop during treatment of infantile spasms consists of sodium restriction and diuretic therapy rather than discontinuation of corticotropin.

## Parenteral Dosage Forms

Note: Bracketed uses in the *Dosage Forms* section refer to categories of use and/or indications that are not included in U.S. product labeling.

### CORTICOTROPIN FOR INJECTION USP

**Usual adult and adolescent dose**
Adrenocortical insufficiency (diagnosis)—
Intravenous infusion, 10 to 25 Units in 500 mL of 5% dextrose in water, infused over an eight-hour period.

**Usual pediatric dose**
Adrenocortical insufficiency (diagnosis)—
Use is not recommended. The synthetic fragment of corticotropin, cosyntropin, is the recommended diagnostic agent.
[Seizures, myoclonic, infantile (treatment)][1]—
Use is not recommended. Repository corticotropin injection USP is the preferred product.

**Size(s) usually available**
U.S.—
25 USP Units per vial (Rx) [*Acthar*].
40 USP Units per vial (Rx) [*ACTH; Acthar* [GENERIC]].
Canada—
40 IU per vial (Rx) [*Acthar Powder*].

**Packaging and storage**
Prior to reconstitution, store between 15 and 30 °C (59 and 86 °F), unless otherwise specified by manufacturer.

**Preparation of dosage form**
Corticotropin for injection should be reconstituted with sterile water or sodium chloride for injection, so that the individual dose is contained in 1 to 2 mL of solution.

**Stability**
After reconstitution, solution should be used immediately.

### REPOSITORY CORTICOTROPIN INJECTION USP

**Usual adult and adolescent dose**
Use is not recommended.

**Usual pediatric dose**
[Seizures, myoclonic, infantile (treatment)][1]—
Intramuscular, 20 to 40 Units per day or 80 Units every other day.

Note: The optimal dose of corticotropin for the treatment of infantile myoclonic seizures has not been established. Another recommended regimen for infantile myoclonic seizures is an initial dose of 150 Units per square meter of body surface area per day administered intramuscularly in two divided doses for one week, followed by 75 Units per square meter of body surface area per day for one week, then 75 Units per square meter of body surface area administered every other day for one week. Corticotropin dosage is then gradually tapered over the subsequent nine weeks.

The optimal duration of therapy is not known.

Dose should be tapered gradually when discontinuing corticotropin therapy.

**Strength(s) usually available**
U.S.—
40 USP Units per mL (Rx) [*H.P. Acthar Gel* [GENERIC]].
80 USP Units per mL (Rx) [*H.P. Acthar Gel* [GENERIC]].

Canada—
40 IU per mL (Rx) [*Acthar Gel (H.P.)*].

**Packaging and storage**
Store between 2 and 8 °C (36 and 46 °F), unless otherwise specified by manufacturer.

[1] Not included in Canadian product labeling.

### Selected Bibliography

Snead OC. Other antiepileptic drugs: adrenocorticotropic hormone (ACTH). In: Levy R, Mattson R, Meldrum B, editors. Antiepileptic drugs. New York: Raven Press, 1995: 941-8.

Revised: 03/25/96

---

**CORTISONE**—See *Corticosteroids—Glucocorticoid Effects (Systemic)*

---

## COSYNTROPIN Systemic

INN: Tetracosactide
VA CLASSIFICATION (Primary/Secondary): DX900/HS701
Commonly used brand name(s): *Cortrosyn*.
Note: For a listing of dosage forms and brand names by country availability, see *Dosage Forms* section(s).

### Category
Diagnostic aid (adrenal-pituitary function).

### Indications

**Accepted**
Adrenocortical insufficiency (diagnosis)—Cosyntropin is indicated as an aid for diagnosing adrenocortical insufficiency.

Cosyntropin is a synthetic subunit of corticotropin (adrenocorticotropic hormone; ACTH). Cosyntropin is preferable to ACTH for diagnosing primary adrenocortical insufficiency because it is less allergenic. Cosyntropin may be tolerated by most patients who have had an allergic reaction to ACTH or those with a history of allergies.

**Unaccepted**
Cosyntropin is not indicated for the treatment of corticosteroid-responsive medical conditions.

### Pharmacology/Pharmacokinetics

**Physicochemical characteristics**
Chemical group—Synthetic polypeptide identical to the first 24 of the 39 amino acids of corticotropin (ACTH).
Molecular weight—2933.46.

**Mechanism of action/Effect**
Cosyntropin combines with a specific receptor in the adrenal cell plasma membrane and, in patients with normal adrenocortical function, stimulates the initial reaction involved in the synthesis of adrenal steroids including cortisol, cortisone, weak androgenic substances, and a limited quantity of aldosterone) from cholesterol by increasing the quantity of the substrate within the mitochondria. Cosyntropin does not significantly increase plasma cortisol concentration in patients with primary or secondary adrenocortical insufficiency.

Cosyntropin has less immunogenic activity than ACTH because the amino acid sequence having most of the antigenic activity of ACTH (i.e., amino acids 25–39) is not present in cosyntropin.

**Time to peak effect**
The maximal increase in plasma cortisol concentration usually occurs approximately 45 to 60 minutes following intravenous or subcutaneous administration of cosyntropin.

### Precautions to Consider

**Cross-sensitivity and/or related problems**
Although most patients allergic to corticotropin do not exhibit allergy to cosyntropin, some of these patients may be allergic to cosyntropin also.

**Carcinogenicity/Mutagenicity**
Long-term animal studies have not been conducted to evaluate the carcinogenic or mutagenic potential of cosyntropin.

**Pregnancy/Reproduction**
Pregnancy—Studies have not been done in humans.
Studies have not been done animals.
FDA Pregnancy Category C.

**Breast-feeding**
It is not known whether cosyntropin is distributed into breast milk. However, problems in humans have not been documented.

**Pediatrics**
Appropriate studies on the relationship of age to the effects of cosyntropin have not been performed in the pediatric population. However, no pediatrics-specific problems have been documented to date.

**Geriatrics**
No information is available on the relationship of age to the effects of cosyntropin in geriatric patients.

**Drug interactions and/or related problems**
The following drug interactions and/or related problems have been selected on the basis of their potential clinical significance (possible mechanism in parentheses where appropriate)—not necessarily inclusive (» = major clinical significance):

Note: Combinations containing any of the following medications, depending on the amount present, may also interact with this medication.

Blood, whole, or
Plasma
(cosyntropin may be inactivated by enzymes)

**Laboratory value alterations**
The following have been selected on the basis of their potential clinical significance (possible effect in parentheses where appropriate)—not necessarily inclusive (» = major clinical significance):
With results of *this* test
*Due to other medications*
Corticosteroids, glucocorticoid effects, especially cortisone or hydrocortisone
(baseline plasma cortisol concentration may be elevated in patients receiving cortisone or hydrocortisone on the test day and may decrease during the test period)
(with the exception of dexamethasone, other glucocorticoids may interfere with plasma cortisol determinations if radioligand assay tests used are not specific for cortisol)
Spironolactone
(because spironolactone metabolites also fluoresce, plasma cortisol concentrations following cosyntropin administration may be falsely elevated in patients receiving spironolactone when the fluorometric procedure is used but not when radioimmunoassay [RIA] or competitive protein-binding methods are used)

*Due to medical problems or conditions*
   Elevated plasma bilirubin concentrations or
   Free hemoglobin in plasma, presence of
     (falsely elevated plasma cortisol concentrations may occur when the fluorometric method is used)

**Medical considerations/Contraindications**
The medical considerations/contraindications included have been selected on the basis of their potential clinical significance (reasons given in parentheses where appropriate)—not necessarily inclusive (» = major clinical significance).

*Risk-benefit should be considered when the following medical problems exist:*
   Allergic disorders or history of
     (increased risk of allergic reactions)
   Allergy to ACTH or cosyntropin

## Side/Adverse Effects
The following side/adverse effects have been selected on the basis of their potential clinical significance (possible signs and symptoms in parentheses where appropriate)—not necessarily inclusive:

**Those indicating need for medical attention**
Incidence rare
   *Anaphylaxis, generalized* (dizziness; lightheadedness; irritability; seizures; skin rash; hives; itching of skin; slow heartbeat; trouble in breathing; wheezing)

**Those indicating need for medical attention only if they continue or are bothersome**
Incidence less frequent or rare
   *Allergic reaction, mild* (mild fever; nausea; vomiting)

## General Dosing Information
A dose of 250 mcg (0.25 mg) of cosyntropin is equivalent to 25 USP Units of corticotropin.

When used as a diagnostic agent in the screening test for adrenocortical insufficiency, cosyntropin may be administered intramuscularly, subcutaneously, or by intravenous injection. If a greater stimulus is needed, cosyntropin may be administered as an intravenous infusion.

The following criteria may be used as guidelines to determine if the patient has a normal response to cosyntropin. Some interlaboratory variation may occur.
1. Morning control plasma cortisol concentration exceeds 5 mcg (0.005 mg) per 100 mL.
2. Thirty-minute cortisol concentration shows an increase of at least 7 mcg (0.007 mg) per 100 mL above the control level.
3. Thirty-minute cortisol concentration exceeds 18 mcg (0.018 mg) per 100 mL.

Patients who fail to respond to a single dose corticotropin stimulation test using a dose of 250 mcg (0.25 mg) of cosyntropin may be diagnosed as having primary or secondary adrenocortical insufficiency.

## Parenteral Dosage Forms
### COSYNTROPIN FOR INJECTION
**Usual adult and adolescent dose**
Diagnostic aid—
   Intramuscular or subcutaneous, 250 mcg (0.25 mg).
   Intravenous, 250 mcg (0.25 mg), administered over a two-minute period.
   Intravenous infusion, 250 mcg (0.25 mg), administered at a rate of 40 mcg (0.04 mg) per hour over a six-hour period.

**Usual pediatric dose**
Diagnostic aid—
   Children up to 2 years of age: Intramuscular, 125 mcg (0.125 mg).
   Children 2 years of age and older: See *Usual adult and adolescent dose*.

**Size(s) usually available**
U.S.—
   250 mcg (0.25 mg) per vial (Rx) [*Cortrosyn* (mannitol 10 mg)].
Canada—
   250 mcg (0.25 mg) per vial (Rx) [*Cortrosyn* (mannitol 10 mg)].

**Packaging and storage**
Prior to reconstitution, store between 15 and 30 °C (59 and 86 °F), unless otherwise specified by manufacturer.

**Preparation of dosage form**
Add 1 mL of diluent provided (0.9% sodium chloride injection) to the vial containing 250 mcg (0.25 mg) of cosyntropin. The resultant solution contains 250 mcg (0.25 mg) of cosyntropin per mL.
For intravenous infusion, cosyntropin may be further diluted with 5% dextrose injection or 0.9% sodium chloride injection.

**Stability**
After reconstitution with 0.9% sodium chloride injection, 250 mcg (0.25 mg)-per-mL-solutions are stable for 24 hours at room temperature or for 21 days when refrigerated at 2 to 8 °C (36 to 46 °F). After further dilution, solutions are stable for 12 hours at room temperature.

Revised: 09/09/92

# COUGH/COLD COMBINATIONS  Systemic

VA CLASSIFICATION (Primary):
   Bromodiphenhydramine and Codeine (Systemic)—RE301
   Bromodiphenhydramine, Diphenhydramine, Codeine, Ammonium Chloride, and Potassium Guaiacolsulfonate (Systemic)—RE301
   Brompheniramine, Phenylephrine, Phenylpropanolamine, and Codeine (Systemic)—RE301
   Brompheniramine, Phenylephrine, Phenylpropanolamine, and Dextromethorphan (Systemic)—RE301
   Brompheniramine, Phenylephrine, Phenylpropanolamine, Codeine, and Guaifenesin (Systemic)—RE301
   Brompheniramine, Phenylephrine, Phenylpropanolamine, and Guaifenesin (Systemic)—RE503
   Brompheniramine, Phenylephrine, Phenylpropanolamine, Hydrocodone, and Guaifenesin (Systemic)—RE301
   Brompheniramine, Phenylpropanolamine, and Codeine (Systemic)—RE301
   Brompheniramine, Phenylpropanolamine, and Dextromethorphan (Systemic)—RE502
   Brompheniramine, Pseudoephedrine, and Dextromethorphan (Systemic)—RE502
   Carbinoxamine, Pseudoephedrine, and Dextromethorphan (Systemic)—RE502
   Chlorpheniramine and Dextromethorphan (Systemic)—RE507
   Chlorpheniramine, Ephedrine, and Guaifenesin (Systemic)—RE503
   Chlorpheniramine, Ephedrine, Phenylephrine, and Carbetapentane (Systemic)— RE502
   Chlorpheniramine, Ephedrine, Phenylephrine, Dextromethorphan, Ammonium Chloride, and Ipecac (Systemic)—RE504
   Chlorpheniramine and Hydrocodone (Systemic)—RE301
   Chlorpheniramine, Phenindamine, Phenylephrine, Dextromethorphan, Acetaminophen, Salicylamide, Caffeine, and Ascorbic Acid (Systemic)—RE506
   Chlorpheniramine, Pheniramine, Pyrilamine, Phenylephrine, Hydrocodone, Salicylamide, Caffeine, and Ascorbic Acid (Systemic)—RE301
   Chlorpheniramine, Phenylephrine, Codeine, and Ammonium Chloride (Systemic)—RE301
   Chlorpheniramine, Phenylephrine, Codeine, and Potassium Iodide (Systemic)—RE301
   Chlorpheniramine, Phenylephrine, and Dextromethorphan (Systemic)—RE502
   Chlorpheniramine, Phenylephrine, Dextromethorphan, Acetaminophen, and Salicylamide (Systemic)—RE506
   Chlorpheniramine, Phenylephrine, Dextromethorphan, and Guaifenesin (Systemic)—RE504
   Chlorpheniramine, Phenylephrine, Dextromethorphan, Guaifenesin, and Ammonium Chloride (Systemic)—RE504
   Chlorpheniramine, Phenylephrine, and Guaifenesin (Systemic)—RE503
   Chlorpheniramine, Phenylephrine, and Hydrocodone (Systemic)—RE301
   Chlorpheniramine, Phenylephrine, Hydrocodone, Acetaminophen, and Caffeine (Systemic)—RE301
   Chlorpheniramine, Phenylephrine, Phenylpropanolamine, Carbetapentane, and Potassium Guaiacolsulfonate (Systemic)—RE504
   Chlorpheniramine, Phenylephrine, Phenylpropanolamine, and Codeine (Systemic)—RE301

Chlorpheniramine, Phenylephrine, Phenylpropanolamine, Dextromethorphan, Potassium Guaiacolsulfonate, and Ipecac (Systemic)—RE504
Chlorpheniramine, Phenylephrine, Phenylpropanolamine, and Dihydrocodeine (Systemic)—RE301
Chlorpheniramine, Phenylpropanolamine, and Caramiphen (Systemic)—RE502
Chlorpheniramine, Phenylpropanolamine, and Dextromethorphan (Systemic)—RE502
Chlorpheniramine, Phenylpropanolamine, Dextromethorphan, and Acetaminophen (Systemic)—RE506
Chlorpheniramine, Phenylpropanolamine, Dextromethorphan, and Aspirin (Systemic)—RE506
Chlorpheniramine, Phenylpropanolamine, and Guaifenesin (Systemic)—RE503
Chlorpheniramine, Phenylpropanolamine, Guaifenesin, and Acetaminophen (Systemic)—RE599
Chlorpheniramine, Phenylpropanolamine, Guaifenesin, Sodium Citrate, and Citric Acid (Systemic)—RE503
Chlorpheniramine, Phenyltoloxamine, Ephedrine, Codeine, and Guaiacol Carbonate (Systemic)—RE301
Chlorpheniramine, Pseudoephedrine, and Codeine (Systemic)—RE301
Chlorpheniramine, Pseudoephedrine, Codeine, and Acetaminophen (Systemic)—RE506
Chlorpheniramine, Pseudoephedrine, Dextromethorphan, and Acetaminophen (Systemic)—RE506
Chlorpheniramine, Pseudoephedrine, and Dextromethorphan (Systemic)—RE502
Chlorpheniramine, Pseudoephedrine, Dextromethorphan, and Guaifenesin (Systemic)—RE504
Chlorpheniramine, Pseudoephedrine, and Guaifenesin (Systemic)—RE503
Chlorpheniramine, Pseudoephedrine, and Hydrocodone (Systemic)—RE301
Codeine, Ammonium Chloride, and Guaifenesin (Systemic)—RE301
Codeine and Calcium Iodide (Systemic)—RE301
Codeine and Guaifenesin (Systemic)—RE301
Codeine and Iodinated Glycerol (Systemic)—RE301
Dexchlorpheniramine, Pseudoephedrine, and Guaifenesin (Systemic)—RE503
Dextromethorphan and Acetaminophen (Systemic)—RE302
Dextromethorphan and Guaifenesin (Systemic)—RE302
Dextromethorphan and Iodinated Glycerol (Systemic)—RE302
Diphenhydramine, Codeine, and Ammonium Chloride (Systemic)—RE301
Diphenhydramine, Dextromethorphan, and Ammonium Chloride (Systemic)—RE502
Diphenylpyraline, Phenylephrine, and Dextromethorphan (Systemic)—RE502
Doxylamine, Codeine, and Acetaminophen (Systemic)—RE509
Doxylamine, Etafedrine, and Hydrocodone (Systemic)—RE502
Doxylamine, Phenylpropanolamine, Dextromethorphan, and Aspirin (Systemic)—RE506
Doxylamine, Pseudoephedrine, Dextromethorphan, and Acetaminophen (Systemic)—RE506
Ephedrine, Carbetapentane, and Guaifenesin (Systemic)—RE513
Ephedrine and Guaifenesin (Systemic)—RE516
Ephedrine and Potassium Iodide (Systemic)—RE516
Hydrocodone and Guaifenesin (Systemic)—RE301
Hydrocodone and Homatropine (Systemic)—RE301
Hydrocodone and Potassium Guaiacolsulfonate (Systemic)—RE301
Hydromorphone and Guaifenesin (Systemic)—RE301
Pheniramine, Codeine, and Guaifenesin (Systemic)—RE301
Pheniramine, Phenylephrine, Codeine, Sodium Citrate, Sodium Salicylate, and Caffeine (Systemic)—RE301
Pheniramine, Phenylephrine, and Dextromethorphan (Systemic)—RE502
Pheniramine, Phenylephrine, Phenylpropanolamine, Hydrocodone, and Guaifenesin (Systemic)—RE301
Pheniramine, Pyrilamine, Hydrocodone, Potassium Citrate, and Ascorbic Acid (Systemic)—RE301
Pheniramine, Pyrilamine, Phenylephrine, Phenylpropanolamine, and Hydrocodone (Systemic)—RE301
Pheniramine, Pyrilamine, Phenylpropanolamine, and Codeine (Systemic)—RE301
Pheniramine, Pyrilamine, Phenylpropanolamine, and Dextromethorphan (Systemic)—RE502
Pheniramine, Pyrilamine, Phenylpropanolamine, Dextromethorphan, and Ammonium Chloride (Systemic)—RE504
Pheniramine, Pyrilamine, Phenylpropanolamine, and Hydrocodone (Systemic)—RE301
Pheniramine, Pyrilamine, Phenylpropanolamine, Hydrocodone, and Guaifenesin (Systemic)—RE301
Phenylephrine and Codeine (Systemic)—RE512
Phenylephrine, Dextromethorphan, and Guaifenesin (Systemic)—RE513
Phenylephrine and Guaifenesin (Systemic)—RE516
Phenylephrine, Guaifenesin, Acetaminophen, Salicylamide, and Caffeine (Systemic)—RE599
Phenylephrine and Hydrocodone (Systemic)—RE512
Phenylephrine, Hydrocodone, and Guaifenesin (Systemic)—RE301
Phenylephrine, Phenylpropanolamine, Carbetapentane, and Potassium Guaiacolsulfonate (Systemic)—RE513
Phenylephrine, Phenylpropanolamine, and Guaifenesin (Systemic)—RE516
Phenylpropanolamine and Caramiphen (Systemic)—RE512
Phenylpropanolamine, Codeine, and Guaifenesin (Systemic)—RE301
Phenylpropanolamine and Dextromethorphan (Systemic)—RE512
Phenylpropanolamine, Dextromethorphan, Guaifenesin, and Acetaminophen (Systemic)—RE514
Phenylpropanolamine, Dextromethorphan, and Acetaminophen (Systemic)—RE515
Phenylpropanolamine, Dextromethorphan, and Guaifenesin (Systemic)—RE513
Phenylpropanolamine and Guaifenesin (Systemic)—RE516
Phenylpropanolamine and Hydrocodone (Systemic)—RE301
Phenylpropanolamine, Hydrocodone, Dextromethorphan, and Acetaminophen (Systemic)—RE515
Phenyltoloxamine and Hydrocodone (Systemic)—RE301
Promethazine and Codeine (Systemic)—RE301
Promethazine, Codeine, and Potassium Guaiacolsulfonate (Systemic)—RE301
Promethazine and Dextromethorphan (Systemic)—RE507
Promethazine and Potassium Guaiacolsulfonate (Systemic)—RE599
Promethazine, Phenylephrine, and Codeine (Systemic)—RE301
Promethazine, Phenylephrine, Codeine, and Potassium Guaiacolsulfonate (Systemic)—RE301
Promethazine, Phenylephrine, and Potassium Guaiacolsulfonate (Systemic)—RE503
Promethazine, Pseudoephedrine, and Dextromethorphan (Systemic)—RE502
Pseudoephedrine and Codeine (Systemic)—RE301
Pseudoephedrine, Codeine, and Guaifenesin (Systemic)—RE301
Pseudoephedrine and Dextromethorphan (Systemic)—RE512
Pseudoephedrine, Dextromethorphan, and Acetaminophen (Systemic)—RE515
Pseudoephedrine, Dextromethorphan, and Guaifenesin (Systemic)—RE513
Pseudoephedrine, Dextromethorphan, Guaifenesin, and Acetaminophen (Systemic)—RE514
Pseudoephedrine and Guaifenesin (Systemic)—RE516
Pseudoephedrine and Hydrocodone (Systemic)—RE301
Pseudoephedrine, Hydrocodone, and Guaifenesin (Systemic)—RE301
Pseudoephedrine, Hydrocodone, and Potassium Guaiacolsulfonate—RE301
Pyrilamine and Codeine (Systemic)—RE301
Pyrilamine, Phenylephrine, and Codeine (Systemic)—RE301
Pyrilamine, Phenylephrine, and Dextromethorphan (Systemic)—RE502
Pyrilamine, Phenylephrine, and Hydrocodone (Systemic)—RE301
Pyrilamine, Phenylephrine, Hydrocodone, and Ammonium Chloride (Systemic)—RE301
Pyrilamine, Phenylpropanolamine, Dextromethorphan, Guaifenesin, Potassium Citrate, and Citric Acid (Systemic)—RE504
Pyrilamine, Pseudoephedrine, Dextromethorphan, and Acetaminophen (Systemic)—RE506
Triprolidine, Pseudoephedrine, and Codeine (Systemic)—RE301
Triprolidine, Pseudoephedrine, Codeine, and Guaifenesin (Systemic)—RE301
Triprolidine, Pseudoephedrine, and Dextromethorphan (Systemic)—RE502

Note: Due to the large number of cough/cold products available and the different ingredients they contain, the listing that normally appears in this section has been omitted to save space. To aid the reader in readily finding the combination(s) and/or product(s) of interest, these have been grouped in the *Category* section and in the *Advice for the Patient* monograph according to the following major categories:

Antihistaminic (H$_1$-receptor)-decongestant-antitussive
Antihistaminic (H$_1$-receptor)-decongestant-expectorant

Antihistaminic (H$_1$-receptor)-decongestant-antitussive-expectorant
Antihistaminic (H$_1$-receptor)-decongestant-antitussive-expectorant-analgesic
Antihistaminic (H$_1$-receptor)-decongestant-antitussive-analgesic
Antihistaminic (H$_1$-receptor)-decongestant-expectorant-analgesic
Antihistaminic (H$_1$-receptor)-antitussive
Antihistaminic (H$_1$-receptor)-antitussive-expectorant
Antihistaminic (H$_1$-receptor)-antitussive-analgesic
Antihistaminic (H$_1$-receptor)-expectorant
Antitussive-expectorant
Antitussive-analgesic
Antitussive-anticholinergic
Decongestant-antitussive
Decongestant-antitussive-expectorant
Decongestant-antitussive-expectorant-analgesic
Decongestant-antitussive-analgesic
Decongestant-expectorant
Decongestant-expectorant-analgesic

Other combination products that are used in the symptomatic treatment of colds, but which do not contain either an antitussive or an expectorant, can be found in *Antihistamines and Decongestants (Systemic)*; *Antihistamines, Decongestants, and Analgesics (Systemic)*; *Antihistamines, Decongestants, and Anticholinergics (Systemic)*; and *Decongestants and Analgesics (Systemic)*.

Note: For a listing of dosage forms and brand names by country availability, see *Dosage Forms* section(s).

## Category

**Antihistaminic (H$_1$-receptor)-decongestant-antitussive**—Brompheniramine, Phenylephrine, Phenylpropanolamine, and Codeine; Brompheniramine, Phenylephrine, Phenylpropanolamine, and Dextromethorphan; Brompheniramine, Phenylpropanolamine, and Codeine; Brompheniramine, Phenylpropanolamine, and Dextromethorphan; Brompheniramine, Pseudoephedrine, and Dextromethorphan; Carbinoxamine, Pseudoephedrine, and Dextromethorphan; Chlorpheniramine, Ephedrine, Phenylephrine, and Carbetapentane; Chlorpheniramine, Phenylephrine, and Dextromethorphan; Chlorpheniramine, Phenylephrine, and Hydrocodone; Chlorpheniramine, Phenylephrine, Phenylpropanolamine, and Codeine; Chlorpheniramine, Phenylephrine, Phenylpropanolamine, and Dihydrocodeine; Chlorpheniramine, Phenylpropanolamine, and Caramiphen; Chlorpheniramine, Phenylpropanolamine, and Dextromethorphan; Chlorpheniramine, Pseudoephedrine, and Codeine; Chlorpheniramine, Pseudoephedrine, and Dextromethorphan; Chlorpheniramine, Pseudoephedrine, and Hydrocodone; Diphenylpyraline, Phenylephrine, and Dextromethorphan; Doxylamine, Etafedrine, and Hydrocodone; Pheniramine, Phenylephrine, and Dextromethorphan; Pheniramine, Pyrilamine, Phenylephrine, Phenylpropanolamine, and Hydrocodone; Pheniramine, Pyrilamine, Phenylpropanolamine, and Codeine; Pheniramine, Pyrilamine, Phenylpropanolamine, and Dextromethorphan; Pheniramine, Pyrilamine, Phenylpropanolamine, and Hydrocodone; Promethazine, Phenylephrine, and Codeine; Promethazine, Pseudoephedrine, and Dextromethorphan; Pyrilamine, Phenylephrine, and Codeine; Pyrilamine, Phenylephrine, and Dextromethorphan; Pyrilamine, Phenylephrine, and Hydrocodone; Triprolidine, Pseudoephedrine, and Codeine; Triprolidine, Pseudoephedrine, and Dextromethorphan.

**Antihistaminic (H$_1$-receptor)-decongestant-expectorant**—Brompheniramine, Phenylephrine, Phenylpropanolamine, and Guaifenesin; Chlorpheniramine, Ephedrine, and Guaifenesin; Chlorpheniramine, Phenylephrine, and Guaifenesin; Chlorpheniramine, Phenylpropanolamine, and Guaifenesin; Chlorpheniramine, Pseudoephedrine, and Guaifenesin; Dexchlorpheniramine, Pseudoephedrine, and Guaifenesin; Promethazine, Phenylephrine, and Potassium Guaiacolsulfonate.

**Antihistaminic (H$_1$-receptor)-decongestant-expectorant-analgesic**—Chlorpheniramine, Phenylpropanolamine, Guaifenesin, and Acetaminophen.

**Antihistaminic (H$_1$-receptor)-decongestant-antitussive-expectorant**—Brompheniramine, Phenylephrine, Phenylpropanolamine, Codeine, and Guaifenesin; Brompheniramine, Phenylephrine, Phenylpropanolamine, Hydrocodone, and Guaifenesin; Chlorpheniramine, Ephedrine, Phenylephrine, Dextromethorphan, Ammonium Chloride, and Ipecac; Chlorpheniramine, Phenylephrine, Codeine, and Ammonium Chloride; Chlorpheniramine, Phenylephrine, Codeine, and Potassium Iodide; Chlorpheniramine, Phenylephrine, Dextromethorphan, and Guaifenesin; Chlorpheniramine, Phenylephrine, Dextromethorphan, Guaifenesin, and Ammonium Chloride; Chlorpheniramine, Phenylephrine, Phenylpropanolamine, Carbetapentane, and Potassium Guaiacolsulfonate; Chlorpheniramine, Phenylephrine, Phenylpropanolamine, Dextromethorphan, Potassium Guaiacolsulfonate, and Ipecac; Chlorpheniramine, Phenyltoloxamine, Ephedrine, Codeine, and Guaiacol Carbonate; Chlorpheniramine, Pseudoephedrine, Dextromethorphan, and Guaifenesin; Pheniramine, Phenylephrine, Phenylpropanolamine, Hydrocodone, and Guaifenesin; Pheniramine, Pyrilamine, Phenylpropanolamine, Dextromethorphan, and Ammonium Chloride; Pheniramine, Pyrilamine, Phenylpropanolamine, Hydrocodone, and Guaifenesin; Promethazine, Phenylephrine, Codeine, and Potassium Guaiacolsulfonate; Pyrilamine, Phenylephrine, Hydrocodone, and Ammonium Chloride; Pyrilamine, Phenylpropanolamine, Dextromethorphan, Guaifenesin, Potassium Citrate, and Citric Acid; Triprolidine, Pseudoephedrine, Codeine, and Guaifenesin.

**Antihistaminic (H$_1$-receptor)-decongestant-antitussive-expectorant-analgesic**—Pheniramine, Phenylephrine, Codeine, Sodium Citrate, Sodium Salicylate, and Caffeine.

**Antihistaminic (H$_1$-receptor)-decongestant-antitussive-analgesic**—Chlorpheniramine, Phenindamine, Phenylephrine, Dextromethorphan, Acetaminophen, Salicylamide, Caffeine, and Ascorbic Acid; Chlorpheniramine, Pheniramine, Pyrilamine, Phenylephrine, Hydrocodone, Salicylamide, Caffeine, and Ascorbic Acid; Chlorpheniramine, Phenylephrine, Dextromethorphan, Acetaminophen, and Salicylamide; Chlorpheniramine, Phenylephrine, Hydrocodone, Acetaminophen, and Caffeine; Chlorpheniramine, Phenylpropanolamine, Dextromethorphan, and Acetaminophen; Chlorpheniramine, Phenylpropanolamine, Dextromethorphan, and Aspirin; Chlorpheniramine, Pseudoephedrine, Codeine, and Acetaminophen; Chlorpheniramine, Pseudoephedrine, Dextromethorphan, and Acetaminophen; Doxylamine, Phenylpropanolamine, Dextromethorphan, and Aspirin; Doxylamine, Pseudoephedrine, Dextromethorphan, and Acetaminophen; Pyrilamine, Pseudoephedrine, Dextromethorphan, and Acetaminophen.

**Antihistaminic (H$_1$-receptor)-antitussive**—Bromodiphenhydramine and Codeine; Chlorpheniramine and Dextromethorphan; Chlorpheniramine and Hydrocodone; Phenyltoloxamine and Hydrocodone; Promethazine and Codeine; Promethazine and Dextromethorphan; Pyrilamine and Codeine.

**Antihistaminic (H$_1$-receptor)-antitussive-expectorant**—Bromodiphenhydramine, Diphenhydramine, Codeine, Ammonium Chloride, and Potassium Guaiacolsulfonate; Diphenhydramine, Codeine, and Ammonium Chloride; Diphenhydramine, Dextromethorphan, and Ammonium Chloride; Pheniramine, Codeine, and Guaifenesin; Pheniramine, Pyrilamine, Hydrocodone, Potassium Citrate, and Ascorbic Acid; Promethazine, Codeine, and Potassium Guaiacolsulfonate.

**Antihistaminic (H$_1$-receptor)-antitussive-analgesic**—Doxylamine, Codeine, and Acetaminophen.

**Antihistaminic (H$_1$-receptor)-expectorant**—Promethazine and Potassium Guaiacolsulfonate.

**Antitussive-expectorant**—Codeine, Ammonium Chloride, and Guaifenesin; Codeine and Calcium Iodide; Codeine and Guaifenesin; Codeine and Iodinated Glycerol; Dextromethorphan and Guaifenesin; Dextromethorphan and Iodinated Glycerol; Hydrocodone and Guaifenesin; Hydrocodone and Potassium Guaiacolsulfonate; Hydromorphone and Guaifenesin.

**Antitussive-analgesic**—Dextromethorphan and Acetaminophen.

**Antitussive-anticholinergic**—Hydrocodone and Homatropine.

**Decongestant-antitussive**—Phenylephrine and Codeine; Phenylephrine and Hydrocodone; Phenylpropanolamine and Caramiphen; Phenylpropanolamine and Dextromethorphan; Phenylpropanolamine and Hydrocodone; Pseudoephedrine and Codeine; Pseudoephedrine and Dextromethorphan; Pseudoephedrine and Hydrocodone.

**Decongestant-antitussive-expectorant**—Ephedrine, Carbetapentane, and Guaifenesin; Phenylephrine, Dextromethorphan, and Guaifenesin; Phenylephrine, Hydrocodone, and Guaifenesin; Phenylephrine, Phenylpropanolamine, Carbetapentane, and Potassium Guaiacolsulfonate; Phenylpropanolamine, Codeine, and Guaifenesin; Phenylpropanolamine, Dextromethorphan, and Guaifenesin; Pseudoephedrine, Codeine, and Guaifenesin; Pseudoephedrine, Dextromethorphan, and Guaifenesin; Pseudoephedrine, Hydrocodone, and Guaifenesin; Pseudoephedrine, Hydrocodone, and Potassium Guaiacolsulfonate.

**Decongestant-antitussive-expectorant-analgesic**—Phenylpropanolamine, Dextromethorphan, Guaifenesin, and Acetaminophen; Pseudoephedrine, Dextromethorphan, Guaifenesin, and Acetaminophen.

**Decongestant-antitussive-analgesic**—Phenylpropanolamine, Dextromethorphan, and Acetaminophen; Pseudoephedrine, Dextromethorphan, and Acetaminophen.

**Decongestant-expectorant**—Ephedrine and Guaifenesin; Ephedrine and Potassium Iodide; Phenylephrine and Guaifenesin; Phenylpropanolamine, and Guaifenesin; Phenylpropanolamine and Guaifenesin; Pseudoephedrine and Guaifenesin.

**Decongestant-expectorant-analgesic**—Phenylephrine, Guaifenesin, Acetaminophen, Salicylamide, and Caffeine.

## Indications

### Accepted
Cough (treatment)—Combination products containing antitussives and/or expectorants may be indicated for the symptomatic relief of cough due to colds and minor upper respiratory infections.

Cough and nasal congestion (treatment)—Combination products containing antitussives and/or expectorants, and nasal decongestants may be indicated for the symptomatic relief of cough and nasal congestion due to the common cold and other respiratory infections. Also, products containing antihistamines may provide relief of the cough, nasal congestion, rhinorrhea, and sneezing associated with allergy and the common cold. However, controlled clinical studies have not demonstrated that antihistamines are significantly more effective than placebo in relieving cold symptoms.

Cold symptoms (treatment)—Combination products containing antihistamines, antitussives or expectorants, nasal decongestants, and analgesics may be indicated for the temporary relief of coughs, nasal congestion, and associated aches, pains, and general discomfort due to colds, flu, or allergy. The antihistamine in these cold combinations may provide relief of nasal congestion, rhinorrhea, and sneezing. It may also serve as an adjunct because of its anticholinergic drying effects. However, in many cough/cold combinations, the dosage level of the antihistamine is below that required to obtain a significant effect. Also, controlled clinical studies have not demonstrated that antihistamines are significantly more effective than placebo in relieving cold symptoms.

### Unaccepted
Cough/cold combination products that contain both an antitussive and an expectorant usually do not offer any advantage over products that contain only one of these agents. In some cases, their combination may be detrimental in the treatment of coughs, since antitussives should be used only in the treatment of dry coughs and not for productive coughs.

Some products containing an anticholinergic have been used to help dry excessive nasal secretions associated with the common cold and allergic rhinitis; however, the efficacy of anticholinergics for this use in these combination products has not been established. In most products, the anticholinergic is included in doses below the therapeutic level in an attempt to prevent abuse by deliberate overdosage (e.g., in combinations containing a narcotic antitussive).

Combination products that contain an analgesic are generally not recommended for regular use for the treatment of cold symptoms during the common cold or acute allergic rhinitis since they may mask fever, which may indicate a secondary bacterial infection.

Ammonium chloride, calcium iodide, citric acid, guaiacol carbonate, iodinated glycerol, ipecac, potassium citrate, potassium guaiacolsulfonate, potassium iodide, and sodium citrate are included as expectorants in these combinations; however, the Food and Drug Administration (FDA) has not found them to be useful for this indication. Therefore, FDA has requested manufacturers to reformulate their products to replace these ingredients with guaifenesin.

## Pharmacology/Pharmacokinetics
Antihistamine-containing—See *Antihistamines (Systemic)*.
Decongestant-containing—See:
   *Ephedrine* in *Bronchodilators, Adrenergic (Systemic)*.
   *Phenylpropanolamine (Systemic)*.
   *Pseudoephedrine (Systemic)*.
Dextromethorphan-containing—See *Dextromethorphan (Systemic)*.
Opioid (narcotic) antitussive–containing—See *Opioid (Narcotic) Analgesics (Systemic)*.
Expectorant-containing—See:
   *Guaifenesin (Systemic)*.
   *Iodinated Glycerol (Systemic)*.
Analgesic-containing—See:
   *Acetaminophen (Systemic)*.
   *Acetaminophen and Salicylates (Systemic)*.
   *Salicylates (Systemic)*.
Homatropine-containing—See *Anticholinergics/Antispasmodics (Systemic)*.

## Precautions to Consider
Antihistamine-containing—See *Antihistamines (Systemic)*.
Antihistamine- and decongestant-containing—See *Antihistamines and Decongestants (Systemic)*.
Decongestant-containing—See:
   *Ephedrine* in *Bronchodilators, Adrenergic (Systemic)*.
   *Phenylpropanolamine (Systemic)*.
   *Pseudoephedrine (Systemic)*.
Dextromethorphan-containing—See *Dextromethorphan (Systemic)*.
Opioid (narcotic) antitussive–containing—See *Opioid (Narcotic) Analgesics (Systemic)*.
Expectorant-containing—See:
   *Guaifenesin (Systemic)*.
   *Iodinated Glycerol (Systemic)*.
Analgesic-containing—See:
   *Acetaminophen (Systemic)*.
   *Acetaminophen and Salicylates (Systemic)*.
   *Salicylates (Systemic)*.
Homatropine-containing—See *Anticholinergics/Antispasmodics (Systemic)*.

### Laboratory value alterations
See *Table 1*, page 1028.

## Side/Adverse Effects
Antihistamine-containing—See *Antihistamines (Systemic)*.
Antihistamine- and decongestant-containing—See *Antihistamines and Decongestants (Systemic)*.
Decongestant-containing—See:
   *Ephedrine* in *Bronchodilators, Adrenergic (Systemic)*.
   *Phenylpropanolamine (Systemic)*.
   *Pseudoephedrine (Systemic)*.
Dextromethorphan-containing—See *Dextromethorphan (Systemic)*.
Opioid (narcotic) antitussive–containing—See *Opioid (Narcotic) Analgesics (Systemic)*.
Expectorant-containing—See:
   *Guaifenesin (Systemic)*.
   *Iodinated Glycerol (Systemic)*.
Analgesic-containing—See:
   *Acetaminophen (Systemic)*.
   *Acetaminophen and Salicylates (Systemic)*.
   *Salicylates (Systemic)*.
Homatropine-containing—See *Anticholinergics/Antispasmodics (Systemic)*.

## Patient Consultation
See *Table 2*, page 1029.

## Oral Dosage Forms
See *Table 3*, page 1032.

---
Revised: 09/03/92
Interim revision: 08/11/95; 08/28/96

## Table 1. Laboratory value alterations

The following have been selected on the basis of their potential clinical significance (possible effect in parentheses where appropriate)—not necessarily inclusive (» = major clinical significance):

Legend:
I = Antihistamine-containing
II = Decongestant-containing
III = Antitussive-containing
IV = Expectorant-containing
V = Analgesic-containing

| | I | II | III | IV | V |
|---|---|---|---|---|---|
| **With diagnostic test results** | | | | | |
| Copper sulfate urine sugar tests (false-positive test results may occur with chronic use of salicylates in doses equivalent in salicylate content to 2.4 grams or more of aspirin a day) | | | | | ✔ |
| Gastric emptying studies (opioids delay gastric emptying, thereby invalidating test results) | | | ✔ | | |
| Gerhardt test for urine aceto-acetic acid (aspirin or sodium salicylate may cause interference because reaction with ferric chloride produces a reddish color that persists after boiling) | | | | | ✔ |
| Glucose, blood (acetaminophen may cause falsely decreased blood glucose values when measured by the glucose oxidase/peroxidase method but probably not when measured by the hexokinase/glucose-6-phosphate dehydrogenase [G6PD] method) (values may be falsely increased when certain instruments are used in glucose analysis if high acetaminophen concentrations are present; consult manufacturer's instruction manual) | | | | | ✔ |
| Glucose enzymatic urine sugar tests (false-negative test results may occur with chronic use of salicylates in doses equivalent in salicylate content to 2.4 grams or more of aspirin a day) | | | | | ✔ |
| Hepatobiliary imaging using technetium Tc 99m disofenin, technetium Tc 99m lidofenin, technetium Tc 99m mebrofenin (delivery of these technetium Tc 99m–labeled radiopharmaceuticals to the small bowel may be prevented because opioids may cause constriction of the sphincter of Oddi and increased biliary tract pressure; these actions result in delayed visualization and thus resemble obstruction of the common bile duct) | | | ✔ | | |
| 5-hydroxyindoleacetic acid (5-HIAA), urine (urinary determinations may be falsely increased when nitrosonaphthol reagent is used because of color interference by guaifenesin metabolites) (acetaminophen may cause false-positive results in qualitative screening tests using nitrosonaphthol reagent; the quantitative test is unaffected) (aspirin may alter results when fluorescent method is used) | | | | | ✔ |
| Pancreatic function determinations using bentiromide (administration of acetaminophen prior to the bentiromide test will invalidate test results because acetaminophen is also metabolized to an arylamine and will thus increase the apparent quantity of para-aminobenzoic acid [PABA] recovered; it is recommended that acetaminophen be discontinued at least 3 days prior to administration of bentiromide) | | | | | ✔ |
| Skin tests using allergen extracts (antihistamines contained in these combinations may inhibit the cutaneous histamine response thus producing false-negative results; it is recommended that antihistamine-containing medication be discontinued at least 72 hours before testing begins) | ✔ | | | | |
| Thyroid function tests (iodides may alter the results of these tests, and a high intake of inorganic iodides has also been shown to interfere with determination of protein bound iodine [PBI]; these effects have not been reported with iodinated glycerol in usual recommended doses, but they should be kept in mind for patients receiving prolonged therapy) | | | | ✔ | |
| Uric acid, serum (acetaminophen may cause falsely increased values when the phosphotungstate uric acid test method is used) | | | | | ✔ |
| Vanillylmandelic acid (VMA), urine (guaifenesin or its metabolites may cause color interference with urinary determinations) (values may be falsely increased or decreased by salicylates, depending on the method used) | | | | | ✔ |
| **With physiology/laboratory test values** | | | | | |
| Amylase activity, plasma, and Lipase activity, plasma (may be increased because opioids can cause contractions of the sphincter of Oddi and increased biliary tract pressure; the diagnostic utility of determinations of these enzymes may be compromised for up to 24 hours after the medication has been given) | | | ✔ | | |
| Bilirubin, serum, and Lactate dehydrogenase (LDH), serum, and Prothrombin time and Transaminase, serum (prothrombin time and concentrations of bilirubin, LDH, and transaminase may be increased indicating acetaminophen-induced hepatotoxicity, especially in alcoholics, patients taking hepatic enzyme–inducing agents, or those with pre-existing hepatic disease, when single toxic doses [> 8–10 grams] are taken or with prolonged use of lower doses [> 3–5 grams a day]) | | | | | ✔ |

## Table 1. Laboratory value alterations *(continued)*

Legend:
 I=Antihistamine-containing
 II=Decongestant-containing
 III=Antitussive-containing
 IV=Expectorant-containing
 V=Analgesic-containing

| The following have been selected on the basis of their potential clinical significance (possible effect in parentheses where appropriate)—not necessarily inclusive (» = major clinical significance): | I | II | III | IV | V |
|---|---|---|---|---|---|
| Bleeding time (may be prolonged by aspirin for 4 to 7 days because of suppressed platelet aggregation; as little as 40 mg of aspirin affects platelet function for at least 96 hours following administration; however, clinical bleeding problems have not been reported with small doses [150 mg or less]) | | | | | ✓ |
| Platelet aggregation (may be transiently decreased by guaifenesin; however, effects on bleeding time are unlikely) | | | | ✓ | |
| Potassium, serum (concentrations may be decreased by aspirin or sodium salicylate because of increased potassium excretion caused by direct effect on renal tubules) | | | | | ✓ |
| Protirelin-induced thyroid-stimulating hormone (TSH) release (TSH response to protirelin may be decreased by aspirin in doses of 2 to 3.6 grams daily; peak TSH concentrations occur at the same time after administration but are reduced) | | | | | ✓ |
| Uric acid, serum (concentrations may be increased with doses of aspirin or sodium salicylate producing plasma salicylate concentrations below 100 to 150 mcg per mL or decreased with doses producing plasma salicylate concentrations above 100 to 150 mcg per mL) | | | | | ✓ |

## Table 2. Patient Consultation

As an aid to patient consultation, refer to *Advice for the Patient, Cough/Cold Combinations (Systemic)*.
In providing consultation, consider emphasizing the following selected information (» = major clinical significance):

Legend:
 I=Antihistamine-containing
 II=Decongestant-containing
 III=Opioid (Narcotic) Antitussive–containing
 IV=Non-opioid Antitussive–containing
 V=Expectorant-containing
 VI=Analgesic-containing[1]
 VII=Anticholinergic-containing

| | I | II | III | IV | V | VI | VII |
|---|---|---|---|---|---|---|---|
| **Before using this medication** | | | | | | | |
| » Conditions affecting use, especially: | | | | | | | |
|     Sensitivity to any of the medications in the combination being taken | ✓ | ✓ | ✓ | ✓ | ✓ | ✓ | ✓ |
|   Pregnancy— | | | | | | | |
|     Concern for the fetus or newborn infant, especially with high-dose and/or long-term usage | ✓ | ✓ | ✓ | ✓ | ✓ | ✓ | ✓ |
|     Psychiatric disorders more likely with use of phenylpropanolamine in postpartum women | | ✓ | | | | | |
|     Physical dependence in the neonate possible with regular use | | | ✓ | | | | |
|     Iodinated glycerol not recommended, because may induce fetal goiter | | | | | ✓ | | |
|   Breast-feeding— | | | | | | | |
|     Antihistamines may cause excitement or irritability in nursing infant | ✓ | | | | | | |
|     High risk for infants from sympathomimetic amines | | ✓ | | | | | |
|     Concern with high doses and chronic use because of high salicylate intake by infant | | | | | | ✓[2] | |
|     Iodinated glycerol not recommended, because may induce skin rash and thyroid suppression in nursing infant | | | | | ✓ | | |

[1] In children the use of combinations containing both acetaminophen and salicylates is controversial. Also, studies have suggested that aspirin usage may be associated with the development of Reye's syndrome in children/adolescents with acute febrile illnesses, especially influenza and varicella. It is recommended that salicylate therapy not be initiated in febrile pediatric or adolescent patients until after the presence of such an illness has been ruled out. Also, it is recommended that chronic salicylate therapy in these patients be discontinued if a fever occurs, and not resumed until it has been determined that an illness that may predispose to Reye's syndrome is not present or has run its course. In addition, pediatric patients, especially those with fever and dehydration, may be more susceptible to the toxic effects of salicylates.

[2] Applies to salicylates only, particularly aspirin.

[3] Applies to iodides (e.g., calcium iodide, iodinated glycerol, potassium iodide) only.

[4] Applies to dextromethorphan.

[5] Danger of overdose of acetaminophen, salicylates, or opioid (narcotic) antitussives; also, acetaminophen may cause liver damage with long-term or high-dose use.

[6] In addition to drowsiness and dizziness, a false sense of well-being may also occur with the opioid (narcotic) antitussives.

[7] The possibility of insomnia may be minimized with preparations containing an antihistamine or an opioid (narcotic) antitussive.

[8] Applies to acetaminophen only.

[9] Caution should be exercised whether alcoholism is active or in remission with all alcohol-containing products.

## Table 2. Patient Consultation (continued)

As an aid to patient consultation, refer to *Advice for the Patient, Cough/Cold Combinations (Systemic)*.
In providing consultation, consider emphasizing the following selected information (» = major clinical significance):

Legend
I = Antihistamine-containing
II = Decongestant-containing
III = Opioid (Narcotic) Antitussive–containing
IV = Non-opioid Antitussive–containing
V = Expectorant-containing
VI = Analgesic-containing[1]
VII = Anticholinergic-containing

| | I | II | III | IV | V | VI | VII |
|---|---|---|---|---|---|---|---|
| Use in children— | | | | | | | |
|   Increased susceptibility to anticholinergic effects | ✓ | | | | | | ✓ |
|   Increased susceptibility to vasopressor effects of sympathomimetic amines | | ✓ | | | | | |
|   Psychiatric disorders more likely with use of phenylpropanolamine in children up to 6 years of age | | ✓ | | | | | |
|   Paradoxical reaction (hyperexcitability) | ✓ | | ✓ | | | | ✓ |
|   Increased susceptibility to toxic effects of salicylates, especially if fever and dehydration present | | | | | | ✓[2] | |
|   Possible association between aspirin usage and Reye's syndrome | | | | | | ✓[2] | |
|   Increased susceptibility to goitrogenic effects of iodides | | | | | ✓[3] | | |
|   Increased susceptibility to respiratory depressant effects of opioids in children up to 2 years of age | | | ✓ | | | | |
| Use in the elderly— | | | | | | | |
|   Anticholinergic effects more likely to occur | ✓ | | | | | | ✓ |
|   Increased sensitivity to CNS and vasopressor effects of sympathomimetic amines | | ✓ | | | | | |
|   Increased susceptibility to toxic effects of salicylates | | | | | | ✓[2] | |
|   Increased susceptibility to respiratory depressant effects of opioids | | | ✓ | | | | |
| Other medications, especially: | | | | | | | |
|   Alcohol | ✓ | | ✓ | ✓[4] | | ✓ | |
|   Alkalizers, urinary | | | | | | ✓[2] | |
|   Anticholinergics | ✓ | | | | | | ✓ |
|   Anticoagulants | | | | | | ✓[2] | |
|   Antidepressants, tricyclic | ✓ | | | | | | |
|   Antidiabetic agents, oral | | | | | | ✓[2] | |
|   Antihypertensives | | ✓ | | | | | |
|   Anti-inflammatory drugs, nonsteroidal | | | | | | ✓[2] | |
|   Antithyroid agents | | | | | ✓[3] | | |
|   Beta-adrenergic blocking agents, oral | | ✓ | | | | | |
|   CNS depressants | ✓ | | ✓ | ✓[4] | | | |
|   CNS stimulants | | ✓ | | | | | |
|   Heparin | | | | | | ✓[2] | |
|   Lithium | | | | | ✓[3] | | |
|   Methotrexate | | | | | | ✓[2] | |
|   Monoamine oxidase (MAO) inhibitors | ✓ | ✓ | | ✓[4] | | | ✓ |
|   Platelet aggregation inhibitors | | | | | | ✓[2] | |
|   Probenecid | | | | | | ✓[2] | |
|   Rauwolfia alkaloids | | ✓ | | | | | |
|   Sulfinpyrazone | | | | | | ✓[2] | |
|   Thrombolytic agents | | | | | | ✓[2] | |
|   Vancomycin | | | | | | ✓[2] | |
|   Zidovudine | | | | | | ✓[2] | |
| Other medical problems, especially: | | | | | | | |
|   Alcoholism, active[9] | | | | | | ✓[8] | |
|   Asthma | | | ✓ | ✓[4] | | ✓[2] | |
|   Bleeding problems | | | | | | ✓[2] | |
|   Cardiovascular disease | | ✓ | | | | | |
|   Diabetes | | ✓ | | | | | |
|   Diarrhea | | | ✓ | | | | |
|   Gastritis or peptic ulcer | | | | | | ✓[2] | |
|   Glaucoma | ✓ | | | | | | ✓ |
|   Hypertension | | ✓ | | | | | |
|   Inflammatory bowel disease | | | ✓ | | | | |
|   Prostatic hypertrophy | ✓ | | | | | | ✓ |
|   Thyroid disease | | ✓ | | | | | |
| **Proper use of this medication** | | | | | | | |
|   Taking with food, water, or milk to minimize gastric irritation | | | | | | ✓[2] | |
| » Importance of drinking a glass of water after each dose of medication to help loosen mucus in lungs | ✓ | ✓ | ✓ | ✓ | ✓ | ✓ | ✓ |
| » Importance of not taking more medication than the amount recommended | ✓ | ✓ | ✓[5] | ✓ | ✓ | ✓[5] | ✓ |
|   Swallowing extended-release dosage form whole | ✓ | ✓ | ✓ | ✓ | ✓ | ✓ | ✓ |
| » Not taking combinations containing aspirin if a strong vinegar-like odor is present | | | | | | ✓ | |
|   Missed dose: If on scheduled dosing regimen—Taking as soon as possible; not taking if almost time for next dose; not doubling doses | ✓ | ✓ | ✓ | ✓ | ✓ | ✓ | ✓ |
| » Proper storage | ✓ | ✓ | ✓ | ✓ | ✓ | ✓ | ✓ |

## Table 2. Patient Consultation *(continued)*

As an aid to patient consultation, refer to *Advice for the Patient, Cough/Cold Combinations (Systemic)*.
In providing consultation, consider emphasizing the following selected information (» = major clinical significance):

Legend
I = Antihistamine-containing
II = Decongestant-containing
III = Opioid (Narcotic) Antitussive–containing
IV = Non-opioid Antitussive–containing
V = Expectorant-containing
VI = Analgesic-containing[1]
VII = Anticholinergic-containing

| | I | II | III | IV | V | VI | VII |
|---|---|---|---|---|---|---|---|
| **Precautions while using this medication** | | | | | | | |
| » Checking with physician if symptoms persist after medication has been used for 7 days or if high fever, skin rash, or continuing headache is present with cough | ✓ | ✓ | ✓ | ✓ | ✓ | ✓ | ✓ |
| Possible interference with skin tests using allergens; need to inform physician of use of medication | ✓ | | | | | | |
| » Avoiding use of alcohol or other CNS depressants | ✓ | | ✓ | | | | |
| » Caution if drowsiness or dizziness occurs | ✓ | | ✓[6] | | | | |
| Lying down if nausea occurs | | | ✓ | | | | |
| Possible dryness of mouth; using sugarless candy or gum, ice, or saliva substitute for relief; checking with physician or dentist if dry mouth continues for more than 2 weeks | ✓ | | | | | | ✓ |
| May mask ototoxic effects of large doses of salicylates | ✓ | | | | | | |
| » Caution if taking phenylpropanolamine-containing appetite suppressants | | ✓ | | | | | |
| » Possible insomnia; taking the medication a few hours before bedtime | | ✓[7] | | | | | |
| » Caution during exercise and hot weather; overheating may result in heat stroke | | | | | | | ✓ |
| Caution when getting up suddenly from a lying or sitting position | | | ✓ | | | | |
| Need to inform physician or dentist of use of medication if any kind of surgery (including dental surgery) or emergency treatment is required | | ✓ | ✓ | | | | |
| » Caution if other medications containing acetaminophen, aspirin, or other salicylates (including diflunisal) are used | | | | | | ✓ | |
| Diabetics: Salicylates present in some of these combinations may cause false urine sugar tablet test results with use of larger doses | | | | | | ✓ | |
| Not taking products containing aspirin for 5 days prior to any kind of surgery, unless otherwise directed by physician | | | | | | ✓ | |
| **Side/adverse effects** | | | | | | | |
| Signs of potential side effects, especially: | | | | | | | |
| Allergic reactions | ✓ | ✓ | ✓ | ✓ | ✓ | ✓ | ✓ |
| Anemia | | | | | | ✓ | |
| Anticholinergic effects | ✓ | | | | | | ✓ |
| Blood dyscrasias | ✓ | | | | | | |
| Gastrointestinal irritation or bleeding | | | | | | ✓[2] | |
| Jaundice | | | | | | ✓[8] | |
| Parotitis, acute | | | | | ✓[3] | | |

[1] In children the use of combinations containing both acetaminophen and salicylates is controversial. Also, studies have suggested that aspirin usage may be associated with the development of Reye's syndrome in children/adolescents with acute febrile illnesses, especially influenza and varicella. It is recommended that salicylate therapy not be initiated in febrile pediatric or adolescent patients until after the presence of such an illness has been ruled out. Also, it is recommended that chronic salicylate therapy in these patients be discontinued if a fever occurs, and not resumed until it has been determined that an illness that may predispose to Reye's syndrome is not present or has run its course. In addition, pediatric patients, especially those with fever and dehydration, may be more susceptible to the toxic effects of salicylates.
[2] Applies to salicylates only, particularly aspirin.
[3] Applies to iodides (e.g., calcium iodide, iodinated glycerol, potassium iodide) only.
[4] Applies to dextromethorphan.
[5] Danger of overdose of acetaminophen, salicylates, or opioid (narcotic) antitussives; also, acetaminophen may cause liver damage with long-term or high-dose use.
[6] In addition to drowsiness and dizziness, a false sense of well-being may also occur with the opioid (narcotic) antitussives.
[7] The possibility of insomnia may be minimized with preparations containing an antihistamine or an opioid (narcotic) antitussive.
[8] Applies to acetaminophen only.
[9] Caution should be exercised whether alcoholism is active or in remission with all alcohol-containing products.

**1032 Cough/Cold Combinations (Systemic)** USP DI

## Table 3. Oral Dosage Forms

Note: Content per capsule, tablet, or 5 mL, unless otherwise stated.

| Brand or generic name [availability] | Antihistamines | Decongestants | Antitussives Opioid | Antitussives Non-opioid | Expectorants | Analgesics | Other content information as per product label | Usual Adult and Adolescent Dose prn‡ | Usual Pediatric Dose prn | Packaging, Storage, and Auxiliary labelings§ |
|---|---|---|---|---|---|---|---|---|---|---|
| Actagen-C Cough Syrup (Schedule V) [U.S.] | Triprolidine HCl 1.25 mg | Pseudoephedrine HCl 30 mg | Codeine PO₄ 10 mg | | | | Alcohol 4.3% | 10 mL q 4–6 hr (max 40 mL/day) | 2–6 yrs: 2.5 mL; 6–12 yrs: 5 mL, q 4–6 hr | b, c, d, e, f |
| Actifed w/Codeine Cough Syrup (Schedule V) [U.S.] | Triprolidine HCl 1.25 mg | Pseudoephedrine HCl 30 mg | Codeine PO₄ 10 mg | | | | Alcohol 4.3% | 10 mL q 4–6 hr (max 4 doses/day) | 2–6 yrs: 2.5 mL; 6–12 yrs: 5 mL, q 4–6 hr (max 4 doses/day) | b, c, d, e, f |
| Actifed DM Oral Solution (OTC) [Canada] | Triprolidine HCl 1.25 mg | Pseudoephedrine HCl 30 mg | | Dextromethorphan HBr 15 mg | | | Alcohol 5% | 10 mL q 8 hr | 6 mos–2 yrs: 1.25 mL, 2–6 yrs: 2.5 mL, 6–11 yrs: 5 mL, q 8 hr | b, c, e |
| Tablets (OTC) [Canada] | Triprolidine HCl 2.5 mg | Pseudoephedrine HCl 60 mg | | Dextromethorphan HBr 30 mg | | | Scored | 1 tab q 4–6 hr (max 4 tabs/day) | 6–11 yrs: ½ tab q 4–6 hr | b, e |
| Alka-Seltzer Plus Cold and Cough Effervescent Tablets (OTC) [U.S.] | Chlorpheniramine maleate 2 mg | Phenylpropanolamine bitartrate 20 mg | | Dextromethorphan HBr 10 mg | | Aspirin 325 mg | Phenylalanine 11.2 mg Sodium 507 mg | 2 tabs dissolved in 120 mL water q 4 hr (max 8 tabs/day) | | a, e |
| Alka-Seltzer Plus Cold & Cough Medicine Liqui-Gels Capsules (OTC) [U.S.] | Chlorpheniramine maleate 2 mg | Pseudoephedrine HCl 30 mg | | Dextromethorphan HBr 10 mg | | Acetaminophen 250 mg | | 2 caps q 4 hr (max 8 caps/day) | 6–12 yrs: 1 cap q 4 hr (max 4 caps/day) | a, e |
| Alka-Seltzer Plus Flu & Body Aches Effervescent Tablets (OTC) [U.S.] | Chlorpheniramine maleate 2 mg | Phenylpropanolamine bitartrate 20 mg | | Dextromethorphan HBr 10 mg | | Acetaminophen 325 mg | Sodium 111 mg Phenylalanine 11.2 mg | 2 tabs dissolved in 120 mL hot water q 4 hr (max 8 tabs/day) | | a, e |
| Alka-Seltzer Plus Flu & Body Aches Medicine Liqui-Gels Capsules (OTC) [U.S.] | | Pseudoephedrine HCl 30 mg | | Dextromethorphan HBr 10 mg | | Acetaminophen 250 mg | | 2 caps q 4 hr (max 8 caps/day) | 6–12 yrs: 1 cap q 4 hr (max 4 caps/day) | a, e |

Table 3. Oral Dosage Forms (continued)

Note: Content per capsule, tablet, or 5 mL, unless otherwise stated.

| Brand or generic name [availability] | Antihistamines | Decongestants | Antitussives Opioid | Antitussives Non-opioid | Expectorants | Analgesics | Other content information as per product label | Usual Adult and Adolescent Dose prn‡ | Usual Pediatric Dose prn | Packaging, Storage, and Auxiliary labeling§ |
|---|---|---|---|---|---|---|---|---|---|---|
| Alka-Seltzer Plus Night Time Cold Effervescent Tablets (OTC) [U.S.] | Doxylamine succinate 6.25 mg | Phenylpropanolamine bitartrate 20 mg | | Dextromethorphan HBR 15 mg | | Aspirin 500 mg | Sodium 506 mg Phenylalanine 16.2 mg | 2 tabs dissolved in 120 mL water hs or q 4 hr (max 8 tabs/day) | | a, e |
| Alka-Seltzer Plus Night-Time Cold Liqui-Gels Capsules (OTC) [U.S.] | Doxylamine succinate 6.25 mg | Pseudoephedrine HCl 30 mg | | Dextromethorphan HBr 10 mg | | Acetaminophen 250 mg | Alcohol free | 2 caps hs or q 4 hr (max 8 caps/day) | Not recommended | b, e |
| Allerfrin w/Codeine Syrup (Schedule V) [U.S.] | Triprolidine HCl 1.25 mg | Pseudoephedrine HCl 30 mg | Codeine PO₄ 10 mg | | | | Alcohol 4.3% | 10 mL q 4–6 hr (max 40 mL/day) | 2–6 yrs: 2.5 mL, 6–12 yrs: 5 mL, q 4–6 hr | b, c, d, e, f |
| All-Nite Cold Formula Oral Solution (OTC) [U.S.] | Doxylamine succinate 1.25 mg | Pseudoephedrine HCl 10 mg | | Dextromethorphan HBr 5 mg | | Acetaminophen 167 mg | Alcohol 25% | 30 mL hs or 30 mL q 6 hr | | a, c, e |
| Ambenyl Cough Syrup (Schedule V) [U.S.] | Bromodiphenhydramine HCl 12.5 mg | | Codeine PO₄ 10 mg | | | | Alcohol 5% | 5–10 mL q 4–6 hr | 6–12 yrs: 2.5–5 mL q 6 hr | a, c, d, e, f |
| Syrup (N) [Canada] | Bromodiphenhydramine HCl 3.75 mg, Diphenhydramine HCl 8.75 mg | | Codeine PO₄ 10 mg | | Ammonium Cl† 80 mg, Potassium guaiacolsulfonate† 80 mg | | Alcohol 5% | 5–10 mL q 4–6 hr (max 60 mL/day) | 2–6 yrs: 1.25–2.5 mL, 6–12 yrs: 2.5–5 mL q 6 hr | a, c, d, e, f |
| Ambenyl-D Decongestant Cough Formula Oral Solution (OTC) [U.S.] | | Pseudoephedrine HCl 30 mg | | Dextromethorphan HBr 15 mg | Guaifenesin 100 mg | | Alcohol 9.5% | 5–10 mL q 4 hr | 2–6 yrs: 2.5 mL, 6–12 yrs: 5 mL q 6 hr | b, c |

*Specific formulations may vary among the different manufacturers, check product labeling.
†Efficacy as expectorant has not been established.
‡Geriatric patients may be more sensitive to effects of usual adult dose.
§For appropriate *Packaging and storage* and *Auxiliary labeling* information refer to designated letters as follows:
    a—Store below 40 °C (104 °F), preferably between 15 and 30 °C (59 and 86 °F), in a tight container, unless otherwise specified by manufacturer.
    a¹—Store below 30 °C (86 °F), unless otherwise specified by manufacturer. Avoid exposure to excessive heat.
    a²—Store below 25 °C (77 °F), unless otherwise specified by manufacturer.
    b—Store below 40 °C (104 °F), preferably between 15 and 30 °C (59 and 86 °F), in a well-closed container, unless otherwise specified by manufacturer.
    c—Protect from freezing.
    d—Protect from light.
    e—Auxiliary labeling: · May cause drowsiness. · Avoid alcoholic beverages.
    f—Auxiliary labeling: · May be habit forming.
    g—Auxiliary labeling: · Shake well.
    h—Dispense in dropper bottle.
    i—Chew well before swallowing.
**Included in subtherapeutic amount to discourage deliberate overdosage.

**Cough/Cold Combinations (Systemic)**

Table 3. Oral Dosage Forms *(continued)*

Note: Content per capsule, tablet, or 5 mL, unless otherwise stated.

| Brand or generic name [availability] | Antihistamines | Decongestants | Antitussives Opioid | Antitussives Non-opioid | Expectorants | Analgesics | Other content information as per product label | Usual Adult and Adolescent Dose prn‡ | Usual Pediatric Dose prn | Packaging, Storage, and Auxiliary labelings§ |
|---|---|---|---|---|---|---|---|---|---|---|
| *Ambophen* Syrup (Schedule V) [U.S.] | Bromodiphen-hydramine HCl 12.5 mg | | Codeine PO₄ 10 mg | | | | Alcohol 5% | 5–10 mL q 4–6 hr | 2–6 yrs: 1.25–2.5 mL, 6–12 yrs: 2.5–5 mL, q 6 hr | b, c, d, e, f |
| *Amgenal Cough* Syrup (Schedule V) [U.S.] | Bromodiphen-hydramine HCl 12.5 mg | | Codeine PO₄ 10 mg | | | | | 5–10 mL q 4–6 hr | | b, c, e, f |
| *Ami-Tex* Capsules (Rx) [U.S.] | | Phenylephrine HCl 5 mg, Phenylpropanolamine HCl 45 mg | | | Guaifenesin 200 mg | | | 1 cap q 6 hr | Not recommended | a¹, d |
| *Ami-Tex LA* Extended-release Tablets (Rx) [U.S.] | | Phenylpropanolamine HCl 75 mg | | | Guaifenesin 400 mg | | Scored | 1 tab q 12 hr | 6–12 yrs: ½ tab q 12 hr | a¹, d |
| *Anaplex HD* Syrup (Schedule III) [U.S.] | Chlorpheniramine maleate 2 mg | Phenylephrine HCl 5 mg | Hydrocodone bitartrate 1.7 mg | | | | Alcohol free Sugar free | 10 mL q 6–8 hr | | b, c, e, f |
| *Anatuss* Syrup (OTC) [U.S.] | | Phenylpropanolamine HCl 25 mg | | Dextromethorphan HBr 15 mg | Guaifenesin 100 mg | | Alcohol free Sugar free | 10 mL q 6 hr (max 4 doses/day) | 6–12 yrs: 5 mL q 6 hr (max 4 doses/day) | b, c, e |
| Tablets (Rx) [U.S.] | | Phenylpropanolamine HCl 25 mg | | Dextromethorphan HBr 15 mg | Guaifenesin 100 mg | Acetaminophen 325 mg | | 2 tabs q 4–6 hr (max 4 doses/day) | 6–12 yrs: 1 tab q 4–6 hr (max 4 doses/day) | b, e |
| *Anatuss DM* Syrup (OTC) [U.S.] | | Pseudoephedrine HCl 30 mg | | Dextromethorphan HBr 10 mg | Guaifenesin 100 mg | | | 10 mL q 4 hr (max 4 doses/day) | 6–12 yrs: 5 mL q 4 hr (max 4 doses/day) | b, c |
| Tablets (OTC) [U.S.] | | Pseudoephedrine HCl 60 mg | | Dextromethorphan HBr 20 mg | Guaifenesin 400 mg | | Film coated Scored | 1 tab q 4 hr (max 4 doses/day) | 6–12 yrs: ½ tab q 4 hr (max 4 doses/day) | b |
| *Anatuss LA* Extended-release Tablets (Rx) [U.S.] | | Pseudoephedrine HCl 120 mg | | | Guaifenesin 400 mg | | Scored | 1 tab q 12 hr | 6–12 yrs: ½ tab q 12 hr | b |

## Table 3. Oral Dosage Forms (continued)

Note: Content per capsule, tablet, or 5 mL, unless otherwise stated.

| Brand or generic name [availability] | Antihistamines | Decongestants | Antitussives Opioid | Antitussives Non-opioid | Expectorants | Analgesics | Other content information as per product label | Usual Adult and Adolescent Dose prn‡ | Usual Pediatric Dose prn | Packaging, Storage, and Auxiliary labeling§ |
|---|---|---|---|---|---|---|---|---|---|---|
| Anti-Tuss DM Expectorant Oral Solution (OTC) [U.S.] | | | | Dextromethorphan HBr 15 mg | Guaifenesin 100 mg | | Alcohol 1.4% | 10 mL q 6–8 hr | 2–6 yrs: 2.5 mL, 6–12 yrs: 5 mL, q 6–8 hr | b, c |
| Aprodine with Codeine Syrup (Schedule V) [U.S.] | Triprolidine HCl 1.25 mg | Pseudoephedrine HCl 30 mg | Codeine PO₄ 10 mg | | | | | 10 mL q 4–6 hr (max 40 mL/day) | | b, c, e, f |
| Atuss DM Syrup (Rx) [U.S.] | Chlorpheniramine maleate 2 mg | Phenylephrine HCl 5 mg | | Dextromethorphan HBr 15 mg | | | Alcohol free | 10 mL q 6 hr | 6–12 yrs: 5 mL q 6 hr | a, d, e |
| Atuss EX Syrup (Schedule III) [U.S.] | | | Hydrocodone bitartrate 5 mg | | Guaifenesin 100 mg | | Alcohol free Sugar free | 5 mL q 4 hr (max 30 mL/day) | 2–12 yrs: 2.5 mL q 4 hr | a, f |
| Atuss HD Oral Solution (Schedule III) [U.S.] | Chlorpheniramine maleate 2 mg | Phenylephrine HCl 5 mg | Hydrocodone bitartrate 2.5 mg | | | | Alcohol free | 10 mL q 4 hr (max 40 mL/day) | 6–12 yrs: 5 mL q 4 hr (max 20 mL/day) | a, d, f |
| Banex-LA Extended-release Tablets (Rx) [U.S.] | | Phenylpropanolamine HCL 75 mg | | | Guaifenesin 400 mg | | | 1 tab q 12 hr | | b |
| Banex Liquid Oral Solution (Rx) [U.S.] | | Phenylephrine HCl 5 mg, Phenylpropanolamine HCl 20 mg | | | Guaifenesin 100 mg | | Alcohol 5% | 10 mL q 6 hr | 2–4 yrs: 2.5 mL, 4–6 yrs: 5 mL, 6–12 yrs: 7.5 mL, q 6 hr | b, c |

*Specific formulations may vary among the different manufacturers, check product labeling.
†Efficacy as expectorant has not been established.
‡Geriatric patients may be more sensitive to effects of usual adult dose.
§For appropriate *Packaging and storage* and *Auxiliary labeling* information refer to designated letters as follows:
 a—Store below 40 °C (104 °F), preferably between 15 and 30 °C (59 and 86 °F), in a tight container, unless otherwise specified by manufacturer.
 a¹—Store below 30 °C (86 °F), unless otherwise specified by manufacturer. Avoid exposure to excessive heat.
 a²—Store below 25 °C (77 °F), unless otherwise specified by manufacturer.
 b—Store below 40 °C (104 °F), preferably between 15 and 30 °C (59 and 86 °F), in a well-closed container, unless otherwise specified by manufacturer.
 c—Protect from freezing.
 d—Protect from light.
 e—Auxiliary labeling: · May cause drowsiness. · Avoid alcoholic beverages.
 f—Auxiliary labeling: · May be habit forming.
 g—Auxiliary labeling: · Shake well.
 h—Dispense in dropper bottle.
 i—Chew well before swallowing.
**Included in subtherapeutic amount to discourage deliberate overdosage.

**1036  Cough/Cold Combinations (Systemic)**  USP DI

## Table 3. Oral Dosage Forms (continued)

Note: Content per capsule, tablet, or 5 mL, unless otherwise stated.

| Brand or generic name [availability] | Antihistamines | Decongestants | Antitussives Opioid | Antitussives Non-opioid | Expectorants | Analgesics | Other content information as per product label | Usual Adult and Adolescent Dose prn‡ | Usual Pediatric Dose prn | Packaging, Storage, and Auxiliary labelings§ |
|---|---|---|---|---|---|---|---|---|---|---|
| *Benylin Codeine D-E Syrup* (N) [Canada] | | Pseudoephedrine HCl 30 mg | Codeine PO₄ 3.3 mg | | Guaifenesin 100 mg | | Alcohol 5% Sodium 25 mg Sugar free | 10 mL q 4 hr (max 40 mL/day) | | b, c, e, f |
| *Benylin DM-D Syrup* (OTC) [Canada] | | Pseudoephedrine HCl 30 mg | | Dextromethorphan HBr 15 mg | | | Alcohol free Sodium 19 mg Sugar free | 10 mL q 6 hr (max 4 doses/day) | 2–5 yrs: 2.5 mL, 6–11 yrs: 5 mL, q 6 hr (max 4 doses/day) | a |
| *Benylin DM-D for Children Syrup* (OTC) [Canada] | | Pseudoephedrine HCl 15 mg | | Dextromethorphan HBr 7.5 mg | | | Alcohol free Sodium 11.04 mg Sugar free | | 2–5 yrs: 5 mL, 6–12 yrs: 10 mL, q 6 hr | a |
| *Benylin DM-D-E Syrup* (OTC) [Canada] | | Pseudoephedrine HCl 30 mg | | Dextromethorphan HBr 15 mg | Guaifenesin 100 mg | | Alcohol 5% Sodium 20.6 mg Sugar free | 10 mL q 6 hr (max 4 doses/day) | 2–5 yrs: 2.5 mL, 6–11 yrs: 5 mL, q 6 hr (max 4 doses/day) | a |
| *Benylin DM-D-E Extra Strength Syrup* (OTC) [Canada] | | Pseudoephedrine HCl 30 mg | | Dextromethorphan HBr 15 mg | Guaifenesin 200 mg | | Alcohol 5% Sodium 19.6 mg Sugar free | 10 mL q 6 hr (max 4 doses/day) | Not recommended | a |
| *Benylin DM-E Syrup* (OTC) [Canada] | | | | Dextromethorphan HBr 15 mg | Guaifenesin 100 mg | | Alcohol 5% Sodium 20.6 mg Sugar free | 10 mL q 6 hr (max 4 doses/day) | 2–5 yrs: 2.5 mL, 6–11 yrs: 5 mL, q 6 hr (max 4 doses/day) | a |
| *Benylin DM-E Extra Strength Syrup* (OTC) [Canada] | | | | Dextromethorphan HBr 15 mg | Guaifenesin 200 mg | | Alcohol Sodium 19.6 mg Sugar free | 10 mL q 6 hr (max 4 doses/day) | Not recommended | a |
| *Benylin Expectorant Oral Solution* (OTC) [U.S.] | | | | Dextromethorphan HBr 5 mg | Guaifenesin 100 mg | | Alcohol free Sugar free | 20 mL q 4 hr (max 6 doses/day) | 2–6 yrs: 5 mL, 6–12 yrs: 10 mL, q 4 hr (max 6 doses/day) | b, c |

USP DI  Cough/Cold Combinations (Systemic) 1037

Table 3. Oral Dosage Forms (continued)

Note: Content per capsule, tablet, or 5 mL, unless otherwise stated.

| Brand or generic name [availability] | Antihistamines | Decongestants | Antitussives — Opioid | Antitussives — Non-opioid | Expectorants | Analgesics | Other content information as per product label | Usual Adult and Adolescent Dose prn‡ | Usual Pediatric Dose prn | Packaging, Storage, and Auxiliary labeling§ |
|---|---|---|---|---|---|---|---|---|---|---|
| *Benylin 4 Flu* Oral Solution (OTC) [Canada] | | Pseudoephedrine HCl 30 mg/15 mL | | Dextromethorphan HBr 15 mg/15 mL | Guaifenesin 100 mg/15 mL | Acetaminophen 500 mg/15 mL | Alcohol 5% Sugar free | 30 mL q 6 hr (max 4 doses/day) | Not recommended | a, c |
| *Benylin Multi-Symptom* Oral Solution (OTC) [U.S.] | | Pseudoephedrine HCl 15 mg | | Dextromethorphan HBr 5 mg | Guaifenesin 100 mg | | Alcohol free Sugar free | 20 mL q 4 hr (max 4 doses/day) | 2–6 yrs: 5 mL, 6–12 yrs: 10 mL, q 4 hr (max 4 doses/day) | b |
| *Biohisdex DM* Oral Solution (OTC) [Canada] | Diphenylpyraline HCl 2 mg | Phenylephrine HCl 20 mg | | Dextromethorphan HBr 10 mg | | | | 10 mL q 4 hr (max 4 doses/day) | 6–12 yrs: 10 mL q 4 hr (max 4 doses/day) | a, e |
| *Biohistine DM* Oral Solution (OTC) [Canada] | Diphenylpyraline HCl 1 mg | Phenylephrine HCl 10 mg | | Dextromethorphan HBr 5 mg | | | | | <1 yr: 2.5 mL, 1–4 yrs: 5 mL, 5–12 yrs: 10 mL, q 4 hr (max 4 doses/day) | a, e |
| *Bromanate DC Cough* Syrup (Schedule V) [U.S.] | Brompheniramine maleate 2 mg | Phenylpropanolamine HCl 12.5 mg | Codeine PO₄ 10 mg | | | | Alcohol 0.95% | 10 mL q 4 hr | 2–6 yrs: 2.5 mL, 6–12 yrs: 5 mL, q 4 hr | a, c, d, e, f |
| *Bromanyl* Syrup (Schedule V) [U.S.] | Bromodiphenhydramine HCl 12.5 mg | | Codeine PO₄ 10 mg | | | | | 5–10 mL q 4–6 hr | | b, c, e, f |

*Specific formulations may vary among the different manufacturers; check product labeling.
†Efficacy as expectorant has not been established.
‡Geriatric patients may be more sensitive to effects of usual adult dose.
§For appropriate *Packaging and storage* and *Auxiliary labeling* information refer to designated letters as follows:
a—Store below 40 °C (104 °F), preferably between 15 and 30 °C (59 and 86 °F), in a tight container, unless otherwise specified by manufacturer.
a¹—Store below 30 °C (86 °F), preferably between 15 and 30 °C (59 and 86 °F), in a tight container, unless otherwise specified by manufacturer. Avoid exposure to excessive heat.
a²—Store below 25 °C (77 °F), unless otherwise specified by manufacturer.
b—Store below 40 °C (104 °F), preferably between 15 and 30 °C (59 and 86 °F), in a well-closed container, unless otherwise specified by manufacturer.
c—Protect from freezing.
d—Protect from light.
e—Auxiliary labeling: • May cause drowsiness. • Avoid alcoholic beverages.
f—Auxiliary labeling: • May be habit forming.
g—Auxiliary labeling: • Shake well.
h—Dispense in dropper bottle.
i—Chew well before swallowing.
**Included in subtherapeutic amount to discourage deliberate overdosage.

## 1038 Cough/Cold Combinations (Systemic)

Table 3. Oral Dosage Forms (continued)

Note: Content per capsule, tablet, or 5 mL, unless otherwise stated.

| Brand or generic name [availability] | Antihistamines | Decongestants | Antitussives Opioid | Antitussives Non-opioid | Expectorants | Analgesics | Other content information as per product label | Usual Adult and Adolescent Dose prn‡ | Usual Pediatric Dose prn | Packaging, Storage, and Auxiliary labeling§ |
|---|---|---|---|---|---|---|---|---|---|---|
| Bromarest DX Cough Syrup (Rx) [U.S.] | Brompheniramine maleate 2 mg | Pseudoephedrine HCl 30 mg | | Dextromethorphan HBr 10 mg | | | Alcohol 0.95% | 10 mL q 4 hr | | b, c, e |
| Bromatane DX Cough Syrup (Rx) [U.S.] | Brompheniramine maleate 2 mg | Pseudoephedrine HCl 30 mg | | Dextromethorphan HBr 10 mg | | | | 10 mL q 4 hr | | b, c, e |
| Bromfed-DM Syrup (Rx) [U.S.] | Brompheniramine maleate 2 mg | Pseudoephedrine HCl 30 mg | | Dextromethorphan HBr 10 mg | | | Alcohol free | 10 mL q 4 hr (max 6 doses/day) | 2–6 yrs: 2.5 mL; 6–12 yrs: 5 mL, q 4 hr (max 6 doses/day) | a, c, d, e |
| Bromodiphenhydramine and Codeine* Syrup (Schedule V) [U.S.] | Bromodiphenhydramine HCl 12.5 mg | | Codeine PO$_4$ 10 mg | | | | May contain alcohol | 5–10 mL q 4–6 hr | | b, c, e, f |
| Bromotuss with Codeine Syrup (Schedule V) [U.S.] | Bromodiphenhydramine HCl 12.5 mg | | Codeine PO$_4$ 10 mg | | | | | 5–10 mL q 4–6 hr | | b, c, e, f |
| Bromphen DC w/Codeine Cough Syrup (Schedule V) [U.S.] | Brompheniramine maleate 2 mg | Phenylpropanolamine HCl 12.5 mg | Codeine PO$_4$ 10 mg | | | | Alcohol 0.95% | 10 mL q 4 hr | 2–6 yrs: 2.5 mL; 6–12 yrs: 5 mL, q 4 hr | a, c, d, e, f |
| Bromphen DX Cough Syrup (Rx) [U.S.] | Brompheniramine maleate 2 mg | Pseudoephedrine HCl 30 mg | | Dextromethorphan HBr 10 mg | | | Alcohol 0.95% | 10 mL q 4 hr | | b, c, e |
| Broncholate Syrup (Rx) [U.S.] | | Ephedrine HCl 6.25 mg | | | Guaifenesin 100 mg | | | 10–20 mL q 4 hr | 2–6 yrs: 2.5–5 mL; 6–12 yrs: 5–10 mL, q 4 hr | a, c, d |
| Bronkotuss Expectorant Oral Solution (Rx) [U.S.] | Chlorpheniramine maleate 4 mg | Ephedrine sulfate 8.2 mg | | | Guaifenesin 100 mg | | Alcohol 5% | 5 mL q 3–4 hr | 6–12 yrs: 2.5 mL q 3–4 hr | b, c, e |
| Brontex Oral Solution (Schedule V) [U.S.] | | | Codeine PO$_4$ 2.5 mg | | Guaifenesin 75 mg | | | 20 mL q 4 hr (max 120 mL/day) | 6–12 yrs: 10 mL q 4 hr | b, e, f |
| Tablets (Schedule III) [U.S.] | | | Codeine PO$_4$ 10 mg | | Guaifenesin 300 mg | | | 1 tab q 4 hr | Not recommended | b, e, f |

**Cough/Cold Combinations (Systemic) 1039**

Table 3. Oral Dosage Forms (*continued*)

Note: Content per capsule, tablet, or 5 mL, unless otherwise stated.

| Brand or generic name [availability] | Antihistamines | Decongestants | Antitussives — Opioid | Antitussives — Non-opioid | Expectorants | Analgesics | Other content information as per product label | Usual Adult and Adolescent Dose prn‡ | Usual Pediatric Dose prn | Packaging, Storage, and Auxiliary labeling§ |
|---|---|---|---|---|---|---|---|---|---|---|
| *Brotane DX Cough Syrup* (Rx) [U.S.] | Brompheniramine maleate 2 mg | Pseudoephedrine HCl 30 mg | | Dextromethorphan HBr 10 mg | | | Alcohol 0.95% | 10 mL q 4 hr | 2–6 yrs: 2.5 mL; 6–12 yrs: 5 mL, q 4 hr | a, c, d, e |
| *Buckley's DM Oral Solution* [Canada] | | Pseudoephedrine HCl 30 mg | | Dextromethorphan HBr 12.5 mg | | | Alcohol free Sugar free | 10 mL q 6 hr (max 4 doses/day) | 6–12 yrs: 5 mL q 6 hr (max 4 doses/day) | a, g |
| *Calcidrine Syrup* (Schedule V) [U.S.] | | | Codeine 8.4 mg | | Calcium iodide† 152 mg | | Alcohol 6% | 5–10 mL q 4 hr | 2–6 yrs: 2.5 mL; 6–10 yrs: 2.5–5 mL, q 4 hr | a, c, d, e, f |
| *Caldomine-DH Forte Oral Solution* (N) [Canada] | Pheniramine maleate 12.5 mg Pyrilamine maleate 12.5 mg | Phenylpropanolamine HCl 25 mg | Hydrocodone bitartrate 5 mg | | | | | 5 mL q 4 hr | 2–6 yrs: 1.25 mL; 6–12 yrs: 2.5 mL, q 4–6 hr See also *Caldomine-DH Pediatric Oral Solution* | b, c, e, f |
| *Caldomine-DH Pediatric Oral Solution* (N) [Canada] | Pheniramine maleate 6.25 mg Pyrilamine maleate 6.25 mg | Phenylpropanolamine HCl 12.5 mg | Hydrocodone bitartrate 1.66 mg | | | | | Intended for pediatric use. See *Caldomine-DH Forte Oral Solution* | 1–6 yrs: 2.5 mL; 6–12 yrs: 5 mL, q 4 hr | b, c, e, f |

*Specific formulations may vary among the different manufacturers, check product labeling.
†Efficacy as expectorant has not been established.
‡Geriatric patients may be more sensitive to effects of usual adult dose.
§For appropriate *Packaging and storage* and *Auxiliary labeling* information refer to designated letters as follows:
  a—Store below 40 °C (104 °F), preferably between 15 and 30 °C (59 and 86 °F), in a tight container, unless otherwise specified by manufacturer.
  a¹—Store below 30 °C (86 °F), unless otherwise specified by manufacturer. Avoid exposure to excessive heat.
  a²—Store below 25 °C (77 °F), unless otherwise specified by manufacturer.
  b—Store below 40 °C (104 °F), preferably between 15 and 30 °C (59 and 86 °F), in a well-closed container, unless otherwise specified by manufacturer.
  c—Protect from freezing.
  d—Protect from light.
  e—Auxiliary labeling: · May cause drowsiness. · Avoid alcoholic beverages.
  f—Auxiliary labeling: · May be habit forming.
  g—Auxiliary labeling: · Shake well.
  h—Dispense in dropper bottle.
  i—Auxiliary labeling: · Chew well before swallowing.
**Included in subtherapeutic amount to discourage deliberate overdosage.

## Table 3. Oral Dosage Forms (continued)

Note: Content per capsule, tablet, or 5 mL, unless otherwise stated.

| Brand or generic name [availability] | Antihistamines | Decongestants | Antitussives Opioid | Antitussives Non-opioid | Expectorants | Analgesics | Other content information as per product label | Usual Adult and Adolescent Dose prn‡ | Usual Pediatric Dose prn | Packaging, Storage, and Auxiliary labeling§ |
|---|---|---|---|---|---|---|---|---|---|---|
| *Calmydone* Syrup (N) [Canada] | Doxylamine succinate 1.2 mg/mL | Etafedrine HCl 3.33 mg/mL | Hydrocodone bitartrate 0.33 mg/mL | | | | Alcohol 5% Sodium citrate 45.60 mg/mL | 5 mL q 3–5 hr (max 6 doses/day) | 1–6 yrs: 1.25–2.5 mL, 6–12 yrs: 2.5–5 mL, q 3–5 hr (max 3 doses/day) | a, e, f |
| *Calmylin #2* Syrup (OTC) [Canada] | | Pseudoephedrine HCl 30 mg | | Dextromethorphan HBr 15 mg | | | Alcohol free Sugar free | 5–10 mL q 6–8 hr | 2–5 yrs: 2.5 mL, 6–12 yrs: 5 mL, q 6–8 hr | a, c, e |
| *Calmylin #3* Syrup (OTC) [Canada] | | Pseudoephedrine HCl 30 mg | | Dextromethorphan HBr 15 mg | Guaifenesin 100 mg | | Alcohol 5% Sugar free | 10 mL q 6–8 hr | 2–5 yrs: 2.5 mL, 6–12 yrs: 5 mL, q 6–8 hr | a, c, e |
| *Calmylin #4* Syrup (OTC) [Canada] | Diphenhydramine HCl 12.5 mg | | | Dextromethorphan HBr 15 mg | Ammonium chloride† 125 mg | | Alcohol 5% | 5–10 mL q 6–8 hr | 2–3 yrs: 1.25 mL, 4–12 yrs: 2.5–5 mL, q 6–8 hr | a, c, e |
| *Calmylin Codeine D-E* Oral Solution (N) [Canada] | | Pseudoephedrine HCl 30 mg | Codeine PO₄ 3.33 mg | | Guaifenesin 100 mg | | Sugar free | 10 mL q 4 hr (max 40 mL/day) | | a, e |
| *Calmylin Cough & Flu* Syrup (OTC) [Canada] | | Pseudoephedrine HCl 30 mg/ 15 mL | | Dextromethorphan HBr 15 mg/15 mL | Guaifenesin 100 mg/ 15 mL | Acetaminophen 325 mg/ 15 mL | Alcohol free Sugar free | 15–30 mL q 6–8 hr (max 120 mL/day) | Not recommended | a, c |
| *Calmylin DM-D-E Extra Strength* Syrup (OTC) [Canada] | | Pseudoephedrine HCl 30 mg | | Dextromethorphan HBr 15 mg | Guaifenesin 200 mg | | Alcohol 5% Sugar free | 10 mL q 6 hr | Not recommended | a, c |
| *Calmylin DM-E* Syrup (OTC) [Canada] | | | | Dextromethorphan HBr 15 mg | Guaifenesin 100 mg | | Alcohol 5% Sugar free | 10 mL q 6 hr max 4 doses/day | 2–5 yrs: 2.5 mL, 6–11 yrs: 5 mL, q 6 hr max 4 doses/day | a, c |
| *Calmylin Original with Codeine* Syrup (N) [Canada] | Diphenhydramine HCl 12.5 mg | | Codeine PO₄ 3.33 mg | | Ammonium chloride† 125 mg | | Alcohol 2.9% | 5–10 mL q 3–4 hr | | b, c, e, f |

Table 3. Oral Dosage Forms *(continued)*

Note: Content per capsule, tablet, or 5 mL, unless otherwise stated.

| Brand or generic name [availability] | Antihistamines | Decongestants | Antitussives Opioid | Antitussives Non-opioid | Expectorants | Analgesics | Other content information as per product label | Usual Adult and Adolescent Dose prn‡ | Usual Pediatric Dose prn | Packaging, Storage, and Auxiliary labeling§ |
|---|---|---|---|---|---|---|---|---|---|---|
| *Calmylin Pediatric Syrup* (OTC) [Canada] | | Pseudoephedrine HCl 15 mg | | Dextromethorphan HBr 7.5 mg | | | Alcohol free Sugar free | | 1–2 yrs: 2.5 mL, 2–6 yrs: 5 mL, 6–12 yrs: 10 mL, q 6–8 hr | a, c |
| *Carbinoxamine Compound Syrup* (Rx) [U.S.] | Carbinoxamine maleate 4 mg | Pseudoephedrine HCl 60 mg | | Dextromethorphan HBr 15 mg | | | Alcohol <0.2% | 5 mL q 6 hr | 18 mos–6 yrs: 2.5 mL, >6 yrs: 5 mL, q 4–6 hr | a, c, d, e |
| *Carbinoxamine Compound-Drops Oral Solution* (Rx) [U.S.] | Carbinoxamine maleate 2 mg/mL | Pseudoephedrine HCl 25 mg/mL | | Dextromethorphan HBr 4 mg/mL | | | Alcohol <0.2% | | 1–18 mos: 0.25–1 mL q 6 hr | b, c, e |
| *Carbodec DM Syrup* (Rx) [U.S.] | Carbinoxamine maleate 4 mg | Pseudoephedrine HCl 60 mg | | Dextromethorphan HBr 15 mg | | | Alcohol free Sugar free | 5 mL q 6 hr | 18 mos–6 yrs: 2.5 mL, >6 yrs: 5 mL, q 4–6 hr | a, c, d, e |
| *Carbodec DM Drops Oral Solution* (Rx) [U.S.] | Carbinoxamine maleate 2 mg/mL | Pseudoephedrine HCl 25 mg/mL | | Dextromethorphan HBr 4 mg/mL | | | Alcohol free Sugar free | Intended for pediatric use. See *Carbodec DM Syrup* | 1–3 mos: 0.25 mL, 3–6 mos: 0.50 mL, 6–9 mos: 0.75 mL, 9–18 mos: 1 mL, q 6 hr | a, c, e, h |
| *Cardec DM Syrup* (Rx) [U.S.] | Carbinoxamine maleate 4 mg | Pseudoephedrine HCl 60 mg | | Dextromethorphan HBr 15 mg | | | Alcohol <0.6% | 5 mL q 6 hr | | b, c, e |

\*Specific formulations may vary among the different manufacturers, check product labeling.
†Efficacy as expectorant has not been established.
‡Geriatric patients may be more sensitive to effects of usual adult dose.
§For appropriate *Packaging and storage* and *Auxiliary labeling* information refer to designated letters as follows:
  a—Store below 40 °C (104 °F), preferably between 15 and 30 °C (59 and 86 °F), in a tight container, unless otherwise specified by manufacturer.
  a¹—Store below 30 °C (86 °F), unless otherwise specified by manufacturer. Avoid exposure to excessive heat.
  a²—Store below 25 °C (77 °F), unless otherwise specified by manufacturer.
  b—Store below 40 °C (104 °F), preferably between 15 and 30 °C (59 and 86 °F), in a well-closed container, unless otherwise specified by manufacturer.
  c—Protect from freezing.
  d—Protect from light.
  e—Auxiliary labeling: · May cause drowsiness. · Avoid alcoholic beverages.
  f—Auxiliary labeling: · May be habit forming.
  g—Auxiliary labeling: · Shake well.
  h—Dispense in dropper bottle.
  i—Chew well before swallowing.
\*\*Included in subtherapeutic amount to discourage deliberate overdosage.

**1042**  **Cough/Cold Combinations (Systemic)**  *USP DI*

**Table 3. Oral Dosage Forms** *(continued)*
Note: Content per capsule, tablet, or 5 mL, unless otherwise stated.

| Brand or generic name [availability] | Antihistamines | Decongestants | Antitussives - Opioid | Antitussives - Non-opioid | Expectorants | Analgesics | Other content information as per product label | Usual Adult and Adolescent Dose prn‡ | Usual Pediatric Dose prn | Packaging, Storage, and Auxiliary labeling§ |
|---|---|---|---|---|---|---|---|---|---|---|
| *Cardec DM Drops* Oral Solution (Rx) [U.S.] | Carbinoxamine maleate 2 mg/mL | Pseudoephedrine HCl 25 mg/mL | | Dextromethorphan HBr 4 mg/mL | | | May contain alcohol | Intended for pediatric use | 1–18 mos: 0.25–1 mL q 6 hr | b, c, e |
| *Cardec DM Pediatric* Syrup (Rx) [U.S.] | Carbinoxamine maleate 4 mg | Pseudoephedrine HCl 60 mg | | Dextromethorphan HBr 15 mg | | | Alcohol <0.6% | Intended for pediatric use | 2.5–5 mL q 6 hr | b, c |
| *Cerose-DM* Oral Solution (OTC) [U.S.] | Chlorpheniramine maleate 4 mg | Phenylephrine HCl 10 mg | | Dextromethorphan HBr 15 mg | | | Alcohol 2.4% Sugar free | 5 mL q 4 hr (max 30 mL/day) | 6–12 yrs: 2.5 mL q 4 hr (max 15 mL/day) | a, c, e |
| *Cheracol* Syrup USP (Schedule V) [U.S.] | | | Codeine PO₄ 10 mg | | Guaifenesin 100 mg | | Alcohol 4.75% | 10 mL q 4–6 hr | 6–12 yrs: 5 mL q 4–6 hr | a, d, e, f |
| Syrup (N) [Canada] | | | Codeine PO₄ 10 mg | | Ammonium Cl† 91 mg, Guaifenesin 100 mg | | Alcohol 3% | 5–15 mL q 2–4 hr as needed | 1 month: 2–3 drops, 3 mos: 4–6 drops, >1 yr: 2.5–5 mL according to age | b, c, e, f |
| *Cheracol D Cough* Oral Solution (OTC) [U.S.] | | | | Dextromethorphan HBr 10 mg | Guaifenesin 100 mg | | Alcohol 4.75% | 10 mL q 4 hr (max 60 mL/day) | 22.5 mL (max 15 mL/day) 6–12 yrs: 5 mL (max 30 mL/day) q 4 hr | b, c |
| *Cheracol Plus* Syrup (OTC) [U.S.] | Chlorpheniramine maleate 4 mg/15 mL | Phenylpropanolamine HCl 25 mg/15 mL | | Dextromethorphan HBr 20 mg/15 mL | | | Alcohol 8% | 15 mL q 4 hr (max 90 mL/day) | | b, c, e |
| *Children's Formula Cough* Syrup (OTC) [U.S.] | | | | Dextromethorphan HBr 5 mg | Guaifenesin 50 mg | | Alcohol free | 20 mL q 6 hr (max 4 doses/day) | 2–6 yrs: 5 mL, 6–12 yrs: 10 mL, q 6 hr (max 4 doses/day) | b, c |

USP DI  Cough/Cold Combinations (Systemic) 1043

Table 3. Oral Dosage Forms (continued)

Note: Content per capsule, tablet, or 5 mL, unless otherwise stated.

| Brand or generic name [availability] | Antihistamines | Decongestants | Antitussives Opioid | Antitussives Non-opioid | Expectorants | Analgesics | Other content information as per product label | Usual Adult and Adolescent Dose prn‡ | Usual Pediatric Dose prn | Packaging, Storage, and Auxiliary labelings§ |
|---|---|---|---|---|---|---|---|---|---|---|
| *Children's Tylenol Cold Plus Cough Multi Symptom* Oral Solution (OTC) [U.S.] | Chlorpheniramine maleate 1 mg | Pseudoephedrine HCl 15 mg | | Dextromethorphan HBr 5 mg | | Acetaminophen 160 mg | Alcohol free | Intended for pediatric use | 2–5 yrs: 5 mL, 6–11 yrs: 10 mL, q 4–6 hr (max 4 doses/day) | b, c, e |
| Chewable Tablets (OTC) [U.S.] | Chlorpheniramine maleate 0.5 mg | Pseudoephedrine HCl 7.5 mg | | Dextromethorphan HBr 2.5 mg | | Acetaminophen 80 mg | | Intended for pediatric use | 2–5 yrs: 2 tabs, 6–11 yrs: 4 tabs, q 4–6 hr (max 4 doses/day) | b, e, i |
| *Chlorgest-HD* Oral Solution (Schedule III) [U.S.] | Chlorpheniramine maleate 4 mg | Phenylephrine HCl 5 mg | Hydrocodone bitartrate 1.67 mg | | | | Alcohol free Sugar free | 10 mL q 6–8 hr | | b, c, e, f |
| *Citra Forte* Capsules (Schedule III) [U.S.] | Chlorpheniramine maleate 1 mg, Pheniramine maleate 6.25 mg, Pyrilamine maleate 8.33 mg | Phenylephrine HCl 10 mg | Hydrocodone bitartrate 5 mg | | | Salicylamide 227 mg | Ascorbic acid 50 mg, Caffeine 30 mg | 1–2 caps q 3–4 hr | Pediatric strength not available | b, e, f |
| Syrup (Schedule III) [U.S.] | Pheniramine maleate 2.5 mg, Pyrilamine maleate 3.33 mg | | Hydrocodone bitartrate 5 mg | | Potassium citrate† 150 mg | | Alcohol 2%, Ascorbic acid 30 mg | 5–10 mL q 3–4 hr | 6–12 yrs: 2.5–5 mL q 3–4 hr | b, c, d, e, f |
| *CoActifed* Oral Solution (N) [Canada] | Triprolidine HCl 2 mg | Pseudoephedrine HCl 30 mg | Codeine PO₄ 10 mg | | | | Alcohol free | 10 mL q 4–6 hr | <6 yrs: 2.5 mL, 6–12 yrs: 5 mL, q 4–6 hr | b, c, d, e, f |

*Specific formulations may vary among the different manufacturers, check product labeling.
†Efficacy as expectorant has not been established.
‡Geriatric patients may be more sensitive to effects of usual adult dose.
§For appropriate *Packaging and storage* and *Auxiliary labeling* information refer to designated letters as follows:
  a¹—Store below 40 °C (104 °F), preferably between 15 and 30 °C (59 and 86 °F), in a tight container, unless otherwise specified by manufacturer.
  a²—Store below 30 °C (86 °F), unless otherwise specified by manufacturer. Avoid exposure to excessive heat.
  a³—Store below 25 °C (77 °F), unless otherwise specified by manufacturer.
  b—Store below 40 °C (104 °F), preferably between 15 and 30 °C (59 and 86 °F), in a well-closed container, unless otherwise specified by manufacturer.
  c—Protect from freezing.          f—Auxiliary labeling: · May be habit forming.     h—Dispense in dropper bottle.
  d—Protect from light.             g—Auxiliary labeling: · Shake well.                i—Chew well before swallowing.
  e—Auxiliary labeling: · May cause drowsiness. · Avoid alcoholic beverages.
**Included in subtherapeutic amount to discourage deliberate overdosage.

**Table 3. Oral Dosage Forms** *(continued)*

Note: Content per capsule, tablet, or 5 mL, unless otherwise stated.

| Brand or generic name [availability] | Antihistamines | Decongestants | Antitussives - Opioid | Antitussives - Non-opioid | Expectorants | Analgesics | Other content information as per product label | Usual Adult and Adolescent Dose prn‡ | Usual Pediatric Dose prn | Packaging, Storage, and Auxiliary labeling§ |
|---|---|---|---|---|---|---|---|---|---|---|
| *CoActifed (continued)* Tablets (N) [Canada] | Triprolidine HCl 4 mg | Pseudoephedrine HCl 60 mg | Codeine PO₄ 20 mg | | | | Scored | 1 tab q 4–6 hr | <6 yrs: See CoActifed Syrup 6–12 yrs: ½ tab q 4–6 hr | b, d, e, f |
| *CoActifed Expectorant* Oral Solution (N) [Canada] | Triprolidine HCl 2 mg | Pseudoephedrine HCl 30 mg | Codeine PO₄ 10 mg | | Guaifenesin 100 mg | | Alcohol free | 10 mL q 4–6 hr | <6 yrs: 2.5 mL, 6–12 yrs: 5 mL, q 4–6 hr | b, c, d, e, f |
| *Co-Apap* Tablets (OTC) [U.S.] | Chlorpheniramine maleate 2 mg | Pseudoephedrine HCl 30 mg | | Dextromethorphan HBr 15 mg | | Acetaminophen 325 mg | | 2 tabs q 6 hr | 6–12 yrs: 1 tab q 6 hr | b, e |
| *Co-Complex DM Caplets* Tablets (OTC) [U.S.] | | Pseudoephedrine HCl 30 mg | | Dextromethorphan HBr 15 mg | | Acetaminophen 500 mg | Dye free | 2 tabs q 6 hr (max 8 tabs/day) | Not recommended | b |
| *Codamine* Syrup (Schedule III) [U.S.] | | Phenylpropanolamine HCl 25 mg | Hydrocodone bitartrate 5 mg | | | | | 5 mL q 6 hr | 6–12 yrs: 2.5 mL q 4–6 hr | b, c, d, e, f |
| *Codamine Pediatric* Syrup (Schedule III) [U.S.] | | Phenylpropanolamine HCl 12.5 mg | Hydrocodone bitartrate 2.5 mg | | | | | Intended for pediatric use. See *Codamine Syrup* | 2–6 yrs: 2.5 mL, 6–12 yrs: 5 mL, q 4–6 hr | b, c, d, e, f |
| *Codan* Syrup (Schedule III) [U.S.] | | | Hydrocodone bitartrate 5 mg | | | | Homatropine MBr 1.5 mg** | 5 mL q 4–6 hr | <2 yrs: 1.25 mL, 2–12 yrs: 2.5 mL, q 4–6 hr | b, c, d, e, f |
| *Codegest Expectorant* Oral Solution (Schedule V) [U.S.] | | Phenylpropanolamine HCl 12.5 mg | Codeine PO₄ 10 mg | | Guaifenesin 100 mg | | Alcohol free Sugar free Dye free | 5–10 mL q 4–6 hr | | b, c, e, f |
| *Codehist DH* Elixir (Schedule V) [U.S.] | Chlorpheniramine maleate 2 mg | Pseudoephedrine HCl 30 mg | Codeine PO₄ 10 mg | | | | Alcohol 5.7% | 10 mL q 4 hr (max 40 mL/day) | 2–6 yrs: 1.25–2.5 mL, 6–12 yrs: 2.5–5 mL, q 4 hr | a, c, d, e, f |
| *Codiclear DH* Syrup (Schedule III) [U.S.] | | | Hydrocodone bitartrate 5 mg | | Guaifenesin 100 mg | | Alcohol free Sugar free Dye free | 5–7.5 mL q 4–6 hr (max 30 mL/day) | 3–6 yrs: 1.25–2.5 mL, 6–12 yrs: 2.5–5 mL, q 4–6 hr | b, c, d, e, f |

Table 3. Oral Dosage Forms (continued)

Note: Content per capsule, tablet, or 5 mL, unless otherwise stated.

| Brand or generic name [availability] | Antihistamines | Decongestants | Antitussives Opioid | Antitussives Non-opioid | Expectorants | Analgesics | Other content information as per product label | Usual Adult and Adolescent Dose prn‡ | Usual Pediatric Dose prn | Packaging, Storage, and Auxiliary labelings§ |
|---|---|---|---|---|---|---|---|---|---|---|
| Codimal DH Syrup (Schedule III) [U.S.] | Pyrilamine maleate 8.33 mg | Phenylephrine HCl 5 mg | Hydrocodone bitartrate 1.66 mg | | | | Alcohol free | 5–10 mL q 4 hr | 6 mos–2 yrs: 1.25 mL q 6 hr; 2–6 yrs: 2.5 mL, 6–12 yrs: 5 mL, q 4 hr | b, c, d, e, f |
| Codimal DM Syrup (OTC) [U.S.] | Pyrilamine maleate 8.33 mg | Phenylephrine HCl 5 mg | | Dextromethorphan HBr 10 mg | | | Alcohol free Sugar free Dye free | 10 mL q 4 hr | 6–12 yrs: 5 mL q 4 hr | b, c, e |
| Codimal PH Syrup (Schedule V) [U.S.] | Pyrilamine maleate 8.33 mg | Phenylephrine HCl 5 mg | Codeine PO$_4$ 10 mg | | | | Alcohol free | 5–10 mL q 4–6 hr | 6–12 yrs: 5 mL q 4 hr | b, c, e, f |
| Comtrex Cough Formula Oral Solution (OTC) [U.S.] | | Pseudoephedrine HCl 15 mg | | Dextromethorphan HBr 7.5 mg | Guaifenesin 50 mg | Acetaminophen 125 mg | Alcohol 20% | 20 mL q 4 hr (max 80 mL/day) | | b, c |
| Comtrex Daytime Caplets Tablets (OTC) [U.S.] | | Pseudoephedrine HCl 30 mg | | Dextromethorphan HBr 10 mg | | Acetaminophen 325 mg | | 2 tabs q 4 hr | Intended for adult use | b |
| Comtrex Daytime Maximum Strength Cold, Cough and Flu Relief Tablets (OTC) [U.S.] | | Pseudoephedrine HCl 30 mg | | Dextromethorphan HBr 15 mg | | Acetaminophen 500 mg | Available in a dual package that also contains Comtrex Nighttime Maximum Strength Cold, Cough and Flu Relief | 2 tabs q 6 hr (max 4 tabs/day) | | b |

*Specific formulations may vary among the different manufacturers, check product labeling.
†Efficacy as expectorant has not been established.
‡Geriatric patients may be more sensitive to effects of usual adult dose.
§For appropriate *Packaging and storage* and *Auxiliary labeling* information refer to designated letters as follows:
  a—Store below 40 °C (104 °F), preferably between 15 and 30 °C (59 and 86 °F), in a tight container, unless otherwise specified by manufacturer.
  a¹—Store below 30 °C (86 °F), unless otherwise specified by manufacturer. Avoid exposure to excessive heat.
  a²—Store below 25 °C (77 °F), unless otherwise specified by manufacturer.
  b—Store below 40 °C (104 °F), preferably between 15 and 30 °C (59 and 86 °F), in a well-closed container, unless otherwise specified by manufacturer.
  c—Protect from freezing.                                     f—Auxiliary labeling: · May be habit forming.      h—Dispense in dropper bottle.
  d—Protect from light.                                        g—Auxiliary labeling: · Shake well.                 i—Chew well before swallowing.
  e—Auxiliary labeling: · May cause drowsiness. · Avoid alcoholic beverages.
**Included in subtherapeutic amount to discourage deliberate overdosage.

# Cough/Cold Combinations (Systemic)

**Table 3. Oral Dosage Forms** *(continued)*

Note: Content per capsule, tablet, or 5 mL, unless otherwise stated.

| Brand or generic name [availability] | Antihistamines | Decongestants | Antitussives Opioid | Antitussives Non-opioid | Expectorants | Analgesics | Other content information as per product label | Usual Adult and Adolescent Dose prn‡ | Usual Pediatric Dose prn | Packaging, Storage, and Auxiliary labeling§ |
|---|---|---|---|---|---|---|---|---|---|---|
| *Comtrex Daytime Maximum Strength Cold and Flu Relief* Tablets (OTC) [U.S.] | | Pseudoephedrine HCl 30 mg | | Dextromethorphan HBr 15 mg | | Acetaminophen 500 mg | Available in a dual package that also contains *Comtrex Nighttime Maximum Strength Cold and Flu Relief* | 2 tabs q 6 hr (max 4 tabs/day) | | b |
| *Comtrex Maximum Strength Multi-Symptom Liqui-Gels* Capsules (OTC) [U.S.] | Chlorpheniramine maleate 2 mg | Phenylpropanolamine HCl 12.5 mg | | Dextromethorphan HBr 15 mg | | Acetaminophen 500 mg | | 2 caps q 6 hr (max 8 caps/day) | | b, c, e |
| *Comtrex Multi-Symptom Cold Reliever* Capsules (OTC) [U.S.] | Chlorpheniramine maleate 1 mg | Phenylpropanolamine HCl 12.5 mg | | Dextromethorphan HBr 10 mg | | Acetaminophen 325 mg | | 2 caps q 4 hr | 6–12 yrs: 1 cap q 4 hr | b, e |
| Oral Solution (OTC) [U.S.] | Chlorpheniramine maleate 0.33 mg | Phenylpropanolamine HCl 4.2 mg | | Dextromethorphan HBr 3.3 mg | | Acetaminophen 108.3 mg | Alcohol 20% | 30 mL q 4 hr | 6–12 yrs: 15 mL q 4 hr | b, c, e |
| Tablets (OTC) [U.S.] | Chlorpheniramine maleate 1 mg | Phenylpropanolamine HCl 12.5 mg | | Dextromethorphan HBr 10 mg | | Acetaminophen 325 mg | | 2 tabs q 4 hr | 6–12 yrs: 1 tab q 4 hr | b, e |
| *Comtrex Multi-Symptom Maximum Strength Non-Drowsy* Caplets Tablets (OTC) [U.S.] | | Pseudoephedrine HCl 30 mg | | Dextromethorphan HBr 15 mg | | Acetaminophen 500 mg | | 2 tabs q 6 hr (max 8 tabs/day) | Intended for adult use | b |
| *Comtrex Nighttime* Tablets (OTC) [U.S.] | Chlorpheniramine maleate 2 mg | Pseudoephedrine HCl 30 mg | | Dextromethorphan HBr 10 mg | | Acetaminophen 325 mg | | 2 tabs hs | Intended for adult use | b, e |
| *Comtrex Nighttime Maximum Strength Cold, Cough and Flu Relief* Oral Solution (OTC) [U.S.] | Chlorpheniramine maleate 4 mg/ 30 mL | Pseudoephedrine HCl 60 mg/ 30 mL | | Dextromethorphan HBr 30 mg/ 30 mL | | Acetaminophen 1000 mg/ 30 mL | Alcohol 10% Available in a dual package that also contains *Comtrex Daytime Maximum Strength Cold, Cough and Flu Relief* | 30 mL hs | | b, c, e |

Table 3. Oral Dosage Forms (continued)

Note: Content per capsule, tablet, or 5 mL, unless otherwise stated.

| Brand or generic name [availability] | Antihistamines | Decongestants | Antitussives Opioid | Antitussives Non-opioid | Expectorants | Analgesics | Other content information as per product label | Usual Adult and Adolescent Dose prn‡ | Usual Pediatric Dose prn | Packaging, Storage, and Auxiliary labeling§ |
|---|---|---|---|---|---|---|---|---|---|---|
| *Comtrex Nighttime Maximum Strength Cold and Flu Relief* Tablets (OTC) [U.S.] | Chlorpheniramine maleate 2 mg | Pseudoephedrine HCl 30 mg | | Dextromethorphan HBr 15 mg | | Acetaminophen 500 mg | Available in a dual package that also contains *Comtrex Daytime Maximum Strength Cold and Flu Relief* | 2 tabs hs | | b, e |
| *Concentrin* Capsules USP (OTC) [U.S.] | | Pseudoephedrine HCl 30 mg | | Dextromethorphan HBr 15 mg | Guaifenesin 100 mg | | | 2 caps q 6 hr | 6–12 yrs: 1 cap q 6 hr | a, d |
| *Conex* Syrup (OTC) [U.S.] | | Phenylpropanolamine HCl 12.5 mg | | | Guaifenesin 100 mg | | | 5–10 mL q 4 hr (max 50 mL/day) | 2–6 yrs: 2.5 mL, 6–12 yrs: 5 mL, q 4–6 hr | b, c |
| *Conex with Codeine Liquid* Syrup (Schedule V) [U.S.] | | Phenylpropanolamine HCl 12.5 mg | Codeine PO₄ 10 mg | | Guaifenesin 100 mg | | | 5–10 mL q 4–6 hr (max 60 mL/day) | 2–12 yrs: 2.5–5 mL q 4–6 hr | b, c, e, f |
| *Congess JR* Extended-release Capsules (Rx) [U.S.] | | Pseudoephedrine HCl 60 mg (extended-release) | | | Guaifenesin 125 mg (immediate release) | | | Intended for pediatric use. See *Congess SR* Extended-release Capsules | 6–12 yrs: 1 cap q 12 hr | a¹, d |
| *Congess SR* Extended-release Capsules (Rx) [U.S.] | | Pseudoephedrine HCl 120 mg (extended-release) | | | Guaifenesin 250 mg (immediate release) | | | 1 cap q 12 hr | Intended for adult use. See *Congess JR* Extended-release Capsules | a¹, d |

*Specific formulations may vary among the different manufacturers, check product labeling.
†Efficacy as expectorant has not been established.
‡Geriatric patients may be more sensitive to effects of usual adult dose.
§For appropriate *Packaging and storage* and *Auxiliary labeling* information refer to designated letters as follows:
 a—Store below 40 °C (104 °F), preferably between 15 and 30 °C (59 and 86 °F), in a tight container, unless otherwise specified by manufacturer.
 a¹—Store below 30 °C (86 °F), unless otherwise specified by manufacturer. Avoid exposure to excessive heat.
 a²—Store below 25 °C (77 °F), unless otherwise specified by manufacturer.
 b—Store below 40 °C (104 °F), preferably between 15 and 30 °C (59 and 86 °F), in a well-closed container, unless otherwise specified by manufacturer.
 c—Protect from freezing.
 d—Protect from light.
 e—Auxiliary labeling: · May cause drowsiness. · Avoid alcoholic beverages.
 f—Auxiliary labeling: · May be habit forming.
 g—Auxiliary labeling: · Shake well.
 h—Dispense in dropper bottle.
 i—Chew well before swallowing.
**Included in subtherapeutic amount to discourage deliberate overdosage.

1048    Cough/Cold Combinations (Systemic)    USP DI

Table 3. Oral Dosage Forms (continued)

Note: Content per capsule, tablet, or 5 mL, unless otherwise stated.

| Brand or generic name [availability] | Antihistamines | Decongestants | Antitussives Opioid | Antitussives Non-opioid | Expectorants | Analgesics | Other content information as per product label | Usual Adult and Adolescent Dose prn‡ | Usual Pediatric Dose prn | Packaging, Storage, and Auxiliary labeling§ |
|---|---|---|---|---|---|---|---|---|---|---|
| *Congestac Caplets* Tablets (OTC) [U.S.] | | Pseudoephedrine HCl 60 mg | | | Guaifenesin 400 mg | | | 1 tab q 4 hr (max 4 tabs/day) | | b |
| *Contac Cold/Flu Day Caplets* Tablets (OTC) [U.S.] | | Pseudoephedrine HCl 60 mg | | Dextromethorphan HBr 30 mg | | Acetaminophen 650 mg | Available in a dual package that also contains *Contac Cold/Flu Night Caplets* | 1 tab q 6 hr (max 4 tabs/day of any combination of Day or Night caplets) | | b |
| *Contac Severe Cold & Flu Caplets* Tablets (OTC) [U.S.] | Chlorpheniramine maleate 2 mg | Phenylpropanolamine HCl 12.5 mg | | Dextromethorphan HBr 15 mg | | Acetaminophen 500 mg | | 2 tabs q 6 hr (max 8 tabs/day) | | b, c, e |
| *Contac Severe Cold & Flu Non-Drowsy Caplets* Tablets (OTC) [U.S.] | | Pseudoephedrine HCl 30 mg | | Dextromethorphan HBr 15 mg | | Acetaminophen 325 mg | | 2 tabs q 6 hr (max 8 tabs/day) | | b |
| *Contuss* Oral Solution (Rx) [U.S.] | | Phenylephrine HCl 5 mg, Phenylpropanolamine HCl 20 mg | | | Guaifenesin 100 mg | | Alcohol 5% | 10 mL q 6 hr | | b, c |
| *Cophene-S* Syrup (Schedule V) [U.S.] | Chlorpheniramine maleate 5 mg | Phenylephrine HCl 20 mg, Phenylpropanolamine HCl 20 mg | Dihydrocodeine bitartrate 3 mg | | | | | 5 mL q 4–6 hr | 2–6 yrs: 0.625–1.25 mL, 6–12 yrs: 1.25–2.5 mL, q 4–6 hr | b, c, e, f |
| *Cophene-X* Capsules (Rx) [U.S.] | | Phenylephrine HCl 10 mg, Phenylpropanolamine HCl 10 mg | | Carbetapentane citrate 20 mg | Potassium guaiacolsulfonate† 45 mg | | | 1–2 caps q 4–6 hr | Pediatric strength not available. See *Cophene-XP* Syrup | b |
| *Cophene XP* Oral Solution (Schedule III) [U.S.] | | Pseudoephedrine HCl 60 mg | Hydrocodone bitartrate 5 mg | | Guaifenesin 200 mg | | Alcohol 12.5% | 5 mL q 6 hr | | b, c, e, f |
| *Cophene-XP* Syrup (Rx) [U.S.] | Chlorpheniramine maleate 2.5 mg | Phenylephrine HCl 10 mg, Phenylpropanolamine HCl 10 mg | | Carbetapentane citrate 20 mg | Potassium guaiacolsulfonate† 45 mg | | | 10 mL q 4–6 hr | 2–6 yrs: 1.25–2.5 mL, 6–12 yrs: 2.5–5 mL, q 6 hr | b, c, e |
| *Coristex-DH* Oral Solution (N) [Canada] | | Phenylephrine HCl 20 mg | Hydrocodone bitartrate 5 mg | | | | Alcohol 4.25% Sucrose 33% | 5 mL q 4 hr | 6–12 yrs: 2.5 mL q 4 hr | a, c, d, e, f |

USP DI  Cough/Cold Combinations (Systemic) 1049

Table 3. Oral Dosage Forms (continued)

Note: Content per capsule, tablet, or 5 mL, unless otherwise stated.

| Brand or generic name [availability] | Antihistamines | Decongestants | Antitussives - Opioid | Antitussives - Non-opioid | Expectorants | Analgesics | Other content information as per product label | Usual Adult and Adolescent Dose prn‡ | Usual Pediatric Dose prn | Packaging, Storage, and Auxiliary labeling§ |
|---|---|---|---|---|---|---|---|---|---|---|
| *Coristine-DH* Oral Solution (N) [Canada] | | Phenylephrine HCl 10 mg | Hydrocodone bitartrate 1.7 mg | | | | Alcohol 4.3% Sucrose 33% | 10 mL q 4 hr | 6 mos–1 yr: 1.25–2.5 mL, 1–12 yrs: 2.5–5 mL, q 4 hr | a, c, d, e, f |
| *CoSudafed* Syrup (N) [Canada] | | Pseudoephedrine HCl 30 mg | Codeine PO₄ 10 mg | | | | | 10 mL q 4–6 hr (max 40 mL/day) | 2–5 yrs: 2.5 mL (max 10 mL/day), 6–11 yrs: 5 mL (max 20 mL/day), q 4–6 hr | a, d, e, f |
| Tablets (N) [Canada] | | Pseudoephedrine HCl 60 mg | Codeine PO₄ 20 mg | | | | Scored | ½–1 tab q 4–6 hr (max 4 tabs/day) | | b, d, e, f |
| *CoSudafed Expectorant* Syrup (N) [Canada] | | Pseudoephedrine HCl 30 mg | Codeine PO₄ 10 mg | | Guaifenesin 100 mg | | | 10 mL q 4–6 hr (max 40 mL/day) | 2–5 yrs: 2.5 mL (max 10 mL/day), 6–11 yrs: 5 mL (max 20 mL/day), q 4–6 hr | a, d, e, f |
| *Cotridin* Oral Solution (N) [Canada] | Triprolidine HCl 2 mg | Pseudoephedrine HCl 30 mg | Codeine PO₄ 10 mg | | | | Alcohol free | 10 mL q 4–6 hr (max 4 doses/day) | 2–6 yrs: 2.5 mL, 6–12 yrs: 5 mL, q 4–6 hr (max 4 doses/day) | a, d, e, f |

*Specific formulations may vary among the different manufacturers, check product labeling.
†Efficacy as expectorant has not been established.
‡Geriatric patients may be more sensitive to effects of usual adult dose.
§For appropriate *Packaging and storage* and *Auxiliary labeling* information refer to designated letters as follows:

  a—Store below 40 °C (104 °F), preferably between 15 and 30 °C (59 and 86 °F), in a tight container, unless otherwise specified by manufacturer.
  a¹—Store below 30 °C (86 °F), unless otherwise specified by manufacturer. Avoid exposure to excessive heat.
  a²—Store below 25 °C (77 °F), unless otherwise specified by manufacturer.
  b—Store below 40 °C (104 °F), preferably between 15 and 30 °C (59 and 86 °F), in a well-closed container, unless otherwise specified by manufacturer.
  c—Protect from freezing.          f—Auxiliary labeling: · May be habit forming.          h—Dispense in dropper bottle.
  d—Protect from light.              g—Auxiliary labeling: · Shake well.                     i—Chew well before swallowing.
  e—Auxiliary labeling: · May cause drowsiness. · Avoid alcoholic beverages.
**Included in subtherapeutic amount to discourage deliberate overdosage.

## Table 3. Oral Dosage Forms (continued)

Note: Content per capsule, tablet, or 5 mL, unless otherwise stated.

| Brand or generic name [availability] | Antihistamines | Decongestants | Antitussives Opioid | Antitussives Non-opioid | Expectorants | Analgesics | Other content information as per product label | Usual Adult and Adolescent Dose prn‡ | Usual Pediatric Dose prn | Packaging, Storage, and Auxiliary labeling§ |
|---|---|---|---|---|---|---|---|---|---|---|
| *Corridin Expectorant* Oral Solution (N) [Canada] | Triprolidine HCl 2 mg | Pseudoephedrine HCl 30 mg | Codeine PO₄ 10 mg | | Guaifenesin 100 mg | | Alcohol free | 10 mL q 6 hr (max 4 doses/day) | 2–5 yrs: 2.5 mL, 6–11 yrs: 5 mL, q 6 hr (max 4 doses/day) | a, d, e, f |
| *Co-Tuss V* Oral Solution (Schedule III) [U.S.] | | | Hydrocodone bitartrate 5 mg | | Guaifenesin 100 mg | | | 5 mL q 4 hr | | b, c, e, f |
| *C-Tussin Expectorant* Syrup (Schedule V) [U.S.] | | Phenylpropanolamine HCl 12.5 mg | Codeine PO₄ 10 mg | | Guaifenesin 200 mg | | Alcohol 7.5% | 10 mL q 4 hr | 2–6 yrs: 2.5 mL, 6–12 yrs: 5 mL, q 4 hr | a, c, d, e, f |
| *Decohistine DH* Oral Solution (Schedule V) [U.S.] | Chlorpheniramine maleate 2 mg | Pseudoephedrine HCl 30 mg | Codeine PO₄ 10 mg | | | | Alcohol 5.8% | 5–10 mL q 4–6 hr (max 40 mL/day) | | b, c, e, f |
| *Deconamine CX* Oral Solution (Schedule III) [U.S.] | | Pseudoephedrine HCl 60 mg | Hydrocodone bitartrate 5 mg | | Guaifenesin 200 mg | | Alcohol 12.5% | 5 mL q 6 hr (max 4 doses/day) | 25–50 lbs: 1.25 mL, 50–90 lbs: 2.5 mL, q 6 hours (max 4 doses/day) | a, d, e, f |
| Tablets (Schedule III) [U.S.] | | Pseudoephedrine HCl 30 mg | Hydrocodone bitartrate 5 mg | | Guaifenesin 300 mg | | Scored | 1–1½ tabs q 6 hr (max 4 doses/day) | 6–12 yrs: ½–1 tab q 6 hours (max 4 doses/day) | a, e, f |
| *Deconsal II* Extended-release Tablets (Rx) [U.S.] | | Pseudoephedrine HCl 60 mg | | | Guaifenesin 600 mg | | Scored | 1–2 tabs q 12 hr (max 4 tabs/day) | 2–6 yrs: ½ tab (max 1 tab/day), 6–12 yrs: 1 tab (max 2 tabs/day), q 12 hr | b |

USP DI — Cough/Cold Combinations (Systemic) 1051

Table 3. Oral Dosage Forms (continued)

Note: Content per capsule, tablet, or 5 mL, unless otherwise stated.

| Brand or generic name [availability] | Antihistamines | Decongestants | Antitussives Opioid | Antitussives Non-opioid | Expectorants | Analgesics | Other content information as per product label | Usual Adult and Adolescent Dose prn[‡] | Usual Pediatric Dose prn | Packaging, Storage, and Auxiliary labeling[§] |
|---|---|---|---|---|---|---|---|---|---|---|
| *Deconsal Pediatric* Extended-release Capsules (Rx) [U.S.] | | Phenylephrine HCl 7.5 mg | | | Guaifenesin 300 mg | | | 2–3 caps q 12 hr | 2–6 yrs: 1 cap (max 2 caps/day), 6–12 yrs: 1–2 caps (max 4 caps/day), q 12 hr | b |
| *Deproist Expectorant with Codeine* Oral Solution (Schedule V) [U.S.] | | Pseudoephedrine HCl 30 mg | Codeine PO$_4$ 10 mg | | Guaifenesin 100 mg | | Alcohol 8.2% | 10 mL q 4 hr (max 40 mL/day) | 2–6 yrs: 2.5 mL, 6–12 yrs: 5 mL, q 4 hr | a, c, d, e, f |
| *Despec* Oral Solution (Rx) [U.S.] | | Phenylephrine HCl 5 mg, Phenylpropanolamine HCl 20 mg | | | Guaifenesin 100 mg | | Alcohol 5% | 10 mL q 6 hr | 2–4 yrs: 2.5 mL, 4–6 yrs: 5 mL, 6–12 yrs: 7.5 mL, q 6 hr | b, c |
| *Despec SF* Oral Solution (Rx) [U.S.] | | Phenylephrine HCl 5 mg, Phenylpropanolamine HCl 20 mg | | | Guaifenesin 100 mg | | Alcohol free Dye free Sugar free | 10 mL q 6 hr | 2–4 yrs: 2.5 mL, 4–6 yrs: 5 mL, 6–12 yrs: 7.5 mL, q 6 hr | b, c |
| *Despec-SR Caplets* Extended-release Tablets (Rx) [U.S.] | | Phenylpropanolamine HCl 75 mg | | | Guaifenesin 600 mg | | Scored | 1 tab q 12 hr | 6–12 yrs: ½ tab q 12 hr | a, d |

*Specific formulations may vary among the different manufacturers, check product labeling.
†Efficacy as expectorant has not been established.
‡Geriatric patients may be more sensitive to effects of usual adult dose.
§For appropriate *Packaging and storage* and *Auxiliary labeling* information refer to designated letters as follows:
  a — Store below 40 °C (104 °F), preferably between 15 and 30 °C (59 and 86 °F), in a tight container, unless otherwise specified by manufacturer.
  a¹ — Store below 30 °C (86 °F), unless otherwise specified by manufacturer. Avoid exposure to excessive heat.
  a² — Store below 25 °C (77 °F), unless otherwise specified by manufacturer.
  b — Store below 40 °C (104 °F), preferably between 15 and 30 °C (59 and 86 °F), in a well-closed container, unless otherwise specified by manufacturer.
  c — Protect from freezing.
  d — Protect from light.
  e — Auxiliary labeling: · May cause drowsiness. · Avoid alcoholic beverages.
  f — Auxiliary labeling: · May be habit forming.
  g — Auxiliary labeling: · Shake well.
  h — Dispense in dropper bottle.
  i — Chew well before swallowing.
**Included in subtherapeutic amount to discourage deliberate overdosage.

**Table 3. Oral Dosage Forms** *(continued)*

Note: Content per capsule, tablet, or 5 mL, unless otherwise stated.

| Brand or generic name [availability] | Antihistamines | Decongestants | Antitussives Opioid | Antitussives Non-opioid | Expectorants | Analgesics | Other content information as per product label | Usual Adult and Adolescent Dose prn‡ | Usual Pediatric Dose prn | Packaging, Storage, and Auxiliary labeling§ |
|---|---|---|---|---|---|---|---|---|---|---|
| *De-Tuss* Syrup (Schedule III) [U.S.] | | Pseudoephedrine HCl 60 mg | Hydrocodone bitartrate 5 mg | | | | Alcohol 5% | 5 mL q 4–6 hr | 2–6 yrs: 1.25 mL, 6–12 yrs: 2.5 mL, q 4–6 hr | b, c, d, e, f |
| *Detussin Expectorant* Oral Solution (Schedule III) [U.S.] | | Pseudoephedrine HCl 60 mg | Hydrocodone bitartrate 5 mg | | Guaifenesin 200 mg | | Alcohol 12.5% | 5 mL q 4–6 hr | | b, c, e, f |
| *Detussin Liquid* Oral Solution (Schedule III) [U.S.] | | Pseudoephedrine HCl 60 mg | Hydrocodone bitartrate 5 mg | | | | Alcohol 5% | 5 mL q 6 hr | 2–6 yrs: 1.25 mL, 6–12 yrs: 2.5 mL, q 4–6 hr | b, c, d, e, f |
| *Dexafed Cough* Syrup (OTC) [U.S.] | | Phenylephrine HCl 5 mg | | Dextromethorphan HBr 10 mg | Guaifenesin 100 mg | | Alcohol free Sugar free | 10 mL q 4 hr (max 6 doses/day) | | b, c |
| *Diabetic Tussin DM* Oral Solution (OTC) [U.S.] | | | | Dextromethorphan HBr 10 mg | Guaifenesin 100 mg | | Alcohol free Sugar free Dye free | 10 mL q 4 hr | | b, c |
| *Dihistine DH* Oral Solution (Schedule V) [U.S.] | Chlorpheniramine maleate 2 mg | Pseudoephedrine HCl 30 mg | Codeine PO₄ 10 mg | | | | Alcohol 5% | 10 mL q 4–6 hr (max 40 mL/day) | 2–6 yrs: 1.25–2.5 mL, 6–12 yrs: 2.5–5 mL, q 6 hr | a, c, e, f |
| *Dihistine Expectorant* Oral Solution (Schedule V) [U.S.] | | Pseudoephedrine HCl 30 mg | Codeine PO₄ 10 mg | | Guaifenesin 100 mg | | Alcohol 7.5% | 10 mL q 4 hr (max 40 mL/day) | | b, c, e, f |
| *Dilaudid Cough* Syrup (Schedule II) [U.S.] | | | Hydromorphone HCl 1 mg | | | | Alcohol 5% Tartrazine | 5 mL q 3–4 hr | Not recommended | b, c, e, f |
| *Dimacol Caplets* Tablets (OTC) [U.S.] | | Pseudoephedrine HCl 30 mg | | Dextromethorphan HBr 10 mg | Guaifenesin 100 mg | | | 2 tabs q 4 hr (max 4 doses/day) | 6–12 yrs: 1 tab q 4 hr | b |
| *Dimetane-DC Cough* Syrup (Schedule V) [U.S.] | Brompheniramine maleate 2 mg | Phenylpropanolamine HCl 12.5 mg | Codeine PO₄ 10 mg | | | | Alcohol 0.95% Sugar free | 10 mL q 4 hr | 2–6 yrs: 2.5 mL, 6–12 yrs: 5 mL, q 4 hr | a, c, d, e, f |
| *Dimetane-DX Cough* Syrup (Rx) [U.S.] | Brompheniramine maleate 2 mg | Pseudoephedrine HCl 30 mg | | Dextromethorphan HBr 10 mg | | | Alcohol 0.95% Sugar free | 10 mL q 4 hr | 2–6 yrs: 2.5 mL, 6–12 yrs: 5 mL, q 4 hr | a, c, d, e |

Table 3. Oral Dosage Forms (*continued*)

Note: Content per capsule, tablet, or 5 mL, unless otherwise stated.

| Brand or generic name [availability] | Antihistamines | Decongestants | Antitussives - Opioid | Antitussives - Non-opioid | Expectorants | Analgesics | Other content information as per product label | Usual Adult and Adolescent Dose prn‡ | Usual Pediatric Dose prn | Packaging, Storage, and Auxiliary labeling§ |
|---|---|---|---|---|---|---|---|---|---|---|
| *Dimetane Expectorant* Oral Solution (OTC) [Canada] | Brompheniramine maleate 2 mg | Phenylephrine HCl 5 mg, Phenylpropanolamine HCl 5 mg | | | Guaifenesin 100 mg | | Alcohol 3.5% | 5–10 mL q 6 hr | 2–6 yrs: 1.25–2.5 mL, 6–12 yrs: 2.5–5 mL, q 6–8 hr | a, c, e |
| *Dimetane Expectorant-C* Oral Solution (N) [Canada] | Brompheniramine maleate 2 mg | Phenylephrine HCl 5 mg, Phenylpropanolamine HCl 5 mg | Codeine PO₄ 10 mg | | Guaifenesin 100 mg | | Alcohol 3.5% | 5–10 mL q 6 hr | 2–6 yrs: 1.25–2.5 mL, 6–12 yrs: 2.5–5 mL, q 6–8 hr | a, c, d, e, f |
| *Dimetane Expectorant-DC* Oral Solution (N) [Canada] | Brompheniramine maleate 2 mg | Phenylephrine HCl 5 mg, Phenylpropanolamine HCl 5 mg | Hydrocodone bitartrate 1.8 mg | | Guaifenesin 100 mg | | Alcohol 3.5% | 5–10 mL q 6 hr | 2–6 yrs: 1.25–2.5 mL, 6–12 yrs: 2.5–5 mL, q 6–8 hr | b, c, e, f |
| *Dimetapp-C* Syrup (N) [Canada] | Brompheniramine maleate 2 mg | Phenylephrine HCl 5 mg, Phenylpropanolamine HCl 5 mg | Codeine PO₄ 10 mg | | | | Alcohol Sodium 3.1 mg Sugar free | 10 mL q 4 hr | 2–6 yrs: 2.5 mL, 6–12 yrs: 5 mL, q 4 hr | a |
| *Dimetapp DM* Elixir (OTC) [U.S.] | Brompheniramine maleate 2 mg | Phenylpropanolamine HCl 12.5 mg | | Dextromethorphan HBr 10 mg | | | Alcohol free | 10 mL q 4 hr (max 60 mL/day) | 6–12 yrs: 5 mL q 4 hr (max 30 mL/day) | b, c, e |
| *Dimetapp-DM* Elixir (OTC) [Canada] | Brompheniramine maleate 4 mg | Phenylephrine HCl 5 mg, Phenylpropanolamine HCl 5 mg | | Dextromethorphan HBr 15 mg | | | Alcohol 3% Sugar free | 5–10 mL q 6–8 hr | 2–6 yrs: 2.5 mL, 6–12 yrs: 5 mL, q 6–8 hr | b, c, e |
| Tablets (OTC) [Canada] | Brompheniramine maleate 4 mg | Phenylephrine HCl 5 mg, Phenylpropanolamine HCl 5 mg | | Dextromethorphan HBr 15 mg | | | Scored | 1–2 tabs q 6–8 hr | 2–6 yrs: ½ tab, 6–12 yrs: 1 tab, q 6–8 hr | b, e |

*Specific formulations may vary among the different manufacturers, check product labeling.
†Efficacy as expectorant has not been established.
‡Geriatric patients may be more sensitive to effects of usual adult dose.
§For appropriate *Packaging and storage* and *Auxiliary labeling* information refer to designated letters as follows:

a—Store below 40 °C (104 °F), preferably between 15 and 30 °C (59 and 86 °F), in a tight container, unless otherwise specified by manufacturer. Avoid exposure to excessive heat.
a¹—Store below 30 °C (86 °F), unless otherwise specified by manufacturer.
a²—Store below 25 °C (77 °F), unless otherwise specified by manufacturer.
b—Store below 40 °C (104 °F), preferably between 15 and 30 °C (59 and 86 °F), in a well-closed container, unless otherwise specified by manufacturer.
c—Protect from freezing.
d—Protect from light.
e—Auxiliary labeling: · May cause drowsiness. · Avoid alcoholic beverages.
f—Auxiliary labeling: · May be habit forming.
g—Auxiliary labeling: · Shake well.
h—Dispense in dropper bottle.
i—Chew well before swallowing.
**Included in subtherapeutic amount to discourage deliberate overdosage.

**1054  Cough/Cold Combinations (Systemic)**  USP DI

Table 3. Oral Dosage Forms (continued)

Note: Content per capsule, tablet, or 5 mL, unless otherwise stated.

| Brand or generic name [availability] | Antihistamines | Decongestants | Antitussives Opioid | Antitussives Non-opioid | Expectorants | Analgesics | Other content information as per product label | Usual Adult and Adolescent Dose prn‡ | Usual Pediatric Dose prn | Packaging, Storage, and Auxiliary labelings§ |
|---|---|---|---|---|---|---|---|---|---|---|
| *Dimetapp DM Cold & Cough Elixir* (OTC) [U.S.] | Brompheniramine maleate 2 mg | Phenylpropanolamine HCl 12.5 mg | | Dextromethorphan HBr 10 mg | | | Alcohol free | 10 mL q 4 hr (max 6 doses/day) | 6–12 yrs: 5 mL q 4 hr (max 6 doses/day) | b, c, e |
| *Dimetapp Maximum Strength Cold & Cough Liqui-Gels Capsules* (OTC) [U.S.] | Brompheniramine maleate 4 mg | Phenylpropanolamine HCl 25 mg | | Dextromethorphan HBr 20 mg | | | | 1 cap q 4 hr (max 6 caps/day) | | a, e |
| *Donatussin Syrup* (Rx) [U.S.] | Chlorpheniramine maleate 2 mg | Phenylephrine HCl 10 mg | | Dextromethorphan HBr 7.5 mg | Guaifenesin 100 mg | | Alcohol free | 5 mL q 4–6 hr (max 6 doses/day) | 2–6 yrs: 1.25 mL, 6–12 yrs: 2.5 mL, q 4–6 hr | b, c, e |
| *Donatussin DC Syrup* (Schedule III) [U.S.] | | Phenylephrine HCl 7.5 mg | Hydrocodone bitartrate 2.5 mg | | Guaifenesin 50 mg | | Alcohol free | 10 mL q 4–6 hr (max 6 doses/day) | 3–6 yrs: 2.5 mL, 6–12 yrs: 5 mL, q 4–6 hr | b, c, d, e, f |
| *Donatussin Drops Oral Solution* (Rx) [U.S.] | Chlorpheniramine maleate 5 mg (1 mg/mL) | Phenylephrine HCl 10 mg (2 mg/mL) | | | Guaifenesin 100 mg (20 mg/mL) | | Alcohol free | Intended for pediatric use | <3 mos: 2–3 drops/mo of age, 3–6 mos: 0.3–0.6 mL, 6 mos–1 yr: 0.6–1 mL, 1–2 yrs: 1–2 mL, q 4–6 hr | b, c, e, h |
| *Dondril Tablets* (OTC) [U.S.] | Chlorpheniramine maleate 1 mg | Phenylephrine HCl 5 mg | | Dextromethorphan HBr 10 mg | | | | 2 tabs q 4 hr | 6–12 yrs: 1 tab q 4 hr | b, e |
| *Dorcol Children's Cough Syrup* (OTC) [U.S.] | | Pseudoephedrine HCl 15 mg | | Dextromethorphan HBr 5 mg | Guaifenesin 50 mg | | Alcohol free | Intended for pediatric use | 2–6 yrs: 5 mL, 6–12 yrs: 10 mL, q 4 hr (max 4 doses/day) | b, c |
| *Drixoral Cough & Congestion Liquid Caps* (OTC) [U.S.] | | Pseudoephedrine HCl 60 mg | | Dextromethorphan HBr 30 mg | | | | 1 cap q 6 hr (max 4 caps/day) | Not recommended | a[1], c |

USP DI — Cough/Cold Combinations (Systemic) 1055

Table 3. Oral Dosage Forms *(continued)*

Note: Content per capsule, tablet, or 5 mL, unless otherwise stated.

| Brand or generic name [availability] | Antihistamines | Decongestants | Antitussives Opioid | Antitussives Non-opioid | Expectorants | Analgesics | Other content information as per product label | Usual Adult and Adolescent Dose prn‡ | Usual Pediatric Dose prn | Packaging, Storage, and Auxiliary labeling§ |
|---|---|---|---|---|---|---|---|---|---|---|
| *Drixoral Cough & Sore Throat Liquid Caps* Capsules (OTC) [U.S.] | | | | Dextromethorphan HBr 15 mg | | Acetaminophen 325 mg | | 2 caps q 6–8 hr (max 8 caps/day) | 6–12 yrs: 1 cap q 6–8 hr (max 4 caps/day) | a[1], c |
| *Dura-Gest* Capsules (Rx) [U.S.] | | Phenylephrine HCl 5 mg, Phenylpropanolamine HCl 45 mg | | | Guaifenesin 200 mg | | | 1 cap q 6 hr | Not recommended | a[2], d |
| *Duratex* Capsules (Rx) [U.S.] | | Phenylephrine HCl 5 mg, Phenylpropanolamine HCl 45 mg | | | Guaifenesin 200 mg | | | 1 cap q 6 hr | Not recommended | a[1] |
| *Duratuss* Extended-release Tablets (Rx) [U.S.] | | Pseudoephedrine HCl 120 mg | | | Guaifenesin 600 mg | | Scored Dye free Film-coated | 1 tab q 12 hr | 6–12 yrs: ½ tab q 12 hr | b |
| *Duratuss HD* Elixir (Schedule III) [U.S.] | | Pseudoephedrine HCl 30 mg | Hydrocodone bitartrate 2.5 mg | | Guaifenesin 100 mg | | Alcohol 5% | 10 mL q 4–6 hr (max 4 doses/day) | 6–12 yrs: 5 mL q 4–6 hr (max 4 doses/day) | b, c, e, f |
| *Dura-Vent* Extended-release Tablets (Rx) [U.S.] | | Phenylpropanolamine HCl 75 mg | | | Guaifenesin 600 mg | | Dye free Scored | 1 tab q 12 hr | <6 yrs: Not recommended 6–12 yrs: ½ tab q 12 hr | a[2], d |
| *ED-TLC* Oral Solution (Schedule III) [U.S.] | Chlorpheniramine maleate 2 mg | Phenylephrine HCl 5 mg | Hydrocodone bitartrate 1.67 mg | | | | | 10 mL q 6–8 hr | 6–12 yrs: 5 mL q 6–8 hr | b, c, e, f |

*Specific formulations may vary among the different manufacturers, check product labeling.
†Efficacy as expectorant has not been established.
‡Geriatric patients may be more sensitive to effects of usual adult dose.
§For appropriate *Packaging and storage* and *Auxiliary labeling* information refer to designated letters as follows:
  a—Store below 40 °C (104 °F), preferably between 15 and 30 °C (59 and 86 °F), in a tight container, unless otherwise specified by manufacturer.
  a[1]—Store below 30 °C (86 °F), unless otherwise specified by manufacturer. Avoid exposure to excessive heat.
  a[2]—Store below 25 °C (77 °F), unless otherwise specified by manufacturer.
  b—Store below 40 °C (104 °F), preferably between 15 and 30 °C (59 and 86 °F), in a well-closed container, unless otherwise specified by manufacturer.
  c—Protect from freezing.
  d—Protect from light.
  e—Auxiliary labeling: · May cause drowsiness. · Avoid alcoholic beverages.
  f—Auxiliary labeling: · May be habit forming.
  g—Auxiliary labeling: · Shake well.
  h—Dispense in dropper bottle.
  i—Chew well before swallowing.
**Included in subtherapeutic amount to discourage deliberate overdosage.

**1056    Cough/Cold Combinations (Systemic)**                                                                                                                                  *USP DI*

**Table 3. Oral Dosage Forms** *(continued)*

Note: Content per capsule, tablet, or 5 mL, unless otherwise stated.

| Brand or generic name [availability] | Antihistamines | Decongestants | Antitussives - Opioid | Antitussives - Non-opioid | Expectorants | Analgesics | Other content information as per product label | Usual Adult and Adolescent Dose prn‡ | Usual Pediatric Dose prn | Packaging, Storage, and Auxiliary labeling§ |
|---|---|---|---|---|---|---|---|---|---|---|
| *ED Tuss HC* Oral Solution (Schedule III) [U.S.] | Chlorpheniramine maleate 4 mg | Phenylephrine HCl 10 mg | Hydrocodone bitartrate 2.5 mg | | | | Alcohol 5% | 5 mL q 6 hr | 2–6 yrs: 1.25 mL, 6–12 yrs: 2.5 mL, q 4–6 hr | b, c, e, f |
| *Effective Strength Cough Formula* Oral Solution (OTC) [U.S.] | Chlorpheniramine maleate 2 mg | | | Dextromethorphan HBr 15 mg | | | Alcohol 10% | 10 mL q 6 hr | | b, c, e |
| *Effective Strength Cough Formula with Decongestant* Oral Solution (OTC) [U.S.] | | Pseudoephedrine HCl 20 mg | | Dextromethorphan HBr 10 mg | | | Alcohol 10% | 15 mL q 6 hr | | b, c, e |
| *Endagen-HD* Oral Solution (Schedule III) [U.S.] | Chlorpheniramine maleate 2 mg | Phenylephrine HCl 5 mg | Hydrocodone bitartrate 1.7 mg | | | | Alcohol free | 10 mL q 6–8 hr | 6–12 yrs: 5 mL q 6–8 hr | b, c, e, f |
| *Endal* Extended-release Tablets (Rx) [U.S.] | | Phenylephrine HCl 20 mg | | | Guaifenesin 300 mg | | | 1 or 2 tabs q 12 hr | | b |
| *Endal Expectorant* Syrup (Schedule V) [U.S.] | | Phenylpropanolamine HCl 12.5 mg | Codeine PO₄ 10 mg | | Guaifenesin 100 mg | | Alcohol 5% Sugar free Dye free | 5–10 mL q 6–8 hr | 2–6 yrs: 2.5 mL, 6–12 yrs: 5 mL, q 6–8 hr | b, c, e, f |
| *Endal-HD* Syrup (Schedule III) [U.S.] | Chlorpheniramine maleate 2 mg | Phenylephrine HCl 5 mg | Hydrocodone bitartrate 1.67 mg | | | | | 10 mL q 6–8 hr (max 40 mL/day) | 6–12 yrs: 5 mL q 6–8 hr | b, c, e, f |
| *Endal-HD Plus* Oral Solution (Schedule III) [U.S.] | Chlorpheniramine maleate 2 mg | Phenylephrine HCl 5 mg | Hydrocodone bitartrate 2.5 mg | | | | Alcohol free Dye free | 10 mL q 4 hr (max 40 mL/day) | | b, c, e, f |
| *Enomine* Capsules (Rx) [U.S.] | | Phenylephrine HCl 5 mg, Phenylpropanolamine HCl 45 mg | | | Guaifenesin 200 mg | | | 1 cap q 6 hr | | b |
| *Entex* Capsules (Rx) [U.S.] | | Phenylephrine HCl 5 mg, Phenylpropanolamine HCl 45 mg | | | Guaifenesin 200 mg | | | 1 cap q 6 hr | Not recommended | b |
| *Entex LA* Extended-release Tablets (Rx) [U.S.] | | Phenylpropanolamine HCl 75 mg | | | Guaifenesin 400 mg | | Scored | 1 tab q 12 hr | 6–12 yrs: ½ tab q 12 hr | b |

USP DI          Cough/Cold Combinations (Systemic)   1057

Table 3. Oral Dosage Forms (continued)

Note: Content per capsule, tablet, or 5 mL, unless otherwise stated.

| Brand or generic name [availability] | Antihistamines | Decongestants | Antitussives Opioid | Antitussives Non-opioid | Expectorants | Analgesics | Other content information as per product label | Usual Adult and Adolescent Dose prn‡ | Usual Pediatric Dose prn | Packaging, Storage, and Auxiliary labeling§ |
|---|---|---|---|---|---|---|---|---|---|---|
| *Entex LA* (continued) Extended-release Tablets (Rx) [Canada] | | Phenylpropanolamine HCl 75 mg | | | Guaifenesin 600 mg | | Scored | 1 tab q 12 hr | 6–12 yrs: ½ tab q 12 hr | b |
| *Entex Liquid* Oral Solution (Rx) [U.S.] | | Phenylephrine HCl 5 mg, Phenylpropanolamine HCl 20 mg | | | Guaifenesin 100 mg | | Alcohol 5% | 10 mL q 6 hr (max 4 doses/day) | 2–4 yrs: 2.5 mL, 4–6 yrs: 5 mL, 6–12 yrs: 7.5 mL q 6 hr (max 4 doses/day) | b, c |
| *Entex PSE* Extended-release Tablets (Rx) [U.S.] | | Pseudoephedrine HCl 120 mg | | | Guaifenesin 600 mg | | Scored | 1 tab q 12 hr | 6–12 yrs: ½ tab q 12 hr | b |
| *Entuss-D* Oral Solution (Schedule III) [U.S.] | | Pseudoephedrine HCl 30 mg | Hydrocodone bitartrate 5 mg | | Potassium guaiacolsulfonate 300 mg | | Alcohol free Sugar free Dye free | 5–7.5 mL q 6 hr (max 4 doses/day) | 2–6 yrs: 1.25–2.5 mL, 6–12 yrs: 2.5–5 mL q 6 hr (max 4 doses/day) | b, c, d, e, f |
| Tablets (Schedule III) [U.S.] | | Pseudoephedrine HCl 30 mg | Hydrocodone bitartrate 5 mg | | Guaifenesin 300 mg | | Scored Dye free | 1–1½ tabs q 4–6 hr | 6–12 yrs: ½–1 tab q 4–6 hr | b, d, e, f |

*Specific formulations may vary among the different manufacturers; check product labeling.
†Efficacy as expectorant has not been established.
‡Geriatric patients may be more sensitive to effects of usual adult dose.
§For appropriate *Packaging and storage* and *Auxiliary labeling* information refer to designated letters as follows:
a—Store below 40 °C (104 °F), preferably between 15 and 30 °C (59 and 86 °F), in a tight container, unless otherwise specified by manufacturer.
a¹—Store below 30 °C (86 °F), unless otherwise specified by manufacturer. Avoid exposure to excessive heat.
a²—Store below 25 °C (77 °F), unless otherwise specified by manufacturer.
b—Store below 40 °C (104 °F), preferably between 15 and 30 °C (59 and 86 °F), in a well-closed container, unless otherwise specified by manufacturer.
c—Protect from freezing.
d—Protect from light.
e—Auxiliary labeling: • May cause drowsiness. • Avoid alcoholic beverages.
f—Auxiliary labeling: • May be habit forming.
g—Auxiliary labeling: • Shake well.
h—Dispense in dropper bottle.
i—Chew well before swallowing.
**Included in subtherapeutic amount to discourage deliberate overdosage.

## Table 3. Oral Dosage Forms (continued)

Note: Content per capsule, tablet, or 5 mL, unless otherwise stated.

| Brand or generic name [availability] | Antihistamines | Decongestants | Antitussives Opioid | Antitussives Non-opioid | Expectorants | Analgesics | Other content information as per product label | Usual Adult and Adolescent Dose prn‡ | Usual Pediatric Dose prn | Packaging, Storage, and Auxiliary labeling§ |
|---|---|---|---|---|---|---|---|---|---|---|
| *Entuss-D Jr.* Oral Solution (Schedule III) [U.S.] | | Pseudoephedrine HCl 30 mg | Hydrocodone bitartrate 2.5 mg | | Guaifenesin 100 mg | | Alcohol 5% | 10 mL q 6 hr (max 4 doses/day) | 2–6 yrs: 2.5 mL, 6–12 yrs: 5 mL, q 6 hr (max 4 doses/day) | b, c, d, e, f |
| *Entuss Expectorant* Oral Solution (Schedule III) [U.S.] | | | Hydrocodone bitartrate 5 mg | | Potassium guaiacol-sulfonate† 300 mg | | Alcohol free Sugar free | 5–7.5 mL q 4–6 hr | 3–6 yrs: 1.25–2.5 mL, 6–12 yrs: 2.5–5 mL, q 4–6 hr | b, c, d, e, f |
| Tablets (Schedule III) [U.S.] | | | Hydrocodone bitartrate 5 mg | | Guaifenesin 300 mg | | Scored | 1–1½ tabs q 4–6 hr | Pediatric strength not available | b, e, f |
| *Eudal-SR* Extended-release Tablets (Rx) [U.S.] | | Pseudoephedrine HCl 120 mg | | | Guaifenesin 400 mg | | Scored | 1 tab q 12 hr | | b |
| *Exgest LA* Extended-release Tablets (Rx) [U.S.] | | Phenylpropanolamine HCl 75 mg | | | Guaifenesin 400 mg | | Scored | 1 tab q 12 hr | –6–12 yrs: ½ tab q 12 hr | b |
| *Expressin 400* Caplets Tablets (OTC) [U.S.] | | Pseudoephedrine HCl 60 mg | | | Guaifenesin 400 mg | | Dye free | 1 tab q 4 hr (max 4 tabs/day) | 6–12 yrs: ½ tab q 4 hr (max 2 tabs/day) | b |
| *Extra Action Cough* Syrup (OTC) [U.S.] | | | | Dextromethorphan HBr 10 mg | Guaifenesin 100 mg | | Alcohol 1.4% | 10 mL q 6–8 hr | 2–6 yrs: 2.5 mL, 6–12 yrs: 5 mL, q 6–8 hr | b, c |
| *Father John's Medicine Plus* Oral Solution (OTC) [U.S.] | Chlorpheniramine maleate 1 mg | Phenylephrine HCl 2.5 mg | | Dextromethorphan HBr 7.5 mg | Guaifenesin 30 mg, Ammonium Cl† 83.3 mg | | Alcohol free | 5–10 mL q 3–4 hr | 2–6 yrs: 5 mL, 6–12 yrs: 5–10 mL, q 6–8 hr | b, c, e |
| *Fendol* Tablets (OTC) [U.S.] | | Phenylephrine HCl 5 mg | | | Guaifenesin 100 mg | Acetaminophen 355 mg, Salicylamide 65 mg | Caffeine 32 mg | 2 tabs q 4 hr | Pediatric strength not available | a |

Table 3. Oral Dosage Forms (*continued*)

Note: Content per capsule, tablet, or 5 mL, unless otherwise stated.

| Brand or generic name [availability] | Antihistamines | Decongestants | Antitussives Opioid | Antitussives Non-opioid | Expectorants | Analgesics | Other content information as per product label | Usual Adult and Adolescent Dose prn‡ | Usual Pediatric Dose prn | Packaging, Storage, and Auxiliary labeling§ |
|---|---|---|---|---|---|---|---|---|---|---|
| *Fenesin DM* Extended-release Tablets (Rx) [U.S.] | | | | Dextromethorphan HBr 30 mg | Guaifenesin 600 mg | | Scored | 1–2 tabs q 12 hr | 2–6 yrs: ½ tab, 6–12 yrs: 1 tab, q 12 hr | a², d |
| *Gelpirin-CCF* Tablets (OTC) [U.S.] | Chlorpheniramine maleate 1 mg | Phenylpropanolamine HCl 12.5 mg | | | Guaifenesin 25 mg | Acetaminophen 325 mg | | 2 tabs q 4 hr (max 12 tabs/day) | 6–12 yrs: 1 tab q 4 hr (max 6 tabs/day) | b, e |
| *Genatuss DM* Syrup (OTC) [U.S.] | | | | Dextromethorphan HBr 10 mg | Guaifenesin 100 mg | | Alcohol free | 10 mL q 4 hr | | b, c |
| *Genite* Oral Solution (OTC) [U.S.] | Doxylamine succinate 1.25 mg | Pseudoephedrine HCl 10 mg | | Dextromethorphan HBr 5 mg | | Acetaminophen 167 mg | Alcohol 25% Tartrazine | 30 mL hs or q 6 hr | | b, c |
| *Glycofed* Tablets (OTC) [U.S.] | | Pseudoephedrine HCl 30 mg | | | Guaifenesin 100 mg | | Scored | 1–2 tabs q 6 hr | | b |
| *Glycotuss-dM* Tablets (OTC) [U.S.] | | | | Dextromethorphan HBr 10 mg | Guaifenesin 100 mg | | | 1–2 tabs q 4 hr | 6–12 yrs: 1 tab q 4 hr | b |
| *Glydeine Cough* Syrup USP (Schedule V) [U.S.] | | | Codeine PO₄ 10 mg | | Guaifenesin 100 mg | | Alcohol 3.5% | 5–10 mL q 4 hr | 2–6 yrs: 2.5 mL, 6–12 yrs: 5 mL, q 4 hr | a, d, e, f |
| *GP-500* Extended-release Tablets (Rx) [U.S.] | | Pseudoephedrine HCl 120 mg | | | Guaifenesin 500 mg | | Scored | 1 tab q 12 hr | 6–12 yrs: ½ tab q 12 hr | a, d |

*Specific formulations may vary among the different manufacturers, check product labeling.
†Efficacy as expectorant has not been established.
‡Geriatric patients may be more sensitive to effects of usual adult dose.
§For appropriate *Packaging and storage* and *Auxiliary labeling* information refer to designated letters as follows:

a—Store below 40 °C (104 °F), preferably between 15 and 30 °C (59 and 86 °F), in a tight container, unless otherwise specified by manufacturer.
a¹—Store below 30 °C (86 °F), unless otherwise specified by manufacturer. Avoid exposure to excessive heat.
a²—Store below 25 °C (77 °F), unless otherwise specified by manufacturer.
b—Store below 40 °C (104 °F), preferably between 15 and 30 °C (59 and 86 °F), in a well-closed container, unless otherwise specified by manufacturer.
c—Protect from freezing.
d—Protect from light.
e—Auxiliary labeling: · May cause drowsiness. · Avoid alcoholic beverages.
f—Auxiliary labeling: · May be habit forming.
g—Auxiliary labeling: · Shake well.
h—Dispense in dropper bottle.
i—Chew well before swallowing.

**Included in subtherapeutic amount to discourage deliberate overdosage.

**Table 3. Oral Dosage Forms** *(continued)*

Note: Content per capsule, tablet, or 5 mL, unless otherwise stated.

| Brand or generic name [availability] | Antihistamines | Decongestants | Antitussives Opioid | Antitussives Non-opioid | Expectorants | Analgesics | Other content information as per product label | Usual Adult and Adolescent Dose prn‡ | Usual Pediatric Dose prn | Packaging, Storage, and Auxiliary labeling§ |
|---|---|---|---|---|---|---|---|---|---|---|
| *Guaifed* Extended-release Capsules (Rx) [U.S.] | | Pseudoephedrine HCl 120 mg (extended-release) | | | Guaifenesin 250 mg (immediate release) | | | 1 cap q 12 hr | Pediatric strength not available | a |
| Syrup (OTC) [U.S.] | | Pseudoephedrine HCl 30 mg | | | Guaifenesin 200 mg | | Sugar free | 10 mL q 4–6 hr (max 4 doses/day) | 2–6 yrs: 2.5 mL, 6–12 yrs: 5 mL, q 4–6 hr (max 4 doses/day) | b |
| *Guaifed-PD* Extended-release Capsules (Rx) [U.S.] | | Pseudoephedrine HCl 60 mg (extended-release) | | | Guaifenesin 300 mg (immediate release) | | | 1–2 caps q 12 hr | 6–12 yrs: 1 cap q 12 hr | a |
| *Guaifenesin and Codeine*\* Syrup USP (Schedule V) [U.S.] | | | Codeine PO$_4$ 10 mg | | Guaifenesin 100 mg | | | 10 mL q 4 hr | | a, d, e, f |
| *Guaifenesin, Codeine, and Pseudoephedrine*\* Oral Solution (Schedule V) [U.S.] | | Pseudoephedrine HCl 30 mg | Codeine PO$_4$ 10 mg | | Guaifenesin 100 mg | | May contain alcohol | 10 mL q 4 hr (max 40 mL/day) | | a, d, e, f |
| Syrup (Schedule V) [U.S.] | | Pseudoephedrine HCl 30 mg | Codeine PO$_4$ 10 mg | | Guaifenesin 100 mg | | May contain alcohol | 10 mL q 4 hr (max 40 mL/day) | | a, d, e, f |
| Syrup (N) [Canada] | | Pseudoephedrine HCl 30 mg | Codeine PO$_4$ 3.3 mg | | Guaifenesin 100 mg | | Alcohol | 10 mL q 4 hr (max 4 doses/day) | | a, d, e, f |
| *Guaifenex PPA 75* Extended-release Tablets (Rx) [U.S.] | | Phenylpropanolamine HCl 75 mg | | | Guaifenesin 600 mg | | | 1 tab q 12 hr | 6–12 yrs: ½ tab q 12 hr | a, d |
| *Guaifenex PSE 60* Extended-release Tablets (Rx) [U.S.] | | Pseudoephedrine HCl 60 mg | | | Guaifenesin 600 mg | | Scored | 1–2 tabs q 12 hr (max 4 tabs/day) | 2–6 yrs: ½ tab (max 1 tab/day), 6–12 yrs: 1 tab (max 2 tabs/day), q 12 hr | a, d |

Table 3. Oral Dosage Forms (continued)

Note: Content per capsule, tablet, or 5 mL, unless otherwise stated.

| Brand or generic name [availability] | Antihistamines | Decongestants | Antitussives Opioid | Antitussives Non-opioid | Expectorants | Analgesics | Other content information as per product label | Usual Adult and Adolescent Dose prn[‡] | Usual Pediatric Dose prn | Packaging, Storage, and Auxiliary labeling[§] |
|---|---|---|---|---|---|---|---|---|---|---|
| *Guaifenex PSE 120* Extended-release Tablets (Rx) [U.S.] | | Pseudoephedrine HCl 120 mg | | | Guaifenesin 600 mg | | Scored | 1 tab q 12 hr | 6–12 yrs: ½ tab q 12 hr | a, d |
| *GuaiMAX-D* Extended-release Tablets (Rx) [U.S.] | | Pseudoephedrine HCl 120 mg | | | Guaifenesin 600 mg | | Scored | 1 tab q 12 hr | 6–12 yrs: ½ tab q 12 hr | b |
| *Guaipax* Extended-release Tablets (Rx) [U.S.] | | Phenylpropanolamine HCl 75 mg | | | Guaifenesin 400 mg | | | 1 tab q 12 hr | 6–12 yrs: ½ tab q 12 hr | b |
| *Guaitab* Tablets (OTC) [U.S.] | | Pseudoephedrine HCl 60 mg | | | Guaifenesin 400 mg | | Scored | 1 tab q 4–6 hr (max 4 tabs/day) | 6–12 yrs: ½ tab q 4–6 hr (max 2 tabs/day) | b |
| *Guaivent* Extended-release Capsules (Rx) [U.S.] | | Pseudoephedrine HCl 120 mg (extended-release) | | | Guaifenesin 250 mg (immediate-release) | | | 1 cap q 12 hr | 6–12 yrs: 1 cap q 12 hr | a |
| *Guaivent PD* Extended-release Capsules (Rx) [U.S.] | | Pseudoephedrine HCl 60 mg (extended-release) | | | Guaifenesin 300 mg (immediate-release) | | | 1–2 caps q 12 hr | 6–12 yrs: 1 cap q 12 hr | a |
| *Guai-Vent/PSE* Extended-release Tablets (Rx) [U.S.] | | Pseudoephedrine HCl 120 mg | | | Guaifenesin 600 mg | | Scored | 1 tab q 12 hr | 6–12 yrs: ½ tab q 12 hr | a[2], d |
| *GuiaCough CF* Oral Solution (OTC) [U.S.] | | Phenylpropanolamine HCl 12.5 mg | | Dextromethorphan HBr 10 mg | Guaifenesin 100 mg | | Alcohol 4.75% | 10 mL q 4 hr | | b, c |

\*Specific formulations may vary among the different manufacturers, check product labeling.
†Efficacy as expectorant has not been established.
‡Geriatric patients may be more sensitive to effects of usual adult dose.
§For appropriate *Packaging and storage* and *Auxiliary labeling* information refer to designated letters as follows:
  a—Store below 40 °C (104 °F), preferably between 15 and 30 °C (59 and 86 °F), in a tight container, unless otherwise specified by manufacturer.
  a[1]—Store below 30 °C (86 °F), unless otherwise specified by manufacturer. Avoid exposure to excessive heat.
  a[2]—Store below 25 °C (77 °F), unless otherwise specified by manufacturer.
  b—Store below 40 °C (104 °F), preferably between 15 and 30 °C (59 and 86 °F), in a well-closed container, unless otherwise specified by manufacturer.
  c—Protect from freezing.  f—Auxiliary labeling: · May be habit forming.  h—Dispense in dropper bottle.
  d—Protect from light.  g—Auxiliary labeling: · Shake well.  i—Chew well before swallowing.
  e—Auxiliary labeling: · May cause drowsiness. · Avoid alcoholic beverages.
\*\*Included in subtherapeutic amount to discourage deliberate overdosage.

Table 3. Oral Dosage Forms (continued)

Note: Content per capsule, tablet, or 5 mL, unless otherwise stated.

| Brand or generic name [availability] | Antihistamines | Decongestants | Antitussives Opioid | Antitussives Non-opioid | Expectorants | Analgesics | Other content information as per product label | Usual Adult and Adolescent Dose prn‡ | Usual Pediatric Dose prn | Packaging, Storage, and Auxiliary labeling§ |
|---|---|---|---|---|---|---|---|---|---|---|
| *GuiaCough PE* Oral Solution (OTC) [U.S.] | | Pseudoephedrine HCl 30 mg | | | Guaifenesin 100 mg | | Alcohol 1.4% | 10 mL q 4 hr (max 40 mL/day) | | b, c |
| *Guiamid D.M. Liquid* Oral Solution (OTC) [U.S.] | | | | Dextromethorphan HBr 15 mg | Guaifenesin 100 mg | | Alcohol 1.4% | 10 mL q 6–8 hr | 2–6 yrs: 2.5 mL, 6–12 yrs: 5 mL, q 6–8 hr | b, c |
| *Guiatuss A.C.* Syrup USP (Schedule V) [U.S.] | | | Codeine PO₄ 10 mg | | Guaifenesin 100 mg | | Alcohol 3.5% | 10 mL q 4 hr | 2–6 yrs: 1.25–2.5 mL, 6–12 yrs: 2.5–5 mL, q 4–6 hr | a, d, e, f |
| *Guiatuss CF* Oral Solution (OTC) [U.S.] | | Phenylpropanolamine HCl 12.5 mg | | Dextromethorphan HBr 10 mg | Guaifenesin 100 mg | | Alcohol free | 10 mL q 4 hr | | b, c |
| *Guiatuss DAC* Oral Solution (Schedule V) [U.S.] | | Pseudoephedrine HCl 30 mg | Codeine PO₄ 10 mg | | Guaifenesin 100 mg | | Alcohol 1.9% | 10 mL q 4 hr (max 40 mL/day) | | b, c, e, f |
| *Guiatuss-DM* Oral Solution (OTC) [U.S.] | | | | Dextromethorphan HBr 10 mg | Guaifenesin 100 mg | | | 10 mL q 4 hr | | b, c |
| Syrup (OTC) [U.S.] | | | Codeine PO₄ 10 mg | Dextromethorphan HBr 10 mg | Guaifenesin 100 mg | | Alcohol 1.4% | 10 mL q 6–8 hr | 2–6 yrs: 2.5 mL, 6–12 yrs: 5 mL, q 6–8 hr | b, c |
| *Guiatussin with Codeine Liquid* Oral Solution (Schedule V) [U.S.] | | | Codeine PO₄ 10 mg | | Guaifenesin 100 mg | | Alcohol 3.5% | 10 mL q 4 hr | 2–6 yrs: 1.25–2.5 mL, 6–12 yrs: 2.5–5 mL, q 4–6 hr | b, c, e, f |
| *Guiatussin DAC* Syrup (Schedule V) [U.S.] | | Pseudoephedrine HCl 30 mg | Codeine PO₄ 10 mg | | Guaifenesin 100 mg | | Alcohol 1.6% Sugar free | 10 mL q 4 hr (max 40 mL/day) | | b, c, e, f |
| *Guiatussin w/Dextromethorphan* Oral Solution (OTC) [U.S.] | | | | Dextromethorphan HBr 15 mg | Guaifenesin 100 mg | | Alcohol 1.4% | 10 mL q 6–8 hr | | b, c |
| *Guiatuss PE* Syrup (OTC) [U.S.] | | Pseudoephedrine HCl 30 mg | | | Guaifenesin 100 mg | | Alcohol free | 10 mL q 4 hr (max 40 mL/day) | | b, c |

USP DI  Cough/Cold Combinations (Systemic) 1063

Table 3. Oral Dosage Forms (continued)

Note: Content per capsule, tablet, or 5 mL, unless otherwise stated.

| Brand or generic name [availability] | Antihistamines | Decongestants | Antitussives Opioid | Antitussives Non-opioid | Expectorants | Analgesics | Other content information as per product label | Usual Adult and Adolescent Dose prn‡ | Usual Pediatric Dose prn | Packaging, Storage, and Auxiliary labeling§ |
|---|---|---|---|---|---|---|---|---|---|---|
| *Halotussin-DM* Oral Solution (OTC) [U.S.] | | | | Dextromethorphan HBr 10 mg | Guaifenesin 100 mg | | Alcohol free With or without sugar | 10 mL q 6–8 hr | 2–6 yrs: 2.5 mL, 6–12 yrs: 5 mL, q 6–8 hr | b, c |
| *Histenol* Tablets (OTC) [Canada] | | Pseudoephedrine HCl 30 mg | | Dextromethorphan HBr 10 mg | | Acetaminophen 325 mg | | 1–2 tabs q 4 hr (max 8 tabs/day) | 6–12 yrs: ½–1 tab q 4 hr | a |
| *Histinex DM* Syrup (Rx) [U.S.] | Brompheniramine maleate 2 mg | Phenylpropanolamine HCl 12.5 mg | | Dextromethorphan HBr 10 mg | | | | 10 mL q 4 hr | | b, c, e |
| *Histinex HC* Syrup (Schedule III) [U.S.] | Chlorpheniramine maleate 2 mg | Phenylephrine HCl 5 mg | Hydrocodone bitartrate 2.5 mg | | | | Alcohol free Sugar free | 10 mL q 4 hr (max 40 mL/day) | 6–12 yrs: 5 mL q 4 hr (max 20 mL/day) | a, d, e, f |
| *Histinex PV* Syrup (Schedule III) [U.S.] | Chlorpheniramine maleate 2 mg | Pseudoephedrine HCl 30 mg | Hydrocodone bitartrate 2.5 mg | | | | Alcohol free Sugar free | 10 mL q 4–6 hr (max 4 doses/day) | 2–6 yrs: 2.5 mL, 6–12 yrs: 5 mL q 4–6 hr (max 4 doses/day) | a, d, f |
| *Histussin HC* Syrup (Schedule III) [U.S.] | Chlorpheniramine maleate 2 mg | Phenylephrine HCl 5 mg | Hydrocodone bitartrate 2.5 mg | | | | Alcohol free Sugar free | 10 mL q 4 hr | 6–12 yrs: 5 mL q 4 hr | b, c, e, f |
| *Humibid DM* Extended-release Tablets (Rx) [U.S.] | | | | Dextromethorphan HBr 30 mg | Guaifenesin 600 mg | | Scored | 1–2 tabs q 12 hr (max 4 tabs/day) | 2–6 yrs: ½ tab, 6–12 yrs: 1 tab, q 12 hr (max 2 doses/day) | b |

*Specific formulations may vary among the different manufacturers, check product labeling.
†Efficacy as expectorant has not been established.
‡Geriatric patients may be more sensitive to effects of usual adult dose.
§For appropriate *Packaging and storage* and *Auxiliary labeling* information refer to designated letters as follows:

a—Store below 40 °C (104 °F), preferably between 15 and 30 °C (59 and 86 °F), in a tight container, unless otherwise specified by manufacturer.
a¹—Store below 30 °C (86 °F), unless otherwise specified by manufacturer. Avoid exposure to excessive heat.
a²—Store below 25 °C (77 °F), unless otherwise specified by manufacturer.
b—Store below 40 °C (104 °F), preferably between 15 and 30 °C (59 and 86 °F), in a well-closed container, unless otherwise specified by manufacturer.
c—Protect from freezing.
d—Protect from light.
e—Auxiliary labeling: · May cause drowsiness. · Avoid alcoholic beverages.
f—Auxiliary labeling: · May be habit forming.
g—Auxiliary labeling: · Shake well.
h—Dispense in dropper bottle.
i—Chew well before swallowing.

**Included in subtherapeutic amount to discourage deliberate overdosage.

1064    Cough/Cold Combinations (Systemic)                                                                                                          USP DI

Table 3. Oral Dosage Forms (continued)

Note: Content per capsule, tablet, or 5 mL, unless otherwise stated.

| Brand or generic name [availability] | Antihistamines | Decongestants | Antitussives - Opioid | Antitussives - Non-opioid | Expectorants | Analgesics | Other content information as per product label | Usual Adult and Adolescent Dose prn‡ | Usual Pediatric Dose prn | Packaging, Storage, and Auxiliary labeling§ |
|---|---|---|---|---|---|---|---|---|---|---|
| *Humibid DM Pediatric* Extended-release Capsules (Rx) [U.S.] | | | | Dextromethorphan HBr 15 mg | Guaifenesin 300 mg | | | 2–4 caps q 12 hr (max 8 caps/day) | 2–6 yrs: 1 cap, 6–12 yrs: 1–2 caps, q 12 hr (max 2 doses/day) | b |
| *Humibid Guaifenesin Plus* Tablets (OTC) [U.S.] | | Pseudoephedrine HCl 60 mg | | | Guaifenesin 400 mg | | | 1 tab q 4–6 hrs (max 4 tabs/day) | 6–12 yrs: ½ tab q 4–6 hr (max 2 tabs/day) | b |
| *Hycodan* Syrup (Schedule III) [U.S.] | | | Hydrocodone bitartrate 5 mg | | | | Homatropine MBr 1.5 mg** | 5 mL q 4–6 hr (max 30 mL/day) | 6–12 yrs: 2.5 mL q 4–6 hr (max 15 mL/day) | b, c, e, f |
| Syrup (N) [Canada] | | | Hydrocodone bitartrate 5 mg | | | | Alcohol free | 5 mL at intervals ≥4 hr (max 30 mL/day) | <2 yrs: 1.25 mL (max 7.5 mL/day), 2–12 yrs: 2.5 mL (max 15 mL/day) at intervals ≥4 hr | b, c, d, e, f |
| Tablets (Schedule III) [U.S.] | | | Hydrocodone bitartrate 5 mg | | | | Homatropine MBr 1.5 mg** Scored | 1 tab q 4–6 hr (max 6 tabs/day) | 6–12 yrs: ½ tab q 4–6 hr (max 3 tabs/day). See also *Hycodan* Syrup | b, e, f |
| Tablets (N) [Canada] | | | Hydrocodone bitartrate 5 mg | | | | Scored | 1 tab at intervals ≥4 hr (max 6 tabs/day) | <2 yrs: ¼ tab (max 1½ tabs/day), 2–12 yrs: ½ tab (max 3 tabs/day), at intervals ≥4 hr. See also *Hycodan* Syrup | b, d, e, f |
| *Hycomine* Syrup (Schedule III) [U.S.] | | Phenylpropanolamine HCl 25 mg | Hydrocodone bitartrate 5 mg | | | | Alcohol free Sugar free | 5 mL q 4 hr (max 30 mL/day) | See *Hycomine Pediatric Syrup* | b, c, e, f |

USP DI    Cough/Cold Combinations (Systemic) 1065

Table 3. Oral Dosage Forms (continued)

Note: Content per capsule, tablet, or 5 mL, unless otherwise stated.

| Brand or generic name [availability] | Antihistamines | Decongestants | Antitussives Opioid | Antitussives Non-opioid | Expectorants | Analgesics | Other content information as per product label | Usual Adult and Adolescent Dose prn‡ | Usual Pediatric Dose prn | Packaging, Storage, and Auxiliary labeling§ |
|---|---|---|---|---|---|---|---|---|---|---|
| *Hycomine (continued)* Syrup (N) [Canada] | Pyrilamine maleate 12.5 mg | Phenylephrine HCl 10 mg | Hydrocodone bitartrate 5 mg | | Ammonium Cl† 60 mg | | Alcohol free | 5 mL at intervals ≥4 hr (max 30 mL/day) | See *Hycomine-S Pediatric* Syrup | b, c, d, e, f |
| *Hycomine Compound* Tablets (Schedule III) [U.S.] | Chlorpheniramine maleate 2 mg | Phenylephrine HCl 10 mg | Hydrocodone bitartrate 5 mg | | | Acetaminophen 250 mg | Caffeine 30 mg Scored | 1 tab 4 times/day (at intervals ≥4 hr) | 6–12 yrs: ½ tab 4 times/day (at intervals ≥4 hr) | b, e, f |
| *Hycomine Pediatric* Syrup (Schedule III) [U.S.] | | Phenylpropanolamine HCl 12.5 mg | Hydrocodone bitartrate 2.5 mg | | | | Alcohol free Sugar free | Intended for pediatric use. See *Hycomine* Syrup | 6–12 yrs: 5 mL q 4 hr (max 30 mL/day) | b, c, f |
| *Hycomine-S Pediatric* Syrup (N) [Canada] | Pyrilamine maleate 6.25 mg | Phenylephrine HCl 5 mg | Hydrocodone bitartrate 2.5 mg | | Ammonium Cl† 30 mg | | Alcohol free | 10 mL at intervals ≥4 hr (max 60 mL/day) | <2 yrs: 0.3 mg of hydrocodone bitartrate/kg/day in 4 divided doses; 3–6 yrs: 2.5 mL (max 15 mL/day), 6–12 yrs: 5 mL (max 40 mL/day), at intervals ≥4 hrs | b, c, d, e, f, h |

*Specific formulations may vary among the different manufacturers, check product labeling.
†Efficacy as expectorant has not been established.
‡Geriatric patients may be more sensitive to effects of usual adult dose.
§For appropriate *Packaging and storage* and *Auxiliary labeling* information refer to designated letters as follows:
 a—Store below 40 °C (104 °F), preferably between 15 and 30 °C (59 and 86 °F), in a tight container, unless otherwise specified by manufacturer.
 a¹—Store below 30 °C (86 °F), unless otherwise specified by manufacturer. Avoid exposure to excessive heat.
 a²—Store below 25 °C (77 °F), unless otherwise specified by manufacturer.
 b—Store below 40 °C (104 °F), preferably between 15 and 30 °C (59 and 86 °F), in a well-closed container, unless otherwise specified by manufacturer.
 c—Protect from freezing.                      f—Auxiliary labeling: • May be habit forming.     h—Dispense in dropper bottle.
 d—Protect from light.                          g—Auxiliary labeling: • Shake well.               i—Chew well before swallowing.
 e—Auxiliary labeling: • May cause drowsiness. • Avoid alcoholic beverages.
**Included in subtherapeutic amount to discourage deliberate overdosage.

**1066 Cough/Cold Combinations (Systemic)**

Table 3. Oral Dosage Forms *(continued)*
Note: Content per capsule, tablet, or 5 mL, unless otherwise stated.

| Brand or generic name [availability] | Antihistamines | Decongestants | Antitussives Opioid | Antitussives Non-opioid | Expectorants | Analgesics | Other content information as per product label | Usual Adult and Adolescent Dose prn‡ | Usual Pediatric Dose prn | Packaging, Storage, and Auxiliary labeling§ |
|---|---|---|---|---|---|---|---|---|---|---|
| *Hycotuss Expectorant* Syrup (Schedule III) [U.S.] | | | Hydrocodone bitartrate 5 mg | | Guaifenesin 100 mg | | Alcohol 10% | 5 mL after meals and hs (at intervals ≥4 hr) (max single dose 10 mL, max 30 mL/day) | 6–12 yrs: 2.5 mL (at intervals ≥4 hr) (max single dose 5 mL, max 15 mL/day) | b, c, e, f |
| Hydrocodone and Guaifenesin* Oral Solution (Schedule III) [U.S.] | | | Hydrocodone bitartrate 5 mg | | Guaifenesin 100 mg | | Alcohol free Sugar free Dye free | 5 mL q 4 hr (max 30 mL/day) | 2–12 yrs: 2.5 mL q 4 hr | a, e, f |
| Hydrocodone and Homatropine* Syrup (Schedule III) [U.S.] | | | Hydrocodone bitartrate 5 mg | | | | Homatropine MBr 1.5 mg** | 5 mL q 4–6 hr | <2 yrs: 1.25 mL, 2–12 yrs: 2.5 mL, q 4–6 hr | b, c, d, e, f |
| *Hydromet* Syrup (Schedule III) [U.S.] | | | Hydrocodone bitartrate 5 mg | | | | Homatropine MBr 1.5 mg** | 5 mL q 4–6 hr | | b, c, e, f |
| *Hydromine* Syrup (Schedule III) [U.S.] | | Phenylpropanolamine HCl 25 mg | Hydrocodone bitartrate 5 mg | | | | | 5 mL q 4 hr | Not intended for pediatric use. See *Hydromine Pediatric* | a, c, d, e, f |
| *Hydromine Pediatric* Syrup (Schedule III) [U.S.] | | Phenylpropanolamine HCl 12.5 mg | Hydrocodone bitartrate 2.5 mg | | | | | Intended for pediatric use | 6–12 yrs: 5 mL q 4 hr | a, c, d, e, f |
| *Hydropane* Syrup (Schedule III) [U.S.] | | | Hydrocodone bitartrate 5 mg | | | | Homatropine MBr 1.5 mg** | 5 mL q 4–6 hr | <2 yrs: 1.25 mL, 2–12 yrs: 2.5 mL, q 4–6 hr | b, c, d, e, f |
| *Hydrophen* Oral Solution (Schedule III) [U.S.] | | Phenylpropanolamine HCl 25 mg | Hydrocodone bitartrate 5 mg | | | | | 5 mL q 4–6 hr | 6–12 yrs: 2.5 mL q 4–6 hr | b, c, d, e, f |
| *Improved Sino-Tuss* Tablets (OTC) [U.S.] | Chlorpheniramine maleate 2 mg | Phenylephrine HCl 5 mg | | Dextromethorphan HBr 10 mg | | Acetaminophen 100 mg, Salicylamide 227 mg | | 1 tab q 4 hr | Pediatric strength not available | b, e |

Table 3. Oral Dosage Forms *(continued)*

Note: Content per capsule, tablet, or 5 mL, unless otherwise stated.

| Brand or generic name [availability] | Antihistamines | Decongestants | Antitussives - Opioid | Antitussives - Non-opioid | Expectorants | Analgesics | Other content information as per product label | Usual Adult and Adolescent Dose prn‡ | Usual Pediatric Dose prn | Packaging, Storage, and Auxiliary labeling§ |
|---|---|---|---|---|---|---|---|---|---|---|
| *Iobid DM* Extended-release Tablets (Rx) [U.S.] | | | | Dextromethorphan HBr 30 mg | Guaifenesin 600 mg | | | 1–2 tabs q 12 hr (max 4 tabs/day) | 2–6 yrs: ½ tab, 6–12 yrs: 1 tab, q 12 hr (max 2 doses/day) | a, d |
| *Iodal HD* Oral Solution (Schedule III) [U.S.] | Chlorpheniramine maleate 2 mg | Phenylephrine HCl 5 mg | Hydrocodone bitartrate 1.67 mg | | | | | 10 mL q 4 hr (max 40 mL/day) | 6–12 yrs: 5 mL q 4 hr (max 20 mL/day) | a, d, e, f |
| *Iohist DM* Oral Solution (Rx) [U.S.] | Brompheniramine maleate 2 mg | Phenylpropanolamine HCl 12.5 mg | | Dextromethorphan HBr 10 mg | | | | 10 mL q 4 hr (max 6 doses/day) | 2–6 yrs: 2.5 mL, 6–12 yrs: 5 mL, q 4 hr (max 6 doses/day) | a, d, e |
| *Iophen-C Liquid* Oral Solution (Schedule V) [U.S.] | | | Codeine PO₄ 10 mg | | Iodinated glycerol† 30 mg | | | 5–10 mL q 4 hr | 2–6 yrs: 1.25–2.5 mL, 6–12 yrs: 2.5–5 mL, q 4–6 hr | b, c, e, f |
| *Iophen DM* Oral Solution (Rx) [U.S.] | | | | Dextromethorphan HBr 10 mg | Iodinated glycerol† 30 mg | | | 5–10 mL q 4 hr | | b, c |
| *Iosal II* Extended-release Tablets (Rx) [U.S.] | | Pseudoephedrine HCl 60 mg | | | Guaifenesin 600 mg | | | 1–2 tabs q 12 hr (max 4 tabs/day) | 2–5 yrs: ½ tab, 6–12 yrs: 1 tab, q 12 hr (max 2 doses/day) | a, d |

*Specific formulations may vary among the different manufacturers, check product labeling.
†Efficacy as expectorant has not been established.
‡Geriatric patients may be more sensitive to effects of usual adult dose.
§For appropriate *Packaging and storage* and *Auxiliary labeling* information refer to designated letters as follows:
 a—Store below 40 °C (104 °F), preferably between 15 and 30 °C (59 and 86 °F), in a tight container, unless otherwise specified by manufacturer.
 a¹—Store below 30 °C (86 °F), in a tight container, unless otherwise specified by manufacturer. Avoid exposure to excessive heat.
 a²—Store below 25 °C (77 °F), unless otherwise specified by manufacturer.
 b—Store below 40 °C (104 °F), preferably between 15 and 30 °C (59 and 86 °F), in a well-closed container, unless otherwise specified by manufacturer.
 c—Protect from freezing.
 d—Protect from light.
 e—Auxiliary labeling: · May cause drowsiness. · Avoid alcoholic beverages.
 f—Auxiliary labeling: · May be habit forming.
 g—Auxiliary labeling: · Shake well.
 h—Dispense in dropper bottle.
 i—Chew well before swallowing.
**Included in subtherapeutic amount to discourage deliberate overdosage.

## Table 3. Oral Dosage Forms (continued)

Note: Content per capsule, tablet, or 5 mL, unless otherwise stated.

| Brand or generic name [availability] | Antihistamines | Decongestants | Antitussives Opioid | Antitussives Non-opioid | Expectorants | Analgesics | Other content information as per product label | Usual Adult and Adolescent Dose prn‡ | Usual Pediatric Dose prn | Packaging, Storage, and Auxiliary labelings§ |
|---|---|---|---|---|---|---|---|---|---|---|
| *Iotussin HC* Oral Solution (Schedule III) [U.S.] | Chlorpheniramine maleate 2 mg | Phenylephrine HCl 5 mg | Hydrocodone bitartrate 2.5 mg | | | | | 10 mL q 4 hr (max 40 mL/day) | 6–12 yrs: 5 mL q 4 hr (max 20 mL/day) | a, d, e, f |
| *Ipsatol Cough Formula for Children and Adults* Syrup (OTC) [U.S.] | | Phenylpropanolamine HCl 9 mg | | Dextromethorphan HBr 10 mg | Guaifenesin 100 mg | | Alcohol free | 10 mL q 4 hr (max 6 doses/day) | 2–6 yrs: 2.5 mL, 6–12 yrs: 5 mL, q 4 hr (max 6 doses/day) | b, c |
| *Kiddy Koff* Syrup (OTC) [U.S.] | | Phenylpropanolamine HCl 6.25 mg | | Dextromethorphan HBr 5 mg | Guaifenesin 50 mg | | Alcohol 5% | Intended for pediatric use | 2–6 yrs: 5 mL, 6–12 yrs: 10 mL, q 4 hr | b, c |
| *KIE* Syrup (Rx) [U.S.] | | Ephedrine HCl 8 mg | | | Potassium iodide† 150 mg | | Alcohol free | 10–15 mL q 4–6 hr | 6–12 yrs: 5 mL q 4 hr | b, c |
| *Kolephrin/DM Cough and Cold Medication* Tablets (OTC) [U.S.] | Chlorpheniramine maleate 2 mg | Pseudoephedrine HCl 30 mg | | Dextromethorphan HBr 10 mg | | Acetaminophen 325 mg | | 2 tab q 4–6 hr (max 8 tabs/day) | 6–12 yrs: 1 tab q 4–6 hr (max 4 tabs/day) | b, e |
| *Kolephrin GG/DM* Oral Solution (OTC) [U.S.] | | | | Dextromethorphan HBr 10 mg | Guaifenesin 150 mg | | Alcohol free | 10 mL q 4 hr | 2–6 yrs: 2.5 mL, 6–12 yrs: 5 mL, q 4 hr | b, c |
| *Kophane Cough and Cold Formula* Oral Solution (OTC) [U.S.] | Chlorpheniramine maleate 2 mg | Phenylpropanolamine HCl 12.5 mg | | Dextromethorphan HBr 10 mg | | | Alcohol free | 10 mL q 4 hr | 6–12 yrs: 5 mL q 4 hr | b, c, e |
| *Kwelcof Liquid* Oral Solution (Schedule III) [U.S.] | | | Hydrocodone bitartrate 5 mg | | Guaifenesin 100 mg | | Alcohol free Sugar free Dye free | 5 mL q 4–6 hr | 2–12 yrs: 2.5–5 mL q 4–6 hr | b, c, e, f |
| *Lanatuss Expectorant* Oral Solution (OTC) [U.S.] | Chlorpheniramine maleate 2 mg | Phenylpropanolamine HCl 5 mg | | | Guaifenesin 100 mg, Sodium citrate† 197 mg, Citric acid† 60 mg | | Sugar free | 5 mL q 6–8 hr | 2–6 yrs: 1.25–2.5 mL, 6–12 yrs: 2.5–5 mL, q 6–8 hr | b, c, e |

## Table 3. Oral Dosage Forms (continued)

Note: Content per capsule, tablet, or 5 mL, unless otherwise stated.

| Brand or generic name [availability] | Antihistamines | Decongestants | Antitussives Opioid | Antitussives Non-opioid | Expectorants | Analgesics | Other content information as per product label | Usual Adult and Adolescent Dose prn‡ | Usual Pediatric Dose prn | Packaging, Storage, and Auxiliary labeling§ |
|---|---|---|---|---|---|---|---|---|---|---|
| Liqui-Histine DM Syrup (Rx) [U.S.] | Brompheniramine maleate 2 mg | Phenylpropanolamine HCl 12.5 mg | | Dextromethorphan HBr 10 mg | | | Alcohol free Sugar free | 10 mL q 4 hr (max 6 doses/day) | 2–6 yrs: 2.5 mL, 6–12 yrs: 5 mL, q 4 hr (max 6 doses/day) | a, d, e |
| Mapap Cold Formula Tablets (OTC) [U.S.] | Chlorpheniramine maleate 2 mg | Pseudoephedrine HCl 30 mg | | Dextromethorphan HBr 15 mg | | Acetaminophen 325 mg | | 2 tabs q 6 hr | 6–12 yrs: 1 tab q 6 hr | b, e |
| Marcof Expectorant Syrup (Schedule III) [U.S.] | | | Hydrocodone bitartrate 5 mg | | Potassium guaiacolsulfonate† 300 mg | | Alcohol free Sugar free | 5–7.5 mL q 6 hr | 3–6 yrs: 1.25–2.5 mL, 6–12 yrs: 2.5–5 mL, q 6 hr | a, c, e, f |
| Med-Hist Exp Oral Solution (Schedule III) [U.S.] | | Pseudoephedrine HCl 60 mg | Hydrocodone bitartrate 5 mg | | Guaifenesin 200 mg | | Alcohol 12.5% | 5 mL q 6 hr | 25–50 lbs: 1.25 mL, 50–90 lbs: 2.5 mL, q 6 hr | a, d, e, f |
| Med-Hist HC Oral Solution (Schedule III) [U.S.] | Chlorpheniramine maleate 2 mg | Phenylephrine HCl 5 mg | Hydrocodone bitartrate 2.5 mg | | | | Alcohol 5% | 10 mL q 6–8 hr | 6–12 yrs: 5 mL q 6–8 hr | a, d, e, f |
| Mercodol with Decapryn Syrup (N) [Canada] | Doxylamine succinate 6 mg | Etafedrine HCl 16.65 mg | Hydrocodone bitartrate 1.65 mg | | | | Alcohol, Sodium citrate 200 mg | 5 mL q 3–5 hr (max 30 mL/day) | 1–6 yrs: 1.25–2.5 mL (max 7.5 mL/day), 6–12 yrs: 2.5–5 mL (max 15 mL/day) | a, e, f |

*Specific formulations may vary among the different manufacturers, check product labeling.
†Efficacy as expectorant has not been established.
‡Geriatric patients may be more sensitive to effects of usual adult dose.
§For appropriate *Packaging and storage* and *Auxiliary labeling* information refer to designated letters as follows:

a—Store below 40 °C (104 °F), preferably between 15 and 30 °C (59 and 86 °F), in a tight container, unless otherwise specified by manufacturer.
a¹—Store below 30 °C (86 °F), unless otherwise specified by manufacturer. Avoid exposure to excessive heat.
a²—Store below 25 °C (77 °F), unless otherwise specified by manufacturer.
b—Store below 40 °C (104 °F), preferably between 15 and 30 °C (59 and 86 °F), in a well-closed container, unless otherwise specified by manufacturer.
c—Protect from freezing.
d—Protect from light.
e—Auxiliary labeling: • May cause drowsiness. • Avoid alcoholic beverages.
f—Auxiliary labeling: • May be habit forming.
g—Auxiliary labeling: • Shake well.
h—Dispense in dropper bottle.
i—Chew well before swallowing.

**Included in subtherapeutic amount to discourage deliberate overdosage.

Table 3. Oral Dosage Forms *(continued)*

Note: Content per capsule, tablet, or 5 mL, unless otherwise stated.

| Brand or generic name [availability] | Antihistamines | Decongestants | Antitussives Opioid | Antitussives Non-opioid | Expectorants | Analgesics | Other content information as per product label | Usual Adult and Adolescent Dose prn‡ | Usual Pediatric Dose prn | Packaging, Storage, and Auxiliary labeling§ |
|---|---|---|---|---|---|---|---|---|---|---|
| *Mersyndol with Codeine* Tablets (N) [Canada] | Doxylamine succinate 5 mg | | Codeine PO₄ 8 mg | | | Acetaminophen 325 mg | | 1–2 tabs q 4 hr (max 12 tabs/day) | | a, e, f |
| *Midahist DH* Elixir (Schedule V) [U.S.] | Chlorpheniramine maleate 2 mg | Pseudoephedrine HCl 30 mg | Codeine PO₄ 10 mg | | | | Alcohol 5% | 10 mL q 4 hr | 2–6 yrs: 1.25–2.5 mL, 6–12 yrs: 2.5–5 mL, q 6 hr | a, c, e, f |
| *Muco-Fen DM* Extended-release Tablets (Rx) [U.S.] | | | | Dextromethorphan HBr 30 mg | Guaifenesin 600 mg | | Scored Dye free | 1–2 tabs q 12 hr (max 4 tabs/day) | 2–6 yrs: ½ tab (max 1 tab /day), 6–12 yrs: 1 tab (max 2 tabs/day), q 12 hr | a |
| *Myminic Expectorant* Oral Solution (OTC) [U.S.] | | Phenylpropanolamine HCl 6.25 mg | | | Guaifenesin 50 mg | | Alcohol free | 10 mL q 4 hr | | b, c |
| *Myminicol* Oral Solution (OTC) [U.S.] | Chlorpheniramine maleate 2 mg | Phenylpropanolamine HCl 6.25 mg | | Dextromethorphan HBr 5 mg | | | Alcohol free | 10 mL q 4 hr | | b, c, e |
| *Myphetane DC Cough* Syrup (Schedule V) [U.S.] | Brompheniramine maleate 2 mg | Phenylpropanolamine HCl 12.5 mg | Codeine PO₄ 10 mg | | | | Alcohol 1.2% | 10 mL q 4 hr | 2–6 yrs: 2.5 mL, 6–12 yrs: 5 mL, q 4 hr | a, c, d, e, f |
| *Myphetane DX Cough* Syrup (Rx) [U.S.] | Brompheniramine maleate 2 mg | Pseudoephedrine HCl 30 mg | | Dextromethorphan HBr 10 mg | | | Alcohol 1% | 10 mL q 4 hr | | b, c, e |
| *Mytussin AC* Syrup USP (Schedule V) [U.S.] | | | Codeine PO₄ 10 mg | | Guaifenesin 100 mg | | Alcohol 3.5% | 10 mL q 4 hr | 2–6 yrs: 2.5 mL, 6–12 yrs: 5 mL, q 4 hr | b, c, e, f |

USP DI — Cough/Cold Combinations (Systemic) — 1071

Table 3. Oral Dosage Forms (continued)

Note: Content per capsule, tablet, or 5 mL, unless otherwise stated.

| Brand or generic name [availability] | Antihistamines | Decongestants | Antitussives Opioid | Antitussives Non-opioid | Expectorants | Analgesics | Other content information as per product label | Usual Adult and Adolescent Dose prn‡ | Usual Pediatric Dose prn | Packaging, Storage, and Auxiliary labeling§ |
|---|---|---|---|---|---|---|---|---|---|---|
| Mytussin DAC Oral Solution (Schedule V) [U.S.] | | Pseudoephedrine HCl 30 mg | Codeine PO₄ 10 mg | | Guaifenesin 100 mg | | Alcohol 1.7% Sugar free | 10 mL q 4 hr (max 40 mL/day) | 2–6 yrs: 2.5 mL, 6–12 yrs: 5 mL, q 4 hr | a, c, e, f |
| Mytussin DM Oral Solution (OTC) [U.S.] | | | | Dextromethorphan HBr 10 mg | Guaifenesin 100 mg | | Alcohol free | 10 mL q 4 hr | 2–6 yrs: 2.5 mL, 6–12 yrs: 5 mL, q 6–8 hr | a, c, d, e |
| Naldecon-CX Adult Liquid Oral Solution (Schedule V) [U.S.] | | Phenylpropanolamine HCl 12.5 mg | Codeine PO₄ 10 mg | | Guaifenesin 200 mg | | Alcohol free Sugar free | 10 mL q 4 hr | 2–6 yrs: 1.25–2.5 mL, 6–12 yrs: 2.5–5 mL, q 4–6 hr | b, c, e, f, g |
| Naldecon-DX Adult Liquid Oral Solution (OTC) [U.S.] | | Phenylpropanolamine HCl 12.5 mg | | Dextromethorphan HBr 5 mg | Guaifenesin 200 mg | | Alcohol free Sugar free | 10 mL q 4 hr (max 6 doses/day) | Not intended for pediatric use | b, c |
| Naldecon-DX Children's Syrup Syrup (OTC) [U.S.] | | Phenylpropanolamine HCl 6.25 mg | | Dextromethorphan HBr 5 mg | Guaifenesin 100 mg | | Alcohol 0.6% | Intended for pediatric use | 2–6 yrs: 5 mL, >6 yrs: 10 mL, q 4 hr (max 6 doses/day) | b, c |
| Naldecon-DX Pediatric Drops Oral Solution (OTC) [U.S.] | | Phenylpropanolamine HCl 6.25 mg/mL | | Dextromethorphan HBr 5 mg/mL | Guaifenesin 50 mg/mL | | Alcohol free Sugar free | Intended for pediatric use | 2–6 yrs: 1 mL q 4 hr (max 6 doses/day) | b, c |

*Specific formulations may vary among the different manufacturers, check product labeling.
†Efficacy as expectorant has not been established.
‡Geriatric patients may be more sensitive to effects of usual adult dose.
§For appropriate Packaging and storage and Auxiliary labeling information refer to designated letters as follows:
  a¹—Store below 40 °C (104 °F), preferably between 15 and 30 °C (59 and 86 °F), in a tight container, unless otherwise specified by manufacturer.
  a²—Store below 30 °C (86 °F), unless otherwise specified by manufacturer. Avoid exposure to excessive heat.
  a³—Store below 25 °C (77 °F), unless otherwise specified by manufacturer.
  b—Store below 40 °C (104 °F), preferably between 15 and 30 °C (59 and 86 °F), in a well-closed container, unless otherwise specified by manufacturer.
  c—Protect from freezing.
  d—Protect from light.
  e—Auxiliary labeling: · May cause drowsiness. · Avoid alcoholic beverages.
  f—Auxiliary labeling: · May be habit forming.
  g—Auxiliary labeling: · Shake well.
  h—Dispense in dropper bottle.
  i—Chew well before swallowing.
**Included in subtherapeutic amount to discourage deliberate overdosage.

1072 Cough/Cold Combinations (Systemic) USP DI

Table 3. Oral Dosage Forms (continued)

Note: Content per capsule, tablet, or 5 mL, unless otherwise stated.

| Brand or generic name [availability] | Antihistamines | Decongestants | Antitussives Opioid | Antitussives Non-opioid | Expectorants | Analgesics | Other content information as per product label | Usual Adult and Adolescent Dose prn‡ | Usual Pediatric Dose prn | Packaging, Storage, and Auxiliary labeling§ |
|---|---|---|---|---|---|---|---|---|---|---|
| Naldecon-EX Children's Syrup (OTC) [U.S.] | | Phenylpropanolamine HCl 6.25 mg | | | Guaifenesin 100 mg | | Alcohol free Sugar free | Intended for pediatric use | 2–6 yrs: 5 mL; 6–12 yrs: 10 mL, q 4 hr (max 6 doses/day) | b, c |
| Naldecon-EX Pediatric Drops Oral Solution (OTC) [U.S.] | | Phenylpropanolamine HCl 6.25 mg/mL | | | Guaifenesin 50 mg/mL | | Alcohol free Sugar free | Intended for pediatric use | 2–6 yrs: 1 mL q 4 hr (max 6 doses/day) | b, c, h |
| Naldecon Senior DX Oral Solution (OTC) [U.S.] | | | | Dextromethorphan HBr 10 mg | Guaifenesin 200 mg | | Alcohol free | 10 mL q 4 hr (max 6 doses/day) | | b, c |
| Nalex Extended-release Capsules (Rx) [U.S.] | | Pseudoephedrine HCl 120 mg | | | Guaifenesin 250 mg (immediate release) | | | 1 cap q 12 hr | | a |
| Nalex DH Elixir (Schedule III) [U.S.] | | Phenylephrine HCl 5 mg | Hydrocodone bitartrate 1.67 mg | | | | Alcohol 5% | 10 mL q 4–6 hr (max 4 doses/day) | 2–6 yrs: 2.5–5 mL; 6–12 yrs: 5 mL, q 4–6 hr (max 4 doses/day) | a, c, d, f |
| Nalex Jr. Extended-release Capsules (Rx) [U.S.] | | Pseudoephedrine HCl 60 mg | | | Guaifenesin 300 mg | | | 1–2 caps q 12 hr | 6–12 yrs: 1 cap q 12 hr | a |
| Nasabid Extended-release Capsules (Rx) [U.S.] | | Pseudoephedrine HCl 90 mg | | | Guaifenesin 250 mg | | | 1 cap q 12 hr | Not recommended | a, d |
| Nasatab LA Extended-release Tablets (Rx) [U.S.] | | Pseudoephedrine HCl 120 mg | | | Guaifenesin 500 mg | | Scored Dye free | 1 tab q 12 hr | | b, c |
| Nasatuss Syrup (Schedule III) [U.S.] | | Phenylephrine HCl 5 mg | Hydrocodone bitartrate 2.5 mg | | | | Alcohol free Sugar free | 10 mL q 4 hr | 6–12 yrs: 5 mL q 4 hr | b, c, e, f |
| Neo Citran Day Caps Extra Strength Caplets (OTC) [Canada] | Chlorpheniramine maleate 2 mg | Pseudoephedrine HCl 30 mg | | Dextromethorphan HBr 15 mg | | Acetaminophen 500 mg | | 2 tabs q 8 hr (max 6 tabs/day) | | b |

**Table 3. Oral Dosage Forms** *(continued)*

Note: Content per capsule, tablet, or 5 mL, unless otherwise stated.

| Brand or generic name [availability] | Antihistamines | Decongestants | Antitussives Opioid | Antitussives Non-opioid | Expectorants | Analgesics | Other content information as per product label | Usual Adult and Adolescent Dose prn‡ | Usual Pediatric Dose prn | Packaging, Storage, and Auxiliary labeling§ |
|---|---|---|---|---|---|---|---|---|---|---|
| *Neo Citran DM Coughs and Colds* for Oral Solution (OTC) [Canada] | Pheniramine maleate 20 mg/pouch | Phenylephrine HCl 10 mg/pouch | | Dextromethorphan HBr 30 mg/pouch | | | Vitamin C 50 mg, Tartrazine | 1 pouch dissolved in 8 oz boiling water q 6–8 hr (max 3 pouches/day) | | e |
| *Norel* Capsules (Rx) [U.S.] | | Phenylephrine HCl 5 mg, Phenylpropanolamine HCl 45 mg | | | Guaifenesin 200 mg | | | 1 cap q 6 hr | Not recommended | a, d |
| *Novagest Expectorant w/Codeine* Oral Solution (Schedule V) [U.S.] | | Pseudoephedrine HCl 30 mg | Codeine PO₄ 10 mg | | Guaifenesin 100 mg | | Alcohol 1.4% | 10 mL q 4 hr | | b, c, e, f |
| *Novahistex C* Oral Solution (N) [Canada] | | Phenylephrine HCl 20 mg | Codeine PO₄ 15 mg | | | | Alcohol free | 5 mL q 4–6 hr | 6–12 yrs: 2.5 mL q 4–6 hr | b, c, e, f |
| *Novahistex DH* Oral Solution (N) [Canada] | | Phenylephrine HCl 20 mg | Hydrocodone bitartrate 5 mg | | | | Alcohol free | 5 mL q 4 hr | | b, c, e, f |
| *Novahistex DH Expectorant* Oral Solution (N) [Canada] | | Phenylephrine HCl 20 mg | Hydrocodone bitartrate 5 mg | | Guaifenesin 200 mg | | Alcohol free Fructose 10%, Glucose 14.3% | 5 mL q 4 hr | | b, c, e, f |
| *Novahistex DM w/Decongestant* Oral Solution (OTC) [Canada] | | Pseudoephedrine HCl 30 mg | | Dextromethorphan HBr 15 mg | | | Alcohol free | 10 mL q 4–6 hr (max 40 mL/day) | 6–12 yrs: 5 mL q 6 hr | b, c, e |
| *Novahistex DM Expectorant w/Decongestant* Oral Solution (OTC) [Canada] | | Pseudoephedrine HCl 30 mg | | Dextromethorphan HBr 15 mg | Guaifenesin 100 mg | | Alcohol free | 10 mL q 4–6 hr (max 40 mL/day) | | b |

*Specific formulations may vary among the different manufacturers, check product labeling.
†Efficacy as expectorant has not been established.
‡Geriatric patients may be more sensitive to effects of usual adult dose.
§For appropriate *Packaging and storage* and *Auxiliary labeling* information refer to designated letters as follows:
  a—Store below 40 °C (104 °F), preferably between 15 and 30 °C (59 and 86 °F), in a tight container, unless otherwise specified by manufacturer.
  a¹—Store below 30 °C (86 °F), unless otherwise specified by manufacturer. Avoid exposure to excessive heat.
  a²—Store below 25 °C (77 °F), unless otherwise specified by manufacturer.
  b—Store below 40 °C (104 °F), preferably between 15 and 30 °C (59 and 86 °F), in a well-closed container, unless otherwise specified by manufacturer.
  c—Protect from freezing.
  d—Protect from light.
  e—Auxiliary labeling: · May cause drowsiness. · Avoid alcoholic beverages.
  f—Auxiliary labeling: · May be habit forming.
  g—Auxiliary labeling: · Shake well.
  h—Dispense in dropper bottle.
  i—Chew well before swallowing.
**Included in subtherapeutic amount to discourage deliberate overdosage.

## Table 3. Oral Dosage Forms (continued)

Note: Content per capsule, tablet, or 5 mL, unless otherwise stated.

| Brand or generic name [availability] | Antihistamines | Decongestants | Antitussives — Opioid | Antitussives — Non-opioid | Expectorants | Analgesics | Other content information as per product label | Usual Adult and Adolescent Dose prn‡ | Usual Pediatric Dose prn | Packaging, Storage, and Auxiliary labeling§ |
|---|---|---|---|---|---|---|---|---|---|---|
| *Novahistex Expectorant w/Decongestant* Oral Solution (OTC) [Canada] | | Pseudoephedrine HCl 30 mg | | | Guaifenesin 100 mg | | Alcohol free | 10 mL q 4–6 hr (max 40 mL/day) | | b |
| *Novahistine DH* Oral Solution (N) [Canada] | | Phenylephrine HCl 10 mg | Hydrocodone bitartrate 1.7 mg | | | | Alcohol free | 10 mL q 4 hr | 6 mos–1 yr: 1.25–2.5 mL, 1–12 yrs: 2.5–5 mL, q 4 hr | b, c, e, f |
| *Novahistine DH Liquid* Oral Solution (Schedule V) [U.S.] | Chlorpheniramine maleate 2 mg | Pseudoephedrine HCl 30 mg | Codeine PO₄ 10 mg | | | | Alcohol 5% | 10 mL q 4–6 hr (max 40 mL/day) | 6–12 yrs: 5 mL q 4–6 hr (max 20 mL/day) | a, c, d, e, f |
| *Novahistine DM w/Decongestant* Oral Solution (OTC) [Canada] | | Pseudoephedrine HCl 15 mg | | Dextromethorphan HBr 7.5 mg | | | Alcohol free | | 2–5 yrs: 5 mL (max 20 mL/day), 6–12 yrs: 10 mL (max 40 mL/day), q 4–6 hr | a |
| *Novahistine DM Expectorant w/Decongestant* Oral Solution (OTC) [Canada] | | Pseudoephedrine HCl 15 mg | | Dextromethorphan HBr 7.5 mg | Guaifenesin 50 mg | | Alcohol free | | 2–5 yrs: 5 mL (max 20 mL/day), 6–12 yrs: 10 mL (max 40 mL/day), q 4–6 hr | a |
| *Novahistine DMX Liquid* Oral Solution (OTC) [U.S.] | | Pseudoephedrine HCl 30 mg | | Dextromethorphan HBr 10 mg | Guaifenesin 100 mg | | Alcohol 5% | 10 mL q 4 hr (max 40 mL/day) | 6–12 yrs: 5 mL q 4 hr (max 20 mL/day) | b, c |
| *Novahistine Expectorant* Oral Solution (Schedule V) [U.S.] | | Pseudoephedrine HCl 30 mg | Codeine PO₄ 10 mg | | Guaifenesin 100 mg | | Alcohol 7.5% | 10 mL q 4 hr (max 40 mL/day) | 6–12 yrs: 5 mL q 4 hr (max 20 mL/day) | a, c, e, f |

USP DI — Cough/Cold Combinations (Systemic) 1075

Table 3. Oral Dosage Forms (continued)

Note: Content per capsule, tablet, or 5 mL, unless otherwise stated.

| Brand or generic name [availability] | Antihistamines | Decongestants | Antitussives Opioid | Antitussives Non-opioid | Expectorants | Analgesics | Other content information as per product label | Usual Adult and Adolescent Dose prn‡ | Usual Pediatric Dose prn | Packaging, Storage, and Auxiliary labeling§ |
|---|---|---|---|---|---|---|---|---|---|---|
| *Nucochem Expectorant* Syrup (Schedule III) [U.S.] | | Pseudoephedrine HCl 60 mg | Codeine PO₄ 20 mg | | Guaifenesin 200 mg | | Alcohol 12.5% | 5 mL q 6 hr | 2–6 yrs: 1.25 mL, 6–12 yrs: 2.5 mL, q 6 hr | b, c, e, f |
| *Nucochem Pediatric Expectorant* Syrup (Schedule V) [U.S.] | | Pseudoephedrine HCl 30 mg | Codeine PO₄ 10 mg | | Guaifenesin 100 mg | | Alcohol 6% | 10 mL q 6 hr | 2–6 yrs: 2.5 mL, 6–12 yrs: 5 mL, q 6 hr | b, c, e, f |
| *Nucofed* Capsules (Schedule III) [U.S.] | | Pseudoephedrine HCl 60 mg | Codeine PO₄ 20 mg | | | | | 1 cap q 6 hr (max 4 caps/day) | Pediatric strength not available. See *Nucofed* Syrup | b, e, f |
| Syrup (Schedule III) [U.S.] | | Pseudoephedrine HCl 60 mg | Codeine PO₄ 20 mg | | | | Alcohol free, Sucrose 2.25 gm | 5 mL q 6 hr (max 4 doses/day) | 2–6 yrs: 1.25 mL, 6–12 yrs: 2.5 mL, q 6 hr (max 4 doses/day) | b, c, e, f |
| *Nucofed Expectorant* Syrup (Schedule III) [U.S.] | | Pseudoephedrine HCl 60 mg | Codeine PO₄ 20 mg | | Guaifenesin 200 mg | | Alcohol 12.5% | 5 mL q 6 hr (max 4 doses/day) | 2–6 yrs: 1.25 mL, 6–12 yrs: 2.5 mL, q 6 hr (max 4 doses/day) | b, c, e, f |

*Specific formulations may vary among the different manufacturers; check product labeling.
†Efficacy as expectorant has not been established.
‡Geriatric patients may be more sensitive to effects of usual adult dose.
§For appropriate *Packaging and storage* and *Auxiliary labeling* information refer to designated letters as follows:
 a— Store below 40 °C (104 °F), preferably between 15 and 30 °C (59 and 86 °F), in a tight container, unless otherwise specified by manufacturer.
 a¹— Store below 30 °C (86 °F), unless otherwise specified by manufacturer. Avoid exposure to excessive heat.
 a²— Store below 25 °C (77 °F), unless otherwise specified by manufacturer.
 b— Store below 40 °C (104 °F), preferably between 15 and 30 °C (59 and 86 °F), in a well-closed container, unless otherwise specified by manufacturer.
 c— Protect from freezing.
 d— Protect from light.
 e— Auxiliary labeling: • May cause drowsiness. • Avoid alcoholic beverages.
 f— Auxiliary labeling: • May be habit forming.
 g— Auxiliary labeling: • Shake well.
 h— Dispense in dropper bottle.
 i— Chew well before swallowing.
**Included in subtherapeutic amount to discourage deliberate overdosage.

Table 3. Oral Dosage Forms *(continued)*

Note: Content per capsule, tablet, or 5 mL, unless otherwise stated.

| Brand or generic name [availability] | Antihistamines | Decongestants | Antitussives Opioid | Antitussives Non-opioid | Expectorants | Analgesics | Other content information as per product label | Usual Adult and Adolescent Dose prn‡ | Usual Pediatric Dose prn | Packaging, Storage, and Auxiliary labeling§ |
|---|---|---|---|---|---|---|---|---|---|---|
| *Nucofed Pediatric Expectorant* Syrup (Schedule V) [U.S.] | | Pseudoephedrine HCl 30 mg | Codeine PO₄ 10 mg | | Guaifenesin 100 mg | | Alcohol 6% | 10 mL q 6 hr (max 4 doses/day) | 2–6 yrs: 2.5 mL, 6–12 yrs: 5 mL, q 6 hr (max 4 doses/day) | a, c, e, f |
| *Nucotuss Expectorant* Syrup (Schedule III) [U.S.] | | Pseudoephedrine HCl 60 mg | Codeine PO₄ 20 mg | | Guaifenesin 200 mg | | Alcohol 12.5% | 5 mL q 6 hr | | b, c, e, f |
| *Nucotuss Pediatric Expectorant* Syrup (Schedule V) [U.S.] | | Pseudoephedrine HCl 30 mg | Codeine PO₄ 10 mg | | Guaifenesin 100 mg | | Alcohol 6% | | 2–<12 yrs: 2.5–5 mL q 6 hr | b, c, e, f |
| *Nytcold Medicine* Oral Solution (OTC) [U.S.] | Doxylamine succinate 1.25 mg | Pseudoephedrine HCl 10 mg | | Dextromethorphan HBr 5 mg | | Acetaminophen 167 mg | Alcohol 25% | 30 mL hs or 30 mL q 6 hr | | b, c, e |
| *Nytime Cold Medicine Liquid* Oral Solution (OTC) [U.S.] | Doxylamine succinate 1.2 mg (7.5 mg/30 mL) | Pseudoephedrine HCl 10 mg (60 mg/30 mL) | | Dextromethorphan HBr 5 mg (30 mg/30 mL) | | Acetaminophen 166.6 mg (1000 mg/30 mL) | Alcohol 25% | 30 mL hs or q 6 hr | Not recommended | b, c, e |
| *Omnicol* Tablets (Rx) [U.S.] | Chlorpheniramine maleate 4 mg, Phenindamine tartrate 4 mg | Phenylephrine HCl 5 mg | | Dextromethorphan HBr 15 mg | | Acetaminophen 100 mg, Salicylamide 227 mg | Caffeine 10 mg, Ascorbic acid 25 mg Sugar coated | 1 tab q 4 hr | Pediatric strength not available | b, e |
| *Omni-Tuss* Oral Suspension (N) [Canada] | Chlorpheniramine 3 mg, Phenyltoloxamine 5 mg (as cation exchange resin complexes) | Ephedrine 25 mg (as cation exchange resin complex) | Codeine 10 mg (as cation exchange resin complex) | | Guaiacol carbonate† 20 mg | | Alcohol free Sodium 20 mg | 5 mL q 12 hr | 6–12 yrs: 2.5 mL, q 12 hr | b, c, e, f, g |
| *Ordrine AT* Extended-release Capsules (Rx) [U.S.] | | Phenylpropanolamine HCl 75 mg | | Caramiphen edisylate 40 mg | | | | 1 cap q 12 hr | | b |
| *Ornade-DM 10* Oral Solution (OTC) [Canada] | Chlorpheniramine maleate 2 mg | Phenylpropanolamine HCl 15 mg | | Dextromethorphan HBr 10 mg | | | Alcohol 4.7% Sugar free | Intended for pediatric use. See *Ornade DM 15* and *Ornade DM 30* Oral Solution | 1–5 yrs: 2.5 mL, 6–12 yrs: 5 mL, q 6 hr | b, c, e |

USP DI                                                                                                                    Cough/Cold Combinations (Systemic)    1077

Table 3. Oral Dosage Forms (continued)

Note: Content per capsule, tablet, or 5 mL, unless otherwise stated.

| Brand or generic name [availability] | Antihistamines | Decongestants | Antitussives — Opioid | Antitussives — Non-opioid | Expectorants | Analgesics | Other content information as per product label | Usual Adult and Adolescent Dose prn‡ | Usual Pediatric Dose prn | Packaging, Storage, and Auxiliary labeling§ |
|---|---|---|---|---|---|---|---|---|---|---|
| Ornade-DM 15 Oral Solution (OTC) [Canada] | Chlorpheniramine maleate 2 mg | Phenylpropanolamine HCl 15 mg | | Dextromethorphan HBr 15 mg | | | Alcohol 3.8% Sugar free | 5–10 mL q 6–8 hr | 2–4 yrs: 1.25 mL, 4–9 yrs: 2.5 mL, 9–12 yrs: 2.5–5 mL, q 6–8 hr | b, c, e |
| Ornade-DM 30 Oral Solution (OTC) [Canada] | Chlorpheniramine maleate 2 mg | Phenylpropanolamine HCl 15 mg | | Dextromethorphan HBr 30 mg | | | Alcohol free Sugar free | 5 mL q 6–8 hr | Not intended for pediatric use. See Ornade-DM 10 and Ornade-DM 15 Oral Solution | b, c, e |
| Ornade Expectorant Oral Solution (OTC) [Canada] | Chlorpheniramine maleate 2 mg | Phenylpropanolamine HCl 15 mg | | | Guaifenesin 100 mg | | Alcohol 7% Sugar free | 5–10 mL q 6–8 hr | 1–6 yrs: 2.5 mL, 6–12 yrs: 5 mL, q 6–8 hr | b, c, e |
| Ornex Severe Cold No Drowsiness Caplets Tablets (OTC) [U.S.] | | Pseudoephedrine HCl 30 mg | | Dextromethorphan HBr 15 mg | | Acetaminophen 500 mg | | 2 tabs q 6 hr (max 8 tabs/day) | | b |
| PanMist-JR Extended-release Tablets (Rx) [U.S.] | | Pseudoephedrine HCl 45 mg | | | Guaifenesin 600 mg | | | 1–2 tabs q 12 hrs (max 4 tabs/day) | 6–12 yrs: 1 tab q 12 hrs (max 2 tabs/day) | b, d |
| Para-Hist HD Oral Solution (Schedule III) [U.S.] | Chlorpheniramine maleate 2 mg | Phenylephrine HCl 5 mg | Hydrocodone bitartrate 1.67 mg | | | | | 10 mL q 6–8 hr | | b, c, e, f |
| Partuss LA Extended-release Tablets (Rx) [U.S.] | | Phenylpropanolamine HCl 75 mg | | | Guaifenesin 400 mg | | | 1 tab q 12 hr | | b |

*Specific formulations may vary among the different manufacturers, check product labeling.
†Efficacy as expectorant has not been established.
‡Geriatric patients may be more sensitive to effects of usual adult dose.
§For appropriate Packaging and storage and Auxiliary labeling information refer to designated letters as follows:
  a—Store below 40 °C (104 °F), preferably between 15 and 30 °C (59 and 86 °F), in a tight container, unless otherwise specified by manufacturer.
  a¹—Store below 30 °C (86 °F), unless otherwise specified by manufacturer. Avoid exposure to excessive heat.
  a²—Store below 25 °C (77 °F), unless otherwise specified by manufacturer.
  b—Store below 40 °C (104 °F), preferably between 15 and 30 °C (59 and 86 °F), in a well-closed container, unless otherwise specified by manufacturer.
  c—Protect from freezing.                                                f—Auxiliary labeling: · May be habit forming.      h—Dispense in dropper bottle.
  d—Protect from light.                                                    g—Auxiliary labeling: · Shake well.                i—Chew well before swallowing.
  e—Auxiliary labeling: · May cause drowsiness. · Avoid alcoholic beverages.
**Included in subtherapeutic amount to discourage deliberate overdosage.

**1078  Cough/Cold Combinations (Systemic)**  USP DI

### Table 3. Oral Dosage Forms (continued)

Note: Content per capsule, tablet, or 5 mL, unless otherwise stated.

| Brand or generic name [availability] | Antihistamines | Decongestants | Antitussives Opioid | Antitussives Non-opioid | Expectorants | Analgesics | Other content information as per product label | Usual Adult and Adolescent Dose prn‡ | Usual Pediatric Dose prn | Packaging, Storage, and Auxiliary labeling§ |
|---|---|---|---|---|---|---|---|---|---|
| *PediaCare Cough-Cold* Oral Solution (OTC) [U.S.] | Chlorpheniramine maleate 1 mg | Pseudoephedrine HCl 15 mg | | Dextromethorphan HBr 5 mg | | | Alcohol free | Intended for pediatric use | 2–3 yrs: 5 mL, 4–5 yrs: 7.5 mL, 6–8 yrs: 10 mL, 9–10 yrs: 12.5 mL, 11 yrs: 15 mL, q 4–6 hr | b, c, e |
| Chewable Tablets (OTC) [U.S.] | Chlorpheniramine maleate 1 mg | Pseudoephedrine HCl 15 mg | | Dextromethorphan HBr 5 mg | | | Phenylalanine 6 mg | Intended for pediatric use | 2–3 yrs: 1 tab, 4–5 yrs: 1½ tabs, 6–8 yrs: 2 tabs, 9–10 yrs: 2½ tabs, 11 yrs: 3 tabs, q 6–8 hr | b, e, i |
| *PediaCare NightRest Cough-Cold Liquid* Oral Solution (OTC) [U.S.] | Chlorpheniramine maleate 1 mg | Pseudoephedrine HCl 15 mg | | Dextromethorphan HBr 7.5 mg | | | Alcohol free | Intended for pediatric use | 2–3 yrs: 5 mL, 4–5 yrs: 7.5 mL, 6–8 yrs: 10 mL, 9–10 yrs: 12.5 mL, 11 yrs: 15 mL, q 6–8 hr | b, c, e |
| *Pediacof Cough* Syrup (Schedule V) [U.S.] | Chlorpheniramine maleate 0.75 mg | Phenylephrine HCl 2.5 mg | Codeine PO₄ 5 mg | | Potassium iodide† 75 mg | | Alcohol 5% | Intended for pediatric use | 6 mos–1 yr: 1.25 mL, 1–3 yrs: 2.5–5 mL, 3–6 yrs: 5–10 mL, 6–12 yrs: 10 mL, q 4–6 hr | b, c, e, f |
| *PediaPressin Pediatric Drops* Oral Solution (OTC) [U.S.] | | Pseudoephedrine HCl 15 mg/mL | | Dextromethorphan HBr 5 mg/mL | Guaifenesin 50 mg/mL | | Alcohol free Dye free Sugar free | Intended for pediatric use | 2–6 yrs: 1 mL q 4 hr (max 4 doses/day) | b |

Table 3. Oral Dosage Forms (continued)

Note: Content per capsule, tablet, or 5 mL, unless otherwise stated.

| Brand or generic name [availability] | Antihistamines | Decongestants | Antitussives Opioid | Antitussives Non-opioid | Expectorants | Analgesics | Other content information as per product label | Usual Adult and Adolescent Dose prn‡ | Usual Pediatric Dose prn | Packaging, Storage, and Auxiliary labeling§ |
|---|---|---|---|---|---|---|---|---|---|---|
| *Pedituss Cough* Syrup (Schedule V) [U.S.] | Chlorpheniramine maleate 0.75 mg | Phenylephrine HCl 2.5 mg | Codeine PO₄ 5 mg | | Potassium iodide† 75 mg | | | 6 mos–12 yrs: 1.25–10 mL q 4–6 hr | | b, c, e, f |
| *Penntuss* Oral Suspension (N) [Canada] | Chlorpheniramine maleate 4 mg (as polistirex) | | Codeine 10 mg (as polistirex) | | | | Alcohol free, Sodium 4.6 mg | 10–15 mL q 12 hr (max 30 mL/day) | 2–5 yrs: 2.5 mL (max 5 mL/day), 6–12 yrs: 5 mL (max 10 mL/day), q 12 hr | b, e, f, g |
| *Pentazine VC w/Codeine* Oral Solution (Schedule V) [U.S.] | Promethazine HCl 6.25 mg | | Codeine PO₄ 10 mg | | | | | 5 mL q 4–6 hr | | b, c, e, f |
| *Phanatuss* Syrup (OTC) [U.S.] | | | | Dextromethorphan HBr 10 mg | Guaifenesin 100 mg | | Alcohol free Sugar free | 10 mL q 3–4 hr (max 8 doses/day) | 2–6 yrs: 2.5 mL q 4 hr, 6–12 yrs: 5 mL, q 3–4 hr (max 6 doses/day) | b, c |
| *Phanatussin* Syrup (OTC) [U.S.] | Pyrilamine maleate 40 mg | Phenylpropanolamine HCl 25 mg | | Dextromethorphan HBr 15 mg | Guaifenesin 100 mg, Potassium citrate† 75 mg, Citric acid† 35 mg | | Alcohol free Sodium free | 10 mL q 4–8 hr (max 4 doses/day) | 2–6 yrs: 2.5 mL, 6–12 yrs: 5 mL, q 4–6 hr | b, c |

*Specific formulations may vary among the different manufacturers, check product labeling.
†Efficacy as expectorant has not been established.
‡Geriatric patients may be more sensitive to effects of usual adult dose.
§For appropriate *Packaging and storage* and *Auxiliary labeling* information refer to designated letters as follows:

a¹—Store below 40 °C (104 °F), preferably between 15 and 30 °C (59 and 86 °F), in a tight container, unless otherwise specified by manufacturer. Avoid exposure to excessive heat.
a²—Store below 25 °C (77 °F), unless otherwise specified by manufacturer.
b—Store below 40 °C (104 °F), preferably between 15 and 30 °C (59 and 86 °F), in a well-closed container, unless otherwise specified by manufacturer.
c—Protect from freezing.
d—Protect from light.
e—Auxiliary labeling: · May cause drowsiness. · Avoid alcoholic beverages.
f—Auxiliary labeling: · May be habit forming.
g—Auxiliary labeling: · Shake well.
h—Dispense in dropper bottle.
i—Chew well before swallowing.

**Included in subtherapeutic amount to discourage deliberate overdosage.

**1080** Cough/Cold Combinations (Systemic) — USP DI

## Table 3. Oral Dosage Forms (continued)

Note: Content per capsule, tablet, or 5 mL, unless otherwise stated.

| Brand or generic name [availability] | Antihistamines | Decongestants | Antitussives Opioid | Antitussives Non-opioid | Expectorants | Analgesics | Other content information as per product label | Usual Adult and Adolescent Dose prn‡ | Usual Pediatric Dose prn | Packaging, Storage, and Auxiliary labeling§ |
|---|---|---|---|---|---|---|---|---|---|
| *Pharmasave Children's Cough Syrup* (OTC) [Canada] | | Pseudoephedrine HCl 15 mg | | Dextromethorphan HBr 7.5 mg | | | Alcohol free Sugar free | | 2–5 yrs: 5 mL, 6–11 yrs: 10 mL, q 6–8 hr (max 4 doses/day) | a, d |
| *Pharmasave DM + Decongestant/Expectorant Syrup* (OTC) [Canada] | | Pseudoephedrine HCl 15 mg | | Dextromethorphan HBr 15 mg | Guaifenesin 100 mg | | Alcohol Sugar free | 10 mL q 6 hr (max 4 doses/day) | 2–5 yrs: 2.5 mL, 6–11 yrs: 5 mL, q 6 hr (max 4 doses/day) | a, d |
| *Pharmasave DM + Expectorant Syrup* (OTC) [Canada] | | | | Dextromethorphan HBr 15 mg | Guaifenesin 100 mg | | Alcohol Sugar free | 10 mL q 6 hr (max 4 doses/day) | 2–5 yrs: 2.5 mL, 6–11 yrs: 5 mL, q 6 hr (max 4 doses/day) | a, d |
| *Phenameth DM Syrup* (Rx) [U.S.] | Promethazine HCl 6.25 mg | | | Dextromethorphan HBr 15 mg | | | Alcohol | 5 mL q 4–6 hr | | b, c, e |
| *Phenameth VC with Codeine Syrup* (Schedule V) [U.S.] | Promethazine HCl 6.25 mg | Phenylephrine HCl 5 mg | Codeine PO₄ 10 mg | | | | Alcohol 7% | 5 mL q 4–6 hr | 2–6 yrs: 1.25–5 mL, 6–12 yrs: 2.5–5 mL, q 4–6 hr | a, c, d, e, f |
| *Phenergan with Codeine Syrup* (Schedule V) [U.S.] | Promethazine HCl 6.25 mg | | Codeine PO₄ 10 mg | | | | Alcohol 7% | 5 mL q 4–6 hr (max 30 mL/day) | 2–6 yrs: 1.25–2.5 mL, 6–12 yrs: 2.5–5 mL, q 4–6 hr | a, c, d, e, f |
| *Phenergan with Dextromethorphan Syrup* (Rx) [U.S.] | Promethazine HCl 6.25 mg | | | Dextromethorphan HBr 15 mg | | | Alcohol 7% | 5 mL q 4–6 hr (max 30 mL/day) | 2–6 yrs: 1.25–2.5 mL (max 10 mL/day), 6–12 yrs: 2.5–5 mL (max 20 mL/day) q 4–6 hr | a, c, d, e |

Table 3. Oral Dosage Forms (*continued*)

Note: Content per capsule, tablet, or 5 mL, unless otherwise stated.

| Brand or generic name [availability] | Antihistamines | Decongestants | Antitussives Opioid | Antitussives Non-opioid | Expectorants | Analgesics | Other content information as per product label | Usual Adult and Adolescent Dose prn‡ | Usual Pediatric Dose prn | Packaging, Storage, and Auxiliary labeling§ |
|---|---|---|---|---|---|---|---|---|---|---|
| *Phenergan Expectorant Syrup* (OTC) [Canada] | Promethazine HCl 5.65 mg | | | | Potassium guaiacolsulfonate† 40 mg | | | 5–10 mL q 4–6 hr | >2 yrs: 2.5–5 mL q 4–6 hr | a, d, e |
| *Phenergan Expectorant w/Codeine Syrup* (N) [Canada] | Promethazine HCl 5.65 mg | | Codeine PO₄ 10 mg | | Potassium guaiacolsulfonate† 40 mg | | | 5–10 mL q 4–6 hr | >2 yrs: 2.5–5 mL q 4–6 hr | a, d, e, f, g |
| *Phenergan VC with Codeine Syrup* (Schedule V) [U.S.] | Promethazine HCl 6.25 mg | Phenylephrine HCl 5 mg | Codeine PO₄ 10 mg | | | | Alcohol 7% | 5 mL q 4–6 hr (max 30 mL/day) | 2–6 yrs: 1.25–2.5 mL (max 6–9 mL/day), 6–12 yrs: 2.5–5 mL (max 15 mL/day), q 4–6 hr | a, c, d, e, f |
| *Phenergan VC Expectorant Syrup* (OTC) [Canada] | Promethazine HCl 5 mg | Phenylephrine HCl 5 mg | | | Potassium guaiacolsulfonate† 44 mg | | Alcohol | 5–10 mL q 4–6 hr | >2 yrs: 2.5–5 mL q 4–6 hr | a, d, e |
| *Phenergan VC Expectorant w/Codeine Syrup* (N) [Canada] | Promethazine HCl 5 mg | Phenylephrine HCl 5 mg | Codeine PO₄ 10 mg | | Potassium guaiacolsulfonate† 44 mg | | | 5–10 mL q 4–6 hr | >2 yrs: 2.5–5 mL q 4–6 hr | a, d, e, f |
| *Phenhist DH w/Codeine Oral Solution* (Schedule V) [U.S.] | Chlorpheniramine maleate 2 mg | Pseudoephedrine HCl 30 mg | Codeine PO₄ 10 mg | | | | Alcohol 5% | 10 mL q 4 hr (max 40 mL/day) | | b, c, e, f |
| *Phenhist Expectorant Oral Solution* (Schedule V) [U.S.] | | Pseudoephedrine HCl 30 mg | Codeine PO₄ 10 mg | | Guaifenesin 100 mg | | Alcohol 7.5% | 10 mL q 4 hr (max 40 mL/day) | 2–6 yrs: 1.25–2.5 mL, 6–12 yrs: 2.5–5 mL q 4–6 hr | a, c, e, f |

*Specific formulations may vary among the different manufacturers, check product labeling.
†Efficacy as expectorant has not been established.
‡Geriatric patients may be more sensitive to effects of usual adult dose.
§For appropriate *Packaging and storage* and *Auxiliary labeling* information refer to designated letters as follows:
 a—Store below 40 °C (104 °F), preferably between 15 and 30 °C (59 and 86 °F), in a tight container, unless otherwise specified by manufacturer.
 a¹—Store below 30 °C (86 °F), unless otherwise specified by manufacturer. Avoid exposure to excessive heat.
 a²—Store below 25 °C (77 °F), unless otherwise specified by manufacturer.
 b—Store below 40 °C (104 °F), preferably between 15 and 30 °C (59 and 86 °F), in a well-closed container, unless otherwise specified by manufacturer.
 c—Protect from freezing.
 d—Protect from light.
 e—Auxiliary labeling: · May cause drowsiness. · Avoid alcoholic beverages.
 f—Auxiliary labeling: · May be habit forming.
 g—Auxiliary labeling: · Shake well.
 h—Dispense in dropper bottle.
 i—Chew well before swallowing.
**Included in subtherapeutic amount to discourage deliberate overdosage.

**1082  Cough/Cold Combinations (Systemic)**  USP DI

Table 3. Oral Dosage Forms *(continued)*

Note: Content per capsule, tablet, or 5 mL, unless otherwise stated.

| Brand or generic name [availability] | Antihistamines | Decongestants | Antitussives Opioid | Antitussives Non-opioid | Expectorants | Analgesics | Other content information as per product label | Usual Adult and Adolescent Dose prn‡ | Usual Pediatric Dose prn | Packaging, Storage, and Auxiliary labeling§ |
|---|---|---|---|---|---|---|---|---|---|---|
| *Phenylfenesin L.A. Extended-release Tablets (Rx)* [U.S.] | | Phenylpropanolamine HCl 75 mg | | | Guaifenesin 400 mg | | Scored | 1 tab q 12 hr | 6–12 yrs: ½ tab q 12 hr | b |
| *Phenylpropanolamine and Guaifenesin* Extended-release Tablets (Rx)* [U.S.] | | Phenylpropanolamine HCl 75 mg | | | Guaifenesin 400 mg | | May be scored | 1 tab q 12 hr | 6–12 yrs: ½ tab q 12 hr | a, d |
| *Phenylpropanolamine and Hydrocodone* Syrup (Schedule III)* [U.S.] | | Phenylpropanolamine HCl 25 mg | Hydrocodone bitartrate 5 mg | | | | | 5 mL q 6 hr | | b, c, d, e, f |
| *Pherazine w/Codeine Syrup (Schedule V)* [U.S.] | Promethazine HCl 6.25 mg | | Codeine PO₄ 10 mg | | | | Alcohol 7% | 5 mL q 4–6 hr | | b, c, e, f |
| *Pherazine DM Syrup (Rx)* [U.S.] | Promethazine HCl 6.25 mg | | | Dextromethorphan HBr 15 mg | | | Alcohol 7% | 5 mL q 4–6 hr | | b, c, e |
| *Pherazine VC with Codeine Syrup (Schedule V)* [U.S.] | Promethazine HCl 6.25 mg | Phenylephrine HCl 5 mg | Codeine PO₄ 10 mg | | | | Alcohol 7% | 5 mL q 4–6 hr | 2–6 yrs: 1.25–2.5 mL; 6–12 yrs: 2.5–5 mL; q 4–6 hr | a, c, d, e, f |
| *Pneumotussin HC Syrup (Schedule III)* [U.S.] | | | Hydrocodone bitartrate 5 mg | | Guaifenesin 100 mg | | Alcohol free Sugar free | 5 mL q 4 hr | | b, c, e, f |
| *Polaramine Expectorant Oral Solution (Rx)* [U.S.] | Dexchlorpheniramine maleate 2 mg | Pseudoephedrine sulfate 20 mg | | | Guaifenesin 100 mg | | Alcohol 7.2% | 5–10 mL q 6–8 hr | 2–6 yrs: 1.25–2.5 mL; 6–12 yrs: 2.5–5 mL; q 6–8 hr | a, c, d, e |
| *Poly-Histine-CS Syrup (Schedule V)* [U.S.] | Brompheniramine maleate 2 mg | Phenylpropanolamine HCl 12.5 mg | Codeine PO₄ 10 mg | | | | Alcohol free | 10 mL q 4 hr | 2–6 yrs: 1.25–2.5 mL; 6–12 yrs: 2.5–5 mL; q 4–6 hr | b, c, e, f |
| *Poly-Histine-DM Syrup (Rx)* [U.S.] | Brompheniramine maleate 2 mg | Phenylpropanolamine HCl 12.5 mg | | Dextromethorphan HBr 10 mg | | | Alcohol free Sugar free | 10 mL q 4 hr | 2–6 yrs: 1.25–2.5 mL; 6–12 yrs: 2.5–5 mL; q 4–6 hr | b, c, e, f |

Table 3. Oral Dosage Forms (continued)

Note: Content per capsule, tablet, or 5 mL, unless otherwise stated.

| Brand or generic name [availability] | Antihistamines | Decongestants | Antitussives Opioid | Antitussives Non-opioid | Expectorants | Analgesics | Other content information as per product label | Usual Adult and Adolescent Dose prn‡ | Usual Pediatric Dose prn | Packaging, Storage, and Auxiliary labeling§ |
|---|---|---|---|---|---|---|---|---|---|---|
| Primatuss Cough Mixture 4 Oral Solution (OTC) [U.S.] | Chlorpheniramine maleate 2 mg | | | Dextromethorphan HBr 15 mg | | | Alcohol 10% | 10 mL q 8 hr | | b, c, e |
| Primatuss Cough Mixture 4D Oral Solution (OTC) [U.S.] | | Pseudoephedrine HCl 20 mg | | Dextromethorphan HBr 10 mg | Guaifenesin 67 mg | | Alcohol 10% | 15 mL q 6 hr | | b, c |
| Profen II Extended-release Tablets (Rx) [U.S.] | | Phenylpropanolamine HCl 37.5 mg | | | Guaifenesin 600 mg | | Scored Dye free | 1–2 tabs q 12 hr (max 4 tabs/day) | 2–6 yrs: ½ tab (max 1 tab/day), 6–12 yrs: 1 tab (max 2 tabs/day), q 12 hr | b |
| Profen-LA Extended-release Tablets (Rx) [U.S.] | | Phenylpropanolamine HCl 75 mg | | | Guaifenesin 600 mg | | Scored Dye free | 1 tab q 12 hr | 6–12 yrs: ½ tab q 12 hr | b |
| Promatussin DM Syrup (OTC) [Canada] | Promethazine HCl 6.25 mg | Pseudoephedrine HCl 60 mg | | Dextromethorphan HBr 15 mg | | | Alcohol 0.2% Bisulfites | 5 mL q 6 hr (max 4 doses/day) | 6–12 yrs: 2.5 mL q 6 hr (max 4 doses/day) | a, d, e |
| Promatussin DM Children's Syrup [Canada] | Promethazine HCl 3.125 mg | Pseudoephedrine HCl 30 mg | | Dextromethorphan HBr 7.5 mg | | | Alcohol 0.2% Bisulfites | Intended for pediatric use | 2–6 yrs: 2.5 mL, 6–12 yrs: 5 mL, q 6 hr (max 4 doses/day) | a, d, e |

*Specific formulations may vary among the different manufacturers, check product labeling.
†Efficacy as expectorant has not been established.
‡Geriatric patients may be more sensitive to effects of usual adult dose.
§For appropriate *Packaging and storage* and *Auxiliary labeling* information refer to designated letters as follows:
   a—Store below 40 °C (104 °F), preferably between 15 and 30 °C (59 and 86 °F), in a tight container, unless otherwise specified by manufacturer.
   a¹—Store below 30 °C (86 °F), unless otherwise specified by manufacturer. Avoid exposure to excessive heat.
   a²—Store below 25 °C (77 °F), unless otherwise specified by manufacturer.
   b—Store below 40 °C (104 °F), preferably between 15 and 30 °C (59 and 86 °F), in a well-closed container, unless otherwise specified by manufacturer.
   c—Protect from freezing.
   d—Protect from light.
   e—Auxiliary labeling: · May cause drowsiness. · Avoid alcoholic beverages.
   f—Auxiliary labeling: · May be habit forming.
   g—Auxiliary labeling: · Shake well.
   h—Dispense in dropper bottle.
   i—Chew well before swallowing.
**Included in subtherapeutic amount to discourage deliberate overdosage.

## Cough/Cold Combinations (Systemic)

### Table 3. Oral Dosage Forms (continued)

Note: Content per capsule, tablet, or 5 mL, unless otherwise stated.

| Brand or generic name [availability] | Antihistamines | Decongestants | Antitussives (Opioid) | Antitussives (Non-opioid) | Expectorants | Analgesics | Other content information as per product label | Usual Adult and Adolescent Dose prn‡ | Usual Pediatric Dose prn | Packaging, Storage, and Auxiliary labeling§ |
|---|---|---|---|---|---|---|---|---|---|---|
| Promethazine and Codeine* Syrup (Schedule V) [U.S.] | Promethazine HCl 6.25 mg | | Codeine PO₄ 10 mg | | | | May contain alcohol | 5 mL q 4–6 hr | 2–6 yrs: 1.25–2.5 mL, 6–12 yrs: 2.5–5 mL, q 4–6 hr | a, c, d, e, f |
| Promethazine DM Oral Solution (Rx) [U.S.] | Promethazine HCl 6.25 mg | | | Dextromethorphan HBr 15 mg | | | Alcohol | 5 mL q 4–6 hr | | b, c, e |
| Promethazine VC w/Codeine Oral Solution (Schedule V) [U.S.] | Promethazine HCl 6.25 mg | Phenylephrine HCl 5 mg | Codeine PO₄ 10 mg | | | | Alcohol | 5 mL q 4–6 hr | | b, c, e, f |
| Prometh w/Dextromethorphan Syrup (Rx) [U.S.] | Promethazine HCl 6.25 mg | | | Dextromethorphan HBr 15 mg | | | Alcohol 7% | 5 mL q 4–6 hr | | b, c, e |
| Promethist w/Codeine Syrup (Schedule V) [U.S.] | Promethazine HCl 6.25 mg | Phenylephrine HCl 5 mg | Codeine PO₄ 10 mg | | | | Alcohol | 5 mL q 4–6 hr | | b, c, e, f |
| Prometh VC with Codeine Oral Solution (Schedule V) [U.S.] | Promethazine HCl 6.25 mg | Phenylephrine HCl 5 mg | Codeine PO₄ 10 mg | | | | Alcohol 7% | 5 mL q 4–6 hr | 2–6 yrs: 1.25–2.5 mL, 6–12 yrs: 2.5–5 mL, q 4–6 hr | a, c, d, e, f |
| Prominic Expectorant Oral Solution (OTC) [U.S.] | | Phenylpropanolamine HCl 12.5 mg | | | Guaifenesin 100 mg | | Alcohol 5% | 10 mL q 4 hr | 2–6 yrs: 2.5 mL, 6–12 yrs: 5 mL, q 4 hr | b, c |
| Prominicol Cough Syrup (OTC) [U.S.] | Pheniramine maleate 6.25 mg, Pyrilamine maleate 6.25 mg | Phenylpropanolamine HCl 12.5 mg | | Dextromethorphan HBr 15 mg | | | Ammonium Cl† 90 mg | 10 mL q 4 hr | 2–6 yrs: 2.5 mL, 6–12 yrs: 5 mL, q 6–8 hr | b, c, e |
| Promist HD Liquid Oral Solution (Schedule III) [U.S.] | Chlorpheniramine maleate 2 mg | Pseudoephedrine HCl 30 mg | Hydrocodone bitartrate 2.5 mg | | | | Alcohol 5% | 10 mL q 6–8 hr | 2–6 yrs: 2.5 mL, 6–12 yrs: 5 mL, q 6–8 hr | b, c, d, e, f |

USP DI  Cough/Cold Combinations (Systemic) 1085

Table 3. Oral Dosage Forms (continued)

Note: Content per capsule, tablet, or 5 mL, unless otherwise stated.

| Brand or generic name [availability] | Antihistamines | Decongestants | Antitussives (Opioid) | Antitussives (Non-opioid) | Expectorants | Analgesics | Other content information as per product label | Usual Adult and Adolescent Dose prn‡ | Usual Pediatric Dose prn | Packaging, Storage, and Auxiliary labeling§ |
|---|---|---|---|---|---|---|---|---|---|---|
| *Protuss-D* Oral Solution (Schedule III) [U.S.] | | Pseudoephedrine HCl 30 mg | Hydrocodone bitartrate 5 mg | | Potassium guaiacolsulfonate† 300 mg | | Alcohol free Dye free Sugar free | 5–7.5 mL q 6 hr | 3–6 yrs: 1.25–2.5 mL, 6–12 yrs: 2.5–5 mL, q 6 hr | a, e, f |
| *Pseudo-Car DM* Syrup (Rx) [U.S.] | Carbinoxamine maleate 4 mg | Pseudoephedrine HCl 60 mg | | Dextromethorphan HBr 15 mg | | | Alcohol 0.19% | 5 mL q 6 hr | 18 mos–6 yrs: 2.5 mL, >6 yrs: 5 mL, q 6 hr | a, c, d, e |
| Pseudoephedrine and Guaifenesin* Extended-release Tablets (Rx) [U.S.] | | Pseudoephedrine HCl 120 mg | | | Guaifenesin 600 mg | | May be scored | 1 tab q 12 hr | 6–12 yrs: ½ tab q 12 hr | a, d |
| *P-V-Tussin* Syrup (Schedule III) [U.S.] | Chlorpheniramine maleate 2 mg | Pseudoephedrine HCl 30 mg | Hydrocodone bitartrate 2.5 mg | | | | Alcohol 5% | 10 mL q 4–6 hr (max 4 doses/day) | 2–6 yrs: 2.5 mL, 6–12 yrs: 5 mL, q 4–6 hr (max 4 doses/day) | a, c, e, f |
| Tablets (Schedule III) [U.S.] | | Pseudoephedrine 60 mg | Hydrocodone bitartrate 5 mg | | | | Scored | 1 tab q 4–6 hr (max 4 doses/day) | | a, d, e, f |
| *Quelidrine Cough* Syrup (OTC) [U.S.] | Chlorpheniramine maleate 2 mg | Ephedrine HCl 5 mg, Phenylephrine HCl 5 mg | | Dextromethorphan HBr 10 mg | Ammonium Cl† 40 mg, Ipecac fluidextract† 0.005 mL | | Alcohol 2% | 5 mL q 4–6 hr | 2–6 yrs: 1.25 mL, 6–12 yrs: 2.5 mL, q 4–6 hr | a², c, e |

*Specific formulations may vary among the different manufacturers, check product labeling.
†Efficacy as expectorant has not been established.
‡Geriatric patients may be more sensitive to effects of usual adult dose.
§For appropriate *Packaging and storage* and *Auxiliary labeling* information refer to designated letters as follows:
 a—Store below 40 °C (104 °F), preferably between 15 and 30 °C (59 and 86 °F), in a tight container, unless otherwise specified by manufacturer.
 a¹—Store below 30 °C (86 °F), unless otherwise specified by manufacturer. Avoid exposure to excessive heat.
 a²—Store below 25 °C (77 °F), unless otherwise specified by manufacturer.
 b—Store below 40 °C (104 °F), preferably between 15 and 30 °C (59 and 86 °F), in a well-closed container, unless otherwise specified by manufacturer.
 c—Protect from freezing.     f—Auxiliary labeling: · May be habit forming.     h—Dispense in dropper bottle.
 d—Protect from light.         g—Auxiliary labeling: · Shake well.                i—Chew well before swallowing.
 e—Auxiliary labeling: · May cause drowsiness. · Avoid alcoholic beverages.
**Included in subtherapeutic amount to discourage deliberate overdosage.

Cough/Cold Combinations (Systemic)

Table 3. Oral Dosage Forms (continued)

Note: Content per capsule, tablet, or 5 mL, unless otherwise stated.

| Brand or generic name [availability] | Antihistamines | Decongestants | Antitussives Opioid | Antitussives Non-opioid | Expectorants | Analgesics | Other content information as per product label | Usual Adult and Adolescent Dose prn‡ | Usual Pediatric Dose prn | Packaging, Storage, and Auxiliary labeling§ |
|---|---|---|---|---|---|---|---|---|---|---|
| Rentamine Pediatric Oral Suspension (Rx) [U.S.] | Chlorpheniramine tannate 4 mg | Ephedrine tannate 5 mg, Phenylephrine tannate 5 mg | | Carbetapentane tannate 30 mg | | | | Intended for pediatric use | 2–6 yrs: 2.5–5 mL, 6–12 yrs: 5–10 mL, q 12 hr | b, c, e, g |
| Rescaps-D S.R. Extended-release Capsules (Rx) [U.S.] | | Phenylpropanolamine HCl 75 mg | | Caramiphen edisylate 40 mg | | | | 1 cap q 12 hr | Pediatric strength not available | a, d |
| Rescon-DM Oral Solution (OTC) [U.S.] | Chlorpheniramine maleate 2 mg | Pseudoephedrine HCl 30 mg | | Dextromethorphan HBr 10 mg | | | Alcohol free Sugar free Dye free | 10 mL q 4–6 hr | | b, c, e |
| Rescon-GG Oral Solution (OTC) [U.S.] | | Phenylephrine HCl 5 mg | | | Guaifenesin 100 mg | | Alcohol free Sugar free | 10 mL q 4–6 hr | | b, c |
| Respa-1st Extended-release Tablets (Rx) [U.S.] | | Pseudoephedrine HCl 60 mg | | | Guaifenesin 600 mg | | Scored | 1–2 tabs q 12 hr | 6–12 yrs: 1 tab q 12 hr | b |
| Respa-DM Extended-release Tablets (Rx) [U.S.] | | | | Dextromethorphan HBr 30 mg | Guaifenesin 600 mg | | Scored | 1–2 tabs q 12 hr | 6–12 yrs: 1 tab q 12 hr | b |
| Respaire-60 SR Extended-release Capsules (Rx) [U.S.] | | Pseudoephedrine HCl 60 mg (extended-release) | | | Guaifenesin 200 mg (immediate-release) | | | 2 caps q 12 hr | 6–12 yrs: 1 cap q 12 hr | b |
| Respaire-120 SR Extended-release Capsules (Rx) [U.S.] | | Pseudoephedrine HCl 120 mg (extended-release) | | | Guaifenesin 250 mg (immediate-release) | | | 1 cap q 12 hr | Intended for adult use. See Respaire-60 SR | b |
| Rhinosyn-DM Oral Solution (OTC) [U.S.] | Chlorpheniramine maleate 2 mg | Pseudoephedrine HCl 30 mg | | Dextromethorphan HBr 15 mg | | | Alcohol 1.4% Dye free | 10 mL q 6 hr | 2–6 yrs: 2.5 mL, 6–12 yrs: 5 mL q 6 hr | b, c, e |
| Rhinosyn-DMX Expectorant Syrup (OTC) [U.S.] | | | | Dextromethorphan HBr 15 mg | Guaifenesin 100 mg | | Alcohol 6% Dye free | 10 mL q 6 hr | 2–6 yrs: 2.5 mL, 6–12 yrs: 5 mL, q 6 hr | a, c, d |

## Table 3. Oral Dosage Forms (continued)

Note: Content per capsule, tablet, or 5 mL, unless otherwise stated.

| Brand or generic name [availability] | Antihistamines | Decongestants | Antitussives Opioid | Antitussives Non-opioid | Expectorants | Analgesics | Other content information as per product label | Usual Adult and Adolescent Dose prn‡ | Usual Pediatric Dose prn | Packaging, Storage, and Auxiliary labeling§ |
|---|---|---|---|---|---|---|---|---|---|---|
| *Rhinosyn-X* Oral Solution (OTC) [U.S.] | | Pseudoephedrine HCl 30 mg | | Dextromethorphan HBr 10 mg | Guaifenesin 100 mg | | Alcohol 7.5% Dye free | 10 mL q 4 hr | 2–6 yrs: 2.5 mL, 6–12 yrs: 5 mL, q 4 hr | b, c, d |
| *Robafen AC Cough* Syrup USP (Schedule V) [U.S.] | | | Codeine PO$_4$ 10 mg | | Guaifenesin 100 mg | | Alcohol 3.5% | 5–10 mL q 4–6 hr | | a, c, d, e, f |
| *Robafen CF* Oral Solution (OTC) [U.S.] | | Phenylpropanolamine HCl 12.5 mg | | Dextromethorphan HBr 10 mg | Guaifenesin 100 mg | | | 10 mL q 4 hr | | b, c |
| *Robafen DAC* Syrup (Schedule V) [U.S.] | | Pseudoephedrine HCl 30 mg | Codeine PO$_4$ 10 mg | | Guaifenesin 100 mg | | Alcohol 1.4% | 10 mL q 4 hr (max 40 mL/day) | | b, c, e, f |
| *Robafen DM* Syrup (OTC) [U.S.] | | | | Dextromethorphan HBr 10 mg | Guaifenesin 100 mg | | Alcohol 1.4% | 5–10 mL q 4 hr | | b, c |
| *Robitussin A-C* Syrup USP (Schedule V) [U.S.] | | | Codeine PO$_4$ 10 mg | | Guaifenesin 100 mg | | Alcohol 3.5% Sugar free | 10 mL q 4 hr (max 6 doses/day) | 6–12 yrs: 5 mL q 4 hr (max 6 doses/day) | a, c, d, e, f |
| Syrup (N) [Canada] | Pheniramine maleate 7.5 mg | | Codeine PO$_4$ 10 mg | | Guaifenesin 100 mg | | Alcohol 3.5% | 5–10 mL q 4–6 hr | 6–12 yrs: 2.5–5 mL q 4–6 hr | b, c, e, f |
| *Robitussin-CF* Oral Solution (OTC) [U.S.] | | Phenylpropanolamine HCl 12.5 mg | | Dextromethorphan HBr 10 mg | Guaifenesin 100 mg | | Alcohol free | 10 mL q 4 hr (max 60 mL/day) | 2–6 yrs: 2.5 mL (max 15 mL/day), 6–12 yrs: 5 mL (max 30 mL/day), q 4 hr | b, c |

*Specific formulations may vary among the different manufacturers, check product labeling.
†Efficacy as expectorant has not been established.
‡Geriatric patients may be more sensitive to effects of usual adult dose.
§For appropriate *Packaging and storage* and *Auxiliary labeling* information refer to designated letters as follows:
  a—Store below 40 °C (104 °F), preferably between 15 and 30 °C (59 and 86 °F), in a tight container, unless otherwise specified by manufacturer.
  a¹—Store below 30 °C (86 °F), unless otherwise specified by manufacturer. Avoid exposure to excessive heat.
  a²—Store below 25 °C (77 °F), unless otherwise specified by manufacturer.
  b—Store below 40 °C (104 °F), preferably between 15 and 30 °C (59 and 86 °F), in a well-closed container, unless otherwise specified by manufacturer.
  c—Protect from freezing.
  d—Protect from light.
  e—Auxiliary labeling: · May cause drowsiness. · Avoid alcoholic beverages.
  f—Auxiliary labeling: · May be habit forming.
  g—Auxiliary labeling: · Shake well.
  h—Dispense in dropper bottle.
  i—Chew well before swallowing.
**Included in subtherapeutic amount to discourage deliberate overdosage.

Table 3. Oral Dosage Forms *(continued)*

Note: Content per capsule, tablet, or 5 mL, unless otherwise stated.

| Brand or generic name [availability] | Antihistamines | Decongestants | Antitussives Opioid | Antitussives Non-opioid | Expectorants | Analgesics | Other content information as per product label | Usual Adult and Adolescent Dose prn‡ | Usual Pediatric Dose prn | Packaging, Storage, Auxiliary labelings§ |
|---|---|---|---|---|---|---|---|---|---|---|
| *Robitussin-CF (continued)* Syrup (OTC) [Canada] | | Phenylpropanolamine HCl 12.5 mg | | Dextromethorphan HBr 10 mg | Guaifenesin 100 mg | | Alcohol | 15 mL q 6–8 hr | 2–6 yrs: 3.75 mL, 6–12 yrs: 7.5 mL, q 6–8 hr | b, c |
| *Robitussin with Codeine* Syrup (N) [Canada] | Pheniramine maleate 7.5 mg | | Codeine PO₄ 3.3 mg | | Guaifenesin 100 mg | | Alcohol 3.5% | 15 mL q 4–6 hr | 6–12 yrs: 7.5 mL q 4–6 hr | b, c, e, f |
| *Robitussin Cold and Cough Liqui-Gels* Capsules USP (OTC) [U.S.] | | Pseudoephedrine HCl 30 mg | | Dextromethorphan HBr 10 mg | Guaifenesin 200 mg | | | 2 caps q 4 hr (max 8 caps/day) | 6–12 yrs: 1 cap q 4 hr (max 4 caps/day) | a, d |
| *Robitussin Cold, Cough & Flu Liqui-Gels* Capsules (OTC) [U.S.] | | Pseudoephedrine HCl 30 mg | | Dextromethorphan HBr 10 mg | Guaifenesin 100 mg | Acetaminophen 250 mg | | 2 caps q 4 hr (max 8 caps/day) | 6–12 yrs: 1 cap q 4 hr (max 4 caps/day) | b |
| *Robitussin Cough & Cold* Oral Solution (OTC) [Canada] | | Pseudoephedrine HCl 30 mg | | Dextromethorphan HBr 15 mg | Guaifenesin 100 mg | | Alcohol | 10 mL q 6–8 hr (max 4 doses/day) | 2–6 yrs: 2.5 mL, 6–12 yrs: 5 mL, q 6–8 hr (max 4 doses/day) | b, c |
| *Robitussin Cough & Cold Liqui-Fills* Capsules USP (OTC) [Canada] | | Pseudoephedrine HCl 30 mg | | Dextromethorphan HBr 10 mg | Guaifenesin 200 mg | | | 2 caps q 6 hr (max 4 doses/day) | 6–12 yrs: 1 cap q 6 hr (max 4 doses/day) | a |
| *Robitussin-DAC* Syrup (Schedule V) [U.S.] | | Pseudoephedrine HCl 30 mg | Codeine PO₄ 10 mg | | Guaifenesin 100 mg | | Alcohol 1.9% Sugar free | 10 mL q 4 hr (max 40 mL/day) | 6–12 yrs: 5 mL q 4 hr | a, c, e, f |
| *Robitussin-DM* Oral Solution (OTC) [U.S] | | | | Dextromethorphan HBr 10 mg | Guaifenesin 100 mg | | Alcohol free | 10 mL q 4 hr (max 60 mL/day) | 2–6 yrs: 2.5 mL (max 15 mL/day), 6–12 yrs: 5 mL (max 30 mL/day), q 4 hr | b, c |
| Syrup (N) [Canada] | | | | Dextromethorphan HBr 15 mg | Guaifenesin 100 mg | | Alcohol 1.4% | 10 mL q 6–8 hr | 2–6 yrs: 2.5 mL, 6–12 yrs: 5 mL, q 6–8 hr | b, c |

Table 3. Oral Dosage Forms (continued)

Note: Content per capsule, tablet, or 5 mL, unless otherwise stated.

| Brand or generic name [availability] | Antihistamines | Decongestants | Antitussives Opioid | Antitussives Non-opioid | Expectorants | Analgesics | Other content information as per product label | Usual Adult and Adolescent Dose prn‡ | Usual Pediatric Dose prn | Packaging, Storage, and Auxiliary labeling§ |
|---|---|---|---|---|---|---|---|---|---|---|
| Robitussin Maximum Strength Cough and Cold Oral Solution (OTC) [U.S.] | | Pseudoephedrine HCl 30 mg | | Dextromethorphan HBr 15 mg | | | Alcohol 1.4% | 10 mL q 6 hr (max 40 mL/day) | | b, c |
| Robitussin Night Relief Oral Solution (OTC) [U.S.] | Pyrilamine maleate 50 mg/30 mL | Pseudoephedrine HCl 60 mg/30 mL | | Dextromethorphan HBr 30 mg/30 mL | | Acetaminophen 650 mg/30 mL | Alcohol free | 30 mL hs or q 6 hr | | b, e |
| Robitussin Night-Time Cold Formula Capsules (OTC) [U.S.] | Doxylamine succinate 6.25 mg | Pseudoephedrine HCl 30 mg | | Dextromethorphan HBr 15 mg | | Acetaminophen 325 mg | | 2 caps q 6 hr | Not recommended | b |
| Robitussin-PE Oral Solution (OTC) [U.S.] | | Pseudoephedrine HCl 30 mg | | | Guaifenesin 100 mg | | Alcohol free | 10 mL q 4 hr (max 40 mL/day) | 2–6 yrs: 2.5 mL (max 10 mL/day), 6–12 yrs: 5 mL (max 20 mL/day), q 4 hr | b, c |
| Syrup (OTC) [Canada] | | Pseudoephedrine HCl 30 mg | | | Guaifenesin 100 mg | | Alcohol | 10 mL q 6 hr | 2–6 yrs: 2.5 mL, 6–12 yrs: 5 mL, q 6 hr | b, c |

*Specific formulations may vary among the different manufacturers, check product labeling.
†Efficacy as expectorant has not been established.
‡Geriatric patients may be more sensitive to effects of usual adult dose.
§For appropriate *Packaging and storage* and *Auxiliary labeling* information refer to designated letters as follows:
  a—Store below 40 °C (104 °F), preferably between 15 and 30 °C (59 and 86 °F), in a tight container, unless otherwise specified by manufacturer.
  a¹—Store below 30 °C (86 °F), unless otherwise specified by manufacturer. Avoid exposure to excessive heat.
  a²—Store below 25 °C (77 °F), unless otherwise specified by manufacturer.
  b—Store below 40 °C (104 °F), preferably between 15 and 30 °C (59 and 86 °F), in a well-closed container, unless otherwise specified by manufacturer.
  c—Protect from freezing.
  d—Protect from light.
  e—Auxiliary labeling: · May cause drowsiness. · Avoid alcoholic beverages.
  f—Auxiliary labeling: · May be habit forming.
  g—Auxiliary labeling: · Shake well.
  h—Dispense in dropper bottle.
  i—Chew well before swallowing.
**Included in subtherapeutic amount to discourage deliberate overdosage.

**Table 3. Oral Dosage Forms** *(continued)*

Note: Content per capsule, tablet, or 5 mL, unless otherwise stated.

| Brand or generic name [availability] | Antihistamines | Decongestants | Antitussives - Opioid | Antitussives - Non-opioid | Expectorants | Analgesics | Other content information as per product label | Usual Adult and Adolescent Dose prn‡ | Usual Pediatric Dose prn | Packaging, Storage, and Auxiliary labeling§ |
|---|---|---|---|---|---|---|---|---|---|---|
| *Robitussin Pediatric Cough & Cold* Oral Solution (OTC) [U.S.] | | Pseudoephedrine HCl 15 mg | | Dextromethorphan HBr 7.5 mg | | | Alcohol free | 20 mL q 6 hr (max 80 mL/day) | 2–6 yrs: 5 mL (max 20 mL/day), 6–12 yrs: 10 mL (max 40 mL/day), q 6 hr | b, c |
| *Syrup* (OTC) [Canada] | | Pseudoephedrine HCl 15 mg | | Dextromethorphan HBr 7.5 mg | | | Alcohol free | 20 mL q 6–8 hr | 2–6 yrs: 5 mL, 6–12 yrs: 10 mL, q 6–8 hr | b, c |
| *Robitussin Severe Congestion Liqui-Gels* Capsules USP (OTC) [U.S.] | | Pseudoephedrine HCl 30 mg | | | Guaifenesin 200 mg | | | 2 caps q 4 hr (max 8 caps/day) | 6–12 yrs: 1 cap q 4 hr (max 4 caps/day) | a, d |
| *Rolatuss Expectorant* Oral Solution (Schedule V) [U.S.] | Chlorpheniramine maleate 2 mg | Phenylephrine HCl 5 mg | Codeine PO₄ 9.85 mg | | Ammonium Cl† 33.3 mg | | Alcohol 5% | 5–10 mL q 6–8 hr | | b, c, e, f |
| *Rolatuss w/Hydrocodone* Oral Solution (Schedule III) [U.S.] | Pheniramine maleate 3.3 mg, Pyrilamine maleate 3.3 mg | Phenylephrine HCL 5 mg, Phenylpropanolamine HCl 3.3 mg | Hydrocodone bitartrate 1.7 mg | | | | | 10 mL q 6 hr | | b, c, e, f |
| *Rondamine-DM Drops* Oral Solution (Rx) [U.S.] | Carbinoxamine maleate 2 mg/mL | Pseudoephedrine HCl 25 mg/mL | | Dextromethorphan HBr 4 mg/mL | | | | | 1–18 mos: 0.25–1 mL q 6 hr | b, c, e |
| *Rondec-DM Syrup* (Rx) [U.S.] | Carbinoxamine maleate 4 mg | Pseudoephedrine HCl 60 mg | | Dextromethorphan HBr 15 mg | | | Alcohol free Sugar free | 5 mL q 6 hr | 18 mos–6 yrs: 2.5 mL, >6 yrs: 5 mL, q 6 hr | a¹, c, d, e |
| *Rondec-DM Drops* Oral Solution (Rx) [U.S.] | Carbinoxamine maleate 2 mg/mL | Pseudoephedrine HCl 25 mg/mL | | Dextromethorphan HBr 4 mg/mL | | | Alcohol free Sugar free | Intended for pediatric use. See *Rondec-DM* Syrup | 1–3 mos: 0.25 mL, 3–6 mos: 0.50 mL, 6–9 mos: 0.75 mL, 9–18 mos: 1 mL, q 6 hr >18 mos: See *Rondec-DM* Syrup | a¹, c, e, h |

Table 3. Oral Dosage Forms (continued)

Note: Content per capsule, tablet, or 5 mL, unless otherwise stated.

| Brand or generic name [availability] | Antihistamines | Decongestants | Antitussives Opioid | Antitussives Non-opioid | Expectorants | Analgesics | Other content information as per product label | Usual Adult and Adolescent Dose prn‡ | Usual Pediatric Dose prn | Packaging, Storage, and Auxiliary labeling§ |
|---|---|---|---|---|---|---|---|---|---|---|
| Ru-Tuss DE Extended-release Tablets (Rx) [U.S.] | | Pseudoephedrine HCl 120 mg | | | Guaifenesin 600 mg | | Scored | 1 tab q 12 hr | 6–12 yrs: ½ tab q 12 hr | b |
| Ru-Tuss Expectorant Oral Solution (OTC) [U.S.] | | Pseudoephedrine HCl 30 mg | | Dextromethorphan HBr 10 mg | Guaifenesin 100 mg | | Alcohol 10% | 10 mL q 4–6 hr (max 40 mL/day) | 2–6 yrs: 2.5 mL, 6–12 yrs: 5 mL, q 4–6 hr (max 4 doses/day) | b, c, e, f |
| Ru-Tuss with Hydrocodone Liquid Oral Solution (Schedule III) [U.S.] | Pheniramine maleate 3.3 mg Pyrilamine maleate 3.3 mg | Phenylephrine HCl 5 mg Phenylpropanolamine HCl 3.3 mg | Hydrocodone bitartrate 1.7 mg | | | | Alcohol 5% | 10 mL q 4–6 hr (max 40 mL/day) | 2–6 yrs: 2.5–5 mL, 6–12 yrs: 5 mL, q 4–6 hr (max 4 doses/day) | b, c, d, e, f |
| Rymed Capsules USP (Rx) [U.S.] | | Pseudoephedrine HCl 30 mg | | | Guaifenesin 250 mg | | | 1 cap q 6 hr | Pediatric strength not available. See Rymed Liquid Oral Solution | b |
| Rymed Liquid Oral Solution (OTC) [U.S.] | | Pseudoephedrine HCl 30 mg | | | Guaifenesin 100 mg | | Alcohol 1.4% Sugar free | 10 mL q 4 hr | 2–6 yrs: 2.5 mL, 6–12 yrs: 5 mL, q 4 hr | b, c |
| Rymed-TR Caplets Extended-release Tablets (Rx) [U.S.] | | Phenylpropanolamine HCl 75 mg | | | Guaifenesin 400 mg | | | 1 tab q 12 hr | Pediatric strength not available | b |

*Specific formulations may vary among the different manufacturers, check product labeling.
†Efficacy as expectorant has not been established.
‡Geriatric patients may be more sensitive to effects of usual adult dose.
§For appropriate *Packaging and storage* and *Auxiliary labeling* information refer to designated letters as follows:
a—Store below 40 °C (104 °F), preferably between 15 and 30 °C (59 and 86 °F), in a tight container, unless otherwise specified by manufacturer.
a¹—Store below 30 °C (86 °F), unless otherwise specified by manufacturer. Avoid exposure to excessive heat.
a²—Store below 25 °C (77 °F), unless otherwise specified by manufacturer.
b—Store below 40 °C (104 °F), preferably between 15 and 30 °C (59 and 86 °F), in a well-closed container, unless otherwise specified by manufacturer.
c—Protect from freezing.
d—Protect from light.
e—Auxiliary labeling: · May cause drowsiness. · Avoid alcoholic beverages.
f—Auxiliary labeling: · May be habit forming.
g—Auxiliary labeling: · Shake well.
h—Dispense in dropper bottle.
i—Chew well before swallowing.
**Included in subtherapeutic amount to discourage deliberate overdosage.

## Table 3. Oral Dosage Forms (continued)

Note: Content per capsule, tablet, or 5 mL, unless otherwise stated.

| Brand or generic name [availability] | Antihistamines | Decongestants | Antitussives — Opioid | Antitussives — Non-opioid | Expectorants | Analgesics | Other content information as per product label | Usual Adult and Adolescent Dose prn‡ | Usual Pediatric Dose prn | Packaging, Storage, and Auxiliary labeling§ |
|---|---|---|---|---|---|---|---|---|---|---|
| *Ryna-C Liquid* Oral Solution (Schedule V) [U.S.] | Chlorpheniramine maleate 2 mg | Pseudoephedrine HCl 30 mg | Codeine PO₄ 10 mg | | | | Alcohol free Dye free Sugar free | 10 mL q 6 hr (max 40 mL/day) | 6–12 yrs: 5 mL q 6 hr | b, c, e, f |
| *Ryna-CX Liquid* Oral Solution (Schedule V) [U.S.] | | Pseudoephedrine HCl 30 mg | Codeine PO₄ 10 mg | | Guaifenesin 100 mg | | Alcohol free Dye free Sugar free | 10 mL q 6 hr (max 40 mL/day) | 6–12 yrs: 5 mL q 6 hr | b, c, e, f |
| *Rynatuss* Tablets (Rx) [U.S.] | Chlorpheniramine tannate 5 mg | Ephedrine tannate 10 mg, Phenylephrine tannate 10 mg | | Carbetapentane tannate 60 mg | | | Scored | 1–2 tabs q 12 hr | 6–12 yrs: ½–1 tab q 12 hr | b, e |
| *Rynatuss Pediatric* Oral Suspension (Rx) [U.S.] | Chlorpheniramine tannate 4 mg | Ephedrine tannate 5 mg, Phenylephrine tannate 5 mg | | Carbetapentane tannate 30 mg | | | | Intended for pediatric use. See *Rynatuss* Tablets | 2–6 yrs: 2.5–5 mL, q 12 yrs: 5–10 mL, q 12 hr | b, c, e, g |
| *Safe Tussin 30* Oral Solution (OTC) [U.S.] | | | | Dextromethorphan HBr 30 mg | Guaifenesin 200 mg | | Alcohol free Sodium free Sugar free Dye free | 10 mL q 6 hr (max 4 doses/day) | 2–6 yrs: 2.5 mL, 6–12 yrs: 5 mL, q 6 hr (max 4 doses/day) | b, c |
| *Saleto-CF* Tablets (OTC) [U.S.] | | Phenylpropanolamine HCl 12.5 mg | | Dextromethorphan HBr 10 mg | | Acetaminophen 325 mg | | 2 tabs q 4 hr | 6–12 yrs: 1 tab q 4 hr | b |
| *Scot-Tussin DM* Oral Solution (OTC) [U.S.] | Chlorpheniramine maleate 2 mg | | | Dextromethorphan HBr 15 mg | | | Alcohol free Sugar free | 5 mL q 4 hr or 10 mL q 6–8 hr | | b, c, e |
| *Scot-Tussin Senior Clear* Oral Solution (OTC) [U.S.] | | | | Dextromethorphan HBr 15 mg | Guaifenesin 200 mg | | Phenylalanine Alcohol free Sugar free | 5 mL q 4 hr (max 30 mL/day) | | a |
| *Silaminic Expectorant* Oral Solution (OTC) [U.S.] | | Phenylpropanolamine HCl 12.5 mg | | | Guaifenesin 100 mg | | | 10 mL q 4 hr (max 6 doses/day) | 2–6 yrs: 2.5 mL, 6–12 yrs: 5 mL, q 4 hr (max 6 doses/day) | a |
| *Sildec-DM* Syrup (Rx) [U.S.] | Carbinoxamine maleate 4 mg | Pseudoephedrine HCl 60 mg | | Dextromethorphan HBr 15 mg | | | Alcohol free | 5 mL q 6 hr | 18 mos–6 yrs: 2.5 mL, >6 yrs: 5 mL, q 6 hr | a, d, e |

Table 3. Oral Dosage Forms (*continued*)

Note: Content per capsule, tablet, or 5 mL, unless otherwise stated.

| Brand or generic name [availability] | Antihistamines | Decongestants | Antitussives - Opioid | Antitussives - Non-opioid | Expectorants | Analgesics | Other content information as per product label | Usual Adult and Adolescent Dose prn‡ | Usual Pediatric Dose prn | Packaging, Storage, and Auxiliary labeling§ |
|---|---|---|---|---|---|---|---|---|---|---|
| *Sildec-DM Oral Drops* Oral Solution (Rx) [U.S.] | Carbinoxamine maleate 2 mg/mL | Pseudoephedrine HCl 25 mg/mL | | Dextromethorphan HBr 4 mg/mL | | | Alcohol free Sugar free | Intended for pediatric use | 1–3 mos: ¼ mL; 3–6 mos: ½ mL; 6–9 mos: ¾ mL; 9–18 mos: 1 mL, q 6 hr | a, d, e, h |
| *Sildicon-E Pediatric Drops* Oral Solution (OTC) [U.S.] | | Phenylpropanolamine HCl 6.25 mg/mL | | | Guaifenesin 30 mg/mL | | Alcohol 0.6% | | 2–6 yrs: 1 mL q 4 hr (max 6 doses/day) | a, d, h |
| *Silexin Cough* Syrup (OTC) [U.S.] | | | | Dextromethorphan HBr 30 mg | Guaifenesin 200 mg | | Alcohol free Sugar free | 20 mL q 6–8 hr | 6–12 yrs: 10 mL q 6–8 hr | b, c |
| *Siltapp w/Dextromethorphan Cough & Cold Elixir* (OTC) [U.S.] | Brompheniramine maleate 2 mg | Phenylpropanolamine HCl 12.5 mg | | Dextromethorphan HBr 10 mg | Guaifenesin 100 mg | | Alcohol 2.3% | 10 mL q 4 hr (max 6 doses/day) | 6–12 yrs: 5 mL q 4 hr (max 6 doses/day) | a, e |
| *Sil-Tex* Oral Solution (Rx) [U.S.] | | Phenylephrine HCl 5 mg, Phenylpropanolamine HCl 20 mg | | | Guaifenesin 100 mg | | Alcohol 5% | 10 mL q 6 hr | 2–4 yrs: 2.5 mL; 4–6 yrs: 5 mL; 6–12 yrs: 7.5 mL, q 6 hr | a[1] |
| *Siltussin-CF* Oral Solution (OTC) [U.S.] | | Phenylpropanolamine HCl 12.5 mg | | Dextromethorphan HBr 10 mg | Guaifenesin 100 mg | | Alcohol 4.75% | 10 mL q 4 hr (max 6 doses/day) | 2–6 yrs: 2.5 mL; 6–12 yrs: 5 mL, q 4 hr (max 6 doses/day) | a |

*Specific formulations may vary among the different manufacturers, check product labeling.
†Efficacy as expectorant has not been established.
‡Geriatric patients may be more sensitive to effects of usual adult dose.
§For appropriate *Packaging and storage* and *Auxiliary labeling* information refer to designated letters as follows:
 a—Store below 40 °C (104 °F), preferably between 15 and 30 °C (59 and 86 °F), in a tight container, unless otherwise specified by manufacturer.
 a[1]—Store below 30 °C (86 °F), unless otherwise specified by manufacturer. Avoid exposure to excessive heat.
 a[2]—Store below 25 °C (77 °F), unless otherwise specified by manufacturer.
 b—Store below 40 °C (104 °F), preferably between 15 and 30 °C (59 and 86 °F), in a well-closed container, unless otherwise specified by manufacturer.
 c—Protect from freezing.
 d—Protect from light.
 e—Auxiliary labeling: · May cause drowsiness. · Avoid alcoholic beverages.
 f—Auxiliary labeling: · May be habit forming.
 g—Auxiliary labeling: · Shake well.
 h—Dispense in dropper bottle.
 i—Chew well before swallowing.
**Included in subtherapeutic amount to discourage deliberate overdosage.

1094 Cough/Cold Combinations (Systemic) USP DI

Table 3. Oral Dosage Forms (continued)

Note: Content per capsule, tablet, or 5 mL, unless otherwise stated.

| Brand or generic name [availability] | Antihistamines | Decongestants | Antitussives Opioid | Antitussives Non-opioid | Expectorants | Analgesics | Other content information as per product label | Usual Adult and Adolescent Dose prn‡ | Usual Pediatric Dose prn | Packaging, Storage, and Auxiliary labelings§ |
|---|---|---|---|---|---|---|---|---|---|---|
| *Siltussin DM* Syrup (OTC) [U.S.] | | | | Dextromethorphan HBr 10 mg | Guaifenesin 100 mg | | Alcohol free | 5–10 mL q 4 hr | | b, c |
| *Sinufed Timecelles* Extended-release Capsules (Rx) [U.S.] | | Pseudoephedrine HCl 60 mg | | | Guaifenesin 300 mg | | | 1–2 caps q 12 hr | 6–12 yrs: 1 cap q 12 hr | b |
| *Sinupan* Extended-release Capsules (Rx) [U.S.] | | Phenylephrine HCl 40 mg | | | Guaifenesin 200 mg | | Dye free | 1 cap q 12 hr | | b |
| *Sinutab with Codeine* Tablets (N) [Canada] | Chlorpheniramine maleate 2 mg | Pseudoephedrine HCl 30 mg | Codeine 8 mg | | | Acetaminophen 325 mg | | 1–2 tabs q 4–6 hr (max 8 tabs/day) | | b, e, f |
| *Sinutab Non-Drying No Drowsiness Liquid Caps* Capsules USP (OTC) [U.S.] | | Pseudoephedrine HCl 30 mg | | | Guaifenesin 200 mg | | | 2 caps q 4 hr (max 8 caps/day) | | a² |
| *SINUvent* Extended-release Tablets (Rx) [U.S.] | | Phenylpropanolamine HCl 75 mg | | | Guaifenesin 600 mg | | Scored | 1 tab q 12 hr | 6–12 yrs: ½ tab q 12 hr | b |
| *Snaplets-DM* Granules (OTC) [U.S.] | | Phenylpropanolamine HCl 6.25 mg/pack | | Dextromethorphan HBr 5 mg/pack | | | | Intended for pediatric use | 2–6 yrs: 1 pack, 6–12 yrs: 2 packs, sprinkled on soft food q 4 hr | b |
| *Snaplets-EX* Granules (OTC) [U.S.] | | Phenylpropanolamine HCl 6.25 mg/pack | | | Guaifenesin 50 mg/pack | | | Intended for pediatric use | 2–6 yrs: 1 pack, 6–12 yrs: 2 packs, sprinkled on soft food q 4 hr | b |
| *Snaplets-Multi* Granules (OTC) [U.S.] | Chlorpheniramine maleate 1 mg/pack | Phenylpropanolamine HCl 6.25 mg/pack | | Dextromethorphan HBr 5 mg/pack | | | | Intended for pediatric use | 2–6 yrs: 1 pack, 6–12 yrs: 2 packs, sprinkled on soft food q 4 hr | b, e |

USP DI  Cough/Cold Combinations (Systemic) 1095

Table 3. Oral Dosage Forms (continued)

Note: Content per capsule, tablet, or 5 mL, unless otherwise stated.

| Brand or generic name [availability] | Antihistamines | Decongestants | Antitussives Opioid | Antitussives Non-opioid | Expectorants | Analgesics | Other content information as per product label | Usual Adult and Adolescent Dose prn‡ | Usual Pediatric Dose prn | Packaging, Storage, and Auxiliary labeling§ |
|---|---|---|---|---|---|---|---|---|---|---|
| *SRC Expectorant* Oral Solution (Schedule III) [U.S.] | | Pseudoephedrine HCl 60 mg | Hydrocodone bitartrate 5 mg | | Guaifenesin 200 mg | | Alcohol 12.5% | 5 mL q 4–6 hr (max 20 mL/day) | Not recommended | b, c, e, f |
| *Stamoist E* Extended-release Tablets (Rx) [U.S.] | | Pseudoephedrine HCl 120 mg | | | Guaifenesin 500 mg | | Dye free Scored | 1 tab q 12 hr | | b |
| *Stamoist LA* Extended-release Tablets (Rx) [U.S.] | | Phenylpropanolamine HCl 75 mg | | | Guaifenesin 400 mg | | Scored | 1 tab q 12 hr | | b |
| *Statuss Expectorant* Oral Solution (Schedule V) [U.S.] | | Phenylpropanolamine HCl 12.5 mg | Codeine PO₄ 10 mg | | Guaifenesin 100 mg | | Alcohol 5% Dye free | 5–10 mL q 6–8 hr | 2–6 yrs: 2.5 mL, 6–12 yrs: 5 mL, q 6–8 hr | a, e, f |
| *Statuss Green* Oral Solution (Schedule III) [U.S.] | Pheniramine maleate 3.3 mg, Pyrilamine maleate 3.3 mg | Phenylephrine HCl 5 mg, Phenylpropanolamine HCl 3.3 mg | Hydrocodone bitartrate 1.67 mg | | | | Alcohol 5% | 10 mL q 4–6 hr | | b, c, e, f |
| *S-T Forte* Oral Solution (Schedule III) [U.S.] | Pheniramine maleate 13.33 mg | Phenylephrine HCl 5 mg, Phenylpropanolamine HCl 5 mg | Hydrocodone bitartrate 2.5 mg | | Guaifenesin 80 mg | | Alcohol 5% Sugar free | 5 mL q 6–8 hr (max 20 mL/day) | 6 mos–1 yr: 10 drops, 1–3 yrs: 20 drops, 3–12 yrs: 2.5 mL, q 6–8 hr | b, c, e, f |

*Specific formulations may vary among the different manufacturers, check product labeling.
†Efficacy as expectorant has not been established.
‡Geriatric patients may be more sensitive to effects of usual adult dose.
§For appropriate *Packaging and storage* and *Auxiliary labeling* information refer to designated letters as follows:
  a—Store below 40 °C (104 °F), preferably between 15 and 30 °C (59 and 86 °F), in a tight container, unless otherwise specified by manufacturer.
  a¹—Store below 30 °C (86 °F), unless otherwise specified by manufacturer. Avoid exposure to excessive heat.
  a²—Store below 25 °C (77 °F), unless otherwise specified by manufacturer.
  b—Store below 40 °C (104 °F), preferably between 15 and 30 °C (59 and 86 °F), in a well-closed container, unless otherwise specified by manufacturer.
  c—Protect from freezing.              f—Auxiliary labeling: · May be habit forming.        h—Dispense in dropper bottle.
  d—Protect from light.                  g—Auxiliary labeling: · Shake well.                  i—Chew well before swallowing.
  e—Auxiliary labeling: · May cause drowsiness. · Avoid alcoholic beverages.
**Included in subtherapeutic amount to discourage deliberate overdosage.

Table 3. Oral Dosage Forms (continued)

Note: Content per capsule, tablet, or 5 mL, unless otherwise stated.

| Brand or generic name [availability] | Antihistamines | Decongestants | Antitussives Opioid | Antitussives Non-opioid | Expectorants | Analgesics | Other content information as per product label | Usual Adult and Adolescent Dose prn‡ | Usual Pediatric Dose prn | Packaging, Storage, and Auxiliary labeling§ |
|---|---|---|---|---|---|---|---|---|---|---|
| S-T Forte (continued) Syrup (Schedule III) [U.S.] | Pheniramine maleate 13.33 mg | Phenylephrine HCl 5 mg, Phenylpropanolamine HCl 5 mg | Hydrocodone bitartrate 2.5 mg | | Guaifenesin 80 mg | | Alcohol 5% | 5 mL q 6–8 hr (max 20 mL/day) | 6 mos–1 yr: 10 drops, 1–3 yrs: 20 drops, 3–12 yrs: 2.5 mL, q 6–8 hr | b, c, e, f |
| S-T Forte 2 Oral Solution (Schedule III) [U.S.] | Chlorpheniramine maleate 2 mg | | Hydrocodone bitartrate 2.5 mg | | | | Glycerin 99.7% Alcohol free Sugar free Dye free | 5 mL q 6–8 hr (max 20 mL) | 6 mos–1 yr: 10 drops, 1–3 yrs: 20 drops, 3–12 yrs: 2.5 mL, q 6–8 hr | b, c, e, f |
| Sudafed Children's Cold & Cough Syrup (OTC) [U.S.] | | Pseudoephedrine HCl 15 mg | | Dextromethorphan HBr 5 mg | Guaifenesin 100 mg | | Alcohol free Sugar free | 20 mL q 4 hr (max 4 doses/day) | 2–6 yrs: 5 mL, 6–12 yrs: 10 mL, q 4 hr (max 4 doses/day) | b, c, d |
| Sudafed Children's Non-Drowsy Cold & Cough Oral Solution (OTC) [U.S.] | | Pseudoephedrine HCl 15 mg | | Dextromethorphan HBr 5 mg | Guaifenesin 100 mg | | Alcohol Free Sugar free | 20 mL q 4 hr (max 4 doses/day) | 2–6 yrs: 5 mL, 6–12 yrs: 10 mL, q 4 hr (max 4 doses/day) | b, c, d |
| Sudafed Cold & Cough Liquid Caps Capsules (OTC) [U.S.] | | Pseudoephedrine HCl 30 mg | | Dextromethorphan HBr 10 mg | Guaifenesin 100 mg | Acetaminophen 250 mg | | 2 caps q 4 hr (max 8 caps/day) | Not recommended | b, c, d |
| Sudafed Cold & Flu Gelcaps Capsules (OTC) [Canada] | | Pseudoephedrine HCl 30 mg | | Dextromethorphan HBr 10 mg | Guaifenesin 100 mg | Acetaminophen 250 mg | | 2 caps q 4 hr | | b, d |
| Sudafed Cough & Cold Extra Strength Caplets Tablets (OTC) [Canada] | | Pseudoephedrine HCl 60 mg | | Dextromethorphan HBr 30 mg | | Acetaminophen 500 mg | Scored | 1 tab q 4–6 hr (max 4 tabs/day) | | b, d |

USP DI  Cough/Cold Combinations (Systemic) 1097

Table 3. Oral Dosage Forms (continued)

Note: Content per capsule, tablet, or 5 mL, unless otherwise stated.

| Brand or generic name [availability] | Antihistamines | Decongestants | Antitussives Opioid | Antitussives Non-opioid | Expectorants | Analgesics | Other content information as per product label | Usual Adult and Adolescent Dose prn‡ | Usual Pediatric Dose prn | Packaging, Storage, and Auxiliary labeling§ |
|---|---|---|---|---|---|---|---|---|---|---|
| Sudafed DM Oral Solution (OTC) [Canada] | | Pseudoephedrine HCl 30 mg | | Dextromethorphan HBr 15 mg | | | Alcohol | 10 mL q 4–6 hr (max 40 mL/day) | 4 mos–2 yr: 1.25 mL; 2–5 yrs: 2.5 mL; 6–11 yrs: 5 mL; q 4–6 hr (max 4 doses/day) | b, c |
| Sudafed Non-Drowsy Non-Drying Sinus Liquid Caps Capsules USP (OTC) [U.S.] | | Pseudoephedrine HCl 30 mg | | | Guaifenesin 200 mg | | | 2 caps q 4 hr (max 8 caps/day) | | a, d |
| Sudafed Severe Cold Formula Tablets (OTC) [U.S.] | | Pseudoephedrine HCl 30 mg | | Dextromethorphan HBr 15 mg | | Acetaminophen 500 mg | | 2 tabs q 6 hr (max 8 tabs/day) | Intended for adult use | a[2] |
| Sudafed Severe Cold Formula Caplets Tablets (OTC) [U.S.] | | Pseudoephedrine HCl 30 mg | | Dextromethorphan HBr 15 mg | | Acetaminophen 500 mg | | 2 tabs q 6 hr (max 8 tabs/day) | Intended for adult use | a[2] |
| Sudal 60/500 Extended-release Tablets (Rx) [U.S.] | | Pseudoephedrine HCl 60 mg | | | Guaifenesin 500 mg | | Scored | 1–2 tabs q 12 hr | 6–12 yrs: ½ – 1 tab q 12 hr | a, d |
| Sudal 120/600 Extended-release Tablets (Rx) [U.S.] | | Pseudoephedrine HCl 120 mg | | | Guaifenesin 600 mg | | Scored | 1 tab q 12 hr | 6–12 yrs: ½ tab q 12 hr | a, d |

*Specific formulations may vary among the different manufacturers, check product labeling.
†Efficacy as expectorant has not been established.
‡Geriatric patients may be more sensitive to effects of usual adult dose.
§For appropriate *Packaging and storage* and *Auxiliary labeling* information refer to designated letters as follows:
  a—Store below 40 °C (104 °F), preferably between 15 and 30 °C (59 and 86 °F), in a tight container, unless otherwise specified by manufacturer.
  a[1]—Store below 30 °C (86 °F), unless otherwise specified by manufacturer. Avoid exposure to excessive heat.
  a[2]—Store below 25 °C (77 °F), unless otherwise specified by manufacturer.
  b—Store below 40 °C (104 °F), preferably between 15 and 30 °C (59 and 86 °F), in a well-closed container, unless otherwise specified by manufacturer.
  c—Protect from freezing.
  d—Protect from light.
  e—Auxiliary labeling: • May cause drowsiness. • Avoid alcoholic beverages.
  f—Auxiliary labeling: • May be habit forming.
  g—Auxiliary labeling: • Shake well.
  h—Dispense in dropper bottle.
  i—Chew well before swallowing.
**Included in subtherapeutic amount to discourage deliberate overdosage.

1098 Cough/Cold Combinations (Systemic)  USP DI

Table 3. Oral Dosage Forms (continued)

Note: Content per capsule, tablet, or 5 mL, unless otherwise stated.

| Brand or generic name [availability] | Antihistamines | Decongestants | Antitussives Opioid | Antitussives Non-opioid | Expectorants | Analgesics | Other content information as per product label | Usual Adult and Adolescent Dose prn‡ | Usual Pediatric Dose prn | Packaging, Storage, and Auxiliary labelings§ |
|---|---|---|---|---|---|---|---|---|---|---|
| *Suppressin DM* Oral Solution (OTC) [U.S.] | | | | Dextromethorphan HBr 10 mg | Guaifenesin 100 mg | | Alcohol free Dye free Sugar free | 10 mL q 4 hr (max 6 doses/day) | 2–6 yrs: 2.5 mL, 6–12 yrs: 5 mL, q 4 hr (max 6 doses/day) | b |
| *Suppressin DM Caplets* Tablets (OTC) [U.S.] | | | | Dextromethorphan HBr 15 mg | Guaifenesin 200 mg | | Dye free | 2 tabs q 6 hr (max 8 tabs/day) | Not recommended | b |
| *Suppressin DM Plus* Oral Solution (OTC) [U.S.] | | Phenylephrine HCl 5 mg | | Dextromethorphan HBr 10 mg | Guaifenesin 100 mg | | Alcohol free Dye free Sugar free | 10 mL q 4 hr (max 6 doses/day) | 2–6 yrs: 2.5 mL, 6–12 yrs: 5 mL, q 4 hr (max 6 doses/day) | b |
| *Syracol CF* Tablets (OTC) [U.S.] | | | | Dextromethorphan HBr 15 mg | Guaifenesin 200 mg | | | 2 tabs q 6–8 hr (max 8 tabs/day) | 2–6 yrs: ½ tab, 6–12 yrs: 1 tab, q 6–8 hr | b |
| *Tantacol DM* Syrup (OTC) [Canada] | Pheniramine maleate 6.25 mg, Pyrilamine maleate 6.25 mg | Phenylpropanolamine HCl 12.5 mg | | Dextromethorphan HBr 15 mg | | | | 5–10 mL q 6–8 hr | 2–6 yrs: 2.5 mL, 6–12 yrs: 5 mL, q 6–8 hr | a |
| *Tanta Cough Syrup* Syrup (OTC) [Canada] | | | | Dextromethorphan HBr 15 mg | Guaifenesin 100 mg | | Alcohol 1.4% | 10 mL q 6–8 hr (max 4 doses/day) | 2–6 yrs: 2.5 mL, 6–12 yrs: 5 mL, q 6–8 hr (max 4 doses/day) | a |
| *TheraFlu Flu, Cold & Cough Medicine* for Oral Solution (OTC) [U.S.] | Chlorpheniramine maleate 4 mg/packet | Pseudoephedrine HCl 60 mg/packet | | Dextromethorphan HBr 20 mg/packet | | Acetaminophen 650 mg packet | | 1 packet dissolved in 6-oz cup of hot water q 4 hr (max 4 packets/day) | | b, e |

Table 3. Oral Dosage Forms (*continued*)

Note: Content per capsule, tablet, or 5 mL, unless otherwise stated.

| Brand or generic name [availability] | Antihistamines | Decongestants | Antitussives - Opioid | Antitussives - Non-opioid | Expectorants | Analgesics | Other content information as per product label | Usual Adult and Adolescent Dose prn‡ | Usual Pediatric Dose prn | Packaging, Storage, and Auxiliary labeling§ |
|---|---|---|---|---|---|---|---|---|---|---|
| *TheraFlu Maximum Strength Non-Drowsy Formula Flu, Cold & Cough Medicine for Oral Solution* (OTC) [U.S.] | | Pseudoephedrine HCl 60 mg/packet | | Dextromethorphan HBr 30 mg/packet | | Acetaminophen 1000 mg/packet | | 1 packet dissolved in 6-oz cup of hot water q 6 hr (max 4 packets/day) | Not recommended | b |
| *TheraFlu Maximum Strength Non-Drowsy Formula Flu, Cold & Cough Medicine Caplets Tablets* (OTC) [U.S.] | | Pseudoephedrine HCl 30 mg | | Dextromethorphan HBr 15 mg | | Acetaminophen 500 mg | | 2 tabs q 6 hr (max 8 tabs/day) | | b |
| *TheraFlu Nighttime Maximum Strength Flu, Cold & Cough for Oral Solution* (OTC) [U.S.] | Chlorpheniramine maleate 4 mg/packet | Pseudoephedrine HCl 60 mg/packet | | Dextromethorphan HBr 30 mg/packet | | Acetaminophen 1000 mg/packet | | 1 packet dissolved in 6-oz cup of hot water q 6 hr (max 4 packets/day) | | b, e |
| *Threamine DM Syrup* (OTC) [U.S.] | Chlorpheniramine maleate 2 mg | Phenylpropanolamine HCl 12.5 mg | | Dextromethorphan HBr 10 mg | | | | 10 mL q 4–6 hr | | b, c, e |
| *T-Koff Oral Solution* (Schedule V) [U.S.] | Chlorpheniramine maleate 5 mg | Phenylephrine HCl 20 mg, Phenylpropanolamine HCl 20 mg | Codeine PO$_4$ 10 mg | | | | | 5 mL q 4–6 hr | 2–6 yrs: 1.25–2.5 mL; 6–12 yrs: 2.5–5 mL; q 4–6 hr | b, c, e, f |
| *Tolu-Sed Cough Syrup USP* (Schedule V) [U.S.] | | | Codeine PO$_4$ 10 mg | | Guaifenesin 100 mg | | Alcohol 10% Sugar free | 10 mL q 4 hr | 1–6 yrs: 1.25–2.5 mL; 6–12 yrs: 2.5–5 mL; q 4–6 hr | a, c, d, e, f |

*Specific formulations may vary among the different manufacturers, check product labeling.
†Efficacy as expectorant has not been established.
‡Geriatric patients may be more sensitive to effects of usual adult dose.
§For appropriate *Packaging and storage* and *Auxiliary labeling* information refer to designated letters as follows:
 a—Store below 40 °C (104 °F), preferably between 15 and 30 °C (59 and 86 °F), in a tight container, unless otherwise specified by manufacturer.
 a¹—Store below 30 °C (86 °F), unless otherwise specified by manufacturer. Avoid exposure to excessive heat.
 a²—Store below 25 °C (77 °F), unless otherwise specified by manufacturer.
 b—Store below 40 °C (104 °F), preferably between 15 and 30 °C (59 and 86 °F), in a well-closed container, unless otherwise specified by manufacturer.
 c—Protect from freezing.
 d—Protect from light.
 e—Auxiliary labeling: · May cause drowsiness. · Avoid alcoholic beverages.
 f—Auxiliary labeling: · May be habit forming.
 g—Auxiliary labeling: · Shake well.
 h—Dispense in dropper bottle.
 i—Chew well before swallowing.
**Included in subtherapeutic amount to discourage deliberate overdosage.

# Table 3. Oral Dosage Forms (continued)

Note: Content per capsule, tablet, or 5 mL, unless otherwise stated.

| Brand or generic name [availability] | Antihistamines | Decongestants | Antitussives Opioid | Antitussives Non-opioid | Expectorants | Analgesics | Other content information as per product label | Usual Adult and Adolescent Dose prn‡ | Usual Pediatric Dose prn | Packaging, Storage, and Auxiliary labelings§ |
|---|---|---|---|---|---|---|---|---|---|---|
| *Tolu-Sed DM* Syrup (OTC) [U.S.] | | | | Dextromethorphan HBr 10 mg | Guaifenesin 100 mg | | Alcohol 10% Sugar free | 10 mL q 4 hr | 1–6 yrs: 1.25–2.5 mL, 6–12 yrs: 2.5–5 mL, q 4 hr | b, c |
| *Touro DM* Extended-release Tablets (Rx) [U.S.] | | | | Dextromethorphan HBr 30 mg | Guaifenesin 575 mg | | | 1–2 tabs q 12 hrs (max 4 tabs/day) | 2–6 yrs: ½ tab q 12 hrs (max 1 tab/day) 6–12 yrs: 1 tab q 12 hrs (max 2 tabs/day) | b, d |
| *Touro LA Caplets* Extended-release Tablets (Rx) [U.S.] | | Pseudoephedrine HCl 120 mg | | | Guaifenesin 500 mg | | Scored | 1 tab q 12 hr | | b |
| *Triacin C Cough* Syrup (Schedule V) [U.S.] | Triprolidine HCl 1.25 mg | Pseudoephedrine HCl 30 mg | Codeine PO₄ 10 mg | | | | Alcohol 4.3% | 10 mL q 4–6 hr (max 40 mL/day) | 2–6 yrs: 2.5 mL, 6–12 yrs: 5 mL, q 4–6 hr | b, c, d, e, f |
| *Triafed w/Codeine* Syrup (Schedule V) [U.S.] | Triprolidine HCl 1.25 mg | Pseudoephedrine HCl 30 mg | Codeine PO₄ 10 mg | | | | | 10 mL q 4–6 hr (max 40 mL/day) | | b, c, e, f |
| *Triaminic AM Non-Drowsy Cough and Decongestant* Oral Solution (OTC) [U.S.] | | Pseudoephedrine HCl 15 mg | | Dextromethorphan HBr 7.5 mg | | | Alcohol free Dye free | 20 mL q 6 hr (max 80 mL/day) | 2–6 yrs: 5 mL (max 20 mL/day), 6–12 yrs: 10 mL (max 40 mL/day), q 6 hr | b |
| *Triaminic-DM Cough Relief* Syrup (OTC) [U.S.] | | Phenylpropanolamine HCl 6.25 mg | | Dextromethorphan HBr 5 mg | | | Alcohol free | 20 mL q 4 hr (max 6 doses/day) | 3 mos–1 yr: 1.25 mL, 1–2 yrs: 2.5 mL, 2–6 yrs: 5 mL, 6–12 yrs: 10 mL, q 4 hr | b, c |
| *Triaminic DM DayTime for Children* Syrup (OTC) [Canada] | | Phenylpropanolamine HCl 8.75 mg | | Dextromethorphan HBr 7.5 mg | Guaifenesin 37.5 mg | | Alcohol 5.5% | | 2–6 yrs: 5 mL, 6–12 yrs: 10 mL, q 6–8 hr | a, e |
| *Triaminic-DM Expectorant* Oral Solution (OTC) [Canada] | Chlorpheniramine maleate 2 mg | Pseudoephedrine HCl 30 mg | | Dextromethorphan HBr 15 mg | Guaifenesin 100 mg | | Alcohol 7.1% | 10 mL q 6 hr | 2–6 yrs: 2.5 mL, 6–12 yrs: 5 mL, q 4 hr | b, c, e |

USP DI  Cough/Cold Combinations (Systemic) 1101

Table 3. Oral Dosage Forms (continued)

Note: Content per capsule, tablet, or 5 mL, unless otherwise stated.

| Brand or generic name [availability] | Antihistamines | Decongestants | Antitussives — Opioid | Antitussives — Non-opioid | Expectorants | Analgesics | Other content information as per product label | Usual Adult and Adolescent Dose prn‡ | Usual Pediatric Dose prn | Packaging, Storage, and Auxiliary labeling§ |
|---|---|---|---|---|---|---|---|---|---|---|
| Triaminic DM NightTime for Children Syrup (OTC) [Canada] | Chlorpheniramine maleate 1 mg | Pseudoephedrine HCl 15.0 mg | | Dextromethorphan HBr 7.5 mg | | | Alcohol free | 20 mL q 6–8 hr | 2–6 yrs: 5 mL, 6–12 yrs: 10 mL, q 6–8 hr | a, d, e |
| Triaminic Expectorant Oral Solution (OTC) [U.S.] | | Phenylpropanolamine HCl 6.25 mg | | | Guaifenesin 50 mg | | Alcohol free | 20 mL q 4 hr (max 6 doses/day) | 3 mos–1 yr: 1.25 mL, 1–2 yrs: 2.5 mL, 2–6 yrs: 5 mL, 6–12 yrs: 10 mL, q 4 hr (max 6 doses/day) | b, c |
| Oral Solution (OTC) [Canada] | Chlorpheniramine maleate 2 mg | Pseudoephedrine HCl 30 mg | | | Guaifenesin 100 mg | | Alcohol 7.8% Sodium 13.68 mg | 10 mL q 6 hr | 2–6 yrs: 2.5 mL, 6–12 yrs: 5 mL, q 6 hr | b, c, e |
| Triaminic Expectorant w/Codeine Oral Solution (Schedule V) [U.S.] | | Phenylpropanolamine HCl 12.5 mg | Codeine PO₄ 10 mg | | Guaifenesin 100 mg | | Alcohol 5% | 10 mL q 4 hr (max 6 doses/day) | 3 mos–2 yrs: 2 drops/kg body weight, 2–6 yrs: 2.5 mL, 6–12 yrs: 5 mL, q 4 hr (max 6 doses/day) | b, c, e, f |

*Specific formulations may vary among the different manufacturers, check product labeling.
†Efficacy as expectorant has not been established.
‡Geriatric patients may be more sensitive to effects of usual adult dose.
§For appropriate *Packaging and storage* and *Auxiliary labeling* information refer to designated letters as follows:
  a — Store below 40 °C (104 °F), preferably between 15 and 30 °C (59 and 86 °F), in a tight container, unless otherwise specified by manufacturer.
    a¹ — Store below 30 °C (86 °F), unless otherwise specified by manufacturer. Avoid exposure to excessive heat.
    a² — Store below 25 °C (77 °F), unless otherwise specified by manufacturer.
  b — Store below 40 °C (104 °F), preferably between 15 and 30 °C (59 and 86 °F), in a well-closed container, unless otherwise specified by manufacturer.
  c — Protect from freezing.                                f — Auxiliary labeling: · May be habit forming.    h — Dispense in dropper bottle.
  d — Protect from light.                                    g — Auxiliary labeling: · Shake well.            i — Chew well before swallowing.
  e — Auxiliary labeling: · May cause drowsiness. · Avoid alcoholic beverages.
**Included in subtherapeutic amount to discourage deliberate overdosage.

**Table 3. Oral Dosage Forms** (*continued*)

Note: Content per capsule, tablet, or 5 mL, unless otherwise stated.

| Brand or generic name [availability] | Antihistamines | Decongestants | Antitussives - Opioid | Antitussives - Non-opioid | Expectorants | Analgesics | Other content information as per product label | Usual Adult and Adolescent Dose prn‡ | Usual Pediatric Dose prn | Packaging, Storage, and Auxiliary labeling§ |
|---|---|---|---|---|---|---|---|---|---|---|
| *Triaminic Expectorant DH* Elixir (N) [Canada] | Pheniramine maleate 6.25 mg, Pyrilamine maleate 6.25 mg | Phenylpropanolamine HCl 12.5 mg | Hydrocodone bitartrate 1.67 mg | | Guaifenesin 100 mg | | Alcohol 5% | 10 mL q 4 hr | 2–6 yrs: 2.5 mL, 6–12 yrs: 5 mL, q 4 hr | b, c, e, f |
| Oral Solution (Schedule III) [U.S.] | Pheniramine maleate 6.25 mg, Pyrilamine maleate 6.25 mg | Phenylpropanolamine HCl 12.5 mg | Hydrocodone bitartrate 1.67 mg | | Guaifenesin 100 mg | | Alcohol 5% | 10 mL q 4 hr | 1–6 yrs: 2.5 mL, 6–12 yrs: 5 mL, q 4 hr | b, c, e, f |
| *Triaminic Night Time* Oral Solution (OTC) [U.S.] | Chlorpheniramine maleate 1 mg | Pseudoephedrine HCl 15 mg | | Dextromethorphan HBr 7.5 mg | | | Alcohol free | 20 mL q 6 hr (max 4 doses/day) | 6–12 yrs: 10 mL q 6 hr (max 4 doses/day) | b, c, e |
| *Triaminicol DM* Syrup (OTC) [Canada] | Chlorpheniramine maleate 2 mg | Pseudoephedrine HCl 30 mg | | Dextromethorphan HBr 15 mg | | | Alcohol free | 10 mL q 6 hr | 2–6 yrs: 2.5 mL, 6–12 yrs: 5 mL, q 6 hr | b, c, e |
| *Triaminicol Multi-Symptom Cold and Cough Medicine* Tablets (OTC) [U.S.] | Chlorpheniramine maleate 2 mg | Phenylpropanolamine HCl 12.5 mg | | Dextromethorphan HBr 10 mg | | Acetaminophen 160 mg | | 2 tabs q 4 hr (max 12 tabs/day) | 6–12 yrs: 1 tab q 4 hr (max 6 tabs/day) | b |
| *Triaminic Sore Throat Formula* Oral Solution (OTC) [U.S.] | | Pseudoephedrine HCl 15 mg | | Dextromethorphan HBr 7.5 mg | | | Alcohol free | 20 mL q 6 hr (max 4 doses/day) | 2–6 yrs: 5 mL, 6–12 yrs: 10 mL, q 6 hr (max 4 doses/day) | b, c |
| *Triaminic Triaminicol* Oral Solution (OTC) [U.S.] | Chlorpheniramine maleate 1 mg | Phenylpropanolamine HCl 6.25 mg | | Dextromethorphan HBr 5 mg | | | Alcohol free | 20 mL q 4–6 hr (max 6 doses/day) | 6–12 yrs: 10 mL q 4–6 hr (max 6 doses/day) | b, c, e |
| *Tricodene* Oral Solution (Schedule V) [U.S.] | Pyrilamine maleate 12.5 mg | | Codeine PO₄ 8.2 mg | | | | Alcohol free | 10 mL q 6–8 hr (max 60 mL/day) | 6–12 yrs: 5 mL q 6–8 hr (max 30 mL/day) | b, c, e, f |

## Table 3. Oral Dosage Forms (continued)

Note: Content per capsule, tablet, or 5 mL, unless otherwise stated.

| Brand or generic name [availability] | Antihistamines | Decongestants | Antitussives Opioid | Antitussives Non-opioid | Expectorants | Analgesics | Other content information as per product label | Usual Adult and Adolescent Dose prn‡ | Usual Pediatric Dose prn | Packaging, Storage, and Auxiliary labeling§ |
|---|---|---|---|---|---|---|---|---|---|---|
| *Tussaminic DH Forte* Syrup (N) [Canada] | Pheniramine maleate 12.5 mg, Pyrilamine maleate 12.5 mg | Phenylpropanolamine HCl 25 mg | Hydrocodone bitartrate 5 mg | | | | Alcohol free | 5 mL q 4 hr | Intended for adult use | b, c, e, f |
| *Tussaminic DH Pediatric* Syrup (N) [Canada] | Pheniramine maleate 6.25 mg, Pyrilamine maleate 6.25 mg | Phenylpropanolamine HCl 12.5 mg | Hydrocodone bitartrate 1.67 mg | | | | Alcohol free | Intended for pediatric use. See *Tussaminic DH Forte* Oral Solution | 2–6 yrs: 2.5 mL, 6–12 yrs: 5 mL, q 4 hr | b, c, e, f |
| *Tussar-2* Syrup (Schedule V) [U.S.] | | Pseudoephedrine HCl 30 mg | Codeine PO₄ 10 mg | | Guaifenesin 100 mg | | Alcohol 2.5% | 10 mL q 4 hr (max 40 mL/ day) | 1.25–2.5 mL, 6–12 yrs: 2.5–5 mL, q 4–6 hr | b, c, e, f |
| *Tussar DM* Syrup (OTC) [U.S.] | Chlorpheniramine maleate 2 mg | Pseudoephedrine HCl 30 mg | | Dextromethorphan HBr 15 mg | | | Alcohol free | 10 mL q 6 hr | 6–12 yrs: 5 mL q 6 hrs | b, c, e |
| *Tussar SF* Syrup (Schedule V) [U.S.] | | Pseudoephedrine HCl 30 mg | Codeine PO₄ 10 mg | | Guaifenesin 100 mg | | Alcohol 2.5% Sugar free | 10 mL q 4 hr (max 40 mL/ day) | Not recommended | b, c, e, f |
| *Tuss-DA* Syrup (Rx) [U.S.] | | Pseudoephedrine HCl 30 mg | | Dextromethorphan HBr 20 mg | | | Alcohol free | 2.5–5 mL q 4 hr or 7.5 mL q 6–8 hr (max 30 mL/ day) | 2–6 yrs: 0.63–1.25 mL q 4 hr or 1.7 mL q 6–8 hr (max 7.5 mL/ day) 6–12 yrs: 1.25–2.5 mL q 4 hr or 3.75 mL q 6–8 hr (max 15 mL/ day) | b, c |

*Specific formulations may vary among the different manufacturers, check product labeling.
†Efficacy as expectorant has not been established.
‡Geriatric patients may be more sensitive to effects of usual adult dose.
§For appropriate *Packaging and storage* and *Auxiliary labeling* information refer to designated letters as follows:
 a—Store below 40 °C (104 °F), preferably between 15 and 30 °C (59 and 86 °F), in a tight container, unless otherwise specified by manufacturer.
 a¹—Store below 30 °C (86 °F), unless otherwise specified by manufacturer. Avoid exposure to excessive heat.
 a²—Store below 25 °C (77 °F), unless otherwise specified by manufacturer.
 b—Store below 40 °C (104 °F), preferably between 15 and 30 °C (59 and 86 °F), in a well-closed container, unless otherwise specified by manufacturer.
 c—Protect from freezing.                                f—Auxiliary labeling: • May be habit forming.        h—Dispense in dropper bottle.
 d—Protect from light.                                    g—Auxiliary labeling: • Shake well.                        i—Chew well before swallowing.
 e—Auxiliary labeling: • May cause drowsiness. • Avoid alcoholic beverages.
**Included in subtherapeutic amount to discourage deliberate overdosage.

**Table 3. Oral Dosage Forms** *(continued)*

Note: Content per capsule, tablet, or 5 mL, unless otherwise stated.

| Brand or generic name [availability] | Antihistamines | Decongestants | Antitussives Opioid | Antitussives Non-opioid | Expectorants | Analgesics | Other content information as per product label | Usual Adult and Adolescent Dose prn‡ | Usual Pediatric Dose prn | Packaging, Storage, and Auxiliary labeling§ |
|---|---|---|---|---|---|---|---|---|---|---|
| *Tuss-DM* Tablets (OTC) [U.S.] | | | | Dextromethorphan HBr 10 mg | Guaifenesin 200 mg | | | 1–2 tabs q 4 hr | 6–12 yrs: ½–1 tab q 4 hr | b |
| *Tussex Cough* Syrup (OTC) [U.S.] | | Phenylephrine HCl 5 mg | | Dextromethorphan HBr 10 mg | Guaifenesin 100 mg | | | 10 mL q 4 hr | | b |
| *Tussigon* Tablets (Schedule III) [U.S.] | | | Hydrocodone bitartrate 5 mg | | | | Homatropine MBr** 1.5 mg Scored | 1 tab q 4–6 hr | 6–12 yrs: ½ tab q 4–6 hr | b, d, e, f |
| *Tussilyn DM* Syrup (OTC) [Canada] | Chlorpheniramine maleate 2.5 mg | Pseudoephedrine HCl 30 mg | | Dextromethorphan HBr 15 mg | | | | 10 mL q 8 hr | 2–6 yrs: 2.5 mL, 6–12 yrs: 5 mL, q 8 hr | a |
| *Tussionex* Oral Suspension (N) [Canada] | Phenyltoloxamine as resin complex 10 mg | | Hydrocodone as resin complex 5 mg | | | | Sugar free | 5 mL q 8–12 hr (max 2 doses/day) | 1–5 yrs: 2.5 mL, >5 yrs: 5 mL, q 12 hr (max 2 doses/day) | b, c, e, f, g |
| Tablets (N) [Canada] | Phenyltoloxamine as resin complex 10 mg | | Hydrocodone as resin complex 5 mg | | | | Scored | 1 tab q 8–12 hr (max 2 tabs/day) | | b, e, f |
| *Tussionex Pennkinetic* Oral Suspension (Schedule III) [U.S.] | Chlorpheniramine maleate 8 mg (as polistirex) | | Hydrocodone bitartrate 10 mg (as polistirex) | | | | Alcohol free | 5 mL q 12 hr | >6 yrs: 2.5 mL q 12 hr | b, c, e, f, g |
| *Tussi-Organidin DM NR Liquid* Oral Solution (Rx) [U.S.] | | | | Dextromethorphan HBr 10 mg | Guaifenesin 100 mg | | Alcohol free Sugar free | 10 mL q 4 hr (max 6 doses/day) | 6 mos–2 yrs: 0.6–1.25 mL, 2–6 yrs: 2.5 mL, 6–12 yrs: 5 mL, q 4 hr (max 6 doses/day) | a, c, d |

Table 3. Oral Dosage Forms (continued)

Note: Content per capsule, tablet, or 5 mL, unless otherwise stated.

| Brand or generic name [availability] | Antihistamines | Decongestants | Antitussives Opioid | Antitussives Non-opioid | Expectorants | Analgesics | Other content information as per product label | Usual Adult and Adolescent Dose prn‡ | Usual Pediatric Dose prn | Packaging, Storage, and Auxiliary labeling§ |
|---|---|---|---|---|---|---|---|---|---|---|
| *Tricodene Forte* Oral Solution (OTC) [U.S.] | Chlorpheniramine maleate 2 mg | Phenylpropanolamine HCl 12.5 mg | | Dextromethorphan HBr 10 mg | | | Alcohol free | 10 mL q 4 hr (max 60 mL/day) | 6–12 yrs: 5 mL q 4 hr (max 30 mL/day) | b, c, e |
| *Tricodene NN* Oral Solution (OTC) [U.S.] | Chlorpheniramine maleate 2 mg | Phenylpropanolamine HCl 12.5 mg | | Dextromethorphan HBr 10 mg | | | Alcohol free | 10 mL q 4 hr (max 60 mL/day) | 6–12 yrs: 5 mL q 4 hr (max 30 mL/day) | b, c, e |
| *Tricodene Pediatric* Oral Solution (OTC) [U.S.] | | Phenylpropanolamine HCl 12.5 mg | | Dextromethorphan HBr 10 mg | | | Alcohol free | Intended for pediatric use | 2–6 yrs: 2.5 mL (max 15 mL/day), 6–12 yrs: 5 mL (max 30 mL/day), q 4 hr | b, c |
| *Tricodene Sugar Free* Oral Solution (OTC) [U.S.] | Chlorpheniramine maleate 2 mg | | | Dextromethorphan HBr 10 mg | | | Alcohol free | 10 mL q 4–6 hr (max 60 mL/day) | 6–12 yrs: 5 mL q 4–6 hr | b, c, e |
| *Trifed-C Cough* Syrup (Schedule V) [U.S.] | Triprolidine HCl 1.25 mg | Pseudoephedrine HCl 30 mg | Codeine PO₄ 10 mg | | | | Alcohol 4.4% | 10 mL q 4–6 hr (max 40 mL/day) | 2–6 yrs: 2.5 mL, 6–12 yrs: 5 mL, q 4–6 hr | b, c, d, e, f |
| *Triminol Cough* Syrup (OTC) [U.S.] | Chlorpheniramine maleate 2 mg | Phenylpropanolamine HCl 12.5 mg | | Dextromethorphan HBr 10 mg | | | | 10 mL q 4 hr | | b, c, e |

*Specific formulations may vary among the different manufacturers; check product labeling.
†Efficacy as expectorant has not been established.
‡Geriatric patients may be more sensitive to effects of usual adult dose.
§For appropriate *Packaging and storage* and *Auxiliary labeling* information refer to designated letters as follows:
 a—Store below 40 °C (104 °F), preferably between 15 and 30 °C (59 and 86 °F), in a tight container, unless otherwise specified by manufacturer.
 a¹—Store below 30 °C (86 °F), unless otherwise specified by manufacturer. Avoid exposure to excessive heat.
 a²—Store below 25 °C (77 °F), unless otherwise specified by manufacturer.
 b—Store below 40 °C (104 °F), preferably between 15 and 30 °C (59 and 86 °F), in a well-closed container, unless otherwise specified by manufacturer.
 c—Protect from freezing.
 d—Protect from light.
 e—Auxiliary labeling: · May cause drowsiness. · Avoid alcoholic beverages.
 f—Auxiliary labeling: · May be habit forming.
 g—Auxiliary labeling: · Shake well.
 h—Dispense in dropper bottle.
 i—Chew well before swallowing.
**Included in subtherapeutic amount to discourage deliberate overdosage.

**1104** Cough/Cold Combinations (Systemic) USP DI

**Table 3. Oral Dosage Forms** *(continued)*

Note: Content per capsule, tablet, or 5 mL, unless otherwise stated.

| Brand or generic name [availability] | Antihistamines | Decongestants | Antitussives — Opioid | Antitussives — Non-opioid | Expectorants | Analgesics | Other content information as per product label | Usual Adult and Adolescent Dose prn‡ | Usual Pediatric Dose prn | Packaging, Storage, and Auxiliary labelings§ |
|---|---|---|---|---|---|---|---|---|---|---|
| *Triphenyl Expectorant Oral Solution* (OTC) [U.S.] | | Phenylpropanolamine HCl 12.5 mg | | | Guaifenesin 100 mg | | Alcohol 5% | 10 mL q 4 hr | 2–6 yrs: 2.5 mL, 6–12 yrs: 5 mL, q 4 hr | b, c |
| *Tri-Tannate Plus Pediatric Oral Suspension* (Rx) [U.S.] | Chlorpheniramine tannate 4 mg | Ephedrine tannate 5 mg, Phenylephrine tannate 5 mg | | Carbetapentane tannate 30 mg | | | | | 2–<6 yrs: 2.5–10 mL q 12 hr | b, c, e |
| *Tusquelin Syrup* (Rx) [U.S.] | Chlorpheniramine maleate 2 mg | Phenylephrine HCl 5 mg, Phenylpropanolamine HCl 5 mg | | Dextromethorphan HBr 15 mg | | | Alcohol 5% | 5–10 mL q 6 hr | 2–6 yrs: 1.25–2.5 mL, 6–12 yrs: 2.5–5 mL, q 6 hr | b, c, e |
| *Tuss-Ade Extended-release Capsules* (Rx) [U.S.] | | Phenylpropanolamine HCl 75 mg | | Caramiphen edisylate 40 mg | | | | 1 cap q 12 hr | Pediatric strength not available | b |
| *Tussafed Syrup* (Rx) [U.S.] | Carbinoxamine maleate 4 mg | Pseudoephedrine HCl 60 mg | | Dextromethorphan HBr 15 mg | | | Alcohol free Sugar free | 5 mL q 4–6 hr | 18 mos–6 yrs: 2.5 mL, >6 yrs: 5 mL, q 4–6 hr | a, c, d, e |
| *Tussafed Drops Oral Solution* (Rx) [U.S.] | Carbinoxamine maleate 2 mg/mL | Pseudoephedrine HCl 25 mg/mL | | Dextromethorphan HBr 4 mg/mL | | | Alcohol free Sugar free | | 1–18 mos: 0.25–1 mL q 6 hr | b, c, e |
| *Tussafin Expectorant Oral Solution* (Schedule III) [U.S.] | | Pseudoephedrine HCl 60 mg | Hydrocodone bitartrate 5 mg | | Guaifenesin 200 mg | | Alcohol 12.5% | 5 mL q 4–6 hr (max 20 mL/day) | | b, c, e, f |
| *Tuss-Allergine Modified T.D. Extended-release Capsules* (Rx) [U.S.] | | Phenylpropanolamine HCl 75 mg | | Caramiphen edisylate 40 mg | | | | 1 cap q 12 hr | Pediatric strength not available | b |
| *Tussaminic C Forte Syrup* (N) [Canada] | Pheniramine maleate 12.5 mg, Pyrilamine maleate 12.5 mg | Phenylpropanolamine HCl 25 mg | Codeine PO₄ 15 mg | | | | Alcohol free | 5 mL q 4 hr | Intended for adult use | b, c, e, f |
| *Tussaminic C Pediatric Syrup* (N) [Canada] | Pheniramine maleate 6.25 mg, Pyrilamine maleate 6.25 mg | Phenylpropanolamine HCl 12.5 mg | Codeine PO₄ 5 mg | | | | Alcohol free | Intended for pediatric use | 2–6 yrs: 2.5 mL, 6–12 yrs: 5 mL, q 4 hr | b, c, e, f |

Table 3. Oral Dosage Forms (*continued*)

Note: Content per capsule, tablet, or 5 mL, unless otherwise stated.

| Brand or generic name [availability] | Antihistamines | Decongestants | Antitussives - Opioid | Antitussives - Non-opioid | Expectorants | Analgesics | Other content information as per product label | Usual Adult and Adolescent Dose prn‡ | Usual Pediatric Dose prn | Packaging, Storage, and Auxiliary labeling§ |
|---|---|---|---|---|---|---|---|---|---|---|
| *Tussi-Organidin DM-S NR Liquid* Oral Solution (Rx) [U.S.] | | | | Dextromethorphan HBr 10 mg | Guaifenesin 100 mg | | Alcohol free Sugar free | 10 mL q 4 hr (max 6 doses/day) | 6 mos–2 yrs: 0.6–1.25 mL, 2–6 yrs: 2.5 mL, 6–12 yrs: 5 mL, q 4 hr (max 6 doses/day) | a, c, d |
| *Tussi-Organidin NR Liquid* Oral Solution (Schedule V) [U.S.] | | | Codeine PO$_4$ 10 mg | | Guaifenesin 100 mg | | Alcohol free Sugar free | 10 mL q 4 hr (max 6 doses/day) | 2–6 yrs: 1 mg/kg/day of codeine given in 4 divided doses 6–12 yrs: 5 mL q 4 hr (max 6 doses/day) | a, c, d, e, f |
| *Tussi-Organidin-S NR Liquid* Oral Solution (Schedule V) [U.S.] | | | Codeine PO$_4$ 10 mg | | Guaifenesin 100 mg | | Alcohol free Sugar free | 10 mL q 4 hr (max 6 doses/day) | 2–6 yrs: 1 mg/kg/day of codeine given in 4 divided doses 6–12 yrs: 5 mL q 4 hr (max 6 doses/day) | a, c, d, e, f |
| *Tussirex* Oral Solution (Schedule V) [U.S.] | Pheniramine maleate 13.3 mg | Phenylephrine HCl 4.2 mg | Codeine PO$_4$ 10 mg | | Sodium citrate† 83.3 mg | Sodium salicylate 83.3 mg | Caffeine citrate 25 mg Alcohol free With or without sugar | 5 mL q 8 hr | | b, c, e, f |

*Specific formulations may vary among the different manufacturers, check product labeling.
†Efficacy as expectorant has not been established.
‡Geriatric patients may be more sensitive to effects of usual adult dose.
§For appropriate *Packaging and storage* and *Auxiliary labeling* information refer to designated letters as follows:
 a—Store below 40 °C (104 °F), preferably between 15 and 30 °C (59 and 86 °F), in a tight container, unless otherwise specified by manufacturer.
 a¹—Store below 30 °C (86 °F), unless otherwise specified by manufacturer. Avoid exposure to excessive heat.
 a²—Store below 25 °C (77 °F), unless otherwise specified by manufacturer.
 b—Store below 40 °C (104 °F), preferably between 15 and 30 °C (59 and 86 °F), in a well-closed container, unless otherwise specified by manufacturer.
 c—Protect from freezing.　　　　　　　　　　　f—Auxiliary labeling: · May be habit forming.　　h—Dispense in dropper bottle.
 d—Protect from light.　　　　　　　　　　　　g—Auxiliary labeling: · Shake well.　　　　　　i—Chew well before swallowing.
 e—Auxiliary labeling: · May cause drowsiness. · Avoid alcoholic beverages.
**Included in subtherapeutic amount to discourage deliberate overdosage.

Table 3. Oral Dosage Forms (continued)

Note: Content per capsule, tablet, or 5 mL, unless otherwise stated.

| Brand or generic name [availability] | Antihistamines | Decongestants | Antitussives Opioid | Antitussives Non-opioid | Expectorants | Analgesics | Other content information as per product label | Usual Adult and Adolescent Dose prn‡ | Usual Pediatric Dose prn | Packaging, Storage, and Auxiliary labeling§ |
|---|---|---|---|---|---|---|---|---|---|---|
| *Tuss-LA* Extended-release Tablets (Rx) [U.S.] | | Pseudoephedrine HCl 120 mg | | | Guaifenesin 500 mg | | Scored | 1 tab q 12 hr | 2–6 yrs: Not recommended; 6–12 yrs: ½ tab q 12 hr | b |
| *Tusso-DM* Oral Solution (Rx) [U.S.] | | | | Dextromethorphan HBr 10 mg | Iodinated glycerol† 30 mg | | Alcohol free Sugar free | 5–10 mL q 4 hr | 2–6 yrs: 1.25–2.5 mL, 6–12 yrs: 5 mL, q 4 hr | a, c |
| *Tussogest* Extended-release Capsules (Rx) [U.S.] | | Phenylpropanolamine HCl 75 mg | | Caramiphen edisylate 40 mg | | | | 1 cap q 12 hr | Pediatric strength not available | b |
| *Tuss-Ornade Spansules* Extended-release Capsules (Rx) [Canada] | | Phenylpropanolamine HCl 50 mg | | Caramiphen edisylate 20 mg | | | | 1 cap q 12 hr | Pediatric strength not available | b |
| *Tylenol Children's Cold DM Medication* Oral Solution (OTC) [Canada] | Chlorpheniramine maleate 1 mg | Pseudoephedrine HCl 15 mg | | Dextromethorphan HBr 7.5 mg | | Acetaminophen 160 mg | Alcohol free | Intended for pediatric use | 2–5 yrs: 5 mL, 6–12 yrs: 10 mL, q 4–6 hr (max 4 doses/day) | a |
| Chewable Tablets (OTC) [Canada] | Chlorpheniramine maleate 0.5 mg | Pseudoephedrine HCl 7.5 mg | | Dextromethorphan HBr 3.75 mg | | Acetaminophen 80 mg | Phenylalanine | Intended for pediatric use | 2–5 yrs: 2 tabs, 6–12 yrs: 4 tabs, q 4–6 hr (max 4 doses/day) | b, i |
| *Tylenol Cold and Flu* for Oral Solution (OTC) [Canada] | Chlorpheniramine maleate 4 mg/pouch | Pseudoephedrine HCl 60 mg/pouch | | Dextromethorphan HBr 30 mg/pouch | | Acetaminophen 650 mg/pouch | Phenylalanine, Sugar 19 grams/pouch | 1 pouch dissolved in 225 mL of hot water q 4–6 hr (max 3 pouches/day) | Intended for adult use | b, e |
| *Tylenol Cold and Flu No Drowsiness Powder* for Oral Solution (OTC) [U.S.] | | Pseudoephedrine HCl 60 mg/packet | | Dextromethorphan HBr 30 mg/packet | | Acetaminophen 650 mg/packet | Phenylalanine 11 mg/packet | 1 packet dissolved in 180 mL of hot water q 6 hr | | b, c |

USP DI — Cough/Cold Combinations (Systemic) 1109

Table 3. Oral Dosage Forms (continued)

Note: Content per capsule, tablet, or 5 mL, unless otherwise stated.

| Brand or generic name [availability] | Antihistamines | Decongestants | Antitussives Opioid | Antitussives Non-opioid | Expectorants | Analgesics | Other content information as per product label | Usual Adult and Adolescent Dose prn‡ | Usual Pediatric Dose prn | Packaging, Storage, and Auxiliary labeling§ |
|---|---|---|---|---|---|---|---|---|---|---|
| *Tylenol Cold Medication Oral Solution* (OTC) [U.S.] | Chlorpheniramine maleate 0.66 mg (2 mg/15 mL) | Pseudoephedrine HCl 10 mg (30 mg/15 mL) | | Dextromethorphan HBr 5 mg (15 mg/15 mL) | | Acetaminophen 108.3 mg (325 mg/15 mL) | Alcohol 7% | 15–30 mL q 6 hr | Intended for adult use | b, c, e |
| Tablets (OTC) [U.S.] | Chlorpheniramine maleate 2 mg | Pseudoephedrine HCl 30 mg | | Dextromethorphan HBr 15 mg | | Acetaminophen 325 mg | | 2 tabs q 6 hr (max 8 tabs/day) | 6–11 yrs: 1 tab q 6 hr (max 4 tabs/day) | b, e |
| *Tylenol Cold Medication Caplets* Tablets (OTC) [U.S.] | Chlorpheniramine maleate 2 mg | Pseudoephedrine HCl 30 mg | | Dextromethorphan HBr 15 mg | | Acetaminophen 325 mg | | 2 tabs q 6 hr (max 8 tabs/day) | 6–11 yrs: 1 tab q 6 hr (max 4 tabs/day) | b, e |
| *Tylenol Cold Medication Extra Strength Daytime Caplets* Tablets (OTC) [Canada] | | Pseudoephedrine HCl 30 mg | | Dextromethorphan HBr 15 mg | | Acetaminophen 500 mg | | 1–2 tabs q 6 hr (max 8 tabs/day) | Intended for adult use | b |
| *Tylenol Cold Medication Extra Strength Nighttime Caplets* Tablets (OTC) [Canada] | Chlorpheniramine maleate 2 mg | Pseudoephedrine HCl 30 mg | | Dextromethorphan HBr 15 mg | | Acetaminophen 500 mg | | 1–2 tabs q 6 hr (max 8 tabs/day) | Intended for adult use | b, e |
| *Tylenol Cold Medication, Non-Drowsy Caplets* Tablets (OTC) [U.S.] | | Pseudoephedrine HCl 30 mg | | Dextromethorphan HBr 15 mg | | Acetaminophen 325 mg | | 2 tabs q 6 hr (max 8 tabs/day) | 6–11 yrs: 1 tab q 6 hr (max 4 tabs/day) | b, e |
| *Tylenol Cold Medication, Non-Drowsy Gelcaps* Tablets (OTC) [U.S.] | | Pseudoephedrine HCl 30 mg | | Dextromethorphan HBr 15 mg | | Acetaminophen 325 mg | | 2 tabs q 6 hr (max 8 tabs/day) | 6–11 yrs: 1 tab q 6 hr (max 4 tabs/day) | b, e |
| *Tylenol Cold Medication Regular Strength Daytime Caplets* Tablets (OTC) [Canada] | | Pseudoephedrine HCl 30 mg | | Dextromethorphan HBr 15 mg | | Acetaminophen 325 mg | | 1–2 tabs q 6 hr (max 8 tabs/day) | Intended for adult use | b |

*Specific formulations may vary among the different manufacturers, check product labeling.
†Efficacy as expectorant has not been established.
‡Geriatric patients may be more sensitive to effects of usual adult dose.
§For appropriate *Packaging and storage* and *Auxiliary labeling* information refer to designated letters as follows:
  a—Store below 40 °C (104 °F), preferably between 15 and 30 °C (59 and 86 °F), in a tight container, unless otherwise specified by manufacturer.
  a[1]—Store below 30 °C (86 °F), unless otherwise specified by manufacturer. Avoid exposure to excessive heat.
  a[2]—Store below 25 °C (77 °F), unless otherwise specified by manufacturer.
  b—Store below 40 °C (104 °F), preferably between 15 and 30 °C (59 and 86 °F), in a well-closed container, unless otherwise specified by manufacturer.
  c—Protect from freezing.
  d—Protect from light.
  e—Auxiliary labeling: · May cause drowsiness. · Avoid alcoholic beverages.
  f—Auxiliary labeling: · May be habit forming.
  g—Auxiliary labeling: · Shake well.
  h—Dispense in dropper bottle.
  i—Chew well before swallowing.
***Included in subtherapeutic amount to discourage deliberate overdosage.

1110  Cough/Cold Combinations (Systemic)  USP DI

Table 3. Oral Dosage Forms (continued)

Note: Content per capsule, tablet, or 5 mL, unless otherwise stated.

| Brand or generic name [availability] | Antihistamines | Decongestants | Antitussives Opioid | Antitussives Non-opioid | Expectorants | Analgesics | Other content information as per product label | Usual Adult and Adolescent Dose prn‡ | Usual Pediatric Dose prn | Packaging, Storage, and Auxiliary labeling§ |
|---|---|---|---|---|---|---|---|---|---|---|
| Tylenol Cold Medication Regular Strength Nighttime Caplets (OTC) [Canada] | Chlorpheniramine maleate 2 mg | Pseudoephedrine HCl 30 mg | | Dextromethorphan HBr 15 mg | | Acetaminophen 325 mg | | 1–2 tabs q 6 hr (max 8 tabs/day) | Intended for adult use | b, e |
| Tylenol Cold Multi-Symptom for Oral Solution (OTC) [U.S.] | Chlorpheniramine maleate 4 mg/packet | Pseudoephedrine HCl 60 mg/packet | | Dextromethorphan HBr 30 mg/packet | | Acetaminophen 650 mg/packet | Phenylalanine 11 mg/packet | 1 packet dissolved in 180 mL of hot water q 6 hr | Intended for adult use | b, e |
| Tylenol Cough Extra Strength Caplets Tablets (OTC) [Canada] | | | | Dextromethorphan HBr 15 mg | | Acetaminophen 500 mg | | 2 tabs q 6–8 hr (max 8 tabs/day) | | b |
| Tylenol Cough Medication with Decongestant, Regular Strength Oral Suspension (OTC) [Canada] | | Pseudoephedrine HCl 60 mg/15 mL | | Dextromethorphan HBr 30 mg/15 mL | | Acetaminophen 650 mg/15 mL | | 15 mL q 6–8 hr (max 60 mL/day) | | a, c |
| Tylenol Cough Medication Regular Strength Oral Suspension (OTC) [Canada] | | | | Dextromethorphan HBr 30 mg/15 mL | | Acetaminophen 650 mg/15 mL | | 15 mL q 6–8 hr (max 60 mL/day) | Intended for adult use | a, c |
| Tylenol Extra Strength Cold and Flu Medication Powder for Oral Solution (OTC) [Canada] | Chlorpheniramine maleate 4 mg/pouch | Pseudoephedrine HCl 60 mg/pouch | | Dextromethorphan HBr 30 mg/pouch | | Acetaminophen 1000 mg/pouch | Sugar 17.5 grams/pouch (honey/lemon flavor) Sodium 1.2 grams/pouch (chicken soup flavor) | 1 pouch dissolved in 225 mL of hot water q 4–6 hr (max 3 pouches/day) | | b, e |
| Tylenol Junior Strength Cold DM Medication Chewable Tablets (OTC) [Canada] | Chlorpheniramine maleate 1 mg | Pseudoephedrine HCl 15 mg | | Dextromethorphan HBr 7.5 mg | | Acetaminophen 160 mg | Phenylalanine Scored | | 2–5 yrs: 1 tab, 6–11 yrs: 2 tabs, q 4–6 hr (max 4 doses/day) | b, i |
| Tylenol Maximum Strength Flu Gelcaps Tablets (OTC) [U.S.] | | Pseudoephedrine HCl 30 mg | | Dextromethorphan HBr 15 mg | | Acetaminophen 500 mg | | 2 tabs q 6 hr (max 8 tabs/day) | Not recommended | b |

USP DI    Cough/Cold Combinations (Systemic)    1111

Table 3. Oral Dosage Forms (continued)

Note: Content per capsule, tablet, or 5 mL, unless otherwise stated.

| Brand or generic name [availability] | Antihistamines | Decongestants | Antitussives Opioid | Antitussives Non-opioid | Expectorants | Analgesics | Other content information as per product label | Usual Adult and Adolescent Dose prn‡ | Usual Pediatric Dose prn | Packaging, Storage, and Auxiliary labeling§ |
|---|---|---|---|---|---|---|---|---|---|---|
| *Tylenol Multi-Symptom Cough* Oral Solution (OTC) [U.S.] | | | | Dextromethorphan HBr 10 mg | | Acetaminophen 217 mg | Alcohol 5% | 15 mL q 6–8 hr (max 4 doses/day) | 6–11 yrs: 7.5 mL q 6–8 hr (max 4 doses/day) | b, c |
| *Tylenol Multi-Symptom Cough with Decongestant* Oral Solution (OTC) [U.S.] | | Pseudoephedrine HCl 20 mg | | Dextromethorphan HBr 10 mg | | Acetaminophen 217 mg | Alcohol 5% | 15 mL q 6–8 hr (max 4 doses/day) | 6–11 yrs: 7.5 mL q 6–8 hr (max 4 doses/day) | b, c |
| *Tyrodone* Oral Solution (Schedule III) [U.S.] | | Pseudoephedrine HCl 60 mg | Hydrocodone bitartrate 5 mg | | | | Alcohol 5% | 5 mL q 4–6 hr | | a, c, e, f |
| *ULR-LA* Extended-release Tablets (Rx) [U.S.] | | Phenylpropanolamine HCl 75 mg | | | Guaifenesin 400 mg | | | 1 tab q 12 hr | | b |
| *Unituss HC* Syrup (Schedule III) [U.S.] | Chlorpheniramine maleate 2 mg | Phenylephrine HCl 5 mg | Hydrocodone bitartrate 2.5 mg | | | | Alcohol free Dye free Sugar free | 10 mL q 4 hr (max 40 mL/day) | 6–12 yrs: 5 mL q 4 hr (max 20 mL/day) | a, c, d, e, f |
| *Uni-tussin DM* Syrup (OTC) [U.S.] | | | | Dextromethorphan HBr 10 mg | Guaifenesin 100 mg | | Alcohol free | 10 mL q 4 hr | | b, c |
| *Unproco* Capsules (Rx) [U.S.] | | | | Dextromethorphan HBr 30 mg | Guaifenesin 200 mg | | | 1 cap q 4 hr | Pediatric strength not available | a, d |
| *Vanex Expectorant* Oral Solution (Schedule III) [U.S.] | | Pseudoephedrine HCl 30 mg | Hydrocodone bitartrate 2.5 mg | | Guaifenesin 100 mg | | Alcohol 5% Dye free | 10 mL q 4–6 hr | 6–12 yrs: 5 mL q 4–6 hr | b, c, d, e, f |

*Specific formulations may vary among the different manufacturers, check product labeling.
†Efficacy as expectorant has not been established.
‡Geriatric patients may be more sensitive to effects of usual adult dose.
§For appropriate *Packaging and storage* and *Auxiliary labeling* information refer to designated letters as follows:
 a—Store below 40 °C (104 °F), preferably between 15 and 30 °C (59 and 86 °F), in a tight container, unless otherwise specified by manufacturer.
 a¹—Store below 30 °C (86 °F), unless otherwise specified by manufacturer. Avoid exposure to excessive heat.
 a²—Store below 25 °C (77 °F), unless otherwise specified by manufacturer.
 b—Store below 40 °C (104 °F), preferably between 15 and 30 °C (59 and 86 °F), in a well-closed container, unless otherwise specified by manufacturer.
 c—Protect from freezing.   f—Auxiliary labeling: · May be habit forming.   h—Dispense in dropper bottle.
 d—Protect from light.   g—Auxiliary labeling: · Shake well.   i—Chew well before swallowing.
 e—Auxiliary labeling: · May cause drowsiness. · Avoid alcoholic beverages.
**Included in subtherapeutic amount to discourage deliberate overdosage.

## Table 3. Oral Dosage Forms (continued)

Note: Content per capsule, tablet, or 5 mL, unless otherwise stated.

| Brand or generic name [availability] | Antihistamines | Decongestants | Antitussives – Opioid | Antitussives – Non-opioid | Expectorants | Analgesics | Other content information as per product label | Usual Adult and Adolescent Dose prn‡ | Usual Pediatric Dose prn | Packaging, Storage, and Auxiliary labeling§ |
|---|---|---|---|---|---|---|---|---|---|---|
| *Vanex Grape* Oral Solution (Schedule V) [U.S.] | Chlorpheniramine maleate 5 mg | Phenylephrine HCl 20 mg, Phenylpropanolamine HCl 20 mg | Dihydrocodeine bitartrate 3 mg | | | | Alcohol free Sugar free | 5 mL q 4–5 hr | 6–12 yrs: 2.5 mL q 4–5 hr | a, e, f |
| *Vanex-HD* Oral Solution (Schedule III) [U.S.] | Chlorpheniramine maleate 2 mg | Phenylephrine HCl 5 mg | Hydrocodone bitartrate 1.7 mg | | | | Alcohol free Dye free | 10 mL q 6–8 hr | 6–12 yrs: 5 mL q 6–8 hr | b, c, e, f |
| *V-Dec-M* Extended-release Tablets (Rx) [U.S.] | | Pseudoephedrine HCl 120 mg | | | Guaifenesin 500 mg | | Scored | 1 tab q 12 hr | | b |
| *Versacaps* Extended-release Capsules (Rx) [U.S.] | | Pseudoephedrine HCl 60 mg | | | Guaifenesin 300 mg | | | 1–2 caps q 12 hr | | b |
| *Vicks Children's NyQuil* Oral Solution (OTC) [Canada] | Chlorpheniramine maleate 2 mg/15 mL | Pseudoephedrine HCl 30 mg/15 mL | | Dextromethorphan HBr 15 mg/15 mL | | | Alcohol free | Intended for pediatric use | 1–5 yrs: 7.5 mL; 6–11 yrs: 15 mL hs | b, c, e |
| *Vicks Children's NyQuil Cold/ Cough Relief* Oral Solution (OTC) [U.S.] | Chlorpheniramine maleate 2 mg/15 mL | Pseudoephedrine HCl 30 mg/15 mL | | Dextromethorphan HBr 15 mg/15 mL | | | Alcohol free | 30 mL q 6 hr (max 4 doses/day) | 6–11 yrs: 15 mL q 6 hr (max 4 doses/day) | b, c, e |
| *Vicks 44 Cough and Cold Relief Non-Drowsy LiquiCaps* Capsules (OTC) [U.S.] | | Pseudoephedrine HCl 60 mg | | Dextromethorphan HBr 30 mg | | | Alcohol free | 1 cap q 6 hr (max 4 caps/day) | Not recommended | b |
| *Vicks 44D Cough and Head Congestion* Oral Solution (OTC) [U.S.] | | Pseudoephedrine HCl 20 mg (60 mg/15 mL) | | Dextromethorphan HBr 10 mg (30 mg/15 mL) | | | Alcohol 10% | 15 mL q 6 hr | | b, c |
| *Vicks Cough Syrup* Syrup (OTC) [Canada] | | Ephedrine 2.7 mg | | Carbetapentane citrate 5 mg | Guaifenesin 66.7 mg | | Alcohol Sugar | 15 mL q 4 hr (max 4 doses/day) | 2–4 yrs: 2.5 mL, 5–9 yrs: 3.75 mL, 10–14 yrs: 7.5 mL, q 4 hr (max 4 doses/day) | b, c |

USP DI — Cough/Cold Combinations (Systemic) 1113

Table 3. Oral Dosage Forms (continued)

Note: Content per capsule, tablet, or 5 mL, unless otherwise stated.

| Brand or generic name [availability] | Antihistamines | Decongestants | Antitussives Opioid | Antitussives Non-opioid | Expectorants | Analgesics | Other content information as per product label | Usual Adult and Adolescent Dose prn‡ | Usual Pediatric Dose prn | Packaging, Storage, and Auxiliary labelings§ |
|---|---|---|---|---|---|---|---|---|---|---|
| Vicks DayQuil Liquicaps Capsules (OTC) [Canada] | | Pseudoephedrine HCl 30 mg | | Dextromethorphan HBr 10 mg | Guaifenesin 100 mg | Acetaminophen 250 mg | Alcohol free | 2 caps q 4–6 hr (max 8 caps/day) | | a |
| Vicks DayQuil Multi-Symptom Cold/Flu LiquiCaps Capsules (OTC) [U.S.] | | Pseudoephedrine HCl 30 mg | | Dextromethorphan HBr 10 mg | Guaifenesin 100 mg | Acetaminophen 250 mg | | 2 caps q 4 hr (max 8 caps/day) | 6–11 yrs: 1 cap q 4 hr (max 4 caps/day) | b, c |
| Vicks DayQuil Multi-Symptom Cold/Flu Relief Oral Solution (OTC) [U.S.] | | Pseudoephedrine HCl 30 mg/15 mL | | Dextromethorphan HBr 10 mg/15 mL | Guaifenesin 100 mg/15 mL | Acetaminophen 325 mg/15 mL | Alcohol free | 30 mL q 4 hr (max 4 doses/day) | 6–11 yrs: 15 mL q 4 hr (max 4 doses/day) | b, c |
| Vicks DayQuil Sinus Pressure and Congestion Relief Caplets Tablets (OTC) [U.S.] | | Phenylpropanolamine HCl 25 mg | | | Guaifenesin 200 mg | | | 1 tab q 4 hr (max 6 tabs/day) | | b |
| Vicks 44E Cough & Chest Congestion Oral Solution (OTC) [U.S.] | | | | Dextromethorphan HBr 6.67 mg (20 mg/15 mL) | Guaifenesin 66.7 mg (200 mg/15 mL) | | Alcohol 10% | 15 mL q 4 hr (max 90 mL/day) | | b |
| Vicks Formula 44-D Syrup (OTC) [Canada] | | Pseudoephedrine HCl 60 mg/15 mL | | Dextromethorphan HBr 30 mg/15 mL | | | Alcohol | 15 mL q 6–8 hr (max 60 mL/day) | | b, d, g |
| Vicks Formula 44-d Pediatric Syrup (OTC) [Canada] | | Pseudoephedrine HCl 10 mg (30 mg/15 mL) | | Dextromethorphan HBr 5 mg (15 mg/15 mL) | | | Alcohol free | | 1–5 yrs: 7.5 mL, 6–11 yrs: 15 mL, q 6–8 hr (max 4 doses/day) | b, d, g |
| Vicks Formula 44E Syrup (OTC) [Canada] | | | | Dextromethorphan HBr 20 mg/15 mL | Guaifenesin 200 mg/15 mL | | Alcohol | 15 mL q 4 hr (max 90 mL/day) | | b, d, g |

*Specific formulations may vary among the different manufacturers; check product labeling.
†Efficacy as expectorant has not been established.
‡Geriatric patients may be more sensitive to effects of usual adult dose.
§For appropriate Packaging and storage and Auxiliary labeling information refer to designated letters as follows:
  a—Store below 40 °C (104 °F), preferably between 15 and 30 °C (59 and 86 °F), in a tight container, unless otherwise specified by manufacturer.
  a¹—Store below 30 °C (86 °F), unless otherwise specified by manufacturer. Avoid exposure to excessive heat.
  a²—Store below 25 °C (77 °F), unless otherwise specified by manufacturer.
  b—Store below 40 °C (104 °F), preferably between 15 and 30 °C (59 and 86 °F), in a well-closed container, unless otherwise specified by manufacturer.
  c—Protect from freezing.
  d—Protect from light.
  e—Auxiliary labeling: · May cause drowsiness. · Avoid alcoholic beverages.
  f—Auxiliary labeling: · May be habit forming.
  g—Auxiliary labeling: · Shake well.
  h—Dispense in dropper bottle.
  i—Chew well before swallowing.
**Included in subtherapeutic amount to discourage deliberate overdosage.

1114  Cough/Cold Combinations (Systemic)  USP DI

Table 3. Oral Dosage Forms (*continued*)

Note: Content per capsule, tablet, or 5 mL, unless otherwise stated.

| Brand or generic name [availability] | Antihistamines | Decongestants | Antitussives Opioid | Antitussives Non-opioid | Expectorants | Analgesics | Other content information as per product label | Usual Adult and Adolescent Dose prn‡ | Usual Pediatric Dose prn | Packaging, Storage, and Auxiliary labeling§ |
|---|---|---|---|---|---|---|---|---|---|---|
| *Vicks Formula 44e Pediatric Syrup* (OTC) [Canada] | | | | Dextromethorphan HBr 3.3 mg (10 mg/15 mL) | Guaifenesin 33.3 mg (100 mg/15 mL) | | Alcohol free | | 1–5 yrs: 7.5 mL; 6–11 yrs: 15 mL, q 4 hr (max 6 doses/day) | b, d, g |
| *Vicks Formula 44 Syrup* (OTC) [Canada] | Chlorpheniramine maleate 1 mg (4 mg/20 mL) | Pseudoephedrine HCl 15 mg (60 mg/20 mL) | | Dextromethorphan HBr 7.5 mg (30 mg/20 mL) | | Acetaminophen 162.5 mg (650 mg/20 mL) | Alcohol | 20 mL q 6–8 hr (max 80 mL/day) | | b, d, e, g |
| *Vicks 44M Cough, Cold and Flu Relief Oral Solution* (OTC) [U.S.] | Chlorpheniramine maleate 1 mg (4 mg/20 mL) | Pseudoephedrine HCl 15 mg (60 mg/20 mL) | | Dextromethorphan HBr 7.5 mg (30 mg/20 mL) | | Acetaminophen 162.5 mg (650 mg/20 mL) | Alcohol 10% | 20 mL q 6 hr (max 80 mL/day) | | b, c |
| *Vicks 44M Cough, Cold and Flu Relief LiquiCaps Capsules* (OTC) [U.S.] | Chlorpheniramine maleate 2 mg | Pseudoephedrine HCl 30 mg | | Dextromethorphan HBr 10 mg | | Acetaminophen 250 mg | Alcohol free Sugar free | 2 caps q 4 hr (max 8 caps/day) | 6–12 yrs: 1 cap q 4 hr (max 4 caps/day) | b, e |
| *Vicks NyQuil Oral Solution* (OTC) [Canada] | Doxylamine succinate 12.5 mg/30 mL | Pseudoephedrine HCl 60 mg/30 mL | | Dextromethorphan HBr 30 mg/30 mL | | Acetaminophen 1000 mg/30 mL | Alcohol | 30 mL hs or q 6–8 hr (max 90 mL/day) | | b, c, e |
| *Vicks NyQuil Hot Therapy for Oral Solution* (OTC) [U.S.] | Doxylamine succinate 12.5 mg/packet | Pseudoephedrine HCl 60 mg/packet | | Dextromethorphan HBr 30 mg/packet | | Acetaminophen 1000 mg/packet | | 1 packet dissolved in 6-oz cup of hot water hs or q 6 hr | Intended for adult use | b, e |
| *Vicks NyQuil LiquiCaps Capsules* (OTC) [Canada] | Doxylamine succinate 6.25 mg | Pseudoephedrine HCl 30 mg | | Dextromethorphan HBr 10 mg | | Acetaminophen 250 mg | Sugar free | 2 caps hs or q 4–6 hr (max 8 caps/day) | | b, e |
| *Vicks NyQuil Multi-Symptom Cold/Flu LiquiCaps Capsules* (OTC) [U.S.] | Doxylamine succinate 6.25 mg | Pseudoephedrine HCl 30 mg | | Dextromethorphan HBr 10 mg | | Acetaminophen 250 mg | | 2 caps q 4 hr (max 8 caps/day) | Intended for adult use | b, e |
| *Vicks NyQuil Multi-Symptom Cold/Flu Relief Oral Solution* (OTC) [U.S.] | Doxylamine succinate 2 mg (12.5 mg/30 mL) | Pseudoephedrine HCl 10 mg (60 mg/30 mL) | | Dextromethorphan HBr 5 mg (30 mg/30 mL) | | Acetaminophen 166.6 mg (1000 mg/30 mL) | Alcohol 10% | 30 mL hs or q 6 hr (max 4 doses/day) | Not recommended | b, c, e |

USP DI — Cough/Cold Combinations (Systemic) 1115

Table 3. Oral Dosage Forms (continued)

Note: Content per capsule, tablet, or 5 mL, unless otherwise stated.

| Brand or generic name [availability] | Antihistamines | Decongestants | Antitussives Opioid | Antitussives Non-opioid | Expectorants | Analgesics | Other content information as per product label | Usual Adult and Adolescent Dose prn‡ | Usual Pediatric Dose prn | Packaging, Storage, and Auxiliary labelings§ |
|---|---|---|---|---|---|---|---|---|---|---|
| Vicks Pediatric 44D Cough & Head Decongestion Oral Solution (OTC) [U.S.] | | Pseudoephedrine HCl 10 mg | | Dextromethorphan HBr 5 mg | | | Alcohol free | 30 mL q 6 hr (max 4 doses/day) | 2–5 yrs: 7.5 mL, 6–11 yrs: 15 mL, q 6 hr (max 4 doses/day) | b, c |
| Vicks Pediatric 44E Oral Solution (OTC) [U.S.] | | | | Dextromethorphan HBr 3.3 mg | Guaifenesin 33.3 mg | | Alcohol free | 30 mL q 4 hr (max 6 doses/day) | 2–5 yrs: 7.5 mL, 6–11 yrs: 15 mL, q 4 hr (max 6 doses/day) | b, c |
| Vicks Pediatric 44M Multi-Symptom Cough & Cold Oral Solution (OTC) [U.S.] | Chlorpheniramine maleate 0.67 mg | Pseudoephedrine HCl 10 mg | | Dextromethorphan HBr 5 mg | | | Alcohol free | 30 mL q 6 hr (max 4 doses/day) | 6–11 yrs: 15 mL q 6 hr (max 4 doses/day) | b, c, e |
| Vicodin Tuss Syrup (Schedule III) [U.S.] | | | Hydrocodone bitartrate 5 mg | | Guaifenesin 100 mg | | Alcohol free Sugar free Dye free | 5 mL q 4 hr (max 6 doses/day) | 6–12 yrs: 2.5–5 mL q 4 hr (max 6 doses/day) | b, c, e, f |
| Zephrex Tablets (Rx) [U.S.] | | Pseudoephedrine HCl 60 mg | | | Guaifenesin 400 mg | | | 1 tab q 6 hr | Pediatric strength not available | b |
| Zephrex-LA Extended-release Tablets (Rx) [U.S.] | | Pseudoephedrine HCl 120 mg | | | Guaifenesin 600 mg | | Scored | 1 tab q 12 hr | Pediatric strength not available | b |

*Specific formulations may vary among the different manufacturers, check product labeling.
†Efficacy as expectorant has not been established.
‡Geriatric patients may be more sensitive to effects of usual adult dose.
§For appropriate *Packaging and storage* and *Auxiliary labeling* information refer to designated letters as follows:
  a—Store below 40 °C (104 °F), preferably between 15 and 30 °C (59 and 86 °F), in a tight container, unless otherwise specified by manufacturer.
  a¹—Store below 30 °C (86 °F), unless otherwise specified by manufacturer. Avoid exposure to excessive heat.
  a²—Store below 25 °C (77 °F), unless otherwise specified by manufacturer.
  b—Store below 40 °C (104 °F), preferably between 15 and 30 °C (59 and 86 °F), in a well-closed container, unless otherwise specified by manufacturer.
  c—Protect from freezing.
  d—Protect from light.
  e—Auxiliary labeling: • May cause drowsiness. • Avoid alcoholic beverages.
  f—Auxiliary labeling: • May be habit forming.
  g—Auxiliary labeling: • Shake well.
  h—Dispense in dropper bottle.
  i—Chew well before swallowing.
**Included in subtherapeutic amount to discourage deliberate overdosage.

# CROMOLYN Inhalation-Local

INN: Cromoglicic acid
BAN: Cromoglycic acid
JAN: Sodium cromoglicate

VA CLASSIFICATION (Primary/Secondary): RE101/RE106

Commonly used brand name(s): *Intal; Novo-cromolyn; PMS-Sodium Cromoglycate.*

Other commonly used names are cromoglicic acid, cromoglycic acid, sodium cromoglicate, and sodium cromoglycate.

Note: For a listing of dosage forms and brand names by country availability, see *Dosage Forms* section(s).

## Category

Anti-inflammatory, nonsteroidal (inhalation); mast cell stabilizer; asthma prophylactic; antiallergic (inhalation).

## Indications

**Accepted**

Asthma (prophylaxis)—Cromolyn inhalation is indicated as first-line anti-inflammatory medication, either alone or as an adjunct to bronchodilator therapy, for the prevention of airway inflammation and bronchoconstriction in patients with mild to moderate asthma who require daily therapy.

Bronchospasm (prophylaxis)—Cromolyn inhalation is indicated to prevent acute bronchospasm induced by exercise, or by exposure to allergens, cold dry air, environmental pollutants, or other known precipitating factors, whether exposure is episodic or continuous.

**Unaccepted**

Cromolyn inhalation is not indicated for the reversal or relief of acute asthma attacks, especially in status asthmaticus; cromolyn has no immediate bronchodilating activity.

## Pharmacology/Pharmacokinetics

**Physicochemical characteristics**
Molecular weight—512.34.

**Mechanism of action/Effect**

The exact mechanism by which cromolyn prevents immediate-onset and delayed-onset asthmatic reactions following inhaled allergens or non-immunological stimuli is not completely known. Cromolyn inhibits the release of mediators, such as histamine and leukotrienes, from mast cells. Prevention of mediator release is thought to result from indirect blockade of the entry of calcium ions into the cells. Cromolyn has also been shown to inhibit the movement of other inflammatory cells such as neutrophils, eosinophils, and monocytes. Additionally, cromolyn has been shown in animal studies to inhibit neuronal reflexes within the lung, prevent down-regulation of beta-2-adrenergic receptors on lymphocytes, and to inhibit bronchospasm caused by tachykinins.

Cromolyn has no intrinsic bronchodilator, glucocorticoid, or antihistaminic action.

**Absorption**

Following administration of cromolyn by inhalation, approximately 8 to 10% of the radioactively labeled dose of cromolyn penetrates the lungs from which it is readily absorbed into systemic circulation. The remainder is either exhaled or swallowed and excreted via the alimentary tract, with very little medication absorbed.

**Onset of action**

Cromolyn inhibits a decrease in forced expiratory volume in one second ($FEV_1$) when inhaled 1 minute before antigen challenge. When cromolyn is used as maintenance therapy, clinical improvement in symptoms and lung function usually occurs within 4 weeks of beginning treatment. However, in some patients, improvement may occur almost immediately.

**Duration of action**
Protection against antigen or exercise challenge—Up to 2 hours.

**Elimination**
Unchanged, approximately equally divided between urine and bile.

## Precautions to Consider

**Carcinogenicity**

Long-term studies in mice (12 months intraperitoneal treatment followed by 6 months observation), hamsters (12 months intraperitoneal treatment followed by 12 months observation), and rats (18 months subcutaneous treatment) showed that cromolyn has no neoplastic effect.

**Mutagenicity**

In various mutagenicity studies, there was no evidence of chromosomal damage or cytotoxicity.

**Pregnancy/Reproduction**

Fertility—In animal reproduction studies with cromolyn, there was no evidence of impaired fertility.

Pregnancy—Although extensive studies in humans have not been done, some limited data suggest that cromolyn is not associated with an increased incidence of fetal anomalies. Poorly controlled asthma and loss of pulmonary function present a greater risk to the mother and may result in placental hypoxemia and increased perinatal mortality, increased prematurity, and low birth weight.

Reproduction studies in mice, rats, and rabbits with cromolyn administered parenterally in doses of up to 338 times the human clinical dose showed no evidence of fetal malformations. Adverse fetal effects (increased resorptions and decreased fetal weight) were noted only with very high parenteral doses that produced maternal toxicity.

Studies in pregnant mice have shown that the addition of cromolyn (338 times the human dose) to isoproterenol (90 times the human dose) appears to increase the incidence of both resorptions and malformations.

FDA Pregnancy Category B.

**Breast-feeding**

It is not known whether cromolyn is distributed into human breast milk; however, problems have not been documented. Since cromolyn reaches very low concentrations in maternal serum, it would be expected to reach even lower and probably undetectable concentrations in breast milk.

In monkeys given intravenous cromolyn, concentrations in breast milk measured less than 0.001% of the administered dose.

**Pediatrics**

Appropriate studies performed to date have not demonstrated pediatrics-specific problems that would limit the usefulness of cromolyn in children.

**Geriatrics**

Although appropriate studies on the relationship of age to the effects of cromolyn inhalation have not been performed in the geriatric population, no geriatrics-specific problems have been documented to date.

**Laboratory value alterations**

The following have been selected on the basis of their potential clinical significance (possible effect in parentheses where appropriate)—not necessarily inclusive (» = major clinical significance):

With diagnostic test results
Bronchial airway hyperreactivity assessment
(cromolyn alters bronchial airway hyperreactivity over time by its proposed anti-inflammatory effect; this may lead to a lessened response to methacholine challenge in some patients)

**Medical considerations/Contraindications**

The medical considerations/contraindications included have been selected on the basis of their potential clinical significance (reasons given in parentheses where appropriate)—not necessarily inclusive (» = major clinical significance).

*Risk-benefit should be considered when the following medical problem exists:*
Sensitivity to cromolyn

## Side/Adverse Effects

Note: Adverse reactions to cromolyn sodium are uncommon. Angioedema, bronchospasm, cough, dizziness, dysuria and urinary frequency, headache, joint swelling and pain, laryngeal edema, lacrimation, nausea, nasal congestion, rash, swollen parotid glands, and urticaria attributed to cromolyn have been reported to occur in less than 1 in 10,000 patients. Anemia, exfoliative dermatitis, hemoptysis, hoarseness, myalgia, nephrosis, periarteritic vasculitis, pericarditis, peripheral neuritis, photodermatitis, polymyositis, pulmonary infiltrates with eosinophilia, and vertigo have been reported in less than 1 in 100,000 patients. In all cases the causal relationship is unclear.

The following side/adverse effects have been selected on the basis of their potential clinical significance (possible signs and symptoms in parentheses where appropriate)—not necessarily inclusive:

Those indicating need for medical attention
Incidence rare
   *Anaphylactic reaction* (difficulty in swallowing; hives; itching of skin; swelling of face, lips, or eyelids; increased wheezing or difficulty in breathing; low blood pressure)—reported in less than 1 in 100,000 patients

Those indicating need for medical attention only if they continue or are bothersome
Incidence more frequent
   *Bad taste in mouth*—for metered dose inhaler; *throat irritation or dryness*

## Patient Consultation

As an aid to patient consultation, refer to *Advice for the Patient, Cromolyn (Inhalation).*

In providing consultation, consider emphasizing the following selected information (» = major clinical significance):

**Before using this medication**
» Conditions affecting use, especially:
   Sensitivity to cromolyn

**Proper use of this medication**
» Helps prevent, but does not relieve, acute attacks of asthma or bronchospasm
» Importance of not using more medication than the amount prescribed
   Reading patient instructions carefully before using
   Checking periodically with health care professional for proper use of inhaler to prevent incorrect dosage
» Proper dosing
   Missed dose: If used regularly, using as soon as possible; using any remaining doses for that day at regularly spaced intervals
» Proper storage
*For inhalation aerosol dosage form*
   Keeping record of number of sprays used, if possible; not floating canister in water to test fullness
   Testing or priming inhaler before using first time or if not used for a while
   Proper administration technique
   Proper administration technique with spacer device
   Proper cleaning procedure for inhaler
*For inhalation capsule dosage form*
» Not swallowing capsules; medication not effective if swallowed
   Using with Spinhaler or Halermatic inhaler
   Proper loading technique for inhaler
   Proper administration technique
   Proper cleaning procedure for inhaler
*For inhalation solution dosage form*
   Not using if solution cloudy or contains particles
   Proper breaking of ampul
   Using in a power-operated nebulizer with an adequate flow rate and equipped with face mask or mouthpiece; not using hand-squeezed bulb nebulizers
*For patients on scheduled dosing regimen*
» Compliance with therapy; may require up to 4 weeks for full benefit

**Precautions while using this medication**
» Checking with physician if symptoms do not improve within first 4 weeks; checking with physician immediately if condition becomes worse
» Importance of not discontinuing concurrent systemic corticosteroid or bronchodilator therapy without physician's advice
   Possible throat irritation or dryness; gargling and rinsing mouth or taking drink of water after each dose to help prevent these effects

**Side/adverse effects**
   Signs of potential side effects, especially anaphylactic reaction
   Cromolyn inhalation aerosol may cause an unpleasant taste

## General Dosing Information

When cromolyn is introduced into the patient's therapeutic regimen after an acute episode, the episode must be under control, the airway clear, and the patient able to inhale adequately.

A decrease in severity of clinical symptoms or in the need for concomitant therapy is a sign of improvement that will be evident in the first 4 weeks of therapy if patient responds to cromolyn therapy.

In asthmatic patients receiving systemic corticosteroids and/or bronchodilators prior to institution of cromolyn, the corticosteroid and/or bronchodilator should be continued following initiation of cromolyn therapy. However, an attempt should be made to reduce the dosage of the systemic corticosteroid and/or institute an alternate-day regimen. The dosage of the corticosteroid should be reduced gradually to avoid an exacerbation of asthma.

*For inhalation solution dosage form only*—Cromolyn solution should be administered from a power-operated nebulizer having an adequate flow rate (6 to 8 liters per minute) and equipped with a suitable face mask or mouthpiece. Hand-squeezed bulb nebulizers are not suitable for administration of cromolyn solution.

## Inhalation Dosage Forms

### CROMOLYN SODIUM INHALATION AEROSOL

**Usual adult and adolescent dose**
Asthma (prophylaxis)—
   Oral inhalation, 2 inhalations (1.6 or 2 mg) four times a day at regular intervals of four to six hours.
   Note: When the patient is stabilized on a maintenance regimen of four times a day, the dosing frequency may be gradually reduced to three times a day, then to two times a day in some patients.
Bronchospasm (prophylaxis)—
   Oral inhalation, 2 inhalations (1.6 or 2 mg) as a single dose administered at least ten to fifteen (but not more than sixty) minutes before exercise or exposure to any precipitating factor.

**Usual adult prescribing limits**
Up to 16 puffs (12.8 or 16 mg) daily.

**Usual pediatric dose**
Children up to 5 years of age—Dosage has not been established.
Children 5 years of age and over—See *Usual adult and adolescent dose*.

**Usual geriatric dose**
See *Usual adult and adolescent dose*.

**Strength(s) usually available**
U.S.—
   800 mcg (0.8 mg) per metered spray (Rx) [*Intal*].
Canada—
   1 mg per metered spray (Rx) [*Intal*].
Note: In Canada, metered dose inhalers are labeled according to the amount of cromolyn delivered at the valve; in the U.S., metered dose inhalers are labeled according to the amount of cromolyn delivered at the mouthpiece or actuator. Therefore, 1 mg of cromolyn delivered at the valve is equivalent to 800 mcg delivered at the mouthpiece.

**Packaging and storage**
Store between 15 and 30 °C (59 and 86 °F), unless otherwise specified by manufacturer. Protect from freezing.

**Auxiliary labeling**
• For oral inhalation only.
• Shake well before using.
• Store away from heat and direct sunlight.

**Note**
Include patient instructions when dispensing.
Demonstrate inhalation technique to patient when dispensing.

**Additional information**
U.S.—Each 8.1-gram canister delivers at least 112 metered sprays; each 14.2-gram canister delivers at least 200 metered sprays.
Canada—Each canister delivers either 112 or 200 metered sprays.

### CROMOLYN SODIUM FOR INHALATION (CAPSULES) USP

**Usual adult and adolescent dose**
Asthma (prophylaxis)—
   Oral inhalation, 20 mg (1 capsule) four times a day at regular intervals of four to six hours.
   Note: When the patient is stabilized on a maintenance regimen of four times a day, the dosing frequency may be gradually reduced to three times a day, then to two times a day in some patients.
Bronchospasm (prophylaxis)—
   Oral inhalation, 20 mg (1 capsule) as a single dose administered at least ten to fifteen (but not more than sixty) minutes before exercise or exposure to the precipitating factor.

**Usual adult prescribing limits**
Up to 160 mg (8 capsules) daily.

**Usual pediatric dose**
Children up to 2 years of age—Dosage has not been established.
Children 2 years of age and over—See *Usual adult and adolescent dose*.

**Usual geriatric dose**
See *Usual adult and adolescent dose*.

# Cromolyn (Inhalation-Local)

**Strength(s) usually available**
U.S.—
 Not commercially available.
Canada—
 20 mg per inhalation capsule (Rx) [*Intal*].

**Packaging and storage**
Store below 40 °C (104 °F), preferably between 15 and 30 °C (59 and 86 °F), unless otherwise specified by manufacturer. Store in a tight, light-resistant container.

**Auxiliary labeling**
• For inhalation only—Do not swallow capsules.

**Note**
Include patient instructions when dispensing.
Demonstrate administration technique to patient when dispensing.
Demonstration kits may be available.

## CROMOLYN SODIUM INHALATION SOLUTION USP

**Usual adult and adolescent dose**
Asthma (prophylaxis)—
 Oral inhalation, 20 mg four times a day at regular intervals of four to six hours.
 Note: When the patient is stabilized on a maintenance regimen of four times a day, the dosing frequency may be gradually reduced to three times a day, then to two times a day in some patients.
Bronchospasm (prophylaxis)—
 Oral inhalation, 20 mg as a single dose administered at least ten to fifteen (but not more than sixty) minutes before exercise or exposure to the precipitating factor.

**Usual adult prescribing limits**
Up to 160 mg daily.

**Usual pediatric dose**
Children up to 2 years of age—Dosage has not been established.
Children 2 years of age and over—See *Usual adult and adolescent dose*.

**Usual geriatric dose**
See *Usual adult and adolescent dose*.

**Strength(s) usually available**
U.S.—
 20 mg per 2-ml ampul (Rx) [*Intal*; GENERIC].
Canada—
 20 mg per 2-ml ampul (Rx) [*Intal*; *Novo-cromolyn*; *PMS-Sodium Cromoglycate*].

**Packaging and storage**
Store below 40 °C (104 °F), preferably between 15 and 30 °C (59 and 86 °F), unless otherwise specified by manufacturer. Protect from freezing. Protect from light.

**Stability**
Solution should not be used if it is cloudy or contains a precipitate.
Any solution remaining in the nebulizer should be discarded.
Cromolyn sodium inhalation solution has been shown to be physically and chemically compatible with acetylcysteine, albuterol, epinephrine, isoetharine, isoproterenol, metaproterenol, and terbutaline solutions for up to 60 minutes.
When combining cromolyn and ipratropium inhalation solutions, it is recommended that only *preservative-free* ipratropium solution be used. Mixing cromolyn inhalation solution with ipratropium inhalation solution containing the preservative benzalkonium chloride is not recommended because mixing results in cloudiness of the solution, which is due to complexation between cromolyn sodium and benzalkonium chloride, although no precipitation or significant decrease in the concentration of cromolyn or ipratropium occurs.
Cromolyn should not be mixed with bitolterol inhalation solution, since mixing results in cloudiness of the solution.

**Auxiliary labeling**
• For inhalation only.

**Note**
Include patient information when dispensing.
Demonstrate opening and emptying of ampul when dispensing.

## Selected Bibliography

Murphy S. Cromolyn sodium: basic mechanisms and clinical usage. Pediatr Asthma Allergy Immunol 1988; 2: 237-54.
Murphy S, Kelly HW. Cromolyn sodium: a review of mechanisms and clinical use in asthma. DICP 1987; 21: 22-35.

Revised: 04/23/96

---

# CROMOLYN  Nasal

VA CLASSIFICATION (Primary): NT900
Commonly used brand name(s): *Nasalcrom*; *Rynacrom*.
Another commonly used name is sodium cromoglycate.
Note: For a listing of dosage forms and brand names by country availability, see *Dosage Forms* section(s).

## Category
Mast cell stabilizer (nasal); antiallergic (nasal).

## Indications

**Accepted**
Rhinitis, allergic (prophylaxis and treatment)—Cromolyn sodium nasal solution is indicated for the prophylaxis and treatment of the symptoms of perennial and seasonal allergic rhinitis.
Cromolyn sodium for nasal insufflation is indicated for the prophylaxis of seasonal allergic rhinitis.

## Pharmacology/Pharmacokinetics

**Physicochemical characteristics**
Molecular weight—512.34.
pH—4.5 to 6.5.

**Mechanism of action/Effect**
Cromolyn is a mast cell stabilizer that inhibits the Type I immediate hypersensitivity reaction by preventing the antigen-stimulated release of histamine. Cromolyn also prevents the release of leukotrienes and inhibits eosinophil chemotaxis.
*In vitro* and *in vivo* animal studies have shown that cromolyn inhibits the degranulation of sensitized mast cells that occurs after exposure to specific antigens. Some *in vitro* studies have shown that cromolyn inhibits the degranulation of nonsensitized rat mast cells by phospholipase A and the subsequent release of chemical mediators.

**Other actions/effects**
Cromolyn has no intrinsic bronchodilator, antihistaminic, or anti-inflammatory action.

**Absorption**
Poorly absorbed from the gastrointestinal tract. After instillation of cromolyn nasal solution, less than 7% of the total dose administered is absorbed.

**Onset of therapeutic effect**
Seasonal allergic rhinitis—Results are usually noticeable in less than 1 week.

**Time to peak effect**
Perennial allergic rhinitis—Results are usually noticeable in approximately 1 week; however, in some cases up to 4 weeks may be required.

**Elimination**
Nasal solution—The portion of the dose that is absorbed (7%) is rapidly excreted unchanged in the bile and urine; the remainder of the dose is expelled from the nose, or swallowed and excreted via the alimentary tract.

## Precautions to Consider

**Carcinogenicity**
Long-term studies with cromolyn in mice (12 months intraperitoneal treatment followed by 6 months observation), hamsters (12 months intraperitoneal treatment followed by 12 months observation), and rats (18 months subcutaneous treatment) did not show any neoplastic effect.

**Mutagenicity**
In various mutagenicity studies, there was no evidence of chromosomal damage or cytotoxicity.

**Pregnancy/Reproduction**
Fertility—Animal reproduction studies with cromolyn showed no evidence of impaired fertility.
Pregnancy—Adequate and well-controlled studies in humans have not been done.

A ten year study of 296 pregnant asthmatic women in Sri Lanka administered cromolyn by oral inhalation during part or all of their pregnancies resulted in 4 infants (1.35%) with malformations. However, epidemiological studies suggest that the usual incidence of fetal abnormalities in the Sri Lanka population is 2 to 3%.

Reproduction studies in mice, rats, and rabbits with cromolyn administered parenterally in doses up to 338 times the human clinical doses showed no evidence of fetal malformations. (Adverse fetal effects [increased resorptions and decreased fetal weight] were noted only at very high parenteral doses that produced maternal toxicity.)

FDA Pregnancy Category B.

**Breast-feeding**
It is not known whether cromolyn is distributed into breast milk; however, cromolyn reaches very low concentrations in maternal serum. Problems in humans have not been documented.

**Pediatrics**
Appropriate studies on the relationship of age to the effects of nasal cromolyn have not been performed in the U.S. in children up to 6 years of age (in Canada, up to 5 years of age). In older children, no pediatrics-specific problems have been documented to date.

**Geriatrics**
Appropriate studies on the relationship of age to the effects of nasal cromolyn have not been performed in the geriatric population. However, no geriatrics-specific problems have been documented to date.

**Drug interactions and/or related problems**
The following drug interactions and/or related problems have been selected on the basis of their potential clinical significance (possible mechanism in parentheses where appropriate)—not necessarily inclusive (» = major clinical significance):

Methacholine, for inhalation
(cromolyn may decrease slightly, but inconsistently, the response to methacholine challenge in the diagnosis of bronchial airway hyperreactivity; however, cromolyn generally does not cause false-negative tests)

**Medical considerations/Contraindications**
The medical considerations/contraindications included have been selected on the basis of their potential clinical significance (reasons given in parentheses where appropriate)—not necessarily inclusive (» = major clinical significance):

*Risk-benefit should be considered when the following medical problems exist:*

Polyps, nasal
(medication may not be effective if nasal passage obstruction exists)
Sensitivity to cromolyn

## Side/Adverse Effects

Note: Eosinophilic pneumonia has been reported rarely with cromolyn nasal products.

Although not reported for cromolyn nasal solution, some side/adverse effects that have occurred with cromolyn formulations for inhalation include joint pain and swelling, and, reported rarely, serum sickness, periarteritic vasculitis, polymyositis, pericarditis, photodermatitis, exfoliative dermatitis, peripheral neuritis, pneumonitis, heart failure, and nephrosis.

The following side/adverse effects have been selected on the basis of their potential clinical significance (possible signs and symptoms in parentheses where appropriate)—not necessarily inclusive:

**Those indicating need for medical attention**
Incidence rare
*Anaphylactic reaction* (coughing; difficulty in swallowing; hives; itching of skin; swelling of face, lips, or eyelids; wheezing or difficulty in breathing); *epistaxis* (nosebleeds); *skin rash*

**Those indicating need for medical attention only if they continue or are bothersome**
Incidence more frequent
*Burning, stinging, or irritation inside of nose; increase in sneezing*
Incidence less frequent
*Cough; headache; postnasal drip; unpleasant taste*

## Patient Consultation

As an aid to patient consultation, refer to *Advice for the Patient, Cromolyn (Nasal)*.

In providing consultation, consider emphasizing the following selected information (» = major clinical significance):

**Before using this medication**
» Conditions affecting use, especially:
Sensitivity to cromolyn
Use in children—Safety and efficacy have not been established in the U.S. in children up to 6 years of age (in Canada, up to 5 years of age)

**Proper use of this medication**
Reading patient directions carefully
Clearing nasal passages before use
For *cromolyn nasal solution:* Using with a special spray device; wiping nosepiece with a clean tissue and replacing dust cap after use to keep unit clean
For *cromolyn for nasal insufflation:* Using with a special inhaler; understanding exactly how to use inhaler; wiping nosepiece with a clean tissue and replacing dust cap after use; washing only nosepiece in warm water, drying thoroughly; not washing bulb or dampening bulb interior
» Importance of not using more medication than the amount prescribed
» Using every day in regularly spaced doses in order for medication to work properly; results are usually noticeable in approximately 1 week; however in perennial allergic rhinitis, up to 4 weeks may be required for full benefit
» Proper dosing
Missed dose: Using as soon as possible; using any remaining doses for that day at regularly spaced intervals; not doubling doses
» Proper storage

**Precautions while using this medication**
» Checking with physician if symptoms do not improve or if condition becomes worse

**Side/adverse effects**
Signs of potential side effects, especially anaphylactic reaction, epistaxis, and skin rash

## General Dosing Information

Prior to administration of cromolyn nasal solution or cromolyn for nasal insufflation, the nasal passages should be cleared. During administration, patient should inhale through the nose.

In the management of seasonal allergic rhinitis (pollinosis) and for the prevention of rhinitis caused by other types of specific airborne allergens, treatment with nasal cromolyn is more effective if started prior to exposure to the offending allergen. Therapy should be continued throughout the period of exposure (i.e., until the pollen season is over or until the patient is no longer exposed to the offending allergen).

In the management of perennial allergic rhinitis, improvement of condition may not become apparent for up to 2 to 4 weeks. Concurrent use of an antihistamine and/or a nasal decongestant may be necessary during this time; however, the need for these medications should decrease and these medications may be discontinued when the full effect of nasal cromolyn is achieved.

## Nasal Dosage Forms

### CROMOLYN SODIUM FOR NASAL INSUFFLATION

**Usual adult and adolescent dose**
Allergic rhinitis, seasonal (prophylaxis)—
Initial: Nasal insufflation, 10 mg in each nostril four times a day at four- to six-hour intervals.
Maintenance: Nasal insufflation, 10 mg in each nostril every eight to twelve hours.

**Usual pediatric dose**
Allergic rhinitis, seasonal (prophylaxis)—
Children up to 5 years of age: Dosage has not been established.
Children 5 years of age and over: See *Usual adult and adolescent dose*.

**Usual geriatric dose**
See *Usual adult and adolescent dose*.

**Strength(s) usually available**
U.S.—
Not commercially available.
Canada—
10 mg per cartridge (Rx) [*Rynacrom* (lactose 10 mg)].

**Packaging and storage**
Store below 30 °C (86 °F), in the original container, in a dry place, unless otherwise specified by manufacturer.

**Stability**
Storage in a damp atmosphere may cause the contents to absorb moisture and render the powder unusable.

### Auxiliary labeling
- For the nose.

### Note
Dispense with nasal insufflator.
Include patient instructions when dispensing.
Explain administration technique.

## CROMOLYN SODIUM NASAL SOLUTION USP

### Usual adult and adolescent dose
Allergic rhinitis, perennial or seasonal (prophylaxis and treatment)—
Intranasal, 5.2 mg in each nostril three or four times a day at regular intervals. Alternatively, 2.6 mg in each nostril six times a day; when an adequate response has been obtained, the dosage may be reduced to 2.6 mg in each nostril two or three times a day.

### Usual adult prescribing limits
Up to 5.2 mg in each nostril six times a day.

### Usual pediatric dose
Allergic rhinitis, perennial or seasonal (prophylaxis and treatment)—
Children up to 6 years of age (in Canada, up to 5 years of age): Safety and efficacy have not been established.
Children 6 years of age (in Canada, 5 years of age) and over: See *Usual adult and adolescent dose*.

### Usual geriatric dose
See *Usual adult and adolescent dose*.

### Strength(s) usually available
U.S.—
40 mg per mL (5.2 mg per metered spray) (Rx) [*Nasalcrom* (benzalkonium chloride 0.01%; edetate disodium 0.01%)].
Canada—
20 mg per mL (2.6 mg per metered spray) (Rx) [*Rynacrom* (benzalkonium chloride 0.01%)].

### Packaging and storage
Store below 40 °C (104 °F), preferably between 15 and 30 °C (59 and 86 °F), unless otherwise specified by manufacturer. Store in a tight, light-resistant container. Protect from freezing.

### Auxiliary labeling
- For the nose.

### Note
Include patient instructions when dispensing.
Explain administration technique.

### Additional information
The nasal spray bottle containing 520 mg/13 mL delivers at least 100 sprays.

Revised: 04/20/94

# CROMOLYN Ophthalmic

INN: Cromoglicic acid.
BAN: Cromoglycic acid.

VA CLASSIFICATION (Primary): OP900

Commonly used brand name(s): *Crolom; Opticrom; Vistacrom*.

Another commonly used name is sodium cromoglycate.

Note: For a listing of dosage forms and brand names by country availability, see *Dosage Forms* section(s).

## Category
Mast cell stabilizer (ophthalmic); antiallergic (ophthalmic).

## Indications
Note: Bracketed information in the *Indications* section refers to uses that are not included in U.S. product labeling.

### Accepted
[Conjunctivitis, seasonal allergic (treatment)]
Conjunctivitis, vernal (treatment)[1]
Keratitis, vernal (treatment)[1] or
Keratoconjunctivitis, vernal (treatment)—Cromoryn ophthalmic solution is indicated in the treatment of certain allergic ocular disorders, specifically, seasonal allergic conjunctivitis, vernal conjunctivitis, vernal keratitis, and vernal keratoconjunctivitis.

[1]Not included in Canadian product labeling.

## Pharmacology/Pharmacokinetics

### Physicochemical characteristics
Molecular weight—512.34.
pH—4.0 to 7.0.

### Mechanism of action/Effect
Cromolyn is a mast cell stabilizer that inhibits the Type I immediate hypersensitivity reaction by preventing the antigen-stimulated release of histamine. Cromolyn also prevents the release of leukotrienes and inhibits eosinophil chemotaxis.

*In vitro* and *in vivo* animal studies have shown that cromolyn inhibits the degranulation of sensitized mast cells that occurs after exposure to specific antigens. Some *in vitro* studies have shown that cromolyn inhibits the degranulation of nonsensitized rat mast cells by phospholipase A and the subsequent release of chemical mediators. One study has shown that cromolyn does not inhibit the enzymatic action of released phospholipase A on its specific substrate.

### Absorption
Poorly absorbed.
In normal individuals, approximately 0.03% of cromolyn is absorbed systemically following ophthalmic administration.
Studies in rabbits have shown that less than 0.07% of the administered dose is absorbed systemically following multiple doses. Also, trace amounts (less than 0.01%) of the administered dose penetrate into the aqueous humor, and clearance from this chamber is almost complete within 24 hours following discontinuation of treatment.

### Onset of therapeutic effect
Usually within a few days.

## Precautions to Consider

### Carcinogenicity
Long-term studies in mice (12 months of intraperitoneal treatment followed by 6 months of observation), hamsters (12 months of intraperitoneal treatment followed by 12 months of observation), and rats (18 months of subcutaneous treatment) did not show any neoplastic effect associated with administration of cromolyn.

### Mutagenicity
In various mutagenicity studies, there was no evidence of chromosomal damage or cytotoxicity.

### Pregnancy/Reproduction
Fertility—In animal reproduction studies with cromolyn, there was no evidence of impaired fertility.

Pregnancy—Adequate and well-controlled studies in humans have not been done.
Reproduction studies in mice, rats, and rabbits with cromolyn administered parenterally in doses up to 338 times the human clinical doses showed no evidence of fetal malformations. Adverse fetal effects (increased resorptions and decreased fetal weight) were noted only at very high parenteral doses that produced maternal toxicity.

FDA Pregnancy Category B.

### Breast-feeding
It is not known whether cromolyn is distributed into breast milk. However, problems in humans have not been documented. Since cromolyn reaches very low concentrations in maternal serum, it would be expected to reach even lower and probably undetectable concentrations in breast milk.

### Pediatrics
Appropriate studies on the relationship of age to the effects of ophthalmic cromolyn have not been performed in children up to 4 years of age. Safety and efficacy have not been established. In older children, no pediatrics-specific problems have been documented to date.

### Geriatrics
Appropriate studies on the relationship of age to the effects of cromolyn have not been performed in the geriatric population. However, geriatrics-specific problems that would limit the usefulness of this medication in the elderly are not expected.

### Medical considerations/Contraindications
The medical considerations/contraindications included have been selected on the basis of their potential clinical significance (reasons given in

parentheses where appropriate)—not necessarily inclusive (» = major clinical significance).

***Risk-benefit should be considered when the following medical problem exists:***
Sensitivity to cromolyn

## Side/Adverse Effects

The following side/adverse effects have been selected on the basis of their potential clinical significance (possible signs and symptoms in parentheses where appropriate)—not necessarily inclusive:

**Those indicating need for medical attention**
Incidence rare
*Chemosis* (swelling of the membrane covering the white part of the eye); *conjunctival injection* (redness of the white part of the eye); *styes, or other signs of eye irritation not present before therapy; contact dermatitis* (rash or redness around the eyes)

**Those indicating need for medical attention only if they continue or are bothersome**
Incidence more frequent
*Burning or stinging of eye, mild, temporary*
Incidence less frequent or rare
*Dryness or puffiness around the eye; watering or itching of eye, increased*

## Patient Consultation

As an aid to patient consultation, refer to *Advice for the Patient, Cromolyn (Ophthalmic)*.
In providing consultation, consider emphasizing the following selected information (» = major clinical significance):

**Before using this medication**
» Conditions affecting use, especially:
   Sensitivity to cromolyn
   Use in children—Safety and efficacy have not been established in children up to 4 years of age

**Proper use of this medication**
Proper administration technique; not touching applicator tip to any surface; keeping container tightly closed
» Importance of not using more medication than the amount prescribed
» Compliance with therapy; symptomatic response usually occurs within a few days
» Proper dosing
   Missed dose: Using as soon as possible
» Proper storage

**Precautions while using this medication**
» Checking with physician if symptoms do not improve or if condition becomes worse

**Side/adverse effects**
Signs of potential side effects, especially chemosis, conjunctival injection, styes, or other signs of eye irritation not present before therapy; or contact dermatitis

## General Dosing Information

Symptomatic response to therapy (decreased itching, redness, watering, and discharge) usually occurs within a few days; however, treatment may be required for up to 6 weeks.

Corticosteroids may be used concurrently with cromolyn, if required.
Although the manufacturer recommends that patients not wear soft contact lenses during treatment with cromolyn ophthalmic solution, medical experts do not believe this precaution is necessary unless the patient has corneal epithelial problems and the medication is to be used more often than once every 1 to 2 hours. No significant problems have been documented with ophthalmic solutions containing 0.03% or less of benzalkonium chloride as a preservative, and used as eyedrops in patients with no significant corneal surface problems.

## Ophthalmic Dosage Forms

Note: Bracketed uses in the *Dosage Forms* section refer to categories of use and/or indications that are not included in U.S. product labeling.

### CROMOLYN SODIUM OPHTHALMIC SOLUTION USP

**Usual adult and adolescent dose**
[Conjunctivitis, seasonal allergic]
Conjunctivitis, vernal[1]
Keratitis, vernal or[1]
Keratoconjunctivitis, vernal—
   Topical, to the conjunctiva, 1 drop four to six times a day at regular intervals.

**Usual adult prescribing limits**
Up to 12.8 mg.

**Usual pediatric dose**
[Conjunctivitis, seasonal allergic]
Conjunctivitis, vernal[1]
Keratitis, vernal[1] or
Keratoconjunctivitis, vernal—
   Children up to 4 years of age: Safety and efficacy have not been established.
   Children 4 years of age and older: See *Usual adult and adolescent dose*.

**Usual geriatric dose**
See *Usual adult and adolescent dose*.

**Strength(s) usually available**
U.S.—
   4% (Rx) [*Crolom* (benzalkonium chloride; edetate disodium; hydrochloric acid; sodium hydroxide)].
Canada—
   2% (Rx) [*Opticrom* (benzalkonium chloride); *Vistacrom* (benzalkonium chloride 0.01%; edetate disodium)].
Note: One drop of cromolyn sodium ophthalmic solution 2% contains approximately 0.8 mg of cromolyn sodium; and one drop of cromolyn sodium ophthalmic solution 4% contains approximately 1.6 mg of cromolyn sodium.

**Packaging and storage**
Store below 40 °C (104 °F), preferably between 15 and 30 °C (59 and 86 °F), unless otherwise specified by manufacturer. Store in a tight, light-resistant container. Protect from freezing.

**Auxiliary labeling**
• For the eye.

[1]Not included in Canadian product labeling.

Revised: 04/19/94
Interim revision: 07/10/95

---

# CROMOLYN  Systemic/Oral-Local

VA CLASSIFICATION (Primary): IM900
Commonly used brand name(s): *Gastrocrom; Nalcrom*.
Another commonly used name is sodium cromoglycate.
Note: For a listing of dosage forms and brand names by country availability, see *Dosage Forms* section(s).

## Category

Mast cell stabilizer; antiallergic (systemic).

## Indications

**Accepted**
Mastocytosis (treatment)[1]—Cromolyn administered orally is indicated in the treatment of mastocytosis. It has been shown to improve the symptoms of mastocytosis, such as diarrhea, flushing, headache, vomiting, urticaria, abdominal pain, nausea, and itching.

Note: Although oral cromolyn is approved in Canada for gastrointestinal allergy, the USP DI Advisory Panels believe there is insufficient evidence to support the effectiveness of cromolyn in the prophylaxis of food allergy and the prophylaxis and treatment of chronic inflammatory bowel disease. Further studies are needed to determine the efficacy of oral cromolyn in these conditions. The preferred therapy for gastrointestinal allergy to food is avoidance of those foods to which the patient is allergic. In the prophylaxis and treatment of chronic inflammatory bowel disease, agents that have been proven effective in this condition should be used.

[1]Not included in Canadian product labeling.

## Pharmacology/Pharmacokinetics

**Physicochemical characteristics**
Molecular weight—512.34.

**Mechanism of action/Effect**
Cromolyn inhibits mast cell release of histamine, leukotrienes, and other substances that cause hypersensitivity reactions, probably by interfering with calcium transport across the mast cell membrane. Cromolyn does not possess any intrinsic antihistamine, anti-inflammatory, glucocorticoid, or vasoconstrictive activity.

*In vitro* and *in vivo* animal studies have shown that cromolyn inhibits degranulation of sensitized mast cells that occurs after exposure to specific antigens. Some *in vitro* studies have shown that cromolyn inhibits both degranulation of nonsensitized rat mast cells stimulated by phospholipase A and the subsequent release of chemical mediators.

**Absorption**
Poorly absorbed from the gastrointestinal tract; only about 1% of an oral dose is absorbed.

**Half-life**
Approximately 80 minutes.

**Elimination**
Renal/biliary; unchanged.

## Precautions to Consider

**Carcinogenicity**
Long-term studies in mice (12 months intraperitoneal treatment followed by 6 months observation), hamsters (12 months intraperitoneal treatment followed by 12 months observation), and rats (18 months subcutaneous treatment) showed that cromolyn has no neoplastic effect.

**Mutagenicity**
In various mutagenicity studies, there was no evidence of chromosomal damage or cytotoxicity.

**Pregnancy/Reproduction**
Fertility—In animal reproduction studies with cromolyn, there was no evidence of impaired fertility.

Pregnancy—Adequate and well-controlled studies in humans have not been done.

Studies in mice, rats, and rabbits with cromolyn administered parenterally in doses up to 338 times the human clinical doses showed no evidence of fetal malformations. Adverse fetal effects (increased resorptions and decreased fetal weight) were noted only at very high parenteral doses that produced maternal toxicity.

Studies in pregnant mice have shown that cromolyn alone, administered subcutaneously in doses of 60 to 540 mg per kg of body weight (mg/kg) (38 to 338 times the human dose), does not cause significant increases in resorptions or major malformations; however, the addition of cromolyn (338 times the human dose) to isoproterenol (90 times the human dose) appears to increase the incidence of both resorptions and malformations.

FDA Pregnancy Category B.

**Breast-feeding**
It is not known whether cromolyn is distributed into breast milk. However, problems in humans have not been documented. Since cromolyn reaches very low concentrations in maternal serum, it would be expected to reach even lower and probably undetectable concentrations in breast milk.

**Pediatrics**
Appropriate studies on the relationship of age to the effects of oral cromolyn have not been performed in the pediatric population. However, no pediatrics-specific problems have been documented to date.

Studies in animals have suggested an increased risk of toxicity in premature animals when cromolyn was administered in doses much higher than those clinically recommended for human use.

Use of oral cromolyn is not recommended in premature to term infants.

Use of oral cromolyn in children younger than 2 years of age should be reserved for patients with severe, incapacitating disease.

**Geriatrics**
Appropriate studies performed to date have not demonstrated geriatrics-specific problems that would limit the usefulness of cromolyn in the elderly. However, elderly patients are more likely to have age-related hepatic function impairment and renal function impairment, which may require reduction of dosage in patients receiving cromolyn.

**Medical considerations/Contraindications**
The medical considerations/contraindications included have been selected on the basis of their potential clinical significance (reasons given in parentheses where appropriate)—not necessarily inclusive (» = major clinical significance).

*Risk-benefit should be considered when the following medical problems exist:*

Hepatic function impairment
  (excretion via biliary route; dosage reduction may be necessary )
Renal function impairment
  (excretion via renal route; dosage reduction may be necessary)
Sensitivity to cromolyn

## Side/Adverse Effects

Note: Although not reported with oral use of cromolyn, some side/adverse effects that have occurred with cromolyn formulations for inhalation include angioedema, swelling of joints, and, reported rarely, serum sickness, periarteritic vasculitis, polymyositis, pericarditis, photodermatitis, exfoliative dermatitis, peripheral neuritis, and nephrosis.

The following side/adverse effects have been selected on the basis of their potential clinical significance (possible signs and symptoms in parentheses where appropriate)—not necessarily inclusive:

**Those indicating need for medical attention**
Incidence less frequent
  *Skin rash*

Incidence rare
  *Anaphylactic reaction, severe* (coughing; difficulty in swallowing; hives; itching of skin; swelling of face, lips, or eyelids; wheezing or difficulty in breathing)

**Those indicating need for medical attention only if they continue or are bothersome**
Incidence more frequent
  *Diarrhea; headache*

Incidence less frequent or rare
  *Abdominal pain; irritability; myalgia* (muscle pain); *nausea; trouble in sleeping*

  Note: The above side/adverse effects occurring in patients with mastocytosis are usually transient and could represent symptoms of the disease.

## Patient Consultation

As an aid to patient consultation, refer to *Advice for the Patient, Cromolyn (Oral)*.

In providing consultation, consider emphasizing the following selected information (» = major clinical significance):

**Before using this medication**
» Conditions affecting use, especially:
    Sensitivity to cromolyn
    Use in children—In premature to term infants, use of oral cromolyn is not recommended; in children younger than 2 years of age, use of oral cromolyn should be reserved for patients with severe, incapacitating disease

**Proper use of this medication**
Proper administration:
  Capsules—
    For optimal results, dissolving contents of capsule(s) in one-half glass (4 ounces) of hot water and stirring until the medication is completely dissolved (solution will become clear) and then adding and stirring in an equal amount (4 ounces) of cold water
    Drinking all of liquid to receive full dose
    Not mixing medication with fruit juice, milk, or foods
  Ampuls—
    Breaking open ampul(s) and squeezing all contents into a glass of water and then stirring the solution well
    Drinking all of liquid to receive full dose
» Importance of not using more medication than the amount prescribed
» Importance of taking medication at regular intervals for optimum therapeutic effect
» Proper dosing
    Missed dose: Taking as soon as possible; taking any remaining doses for that day at regularly spaced intervals
» Proper storage

**Precautions while using this medication**
» Checking with physician if symptoms do not improve or if condition becomes worse

**Side/adverse effects**
Signs of potential side effects, especially skin rash and severe anaphylactic reaction

## General Dosing Information

For optimal results, the contents of the capsules should be dissolved in warm water only and taken as a solution. The powder should not be mixed with fruit juice, milk, or food. Ampul(s) should be broken and the contents squeezed into a glass of water which is then stirred well. The entire glass of water, containing the medication, should be consumed for the patient to receive the full dose.

If hepatic or renal impairment is present, the cromolyn dose should be reduced as neccessary.

After the desired therapeutic response has been obtained, the dose may be reduced to the lowest level at which there is a reduction in the severity of the patient's symptoms.

## Oral Dosage Forms

### CROMOLYN SODIUM CAPSULES

**Usual adult and adolescent dose**
Mastocytosis[1]—
  Oral, 200 mg four times a day, thirty minutes before meals and at bedtime.

**Usual pediatric dose**
Mastocytosis[1]—
  Premature to term infants:
    Use is not recommended.
  Term infants and children up to 2 years of age:
    Oral, 20 mg per kg of body weight per day in four divided doses. If control of symptoms is not achieved within two to three weeks in children six months to two years of age, dosage may be increased, if necessary, up to 30 mg per kg of body weight per day.
Note: Use of oral cromolyn in children younger than 2 years of age should be reserved for patients with severe, incapacitating disease.
  Children 2 to 12 years of age:
    Oral, 100 mg four times a day, thirty minutes before meals and at bedtime. If control of symptoms is not achieved within two to three weeks, dosage may be increased, if necessary, up to 40 mg per kg of body weight per day.
  Children 12 years of age and older:
    See *Usual adult and adolescent dose.*

**Usual geriatric dose**
See *Usual adult and adolescent dose.*

**Strength(s) usually available**
U.S.—
  100 mg (Rx) [*Gastrocrom*].
Canada—
  100 mg (Rx) [*Nalcrom*].

**Packaging and storage**
Store at temperatures between 15 and 30 °C (59 and 86 °F), unless otherwise specified by manufacturer. Store in a tight container. Keep out of the reach of children.

**Preparation of dosage form**
For optimal results, the contents of the capsule should be dissolved in one-half glass (4 ounces) of hot water, and stirred until completely dissolved. Then, one-half glass (4 ounces) of cold water is added to the solution.

**Auxiliary labeling**
- Do not swallow capsule whole.
- Mix with water only. Do not mix with fruit juice, milk, or food.

### CROMOLYN SODIUM ORAL CONCENTRATE

**Usual adult and adolescent dose**
Mastocytosis—
  Oral, 200 mg four times a day, thirty minutes before meals and at bedtime.

**Usual pediatric dose**
Mastocytosis—
  Premature to term infants:
    Use is not recommended.
  Term infants and children up to 2 years of age:
    Oral, 20 mg per kg of body weight per day in four divided doses. If control of symptoms is not achieved within two or three weeks in children six months to two years of age, the dosage may be increased, if neccessary, up to a maximum of 40 mg per kg per day.
Note: Use of oral cromolyn in children younger than two years of age should be reserved for patients with severe, incapacitating disease.
  Children 2 to 12 years of age:
    Oral, 100 mg four times a day, thirty minutes before meals and at bedtime.
  Children 12 years of age and older:
    See *Usual adult and adolescent dose.*

**Usual geriatric dose**
See *Usual adult and adolescent dose.*
U.S.—
  100 mg per 5 mL (Rx) [*Gastrocrom* (for oral use only)].
Note: The oral concentrate is available as unit dose ampuls.
Canada—
  Not commercially available.

**Packaging and storage**
Store between 15 and 30 °C (59 and 86 °F), unless otherwise specified by manufacturer. Keep out of the reach of children. Store ampuls in foil pouch until ready for use. Protect ampuls from light. Do not use if solution becomes cloudy or discolored.

**Preparation of dosage form**
Ampul(s) should be broken and the contents squeezed into a glass of water which is then stirred well.

Note: Not for inhalation or injection.

---
[1]Not included in Canadian product labeling.

---

Revised: 08/14/98

---

**CROTAMITON**—The *Crotamiton (Topical)* monograph is not included in this published version of the USP DI database. Copies of the monograph are available on request from Micromedex, Inc. - Reprint Requests, 6200 S. Syracuse Way, Suite 300, Englewood, CO 80111; telephone (303) 486-6400; telefax (303) 486-6464; Email: USPDI@MDX.COM.

---

**CUPRIC SULFATE**—See *Copper Supplements (Systemic)*

---

**CYANOCOBALAMIN**—See *Vitamin B$_{12}$ (Systemic)*

---

# CYANOCOBALAMIN CO 57   Systemic

**VA CLASSIFICATION (Primary):** DX201

Commonly used brand name(s): *Dicopac; Rubratrope-57.*

Note: For a listing of dosage forms and brand names by country availability, see *Dosage Forms* section(s).

## Category

Diagnostic aid, radioactive (cyanocobalamin malabsorption syndromes).

## Indications

**Accepted**

Anemia (diagnosis)—Cyanocobalamin Co 57 is indicated in the diagnosis of pernicious anemia.

Vitamin B$_{12}$ deficiency (diagnosis adjunct)—Cyanocobalamin Co 57 is indicated as an adjunct in diagnosing intestinal cyanocobalamin malabsorption syndromes due to lack of intrinsic factor (IF) or other defects in intestinal absorption (e.g., blind loop syndrome and diverticulitis, celiac disease, Crohn's disease, lesions in the small intestine, severe pancreatitis, tropical sprue).

Cyanocobalamin Co 57 may be used either in fecal excretion determinations of unabsorbed cyanocobalamin or urinary excretion determinations (Schilling test) of absorbed cyanocobalamin. However, a normal Schilling test does not rule out the possibility of vitamin B$_{12}$ deficiency.

# Cyanocobalamin Co 57 (Systemic)

## Physical Properties

### Nuclear Data

| Radionuclide (half-life) | Mode of decay | Principal emissions (keV) | Mean number of emissions/ disintegration |
|---|---|---|---|
| Co 57 (270.9 days) | Electron capture | Gamma (122) | 0.86 |
| Co 58 (71.3 days) | Electron capture 85% | Gamma 99% (810.5) | 0.84 |
|  | Positron emission 15% | Annihilation 200% (511) | 0.30 |

## Pharmacology/Pharmacokinetics

### Mechanism of action/Effect
The action of cyanocobalamin Co 57 in the body is identical to that of dietary cyanocobalamin. In order to be readily absorbed from the gastrointestinal tract, it must form a complex with intrinsic factor (IF). The absorption or lack of absorption of radiolabeled cyanocobalamin is determined by the measurement of samples of urine or feces with scintillation counting devices. In patients with pernicious anemia, absorption of cyanocobalamin is less than normal, but it may be normalized by the concurrent administration of IF with cyanocobalamin. Thus, if normal absorption is not obtained, repeat studies may be performed administering IF along with the test dose of cyanocobalamin Co 57 to differentiate pernicious anemia from other causes of cyanocobalamin malabsorption.

### Absorption
Oral—30 to 97% of doses up to 2 micrograms of cyanocobalamin (complexed to IF) are absorbed from the gastrointestinal tract in the distal ileum. At doses greater than 2 micrograms, the IF-dependent absorption process becomes saturated, and the percentage absorbed significantly decreases.

### Protein binding
High (>90%, primarily to the specific transcobalamin II vitamin $B_{12}$-binding protein).

### Half-life
For cyanocobalamin—Biological (in liver): Approximately 500 days.

### Time to peak concentration
6 to 14 hours.

### Radiation dosimetry:

**Co 57 Estimated absorbed radiation dose**

| Organ | Without flushing mGy/MBq | Without flushing rad/microcurie | With flushing* mGy/MBq | With flushing* rad/microcurie |
|---|---|---|---|---|
| Liver | 36 | 0.13 | 24 | 0.089 |
| Adrenals | 3.8 | 0.014 | 2.5 | 0.0093 |
| Pancreas | 3.8 | 0.014 | 2.6 | 0.0096 |
| Kidneys | 3.5 | 0.013 | 2.3 | 0.0085 |
| Large intestine (upper) | 2.6 | 0.0096 | 1.8 | 0.0067 |
| Lungs | 2.4 | 0.0088 | 1.6 | 0.0059 |
| Red marrow | 2.3 | 0.0085 | 1.5 | 0.0055 |
| Small intestine | 2.0 | 0.0074 | 1.4 | 0.0052 |
| Stomach wall | 2.0 | 0.0074 | 1.4 | 0.0052 |
| Bone surfaces | 1.8 | 0.0067 | 1.2 | 0.0044 |
| Breast | 1.5 | 0.0055 | 0.98 | 0.0036 |
| Spleen | 1.4 | 0.0052 | 0.97 | 0.0036 |
| Large intestine (lower) | 1.3 | 0.0048 | 0.97 | 0.0036 |
| Ovaries | 1.2 | 0.0044 | 0.83 | 0.0031 |
| Uterus | 1.2 | 0.0044 | 0.84 | 0.0031 |
| Bladder wall | 0.95 | 0.0035 | 0.64 | 0.0024 |
| Testes | 0.69 | 0.0025 | 0.46 | 0.0017 |

**Co 57 Estimated absorbed radiation dose (continued)**

| Organ | Without flushing mGy/MBq | Without flushing rad/microcurie | With flushing* mGy/MBq | With flushing* rad/microcurie |
|---|---|---|---|---|
| Thyroid | 0.66 | 0.0024 | 0.44 | 0.0016 |
| Other tissue | 1.4 | 0.0052 | 0.95 | 0.0035 |
| Effective dose | 4.0 mSv/MBq | 0.015 rem/microcurie | 2.7 mSv/MBq | 0.010 rem/microcurie |

*The administration of a flushing dose of nonradioactive cyanocobalamin decreases the absorbed radiation dose.

**Co 58 Estimated absorbed radiation dose**

| Organ | Without flushing mGy/MBq | Without flushing rad/microcurie | With flushing* mGy/MBq | With flushing* rad/microcurie |
|---|---|---|---|---|
| Liver | 54 | 0.20 | 36 | 0.13 |
| Adrenals | 10 | 0.037 | 6.7 | 0.025 |
| Pancreas | 9.1 | 0.034 | 6.1 | 0.023 |
| Kidneys | 7.9 | 0.029 | 5.3 | 0.020 |
| Large intestine (upper) | 6.3 | 0.023 | 4.4 | 0.016 |
| Lungs | 5.5 | 0.020 | 3.6 | 0.013 |
| Stomach wall | 4.9 | 0.018 | 3.3 | 0.012 |
| Small intestine | 4.7 | 0.017 | 3.2 | 0.012 |
| Breast | 3.7 | 0.014 | 2.5 | 0.0093 |
| Spleen | 3.5 | 0.013 | 2.4 | 0.0088 |
| Large intestine (lower) | 3.4 | 0.013 | 2.7 | 0.010 |
| Red marrow | 3.3 | 0.012 | 2.2 | 0.0081 |
| Uterus | 2.8 | 0.010 | 1.9 | 0.0070 |
| Bone surfaces | 2.6 | 0.0096 | 1.8 | 0.0067 |
| Ovaries | 2.5 | 0.0093 | 1.8 | 0.0067 |
| Bladder wall | 2.4 | 0.0088 | 1.6 | 0.0059 |
| Testes | 2.1 | 0.0078 | 1.4 | 0.0052 |
| Thyroid | 1.8 | 0.0067 | 1.2 | 0.0044 |
| Other tissue | 3.3 | 0.012 | 2.2 | 0.0081 |
| Effective dose | 7.5 mSv/MBq | 0.028 rem/microcurie | 5.1 mSv/MBq | 0.019 rem/microcurie |

*The administration of a flushing dose of nonradioactive cyanocobalamin decreases the absorbed radiation dose.

### Elimination
In normal patients—Renal (7 to 10% or more); fecal (50% or less).
In patients with reduced absorption—Renal (0 to 7%); fecal (70 to 100%).

Note: Diagnosis of pernicious anemia in patients with reduced absorption is confirmed if abnormal results become normal when IF is administered with the test dose of cyanocobalamin Co 57.
Cyanocobalamin Co 57 is also eliminated in breast milk.

## Precautions to Consider

### Carcinogenicity/Mutagenicity
Long-term animal studies to evaluate carcinogenic or mutagenic potential of cyanocobalamin Co 57 have not been performed.

### Pregnancy/Reproduction
Pregnancy—Adequate and well-controlled studies have not been done in humans. Diagnostic testing should be postponed, if possible, until after delivery since cyanocobalamin Co 57 crosses the placenta and is taken up by the fetus.
To avoid the possibility of radiation exposure to the fetus, in those circumstances where the patient's pregnancy status is uncertain, a pregnancy test will help to prevent inadvertent administration of this preparation during pregnancy.
Studies have not been done in animals.
FDA Pregnancy Category C.

### Breast-feeding
Cyanocobalamin Co 57 is excreted in breast milk in very small concentrations. Although discontinuation of breast-feeding is not essential, because of the potential risk to the infant from radiation exposure, tempo-

rary discontinuation of nursing is recommended for a short period of time.

**Pediatrics**

Although cyanocobalamin Co 57 is used in children, there have been no specific studies evaluating safety and efficacy. When used in children, the diagnostic benefit should be judged to outweigh the potential risk of radiation.

**Geriatrics**

Appropriate studies performed to date have not demonstrated geriatrics-specific problems that would limit the usefulness of cyanocobalamin Co 57 in the elderly. However, elderly patients are more likely to have age-related renal function impairment which may falsely depress Schilling test results; a 48-hour urine collection period (instead of the usual 24-hour period) is recommended in patients with impaired renal function.

Also, in geriatric patients with gastric atrophy that is severe enough to cause a lack of gastric acid and enzymes, the splitting of vitamin $B_{12}$ from its peptide linkages in food cannot be accomplished, thus causing vitamin $B_{12}$ deficiency. However, the gastric atrophy may not be severe enough to cause a lack of gastric intrinsic factor and thus the results of the Schilling test may be normal, unless cyanocobalamin Co 57 is given after incubation with serum protein (e.g., chicken serum).

**Drug interactions and/or related problems**

See *Laboratory value alterations*.

**Laboratory value alterations**

The following have been selected on the basis of their potential clinical significance (possible effect in parentheses where appropriate)—not necessarily inclusive (» = major clinical significance):

With result of *this* test
Due to other medications
  Alcohol, excessive intake for longer than 2 weeks or
  Aminosalicylates or
  Antibiotics, especially oral neomycin or
  Anticonvulsants, especially phenobarbital, phenytoin, and primidone or
  Calcium-chelating agents, such as edetate disodium and penicillamine or
  Cholestyramine, prolonged use or
  Colchicine or
  Potassium, extended-release
    (may impair absorption of radioactive cyanocobalamin )
  Cyanocobalamin, nonradioactive
    (prior administration may impair absorption and excretion of cyanocobalamin Co 57; it is recommended that 24 hours elapse before the administration of cyanocobalamin Co 57)
Due to medical problems or conditions
  Renal function impairment
    (Schilling test results may be falsely depressed)
With results of *other* tests
  Bone marrow studies and
  Cyanocobalamin determinations, serum and
  Reticulocyte counts
    (values may be altered because of hematopoietic response resulting from administration of large parenteral doses of cyanocobalamin given in conjunction with Schilling test; it is recommended that these tests be done prior to Schilling test)

**Medical considerations/Contraindications**

The medical considerations/contraindications included have been selected on the basis of their potential clinical significance (reasons given in parentheses where appropriate)—not necessarily inclusive (» = major clinical significance).

See also *Laboratory value alterations*.

*Risk-benefit should be considered when the following medical problem exists:*

Sensitivity to cyanocobalamin

## Side/Adverse Effects

Note: Presently, there are no known side/adverse effects associated with cyanocobalamin Co 57 used orally as a diagnostic aid. However, side/adverse effects, such as anaphylactic shock, have been reported with the parenteral use of nonradioactive cyanocobalamin.

## Patient Consultation

As an aid to patient consultation, refer to *Advice for the Patient, Radiopharmaceuticals (Diagnostic)*.

In providing consultation, consider emphasizing the following selected information (» = major clinical significance):

Description of use
  Action in the body: Identical to dietary cyanocobalamin
  Absorption of radioactive cyanocobalamin determined by measurement of radioactivity in urine or fecal samples
  Small amounts used in diagnosis; radiation exposure is considered low
Before having this test
» Conditions affecting use, especially:
    Sensitivity to cyanocobalamin
      Pregnancy—Crosses the placenta; risk to fetus from radiation exposure as opposed to benefit derived from use should be considered
      Breast-feeding—Excreted in breast milk; temporary discontinuation of nursing recommended because of risk of radiation exposure to infant
      Use in children—Risk of radiation exposure
Preparation for this test
  Special preparatory instructions may be given; patient should inquire in advance:
    Avoiding oral or parenteral cyanocobalamin for at least 24 hours prior to administration of cyanocobalamin Co 57
    Fasting for at least 8 to 12 hours prior to administration of cyanocobalamin Co 57
Precautions after having this test
  No special precautions when used for diagnosis
Side/adverse effects
  No side effects reported with diagnostic doses

## General Dosing Information

Radiopharmaceuticals are to be administered only by or under the supervision of physicians who have had extensive training in the safe use and handling of radionuclides and who are approved by the appropriate State agency or, outside the U.S., the appropriate authority.

Fasting is recommended for at least 8 to 12 hours prior to the administration of the test dose of cyanocobalamin Co 57. Two hours after the ingestion of the test dose, a light breakfast may be given.

Voiding is recommended immediately prior to the administration of the test dose of cyanocobalamin Co 57. Also, radioactivity measurement of a pre-test urine sample should be obtained prior to starting the study to establish the absence of any potentially interfering radioisotope.

To prevent interference with absorption and elimination, at least 24 hours should elapse prior to the administration of cyanocobalamin Co 57 if a flushing dose for the Schilling test or a therapeutic injection of cyanocobalamin has previously been administered.

In the Schilling test, a flushing dose of 1 mg of nonradioactive cyanocobalamin must be intramuscularly injected within 2 hours following the administration of cyanocobalamin Co 57. A second flushing dose may be injected 24 hours later to help reduce the amount of radioactivity retained by the body.

Manufacturer's package insert or other appropriate literature should be consulted for specific test procedure.

**Safety considerations for handling this radiopharmaceutical**

Improper handling of this radiopharmaceutical may cause radioactive contamination. Guidelines for handling radioactive material have been prepared by scientific, professional, state, federal, and international bodies and are available to the specially qualified and authorized users who have access to radiopharmaceuticals.

## Oral Dosage Forms

### CYANOCOBALAMIN Co 57 CAPSULES USP

**Usual adult and adolescent administered activity**

Diagnosis of cyanocobalamin malabsorption syndromes—
  Oral, 0.02 to 0.037 megabecquerel (0.5 to 1 microcurie).

  Note: If the test kit containing both the cyanocobalamin Co 57 (bound to intrinsic factor [IF]) and the cyanocobalamin Co 58 capsules is used, both capsules are administered simultaneously. The test is performed in a manner similar to the Schilling test, except that both vitamin $B_{12}$ absorption and response to IF are measured simultaneously.

**Usual pediatric administered activity**

See *Usual adult and adolescent administered activity*.

**Usual geriatric administered activity**

See *Usual adult and adolescent administered activity*.

## Cyanocobalamin Co 57 (Systemic)

### Strength(s) usually available
U.S.—
- 0.02 megabecquerel (0.5 microcurie), with a specific activity ranging from 0.02 to 0.037 megabecquerel (0.5 to 1 microcurie) per microgram of cyanocobalamin, per capsule, at time of calibration (Rx) [GENERIC].
- 0.02 to 0.037 megabecquerel (0.5 to 1 microcurie), nominal activity per capsule, at time of calibration (Rx) [*Rubratrope-57*].
- 0.02 megabecquerel (0.5 microcurie), nominal activity per capsule, at time of calibration (Rx) [*Dicopac*].

Note: The *Dicopac* test kit also contains a capsule of cyanocobalamin Co 58 with 0.03 megabecquerel (0.8 microcurie), nominal activity at time of calibration.

Canada—
- 0.02 megabecquerel (0.5 microcurie) per capsule, at time of calibration (Rx) [GENERIC].

### Packaging and storage
Store below 40 °C (104 °F), preferably between 15 and 30 °C (59 and 86 °F), unless otherwise specified by manufacturer. Store in a well-closed, light-resistant container.

Note: The *Dicopac* test kit should be stored between 2 and 4 °C (36 and 40 °F).

### Stability
Deteriorates in presence of strong light, traces of reducing agents, or microorganisms. Decomposes when autoclaved at 115 °C (239 °F) for 30 minutes.

### Note
Caution—Radioactive material.

### Selected Bibliography
Zuckier LS, Chervu LR. Schilling evaluation of pernicious anemia: current status. J Nucl Med 1984; 25(9): 1032-9.

Revised: 08/08/92
Interim revision: 08/02/94

---

**CYCLANDELATE**—The *Cyclandelate (Systemic)* monograph is not included in this published version of the USP DI database. Copies of the monograph are available on request from Micromedex, Inc. - Reprint Requests, 6200 S. Syracuse Way, Suite 300, Englewood, CO 80111; telephone (303) 486-6400; telefax (303) 486-6464; Email: USPDI@MDX.COM.

---

**CYCLIZINE**—The *Cyclizine (Systemic)* monograph is not included in this published version of the USP DI database. Copies of the monograph are available on request from Micromedex, Inc. - Reprint Requests, 6200 S. Syracuse Way, Suite 300, Englewood, CO 80111; telephone (303) 486-6400; telefax (303) 486-6464; Email: USPDI@MDX.COM.

---

# CYCLOBENZAPRINE  Systemic

VA CLASSIFICATION (Primary): MS200
Commonly used brand name(s): *Cycoflex*; *Flexeril*.

Note: For a listing of dosage forms and brand names by country availability, see *Dosage Forms* section(s).

## Category
Skeletal muscle relaxant.

## Indications
Note: Bracketed information in the *Indications* section refers to uses that are not included in U.S. product labeling.

### Accepted
Spasm, skeletal muscle (treatment)—Cyclobenzaprine is indicated as an adjunct to other measures, such as rest and physical therapy, for the relief of muscle spasm associated with acute, painful musculoskeletal conditions. It is not effective in relieving muscle spasm or spasticity caused by central nervous system (CNS) disorders.

[Fibromyalgia syndrome][1]—Cyclobenzaprine is indicated in the treatment of fibromyalgia syndrome (fibrositis, fibrositis syndrome). It has been shown to decrease pain, reduce muscle tightness and the number of tender points, and improve sleep in patients with this condition.

[1] Not included in Canadian product labeling.

## Pharmacology/Pharmacokinetics

### Physicochemical characteristics
Molecular weight—311.85.
pKa—8.47 (25 °C).

### Mechanism of action/Effect
The precise mechanism of action has not been fully determined. Cyclobenzaprine acts primarily at the brain stem to reduce tonic somatic motor activity influencing both gamma and alpha motoneurons. Actions at spinal cord sites may also be involved.

### Other actions/effects
Cyclobenzaprine is structurally related to, and may have actions similar to, the tricyclic antidepressants. These possible effects include central and peripheral anticholinergic actions, a sedative effect, and an increase in heart rate.

### Absorption
Well (but slowly) absorbed following oral administration.

### Protein binding
Very high (93%), with plasma concentrations ranging from 0.1 to 1 mcg per mL (0.32 to 3.21 micromoles per L).

### Biotransformation
Gastrointestinal and hepatic.

### Half-life
1 to 3 days.

### Onset of action
Within 1 hour.

### Time to peak concentration
3 to 8 hours.

### Peak serum concentration
15 to 25 nanograms per mL (0.048 to 0.08 micromoles per L) following a single 10-mg oral dose; subject to large interpatient variation.

### Therapeutic plasma concentration
20 to 30 nanograms per mL (0.064 to 0.096 micromoles per L).

### Time to peak effect
1 to 2 weeks.

### Duration of action
Single dose—12 to 24 hours.

### Elimination
Renal, primarily as conjugated metabolites (<1% of a dose is excreted unchanged); 51% of a single 10-mg dose is excreted within 5 days. Cyclobenzaprine undergoes enterohepatic circulation. Some unchanged cyclobenzaprine is also eliminated via the bile and feces.

## Precautions to Consider

### Carcinogenicity
Cyclobenzaprine did not show evidence of carcinogenicity in an 81-week study in mice or a 105-week study in rats.

### Mutagenicity
No evidence of mutagenicity occurred in male mice receiving up to 20 times the human dose of cyclobenzaprine.

### Pregnancy/Reproduction
Fertility—No evidence of impaired fertility occurred in male or female rats receiving up to 10 times the human dose of cyclobenzaprine.

Pregnancy—Adequate and well-controlled studies in humans have not been done.

Studies in rats, mice, and rabbits have not shown that cyclobenzaprine has adverse effects on the fetus when given in doses up to 20 times the human dose.

FDA Pregnancy Category B.

### Breast-feeding
Problems in humans have not been documented. It is not known whether cyclobenzaprine is distributed into breast milk; however, it is known

that some of the structurally related tricyclic antidepressants are distributed into breast milk.

**Pediatrics**
No information is available on the relationship of age to the effects of cyclobenzaprine in pediatric patients. Safety and efficacy have not been established.

**Adolescents**
No information is available on the relationship of age to the effects of cyclobenzaprine in adolescents up to 15 years of age. Safety and efficacy have not been established.

**Geriatrics**
No information is available on the relationship of age to the effects of cyclobenzaprine in geriatric patients. However, it is known that geriatric patients exhibit increased sensitivity to other medications with anticholinergic activity and are more likely than younger adults to experience adverse reactions to the tricyclic antidepressants, which are structurally related to cyclobenzaprine.

**Dental**
The peripheral anticholinergic effects of cyclobenzaprine may inhibit salivary flow, thus contributing to the development of caries, periodontal disease, oral candidiasis, and discomfort.

**Drug interactions and/or related problems**
The following drug interactions and/or related problems have been selected on the basis of their potential clinical significance (possible mechanism in parentheses where appropriate)—not necessarily inclusive (» = major clinical significance):

Note: Combinations containing any of the following medications, depending on the amount present, may also interact with this medication.
In addition to the documented interactions listed below, the possibility should be considered that other interactions applying to tricyclic antidepressants may also apply to cyclobenzaprine because they are all chemically related.

» Alcohol or
» Antidepressants, tricyclic or
» CNS depression–producing medications, other (See *Appendix II*)
(concurrent use with cyclobenzaprine may result in additive CNS depressant effects; caution is recommended, and dosage of one or both agents should be reduced)
(concurrent use of a tricyclic antidepressant with cyclobenzaprine may also increase the risk of other side effects, such as anticholinergic effects and increased heart rate)

Antidyskinetics or
Anticholinergics or other medications with anticholinergic activity (See *Appendix II*)
(cyclobenzaprine may potentiate the anticholinergic actions of these medications; patients should be advised to report occurrence of gastrointestinal problems promptly, since paralytic ileus may occur)

Guanadrel or
Guanethidine
(cyclobenzaprine may decrease or block the antihypertensive effects of these medications)

» Monoamine oxidase (MAO) inhibitors, including furazolidone, procarbazine, and selegiline
(concurrent use with cyclobenzaprine is not recommended on an outpatient basis, as hyperpyretic crises, severe seizures, and death have resulted when MAO inhibitors were used concurrently with tricyclic antidepressants; a minimum of 14 days should elapse between discontinuance of MAO inhibitors and initiation of cyclobenzaprine therapy, unless the patient is hospitalized; a minimum of 5 to 7 days should elapse between discontinuance of cyclobenzaprine and initiation of MAO inhibitor therapy)

**Medical considerations/Contraindications**
The medical considerations/contraindications included have been selected on the basis of their potential clinical significance (reasons given in parentheses where appropriate)—not necessarily inclusive (» = major clinical significance).

*Except under special circumstances, this medication should not be used when the following medical problems exist:*
» Acute recovery phase of myocardial infarction or
» Cardiac arrhythmias or
» Congestive heart failure or
» Heart block or other conduction disturbances
(possible adverse cardiovascular effects)

» Hyperthyroidism
(increased risk of cardiac arrhythmias; also, tachycardia associated with hyperthyroidism may be exacerbated)

*Risk-benefit should be considered when the following medical problems exist:*
Glaucoma or predisposition to or
Urinary retention or history of
(cyclobenzaprine's anticholinergic effects may be detrimental to patients with these conditions)
Sensitivity to cyclobenzaprine

## Side/Adverse Effects

The following side/adverse effects have been selected on the basis of their potential clinical significance (possible signs and symptoms in parentheses where appropriate)—not necessarily inclusive:

**Those indicating need for medical attention**
Incidence rare
*Anaphylaxis* (changes in facial skin color; skin rash, hives, and/or itching; fast or irregular breathing; puffiness or swelling of the eyelids or the area around the eyes; shortness of breath, troubled breathing, tightness in chest, and/or wheezing); *angioedema* (large, hive-like swellings on face, eyelids, mouth, lips, and/or tongue); *anticholinergic effect* (problems in urinating); *CNS toxicity* (abnormal thinking and dreaming; clumsiness or unsteadiness; severe confusion or disorientation; mental depression; ringing or buzzing in ears); *dermatitis, allergic* (skin rash, hives, or itching); *hepatitis/cholestasis* (yellow eyes or skin); *syncope* (fainting)

Note: *Mania* has also been reported in a few patients with pre-existing psychiatric illness.

**Those indicating need for medical attention only if they continue or are bothersome**
Incidence more frequent
*Anticholinergic effects* (dryness of mouth [7 to 27%] blurred vision [<3%]); *dizziness or lightheadedness*—3 to 11%; *drowsiness*—16 to 39%

Note: *Dizziness, lightheadedness,* and *drowsiness* may be caused by cyclobenzaprine's anticholinergic, as well as its CNS, effects.

Incidence less frequent or rare (<3%)
*CNS effects* (headache; confusion; excitement or nervousness; general feeling of discomfort or illness; numbness, tingling, pain, or weakness in hands or feet; muscle twitching; trembling; trouble in sleeping; unusual tiredness); *constipation; frequent urination; gastrointestinal irritation* (stomach cramps or pain; bloated feeling or gas; diarrhea; indigestion; nausea; vomiting); *pounding heartbeat; problems in speaking; unpleasant taste or other taste changes; unusual muscle weakness*

## Overdose

For specific information on the agents used in the management of cyclobenzaprine overdose, see:
*Benzodiazepines (Systemic)* monograph;
*Charcoal, Activated (Oral-Local)* monograph;
*Neostigmine* in *Antimyasthenics (Systemic)* monograph;
*Physostigmine (Systemic)* monograph;
*Propranolol* in *Beta-adrenergic Blocking Agents (Systemic)* monograph; and/or
*Pyridostigmine* in *Antimyasthenics (Systemic)* monograph.

For more information on the management of overdose or unintentional ingestion, **contact a Poison Control Center** (see *Poison Control Center Listing*).

**Clinical effects of overdose**
The following effects have been on the basis of their potential clinical significance (possible signs and symptoms in parentheses where appropriate)—not necessarily inclusive:

Acute and chronic
*Cardiotoxicity* (fast or irregular heartbeat; low blood pressure; troubled breathing)—may include bundle branch block or other arrhythmias and congestive heart failure; *CNS toxicity* (severe confusion; delirium; convulsions; severe drowsiness; hallucinations; severe nervousness or restlessness); *dry, hot, flushed skin*—a few cases of paradoxical diaphoresis have also been reported; *increase or decrease in body temperature; unexplained muscle stiffness; vomiting*

**Treatment of overdose**
To decrease absorption—Emptying the stomach via induction of emesis, gastric lavage, or activated charcoal.

**Cyclobenzaprine (Systemic)**

Monitoring—Taking an electrocardiogram (ECG) and monitoring cardiac function if any signs of dysrhythmia are evident.

Careful monitoring of the patient.

Specific treatment—

Use of physostigmine salicylate for severe or life-threatening anticholinergic effects. Repeating dose as required if life-threatening symptoms (e.g., arrhythmias, convulsions, coma) persist or recur. Because of its toxicity, physostigmine is recommended only in severe cases. See the package insert or *Physostigmine (Systemic)* for specific dosing guidelines for use of this product.

Use of neostigmine, pyridostigmine, or propranolol for cardiac arrhythmias. See the package insert or *Neostigmine* or *Pyridostigmine* in *Antimyasthenics (Systemic)* or *Propranolol* in *Beta-adrenergic Blocking Agents (Systemic)* for specific dosing guidelines for use of this product.

Use of a short-acting digitalis preparation for cardiac failure should be considered. Close monitoring of cardiac function for at least 5 days is recommended. See the package insert or *Digitalis Glycosides (Systemic)* for specific dosing guidelines for use of this product.

Use of an appropriate anticonvulsant for convulsions. Benzodiazepines are most often used. However, because intravenously administered benzodiazepines may cause respiratory and circulatory depression, especially when administered rapidly, medications and equipment needed for support of respiration and for resuscitation must be immediately available. See the package insert or *Benzodiazepines (Systemic)* for specific dosing guidelines for use of this product.

Supportive—May include maintaining an open airway, maintaining adequate fluid intake, regulating body temperature, and treating circulatory shock, convulsions, and metabolic acidosis, if necessary. Patients in whom intentional overdose is known or suspected should be referred for psychiatric consultation.

Note: Dialysis is probably of no value in removing cyclobenzaprine from the body.

## Patient Consultation

As an aid to patient consultation, refer to *Advice for the Patient, Cyclobenzaprine (Systemic)*.

In providing consultation, consider emphasizing the following selected information (» = major clinical significance):

### Before using this medication
» Conditions affecting use, especially:
   Sensitivity to cyclobenzaprine
   Other medications, especially other CNS depression–producing medications, monoamine oxidase inhibitors, and tricyclic antidepressants
   Other medical problems, especially cardiac arrhythmias, congestive heart failure, heart block or other conduction disturbances, hyperthyroidism, and myocardial infarction (acute recovery phase)

### Proper use of this medication
Not taking more medication than the amount prescribed, to minimize possibility of side effects
» Proper dosing
   Missed dose: Taking if remembered within an hour; not taking if not remembered until later; not doubling doses
» Proper storage

### Precautions while using this medication
» Avoiding alcohol or other CNS depressants unless prescribed or otherwise approved by physician
» Caution if blurred vision, drowsiness, or dizziness occurs

Possible dryness of mouth; using sugarless gum or candy, ice, or saliva substitute for relief; checking with dentist if dry mouth continues for more than 2 weeks

### Side/adverse effects
Signs and symptoms of potential side effects, especially anaphylaxis, angioedema, allergic dermatitis, hepatitis, and syncope

## General Dosing Information

It is recommended that cyclobenzaprine therapy for acute, painful musculoskeletal conditions be discontinued after 2 to 3 weeks, because evidence of its effectiveness for longer periods is not available. However, studies of the usefulness of cyclobenzaprine in fibromyalgia syndrome have indicated that the medication remains effective for at least 12 weeks.

Cyclobenzaprine is closely related to the tricyclic antidepressants and shares many of their adverse reactions and drug interactions.

## Oral Dosage Forms

Note: Bracketed uses in the *Dosage Forms* section refer to categories of use and/or indications that are not included in U.S. product labeling.

### CYCLOBENZAPRINE HYDROCHLORIDE TABLETS USP

**Usual adult dose**
Acute musculoskeletal conditions—Oral, 20 to 40 mg a day in two to four divided doses, usually 10 mg three times a day.
[Fibromyalgia syndrome][1]—Oral, 5 to 40 mg at bedtime.

**Usual adult prescribing limits**
Not to exceed 60 mg daily.

**Usual pediatric and adolescent dose**
Children up to 15 years of age—Dosage has not been established.
Patients 15 years of age and older—See *Usual adult dose*

**Strength(s) usually available**
U.S.—
  10 mg (Rx) [*Cycoflex; Flexeril;* GENERIC].
Canada—
  10 mg (Rx) [*Flexeril*].

**Packaging and storage**
Store below 40 °C (104 °F), preferably between 15 and 30 °C (59 and 86 °F). Store in a well-closed container.

**Auxiliary labeling**
- May cause drowsiness.
- Avoid alcoholic beverages.

[1]Not included in Canadian product labeling.

## Selected Bibliography

Katz WA, Dube J. Cyclobenzaprine in the treatment of acute muscle spasm: review of a decade of clinical experience. Clin Ther 1988; 10: 216-28.

Revised: 07/28/94

---

**CYCLOPENTOLATE**—The *Cyclopentolate (Ophthalmic)* monograph is not included in this published version of the USP DI database. Copies of the monograph are available on request from Micromedex, Inc. - Reprint Requests, 6200 S. Syracuse Way, Suite 300, Englewood, CO 80111; telephone (303) 486-6400; telefax (303) 486-6464; Email: USPDI@MDX.COM.

---

# CYCLOPHOSPHAMIDE  Systemic

VA CLASSIFICATION (Primary/Secondary): AN100/DE801; IM600; MS105

Commonly used brand name(s): *Cytoxan; Neosar; Procytox*.

Note: For a listing of dosage forms and brand names by country availability, see *Dosage Forms* section(s).

## Category
Antineoplastic; immunosuppressant.

## Indications
Note: Bracketed information in the *Indications* section refers to uses that are not included in U.S. product labeling.

### Accepted
Leukemia, acute lymphocytic (treatment) or
Leukemia, acute nonlymphocytic (treatment)—Cyclophosphamide is indicated for treatment of acute lymphoblastic (stem-cell) leukemia in children (including during remission to prolong the duration), and for treatment of acute nonlymphocytic leukemia.

Leukemia, chronic myelocytic (treatment) or
Leukemia, chronic lymphocytic (treatment)—Cyclophosphamide is indicated for treatment of chronic granulocytic leukemia (it is usually ineffective in acute blastic crisis) and chronic lymphocytic leukemia.
Carcinoma, ovarian, epithelial (treatment)
Carcinoma, breast (treatment)
Neuroblastoma (treatment)
Retinoblastoma (treatment)
[Carcinoma, lung, non-small cell (treatment)]
[Carcinoma, lung, small cell (treatment)]
[Carcinoma, cervical (treatment)][1]
[Carcinoma, endometrial (treatment)][1]
[Carcinoma, bladder (treatment)][1]
[Carcinoma, prostatic (treatment)][1]
[Carcinoma, testicular (treatment)][1] or
[Wilms' tumor (treatment)][1]—Cyclophosphamide is indicated for treatment of adenocarcinoma of the ovary, breast carcinoma, neuroblastoma [in patients with disseminated disease], retinoblastoma, small-cell and non–small-cell lung carcinoma, cervical carcinoma, and for endometrial carcinoma, bladder carcinoma, prostatic carcinoma, testicular carcinoma, and Wilms' tumor.
Lymphomas, Hodgkin's (treatment) or
Lymphomas, non-Hodgkin's (treatment)—Cyclophosphamide is indicated for treatment of Stage III and IV (Ann Arbor or Peter's Staging System) Hodgkin's disease and non-Hodgkin's lymphomas including nodular or diffuse lymphocytic lymphoma, mixed-cell type lymphoma, histiocytic lymphoma, Burkitt's lymphoma, and [lymphoblastic lymphosarcoma].
Multiple myeloma (treatment)—Cyclophosphamide is indicated for treatment of multiple myeloma.
Mycosis fungoides (treatment)—Cyclophosphamide is indicated for treatment of advanced mycosis fungoides.
Nephrotic syndrome (treatment)[1]—Cyclophosphamide is indicated as an immunosuppressant in the treatment of steroid-resistant or frequently relapsing steroid-sensitive biopsy-proven minimal-change nephrotic syndrome in children [and adults].
[Ewing's sarcoma (treatment)][1]
[Osteosarcoma, (treatment)][1]or
[Sarcomas, soft tissue (treatment)][1]—Cyclophosphamide is indicated for treatment of various sarcomas, including Ewing's sarcoma, osteosarcoma, and soft-tissue sarcomas.
[Tumors, germ cell, ovarian (treatment)][1]
[Tumors, brain, primary][1] or
[Tumors, trophoblastic, gestational][1]—Cyclophosphamide is indicated for treatment of germ cell ovarian, primary brain, and gestational trophoblastic tumors.
[Thymoma][1]—Cyclophosphamide is indicated for treatment of thymoma.
[Waldenström's macroglobulinemia][1]—Cyclophosphamide is indicated for treatment of Waldenström's macroglobulinemia.
[Transplant rejection, organ (prophylaxis)][1]—Cyclophosphamide is used for its immunosuppressant activity, for prevention of rejection in homotransplantation.
[Arthritis, rheumatoid (treatment)][1]
[Wegener's granulomatosis (treatment)][1]
[Lupus erythematosus, systemic][1]
[Dermatomyositis, systemic (treatment)][1] or
[Multiple sclerosis (treatment)][1]—Cyclophosphamide is used as an immunosuppressant in the treatment of rheumatoid arthritis and other autoimmune diseases such as polymyositis (systemic dermatomyositis), multiple sclerosis, Wegener's granulomatosis, systemic lupus erythematosus (SLE), and other types of vasculitis.
Extreme caution is recommended in use of cyclophosphamide for non-neoplastic conditions because of potential carcinogenicity with long-term use of this agent.

[1]Not included in Canadian product labeling.

## Pharmacology/Pharmacokinetics

**Physicochemical characteristics**
Molecular weight—279.10.

**Mechanism of action/Effect**
Cyclophosphamide is classed as an alkylating agent of the nitrogen mustard type. An activated form of cyclophosphamide, phosphoramide mustard, alkylates or binds with many intracellular molecular structures, including nucleic acids. Its cytotoxic action is primarily due to cross-linking of strands of DNA and RNA, as well as inhibition of protein synthesis.

**Other actions/effects**
Cyclophosphamide is a potent immunosuppressant. It also causes marked and persistent inhibition of cholinesterase activity.

**Absorption**
Well absorbed after oral administration (bioavailability greater than 75%).

**Distribution**
Crosses blood-brain barrier to limited extent.

**Protein binding**
Very low (some active metabolites—greater than 60%).

**Biotransformation**
Hepatic (including initial activation and subsequent degradation).

**Half-life**
Unchanged drug—3 to 12 hours.

**Time to peak concentration**
Plasma—Metabolites: 2 to 3 hours after intravenous administration.

**Elimination**
Renal, 5 to 25% unchanged.
In dialysis—Cyclophosphamide is dialyzable.

## Precautions to Consider

**Carcinogenicity/Mutagenicity**
Secondary malignancies are potential delayed effects of many antineoplastic agents, although it is not clear whether the effect is related to their mutagenic or immunosuppressive action. The effect of dose and duration of therapy is also unknown, although risk seems to increase with long-term use. Although information is limited, available data seem to indicate that the carcinogenic risk is greatest with the alkylating agents.
Cyclophosphamide is a potent carcinogen in animals. In humans, it has been associated with development of myeloproliferative and lymphoproliferative carcinomas as well as urinary bladder carcinoma (especially in patients who developed hemorrhagic cystitis while receiving cyclophosphamide) up to several years after administration. One case of carcinoma of the renal pelvis occurred in a patient who received long-term treatment with cyclophosphamide for cerebral vasculitis.

**Pregnancy/Reproduction**
Fertility—Gonadal suppression, resulting in amenorrhea or azoospermia, may occur in patients taking antineoplastic therapy, especially with the alkylating agents. In general, these effects appear to be related to dose and length of therapy and may be irreversible. Prediction of the degree of testicular or ovarian function impairment is complicated by the common use of combinations of several antineoplastics, which makes it difficult to assess the effects of individual agents.
However, there have been numerous reports of gonadal suppression with use of cyclophosphamide, which seems to depend on dose, duration, and state of gonadal function at the time of therapy; sterility may be irreversible in some patients.
Paternal use of cyclophosphamide prior to conception has been associated with cardiac and limb abnormalities in an infant.
Pregnancy—Cyclophosphamide crosses the placenta. Use in humans has resulted in both normal and malformed (missing fingers and/or toes, cardiac anomalies, hernias) newborns; risk seems to be less in the second and third trimesters. Low birth weight is also a risk with exposure of the fetus to antineoplastics.
First trimester: It is usually recommended that use of antineoplastics, especially combination chemotherapy, be avoided whenever possible, especially during the first trimester. Although information is limited because of the relatively few instances of antineoplastic administration during pregnancy, the mutagenic, teratogenic, and carcinogenic potential of these medications must be considered.
Other hazards to the fetus include adverse reactions seen in adults.
In general, use of a contraceptive is recommended during cytotoxic drug therapy.
Studies in animals have shown that cyclophosphamide is teratogenic in mice, rats, rabbits, and monkeys given 0.02, 0.08, 0.5, and 0.07 times the human dose, respectively.
FDA Pregnancy Category D.

**Breast-feeding**
Cyclophosphamide is distributed into breast milk. Breast-feeding is not recommended during chemotherapy because of the risks to the infant (adverse effects, mutagenicity, carcinogenicity).

**Pediatrics**
Appropriate studies performed to date have not demonstrated pediatrics-specific problems that would limit the usefulness of cyclophosphamide in children.
Prepubescent girls treated with cyclophosphamide usually develop secondary sexual characteristics normally, have regular menses, and subse-

quently conceive; however, ovarian fibrosis and apparent complete loss of germ cells after prolonged treatment in late prepubescence have been reported. Prepubescent boys treated with cyclophosphamide develop secondary sexual characteristics normally, but may have oligospermia or azoospermia, increased gonadotropin secretion, and some degree of testicular atrophy; azoospermia may be reversible, although possibly not for several years after the end of cyclophosphamide therapy.

### Geriatrics
Although appropriate studies on the relationship of age to the effects of cyclophosphamide have not been performed in the geriatric population, geriatrics-specific problems are not expected to limit the usefulness of this medication in the elderly. However, elderly patients are more likely to have age-related renal function impairment, which may require caution in patients receiving cyclophosphamide.

### Dental
The bone marrow depressant effects of cyclophosphamide may result in an increased incidence of microbial infection, delayed healing, and gingival bleeding. Dental work, whenever possible, should be completed prior to initiation of therapy or deferred until blood counts have returned to normal. Patients should be instructed in proper oral hygiene during treatment, including caution in use of regular toothbrushes, dental floss, and toothpicks.

Cyclophosphamide may also rarely cause stomatitis associated with considerable discomfort.

### Drug interactions and/or related problems
The following drug interactions and/or related problems have been selected on the basis of their potential clinical significance (possible mechanism in parentheses where appropriate)—not necessarily inclusive (» = major clinical significance):

Note: Combinations containing any of the following medications, depending on the amount present, may also interact with this medication.

Allopurinol or
Colchicine or
» Probenecid or
» Sulfinpyrazone
(cyclophosphamide may raise the concentration of blood uric acid; dosage adjustment of antigout agents may be necessary to control hyperuricemia and gout; uricosuric antigout agents may increase risk of uric acid nephropathy)
(concurrent use with allopurinol may enhance the bone marrow toxicity of cyclophosphamide; if concurrent use is required, close observation for toxic effects should be considered)

Anticoagulants, oral
(cyclophosphamide may increase anticoagulant activity as a result of decreased hepatic synthesis of procoagulant factors and interference with platelet formation, but may also decrease anticoagulant activity by an unknown mechanism)

Blood dyscrasia–causing medications (see *Appendix II*)
(leukopenic and/or thrombocytopenic effects of cyclophosphamide may be increased with concurrent or recent therapy if these medications cause the same effects; dosage adjustment of cyclophosphamide, if necessary, should be based on blood counts)

» Bone marrow depressants, other (see *Appendix II*) or
» Radiation therapy
(additive bone marrow depression may occur; dosage reduction may be required when two or more bone marrow depressants, including radiation, are used concurrently or consecutively)

» Cocaine
(inhibition of cholinesterase activity by cyclophosphamide reduces or slows cocaine metabolism, thereby increasing and/or prolonging its effects and increasing the risk of toxicity)

» Cytarabine
(concurrent use of high-dose cytarabine with cyclophosphamide for bone marrow transplant preparation has been reported to result in an increase in cardiomyopathy with subsequent death)

Daunorubicin or
Doxorubicin
(concurrent use with cyclophosphamide may result in increased cardiotoxicity; it is recommended that the total dose of daunorubicin or doxorubicin not exceed 400 mg per square meter of body surface)

Hepatic enzyme inducers (see *Appendix II*)
(these agents may induce microsomal metabolism to increase formation of alkylating metabolites of cyclophosphamide, thereby reducing the half-life and increasing the activity of cyclophosphamide)

» Immunosuppressants, other, such as:
Azathioprine
Chlorambucil
Corticosteroids, glucocorticoid
Cyclosporine
Mercaptopurine
Muromonab-CD3
(concurrent use with cyclophosphamide may increase the risk of infection and development of neoplasms)

Lovastatin
(concurrent use in cardiac transplant patients may be associated with an increased risk of rhabdomyolysis and acute renal failure)

Succinylcholine
(cyclophosphamide may decrease plasma concentrations or activity of pseudocholinesterase, the enzyme that metabolizes succinylcholine, thereby enhancing the neuromuscular blockade of succinylcholine. Increased or prolonged respiratory depression or paralysis [apnea] may occur but is of minor clinical significance while the patient is being mechanically ventilated; however, caution and careful monitoring of the patient are recommended during and following concurrent or sequential use, especially if there is a possibility of incomplete reversal of neuromuscular blockade postoperatively)

Vaccines, killed virus
(because normal defense mechanisms may be suppressed by cyclophosphamide therapy, the patient's antibody response to the vaccine may be decreased. The interval between discontinuation of medications that cause immunosuppression and restoration of the patient's ability to respond to the vaccine depends on the intensity and type of immunosuppression-causing medication used, the underlying disease, and other factors; estimates vary from 3 months to 1 year)

» Vaccines, live virus
(because normal defense mechanisms may be suppressed by cyclophosphamide therapy, concurrent use with a live virus vaccine may potentiate the replication of the vaccine virus, may increase the side/adverse effects of the vaccine virus, and/or may decrease the patient's antibody response to the vaccine; immunization of these patients should be undertaken only with extreme caution after careful review of the patient's hematologic status and only with the knowledge and consent of the physician managing the cyclophosphamide therapy. The interval between discontinuation of medications that cause immunosuppression and restoration of the patient's ability to respond to the vaccine depends on the intensity and type of immunosuppression-causing medication used, the underlying disease, and other factors; estimates vary from 3 months to 1 year. Patients with leukemia in remission should not receive live virus vaccine until at least 3 months after their last chemotherapy. In addition, immunization with oral poliovirus vaccine should be postponed in persons in close contact with the patient, especially family members)

### Laboratory value alterations
The following have been selected on the basis of their potential clinical significance (possible effect in parentheses where appropriate)—not necessarily inclusive (» = major clinical significance):

With diagnostic test results
Candida skin test and
Mumps skin test and
Trichophyton skin test and
Tuberculin PPD skin test
(positive reactions may be suppressed)

Papanicolaou (PAP) test
(false-positive results may be produced)

With physiology/laboratory test values
Pseudocholinesterase
(serum concentrations may be decreased)

Uric acid
(blood and urine concentrations may be increased)

### Medical considerations/Contraindications
The medical considerations/contraindications included have been selected on the basis of their potential clinical significance (reasons given in parentheses where appropriate)—not necessarily inclusive (» = major clinical significance).

### Risk-benefit should be considered when the following medical problems exist:
Adrenalectomy
(toxic effects of cyclophosphamide may be increased; dosage ad-

justment of both replacement steroids and cyclophosphamide may be necessary)
» Bone marrow depression
» Chickenpox, existing or recent (including recent exposure) or
» Herpes zoster
(risk of severe generalized disease)
Gout, history of or
Urate renal stones, history of
(risk of hyperuricemia)
» Hepatic function impairment
(effect of cyclophosphamide may be reduced because of its dependence on hepatic microsomal enzyme activation)
» Infection
» Renal function impairment
(reduced elimination; dosage reduction usually not necessary)
Sensitivity to cyclophosphamide
» Tumor cell infiltration of bone marrow
(a reduction by one-third to one-half in cyclophosphamide dosage for induction is recommended for patients with bone marrow depression due to tumor cell infiltration)
» Caution should be used also in patients who have had previous cytotoxic drug therapy or radiation therapy; a reduction by one-third to one-half in cyclophosphamide dosage for induction is recommended for patients with bone marrow depression due to cytotoxic or radiation therapy.

**Patient monitoring**
The following may be especially important in patient monitoring (other tests may be warranted in some patients, depending on condition; » = major clinical significance):

Alanine aminotransferase (ALT [SGPT]) values, serum and
Aspartate aminotransferase (AST [SGOT]) values, serum and
Bilirubin values, serum and
Lactate dehydrogenase (LDH) values, serum
(determinations recommended prior to initiation of therapy and at periodic intervals during therapy; frequency varies according to clinical state, agent, dose, and other agents being used concurrently)

Blood urea nitrogen (BUN) concentrations and
Creatinine concentrations, serum
(determinations recommended prior to initiation of therapy and at periodic intervals during therapy; frequency varies according to clinical state, agent, dose, and other agents being used concurrently)

» Examination of urine for microscopic hematuria
(recommended at periodic intervals during therapy, as well as for several hours following a large intravenous dose)
» Hematocrit or hemoglobin and
» Leukocyte count, total and, if appropriate, differential and
» Platelet count
(determinations recommended prior to initiation of therapy and at periodic intervals during therapy; frequency varies according to clinical state, agent, dose, and other agents being used concurrently)

Uric acid concentrations, serum
(determinations recommended prior to initiation of therapy and at periodic intervals during therapy; frequency varies according to clinical state, agent, dose, and other agents being used concurrently)

Urinary output and
Urinary specific gravity
(determinations recommended following high-dose intravenous administration to detect possible syndrome of inappropriate antidiuretic hormone [SIADH])

## Side/Adverse Effects

Note: Many "side effects" of antineoplastic therapy are unavoidable and represent the medication's pharmacologic action. Some of these (for example, leukopenia and thrombocytopenia) are actually used as parameters to aid in individual dosage titration.

The following side/adverse effects have been selected on the basis of their potential clinical significance (possible signs and symptoms in parentheses where appropriate)—not necessarily inclusive:

**Those indicating need for medical attention**
Incidence more frequent
*Gonadal suppression* (missing menstrual periods); *leukopenia or infection* (less frequently, fever or chills; cough or hoarseness; lower back or side pain; painful or difficult urination)—usually asymptomatic
Note: With *gonadal suppression*, regular menses usually resume within a few months after the end of cyclophosphamide therapy.

A marked *leukopenia* usually occurs, with the nadir of the leukocyte count occurring 7 to 12 days after administration and recovery after 17 to 21 days.
With high-dose and/or long-term therapy
*Cardiotoxicity, including acute myopericarditis* (fast heartbeat; fever or chills; shortness of breath); *condition resembling syndrome of inappropriate antidiuretic hormone (SIADH)* (dizziness, confusion, or agitation; unusual tiredness or weakness); *hemorrhagic cystitis* (blood in urine; painful urination); *hyperuricemia, uric acid nephropathy, nonhemorrhagic cystitis, or nephrotoxicity* (joint pain; lower back or side pain; swelling of feet or lower legs); *pneumonitis or interstitial pulmonary fibrosis* (cough, shortness of breath)
Note: *Cardiotoxicity* is most severe with use of doses of 180 to 270 mg per kg of body weight (mg/kg) within four to six days.
A few cases of severe and sometimes fatal *congestive heart failure* have occurred within a few days after the first dose of a high-dose course of cyclophosphamide; histopathologic examination primarily revealed *hemorrhagic myocarditis*. Hemopericardium has occurred secondary to hemorrhagic myocarditis and myocardial necrosis. Pericarditis has been reported independent of any hemopericardium.
*Hemorrhagic cystitis* may occur within a few hours or be delayed several weeks; thought to be caused by metabolites of cyclophosphamide (chloroacetic acid, acrolein) excreted in the urine. Usually resolves a few days after withdrawal of cyclophosphamide, but may persist; may be fatal. Fibrosis of the urinary bladder, with or without cystitis, may also occur and may be extensive. Atypical urinary bladder epithelial cells may be found in urine. Hemorrhagic ureteritis and renal tubular necrosis, which usually resolve after withdrawal of cyclophosphamide, have also been reported.
*Hyperuricemia* with uric acid nephropathy occurs most commonly during initial treatment of patients with leukemia or lymphoma, as a result of rapid cell breakdown which leads to elevated serum uric acid concentrations.
Incidence less frequent
*Anemia; thrombocytopenia* (unusual bleeding or bruising; black, tarry stools; blood in urine or stools; pinpoint red spots on skin)—usually asymptomatic
Incidence rare
*Anaphylactic reaction* (sudden shortness of breath); *hemorrhagic colitis* (black, tarry stools); *hepatitis* (yellow eyes or skin); *hyperglycemia* (frequent urination; unusual thirst); *redness, swelling, or pain at site of injection; stomatitis* (sores in mouth and on lips)
Note: *Anaphylaxis* has resulted in death.

**Those indicating need for medical attention only if they continue or are bothersome**
Incidence more frequent
*Darkening of skin and fingernails; loss of appetite; nausea or vomiting*—especially with high oral doses
Incidence less frequent
*Diarrhea or stomach pain; flushing or redness of face; headache; increased sweating; myxedema* (swollen lips); *skin rash, hives, or itching*

**Those not indicating need for medical attention**
Incidence more frequent
*Loss of hair*
Note: Normal *hair growth* usually returns after treatment has ended, although it may be slightly different in color or texture.

**Those indicating the need for medical attention if they occur after medication is discontinued**
*Hemorrhagic cystitis* (blood in urine)

## Patient Consultation

As an aid to patient consultation, refer to *Advice for the Patient, Cyclophosphamide (Systemic)*.
In providing consultation, consider emphasizing the following selected information (» = major clinical significance):

**Before using this medication**
» Conditions affecting use, especially:
Sensitivity to cyclophosphamide
Pregnancy—Use not recommended because of mutagenic, teratogenic, and carcinogenic potential; advisability of using contraception; telling physician immediately if pregnancy is suspected
Breast-feeding—Not recommended because of risk of serious side effects

Other medications, especially probenecid, sulfinpyrazone, other bone marrow depressants, other immunosuppressants, or cytotoxic drug or radiation therapy

Other medical problems, especially chickenpox, herpes zoster, hepatic function impairment, other infections, or renal function impairment

**Proper use of this medication**
» Importance of not taking more or less medication than the amount prescribed

Caution in taking combination therapy; taking each medication at the right time
» Importance of ample fluid intake and subsequent increase in urine output, as well as frequent voiding (including at least once during night), to prevent hemorrhagic cystitis and aid in excretion of uric acid; following physician instructions for recommended fluid intake; some patients may require up to 3000 mL (3 quarts) per day

Usually best if taken in the morning to reduce risk of hemorrhagic cystitis; however, physician may recommend taking in small doses throughout day to lessen stomach upset; following physician's instructions for timing of doses
» Probability of nausea, vomiting, and loss of appetite; importance of continuing medication despite stomach upset; checking with physician before discontinuing medication

Checking with physician if vomiting occurs shortly after dose is taken
» Proper dosing

Missed dose: Not taking at all; not doubling doses; checking with physician
» Proper storage

**Precautions while using this medication**
» Importance of close monitoring by physician
» Avoiding immunizations unless approved by physician; other persons in patient's household should avoid immunizations with oral poliovirus vaccine; avoiding persons who have taken oral poliovirus vaccine or wearing a protective mask that covers nose and mouth

Caution if any kind of surgery, including dental surgery, or emergency treatment with general anesthesia is required within 10 days of treatment

*Caution if bone marrow depression occurs*
» Avoiding exposure to persons with infections, especially during periods of low blood counts; checking with physician immediately if fever or chills, cough or hoarseness, lower back or side pain, or painful or difficult urination occurs
» Checking with physician immediately if unusual bleeding or bruising; black, tarry stools; blood in urine; or pinpoint red spots on skin occur

Caution in use of regular toothbrush, dental floss, or toothpick; physician, dentist, or nurse may suggest alternatives; checking with physician before having dental work done

Not touching eyes or inside of nose unless hands washed immediately before

Using caution to avoid accidental cuts with use of sharp objects such as safety razor or fingernail or toenail cutters

Avoiding contact sports or other situations where bruising or injury could occur

Caution if any laboratory tests required; possible interference with test results

**Side/adverse effects**
Signs of potential side effects, especially gonadal suppression, leukopenia, infection, SIADH, cardiotoxicity, hemorrhagic cystitis, hyperuricemia, uric acid nephropathy, nonhemorrhagic cystitis, nephrotoxicity, pneumonitis, interstitial pulmonary fibrosis, anemia, thrombocytopenia, anaphylactic reaction, hemorrhagic colitis, hepatitis, hyperglycemia, redness or swelling or pain at site of injecton, and stomatitis

Physician or nurse can help in dealing with side effects

Possibility of hair loss; normal hair growth should return after treatment has ended; new hair may be slightly different in color or texture

# General Dosing Information

Patients receiving cyclophosphamide should be under supervision of a physician experienced in cancer chemotherapy or immunosuppressive therapy.

A variety of dosage schedules and regimens of cyclophosphamide, alone or in combination with other antitumor agents, are used. The prescriber may consult the medical literature as well as the manufacturer's literature in choosing a specific dosage.

Dosage must be adjusted to meet the individual requirements of each patient, based on clinical response and appearance or severity of toxicity.

Development of uric acid nephropathy in patients with leukemia or lymphoma may be prevented by adequate oral hydration and, in some cases, administration of allopurinol. Alkalinization of urine may be necessary if serum uric acid concentrations are elevated.

To reduce the risk of hemorrhagic cystitis, adequate hydration is recommended prior to cyclophosphamide treatment and for at least 72 hours following treatment to ensure ample urine output. In addition, the patient should be encouraged to take cyclophosphamide in the morning so that the majority of the metabolites have been excreted by bedtime and to void frequently, to prevent prolonged contact of irritating metabolites with bladder mucosa.

Cyclophosphamide should be discontinued at the first sign of hemorrhagic cystitis. In severe cases, blood replacement may be necessary. Electrocautery diversion of urine flow, cryosurgery, and formaldehyde bladder instillations have been used. Resumption of therapy should be undertaken with caution since recurrence is common.

Initiation of planned maintenance antineoplastic therapy is recommended as soon as the leukocyte count returns to adequate levels following induction.

If marked leukopenia (particularly granulocytopenia) or thrombocytopenia occurs, cyclophosphamide therapy should be withdrawn until leukocyte and platelet counts return to satisfactory levels. Then therapy may be reinstituted, possibly at a lower dose.

In acute leukemia, cyclophosphamide may be administered despite the presence of thrombocytopenia and bleeding; cessation of bleeding and increase in platelet count have occurred in some cases during treatment and platelet transfusions are useful in others.

Special precautions are recommended in patients who develop thrombocytopenia as a result of administration of cyclophosphamide. These may include extreme care in performing invasive procedures; regular inspection of intravenous sites, skin (including perirectal area), and mucous membrane surfaces for signs of bleeding or bruising; limiting frequency of venipuncture and avoiding intramuscular injections; testing urine, emesis, stool, and secretions for occult blood; care in use of regular toothbrushes, dental floss, toothpicks, safety razors, and fingernail and toenail cutters; avoiding constipation; and using caution to prevent falls and other injuries. Such patients should avoid alcohol and aspirin intake because of the risk of gastrointestinal bleeding. Platelet transfusions may be required.

Patients who develop leukopenia should be observed carefully for signs of infection. Antibiotic support may be required. In neutropenic patients who develop fever, broad-spectrum antibiotic coverage should be initiated empirically, pending bacterial cultures and appropriate diagnostic tests.

**For parenteral dosage forms only**
Cyclophosphamide may be administered by intravenous push or infusion, intramuscularly, intraperitoneally, or intrapleurally.

**Diet/Nutrition**
Oral cyclophosphamide should usually be taken on an empty stomach; however, if stomach upset occurs, doses may be divided and given with meals.

**Safety considerations for handling this medication**
There is limited but increasing evidence and concern that personnel involved in preparation and administration of parenteral antineoplastics may be at some risk because of the potential mutagenicity, teratogenicity, and/or carcinogenicity of these agents, although the actual risk is unknown. USP advisory panels recommend cautious handling both in preparation and disposal of antineoplastic agents. Precautions that have been suggested include:
• Use of a biological containment cabinet during reconstitution and dilution of parenteral medications and wearing of disposable surgical gloves and masks.
• Use of proper technique to prevent contamination of the medication, work area, and operator during transfer between containers (including proper training of personnel in this technique).
• Cautious and proper disposal of needles, syringes, vials, ampuls, and unused medication.

A number of medical centers have developed detailed guidelines for handling of antineoplastic agents.

**Combination chemotherapy**
Cyclophosphamide may be used in combination with other agents in various regimens. As a result, incidence and/or severity of side effects may be altered and different dosages (usually reduced) may be used. For example, cyclophosphamide is part of the following chemotherapeutic combinations (some commonly used acronyms are in parentheses):
—carmustine, cyclophosphamide, vinblastine, procarbazine, and prednisone (BCVPP).
—cyclophosphamide, doxorubicin, and fluorouracil (CAF).

—cyclophosphamide, doxorubicin, methotrexate, and procarbazine (CAMP).
—cyclophosphamide, doxorubicin, and cisplatin (CAP).
—cyclophosphamide, doxorubicin, vincristine, and prednisone (CHOP).
—cyclophosphamide, doxorubicin, and cisplatin (CISCA).
—cyclophosphamide, methotrexate, and lomustine (CMC).
—cyclophosphamide, methotrexate, and fluorouracil (CMF).
—cyclophosphamide, methotrexate, fluorouracil, vincristine, and prednisone (CMFVP).
—cyclophosphamide, vincristine, and prednisone (COP or CVP).
—cyclophosphamide, vincristine, doxorubicin, and dacarbazine (CyVADIC).
—vincristine, dactinomycin, and cyclophosphamide (VAC).

For specific dosages and schedules, consult the literature. For information regarding each agent, consult the individual monographs.

## Oral Dosage Forms

Note: Bracketed uses in the *Dosage Forms* section refer to categories of use and/or indications that are not included in U.S. product labeling.

### CYCLOPHOSPHAMIDE ORAL SOLUTION

Note: In the U.S. and Canada, Cyclophosphamide Injection USP [*Cytoxan; Neosar; Procytox;* GENERIC] is the dosage form being used to prepare the oral solution dosage form.

**Usual adult dose**
Leukemia, acute lymphocytic or
Leukemia, acute nonlymphocytic or
Leukemia, chronic myelocytic or
Leukemia, chronic lymphocytic or
Carcinoma, ovarian, epithelial or
Carcinoma, breast or
Neuroblastoma or
Retinoblastoma or
[Carcinoma, lung, non-small cell] or
[Carcinoma, lung, small cell] or
[Carcinoma, endometrial][1] or
[Carcinoma, bladder][1] or
[Carcinoma, prostatic][1] or
Lymphomas, Hodgkin's or
Lymphomas, non-Hodgkin's or
Multiple myeloma or
Mycosis fungoides or
[Ewing's sarcoma][1] or
[Sarcomas, soft tissue][1] or
[Tumors, germ cell, ovarian][1]—
  Oral, 1 to 5 mg per kg of body weight per day.
[Rheumatoid arthritis][1]—
  Oral, 1.5 to 2 mg per kg of body weight per day, the dosage being increased up to a maximum of 3 mg per kg of body weight per day.
[Wegener's granulomatosis][1]—
  Oral, 1 to 2 mg per kg of body weight per day, administered in combination with prednisone.

**Usual pediatric dose**
Leukemia, acute lymphocytic or
Leukemia, acute nonlymphocytic or
Leukemia, chronic myelocytic or
Leukemia, chronic lymphocytic or
Neuroblastoma or
Retinoblastoma or
Lymphomas, Hodgkin's; or
Lymphomas, non-Hodgkin's—
  Induction: Oral, 2 to 8 mg per kg of body weight or 60 to 250 mg per square meter of body surface a day in divided doses for six or more days.
  Maintenance: Oral, 2 to 5 mg per kg of body weight or 50 to 150 mg per square meter of body surface twice a week.
Nephrotic syndrome—
  Oral, 2.5 to 3 mg per kg of body weight per day.

**Strength(s) usually available**
U.S.—
  Dosage form not commercially available. Compounding required for prescriptions.
Canada—
  Dosage form not commercially available. Compounding required for prescriptions.

**Packaging and storage**
Store between 2 and 8 °C (36 and 46 °F). Protect from freezing. Store in a tight container.

**Preparation of dosage form**
Cyclophosphamide oral solution may be prepared by dissolving Cyclophosphamide for Injection USP in Aromatic Elixir NF to a concentration of 1 to 5 mg of cyclophosphamide per mL.

**Stability**
Stable for up to 14 days when stored in a glass container in the refrigerator.

**Auxiliary labeling**
• For oral use.
• Take on an empty stomach.
• Drink plenty of water with this medicine.

### CYCLOPHOSPHAMIDE TABLETS USP

**Usual adult dose**
Leukemia, acute lymphocytic or
Leukemia, acute nonlymphocytic or
Leukemia, chronic myelocytic or
Leukemia, chronic lymphocytic or
Carcinoma, ovarian, epithelial or
Carcinoma, breast or
Neuroblastoma or
Retinoblastoma or
[Carcinoma, lung, non-small cell] or
[Carcinoma, lung, small cell] or
[Carcinoma, endometrial][1] or
[Carcinoma, bladder][1] or
[Carcinoma, prostatic][1] or
Lymphomas, Hodgkin's or
Lymphomas, non-Hodgkin's or
Multiple myeloma or
Mycosis fungoides or
[Ewing's sarcoma][1] or
[Sarcomas, soft tissue][1] or
[Tumors, germ cell, ovarian][1]—
  Oral, 1 to 5 mg per kg of body weight per day.
[Rheumatoid arthritis][1]—
  Oral, 1 to 2 mg per kg of body weight per day, the dose being adjusted on the basis of leukocyte counts.
[Wegener's granulomatosis][1]—
  Oral, 1.5 to 2 mg per kg of body weight per day, the dosage being increased up to a maximum of 3 mg per kg of body weight per day.

**Usual pediatric dose**
Leukemia, acute lymphocytic or
Leukemia, acute nonlymphocytic or
Leukemia, chronic myelocytic or
Leukemia, chronic lymphocytic or
Neuroblastoma or
Retinoblastoma or
Lymphomas, Hodgkin's or
Lymphomas, non-Hodgkin's—
  Induction: Oral, 2 to 8 mg per kg of body weight or 60 to 250 mg per square meter of body surface a day in divided doses for six or more days.
  Maintenance: Oral, 2 to 5 mg per kg of body weight or 50 to 150 mg per square meter of body surface twice a week.
Nephrotic syndrome[1]—
  Oral, 2.5 to 3 mg per kg of body weight per day.

**Strength(s) usually available**
U.S.—
  25 mg (Rx) [*Cytoxan* (lactose)].
  50 mg (Rx) [*Cytoxan* (lactose)].
Canada—
  25 mg (Rx) [*Cytoxan; Procytox*].
  50 mg (Rx) [*Cytoxan; Procytox*].

**Packaging and storage**
Store between 2 and 25 °C (36 and 77 °F). Store in a tight container.

**Auxiliary labeling**
• Take on an empty stomach.
• Drink plenty of water with this medicine.

## Parenteral Dosage Forms

Note: Bracketed uses in the *Dosage Forms* section refer to categories of use and/or indications that are not included in U.S. product labeling.

1134    Cyclophosphamide (Systemic)    USP DI

## CYCLOPHOSPHAMIDE FOR INJECTION USP
### Usual adult dose
Leukemia, acute lymphocytic or
Leukemia, acute nonlymphocytic or
Leukemia, chronic myelocytic or
Leukemia, chronic lymphocytic or
Carcinoma, ovarian, epithelial or
Carcinoma, breast or
Neuroblastoma or
Retinoblastoma or
[Carcinoma, lung, non-small cell] or
[Carcinoma, lung, small cell] or
[Carcinoma, endometrial][1] or
[Carcinoma, bladder][1] or
[Carcinoma, prostatic][1] or
Lymphomas, Hodgkin's or
Lymphomas, non-Hodgkin's or
Multiple myeloma or
Mycosis fungoides or
[Ewing's sarcoma][1] or
[Sarcomas, soft tissue][1] or
[Tumors, germ cell, ovarian][1]—
    Initial: Intravenous, 40 to 50 mg per kg of body weight in divided doses over a period of two to five days, or 10 to 15 mg per kg of body weight every seven to ten days, or 3 to 5 mg per kg of body weight two times a week, or 1.5 to 3 mg per kg of body weight a day.

### Usual adult prescribing limits
Much higher dosages have been used, depending on the condition being treated. Physicians should consult the medical literature in choosing a specific dosage.

### Usual pediatric dose
Leukemia, acute lymphocytic or
Leukemia, acute nonlymphocytic or
Leukemia, chronic myelocytic or
Leukemia, chronic lymphocytic or
Neuroblastoma or
Retinoblastoma or
Lymphomas, Hodgkin's or
Lymphomas, non-Hodgkin's—
    Induction: Intravenous, 2 to 8 mg per kg of body weight or 60 to 250 mg per square meter of body surface a day in divided doses for six or more days (or total dose for seven days once a week).
    Maintenance: Intravenous, 10 to 15 mg per kg of body weight every seven to ten days, or 30 mg per kg of body weight at three- to four-week intervals or when bone marrow recovery occurs.

### Strength(s) usually available
U.S.—
    Lyophilized
        100 mg (Rx) [*Cytoxan* (mannitol 75 mg)].
        200 mg (Rx) [*Cytoxan* (mannitol 150 mg)].
        500 mg (Rx) [*Cytoxan* (mannitol 375 mg)].
        1 gram (Rx) [*Cytoxan* (mannitol 750 mg)].
        2 grams (Rx) [*Cytoxan* (mannitol 1.5 grams)].
    Nonlyophilized
        100 mg (Rx) [*Cytoxan* (sodium chloride 45 mg [1.9 mmol]); *Neosar* (sodium chloride 45 mg [1.9 mmol]); GENERIC].
        200 mg (Rx) [*Cytoxan* (sodium chloride 90 mg [3.9 mmol]); *Neosar* (sodium chloride 90 mg [3.9 mmol]); GENERIC].
        500 mg (Rx) [*Cytoxan* (sodium chloride 225 mg [9.7 mmol]); *Neosar* (sodium chloride 225 mg [9.7 mmol]); GENERIC].
        1 gram (Rx) [*Cytoxan* (sodium chloride 450 mg [19.5 mmol]); *Neosar* (sodium chloride 450 mg [19.5 mmol]); GENERIC].
        2 grams (Rx) [*Cytoxan* (sodium chloride 900 mg [39 mmol]); *Neosar* (sodium chloride 900 mg [39 mmol])].
Canada—
    Lyophilized
        500 mg (Rx) [*Cytoxan* (mannitol 375 mg)].
        750 mg (Rx) [*Cytoxan* (mannitol 562.5 mg)].
        1 gram (Rx) [*Cytoxan* (mannitol 750 mg)].
        2 grams (Rx) [*Cytoxan* (mannitol 1.5 grams)].
    Nonlyophilized
        200 mg (Rx) [*Procytox* (sodium chloride 90 mg [3.9 mmol])].
        500 mg (Rx) [*Procytox* (sodium chloride 225 mg [9.7 mmol])].
        1 gram (Rx) [*Procytox* (sodium chloride 450 mg [19.5 mmol])].

### Packaging and storage
Store at a temperature not exceeding 25 °C (77 °F).

### Preparation of dosage form
Nonlyophilized cyclophosphamide for injection may be prepared for parenteral use by adding 5 mL (100-mg vial), 10 mL (200-mg vial), 25 mL (500-mg vial), 50 mL (1-gram vial), or 100 mL (2-gram vial) of sterile water for injection or bacteriostatic water for injection (paraben-preserved only) to the vial and shaking to dissolve (may be difficult and take up to 6 minutes) to provide a solution containing 20 mg of cyclophosphamide per mL. The resulting solution may be added to 5% dextrose injection, 5% dextrose and 0.9% sodium chloride injection, 5% dextrose and Ringer's injection, lactated Ringer's injection, 0.45% sodium chloride injection, or sodium lactate injection for administration by intravenous infusion.

Lyophilized cyclophosphamide for injection may be prepared for parenteral use by adding 5 mL (100-mg vial), 10 mL (200-mg vial), 20 to 25 mL (500-mg vial), 50 mL (1-gram vial), or 80 to 100 mL (2-gram vial) of sterile water for injection or bacteriostatic water for injection (paraben-preserved only) to the vial and shaking to dissolve (takes about 45 seconds) to provide a solution containing 20 mg of cyclophosphamide per mL. The resulting solution may be added to 5% dextrose injection, 5% dextrose and 0.9% sodium chloride injection, 5% dextrose and Ringer's injection, lactated Ringer's injection, 0.45% sodium chloride injection, or sodium lactate injection for administration by intravenous infusion.

Caution: Use of diluents containing benzyl alcohol is not recommended for preparation of medications for use in neonates. A fatal toxic syndrome consisting of metabolic acidosis, central nervous system (CNS) depression, respiratory problems, renal failure, hypotension, and possibly seizures and intracranial hemorrhages has been associated with this use.

### Stability
Reconstituted solutions of cyclophosphamide are stable for 24 hours at room temperature, or for 6 days if refrigerated. If bacteriostatic water for injection is not used for reconstitution, it is recommended that the solution be used promptly (preferably within 6 hours).

### Note
Because cyclophosphamide for injection contains no preservative, caution in preparing and storing solutions is required to ensure sterility.

---

[1]Not included in Canadian product labeling.

Revised: 07/11/94
Interim revision: 09/30/97

---

# CYCLOSERINE   Systemic †

VA CLASSIFICATION (Primary): AM500
Commonly used brand name(s): *Seromycin*.
Note: For a listing of dosage forms and brand names by country availability, see *Dosage Forms* section(s).

†Not commercially available in Canada.

## Category
Antibacterial (antimycobacterial).

## Indications
Note: Bracketed information in the *Indications* section refers to uses that are not included in U.S. product labeling.

### Accepted
Tuberculosis (treatment)—Cycloserine is indicated in combination with other antituberculars in the treatment of tuberculosis after failure of the primary medications (pyrazinamide, streptomycin, isoniazid, rifampin, and ethambutol).

[Mycobacterial infections, atypical (treatment)]—Cycloserine is used in the treatment of atypical mycobacterial infections, such as *Mycobacterium avium* complex.

Not all species or strains of a particular organism may be susceptible to cycloserine.

### Unaccepted
Although cycloserine has been used for the treatment of urinary tract infections, it has been superseded by newer, safer, and/or more effective agents (e.g., aminoglycosides, beta-lactams, quinolones, trimethoprim).

## Pharmacology/Pharmacokinetics

**Physicochemical characteristics**
Molecular weight—102.09.

**Mechanism of action/Effect**
Cycloserine, a broad-spectrum antibiotic, may be bactericidal or bacteriostatic, depending on its concentration at the site of infection and the susceptibility of the organism.

Cycloserine is an analog of the amino acid D-alanine. It interferes with an early step in bacterial cell wall synthesis in the cytoplasm by competitive inhibition of 2 enzymes, L-alanine racemase, which forms D-alanine from L-alanine, and D-alanine-D-alanine synthetase, which incorporates D-alanine into the pentapeptide necessary for peptidoglycan formation and bacterial cell wall synthesis.

**Absorption**
Rapidly and almost completely (70 to 90%) absorbed from the gastrointestinal tract following oral administration.

**Distribution**
Wide, to most body fluids and tissues, including cerebrospinal fluid (CSF), breast milk, bile, sputum, lymph tissue, lungs, and ascitic, pleural, and synovial fluids; crosses the placenta.
CSF concentrations of cycloserine approach those found in the serum.
   Urine concentrations—
      —High, 55 to 340 mcg per mL.

**Protein binding**
None.

**Biotransformation**
Up to 35%.

**Half-life**
Normal renal function—
   10 hours.
Impaired renal function—
   Prolonged.

**Time to peak serum concentration**
3 to 4 hours.

**Peak serum concentration**
25 to 30 mcg/mL after a dose of 250 mg every 12 hours.

**Elimination**
Renal, by glomerular filtration; 50% excreted unchanged within 12 hours; 65 to 70% excreted unchanged within 24 to 72 hours; accumulates in patients with impaired renal function.
Fecal, small amounts.
   Dialysis—
      Cycloserine is removed by hemodialysis.

## Precautions to Consider

**Carcinogenicity/Mutagenicity**
Studies have not been performed to determine the carcinogenic potential of cycloserine. The Ames test and unscheduled DNA repair test were negative.

**Pregnancy/Reproduction**
Fertility—A study in 2 generations of rats showed no impairment of fertility relative to controls for the first mating, but somewhat lower fertility for the second mating.
Pregnancy—Cycloserine crosses the placenta; fetal serum concentrations may approach maternal serum concentrations.
A study in 2 generations of rats given doses up to 100 mg per kg of body weight per day demonstrated no teratogenic effect in the offspring.
FDA Pregnancy Category C.

**Breast-feeding**
Cycloserine is distributed into breast milk; concentrations may approach or exceed maternal serum concentrations.

**Pediatrics**
Appropriate studies on the relationship of age to the effects of cycloserine have not been performed in the pediatric population. However, no pediatrics-specific problems have been documented to date.

**Geriatrics**
No information is available on the relationship of age to the effects of cycloserine in geriatric patients. However, elderly patients are more likely to have an age-related decrease in renal function, which may require an adjustment of dosage in patients receiving cycloserine.

**Drug interactions and/or related problems**
The following drug interactions and/or related problems have been selected on the basis of their potential clinical significance (possible mechanism in parentheses where appropriate)—not necessarily inclusive (» = major clinical significance):

Note: Combinations containing any of the following medications, depending on the amount present, may also interact with this medication.

» Alcohol
   (may increase the risk of seizures, especially in chronic alcohol abuse; patients should be advised to avoid concurrent use)
» Ethionamide
   (concurrent use may result in increased incidence of central nervous system [CNS] effects, especially seizures; dosage adjustments may be necessary and patients should be monitored closely for signs of CNS toxicity)
Isoniazid
   (concurrent use may result in increased incidence of CNS effects such as dizziness or drowsiness; dosage adjustments may be necessary, and patients should be monitored closely for signs of CNS toxicity)
Pyridoxine
   (cycloserine may cause anemia or peripheral neuritis by acting as a pyridoxine antagonist or increasing renal excretion of pyridoxine; requirements for pyridoxine may be increased in patients receiving cycloserine)

**Laboratory value alterations**
The following have been selected on the basis of their potential clinical significance (possible effect in parentheses where appropriate)—not necessarily inclusive (» = major clinical significance):

With physiology/laboratory test values
   Alanine aminotransferase (ALT [SGPT]) and
   Aspartate aminotransferase (AST [SGOT])
      (concentrations may be increased—especially in patients with pre-existing liver disease)

**Medical considerations/Contraindications**
The medical considerations/contraindications included have been selected on the basis of their potential clinical significance (reasons given in parentheses where appropriate)—not necessarily inclusive (» = major clinical significance):

*Risk-benefit should be considered when the following medical problems exist:*
» Alcoholism, active or in remission
   (cycloserine may increase the risk of seizures in alcoholics)
Anxiety, severe or
Mental depression or
Psychosis
   (cycloserine may cause anxiety, mental depression, and psychosis, especially at higher doses)
» Hypersensitivity to cycloserine
» Renal function impairment
   (because cycloserine is renally excreted, cycloserine may accumulate in patients with renal function impairment, leading to an increased risk of side effects; the medication should not be given to patients with renal function impairment [creatinine clearance of <50 mL per minute (0.83 mL per second)])
» Seizure disorders, history of
   (cycloserine may increase the risk of seizures in patients with a seizure disorder)

**Patient monitoring**
The following may be especially important in patient monitoring (other tests may be warranted in some patients, depending on condition; » = major clinical significance):

Blood urea nitrogen (BUN) concentrations and
Creatinine concentrations, serum
   (may be required periodically since patients with impaired renal function require a reduction in dose or discontinuation of the medication)
Cycloserine concentrations, serum
   (may be required at least weekly in patients with slightly impaired, but stable, renal function, in patients receiving more than 500 mg daily, or in patients showing signs and symptoms of toxicity; concentrations above 30 mcg/mL should be avoided)
Hemoglobin concentration
   (may be required periodically since administration of cycloserine and other antituberculars has been associated in a few instances with vitamin $B_{12}$ and/or folic acid deficiency, megaloblastic anemia, and sideroblastic anemia)

## Cycloserine (Systemic)

### Side/Adverse Effects

Note: The side effects of cycloserine, particularly CNS toxicity, may be dose-related and more commonly seen with daily doses greater than 500 mg. Acute toxicity may occur if more than 1 gram is ingested by an adult, and chronic toxicity may occur with ingestion of more than 500 mg daily. The ratio of toxic dose to effective dose is small.

Administraton of 200 to 300 mg of pyridoxine daily may help to prevent cycloserine-related neurotoxicity.

The following side/adverse effects have been selected on the basis of their potential clinical significance (possible signs and symptoms in parentheses where appropriate)—not necessarily inclusive:

#### Those indicating need for medical attention
Incidence more frequent
  *CNS toxicity* (anxiety; confusion; dizziness; drowsiness; increased irritability; increased restlessness; mental depression; muscle twitching or trembling; nervousness; nightmares; other mood or mental changes; speech problems; thoughts of suicide)
Incidence less frequent
  *Hypersensitivity* (skin rash); *peripheral neuropathy* (numbness, tingling, burning pain, or weakness in the hands or feet); *seizures*

#### Those indicating need for medical attention only if they continue or are bothersome
Incidence more frequent
  *Headache*

### Patient Consultation

As an aid to patient consultation, refer to *Advice for the Patient, Cycloserine (Systemic)*.

In providing consultation, consider emphasizing the following selected information (» = major clinical significance):

#### Before using this medication
» Conditions affecting use, especially:
    Pregnancy—Cycloserine crosses the placenta and fetal serum concentrations may approach maternal serum concentrations
    Breast-feeding—Cycloserine is distributed into breast milk. Concentrations may approach or exceed maternal serum concentrations
    Other medications, especially alcohol and ethionamide
    Other medical problems, especially alcoholism (active or in remission), a history of seizure disorders, or renal function impairment

#### Proper use of this medication
Taking this medication after meals if gastrointestinal irritation occurs
» Compliance with full course of therapy; in tuberculosis, therapy may take months or years
» Importance of not missing doses and taking at evenly spaced times
» Proper dosing
    Missed dose: Taking as soon as possible; not taking if almost time for next dose; not doubling doses
» Proper storage

#### Precautions while using this medication
Regular visits to physician to check progress
Checking with physician if no improvement within 2 to 3 weeks
» Checking with physician immediately if thoughts of suicide occur
» Caution if dizziness or drowsiness occurs
» Avoiding alcoholic beverages while taking this medication

#### Side/adverse effects
Signs of potential side effects, especially CNS toxicity, hypersensitivity reactions, peripheral neuropathy, and seizures

### General Dosing Information

Cycloserine may be taken after meals if gastrointestinal irritation occurs.

Since bacterial resistance may develop rapidly when cycloserine is administered alone in the treatment of tuberculosis, it should only be administered concurrently with other antituberculars.

Patients receiving more than 500 mg of cycloserine daily should be closely observed for symptoms of CNS toxicity.

In the treatment of tuberculosis, therapy may have to be continued for 1 to 2 years and may even be required for up to several years or indefinitely, although in some patients shorter treatment regimens may also be effective.

Serum concentrations should be monitored where possible. Concentrations should be maintained at approximately 25 to 30 mcg/mL in the treatment of tuberculosis. Concentrations above 30 mcg/mL should be avoided since toxicity is closely related to excessive serum concentrations. In addition, the ratio of toxic dose to effective dose is small.

Patients with severe renal function impairment (creatinine clearance of <50 mL per minute [0.83 mL per second]) should not receive cycloserine because of the increased risk of neurotoxicity.

#### For treatment of adverse effects
Recommended treatment consists of the following:
  • Inducing emesis and/or use of gastric lavage.
  • Administering activated charcoal and cathartic every 4 hours until clinically stable.
  • Providing supportive therapy.
  • Using anticonvulsants to control seizures.
  • Administering 200 to 300 mg of pyridoxine daily to treat neurotoxicity.

### Oral Dosage Forms

#### CYCLOSERINE CAPSULES USP

**Usual adult and adolescent dose**
Tuberculosis—
  In combination with other antituberculars: Oral, 250 mg every twelve hours for the first two weeks, then cautiously increased as necessary and tolerated, up to 250 mg every six to eight hours and monitored by serum determinations.

**Usual adult prescribing limits**
Up to a maximum of 1 gram daily.
Note: Doses up to 1.5 grams daily have been used.

**Usual pediatric dose**
Tuberculosis—
  In combination with other antituberculars: Doses of 10 to 20 mg per kg of body weight per day in divided doses have been used.

**Strength(s) usually available**
U.S.—
  250 mg (Rx) [*Seromycin*].
Canada—
  Not commercially available.

**Packaging and storage**
Store below 40 °C (104 °F), preferably between 15 and 30 °C (59 and 86 °F), unless otherwise specified by manufacturer. Store in a tight container.

**Stability**
Cycloserine maintains its potency in alkaline solutions, but is rapidly destroyed at neutral or acid pH.

**Auxiliary labeling**
• Avoid alcoholic beverages.
• May cause drowsiness, or dizziness.
• Continue medicine for full time of treatment.

Revised: 05/02/94

# CYCLOSPORINE  Systemic

INN: Ciclosporin
VA CLASSIFICATION (Primary/Secondary): IM600/DE801; MS109
Commonly used brand name(s): *Neoral; Sandimmune*.
Another commonly used name is cyclosporin A.

Note: For a listing of dosage forms and brand names by country availability, see *Dosage Forms* section(s).

## Category

Immunosuppressant; antipsoriatic; antirheumatic.

## Indications

Note: Bracketed information in the *Indications* section refers to uses that are not included in U.S. product labeling.

### Accepted

Transplant rejection, organ (prophylaxis)—Cyclosporine is indicated, usually in combination with corticosteroids, for prevention of rejection of renal, hepatic, and cardiac transplants (allografts). [Cyclosporine is also indicated for prevention of rejection of heart-lung and pancreatic transplants.]

Transplant rejection, organ (treatment)—Cyclosporine is indicated for treatment of chronic rejection in patients previously treated with other immunosuppressants.

Arthritis, rheumatoid (treatment)—Cyclosporine is indicated for severe, active, rheumatoid arthritis failing to respond adequately to therapy with methotrexate alone.

Psoriasis, severe (treatment)—Cyclosporine is indicated for severe, recalcitrant, plaque-type psoriasis failing to respond to at least one systemic therapy or in patients unable to tolerate other systemic therapy.

[Graft-versus-host disease (prophylaxis)] or
[Graft-versus-host disease (treatment)]—Cyclosporine is indicated for prophylaxis and treatment of graft-versus-host disease after bone marrow transplantation.

[Nephrotic syndrome (treatment)]—Cyclosporine is indicated to induce and maintain remissions for steroid-dependent and steroid-resistant nephrotic syndrome due to glomerular diseases.

### Acceptance not established

Data are insufficient to prove that cyclosporine is effective for treatment of generalized pustular or erythrodermic psoriasis.

## Pharmacology/Pharmacokinetics

### Physicochemical characteristics

Molecular weight—1202.64.

### Mechanism of action/Effect

The exact mechanism of action is unknown but seems to be related to the inhibition of production and release of interleukin-2, which is a proliferative factor necessary for the induction of cytotoxic T lymphocytes in response to alloantigenic challenge, and which plays a major role in both cellular and humoral immune responses. Cyclosporine does not affect the nonspecific defense system of the host and does not cause significant myelosuppression.

### Absorption

Variable and incomplete from gastrointestinal tract; bioavailability of *Sandimmune®* is about 30% but may increase with increasing dosage and duration of treatment. Absorption may be decreased after liver transplantation or in patients with liver disease or gastrointestinal function impairment (e.g., diarrhea, vomiting, ileus).

Cyclosporine modified capsules and oral solution (i.e., *Neoral®*) have increased bioavailability compared to the standard oral formulations of cyclosporine (i.e., *Sandimmune®*). However, the absorption is still variable and incomplete from the gastrointestinal tract; bioavailability may be less than 10% in some liver transplant patients, but may be as high as 89% in some kidney transplant patients. In studies in kidney transplant, liver transplant, psoriasis, and rheumatoid arthritis patients, the mean area under the serum concentration-versus-time curve (AUC) was 20 to 50% greater following administration of *Neoral®* compared to the AUC following administration of *Sandimmune®*.

### Protein binding

Very high (90%), primarily to lipoproteins.

### Biotransformation

Hepatic, extensive, primarily by cytochrome P450 3A enzymes. Cyclosporine is metabolized to a lesser extent in the gastrointestinal system and in the kidneys.

### Half-life

Biphasic, variable—
  Terminal:
    Children—Approximately 7 hours (range, 7 to 19 hours).
    Adults—Approximately 19 hours (range, 10 to 27 hours).

### Time to peak concentration

Cyclosporine capsules and oral solution (*Sandimmune®*):
  Plasma or blood: 3.5 hours.
Cyclosporine modified capsules and oral solution (*Neoral®*):
  Blood: 1.5 to 2 hours.

### Peak serum concentration

Plasma or blood—Whole blood concentrations may be 2 to 9 times higher than plasma concentrations.

### Elimination

Biliary/fecal; renal, 6% (0.1% unchanged).
In dialysis—Not dialyzable.

## Precautions to Consider

### Cross-sensitivity and/or related problems

Patients sensitive to polyoxyethylated castor oil may be sensitive to the injectable dosage form also, since the injection contains a polyoxyethylated castor oil vehicle.

### Carcinogenicity/Tumorigenicity

A 78-week study in mice at doses of 1, 4, and 16 mg per kg of body weight (mg/kg) a day found a statistically significant trend for lymphocytic lymphomas in females, and the incidence of hepatocellular carcinomas in mid-dose males significantly exceeded the control value. A 24-month study in rats at doses of 0.5, 2, and 8 mg/kg a day found that incidence of pancreatic islet cell adenomas significantly exceeded the control rate in the low dose level. The hepatocellular carcinomas and pancreatic islet cell adenomas were not dose-related.

Lymphomas and skin malignancies have developed in humans treated with cyclosporine. The risk of these malignancies is related to the intensity and duration of immunosuppression. The incidence of malignancies is similar to that in patients receiving other (e.g., tacrolimus-based) regimens.

Psoriasis patients receiving cyclosporine are at increased risk of developing skin malignancies if they were treated previously with psoralen plus ultraviolet light A (PUVA), methotrexate, ultraviolet light B (UVB), coal tar, or radiation therapy. The risk of skin cancer is greatest with previous PUVA treatment.

### Mutagenicity

No evidence of mutagenicity/genotoxicity was found in the Ames test, the V79-HGPRT test, the micronucleus test in mice and Chinese hamsters, the chromosome-aberration tests in Chinese hamster bone marrow, the mouse dominant lethal assay, and the DNA-repair test in sperm from treated mice. However, one study analyzing sister chromatid exchange (SCE) induction by cyclosporine using human lymphocytes *in vitro* gave indication of a positive effect (i.e., induction of SCE) at high concentrations in this system.

### Pregnancy/Reproduction

Fertility—Studies in male and female rats found no evidence of impairment of fertility.

Pregnancy—Adequate and well-controlled studies in humans have not been done.

Cyclosporine crosses the placenta.

In a retrospective study of 116 pregnancies of women who received cyclosporine during (and usually throughout) pregnancy, the only consistent patterns of abnormality were premature birth (gestational period of 28 to 36 weeks) and low birth weight for gestational age. Preterm delivery occurred in 47%. Seven malformations were reported in 5 viable infants and in 2 cases of fetal loss. Neonatal complications occurred in 27%. The exact relationship of cyclosporine to these effects has not been established.

Studies in rats and rabbits have shown that cyclosporine is embryotoxic and fetotoxic at doses 2 to 5 times the human dose. At toxic doses (30 mg/kg a day in rats and 100 mg/kg a day in rabbits), cyclosporine was embryotoxic and fetotoxic, as indicated by increased pre- and postnatal mortality and reduced fetal weight together with related skeletal retardations. No embryolethal or teratogenic effects occurred at normal doses (up to 17 mg/kg a day in rats and up to 30 mg/kg a day in rabbits).

FDA Pregnancy Category C.

### Breast-feeding

Cyclosporine is distributed into breast milk. Mothers taking cyclosporine should not breast-feed their babies because of the potential risk of serious adverse effects (e.g., hypertension, nephrotoxicity, malignancy) in the infant.

### Pediatrics

Appropriate studies performed to date in pediatric patients receiving cyclosporine for organ transplantation have not demonstrated pediatrics-specific problems that would limit the usefulness of cyclosporine in children. Cyclosporine has been used in pediatric patients 1 year of age and older receiving organ transplantations. Pediatric patients have increased clearance of cyclosporine as compared with adult patients. The safety and efficacy of cyclosporine to treat psoriasis and rheumatoid arthritis in pediatric patients have not been established.

### Geriatrics

Geriatric patients were included in the clinical trials of cyclosporine to treat rheumatoid arthritis. Geriatric patients were more likely to experience hypertension and increases in serum creatinine concentrations than younger adult patients.

## Dental

Gingival hyperplasia, a common complication of cyclosporine therapy, usually starts as gingivitis or gum inflammation in the first month of treatment. The incidence is higher in children under 15 years of age than in adults. Gingival tissue changes are similar to those produced by phenytoin, although with less-mature collagen. Tissue overgrowth may be greater anteriorly than posteriorly, creating aesthetic and psychological problems for the young patient. A strict program of teeth cleaning by a professional combined with plaque control by the patient, if begun within 10 days of initiation of cyclosporine therapy, will minimize the growth rate and the severity of gingival enlargement. Periodontal surgery may be indicated, and should be followed by careful plaque control to inhibit recurrence of gum enlargement.

The immunosuppressant effects of cyclosporine may result in an increased incidence of microbial infection and delayed healing. Dental work, whenever possible, should be completed prior to initiation of therapy with cyclosporine. Patients should be instructed in proper oral hygiene during treatment, including caution in use of regular toothbrushes, dental floss, and toothpicks.

## Drug interactions and/or related problems

The following drug interactions and/or related problems have been selected on the basis of their potential clinical significance (possible mechanism in parentheses where appropriate)—not necessarily inclusive (» = major clinical significance):

Note: Combinations containing any of the following medications, depending on the amount present, may also interact with this medication.

» Allopurinol or
» Androgens or
» Bromocriptine or
» Cimetidine or
» Clarithromycin or
» Danazol or
» Diltiazem or
» Erythromycin or
» Estrogens or
» Fluconazole or
» Human immunodeficiency virus (HIV) protease inhibitors or
» Itraconazole or
» Ketoconazole or
Metoclopramide or
Miconazole or
» Nefazodone or
» Nicardipine or
» Verapamil
(may increase blood concentrations of cyclosporine by inhibiting cytochrome P450 3A enzymes, and may increase the risk of hepatotoxicity and nephrotoxicity; because of its similarity to ketoconazole, miconazole may be expected to have the same effect; although concurrent use of HIV protease inhibitors and cyclosporine have not been studied, HIV protease inhibitors are known to inhibit cytochrome P450 3A enzymes; frequent monitoring of blood cyclosporine concentrations and hepatic and renal function may be needed if these drugs are used concurrently with cyclosporine)

Anti-inflammatory drugs, nonsteroidal (NSAIDs)
(concurrent use of NSAIDs, especially indomethacin, with cyclosporine may increase the risk of renal failure; concurrent administration with cyclosporine may also result in hyperkalemia; additive decreases in renal function have been reported with concurrent use of diclofenac or naproxen with cyclosporine)

» Coal tar or
» Methoxsalen or
» Radiation therapy or
» Trioxsalen
(patients with psoriasis receiving cyclosporine are at increased risk of developing skin malignancies if they were previously treated with a psoralen [e.g., methoxsalen or trioxsalen] plus ultraviolet light A [PUVA] or coal tar, or if they received previous radiation therapy)

» Grapefruit or
» Grapefruit juice
(decreased metabolism of cyclosporine, resulting in increased blood concentrations of cyclosporine, may occur; there is an increased risk of toxicity with concurrent use)

Hepatic enzyme inducers (see *Appendix II*)
(may enhance metabolism of cyclosporine by induction of cytochrome P-450 3A enzymes; dosage adjustment may be required)

Hyperkalemia-causing medications, such as:
Angiotensin-converting enzyme (ACE) inhibitors
Beta-adrenergic blocking agents
Digitalis glycosides, with acute overdose
» Diuretics, potassium-sparing
Heparin
Penicillins, potassium-containing, with high doses
Phosphates, potassium-containing
Potassium citrate–containing medications
Potassium iodide
Potassium supplements
Succinylcholine chloride
(concurrent administration with cyclosporine may result in hyperkalemia)

» Immunosuppressants, other, such as:
Azathioprine
Chlorambucil
Corticosteroids, glucocorticoid
Cyclophosphamide
Mercaptopurine
Muromonab-CD3
(concurrent use with cyclosporine may increase the risk of infection and development of lymphoproliferative disorders)

» Lovastatin or
» Simvastatin
(increased risk of rhabdomyolysis and acute renal failure)

Methotrexate
(in one study, concurrent administration of cyclosporine and methotrexate to patients to treat rheumatoid arthritis resulted in higher blood concentrations of methotrexate and lower blood concentrations of the primary metabolite of methotrexate than in patients receiving methotrexate alone; the clinical significance of this interaction is not known; patients with psoriasis receiving cyclosporine are at increased risk of developing skin malignancies if they were previously treated with methotrexate)

Methylprednisolone
(seizures have been observed in patients receiving cyclosporine and high doses of methylprednisolone)

Nephrotoxic medications (see *Appendix II*)
(concurrent use with cyclosporine may result in enhanced nephrotoxicity; dosage reduction or withdrawal of both medications may be necessary if renal impairment occurs)

Nifedipine
(increased risk of gingival hyperplasia)

Vaccines, killed virus
(because normal defense mechanisms may be suppressed by cyclosporine therapy, the patient's antibody response to the vaccine may be decreased. The interval between discontinuation of medications that cause immunosuppression and restoration of the patient's ability to respond to the vaccine depends on the intensity and type of immunosuppression-causing medication used, the underlying disease, and other factors; estimates vary from 3 months to 1 year)

» Vaccines, live virus
(because normal defense mechanisms may be suppressed by cyclosporine therapy, concurrent use with a live virus vaccine may potentiate the replication of the vaccine virus, may increase the side/adverse effects of the vaccine virus, and/or may decrease the patient's antibody response to the vaccine; immunization of these patients should be undertaken only after review of the patient's hematologic status and only with the knowledge and consent of the physician managing the cyclosporine therapy. The interval between discontinuation of medications that cause immunosuppression and restoration of the patient's ability to respond to the vaccine depends on the intensity and type of immunosuppression-causing medication used, the underlying disease, and other factors; estimates vary from 3 months to 1 year. Oral poliovirus vaccine should not be used in persons in close contact with the patient, especially family members)

## Laboratory value alterations

The following have been selected on the basis of their potential clinical significance (possible effect in parentheses where appropriate)—not necessarily inclusive (» = major clinical significance):

With physiology/laboratory test values
Alanine aminotransferase (ALT [SGPT]) values, serum and
Alkaline phosphatase values, serum and
Amylase values, serum and
Aspartate aminotransferase (AST [SGOT]) values, serum and
Bilirubin concentrations, serum
(may be increased in association with hepatotoxicity)

Blood urea nitrogen (BUN) and
Creatinine, serum
(concentrations are commonly increased during first few days of cyclosporine therapy; does not necessarily indicate rejection in renal transplant patients)

Magnesium
(serum concentrations may be decreased; may be related to nephrotoxicity)

Potassium and
Uric acid
(serum concentrations may be increased)

**Medical considerations/Contraindications**

The medical considerations/contraindications included have been selected on the basis of their potential clinical significance (reasons given in parentheses where appropriate)—not necessarily inclusive (» = major clinical significance).

*Except under special circumstances, this medication should not be used when the following medical problems exist:*

» Malignancy, current or
» Premalignant skin lesions
(cyclosporine is associated with an increased susceptibility to malignancies)

*Risk-benefit should be considered when the following medical problems exist:*

» Chickenpox, existing or recent (including recent exposure) or
» Herpes zoster
(risk of severe generalized disease)
» Hepatic function impairment
(reduced biotransformation; reduced absorption; dosage reduction may be necessary)

Hyperkalemia
Hypertension
(cyclosporine may exacerbate hypertension)
» Infection
Malabsorption
(achieving therapeutic plasma concentrations of cyclosporine may be difficult)
» Renal function impairment
(dose reduction may be necessary; cyclosporine should not be used to treat psoriasis in patients with renal function impairment)
» Sensitivity to cyclosporine

**Patient monitoring**

The following may be especially important in patient monitoring (other tests may be warranted in some patients, depending on condition; » = major clinical significance):

Alanine aminotransferase (ALT [SGPT]) values, serum and
Alkaline phosphatase values, serum and
Amylase values, serum and
Aspartate aminotransferase (AST [SGOT]) values, serum and
Bilirubin concentrations, serum
(determinations recommended at periodic intervals to monitor hepatic function)

Blood pressure measurements
(recommended at periodic intervals to detect hypertension)
(blood pressure should be measured every 2 weeks for the first 2 months following the conversion from *Sandimmune®* to *Neoral®*)
» Blood urea nitrogen (BUN) concentrations and
» Creatinine concentrations, serum and
» Uric acid concentrations, serum
(determinations recommended at regular intervals to monitor renal function)
(serum creatinine concentrations should be measured every 2 weeks for the first 2 months following the conversion from *Sandimmune®* to *Neoral®*)

Cholesterol, serum
(values may be increased)
» Cyclosporine concentrations, plasma or blood, trough, by radioimmunoassay (RIA) or high pressure liquid chromatography (HPLC)
(recommended for all patients, especially those receiving oral cyclosporine, because of erratic absorption, or for transplant patients to ensure that the patient is receiving an adequate but not toxic dose; because of extreme variability in results achieved depending on whether plasma or whole blood concentrations are measured, timing of samples, handling of samples, and choice of RIA or HPLC, determinations must be standardized within each individual medical center; trough blood concentrations usually are used to monitor therapy)
(when converting a transplant patient from cyclosporine capsules or cyclosporine oral solution [*Sandimmune®*] to cyclosporine modified capsules or cyclosporine modified oral solution [*Neoral®*], the trough blood concentration should be measured every 4 to 7 days during the conversion; if a patient is suspected of having poor absorption of *Sandimmune®*, the cyclosporine trough blood concentration should be monitored very frequently during the conversion because higher-than-expected trough blood concentrations are possible; the manufacturer recommends measuring the trough blood concentration daily until steady-state is reached for patients who required *Sandimmune®* doses exceeding 10 mg per kg of body weight a day)

» Dental examinations
(recommended at 3-month intervals for teeth cleaning and reinforcement of patient's careful plaque control for inhibition of gingival hyperplasia)

Magnesium concentrations, serum and
Potassium concentrations, serum
(determinations recommended at periodic intervals)

Note: *Neoral®* product labeling gives specific guidance for monitoring patients receiving *Neoral®* for treatment of psoriasis and rheumatoid arthritis. Patients receiving *Neoral®* for treatment of psoriasis should have two baseline serum creatinine measurements. Blood pressure, BUN, cholesterol, complete blood count (CBC), serum magnesium, serum potassium, and uric acid should be measured prior to beginning therapy with *Neoral®*. During the initial 3 months of therapy these parameters should be measured once every 2 weeks. After the first 3 months of therapy, these parameters should be measured once every month in stable patients. Patient condition or changes in dose may necessitate more frequent measurements.

Patients receiving *Neoral®* for treatment of rheumatoid arthritis should have two baseline blood pressure measurements and two baseline serum creatinine measurements. During the initial 3 months of therapy these parameters should be measured once every 2 weeks. After the first 3 months of therapy, these parameters should be measured once every month in stable patients. Addition of increased doses of nonsteroidal anti-inflammatory drug therapy to the regimen may necessitate additional monitoring of blood pressure and serum creatinine. Patients receiving methotrexate in addition to *Neoral®* should have CBC and liver function tests (LFT) monitored each month.

In patients receiving *Neoral®* for treatment of nephrotic syndrome, changes in renal function related to nephrotic syndrome may be difficult to distinguish from cyclosporine-induced renal dysfunction. Renal biopsy should be considered for patients with steroid-dependent minimal change nephropathy maintained on *Neoral®* for more than 1 year.

## Side/Adverse Effects

Note: *Post-transplant lymphoproliferative disorders (PTLD)*, including lymphomas and skin malignancies, have been reported in patients receiving cyclosporine; some have regressed when the medication was discontinued. PTLD results from the degree of immunosuppression, not specifically from the use of cyclosporine. Similarly, *infection* may occur in patients receiving cyclosporine. The occurrence of infections results from the degree of immunosuppression, not specifically from the use of cyclosporine.

*Gingival hyperplasia, hypertension, hirsutism, nephrotoxicity,* and *tremor* are the most significant adverse effects in transplant patients resulting from the use of cyclosporine.

*Gastrointestinal disturbances,* including *abdominal discomfort, dyspepsia,* and *nausea, headache, hirsutism, hypertension,* and *nephrotoxicity* are the most significant adverse effects resulting from the use of cyclosporine in patients with rheumatoid arthritis.

*Gastrointestinal disturbances, headache, hirsutism, hypertension, lethargy, muscle or joint pain, nephrotoxicity,* and *paresthesias* are the most significant adverse effects resulting from the use of cyclosporine in patients with psoriasis.

*Gastrointestinal disturbances, gingival hyperplasia, hirsutism, hypertension, nephrotoxicity, paresthesia,* and *tremor* are the most significant adverse effects resulting from the use of cyclosporine in patients with nephrotic syndrome.

The following side/adverse effects have been selected on the basis of their potential clinical significance (possible signs and symptoms in parentheses where appropriate)—not necessarily inclusive:

**Those indicating need for medical attention**
Incidence more frequent
> *Gingival hyperplasia* (bleeding, tender, or enlarged gums); *hypertension*—usually asymptomatic; *nephrotoxicity*—usually asymptomatic
>
> Note: *Gingival hyperplasia* is usually reversible within 6 months after withdrawal of cyclosporine.
>
> *Hypertension* occurs commonly and may be acute, severe, and dose-related (usually associated with doses of 25 to 50 mg per kg of body weight [mg/kg] a day) or chronic and mild to moderate (usually associated with reduced renal function).
>
> *Nephrotoxicity* has been reported in 25, 37, and 38% of kidney, liver, and heart transplantation patients receiving cyclosporine, respectively. Mild *nephrotoxicity* (presenting as an arrest in the fall of pre-operative elevations of blood urea nitrogen [BUN] and creatinine at a range of 35 to 45 mg per deciliter and 2 to 2.5 mg per deciliter, respectively) usually occurs 2 to 3 months after renal, cardiac, or hepatic transplantation and usually responds to dosage reduction. More overt toxicity, with rapidly rising BUN and creatinine concentrations, occurs early after transplantation and must be differentiated from rejection episodes; toxicity usually responds to dosage reduction. Up to 20% of renal transplant patients may have simultaneous nephrotoxicity and rejection.
>
> A form of chronic progressive *nephrotoxicity*, characterized by serial deterioration in renal function and morphologic changes in the kidneys (interstitial fibrosis with tubular atrophy) may occur; reduction in a rising serum creatinine will fail to occur despite reduction in dose or withdrawal of cyclosporine in 5 to 15% of patients; in addition, toxic tubulopathy, peritubular capillary congestion, arteriolopathy, and a striped form of interstitial fibrosis with tubular atrophy may be present. Development of chronic *nephrotoxicity* may be related to high cumulative doses or persistently high circulating trough concentrations of cyclosporine. Effects may be irreversible.
>
> *Nephrotoxicity* (interstitial fibrosis with tubular atrophy) has been reported in 21% of psoriasis patients receiving cyclosporine for an average period of 23 months, and in 10% of rheumatoid arthritis patients receiving cyclosporine for an average period of 19 months. *Nephrotoxicity* in these patients was established by biopsy. Most patients with *nephrotoxicity* were receiving daily doses in excess of 4 mg per kg of body weight.

Incidence less frequent
> *Hepatotoxicity*—usually asymptomatic; usually seen as elevations of hepatic enzymes and bilirubin; *hypomagnesemia*—usually asymptomatic; *infection* (fever or chills; frequent urge to urinate); *seizures; vomiting*
>
> Note: *Seizures* may be related to nephrotoxicity and hypomagnesemia.
> *Hepatotoxicity* usually responds to dosage reduction.

Incidence rare
> *Anaphylaxis* (flushing of face and neck; wheezing or shortness of breath)—with parenteral use; *hemolytic-uremic syndrome; hyperkalemia* (confusion; irregular heartbeat; numbness or tingling in hands, feet, or lips; shortness of breath or difficult breathing; unexplained nervousness; unusual tiredness or weakness; weakness or heaviness of legs); *pancreatitis* (severe stomach pain with nausea and vomiting); *paresthesia* (tingling); *PTLD* (fever; general feeling of discomfort and illness; weight loss); *renal toxicity* (blood in urine)
>
> Note: *Anaphylaxis* occurs only with intravenous use and may be related to the vehicle. The reaction includes facial flushing, acute respiratory distress, blood pressure changes, and tachycardia. A fatality has been reported. Subsequent oral administration of cyclosporine in patients who have experienced an anaphylactic reaction to intravenous cyclosporine has not produced a reaction.
>
> The *hemolytic-uremic syndrome* can occur in the absence of rejection, but may result in graft failure. It is accompanied by avid platelet consumption within the graft. It usually responds, if detected early, to dosage reduction or withdrawal of cyclosporine.
>
> Irregular heartbeat is usually the earliest clinical indication of *hyperkalemia* and is readily detected by electrocardiogram (ECG). *Hyperkalemia* sometimes may be associated with hyperchloremic metabolic acidosis.

**Those indicating need for medical attention only if they continue or are bothersome**
Incidence more frequent
> *Hirsutism* (increase in hair growth); *tremor* (trembling and shaking of hands)—dose-related

Incidence less frequent
> *Acne or oily skin; gastrointestinal disturbances including abdominal discomfort, dyspepsia, and nausea; headache; leg cramps; lethargy*

## Overdose
For more information on the management of overdose or unintentional ingestion, **contact a Poison Control Center** (see *Poison Control Center Listing*).

**Clinical effects of overdose**
The following effects have been selected on the basis of their potential clinical significance (possible signs and symptoms in parentheses where appropriate)—not necessarily inclusive:

Acute
> *Flushing of face; gum soreness and bleeding; headache; hepatotoxicity* (flu-like symptoms); *hyperesthesia* (tingling in the hands and feet); *nephrotoxicity*—usually asymptomatic

**Treatment of overdose**
In general, treatment is symptomatic and supportive.

To decrease absorption—Forced emesis may be useful for up to 2 hours after oral ingestion of toxic doses of cyclosporine.

To enhance elimination—Cyclosporine is not removable by hemodialysis or charcoal hemoperfusion.

Specific treatment—Transient *hepatotoxicity* and *nephrotoxicity* usually respond to withdrawal of cyclosporine.

Patients in whom intentional overdose is confirmed or suspected should be referred for psychiatric consultation.

## Patient Consultation
As an aid to patient consultation, refer to *Advice for the Patient, Cyclosporine (Systemic)*.

In providing consultation, consider emphasizing the following selected information (» = major clinical significance):

**Before using this medication**
» Conditions affecting use, especially:
  Sensitivity to cyclosporine
  Pregnancy—Crosses the placenta; causes birth defects or fetal death in animals
  Breast-feeding—Distributed into breast milk; breast-feeding not recommended because of risk of serious side effects
  Dental—Dental work should be completed prior to initiation of therapy whenever possible
  Other medications, especially allopurinol, androgens, bromocriptine, cimetidine, clarithromycin, coal tar, danazol, diltiazem, erythromycin, estrogens, fluconazole, human immunodeficiency virus (HIV) protease inhibitors, itraconazole, other immunosuppressants, ketoconazole, lovastatin, methoxsalen, nefazodone, nicardipine, potassium-sparing diuretics, radiation therapy, simvastatin, trioxsalen or verapamil
  Other medical problems, especially chickenpox, current malignancy, hepatic function impairment, herpes zoster, infection, premalignant skin lesions, or renal function impairment

**Proper use of this medication**
» Importance of not taking more or less medication than the amount prescribed
  Getting into the habit of taking at the same time each day and in a consistent relation to the type and timing of the intake of food to help increase compliance and maintain steady blood concentrations; if cyclosporine causes stomach upset, checking with physician before changing relation between cyclosporine intake and type and timing of food intake
  Not drinking grapefruit juice or eating grapefruit
  Taking solution orally; special dropper to be used for accurate measuring
  Mixing oral solution (*Sandimmune®*) with milk, chocolate milk, or orange juice and mixing modified oral solution (*Neoral®*) with apple juice or orange juice (preferably at room temperature) in a glass (not wax-lined or plastic disposable) container to improve palatability; stirring well and drinking immediately, then rinsing glass and drinking to make sure all medication is taken; wiping dropper dry but not rinsing with water (to prevent cloudiness)

» Checking with physician before discontinuing medication; possible need for lifelong therapy
» Proper dosing
  Missed dose: Taking as soon as possible if remembered within 12 hours; not taking if almost time for next dose; not doubling doses
» Proper storage

### Precautions while using this medication
» Importance of close monitoring by physician
» Avoiding immunizations unless approved by physician; other persons in patient's household should avoid immunizations with oral poliovirus vaccine; avoiding persons who have taken oral poliovirus vaccine or wearing a protective mask that covers nose and mouth
» Maintaining good dental hygiene and seeing dentist frequently for teeth cleaning to prevent tenderness, bleeding, and gum enlargement

### Side/adverse effects
Importance of discussing possible effects, including cancer, with physician

Signs of potential side effects, especially gingival hyperplasia, hypertension, nephrotoxicity, hepatotoxicity, hypomagnesemia, infection, seizures, vomiting, anaphylaxis, hemolytic-uremic syndrome, hyperkalemia, pancreatitis, paresthesia, post-transplant lymphoproliferative disorders (PTLD), and renal toxicity

## General Dosing Information

Patients receiving cyclosporine should be under the supervision of a physician experienced in immunosuppressive therapy.

If an infection develops, it must be treated promptly; reduction of dosage or withdrawal of cyclosporine may be necessary.

### For parenteral dosage form
Because of the risk of anaphylaxis, it is recommended that the parenteral dosage form be used only in patients unable to take cyclosporine orally for prophylaxis and treatment of transplant rejection.

Cyclosporine usually should be administered by slow intravenous infusion over a period of 2 to 6 hours; however it may be given over a period of up to 24 hours. Rapid intravenous administration may cause acute nephrotoxicity, as well as less serious side effects such as flushing and nausea.

It is recommended that patients receiving intravenous cyclosporine be under continuous observation for at least the first 30 minutes of the infusion and at frequent intervals after that. Equipment and medications (including epinephrine and oxygen) necessary for treatment of a possible anaphylactic reaction should be immediately available during each administration of cyclosporine.

### For use in prophylaxis and treatment of transplant rejection
The dose of cyclosporine should be adjusted based on the clinical response of the patient, trough blood concentrations of the medicine, and the appearance or severity of toxicity.

If signs of allograft rejection occur, a larger dose may be necessary; other therapy should be considered if they persist.

Cyclosporine usually is used in conjunction with other immunosuppressants (e.g., corticosteroids and azathioprine).

Antiviral prophylaxis, i.e., with acyclovir, ganciclovir, and immune globulins, may be advisable for some patients receiving cyclosporine, especially cytomegalovirus (CMV) prophylaxis in patients who have not been exposed to CMV prior to transplantation and who receive a CMV-positive graft.

Vaccination schedules should be continued, except for live vaccines. Vaccinations against hepatitis A and B are recommended. Inactivated poliovirus vaccine should be used instead of oral poliovirus vaccine for both the patient and for people living in the same household as the patient. Vaccines given to immunosuppressed patients may not result in a protective antibody response. Protective antibody concentrations should be checked after the vaccine has been administered.

If a patient is exposed to measles, mumps, rubella, or varicella for the first time while receiving cyclosporine, the patient should receive prophylactic therapy with immune globulin, i.e., pooled human immune globulin or varicella immune globulin.

Newly transplanted patients usually receive adjunctive treatment with corticosteroids. The corticosteroids are tapered to target doses within a few months of transplantation. A typical dosage schedule may start with the equivalent of prednisone 2 mg/kg a day and taper to 0.15 mg/kg a day by 2 months following transplantation.

### For use in treatment of rheumatoid arthritis
Salicylates, nonsteroidal anti-inflammatory drugs, and corticosteroids may be continued with cyclosporine.

There is little long-term data on the use of cyclosporine in the treatment of rheumatoid arthritis. Recurrence of disease activity is usually seen within 4 weeks after stopping cyclosporine.

### For use in treatment of psoriasis
When cyclosporine is used to treat psoriasis, any skin lesions not typical for psoriatic plaque should be biopsied and assessed for malignant or premalignant status before beginning therapy with cyclosporine. Psoriasis patients receiving psoralen and ultraviolet light A (PUVA), ultraviolet light B (UVB), other radiation therapy, or other immunosuppressants should not receive cyclosporine because of the risk of excessive immunosuppression and malignancies.

Patients usually experience some improvement within 2 weeks of beginning cyclosporine, but satisfactory control may require 12 to 16 weeks of therapy with cyclosporine. After satisfactory control of psoriasis is achieved, the dose of cyclosporine should be decreased to the lowest dose needed to control the disease.

There is little experience with long-term treatment of psoriasis with cyclosporine, and continuous treatment longer than one year is not recommended. Relapse of psoriasis occurs in up to 75% of patients within 16 weeks of stopping treatment with cyclosporine.

### Diet/Nutrition
The rate of absorption of oral cyclosporine is decreased in the presence of food, but the extent of absorption may or may not be affected, depending on the type of food ingested. Cyclosporine should be given consistently in relation to food.

Bioavailability of cyclosporine may be increased by ingestion of grapefruit or grapefruit juice, resulting in toxic blood concentrations of cyclosporine.

Cyclosporine oral solution (*Sandimmune*®) should be mixed with milk, chocolate milk, or orange juice to improve taste. Cyclosporine modified oral solution (*Neoral*®) should be mixed with apple juice or orange juice to improve taste. *Neoral*® should not be mixed with milk because the mixture may be unpalatable. Patients should avoid switching diluents frequently because the absorption may change with different diluents.

### Bioequivalence information
Cyclosporine modified capsules and cyclosporine modified oral solution (*Neoral*®) are not bioequivalent to cyclosporine capsules and cyclosporine oral solution (*Sandimmune*®). For a given trough concentration, the mean area under the serum concentration-versus-time curve (AUC) is larger with *Neoral*® than it is with *Sandimmune*®. When converting from one product to another, frequent monitoring of cyclosporine blood concentrations and patient status are needed to monitor for organ rejection and/or cyclosporine toxicity.

When converting a transplant patient from cyclosporine capsules or cyclosporine oral solution (*Sandimmune*®) to cyclosporine modified capsules or cyclosporine modified oral solution (*Neoral*®), the same daily dose (i.e., a 1-to-1 dose conversion) of *Neoral*® should be started and adjusted based on trough blood concentration. The same target trough concentration should be used. The trough blood concentration should be measured once every 4 to 7 days during the conversion. If a patient is suspected of having poor absorption of *Sandimmune*®, the cyclosporine trough blood concentration should be monitored very frequently during the conversion because higher-than-expected trough blood concentrations are possible. The manufacturer recommends measuring the trough blood concentration daily until steady-state is reached for patients who required *Sandimmune*® doses exceeding 10 mg per kg of body weight a day. Blood pressure and serum creatinine should also be measured frequently (i.e., every 2 weeks) for the first 2 months following the conversion to *Neoral*®.

When converting a rheumatoid arthritis, psoriasis, or nephrotic syndrome patient from oral *Sandimmune*® to *Neoral*®, the initial dose of *Neoral*® should be 70% of the *Sandimmune*® dose (i.e., a 1-to-0.7 dose conversion). The dose should be adjusted based on the trough blood concentration and the clinical condition of the patient.

### For treatment of adverse effects
Recommended treatment consists of the following:

Transplant patients
- Many adverse effects (e.g., gastrointestinal toxicity, hyperkalemia, hypomagnesemia, nephrotoxicity) may respond to a reduction in dose. If adverse effects do not respond to a reduction in dose, it may be advisable to convert the patient to a tacrolimus-based immunosuppressant regimen.

Nephrotic syndrome and rheumatoid arthritis patients
- The dose of cyclosporine should be decreased by 25 to 50% if a patient experiences hypertension, elevations in serum creatinine that are ≥ 30% above baseline, or other laboratory abnormalities. If this does not control the adverse effect, or if the adverse effect is severe, cyclosporine should be discontinued.

Psoriasis patients
- The dose of cyclosporine should be decreased by 25 to 50% if a patient experiences hypertension, elevations in serum creatinine that are ≥ 25% above baseline, or other laboratory abnormalities. If this does not control the adverse effect, or if the adverse effect is severe, cyclosporine should be discontinued.

## Oral Dosage Forms

Note: Bracketed uses in the Dosage Forms section refer to categories of use and/or indications that are not included in U.S. product labeling.

### CYCLOSPORINE CAPSULES USP

**Usual adult and adolescent dose**
Transplant rejection (prophylaxis) or
Transplant rejection (treatment)—
> Initial: Oral, 12 to 15 mg per kg of body weight a day beginning four to twelve hours before surgery and continuing for one to two weeks postoperatively, then reduced, usually by 5% a week, to the maintenance dose.
> Maintenance: Oral, 5 to 10 mg per kg of body weight a day.

**Usual pediatric dose**
See *Usual adult and adolescent dose*. Pediatric patients may require higher or more frequent dosing because of accelerated clearance.

**Strength(s) usually available**
U.S.—
>    25 mg (Rx) [*Sandimmune*].
>    50 mg (Rx) [*Sandimmune*].
>    100 mg (Rx) [*Sandimmune*].

Canada—
>    25 mg (Rx) [*Sandimmune*].
>    100 mg (Rx) [*Sandimmune*].

**Packaging and storage**
Store below 25 °C (77 °F), in a tight container, unless otherwise specified by manufacturer.

### CYCLOSPORINE ORAL SOLUTION USP

**Usual adult and adolescent dose**
See *Cyclosporine Capsules USP*.

**Usual pediatric dose**
See *Cyclosporine Capsules USP*.

**Strength(s) usually available**
U.S.—
>    100 mg per mL (Rx) [*Sandimmune* (ethanol 100 mg per mL)].

Canada—
>    100 mg per mL (Rx) [*Sandimmune* (ethanol 100 mg per mL)].

**Packaging and storage**
Store below 30 °C (86 °F), unless otherwise specified by manufacturer. Store in a tight container. Do not refrigerate (according to manufacturer's labeling).

**Stability**
Contents of opened container must be used within 2 months.

**Note**
When dispensing, include a calibrated liquid measuring device provided by the manufacturer.

### CYCLOSPORINE MODIFIED CAPSULES

**Usual adult and adolescent dose**
Transplant rejection (prophylaxis) or
Transplant rejection (treatment)—
> See *Cyclosporine Capsules USP*.

Rheumatoid arthritis (treatment)—
> Oral, 2.5 mg per kg of body weight a day, in two divided doses. If insufficient clinical benefit has been observed after eight weeks, the dose may be increased by 0.5 to 0.75 mg per kg of body weight a day. The dose may be increased again after four additional weeks of therapy to a maximum dose of 4 mg per kg of body weight a day. If no clinical benefit is evident by sixteen weeks of therapy, treatment with cyclosporine should be discontinued.

Psoriasis (treatment)—
> Oral, 2.5 mg per kg of body weight a day, in two divided doses. If insufficient clinical benefit has been observed after four weeks the dose may be increased by 0.5 mg per kg of body weight a day. The dose may be increased again at two-week intervals to a maximum dose of 4 mg per kg of body weight a day. If no clinical benefit is evident by six weeks of treatment with 4 mg per kg of body weight a day, cyclosporine should be discontinued. After satisfactory control of psoriasis is achieved, the dose of cyclosporine should be decreased to the lowest dose needed to control the disease.

[Graft-versus-host disease (prophylaxis)]—
> Oral, 12.5 mg per kg of body weight a day, in two divided doses. After three to six months of treatment, the cyclosporine dose should be tapered gradually to zero by one year following transplantation.

[Graft-versus-host disease (treatment)]—
> Mild graft-versus-host disease occurring after discontinuation of cyclosporine may be treated by the re-introduction of low-dose *Neoral*®.

[Nephrotic syndrome (treatment)]—
> Initial: Oral, 3.5 mg per kg of body weight a day, in two divided doses. If no clinical benefit is evident by three months of treatment, cyclosporine should be discontinued.
> Maintenance: The dose should be adjusted based on efficacy, as measured by proteinuria, and side effects, but should not exceed 5 mg per kg of body weight a day.

**Usual pediatric dose**
Transplant rejection (prophylaxis)—
> See *Cyclosporine Capsules USP*.

[Nephrotic syndrome (treatment)]—
> Initial: Oral, 4.2 mg per kg of body weight a day, in two divided doses. If no clinical benefit is evident by three months of treatment, cyclosporine should be discontinued.
> Maintenance: The dose should be adjusted based on efficacy, as measured by proteinuria, and side effects, but should not exceed 6 mg per kg of body weight a day.

**Strength(s) usually available**
U.S.—
>    25 mg (Rx) [*Neoral* (ethanol 95 mg per mL)].
>    100 mg (Rx) [*Neoral* (ethanol 95 mg per mL)].

Canada—
>    25 mg (Rx) [*Neoral*].
>    50 mg (Rx) [*Neoral*].
>    100 mg (Rx) [*Neoral*].

**Packaging and storage**
Store between 20 and 25 °C (68 and 77 °F). Store in a tight container. Do not refrigerate.

### CYCLOSPORINE MODIFIED ORAL SOLUTION

**Usual adult and adolescent dose**
See *Cyclosporine Modified Capsules*.

**Usual pediatric dose**
See *Cyclosporine Modified Capsules*.

**Strength(s) usually available**
U.S.—
>    100 mg per mL (Rx) [*Neoral* (ethanol 95 mg per mL)].

Canada—
>    100 mg per mL (Rx) [*Neoral* (ethanol 95 mg per mL)].

**Packaging and storage**
Store between 20 and 25 °C (68 and 77 °F). Store in a tight container. Do not refrigerate.

**Stability**
Contents of opened container must be used within 2 months.

**Note**
When dispensing, include a calibrated liquid measuring device provided by the manufacturer.

## Parenteral Dosage Forms

### CYCLOSPORINE CONCENTRATE FOR INJECTION USP

**Usual adult and adolescent dose**
Transplant rejection (prophylaxis)—
> Initial: Intravenous infusion, 2 to 6 mg per kg of body weight a day beginning four to twelve hours prior to surgery and continuing postoperatively until the patient can tolerate the oral solution.

**Usual pediatric dose**
See *Usual adult and adolescent dose*. Pediatric patients may require higher or more frequent dosing because of accelerated clearance.

**Strength(s) usually available**
U.S.—
>    50 mg per mL (Rx) [*Sandimmune* (polyoxyethylated castor oil 650 mg per mL; ethanol 278 mg per mL)].

Canada—
>    50 mg per mL (Rx) [*Sandimmune* (polyoxyethylated castor oil 650 mg per mL; ethanol 278 mg per mL)].

**Packaging and storage**
Store below 30 °C (86 °F), unless otherwise specified by manufacturer. Protect from freezing.

**Preparation of dosage form**
Cyclosporine Concentrate for Injection USP is prepared for intravenous administration by diluting each mL in 20 to 100 mL of 0.9% sodium chloride injection or 5% dextrose injection. Use of glass containers is recommended because of possible leaching of diethylhexylphthalate (DEHP) from polyvinyl chloride (PVC) bags into cyclosporine solutions.

### Stability
Reconstituted solutions are stable for up to 24 hours in 5% dextrose injection and for 6 hours (in PVC containers) to 12 hours (in glass containers) in 0.9% sodium chloride injection. Significant amounts of cyclosporine are lost when it is administered through PVC tubing.

### Selected Bibliography
Fahey JL, et al. UCLA Conference. Immune interventions in disease. Ann Intern Med 1987; 106: 257-74.
Ptachcinski RJ, Burckart GJ, Venkataramanan R. Cyclosporine. Drug Intell Clin Pharm 1985; 19: 90-100.
Scott JP, Higenbottam TW. Adverse reactions and interactions of cyclosporine. Med Toxicol 1988; 3: 107-27.

Revised: 07/23/98

---

**CYCLOTHIAZIDE** — See *Diuretics, Thiazide (Systemic)*

**CYPROHEPTADINE** — See *Antihistamines (Systemic)*

**CYSTEAMINE** — The *Cysteamine (Systemic)* monograph is not included in this published version of the USP DI database. Copies of the monograph are available on request from Micromedex, Inc. - Reprint Requests, 6200 S. Syracuse Way, Suite 300, Englewood, CO 80111; telephone (303) 486-6400; telefax (303) 486-6464; Email: USPDI@MDX.COM.

---

# CYTARABINE Systemic

VA CLASSIFICATION (Primary): AN300
Commonly used brand name(s): *Cytosar; Cytosar-U*.
Other commonly used names are ara-C and cytosine arabinoside.
Note: For a listing of dosage forms and brand names by country availability, see *Dosage Forms* section(s).

## Category
Antineoplastic.

## Indications
Note: Bracketed information in the *Indications* section refers to uses that are not included in U.S. product labeling.
**Accepted**
Leukemia, acute lymphocytic (treatment)
Leukemia, acute myelocytic (treatment)
Leukemia, meningeal (prophylaxis and treatment)
Erythroleukemia (treatment)
Leukemia, chronic myelocytic (treatment)
Lymphomas, non-Hodgkin's (treatment)
[Lymphomas, Hodgkin's (treatment)][1] or
[Myelodysplastic syndrome (treatment)][1]—Cytarabine is indicated for treatment of acute lymphocytic leukemia, acute myelocytic leukemia, meningeal leukemia (by intrathecal injection), erythroleukemia, chronic myelocytic leukemia (blast phase), non-Hodgkin's lymphomas in children, Hodgkin's disease, and myelodysplastic syndrome.

[1] Not included in Canadian product labeling.

## Pharmacology/Pharmacokinetics
**Physicochemical characteristics**
Molecular weight—243.22.
pKa—4.35 in 60% aqueous ethanol.

**Mechanism of action/Effect**
Cytarabine is an antimetabolite. Cytarabine is cell cycle–specific for the S phase of cell division. Activity occurs as the result of activation to cytarabine triphosphate in the tissues and includes inhibition of DNA synthesis with little effect on RNA and protein synthesis.

**Other actions/effects**
Cytarabine is a potent immunosuppressant.

**Distribution**
Only moderate amounts cross the blood-brain barrier with rapid intravenous administration, although cerebrospinal concentrations of 40 to 50% of steady state plasma concentrations are attained after continuous intravenous infusion.

**Protein binding**
Low (15%).

**Biotransformation**
Rapidly deaminated in blood and tissues, especially the liver, but minimally in the cerebrospinal fluid (CSF).

**Half-life**
Varies between individuals; may relate to cytotoxicity.
Alpha phase—10 to 15 minutes.
Beta phase—1 to 3 hours (about 2 hours after intrathecal administration).

**Time to peak plasma concentration**
Subcutaneous—20 to 60 minutes.

**Elimination**
Renal, less than 10% unchanged.

## Precautions to Consider
**Carcinogenicity**
Secondary malignancies are potential delayed effects of many antineoplastic agents, although it is not clear whether the effect is related to their mutagenic or immunosuppressive action. The effect of dose and duration of therapy is also unknown, although risk seems to increase with long-term use. Although information is limited, available data seem to indicate that the carcinogenic risk is greatest with the alkylating agents.
Antimetabolites have been shown to be carcinogenic in animals and may be associated with an increased risk of development of secondary carcinomas in humans, although the risk appears to be less than with alkylating agents.

**Mutagenicity**
Cytarabine may cause chromosomal damage, including chromatoid breaks, in humans. Malignant transformation of rodent cells in culture has been reported.

**Pregnancy/Reproduction**
Fertility—Gonadal suppression, resulting in amenorrhea or azoospermia, may occur in patients taking antineoplastic therapy, especially with the alkylating agents. In general, these effects appear to be related to dose and length of therapy and may be irreversible. Prediction of the degree of testicular or ovarian function impairment is complicated by the common use of combinations of several antineoplastics, which makes it difficult to assess the effects of individual agents.
Cytarabine has been associated with reversible germ cell toxicity in humans.

Pregnancy—Studies in humans have not been done.
In humans, one case of trisomy, one case of extremity and ear deformities, one case of upper and lower distal limb defects, and one case of enlarged spleen have been reported in infants of mothers who received cytarabine. Other problems reported include pancytopenia; transient depression of leukocyte counts, hematocrit, or platelet counts; electrolyte abnormalities; transient eosinophilia; increased IgM concentrations and hyperpyrexia; fatal gastroenteritis; and prematurity and low birth weight. Several normal births have also been reported.
First trimester: It is usually recommended that use of antineoplastics, especially combination chemotherapy, be avoided whenever possible, especially during the first trimester. Although information is limited because of the relatively few instances of antineoplastic administration during pregnancy, the mutagenic, teratogenic, and carcinogenic potential of these medications must be considered.
Other hazards to the fetus include adverse reactions seen in adults.
In general, use of a contraceptive is recommended during cytotoxic drug therapy.
Cytarabine is teratogenic in some animal species.
FDA Pregnancy Category D.

**Breast-feeding**
Although very little information is available regarding distribution of antineoplastic agents into breast milk, breast-feeding is not recommended while cytarabine is being administered because of the risks to the infant (adverse effects, mutagenicity, carcinogenicity). It is not known whether cytarabine is distributed into breast milk.

## Pediatrics
Appropriate studies on the relationship of age to the effects of cytarabine have not been performed in the pediatric population. However, pediatrics-specific problems that would limit the usefulness of this medication in children are not expected.

## Geriatrics
Although appropriate studies on the relationship of age to the effects of cytarabine have not been performed in the geriatric population, geriatrics-specific problems that would limit the usefulness of this medication in the elderly are not expected. However, elderly patients are more likely to have age-related renal function impairment, which may require reduction of dosage in patients receiving cytarabine.

## Dental
The bone marrow depressant effects of cytarabine may result in an increased incidence of microbial infection, delayed healing, and gingival bleeding. Dental work, whenever possible should be completed prior to initiation of therapy or deferred until blood counts have returned to normal. Patients should be instructed in proper oral hygiene during treatment, including caution in use of regular toothbrushes, dental floss, and toothpicks.

Cytarabine also commonly causes stomatitis associated with considerable discomfort.

## Drug interactions and/or related problems
The following drug interactions and/or related problems have been selected on the basis of their potential clinical significance (possible mechanism in parentheses where appropriate)—not necessarily inclusive (» = major clinical significance):

Note: Combinations containing any of the following medications, depending on the amount present, may also interact with this medication.

Allopurinol or
Colchicine or
» Probenecid or
» Sulfinpyrazone
(cytarabine may raise the concentration of blood uric acid; dosage adjustment of antigout agents may be necessary to control hyperuricemia and gout; allopurinol may be preferred to prevent or reverse cytarabine-induced hyperuricemia because of risk of uric acid nephropathy with uricosuric antigout agents)

Blood dyscrasia–causing medications (See *Appendix II*)
(leukopenic and/or thrombocytopenic effects of cytarabine may be increased with concurrent or recent therapy if these medications cause the same effects; dosage adjustment of cytarabine, if necessary, should be based on blood counts)

» Bone marrow depressants, other (See *Appendix II*) or
Radiation therapy
(additive bone marrow depression may occur; dosage reduction may be required when two or more bone marrow depressants, including radiation, are used concurrently or consecutively)

» Cyclophosphamide
(concurrent use with high-dose cytarabine therapy for bone marrow transplant preparation has been reported to result in an increase in cardiomyopathy with subsequent death; the cardiac toxicity may be schedule dependent)

» Immunosuppressants, other, such as:
Azathioprine
Chlorambucil
Corticosteroids, glucocorticoid
Cyclophosphamide
Cyclosporine
Mercaptopurine
Muromonab CD-3
Tacrolimus
(concurrent use with cytarabine may increase the risk of infection)

Methotrexate
(administration of cytarabine 48 hours before or 10 minutes after initiation of methotrexate therapy may result in a synergistic cytotoxic effect; however, evidence is inconclusive and dosage adjustment based on routine hematologic monitoring is recommended)

Vaccines, killed virus
(because normal defense mechanisms may be suppressed by cytarabine therapy, the patient's antibody response to the vaccine may be decreased. The interval between discontinuation of medications that cause immunosuppression and restoration of the patient's ability to respond to the vaccine depends on the intensity and type of immunosuppression-causing medication used, the underlying disease, and other factors; estimates vary from 3 months to 1 year)

» Vaccines, live virus
(because normal defense mechanisms may be suppressed by cytarabine therapy, concurrent use with a live virus vaccine may potentiate the replication of the vaccine virus, may increase the side/adverse effects of the vaccine virus, and/or may decrease the patient's antibody response to the vaccine; immunization of these patients should be undertaken only with extreme caution after careful review of the patient's hematologic status and only with the knowledge and consent of the physician managing the cytarabine therapy. The interval between discontinuation of medications that cause immunosuppression and restoration of the patient's ability to respond to the vaccine depends on the intensity and type of immunosuppression-causing medication used, the underlying disease, and other factors; estimates vary from 3 months to 1 year. Patients with leukemia in remission should not receive live virus vaccine until at least 3 months after their last chemotherapy. In addition, immunization with oral poliovirus vaccine should be postponed in persons in close contact with the patient, especially family members)

## Laboratory value alterations
The following have been selected on the basis of their potential clinical significance (possible effect in parentheses where appropriate)—not necessarily inclusive (» = major clinical significance):

With physiology/laboratory test values
Alkaline phosphatase values, serum and
Aspartate aminotransferase (AST [SGOT]) values, serum and
Bilirubin concentrations, serum
(may be increased, indicating possible hepatotoxicity)

Uric acid
(concentrations in blood and urine may be increased)

## Medical considerations/Contraindications
The medical considerations/contraindications included have been selected on the basis of their potential clinical significance (reasons given in parentheses where appropriate)—not necessarily inclusive (» = major clinical significance).

*Risk-benefit should be considered when the following medical problems exist:*

» Bone marrow depression
(lower dosage may be necessary)
» Chickenpox, existing or recent (including recent exposure) or
» Herpes zoster
(risk of severe generalized disease)
Gout, history of or
Urate renal stones, history of
(risk of hyperuricemia)
» Hepatic function impairment
(reduced detoxification of cytarabine; lower dosage may be necessary)
» Infection
Renal function impairment
(reduced elimination; lower dosage may be necessary)
Sensitivity to cytarabine
» Tumor cell infiltration of the bone marrow
» Caution should be used also in patients who have had previous cytotoxic drug therapy or radiation therapy.

## Patient monitoring
The following are especially important in patient monitoring (other tests may be warranted in some patients, depending on condition; (» = major clinical significance):

Alanine aminotransferase (ALT [SGPT]) values, serum and
Aspartate aminotransferase (AST [SGOT]) values, serum and
Bilirubin concentrations, serum and
Lactate dehydrogenase (LDH) values, serum
(recommended prior to initiation of therapy and at periodic intervals during therapy; frequency varies according to clinical state, agent, dose, and other agents being used concurrently)

» Bone marrow aspiration
(recommended at 2-week intervals until remission occurs)
» Hematocrit or hemoglobin and
Leukocyte count, total and, if appropriate, differential and
» Platelet count
(determinations recommended prior to initiation of therapy and at periodic intervals during therapy; frequency varies according to clinical state, agent, dose, and other agents being used concurrently)

Uric acid concentrations, serum
(recommended prior to initiation of therapy and at periodic intervals

during therapy; frequency varies according to clinical state, agent, dose, and other agents being used concurrently)

## Side/Adverse Effects

Note: Many "side effects" of antineoplastic therapy are unavoidable and represent the medication's pharmacologic action. Some of these (for example, leukopenia and thrombocytopenia) are actually used as parameters to aid in individual dosage titration.

Incidence of side effects (except nausea and vomiting) is higher with continuous intravenous administration than with rapid intravenous administration.

Intrathecal administration may result in systemic effects.

Acute pancreatitis has been reported in patients previously treated with asparaginase.

High-dose therapy has been associated with severe and potentially fatal toxicity, including reversible corneal toxicity and hemorrhagic conjunctivitis (which may be prevented or reduced by prophylactic administration of a local corticosteroid eye drop), cerebral dysfunction (confusion, tiredness, memory loss, seizures), cerebellar dysfunction (trouble in speaking, standing, or walking; tremors), gastrointestinal ulceration, peritonitis (including pneumatosis cystoides intestinalis leading to peritonitis), sepsis and liver abscess, pulmonary edema, hepatic damage with hyperbilirubinemia, bowel necrosis, necrotizing colitis, skin rash leading to desquamation, fatal cardiomyopathy, a potentially fatal syndrome of sudden respiratory distress progressing to pulmonary edema and cardiomegaly, and peripheral motor and sensory neuropathies.

The following side/adverse effects have been selected on the basis of their potential clinical significance (possible signs and symptoms in parentheses where appropriate)—not necessarily inclusive:

**Those indicating need for medical attention**
Incidence more frequent—occurring in 15 to 100% of patients
*Leukopenia or infection* (usually asymptomatic; less frequently, fever or chills; cough or hoarseness; lower back or side pain; painful or difficult urination); *stomatitis* (sores in mouth and on lips); *thrombocytopenia* (usually asymptomatic; less frequently, unusual bleeding or bruising; black, tarry stools; blood in urine or stools; pinpoint red spots on skin)

Note: With *leukopenia*, leukocyte levels decline in two phases starting in the first 24 hours, with a nadir at days 7 to 9, a brief rise until the twelfth day, and a deeper fall with a nadir at days 15 to 24. Levels rise rapidly to baseline in the next 10 days.

With *thrombocytopenia*, platelet counts fall noticeably by 5 days following a dose, with the nadir at 12 to 15 days and a rise to baseline over the next 10 days.

Incidence less frequent—occurring in 10% or less of patients
*Central nervous system (CNS) toxicity, cerebellar or cerebral* (numbness or tingling in fingers, toes, or face; unusual tiredness)—more frequent with high-dose therapy; *hyperuricemia or uric acid nephropathy* (joint pain; lower back or side pain; swelling of feet or lower legs)

Note: *Hyperuricemia or uric acid nephropathy* occurs most commonly during initial treatment of leukemia or lymphoma, as a result of rapid cell breakdown, which leads to elevated serum uric acid concentrations.

Incidence rare—occurring in 2% or less of patients
*Cellulitis or thrombophlebitis* (pain at injection site); *drug reaction or ara-C syndrome* (bone or muscle pain; chest pain; fever; general feeling of discomfort or illness or weakness; reddened eyes; skin rash); *esophagitis* (difficulty in swallowing; heartburn); *gastrointestinal hemorrhage* (black, tarry stools); *hepatotoxicity* (yellow eyes or skin); *megaloblastic anemia* (fainting spells; irregular heartbeat; unusual tiredness; weakness); *pulmonary edema or diffuse interstitial pneumonitis* (cough; shortness of breath); *urinary retention* (decrease in urination)

Note: The *drug reaction or ara-C syndrome* usually occurs 6 to 12 hours after administration; it may be prevented by or respond to steroid treatment.

**Those indicating need for medical attention only if they continue or are bothersome**
Incidence more frequent—occurring in 15 to 100% of patients
*Loss of appetite; nausea and vomiting*

Note: *Nausea and vomiting* occur more frequently when large intravenous doses are administered quickly than when they are infused.

Incidence less frequent or rare—occurring in 10% or less of patients
*Diarrhea; dizziness; headache, especially after intrathecal administration; itching of skin; skin freckling*

**Those not indicating need for medical attention**
Incidence less frequent or rare
*Loss of hair*

Note: Complete *alopecia* is more frequent with high-dose therapy.

**Those indicating the need for medical attention if they occur after medication is discontinued**
*Bone marrow depression* (black, tarry stools; blood in urine or stools; cough or hoarseness; fever or chills; lower back or side pain; painful or difficult urination; pinpoint red spots on skin; unusual bleeding or bruising)

## Patient Consultation

As an aid to patient consultation, refer to *Advice for the Patient, Cytarabine (Systemic)*.

In providing consultation, consider emphasizing the following selected information (» = major clinical significance):

**Before using this medication**
» Conditions affecting use, especially:
  Sensitivity to cytarabine
  Pregnancy—Use not recommended because of mutagenic, teratogenic, and carcinogenic potential; advisability of using contraception; telling physician immediately if pregnancy is suspected
  Breast-feeding—Not recommended because of risk of serious side effects
  Other medications, especially probenecid, sulfinpyrazone, other bone marrow depressants, other immunosuppressants, or other cytotoxic drug or radiation therapy
  Other medical problems, especially chickenpox, herpes zoster, hepatic function impairment, or infection

**Proper use of this medication**
Caution in taking combination therapy; taking each medication at the right time
Importance of ample fluid intake and subsequent increase in urine output to aid in excretion of uric acid
Frequency of nausea and vomiting; importance of continuing medication despite stomach upset
» Proper dosing

**Precautions while using this medication**
» Importance of close monitoring by the physician
» Avoiding immunizations unless approved by physician; other persons in patient's household should avoid immunizations with oral poliovirus vaccine; avoiding persons who have taken oral poliovirus vaccine or wearing a protective mask that covers nose and mouth
*Caution if bone marrow depression occurs:*
» Avoiding exposure to persons with bacterial infections, especially during periods of low blood counts; checking with physician immediately if fever or chills, cough or hoarseness, lower back or side pain, or painful or difficult urination occur
» Checking with physician immediately if unusual bleeding or bruising; black, tarry stools; blood in urine or stools; or pinpoint red spots on skin occur
Caution in use of regular toothbrush, dental floss, or toothpick; physician, dentist, or nurse may suggest alternatives; checking with physician before having dental work done
Not touching eyes or inside of nose unless hands washed immediately before
Using caution to avoid accidental cuts with use of sharp objects such as safety razor or fingernail or toenail cutters
Avoiding contact sports or other situations where bruising or injury could occur

**Side/adverse effects**
May cause adverse effects such as blood problems; importance of discussing possible effects with physician
Signs of potential side effects, especially leukopenia, infection, stomatitis, thrombocytopenia, CNS toxicity, hyperuricemia, uric acid nephropathy, cellulitis, thrombophlebitis, drug reaction, ara-C syndrome, esophagitis, gastrointestinal hemorrhage, hepatotoxicity, megaloblastic anemia, pulmonary edema, diffuse interstitial pneumonitis, and urinary retention
Physician or nurse can help in dealing with side effects
Possibility of hair loss; normal hair growth should return after treatment has ended

## General Dosing Information

It is recommended that for induction therapy cytarabine be administered in a hospital setting under supervision of a physician experienced in antimetabolite chemotherapy. Intrathecal therapy should be carried out only by a physician familiar with the regimen.

A variety of dosage schedules and regimens of cytarabine, alone or in combination with other antitumor agents, are used. The prescriber may consult the medical literature as well as the manufacturer's literature in choosing a specific dosage.

Dosage must be adjusted to meet the individual requirements of each patient, on the basis of clinical response and degree of bone marrow depression.

Patients generally tolerate higher doses with less hematologic depression when cytarabine is administered by rapid intravenous injection rather than by slow infusion, although nausea and vomiting may be more severe and may persist for several hours after the injection.

Development of uric acid nephropathy in patients with leukemia or lymphoma may be prevented by adequate oral hydration and, in some cases, administration of allopurinol. Alkalinization of urine may be necessary if serum uric acid concentrations are elevated.

It is recommended that an induction program be continued until either response or toxicity occurs, or until it becomes clear that the patient will not respond. Bone marrow improvement may require 7 to 64 days; treatment is stopped when the bone marrow becomes hypocellular and is resumed when it recovers.

If leukocyte counts fall below 1000 per cubic millimeter or platelet counts below 50,000 per cubic millimeter, cytarabine therapy may need to be withdrawn until definite signs of bone marrow recovery occur. The lowest leukocyte and platelet levels are usually reached after 12 to 24 drug-free days. Therapy should be resumed when appropriate leukocyte and platelet levels are reached; these levels may be lower than normal to avoid patient escape from control.

In acute leukemia, cytarabine may be administered despite the presence of thrombocytopenia and bleeding; cessation of bleeding and increase in platelet count have occurred in some cases during treatment and platelet transfusions are useful in others.

Special precautions are recommended in patients who develop thrombocytopenia as a result of administration of cytarabine. These may include extreme care in performing invasive procedures; regular inspection of intravenous sites, skin (including perirectal area), and mucous membrane surfaces for signs of bleeding or bruising; limiting frequency of venipuncture and avoiding intramuscular injections; testing urine, emesis, stool, and secretions for occult blood; care in use of regular toothbrushes, dental floss, toothpicks, safety razors, and fingernail and toenail cutters; avoiding constipation; and using caution to prevent falls and other injuries. Such patients should avoid alcohol and aspirin intake because of the risk of gastrointestinal bleeding. Platelet transfusions may be required.

Patients who develop leukopenia should be observed carefully for signs of infection. Antibiotic support may be required. In neutropenic patients who develop fever, broad-spectrum antibiotic coverage should be initiated empirically, pending bacterial cultures and appropriate diagnostic tests.

**Safety considerations for handling this medication**

There is limited but increasing evidence and concern that personnel involved in preparation and administration of parenteral antineoplastics may be at some risk because of the potential mutagenicity, teratogenicity, and/or carcinogenicity of these agents, although the actual risk is unknown. USP advisory panels recommend cautious handling both in preparation and disposal of antineoplastic agents. Precautions that have been suggested include:
- Use of a biological containment cabinet during reconstitution and dilution of parenteral medications and wearing of disposable surgical gloves and masks.
- Use of proper technique to prevent contamination of the medication, work area, and operator during transfer between containers (including proper training of personnel in this technique).
- Cautious and proper disposal of needles, syringes, vials, ampuls, and unused medication.

A number of medical centers have developed detailed guidelines for handling of antineoplastic agents.

**Combination chemotherapy**

Cytarabine is usually used in combination with other agents in various regimens. As a result, incidence and/or severity of side effects may be altered and different dosages (usually reduced) may be used. For example, cytarabine is part of the following chemotherapeutic combinations (some commonly used acronyms are in parentheses):
— cytarabine and doxorubicin (Ara-C + ADR).
— cytarabine, daunorubicin, prednisolone, and mercaptopurine (Ara-C + DNR + PRED + MP).
— cytarabine and thioguanine (Ara-C + 6-TG).
— cytarabine, thioguanine, and daunorubicin.
— cytarabine, doxorubicin, vincristine, and prednisolone.
— cytarabine, daunorubicin, thioguanine, prednisone, and vincristine.
— cytarabine and daunorubicin.
— cytarabine and mitoxantrone.

For specific dosages and schedules, consult the literature. For information regarding each agent, consult the individual monographs.

## Parenteral Dosage Forms

### CYTARABINE STERILE USP

**Usual adult and adolescent dose**
Acute myelocytic leukemia or
Erythroleukemia—
Induction: Intravenous, 100 to 200 mg per square meter of body surface or 3 mg per kg of body weight per day (as a continuous infusion over twenty-four hours or in divided doses by rapid injection) for five to ten days, with the course repeated approximately every two weeks.
Maintenance: Subcutaneous, 1 mg per kg of body weight one or two times a week.
Note: High-dose cytarabine therapy has been used in selected patients with refractory acute leukemia or lymphomas. One commonly used regimen is 2 to 3 grams per square meter of body surface intravenously (over 1 to 3 hours) every twelve hours for two to six days. High-dose cytarabine therapy should be used with extreme caution and only by clinicians familiar with the procedure.
Meningeal leukemia—
Intrathecal, 5 to 75 mg per square meter of body surface at intervals ranging from once a day for four days to once every four days. A frequently used dosage is 30 mg per square meter of body surface once every four days until CSF findings are normal, followed by one additional dose.

**Usual pediatric dose**
See *Usual adult and adolescent dose*.
Note: Safety of use in infants has not been established.

**Size(s) usually available**
U.S.—
100 mg (Rx) [*Cytosar-U*; GENERIC].
500 mg (Rx) [*Cytosar-U*; GENERIC].
1 gram (Rx) [*Cytosar-U*].
2 grams (Rx) [*Cytosar-U*].
Canada—
100 mg (Rx) [*Cytosar*].
500 mg (Rx) [*Cytosar*].
1 gram (Rx) [*Cytosar*].
2 grams (Rx) [*Cytosar*].

**Packaging and storage**
Store below 40 °C (104 °F), preferably between 15 and 30 °C (59 and 86 °F), unless otherwise specified by manufacturer.

**Preparation of dosage form**
Caution: Use of diluents containing benzyl alcohol is not recommended for preparation of medications for use in neonates. A fatal toxic syndrome consisting of metabolic acidosis, CNS depression, respiratory problems, renal failure, hypotension, and possibly seizures and intracranial hemorrhages has been associated with this use. Diluents containing benzyl alcohol should also be avoided in preparation of high-dose and intrathecal therapy.

Sterile Cytarabine USP is reconstituted for *intravenous* or *subcutaneous* (but *not intrathecal*) use by adding 5 mL of bacteriostatic water for injection (with benzyl alcohol) provided by the manufacturer to the 100-mg vial, producing a solution containing 20 mg of cytarabine per mL, or by adding 10 mL of bacteriostatic water for injection to the 500-mg vial, producing a solution containing 50 mg of cytarabine per mL.

Cytarabine solutions may be further diluted with water for injection, 5% dextrose injection, or 0.9% sodium chloride injection for administration by intravenous infusion.

Sterile Cytarabine USP is reconstituted for *intrathecal* use by adding 5 or 10 mL of an isotonic buffered diluent (without preservatives) such as Elliott's B solution, lactated Ringer's injection, or the patient's cerebrospinal fluid (CSF) to the 100- or 500-mg vial, respectively. The volume administered should correspond to an equal volume of CSF removed.

**Stability**
Reconstituted solutions are stable at room temperature for 48 hours. Solutions that develop a slight haze should be discarded. Infusion solutions containing up to 500 mcg (0.5 mg) of cytarabine per mL are stable at room temperature for 7 days. Solutions for intrathecal use should be used immediately after preparation.

## Selected Bibliography
Bolwell BJ, Cassileth PA, Gale RP. High dose cytarabine. A review. Leukemia 1988 May; 2: 253-60.

Revised: 07/15/94

# DACARBAZINE Systemic

VA CLASSIFICATION (Primary): AN900
Commonly used brand name(s): *DTIC; DTIC-Dome*.
Note: For a listing of dosage forms and brand names by country availability, see *Dosage Forms* section(s).

## Category
Antineoplastic.

## Indications
Note: Bracketed information in the *Indications* section refers to uses that are not included in U.S. product labeling.

**Accepted**
Melanoma, malignant (treatment)—Dacarbazine is indicated for treatment of metastatic malignant melanoma.

Lymphomas, Hodgkin's (treatment)[1]—Dacarbazine is indicated for treatment of Hodgkin's disease as second-line therapy in combination with other effective agents.

[Sarcomas, soft tissue (treatment)][1]—Dacarbazine is used for treatment of some soft-tissue metastatic sarcomas.

[Carcinoma, islet cell (treatment)][1]—Dacarbazine is used for treatment of islet cell carcinoma.

[1]Not included in Canadian product labeling.

## Pharmacology/Pharmacokinetics

**Physicochemical characteristics**
Molecular weight—182.19.
pKa—4.42.

**Mechanism of action/Effect**
Dacarbazine is thought to be an alkylating agent. Major action is believed to be alkylation; dacarbazine is cell cycle–phase-nonspecific. Dacarbazine may inhibit DNA and RNA synthesis via formation of carbonium ions. Some activity and toxicity may occur as the result of activation by hepatic enzymes.

**Distribution**
Crosses the blood-brain barrier only to a limited extent.

**Protein binding**
Very low.

**Biotransformation**
Hepatic, extensive.

**Half-life**
Normal—
 Alpha phase: 19 minutes.
 Beta phase: 5 hours.
Renal or hepatic function impairment—
 Alpha phase: 55 minutes.
 Beta phase: 7.2 hours.

**Elimination**
Renal; 40% of injected dose in 6 hours, one half of that unchanged.

## Precautions to Consider

**Carcinogenicity/Mutagenicity**
Secondary malignancies are potential delayed effects of many antineoplastic agents, although it is not clear whether the effect is related to their mutagenic or immunosuppressive action. The effect of dose and duration of therapy is also unknown, although risk seems to increase with long-term use. Although information is limited, available data seem to indicate that the carcinogenic risk is greatest with the alkylating agents.
Dacarbazine is a potent carcinogen in animals. In rats, dacarbazine produced proliferative endocardial lesions, including fibrosarcomas and sarcomas; in mice, angiosarcomas of the spleen were induced.

**Pregnancy/Reproduction**
Fertility—Gonadal suppression, resulting in amenorrhea or azoospermia, may occur in patients taking antineoplastic therapy, especially with the alkylating agents. In general, these effects appear to be related to dose and length of therapy and may be irreversible. Prediction of the degree of testicular or ovarian function impairment is complicated by the common use of combinations of several antineoplastics, which makes it difficult to assess the effects of individual agents.

Pregnancy—Adequate and well-controlled studies in humans have not been done.
First trimester: It is usually recommended that use of antineoplastics, especially combination chemotherapy, be avoided whenever possible, especially during the first trimester. Although information is limited because of the relatively few instances of antineoplastic administration during pregnancy, the mutagenic, teratogenic, and carcinogenic potential of these medications must be considered.
Other hazards to the fetus include adverse reactions seen in adults.
In general, use of a contraceptive is recommended during cytotoxic drug therapy.
Studies in rats have shown that dacarbazine is teratogenic at doses 20 times the human daily dose given on day 12 of gestation. Administration of 10 times the human daily dose to male rats twice weekly for 9 weeks resulted in an increased incidence of fetal resorptions in female rats mated to them. Dacarbazine caused fetal skeletal anomalies in rabbits given seven times the human daily dose on days 6 to 15 of gestation.
FDA Pregnancy Category C.

**Breast-feeding**
Although very little information is available regarding distribution of antineoplastic agents into breast milk, breast-feeding is not recommended while dacarbazine is being administered because of the risks to the infant (adverse effects, mutagenicity, carcinogenicity). It is not known whether dacarbazine is distributed into breast milk.

**Pediatrics**
Appropriate studies on the relationship of age to the effects of dacarbazine have not been performed in the pediatric population.

**Geriatrics**
No information is available on the relationship of age to the effects of dacarbazine in geriatric patients. However, elderly patients are more likely to have age-related renal function impairment, which may require reduction of dosage in patients receiving dacarbazine.

**Dental**
The bone marrow depressant effects of dacarbazine may result in an increased incidence of microbial infection, delayed healing, and gingival bleeding. Dental work, whenever possible, should be completed prior to initiation of therapy or deferred until blood counts have returned to normal. Patients should be instructed in proper oral hygiene during treatment, including caution in use of regular toothbrushes, dental floss, and toothpicks.
Dacarbazine may also rarely cause stomatitis associated with considerable discomfort.

**Drug interactions and/or related problems**
The following drug interactions and/or related problems have been selected on the basis of their potential clinical significance (possible mechanism in parentheses where appropriate)—not necessarily inclusive (» = major clinical significance):

Note: Combinations containing any of the following medications, depending on the amount present, may also interact with this medication.

Allopurinol
 (dacarbazine-induced inhibition of xanthine oxidase may cause additive hypouricemic effects when used concurrently with allopurinol)

Blood dyscrasia–causing medications (see *Appendix II*)
 (leukopenic and/or thrombocytopenic effects of dacarbazine may be increased with concurrent or recent therapy if these medications cause the same effects; dosage adjustment of dacarbazine, if necessary, should be based on blood counts)

» Bone marrow depressants, other (see *Appendix II*) or
 Radiation therapy
 (additive bone marrow depression may occur; dosage reduction may be required when two or more bone marrow depressants, including radiation, are used concurrently or consecutively)

Hepatic enzyme inducers (see *Appendix II*)
 (may enhance metabolism of dacarbazine by induction of hepatic microsomal enzymes; dosage adjustment may be necessary)

Vaccines, killed virus
 (because normal defense mechanisms may be suppressed by dacarbazine therapy, the patient's antibody response to the vaccine may be decreased. The interval between discontinuation of medications that cause immunosuppression and restoration of the patient's ability to respond to the vaccine depends on the intensity and type of immunosuppression-causing medication used, the underlying disease, and other factors; estimates vary from 3 months to 1 year)

» Vaccines, live virus
(because normal defense mechanisms may be suppressed by dacarbazine therapy, concurrent use with a live virus vaccine may potentiate the replication of the vaccine virus, may increase the side/adverse effects of the vaccine virus, and/or may decrease the patient's antibody response to the vaccine; immunization of these patients should be undertaken only with extreme caution after careful review of the patient's hematologic status and only with the knowledge and consent of the physician managing the dacarbazine therapy. The interval between discontinuation of medications that cause immunosuppression and restoration of the patient's ability to respond to the vaccine depends on the intensity and type of immunosuppression-causing medication used, the underlying disease, and other factors; estimates vary from 3 months to 1 year. In addition, immunization with oral poliovirus vaccine should be postponed in persons in close contact with the patient, especially family members)

### Laboratory value alterations
The following have been selected on the basis of their potential clinical significance (possible effect in parentheses where appropriate)—not necessarily inclusive (» = major clinical significance):

With physiology/laboratory test values
Alanine aminotransferase (ALT [SGPT]) and
Alkaline phosphatase and
Aspartate aminotransferase (AST [SGOT])
(serum values may be transiently increased; may indicate hepatotoxicity)
Blood urea nitrogen (BUN)
(concentrations may be transiently increased)

### Medical considerations/Contraindications
The medical considerations/contraindications included have been selected on the basis of their potential clinical significance (reasons given in parentheses where appropriate)—not necessarily inclusive (» = major clinical significance).

*Risk-benefit should be considered when the following medical problems exist:*
» Bone marrow depression
» Chickenpox, existing or recent (including recent exposure) or
» Herpes zoster
(risk of severe generalized disease)
» Hepatic function impairment
» Infection
» Renal function impairment
(reduced elimination; dosage reduction may be required)
Sensitivity to dacarbazine
» Caution should be used also in patients who have had previous cytotoxic drug therapy or radiation therapy.

### Patient monitoring
The following are especially important in patient monitoring (other tests may be warranted in some patients, depending on condition; (» = major clinical significance):

Blood urea nitrogen (BUN) concentrations and
Creatinine concentrations, serum
(recommended prior to initiation of therapy and at periodic intervals during therapy; frequency varies according to clinical state, agent, dose, and other agents being used concurrently)
» Hematocrit or hemoglobin and
» Leukocyte count, total and, if appropriate, differential and
» Platelet count
(determinations recommended prior to initiation of therapy and at periodic intervals during therapy; frequency varies according to clinical state, agent, dose, and other agents being used concurrently)
Alanine aminotransferase (ALT [SGPT]) values, serum and
Aspartate aminotransferase (AST [SGOT]) values, serum and
Lactate dehydrogenase (LDH) values, serum
(recommended prior to initiation of therapy and at periodic intervals during therapy; frequency varies according to clinical state, agent, dose, and other agents being used concurrently)
Bilirubin concentrations, serum and
Uric acid concentrations, serum
(recommended prior to initiation of therapy and at periodic intervals during therapy; frequency varies according to clinical state, agent, dose, and other agents being used concurrently)

## Side/Adverse Effects
Note: Many "side effects" of antineoplastic therapy are unavoidable and represent the medication's pharmacologic action. Some of these (for example, leukopenia and thrombocytopenia) are actually used as parameters to aid in individual dosage titration.

According to some investigators, photodegradation products of dacarbazine solution may be responsible for some of its adverse effects, including local toxicity (burning and vein pain), nausea and vomiting, and hepatotoxicity.

The following side/adverse effects have been selected on the basis of their potential clinical significance (possible signs and symptoms in parentheses where appropriate)—not necessarily inclusive:

### Those indicating need for medical attention
Incidence more frequent
*Anemia; extravasation and tissue damage or pain in injected vein* (redness, swelling, or pain at site of injection); *leukopenia* (fever or chills; cough or hoarseness; lower back or side pain; painful or difficult urination)—usually asymptomatic; *thrombocytopenia* (unusual bleeding or bruising; black, tarry stools; blood in urine or stools; pinpoint red spots on skin)—usually asymptomatic

Note: The fall in leukocyte count usually begins within 16 to 20 days after administration, with the nadir at 21 to 25 days and recovery 3 to 5 days later. *Leukopenia* may be severe enough to be fatal.
The nadir usually occurs 16 days after administration, with recovery 3 to 5 days later. *Thrombocytopenia* may be severe enough to be fatal.

Incidence rare
*Anaphylaxis* (shortness of breath; swelling of face); *hepatotoxicity, including hepatic vein thrombosis; and hepatocellular necrosis* (fever; stomach pain; yellow eyes or skin); *stomatitis* (sores in mouth and on lips)

Note: *Hepatotoxicity* is uniformly fatal. It has been reported with use of dacarbazine alone and in combination with other agents.

### Those indicating need for medical attention only if they continue or are bothersome
Incidence more frequent—greater than 90%
*Loss of appetite; nausea and vomiting*

Note: *Nausea and vomiting* may last for 1 to 12 hours after administration but usually lessen considerably within 1 to 2 days after treatment is started.

Incidence less frequent
*Flushing of face; influenza-like syndrome* (fever; feelings of uneasiness; joint or muscle pain); *numbness of face*

Note: The *influenza-like syndrome* begins after 7 days and may last 1 to 3 weeks; it may occur with repeated treatments.

### Those not indicating need for medical attention
Incidence less frequent
*Loss of hair*

### Those indicating the need for medical attention if they occur after medication is discontinued
*Bone marrow depression* (black, tarry stools; blood in urine or stools; cough or hoarseness; fever or chills; lower back or side pain; painful or difficult urination; pinpoint red spots on skin; unusual bleeding or bruising)

## Patient Consultation
As an aid to patient consultation, refer to *Advice for the Patient, Dacarbazine (Systemic)*.

In providing consultation, consider emphasizing the following selected information (» = major clinical significance):

### Before using this medication
» Conditions affecting use, especially:
Sensitivity to dacarbazine
Pregnancy—Use not recommended because of mutagenic, teratogenic, and carcinogenic potential; advisability of using contraception; telling physician immediately if pregnancy is suspected
Breast-feeding—Not recommended because of risk of serious side effects
Other medications, especially other bone marrow depressants or previous cytotoxic drug or radiation therapy
Other medical problems, especially chickenpox, herpes zoster, hepatic function impairment, infection, or renal function impairment

### Proper use of this medication
Caution in taking combination therapy; taking each medication at the right time

Frequency of nausea, vomiting, and loss of appetite; importance of continuing medication despite stomach upset; should lessen after 1 or 2 days
» Proper dosing

**Precautions while using this medication**
» Importance of close monitoring by the physician
» Avoiding immunizations unless approved by physician; other persons in patient's household should avoid immunizations with oral poliovirus vaccine; avoiding persons who have taken oral poliovirus vaccine or wearing a protective mask that covers nose and mouth

*Caution if bone marrow depression occurs*
» Avoiding exposure to persons with infections, especially during periods of low blood counts; checking with physician immediately if fever or chills, cough or hoarseness, lower back or side pain, or painful or difficult urination occurs
» Checking with physician immediately if unusual bleeding or bruising; black, tarry stools; blood in urine or stools; or pinpoint red spots on skin occur

Caution in use of regular toothbrush, dental floss, or toothpick; physician, dentist, or nurse may suggest alternatives; checking with physician before having dental work done

Not touching eyes or inside of nose unless hands are washed immediately before

Using caution to avoid accidental cuts with use of sharp objects such as safety razor or fingernail or toenail cutters

Avoiding contact sports or other situations where bruising or injury could occur
» Possibility of local tissue injury and scarring if infiltration of intravenous solution occurs; telling doctor or nurse right away about redness, pain, or swelling at injection site

**Side/adverse effects**
May cause adverse effects such as blood problems, loss of hair, and cancer; importance of discussing possible effects with physician

Signs of potential side effects, especially anemia, extravasation, pain in injected vein, leukopenia, thrombocytopenia, anaphylaxis, hepatotoxicity, and stomatitis

Physician or nurse can help in dealing with side effects

Possibility of hair loss; normal hair growth should return after treatment has ended

## General Dosing Information

Patients receiving dacarbazine should be under supervision of a physician experienced in cancer chemotherapy.

A variety of dosage schedules and regimens of dacarbazine, alone or in combination with other antitumor agents, are used. The prescriber may consult the medical literature as well as the manufacturer's literature in choosing a specific dosage.

Dosage must be adjusted to meet the individual requirements of each patient, on the basis of clinical response and degree of bone marrow depression.

Dacarbazine may be administered into the tubing of a freely running intravenous solution over a 1- to 2-minute period, or by intravenous infusion over a 15- to 30-minute period. Administration by intravenous infusion may prevent pain along the injected vein.

Care should be taken to avoid extravasation of dacarbazine because of the risk of severe pain and tissue necrosis.

If extravasation of dacarbazine occurs during intravenous administration, as indicated by local burning or stinging, the injection and infusion should be stopped immediately and resumed, completing the dose, in another vein.

If marked leukopenia (particularly granulocytopenia) or thrombocytopenia occurs, dacarbazine should be discontinued until leukocyte and platelet counts return to satisfactory levels, usually within a week after the nadir.

Special precautions are recommended in patients who develop thrombocytopenia as a result of administration of dacarbazine. These may include extra care in performing invasive procedures, regular inspection of intravenous sites, skin (including perirectal area), and mucous membrane surfaces for signs of bleeding or bruising; limiting frequency of venipuncture and avoiding intramuscular injections; testing urine, emesis, stool, and secretions for occult blood; care in use of regular toothbrushes, dental floss, toothpicks, safety razors, and fingernail and toenail cutters; avoiding constipation; and using caution to prevent falls and other injuries. Such patients should avoid alcohol and aspirin intake because of the risk of gastrointestinal bleeding. Platelet transfusion may be required.

Patients who develop leukopenia should be observed carefully for signs of infection. Antibiotic support may be required. In neutropenic patients who develop fever, broad-spectrum antibiotic coverage should be initiated empirically, pending bacterial cultures and appropriate diagnostic tests.

**Safety considerations for handling this medication**
There is limited but increasing evidence and concern that personnel involved in preparation and administration of parenteral antineoplastics may be at some risk because of the potential mutagenicity, teratogenicity, and/or carcinogenicity of these agents, although the actual risk is unknown. USP advisory panels recommend cautious handling both in preparation and disposal of antineoplastic agents. Precautions that have been suggested include:
• Use of a biological containment cabinet during reconstitution and dilution of parenteral medications and wearing of disposable surgical gloves and masks.
• Use of proper technique to prevent contamination of the medication, work area, and operator during transfer between containers (including proper training of personnel in this technique).
• Cautious and proper disposal of needles, syringes, vials, ampuls, and unused medication.

A number of medical centers have developed detailed guidelines for handling of antineoplastic agents.

**Combination chemotherapy**
Dacarbazine may be used in combination with other agents in various regimens. As a result, incidence and/or severity of side effects may be altered and different dosages (usually reduced) may be used. For example, dacarbazine is part of the following chemotherapeutic combinations (some commonly used acronyms are in parentheses):
—doxorubicin, bleomycin, vinblastine, and dacarbazine (ABVD),
—cyclophosphamide, vincristine, doxorubicin, and dacarbazine (CY-VADIC).

For specific dosages and schedules, consult the literature. For information regarding each agent, consult the individual monographs.

## Parenteral Dosage Forms

### DACARBAZINE FOR INJECTION USP

**Usual adult dose**
Melanoma, malignant—
   Intravenous, 2 to 4.5 mg per kg of body weight a day for ten days; may be repeated every twenty-eight days, or
   Intravenous, up to 250 mg per square meter of body surface area a day for five days; may be repeated every twenty-one days.
Lymphomas, Hodgkin's[1]—
   Intravenous, 150 mg per square meter of body surface area a day for five days, in combination with other agents; may be repeated every twenty-eight days, or
   Intravenous, 375 mg per square meter of body surface area on day 1, in combination with other agents, repeated every fifteen days.

Note: Dacarbazine may be as effective at the lower dosage as at the higher dosage.
Dacarbazine has also been administered as a single daily dose of 850 mg per square meter of body surface area every twenty-one to forty-two days, with no apparent increase in hematologic toxicity, although extreme nausea and vomiting may occur.

**Usual pediatric dose**
Dosage has not been established.

**Strength(s) usually available**
U.S.—
   100 mg (Rx) [*DTIC-Dome* (mannitol 37.5 mg)] [GENERIC (mannitol)].
   200 mg (Rx) [*DTIC-Dome* (mannitol 75 mg)] [GENERIC (mannitol)].
Canada—
   200 mg [*DTIC*].

**Packaging and storage**
Store below 40 °C (104 °F), preferably between 15 and 30 °C (59 and 86 °F), unless otherwise specified by the manufacturer. Protect from light.

**Preparation of dosage form**
Dacarbazine for Injection USP may be prepared for parenteral use by adding 9.9 mL (100-mg vial), 19.7 mL (200-mg vial), or 49.5 mL (500-mg vial) of sterile water for injection to the vial, producing a colorless or clear yellow solution containing 10 mg of dacarbazine per mL.
Reconstituted solutions may be further diluted with up to 250 mL of 5% dextrose injection or 0.9% sodium chloride injection for administration by intravenous infusion.

## Stability

Reconstituted solutions of dacarbazine are stable for up to 72 hours at 4 °C (39 °F) or for up to 8 hours at normal room conditions (temperature and light). Solutions further diluted for administration by intravenous infusion are stable for up to 24 hours at 4 °C (39 °F) or for up to 8 hours at normal room conditions (temperature and light). A change in color of the solution to pink indicates decomposition.

[1] Not included in Canadian product labeling.

Revised: 07/11/94
Interim revision: 09/30/97

# DACLIZUMAB   Systemic—INTRODUCTORY VERSION

VA CLASSIFICATION (Primary): IM600

Commonly used brand name(s): *Zenapax*.

Another commonly used name is dacliximab.

Note: For a listing of dosage forms and brand names by country availability, see *Dosage Forms* section(s).

## Category

Immunosuppressant; monoclonal antibody.

## Indications

### General considerations

The efficacy of daclizumab was demonstrated in two placebo-controlled, multicenter trials in which daclizumab was administered in conjunction with triple-therapy (cyclosporine, corticosteroids, and azathioprine) or double-therapy (cyclosporine and corticosteroids). The primary end point in the trials was the incidence of biopsy-proven acute rejection within the first 6 months following transplantation. The incidence of biopsy-proven acute rejection was lower in the daclizumab-treated group in both the triple-therapy ($P = 0.03$) and the double-therapy ($P = 0.001$) trials.

A secondary end point in the trials was the incidence of biopsy-proven acute rejection at 1 year following transplantation. Biopsy-proven rejection at 1 year was not significantly different between the placebo-treated group (38%) and the daclizumab-treated group (28%) in the triple-therapy regimen ($P = 0.09$). However, there was a significant difference in this end point in the double-therapy regimen (49% vs 28% incidence of biopsy-proven rejection in the placebo-treated and daclizumab-treated groups, respectively [$P < 0.001$]).

Another secondary end point in the trials was graft survival 1 year following transplantation. There was no significant difference in either the triple-therapy trial ($P = 0.08$) or the double-therapy trial ($P = 0.3$).

The trials also compared patient survival at 1 year following transplantation. Patient survival was not significantly different between the placebo-treated group (96%) and the daclizumab-treated group (98%) in the triple-therapy regimen ($P = 0.51$). However, there was a significant difference in this end point in the double-therapy regimen (94% vs 99% survival in the placebo-treated and daclizumab-treated groups, respectively [$P = 0.01$]).

The incidences of lymphoproliferative disorders and opportunistic infections were not increased in the daclizumab-treated patients in the trials. However, only 336 patients were treated with daclizumab in these trials. Additional experience with daclizumab is needed to evaluate its potential for causing lymphoproliferative disorders and opportunistic infections.

The long-term ability of the immune system to respond to antigens first encountered while being treated with daclizumab is not known.

### Accepted

Transplant rejection, kidney (prophylaxis)—Daclizumab is indicated, in combination with cyclosporine and corticosteroids, for the prevention of acute rejection of transplanted kidneys.

## Pharmacology/Pharmacokinetics

### Physicochemical characteristics

Source—Composite of human (90%) and murine (10%) antibody sequences obtained through recombinant DNA technology.
Molecular weight—Approximately 144,000 daltons.
pH—Adjusted with hydrochloric acid or sodium hydroxide to approximately 6.9.

### Mechanism of action/Effect

Daclizumab is an interleukin-2 (IL-2) receptor antagonist that binds to the alpha subunit of IL-2 receptor complex and inhibits IL-2 binding. By inhibiting IL-2 binding, IL-2–mediated activation of lymphocytes is prevented, and the response of the immune system to antigens is impaired.

### Distribution

The volume of distribution (Vol$_D$) is approximately 0.074 L per kg of body weight (L/kg). The central and peripheral volumes of distribution are estimated to be about 0.031 and 0.0425 L/kg, respectively.

### Half-life

Elimination—
   11 to 38 days.

### Peak serum concentration

The peak serum concentration in the five-dose course of treatment occurs after the fifth dose, and is estimated to be $32 \pm 22$ micrograms per milliliter (mcg/mL).

### Therapeutic serum concentration

5 to 10 mcg/mL.

## Precautions to Consider

### Carcinogenicity

Studies have not been done to evaluate the carcinogenic potential of daclizumab. In the pre-approval trials of daclizumab, there was not an increased incidence of lymphoproliferative disorders in the daclizumab-treated patients. Long-term follow-up studies are not available in these patients. However, it is known that patients receiving immunosuppressive therapy are at increased risk for developing malignancies.

### Mutagenicity

Daclizumab was not mutagenic in the Ames test or the V79 chromosomal aberration assay, with or without activation.

### Pregnancy/Reproduction

Fertility—Adequate and well-controlled studies have not been done.
Pregnancy—Daclizumab crosses the placenta. Adequate and well-controlled studies have not been done in humans.

FDA Pregnancy Category C.

### Breast-feeding

It is not known whether daclizumab is distributed into breast milk. The manufacturer recommends that patients receiving daclizumab discontinue breast-feeding.

### Pediatrics

Appropriate studies on the relationship of age to the effects of daclizumab have not been performed in pediatric patients. Preliminary data from the use of daclizumab in 25 pediatric patients 11 months to 17 years of age suggest that pediatric patients receiving daclizumab may experience more hypertension and dehydration than adult patients. Although pediatric patients receiving the same weight-adjusted dose as adults (i.e., 1 milligram per kilogram of body weight [mg/kg]) had lower serum concentrations than did adult patients, the dose was sufficient to saturate the alpha subunit of the interleukin-2 (IL-2) receptor on lymphocytes.

### Geriatrics

No information is available on the relationship of age to the effects of daclizumab in geriatric patients.

### Dental

The immunosuppressive effects of daclizumab may result in an increased incidence of certain microbial infections and delayed healing. Dental work, whenever possible, should be completed prior to initiation of therapy and undertaken with caution during therapy. Patients should be instructed in proper oral hygiene.

### Drug interactions and/or related problems

Note: In clinical trials, daclizumab was administered to patients receiving other immunosuppressants (antilymphocyte globulin, antithymocyte globulin, azathioprine, corticosteroids, cyclosporine, muromonab-CD3, mycophenolate mofetil, and tacrolimus) and anti-infectives (acyclovir and ganciclovir). No drug interactions have been evaluated or reported with daclizumab.

### Laboratory value alterations

The following have been selected on the basis of their potential clinical significance (possible effect in parentheses where appropriate)—not necessarily inclusive (» = major clinical significance):

With physiology/laboratory test values
Glucose, blood
(concentration may be increased)

### Medical considerations/Contraindications
The medical considerations/contraindications included have been selected on the basis of their potential clinical significance (reasons given in parentheses where appropriate)—not necessarily inclusive (» = major clinical significance).

*Except under special circumstances, this medication should not be used when the following medical problem exists:*
» Allergy to daclizumab, history of
   Note: Anaphylactoid reactions have not been reported following administration of daclizumab. However, anaphylactoid reactions are possible following administration of proteins.

*Risk-benefit should be considered when the following medical problems exist:*
Diabetes mellitus
   (risk of loss of blood glucose control)
Infection
   (immunosuppression may exacerbate infection)
Malignancy, current or history of
   (immunosuppression is associated with an increased incidence of some malignancies)

### Patient monitoring
The following may be especially important in patient monitoring (other tests may be warranted in some patients, depending on condition; » = major clinical significance):
Blood pressure and
Heart rate and
Respiratory rate
   (routine monitoring of vital signs is recommended while daclizumab is administered and for a short period of time following the infusion to monitor for anaphylactoid reaction)
Wound infection
   (daclizumab may cause an increased risk of wound infection)
Note: Although the incidences of malignancies and systemic infection were not increased in the daclizumab-treated group in pre-approval clinical trials, patients receiving daclizumab should be monitored routinely for malignancy and systemic infection.

## Side/Adverse Effects
Note: In clinical trials, the incidence of adverse effects in the daclizumab-treated group was similar to that in the placebo-treated group.

The following side/adverse effects have been selected on the basis of their potential clinical significance (possible signs and symptoms in parentheses where appropriate)—not necessarily inclusive:

### Those indicating need for medical attention
Incidence less frequent
   **Chest pain; dyspnea** (shortness of breath); **fever; hypertension**—usually asymptomatic; **hypotension** (dizziness); **nausea; peripheral edema** (swelling of feet or lower legs); **pulmonary edema** (coughing; shortness of breath); **tachycardia** (rapid heartbeat); **tremor** (trembling or shaking of the hands or feet); **vomiting; weakness; wound infection** (red, tender, or oozing skin at incision)
Incidence rare
   **Hyperglycemia** (frequent urination)

### Those indicating need for medical attention only if they continue or are bothersome
Incidence less frequent
   **Arthralgia** (joint pain); **constipation; diarrhea; dizziness; dyspepsia** (heartburn); **headache; insomnia** (trouble in sleeping); **myalgia** (muscle pain); **slow wound healing**

## Overdose
There is no clinical experience with overdose of daclizumab, and a maximum tolerated dose has not been established. Some bone marrow transplant recipients have received 1.5 mg per kg of body weight without any adverse effects.

## Patient Consultation
As an aid to patient consultation, refer to *Advice for the Patient, Daclizumab (Systemic)—Introductory version.*

In providing consultation, consider emphasizing the following selected information (» = major clinical significance):

### Before using this medication
» Conditions affecting use, especially:
   Allergy to daclizumab
   Carcinogenicity—Use of daclizumab may be associated with an increased risk of malignancy
   Pregnancy—Daclizumab crosses the placenta
   Breast-feeding—Use is not recommended
   Use in children—Children receiving daclizumab may experience higher incidences of hypertension and dehydration than adult patients
   Dental—Dental work should be completed prior to initiation of therapy whenever possible

### Proper use of this medication
» Proper dosing
   Advisability of women of childbearing age using effective contraception before, during, and for several months after receiving daclizumab

### Precautions while receiving this medication
» Importance of close monitoring by a physician

### Side/adverse effects
Signs of potential side effects, especially chest pain, dyspnea, fever, hypertension, hypotension, nausea, peripheral edema, pulmonary edema, tachycardia, tremor, vomiting, weakness, wound infection and hyperglycemia

## General Dosing Information
Daclizumab should be used only by physicians experienced in the management of organ transplant patients. Medications for the treatment of severe hypersensitivity reactions should be immediately available when daclizumab is administered.

Daclizumab must be diluted prior to administration.

Shaking of the vial or prepared solution of daclizumab may cause foaming and should be avoided.

No dosage adjustment is needed for administration to patients with renal function impairment. There are no data for administration to patients with hepatic function impairment.

There is no experience with treating patients with more than one course of therapy with daclizumab.

## Parenteral Dosage Forms

### DACLIZUMAB STERILE CONCENTRATE FOR INJECTION

#### Usual adult and adolescent dose
Transplant rejection, kidney (prophylaxis)—
   Intravenous infusion over fifteen minutes, 1 mg per kg of body weight every fourteen days for five doses beginning no earlier than twenty-four hours prior to transplantation.

#### Usual pediatric dose
See *Usual adult and adolescent dose.*
Note: Although testing has not been completed in pediatric patients, preliminary data suggest that the same weight-adjusted dose used in adults is appropriate for pediatric patients.

#### Usual geriatric dose
See *Usual adult and adolescent dose.*

#### Strength(s) usually available
U.S.—
   5 mg per mL (Rx) [*Zenapax* (sodium phosphate monobasic monohydrate 3.6 mg per mL; sodium phosphate dibasic heptahydrate 11 mg per mL; sodium chloride 4.6 mg per mL; polysorbate 80 0.2 mg per mL)].

#### Packaging and storage
Store between 2 and 8 °C (36 and 46 °F). Protect from light and freezing.

#### Preparation of dosage form
Daclizumab must be diluted prior to infusion. The dose may be diluted in 50 mL of 0.9% sodium chloride injection. When the diluted solution is mixed, the bag should be gently inverted. Care should be taken to avoid shaking vials and prepared solutions of daclizumab.

### Stability
Daclizumab does not contain preservatives. Prepared solutions of daclizumab should be used within 4 hours. If refrigerated at 4 ºC (39 ºF), solutions should be used within 24 hours. The prepared solution should be inspected for particulate matter and clarity before administration to the patient, and should be discarded if particulate matter is present.

### Incompatibilities
There are no data on the compatibility or incompatibility of other drugs or solutions with daclizumab. Until more data are available, other drugs should not be infused simultaneously through the same intravenous line.

Developed: 04/03/98

# DACTINOMYCIN  Systemic

VA CLASSIFICATION (Primary): AN200
Commonly used brand name(s): *Cosmegen*.
Another commonly used name is actinomycin-D.
Note: For a listing of dosage forms and brand names by country availability, see *Dosage Forms* section(s).

## Category
Antineoplastic.

## Indications
Note: Bracketed information in the *Indications* section refers to uses that are not included in U.S. product labeling.

### Accepted
Ewing's sarcoma (treatment) or
Sarcoma botryoides (treatment)—Dactinomycin is indicated as a single agent or in combination with other chemotherapeutic agents for palliative treatment of Ewing's sarcoma and sarcoma botryoides.
Tumors, trophoblastic, gestational (treatment)—Dactinomycin is indicated as a single agent or in combination with other chemotherapeutic agents for treatment of gestational trophoblastic tumors.
Carcinoma, testicular (treatment)
Wilms' tumor (treatment)
Rhabdomyosarcoma (treatment)
[Carcinoma, ovarian (treatment)][1]
[Sarcoma, Kaposi's (treatment)][1] or
[Osteosarcoma (treatment)][1]—Dactinomycin is indicated in combination with other chemotherapeutic agents for treatment of testicular carcinoma, Wilms' tumor, rhabdomyosarcoma, ovarian carcinoma, Kaposi's sarcoma, and osteosarcoma.

### Unaccepted
Although dactinomycin has antibacterial activity, its toxic effects preclude its use in the treatment of infectious diseases.

[1]Not included in Canadian product labeling.

## Pharmacology/Pharmacokinetics

### Physicochemical characteristics
Molecular weight—1255.43.

### Mechanism of action/Effect
Dactinomycin is classified as an antibiotic but is not used as an antimicrobial agent. Dactinomycin is considered to be cell cycle–phase nonspecific. Its antineoplastic action may involve binding to DNA by intercalation between base pairs and inhibition of DNA-dependent RNA synthesis.

### Other actions/effects
Has some bacteriostatic activity on gram-positive and on gram-negative bacteria and on some fungi. Also has some immunosuppressant activity.

### Distribution
Does not cross the blood-brain barrier.

### Protein binding
Extensive tissue binding.

### Biotransformation
Minimal.

### Half-life
36 hours.

### Elimination
Biliary/fecal—50% unchanged.
Renal—10% unchanged.
About 30% of a dose is recoverable in urine and feces in 1 week.

## Precautions to Consider

### Carcinogenicity/Mutagenicity
Secondary malignancies are potential delayed effects of many antineoplastic agents, although it is not clear whether the effect is related to their mutagenic or immunosuppressive action. The effect of dose and duration of therapy is also unknown, although risk seems to increase with long-term use. Although information is limited, available data seem to indicate that the carcinogenic risk is greatest with the alkylating agents.
Dactinomycin is carcinogenic in mice and rats. Repeated subcutaneous or intraperitoneal injections produced local sarcomas in mice and rats. Intraperitoneal injections of 0.05 mg per kg of body weight (mg/kg) two to five times per week for 18 weeks in male F344 rats resulted in mesenchymal tumors, the first tumor appearing at 23 weeks.
Dactinomycin has been shown to be mutagenic in both *in vitro* and *in vivo* tests (human fibroblasts and leukocytes, HELA cells) and causes DNA damage and cytogenetic effects in mice and rats.

### Pregnancy/Reproduction
Fertility—Gonadal suppression, resulting in amenorrhea or azoospermia, may occur in patients taking antineoplastic therapy, especially with the alkylating agents. In general, these effects appear to be related to dose and length of therapy and may be irreversible. Prediction of the degree of testicular or ovarian function impairment is complicated by the common use of combinations of several antineoplastics, which makes it difficult to assess the effects of individual agents.
Pregnancy—Dactinomycin crosses the placenta. Adequate and well-controlled studies in humans have not been done.
First trimester: It is usually recommended that use of antineoplastics, especially combination chemotherapy, be avoided whenever possible, especially during the first trimester. Although information is limited because of the relatively few instances of antineoplastic administration during pregnancy, the mutagenic, teratogenic, and carcinogenic potential of these medications must be considered.
Other hazards to the fetus include adverse reactions seen in adults.
In general, use of a contraceptive is recommended during cytotoxic drug therapy.
Some studies in rats, rabbits, and hamsters have shown that dactinomycin causes malformations and embryotoxicity when given intravenously in doses of 50 to 100 mcg (0.05 to 0.1 mg) per kg of body weight (corresponding to three to seven times the maximum recommended human dose).
FDA Pregnancy Category C.

### Breast-feeding
It is not known whether dactinomycin is distributed into breast milk. However, breast-feeding is not recommended while dactinomycin is being administered because of the risks to the infant (adverse effects, mutagenicity, carcinogenicity).

### Pediatrics
Because of the increased risk of toxicity in infants, dactinomycin should be used only in infants older than 6 to 12 months of age, unless potential benefit outweighs risk.

### Geriatrics
No information is available on the relationship of age to the effects of dactinomycin in geriatric patients.

### Dental
The bone marrow depressant effects of dactinomycin may result in an increased incidence of microbial infection, delayed healing, and gingival bleeding. Dental work, whenever possible, should be completed prior to initiation of therapy or deferred until blood counts have returned to normal. Patients should be instructed in proper oral hygiene during treatment, including caution in use of regular toothbrushes, dental floss, and toothpicks.
Dactinomycin commonly causes ulcerative stomatitis and pharyngitis associated with considerable discomfort. Sores often occur under the tongue.

### Drug interactions and/or related problems
The following drug interactions and/or related problems have been selected on the basis of their potential clinical significance (possible mechanism

# Dactinomycin (Systemic)

in parentheses where appropriate)—not necessarily inclusive (» = major clinical significance):

Note: Combinations containing any of the following medications, depending on the amount present, may also interact with this medication.

Allopurinol or
Colchicine or
» Probenecid or
» Sulfinpyrazone
(dactinomycin may raise the concentration of blood uric acid; dosage adjustment of antigout agents may be necessary to control hyperuricemia and gout; allopurinol may be preferred because of risk of uric acid nephropathy with uricosuric antigout agents)

Blood dyscrasia–causing medications (see *Appendix II*)
(leukopenic and/or thrombocytopenic effects of dactinomycin may be increased with concurrent or recent therapy if these medications cause the same effects; dosage adjustment of dactinomycin, if necessary, should be based on blood counts)

» Bone marrow depressants, other (see *Appendix II*) or
» Radiation therapy
(concurrent use with dactinomycin may potentiate the effects of these medications and radiation therapy, including gastrointestinal toxicity, bone marrow depression, and erythema and tanning of the skin; lower doses of each are recommended. Dactinomycin alone may reactivate erythema from previous radiation therapy)

Doxorubicin
(concurrent or sequential use may result in increased cardiotoxicity; it is recommended that the total dose of doxorubicin not exceed 450 mg per square meter of body surface area)

Vaccines, killed virus
(because normal defense mechanisms may be suppressed by dactinomycin therapy, the patient's antibody response to the vaccine may be decreased. The interval between discontinuation of medications that cause immunosuppression and restoration of the patient's ability to respond to the vaccine depends on the intensity and type of immunosuppression-causing medication used, the underlying disease, and other factors; estimates vary from 3 months to 1 year)

» Vaccines, live virus
(because normal defense mechanisms may be suppressed by dactinomycin therapy, concurrent use with a live virus vaccine may potentiate the replication of the vaccine virus, may increase the side/adverse effects of the vaccine virus, and/or may decrease the patient's antibody response to the vaccine; immunization of these patients should be undertaken only with extreme caution after careful review of the patient's hematologic status and only with the knowledge and consent of the physician managing the dactinomycin therapy. The interval between discontinuation of medications that cause immunosuppression and restoration of the patient's ability to respond to the vaccine depends on the intensity and type of immunosuppression-causing medication used, the underlying disease, and other factors; estimates vary from 3 months to 1 year. In addition, immunization with oral poliovirus vaccine should be postponed in persons in close contact with the patient, especially family members)

## Laboratory value alterations
The following have been selected on the basis of their potential clinical significance (possible effect in parentheses where appropriate)—not necessarily inclusive (» = major clinical significance):

With diagnostic test results
Bioassay procedures for determinations of antibacterial drug concentrations
(may be interfered with)

With physiology/laboratory test values
Hepatic enzymes
(serum values may rarely be increased)
Uric acid concentrations in blood and urine
(may be increased)

## Medical considerations/Contraindications
The medical considerations/contraindications included have been selected on the basis of their potential clinical significance (reasons given in parentheses where appropriate)—not necessarily inclusive (» = major clinical significance).

***Risk-benefit should be considered when the following medical problems exist:***
» Bone marrow depression

» Chickenpox, existing or recent (including recent exposure) or
» Herpes zoster
(risk of severe generalized disease)

Gout, history of or
Urate renal stones, history of
(risk of hyperuricemia)

» Hepatic function impairment
(some clinicians recommend reduction of dosage by one third or one half in patients with hyperbilirubinemia)

» Infection
Sensitivity to dactinomycin

» Caution should be used also in patients who have had previous cytotoxic drug therapy or radiation therapy.

## Patient monitoring
The following are especially important in patient monitoring (other tests may be warranted in some patients, depending on condition; (» = major clinical significance):

Alanine aminotransferase (ALT [SGPT]) values, serum and
Aspartate aminotransferase (AST [SGOT]) values, serum and
Bilirubin concentrations, serum and
Lactate dehydrogenase (LDH) values, serum
(recommended prior to initiation of therapy and at periodic intervals during therapy; frequency varies according to clinical state, agent, dose, and other agents being used concurrently)

» Checking patient's mouth for ulceration
(recommended before administration of each dose)

» Hematocrit or hemoglobin and
» Leukocyte count, total and, if appropriate, differential and
» Platelet count
(determinations recommended prior to initiation of therapy and at periodic intervals during therapy; frequency varies according to clinical state, agent, dose, and other agents being used concurrently)

Uric acid concentrations, serum
(recommended prior to initiation of therapy and at periodic intervals during therapy; frequency varies according to clinical state, agent, dose, and other agents being used concurrently)

# Side/Adverse Effects
Note: Many "side effects" of antineoplastic therapy are unavoidable and represent the medication's pharmacologic action. Some of these (for example, leukopenia and thrombocytopenia) are actually used as parameters to aid in individual dosage titration.

Most side effects appear 2 to 4 days after a course is completed and may not be maximal for 1 to 2 weeks.

Combination therapy with radiation may be associated with more frequent and severe side effects of the radiation, including gastric distress and inflammation of mucous membranes at the irradiated site. Severe reactions may occur if high dosages are used. Hepatotoxicity (hepatomegaly, increased serum aspartate aminotransferase [AST (SGOT)], ascites) has occurred when dactinomycin was used within the first 2 months after radiation therapy for right-sided Wilms' tumor.

Complications associated with use of isolation-perfusion administration are mainly related to how much medication reaches the systemic circulation and may include myelosuppression, absorption of toxic products from massive neoplastic tissue destruction, increased risk of infection, impaired wound healing, and superficial gastric mucosal ulceration. Other potential side/adverse effects include edema of the extremity involved, soft tissue damage in the exposed area, and venous thrombosis.

The following side/adverse effects have been selected on the basis of their potential clinical significance (possible signs and symptoms in parentheses where appropriate)—not necessarily inclusive:

## Those indicating need for medical attention
Incidence more frequent
***Anemia, possibly progressing to aplastic anemia; esophagitis*** (difficulty in swallowing; heartburn); ***gastrointestinal ulceration or proctitis*** (black, tarry stools; continuing diarrhea; continuing stomach pain); ***leukopenia*** (fever or chills; cough or hoarseness; lower back or side pain; painful or difficult urination)—usually asymptomatic; ***thrombocytopenia*** (unusual bleeding or bruising; black, tarry stools; blood in urine or stools; pinpoint red spots on skin)—usually asymptomatic; ***ulcerative stomatitis*** (sores in mouth and on lips)

Note: Bone marrow depression occurs approximately 7 to 10 days after a course of therapy, with the nadir reached at about 3 weeks and recovery within about 3 weeks after nadir. It may be severe and progress to pancytopenia and agranulocytosis, which are potentially fatal.

With *ulcerative stomatitis*, sores often occur under the tongue.

Incidence rare
*Anaphylaxis* (wheezing); ***cellulitis or phlebitis*** (pain at injection site); ***hepatotoxicity, including ascites, hepatomegaly, hepatitis, and hepatic function test abnormalities*** (yellow eyes or skin); ***hyperuricemia or uric acid nephropathy*** (joint pain; lower back or side pain; swelling of feet or lower legs)

Note: *Hepatotoxicity* is usually reversible, but fatalities have been reported.

*Hyperuricemia or uric acid nephropathy* occurs most commonly during initial treatment of patients with leukemia or lymphoma, as a result of rapid cell breakdown which leads to elevated serum uric acid concentrations.

**Those indicating need for medical attention only if they continue or are bothersome**
Incidence more frequent
*Darkening of skin*—if patient has received previous radiation therapy; ***nausea and vomiting; redness of skin; skin rash or acne; unusual tiredness***

Note: *Nausea and vomiting* occur during the first few hours after administration, and may last 4 to 20 hours.

**Those not indicating need for medical attention**
Incidence more frequent
*Loss of hair*

Note: *Loss of hair* usually begins 7 to 10 days after administration and may involve scalp and eyebrows.

**Those indicating the need for medical attention if they occur after medication is discontinued**
***Bone marrow depression*** (black, tarry stools; blood in urine or stools; cough or hoarseness; fever or chills; lower back or side pain; painful or difficult urination; pinpoint red spots on skin; unusual bleeding or bruising); ***gastrointestinal ulceration*** (black, tarry stools; diarrhea; stomach pain); ***hepatotoxicity*** (yellow eyes or skin); ***stomatitis*** (sores in mouth and on lips)

## Patient Consultation

As an aid to patient consultation, refer to *Advice for the Patient, Dactinomycin (Systemic)*.

In providing consultation, consider emphasizing the following selected information (» = major clinical significance):

**Before using this medication**
» Conditions affecting use, especially:
Sensitivity to dactinomycin
Pregnancy—Use not recommended because of mutagenic, teratogenic, and carcinogenic potential; advisability of using contraception; telling physician immediately if pregnancy is suspected
Breast-feeding—Not recommended because of risk of serious side effects
Use in children—Not recommended in infants less than 6 to 12 months of age
Other medications, especially probenecid, sulfinpyrazone, other bone marrow depressants, live virus vaccines, or previous cytotoxic drug or radiation therapy
Other medical problems, especially chickenpox, hepatic function impairment, herpes zoster, or infection

**Proper use of this medication**
Caution in taking combination therapy; taking each medication at the right time
Frequency of nausea and vomiting; importance of continuing medication despite stomach upset
» Proper dosing

**Precautions while using this medication**
» Importance of close monitoring by physician
» Avoiding immunizations unless approved by physician; other persons in patient's household should avoid immunizations with oral poliovirus vaccine; avoiding persons who have taken oral poliovirus vaccine or wearing a protective mask that covers nose and mouth

*Caution if bone marrow depression occurs*
» Avoiding exposure to persons with infections, especially during periods of low blood counts; checking with physician immediately if fever or chills, cough or hoarseness, lower back or side pain, or painful or difficult urination occurs
» Checking with physician immediately if unusual bleeding or bruising; black, tarry stools; blood in urine or stools; or pinpoint red spots on skin occur

Caution in use of regular toothbrush, dental floss, or toothpick; physician, dentist, or nurse may suggest alternatives; checking with physician before having dental work done
Not touching eyes or inside of nose unless hands washed immediately before
Using caution to avoid accidental cuts with use of sharp objects such as safety razor or fingernail or toenail cutters
Avoiding contact sports or other situations where bruising or injury could occur
» Possibility of local tissue injury and scarring if infiltration of intravenous solution occurs; telling physician or nurse right away about redness, pain, or swelling at injection site

**Side/adverse effects**
May cause adverse effects such as blood problems and cancer; importance of discussing possible effects with physician
Signs of potential side effects, especially anemia, esophagitis, gastrointestinal ulceration, proctitis, leukopenia, thrombocytopenia, ulcerative stomatitis, anaphylaxis, cellulitis, phlebitis, hepatotoxicity, hyperuricemia, and uric acid nephropathy
Physician or nurse can help in dealing with side effects
Possibility of hair loss; normal hair growth should return after treatment has ended

## General Dosing Information

It is recommended that dactinomycin be administered only under supervision of a physician experienced in cancer chemotherapy.

A variety of dosage schedules and regimens of dactinomycin, alone or in combination with other antitumor agents, are used. The prescriber may consult the medical literature as well as the manufacturer's literature in choosing a specific dosage.

Dosage must be adjusted to meet the individual requirements of each patient, based on size and location of the neoplasm, clinical response, and appearance or severity of toxicity.

A lower dosage of dactinomycin (based on body surface area) and daily observation for toxicity is recommended for obese patients, especially if they are receiving dactinomycin by regional isolation perfusion; calculation of dosage on the basis of body surface area (i.e., to relate dosage to lean body mass) is recommended. A lower dosage is also recommended for those who are receiving or have received within 3 to 6 weeks other antineoplastic chemotherapy or radiation therapy.

Intravenous fluid therapy and administration of allopurinol for 4 to 5 days may be necessary during a period of severe oral toxicity (i.e., if the patient cannot drink) to prevent hyperuricemia and hyperuricuria resulting from tumor regression.

It is recommended that dactinomycin be given no later than the first 5 to 7 days of radiation therapy because of the risk of severe vesication.

Dactinomycin must be given in short intermittent courses to avoid serious toxicity, which may not appear until 2 to 4 days after the last dose and may not be maximal for 1 to 2 weeks.

Reconstituted solutions of dactinomycin may be injected slowly into the tubing of a running intravenous infusion or diluted for administration by intravenous infusion over 10 to 15 minutes in 5% dextrose injection or 0.9% sodium chloride injection.

Prescribers should consult the medical literature in choosing a dosage and technique for isolation-perfusion administration.

Care should be taken to avoid contact of dactinomycin, which is very corrosive, with soft tissues. In at least one case, extravasation has led to contracture of the arms. If the medication is given directly into the vein rather than by infusion, one sterile needle should be used for reconstituting and withdrawing the dose from the vial and another for administration.

If extravasation of dactinomycin occurs during intravenous administration, the injection or infusion should be stopped immediately and the remaining dose given via another vein, care being taken to avoid soft tissue contact.

Systemic absorption of toxic products from neoplastic tissue destruction during administration of dactinomycin by isolation-perfusion can be minimized by removing the perfusate after the procedure.

If marked leukopenia (particularly granulocytopenia), thrombocytopenia, diarrhea, or stomatitis occurs, dactinomycin therapy should be withdrawn immediately. When leukocyte and platelet counts return to satisfactory levels and the patient has recovered, therapy may be reinstituted.

Special precautions are recommended in patients who develop thrombocytopenia as a result of administration of dactinomycin. These may include extreme care in performing invasive procedures; regular inspection of intravenous sites, skin (including perirectal area), and mu-

## Dactinomycin (Systemic)

cous membrane surfaces for signs of bleeding or bruising; limiting frequency of venipuncture and avoiding intramuscular injections; testing urine, emesis, stool, and secretions for occult blood; care in use of regular toothbrushes, dental floss, toothpicks, safety razors, and fingernail and toenail cutters; avoiding constipation; and using caution to prevent falls and other injuries. Such patients should avoid alcohol and aspirin intake because of the risk of gastrointestinal bleeding. Platelet transfusions may be required.

Patients who develop leukopenia should be observed carefully for signs of infection. Antibiotic support may be required. In neutropenic patients who develop fever, broad-spectrum antibiotic coverage should be initiated empirically, pending bacterial cultures and appropriate diagnostic tests.

### Safety considerations for handling this medication

There is limited but increasing evidence and concern that personnel involved in preparation and administration of parenteral antineoplastics may be at some risk because of the potential mutagenicity, teratogenicity, and/or carcinogenicity of these agents, although the actual risk is unknown. USP advisory panels recommend cautious handling both in preparation and disposal of antineoplastic agents. Precautions that have been suggested include:

- Use of a biological containment cabinet during reconstitution and dilution of parenteral medications and wearing of disposable surgical gloves and masks.
- Use of proper technique to prevent contamination of the medication, work area, and operator during transfer between containers (including proper training of personnel in this technique).
- Cautious and proper disposal of needles, syringes, vials, ampuls, and unused medication.

A number of medical centers have developed detailed guidelines for handling of antineoplastic agents.

### Combination chemotherapy

Dactinomycin may be used in combination with other agents in various regimens. As a result, incidence and/or severity of side effects may be altered and different dosages (usually reduced) may be used. For example, dactinomycin is part of the following chemotherapeutic combinations (some commonly used acronyms are in parentheses):
—methotrexate, dactinomycin, cyclophosphamide (MAC).
—etoposide, methotrexate, dactinomycin, leucovorin, vincristine, cyclophosphamide (EMA-CO).
—vinblastine, dactinomycin, bleomycin, cisplatin, cyclophosphamide (VAB-6).
—vincristine and dactinomycin.
—vincristine, dactinomycin, and cyclophosphamide (VAC).
—doxorubicin, vincristine, dactinomycin, and cyclophosphamide.
—doxorubicin, vinblastine, bleomycin, dacarbazine, vincristine, and dactinomycin.
—high-dose methotrexate, leucovorin, doxorubicin, bleomycin, cyclophosphamide, cisplatin, and dactinomycin.

For specific dosages and schedules, consult the literature. For information regarding each agent, consult the individual monographs.

## Parenteral Dosage Forms

Note: Bracketed uses in the *Dosage Forms* section refer to categories of use and/or indications that are not included in U.S. product labeling.

### DACTINOMYCIN FOR INJECTION USP

**Usual adult dose**
Carcinoma, testicular or
Tumors, trophoblastic, gestational or
Wilms' tumor or
[Carcinoma, ovarian][1] or
Rhabdomyosarcoma or
Ewing's sarcoma or
Sarcoma botryoides—
  Intravenous, 10 to 15 mcg (0.01 to 0.015 mg) per kg of body weight a day for a maximum of five days every four to six weeks or
  Intravenous, 500 mcg (0.5 mg) per square meter of body surface area once a week (maximum 2 mg a week) for three weeks.

Ewing's sarcoma or
Sarcoma botryoides—
  Isolation-perfusion, 50 mcg (0.05 mg) per kg of body weight for lower extremity or pelvis, or 35 mcg (0.035 mg) per kg of body weight for upper extremity.

Note: Dosage should be based on body surface area in obese or edematous patients.

**Usual adult prescribing limits**
15 mcg (0.015 mg) per kg of body weight or 400 to 600 mcg (0.4 to 0.6 mg) per square meter of body surface area per day for five days.

**Usual pediatric dose**
Carcinoma, testicular or
Tumors, trophoblastic, gestational or
Wilms' tumor or
[Carcinoma, ovarian][1] or
Rhabdomyosarcoma or
Ewing's sarcoma or
Sarcoma botryoides—
  Intravenous, 10 to 15 mcg (0.01 to 0.015 mg) per kg of body weight a day or 450 mcg (0.45 mg) per square meter of body surface area per day (up to 500 mcg [0.5 mg] per day) for a maximum of five days, or a total dose of 2.5 mg per square meter of body surface area in divided daily doses over a seven-day period. A second course may be given after four to six weeks, provided all signs of toxicity have disappeared.

Ewing's sarcoma or
Sarcoma botryoides—
  Isolation-perfusion, 50 mcg (0.05 mg) per kg of body weight for lower extremity or pelvis, or 35 mcg (0.035 mg) per kg of body weight for upper extremity.

Note: Because of the increased risk of toxicity in infants, dactinomycin should be used only in infants older than 6 to 12 months of age.

**Usual pediatric prescribing limits**
15 mcg (0.015 mg) per kg of body weight or 400 to 600 mcg (0.4 to 0.6 mg) per square meter of body surface area per day for five days.

**Strength(s) usually available**
U.S.—
  500 mcg (0.5 mg) (Rx) [*Cosmegen* (mannitol 20 mg)].
Canada—
  500 mcg (0.5 mg) (Rx) [*Cosmegen* (mannitol 20 mg)].

**Packaging and storage**
Store at controlled room temperature between 15 and 30 °C (59 and 86 °F). Protect from light, humidity, and excessive heat.

**Preparation of dosage form**
Dactinomycin for Injection USP is reconstituted for use by adding 1.1 mL of sterile water for injection (without preservative) to the vial, producing a clear, gold-colored solution containing 500 mcg (0.5 mg) of dactinomycin per mL. Use of sodium chloride injection or water for injection containing preservatives (benzyl alcohol, parabens) for reconstitution results in precipitation.

Reconstituted solutions of dactinomycin may be diluted in 5% dextrose injection or 0.9% sodium chloride injection for administration by intravenous infusion.

**Stability**
Discard any unused portion of reconstituted dactinomycin solutions.

**Note**
Great care should be taken to prevent inhalation of particles of Dactinomycin for Injection USP and exposure of skin to it. If accidental eye contact occurs, immediate irrigation with copious amounts of water, followed by an ophthalmologic consultation, is recommended; if accidental skin contact occurs, irrigation with water for at least 15 minutes is recommended.

Use of some intravenous in-line filters containing cellulose ester membrane filters has been reported to partially remove dactinomycin from intravenous solution.

---

[1]Not included in Canadian product labeling.

Revised: 07/11/94
Interim revision: 09/30/97

# DALTEPARIN Systemic

VA CLASSIFICATION (Primary): BL111
Commonly used brand name(s): *Fragmin*.
Another commonly used name is tedelparin.

Note: For a listing of dosage forms and brand names by country availability, see *Dosage Forms* section(s).

## Category
Anticoagulant; antithrombotic.

Note: Dalteparin is one of a group of substances known as low molecular weight heparins (LMWHs).

## Indications
Note: Bracketed information in the *Indications* section refers to uses that are not included in U.S. product labeling.

### General considerations
The use of low molecular weight heparins (LMWHs) has several advantages compared to heparin. Improved bioavailability at low doses when administered subcutaneously, a longer plasma half-life, and a more predictable anticoagulant response allow for simpler dosing without laboratory monitoring. Studies in animals show that with doses of equivalent antithrombotic effect, LMWHs produce less bleeding than standard heparin. The clinical importance of this observation is uncertain, but may allow the use of higher anticoagulant doses of LMWHs, thereby improving efficacy without compromising safety. The potential advantage of reduced bleeding has been demonstrated in studies in patients receiving high doses for the treatment of venous thrombosis. However, in studies using prophylactic doses, no difference in bleeding has been demonstrated. This contrasting effect may be due to inappropriate dosage regimens in early studies, and the difficulty of measuring hemorrhagic tendencies in humans. LMWHs are associated with a lower incidence of heparin-induced thrombocytopenia, possibly due to reduced effects on platelet function and binding. These advantages must be weighed against the higher cost of the LMWHs, although the simpler dosing regimens used with LMWHs may allow home treatment in selected patients, thereby reducing overall costs and improving patient satisfaction.

Meta-analyses of randomized, controlled trials comparing various LMWHs to unfractionated heparin in the treatment of deep venous thrombosis (DVT) have shown a trend toward greater efficacy, fewer major hemorrhages, and reduced total mortality with the use of LMWHs.

Unfractionated heparin is routinely used during hemodialysis to prevent thrombosis in the extracorporeal system. However, increased risks of bleeding and, with long-term use, complications such as osteoporosis and altered lipid metabolism make it a less-than-ideal agent for this purpose. Dalteparin may have a lower risk of osteoporosis and a reduced stimulation of lipolytic activity, making it an advantageous alternative to heparin in this setting.

### Accepted
Thromboembolism, pulmonary (prophylaxis); and

Thrombosis, deep venous (prophylaxis)—Dalteparin is indicated for prevention of deep venous thrombosis (DVT), which may lead to pulmonary embolism, in patients undergoing abdominal or [hip] surgery who are at risk for thromboembolic complications.

Patients at risk include patients who are over 40 years of age, obese, undergoing surgery under general anesthesia lasting longer than 30 minutes, or patients who have additional risk factors such as malignancy or a history of DVT or pulmonary embolism.

Note: The use of LMWHs for the above indications has received grade A recommendations (supported by the highest level of evidence) from the Fourth American College of Chest Physicians (ACCP) Consensus Conference on Antithrombotic Therapy. The recommendations are based on the results of studies not only with dalteparin, but with other LMWHs also.

[Thrombosis, deep venous (treatment)]—Dalteparin is used in the treatment of DVT. It has been shown to be as safe and effective as unfractionated heparin when administered subcutaneously or by continuous intravenous infusion.

[Thrombosis of the extracorporeal system during hemodialysis (prophylaxis)]—Dalteparin, given as either a single intravenous injection prior to dialysis, or as a continuous intravenous infusion during dialysis, is used to prevent thrombosis in the extracorporeal system during hemodialysis.

### Acceptance not established
Low molecular weight heparins have been used to *prevent venous thromboembolism in patients who have had an ischemic stroke* and have lower extremity weakness. Pooled data indicate that the incidence of leg DVT is 42% in these patients. Dalteparin has been shown to significantly reduce the incidence of DVT when compared with placebo in one small study. However, another placebo-controlled study failed to show a difference, although the dosing regimens used in the studies were not comparable. The Fourth ACCP Consensus Conference on Antithrombotic Therapy considers both low-dose unfractionated heparin and LMWH effective in this setting and gives the indication a grade A recommendation. The optimal prophylactic regimen for dalteparin has not yet been determined.

There have been reports of the use of dalteparin for other conditions, including:
- *unstable coronary artery disease, to prevent new cardiac events*;
- *long-term anticoagulant therapy following an acute DVT in patients unable to take oral anticoagulants*;
- *prevention of venous thromboembolism following an acute anterior wall myocardial infarction*;
- *maintaining femoropopliteal graft patency*;
- *an alternative to unfractionated heparin in patients with heparin-induced thrombocytopenia (HIT)*;
- *treatment of disseminated intravascular coagulation*; and
- *treatment of proliferative glomerulonephritis*.

These reports were either case reports or single studies; therefore, the utility of dalteparin in these situations still requires confirmation with larger follow-up studies. It should be noted that LMWHs are not indicated for the treatment of HIT because of their potential cross-reactivity with heparin, but may have utility in patients who have a negative platelet aggregation test for the selected LMWH.

In addition, the Fourth ACCP Consensus Conference on Antithrombotic Therapy has stated that LMWHs may be used to prevent venous thromboembolism in patients undergoing *total knee replacement* (a grade A recommendation), patients with *acute spinal cord injury* (a grade B recommendation, supported by the second highest level of evidence), patients with *multiple trauma* (a grade C recommendation, supported by the lowest levels of evidence), and in *general medical* patients with clinical risk factors such as congestive heart failure and/or chest infections (a grade A recommendation). However, dalteparin has not been studied in any of these conditions, and its safety and efficacy for these uses are unknown. Until studies are available, use of dalteparin in these conditions can only be determined on a case-by-case basis.

## Pharmacology/Pharmacokinetics

### Physicochemical characteristics
Source—Obtained by nitrous acid depolymerization of sodium heparin from porcine intestinal mucosa.

Molecular weight—90% of the material is between 2000 and 9000 daltons (average 5000 daltons).

### Mechanism of action/Effect
Dalteparin's antithrombotic properties are achieved by enhancing the inhibition of coagulation factor Xa and thrombin (factor IIa) by binding to antithrombin III (ATIII). Unlike heparin, however, dalteparin preferentially potentiates the inhibition of coagulation factor Xa. It is less able to inhibit thrombin because the inactivation of thrombin requires a minimum chain length of 18 saccharides; this chain length is found in only 25 to 50% of low molecular weight heparin molecules. While the ratio of anti-factor Xa activity to anti-factor IIa activity for heparin is 1:1, the ratio for dalteparin is 2.2:1. Dalteparin does not significantly affect clotting tests such as prothrombin time (PT), thrombin time (TT), or activated partial thromboplastin time (APTT).

### Other actions/effects
Compared to heparin, dalteparin binds less to endothelial cells. Heparin's binding to these cells affects both lipid metabolism and platelet function. Dalteparin, therefore, produces no significant changes in platelet aggregation, fibrinolysis, platelet factor 4, or lipoprotein lipase.

### Absorption
Approximately 90% bioavailable following subcutaneous injection, measured as anti-factor Xa activity.

### Protein binding
Very low (< 10%). The much lower protein binding compared to heparin contributes to dalteparin's greater bioavailability and more predictable anticoagulant response.

### Half-life
Elimination, apparent, based on anti-factor Xa activity—3 to 5 hours after subcutaneous administration; approximately 2 hours following intravenous injection. May be increased to approximately 6 to 7 hours in patients with impaired renal function.

### Time to peak concentration
Approximately 4 hours following subcutaneous injection.

### Peak serum concentration
Dose-related. After single subcutaneous doses of 2500, 5000, and 10,000 International Units (IU), peak concentrations of plasma anti-factor Xa activity were 0.19 ± 0.04, 0.41 ± 0.07, and 0.82 ± 0.10 IU/mL, respectively.

### Therapeutic plasma concentration
As anti-factor Xa activity—0.2 to 1 IU/mL.

## Elimination
Renal.

## Precautions to Consider

### Cross-sensitivity and/or related problems
Patients with known hypersensitivity to heparin or to pork products may be sensitive to dalteparin also.

### Carcinogenicity
No long-term animal studies have been performed with dalteparin to determine its carcinogenic potential.

### Mutagenicity
Dalteparin was not mutagenic in the *in vitro* Ames test, the mouse lymphoma cell forward mutation test, the human lymphocyte chromosomal aberration test, and the *in vivo* mouse micronucleus test.

### Pregnancy/Reproduction
Fertility—In studies of rats, subcutaneous doses up to 1200 International Units per kg of body weight (IU/kg) did not affect fertility.

Pregnancy—Adequate and well-controlled studies in humans have not been done.

Heparin is considered to be the anticoagulant of choice during pregnancy since it does not cross the placenta. There is also evidence that dalteparin does not cross the placenta. The advantages of dalteparin over heparin during pregnancy include the potential for once-daily administration, a lower incidence of heparin-induced thrombocytopenia, and possibly a lower risk of heparin-induced osteoporosis. However, until adequate clinical studies comparing the use of dalteparin to heparin during pregnancy are performed, there is insufficient evidence to support the routine use of dalteparin.

Studies in pregnant rats and rabbits given intravenous doses of dalteparin up to 2400 IU/kg and 4800 IU/kg, respectively, showed no evidence of harm to the fetus.

FDA Pregnancy Category B.

Note: The 25,000-IU-per-mL multi-dose vial contains benzyl alcohol, which is not recommended for use during pregnancy since benzyl alcohol may cross the placenta.

### Breast-feeding
It is not known whether dalteparin is distributed into breast milk. However, problems in humans have not been documented.

### Pediatrics
No information is available on the relationship of age to the effects of dalteparin in pediatric patients. Safety and efficacy have not been established.

Note: The 25,000-IU-per-mL multi-dose vial contains benzyl alcohol, which is not recommended for use in neonates.

### Geriatrics
Appropriate studies performed to date have not demonstrated geriatrics-specific problems that would limit the usefulness of dalteparin in the elderly.

Pharmacokinetic differences requiring dose reductions have not been noted in elderly subjects. Clinical studies performed in elderly patients have not shown an increase in bleeding.

### Drug interactions and/or related problems
The following drug interactions and/or related problems have been selected on the basis of their potential clinical significance (possible mechanism in parentheses where appropriate)—not necessarily inclusive (» = major clinical significance):

Note: Combinations containing any of the following medications, depending on the amount present, may also interact with this medication.

In addition to the interactions listed below, the possibility should be considered that multiple effects leading to further impairment of blood clotting and/or increased risk of bleeding may occur if dalteparin is administered to a patient receiving any medication having a significant potential for causing hypoprothrombinemia, thrombocytopenia, or gastrointestinal ulceration or hemorrhage.

Anticoagulants, coumarin- or indandione-derivative, or
Platelet aggregation inhibitors (see *Appendix II*) such as:
» Anti-inflammatory drugs, nonsteroidal (NSAIDs)
» Aspirin
  Dextran
» Ticlopidine
  (increased risk of bleeding must be considered)

Thrombolytic agents, such as:
  Alteplase (rt-PA)
  Anistreplase (APSAC)
  Streptokinase
  Urokinase
  (concurrent or sequential use may increase the risk of bleeding; however, unfractionated heparin is used concurrently with thrombolytic therapy in patients with acute myocardial infarction, and may be continued post-thrombolysis to prevent further thromboembolism; experience with the use of low molecular weight heparin in this setting is limited; careful monitoring of the patient is recommended if dalteparin is used under these circumstances)

### Laboratory value alterations
The following have been selected on the basis of their potential clinical significance (possible effect in parentheses where appropriate)—not necessarily inclusive (» = major clinical significance):

With physiology/laboratory test values
  Alanine aminotransferase (ALT [SGPT]) and
  Aspartate aminotransferase (AST [SGOT])
    (serum values may be increased during dalteparin therapy and are reversible; the usefulness of these enzymes in the differential diagnosis of myocardial infarction, pulmonary embolism, or liver disease may, therefore, be decreased)

  Free fatty acids and
  Triglycerides
    (initially, plasma triglyceride concentrations may decrease, with a resulting increase in plasma free fatty acids, due to stimulation of lipolytic activity by release of lipoprotein lipase from tissue sites. However, release of lipoprotein lipase is not as pronounced as that seen with heparin. The subsequent increase in plasma triglyceride concentrations that is seen with long-term heparin use due to depletion of lipoprotein lipase has not been seen with dalteparin. Since the increase in triglyceride concentrations is a particular problem in uremic patients who require chronic hemodialysis and the long-term use of heparin, dalteparin may be advantageous in this population due to its reduced stimulation of lipolytic activity)

### Medical considerations/Contraindications
The medical considerations/contraindications included have been selected on the basis of their potential clinical significance (reasons given in parentheses where appropriate)—not necessarily inclusive (» = major clinical significance).

*Except under special circumstances, this medication should not be used when the following medical problems exist:*

» Bleeding, major, active
  (may be exacerbated)
» Hypertension, severe, uncontrolled
  (increased risk of cerebral hemorrhage)
» Stroke, hemorrhagic or
» Stroke, ischemic, large
  (increased risk of uncontrollable hemorrhage; cardioembolic strokes have a risk of secondary hemorrhagic transformation, with large infarcts [i.e., deficits involving the entire middle cerebral distribution] especially prone to worsening; some clinicians recommend waiting 7 days before initiating anticoagulant therapy in patients with large infarcts)
» Thrombocytopenia associated with positive *in vitro* tests for antiplatelet antibody in the presence of dalteparin or
» Thrombocytopenia, dalteparin- or heparin-induced, history of
  (risk of recurrence)

*Risk-benefit should be considered when the following medical problems exist:*

Any medical procedure or condition in which the risk of bleeding or hemorrhage is present, such as:
» Anesthesia, epidural or spinal
  (risk of epidural or spinal hematoma, which can result in long-term or permanent paralysis; this risk is increased with the use of indwelling epidural catheters or by the concomitant use of medications that affect hemostasis, such as nonsteroidal anti-inflammatory drugs, platelet inhibitors, or other anticoagulants; the risk also may be increased by traumatic or repeated epidural or spinal puncture. See *General Dosing Information* for guidelines regarding the use of regional anesthesia in patients receiving perioperative dalteparin.)
» Bleeding disorders, congenital or acquired
» Endocarditis, bacterial
» Hepatic function impairment, severe
» Platelet defects
» Renal function impairment, severe
» Retinopathy, diabetic or hypertensive
» Surgery, brain, ophthalmological, or spinal, recent

» Ulcers, other lesions, or recent bleeding of the gastrointestinal tract, active
Sensitivity to dalteparin or to heparin

**Patient monitoring**
The following may be especially important in patient monitoring (other tests may be warranted in some patients, depending on condition; » = major clinical significance):

» Anti-factor Xa activity
(monitoring of plasma anti-factor Xa activity is considered optional when dalteparin is used therapeutically, and is recommended in patients undergoing acute hemodialysis, with recommended plasma concentrations as follows:
- Treatment of deep venous thrombosis—
    Subcutaneous, > 0.3 International Units anti-factor Xa activity per mL (IU/mL) before injection and < 1.5 IU/mL 3 to 4 hours after injection;
    Intravenous, 0.5 to 1 IU/mL
- Acute hemodialysis—0.2 to 0.4 IU/mL

Note: No special monitoring is needed when dalteparin is used prophylactically. Routine clotting assays such as activated partial thromboplastin time (APTT), prothrombin time (PT), or thrombin time (TT) are unsuitable for monitoring dalteparin's anticoagulant activity since dalteparin does not significantly affect these tests; increased doses intended to prolong the APTT could cause overdosing and bleeding. Prolongation of the APTT should only be used as a criterion of overdose.

Blood counts, complete (CBC), including:
Hematocrit
Hemoglobin
» Platelet count
(recommended prior to the initiation of therapy, then twice weekly for the duration of therapy to detect occult bleeding or any degree of thrombocytopenia)

Blood pressure measurement
(recommended periodically during therapy; an unexplained drop in blood pressure may signal occult bleeding)

» Neurologic status
(monitor for signs and symptoms of neurological impairment such as paresthesias, leg weakness, sensory loss, motor deficit, or bowel/bladder dysfunction, which may indicate a potential epidural or spinal hematoma; if neurologic compromise is noted, urgent intervention is necessary, including radiographic confirmation and decompressive laminectomy; good or partial recovery is more likely if surgery is performed within 8 hours of the development of paraplegia)

» Platelet aggregation test
(recommended prior to the initiation of therapy in patients who have congenital, or a history of drug-induced, thrombocytopenia or platelet defects; if the result is negative, dalteparin therapy may be instituted, with daily monitoring of the platelet count; however, if the result is positive, dalteparin should not be given)

Stool tests for occult blood
(should be performed at regular intervals during therapy)

## Side/Adverse Effects

Note: The occurrence of hemorrhage may be increased with higher doses. Also, other risk factors may be associated with hemorrhage, including a serious concurrent illness, chronic heavy consumption of alcohol, use of platelet inhibiting drugs, renal failure, and female sex.

*Osteoporosis* is associated with the use of long-term, high-dose heparin. Dalteparin has been shown to have a weak osteopenic effect in dogs. However, the effect does not appear to be as great as that seen with heparin; therefore, the risk of heparin-induced osteoporosis may be lower with dalteparin.

The following side/adverse effects have been selected on the basis of their potential clinical significance (possible signs and symptoms in parentheses where appropriate)—not necessarily inclusive:

**Those indicating need for medical attention**
Incidence more frequent
*Hematoma at injection site* (deep, dark purple bruise, pain, or swelling at place of injection)
Incidence less frequent
*Hemorrhage* (bleeding gums; coughing up blood; difficulty in breathing or swallowing; dizziness; headache; increased menstrual flow or vaginal bleeding; nosebleeds; paralysis; prolonged bleeding from cuts; red or dark brown urine; red or black, tarry stools; shortness of breath; unexplained pain, swelling, or discomfort, especially in the chest, abdomen, joints, or muscles; unusual bruising; vomiting of blood or coffee ground–like material; weakness)

Incidence rare
*Allergic reaction* (fever; skin rash, hives, or itching); *anaphylactoid reaction* (bluish discoloration, flushing, or redness of skin; coughing; difficulty in swallowing; dizziness or feeling faint, severe; skin rash, hives [may include giant urticaria], or itching; swelling of eyelids, face, or lips; tightness in chest, troubled breathing, and/or wheezing); *epidural or spinal hematoma* (back pain; bowel/bladder dysfunction; leg weakness; numbness; paralysis; paresthesias)—back pain is not a typical presentation but some patients may experience this symptom; *skin necrosis* (blue-green to black skin discoloration; pain, redness, or sloughing of skin at place of injection); *thrombocytopenia* (bleeding from mucous membranes; rash consisting of pinpoint, purple-red spots, often beginning on the legs; unusual bruising)

Note: If an *epidural* or *spinal hematoma* is suspected, urgent intervention is necessary, including radiographic confirmation and decompressive laminectomy. Good or partial recovery is more likely if surgery is performed within 8 hours of the development of paraplegia.

The syndrome of *thrombocytopenia with thrombosis* is a well-known complication of unfractionated heparin therapy. Low molecular weight heparins (LMWHs) are associated with a lower incidence of heparin-induced thrombocytopenia. However, there have been case reports of this complication with LMWHs. Clinicians should be aware of the possible occurrence of thromboembolic events with the use of LMWHs, and should monitor the platelet count appropriately.

**Those indicating need for medical attention only if they continue or are bothersome**
Incidence less frequent
*Pain at injection site*

## Overdose

For specific information on the agents used in the management of dalteparin overdose, see the *Protamine (Systemic)* monograph.
For more information on the management of overdose, **contact a Poison Control Center** (see *Poison Control Center Listing*).

**Clinical effects of overdose**
The following effects have been selected on the basis of their potential clinical significance (possible signs and symptoms in parentheses where appropriate)—not necessarily inclusive:
Acute effects
*Bleeding complications or hemorrhage* (bleeding gums; coughing up blood; difficulty in breathing or swallowing; dizziness; headache; increased menstrual flow or vaginal bleeding; nosebleeds; paralysis; prolonged bleeding from cuts; red or dark brown urine; red or black, tarry stools; shortness of breath; unexplained pain, swelling, or discomfort, especially in the chest, abdomen, joints, or muscles; unusual bruising; vomiting of blood or coffee ground–like material; weakness)

**Treatment of overdose**
Specific treatment—Administration of protamine, a heparin antagonist, is required. One mg of protamine sulfate (1% solution) per 100 anti-factor Xa International Units (IU) of dalteparin is given as a slow intravenous injection. If the activated partial thromboplastin time (APTT) measured 2 to 4 hours after the first injection remains prolonged, a second injection of 0.5 mg protamine sulfate per 100 anti-factor Xa IU of dalteparin may be administered. However, the APTT may remain more prolonged with dalteparin than with conventional heparin, despite the additional dosing of protamine. In all cases, the anti-factor Xa activity is only neutralized to about 25 to 50%.

Protamine sulfate should be administered with great care to avoid an overdose. Severe hypotensive and anaphylactoid reactions, possibly fatal, may occur with protamine sulfate. It should be administered only when resuscitation techniques and treatment of anaphylactic shock are readily available.

## Patient Consultation

As an aid to patient consultation, refer to *Advice for the Patient, Dalteparin (Systemic)*.
In providing consultation, consider emphasizing the following selected information (» = major clinical significance):

**Before using this medication**
» Conditions affecting use, especially:
    Sensitivity to dalteparin, heparin, or pork products
    Other medications, especially platelet aggregation inhibitors, such as aspirin, nonsteroidal anti-inflammatory drugs, and ticlopidine

Other medical problems, especially bleeding, major, active; bleeding disorders; endocarditis, bacterial; hepatic function impairment, severe; hypertension, severe, uncontrolled; platelet defects; renal function impairment, severe; retinopathy, diabetic or hypertensive; stroke, hemorrhagic or ischemic; surgery, recent; thrombocytopenia; and ulcers, other lesions, or recent bleeding of the gastrointestinal tract

**Proper use of this medication**
» Proper injection technique
» Safe handling and disposal of syringe
» Proper dosing
    Missed dose: Using as soon as possible; not using if almost time for next dose; not doubling doses
» Proper storage

**Precautions while using this medication**
» Need to inform all physicians and dentists that this medicine is being used
» Notifying physician immediately if signs and symptoms of bleeding or epidural/spinal hematoma occur

**Side/adverse effects**
Signs and symptoms of potential side effects, especially hematoma at injection site, hemorrhage, allergic reaction, anaphylactoid reaction, epidural/spinal hematoma, skin necrosis, and thrombocytopenia

## General Dosing Information

Dalteparin cannot be used interchangeably (unit for unit) with unfractionated heparin or other low molecular weight heparins.

Dalteparin is administered by deep subcutaneous injection. It must not be injected intramuscularly.

Injection technique: The patient should be sitting or lying down during the injection. Injection sites include a U-shaped area around the navel, the upper outer side of the thigh, or the upper outer quadrant of the buttock. The site should be varied daily. When giving the injection around the navel or the thigh, a fold of skin must be lifted up with thumb and forefinger, and the entire length of the needle should be inserted at a 45- to 90-degree angle.

If a thromboembolic event occurs during dalteparin prophylaxis, dalteparin should be discontinued and appropriate therapy initiated.

**Guidelines regarding the use of regional anesthesia in patients receiving perioperative dalteparin**

Preoperative dalteparin—A single-dose spinal anesthetic may be the safest neuraxial technique. Needle placement should occur at least 10 to 12 hours after the last dose of dalteparin. Subsequent dosing should be delayed for at least 2 hours after needle placement. The presence of blood during needle placement may justify a delay in the start of postoperative prophylaxis.

Postoperative dalteparin—Patients may safely undergo single-dose and continuous catheter techniques. With a continuous technique, the epidural catheter should be left indwelling overnight and removed the following day, and the first dose of dalteparin should be given 2 hours after catheter removal. Postoperative prophylaxis in the presence of an indwelling catheter must be administered carefully and with close surveillance of the patient's neurologic status. An opioid and/or dilute local anesthetic solution is recommended in these patients to allow intermittent assessment of neurologic function.

The timing of catheter removal is extremely important. Removal should be delayed for at least 10 to 12 hours after a dose of dalteparin. Subsequent dosing should not occur for at least 2 hours following catheter removal.

## Parenteral Dosage Forms

Note: Bracketed uses in the *Dosage Forms* section refer to categories of use and/or indications that are not included in U.S. product labeling.

### DALTEPARIN SODIUM INJECTION

**Usual adult dose**
Thromboembolism, pulmonary (prophylaxis) and
Thrombosis, deep venous (prophylaxis)—
    General surgery: Subcutaneous, 2500 International Units (IU) initially, given one to two hours prior to abdominal surgery, then repeated once a day for five to ten days following surgery, until the patient is mobile.
    General surgery associated with other risk factors, or [hip surgery]: Subcutaneous, 5000 IU given the evening before the operation, then repeated once a day every evening for five to ten days following surgery, until the patient is mobile. Alternatively, 2500 IU given one to two hours prior to surgery and again eight to twelve hours later, followed by 5000 IU each morning for five to ten days following surgery, until the patient is mobile.

[Thrombosis, deep venous (treatment)]—
    Subcutaneous, 200 IU per kg of body weight once a day, or 100 IU per kg of body weight two times a day. Alternatively, it may be administered at a dose of 200 IU per kg of body weight given as a continuous intravenous infusion over twenty-four hours (i.e., 8.33 IU per kg of body weight per hour). Treatment may be guided by monitoring anti-factor Xa activity. Concomitant treatment with a vitamin K antagonist, such as warfarin, should begin at the same time, and dalteparin should be discontinued when the vitamin K antagonist reaches a full therapeutic effect, usually after five or six days of therapy.

[Thrombosis of the extracorporeal system during hemodialysis (prophylaxis)]—
Chronic renal failure in patients with no known bleeding risk—
    Dialysis lasting up to four hours—Intravenous, 5000 IU, as a single injection into the arterial line at the start of dialysis; or dosed as for dialysis procedures of more than four hours' duration.
    Dialysis lasting more than four hours—Intravenous loading dose, 30 to 40 IU per kg of body weight followed by a continuous intravenous infusion of 10 to 15 IU per kg of body weight per hour.
Acute renal failure in patients with a high bleeding risk—
    Intravenous loading dose, 5 to 10 IU per kg of body weight, followed by a continuous intravenous infusion of 4 to 5 IU per kg of body weight per hour. Therapy should be guided by monitoring anti-factor Xa activity.

**Usual pediatric dose**
Safety and efficacy have not been established. A case report described the use of dalteparin in a neonate who developed a proximal deep vein thrombosis following balloon valvuloplasty for pulmonary stenosis. Dalteparin was administered subcutaneously at a dose of 100 IU per kg of body weight two times a day for two days, followed by 200 IU per kg of body weight once a day for twelve weeks (administered by the infant's mother at home). No problems were reported during treatment.
Note: The 10,000- and 25,000-IU-per-mL multi-dose vials contain benzyl alcohol, which is not recommended for use in neonates.

**Strength(s) usually available**
U.S.—
    2500 anti-factor Xa IU (16 mg dalteparin sodium) per 0.2 mL (Rx) [*Fragmin* (in single unit-dose syringes)].
    5000 anti-factor Xa IU (32 mg dalteparin sodium) per 0.2 mL (Rx) [*Fragmin* (in single unit-dose syringes)].
    10,000 anti-factor Xa IU (64 mg dalteparin sodium) per mL (Rx) [*Fragmin* (in 9.5 mL multiple-dose vials; benzyl alcohol 14 mg per mL)].
Canada—
    2500 anti-factor Xa IU (16 mg dalteparin sodium) per 0.2 mL (Rx) [*Fragmin* (in single unit-dose syringes)].
    5000 anti-factor Xa IU (32 mg dalteparin sodium) per 0.2 mL (Rx) [*Fragmin* (in single unit-dose syringes)].
    2500 anti-factor Xa IU (16 mg dalteparin sodium) per mL (Rx) [*Fragmin* (in 4-mL ampuls)].
    10,000 anti-factor Xa IU (64 mg dalteparin sodium) per mL (Rx) [*Fragmin* (in 1-mL ampuls)].
    25,000 anti-factor Xa IU (160 mg dalteparin sodium) per mL (Rx) [*Fragmin* (in 3.8-mL multi-dose vials; benzyl alcohol 14 mg per mL)].

**Packaging and storage**
Store at controlled room temperature, between 20 and 25 °C (68 and 77 °F).

**Preparation of dosage form**
For a continuous intravenous infusion, dalteparin may be diluted in 0.9% sodium chloride injection or 5% dextrose injection in glass or plastic containers. The recommended postdilution concentration is 20 IU per mL, which can be prepared by adding 2500 IU to 125 mL or 10,000 IU to 500 mL of solution. The solution should be used within 24 hours.

**Stability**
The 25,000-IU-per-mL multi-dose vial must be used within two weeks after initial penetration.

**Incompatibilities**
Dalteparin sodium injection should not be mixed with other injections or infusions unless compatibility has been established.

**Additional information**
The 10,000- and 25,000-IU-per-mL multi-dose vials contain benzyl alcohol, which is not recommended for use in neonates. A fatal syndrome consisting of metabolic acidosis, central nervous system depression, respiratory problems, renal failure, hypotension, and possibly seizures and intracranial hemorrhage has been associated with the administration of benzyl alcohol to neonates.

## Selected Bibliography

Dalen JE, Hirsh J, editors. Fourth ACCP Consensus Conference on Antithrombotic Therapy. Chest 1995; 108(Suppl): 225S-522S.

Green D, Hirsh J, Heit J, et al. Low molecular weight heparin: a critical analysis of clinical trials. Pharmacol Rev 1994; 46: 89-109.

Kakkar VV, Cohen AT, Edmonson RA, et al. Low molecular weight versus standard heparin for prevention of venous thromboembolism after major abdominal surgery. Lancet 1993; 341: 259-65.

Developed: 01/06/96
Interim revision: 07/28/98

---

# DANAPAROID  Systemic—INTRODUCTORY VERSION

VA CLASSIFICATION (Primary): BL112

Another commonly used name is ORG 10172.

Note: For a listing of dosage forms and brand names by country availability, see *Dosage Forms* section(s).

## Category

Antithrombotic.

Note: Danaparoid has been categorized as one of a group of substances known as low molecular weight heparins (LMWHs), although it is technically a heparinoid.

## Indications

### Accepted

Thromboembolism, pulmonary (prophylaxis) and

Thrombosis, deep venous (prophylaxis)—Danaparoid is indicated for the prevention of postoperative deep venous thrombosis (DVT), which may lead to pulmonary embolism (PE), in patients undergoing elective hip replacement surgery.

## Pharmacology/Pharmacokinetics

### Physicochemical characteristics

Source—Isolated from porcine intestinal mucosa.

Composition—Depolymerized mixture of low molecular weight sulfated glycosaminoglycans, consisting of approximately 84% heparan sulfate, approximately 12% dermatan sulfate, and approximately 4% chondroitin sulfates.

Molecular weight—Approximately 5500 daltons (average).

### Mechanism of action/Effect

Danaparoid prevents fibrin formation in the coagulation pathway by inhibiting thrombin generation through the inhibition of coagulation factor Xa and thrombin (factor IIa). Unlike heparin, however, danaparoid preferentially potentiates the inhibition of coagulation factor Xa, with a ratio of anti-factor Xa activity to anti-factor IIa activity greater than 22:1. Danaparoid has little effect on clotting assays such as prothrombin time (PT), partial thromboplastin time (PTT), and bleeding time.

### Other actions/effects

Danaparoid has only minor effects on platelet function, platelet aggregability, and fibrinolytic activity.

### Absorption

Approximately 100% bioavailable following subcutaneous injection, measured as anti-factor Xa activity.

### Half-life

Elimination—approximately 24 hours (average).

### Time to peak concentration

Approximately 2 to 5 hours following subcutaneous injection.

### Peak serum concentration

Dose-related. After single subcutaneous doses of 750, 1500, 2250, and 3250 anti-factor Xa units, peak concentrations of plasma anti-factor Xa activity were 102.4, 206.1, 283.9, and 403.4 microunits per mL, respectively.

### Elimination

Renal. In patients with severely impaired renal function, the elimination half-life of plasma anti-factor Xa activity may be prolonged.

## Precautions to Consider

### Cross-sensitivity and/or related problems

Patients hypersensitive to heparin or to pork products may be sensitive to danaparoid also.

### Carcinogenicity

No long-term animal studies have been performed with danaparoid to determine its carcinogenic potential.

### Mutagenicity

Danaparoid was not mutagenic in the Ames test, the *in vitro* CHL/HGPRT forward gene mutation assay, the *in vitro* CHO cell chromosome aberration test, the *in vitro* HeLa cell unscheduled DNA synthesis (UDS) test or the *in vivo* mouse micronucleus test.

### Pregnancy/Reproduction

Fertility—In studies in rats, intravenous doses of up to 1090 anti-factor Xa units per kg of body weight (units/kg) per day (up to 5.9 times the human subcutaneous dose on a body surface area basis) did not affect fertility or reproductive performance.

Pregnancy—Adequate and well-controlled studies in humans have not been done.

Studies in pregnant rats and rabbits given intravenous doses of danaparoid up to 1600 units/kg per day (up to 8.7 times the human dose on a body surface area basis) and up to 780 units/kg per day (up to 6 times the human dose on a body surface area basis), respectively, showed no evidence of harm to the fetus.

FDA Pregnancy Category B.

### Breast-feeding

It is not known whether danaparoid is distributed into breast milk. However, problems in humans have not been documented.

### Pediatrics

No information is available on the relationship of age to the effects of danaparoid in pediatric patients. Safety and efficacy have not been established.

### Geriatrics

No information is available on the relationship of age to the effects of danaparoid in geriatric patients.

### Drug interactions and/or related problems

The following drug interactions and/or related problems have been selected on the basis of their potential clinical significance (possible mechanism in parentheses where appropriate)—not necessarily inclusive (» = major clinical significance):

Note: Combinations containing any of the following medications, depending on the amount present, may also interact with this medication.

Anticoagulants, coumarin- or indandione-derivative or
Platelet aggregation inhibitors
(increased risk of bleeding must be considered; the results of the prothrombin time [PT] and *Thrombotest*™, used for monitoring oral anticoagulant activity, are unreliable within 5 hours following danaparoid administration)

### Medical considerations/Contraindications

The medical considerations/contraindications included have been selected on the basis of their potential clinical significance (reasons given in parentheses where appropriate)—not necessarily inclusive (» = major clinical significance).

*Except under special circumstances, this medication should not be used when the following medical problems exist:*

» Bleeding, major, active
  (may be exacerbated)

» Hypertension, severe, uncontrolled
  (increased risk of cerebral hemorrhage)

» Stroke, hemorrhagic
  (increased risk of uncontrollable hemorrhage)

» Thrombocytopenia associated with positive *in vitro* tests for antiplatelet antibody in the presence of danaparoid
  (risk of recurrence)

  Note: Danaparoid exhibits a low cross-reactivity with antiplatelet antibodies in individuals with Type II heparin-induced thrombocytopenia (HIT).

**1162  Danaparoid (Systemic)—Introductory Version**

*Risk-benefit should be considered when the following medical problems exist:*

Any medical procedure or condition in which the risk of bleeding or hemorrhage is present, such as:
» Anesthesia, epidural or spinal
(risk of epidural or spinal hematoma, which can result in long-term or permanent paralysis; this risk is increased with the use of in-dwelling epidural catheters or by the concomitant use of medications that affect hemostasis, such as nonsteroidal anti-inflammatory drugs, platelet inhibitors, or other anticoagulants; the risk may also be increased by traumatic or repeated epidural or spinal puncture)
» Blood dyscrasias, hemorrhagic, congenital or acquired
» Endocarditis, bacterial
» Renal function impairment, severe
» Stroke, nonhemorrhagic
» Surgery, especially brain, spinal, or ophthalmologic
» Ulceration, other lesions, or recent bleeding of the gastrointestinal tract, active

Sensitivity to danaparoid, heparin, pork products, or sulfites
(patients sensitive to sulfites may be sensitive to danaparoid injection because it contains sodium sulfite; sulfite sensitivity is seen more frequently in asthmatic than in nonasthmatic patients, and may result in allergic-type reactions, including anaphylactic symptoms and life-threatening or less severe asthmatic episodes)

**Patient monitoring**

The following may be especially important in patient monitoring (other tests may be warranted in some patients, depending on condition; » = major clinical significance):

Note: Since danaparoid has only a small effect on factor IIa activity, routine coagulation tests such as prothrombin time (PT), activated partial thromboplastin time (APTT), kaolin cephalin clotting time (KCCT), whole blood clotting time (WBCT), and thrombin time (TT) are unsuitable for monitoring danaparoid activity at recommended doses.

Patients with a serum creatinine ≥ 2 mg per deciliter should be carefully monitored, since danaparoid's activity may be prolonged in these patients.

» Blood counts, complete (CBC), including
Hematocrit
Platelet count
(recommended during treatment to detect occult bleeding or any degree of thrombocytopenia)
Blood pressure measurement
(recommended periodically during therapy; an unexplained drop in blood pressure may signal occult bleeding)
» Neurologic status
(frequent monitoring for signs and symptoms of neurological impairment is recommended; if neurologic compromise is noted, urgent treatment is necessary)
Stool tests for occult blood
(should be performed at regular intervals during therapy)

## Side/Adverse Effects

The following side/adverse effects have been selected on the basis of their potential clinical significance (possible signs and symptoms in parentheses where appropriate)—not necessarily inclusive:

Note: No cases of *white clot syndrome* or *Type II thrombocytopenia* have been reported in clinical studies for the prophylaxis of deep venous thrombosis in patients receiving multiple doses of danaparoid for up to 14 days.

**Those indicating need for medical attention**
Incidence less frequent
*Fever; hemorrhage* (bleeding gums; coughing up blood; difficulty in breathing or swallowing; dizziness; headache; increased menstrual flow or vaginal bleeding; nosebleeds; paralysis; prolonged bleeding from cuts; red or dark brown urine; red or black, tarry stools; shortness of breath; unexplained pain, swelling, or discomfort, especially in the chest, abdomen, joints, or muscles; unusual bruising; vomiting of blood or coffee ground–like material; weakness)
Incidence rare
*Epidural or spinal hematoma* (back pain; bowel/bladder dysfunction; leg weakness; numbness; paralysis; paresthesias)—back pain is not a typical presentation but some patients may experience this symptom; *skin rash*
Note: If an *epidural or spinal hematoma* is suspected, urgent intervention is necessary.

**Those indicating need for medical attention only if they continue or are bothersome**
Incidence more frequent
*Pain at injection site*
Incidence less frequent
*Constipation; nausea*

## Overdose

For specific information on the agents used in the management of danaparoid overdose, see the *Protamine (Systemic)* monograph.
For more information on the management of overdose, **contact a Poison Control Center** (see *Poison Control Center Listing*).

**Clinical effects of overdose**
The following effects have been selected on the basis of their potential clinical significance (possible signs and symptoms in parentheses where appropriate)—not necessarily inclusive:

Acute
*Bleeding complications, which may include blood in urine; bloody or black, tarry stools; bruising; coughing up blood; ecchymosis* (large, non-elevated blue or purplish patches in the skin)*; hematoma; hypochromic anemia* (fatigue; headache; irritability; lightheadedness)*; nosebleed; persistent bleeding or oozing from mucous membranes or surgical wound; shortness of breath; vomiting of blood or material that looks like coffee grounds*

**Treatment of overdose**
The effects of danaparoid on anti-factor Xa activity cannot be antagonized with any known agent at this time. Although protamine sulfate partially neutralizes the anti-factor Xa activity of danaparoid and can be safely coadministered, there is no evidence that protamine sulfate can reduce severe, nonsurgical bleeding during treatment with danaparoid.

Specific treatment—In the event of serious bleeding, danaparoid should be stopped and blood or blood product transfusions should be administered as needed.

## Patient Consultation

As an aid to patient consultation, refer to *Advice for the Patient, Danaparoid (Systemic)—Introductory Version.*
In providing consultation, consider emphasizing the following selected information (» = major clinical significance):

**Before using this medication**
» Conditions affecting use, especially:
Sensitivity to danaparoid, heparin, pork products, or sulfites
Other medical problems, especially bacterial endocarditis; bleeding; hemorrhagic blood dyscrasias; severe renal function impairment; severe, uncontrolled hypertension; stroke; surgery; thrombocytopenia; and ulcers or other lesions of the gastrointestinal tract

**Proper use of this medication**
» Proper dosing

**Precautions while using this medication**
» Need to inform all health care providers of use of medication
» Notifying physician immediately if signs and symptoms of bleeding or epidural/spinal hematoma occur

**Side/adverse effects**
Signs of potential side effects, especially fever, hemorrhage, epidural or spinal hematoma, and skin rash

## General Dosing Information

The anti-factor Xa unit activity of danaparoid is not equivalent to that of heparin or low molecular weight heparins. Therefore, danaparoid cannot be used interchangeably (unit for unit) with unfractionated heparin or any low molecular weight heparin.

Danaparoid is administered by deep subcutaneous injection. **It must not be injected intramuscularly**.

Injection technique: The patient should be lying down during injection. A 25- to 26-gauge needle should be used to minimize tissue trauma. Administration should be alternated between the left and right anterolateral and left and right posterolateral abdominal wall. A fold of skin must be lifted up with thumb and forefinger, and the entire length of the needle should be inserted. The skin fold should be held throughout the injection and should not be pinched or rubbed afterwards.

## Parenteral Dosage Forms

### DANAPAROID SODIUM INJECTION

**Usual adult dose**
Thromboembolism, pulmonary (prophylaxis) and
Thrombosis, deep venous (prophylaxis)—
Subcutaneous, 750 anti-factor Xa units two times a day, beginning one to four hours prior to hip replacement surgery, and then no sooner than two hours after surgery. Treatment should be continued until the risk of deep venous thrombosis has diminished, usually within seven to ten days, but may be continued for up to fourteen days.

**Usual pediatric dose**
Safety and efficacy have not been established.

**Strength(s) usually available**
U.S.—
750 anti-factor Xa units per 0.6 mL (Rx) [*Orgaran* (in single unit-dose syringes; sodium sulfite 0.15% [to prevent discoloration])].
750 anti-factor Xa units per 0.6 mL (Rx) [*Orgaran* (in 0.6-mL ampuls; sodium sulfite 0.15% [to prevent discoloration])].

**Packaging and storage**
Ampuls should be stored between 2 and 30 °C (36 and 86 °F). Syringes should be stored between 2 and 8 °C (36 and 46 °F). Protect from light.

Developed: 04/28/97
Interim revision: 07/10/98

---

# DANAZOL  Systemic

VA CLASSIFICATION (Primary/Secondary): HS109/IM900
Commonly used brand name(s): *Cyclomen; Danocrine*.
Note: For a listing of dosage forms and brand names by country availability, see *Dosage Forms* section(s).

## Category
Gonadotropin inhibitor; angioedema (hereditary) prophylactic.

## Indications
Note: Bracketed information in the *Indications* section refers to uses that are not included in U.S. product labeling.

**Accepted**
Endometriosis (treatment)—Danazol is indicated for the treatment of pain and/or infertility due to endometriosis.
Breast disease, fibrocystic (treatment)—Danazol is indicated for the treatment of fibrocystic breast disease in patients whose symptoms are not relieved by analgesics, the use of well-fitted bras, or other simple methods.
Angioedema, hereditary (prophylaxis)[1]—Danazol is indicated for the prophylactic treatment of hereditary angioedema (cutaneous, abdominal, and laryngeal) in males and females, including prior to surgery.
[Gynecomastia (treatment)][1]
[Menorrhagia (treatment)][1] or
[Puberty, precocious (treatment)][1]—Danazol is being used to treat gynecomastia, menorrhagia, and precocious puberty in females.

[1]Not included in Canadian product labeling.

## Pharmacology/Pharmacokinetics

**Physicochemical characteristics**
Chemical group—Synthetic androgen.
Molecular weight—337.46.

**Mechanism of action/Effect**
Gonadotropin inhibitor—May suppress the pituitary-ovarian axis by inhibiting the output of pituitary gonadotropins. Danazol depresses the preovulatory surge in output of follicle-stimulating hormone (FSH) and luteinizing hormone (LH) and therefore reduces ovarian estrogen production. Danazol may also directly inhibit ovarian steroidogenesis, bind to androgen, progesterone, and glucocorticoid receptors, bind to sex-hormone–binding globulin and corticosteroid-binding globulin, and increase the metabolic clearance rate of progesterone.
Endometriosis—As a consequence of suppression of ovarian function, both normal and ectopic endometrial tissues become inactive and atrophic. As a result, anovulation and associated amenorrhea occur.
Fibrocystic breast disease—Exact mechanism of action is unknown, but may be related to suppressed estrogenic stimulation as a result of decreased ovarian production of estrogen; a direct effect on steroid receptor sites in breast tissue is also possible. Disappearance of nodularity, relief of pain and tenderness, and possibly changes in the menstrual pattern result.
Hereditary angioedema—Correction of the underlying biochemical deficiency: Increases serum levels of C1 esterase inhibitor, resulting in increased serum levels of the C4 component of the complement system.

**Other actions/effects**
Weak androgenic effects.

**Biotransformation**
Hepatic, to inactive metabolites.

**Half-life**
Approximately 4.5 hours (variable).

**Onset of action**
Fibrocystic breast disease—Relief of breast pain and tenderness usually begins within 1 month.

**Peak serum concentration**
Following 100-mg dose twice a day—200 to 800 nanograms per mL.
Following 200-mg dose twice a day for 14 days—250 nanograms to 2 mcg per mL.

**Time to peak effect**
Anovulation and amenorrhea—Usually occur after 6 to 8 weeks of therapy.
Fibrocystic breast disease—Breast pain and tenderness are usually eliminated in 2 to 3 months of therapy. Elimination of nodularity usually requires 4 to 6 months of uninterrupted therapy.

**Duration of action**
Anovulation and amenorrhea—Ovulation and cyclic bleeding usually return within 60 to 90 days after therapy is withdrawn.
Fibrocystic breast disease—Symptoms return to some degree within 1 year after therapy is withdrawn in 50% of patients.

**Elimination**
Renal.

## Precautions to Consider

**Pregnancy/Reproduction**
Pregnancy—Danazol is contraindicated during pregnancy. Continuing treatment may result in an androgenic effect (clitoral hypertrophy, labial fusion of the external genitalia, urogenital sinus defect, vaginal atresia, ambiguous genitalia) on the female fetus.

**Breast-feeding**
Nursing mothers should be advised to contact physician before nursing infants. Use by nursing mothers is not recommended because of possible androgenic effects in the infant, such as precocious sexual development in males and virilization in females.

**Pediatrics**
Caution is recommended in children and growing adolescents who are being treated for hereditary angioedema because of possible androgenic effects, such as precocious sexual development in males and virilization in females. Premature epiphyseal closure may also occur.

**Geriatrics**
No information is available on the relationship of age to the effects of danazol in geriatric patients.
Treatment of geriatric male patients with androgens may cause increased risk of prostatic hypertrophy or prostatic carcinoma.

**Drug interactions and/or related problems**
The following drug interactions and/or related problems have been selected on the basis of their potential clinical significance (possible mechanism in parentheses where appropriate)—not necessarily inclusive (» = major clinical significance):

» Anticoagulants, coumarin- or indandione-derivative
(concurrent use with danazol may enhance effects of anticoagulants because of decreased hepatic synthesis of procoagulant factors, and may cause bleeding)
Antidiabetic agents, oral or
Insulin
(danazol may increase blood glucose concentrations and resistance to insulin due to changes in metabolism of carbohydrates)

## Danazol (Systemic)

Cyclosporine
(danazol has been reported to increase plasma concentrations of cyclosporine and may increase the risk of nephrotoxicity)

**Laboratory value alterations**
The following have been selected on the basis of their potential clinical significance (possible effect in parentheses where appropriate)—not necessarily inclusive (» = major clinical significance):

With physiology/laboratory test values
Alanine aminotransferase (ALT [SGPT]) or
Aspartate aminotransferase (AST [SGOT])
(serum concentrations may be increased early in therapy and decrease toward baseline later in therapy; generally return to baseline within one month following therapy)

Aldosase or
Creatine kinase (CK)
(concentrations may be increased in presence of muscle toxicity or rhabdomyolysis)

Blood pressure
(may be increased as a result of volume expansion)

Cholic acid concentration, serum or
Cholic acid-to-chenodeoxycholic acid serum concentrations ratio
(fasting levels may be increased during therapy; generally return to baseline within one month following therapy)

Glucose, blood concentrations or
Lipoproteins, low-density
(concentrations may be increased)

Glucose tolerance
(may be impaired)

Lipoproteins, high-density
(concentrations may be decreased)

Thyroid function tests
(may decrease total serum thyroxine [$T_4$] and increase triiodothyroxine [$T_3$] uptake; however, free $T_4$ and thyroid-stimulating hormone [TSH] remain normal because of a concomitant decrease in thyroid-binding globulin [TBG])

**Medical considerations/Contraindications**
The medical considerations/contraindications included have been selected on the basis of their potential clinical significance (reasons given in parentheses where appropriate)—not necessarily inclusive (» = major clinical significance).

*Risk-benefit should be considered when the following medical problems exist:*

Cardiac function impairment or
Epilepsy or
Migraine headaches or
Renal function impairment
(may be aggravated by fluid retention induced by danazol)

» Cardiac function impairment, severe
Diabetes mellitus
(possible impairment of glucose tolerance)
» Hepatic function impairment, severe
» Renal function impairment, severe
Sensitivity to anabolic steroids, androgens, or danazol
» Vaginal bleeding, undiagnosed abnormal

**Patient monitoring**
The following may be especially important in patient monitoring (other tests may be warranted in some patients, depending on condition; » = major clinical significance):

Biopsy of cysts or
Mammography
(recommended prior to initiation of treatment for fibrocystic breast disease to rule out carcinoma; recommended during treatment if nodules persist or enlarge)

» Hepatic function determinations
(recommended at periodic intervals during therapy)

Pregnancy test
(recommended if treatment of endometriosis or fibrocystic breast disease not started during menstruation or in patients with irregular cycles)

Semen volume and viscosity determinations and
Sperm count and motility determinations
(recommended every 3 to 4 months, especially in adolescents)

## Side/Adverse Effects

The following side/adverse effects have been selected on the basis of their potential clinical significance (possible signs and symptoms in parentheses where appropriate)—not necessarily inclusive:

**Those indicating need for medical attention**
Incidence more frequent
*In females*
***Amenorrhea*** (stopping of menstrual periods); ***breakthrough bleeding*** (heavier, irregular vaginal bleeding between regular menses); ***spotting*** (lighter, irregular vaginal bleeding between regular menses); ***decreased breast size; irregular menstrual periods; weight gain***

Note: *Amenorrhea* occurs in most patients treated for endometriosis. Also occurs in 50% of patients treated for fibrocystic breast disease with doses of 100 mg or more; anovulation may not occur. Amenorrhea may be prolonged after danazol therapy is discontinued in any patient.

*Breakthrough bleeding* or *spotting* may occur in first few months of therapy for endometriosis; does not necessarily indicate lack of efficacy.

*Irregular menstrual periods* occur in 25% of patients treated for fibrocystic breast disease; anovulation may not occur.

Incidence less frequent
*In both females and males*
***Edema*** (rapid weight gain; swelling of feet or lower legs)—dose-related; ***rhabdomyolysis*** (muscle cramps or spasms; unusual tiredness or weakness); ***virilism*** (acne; oily skin; oily hair)—dose-related

Incidence rare
*In both females and males*
***Bladder telangiectasia*** (blood in urine); ***bleeding gums; carpal tunnel syndrome*** (pain, numbness, tingling or burning in all fingers except smallest finger); ***cataracts*** (gradual blurring or loss of vision); ***cholestatic jaundice***—has occurred during long-term treatment with other 17-alkylated androgens; ***discharge from nipple; eosinophilia*** (general feeling of illness; sudden coughing episodes); ***hepatic dysfunction*** (yellow eyes or skin)—with doses greater than 400 mg of danazol per day; ***intracranial hypertension, benign*** (severe headache; decrease in vision; double vision; vomiting); ***leukocytosis*** (sore throat; headache; general feeling of illness; chills; eye pain; cough; unusual tiredness); ***pancreatitis, acute*** (sudden, severe, continuing pain in upper or middle of abdomen; nausea; vomiting; unusual tiredness; bloating and tenderness of abdomen; fever; fast heartbeat; transient yellow eyes or skin color); ***peliosis hepatis*** (dark-colored urine; hives; light-colored stools; continuing loss of appetite; purple- or red-colored spots on body or inside the mouth or nose; sore throat; fever; nausea; vomiting)—has occurred during long-term treatment with other 17-alkylated androgens; ***polyneuritis, acute idiopathic*** (tingling sensation or weakness in both legs, moving upward to both arms, trunk and face; numbness); ***skin rashes; Stevens-Johnson syndrome*** (lesions on skin and inside the mouth or nose; fever; general feeling of illness; cough; sore throat; chest pain; vomiting; diarrhea; joint pain; muscle aches); ***thrombocytopenia*** (unusual bruising or bleeding; more frequent nosebleeds; heavier menstrual periods)

*In females only*
***Virilism*** (enlarged clitoris; hoarseness or deepening of voice; unnatural hair growth)—dose related

*In males only*
***Testicular atrophy*** (decrease in testicle size)

**Those indicating need for medical attention only if they continue or are bothersome**
Incidence less frequent
*In both females and males*
***Hypoestrogenism*** (flushing or redness of skin; mood or mental changes; nervousness; sweating)

Incidence rare
*In both females and males*
***Photosensitivity***

*In females only*
***Monilial vaginitis*** (burning, dryness, or itching of vagina; vaginal bleeding)—hypoestrogenic effect

## Patient Consultation

As an aid to patient consultation, refer to *Advice for the Patient, Danazol (Systemic)*.

In providing consultation, consider emphasizing the following selected information (» = major clinical significance):

**Before using this medication**
» Conditions affecting use, especially:
  Sensitivity to anabolic steroids, androgens, or danazol
  Pregnancy—Use is not recommended during pregnancy because of possible androgenic effects on female fetus
  Breast-feeding—Use is usually not recommended because of possible androgenic effects in the infant
  Use in children—Caution is recommended because of possible androgenic effects
  Other medications, especially coumarin- or indandione-derivative anticoagulants
  Other medical problems, especially severe cardiac function impairment, undiagnosed abnormal vaginal bleeding, severe hepatic function impairment, or severe renal function impairment

**Proper use of this medication**
» Taking for full time of therapy
» Proper dosing
  Missed dose: Taking as soon as possible; not taking if almost time for next dose; not doubling doses
» Proper storage

**Precautions while using this medication**
Regular visits to physician to check progress during therapy
Diabetics: May alter blood sugar levels
» Possible photosensitivity reactions: caution during exposure to sun or when using sunlamps, tanning booths or beds
*For treatment of endometriosis or fibrocystic breast disease*
  Possibility of amenorrhea or irregular menstrual periods; checking with physician if regular menstruation does not occur within 60 to 90 days after discontinuation of medication
  Advisability of using nonhormonal forms of contraception during therapy; not using oral contraceptives
» Stopping medication and checking with physician if pregnancy is suspected

**Side/adverse effects**
Signs of potential side effects, especially edema, virilism in females, liver dysfunction, peliosis hepatis, polyneuritis, pancreatitis, carpal tunnel syndrome, hematologic disorders, Stevens-Johnson syndrome, cataracts, intracranial hypertension, bladder telangiectasia, testicular atrophy, and irregular menstrual periods

## General Dosing Information

In the treatment of endometriosis and fibrocystic breast disease, it is recommended that therapy begin with the first day of the menstrual cycle after pregnancy has been ruled out.

Development of amenorrhea is usually evidence of a clinical response to danazol in the treatment of endometriosis, although spotting or bleeding from the atrophic endometrium can still occur.

In the treatment of endometriosis, therapy should be continued uninterrupted for 3 to 6 months, and may be continued for 9 months if necessary.

Dosage requirements for continuous treatment of hereditary angioedema should be individualized on the basis of the patient's clinical response.

It is recommended that danazol treatment be discontinued if signs of virilization (which may not be reversible) occur.

## Oral Dosage Forms

### DANAZOL CAPSULES USP

**Usual adult and adolescent dose**
Endometriosis—
  Moderate to severe: Oral, 400 mg two times a day (beginning Day 1 of menstruation, if possible) for at least three to six months, and may be continued for nine months if necessary.
  Mild: Oral, 100 to 200 mg two times a day (beginning Day 1 of menstruation, if possible) for at least three to six months, and may be continued for nine months if necessary.
Note: If symptoms recur after discontinuation of therapy, therapy may be reinstituted.
Fibrocystic breast disease—
  Oral, 50 to 200 mg two times a day (beginning Day 1 of menstruation, if possible).
Note: If symptoms recur within one year of discontinuation of therapy, therapy may be reinstituted.
Angioedema (hereditary) prophylactic[1]—
  Oral, initially 200 mg two or three times a day until the desired initial response is obtained; then the maintenance dosage is determined by decreasing the initial dosage by 50% or less at intervals of one to three months or longer, depending on frequency of attacks prior to treatment.
Note: Daily dosage may be increased by up to 200 mg if condition is not controlled at lower doses.

**Usual adult prescribing limits**
Oral, 800 mg per day.

**Usual pediatric dose**
Dosage has not been established.

**Strength(s) usually available**
U.S.—
  50 mg (Rx) [*Danocrine* (benzyl alcohol; lactose; parabens)].
  100 mg (Rx) [*Danocrine* (benzyl alcohol; lactose; parabens)].
  200 mg (Rx) [*Danocrine* (benzyl alcohol; lactose; parabens); GENERIC].
Canada—
  50 mg (Rx) [*Cyclomen* (lactose)].
  100 mg (Rx) [*Cyclomen* (lactose)].
  200 mg (Rx) [*Cyclomen* (lactose)].

**Packaging and storage**
Store below 40 °C (104 °F), preferably between 15 and 30 °C (59 and 86 °F), unless otherwise specified by manufacturer. Store in a well-closed container.

[1] Not included in Canadian product labeling.

Revised: 06/15/93

# DANTROLENE  Systemic

VA CLASSIFICATION (Primary): MS200
Commonly used brand name(s): *Dantrium; Dantrium Intravenous*.
Note: For a listing of dosage forms and brand names by country availability, see *Dosage Forms* section(s).

## Category

Malignant hyperthermia therapy adjunct; Antispastic; Neuroleptic malignant syndrome therapy adjunct; Muscle phosphorylase deficiency therapy adjunct; Duchenne muscular dystrophy therapy adjunct.

## Indications

Note: Bracketed information in the *Indications* section refers to uses that are not included in U.S. product labeling.

**Accepted**
Hyperthermia, malignant (prophylaxis and treatment adjunct)—Intravenous dantrolene is indicated to reverse the symptoms of the malignant hyperthermic crisis syndrome occurring during or following surgery or anesthesia. However, dantrolene is not a substitute for other measures, including discontinuation of possible triggering agents (such as potent inhalation anesthetics, succinylcholine, or stress), management of increased oxygen requirements and metabolic acidosis, institution of cooling, and correction of fluid and electrolyte imbalances. Oral or intravenous dantrolene is indicated as a follow-up to initial intravenous therapy to prevent recurrence of symptoms, but caution in such use is recommended.

Dantrolene is also indicated for administration prior to surgery or anesthesia to prevent or attenuate the symptoms of the malignant hyperthermic crisis syndrome in patients known or suspected to be at risk for this complication. However, preliminary evidence suggests that prophylactic use of dantrolene is not necessary for most patients, provided that careful patient management procedures are followed (including avoiding known triggering agents during surgery, careful monitoring intra- and postoperatively, and administering intravenous dantrolene if symptoms of malignant hyperthermia develop). Perioperative complications (such as atelectasis, retained secretions, diminished swallow and gag reflexes, impaired postoperative ventilation requiring prolonged endotracheal intubation, and delayed or difficult postoperative ambulation), possibly associated with dantrolene-induced muscle weakness, have been reported following prophylactic use of oral dantrolene and should be considered a possibility following intravenous administration

# Dantrolene (Systemic)

also. Patients with pre-existing myopathy, predisposing neuromuscular disease, or compromised respiratory reserve may be especially at risk for these complications. Although many anesthesiologists advocate prophylactic use of dantrolene, provided that the risk of complications is considered and patients carefully selected, others recommend that dantrolene not be used prophylactically. Patients receiving prophylactic dantrolene should be carefully monitored postoperatively to detect possible prolonged or delayed effects of the medication. The controversy concerning prophylactic use of dantrolene for malignant hyperthermia does *not* extend to its therapeutic use for other indications.

Spasticity (treatment)—Oral dantrolene is indicated to relieve spasticity caused by upper motor neuron disorders such as spinal cord injury, cerebrovascular accident, cerebral palsy, and multiple sclerosis. It may be especially beneficial for patients whose functional rehabilitation is retarded by the sequelae of spasticity. However, baclofen is now more commonly used for this indication.

[Neuroleptic malignant syndrome (treatment)][1]—Dantrolene is used to relieve the symptoms of neuroleptic malignant syndrome, which are similar to those caused by malignant hyperthermia.

[Pain, exercise-induced, in muscle phosphorylase deficiency (treatment)][1]; or

[Pain, exercise-induced, in Duchenne muscular dystrophy (treatment)][1]—Oral dantrolene is used to relieve exercise-induced pain in patients with these conditions.

[Spasms, flexor (treatment)][1]—Oral dantrolene is used in the management of flexor spasms in patients who are confined to bed or a wheelchair.

**Unaccepted**
Dantrolene should not be used in patients who require spasticity to sustain upright posture or balance in locomotion, or to obtain increased function.

Dantrolene is not indicated for relief of skeletal muscle spasm caused by rheumatic disorders.

---

[1]Not included in Canadian product labeling.

## Pharmacology/Pharmacokinetics

**Physicochemical characteristics**
Molecular weight—399.29.

**Mechanism of action/Effect**
Malignant hyperthermia therapy adjunct—
By interfering with the release of calcium ion from the sarcoplasmic reticulum, dantrolene prevents or reduces the increase in myoplasmic calcium ion concentration that activates the acute catabolic processes associated with the malignant hyperthermic crisis syndrome.

Antispastic—
Acts directly on skeletal muscle to dissociate excitation-contraction coupling, probably by interfering with the release of calcium ion from the sarcoplasmic reticulum. Dantrolene reduces muscle contractions mediated via both polysynaptic and monosynaptic reflexes. The extent to which any central nervous system (CNS) actions may contribute to the skeletal muscle relaxant effects is unknown.

**Biotransformation**
Hepatic; probably by hepatic microsomal enzymes.

**Half-life**
Intravenous—4 to 8 hours
Oral—8.7 hours (100-mg dose)

**Onset of action**
Spasticity caused by upper motor neuron disorders—1 week or more.

**Time to peak concentration**
Oral—5 hours

**Peak whole blood concentration**
300 to 1100 nanograms per mL following administration of 25 to 100 mg; subject to interpatient variation.

**Therapeutic serum concentration**
100 to 600 nanograms per mL; subject to interpatient variation.

**Elimination**
Renal, as metabolites. Small amounts may also be excreted unchanged.

## Precautions to Consider

**Carcinogenicity/Tumorigenicity**
An increased incidence of nonmalignant and malignant mammary tumors occurred with chronic (18 months) administration of dantrolene in doses of 15, 30, or 60 mg per kg of body weight (mg/kg) per day to female Sprague-Dawley rats. Also, an increased incidence of hepatic lymphangiomas and angiosarcomas occurred with chronic administration of 60 mg/kg per day. However, dantrolene did not produce these effects in other studies when administered for 2 years to mice or 2½ years to rats. The risk of carcinogenicity in humans is not known; therefore, risk-benefit with chronic therapy must be considered.

**Pregnancy/Reproduction**
Pregnancy—Problems in humans have not been documented.

**Breast-feeding**
Dantrolene should not be used in nursing mothers.

**Pediatrics**
Appropriate studies performed to date have not demonstrated pediatrics-specific problems that would limit the usefulness of dantrolene in children. However, long-term studies have not been done in children <5 years of age.

**Geriatrics**
No information is available on the relationship of age to the effects of dantrolene in geriatric patients.

**Drug interactions and/or related problems**
The following drug interactions and/or related problems have been selected on the basis of their potential clinical significance (possible mechanism in parentheses where appropriate)—not necessarily inclusive (» = major clinical significance):

Note: Combinations containing any of the following medications, depending on the amount present, may also interact with this medication.

*For short-term (up to 3 days) or chronic use*
» CNS depression–producing medications (See *Appendix II*)
(concurrent use with dantrolene may result in increased CNS depressant effects; caution is recommended and dosage of one or both agents should be reduced)

*For chronic oral use only*
» Hepatotoxic medications, other (See *Appendix II*)
(concurrent use of these medications with dantrolene may increase the risk of hepatotoxicity; females over 35 years of age may be especially at risk with concurrent use of estrogens)

*For intravenous use in treating malignant hyperthermia only*
Calcium channel blockers
(concurrent administration of therapeutic doses of verapamil with intravenous dantrolene to halothane/alpha-chloralose anesthetized swine has caused ventricular fibrillation and cardiovascular collapse associated with severe hypokalemia; although the relevance of these findings to humans has not been determined, it is recommended that calcium channel blockers not be used concurrently with intravenous dantrolene in the management of a malignant hyperthermic crisis)

**Laboratory value alterations**
The following have been selected on the basis of their potential clinical significance (possible effect in parentheses where appropriate)—not necessarily inclusive (» = major clinical significance):

With physiology/laboratory test values
Liver function tests
(abnormalities may occur indicating hepatotoxicity)

**Medical considerations/Contraindications**
The medical considerations/contraindications included have been selected on the basis of their potential clinical significance (reasons given in parentheses where appropriate)—not necessarily inclusive (» = major clinical significance).

Note: The following precautions do *not* apply to short-term intravenous use of dantrolene for treatment of a malignant hyperthermic crisis, unless otherwise specified.

*Except under special circumstances, this medication should not be used when the following medical problem exists:*
» Hepatic disease, active, such as hepatitis or cirrhosis
(increased risk of hepatotoxicity)

*Risk-benefit should be considered when the following medical problems exist:*
Cardiac function impairment, especially if due to myocardial disease
(dantrolene may cause pleural effusion and pericarditis)
Hepatic function impairment or history of
(possible increased risk of hepatotoxicity)
Myopathy, pre-existing or
Neuromuscular disease predisposing to respiratory insufficiency
(increased risk of perioperative complications when dantrolene is used as prophylaxis against malignant hyperthermia)

Pulmonary function impairment, especially obstructive pulmonary disease
(dantrolene may cause respiratory depression, possibly associated with muscle weakness, or pleural effusion)

Sensitivity to dantrolene

Caution is also recommended in patients older than 35 years of age, especially females, because of the increased risk of hepatotoxicity.

**Patient monitoring**

The following may be especially important in patient monitoring (other tests may be warranted in some patients, depending on condition; » = major clinical significance):

Blood cell counts and
Renal function determinations
(may be required at periodic intervals during chronic therapy)

» Hepatic function determinations, including:

Alanine aminotransferase (ALT [SGPT]), serum
Alkaline phosphatase
Aspartate aminotransferase (AST [SGOT]), serum
Bilirubin, total
Gammaglutamyl transpeptidase (GGTP)
(may be required before initiation of chronic therapy to determine baseline values and to identify pre-existing hepatic dysfunction or disease and at periodic intervals during chronic therapy)

## Side/Adverse Effects

Note: Dantrolene-induced hepatotoxicity may be caused by an idiosyncratic or allergic reaction to the medication. The risk of hepatotoxicity appears greater with females, patients over 35 years of age, and patients concurrently taking other medications. In particular, females over 35 years of age who are receiving estrogen therapy have an increased frequency of hepatotoxicity. Hepatotoxicity may be less likely to occur in patients taking up to 400 mg per day than in those taking 800 mg or more per day. Even short-term administration of the larger doses within a treatment regimen may increase the risk of hepatotoxicity. Overt hepatitis occurs most frequently between the third and twelfth months of chronic therapy.

The following side/adverse effects have been selected on the basis of their potential clinical significance (possible signs and symptoms in parentheses where appropriate)—not necessarily inclusive:

**Those indicating need for medical attention**
Incidence less frequent
*With short-term (up to 3 days) or chronic oral use*

*Diarrhea, severe; respiratory depression* (shortness of breath or slow or troubled breathing)

Note: *Severe diarrhea* may necessitate temporary discontinuation of therapy. If severe diarrhea recurs when therapy is resumed, therapy should probably be discontinued permanently.

*With chronic oral use only*

*Bloody or dark urine; confusion; constipation, severe*—may cause abdominal distention or other symptoms of bowel obstruction; *convulsions; dermatitis, allergic* (skin rash, hives, or itching); *difficult urination; hepatotoxicity* (yellow eyes or skin)—may be preceded by gastrointestinal symptoms such as nausea, vomiting, anorexia, and abdominal discomfort; *mental depression; phlebitis* (pain, tenderness, changes in skin color, or swelling of foot or leg); *pleural effusion with pericarditis* (chest pain)

**Those indicating need for medical attention only if they continue or are bothersome**
Incidence more frequent
*With short-term (up to 3 days) or chronic oral use*

*Diarrhea, mild; dizziness or lightheadedness; drowsiness; general feeling of discomfort or illness; muscle weakness not affecting muscles of respiration; nausea or vomiting; unusual tiredness*

Incidence less frequent
*Abdominal or stomach cramps or discomfort*

*With chronic oral use only*
Incidence less frequent

*Blurred or double vision or any change in vision; chills and fever; constipation, mild; difficulty in swallowing; frequent urge to urinate or uncontrolled urination; headache; loss of appetite; slurring of speech or other speech problems; sudden decrease in amount of urine; trouble in sleeping; unusual nervousness*

## Overdose

For more information on the management of overdose or unintentional ingestion, **contact a Poison Control Center** (see *Poison Control Center Listing*).

### Treatment of overdose

To decrease absorption—Removing unabsorbed dantrolene (if ingested orally) via induction of emesis or gastric lavage.

Monitoring—May include monitoring the electrocardiogram (ECG), carefully observing the patient, and instituting supportive treatment of observed symptoms.

Supportive care—Administering large quantities of intravenous fluids to prevent crystalluria.

Maintaining an adequate airway, with equipment for artificial resuscitation at hand. Patients in whom intentional overdose is known or suspected should be referred to for psychiatric consultation.

Note: The possible value of dialysis in treating overdosage has not been determined.

## Patient Consultation

As an aid to patient consultation, refer to *Advice for the Patient, Dantrolene (Systemic)*.

In providing consultation, consider emphasizing the following selected information (» = major clinical significance):

### Before using this medication
» Conditions affecting use, especially:
Other medications, especially CNS depression-producing medications and other hepatotoxic medications
Other medical problems, especially hepatic disease

### Proper use of this medication
Mixing contents of capsule with fruit juice or other liquid if unable to swallow capsule; drinking immediately after mixing
» Not taking more medication than the amount prescribed, to minimize risk of hepatotoxicity or other adverse effects
» Proper dosing
Missed dose: Taking if remembered within an hour or so; not taking if not remembered within an hour; not doubling doses
» Proper storage

### Precautions while using this medication
Regular visits to physician to check progress during long-term therapy; possibility of blood tests to check for side effects
» Avoiding alcohol or other CNS depressants during therapy unless prescribed or otherwise approved by physician
» Caution if drowsiness, dizziness or lightheadedness, vision disturbances, or muscle weakness occurs

### Side/adverse effects
Signs of potential side effects, especially bloody or dark urine; confusion; constipation, severe; convulsions; allergic dermatitis; diarrhea, severe; difficult urination; hepatitis; mental depression; phlebitis; pleural effusion with pericarditis; and respiratory depression

## General Dosing Information

Side effects such as drowsiness, dizziness, weakness, tiredness, or gastrointestinal irritation may be minimized by initiating therapy with a low dose and gradually increasing the dosage until maximal benefit is achieved.

If no benefit is observed after 45 days of therapy, the medication should be discontinued.

Dantrolene should be discontinued if a patient develops symptoms of hepatitis during therapy. If hepatic function test abnormalities without symptoms of overt hepatitis occur, the medication should probably be discontinued; however, in some patients, hepatic function test values have returned to normal despite continuation of therapy. Reinstitution or continuation of therapy should be considered only for patients receiving major benefit from the medication. Reinstitution of therapy following dantrolene-induced hepatitis should be attempted only after the symptoms and hepatic function test abnormalities have cleared. The patient should be hospitalized. Therapy should be resumed with very small and gradually increasing doses. Liver function tests should be performed frequently and the medication withdrawn immediately if any abnormalities occur.

### For parenteral dosage form only
Extravasation of the intravenous solution into surrounding tissues should be avoided because of the high pH of the solution.

## Oral Dosage Forms

### DANTROLENE SODIUM CAPSULES

**Usual adult and adolescent dose**
Malignant hyperthermic crisis prophylaxis—
  Oral, 4 to 8 mg per kg of body weight per day in three or four divided doses for one to two days prior to surgery. The last dose should be given three to four hours prior to scheduled surgery with a minimum of water.
Post-malignant hyperthermic crisis treatment (as a follow-up to intravenous therapy)—
  Oral, 4 to 8 mg per kg of body weight per day in four divided doses for one to three days.
Antispastic—
  Oral, 25 mg once a day, initially; total daily dose may be increased by 25 mg every four to seven days until optimal response is achieved or until a dosage of 100 mg four times a day is reached. Medication should be administered in four divided daily doses whenever possible.

**Usual pediatric dose**
Antispastic—
  Oral, 500 mcg (0.5 mg) per kg of body weight two times a day, initially; total daily dose may be increased by 500 mcg (0.5 mg) per kg of body weight every four to seven days until optimal response is achieved or until a dosage of 3 mg per kg of body weight four times a day is reached. Medication should be administered in four divided daily doses whenever possible.
Note: The maximum recommended pediatric dosage is 400 mg a day.

**Strength(s) usually available**
U.S.—
  25 mg (Rx) [*Dantrium* (lactose)].
  50 mg (Rx) [*Dantrium* (lactose)].
  100 mg (Rx) [*Dantrium* (lactose)].
Canada—
  25 mg (Rx) [*Dantrium* (lactose)].
  100 mg (Rx) [*Dantrium* (lactose)].

**Packaging and storage**
Store below 40 °C (104 °F), preferably between 15 and 30 °C (59 and 86 °F), in a well-closed container, unless otherwise specified by manufacturer.

**Preparation of dosage form**
For patients who cannot take oral solids
Single dose: Immediately prior to use, add the contents of the required number of capsules to fruit juice or other liquid and stir to mix.
Multiple dose: Empty 5 capsules (100 mg each) into 50 mL of Syrup NF; add 150 mg of citric acid dissolved in 10 mL of water; add enough Syrup NF to make 100 mL of suspension. This suspension will contain 25 mg of dantrolene sodium per 5 mL. Although the stability of such an extemporaneous preparation is unknown, it is thought to be stable for several days when refrigerated. However, since it contains no preservative, care must be taken to avoid contamination.

**Auxiliary labeling**
• May cause drowsiness.
• Avoid alcoholic beverages.

## Parenteral Dosage Forms

### DANTROLENE SODIUM FOR INJECTION

**Usual adult and adolescent dose**
Malignant hyperthermia therapy adjunct—
  Prophylactic[1]: Intravenous infusion, 2.5 mg per kg of body weight, administered over a one-hour period prior to anesthesia.
  Therapeutic: Intravenous, by continuous rapid push, at least 1 mg per kg of body weight, initially, with administration being continued until the symptoms subside or until the maximum cumulative dose of 10 mg per kg of body weight has been reached. Administration may be repeated if symptoms recur.
  Note: For treatment of a malignant hyperthermic crisis, some anesthesiologists recommend an initial dose of 2.5 to 3 mg per kg of body weight.

**Usual pediatric dose**
See *Usual adult and adolescent dose*.

**Size(s) usually available**
U.S.—
  20 mg (Rx) [*Dantrium Intravenous*].
Canada—
  20 mg (Rx) [*Dantrium Intravenous*].

**Packaging and storage**
Prior to reconstitution, store below 30 °C (86 °F), protected from prolonged exposure to light, unless otherwise specified by manufacturer.

**Preparation of dosage form**
60 mL of sterile water for injection without a bacteriostatic agent should be added to the vial containing 20 mg of dantrolene sodium and shaken until the solution is clear. The solution will contain 333 mcg (0.33 mg) per mL.

**Stability**
After reconstitution, protect from temperatures below 15 °C (59 °F) or above 30 °C (86 °F). Protect from direct light. Use within 6 hours following reconstitution.
Precipitate formation has occurred after transfer of reconstituted dantrolene solutions to large glass bottles for preparation of an intravenous infusion. It is recommended that intravenous infusions be prepared in sterile plastic bags, immediately prior to the time of anticipated use. Also, the prepared infusion should be inspected for cloudiness and/or precipitation prior to use, and discarded if either is present.

**Incompatibilities**
Dantrolene is incompatible with acidic solutions, including 5% dextrose injection and 0.9% sodium chloride injection. Acidic solutions should not be used for reconstituting the medication.

---
[1]Not included in Canadian product labeling.

Revised: 05/10/93

---

# DAPIPRAZOLE  Ophthalmic

VA CLASSIFICATION (Primary): OP900
Commonly used brand name(s): *Rev-Eyes*.
Note: For a listing of dosage forms and brand names by country availability, see *Dosage Forms* section(s).

## Category
Antimydriatic.

## Indications

**Accepted**
Mydriasis, reversal of—Indicated in the treatment of pharmacologically induced mydriasis produced by sympathomimetic (phenylephrine) or parasympatholytic (tropicamide) agents.

**Unaccepted**
Dapiprazole is not indicated for the reduction of intraocular pressure, in the treatment of open angle glaucoma, or for any indication other than reversal of induced mydriasis.

## Pharmacology/Pharmacokinetics

**Physicochemical characteristics**
Molecular weight—361.93.
Description—Dapiprazole hydrochloride is a sterile, white, lyophilized powder soluble in water.
Dapiprazole hydrochloride solution is a clear, colorless, slightly viscous solution.
Other characteristics—Reconstituted solution has a pH between 4.5 and 6 and an osmolarity of approximately 415 mOsm.

**Mechanism of action/Effect**
Dapiprazole is an alpha-adrenergic blocking agent and acts by blocking the alpha-adrenergic receptors in smooth muscle. Dapiprazole produces miosis through an effect on the dilator muscle of the iris.
Dapiprazole has demonstrated safe and rapid reversal of mydriasis produced by phenylephrine and, to a lesser degree, of that produced by tropicamide. It has not been tested against other mydriatics. In patients with decreased accommodative amplitude due to treatment with tropicamide, the miotic effect of dapiprazole may partially increase the accommodative amplitude.

## Other actions/effects
Dapiprazole does not significantly alter intraocular pressure in normotensive eyes or in eyes with elevated intraocular pressure.

Dapiprazole does not have any significant effect on ciliary muscle contraction, and therefore does not induce a significant change in the anterior chamber depth or in the thickness of the lens.

## Onset of action
Eye color affects the rate of pupillary constriction. In individuals with brown irides, the rate of pupillary constriction may be slightly slower than in individuals with blue or green irides. Eye color does not appear to affect the final pupil size.

# Precautions to Consider

## Carcinogenicity
Dapiprazole has been shown to significantly increase the incidence of liver tumors in rats after continuous dietary administration for 104 weeks. This effect was found only in male rats treated with the highest dose administered in the study, i.e., 300 mg per kg of body weight (mg/kg) per day (80,000 times the human dose). The effect was not observed in male and female rats at doses of 30 and 100 mg/kg per day or in female rats at doses of 300 mg/kg per day.

## Mutagenicity
Dapiprazole has not been shown to be mutagenic.

## Pregnancy/Reproduction
Fertility—Studies have not shown that dapiprazole impairs fertility.

Pregnancy—Adequate and well-controlled studies have not been done in pregnant women.

Reproduction studies have been performed in rats and rabbits at doses up to 128,000 and 27,000 times the human ophthalmic dose, respectively, and have revealed no evidence of harm to the fetus due to dapiprazole.

FDA Pregnancy Category B.

## Breast-feeding
It is not known whether dapiprazole is distributed into human milk. However, problems in humans have not been documented.

## Pediatrics
Appropriate studies on the relationship of age to the effects of dapiprazole have not been performed in the pediatric population. Safety and efficacy have not been established.

## Geriatrics
Appropriate studies on the relationship of age to the effects of dapiprazole have not been performed in the geriatric population. However, geriatrics-specific problems that would limit the usefulness of this medication in the elderly are not expected.

## Medical considerations/Contraindications
The medical considerations/contraindications included have been selected on the basis of their potential clinical significance (reasons given in parentheses where appropriate)—not necessarily inclusive (» = major clinical significance).

*Except under special circumstances, this medication should not be used when the following medical problems exist:*
» Iritis, acute, or other conditions where miosis is undesirable

*Risk-benefit should be considered when the following medical problem exists:*
   Sensitivity to dapiprazole

# Side/Adverse Effects

Note: Miosis produced by dapiprazole may cause difficulty in dark adaptation, may reduce the field of vision, or may reduce central visual acuity.

The following side/adverse effects have been selected on the basis of their potential clinical significance (possible signs and symptoms in parentheses where appropriate)—not necessarily inclusive:

**Those indicating need for medical attention**
Incidence less frequent
   *Edema of cornea* (swelling of the clear part of the eye)—incidence 10 to 40%; *punctate keratitis* (severe irritation of the clear part of the eye)—incidence 10 to 40%

**Those indicating need for medical attention only if they continue or are bothersome**
Incidence more frequent
   *Burning of eye upon administration of medication*—incidence 50%; *conjunctival injection, usually lasting 20 minutes* (redness of the white part of the eye)—incidence 80%

Incidence less frequent
   *Blurring of vision*—incidence <10%; *browache*—incidence 10 to 40%; *chemosis* (swelling of the membrane covering the white part of the eye)—incidence 10 to 40%; *dryness of eye*—incidence <10%; *edema of eyelid* (swelling of eyelid)—incidence 10 to 40%; *erythema of eyelid* (redness of eyelid)—incidence 10 to 40%; *headache*—incidence 10 to 40%; *itching of eye*—incidence 10 to 40%; *photophobia* (increased sensitivity of eye to light)—incidence 10 to 40%; *ptosis* (drooping of upper eyelid)—incidence 10 to 40%; *tearing of eye*—incidence <10%

# Patient Consultation
As an aid to patient consultation, refer to *Advice for the Patient, Dapiprazole (Ophthalmic)*.

In providing consultation, consider emphasizing the following selected information (» = major clinical significance):

**Before using this medication**
» Conditions affecting use, especially:
   Other medical problems, especially acute iritis or other conditions where miosis is undesirable

**Proper use of this medication**
» Proper dosing

**Precautions while using this medication**
» Medication causes blurred vision or other vision problems; not driving, using machines, or doing anything else that could be dangerous if unable to see well
Possible eye photosensitivity; wearing sunglasses that block ultra-violet light

**Side/adverse effects**
   Signs of potential side effects, especially edema of cornea and punctate keratitis

# Ophthalmic Dosage Forms

## DAPIPRAZOLE HYDROCHLORIDE FOR OPHTHALMIC SOLUTION

**Usual adult dose**
Antimydriatic—
   Topical, to the conjunctiva, 1 drop, followed by another 1 drop after five minutes; administration to start immediately following the retinal examination, to reverse the diagnostic mydriasis.

**Usual adult prescribing limits**
Dapiprazole should not be used more frequently than once a week.

**Usual pediatric dose**
Safety and efficacy have not been established.

**Strength(s) usually available**
U.S.—
   0.5% (5 mg of dapiprazole HCl per mL when reconstituted) (Rx) [*Rev-Eyes* (hydroxypropyl methylcellulose 0.4%; benzalkonium chloride 0.01%; mannitol 2%; sodium chloride; edetate sodium 0.01%; sodium phosphate dibasic; sodium phosphate monobasic; water for injection)].
Canada—
   0.5% (5 mg of dapiprazole HCl per mL when reconstituted) (Rx) [*Rev-Eyes*].

**Packaging and storage**
Store below 40 °C (104 °F), preferably between 15 and 30 °C (59 and 86 °F), unless otherwise specified by manufacturer.

**Preparation of dosage form**
Dapiprazole is supplied in a kit consisting of one vial of dapiprazole hydrochloride (25 mg), one vial of diluent (5 mL), and one dropper for dispensing.

To prepare the solution, pour diluent into medication vial, attach dropper assembly to vial, and shake vial for several minutes to dissolve powder.

**Stability**
Once the eyedrops have been reconstituted they may be stored at room temperature (15 to 30 °C [59 to 86 °F]) for 21 days. The solution should be discarded if it is not clear and colorless.

**Auxiliary labeling**
• For the eye.

## Selected Bibliography

Nyman N, Keates EU. Effects of dapiprazole on the reversal of pharmacologically induced mydriasis. Optom Vis Sci 1990 Sep; 67(9): 705-9.

Allinson RW et al. Reversal of mydriasis by dapiprazole. Ann Ophthalmol 1990 Apr; 22(4): 131-3, 138.

Revised: 04/13/92
Interim revision: 08/16/93

---

# DAPSONE Systemic

VA CLASSIFICATION (Primary/Secondary): AM900/AP101; AP109; AM700

Commonly used brand name(s): *Avlosulfon*.

Another commonly used name is DDS.

Note: For a listing of dosage forms and brand names by country availability, see *Dosage Forms* section(s).

## Category

Antibacterial (antileprosy agent); dermatitis herpetiformis suppressant; antiprotozoal; antifungal.

## Indications

Note: Bracketed information in the *Indications* section refers to uses that are not included in U.S. product labeling.

### Accepted

Leprosy (treatment)—Dapsone is indicated in combination with other antileprosy agents in the treatment of all types of leprosy (Hansen's disease) caused by *Mycobacterium leprae*.

Dermatitis herpetiformis (treatment)—Dapsone is indicated in the treatment of dermatitis herpetiformis.

[Actinomycotic mycetoma (treatment)][1]—Dapsone is used in the treatment of actinomycotic mycetoma.

[Cicatricial pemphigoid (treatment)][1]—Dapsone is used in the treatment of desquamative gingival lesions caused by cicatricial pemphigoid.

[Dermatosis, subcorneal pustular (treatment)][1]—Dapsone is used in the treatment of subcorneal pustular dermatosis.

[Granuloma annulare (treatment)][1]—Dapsone is used in the treatment of granuloma annulare.

[Lupus erythematosus, systemic (treatment)][1]—Dapsone is used in the treatment of certain skin lesions of systemic lupus erythematosus, including bullous eruptions and urticarial vasculitis.

[Malaria (prophylaxis)][1]—Dapsone is used in combination with pyrimethamine as secondary agents in the prophylaxis of chloroquine-resistant malaria caused by *Plasmodium falciparum*. Dapsone is also used in combination with pyrimethamine and chloroquine in the prophylaxis of malaria caused by *Plasmodium vivax*.

[Pemphigoid (treatment)][1]—Dapsone is used in the treatment of pemphigoid lesions with oral manifestations.

[Pneumonia, *Pneumocystis carinii* (prophylaxis and treatment)][1]—Dapsone is used in combination with trimethoprim in the treatment of mild to moderate pneumonia caused by *Pneumocystis carinii* (PCP). No difference in efficacy was found in a study comparing the dapsone-trimethoprim combination with oral trimethoprim-sulfamethoxazole. However, studies have shown that dapsone alone appeared to have inferior efficacy for treatment of PCP.

Dapsone has also been used alone in the prophylaxis of PCP.

[Polychondritis, relapsing (treatment)][1]—Dapsone is used in the treatment of relapsing polychondritis.

[Pyoderma gangrenosum (treatment)][1]—Dapsone is used in the treatment of pyoderma gangrenosum.

[1]Not included in Canadian product labeling.

## Pharmacology/Pharmacokinetics

### Physicochemical characteristics

Molecular weight—248.30.

### Mechanism of action/Effect

Antibacterial (antileprosy agent)—Dapsone, a sulfone, is bacteriostatic and probably acts by a mechanism similar to that of the sulfonamides, interfering with folate synthesis. Both have a similar range of antibacterial activity and are antagonized by para-aminobenzoic acid.

Dermatitis herpetiformis suppressant—Mechanism is unknown, but not due to dapsone's bacteriostatic effect. Dapsone may act as an enzyme inhibitor or oxidizing agent. In addition, it has numerous immunologic effects (e.g., immunosuppression), which most likely account for its suppression of dermatitis herpetiformis.

### Absorption

Slowly absorbed from the gastrointestinal tract; absorption half-life of 1.1 hours. Overall bioavailability is 70 to 80%; may be less in patients with severe leprosy. An acidic environment is needed for optimal absorption.

### Distribution

Well distributed throughout total body water and is found in all tissues, especially liver, muscle, kidneys, and skin. Saliva concentrations are 18 to 27% of corresponding plasma dapsone concentrations. Dapsone also crosses the placenta.

$Vol_D$—1.5 L per kg (1.9 L per kg when given with pyrimethamine).

### Protein binding

Dapsone—Moderate to high (70–90%).
Monoacetyl dapsone (MADDS)—Very high (99%).

### Biotransformation

Dapsone is acetylated by N-acetyltransferase in the liver to its major metabolite, monoacetyl dapsone (MADDS). MADDS is also deacetylated to dapsone; equilibrium is reached within a few hours. Patients may be divided into slow or fast acetylators. However, unlike with other medications, no relationship has been seen between acetylator type and side effects. There was also no significant difference between the 2 groups in plasma concentrations or pharmacokinetics; therapeutic response was the same in both groups.

Dapsone is also N-hydroxylated to dapsone hydroxylamine in the liver by the mixed oxidase system in the presence of oxygen and NADPH, and appears to be responsible for the drug's hematologic toxicity.

Both major metabolites have very low activity and do not contribute to the therapeutic effect of dapsone.

### Half-life

10 to 50 hours (average, 30 hours) for both dapsone and MADDS.

### Time to peak serum concentration

2 to 6 hours, but variable.

### Peak serum concentration

50 mg (single dose)—0.6 to 0.7 mcg/mL.
100 mg (single dose)—1.7 to 1.9 mcg/mL.
100 mg (steady state)—3.1 to 3.3 mcg/mL.

### Elimination

Renal—70 to 85% slowly excreted in the urine as dapsone and metabolites; 5 to 15% of dapsone dose excreted in urine by active tubular secretion, and the remainder excreted as metabolites. Metabolites are partly conjugated, primarily as glucuronides and sulfates.

Biliary—Enterohepatic circulation following biliary excretion of free drug also occurs. Because of this, dapsone may persist in the plasma for up to several weeks after therapy is discontinued.

## Precautions to Consider

### Cross-sensitivity and/or related problems

Patients allergic to dapsone may be allergic to sulfonamides, although this has not been clearly established.

### Carcinogenicity/Tumorigenicity

Studies in male rats and female mice have shown that dapsone causes mesenchymal tumors of the spleen and peritoneum. Dapsone has been shown to cause thyroid carcinoma in female rats as well.

### Mutagenicity

Dapsone has not been shown to be mutagenic in *Salmonella typhimurium* tester strains 1535, 1537, 1538, 98, or 100, when tested with or without microsomal activation.

### Pregnancy/Reproduction

Pregnancy—Dapsone crosses the placenta. Adequate and well-controlled studies in humans and animals have not been done. However, other studies in humans have not shown that dapsone causes adverse effects on reproductive capacity or on the fetus. Dapsone has been recommended for maintenance therapy of pregnant leprosy and dermatitis herpetiformis patients.

FDA Pregnancy Category C.

### Breast-feeding
Dapsone is distributed into breast milk. In one case report, the concentration of dapsone in breast milk was approximately 67% of the corresponding serum concentration. The serum dapsone concentration in the nursing infant reached 27% of the mother's serum concentration. In addition, dapsone could potentially cause hemolytic anemia in glucose-6-phosphate dehydrogenase (G6PD)–deficient neonates.

### Pediatrics
Appropriate studies on the relationship of age to the effects of dapsone have not been performed in the pediatric population. However, no pediatrics-specific problems have been documented to date. Dapsone is generally not considered to have an effect on the later growth, development, and functional development of the child.

### Geriatrics
No information is available on the relationship of age to the effects of dapsone in geriatric patients.

### Drug interactions and/or related problems
The following drug interactions and/or related problems have been selected on the basis of their potential clinical significance (possible mechanism in parentheses where appropriate)—not necessarily inclusive (» = major clinical significance):

Note: Combinations containing any of the following medications, depending on the amount present, may also interact with this medication.

Aminobenzoates (PABA)
(concurrent use in the treatment of leprosy is not recommended since aminobenzoates may be absorbed by bacteria preferentially over sulfones, thereby antagonizing the bacteriostatic effect of sulfones; however, aminobenzoates do not antagonize the effect of dapsone in the treatment of dermatitis herpetiformis)

Blood dyscrasia–causing medications (See *Appendix II*)
(dapsone may, on rare occasions, cause an idiosyncratic agranulocytosis, aplastic anemia, or other blood dyscrasias; if concurrent use is required, close observation for myelotoxic effects should be considered)

» Didanosine (ddI)
(concurrent administration of dapsone with ddI may decrease the absorption of dapsone; ddI must be given with a buffer to neutralize stomach acidity in order to increase its absorption, and dapsone requires an acidic environment for optimal absorption; until studies are completed that confirm this interaction, dapsone should be administered at least 2 hours before or 2 hours after ddI is given)

» Hemolytics, other (See *Appendix II*)
(concurrent use with dapsone may increase the potential for toxic side effects)

Rifampin
(concurrent use may stimulate hepatic microsomal enzyme activity, resulting in as much as a 7- to 10-fold decrease in dapsone concentrations; however, dapsone dosage adjustments are not required during concurrent rifampin therapy for leprosy since dapsone concentrations are still higher than the MIC, although they may be required in the treatment of other diseases, such as PCP)

Trimethoprim
(concurrent use with dapsone may increase the plasma concentrations of both dapsone and trimethoprim, possibly due to an inhibition in dapsone metabolism, and/or competition for renal secretion between the 2 medications; increased serum dapsone concentrations may increase the frequency and severity of side effects, especially methemoglobinemia and hemolytic anemia)

### Medical considerations/Contraindications
The medical considerations/contraindications included have been selected on the basis of their potential clinical significance (reasons given in parentheses where appropriate)—not necessarily inclusive (» = major clinical significance).

*Risk-benefit should be considered when the following medical problems exist:*

Allergy to dapsone or sulfonamides
» Anemia, severe or
» Glucose-6-phosphate dehydrogenase (G6PD) deficiency or
» Methemoglobin reductase deficiency
(hemolytic anemia may occur)
Hepatic function impairment
(dapsone may cause toxic hepatitis and cholestatic jaundice; alcoholic liver disease may decrease the plasma protein binding of dapsone, increasing the amount of circulating free drug)

### Patient monitoring
The following may be especially important in patient monitoring (other tests may be warranted in some patients, depending on condition; » = major clinical significance):

» Alanine aminotransferase (ALT [SGPT]) and
» Aspartate aminotransferase (AST [SGOT])
(values should be determined prior to and periodically during treatment; dapsone should be discontinued if there is evidence of progressive hepatic damage)

Blood urea nitrogen and
Creatinine, serum
(determinations required periodically during treatment in patients with severely impaired renal function, who may also require a reduction in dose; dapsone should be discontinued in anuric patients)

» Complete blood counts (CBCs) and
» Platelet counts and
» Reticulocyte count
(required prior to treatment, followed by monthly counts for 1 to 3 months, and semi-annually thereafter; in patients with HIV infection, CBCs are recommended every 2 to 3 days for the first 2 to 3 weeks of therapy; if a significant reduction in leukocytes, platelets, or hematocrit occurs, or if there is an increase in the reticulocyte count, dapsone should be discontinued and the patient should be monitored closely)

Glucose-6-phosphate dehydrogenase (G6PD) concentration
(determination recommended in patients at high risk prior to treatment; if a deficiency is found, dapsone should be given with extreme caution since hemolytic effects may be exaggerated; dosage adjustments may be required)

Methemoglobin, serum
(level should be obtained in patients with cyanosis, lightheadedness, fatigue, headache, or shortness of breath; dapsone should be discontinued at a methemoglobin level of > 20%, and treatment with methylene blue should be considered in symptomatic patients with levels > 30%)

## Side/Adverse Effects

Note: When dapsone is used in high doses, peripheral motor weakness may occur more frequently.

Fatalities have occurred due to agranulocytosis, aplastic anemia, and other blood dyscrasias. In addition, serious cutaneous reactions, such as exfoliative dermatitis, toxic erythema, erythema multiforme, toxic epidermal necrolysis, morbilliform and scarlatiniform reactions, and erythema nodosum may occur. Dapsone therapy should be promptly discontinued if new or toxic dermatologic reactions occur. However, leprosy reactional states do not require discontinuation of therapy.

A dose-related hemolysis is seen in all patients, with a slight decrease in hemoglobin and an increase in reticulocyte count. Patients with G6PD-deficiency or a decrease in activity in glutathione reductase are more susceptible to hemolysis. A low level of methemoglobinemia also occurs in all patients at recommended doses.

The following side/adverse effects have been selected on the basis of their potential clinical significance (possible signs and symptoms in parentheses where appropriate)—not necessarily inclusive:

### Those indicating need for medical attention
Incidence more frequent
*Hemolytic anemia* (back, leg, or stomach pains; loss of appetite; pale skin; unusual tiredness or weakness; fever); *hypersensitivity* (skin rash); *methemoglobinemia* (cyanosis—bluish fingernails, lips, or skin; difficult breathing; unusual tiredness or weakness)

Incidence rare
*Blood dyscrasias* (fever and sore throat; unusual bleeding or bruising; unusual tiredness and weakness); *exfoliative dermatitis* (itching, dryness, redness, scaling, or peeling of the skin or loss of hair); *hepatic damage* (yellow eyes or skin); *mood or other mental changes*; *peripheral neuritis* (numbness, tingling, pain, burning, or weakness in hands or feet); *"sulfone syndrome"* (fever; malaise; exfoliative dermatitis; jaundice; lymphadenopathy; methemoglobinemia; anemia)—a hypersensitivity reaction that usually occurs after 6 to 8 weeks of therapy

### Those indicating need for medical attention only if they continue or are bothersome
Incidence rare—usually dose-related
*Central nervous system toxicity* (headache; insomnia; nervousness); *gastrointestinal disturbances* (anorexia; nausea or vomiting)

## Overdose

For more information on the management of overdose or unintentional ingestion, **contact a Poison Control Center** (see *Poison Control Center Listing*).

**Treatment of overdose**
Recommended treatment consists of the following:

To decrease absorption—

Performance of gastric lavage. Gastric emptying of dapsone may be delayed after an overdose, and tablet fragments have been found in stomach returns after lavage as late as 5 to 12 hours post-ingestion.

Administration of activated charcoal (30 grams), concurrently with a cathartic, every 6 hours for at least 48 to 72 hours. Repeated doses of activated charcoal reduce the half-life of dapsone and MADDS by approximately 50% to 12.7 hours.

Specific treatment—

In emergency situations, slow, intravenous administration of methylene blue, 1 to 2 mg per kg of body weight (mg/kg). Methylene blue should not be given to fully expressed G6PD-deficient patients. May be repeated if methemoglobin reaccumulates. A continuous infusion of methylene blue has also been used to prevent toxicity from accidental "over-bolusing" of methylene blue, and permit titration of the infusion to methemoglobin levels. A 0.05% solution in 0.9% sodium chloride is usually started at a rate of 0.1 mg/kg per hour.

Supportive care—Patients in whom intentional overdose is known or suspected should be referred for psychiatric consultation.

## Patient Consultation

As an aid to patient consultation, refer to *Advice for the Patient, Dapsone (Systemic)*.

In providing consultation, consider emphasizing the following selected information (» = major clinical significance):

**Before using this medication**
» Conditions affecting use, especially:
  Allergy to sulfonamides
  Pregnancy—Dapsone crosses the placenta
  Breast-feeding—Dapsone is distributed into breast milk; it may cause hemolytic anemia in G6PD-deficient neonates
  Other medications, especially other hemolytics and didanosine
  Other medical problems, especially severe anemia, G6PD deficiency, or methemoglobin reductase deficiency

**Proper use of this medication**
» Proper dosing
  Missed dose: Taking as soon as possible; not taking if almost time for next dose; not doubling doses
» Proper storage
*For leprosy*
» Compliance with full course of therapy, which may take years
» Importance of not missing doses and taking at same time every day
*For dermatitis herpetiformis*
  Possible need for gluten-free diet
*For Pneumocystis carinii pneumonia*
» Compliance with full course of therapy

**Precautions while using this medication**
Regular visits to physician to check progress
Checking with physician if no improvement within 2 to 3 months (leprosy), within 1 week (PCP), or within a few days (dermatitis herpetiformis)

**Side/adverse effects**
Signs of potential side effects, especially hemolytic anemia, blood dyscrasias, hypersensitivity reactions, methemoglobinemia, exfoliative dermatitis, peripheral neuropathy, hepatic damage, "sulfone syndrome", and mood and other mental changes

## General Dosing Information

Since bacterial resistance may develop when dapsone is administered alone in the treatment of leprosy, for initial treatment, concurrent administration with rifampin is generally recommended. Clofazimine, ethionamide, or prothionamide (investigational) may be used in place of rifampin, but they are considered less effective.

Dapsone therapy should be discontinued promptly if new or toxic dermatologic reactions occur. However, leprosy reactional states do not require discontinuation of therapy. Large doses of corticosteroids should be given if severe "reversal" reactions (type 1) or neuritis occurs during treatment of leprosy.

Depending on the drug regimen used, therapy may have to be continued for 6 months to 3 years or more in indeterminate and tuberculoid leprosy, 2 to 10 years in borderline (dimorphous) leprosy, and 2 years to life in lepromatous leprosy.

In the treatment of dermatitis herpetiformis, a gluten-free diet for 6 months may allow a reduction in dose by approximately 50% or discontinuation of dapsone.

## Oral Dosage Forms

Note: Bracketed uses in the *Dosage Forms* section refer to categories of use and/or indications that are not included in U.S. product labeling.

### DAPSONE TABLETS USP

**Usual adult and adolescent dose**
Leprosy (Hansen's disease)—
  Oral, in combination with one or more other antileprosy agents, 50 to 100 mg of dapsone once a day; or 1.4 mg per kg of body weight once a day.
Dermatitis herpetiformis suppressant—
  Oral, initially 50 mg daily. Doses may be increased up to 300 mg daily if symptoms are not completely controlled. The dose should then be reduced to the lowest effective maintenance dose as soon as possible.
[Actinomycotic mycetoma]—
  Oral, 100 mg twice a day for several months after clinical symptoms have disappeared.
[Dermatosis, subcorneal pustular][1]—
  Oral, initially 100 mg once a day, increasing the dose by 50 mg every one to two weeks until remission occurs. The dose should then be gradually reduced to the lowest effective maintenance dose.
[Granuloma annulare][1]—
  Oral, 100 mg once a day.
[Malaria (prophylaxis)][1]—
  Oral, 100 mg of dapsone in combination with 12.5 mg of pyrimethamine once every seven days.
[Pneumonia, *Pneumocystis carinii*][1]—
  Treatment: Oral, 100 mg of dapsone once a day in combination with 20 mg per kg of body weight per day of trimethoprim, for twenty-one days.
  Prophylaxis: Oral, 50 to 100 mg once a day.
[Polychondritis, relapsing][1]—
  Oral, 100 mg once or twice a day.
[Pyoderma gangrenosum][1]—
  Oral, 50 to 100 mg once a day, in combination with other medications.

**Usual adult prescribing limits**
Leprosy (Hansen's disease)—
  Up to 100 mg daily.
Dermatitis herpetiformis suppressant—
  Up to 300 mg daily.
Polychondritis, relapsing[1]—
  Up to 200 mg daily.

**Usual pediatric dose**
Leprosy (Hansen's disease)—
  Oral, in combination with one or more other antileprosy agents, 1.4 mg of dapsone per kg of body weight once a day.
Dermatitis herpetiformis suppressant—
  Oral, initially 2 mg per kg of body weight daily. Doses may be increased if symptoms are not completely controlled. The dose should then be reduced to the lowest effective maintenance dose as soon as possible.
[Pneumonia, *Pneumocystis carinii* (prophylaxis)][1]—
  In children older than 1 month of age: Oral, 1 mg per kg of body weight, up to 100 mg daily.

**Strength(s) usually available**
U.S.—
  25 mg (Rx) [GENERIC (may be scored)].
  100 mg (Rx) [GENERIC (may be scored)].
Canada—
  100 mg (Rx) [*Avlosulfon* (scored)].

**Packaging and storage**
Store below 40 °C (104 °F), preferably between 15 and 30 °C (59 and 86 °F), unless otherwise specified by manufacturer. Store in a well-closed, light-resistant container.

**Auxiliary labeling**
• Continue medicine for full time of treatment (for leprosy and PCP).

---
[1]Not included in Canadian product labeling.

---
Revised: 06/26/92
Interim revision: 03/17/94

# DAUNORUBICIN Systemic

VA CLASSIFICATION (Primary): AN200
Commonly used brand name(s): *Cerubidine*.
Note: For a listing of dosage forms and brand names by country availability, see *Dosage Forms* section(s).

## Category
Antineoplastic.

## Indications
Note: Bracketed information in the *Indications* section refers to uses that are not included in U.S. product labeling.

**Accepted**
Leukemia, acute lymphocytic (treatment) or
Leukemia, acute nonlymphocytic (treatment)—Daunorubicin is indicated, in combination with other antineoplastics, for treatment of acute lymphocytic leukemia and acute nonlymphocytic leukemia (acute myelocytic leukemia, acute monocytic leukemia[1], erythroleukemia[1]).

[Neuroblastoma (treatment)][1]—Daunorubicin is used for treatment of solid tumors of childhood, such as neuroblastoma.

[Lymphomas, non-Hodgkin's (treatment)]—Daunorubicin is used for treatment of non-Hodgkin's lymphomas such as lymphosarcoma and reticulum cell sarcomas.

[Ewing's sarcoma (treatment)]—Daunorubicin is used for treatment of Ewing's sarcoma.

[Wilms' tumor (treatment)]—Daunorubicin is used for treatment of Wilms' tumor.

[Leukemia, chronic myelocytic (treatment)]—Daunorubicin is used for treatment of chronic myelocytic (myelogenous) leukemia.

[1]Not included in Canadian product labeling.

## Pharmacology/Pharmacokinetics
**Physicochemical characteristics**
Molecular weight—563.99.
pKa—10.3.

**Mechanism of action/Effect**
Daunorubicin is an anthracycline glycoside; it is classified as an antibiotic but is not used as an antimicrobial agent. Daunorubicin is most active in the S phase of cell division, but is not cycle phase–specific. Its exact mechanism of antineoplastic action is unknown but may involve binding to DNA by intercalation between base pairs and inhibition of DNA and RNA synthesis by template disordering and steric obstruction.

**Other actions/effects**
Also has immunosuppressant effects.

**Distribution**
Rapidly distributed throughout the body, especially to the kidneys, spleen, liver, and heart, as unchanged medication and metabolites. It does not cross the blood-brain barrier.

**Biotransformation**
Rapidly (within 1 hour) in the liver to produce an active metabolite, daunorubicinol. Further metabolism—Hepatic.

**Half-life**
Distribution—
  45 minutes.
Elimination—
  Daunorubicin: 18.5 hours.
  Metabolites: 55 hours.
  Daunorubicinol: 26.7 hours.

**Elimination**
In the urine, 25% in an active form; an estimated 40% is eliminated by biliary excretion.

## Precautions to Consider

**Carcinogenicity/Mutagenicity**
Secondary malignancies are potential delayed effects of many antineoplastic agents, although it is not clear whether the effect is related to their mutagenic or immunosuppressive action. The effect of dose and duration of therapy is also unknown, although risk seems to increase with long-term use.
Daunorubicin subcutaneous injection causes fibrosarcomas at the injection site in mice; however, it did not cause a carcinogenic effect within 22 months of observation after oral or intraperitoneal administration in mice. Daunorubicin is potentially carcinogenic in humans.

**Pregnancy/Reproduction**
Fertility—Gonadal suppression, resulting in amenorrhea or azoospermia, may occur in patients taking antineoplastic therapy, especially with the alkylating agents. In general, these effects appear to be related to dose and length of therapy and may be irreversible. Prediction of the degree of testicular or ovarian function impairment is complicated by the common use of combinations of several antineoplastics, which makes it difficult to assess the effects of individual agents.
Daunorubicin causes testicular atrophy in male dogs.

Pregnancy—Adequate and well-controlled studies have not been done in humans.
First trimester: It is usually recommended that use of antineoplastics, especially combination chemotherapy, be avoided whenever possible, especially during the first trimester. Although information is limited because of the relatively few instances of antineoplastic administration during pregnancy, the mutagenic, teratogenic, and carcinogenic potential of these medications must be considered.
Other hazards to the fetus include adverse reactions seen in adults.
In general, use of a contraceptive is recommended during cytotoxic drug therapy.
Studies in rabbits found an increased incidence of fetal abnormalities (parieto-occipital cranioschisis, umbilical hernias, rachischisis) and abortions, and studies in mice showed decreases in fetal birth weight and postdelivery growth rate.
FDA Pregnancy Category D.

**Breast-feeding**
Although very little information is available regarding distribution of antineoplastic agents into breast milk, breast-feeding is not recommended while daunorubicin is being administered because of the risks to the infant (adverse effects, mutagenicity, carcinogenicity).

**Pediatrics**
Appropriate studies on the relationship of age to the effects of daunorubicin have not been performed in the pediatric population.

**Geriatrics**
Although appropriate studies on the relationship of age to the effects of daunorubicin have not been performed in the geriatric population, cardiotoxicity may be more frequent in the elderly. Caution should also be used in patients who have inadequate bone marrow reserves due to old age. In addition, elderly patients are more likely to have age-related renal function impairment, which may require reduction of dosage in patients receiving daunorubicin.

**Dental**
The bone marrow depressant effects of daunorubicin may result in an increased incidence of microbial infection, delayed healing, and gingival bleeding. Dental work, whenever possible, should be completed prior to initiation of therapy or deferred until blood counts have returned to normal. Patients should be instructed in proper oral hygiene during treatment, including caution in use of regular toothbrushes, dental floss, and toothpicks.
Daunorubicin also commonly causes stomatitis which may be associated with considerable discomfort.

**Drug interactions and/or related problems**
The following drug interactions and/or related problems have been selected on the basis of their potential clinical significance (possible mechanism in parentheses where appropriate)—not necessarily inclusive (» = major clinical significance):
Note: Combinations containing any of the following medications, depending on the amount present, may also interact with this medication.

  Allopurinol or
  Colchicine or
» Probenecid or
» Sulfinpyrazone
    (daunorubicin may raise the concentration of blood uric acid; dosage adjustment of antigout agents may be necessary to control hyperuricemia and gout; allopurinol may be preferred to prevent or reverse daunorubicin-induced hyperuricemia because of risk of uric acid nephropathy with uricosuric antigout agents)

  Blood dyscrasia–causing medications (see *Appendix II*)
    (leukopenic and/or thrombocytopenic effects of daunorubicin may be increased with concurrent or recent therapy if these medications cause the same effects; dosage adjustment of daunorubicin, if necessary, should be based on blood counts)

- » Bone marrow depressants, other (see *Appendix II*) or
  Radiation therapy
  (additive bone marrow depression may occur; dosage reduction may be required when two or more bone marrow depressants, including radiation, are used concurrently or consecutively)
- Cyclophosphamide or
  Radiation therapy to mediastinal area
  (concurrent use may result in increased cardiotoxicity; it is recommended that the total dose of daunorubicin not exceed 400 mg per square meter of body surface)
- Doxorubicin
  (use of daunorubicin in a patient who has previously received doxorubicin increases the risk of cardiotoxicity; dosage adjustment is necessary. Daunorubicin should not be used in patients who have previously received complete cumulative doses of doxorubicin or daunorubicin; in patients who have previously received less than a complete cumulative dose of doxorubicin, the total cumulative dose of doxorubicin plus daunorubicin should not exceed 550 mg per square meter of body surface)
- Hepatotoxic medications, other (see *Appendix II*)
  (concurrent use may increase the risk of toxicity; for example, high-dose methotrexate may impair liver function and increase toxicity of subsequently administered daunorubicin)
- Vaccines, killed virus
  (because normal defense mechanisms may be suppressed by daunorubicin therapy, the patient's antibody response to the vaccine may be decreased. The interval between discontinuation of medications that cause immunosuppression and restoration of the patient's ability to respond to the vaccine depends on the intensity and type of immunosuppression-causing medication used, the underlying disease, and other factors; estimates vary from 3 months to 1 year)
- » Vaccines, live virus
  (because normal defense mechanisms may be suppressed by daunorubicin therapy, concurrent use with a live virus vaccine may potentiate the replication of the vaccine virus, may increase the side/adverse effects of the vaccine virus, and/or may decrease the patient's antibody response to the vaccine; immunization of these patients should be undertaken only with extreme caution after careful review of the patient's hematologic status and only with the knowledge and consent of the physician managing the daunorubicin therapy. The interval between discontinuation of medications that cause immunosuppression and restoration of the patient's ability to respond to the vaccine depends on the intensity and type of immunosuppression-causing medication used, the underlying disease, and other factors; estimates vary from 3 months to 1 year. Patients with leukemia in remission should not receive live virus vaccine until at least 3 months after their last chemotherapy. In addition, immunization with oral poliovirus vaccine should be postponed in persons in close contact with the patient, especially family members)

**Laboratory value alterations**
The following have been selected on the basis of their potential clinical significance (possible effect in parentheses where appropriate)—not necessarily inclusive (» = major clinical significance):

With physiology/laboratory test values
  Alkaline phosphatase values, serum and
  Aspartate aminotransferase (AST [SGOT]) values, serum and
  Bilirubin concentrations, serum
    (may be increased transiently)
  Uric acid
    (concentrations in blood and urine may be increased)

**Medical considerations/Contraindications**
The medical considerations/contraindications included have been selected on the basis of their potential clinical significance (reasons given in parentheses where appropriate)—not necessarily inclusive (» = major clinical significance):

*Risk-benefit should be considered when the following medical problems exist:*
- » Bone marrow depression
- » Chickenpox, existing or recent (including recent exposure) or
- » Herpes zoster
  (risk of severe generalized disease)
- Gout, history of or
  Urate renal stones, history of
    (risk of hyperuricemia)
- » Heart disease

- » Hepatic function impairment
  (reduction in dosage is recommended; three quarters of the normal dose is recommended in patients with serum bilirubin concentrations of 1.2 to 3 mg per 100 mL; one half of the normal dose is recommended in patients with serum bilirubin concentrations of greater than 3 mg per 100 mL)
- » Infection
  Renal function impairment
  (reduced elimination; dosage reduction is recommended; one half of the normal dose is recommended in patients with serum creatinine concentrations of greater than 3 mg per 100 mL)
  Sensitivity to daunorubicin
- » Tumor cell infiltration of the bone marrow
- » Caution should be used also in patients with inadequate bone marrow reserves due to previous cytotoxic drug or radiation therapy.

**Patient monitoring**
The following may be especially important in patient monitoring (other tests may be warranted in some patients, depending on condition; » = major clinical significance):

Alanine aminotransferase (ALT [SGPT]) values, serum and
Aspartate aminotransferase (AST [SGOT]) values, serum and
Bilirubin concentrations, serum and
Lactate dehydrogenase (LDH) values, serum
  (recommended prior to initiation of therapy and at periodic intervals during therapy; frequency varies according to clinical state, agent, dose, and other agents being used concurrently)
- » Chest x-ray and
- » Echocardiography and
  Electrocardiogram (ECG) studies and
- » Radionuclide angiography determination of ejection fraction
  (recommended prior to initiation of therapy and at periodic intervals during therapy)
- » Hematocrit or hemoglobin and
- » Leukocyte count, total and, if appropriate, differential and
- » Platelet count
  (determinations recommended prior to initiation of therapy and at periodic intervals during therapy; frequency varies according to clinical state, agent, dose, and other agents being used concurrently)
  Uric acid concentrations, serum
  (recommended prior to initiation of therapy and at periodic intervals during therapy; frequency varies according to clinical state, agent, dose, and other agents being used concurrently)

## Side/Adverse Effects
Note: Many "side effects" of antineoplastic therapy are unavoidable and represent the medication's pharmacologic action. Some of these (for example, leukopenia and thrombocytopenia) are actually used as parameters to aid in individual dosage titration.

The following side/adverse effects have been selected on the basis of their potential clinical significance (possible signs and symptoms in parentheses where appropriate)—not necessarily inclusive:

**Those indicating need for medical attention**
Incidence more frequent
  *Esophagitis or stomatitis* (sores in mouth and on lips); *leukopenia or infection* (fever or chills; cough or hoarseness; lower back or side pain; painful or difficult urination)—usually asymptomatic
  Note: With *esophagitis* or *stomatitis*, sores in mouth and on lips occur 3 to 7 days after administration.
    *Leukopenia* occurs in all patients. The nadir of the leukocyte count occurs 10 to 14 days after a dose. Recovery usually occurs within 21 days after a dose.
    In addition to the risk of *infection*, febrile drug reactions may also occur during or immediately after administration.
Incidence less frequent
  *Cardiotoxicity in the form of congestive heart failure* (irregular heartbeat; shortness of breath; swelling of feet and lower legs); *cellulitis or tissue necrosis* (pain at injection site)—caused by extravasation; *gastrointestinal ulceration* (stomach pain); *hyperuricemia or uric acid nephropathy* (joint pain; lower back or side pain); *thrombocytopenia* (unusual bleeding or bruising; black, tarry stools; blood in urine or stools; pinpoint red spots on skin)—usually asymptomatic
  Note: Incidence of *cardiotoxicity* is more frequent in adults receiving a total cumulative dosage over 550 mg per square meter of body surface (450 mg per square meter of body surface in patients who have received previous chest irradiation), in the elderly,

and in patients with a history of cardiac disease or mediastinal radiation.

*Cardiotoxicity* usually appears within 1 to 6 months after initiation of therapy. It may develop suddenly and may not be detected by routine ECG. It may be irreversible and fatal but responds to treatment if detected early.

*Hyperuricemia or uric acid nephropathy* occurs most commonly during initial treatment of patients with leukemia or lymphoma, as a result of rapid cell breakdown which leads to elevated serum uric acid concentrations.

Incidence rare
> **Allergic reaction** (skin rash or itching); **cardiotoxicity in the form of pericarditis-myocarditis**

**Those indicating need for medical attention only if they continue or are bothersome**
Incidence more frequent
> *Nausea and vomiting*
>
> Note: *Nausea and vomiting* are usually mild and transient, occurring soon after administration and lasting 24 to 48 hours.

Incidence less frequent or rare
> **Darkening or redness of skin**—if patient has received previous radiation therapy; **diarrhea**

**Those not indicating need for medical attention**
Incidence more frequent
> *Loss of hair; reddish urine*
>
> Note: *Loss of hair* occurs in most patients. Growth usually resumes 5 or more weeks after therapy is completed.
>
> *Reddish urine* usually clears within 48 hours.

Those indicating the need for medical attention if they occur after medication is discontinued
> **Cardiotoxicity** (irregular heartbeat; shortness of breath; swelling of feet and lower legs)

## Patient Consultation

As an aid to patient consultation, refer to *Advice for the Patient, Daunorubicin (Systemic)*.

In providing consultation, consider emphasizing the following selected information (» = major clinical significance):

### Before using this medication
» Conditions affecting use, especially:
   Sensitivity to daunorubicin
   Pregnancy—Use not recommended because of mutagenic, teratogenic, and carcinogenic potential; advisability of using a contraceptive; telling physician immediately if pregnancy is suspected
   Breast-feeding—Not recommended because of risk of serious side effects
   Use in the elderly—Increased risk of cardiotoxicity, bone marrow depression
   Other medications, especially probenecid, sulfinpyrazone, other bone marrow depressants, or previous cytotoxic drug or radiation therapy
   Other medical problems, especially chickenpox, herpes zoster, heart disease, hepatic function impairment, or infection

### Proper use of this medication
Caution in taking combination therapy; taking each medication at the right time
Importance of ample fluid intake and subsequent increase in urine output to aid in excretion of uric acid
Frequency of nausea and vomiting; importance of continuing medication despite stomach upset
» Proper dosing

### Precautions while using this medication
» Importance of close monitoring by the physician
» Avoiding immunizations unless approved by physician; other persons in patient's household should avoid immunizations with oral poliovirus vaccine; avoiding persons who have taken oral poliovirus vaccine or wearing a protective mask that covers nose and mouth

*Caution if bone marrow depression occurs*
» Avoiding exposure to persons with infections, especially during periods of low blood counts; checking with physician immediately if fever or chills, cough or hoarseness, lower back or side pain, or painful or difficult urination occurs
» Checking with physician immediately if unusual bleeding or bruising; black, tarry stools; blood in urine or stools; or pinpoint red spots on skin occur

Caution in use of regular toothbrush, dental floss, or toothpick; physician, dentist, or nurse may suggest alternatives; checking with physician before having dental work done
Not touching eyes or inside of nose unless hands washed immediately before
Using caution to avoid accidental cuts with use of sharp objects such as safety razor or fingernail or toenail cutters
Avoiding contact sports or other situations where bruising or injury could occur
» Possibility of local tissue injury and scarring if infiltration of intravenous solution occurs; telling doctor or nurse right away about redness, pain, or swelling at injection site

### Side/adverse effects
May cause adverse effects such as blood problems, loss of hair, heart problems, and cancer; importance of discussing possible effects with physician
Signs of potential side effects, especially esophagitis, stomatitis, leukopenia, infection, cardiotoxicity, cellulitis or tissue necrosis caused by extravasation, gastrointestinal ulceration, hyperuricemia, uric acid nephropathy, thrombocytopenia, and allergic reaction
Physician or nurse can help in dealing with side effects
Reddish urine may be alarming to patient although medically insignificant
Possibility of hair loss; normal hair growth should return after treatment has ended

## General Dosing Information

Patients receiving daunorubicin should be under supervision of a physician experienced in cancer chemotherapy. It is recommended that the patient be hospitalized at least during initial treatment.

A variety of dosage schedules of daunorubicin, alone or in combination with other antitumor agents, are used. The prescriber may consult the medical literature as well as the manufacturer's literature in choosing a specific dosage.

Dosage must be adjusted to meet the individual requirements of each patient, on the basis of clinical response and appearance or severity of toxicity.

The desired dose of daunorubicin is withdrawn from the vial of reconstituted solution into a syringe containing 10 to 15 mL of 0.9% sodium chloride injection and then injected over 2 to 3 minutes into the tubing or side arm of a rapidly running intravenous infusion of 5% dextrose injection or 0.9% sodium chloride injection.

Care must be taken to avoid extravasation during intravenous administration. Facial flushing or erythematous streaking along the vein indicates overly rapid injection.

Administration by intravenous infusion is not recommended because of irritation to the vein and the risk of thrombophlebitis.

If extravasation of daunorubicin occurs during intravenous administration, as indicated by local burning or stinging, the injection and infusion should be stopped immediately and resumed, completing the dose, in another vein.

Because it will cause local tissue necrosis, daunorubicin must not be administered intramuscularly or subcutaneously.

Development of uric acid nephropathy in patients with leukemia or lymphoma may be prevented by adequate oral hydration and, in some cases, administration of allopurinol. Alkalinization of urine may be necessary if serum uric acid concentrations are elevated.

In general, it is recommended that a course of daunorubicin be administered no more frequently than every 21 days to allow the bone marrow to recover.

In acute leukemia, daunorubicin may be administered despite the presence of thrombocytopenia and bleeding; stoppage of bleeding and increase in platelet count have occurred during treatment in some cases and platelet transfusions are useful in others.

Special precautions are recommended in patients who develop thrombocytopenia as a result of administration of daunorubicin. These may include extreme care in performing invasive procedures; regular inspection of intravenous sites, skin (including perirectal area), and mucous membrane surfaces for signs of bleeding or bruising; limiting frequency of venipuncture and avoiding intramuscular injections; testing urine, emesis, stool, and secretions for occult blood; care in use of regular toothbrushes, dental floss, toothpicks, safety razors, and fingernail and toenail cutters; avoiding constipation; and using caution to prevent falls and other injuries. Such patients should avoid alcohol and aspirin intake because of the risk of gastrointestinal bleeding. Platelet transfusions may be required.

Patients who develop leukopenia should be observed carefully for signs of infection. Antibiotic support may be required. In neutropenic patients who develop fever, broad-spectrum antibiotic coverage should be initiated empirically, pending bacterial cultures and appropriate diagnostic tests.

**Safety considerations of handling this medication**
There is limited but increasing evidence and concern that personnel involved in preparation and administration of parenteral antineoplastics may be at some risk because of the potential mutagenicity, teratogenicity, and/or carcinogenicity of these agents, although the actual risk is unknown. USP advisory panels recommend cautious handling both in preparation and disposal of antineoplastic agents. Precautions that have been suggested include:
- Use of a biological containment cabinet during reconstitution and dilution of parenteral medications and wearing of disposable surgical gloves and masks.
- Use of proper technique to prevent contamination of the medication, work area, and operator during transfer between containers (including proper training of personnel in this technique).
- Cautious and proper disposal of needles, syringes, vials, ampuls, and unused medication.

A number of medical centers have developed detailed guidelines for handling of antineoplastic agents.

**Combination chemotherapy**
Daunorubicin may be used in combination with other agents in various regimens. As a result, incidence and/or severity of side effects may be altered and different dosages (usually reduced) may be used. For example, daunorubicin is part of the following chemotherapeutic combination:
—daunorubicin, vincristine, and prednisone.

For specific dosages and schedules, consult the literature. For information regarding each agent, consult the individual monographs.

## Parenteral Dosage Forms

### DAUNORUBICIN HYDROCHLORIDE FOR INJECTION USP

Note: The doses and strengths of the available dosage forms are expressed in terms of the daunorubicin base, not the hydrochloride salt.

**Usual adult dose**
Leukemia, acute lymphocytic—
　Intravenous, 45 mg (base) per square meter of body surface on days 1, 2, and 3 of a thirty-two–day course in combination with vincristine, prednisone, and asparaginase.
Leukemia, acute nonlymphocytic—
　Intravenous, 45 mg (base) per square meter of body surface on days 1, 2, and 3 of the first course and days 1 and 2 of the second course, in combination with cytarabine.

**Usual adult prescribing limits**
Up to a total lifetime dosage of 550 mg (base) per square meter of body surface, 450 mg per square meter of body surface in patients who have received previous chest irradiation (to reduce risk of cardiotoxicity).

**Usual pediatric dose**
Leukemia, acute lymphocytic—
　Intravenous, 25 mg (base) per square meter of body surface once a week, in combination with vincristine and prednisone.
Note: In children less than 2 years of age or below 0.5 square meter of body surface, dosage should be calculated on the basis of mg per kg of body weight rather than body surface area.

**Usual geriatric dose**
For patients 60 years of age and older—
　Leukemia, acute nonlymphocytic:
　　Intravenous, 30 mg (base) per square meter of body surface on days 1, 2, and 3 of the first course and days 1 and 2 of the second course, in combination with cytarabine.
Note: This dose is based on a single study and may not be appropriate if optimal supportive care is available.

**Size(s) usually available**
U.S.—
　20 mg (base) (21.4 mg as HCl) (Rx) [*Cerubidine* (mannitol 100 mg)].
Canada—
　20 mg (base) (21.4 mg as HCl) (Rx) [*Cerubidine*].

**Packaging and storage**
Store below 40 °C (104 °F), preferably between 15 and 30 °C (59 and 86 °F), unless otherwise specified by manufacturer. Protect from light.

**Preparation of dosage form**
Daunorubicin for Injection USP is reconstituted for intravenous administration by adding 4 mL of sterile water for injection to the vial and shaking gently to dissolve, producing a solution containing 5 mg of daunorubicin (base) per mL.

**Stability**
Reconstituted solutions of daunorubicin are stable for 24 hours at room temperature or 48 hours between 2 and 8 °C (36 and 46 °F) when protected from light.

**Note**
Any daunorubicin powder or solution that comes in contact with the skin or mucosa should be washed off thoroughly with soap and water.

### Selected Bibliography
DeVita VT, Hellman S, Rosenberg SA. Cancer principles and practice of oncology. 5th ed. Philadelphia: Lippincott-Raven Publishers; 1997.

Revised: 07/11/94
Interim revision: 09/26/97

---

# DAUNORUBICIN, LIPOSOMAL   Systemic†

VA CLASSIFICATION (Primary): AN200
Commonly used brand name(s): *DaunoXome*.
Note: For a listing of dosage forms and brand names by country availability, see *Dosage Forms* section(s).

†Not commercially available in Canada.

## Category
Antineoplastic.

## Indications

**Accepted**
Kaposi's sarcoma (KS), acquired immunodeficiency syndrome (AIDS)–associated (treatment)—Liposomal daunorubicin is indicated as a first-line cytotoxic therapy for advanced AIDS-associated KS. Liposomal daunorubicin is not recommended in patients with less than advanced AIDS-associated KS.
Note: The treatment of AIDS-associated KS is dependent on the extent and severity of the KS and the patient's clinical condition. For patients with minimal disease, local treatments such as excision, radiotherapy, or intralesional chemotherapy will be adequate. However, for those with severe cutaneous or systemic disease, systemic chemotherapy may be required. Patients with severe debilitation due to their general condition are best served by optimal palliative care.

## Pharmacology/Pharmacokinetics

Note: A human pharmacokinetics study has shown that the pharmacokinetics of liposomal daunorubicin are significantly different from those of conventional daunorubicin, which may account for both its reduced toxicity and its potentially enhanced activity. However, the pharmacokinetics of liposomal daunorubicin have not been evaluated in women, in a variety of ethnic groups, or in patients with renal and hepatic insufficiency.

**Physicochemical characteristics**
Source—Daunorubicin is an anthracycline antibiotic originally obtained from *Streptomyces peucetius*. Daunorubicin also may be isolated from *Streptomyces coeruleorubidus*. Liposomal daunorubicin is an aqueous solution of the citrate salt of daunorubicin encapsulated within lipid vesicles (liposomes) composed of a lipid bilayer of highly purified distearoylphosphatidylcholine (DSPC) and cholesterol in a 2:1 molar ratio.

**Mechanism of action/Effect**
Liposomal daunorubicin is a liposomal preparation of daunorubicin formulated to maximize the selectivity of daunorubicin for solid tumors *in situ*. While in the circulation, the liposomal formulation helps to protect the entrapped daunorubicin from chemical and enzymatic degradation, minimizes protein binding, and generally decreases uptake by normal (nonreticuloendothelial system) tissues. Once within the tumor environment, daunorubicin is released over time, enabling it to exert its antineoplastic activity.
The specific mechanism by which liposomal daunorubicin is able to deliver daunorubicin to solid tumors *in situ* is not known. However, it is be-

lieved to be a function of increased permeability of the tumor neovasculature to some particles in the size range of liposomal daunorubicin.
In animal studies, liposomal daunorubicin has demonstrated improved activity against solid tumors compared with that of conventional daunorubicin.

### Distribution
Limited to vascular fluid.

Volume of distribution (Vol$_D$)—Steady-state: 6.4 liters following intravenous administration of 40 mg per square meter of body surface area (mg/m$^2$), over 30 to 60 minutes.

In animal studies, liposomal daunorubicin appeared to cross the blood-brain barrier and to accumulate selectively in solid tumor tissues to a greater extent than occurs with nonencapsulated daunorubicin.

### Biotransformation
Daunorubicinol, the major active metabolite of daunorubicin, was detected at low concentrations in the plasma following intravenous administration of liposomal daunorubicin.

### Half-life
Distribution—4.41 hours following intravenous administration of a 40 mg/m$^2$ dose over 30 to 60 minutes.

### Elimination
Plasma clearance—17 mL per minute following intravenous administration of a 40 mg/m$^2$ dose over 30 to 60 minutes.

## Precautions to Consider

### Cross-sensitivity and/or related problems
Liposomal daunorubicin is not recommended in patients hypersensitive to daunorubicin or the liposomal components.

### Carcinogenicity
Studies to evaluate the carcinogenic potential of liposomal daunorubicin have not been performed. However, the active ingredient, daunorubicin, was found to increase the incidence of mammary tumors in rats following a single dose of 12.5 mg per kg of body weight (mg/kg) (approximately two times the recommended human dose on a mg per square meter of body surface area [mg/m$^2$] basis).

### Mutagenicity
Studies to evaluate the mutagenic potential of liposomal daunorubicin have not been performed. However, the active ingredient, daunorubicin, was mutagenic in *in vitro* tests (Ames test and V79 hamster cell assay) and clastogenic in *in vitro* (CCRF-CEM human lymphoblasts) and *in vivo* (SCE assay in mouse bone marrow) test systems.

### Pregnancy/Reproduction
Fertility—Studies to evaluate the effects of liposomal daunorubicin on fertility have not been performed; however, the active ingredient, daunorubicin, caused testicular atrophy and total aplasia of spermatocytes in the seminiferous tubules in male dogs administered 0.25 mg/kg per day (approximately eight times the recommended human dose on a mg/m$^2$ basis).

Pregnancy—Adequate and well-controlled studies in humans have not been done. Furthermore, the pharmacokinetics of liposomal daunorubicin have not been evaluated in women.

In general, use of a contraceptive method is recommended during cytotoxic drug therapy.

Liposomal daunorubicin caused severe maternal toxicity and embryolethality in rats administered doses of 2 mg/kg per day (one third of the maximum recommended human dose) on days 6 through 15 of gestation. Studies in rats administered doses of 0.3 mg/kg per day (one twentieth of the maximum recommended human dose) on days 6 through 15 of gestation showed that liposomal daunorubicin caused embryotoxicity (increased embryofetal deaths, reduced numbers of litters, and reduced litter size) and caused fetal malformations (anophthalmia, microphthalmia, incomplete ossification).

FDA Pregnancy Category D.

### Breast-feeding
It is not known whether liposomal daunorubicin is distributed into breast milk. However, breast-feeding is not recommended while liposomal daunorubicin is being administered because of the potential risk of adverse reactions in the infant.

### Pediatrics
No information is available on the relationship of age to the effects of liposomal daunorubicin in pediatric patients. Safety and efficacy have not been established.

### Geriatrics
No information is available on the relationship of age to the effects of liposomal daunorubicin in geriatric patients. However, elderly patients are more likely to have age-related renal function impairment, which may require caution in patients receiving liposomal daunorubicin. Safety and efficacy have not been established.

### Dental
The leukopenic and thrombocytopenic effects of liposomal daunorubicin may result in an increased incidence of certain microbial infections of the mouth, delayed healing, and gingival bleeding. If leukopenia or thrombocytopenia occurs, dental work should be deferred until blood counts have returned to normal. Patients should be instructed in proper oral hygiene, including caution in use of regular toothbrushes, dental floss, and toothpicks.

### Drug interactions and/or related problems
The following drug interactions and/or related problems have been selected on the basis of their potential clinical significance (possible mechanism in parentheses where appropriate)—not necessarily inclusive (» = major clinical significance):

Note: Combinations containing any of the following medications, depending on the amount present, may also interact with this medication.

Allopurinol or
Colchicine or
» Probenecid or
» Sulfinpyrazone
(liposomal daunorubicin may raise the concentration of blood uric acid; dosage adjustment of antigout agents may be necessary to control hyperuricemia and gout; allopurinol may be preferred to prevent or reverse liposomal daunorubicin–induced hyperuricemia because of risk of uric acid nephropathy with uricosuric antigout agents)

» Daunorubicin, prior use of or
» Doxorubicin, prior use of or
» Other anthracycline antineoplastics, prior use of
(use of liposomal daunorubicin in a patient who previously has received anthracenedione antineoplastic agents, daunorubicin, doxorubicin, or other anthracycline antineoplastics increases the risk for cardiotoxicity; dosage adjustment is necessary)

(prior anthracycline use is also significantly associated with short survival)

Blood dyscrasia–causing medications (see *Appendix II*)
(leukopenic and/or thrombocytopenic effects of liposomal daunorubicin may be increased with concurrent or recent therapy if these medications cause the same effects; dosage adjustment of liposomal daunorubicin, if necessary, should be based on blood counts)

» Bone marrow depressants, other (see *Appendix II*) or
Radiation therapy
(additive bone marrow depression may occur; dosage reduction may be required when two or more bone marrow depressants, including radiation, are used concurrently or consecutively)

Cyclophosphamide or
Radiation therapy to mediastinal area
(concurrent use may result in increased cardiotoxicity; it is recommended that the total dose of liposomal daunorubicin not exceed 400 mg/m$^2$)

Hepatotoxic medications, other (see *Appendix II*)
(concurrent use may increase the risk of toxicity; for example, high-dose methotrexate may impair liver function and increase toxicity of subsequently administered liposomal daunorubicin)

Vaccines, killed virus
(because normal defense mechanisms may be suppressed by liposomal daunorubicin therapy, the patient's antibody response to the vaccine may be decreased. The interval between discontinuation of medications that cause immunosuppression and restoration of the patient's ability to respond to the vaccine depends on the intensity and type of immunosuppression-causing medication used, the underlying disease, and other factors; estimates vary from 3 months to 1 year)

» Vaccines, live virus
(because normal defense mechanisms may be suppressed by liposomal daunorubicin therapy, concurrent use with a live virus vaccine may potentiate the replication of the vaccine virus, may increase the side/adverse effects of the vaccine virus, and/or may decrease the patient's antibody response to the vaccine; immunization of these patients should be undertaken only with extreme caution after careful review of the patient's hematologic status and only with the knowledge and consent of the physician managing the liposomal daunorubicin therapy. The interval between discontinuation of medications that cause immunosuppression and restoration of the patient's ability to respond to the vaccine depends on the intensity and type of immunosuppression-causing medication used, the underly-

ing disease, and other factors; estimates vary from 3 months to 1 year. Patients with leukemia in remission should not receive live virus vaccine until at least 3 months after their last chemotherapy. In addition, immunization with oral poliovirus vaccine should be postponed in persons in close contact with the patient, especially family members)

**Laboratory value alterations**
The following have been selected on the basis of their potential clinical significance (possible effect in parentheses where appropriate)—not necessarily inclusive (» = major clinical significance):

With physiology/laboratory test values
» Cardiac function tests
    (left ventricular ejection fraction may be decreased, possibly indicating cardiotoxicity)
  Hematocrit or
  Hemoglobin or
» Leukocyte counts or
  Platelet counts
    (may be decreased)

**Medical considerations/Contraindications**
The medical considerations/contraindications included have been selected on the basis of their potential clinical significance (reasons given in parentheses where appropriate)—not necessarily inclusive (» = major clinical significance).

*Except under special circumstances, this medication should not be used when the following medical problem exists:*
» Previous hypersensitivity reaction to liposomal daunorubicin or its components

*Risk-benefit should be considered when the following medical problems exist:*
» Bone marrow depression
» Cardiac disease, pre-existing
    (may increase risk of cardiotoxicity; monitoring of cardiac function is recommended)
» Chickenpox, existing or recent (including recent exposure) or
» Herpes zoster
    (risk of severe generalized disease)
» Granulocytopenia, severe
    (treatment should be withheld if the absolute granulocyte count is lower than 750 cells per cubic millimeter)
» Hepatic function impairment
    (excretion may be delayed; reduction in dosage is recommended; three fourths of the normal dose is recommended in patients with serum bilirubin concentrations of 1.2 to 3 mg per deciliter; one half of the normal dose is recommended in patients with serum bilirubin concentrations of greater than 3 mg per deciliter)
» Renal function impairment
    (excretion may be delayed; reduction in dosage is recommended; one half of the normal dose is recommended in patients with serum creatinine concentrations greater than 3 mg per deciliter)
» Sensitivity to daunorubicin or to the liposomal components
» Tumor cell infiltration of the bone marrow
» Caution should be used also in patients with inadequate bone marrow reserves due to previous cytotoxic drug or radiation therapy

**Patient monitoring**
The following may be especially important in patient monitoring (other tests may be warranted in some patients, depending on condition; » = major clinical significance):

  Alanine aminotransferase (ALT [SGPT]) values, serum and
  Aspartate aminotransferase (AST [SGOT]) values, serum and
  Bilirubin concentrations, serum and
  Lactate dehydrogenase (LDH) values, serum
    (recommended prior to initiation of therapy and at periodic intervals during therapy; frequently varies according to clinical state, agent, dose, and other agents being used concurrently)
» Cardiac function
    (recommended prior to initiation of therapy and at periodic intervals during therapy)
» Hematocrit or hemoglobin and
» Leukocyte count, total and, if appropriate, differential and
» Platelet count
    (determinations recommended prior to initiation of therapy and at periodic intervals during therapy; frequently varies according to clinical state, agent, dose, and other agents being used concurrently)

» Left ventricular ejection fraction
    (determination recommended at total cumulative doses of 320 mg/m$^2$, 480 mg/m$^2$, and every 240 mg/m$^2$ thereafter)
» Observation for evidence of intercurrent or opportunistic infections

## Side/Adverse Effects
The following side/adverse effects have been selected on the basis of their potential clinical significance (possible signs and symptoms in parentheses where appropriate)—not necessarily inclusive:

**Those indicating need for medical attention**
Incidence more frequent
  *Dyspnea* (shortness of breath; troubled breathing)—less frequently, may be severe or associated with pulmonary infiltrations; *neuropathy* (weakness or numbness in arms or legs); *neutropenia* (cough or hoarseness; fever or chills; lower back or side pain; painful or difficult urination; sore throat)

  Note: Clinical studies have demonstrated that *neutropenia* is the predominant hematologic toxicity following treatment with liposomal daunorubicin. In one study, 36% of patients experienced grade 3 neutropenia (< 1000 cells/mm$^2$), while 15% of patients experienced grade 4 neutropenia (< 500 cells/mm$^2$). Furthermore, patients receiving this medication may experience a higher frequency of opportunistic infections and neutropenic fevers. Acquired immunodeficiency syndrome (AIDS) patients are susceptible to a variety of opportunistic infections, and chemotherapy-associated bone marrow suppression may enhance this risk. It is possible that liposomal daunorubicin may interfere with monocyte-macrophage function, and thus increase susceptibility to opportunistic infections.

Incidence less frequent
  *Anemia* (unusual tiredness or weakness); *cardiotoxicity* (irregular heartbeat; shortness of breath; swelling of the feet and lower legs); *chest pain; edema* (swelling of abdomen, face, fingers, hands, feet, or lower legs; weight gain); *gastrointestinal hemorrhage* (black, tarry stools; bloody stools; bloody vomit); *hemoptysis* (coughing up blood); *hypertension*—usually asymptomatic; *renal effects, including dysuria* (painful or difficult urination); *nocturia* (unusual nighttime urination); *or polyuria* (producing large amounts of pale, dilute urine); *stomatitis* (sores in mouth and on lips); *syncope* (fainting); *tachycardia* (fast heartbeat); *thrombocytopenia* (black, tarry stools; unusual bleeding or bruising; blood in urine or stools; pinpoint red spots on skin)

  Note: Cardiac function should be monitored regularly in patients receiving liposomal daunorubicin because of the potential risk for *cardiotoxicity* and congestive heart failure. Cardiac monitoring is advised especially in those patients who have received prior anthracycline therapy or who have pre-existing cardiac disease. Cardiotoxicity can occur with cumulative doses of greater than 300 mg per square meter of body surface area.

**Those indicating need for medical attention only if they continue or are bothersome**
Incidence more frequent
  *Abdominal pain; allergic reaction* (chills; fever; skin rash or itching)—severe reactions occur less frequently; *diarrhea; headache; infusion-related reaction* (back pain; chest tightness; flushing)—usually mild to moderate in severity; *nausea and vomiting*—severe reactions occur less frequently; *rigors* (feeling unusually cold; shivering)

  Note: An *infusion-related reaction* may occur during the first 5 minutes of the infusion and may be related to the liposomal component of liposomal daunorubicin.

Incidence less frequent
  *Arthralgia or myalgia* (pain in joints or muscles); *conjunctivitis* (dry, irritated, itching, or red eyes); *constipation; dizziness; dry mouth; dysphagia* (difficulty swallowing); *eye pain; folliculitis* (painful, red, hot, or irritated hair follicles); *gingival bleeding* (bleeding gums); *hemorrhoids* (bleeding after defecation; uncomfortable swelling around anus); *injection site inflammation* (red, hot, or irritated skin at site of injection; pain at site of injection; swelling or lump under skin at site of injection)—if extravasation occurs; *insomnia* (sleeplessness); *somnolence* (extreme feeling of sleepiness); *tenesmus* (frequent urge to defecate); *tinnitus* (ringing sound in ears); *tooth caries* (tooth pain); *tremor* (uncontrollable movement of body)

  Note: Local tissue necrosis has not been observed when extravasation occurs.

**Those not indicating need for medical attention**
Incidence less frequent
  *Alopecia* (loss of hair)

  Note: *Alopecia*, a frequent side effect associated with anthracycline therapy, is usually mild to moderate in severity following liposomal daunorubicin therapy. In one study, alopecia occurred in only 8% of patients treated with liposomal daunorubicin.

## Overdose

For specific information on the agents used in the management of liposomal doxorubicin overdose, see:
- *Filgrastim* and/or
- *Sargramostim* in *Colony Stimulating Factors (Systemic)* monograph.

For more information on the management of overdose, **contact a Poison Control Center** (see *Poison Control Center Listing*).

**Clinical effects of overdose**
The following effects have been selected on the basis of their potential clinical significance (possible signs and symptoms in parentheses where appropriate)—not necessarily inclusive:

Acute
*Mucositis* (sores in mouth and on lips); *neutropenia* (cough or hoarseness; fever or chills; lower back or side pain; painful or difficult urination; sore throat)—usually asymptomatic; *thrombocytopenia* (black, tarry stools; blood in urine or stools; pinpoint red spots on skin; unusual bleeding or bruising)—usually asymptomatic

**Treatment of overdose**
Treatment of leukopenia includes antibiotic therapy and administration of colony stimulating factors (filgrastim [rG-CSF] or sargramostim [rGM-CSF]).

Treatment of thrombocytopenia includes hospitalization of the patient and platelet transfusions.

## Patient Consultation

As an aid to patient consultation, refer to *Advice for the Patient, Daunorubicin, Liposomal (Systemic)*.

In providing consultation, consider emphasizing the following selected information (» = major clinical significance):

**Before using this medication**
» Conditions affecting use, especially:
  Hypersensitivity to daunorubicin or the liposomal component
  Pregnancy—Use is not recommended because of embryotoxic and maternotoxic potential; advisability of using contraception
  Breast-feeding—Use is not recommended because of the potential for serious adverse effects in nursing infants
  Other medications, especially daunorubicin, doxorubicin, live virus vaccines, other anthracycline antineoplastics, other bone marrow depressants, previous cytotoxic drug or radiation therapy, probenecid or sulfinpyrazone
  Other medical problems, especially bone marrow depression; cardiac disease, pre-existing; chickenpox; granulocytopenia, severe; hepatic function impairment; herpes zoster; renal function impairment; or tumor cell infiltration of bone marrow

**Proper use of this medication**
Caution in taking combination therapy; taking each medication at the right time
Importance of ample fluid intake and subsequent increase in urine output to aid in excretion of uric acid
Frequency of nausea and vomiting; importance of continuing medication despite stomach upset
» Proper dosing

**Precautions while using this medication**
» Importance of close monitoring by the physician
» Avoiding immunizations unless approved by the physician; other persons in patient's household should avoid immunizations with oral poliovirus vaccine; avoiding persons who have taken oral poliovirus vaccine, or wearing a protective mask that covers nose and mouth
*Caution if bone marrow depression occurs*
» Avoiding exposure to persons with infections, especially during periods of low blood counts; checking with physician immediately if fever or chills, cough or hoarseness, lower back or side pain, or painful or difficult urination occurs
» Checking with physician immediately if unusual bleeding or bruising; black, tarry stools; blood in urine or stools; or pinpoint red spots on skin occur
Caution in use of regular toothbrush, dental floss, or toothpick; physician, dentist, or nurse may suggest alternatives; checking with physician before having dental work done
Not touching eyes or inside of nose unless hands washed immediately before
Using caution to avoid accidental cuts with use of sharp objects such as safety razor or fingernail or toenail cutters
Avoiding contact sports or other situations where bruising or injury could occur

» Possibility of local tissue injury and scarring if infiltration of intravenous solution occurs; telling doctor or nurse right away about redness, pain, or swelling at injection site

**Side/adverse effects**
May cause adverse effects such as blood problems, loss of hair, heart problems, and cancer
Signs of potential side effects, especially dyspnea; neuropathy; neutropenia; anemia; cardiotoxicity; chest pain; edema; gastrointestinal hemorrhage; hemoptysis; hypertension; renal effects, including dysuria, nocturia, or polyuria; stomatitis; syncope; tachycardia; and thrombocytopenia
Physician or nurse can help in dealing with side effects
Reddish urine for 1 to 2 days after administration may be alarming to patient although medically insignificant
Possibility of hair loss; normal hair growth should resume after treatment has ended

## General Dosing Information

Patients receiving liposomal daunorubicin should be under supervision of a physician experienced in cancer chemotherapy.

Liposomal daunorubicin should be administered intravenously over a period of 60 minutes at a dose of 40 mg per square meter of body surface area (mg/m$^2$), with doses repeated every 2 weeks. Blood counts should be performed prior to each dose and therapy should be withheld if the absolute granulocyte count is less than 750 cells/mm$^3$.

Treatment with liposomal daunorubicin should be continued until there is evidence of progressive disease, or until other intercurrent complications of human immunodeficiency virus (HIV) disease preclude continuation of therapy.

Patients may experience an acute reaction following rapid infusion. The reaction usually consists of shortness of breath, facial flushing, back pain, fever, and chills. This reaction is related to the rate of infusion; slowing the infusion rate may eliminate this problem.

If the reaction persists after the infusion rate is decreased, the infusion should be discontinued. After discontinuation of the infusion, intravenous administration of diphenhydramine and hydrocortisone and oxygen administration via facial mask usually helps full recovery with no sequelae.

Dosage should be adjusted for patients with impaired renal function. A dose reduction of 50% is recommended if serum creatinine concentrations are > 3 mg per deciliter (mg/dL).

Dosage should be adjusted for patients with impaired hepatic function. A dose reduction of 25% is recommended if serum bilirubin concentrations are 1.2 to 3 mg/dL. A dose reduction of 50% is recommended if serum bilirubin concentrations are > 3 mg/dL.

**Safety considerations for handling this medication**
There is limited but increasing evidence and concern that personnel involved in preparation and administration of parenteral antineoplastic agents may be at some risk because of the potential mutagenicity, teratogenicity, and/or carcinogenicity of these agents, although the actual risk is unknown. USP advisory panels recommend cautious handling both in preparation and disposal of antineoplastic agents. Precautions that have been suggested include:
- Use of a biological containment cabinet during reconstitution and dilution of parenteral medications and wearing of disposable surgical gloves and masks.
- Use of proper technique to prevent contamination of the medication, work area, and operator during transfer between containers (including proper training of personnel in this technique).
- Cautious and proper disposal of needles, syringes, vials, ampuls, and unused medication.

A number of medical centers have developed detailed guidelines for handling of antineoplastic agents.

## Parenteral Dosage Forms

Note: The dosing and strengths of the dosage forms available are expressed in terms of liposomal daunorubicin base (not the citrate salt).

### DAUNORUBICIN, LIPOSOMAL INJECTION

**Usual adult dose**
AIDS-associated Kaposi's sarcoma—
  Intravenous infusion (over sixty minutes), 40 mg (base) per square meter of body surface area, repeated every two weeks.

  Note: Dosage should be adjusted for patients with impaired renal function. A dose reduction of 50% is recommended if serum creatinine concentrations are > 3 mg per deciliter (mg/dL).

## Daunorubicin, Liposomal (Systemic)

Dosage should be adjusted for patients with impaired hepatic function. A dose reduction of 25% is recommended if serum bilirubin concentrations are 1.2 to 3 mg/dL. A dose reduction of 50% is recommended if serum bilirubin concentrations are > 3 mg/dL.

**Usual pediatric dose**
Safety and efficacy have not been established.

**Usual geriatric dose**
Safety and efficacy have not been established.

**Size(s) usually available**
U.S.—
  2 mg per mL (base) (25-mL, single-dose vial) (Rx) [*DaunoXome*].
Canada—
  Not commercially available.

**Packaging and storage**
Store between 2 and 8 °C (36 and 46 °F). Do not freeze. Protect from light.

**Preparation of dosage form**
Liposomal daunorubicin should be diluted 1:1 with 5% dextrose injection before administration. Each vial of liposomal daunorubicin contains daunorubicin citrate equivalent to 50 mg daunorubicin base at a concentration of 2 mg per mL. The recommended concentration after dilution is 1 mg daunorubicin per mL.
Note: Aseptic techniques should be strictly observed when handling liposomal daunorubicin, since no preservatives or bacteriostatic agents are present in liposomal daunorubicin or in the materials recommended for dilution.

**Stability**
Diluted liposomal daunorubicin is stable for 6 hours when stored between 2 and 8 °C (36 and 46 °F).

**Incompatibilities**
Liposomal daunorubicin should be diluted only in 5% dextrose injection. Liposomal daunorubicin should not be mixed with other medications, other diluents, or bacteriostatic agents. Mixing liposomal daunorubicin with any other diluent may cause precipitation.

**Note**
Liposomal daunorubicin is a red, translucent dispersion. In-line filters should not be used because liposomal daunorubicin is not a clear solution.

Developed: 06/23/98

---

# DECONGESTANTS AND ANALGESICS Systemic

This monograph includes information on the following: 1) Phenylephrine and Acetaminophen; 2) Phenylephrine, Phenylpropanolamine, and Acetaminophen; 3) Phenylpropanolamine and Acetaminophen; 4) Phenylpropanolamine, Acetaminophen, and Aspirin; 5) Phenylpropanolamine, Acetaminophen, and Caffeine; 6) Phenylpropanolamine, Acetaminophen, Salicylamide, and Caffeine; 7) Phenylpropanolamine and Aspirin; 8) Pseudoephedrine and Acetaminophen; 9) Pseudoephedrine and Aspirin; 10) Pseudoephedrine and Ibuprofen.

**VA CLASSIFICATION (Primary):** RE599

**NOTE:** The *Decongestants and Analgesics (Systemic)* monograph is maintained on the USP DI electronic data base. For a printed copy of the most recent revision of the complete monograph, contact Micromedex, Inc. - Reprint Requests, 6200 S. Syracuse Way, Suite 300, Englewood, CO 80111; telephone (303) 486-6400; telefax (303) 486-6464; Email: USPDI@MDX.COM.

For information on the specific components of this combination, see the *USP DI* monographs for *Acetaminophen (Systemic)*, *Anti-inflammatory Drugs, Nonsteroidal (Systemic)*, *Caffeine (Systemic)*, *Phenylpropanolamine (Systemic)*, *Pseudoephedrine (Systemic)*, *Salicylates (Systemic)*, and *Sympathomimetic Agents—Cardiovascular Use (Systemic)*.

The information that follows is selectively abstracted from the complete monograph and is provided to facilitate drug use review and patient counseling.

Note: For a listing of dosage forms and brand names by country availability, see *Dosage Forms* section(s).

## Category
Decongestant-analgesic.

## Indications
**Accepted**
Congestion, nasal (treatment)
Congestion, sinus (treatment) and
Headache, sinus (treatment)—Decongestant and analgesic combinations are indicated for the temporary relief of nasal and sinus congestion and headache pain caused by sinusitis, common colds, allergy, and hay fever.

The therapeutic effectiveness of oral phenylephrine as a nasal decongestant has been questioned, especially at the usual oral dose.

## Patient Consultation
As an aid to patient consultation, refer to *Advice for the Patient, Decongestants and Analgesics (Systemic)*.
In providing consultation, consider emphasizing the following selected information (» = major clinical significance):

**Before using this medication**
» Conditions affecting use, especially:
  Sensitivity to other sympathomimetic amines, salicylates or other nonsteroidal anti-inflammatory drugs
  Pregnancy—Concern with high doses and long-term therapy because of salicylate effects; use of aspirin-containing combinations not recommended during third trimester; use of ibuprofen-containing combinations during second half of pregnancy not recommended because of potential adverse effect on fetal blood flow
  Breast-feeding—High risk for infants from sympathomimetic amines; also, concern with high doses and chronic use because of high salicylate intake by infant
  Use in children—Increased sensitivity to vasopressor and psychiatric effects of sympathomimetic amines; also, increased susceptibility to toxic effects of salicylates, especially if fever and dehydration present; possible association between aspirin usage and Reye's syndrome
  Use in adolescents—Possible association between aspirin usage and Reye's syndrome
  Use in the elderly—Increased susceptibility to effects of sympathomimetic amines and toxic effects of salicylates; increased risk of toxicity with ibuprofen
  Other medications, especially for high blood pressure or depression, CNS depressants or stimulants, and others that may interact with acetaminophen, ibuprofen, and/or salicylates depending on specific ingredients of combination
  Other medical problems, especially hypertension (for all combinations); alcoholism or hepatitis (for acetaminophen-containing combinations); hemophilia or other bleeding problems (for aspirin-containing combinations); asthma, gastritis, or peptic ulcer (with salicylate-containing combinations); clotting defects, peptic ulcer or other gastrointestinal tract disease, or stomatitis (for ibuprofen-containing combinations)

**Proper use of this medication**
» Importance of not taking more medication than the amount recommended
» Proper dosing
  Missed dose: If on scheduled dosing regimen—Taking as soon as possible; not taking if almost time for next dose; not doubling doses
» Proper storage
*For salicylate-containing combinations*
  Taking with food or a full glass (240 mL) of water to minimize gastrointestinal irritation
» Not taking combinations containing aspirin if a strong vinegar-like odor is present
*For ibuprofen-containing combinations*
  Taking with food or antacids (a magnesium- and aluminum-containing antacid may be preferred) to reduce gastrointestinal irritation; not lying down for 15 to 30 minutes after taking

**Precautions while using this medication**
  Checking with physician if symptoms persist or become worse, or if high fever is present
» Caution if taking phenylpropanolamine-containing appetite suppressants

» Possible insomnia; taking the medication a few hours before bedtime
Need to inform physician or dentist of use of medication if any kind of surgery (including dental surgery or emergency treatment is required)
» Caution if other medications containing acetaminophen, aspirin, or other salicylates (including diflunisal) are used
Avoiding use of alcoholic beverages while taking these medications; alcohol consumption may increase risk of ibuprofen- or salicylate-induced gastrointestinal toxicity and acetaminophen-induced liver toxicity
» Suspected overdose: Getting emergency help at once
Not taking products containing aspirin for 5 days prior to any kind of surgery, unless otherwise directed by physician
Diabetics: Aspirin present in some combination formulations may cause false urine sugar test results with prolonged use of 8 or more 325-mg (5-grain) doses per day

*For ibuprofen-containing combinations*
» Caution if drowsiness or dizziness occurs

### Side/adverse effects

Signs of potential side effects, especially allergic reactions, anemia, cardiac effects, CNS stimulation, psychotic episodes, severe dizziness, severe nervousness or restlessness (for all combinations); blood dyscrasias, hepatitis, hepatotoxicity (for acetaminophen-containing); signs of gastrointestinal irritation or bleeding (for ibuprofen- or salicylate-containing); and cutaneous adverse effects, hepatitis, renal impairment (for ibuprofen-containing)

## Oral Dosage Forms

See *Table 1*, page 1181.

Revised: 09/07/94
Interim revision: 07/18/95; 08/28/96

### Table 1. Oral Dosage Forms

Note: Content per capsule, tablet, or 5 mL, unless otherwise stated.

| Brand or generic name [availability] | Decongestants | Analgesics | Other content information as per product label | Usual adult and adolescent dose*(prn) | Usual pediatric dose (prn) | Packaging, storage, and auxiliary labeling |
|---|---|---|---|---|---|---|
| *Actifed Sinus Daytime* Tablets USP (OTC) [U.S.] | Pseudoephedrine HCl 30 mg | Acetaminophen 500 mg | Available in a dual package that also contains *Actifed Sinus Nighttime Tablets* | 2 tabs q 6 hr (max 8 total *Daytime* and *Nighttime* tabs/day) | Not recommended | † |
| *Actifed Sinus Daytime Caplets* Tablets USP (OTC) [U.S.] | Pseudoephedrine HCl 30 mg | Acetaminophen 500 mg | Available in a dual package that also contains *Actifed Sinus Nighttime Caplets* | 2 tabs q 6 hr (max 8 total *Daytime* and *Nighttime* tabs/day) | Not recommended | † |
| *Advil Cold and Sinus* Tablets USP (OTC) [U.S.] | Pseudoephedrine HCl 30 mg | Ibuprofen 200 mg | | 1–2 tabs q 4–6 hr (max 6 tabs/day) | | † |
| *Advil Cold and Sinus Caplets* Tablets USP (OTC) [U.S./Canada] | Pseudoephedrine HCl 30 mg | Ibuprofen 200 mg | | 1–2 tabs q 4–6 hr (max 6 tabs/day) | | † |
| *Alka-Seltzer Plus Sinus Medicine* Effervescent Tablets (OTC) [U.S.] | Phenylpropanolamine bitartrate 20 mg | Aspirin 325 mg | Sodium 504 mg Phenylalanine 12.32 mg | 2 tabs q 4 hr dissolved in 120 mL water (max 8 tabs/day) | | † |
| *Allerest No-Drowsiness Caplets* Tablets USP (OTC) [U.S.] | Pseudoephedrine HCl 30 mg | Acetaminophen 325 mg | | 2 tabs q 4–6 hr (max 8 tabs daily) | 6–12 yrs: 1 tab q 4–6 hr (max 4 tabs/day) | † |
| *Aspirin-Free Bayer Select Sinus Pain Relief Caplets* Tablets USP (OTC) [U.S.] | Pseudoephedrine HCl 30 mg | Acetaminophen 500 mg | | 2 tabs q 4–6 hr (max 8 tabs/day) | | † |
| *BC Cold Powder Non-Drowsy Formula* for Oral Solution (OTC) [U.S.] | Phenylpropanolamine HCl 25 mg/packet | Aspirin 650 mg/packet | Lactose | 1 packet dissolved in water q 3–4 hr (max 4 doses/day) | | † |
| *Coldrine* Tablets USP (OTC) [U.S.] | Pseudoephedrine HCl 30 mg | Acetaminophen 325 mg | Sodium metabisulfate | 2 tabs q 6 hr | | † |
| *Contac Allergy/Sinus Day Caplets* Tablets USP (OTC) [U.S.] | Pseudoephedrine HCl 60 mg | Acetaminophen 650 mg | Available in a dual package that also contains *Contac Allergy/ Sinus Night Caplets* | 1 tab q 6 hr (max 4 tabs/day) | | † |

*Geriatric patients may be more sensitive to the effects of usual adult dose.
†Store below 40 °C (104 °F), preferably between 15 and 30 °C (59 and 86 °F), in a tight container, unless otherwise specified by manufacturer.

## Table 1. Oral Dosage Forms (continued)

Note: Content per capsule, tablet, or 5 mL, unless otherwise stated.

| Brand or generic name [availability] | Decongestants | Analgesics | Other content information as per product label | Usual adult and adolescent dose*(prn) | Usual pediatric dose (prn) | Packaging, storage, and auxiliary labeling |
|---|---|---|---|---|---|---|
| *Contac Non-Drowsy Formula Sinus Caplets* Tablets USP (OTC) [U.S.] | Pseudoephedrine HCl 30 mg | Acetaminophen 500 mg | | 2 tab q 6 hr | | † |
| *Coricidin Non-Drowsy Sinus Formula* Tablets (OTC) [Canada] | Phenylpropanolamine HCl 12.5 mg | Aspirin 325 mg | | 2 tabs q 4 hr (max 8 tabs/day) | | † |
| *Dilotab* Tablets (OTC) [Canada] | Phenylpropanolamine HCl 12.5 mg | Acetaminophen 325 mg | | 2 tabs q 4 hr (max 8 tabs/day) | 6–12 yrs: 1 tab q 4 hr (max 4 tabs/day) | † |
| *Dimetapp-A Sinus* Tablets (OTC) [Canada] | Phenylephrine HCl 5 mg, Phenylpropanolamine HCl 5 mg | Acetaminophen 325 mg | Scored | 1–2 tabs q 4–6 hr (max 8 tabs/day) | | † |
| *Dimetapp Sinus Caplets* Tablets USP (OTC) [U.S.] | Pseudoephedrine HCl 30 mg | Ibuprofen 200 mg | | 1–2 tabs q 4–6 hr (max 6 tabs/day) | | † |
| *Dristan Cold Caplets* Tablets USP (OTC) [U.S.] | Pseudoephedrine HCl 30 mg | Acetaminophen 500 mg | | 2 tabs q 4–6 hr (max 8 tabs/day) | | † |
| *Dristan N.D. Caplets* Tablets USP (OTC) [Canada] | Pseudoephedrine HCl 30 mg | Acetaminophen 325 mg | | 2 tabs q 4 hr (max 8 tabs/day) | 6–12 yrs: 1 tab q 4 hr (max 4 tabs/day) | † |
| *Dristan N.D. Extra Strength Caplets* Tablets USP (OTC) [Canada] | Pseudoephedrine HCl 30 mg | Acetaminophen 500 mg | | 1–2 tabs q 4–6 hr (max 8 tabs/day) | | † |
| *Dristan Sinus Caplets* Tablets USP (OTC) [U.S.] | Pseudoephedrine HCl 30 mg | Ibuprofen 200 mg | | 1–2 tabs q 4–6 hr | | † |
| *Dynafed Maximum Strength* Tablets USP (OTC) [U.S.] | Pseudoephedrine HCl 30 mg | Acetaminophen 500 mg | | 2 tabs q 4–6 hr (max 8 tabs/day) | | † |
| *Emertabs* Tablets (OTC) [Canada] | Phenylpropanolamine HCl 16.2 mg | Acetaminophen 325 mg | Caffeine alkaloid 16.2 mg | 1 tab q 4 hr | | † |
| *Motrin IB Sinus* Tablets USP (OTC) [U.S.] | Pseudoephedrine HCl 30 mg | Ibuprofen 200 mg | | 1–2 tabs q 4–6 hr (max 6 tabs/day) | | † |
| *Motrin IB Sinus Caplets* Tablets USP (OTC) [U.S.] | Pseudoephedrine HCl 30 mg | Ibuprofen 200 mg | | 1–2 tabs q 4–6 hr (max 6 tabs/day) | | † |
| *Neo Citran Extra Strength Sinus* for Oral Solution (OTC) [Canada] | Phenylephrine HCl 10 mg/pouch | Acetaminophen 650 mg/pouch | Vitamin C 50 mg/pouch | Contents of 1 pouch dissolved in 225 mL hot water | | † |
| *Ornex Maximum Strength Caplets* Tablets USP (OTC) [U.S.] | Pseudoephedrine HCl 30 mg | Acetaminophen 500 mg | | 2 tabs q 4–6 hr (max 8 tabs/day) | | † |
| *Ornex No Drowsiness Caplets* Tablets USP (OTC) [U.S.] | Pseudoephedrine HCl 30 mg | Acetaminophen 325 mg | | 2 tabs q 4 hr (max 8 tabs/day) | 6–11 yrs: 1 tab q 4 hr (max 4 tabs/day) | † |
| *PhenAPAP Without Drowsiness* Tablets (OTC) [U.S.] | Pseudoephedrine HCl 30 mg | Acetaminophen 325 mg | | 2 tabs q 4 hr (max 8 tabs/day) | | † |
| *Rhinocaps* Capsules (OTC) [U.S.] | Phenylpropanolamine HCl 20 mg | Acetaminophen 162 mg, Aspirin 162 mg | | 2 caps q 4–6 hr (max 6 caps/day) | | † |

## Table 1. Oral Dosage Forms *(continued)*

Note: Content per capsule, tablet, or 5 mL, unless otherwise stated.

| Brand or generic name [availability] | Decongestants | Analgesics | Other content information as per product label | Usual adult and adolescent dose*(prn) | Usual pediatric dose (prn) | Packaging, storage, and auxiliary labeling |
|---|---|---|---|---|---|---|
| *Saleto D Caplets* Tablets (OTC) [U.S.] | Phenylpropanolamine HCl 18 mg | Acetaminophen 240 mg, Salicylamide 120 mg | Caffeine 16 mg Sodium metabisulfite | 1 tab q 4 hr (max 6 tabs/day) | | † |
| *Sinarest No-Drowsiness Caplets* Tablets USP (OTC) [U.S.] | Pseudoephedrine HCl 30 mg | Acetaminophen 325 mg | | 2 tabs q 4–6 hr (max 8 tabs/day) | 6–12 yrs: 1 tab q 4–6 hr (max 4 tabs/day) | † |
| *Sine-Aid IB Caplets* Tablets USP (OTC) [U.S.] | Pseudoephedrine HCl 30 mg | Ibuprofen 200 mg | | 1–2 tabs q 4–6 hr (max 6 tabs/day) | | † |
| *Sine-Aid Maximum Strength Tablets* Tablets USP (OTC) [U.S.] | Pseudoephedrine HCl 30 mg | Acetaminophen 500 mg | | 2 tabs q 4–6 hr (max 8 tabs/day) | Not recommended | † |
| *Sine-Aid Maximum Strength Caplets* Tablets USP (OTC) [U.S.] | Pseudoephedrine HCl 30 mg | Acetaminophen 500 mg | | 2 tabs q 4–6 hr (max 8 tabs/day) | Not recommended | † |
| *Sine-Aid Maximum Strength Gelcaps* Tablets USP (OTC) [U.S.] | Pseudoephedrine HCl 30 mg | Acetaminophen 500 mg | | 2 tabs q 4–6 hr (max 8 tabs/day) | Not recommended | † |
| *Sine-Off Maximum Strength No Drowsiness Formula Caplets* Tablets USP (OTC) [U.S.] | Pseudoephedrine HCl 30 mg | Acetaminophen 500 mg | | 2 tabs q 6 hr (max 8 tabs/day) | | † |
| *Sinus Excedrin Extra Strength Tablets* USP (OTC) [U.S.] | Pseudoephedrine HCl 30 mg | Acetaminophen 500 mg | | 2 tabs q 6 hr (max 8 tabs/day) | | † |
| *Sinus Excedrin Extra Strength Caplets* Tablets USP (OTC) [U.S.] | Pseudoephedrine HCl 30 mg | Acetaminophen 500 mg | | 2 tabs q 6 hr (max 8 tabs/day) | | † |
| *Sinus-Relief* Tablets USP (OTC) [U.S.] | Pseudoephedrine HCl 30 mg | Acetaminophen 325 mg | | 2 tabs q 4 hr (max 8 tabs/day) | | † |
| *Sinutab No Drowsiness Caplets* Tablets USP (OTC) [Canada] | Pseudoephedrine HCl 30 mg | Acetaminophen 325 mg | Scored Tartrazine free | 2 tabs q 4–6 hr (max 8 tabs/day) | >6 yrs: 1 tab q 4–6 hr (max 4 tabs/day) | † |
| *Sinutab No Drowsiness Extra Strength Caplets* Tablets USP (OTC) [Canada] | Pseudoephedrine HCl 30 mg | Acetaminophen 500 mg | Tartrazine free | 1–2 tabs q 4–6 hr (max 8 tabs/day) | | † |
| *Sinutab Sinus Maximum Strength Without Drowsiness* Tablets USP (OTC) [U.S.] | Pseudoephedrine HCl 30 mg | Acetaminophen 500 mg | | 2 tabs q 6 hr (max 8 tabs/24 hr) | | † |
| *Sinutab Sinus Maximum Strength Without Drowsiness Caplets* Tablets USP (OTC) [U.S.] | Pseudoephedrine HCl 30 mg | Acetaminophen 500 mg | | 2 tabs q 6 hr (max 8 tabs/24 hr) | | † |
| *Sinutrol 500 Caplets* Tablets USP (OTC) [U.S.] | Pseudoephedrine HCl 30 mg | Acetaminophen 500 mg | Dye free | 2 tabs q 4–6 hr (max 8 tabs/day) | | † |
| *Sudafed Head Cold and Sinus Extra Strength Caplets* Tablets USP (OTC) [Canada] | Pseudoephedrine HCl 60 mg | Acetaminophen 500 mg | | 1 tab q 4–6 hr (max 4 tabs/day) | | † |

*Geriatric patients may be more sensitive to the effects of usual adult dose.
†Store below 40 °C (104 °F), preferably between 15 and 30 °C (59 and 86 °F), in a tight container, unless otherwise specified by manufacturer.

## Table 1. Oral Dosage Forms (continued)

Note: Content per capsule, tablet, or 5 mL, unless otherwise stated.

| Brand or generic name [availability] | Decongestants | Analgesics | Other content information as per product label | Usual adult and adolescent dose*(prn) | Usual pediatric dose (prn) | Packaging, storage, and auxiliary labeling |
|---|---|---|---|---|---|---|
| *Sudafed Sinus Maximum Strength Without Drowsiness* Tablets USP (OTC) [U.S.] | Pseudoephedrine HCl 30 mg | Acetaminophen 500 mg | | 2 tabs q 6 hr (max 8 tabs/day) | Not recommended | † |
| *Sudafed Sinus Maximum Strength Without Drowsiness Caplets* Tablets USP (OTC) [U.S.] | Pseudoephedrine HCl 30 mg | Acetaminophen 500 mg | | 2 tabs q 6 hr (max 8 tabs/day) | Not recommended | † |
| *TheraFlu Sinus Maximum Strength Caplets* Tablets USP (OTC) [U.S.] | Pseudoephedrine HCl 30 mg | Acetaminophen 500 mg | | 2 tabs q 6 hr (max 8 tabs/day) | | † |
| *Tylenol Sinus Maximum Strength* Tablets USP (OTC) [U.S.] | Pseudoephedrine HCl 30 mg | Acetaminophen 500 mg | | 2 tabs q 4–6 hr (max 8 tabs/day) | Not recommended | † |
| *Tylenol Sinus Maximum Strength Caplets* Tablets USP (OTC) [U.S.] | Pseudoephedrine HCl 30 mg | Acetaminophen 500 mg | | 2 tabs q 4–6 hr (max 8 tabs/day) | Not recommended | † |
| *Tylenol Sinus Maximum Strength Gelcaps* Capsules USP (OTC) [U.S.] | Pseudoephedrine HCl 30 mg | Acetaminophen 500 mg | | 2 caps q 4–6 hr (max 8 caps/day) | Not recommended | † |
| *Tylenol Sinus Maximum Strength Geltabs* Tablets USP (OTC) [U.S.] | Pseudoephedrine HCl 30 mg | Acetaminophen 500 mg | | 2 tabs q 4–6 hr (max 8 tabs/day) | Not recommended | † |
| *Tylenol Sinus Medication Regular Strength Caplets* Tablets USP (OTC) [Canada] | Pseudoephedrine HCl 30 mg | Acetaminophen 325 mg | Tartrazine free | 1–2 tabs q 4–6 hr (max 8 tabs/day) | | † |
| *Tylenol Sinus Medication Extra Strength Caplets* Tablets USP (OTC) [Canada] | Pseudoephedrine HCl 30 mg | Acetaminophen 500 mg | Tartrazine free | 1–2 tabs q 4–6 hr (max 8 tabs/day) | | † |
| *Ursinus Inlay* Tablets (OTC) [U.S.] | Pseudoephedrine HCl 30 mg | Aspirin 325 mg | | 2 tabs q 4 hr (max 8 tabs/day) | | † |
| *Vicks DayQuil Sinus Pressure & Pain Relief Caplets* Tablets USP (OTC) [U.S.] | Pseudoephedrine HCl 30 mg | Ibuprofen 200 mg | | 1–2 tabs q 4–6 hr (max 6 tabs/day) | | † |

*Geriatric patients may be more sensitive to the effects of usual adult dose.
†Store below 40 °C (104 °F), preferably between 15 and 30 °C (59 and 86 °F), in a tight container, unless otherwise specified by manufacturer.

**DEFEROXAMINE**—The *Deferoxamine (Systemic)* monograph is not included in this published version of the USP DI database. Copies of the monograph are available on request from Micromedex, Inc. - Reprint Requests, 6200 S. Syracuse Way, Suite 300, Englewood, CO 80111; telephone (303) 486-6400; telefax (303) 486-6464; Email: USPDI@MDX.COM.

# DELAVIRDINE  Systemic—INTRODUCTORY VERSION†

VA CLASSIFICATION (Primary): AM804
Commonly used brand name(s): *Rescriptor*.
Note: For a listing of dosage forms and brand names by country availability, see *Dosage Forms* section(s).

†Not commercially available in Canada.

## Category
Antiviral (systemic).

## Indications

**General considerations**
Delavirdine is a non-nucleoside reverse transcriptase inhibitor. Delavirdine used alone or in combination with other antiretroviral agents may confer cross-resistance to other non-nucleoside reverse transcriptase inhibitors. However, the potential for cross-resistance between delavirdine and nucleoside analog reverse transcriptase inhibitors is low because of the different sites of binding on the viral enzyme and distinct mechanisms of action. Also, the potential for cross-resistance between delavirdine

and protease inhibitors is low because of the different enzyme targets involved.

Reduced sensitivity to delavirdine develops rapidly when it is administered as monotherapy.

**Accepted**

Human immunodeficiency virus (HIV) infection (treatment)—Delavirdine is indicated in the treatment of human immunodeficiency virus type 1 (HIV-1) infection in combination with other appropriate antiretroviral therapy.

## Pharmacology/Pharmacokinetics

**Physicochemical characteristics**
Molecular weight—Delavirdine mesylate: 552.68.

**Mechanism of action/Effect**
Delavirdine binds directly to HIV-1 reverse transcriptase and blocks RNA-dependent and DNA-dependent DNA polymerase activities. HIV-1 group 0, a group of highly divergent strains that are uncommon in North America, may not be inhibited by delavirdine. Human DNA polymerase activities are not affected.

**Absorption**
Delavirdine is rapidly absorbed following its oral administration. The bioavailability of delavirdine tablets is increased by approximately 20% when the medication is dissolved in water prior to administration.

**Distribution**
Delavirdine is distributed predominantly into blood plasma.

**Protein binding**
Very high (approximately 98%); primarily to albumin.

**Biotransformation**
Delavirdine is extensively converted to several inactive metabolites, primarily by the enzyme cytochrome P450 3A (CYP3A). Delavirdine reduces the activity of CYP3A, thereby inhibiting the metabolism of delavirdine. Inhibition of CYP3A by delavirdine is reversible within 1 week after discontinuation of therapy.

The major metabolic pathways for delavirdine are *N*-desalkylation and pyridine hydroxylation.

**Half-life**
Elimination from plasma—Mean, 5.8 hours (range, 2 to 11 hours) following treatment with 400 mg three times a day. The apparent half-life increases with dose.

**Time to peak plasma concentration**
Approximately 1 hour.

**Peak plasma concentration**
Mean ± SD steady-state concentration in plasma, approximately 16.1 ± 9.2 mcg/mL (35 ± 20 micromoles per L [micromoles/L]) (range, 0.92 to 46 mcg/mL [2 to 100 micromoles/L]) following doses of 400 mg three times a day; systemic exposure as measured by the area under the plasma concentration–time curve (AUC) is 82.8 ± 46 mcg/mL (180 ± 100 micromoles/L) per hour (range, 2.3 to 236 mcg/mL [5 to 513 micromoles/L] per hour); trough concentration is 6.9 ± 4.6 mcg/mL (15 ± 10 micromoles/L) (range, 0.046 to 20.7 mcg/mL [0.1 to 45 micromoles/L]).

The median AUC in female patients is 31% higher than in male patients following doses of 400 mg every 8 hours.

**Elimination**
Fecal—44%, following multiple doses of 330 mg three times a day in healthy volunteers.

Renal—51%, following multiple doses of 330 mg three times a day in healthy volunteers. Less than 5% of the dose is recovered unchanged in urine.

## Precautions to Consider

**Carcinogenicity**
Long-term carcinogenicity studies have not been completed.

**Mutagenicity**
Delavirdine is not mutagenic *in vitro* in the Ames test, unscheduled DNA synthesis test, chromosome aberration assay in human lymphocytes, or mammalian cell mutation assay in Chinese hamster ovary cells, or *in vivo* in the mouse micronucleus assay.

**Pregnancy/Reproduction**
Fertility—Dosages of 20, 100, and 200 mg of delavirdine per kg of body weight (mg/kg) per day did not impair fertility in male or female rats.

Pregnancy—Adequate and well-controlled studies have not been done in humans.

Delavirdine is teratogenic in rats. Dosages of 50, 100, and 200 mg/kg per day in pregnant rats during organogenesis caused ventricular septal defects. Exposure of rats to doses approximately five times higher than the expected human exposure resulted in marked maternal toxicity, embryotoxicity, fetal development delay, and reduced pup survival. Delavirdine also has been studied in rabbits. Dosages of 200 and 400 mg/kg per day in pregnant rabbits during organogenesis resulted in abortions, embryotoxicity, and maternal toxicity. The lowest dose of delavirdine that caused these toxic effects produced systemic exposures in pregnant rabbits approximately six times higher than that expected in humans at the recommended dose. Although malformations were not apparent at these dosages, only a limited number of fetuses were available for examination due to maternal and embryo death. The no-observed-adverse-effect dose in pregnant rabbits was 100 mg/kg per day, a dosage that exposed rabbits to a lower plasma concentration of delavirdine than would be expected in humans at the recommended clinical dose.

FDA Pregnancy Category C.

**Breast-feeding**
It is not known whether delavirdine is distributed into breast milk. However, breast-feeding is not recommended for HIV-infected mothers because of the potential for postnatal transmission of HIV to uninfected infants.

Delavirdine is distributed into milk in rats.

**Pediatrics**
Appropriate studies on the relationship of age to the effects of delavirdine have not been performed in children up to 16 years of age. Safety and efficacy have not been established.

**Geriatrics**
No information is available on the relationship of age to the pharmacokinetics of delavirdine in patients older than 65 years of age. Safety and efficacy have not been established.

**Drug interactions and/or related problems**
The following drug interactions and/or related problems have been selected on the basis of their potential clinical significance (possible mechanism in parentheses where appropriate)—not necessarily inclusive (» = major clinical significance):

Note: Combinations containing any of the following medications, depending on the amount present, may also interact with this medication.

» Amphetamines or
» Astemizole or
» Benzodiazepines or
» Calcium channel blocking agents or
» Cisapride or
» Ergot derivatives or
» Terfenadine
  (concurrent administration of amphetamines, astemizole, benzodiazepines, calcium channel blocking agents, cisapride, ergot derivatives, or terfenadine with delavirdine may result in potentially serious and/or life-threatening adverse events as a result of the inhibitory effect of delavirdine on CYP isoenzymes 3A and 2C9; it is recommended that dosage adjustments be made for these medications, or that alternative medications be used, while patients are taking delavirdine)

Antacids
  (concurrent administration of delavirdine 300 mg with aluminum and magnesium oral suspension decreases the area under the plasma concentration–time curve [AUC] for delavirdine by 41 ± 19%; patients should be advised not to take antacids within 1 hour of taking delavirdine)

» Carbamazepine or
» Phenobarbital or
» Phenytoin
  (concurrent use of delavirdine with carbamazepine, phenobarbital, or phenytoin substantially decreases the trough plasma concentration of delavirdine; concurrent use is not recommended)

» Cimetidine or
» Famotidine or
» Nizatidine or
» Ranitidine
  (cimetidine, famotidine, nizatidine, and ranitidine increase gastric pH and may reduce absorption of delavirdine; long-term use of these medications with delavirdine is not recommended)

» Clarithromycin
  (concurrent administration of delavirdine 300 mg three times a day with clarithromycin 500 mg two times a day increases the AUC for delavirdine by 44 ± 50%; the AUC for clarithromycin increases by approximately 100%)

Didanosine
(concurrent administration of delavirdine 400 mg three times a day with didanosine 125 or 250 mg two times a day, for 2 weeks, decreases the AUCs for delavirdine and didanosine by approximately 20% as compared with administration of delavirdine and didanosine at least 1 hour apart; patients should be advised not to take didanosine within 1 hour of taking delavirdine)

Fluoxetine or
Ketoconazole
(concurrent administration increases the trough plasma concentration of delavirdine by approximately 50%)

» Indinavir
(delavirdine inhibits the metabolism of indinavir; concurrent administration of delavirdine 400 mg three times a day with a single 400-mg dose of indinavir results in AUC values for indinavir that are slightly less than those observed following administration of a single 800-mg dose of indinavir alone; it is recommended that the dose of indinavir be reduced to 600 mg three times a day when used concurrently with delavirdine; however, safety and efficacy of this combination have not been established)

» Rifabutin
(concurrent administration of delavirdine 400 mg three times a day with rifabutin 300 mg once a day decreases the AUC for delavirdine by 80 ± 10%; the AUC for rifabutin increases by at least 100%; concurrent use is not recommended)

» Rifampin
(concurrent administration of delavirdine 400 mg three times a day with rifampin 600 mg once a day decreases the AUC for delavirdine by 96 ± 4%; concurrent use is not recommended)

Saquinavir
(concurrent administration of delavirdine 400 mg three times a day with saquinavir 600 mg three times a day decreases the AUC for delavirdine by 15 ± 16%; the AUC for saquinavir increases fivefold; safety and efficacy of this combination have not been established)

**Laboratory value alterations**
The following have been selected on the basis of their potential clinical significance (possible effect in parentheses where appropriate)—not necessarily inclusive (» = major clinical significance):

With physiology/laboratory test values
Alanine aminotransferase (ALT [SGPT]) and
Aspartate aminotransferase (AST [SGOT])
(serum values may be increased)
Neutrophil count
(may be reduced)

**Medical considerations/Contraindications**
The medical considerations/contraindications included have been selected on the basis of their potential clinical significance (reasons given in parentheses where appropriate)—not necessarily inclusive (» = major clinical significance).

*Risk-benefit should be considered when the following medical problem exists:*
» Hepatic function impairment
(delavirdine is metabolized primarily by the liver)

## Side/Adverse Effects
The following side/adverse effects have been selected on the basis of their potential clinical significance (possible signs and symptoms in parentheses where appropriate)—not necessarily inclusive:

**Those indicating need for medical attention**
Incidence more frequent
*Skin rash, severe, with itching*
Incidence less frequent
*Blisters; conjunctivitis* (eye inflammation); *fever; joint aches; muscle aches; oral lesions* (sores in mouth); *swelling*
Incidence rare
*Dyspnea* (difficulty in breathing)

**Those indicating need for medical attention only if they continue or are bothersome**
Incidence more frequent
*Diarrhea; fatigue* (unusual tiredness or weakness); *headache; nausea*
Incidence less frequent
*Vomiting*

## Overdose
For more information on the management of overdose or unintentional ingestion, **contact a Poison Control Center** (see *Poison Control Center Listing*).
No cases of overdose have been reported in humans. However, doses of up to 850 mg three times a day for up to 6 months have been taken without serious medication-related events.

**Treatment of overdose**
To decrease absorption—Unabsorbed delavirdine should be removed by emesis or gastric lavage.
Monitoring—Vital signs should be monitored.
Supportive care—Patients should receive supportive therapy. Patients in whom intentional overdose is confirmed or suspected should be referred for psychiatric consultation.

## Patient Consultation
As an aid to patient consultation, refer to *Advice for the Patient, Delavirdine (Systemic)—Introductory Version*.
In providing consultation, consider emphasizing the following selected information (» = major clinical significance):

**Before using this medication**
» Conditions affecting use, especially:
Hypersensitivity to delavirdine
Breast-feeding—It is not known whether delavirdine is distributed into breast milk; however, breast-feeding is not recommended for HIV-infected mothers
Other medications, especially amphetamines, astemizole, benzodiazepines, calcium channel blocking agents, carbamazepine, cimetidine, cisapride, clarithromycin, ergot derivatives, famotidine, indinavir, nizatidine, phenobarbital, phenytoin, ranitidine, rifabutin, rifampin, and terfenadine
Other medical problems, especially hepatic function impairment

**Proper use of this medication**
Taking with or without food
Taking tablets whole or after dispersion in water
Not taking within 1 hour of antacids
» Importance of not taking more medication than prescribed; importance of not discontinuing medication without checking with physician
» Compliance with full course of therapy
» Proper dosing
Missed dose: Taking as soon as possible; not taking if almost time for next dose; not doubling doses
» Proper storage

**Precautions while using this medication**
» Regular visits to physician to check progress

**Side/adverse effects**
Signs of potential side effects, especially severe skin rash with itching, blisters, conjunctivitis, fever, joint aches, muscle aches, oral lesions, swelling, or dyspnea.

## General Dosing Information
Delavirdine should be used in combination with other antiretroviral agents.
Patients with achlorhydria should take delavirdine with an acidic beverage such as orange juice or cranberry juice.
Delavirdine should be taken at least 1 hour before or after taking antacids or didanosine.

**For treatment of adverse effects**
Recommended treatment consists of the following:
• Symptomatic relief of skin rash with diphenhydramine hydrochloride, hydroxyzine hydrochloride, and/or topical corticosteroids.

## Oral Dosage Forms

### DELAVIRDINE MESYLATE TABLETS
**Usual adult dose**
Human immunodeficiency virus (HIV) infection—
Oral, 400 mg three times a day.

**Usual pediatric dose**
Safety and efficacy have not been established in children up to 16 years of age.

**Usual geriatric dose**
Safety and efficacy have not been established in patients older than 65 years of age.

**Strength(s) usually available**
U.S.—
100 mg (Rx) [*Rescriptor* (lactose)].

**Packaging and storage**
Store between 20 and 25 °C (68 and 77 °F) in a tight container. Protect from high humidity.

**Preparation of dosage form**
Delavirdine tablets may be dispersed in water prior to consumption. To prepare a dispersion, four 100-mg tablets should be added to at least three ounces of water and allowed to stand for a few minutes. The mixture should then be stirred until a uniform dispersion occurs. This dispersion should be consumed promptly. The glass should be rinsed and the rinse swallowed to ensure that the entire dose is consumed.

Developed: 10/17/97

---

**DEHYDROCHOLIC ACID** — See *Laxatives (Local)*

---

**DEMECARIUM** — See *Antiglaucoma Agents, Cholinergic, Long-acting (Ophthalmic)*

---

**DEMECLOCYCLINE** — See *Tetracyclines (Systemic)*

---

**DESERPIDINE** — See *Rauwolfia Alkaloids (Systemic)*

---

**DESFLURANE** — The *Desflurane (Inhalation-Systemic)* monograph is not included in this published version of the USP DI database. Copies of the monograph are available on request from Micromedex, Inc. - Reprint Requests, 6200 S. Syracuse Way, Suite 300, Englewood, CO 80111; telephone (303) 486-6400; telefax (303) 486-6464; Email: USPDI@MDX.COM.

---

**DESIPRAMINE** — See *Antidepressants, Tricyclic (Systemic)*

---

# DESMOPRESSIN  Systemic

VA CLASSIFICATION (Primary/Secondary): HS702/CV900; BL116

Commonly used brand name(s): *DDAVP; DDAVP Nasal Spray; DDAVP Rhinal Tube; DDAVP Rhinyle Nasal Solution; DDAVP Spray; Octostim; Stimate; Stimate Nasal Spray.*

Note: For a listing of dosage forms and brand names by country availability, see *Dosage Forms* section(s).

## Category

Antidiuretic (central diabetes insipidus)—Desmopressin Acetate Nasal Solution; Desmopressin Acetate Injection.
Antidiuretic (primary nocturnal enuresis)—Desmopressin Acetate Nasal Solution.
Antihemorrhagic—Desmopressin Acetate Injection.

## Indications

**Accepted**

Diabetes insipidus, central (treatment)—Desmopressin is indicated for the prevention or control of polydipsia, polyuria, and dehydration associated with central diabetes insipidus caused by insufficient antidiuretic hormone. Its efficacy, ease of administration, long duration of action, and relative lack of side effects make desmopressin the drug of choice for central diabetes insipidus.

Desmopressin is preferred to vasopressin injection and oral antidiuretics for use in children. Children have been found to respond well to desmopressin therapy.

Desmopressin is also indicated to manage temporary polydipsia and polyuria associated with trauma to, or surgery in, the pituitary region.

Desmopressin is ineffective in the treatment of nephrogenic diabetes insipidus or polyuria associated with psychogenic diabetes insipidus, renal disease, hypokalemia, hypercalcemia, or the administration of demeclocycline or lithium.

Enuresis, primary nocturnal (treatment)—Desmopressin nasal solution is indicated in the treatment of primary nocturnal enuresis.

Hemophilia A (treatment) or
von Willebrand's disease (treatment)—The injectable form of desmopressin is indicated for patients with mild hemophilia A or mild to moderate classic von Willebrand's disease (Type I), with factor VIII concentrations greater than 5%. It is useful when administered 15 to 30 minutes before surgery to maintain hemostasis. Desmopressin will usually stop the bleeding in these patients with episodes of spontaneous or trauma-induced hemarthroses, intramuscular hematomas, or mucosal bleeding.

Desmopressin is not indicated for patients with factor VIII concentrations of 5% or less (except in certain clinical situations with careful monitoring), or in patients who have factor VIII antibodies. Desmopressin is not indicated for treatment of severe classic von Willebrand's disease (Type III) and when there is evidence of an abnormal molecular form of von Willebrand antigen. In patients with Type IIB von Willebrand's disease, desmopressin may induce platelet aggregation, and use is not recommended.

## Pharmacology/Pharmacokinetics

**Physicochemical characteristics**
Source—Synthetic polypeptide structurally related to the posterior pituitary hormone arginine vasopressin (antidiuretic hormone).
Molecular weight—1183.32.

**Mechanism of action/Effect**
Antidiuretic—Increases water reabsorption in the kidney by increasing the cellular permeability of the collecting ducts, resulting in an increase in urine osmolality with a concurrent decrease in urine output.
Antihemorrhagic—Increases plasma levels of clotting factor VIII (antihemophilic factor) and von Willebrand's factor activity as well as a possible direct effect on the blood vessel wall.

**Other actions/effects**
Much less pressor activity than vasopressin and less action on visceral smooth muscle.

**Absorption**
10 to 20% from nasal mucosa. An intravenous dose of desmopressin possesses antidiuretic activity approximately 10 times that of the same nasal desmopressin dose.

**Biotransformation**
Renal.

**Half-life**
Fast phase—7.8 minutes.
Slow phase—75.5 minutes.

**Onset of action**
Antidiuretic—Intranasal: Within 1 hour.
Antihemorrhagic—Increased factor VIII activity and von Willebrand factor levels: Intravenous—15 to 30 minutes.

**Time to peak serum concentration**
Intranasal—1 to 5 hours.

**Time to peak effect**
Antidiuretic—Intranasal: 1 to 5 hours.
Antihemorrhagic—Increased factor VIII activity and von Willebrand factor levels: Intravenous—90 minutes to 2 hours.

**Duration of action**
Antidiuretic—
  Intranasal:
    Variable, 8 to 20 hours; long duration of action is due to the medication's rate of absorption from nasal mucosa, persistence in plasma, and effect on renal tubules. Effect ends abruptly, over a period of 60 to 90 minutes.
Antihemorrhagic—
  Mild hemophilia A: Intravenous—4 to 24 hours.
  von Willebrand's disease: Intravenous—Approximately 3 hours.

## Precautions to Consider

### Carcinogenicity/Mutagenicity
Studies have not been done in either animals or humans.

### Pregnancy/Reproduction
Pregnancy—Controlled studies in humans have not been done.

Clinical use of desmopressin in pregnant women has been reported, with no adverse effects in the fetus. Desmopressin does not appear to have uterotonic activity.

Studies in rats and rabbits have not shown that desmopressin causes adverse effects on the fetus.

FDA Pregnancy Category B.

### Breast-feeding
In a study conducted in one woman, desmopressin was distributed into breast milk in minimal amounts, following a 10 mcg intranasal dose. However, problems in humans have not been documented.

### Pediatrics
Use of desmopressin as an antihemorrhagic in infants less than 3 months of age is not recommended, because of an increased tendency to fluid balance problems in neonates. However, desmopressin may be the drug of choice for use as an antidiuretic in older children because of its low incidence of side effects.

Caution and careful restriction of fluid intake are recommended with use in infants because of the increased risk of hyponatremia and water intoxication.

### Geriatrics
Although appropriate studies have not been performed in the geriatric population, caution and careful restriction of fluid intake are recommended with use in the elderly because of the increased risk of hyponatremia and water intoxication.

### Drug interactions and/or related problems
The following drug interactions and/or related problems have been selected on the basis of their potential clinical significance (possible mechanism in parentheses where appropriate)—not necessarily inclusive (» = major clinical significance):

Note: Combinations containing any of the following medications, depending on the amount present, may also interact with this medication.

Carbamazepine or
Chlorpropamide or
Clofibrate
(may potentiate the antidiuretic effect of desmopressin when used concurrently)

Demeclocycline or
Lithium or
Norepinephrine
(may decrease the antidiuretic effect of desmopressin when used concurrently)

### Medical considerations/Contraindications
The medical considerations/contraindications included have been selected on the basis of their potential clinical significance (reasons given in parentheses where appropriate)—not necessarily inclusive (» = major clinical significance).

*Risk-benefit should be considered when the following medical problems exist:*

Allergic rhinitis or
Nasal congestion or edema or
Upper respiratory infection
(nasal absorption of desmopressin may be erratic)

Allergy to desmopressin

Coronary artery disease or
Hypertensive cardiovascular disease
(large doses of desmopressin may rarely produce a slight increase in blood pressure)

Cystic fibrosis or
Dehydration
(risk of hyponatremia may be increased)

Thrombosis, predisposition to
(rarely, myocardial infarction and strokes have been reported to occur following the use of desmopressin in patients predisposed to thrombus formation; although it is not known whether these events were related to the use of desmopressin, caution is recommended in the use of desmopressin in this patient population)

### Patient monitoring
The following may be especially important in patient monitoring (other tests may be warranted in some patients, depending on condition; » = major clinical significance):

*For use as an antidiuretic*
Electrolytes
(measurement of serum concentrations is recommended if therapy is continued beyond 7 days or as determined by physician)

Urine osmolality and/or
Urine volume
(determinations recommended at appropriate intervals to monitor response and aid in dosage adjustment; in some cases, plasma osmolality determinations may be necessary)

*For use in hemophilia A*
Factor VIII coagulant concentration
(determinations recommended at appropriate intervals to monitor response)

*For use in von Willebrand's disease*
Bleeding times and
Factor VIII coagulant and
Ristocetin cofactor (von Willebrand factor) and
von Willebrand factor (factor VIII–related antigen)
(determinations recommended at appropriate intervals to monitor response)

## Side/Adverse Effects

Note: Rarely, thrombotic events (myocardial infarction and strokes) have been reported to occur following the use of desmopressin in patients predisposed to thrombus formation. Although it is not known whether these events were related to the use of desmopressin, caution is recommended in the use of desmopressin in this patient population.

The following side/adverse effects have been selected on the basis of their potential clinical significance (possible signs and symptoms in parentheses where appropriate)—not necessarily inclusive:

### Those indicating need for medical attention
Incidence rare—dose-related
*Slight hypertension*—with intravenous use; *hyponatremia or water intoxication* (coma; confusion; continuing headache; decreased urination; drowsiness; rapid weight gain; seizures)

Note: *Hypotension* may be caused by rapid intravenous administration.

### Those indicating need for medical attention only if they continue or are bothersome
Incidence less frequent or rare—dose-related
*Abdominal or stomach cramps; flushing or redness of skin; pain in vulva*

With high doses
*Headache; nausea*

With intranasal use
*Runny or stuffy nose*

With intravenous use
*Pain, redness, or swelling at site of injection*

## Overdose
For more information on the management of overdose or unintentional ingestion, **contact a Poison Control Center** (see *Poison Control Center Listing*).

### Treatment of overdose
Treatment of overdose consists of reduction of dosage and, if fluid overload is severe, administration of furosemide.

## Patient Consultation
As an aid to patient consultation, refer to *Advice for the Patient, Desmopressin (Systemic)*.

In providing consultation, consider emphasizing the following selected information (» = major clinical significance):

### Before using this medication
» Conditions affecting use, especially:
  Allergy to desmopressin
  Breast-feeding—Distributed into breast milk in minimal amounts
  Use in children—Infants may be more sensitive to effects
  Use in the elderly—Increased risk of hyponatremia and water intoxication

**Proper use of this medication**
» Proper dosing
» Proper storage
*For intranasal use only*
» Importance of not using more medication than the amount prescribed
  Proper administration technique; following patient instructions
*Missed dose*
  If dosing schedule is once a day—Using as soon as possible if remembered same day; if not remembered until next day, not using at all and not doubling dose, but going back to regular schedule
  If dosing schedule is more than once a day—Using as soon as possible; not using at all if almost time for next dose; not doubling doses

**Side/adverse effects**
Signs of potential side effects, especially water intoxication and hyponatremia

## General Dosing Information

Fluid intake should be adjusted to decrease the potential for water intoxication and hyponatremia, especially in very young and geriatric patients.

Tolerance may develop with long-term intranasal use or tachyphylaxis may occur when intravenous doses are administered more frequently than every 24 to 48 hours.

**For use in central diabetes insipidus**
Initially, therapy should be directed to control nocturia.
The dosage of desmopressin should be adjusted according to the diurnal pattern of response, with the morning and evening doses being separately adjusted.
Response to therapy can be measured by the volume and frequency of urination and an adequate duration of sleep.

**For intranasal dosage forms**
Desmopressin is administered intranasally as a spray or through a flexible, calibrated catheter known as a rhinyle.
The nasal spray delivery unit should not be used beyond the labeled number of sprays; if it is, the accuracy of the dose delivered cannot be assured.

## Nasal Dosage Forms

### DESMOPRESSIN ACETATE NASAL SOLUTION

**Usual adult and adolescent dose**
Central diabetes insipidus—
  Initial: Intranasal, 10 mcg at bedtime; this dose may be increased nightly in increments of 2.5 mcg until a satisfactory sleep response is obtained. If urine volume is still large, a 10-mcg morning dose may be added and adjusted to obtain the desired response.
  Maintenance: Intranasal, 10 to 40 mcg per day, as a single dose or in two or three divided doses per day.
  Note: In one-quarter to one-third of patients, adequate control is maintained with a single daily dose; however, in some patients, three doses per day are necessary.
Nocturnal enuresis—
  Initial: Intranasal, 10 mcg into each nostril at bedtime (total dose per day of 20 mcg).
  Maintenance: Dosage is adjusted according to patient response; total dose per day may range from 10 to 40 mcg.

**Usual pediatric dose**
Central diabetes insipidus—
  Children up to 3 months of age:
    Dosage has not been established.
  Children 3 months to 12 years of age:
    Initial—Intranasal, 5 mcg at bedtime; this dose may be increased nightly in increments of 2.5 mcg until a satisfactory sleep response is obtained. If urine volume is still large, a 5-mcg morning dose may be added and adjusted to obtain the desired response.
    Maintenance—Intranasal, 2 to 4 mcg per kg of body weight per day or 5 to 30 mcg per day, as a single dose or in two divided doses per day.
Nocturnal enuresis—
  Children up to 6 years of age:
    Dosage has not been established.
  Children 6 years of age and older:
    Initial—Intranasal, 10 mcg into each nostril at bedtime (total dose per day of 20 mcg).
    Maintenance—Dosage is adjusted according to patient response; total dose per day may range from 10 to 40 mcg.

**Strength(s) usually available**
U.S.—
  10 mcg per 0.1 mL metered spray (0.01%) (Rx) [*DDAVP Nasal Spray*].
  100 mcg per mL (0.01%) (Rx) [*DDAVP Rhinal Tube*; GENERIC].
  150 mcg per 0.1 mL metered spray (0.15%) (Rx) [*Stimate Nasal Spray*].
Canada—
  10 mcg per 0.1 mL metered spray (0.01%) (Rx) [*DDAVP Spray*].
  100 mcg per mL (0.01%) (Rx) [*DDAVP Rhinyle Nasal Solution*].

**Packaging and storage**
Store at about 4 °C (39 °F), unless otherwise specified by manufacturer. Protect from freezing.

**Auxiliary labeling**
• Refrigerate.

**Note**
Include patient instructions when dispensing.

## Parenteral Dosage Forms

### DESMOPRESSIN ACETATE INJECTION

**Usual adult and adolescent dose**
Antidiuretic—
  Intravenous (direct) or subcutaneous, 2 to 4 mcg per day, usually in two divided doses in the morning and evening.
Antihemorrhagic—
  Intravenous, 0.3 mcg per kg of body weight diluted in 50 mL of 0.9% sodium chloride injection and infused slowly over fifteen to thirty minutes; repeated as needed.

**Usual pediatric dose**
Antihemorrhagic—
  Infants less than 3 months of age:
    Use is not recommended.
  Children 3 months of age and over:
    For children weighing 10 kg or less—Intravenous, 0.3 mcg per kg of body weight diluted in 10 mL of 0.9% sodium chloride injection and infused slowly over fifteen to thirty minutes; repeated as needed.
    For children weighing more than 10 kg—Intravenous, 0.3 mcg per kg of body weight diluted in 50 mL of 0.9% sodium chloride injection and infused slowly over fifteen to thirty minutes; repeated as needed.

**Strength(s) usually available**
U.S.—
  4 mcg per mL (Rx) [*DDAVP; Stimate* [GENERIC].
  15 mcg per mL (Rx) [*DDAVP*].
Canada—
  4 mcg per mL (Rx) [*DDAVP*].
  15 mcg per mL (Rx) [*Octostim*].

**Packaging and storage**
Store at about 4 °C (39 °F), unless otherwise specified by manufacturer. Protect from freezing.

## Selected Bibliography

Aledort LM. Treatment of von Willebrand's disease [review]. Mayo Clin Proceed 1991; 66: 841-6.
Blevins LS, Jr. Wand GS. Diabetes insipidus [review]. Crit Care Med 1992; 20(1): 69-79.
Miller K, Klauber GT. Desmopressin acetate in children with primary nocturnal enuresis. Clin Ther 1990; 12(4): 357-66.
Salva KM, Kim HC, Nahum K, et al. DDAVP in the treatment of bleeding disorders. Pharmacother 1988; 8(2): 94-9.

Revised: 10/26/92
Interim revision: 06/02/94; 07/19/96

**DESONIDE**—See *Corticosteroids (Topical)*

**DESOXIMETASONE**—See *Corticosteroids (Topical)*

**DEXAMETHASONE**—See *Corticosteroids—Glucocorticoid Effects (Systemic); Corticosteroids (Inhalation-Local); Corticosteroids (Nasal); Corticosteroids (Ophthalmic); Corticosteroids (Otic); Corticosteroids (Topical)*

**DEXCHLORPHENIRAMINE**—See *Antihistamines (Systemic)*

# DEXRAZOXANE Systemic—INTRODUCTORY VERSION

VA CLASSIFICATION (Primary): AN700
Commonly used brand name(s): *Zinecard*.
Note: For a listing of dosage forms and brand names by country availability, see *Dosage Forms* section(s).

## Category
Chelating agent.

## Indications

**Accepted**

Cardiomyopathy (prophylaxis)—Dexrazoxane is indicated for reducing the incidence and severity of cardiomyopathy associated with the administration of doxorubicin in women with metastatic breast cancer who have received a cumulative doxorubicin dose of 300 mg per square meter of body surface (mg/m$^2$) and who would benefit from continued therapy with doxorubicin.

Dexrazoxane is not indicated for use at the time of initiation of doxorubicin therapy. Concurrent use of dexrazoxane with the initiation of fluorouracil, doxorubicin, and cyclophosphamide (FAC) therapy is not recommended because of possible interference with the antitumor efficacy of the regimen.

## Pharmacology/Pharmacokinetics

**Physicochemical characteristics**
Molecular weight—268.28.
pKa—2.1.

**Mechanism of action/Effect**
The mechanism of action of dexrazoxane's cardioprotective activity is not fully understood. Dexrazoxane is a cyclic derivative of ethylenediamine tetra-acetic acid (EDTA) that readily penetrates cell membranes. Laboratory studies suggest that dexrazoxane is converted intracellularly to a ring-opened chelating agent that interferes with iron-mediated free radical generation thought to be responsible, in part, for anthracycline-induced cardiomyopathy. Dexrazoxane does not affect the pharmacokinetics of doxorubicin.

**Distribution**
Following a rapid distributive phase (0.2 to 0.3 hours), dexrazoxane reaches post-distributive equilibrium within 2 to 4 hours, primarily in total body water.
Volume of distribution—Steady-state: 25 liters per square meter of body surface.

**Protein binding**
Not bound to plasma proteins.

**Biotransformation**
Metabolic products include the unchanged drug, a diacid-diamide cleavage product, and two monoacid-monoamide ring products of unknown concentrations.

**Half-life**
Elimination—2.5 hours.

**Peak concentration**
Plasma—After administration of a dose of 500 mg per square meter of body surface (mg/m$^2$): 36.5 mcg per mL.

**Elimination**
Renal—42%.
In dialysis—It is not known whether dexrazoxane is removable by dialysis. However, because a significant dose fraction (greater than 0.4) of unchanged drug is retained in the plasma pool, minimal tissue partitioning or binding occurs, and systemic drug availability in the unbound form is greater than 90%, it is possible that dexrazoxane is removable by conventional peritoneal dialysis or hemodialysis.

## Precautions to Consider

**Carcinogenicity**
Carcinogenicity studies have not been done in animals or humans.

**Mutagenicity**
Dexrazoxane was not mutagenic in the Ames test but was found to be clastogenic to human lymphocytes *in vitro* and to mouse bone marrow erythrocytes *in vivo* (micronucleus test).

**Pregnancy/Reproduction**
Fertility—Dexrazoxane produced testicular atrophy in rats and dogs at doses as low as 30 mg per kg of body weight (mg/kg) weekly for 6 weeks (1/3 the human dose on a mg per square meter of body surface [mg/m$^2$] basis) and 20 mg/kg weekly for 13 weeks (approximately equal to the human dose on a mg/m$^2$ basis), respectively.

Pregnancy—Adequate and well-controlled studies in humans have not been done.
Studies in pregnant rats, at doses of 2 mg/kg (1/40 the human dose on a mg/m$^2$ basis) given daily during the period of organogenesis, found dexrazoxane to be maternotoxic; dexrazoxane was embryotoxic and teratogenic at doses of 8 mg/kg (1/10 the human dose on a mg/m$^2$ basis) and also impaired fertility at maturity in both males and females. Teratogenic effects in rats included imperforate anus, microphthalmia, and anophthalmia. Studies in pregnant rabbits, at doses of 5 mg/kg (1/10 the human dose on a mg/m$^2$ basis), found dexrazoxane to be maternotoxic; dexrazoxane was embryotoxic and teratogenic at doses of 20 mg/kg (1/2 the human dose on a mg/m$^2$ basis). Teratogenic effects in rabbits included several skeletal malformations such as short tail, rib and thoracic malformations, and soft tissue variations including subcutaneous, eye, and cardiac hemorrhagic areas, as well as agenesis of the gallbladder and of the intermediate lobe of the lung.

FDA Pregnancy Category C.

**Breast-feeding**
It is not known whether dexrazoxane is distributed into breast milk.

**Pediatrics**
No information is available on the relationship of age to the effects of dexrazoxane in pediatric patients. Safety and efficacy have not been established.

**Geriatrics**
No information is available on the relationship of age to the effects of dexrazoxane in geriatric patients.

**Drug interactions and/or related problems**
The following drug interactions and/or related problems have been selected on the basis of their potential clinical significance (possible mechanism in parentheses where appropriate)—not necessarily inclusive (» = major clinical significance):

Note: Combinations containing any of the following medications, depending on the amount present, may also interact with this medicine.

» Bone marrow depressants (See *Appendix II*)
(enhanced bone marrow depression may occur)

**Patient monitoring**
The following may be especially important in patient monitoring (other tests may be warranted in some patients, depending on condition; » = major clinical significance):

» Cardiac function tests
(recommended at periodic intervals because dexrazoxane reduces, but does not eliminate, the risk of doxorubicin cardiotoxicity, especially in patients who have already received a cumulative doxorubicin dose of 300 mg/m$^2$)

» Complete blood count (CBC)
(frequent determinations are recommended because of the risk of increased bone marrow depression with concurrent use of cytotoxic medications)

USP DI                                    Dexrazoxane (Systemic)—Introductory Version    1191

## Side/Adverse Effects

Note: Most adverse experiences encountered with the administration of dexrazoxane are probably the result of the FAC (fluorouracil, doxorubicin, and cyclophosphamide) chemotherapy regimen, with the exception of pain at the injection site.

Severity of leukopenia and thrombocytopenia at nadir with the FAC regimen was greater in patients receiving dexrazoxane, but recovery was similar with or without dexrazoxane.

The following side/adverse effects have been selected on the basis of their potential clinical significance (possible signs and symptoms in parentheses where appropriate)—not necessarily inclusive:

**Those indicating need for medical attention**
Incidence less frequent
*Pain at injection site*

## Patient Consultation

As an aid to patient consultation, refer to *Advice for the Patient, Dexrazoxane (Systemic)—Introductory Version.*

**Before using this medication**
» Conditions affecting use, especially:
    Pregnancy—Teratogenic effects in animals
    Breast-feeding—Not recommended
    Other medications, especially bone marrow depressants

**Proper use of this medication**
» Proper dosing

**Side/adverse effects**
Signs of potential side effects, especially pain at injection site

## General Dosing Information

Dexrazoxane solution should be given by slow intravenous injection or rapid-drip intravenous infusion from a bag. The intravenous injection of doxorubicin should be administered within 30 minutes after the beginning of the infusion of dexrazoxane. Doxorubicin should not be administered prior to dexrazoxane.

**Safety considerations for handling this medication**

It is suggested that dexrazoxane be handled with the same caution as antineoplastic agents.

There is limited but increasing evidence and concern that personnel involved in preparation and administration of parenteral antineoplastics may be at some risk because of the potential mutagenicity, teratogenicity, and/or carcinogenicity of these agents, although the actual risk is unknown. USP advisory panels recommend cautious handling both in preparation and disposal of antineoplastic agents. Precautions that have been suggested include:
• Use of a biological containment cabinet during reconstitution and dilution of parenteral medications and wearing of disposable surgical gloves and masks.
• Use of proper technique to prevent contamination of the medication, work area, and operator during transfer between containers (including proper training of personnel in this technique).
• Cautious and proper disposal of needles, syringes, vials, ampuls, and unused medication.
A number of medical centers have developed detailed guidelines for handling of antineoplastic agents.

## Parenteral Dosage Forms

### DEXRAZOXANE FOR INJECTION

Note: Dexrazoxane for injection contains dexrazoxane hydrochloride, but strength and dosage are expressed in terms of dexrazoxane.

**Usual adult dose**
Cardiomyopathy—
Intravenous, in a dosage ratio of 10 parts dexrazoxane to 1 part doxorubicin (10:1), or 500 mg of dexrazoxane per square meter of body surface (mg/m$^2$) for every 50 mg/m$^2$ of doxorubicin, repeated every three weeks, providing recovery has occurred.

Note: Administer solution by slow intravenous injection or by rapid-drip intravenous infusion from a bag. Doxorubicin should be administered within thirty minutes after the *beginning* of the dexrazoxane infusion.

**Usual pediatric dose**
Safety and efficacy have not been established.

**Size(s) usually available**
U.S.—
    250 mg (base) (single-dose vial) (Rx) [*Zinecard*].
    500 mg (base) (single-dose vial) (Rx) [*Zinecard*].

**Packaging and storage**
Store at controlled room temperature between 15 and 30 °C (59 and 86 °F). Store reconstituted solution up to six hours at controlled room temperature or under refrigeration between 2 and 8 °C (36 and 46 °F).

**Preparation of dosage form**
Dexrazoxane for injection is prepared for intravenous administration by adding 25 or 50 mL of 0.167 molar (M/6) sodium lactate injection (provided by the manufacturer) to the 250- or 500-mg vial, respectively, to produce a solution containing 10 mg per mL (mg/mL).
The reconstituted solution may be further diluted with either 0.9% sodium chloride injection or 5% dextrose injection to a concentration ranging from 1.3 to 5.0 mg/mL in intravenous infusion bags.

**Stability**
After reconstitution or further dilution, dexrazoxane solution is stable for 6 hours at controlled room temperature (between 15 and 30 °C [59 and 86 °F]) or under refrigeration (between 2 and 8 °C [36 and 46 °F]). Any unused solution should be discarded.

**Incompatibilities**
Dexrazoxane should not be mixed with other medications.

**Auxiliary labeling**
• Discard unused solution.

**Note**
If accidental contamination of the skin or mucosae with dexrazoxane occurs, the area should be immediately and thoroughly washed with soap and water.

Developed: 09/28/95

---

**DEXTROAMPHETAMINE**—See *Amphetamines (Systemic)*

---

# DEXTROMETHORPHAN   Systemic

VA CLASSIFICATION (Primary): RE302

Commonly used brand name(s): *Balminil D.M.; Benylin Adult; Benylin Pediatric; Broncho-Grippol-DM; Calmylin #1; Children's Hold; Cough-X; Creo-Terpin; DM Syrup; Delsym; Drixoral Cough Liquid Caps; Hold; Koffex; Mediquell; Neo-DM; Ornex•DM 15; Ornex•DM 30; Pertussin CS; Pertussin Cough Suppressant; Pertussin ES; Robidex; Robitussin Cough Calmers; Robitussin Maximum Strength Cough Suppressant; Robitussin Pediatric; Sedatuss; St. Joseph Cough Suppressant for Children; Sucrets Cough Control Formula; Trocal; Vicks Formula 44 Pediatric Formula.*

Note: For a listing of dosage forms and brand names by country availability, see *Dosage Forms* section(s).

## Category
Antitussive.

## Indications

**Accepted**
Cough (treatment)—Dextromethorphan is indicated for the symptomatic relief of nonproductive cough due to minor throat and bronchial irritation occurring with colds or inhaled irritants.

## Pharmacology/Pharmacokinetics

**Mechanism of action/Effect**
Suppresses the cough reflex by a direct action on the cough center in the medulla of the brain.

**Biotransformation**
Hepatic. Rapidly and extensively metabolized to dextrorphan (active metabolite).

**Onset of action**
Usually within one-half hour.

## Dextromethorphan (Systemic)

**Duration of action**
Up to 6 hours.

Note: The extended-release oral suspension delivers dextromethorphan from an ion-exchange complex over a period of 9 to 12 hours.

**Elimination**
Primarily renal (excreted as unchanged dextromethorphan and demethylated metabolites, including dextrorphan).

## Precautions to Consider

**Pregnancy/Reproduction**
Pregnancy—Problems in humans have not been documented.

**Breast-feeding**
It is not known whether dextromethorphan is distributed into breast milk. However, problems in humans have not been documented.

**Pediatrics**
Appropriate studies on the relationship of age to the effects of dextromethorphan have not been performed in the pediatric population. However, no pediatrics-specific problems have been documented to date.

**Geriatrics**
No information is available on the relationship of age to the effects of dextromethorphan in geriatric patients.

**Drug interactions and/or related problems**
The following drug interactions and/or related problems have been selected on the basis of their potential clinical significance (possible mechanism in parentheses where appropriate)—not necessarily inclusive (» = major clinical significance):

Note: Combinations containing any of the following medications, depending on the amount present, may also interact with this medication.

» Central nervous system (CNS) depression–producing medications, other (see *Appendix II*)
(concurrent use may potentiate the CNS depressant effects of these medications or dextromethorphan)

» Monoamine oxidase (MAO) inhibitors, including furazolidone and procarbazine
(concurrent use with dextromethorphan may cause adrenergic crisis, collapse, coma, dizziness, excitation, hypertension, hyperpyrexia, intracerebral bleeding, lethargy, nausea, psychotic behavior, spasms, and tremors )

Quinidine
(inhibition of the cytochrome P4502D6 enzyme system by quinidine may cause a decrease in the hepatic metabolism of dextromethorphan, which may result in increased dextromethorphan serum concentrations; higher concentrations of dextromethorphan have been associated with an increased incidence of side effects)

**Medical considerations/Contraindications**
The medical considerations/contraindications included have been selected on the basis of their potential clinical significance (reasons given in parentheses where appropriate)—not necessarily inclusive (» = major clinical significance):

*Risk-benefit should be considered when the following medical problems exist:*

» Asthma
(dextromethorphan may impair expectoration and thus increase airway resistance)

» Cough, productive
(inhibition of cough reflex may lead to retention of secretions)

Hepatic function impairment
(metabolism of dextromethorphan may be impaired)

Sensitivity to dextromethorphan

## Side/Adverse Effects

Note: Toxic psychosis (hyperactivity, visual and auditory hallucinations) has been reported after ingestion of 300 mg or more of dextromethorphan.

Respiratory depression has been reported to occur with very high doses.

Dextromethorphan abuse and dependence may occur rarely, especially following prolonged use of high doses.

The following side/adverse effects have been selected on the basis of their potential clinical significance (possible signs and symptoms in parentheses where appropriate)—not necessarily inclusive:

Those indicating need for medical attention only if they continue or are bothersome
Incidence less frequent or rare
*Mild dizziness; mild drowsiness; nausea or vomiting; stomach pain*

## Overdose

For more information on the management of overdose or unintentional ingestion, **contact a Poison Control Center** (see *Poison Control Center Listing*).

**Clinical effects of overdose**
The following effects have been selected on the basis of their potential clinical significance (possible signs and symptoms in parentheses where appropriate—not necessarily inclusive:

Symptoms of overdose
*Confusion; drowsiness or dizziness; severe nausea or vomiting; severe unusual excitement, nervousness, restlessness, or irritability*

## Patient Consultation

As an aid to patient consultation, refer to *Advice for the Patient, Dextromethorphan (Systemic)*.

In providing consultation, consider emphasizing the following selected information (» = major clinical significance):

**Before using this medication**
» Conditions affecting use, especially:
Sensitivity to dextromethorphan
Other medications, especially other CNS depressants and MAO inhibitors
Other medical problems, especially asthma and productive cough

**Proper use of this medication**
» Importance of not using more medication than the amount prescribed because of habit-forming potential
» Proper dosing
Missed dose: If on a scheduled dosing regimen—Taking as soon as possible; not taking if almost time for next dose; not doubling doses
» Proper storage

**Precautions while using this medication**
Checking with physician if cough persists after medication has been used for 7 days or if high fever, skin rash, or continuing headache is present with cough

## Oral Dosage Forms

### DEXTROMETHORPHAN HYDROBROMIDE CAPSULES

**Usual adult and adolescent dose**
Antitussive—
Oral, 10 to 20 mg every four hours or 30 mg every six to eight hours, as needed.

**Usual adult prescribing limits**
Up to 120 mg per day.

**Usual pediatric dose**
Antitussive—
Children up to 2 years of age: Use is not recommended.
Children 2 to 6 years of age: Oral, 2.5 to 5 mg every four hours or 7.5 mg every six to eight hours, as needed, not to exceed 30 mg per day.
Children 6 to 12 years of age: Oral, 5 to 10 mg every four hours or 15 mg every six to eight hours, as needed, not to exceed 60 mg per day.

Note: Administration of a specific product to a pediatric patient depends upon the ability to achieve suitable dosage for the age of the child.

**Usual geriatric dose**
See *Usual adult and adolescent dose*

**Strength(s) usually available**
U.S.—
30 mg (OTC) [*Drixoral Cough Liquid Caps*].
Canada—
30 mg (OTC) [*Ornex•DM 30*].

**Packaging and storage**
Store below 40 °C (104 °F), preferably between 15 and 30 °C (59 and 86 °F), in a well-closed container, unless otherwise specified by manufacturer.

### DEXTROMETHORPHAN HYDROBROMIDE LOZENGES

**Usual adult and adolescent dose**
See *Dextromethorphan Hydrobromide Capsules*.

**Usual adult prescribing limits**
Up to 120 mg per day.

**Usual pediatric dose**
See *Dextromethorphan Hydrobromide Capsules.*

Note: Administration of a specific product to a pediatric patient depends upon the ability to achieve suitable dosage for the age of the child.

**Usual geriatric dose**
See *Dextromethorphan Hydrobromide Capsules.*

**Strength(s) usually available**
U.S.—
  5 mg (OTC) [*Children's Hold; Cough-X* (benzocaine 2 mg); *Hold; Pertussin Cough Suppressant; Robitussin Cough Calmers; Sucrets Cough Control Formula*].
  7.5 mg (OTC) [*Trocal*].
Canada—
  Not commercially available.

**Packaging and storage**
Store below 40 °C (104 °F), preferably between 15 and 30 °C (59 and 86 °F), in a well-closed container, unless otherwise specified by manufacturer.

## DEXTROMETHORPHAN HYDROBROMIDE SYRUP USP

**Usual adult and adolescent dose**
See *Dextromethorphan Hydrobromide Capsules.*

**Usual adult prescribing limits**
Up to 120 mg per day.

**Usual pediatric dose**
Children up to 2 years of age: Dosage must be individualized by physician.
Children 2 to 12 years of age: See *Dextromethorphan Hydrobromide Capsules.*

**Usual geriatric dose**
See *Dextromethorphan Hydrobromide Capsules.*

**Strength(s) usually available**
U.S.—
  3.5 mg per 5 mL (OTC) [*Pertussin CS* (alcohol free)].
  7.5 mg per 5 mL (OTC) [*Benylin Pediatric* (alcohol free; sugar free); *Robitussin Pediatric* (alcohol free); *St. Joseph Cough Suppressant for Children* (alcohol free)].
  10 mg per 15 mL (OTC) [*Creo-Terpin* (alcohol 25%)].
  15 mg per 5 mL (OTC) [*Benylin Adult* (alcohol free; sugar free); *Pertussin ES* (alcohol 9.5%); *Robitussin Maximum Strength Cough Suppressant* (alcohol 1.4%); *Vicks Formula 44 Pediatric Formula*].
Canada—
  7.5 mg per 5 mL (OTC) [*Robitussin Pediatric* (alcohol free)].
  10 mg per 5 mL (OTC) [*Sedatuss*].
  15 mg per 5 mL (OTC) [*Balminil D.M.; Broncho-Grippol-DM; Calmylin #1* (alcohol free; sugar free); *DM Syrup; Koffex; Neo-DM; Ornex•DM 15; Robidex* (alcohol 3.5%)].

**Packaging and storage**
Store between 15 and 30 °C (59 and 86 °F), unless otherwise specified by manufacturer. Store in a tight, light-resistant container. Protect from freezing.

## DEXTROMETHORPHAN HYDROBROMIDE CHEWABLE TABLETS

**Usual adult and adolescent dose**
See *Dextromethorphan Hydrobromide Capsules.*

**Usual adult prescribing limits**
Up to 120 mg per day.

**Usual pediatric dose**
See *Dextromethorphan Hydrobromide Capsules.*

Note: Administration of a specific product to a pediatric patient depends upon the ability to achieve suitable dosage for the age of the child.

**Usual geriatric dose**
See *Dextromethorphan Hydrobromide Capsules.*

**Strength(s) usually available**
U.S.—
  15 mg (OTC) [*Mediquell*].
Canada—
  Not commercially available.

**Packaging and storage**
Store below 40 °C (104 °F), preferably between 15 and 30 °C (59 and 86 °F), in a well-closed container, unless otherwise specified by manufacturer.

**Auxiliary labeling**
• Chew well before swallowing.

## DEXTROMETHORPHAN POLISTIREX EXTENDED-RELEASE ORAL SUSPENSION

**Usual adult and adolescent dose**
Antitussive—
  Oral, 60 mg every twelve hours, as needed.

**Usual adult prescribing limits**
Up to 120 mg per day.

**Usual pediatric dose**
Antitussive—
  Children up to 2 years of age: Dosage must be individualized by physician.
  Children 2 to 6 years of age: Oral, 15 mg every twelve hours, as needed, not to exceed 30 mg per day.
  Children 6 to 12 years of age: Oral, 30 mg every twelve hours, as needed, not to exceed 60 mg per day.

**Usual geriatric dose**
See *Usual adult and adolescent dose*

**Strength(s) usually available**
U.S.—
  30 mg (equivalent of dextromethorphan hydrobromide) per 5 mL (OTC) [*Delsym* (alcohol free)].
Canada—
  30 mg (equivalent of dextromethorphan hydrobromide) per 5 mL (OTC) [*Delsym* (alcohol free)].

**Packaging and storage**
Store below 40 °C (104 °F), preferably between 15 and 30 °C (59 and 86 °F), in a well-closed container, unless otherwise specified by manufacturer. Protect from freezing.

**Auxiliary labeling**
• Shake well.

## Selected Bibliography
Irwin RS, Curley FJ, Bennett FM. Appropriate use of antitussives and protussives. Drugs 1993; 46(1): 80-91.
Segal S, et al. Use of codeine- and dextromethorphan-containing cough syrups in pediatrics. Pediatrics 1978; 62(1): 118-22.

Revised: 06/23/94
Interim revision: 06/13/95

---

# DEXTROSE AND ELECTROLYTES — See *Carbohydrates and Electrolytes (Systemic)*

---

# DEXTROTHYROXINE — The *Dextrothyroxine (Systemic)* monograph is not included in this published version of the USP DI database. Copies of the monograph are available on request from Micromedex, Inc. - Reprint Requests, 6200 S. Syracuse Way, Suite 300, Englewood, CO 80111; telephone (303) 486-6400; telefax (303) 486-6464; Email: USPDI@MDX.COM.

---

# DEZOCINE Systemic†

**VA CLASSIFICATION (Primary):** CN101
Commonly used brand name(s): *Dalgan*.
Note: For a listing of dosage forms and brand names by country availability, see *Dosage Forms* section(s).

†Not commercially available in Canada.

## Category
Analgesic.

# Dezocine (Systemic)

## Indications

**Accepted**

Pain (treatment)—Dezocine is indicated for the short-term relief of pain. Dezocine's antagonist activity must be considered prior to administration because it may precipitate withdrawal symptoms if the patient is physically dependent on a mu-receptor opioid analgesic. A patient who has developed a significant degree of tolerance to other opioids during long-term treatment is probably not a suitable candidate for dezocine treatment.

**Unaccepted**

Dezocine has not been adequately studied, and is not currently recommended, for treatment of chronic pain.

## Pharmacology/Pharmacokinetics

**Physicochemical characteristics**

Chemical group—An opioid agonist/antagonist analgesic of the aminotetralin series.
Molecular weight—245.36.
 $n$–Octanol: Water partition coefficient—1.7

**Mechanism of action/Effect**

Analgesic—
Opioid analgesics bind with stereospecific receptors at many sites within the central nervous system (CNS) to alter processes affecting both the perception of pain and the emotional response to pain. Although precise sites and mechanisms of action have not been fully determined, opioids have been shown to cause alterations in release of various neurotransmitters from afferent nerves sensitive to painful stimuli.

It has been proposed that there are multiple subtypes of opioid receptors, each mediating various therapeutic and/or side effects of opioid drugs. The actions of an opioid analgesic may therefore depend upon its binding affinity for each type of receptor and whether it acts as a full agonist or a partial agonist or is inactive at each type of receptor. At least 2 of these types of receptors (mu and kappa) mediate analgesia. Mu receptors are widely distributed throughout the CNS, especially in the limbic system (frontal cortex, temporal cortex, amygdala, and hippocampus), thalamus, striatum, hypothalamus, and midbrain as well as laminae I, II, IV, and V of the dorsal horn in the spinal cord. Kappa receptors are localized primarily in the spinal cord and in the cerebral cortex. A third type of receptor (sigma) does not mediate analgesia; actions at this receptor may produce the subjective and psychotomimetic effects characteristic of most opioids having mixed agonist/antagonist activity. Dezocine may act primarily as a partial agonist at the mu receptor. Dezocine has relatively low activity (compared with pentazocine) at the sigma receptor, but psychotomimetic-like effects have been reported after administration of high doses.

Antagonist—
Dezocine may displace other mu-receptor opioid agonists from their receptor binding sites and competitively inhibit their actions. It may therefore precipitate withdrawal symptoms in physically dependent patients who are chronically receiving these agonists. If administered first, dezocine may also reduce or block the effects of subsequently administered mu-receptor agonists. The antagonist actions of dezocine may impose a ceiling on its analgesic effects.

**Other actions/effects**

Dezocine shares the CNS depressant and respiratory depressant effects of opioid analgesics. The respiratory depressant effect of dezocine is subject to a ceiling effect, with maximal respiratory depression occurring at a total cumulative dose of about 30 mg per kg of body weight (mg/kg). Respiratory depression induced by dezocine occurs more rapidly, is more pronounced for about the first 1to 2 hours, and persists for approximately the same time as that induced by equianalgesic doses of morphine.

Dezocine has not been shown to produce clinically significant cardiovascular adverse effects. However, although cardiac or respiratory performance and systolic and diastolic blood pressures were not significantly altered, increases in cardiac index, stroke volume index, left ventricular stroke work index, and pulmonary vascular resistance occurred in one study when a single dose of 125 mcg per kg of body weight was administered intravenously to patients with stable coronary artery disease. Dezocine has not been studied in patients with severe and/or unstable cardiovascular disease.

Because of its antagonist activity, dezocine may have less potential for causing dependence or abuse than strong opioid analgesics having only agonist activity. However, when dezocine was administered to subjects with a history of opioid abuse, they reported typical subjective opioid effects (e.g., liking, euphoria) and identified the medication as "dope". Also, the medication substituted for morphine in abuse-liability testing in animals. Therefore, dezocine has the potential to be abused, especially by individuals with a history of opioid abuse or dependence.

Although studies in humans have not been done, dezocine did not cause histamine release or bronchoconstriction in an animal study.

Although specific studies with dezocine have not been done, the probability exists that the medication, like other opioid analgesics, may decrease gastrointestinal motility. Also, studies have not been done to determine whether dezocine, like most other opioids, has antitussive or antidiuretic activity or increases biliary tract pressure.

**Absorption**

Intramuscular—Rapid and complete.

**Biotransformation**

Hepatic, via conjugation (glucuronidation).

**Half-life**

Elimination—
Intramuscular: Average 2.2 hours
Intravenous:
5-mg dose—Average 1.7 to 2.6 hours (range 0.6 to 4.4 hours)
10-mg dose (infused over 5 minutes)—Average 2.4 to 2.6 hours (range 1.2 to 7.4 hours). In patients with hepatic cirrhosis, the half-life is increased by 30 to 50%, probably due to the 30 to 50% expansion of dezocine's volume of distribution in these patients.
20-mg dose—Average 2.4 to 2.8 hours (range 1.4 to 6.5 hours)

**Onset of action**

Intramuscular—Within 30 minutes.
Intravenous—Within 15 minutes.

**Time to peak concentration**

Intramuscular—10 to 90 minutes; average about 35 minutes.

**Therapeutic plasma concentration**

Steady-state—5 to 9 nanograms per mL.

**Peak serum concentration**

Intramuscular (10-mg single dose)—10 to 38 (average 19) nanograms per mL (0.03 to 0.11 [average 0.55] micromoles per L).

**Time to peak effect**

Intramuscular—0.6 to 2.5 hours (average 1 to 2 hours).

**Elimination**

Renal (66% of a dose), about 1% as unchanged dezocine and the remainder as the glucuronide conjugate. The effect of renal function impairment on clearance has not been studied. Also, in healthy subjects, the total body clearance is greater than the sum of hepatic and renal blood flow, suggesting additional mechanisms of excretion (e.g., biliary).

Total body clearance—
5-mg intravenous dose: 3.52 (range 2.1–6.2) L per hour per kg of body weight (L/hr/kg).
10-mg intravenous dose: 3.33 (range 1.7–7.2) L/hr/kg.
20-mg intravenous dose: 2.76 (range 1.7–4.1) L/hr/kg.

## Precautions to Consider

**Pregnancy/Reproduction**

Pregnancy—Adequate and well-controlled studies have not been done in pregnant women. Although there is no experience with long-term administration of dezocine to pregnant women, the possibility must be considered that regular use during pregnancy may cause physical dependence in the fetus, leading to withdrawal symptoms (convulsions, irritability, excessive crying, tremors, hyperactive reflexes, fever, vomiting, diarrhea, sneezing, and yawning) in the neonate.

Studies in mice, rats, and rabbits did not show evidence of teratogenicity. However, intramuscular or intravenous administration of dezocine to rats produced a dose-related decrease in food consumption and body weight in the parental generation and a resultant decrease in pup body weight.

FDA Pregnancy Category C.

Labor and delivery—The safety of dezocine administration during labor has not been established.

**Breast-feeding**

It is not known whether dezocine is distributed into breast milk. However, problems in humans have not been documented.

**Pediatrics**

No information is available on the relationship of age to the effects of dezocine in pediatric patients. Safety and efficacy in patients up to 18 years of age have not been established.

**Geriatrics**

No information is available on the relationship of age to the effects of dezocine in geriatric patients. However, geriatric patients are more susceptible to the effects, especially the respiratory depressant effects, of other opioid analgesics. Also, geriatric patients have been shown to metabolize or eliminate some opioid analgesics more slowly, and/or to be more sensitive to the analgesic effects of opioid analgesics, than younger adults. Therefore, lower doses and/or a longer interval between doses may be sufficient to provide effective analgesia. It is recommended that dezocine therapy in geriatric patients be initiated with lower doses than would be used for younger adults, and that subsequent doses be individualized according to patient tolerance and response.

**Drug interactions and/or related problems**
The following drug interactions and/or related problems have been selected on the basis of their potential clinical significance (possible mechanism in parentheses where appropriate)—not necessarily inclusive (» = major clinical significance):

Note: Combinations containing any of the following medications, depending on the amount present, may also interact with this medication.

Other interactions applying to opioid analgesics may apply to dezocine also, although documentation is currently not available.

Antidiarrheals, antiperistaltic, such as:
  Difenoxin and atropine
  Diphenoxylate and atropine
  Kaolin, pectin, belladonna alkaloids and opium
  Loperamide
  Opium tincture
  Paregoric
    (repeated administration of both dezocine and any of these antidiarrheals may increase the risk of severe constipation as well as CNS depression)

» CNS depression–producing medications, other (See *Appendix II*) or Monoamine oxidase (MAO) inhibitors, including furazolidone, procarbazine, and selegiline
    (concurrent use may increase the CNS depressant, respiratory depressant, and hypotensive effects of these medications and/or dezocine; caution and a reduction in dosage of either or both medications are recommended)

Hydroxyzine
    (concurrent use with dezocine may result in increased analgesia as well as increased CNS depressant and hypotensive effects)

Naloxone
    (antagonizes the analgesic, CNS, and respiratory depressant effects of dezocine; however, because naloxone may precipitate withdrawal symptoms in physically dependent patients, dosage of naloxone should be carefully titrated when used to treat opioid overdosage in dependent patients)

» Naltrexone
    (although not documented, the possibility must be considered that usual doses of dezocine will be ineffective if administered to a patient receiving naltrexone therapy [because naltrexone blocks the therapeutic effects of other potent opioids] and that administration of increased doses of dezocine to override naltrexone-induced blockade of opioid receptors may increase the risk of adverse effects)

» Opioid analgesics, other
    (if administered prior to another mu-receptor agonist, dezocine may reduce the therapeutic effects of the other opioid)
    (dezocine may precipitate withdrawal symptoms in physically dependent patients who are chronically receiving potent mu-receptor agonists such as morphine)

**Laboratory value alterations**
The following have been selected on the basis of their potential clinical significance (possible effect in parentheses where appropriate)—not necessarily inclusive (» = major clinical significance):

With diagnostic test results
  Amylase activity, in plasma and
  Lipase activity, in plasma
    (increases associated with opioid-induced contractions of the sphincter of Oddi and increased biliary tract pressure have been reported with most other opioid analgesics; although these effects have not been reported with dezocine, the possibility should be considered that the diagnostic utility of determinations of these enzymes may be compromised after dezocine administration)
  Gastric emptying studies
    (opioid analgesics such as dezocine may delay gastric emptying, thereby invalidating test results)
  Hepatobiliary imaging, radionuclide
    (like most other opioid analgesics, dezocine may prevent or delay delivery of the radionuclide to the small bowel, resulting in delayed visualization and in results resembling obstruction of the common bile duct)

With physiology/laboratory test values
  Alkaline phosphatase activity and
  Aspartate aminotransferase (AST [SGOT]) activity
    (may be increased [incidences <1%])
  Cerebrospinal fluid (CSF) pressure
    (may be increased; effect is secondary to respiratory depression–induced carbon dioxide retention)
  Hemoglobin
    (concentrations may be decreased [incidence <1%])

**Medical considerations/Contraindications**
The medical considerations/contraindications included have been selected on the basis of their potential clinical significance (reasons given in parentheses where appropriate)—not necessarily inclusive (» = major clinical significance):

*Except under special circumstances, this medication should not be used when the following medical problem exists:*
» Respiratory depression, acute
    (may be exacerbated)

*Risk-benefit should be considered when the following medical problems exist:*
  Abdominal conditions, acute
    (diagnosis or clinical course may be obscured)
» Asthma, acute attack or
» Respiratory impairment or disease, chronic
    (opioid analgesics may decrease respiratory drive and increase airway resistance; a reduction in dosage is recommended)
  Cardiovascular disease, severe and/or unstable
    (although clinically significant cardiovascular adverse effects have not been reported to date with dezocine, the opioid has not been studied in patients with severe and/or unstable cardiovascular disease; caution is recommended if dezocine is to be administered to patients with angina pectoris or compromised cardiac function, following cardiac or cardiovascular surgery, or to relieve pain due to acute myocardial infarction)
» Dependence on opioid analgesics, current, confirmed or
  Dependence on opioid analgesics, current, suspected
    (because of the risk of precipitating withdrawal symptoms, dezocine should be administered only after a suitable period of withdrawal from other opioids)
  Diarrhea associated with pseudomembranous colitis caused by cephalosporins, lincomycins (possibly including topical clindamycin) or penicillins or
  Diarrhea caused by poisoning, until toxic material has been eliminated from the gastrointestinal tract
    (possibility should be considered that dezocine, like other opioid analgesics, may slow elimination of toxic material, thereby worsening and/or prolonging the diarrhea, when administered repeatedly)
  Drug abuse or dependence, history of, including acute alcoholism or
  Emotional instability or
  Suicidal ideation or attempts
    (risk of abuse, especially relapse by patients recovering from a drug dependency; it is recommended that dezocine be administered to patients with such problems only in a medically controlled environment)
  Gallbladder disease or gallstones
    (possibility should be considered that dezocine, like other opioid analgesics, may cause biliary contraction)
  Gastrointestinal surgery, recent or
  Inflammatory bowel disease, severe
    (possibility should be considered that dezocine, like other opioid analgesics, may alter gastrointestinal motility; in patients with severe inflammatory bowel disease, an increased risk of toxic megacolon may result)
  Head injury or
  Increased intracranial pressure, pre-existing or
  Intracranial lesions
    (risk of respiratory depression and further elevation of cerebrospinal fluid pressure may be increased; also, opioid analgesics may cause sedation and pupillary changes that may obscure clinical course of head injury)
  Hepatic function impairment
    (the elimination half-life of dezocine may be prolonged by up to 50% in patients with hepatic cirrhosis, probably because of an in-

crease in the medication's volume of distribution; although any effect of other forms of hepatic function impairment on the pharmacokinetics of dezocine has not been determined, caution and a reduction in dosage are recommended)

Hypothyroidism
(risk of respiratory depression and prolonged CNS depression is greatly increased)

Prostatic hypertrophy or obstruction or
Urethral stricture or
Urinary tract surgery, recent
(possibility must be considered that dezocine, like other opioid analgesics, may cause urinary retention, which may be detrimental to the patient)

Renal function impairment
(although the effect of renal function impairment on the elimination of dezocine has not been determined, caution and a reduction in dose are recommended)

Sensitivity to dezocine, history of

Caution is also advised in administration to geriatric or very ill or debilitated patients, who may be more sensitive to the effects, especially the respiratory depressant effects, of opioid analgesics.

## Side/Adverse Effects

Note: Side effects are more frequent when the dezocine plasma concentration is 45 nanograms per mL (0.13 micromoles per L) or higher. The highest dose administered to nontolerant healthy adults without toxicity is 30 mg per 70 kg of body weight.

Dezocine appears less likely than pentazocine to cause the subjective and psychotomimetic effects characteristic of sigma-receptor agonists. These effects may include several or all of the following, occurring as a group: confusion, delusions, feelings of depersonalization or unreality, hallucinations (usually visual), dysphoria, nightmares, and nervousness or anxiety. However, psychotomimetic-like effects have been reported with high doses of dezocine.

Dezocine may have less dependence or abuse liability than other potent opioid analgesics (i.e., potent mu-receptor agonists). However, the medication has the potential for abuse, especially by individuals with a history of opioid abuse.

The following side/adverse effects have been selected on the basis of their potential clinical significance (possible signs and symptoms in parentheses where appropriate)—not necessarily inclusive:

**Those indicating need for medical attention, unless otherwise referenced**
Incidence rare (<1%)
*Atelectasis* (coughing; difficult breathing); ***chest pain; CNS toxicity*** (delirium; delusions; mental depression); ***dermatitis*** (skin rash; itching); ***difficult, decreased, or frequent urination; edema*** (swelling of face, fingers, lower legs, or feet; weight gain); ***hypertension; hypotension*** (if severe—dizziness, tiredness); ***irregular heartbeat; respiratory depression*** (slow, shallow, or difficult breathing); ***thrombophlebitis***

**Those indicating need for medical attention only if they continue or are bothersome**
Incidence more frequent (3–9%)
*Drowsiness; gastric upset* (nausea; vomiting)
Incidence less frequent (1–3%) or rare (<1%)
*CNS effects* (anxiety; blurred or double vision; confusion; crying; dizziness or lightheadedness; slurred speech); *flushing or redness of skin; gastrointestinal effects* (abdominal pain or distress; constipation; diarrhea)

**Those indicating possible withdrawal and the need for medical attention if they occur after medication is discontinued**
*Body aches; diarrhea; fast heartbeat; fever, runny nose, or sneezing; gooseflesh; increased sweating; loss of appetite; nausea or vomiting; nervousness, restlessness, or irritability; shivering or trembling; stomach cramps; trouble in sleeping; unusually large pupils of eyes; weakness; yawning*

## Overdose

For specific information on the agents used in the management of dezocine overdose, see *Naloxone (Systemic)* monograph.

For more information on the management of overdose or unintentional ingestion, **contact a Poison Control Center** (see *Poison Control Center Listing*).

### Clinical effects of overdose

The following effects have been selected on the basis of their potential clinical significance (possible signs and symptoms in parentheses where appropriate)—not necessarily inclusive:

Acute and chronic
*Cold, clammy skin; confusion, nervousness, or restlessness, severe; convulsions; dizziness, severe; drowsiness, severe; low blood pressure; pinpoint pupils of eyes; slow heartbeat; slow or troubled breathing; unconsciousness; weakness, severe*

### Treatment of overdose

Although there is no experience with dezocine overdose, recommended treatment of overdose of opioid analgesics consists of the following:

Specific treatment—Use of the opioid antagonist naloxone. See the package insert or *Naloxone (Systemic)* monograph for specific dosing guidelines for use of this product. The fact that naloxone may also antagonize the analgesic actions of opioid analgesics and may precipitate withdrawal symptoms in physically dependent patients must be kept in mind.

Monitoring—Continue to monitor the patient (mandatory because the duration of action of the opioid analgesic may exceed that of the antagonist) and administer additional naloxone as needed. Alternatively, initial treatment may be followed by continuous intravenous infusion of naloxone, with the rate of infusion being adjusted according to patient response.

Supportive care—May include establishing adequate respiratory exchange through provision of a patent airway and institution of assisted or controlled respiration.

May also include administering intravenous fluids and/or vasopressors and using other supportive measures as needed. Patients in whom intentional overdose is confirmed or suspected should be referred for psychiatric consultation.

## Patient Consultation

As an aid to patient consultation, refer to *Advice for the Patient, Dezocine (Systemic)*.

In providing consultation, consider emphasizing the following selected information (» = major clinical significance):

### Before using this medication
» Conditions affecting use, especially:
   Sensitivity to dezocine, history of
   Use in the elderly—Increased risk of respiratory depression or other adverse effects
   Other medications, especially other CNS depression-producing medications, other opioids, and naltrexone
   Other medical problems, especially asthma or other acute or chronic respiratory problems

### Proper use of this medication
Proper administration technique (if dispensed for home use)
» Importance of not taking more medication than the amount prescribed because of danger of overdose and habit-forming potential
» Proper dosing
Missed dose (if on scheduled dosing): Using as soon as possible; not using if almost time for next dose; not doubling doses
» Proper storage

### Precautions while using this medication
» Avoiding alcohol or other CNS depressants during therapy
» Caution if dizziness, drowsiness, or lightheadedness occurs
Caution when getting up suddenly from a lying or sitting position
Lying down if nausea, vomiting, dizziness, or lightheadedness occurs
Caution if any kind of surgery (including dental surgery) or emergency treatment is required
» Suspected overdose: Getting emergency help at once

### Side/adverse effects
Signs and symptoms of potential side effects, especially atelectasis; chest pain; CNS toxicity; dermatitis; difficult, decreased, or frequent urination; edema; hypertension; hypotension; irregular heartbeat; respiratory depression; and thrombophlebitis

## General Dosing Information

In recommended doses, dezocine is equipotent with morphine on a mg-per-mg basis.

Dosage and dosing intervals should be adjusted according to the patient's age, weight, and physical status, as well as the severity of pain, other medications given concurrently, and patient response to initial doses.

Dezocine is administered intravenously or intramuscularly. Subcutaneous administration is not recommended. In animal studies, repeated injection at a single site has caused subcutaneous inflammation, vascular irritation, and venous thrombosis.

Opioid analgesics may depress respiration, especially in geriatric, very ill, or debilitated patients and patients with respiratory problems. It is recommended that dosage of dezocine for these patients be reduced initially, then adjusted as required and tolerated. However, geriatric patients may also be more sensitive to the analgesic effects of opioid analgesics so that lower doses and/or a longer interval between doses may be sufficient to provide effective analgesia.

Concurrent administration of a non-opioid analgesic (such as aspirin or other salicylates, other nonsteroidal anti-inflammatory drugs, or acetaminophen) with an opioid analgesic provides additive analgesia and may permit lower doses of the opioid analgesic to be utilized.

Rapid intravenous injection of other strong opioid analgesics has caused anaphylactoid reactions, severe respiratory depression, hypotension, peripheral circulatory collapse, and cardiac arrest. Although these effects have not been documented with dezocine, precautions applying to other opioid analgesics may apply, i.e., administering the medication slowly, with an opioid antagonist and equipment for artificial ventilation available.

When an opioid analgesic is administered parenterally, the patient usually should be lying down and should remain recumbent for a period of time to minimize side effects such as hypotension, dizziness, lightheadedness, nausea, and vomiting. If these side effects occur in an ambulatory patient, they may be relieved if the patient lies down.

In patients with shock, impaired perfusion may prevent complete absorption following intramuscular injection. Repeated administration may result in overdose due to an excessive amount suddenly being absorbed when circulation is restored.

## Parenteral Dosage Forms

### DEZOCINE INJECTION

**Usual adult dose**
Analgesic—
  Intramuscular, 5 to 20 mg (usually 10 mg, initially). May be repeated every three to six hours as needed.
  Intravenous, 2.5 to 10 mg (usually 5 mg, initially). May be repeated every two to four hours as needed.

Note: Lower doses may be required for geriatric, very ill, or debilitated patients and patients with respiratory problems.

**Usual adult prescribing limits**
Single intramuscular dose—20 mg, although there is some evidence that, because of dezocine's antagonist activity, 15 mg may be the maximally effective dose.
Total daily dose—120 mg.

**Usual pediatric and adolescent dose**
Patients up to 18 years of age—Safety and efficacy have not been established.

**Strength(s) usually available**
U.S.—
  5 mg per mL (Rx) [*Dalgan* (sodium metabisulfite)].
  10 mg per mL (Rx) [*Dalgan* (sodium metabisulfite)].
  15 mg per mL (Rx) [*Dalgan* (sodium metabisulfite)].
Canada—
  Not commercially available.

**Packaging and storage**
Store below 40 °C (104 °F), preferably between 15 and 30 °C (59 and 86 °F), protected from light, unless otherwise specified by manufacturer.

**Auxiliary labeling**
- May cause drowsiness.
- Avoid alcoholic beverages.
- May be habit-forming.

**Note**
Although a potent opioid (narcotic) analgesic, dezocine is not a controlled substance in the U.S.

### Selected Bibliography
O'Brien JJ, Benfield P. Dezocine. A preliminary review of its pharmacodynamic and pharmacokinetic properties, and therapeutic efficacy. Drugs 1989; 38: 226-48.
Stanbaugh JE, McAdams J. Comparison of intramuscular dezocine with butorphanol and placebo in chronic cancer pain: A method to evaluate analgesia after both single and repeated doses. Clin Pharmacol Ther 1987; 42: 210-9.
Galloway FM, Varma S. Double-blind comparison of intravenous doses of dezocine, butorphanol, and placebo for relief of postoperative pain. Anesth Analg 1986; 65: 283-7.

Revised: 08/29/94

---

**DIATRIZOATE AND IODIPAMIDE**—The *Diatrizoate and Iodipamide (Local)* monograph is not included in this published version of the USP DI database. Copies of the monograph are available on request from Micromedex, Inc. - Reprint Requests, 6200 S. Syracuse Way, Suite 300, Englewood, CO 80111; telephone (303) 486-6400; telefax (303) 486-6464; Email: USPDI@MDX.COM.

---

**DIATRIZOATES**—The *Diatrizoates (Local)* monograph is not included in this published version of the USP DI database. Copies of the monograph are available on request from Micromedex, Inc. - Reprint Requests, 6200 S. Syracuse Way, Suite 300, Englewood, CO 80111; telephone (303) 486-6400; telefax (303) 486-6464; Email: USPDI@MDX.COM.

---

**DIATRIZOATES**—The *Diatrizoates (Systemic)* monograph is not included in this published version of the USP DI database. Copies of the monograph are available on request from Micromedex, Inc. - Reprint Requests, 6200 S. Syracuse Way, Suite 300, Englewood, CO 80111; telephone (303) 486-6400; telefax (303) 486-6464; Email: USPDI@MDX.COM.

---

**DIAZEPAM**—See *Benzodiazepines (Systemic)*

---

# DIAZOXIDE   Oral-Systemic

VA CLASSIFICATION (Primary/Secondary): HS508/GA900
Commonly used brand name(s): *Proglycem*.
Note: For a listing of dosage forms and brand names by country availability, see *Dosage Forms* section(s).

## Category
Antihypoglycemic.

## Indications

### Accepted
Hypoglycemia (treatment)—Diazoxide is indicated orally for the management of hypoglycemia due to hyperinsulinism associated with inoperable islet cell adenoma or carcinoma, or extrapancreatic malignancy; leucine sensitivity; islet cell hyperplasia; nesidioblastosis; or adenomatosis. Diazoxide should only be used in hypoglycemia that is confirmed to be caused by hyperinsulinism unresponsive to other treatment.

### Unaccepted
Although oral diazoxide reduces blood pressure gradually, it is not used in the chronic treatment of hypertension because of its side effects.

Diazoxide is not recommended for use in the treatment of functional hypoglycemia.

## Pharmacology/Pharmacokinetics

### Physicochemical characteristics
Chemical group—Diazoxide is a nondiuretic thiazide derivative.
Molecular weight—230.67.
pKa—8.5.

### Mechanism of action/Effect
Hyperglycemic effect is due primarily to inhibition of insulin release from the pancreas, as well as an extrapancreatic (catecholamine-induced) effect.

### Absorption
Readily absorbed following oral administration; the suspension may produce higher blood concentrations than the capsule form in some patients.

### Protein binding
Very high (more than 90%) to serum proteins; reduced in uremia.

### Biotransformation
Hepatic.

### Half-life
Normal renal function—28 ±8.3 hours.
Anuria—20 to 53 hours; may also be prolonged with overdosage.

### Onset of action
1 hour.

### Duration of action
Normal renal function— 8 hours or less.

### Elimination
Renal; approximately 50% unchanged.
In dialysis—Diazoxide is dialyzable; a higher dose or additional doses may be required when patients are being dialyzed.

## Precautions to Consider

### Cross-sensitivity and/or related problems
Patients sensitive to thiazide diuretics or other sulfonamide-type medications may be sensitive to this medication also.

### Carcinogenicity/Mutagenicity
Studies have not been done in either animals or humans.

### Pregnancy/Reproduction
Pregnancy—Diazoxide crosses the placenta. Adequate studies in humans have not been done. Possible adverse effects in infants of mothers who received diazoxide include transient hyperglycemia, hyperbilirubinemia, alopecia, hypertrichosis, and thrombocytopenia.
In rats, increased fetal resorptions, fetal skeletal abnormalities, and delayed parturition were seen. In rabbits, some teratogenic (skeletal, pancreatic, and cardiac) effects have been observed.

FDA Pregnancy Category C.

Labor—Diazoxide may inhibit labor, although oxytocin will reverse this effect.

### Breast-feeding
It is not known whether diazoxide is distributed into breast milk. However, problems in humans have not been documented.

### Pediatrics
Diazoxide-induced edema occurs most frequently in infants. In susceptible patients, this may lead to congestive heart failure.
The development of abnormal facial features has been reported in 4 children who were treated chronically (more than 4 years) with diazoxide for hypoglycemia due to hyperinsulinism.

### Geriatrics
No information is available on the relationship of age to the effects of diazoxide in geriatric patients. However, elderly patients are more likely to have age-related renal function impairment, which may require a reduction in dosage and/or a longer dosing interval.

### Drug interactions and/or related problems
The following drug interactions and/or related problems have been selected on the basis of their potential clinical significance (possible mechanism in parentheses where appropriate)—not necessarily inclusive (» = major clinical significance):

Note: Combinations containing any of the following medications, depending on the amount present, may also interact with this medication.

Alpha-adrenergic blocking agents, such as:
  Labetalol
  Phenoxybenzamine
  Phentolamine
  Prazosin
  Tolazoline or
Other medications with alpha-adrenergic blocking action, such as:
  Dihydroergotamine
  Ergoloid mesylates
  Ergotamine
  Haloperidol
  Loxapine
  Phenothiazines
  Thioxanthenes
    (concurrent use antagonizes the inhibition of insulin release by diazoxide)

Anticoagulants, coumarin- or indandione-derivative
  (increased anticoagulant effects may occur because of displacement of the anticoagulant from protein-binding sites; adjustment of anticoagulant dosage may be necessary)
» Anticonvulsants, hydantoin
  (concurrent use is generally not recommended since it may result in decreased efficacy of either medication)
Antigout medications
  (diazoxide may raise the concentration of blood uric acid; dosage adjustment of antigout medications may be necessary)
Beta-adrenergic blocking agents, ophthalmic, if significant systemic absorption occurs or
Beta-adrenergic blocking agents, systemic
  (concurrent use prevents diazoxide-induced tachycardia; however, risk of hypotension may be increased)
Diuretics, loop or
Diuretics, thiazide or
Indapamide
  (may potentiate the antihypertensive, hyperglycemic, and hyperuricemic actions of diazoxide; when used concurrently, adjustment of diazoxide dosage may be necessary)
» Hypotension-producing medications, other, (See *Appendix II*) or
» Vasodilators, peripheral, for example, cyclandelate, hydralazine, isoxsuprine, nicotinyl alcohol, nylidrin, papaverine
  (concurrent use with diazoxide may result in an additive hypotensive effect, which may be severe; dosage adjustments may be necessary, and patients should be continuously observed for excessive fall in blood pressure for several hours after concurrent administration)

### Laboratory value alterations
The following have been selected on the basis of their potential clinical significance (possible effect in parentheses where appropriate)—not necessarily inclusive (» = major clinical significance):

With diagnostic test results
  Insulin response to glucagon
    (false-negative results)

With physiology/laboratory test values
  Alkaline phosphatase and
  Aspartate aminotransferase (AST [SGOT]) and
  Free fatty acid and
  Sodium and
  Uric acid
    (serum concentrations may be increased)
  Blood pressure
    (may be increased)
  Creatinine clearance and
  Electrolytes, urine, such as chloride, bicarbonate, potassium, and sodium and
  Hematocrit and
  Hemoglobin and
  Immunoglobulin G (IgG), plasma
    (may be decreased)
  Glucose and
  Urea nitrogen (BUN)
    (blood concentrations may be increased)
  Heart rate
    (may be transiently increased)

### Medical considerations/Contraindications
The medical considerations/contraindications included have been selected on the basis of their potential clinical significance (reasons given in parentheses where appropriate)—not necessarily inclusive (» = major clinical significance).

*Risk-benefit should be considered when the following medical problems exist:*

» Acute aortic dissection
» Compensatory hypertension, such as that associated with aortic coarctation or arteriovenous shunt
» Coronary or cerebral insufficiency
Gout, history of or
Hyperuricemia
  (may be exacerbated)
Hepatic function impairment
Hypokalemia
  (hyperglycemic effects are potentiated)

» Inadequate cardiac reserve, such as uncompensated congestive heart failure
Renal function impairment
(half-life of diazoxide may be prolonged; reduced dosage may be necessary with frequent use)
Sensitivity to diazoxide, sulfonamides, or thiazides

**Patient monitoring**
The following may be especially important in patient monitoring (other tests may be warranted in some patients, depending on condition; » = major clinical significance):
Aspartate aminotransferase (AST [SGOT]), serum and
Creatinine clearance and
Hematocrit and
Leukocyte count, differential and total and
Platelet count and
Urea nitrogen, blood, (BUN) and
Uric acid, serum
(determinations recommended at periodic intervals during prolonged therapy)
» Glucose
(measurement of blood or urine concentrations is recommended at periodic intervals in patients taking diazoxide until hypoglycemia is corrected and stabilized)
» Ketones
(results of monitoring for ketones in urine reported by the patient to the physician provides frequent and relatively inexpensive monitoring of the condition)

## Side/Adverse Effects

The following side/adverse effects have been selected on the basis of their potential clinical significance (possible signs and symptoms in parentheses where appropriate)—not necessarily inclusive:

**Those indicating need for medical attention**
Incidence more frequent
*Edema* (decreased urination; rapid weight gain; swelling of feet or lower legs)
Note: *Edema* occurs most commonly in young infants and adults and may lead to congestive heart failure in susceptible patients.
Incidence less frequent
*Tachycardia* (fast heartbeat)
Incidence rare
*Allergic reaction* (fever; skin rash); ***angina pectoris, myocardial infarction, or myocardial ischemia*** (chest pain; unexplained shortness of breath)—most commonly occurring during physical exertion; ***thrombocytopenia*** (unusual bleeding or bruising); ***transient focal cerebral ischemic attacks*** (confusion; numbness of the hands)
With long-term use
*Extrapyramidal effects* (stiffness of limbs; trembling and shaking of hands and fingers)

**Those indicating need for medical attention only if they continue or are bothersome**
Incidence less frequent
*Changes in ability to taste; ileus* (constipation); *loss of appetite; nausea; stomach pain; vomiting*
With long-term use
*Hypertrichosis* (increased hair growth on forehead, back, arms, and legs)

## Overdose

For specific information on the agents used in the management of diazoxide overdose, see *Insulin (Systemic)* monograph.
For more information on the management of overdose or unintentional ingestion, **contact a Poison Control Center** (see *Poison Control Center Listing*).

**Clinical effects of overdose**
The following effects have been selected on the basis of their potential clinical significance (possible signs and symptoms in parentheses where appropriate)—not necessarily inclusive:
***Hyperglycemia or ketoacidosis*** (continuing loss of appetite; drowsiness; flushed, dry skin; fruit-like breath odor; increased urination; unusual thirst)—more likely when administered during intercurrent illness

**Treatment of overdose**
Specific treatment—Administration of insulin to treat hyperglycemia and prevent ketoacidosis.

Monitoring—Monitoring the patient for up to 7 days, especially if severe hyperglycemia occurs.
Supportive care—Restoration of fluid and electrolyte balance. Patients in whom intentional overdose is known or suspected should be referred for psychiatric consultation.

## Patient Consultation

As an aid to patient consultation, refer to *Advice for the Patient, Diazoxide (Oral)*.
In providing consultation, consider emphasizing the following selected information (» = major clinical significance):

**Before using this medication**
» Conditions affecting use, especially:
Sensitivity to diazoxide, thiazide diuretics, or other sulfonamide-type medications
Pregnancy—Studies in animals have demonstrated teratogenicity; effects on infants born to mothers who received diazoxide may include hyperglycemia, hyperbilirubinemia, alopecia, hypertrichosis, and thrombocytopenia
Labor—May inhibit labor
Other medications, especially hydantoin anticonvulsants, other hypotension-producing medications, or peripheral vasodilators
Other medical problems, especially acute aortic dissection, compensatory hypertension, coronary or cerebral insufficiency, or inadequate cardiac reserve

**Proper use of this medication**
» Not taking more or less medication than the amount prescribed; taking at same time each day
» Importance of diet in helping control condition
» Testing for sugar in urine or blood, and ketones in urine
» Proper dosing
Missed dose: Taking as soon as possible; not taking if almost time for next dose; not doubling doses
» Proper storage

**Precautions while using this medication**
» Regular visits to physician to check progress, especially during the first few weeks of treatment
» Caution if any kind of surgery (including dental surgery) or emergency treatment is required
» Not taking other medications, especially OTC sympathomimetics, unless discussed with physician
» Symptoms of hyperglycemia or ketoacidosis
Symptoms of hypoglycemia

**Side/adverse effects**
Possibility of excessive hair growth, which is reversible in several weeks or months when medication is withdrawn
Signs of potential side effects, especially edema, tachycardia, allergic reaction, angina pectoris, myocardial infarction or ischemia, thrombocytopenia, transient focal cerebral ischemic attacks, and extrapyramidal effects

## General Dosing Information

Diazoxide is often administered concurrently with a diuretic to prevent congestive heart failure due to fluid retention.
In some patients, the oral suspension dosage form of diazoxide produces higher blood concentrations than the capsule form; caution is recommended when a patient is switched from one dosage form to another.
Hyperglycemia is usually transient after intravenous administration of diazoxide (persisting 24 to 48 hours), but may be more persistent after prolonged oral administration and may rarely progress to ketoacidosis or hyperosmolar coma.
If diazoxide is not effective within 2 to 3 weeks in the treatment of hypoglycemia, it is recommended that therapy with the medication be re-evaluated.

## Oral Dosage Forms

### DIAZOXIDE CAPSULES USP
**Usual adult and adolescent dose**
Antihypoglycemic—
Initial: Oral, 1 mg per kg of body weight every eight hours, adjusted according to clinical response.
Maintenance: Oral, 3 to 8 mg per kg of body weight a day, divided into two or three equal doses every twelve or eight hours, respectively.

**Usual adult prescribing limits**
Oral, up to 15 mg per kg of body weight a day.

# Diazoxide (Oral-Systemic)

**Usual pediatric dose**
Antihypoglycemic—
  Neonates and infants:
    Initial—Oral, 3.3 mg per kg of body weight every eight hours, adjusted according to clinical response.
    Maintenance—Oral, 8 to 15 mg per kg of body weight a day, divided into two or three equal doses every twelve or eight hours, respectively.
  Children:
    See *Usual adult and adolescent dose*.

**Strength(s) usually available**
U.S.—
  50 mg (Rx) [*Proglycem*].
Canada—
  50 mg (Rx) [*Proglycem* (lactose)].
  100 mg (Rx) [*Proglycem* (lactose)].

**Packaging and storage**
Store below 40 °C (104 °F), preferably between 15 and 30 °C (59 and 86 °F), unless otherwise specified by manufacturer. Store in a well-closed container.

## DIAZOXIDE ORAL SUSPENSION USP

**Usual adult and adolescent dose**
See *Diazoxide Capsules USP*.

**Usual pediatric dose**
See *Diazoxide Capsules USP*.

**Strength(s) usually available**
U.S.—
  50 mg per mL (Rx) [*Proglycem* (alcohol 7.25%)].
Canada—
  50 mg per mL (Rx) [*Proglycem* (alcohol 7.25%; parabens)].

**Packaging and storage**
Store below 40 °C (104 °F), preferably between 15 and 30 °C (59 and 86 °F), unless otherwise specified by manufacturer. Store in a tight container. Protect from light. Protect from freezing.

**Auxiliary labeling**
• Shake well before using.

Revised: 12/15/92
Interim revision: 05/24/94

---

# DIAZOXIDE  Parenteral-Systemic

VA CLASSIFICATION (Primary): CV409

Commonly used brand name(s): *Hyperstat*.

Note: For a listing of dosage forms and brand names by country availability, see *Dosage Forms* section(s).

## Category
Antihypertensive.

## Indications

**Accepted**

Hypertension (treatment)—Diazoxide is indicated intravenously for the emergency reduction of blood pressure in malignant hypertension or hypertensive crisis. Diazoxide is ineffective against hypertension associated with monoamine oxidase (MAO) inhibitor therapy or pheochromocytoma, but has been used investigationally by intravenous infusion to treat chronic hypertension in nonemergency situations.

**Unaccepted**

Parenteral diazoxide has only a transient hyperglycemic effect; oral diazoxide is more appropriate for treatment of hypoglycemia.

## Pharmacology/Pharmacokinetics

**Physicochemical characteristics**
Molecular weight—230.67.
pKa—8.5.

**Mechanism of action/Effect**
Exact mechanism of antihypertensive action is unknown. Diazoxide produces arteriolar vasodilation and decreased peripheral resistance.

**Other actions/effects**
Diazoxide has a hyperglycemic effect that is due primarily to inhibition of insulin release from the pancreas, as well as an extrapancreatic (catecholamine-induced) effect.

**Protein binding**
High to very high (more than 90%) to albumin; reduced in uremia.

**Biotransformation**
Hepatic.

**Half-life**
Normal—21 to 36 hours (average, 28 hours).
Anuric—20 to 53 hours.
Note: The plasma half-life is much longer than the hypotensive effect; accumulation occurs with repeated doses.

**Onset of action**
1 minute (after intravenous push).

**Time to peak effect**
2 to 5 minutes (after intravenous push).

**Duration of action**
2 to 12 hours.

**Elimination**
Renal; approximately 50% unchanged.
In dialysis—Diazoxide is dialyzable; a higher dose or additional doses may be required when patients are being dialyzed.

## Precautions to Consider

**Cross-sensitivity and/or related problems**
Patients sensitive to thiazide diuretics or other sulfonamide-type medications, including bumetanide, furosemide, and carbonic anhydrase inhibitors, may be sensitive to this medication also.

**Pregnancy/Reproduction**
Pregnancy—Diazoxide crosses the placenta. Studies in humans have not been done. However, possible adverse effects in infants of mothers who receive diazoxide include hyperglycemia, hyperbilirubinemia, alopecia or increased hair growth, and thrombocytopenia.
Increased fetal resorptions, delayed parturition, and some teratogenic (skeletal, pancreatic, and cardiac) effects have been observed in animals.
Labor—Diazoxide may also inhibit labor, although oxytocin will reverse this effect.

**Breast-feeding**
It is not known if diazoxide is distributed into breast milk. However, problems in humans have not been documented.

**Pediatrics**
Studies performed to date have not demonstrated pediatrics-specific problems that would limit the usefulness of parenteral diazoxide in children.

**Geriatrics**
No information is available on the relationship of age to the effects of parenteral diazoxide in geriatric patients. However, elderly patients are more likely to have age-related renal function impairment, which may require reduction of dose in patients receiving parenteral diazoxide.

**Drug interactions and/or related problems**
The following drug interactions and/or related problems have been selected on the basis of their potential clinical significance (possible mechanism in parentheses where appropriate)—not necessarily inclusive (» = major clinical significance):

Note: Combinations containing any of the following medications, depending on the amount present, may also interact with this medication.

Allopurinol or
Colchicine or
Probenecid or
Sulfinpyrazone
  (diazoxide may raise the concentration of blood uric acid; dosage adjustment of antigout medications may be necessary to control hyperuricemia and gout)

Anticoagulants, coumarin- or indandione-derivative
  (concurrent use with diazoxide may result in increased anticoagulant effects because of displacement of the anticoagulant from protein-binding sites; anticoagulant dosage adjustments may be necessary)

Antidiabetic agents, oral or
Insulin
(concurrent or consecutive use reverses the hyperglycemic effects of diazoxide; in addition, dosage adjustments of hypoglycemic medications may be necessary if diazoxide is administered to diabetics)

Anti-inflammatory drugs, nonsteroidal (NSAIDs), especially indomethacin or
Estrogens or
Sympathomimetics
(concurrent use antagonizes the hypotensive effects of diazoxide; indomethacin and possibly other NSAIDs may antagonize the hypotensive effect by inhibiting renal prostaglandin synthesis and/or by causing sodium and fluid retention; estrogen-induced fluid retention tends to increase blood pressure)

Beta-adrenergic blocking agents, ophthalmic
(if significant systemic absorption of ophthalmic beta-blockers occurs, concurrent use may increase the hypotensive effect of diazoxide)

Beta-adrenergic blocking agents, systemic
(concurrent use prevents the tachycardia produced by diazoxide but may also increase the hypotensive effect)

Diuretics, loop or
Diuretics, thiazide or
Indapamide
(may potentiate the antihypertensive, hyperglycemic, and hyperuricemic actions of diazoxide; when used concurrently, dosage adjustments may be necessary)

» Hypotension-producing medications, other (see *Appendix II*) or
Ritodrine, intravenous or
» Vasodilators, peripheral, such as cyclandelate, isoxsuprine, nicotinyl alcohol, nylidrin, papaverine
(concurrent use with diazoxide may result in an additive hypotensive effect, which may be severe; dosage adjustments may be necessary, and patients should be continuously observed for excessive fall in blood pressure for several hours after concurrent administration)

**Laboratory value alterations**
The following have been selected on the basis of their potential clinical significance (possible effect in parentheses where appropriate)—not necessarily inclusive (» = major clinical significance):

With diagnostic test results
Insulin response to glucagon
(false-negative results)

With physiology/laboratory test values
Alkaline phosphatase values and
Aspartate aminotransferase (AST [SGOT]) values and
Blood urea nitrogen (BUN) concentrations and
Free fatty acid concentrations, serum and
Glucose concentrations, blood and
Sodium concentrations, serum (excretion decreased) and
Uric acid concentrations, serum
(may be increased)

Creatinine clearance and
Hematocrit and
Hemoglobin concentrations and
Immunoglobulin G (IgG) concentrations in plasma and
Urinary excretion of potassium, chloride, and bicarbonate
(may be decreased)

**Medical considerations/Contraindications**
The medical considerations/contraindications included have been selected on the basis of their potential clinical significance (reasons given in parentheses where appropriate)—not necessarily inclusive (» = major clinical significance).

***Risk-benefit should be considered when the following medical problems exist:***

» Acute aortic dissection
» Compensatory hypertension, such as that associated with aortic coarctation or arteriovenous shunt
(decrease in blood pressure may exacerbate this condition)
» Coronary or cerebral insufficiency or
Gout, history of
(conditions may be exacerbated)
» Diabetes mellitus
(hyperglycemic effects of diazoxide may require management measures in these patients)
Hepatic function impairment
Hypokalemia
(hyperglycemic effects potentiated)
» Poor cardiac reserve, such as uncompensated congestive heart failure
(diazoxide-induced sodium retention may precipitate edema in these patients)
Renal function impairment
(reduced dosage of diazoxide may be necessary if it is administered repeatedly to patients with renal function impairment, since protein binding is reduced in uremia and the half-life of the medication may be prolonged)
Sensitivity to diazoxide

**Patient monitoring**
The following may be especially important in patient monitoring (other tests may be warranted in some patients, depending on condition; » = major clinical significance):

Blood glucose determinations
(recommended at periodic intervals after parenteral administration to monitor hyperglycemia, especially in diabetics or patients with renal or hepatic function impairment)

» Blood pressure determinations
(recommended at frequent intervals after parenteral administration until blood pressure has stabilized, then at hourly intervals until the medication is withdrawn)

## Side/Adverse Effects

The following side/adverse effects have been selected on the basis of their potential clinical significance (possible signs and symptoms in parentheses where appropriate)—not necessarily inclusive:

**Those indicating need for medical attention**
Incidence more frequent
***Sodium and water retention and edema*** (decrease in urination; swelling of hands, feet, or lower legs)
Note: *Sodium and water retention* occurs most commonly in young infants and adults after repeated injections and may lead to congestive heart failure in susceptible patients.

Incidence less frequent
***Hyperglycemia*** (drowsiness; fruit-like breath odor; increased urination; unusual thirst); ***hypotension; tachycardia*** (fast heartbeat)
Note: *Hyperglycemia* is usually transient after intravenous administration of diazoxide (persisting 24 to 48 hours), but may be more persistent after more than three parenteral doses within a short period (up to 24 hours) and may rarely progress to ketoacidosis and hyperosmolar coma.

Incidence rare
***Allergic reaction or thrombocytopenia*** (fever; skin rash; unusual bleeding or bruising); ***cerebral ischemia or thrombosis*** (confusion; numbness of hands); ***hyperosmolar coma*** (confusion); ***myocardial ischemia, angina pectoris, or myocardial infarction*** (chest pain)

**Those indicating need for medical attention only if they continue or are bothersome**
Incidence less frequent
***Changes in ability to taste; constipation; loss of appetite; nausea and vomiting; stomach pain***

Occurring with intravenous use
***Back pain; ringing in ears; vasodilation*** (flushing or redness of face; headache; weakness); ***warmth or pain along injected vein***

Incidence rare
***Orthostatic hypotension*** (dizziness or lightheadedness, especially when getting up from a lying or sitting position)

## Overdose

For more information on the management of overdose or unintentional ingestion, **contact a Poison Control Center** (see *Poison Control Center Listing*).

**Treatment of overdose**
Severe hypotension usually responds to treatment with a vasopressor such as norepinephrine or metaraminol.

## General Dosing Information

It is recommended that diazoxide be administered only into a peripheral vein via an established intravenous line, to prevent cardiac arrhythmia.

Intramuscular, intracavitary, or subcutaneous administration is not recommended since pain may occur at the site of injections.

Diazoxide has been thought to be most effective in reducing blood pressure when intravenous administration is completed within 10 to 30 seconds.

Slower administration supposedly reduces or shortens the response because of extensive protein binding. However, recent studies have suggested that administration of diazoxide by intravenous infusion may produce a similar (although usually smaller) but more gradual fall in blood pressure in both chronic hypertension and hypertensive crisis, reducing the risk of impaired perfusion of vital organs that may occur with a sudden fall in blood pressure. One study used a dose of 5 mg per kg of body weight (mg/kg) (15 mg per mL of intravenous infusion) administered at a rate of 15 mg per minute over 20 to 30 minutes. Other studies have found no effect when diazoxide is administered by intravenous infusion; further study is necessary to resolve this controversy.

Care must be taken to avoid extravasation during intravenous administration since cellulitis and pain (but not necrosis) may result. If extravasation occurs, conservative treatment with cold packs is recommended.

It is recommended that diazoxide injection be administered with the patient recumbent during and for 15 to 30 minutes after administration.

Tolerance to the antihypertensive effects of diazoxide may develop unless expansion of plasma and extracellular fluid volume is prevented by use of a diuretic.

Diazoxide is often administered with a diuretic to obtain maximum antihypertensive effect and prevent congestive heart failure due to sodium and water retention. Loop diuretics such as furosemide or ethacrynic acid may be the most useful. Administration of 40 to 80 mg of furosemide intravenously 30 to 60 minutes prior to intravenous diazoxide has been recommended.

Because of the long half-life of diazoxide, patients who develop marked hyperglycemia as a result of overdosage require prolonged monitoring (up to 7 days) while blood sugar concentrations stabilize.

## Parenteral Dosage Forms

### DIAZOXIDE INJECTION USP

**Usual adult and adolescent dose**
Antihypertensive—
Intravenous, up to 150 mg, or 1 to 3 mg per kg of body weight, repeated every five to fifteen minutes if necessary to obtain the desired response. Further doses may be administered every four to twenty-four hours as needed to maintain the desired blood pressure until oral antihypertensive medication is effective, usually within four to five days.

**Usual adult prescribing limits**
1.2 grams per day.

**Usual pediatric dose**
Antihypertensive—
Intravenous, 1 to 3 mg per kg of body weight or 30 to 90 mg per square meter of body surface, repeated in five to fifteen minutes if necessary to obtain the desired response. Further doses may be administered every four to twenty-four hours as needed to maintain the desired blood pressure until oral antihypertensive medication is effective.

**Strength(s) usually available**
U.S.—
15 mg per mL (Rx) [*Hyperstat* (sodium bisulfite 0.24 mg per mL); GENERIC].
Canada—
15 mg per mL (Rx) [*Hyperstat*].

**Packaging and storage**
Store below 40 °C (104 °F), preferably between 15 and 30 °C (59 and 86 °F), unless otherwise specified by manufacturer. Protect from light. Protect from freezing.

Revised: 05/14/93
Interim revision: 08/12/98

---

**DIBUCAINE**—See *Anesthetics (Mucosal-Local)*; *Anesthetics (Topical)*

---

**DICHLORPHENAMIDE**—See *Carbonic Anhydrase Inhibitors (Systemic)*

---

**DICLOFENAC**—See *Anti-inflammatory Drugs, Nonsteroidal (Ophthalmic)*; *Anti-inflammatory Drugs, Nonsteroidal (Systemic)*

---

# DICLOFENAC AND MISOPROSTOL Systemic—INTRODUCTORY VERSION

VA CLASSIFICATION (Primary): MS109
Note: For a listing of dosage forms and brand names by country availability, see *Dosage Forms* section(s).

## Category
Antirheumatic (nonsteroidal anti-inflammatory).

## Indications
**Accepted**
Arthritis, rheumatoid (treatment) or
Osteoarthritis (treatment)—Diclofenac and misoprostol combination is indicated for treatment of the signs and symptoms of rheumatoid arthritis and osteoarthritis in patients at high risk of developing nonsteroidal anti-inflammatory drug (NSAID)–induced gastric and duodenal ulcers.

## Pharmacology/Pharmacokinetics
**Physicochemical characteristics**
Molecular weight—Diclofenac sodium: 318.14.
Misoprostol: 382.54.

**Mechanism of action/Effect**
Diclofenac—Diclofenec is a nonsteroidal anti-inflammatory drug (NSAID). Results of pharmacological studies show that diclofenac has anti-inflammatory, analgesic, and antipyretic therapeutic effects. The exact mechanism of action has not been determined. A deficiency of prostaglandins within the gastric and duodenal mucosa may lead to a decrease in bicarbonate and mucus secretion, resulting in possible mucosal damage caused by NSAIDs.
Misoprostol—
Cytoprotective:
Misoprostol enhances natural gastromucosal defense mechanisms and healing in acid-related disorders, probably by increasing production of gastric mucus and mucosal secretion of bicarbonate.
Antisecretory:
Misoprostol inhibits basal and nocturnal gastric acid secretion by direct action on parietal cells; also inhibits gastric acid secretion stimulated by coffee, food, histamine, and pentagastrin. It decreases pepsin secretion under basal, but not histamine, stimulation. Misoprostol has no significant effect on fasting or postprandial gastrin or intrinsic factor output.

**Absorption**
Diclofenac—Rapidly absorbed following oral administration.
Misoprostol—Rapidly absorbed following oral administration.
Following oral administration of diclofenac and misoprostol combination (50 mg/200 mcg and 75 mg/200 mcg doses, respectively), a similar rate and extent of absorption for diclofenac and misoprostol administered alone were observed. Food decreases the bioavailability of the combination of diclofenac and misoprostol.

**Protein binding**
Diclofenac—Very high (99%).
Misoprostol acid (active metabolite)—High (< 90%).

**Biotransformation**
Diclofenac—Hepatic; almost 50% eliminated via first-pass metabolism; some active metabolites.
Misoprostol—Rapidly de-esterified to misoprostol acid (primary biologically active metabolite).

**Half-life**
Elimination—
Diclofenac: 120 minutes.
Misoprostol acid metabolite: Approximately 30 minutes.

**Onset of action**
Misoprostol—Within 30 minutes.

**Time to peak concentration**
Diclofenac—2 hours.
Misoprostol acid—Approximately 20 minutes.

**Peak serum concentration**
Diclofenac—1.5 and 2 mcg/mL (50- and 75-mg doses, respectively).

**Duration of action**
Misoprostol—Approximately 3 hours.

**Elimination**
Diclofenac—
   Renal:
      Approximately 65% (little or none unchanged).
   Biliary:
      Approximately 35% (little or none unchanged).
Misoprostol—
   Renal:
      70%.

## Precautions to Consider

### Cross-sensitivity and/or related problems
Patients sensitive to diclofenac or other nonsteroidal anti-inflammatory drugs (NSAIDs), misoprostol or other prostaglandins, or prostaglandin analogs may be sensitive to diclofenac and misoprostol combination.

Diclofenac and misoprostol combination may cause bronchoconstriction or anaphylaxis in aspirin-sensitive asthmatics, especially those with aspirin-induced nasal polyps, asthma, and other allergic reactions (the "aspirin triad").

### Carcinogenicity/Tumorigenicity
*Diclofenac*—No evidence of tumorigenicity was found in rats receiving oral doses of diclofenac of up to 2 mg per kilogram of body weight (mg/kg) per day (approximately 12 mg per square meter of body surface area [mg/m$^2$] per day) for 24 months. Studies in male and female mice receiving doses of diclofenac of up to 0.3 mg/kg per day (approximately 0.006 times the maximum recommended human dose [MRHD] on a mg/m$^2$ basis) and 1 mg/kg per day (approximately 0.02 times the MRHD on a mg/m$^2$ basis) for 24 months, respectively, showed no carcinogenic potential.

*Misoprostol*—No evidence of carcinogenicity was found in rats and mice receiving oral doses of misoprostol of up to 2.4 mg/kg per day (approximately 24 times the MRHD on a mg/m$^2$ basis) for 24 months and doses of up to 16 mg/kg per day (approximately 80 times the MRHD on a mg/m$^2$ basis) for 21 months, respectively.

### Mutagenicity
Diclofenac and misoprostol combination was not genotoxic in the Ames test, Chinese hamster ovary cell (CHO/HGPRT) forward mutation test, rat lymphocyte chromosome aberration test, or in a mouse micronucleus test.

### Pregnancy/Reproduction
Fertility—*Diclofenac*: Studies in male and female rats receiving doses of diclofenac of up to 4 mg/kg per day (approximately 0.16 times the MRHD on a mg/m$^2$ basis) found no effect on fertility and reproductive performance.

*Misoprostol*: Fertility studies done in male and female rats receiving oral doses from 0.1 to 10 mg/kg per day (approximately 1 to 100 times the MRHD on a mg/m$^2$ basis) found dose-related preimplantation and postimplantation losses. In addition, a significant decrease in the number of live pups born was observed at the highest dose. These results suggest that misoprostol may have adverse effects on fertility.

Pregnancy—**Diclofenac and misoprostol combination is contraindicated in pregnancy.**

Diclofenac and misoprostol combination was not teratogenic in reproductive studies in rabbits receiving oral doses of up to 10 mg/kg per day (approximately 0.8 times the MRHD on a mg/m$^2$ basis) of diclofenac and 0.04 mg/kg per day (approximately 0.8 times the MRHD on a mg/m$^2$ basis) of misoprostol.

FDA Pregnancy Category X.

Patients of childbearing potential may use diclofenac and misoprostol combination if nonsteroidal anti-inflammatory drug (NSAID) therapy is required and patient is at high risk of complications from gastric ulcers associated with the use of NSAIDs, or is at high risk of developing gastric ulceration. Such patients must comply with effective contraceptive measures, must have had a negative serum pregnancy test within 2 weeks prior to initiation of therapy, and must start diclofenac and misoprostol combination only on the second or third day of the next normal menstrual period. Additionally, patients must receive both oral and written warnings of the hazards of misoprostol, such as the risk of possible contraception failure and the danger to other women of childbearing potential should the drug be taken by mistake.

*Diclofenac*: Diclofenac may cause premature closure of the ductus arteriosus, which may affect the fetal cardiovascular system. Also, diclofenac, like other NSAIDs, may inhibit uterine contractions.

No teratogenicity was demonstrated in reproductive studies in rabbits receiving oral doses of diclofenac of up to 10 mg/kg per day (approximately 0.8 times the MRHD on a mg/m$^2$ basis) per day, in mice receiving oral doses of up to 20 mg/kg per day (approximately 0.4 times the MRHD on a mg/m$^2$ basis), or in rats receiving oral doses of up to 10 mg/kg per day (approximately 4 times the MRHD on a mg/m$^2$ basis).

*Misoprostol*: Studies in humans have shown that misoprostol causes an increase in the frequency and intensity of uterine contractions. Misoprostol administration has also been associated with a higher incidence of uterine bleeding and expulsion of uterine contents. Miscarriages caused by misoprostol may be incomplete.

No teratogenicity was demonstrated in reproductive studies in rats receiving oral doses of misoprostol of up to 1.6 mg/kg per day (approximately 16 times the MRHD on a mg/m$^2$ basis) or in rabbits receiving oral doses of up to 1 mg/kg per day (approximately 20 times the MRHD on a mg/m$^2$ basis).

### Breast-feeding
Diclofenac and misoprostol combination is not recommended for use in nursing mothers.

*Diclofenac*—Diclofenac is distributed into breast milk.

*Misoprostol*—It is not known whether misoprostol is distributed into breast milk. Since misoprostol is rapidly metabolized, it is unlikely to be distributed into breast milk. Although studies have not been done, it is possible that the active metabolite (misoprostol acid) may be distributed into breast milk.

### Pediatrics
Appropriate studies on the relationship of age to the effects of diclofenac and misoprostol combination have not been performed in children up to 18 years of age. Safety and efficacy have not been established.

### Geriatrics
Studies in approximately 500 patients 65 years of age or older have not demonstrated geriatrics-specific problems that would limit the use of diclofenac and misoprostol combination in the elderly. However, nonsteroidal anti-inflammatory drug (NSAID)–induced adverse effects may be less tolerable in geriatric patients than in younger patients. Also, elderly patients are more likely to have age-related renal function impairment, which may require close monitoring in patients receiving diclofenac and misoprostol combination.

### Drug interactions and/or related problems
The following drug interactions and/or related problems have been selected on the basis of their potential clinical significance (possible mechanism in parentheses where appropriate)—not necessarily inclusive (» = major clinical significance):

Note: Combinations containing any of the following medications, depending on the amount present, may also interact with this medication.

Antacids, especially magnesium-containing
   (concurrent use of diclofenac may delay the absorption of diclofenac)
   (concurrent use with misoprostol may aggravate misoprostol-induced diarrhea)

» Anticoagulants, coumarin- or indandione-derivative or
» Corticosteroids, glucocorticoid
   (concurrent use of diclofenac may result in increased risk of gastrointestinal bleeding)

Antidiabetic agents, oral or
Insulin
   (diclofenac may cause changes in the effects of insulin or oral hypoglycemic agents; dosage adjustment of the antidiabetic agent may be necessary)

Antihypertensives, such as:
Angiotensin-converting enzyme (ACE) inhibitors
Diuretics, especially
» Potassium-sparing diuretics
   (increased monitoring of the response to antihypertensive agents is advisable when diclofenac is used concurrently because diclofenac has been shown to inhibit the effects of antihypertensives; caution is recommended)
   (concurrent use of potassium-sparing diuretics with diclofenac may increase the risk of hyperkalemia)
   (concurrent use of diuretics and ACE inhibitors with diclofenac may increase the risk of renal failure secondary to the decrease in renal blood flow caused by inhibition of renal prostaglandin synthesis)

» Aspirin
(concurrent use with diclofenac is not recommended; use with aspirin may result in a lower plasma concentration, peak plasma levels, and area under the plasma concentration–time curve of diclofenac)

» Cyclosporine
(inhibition of renal prostaglandin activity by diclofenac may increase the plasma concentration of cyclosporine and/or the risk of cyclosporine-induced nephrotoxicity; patients should be monitored carefully during concurrent use)

» Digitalis glycosides
(diclofenac has been shown to increase serum digoxin concentrations leading to an increased risk of digitalis toxicity; increased monitoring for digitalis toxicity is recommended during concurrent use with diclofenac and misoprostol combination)

» Lithium
(inhibition of renal prostaglandin activity by diclofenac may result in an increase in the plasma concentration of lithium and a decrease in its renal clearance; patients should be monitored carefully for signs of lithium toxicity)

» Methotrexate
(diclofenac may decrease protein binding and/or renal elimination of methotrexate, resulting in increased and prolonged methotrexate plasma concentrations and an increased risk of toxicity; close monitoring is recommended, especially in patients with renal function impairment)

**Laboratory value alterations**
The following have been selected on the basis of their potential clinical significance (possible effect in parentheses where appropriate)—not necessarily inclusive (» = major clinical significance):

With physiology/laboratory test values
Alanine aminotransferase (ALT [SGPT]), serum or
Aspartate aminotransferase (AST [SGOT]), serum
(values may be increased; liver function test abnormalities may return to normal despite continued use; however, if significant abnormalities occur, clinical signs and symptoms consistent with liver disease develop, or systemic manifestations such as eosinophilia or rash occur, the medication should be discontinued)
(in clinical trials with diclofenac, elevations of AST of more than 3 times the upper limit of normal occurred with overall rates of 2% in patients treated for 2 months and of ALT and/or AST in 4% of patients treated for 2 to 6 months; values in excess of 8 times the upper limit of normal occurred in approximately 1% of the patients)
Platelet aggregation
(may be decreased with diclofenac)

**Medical considerations/Contraindications**
The medical considerations/contraindications included have been selected on the basis of their potential clinical significance (reasons given in parentheses where appropriate)—not necessarily inclusive (» = major clinical significance).

*Except under special circumstances, this medication should not be used when the following medical problems exist:*

» Allergic reaction, severe, such as anaphylaxis or angioedema, induced by aspirin, or other nonsteroidal anti-inflammatory drugs (NSAIDs), history of or

» Nasal polyps associated with bronchospasm, aspirin-induced
(high risk of severe allergic reaction because of cross-sensitivity)

» Renal disease, severe
(use is not recommended)

» Sensitivity to diclofenac or other NSAIDs, misoprostol, or other prostaglandins

*Risk-benefit should be considered when the following medical problems exist:*

Anemia or
Asthma
(may be exacerbated)
Bleeding problems, including:
» Coagulation disorders
» Platelet disorders
(increased risk of bleeding due to the inhibition of platelet aggregation; diclofenac and misoprostol combination does not generally affect platelet counts, prothrombin time, or partial thromboplastin time; careful monitoring is recommended)
Conditions predisposing to and/or exacerbated by fluid retention, such as:
Compromised cardiac function
Congestive heart disease
Edema, pre-existing
Hypertension
Renal function impairment or failure
(diclofenac and misoprostol combination may cause fluid retention and edema)
Conditions predisposing to gastrointestinal toxicity, such as:
Alcoholism, active
» Gastrointestinal bleeding, history of
*Helicobacter pylori*–positive status
» Peptic ulcer disease, history of
Tobacco use, or recent history of
(diclofenac and misoprostol combination should be used with extreme caution in patients with peptic ulcer disease or gastrointestinal bleeding; dosage adjustment is recommended to minimize potential risk of gastrointestinal bleeding)
Congestive heart failure or
Extracellular volume depletion or
» Hepatic function impairment or
» Renal function impairment
(increased risk of renal failure secondary to the decrease in renal blood flow caused by inhibition of renal prostaglandin synthesis)
(diclofenac and its metabolites are excreted primarily via the kidney; therefore, the risk of toxicity associated with the accumulation of diclofenac may be increased; close monitoring is recommended)
Porphyria, hepatic
(diclofenac may precipitate an acute attack)
Systemic lupus erythematosus
(patient may be predisposed to aseptic meningitis)
» Caution is also recommended in geriatric patients, who may be more likely to develop adverse hepatic or renal effects with diclofenac and in whom gastrointestinal ulceration or bleeding is more likely to cause serious consequences

**Patient monitoring**
The following may be especially important in patient monitoring (other tests may be warranted in some patients, depending on condition; » = major clinical significance):

Blood counts, complete (CBC) and
Chemistry profile, blood
(routine monitoring is recommended)
Hemoglobin determinations and/or
Hematocrit determinations
(although routine monitoring is not necessary for most patients during therapy, appropriate tests should be performed if symptoms of anemia occur)
Liver function tests, especially determination of transaminase (AST [SGOT]; ALT [SGPT]) serum values
(it is recommended that hepatic function tests be performed within 4 to 8 weeks following initiation of diclofenac and misoprostol combination therapy and periodically thereafter)

# Side/Adverse Effects

The following side/adverse effects have been selected on the basis of their potential clinical significance (possible signs and symptoms in parentheses where appropriate)—not necessarily inclusive:

**Those indicating need for medical attention**
Incidence less frequent
*Cardiovascular effects, including arrhythmias* (irregular heartbeat); *hypertension* (increased blood pressure); *hypotension* (lightheadedness or dizziness); *palpitations* (pounding heartbeat); *syncope* (fainting); *and tachycardia* (increased heart rate); *central nervous system effects, including confusion; hallucinations* (seeing, hearing, or feeling things that are not there); *meningitis, aseptic* (severe headache; drowsiness; confusion; stiff neck and/or back; general feeling of illness or nausea); *fluid retention; gastrointestinal bleeding; gastrointestinal ulceration, including; esophageal; gastric; or peptic ulceration* (severe stomach pain, cramping, or burning; bloody, or black tarry stools; vomiting of material that looks like coffee grounds; severe and continuing nausea; heartburn and/or indigestion); *hematologic effects, including agranulocytosis* (fever with or without chills; sores, ulcers, or white spots on lips or in mouth; sore throat); *aplastic anemia* (shortness of breath, troubled breathing, tightness in chest, and/or wheezing; sores, ulcers, or white spots on lips or in mouth; sore throat); *ecchymosis* (large, nonelevated blue or purplish patches in the skin); *hemolytic anemia* (troubled breathing, exertional; unusual tiredness or weakness); *leukopenia* (rarely, fever or chills; cough or hoarseness; lower back or side pain; painful or difficult urination); *purpura* (bruises and/or red spots on skin); *thrombocytopenia* (rarely, unusual bleeding or bruising;

black, tarry stools; blood in urine or stools; pinpoint red spots on skin)—usually asymptomatic; *hepatitis or jaundice* (chills; fever; itching of the skin; nausea; yellow eyes or skin; stomach pain; unusual tiredness); *intestinal perforation* (severe pain, cramping, or burning; bloody, or black tarry stools; vomiting of material that looks like coffee grounds; severe and continuing nausea; heartburn and/or indigestion); *mood or mental changes, including disorientation; mental depression; psychotic reaction; pancreatitis* (fever with or without chills; stomach pain; swelling and/or tenderness in upper stomach); *rectal bleeding; renal failure* (increased blood pressure; shortness of breath, troubled breathing, tightness in chest and/or wheezing; sudden decrease in the amount of urine; swelling of face, fingers, feet, and/or lower legs; continuing thirst; unusual tiredness or weakness; weight gain); *seizures; Steven-Johnson syndrome* (bleeding or crusting sores on lips; chest pain; fever with or without chills; muscle cramps or pain; skin rash; sores, ulcers, or white spots on mouth; sore throat)

Note: A 6-week study in 572 patients with osteoarthritis receiving diclofenac and misoprostol combination (50 mg of diclofenac and 200 mcg of misoprostol three times daily or 75 mg of diclofenac and 200 mcg of misoprostol twice daily) found a statistically significant lower incidence of *gastric ulcers* compared to patients receiving diclofenac 75 mg twice daily.

Rare

*Anaphylaxis or anaphylactoid reactions* (changes in facial skin color; skin rash, hives, and/or itching; fast or irregular breathing; puffiness or swelling of the eyelids or around the eyes; shortness of breath, troubled breathing, tightness in chest, and/or wheezing); *severe hepatic reactions* (chills; fever; itching of the skin; nausea; yellow eyes or skin; stomach pain; unusual tiredness)

**Those indicating need for medical attention only if they continue or are bothersome**

Incidence more frequent

*Abdominal pain; diarrhea; dyspepsia* (heartburn); *flatulence* (gas)

Note: *Diarrhea* is dose-related, usually developing early in the course of therapy, and self-limiting, often resolving in 2 to 7 days.

Incidence less frequent

*Abnormal vision; acne; alopecia* (loss of hair); *anorexia* (decreased appetite); *central nervous system effects, including drowsiness; irritability or nervousness; dry mouth; dysphagia* (trouble in swallowing); *impotence* (decrease in sexual ability); *migraine* (headache, severe and throbbing; sometimes with nausea or vomiting); *myalgia* (muscle pain); *paresthesias* (tingling, burning, or prickling sensations); *taste perversion* (change in sense of taste); *tremor* (trembling or shaking); *vaginal bleeding*

## Overdose

For specific information on the agents used in the management of diclofenac and misoprostol combination overdose, see the *Charcoal, Activated (Oral-Local)* monograph.

For more information on the management of overdose or unintentional ingestion, **contact a Poison Control Center** (see *Poison Control Center Listing*).

### Clinical effects of overdose

The following effects have been selected on the basis of their potential clinical significance (possible signs and symptoms in parentheses where appropriate)—not necessarily inclusive:

Acute and/or chronic

*Bradycardia* (slow heartbeat); *confusion; drowsiness; dyspnea* (shortness of breath); *fever; gastrointestinal effects* (diarrhea; nausea and/or vomiting; stomach pain); *hypotension* (decrease in blood pressure); *palpitations* (pounding heartbeat); *tremor* (trembling or shaking); *seizures*

### Treatment of overdose

To decrease absorption—Emptying the stomach via gastric lavage.

To enhance elimination—Inducing diuresis.

Administering activated charcoal.

Supportive care—Monitoring and supporting vital functions. Patients in whom intentional overdose is confirmed or suspected should be referred for psychiatric consultation.

## Patient Consultation

As an aid to patient consultation, refer to *Advice for the Patient Diclofenac and Misoprostol (Systemic)—Introductory version*.

In providing consultation, consider emphasizing the following selected information (» = major clinical significance):

### Before using this medication

» Conditions affecting use, especially:

Sensitivity to diclofenac or misoprostol

Allergies to aspirin or any other nonsteroidal anti-inflammatory drugs (NSAIDs), or other prostaglandins or prostaglandin analogs

Pregnancy—Use of diclofenac and misoprostol combination is contraindicated during pregnancy; patients of childbearing potential must take measures to assure they are not pregnant prior to therapy and to prevent pregnancy during therapy

Breast-feeding—Diclofenac is distributed into breast milk

Use in the elderly—Increased risk of toxicity

Other medications, especially anticoagulants, coumarin- or indandione-derivative, corticosteroids, aspirin, cyclosporine, digitalis glycosides, lithium, methotrexate, potassium-sparing diuretics

Other medical problems, especially allergic reaction (severe), aspirin-induced nasal polyps associated with bronchospasm, coagulation disorders, gastrointestinal bleeding or history of, hepatic function impairment, peptic ulcer disease or history of, platelet disorders, renal disease (severe) or history of, or renal function impairment

### Proper use of this medication

» Not taking more medication than prescribed

Not taking with magnesium-containing antacids

Not chewing, crushing, or dissolving tablets

Not giving medication to another person

Taking with or after meals

» Proper dosing

Missed dose: Taking as soon as possible; not taking if almost time for next dose; not doubling doses

» Proper storage

### Precautions while using this medication

» Stopping medication and checking with physician immediately if pregnancy is suspected

Consulting physician if diarrhea develops and continues for more than a week

Regular visits to physician during prolonged therapy

» Possibility of gastrointestinal ulceration or bleeding

» Possibility that alcohol may increase the risk of ulceration

Not taking NSAIDs, including ketorolac, concurrently, and not taking acetaminophen or aspirin or other salicylates for more than a few days while receiving diclofenac and misoprostol combination, unless concurrent use is prescribed by, and patient remains under the care of, a physician or dentist

### Side/adverse effects

Signs of potential side effects, especially cardiovascular effects, central nervous system effects, fluid retention, gastrointestinal bleeding, gastrointestinal ulceration, hematologic effects, hepatic effects, intestinal perforation, mood or mental changes, pancreatitis, rectal bleeding, renal effects, seizures, Steven-Johnson syndrome, anaphylaxis or anaphylactoid reactions

## General Dosing Information

Diclofenac and misoprostol combination should be prescribed with extreme caution in patients with a prior history of ulcer disease or gastrointestinal bleeding. To minimize the risk for potential adverse events, the lowest effective dose should be used for the shortest possible duration.

Diclofenac and misoprostol combination is not recommended for patients who would not receive the appropriate dose of both ingredients.

## Oral Dosage Forms

### DICLOFENAC AND MISOPROSTOL TABLETS

**Usual adult dose**

Osteoarthritis—

Oral, 50 mg of diclofenac and 200 mcg of misoprostol three times a day.

Rheumatoid arthritis—

Oral, 50 mg of diclofenac and 200 mcg of misoprostol three to four times a day.

Rheumatoid arthritis and osteoarthritis (for patients who experience intolerance)—

Oral, 50 mg of diclofenac and 200 mcg of misoprostol two times a day or 75 mg of diclofenac and 200 mcg of misoprostol two times a day.

Note: Dosage may also be individualized using separate products of diclofenac and misoprostol. Thereafter, the patient may be changed to the appropriate diclofenac and misoprostol combination dose. If clinically indicated, misoprostol may be used with diclofenac and misoprostol combination to optimize the misoprostol drug regimen.

**Usual adult prescribing limits**
In osteoarthritis—150 mg of diclofenac and 800 mcg of misoprostol.
In rheumatoid arthritis—225 mg of diclofenac and 800 mcg of misoprostol.

**Usual pediatric dose**
Safety and efficacy have not been established in persons younger than 18 years of age.

**Usual geriatric dose**
See *Usual adult dose*.

**Strength(s) usually available**
U.S.—
  50 mg of diclofenac and 200 micrograms of misoprostol (Rx) [*Arthrotec 50* (colloidal silicon dioxide; corn starch; crospovidone; hydrogenated castor oil; hydroxypropyl methylcellulose; lactose; magnesium stearate; methacrylic acid copolymer; micro-crystalline cellulose; povidone (polyvidone) K-30; sodium hydroxide; talc; triethyl citrate)].
  75 mg of diclofenac and 200 micrograms of misoprostol (Rx) [*Arthrotec 75* (colloidal silicon dioxide; corn starch; crospovidone; hydrogenated castor oil; hydroxypropyl methylcellulose; lactose; magnesium stearate; methacrylic acid copolymer; micro-crystalline cellulose; povidone (polyvidone) K-30; sodium hydroxide; talc; triethyl citrate)].

**Packaging and storage**
Store at or below 25 °C (77 °F).

**Auxiliary labeling**
- Avoid alcoholic beverages.
- Take with food

Developed: 05/27/98

---

## DICLOXACILLIN—See *Penicillins (Systemic)*

## DICUMAROL—See *Anticoagulants (Systemic)*

## DICYCLOMINE—See *Anticholinergics/Antispasmodics (Systemic)*

---

# DIDANOSINE  Systemic

VA CLASSIFICATION (Primary): AM804
Commonly used brand name(s): *Videx*.
Other commonly used names are ddI and 2,3-dideoxyinosine.
Note:  For a listing of dosage forms and brand names by country availability, see *Dosage Forms* section(s).

## Category
Antiviral (systemic).

## Indications
Note:  Bracketed information in the *Indications* section refers to uses that are not included in U.S. product labeling.

**Accepted**
Human immunodeficiency virus (HIV) infection, advanced (treatment) or Immunodeficiency syndrome, acquired (AIDS) (treatment)—Didanosine is indicated in the treatment of adults and children over 6 months of age with advanced HIV infection who are intolerant of zidovudine therapy or who have demonstrated significant clinical or immunologic deterioration during zidovudine therapy; didanosine is also indicated in the treatment of adults with advanced HIV infection who have received prior zidovudine therapy. [Didanosine is also used in combination with zidovudine.][1]

[1]Not included in Canadian product labeling.

## Pharmacology/Pharmacokinetics

**Physicochemical characteristics**
Molecular weight—236.2.

**Mechanism of action/Effect**
Didanosine (ddI) is metabolized intracellularly by a series of cellular enzymes to its active moiety, 2,3–dideoxyadenosine-5-triphosphate (ddA-TP), which inhibits HIV DNA polymerase (reverse transcriptase). HIV replication is suppressed by chain termination, competitive inhibition of reverse transcriptase, or both. The intracellular half-life of ddA-TP is greater than 12 hours.

**Absorption**
Didanosine is acidlabile; all oral formulations contain or are compounded with buffering agents to increase the gastric pH; this results in a decreased breakdown of didanosine and a subsequent increase in absorption. All formulations should be taken on an empty stomach. Administration within 5 minutes of a meal decreases the peak plasma concentration ($C_{max}$) and mean area under the plasma concentration versus time curve (AUC) by approximately 50%. If didanosine is not buffered in the stomach, it forms 2,3–dideoxyribose and hypoxanthine, a precursor of uric acid.
Bioavailability was extremely variable in both adults and children after ingestion of a lyophilized formulation similar to the pediatric product for oral solution:
  Adults—Approximately 33% after a single dose and approximately 37% after 4 weeks of therapy in adults receiving 7 mg per kg of body weight (mg/kg) or less.
  Children (7 months to 19 years of age)—Average 19 to 42% (range, 2 to 89%).
  The chewable/dispersible buffered tablets were found to be 20 to 25% more bioavailable than the buffered powder for oral solution when studied in 18 asymptomatic HIV-seropositive adults.

**Distribution**
Crosses blood-brain barrier and distributes into the cerebrospinal fluid (CSF)—
  Adults: Approximately 19 to 21% of the simultaneous plasma concentration 1 hour after an intravenous dose.
  Children (8 months to 18 years of age): In one study, didanosine distribution into the CSF of 7 children was approximately 46% (range, 12 to 85%) of the simultaneous plasma concentration 1.5 to 3.5 hours after a single dose; however, studies done in rhesus monkeys showed poor CSF penetration, and another study done in children found that didanosine was not detectable in 17 of 20 CSF samples, and penetration into the CSF was limited.
$Vol_D$—
  Adults: Average 0.7 to 1 L per kg.
  Children (8 months to 18 years of age): Approximately 35.6 L per square meter of body surface ($L/m^2$) [range, 18.4 to 60.7 $L/m^2$].

**Protein binding**
Low (<5%).

**Biotransformation**
Rapidly metabolized intracellularly to its active moiety, 2,3–dideoxyadenosine-5-triphosphate (ddA-TP). However, the metabolism of didanosine has not been fully evaluated in humans. Extensive metabolism occurred in dogs administered oral, radiolabeled didanosine; identified urinary metabolites include allantoin, which accounted for approximately 61% of the dose, hypoxanthine, xanthine, and uric acid.

**Half-life**
Adults—Approximately 1.5 hours (range, 0.8 to 2.7 hours).
Children (8 months to 18 years of age)—Approximately 0.8 hour (range, 0.5 to 1.2 hours).
Severe renal failure—Approximately 4.5 hours.
Intracellular half-life of ddA-TP is 8 to 24 hours *in vitro*.

**Time to peak concentration**
0.5 to 1 hour.

**Peak serum concentration**
Adults—
  Approximately 1.6 mcg per mL (range, 0.6 to 2.9 mcg per mL) after a single 375-mg dose of buffered powder for oral solution.
  Approximately 1.6 mcg per mL (range, 0.5 to 2.6 mcg per mL) after a single 300-mg dose of the buffered chewable/dispersible tablet.
Children (8 months to 18 years of age)—
  Steady state values after oral administration of 80, 120, and 180 mg per square meter of body surface were 0.8, 1.4, and 1.7 mcg per mL, respectively.

## Elimination
Renal clearance by glomerular filtration and active tubular secretion makes up approximately 50% of the total body clearance; urinary recovery was approximately 20% (range, 3 to 31%) after a single oral dose in adults and approximately 17% (range, 5 to 30%) at steady state in children. No accumulation was evident in either adults or children.

Dialysis—A 4-hour hemodialysis session reduces the serum didanosine concentration by approximately 20%.

## Precautions to Consider

### Carcinogenicity
Long-term carcinogenicity studies in animals have not been completed.

### Mutagenicity
No evidence of mutagenicity was observed in either the Ames *Salmonella* mutagenicity assays (with or without metabolic activation) or a mutagenicity assay conducted with *Escherichia coli* tester strain WP2 uvrA, where only a slight increase in revertants was observed. In a mammalian cell gene mutation assay conducted in L5178Y/YK+/− mouse lymphoma cells, didanosine was weakly positive in both the presence and absence of metabolic activation at concentrations of approximately 2000 mcg per mL and above. High concentrations of didanosine (≥ 5000 mcg per mL) elevated the frequency of cells bearing chromosome aberrations in an *in vitro* cytogenic study performed in cultured human peripheral lymphocytes. Another *in vitro* mammalian cell chromosome aberrations study using Chinese Hamster Lung cells produced chromosomal aberrations at ≥ 500 mcg per mL after 48 hours of exposure; however, no significant elevations in the frequency of cells with chromosomal aberrations were seen at concentrations up to 250 mcg per mL. In a BALB/c 3T3 *in vitro* transformation assay, didanosine was considered positive only at concentrations of 3000 mcg per mL and above. No evidence of genotoxicity was observed in rat and mouse micronucleus assays.

### Pregnancy/Reproduction
Fertility—No evidence of impaired fertility has been found in rats and rabbits receiving 12 and 14.2 times the estimated human dose of didanosine, based on plasma levels.

Pregnancy—Didanosine crosses the placenta. However, studies in humans have not been done. Unlike zidovudine, it is not known whether didanosine reduces perinatal transmission of HIV infection.

No evidence of harm to the fetus has been found in rats and rabbits receiving 12 and 14.2 times the estimated human dose of didanosine, based on plasma levels. At approximately 12 times the estimated human dose, didanosine was slightly toxic to female rats and their pups during mid and late lactation. The rats showed reduced body weight gains and food intake, but the physical and functional development of the offspring was not impaired and there were no major changes in the F2 generation.

FDA Pregnancy Category B.

### Breast-feeding
It is not known whether didanosine is distributed into breast milk.

There have been case reports of HIV being transmitted from an infected mother to her nursing infant through breast milk. Therefore, breast-feeding is not recommended in HIV-infected mothers where safe infant formula is available and affordable.

### Pediatrics
Data in children over 3 months of age with symptomatic HIV infection suggest that didanosine is well tolerated and may produce an improvement in neuropsychological function, immunological function, p24 antigen levels, and weight gain. However, these data are preliminary. As with adults, the major serious side effect to date in children has been pancreatitis, which usually occurred at doses above 300 mg per square meter of body surface (mg/m$^2$) per day. Retinal depigmentation has been reported in approximately 7% of children treated with didanosine, especially at doses above 300 mg/m$^2$ per day.

### Geriatrics
No information is available on the relationship of age to the effects of didanosine in geriatric patients. However, elderly patients are more likely to have an age-related decrease in renal function, which may require a reduction in dose.

### Drug interactions and/or related problems
The following drug interactions and/or related problems have been selected on the basis of their potential clinical significance (possible mechanism in parentheses where appropriate)—not necessarily inclusive (» = major clinical significance):

Note: Combinations containing any of the following medications, depending on the amount present, may also interact with this medication.

» Alcohol or
» Asparaginase or
» Azathioprine or
» Estrogens or
» Furosemide or
» Methyldopa or
» Nitrofurantoin or
» Pentamidine, intravenous or
» Sulfonamides or
» Sulindac or
» Tetracyclines or
» Thiazide diuretics or
» Valproic acid or
  Other drugs associated with pancreatitis
  (medications associated with the development of pancreatitis should be avoided during didanosine therapy or, if concurrent use is necessary, used with caution since didanosine may cause pancreatitis, which, on rare occasion, has been fatal)

» Chloramphenicol or
» Cisplatin or
» Dapsone or
» Ethambutol or
» Ethionamide or
» Hydralazine or
» Isoniazid or
» Lithium or
» Metronidazole or
» Nitrofurantoin or
» Nitrous oxide or
» Phenytoin or
» Stavudine or
» Vincristine or
» Zalcitabine or
  Other drugs associated with peripheral neuropathy
  (since didanosine has been shown to cause peripheral neuropathy, medications associated with the development of neuropathy should be avoided during didanosine therapy or, if concurrent use is necessary, used with caution)

» Dapsone or
» Itraconazole or
» Ketoconazole
  (concurrent administration of dapsone with didanosine may decrease the absorption of dapsone; didanosine is combined with a buffer to neutralize stomach acidity in order to increase its absorption, while dapsone requires an acidic environment for optimal absorption; dapsone and any other medications that also depend on the gastric acidity for optimal absorption, such as itraconazole and ketoconazole, should be administered at least 2 hours before or 2 hours after didanosine is given)

» Fluoroquinolone antibiotics, such as ciprofloxacin, enoxacin, lomefloxacin, norfloxacin, and ofloxacin or
» Tetracyclines
  (concurrent administration of the didanosine chewable/dispersible tablets or pediatric powder for oral solution with fluoroquinolone antibiotics or tetracyclines may cause a decrease in the plasma concentrations of these antibiotics; these 2 didanosine products contain magnesium- and aluminum-containing antacids, which will reduce the absorption of these antibiotics by chelation; fluoroquinolone antibiotics and tetracyclines should be administered at least 2 hours before or 2 hours after didanosine chewable/dispersible tablets or pediatric powder for oral solution is given; buffered didanosine powder for oral solution contains a citrate-phosphate buffer, which will not interact with the fluoroquinolone antibiotics or tetracyclines)

### Laboratory value alterations
The following have been selected on the basis of their potential clinical significance (possible effect in parentheses where appropriate)—not necessarily inclusive (» = major clinical significance):

With physiology/laboratory test values
  Alanine aminotransferase (ALT [SGPT]) and
  Alkaline phosphatase and
  Aspartate aminotransferase (AST [SGOT]) and
  Bilirubin, serum
    (values may be increased to greater than 5 times the upper normal limit; the incidence of laboratory abnormalities occurs more frequently in patients with abnormal baseline values)

» Amylase, serum and
Lipase, serum and
Triglycerides, serum
(values may be increased)
Potassium, serum
(concentrations may be decreased; decrease may be secondary to diarrhea from the buffer rather than to didanosine itself)
» Uric acid, serum
(didanosine may cause an asymptomatic increase in uric acid concentrations; may be dose-related; uric acid levels fall with hydration and/or a decrease in dose)

**Medical considerations/Contraindications**
The medical considerations/contraindications included have been selected on the basis of their potential clinical significance (reasons given in parentheses where appropriate)—not necessarily inclusive (» = major clinical significance).

*Risk-benefit should be considered when the following medical problems exist:*
» Alcoholism, active or
» Hypertriglyceridemia, or history of or
» Pancreatitis, or history of
(didanosine has caused pancreatitis, which, on rare occasion, has been fatal; patients who have pancreatitis or a history of pancreatitis, or are at risk for pancreatitis should either not take didanosine or should take it with extreme caution)
» Conditions requiring sodium-restriction, such as cardiac failure, cirrhosis of the liver or severe hepatic disease, peripheral or pulmonary edema, hypernatremia, hypertension, renal function impairment, or toxemia of pregnancy
(each 2-tablet dose of didanosine chewable/dispersible tablets contains 529 mg of sodium, and each single-dose packet of buffered didanosine powder for oral solution contains 1380 mg of sodium)
Gouty arthritis
(didanosine may cause an increase in uric acid levels, especially in patients who already have an abnormally high baseline before the didanosine therapy is initiated)
Hepatic function impairment
(patients with hepatic function impairment may be at increased risk of toxicity due to altered metabolism; this may require a reduction in dose)
Phenylketonuria
(didanosine chewable/dispersible tablets contain 45 mg or 67.4 mg of phenylalanine per 2-tablet dose, depending on the strength used)
» Peripheral neuropathy
(didanosine may cause peripheral neuropathy, which may require a reduction in dose)
Renal function impairment
(patients with renal function impairment may be at increased risk of toxicity due to decreased clearance through the kidneys, especially patients with a serum creatinine concentration of > 1.5 mg/dL or a creatinine clearance of < 60 mL/min; this may require a reduction in dose; also, each didanosine chewable/dispersible tablet contains 15.7 mEq of magnesium hydroxide, which may lead to a magnesium overload in patients with severe renal disease, especially after prolonged dosing)

**Patient monitoring**
The following may be especially important in patient monitoring (other tests may be warranted in some patients, depending on condition; » = major clinical significance):
» Amylase, serum and
» Lipase, serum and
Triglycerides, serum
(didanosine administration has been associated with pancreatitis; patients should be monitored for laboratory changes consistent with pancreatitis, such as elevated amylase, lipase, and triglyceride concentrations; didanosine should be discontinued if amylase concentration is elevated by 1.5 to 2 times normal limits and/or the patient has symptoms consistent with pancreatitis)
» Ophthalmologic examinations
(dilated ophthalmoscopy should be performed in children every 3 to 6 months, or if there is a change in vision, to monitor for the development and progression of retinal depigmentation; the lesions appear initially in the midperiphery of the fundus; therefore, central vision is not immediately threatened. If retinal lesions are observed, the patient should be re-examined monthly to assess progression; treatment with didanosine may need to be discontinued)

Potassium, serum
(serum potassium should be monitored regularly since hypokalemia has been associated with didanosine administration; however, this may be secondary to diarrhea from the buffer)
Uric acid, serum
(serum uric acid concentrations should be monitored regularly since didanosine may cause an asymptomatic hyperuricemia due to the catabolism of the drug; hyperuricemia occurs more frequently in patients who begin therapy with an abnormal baseline uric acid concentration)

## Side/Adverse Effects

Note: Some side effects, such as pancreatitis, peripheral neuropathy, hepatotoxicity, myalgias, hematologic abnormalities, and elevations in uric acid, may be seen with severe HIV disease; therefore, differentiation between the side effects of didanosine therapy and the complications of HIV disease may be difficult.

The incidence of pancreatitis associated with didanosine administration was 5 to 13% in adults in phase I studies, a controlled trial, and the expanded access program, and approximately 6% in children; the fatality rate of pancreatitis in adults was approximately 0.35%. An increased risk has been found to be associated with higher doses in both adults and children ($\geq$ 12.5 mg/kg per day in adults, $\geq$ 300 mg/m$^2$ per day in children); other risk factors include a history of pancreatitis, renal function impairment (without a dose adjustment), alcoholism, a very low CD4 count, and elevated triglycerides. Pancreatitis usually resolves when didanosine is discontinued.

Peripheral neuropathy also appears to be related to higher daily doses. It has occurred more frequently in adults (34% of patients receiving $\leq$ 12.5 mg/kg per day in phase I trials and 13 to 14% in a controlled trial) than in children (3%), and usually resolves over time, but may persist.

Hematologic abnormalities, such as anemia (hemoglobin < 8.0 grams/dL), granulocytopenia (< 1000/microliter), leukopenia (< 2000/microliter), and thrombocytopenia (< 50,000/microliter) have occurred in 5% or less of patients who started therapy with normal baseline values; however, if the patient began didanosine therapy with abnormal baseline values, the incidence of anemia, granulocytopenia, leukopenia, and thrombocytopenia was 0%, 56%, 37%, and 25%, respectively, in adults, and 27%, 62%, 36%, and 67%, respectively, in children.

Peripheral atrophy of the retinal pigment epithelium has occurred in 3 children receiving high doses of didanosine (> 300 mg/m$^2$ per day) and one child receiving a lower dose. The lesions are described as mottling and atrophy of retinal-pigment epithelium, and later become well circumscribed with hyperpigmented borders in the midperiphery of the fundus. Central visual acuity is not affected. The lesions appear to progress with continued didanosine therapy. When the drug is discontinued, the lesions remain with no progression.

The following side/adverse effects have been selected on the basis of their potential clinical significance (possible signs and symptoms in parentheses where appropriate)—not necessarily inclusive:

### Those indicating need for medical attention
Incidence more frequent
*Peripheral neuropathy* (tingling, burning, numbness, and pain in hands or feet)

Incidence less frequent
*Pancreatitis* (abdominal pain; nausea and vomiting)

Incidence rare
*Cardiomyopathy* (shortness of breath; swelling of feet or lower legs); *hematologic toxicity, specifically anemia, granulocytopenia or leukopenia, or thrombocytopenia* (unusual tiredness and weakness; fever, chills, or sore throat; unusual bleeding or bruising); *hepatitis* (yellow skin and eyes); *hypersensitivity* (fever and chills; skin rash and itching); *retinal depigmentation; seizures* (convulsions)

### Those indicating need for medical attention only if they continue or are bothersome
Incidence more frequent
*CNS toxicity* (anxiety; headache; irritability; insomnia; restlessness); *dryness of mouth; gastrointestinal disturbances* (abdominal pain; nausea; diarrhea)

Note: Diarrhea occurs frequently and may be related to the buffering agent; if the diarrhea becomes severe, the patient may require medical attention.

## Patient Consultation

As an aid to patient consultation, refer to *Advice for the Patient, Didanosine (Systemic)*.

In providing consultation, consider emphasizing the following selected information (» = major clinical significance):

### Before using this medication
» Conditions affecting use, especially:
Use in children—May cause retinal depigmentation, which is more likely to occur in children receiving doses above 300 mg/m² per day
Other medications, especially other drugs associated with pancreatitis and peripheral neuropathy, dapsone or medications that require an acidic environment for absorption, tetracyclines, or fluoroquinolone antibiotics
Other medical problems, especially alcoholism, hypertriglyceridemia, pancreatitis or a history of pancreatitis, conditions requiring sodium-restriction, or peripheral neuropathy

### Proper use of this medication
» Importance of not taking more medication than prescribed; importance of not discontinuing medication without checking with physician; discontinuing medication and calling physician at first signs and symptoms of pancreatitis
» Importance of not missing doses and of taking at evenly spaced times
» Proper administration:
*For buffered didanosine for oral solution*
Preparing by opening the packet and dissolving its contents in 1/2 glass (4 ounces) of water. The powder should not be mixed with fruit juice or other acid-containing liquid
Stirring the mixture for approximately 2 to 3 minutes until the powder is completely dissolved
Swallowing the entire solution immediately
*For tablets*
Patients older than 1 year of age must take 2 tablets at each dose to provide adequate buffering and to prevent gastric acid degradation of didanosine
Children under 1 year of age should receive a 1-tablet dose. The recommended dose for children is based on body surface area and, for adults, on body weight
Thoroughly chewing, manually crushing, or dispersing in at least 1 ounce of water prior to consumption. Because the tablets are hard, they may be difficult to chew for some patients; manually crushing or dispersing the tablets may be preferable. To disperse tablets, 2 tablets should be added to at least 1 ounce of drinking water. The mixture should be stirred until a uniform dispersion forms and consumed immediately
» Proper dosing
Missed dose: Taking as soon as possible; not taking if almost time for next dose; not doubling doses
» Proper storage

### Precautions while using this medication
» Regular visits to physician for blood tests
» Importance of not taking other medications concurrently without checking with physician
» Using a condom to help prevent transmission of the AIDS virus to others; not sharing needles or injectable equipment with anyone

### Side/adverse effects
Signs of potential side effects, especially peripheral neuropathy, pancreatitis, cardiomyopathy, hematologic toxicities, hepatitis, hypersensitivity, retinal depigmentation, and seizures

## General Dosing Information

Two tablets must be taken at each dose by patients older than 1 year of age to provide adequate buffering and to prevent gastric acid degradation of didanosine. Children under 1 year of age should receive a 1-tablet dose. The recommended dose for children is based on body surface area and, for adults, on body weight.

It is recommended that patients on hemodialysis receive their dose of didanosine after dialysis.

### Diet/Nutrition
All didanosine formulations should be taken on an empty stomach. Administration with food decreases absorption by approximately 50%.

Patients on sodium-restricted diets should be made aware that each 2-tablet dose of didanosine tablets contains 529 mg (23 mEq) of sodium, and each single-dose packet of buffered didanosine for oral solution contains 1380 mg (60 mEq) of sodium.

Patients with phenylketonuria should be made aware that each 2-tablet dose of didanosine tablets contains 45 mg or 67.4 mg of phenylalanine, depending on the strength of tablets used.

### Bioequivalence information
Didanosine tablets are 20 to 25% more bioavailable than the buffered powder for oral solution. Because of this, the dose of the tablets is correspondingly lower and the dosing of the 2 products cannot be interchanged.

## Oral Dosage Forms

### BUFFERED DIDANOSINE FOR ORAL SOLUTION

#### Usual adult and adolescent dose
Antiviral—
Oral:
Patients weighing less than 60 kg—167 mg every twelve hours.
Patients weighing ≥60 kg—250 mg every twelve hours.

#### Usual pediatric dose
This product is usually not prescribed for small children. See *Didanosine for Buffered Oral Suspension* or *Didanosine Tablets*.

#### Strength(s) usually available
U.S.—
100 mg per packet (Rx) [*Videx* (citrate-phosphate buffer; sodium 1380 mg; sucrose)].
167 mg per packet (Rx) [*Videx* (citrate-phosphate buffer; sodium 1380 mg; sucrose)].
250 mg per packet (Rx) [*Videx* (citrate-phosphate buffer; sodium 1380 mg; sucrose)].
375 mg per packet (Rx) [*Videx* (citrate-phosphate buffer; sodium 1380 mg; sucrose)].
Canada—
Not commercially available.

#### Packaging and storage
Store below 40 °C (104 °F), preferably between 15 and 30 °C (59 and 86 °F), unless otherwise specified by manufacturer.

#### Stability
After preparation, the solution may be stored at room temperature for up to 4 hours.

#### Incompatibilities
Didanosine is unstable in acidic solutions and should not be mixed with fruit juice or other acid-containing liquid.

#### Auxiliary labeling
• Dissolve contents of packet in one-half glass (4 ounces) of water.
• Continue medicine for full time of treatment.
• Take on empty stomach.

### DIDANOSINE FOR BUFFERED ORAL SUSPENSION

#### Usual adult and adolescent dose
This product is usually not used by adults and adolescents. See *Buffered Didanosine for Oral Solution* and *Didanosine Tablets*.

#### Usual pediatric dose
Antiviral—
Oral:
Body surface area up to 0.4 square meters—31 mg (3 mL) every eight to twelve hours.
Body surface area 0.5 to 0.7 square meters—62 mg (6 mL) every eight to twelve hours.
Body surface area 0.8 to 1.0 square meters—94 mg (9.5 mL) every eight to twelve hours.
Body surface area 1.1 to 1.4 square meters—125 mg (12.5 mL) every eight to twelve hours.

#### Strength(s) usually available
U.S.—
2000 mg per 200 mL (when reconstituted according to manufacturer's instructions) (Rx) [*Videx* (aluminum hydroxide; magnesium hydroxide)].
4000 mg per 400 mL (when reconstituted according to manufacturer's instructions) (Rx) [*Videx* (aluminum hydroxide; magnesium hydroxide)].
Canada—
2000 mg per 200 mL (when reconstituted according to manufacturer's instructions) (Rx) [*Videx* (aluminum hydroxide; magnesium hydroxide)].
4000 mg per 400 mL (when reconstituted according to manufacturer's instructions) (Rx) [*Videx* (aluminum hydroxide; magnesium hydroxide)].

#### Packaging and storage
Prior to reconstitution, store below 40 °C (104 °F), preferably between 15 and 30 °C (59 and 86 °F), unless otherwise specified by manufacturer.

# 1210  Didanosine (Systemic)

**Preparation of dosage form**
Didanosine pediatric powder must initially be diluted by adding 100 mL or 200 mL of purified water to the 2000 mg or 4000 mg bottle of powder, respectively. This produces an initial concentration of 20 mg per mL. This solution must be further diluted as follows: One part of the 20 mg per mL solution should be mixed immediately with one part of an aluminum- and magnesium-containing antacid (e.g., Mylanta Double Strength Liquid [formerly Mylanta II] or Maalox TC Suspension). This provides a final dispensing concentration of 10 mg per mL.
For home use, the solution should be dispensed in an appropriately sized, flint-glass bottle with a child-resistant closure.

**Stability**
After reconstitution, the solution may be stored up to 30 days in the refrigerator (2 to 8 °C [36 to 46 °F]). Unused portion should be discarded after 30 days.

**Auxiliary labeling**
- Refrigerate.
- Shake well.
- Continue medicine for full time of treatment.
- Beyond-use date.
- Take on empty stomach.

**Note**
When dispensing, include a calibrated liquid-measuring device.

## DIDANOSINE TABLETS

**Usual adult and adolescent dose**
Antiviral—
   Oral:
      Patients weighing less than 60 kg—125 mg every twelve hours.
      Patients weighing ≥60 kg—200 mg every twelve hours

**Usual pediatric dose**
Antiviral—
   Oral:
      Body surface area up to 0.4 square meters—25 mg every eight to twelve hours.
      Body surface area 0.5 to 0.7 square meters—50 mg every eight to twelve hours.
      Body surface area 0.8 to 1.0 square meters—75 mg every eight to twelve hours.
      Body surface area 1.1 to 1.4 square meters—100 mg every eight to twelve hours.

**Strength(s) usually available**
U.S.—
   25 mg (Rx) [*Videx* (dihydroxyaluminum sodium carbonate; magnesium hydroxide 15.7 mEq; phenylalanine 22.5 mg; sodium 264.5 mg)].
   50 mg (Rx) [*Videx* (dihydroxyaluminum sodium carbonate; magnesium hydroxide 15.7 mEq; phenylalanine 22.5 mg; sodium 264.5 mg)].
   100 mg (Rx) [*Videx* (dihydroxyaluminum sodium carbonate; magnesium hydroxide 15.7 mEq; phenylalanine 22.5 mg; sodium 264.5 mg)].
   150 mg (Rx) [*Videx* (dihydroxyaluminum sodium carbonate; magnesium hydroxide 15.7 mEq; phenylalanine 33.7 mg; sodium 264.5 mg)].
Canada—
   25 mg (Rx) [*Videx* (dihydroxyaluminum sodium carbonate; magnesium hydroxide 15.7 mEq; phenylalanine 22.5 mg; sodium 264.5 mg)].
   50 mg (Rx) [*Videx* (dihydroxyaluminum sodium carbonate; magnesium hydroxide 15.7 mEq; phenylalanine 22.5 mg; sodium 264.5 mg)].
   100 mg (Rx) [*Videx* (dihydroxyaluminum sodium carbonate; magnesium hydroxide 15.7 mEq; phenylalanine 22.5 mg; sodium 264.5 mg)].
   150 mg (Rx) [*Videx* (dihydroxyaluminum sodium carbonate; magnesium hydroxide 15.7 mEq; phenylalanine 33.7 mg; sodium 264.5 mg)].

**Packaging and storage**
Store below 40 °C (104 °F), preferably between 15 and 30 °C (59 and 86 °F), unless otherwise specified by manufacturer.

**Stability**
If dispersed in water, the solution may be stored for up to 1 hour at room temperature.

**Auxiliary labeling**
- Continue medicine for full time of treatment.
- Do not swallow tablets whole.
- Take on empty stomach.

Revised: 06/22/94
Interim revision: 01/11/95

## DIENESTROL—See *Estrogens (Vaginal)*

## DIETHYLCARBAMAZINE—The *Diethylcarbamazine (Systemic)* monograph is not included in this published version of the USP DI database. Copies of the monograph are available on request from Micromedex, Inc. - Reprint Requests, 6200 S. Syracuse Way, Suite 300, Englewood, CO 80111; telephone (303) 486-6400; telefax (303) 486-6464; Email: USPDI@MDX.COM.

## DIETHYLPROPION—See *Appetite Suppressants (Systemic)*

## DIETHYLSTILBESTROL—See *Estrogens (Systemic)*

## DIETHYLTOLUAMIDE—The *Diethyltoluamide (Topical)* monograph is not included in this published version of the USP DI database. Copies of the monograph are available on request from Micromedex, Inc. - Reprint Requests, 6200 S. Syracuse Way, Suite 300, Englewood, CO 80111; telephone (303) 486-6400; telefax (303) 486-6464; Email: USPDI@MDX.COM.

# DIFENOXIN AND ATROPINE   Systemic†

VA CLASSIFICATION (Primary): GA208

Note: Controlled substance classification—
   U.S.—Schedule IV.

Commonly used brand name(s): *Motofen*.

Note: For a listing of dosage forms and brand names by country availability, see *Dosage Forms* section(s).

†Not commercially available in Canada.

## Category
Antidiarrheal (antiperistaltic).

## Indications

Note: The efficacy of any antidiarrheal medication for treatment of most cases of nonspecific diarrhea is questionable, especially in children. **Preferred treatment for acute, nonspecific diarrhea consists of fluid and electrolyte replacement, nutritional therapy, and, if possible, elimination of the underlying cause of the diarrhea.**

**Accepted**
Diarrhea (treatment adjunct)—Difenoxin and atropine combination is indicated in adults, as an adjunct to fluid and electrolyte therapy, in the symptomatic treatment of acute nonspecific diarrhea and acute exacerbations of chronic functional diarrhea.

**Unaccepted**
Difenoxin and atropine combination is not recommended for treatment of diarrhea in children.

## Pharmacology/Pharmacokinetics

**Physicochemical characteristics**
Molecular weight—Atropine sulfate: 694.84.
Difenoxin: 424.54.

### Mechanism of action/Effect
Difenoxin—Probably acts both locally and centrally to reduce intestinal motility. Antidiarrheal activity is about 5 times that of diphenoxylate.
Atropine—Has anticholinergic activity. However, in this preparation atropine is included in doses below the therapeutic level in an attempt to prevent abuse by deliberate overdosage.

### Biotransformation
Hepatic.

### Half-life
Atropine—2.5 hours.
Difenoxin—4.5 hours.

### Time to peak concentration
Difenoxin—40 to 60 minutes.

### Peak serum concentration
Difenoxin—2-mg dose produces a serum concentration of 160 nanograms per mL.

### Elimination
Atropine—Renal; 30 to 50% excreted unchanged.
Difenoxin—Renal/fecal.

## Precautions to Consider

### Carcinogenicity
Long-term studies in rats with difenoxin and atropine have not shown any evidence of carcinogenesis.

### Mutagenicity
Studies to evaluate mutagenic potential of difenoxin and atropine have not been performed.

### Pregnancy/Reproduction
Pregnancy—Studies in humans have not been done.
Reproduction studies in rats and rabbits have not shown evidence of teratogenicity with doses of difenoxin and atropine up to 75 times the human therapeutic dose. However, studies in rats have shown that difenoxin and atropine combination causes an increase in delivery time and a significant increase in the percent of stillbirths when given in doses of 20 times the maximum human dose.
FDA Pregnancy Category C.

### Breast-feeding
Problems in humans have not been documented. However, risk-benefit must considered since both difenoxin and atropine are distributed into breast milk and have the potential to cause serious adverse effects in the nursing infant. There is no information concerning the concentration of these drugs in breast milk.

### Pediatrics
Difenoxin and atropine combination is not recommended for treatment of diarrhea in children. Recommended treatment consists of oral rehydration therapy to prevent loss of fluids and electrolytes, nutritional therapy, and, if possible, elimination of the underlying cause of the diarrhea.
Infants and young children exhibit increased sensitivity to the toxic effects of atropine. Children may also be more susceptible to the respiratory depressant effects of difenoxin.

### Geriatrics
No information is available on the relationship of age to the effects of difenoxin and atropine in geriatric patients. However, elderly patients may be more susceptible to the respiratory depressant effects of difenoxin, and to the mild anticholinergic effects and confusion caused by atropine.
In geriatric patients with diarrhea, caution is recommended because of the risk of fluid and electrolyte loss.

### Drug interactions and/or related problems
The following drug interactions and/or related problems have been selected on the basis of their potential clinical significance (possible mechanism in parentheses where appropriate)—not necessarily inclusive (» = major clinical significance):

Note: Combinations containing any of the following medications, depending on the amount present, may also interact with this medication.

Addictive medications, other, especially central nervous system (CNS) depressants with habituating potential
(concurrent use with difenoxin may increase the risk of habituation; caution is recommended)

» Alcohol or
» CNS depression–producing medications, other (See *Appendix II*)
(concurrent use with difenoxin may increase the CNS depressant effects of either difenoxin or these medications; also, when tricyclic antidepressants are used concurrently with atropine, their anticholinergic effects may be intensified; dosage adjustment may be required)

» Anticholinergics or other medications with anticholinergic activity (See *Appendix II*)
(these medications may enhance the effects of atropine during concurrent use; significant interaction is unlikely with usual doses of difenoxin and atropine combination, but may occur with its abuse)

» Monoamine oxidase (MAO) inhibitors, including furazolidone and procarbazine
(concurrent use with difenoxin may precipitate hypertensive crisis; MAO inhibitors may block detoxification of atropine, thus potentiating its action)

» Naltrexone
(administration of naltrexone to a patient physically dependent on opioid drugs, such as difenoxin, will precipitate withdrawal symptoms; symptoms may appear within 5 minutes of naltrexone administration, persist for up to 48 hours, and be difficult to reverse)
(naltrexone blocks the therapeutic effects of opioids, including antidiarrheal effects; naltrexone therapy should not be initiated in patients receiving difenoxin; also, patients receiving naltrexone should be advised to use alternative antidiarrheals when necessary)

Opioid (narcotic) analgesics
(concurrent use with difenoxin may result in increased risk of severe constipation and additive CNS depressant effects)

### Laboratory value alterations
The following have been selected on the basis of their potential clinical significance (possible effect in parentheses where appropriate)—not necessarily inclusive (» = major clinical significance):

With diagnostic test results
» Phenolsulfonphthalein (PSP) excretion test
(atropine utilizes the same tubular mechanism of excretion as PSP, resulting in decreased urinary excretion of PSP; concurrent use of atropine is not recommended in patients receiving a PSP excretion test)

With physiology/laboratory test values
Amylase, serum
(values may be increased as a result of spasm of the sphincter of Oddi)

### Medical considerations/Contraindications
The medical considerations/contraindications included have been selected on the basis of their potential clinical significance (reasons given in parentheses where appropriate)—not necessarily inclusive (» = major clinical significance).

*Except under special circumstances, this medication should not be used when the following medical problems exist:*

» Colitis, severe
(patient may develop toxic megacolon)

» Diarrhea associated with pseudomembranous colitis resulting from treatment with broad-spectrum antibiotics
(inhibition of peristalsis may delay the removal of toxin from the colon, thereby prolonging and/or worsening the diarrhea)

*Risk-benefit should be considered when the following medical problems exist:*

Alcoholism, active or in remission or
Drug abuse or dependence, history of
(difenoxin content may increase chances of drug abuse in patient already predisposed to dependence)

Cardiovascular instability
(possible increase in heart rate may be undesirable)

» Dehydration
(may predispose to delayed difenoxin intoxication; inhibition of peristalsis may result in fluid retention in colon and may further aggravate dehydration; discontinuation of medication and rehydration therapy is essential if symptoms of dehydration, such as dryness of mouth, excessive thirst, wrinkled skin, decreased urination, and dizziness or lightheadedness, are present; fluid loss may have serious consequences, such as circulatory collapse and renal failure)

Diarrhea caused by infectious organisms
(bacterial diarrhea may worsen due to the increased contact time between the mucosa and the penetrating microorganism; however, there is no evidence of this occurring in actual practice)

» Diarrhea caused by poisoning, until toxic material has been eliminated from gastrointestinal tract

Down's syndrome
(atropine may cause abnormal increase in pupillary dilation and acceleration of heart rate)
» Dysentery, acute, characterized by bloody stools and elevated temperature
(sole treatment with antiperistaltic antidiarrheals may be inadequate; antibiotic therapy may be required)
Gallbladder disease or gallstones
(difenoxin may cause biliary tract spasm)
» Gastrointestinal tract obstruction
(use of atropine and difenoxin combination may result in pseudo-obstruction, or dilation of the large or small bowel)
Glaucoma, angle-closure
(although unlikely with usual doses of this combination, atropine may precipitate an acute attack of angle-closure glaucoma)
» Hepatic function impairment or jaundice
(difenoxin may precipitate hepatic coma; it is recommended that dosage be reduced in patients with impaired hepatic function)
Hiatal hernia associated with reflux esophagitis or
Hypertension
(although unlikely with usual doses of this combination, atropine may aggravate these conditions)
Hyperthyroidism
(characterized by tachycardia, which may be increased by atropine)
Hypothyroidism
(difenoxin may increase risk of respiratory depression)
Incontinence, overflow
(secondary to constipation, but often mistaken for diarrhea; use of difenoxin and atropine may worsen constipation and/or result in pseudo-obstruction of the colon)
Intestinal atony in the elderly or debilitated
(although unlikely with usual doses of this combination, use of atropine may result in obstruction)
Myasthenia gravis
(although unlikely with usual doses of this combination, atropine may aggravate condition because of inhibition of acetylcholine action)
Prostatic hypertrophy or
Urethral stricture, acute or
Urinary retention
(reduction in tone of urinary bladder may aggravate or lead to complete urinary retention)
Renal function impairment
(decreased elimination of atropine may increase the risk of side effects)
Respiratory disease or impairment
(increased risk of respiratory depression)
Sensitivity to atropine or difenoxin

**Patient monitoring**

The following may be especially important in patient monitoring (other tests may be warranted in some patients, depending on condition; » = major clinical significance):
» Hepatic function determinations
(recommended at periodic intervals during long-term therapy, especially for patients with hepatic function impairment)

## Side/Adverse Effects

The following side/adverse effects have been selected on the basis of their potential clinical significance (possible signs and symptoms in parentheses where appropriate)—not necessarily inclusive:

**Those indicating need for medical attention**
Incidence less frequent or rare
*Paralytic ileus or toxic megacolon* (bloating; constipation; loss of appetite; severe stomach pain with nausea and vomiting)

**Those indicating need for medical attention only if they continue, worsen, or are bothersome**
Incidence less frequent or rare
*Anticholinergic effects, mild* (blurred vision; difficult urination; dryness of skin and mouth; fever); *confusion; dizziness or lightheadedness; drowsiness; headache; trouble in sleeping; unusual tiredness or weakness*
Note: Since atropine is present in a subtherapeutic dose, symptoms of *mild anticholinergic effects* probably indicate overdosage, although in children they may occur at therapeutic doses.

**Those indicating possible withdrawal and the need for medical attention if they occur after discontinuation of prolonged high-dose therapy**
Incidence rare
*Increased sweating; muscle cramps; nausea or vomiting; shivering or trembling; stomach cramps*

## Overdose

For specific information on the agents used in the management of difenoxin and atropine overdose, see:
• *Naloxone (Systemic)* monograph.
For more information on the management of overdose or unintentional ingestion, **contact a Poison Control Center** (see *Poison Control Center Listing*).

**Clinical effects of overdose**
The following effects have been selected on the basis of their potential clinical significance (possible signs and symptoms in parentheses where appropriate)—not necessarily inclusive:
*Anticholinergic effects, severe* (continuing blurred vision or changes in near vision; fast heartbeat; severe drowsiness; severe dryness of mouth, nose, and throat; unusual warmth, dryness, and flushing of skin); *coma; respiratory depression* (severe shortness of breath or troubled breathing); *unusual excitement, nervousness, restlessness, or irritability*
Note: *Respiratory depression* may occur as late as 12 to 30 hours after ingestion.

**Treatment of overdose**
Treatment of overdose with difenoxin and atropine is the same as treatment for meperidine or morphine overdosage and involves the following:
To decrease absorption—Gastric lavage if vomiting has not occurred.
Specific treatment—Intravenous administration of 0.4 mg of naloxone, which may be repeated at 2- to 3-minute intervals, for respiratory depression.
Monitoring—Prolonged and careful monitoring for 48 to 72 hours.
Supportive care—Support of respiration. Patients in whom intentional overdose is confirmed or suspected should be referred for psychiatric consultation.

## Patient Consultation

As an aid to patient consultation, refer to *Advice for the Patient, Difenoxin and Atropine (Systemic)*.
In providing consultation, consider emphasizing the following selected information (» = major clinical significance):

**Before using this medication**
» Conditions affecting use, especially:
Sensitivity to atropine or difenoxin
Pregnancy—Studies in rats show increased delivery time and stillbirth at doses 20 times maximum human dose
Breast-feeding—Difenoxin and atropine distributed into breast milk; potential for serious adverse effects in nursing infant
Use in children—Not recommended for use in children; increased susceptibility to toxic effects of atropine and respiratory depressant effects of difenoxin; risk of dehydration
Use in the elderly—Increased risk of respiratory depression; risk of dehydration
Other medications, especially other anticholinergics, CNS depressants, MAO inhibitors, or naltrexone
Other medical problems, especially acute dysentery; dehydration; diarrhea caused by antibiotics or poisoning; gastrointestinal tract obstruction; hepatic function impairment or jaundice; or severe colitis

**Proper use of this medication**
Taking with food or meals if gastric irritation occurs
» Importance of not taking more medication than the amount prescribed because of habit-forming potential
» Importance of maintaining adequate hydration and proper diet
» Proper dosing
Missed dose: If on scheduled dosing regimen—Taking as soon as possible; not taking if almost time for next dose; not doubling doses
» Proper storage

**Precautions while using this medication**
Regular visits to physician to check progress during prolonged therapy
» Consulting physician if diarrhea is not controlled within 48 hours and/or fever develops
» Avoiding use of alcohol or other CNS depressants during therapy
» Suspected overdose: Getting emergency help at once

Need to inform physician or dentist of use of medication if any kind of surgery (including dental surgery) or emergency treatment is required
» Caution if dizziness or drowsiness occurs

### Side/adverse effects
Signs of potential side effects, especially paralytic ileus or toxic megacolon

## General Dosing Information

If clinical improvement is not observed within 48 hours, treatment with difenoxin and atropine should be discontinued.

Inhibition of peristalsis may produce fluid retention in the bowel, which may aggravate dehydration and depletion of electrolytes, and may also increase variability of response to the medication. If dehydration or electrolyte imbalance occurs, difenoxin and atropine therapy should be withheld until appropriate corrective therapy has begun.

To prevent development of toxic megacolon in patients with acute ulcerative colitis, treatment with difenoxin and atropine should be discontinued promptly if abdominal pain or distention or other specific gastrointestinal symptoms such as anorexia, bloating, constipation, nausea, or vomiting occur.

Prolonged use of larger-than-usual therapeutic doses may result in physical dependence.

Tolerance to the antidiarrheal effects of difenoxin and atropine may develop with prolonged use.

This medication may suppress respiration, especially in the elderly, the very ill, and patients with respiratory problems. Lower doses may be required for these patients.

## Oral Dosage Forms

### DIFENOXIN HYDROCHLORIDE AND ATROPINE SULFATE TABLETS

#### Usual adult and adolescent dose
Antidiarrheal (antiperistaltic)—
Oral, the equivalent of difenoxin hydrochloride, 2 mg initially, then 1 mg after each loose stool or every three or four hours as needed.

#### Usual adult prescribing limits
Up to the equivalent of 8 mg of difenoxin hydrochloride daily.

#### Usual pediatric dose
Use is not recommended.

#### Usual geriatric dose
See *Usual adult and adolescent dose.*

Note: Geriatric patients may be more sensitive to the effects of the usual adult dose.

### Strength(s) usually available
U.S.—
1 mg of difenoxin hydrochloride and 25 mcg (0.025 mg) of atropine sulfate (Rx) [*Motofen* (scored; calcium stearate; cellulose; lactose; corn starch)].
Canada—
Not commercially available.

### Packaging and storage
Store below 40 °C (104 °F), preferably between 15 and 30 °C (59 and 86 °F), in a well-closed container, unless otherwise specified by manufacturer.

### Auxiliary labeling
- May cause drowsiness.
- Avoid alcoholic beverages.
- Keep out of reach of children.
- May be habit-forming.

### Note
Controlled substance in the U.S.

### Selected Bibliography
Binder HJ. Net fluid and electrolyte secretion: the pathophysiologic basis of diarrhea. In: Binder HJ, editor. Mechanism of intestinal secretion. New York: Alan R Liss Inc., 1979: 1-15.
Brownlee HJ, editor. Proceedings of a symposium: Management of acute nonspecific diarrhea. Am J Med 1990; 88 (Suppl 6A).

Revised: 07/15/94

---

**DIFLORASONE**—See *Corticosteroids (Topical)*

---

**DIFLUCORTOLONE**—See *Corticosteroids (Topical)*

---

**DIFLUNISAL**—See *Anti-inflammatory Drugs, Nonsteroidal (Systemic)*

---

# DIGITALIS GLYCOSIDES   Systemic

This monograph includes information on the following: 1) Digitoxin; 2) Digoxin.
VA CLASSIFICATION (Primary/Secondary): CV050/CV300; CV900
Commonly used brand name(s): *Crystodigin*[1]; *Digitaline*[1]; *Lanoxicaps*[2]; *Lanoxin*[2].
Note: For a listing of dosage forms and brand names by country availability, see *Dosage Forms* section(s).

## Category
Antiarrhythmic; cardiotonic.

## Indications

### Accepted
Arrhythmias, cardiac (prophylaxis and treatment)—Digitalis glycosides are indicated for the control of ventricular response rates in atrial fibrillation and atrial flutter. Digitalis glycosides are also indicated for the control of paroxysmal atrioventricular (AV) nodal reentrant tachycardia; digitalis glycosides may convert paroxysmal AV nodal reentrant tachycardia to normal sinus rhythm.

Congestive heart failure (treatment)—Digitalis glycosides are indicated for the treatment of all degrees of congestive heart failure. They are generally most effective in "low output" failure associated with depressed left ventricular function and much less effective in "high output" failure (bronchopulmonary insufficiency, arteriovenous fistula, anemia, beriberi, infection, hyperthyroidism). Their positive inotropic action results in improved cardiac output and an improvement in the signs and symptoms of hemodynamic insufficiency such as dyspnea, edema, and/or venous congestion.

### Unaccepted
The use of digitalis glycosides in the treatment of obesity has been determined unwarranted and dangerous, since these drugs may cause potentially fatal arrhythmias or other adverse effects.

## Pharmacology/Pharmacokinetics
See *Table 1*, page 1219.

### Physicochemical characteristics
Molecular weight—
Digitoxin: 764.95.
Digoxin: 780.95.

### Mechanism of action/Effect
Two major actions are produced by therapeutic doses of digitalis glycosides—
(1) Force and velocity of myocardial contraction are increased (positive inotropic effect). This effect is thought to result from inhibition of movement of sodium and potassium ions across myocardial cell membranes by complexing with adenosine triphosphatase. As a result, there is enhancement of calcium influx and an augmented release of free calcium ions within the myocardial cells to subsequently potentiate the activity of the contractile muscle fibers of the heart.
(2) A decrease in the conduction rate and increase in the effective refractory period of the atrioventricular (AV) node is predominantly due to an indirect effect caused by enhancement of parasympathetic tone and decrease in sympathetic tone.

### Absorption

**Digitoxin**—Highly lipophilic; almost completely absorbed after oral administration.

**Digoxin**—Bioavailability is 60 to 80% (tablets), 70 to 85% (oral elixir or intramuscular injection), or 90 to 100% (capsules). The rate, but not the extent, of oral absorption is reduced when the tablets or capsules are taken after meals. In some patients, digoxin is converted to inactive products by colonic bacteria in the gut.

## Precautions to Consider

### Cross-sensitivity and/or related problems
Allergic reactions to a digitalis glycoside preparation occur rarely. Such reactions do not necessarily encompass all digitalis glycosides and therefore may not preclude the trial of another digitalis glycoside.

### Carcinogenicity
Studies have not been done.

### Pregnancy/Reproduction
**Pregnancy**—Studies have not been done in humans. Digitalis glycosides cross the placenta; at delivery the neonatal serum digoxin concentration is similar to the maternal concentration. Maternal dosage requirements of digitalis glycosides often increase in the final weeks of pregnancy. Studies have not been done in animals.

FDA Pregnancy Category C.

**Postpartum**—Following delivery, and for up to 6 weeks thereafter, the maternal dosage often must be reduced to maintain acceptable serum concentrations.

### Breast-feeding
Digoxin is excreted in breast milk. The total amount received daily by the infant is estimated to be less than the usual daily maintenance dose. However, problems in humans have not been documented. It is not known whether digitoxin is excreted in breast milk.

### Pediatrics
Digitalis glycosides are a major cause of accidental poisoning in children. The tolerance of newborn infants to digitalis glycosides is variable, since their renal clearance of the medication is reduced. Premature and immature infants are especially sensitive. Dosage should be reduced and individualized according to the infant's degree of maturity, since renal clearance increases as the infant matures. Children older than 1 month of age generally require proportionally larger doses than adults on the basis of body weight or body surface area.

### Geriatrics
Appropriate studies on the relationship of age to the effects of digitalis glycosides have not been performed in the geriatric population. However, elderly patients are more likely to have age-related hepatic or renal function impairment, which may require lower doses of digitalis glycosides. In addition, elderly patients may also have a decreased volume of distribution for digitalis glycosides and electrolyte imbalances (e.g., hypokalemia), which may require lower doses of digitalis glycosides in order to avoid toxicity. (Digoxin clearance is less affected by hepatic function impairment, while digitoxin clearance is less affected by renal function impairment.)

Digoxin-induced loss of appetite is a significant risk in frail elderly patients.

### Dental
An increased gag reflex may increase the difficulty of taking a dental impression.

### Drug interactions and/or related problems
The following drug interactions and/or related problems have been selected on the basis of their potential clinical significance (possible mechanism in parentheses where appropriate)—not necessarily inclusive (» = major clinical significance):

Note: Combinations containing any of the following medications, depending on the amount present, may also interact with this medication.

» Amiodarone
  (amiodarone increases serum concentrations of digoxin and probably other digitalis glycosides, possibly to toxic levels; when amiodarone therapy is initiated, the digitalis glycoside should be withdrawn or the dose reduced by 50%; if digitalis glycoside therapy is continued, serum concentrations should be carefully monitored; amiodarone and digitalis glycosides may also produce additive effects on sinoatrial [SA] and atrioventricular [AV] nodes)

Antacids
  (aluminum- and magnesium-containing antacids may inhibit absorption of digitalis glycosides, resulting in decreased plasma concentrations)

» Antiarrhythmics, other, including other digitalis preparations or
» Calcium salts, parenteral or
  Cocaine or
  Pancuronium or
  Rauwolfia alkaloids or
» Succinylcholine or
» Sympathomimetics
  (concurrent use with digitalis glycosides may increase the risk of cardiac arrhythmias; caution and close electrocardiographic [ECG] monitoring are very important if concurrent use is necessary)

» Antidiarrheal adsorbents (e.g., kaolin and pectin) or
» Cholestyramine or
» Colestipol or
  Dietary fiber, such as bran (large quantities) or
  Laxatives, bulk or
  Neomycin, oral or
  Sulfasalazine
  (concurrent use may inhibit digitalis glycosides absorption, resulting in decreased therapeutic effect of the glycoside; patients should be monitored closely for evidence of altered digitalis effect)

» Calcium channel blocking agents
  (serum digitalis glycoside concentrations may be increased during concurrent use, especially with verapamil and, to a lesser extent, diltiazem; nicardipine and nifedipine do not appear to have a significant effect. Concurrent use of digitalis glycosides with diltiazem and verapamil may result in excessive bradycardia because of additive depression of AV nodal conduction; nicardipine and nifedipine do not produce this effect. Digitalis glycoside dosage may need to be reduced and the patient carefully monitored for digitalis toxicity)

» Diuretics, potassium-depleting (such as bumetanide, ethacrynic acid, furosemide, indapamide, mannitol, or thiazides) or
» Hypokalemia-causing medications, other (See *Appendix II*)
  (hypokalemia caused by these medications may enhance the possibility of digitalis toxicity; frequent potassium determinations are recommended)

Edrophonium
  (when digitalis glycosides are used concurrently with edrophonium, the additive vagomimetic effects may cause excessive slowing of the heart rate)

Erythromycin or
Neomycin or
Tetracycline
  (although there have been no reported cases of clinical toxicity, concurrent use of oral antibiotics may increase serum digoxin concentrations in some individuals; in these individuals, altering the bowel flora with antibiotics may diminish digoxin conversion to inactive metabolites, resulting in increased serum digoxin concentrations; although there are limited data, this interaction has been reported with oral use of erythromycin, neomycin, and tetracycline)

Hepatic enzyme inducers (See *Appendix II*)
  (concurrent use may increase the metabolism of digitalis glycosides; may require dosage adjustment of digitalis glycosides, with the possible exception of digoxin)

Indomethacin
  (when indomethacin is administered concurrently with digitalis glycosides to the premature neonate, renal clearance of the digitalis glycoside may be decreased, leading to increased plasma concentrations, elimination half-lives, and risk of digitalis toxicity; it is recommended that digitalis dosage be reduced by 50% when indomethacin therapy is initiated and that further digitalis dosage adjustment be based on monitoring of ECG and digitalis concentration)
  (although not documented, the possibility should be considered that indomethacin may also increase digitalis concentration in adults and that digitalis dosage adjustment may be required)

» Magnesium sulfate, parenteral
  (parenteral magnesium sulfate must be administered with extreme caution in digitalized patients, especially if intravenous calcium salts are also employed; cardiac conduction changes and heart block may occur)

» Potassium salts
  (not recommended for concurrent use with digitalis glycosides in digitalized patients with severe or complete heart block; however, potassium supplements are often used to prevent or correct hypokalemia, especially when potassium-depleting diuretics such as the thiazides are administered concurrently with digitalis glycosides. Careful monitoring of serum potassium during use of supplemental

potassium is extremely important in order to avoid hyperkalemia, which is very dangerous in digitalized patients)
» Propafenone
(concurrent use with digoxin results in an increase in serum digoxin concentrations ranging from 35 to 85%, which appears to be unrelated to digoxin renal clearance but may be related to a decrease in volume of distribution and nonrenal clearance; careful monitoring of digoxin concentrations and dosage reduction of digoxin are recommended when propafenone is initiated; subsequent dosage adjustments should be based on serum digoxin concentrations)
» Quinidine or
Quinine
(concurrent use may result in substantially increased serum concentrations of digoxin; studies with digitoxin indicate a similar change; serum concentrations should be monitored and dosage adjusted as indicated)
» Spironolactone
(spironolactone may increase the half-life of digoxin; dosage reduction or increased dosing intervals of digoxin may be necessary and careful monitoring is recommended)
Succinylcholine
(may cause sudden release of potassium from muscle cells, increasing the risk of digitalis-induced arrhythmias)
» Sucralfate
(concurrent use with digoxin may decrease the absorption of digoxin; patients should be advised not to take sucralfate within 2 hours of digoxin)
Thallous chloride Tl 201
(in animal studies, concurrent use of digitalis glycosides decreased myocardial uptake of thallous chloride Tl 201; human data are not available)

**Laboratory value alterations**
The following have been selected on the basis of their potential clinical significance (possible effect in parentheses where appropriate)—not necessarily inclusive (» = major clinical significance):
With diagnostic test results
Electrocardiogram
(digitalis glycosides may produce false-positive ST-T changes during exercise testing)

**Medical considerations/Contraindications**
The medical considerations/contraindications included have been selected on the basis of their potential clinical significance (reasons given in parentheses where appropriate)—not necessarily inclusive (» = major clinical significance).

***Except under special circumstances, these medications should not be used when the following medical problems exist:***
» Toxic effects present from prior administration of any digitalis preparation
» Ventricular fibrillation

***Risk-benefit should be considered when the following medical problems exist:***
*For all digitalis glycosides*
» Atrioventricular (AV) block, incomplete, especially in patients with Stokes-Adams attacks
(may progress to complete block)
» Carotid sinus hypersensitivity
(digitalis glycosides may cause an increase in vagal tone)
» Glomerulonephritis, acute, accompanied by heart failure
(use of a low total daily dose is recommended, administered in divided doses, with constant ECG monitoring; use of antihypertensives and diuretics is also recommended and the digitalis glycoside should be withdrawn as soon as possible)
Hepatic function impairment, especially with digitoxin
(reduced metabolism; dosage reduction may be necessary)
» Hypercalcemia or
» Hyperkalemia
(increased risk of digitalis-induced arrhythmias, primarily heart block)
» Hypocalcemia
(digitalis glycosides may be ineffective; administration of calcium may be necessary)
» Hypokalemia (including that resulting from drugs, dialysis, mechanical suction of gastrointestinal secretions, malnutrition, diarrhea, prolonged vomiting, old age, and long-standing heart failure) or
» Hypomagnesemia
(increased risk of digitalis toxicity)
Hypothyroidism or
Hyperthyroidism
(altered sensitivity to digitalis; hyperthyroid patients may be less sensitive to digitalis and require larger doses, while hypothyroid patients may be more sensitive and require smaller doses; dosage adjustment may be necessary as patients become euthyroid)
» Idiopathic hypertrophic subaortic stenosis
(aggravated left ventricular outflow restrictions)
» Ischemic heart disease or
» Myocardial infarction, acute or
» Myocarditis, acute, including rheumatic carditis or viral myocarditis or
» Myxedema or
» Pulmonary disease, severe
(increased sensitivity of the myocardium to the effects of digitalis glycosides and increased risk of digitalis-induced arrhythmias)
Pericarditis, chronic constrictive
(patients may fail to respond to digitalis glycosides, and slowing of the heart rate may further reduce cardiac output)
» Premature ventricular contractions or
» Ventricular tachycardia
(risk of exacerbation; digitalis glycosides should not be used unless congestive heart failure supervenes after a protracted episode not due to digitalis)
Sensitivity to the digitalis glycoside prescribed
» Sick sinus syndrome
(possible worsening of sinus bradycardia or sinoatrial [SA] block)
» Wolff-Parkinson-White syndrome, especially when associated with atrial fibrillation
(possibility of fatal ventricular arrhythmias)
» Caution is also recommended in debilitated patients and patients using electronic cardiac pacemakers; these patients require careful dosage titration, as they may exhibit toxic responses at doses and serum concentrations generally tolerated by other patients.
*For digoxin only*
Renal function impairment
(reduced excretion and potential toxicity; dosage reduction may be required; in addition, time to achieve a new or steady-state concentration is increased; although digitoxin excretion is also reduced, no dosage reduction is necessary because metabolism and half-life are not affected)

**Patient monitoring**
The following may be especially important in patient monitoring (other tests may be warranted in some patients, depending on condition; » = major clinical significance):
Cardioglycoside, steady-state, trough
(serum concentrations may be required at periodic intervals, especially in patients with renal function impairment or if digitalis intoxication is suspected; toxicity to digitoxin and digoxin usually occurs at serum concentrations of > 35 and > 2 nanograms per mL, respectively. Individual tolerance and requirements vary; toxicity may occur with < 2 nanograms of digoxin per mL in some patients; others may require > 2 nanograms per mL for effective therapy. Digoxin-like immunoreactive substances have been reported to cause falsely increased serum digitalis glycoside concentration results, especially in infants and neonates, pregnant women, and in patients with hepatic or renal function impairment)
» Electrocardiogram (ECG) monitoring
(recommended at periodic intervals; if paroxysmal atrial tachycardias with atrioventricular (AV) block or ventricular tachycardia occurs, the digitalis glycoside should be withdrawn and the patient's digitalization and electrolyte status should be evaluated)
Electrolyte, especially potassium, calcium, and magnesium concentrations, serum
(recommended at periodic intervals, especially in patients also receiving diuretics, to detect possible electrolyte imbalance, which may increase the chance of digitalis toxicity, particularly with regard to arrhythmias, and may affect dosage requirements)
Hepatic function determinations and
Renal function determinations
(recommended at periodic intervals)
Pulse (apical) check
(recommended at periodic intervals, especially in patients with atrial fibrillation or when dosage change is made; dosage alteration may be necessary if the pulse rate falls below 60 beats per minute)

## Side/Adverse Effects

Note: Some side/adverse affects, including nausea and vomiting and some arrhythmias, may also be symptoms of toxicity. If there is any doubt about the cause of these symptoms, the digitalis glycoside should be withdrawn until the cause is determined.

The first signs of toxicity in infants and small children are usually cardiac arrhythmias, while in adults and older children, the first symptoms of overdose may be stomach upset, abdominal pain, loss of appetite, or unusually slow heart rate.

In adults, the most common arrhythmia is premature ventricular beats (extrasystoles); paroxysmal and nonparoxysmal nodal rhythms, atrioventricular (AV) (interference) dissociation, and paroxysmal atrial tachycardia with block are also common; increasing AV block may occur; death may occur from ventricular fibrillation. In children, premature ventricular systoles are rare, while nodal and atrial systoles are more frequent; atrial arrhythmias, atrial ectopic rhythms, and paroxysmal atrial tachycardia (particularly with AV block) are more common; ventricular arrhythmias are rare. An increase in PR interval may occur in newborns.

The following side/adverse effects have been selected on the basis of their potential clinical significance (possible signs and symptoms in parentheses where appropriate)—not necessarily inclusive:

**Those indicating need for medical attention**
Incidence rare
  *Allergic reaction* (skin rash or hives)
Signs and/or symptoms of toxicity or intolerance (in order of occurrence)
  *Stimulation of medullary centers* (loss of appetite; nausea or vomiting); *lower stomach pain; diarrhea; electrolyte imbalance, possible* (unusual tiredness or weakness, extreme); *slow or irregular heartbeat*—may be fast heartbeat in children; *blurred vision or other visual disturbances such as colored halos seen around objects*—"yellow," "green," or "white vision"; *drowsiness; confusion or mental depression; headache; fainting*

Note: Large doses may also have a local irritating emetic action.

## Overdose

For more information on the management of overdose or unintentional ingestion, **contact a Poison Control Center** (see *Poison Control Center Listing*).

**Treatment of overdose**
Discontinuation of digitalis medication is often all that is required if symptoms are not severe and occur near the expected time for peak medication effect.

Administration of activated charcoal, cholestyramine, or colestipol may be useful to accelerate clearance of the glycoside.

Potassium salts may be administered if hypokalemia is present and renal function is adequate, but should not be used if hyperkalemia or complete heart block exists unless those conditions are related primarily to supraventricular tachycardia.

For correction of hypokalemia, potassium may be administered:
  Orally in divided doses—
    Adults: 40 to 80 mEq (mmol).
    Children: 1 to 1.5 mEq (mmol) per kg of body weight.
  Intravenously when correction is urgent—
    Adults: 40 to 80 mEq (mmol) (diluted to 40 mEq [mmol] per 500 mL of 5% dextrose injection) at a rate not exceeding 20 mEq (mmol) per hour and adjusted as indicated by monitoring.
    Children: 1 to 1.5 mEq (mmol) per kg of body weight (diluted in appropriate volume of 5% dextrose injection for patient size) at a rate not exceeding 0.5 mEq (mmol) per kg of body weight per hour and adjusted as indicated by monitoring.

Other agents that have been used to correct arrhythmias caused by digitalis toxicity are lidocaine, procainamide, propranolol, and phenytoin. Ventricular pacing may be temporarily beneficial in cases of advanced heart block.

A chelating agent (e.g., EDTA) may be useful to bind calcium for treatment of arrhythmias caused by digitalis toxicity, hypokalemia, or hypercalcemia.

For life-threatening digoxin or digitoxin overdose—Intravenous administration of digoxin immune Fab (ovine) through a membrane filter. A vial containing 40 mg of digoxin immune Fab (ovine) will bind approximately 0.6 mg of digoxin or digitoxin. See the package insert or *Digoxin Immune Fab (Ovine) (Systemic)* for specific dosing guidelines and precautions in use of the product.

## Patient Consultation

As an aid to patient consultation, refer to *Advice for the Patient, Digitalis Medicines (Systemic)*.

In providing consultation, consider emphasizing the following selected information (» = major clinical significance):

**Before using this medication**
» Conditions affecting use, especially:
    Sensitivity to the digitalis glycoside prescribed
    Pregnancy—Cross placenta
    Use in children—Infant responses vary; careful dosage adjustment required
    Use in the elderly—Increased sensitivity to effects
    Other medications, especially potassium-depleting diuretics or other hypokalemia-causing medications, amiodarone, other antiarrhythmics, sympathomimetics, antidiarrheal adsorbents, calcium channel blocking agents, cholestyramine, colestipol, potassium-containing medications or supplements, quinidine, spironolactone, or sucralfate
    Other medical problems, especially severe pulmonary disease, conduction disturbance, ventricular arrhythmias, ischemic heart disease, recent myocardial infarction, or myocarditis

**Proper use of this medication**
» Compliance with therapy; taking exactly as directed, not taking more or less
    Proper administration of elixir: Taking orally; special dropper to be used for accurate measuring
    Taking medication at the same time each day to help increase compliance
    Checking apical pulse as directed (checking with physician if less than 60 beats per minute)
» Proper dosing
    Missed dose: Taking as soon as remembered if within 12 hours of scheduled dose; not taking if remembered later; not doubling doses; checking with doctor if dose missed for 2 days or more
» Proper storage

**Precautions while using this medication**
    Regular visits to physician to check progress
» Checking with physician before discontinuing medication
» Keeping medication out of reach of children
» Reporting to physician any nausea, vomiting, diarrhea, loss of appetite, or extremely slow pulse as possible signs of overdose
» Caution if medical or dental surgery or emergency treatment is required
    Carrying medical identification card
» Avoiding other medications unless prescribed by physician
    Caution in using medications of similar appearance

**Side/adverse effects**
    Signs of potential side effects, especially allergic reaction, and signs and symptoms of overdose

## General Dosing Information

Recommended doses are averages only; each dose must be adjusted to meet the individual patient's requirements.

Before a loading dose of a digitalis preparation is administered, it is extremely important to determine whether the patient has taken any form of digitalis during the previous 2 or 3 weeks, since some residual effect may require a reduced dosage to avoid toxicity.

Dosage calculations should be based on ideal (lean) body weight, since digitalis glycosides are not taken up by adipose tissue.

Digoxin may be the preferred cardioglycoside in some patients with liver function impairment because it does not undergo extensive hepatic metabolism.

Reduction of digitalis glycoside dosage prior to cardioversion may be desirable to avoid induction of ventricular arrhythmias; however, the benefit must be weighed against the risk of rapid increase in ventricular response to atrial fibrillation if the digitalis glycoside is withheld 1 to 2 days prior to cardioversion. If digitalis glycoside toxicity is suspected, electrical cardioversion of arrhythmias should be delayed, if possible. When it is considered absolutely necessary, use of the lowest possible energy level and/or pretreatment with lidocaine is recommended.

**For parenteral dosage forms only**
The intravenous route is preferred when parenteral administration is indicated. Intramuscular use involves greater local discomfort, slower effect, and erratic bioavailability. Intravenous injections should be administered over a period of at least 5 minutes.

Intramuscular injections are used only when the oral or intravenous routes cannot be used. The injection should be administered deeply into the muscle and preferably should not exceed 2 mL at any one injection site.

Following the injection, each site should be massaged well to reduce painful local reactions.

When a patient is transferred from a parenteral digitalis glycoside to an oral digitalis dosage form, dosage adjustments may be necessary to compensate for the pharmacokinetic differences among the medications. One exception is the transfer from digoxin injection to the liquid-filled, soft capsules of digoxin, because both dosage forms have the same bioavailability.

## DIGITOXIN

## Summary of Differences
Pharmacology/pharmacokinetics:
    Hepatically metabolized; renal excretion of inactive metabolites has little effect on digitoxin action.
    Protein binding—Very high.
    Half-life—120 to 216 hours.
    Onset of action—1 to 4 hours.
    Time to peak effect—8 to 14 hours.
    Duration of action—Approximately 14 days.
Precautions:
    Medical considerations/Contraindications—Dosage reduction not necessary in renal function impairment.

## Oral Dosage Forms
### DIGITOXIN TABLETS USP
**Usual adult dose**
Antiarrhythmic or
Cardiotonic—
    Digitalization:
        Rapid—Oral, 600 mcg (0.6 mg) initially, then 400 mcg (0.4 mg) after four to six hours and 200 mcg (0.2 mg) after another four- to six-hour period, followed by a daily maintenance dose as needed and tolerated, or
        Slow—Oral, 200 mcg (0.2 mg) two times a day for four days, followed by a daily maintenance dose as needed and tolerated.
    Maintenance:
        Oral, 50 to 300 mcg (0.05 to 0.3 mg) once a day, the dosage being adjusted as needed and tolerated.
Note:  Geriatric patients, debilitated patients, and patients using electronic cardiac pacemakers require careful dosage titration, as they may exhibit toxic responses at doses and serum concentrations generally tolerated by other patients.

**Usual adult prescribing limits**
Digitalization—Up to a total of 1.6 mg over one or two days.

**Usual pediatric dose**
Prepared oral digitoxin dosage forms are limited and may not be suitable for small children. Other digitalis glycosides may be considered.

**Strength(s) usually available**
U.S.—
    100 mcg (0.1 mg) (Rx) [*Crystodigin* (scored); GENERIC].
    200 mcg (0.2 mg) (Rx) [GENERIC].
Canada—
    100 mcg (0.1 mg) (Rx) [*Digitaline*].

**Packaging and storage**
Store below 40 °C (104 °F), preferably between 15 and 30 °C (59 and 86 °F), unless otherwise specified by manufacturer. Store in a well-closed container.

**Auxiliary labeling**
- Keep out of reach of children.
- Do not take other medicines without advice from your doctor.

## DIGOXIN

## Summary of Differences
Pharmacology/pharmacokinetics:
    Bioavailability—60 to 80% (tablets), 70 to 85% (oral elixir or intramuscular injection), or 90 to 100% (capsules).
    Protein binding—Low.
    Biotransformation—Minimal hepatic metabolism; excretion and half-life determined by renal function.
    Half-life—36 to 48 hours.
    Onset of action—5 to 30 minutes (intravenous) or 30 minutes to 2 hours (oral).
    Time to peak effect—1 to 4 hours (intravenous) or 2 to 6 hours (oral).
    Duration of action—Approximately 6 days.
Precautions:
    Medical considerations/Contraindications—Dosage reduction may be required in renal function impairment.

## Additional Dosing Information
**Bioequivalence information**
Bioavailability differences exist among dosage forms of digoxin. Changing therapy from one dosage form to another may require dosage adjustments. A 100-mcg (0.1-mg) dose of the injection or of the digoxin-solution capsule is bioequivalent to a 125-mcg (0.125-mg) dose of the tablet or elixir.
For digoxin tablets—
    Variability in the bioavailability of digoxin tablets was recognized as a clinical problem in the early 1970's. These differences in bioavailability were reported among different brands of digoxin tablets as well as among different lots of digoxin tablets produced by the same manufacturer. In response to the problems of bio-inequivalence, official dissolution standards were established. Problems have not been reported following establishment of these standards. However, because bioavailability from any digoxin tablet is incomplete ($\leq$ 80%), clinicians should consider this as a possible source of the problem when unexplained difficulty is encountered in the digitalization or maintenance therapy of patients with digoxin tablets.

## Oral Dosage Forms
### DIGOXIN CAPSULES
**Usual adult dose**
Antiarrhythmic or
Cardiotonic—
    Digitalization:
        Rapid—Oral, initially, 400 to 600 mcg (0.4 to 0.6 mg) with additional doses of 100 to 300 mcg (0.1 to 0.3 mg) administered every six to eight hours as needed and tolerated until the desired effect is clinically evident.
        Slow—Oral, a total of 50 to 350 mcg (0.05 to 0.35 mg) per day *divided* and administered in two doses, the dosage being repeated for seven to twenty-two days as needed to reach steady-state serum concentrations.
    Maintenance:
        Oral, 50 to 350 mcg (0.05 to 0.35 mg) administered as one or two doses per day as needed and tolerated.
Note:  Patients with impaired renal function, geriatric patients, debilitated patients, and patients using electronic cardiac pacemakers require careful dosage titration, as they may exhibit toxic responses at doses and serum concentrations generally tolerated by other patients.

**Usual pediatric dose**
Antiarrhythmic or
Cardiotonic—
    Digitalization:
        The following total amounts *divided* into three or more doses, with the initial portion representing approximately one-half the total, doses then being administered every four to eight hours.
        Premature neonates—
            Oral, 15 to 25 mcg (0.015 to 0.025 mg) per kg of body weight.
        Full-term neonates—
            Oral, 20 to 30 mcg (0.02 to 0.03 mg) per kg of body weight.
        Infants 1 month to 2 years of age—
            Oral, 30 to 50 mcg (0.03 to 0.05 mg) per kg of body weight.
        Children 2 to 5 years of age—
            Oral, 25 to 35 mcg (0.025 to 0.035 mg) per kg of body weight.
        Children 5 to 10 years of age—
            Oral, 15 to 30 mcg (0.015 to 0.03 mg) per kg of body weight.
        Children over 10 years of age—
            Oral, 8 to 12 mcg (0.008 to 0.012 mg) per kg of body weight.
    Maintenance:
        Premature neonates: Oral, 20 to 30% of the total digitalizing dose, divided and administered in two or three equal portions per day.
        Full-term neonates, infants, and children up to 10 years of age: Oral, 25 to 35% of the total digitalizing dose, divided and administered in two or three equal portions per day.
        Children 10 years of age and over: Oral, 25 to 35% of the total digitalizing dose administered once a day.
Note:  In small children (especially premature and immature infants), careful titration of dosage is required with close monitoring of patient's serum concentrations and ECG readings.

**Strength(s) usually available**
U.S.—
   50 mcg (0.05 mg) (Rx) [*Lanoxicaps* (ethyl alcohol 8%)].
   100 mcg (0.1 mg) (Rx) [*Lanoxicaps* (ethyl alcohol 8%)].
   200 mcg (0.2 mg) (Rx) [*Lanoxicaps* (ethyl alcohol 8%)].
   Note: Digoxin capsules consist of a stable digoxin solution enclosed in a soft gelatin capsule.
Canada—
   Not commercially available.

**Packaging and storage**
Store between 15 and 30 °C (59 and 86 °F) unless otherwise specified by manufacturer. Store in a tight container.

**Auxiliary labeling**
• Keep out of reach of children.
• Keep container tightly closed.
• Do not take other medicines without advice from your doctor.

**Note**
When patients are switched from digoxin tablets to digoxin capsules, or vice versa, the difference in bioavailability must be kept in mind.

## DIGOXIN ELIXIR USP

**Usual adult dose**
Digitalization:
   Rapid: Oral, a total of 0.75 to 1.25 mg *divided* into two or more doses, each then being administered every six to eight hours.
   Slow: Oral, 125 to 500 mcg (0.125 to 0.5 mg) once a day for seven days.
Maintenance:
   Oral, 125 to 500 mcg (0.125 to 0.5 mg) once a day.
Note: Patients with impaired renal function, geriatric patients, debilitated patients, and patients using electronic cardiac pacemakers require careful dosage titration, as they may exhibit toxic responses at doses and serum concentrations generally tolerated by other patients.

**Usual pediatric dose**
Digitalization—
   The following total amounts *divided* into two or more doses, administered at six- to eight-hour intervals:
   Premature and newborn infants up to 1 month of age—
      Oral, 20 to 35 mcg (0.02 to 0.035 mg) per kg of body weight.
   Infants 1 month to 2 years of age—
      Oral, 35 to 60 mcg (0.035 to 0.06 mg) per kg of body weight.
   Children 2 to 5 years of age—
      Oral, 30 to 40 mcg (0.03 to 0.04 mg) per kg of body weight.
   Children 5 to 10 years of age—
      Oral, 20 to 35 mcg (0.02 to 0.035 mg) per kg of body weight.
   Children over 10 years of age—
      Rapid: Oral, a total of 0.75 to 1.25 mg *divided* into two or more doses, each then being administered every six to eight hours.
      Slow: Oral, 125 to 500 mcg (0.125 to 0.5 mg) once a day for seven days.
Maintenance—
   Oral, one-fifth to one-third of the total digitalizing dose administered once a day.
Note: Alternative pediatric dosage (the "small-dose" method)—Oral, 17 mcg (0.017 mg) per kg of body weight per day. This dosage method has the advantage of easier control and therefore less chance for toxicity.
   In small children (especially premature and immature infants) careful titration of dosage is required with close monitoring of patient's serum concentrations and ECG readings.

**Strength(s) usually available**
U.S.—
   50 mcg (0.05 mg) per mL (Rx) [*Lanoxin* (alcohol 10%); GENERIC].
Canada—
   50 mcg (0.05 mg) per mL (Rx) [*Lanoxin* (alcohol 11.5%; tartrazine)].

**Packaging and storage**
Store below 40 °C (104 °F), preferably between 15 and 30 °C (59 and 86 °F), unless otherwise specified by manufacturer. Store in a tight container.

**Auxiliary labeling**
• Keep out of reach of children.
• Keep container tightly closed.
• Do not take other medicines without advice from your doctor.

## DIGOXIN TABLETS USP

Note: Variability in the bioavailability of digoxin tablets was recognized as a clinical problem in the early 1970's. These differences in bioavailability were reported among different brands of digoxin tablets as well as among different lots of digoxin tablets produced by the same manufacturer. In response to the problems of bio-inequivalence, official dissolution standards were established. Problems have not been reported following establishment of these standards. However, because bioavailability from any digoxin tablet is incomplete (≤ 80%), clinicians should consider this as a possible source of the problem when unexplained difficulty is encountered in the digitalization or maintenance therapy of patients with digoxin tablets.

**Usual adult dose**
Digitalization:
   Rapid: Oral, a total of 0.75 to 1.25 mg *divided* into two or more doses, each then being administered every six to eight hours.
   Slow: Oral, 125 to 500 mcg (0.125 to 0.5 mg) once a day for seven days.
Maintenance:
   Oral, 125 to 500 mcg (0.125 to 0.5 mg) once a day.
Note: Patients with impaired renal function, geriatric patients, debilitated patients, and patients using electronic cardiac pacemakers require careful dosage titration, as they may exhibit toxic responses at doses and serum concentrations generally tolerated by other patients.

**Usual pediatric dose**
Digitalization—
   The following total amounts *divided* into two or more doses, administered at six- to eight-hour intervals:
   Premature and newborn infants up to 1 month of age—
      Oral, 20 to 35 mcg (0.02 to 0.035 mg) per kg of body weight.
   Infants 1 month to 2 years of age—
      Oral, 35 to 60 mcg (0.035 to 0.06 mg) per kg of body weight.
   Children 2 to 5 years of age—
      Oral, 30 to 40 mcg (0.03 to 0.04 mg) per kg of body weight.
   Children 5 to 10 years of age—
      Oral, 20 to 35 mcg (0.02 to 0.035 mg) per kg of body weight.
   Children over 10 years of age—
      Rapid: Oral, a total of 0.75 to 1.25 mg *divided* into two or more doses, each then being administered every six to eight hours.
      Slow: Oral, 125 to 500 mcg (0.125 to 0.5 mg) once a day for seven days.
Maintenance—
   Oral, one-fifth to one-third of the total digitalizing dose administered once a day.
Note: Alternative pediatric dosage (the "small-dose" method)—Oral, 17 mcg (0.017 mg) per kg of body weight per day. This dosage method has the advantage of easier control and therefore less chance for toxicity.
   In small children (especially premature and immature infants) careful titration of dosage is required with close monitoring of patient's serum concentrations and ECG readings.

**Strength(s) usually available**
U.S.—
   125 mcg (0.125 mg) (Rx) [*Lanoxin* (scored); GENERIC].
   250 mcg (0.25 mg) (Rx) [*Lanoxin* (scored); GENERIC].
   500 mcg (0.5 mg) (Rx) [*Lanoxin* (scored)].
Canada—
   62.5 mcg (0.0625 mg) (Rx) [*Lanoxin*].
   125 mcg (0.125 mg) (Rx) [*Lanoxin* (scored)].
   250 mcg (0.25 mg) (Rx) [*Lanoxin* (scored)].

**Packaging and storage**
Store below 40 °C (104 °F), preferably between 15 and 30 °C (59 and 86 °F), unless otherwise specified by manufacturer. Store in a tight container.

**Auxiliary labeling**
• Keep out of reach of children.
• Do not take other medicines without advice from your doctor.

**Note**
Caution—The small, white tablets of digoxin 0.25 mg have been confused by numerous patients with other, similar-looking medications such as furosemide, with resultant serious dosage accidents. To reduce this hazard, the dispenser may:
   —check with the prescriber; suggest digoxin capsules be used instead of tablets.
   —caution the patient about the potential hazard.
   —apply auxiliary "Heart medicine" labels to digoxin tablet container.
   —use containers of different size or appearance for similar-looking medications.
   —suggest that patient not use tablets from both containers at same time.
   —suggest that patient never transfer digoxin from original to other containers.

## Parenteral Dosage Forms
### DIGOXIN INJECTION USP
**Usual adult dose**
Digitalization—Intravenous, initially, 400 to 600 mcg (0.4 to 0.6 mg) with additional doses of 100 to 300 mcg (0.1 to 0.3 mg) administered every four to eight hours as needed and tolerated until the desired effect is clinically evident.

Maintenance—Intravenous, 125 to 500 mcg (0.125 to 0.5 mg) per day in divided doses or as a single dose.

Note: Patients with impaired renal function, geriatric patients, debilitated patients, and patients using electronic cardiac pacemakers require careful dosage titration, as they may exhibit toxic responses at doses and serum concentrations generally tolerated by other patients.

**Usual pediatric dose**
Digitalization—
The following total amounts *divided* into three or more doses, with the initial portion representing approximately one-half the total, doses then being administered every four to eight hours:
Premature neonates—
Intravenous, 15 to 25 mcg (0.015 to 0.025 mg) per kg of body weight.
Full-term neonates—
Intravenous, 20 to 30 mcg (0.02 to 0.03 mg) per kg of body weight.
Infants 1 month to 2 years of age—
Intravenous, 30 to 50 mcg (0.03 to 0.05 mg) per kg of body weight.
Children 2 to 5 years of age—
Intravenous, 25 to 35 mcg (0.025 to 0.035 mg) per kg of body weight.
Children 5 to 10 years of age—
Intravenous, 15 to 30 mcg (0.015 to 0.03 mg) per kg of body weight.
Children over 10 years of age—
Intravenous, 8 to 12 mcg (0.008 to 0.012 mg) per kg of body weight.

Maintenance (begun within 24 hours after digitalization)—
Premature neonates—Intravenous, 20 to 30% of the total digitalizing dose, divided and administered in two or three equal portions per day.
Full-term neonates, infants, and children up to 10 years of age—Intravenous, 25 to 35% of the total digitalizing dose, divided and administered in two or three equal portions per day.
Children over 10 years of age—Intravenous, 25 to 35% of the total digitalizing dose administered once a day.

Note: In small children (especially premature and immature infants) careful titration of dosage is required with close monitoring of patient's serum concentrations and ECG readings.

If parenteral administration is necessary and the intravenous route is not possible, the intravenous dose may be given by the intramuscular route, although this is quite painful and has inconsistent absorption.

**Strength(s) usually available**
U.S.—
100 mcg (0.1 mg) per mL (Rx) [*Lanoxin* (alcohol 10%)].
250 mcg (0.25 mg) per mL (Rx) [*Lanoxin* (alcohol 10%); GENERIC].
Canada—
50 mcg (0.05 mg) per mL (Rx) [*Lanoxin* (alcohol 10%)].
250 mcg (0.25 mg) per mL (Rx) [*Lanoxin* (alcohol 10%)].

**Packaging and storage**
Store below 40 °C (104 °F), preferably between 15 and 30 °C (59 and 86 °F), unless otherwise specified by manufacturer. Protect from freezing.

**Preparation of dosage form**
Digoxin Injection USP may be administered undiluted or may be diluted with a 4-fold or greater volume (to reduce the risk of precipitation) of sterile water for injection, 0.9% sodium chloride injection, or 5% dextrose injection for intravenous administration.

**Stability**
Do not use if markedly discolored or if a precipitate is present. Immediate use of diluted Digoxin Injection USP is recommended.

## Selected Bibliography
Epstein FH. Digitalis. Mechanisms of action and clinical use. N Engl J Med 1988 Feb 11; 318: 358-65.

Revised: 03/10/93
Interim revision: 04/25/95; 08/15/95; 08/19/97

## Table 1. Pharmacology/Pharmacokinetics

| Drug and Route | Protein Binding | Biotransformation | Half-life (hr) | Onset of Action | Time to Peak Effect (hr) | Therapeutic Serum Concentration (nanograms/mL) | Duration of Action (approx. days) | Elimination* |
|---|---|---|---|---|---|---|---|---|
| Digitoxin Oral | Very high (>90%) | Hepatic | 120–216 | 1–4 hr | 8–14 | 13–25 | 14 | Renal (metabolites) |
| Digoxin IV | Low (20–25%) | Hepatic (slight) | 36–48 (4–6 days in anuria) | 5–30 min | 1–4 | 0.5–2.0 | 6 | Renal (50–70% unchanged)† |
| Digoxin Oral | | | | ½–2 hr | 2–6 | | 6 | |

*Digitalis glycosides are not effectively removed from the body by dialysis, exchange transfusion, or cardiopulmonary bypass.
†The breast milk to plasma ratio of digoxin administered to breast-feeding women is 0.6 to 0.9.

---

**DIGITOXIN**—See *Digitalis Glycosides (Systemic)*

**DIGOXIN**—See *Digitalis Glycosides (Systemic)*

---

# DIGOXIN IMMUNE FAB (OVINE) Systemic

VA CLASSIFICATION (Primary): AD900
Commonly used brand name(s): *Digibind*.
Note: For a listing of dosage forms and brand names by country availability, see *Dosage Forms* section(s).

## Category
Antidote, to digitalis glycoside toxicity.

## Indications
**Accepted**
Toxicity, digitalis glycoside (treatment)—Digoxin immune Fab (ovine) is indicated for treatment of potentially life-threatening digoxin or digitoxin overdose (i.e., with severe arrhythmias or hyperkalemia).

## Pharmacology/Pharmacokinetics
**Physicochemical characteristics**
Source—Produced by a process involving immunization of sheep with digoxin that has been coupled as a hapten to human serum albumin, to

stimulate production of digoxin-specific antibodies. After papain digestion of the antibody, digoxin-specific antigen binding (Fab) fragments (molecular weight 46,200 daltons) are isolated and purified by affinity chromatography.
Molecular weight—46,200.

### Mechanism of action/Effect
Preferentially binds molecules of digoxin or digitoxin, and the complex is then excreted by the kidneys. As free serum digoxin is removed, tissue-bound digoxin is also released into the serum to maintain the equilibrium and is bound and removed by digoxin immune Fab. The net result is a reduction in serum and tissue digoxin.

### Half-life
15 to 20 hours.

### Onset of action
Reduction of free active serum digoxin or digitoxin—Less than 1 minute.
Improvement in signs and symptoms of digitalis toxicity—15 to 30 minutes after administration (reversal of inotropic effect is usually slower than reversal of arrhythmias and hyperkalemia and may take several hours).

### Elimination
Renal.

## Precautions to Consider

### Cross-sensitivity and/or related problems
Patients sensitive to sheep or any product of ovine origin may be sensitive to digoxin immune Fab (ovine) also.

### Carcinogenicity
Studies have not been done in either animals or humans.

### Pregnancy/Reproduction
Pregnancy—Studies have not been done in humans.
Studies have not been done in animals.
FDA Pregnancy Category C.

### Breast-feeding
It is not known whether digoxin immune Fab (ovine) passes into breast milk. Problems in humans have not been documented.

### Pediatrics
Studies performed to date have not demonstrated pediatrics-specific problems that would limit the usefulness of digoxin immune Fab (ovine) in children.

### Geriatrics
No information is available on the relationship of age to the effects of digoxin immune Fab (ovine) in geriatric patients. However, elderly patients are more likely to have age-related renal function impairment, which may require caution in patients receiving this medication.

### Laboratory value alterations
The following have been selected on the basis of their potential clinical significance (possible effect in parentheses where appropriate)—not necessarily inclusive (» = major clinical significance):

With diagnostic test results
   Digitalis concentration determinations by immunoassay
     (may be interfered with)

With physiology/laboratory test values
   Digoxin or digitoxin concentrations, serum
     (free active concentrations rapidly fall to undetectable levels)
     (total serum concentrations rise suddenly after administration of Fab antibody but are almost totally bound to the Fab fragment and are inactive; these concentrations decline to undetectable levels several days later as Fab-digoxin complexes are excreted)
   Potassium concentrations, serum
     (may decrease rapidly from high concentrations associated with digitalis toxicity)

### Medical considerations/Contraindications
The medical considerations/contraindications included have been selected on the basis of their potential clinical significance (reasons given in parentheses where appropriate)—not necessarily inclusive (» = major clinical significance).

*Risk-benefit should be considered when the following medical problems exist:*
   Allergy, history of
     (risk of allergic reaction to Fab antibody may be increased)
   Renal function impairment
     (elimination of Fab-digoxin complexes may be delayed since the complex is eliminated renally. In patients who are functionally anephric, glomerular filtration and renal excretion would not be expected to occur; instead, the complex may be eliminated by the reticuloendothelial system; because it is not clear whether reintoxication would result, prolonged monitoring for digitalis toxicity is recommended in these patients)
» Sensitivity to digoxin immune Fab (ovine)

### Patient monitoring
The following may be especially important in patient monitoring (other tests may be warranted in some patients, depending on condition; » = major clinical significance):

Body temperature and
Electrocardiogram (ECG)
   (monitoring recommended during treatment)
» Digoxin or digitoxin concentrations, serum
   (recommended prior to administration of Fab antibody to aid in dosage calculation, but not useful for at least 5 to 7 days after Fab antibody treatment is begun because of interference by the antibody with the test)
» Potassium concentrations, serum
   (recommended at frequent intervals during treatment; hypokalemia should be treated promptly)

## Side/Adverse Effects

Allergic or febrile reactions to digoxin immune Fab (ovine) have been reported rarely. Patients previously treated with the product or allergic to ovine proteins appear to be especially at risk.

Side/adverse effects are related more to withdrawal of digitalis effects than to a direct effect of the antibody fragment. Low cardiac output, including congestive heart failure, may be exacerbated as a result of withdrawal of the inotropic effects of digitalis. Ventricular rate may increase as a result of withdrawal of digitalis being used for atrial fibrillation. Hypokalemia may occur as elevated serum potassium concentrations fall rapidly.

## General Dosing Information

It is recommended that equipment and medications necessary for cardiopulmonary resuscitation be immediately available during administration of digoxin immune Fab (ovine). If necessary, in patients who respond poorly to withdrawal of digoxin's inotropic effect, other intravenous inotropes such as dopamine or dobutamine or cardiac load–reducing agents may be used. Caution is necessary in use of catecholamines because of the risk of aggravation of digitalis toxicity–associated arrhythmias.

Skin-testing for allergy to digoxin immune Fab (ovine) may be performed prior to administration in high-risk patients (i.e., those previously treated with the Fab antibody or with known allergy, especially to sheep proteins). One of two methods may be used:
- Intradermal test: Dilute 0.1 mL of the reconstituted solution (containing 9.5 mg of the Fab antibody per mL) in 9.9 mL of 0.9% sodium chloride injection to produce 10 mL of a solution containing 95 mcg (0.095 mg) per mL; then inject 0.1 mL (9.5 mcg or 0.0095 mg) intradermally. After 20 minutes, inspect the injection site for presence of an urticarial wheal surrounded by a zone of erythema.
- Scratch test: Dilute 0.1 mL of the reconstituted solution (containing 9.5 mg of the Fab antibody per mL) in 9.9 mL of 0.9% sodium chloride injection to produce 10 mL of a solution containing 95 mcg (0.095 mg) per mL; then place 1 drop of the solution on the skin and make a ¼-inch scratch through the drop with a sterile needle. After 20 minutes, inspect the site for presence of an urticarial wheal surrounded by a zone of erythema.

If a positive skin test occurs, use of digoxin immune Fab (ovine) should be avoided unless absolutely necessary.
If a systemic reaction occurs, measures to treat anaphylaxis should be used.

After reconstitution, digoxin immune Fab (ovine) is administered by intravenous infusion, through a 0.22-micron membrane filter, over 30 minutes. However, it may be given by rapid direct intravenous injection if cardiac arrest is imminent.

Redigitalization of the patient, if necessary, should be delayed until elimination of Fab fragments from the body is complete, usually after several days but may be up to a week or longer in patients with renal function impairment.

## Parenteral Dosage Forms

### DIGOXIN IMMUNE FAB (OVINE) FOR INJECTION

#### Usual adult and adolescent dose
Antidote, to digitalis glycoside toxicity—
   Intravenous, in an amount equimolar to the amount of digoxin or digitoxin in the patient's body (total body load [TBL]). A dose of 38 mg of digoxin immune Fab (ovine) binds approximately 0.5 mg of digoxin or digitoxin.

Dosage may be calculated using one of the following formulas:
1) Based on dose of digoxin or digitoxin ingested:
   For digoxin tablets, oral solution, or intramuscular injection—
   Dose (mg) = (Dose ingested [mg] × 0.8)/0.5 × 38
   For digitoxin tablets, digoxin capsules, or intravenous injection of digoxin or digitoxin—
   Dose (mg) = [Dose ingested (mg)/0.5] × 38

Table 1. Approximate dose of digoxin immune Fab (ovine) when amount of digoxin ingested is known.

| Number of digoxin tablets or capsules ingested* | Dose of digoxin immune Fab (ovine) | |
|---|---|---|
| | mg | Number of 38-mg vials |
| 25 | 380 | 10 |
| 50 | 760 | 20 |
| 75 | 1140 | 30 |
| 100 | 1520 | 40 |
| 150 | 2280 | 60 |
| 200 | 3040 | 80 |

*0.25-mg tablets with 80% bioavailability, or 0.2-mg capsules.

2) Based on steady-state serum digoxin or digitoxin concentration (SDC):
   For digoxin—
   Dose (mg) = (SDC [nanograms/mL] × body weight [kg])/100 × 38
   For digitoxin—
   Dose (mg) = (SDC [nanograms/mL] × body weight [kg])/1000 × 38

Table 2. Approximate *adult and adolescent* dose *(number of 38-mg vials)* of digoxin immune Fab (ovine) when serum digoxin concentration (SDC) is known.

| SDC (ng/mL) | Patient weight (kg) | | | | |
|---|---|---|---|---|---|
| | 40 | 60 | 70 | 80 | 100 |
| 1 | 0.5 | 0.5 | 1 | 1 | 1 |
| 2 | 1 | 1 | 2 | 2 | 2 |
| 4 | 2 | 3 | 3 | 3 | 4 |
| 8 | 3 | 5 | 6 | 7 | 8 |
| 12 | 5 | 7 | 9 | 10 | 12 |
| 16 | 7 | 10 | 11 | 13 | 16 |
| 20 | 8 | 12 | 14 | 16 | 20 |

Note: Dosage of digoxin immune Fab (ovine) is approximate, since total body digitalis load can be difficult to estimate. After the initial dose, need for and amount of additional dosing should be determined using clinical judgment.

If neither an estimated ingestion amount of digitalis nor the SDC is available, 760 mg of digoxin immune Fab (ovine) may be administered, which will be adequate to treat most life-threatening ingestions.

### Usual pediatric dose
See *Usual adult and adolescent dose* (including Note).

Note: In small children, monitoring for volume overload is important.

For infants, who can have much smaller dosage requirements, it is recommended that digoxin immune Fab (ovine) be reconstituted as directed and administered with a tuberculin syringe. For very small doses, a reconstituted 38-mg vial can be diluted with 34 mL of 0.9% sodium chloride injection to produce a solution containing 1 mg per mL.

For approximate dose when amount of digoxin ingested is known, see *Usual adult and adolescent dose—Table 1*.

Table 3. Approximate *pediatric* dose *(mg)* of digoxin immune Fab (ovine) when serum digoxin concentration (SDC) is known.

| SDC (ng/mL) | Patient weight (kg) | | | | |
|---|---|---|---|---|---|
| | 1 | 3 | 5 | 10 | 20 |
| 1 | 0.4 | 1 | 2 | 4 | 8 |
| 2 | 1 | 2 | 4 | 8 | 15 |
| 4 | 1.5 | 5 | 8 | 15 | 30 |
| 8 | 3 | 9 | 15 | 30 | 61 |
| 12 | 5 | 14 | 23 | 46 | 91 |
| 16 | 6 | 18 | 30 | 61 | 122 |
| 20 | 8 | 23 | 38 | 76 | 152 |

### Size(s) usually available
U.S.—
  38 mg (Rx) [*Digibind* (preservative-free)].
Canada—
  38 mg (Rx) [*Digibind* (preservative-free)].

### Packaging and storage
Store between 2 and 8 °C (36 and 46 °F). Unreconstituted vials may be stored at up to 30 °C (86 °F) for up to 30 days.

### Preparation of dosage form
Digoxin immune Fab (ovine) for injection is reconstituted for intravenous administration by dissolving 38 mg in 4 mL of sterile water for injection and mixing gently, to produce a solution containing 9.5 mg per mL. The resulting solution may be further diluted with 0.9% sodium chloride injection to a convenient volume for administration by intravenous infusion.

### Stability
Reconstituted solution should be used immediately, but may be stored for up to 4 hours between 2 and 8 °C (36 and 46 °F).

## Selected Bibliography
Antman EM, Wenger TL, Butler VP, Haber E, Smith TW. Treatment of 150 cases of life-threatening digitalis intoxication with digoxin-specific Fab antibody fragments. Circulation 1990; 81: 1744-52.

Stolshek BS, Osterhout SK, Dunham G. The role of digoxin-specific antibodies in the treatment of digitalis poisoning. Med Toxicol 1988; 3: 167-71.

Hickey AR, Wenger TL, Carpenter V, et al. Digoxin immune Fab therapy in the management of digitalis intoxication: safety and efficacy results of an observational study. J Am Coll Cardiol 1991; 17: 590-8.

Revised: 08/17/95

---

**DIHYDROERGOTAMINE**—See *Vascular Headache Suppressants, Ergot Derivative–containing (Systemic)*

---

# DIHYDROERGOTAMINE  Nasal-Systemic—INTRODUCTORY VERSION

JAN: Dihydroergotamine Mesilate.
VA CLASSIFICATION (Primary): CN105
Note: For a listing of dosage forms and brand names by country availability, see *Dosage Forms* section(s).

## Category
Antimigraine agent.

## Indications
### Accepted
Headache, migraine (treatment)—Intranasal dihydroergotamine is indicated to relieve (abort) acute migraine headaches (with or without aura).

### Unaccepted
Intranasal dihydroergotamine is not recommended for treatment of basilar artery migraine or hemiplegic migraine.

## Pharmacology/Pharmacokinetics
### Physicochemical characteristics
Source—Synthetic.
Molecular weight—679.8.

### Mechanism of action/Effect
Dihydroergotamine is an ergot derivative that interacts with several neurotransmitter receptors, including alpha-adrenergic, serotonergic (tryptaminergic), and dopaminergic receptors. The dihydroergotamine-induced decreases in the firing of serotonergic (5-hydroxytryptaminergic, 5-HT) neurons may be responsible for relief of migraine headache. Specifically, it is thought that agonist activity at the 5-HT$_{1D}$ receptor

subtype provides relief of acute headache. It has been proposed that constriction of cerebral blood vessels by the ergot derivative (resulting from alpha-adrenergic stimulation as well as from activity at 5-HT receptors) reduces the pulsation in cerebral arteries that may be responsible for the pain of migraine headaches. It has also been proposed that dihydroergotamine may relieve vascular headaches by decreasing the release of pro-inflammatory neuropeptide release.

### Other actions/effects
Dihydroergotamine stimulates uterine smooth muscle.

### Absorption
Following intranasal administration, the bioavailability of dihydroergotamine is 32%. The rate of absorption of intranasal dihydroergotamine demonstrates interpatient variability, which may be dependent on the administration technique.

### Protein binding
Very high (93%).

### Biotransformation
Hepatic; extensive. The principal metabolite, 8′-hydroxy-dihydroergotamine, is pharmacologically active. Following intranasal administration of dihydroergotamine, the metabolites represent 20 to 30% of the area under the plasma concentration–time curve (AUC).

### Half-life
Approximately 10 hours.

### Elimination
Primarily fecal (biliary). Following intranasal administration of dihydroergotamine, 2% of the dose is excreted in the urine.

## Precautions to Consider

### Carcinogenicity
Long-term studies in mice and rabbits are currently being done to evaluate the carcinogenic potential of dihydroergotamine.

### Mutagenicity
Dihydroergotamine demonstrated no mutagenic effects in presence or absence of metabolic activation in the Ames test or the *in vitro* mammalian Chinese hamster gene mutation assays, or in the rat hepatocyte unscheduled DNA synthesis test assay. There was evidence of clastogenic activity in the V79 Chinese hamster cell assay with metabolic activation and the cultured human peripheral blood lymphocyte *in vitro* chromosomal aberration assays. However, there was no evidence of clastogenic activity in the *in vivo* mouse and hamster micronucleus tests.

### Pregnancy/Reproduction
Fertility—There was no evidence of impairment of fertility in rats receiving doses of intranasal dihydroergotamine of up to 1.6 mg per kg of body weight (mg/kg) per day (area under the plasma concentration–time curve [AUC] exposure approximately 9 to 11 times the maximum recommended human dose [MRHD]).

Pregnancy—Adequate and well-controlled studies in humans have not been done. However, **use during pregnancy is contraindicated** because of intranasal dihydroergotamine's oxytocic activity, which may result in fetal harm. Therefore, if intranasal dihydroergotamine should be used by a pregnant woman, or if a woman becomes pregnant during treatment, she should be advised that this medication may harm the fetus.

An embryofetal developmental study during the organogenesis period in pregnant rabbits showed that intranasal dihydroergotamine doses of up to 0.16 mg per day or greater (AUC exposure approximately 0.4 to 1.2 times the exposure in humans receiving the MRHD) resulted in decreased fetal body weight and/or skeletal ossification. In rabbits receiving doses of intranasal dihydroergotamine of up to 3.6 mg per day during the organogenesis period (equivalent to maternal concentration of approximately 7 times the MRHD), a delay in skeletal ossification was observed in the fetuses. However, in rabbits receiving doses of up to 1.2 mg per day (equivalent to maternal concentrations of 2.5 times the MRHD), no delay in ossification was observed. In female rats receiving doses of intranasal dihydroergotamine of up to 0.16 mg per day or greater during pregnancy and lactation, decreased body weights and impaired reproductive function were observed in the offspring. Intranasal dihydroergotamine doses that produced developmental effects in these studies were below those that demonstrated evidence of any maternal toxicity. In addition, the prolonged vasoconstriction of the uterine vessels and/or increased myometrial tone resulted in a reduction in the uteroplacental blood flow, which is presumed to be the cause for dihydroergotamine-induced intrauterine growth retardation.

FDA Pregnancy Category X.

### Breast-feeding
It is expected that intranasal dihydroergotamine would be distributed into human breast milk. However, there is currently no data on the concentration of dihydroergotamine distributed into human breast milk.

Ergot alkaloids are distributed into human breast milk and have the potential to cause adverse effects, such as vomiting, diarrhea, weak pulse, and unstable blood pressure. These medications may also inhibit lactation.

Due to intranasal dihydroergotamine's potential to cause serious adverse effects, use of this medicine is not recommended for nursing mothers.

### Pediatrics
No information is available on the relationship of age to the effects of intranasal dihydroergotamine in pediatric patients. Safety and efficacy have not been established.

### Geriatrics
No information is available on the relationship of age to the effects of intranasal dihydroergotamine in geriatric patients.

### Drug interactions and/or related problems
The following drug interactions and/or related problems have been selected on the basis of their potential clinical significance (possible mechanism in parentheses where appropriate)—not necessarily inclusive (» = major clinical significance):

Note: Combinations containing any of the following medications, depending on the amount present, may also interact with this medication.

Antibiotics, macrolide, especially, such as:
  Erythromycin
  Troleandomycin
    (these antibiotics may inhibit the metabolism of intranasal dihydroergotamine and increase the risk of vasospasm)

Beta-adrenergic blocking agents
  (these medications may potentiate vasoconstriction)

» Ergot alkaloids, other or
» Vasoconstrictors, systemic, other, such as:
  Cocaine
  Epinephrine, parenteral
  Metaraminol
  Methoxamine
  Norepinephrine
  Phenylephrine, parenteral
    (concurrent use with intranasal dihydroergotamine may result in additive increases of blood pressure)

» 5-hydroxytryptamine agonists, such as:
  Sumatriptan
    (a delay of 24 hours between administration of sumatriptan and intranasal dihydroergotamine is recommended because of the possibility of additive and/or prolonged vasoconstriction)

Nicotine
  (this medication may potentiate vasoconstriction)

### Medical considerations/Contraindications
The medical considerations/contraindications included have been selected on the basis of their potential clinical significance (reasons given in parentheses where appropriate)—not necessarily inclusive (» = major clinical significance).

*Except under special circumstances, this medication should not be used when the following medical problems exist:*

» Coronary artery disease, especially:
  Angina pectoris
  Myocardial infarction, history of
  Myocardial ischemia, silent, documented
  Prinzmetal's angina

» Other conditions in which coronary vasoconstriction would be detrimental
  (intranasal dihydroergotamine may cause coronary vasospasms)

» Hepatic function impairment, severe
» Hypertension, severe, uncontrolled
  (may be exacerbated)

» Renal function impairment, severe
» Vascular surgery

*Risk-benefit should be considered when the following medical problems exist:*

Coronary artery disease, predisposition to
  (intranasal dihydroergotamine may cause serious coronary adverse effects; patients in whom coronary artery disease is a possibility on the basis of age or the presence of other risk factors, such as dia-

betes, hypercholesterolemia, obesity, a strong family history of coronary artery disease, or tobacco smoking, should be evaluated for the presence of cardiovascular disease before intranasal dihydroergotamine is prescribed; even after a satisfactory evaluation, the advisability of administering the patient's first dose under medical supervision should be considered)

Hypersensitivity to ergot alkaloids

Hypertension, controlled
   (may precipitate an increase in blood pressure)

» Sepsis

**Patient monitoring**

The following may be especially important in patient monitoring (other tests may be warranted in some patients, depending on condition; » = major clinical significance):

Electrocardiogram (ECG)
   (monitoring is recommended for long-term intermittent users of intranasal dihydroergotamine)

## Side/Adverse Effects

The following side/adverse effects have been selected on the basis of their potential clinical significance (possible signs and symptoms in parentheses where appropriate)—not necessarily inclusive:

**Those indicating need for medical attention**

Incidence less frequent or rare

*Cardiovascular effects, including angina pectoris; arrythmias* (irregular heartbeat); *coronary vasospasm–induced* (chest pain); *myocardial infarction or ischemia* (feeling of heaviness in chest; pain in back, chest, or left arm; shortness of breath or troubled breathing); *peripheral ischemia* (itching of skin; numbness and tingling of face, fingers, or toes; pain in arms legs, or lower back, especially pain in calves and/or heels upon exertion; pale, bluish-colored, or cold hands or feet; weak or absent pulses in legs); *upper respiratory tract infection* (cough, fever, sneezing, or sore throat)

**Those indicating need for medical attention only if they continue or are bothersome**

Incidence more frequent

*Asthenia* (unusual tiredness or weakness); *diarrhea; dizziness; dry mouth; fatigue* (unusual feeling of tiredness); *hot flashes* (sudden sweatings and feelings of warmth); *irritation in the nose* (burning or tingling sensation, dryness, soreness or pain in the nose; runny and/or stuffy nose; unexplained nosebleeds); *increased sweating; muscle stiffness; nausea and/or vomiting; paresthesia* (sensation of burning, warmth, heat, numbness, tightness, or tingling); *pharyngitis* (sore throat); *sinusitis* (runny or stuffy nose; headache); *somnolence* (sleepiness); *taste perversion* (change in sense of taste)

Note: *Irritation in the nose* was found to be mild to moderate. In most cases, the symptoms resolved within four hours of the administration of intranasal dihydroergotamine.

Incidence less frequent or rare

*Anorexia* (decreased appetite); *bronchitis* (congestion in chest; cough; difficult and/or painful breathing); *central nervous system (CNS) effects, including anxiety; confusion; depression; euphoria* (unusual feeling of well being); *insomnia* (trouble in sleeping); *nervousness; cold, clammy skin; dyspepsia* (heartburn); *dysphagia* (difficulty swallowing); *dyspnea* (shortness of breath); *edema* (swelling of face, fingers, feet or lower legs); *ear pain; eye problems, including blurred vision; conjunctivitis* (red or irritated eyes); *eye pain; increased watering of the eyes; fever; hypotension* (dizziness or lightheadedness when getting up from a lying or sitting position; sudden fainting); *increased salivation* (increased watering of the mouth); *increased yawning; palpitations* (pounding heartbeat); *pruritus* (itching of the skin); *muscle weakness; petechia* (pinpoint red spots on skin); *skin rash; tinnitus* (ringing or buzzing in the ears); *stomach pain; tremors* (trembling or shaking of hands or feet)

## Overdose

For more information on the management of overdose or unintentional ingestion, **contact a Poison Control Center** (see *Poison Control Center Listing*).

**Clinical effects of overdose**

The following effects have been selected on the basis of their potential clinical significance (possible signs and symptoms in parentheses where appropriate)—not necessarily inclusive:

Acute and/or chronic

*Confusion; convulsions; delirium; hypertension* (dizziness); headaches, severe or continuing; increase in blood pressure); *nausea and/or vomiting; numbness, tingling, and/or pain in the legs or arms; respiratory depression* (shortness of breath); *stomach pain*

**Treatment of overdose**

Specific treatment—
   For peripheral vasospasm: Warmth should be applied to ischemic extremities. If necessary a vasodilator may be administered. Nursing measures designed to prevent tissue damage should be instituted.

Supportive care—
   Patients in whom intentional overdose is confirmed or suspected should be referred for psychiatric consultation.

## Patient Consultation

As an aid to patient consultation, refer to *Advice for the Patient, Dihydroergotamine (Nasal-Systemic)—Introductory Version*.

In providing consultation, consider emphasizing the following selected information (» = major clinical significance):

**Before using this medication**

» Conditions affecting use, especially:
   Hypersensitivity to ergot alkaloids
   Pregnancy—Use of intranasal dihydroergotamine is contraindicated during pregnancy because of its potential oxytocic activity, which may result in fetal harm
   Breast-feeding—Use of intranasal dihydroergotamine is not recommended for nursing mothers. Intranasal dihydroergotamine may be distributed into breast milk and cause adverse effects, such as vomiting, diarrhea, weak pulse, unstable blood pressure, seizures in the infant. Also, intranasal dihydroergotamine may inhibit lactation
   Other medications, especially 5-hydroxytryptamine agonists and vasoconstrictors
   Other medical problems, especially coronary artery disease, or other conditions that may be adversely affected by coronary artery constriction; hypertension, severe, uncontrolled

**Proper use of this medication**

» Proper administration technique; reading patient directions carefully before use
» Not administering if atypical headache symptoms are present; checking with physician instead
» Administering after onset of headache pain
   Additional benefit may be obtained if the patient lies down in a quiet, dark room after administering medication
   Using additional doses, if needed, for return of migraine headache after initial relief was obtained, provided that prescribed limits (quantity used and frequency of administration) are not exceeded
   Compliance with prophylactic therapy, if prescribed
» Proper dosing
» Proper storage

**Precautions while using this medication**

Avoiding alcohol, which aggravates headache
Caution when driving or doing anything else requiring alertness because of possible drowsiness, dizziness, lightheadedness, impairment of physical or mental abilities

**Side/adverse effects**

Signs of potential side effects, especially cardiovascular effects, peripheral ischemia, or upper respiratory tract infection

## Nasal Dosage Form

### DIHYDROERGOTAMINE MESYLATE NASAL SOLUTION USP

**Usual adult dose**

Antimigraine agent—
   Nasal, 0.5 mg (one spray) in each nostril. Followed by another 0.5 mg (one spray) dose in each nostril fifteen minutes later.

**Usual adult prescribing limits**

Nasal, 3 mg (6 sprays) per day; or 4 mg (8 sprays) per week.

**Usual pediatric dose**

Safety and efficacy have not been established in patients younger than 18 years of age.

**Usual geriatric dose**

See *Usual adult dose*.

**Strength(s) usually available**
U.S.—
 0.5 mg per metered spray (Rx) [*Migranal* (caffeine; dextrose; carbon dioxide)].

**Packaging and storage**
Store below 25 °C (77 °F).

Developed: 07/08/98

# DIHYDROTACHYSTEROL — See *Vitamin D and Analogs (Systemic)*

# DIHYDROXYALUMINUM AMINOACETATE — See *Antacids (Oral-Local)*

# DIHYDROXYALUMINUM SODIUM CARBONATE — See *Antacids (Oral-Local)*

# DILOXANIDE — The *Diloxanide (Systemic)* monograph is not included in this published version of the USP DI database. Copies of the monograph are available on request from Micromedex, Inc. - Reprint Requests, 6200 S. Syracuse Way, Suite 300, Englewood, CO 80111; telephone (303) 486-6400; telefax (303) 486-6464; Email: USPDI@MDX.COM.

# DILTIAZEM — See *Calcium Channel Blocking Agents (Systemic)*

# DIMENHYDRINATE — See *Antihistamines (Systemic)*

# DIMERCAPROL Systemic

VA CLASSIFICATION (Primary): AD300
Commonly used brand name(s): *BAL in Oil*.
Other commonly used names are British Anti-Lewisite and dimercaptopropanol.
Note: For a listing of dosage forms and brand names by country availability, see *Dosage Forms* section(s).

## Category
Chelating agent.

## Indications
**Accepted**
Toxicity, arsenic (treatment)
Toxicity, gold (treatment) or
Toxicity, mercury (treatment)—Dimercaprol is indicated as a chelating agent in arsenic, gold, and mercury (soluble inorganic compounds) poisoning following ingestion, inhalation, or absorption through the skin of these metals or their salts, or following overdose of therapeutic agents containing the metals.

In arsenic (except for arsine gas) toxicity, early administration of dimercaprol may help reverse the acute and some of the chronic manifestations of poisoning, although polyneuropathy may be refractory. Chelation therapy is recommended if urine arsenic levels are consistently above 200 mcg per liter.

In gold toxicity resulting from therapeutic uses of gold compounds for arthritis, dimercaprol may be effective in enhancing the excretion of accumulated gold salts. In patients with severe renal, hematologic, pulmonary, or enterocolitic complications who do not improve with high-dose corticosteroid treatment or who develop steroid-related adverse reactions, dimercaprol may be considered and has been used successfully. However, patients must be carefully monitored because of the adverse reactions that accompany its use.

In acute inorganic and aryl organic mercury toxicity, dimercaprol therapy is most effective when begun within 1 or 2 hours after ingestion, and ceases to be effective after about 6 hours. Dimercaprol is of questionable efficacy in elemental mercury poisoning.

Toxicity, lead (treatment adjunct)—Dimercaprol is indicated for treatment of acute and chronic lead poisoning when administered in conjunction with edetate calcium disodium (calcium EDTA). When administered promptly, dimercaprol complements edetate calcium disodium by more rapidly removing lead from red blood cells and the central nervous system (CNS) than does edetate calcium disodium alone, and by assisting in mobilization of lead from skeletal stores. This combination is less toxic than edetate calcium disodium alone because lower doses of each can be used. The rate of lead excretion is doubled when the combination is used, thus decreasing the mortality rate and the likelihood of permanent neurologic deficits from lead poisoning.

Signs and symptoms of severe, symptomatic lead poisoning include anemia, gastrointestinal complaints (abdominal pain and vomiting), nephropathy, and encephalopathy. Signs and symptoms of lead encephalopathy include headache and insomnia; persistent vomiting, sometimes projectile; visual disturbances; irritability, restlessness, delirium, hallucinations; ataxia; convulsions and coma; and characteristically high intracranial pressure. Recovery is slow and often incomplete, with residual neurological deficits.

Clinical signs suggesting lead poisoning in children and adults that should be treated with the dimercaprol, edetate calcium disodium combination include the following:
• Patient is severely symptomatic (with or without encephalopathy).
• Blood lead concentrations are greater than or equal to 70 mcg per deciliter.

**Unaccepted**
Dimercaprol should not be used in iron, cadmium, selenium, silver, or uranium poisoning because the dimercaprol-metal complexes are more toxic, especially to the kidneys, than the metal alone.

In methylmercury or other short-chain alkyl organic mercury intoxication, dimercaprol enhances the distribution of mercury into the brain, and is contraindicated.

Dimercaprol is of questionable value in poisoning by the heavy metals antimony and bismuth.

Dimercaprol is contraindicated in poisoning from arsine gas ($AsH_3$).

## Pharmacology/Pharmacokinetics

**Physicochemical characteristics**
Molecular weight—124.22.

**Mechanism of action/Effect**
Chelating agent—
 Certain heavy metals, especially arsenic, gold, lead, and mercury, form ligands in the body with the sulfhydryl (-SH) groups of the pyruvate-oxidase enzyme system, and inhibit the normal functioning of the enzymes that are dependent on free sulfhydryl groups for their activity. Dimercaprol, having a greater affinity for the metal than does the protein, reverses the enzyme inhibition by chelating the metal and preventing or reversing its toxic effects by regeneration of free sulfhydryl groups. The resulting dimercaprol-metal complex is relatively stable and rapidly excreted.
 In addition, in lead toxicity, dimercaprol causes a fast but short-lived reduction in lead concentrations in red blood cells and CNS, and effects a greater total lead excretion (urinary and fecal) than edetate calcium disodium because of its high fecal lead output. The addition of equimolar amounts of dimercaprol to edetate calcium disodium doubles the ratio of chelants to lead, thus providing the molar excess of chelating agent that is necessary for significant heavy metal excretion.

**Distribution**
All tissues, including the brain, but mainly in the intracellular space. The highest concentrations are in the liver and kidneys.

**Biotransformation**
About 50% rapidly metabolized to inactive metabolites.

**Onset of action**
30 minutes.

**Time to peak concentration**
30 to 60 minutes after intramuscular administration.

**Duration of action**
About 4 hours. Frequent doses at 3- to 4-hour intervals over prolonged periods are necessary to maintain therapeutic effect.

**Elimination**
50% as the dimercaprol-metal complex, via the renal and biliary tracts; as metabolites, in the urine; metabolism and excretion are usually complete within 6 to 24 hours.

## Precautions to Consider

### Cross-sensitivity and/or related problems
Dimercaprol injection should not be used in patients who are allergic to peanuts or peanut products.

### Pregnancy/Reproduction
Pregnancy—Adequate and well-controlled studies have not been done in humans.
Studies have not been done in animals.
FDA Pregnancy Category C.

### Breast-feeding
It is not known whether dimercaprol is distributed into breast milk.

### Pediatrics
Fever, which appears after the second or third dose of dimercaprol, persists throughout therapy, and disappears upon withdrawal of therapy, is more likely to occur in children than in adults. A transient reduction of polymorphonuclear leukocytes may also be seen.

### Geriatrics
No information is available on the relationship of age to the effects of dimercaprol in geriatric patients.

### Drug interactions and/or related problems
The following drug interactions and/or related problems have been selected on the basis of their potential clinical significance (possible mechanism in parentheses where appropriate)—not necessarily inclusive (» = major clinical significance):

» Iron salts
(concurrent administration of medicinal iron with dimercaprol results in the formation of a toxic complex; if iron deficiency is present, its treatment should be postponed until therapy with dimercaprol has been discontinued for at least twenty-four hours; however, severe iron deficiency anemia occurring during dimercaprol therapy should be managed with blood transfusion)

### Laboratory value alterations
The following have been selected on the basis of their potential clinical significance (possible effect in parentheses where appropriate)—not necessarily inclusive (» = major clinical significance):

With diagnostic test results
Thyroid tests
(when test is done during or immediately after dimercaprol therapy, iodine I 131 thyroidal uptake values may be decreased because of dimercaprol interference with normal accumulation of iodine in the thyroid gland)

With physiology/laboratory test values
Alanine aminotransferase (ALT [SGPT]) and
Aspartate aminotransferase (AST [SGOT])
(values may be temporarily elevated)
Polymorphonuclear leukocyte count
(a transient reduction may be seen in children)

### Medical considerations/Contraindications
The medical considerations/contraindications included have been selected on the basis of their potential clinical significance (reasons given in parentheses where appropriate)—not necessarily inclusive (» = major clinical significance).

*Except under special circumstances, this medication should not be used when the following medical problems exist:*

» Arsine gas poisoning
(chelation with dimercaprol is not useful in acute poisoning because it does not prevent hemolysis)

» Hepatic function impairment
(except in postarsenical jaundice, which may only require a reduction in dosage, metabolism may be reduced)

» Iron, cadmium, selenium, silver, or uranium poisoning
(dimercaprol-metal complexes of these metals are more toxic than the metal alone, and may cause nephrotoxicity)

» Organic (short-chain alkyl) mercury poisoning
(distribution of mercury to the brain is enhanced by dimercaprol)

*Risk-benefit should be considered when the following medical problems exist:*

Glucose-6-phosphate dehydrogenase (G6PD) deficiency
(dimercaprol may induce hemolysis and should be used only in life-threatening situations in patients with this deficiency)
Hypertension
(may be exacerbated)
Renal function impairment or
» Renal insufficiency, acute
(dimercaprol should be used cautiously if acute renal insufficiency develops during therapy because accumulation of dimercaprol may result in toxic serum concentrations; if oliguria is present, dimercaprol should be used with caution and/or in reduced dosage)
Sensitivity to dimercaprol

### Patient monitoring
The following may be especially important in patient monitoring (other tests may be warranted in some patients, depending on condition; » = major clinical significance):

Alkaline phosphatase concentrations, serum and
Blood urea nitrogen (BUN) concentrations and
Calcium concentrations, serum and
Creatinine concentrations, serum and
Electrolyte concentrations, serum and
Phosphorus concentrations, serum
(determinations recommended to detect evidence of renal function impairment; hemodialysis may be necessary)
Blood pressure and
Heart rate
(recommended periodically during therapy, since both may be increased)
Fluid balance
(recommended for determination of dehydration or impending renal insufficiency; parenteral fluids should be administered, at least during the first 2 or 3 days of dimercaprol therapy, to replace oral feedings that may not be tolerated or to minimize nausea and vomiting caused by either dimercaprol or the toxic agent or both)
Heavy metal concentration in blood and
24-hour urine excretion
(recommended to determine dosage and duration of therapy)
Hemoglobin
(recommended periodically in mercury toxicity)
Urinary pH
(recommended periodically; maintenance of an alkaline pH decreases the risk of nephrotoxicity, which may occur because of dissociation of the dimercaprol-metal complex in acidic urine)

## Side/Adverse Effects

The following side/adverse effects have been selected on the basis of their potential clinical significance (possible signs and symptoms in parentheses where appropriate)—not necessarily inclusive:

### Those indicating need for medical attention
Incidence more frequent
*Fast heartbeat; fever*—especially in children; *increased blood pressure*—both systolic and diastolic, roughly dose related
Incidence less frequent
*Abscesses, usually sterile, at injection site* (painful, red, and pus-containing sores)

### Those indicating need for medical attention only if they continue or are bothersome
Incidence more frequent
*Burning feeling in lips, mouth, throat, and penis; conjunctivitis; eyelid twitching; feeling of constriction or pain in throat, chest, or hands; headache; nausea and sometimes vomiting; pain at injection site; runny nose; sweating of forehead and hands; tingling of hands; unpleasant breath odor; watery eyes and mouth*
Note: All of the effects listed above, except *pain at injection site* and *unpleasant breath odor*, may occur with doses above the recommended dose, may be mild and temporary, and are often accompanied by feelings of anxiety, weakness, and unrest.
Incidence less frequent
*Abdominal pain; lower back pain; tremors*

## Overdose

For more information on the management of overdose or unintentional ingestion, **contact a Poison Control Center** (see *Poison Control Center Listing*).

### Clinical effects of overdose
*Convulsions; severe drowsiness; severe vomiting*

Note: These symptoms may be seen at doses above 5 mg per kg of body weight (mg/kg), beginning within 30 minutes and usually subsiding within 6 hours following injection.

## General Dosing Information

In any heavy metal poisoning, supportive therapy is as important to survival as chelation therapy. Removal of patient from exposure is the primary therapy for exposed patients. Depending on the metal, supportive treatment may include removal of the residual metal from the body with emesis or gastric lavage; intravenous fluids to correct dehydration and electrolyte deficiencies; bed rest; preservation of body heat; exchange transfusions; abdominal radiographs; and analgesics.

Since dimercaprol is better able to prevent inhibition of sulfhydryl enzymes than to reactivate them, dimercaprol therapy is most effective when begun immediately after exposure. The toxic metal ion is inactivated and its incorporation into binding sites in blood and tissue is prevented. If reactivation of enzymes is necessary, prolonged therapy may be required.

Dimercaprol is always administered by deep intramuscular injection, never by intravenous or subcutaneous injection. Rotating injection sites may minimize development of abscesses.

The dosage of dimercaprol must be repeated frequently for several days. This maintains a plasma concentration of free dimercaprol in the body fluids that enhances the continuous formation of a rapidly excreted stable complex of 2:1 (dimercaprol:metal) until a significant portion of the metal is eliminated from the body.

Because the dimercaprol-metal chelation is reversible and can rapidly dissociate in an acid medium, alkalinization of the urine is necessary to prevent dissociation into the toxic metal and potentially nephrotoxic dimercaprol. After assuring adequate urine volume, a less acid urine may be achieved by oral administration of sodium bicarbonate, with the dosage and frequency being determined by monitoring urinary pH. If patients are placed on parenteral fluids, adjustment of the composition of the solutions may provide a neutral urine, or alkalization of the urine may be achieved by intravenous infusion of sodium bicarbonate over 4 to 8 hours. Such patients may be advanced cautiously to clear oral liquids or oral rehydration solutions.

### For acute lead encephalopathy

Dimercaprol is combined with edetate calcium disodium because the maximum safe dose of edetate calcium disodium alone may cause a shift of lead into the central nervous system (CNS). The preferred route of administration for edetate calcium disodium is intravenous, and dimercaprol is given by deep intramuscular injection, in divided doses every 4 hours for 5 days. If both medications are given by intramuscular injection, they must be given at separate sites. Dimercaprol is given alone for the first dose 4 hours before the combination is begun. In asymptomatic or mildly symptomatic patients, dimercaprol may be discontinued after 72 hours, with edetate calcium disodium being continued for an additional 48 to 72 hours at reduced dosage.

Oral penicillamine is used for long-term chelation therapy after initial therapy with edetate calcium disodium or combined dimercaprol and edetate calcium disodium, especially if long-bone radiographs show lead lines. The oral chelating agent succimer is used for treatment of children with blood lead concentrations greater than 45 micrograms per deciliter. Although use to date has been limited, toxicity with succimer appears to be less than with other agents.

### For prevention or treatment of adverse effects

• For histaminic effects, mild and temporary—Recommended treatment may include administration of diphenhydramine in doses up to 1.5 mg per kg intramuscularly or orally every 6 hours.

• For nausea or vomiting—May be prevented by giving patient nothing orally and hydrating initially with parenteral fluids. After clinical improvement occurs, clear liquids may be administered orally as parenteral fluids are phased out.

• For sterile abscesses—May be prevented by rotating sites of injection and always administering *deep* intramuscular injections. If existing abscess does not subside spontaneously, aspiration and drainage may be necessary.

## Parenteral Dosage Forms

### DIMERCAPROL INJECTION USP

**Usual adult and adolescent dose**
Arsenic or gold toxicity—
  Severe: Intramuscular (deep), 3 mg per kg of body weight every four hours for two days, four times on the third day, then twice a day for ten days; or 3 mg per kg of body weight every four hours on the first day, 2 mg per kg of body weight every four hours on the second day, 3 mg per kg of body weight every six hours on the third day, and 3 mg per kg of body weight every twelve hours on each of the following ten days or until recovery.
  Mild: Intramuscular (deep), 2.5 mg per kg of body weight every six hours for two days, every twelve hours on the third day, and once a day on each of the following ten days or until recovery.
Mercury toxicity—
  Intramuscular (deep), 3 to 5 mg per kg of body weight every four hours for two days, then 2.5 to 3 mg per kg of body weight every six hours for two days, then 2.5 to 3 mg per kg of body weight every twelve hours for seven days.
Lead toxicity—
  Severe (encephalopathy): Intramuscular, 4 mg per kg of body weight for the first dose, repeated at four-hour intervals in conjunction with edetate calcium disodium (calcium EDTA) injection, which is usually administered intravenously, but may be administered intramuscularly at a separate site. This treatment is maintained for two to seven days. If the blood lead concentration after this first course of therapy exceeds 100 mcg per deciliter, treatment may be resumed for an additional five days, following an interval of at least two days without treatment.
  Mild: Intramuscular, 4 mg per kg of body weight for the first dose, the dose then being reduced to 3 mg per kg of body weight and administered at four-hour intervals in conjunction with edetate calcium disodium injection, which is administered at a separate site.

**Usual adult prescribing limits**
5 mg per kg of body weight.

**Usual pediatric dose**
Lead toxicity—
  Symptomatic children
    Acute (with or without encephalopathy)—Intramuscular (deep), 75 mg per square meter of body surface area every four hours (up to 450 mg per square meter per twenty-four hours). After four hours, calcium EDTA injection, 1500 mg per square meter of body surface area per twenty-four hours, should be administered on a four-hour schedule, intravenously or intramuscularly at a separate site. This treatment is maintained for five days. If the blood lead concentration after this first course of therapy exceeds 70 mcg per deciliter, treatment may be resumed for an additional five days, following an interval of at least two days without treatment. The cycle may be repeated, depending on the clinical response.
  Asymptomatic children
    Intramuscular (deep), 50 mg per square meter of body surface area every four hours. After four hours, calcium EDTA injection, 1000 mg per square meter of body surface area per twenty-four hours, should be administered on a four-hour schedule simultaneously intravenously or intramuscularly at a separate site. This treatment is maintained for five days. Dimercaprol may be discontinued after three days if blood lead concentrations are less than 50 mcg per deciliter. If the blood lead concentration after this first course of therapy exceeds 70 mcg per deciliter, treatment may be resumed for an additional five days, following an interval of at least two days without treatment. Calcium EDTA injection should be continued for five more days. The cycle may be repeated depending on the clinical response.

**Strength(s) usually available**
U.S.—
  100 mg per mL (Rx) [*BAL in Oil* (benzyl benzoate 200 mg; peanut oil 700 mg)].
Canada—
  100 mg per mL (Rx) [*BAL in Oil* (benzyl benzoate 200 mg; peanut oil 700 mg)].

**Packaging and storage**
Store below 40 °C (104 °F), preferably between 15 and 30 °C (59 and 86 °F), unless otherwise specified by manufacturer.

Revised: 11/11/94

# DIMETHYL SULFOXIDE  Mucosal-Local

VA CLASSIFICATION (Primary): GU900

Commonly used brand name(s): *Rimso-50*.

Another commonly used name is DMSO.

Note: For a listing of dosage forms and brand names by country availability, see *Dosage Forms* section(s).

## Category

Anti-inflammatory, local (interstitial cystitis).

## Indications

### Accepted

Cystitis, interstitial (treatment)—Dimethyl sulfoxide is indicated for the symptomatic relief of interstitial cystitis.

### Unaccepted

Dimethyl sulfoxide has *not* been shown to be effective in the treatment of bacterial infections of the urinary tract.

Also, topical use of dimethyl sulfoxide as a vehicle for enhancing the percutaneous absorption of other drugs has *not* been shown to be effective.

In addition, dimethyl sulfoxide administered topically, orally, or intravenously has *not* been proven to be effective in the treatment of musculoskeletal disorders; diseases of connective tissue (e.g., osteoarthritis, rheumatoid arthritis, cutaneous manifestations of scleroderma, gout, ankylosing spondylitis); viral, bacterial, fungal, or parasitic infections of the skin; burns; postoperative pain; wounds (to promote healing); or mental conditions.

However, investigational studies are being conducted on the transcutaneous carrier properties of dimethyl sulfoxide and on the efficacy of dimethyl sulfoxide in scleroderma, head injury, stroke, spinal cord trauma, arthritis, trauma of acute injuries, such as sprains and strains, and other disorders.

## Pharmacology/Pharmacokinetics

### Physicochemical characteristics

Molecular weight—78.13.

### Mechanism of action/Effect

The mechanism by which dimethyl sulfoxide produces anti-inflammatory effects in interstitial cystitis is not known.

### Absorption

Dimethyl sulfoxide is absorbed systemically following topical application.

### Biotransformation

Metabolized to dimethyl sulfone and dimethyl sulfide.

### Elimination

Dimethyl sulfoxide and one of its metabolites, dimethyl sulfone, are excreted in the urine and feces. The other metabolite, dimethyl sulfide, is eliminated via breath and through the skin.

## Precautions to Consider

### Pregnancy/Reproduction

Pregnancy—Studies in humans have not been done.

Studies in hamsters, rats, and mice have shown that dimethyl sulfoxide causes teratogenic effects when administered intraperitoneally at high doses of 2.5 to 12 grams per kg of body weight. In addition, studies in rabbits have shown that dimethyl sulfoxide causes teratogenic effects when administered topically at doses of 5 grams per kg of body weight for the first 2 days, then 2.5 grams per kg of body weight for the last 8 days. However, in another study using rabbits, dimethyl sulfoxide was not shown to cause any abnormalities when administered topically at doses of 1.1 grams per kg of body weight on Days 3 through 16 of gestation. Furthermore, dimethyl sulfoxide was not shown to cause reproductive problems in hamsters, rats, and mice when administered in oral or topical doses.

FDA Pregnancy Category C.

### Breast-feeding

It is not known whether dimethyl sulfoxide is excreted in breast milk and problems in humans have not been documented; however, dimethyl sulfoxide is systemically absorbed.

### Pediatrics

Appropriate studies on the relationship of age to the effects of this medicine have not been performed in the pediatric population.

### Geriatrics

Appropriate studies on the relationship of age to the effects of this medicine have not been performed in the geriatric population. However, no geriatrics-specific problems have been documented to date.

### Drug interactions and/or related problems

The following drug interactions and/or related problems have been selected on the basis of their potential clinical significance (possible mechanism in parentheses where appropriate)—not necessarily inclusive (» = major clinical significance):

Note: Combinations containing any of the following medications, depending on the amount present, may also interact with this medication.

Medications, intravesical, other
(effects may be increased when these medications are used concurrently with dimethyl sulfoxide)

### Medical considerations/Contraindications

The medical considerations/contraindications included have been selected on the basis of their potential clinical significance (reasons given in parentheses where appropriate)—not necessarily inclusive (» = major clinical significance).

*Risk-benefit should be considered when the following medical problems exist:*

Sensitivity to dimethyl sulfoxide

Urinary tract malignancy
(use of dimethyl sulfoxide may be harmful because of drug-induced vasodilation)

### Patient monitoring

The following may be especially important in patient monitoring (other tests may be warranted in some patients, depending on condition; » = major clinical significance):

Biochemical screening, particularly liver and renal function tests and Blood cell counts, complete
(recommended approximately every 6 months during therapy)

Ophthalmologic examinations, complete
(recommended prior to and at periodic intervals during therapy, since changes in the refractive index and lens opacities have been documented in animal studies when dimethyl sulfoxide was given chronically)

## Side/Adverse Effects

The following side/adverse effects have been selected on the basis of their potential clinical significance (possible signs and symptoms in parentheses where appropriate)—not necessarily inclusive:

### Those indicating need for medical attention

*Anaphylactoid reaction* (nasal congestion; shortness of breath or troubled breathing; skin rash, hives, or itching; swelling of face)

### Those not indicating need for medical attention

*Discomfort, moderate to severe, during administration; garlic-like odor on breath and skin; garlic-like taste*

## Overdose

For information on the management of overdose or unintentional ingestion, **contact a Poison Control Center** (see *Poison Control Center Listing*).

### Treatment of overdose

If dimethyl sulfoxide is accidently ingested:

To decrease absorption—
Emesis should be induced. Measures that may be considered include gastric lavage and administration of activated charcoal.

To enhance elimination—
Forced diuresis should be considered.

## Patient Consultation

As an aid to patient consultation, refer to *Advice for the Patient, Dimethyl Sulfoxide (Mucosal)*.

In providing consultation, consider emphasizing the following selected information (» = major clinical significance):

### Before using this medication

» Conditions affecting use, especially:
Allergy to dimethyl sulfoxide

### Proper use of this medication

» Proper dosing

### Side/adverse effects
Moderately severe discomfort may occur during administration, but usually lessens with repeated instillations

A garlic-like taste, which may occur within a few minutes after instillation and last for several hours, and a garlic-like odor on the breath and skin, which may last for 72 hours, may be alarming to patient although medically insignificant

Signs of potential side effects, especially anaphylactoid reaction

## General Dosing Information
Dimethyl sulfoxide irrigation is not for intramuscular or intravenous injection or for cutaneous application. It is to be instilled directly into the bladder using a catheter or an asepto syringe.

Prior to inserting the catheter, application of an analgesic lubricant such as lidocaine jelly to the urethra is recommended to avoid spasm.

The medication is expelled by spontaneous voiding.

When symptomatic relief is not complete, 500 mL of a solution containing 1 part of dimethyl sulfoxide and 1 part of sterile water may be used to distend the bladder prior to instillation of the 50-mL dose.

Dimethyl sulfoxide solution 99% is used as a cryopreservative and should not be used for bladder irrigation.

## Topical Dosage Forms

### DIMETHYL SULFOXIDE IRRIGATION USP

**Usual adult and adolescent dose**
Intravesical instillation, 50 mL of a 50% solution, retained in the bladder for fifteen minutes; treatment repeated every two weeks until maximum symptomatic relief is obtained, then time intervals between treatments increased appropriately.

**Usual pediatric dose**
Dosage has not been established.

**Strength(s) usually available**
U.S.—
50% [*Rimso-50;* GENERIC].
Canada—
50% [*Rimso-50*].

**Packaging and storage**
Store between 15 and 30 °C (59 and 86 °F), unless otherwise specified by manufacturer. Protect from strong light.

Revised: 03/04/92
Interim revision: 03/28/94

---

**DINOPROST**—The *Dinoprost (Parenteral-Local)* monograph is not included in this published version of the USP DI database. Copies of the monograph are available on request from Micromedex, Inc. - Reprint Requests, 6200 S. Syracuse Way, Suite 300, Englewood, CO 80111; telephone (303) 486-6400; telefax (303) 486-6464; Email: USPDI@MDX.COM.

---

# DINOPROSTONE  Cervical/Vaginal

Note: This monograph contains information on both the dinoprostone vaginal suppositories and the vaginal system (a suppository within a retrieval device). Each may be inappropriately referred to as dinoprostone vaginal insert in other types of information. It is important to avoid confusing the two dosage forms, since each has a different use and strength.

VA CLASSIFICATION (Primary/Secondary): HS200/GU600; GU900

Commonly used brand name(s): *Cervidil; Prepidil; Prostin E2.*

Some other commonly used names are prostaglandin $E_2$ or $PGE_2$.

Note: For a listing of dosage forms and brand names by country availability, see *Dosage Forms* section(s).

## Category
Prostaglandin; oxytocic; abortifacient; antihemorrhagic (postabortion uterine bleeding; postpartum uterine bleeding).

## Indications
Note: Bracketed information in the *Indications* section refers to uses that are not included in U.S. product labeling.

**Accepted**
Abortion, elective—Dinoprostone vaginal suppositories are used for aborting midtrimester pregnancy (from the twelfth through the twentieth week of gestation as calculated from the first day of the last normal menstrual period).

Abortion, missed (treatment) or

Abortion, therapeutic—Dinoprostone vaginal suppositories are indicated for evacuation of the uterine contents in management of missed abortion or for therapeutic abortion in cases of intrauterine fetal death up to 28 weeks of gestational age as calculated from the first day of the last normal menstrual period. Dinoprostone vaginal gel or suppository is not approved for use as an abortifacient in cases of intrauterine fetal death at more than 28 weeks' gestation because it is associated with an increased risk of uterine rupture. Confirmation of intrauterine fetal death should be made prior to use of dinoprostone for missed abortion or intrauterine fetal death.

Cervical ripening—Prior to induction of labor when medically indicated, dinoprostone cervical gel or dinoprostone vaginal system is used to initiate or continue ripening an unfavorable cervix in pregnant patients at or near term. The vaginal system is removed when active labor begins. [Extemporaneously prepared dinoprostone gels have also been used in cervical ripening prior to induction of labor and prior to abortion procedures, such as vacuum curettage].

[Hemorrhage, postpartum (treatment)] or

[Hemorrhage, postabortion (treatment)]—Dinoprostone vaginal suppositories are used to reduce blood loss and correct uterine atony postpartum and postabortion in patients unresponsive to conventional treatment such as oxytocin, ergonovine, or methylergonovine.

Hydatidiform mole, benign (treatment)—Although vacuum curettage is preferred, dinoprostone vaginal suppositories are indicated for evacuation of the uterine contents in the treatment of nonmetastatic benign hydatidiform mole.

Labor, induction of—Dinoprostone vaginal gel is used for induction of labor at or near term.

**Unaccepted**
Dinoprostone vaginal suppository is not indicated for use to terminate a pregnancy of greater than 28 weeks gestation or when a fetus *in utero* has reached a stage of viability. Also, the vaginal suppository or vaginal gel should not be used for cervical ripening.

## Pharmacology/Pharmacokinetics

**Physicochemical characteristics**
Description—Dinoprostone vaginal system: The system includes a flat suppository contained within a retrieval device (polyester pouch with string). The suppository in the vaginal system (polyethylene oxide and urethane copolymer) measures 29 mm by 9.5 mm with a thickness of 0.8 mm.

Chemical group—Dinoprostone is the naturally occurring prostaglandin $E_2$.

Molecular weight—352.47.

**Mechanism of action/Effect**
For uterine stimulation—
Dinoprostone appears to act directly on the myometrium, but this has not been completely established. It stimulates myometrial contractions in the gravid uterus that are similar to the contractions that occur in the term uterus during natural labor. These contractions are usually sufficient to cause abortion. Uterine response to prostaglandins increases gradually throughout pregnancy. Dinoprostone does not act directly on the fetoplacental unit and is not considered a fetocidal agent.

For cervical ripening—
Dinoprostone softens the cervix and facilitates cervical dilation and effacement. Dinoprostone stimulates collagenase secretion, and thus reduces the collagen network within the cervix. By favorably changing the cervical score, dinoprostone reduces the number of failed inductions or instrumental deliveries, shortens the induction-to-delivery interval, and reduces the amount of oxytocin that may be needed. The dose of dinoprostone used locally to ripen the cervix

is lower than that used to stimulate the uterus. Although not prominent with low local doses, uterine stimulation may occur with the dinoprostone vaginal system or cervical gel.

**Other actions/effects**
Dinoprostone stimulates the smooth muscle of the gastrointestinal tract. It may also cause bronchodilation or bronchoconstriction and vasodilation. Dinoprostone can elevate body temperature due to its effect on hypothalamic thermoregulation.

**Absorption**
Dinoprostone vaginal system for cervical ripening—Absorbed at a rate of 0.3 mg per hour over 12 hours while the vaginal system is in place. Systemic effects are seen rarely, although the systemic contributions of dinoprostone and its metabolites are difficult to assess due to the prostaglandins endogenously produced during labor.

**Protein binding**
73%, to albumin.

**Biotransformation**
Rapid metabolism of dinoprostone occurs primarily in the local tissues; any systemic absorption of the medication is cleared mainly in the maternal lungs and, secondarily, at sites such as the liver and kidneys.

**Half-life**
Less than 5 minutes.

**Onset of action**
Uterine stimulation—Contractions begin within 10 minutes following insertion of a dinoprostone vaginal suppository.

**Time to peak effect**
Uterine stimulation—The mean abortion time with dinoprostone is about 17 hours (range, 12 to 24 hours).

**Duration of action**
Uterine stimulation—Contractions persist for 2 to 6 hours following insertion of a 20-mg dinoprostone vaginal suppository.
Cervical ripening—Continues, while in place, for up to 12 hours per dinoprostone vaginal system. On removal, action lasts 2 to 13 minutes.

**Elimination**
Primarily renal as metabolites, with a small amount excreted in the feces.

## Precautions to Consider

### Cross-sensitivity and/or related problems
Patients hypersensitive to oxytocin or other oxytocics may be hypersensitive to dinoprostone, even when it is used only for cervical ripening. Also, patients allergic to other prostaglandins, such as misoprostol, may be allergic to dinoprostone.

### Carcinogenicity
Studies have not been done in animals or humans on the carcinogenicity of dinoprostone.

### Mutagenicity
The micronucleus test, Ames assay, and unscheduled DNA synthesis assay revealed no evidence of mutagenicity with dinoprostone.

### Pregnancy/Reproduction
Pregnancy—Any pregnancy termination that fails with dinoprostone should be completed by another method.
Proliferation of bone has been reported with clinical use of prostaglandin E$_1$ during prolonged therapy. There is no evidence to date that the short-term use of dinoprostone (prostaglandin E$_2$) causes proliferation of bone in the fetus and is unlikely since it is administered after the period of organogenesis.
Although animal studies with dinoprostone did not reveal teratogenic properties, dinoprostone has been shown to be embryotoxic in rats and rabbits. In animal studies, prostaglandins of the E and F series have caused proliferation of bone with high doses.
FDA Pregnancy Category C.
Labor and delivery—Use of high doses may result in excessive uterine tone, causing decreased uterine blood flow and fetal distress.

### Drug interactions and/or related problems
The following drug interactions and/or related problems have been selected on the basis of their potential clinical significance (possible mechanism in parentheses where appropriate)—not necessarily inclusive (» = major clinical significance):

» Oxytocin or other oxytocics
(concurrent or sequential use with dinoprostone potentiates the effects of endogenous and exogenous oxytocin and can produce uterine hypertonus, uterine rupture, cervical laceration, or fetal distress, especially in the absence of adequate cervical dilation. Although oxytocin is used sequentially with dinoprostone for therapeutic advantage, a delay between administering oxytocin and dinoprostone is recommended: oxytocin may be administered 30 minutes after removal of the dinoprostone vaginal system, 6 to 12 hours after insertion of cervical gel or vaginal suppository, or 12 to 24 hours after insertion of vaginal gel. The patient should be continuously monitored)
(dinoprostone should not be used for cervical ripening or uterine stimulation if the patient is already receiving oxytocin or any other oxytocic agent)

### Laboratory value alterations
The following have been selected on the basis of their potential clinical significance (possible effect in parentheses where appropriate)—not necessarily inclusive (» = major clinical significance):

With physiology/laboratory test values
Blood pressure, maternal or
Heart rate, maternal or fetal
(may be decreased or increased, especially with large doses; a decrease in diastolic blood pressure of greater than 20 mm of Hg has been reported in approximately 10% of patients receiving dinoprostone)

Body temperature
(a temperature increase of greater than 1.1 °C [2 °F] usually occurs within 15 to 45 minutes following insertion of suppository; this effect has not been seen with the doses of the cervical gel used for cervical ripening. Body temperature returns to normal within 2 to 6 hours after discontinuation of medication or removal of suppository from vagina)

### Medical considerations/Contraindications
The medical considerations/contraindications included have been selected on the basis of their potential clinical significance (reasons given in parentheses where appropriate)—not necessarily inclusive (» = major clinical significance).

*Except under special circumstances, this medication should not be used when the following medical problems exist:*

» Allergy to dinoprostone or other prostaglandin E2 analogs, such as misoprostol

» Conditions that contraindicate vaginal delivery or induction of labor, including
Actively contracting or hypertonic uterus
Cephalopelvic disproportion, significant or
Fetal distress without imminent delivery
Fetal malpresentation
Multiparity greater than six, history of
Pelvic inflammatory disease, acute
Uterine or vaginal bleeding, unexplained
(induction of labor, vaginal delivery, or prolonged contractions are not generally recommended)

*Risk-benefit should be considered when the following medical problems exist:*

Anemia, or history of
(increased incidence of excessive uterine bleeding postabortion or postpartum with use of dinoprostone in doses that induce cervical ripening or stimulate the uterus)

Asthma, or history of
(increased risk of bronchoconstriction when dinoprostone is used in doses that induce uterine stimulation, including use in patients with a history of childhood asthma without adult asthma)

» Cardiac disease, active, including Eisenmenger complex
(when dinoprostone is used in doses that stimulate the uterus, a decrease in blood pressure and bradycardia may result in cardiovascular collapse and angina pectoris)

Cardiovascular disease, history of or
Hypertension, or history of or
Hypotension, history of or
Preeclampsia
(condition may be aggravated by possible vasoconstriction or decreased blood pressure; two cases of myocardial infarction have occurred in patients with a history of cardiovascular disease with use of dinoprostone in doses that stimulate the uterus)

Cervical stenosis or
Uterine surgery, history of
(increased risk of uterine rupture with use of dinoprostone in doses that stimulate the uterus)

Cervicitis or
Endocervical lesions, infected or
Vaginitis, acute
(in some cases, medically induced cervical ripening may increase risk of cervical injury or chronic cervicitis)

Epilepsy, or history of
(rarely, when used in doses that stimulate the uterus, dinoprostone has been reported to cause seizures in patients with epilepsy whose seizures were poorly controlled prior to its use)

Glaucoma
(increases in intraocular pressure and miosis have been reported rarely during the use of prostaglandins; dinoprostone may have similar effects when used in doses that stimulate the uterus)

Hepatic disease, active or
Renal disease, active
(metabolism and elimination of dinoprostone may be impaired, resulting in prolonged half-life)

» Hypersensitivity to dinoprostone or other oxytocics, history of
Hypertonus, uterine, history of
(excessive dosage, use of dinoprostone in doses that stimulate the uterus, or, to a lesser extent, sequential use of dinoprostone with oxytocin at doses that induce cervical ripening may cause uterine hypertonicity with spasm and tetanic contraction that can lead to posterior cervical perforations, cervical lacerations, uterine rupture, and hemorrhage)

Pulmonary disease, active
(use of dinoprostone in doses that stimulate the uterus may decrease pulmonary blood flow and increase pulmonary arterial pressure)

**Patient monitoring**
The following may be especially important in patient monitoring (other tests may be warranted in some patients, depending on condition; » = major clinical significance):

Blood pressure, maternal and
Contractions, frequency, duration, and force of and
Heart rate, fetal and maternal and
Temperature, maternal and
Uterine tone
(monitoring of these parameters is recommended at frequent intervals during abortion procedure or labor and delivery; well-hydrating patient with an electrolyte solution counteracts the decreased peripheral-resistance and induced vasodilatation)

(continuous monitoring of uterine activity and fetal state is especially recommended for patients with known history of hypertonic contractility or tetanic uterine contractions)

(maternal temperature increases of greater than 2° F (1.1° C) occurs in 50% of patients 15 to 45 minutes after vaginal suppository administration and normalizes within 2 to 6 hours after therapy is discontinued; differentiation between endometritis pyrexia and dinoprostone-induced pyrexia should be considered)

Vaginal examination
(recommended prior to each dose and after delivery or abortion to monitor cervical response and to check for signs of cervical trauma)

## Side/Adverse Effects

The following side/adverse effects have been selected on the basis of their potential clinical significance (possible signs and symptoms in parentheses where appropriate)—not necessarily inclusive:

**Those indicating need for medical attention**
Incidence less frequent or rare
*Anaphylaxis, generalized* (swelling of face, inside the nose, and eyelids; hives; shortness of breath; trouble in breathing; tightness in chest; wheezing); *bradycardia* (slow heartbeat); *bronchoconstriction* (wheezing; troubled breathing; tightness in chest)—especially in asthmatics; *increased uterine pain accompanying abortion*—correlates with efficacy; *peripheral vasoconstriction* (pale, cool, or blotchy skin on arms or legs; weak or absent pulse in arms or legs)—possibly severe; *substernal pressure or pain* (pressing or painful feeling in chest); *tachycardia* (fast heartbeat); *uterine hypertonus* (severe cramping of the uterus)

Note: If *uterine hypertonus* occurs with dinoprostone at any dose, fetal distress or uterine rupture can result. Uterine rupture has occurred with use of the cervical gel to cause cervical ripening.
Systemic effects of *bradycardia, bronchoconstriction, substernal pressure or pain,* and *tachycardia* are seen rarely when dinoprostone is used for cervical ripening.

**Those indicating need for medical attention only if they continue or are bothersome**
Incidence more frequent
*Abdominal or stomach cramps; diarrhea*—about 40% with use of 20-mg suppositories; 1% with use of cervical gel or vaginal system; *fever, transient*—about 50% with use of 20-mg suppositories; 1% with use of cervical gel or vaginal system; *nausea*—about 33% with use of 20-mg suppositories; 1% with use of cervical gel or vaginal system; *vomiting*—about 67% with use of vaginal suppository or vaginal gel; 1% with use of cervical gel or vaginal system

Incidence less frequent—for vaginal suppositories or vaginal gel, about 10% with use of 20-mg suppositories
*Chills or shivering; headache*

Incidence rare—for vaginal suppositories or vaginal gel
*Flushing; ileus, adynamic* (constipation, tender or mildly bloated abdomen); *vulvar edema*

**Those indicating possible postabortion complications and the need for medical attention if they occur after medication is discontinued**
*Endometritis* (continuing chills; shivering; continuing fever—usually on third day post-abortion; foul-smelling vaginal discharge; pain in lower abdomen); *unusual increase in uterine bleeding*

## Patient Consultation

As an aid to patient consultation, refer to *Advice for the Patient, Dinoprostone (Cervical/Vaginal)*.

In providing consultation, consider emphasizing the following selected information (» = major clinical significance):

**Before using this medication**
» Conditions affecting use, especially:
Allergies to dinoprostone or other prostaglandins or hypersensitivity to dinoprostone, oxytocin, or other oxytocics
Pregnancy—Any pregnancy termination that fails with dinoprostone should be completed by another method
Other medical problems, especially cardiac disease or conditions that contraindicate vaginal delivery or induction of labor

**Proper use of this medication**
» Remaining in supine position for 10 minutes following insertion of suppository, 10 to 30 minutes following application of cervical gel, 30 minutes following application of vaginal gel, and 2 hours following insertion of vaginal system
» Proper dosing
» Proper storage

**Side/adverse effects**
Signs of potential side effects, especially anaphylaxis, bradycardia, bronchoconstriction, increased uterine pain accompanying abortion, peripheral vasoconstriction, substernal pressure or pain, tachycardia, uterine hypertonus
Fetal distress can result if maternal uterine hypertonus occurs at any dose of dinoprostone
Signs of postabortion complications, such as endometritis or unusual increase in uterine bleeding, after medication has been discontinued

## General Dosing Information

Patients receiving dinoprostone should be hospitalized and under the supervision of a physician experienced in its use.

Procedures for applying dinoprostone should be carefully followed. Amnionitis and intrauterine fetal sepsis have been associated with extra-amniotic intrauterine administration of dinoprostone.

When it is used in doses that stimulate the uterus, experts recommend that antiemetic and antidiarrheal medications be administered prior to or concurrently with dinoprostone to decrease the possibility of gastrointestinal side effects. Narcotic analgesics may be given for uterine pain.

In those patients with profuse vaginal bleeding or ruptured membranes, blood or fluid present in the cervix and vagina may cause expulsion of dinoprostone, thereby interfering with the absorption and efficacy of dinoprostone.

**For cervical ripening**
When using a water-miscible lubricant to aid the insertion of dinoprostone vaginal system, avoid applying excessive amounts; otherwise, premature release of dinoprostone can occur.

Avoid applying the dinoprostone cervical gel above the cervical os because of the greater possibility of causing uterine hyperstimulation. Select the proper catheter for cervical application of the cervical gel, depending on whether the cervix is effaced: use the 10-mm catheter with no effacement, and the 20-mm catheter with 50% effacement.

**For uterine stimulation**
Confirmation of intrauterine fetal death should be made prior to use of dinoprostone for missed abortion or intrauterine fetal death.
Dinoprostone is not feticidal and may result in delivery of a live fetus.

**Safety considerations for handling this medication**
Dinoprostone should be handled cautiously. Suggested precautions for handling, preparing, and disposing of dinoprostone include the following:
- Avoid skin contact with dinoprostone, washing hands immediately with soap and water after administration.
- Use proper technique to prevent contamination of the medication, work area, and operator during transfer to patient.
- Cautiously and properly dispose of catheters, vaginal retrieval system, and unused medication.

**For treatment of adverse effects**
Treatment is primarily symptomatic, conservative, and supportive and may include the following:
- Repositioning the patient and giving oxygen may be adequate to ease transient abnormal uterine contractions, especially if dinoprostone was used for cervical ripening. Removing the vaginal system reverses uterine hyperstimulation within 2 to 13 minutes without need for tocolytic therapy in most cases.
- Sponging or irrigation with sterile saline of upper vagina to remove residual dinoprostone or removing vaginal suppository or system to prevent further absorption.
- Using tocolytic therapy, such as ritodrine, terbutaline, or magnesium sulfate, to treat uterine hyperstimulation. Data on treating dinoprostone-induced adverse effects with prostaglandin antagonists are presently insufficient.

## Cervical Dosage Forms

### DINOPROSTONE CERVICAL GEL

**Usual adult and adolescent dose**
Cervical ripening—
Intracervical, 0.5 mg placed into the cervical canal, just below the internal cervical os, using the syringe and catheter provided. Patient should remain in supine position for at least fifteen to thirty minutes following administration. A need for an additional dose is determined by the physician and ensuing clinical events.

**Usual adult prescribing limits**
Cervical ripening—
Maximum cumulative dose is 1.5 mg (7.5 mL) in 24 hours.

**Strength(s) usually available**
U.S.—
0.5 mg per 2.5 mL (3 grams) prefilled single-use syringe (Rx) [*Prepidil*].
Canada—
0.5 mg per 2.5 mL (3 grams) prefilled single-use syringe (Rx) [*Prepidil*].

Note: Packaging contains two catheter tips (10 and 20 mm).

**Packaging and storage**
Store between 2 and 8° C (36 and 46° F).

**Preparation of dosage form**
Bring medication to room temperature just prior to administration. Do not force warming by use of external heat source, such as water bath or microwave oven.
Each application is for single use and unused contents should be discarded, including the small amount of gel remaining in the catheter.

## Vaginal Dosage Forms

### DINOPROSTONE VAGINAL GEL

**Usual adult and adolescent dose**
Induction of labor—
Intravaginal, 1 mg placed into the posterior fornix of the vaginal canal. The patient should remain in supine position for at least fifteen to thirty minutes after administration. A dose of 1 or 2 mg may be repeated once, six hours later, if needed.

**Strength(s) usually available**
U.S.—
Not commercially available.
Canada—
1 mg per 2.5 mL (3 grams) applicatorful (Rx) [*Prostin E_2*].
2 mg per 2.5 mL (3 grams) applicatorful (Rx) [*Prostin E_2*].

**Packaging and storage**
Store below 2 and 8 °C (36 and 46 °F).

**Preparation of dosage form**
Bring medication to room temperature just prior to administration. Do not force warming by use of external heat source, such as water bath or microwave oven.

### DINOPROSTONE VAGINAL SUPPOSITORIES

**Usual adult and adolescent dose**
Abortifacient—
Intravaginal, 20 mg, repeated every three to five hours, adjusted according to patient response until abortion occurs. Patient should remain in supine position for at least ten minutes following insertion.

**Usual adult prescribing limits**
Abortifacient—
Maximum cumulative dose is 240 mg; continuous administration of dinoprostone for more than 2 days is not recommended.

**Strength(s) usually available**
U.S.—
20 mg (Rx) [*Prostin E_2*].
Canada—
Not commercially available.

**Packaging and storage**
Store below −20 °C (−4 °F), unless otherwise specified by manufacturer.

**Preparation of dosage form**
Bring medication to room temperature just prior to administration. Do not force warming by use of external heat source, such as water bath or microwave oven.

### DINOPROSTONE VAGINAL SYSTEM

Note: This monograph contains information on both the dinoprostone vaginal suppositories and the vaginal system (a suppository within a retrieval device). Each may be inappropriately referred to as dinoprostone vaginal insert in other types of information. It is important to avoid confusing the two dosage forms, since each has a different use and strength.

**Usual adult and adolescent dose**
Cervical ripening—
Intravaginal, 10 mg (one system delivering 0.3 mg per hour) placed transversely into the posterior fornix of the vaginal canal and removed upon onset of active labor or twelve hours after insertion, whichever occurs first. The patient should remain in supine position for at least two hours after administration.

Note: A minimal amount of lubricant should be used to aid system insertion.

**Strength(s) usually available**
U.S.—
10 mg (Rx) [*Cervidil*].
Canada—
Not commercially available.

**Packaging and storage**
Store below 2 and 8 °C (36 and 46 °F), unless otherwise specified by manufacturer.

**Preparation of dosage form**
Warming is not necessary.

## Selected Bibliography

Rayburn WF. Prostaglandin E2 gel for cervical ripening and induction of labor: a critical analysis. Am J Obstet Gynecol 1989; 160(3): 529-34.
Castadot RG. Pregnancy termination: techniques, risks, and complications and their management. Fertil Steril 1986; 45(1): 5-17.

Revised: 08/20/97

---

**DIPHENHYDRAMINE**—See *Antihistamines (Systemic)*

# DIPHENIDOL Systemic†

INN: Difenidol
VA CLASSIFICATION (Primary/Secondary): CN550/GA605
Commonly used brand name(s): *Vontrol*.
Note: For a listing of dosage forms and brand names by country availability, see *Dosage Forms* section(s).

†Not commercially available in Canada.

## Category
Antiemetic; antivertigo agent.

## Indications
**Accepted**
Vertigo (prophylaxis and treatment)—Diphenidol is indicated in the prevention and symptomatic treatment of peripheral (labyrinthine) vertigo and associated nausea and vomiting that occur in such conditions as Meniere's disease and surgery of the middle and inner ear.

Nausea and vomiting (prophylaxis and treatment) and

Nausea and vomiting, cancer chemotherapy–induced (prophylaxis and treatment)—Diphenidol is indicated also for the control of nausea and vomiting associated with postoperative states, malignant neoplasms, labyrinthine disturbances, antineoplastic agent therapy, radiation sickness, and infectious diseases.

**Unaccepted**
Diphenidol has been used in the treatment of ventricular tachyarrhythmias; however, the use of diphenidol as an antiarrhythmic is unwarranted because of the frequency and severity of adverse central nervous system (CNS) effects.

Diphenidol is *not* indicated for use in the nausea and vomiting of pregnancy.

## Pharmacology/Pharmacokinetics
**Physicochemical characteristics**
Molecular weight—Diphenidol hydrochloride: 345.91.

**Mechanism of action/Effect**
The mechanism by which diphenidol exerts its antiemetic and antivertigo effects is not precisely known. It is thought to diminish vestibular stimulation and depress labyrinthine function. An action on the medullary chemoreceptive trigger zone may also be involved in the antiemetic effect.

**Other actions/effects**
Diphenidol has no significant sedative, tranquilizing, or antihistaminic action. It has a weak peripheral anticholinergic effect.

**Absorption**
Well absorbed from gastrointestinal tract after oral administration.

**Half-life**
4 hours.

**Time to peak concentration**
1½ to 3 hours.

**Elimination**
Primarily renal (about 90% of drug). Most of an oral dose is excreted within 3 to 4 days.

## Precautions to Consider
**Pregnancy/Reproduction**
Pregnancy—Studies in humans and animals have not shown a significant difference in conception rate, litter size, live birth or viability, or birth abnormalities between diphenidol-treated and untreated control groups.

**Breast-feeding**
Problems in humans have not been documented.

**Pediatrics**
Appropriate studies on the relationship of age to the effects of diphenidol used in the prophylaxis or treatment of vertigo have not been performed in the pediatric population. Also, appropriate studies with diphenidol used in the prophylaxis or treatment of nausea and vomiting in children weighing less than 22.8 kg have not been performed; use in these children is not recommended.

**Geriatrics**
No information is available on the relationship of age to the effects of diphenidol in geriatric patients.

**Drug interactions and/or related problems**
The following drug interactions and/or related problems have been selected on the basis of their potential clinical significance (possible mechanism in parentheses where appropriate)—not necessarily inclusive (» = major clinical significance):

Note: Combinations containing any of the following medications, depending on the amount present, may also interact with this medication.

Anticholinergics or other medications with anticholinergic activity (See *Appendix II*)
(anticholinergic effects may be potentiated when these medications are used concurrently with diphenidol)

Apomorphine
(prior ingestion of diphenidol may decrease the emetic response to apomorphine in the treatment of poisoning)

» CNS depression–producing medications (See *Appendix II*)
(concurrent use may potentiate the effects of either these medications or diphenidol)

**Medical considerations/Contraindications**
The medical considerations/contraindications included have been selected on the basis of their potential clinical significance (reasons given in parentheses where appropriate)—not necessarily inclusive (» = major clinical significance).

*Except under special circumstances, this medication should not be used when the following medical problem exists:*

» Anuria
(renal shut-down may increase risk of systemic accumulation of diphenidol)

*Risk-benefit should be considered when the following medical problems exist:*

Gastrointestinal tract obstructive disease, such as stenosing peptic ulcer and pyloric or duodenal obstruction
(decrease in motility and tone may occur, resulting in obstruction and gastric retention)

Genitourinary tract obstructive disease, such as prostatic hypertrophy
(use may precipitate urinary retention)

Glaucoma
(use may increase intraocular pressure)

» Hypotension
(may be exacerbated)

» Renal function impairment
(decreased excretion may increase the risk of side effects)

Sensitivity to diphenidol

Caution is recommended when diphenidol is used, since signs of intestinal obstruction, brain tumor, or overdosage of toxic drugs may be obscured by its antiemetic action.

## Side/Adverse Effects
Note: Hallucinations, disorientation, and confusion have been reported with usual doses of diphenidol within the first 3 days of therapy. Upon cessation of therapy, symptoms disappeared within 3 days.

The following side/adverse effects have been selected on the basis of their potential clinical significance (possible signs and symptoms in parentheses where appropriate)—not necessarily inclusive:

**Those indicating need for medical attention**
Incidence rare—less than 0.5%
*Confusion; hallucinations*

**Those indicating need for medical attention only if they continue or are bothersome**
Incidence more frequent
*Drowsiness*

Incidence less frequent or rare
*Blurred vision; dizziness; dryness of mouth; headache; heartburn; nervousness, restlessness, or trouble in sleeping; skin rash; stomach upset or pain; unusual tiredness or weakness*

## Overdose
For more information on the management of overdose or unintentional ingestion, **contact a Poison Control Center** (see *Poison Control Center Listing*).

### Clinical effects of overdose
The following effects have been selected on the basis of their potential clinical significance (possible signs and symptoms in parentheses where appropriate)–not necessarily inclusive:

**Drowsiness, severe; hypotension** (severe unusual tiredness or weakness); **respiratory depression** (shortness of breath or troubled breathing)

### Treatment of overdose
Treatment of overdosage is essentially supportive, including the following:
To decrease absorption—Early gastric lavage.
Supportive care—Maintenance of blood pressure and respiration. Patients in whom intentional overdose is confirmed or suspected should be referred for psychiatric consultation.

## Patient Consultation
As an aid to patient consultation, refer to *Advice for the Patient, Diphenidol (Systemic).*
In providing consultation, consider emphasizing the following selected information (» = major clinical significance):

**Before using this medication**
» Conditions affecting use, especially:
  Sensitivity to diphenidol
  Use in children—Not recommended for prophylaxis or treatment of nausea and vomiting in children weighing less than 22.8 kg
  Other medications, especially CNS depressants
  Other medical problems, especially anuria, hypotension, renal function impairment

**Proper use of this medication**
Taking with food, water, or milk to minimize gastric irritation
» Importance of not taking more medication than the amount prescribed
» Proper dosing
  Missed dose: If on a regular dosing schedule—using as soon as possible; if almost time for next dose, not using at all; not doubling doses
» Proper storage

**Precautions while using this medication**
» Avoiding use of alcohol or other CNS depressants
» Caution if drowsiness or blurred vision occurs

**Side/adverse effects**
Signs of potential side effects, especially confusion and hallucinations

## General Dosing Information
Because of its potential to cause hallucinations, disorientation, or confusion, use of diphenidol should be limited to patients who are hospitalized or under comparable continuous close professional supervision.

### Diet/Nutrition
In the preventive treatment of vertigo and associated nausea and vomiting, diphenidol may be taken with food, water, or milk to minimize gastric irritation. However, if nausea and vomiting are present, the further intake of liquids or food may aggravate the condition.

## Oral Dosage Forms

### DIPHENIDOL HYDROCHLORIDE TABLETS

**Usual adult and adolescent dose**
Antiemetic and
Antivertigo—
  Oral, 25 to 50 mg every four hours as needed.

**Usual adult prescribing limits**
300 mg a day.

**Usual pediatric dose**
Antiemetic—
  Oral, 880 mcg (0.88 mg) per kg of body weight or 25 mg per square meter of body surface every four hours as needed. If symptoms persist, dose may be repeated in one hour after initial dose; subsequent doses should be spaced four hours apart; or,
  For children weighing 22.8 to 45.6 kg: Oral, 25 mg every four hours as needed.
Note: Children weighing up to 22.8 kg—Use is not recommended.

**Usual pediatric prescribing limits**
For children weighing 22.8 kg and over: 5.5 mg per kg of body weight a day.

**Strength(s) usually available**
U.S.—
  25 mg (Rx) [*Vontrol* (acacia; calcium sulfate; cellulose; FD&C No. 5 [tartrazine]; FD&C Yellow No. 6; magnesium stearate; starch)].
Canada—
  Not commercially available.

**Packaging and storage**
Store below 40 °C (104 °F), preferably between 15 and 30 °C (59 and 86 °F), in a tight, light-resistant container, unless otherwise specified by manufacturer.

**Auxiliary labeling**
• May cause drowsiness.
• Avoid alcoholic beverages.

Revised: 04/16/93

---

# DIPHENOXYLATE AND ATROPINE  Systemic

VA CLASSIFICATION (Primary): GA208
Note: Controlled substance classification—
  U.S.: V
  Canada: N
Commonly used brand name(s): *Lofene; Logen; Lomocot; Lomotil; Lonox; Vi-Atro.*
Note: For a listing of dosage forms and brand names by country availability, see *Dosage Forms* section(s).

## Category
Antidiarrheal (antiperistaltic).

## Indications
Note: The efficacy of any antidiarrheal medication for treatment of most cases of nonspecific diarrhea is questionable, especially in children. **Preferred treatment for acute, nonspecific diarrhea consists of fluid and electrolyte replacement, nutritional therapy, and, if possible, elimination of the underlying cause of the diarrhea.**

**Accepted**
Diarrhea (treatment adjunct)—Diphenoxylate and atropine combination is indicated in adults, as an adjunct to fluid and electrolyte therapy, in the symptomatic treatment of acute and chronic diarrhea.

**Unaccepted**
Diphenoxylate and atropine combination is not recommended for treatment of diarrhea in children.

## Pharmacology/Pharmacokinetics

**Physicochemical characteristics**
Molecular weight—Atropine sulfate: 694.84.
Diphenoxylate hydrochloride: 489.06.

**Mechanism of action/Effect**
Diphenoxylate—Probably acts both locally and centrally to reduce intestinal motility.
Atropine—Has anticholinergic activity. However, in this preparation atropine is included in doses below the therapeutic level in an attempt to prevent abuse by deliberate overdosage.

**Duration of effect**
3 to 4 hours.

**Biotransformation**
Diphenoxylate—Hepatic; the major metabolite difenoxin (diphenoxylic acid) has similar activity.

**Half-life**
Atropine—2.5 hours.
Diphenoxylate—2.5 hours.
Diphenoxylic acid—4.5 hours.

**Onset of effect**
45 to 60 minutes.

**Elimination**
Atropine—Renal; 30 to 50% excreted unchanged.
Diphenoxylate—Fecal/renal; less than 1% eliminated unchanged in urine.

## Precautions to Consider

### Pregnancy/Reproduction
Pregnancy—Adequate and well-controlled studies in humans have not been done.

Although studies in animals with diphenoxylate and atropine have not shown any evidence of teratogenicity, risk-benefit must be considered since a study in rats showed that maternal weight gain was reduced when diphenoxylate was given at doses of 20 mg per kg per day. Also, at the same dosage, fertility was decreased, and out of 27 matings only 4 rats conceived and bore 25 normal young. Studies in rabbits showed no embryotoxic, teratogenic, or contraceptive effects.

FDA Pregnancy Category C.

### Breast-feeding
Problems in humans have not been documented. However, both diphenoxylate's metabolite, diphenoxylic acid, and atropine are distributed into breast milk.

### Pediatrics
Diphenoxylate and atropine combination is not recommended for treatment of diarrhea in children. Recommended treatment consists of oral rehydration therapy to prevent loss of fluids and electrolytes, nutritional therapy, and, if possible, elimination of the underlying cause of the diarrhea.

Infants and young children are especially susceptible to the toxic effects of atropine.

Children may also be more susceptible to the respiratory depressant effects of diphenoxylate.

### Geriatrics
No information is available on the relationship of age to the effects of diphenoxylate and atropine in geriatric patients. However, elderly patients may be more susceptible to the respiratory depressant effects of diphenoxylate, and to the mild anticholinergic effects and confusion caused by atropine.

In geriatric patients with diarrhea, caution is recommended because of the risk of fluid and electrolyte loss.

### Drug interactions and/or related problems
The following drug interactions and/or related problems have been selected on the basis of their potential clinical significance (possible mechanism in parentheses where appropriate)—not necessarily inclusive (» = major clinical significance):

Note: Combinations containing any of the following medications, depending on the amount present, may also interact with this medication.

Addictive medications, other, especially central nervous system (CNS) depressants with habituating potential
(concurrent use with diphenoxylate may increase the risk of habituation; caution is recommended)

» Alcohol or
» CNS depression–producing medications, other (See *Appendix II*)
(concurrent use with diphenoxylate may increase the CNS depressant effects of either diphenoxylate or these medications; also, when tricyclic antidepressants are used concurrently with atropine, their anticholinergic effects may be intensified; dosage adjustment may be required)

» Anticholinergics or other medications with anticholinergic action (See *Appendix II*)
(these medications may enhance the effects of atropine during concurrent use; significant interaction is unlikely with usual doses of diphenoxylate and atropine combination, but may occur with its abuse)

» Monoamine oxidase (MAO) inhibitors, including furazolidone, procarbazine, and selegiline
(concurrent use with diphenoxylate may precipitate hypertensive crisis; MAO inhibitors may block detoxification of atropine, thus potentiating its action)

» Naltrexone
(administration of naltrexone to a patient physically dependent on opioid drugs, such as diphenoxylate, will precipitate withdrawal symptoms; symptoms may appear within 5 minutes of naltrexone administration, persist for up to 48 hours, and be difficult to reverse)

(naltrexone blocks the therapeutic effects of opioids, including the antidiarrheal effects; also, patients receiving naltrexone should be advised to use alternative antidiarrheals when necessary)

Opioid (narcotic) analgesics
(concurrent use with diphenoxylate may result in increased risk of severe constipation and additive CNS depressant effects)

### Laboratory value alterations
The following have been selected on the basis of their potential clinical significance (possible effect in parentheses where appropriate)—not necessarily inclusive (» = major clinical significance):

With diagnostic test results
» Phenolsulfonphthalein (PSP) excretion test
(atropine utilizes the same tubular mechanism of excretion as PSP, resulting in decreased urinary excretion of PSP; concurrent use of atropine is not recommended in patients receiving PSP excretion test)

With physiology/laboratory test values
Amylase, serum
(values may be increased as a result of spasm of the sphincter of Oddi)

### Medical considerations/Contraindications
The medical considerations/contraindications included have been selected on the basis of their potential clinical significance (reasons given in parentheses where appropriate)—not necessarily inclusive (» = major clinical significance):

*Except under special circumstances, this medication should not be used when the following medical problems exist:*

» Colitis, severe
(patient may develop toxic megacolon)

» Diarrhea associated with pseudomembranous colitis resulting from treatment with broad-spectrum antibiotics
(inhibition of peristalsis may delay the removal of toxins from the colon, thereby prolonging and/or worsening the diarrhea)

*Risk-benefit should be considered when the following medical problems exist:*

Alcoholism, active or in remission, or
Drug abuse or dependence, history of
(diphenoxylate content may increase chances of drug abuse in patient already predisposed to dependence)

Cardiovascular instability
(possible increase in heart rate may be undesirable)

» Dehydration
(may predispose to delayed diphenoxylate intoxication; inhibition of peristalsis may result in fluid retention in colon and may further aggravate dehydration; discontinuation of medication and rehydration therapy is essential if signs or symptoms of dehydration, such as dryness of mouth, excessive thirst, wrinkled skin, decreased urination, and dizziness or lightheadedness, are present; fluid loss may have serious consequences, such as circulatory collapse and renal failure)

Diarrhea caused by infectious organisms
(bacterial diarrhea may worsen due to the increased contact time between the mucosa and the penetrating microorganism; however, there is no evidence of this occurring in actual practice)

» Diarrhea caused by poisoning, until toxic material has been eliminated from gastrointestinal tract

Down's syndrome
(atropine may cause abnormal increase in pupillary dilation and acceleration of heart rate)

» Dysentery, acute, characterized by bloody stools and elevated temperature
(sole treatment with antiperistaltic antidiarrheals may be inadequate; antibiotic therapy may be required)

Gallbladder disease or gallstones
(diphenoxylate may cause biliary tract spasm)

» Gastrointestinal tract obstruction
(may result in pseudo-obstruction, or in dilation of the large or small bowel)

Glaucoma, angle-closure
(although unlikely with usual doses of this combination, atropine may precipitate an acute attack of angle-closure glaucoma)

» Hepatic function impairment or jaundice
(diphenoxylate may precipitate hepatic coma; it is recommended that dosage be reduced in patients with impaired hepatic function)

Hiatal hernia associated with reflux esophagitis
(although unlikely with usual doses of this combination, atropine may aggravate condition)

Hypertension
(although unlikely with usual doses of this combination, atropine may aggravate condition)

Hyperthyroidism
(characterized by tachycardia, which may be increased by atropine)
Hypothyroidism
(diphenoxylate may increase risk of respiratory depression)
Incontinence, overflow
(secondary to constipation, but often mistaken for diarrhea; use of diphenoxylate and atropine may worsen constipation and/or cause dilation or pseudo-obstruction of the colon)
Intestinal atony of the elderly or debilitated
(although unlikely with usual doses of this combination, use of atropine may result in obstruction)
Myasthenia gravis
(although unlikely with usual doses of this combination, atropine may aggravate condition because of inhibition of acetylcholine action)
Prostatic hypertrophy or
Urethral stricture, acute or
Urinary retention
(reduction in tone of urinary bladder may aggravate or lead to complete urinary retention)
Renal function impairment
(decreased elimination of atropine may increase the risk of side effects)
Respiratory disease or impairment
(increased risk of respiratory depression)
Sensitivity to atropine or diphenoxylate

**Patient monitoring**
The following may be especially important in patient monitoring (other tests may be warranted in some patients, depending on condition; » = major clinical significance):
» Hepatic function determinations
(recommended at periodic intervals during long-term therapy, especially for patients with hepatic function impairment)

## Side/Adverse Effects

The following side/adverse effects have been selected on the basis of their potential clinical significance (possible signs and symptoms in parentheses where appropriate)—not necessarily inclusive:

**Those indicating need for medical attention**
Incidence less frequent or rare
*Paralytic ileus or toxic megacolon* (bloating; constipation; loss of appetite; severe stomach pain with nausea and vomiting)

**Those indicating need for medical attention only if they continue, worsen, or are bothersome**
Incidence less frequent or rare
*Anticholinergic effects, mild* (blurred vision; difficult urination; dryness of skin and mouth; fever); *CNS depression* (dizziness or light-headedness; drowsiness; mental depression); *confusion; headache; numbness of hands or feet; skin rash or itching; swelling of the gums*
Note: Since atropine is present in a subtherapeutic dose, the appearance of these symptoms probably indicates overdosage.

**Those indicating possible withdrawal and the need for medical attention if they occur after discontinuation of prolonged high-dose therapy**
Incidence rare
*Increased sweating; muscle cramps; nausea or vomiting; shivering or trembling; stomach cramps*

## Overdose

For specific information on the agents used in the management of diphenoxylate and atropine overdose, see:
- *Charcoal, Activated (Oral-Local)* monograph; and/or
- *Naloxone (Systemic)* monograph.

For more information on the management of overdose or unintentional ingestion, **contact a Poison Control Center** (see *Poison Control Center Listing*).

**Clinical effects of overdose**
The following effects have been selected on the basis of their potential clinical significance (possible signs and symptoms in parentheses where appropriate)–not necessarily inclusive:

*Anticholinergic effects, severe* (continuing blurred vision or changes in near vision; fast heartbeat; severe drowsiness; severe dryness of mouth, nose, and throat; unusual warmth, dryness, and flushing of skin); *coma; respiratory depression* (severe shortness of breath or troubled breathing); *unusual excitement, nervousness, restlessness, or irritability*

Note: *Respiratory depression* may occur as late as 12 to 30 hours after ingestion.

Possible symptoms of overdose
*Anticholinergic effects, mild* (blurred vision; difficult urination; dryness of skin and mouth; fever); *CNS depression* (dizziness or light-headedness; drowsiness; mental depression); *confusion; headache; numbness of hands or feet; skin rash or itching; swelling of the gums*
Note: Since atropine is present in a subtherapeutic dose, the appearance of these symptoms probably indicates overdosage.

**Treatment of overdose**
Treatment of overdose with diphenoxylate and atropine is the same as treatment for meperidine or morphine overdosage and involves the following:
To decrease absorption—Induction of vomiting, or gastric lavage, if vomiting has not occurred; administration of a slurry of 100 grams of activated charcoal, after induction of vomiting or gastric lavage, in non-comatose patients.
Specific treatment—Intravenous administration of 0.4 mg (0.01 mg per kg of body weight in children) of narcotic antagonist naloxone, which may be repeated at 2- to 3-minute intervals, for respiratory depression.
Monitoring—Careful monitoring for 48 to 72 hours.
Supportive care—Support of respiration. Patients in whom intentional overdose is confirmed or suspected should be referred for psychiatric consultation.

## Patient Consultation

As an aid to patient consultation, refer to *Advice for the Patient, Diphenoxylate and Atropine (Systemic)*.
In providing consultation, consider emphasizing the following selected information (» = major clinical significance):

**Before using this medication**
» Conditions affecting use, especially:
Sensitivity to atropine or diphenoxylate
Pregnancy—Studies in rats show decreased fertility and decreased maternal weight gain
Breast-feeding—Diphenoxylate and atropine distributed into breast milk; potential for serious adverse effects in nursing infant
Use in children—Not recommended for use in children; increased susceptibility to toxic effects of atropine and respiratory depressant effects of diphenoxylate; risk of dehydration
Use in the elderly—Increased risk of respiratory depression, anticholinergic effects, and confusion; risk of dehydration
Other medications, especially other anticholinergics, CNS depressants, MAO inhibitors, or naltrexone
Other medical problems, especially acute dysentery; dehydration; diarrhea caused by antibiotics or poisoning; gastrointestinal tract obstruction; hepatic function impairment or jaundice; or severe colitis

**Proper use of this medication**
Taking with food or meals if gastric irritation occurs
» Importance of not taking more medication than the amount prescribed because of habit-forming potential
» Importance of maintaining adequate hydration and proper diet
» Proper dosing
Missed dose: If on a scheduled dosing regimen—Taking as soon as possible; not taking if almost time for next dose; not doubling doses
» Proper storage
*For liquid dosage form*
Proper administration technique: Measuring amount with dropper and taking by mouth

**Precautions while using this medication**
Regular visits to physician to check progress during prolonged therapy
» Consulting physician if diarrhea is not controlled within 48 hours and/or fever develops
» Avoiding use of alcohol or other CNS depressants during therapy
» Suspected overdose: Getting emergency help at once
Need to inform physician or dentist of use of medication if any kind of surgery (including dental surgery) or emergency treatment is required
» Caution if dizziness or drowsiness occurs

**Side/adverse effects**
Signs of potential side effects, especially paralytic ileus or toxic megacolon

## General Dosing Information

Treatment with diphenoxylate and atropine should be continued for 24 to 48 hours before it is considered ineffective in acute diarrhea. If clinical

# Diphenoxylate and Atropine (Systemic)

improvement of chronic diarrhea after treatment with a maximum daily dose of 20 mg of diphenoxylate is not observed within 10 days, treatment should be discontinued.

Inhibition of peristalsis may produce fluid retention in the bowel, which may aggravate dehydration and depletion of electrolytes, and may also increase variability of response to the medication. If dehydration or electrolyte imbalance occurs, diphenoxylate and atropine therapy should be withheld until appropriate corrective therapy has begun.

To prevent development of toxic megacolon in patients with acute ulcerative colitis, treatment with diphenoxylate and atropine should be discontinued promptly if abdominal distention or other specific gastrointestinal symptoms such as anorexia, bloating, constipation, nausea, vomiting, or abdominal pain occur.

Prolonged use of larger than usual therapeutic doses may result in physical dependence.

Tolerance to the antidiarrheal effects of diphenoxylate and atropine may develop with prolonged use.

This medication may suppress respiration, especially in the elderly, the very ill, and patients with respiratory problems. Lower doses may be required for these patients.

## Oral Dosage Forms

### DIPHENOXYLATE HYDROCHLORIDE AND ATROPINE SULFATE ORAL SOLUTION USP

**Usual adult and adolescent dose**
Antidiarrheal (antiperistaltic)—
  Initial: Oral, 5 mg of diphenoxylate hydrochloride and 50 mcg (0.05 mg) of atropine sulfate three or four times a day.
  Maintenance: Oral, 5 mg of diphenoxylate hydrochloride and 50 mcg (0.05 mg) of atropine sulfate once a day, as needed.

**Usual adult prescribing limits**
20 mg per day.

**Usual pediatric dose**
Antidiarrheal (antiperistaltic)—
  Children up to 12 years of age: Use is not recommended.
  Children 12 years of age and older: See *Usual adult and adolescent dose*.

**Usual geriatric dose**
See *Usual adult and adolescent dose*.

Note: Geriatric patients may be more sensitive to the effects of the usual adult dose.

**Strength(s) usually available**
U.S.—
  2.5 mg of diphenoxylate hydrochloride and 25 mcg (0.025 mg) of atropine sulfate, per 5 mL (Rx) [*Lomotil* (alcohol 15%); GENERIC].
Canada—
  Not commercially available.

**Packaging and storage**
Store below 40 °C (104 °F), preferably between 15 and 30 °C (59 and 86 °F), unless otherwise specified by manufacturer. Store in a tight, light-resistant container. Protect from freezing.

**Auxiliary labeling**
• May cause drowsiness.
• Avoid alcoholic beverages.
• Keep out of reach of children.

**Note**
Controlled substance in the U.S.

### DIPHENOXYLATE HYDROCHLORIDE AND ATROPINE SULFATE TABLETS USP

**Usual adult and adolescent dose**
See *Diphenoxylate Hydrochloride and Atropine Sulfate Oral Solution USP*.

**Usual pediatric dose**
Antidiarrheal (antiperistaltic)—
  Children up to 12 years of age: Use is not recommended.
  Children 12 years of age and older: See *Usual adult and adolescent dose*.

**Usual geriatric dose**
See *Usual adult and adolescent dose*.

Note: Geriatric patients may be more sensitive to the effects of the usual adult dose.

**Strength(s) usually available**
U.S.—
  2.5 mg of diphenoxylate hydrochloride and 25 mcg (0.025 mg) of atropine sulfate (Rx) [*Lofene; Logen; Lomocot; Lomotil; Lonox; Vi-Atro;* GENERIC].
Canada—
  2.5 mg of diphenoxylate hydrochloride and 25 mcg (0.025 mg) of atropine sulfate (Rx) [*Lomotil*].

**Packaging and storage**
Store below 40 °C (104 °F), preferably between 15 and 30 °C (59 and 86 °F), in a well-closed container, unless otherwise specified by manufacturer. Store in a light-resistant container.

**Auxiliary labeling**
• May cause drowsiness.
• Avoid alcoholic beverages.
• Keep out of reach of children.
• May be habit-forming.

**Note**
Controlled substance in the U.S. and Canada.

### Selected Bibliography

Brownlee HJ, editor. Proceedings of a symposium: Management of acute nonspecific diarrhea. Am J Med 1990; 88(Suppl 6A).
Gaginella TS. Diarrhea: some new aspects of pharmacotherapy. Drug Intell Clin Pharm 1983; 17: 914-6.

Revised: 08/22/94

---

**DIPHENYLPYRALINE**—See *Antihistamines (Systemic)*

---

**DIPHTHERIA ANTITOXIN**—The *Diphtheria Antitoxin (Systemic)* monograph is not included in this published version of the USP DI database. Copies of the monograph are available on request from Micromedex, Inc. - Reprint Requests, 6200 S. Syracuse Way, Suite 300, Englewood, CO 80111; telephone (303) 486-6400; telefax (303) 486-6464; Email: USPDI@MDX.COM.

---

**DIPHTHERIA AND TETANUS TOXOIDS DT**—See *Diphtheria and Tetanus Toxoids (Systemic)*

---

# DIPHTHERIA AND TETANUS TOXOIDS  Systemic

This monograph includes information on the following: 1) Diphtheria and Tetanus Toxoids for Pediatric Use (DT); 2) Tetanus and Diphtheria Toxoids for Adult Use (Td).

Note: There are some differences in terminology with respect to the use of the terms "primary" and "reinforcing" in some of the manufacturers' labeling used for this monograph. In this monograph, the term "primary immunizing series" will be used to denote the initial doses that are usually given 4 to 8 weeks apart as well as the "reinforcing" dose that is usually given 6 to 12 months thereafter. The dose usually given at 4 to 6 years of age and the doses given every 10 years will be called booster doses.

VA CLASSIFICATION (Primary): IM200

Other commonly used names are: DT [Diphtheria and Tetanus Toxoids]; Td [Tetanus and Diphtheria Toxoids].

Note: For a listing of dosage forms and brand names by country availability, see *Dosage Forms* section(s).

## Category
Immunizing agent (active).

## Indications

**Accepted**
Diphtheria and tetanus (prophylaxis)—Diphtheria and tetanus toxoid combination is indicated for immunization against diphtheria and tetanus.

Diphtheria and tetanus toxoids for pediatric use (DT) is indicated for immunization of infants and children 6 weeks up to 7 years of age who, because of a contraindication to pertussis vaccine, cannot receive diphtheria and tetanus toxoids and pertussis vaccine (DTP) combination. If there is no contraindication to pertussis vaccine, DTP is the vaccine of choice for this age group.

Tetanus and diphtheria toxoids for adult use (Td) is indicated for immunization of adults and children 7 years of age and older.

## Pharmacology/Pharmacokinetics

### Physicochemical characteristics
Source—
Diphtheria toxoid is prepared by first cultivating a suitable strain of *Corynebacterium diphtheriae*. Tetanus toxoid is prepared by first cultivating a suitable strain of *Clostridium tetani*. The resulting toxins are detoxified with formaldehyde. The detoxified toxins (toxoids) are adsorbed onto an aluminum salt. This prolongs and enhances the antigenic properties by retarding the rate of absorption of the injected toxoid in the body.

### Mechanism of action/Effect
Following intramuscular injection, diphtheria toxoid and tetanus toxoid induce the formation of diphtheria antitoxin and tetanus antitoxin, respectively.

### Protective effect
Diphtheria antitoxin—
The protective level in serum is 0.01 unit per mL.
Tetanus antitoxin—
The protective level in serum is 0.01 unit per mL.

### Time to protective effect
For diphtheria and tetanus toxoids for pediatric use (DT)—
In a study of 20 children under 1 year of age, protective levels of diphtheria and tetanus antitoxins were detected in 100% of the children after administration of 3 doses of DT. In addition, protective levels of diphtheria and tetanus antitoxins were detected in 100% of the children after administration of 2 doses of DT, but maternal antibody may have contributed to the total neutralizing antibody in some of these children.
For tetanus and diphtheria toxoids for adult use (Td)—
Response to primary immunization—
Diphtheria—In a study of 10 adults who had less than 0.001 unit per mL of diphtheria antitoxin in pre-immunization serum, protective levels of diphtheria antitoxin were detected in 50% of the adults after administration of 2 doses of Td, each containing 2 Lf units of diphtheria toxoid. In a similar study of 6 adults, protective levels of diphtheria antitoxin were detected in 100% of the adults after administration of 3 doses of Td.
Tetanus—In a study of 20 adults who had less than 0.0025 unit per mL of tetanus antitoxin in pre-immunization serum, protective levels of tetanus antitoxin were detected in 70% of the adults after administration of 2 doses, and in 100% of the adults after administration of 3 doses, of Td, each containing 2 Lf units of tetanus toxoid.
Response to booster doses—
Booster doses of Td given as long as 25 to 30 years after primary immunization series have produced rapid and significant increases in the levels of both tetanus and diphtheria antitoxins.
Diphtheria—In a study of 140 adolescent males, protective levels of diphtheria antitoxin were detected in 100% of the males after administration of a single booster dose of Td containing 1 Lf unit of diphtheria toxoid.
Tetanus—In a study of 36 adults, protective levels of tetanus antitoxin were detected in 100% of the adults after administration of a single booster dose of Td containing 1 Lf unit of tetanus toxoid.

### Duration of protective effect
At least 10 years for both diphtheria toxoid and tetanus toxoid following a completed primary immunizing series of injections.

## Precautions to Consider

### Cross-sensitivity and/or related problems
Patients sensitive to diphtheria toxoid or tetanus toxoid may be sensitive to diphtheria and tetanus toxoids for pediatric use (DT) or tetanus and diphtheria toxoids for adult use (Td) also.

### Carcinogenicity/Mutagenicity
Studies have not been done.

### Pregnancy/Reproduction
Fertility—Studies have not been done.
Pregnancy—There is no evidence that diphtheria and tetanus toxoid combination is teratogenic.
For DT: Use of DT is not recommended in females of child-bearing age.
For Td: Unimmunized pregnant women should receive 2 properly spaced doses of Td before delivery, preferably during the last 2 trimesters. Incompletely immunized pregnant women should complete the primary immunizing series of Td. Those fully immunized more than 10 years ago should receive a booster dose of Td.
Studies have not been done in animals.
FDA Pregnancy Category C.

### Breast-feeding
Diphtheria and tetanus toxoids have not been isolated from breast milk.
For DT—Use of DT is not recommended in females of child-bearing age.
For Td—There is no evidence that breast milk from women who have received Td is harmful to infants.

### Pediatrics
For DT—
Infants up to 6 weeks of age: Use of DT is not recommended.
Infants and children up to 7 years of age: Pediatrics-specific problems that would limit the usefulness of DT in these children are not expected.
Children 7 years of age and older: Use of DT is not recommended in this age group.
For Td—
Infants and children up to 7 years of age: Use of Td is not recommended in this age group.
Children 7 years of age and older: Pediatrics-specific problems that would limit the usefulness of Td in these children are not expected.

### Geriatrics
For DT—Use of DT is not recommended in this age group.
For Td—Although appropriate studies on the relationship of age to the effects of Td have not been performed in the geriatric population, geriatrics-specific problems are not expected to limit the usefulness of Td in the elderly. However, the immune response in the elderly may be slightly diminished.

### Drug interactions and/or related problems
The following drug interactions and/or related problems have been selected on the basis of their potential clinical significance (possible mechanism in parentheses where appropriate)—not necessarily inclusive (» = major clinical significance):

Note: Combinations containing any of the following medications, depending on the amount present, may also interact with this medication.

Immunosuppressants or
Radiation therapy
(because normal defense mechanisms are suppressed, the patient's antibody response to DT or Td may be decreased during therapy and deferral of routine DT or Td administration may be considered. The precaution does not apply to corticosteroids used as replacement therapy, for short-term [less than 2 weeks] systemic therapy, or by other routes of administration that do not cause immunosuppression. Where possible, immunosuppressive therapy should be interrupted when immunization is required because of a tetanus-prone wound)

### Medical considerations/Contraindications
The medical considerations/contraindications included have been selected on the basis of their potential clinical significance (reasons given in parentheses where appropriate)—not necessarily inclusive (» = major clinical significance).

*Except under special circumstances, this medication should not be used when the following medical problems exist:*
» Febrile illness or
» Infection, acute
(routine primary or booster immunization should not be administered until the acute symptoms of the patient's illness have abated; however, emergency tetanus prophylaxis for wounds should be administered as usual. A minor afebrile illness, such as an upper respiratory infection, usually does not preclude administration of DT or Td)
» Sensitivity to DT or Td
» Tetanus infection
(products containing tetanus toxoid should not be used to treat a tetanus infection; tetanus antitoxin, preferably tetanus immune globulin [TIG], should be used instead; after recovery, the primary immunizing series should be initiated or continued, since a tetanus infection does not confer immunity)

*Risk-benefit should be considered when the following medical problem exists:*
» Sensitivity to thimerosal

## Side/Adverse Effects

Note: Although both the diphtheria toxoid and the tetanus toxoid components may evoke local and systemic allergic responses, it has been suggested that the tetanus toxoid component may be the more common cause.

If an Arthus-type hypersensitivity reaction or a fever over 39.4 °C (103 °F) occurs following a dose of diphtheria and tetanus toxoid combination, the patient usually has a very high serum tetanus antitoxin level and no additional doses of tetanus toxoid should be given for any reason, including wound management, more frequently than every 10 years.

Neurological reactions, such as convulsions, encephalopathy, and various mono- and polyneuropathies, have been reported following administration of preparations containing diphtheria toxoid and/or tetanus toxoid. Pallor, coldness, and hyporesponsiveness were reported in 1 child. In the differential diagnosis of polyradiculoneuropathies, previous administration of tetanus toxoid should be considered as a possible cause. If a neurologic reaction or a severe systemic allergic reaction occurs following a dose of diphtheria and tetanus toxoids for pediatric use (DT) or tetanus and diphtheria toxoids for adult use (Td), the person should not be further immunized with DT or Td.

Booster doses of tetanus toxoid administered more frequently than every 10 years have been reported to result in increased occurrence and severity of adverse reactions.

Generally, a history of hypersensitivity reactions other than anaphylaxis, such as delayed-type, cell-mediated allergic reaction (contact dermatitis), does not preclude immunization.

Sterile abscesses have been reported rarely following administration of DT or Td. These are thought to be caused by inadvertent subcutaneous injection of the aluminum adjuvant in the product.

Use of jet injectors, which deposit some toxoid in the subcutaneous tissue, has been associated with a higher frequency of local reactions than has intramuscular injection by needle.

The following side/adverse effects have been selected on the basis of their potential clinical significance (possible signs and symptoms in parentheses where appropriate)—not necessarily inclusive:

**Those indicating need for medical attention**
Incidence rare
*For DT and Td*
**Anaphylactic reaction** (difficulty in breathing or swallowing; hives; itching, especially of soles or palms; reddening of skin, especially around ears; swelling of eyes, face, or inside of nose; unusual tiredness or weakness, sudden and severe); *arthralgias* (joint aches or pain); *neurologic reaction* (confusion; excessive sleepiness; fever over 39.4 °C [103 °F]; headache, severe or continuing; seizures; unusual irritability; vomiting, severe or continuing); *pruritus* (itching); *skin rash; urticaria* (hives)

**Additional side/adverse effects that may occur because of very high serum tetanus antitoxin levels and may indicate a need for medical attention**
*Incidence rare*
**Arthus-type reaction** (swelling, blistering, pain, or other severe local reaction at injection site); *fever over 39.4 °C (103 °F)*
Note: *Arthus-type reaction* and *fever over 39.4 °C* usually occur only in patients old enough to receive Td, i.e., persons old enough to have received multiple booster doses of a tetanus toxoid–containing product. An *Arthus-type reaction* generally starts within 2 to 8 hours after the injection and may be severe and extensive.

**Those indicating need for medical attention only if they continue or are bothersome**
Incidence more frequent
*For DT and Td*
**Redness or hard lump at injection site**—may persist for a few days
*For DT only*
**Fever under 39.4 °C (103 °F); swelling, pain, or tenderness at injection site**—may persist for a few days
Incidence less frequent
*For DT and Td*
**Nodule (hard lump) at injection site; subcutaneous atrophy (dent or indentation) at injection site**
Note: *Nodule (hard lump) at injection site* probably is caused by the aluminum content of the toxoids and may persist for a few weeks

*For DT only*
**Anorexia** (loss of appetite); *drowsiness; fretfulness; persistent crying; vomiting*
*For Td only*
**Axillary lymphadenopathy** (swelling of glands in armpit); *chills; fever under 39.4 °C (103 °F); headache; hypotension* (unusual tiredness or weakness); *malaise* (general feeling of discomfort or illness); *muscle aches; tachycardia* (fast heartbeat)

## Patient Consultation

As an aid to patient consultation, refer to *Advice for the Patient, Diphtheria and Tetanus Toxoids (Systemic)*.
In providing consultation, consider emphasizing the following selected information (» = major clinical significance):

**Before receiving this vaccine**
» Conditions affecting use, especially:
 Sensitivity to diphtheria toxoid, tetanus toxoid, or thimerosal
 Use in children—Not recommended for infants up to 6 weeks of age; only diphtheria and tetanus toxoids for pediatric use (DT) is recommended for infants and children 6 weeks to 7 years of age; only tetanus and diphtheria toxoids for adult use (Td) is recommended for children 7 years of age and older
 Use in the elderly—Only tetanus and diphtheria toxoids for adult use (Td) is recommended; the immune response in the elderly may be slightly diminished
 Other medical problems, especially acute infection, febrile illness, or tetanus infection

**Proper use of this vaccine**
» Proper dosing

**Side/adverse effects**
Notifying physician of any side effect that occurs after a dose of DT or Td, even if the side effect has gone away without treatment
Signs of potential side effects, especially anaphylactic reaction; arthralgias; neurologic reaction; pruritus; skin rash; urticaria; Arthus-type reaction; and fever over 39.4 °C (103 °F)

## General Dosing Information

Diphtheria and tetanus toxoid combination is administered by deep intramuscular injection into the deltoid (for adults and older children) or into the area of the midlateral muscles (vastus lateralis) of the thigh (for infants and younger children). The same muscle site should not be used more than once during the course of the primary immunizing series. The vaccine should not be injected subcutaneously or intravenously.

Before each additional dose of diphtheria and tetanus toxoids for pediatric use (DT) or tetanus and diphtheria toxoids for adult use (Td), the health status of the patient should be assessed. In addition, information should be obtained regarding any symptom and/or sign of an adverse reaction that occurred after the previous dose.

Routine immunization of adults and children over 6 months of age should be deferred during an outbreak of poliomyelitis in the community, unless there is also an outbreak of diphtheria. In either case, emergency tetanus prophylaxis for wounds should be administered as usual.

Persons with impaired immune response may be immunized, but may have reduced antibody response to DT or Td. Persons infected with human immunodeficiency virus (HIV) may receive DT or Td whether they have asymptomatic or symptomatic HIV infection.

Diphtheria infection may not (and tetanus infection does not) confer immunity; therefore, initiation or completion of active immunization with DT or Td is indicated at the time of recovery from either of these infections.

Interruption of the recommended schedule for the primary immunizing series of DT or Td by a delay between doses does not interfere with the final immunity achieved and does not necessitate starting the series over again, regardless of the length of time that elapsed between doses.

**Emergency tetanus prophylaxis of wounds**
Patients who were unimmunized or inadequately immunized with a tetanus toxoid–containing product prior to a wound should complete their primary immunizing series as soon as possible.

For routine wound management in children under 7 years of age who have not received the primary immunizing series against tetanus, DT (or DTP, if appropriate) should be used instead of single-antigen tetanus toxoid. In addition, children whose wounds are considered to be prone to tetanus infection and who have had fewer than 3 doses (or an unknown number of doses) of a tetanus toxoid–containing product also should be administered tetanus antitoxin, preferably tetanus immune globulin (TIG). A separate syringe and site of administration should be used for DT and TIG.

The decision to administer Td for wound management with or without concomitant passive immunization using tetanus immune globulin (TIG) depends on the condition of the wound and the patient's immunization history. Examples of wounds that are not clean, minor wounds are: wounds contaminated with dirt, feces, soil, or saliva; puncture wounds; wounds caused by tearing; and wounds resulting from missiles, crushing, burns, or frostbite. Tetanus has rarely occurred in persons who have received a documented primary immunizing series of a tetanus toxoid–containing product. Persons who have received the primary immunizing series and whose wounds are minor and uncontaminated should receive a booster dose of a tetanus toxoid–containing product, such as Td, only if they have not received a tetanus toxoid booster dose within the past 10 years. Persons who have received the primary immunizing series and who have wounds that are not minor and uncontaminated should receive a booster dose of a tetanus toxoid–containing product, such as Td, only if they have not received a tetanus toxoid booster dose within the past 5 years. Persons who have not received the primary immunizing series against tetanus (or whose immunization history is unknown) should be immunized with a tetanus toxoid–containing product, such as Td. If persons who have not received the primary immunizing series against tetanus (or whose immunization history is unknown) have wounds that are considered to be prone to tetanus infection, tetanus antitoxin (preferably TIG) should be administered in addition to Td. A separate syringe and site of administration should be used for Td and TIG.

### Emergency diphtheria prophylaxis

Immunization with diphtheria toxoid reduces the risk of developing diphtheria and lessens the severity of clinical illness. However, it does not eliminate *Corynebacterium diphtheriae* from the pharynx or the skin.

Household and other close contacts of persons with diphtheria infection who have received fewer than 3 doses of a diphtheria toxoid–containing product should receive an immediate dose of a diphtheria toxoid–containing product, such as DT or Td (according to their age requirement), and should complete the primary immunizing series according to schedule. Household and other close contacts who have received 3 or more doses of a diphtheria toxoid–containing product and who have not received an additional dose within 5 years should receive a booster dose of a diphtheria toxoid–containing product, such as DT or Td (according to their age requirement).

### For treatment of adverse effects

Recommended treatment includes:
- For mild hypersensitivity reaction—Administering antihistamines and, if necessary, corticosteroids.
- For severe hypersensitivity or anaphylactic reaction—Administering epinephrine. Antihistamines or corticosteroids may also be administered as required.

---

## DIPHTHERIA AND TETANUS TOXOIDS (DT)

## Summary of Differences

Indications: Diphtheria and tetanus toxoids for pediatric use (DT) is indicated for immunization of infants and children 6 weeks up to 7 years of age.

Strength(s) usually available: DT contains 6.6 to 25 Lf units of diphtheria toxoid and 5 to 10 Lf units of tetanus toxoid, per dose.

## Additional Dosing Information

Diphtheria toxoid of the strength used in DT is not recommended for adults and children 7 years of age and older, because of the increased risk of side/adverse effects associated with the use of higher doses of diphtheria toxoid in this age group.

It is recommended that infants and children up to 7 years of age receive diphtheria and tetanus toxoids as part of Diphtheria and Tetanus Toxoids and Pertussis Vaccine Adsorbed (DTP). In those cases in which the pertussis vaccine is contraindicated, it is recommended that DT be administered instead.

The primary immunizing series of DT consists of 4 doses (3 initial and 1 reinforcing) for children 6 weeks up to 1 year of age (in Canada, 2 months up to 7 years of age) or 3 doses (2 initial and 1 reinforcing) for children 1 to 7 years of age.

Preterm infants should be immunized according to their chronological age from birth.

DT can be administered concurrently with the following, using separate body sites and separate syringes (for parenterals), and the precautions that apply to each immunizing agent:

- Hepatitis B recombinant or plasma-derived vaccine.
- Polysaccharide vaccines, such as haemophilus b polysaccharide vaccine, haemophilus b conjugate vaccine, or pneumococcal polyvalent vaccine.
- Live virus vaccines, such as measles, mumps, and rubella (MMR) or oral polio vaccine (OPV).
- Inactivated poliovirus vaccine (IPV) or enhanced-potency inactivated vaccine (enhanced-potency IPV).

## Parenteral Dosage Forms

### (FOR PEDIATRIC USE) USP DIPHTHERIA AND TETANUS TOXOIDS ADSORBED (DT)

Note: DT is indicated for immunization of infants and children 6 weeks up to 7 years of age who cannot receive diphtheria and tetanus toxoids and pertussis vaccine (DTP) combination, because of a contraindication to pertussis vaccine. If there is no contraindication to pertussis vaccine, DTP is the vaccine of choice for this age group.

### Usual adult and adolescent dose

Use is not recommended. Tetanus and diphtheria toxoids for adult use (Td) should be administered instead.

### Usual pediatric dose

Diphtheria and tetanus (prophylaxis)—
Intramuscular, preferably into the deltoid or the midlateral muscles of the thigh
U.S.:
Children 6 weeks to 1 year of age: 0.5 mL at four- to eight-week intervals for a total of three doses. A fourth dose of 0.5 mL is administered six to twelve months after the third dose. A booster (fifth) dose of 0.5 mL is usually administered at four through six years of age (i.e., preferably prior to school entry); however, if the fourth dose of the primary immunizing series was administered after the fourth birthday, a booster (fifth) dose is not necessary.
Children 1 to 7 years of age: 0.5 mL followed by 0.5 mL four to eight weeks later for a total of two doses. A third dose of 0.5 mL is administered six to twelve months after the second dose. A booster (fourth) dose of 0.5 mL is usually administered at four through six years of age (i.e., preferably prior to school entry); however, if the third dose of the primary immunizing series was administered after the fourth birthday, a booster (fourth) dose is not necessary.
Children 7 years of age and older: Use is not recommended. Td should be administered instead.
Canada:
Children 2 months to 7 years of age: 0.5 mL at eight-week intervals for a total of three doses. A fourth dose of 0.5 mL is administered twelve months after the third dose. A booster (fifth) dose of 0.5 mL is usually administered at four through six years of age (i.e., preferably prior to school entry); however, if the fourth dose of the primary immunizing series was administered after the fourth birthday, a booster (fifth) dose is not necessary.
Children 7 years of age and older: Use is not recommended. Td should be administered instead.

### Strength(s) usually available

U.S.—
6.6 Lf units of diphtheria toxoid and 5 Lf units of tetanus toxoid per 0.5 mL dose (Rx) [GENERIC (may contain thimerosal)].
7.5 Lf units of diphtheria toxoid and 7.5 Lf units of tetanus toxoid per 0.5 mL dose (Rx) [GENERIC (may contain thimerosal)].
10 Lf units of diphtheria toxoid and 5 Lf units of tetanus toxoid per 0.5 mL dose (Rx) [GENERIC (may contain thimerosal)].
12.5 Lf units of diphtheria toxoid and 5 Lf units of tetanus toxoid per 0.5 mL dose (Rx) [GENERIC (may contain thimerosal)].
15 Lf units of diphtheria toxoid and 10 Lf units of tetanus toxoid per 0.5 mL dose (Rx) [GENERIC (may contain thimerosal)].
Canada—
25 Lf units of diphtheria toxoid and 5 Lf units of tetanus toxoid in each 0.5 mL dose (Rx) [GENERIC (may contain thimerosal)].

Note: Lf is the quantity of toxoid as assessed by flocculation.

### Packaging and storage

Store between 2 and 8 °C (36 and 46 °F), unless otherwise specified by manufacturer. Store away from the freezer compartment. Protect from freezing.

### Stability

Freezing destroys activity. The product should not be used if it has been exposed to freezing. In addition, the product should not be left out at room temperature (e.g., between patients).

## Auxiliary labeling
- Shake the vial vigorously immediately before each dose is withdrawn in order to resuspend the contents.
- Protect from freezing.

---

### TETANUS AND DIPHTHERIA TOXOIDS (Td)

## Summary of Differences
Indications: Tetanus and diphtheria toxoids for adult use (Td) is indicated for immunization of adults and children 7 years of age and older.

Side/adverse effects: Arthus-type reaction and fever over 39.4 °C usually occur only in patients old enough to receive Td, i.e., persons old enough to have received multiple booster doses of a tetanus toxoid–containing product.

Strength(s) usually available: Td contains 2 Lf units of diphtheria toxoid and 2 to 10 Lf units of tetanus toxoid, per dose.

## Additional Dosing Information
The concentration of diphtheria toxoid in Td, which is intended for use in persons 7 years of age and older, is lower than that of the concentration of diphtheria toxoid in diphtheria and tetanus toxoids for pediatric use (DT).

It is recommended that adults and children 7 years of age and older receive Td rather than the single-entity tetanus toxoid for the primary immunizing series, all booster doses, and active tetanus immunization in wound management. This is to help ensure protection against diphtheria infection, since a large proportion of adults is susceptible to diphtheria infection.

The primary immunizing series of Td consists of 3 doses (2 initial and 1 reinforcing) for adults and children 7 years of age and older.

## Parenteral Dosage Forms

### TETANUS AND DIPHTHERIA TOXOIDS ADSORBED FOR ADULT USE (Td) USP

**Usual adult and adolescent dose**
Diphtheria and tetanus (prophylaxis)—Intramuscular, preferably into the deltoid: 0.5 mL followed by 0.5 mL four to eight weeks later (in Canada, eight weeks later) for a total of two doses. A third dose of 0.5 mL is administered six to twelve months after the second dose. A booster dose of 0.5 mL is administered every ten years thereafter.

Note: If a booster dose of Td is administered less than ten years after the previous booster dose (e.g., as part of wound management or after exposure to diphtheria), the next booster dose should be administered ten years after the interim dose.

**Usual pediatric dose**
Diphtheria and tetanus (prophylaxis)—Intramuscular, preferably into the deltoid or the midlateral muscles of the thigh—
  Children up to 7 years of age—Use is not recommended. Diphtheria and tetanus toxoids for pediatric use (DT) should be administered instead.
  Children 7 years of age and older—See *Usual adult and adolescent dose.*

**Strength(s) usually available**
U.S.—
  2 Lf units of tetanus toxoid and 2 Lf units of diphtheria toxoid per 0.5 mL dose (Rx) [GENERIC (may contain thimerosal)].
  5 Lf units of tetanus toxoid and 2 Lf units of diphtheria toxoid per 0.5 mL dose (Rx) [GENERIC (may contain thimerosal)].
  10 Lf units of tetanus toxoid and 2 Lf units of diphtheria toxoid per 0.5 mL dose (Rx) [GENERIC (may contain thimerosal)].
Canada—
  5 Lf units of tetanus toxoid and 2 Lf units of diphtheria toxoid per 0.5 mL dose (Rx) [GENERIC (may contain thimerosal)].

Note: Lf is the quantity of toxoid as assessed by flocculation.

**Packaging and storage**
Store between 2 and 8 °C (36 and 46 °F), unless otherwise specified by manufacturer. Store away from the freezer compartment. Protect from freezing.

**Stability**
Freezing destroys activity. The product should not be used if it has been exposed to freezing. In addition, the product should not be left out at room temperature (e.g., between patients).

**Auxiliary labeling**
- Shake the vial vigorously immediately before each dose is withdrawn in order to resuspend the contents.
- Protect from freezing.

## Selected Bibliography
Centers for Disease Control and Prevention. Diphtheria, tetanus, and pertussis: recommendations for vaccine use and other preventive measures: recommendations of the Immunization Practices Advisory Committee (ACIP). MMWR 1991 Aug 8; 40(RR-10): 1-28.

Developed: 04/26/95

---

# DIPHTHERIA AND TETANUS TOXOIDS AND PERTUSSIS VACCINE ADSORBED Systemic

Note: This monograph describes diphtheria and tetanus toxoids combined with either whole-cell pertussis vaccine or acellular pertussis vaccine. The acellular pertussis-containing vaccine is indicated by the term DTaP or acellular DTP. The whole-cell pertussis-containing vaccine is indicated by the term DTwP or whole-cell DTP. For general statements, the term DTP will be used.

VA CLASSIFICATION (Primary): IM900

Commonly used brand name(s): *Acel-Imune; Tri-Immunol; Tripedia.*

Other commonly used names are acellular DTP, DTaP, DTP, DTwP, and whole-cell DTP.

Note: For a listing of dosage forms and brand names by country availability, see *Dosage Forms* section(s).

## Category
Immunizing agent (active).

## Indications
**Accepted**
Diphtheria, tetanus, and pertussis (prophylaxis)—Whole-cell DTP (DTwP) is indicated for immunization against diphtheria, tetanus, and pertussis. The Immunization Practices Advisory Committee (ACIP) recommends the use of acellular DTP (DTaP) instead of whole-cell DTP for the fourth or fifth dose of the immunization series because of a decreased incidence of side/adverse effects associated with DTaP. The main objective of DTP immunization is to prevent the severe complications, including death, that may arise from the toxins or infections associated with diphtheria, tetanus, and pertussis.

Unless otherwise contraindicated, all children from 2 months up to 7 years of age should be immunized against diphtheria, tetanus, and pertussis, including:
- Those recovering from diphtheria or tetanus. Since a diphtheria or tetanus infection may not confer immunity, active immunization should be initiated or continued at the time of recovery from the illness and the remaining doses of the primary series administered as early as possible according to the schedule of doses.
- Those recovering from a pertussis-like syndrome. Unless a pertussis diagnosis is confirmed by a culture, DTP immunization should be initiated or continued because a pertussis-like syndrome may be caused by another *Bordetella* species, a chlamydia, or a virus. Children who have recovered from a culture-confirmed pertussis infection no longer require pertussis vaccine and should be immunized with diphtheria and tetanus toxoids for pediatric use (DT) according to current labeling.
- Those who have not yet received the recommended number of doses of pertussis vaccine. DTP may be used to immunize these children as long as the total number of doses that the child receives of either the diphtheria or tetanus toxoid does not exceed 6 doses before 7 years of age. Alternatively, a single-antigen pertussis vaccine may be used to complete immunization against pertussis. In the U.S., single-antigen whole-cell pertussis vaccine is currently available only from the Biologics Products Program of the Michigan State Health Department for use within Michigan; however, the vaccine may be available for use outside Michigan under special circumstances as determined by the program.

- Close contacts, household or other, of persons with pertussis. Children who have not completed the 4-dose primary series of DTP should receive an immediate dose of DTP and should subsequently complete the primary series with the minimum recommended intervals between doses. Children who have completed the 4-dose primary series but have not received a dose of DTP within the last 3 years should receive an immediate dose of DTP.

Although some health-care providers inappropriately consider certain conditions as contraindications, the following conditions are *not* contraindications to immunization with DTP:
- Stable neurologic conditions, including well-controlled seizures.
- Resolved or corrected neurologic disorders. DTP is recommended for infants with certain neurologic problems, such as neonatal hypocalcemic tetany or hydrocephalus (following placement of shunt and without seizures), that have been corrected or have subsided without residua.
- A family history of convulsions or other CNS disorders.
- A family history of sudden-infant-death syndrome (SIDS).
- A family history of an adverse reaction to DTP.
- Premature birth. The chronological age from birth should be used for initiating immunization.

Because the incidence and severity of pertussis infection decrease with age, while the chance of side/adverse effects from the pertussis vaccine in DTP still exists, and because the chance of side/adverse effects associated with the strength of diphtheria toxoid used in DTP increases with age, immunization with DTP is not recommended for children 7 years of age and older and adults. Instead, these persons should receive periodic immunizations with tetanus and diphtheria toxoids for adult use (Td) according to current labeling.

## Pharmacology/Pharmacokinetics

### Physicochemical characteristics
Source—Whole-cell DTP vaccine consists of a mixture of the detoxified toxins (toxoids) of diphtheria and tetanus and inactivated *B. pertussis* bacteria that have been adsorbed onto an aluminum salt. The DTaP vaccine consists of a mixture of the detoxified toxins (toxoids) of diphtheria and tetanus and a detoxified acellular pertussis vaccine component, prepared from *B. pertussis* bacteria, that have been adsorbed onto an aluminum salt.

### Mechanism of action/Effect
Diphtheria—Following intramuscular injection, diphtheria toxoid induces the formation of antitoxin.
Tetanus—Following intramuscular injection, tetanus toxoid induces the formation of antitoxin.
Pertussis—Following intramuscular injection, acellular or whole-cell pertussis vaccine induces the formation of several antibodies thought to be clinically protective. The exact mechanism of protection is not known.

### Protective efficacy
Diphtheria—A serum level of antibody greater than approximately 0.01 to 0.1 diphtheria toxin neutralization unit per mL is generally considered protective.
Tetanus—Tetanus toxoid is highly effective, with a failure rate in fully immunized persons of less than 4 per 100 million. Protective levels of serum antitoxin greater than or equal to 0.01 tetanus toxin neutralization unit per mL are achieved after primary immunization with DTP.
Pertussis—Immunization with 3 or more doses of DTP induces immunity against clinical pertussis disease in 80 to 90% of susceptible persons.

### Duration of protective effect
Diphtheria—Primary immunization with DTP protects more than 95% of persons for at least 10 years.
Tetanus—Primary immunization with DTP protects 95% of persons for at least 10 years.
Pertussis—Following primary immunization with DTP vaccine, immunity to pertussis usually persists through childhood, but is thought to decrease over time. Lifelong immunity is probably attained through subsequent mild pertussis infection.

## Precautions to Consider

### Cross-sensitivity and/or related problems
Patients sensitive to diphtheria toxoid, tetanus toxoid, or acellular or whole-cell pertussis vaccine will be sensitive to DTP also.

### Pediatrics
Whole-cell DTP is recommended for children from 2 months up to 7 years of age. The Immunization Practices Advisory Committee (ACIP) recommends the use of DTaP instead of whole-cell DTP for the fourth or fifth dose of the immunization series because of a decreased incidence of side/adverse effects associated with DTaP.

The highest fatality rates from diphtheria and pertussis occur in the very young.
A history of prematurity is not a reason to defer vaccination with DTP.
If a previous dose of DTP caused an immediate anaphylactic reaction, further doses of DTP should not be administered. Because of uncertainty as to which component of the vaccine may be responsible, it is recommended that no further immunization be carried out with any of the three antigens in DTP. Alternatively, because of the importance of tetanus immunization, individuals who had this reaction should be referred for evaluation by an allergist and desensitized to tetanus toxoid if specific allergy can be demonstrated.
If a previous dose of DTP caused any of the following effects (which are most frequently assumed to be attributable to the pertussis vaccine component), subsequent immunization of children up to 7 years of age should consist of only diphtheria and tetanus toxoids for pediatric use (DT) instead of DTP:
- Collapse or shock-like state (hypotonic-hyporesponsive episode), occurring within 48 hours.
- Convulsions, with or without fever, occurring within 3 days.
- Crying, persistent and inconsolable, lasting 3 or more hours and occurring within 48 hours.
- Encephalopathy, not due to another identifiable cause. A causal relationship between DTP and permanent brain damage has not been demonstrated according to ACIP. Encephalopathy is defined as an acute, severe CNS disorder occurring within 7 days following immunization, consisting of major alterations in consciousness, unresponsiveness, generalized or focal seizures that persist more than a few hours, and failure to recover within 24 hours. Even though causation by DTP cannot be established, subsequent doses of pertussis vaccine should not be given. In addition, it may be desirable to delay administering the balance of the doses of DT necessary to complete the primary schedule so that the child's neurological status can clarify.
- Fever of 40.5 °C (105 °F) or more, occurring within 48 hours and not due to other causes.

Because the incidence and severity of pertussis infection decrease with age while the chance of side/adverse effects from the pertussis vaccine in DTP still exists, and because the chance of side/adverse effects associated with the strength of diphtheria toxoid used in DTP increases with age, immunization with DTP is not recommended for children 7 years of age and older and adults. Instead, these persons should receive periodic immunizations with tetanus and diphtheria toxoids for adult use (Td) according to current labeling.

### Drug interactions and/or related problems
The following drug interactions and/or related problems have been selected on the basis of their potential clinical significance (possible mechanism in parentheses where appropriate)—not necessarily inclusive (» = major clinical significance):

Note: Combinations containing any of the following medications, depending on the amount present, may also interact with this medication.

Immunosuppressive agents or
Radiation therapy
(because normal defense mechanisms are suppressed, concurrent use of immunosuppressive agents or radiation therapy with DTP may decrease the patient's antibody response to DTP or may result in aberrant responses to active immunization procedures. The precaution does not apply to corticosteroids used as replacement therapy, for short-term [less than 2 weeks] systemic therapy, or by other routes of administration that do not cause immunosuppression. If immunosuppressive therapy will be discontinued shortly, immunization with DTP should be deferred until the patient has discontinued therapy for 1 month; otherwise, the patient should be immunized with DTP while still undergoing therapy)

Influenza vaccine, whole or split virus
(influenza vaccine and DTP should not be administered within 3 days of one another, so that the cause of any adverse effect is clear)

### Medical considerations/Contraindications
The medical considerations/contraindications included have been selected on the basis of their potential clinical significance (reasons given in parentheses where appropriate)—not necessarily inclusive (» = major clinical significance).

*Except under special circumstances, this medication should not be used when the following medical problems exist:*
» Central nervous system (CNS) disorders, evolving or changing, whether or not the disorder is associated with seizure activity or
» Encephalopathy, progressive or
» Epilepsy, uncontrolled
(increased risk of side/adverse effects)

» Febrile illness, severe
  (to avoid confusing manifestations of illness with possible side/adverse effects of vaccine; minor illnesses, such as upper respiratory infection, do not preclude administration of vaccine)

*Risk-benefit should be considered when the following medical problems exist:*
Neurological disease, suspected
  (initiation of DTP should be delayed until there is clarification of the child's neurological status; however, the decision whether or not to commence immunization with DTP should be made by the child's first birthday. When making the decision, it should be recognized that children with severe neurological disorders may be at increased risk of pertussis because of their attendance at special schools or clinics where many of the other children attending may not be immunized. In addition, children with neurological disorders may be at increased risk from complications of pertussis)
Seizures, or family history of
  (children who have had seizures previously, either febrile or non-febrile, or who have a family history of seizures, are more likely to have seizures following DTP administration than children without such histories; however, data do not indicate that seizures that occur in the absence of other neurological reactions and that are temporally associated with DTP administration induce permanent brain damage in these children. All children with seizures should be fully evaluated to clarify their medical and neurological status before a decision is made to initiate vaccination with DTP. In addition, acetaminophen, 15 mg/kg, should be administered at the time of immunization and every 4 hours thereafter for 24 hours)
Sensitivity to diphtheria or tetanus toxoids or to pertussis vaccine

## Side/Adverse Effects

Note: DTaP causes fever less often than whole-cell DTP, and it is anticipated that adverse reactions precipitated by fever, such as febrile convulsions, will occur less often in children receiving DTaP.

Although the occurrence of sudden-infant-death syndrome (SIDS) has been related temporally to administration of DTP, studies have not found a causal relationship between DTP immunization and the syndrome.

Claims that DTP may be responsible for transverse myelitis, hyperactivity, learning disorders, infantile autism, and progressive degenerative CNS conditions have no scientific basis. In addition there is no evidence for a causal relationship between DTP immunization and hemolytic anemia or thrombocytopenic purpura.

Children who have had seizures previously, either febrile or non-febrile, or who have a family history of seizures, are more likely to have seizures following DTP administration than children without such histories. In addition, data do not indicate that seizures that occur in the absence of other neurological reactions and that are temporally associated with DTP administration induce permanent brain damage in these children.

The frequency of fever or local reactions following DTP vaccination is significantly higher with increasing numbers of doses of DTP, whereas other mild to moderate systemic reactions (e.g., vomiting or fretfulness) are significantly less frequent with increasing numbers of doses.

The following side/adverse effects have been selected on the basis of their potential clinical significance (possible signs and symptoms in parentheses where appropriate)—not necessarily inclusive:

**Those indicating need for medical attention**
Incidence rare
  *Anaphylactic reaction* (difficulty in breathing or swallowing; hives; itching, especially of soles or palms; reddening of skin, especially around ears; swelling of eyes, face, or inside of nose; unusual tiredness or weakness, sudden and severe); *convulsions, with or without fever, occurring within 3 days; crying, persistent and inconsolable, occurring within 48 hours and lasting 3 or more hours; encephalopathy, occurring within 7 days* (severe alterations in consciousness, with generalized or focal neurological signs; confusion; severe or continuing headache; unusual irritability; excessive sleepiness; severe or continuing vomiting); *fever of 40.5 °C (105 °F) or more, occurring within 48 hours; or hypotonic-hyporesponsive episode, occurring within 48 hours* (collapse or shock-like state)

**Those indicating need for medical attention only if they continue or are bothersome**
Incidence more frequent
  *Abscess or local reaction* (redness, swelling, tenderness, or pain at injection site); *fever between 38 and 39 °C (100.4 and 102.2 °F)*—usually lasting up to, but no longer than, 48 hours; may be accompanied by fretfulness, drowsiness, vomiting, and anorexia; *lump at injection site*—may be present for a few weeks after injection
Incidence less frequent
  *Fever between 39 and 40 °C (102.2 and 104 °F)*—usually lasting up to, but no longer than, 48 hours; may be accompanied by fretfulness, drowsiness, vomiting, and anorexia
Incidence rare
  *Cervical lymphadenopathy* (swollen glands on side of neck following DTP injections into arm); *fever between 40 and 40.5 °C (104 and 105 °F)*—usually lasting up to, but no longer than, 48 hours; may be accompanied by fretfulness, drowsiness, vomiting, and anorexia; *Skin rash*

## Patient Consultation

As an aid to patient consultation, refer to *Advice for the Patient, Diphtheria and Tetanus Toxoids and Pertussis Vaccine Adsorbed (Systemic)*.
In providing consultation, consider emphasizing the following selected information (» = major clinical significance):

**Before receiving this vaccine**
» Conditions affecting use, especially:
  Sensitivity to diphtheria or tetanus toxoids, pertussis vaccine, or DTP
  Other medical problems, especially evolving or changing central nervous system (CNS) disorders, whether or not the disorder is associated with seizure activity; progressive encephalopathy; uncontrolled epilepsy; or severe febrile illness

**Proper use of this vaccine**
» Proper dosing

**After receiving this vaccine**
Possibly receiving acetaminophen at time of injection; possibly continuing acetaminophen every four hours for twenty-four hours following injection; checking with physician if there are questions

**Side/adverse effects**
Notifying physician of any side effect that occurs after a dose of DTP, even though the side effect may have gone away without treatment
Signs of potential side effects, especially anaphylactic reaction; convulsions, with or without fever, occurring within 3 days; crying, persistent and inconsolable, occurring within 48 hours and lasting 3 or more hours; encephalopathy occurring within 7 days; fever of 40.5 °C (105 °F) or more, occurring within 48 hours; or hypotonic-hyporesponsive episode occurring within 48 hours

## General Dosing Information

The usual primary immunization against diphtheria, tetanus, and pertussis consists of four 0.5-mL doses of DTP. In addition, a booster dose of DTP is usually administered at 4 through 6 years of age. Either whole-cell DTP or DTaP may be used for the fourth and fifth doses. However, the Immunization Practices Advisory Committee (ACIP) recommends the use of DTaP, because it causes fewer local reactions, less fever, and fewer other common systemic adverse reactions than does the whole-cell DTP.

It is recommended that only full doses (0.5 mL) of DTP be administered. Concern about adverse reactions have led some health care professionals to administer reduced doses of DTP. However, no evidence indicates that decreased doses will decrease the frequency of severe adverse effects. In addition, protection may be compromised.

It is usually recommended that immunization against diphtheria, tetanus, and pertussis be initiated at 2 months of age. However, some sources recommend initiating the DTP series at the infant's 6-week checkup. In addition, pertussis outbreaks may warrant administering the first 3 doses at 6, 10, and 14 weeks of age to provide protection as early as possible.

DTP should be administered by deep intramuscular injection, preferably into the midlateral muscles of the thigh in infants or into the deltoid in children. Each of the 4 primary immunizing doses of DTP should be injected at a different site.

Before each additional dose of DTP, the health status of the child should be reassessed. In addition, information should be obtained regarding any symptom and/or sign of an adverse reaction after the previous dose.

Delay, of any length, in the recommended interval of doses does not interfere with the final immunity achieved and does not require starting the series over again. If a delay occurs, series should be resumed as soon as possible and the doses continued at the recommended intervals, until the total number of doses required is administered.

Although the fourth dose of DTP and the third dose of oral polio vaccine (OPV) have traditionally been administered to children 18 months of age and measles, mumps, and rubella vaccine (MMR) has traditionally been administered to children 15 months of age, it is now recommended that DTP, OPV, and MMR be administered concurrently to children 15 months of age. MMR should not be postponed in order to administer these vaccines concurrently at 18 months of age. In addition, the traditional method is still an acceptable alternative.

Persons infected with human immunodeficiency virus (HIV) may receive DTP whether they have asymptomatic or symptomatic HIV infection.

Diphtheria toxoid, tetanus toxoid, and pertussis vaccine (whole-cell DTP or DTaP), can be administered concurrently with the following, using separate body sites and separate syringes (for parenterals), and the precautions that apply to each immunizing agent:
- Polysaccharide vaccines, such as haemophilus b polysaccharide vaccine, haemophilus b conjugate vaccine, meningococcal polysaccharide vaccine, or pneumococcal polyvalent vaccine.
- Live virus vaccines, such as measles, mumps, rubella, and/or oral polio vaccine (OPV).
- Inactivated poliovirus vaccine (IPV) or enhanced-potency inactivated vaccine (enhanced-potency IPV).
- Hepatitis B recombinant or plasma-derived vaccine.
- Inactivated vaccines, other, except cholera, typhoid (parenteral), and plague. It is recommended that cholera, typhoid (parenteral), and plague vaccines be administered on separate occasions because of these vaccines' propensity to cause side/adverse effects.

Continued use of this medication is contraindicated, according to ACIP, when the following medical problems occur:
- Anaphylactic reaction, immediate (because of uncertainty as to which component of the vaccine may be responsible, it is recommended that no further immunization be carried out with any of the three antigens in DTP. Alternatively, because of the importance of tetanus immunization, such individuals should be referred for evaluation by an allergist and desensitized to tetanus toxoid if specific allergy can be demonstrated).
- Encephalopathy, not due to another identifiable cause (a causal relation between DTP and permanent brain damage has not been demonstrated according to ACIP. Encephalopathy is defined as an acute, severe CNS disorder occurring within 7 days following immunization, consisting of major alterations in consciousness, unresponsiveness, generalized or focal seizures that persist more than a few hours, and failure to recover within 24 hours. Even though causation by DTP cannot be established, subsequent doses of pertussis vaccine should not be given. In addition, it may be desirable to delay administering the balance of the doses of DT necessary to complete the primary schedule so that the child's neurological status can clarify).

Continued use of the pertussis component of this medication, either whole-cell or acellular, should be carefully considered when the following medical problems occur in temporal relation to administration of DTP:
- Convulsions, with or without fever, occurring within 3 days.
- Crying, persistent and inconsolable, lasting 3 or more hours and occurring within 48 hours.
- Fever ≥ 40.5 °C (105 °F) occurring within 48 hours and not due to other causes.
- Hypotonic-hyporesponsive episode (collapse or shock-like state) occurring within 48 hours.

Continued use of this medication should be carefully considered when the following medical problem occurs:
- Neurological event occurring between doses of DTP but not temporally associated (if the child is under 1 year of age and has not received all 3 doses of the primary series, further doses of DTP should be deferred until there is clarification of the child's neurological status; however, the decision whether or not to continue immunization with DTP should be made no later than the child's first birthday and should be based on the nature of the neurological event and the risk/benefit associated with the vaccine. If the child is over 1 year of age, the child's neurological status should be evaluated to ensure that the disorder is stable before immunization with DTP is continued).

### For treatment of adverse effects
Recommended treatment includes:
- For mild hypersensitivity reaction—Administering antihistamines, and, if necessary, glucocorticoids.
- For severe hypersensitivity or anaphylactic reaction—Administering epinephrine. Antihistamines or glucocorticoids may also be administered as required.

## Parenteral Dosage Forms

### DIPHTHERIA AND TETANUS TOXOIDS AND ACELLULAR PERTUSSIS VACCINE ADSORBED

**Usual adult and adolescent dose**
Use is not recommended.

Note: Diphtheria toxoid of the strength used in DTP is not recommended for adults, because of the increased risk of side/adverse effects associated with the use of higher doses of diphtheria toxoid in adults. In addition, at the present time, acellular pertussis vaccine is not recommended for adults. Instead, tetanus and diphtheria toxoids for adult use (Td) should be administered according to its current labeling.

**Usual pediatric dose**
Children 2 to 15 months of age—
Use is not recommended. Whole-cell DTP should be administered instead.

Children 15 months up to 7 years of age who have previously been immunized with three or four doses of whole-cell DTP vaccine—
Intramuscular, 0.5 mL, preferably into the midlateral muscles of the thigh or deltoid, according to one of the following schedules:
If three previous doses of whole-cell DTP have been administered:
One dose at fifteen to eighteen months of age, but not less than six months after the previous dose, followed by another dose at four to six years of age.
If four previous doses of whole-cell DTP have been administered and the fourth dose was administered before the fourth birthday:
One dose at four to six years of age.
Note: If the fourth dose of whole-cell DTP was administered after the fourth birthday, no additional dose is necessary.
If pertussis vaccine is contraindicated in a child under seven years of age, DTP should not be administered. Instead, diphtheria and tetanus toxoids for pediatric use (DT) should be administered according to its current labeling.

Children 7 years of age and older—
Use is not recommended.

Note: Diphtheria toxoid of the strength used in DTP is not recommended for children seven years of age and older, because of the increased risk of side/adverse effects associated with the use of higher doses of diphtheria toxoid in older children. In addition, at the present time, acellular pertussis vaccine is not recommended for children seven years of age and older. Instead, tetanus and diphtheria toxoids for adult use (Td) should be administered according to its current labeling.

**Strength(s) usually available**
U.S.—
6.7 Lf of diphtheria toxoid, 5 Lf of tetanus toxoid, 23.4 mcg protein of filamentous hemagglutinin (FHA), and 23.4 mcg protein of inactivated pertussis toxin (PT) (toxoid), in each 0.5-mL dose. Each 0.5-mL dose contains aluminum present as aluminum potassium sulfate (Rx) [*Tripedia* (thimerosal 1:10,000)].
7.5 Lf of diphtheria toxoid, 5 Lf of tetanus toxoid, and 300 hemagglutinating (HA) units of acellular pertussis vaccine, in each 0.5-mL dose. The acellular pertussis vaccine component contains approximately 40 mcg of pertussis antigens (approximately 86% filamentous hemagglutinin [FHA], approximately 8% lymphocytosis-promoting factor [LPF], approximately 4% 69-kilodalton [69kd] outer membrane protein, and approximately 2% type 2 fimbriae [pertussis-specific agglutinogen]), in each 0.5-mL dose. Each 0.5-mL dose contains not more than 850 mcg (0.85 mg) of aluminum present as aluminum hydroxide and aluminum phosphate (Rx) [*Acel-Imune* (thimerosal 1:10,000)].

Canada—
Not commercially available.

Note: Lf is the quantity of toxoid as assessed by flocculation.
A hemagglutinating (HA) unit is that amount of material that completely agglutinates chicken red blood cells as measured by the HA assay.

**Packaging and storage**
Store between 2 and 8 °C (36 and 46 °F), unless otherwise specified by manufacturer. Protect from freezing.

**Preparation of dosage form**
The product should be shaken well immediately before withdrawing each dose, to obtain a uniform suspension. The product should be discarded if it has remaining clumps after vigorous agitation.

**Stability**
The vaccine should be kept refrigerated, but should not be frozen, exposed to freezing temperatures, or stored near freezing surfaces.

**Auxiliary labeling**
- Shake well.
- Do not freeze.

# DIPHTHERIA AND TETANUS TOXOIDS AND PERTUSSIS VACCINE ADSORBED USP

**Usual adult and adolescent dose**
Use is not recommended.

Note: Diphtheria toxoid of the strength used in DTP is not recommended for adults, because of the increased risk of side/adverse effects associated with the use of higher doses of diphtheria toxoid in adults. In addition, whole-cell pertussis vaccine is not recommended for adults, because the incidence and severity of pertussis infection decrease with age, while the chance of side/adverse effects from the pertussis vaccine still exists. Instead, tetanus and diphtheria toxoids for adult use (Td) should be administered according to its current labeling.

**Usual pediatric dose**
Children 2 months up to 7 years of age—
Intramuscular, preferably into the midlateral muscles of the thigh or deltoid, 0.5 mL at four- to eight-week intervals for three doses, followed by a fourth dose of 0.5 mL six to twelve months after the third dose. A booster (fifth) dose of 0.5 mL is usually administered at four through six years of age; however, if the fourth dose of the basic immunizing series was administered after the fourth birthday, a booster (fifth) dose is not necessary.

Note: Pertussis outbreaks may warrant administering the first three doses at six, ten, and fourteen weeks of age to provide protection as early as possible.

If the child is over one year of age at the time the third dose is due, the third dose should be administered six to twelve months (instead of the usual four to eight weeks) after the second dose, and the fourth dose should be omitted. The booster dose should be administered as usual.

DTaP is recommended for use instead of whole-cell DTP for the fourth or fifth dose of the immunization series.

If pertussis vaccine is contraindicated in a child under seven years of age, DTP should not be used. Instead, diphtheria and tetanus toxoids for pediatric use (DT) should be administered according to its current labeling.

Children 7 years of age and older—
Use is not recommended.

Note: Diphtheria toxoid of the strength used in DTP is not recommended for children seven years of age and older, because of the increased risk of side/adverse effects associated with the use of higher doses of diphtheria toxoid in older children. In addition, whole-cell pertussis vaccine is not recommended for children seven years of age and older, because the incidence and severity of pertussis infection decrease with age, while the chance of side/adverse effects from the pertussis vaccine still exists. Instead, tetanus and diphtheria toxoids for adult use (Td) should be administered according to its current labeling.

**Strength(s) usually available**
U.S.—
- 12.5 Lf of diphtheria toxoid aluminum phosphate adsorbed, 5 Lf of tetanus toxoid aluminum phosphate adsorbed, and 4 Protective Units of pertussis vaccine, in each 0.5-mL dose. Each 0.5-mL dose contains not more than 800 mcg (0.8 mg) of aluminum (Rx) [*Tri-Immunol* (thimerosal 1:10,000)].
- 6.7 Lf of diphtheria toxoid aluminum potassium sulfate adsorbed, 5 Lf of tetanus toxoid aluminum potassium sulfate adsorbed, and 4 Protective Units of pertussis vaccine, in each 0.5-mL dose. Each 0.5-mL dose may contain not more than 250 mcg (0.25 mg) of aluminum in the form of aluminum potassium sulfate (Rx) [GENERIC (may contain thimerosal)].

Canada—
- 12.5 Lf of diphtheria toxoid aluminum phosphate adsorbed, 5 Lf of tetanus toxoid aluminum phosphate adsorbed, and 4 Protective Units of pertussis vaccine, in each 0.5-mL dose. Each 0.5-mL dose contains not more than 800 mcg (0.8 mg) of aluminum (Rx) [*Tri-Immunol* (thimerosal 1:10,000)].
- 25 Lf of diphtheria toxoid aluminum phosphate adsorbed, 5 Lf of tetanus toxoid aluminum phosphate adsorbed, and 4 to 12 Protective Units of pertussis vaccine, in each 0.5-mL dose. Each 0.5-mL dose may contain 1.5 mg of aluminum phosphate (Rx) [GENERIC (may contain thimerosal)].

Note: Lf is the quantity of toxoid as assessed by flocculation.

**Packaging and storage**
Store between 2 and 8 °C (36 and 46 °F), unless otherwise specified by manufacturer. Protect from freezing.

**Preparation of dosage form**
The product should be shaken well immediately before withdrawing each dose, since product contains a bacterial suspension and vigorous agitation may be necessary to resuspend the contents of the vial. The product should be discarded if it has remaining clumps after vigorous agitation.

**Stability**
The vaccine should be refrigerated, but should not be frozen, exposed to freezing temperatures, or stored near freezing surfaces. If the vaccine is stored at temperatures below 2 °C (36 °F) or above 25 °C (77 °F) for as little as 24 hours, or if the vaccine is exposed to freezing temperatures or stored near freezing surfaces, subsequent resuspension of the vaccine may be difficult or impossible. Vaccine should not be used if resuspension without any visible clumps cannot be achieved by vigorous shaking.

**Auxiliary labeling**
- Shake well.
- Do not freeze.

Revised: 06/09/93
Interim revision: 03/29/94

---

# DIPHTHERIA AND TETANUS TOXOIDS AND PERTUSSIS VACCINE ADSORBED AND HAEMOPHILUS B CONJUGATE VACCINE   Systemic

This monograph includes information on the following: 1) Diphtheria and tetanus toxoids combined with whole-cell pertussis vaccine and Haemophilus b conjugate vaccine (HbOC—diphtheria CRM197 protein conjugate); 2) Diphtheria and tetanus toxoids combined with whole-cell pertussis vaccine and Haemophilus b conjugate vaccine (PRP-D—diphtheria toxoid conjugate)*.

VA CLASSIFICATION (Primary): IM900

Commonly used brand name(s): *DPT-Hib; Tetramune.*

Other commonly used names are:
DTP-HbOC [Diphtheria and tetanus toxoids combined with whole-cell pertussis vaccine and Haemophilus b conjugate vaccine (HbOC—diphtheria CRM$_{197}$ protein conjugate)]
DTP-Hib [Diphtheria and tetanus toxoids combined with whole-cell pertussis vaccine and Haemophilus b conjugate vaccine (HbOC—diphtheria CRM$_{197}$ protein conjugate)] or [Diphtheria and tetanus toxoids combined with whole-cell pertussis vaccine and Haemophilus b conjugate vaccine (PRP-D—diphtheria toxoid conjugate)]
DTP-PRP-D [Diphtheria and tetanus toxoids combined with whole-cell pertussis vaccine and Haemophilus b conjugate vaccine (PRP-D—diphtheria toxoid conjugate)]

Note: For a listing of dosage forms and brand names by country availability, see *Dosage Forms* section(s).

*Not commercially available in U.S.

## Category
Immunizing agent (active).

## Indications

**Accepted**
Diphtheria, tetanus, pertussis, and *Haemophilus influenzae* type b diseases (prophylaxis)—Diphtheria and tetanus toxoids and pertussis vaccine adsorbed and Haemophilus b conjugate vaccine combination (DTP-Hib) is indicated for immunization against the diseases caused by diphtheria, tetanus, pertussis, and *Haemophilus influenzae* type b organisms in infants and children up to 5 years of age when the schedules for immunization with the separate vaccines, diphtheria and tetanus toxoids and pertussis vaccine (DTP) and Haemophilus b conjugate vaccine (Hib), coincide.

## Pharmacology/Pharmacokinetics

### Physicochemical characteristics
Source—
  Diphtheria and tetanus: Diphtheria toxoid is prepared from *Corynebacterium diphtheriae* toxin and tetanus toxoid is prepared from *Clostridium tetani* toxin. Both toxins are detoxified with formaldehyde. The toxoids are adsorbed onto aluminum phosphate.
  Pertussis: Pertussis vaccine is prepared from *Bordetella pertussis* bacteria, which are inactivated with thimerosal.
  Haemophilus b: Purified capsular polysaccharide, a polymer of ribose, ribitol, and phosphate (PRP), is derived from the bacterium *Haemophilus influenzae* type b. It is conjugated in one of the following ways
    For the diphtheria $CRM_{197}$ protein conjugate: Oligosaccharides are derived from the polysaccharide and bound directly to $CRM_{197}$ (a nontoxic variant of diphtheria toxin) by reductive amination.
    For the diphtheria toxoid conjugate: The polysaccharide is conjugated to the diphtheria toxoid via a 6-carbon linker molecule.

### Mechanism of action/Effect
Diphtheria—Following intramuscular injection, diphtheria toxoid induces the formation of diphtheria antitoxin.
Tetanus—Following intramuscular injection, tetanus toxoid induces the formation of tetanus antitoxin.
Pertussis—Following intramuscular injection, pertussis vaccine induces the formation of several antibodies thought to be clinically protective. The exact mechanism of protection is not known.
Haemophilus b—*Haemophilus influenzae* type b (Hib) bacteria are surrounded by polysaccharide capsules, which make these bacteria resistant to attack by white blood cells. The vaccine, which is derived from the purified polysaccharide from Hib cells, stimulates production of anticapsular antibodies and provides active immunity to the Hib bacteria. Whereas the nonconjugated polysaccharide vaccine predominantly stimulates B-cells to produce antibodies (known as being T-cell independent), Haemophilus b conjugate vaccine stimulates T-cells also. The additional stimulation of T-cells (known as being T-cell dependent) is particularly important in young children to ensure an adequate and persistent antibody response. Stimulation of T-cells also results in an anamnestic response to future doses of the conjugate or nonconjugate vaccine and to future natural exposure to Hib, resulting in elevated antibody titers.

### Protective effect
Diphtheria—The protective titer of diphtheria antitoxin in serum is considered to be 0.01 unit per mL.
Tetanus—The protective titer of tetanus antitoxin in serum is considered to be 0.01 unit per mL.
Pertussis—The potency of the inactivated *B. pertussis* cells in the vaccine is assayed by comparison with the U.S. standard pertussis vaccine in the intracerebral mouse protection test. The protective efficacy of pertussis vaccines for humans has been shown to correlate with the measure of vaccine potency.
Haemophilus b—Antibody response to Haemophilus b conjugate vaccine is age related in children, with the immune response improving with increasing age. The titer of antibody from Haemophilus b conjugate vaccine required for protection against invasive disease has not been clearly established. However, in studies using Haemophilus b polysaccharide vaccine, a geometric mean titer (GMT) of 1 mcg per mL of serum 3 weeks after immunization correlated with protection and suggests long-term protection from invasive disease.

### Duration of protective effect
Diphtheria—At least 10 years for diphtheria toxoid following a completed primary immunizing series of injections.
Tetanus—At least 10 years for tetanus toxoid following a completed primary immunizing series of injections.
Pertussis—Following a completed primary immunizing series of injections, immunity to pertussis usually persists throughout childhood, but is thought to decrease over time. Lifelong immunity is probably attained through subsequent mild pertussis infection.
Haemophilus b—The duration of immunity is unknown.

## Precautions to Consider

### Cross-sensitivity and/or related problems
Patients sensitive to diphtheria or tetanus toxoid, whole cell or acellular pertussis vaccine, Haemophilus b polysaccharide vaccine, or any type of Haemophilus b conjugate vaccine may be sensitive to diphtheria and tetanus toxoids and pertussis vaccine adsorbed and Haemophilus b conjugate vaccine combination (DTP-Hib) also.

### Carcinogenicity/Mutagenicity
Studies have not been done.

### Pregnancy/Reproduction
Fertility—Studies have not been done.
Pregnancy—Studies have not been done in humans. DTP-Hib is not recommended for use in persons 7 years of age or older.
Studies have not been done in animals.
FDA Pregnancy Category C.

### Pediatrics
Safety and efficacy have not been established for children younger than 6 weeks of age for DTP-Hib (HbOC—diphtheria $CRM_{197}$ protein conjugate) or younger than 18 months of age for DTP-Hib (PRP-D—diphtheria toxoid conjugate). DTP-Hib is not recommended for use in children 7 years of age or older. (The DTP component is not recommended for use in persons 7 years of age or older, because of the increased risk of side/adverse reactions; the Hib component is not recommended for use in persons 5 years of age or older, except for patients with certain chronic conditions associated with an increased risk of Hib disease.)
Immunization with DTP-Hib is *contraindicated* if a previous immunization with a DTP- or pertussis-containing vaccine was temporally related to an immediate anaphylactic reaction or encephalopathy occurring within 7 days after immunization. See also *General Dosing Information*.
Although the following events *were* considered contraindications in previous recommendations of the Advisory Committee of Immunization Practices (ACIP) of the Centers for Disease Control and Prevention (CDC), they are now considered *precautions*. Immunization with DTP-Hib should be carefully considered if a previous immunization with a DTP- or pertussis-containing vaccine was temporally related to fever of ≥ 40.5 °C (105 °F) occurring within 48 hours; hypotonic-hyporesponsive episode (collapse or shock-like state) occurring within 48 hours; persistent and inconsolable crying lasting 3 or more hours and occurring within 48 hours; or seizures with or without fever occurring within 3 days. See also *General Dosing Information*.

### Drug interactions and/or related problems
The following drug interactions and/or related problems have been selected on the basis of their potential clinical significance (possible mechanism in parentheses where appropriate)—not necessarily inclusive (» = major clinical significance):

Note:  Combinations containing any of the following medications, depending on the amount present, may also interact with this vaccine.

Immunosuppressive agents
Radiation therapy
  (because normal defense mechanisms are suppressed by immunosuppressive agents or radiation treatment, the patient's antibody response to DTP-Hib may be decreased. If possible, children who are to undergo therapy with agents that cause immunosuppression, including treatment for Hodgkin's disease, should receive the vaccine at least 10 days, and preferably more than 14 days, before receiving the immunosuppressive agent; otherwise, it may be preferable to postpone the immunization until after the immunosuppressive therapy is completed. The interval between discontinuation of therapy that causes immunosuppression and the restoration of the patient's ability to respond to an active immunizing agent depends on the intensity and type of immunosuppressive therapy used, the underlying disease, and other factors; estimates vary from 3 months to 1 year. The precaution does not apply to corticosteroids used as replacement therapy, for short-term [less than 2 weeks] systemic therapy, or by other routes of administration that do not cause immunosuppression)

### Laboratory value alterations
The following have been selected on the basis of their potential clinical significance (possible effect in parentheses where appropriate)—not necessarily inclusive (» = major clinical significance):

With diagnostic test results
  Antigen detection tests
    (there is a possibility that the conjugate vaccine may interfere with interpretation of antigen detection tests, such as latex agglutination and countercurrent immunoelectrophoresis, that are used for diagnosis of systemic Hib disease. For example, purified capsular polysaccharide [a polymer of ribose, ribitol, and phosphate (PRP)], which is associated with Haemophilus b vaccines, was detected in the urine of some persons for up to 7 days following immunization with an Haemophilus b vaccine conjugated with meningococcal protein [PRP-OMP])

### Medical considerations/Contraindications
The medical considerations/contraindications included have been selected on the basis of their potential clinical significance (reasons given in parentheses where appropriate)—not necessarily inclusive (» = major clinical significance).

*Except under special circumstances, this vaccine should not be used when the following medical problems exist:*

» Central nervous system (CNS) disorders, evolving or changing, whether or not the disorder is associated with seizure activity
(there appears to be an increased risk of the appearance of manifestations of the underlying neurological disorder within 2 or 3 days after immunization. This may lead to confusion in interpretation of the neurological disorder. However, prolonged manifestations, increased progression, or exacerbation of the disorder has not been identified)

» Febrile illness or
» Infection, acute
(administration of DTP-Hib should be postponed until the acute symptoms of the patient's illness have abated to avoid confusing the symptoms of the illness with the side effects of the vaccine; however, minor illnesses, such as mild upper-respiratory infections with or without low-grade fever are not contraindications)

» Sensitivity to DTP-Hib

*Risk-benefit should be considered when the following medical problems exist:*

Neurological disease, suspected
(initiation of DTP, but not other childhood vaccines, should be delayed until there is clarification of the child's neurological status; however, the decision whether or not to commence immunization with DTP should be made by the child's first birthday. When making the decision, it should be recognized that neurologically disabled children may be at increased risk of pertussis because of their attendance at special schools or clinics where many of the other children attending may not be immunized. In addition, neurologically disabled children may be at increased risk from complications of pertussis)
(See also *General Dosing Information*.)

Seizures
(children who have had seizures prior to DTP administration, whether febrile or afebrile, appear to be more likely to have seizures following DTP immunization than children without such histories. However, current evidence indicates that seizures following DTP immunization do not cause permanent brain damage. A seizure occurring within 3 days of DTP immunization in a child with a history of seizures may be initiated by vaccine-induced fever in a child prone to febrile seizures, induced by the pertussis component, or unrelated to the vaccine. Therefore, it is prudent to delay DTP immunization in infants and children with a history of seizures until the child's status has been fully assessed and the condition has been stabilized. However, it should be noted that delaying DTP immunization until the second 6 months of life will increase the risk of febrile seizures among predisposed children. Children with a history of seizures should be given acetaminophen, 15 mg per kg of body weight (mg/kg), at the time of immunization and every 4 hours for the next 24 hours)
(See also *General Dosing Information*.)

Seizures or other CNS disorders, family history of
(children with a family history of seizures or other CNS disorders appear to be more likely to have seizures following DTP immunization than do children without such histories; however, these seizures are usually caused by fever. Acetaminophen, 15 mg/kg, should be given to these children at the time of immunization and every 4 hours for the next 24 hours)

Sensitivity to thimerosal

## Side/Adverse Effects

Note: Children who have had seizures previously, whether febrile or afebrile, appear to be more likely to have seizures following a diphtheria and tetanus toxoids and pertussis vaccine (DTP)–containing immunization than children without such histories. However, current evidence indicates that seizures following a DTP-containing immunization do not cause permanent brain damage. See also *General Dosing Information*.

Fever that does not begin until 24 or more hours after immunization or persists for more than 24 hours after immunization should not be assumed to be due to a DTP-containing immunization.

The following side/adverse effects have been selected on the basis of their potential clinical significance (possible signs and symptoms in parentheses where appropriate)—not necessarily inclusive:

**Those indicating need for medical attention**
Incidence rare
*Anaphylactic reaction* (difficulty in breathing or swallowing; hives; itching, especially of soles or palms; reddening of skin, especially around ears; swelling of eyes, face, or inside of nose; unusual tiredness or weakness, sudden and severe); *convulsions, with or without fever, occurring within 3 days; crying, persistent and inconsolable, occurring within 48 hours and lasting 3 or more hours; encephalopathy, occurring within 7 days* (severe alterations in consciousness, with generalized or focal neurological signs; confusion; severe or continuing headache; unusual and continuing irritability; excessive sleepiness; severe or continuing vomiting); *fever of 40.5 °C (105 °F) or more, occurring within 48 hours; hypotonic-hyporesponsive episode, occurring within 48 hours* (collapse or shock-like state)

**Those indicating need for medical attention only if they continue or are bothersome**
Incidence more frequent
*Drowsiness; erythema, swelling, or warm feeling at injection site* (redness, swelling, or warm feeling at place of injection); *fever up to 39 °C (102.2 °F)*—usually lasting up to, but no longer than, 48 hours; may be accompanied by fretfulness, drowsiness, vomiting, and anorexia; *fretfulness; irritability; lump at injection site*—may be present for a few weeks after injection; *pain or tenderness at injection site*

Incidence less frequent
*Anorexia* (loss of appetite); *diarrhea; fever between 39 and 40 °C (102.2 and 104 °F)*—usually lasting up to, but no longer than, 48 hours; may be accompanied by fretfulness, drowsiness, vomiting, and anorexia; *induration at injection site* (hard lump)—may be present for a few days after injection; *vomiting*

Incidence rare
*Abscess, sterile* (redness, swelling, tenderness, or pain at injection site); *fever between 40 and 40.4 °C (104 and 104.8 °F)*—usually lasting up to, but no longer than, 48 hours; may be accompanied by fretfulness, drowsiness, vomiting, and anorexia; incidence 1 to 5%; *lethargy* (lack of interest; reduced physical activity); *skin rash*

## Patient Consultation

As an aid to patient consultation, refer to *Advice for the Patient, Diphtheria and Tetanus Toxoids and Pertussis Vaccine Adsorbed and Haemophilus b Conjugate Vaccine (Systemic)*.

In providing consultation, consider emphasizing the following selected information (» = major clinical significance):

**Before receiving this vaccine**
» Conditions affecting use, especially:
Sensitivity to diphtheria or tetanus toxoid, whole cell or acellular pertussis vaccine, Haemophilus b polysaccharide vaccine, any type of Haemophilus b conjugate vaccine, or thimerosal
Use in children—Safety and efficacy have not been established for children younger than 6 weeks of age (administration usually begins at 2 months of age); not recommended for use in children 7 years of age or older
Other medical problems, especially acute infection; evolving or changing central nervous system (CNS) disorders, whether or not the disorder is associated with seizure activity; or febrile illness

**Proper use of this vaccine**
» Proper dosing

**After receiving this vaccine**
Possibly receiving acetaminophen at time of injection; possibly continuing acetaminophen every 4 hours for 24 hours following injection; checking with physician if there are questions
Possibility of vaccine interfering with laboratory tests that check for Hib disease; informing physician of recent DTP-Hib vaccination if treated for a severe infection within 2 weeks after administration

**Side/adverse effects**
Signs of potential side effects, especially anaphylactic reaction; convulsions, with or without fever, occurring within 3 days; crying, persistent and inconsolable, occurring within 48 hours and lasting 3 or more hours; encephalopathy, occurring within 7 days; fever of 40.5 °C (105 °F) or more, occurring within 48 hours; and hypotonic-hyporesponsive episode, occurring within 48 hours

## General Dosing Information

Diphtheria and tetanus toxoids and pertussis vaccine adsorbed and Haemophilus b conjugate vaccine combination (DTP-Hib) is not recommended for use in persons 7 years of age or older. (The DTP component is not recommended for use in persons 7 years of age or older, because of the increased risk of side/adverse reactions; the Hib component is not recommended for use in persons 5 years of age or older, except for patients with certain chronic conditions associated with an increased risk of Hib disease.)

DTP-Hib vaccine may be administered concurrently with the following, using separate body sites and syringes for the parenterals, and the precautions that apply to each immunizing agent:
- Hepatitis B recombinant or plasma-derived vaccine.
- Influenza virus vaccine. In the past it was recommended that influenza virus vaccine and a pertussis-containing vaccine should not be administered within 3 days of one another. Since both influenza virus vaccine and pertussis vaccine may cause febrile reactions in young children, the time interval was recommended so that the cause of any adverse effect was clear. However, the American Academy of Pediatrics (AAP) now accepts concurrent administration of these vaccines.
- Measles, mumps, and rubella vaccine (MMR).
- Poliovirus vaccines (oral [OPV], inactivated [IPV], or enhanced-potency inactivated [enhanced-potency IPV]).

Preterm infants should be immunized according to their chronological age from birth.

Continued use of this vaccine is *contraindicated because of its DTP component*, according to the Advisory Committee Immunization Practices (ACIP), when the following medical problems occur:
- Anaphylactic reaction, immediate. Because of uncertainty as to which component of the vaccine may be responsible, it is recommended that no further immunization be carried out with any of the three antigens in DTP. Alternatively, because of the importance of tetanus immunization, such individuals should be referred to an allergist for evaluation and desensitized to tetanus toxoid if specific allergy can be demonstrated.
- Encephalopathy, not due to another identifiable cause. Encephalopathy is defined as an acute, severe CNS disorder occurring within 7 days following immunization and generally consisting of major alterations in consciousness, unresponsiveness, generalized or focal seizures that persist more than a few hours, and failure to recover within 24 hours. Even though causation by DTP cannot be established, subsequent doses of the pertussis component should not be given. In addition, it may be desirable to delay for a period of months so that the child's neurological status can clarify before continuing the immunization series with diphtheria and tetanus toxoids combination (DT) instead of DTP.

Although the following events *were* considered contraindications to continued use of pertussis vaccine, in previous ACIP recommendations, they are now considered *precautions*. There may be circumstances, such as a high incidence of pertussis in the community, in which the potential benefits outweigh possible risks, particularly since these events are not associated with permanent sequelae. Therefore, continued use of this vaccine should be *carefully considered because of its pertussis component* when the following medical problems occur:
- Fever ≥ 40.5 °C (105 °F) occurring within 48 hours and not due to other causes. This is considered a precaution because of the likelihood that fever following a subsequent dose of DTP vaccine also will be high. Because such febrile reactions are usually attributed to the pertussis component, the immunization series should be continued with DT.
- Hypotonic-hyporesponsive episode (collapse or shock-like state) occurring within 48 hours. Although these uncommon events have not been recognized to cause death or to induce permanent neurological sequelae, it is prudent to omit the pertussis component and continue the immunization series with DT.
- Persistent and inconsolable crying lasting 3 or more hours and occurring within 48 hours. Follow-up of infants who have cried inconsolably following DTP immunization has indicated that this reaction is without long-term sequelae and is not associated with other reactions of greater significance. Inconsolable crying occurs most frequently following the first dose of DTP. However, crying for longer than 30 minutes following a DTP injection can be a predictor of increased likelihood of persistent crying following subsequent doses. Children who react with persistent crying have had a higher rate of substantial local reactions than did children who had other DTP-associated reactions (including high fever, seizures, and hypotonic-hyporesponsive episodes), suggesting that prolonged crying was really a pain reaction.
- Seizures, with or without fever, occurring within 3 days. Short-lived seizures, with or without fever, have not been shown to cause permanent sequelae. Furthermore, the occurrence of prolonged febrile seizures (i.e., status epilepticus, defined as any seizure lasting longer than 30 minutes or recurrent seizures lasting a total of 30 minutes without the child fully regaining consciousness), irrespective of their cause, involving an otherwise normal child does not substantially increase the risk for subsequent febrile (brief or prolonged) or afebrile seizures. The risk is significantly increased only among those children who are neurologically abnormal before their episode of status epilepticus. Accordingly, although a seizure following DTP immunization previously has been considered a contraindication to further doses of the pertussis component, under certain circumstances subsequent doses may be indicated, particularly if the risk of pertussis in the community is high. If a child has a seizure following the first or second dose of DTP, it is desirable to delay subsequent doses until the child's neurologic status is better defined. By the child's first birthday, the presence of an underlying neurologic disorder has usually been determined. A decision should be made whether to continue with DTP instead of automatically switching to DT. Regardless of whether DTP or DT is chosen, acetaminophen, 15 mg per kg of body weight (mg/kg), should be given at the time of immunization and every 4 hours for the next 24 hours.

Continued use of this vaccine *should be carefully considered because of its DTP component* if a neurological event (e.g., seizure) occurs between doses of, but not temporally associated with, this vaccine. If the event occurs before the child's first birthday and the child has not received all 3 doses of the primary DTP series, further doses of DTP, but not other childhood vaccines, should be deferred until there is clarification of the child's neurological status; however, the decision whether or not to continue immunization with DTP should be made no later than the child's first birthday and should be based on the nature of the neurological event and the risk/benefit associated with the vaccine. If the event occurs after the child's first birthday, the child's neurological status should be evaluated to ensure that the disorder is stable before immunization with DTP is continued. See also *Medical considerations/Contraindications*.

Children with stable neurologic conditions, including well-controlled seizures, may be immunized with a DTP-containing vaccine. The occurrence of a single seizure that is not temporally associated with DTP does not contraindicate DTP immunization, particularly if the seizure can be explained. Parents of children with histories of seizures should be informed of the increased risk of postimmunization seizures. In addition, acetaminophen, 15 mg/kg, should be given at the time of immunization and every 4 hours for the next 24 hours to reduce the possibility of postimmunization fever. See also *Medical considerations/Contraindications*.

Immunization with a DTP-containing vaccine is recommended for children with certain neurologic problems, such as hydrocephalus (following placement of a shunt and if the child is without seizures) or neonatal hypocalcemic tetany, that have been corrected or have clearly subsided without residua.

Before each additional dose of DTP-Hib, the health status of the patient should be assessed. In addition, information should be obtained regarding any symptom or sign of an adverse reaction that occurred after the previous dose.

If tetanus immune globulin (TIG) or diphtheria antitoxin is being administered at the same time as DTP-Hib, separate body sites and separate syringes should be used.

**For treatment of adverse effects**
Recommended treatment includes:
- For mild hypersensitivity reaction—Administering antihistamines, and, if necessary, glucocorticoids.
- For severe hypersensitivity or anaphylactic reaction—Administering epinephrine. Antihistamines or glucocorticoids may also be administered as required.

---

### DIPHTHERIA AND TETANUS TOXOIDS AND PERTUSSIS VACCINE ADSORBED AND HAEMOPHILUS B CONJUGATE VACCINE (HbOC—DIPHTHERIA CRM$_{197}$ PROTEIN CONJUGATE)

## Parenteral Dosage Forms

### DIPHTHERIA AND TETANUS TOXOIDS AND PERTUSSIS VACCINE ADSORBED AND HAEMOPHILUS B CONJUGATE VACCINE (HbOC—diphtheria CRM$_{197}$ protein conjugate)—INJECTION

Note: Diphtheria and tetanus toxoids and pertussis vaccine adsorbed and Haemophilus b conjugate vaccine combination (DTP-Hib) may be used whenever the schedules for immunization with the separate vaccines, diphtheria and tetanus toxoids and pertussis vaccine (DTP) and Haemophilus b conjugate vaccine (Hib), coincide.

**Usual adult and adolescent dose**
Use is not recommended.

**Usual pediatric dose**
Active immunizing agent—
  Intramuscular, 0.5 mL into the outer aspect of the upper arm (deltoid) or into the lateral mid thigh (vastus lateralis)
  Children up to 2 months of age—Use is not recommended.

Children 2 to 6 months of age at the first dose—Three doses, at least two months apart. Then, a fourth dose at 12 to 18 months of age after at least a 6-month interval following the third dose.

Note: Alternatively, Hib vaccine and either acellular DTP (DTaP) or whole-cell DTP may be administered as separate injections for the fourth dose at 12 to 18 months of age. (DTaP is preferred for doses four and five of the five-dose DTP series in order to reduce the chance of side effects.)

Children 7 to 11 months of age at the first dose—Two doses, at least two months apart, followed by appropriate doses of DTP or Hib (or DTP-Hib, where use of the two vaccines coincides) to complete each vaccine's immunization schedule. (A child 7 to 11 months of age should receive a total of 3 doses of a product containing HbOC.)

Children 12 to 14 months of age at the first dose—One dose, followed by appropriate doses of DTP or Hib (or DTP-Hib, when use of the two vaccines coincides) to complete each vaccine's immunization schedule. (A child 12 to 14 months of age should receive a total of 2 doses of a product containing HbOC.)

Children 15 to 59 months of age at the first dose—One dose, followed by appropriate doses of DTP to complete the immunization schedule for DTP. (A child 15 to 59 months of age should receive a single dose of a product containing HbOC.)

Note: The above dosage schedules do not negate the necessity of any additional doses or boosters of DTP or Hib that are required.

The above doses assume that neither DTP nor Hib vaccine has been administered previously.

DTP-Hib vaccine may be used also to complete an immunization series already initiated with any Hib vaccine and/or any DTP vaccine in those instances where the two vaccine schedules coincide.

Although any Hib vaccine type (licensed for use in that particular age group) may be used where the individual vaccine is required, use of the same Hib vaccine type throughout a primary immunization series is preferable.

**Strength(s) usually available**

U.S.—
12.5 Lf of diphtheria toxoid, 5 Lf of tetanus toxoid, 4 protective units of pertussis vaccine, 10 mcg (0.01 mg) of purified Haemophilus b saccharide, and approximately 25 mcg (0.025 mg) of CRM$_{197}$ protein (a nontoxic variant of diphtheria toxin), per 0.5 mL dose. Each 0.5-mL dose contains not more than 850 mcg (0.85 mg) of aluminum (Rx) [*Tetramune* (thimerosal 1:10,000)].

Canada—
12.5 Lf of diphtheria toxoid, 5 Lf of tetanus toxoid, 4 protective units of pertussis vaccine, 10 mcg (0.01 mg) of purified Haemophilus b saccharide, and approximately 25 mcg (0.025 mg) of CRM$_{197}$ protein (a nontoxic variant of diphtheria toxin), per 0.5 mL dose. Each 0.5-mL dose contains not more than 850 mcg (0.85 mg) of aluminum (Rx) [*Tetramune* (thimerosal 1:10,000)].

Note: Lf is the quantity of toxoid as assessed by flocculation.

**Packaging and storage**
Store between 2 and 8 °C (36 and 46 °F), unless otherwise specified by manufacturer. Protect from freezing.

**Preparation of dosage form**
The product should be shaken well immediately before withdrawing each dose. The product should be discarded if clumps remain after vigorous agitation.

**Stability**
The vaccine should be refrigerated, but kept away from the freezer compartment. Vaccine that has been frozen should be discarded.

**Auxiliary labeling**
- Shake well.
- Do not freeze.

---

*DIPHTHERIA AND TETANUS TOXOIDS AND PERTUSSIS VACCINE ADSORBED AND HAEMOPHILUS B CONJUGATE VACCINE (PRP-D—DIPHTHERIA TOXOID CONJUGATE)*

## Parenteral Dosage Forms

**DIPHTHERIA AND TETANUS TOXOIDS AND PERTUSSIS VACCINE ADSORBED AND HAEMOPHILUS B CONJUGATE VACCINE (PRP-D— diphtheria toxoid conjugate)—INJECTION**

**Usual adult and adolescent dose**
Use is not recommended.

**Usual pediatric dose**
Active immunizing agent—
Intramuscular, 0.5 mL into the outer aspect of the upper arm (deltoid) or into the lateral mid thigh (vastus lateralis):
Children up to 18 months of age—Use is not recommended.
Children 18 to 59 months of age—DTP-Hib may be administered when the single dose of Hib coincides with the fourth or fifth scheduled dose of DTP.

**Strength(s) usually available**

U.S.—
Not commercially available.

Canada—
25 Lf of diphtheria toxoid, 5 Lf of tetanus toxoid, 4 to 12 protective units of pertussis vaccine, 25 mcg (0.025 mg) of purified Haemophilus b capsular polysaccharide, and 18 mcg (0.018 mg) of diphtheria toxoid protein, per 0.5 mL dose. Each 0.5-mL dose contains 1.5 mg of aluminum phosphate (Rx) [*DPT-Hib* (thimerosal 0.01%)].

Note: Lf is the quantity of toxoid as assessed by flocculation.

**Packaging and storage**
Store between 2 and 8 °C (36 and 46 °F), unless otherwise specified by manufacturer. Protect from freezing.

**Preparation of dosage form**
The product should be shaken well immediately before withdrawing each dose. The product should be discarded if clumps remain after vigorous agitation.

**Stability**
The vaccine should be refrigerated, but kept away from the freezer compartment. Vaccine that has been frozen should be discarded.

**Auxiliary labeling**
- Shake well.
- Do not freeze.

## Selected Bibliography

Centers for Disease Control and Prevention. Recommendations for use of Haemophilus b conjugate vaccines and a combined diphtheria, tetanus, pertussis, and Haemophilus b vaccine. Recommendations of the Advisory Committee on Immunization Practices (ACIP). MMWR 1993 Sep 17; 42(RR-13): 1-15.

Centers for Disease Control and Prevention. Diphtheria, tetanus, and pertussis: recommendations for vaccine use and other preventive measures: recommendations of the Immunization Practices Advisory Committee (ACIP). MMWR 1991 Aug 8; 40(RR-10): 1-28.

Centers for Disease Control and Prevention. Haemophilus b conjugate vaccines for prevention of Haemophilus influenzae type b disease among infants and children two months of age and older: recommendation of the Immunization Practices Advisory Committee (ACIP). MMWR 1991 Jan 11: 40 (RR-1).

Developed: 11/27/96

---

**DIPHTHERIA AND TETANUS TOXOIDS AND PERTUSSIS VACCINE ADSORBED AND HAEMOPHILUS B CONJUGATE VACCINE (HBOC—DIPHTHERIA CRM$_{197}$ PROTEIN CONJUGATE)**—See *Diphtheria and Tetanus Toxoids and Pertussis Vaccine Adsorbed and Haemophilus B Conjugate Vaccine (Systemic)*

---

**DIPHTHERIA AND TETANUS TOXOIDS AND PERTUSSIS VACCINE ADSORBED AND HAEMOPHILUS B CONJUGATE VACCINE (PRP-D—DIPHTHERIA TOXOID CONJUGATE)**—
See *Diphtheria and Tetanus Toxoids and Pertussis Vaccine Adsorbed and Haemophilus b Conjugate Vaccine (Systemic)*

# DIPIVEFRIN Ophthalmic

INN: Dipivefrine
VA CLASSIFICATION (Primary): OP114
Commonly used brand name(s): *Ophtho-Dipivefrin; Propine C Cap B.I.D.*
Note: For a listing of dosage forms and brand names by country availability, see *Dosage Forms* section(s).

## Category

Antiglaucoma agent (ophthalmic).

Note: Dipivefrin belongs to a group of drugs known as prodrugs. Prodrugs are usually not active in themselves, but require biotransformation to the parent compound before being therapeutically active. Dipivefrin is a prodrug of epinephrine.

## Indications

Note: Bracketed information in the *Indications* section refers to uses that are not included in U.S. product labeling.

**Accepted**
Glaucoma, open-angle (treatment)—Indicated as initial therapy for the control of intraocular pressure in chronic open-angle glaucoma. Also, for open-angle glaucoma that is difficult to control, the addition of dipivefrin to other antiglaucoma agents, such as pilocarpine, carbachol, echothiophate, timolol, or acetazolamide, has been shown to be effective.

[Glaucoma, secondary (treatment)][1]—Dipivefrin is used in the treatment of secondary glaucoma.

[1]Not included in Canadian product labeling.

## Pharmacology/Pharmacokinetics

**Physicochemical characteristics**
Source—Dipivefrin is a prodrug formed by the diesterification of epinephrine and pivalic acid.
Molecular weight—387.90.

**Mechanism of action/Effect**
Dipivefrin is converted to epinephrine inside the eye by enzyme hydrolysis. The liberated epinephrine, an adrenergic agonist, appears to exert its action by decreasing aqueous production and enhancing aqueous outflow facility.

**Onset of action**
About 30 minutes.

**Time to peak effect**
About 1 hour.

## Precautions to Consider

**Cross-sensitivity and/or related problems**
Patients sensitive to epinephrine may be sensitive to dipivefrin also, since ophthalmic dipivefrin is converted to epinephrine inside the eye by enzyme hydrolysis.

**Tumorigenicity**
Studies in rabbits have indicated a dose-related incidence of meibomian gland retention cysts following topical administration of both dipivefrin and epinephrine.

**Pregnancy/Reproduction**
Pregnancy—Adequate and well-controlled studies in humans have not been done.
Studies in rats and rabbits at daily oral doses of up to 10 mg per kg of body weight (mg/kg) (5 mg/kg in teratogenicity studies) have not shown that dipivefrin causes impaired fertility or harm to the fetus.
FDA Pregnancy Category B.

**Breast-feeding**
It is not known whether dipivefrin is distributed into breast milk; however, dipivefrin may be systemically absorbed.

**Pediatrics**
Appropriate studies on the relationship of age to the effects of this medicine have not been performed in the pediatric population. However, no pediatrics-specific problems have been documented to date.

**Geriatrics**
Appropriate studies on the relationship of age to the effects of this medicine have not been performed in the geriatric population. However, no geriatrics-specific problems have been documented to date.

**Drug interactions and/or related problems**
The following drug interactions and/or related problems have been selected on the basis of their potential clinical significance (possible mechanism in parentheses where appropriate)—not necessarily inclusive (» = major clinical significance):

Note: Combinations containing any of the following medications, depending on the amount present, may also interact with this medication.
Dipivefrin is converted to epinephrine inside the eye by enzyme hydrolysis.

Anesthetics, hydrocarbon inhalation, such as:
Chloroform
Cyclopropane
Enflurane
Halothane
Isoflurane
Methoxyflurane
Trichloroethylene
(if significant systemic absorption of ophthalmic epinephrine occurs, concurrent use of cyclopropane, halothane, or possibly chloroform may increase the risk of severe ventricular arrhythmias because these anesthetics greatly sensitize the myocardium to the effects of sympathomimetics; therapy with dipivefrin should be interrupted prior to general anesthesia in patients receiving these anesthetics)
(enflurane, isoflurane, methoxyflurane, or especially trichloroethylene may also cause some sensitization of the myocardium to the effects of sympathomimetics; caution is recommended during concurrent use with dipivefrin)

Antidepressants, tricyclic or
Maprotiline or
Nomifensine
(if significant systemic absorption of ophthalmic epinephrine occurs, concurrent use of these medications may potentiate the cardiovascular effects of the epinephrine, possibly resulting in arrhythmias, hypertension, or tachycardia)

Beta-adrenergic blocking agents, ophthalmic
(concurrent use of ophthalmic betaxolol, levobunolol, or timolol with ophthalmic dipivefrin may provide a beneficial additive effect in lowering intraocular pressure)

Digitalis glycosides
(if significant systemic absorption of ophthalmic epinephrine occurs, concurrent use of digitalis glycosides may increase the risk of cardiac arrhythmias; caution is recommended if concurrent use is necessary)

Sympathomimetics, systemic
(if significant systemic absorption of ophthalmic epinephrine occurs, concurrent use of systemic sympathomimetics may result in additive toxic effects)

**Medical considerations/Contraindications**
The medical considerations/contraindications included have been selected on the basis of their potential clinical significance (reasons given in parentheses where appropriate)—not necessarily inclusive (» = major clinical significance).

*Except under special circumstances, this medication should not be used when the following medical problem exists:*
» Glaucoma, angle-closure, predisposition to
(dilation of pupil may predispose patient to an attack of angle-closure glaucoma)

*Risk-benefit should be considered when the following medical problems exists:*
Aphakic eyes
(macular edema may occur)
Sensitivity to dipivefrin

**Patient monitoring**
The following may be especially important in patient monitoring (other tests may be warranted in some patients, depending on condition; » = major clinical significance):

Fundus examinations and
Visual acuity determinations
(recommended at periodic intervals during therapy in aphakic patients)

Intraocular pressure determinations
(recommended at periodic intervals during therapy)

## Side/Adverse Effects

Note: Therapy with epinephrine (or its prodrug dipivefrin) can lead to adrenochrome deposits in the conjunctiva and cornea.

The following side/adverse effects have been selected on the basis of their potential clinical significance (possible signs and symptoms in parentheses where appropriate)—not necessarily inclusive:

**Those indicating need for medical attention**
Incidence rare
*Systemic absorption* (faster irregular heartbeat or increase in blood pressure)

**Those indicating need for medical attention only if they continue or are bothersome**
Incidence less frequent
*Burning, stinging, or other eye irritation; increased sensitivity of eyes to light*

## Patient Consultation

As an aid to patient consultation, refer to *Advice for the Patient, Dipivefrin (Ophthalmic)*.
In providing consultation, consider emphasizing the following selected information (» = major clinical significance):

**Before using this medication**
» Conditions affecting use, especially:
Sensitivity to dipivefrin or epinephrine
Other medical problems, especially predisposition to angle-closure glaucoma

**Proper use of this medication**
» Importance of not using more medication than the amount prescribed
Proper administration technique
Washing hands immediately after applying eye drops
Preventing contamination: Not touching applicator tip to any surface; keeping container tightly closed
» Proper dosing
Missed dose: Applying as soon as possible; if almost time for next dose, skipping missed dose and going back to regular dosing schedule; not doubling doses
» Proper storage

**Precautions while using this medication**
Regular visits to physician to check eye pressure during therapy

**Side/adverse effects**
Signs of potential side effects, especially fast or irregular heartbeat or increase in blood pressure

## General Dosing Information

Although some manufacturers recommend a dose of 2 drops of an ophthalmic solution at appropriate intervals, the conjunctival sac will usually hold only 1 drop.

When used to replace epinephrine, the epinephrine should be discontinued when dipivefrin therapy is started.
When used to replace an antiglaucoma agent other than epinephrine, the other antiglaucoma agent should be continued on the first day that dipivefrin is used but discontinued on the second day.
When used in addition to other antiglaucoma agents, dipivefrin should be administered at the usual adult dose.

## Ophthalmic Dosage Forms

### DIPIVEFRIN HYDROCHLORIDE OPHTHALMIC SOLUTION USP

**Usual adult and adolescent dose**
Antiglaucoma agent (ophthalmic)—
Topical, to the conjunctiva, 1 drop of a 0.1% solution every twelve hours.

**Usual pediatric dose**
See *Usual adult and adolescent dose*.

**Usual geriatric dose**
See *Usual adult and adolescent dose*.

**Strength(s) usually available**
U.S.—
0.1% (1 mg per mL as the hydrochloride) (Rx) [*Propine C Cap B.I.D.* (benzalkonium chloride 0.005%); GENERIC].
Canada—
0.1% (1 mg per mL as the hydrochloride) (Rx) [*Ophtho-Dipivefrin; Propine C Cap B.I.D.* (benzalkonium chloride 0.004%; sodium metabisulfite); GENERIC].

**Packaging and storage**
Store below 40 °C (104 °F), preferably between 15 and 30 °C (59 and 86 °F), unless otherwise specified by manufacturer. Store in a tight, light-resistant container. Protect from freezing.

**Auxiliary labeling**
• For the eye.
• Keep container tightly closed.

Revised: 05/14/92
Interim revision: 08/16/93; 10/19/93; 12/14/93

---

**DIPYRIDAMOLE**—The *Dipyridamole (Systemic)* monograph is not included in this published version of the USP DI database. Copies of the monograph are available on request from Micromedex, Inc. - Reprint Requests, 6200 S. Syracuse Way, Suite 300, Englewood, CO 80111; telephone (303) 486-6400; telefax (303) 486-6464; Email: USPDI@MDX.COM.

# DIRITHROMYCIN Systemic†

VA CLASSIFICATION (Primary): AM200

Commonly used brand name(s): *Dynabac*.

Note: For a listing of dosage forms and brand names by country availability, see *Dosage Forms* section(s).

†Not commercially available in Canada.

## Category

Antibacterial (systemic).

## Indications

### General considerations

Dirithromycin is an oral macrolide antibiotic with *in vitro* activity similar to that of erythromycin. Dirithromycin has a longer elimination half-life than erythromycin does and also achieves a higher concentration in some tissues. The *in vitro* activity of dirithromycin against gram-positive bacteria is similar to that of erythromycin and azithromycin, and generally less than that of clarithromycin. Penicillin-sensitive and methicillin-sensitive *Staphylococcus aureus* are susceptible to dirithromycin; however, methicillin-resistant *S. aureus* is resistant. Dirithromycin is also active against *Streptococcus pyogenes*, *S. pneumoniae*, and *Listeria monocytogenes*. *Enterococcus faecalis* and *E. faecium* are generally resistant. Gram-positive organisms that are resistant to erythromycin are also resistant to dirithromycin.

Gram-negative bacteria that are sensitive to dirithromycin include *Helicobacter pylori*, *H. jejuni*, *Moraxella catarrhalis*, *Bordetella pertussis*, and some strains of *Neisseria gonorrhoeae*. Dirithromycin is not active against *Brucella* species, some strains of *Haemophilus influenzae*, or Enterobacteriaceae. Dirithromycin and erythromycin have comparable activity against *Legionella pneumophila*.

*Chlamydia trachomatis* is moderately susceptible to dirithromycin. It has little *in vitro* activity against most anaerobes and is inactive against *Toxoplasma gondii*; however, like erythromycin, dirithromycin has good activity against *Mycoplasma pneumoniae*.

### Accepted

Bronchitis, bacterial exacerbations (treatment)
Legionnaires' disease (treatment)
Pharyngitis, streptococcal (treatment)
Pneumonia, mycoplasmal (treatment)
Pneumonia, *Streptococcus pneumoniae* (treatment) or
Skin and soft tissue infections (treatment)—Dirithromycin is indicated in the treatment of these disease states when they are caused by susceptible organisms.

#### Unaccepted
Dirithromycin should not be used for the treatment of known, suspected, or potential *bacteremia* because serum concentrations are not high enough to provide antibacterial coverage of the blood stream.

## Pharmacology/Pharmacokinetics

### Physicochemical characteristics
Molecular weight—Dirithromycin: 835.09.
Erythromycylamine: 743.97.

### Mechanism of action/Effect
Dirithromycin binds to the 50 S subunit of the 70 S ribosome of susceptible organisms, thereby inhibiting bacterial RNA-dependent protein synthesis. Macrolide antibiotics are more active at an alkaline pH, which allows the un-ionized form to penetrate the bacterial cell wall to a greater extent.

### Absorption
Dirithromycin is rapidly absorbed and converted to the active compound, erythromycylamine, by nonenzymatic hydrolysis. Dirithromycin should be administered with food or within one hour of having eaten a meal. When dirithromycin was administered with food, there was a slight increase in absorption; in addition, there was a significant decrease in peak plasma concentration (33%) when dirithromycin was administered one hour before food. Dietary fat had little or no effect on bioavailability. Absolute bioavailability of dirithromycin is 6 to 14%.

### Distribution
Rapidly and extensively distributed into extravascular tissues. Dirithromycin concentrates in alveolar macrophages and phagocytes; higher concentrations are found in tissues, such as prostate, tonsils, healthy lung, infected lung, and bronchial mucosa, than are found in serum or plasma. Tissue concentrations may be 20 to 30 times higher than simultaneously obtained serum concentrations. No information is available on penetration into the cerebrospinal fluid. Mean apparent volume of distribution is approximately 800 liters (L).

### Protein binding
Erythromycylamine—Low (15 to 30%).

### Biotransformation
Dirithromycin is converted by nonenzymatic hydrolysis during absorption to the active compound, erythromycylamine. Sixty to 90% of a dose is hydrolyzed to erythromycylamine within 35 minutes after dosing, and conversion is nearly complete after 1.5 hours. Erythromycylamine undergoes little or no hepatic biotransformation. No other metabolites of dirithromycin have been detected in the serum.

### Half-life
Erythromycylamine—30 to 50 hours.

### Time to peak concentration
Erythromycylamine—Approximately 4 to 5 hours.

### Peak serum concentration
A single 500-mg dose of dirithromycin produces an erythromycylamine concentration of 0.3 to 0.48 mcg per mL (0.4 to 0.64 micromole per L).

### Elimination
Fecal; 81 to 97% of an administered dose of erythromycylamine is eliminated in the bile.
Renal; approximately 1.2 to 2.9% of an administered dose is excreted renally within 36 hours.
In dialysis—Hemodialysis, forced diuresis, peritoneal dialysis, and hemoperfusion have not been established as being beneficial for an overdose of dirithromycin. Hemodialysis is not effective in the removal of erythromycylamine in patients with chronic renal failure.

## Precautions to Consider

### Cross-sensitivity and/or related problems
Patients hypersensitive to erythromycin or other macrolide antibiotics may be sensitive to dirithromycin.

### Carcinogenicity
Studies in animals have not been done.

### Mutagenicity
No mutagenic potential was found when dirithromycin was used in standard tests of genotoxocity, which included *in vitro* and *in vivo* bacterial mutation tests. These tests included the bacterial reverse-mutation test (Ames test), DNA repair (UDS) in rat hepatocytes, Chinese hamster lung fibroblast (V79) test, micronucleus test in mice, sister-chromatid exchange in human lymphocytes, sister-chromatid exchange in Chinese hamsters, and the mouse lymphoma assay.

### Pregnancy/Reproduction
Fertility—Studies done in rats given doses of dirithromycin up to 21 times the maximum recommended human dose (MRHD) on a mg per square meter of body surface area (mg/m$^2$) basis and in rabbits at doses up to 4 times the MRHD on a mg/m$^2$ basis revealed no evidence of impaired fertility.

Pregnancy—Adequate and well-controlled studies have not been done in humans.

Studies in rats given doses of dirithromycin up to 21 times the MRHD on a mg/m$^2$ basis and in rabbits at doses up to 4 times the MRHD on a mg/m$^2$ basis revealed no evidence of harm to the fetus. A study in CD-1 mice showed that fetal weight was significantly depressed at a dose of 1000 mg per kg of body weight (mg/kg) (8 times the MRHD on a mg/m$^2$ basis). There was also developmental retardation and increased occurrences of incomplete ossification among these fetuses. The decrease in ossification was also seen in rats given 1000 mg/kg per day for 2 weeks prior to mating, throughout the mating period, and throughout gestation.

FDA Pregnancy Category C.

Labor and delivery—Dirithromycin has not been studied for use during labor and delivery.

### Breast-feeding
It is not known whether dirithromycin and its metabolite, erythromycylamine, are distributed into breast milk. However, dirithromycin is distributed into the milk of rodents, and other macrolide antibiotics are distributed into human breast milk.

### Pediatrics
No information is available on the relationship of age to the effects of dirithromycin in children up to 12 years of age. Safety and effectiveness have not been established.

### Geriatrics
Appropriate studies performed to date have not demonstrated geriatrics-specific problems that would limit the usefulness of dirithromycin in the elderly.

### Drug interactions and/or related problems
The following drug interactions and/or related problems have been selected on the basis of their potential clinical significance (possible mechanism in parentheses where appropriate)—not necessarily inclusive (» = major clinical significance):

Note: Combinations containing any of the following medications, depending on the amount present, may also interact with this medication.

Unlike erythromycin and some other macrolide antibiotics, dirithromycin and erythromycylamine have not been found to interact with the cytochrome P-450 system and they do not have a significant effect on oxidative drug metabolism.

Antacids, aluminum-, calcium-, and/or magnesium-containing or
Histamine H$_2$-receptor antagonists
(the absorption of dirithromycin is slightly enhanced when administered concurrently with antacids or H$_2$-receptor antagonists due to increased and faster absorption in the presence of lower gastric acidity)

Astemizole or
Terfenadine
(in a prospective study done in six healthy volunteers, dirithromycin did not affect the metabolism of terfenadine; however, serious cardiac arrhythmias, some resulting in death, have occurred in patients taking terfenadine and other macrolide antibiotics; until further studies are completed, astemizole or terfenadine and dirithromycin should be used with caution)

Contraceptives, estrogen-containing, oral
(concurrent administration of dirithromycin with an estrogen-containing oral contraceptive was found to increase the clearance of the ethinyl estradiol component of an oral contraceptive; however, ovulation was not found to have occurred)

Theophylline
(concurrent use of theophylline and dirithromycin in 12 healthy volunteers resulted in a small, nonsignificant change in the steady-state plasma concentration of theophylline; in patients with chronic obstructive pulmonary disease [COPD], there was also no significant change in steady-state theophylline pharmacokinetics; other macrolide antibiotics have been found to increase the plasma concentration of theophylline; therefore, monitoring of theophylline serum concentrations is recommended)

## Dirithromycin (Systemic)

**Laboratory value alterations**
The following have been selected on the basis of their potential clinical significance (possible effect in parentheses where appropriate)—not necessarily inclusive (» = major clinical significance):

With physiology/laboratory test values
  Creatine kinase (CK) and
  Potassium, serum
    (values may be increased)
  Platelets
    (counts may be increased)

**Medical considerations/Contraindications**
The medical considerations/contraindications included have been selected on the basis of their potential clinical significance (reasons given in parentheses where appropriate)—not necessarily inclusive (» = major clinical significance).

*Risk-benefit should be considered when the following medical problems exist:*
  Hepatic function impairment
    (because dirithromycin and erythromycylamine are hepatically eliminated, dirithromycin should be used with caution in patients with moderate to severe hepatic function impairment; no change in dosing is necessary in patients with mildly impaired hepatic function)
  Hypersensitivity to dirithromycin, erythromycin, or other macrolide antibiotics

### Side/Adverse Effects
The following side/adverse effects have been selected on the basis of their potential clinical significance (possible signs and symptoms in parentheses where appropriate)—not necessarily inclusive:

**Those indicating need for medical attention**
Incidence rare
  *Clostridium difficile* colitis (severe abdominal or stomach cramps and pain; abdominal tenderness; watery and severe diarrhea, which may also be bloody; fever)

**Those indicating need for medical attention only if they continue or are bothersome**
Incidence less frequent
  *Dizziness; gastrointestinal disturbances* (abdominal discomfort or pain; diarrhea; nausea; vomiting); **headache; weakness**

### Overdose
There is no specific information on the overdose of dirithromycin. Symptoms of toxicity after an overdose of other macrolide antibiotics include nausea, epigastric pain, and diarrhea. Forced diuresis, peritoneal dialysis, hemodialysis, or hemoperfusion have not been established as being beneficial in the treatment of an overdose of dirithromycin; hemodialysis is ineffective in increasing the elimination of erythromycylamine from the plasma in patients with chronic renal failure.
For more information on the management of overdose or unintentional ingestion, **contact a Poison Control Center** (see *Poison Control Center Listing*).

### Patient Consultation
As an aid to patient consultation, refer to *Advice for the Patient, Dirithromycin (Systemic)*.
In providing consultation, consider emphasizing the following selected information (» = major clinical significance):

**Before using this medication**
» Conditions affecting use, especially:
    Hypersensitivity to dirithromycin or other macrolide antibiotics
    Pregnancy—Birth defects were found in animal fetuses in some studies in which high dosages of dirithromycin were used

**Proper use of this medication**
  Dirithromycin should be taken with food or within 1 hour after eating
» Compliance with full course of therapy
» Do not cut, crush, or chew tablets
» Proper dosing
  Missed dose: Taking as soon as possible; not taking if almost time for next dose; not doubling doses
» Proper storage

**Precautions while using this medication**
  Checking with physician if no improvement within a few days

**Side/adverse effects**
  Signs of potential side effects, especially *Clostridium difficile* colitis

### General Dosing Information
Dirithromycin should be taken with food or within one hour after eating.
Tablets should not be cut, chewed, or crushed.

### Oral Dosage Forms

#### DIRITHROMYCIN TABLETS

**Usual adult and adolescent dose**
Antibacterial—
  Bronchitis, acute bacterial exacerbations and secondary bacterial infections due to *Moraxella catarrhalis* or *Streptococcus pneumoniae* or Skin and soft tissue infections due to methicillin-susceptible *Staphylococcus aureus*: Oral, 500 mg once a day for seven days.
  Pharyngitis, streptococcal: Oral, 500 mg once a day for ten days.
  Pneumonia due to *S. pneumoniae*, *Legionella pneumophila*, or *Mycoplasma pneumoniae*: Oral, 500 mg once a day for fourteen days.

**Usual pediatric dose**
Antibacterial—
  Children up to 12 years of age: Safety and effectiveness have not been established.
  Children 12 years of age and older: See *Usual adult and adolescent dose*.

**Usual geriatric dose**
See *Usual adult and adolescent dose*.

**Strength(s) usually available**
U.S.—
  250 mg (Rx) [*Dynabac*].
Canada—
  Not commercially available.

**Packaging and storage**
Store between 15 and 30 °C (59 and 86 °F).

**Auxiliary labeling**
• Continue medicine for full time of treatment.
• Do not cut, crush, or chew tablets.
• Take with food.

Developed: 06/24/96

---

# DISOPYRAMIDE Systemic

VA CLASSIFICATION (Primary): CV300
Commonly used brand name(s): *Norpace; Norpace CR; Rythmodan; Rythmodan-LA*.
Note: For a listing of dosage forms and brand names by country availability, see *Dosage Forms* section(s).

## Category
Antiarrhythmic.

## Indications
Note: Bracketed information in the *Indications* section refers to uses that are not included in U.S. product labeling.

**Accepted**
Arrhythmias, ventricular (treatment)—Disopyramide is indicated for the treatment of documented, life-threatening ventricular arrhythmias, such as ventricular tachycardia.
[Tachycardia, supraventricular (prophylaxis and treatment)][1]—Disopyramide is used for prophylaxis and treatment of some supraventricular tachycardias.

[1]Not included in Canadian product labeling.

## Pharmacology/Pharmacokinetics

**Physicochemical characteristics**
Molecular weight—Disopyramide phosphate: 437.47.
pKa—8.4.

### Mechanism of action/Effect
Disopyramide depresses myocardial responsiveness and the electrophysiological conduction rate with the exception of the atrioventricular (AV) nodal and the His-Purkinje rates, which are essentially unchanged. Diastolic depolarization is slowed in those tissues having augmented automaticity, and the effective refractory period of the atrium and the ventricles is increased. However, conduction in accessory pathways is prolonged. In the Vaughan Williams classification of antiarrhythmics, disopyramide is considered to be a class I agent.

### Other actions/effects
Disopyramide has a negative inotropic effect. It possesses anticholinergic activity but no noticeable alpha- or beta-adrenergic effects.

### Absorption
Rapid and nearly complete.

### Protein binding
Moderate (approximately 50% at therapeutic concentrations but may range from 35 to 95% depending largely on serum concentration).

### Biotransformation
Hepatic; primary metabolite has antiarrhythmic and anticholinergic activity.

### Half-life
Normal—7 hours (range 4 to 10 hours in healthy adults).
Renal function impairment (creatinine clearance less than 40 mL per minute)—8 to 18 hours.

### Onset of therapeutic effect
A 300-mg oral loading dose with regular capsules will usually produce a therapeutic effect in 30 minutes to 3.5 hours.

### Time to peak concentration
30 minutes to 3 hours.

### Therapeutic serum concentration
2 to 4 mcg per mL; however, because of variable protein binding and potential toxicity of free unbound drug, serum concentrations should not be used for dosage adjustment.

### Duration of action
After 300-mg oral dose with regular capsules—1.5 to 8.5 hours.

### Elimination
Renal—Approximately 80% (about 50% unchanged and 30% metabolites).
Biliary—Approximately 15%.
In dialysis—Disopyramide is rapidly removed from general circulation during hemodialysis; dialysis patients may require additional dosage following dialysis and should remain under observation until condition is stabilized.

## Precautions to Consider

### Carcinogenicity
No evidence of carcinogenic potential was found in rats given oral disopyramide for 18 months at doses up to 30 times the usual human dose by weight.

### Mutagenicity
The Ames test for mutagenic potential was negative.

### Pregnancy/Reproduction
Fertility—No adverse effect on fertility was found in rats given disopyramide at doses up to 250 mg per kg of body weight (mg/kg) per day.
Pregnancy—Adequate and well-controlled studies in humans have not been done. However, disopyramide has been found in human fetal blood and has been reported to stimulate uterine contractions in pregnant women.
Administration of disopyramide to pregnant rats at doses 20 times the usual daily human dose by weight was associated with decreased numbers of implantation sites and decreased growth and survival of pups. Increased resorption rates were observed in rabbits given disopyramide 60 mg/kg per day.
FDA Pregnancy Category C.

### Breast-feeding
Disopyramide is distributed into human breast milk at a concentration less than that in plasma.

### Pediatrics
Studies performed to date have not demonstrated pediatrics-specific problems that would limit the usefulness of disopyramide in children.

### Geriatrics
Although appropriate studies on the relationship of age to the effects of disopyramide have not been performed in the geriatric population, the elderly may exhibit increased sensitivity to the anticholinergic effects such as urinary retention and dry mouth. In addition, elderly patients are more likely to have age-related renal function impairment, which may require caution and reduction of dosage in patients receiving disopyramide.

### Dental
The secondary anticholinergic effects of disopyramide may decrease or inhibit salivary flow, especially in middle-aged or elderly patients, thus contributing to the development of caries, periodontal disease, oral candidiasis, and discomfort.

### Drug interactions and/or related problems
The following drug interactions and/or related problems have been selected on the basis of their potential clinical significance (possible mechanism in parentheses where appropriate)—not necessarily inclusive (» = major clinical significance):

Note: Combinations containing any of the following medications, depending on the amount present, may also interact with this medication.

Alcohol
(concurrent use of moderate to excessive quantities with disopyramide may enhance the development of hypoglycemia and/or hypotension because of additive effects)

» Antiarrhythmics, other, especially:
Diltiazem or
Encainide or
Flecainide or
Lidocaine or
Procainamide or
Propranolol and other beta-adrenergic blocking agents or
Quinidine or
Tocainide or
Verapamil
(caution is advised when used concurrently with disopyramide, as such usage may result in excessively prolonged electrocardial conduction with decreased cardiac output)
(close monitoring is essential, as clinical heart failure may worsen during use of disopyramide with beta-adrenergic blocking agents in patients with decreased ventricular performance)
(disopyramide should not be administered within 48 hours before or 24 hours following verapamil; deaths have been reported)

Anticholinergics or other medications with anticholinergic activity (See *Appendix II*)
(anticholinergic effects may be intensified when these medications are used concurrently with disopyramide because of secondary anticholinergic activity of disopyramide)

Anticoagulants, coumarin- or indandione-derivative
(concurrent use of warfarin and disopyramide has been reported to increase or decrease the anticoagulant effect; although clinical significance has not been determined, caution is recommended)

Antidiabetic agents, oral or
Insulin
(hypoglycemic effects may be intensified in rare cases by the concurrent use of disopyramide because of additive hypoglycemic effects; patients prone to hypoglycemia should be closely monitored)

Hepatic enzyme inducers (See *Appendix II*)
(concurrent use may reduce serum disopyramide to ineffective concentrations; therefore monitoring of its serum concentrations is necessary during concurrent therapy)

Hypotension-producing medications, other (See *Appendix II*)
(concurrent use with disopyramide may increase the hypotensive effects)

» Pimozide
(concurrent use with disopyramide may potentiate cardiac arrhythmias, which are seen on electrocardiogram [ECG] as prolongation of QT interval)

### Laboratory value alterations
The following have been selected on the basis of their potential clinical significance (possible effect in parentheses where appropriate)—not necessarily inclusive (» = major clinical significance):

With physiology/laboratory test values
Blood glucose concentrations
(may be decreased by an undetermined mechanism)
ECG changes, such as:
QRS widening
QT prolongation
(may occur with overdose)

### Medical considerations/Contraindications
The medical considerations/contraindications included have been selected on the basis of their potential clinical significance (reasons given in

parentheses where appropriate)—not necessarily inclusive (» = major clinical significance).

*Except under special circumstances, this medication should not be used when the following medical problems exist:*
- » Atrioventricular (AV) block, pre-existing second or third degree without pacemaker
- » Cardiogenic shock

*Risk-benefit should be considered when the following medical problems exist:*
- Bladder neck obstruction
  (anticholinergic activity of disopyramide may cause urinary retention)
- » Cardiac conduction abnormalities, such as sick sinus syndrome, Wolff-Parkinson-White syndrome, or bundle branch block
  (disopyramide may produce additive cardiac depression)
- » Cardiomyopathies
  (risk of congestive heart failure and hypotension with disopyramide; patient should not receive loading dose and dose reduction may be indicated)
- » Congestive heart failure, uncompensated or poorly compensated
  (possible aggravation and risk of hypotension)
  (caution use of disopyramide in patients with a very low left ventricular ejection fraction, especially < 30%, because of its cardiodepressant effects)
- » Diabetes mellitus
  (disopyramide may significantly lower blood glucose levels)
- » Glaucoma, closed-angle, history of
  (anticholinergic activity of disopyramide may result in precipitation of acute condition)
- » Hepatic function impairment
  (possible accumulation of disopyramide; dosage reduction may be required)
- » Hyperkalemia
  (risk of serious arrhythmias)
- » Hypokalemia
  (may reduce efficacy of disopyramide)
- » Myasthenia gravis
  (anticholinergic effect of disopyramide may result in myasthenic crisis)
- » Prostatic enlargement
  (possible urinary retention; may be exacerbated by anticholinergic effect)
- » Renal function impairment
  (accumulation of disopyramide because of reduced excretion; dosage reduction may be required; disopyramide extended-release capsules are not recommended for patients with severe renal insufficiency [creatinine clearance of 40 mL per minute (0.67 mL per second) or less])
- Sensitivity to disopyramide

**Patient monitoring**
The following may be especially important in patient monitoring (other tests may be warranted in some patients, depending on condition; » = major clinical significance):
- Blood glucose concentrations
  (recommended at periodic intervals in patients at risk of developing hypoglycemia, e.g., those with congestive heart failure, chronic malnutrition, or hepatic or renal function impairment, or those taking medications such as beta-blockers)
- Blood pressure determinations
  (recommended at periodic intervals during therapy; if hypotension occurs and is not caused by an arrhythmia, disopyramide should be withdrawn and reinstituted at a lower dose only after adequate cardiac compensation is established)
- » ECG monitoring
  (recommended at periodic intervals during therapy; if significant QRS widening [> 25%] occurs, disopyramide should be withdrawn; if significant QT prolongation [> 25%] occurs, the patient requires dose monitoring and possible discontinuation of disopyramide)
- Hepatic function and
- Intraocular pressure and
- Potassium concentrations, serum, and
- Renal function
  (determinations recommended prior to initiation of therapy and, if necessary, at periodic intervals during therapy)

## Side/Adverse Effects

Note: Overdose may lead to apnea, loss of consciousness, cardiac arrhythmias, loss of spontaneous respiration, and death. Toxic plasma concentrations are associated with excessive widening of the QRS complex and QT interval, worsening of congestive heart failure, hypotension, conduction disturbances, bradycardia, and ultimately asystole; obvious anticholinergic effects also occur.

In the National Heart, Lung, and Blood Institute's Cardiac Arrhythmias Suppression Trial (CAST), treatment with encainide or flecainide was found to be associated with excessive mortality or increased nonfatal cardiac arrest rate, as compared with placebo, in patients with asymptomatic, non–life-threatening arrhythmias who had had a recent myocardial infarction. The implications of these results for other patient populations or other antiarrhythmic agents are uncertain.

The following side/adverse effects have been selected on the basis of their potential clinical significance (possible signs and symptoms in parentheses where appropriate)—not necessarily inclusive:

**Those indicating need for medical attention**
Incidence more frequent— 10 to 20%
  *Anticholinergic effect* (difficult urination)
Incidence less frequent—1 to 10%
  *Chest pain; confusion; congestive heart failure, possible, or fluid retention* (fast or slow heartbeat; unexplained shortness of breath; swelling of feet or lower legs; rapid weight gain); *hypotension* (dizziness, lightheadedness, or fainting); *muscle weakness*
Incidence rare—<1%
  *Aggravation of glaucoma, possible* (eye pain); *agranulocytosis* (sore throat and fever); *cholestatic jaundice* (yellow eyes or skin); *hypoglycemia* (anxious feeling; chills; cold sweats; confusion; cool, pale skin; drowsiness; fast heartbeat; headache; hunger, excessive; nausea; nervousness; shakiness; unsteady walk; or unusual tiredness or weakness); *mental depression*

**Those indicating need for medical attention only if they continue or are bothersome**
Incidence more frequent—40%
  *Anticholinergic effect* (dryness of mouth and throat)
Incidence less frequent—1 to 10%
  *Anorexia* (loss of appetite); *anticholinergic effect* (blurred vision; constipation; dry eyes and nose); *bloating or stomach pain; decreased sexual ability; urinary frequency or urgency* (frequent urge to urinate)

## Overdose

For more information on the management of overdose or unintentional ingestion, **contact a Poison Control Center** (see *Poison Control Center Listing*).

**Treatment of overdose**
There is no specific antidote for disopyramide; treatment should be symptomatic and supportive, and may include mechanical respirator and endocardial pacer when indicated or use of cardiac glycosides, diuretics, dopamine, isoproterenol, or neostigmine when indicated. ECG monitoring is essential.

Hemodialysis or charcoal hemoperfusion has been used successfully.

## Patient Consultation

As an aid to patient consultation, refer to *Advice for the Patient, Disopyramide (Systemic)*.

In providing consultation, consider emphasizing the following selected information (» = major clinical significance):

**Before using this medication**
- » Conditions affecting use, especially:
  - Sensitivity to disopyramide
  - Pregnancy—May initiate uterine contractions
  - Breast-feeding—Passes into breast milk
  - Use in the elderly—Increased sensitivity to anticholinergic effects
  - Other medications, especially other antiarrhythmics or pimozide
  - Other medical problems, especially second or third degree atrioventricular (AV) block, cardiogenic shock, cardiac conduction abnormalities, cardiomyopathies, uncompensated or poorly compensated congestive heart failure, diabetes mellitus, history of closed-angle glaucoma, hepatic function impairment, hyperkalemia or hypokalemia, myasthenia gravis, prostatic enlargement, or renal function impairment

### Proper use of this medication
» Compliance with therapy; not taking more medication than directed
   Proper administration of extended-release capsules: Swallowing capsule whole, without breaking, crushing, or chewing
   Proper administration of extended-release tablets: Not crushing or chewing
» Importance of not missing doses and taking at evenly spaced intervals
» Proper dosing
   Missed dose: Taking as soon as possible, unless within 4 hours of next dose; not doubling doses
» Proper storage

### Precautions while using this medication
» Regular visits to physician to check progress
» Checking with physician before stopping medication because of adverse cardiac effects with sudden withdrawal
» Caution when driving or doing things requiring alertness because of possible dizziness, lightheadedness, or fainting, especially when getting up suddenly from lying or sitting position
» Avoiding alcoholic beverages
» Notifying physician and taking sugar if symptoms of hypoglycemia occur
» Possible blurred vision; avoiding driving, using machines, or doing other things requiring clear vision if blurred vision occurs
   Possible dryness of eyes, mouth, and nose; using sugarless candy or gum, ice, or saliva substitute for relief of dry mouth; checking with physician or dentist if dry mouth continues for more than 2 weeks
» Caution during exercise or hot weather because of possible reduced sweating and impaired heat tolerance

### Side/adverse effects
Signs of potential side effects, especially difficult urination, chest pains, confusion, congestive heart failure, fluid retention, hypotension, muscle weakness, aggravation of glaucoma, agranulocytosis, cholestatic jaundice, mental depression, and hypoglycemia

## General Dosing Information
The dosage for all patients should be individualized within limits of response and tolerance, with required dosage adjustments being made gradually.

Patients of small body size (less than 50 kg body weight) may require reduced dosage.

When a loading dose is used, close monitoring is required for possible development of hypotension and/or congestive heart failure.

Patients receiving quinidine sulfate or procainamide may be changed to disopyramide therapy by starting the regular maintenance dose of disopyramide 6 to 12 hours after the last quinidine sulfate dose or 3 to 6 hours after the last dose of procainamide.

Patients with atrial flutter or fibrillation should be digitalized prior to disopyramide treatment to ensure that drug-induced enhancement of atrioventricular (AV) conduction does not increase the ventricular rate beyond acceptable limits.

Because disopyramide is removed by hemodialysis, additional dosage may be required following dialysis.

If first-degree AV block develops, dosage of disopyramide should be reduced. If block persists or worsens, the medication may have to be withdrawn.

## Oral Dosage Forms
Note: The dosing and strengths of the dosage forms available are expressed in terms of disopyramide base.

### DISOPYRAMIDE CAPSULES
**Usual adult dose**
Antiarrhythmic—
   Loading dose (for rapid control of ventricular arrhythmia):
      Oral, 300 mg (base) (200 mg for body weight less than 50 kg).
      Note: A loading dose is not recommended for patients with cardiomyopathy or possible cardiac decompensation.
   Maintenance:
      Oral, 150 mg (base) every six hours (or 100 mg [base] every six to eight hours for body weight less than 50 kg or in patients with cardiomyopathy or possible cardiac decompensation), the dosage being adjusted as needed and tolerated.
      Note: Geriatric patients may be more sensitive to the effects of the usual adult dose.
         Creatinine clearance is used to determine adjustment of dosing interval in cases of renal insufficiency:

| Creatinine Clearance (mL/min) | (mL/s) | Approximate Maintenance Dosing Interval |
|---|---|---|
| 30–40 | 0.5–0.67 | Every 8 hr |
| 15–30 | 0.25–0.5 | Every 12 hr |
| <15 | <0.25 | Every 24 hr |

**Usual adult prescribing limits**
Up to 800 mg (base) daily.
Note: Although total daily doses of up to 1.6 grams (base) have been used in patients with severe refractory ventricular tachycardia, such high doses are restricted to the hospitalized patient.

**Usual pediatric dose**
Antiarrhythmic—
   Oral, the following doses equally divided and administered every six hours (or at other individually appropriate intervals):
      Children up to 1 year of age:
         10 to 30 mg (base) per kg of body weight per day.
      Children 1 to 4 years of age:
         10 to 20 mg (base) per kg of body weight per day.
      Children 4 to 12 years of age:
         10 to 15 mg (base) per kg of body weight per day.
      Children 12 to 18 years of age:
         6 to 15 mg (base) per kg of body weight per day.
Note: Children should be hospitalized during the initial period of therapy to allow close monitoring until a maintenance dose is established.

**Strength(s) usually available**
U.S.—
   Not commercially available.
Canada—
   100 mg (Rx) [*Rythmodan*].
   150 mg (Rx) [*Rythmodan*].

**Packaging and storage**
Store between 15 and 30 °C (59 and 86 °F), in a well-closed container, unless otherwise specified by manufacturer.

**Auxiliary labeling**
• Avoid alcoholic beverages.
• May cause blurred vision.
• Do not take other medicines without advice from your doctor.

### DISOPYRAMIDE PHOSPHATE CAPSULES USP
**Usual adult dose**
See *Disopyramide Capsules*.

**Usual adult prescribing limits**
See *Disopyramide Capsules*.

**Usual pediatric dose**
See *Disopyramide Capsules*.

**Strength(s) usually available**
U.S.—
   100 mg (base) (Rx) [*Norpace* (lactose); GENERIC].
   150 mg (base) (Rx) [*Norpace* (lactose); GENERIC].
Canada—
   100 mg (base) [*Norpace* (lactose)].
   150 mg (base) [*Norpace* (lactose)].

**Packaging and storage**
Store between 15 and 30 °C (59 and 86 °F), unless otherwise specified by manufacturer. Store in a well-closed container.

**Preparation of dosage form**
For patients who cannot take oral solids—Prepare a liquid suspension for oral use by adding the entire contents from the required number of 100-mg (base) regular Disopyramide Phosphate Capsules USP (do not use extended-release capsules) to an appropriate quantity of Cherry Syrup NF to make a suitable concentration of 1 to 10 mg per mL. Add accessory 'Shake' and 'Refrigerate' labels and dispense in amber glass bottles with child-proof caps.

**Stability**
The extemporaneously prepared oral suspension of disopyramide is stable for one month when refrigerated.

**Auxiliary labeling**
• Avoid alcoholic beverages.
• May cause blurred vision.
• Do not take other medicines without advice from your doctor.
For oral suspension—
   • Avoid alcoholic beverages.
   • May cause blurred vision.
   • Shake well.

## DISOPYRAMIDE PHOSPHATE EXTENDED-RELEASE CAPSULES USP

**Usual adult dose**
Antiarrhythmic—
   Oral, 300 mg (base) every twelve hours (200 mg every twelve hours for body weight less than 50 kg).
   Note: Extended-release dosage form is not recommended for initial dosage, but for maintenance dosage only.
   When transferring from the regular oral dosage form, it is recommended that the first dose of the extended-release dosage form be given six hours after the last regular dose.

**Usual adult prescribing limits**
Up to 800 mg (base) daily.
   Note: Although total daily doses of up to 1.6 grams (base) have been used in patients with severe refractory ventricular tachycardia, such high doses are restricted to the hospitalized patient.

**Usual pediatric dose**
Use is not recommended.

**Strength(s) usually available**
U.S.—
   100 mg (base) (Rx) [*Norpace CR;* GENERIC].
   150 mg (base) (Rx) [*Norpace CR;* GENERIC].
Canada—
   Not commercially available.

**Packaging and storage**
Store between 15 and 30 °C (59 and 85 °F), unless otherwise specified by manufacturer. Store in a well-closed container.

**Auxiliary labeling**
- Avoid alcoholic beverages.
- May cause blurred vision.
- Do not take other medicines without advice from your doctor.
- Swallow capsule whole.

## DISOPYRAMIDE PHOSPHATE EXTENDED-RELEASE TABLETS

**Usual adult dose**
See *Disopyramide Phosphate Extended-release Capsules USP*.

**Usual pediatric dose**
Use is not recommended.

**Strength(s) usually available**
U.S.—
   Not commercially available.
Canada—
   150 mg (base) (Rx) [*Norpace CR; Rythmodan-LA* (scored)].

**Packaging and storage**
Store between 15 and 30 °C (59 and 86 °F), in a well-closed container, unless otherwise specified by manufacturer.

**Auxiliary labeling**
- Avoid alcoholic beverages.
- May cause blurred vision.
- Swallow tablet whole.
- Do not take other medicines without advice from your doctor.

## Parenteral Dosage Forms

### DISOPYRAMIDE INJECTION

Note: Use of the parenteral dosage form may be accompanied by a hypotensive response. This route should be limited to emergencies and the medication should be given in a hospital where intensive coronary care unit facilities are available.

**Usual adult dose**
Antiarrhythmic—
   Loading dose—
      Intravenous—2 mg (base) per kg of body weight (1 mg [base] per kg of body weight for patients with compromised left ventricular function) administered in three equally divided doses; each dose should be injected slowly over a period of three minutes with an interval of three minutes between each dose.
      Intravenous infusion—2 mg (base) per kg of body weight (1 mg [base] per kg of body weight for patients with compromised left ventricular function) administered over fifteen minutes.
      Note: An additional 1 to 2 mg (base) per kg of body weight may be administered by slow infusion over the next forty-five minutes if adequate control of the arrhythmia is not achieved. Careful monitoring of the patient is recommended.
   Maintenance—
      Intravenous infusion, 0.4 mg (400 mcg) (base) per kg of body weight per hour given for up to twenty-four hours.
   Note: Total intravenous administration during the first hour should not exceed 300 mg (base) and the total administration during the first twenty-four hours should not exceed 800 mg (base).

**Usual pediatric dose**
Safety and efficacy have not been established.

**Strength(s) usually available**
U.S.—
   Not commercially available.
Canada—
   10 mg (base) per mL (Rx) [*Rythmodan* (benzyl alcohol 10 mg per mL)].

**Packaging and storage**
Store below 40 °C (104 °F), preferably between 15 and 30 °C (59 and 86 °F), unless otherwise specified by manufacturer. Protect from freezing.

**Preparation of dosage form**
Rythmodan injection is physically compatible with dextrose injection BP, sodium chloride injection BP, compound sodium chloride injection BP, and compound sodium lactate injection BP.
Caution—Use of diluents containing benzyl alcohol is not recommended for preparation of medications for use in neonates. A fatal toxic syndrome consisting of metabolic acidosis, CNS depression, respiratory problems, renal failure, hypotension, and possibly seizures and intracranial hemorrhages has been associated with this use.

### Selected Bibliography

Taylor EH, Pappas AA. Disopyramide: clinical indications, pharmacokinetics and laboratory assessment. Ann Clin Lab Sci 1986 Jul-Aug; 16(4): 289-95.

Siddoway LA, Woosley RL. Clinical pharmacokinetics of disopyramide. Clin Pharmacokinet 1986 May-Jun; 11(3): 214-22.

Revised: 05/14/93
Interim revision: 04/13/95

---

# DISULFIRAM Systemic

VA CLASSIFICATION (Primary): AD100
Commonly used brand name(s): *Antabuse*.
Note: For a listing of dosage forms and brand names by country availability, see *Dosage Forms* section(s).

## Category
Alcohol-abuse deterrent.

## Indications

**Accepted**
Alcoholism (treatment)—Disulfiram is used to help maintain sobriety in the treatment of chronic alcoholism in conjunction with supportive and psychotherapeutic measures.

## Pharmacology/Pharmacokinetics

**Physicochemical characteristics**
Molecular weight—296.52.

**Mechanism of action/Effect**
Produces irreversible inhibition of the enzyme responsible for oxidation of the ethanol metabolite acetaldehyde. The resultant accumulation of acetaldehyde may be responsible for most of the signs and symptoms occurring after ethanol ingestion in disulfiram-treated patients. The hypotensive response may be due to inhibition of norepinephrine synthesis by the major disulfiram metabolite diethyldithiocarbamate.

**Absorption**
Slow. 80 to 90% of an oral dose is absorbed.

**Biotransformation**
Hepatic.

**Onset of action**
A single dose of disulfiram will begin to affect ethanol metabolism within 1 to 2 hours.

**Duration of action**
Disulfiram-alcohol reactions may occur up to 14 days following last dose of disulfiram.

**Elimination**
Primarily renal, as metabolites. Some of the metabolites are also exhaled as carbon disulfide. Up to 20% of a dose may remain in the body for 1 week or longer. About 5 to 20% of a dose is eliminated unchanged in the feces.

## Precautions to Consider

### Cross-sensitivity and/or related problems
Patients sensitive to other thiuram derivatives (used in rubber, pesticides, or fungicides) may be sensitive to disulfiram also.

### Pregnancy/Reproduction
Pregnancy—Adequate and well-controlled studies in humans have not been done. However, there have been a few reports of congenital defects in infants whose mothers received disulfiram during pregnancy. Further study is needed to determine the relationship between disulfiram and congenital malformations.
Disulfiram is reported to be embryotoxic in animals.

### Breast-feeding
Problems in humans have not been documented.

### Pediatrics
No information is available on the relationship of age to the effects of disulfiram in pediatric patients. Safety and efficacy have not been established.

### Geriatrics
No information is available on the relationship of age to the effects of disulfiram in geriatric patients. However, elderly patients are more likely to have age-related renal function impairment, which may require caution in patients receiving this medication. In addition, elderly patients with cardiac or cerebrovascular disease may not tolerate the hypotension that accompanies the disulfiram-alcohol reaction as well as younger patients.

### Drug interactions and/or related problems
The following drug interactions and/or related problems have been selected on the basis of their potential clinical significance (possible mechanism in parentheses where appropriate)—not necessarily inclusive (» = major clinical significance):

Note: Combinations containing any of the following medications, depending on the amount present, may also interact with this medication.

» Alcohol
  (use of alcohol or alcohol-containing products within 14 days of disulfiram therapy will result in a disulfiram-alcohol reaction)

» Alfentanil
  (chronic preoperative administration or perioperative use of hepatic enzyme inhibitors, such as disulfiram, may decrease plasma clearance and prolong the duration of action of alfentanil)

Amoxicillin and clavulanate combination or
Bacampicillin
  (metabolism of bacampicillin produces low plasma concentrations of alcohol and acetaldehyde; although the risk of a disulfiram-alcohol interaction appears minimal, caution is recommended if concurrent use is unavoidable)
  (a similar reaction is thought to occur with amoxicillin and clavulanate combination)

» Anticoagulants, coumarin- or indandione-derivative
  (anticoagulant effect may be increased during concurrent use with disulfiram because of inhibition of the enzymatic metabolism of the anticoagulant; also, disulfiram may act directly in the liver to increase the hypoprothrombinemia-inducing activity of coumarin derivatives; anticoagulant dosage adjustments based on prothrombin time determinations may be necessary during and following concurrent use)

» Anticonvulsants, hydantoin, especially phenytoin
  (concurrent use with disulfiram may increase the serum concentrations of hydantoins, possibly leading to hydantoin toxicity; hydantoin serum concentrations should be obtained prior to and during concurrent therapy with disulfiram and dosage adjustments made accordingly)

Antidepressants, tricyclic, especially amitriptyline
  (concurrent use with disulfiram may cause transient delirium)

Ascorbic acid
  (may interfere with the disulfiram-alcohol reaction, especially with chronic use or high doses of ascorbic acid; although controversial, this effect has been used beneficially by some clinicians in the management of disulfiram-alcohol reactions)

Central nervous system (CNS) depression–producing medications (See *Appendix II*)
  (concurrent use may enhance the CNS depressant effects of either these medications or disulfiram)

Ethylene dibromide
  (exposure to ethylene dibromide or its vapors concurrently with disulfiram treatment may result in a toxic reaction)

Hepatic enzyme inhibitors (See *Appendix II*)
  (concurrent use of disulfiram with other hepatic enyzme inhibitors may potentiate the effect )

Hepatotoxic medication, other (See *Appendix II*)
  (concurrent use of disulfiram with other hepatotoxic medications may increase the potential for hepatotoxicity)

» Isoniazid
  (concurrent use may result in increased incidence of CNS effects, such as dizziness, incoordination, irritability, or insomnia; a reduction of dosage or discontinuation of disulfiram may be necessary)

» Metronidazole
  (concurrent use with disulfiram may result in confusion and psychotic reactions because of combined toxicity; metronidazole is not recommended concurrently with, and for 2 weeks following, disulfiram)

Midazolam
  (concurrent use may decrease first-pass metabolism and elimination of midazolam in the liver, probably by competitive inhibition at the cytochrome P-450 binding sites, thereby increasing steady-state plasma concentrations of midazolam)

Neurotoxic medications (See *Appendix II*)
  (concurrent use of disulfiram with other neurotoxic medications may increase the potential for neurotoxicity)

» Organic solvents
  (exposure to organic solvents, ingested or inhaled, which may contain alcohol, acetaldehyde, paraldehyde, or structural analogs, may result in a disulfiram-alcohol reaction)

» Paraldehyde
  (concurrent use with disulfiram is not recommended, because inhibition of acetaldehyde dehydrogenase may occur, resulting in decreased metabolism of paraldehyde and increased blood concentrations of paraldehyde and acetaldehyde)

### Laboratory value alterations
The following have been selected on the basis of their potential clinical significance (possible effect in parentheses where appropriate)—not necessarily inclusive (» = major clinical significance):

With physiology/laboratory test values
  Cholesterol concentrations, serum
    (may be increased with doses of 500 mg a day)
  Vanillylmandelic acid (VMA) concentrations, urine
    (may be decreased)

### Medical considerations/Contraindications
The medical considerations/contraindications included have been selected on the basis of their potential clinical significance (reasons given in parentheses where appropriate)—not necessarily inclusive (» = major clinical significance).

*Risk-benefit should be considered when the following medical problems exist:*

Allergic eczematous contact dermatitis
  (may be exacerbated)
Cardiovascular disorders
  (disulfiram-alcohol reaction may exacerbate condition)
Depression
  (behavioral toxicity may be precipitated)
Diabetes mellitus
  (disulfiram-alcohol reaction may exacerbate condition)
Epilepsy or other seizure disorder, or history of
  (disulfiram-alcohol reaction may exacerbate condition)
Hepatic function impairment or cirrhosis
  (increased potential for hepatotoxicity)

Hypothyroidism
(disulfiram-alcohol reaction may exacerbate condition)
Psychoses
(behavioral toxicity may be precipitated)
Pulmonary insufficiency, severe
(disulfiram-alcohol reaction may exacerbate condition)
Renal function impairment
(disulfiram elimination may be inhibited)
Sensitivity to disulfiram, rubber, pesticides, or fungicides

**Patient monitoring**
The following may be especially important in patient monitoring (other tests may be warranted in some patients, depending on condition; » = major clinical significance):

Blood cell counts and
Blood chemistry profiles
(recommended at 6-month intervals during therapy)
Hepatic function determinations
(baseline studies are recommended, followed by transaminase tests after 10 to 14 days of therapy; additional liver function tests may also be required at periodic intervals during therapy)

## Side/Adverse Effects

The following side/adverse effects have been selected on the basis of their potential clinical significance (possible signs and symptoms in parentheses where appropriate)—not necessarily inclusive:

**Those indicating need for medical attention**
Incidence less frequent
*Neurotoxicity, including optic neuritis* (eye pain or tenderness or any change in vision); *peripheral neuritis or polyneuritis* (numbness, pain, tingling, or weakness in hands or feet); *psychotic reaction* (mood or mental changes)
Note: *Neurotoxicity* is usually reversible if disulfiram is discontinued.
Incidence rare
*Encephalopathy* (mental changes); *hepatitis* (yellow eyes or skin; darkening of urine; light gray–colored stools; severe stomach pain)
Note: Fulminant hepatic necrosis occurs rarely. Although it cannot be predicted which patients will develop this potentially fatal hepatitis, published experience suggests that the chance of survival is markedly improved if disulfiram is stopped as soon as jaundice is detected. Careful clinical monitoring with discontinuation of disulfiram and laboratory (bilirubin and hepatic enzyme) determinations is recommended when hepatitis is suspected.

**Those indicating need for medical attention only if they continue or are bothersome**
Incidence more frequent
*Drowsiness*
Incidence less frequent or rare
*Headache; impotence* (decreased sexual ability in males); *metallic or garlic-like taste in mouth; skin rash; unusual tiredness*

## Patient Consultation

As an aid to patient consultation, refer to *Advice for the Patient, Disulfiram (Systemic)*.
In providing consultation, consider emphasizing the following selected information (» = major clinical significance):

**Before using this medication**
» Conditions affecting use, especially:
Sensitivity to disulfiram, rubber, pesticides, or fungicides
Other medications, especially alcohol; alfentanil; coumarin- or indandione-derivative anticoagulants; hydantoin anticonvulsants, especially phenytoin; isoniazid; metronidazole; organic solvents; or paraldehyde

**Proper use of this medication**
» Not taking this medication within 12 hours of using any alcohol-containing preparation or medication, or if the blood alcohol level is not zero
» Compliance with therapy
» Proper dosing
» Proper storage

**Precautions while using this medication**
» Not drinking or using any alcohol-containing products or medications while taking this medication and for 14 days after discontinuing this medication
Symptoms of disulfiram-alcohol reaction
Blurred vision
Chest pain
Confusion
Dizziness or fainting
Fast or pounding heartbeat
Flushing or redness of face
Increased sweating
Nausea and vomiting
Throbbing headache
Troubled breathing
Weakness, severe
Rarely, seizures, heart attack, unconsciousness, or death if reaction is severe
Carrying medical identification card during therapy
Regular visits to physician to check progress during long-term therapy
» Checking all liquid medications for presence of alcohol
» Caution if drowsiness occurs
» Checking with physician before using other CNS depressants

**Side/adverse effects**
Signs of potential side effects, especially optic neuritis, peripheral neuritis, polyneuritis, or psychotic reaction

## General Dosing Information

The patient should be made fully aware of the nature of this medicine and the disulfiram-alcohol reaction and its consequences.

Disulfiram should not be administered until the patient has abstained from alcohol for at least 12 hours and the blood alcohol level is zero.

The duration of the disulfiram-alcohol reaction is dependent upon the dose of disulfiram and on the quantity of alcohol ingested; it may persist from 30 minutes to several hours.

Reactions to alcohol may occur for up to 2 weeks following withdrawal of disulfiram therapy.

**For treatment of disulfiram-alcohol reaction**
In severe reactions, supportive measures to restore blood pressure and treat shock should be instituted. Other recommendations include:
• Administration of supplemental oxygen.
• Monitoring of serum potassium levels.
• Monitoring of ECG tracings.
Although controversial, administration of intravenous ascorbic acid or intravenous antihistamines has been advocated by some clinicians. Phenothiazines should not be used as they may exacerbate hypotension.

## Oral Dosage Forms

### DISULFIRAM TABLETS USP

**Usual adult and adolescent dose**
Alcohol-abuse deterrent—
Initial: Oral, up to 500 mg once a day for one or two weeks.
Maintenance: Oral, 125 to 500 mg (average of 250 mg) once a day.
Note: Some clinicians recommend the dose be administered at bedtime to reduce daytime drowsiness.

**Usual pediatric dose**
Safety and efficacy have not been established.

**Usual geriatric dose**
See *Usual adult and adolescent dose*.
Note: Geriatric patients may be more sensitive to the effects of the usual adult dose.

**Strength(s) usually available**
U.S.—
250 mg (Rx) [*Antabuse* (scored); GENERIC].
500 mg (Rx) [*Antabuse* (scored); GENERIC].
Canada—
250 mg (Rx) [*Antabuse* (scored)].
500 mg (Rx) [*Antabuse* (scored)].

**Packaging and storage**
Store below 40 °C (104 °F), preferably between 15 and 30 °C (59 and 86 °F), in a tight, light-resistant container.

**Note**
Patient identification cards may be available from the manufacturer.

## Selected Bibliography

Wright C, Moore RD. Disulfiram treatment of alcoholism. Am J Med 1990; 88: 647-55.

Revised: 01/27/92
Interim revision: 07/20/94

# DIURETICS, LOOP  Systemic

This monograph includes information on the following: 1) Bumetanide†; 2) Etacrynic Acid; 3) Furosemide.

INN:  Ethacrynic Acid—Etacrynic acid
JAN:  Ethacrynic Acid—Etacrynic acid
VA CLASSIFICATION (Primary/Secondary): CV702/CV409; TN900
Commonly used brand name(s): *Apo-Furosemide*[3]; *Bumex*[1]; *Edecrin*[2]; *Furoside*[3]; *Lasix*[3]; *Lasix Special*[3]; *Myrosemide*[3]; *Novosemide*[3]; *Uritol*[3].

Note: For a listing of dosage forms and brand names by country availability, see *Dosage Forms* section(s).

†Not commercially available in Canada.

## Category

Diagnostic aid adjunct (renal disease)—Furosemide.
Diuretic—Bumetanide; Ethacrynic Acid; Furosemide.
Antihypertensive—Bumetanide; Ethacrynic Acid; Furosemide.
Antihypercalcemic—Bumetanide; Ethacrynic Acid; Furosemide.

## Indications

Note: Bracketed information in the *Indications* section refers to uses that are not included in U.S. product labeling.

### Accepted

Edema (treatment)—Bumetanide, ethacrynic acid, and furosemide are indicated in the treatment of edema associated with congestive heart failure, hepatic cirrhosis, and renal disease (including nephrotic syndrome).

Bumetanide, ethacrynic acid, and furosemide are indicated as adjuncts in the treatment of acute pulmonary edema.

Ethacrynic acid is indicated in the short-term management of ascites due to malignancy, idiopathic edema, and lymphedema; and in the short-term management of hospitalized pediatric patients with congenital heart disease or nephrotic syndrome.

Bumetanide, ethacrynic acid, and furosemide are especially useful in patients refractory to other diuretics or with existing acid-base disorders, congestive heart failure, or renal disease.

Hypertension (treatment)—[Bumetanide], [ethacrynic acid][1], and furosemide are indicated in the treatment of mild to moderate hypertension, usually in combination with other antihypertensive agents, and as adjuncts in the treatment of hypertensive crisis.

Bumetanide, ethacrynic acid, and furosemide are not considered to be primary agents in the treatment of essential hypertension. However, they may be indicated in combination with other antihypertensives in the treatment of hypertension associated with impaired renal function. In the stepped-care approach to antihypertensive treatment, bumetanide, ethacrynic acid, or furosemide may be substituted for a thiazide diuretic in patients with renal function impairment.

Hypercalcemia (treatment)—[Bumetanide], [ethacrynic acid][1], and [furosemide][1] are used in the treatment of hypercalcemia.

[Renography, adjunct][1] and
[Renal imaging, radionuclide, adjunct][1]—Furosemide augments radionuclide renography and renal scintigraphy by stimulating the flow of urine and thereby aiding in the differentiation of mechanical obstruction from nonobstructive dilatation in patients with hydroureteronephrosis.

[1]Not included in Canadian product labeling.

## Pharmacology/Pharmacokinetics

### Physicochemical characteristics

Molecular weight—
  Bumetanide: 364.42.
  Ethacrynic acid: 303.14.
  Furosemide: 330.74.
pKa—
  Ethacrynic acid: 3.5.
  Furosemide: 3.9.

### Mechanism of action/Effect

Diuretic—Bumetanide, ethacrynic acid, and furosemide inhibit reabsorption of sodium and water in the ascending limb of the loop of Henle by interfering with the chloride binding site of the $1Na^+$, $1K^+$, $2Cl^-$ cotransport system. Loop diuretics increase the rate of delivery of tubular fluid and electrolytes to the distal sites of hydrogen and potassium ion secretion, while plasma volume contraction increases aldosterone production. The increased delivery and high aldosterone levels promote sodium reabsorption at the distal tubules, thus increasing the loss of potassium and hydrogen ions. Bumetanide may have a small additional action on sodium reabsorption in the proximal tubule since phosphate reabsorption is reduced.

Antihypertensive—Diuretics lower blood pressure initially by reducing plasma and extracellular fluid volume; cardiac output also decreases. Eventually, cardiac output returns to normal with an accompanying decrease in peripheral resistance.

Antihypercalcemic—Loop diuretics increase the urinary excretion of calcium.

### Absorption

Bumetanide—Almost completely absorbed from gastrointestinal tract. Absorption is probably reduced in patients with edematous bowel caused by congestive heart failure or nephrotic syndrome; parenteral administration may be preferable in these patients.

Furosemide—Approximately 60 to 70% of an oral dose of furosemide is absorbed. Food may slow the rate of absorption but does not appear to alter the bioavailability or diuretic effect. Absorption is reduced to 43 to 46% in patients with end-stage renal disease, and is probably reduced also in patients with edematous bowel caused by congestive heart failure or nephrotic syndrome; parenteral administration may be preferable in these patients.

### Protein binding

Bumetanide—Very high (94 to 96%).
Ethacrynic acid—High.
Furosemide—Very high (91 to 97%; almost totally to albumin).

### Biotransformation

Hepatic; metabolism of bumetanide is limited and produces inactive metabolites.

### Half-life

Bumetanide—
  1 to 1½ hours.
Furosemide—
  Wide variation among individuals.
    Normal:
      ½ to 1 hour.
    Anuric:
      75 to 155 minutes.
      In patients with both renal and hepatic insufficiency, half-lives of 11 to 20 hours have been reported.
      In neonates, reported half-lives are prolonged, probably due to low renal and hepatic clearance.

### Onset of action

Diuretic—
  Bumetanide:
    Oral—30 to 60 minutes.
    Intravenous—Within minutes.
  Ethacrynic acid:
    Oral—30 minutes.
    Intravenous—5 minutes.
  Furosemide:
    Oral—20 to 60 minutes.
    Intravenous—5 minutes.

### Time to peak effect

Diuretic—
  Bumetanide:
    Oral—1 to 2 hours.
    Intravenous—15 to 30 minutes.
  Ethacrynic acid:
    Oral—2 hours.
    Intravenous—15 to 30 minutes.
  Furosemide:
    Oral—1 to 2 hours.
    Intravenous—Within 30 minutes.

Note: The maximum antihypertensive effect may not occur until several days after initiation of loop diuretic therapy.

### Duration of action

Diuretic—
  Bumetanide:
    Oral—4 hours with usual doses (1 to 2 mg); 4 to 6 hours with higher doses.
    Intravenous—3.5 to 4 hours.
  Ethacrynic acid:
    Oral—6 to 8 hours.
    Intravenous—2 hours.

Furosemide:
  Oral—6 to 8 hours.
  Intravenous—2 hours.

**Elimination**
Bumetanide—
  Renal (81%; 45% unchanged); biliary/fecal (2%).
Ethacrynic acid—
  Renal (67%); biliary/fecal (33%); 20% excreted unchanged.
Furosemide—
  Renal (88%); biliary/fecal (12%).
In patients with severe renal impairment, renal clearance is reduced but overall plasma clearance may be unchanged because nonrenal clearance is increased. In patients with uremia, both renal and nonrenal clearance are reduced, and elimination is delayed.
In dialysis: Not dialyzable.

## Precautions to Consider

### Cross-sensitivity and/or related problems
Patients sensitive to sulfonamides (including thiazide diuretics) may be sensitive to bumetanide or furosemide also.

### Carcinogenicity/Tumorigenicity
*Bumetanide*—One study in female rats given 60 mg per kg of body weight (mg/kg) of bumetanide for 18 months found an increase in mammary adenomas; repetition of the same study did not result in the same findings.

*Ethacrynic acid*—A 79-week study in rats at doses up to 45 times the human dose revealed no evidence of a tumorigenic effect.

### Mutagenicity
*Bumetanide*—Studies with bumetanide in various strains of *Salmonella typhimurium* in the presence or absence of an *in vitro* metabolic activation system found no evidence of mutagenicity.
*Furosemide*—Mutagenicity studies have not been conducted.

### Pregnancy/Reproduction
Pregnancy—Pregnant women should be advised to contact physician before taking this medication, since routine use of diuretics during normal pregnancy is inappropriate and exposes mother and fetus to unnecessary hazard. Diuretics do not prevent development of toxemia of pregnancy, and there is no satisfactory evidence that they are useful in the treatment of toxemia. Diuretics are indicated only in the treatment of edema due to pathologic causes or as a short course of treatment in patients with severe hypervolemia.

*Bumetanide*—
  Adequate and well-controlled studies in humans have not been done.
  Some studies in animals have shown that bumetanide may cause adverse effects on the fetus. Bumetanide has not been shown to be teratogenic in mice or hamsters; however, one study in rats showed moderate growth retardation and increased incidence of delayed ossification of sternebrae at doses 3400 times the maximum human therapeutic dose. These effects in the rat were associated with maternal weight reductions during dosing and were not observed at doses 1000 times the maximum human therapeutic dose. Delayed ossification of sternebrae was also noted in rabbits at doses 10 times the maximum human therapeutic dose. A slight embryocidal effect in rats and rabbits was evident at doses 3400 and 3.4 times the maximum human therapeutic dose, respectively. In rabbits, a dose-related decrease in litter size and an increase in resorption rate were noted at doses of 3.4 and 10 times the maximum human therapeutic dose.
  FDA Pregnancy Category C.

*Ethacrynic acid*—
  Adequate and well-controlled studies in humans have not been done.
  Studies in mice and rabbits using doses up to 50 times the human dose have not shown evidence of external abnormalities of the fetus. In rats, a decrease in mean body weights of the fetuses was noted at doses 50 times the maximum human dose.
  FDA Pregnancy Category B.

*Furosemide*—
  Furosemide crosses the placenta. Studies in humans have not been done.
  Studies in rabbits and mice have shown that furosemide causes an increased incidence of hydronephrosis in the fetus. In rabbits, unexplained maternal deaths and abortions have occurred at doses 2 to 8 times the maximum recommended human dose.
  FDA Pregnancy Category C.

### Breast-feeding
Furosemide is distributed into breast milk; it is not known whether bumetanide or ethacrynic acid is distributed into breast milk.

### Pediatrics
Caution is required in neonates because of the prolonged half-life of furosemide. Usual pediatric doses may be used, but the dosing interval should be extended.

### Geriatrics
Although appropriate studies on the relationship of age to the effects of loop diuretics have not been performed in the geriatric population, the elderly may be more sensitive to the hypotensive and electrolyte effects. In addition, elderly patients are at greater risk of developing circulatory collapse and thromboembolic episodes. Elderly patients are also more likely to have age-related renal function impairment, which may require adjustment of dosage or dosing interval in patients receiving loop diuretics.

### Drug interactions and/or related problems
The following drug interactions and/or related problems have been selected on the basis of their potential clinical significance (possible mechanism in parentheses where appropriate)—not necessarily inclusive (» = major clinical significance):

Note: Combinations containing any of the following medications, depending on the amount present, may also interact with this medication.

Alcohol or
Hypotension-producing medications, other (See *Appendix II*)
  (hypotensive and/or diuretic effects may be potentiated when these medications are used concurrently with loop diuretics; although some antihypertensive and/or diuretic combinations are frequently used for therapeutic advantage, when used concurrently dosage adjustments may be necessary)

Amiodarone
  (concurrent use of loop diuretics with amiodarone may lead to an increased risk of arrhythmias associated with hypokalemia)

» Amphotericin B, parenteral
  (concurrent and/or sequential administration with loop diuretics should be avoided since the potential for ototoxicity and nephrotoxicity may be increased, especially in the presence of renal function impairment; in addition, concurrent use with loop diuretics may intensify electrolyte imbalance, particularly hypokalemia; frequent electrolyte determinations are recommended and potassium supplementation may be required)

Angiotensin-converting enzyme (ACE) inhibitors
  (sudden and severe hypotension may occur within the first 1 to 5 hours after the initial dose of captopril, enalapril, or lisinopril, particularly in patients who are sodium- and volume-depleted as a result of diuretic therapy. Withdrawal of the diuretic or increase of salt intake approximately 1 week before start of captopril therapy or 2 to 3 days before start of benazepril, enalapril, fosinopril, lisinopril, quinapril, or ramipril therapy, or initiating ACE inhibitor therapy in lower doses, will minimize the reaction; this reaction does not usually recur with subsequent doses, although caution in increasing doses is recommended; diuretics may be reinstituted as necessary)
  (risk of renal failure may be increased in patients who are sodium- and volume-depleted as a result of diuretic therapy)
  (ACE inhibitors may reduce the secondary aldosteronism and hypokalemia caused by diuretics)

» Anticoagulants, coumarin- or indandione-derivative or
Heparin or
Streptokinase or
Urokinase
  (anticoagulant effects may be decreased when these medications are used concurrently with loop diuretics, as a result of reduction of plasma volume leading to concentration of procoagulant factors in the blood; in addition, diuretic-induced improvement of hepatic congestion may lead to improved hepatic function, resulting in increased procoagulant factor synthesis; dosage adjustments may be necessary)
  (anticoagulant effects may be potentiated when these medications are used concurrently with ethacrynic acid as a result of displacement of anticoagulant from protein-binding sites; dosage adjustments of the anticoagulant may be necessary during and after ethacrynic acid therapy or, alternatively, use of furosemide is recommended)
  (gastrointestinal ulcerative or hemorrhagic potential of ethacrynic acid may increase the risk of hemorrhage in patients receiving an-

ticoagulant or thrombolytic therapy; use of a different diuretic is recommended)

Antidiabetic agents, oral or
Insulin
(furosemide, and possibly bumetanide or ethacrynic acid, may rarely raise blood glucose concentrations or interfere with the hypoglycemic effects of these agents; for adult-onset diabetics, dosage adjustment of hypoglycemic medications may be necessary during and after therapy)

Anti-inflammatory drugs, nonsteroidal (NSAIDs), especially indomethacin
(may antagonize the natriuresis and increase in plasma renin activity [PRA] caused by loop diuretics; indomethacin, and possibly other NSAIDs with the exception of diflunisal, may also reduce the increase in urine volume caused by loop diuretics, possibly by inhibiting renal prostaglandin synthesis and/or by causing sodium and fluid retention)

(in addition, concurrent use of NSAIDs with a diuretic may increase the risk of renal failure secondary to a decrease in renal blood flow caused by inhibition of renal prostaglandin synthesis)

(in the premature neonate, administration of 1 mg/kg of furosemide immediately following indomethacin has been shown to prevent or reduce indomethacin-induced adverse renal effects without interfering with ductus arteriosus closure)

Digitalis glycosides
(concurrent use with loop diuretics may enhance the possibility of digitalis toxicity associated with hypokalemia and hypomagnesemia)

» Hypokalemia-causing medications, other (See *Appendix II*)
(risk of severe hypokalemia due to other hypokalemia-causing medications may be increased; monitoring of serum potassium concentrations and cardiac function and potassium supplementation may be required)

» Lithium
(concurrent use with loop diuretics may provoke lithium toxicity because of reduced renal clearance and is not recommended unless patient can be closely monitored)

» Nephrotoxic medications, other (See *Appendix II*) or
Ototoxic medications, other (See *Appendix II*)
(concurrent and/or sequential administration with loop diuretics should be avoided since the potential for ototoxicity and nephrotoxicity may be increased, especially in the presence of renal function impairment)

Neuromuscular blocking agents, nondepolarizing
(loop diuretics may induce hypokalemia, which may enhance the blockade of nondepolarizing neuromuscular blocking agents; serum potassium determinations may be necessary prior to administration of nondepolarizing neuromuscular blocking agents; careful postoperative monitoring of the patient may be necessary following concurrent or sequential use, especially if there is a possibility of incomplete reversal of neuromuscular blockade)

Sympathomimetics
(concurrent use may reduce the antihypertensive effects of the loop diuretics; the patient should be carefully monitored to confirm that the desired effect is being obtained)

*For furosemide only (in addition to those listed above)*
Chloral hydrate
(administration of chloral hydrate followed by intravenous furosemide may result in diaphoresis, hot flashes, and variable blood pressure, including hypertension due to a hypermetabolic state caused by displacement of thyroxine from its bound state)

Probenecid
(probenecid has been found to increase serum concentrations of furosemide by inhibiting active renal tubular secretion)

## Laboratory value alterations
The following have been selected on the basis of their potential clinical significance (possible effect in parentheses where appropriate)—not necessarily inclusive (» = major clinical significance):

With physiology/laboratory test values
*For bumetanide, ethacrynic acid, and furosemide*
Blood glucose concentrations and
Urine glucose concentrations
(may be increased; ethacrynic acid increases blood glucose only rarely, especially in diabetics, prediabetics, or patients with compensated cirrhosis; in patients with uremia, large doses of ethacrynic acid may cause severe hypoglycemia; the effect of bumetanide is controversial and possibly variable)

Blood urea nitrogen (BUN) and
Uric acid, serum
(concentrations may be increased)

Calcium and
Chloride and
Magnesium and
Potassium and
Sodium
(serum concentrations may be decreased)

*For bumetanide only (in addition to the above)*
Phosphate
(urinary concentrations may be increased)

## Medical considerations/Contraindications
The medical considerations/contraindications included have been selected on the basis of their potential clinical significance (reasons given in parentheses where appropriate)—not necessarily inclusive (» = major clinical significance).

### Risk-benefit should be considered when the following medical problems exist:

*For bumetanide, ethacrynic acid, and furosemide*
» Anuria or
» Renal function impairment, severe
(impaired effectiveness and possible delayed excretion with increased risk of toxicity. Although bumetanide, ethacrynic acid, and furosemide are effective diuretics in patients with renal function impairment, reduced clearance may necessitate use of higher doses combined with more prolonged dosing intervals to prevent accumulation and reduce the risk of ototoxicity)

Diabetes mellitus
(loop diuretics cause impaired glucose tolerance)

Gout, history of or
Hyperuricemia
(loop diuretics may elevate serum uric acid concentrations)

Hearing function impairment

Hepatic function impairment, including cirrhosis and ascites
(risk of dehydration and electrolyte imbalance, which may precipitate hepatic coma and death; hospitalization during initiation of therapy is recommended)

Myocardial infarction, acute
(excessive diuresis should be avoided because of the danger of precipitating shock)

Pancreatitis, or history of
(pancreatitis has been reported with bumetanide, ethacrynic acid, and furosemide)

Sensitivity to loop diuretic prescribed

Caution is recommended also in patients who are at increased risk if hypokalemia occurs, including those taking digitalis and diuretics and those with:
Certain diarrheal states
Congestive heart failure
Hepatic cirrhosis and ascites
History of ventricular arrhythmias
Potassium-losing nephropathy
States of aldosterone excess with normal renal function

*For ethacrynic acid and furosemide only (in addition to the above)*
Lupus erythematosus, history of
(exacerbation or activation by ethacrynic acid and furosemide has been reported)

## Patient monitoring
The following may be especially important in patient monitoring (other tests may be warranted in some patients, depending on condition; » = major clinical significance):

Blood pressure measurements
(recommended at periodic intervals in patients being treated for hypertension; selected patients may be taught to monitor their blood pressure at home and report the results at regular physician visits)

Blood urea nitrogen (BUN) and
Carbon dioxide ($CO_2$)
(determinations recommended at periodic intervals during therapy)

Electrolyte concentrations
(determinations recommended at periodic intervals, especially if patients are also taking cardiac glycosides or systemic steroids, or when severe hepatic cirrhosis is present)

Glucose, serum and
Hepatic function and
Renal function and

## Diuretics, Loop (Systemic)

Uric acid, serum
(determinations recommended at periodic intervals)

Hearing examinations
(recommended at periodic intervals in patients receiving prolonged high-dose intravenous therapy)

Weight measurement
(recommended prior to initiation of therapy and at periodic intervals during therapy to monitor water loss)

## Side/Adverse Effects
See *Table 1*, page 1265.

## Patient Consultation
As an aid to patient consultation, refer to *Advice for the Patient, Diuretics, Loop (Systemic)*.

In providing consultation, consider emphasizing the following selected information (» = major clinical significance):

**Before using this medication**
» Conditions affecting use, especially:
 Sensitivity to the loop diuretic prescribed, or to sulfonamides (for bumetanide and furosemide)
 Pregnancy—Not recommended for routine use; reported to cause harmful effects, including birth defects, in animals
 Breast-feeding—Furosemide distributed into breast milk
 Use in the elderly—Elderly patients may be more sensitive to hypotensive and electrolyte effects, and may be at greater risk of developing circulatory collapse and thromboembolic episodes
 Other medications, especially parenteral amphotericin B, oral anticoagulants, other hypokalemia-causing medications, lithium, or other nephrotoxic medications
 Other medical problems, especially anuria or severe renal function impairment

**Proper use of this medication**
 Diuretic effects of the medication and timing of doses to minimize inconvenience of diuresis
 Compliance with therapy; taking medication at the same time(s) each day to maintain the therapeutic effect
 Taking with food or milk to reduce gastrointestinal irritation
» Proper dosing
 Missed dose: Taking as soon as possible; not taking if almost time for next dose; not doubling doses
» Proper storage

*For use as an antihypertensive*
 Possible need for control of weight and diet, especially sodium intake
» Patient may not experience symptoms of hypertension; importance of taking medication even if feeling well
» Does not cure, but controls hypertension; possible need for lifelong therapy; serious consequences of untreated hypertension

*For oral solution dosage form of furosemide (in addition to the above)*
 Taking orally, even if in dropper bottle; importance of accurate measurement

**Precautions while using this medication**
 Making regular visits to physician to check progress
» Possibility of hypokalemia; possible need for additional potassium in diet; not changing diet without first checking with physician
 To prevent dehydration, notifying physician if severe nausea, vomiting, or diarrhea occurs and continues
 Caution if any kind of surgery (including dental surgery) is required
» Caution when getting up suddenly from a lying or sitting position
» Caution in using alcohol, while standing for long periods or exercising, and during hot weather because of enhanced orthostatic hypotensive effects
 Diabetics: May increase blood sugar levels

*For use as an antihypertensive*
» Not taking other medications, especially nonprescription sympathomimetics, unless discussed with physician

*For furosemide (in addition to the above)*
» Possible skin photosensitivity; avoiding unprotected exposure to sun; using protective clothing; using a sun block product that includes protection against both UVA-caused photosensitivity reactions and UVB-caused sunburn reactions; avoiding use of sunlamp, tanning bed, or tanning booth

**Side/adverse effects**
 Signs of potential side effects, especially allergic reaction, blood in urine, electrolyte imbalance, gastrointestinal bleeding, gout, hepatic dysfunction, leukopenia, agranulocytosis, ototoxicity, pancreatitis, thrombocytopenia, and xanthopsia

## General Dosing Information
Dosage must be adjusted to meet the individual requirements of each patient, on the basis of clinical response. The lowest effective dosage should be utilized to minimize potential fluid and electrolyte imbalance.

When loop diuretics are used to promote diuresis, intermittent dosage schedules may reduce the possibility of electrolyte imbalance or hyperuricemia resulting from therapy.

Concurrent administration of potassium supplements or potassium-sparing diuretics may be indicated in patients considered to be at higher risk for developing hypokalemia.

If a single daily dose is indicated, it is preferably taken on arising in order to minimize the effect of increased frequency of urination on sleep.

When bumetanide, ethacrynic acid, or furosemide is added to an antihypertensive regimen, the dose of other antihypertensive agents may have to be reduced in order to prevent an excessive drop in blood pressure.

It is recommended that bumetanide, ethacrynic acid, and furosemide be discontinued if oliguria persists for more than 24 hours at maximal dosage.

---

### BUMETANIDE

## Summary of Differences
Pharmacology/pharmacokinetics:
 Mechanism of action/effect—May have additional action on proximal tubule.
 Biotransformation and elimination—Excreted largely unchanged.
Side/adverse effects:
 Muscle pain may occur with large doses. Chest pain, premature ejaculation, and difficulty in keeping an erection have also been reported.

## Additional Dosing Information
See also *General Dosing Information*.

**For parenteral dosage forms only**
Intravenous administration is generally preferred over intramuscular administration.
Intravenous administration should be at a slow, controlled rate over a 2-minute period.

## Oral Dosage Forms
Note: Bracketed uses in the *Dosage Forms* section refer to categories of use and/or indications that are not included in U.S. product labeling.

### BUMETANIDE TABLETS USP

**Usual adult dose**
[Antihypertensive or]
Diuretic—
 Oral, 500 mcg (0.5 mg) to 2 mg a day as a single daily dose. The dose may be increased, if necessary, by addition of a second or third daily dose with intervals of four to five hours between doses. An intermittent dosage schedule (administration on alternate days for three or four days, with one or two days in between) may also be used.

Note: Geriatric patients may be more sensitive to the effects of the usual adult dose.

**Usual adult prescribing limits**
10 mg a day.

**Usual pediatric dose**
Dosage has not been established.

**Strength(s) usually available**
U.S.—
 500 mcg (0.5 mg) (Rx) [*Bumex* (lactose); GENERIC].
 1 mg (Rx) [*Bumex* (lactose); GENERIC].
 2 mg (Rx) [*Bumex* (lactose); GENERIC].
Canada—
 Not commercially available.

**Packaging and storage**
Store below 40 °C (104 °F), preferably between 15 and 30 °C (59 and 86 °F), unless otherwise specified by manufacturer. Store in a tight, light-resistant container.

**Auxiliary labeling**
• Do not take other medicines without your doctor's advice.

## Parenteral Dosage Forms

Note: Bracketed uses in the *Dosage Forms* section refer to categories of use and/or indications that are not included in U.S. product labeling.

### BUMETANIDE INJECTION USP

**Usual adult dose**
[Antihypertensive or]
Diuretic—
Intravenous or intramuscular, 500 mcg (0.5 mg) to 1 mg, repeated at intervals of two to three hours, if necessary.

**Usual adult prescribing limits**
10 mg a day.

**Usual pediatric dose**
Dosage has not been established.

**Strength(s) usually available**
U.S.—
250 mcg (0.25 mg) per mL (Rx) [*Bumex* (benzyl alcohol 1%)].
Canada—
Not commercially available.

**Packaging and storage**
Store below 40 °C (104 °F), preferably between 15 and 30 °C (59 and 86 °F), unless otherwise specified by manufacturer. Protect from freezing. Protect from light.

**Stability**
Infusion solutions should be freshly prepared and used within a 24-hour period.

---

### ETHACRYNIC ACID

## Summary of Differences

Indications:
Also indicated for short-term management of ascites due to malignancy, idiopathic edema, and lymphedema, and for treatment of hypercalcemia.
Side/adverse effects:
Greatest risk of ototoxicity. Gastrointestinal bleeding and blood in urine may occur with parenteral use. Higher incidence of gastrointestinal upset. Confusion, loss of appetite, and nervousness were reported more often than with other loop diuretics.

## Additional Dosing Information

See also *General Dosing Information*.

Concurrent administration of ammonium chloride or arginine chloride may be indicated in patients considered to be at higher risk of developing metabolic alkalosis as a result of the chloruretic effect.

Because of the profound effect of ethacrynic acid on sodium excretion, rigid dietary salt restriction is not necessary in most patients and may in fact increase the risk of adverse effects due to hyponatremia.

In patients with renal edema, administration of salt-poor albumin may be helpful in preventing reduced response to ethacrynic acid because of hypoproteinemia.

If severe, watery diarrhea occurs, it is recommended that ethacrynic acid be permanently withdrawn.

For parenteral dosage forms only
Intramuscular or subcutaneous administration is not recommended because of local pain and irritation.
Intravenous administration should be at a slow, controlled rate over a period of about 30 minutes.
If a second injection is required, use of a different injection site is recommended to prevent thrombophlebitis.

## Oral Dosage Forms

### ETHACRYNIC ACID ORAL SOLUTION

**Usual adult dose**
Diuretic—
Initial: Oral, 50 to 100 mg a day, in single or divided daily doses with increments of 25 to 50 mg a day as needed.
Maintenance: Oral, reduced to meet individual requirements once dry weight is achieved; usually 50 to 200 mg a day.
Note: Geriatric patients may be more sensitive to the effects of the usual adult dose.

**Usual adult prescribing limits**
400 mg a day.

**Usual pediatric dose**
Diuretic—
Initial: Oral, 25 mg a day, with increments of 25 mg a day as needed.
Maintenance: Oral, adjusted to meet individual requirements.
Note: Use in infants is not recommended.

**Strength(s) usually available**
U.S.—
Dosage form not commercially available in the U.S. Compounding required for prescriptions.
Canada—
Dosage form not commercially available in Canada. Compounding required for prescriptions.

**Packaging and storage**
Store at or below 24 °C (75 °F). Protect from freezing.

**Preparation of dosage form**
An oral liquid dosage form of ethacrynic acid has been prepared by dissolving ethacrynic acid powder in 10% alcohol in water, then bringing it to volume (to produce a solution containing 1 mg of ethacrynic acid per mL) with a 50% aqueous sorbitol solution (with added 0.005% methylparaben and 0.002% propylparaben as preservatives), and adjusting the pH to 7 with sodium hydroxide.

**Stability**
This product was found to be stable for several weeks when stored at 24 °C (75 °F).

**Auxiliary labeling**
• Take with meals or milk.
• Do not take other medicines without your doctor's advice.

**Note**
Check refill frequency to determine compliance in hypertensive patients.

### ETHACRYNIC ACID TABLETS USP

**Usual adult dose**
See *Ethacrynic Acid Oral Solution*.

**Usual adult prescribing limits**
400 mg a day.

**Usual pediatric dose**
See *Ethacrynic Acid Oral Solution*.

**Strength(s) usually available**
U.S.—
25 mg (Rx) [*Edecrin* (lactose)].
50 mg (Rx) [*Edecrin* (lactose)].
Canada—
50 mg (Rx) [*Edecrin* (scored; lactose)].

**Packaging and storage**
Store below 40 °C (104 °F), preferably between 15 and 30 °C (59 and 86 °F), unless otherwise specified by manufacturer. Store in a well-closed container.

**Auxiliary labeling**
• Take with meals or milk.
• Do not take other medicines without your doctor's advice.

**Note**
Check refill frequency to determine compliance in hypertensive patients.

## Parenteral Dosage Forms

### ETHACRYNATE SODIUM FOR INJECTION USP

**Usual adult dose**
Diuretic—
Intravenous, 50 mg (base), or 500 mcg (0.5 mg) to 1 mg per kg of body weight; may be repeated in two to four hours if necessary, then every four to six hours if the patient is responsive. In some emergency situations, the injection may be repeated every hour.
Note: Geriatric patients may be more sensitive to the effects of the usual adult dose.

**Usual adult prescribing limits**
100 mg (base).

**Usual pediatric dose**
Diuretic—
Intravenous, 1 mg (base) per kg of body weight.

**Size(s) usually available**
U.S.—
50 mg (base) (Rx) [*Edecrin* (mannitol 62.5 mg)].
Canada—
50 mg (base) (Rx) [*Edecrin* (mannitol 62.5 mg)].

## 1264 Diuretics, Loop (Systemic)

**Packaging and storage**
Store below 40 °C (104 °F), preferably between 15 and 30 °C (59 and 86 °F), unless otherwise specified by manufacturer.

**Preparation of dosage form**
Infusion solutions can be prepared using 0.9% sodium chloride injection or 5% dextrose injection, after pH has been adjusted when necessary.

**Stability**
A hazy or opalescent solution may result from use of a diluent with a low pH (below 5); use of such a solution is not recommended.
Unused, reconstituted solution should be discarded after 24 hours at room temperature.

**Incompatibilities**
The solution is physically incompatible with whole blood or its derivatives.

---

### FUROSEMIDE

## Summary of Differences

Category:
   Furosemide is used as a diagnostic aid adjunct in renal disease.
Precautions:
   Breast-feeding—Distributed into breast milk.
   Pediatrics—Prolonged half-life in neonates.
   Drug interactions and/or related problems—Also interacts with chloral hydrate and probenecid.
Side/adverse effects:
   Also causes xanthopsia and increased sensitivity of skin to sunlight.

## Additional Dosing Information

See also *General Dosing Information*.

When furosemide is used as an antihypercalcemic, body fluid and sodium chloride should be replaced in order to maintain extracellular fluid volume and increase calcium excretion effectively.

**For parenteral dosage forms only**
Intravenous administration is generally preferred over intramuscular administration.
Intravenous administration should be at a slow, controlled rate over a 1- to 2-minute period.
If high-dose parenteral therapy is indicated, administration should be by controlled intravenous infusion at a rate not exceeding 4 mg per minute.

## Oral Dosage Forms

Note: Bracketed uses in the *Dosage Forms* section refer to categories of use and/or indications that are not included in U.S. product labeling.

### FUROSEMIDE ORAL SOLUTION

**Usual adult dose**
Diuretic—
   Oral, initially 20 to 80 mg as a single dose, the dosage then being increased by an additional 20 to 40 mg at six- to eight-hour intervals, until the desired response is obtained. The maintenance dose as determined by titration is then given daily as a single dose or divided into two or three doses, given once a day every other day, or given once a day for two to four consecutive days out of each week.
Antihypertensive—
   Oral, initially 40 mg two times a day, the dosage then being adjusted according to patient response.
[Antihypercalcemic][1]—
   Oral, 120 mg a day as a single dose or divided into two or three doses.
Note: Geriatric patients may be more sensitive to the effects of the usual adult dose.

**Usual adult prescribing limits**
600 mg a day.
Note: In chronic renal failure, doses of up to 4 grams a day have been used.

**Usual pediatric dose**
Diuretic—
   Oral, initially 2 mg per kg of body weight as a single dose, the dosage then being increased by an additional 1 to 2 mg per kg of body weight at six- to eight-hour intervals, until the desired response is obtained.
Note: Doses as large as 5 mg per kg of body weight may be required in some children with nephrotic syndrome.
   Doses greater than 6 mg per kg of body weight are not recommended.
   Dosing interval should be extended in neonates because of prolonged half-life.

**Strength(s) usually available**
U.S.—
   8 mg per mL (Rx) [GENERIC].
   10 mg per mL (Rx) [*Lasix* (alcohol 11.5%); *Myrosemide* (alcohol 11.5%); GENERIC].
Canada—
   10 mg per mL (Rx) [*Lasix* (sugar-free)].

**Packaging and storage**
Store below 40 °C (104 °F), preferably between 15 and 30 °C (59 and 86 °F), in a well-closed container, unless otherwise specified by manufacturer. Protect from light. Protect from freezing.

**Auxiliary labeling**
• Take by mouth only (when dispensed with graduated dropper).
• Do not take other medicines without your doctor's advice.

**Note**
Do not dispense discolored solution.
When dispensing, include the manufacturer-provided graduated dropper or measuring spoon.
Explain administration technique when dispensed with graduated dropper.
Check refill frequency to determine compliance in hypertensive patients.

### FUROSEMIDE TABLETS USP

**Usual adult dose**
See *Furosemide Oral Solution*.

**Usual adult prescribing limits**
600 mg a day.
Note: In chronic renal failure, doses of up to 4 grams a day have been used.

**Usual pediatric dose**
See *Furosemide Oral Solution*.

**Strength(s) usually available**
U.S.—
   20 mg (Rx) [*Lasix;* GENERIC (may be scored)].
   40 mg (Rx) [*Lasix* (scored); GENERIC (may be scored)].
   80 mg (Rx) [*Lasix;* GENERIC (may be scored)].
Canada—
   20 mg (Rx) [*Apo-Furosemide; Furoside* (scored); *Lasix; Novosemide* (scored); *Uritol* (scored)].
   40 mg (Rx) [*Apo-Furosemide* (scored); *Furoside* (scored); *Lasix* (scored); *Novosemide* (scored); *Uritol* (scored)].
   80 mg (Rx) [*Apo-Furosemide* (scored); *Novosemide* (scored); *Lasix* (scored)].
   500 mg (Rx) [*Lasix Special* (scored)].

**Packaging and storage**
Store below 40 °C (104 °F), preferably between 15 and 30 °C (59 and 86 °F), unless otherwise specified by manufacturer. Store in a well-closed container. Protect from light.

**Stability**
Exposure to light may cause discoloration. Do not dispense discolored tablets.

**Auxiliary labeling**
• Do not take other medicines without your doctor's advice.

**Note**
Since variations in bioavailability have been found among brands, try to avoid switching brands when dispensing refills.
Check refill frequency to determine compliance in hypertensive patients.

## Parenteral Dosage Forms

Note: Bracketed uses in the *Dosage Forms* section refer to categories of use and/or indications that are not included in U.S. product labeling.

### FUROSEMIDE INJECTION USP

**Usual adult dose**
Diuretic—
   Intramuscular or intravenous, initially 20 to 40 mg as a single dose, the dosage then being increased by an additional 20 mg at two-hour intervals until the desired response is obtained. The maintenance dose as determined by titration is then given one or two times a day.
Note: In acute pulmonary edema (not accompanied by hypertensive crisis), the usual initial dose is 40 mg intravenously, followed by 80 mg in one hour if a satisfactory response is not obtained.
Antihypertensive—
   Hypertensive crisis in patients with normal renal function: Intravenous, 40 to 80 mg.

Hypertensive crisis accompanied by pulmonary edema or acute renal failure: Intravenous, 100 to 200 mg.

[Antihypercalcemic][1]—
Intramuscular or intravenous, 80 to 100 mg in severe cases, the dosage being repeated if necessary every one to two hours until the desired response is obtained. In less severe cases, smaller doses may be given every two to four hours.

[Diagnostic aid adjunct (renal disease)]—
Intravenous, 0.3 to 0.5 mg per kg of body weight to a maximum of 40 mg.

Note: Geriatric patients may be more sensitive to the effects of the usual adult dose.

**Usual adult prescribing limits**
Although controversial, doses of up to 6 grams a day administered by slow intravenous infusion have been used in acute renal failure by some clinicians.

**Usual pediatric dose**
Diuretic—
Intramuscular or intravenous, initially 1 mg per kg of body weight as a single dose, the dosage then being increased by an additional 1 mg per kg of body weight at two-hour intervals until the desired response is obtained.

[Antihypercalcemic][1]—
Intramuscular or intravenous, 25 to 50 mg, the dosage being repeated if necessary every four hours until the desired response is obtained.

Note: Doses greater than 6 mg per kg of body weight are not recommended.

Dosing interval should be extended in neonates because of prolonged half-life.

**Strength(s) usually available**
U.S.—
10 mg per mL (Rx) [*Lasix;* GENERIC].
Canada—
10 mg per mL (Rx) [*Lasix* (benzyl alcohol); *Lasix Special; Uritol;* GENERIC].

**Packaging and storage**
Store below 40 °C (104 °F), preferably between 15 and 30 °C (59 and 86 °F), unless otherwise specified by manufacturer. Protect from light. Protect from freezing.

**Preparation of dosage form**
Infusion solutions can be prepared using 0.9% sodium chloride injection, lactated Ringer's injection, or 5% dextrose injection, after pH has been adjusted when necessary.

**Stability**
Infusion solutions should be freshly prepared and used within a 24-hour period.

**Incompatibilities**
Furosemide Injection USP is a mildly buffered alkaline solution and should not be mixed with highly acidic solutions.

[1]Not included in Canadian product labeling.

## Selected Bibliography
The fifth report of the Joint National Committee on Detection, Evaluation, and Treatment of High Blood Pressure (JNC V). Arch Intern Med 1993; 153(2): 154-83.

Revised: 08/02/94
Interim revision: 04/24/95; 08/19/97; 08/13/98

## Table 1. Side/Adverse Effects*

Note: Nephrocalcinosis or nephrolithiasis may occur with furosemide administration if hypercalciuria is present.
Ethacrynic acid appears to be more likely to cause ototoxicity than bumetanide or furosemide and less likely to cause hyperglycemia than furosemide.

The following side/adverse effects have been selected on the basis of their potential clinical significance (possible signs and symptoms in parentheses where appropriate)—not necessarily inclusive:

Legend
I = Bumetanide
II = Ethacrynic acid
III = Furosemide

| | I | II | III |
|---|---|---|---|
| **Those indicating need for medical attention** | | | |
| *Allergic reaction* (skin rash) | R | R | R |
| *Blood in urine*—associated with parenteral use | U | R | U |
| *Electrolyte imbalance such as hyponatremia, hypochloremic alkalosis, and hypokalemia*—occurs frequently, up to 10 to 15% of patients receiving ethacrynic acid (usually not symptomatic; symptoms include dry mouth, increased thirst, irregular heartbeat, mood or mental changes, muscle cramps or pain, nausea or vomiting, unusual tiredness or weakness, weak pulse) | L | L | L |
| *Gastrointestinal bleeding* (black, tarry stools)—associated with parenteral use | U | R | U |
| *Gout* (joint pain, lower back or side pain) | R | R | R |
| *Hepatic dysfunction* (yellow eyes or skin) | R | R | R |
| *Leukopenia or agranulocytosis* (fever or chills, cough or hoarseness, lower back or side pain, painful or difficult urination) | R | R | R |
| *Ototoxicity*—more frequent with renal function impairment and in rapid parenteral administration of large doses (ringing or buzzing in ears or any loss of hearing; usually transient, but permanent deafness has occurred, especially in patients receiving other ototoxic drugs) | R | L† | R |
| *Pancreatitis* (severe stomach pain with nausea and vomiting) | R | R | R |
| *Thrombocytopenia* (unusual bleeding or bruising; black, tarry stools; blood in urine or stools; pinpoint red spots on skin) | R | R | R |
| *Xanthopsia* (yellow vision) | U | U | R |
| **Those indicating need for medical attention only if they continue or are bothersome** | | | |
| *Blurred vision* | L | L | L |
| *Chest pain* | L | U | U |
| *Confusion* | U | L | U |

*Differences in frequency of occurrence may reflect either lack of clinical-use data or actual pharmacologic distinctions among agents (although their basic pharmacologic similarity suggests that side effects occurring with one may occur with the others). M = more frequent; L = less frequent; R = rare; U = unknown.
†Dose-related.

## Table 1. Side/Adverse Effects* (continued)

Note: Nephrocalcinosis or nephrolithiasis may occur with furosemide administration if hypercalciuria is present.
Ethacrynic acid appears to be more likely to cause ototoxicity than bumetanide or furosemide and less likely to cause hyperglycemia than furosemide.

| The following side/adverse effects have been selected on the basis of their potential clinical significance (possible signs and symptoms in parentheses where appropriate)—not necessarily inclusive: | Legend I=Bumetanide II=Ethacrynic acid III=Furosemide | | |
|---|---|---|---|
| | I | II | III |
| *Diarrhea* | L | M† | L |
| *Headache* | L | L | L |
| *Increased sensitivity of skin to sunlight* | U | U | L |
| *Local irritation* (redness or pain at site of injection) | R | R | R |
| *Loss of appetite* | L | M† | L |
| *Nervousness* | U | L | U |
| *Orthostatic hypotension as a result of massive diuresis* (dizziness or lightheadedness when getting up from a lying or sitting position) | M | M | M |
| *Premature ejaculation or difficulty in keeping an erection* | L | U | U |
| *Stomach cramps or pain* | L | L | L |

*Differences in frequency of occurrence may reflect either lack of clinical-use data or actual pharmacologic distinctions among agents (although their basic pharmacologic similarity suggests that side effects occurring with one may occur with the others). M = more frequent; L = less frequent; R = rare; U = unknown.
†Dose-related.

# DIURETICS, POTASSIUM-SPARING Systemic

This monograph includes information on the following: 1) Amiloride; 2) Spironolactone; 3) Triamterene.

VA CLASSIFICATION (Primary/Secondary):
Amiloride—CV704/CV490; TN900
Spironolactone—CV704/CV490; TN900; HS900
Triamterene—CV704/CV490; TN900

Commonly used brand name(s): *Aldactone*[2]; *Dyrenium*[3]; *Midamor*[1]; *Novospiroton*[2].

Note: For a listing of dosage forms and brand names by country availability, see *Dosage Forms* section(s).

## Category

Diuretic—Amiloride; Spironolactone; Triamterene.
Antihypertensive—Amiloride; Spironolactone; Triamterene.
Aldosterone antagonist—Spironolactone.
Diagnostic aid (primary hyperaldosteronism)—Spironolactone.
Antihypokalemic—Amiloride; Spironolactone; Triamterene.

## Indications

Note: Bracketed information in the *Indications* section refers to uses that are not included in U.S. product labeling.

### Accepted

Edema (treatment)—Amiloride, spironolactone, and triamterene are indicated as adjuncts in the management of edematous states, especially when a potassium-sparing diuretic effect is desired. These may include congestive heart failure, hepatic cirrhosis, and nephrotic syndrome, which often involve secondary hyperaldosteronism, as well as idiopathic edema.

Hypertension (treatment adjunct)—Amiloride, spironolactone, and [triamterene][1] are indicated as adjuncts in the treatment of hypertension (for spironolactone, with or without accompanying hyperaldosteronism), especially when a potassium-sparing diuretic effect is desired.

For additional information on initial therapeutic guidelines related to the treatment of hypertension, see *Appendix III*.

Hyperaldosteronism, primary (diagnosis and treatment)—Spironolactone is indicated for diagnosis and short- or long-term management of primary hyperaldosteronism.

Hypokalemia (prophylaxis and treatment)—[Amiloride][1], spironolactone, and [triamterene][1] are indicated for prevention and treatment of hypokalemia in patients for whom other measures are inappropriate or inadequate.

[Polycystic ovary syndrome (treatment)][1]—Spironolactone is also used with some success in the treatment of polycystic ovary syndrome.

[Hirsutism, female (treatment)][1]—Spironolactone has been used in the treatment of female hirsutism.

[1]Not included in Canadian product labeling.

## Pharmacology/Pharmacokinetics

### Physicochemical characteristics

Molecular weight—
Amiloride hydrochloride: 302.12.
Spironolactone: 416.57.
Triamterene: 253.27.

pKa—
Amiloride: 8.7.
Triamterene: 6.2.

### Mechanism of action/Effect

Diuretic or Antihypokalemic—Potassium-sparing diuretics interfere with sodium reabsorption in the distal convoluted tubule, thereby promoting excretion of sodium and water and retention of potassium. Amiloride and triamterene have a direct inhibiting effect on the entry of sodium into the cells, while spironolactone competitively inhibits the action of aldosterone.

Antihypertensive—Diuretics lower blood pressure initially by reducing plasma and extracellular fluid volume; cardiac output also decreases. Eventually, the extracellular fluid volume and the cardiac output return to normal with an accompanying decrease in peripheral resistance.

Aldosterone antagonist or Diagnostic aid (primary hyperaldosteronism)—Spironolactone is a competitive inhibitor of aldosterone; neither amiloride nor triamterene has this effect.

Hirsutism or Polycystic ovary syndrome—May be due to an antiandrogenic effect of spironolactone.

### Absorption

Amiloride—Incompletely (15 to 20%) absorbed from gastrointestinal tract; rate, but not necessarily extent, of absorption is increased after 4 hours of fasting.

Spironolactone—Well absorbed following oral administration; bioavailability is greater than 90%. Absorption is enhanced by concomitant intake of food.

Triamterene—Rapidly but incompletely (30 to 70%) absorbed from the gastrointestinal tract.

### Protein binding

Amiloride—Minimal.
Spironolactone and canrenone—Very high (more than 90%).
Triamterene—Moderate (67%).

**Biotransformation**
Amiloride—Not metabolized.
Spironolactone—Hepatic; approximately 25 to 30% converted to canrenone.
Triamterene—Hepatic.

**Half-life**
Amiloride—
  6 to 9 hours.
Spironolactone—
  Canrenone: 13 to 24 hours (average 19 hours) when administered once or twice daily; 9 to 16 hours (average 12.5 hours) when administered 4 times daily.
Triamterene—
  Normal, 90 to 120 minutes; anuric, 10 hours. Some active metabolites have a normal half-life of up to 12 hours.
  Terminal half-life: 5 to 7 hours.

**Onset of action**
Diuretic—
  Amiloride: Single dose—Within 2 hours.
  Triamterene: Single dose—2 to 4 hours.

**Time to peak concentration**
Amiloride—3 to 4 hours.
Triamterene—2 to 4 hours.

**Time to peak effect**
Diuretic—
  Amiloride: Single dose—6 to 10 hours.
  Spironolactone: Multiple doses—2 to 3 days.
  Triamterene: Multiple doses—1 day to several days.

**Duration of action**
Diuretic—
  Amiloride: Single dose—24 hours.
  Spironolactone: Multiple doses—2 to 3 days.
  Triamterene: Single dose—7 to 9 hours.

**Elimination**
Amiloride—Renal, 20 to 50% (unchanged); fecal, 40% (unchanged).
Spironolactone—Metabolites: Primary route, renal (less than 10% unchanged); secondary route, biliary/fecal.
Triamterene—Primary route, biliary/fecal; secondary route, renal.

## Precautions to Consider

**Carcinogenicity/Tumorigenicity**
*Amiloride—*
  One study in mice at doses up to 25 times the maximum daily human dose and another in male and female rats at doses up to 15 and 20 times the maximum daily human dose for 104 weeks showed no evidence of carcinogenicity or tumorigenicity.
*Spironolactone—*
  Breast carcinoma has been reported in men and women taking this medication, but a direct causal relationship has not yet been established.
  Spironolactone has been found to be tumorigenic in rats, mainly in endocrine organs and the liver. A statistically significant dose-related increase in benign adenomas of the thyroid and testes was found in male rats given spironolactone in doses up to 250 times the usual daily human dose of 2 mg per kg of body weight (mg/kg). In addition, a dose-related increase in proliferative liver changes was revealed in male rats. Hepatocytomegaly, hyperplastic nodules, and hepatocellular carcinoma were evident at the highest dosage level of 500 mg/kg. In female rats, a statistically significant increase in malignant mammary tumors was seen at the mid-dose level.
*Triamterene—*
  Studies evaluating the carcinogenic potential of triamterene have not been done.

**Mutagenicity**
*Amiloride—*In Ames tests, no evidence of mutagenicity was found.

**Pregnancy/Reproduction**
Fertility—*Amiloride:* Studies in rats given amiloride at 20 times the expected maximum human daily dose revealed no evidence of fertility impairment. However, some toxicity in adult rats and rabbits and a decrease in rat pup growth and survival were seen at doses of 5 or more times the expected maximum daily human dose.

Pregnancy—Pregnant women should be advised to contact physician before taking these medications, since routine use of diuretics during normal pregnancy is inappropriate and exposes mother and fetus to unnecessary hazard. Diuretics do not prevent development of toxemia of pregnancy, and there is no satisfactory evidence that they are useful in the treatment of toxemia. Diuretics are indicated only in the treatment of edema due to pathologic causes or as a short course of treatment in patients with severe hypervolemia.
*Amiloride—*
  Adequate and well-controlled studies in humans have not been done.
  Amiloride crosses the placenta in modest amounts in rabbits and mice. However, teratogenicity studies in rabbits and mice given 20 and 25 times the maximum human dose, respectively, revealed no evidence of fetal harm.
  FDA Pregnancy Category B.
*Spironolactone—*
  Spironolactone may cross the placenta. However, problems in humans have not been documented.
*Triamterene—*
  Adequate and well-controlled studies in humans have not been done.
  Triamterene crosses the placenta and appears in the cord blood of ewes. Studies in rats given triamterene in doses up to 30 times the human dose have revealed no evidence of harm to the fetus.
  FDA Pregnancy Category B.

**Breast-feeding**
*Amiloride*—It is not known whether amiloride is distributed into human breast milk. However, problems in humans have not been documented. Amiloride has been shown to be distributed into rat's milk.
*Spironolactone*—Problems in humans have not been documented. However, canrenone (an active metabolite of spironolactone) is distributed into breast milk.
*Triamterene*—It is not known whether triamterene is distributed into human breast milk. However, problems in humans have not been documented. Triamterene has been shown to be distributed into animal milk.

**Pediatrics**
Studies performed to date have not demonstrated pediatrics-specific problems that would limit the usefulness of potassium-sparing diuretics in children.

**Geriatrics**
Although appropriate studies on the relationship of age to the effects of potassium-sparing diuretics have not been performed in the geriatric population, the elderly may be at increased risk of developing hyperkalemia. In addition, elderly patients are more likely to have age-related renal function impairment, which may require caution in patients receiving potassium-sparing diuretics.

**Drug interactions and/or related problems**
The following drug interactions and/or related problems have been selected on the basis of their potential clinical significance (possible mechanism in parentheses where appropriate)—not necessarily inclusive (» = major clinical significance):

Note: Combinations containing any of the following medications, depending on the amount present, may also interact with this medication.

*For all potassium-sparing diuretics*
  Allopurinol or
  Colchicine or
  Probenecid or
  Sulfinpyrazone
    (triamterene may raise the concentration of blood uric acid, but to a lesser extent than thiazide diuretics or ethacrynic acid or furosemide; dosage adjustment of antigout medications may be necessary to control hyperuricemia and gout)

» Anticoagulants, coumarin- or indandione-derivative or
» Heparin
    (anticoagulant effects may be decreased when these medications are used concurrently with potassium-sparing diuretics, as a result of reduction of plasma volume leading to concentration of procoagulant factors in the blood; in addition, diuretic-induced improvement of hepatic congestion may lead to improved hepatic function, resulting in increased procoagulant factor synthesis; dosage adjustments may be necessary)

Anti-inflammatory drugs, nonsteroidal (NSAIDs), especially indomethacin
    (may reduce the antihypertensive effects of the potassium-sparing diuretics; indomethacin may also reduce the natriuretic and diuretic effects of potassium-sparing diuretics, possibly because of renal prostaglandin synthesis inhibition and/or sodium and fluid retention; the patient should be carefully monitored to confirm that the desired effect is being obtained)

- » Angiotensin-converting enzyme (ACE) inhibitors or
  Anti-inflammatory drugs, nonsteroidal (NSAIDs), especially indomethacin or
  (concurrent use of NSAIDs with a diuretic may increase the risk of renal failure secondary to a decrease in renal blood flow caused by inhibition of renal prostaglandin synthesis)
- » Blood from blood bank (may contain up to 30 mEq [mmol] of potassium per liter of plasma or up to 65 mEq [mmol] per liter of whole blood when stored for more than 10 days) or
- » Cyclosporine or
- » Diuretics, potassium-sparing, other or
  Heparin or
- » Low-salt milk (may contain up to 60 mEq [mmol] of potassium per liter) or
- » Potassium-containing medications or
- » Potassium supplements or substances containing high levels of potassium or
  Salt substitutes (most contain substantial amounts of potassium)
  (concurrent administration with potassium-sparing diuretics tends to promote serum potassium accumulation; hyperkalemia may result, especially in patients with renal insufficiency)
  Exchange resins, sodium cycle (such as sodium polystyrene sulfonate)
  (whether administered orally or rectally, these medications reduce serum potassium levels by replacing potassium with sodium; fluid retention may occur in some patients because of the increased sodium intake)
  Hypotension-producing medications, other (See *Appendix II*)
  (antihypertensive and/or diuretic effects may be potentiated when these medications are used concurrently with potassium-sparing diuretics; although some antihypertensive and/or diuretic combinations are frequently used for therapeutic advantage, dosage adjustments may be necessary during concurrent use)
- » Lithium
  (concurrent use with potassium-sparing diuretics is not recommended, as they may provoke lithium toxicity by reducing renal clearance)
  Sympathomimetics
  (may reduce the antihypertensive effects of potassium-sparing diuretics; the patient should be carefully monitored to confirm that the desired effect is being obtained)

*For spironolactone only (in addition to those listed for all potassium-sparing diuretics)*
- » Digoxin
  (spironolactone may increase the half-life of digoxin; dosage reduction or increased dosing intervals of digoxin may be necessary and careful monitoring is recommended)

*For triamterene only (in addition to those listed for all potassium-sparing diuretics)*
  Amantadine
  (triamterene may reduce the renal clearance of amantadine, resulting in increased plasma concentrations and possible amantadine toxicity)
  Folic acid
  (triamterene may act as a folate antagonist by inhibiting dihydrofolate reductase; most significant with high doses and/or prolonged triamterene use; leucovorin calcium must be used instead of folic acid in patients receiving triamterene)

**Laboratory value alterations**
The following have been selected on the basis of their potential clinical significance (possible effect in parentheses where appropriate)—not necessarily inclusive (» = major clinical significance):

With diagnostic test results
*For spironolactone only*
  Digoxin radioimmunoassays
  (results may be falsely elevated)
  Plasma cortisol concentration determination by Mattingly (fluorometric) assay
  (concentration may be falsely increased; withdrawal of spironolactone 4 to 7 days prior to determinations, or substitution of Ertel, Peterson, or Norymberski method, is recommended)

*For triamterene only*
  Fluorescent measurement of quinidine
  (similar fluorescence spectra)

With physiology/laboratory test values
*For amiloride, spironolactone, and triamterene*
  Blood urea nitrogen (BUN) concentrations (especially in patients with pre-existing renal impairment) and
  Calcium excretion, urinary and
  Creatinine concentrations, serum and
  Magnesium concentrations, serum and
  Plasma renin activity (PRA) and
  Potassium concentrations, serum and
  Uric acid concentrations, serum
  (may be increased)
  Sodium
  (serum concentrations may be decreased)

**Medical considerations/Contraindications**
The medical considerations/contraindications included have been selected on the basis of their potential clinical significance (reasons given in parentheses where appropriate)—not necessarily inclusive (» = major clinical significance).

*Except under special circumstances, this medication should not be used when the following medical problem exists:*
- » Hyperkalemia
  (potassium-sparing diuretics may further increase serum potassium concentrations)

*Risk-benefit should be considered when the following medical problems exist:*

For amiloride, spironolactone, and triamterene
- » Anuria or
- » Renal function impairment
  (potassium-sparing diuretics may aggravate electrolyte imbalance; risk of developing hyperkalemia is increased)
  Diabetes mellitus, especially in patients with confirmed or suspected renal insufficiency or
- » Diabetic nephropathy
  (increased risk of hyperkalemia; potassium-sparing diuretic should be discontinued at least 3 days prior to a glucose tolerance test because of the risk of severe hyperkalemia)
- » Hepatic function impairment
  (increased sensitivity to electrolyte changes)
  Hyponatremia
  Metabolic or respiratory acidosis, predisposition to
  (acidosis potentiates hyperkalemic effects of potassium-sparing diuretics; potassium-sparing diuretics may potentiate acidosis)
  Sensitivity to the potassium-sparing diuretic prescribed
- » Caution is also required in severely ill patients and those with relatively small urine volumes, who are at greater risk of developing hyperkalemia.

*For spironolactone only (in addition to those listed above for all potassium-sparing diuretics)*
  Menstrual abnormalities or breast enlargement

*For triamterene only (in addition to those listed above for all potassium-sparing diuretics)*
  Hyperuricemia or gout
  Nephrolithiasis, history of
  (increased risk of forming triamterene stones)

**Patient monitoring**
The following may be especially important in patient monitoring (other tests may be warranted in some patients, depending on condition; » = major clinical significance):

*For amiloride, spironolactone, and triamterene*
- » Blood pressure measurements
  (recommended at periodic intervals in patients being treated for hypertension; selected patients may be trained to perform blood pressure measurements at home and report the results at regular physician visits)
  Blood urea nitrogen (BUN) determinations and/or
  Creatinine concentrations, serum
  (determinations recommended prior to initiation of therapy and at periodic intervals during therapy)
  Electrocardiograms (ECG) and
- » Electrolyte concentrations, serum, especially serum potassium determinations
  (may be required at periodic intervals for patients on long-term therapy, especially if they are also taking systemic steroids, or when congestive heart failure or severe cirrhosis is present)

*For triamterene only*
  Platelet count and
  Total and differential leukocyte count
  (recommended prior to initiation of therapy and at periodic intervals during therapy, especially in patients with impaired hepatic function)

## Side/Adverse Effects
See *Table 1*, page 1271.

## Overdose
For more information on the management of overdose or unintentional ingestion, **contact a Poison Control Center** (see *Poison Control Center Listing*).

**Treatment of overdose**
Overdose should be treated by immediate evacuation of the stomach followed by supportive, symptomatic treatment and monitoring of serum electrolyte concentrations and renal function.

## Patient Consultation
As an aid to patient consultation, refer to *Advice for the Patient, Diuretics, Potassium-sparing (Systemic)*.
In providing consultation, consider emphasizing the following selected information (» = major clinical significance):

**Before using this medication**
» Conditions affecting use, especially:
 Sensitivity to the potassium-sparing diuretic prescribed
 Pregnancy—Not recommended for routine use; triamterene crosses placenta; spironolactone may cross placenta
 Breast-feeding—All potassium-sparing diuretics may be distributed into breast milk
 Use in the elderly—Increased risk of hyperkalemia
 Other medications, especially angiotensin-converting enzyme (ACE) inhibitors, cyclosporine, digoxin, other potassium-sparing diuretics, potassium-containing medications or supplements, or lithium
 Other medical problems, especially diabetic nephropathy, hyperkalemia, renal function impairment or hepatic function impairment

**Proper use of this medication**
 Diuretic effects of the medication and timing of doses to minimize inconvenience of diuresis
 Getting into habit of taking at same time each day to help increase compliance
 Taking with meals or milk to reduce gastrointestinal irritation
» Proper dosing
 Missed dose: Taking as soon as possible; not taking if almost time for next dose; not doubling doses
» Proper storage

*For use as an antihypertensive (amiloride and spironolactone only)*
 Possible need for control of weight and diet, especially sodium intake
» Patient may not experience symptoms of hypertension; importance of taking medication even if feeling well
» Does not cure, but helps control hypertension; possible need for lifelong therapy; checking with physician before discontinuing medication; serious consequences of untreated hypertension

**Precautions while using this medication**
 Regular visits to physician to check progress
 Avoiding excessive ingestion of foods high in potassium or use of salt substitutes or other potassium supplements
 To prevent dehydration, checking with physician if severe nausea, vomiting, or diarrhea occurs and continues
 Caution if any kind of surgery or emergency treatment is required
 Caution if any laboratory tests required; possible interference with test results

*For use as an antihypertensive (amiloride and spironolactone only)*
» Not taking other medications, especially nonprescription sympathomimetics, unless discussed with physician

*For triamterene only*
 Possible photosensitivity; avoiding unprotected exposure to sun; using protective clothing and sun block product; avoiding use of sunlamp, tanning bed, or tanning booth

**Side/adverse effects**
 Signs of potential side effects, especially agranulocytosis, allergic reaction, anaphylaxis, and hyperkalemia (for all potassium-sparing diuretics); megaloblastosis, nephrolithiasis, and thrombocytopenia (for triamterene)

*For spironolactone only (in addition to the above):*
 Possibility of enlargement of breasts in males; usually reversible within several months

## General Dosing Information
Dosage must be adjusted to meet the individual requirements of each patient, on the basis of clinical response. The lowest effective dose should be utilized to minimize potential electrolyte imbalance.

If a single daily dose is indicated, it is preferably taken on arising in order to minimize the effect of increased frequency of urination on sleep, although the diuretic effect of potassium-sparing diuretics alone is mild.

The normal adult concentration of plasma potassium is 3.5 to 5.0 mEq (mmol) per liter, with 4.5 mEq (mmol) often being used as a reference point. Potassium concentrations exceeding 6 mEq (mmol) per liter are dangerous because of possible initiation of cardiac arrhythmias. Normal potassium concentrations tend to be higher in neonates (7.7 mEq [mmol] per liter) than in adults.

Plasma potassium concentrations do not necessarily indicate the true body potassium concentration. A rise in serum pH may cause a decrease in serum potassium concentration and an increase in the intracellular potassium concentration.

It is recommended that potassium-sparing diuretic therapy be withdrawn if hyperkalemia occurs. If hyperkalemia is associated with ECG changes, prompt additional therapy with intravenous sodium bicarbonate, calcium gluconate, or calcium chloride; with oral or rectal sodium polystyrene sulfonate; or with parenteral glucose and insulin may be indicated. It is important to remember that severe hyperkalemia may occur suddenly and may not be preceded by any warning signs.

Recent evidence suggests that withdrawal of antihypertensive therapy prior to surgery is not necessary, but that the anesthesiologist must be aware of such therapy.

**Diet/Nutrition**
It is recommended that oral potassium-sparing diuretics be taken with or after meals to minimize stomach upset, and possibly also to enhance bioavailability.

---
### AMILORIDE
---

## Summary of Differences
Pharmacology/pharmacokinetics:
 Protein binding—Minimal.
 Biotransformation—None; excreted unchanged.
 Duration of action—Diuretic: Single dose—24 hours.
Side/adverse effects:
 No reported cases of agranulocytosis. Amiloride has been reported to cause constipation and muscle cramps.

## Oral Dosage Forms
### AMILORIDE HYDROCHLORIDE TABLETS USP
**Usual adult dose**
Diuretic or
Antihypertensive—
 Oral, 5 to 10 mg per day as a single dose.

Note: Geriatric patients may be more sensitive to the effects of the usual adult dose.

**Usual adult prescribing limits**
Up to 20 mg per day.

**Usual pediatric dose**
Dosage has not been established.

**Strength(s) usually available**
U.S.—
 5 mg (Rx) [*Midamor*; GENERIC].
Canada—
 5 mg (Rx) [*Midamor*].

**Packaging and storage**
Store below 40 °C (104 °F), preferably between 15 and 30 °C (59 and 86 °F), unless otherwise specified by manufacturer. Store in a well-closed container.

**Auxiliary labeling**
• Take with meals or milk.
• Do not take other medicines without your doctor's advice.

**Note**
Check refill frequency to determine compliance in hypertensive patients.

## SPIRONOLACTONE

### Summary of Differences
Indications:
    Diagnosis and treatment of primary hyperaldosteronism. Treatment of polycystic ovary syndrome and female hirsutism.
Pharmacology/pharmacokinetics:
    Mechanism of action/effect—Aldosterone antagonist.
    Protein binding—Very high (more than 90%).
    Biotransformation—Hepatic, extensive, to active metabolite (canrenone).
    Duration of action—Diuretic: Multiple doses—2 to 3 days.
Precautions:
    Carcinogenicity—Tumorigenic in rats and possibly associated with breast carcinoma in humans.
    Drug interactions and/or related problems—Use with digoxin may increase digoxin half-life.
    Laboratory value alterations—May falsely increase plasma cortisol determinations by Mattingly (fluorometric) assay. May falsely elevate digoxin radioimmunoassays.
    Medical considerations/contraindications—Menstrual abnormalities or breast enlargement.
Side/adverse effects:
    Endocrine or antiandrogenic effects more common at doses exceeding 100 mg per day. May cause CNS effects and causes more frequent gastrointestinal irritation.

### Additional Dosing Information
See also *General Dosing Information*.

To reduce delay in onset of effect, a loading dose of 2 to 3 times the daily dose may be administered on the first day of therapy.

When spironolactone is added to therapy with another diuretic or antihypertensive agent, it is recommended that the dosage of the other drug (especially ganglionic blocking agents) be reduced by at least 50% and then adjusted as required.

It is recommended that spironolactone be discontinued several days prior to adrenal vein catheterization for measurement of aldosterone concentrations, for the purpose of attempting lateralization in primary hyperaldosteronism, and for measurements of plasma renin activity.

When high doses of spironolactone are required for treatment of edema due to hepatic cirrhosis, drug dosage may be reduced prior to completion of diuresis to avoid dehydration and precipitation of hepatic coma, although dry weight may be achieved.

### Oral Dosage Forms
Note: Bracketed uses in the *Dosage Forms* section refer to categories of use and/or indications that are not included in U.S. product labeling.

#### SPIRONOLACTONE TABLETS USP
**Usual adult dose**
Edema due to congestive heart failure, hepatic cirrhosis, or nephrotic syndrome—
    Initial: Oral, 25 to 200 mg a day in two to four divided doses for at least five days.
    Maintenance: Oral, 75 to 400 mg a day in two to four divided doses.
Antihypertensive—
    Initial: Oral, 50 to 100 mg a day as a single daily dose or in two to four divided doses for at least two weeks, followed by gradual dosage adjustment every two weeks as necessary up to 200 mg a day.
    Maintenance: Oral, adjusted to meet individual requirements.
Primary hyperaldosteronism—
    Maintenance: Oral, 100 to 400 mg per day in two to four divided daily doses prior to surgery; smaller doses may be used for long-term maintenance in patients unsuitable for surgery.
[Polycystic ovary disease]—
    Oral, 100 to 200 mg per day in two divided daily doses.
[Hirsutism, female]—
    Oral, 100 mg two times a day.
Diagnostic aid (primary hyperaldosteronism)—
    Long test: Oral, 400 mg per day in two to four divided daily doses for three to four weeks.
    Short test: Oral, 400 mg per day in two to four divided daily doses for four days.
Antihypokalemic—
    Diuretic-induced hypokalemia: Oral, 25 to 100 mg per day as a single daily dose or in two to four divided doses.
Note: Geriatric patients may be more sensitive to the effects of the usual adult dose.

**Usual adult prescribing limits**
Dose may be increased up to three times the initial dose or up to a maximum of 400 mg a day.

**Usual pediatric dose**
Edema
Ascites or
Hypertension—
    Initial: Oral, 1 to 3 mg per kg of body weight or 30 to 90 mg per square meter of body surface a day as a single daily dose or in two to four divided doses, the dosage being readjusted after five days. Dosage may be increased up to three times the initial dose.

**Strength(s) usually available**
U.S.
    25 mg (Rx) [*Aldactone*; GENERIC (may be scored)].
    50 mg (Rx) [*Aldactone* (scored)].
    100 mg (Rx) [*Aldactone* (scored)].
Canada
    25 mg (Rx) [*Aldactone* (scored); *Novospiroton* (scored)].
    100 mg (Rx) [*Aldactone* (scored); *Novospiroton* (scored)].

**Packaging and storage**
Store below 40 °C (104 °F), preferably between 15 and 30 °C (59 and 86 °F), unless otherwise specified by manufacturer. Store in a tight, light-resistant container.

**Preparation of dosage form**
For patients who cannot take oral solids—For small children or patients unable to swallow the tablets, Spironolactone Tablets USP may be crushed and dispensed as a suspension in Cherry Syrup NF. This suspension is stable in a refrigerator for 1 month.

**Auxiliary labeling**
• Take with meals or milk.
• Do not take other medicines without your doctor's advice.

**Note**
Check refill frequency to determine compliance in hypertensive patients.

## TRIAMTERENE

### Summary of Differences
Pharmacology/pharmacokinetics:
    Biotransformation—Hepatic.
    Duration of action—Diuretic: Single dose—7 to 9 hours.
Precautions:
    Drug interactions and/or related problems—Triamterene may increase blood uric acid and antagonize allopurinol, colchicine, probenecid, or sulfinpyrazone.
    Laboratory value alterations—May interfere with fluorescent measurement of quinidine.
    Medical considerations/contraindications—Hyperuricemia or gout; history of nephrolithiasis.
Side/adverse effects:
    Nephrolithiasis; megaloblastosis; photosensitivity; thrombocytopenia. No decrease in sexual ability reported.

### Additional Dosing Information
See also *General Dosing Information*.

Since triamterene is a weak folic acid antagonist, it may contribute to development of megaloblastosis in patients who have depleted folic acid stores (e.g., in pregnancy, hepatic cirrhosis).

When triamterene is combined with another diuretic, it is recommended that the initial dosage of each be reduced and then adjusted as required.

### Oral Dosage Forms
#### TRIAMTERENE CAPSULES USP
**Usual adult dose**
Diuretic—
    Initial: Oral, 25 to 100 mg a day.
    Maintenance: Oral, adjusted to meet individual requirements.
Note: Geriatric patients may be more sensitive to the effects of the usual adult dose.

**Usual adult prescribing limits**
Up to 300 mg daily.

**Usual pediatric dose**
Diuretic—
    Initial: Oral, 2 to 4 mg per kg of body weight or 120 mg per square meter of body surface a day or on alternate days in divided doses.

Maintenance: Oral, increased to 6 mg per kg of body weight a day according to individual requirements up to a maximum of 300 mg a day in divided doses.

**Strength(s) usually available**
U.S.—
    50 mg (Rx) [*Dyrenium* (lactose)].
    100 mg (Rx) [*Dyrenium* (lactose)].
Canada—
    Not commercially available.

**Packaging and storage**
Store below 40 °C (104 °F), preferably between 15 and 30 °C (59 and 86 °F), unless otherwise specified by manufacturer. Store in a tight, light-resistant container.

**Auxiliary labeling**
- Take with meals or milk.
- Avoid overexposure to sun or use of sunlamp.
- Do not take other medicines without your doctor's advice.

## TRIAMTERENE TABLETS
**Usual adult dose**
Diuretic—
    Initial: Oral, 25 to 100 mg a day.
    Maintenance: Oral, adjusted to meet individual requirements.
Note: Geriatric patients may be more sensitive to the effects of the usual adult dose.

**Usual adult prescribing limits**
Up to 300 mg daily.

**Usual pediatric dose**
Diuretic—
    Initial: Oral, 2 to 4 mg per kg of body weight or 120 mg per square meter of body surface a day or on alternate days in divided doses.
    Maintenance: Oral, increased to 6 mg per kg of body weight a day according to individual requirements up to a maximum of 300 mg a day in divided doses.

**Strength(s) usually available**
U.S.—
    Not commercially available.
Canada—
    50 mg (Rx) [*Dyrenium*].
    100 mg (Rx) [*Dyrenium* (scored)].

**Packaging and storage**
Store below 40 °C (104 °F), preferably between 15 and 30 °C (59 and 86 °F), unless otherwise specified by manufacturer. Store in a tight, light-resistant container.

**Auxiliary labeling**
- Take with meals or milk.
- Avoid overexposure to sun or use of sunlamp.
- Do not take other medicines without your doctor's advice.

Revised: 10/15/92
Interim revision: 05/18/94

## Table 1. Side/Adverse Effects*

The following side/adverse effects have been selected on the basis of their potential clinical significance (possible signs and symptoms in parentheses where appropriate)—not necessarily inclusive:

Legend:
I = Amiloride
II = Spironolactone
III = Triamterene

| | I | II | III |
|---|---|---|---|
| **Those indicating need for medical attention** | | | |
| *Agranulocytosis* (fever or chills, cough or hoarseness, lower back or side pain, painful or difficult urination) | U | R | R |
| *Allergic reaction or anaphylaxis* (shortness of breath, skin rash or itching) | R | R | R |
| *Hyperkalemia* (confusion; irregular heartbeat; nervousness; numbness or tingling in hands, feet, or lips; shortness of breath or difficult breathing; unusual tiredness or weakness; weakness or heaviness of legs)<br>Note: *Irregular heartbeat* is usually the earliest clinical indication of hyperkalemia and is readily detected by electrocardiogram (ECG). | M† | M† | M† |
| *Megaloblastosis or overdose* (burning, inflamed, or bright red tongue or cracked corners of mouth; weakness) | U | U | R |
| *Nephrolithiasis* (severe lower back or side pain) | U | U | R |
| *Thrombocytopenia* (unusual bleeding or bruising; black, tarry stools; blood in urine or stools; pinpoint red spots on skin) | U | U | R |
| **Those indicating need for medical attention only if they continue or are bothersome** | | | |
| *Antiandrogenic or endocrine effect* (breast tenderness in females, deepening of voice in females, enlargement of breasts in males, inability to have or keep an erection, increased hair growth in females, irregular menstrual periods, sweating)<br>Note: *Gynecomastia* occurs frequently after several months of treatment at doses of spironolactone greater than 100 mg per day and rarely may persist even after spironolactone is discontinued. | U | L‡ | U |
| *Central nervous system (CNS) effect* (clumsiness) | U | L‡ | U |
| *CNS effect* (headache) | L | L‡ | L |
| *Constipation* | L | U | U |
| *Decreased sexual ability* | L | L | U |
| *Dizziness* | L | L | L |
| *Gastrointestinal irritation* (nausea or vomiting, stomach cramps and diarrhea) | L | M | L |
| *Hyponatremia* (drowsiness, dryness of mouth, increased thirst, lack of energy) | L | L | L |
| *Increased sensitivity of skin to sunlight* | U | U | L |
| *Muscle cramps* | L | U | U |

*Differences in frequency of occurrence may reflect either lack of clinical-use data or actual pharmacologic distinctions among agents. M = more frequent; L = less frequent; R = rare; U = unknown.

†Signs and symptoms of hyperkalemia may occur even when potassium-sparing diuretics are combined with thiazide diuretics. Hyperkalemia occurs in approximately 10% of patients when amiloride is used alone and may occur in up to 26% of patients receiving spironolactone even when combined with thiazide diuretics.

‡Incidence related to dose and/or duration of therapy.

# DIURETICS, POTASSIUM-SPARING, AND HYDROCHLOROTHIAZIDE   Systemic

This monograph includes information on the following: 1) Amiloride and Hydrochlorothiazide; 2) Spironolactone and Hydrochlorothiazide; 3) Triamterene and Hydrochlorothiazide.

VA CLASSIFICATION (Primary/Secondary): CV704/CV490; TN900

**NOTE:** The *Diuretics, Potassium-sparing, and Hydrochlorothiazide (Systemic)* monograph is maintained on the USP DI electronic data base. For a printed copy of the most recent revision of the complete monograph, contact Micromedex, Inc. - Reprint Requests, 6200 S. Syracuse Way, Suite 300, Englewood, CO 80111; telephone (303) 486-6400; telefax (303) 486-6464; Email: USPDI@MDX.COM.

For information on the specific components of this combination, see the USP DI monographs for *Diuretics, Potassium-sparing (Systemic)* and *Diuretics, Thiazide (Systemic)*.

The information that follows is selectively abstracted from the complete monograph and is provided to facilitate drug use review and patient counseling.

Note: For a listing of dosage forms and brand names by country availability, see *Dosage Forms* section(s).

## Category
Antihypertensive; antihypokalemic; diuretic.

## Indications

### Accepted
Edema (treatment)—These combinations are indicated as adjuncts in the management of edematous states such as congestive heart failure, hepatic cirrhosis, and nephrotic syndrome, as well as in corticosteroid- and estrogen-induced edema and idiopathic edema.

Hypertension (treatment)—Spironolactone and hydrochlorothiazide, triamterene and hydrochlorothiazide, and amiloride and hydrochlorothiazide[1] are also indicated in the treatment of hypertension, especially when a potassium-sparing diuretic effect is desired.

Fixed-dosage combinations are generally not recommended in initial therapy and are useful in subsequent therapy only when the proportion of the component agents corresponds to the dose of the individual agents, as determined by titration.

For additional information on initial therapeutic guidelines related to the treatment of hypertension, see *Appendix III*.

Hypokalemia (treatment)[1]—Amiloride and hydrochlorothiazide, triamterene and hydrochlorothiazide, and spironolactone and hydrochlorothiazide combinations are also indicated for treatment of diuretic-induced hypokalemia in hypertensive patients in whom other measures are inappropriate or inadequate.

[1]Not included in Canadian product labeling.

## Patient Consultation
As an aid to patient consultation, refer to *Advice for the Patient, Diuretics, Potassium-sparing, and Hydrochlorothiazide (Systemic)*.

In providing consultation, consider emphasizing the following selected information (» = major clinical significance):

### Before using this medication
» Conditions affecting use, especially:
   Sensitivity to the potassium-sparing diuretic prescribed, hydrochlorothiazide or other thiazide diuretics, other sulfonamide-type medications, bumetanide, furosemide, or carbonic anhydrase inhibitors
   Pregnancy—Diuretics not recommended for routine use
   Breast-feeding—Hydrochlorothiazide distributed into breast milk; spironolactone may be distributed into breast milk
   Use in the elderly—Elderly patients may be more sensitive to hypotensive and electrolyte-depleting effects
   Other medications, especially angiotensin-converting enzyme inhibitors, cholestyramine, colestipol, coumarin or indandione anticoagulants, cyclosporine, digitalis glycosides, heparin, lithium, low-salt milk, other potassium-sparing diuretics, potassium-containing medications or supplements, or stored blood from a blood bank
   Other medical problems, especially diabetic nephropathy, hepatic function impairment, renal function impairment or anuria

### Proper use of this medication
Diuretic effects of the medication and timing of doses to minimize inconvenience of diuresis
Getting into habit of taking at same time each day to help increase compliance
Taking with meals or milk to reduce stomach upset
» Proper dosing
   Missed dose: Taking as soon as possible; not taking if almost time for next dose; not doubling doses
» Proper storage

*For use as an antihypertensive*
Possible need for control of weight and diet, especially sodium intake
» Patient may not experience symptoms of hypertension; importance of taking medication even if feeling well
» Does not cure, but helps control hypertension; possible need for lifelong therapy; checking with physician before discontinuing medication; serious consequences of untreated hypertension

### Precautions while using this medication
Regular visits to physician to check progress
» Possibility of hypokalemia or hyperkalemia; possible need for monitoring potassium in diet; not changing diet without first checking with physician
To prevent dehydration, checking with physician if severe nausea, vomiting, or diarrhea occurs and continues
Diabetics: May increase blood sugar levels
Possible photosensitivity; avoiding too much sun; using protective clothing and sun block product; avoiding use of sunlamp, tanning bed, or tanning booth
Caution if any kind of surgery or emergency treatment is required
Caution if any laboratory tests required; possible interference with test results

*For triamterene and hydrochlorothiazide combination*
Not changing brands of triamterene and hydrochlorothiazide combination without checking with physician

*For use an an antihypertensive*
» Not taking other medications, especially nonprescription sympathomimetics, unless discussed with physician

### Side/adverse effects
Signs of potential side effects, especially electrolyte imbalance, agranulocytosis, allergic reaction, cholecystitis or pancreatitis, gout or hyperuricemia, hepatic function impairment, thrombocytopenia, megaloblastosis (for triamterene)

*For spironolactone:*
Possibility of enlargement of breasts in males and irregular menstrual periods in females; usually reversible within several months

---

## AMILORIDE AND HYDROCHLOROTHIAZIDE

## Oral Dosage Forms

### AMILORIDE HYDROCHLORIDE AND HYDROCHLOROTHIAZIDE TABLETS USP

**Usual adult dose**
Diuretic or
Antihypertensive[1]—
   Oral, 1 or 2 tablets a day.

Note: Geriatric patients may be more sensitive to the effects of the usual adult dose.

**Usual pediatric dose**
Dosage has not been established.

**Strength(s) usually available**
U.S.—
   5 mg of amiloride hydrochloride and 50 mg of hydrochlorothiazide (Rx) [*Moduretic* (scored); GENERIC (may be scored)].
Canada—
   5 mg of amiloride hydrochloride and 50 mg of hydrochlorothiazide (Rx) [*Moduret* (scored)].

**Auxiliary labeling**
- Take with meals or milk.
- Avoid overexposure to the sun or use of sunlamp.
- Do not take other medicines without your doctor's advice.

[1]Not included in Canadian product labeling.

## SPIRONOLACTONE AND HYDROCHLOROTHIAZIDE

### Oral Dosage Forms

#### SPIRONOLACTONE AND HYDROCHLOROTHIAZIDE TABLETS USP

**Usual adult dose**
Diuretic—Edema due to congestive heart failure, hepatic cirrhosis, or nephrotic syndrome:—
  Maintenance—Oral, 1 to 4 tablets a day, taken as a single dose or in divided doses.
Antihypertensive—
  Maintenance: Oral, 2 to 4 tablets a day in divided doses.
Note: Geriatric patients may be more sensitive to the effects of the usual adult dose.

**Usual pediatric dose**
Diuretic—
  Maintenance: Oral, 1.65 to 3.3 mg of spironolactone and of hydrochlorothiazide per kg of body weight a day in divided doses.

**Strength(s) usually available**
U.S.—
  25 mg of spironolactone and 25 mg of hydrochlorothiazide (Rx) [Aldactazide; Spirozide; GENERIC (may be scored)].
  50 mg of spironolactone and 50 mg of hydrochlorothiazide (Rx) [Aldactazide (scored)].
Canada—
  25 mg of spironolactone and 25 mg of hydrochlorothiazide (Rx) [Aldactazide (scored); Novo-Spirozine (scored)].
  50 mg of spironolactone and 50 mg of hydrochlorothiazide (Rx) [Aldactazide (scored); Novo-Spirozine (scored)].

**Auxiliary labeling**
• Take with meals or milk.
• Avoid overexposure to the sun or use of sunlamp.
• Do not take other medicines without your doctor's advice.

## TRIAMTERENE AND HYDROCHLOROTHIAZIDE

### Oral Dosage Forms

#### TRIAMTERENE AND HYDROCHLOROTHIAZIDE CAPSULES USP

**Usual adult dose**
Diuretic or
Antihypertensive—
  Oral, 1 or 2 capsules once a day, as determined by individual titration with the component agents; some patients may be maintained on 1 capsule a day or every other day.
Note: Geriatric patients may be more sensitive to the effects of the usual adult dose.

**Usual adult prescribing limits**
Up to 4 capsules daily.

**Usual pediatric dose**
Dosage has not been established.

**Strength(s) usually available**
U.S.—
  37.5 mg of triamterene and 25 mg of hydrochlorothiazide (Rx) [Dyazide (lactose)].
  50 mg of triamterene and 25 mg of hydrochlorothiazide (Rx) [GENERIC].
  75 mg of triamterene and 50 mg of hydrochlorothiazide (Rx) [GENERIC].
Canada—
  Not commercially available.

**Auxiliary labeling**
• Take with meals or milk.
• Avoid overexposure to the sun or use of sunlamp.
• Do not take other medicines without your doctor's advice.

#### TRIAMTERENE AND HYDROCHLOROTHIAZIDE TABLETS USP

**Usual adult dose**
Antihypertensive or
Diuretic—
  Maxzide:
    Oral, 1 tablet per day, as determined by individual titration.
  Apo-Triazide; Dyazide (Canada); Novotriamzide:
    Oral, 1 or 2 tablets two times a day, as determined by individual titration with the component agents; some patients may be maintained on 1 tablet a day or every other day.
Note: Geriatric patients may be more sensitive to the effects of the usual adult dose.

**Usual pediatric dose**
Dosage has not been established.

**Strength(s) usually available**
U.S.—
  37.5 mg of triamterene and 25 mg of hydrochlorothiazide (Rx) [Maxzide (scored)].
  75 mg of triamterene and 50 mg of hydrochlorothiazide (Rx) [Maxzide (scored); GENERIC (may be scored; may contain lactose)].
Canada—
  50 mg of triamterene and 25 mg of hydrochlorothiazide (Rx) [Apo-Triazide (scored); Dyazide (scored); Novo-Triamzide (scored)].

**Auxiliary labeling**
• Take with meals or milk.
• Avoid overexposure to the sun or use of sunlamp.
• Do not take other medicines without your doctor's advice.

Revised: 08/03/94

---

# DIURETICS, THIAZIDE  Systemic

This monograph includes information on the following: 1) Bendroflumethiazide; 2) Chlorothiazide†; 3) Chlorthalidone; 4) Hydrochlorothiazide; 5) Hydroflumethiazide†; 6) Methyclothiazide; 7) Metolazone; 8) Polythiazide†; 9) Quinethazone†; 10) Trichlormethiazide†.

INN: Chlorthalidone—Chlortalidone

VA CLASSIFICATION (Primary/Secondary): CV701/CV409; GU900

Commonly used brand name(s): Apo-Chlorthalidone[3]; Apo-Hydro[4]; Aquatensen[6]; Diucardin[5]; Diuchlor H[4]; Diulo[7]; Diuril[2]; Duretic[6]; Enduron[6]; Esidrix[4]; Hydro-D[4]; Hydro-chlor[4]; HydroDIURIL[4]; Hydromox[9]; Hygroton[3]; Metahydrin[10]; Microzide[4]; Mykrox[7]; Naqua[10]; Naturetin[1]; Neo-Codema[4]; Novo-Hydrazide[4]; Novo-Thalidone[3]; Oretic[4]; Renese[8]; Saluron[5]; Thalitone[3]; Trichlorex[10]; Uridon[3]; Urozide[4]; Zaroxolyn[7].

Note: For a listing of dosage forms and brand names by country availability, see Dosage Forms section(s).

†Not commercially available in Canada.

### Category
Diuretic; antihypertensive; antidiuretic (central and nephrogenic diabetes insipidus); antiurolithic (calcium calculi).

### Indications
Note: Bracketed information in the Indications section refers to uses that are not included in U.S. product labeling.

**Accepted**
Edema (treatment)—Indications include edema associated with congestive heart failure, hepatic cirrhosis with ascites, corticosteroid and estrogen therapy, and some forms of renal function impairment including nephrotic syndrome, acute glomerulonephritis, and chronic renal failure. However, prompt metolazone tablets are not indicated for treatment of edema because a safe and effective diuretic dosage has not been established.

Hypertension (treatment)—Thiazide diuretics are indicated either alone or as adjunctive therapy in the treatment of hypertension.

[Diabetes insipidus, central or nephrogenic (treatment)][1]—Thiazide diuretics are used in the treatment of central and nephrogenic diabetes insipidus.

[Renal calculi, calcium (prophylaxis)][1]—Thiazide diuretics are also used for prevention of calcium-containing renal stones.

[1]Not included in Canadian product labeling.

## Pharmacology/Pharmacokinetics

Note: Although they are not chemically the same, chlorthalidone, metolazone, and quinethazone have the same actions as the thiazide diuretics.

**Physicochemical characteristics**
Molecular weight—
    Bendroflumethiazide: 421.41.
    Chlorothiazide: 295.72.
    Chlorthalidone: 338.76.
    Hydrochlorothiazide: 297.73.
    Hydroflumethiazide: 331.28.
    Methyclothiazide: 360.23.
    Metolazone: 365.83.
    Polythiazide: 439.87.
    Quinethazone: 289.74.
    Trichlormethiazide: 380.65.
pKa—
    Bendroflumethiazide: 8.5.
    Chlorothiazide: 6.7 and 9.5.
    Chlorthalidone: 9.4.
    Hydrochlorothiazide: 7.9 and 9.2.
    Hydroflumethiazide: 8.9 and 10.7.
    Methyclothiazide: 9.4.
    Metolazone: 9.7.
    Quinethazone: 9.3 and 10.7.
    Trichlormethiazide: 8.6.

**Mechanism of action/Effect**
Diuretic—Thiazide diuretics increase urinary excretion of sodium and water by inhibiting sodium reabsorption in the early distal tubules. They increase the rate of delivery of tubular fluid and electrolytes to the distal sites of hydrogen and potassium ion secretion, while plasma volume contraction increases aldosterone production. The increased delivery and increase in aldosterone levels promote sodium reabsorption at the distal tubules, thus increasing the loss of potassium and hydrogen ions.

Antihypertensive—Diuretics lower blood pressure initially by reducing plasma and extracellular fluid volume; cardiac output also decreases. Eventually, cardiac output returns to normal. Thiazide diuretics decrease peripheral resistance by a direct peripheral effect on blood vessels.

Antidiuretic—The antidiuretic effect of thiazide diuretics is a result of mild sodium and water depletion leading to increased reabsorption of glomerular filtrate in the proximal renal tubule and reduced delivery of tubular fluid available for excretion.

Antiurolithic (calcium calculi)—Thiazide diuretics decrease urinary calcium excretion by a direct action on the distal tubule, which may prevent recurrence of calcium-containing renal calculi.

**Absorption**
Thiazide diuretics are absorbed relatively rapidly after oral administration.
Metolazone—The time to peak concentration is 8 hours for extended metolazone tablets and 2 to 4 hours for prompt metolazone tablets. In addition, prompt metolazone tablets have higher bioavailability.

**Protein binding**
Bendroflumethiazide—Very high (94%).
Chlorothiazide—Low to high (20 to 80%).
Chlorthalidone—High (75% [58% to albumin]); increased affinity to carbonic anhydrase in red blood cells.
Hydroflumethiazide—High (74%).
Metolazone—Very high (95%; 50 to 70% to red blood cells).
Polythiazide—High (84%).

**Elimination**
Unchanged; almost totally via the kidneys, with minute quantities in the bile; metolazone undergoes some enterohepatic recycling and slightly greater amounts are excreted in the bile.

| Drug | Half-life (hr) | Onset | Peak | Duration |
|---|---|---|---|---|
| Bendroflumethiazide | 8.5 | 1–2 | 4 | 6–12 |
| Chlorothiazide | 1–2 | 2 | 4 | 6–12 |
| Chlorthalidone | 35 to 50 | 2 | 2 | 48–72 |
| Hydrochlorothiazide | 5.6–14.8 | 2 | 4 | 6–12 |
| Hydroflumethiazide | 17 | 1–2 | 3–4 | 18–24 |
| Methyclothiazide | | 2 | 6 | >24 |
| Metolazone | 14 | 1* | 2* | 12–24* |
| Polythiazide | | 2 | 6 | 24–48 |
| Quinethazone | | 2 | 6 | 18–24 |
| Trichlormethiazide | | 2 | 6 | ≤24 |

*Information on diuretic effect applies to extended metolazone tablets.

Note: In the absence of edema, negative sodium balance induced by thiazide diuretics lasts for 3 days to 4 weeks with chronic administration. Extracellular fluid volumes remain steady thereafter, although at a lower concentration and volume than before initiation of therapy.

The antihypertensive effects of the thiazide diuretics may be noted after 3 to 4 days of therapy, although up to 3 to 4 weeks may be required for optimal effect. Antihypertensive effects persist for up to 1 week after withdrawal of therapy.

## Precautions to Consider

**Cross-sensitivity and/or related problems**
Patients sensitive to other sulfonamide-type medications, bumetanide, furosemide, or carbonic anhydrase inhibitors may be sensitive to this medication also.

**Carcinogenicity/Mutagenicity**
*Bendroflumethiazide*—Studies have not been done in either animals or humans.
*Chlorothiazide*—Carcinogenicity studies have not been done in either animals or humans. Chlorothiazide was not found to be mutagenic in the Ames microbial mutation test, dominant lethal assay, or a test in *Aspergillus nidulans*.
*Hydrochlorothiazide*—Carcinogenicity studies have not been done in either animals or humans. Hydrochlorothiazide was not found to be mutagenic *in vitro* in the Ames microbial mutation test or on examination of urine from patients who received hydrochlorothiazide; however, it did induce nondisjunction in *Aspergillus nidulans*.
*Hydroflumethiazide*—Studies have not been done in either animals or humans.
*Methyclothiazide*—Studies have not been done in either animals or humans.
*Metolazone*—Studies in mice and rats for 1½ to 2 years at doses of 2, 10, and 50 mg per kg of body weight (mg/kg) per day (100, 500, and 2500 times the maximum recommended human dose [MRHD]) found no evidence of carcinogenicity.
*Trichlormethiazide*—Studies have not been done in either animals or humans.

**Pregnancy/Reproduction**
Fertility—*Hydrochlorothiazide*: No adverse effects on fertility were found in rats given doses up to 2 times the maximum recommended human dose of hydrochlorothiazide.
*Methyclothiazide*: No adverse effects on fertility were found in rats given methyclothiazide in doses up to 4 mg per kg of body weight (mg/kg) per day (at least 20 times the maximum recommended human dose).
*Metolazone*: A study in which male rats were given metolazone at doses of 2, 10, and 50 mg/kg for 127 days prior to mating with untreated female rats revealed an increase in the number of resorption sites in dams mated with males given the 50 mg/kg dose. Furthermore, decreased fetal weight and reduced pregnancy rate were observed in dams mated with males from the 10 and 50 mg/kg groups. In mice, there was no evidence that metolazone alters reproductive capacity.

Pregnancy—Thiazide diuretics cross the placenta and appear in cord blood. Although studies in humans have not been done, thiazide diuretics can cause fetal harm when given to pregnant women. Fetal or neonatal jaundice has been reported.

Pregnant women should be advised to contact their physician before taking this medication, since routine use of diuretics during normal pregnancy is inappropriate and exposes mother and fetus to unnecessary hazard. Thiazide diuretics do not prevent development of toxemia of pregnancy, and there is no satisfactory evidence that they are useful in the treatment of toxemia. Thiazide diuretics are indicated only in the treatment of edema due to pathologic causes or as a short course of treatment in patients with severe hypervolemia. Possible hazards include fetal or neonatal jaundice, thrombocytopenia, or other adverse reactions seen in adults.

Studies in animals have not shown that thiazide diuretics cause adverse effects on the fetus at several times the human dose.
    *Bendroflumethiazide*—
        Adequate and well-controlled studies in humans and animals have not been done.
    FDA Pregnancy Category C.
    *Chlorothiazide*—
        Adequate and well-controlled studies in humans have not been done.
        Studies in rabbits, mice, and rats at doses up to 500 mg/kg per day (25 times the MRHD) have not shown that chlorothiazide causes adverse effects on the fetus.
    FDA Pregnancy Category B.

*Chlorthalidone—*
    Adequate and well-controlled studies in humans have not been done.
    Studies in rats and rabbits at doses up to 420 times the human dose have not shown that chlorthalidone causes adverse effects on the fetus.
    FDA Pregnancy Category B.

*Hydrochlorothiazide—*
    Adequate and well-controlled studies in humans have not been done.
    A study in rats at dosages up to 250 mg/kg per day (62.5 times the MRHD) has not shown that hydrochlorothiazide causes adverse effects on the fetus.
    Studies in mice and rabbits with doses up to 100 mg/kg per day (50 times the maximum human dose) revealed no evidence of external abnormalities of the fetus.
    FDA Pregnancy Category B.

*Hydroflumethiazide—*
    Studies have not been done in humans.
    Studies have not been done in animals.
    FDA Pregnancy Category C.

*Methyclothiazide—*
    Studies have not been done in humans.
    Studies in rats and rabbits given methyclothiazide at doses up to 4 mg/kg per day have revealed no evidence of harm to the fetus.
    FDA Pregnancy Category B.

*Metolazone—*
    Adequate and well-controlled studies in humans have not been done.
    Studies in mice, rabbits, and rats at doses up to 50 mg/kg per day (333 times the MRHD) have not shown that metolazone causes adverse effects on the fetus.
    FDA Pregnancy Category B.

*Trichlormethiazide—*
    Adequate and well-controlled studies in humans have not been done.
    Studies in rats at doses 250 to 1250 times the recommended human daily dose have not shown that trichlormethiazide causes adverse effects on the fetus.
    FDA Pregnancy Category C.

**Breast-feeding**
Thiazide diuretics are distributed into breast milk. The American Academy of Pediatrics recommends that nursing mothers avoid thiazide diuretics during the first month of lactation because of reports of suppression of lactation.

**Pediatrics**
Although appropriate studies on the relationship of age to the effects of thiazide diuretics have not been performed in the pediatric population, pediatrics-specific problems that would limit the usefulness of this medication in children are not expected. However, caution is required in jaundiced infants because of the risk of hyperbilirubinemia.

**Geriatrics**
Although appropriate studies on the relationship of age to the effects of thiazide diuretics have not been performed in the geriatric population, the elderly may be more sensitive to the hypotensive and electrolyte effects. In addition, elderly patients are more likely to have age-related renal function impairment, which may require caution in patients receiving thiazide diuretics.

**Drug interactions and/or related problems**
The following drug interactions and/or related problems have been selected on the basis of their potential clinical significance (possible mechanism in parentheses where appropriate)—not necessarily inclusive (» = major clinical significance):

Note:  Combinations containing any of the following medications, depending on the amount present, may also interact with this medication.

  Amantadine
    (hydrochlorothiazide may reduce the renal clearance of amantadine, resulting in increased plasma concentrations and possible amantadine toxicity)

  Amiodarone
    (concurrent use of thiazide diuretics with amiodarone may lead to an increased risk of arrhythmias associated with hypokalemia)

  Anticoagulants, coumarin- or indandione-derivative
    (effects may be decreased when used concurrently with thiazide diuretics as a result of reduction of plasma volume leading to concentration of procoagulant factors in the blood; in addition, diuretic-induced improvement of hepatic congestion may lead to improved hepatic function resulting in increased procoagulant factor synthesis; dosage adjustments may be necessary)

  Antidiabetic agents, oral or
  Insulin
    (thiazide diuretics may raise blood glucose concentrations; for adult-onset diabetics, dosage adjustment of hypoglycemic medications may be necessary during and after thiazide diuretic therapy; insulin requirements may be increased, decreased, or unchanged)

  Anti-inflammatory drugs, nonsteroidal (NSAIDs), especially indomethacin
    (may antagonize the natriuresis and increase in plasma renin activity [PRA] caused by thiazide diuretics; they may also reduce the antihypertensive effect and increase in urine volume caused by thiazide diuretics, possibly by inhibiting renal prostaglandin synthesis and/or by causing sodium and fluid retention; the patient should be carefully monitored to confirm that the desired effect is being obtained)
    (in addition, concurrent use of NSAIDs with a diuretic may increase the risk of renal failure secondary to a decrease in renal blood flow caused by inhibition of renal prostaglandin synthesis)

  Calcium-containing medications
    (concurrent use of thiazide diuretics with large doses of calcium may result in hypercalcemia because of reduced calcium excretion)

» Cholesteramine or
» Colestipol
    (may inhibit gastrointestinal absorption of the thiazide diuretics; administration of thiazide diuretics 1 hour before or 4 hours after cholestyramine or colestipol is recommended)

  Diazoxide
    (concurrent use with thiazide diuretics may enhance hyperglycemic effects; monitoring of blood glucose levels and/or dosage adjustment of one or both agents may be necessary)
    (in addition, concurrent use with thiazide diuretics may enhance hyperuricemic and antihypertensive effects)

  Diflunisal
    (concurrent use of hydrochlorothiazide with diflunisal produces significantly increased plasma concentrations of hydrochlorothiazide; in addition, the hyperuricemic effect of hydrochlorothiazide is decreased)

» Digitalis glycosides
    (concurrent use with thiazide diuretics may enhance the possibility of digitalis toxicity associated with hypokalemia or hypomagnesemia)

  Dopamine
    (concurrent use may increase the diuretic effect of either thiazide diuretics or dopamine, as a result of dopamine's direct effect on dopaminergic receptors to produce vasodilation of renal vasculature and increase renal blood flow; dopamine also has a direct natriuretic effect)

  Hypokalemia-causing medications, other (see *Appendix II*)
    (risk of severe hypokalemia due to other hypokalemia-causing medications may be increased; monitoring of serum potassium concentrations and cardiac function and potassium supplementation may be necessary)

  Hypotension-producing medications, other (see *Appendix II*)
    (antihypertensive and/or diuretic effects may be potentiated when these medications are used concurrently with thiazide diuretics; although some antihypertensive and/or diuretic combinations are frequently used for therapeutic advantage, when used concurrently dosage adjustments may be necessary)

» Lithium
    (concurrent use with thiazide diuretics is not recommended, as they may provoke lithium toxicity because of reduced renal clearance; in addition, lithium has nephrotoxic effects)

  Neuromuscular blocking agents, nondepolarizing
    (thiazide diuretics may induce hypokalemia, which may enhance the blockade of nondepolarizing neuromuscular blocking agents; serum potassium determinations may be necessary prior to administration of nondepolarizing neuromuscular blocking agents; careful postoperative monitoring of the patient may be necessary following concurrent or sequential use, especially if there is a possibility of incomplete reversal of neuromuscular blockade)

  Sympathomimetics
    (may antagonize the antihypertensive effect of the thiazide diuretics; the patient should be carefully monitored to confirm that the desired effect is being obtained)

**Laboratory value alterations**
The following have been selected on the basis of their potential clinical significance (possible effect in parentheses where appropriate)—not necessarily inclusive (» = major clinical significance):

With diagnostic test results
  Bentiromide
    (administration of thiazide diuretics during a bentiromide test period will invalidate test results since thiazide diuretics are also metabolized to arylamines and will thus increase the percent of para-aminobenzoic acid [PABA] recovered; discontinuation of thiazide diuretics at least 3 days prior to the administration of bentiromide is recommended)
  Phenolsulfonphthalein (PSP) excretion test
    (bendroflumethiazide and trichlormethiazide may interfere with PSP excretion)
  Phentolamine and tyramine tests
    (bendroflumethiazide and trichlormethiazide may produce false negative results)

With physiology/laboratory test values
  Bilirubin
    (serum concentrations may be increased by displacement from albumin binding)
  Calcium
    (serum concentrations may be increased; thiazide diuretics should be discontinued before parathyroid function tests are carried out)
  Cholesterol, low-density lipoprotein, and triglyceride and
  Creatinine
    (serum concentrations may be increased)
  Glucose, blood and urine
    (concentrations may be increased, usually only in patients with a predisposition to glucose intolerance)
  Magnesium and
  Potassium and
  Sodium
    (serum concentrations may be decreased; serum magnesium concentrations may increase in uremic patients; a fall in sodium can be life-threatening)
  Protein-bound iodine (PBI)
    (serum concentrations may be decreased)
  Uric acid
    (serum concentrations may be increased)
  Urinary calcium concentrations
    (may be decreased)

**Medical considerations/Contraindications**
The medical considerations/contraindications included have been selected on the basis of their potential clinical significance (reasons given in parentheses where appropriate)—not necessarily inclusive (» = major clinical significance).

*Risk-benefit should be considered when the following medical problems exist:*
» Anuria or severe renal function impairment
    (ineffective; may precipitate azotemia; may produce cumulative effects)
  Diabetes mellitus
    (hypoglycemic medication requirements may be altered)
  Gout, history of or
  Hyperuricemia
    (serum uric acid concentrations may be elevated)
  Hepatic function impairment
    (risk of dehydration which may precipitate hepatic coma and death; plasma half-life is unaltered)
  Hypercalcemia or
  Hypercholesterolemia or
  Hypertriglyceridemia or
  Hyponatremia
    (conditions may be exacerbated; onset of hyponatremia can be sudden and life-threatening)
  Lupus erythematosus, history of
    (exacerbation or activation by thiazide diuretics has been reported)
  Pancreatitis
  Sensitivity to thiazide diuretics or other sulfonamide-derived medications
  Sympathectomy
    (antihypertensive effects may be enhanced)

» Caution is required also in jaundiced infants because of the risk of hyperbilirubinemia.

**Patient monitoring**
The following may be especially important in patient monitoring (other tests may be warranted in some patients, depending on condition; » = major clinical significance):

  Blood glucose and
  Blood urea nitrogen (BUN) and
  Creatinine, serum and
  Uric acid, serum
    (determinations recommended prior to initiation of therapy and if clinical signs of a significant increase occur)
» Blood pressure measurements
    (recommended at periodic intervals in patients being treated for hypertension; selected patients may be trained to perform blood pressure measurements at home and report the results at regular physician visits)
  Cholesterol, serum and
  Triglycerides, serum
    (determinations recommended after 6 months of therapy and annually thereafter)
  Electrolyte, serum, concentrations
    (determinations may be required for patients on long-term therapy, especially if they are also taking cardiac glycosides or systemic steroids, or when severe cirrhosis is present)

## Side/Adverse Effects

Note: Most side effects are dose-related.

The following side/adverse effects have been selected on the basis of their potential clinical significance (possible signs and symptoms in parentheses where appropriate)—not necessarily inclusive:

**Those indicating need for medical attention**
Incidence more frequent
    *Electrolyte imbalance such as hyponatremia* (confusion; convulsions; decreased mentation; fatigue; irritability; muscle cramps); *hypochloremic alkalosis, and hypokalemia* (dryness of mouth; increased thirst; irregular heartbeat; mood or mental changes; muscle cramps or pain; nausea or vomiting; unusual tiredness or weakness; weak pulse)
    Note: *Hyponatremia* as a complication is rare, but constitutes a medical emergency as onset may be rapid.
Incidence rare
    *Agranulocytosis* (fever or chills; cough or hoarseness; lower back or side pain; painful or difficult urination); *allergic reaction* (skin rash or hives); *cholecystitis or pancreatitis* (severe stomach pain with nausea and vomiting); *gout or hyperuricemia* (joint pain, lower back or side pain); *hepatic function impairment* (yellow eyes or skin); *thrombocytopenia* (unusual bleeding or bruising; black, tarry stools; blood in urine or stools; pinpoint red spots on skin)

**Those indicating need for medical attention only if they continue or are bothersome**
Incidence less frequent
    *Anorexia* (loss of appetite); *decreased sexual ability; diarrhea; orthostatic hypotension* (dizziness or lightheadedness when getting up from a lying or sitting position); *photosensitivity* (increased sensitivity of skin to sunlight); *upset stomach*

## Overdose

For more information on the management of overdose or unintentional ingestion, **contact a Poison Control Center** (see *Poison Control Center Listing*).

**Treatment of overdose**
Thiazide diuretic overdose should be treated by immediate evacuation of the stomach followed by supportive, symptomatic treatment and monitoring of serum electrolyte concentrations and renal function.

## Patient Consultation

As an aid to patient consultation, refer to *Advice for the Patient, Diuretics, Thiazide (Systemic)*.
In providing consultation, consider emphasizing the following selected information (» = major clinical significance):

**Before using this medication**
» Conditions affecting use, especially:
    Sensitivity to thiazide diuretics, other sulfonamide-type medications, bumetanide, furosemide, or carbonic anhydrase inhibitors
    Pregnancy—Not recommended for routine use; may cause jaundice, thrombocytopenia, hypokalemia in infant

Breast-feeding—Distributed into breast milk; recommended that nursing mothers avoid thiazides during first month of breast-feeding because of reports of suppression of lactation
Use in children—Caution if giving to infants with jaundice
Use in the elderly—Elderly patients may be more sensitive to hypotensive and electrolyte effects
Other medications, especially cholestyramine, colestipol, digitalis glycosides, or lithium
Other medical problems, especially anuria or severe renal function impairment or infants with jaundice

**Proper use of this medication**
Diuretic effects of the medication and timing of doses to minimize inconvenience of diuresis (except in diabetes insipidus)
Compliance with therapy; taking medication at the same time each day to maintain the therapeutic effect
Proper administration of concentrated oral hydrochlorothiazide solution: Taking orally; special dropper to be used for accurate measuring
» Proper dosing
Missed dose: Taking as soon as possible; not taking if almost time for next dose; not doubling doses
» Proper storage
*For use as an antihypertensive*
Importance of diet; possible need for sodium restriction and/or weight reduction
» Patient may not experience symptoms of hypertension; importance of taking medication even if feeling well
» Does not cure, but helps control hypertension; possible need for lifelong therapy; checking with physician before discontinuing medication; serious consequences of untreated hypertension

**Precautions while using this medication**
Making regular visits to physician to check progress
» Possibility of hypokalemia; possible need for additional potassium in diet; not changing diet without first checking with physician
To prevent dehydration, checking with physician if severe nausea, vomiting, or diarrhea occurs and continues
Diabetics: May increase blood sugar levels
Possible photosensitivity; avoiding unprotected exposure to sun; using protective clothing and sun block product; avoiding use of sunlamp, tanning bed, or tanning booth
*For use as an antihypertensive*
» Not taking other medications, especially nonprescription sympathomimetics, unless discussed with physician

**Side/adverse effects**
Signs of potential side effects, especially electrolyte imbalance, agranulocytosis, allergic reaction, cholecystitis, pancreatitis, hepatic function impairment, hyperuricemia, gout, and thrombocytopenia

## General Dosing Information

The lowest effective dosage should be utilized to minimize potential electrolyte imbalance and the reflex increase in renin and aldosterone levels.

A single daily dose is preferably taken on arising in order to minimize the effect of increased frequency of urination on sleep. When used to promote diuresis, intermittent dosage schedules (drug-free days) may reduce the possibility of electrolyte imbalance or hyperuricemia resulting from therapy.

Concurrent administration of potassium supplements or potassium-sparing diuretics may be indicated in patients considered to be at higher risk for developing hypokalemia. Caution in administering potassium supplements is recommended, however, since loss of potassium is not clinically significant in most patients, and supplementation leads to a risk of development of hyperkalemia.

Recent evidence suggests that withdrawal of antihypertensive therapy prior to surgery is not necessary, but that the anesthesiologist must be aware of such therapy.

**For hypertension**
Low dose thiazide therapy has been found to be effective in the treatment of hypertension.

---
### BENDROFLUMETHIAZIDE
---

## Summary of Differences
Pharmacology/pharmacokinetics:
    Protein binding—Very high.
    Half-life—Normal: 8.5 hours.
    Onset of action—Diuretic: 1 to 2 hours.
    Time to peak effect—Diuretic: 4 hours.
    Duration of action—Diuretic: 6 to 12 hours.
Laboratory value alterations:
    May produce false-negative results in phentolamine, phenolsulfonphthalein, and tyramine tests.

## Oral Dosage Forms

Note: Bracketed uses in the *Dosage Forms* section refer to categories of use and/or indications that are not included in U.S. product labeling.

### BENDROFLUMETHIAZIDE TABLETS USP

**Usual adult dose**
Diuretic or
[Antidiuretic (central or nephrogenic diabetes insipidus)][1]—
    Initial: Oral, 2.5 to 10 mg one or two times a day, once every other day, or once a day for three to five days a week.
    Maintenance: Oral, 2.5 to 5 mg once a day, once every other day, or once a day for three to five days a week.
Antihypertensive—
    Oral, 2.5 to 20 mg per day, as a single dose or in two divided daily doses, the dosage being adjusted according to response.
Note: Geriatric patients may be more sensitive to the effects of the usual adult dose.

**Usual pediatric dose**
Diuretic or
[Antidiuretic (central or nephrogenic diabetes insipidus)][1]—
    Initial: Oral, up to 400 mcg (0.4 mg) per kg of body weight or 12 mg per square meter of body surface a day, as a single dose or in two divided daily doses.
    Maintenance: Oral, 50 to 100 mcg (0.05 to 0.1 mg) per kg of body weight or 1.5 to 3 mg per square meter of body surface once a day.
Antihypertensive—
    Oral, 50 to 400 mcg (0.05 to 0.4 mg) per kg of body weight or 1.5 to 12 mg per square meter of body surface per day, as a single dose or in two divided daily doses, the dosage being adjusted according to response.

**Strength(s) usually available**
U.S.—
    5 mg (Rx) [*Naturetin* (scored; lactose)].
    10 mg (Rx) [*Naturetin* (scored; lactose)].
Canada—
    5 mg (Rx) [*Naturetin* (scored; tartrazine)].

**Packaging and storage**
Store below 40 °C (104 °F), preferably between 15 and 30 °C (59 and 86 °F), unless otherwise specified by manufacturer. Store in a tight container.

**Auxiliary labeling**
• Avoid overexposure to the sun or use of sunlamp.
• Do not take other medicines without your doctor's advice.

**Note**
Check refill frequency to determine compliance in hypertensive patients.

[1]Not included in Canadian product labeling.

---
### CHLOROTHIAZIDE
---

## Summary of Differences
Pharmacology/pharmacokinetics:
    Protein binding—Low to high.
    Half-life—Normal: 13 hours.
    Onset of action—Diuretic: 2 hours.
    Time to peak effect—Diuretic: 4 hours.
    Duration of action—Diuretic: 6 to 12 hours.

## Additional Dosing Information
See also *General Dosing Information*.
For parenteral dosage forms only
    • Care must be taken to avoid extravasation during intravenous administration.
    • Chlorothiazide should not be administered intramuscularly or subcutaneously.

## Oral Dosage Forms

Note: Bracketed uses in the *Dosage Forms* section refer to categories of use and/or indications that are not included in U.S. product labeling.

## CHLOROTHIAZIDE ORAL SUSPENSION USP
**Usual adult dose**
Diuretic or
[Antidiuretic (central or nephrogenic diabetes insipidus)]—
   Oral, 250 mg every six to twelve hours.
Antihypertensive—
   Oral, 250 mg to 1 gram per day, as a single dose or in divided daily doses, the dosage being adjusted according to response.
Note: Geriatric patients may be more sensitive to the effects of the usual adult dose.

**Usual pediatric dose**
Children up to 6 months of age—Oral, 10 to 30 mg per kg of body weight per day, as a single dose or in two divided daily doses, the dosage being adjusted according to response.
Children 6 months of age and over—Oral, 10 to 20 mg per kg of body weight per day, as a single dose or in two divided daily doses, the dosage being adjusted according to response.

**Strength(s) usually available**
U.S.—
   50 mg per mL (Rx) [*Diuril* (alcohol 0.5%; glycerin; methylparaben 0.12%; sodium saccharin; sucrose)].
Canada—
   Not commercially available.

**Packaging and storage**
Store below 40 °C (104 °F), preferably between 15 and 30 °C (59 and 86 °F), unless otherwise specified by manufacturer. Store in a tight container. Protect from freezing.

**Auxiliary labeling**
• Shake well.
• Avoid overexposure to the sun or use of sunlamp.
• Do not take other medicines without your doctor's advice.

**Note**
Check refill frequency to determine compliance in hypertensive patients.

## CHLOROTHIAZIDE TABLETS USP
**Usual adult dose**
Diuretic or
[Antidiuretic (central or nephrogenic diabetes insipidus)]—
   Oral, 250 mg every six to twelve hours.
Antihypertensive—
   Oral, 250 mg to 1 gram per day, as a single dose or in divided daily doses, the dosage being adjusted according to response.
Note: Geriatric patients may be more sensitive to the effects of the usual adult dose.

**Usual pediatric dose**
Children up to 6 months of age—Oral, 10 to 30 mg per kg of body weight per day, as a single dose or in two divided daily doses, the dosage being adjusted according to response.
Children 6 months of age and over—Oral, 10 to 20 mg per kg of body weight per day, as a single dose or in two divided daily doses, the dosage being adjusted according to response.

**Strength(s) usually available**
U.S.—
   250 mg (Rx) [*Diuril* (scored); GENERIC (may be scored)].
   500 mg (Rx) [*Diuril* (scored); GENERIC (may be scored)].
Canada—
   Not commercially available.

**Packaging and storage**
Store below 40 °C (104 °F), preferably between 15 and 30 °C (59 and 86 °F), in a well-closed container, unless otherwise specified by manufacturer.

**Auxiliary labeling**
• Avoid overexposure to the sun or use of sunlamp.
• Do not take other medicines without your doctor's advice.

**Note**
Check refill frequency to determine compliance in hypertensive patients.

# Parenteral Dosage Forms

Note: Bracketed uses in the *Dosage Forms* section refer to categories of use and/or indications that are not included in U.S. product labeling.

## CHLOROTHIAZIDE SODIUM FOR INJECTION USP
**Usual adult dose**
Diuretic or
[Antidiuretic (central or nephrogenic diabetes insipidus)]—
   Intravenous, 250 mg (base) every six to twelve hours.
Antihypertensive—
   Intravenous, 500 mg to 1 gram (base) of chlorothiazide a day, as a single dose or in two divided daily doses.
Note: Geriatric patients may be more sensitive to the effects of the usual adult dose.

**Usual pediatric dose**
Safety and efficacy have not been established.

**Size(s) usually available**
U.S.—
   500 mg (base) (Rx) [*Diuril* (mannitol 250 mg)].
Canada—
   Not commercially available.

**Packaging and storage**
Store below 40 °C (104 °F), preferably between 15 and 30 °C (59 and 86 °F), unless otherwise specified by manufacturer.

**Stability**
Reconstituted solution may be stored at room temperature for 24 hours, after which it must be discarded.

**Incompatibilities**
Solutions of chlorothiazide are not compatible with whole blood or its derivatives.

**Additional information**
Chlorothiazide Sodium for Injection USP is reconstituted for intravenous administration by adding no less than 18 mL of sterile water for injection to the vial and shaking to dissolve, producing a solution containing 25 mg (base) per mL.
Reconstituted solutions may be further diluted with dextrose injection or 0.9% sodium chloride injection for administration by intravenous infusion.

---

## CHLORTHALIDONE

# Summary of Differences
Pharmacology/pharmacokinetics:
   Although not chemically the same, chlorthalidone has the same actions as the thiazide diuretics.
   Protein binding—Very high to carbonic anhydrase in red blood cells.
   Half-life—Normal: 35 to 50 hours.
   Onset of action—Diuretic: 2 hours.
   Time to peak effect—Diuretic: 2 hours.
   Duration of action—Diuretic: 48 to 72 hours.

# Oral Dosage Forms
## CHLORTHALIDONE TABLETS USP
**Usual adult dose**
Diuretic—
   Oral, 25 to 100 mg once a day, or 100 to 200 mg once every other day, or once a day for three days a week.
Antihypertensive—
   Oral, 25 to 100 mg once a day, the dosage being adjusted according to response.
Note: Geriatric patients may be more sensitive to the effects of the usual adult dose.

**Usual pediatric dose**
Oral, 2 mg per kg of body weight or 60 mg per square meter of body surface once a day for three days a week, the dosage being adjusted according to response.

**Strength(s) usually available**
U.S.—
   25 mg (Rx) [*Hygroton; Thalitone;* GENERIC (may be scored)].
   50 mg (Rx) [*Hygroton*; GENERIC (may be scored)].
   100 mg (Rx) [*Hygroton* (scored); GENERIC (may be scored)].
Canada—
   50 mg (Rx) [*Apo-Chlorthalidone* (scored); *Hygroton* (scored); *Novo-Thalidone* (scored); *Uridon* (scored)].
   100 mg (Rx) [*Apo-Chlorthalidone* (scored); *Hygroton* (scored); *Novo-Thalidone* (scored); *Uridon* (scored)].

**Packaging and storage**
Store below 40 °C (104 °F), preferably between 15 and 30 °C (59 and 86 °F), unless otherwise specified by manufacturer. Store in a well-closed container.

USP DI

Diuretics, Thiazide (Systemic) 1279

**Auxiliary labeling**
- Avoid overexposure to the sun or use of sunlamp.
- Do not take other medicines without your doctor's advice.

**Note**
Check refill frequency to determine compliance in hypertensive patients.

---

## HYDROCHLOROTHIAZIDE

## Summary of Differences
Pharmacology/pharmacokinetics:
    Half-life—Normal: 15 hours.
    Onset of action—Diuretic: 2 hours.
    Time to peak effect—Diuretic: 4 hours.
    Duration of action—Diuretic: 6 to 12 hours.

## Oral Dosage Forms
Note: Bracketed uses in the *Dosage Forms* section refer to categories of use and/or indications that are not included in U.S. product labeling.

### HYDROCHLOROTHIAZIDE CAPSULES

**Usual adult dose**
Antihypertensive—
    Oral, initially, 12.5 once a day, administered alone or in combination with other antihypertensive agents.
Note: This lower-dose product is recommended for patients in whom the development of hyperkalemia cannot be risked, including patients taking angiotensin-converting enzyme (ACE) inhibitors.
Note: Geriatric patients may be more sensitive to the effects of the usual adult dose.

**Usual pediatric dose**
See *Hydrochlorothiazide Oral Solution*.

**Strength(s) usually available**
U.S.—
    12.5 mg (Rx) [*Microzide*].
Canada—
    Not commercially available.

**Packaging and storage**
Store between 15 and 30 °C (59 and 86 °F). Store in a well-closed container. Protect from light, moisture, and freezing.

**Auxiliary labeling**
- Avoid overexposure to the sun or use of sunlamp.
- Do not take other medicines without your doctor's advice.

**Note**
Check refill frequency to determine compliance in hypertensive patients.

### HYDROCHLOROTHIAZIDE ORAL SOLUTION

**Usual adult dose**
Diuretic or
[Antidiuretic (central or nephrogenic diabetes insipidus)]—
    Oral, 25 to 100 mg one or two times a day, once every other day, or once a day for three to five days a week.
Antihypertensive—
    Oral, 25 to 100 mg a day, as a single dose or in two divided daily doses, the dosage being adjusted according to response.
Note: Geriatric patients may be more sensitive to the effects of the usual adult dose.

**Usual pediatric dose**
Oral, 1 to 2 mg per kg of body weight or 30 to 60 mg per square meter of body surface per day, as a single dose or in two divided daily doses, the dosage being adjusted according to response.
Note: Infants under 6 months of age may receive up to 3 mg per kg of body weight per day.

**Strength(s) usually available**
U.S.—
    10 mg per mL (Rx) [GENERIC].
    100 mg per mL (Rx) [GENERIC].
Canada—
    Not commercially available.

**Packaging and storage**
Store below 40 °C (104 °F), preferably between 15 and 30 °C (59 and 86 °F), in a well-closed container, unless otherwise specified by manufacturer. Protect from freezing.

**Auxiliary labeling**
- Avoid overexposure to the sun or use of sunlamp.
- Do not take other medicines without your doctor's advice.

**Note**
Check refill frequency to determine compliance in hypertensive patients.
Be careful not to confuse oral solution with concentrated oral solution.
Make sure patient understands how to measure dose of concentrated oral solution with calibrated dropper.

### HYDROCHLOROTHIAZIDE TABLETS USP

**Usual adult dose**
Diuretic or
[Antidiuretic (central or nephrogenic diabetes insipidus)][1]—
    Oral, 25 to 100 mg one or two times a day, once every other day, or once a day for three to five days a week.
Antihypertensive—
    Oral, 25 to 100 mg a day, as a single dose or in two divided daily doses, the dosage being adjusted according to response.
Note: Geriatric patients may be more sensitive to the effects of the usual adult dose.

**Usual pediatric dose**
Oral, 1 to 2 mg per kg of body weight or 30 to 60 mg per square meter of body surface per day, as a single dose or in two divided daily doses, the dosage being adjusted according to response.
Note: Infants under 6 months of age may receive up to 3 mg per kg of body weight per day.

**Strength(s) usually available**
U.S.—
    25 mg (Rx) [*Esidrix* (scored); *HydroDIURIL* (scored); *Oretic* (scored); GENERIC (scored)].
    50 mg (Rx) [*Esidrix* (scored); *Hydro-chlor*; *Hydro-D*; *HydroDIURIL* (scored); *Oretic* (scored); GENERIC (scored)].
    100 mg (Rx) [*Esidrix* (scored); *HydroDIURIL* (scored); GENERIC (scored)].
Canada—
    25 mg (Rx) [*Apo-Hydro* (scored); *HydroDIURIL* (scored); *Neo-Codema* (scored); *Novo-Hydrazide* (scored); *Urozide* (scored)].
    50 mg (Rx) [*Apo-Hydro* (scored); *Diuchlor H* (scored); *HydroDIURIL* (scored); *Neo-Codema* (scored); *Novo-Hydrazide* (scored); *Urozide* (scored)].
    100 mg (Rx) [*Apo-Hydro* (scored); *HydroDIURIL* (scored); *Urozide* (scored)].

**Packaging and storage**
Store below 40 °C (104 °F), preferably between 15 and 30 °C (59 and 86 °F), unless otherwise specified by manufacturer. Store in a well-closed container.

**Auxiliary labeling**
- Avoid overexposure to the sun or use of sunlamp.
- Do not take other medicines without your doctor's advice.

**Note**
Check refill frequency to determine compliance in hypertensive patients.

[1]Not included in Canadian product labeling.

---

## HYDROFLUMETHIAZIDE

## Summary of Differences
Pharmacology/pharmacokinetics:
    Protein binding—High.
    Onset of action—Diuretic: 1 to 2 hours.
    Time to peak effect—Diuretic: 3 to 4 hours.
    Duration of action—Diuretic: 18 to 24 hours.

## Oral Dosage Forms
Note: Bracketed uses in the *Dosage Forms* section refer to categories of use and/or indications that are not included in U.S. product labeling.

### HYDROFLUMETHIAZIDE TABLETS USP

**Usual adult dose**
Diuretic or
[Antidiuretic (central or nephrogenic diabetes insipidus)]—
    Oral, 25 to 100 mg one or two times a day, once every other day, or once a day for three to five days a week.

Antihypertensive—
  Oral, 50 to 100 mg per day, as a single dose or in two divided daily doses, the dosage being adjusted according to response.
Note: Geriatric patients may be more sensitive to the effects of the usual adult dose.

**Usual adult prescribing limits**
Up to 200 mg per day in divided doses.

**Usual pediatric dose**
Oral, 1 mg per kg of body weight or 30 mg per square meter of body surface once a day, the dosage adjusted according to response.

**Strength(s) usually available**
U.S.—
  50 mg (Rx) [*Diucardin* (scored); *Saluron* (scored); GENERIC (may be scored)].
Canada—
  Not commercially available.

**Packaging and storage**
Store below 40 °C (104 °F), preferably between 15 and 30 °C (59 and 86 °F), unless otherwise specified by manufacturer. Store in a tight container.

**Auxiliary labeling**
• Avoid overexposure to the sun or use of sunlamp.
• Do not take other medicines without your doctor's advice.

**Note**
Check refill frequency to determine compliance in hypertensive patients.

## METHYCLOTHIAZIDE

## Summary of Differences
Pharmacology/pharmacokinetics:
  Onset of action—Diuretic: 2 hours.
  Time to peak effect—Diuretic: 6 hours.
  Duration of action—Diuretic: More than 24 hours.

## Oral Dosage Forms
Note: Bracketed uses in the *Dosage Forms* section refer to categories of use and/or indications that are not included in U.S. product labeling.

### METHYCLOTHIAZIDE TABLETS USP
**Usual adult dose**
Diuretic or
[Antidiuretic (central or nephrogenic diabetes insipidus)][1]—
  Oral, 2.5 to 10 mg once a day, once every other day, or once a day for three to five days a week.
Antihypertensive—
  Oral, 2.5 to 5 mg once a day, the dosage being adjusted according to response.
Note: Doses beyond 5 mg once a day will usually not result in further lowering of blood pressure.
Note: Geriatric patients may be more sensitive to the effects of the usual adult dose.

**Usual pediatric dose**
Oral, 50 to 200 mcg (0.05 to 0.2 mg) per kg of body weight or 1.5 to 6 mg per square meter of body surface once a day, the dosage being adjusted according to response.

**Strength(s) usually available**
U.S.—
  2.5 mg (Rx) [*Enduron*; GENERIC (may be scored)].
  5 mg (Rx) [*Aquatensen*; *Enduron*; GENERIC (may be scored)].
Canada—
  5 mg (Rx) [*Duretic*].

**Packaging and storage**
Store below 40 °C (104 °F), preferably between 15 and 30 °C (59 and 86 °F), unless otherwise specified by manufacturer. Store in a well-closed container.

**Auxiliary labeling**
• Avoid overexposure to the sun or use of sunlamp.
• Do not take other medicines without your doctor's advice.

**Note**
Check refill frequency to determine compliance in hypertensive patients.

[1] Not included in Canadian product labeling.

## METOLAZONE

## Summary of Differences
Pharmacology/pharmacokinetics:
  Although not chemically the same, metolazone has actions similar to the thiazide diuretics.
  Absorption—More rapid and more complete with prompt metolazone tablets than with extended metolazone tablets.
  Protein binding—Very high (50 to 70% to red blood cells).
  Half-life—Normal: 8 hours.
  Onset of action—Diuretic: 1 hour.
  Time to peak effect—Diuretic: 2 hours.
  Duration of action—Diuretic: 12 to 24 hours.
  Elimination—Metolazone undergoes some enterohepatic recycling, and slightly greater amounts are excreted in the bile.

## Additional Dosing Information
*Extended metolazone tablets and prompt metolazone tablets should not be substituted for one another* because of significant differences in rate of absorption and bioavailability.

Absorption of metolazone after oral administration is reduced in patients with cardiac disease (65% in normal subjects as compared with 40% in cardiac disease patients).

Plasma clearance of metolazone is 20 mL per minute in patients with renal failure as compared with 110 mL per minute in healthy subjects.

Duration of diuretic effect is dose-related.

Metolazone may be more effective as a diuretic than other thiazides in patients with severe renal failure. Because of this, metolazone has been added to furosemide therapy in resistant patients; however, caution is necessary because of the risk of severe electrolyte imbalance.

## Oral Dosage Forms

### EXTENDED METOLAZONE TABLETS
**Usual adult dose**
Diuretic—
  Oral, 5 to 20 mg once a day.
Antihypertensive—
  Oral, 2.5 to 5 mg once a day, the dosage being adjusted according to response.
Note: Geriatric patients may be more sensitive to the effects of the usual adult dose.

**Usual pediatric dose**
Dosage has not been established.

**Strength(s) usually available**
U.S.—
  2.5 mg (Rx) [*Diulo*; *Zaroxolyn*].
  5 mg (Rx) [*Diulo*; *Zaroxolyn*].
  10 mg (Rx) [*Diulo*; *Zaroxolyn*].
Canada—
  2.5 mg (Rx) [*Zaroxolyn*].
  5 mg (Rx) [*Zaroxolyn*].
  10 mg (Rx) [*Zaroxolyn*].

**Packaging and storage**
Store below 40 °C (104 °F), preferably between 15 and 30 °C (59 and 86 °F), in a well-closed container, unless otherwise specified by manufacturer.

**Auxiliary labeling**
• Avoid overexposure to the sun or use of sunlamp.
• Do not take other medicines without your doctor's advice.

**Note**
Extended and prompt metolazone tablets are not bioequivalent. *One product should not be substituted for the other*. If patients are to be transferred from one to the other, retitration and appropriate changes in dosage may be necessary.

Check refill frequency to determine compliance in hypertensive patients.

### PROMPT METOLAZONE TABLETS
**Usual adult dose**
Antihypertensive—
  Initial: Oral, 500 mcg (0.5 mg) once a day, the dosage being adjusted according to response.
  Maintenance: Oral, 500 mcg (0.5 mg) to 1 mg once a day.

**Usual adult prescribing limits**
Up to 1 mg per day.

**Usual pediatric dose**
Dosage has not been established.

**Strength(s) usually available**
U.S.—
   500 mcg (0.5 mg) (Rx) [*Mykrox*].
Canada—
   Not commercially available.

**Packaging and storage**
Store below 40 °C (104 °F), preferably between 15 and 30 °C (59 and 86 °F), in a well-closed container, unless otherwise specified by manufacturer.

**Auxiliary labeling**
• Avoid overexposure to the sun or use of sunlamp.
• Do not take other medicines without your doctor's advice.

**Note**
Extended and prompt metolazone tablets are not bioequivalent. *One product should not be substituted for the other.* If patients are to be transferred from one to the other, retitration and appropriate changes in dosage may be necessary.
Check refill frequency to determine compliance in hypertensive patients.

---

## POLYTHIAZIDE

## Summary of Differences
Pharmacology/pharmacokinetics:
   Protein binding—High.
   Onset of action—Diuretic: 2 hours.
   Time to peak effect—Diuretic: 6 hours.
   Duration of action—Diuretic: 24 to 48 hours.

## Oral Dosage Forms
Note: Bracketed uses in the *Dosage Forms* section refer to categories of use and/or indications that are not included in U.S. product labeling.

### POLYTHIAZIDE TABLETS USP
**Usual adult dose**
Diuretic or
[Antidiuretic (central or nephrogenic diabetes insipidus)]—
   Oral, 1 to 4 mg once a day, once every other day, or once a day for three to five days a week.
Antihypertensive—
   Oral, 2 to 4 mg once a day, the dosage being adjusted according to response.
Note: Geriatric patients may be more sensitive to the effects of the usual adult dose.

**Usual pediatric dose**
Oral, 20 to 80 mcg (0.02 to 0.08 mg) per kg of body weight or 500 mcg (0.5 mg) to 2.5 mg per square meter of body surface once a day, the dosage being adjusted according to response.

**Strength(s) usually available**
U.S.—
   1 mg (Rx) [*Renese* (scored; lactose)].
   2 mg (Rx) [*Renese* (scored; lactose)].
   4 mg (Rx) [*Renese* (scored; lactose)].
Canada—
   Not commercially available.

**Packaging and storage**
Store below 40 °C (104 °F), preferably between 15 and 30 °C (59 and 86 °F), unless otherwise specified by manufacturer. Store in a tight, light-resistant container.

**Auxiliary labeling**
• Avoid overexposure to the sun or use of sunlamp.
• Do not take other medicines without your doctor's advice.

**Note**
Check refill frequency to determine compliance in hypertensive patients.

---

## QUINETHAZONE

## Summary of Differences
Pharmacology/pharmacokinetics:
   Although not chemically the same, quinethazone has the same actions as the thiazide diuretics.
   Onset of action—Diuretic: 2 hours.
   Time to peak effect—Diuretic: 6 hours.
   Duration of action—Diuretic: 18 to 24 hours.

## Oral Dosage Forms
### QUINETHAZONE TABLETS USP
**Usual adult dose**
Diuretic or
Antihypertensive—
   Oral, 50 to 200 mg per day, as a single dose or in two divided daily doses, adjusted according to response.
Note: Geriatric patients may be more sensitive to the effects of the usual adult dose.

**Usual adult prescribing limits**
Up to 200 mg daily in divided doses.

**Usual pediatric dose**
Dosage has not been established.

**Strength(s) usually available**
U.S.—
   50 mg (Rx) [*Hydromox* (scored)].
Canada—
   Not commercially available.

**Packaging and storage**
Store below 40 °C (104 °F), preferably between 15 and 30 °C (59 and 86 °F), unless otherwise specified by manufacturer. Store in a tight container.

**Auxiliary labeling**
• Avoid overexposure to the sun or use of sunlamp.
• Do not take other medicines without your doctor's advice.

**Note**
Check refill frequency to determine compliance in hypertensive patients.

---

## TRICHLORMETHIAZIDE

## Summary of Differences
Pharmacology/pharmacokinetics:
   Onset of action—Diuretic: 2 hours.
   Time to peak effect—Diuretic: 6 hours.
   Duration of action—Diuretic: Up to 24 hours.
Laboratory value alterations:
   May produce false-negative results in phentolamine, phenolsulfonphthalein, and tyramine tests.

## Oral Dosage Forms
Note: Bracketed uses in the *Dosage Forms* section refer to categories of use and/or indications that are not included in U.S. product labeling.

### TRICHLORMETHIAZIDE TABLETS USP
**Usual adult dose**
Diuretic or
[Antidiuretic (central or nephrogenic diabetes insipidus)]—
   Oral, 1 to 4 mg once a day, once every other day, or once a day for three to five days a week.
Antihypertensive—
   Oral, 2 to 4 mg once a day, the dosage being adjusted according to response.
Note: Geriatric patients may be more sensitive to the effects of the usual adult dose.

**Usual pediatric dose**
For children over 6 months of age—Oral, 70 mcg (0.07 mg) per kg of body weight or 2 mg per square meter of body surface per day, as a single dose or in two divided daily doses, the dosage being adjusted according to response.

**Strength(s) usually available**
U.S.—
   2 mg (Rx) [*Metahydrin*; *Naqua* (scored); GENERIC].
   4 mg (Rx) [*Metahydrin*; *Naqua* (scored); *Trichlorex*; GENERIC].
Canada—
   Not commercially available.

**Packaging and storage**
Store below 40 °C (104 °F), preferably between 15 and 30 °C (59 and 86 °F), unless otherwise specified by manufacturer. Store in a tight container.

# Diuretics, Thiazide (Systemic)

**Auxiliary labeling**
- Avoid overexposure to the sun or use of sunlamp.
- Do not take other medicines without your doctor's advice.

**Note**
Check refill frequency to determine compliance in hypertensive patients.

## Selected Bibliography
The fifth report of the Joint National Committee on Detection, Evaluation, and Treatment of High Blood Pressure (JNC V). Arch Intern Med 1993; 153(2): 154-83.

Freis ED. The cardiovascular risks of thiazide diuretics. Clin Pharmacol Ther 1986 Mar; 39: 239-44.

Brater DC. Clinical use of thiazide diuretics. Hosp Form 1983; 18: 788-93.

Revised: 06/07/92
Interim revision: 06/30/94; 07/01/98

---

**DIVALPROEX**—See *Valproic Acid (Systemic)*

---

**DOBUTAMINE**—See *Sympathomimetic Agents—Cardiovascular Use (Parenteral-Systemic)*

---

# DOCETAXEL  Systemic

VA CLASSIFICATION (Primary): AN900
Commonly used brand name(s): *Taxotere*.
Note: For a listing of dosage forms and brand names by country availability, see *Dosage Forms* section(s).

## Category
Antineoplastic.

## Indications
Note: Bracketed information in the *Indications* section refers to uses that are not included in U.S. product labeling.

**Accepted**

Carcinoma, breast (treatment)—Docetaxel is indicated for treatment of locally advanced or metastatic breast cancer that has progressed or relapsed despite anthracycline-based chemotherapy. [Docetaxel is also accepted as first-line chemotherapy for locally advanced or metastatic breast cancer, based on reports of objective tumor response rates (mostly partial but some complete) in phase II clinical trials.][1]

[Carcinoma, lung, non–small cell (treatment)]—Docetaxel is indicated for treatment of locally advanced or metastatic non–small cell lung carcinoma after platinum-based chemotherapy has failed. It is also accepted as first-line treatment for non–small cell lung carcinoma, based on reports of objective tumor response rates in phase II clinical trials.[1]

[Carcinoma, lung, small cell (treatment)][1]—Docetaxel is accepted for treatment of small-cell lung carcinoma after first-line chemotherapy has failed, based on reports of objective tumor response rates in phase II clinical trials.

[Carcinoma, ovarian (treatment)][1]—Docetaxel is accepted for treatment of ovarian carcinoma after prior platinum-based therapy has failed, based on reports of objective tumor response rates in phase II clinical trials.

[1] Not included in Canadian product labeling.

## Pharmacology/Pharmacokinetics

**Physicochemical characteristics**
Source—Semisynthetic, starting with a precursor extracted from the needles of the European yew, *Taxus baccata*.
Chemical group—Docetaxel is a member of the taxoid family; chemically related to paclitaxel.
Molecular weight—861.94.
Practically insoluble in water; highly lipophilic.

**Mechanism of action/Effect**
Docetaxel is an antimitotic agent. It binds to free tubulin, then promotes the polymerization of tubulin into stable microtubules and inhibits microtubule disassembly, resulting in blockade of cellular mitotic and interphase functions and, consequently, in inhibition of cell division. Unlike paclitaxel and other spindle poisons in clinical use, docetaxel does not alter the number of protofilaments in the bound microtubules.

The mechanisms by which resistance to docetaxel occurs are not completely understood. Studies have shown that docetaxel is active against several tumor cell lines overexpressing the multidrug resistance gene. Also, cross-resistance between docetaxel and paclitaxel does not occur consistently.

**Other actions/effects**
Several *in vitro* and *in vivo* studies have shown that docetaxel has only moderate immunosuppressive activity.

**Distribution**
Volume of distribution at steady-state—Mean, 113 liters (L).
In animal studies, docetaxel was widely distributed to all tissues and organs other than the brain, in which very low concentrations were attained.

**Protein binding**
Very high (97%), primarily to alpha$_1$-acid glycoprotein, albumin, and lipoproteins.

**Biotransformation**
Hepatic; extensively metabolized by cytochrome P450 subfamily 3A (CYP 3A) isoenzymes to one major and three minor metabolites.

**Half-life**
Dose-dependent. Doses of 70 mg per square meter of body surface area (mg/m$^2$) or higher produce a triphasic elimination profile. With lower doses, assay limitations precluded detection of the terminal elimination phase.
*Alpha* (distribution)—
   4 minutes.
*Beta*—
   36 minutes.
*Gamma* (terminal)—
   11.1 hours. The prolonged terminal elimination half-life is caused, in part, by relatively slow efflux from the peripheral compartment.
Note: A preliminary study in pediatric patients receiving 55 mg/m$^2$ of docetaxel reported bi-exponential elimination and a terminal half-life of 2.4 ± 1.8 hours.

**Peak serum concentration**
2.57 to 3.67 mcg per mL (mcg/mL), with doses of 70 to 100 mg/m$^2$.
Note: The area under the docetaxel concentration–time curve (AUC) is 3.13 to 4.83 mcg/mL per hour with doses of 70 to 100 mg/m$^2$. Values may be increased in patients with hepatic function impairment.

**Elimination**
Primarily biliary/fecal. Following administration of radiolabeled docetaxel, fecal and urinary recovery over the next 7 days accounted for approximately 75% and 6%, respectively, of the administered radioactivity. Approximately 80% of the radioactivity that appeared in the feces was excreted during the first 2 days as one major and three minor metabolites; < 8% was unchanged docetaxel.

Total body clearance is approximately 21 L per hour per square meter of body surface area (L/hr/m$^2$) and is not dose-dependent. Values are decreased by an average of 27 to 30%, but with substantial interpatient variability, in patients with hepatic function test abnormalities suggestive of mild to moderate hepatic function impairment.

Note: In a preliminary study in pediatric patients, total body clearance was approximately 9.3 L/hr/m$^2$.

## Precautions to Consider

**Cross-sensitivity and/or related problems**
Patients hypersensitive to paclitaxel may be hypersensitive to docetaxel also.

**Carcinogenicity**
Carcinogenicity studies in animals have not been done.
Secondary malignancies are potential delayed effects of many antineoplastic agents, although it is not clear whether the effect is related to their mutagenic or immunosuppressive action. The effect of dose and duration of therapy is also unknown, although the risk seems to increase with long-term use. The risk of secondary malignancies developing after docetaxel therapy is not known.

**Mutagenicity**
Docetaxel was clastogenic in the *in vitro* chromosome aberration test in Chinese hamster ovary K$_1$ cells and in the *in vivo* mouse micronucleus test. No mutagenicity was observed in the Ames test or the Chinese hamster ovary/hypoxanthine-guanine phosphoribosyltransferase gene mutation assay.

### Pregnancy/Reproduction
Fertility—Decrease in testicular weight, but no overt impairment of fertility, occurred in rats given multiple doses of up to 0.3 mg per kg of body weight (mg/kg) intravenously (approximately one-fiftieth the recommended human dose on a mg per square meter of body surface area [mg/m²] basis). Testicular atrophy or degeneration also occurred in a 10-cycle study (in which the medication was given intravenously at 21-day intervals for 6 months) in rats given 5 mg/kg and dogs given 0.375 mg/kg (approximately one-third and one-fifteenth the recommended human dose on a mg/m² basis, respectively). Similar effects also occurred in rats given lower doses at an increased frequency of administration.

Pregnancy—Adequate and well-controlled studies have not been done in humans.

It is usually recommended that use of antineoplastics, especially combination chemotherapy, be avoided whenever possible, especially during the first trimester. Although information is limited because of the relatively few instances of antineoplastic administration during pregnancy, the mutagenic, teratogenic, and carcinogenic potential of these medications must be considered.

Other hazards to the fetus include adverse reactions seen in adults.

In general, use of contraception is recommended during cytotoxic drug therapy.

Animal studies have shown that docetaxel is distributed to the fetus. Maternal toxicity resulting in embryo- and fetotoxicity occurred in rats given 0.3 mg/kg or more per day and in rabbits given 0.03 mg/kg or more per day (equivalent to or higher than one-fiftieth and one-three hundredth, respectively, the maximum recommended human dose on a mg/m² basis) during the period of organogenesis. Embryotoxic and fetotoxic effects were characterized by increased intrauterine deaths, increased resorptions, decreased fetal weights, and delayed fetal ossification. However, no teratogenicity was apparent in rats and rabbits given doses of 1.8 and 1.2 mg/kg per day, respectively.

FDA Pregnancy Category D.

### Breast-feeding
Although very little information is available regarding distribution of antineoplastic agents into breast milk, breast-feeding is not recommended during chemotherapy because of the potential risks to the infant (adverse effects, mutagenicity, carcinogenicity). It is not known whether docetaxel is distributed into human breast milk, but it is distributed into the milk of lactating animals.

### Pediatrics
Docetaxel has been studied in a limited number of children with refractory cancer. Dose-ranging studies have shown the maximum tolerated dose to be lower in pediatric patients (especially if treated with several prior courses of chemotherapy) than in adults, unless a colony-stimulating factor is used to reduce the occurrence of severe neutropenia. However, safety and efficacy in children younger than 16 years of age have not been established.

### Geriatrics
Several clinical trials with docetaxel have included patients older than 65 years of age. These studies did not show any differences between elderly patients and younger adults in the efficacy, toxicity, or pharmacokinetics of docetaxel. Adjustment of dosage on the basis of age is not needed in geriatric patients.

### Pharmacogenetics
A pharmacokinetic study showed no significant differences in total body clearance of docetaxel between Japanese patients and American or European patients.

### Dental
Docetaxel commonly causes neutropenia, and, less commonly, thrombocytopenia, which may result in an increased incidence of microbial infection, delayed healing, and gingival bleeding. If severe neutropenia occurs, dental work should be deferred until blood counts have returned to normal. Also, patients should be instructed in proper oral hygiene, including caution in use of regular toothbrushes, dental floss, and toothpicks.

Docetaxel commonly causes stomatitis (ulceration of the lips, tongue, and oral cavity), which is usually mild but in some patients may be severe. There is some evidence that severe stomatitis tends to occur at the nadir of the neutrophil count and may contribute to the occurrence of neutropenic fever by providing an entry for pathogens into the body.

### Drug interactions and/or related problems
The following drug interactions and/or related problems have been selected on the basis of their potential clinical significance (possible mechanism in parentheses where appropriate)—not necessarily inclusive (» = major clinical significance):

Note: Combinations containing any of the following medications, depending on the amount present, may also interact with this medication.

Blood dyscrasia–causing medications (see *Appendix II*)
(leukopenic and/or thrombocytopenic effects of docetaxel may be increased with concurrent or recent therapy if these medications cause the same effects; dosage adjustment of docetaxel, if necessary, should be based on blood counts)

» Bone marrow depressants, other (see *Appendix II*) or
Radiation therapy
(additive bone marrow depression may occur; dosage reduction may be required when two or more bone marrow depressants, including radiation, are used concurrently or consecutively)

» Enzyme inhibitors, hepatic, of the cytochrome P450 3A (CYP 3A) isoenzyme, such as:
Erythromycin
Ketoconazole
Midazolam
Orphenadrine
Testosterone
(caution in concurrent use is recommended because *in vitro* studies have shown that inhibitors of the CYP 3A isoenzyme [but not inhibitors of other cytochrome P450 isoenzymes] significantly inhibit docetaxel metabolism)

» Immunosuppressants, other, such as:
Azathioprine
Chlorambucil
Corticosteroids, glucocorticoid
Cyclophosphamide
Cyclosporine
Mercaptopurine
Muromonab CD-3
Tacrolimus
(concurrent use with docetaxel may increase the risk of infection)

Paclitaxel and
Other medications metabolized by the CYP 3A isoenzyme
(*in vitro* studies have shown that paclitaxel, which is partially metabolized by the CYP 3A isoenzyme, significantly inhibits docetaxel metabolism; also, docetaxel inhibits formation of the minor paclitaxel metabolite M4 via CYP 3A [but not formation of the major paclitaxel metabolite M5 via the cytochrome P450 2C isoenzyme]. The possibility should be considered that other medications that are metabolized by the CYP 3A isoenzyme may also alter docetaxel metabolism)

Vaccines, killed virus
(because normal defense mechanisms may be suppressed by docetaxel therapy, the patient's antibody response to the vaccine may be decreased. The interval between discontinuation of medications that cause immunosuppression and restoration of the patient's ability to respond to the vaccine depends on the intensity and type of immunosuppression-causing medication used, the underlying disease, and other factors; estimates vary from 3 months to 1 year)

» Vaccines, live virus
(because normal defense mechanisms may be suppressed by docetaxel therapy, concurrent use with a live virus vaccine may potentiate the replication of the vaccine virus, may increase the side/adverse effects of the vaccine virus, and/or may decrease the patient's antibody response to the vaccine; immunization of these patients should be undertaken only with extreme caution after careful review of the patient's hematologic status and only with the knowledge and consent of the physician managing the docetaxel therapy. The interval between discontinuation of medications that cause immunosuppression and restoration of the patient's ability to respond to the vaccine depends on the intensity and type of immunosuppression-causing medication used, the underlying disease, and other factors; estimates vary from 3 months to 1 year. In addition, immunization with oral poliovirus vaccine should be postponed in persons in close contact with the patient, especially family members)

### Laboratory value alterations
The following have been selected on the basis of their potential clinical significance (possible effect in parentheses where appropriate)—not necessarily inclusive (» = major clinical significance):

With physiology/laboratory test values
Alanine aminotransferase (ALT [SGPT]) and
Alkaline phosphatase and
Aspartate aminotransferase (AST [SGOT]) and
Bilirubin concentrations, serum
(values may be increased; in clinical trials, bilirubin concentrations higher than the upper limit of normal, aminotransferase values >

1.5 times the upper limit of normal, alkaline phosphatase values > 2.5 times the upper limit of normal, and concomitant increases in aminotransferase and alkaline phosphatase values occurred in approximately 9%, 18%, 7.5%, and 4.5% of patients with normal pretreatment values, respectively. However, whether these changes were caused by docetaxel or the underlying disease has not been established)

Hematocrit/hemoglobin values and
Leukocyte, especially neutrophil, count and
Platelet count
(may be decreased; the neutrophil count usually reaches a nadir at a median of 8 days after a treatment and generally returns to pretreatment or near-pretreatment values within the next 1 or 2 weeks)

**Medical considerations/Contraindications**
The medical considerations/contraindications included have been selected on the basis of their potential clinical significance (reasons given in parentheses where appropriate)—not necessarily inclusive (» = major clinical significance).

*Except under special circumstances, this medication should not be used when the following medical problem exists:*
» Hepatic function impairment
(docetaxel clearance will be decreased, resulting in an increased risk of toxic effects, including severe stomatitis, dermatological reactions, and thrombocytopenia as well as severe neutropenia, febrile neutropenia, infections, and toxic death, even if dosage is decreased. Docetaxel is therefore not recommended for patients with hepatic function impairment, especially if bilirubin concentrations are elevated or when transaminase values are > 1.5 times the upper limit of normal and alkaline phosphastase values are > 2.5 times the upper limit of normal. If docetaxel is considered essential for a patient with mild hepatic function impairment, extreme caution and lower doses are recommended)

*Risk-benefit should be considered when the following medical problems exist:*
Alcohol abuse or history of
(risk of severe neurotoxic reactions to docetaxel may be increased)
» Bone marrow depression
(will be exacerbated; treatment should be delayed until the neutrophil count recovers to > 1500 cells per cubic millimeter and the platelet count returns to > 100,000 cells per cubic millimeter)
» Chickenpox, existing or recent (including recent exposure) or
» Herpes zoster
(risk of severe, generalized disease)
Conditions that may predispose to pleural effusion, such as:
Chest radiotherapy, prior or
» Pleural effusion, pre-existing or
Pleural tumor or
Thoracotomy, prior
(increased risk of pleural effusion associated with docetaxel-induced fluid retention)
» Hypersensitivity reaction, severe, history of, to docetaxel, paclitaxel, or other medications formulated with polysorbate 80
» Infection, pre-existing
(recovery may be impaired)
» Caution should also be used in patients who have had previous cytotoxic drug therapy or radiation therapy

**Patient monitoring**
The following may be especially important in patient monitoring (other tests may be warranted in some patients, depending on condition; » = major clinical significance):
Hematocrit or hemoglobin and
» Leukocyte count, total and differential and
Platelet count
(determinations recommended prior to initiation of therapy and at frequent intervals during therapy; administration of docetaxel should be delayed if the neutrophil count is lower than 1500 cells per cubic millimeter and/or the platelet count is lower than 100,000 cells per cubic millimeter . If severe neutropenia [fewer than 500 cells per cubic millimeter] persists for 7 days or more, a reduction in dose is recommended for subsequent courses of therapy)
» Hepatic function studies
(recommended prior to each treatment cycle; it is recommended that docetaxel not be given if abnormalities indicative of hepatic function impairment are present [e.g., bilirubin concentrations higher than the upper limit of normal or transaminase values > 1.5 times the upper limit of normal and alkaline phosphastase values > 2.5 times the upper limit of normal])

» Skin appearance and
» Vital signs
(should be monitored during, and for approximately 1 hour following, an infusion, especially during the first two treatment cycles, to detect signs of a severe hypersensitivity reaction, e.g., dyspnea, hypotension, generalized urticaria, or other signs of angioedema)

## Side/Adverse Effects

Note: Many "side effects" of antineoplastic therapy are unavoidable and represent the medication's pharmacologic action. Some of these (for example, leukopenia and thrombocytopenia) are actually used as parameters to aid in individual dosage titration.

Bone marrow depression (primarily neutropenia) is the major dose-limiting toxicity.

Significant endocrine, hepatic, or renal toxicity clearly attributable to docetaxel has not been reported.

In addition to the side/adverse effects reported below, the following have been reported, but a causal relationship has not been established: cardiovascular—atrial fibrillation, deep vein thrombosis, electrocardiographic abnormalities, pulmonary embolism, syncope, tachycardia, thrombophlebitis; gastrointestinal—constipation, duodenal ulcer, esophagitis, intestinal obstruction, ileus; nervous system—confusion, pain; respiratory—acute pulmonary edema, acute respiratory distress syndrome; urogenital—renal insufficiency.

The following side/adverse effects have been selected on the basis of their potential clinical significance (possible signs and symptoms in parentheses where appropriate)—not necessarily inclusive:

**Those indicating need for medical attention**
Incidence more frequent (> 30%)
*Anemia* (unusual tiredness or weakness); *fever*—not always associated with infection; *fluid retention* (more commonly, swelling of fingers, hands, feet, or lower legs; less commonly, swelling of abdomen or face; noisy, rattling breathing or troubled breathing while at rest; weight gain); *leukopenia or neutropenia*—usually asymptomatic

Note: Although *anemia* occurs very frequently, severe anemia (hemoglobin < 8 grams per deciliter) is relatively infrequent in patients with normal hepatic function. However, the incidence of severe anemia is significantly increased in patients with mild to moderate hepatic function impairment.

*Fluid retention* usually begins in the lower extremities, but may become generalized and, less frequently, lead to pleural effusions, pericardial effusions, or ascites. Prophylactic corticosteroid administration decreases the incidence and severity of this complication and increases the median cumulative dose at which moderate or severe edema occurs (from 400 to 705 [mg/m$^2$]). However, even with recommended prophylaxis, docetaxel causes fluid retention in almost 50% of patients with normal hepatic function; moderate or severe fluid retention requiring medical treatment occurs in approximately 17% and 6%, respectively, of these patients. The incidence and severity of fluid retention are significantly higher in patients with hepatic function impairment. Fluid accumulation is due to increased capillary permeability rather than hypoalbuminemia or cardiac, hepatic, or renal damage. Fluid retention is slowly reversible after treatment is discontinued (median 29 [range, 0 to > 42] weeks to complete reversal).

*Leukopenia* and *neutropenia* occur in > 96% of patients receiving docetaxel; severe neutropenia (neutrophil count below 500 cells per cubic millimeter) is also very common. In most patients, the neutropenia is reversible, noncumulative, and short-lasting. The nadir of the neutrophil count usually occurs 8 days after an infusion. The median duration of severe neutropenia is 7 days, and neutrophil counts usually return to pretreatment or near-pretreatment values in 1 to 2 weeks. *Febrile neutropenia* (severe neutropenia with fever > 38 °C [100.4 °F] and infection requiring intravenous antibiotic therapy and/or hospitalization) occurs less frequently, and deaths due to sepsis are uncommon, in patients with normal hepatic function. Hepatic function impairment significantly increases the risk of severe neutropenia, febrile neutropenia, and septic deaths.

Incidence less frequent (5 to 29%)
***Cutaneous reaction, severe*** (red, scaly, swollen, or peeling areas of skin)—especially likely to occur on the hands and/or feet; ***febrile neutropenia or other infection*** (fever with or without chills; cough or hoarseness; difficult or painful urination; lower back or side pain); ***hypersensitivity reaction, mild*** (back pain; flushing; skin rash or itching, localized; troubled breathing, mild); ***thrombocytopenia*** (rarely, unusual

bleeding or bruising; black, tarry stools; blood in urine or stools; pinpoint red spots on skin)—usually asymptomatic

Note: *Infections* have also been reported in the absence of *febrile neutropenia.*

Fatalities have occurred with docetaxel therapy at doses of 100 mg/m$^2$ (34 of 1435 patients with normal liver function and 6 of 55 patients with hepatic function impairment) and doses of 60 mg/m$^2$ (3 of 481 patients with normal liver function and 3 of 7 patients with hepatic function impairment). Most of the fatalities resulted from sepsis associated with *neutropenia.*

*Hypersensitivity reactions* are most likely to occur during the first two cycles of docetaxel treatment, generally within the first few minutes after the infusion is started. Signs and symptoms usually abate within 15 minutes after the infusion is stopped. After a mild reaction, treatment can usually be reinstituted without further difficulty. However, if a severe reaction (characterized by angioedema, hypotension, bronchospasm, and/or generalized erythema, urticaria, or skin rash) occurs, the infusion should be discontinued immediately and aggressive treatment instituted.

Incidence rare (< 5%)
*Cardiovascular effects, including angina, unstable* (chest pain); *arrhythmia, such as sinus tachycardia, atrial flutter, or paroxysmal atrial tachycardia* (fast or irregular heartbeat); *heart failure* (shortness of breath; swelling of face, fingers, feet, or lower legs); *hypertension* (increase in blood pressure; dizziness; headaches); *and hypotension* (dizziness; fainting)—usually asymptomatic; *hypersensitivity reaction, severe* (decrease in blood pressure, sudden and severe; shortness of breath, troubled breathing, tightness in chest, or wheezing; hives, skin rash, or redness, generalized)

**Those indicating need for medical attention only if they continue or are bothersome**
Incidence more frequent (> 30%)
*Cutaneous reaction, mild* (skin rash or redness); *diarrhea; nausea; neurologic effects, including asthenia* (weakness); *and paresthesias or dysesthesias* (burning, numbness, tingling, or painful sensations); *stomatitis* (sores or ulcers on lips or tongue or inside the mouth)

Note: Rarely, *neurologic effects* may result in moderate to severe neuropathy, leading to decreased dexterity and/or disturbances in gait, usually after cumulative doses of 600 mg/m$^2$ have been given.

Severe *stomatitis* may contribute to the occurrence of febrile neutropenia by providing a portal for entry of pathogens into the body.

Incidence less frequent (5 to 29%)
*Arthralgias or myalgias* (pain in joints or muscles); *headache; infusion site reactions* (dry, red, hot, or irritated skin; pain; or swelling or lump under the skin at place of injection); *nail disorder* (discoloration of fingernails or toenails; rarely, loosening or loss of nails and pain); *vomiting*

**Those not indicating need for medical attention**
Incidence more frequent
*Alopecia* (loss of hair)—occurs in 80% of patients, but is fully reversible after therapy has ended

## Overdose

For more information on the management of overdose or unintentional ingestion, **contact a Poison Control Center** (see *Poison Control Center Listing*).

**Clinical effects of overdose**
The following effects have been selected on the basis of their potential clinical significance (possible signs and symptoms in parentheses where appropriate)—not necessarily inclusive:

Acute and chronic
*Bone marrow suppression, including anemia* (unusual tiredness or weakness)*; leukopenia or neutropenia, with or without infection* (fever with or without chills; cough or hoarseness; lower back or side pain; painful or difficult urination)*; and/or thrombocytopenia* (black, tarry stools; blood in urine or stools; pinpoint red spots on skin; unusual bleeding or bruising); *stomatitis* (sores or ulcers on lips or tongue or inside the mouth); *peripheral neuropathy* (burning, numbness, tingling, or painful sensations; weakness in arms, hands, legs, or feet)

**Treatment of overdose**
It is recommended that the patient be hospitalized for close monitoring of vital functions and treatment of observed effects. Severe bone marrow depression may require transfusion of required blood components. Febrile neutropenia should be treated empirically with broad-spectrum antibiotics, pending bacterial cultures and appropriate diagnostic tests.

## Patient Consultation

As an aid to patient consultation, refer to *Advice for the Patient, Docetaxel (Systemic).*

In providing consultation, consider emphasizing the following selected information (» = major clinical significance):

**Before using this medication**
» Conditions affecting use, especially:
Hypersensitivity to docetaxel, paclitaxel, or polysorbate 80
Pregnancy—Use is not recommended because of embryotoxic, fetotoxic, and carcinogenic potential; advisability of using contraception; informing physician immediately if pregnancy is suspected
Breast-feeding—Not recommended because of potential serious adverse effects
Other medications, especially other bone marrow depressants, other immunosuppressants, inhibitors of the cytochrome P450 3A isoenzyme, such as erythromycin, ketoconazole, midazolam, orphenadrine, and testosterone, and radiation therapy
Other medical problems, especially hepatic function impairment, chickenpox, herpes zoster, infection, or pleural effusion

**Proper use of this medication**
Frequency of nausea and vomiting and/or neuropathy; importance of continuing treatment despite feeling ill
» Importance of compliance with peritreatment corticosteroid regimen
» Proper dosing

**Precautions while using this medication**
» Importance of close monitoring by the physician
» Avoiding immunizations unless approved by physician; other persons in patient's household should avoid immunizations with oral poliovirus vaccine; avoiding other persons who have taken oral poliovirus vaccine or wearing a protective mask that covers nose and mouth

*Caution if bone marrow depression occurs*
» Avoiding exposure to persons with infections, especially during periods of low blood cell counts; checking with physician immediately if fever with or without chills, cough or hoarseness, lower back or side pain, or painful or difficult urination occurs
» Checking with physician immediately if unusual bleeding or bruising; black, tarry stools; blood in urine or stools; or pinpoint red spots on skin occur
Caution in use of regular toothbrush, dental floss, or toothpick; physician, dentist, or nurse may suggest alternatives; checking with physician before having dental work done
Not touching eyes or inside of nose unless hands washed immediately before
Using caution to avoid accidental cuts when using sharp objects such as safety razor or fingernail or toenail cutters
Avoiding contact sports or other situations where bruising or injury could occur

**Side/adverse effects**
May cause adverse effects such as blood problems; importance of discussing possible effects with physician
Signs of potential side effects, especially anemia, fever, fluid retention, severe cutaneous reactions, febrile neutropenia, thrombocytopenia, and cardiovascular effects
» Possibility of hypersensitivity; notifying physician or nurse immediately if back pain, breathing problems, or itching occurs during infusion; physician or nurse will monitor for other signs of allergic reaction and be prepared to institute treatment
Some side effects may be asymptomatic, including anemia, leukopenia or neutropenia, thrombocytopenia, and cardiovascular effects
Physician or nurse can help in dealing with side effects
Probability of hair loss; regrowth should return after treatment has ended

## General Dosing Information

Docetaxel should be administered only under the supervision of a physician experienced in cancer chemotherapy. Adequate facilities and medications for diagnosis and treatment of complications should be readily available.

Peritreatment administration of an oral corticosteroid is recommended to decrease the frequency and severity and delay the onset of docetaxel-induced fluid retention. Aggressive, early diuretic treatment may also be required.

Peritreatment administration of an oral corticosteroid, with or without antihistamines (both $H_1$- and $H_2$-receptor antagonists), also reduces the severity of docetaxel-induced hypersensitivity reactions and cutaneous toxicity. A commonly used regimen consists of 8 mg of dexamethasone orally two times a day for 5 days, beginning 1 day before the docetaxel infusion; the antihistamines, if used, are given intravenously 30 minutes prior to the start of the docetaxel infusion. A recent study has shown that administering 8 mg of dexamethasone orally two times a day for only 3 days, beginning 1 day before the docetaxel infusion, is as effective as the 5-day regimen in reducing the severity of hypersensitivity reactions and fluid retention and also decreases the occurrence of severe stomatitis and infection. Palmar-plantar erythrodysesthesias that occur despite prophylaxis may respond to administration of 50 mg three times a day of pyridoxine.

Docetaxel is not highly emetogenic; routine prophylaxis with antiemetics is generally not required.

Docetaxel is administered by intravenous infusion. *Docetaxel for injection concentrate must be diluted before use.* The needle or catheter should be properly positioned to prevent leakage into surrounding tissue, which may result in irritation, local tissue necrosis, and thrombophlebitis. If extravasation occurs, the infusion should be stopped immediately and the remainder of the dose administered into another vein.

Mild hypersensitivity reactions (flushing, localized skin reactions, back pain, fever, chills, mild dyspnea) do not require interruption of docetaxel therapy. However, severe reactions (angioedema, hypotension requiring treatment, severe dyspnea, bronchospasm, or generalized rash, urticaria, or erythema) require immediate discontinuation of the infusion and aggressive treatment. It is generally recommended that docetaxel not be readministered to patients who experience a severe hypersensitivity reaction despite adequate premedication. However, in patients with objective tumor responses and without other options to docetaxel therapy, re-treatment may be attempted with extreme caution and aggressive premedication by experienced practitioners It is recommended that a slower rate of infusion be used. One patient who experienced major hypersensitivity symptoms during the first two cycles of docetaxel therapy despite prophylaxis with a corticosteroid and a histamine H$_1$-blocking antagonist was able to continue treatment without further difficulty after cromolyn (400 mg four times a day, orally, starting immediately after the second cycle) was added to the prophylactic regimen.

A reduction in subsequent doses is recommended for patients who develop severe neutropenia (neutrophil count < 500 cells per cubic millimeter) that persists for 7 days or more, febrile neutropenia, severe (grade 4) infection, severe peripheral neuropathy, or severe or cumulative cutaneous reactions.

Patients who develop leukopenia should be observed carefully for signs and symptoms of infection. Antibiotic support may be required. In neutropenic patients who develop fever, broad-spectrum antibiotic coverage should be initiated empirically, pending bacterial cultures and appropriate diagnostic tests.

Special precautions are recommended for patients who develop thrombocytopenia as a result of docetaxel therapy. These may include extreme care in performing invasive procedures; regular inspection of intravenous sites, skin (including perirectal area), and mucous membrane surfaces for signs of bleeding or bruising; testing urine, emesis, stool, and secretions for occult blood; care in use of regular toothbrushes, dental floss, toothpicks, safety razors, and fingernail and toenail cutters; avoiding constipation; and using caution to prevent falls and other injuries. Such patients should avoid alcohol and aspirin intake because of the risk of gastrointestinal bleeding. Platelet transfusions may be required.

### Safety considerations for handling this medication

There is limited but increasing evidence and concern that personnel involved in preparation and administration of parenteral antineoplastics may be at some risk because of the potential mutagenicity, teratogenicity, and/or carcinogenicity of these agents, although the actual risk is unknown. USP advisory panels recommend cautious handling both in preparation and disposal of antineoplastic agents. Precautions that have been suggested include:

- Use of a biological containment cabinet during reconstitution and dilution of parenteral medications and wearing of disposable surgical gloves and masks.
- Use of proper technique to prevent contamination of the medication, work area, and operator during transfer between containers (including proper training of personnel in this technique).
- Cautious and proper disposal of needles, syringes, vials, ampuls, and unused medication.
- A number of medical centers and organizations have developed detailed guidelines for handling of antineoplastic agents.

If docetaxel comes into contact with the skin, the skin should be washed immediately and thoroughly with soap and water. If the medication comes into contact with a mucous membrane, the area should be immediately and thoroughly flushed with water.

## Parenteral Dosage Forms

Note: Bracketed uses in the Dosage Forms section refer to categories of use and/or indications that are not included in U.S. product labeling.

### DOCETAXEL FOR INJECTION CONCENTRATE

#### Usual adult dose
Carcinoma, breast —
    Intravenous infusion, 60 to 100 mg per square meter of body surface area, administered as a one-hour infusion every three weeks.

[Carcinoma, lung, non–small cell or]
[Carcinoma, lung, small cell or ][1]
[Carcinoma, ovarian][1]—
    Intravenous, 100 mg per square meter of body surface area, administered as a one-hour infusion every three weeks.

Note: Docetaxel administration should be delayed if the neutrophil count is lower than 1500 cells per cubic millimeter and/or the platelet count is lower than 100,000 cells per cubic millimeter.

A reduction in subsequent doses is recommended for patients who develop severe neutropenia (neutrophil count < 500 cells per cubic millimeter) that persists for 7 days or more, febrile neutropenia, severe (grade 4) infection, severe peripheral neuropathy, or severe or cumulative cutaneous reactions. Dosage in patients originally receiving 100 mg per square meter of body surface area should be decreased by 25%, to 75 mg per square meter of body surface area. If these complications persist or recur, dosage should be further decreased to 55 mg per square meter of body surface area or treatment discontinued.

Docetaxel is not recommended for patients with hepatic function impairment, especially moderate to severe impairment, because of the considerably higher risk of severe toxicity. If docetaxel is considered essential for a patient with mild hepatic function impairment, initial doses of 60 to 75 mg per square meter of body surface area should be used. However, the risk of severe toxicity and septic death will still be significantly higher than for patients with normal hepatic function.

Patients who originally receive 60 mg per square meter of body surface area and who do not develop severe neutropenia, cutaneous reactions, or peripheral neuropathy may tolerate higher doses.

#### Usual pediatric dose
Safety and efficacy in patients up to 16 years of age have not been established.

#### Usual geriatric dose
See *Usual adult dose*.

#### Strength(s) usually available
U.S.—
    20 mg per 0.5 mL (single-dose vial) (Rx) [*Taxotere* (polysorbate 80 1040 mg per mL)].
    80 mg per 2 mL (single-dose vial) (Rx) [*Taxotere* (polysorbate 80 1040 mg per mL)].

Note: Product is packaged together with accompanying diluent (0.5 mL for the 20-mg-per-0.5–mL vial; 2 mL for the 80-mg-per-2–mL vial). The diluent contains 13% of alcohol. The vials contain overfills of docetaxel and diluent to allow for loss due to foaming, adhesion to vial walls, and dead space during initial dilution of the concentrate.

Canada—
    20 mg per 0.5 mL (single-dose vial) (Rx) [*Taxotere* (polysorbate 80 1040 mg per mL)].
    80 mg per 2 mL (single-dose vial) (Rx) [*Taxotere* (polysorbate 80 1040 mg per mL)].

Note: Product is packaged together with accompanying diluent (0.5 mL for the 20-mg-per-0.5–mL vial; 2 mL for the 80-mg-per-2–mL vial). The diluent contains 13% of alcohol. The vials contain overfills of docetaxel and diluent to allow for loss due to foaming, adhesion to vial walls, and dead space during initial dilution of the concentrate.

#### Packaging and storage
Store between 2 and 8 °C (36 and 46 °F). Protect from bright light.

Note: Docetaxel for injection concentrate is not adversely affected by freezing.

### Preparation of dosage form
*Docetaxel for injection concentrate must be diluted, using the following procedure—*
To prepare premix solution:
Remove docetaxel and diluent from the refrigerator and allow to stand for approximately 5 minutes at room temperature. Using aseptic technique and a syringe, transfer the entire contents of the diluent vial to the vial containing docetaxel. Rotate the vial gently for approximately 15 seconds to assure complete mixture of the medication and diluent. The final concentration of docetaxel will be 10 mg per mL. Allow the solution to stand for a few minutes to allow any foam to dissipate. However, the foam need not dissipate completely before the preparation process is continued. Discard the premix solution if it is not clear or contains a precipitate.
To prepare the infusion:
Using aseptic technique and a calibrated syringe, transfer the required quantity of premix solution into a 250-mL infusion bag or bottle containing 5% dextrose injection or 0.9% sodium chloride injection to achieve a final concentration of 0.3 to 0.9 mg per mL. If a dose greater than 240 mg of docetaxel is required, a larger volume of vehicle should be used so that the concentration does not exceed 0.9 mg per mL. Thoroughly mix by manual rotation of the container. Discard the infusion if it is not clear or contains a precipitate.

### Stability
The premix solution is stable for up to 8 hours at room temperature (15 to 25 °C [59 to 77 °F]) or in a refrigerator (2 to 8 °C [36 to 46 °F]). However, it is recommended that the solution be used as soon as possible after preparation.

### Incompatibilities
Contact of undiluted docetaxel with plasticized polyvinyl equipment is not recommended because such contact may cause leaching of the plasticizer, di-2-ethylhexyl phthalate (DEHP). It is recommended that glass bottles or polypropylene or polyolefin plastic products be used for preparation and storage of the infusion, and that the infusion be administered through polyethylene-lined administration sets.

### Auxiliary labeling
- Must be diluted prior to administration.

[1]Not included in Canadian product labeling.

## Selected Bibliography
Hudis CA, Seidman AD, Crown JPA, et al. Phase II and pharmacologic study of docetaxel as initial chemotherapy for metastatic breast cancer. J Clin Oncol 1996; 14: 58-65.

Pronk LC, Stoter G, Verweij J. Docetaxel (Taxotere): single agent activity, development of combination treatment, and reducing side effects. Cancer Treatment Reviews 1995; 21: 463-78.

van Oosterom AT, Schriivers D. Docetaxel (Taxotere), a review of preclinical and clinical experience. Part II: clinical experience. Anti-Cancer Drugs 1995; 6: 356-68.

Developed: 09/17/97

**DOCUSATE**—See *Laxatives (Local)*

# DOLASETRON    Systemic—INTRODUCTORY VERSION

VA CLASSIFICATION (Primary): GA605
Commonly used brand name(s): *Anzemet*.
Note: For a listing of dosage forms and brand names by country availability, see *Dosage Forms* section(s).

## Category
Antiemetic.

## Indications
### Accepted
*Nausea and vomiting, cancer chemotherapy–induced (prophylaxis)*—Dolasetron injection is indicated for the prevention of nausea and vomiting associated with initial and repeat courses of emetogenic cancer chemotherapy, including high-dose cisplatin. Dolasetron tablets are indicated for the prevention of nausea and vomiting associated with moderately-emetogenic cancer chemotherapy, including initial and repeat courses.

*Nausea and vomiting, postoperative (prophylaxis)*—Dolasetron injection and tablets are indicated for the prevention of postoperative nausea and/or vomiting. Routine prophylaxis is not recommended when there is little risk of nausea and/or vomiting developing postoperatively, except in patients in whom nausea and/or vomiting must be avoided.

*Nausea and vomiting, postoperative (treatment)*—Dolasetron injection is indicated for the treatment of postoperative nausea and/or vomiting.

## Pharmacology/Pharmacokinetics

### Physicochemical characteristics
Molecular weight—438.5.
pH—Reconstituted solution: 3.2 to 3.8.
Solubility—Freely soluble in water and propylene glycol; slightly soluble in ethanol; slightly soluble in normal saline.

### Mechanism of action/Effect
Dolasetron, and its active metabolite hydrodolasetron, are highly specific and selective antagonists of serotonin subtype 3 (5-HT$_3$) receptors. 5-HT$_3$ receptors are present peripherally on vagal nerve terminals and centrally in the area postrema of the brain. Chemotherapeutic medications appear to precipitate release of serotonin from the enterochromaffin cells of the small intestine, which then activates 5-HT$_3$ receptors on vagal efferents to initiate the vomiting reflex.

Dolasetron has not been shown to have activity at other known serotonin receptors, and has low affinity for dopamine receptors.

### Other actions/effects
Dolasetron causes dose-related acute, and usually reversible, electrocardiogram (ECG) changes including QRS widening and PR, QT$_c$, and JT prolongation; QT$_c$ prolongation is caused primarily by QRS widening. Dolasetron seems to prolong both depolarization and, to a lesser extent, repolarization time, and its active metabolites may block sodium channels.

Multiple daily doses of dolasetron have not been found to slow colonic transit time. Plasma prolactin concentrations are unaffected by dolasetron.

### Pharmacokinetics
Note: The pharmacokinetics of dolasetron tablets have not been studied in the pediatric population. Data provided in the following sections are based on dolasetron injection administered orally to children.

### Absorption
Orally-administered dolasetron is well absorbed, but the parent drug is rarely detected in plasma due to rapid and complete metabolism to hydrodolasetron.

The apparent absolute bioavailability of oral dolasetron is approximately 75%. Food does not affect the bioavailability of dolasetron taken by mouth.

Orally-administered dolasetron intravenous solution and tablets are bioequivalent.

### Distribution
*Dolasetron*—Radiolabeled dolasetron was not found to be distributed extensively to blood cells.

*Hydrodolasetron*—Mean apparent volume of distribution is 5.8 liters per kg of body weight (L/kg).

### Protein binding
High (69 to 77%). Binding to alpha$_1$-acid glycoprotein is approximately 50%.

### Biotransformation
Hepatic, complete, mainly to the active metabolite hydrodolasetron (by means of the ubiquitous enzyme, carbonyl reductase). Further hydroxylation is mediated by cytochrome P450 CYP2D6 and further *N*-oxidation by both CYP3A and flavin monooxygenase.

### Half-life
Elimination—
Following oral administration:
Hydrodolasetron—8.1 hours (mean).
Note: The apparent clearance of hydrodolasetron in adults is 13.4 mL per minute per kg of body weight (mL/min/kg). In one study, the apparent clearance of hydrodolasetron in children aged 2 to 12 years

receiving dolasetron doses of 1.2 mg per kg of body weight (mg/kg) was approximately 1.6- to 3.4-fold higher than in adults. In a study of pediatric and adolescent cancer patients receiving 0.6, 1.2, or 1.8 mg of dolasetron, mean apparent clearances were 3 times greater for children and 1.8 times greater for adolescents than clearances observed in healthy adults receiving similar doses.

Apparent oral clearance decreases 42% in patients with severe hepatic impairment, and 44% in patients with severe renal impairment. No dosage adjustments appear necessary for these patients.

The pharmacokinetics of hydrodolasetron are linear, and similar in men and women.

Following intravenous injection:
Dolasetron—Less than 10 minutes after intravenous administration.
Hydrodolasetron—7.3 hours.

Note: The apparent clearance of hydrodolasetron is 9.4 mL/min/kg. In one study of children 2 to 11 years of age who received a single 1.2 mg/kg intravenous dose of dolasetron, mean apparent clearance was 40% greater than in healthy adults receiving the same dose. The terminal half-life in these children was 36% shorter than in healthy adults receiving the same dose. The apparent clearance of hydrodolasetron in pediatric and adolescent cancer patients was 1.4- to 2-fold higher than in adult cancer patients.

Following intravenous administration, apparent clearance of hydrodolasetron was unchanged in patients with severe hepatic impairment, and decreased 47% in patients with severe renal impairment. No dosage adjustments appear necessary for these patients.

The pharmacokinetics of hydrodolasetron are linear and independent of infusion rate.

**Time to peak concentration**
Hydrodolasetron—Following oral administration: Approximately 1 hour.
Following intravenous injection: 0.6 hour.

**Peak plasma concentration**
In a study of children aged 3 to 17 years, maximum plasma concentrations were 0.6 to 0.7 times those observed in healthy adults receiving similar dosages.

**Elimination**
Hydrodolasetron—Renal, 67% (53% unchanged and, to a lesser extent, as hydroxylated glucuronides and N-oxide metabolites).
Fecal, 33%, as metabolites.

In dialysis—
It is not known if dolasetron is removable by hemodialysis or peritoneal dialysis.

## Precautions to Consider

### Carcinogenicity
A study in male mice at oral doses of 75, 150, or 300 mg per kg of body weight per day (mg/kg/day) (225, 450, or 900 mg per square meter of body surface area (mg/m$^2$), respectively; 3.4, 6.8, and 13.5 times the recommended human intravenous dose of 66.6 mg/m$^2$ or 3, 6, and 12 times the recommended human oral dose of 74 mg/m$^2$, respectively, for a 50-kg person of average height [1.46 square meters of body surface area]) found a statistically significant ($p < 0.001$) increase in the incidence of combined hepatocellular adenomas and carcinomas at doses of 150 mg/kg/day and above. No increased incidence of hepatic tumors was found at the dose of 75 mg/kg/day in male mice or at doses of up to 300 mg/kg/day in female mice.

### Tumorigenicity
A 24-month study in Sprague-Dawley rats at oral doses of up to 150 mg/kg/day (900 mg/m$^2$; 13.5 times the recommended intravenous dose or 12 times the recommended oral human dose, based on body surface area) in males and up to 300 mg/kg/day (1800 mg/m$^2$; 27 times the recommended intravenous dose or 24 times the recommended oral human dose, based on body surface area) in females found no evidence of tumorigenicity.

### Mutagenicity
Dolasetron was not found to be genotoxic in the Ames test, the rat lymphocyte chromosomal aberration test, the Chinese hamster ovary (CHO) cell (HGPRT) forward mutation test, the rat hepatocyte unscheduled DNA synthesis (UDS) test, and the mouse micronucleus test.

### Pregnancy/Reproduction
Fertility—Studies in female rats at oral doses of up to 100 mg per kg of body weight per day (mg/kg/day) (600 mg/m$^2$ per day; 9 times the recommended human dose based on body surface area) and in male rats at oral doses of up to 400 mg/kg/day (2400 mg/m$^2$ per day; 36 times the recommended human dose based on body surface area) found no effect on fertility or reproductive performance.

Pregnancy—Adequate and well-controlled studies in humans have not been done.

Studies in pregnant rats at intravenous doses of up to 60 mg/kg/day (5.4 times the recommended human dose based on body surface area) or oral doses of up to 100 mg/kg/day (8 times the recommended human dose based on body surface area) and pregnant rabbits at intravenous doses of up to 20 mg/kg/day (3.2 times the recommended human dose based on body surface area) or oral doses of up to 100 mg/kg/day (16 times the recommended human dose based on body surface area) found no evidence of teratogenicity.

It is recommended that dolasetron be used during pregnancy only if clearly needed, since animal reproductive studies may not be predictive of human response.

FDA Pregnancy Category B.

### Breast-feeding
It is not known whether dolasetron is distributed into human breast milk. However, risk-benefit should be considered before administering dolasetron to a nursing woman.

### Pediatrics
Safety and efficacy studies have not been performed in pediatric patients. However, in four open-label, noncomparative pharmacokinetic studies, a total of 108 pediatric patients (between the ages of 2 and 17 years of age) being treated with emetogenic chemotherapy or undergoing surgery with general anesthesia received intravenous dolasetron doses of 0.6, 1.2, 1.8, or 2.4 mg/kg or oral doses of 0.6, 1.2, or 1.8 mg/kg. Overall, dolasetron was well-tolerated. Efficacy in pediatric patients receiving chemotherapy appeared to be consistent with that in adults; there is no efficacy information with regard to postoperative nausea and vomiting. Studies have not been performed in children younger than 2 years of age.

It is expected that the oral tablets of dolasetron will be as safe and effective as dolasetron injection given orally.

### Geriatrics
Efficacy for prevention of nausea and vomiting appears to be the same in geriatric patients as in younger age groups. No dosage adjustment is recommended.

### Drug interactions and/or related problems
The following drug interactions and/or related problems have been selected on the basis of their potential clinical significance (possible mechanism in parentheses where appropriate)—not necessarily inclusive (» = major clinical significance):

Note: Combinations containing any of the following medications, depending on the amount present, may also interact with this medication.

Atenolol
(concurrent use of intravenous dolasetron and atenolol has been found to result in a 27% decrease in clearance of hydrodolasetron)

Cimetidine
(concurrent use of cimetidine, which is a nonselective cytochrome P450 enzyme inhibitor, with dolasetron for 7 days has been found to result in a 24% increase in hydrodolasetron blood concentrations)

» Drugs causing QT$_c$ interval prolongation
(caution is recommended)

Rifampin
(concurrent use of rifampin, which is a potent cytochrome P450 enzyme inducer, with dolasetron has been found to result in a 28% decrease in hydrodolasetron blood concentrations)

### Laboratory value alterations
The following have been selected on the basis of their potential clinical significance (possible effect in parentheses where appropriate)—not necessarily inclusive (» = major clinical significance):

With physiology/laboratory test values
Alanine aminotransferase (ALT [SGPT]), serum and
Aspartate aminotransferase (AST [SGOT]), serum
(values may be increased; increases reportedly are transient and unrelated to dose or duration of therapy)

Electrocardiogram (ECG)
(dolasetron produces a number of ECG changes, including QRS widening and PR, QT$_c$, and JT prolongation; the magnitude of the effect is dose-related; the effect tends to disappear as blood concentrations decline but may persist for 24 hours or longer)

### Medical considerations/Contraindications
The medical considerations/contraindications included have been selected on the basis of their potential clinical significance (reasons given in parentheses where appropriate)—not necessarily inclusive (» = major clinical significance).

*Risk-benefit should be considered when the following medical problems exist:*

» Conditions associated with a risk of development of prolongation of cardiac conduction intervals (especially $QT_c$), including:
  Antiarrhythmic therapy or therapy with other drugs that may cause QT interval prolongation
  Congenital QT syndrome
  Cumulative high-dose anthracycline therapy
  Diuretic treatment with the potential for inducing electrolyte abnormalities
  Hypokalemia
  Hypomagnesemia
    (caution is recommended)
» Sensitivity to dolasetron

## Side/Adverse Effects

The following side/adverse effects have been selected on the basis of their potential clinical significance (possible signs and symptoms in parentheses where appropriate)—not necessarily inclusive:

**Those indicating need for medical attention**
Incidence less frequent
  *Hypertension or hypotension* (asymptomatic)

Incidence rare
  *Anaphylactic reaction* (skin rash, hives, and/or itching; troubled breathing); *bradycardia or palpitations* (slow or irregular heartbeat); *bronchospasm* (troubled breathing); *chest pain; edema* (swelling of face; swelling of feet or lower legs); *hematuria* (blood in urine); *oliguria* (decrease in amount of urine); *pain; pancreatitis* (severe stomach pain with nausea and vomiting); *tachycardia* (fast heartbeat); *urinary retention* (painful urination or trouble in urinating)

  Note: Bradycardia may be associated with electrocardiogram (ECG) changes including QRS widening and PR, $QT_c$, and JT prolongation.

**Those indicating need for medical attention only if they continue or are bothersome**
Incidence more frequent
  *Diarrhea; headache*

Incidence less frequent
  *Abdominal or stomach pain; dizziness or lightheadedness; fatigue* (unusual tiredness); *fever or chills*

## Overdose

For more information on the management of overdose or unintentional ingestion, **contact a Poison Control Center** (see *Poison Control Center Listing*).

**Clinical effects of overdose**
The following effects have been selected on the basis of their potential clinical significance (possible signs and symptoms in parentheses where appropriate)—not necessarily inclusive:

Acute
  *ECG effects, including QRS widening and PR and $QT_c$ prolongation*
  Note: Doses of up to 5 mg per kg of body weight (mg/kg) intravenously or 400 mg orally have been administered safely to both healthy volunteers and cancer patients.
    One patient, a 59-year-old male melanoma patient who developed severe hypotension and dizziness 40 minutes after receiving a dose of 13 mg/kg for 15 minutes, was treated by infusion of a plasma expander, dopamine, and atropine and recovered completely within several hours.
    A 7-year-old boy who received an oral dose of 6 mg/kg before surgery developed no symptoms and required no treatment.

**Treatment of overdose**
If a patient exhibits signs of second-degree or higher atrioventricular (AV) conduction block following a suspected overdose of dolasetron, cardiac telemetry monitoring is recommended.

There is no known specific antidote for dolasetron. Supportive therapy is recommended.

## Patient Consultation

In providing consultation, consider emphasizing the following selected information (» = major clinical significance):

**Before using this medication**
» Conditions affecting use, especially:
    Sensitivity to dolasetron
    Other medications, especially medications causing $QT_c$ interval prolongation
  Other medical problems, especially conditions associated with a risk of prolonged cardiac conduction intervals

**Proper use of this medication**
» Proper dosing

**Side/adverse effects**
  Signs of potential side effects, especially hypertension or hypotension, anaphylactic reaction, bradycardia or palpitations, bronchospasm, chest pain, edema, hematuria, oliguria, pain, pancreatitis, tachycardia, and urinary retention

## General Dosing Information

**For oral dosage forms only**
For children unable to swallow the tablet form of dolasetron, an oral solution may be prepared using dolasetron injection diluted in apple or apple-grape juice.

**For parenteral dosage forms only**
Dolasetron injection may be administered intravenously at a rate of up to 100 mg per thirty seconds, or may be diluted in a compatible intravenous solution to 50 mL and infused over a period of up to fifteen minutes.

## Oral Dosage Forms

### DOLASETRON MESYLATE TABLETS

**Usual adult dose**
Nausea and vomiting, cancer chemotherapy–induced (prophylaxis)—
  Oral, 100 mg given within one hour before chemotherapy
Nausea and vomiting, postoperative (prophylaxis)—
  Oral, 100 mg given within two hours before surgery.

**Usual pediatric dose**
Nausea and vomiting, cancer chemotherapy–induced (prophylaxis)—
  Children 2 to 16 years of age: Oral, 1.8 mg per kg of body weight, up to a maximum of 100 mg, given within one hour before chemotherapy.
  Children up to 2 years of age: Safety and efficacy have not been established.
Nausea and vomiting, postoperative (prophylaxis)—
  Children 2 to 16 years of age: Oral, 1.2 mg per kg of body weight, up to a maximum of 100 mg, given within two hours before surgery.
  Children up to 2 years of age: Safety and efficacy have not been established.

**Usual pediatric prescribing limits**
100 mg.

**Usual geriatric dose**
See *Usual adult dose*.

U.S.—
  50 mg (Rx) [*Anzemet* (carnauba wax; croscarmellose sodium; hydroxypropyl methylcellulose; lactose; magnesium stearate; polyethylene glycol; polysorbate 80; pregelatinized starch; synthetic red iron oxide; titanium dioxide; white wax)].
  100 mg (Rx) [*Anzemet* (carnauba wax; croscarmellose sodium; hydroxypropyl methylcellulose; lactose; magnesium stearate; polyethylene glycol; polysorbate 80; pregelatinized starch; synthetic red iron oxide; titanium dioxide; white wax)].

**Packaging and storage**
Store between 20 and 25 °C (68 and 77 °F). Protect from light.

## Parenteral Dosage Forms

### DOLASETRON MESYLATE INJECTION

**Usual adult dose**
Nausea and vomiting, cancer chemotherapy–induced (prophylaxis)—
  Intravenous, 1.8 mg per kg of body weight as a single dose approximately thirty minutes before chemotherapy or
  Intravenous, 100 mg as a single dose approximately thirty minutes before chemotherapy.
Nausea and vomiting, postoperative (prophylaxis)—
  Intravenous, 12.5 mg as a single dose approximately fifteen minutes before the cessation of anesthesia.
Nausea and vomiting, postoperative (treatment)—
  Intravenous, 12.5 mg as a single dose as soon as nausea or vomiting presents.
Note: Dolasetron mesylate injection may be administered intravenously at a rate of up to 100 mg per thirty seconds, or may be diluted in a compatible intravenous solution to 50 mL and infused over a period of up to fifteen minutes.

**Usual pediatric dose**
Nausea and vomiting, cancer chemotherapy–induced (prophylaxis)—
  Children 2 to 16 years of age: Intravenous, 1.8 mg per kg of body weight as a single dose approximately thirty minutes before chemotherapy, to a maximum of 100 mg per dose.
  Note: Dolasetron mesylate injection also may be administered orally, diluted in apple or apple-grape juice, at a dose of 1.8 mg per kg of body weight (up to a maximum of 100 mg) given within one hour before chemotherapy.
  Children up to 2 years of age: Safety and efficacy have not been established.
Nausea and vomiting, postoperative (prophylaxis)—
  Children 2 to 16 years of age: Intravenous, 0.35 mg per kg of body weight as a single dose approximately fifteen minutes before the cessation of anesthesia, to a maximum of 12.5 mg per dose.
  Note: Dolasetron mesylate injection also may be administered orally, diluted in apple or apple-grape juice, at a dose of 1.2 mg per kg of body weight (up to a maximum of 100 mg) given within two hours before surgery.
  Children up to 2 years of age: Safety and efficacy have not been established.
Nausea and vomiting, postoperative (treatment)—
  Children 2 to 16 years of age: Intravenous, 0.35 mg per kg of body weight as a single dose as soon as nausea or vomiting presents, to a maximum of 12.5 mg per dose.
  Children up to 2 years of age: Safety and efficacy have not been established.
Note: Dolasetron mesylate injection may be administered intravenously at a rate of up to 100 mg per thirty seconds, or may be diluted in a compatible intravenous solution to 50 mL and infused over a period of up to fifteen minutes.

**Usual pediatric prescribing limits**
100 mg.

**Usual geriatric dose**
See *Usual adult dose*.

**Strength(s) usually available**
U.S.—
  20 mg per mL (Rx) [*Anzemet* (mannitol 38.2 mg per mL; acetate buffer)].

**Packaging and storage**
Store between 20 and 25 °C (68 and 77 °F). Protect from light.

**Preparation of dosage form**
Dolasetron mesylate injection may be diluted in 0.9% sodium chloride injection, 5% dextrose injection, 5% dextrose and 0.45% sodium chloride injection, 5% dextrose and Lactated Ringer's injection, Lactated Ringer's injection, or 10% mannitol injection for administration by intravenous infusion.
Dolasetron mesylate injection may be mixed in apple or apple-grape juice for oral administration to pediatric patients.

**Stability**
Because the intravenous solutions recommended for administration by intravenous infusion do not contain preservatives, it is recommended that diluted dolasetron mesylate injection not be used after 24 hours (48 hours if refrigerated).
The solution of dolasetron mesylate in apple or apple-grape juice may be kept for up to 2 hours at room temperature before use.

**Incompatibilities**
Dolasetron mesylate injection should not be mixed with other medications. The intravenous infusion line should be flushed both before and after administration.

Developed: 11/17/97

# DONEPEZIL  Systemic—INTRODUCTORY VERSION

VA CLASSIFICATION (Primary): CN900
Commonly used brand name(s): *Aricept*.
Another commonly used name is E2020.
Note: For a listing of dosage forms and brand names by country availability, see *Dosage Forms* section(s).

## Category
Dementia symptoms treatment adjunct.

## Indications
**Accepted**
Dementia, Alzheimer's type, mild to moderate (treatment)—Donepezil is indicated for the treatment of mild to moderate dementia of the Alzheimer's type. There is no evidence that donepezil alters the underlying process that results in dementia, and donepezil's effectiveness may be decreased as the disease progresses.

## Pharmacology/Pharmacokinetics
**Physicochemical characteristics**
Chemical group—Piperidine derivative.
Molecular weight—415.96.

**Mechanism of action/Effect**
Donepezil is a reversible inhibitor of acetylcholinesterase, and appears to exert its therapeutic effect by enhancing cholinergic function. By inhibiting the hydrolysis of acetylcholine by acetylcholinesterase, donepezil increases acetylcholine concentrations and enhances cholinergic function. As the dementia progresses, fewer cholinergic neurons remain functionally intact, and the effects of donepezil may be lessened.

**Absorption**
Well absorbed, with a relative oral bioavailability of 100%. The rate and extent of absorption are not influenced by food intake or the time of administration.

**Distribution**
Steady-state volume of distribution (Vol$_D$) is 12 liters per kg of body weight (L/kg).

**Protein binding**
Very high (approximately 96%, mainly to albumins [about 75%] and alpha$_1$-acid glycoprotein [about 21%] over the concentration range of 2 to 1000 nanograms per mL).

**Biotransformation**
Donepezil is extensively metabolized to four major metabolites, two of which are known to be active, and a number of minor metabolites. Donepezil is metabolized by cytochrome P450 isoenzymes CYP2D6 and CYP3A4, and undergoes glucuronidation. Following administration of radiolabeled donepezil, plasma radioactivity was present primarily as intact donepezil (53%) and as 6-*O*-desmethyl donepezil (11%); this metabolite has been reported to inhibit acetylcholinesterase to the same extent as donepezil *in vitro* and was found in plasma at concentrations equal to about 20% of donepezil.
In a study of 10 patients with stable alcoholic cirrhosis, the clearance of donepezil was decreased by 20% relative to that in 10 healthy age- and sex-matched subjects.

**Half-life**
Elimination—
  About 70 hours.

**Time to peak concentration**
3 to 4 hours.

**Time to steady-state concentration**
Pharmacokinetics are linear over a dose range of 1 to 10 mg given once a day. Following multiple-dose administration, donepezil accumulates in plasma by four- to sevenfold, and steady-state is reached within 15 days.

**Elimination**
Following administration of radiolabeled donepezil, total radioactivity recovered over a period of 10 days was approximately 57% in urine (17% as unchanged drug) and 15% in feces; 28% remained unrecovered.

## Precautions to Consider
**Cross-sensitivity and/or related problems**
Patients sensitive to other piperidine derivatives may be sensitive to donepezil also.

**Carcinogenicity**
Carcinogenicity studies of donepezil have not been completed.

**Mutagenicity**
Donepezil was not mutagenic in the Ames test (bacterial reverse mutation assay). In the chromosome aberration test in cultures of Chinese hamster lung (CHL) cells, some clastogenic effects were observed. Donepezil was not clastogenic in the *in vivo* mouse micronucleus test.

**Pregnancy/Reproduction**
Fertility—Donepezil demonstrated no effect on fertility in rats given doses approximately eight times the maximum recommended human dose.

Pregnancy—Studies have not been done in humans.

Studies in pregnant rats and rabbits at doses approximately 13 and 16 times the maximum recommended human dose, respectively, showed no evidence for teratogenic potential. However, in a study of pregnant rats administered approximately eight times the maximum recommended human dose from day 17 of gestation through day 20 postpartum, a slight increase in stillbirths and a slight decrease in pup survival through day 4 postpartum were observed.

FDA Pregnancy Category C.

**Breast-feeding**
It is not known whether donepezil is distributed into breast milk; however, use of donepezil is not recommended in breast-feeding women.

**Pediatrics**
Appropriate studies on the relationship of age to the effects of donepezil have not been performed in the pediatric population. Safety and efficacy have not been established.

**Geriatrics**
Mean plasma donepezil concentrations measured during therapeutic monitoring of elderly patients with Alzheimer's disease were comparable to those observed in young healthy volunteers.

**Pharmacogenetics**
No specific pharmacokinetic study was conducted to investigate the effects of gender and race on the disposition of donepezil. However, retrospective pharmacokinetic analysis suggests that gender and race (Japanese and Caucasian) do not affect the clearance of donepezil.

**Surgical**
Because donepezil is a cholinesterase inhibitor, it is likely to exaggerate succinylcholine-type muscle relaxation during anesthesia.

**Drug interactions and/or related problems**
The following drug interactions and/or related problems have been selected on the basis of their potential clinical significance (possible mechanism in parentheses where appropriate)—not necessarily inclusive (» = major clinical significance):

Note: *In vitro* studies of donepezil and other highly protein-bound medications have shown no displacement of or by digoxin, furosemide, and warfarin. Other *in vitro* studies indicate little probability that donepezil interferes with the clearance of other drugs metabolized by CYP3A4 isoenzymes (e.g., cisapride, terfenadine) or by CYP2D6 isoenzymes (e.g., imipramine). It is not known if donepezil has any potential for enzyme induction.

Formal pharmacokinetic studies showed no significant effects of donepezil on the pharmacokinetics of cimetidine, digoxin, theophylline, or warfarin. Similarly, metabolism of donepezil is not significantly affected by concurrent administration of cimetidine or digoxin.

Combinations containing any of the following medications, depending on the amount present, may also interact with this medication.

Anticholinergics (see *Appendix II*)
(cholinesterase inhibitors such as donepezil have the potential to interfere with the activity of these medications)

Anti-inflammatory drugs, nonsteroidal (NSAIDs)
(donepezil may increase gastric acid secretion due to increased cholinergic activity; patients should be monitored closely for symptoms of active or occult gastrointestinal bleeding)

Carbamazepine or
Dexamethasone or
Phenobarbital or
Phenytoin or
Rifampin
(these medications may induce the isoenzymes CYP2D6 and CYP3A4, thus increasing the rate of elimination of donepezil)

Cholinergic agonists (e.g., bethanechol) or
Neuromuscular blocking agents metabolized by plasma cholinesterase (e.g., succinylcholine, mivacurium)
(a synergistic effect may be expected with concurrent use of these medications and donepezil)

Ketoconazole
(as an inhibitor of the CYP3A4 isoenzyme, ketoconazole has been shown to inhibit the metabolism of donepezil *in vitro*; clinical effect is unknown)

Quinidine
(as an inhibitor of the CYP2D6 isoenzyme, quinidine has been shown to inhibit the metabolism of donepezil *in vitro*; clinical effect is unknown)

**Medical considerations/Contraindications**
The medical considerations/contraindications included have been selected on the basis of their potential clinical significance (reasons given in parentheses where appropriate)—not necessarily inclusive (» = major clinical significance).

*Risk-benefit should be considered when the following medical problems exist:*

Asthma, history of or
Chronic obstructive pulmonary disease
(cholinomimetic actions of cholinesterase inhibitors may aggravate the condition)

» Cardiovascular conditions, such as:
Sick sinus syndrome
Supraventricular conduction problems
(cholinesterase inhibitors such as donepezil may have vagotonic effects on heart rate [e.g., bradycardia]; syncopal episodes have been reported)

Hepatic function impairment
(metabolism of donepezil may be impaired)

» Peptic ulcer disease, or history of
(cholinesterase inhibitors may increase gastric acid secretion due to increased cholinergic activity; condition may be exacerbated)

Seizures, history of
(cholinomimetics are believed to have the potential to cause generalized seizures; however, seizure activity also may be a manifestation of the Alzheimer's disease state)

Sensitivity to donepezil or to other piperidine derivatives

Urinary tract obstruction
(cholinomimetics may cause bladder outflow obstruction)

## Side/Adverse Effects

The following side/adverse effects have been selected on the basis of their potential clinical significance (possible signs and symptoms in parentheses where appropriate)—not necessarily inclusive:

**Those indicating need for medical attention**
Incidence more frequent
*Diarrhea; insomnia* (trouble in sleeping); *muscle cramps; nausea; vomiting*

Incidence less frequent
*Abnormal dreams; anorexia* (loss of appetite); *arthritis* (joint pain, stiffness, or swelling); *dizziness; ecchymosis* (unusual bleeding or bruising); *fatigue; frequent urination; headache; mental depression; pain; somnolence* (drowsiness); *syncope* (fainting); *weight loss*

Incidence rare
*Aphasia* (problems with speech); *ataxia* (clumsiness or unsteadiness); *atrial fibrillation* (irregular heartbeat; dizziness; fainting); *bloating; blurred vision; bronchitis; cataract; chest or epigastric pain* (pain in chest, upper stomach, or throat); *dehydration; diaphoresis* (increased sweating); *dyspnea* (troubled breathing); *eye irritation; fecal incontinence* (loss of bowel control); *gastrointestinal bleeding* (black, tarry stools); *hot flashes; hypertension or hypotension* (high or low blood pressure); *increased libido* (increase in sexual desire or performance); *mood or mental changes, including abnormal crying, aggression, delusions, irritability, nervousness, or restlessness; nocturia* (increased urge to urinate during the night); *paresthesia* (burning, prickling, or tingling sensations); *pruritus* (itching); *tremor; urinary incontinence* (loss of bladder control); *urticaria* (hives); *vasodilation* (flushing of skin); *vertigo*

## Overdose

For specific information on the agents used in the management of donepezil overdose, see *Atropine* in the *Anticholinergics/Antispasmodics (Systemic)* monograph.

For more information on the management of overdose or unintentional ingestion, **contact a Poison Control Center** (see *Poison Control Center Listing*).

**1292    Donepezil (Systemic)—Introductory Version**

**Clinical effects of overdose**
The following effects have been selected on the basis of their potential clinical significance (possible signs and symptoms in parentheses where appropriate)—not necessarily inclusive:

Overdosage with cholinesterase inhibitors may result in cholinergic crisis characterized by: *Bradycardia* (slow heartbeat); *hypotension* (low blood pressure); *muscle weakness, increasing*—may result in death if respiratory muscles are involved; *nausea, severe; respiratory depression* (troubled breathing); *salivation, increased* (increased watering of mouth); *seizures; sweating, increased; vomiting, severe*

**Treatment of overdose**
To enhance elimination—It is not known whether donepezil and/or its metabolites can be removed by hemodialysis, peritoneal dialysis, or hemofiltration.

Specific treatment—Tertiary anticholinergics such as atropine may be used as an antidote. Intravenous atropine sulfate titrated to effect is recommended; initially, an intravenous dose of 1 to 2 mg is given, with subsequent doses based upon clinical response. Atypical responses in blood pressure and heart rate have been reported with other cholinomimetics when coadministered with quaternary anticholinergics such as glycopyrrolate.

Supportive care—General supportive measures should be utilized. Patients in whom intentional overdose is confirmed or suspected should be referred for psychiatric consultation.

## Patient Consultation

In providing consultation, consider emphasizing the following selected information (» = major clinical significance):

**Before using this medication**
- » Conditions affecting use, especially:
  - Sensitivity to donepezil or other piperidine derivatives
  - Breast-feeding—Use is not recommended
  - Other medical problems, especially cardiovascular conditions and peptic ulcer disease
  - Surgical—A synergistic effect occurs when donepezil is used concurrently with neuromuscular blocking agents metabolized by plasma cholinesterase (e.g., succinylcholine)

**Proper use of this medication**
- Taking medication exactly as directed; not taking more medication than the amount prescribed because of increased risk of adverse effects
- Taking donepezil at bedtime
- » Proper dosing
- Missed dose: Skipping the missed dose and returning to regular dosing schedule; not doubling doses
- » Proper storage

**Precautions while using this medication**
- Importance of keeping regular appointments with physician
- Caution if any kind of surgery or emergency treatment is required; informing physician or dentist in charge that donepezil is being taken
- Caution if dizziness, drowsiness, or clumsiness or unsteadiness occurs
- » Suspected overdose—Getting emergency help at once

**Side/adverse effects**
Signs of potential side effects, especially diarrhea, insomnia, muscle cramps, nausea, vomiting, abnormal dreams, anorexia, arthritis, dizziness, ecchymosis, fatigue, frequent urination, headache, mental depression, pain, somnolence, syncope, weight loss, aphasia, ataxia, atrial fibrillation, bloating, blurred vision, bronchitis, cataract, chest or epigastric pain, dehydration, diaphoresis, dyspnea, eye irritation, fecal incontinence, gastrointestinal bleeding, hot flashes, hypertension or hypotension, increased libido, mood or mental changes, nocturia, paresthesia, pruritus, tremor, urinary incontinence, urticaria, vasodilation, and vertigo

## General Dosing Information

Donepezil should be taken in the evening, just prior to retiring. It may be taken with or without food.

## Oral Dosage Forms

### DONEPEZIL HYDROCHLORIDE TABLETS

**Usual adult dose**
Alzheimer's dementia—
Oral, initially 5 mg once a day, taken in the evening just prior to retiring. Although a higher dose of 10 mg did not provide a statistically significant greater clinical benefit than the 5-mg dose, a daily dose of 10 mg may provide additional benefit for some patients. However, the 10-mg dose is likely to be associated with a higher incidence of cholinergic side effects than the 5-mg dose. If a trial of the 10-mg dose is desired, dosage should not be increased until patients have been on a daily dose of 5 mg for four to six weeks because steady-state is not achieved for fifteen days and because the rate of adverse effects may be influenced by the rate of dose escalation.

**Usual pediatric dose**
Safety and efficacy have not been established.

**Usual geriatric dose**
See *Usual adult dose*.

**Strength(s) usually available**
U.S.—
- 5 mg (Rx) [*Aricept* (film-coated; corn starch; hydroxypropyl cellulose; hydroxypropyl methylcellulose; lactose monohydrate; magnesium stearate; microcrystalline cellulose; polyethylene glycol; talc; titanium dioxide)].
- 10 mg (Rx) [*Aricept* (film-coated; corn starch; hydroxypropyl cellulose; hydroxypropyl methylcellulose; lactose monohydrate; magnesium stearate; microcrystalline cellulose; polyethylene glycol; talc; titanium dioxide; yellow iron oxide)].

**Packaging and storage**
Store between 15 and 30 °C (59 and 86 °F).

**Auxiliary labeling**
- May cause dizziness.
- May cause drowsiness.

Developed: 11/12/97

---

**DOPAMINE**—See *Sympathomimetic Agents—Cardiovascular Use (Parenteral-Systemic)*

---

# DORNASE ALFA    Inhalation-Local

VA CLASSIFICATION (Primary): RE900
Commonly used brand name(s): *Pulmozyme*.
Other commonly used names are: recombinant human deoxyribonuclease I (rhDNase) and DNase I.
Note: For a listing of dosage forms and brand names by country availability, see *Dosage Forms* section(s).

## Category
Cystic fibrosis therapy adjunct.

## Indications

**Accepted**
Cystic fibrosis (treatment adjunct)—Dornase alfa is indicated in the management of cystic fibrosis patients to improve pulmonary function when it is administered daily and in conjunction with standard therapies. Also, in patients with a forced vital capacity (FVC) greater than 40% of predicted value, daily administration of dornase alfa has been shown to reduce the frequency of respiratory infections requiring parenteral antibiotics.

No studies have been performed with dornase alfa for longer than 12 months.

## Pharmacology/Pharmacokinetics

**Physicochemical characteristics**
Source—Produced by genetically engineered Chinese hamster ovary cells containing deoxyribonucleic acid (DNA) encoding for deoxyribonuclease (DNase).
Chemical group—A purified glycoprotein containing 260 amino acids in primary sequence identical to that of the native human enzyme, DNase.
Molecular weight—29,250.18 daltons.

### Mechanism of action/Effect
The bronchial secretions of cystic fibrosis patients contain high levels of extracellular, polyanionic DNA, which is released by disintegrating inflammatory cells, especially polymorphonuclear neutrophils, present after lung infections. The excess DNA causes the already abnormal sputum to thicken. The viscous, dehydrated mucus is difficult to expectorate, obstructs airways, and contributes to reduced lung volumes and expiratory flow rates. The accumulation of purulent secretions in the airways provides a continuing growth medium for bacteria, causing chronic pulmonary infections, which are the major cause of morbidity and mortality in patients with cystic fibrosis.

*In vitro* studies have shown that DNase, an enzyme normally produced in small quantities in the pancreas and salivary glands, reduces the viscoelasticity of sputum in patients with cystic fibrosis by breaking the long extracellular DNA molecules into smaller fragments.

### Onset of action
Significant improvement in lung function—Within 3 to 8 days.
Reduction in respiratory tract infections—Up to several months.

### Duration of action
Lung function gradually returns to baseline after the drug is discontinued. In one study, 12 to 14% of patients treated with dornase alfa had a forced expiratory volume in one second ($FEV_1$) 15% above baseline 32 days after therapy was discontinued, as compared with 6% of placebo-treated patients. In another study, the time to baseline was shorter; the mean improvement in $FEV_1$ was 7.5% in the patients treated with dornase alfa and 2.2% for the placebo-treated patients 4 days after the last dose.

## Precautions to Consider

### Carcinogenicity
Studies conducted over the lifetime of rats at doses of up to 246 mcg per kg (mcg/kg) of body weight per day, showed no carcinogenic effect. No increase in the development of benign or malignant neoplasms was seen, and no unusual tumor types appeared.

### Mutagenicity
Ames tests using six different strains of bacteria at concentrations of up to 5000 mcg per plate, a cytogenetic assay using human peripheral blood lymphocytes at concentrations of up to 2000 mcg per plate, and a mouse lymphoma assay at concentrations of up to 1000 mcg per plate, with and without metabolic activation, showed no evidence of mutagenic potential.

A micronucleus assay in bone marrow cells of mice, conducted after administration of a bolus intravenous dose of 10 mg per kg of body weight (mg/kg) of dornase alfa on two consecutive days, showed no evidence of chromosomal damage.

### Pregnancy/Reproduction
Fertility—Studies in rats and rabbits given intravenous doses of dornase alfa of up to 10 mg/kg per day (more than 600 times the exposure expected following the recommended human dose) showed no evidence of impairment of fertility in males or females.

Pregnancy—Adequate and well-controlled studies in humans have not been done.

Studies in rats and rabbits given intravenous doses of up to 10 mg/kg per day (more than 600 times the exposure expected following the recommended human dose) showed no evidence of harm or effects on development of the fetus.

FDA Pregnancy Category B.

### Breast-feeding
It is not known whether dornase alfa is distributed into the breast milk of humans; however, little or no measurable concentrations of dornase alfa are expected in human breast milk after long-term administration of recommended doses.

Small amounts of dornase alfa were detected in the milk of monkeys after administration of an intravenous bolus of 100 mg/kg followed by a 6-hour infusion at a dosage of 80 mg/kg per hour.

### Pediatrics
Dornase alfa should be used in patients younger than 5 years of age only if there is potential for improved pulmonary function or for decreasing the risk of respiratory infections, due to limited clinical experience in this population. The safety of dornase alfa was studied over a 2-week period in two groups, children 3 months to 5 years of age, and children 5 to 10 years of age. The PARI BABY reusable nebulizer with its tight-fitting face mask was used for patients unable to inhale and exhale orally throughout the entire treatment. Incidence of cough, rhinitis, and skin rash was slightly higher for the younger group.

### Geriatrics
No information is available on the relationship of age to the effects of dornase alfa in geriatric patients.

### Drug interactions and/or related problems
Possible drug interactions with dornase alfa have not been studied. However, the medication has been used safely and effectively in conjunction with other medications commonly given orally, parenterally, or via inhalation to patients with cystic fibrosis, including analgesics, antibiotics, bronchodilators, corticosteroids, enzymes, and vitamins.

### Medical considerations/Contraindications
The medical considerations/contraindications included have been selected on the basis of their potential clinical significance (reasons given in parentheses where appropriate)—not necessarily inclusive (» = major clinical significance).

*Risk-benefit should be considered when the following medical problem exists:*

Sensitivity to dornase alfa or Chinese hamster ovary cell products

## Side/Adverse Effects
The following side/adverse effects have been selected on the basis of their potential clinical significance (possible signs and symptoms in parentheses where appropriate)—not necessarily inclusive:

**Those indicating need for medical attention only if they continue or are bothersome**
Incidence more frequent
*Chest pain or discomfort; hoarseness; sore throat*
Incidence less frequent
*Conjunctivitis* (redness, itching, pain, swelling, or other irritation of eyes); *decrease in forced vital capacity (FVC)*—≥ 10% decrease as compared with predicted value; *dyspepsia* (upset stomach); *dyspnea* (difficulty breathing); *fever; rhinitis* (runny or stuffy nose); *skin rash*

## Patient Consultation
As an aid to patient consultation, refer to *Advice for the Patient, Dornase Alfa (Inhalation)*.
In providing consultation, consider emphasizing the following selected information (» = major clinical significance):

**Before using this medication**
» Conditions affecting use, especially:
  Sensitivity to dornase alfa

**Proper use of this medication**
Reading patient instructions carefully
» Not using ampul that has been previously opened; not using medication if out of date
» Not using if medication is cloudy or discolored
» Using only with power-operated nebulizer and compressor recommended by manufacturer of medication
» Importance of knowing how to use the medication in the nebulizer; using only with the mouthpiece provided with the nebulizer; not using a face mask
» Compliance with therapy; using at same time every day; some improvement may occur within 1 week; some patients may require weeks to months for full benefits
» Importance of continuing other cystic fibrosis medications as before; not mixing any other medication with dornase alfa in nebulizer; using other medications, such as inhalation bronchodilators, before or after dornase alfa treatment
Preparation of nebulizer for use
Preparation of medication for use in nebulizer; method of opening ampul and emptying ampul contents into nebulizer cup; using all medication in ampul
Proper administration technique
Proper care of nebulizer and compressor after use
» Proper dosing
Missed dose: Taking missed dose as soon as possible; if almost time for next dose, skipping missed dose and going back to regular dosing schedule
» Proper storage: Keeping ampuls in refrigerator in foil pouches at all times; not freezing; not leaving out of refrigerator for more than a total of 24 hours

**Precautions while using this medication**
» Checking with physician if condition becomes worse

**Side/adverse effects**
Signs of potential side effects, especially chest pain or discomfort, hoarseness, sore throat, conjunctivitis, decrease in forced vital capacity, dyspepsia, dyspnea, fever, rhinitis, or skin rash

## General Dosing Information

Dornase alfa inhalation solution is administered by nebulization. The only nebulizers and compressors that should be used are the Hudson T Updraft II disposable jet nebulizer with the Pulmo-Aide compressor, the Marquest Acorn II disposable jet nebulizer with the Pulmo-Aide compressor, and the reusable PARI LC Jet+ nebulizer with the PARI PRONEB compressor. The reusable PARI BABY nebulizer with its tight-fitting face mask may be used in pediatric patients who are unable to inhale and exhale orally throughout the entire course of treatment. The PARI BABY nebulizer should be used with the PARI PRONEB compressor. Safety and efficacy have not been studied with other systems. Therefore, battery-operated systems and ultrasonic nebulizers are not recommended for dornase alfa administration.

A mouthpiece is provided with each nebulizer. A face mask is not recommended, except in certain pediatric patients who are unable to use a mouthpiece, because it may reduce delivery of the medication to the lungs.

Wash hands thoroughly before assembling the nebulizer and adding the medication. The surface used for assembling the nebulizer also must be clean. The nebulizer and its parts must be kept clean at all times, according to the manufacturer's directions.

Dornase alfa solution should not be mixed or diluted with any other medication in the nebulizer cup because of possible physicochemical incompatibilities. However, other concurrently used medications, such as inhaled bronchodilators, may be administered before or after dornase alfa treatment.

## Inhalation Dosage Forms

### DORNASE ALFA INHALATION SOLUTION

**Usual adult and adolescent dose**
Cystic fibrosis therapy adjunct—
    Oral inhalation, 2.5 mg per day via nebulization, the dosage being increased to 2.5 mg two times a day if necessary.

**Usual pediatric dose**
Cystic fibrosis therapy adjunct—
    Children up to 3 months of age: Safety and efficacy have not been established.
    Children 3 months to 5 years of age: Oral inhalation, 2.5 mg per day via nebulization.
    Children 5 years of age and over: See *Usual adult and adolescent dose*.

**Strength(s) usually available**
U.S.—
    1 mg per mL (2.5-mL single-use ampul) (Rx) [*Pulmozyme*].
Canada—
    1 mg per mL (2.5-mL single-use ampul) (Rx) [*Pulmozyme*].

**Packaging and storage**
Store between 2 and 8 °C (36 and 46 °F). Protect from light.

**Stability**
Ampul should be discarded if contents are cloudy or discolored.
Unopened ampuls should not be exposed to temperatures over 30 °C (86 °F) for longer than 24 hours.
Opened ampul must be used at once or discarded.

**Incompatibilities**
Dornase alfa solution should not be mixed or diluted with any other medication in the nebulizer cup due to possible physicochemical incompatibilities.

**Auxiliary labeling**
• For oral inhalation only.

## Selected Bibliography

Bryson HM, Sorkin EM. Dornase alfa, a review of its pharmacological properties and therapeutic potential in cystic fibrosis. Drugs 1994; 48: 894-906.

Witt DM, Anderson L. Dornase alfa: a new option in the management of cystic fibrosis. Pharmacotherapy 1996; 16: 40-8.

Revised: 07/24/97
Interim revision: 07/29/98

---

# DORZOLAMIDE    Ophthalmic†

VA CLASSIFICATION (Primary): OP112
Commonly used brand name(s): *Trusopt*.
Note: For a listing of dosage forms and brand names by country availability, see *Dosage Forms* section(s).

†Not commercially available in Canada.

## Category

Antiglaucoma agent (ophthalmic).

## Indications

**Accepted**
Glaucoma, open-angle (treatment) or
Hypertension, ocular (treatment)—Dorzolamide is indicated in the treatment of elevated intraocular pressure in patients with ocular hypertension or open-angle glaucoma.

## Pharmacology/Pharmacokinetics

**Physicochemical characteristics**
Chemical group—Sulfonamide.
Molecular weight—360.91.
pH—Dorzolamide hydrochloride ophthalmic solution: Approximately 5.6.

**Mechanism of action/Effect**
Dorzolamide is a sulfonamide and a carbonic anhydrase inhibitor. Carbonic anhydrase is an enzyme found in many tissues of the body, including the eye. Carbonic anhydrase catalyzes the reversible reaction involving the hydration of carbon dioxide and the dehydration of carbonic acid. In humans, carbonic anhydrase exists as a number of isoenzymes, the most active of which is carbonic anhydrase II. Carbonic anhydrase II is found primarily in red blood cells, but it also appears in other tissues.
Antiglaucoma agent—Dorzolamide inhibits human carbonic anhydrase II. Inhibition of carbonic anhydrase in the ciliary processes of the eye decreases aqueous humor secretion, presumably by slowing the formation of bicarbonate ions, with subsequent reduction in sodium and fluid transport. The result is a reduction in intraocular pressure. In clinical studies of up to 1 year in duration in patients with glaucoma or ocular hypertension who had baseline intraocular pressure (IOP) of ≥ 23 mm of mercury (mm Hg), dorzolamide had an IOP-lowering effect of approximately 3 to 5 mm Hg throughout the day.

**Other actions/effects**
When dorzolamide was administered orally in doses of 2 mg twice a day for up to 20 weeks to 8 healthy volunteers, inhibition of both carbonic anhydrase II activity and total carbonic anhydrase activity was less than the degree of inhibition considered to be necessary for a pharmacological effect on renal function and respiration in healthy persons. (The oral dose of 2 mg twice a day closely approximates the amount of medication delivered systemically by ophthalmic administration of 2% dorzolamide 3 times a day.)

**Absorption**
Dorzolamide is systemically absorbed when applied to the eye. In a study designed to simulate systemic absorption during long-term ophthalmic administration, 8 healthy subjects were given 2 mg of oral dorzolamide twice a day for up to 20 weeks. (The oral dose of 2 mg twice a day closely approximates the amount of medication delivered systemically by ophthalmic administration of 2% dorzolamide 3 times a day.) Steady state was reached within 8 weeks.

**Distribution**
During chronic dosing, dorzolamide accumulates in red blood cells by binding to carbonic anhydrase II. The N-desethyl metabolite also accumulates in red blood cells by binding primarily to carbonic anhydrase I. Plasma concentrations of dorzolamide and the N-desethyl metabolite are generally below the minimum assay limit of 15 nanomoles.

**Protein binding**
Moderate (approximately 33%).

**Biotransformation**
The only metabolite is the active N-desethyl derivative, which inhibits carbonic anhydrase II to a lesser extent than does dorzolamide. The N-desethyl metabolite also inhibits carbonic anhydrase I.

**Half-life**
After therapy is discontinued, dorzolamide washes out of red blood cells in a nonlinear fashion, resulting in a rapid initial decline in blood con-

centration, followed by a slower elimination phase having a half-life of about 4 months.

**Time to peak effect**
Approximately 2 hours.

**Elimination**
Primarily renal, as unchanged dorzolamide and the *N*-desethyl metabolite.

## Precautions to Consider

### Cross-sensitivity and/or related problems
Patients sensitive to other carbonic anhydrase inhibitors or other sulfonamides, including furosemide, thiazide diuretics, and oral antidiabetic agents, may be sensitive to dorzolamide also.

### Tumorigenicity
In a 21-month study in female and male mice, dorzolamide administered orally in doses of up to 75 mg per kg of body weight (mg/kg) a day (greater than 900 times the recommended human ophthalmic dose) did not result in any treatment-related tumors. In addition, no changes in bladder urothelium were seen in dogs given dorzolamide orally for 1 year at a dose of 2 mg/kg a day (25 times the recommended human ophthalmic dose) or monkeys given dorzolamide topically to the eye for 1 year at a dose of 0.4 mg/kg a day (greater than 5 times the recommended human ophthalmic dose). However, in a 2-year study in male and female Sprague-Dawley rats, dorzolamide administered orally at the highest dose of 20 mg/kg a day (250 times the recommended human ophthalmic dose) produced urinary bladder papillomas in the male rats. Papillomas were not seen in the rats that received the lower oral doses, equivalent to approximately 12 times the recommended human ophthalmic dose. The increased incidence of urinary bladder papillomas seen in the male rats given the highest dose of dorzolamide is also seen in rats given other medications of the carbonic anhydrase inhibitor class. Rats are particularly prone to develop papillomas in response to foreign bodies, compounds causing crystalluria, or diverse sodium salts.

### Mutagenicity
The *in vivo* (mouse) cytogenetic assay, *in vitro* chromosomal aberration assay, alkaline elution assay, V-79 assay, and Ames test were negative for mutagenic potential.

### Pregnancy/Reproduction
Fertility—There were no adverse effects on the reproductive capacity of either male or female rats given oral doses of dorzolamide of up to 188 or 94 times, respectively, the recommended human ophthalmic dose.

Pregnancy—Adequate and well-controlled studies in humans have not been done.
Developmental toxicity studies in rabbits given dorzolamide orally in doses ≥ 2.5 mg/kg a day (31 times the recommended human ophthalmic dose) revealed malformations of the vertebral bodies of the fetuses. Administration of dorzolamide at these doses also caused metabolic acidosis with reduction in body weight gain in dams and decreased weight in fetuses. No treatment-related fetal malformations were seen in rabbits given dorzolamide at a dose of 1 mg/kg a day (13 times the recommended human ophthalmic dose). In addition, there were no treatment-related fetal malformations in developmental toxicity studies in rats given dorzolamide orally at doses of up to 10 mg/kg a day (125 times the recommended human ophthalmic dose).

FDA Pregnancy Category C.

### Breast-feeding
It is not known whether ophthalmic dorzolamide is distributed into breast milk. However, since there is the potential for serious adverse reactions with systemically absorbed carbonic anhydrase inhibitors, including ophthalmic dorzolamide, a decision should be made whether to discontinue breast-feeding or discontinue the medication.

In a study in lactating rats, dorzolamide administered orally at a dose of 7.5 mg/kg a day (94 times the recommended human ophthalmic dose) caused a reduction in body weight gain of 5 to 7% in the pups. In addition, a slight delay in postnatal development (incisor eruption, vaginal canalization, and eye opening) secondary to lower fetal body weight was noted.

### Pediatrics
Appropriate studies on the relationship of age to the effects of dorzolamide have not been performed in the pediatric population. Safety and efficacy have not been established.

### Geriatrics
In clinical studies, 44 and 10% of the total number of patients were 65 and 75 years of age and over, respectively, and no overall differences in effectiveness or safety were observed between these patients and younger patients. Geriatrics-specific problems that would limit the usefulness of this medication in the elderly are not expected.

### Drug interactions and/or related problems
The following drug interactions and/or related problems have been selected on the basis of their potential clinical significance (possible mechanism in parentheses where appropriate)—not necessarily inclusive (» = major clinical significance):

Note: Combinations containing any of the following medications, depending on the amount present, may also interact with this medication.

Amphetamines or
Mecamylamine or
Quinidine
(when amphetamines, mecamylamine, or quinidine are used concurrently with systemic carbonic anhydrase inhibitors, especially acetazolamide, therapeutic and/or side effects may be enhanced or prolonged as a result of decreased elimination caused by alkalinization of urine. A study has shown that ophthalmic dorzolamide does not cause alkalinization of urine when administered in normal therapeutic doses (see *Pharmacology, Other actions/effects*); nonetheless, medical experts suggest that dosage adjustments of amphetamines or quinidine may be needed when ophthalmic dorzolamide therapy is initiated or discontinued. In addition, some medical experts suggest that concurrent use with mecamylamine is not recommended, whereas other medical experts suggest that dosage adjustments of mecamylamine may be needed when ophthalmic dorzolamide therapy is initiated or discontinued)

» Silver preparations, ophthalmic, such as silver nitrate
(topical sulfonamides are incompatible with silver salts; since ophthalmic dorzolamide is a sulfonamide, concurrent use with ophthalmic silver preparations is not recommended)

### Medical considerations/Contraindications
The medical considerations/contraindications included have been selected on the basis of their potential clinical significance (reasons given in parentheses where appropriate)—not necessarily inclusive (» = major clinical significance):

*Except under special circumstances, this medication should not be used when the following medical problem exists:*

» Sensitivity to dorzolamide

*Risk-benefit should be considered when the following medical problems exist:*

Hepatic function impairment
(dorzolamide has not been studied in patients with hepatic impairment; caution should be used if the medication is used in these patients, since dorzolamide is metabolized by the liver)

» Renal calculi or history of
(may be exacerbated or induced during therapy)

Renal function impairment, severe
(dorzolamide and its metabolite are excreted primarily by the kidney; use of dorzolamide is not recommended in patients with a creatinine clearance of less than 30 mL per minute)

## Side/Adverse Effects

Note: Since dorzolamide is a sulfonamide, the same types of adverse reactions that may occur with other sulfonamides may occur with dorzolamide also. With other sulfonamides, fatalities have occurred rarely because of severe reactions, including Stevens-Johnson syndrome, toxic epidermal necrolysis, fulminant hepatic necrosis, agranulocytosis, aplastic anemia, and other blood dyscrasias. If signs of serious reaction or hypersensitivity occur, *use of dorzolamide should be discontinued*.

In clinical studies, local ocular adverse effects, primarily conjunctivitis and eyelid reactions, were reported with chronic administration of dorzolamide. Many of these reactions had the clinical appearance and course of an allergic-type reaction that resolved upon discontinuation of the medication. If local ocular adverse effects such as conjunctivitis and eyelid reactions occur, *use of dorzolamide should be discontinued and the patient evaluated* before a decision is made whether to restart the medication.

Although acid-base and electrolyte disturbances were not reported in the clinical trials of dorzolamide, they have been reported with use of oral carbonic anhydrase inhibitors and have, in some instances, resulted in drug interactions (e.g., toxicity associated with high-dose salicylate therapy).

Carbonic anhydrase activity has been observed in the cytoplasm and around the plasma membranes of the corneal endothelium. However, the effect of continued administration of dorzolamide on the corneal endothelium has not been evaluated fully.

## Dorzolamide (Ophthalmic)

The following side/adverse effects have been selected on the basis of their potential clinical significance (possible signs and symptoms in parentheses where appropriate)—not necessarily inclusive:

**Those indicating need for medical attention**
Incidence more frequent
  *Allergic reaction, ocular* (itching, redness, swelling, or other sign of eye or eyelid irritation)—incidence 10%
Incidence rare
  *Iridocyclitis* (eye pain, tearing, and blurred vision); *skin rash*; *urolithiasis* (blood in urine; nausea or vomiting; pain in side, back, or abdomen)

**Those indicating need for medical attention only if they continue or are bothersome**
Incidence more frequent
  *Bitter taste*—incidence approximately 25%; *burning, stinging, or discomfort when medicine is applied*—incidence 33%; *superficial punctate keratitis* (feeling of something in eye; sensitivity of eyes to light)—incidence 10 to 15%
Incidence less frequent
  *Asthenia* (unusual tiredness or weakness)—infrequently; *blurred vision*—incidence 1 to 5%; *dryness of eyes*—incidence 1 to 5%; *fatigue* (unusual tiredness or weakness)—infrequently; *headache*—infrequently; *nausea*—infrequently; *photophobia* (sensitivity of eye to light)—incidence 1 to 5%; *tearing*—incidence 1 to 5%

## Patient Consultation

As an aid to patient consultation, refer to *Advice for the Patient, Dorzolamide (Ophthalmic)*.
In providing consultation, consider emphasizing the following selected information (≫ = major clinical significance):

**Before using this medication**
≫ Conditions affecting use, especially:
    Sensitivity to dorzolamide, other carbonic anhydrase inhibitors, or other sulfonamides
    Pregnancy—One study in animals has shown maternal toxicity and fetal birth defects at very high doses
    Breast-feeding—Carbonic anhydrase inhibitors (including ophthalmic dorzolamide) have the potential for serious adverse reactions; a decision should be made whether to discontinue breast-feeding or discontinue the medication
    Use in children—Safety and efficacy have not been established
    Other medications, especially ophthalmic silver preparations such as silver nitrate
    Other medical problems, especially renal calculi or history of

**Proper use of this medication**
    Proper administration technique for ophthalmic solution
≫ Importance of using medication only as directed
    Waiting 10 minutes between the use of 2 different ophthalmic preparations to prevent "washing out" of the first one
≫ Proper dosing
    Missed dose: Using as soon as possible; not using if almost time for next dose; not doubling doses
≫ Proper storage

**Precautions while using this medication**
    Regular visits to physician to check progress during therapy
    Checking with physician if signs of ocular allergic reaction, such as itching, redness, swelling, or other sign of eye or eyelid irritation, occur

≫ Caution if blurred vision occurs temporarily; checking with physician if blurred vision continues, since it may be sign of adverse effect
    Possible sensitivity of eyes to sunlight or bright light; wearing sunglasses and avoiding exposure to bright light; checking with physician if discomfort continues

**Side/adverse effects**
    Signs of potential side effects, especially ocular allergic reaction, iridocyclitis, skin rash, and urolithiasis

## General Dosing Information

The efficacy of dorzolamide administered less frequently than 3 times a day (whether alone or in combination with other products) has not been established.

Because of the preservative, benzalkonium chloride, the manufacturer recommends that patients not wear soft contact lenses during treatment with dorzolamide ophthalmic solution. However, medical experts do not believe this precaution is necessary unless the patient has corneal epithelial problems and the medication is to be used more often than once every 1 to 2 hours. No significant problems have been documented with the use of ophthalmic solutions containing 0.03% or less of benzalkonium chloride as a preservative in patients with no significant corneal surface problems.

Dorzolamide may be used concurrently with other medications instilled in the eye to lower intraocular pressure. However, the medications should be administered at least 10 minutes apart.

## Ophthalmic Dosage Forms

### DORZOLAMIDE HYDROCHLORIDE OPHTHALMIC SOLUTION

**Usual adult and adolescent dose**
Antiglaucoma agent (ophthalmic)—
  Topical to the conjunctiva, 1 drop three times a day.

**Usual pediatric dose**
Safety and efficacy have not been established.

**Strength(s) usually available**
U.S.—
  2% (20 mg base) (22.3 mg as the hydrochloride) (Rx) [*Trusopt* (benzalkonium chloride 0.0075%; hydroxyethyl cellulose; mannitol; sodium citrate dihydrate; sodium hydroxide; water for injection)].
Canada—
  Not commercially available.

**Packaging and storage**
Store between 15 and 30 °C (59 and 86 °F), unless otherwise specified by manufacturer. Protect from light and freezing.

**Auxiliary labeling**
• For the eye.

## Selected Bibliography

Serle JB. Pharmacological advances in the treatment of glaucoma. Drugs Aging 1994 Sep; 5(3): 156-70.
Wilkerson M, Cyrlin M, Lippa EA, et al. Four-week safety and efficacy study of dorzolamide, a novel, active topical carbonic anhydrase inhibitor. Arch Ophthalmol 1993 Oct; 111(10): 1343-50.

Developed: 01/31/96

---

# DOXACURIUM   Systemic†

VA CLASSIFICATION (Primary): MS300
Commonly used brand name(s): *Nuromax*.
Note:  For a listing of dosage forms and brand names by country availability, see *Dosage Forms* section(s).

†Not commercially available in Canada.

## Category
Neuromuscular blocking agent.

## Indications

**Accepted**
Muscle (skeletal) relaxation, for surgery—Doxacurium is indicated as an adjunct to anesthesia to facilitate endotracheal intubation and to induce skeletal muscle relaxation in the surgical field. Doxacurium has a long duration of action in adults; use of doses sufficient to facilitate endotracheal intubation should be considered only for procedures expected to last 90 minutes or longer.

**Unaccepted**
Doxacurium has not been adequately studied for facilitating prolonged mechanical ventilation in intensive-care patients.

## Pharmacology/Pharmacokinetics

**Physicochemical characteristics**
Molecular weight—1106.15.

**Mechanism of action/Effect**
Doxacurium is a nondepolarizing (competitive) neuromuscular blocking agent. Nondepolarizing neuromuscular blocking agents inhibit neuro-

muscular transmission by competing with acetylcholine for the cholinergic receptors of the motor end plate, thereby reducing the response of the end plate to acetylcholine. This type of neuromuscular block is usually antagonized by anticholinesterase agents. The paralysis is selective initially and usually appears in the following muscles consecutively: levator muscles of eyelids, muscles of mastication, limb muscles, abdominal muscles, muscles of the glottis, and finally, the intercostal muscles and the diaphragm. Neuromuscular blocking agents have no clinically significant effect on consciousness or the pain threshold.

**Distribution**
Volume of distribution (steady-state)—
   Normal renal function: About 0.22 L per kg of body weight (L/kg) (range, 0.11–0.43 L/kg), in nongeriatric patients. Values within this range have also been reported for geriatric patients (about 0.22 [range, 0.14 to 0.40] L/kg) and for patients with hepatic failure undergoing hepatic transplantation (about 0.29 [range, 0.17 to 0.35] L/kg).
   Renal function impairment: About 0.27 (range, 0.17 to 0.55) L/kg, determined in patients with end-stage renal failure undergoing renal transplantation.

**Protein binding**
Low (about 30%).

**Biotransformation**
Metabolites have not been detected in studies performed to date.

**Half-life**
Elimination—
   Normal renal function: About 86 to 123 (range, 25 to 193) minutes, with doses ranging between 15 and 80 mcg per kg of body weight (mcg/kg). Values within this range have also been reported for geriatric patients (about 96 [range, 50 to 114] minutes) and patients undergoing hepatic transplantation (about 115 [range, 69 to 148] minutes).
   Renal function impairment: About 221 (range, 84 to 592) minutes, determined following administration to patients with end-stage renal failure undergoing kidney transplantation.

**Onset of action**
Time to achieve intubating conditions—

Note: The onset of action of each dose of doxacurium is dependent on dosage and on the age of the patient. The $ED_{95}$ (dose of a neuromuscular blocking agent required to produce 95% suppression of the adductor pollicis muscle twitch response to ulnar nerve stimulation) is lower after establishment of steady-state anesthesia with a potent volatile inhalation agent (e.g., enflurane, halothane, isoflurane) than during other types of anesthesia. The following values were not obtained during steady-state anesthesia with a volatile agent.
   50 mcg/kg: About 5 minutes.
   80 mcg/kg: About 4 minutes.

Note: Information on the time to achieve intubating conditions with lower doses of doxacurium has not been published; however, when a dose of 25 mcg/kg is administered after succinylcholine-assisted intubation, 90% suppression of the response to peripheral nerve stimulation occurs in about 6 minutes.

**Time to peak concentration**
About 2 minutes following administration of an initial dose of 30 mcg/kg or a supplemental dose of 5 mcg/kg administered after 25% recovery from the initial dose.

**Peak serum concentration**
30 mcg/kg—About 340 nanograms per mL (0.31 micromoles/L).
5 mcg/kg (supplemental dose)—90 to 100 nanograms per mL (0.08 to 0.09 micromoles/L); values are consistent for all supplemental doses given at 25% recovery from the previous initial (30 mcg/kg) or supplemental (5 mcg/kg) dose, when the doxacurium concentration has decreased to about 44.75 nanograms per mL (0.04 micromoles/L).

**Time to peak effect**
Note: The time to peak effect is dependent on dosage and the age of the patient. Also, it is shorter during anesthesia with a volatile inhalation agent (specified below when applicable) than during other types of anesthesia. However, the time to peak effect is not altered by prior administration of an intubating dose (1 mg per kg of body weight [mg/kg]) of succinylcholine, provided that doxacurium is administered after recovery of the twitch response to 10% or more of the control value.

In most patients, recommended doses of doxacurium produce maximal responses of 90 to 95% (or even higher) inhibition of the twitch response to peripheral nerve stimulation. However, patients with hepatic failure may be somewhat resistant to the effects of doxacurium; a maximal response of only 70% inhibition of the twitch response was achieved in these patients by a dose that produced higher maximal responses in patients with normal hepatic function.

Time to maximal suppression of the twitch response to peripheral nerve stimulation—
   Children 2 to 12 years of age (halothane anesthesia):
      30 mcg/kg—About 7 minutes.
      50 mcg/kg—About 4 minutes.
   Adults up to 50 years of age with normal hepatic and renal function:
      25 mcg/kg—About 8 to 10 (range, 5.4 to 16) minutes.
      50 mcg/kg—About 4 to 5 (range, 2.5 to 13) minutes.
      80 mcg/kg—About 3.5 (range, 2.4 to 5) minutes.
   Adults up to 55 years of age with end-stage renal failure undergoing renal transplantation:
      Tends to be longer than in nongeriatric adults with normal renal function.
   Adults up to 55 years of age with hepatic failure undergoing hepatic transplantation:
      Tends to be longer than in nongeriatric adults with normal hepatic function.
   Adults older than 65 years of age with normal hepatic and renal function:
      25 mcg/kg (isoflurane anesthesia)—About 11 minutes; slightly more prolonged than in nongeriatric patients with normal hepatic and renal function.

**Duration of action**
Note: Doxacurium's duration of action (for both initial and supplemental doses) is dependent on dosage, the age of the patient, and the clearance rate from plasma (which is at least partially dependent on the patient's renal function), as well as being subject to substantial interpatient variability. The duration of action is more prolonged during anesthesia with a volatile anesthetic (specified below when applicable) than during other types of anesthesia. However, cumulative effects on the duration or depth of neuromuscular blockade do not occur when supplemental doses of doxacurium are given after 25% recovery from an initial dose. Also, the duration of action is not significantly altered by prior administration of an intubating dose (1 mg/kg) of succinylcholine, provided that doxacurium is administered after the twitch response has returned to 10% or more of the control value.

Duration of clinical effect (time for spontaneous recovery of the twitch response to peripheral nerve stimulation to 25% of the control value)—
   Children 2 to 12 years of age (halothane anesthesia):
      30 mcg/kg—About 25 to 30 minutes.
      50 mcg/kg—About 45 to 50 minutes.
   Adults up to 50 years of age with normal renal and hepatic function:
      Initial dose—
         25 mcg/kg: About 55 (range, 9 to 145) minutes.
         40 mcg/kg: About 70 to 85 minutes.
         50 mcg/kg: About 100 (range, 39 to 232) minutes.
         60 mcg/kg: About 123 minutes.
         80 mcg/kg: About 160 (range, 110 to 338) minutes.
      Supplemental dose, administered after 25% recovery from an initial 25 mcg/kg dose—
         5 mcg/kg: About 30 (range, 9 to 57) minutes.
         10 mcg/kg: About 45 (range, 14 to 108) minutes.
   Adults older than 65 years of age with normal renal and hepatic function:
      25 mcg/kg (isoflurane anesthesia)—About 97 (range, 36 to 179) minutes; more variable and more prolonged than in younger adults.
   Adults up to 55 years of age with end-stage renal failure undergoing renal transplantation:
      Values tend to be more variable, as well as more prolonged, than in patients with normal renal function.
      Halothane anesthesia—
         25 mcg/kg initial dose: About 120 minutes.
         5 mcg/kg supplemental dose, administered after 25% recovery from the initial dose: About 27.5 minutes.
      Isoflurane anesthesia—
         15 mcg/kg—About 80 (range, 29 to 133) minutes.
   Adults up to 55 years of age with hepatic failure undergoing hepatic transplantation:
      15 mcg/kg (isoflurane anesthesia)—About 52 (range, 20 to 91) minutes; longer than in patients with normal hepatic function.

Recovery index (time for the twitch response to peripheral stimulation to increase, spontaneously, from 25% to 75% of the control value—)
  Children 2 to 12 years of age (halothane anesthesia):
    About 27 to 34 minutes (range, 11.2 to 57.5) minutes, with doxacurium doses ranging from 27.5 to 50 mcg/kg.
  Adults up to 50 years of age with normal renal and hepatic function:
    25 mcg/kg—About 51 minutes.
    50 mcg/kg—About 84 (range, 40 to 128) minutes.
Time to spontaneous 95% recovery of the twitch response to peripheral stimulation—Determined in adults up to 50 years of age with normal renal and hepatic function—
  25 mcg/kg—Average 74 minutes, but up to 4 hours in some patients.
  40 mcg/kg—Average 126 minutes.
  50 mcg/kg—Average 204 minutes.

**Elimination**
Renal and biliary, as unchanged doxacurium; 24 to 38% of a dose is eliminated in the urine within 6 to 12 hours. The overall extent of biliary excretion is unknown.
  Plasma clearance rate—
    Adults:
      Normal renal function—About 2.2 to 2.6 (range, 1 to 6.6) mL/minute/kg. Values determined over a dose range of 15 to 80 mcg/kg in nongeriatric adults, with 25 mcg/kg in geriatric patients, and with 15 mcg/kg in patients undergoing hepatic transplantation are all within this range.
      Renal failure (patients undergoing transplantation)—About 1.23 (range, 0.48 to 2.4) mL/minute/kg.

## Precautions to Consider

**Carcinogenicity**
Carcogenicity studies have not been done.

**Mutagenicity**
No mutagenicity was detected in the Ames *Salmonella* assay, mouse lymphoma assay, and human lymphocyte assay. However, statistically significant increases in the incidence of structural abnormalities, relative to vehicle controls, occurred in the *in vivo* rat bone marrow cytogenic assay in male rats receiving 0.1 mg per kg of body weight (mg/kg) (0.625 mg per square meter of body surface area [mg/m$^2$]) when the animals were sacrificed 6 hours, but not 24 or 48 hours, after administration. Structural abnormalities also occurred in female rats administered 0.2 mg/kg (1.25 mg/m$^2$) when the animals were sacrificed 24 hours, but not 6 or 48 hours, after administration. Abnormalities did not occur in male or female rats receiving 0.3 mg/kg (1.875 mg/m$^2$) at any time after administration. Because of the lack of a dose-dependent effect, the likelihood that the abnormalities found in this study were treatment-related or are clinically significant is low.

**Pregnancy/Reproduction**
Fertility—Studies have not been done.
Pregnancy—Adequate and well-controlled studies have not been done in pregnant women.
No maternal or fetal toxicity or teratogenicity was found in animal studies performed in nonventilated mice and rats receiving subcutaneous injections of subparalyzing doses.
FDA Pregnancy Category C.
Labor and delivery—Doxacurium has not been studied in obstetrics (labor, vaginal delivery, or Cesarean section). Doxacurium is not recommended for Cesarean section because its duration of action exceeds the expected duration of the surgical procedure.

**Breast-feeding**
It is not known whether doxacurium is distributed into breast milk.

**Pediatrics**
Neonates—Doxacurium injection contains benzyl alcohol, which is not recommended for administration to neonates. A fatal toxic syndrome consisting of metabolic acidosis, CNS depression, respiratory problems, renal failure, hypotension, and possibly seizures and intracranial hemorrhages has been associated with use of this preservative in neonates.
Children 2 to 12 years of age—These patients are less sensitive to the effects of doxacurium than are adults. Higher doses (on a mcg/kg basis) are required to achieve comparable levels of neuromuscular blockade. Even with higher doses, the onset of action, the duration of clinical effect (time for the twitch response to peripheral stimulation to return to 25% of the control value), and the recovery index (time for the spontaneous recovery from 25% to 75% of the twitch response to peripheral stimulation) are all significantly shorter in children than in adults.

**Geriatrics**
Appropriate studies performed to date have shown that elderly patients may be more sensitive than younger adults to the neuromuscular blocking effect of doxacurium. However, the time to maximum block is longer in elderly patients. The duration of clinical effect tends to be longer and more variable in elderly patients. Also, elderly patients are more likely to have age-related renal function impairment, which may also increase sensitivity to, and the duration of action of, doxacurium. The risk of an undesirably prolonged duration of effect in geriatric patients may be reduced by reducing initial dosage and titrating additional doses to achieve the desired response.

**Drug interactions and/or related problems**
The following drug interactions and/or related problems have been selected on the basis of their potential clinical significance (possible mechanism in parentheses where appropriate)—not necessarily inclusive (» = major clinical significance):

Note: Combinations containing any of the following medications, depending on the amount present, may also interact with this medication.
  Some of the following interactions have not been documented with doxacurium. However, because they have been reported to occur with other nondepolarizing neuromuscular blocking agents, the possibility of a significant interaction with doxacurium must be considered.

» Aminoglycosides, possibly including oral neomycin (if significant quantities are absorbed in patients with renal function impairment) or
Anesthetics, parenteral-local (large doses leading to significant plasma concentrations) or
Bacitracin or
» Capreomycin or
» Citrate-anticoagulated blood (massive transfusions) or
» Clindamycin or
Colistin or
Colistimethate sodium or
Lidocaine (intravenous doses > 5 mg/kg) or
» Lincomycin or
» Polymyxins or
Procaine (intravenous) or
Tetracyclines or
Trimethaphan (large doses)
  (neuromuscular blocking activity of these medications may be additive to that of neuromuscular blocking agents; increased or prolonged respiratory depression or paralysis [apnea] may occur, but is of minor clinical significance while the patient is being mechanically ventilated; however, reversal agents have sometimes been ineffective in reversing neuromuscular blockade potentiated by aminoglycosides, clindamycin, lincomycin, or polymyxins; caution and careful monitoring of the patient are recommended during and following concurrent or sequential use, especially if there is a possibility of incomplete reversal of neuromuscular blockade postoperatively)

Analgesics, opioid (narcotic), especially those commonly used as adjuncts to anesthesia
  (central respiratory depressant effects of opioid analgesics may be additive to the respiratory depressant effects of neuromuscular blocking agents; increased or prolonged respiratory depression or paralysis [apnea] may occur, but is of minor clinical significance while the patient is being mechanically ventilated; however, caution and careful monitoring of the patient are recommended during and following concurrent or sequential use, especially if there is a possibility of incomplete reversal of neuromuscular blockade postoperatively)
  (concurrent use of a neuromuscular blocking agent prevents or reverses muscle rigidity induced by sufficiently high doses of most opioid analgesics, especially alfentanil, fentanyl, or sufentanil)

Anesthetics, hydrocarbon inhalation, such as:
  Chloroform
  Cyclopropane
  Enflurane
  Ether
  Halothane
  Isoflurane
  Methoxyflurane
  Trichloroethylene
    (neuromuscular blocking activity of inhalation hydrocarbon anesthetics, especially enflurane or isoflurane, may be additive to that of nondepolarizing neuromuscular blocking agents; a reduction of doxacurium dosage may be necessary when it is given after steady-state anesthesia with one of these anesthetics has been established)

Antihypertensives or other hypotension-inducing medications or
Bradycardia-inducing medications
  (doxacurium does not counteract hypotension or bradycardia in-

duced by other medications or vagal stimulation; the incidence and/or severity of these effects may be increased, especially in patients with compromised cardiac function and in patients receiving 2 or more medications that may decrease heart rate and/or blood pressure [e.g., benzodiazepines, beta-adrenergic blocking agents, calcium channel blocking agents, opioid analgesics] prior to and/or during surgery)

Antimyasthenics or
Edrophonium
(these agents antagonize the effects of nondepolarizing neuromuscular blocking agents; parenteral neostigmine or pyridostigmine are indicated to reverse neuromuscular blockade following surgery; edrophonium in a dose of 1 mg/kg is not recommended for reversal of moderate to deep levels of doxacurium-induced blockade because it has been reported to be less effective than neostigmine [dose of 60 or 80 mcg/kg (0.06 or 0.08 mg/kg)]; use of pyridostigmine for reversal of doxacurium-induced blockade has not been studied)

(neuromuscular blocking agents may antagonize the effects of antimyasthenics on skeletal muscle; temporary dosage adjustment may be required to control symptoms of myasthenia gravis following surgery)

Calcium channel blocking agents
(although an interaction with doxacurium has not been documented, verapamil and nifedipine have been shown to potentiate the effects of several other neuromuscular blocking agents; also, difficulty in reversing verapamil-potentiated neuromuscular blockade with a single dose of neostigmine has been reported)

Calcium salts
(calcium salts may reverse the effects of nondepolarizing neuromuscular blocking agents)

Carbamazepine and/or
Phenytoin
(resistance to the effects of doxacurium, leading to a lengthening of the time needed to achieve adequate skeletal muscle relaxation and to significantly accelerated recovery from an initial or supplemental dose, may occur in patients receiving chronic carbamazepine and/or phenytoin therapy)

Lithium or
Magnesium salts, parenteral or
» Procainamide or
» Quinidine
(these medications may enhance the blockade of the neuromuscular blocking agents; increased or prolonged respiratory depression or paralysis [apnea] may occur but is of minor clinical significance while the patient is being mechanically ventilated; however, caution and careful monitoring of the patient are recommended during and following concurrent or sequential use, especially if there is a possibility of incomplete reversal of neuromuscular blockade postoperatively)

Neuromuscular blocking agents, other
(prior administration of succinylcholine [for endotracheal intubation] does not potentiate the effects of doxacurium, provided that doxacurium is administered after recovery from the effects of succinylcholine has begun)

(administration of doxacurium in conjunction with other nondepolarizing neuromuscular blocking agents has not been studied)

**Medical considerations/Contraindications**
The medical considerations/contraindications included have been selected on the basis of their potential clinical significance (reasons given in parentheses where appropriate)—not necessarily inclusive (» = major clinical significance).

***Risk-benefit should be considered when the following medical problems exist:***
Burns
(doxacurium has not been studied in burn patients; the possibility of resistance, depending on the age and size of the burn, should be considered)

Carcinoma, bronchogenic
(duration of action of neuromuscular blocking agents may be prolonged)

Dehydration or
Electrolyte or acid-base imbalance, especially
Hypokalemia
(action of neuromuscular blocking agents may be altered; neuromuscular blockade is usually counteracted by alkalosis and enhanced by acidosis, but mixed imbalances may be present, leading to unpredictable responses)

(serum potassium determinations may be advisable prior to administration of a nondepolarizing neuromuscular blocking agent, because hypokalemia tends to enhance the blockade produced by these medications; adjustment of dosage of the neuromuscular blocking agent, or correction of potassium concentration prior to administration, may be needed; increased or prolonged respiratory depression or paralysis [apnea] may occur but is of minor clinical significance while the patient is being mechanically ventilated; however, caution and careful monitoring of the patient are recommended during and following concurrent or sequential use, especially if there is a possibility of incomplete reversal of neuromuscular blockade postoperatively)

Hepatic function impairment
(patients with hepatic failure undergoing hepatic transplantation appear less sensitive to the effects of doxacurium than patients with normal hepatic function; a comparative study [in which the same dose was administered under the same type of anesthesia] indicated a tendency toward a slower onset of action and achievement of less intense neuromuscular blockade [maximum block of only 70% and an unusually high incidence of failure to produce more than 50% block] in the hepatic failure patients; however, there was also a tendency toward a prolonged duration of clinical effect in those patients with hepatic failure in whom more than 50% block was achieved)

(doxacurium has not been studied in patients with lesser degrees of hepatic function impairment; caution is recommended)

Hypothermia
(intensity and duration of action of nondepolarizing neuromuscular blocking agents may be increased)

Myasthenia gravis or
Myasthenic syndrome (Eaton-Lambert syndrome)
(increased risk of severe and prolonged muscle paralysis or weakness; a neuromuscular blocking agent with a shorter duration of action may be preferable [although caution is required even with shorter-acting agents])

Pulmonary function impairment or
Respiratory depression
(risk of additive respiratory depression or impairment)

» Renal function impairment
(clearance of doxacurium is decreased, leading to a prolonged elimination half-life and duration of action, in patients with end-stage renal disease undergoing renal transplantation; clearance continues to be decreased after the transplanted kidney begins functioning; these patients may also be more sensitive to the effects of doxacurium than patients with normal renal function; use of a neuromuscular blocking agent with a more predictable duration of action in patients with renal function impairment, i.e., atracurium or vecuronium, may be preferred)

Sensitivity to doxacurium

Caution is also advised if a long-acting neuromuscular blocking agent such as doxacurium is used to assist endotracheal intubation in a patient with a potentially difficult airway; some anesthesiologists recommend that an endotracheal tube be inserted (with the assistance of a short-acting agent) before a long-acting agent is given to such a patient.

## Side/Adverse Effects

Note: Unlike gallamine and pancuronium, doxacurium has no vagolytic activity. Also, histamine release following administration of doxacurium appears minimal, although isolated cases of increased serum histamine or symptoms possibly associated with histamine release (hypotension, cutaneous flushing, urticaria, bronchospasm, or wheezing) have been reported. Therefore, doxacurium causes minimal hemodynamic disturbance, although bradycardia and/or hypotension may occur because doxacurium does not counteract the bradycardia and/or hypotension induced by other medications (e.g., anesthetics, opioid analgesics) or vagal stimulation.

Doxacurium failed to trigger malignant hyperthermia in one study in malignant hyperthermia–susceptible swine (in doses up to 4 times the $ED_{95}$).

The following side/adverse effects have been selected on the basis of their potential clinical significance (possible signs and symptoms in parentheses where appropriate)—not necessarily inclusive:

**Those indicating need for medical attention**
Incidence rare ($< 0.1\%$–$0.3\%$)
***Cardiovascular effects*** (flushing; hypotension); ***double vision; fever; injection site reaction; respiratory effects*** (bronchospasm; wheezing); ***urticaria***

# Doxacurium (Systemic)

## Overdose

For specific information on the agents used in the management of doxacurium overdose see:
- *Atropine* in *Anticholinergics/Antispasmodics (Systemic)* monograph;
- *Glycopyrrolate* in *Anticholinergics/Antispasmodics (Systemic)* monograph; and/or
- *Neostigmine* in *Antimyasthenics (Systemic)* monograph.

For more information on the management of overdose or unintentional ingestion, **contact a Poison Control Center** (see *Poison Control Center Listing*).

### For treatment of overdose

Specific treatment—
- Administering an anticholinesterase agent, e.g., neostigmine (40 to 80 mcg/kg, depending on the dose of doxacurium) to antagonize the action of doxacurium. It is recommended that reversal of doxacurium-induced neuromuscular blockade be attempted only after some spontaneous recovery, as demonstrated using a peripheral nerve stimulator, has taken place. Recovery will not occur as rapidly if the antagonist is administered earlier. Also, higher doses of the anticholinesterase may be needed when more profound levels of block are present (3 or fewer responses to train-of-four stimulation) at the time of reversal. Recovery of the single twitch response to 80% of the control value with recommended doses of neostigmine, when administered after 25% spontaneous recovery has occurred, usually occurs in about 5 minutes; 90 to 95% recovery usually occurs within 20 (range, 7 to 55) minutes. However, recovery of the response to train-of-four stimulation ($T_4$:$T_1$ ratio) is slower than recovery of the response to single twitch stimulation. A $T_4$:$T_1$ ratio of 0.7 generally indicates 90 to 95% recovery. Edrophonium (1 mg per kg of body weight) does not antagonize the effects of doxacurium as rapidly as neostigmine, even when given after $>$ 25% spontaneous recovery has occurred, and is not recommended for reversing moderate to deep levels of block ($<$ 60% recovery). Use of pyridostigmine for antagonism of doxacurium has not been studied. It is recommended that a suitable antimuscarinic agent (e.g., atropine, glycopyrrolate) be administered prior to or concurrently with the antagonist to counteract its muscarinic side effects. However, use of an antagonist is merely an adjunct to, and not to be substituted for, the institution of measures to ensure adequate ventilation.

Monitoring—
- Determining the degree of the neuromuscular blockade, using a peripheral nerve stimulator. Monitoring of vital organ function for the period of paralysis and for an extended period post-recovery. Monitoring the patient following successful antagonism, because the duration of action of doxacurium may exceed that of the antagonist.

Supportive care for apnea or prolonged paralysis—
- Maintaining an adequate airway and assisting or controlling ventilation. Ventilatory assistance should be continued until adequate spontaneous ventilation can be maintained. Ventilatory assistance must be continued until the patient can maintain an adequate ventilatory exchange unassisted. Administration of a sedative or an anxiolytic may be needed if paralysis continues or recurs and/or mechanical ventilation is maintained after the patient is awake.

## General Dosing Information

Neuromuscular blocking agents have no clinically significant effect on consciousness or the pain threshold; therefore, when used as an adjunct to surgery, the neuromuscular blocking agent should always be used with adequate anesthesia or sedation.

Since neuromuscular blocking agents may cause respiratory depression, they should be used only by those individuals experienced in the techniques of tracheal intubation, artificial respiration, and the administration of oxygen under positive pressure; facilities for these procedures should be immediately available.

Doxacurium is intended for intravenous administration only.

The stated doses are intended as a guideline. Actual dosage must be individualized. It is recommended that a peripheral nerve stimulator be used to monitor response, need for additional doses, and reversal.

The $ED_{95}$ (dose required to produce maximum [95%] suppression of the adductor pollicis muscle twitch response to ulnar nerve stimulation) is about 25 (range, 20 to 33) mcg per kg of body weight (mcg/kg). The $ED_{95}$ may be higher in patients with hepatic failure than in patients with normal hepatic function.

When nondepolarizing neuromuscular blocking agents are administered after anesthesia with a volatile inhalation anesthetic has been established, a reduction in dosage, as determined using a peripheral nerve stimulator, may be required. Halothane may cause less potentiation of doxacurium than either enflurane or isoflurane. However, in one study, administration of 15 mcg/kg of doxacurium with isoflurane (the dose having been selected as approximating the $ED_{95}$ for that anesthetic) produced maximum neuromuscular blockade of only 70% in patients undergoing hepatic transplantation and only 86% in patients with normal hepatic function.

The $ED_{95}$ in children 2 to 12 years of age (halothane anesthesia) is about 30 (range, 12 to 52) mcg/kg.

A reduction of initial dosage may be advisable in geriatric, very ill, or debilitated patients; patients with impaired renal function, neuromuscular disease, severe electrolyte abnormalities, or carcinomatosis; and other patients in whom there is a risk of potentiation of neuromuscular blockade or difficulty with reversal. Supplemental doses should be titrated according to patient response.

Higher initial doses may be needed in burn patients and in patients with hepatic failure. However, clinically effective block, once attained in patients with hepatic failure, may persist somewhat longer than in patients with normal hepatic function.

For obese patients ($>$ 30% above ideal body weight for height), dosage of doxacurium should be calculated on the basis of ideal body weight.

## Parenteral Dosage Forms

Note: The dosing and the strength of the dosage form available are expressed in terms of doxacurium base.

### DOXACURIUM CHLORIDE INJECTION

**Usual adult dose**
Neuromuscular blocking agent—
  Initial:
    For endotracheal intubation and surgical relaxation—
      Intravenous, 50 mcg (0.05 mg) (base) per kg of body weight, to provide adequate intubating conditions in about five minutes and about one hundred minutes of relaxation, or
      Intravenous, 80 mcg (0.08 mg) per kg of body weight, to provide adequate intubating conditions in about four minutes and an average of one hundred sixty minutes of relaxation.
    Note: Satisfactory intubating conditions are attained more slowly when initial doses lower than 50 mcg (0.05 mg) are administered.
    For surgical relaxation only, following succinylcholine-assisted endotracheal intubation—
      Intravenous, 25 mcg (0.025 mg) per kg of body weight, to provide an average of sixty minutes of relaxation. Higher doses may be used if a longer duration of relaxation is required.
  Maintenance:
    Intravenous, to be administered after the twitch response to an initial dose has returned to about 25% of the control value or after reappearance of the second twitch response to train-of-four stimulation—
      5 mcg (0.005 mg) per kg of body weight, to provide about thirty minutes of relaxation, or
      10 mcg (0.01 mg) per kg of body weight, to provide about forty-five minutes of relaxation.
    Note: Higher or lower maintenance doses may be given, depending on the desired duration of action.
      The interval between maintenance doses is subject to considerable interindividual variability.

**Usual pediatric dose**
Neuromuscular blocking agent—
  Children up to 2 years of age: Dosage has not been established.
  Children 2 to 12 years of age (inhalation [halothane] anesthesia): Intravenous, 30 mcg (0.03 mg) (base) per kg of body weight, to provide maximum block in about seven minutes and about thirty minutes of relaxation, or
  Intravenous, 50 mcg (0.05 mg) per kg of body weight, to provide maximum block in about four minutes and about forty-five minutes of relaxation.
Note: Maintenance doses are generally required more frequently than in adults.

**Strength(s) usually available**
U.S.—
  1 mg per mL (Rx) [*Nuromax* (0.9% benzyl alcohol)].
Canada—
  Not commercially available.

**Packaging and storage**
Store between 15 and 25 °C (59 and 77 °F), unless otherwise specified by manufacturer. Protect from freezing.

**Preparation of dosage form**
If necessary, doxacurium chloride injection may be diluted up to 1 in 10 with 5% dextrose injection or 0.9% sodium chloride injection.

**Stability**
Doxacurium chloride injection is stable when diluted up to 1 in 10 with 5% dextrose injection or 0.9% sodium chloride injection, when the diluted product is stored in polypropylene syringes and kept at a temperature of 5 to 25 °C (41 to 77 °F) for up to 24 hours.

Diluting the injection diminishes the effectiveness of the preservative in the formulation. Careful attention to aseptic technique is required. It is recommended that the injection be administered immediately after dilution, and that any unused portion of the diluted injection be discarded after 8 hours.

Doxacurium chloride injection is compatible (for Y-site administration) with 5% dextrose injection, 0.9% sodium chloride injection, 5% dextrose and 0.9% sodium chloride injection, and lactated Ringer's injection, and, when the following are diluted as recommended by the manufacturer, with alfentanil hydrochloride injection, fentanyl citrate injection, and sufentanil citrate injection.

**Incompatibilities**
Doxacurium chloride injection is acidic and may not be compatible with alkaline solutions having a pH > 8.5 (e.g., barbiturate injections).

## Selected Bibliography
Estafanous GF, ed. Clinical experience with a new long-acting neuromuscular blocking agent. Proceedings of a symposium. J Cardiothoracic Anesthesia 1990; 4 (Suppl 4): 1-42.

Sarner JB, Brandom BW, Cook DR, et al. Clinical pharmacology of doxacurium chloride (BW A938U) in children. Anesth Analg 1988; 67: 303-6.

Revised: 05/21/92

---

# DOXAPRAM Systemic

VA CLASSIFICATION (Primary): RE900
Commonly used brand name(s): *Dopram*.

Note: For a listing of dosage forms and brand names by country availability, see *Dosage Forms* section(s).

## Category
Respiratory stimulant.

## Indications
**Accepted**
Respiratory depression (treatment)
Doxapram is indicated as a respiratory stimulant in the following conditions—Drug-induced post-anesthesia respiratory depression or apnea not associated with muscle relaxant medications.

Postoperative patients to stimulate deep breathing.

Acute respiratory insufficiency occurring in patients with chronic obstructive pulmonary disease (COPD). Used (only for about 2 hours) as an aid in the prevention of arterial $CO_2$ tension elevation during the administration of oxygen. Doxapram should not be used in conjunction with mechanical ventilation.

**Unaccepted**
Since doxapram hydrochloride injection available in the U.S. contains benzyl alcohol (or chlorobutanol in Canada), its use is contraindicated in newborns and immature infants. The use of benzyl alcohol in the newborn has been associated with a fatal toxic syndrome consisting of metabolic acidosis and central nervous system (CNS), respiratory, circulatory, and renal function impairment.

Although doxapram has been used to treat respiratory and CNS depression (mild to moderate) resulting from drug overdosage, its use for this indication is no longer recommended.

## Pharmacology/Pharmacokinetics
**Physicochemical characteristics**
Molecular weight—432.99.

**Mechanism of action/Effect**
Doxapram stimulates respiration by an action on peripheral carotid chemoreceptors. As the dosage is increased, the central respiratory centers in the medulla are stimulated with progressive stimulation of other parts of the brain and spinal cord. The respiratory stimulant action is manifested by an increase in tidal volume associated with a slight increase in respiratory rate.

**Other actions/effects:**
A pressor response may result from doxapram administration due to the improved cardiac output, rather than from peripheral vasoconstriction. An increased release of catecholamines has been noted.

**Onset of action**
20 to 40 seconds.

**Time to peak effect**
1 to 2 minutes.

**Duration of action:**
5 to 12 minutes.

**Elimination**
Primarily fecal (55%); some renal.

## Precautions to Consider
**Carcinogenicity/Mutagenicity**
Studies have not been done.

**Pregnancy/Reproduction**
Pregnancy—Adequate and well-controlled studies in humans have not been done.

Studies in animals have not shown that doxapram causes adverse effects on the fetus or impairs fertility.

FDA Pregnancy Category B.

**Breast-feeding**
It is not known whether doxapram is distributed into breast milk. However, problems in humans have not been documented.

**Pediatrics**
In addition to the adverse effects of benzyl alcohol in the neonate, potential side effects of doxapram when used in neonatal apnea include central neural stimulation, seizures, and possibly hypertension. If use is absolutely necessary, dosages should be kept at a minimum.

**Geriatrics**
No geriatrics-specific problems have been documented in studies done to date that have included geriatric patients. However, risk-benefit must be considered in elderly patients with significant cardiac impairment, liver function impairment, or renal insufficiency.

**Drug interactions and/or related problems**
The following drug interactions and/or related problems have been selected on the basis of their potential clinical significance (possible mechanism in parentheses where appropriate)—not necessarily inclusive (» = major clinical significance):

Note: Combinations containing any of the following medications, depending on the amount present, may also interact with this medication.

Anesthetics, hydrocarbon inhalation such as:
Chloroform
Cyclopropane
Enflurane
Halothane
Isoflurane
Methoxyflurane
Trichloroethylene
(following discontinuation of anesthetics known to sensitize the myocardium to catecholamines, it is recommended that initiation of doxapram therapy be delayed for at least 10 minutes, since an increase in catecholamine release may occur with doxapram)

CNS stimulation–producing medications, other (See *Appendix II*)
(concurrent use with doxapram may result in additive CNS stimulation to excessive levels, causing nervousness, irritability, insomnia, or possibly convulsions or cardiac arrhythmias; close observation is recommended)

» Monoamine oxidase (MAO) inhibitors, including furazolidone, procarbazine, and selegiline or

» Sympathomimetic agents
(concurrent use may increase the pressor effects of either these medications or doxapram)

**Medical considerations/Contraindications**
The medical considerations/contraindications included have been selected on the basis of their potential clinical significance (reasons given in

parentheses where appropriate)—not necessarily inclusive (» = major clinical significance).

*Except under special circumstances, this medicine should not be used when the following medical problems exist:*
- » Cerebrovascular accidents or
- » Coronary artery disease or
- » Epilepsy or other seizure disorders or
- » Head injury, evidence of or
- » Heart failure, frank, uncompensated or
- » Hypertension, severe
    (doxapram-induced release of catecholamines may exacerbate condition)
- » Incompetence of ventilatory mechanism due to:
    Airway obstruction
    Dyspnea, extreme
    Flail chest
    Muscle paresis
    Pneumothorax
        (may be exacerbated)
- » Pulmonary diseases such as:
    Asthma, bronchial, acute
    Pulmonary embolism
    Respiratory failure due to neuromuscular disorders
    Restrictive respiratory diseases such as pulmonary fibrosis
        (may be exacerbated)

*Risk-benefit should be considered when the following medical problems exist:*
- » Asthma, bronchial, history of
    (may be exacerbated)
- » Cardiac arrhythmia (including severe tachycardia) or
- » Cardiac disease or
- » Edema, cerebral or
- » Hyperthyroidism or
- » Pheochromocytoma
    (doxapram-induced release of catecholamines may exacerbate condition)
- » Liver function impairment
    (metabolism may be altered)
- » Renal function impairment
    (benzyl alcohol, which is excreted in the kidneys, contained in doxapram injection, may be toxic in patients with renal insufficiency)

**Patient monitoring**
The following may be especially important in patient monitoring (other tests may be warranted in some patients, depending on condition; » = major clinical significance):

Blood pressure determinations and
Deep tendon reflexes and
Pulse rate determinations
    (recommended at periodic intervals to prevent overdosage)
Determinations of arterial blood gases
    (recommended prior to administration of doxapram and at least every half hour during the two-hour period of infusion to prevent development of $CO_2$ retention and acidosis when doxapram is used in chronic obstructive pulmonary disease associated with acute hypercapnia; doxapram should be discontinued if the arterial blood gases deteriorate or whenever mechanical ventilation is initiated)

## Side/Adverse Effects

The following side/adverse effects have been selected on the basis of their potential clinical significance (possible signs and symptoms in parentheses where appropriate)—not necessarily inclusive:

**Those indicating need for medical attention**
Incidence less frequent or rare
    *Cardiovascular effects* (chest pain; fast or irregular heartbeat; tightness in chest); *hemolysis*—excessive rate of infusion; *thrombophlebitis* (redness, swelling, or pain at injection site); *wheezing, or troubled or unusually fast breathing*

**Those indicating need for medical attention only if they continue or are bothersome**
Incidence less frequent
    *Confusion; coughing; diarrhea; dizziness or lightheadedness; feeling of unusual warmth; headache; increased sweating; nausea or vomiting; urination problems*

## Overdose

**Clinical effects of overdose**
The following effects have been selected on the basis of their potential clinical significance (possible signs and symptoms in parentheses where appropriate)—not necessarily inclusive:

*Convulsions; fast heartbeat; increased blood pressure; increase in deep tendon reflexes; trembling or uncontrolled movements of the body*

## General Dosing Information

Rapid infusion of doxapram at a rate faster than that recommended may result in hemolysis.

Vascular extravasation or use of a single injection site over an extended period of time should be avoided since either of these may result in thrombophlebitis or local skin irritation.

## Parenteral Dosage Forms

### DOXAPRAM HYDROCHLORIDE INJECTION USP

**Usual adult and adolescent dose**
Post-anesthesia respiratory depression—
    Intravenous, 500 mcg (0.5 mg) to 1 mg per kg of body weight, not to exceed 1.5 mg per kg of body weight, as a single dose; dose may be repeated, if necessary, at five-minute intervals up to a maximum total dose of 2 mg per kg of body weight.
    Intravenous infusion, administered initially at a rate of 5 mg per minute until the desired response is obtained, then reduced to a rate of 1 to 3 mg per minute; the recommended maximum total dose is 4 mg per kg of body weight, or approximately 300 mg.
Acute respiratory insufficiency in chronic obstructive pulmonary disease (COPD)—
    Intravenous infusion, administered initially at a rate of 1 to 2 mg per minute, the rate of administration being increased up to a maximum of 3 mg per minute if necessary; the maximum time period of infusion should not exceed two hours and additional infusions are not recommended.
Note: The rate of infusion should not be increased in severely ill patients because of the associated increased work in breathing.

**Usual pediatric dose**
Post-anesthesia respiratory depression—
    Children up to 12 years of age: Use is not recommended.

**Strength(s) usually available**
U.S.—
    20 mg per mL (Rx) [*Dopram* (benzyl alcohol 0.9%); GENERIC].
Canada—
    20 mg per mL (Rx) [*Dopram* (chlorobutanol 0.5%)].

**Packaging and storage**
Store below 40 °C (104 °F), preferably between 15 and 30 °C (59 and 86 °F), unless otherwise specified by manufacturer. Protect from freezing.

**Preparation of dosage form**
Post-anesthetic CNS depression—Add 250 mg of doxapram hydrochloride to 250 mL of 5 or 10% dextrose injection or 0.9% sodium chloride injection.
Acute respiratory insufficiency—Add 400 mg of doxapram hydrochloride to 180 mL of 5 or 10% dextrose injection or 0.9% sodium chloride injection.

**Incompatibilities**
Doxapram is incompatible with alkaline solutions such as 2.5% thiopental sodium, aminophylline, or sodium bicarbonate. Precipitation or gas formation will result from these admixtures.

**Additional information**
Doxapram hydrochloride injection that contains benzyl alcohol (in Canada, chlorobutanol) as a preservative must not be used in newborns and immature infants. The use of benzyl alcohol in neonates has been associated with a fatal toxic syndrome consisting of metabolic acidosis and CNS, respiratory, circulatory, and renal function impairment.

Revised: 04/16/93

# DOXAZOSIN Systemic

VA CLASSIFICATION (Primary/Secondary): CV150/CV409; GU900

Commonly used brand name(s): *Cardura*.

Note: For a listing of dosage forms and brand names by country availability, see *Dosage Forms* section(s).

## Category

Antihypertensive; benign prostatic hyperplasia therapy agent.

## Indications

### Accepted

Hypertension (treatment)—Doxazosin is indicated in the treatment of hypertension.

Benign prostatic hyperplasia (treatment)[1]—Doxazosin is indicated for the treatment of both the urinary outflow obstruction and the obstructive and irritative symptoms associated with benign prostatic hyperplasia (BPH). Doxazosin may be used in normotensive or hypertensive patients. In normotensive patients with BPH, doxazosin does not appear to significantly lower blood pressure. In hypertensive patients with BPH, both conditions are effectively treated with doxazosin. The long-term effects of doxazosin on the incidence of acute urinary obstruction or other complications of BPH or on the need for surgery have not yet been determined.

[1]Not included in Canadian product labeling.

## Pharmacology/Pharmacokinetics

### Physicochemical characteristics
Molecular weight—547.58.

### Mechanism of action/Effect
Doxazosin has a selective alpha$_1$-adrenergic blocking action, which is thought to account primarily for its effects.

Hypertension—
 Blockade of alpha$_1$-adrenergic receptors by doxazosin results in peripheral vasodilation, which produces a fall in blood pressure because of decreased peripheral vascular resistance.

Benign prostatic hyperplasia—
 Relaxation of smooth muscle in the bladder neck, prostate, and prostate capsule produced by alpha$_1$-adrenergic blockade results in a reduction in urethral resistance and pressure, bladder outlet resistance, and urinary symptoms.

### Other actions/effects
Doxazosin slightly lowers the levels of total cholesterol, low density lipoprotein (LDL) cholesterol, and triglycerides. In addition, doxazosin slightly increases high density lipoprotein (HDL) cholesterol and the HDL/total cholesterol ratio. These lipid effects appear to be the result of doxazosin's effect on lipid metabolism (i.e., increasing LDL receptor activity, decreasing intracellular LDL cholesterol synthesis, decreasing synthesis and secretion of very low density lipoprotein [VLDL] cholesterol, stimulation of lipoprotein lipase activity, and decreasing the rate of cholesterol absorption). However, the implications of these changes are unclear.

### Absorption
Well-absorbed from gastrointestinal tract; bioavailability is about 65%.

### Protein binding
Very high (98 to 99%).

### Biotransformation
Metabolized extensively in the liver. Although several active and inactive metabolites have been identified (2-piperazinyl, 6' and 7'-hydroxy, 6' and 7'-O-desmethyl, and 2-amino), there is no evidence that they are present in substantial amounts.

### Half-life
Elimination—19 to 22 hours; does not appear to be significantly influenced by age or mild to moderate renal impairment.

### Onset of action
Hypertension—1 to 2 hours; there is a slight initial fall in blood pressure within the first hour, but the main hypotensive effect is apparent from 2 hours onwards.

Benign prostatic hyperplasia (BPH)—Within 1 to 2 weeks.

### Time to peak concentration
1.5 to 3.6 hours.

### Peak serum concentration
At steady state, there is a positive linear relationship between peak serum concentration and dose of doxazosin. Following a 1 mg oral dose of doxazosin, the standardized peak serum concentration was 9.6 mcg per L.

### Time to peak effect
Antihypertensive—Single dose: 5 to 6 hours.

### Duration of action
Antihypertensive—Single dose: 24 hours.

### Elimination
Fecal— Unchanged drug, about 5%; metabolites, 63 to 65%.
Renal—9%.
In dialysis—Doxazosin is not removed by hemodialysis.

## Precautions to Consider

### Cross-sensitivity and/or related problems
Patients sensitive to other quinazolines (prazosin, terazosin) may also be sensitive to doxazosin.

### Carcinogenicity
In one 24-month chronic dietary administration study in rats, doxazosin (given at 150 times the maximum recommended human dose) produced no evidence of carcinogenicity. In another similarly conducted study done in mice, up to 18 months of dietary administration produced no evidence of carcinogenicity. The latter study, however, did not use a maximally tolerated dose of doxazosin.

### Mutagenicity
There is no evidence of drug- or metabolic-related effects at either chromosomal or subchromosomal levels.

### Pregnancy/Reproduction
Fertility—Studies in rats given oral doses of 20 mg per kg of body weight (mg/kg) per day (about 75 times the maximum recommended human dose) have shown that doxazosin reduces fertility in male rats.

Pregnancy—Adequate and well-controlled studies in humans have not been done.

Studies in rabbits and rats given daily oral doses of 40 and 20 mg/kg, respectively, have shown no evidence of harm to the fetus. The rabbit study, however, did not use a maximally tolerated dose of doxazosin. Reduced fetal survival was associated with a dosage regimen of 82 mg/kg in rabbits. Following oral administration of labeled doxazosin to pregnant rats, radioactivity was found to cross the placenta.

Studies in peri- and postnatal rats, given 40 or 50 mg/kg per day of doxazosin, revealed evidence of delayed postnatal development manifested by slower body weight gain and slightly later appearance of anatomical features and reflexes.

FDA Pregnancy Category C.

### Breast-feeding
It is not known whether doxazosin is distributed into breast milk. Problems in humans have not been documented. However, in rats given a single oral dose of 1 mg/kg, doxazosin accumulates in rat breast milk with a maximum concentration about 20 times greater than the maternal plasma concentration.

### Pediatrics
No information is available on the relationship of age to the effects of doxazosin in pediatric patients. Safety and efficacy have not been established.

### Geriatrics
A study performed in approximately 2000 hypertensive patients older than 65 years of age did not demonstrate geriatrics-specific problems that would limit the usefulness of doxazosin in the elderly. However, the hypotensive effect of doxazosin may be more pronounced in elderly hypertensive individuals, and lower daily maintenance doses may be required.

Experience with use of doxazosin in elderly patients with benign prostatic hyperplasia (BPH) has shown that the safety profile of doxazosin is similar to that in younger patients.

### Drug interactions and/or related problems
The following drug interactions and/or related problems have been selected on the basis of their potential clinical significance (possible mechanism in parentheses where appropriate)—not necessarily inclusive (» = major clinical significance):

Note: Combinations containing any of the following medications, depending on the amount present, may also interact with this medication.

Anti-inflammatory drugs, nonsteroidal (NSAIDs), especially indomethacin
  (antihypertensive effects of doxazosin may be reduced when the medication is used concurrently with these agents; indomethacin, and possibly other NSAIDs, may antagonize the antihypertensive effect by inhibiting renal prostaglandin synthesis and/or by causing sodium and fluid retention; the patient should be carefully monitored to confirm that the desired effect is being obtained)
Cimetidine
  (concurrent use may slightly increase the serum concentration of doxazosin; however, the clinical significance of this increase is not known)
Hypotension-producing medications, other (See *Appendix II*)
  (antihypertensive effects may be potentiated when these medications are used concurrently with doxazosin; although some antihypertensive and/or diuretic combinations are frequently used to therapeutic advantage, dosage adjustments are necessary during concurrent use)
Sympathomimetics
  (antihypertensive effects of doxazosin may be reduced when it is used concurrently with these agents; the patient should be carefully monitored to confirm that the desired effect is being obtained)
  (concurrent use of doxazosin antagonizes the peripheral vasoconstriction produced by high doses of dopamine)
  (concurrent use of doxazosin may decrease the pressor response to ephedrine)
  (concurrent use of doxazosin may block the alpha-adrenergic effects of epinephrine, possibly resulting in severe hypotension and tachycardia)
  (concurrent use of doxazosin usually decreases, but does not reverse or completely block, the pressor effect of metaraminol)
  (prior administration of doxazosin may decrease the pressor effect and shorten the duration of action of methoxamine and phenylephrine)

## Medical considerations/Contraindications
The medical considerations/contraindications included have been selected on the basis of their potential clinical significance (reasons given in parentheses where appropriate)—not necessarily inclusive (» = major clinical significance).

***Risk-benefit should be considered when the following medical problems exist:***
Hepatic function impairment
  (although studies in patients with impaired hepatic function have not been done, doxazosin is primarily metabolized in the liver, and, therefore, increased sensitivity or prolonged doxazosin effect may occur)
Renal function impairment
  (small incidence of increased risk of first-dose orthostatic hypotensive reaction and prolonged hypotensive effect)
Sensitivity to doxazosin

## Patient monitoring
The following may be especially important in patient monitoring (other tests may be warranted in some patients, depending on condition; » = major clinical significance):
» Blood pressure measurements
  (recommended at 2 to 6 hours postdose following first dose and with each dosage increase, since postural effects are most likely to occur during this time; dosage to be increased as necessary and tolerated based on individual standing blood pressures taken at 2 to 6 hours and 24 hours postdose)

## Side/Adverse Effects
Note: A "first-dose orthostatic hypotensive reaction" sometimes occurs with the initial dose of doxazosin, especially when the patient is in the upright position. Syncope or other postural symptoms such as dizziness may occur. Subsequent occurrence with dosage increases is also possible. Incidence appears to be dose-related, thus, it is important that therapy be initiated with the 1-mg dose. Patients who are volume-depleted or sodium-restricted may be more sensitive to the orthostatic hypotensive effects of doxazosin, and the effect may be exaggerated after exercise.
Hypotensive side effects are more likely to occur in geriatric patients.

The following side/adverse effects have been selected on the basis of their potential clinical significance (possible signs and symptoms in parentheses where appropriate)—not necessarily inclusive:

**Those indicating need for medical attention**
Incidence more frequent
  *Dizziness; vertigo* (dizziness or lightheadedness)
Incidence less frequent
  *Arrhythmias* (irregular heartbeat); *dyspnea* (shortness of breath); *orthostatic hypotension* (dizziness or lightheadedness when getting up from a lying or sitting position; sudden fainting); *palpitations* (pounding heartbeat); *peripheral edema* (swelling of feet or lower legs); *tachycardia* (fast heartbeat)

**Those indicating need for medical attention only if they continue or are bothersome**
Incidence more frequent
  *Headache; unusual tiredness*
Incidence less frequent
  *Nausea; nervousness, restlessness, or unusual irritability; rhinitis* (runny nose); *somnolence* (sleepiness or unusual drowsiness)

## Overdose
For more information on the management of overdose or unintentional ingestion, **contact a Poison Control Center** (see *Poison Control Center Listing*).

**Treatment of overdose**
Treatment of circulatory failure, either by placing the patient in the supine position and elevating the legs or by using additional measures if shock is present, is most important. Volume expanders may be used to treat shock, followed, if necessary, by administration of a vasopressor.
Symptomatic, supportive treatment and monitoring of fluid and electrolyte status.

## Patient Consultation
As an aid to patient consultation, refer to *Advice for the Patient, Doxazosin (Systemic)*.
In providing consultation, consider emphasizing the following selected information (» = major clinical significance):

**Before using this medication**
» Conditions affecting use, especially:
  Sensitivity to quinazolines
  Use in the elderly—Increased sensitivity to hypotensive effects

**Proper use of this medication**
  Compliance with therapy; taking medication at the same time each day to maintain the therapeutic effect
» Proper dosing
  Missed dose: Taking as soon as possible; not taking if almost time for next dose; not doubling doses
» Proper storage
*For use as an antihypertensive*
  Possible need for control of weight and diet, especially sodium intake
» Patient may not experience symptoms of hypertension; importance of taking medication even if feeling well
» Does not cure, but helps control hypertension; possible need for lifelong therapy; serious consequences of untreated hypertension
*For use in benign prostatic hyperplasia (BPH)*
  Relieves symptoms of BPH but does not change the size of the prostate; may not prevent the need for surgery in the future
  May require 1 to 2 weeks of therapy before patient experiences improvement of symptoms

**Precautions while using this medication**
  Making regular visits to physician to check progress
» Not taking other medications, especially nonprescription sympathomimetics, unless discussed with physician
» Caution if dizziness, lightheadedness, or sudden fainting occurs, especially after initial dose; taking first dose at bedtime
» Caution when getting up suddenly from a lying or sitting position
» Caution in using alcohol, while standing for long periods or exercising, and during hot weather, because of enhanced orthostatic hypotensive effects
» Possibility of drowsiness
» Caution when driving or doing anything else requiring alertness because of possible drowsiness, dizziness, or lightheadedness

**Side/adverse effects**
  Signs of potential side effects, especially arrhythmias, dizziness, dyspnea, orthostatic hypotension, palpitations, peripheral edema, tachycardia, and vertigo

## General Dosing Information
In order to minimize the "first-dose orthostatic hypotensive reaction," an initial dose of 1 mg is recommended, with gradual increases in dose

every 2 weeks as needed. Administration of the initial dose at bedtime is recommended, as well as the initial dose of each increment.

**For use as an antihypertensive**
Dosage of doxazosin should be adjusted to meet the individual requirements of each patient, on the basis of blood pressure response.

Doxazosin may be used alone or in combination with a thiazide diuretic or beta-adrenergic blocking agent, both of which reduce the tendency for sodium and water retention, although they also produce additive hypotension. If combination therapy is indicated, individual titration is required to ensure the lowest possible therapeutic dose of each medication.

Increases in dose beyond 4 mg increase the likelihood of excessive postural effects including syncope, postural dizziness/vertigo, and postural hypotension.

When a diuretic or another antihypertensive agent is added to doxazosin therapy, the dose of doxazosin may be reduced, followed by slow dosage titration of the combination. When doxazosin is added to existing diuretic or antihypertensive therapy, the dose of the other agent may be reduced and doxazosin started at a dose of 1 mg once a day.

**For use in benign prostatic hyperplasia**
Prior to initiation of doxazosin therapy, the presence of prostate carcinoma should be ruled out, since prostate carcinoma can present with symptoms similar to those associated with BPH.

## Oral Dosage Forms

Note: The dosing and strengths of the dosage forms available are expressed in terms of doxazosin base (not the mesylate salt).

### DOXAZOSIN MESYLATE TABLETS

**Usual adult dose**
Antihypertensive—
  Initial: Oral, 1 mg (base) once a day, at bedtime.
  Maintenance: Oral, the dosage being increased gradually to meet individual requirements; depending on periodic blood pressure measurements, dosage may be increased every two weeks, titrating upwards to 2, 4, 8, and 16 mg (base) once a day as needed and tolerated.
Note: Increases in dose beyond 4 mg (base) increase the likelihood of excessive postural effects including syncope, postural dizziness/vertigo, and postural hypotension.
  Geriatric patients may be more sensitive to the effects of the usual adult dose.
Benign prostatic hyperplasia[1]—
  Initial: Oral, 1 mg (base) once a day, at bedtime.
  Maintenance: Oral, 1 to 8 mg (base) once a day.

**Usual adult prescribing limits**
16 mg once a day.

**Usual pediatric dose**
Safety and efficacy have not been established.

**Strength(s) usually available**
U.S.—
  1 mg (base) (Rx) [*Cardura*].
  2 mg (base) (Rx) [*Cardura*].
  4 mg (base) (Rx) [*Cardura*].
  8 mg (base) (Rx) [*Cardura*].
Canada—
  1 mg (base) (Rx) [*Cardura*].
  2 mg (base) (Rx) [*Cardura*].
  4 mg (base) (Rx) [*Cardura*].

**Packaging and storage**
Store below 30 °C (86 °F), in a well-closed container, unless otherwise specified by manufacturer.

**Auxiliary labeling**
• Do not take other medicines without your doctor's advice.
• May cause dizziness.

**Note**
Check refill frequency to determine compliance in hypertensive patients.

[1]Not included in Canadian product labeling.

## Selected Bibliography

Cubeddu LX, Fuenmayor N, Caplan N, Ferry D. Clinical pharmacology of doxazosin in patients with essential hypertension. Clin Pharmacol Ther 1987; 41: 439-49.

Talseth T, Westlie L, Daae L. Doxazosin and atenolol as monotherapy in mild and moderate hypertension: A randomized, parallel study with a three year follow-up. Am Heart J 1991; 121: 280-5.

The fifth report of the Joint National Committee on Detection, Evaluation, and Treatment of High Blood Pressure. Arch Intern Med 1993; 153: 154-83.

Revised: 08/02/94
Interim revision: 05/12/95; 08/13/98

---

**DOXEPIN**—See *Antidepressants, Tricyclic (Systemic)*

---

# DOXEPIN Topical

VA CLASSIFICATION (Primary): DE900
Commonly used brand name(s): *Zonalon*.
Note: For a listing of dosage forms and brand names by country availability, see *Dosage Forms* section(s).

## Category

Antipruritic (topical).

## Indications

**Accepted**
Pruritus associated with eczema (treatment)—Doxepin is indicated for the short-term (up to 8 days) topical treatment of moderate pruritus in adult patients with eczematous dermatitis, e.g., atopic dermatitis and lichen simplex chronicus.

## Pharmacology/Pharmacokinetics

**Physicochemical characteristics**
Chemical group—A dibenzoxepin tricyclic antidepressant.
Molecular weight—316.

**Mechanism of action/Effect**
The exact mechanism by which topical doxepin exerts its antipruritic effect is unknown. However, doxepin has potent antihistaminic ($H_1$- and $H_2$- receptor) activity. As a histamine-blocking agent, doxepin appears to bind to histamine receptor sites and competitively inhibits the biological activation of histamine receptors. Because topical doxepin produces drowsiness in significant numbers of patients, it is believed that this sedative property may also have an effect on certain pruritic symptoms.

**Other actions/effects**
Topical doxepin may be absorbed into the systemic circulation and, therefore, may have the potential for causing peripheral and central anticholinergic effects due to its potent and high binding affinity for muscarinic receptors. It may also have the potential to produce prominent cardiovascular effects as a result of its anticholinergic activity on the heart and a 'quinidine-like' myocardial depressant action, as well as inhibition of norepinephrine uptake at adrenergic synapses.

**Absorption**
Doxepin applied topically is absorbed through the skin. As with most topical agents, occlusive dressings may increase the absorption of topical doxepin.

**Distribution**
Once absorbed, doxepin may be distributed in body tissues including lungs, heart, brain, and liver.

**Biotransformation**
Once absorbed into the systemic circulation, doxepin undergoes hepatic metabolism that results in the conversion to the pharmacologically active metabolite, desmethyldoxepin. The parent compound and its metabolite also undergo glucuronidation.

**Half-life**
Desmethyldoxepin—Ranges from 28 to 52 hours.

**Peak plasma concentration**
For both doxepin and its active metabolite, desmethyldoxepin, plasma concentrations are highly variable and are poorly correlated with dosage. In 19 patients with pruritic eczema treated with topical doxepin, plasma doxepin concentrations ranged from nondetectable to 47 nanograms per mL (168.2 nanomoles per L) with a mean of 10.8 nanograms per mL, (38.6 nanomoles per L) after percutaneous absorption. (For oral doxepin, the target therapeutic plasma concentrations for the treatment of

depression range from 30 to 150 nanograms per mL [107.3 to 536.8 nanomoles per L]).

**Elimination**
Renal for both the parent compound and its metabolites.

## Precautions to Consider

**Cross-sensitivity and/or related problems**
Patients sensitive to other dibenzoxepines (tricyclic antidepressants) may also be sensitive to doxepin.

**Carcinogenicity**
Studies on carcinogenicity have not been conducted with topical doxepin.

**Mutagenicity**
Studies on mutagenicity have not been conducted with topical doxepin.

**Pregnancy/Reproduction**
*Fertility*—Studies have not been conducted with topical doxepin in humans.
Studies in rats and rabbits given oral doses of doxepin up to 8 times the topical human dose (on a milligram per kilogram of body weight [mg/kg] basis) have shown no evidence of impaired fertility.
*Pregnancy*—Adequate and well-controlled studies in humans have not been done.
Studies in rats and rabbits given oral doses of doxepin up to 8 times the topical human dose (on a milligram per kilogram of body weight [mg/kg] basis) have shown no evidence of harm to the fetus.
FDA Pregnancy Category B.

**Breast-feeding**
No studies have been done to determine if doxepin is distributed into human milk following topical administration. However, doxepin is distributed into human milk after oral administration. Because significant systemic concentrations of doxepin are obtained when this agent is applied topically, it is possible that this medication could be distributed into human milk after topical administration.
Apnea and drowsiness have been reported in 1 nursing infant whose mother was taking an oral dosage form of doxepin.

**Pediatrics**
Appropriate studies on the relationship of age to the effects of topical doxepin have not been performed in the pediatric population. Safety and efficacy have not been established.

**Geriatrics**
Appropriate studies on the relationship of age to the effects of topical doxepin have not been performed in the geriatric population. However, no geriatrics-specific problems have been documented to date.

**Drug interactions and/or related problems**
The following drug interactions and/or related problems have been selected on the basis of their potential clinical significance (possible mechanism in parentheses where appropriate)—not necessarily inclusive (» = major clinical significance):
Note: Combinations containing any of the following medications, depending on the amount present, may also interact with this medication. (See also *Antidepressants, Tricyclic [Systemic]* monograph for oral doxepin drug interactions).

» Alcohol or
» CNS depression-producing medications, other (See *Appendix II*)
(concurrent use with tricyclic antidepressants may result in serious potentiation of CNS depression, respiratory depression, and hypotensive effects; caution is recommended, and dosage of one or both agents should be reduced)

» Cimetidine
(cimetidine may inhibit the metabolism and increase the plasma concentration of doxepin, leading to toxicity; serious anticholinergic effects have been associated with concurrent use of cimetidine and tricyclic antidepressants)

» Medications metabolized by cytochrome $P_{450}$ isoenzyme $P_{450}IID_6$ such as
Antiarrhythmic agents, Type 1C, including encainide, flecainide, and propafenone
Antidepressants, other
Carbamazepine
Debrisoquine
Dextromethorphan
Phenothiazines
Quinidine
(although no studies have been done on the use of topical doxepin with these medications, caution is recommended because experience with oral tricyclic antidepressants has shown that concurrent use with other medications that are metabolized via the cytochrome $P_{450}$ isoenzyme $P_{450}IID_6$ may result in mutual inhibition of metabolism and in toxicity of either or both medications, especially in patients known to have genetically determined defects in oxidative metabolism involving this enzyme, if dosage of either or both medications is not reduced; the risk may be particularly high with quinidine and with other tricyclic antidepressants because of additive toxicities)

» Monoamine oxidase (MAO) inhibitors
(concurrent use with orally administered tricyclic antidepressants has resulted in serious side effects [convulsions, excitation, hyperpyrexia, and mania] and even death [although there have been patients who have received combinations of these medications without ill effects]; MAO inhibitors should be discontinued at least 2 weeks prior to the initiation of treatment with topical doxepin)

**Medical considerations/Contraindications**
The medical considerations/contraindications included have been selected on the basis of their potential clinical significance (reasons given in parentheses where appropriate)—not necessarily inclusive (» = major clinical significance).

*Risk-benefit should be considered when the following medical problems exist:*

» Glaucoma, narrow-angle, untreated or
» Urinary retention
(doxepin may aggravate these conditions)
Sensitivity to doxepin or other ingredients of the preparation, or history of

## Side/Adverse Effects

The following side/adverse effects have been selected on the basis of their potential clinical significance (possible signs and symptoms in parentheses where appropriate)—not necessarily inclusive:

**Those indicating need for medical attention**
Incidence more frequent—approximately 1 to 10%
*Edema at site of application* (swelling at site of application); *exacerbation of pruritus* (worsening of itching); *exacerbation of eczema* (worsening of eczema); *paresthesias* (burning, crawling, or tingling sensation of the skin)

Incidence rare—less than 1%
*Fever*

**Those indicating need for medical attention only if they continue or are bothersome**
Incidence more frequent—1 to 10%, or as specified
*Burning and/or stinging at the site of application*—approximately 21%; *changes in taste; dizziness; drowsiness*—22%; *dryness and tightness of skin; dryness of mouth and/or lips; emotional changes; fatigue* (unusual tiredness or weakness); *headache; thirst*

Note: *Drowsiness* is the most common adverse effect reported with the use of topical doxepin, especially in those patients receiving treatment over more than 10% of their body surface area. However, this effect was observed to be mild and temporary, usually lasting 1 or 2 days, as reported by the vast majority of patients who experienced drowsiness during the clinical trials. *Burning and/or stinging at the site of application* is the second most common adverse effect reported. In clinical trials, most patients characterized this reaction as mild and about 25% reported it as severe.

Incidence less frequent or rare—less than 1%
*Anxiety; irritation, tingling, scaling, or cracking of skin; nausea*

## Overdose

For specific information on the agent used in the management of doxepin overdose, see:
• *Physostigmine (Systemic)* monograph.

For more information on the management of overdose or unintentional ingestion, **contact a Poison Control Center** (see *Poison Control Center Listing*).

**Clinical effects of overdose**
The following effects have been selected on the basis of their potential clinical significance (possible signs and symptoms in parentheses where appropriate)—not necessarily inclusive:
Note: Signs and symptoms of overdose are generally related to the anticholinergic effects of this medication.

Mild effects
*Blurred vision; drowsiness; dryness of mouth, excessive; stupor* (decreased awareness or responsiveness)

Severe effects
  *Cardiac arrhythmias* (irregular heartbeat); *coma* (unconsciousness); *dilated pupils* (enlarged pupils); *hyperactive reflexes* (increased or excessive unconscious or jerking movements); *hypertension* (increased blood pressure); *hyperthermia* (extremely high fever or body temperature); *hypotension* (dizziness, fainting, or lightheadedness); *hypothermia* (extremely low body temperature; weak or feeble pulse); *paralytic ileus* (abdominal pain and swelling; intractable constipation; vomiting)—may lead to intestinal obstruction; *respiratory depression* (difficulty in breathing); *seizures* (convulsions); *tachycardia* (fast heartbeat); *urinary retention due to bladder atony* (difficulty in passing urine)

**Treatment of overdose**
For mild effects, observation and supportive therapy are recommended. It may be necessary to reduce the percent of body surface area treated or the frequency of application. A thinner layer of cream should be applied.

For severe effects, medical management should consist of aggressive supportive therapy.

To decrease absorption—The area of skin covered with topical doxepin should be thoroughly washed with soap and water.

To enhance elimination—Enhancing elimination of absorbed doxepin through dialysis and forced diuresis have not been successful due to the high tissue and protein binding, large volume of distribution, and limited water solubility of this agent.

Specific treatment—Cardiac arrythmias should be treated with the appropriate antiarrhythmic agents. It has been reported that many of the anticholinergic effects (cardiovascular and central nervous system [CNS] symptoms) of tricyclic antidepressant overdose in adults may be reversed by the slow intravenous administration of physostigmine. The dose should be repeated as required because physostigmine is rapidly metabolized. However, physostigmine should be used with caution because this agent may also increase the risk of cardiac toxicity if used indiscriminately. (See the package insert or *Physostigmine [Systemic]* monograph for specific dosing guidelines for use of this product.) Convulsions may be treated with anticonvulsant agents, such as diazepam or lorazepam; however, barbiturates are not recommended because they may potentiate respiratory depression. If there is any suspicion that the patient may have taken a benzodiazepine in addition to doxepin, flumazenil should not be used to reverse the effects of the benzodiazepine. Administration of flumazenil in such cases has been shown to increase the risk of seizures and/or cardiac arrhythmias.

Monitoring—Vital signs, especially cardiovascular and respiratory functions, should be constantly monitored. Because relapse after apparent recovery has been reported with oral doxepin, electrocardiogram (ECG) monitoring may be required for several days.

Supportive care—For comatose patients, an adequate airway should be established and assisted ventilation should be used if necessary. Patients in whom intentional overdose is known or suspected should be referred for psychiatric consultation.

## Patient Consultation

As an aid to patient consultation, refer to *Advice for the Patient, Doxepin (Topical)*.

In providing consultation, consider emphasizing the following selected information (» = major clinical significance):

**Before using this medication**
» Conditions affecting use, especially:
  Sensitivity to doxepin or other ingredients of the preparation
  Breast-feeding—May be distributed into breast milk
  Other medications, especially alcohol and other CNS depression-producing medications, cimetidine, medications metabolized by cytochrome $P_{450}$ isoenzyme $P_{450}11D_6$, and monoamine oxidase (MAO) inhibitors
  Other medical problems, especially untreated narrow-angle glaucoma and urinary retention

**Proper use of this medication**
» For external use only; not for ophthalmic, oral, or intravaginal use
» Using this medication exactly as directed; not using more of it, not using it more often, and not using it for more than 8 days; not applying medication to an area of skin larger than recommended by physician
  Applying a thin film of doxepin cream to only affected area(s) of skin and rubbing in gently
  Compliance with full course of therapy

» Not using occlusive dressings, which may increase absorption of medication
» Proper dosing
  Missed dose
» Proper storage

**Precautions while using this medication**
  Checking with physician if skin problem does not improve after 8 days or if it becomes worse
» Avoiding alcoholic beverages or other alcohol-containing preparations while using topical doxepin; not taking other medications unless prescribed by physician
» Caution if drowsiness occurs; not driving, using machines, or doing anything else that requires alertness while using topical doxepin; if excessive drowsiness occurs, reducing the number of applications per day, the amount of cream applied, and/or the percentage of body surface area treated, or discontinuing medication after checking with physician
» Possible dryness of mouth; using sugarless gum or candy, ice, or saliva substitute for relief; checking with physician or dentist if dry mouth continues for more than 2 weeks

**Side/adverse effects**
  Signs of potential side effects, especially edema at site of application, exacerbation of pruritus, exacerbation of eczema, paresthesias, and fever

## General Dosing Information

Topical doxepin is for external use only. It is not for ophthalmic, oral, or intravaginal use.

A thin film of doxepin cream should be applied to the affected area(s) of skin.

Drowsiness may occur, especially in patients receiving treatment over more than 10% of their body surface area. Patients should be warned of this possibility and cautioned against driving a motor vehicle or operating hazardous machinery while being treated with topical doxepin. If excessive drowsiness occurs, it may be necessary to reduce the body surface area treated, reduce the number of applications per day, reduce the amount of cream applied, or discontinue the medication.

Topical doxepin should not be used for more than 8 days. Chronic use beyond 8 days may result in higher systemic concentrations of the medication because of increased absorption.

## Topical Dosage Forms

### DOXEPIN HYDROCHLORIDE CREAM

**Usual adult dose**
Antipruritic (topical)—
  Topical, a thin film applied to the affected area(s) of skin four times a day, with an interval of at least three to four hours between applications. Treatment may be continued for up to eight days.

**Usual pediatric dose**
Safety and efficacy have not been established.

**Strength(s) usually available**
U.S.—
  5% (Rx) [*Zonalon* (benzyl alcohol; cetyl alcohol; glyceryl stearate; isopropyl myristate; petrolatum; PEG-100 stearate; purified water; sorbitol; titanium dioxide)].
Canada—
  5% (Rx) [*Zonalon*].

**Packaging and storage**
Store at or below 27 °C (80 °F).

**Auxiliary labeling**
- For external use only.
- May cause drowsiness.
- Avoid alcoholic beverages.

## Selected Bibliography

Drake LA, Fallon JD, Sober A, et al. Relief of pruritus in patients with atopic dermatitis after treatment with topical doxepin cream. J Am Acad Dermatol 1994; 31(4): 613-6.

Developed: 05/26/95

# DOXORUBICIN  Systemic

VA CLASSIFICATION (Primary): AN200

Commonly used brand name(s): *Adriamycin PFS*; *Adriamycin RDF*; *Rubex*.

Note: For a listing of dosage forms and brand names by country availability, see *Dosage Forms* section(s).

## Category
Antineoplastic.

## Indications

Note: Bracketed information in the *Indications* section refers to uses that are not included in U.S. product labeling.

**Accepted**

Leukemia, acute lymphocytic (treatment) or
Leukemia, acute nonlymphocytic (treatment)—Doxorubicin is indicated for treatment of acute lymphocytic (lymphoblastic) leukemia and acute nonlymphocytic (myeloblastic) leukemia.

Carcinoma, bladder (treatment)
Carcinoma, breast (treatment)
Carcinoma, gastric (treatment)
Carcinoma, lung, small cell (treatment)
Carcinoma, ovarian, epithelial (treatment)
Carcinoma, thyroid (treatment)
Neuroblastoma (treatment) or
Wilms' tumor (treatment)—Doxorubicin is indicated for treatment of transitional bladder cell carcinoma, breast carcinoma, gastric carcinoma, small cell lung carcinoma, epithelial ovarian carcinoma, thyroid carcinoma, neuroblastoma, and Wilms' tumor.

[Leukemia, chronic lymphocytic (treatment)][1]—Doxorubicin is indicated for treatment of chronic lymphocytic leukemia.

[Carcinoma, cervical (treatment)]
[Carcinoma, endometrial (treatment)]
[Carcinoma, head and neck (treatment)]
[Carcinoma, hepatocellular, primary (treatment)][1]
[Carcinoma, lung, non–small cell (treatment)]
[Carcinoma, pancreatic (treatment)][1]
[Carcinoma, prostatic (treatment)][1]
[Hepatoblastoma (treatment)][1]
[Thymoma (treatment)][1]
[Tumors, ovarian, germ cell (treatment)] or
[Tumors, trophoblastic, gestational (treatment)][1]—Doxorubicin is indicated for treatment of cervical carcinoma, endometrial carcinoma, squamous cell carcinoma of the head and neck, primary hepatocellular carcinoma, non–small cell lung carcinoma, pancreatic carcinoma, prostatic carcinoma, hepatoblastoma, thymoma, germ cell tumors of the ovary, and gestational trophoblastic tumors.

Lymphoma, Hodgkin's (treatment) or
Lymphoma, non-Hodgkin's (treatment)—Doxorubicin is indicated for treatment of Hodgkin's and non-Hodgkin's lymphomas.

[Ewing's sarcoma (treatment)][1]
[Kaposi's sarcoma, acquired immunodeficiency syndrome (AIDS)–associated (treatment)][1]
Osteosarcoma (treatment) or
Sarcoma, soft tissue (treatment)—Doxorubicin is indicated for treatment of Ewing's sarcoma, AIDS–associated Kaposi's sarcoma, osteosarcoma, and soft tissue sarcoma.

[Multiple myeloma (treatment)][1]—Doxorubicin is indicated for treatment of multiple myeloma.

Note: Although doxorubicin is approved in Canada for treatment of testicular carcinoma, the USP Division of Information Development Hematology-Oncology Advisory Panel believes there is insufficient evidence to support the effectiveness of doxorubicin in the treatment of testicular carcinoma.

[1] Not included in Canadian product labeling.

## Pharmacology/Pharmacokinetics

**Physicochemical characteristics**
Molecular weight—543.53.
Other characteristics—Unstable in solutions with a pH of less than 3 or greater than 7.

**Mechanism of action/Effect**
Doxorubicin is an anthracycline glycoside; it is classified as an antibiotic but is not used as an antimicrobial agent. Doxorubicin is cell cycle–specific for the S phase of cell division. Its exact mechanism of antineoplastic activity is unknown but may involve binding to DNA by intercalation between base pairs and inhibition of DNA and RNA synthesis by template disordering and steric obstruction. Other possible mechanisms of antineoplastic activity include binding to cell membrane lipids, thus altering a variety of cellular functions and interacting with topoisomerase II to form DNA-cleavable complexes.

**Distribution**
$Vol_D$—Steady state: > 20 to 30 L per kg, indicating extensive uptake into tissues.
Does not cross the blood-brain barrier.

**Protein binding**
High (74 to 76%); independent of plasma concentration of doxorubicin.

**Biotransformation**
Occurs rapidly (within 1 hour) in the liver to produce an active metabolite, doxorubicinol. Enzymatic reduction of doxorubicin by oxidases, reductases, and dehydrogenases results in the production of free radicals, which may contribute to cardiotoxicity.

**Half-life**
Distribution—
  Approximately 5 minutes.
Elimination—
  20 to 48 hours for doxorubicin and doxorubicinol.

**Elimination**
Biliary—
  40% unchanged, over 5 days.
Renal—
  5 to 12% of doxorubicin and metabolites appear in urine over 5 days.

## Precautions to Consider

**Carcinogenicity/Mutagenicity**
Secondary malignancies are potential delayed effects of many antineoplastic agents, although it is not clear whether the effect is related to their mutagenic or immunosuppressive action. The effect of dose and duration of therapy is also unknown, although the risk seems to increase with long-term use. Although information is limited, available data seem to indicate that the carcinogenic risk is greatest with the alkylating agents.

Doxorubicin is carcinogenic in animals and is potentially carcinogenic in humans.

**Pregnancy/Reproduction**
Fertility—Gonadal suppression, resulting in amenorrhea or azoospermia, may occur in patients taking antineoplastic therapy, especially with the alkylating agents. In general, these effects appear to be related to dose and length of therapy and may be irreversible. Prediction of the degree of testicular or ovarian function impairment is complicated by the common use of combinations of several antineoplastics, which makes it difficult to assess the effects of individual agents.

Doxorubicin affects gonadal function but has a weaker effect on humans than that seen in experiments with mice.

Pregnancy—Some studies indicate that doxorubicin may cross the placenta in humans.

First trimester: It is usually recommended that use of antineoplastics, especially combination chemotherapy, be avoided whenever possible, especially during the first trimester. Although information is limited because of the relatively few instances of antineoplastic administration during pregnancy, the mutagenic, teratogenic, and carcinogenic potential of these medications must be considered.

Other hazards to the fetus include adverse reactions seen in adults.

In general, use of a contraceptive is recommended during cytotoxic drug therapy.

Doxorubicin is embryotoxic and teratogenic in rats and embryotoxic and abortifacient in rabbits.

**Breast-feeding**
Although very little information is available regarding distribution of antineoplastic agents into breast milk, breast-feeding is not recommended while doxorubicin is being administered because of the risks to the infant (adverse effects, mutagenicity, carcinogenicity).

### Pediatrics
Although appropriate studies on the relationship of age to the effects of doxorubicin have not been performed in the pediatric population, cardiotoxicity may be more frequent in children up to 2 years of age.

### Geriatrics
Although appropriate studies on the relationship of age to the effects of doxorubicin have not been performed in the geriatric population, cardiotoxicity may be more frequent in patients 70 years of age or older. Caution should also be used in patients who have inadequate bone marrow reserves due to old age.

### Dental
The bone marrow depressant effects of doxorubicin may result in an increased incidence of microbial infection, delayed healing, and gingival bleeding. Dental work, whenever possible, should be completed prior to initiation of therapy or deferred until blood counts have returned to normal. Patients should be instructed in proper oral hygiene during treatment, including caution in use of regular toothbrushes, dental floss, and toothpicks.

Doxorubicin also commonly causes stomatitis, which may be associated with considerable discomfort.

### Drug interactions and/or related problems
The following drug interactions and/or related problems have been selected on the basis of their potential clinical significance (possible mechanism in parentheses where appropriate)—not necessarily inclusive (» = major clinical significance):

Note: Combinations containing any of the following medications, depending on the amount present, may also interact with this medication.

Allopurinol or
Colchicine or
» Probenecid or
» Sulfinpyrazone
(doxorubicin may raise the concentration of blood uric acid; dosage adjustment of antigout agents may be necessary to control hyperuricemia and gout; allopurinol may be preferred to prevent or reverse doxorubicin-induced hyperuricemia because of risk of uric acid nephropathy with uricosuric antigout agents)

Blood dyscrasia–causing medications (see *Appendix II*)
(leukopenic and/or thrombocytopenic effects of doxorubicin may be increased with concurrent or recent therapy if these medications cause the same effects; dosage adjustment of doxorubicin, if necessary, should be based on blood counts)

» Bone marrow depressants, other (see *Appendix II*) or
Radiation therapy
(additive bone marrow depression, including severe dermatitis and/or mucositis, may occur; dosage reduction may be required when two or more bone marrow depressants, including radiation, are used concurrently or consecutively)

Cyclophosphamide or
Dactinomycin or
Mitomycin or
Radiation therapy to mediastinal area
(concurrent use may result in increased cardiotoxicity; it is recommended that the total dose of doxorubicin not exceed 400 mg per square meter of body surface area)

(concurrent use of cyclophosphamide with doxorubicin may potentiate cyclophosphamide-induced hemorrhagic cystitis)

» Daunorubicin
(use of doxorubicin in a patient who has previously received daunorubicin increases the risk of cardiotoxicity; dosage adjustment is necessary. Doxorubicin should not be used in patients who have previously received complete cumulative doses of daunorubicin or doxorubicin)

Hepatotoxic medications (see *Appendix II*)
(concurrent use may increase the risk of toxicity; for example, high-dose methotrexate may impair liver function and increase toxicity of subsequently administered doxorubicin)

Streptozocin
(may prolong the half-life of doxorubicin when used concurrently; dosage reduction of doxorubicin is recommended)

Vaccines, killed virus
(because normal defense mechanisms may be suppressed by doxorubicin therapy, the patient's antibody response to the vaccine may be decreased. The interval between discontinuation of medications that cause immunosuppression and restoration of the patient's ability to respond to the vaccine depends on the intensity and type of immunosuppression-causing medication used, the underlying disease, and other factors; estimates vary from 3 months to 1 year)

» Vaccines, live virus
(because normal defense mechanisms may be suppressed by doxorubicin therapy, concurrent use with a live virus vaccine may potentiate the replication of the vaccine virus, may increase the side/adverse effects of the vaccine virus, and/or may decrease the patient's antibody response to the vaccine; immunization of these patients should be undertaken only with extreme caution after careful review of the patient's hematologic status and only with the knowledge and consent of the physician managing the doxorubicin therapy. The interval between discontinuation of medications that cause immunosuppression and restoration of the patient's ability to respond to the vaccine depends on the intensity and type of immunosuppression-causing medication used, the underlying disease, and other factors; estimates vary from 3 months to 1 year. Patients with leukemia in remission should not receive live virus vaccine until at least 3 months after their last chemotherapy. In addition, immunization with oral poliovirus vaccine should be postponed in persons in close contact with the patient, especially family members)

### Laboratory value alterations
The following have been selected on the basis of their potential clinical significance (possible effect in parentheses where appropriate)—not necessarily inclusive (» = major clinical significance):

With physiology/laboratory test values
Electrocardiogram (ECG) changes, transient, including:
Arrhythmias
ST depression
T-wave flattening
(may last up to 2 weeks after a dose or course; withdrawal of doxorubicin is usually not necessary)
QRS reduction
(may be a sign of cardiomyopathy; withdrawal of doxorubicin should be considered)
Uric acid
(concentrations in blood and urine may be increased)

### Medical considerations/Contraindications
The medical considerations/contraindications included have been selected on the basis of their potential clinical significance (reasons given in parentheses where appropriate)—not necessarily inclusive (» = major clinical significance).

*Risk-benefit should be considered when the following medical problems exist:*

» Bone marrow depression
» Chickenpox, existing or recent (including recent exposure) or
» Herpes zoster
(risk of severe generalized disease)
Gout, history of or
Urate renal stones, history of
(risk of hyperuricemia)
» Heart disease
(cardiotoxicity may occur at lower cumulative doses)
» Hepatic function impairment
(slowed excretion. Reduction in dosage is recommended; one half of the normal dose is recommended in patients with serum bilirubin concentrations of 1.2 to 3 mg per 100 mL; one quarter of the normal dose is recommended in patients with serum bilirubin concentrations of 3 to 5 mg per 100 mL)
Sensitivity to doxorubicin
» Tumor cell infiltration of the bone marrow
» Caution should be used also in patients with inadequate bone marrow reserves due to previous cytotoxic drug or radiation therapy.

### Patient monitoring
The following are especially important in patient monitoring (other tests may be warranted in some patients, depending on condition; » = major clinical significance):

Alanine aminotransferase (ALT [SGPT]) values and
Alkaline phosphatase values and
Aspartate aminotransferase (AST [SGOT]) values and
Bilirubin concentrations, serum and
Lactate dehydrogenase (LDH) values
(recommended prior to initiation of therapy and at periodic intervals during therapy; frequency varies according to clinical state, agent, dose, and other agents being used concurrently)

Chest radiograph and
» Echocardiography and
Electrocardiogram (ECG) studies and

» Radionuclide angiography determination of ejection fraction
    (recommended prior to initiation of therapy and at periodic intervals during therapy)
» Examination of patient's mouth for ulceration
    (recommended before administration of each dose)
» Hematocrit or hemoglobin and
» Leukocyte count, total and, if appropriate, differential and
» Platelet count
    (determinations recommended prior to initiation of therapy and at periodic intervals during therapy; frequency varies according to clinical state, agent, dose, and other agents being used concurrently)
   Uric acid concentrations, serum
    (recommended prior to initiation of therapy and at periodic intervals during therapy; frequency varies according to clinical state, agent, dose, and other agents being used concurrently)

## Side/Adverse Effects

Note: Many "side effects" of antineoplastic therapy are unavoidable and represent the medication's pharmacologic action. Some of these (for example, leukopenia and thrombocytopenia) are actually used as parameters to aid in individual dosage titration.

A necrotizing colitis (cecal inflammation, bloody stools, severe and sometimes fatal infections) has been associated with a combination regimen of doxorubicin and cytarabine.

Excessively rapid intravenous administration may produce facial flushing.

The following side/adverse effects have been selected on the basis of their potential clinical significance (possible signs and symptoms in parentheses where appropriate)—not necessarily inclusive:

**Those indicating need for medical attention**
Incidence more frequent
   *Leukopenia or infection* (fever or chills; cough or hoarseness; lower back or side pain; painful or difficult urination)—usually asymptomatic; *stomatitis or esophagitis* (sores in mouth and on lips)
   Note: With *leukopenia*, the nadir of leukocyte count occurs 10 to 14 days after a dose. Recovery usually occurs within 21 days after a dose.
      *Stomatitis or esophagitis* occurs 5 to 10 days after administration. It may be severe and lead to ulceration and the potential for severe infections. It is more severe with a dosage regimen of 3 successive days.
Incidence less frequent
   *Cardiotoxicity, usually in the form of congestive heart failure* (shortness of breath; swelling of feet and lower legs; fast or irregular heartbeat); *extravasation, cellulitis, or tissue necrosis* (pain at injection site); *gastrointestinal ulceration* (stomach pain); *hyperuricemia or uric acid nephropathy* (joint pain; lower back or side pain); *local reaction* (red streaks along injected vein); *phlebosclerosis* (pain at injection site); *postirradiation erythema, recall* (darkening or redness of skin); *thrombocytopenia* (unusual bleeding or bruising; black, tarry stools; blood in urine or stools; pinpoint red spots on skin)—usually asymptomatic
   Note: Incidence of *cardiotoxicity* is more frequent in patients receiving total dosages of over 550 mg per square meter of body surface area (400 mg per square meter of body surface area in patients who have previously received chest irradiation or medications increasing cardiotoxicity) and in patients with a history of cardiac disease or mediastinal radiation, and may be more frequent in children up to 2 years of age and in the elderly.
      *Cardiotoxicity* usually appears within 1 to 6 months after initiation of therapy. Cardiomyopathy has been reported to be associated with persistent voltage reduction in the QRS wave, systolic interval prolongation, and reduction of ejection fraction. It may develop suddenly and may not be detected by routine ECG. It may be irreversible and fatal but responds to treatment if detected early.
      Acute life-threatening arrhythmias have been reported during or within a few hours after administration.
      *Extravasation* may also occur without accompanying stinging or burning and even if blood returns well on aspiration of the infusion needle.
      *Hyperuricemia or uric acid nephropathy* occurs most commonly during initial treatment of patients with leukemia or lymphoma, as a result of rapid cell breakdown that leads to elevated serum uric acid concentrations.
      A *local reaction* may indicate excessively rapid intravenous administration.
      *Phlebosclerosis* occurs especially when small veins are used or a single vein is used repeatedly.
      *Recall postirradiation erythema* occurs if patient has previously received radiation therapy; severe dermatitis and/or mucositis in the irradiated area may occur with concurrent use.
Incidence rare
   *Allergic reaction* (skin rash or itching; fever; chills); *anaphylaxis* (wheezing)

**Those indicating need for medical attention only if they continue or are bothersome**
Incidence more frequent
   *Nausea and vomiting*—may be severe
Incidence less frequent
   *Darkening of soles, palms, or nails*—especially in children and black patients; *diarrhea*

**Those not indicating need for medical attention**
Incidence more frequent
   *Loss of hair; reddish-colored urine*
   Note: *Loss of hair* is complete and reversible. It occurs in most cases.
      *Reddish-colored urine* clears within 48 hours.

**Those indicating the need for medical attention if they occur after medication is discontinued**
   *Cardiotoxicity* (fast or irregular heartbeat; shortness of breath; swelling of feet and lower legs)

## Patient Consultation

As an aid to patient consultation, refer to Advice for the Patient, Doxorubicin (Systemic).
In providing consultation, consider emphasizing the following selected information (» = major clinical significance):

**Before using this medication**
» Conditions affecting use, especially:
   Sensitivity to doxorubicin
   Pregnancy—Use not recommended because of mutagenic, teratogenic, and carcinogenic potential; advisability of using contraception; telling physician immediately if pregnancy is suspected
   Breast-feeding—Not recommended because of risk of serious side effects
   Use in children—Cardiotoxicity more frequent in children up to 2 years of age
   Use in the elderly—Cardiotoxicity may be more frequent in patients 70 years of age and over
   Other medications, especially probenecid, sulfinpyrazone, other bone marrow depressants, daunorubicin, live virus vaccines, or previous cytotoxic drug or radiation therapy
   Other medical problems, especially chickenpox, herpes zoster, heart disease, hepatic function impairment, or tumor cell infiltration of bone marrow

**Proper use of this medication**
   Caution in taking combination therapy; taking each medication at the right time
   Importance of ample fluid intake and subsequent increase in urine output to aid in excretion of uric acid
   Frequency of nausea and vomiting; importance of continuing medication despite stomach upset
» Proper dosing

**Precautions while using this medication**
» Importance of close monitoring by the physician
» Avoiding immunizations unless approved by physician; other persons in patient's household should avoid immunizations with oral poliovirus vaccine; avoiding persons who have taken oral poliovirus vaccine, or wearing a protective mask that covers nose and mouth
*Caution if bone marrow depression occurs*
» Avoiding exposure to persons with infections, especially during periods of low blood counts; checking with physician immediately if fever or chills, cough or hoarseness, lower back or side pain, or painful or difficult urination occurs
» Checking with physician immediately if unusual bleeding or bruising; black, tarry stools; blood in urine or stools; or pinpoint red spots on skin occur
   Caution in use of regular toothbrush, dental floss, or toothpick; physician, dentist, or nurse may suggest alternatives; checking with physician before having dental work done
   Not touching eyes or inside of nose unless hands washed immediately before
   Using caution to avoid accidental cuts with use of sharp objects such as safety razor or fingernail or toenail cutters

Avoiding contact sports or other situations where bruising or injury could occur

» Possibility of local tissue injury and scarring if infiltration of intravenous solution occurs; telling doctor or nurse right away about redness, pain, or swelling at injection site

### Side/adverse effects

May cause adverse effects such as blood problems, loss of hair, heart problems, and cancer

Signs of potential side effects, especially leukopenia, infection, stomatitis, esophagitis, cardiotoxicity, extravasation, cellulitis, tissue necrosis, gastrointestinal ulceration, hyperuricemia, uric acid nephropathy, local reaction, phlebosclerosis, recall of postirradiation erythema, thrombocytopenia, allergic reaction, and anaphylaxis

Physician or nurse can help in dealing with side effects

Reddish urine for 1 to 2 days after administration may be alarming to patient although medically insignificant

Possibility of hair loss; normal hair growth should resume after treatment has ended

## General Dosing Information

Patients receiving doxorubicin should be under supervision of a physician experienced in cancer chemotherapy. It is recommended that the patient be hospitalized at least during initial treatment.

Doxorubicin should not be used in patients who have previously received the maximum acceptable cumulative doses of doxorubicin and/or daunorubicin.

A variety of dosage schedules of doxorubicin, alone or in combination with other antitumor agents, are used. The prescriber may consult the medical literature as well as the manufacturer's literature in choosing a specific dosage.

Dosage must be adjusted to meet the individual requirements of each patient, on the basis of clinical response and appearance or severity of toxicity.

Use of a weekly dosage of doxorubicin may be associated with a reduced risk of cardiotoxicity and hematologic toxicity.

It is recommended that doxorubicin be administered slowly into the tubing of a freely running intravenous infusion of 0.9% sodium chloride injection or 5% dextrose injection (over not less than 3 to 5 minutes). If possible, veins over joints or in extremities with compromised venous or lymphatic drainage should be avoided.

Care must be taken to avoid extravasation during intravenous administration because of the risk of severe ulceration and necrosis. Facial flushing indicates too-rapid injection.

If extravasation of doxorubicin occurs during intravenous administration, as indicated by local swelling at the tip of the needle and local burning or stinging (may also be painless), the injection and infusion should be stopped immediately and resumed, completing the dose, in another vein. Local infiltration of antidotes is not recommended. Use of ice packs and elevation of the extremity to reduce swelling are recommended. Surgical excision of the involved area may be necessary.

Because it will cause local tissue necrosis, doxorubicin must not be administered intramuscularly or subcutaneously.

Doxorubicin has also been administered intra-arterially and as a topical bladder instillation.

Development of uric acid nephropathy in patients with leukemia or lymphoma may be prevented by adequate oral hydration and, in some cases, administration of allopurinol. Alkalinization of urine may be necessary if serum uric acid concentrations are elevated.

In acute leukemia, doxorubicin may be administered despite the presence of thrombocytopenia and bleeding; stoppage of bleeding and increase in platelet count have occurred during treatment in some cases and platelet transfusions are useful in others.

Special precautions are recommended in patients who develop thrombocytopenia as a result of administration of doxorubicin. These may include extreme care in performing invasive procedures; regular inspection of intravenous sites, skin (including perirectal area), and mucous membrane surfaces for signs of bleeding or bruising; limiting frequency of venipuncture and avoiding intramuscular injections; testing urine, emesis, stool, and secretions for occult blood; care in the use of regular toothbrushes, dental floss, toothpicks, safety razors, and fingernail and toenail cutters; avoiding constipation; and using caution to prevent falls and other injuries. Such patients should avoid alcohol and aspirin intake because of the risk of gastrointestinal bleeding. Platelet transfusions may be required.

Patients who develop leukopenia should be observed carefully for signs of infection. Antibiotic support may be required. In neutropenic patients who develop fever, broad-spectrum antibiotic coverage should be initiated empirically, pending bacterial cultures and appropriate diagnostic tests.

### Safety considerations for handling this medication

There is limited but increasing evidence and concern that personnel involved in preparation and administration of parenteral antineoplastic agents may be at some risk because of the potential mutagenicity, teratogenicity, and/or carcinogenicity of these agents, although the actual risk is unknown. USP advisory panels recommend cautious handling both in preparation and disposal of antineoplastic agents. Precautions that have been suggested include:

• Use of a biological containment cabinet during reconstitution and dilution of parenteral medications and wearing of disposable surgical gloves and masks.

• Use of proper technique to prevent contamination of the medication, work area, and operator during transfer between containers (including proper training of personnel in this technique).

• Cautious and proper disposal of needles, syringes, vials, ampuls, and unused medication.

A number of medical centers have developed detailed guidelines for handling of antineoplastic agents.

### Combination chemotherapy

Doxorubicin may be used in combination with other agents in various regimens. As a result, incidence and/or severity of side effects may be altered and different dosages (usually reduced) may be used.

## Parenteral Dosage Forms

Note: Bracketed uses in the *Dosage Forms* section refer to categories of use and/or indications that are not included in U.S. product labeling.

### DOXORUBICIN HYDROCHLORIDE INJECTION USP

**Usual adult dose**

Leukemia, acute lymphocytic or
Leukemia, acute nonlymphocytic or
Carcinoma, bladder or
Carcinoma, breast or
Carcinoma, gastric or
Carcinoma, lung, small cell or
Carcinoma, ovarian, epithelial or
Carcinoma, thyroid or
Neuroblastoma or
Wilms' tumor or
[Carcinoma, cervical] or
[Carcinoma, endometrial] or
[Carcinoma, head and neck] or
Carcinoma, lung, non–small cell or
[Carcinoma, pancreatic][1] or
[Carcinoma, prostatic][1] or
[Tumors, ovarian, germ cell] or
Lymphoma, Hodgkin's or
Lymphoma, non-Hodgkin's or
Sarcoma, soft tissue or
Osteosarcoma or
[Ewing's sarcoma][1] or
[Multiple myeloma][1]—

Intravenous, 60 to 75 mg per square meter of body surface area, repeated every twenty-one days or

Intravenous, 25 to 30 mg per square meter of body surface area a day on two or three successive days, repeated every three to four weeks or

Intravenous, 20 mg per square meter of body surface area once a week. When used in combination with other chemotherapy agents: Intravenous, 40 to 60 mg per square meter of body surface area, repeated every twenty-one to twenty-eight days.

[Leukemia, chronic lymphocytic (treatment)][1] or
[Carcinoma, hepatocellular, primary (treatment)][1] or
[Hepatoblastoma (treatment)][1] or
[Thymoma (treatment)][1] or
[Tumors, trophoblastic, gestational (treatment)][1] or
[Kaposi's sarcoma, acquired immunodeficiency syndrome (AIDS)–associated (treatment)][1]—

Consult medical literature and manufacturer's literature for specific dosage.

**Usual adult prescribing limits**

The risk of developing congestive heart failure is estimated to be 1 to 2% at a total cumulative dosage of 300 mg per square meter of body surface area, 3 to 5% at a total cumulative dosage of 400 mg per square meter of body surface area, 5 to 8% at a total cumulative dosage of 450 mg per square meter of body surface area, and 6 to 20% at a total cumulative dosage of 500 mg per square meter of body surface area. This toxicity may develop at lower cumulative dosages in patients who have previously received chest irradiation, patients who have received medications increasing cardiotoxicity, or patients with pre-existing heart disease.

**Usual pediatric dose**
Intravenous, 30 mg per square meter of body surface area a day on three successive days every four weeks.

**Strength(s) usually available**
U.S.—
   2 mg per mL (5-, 10-, 25-, and 37.5-mL single-dose vials, and 100-mL multidose vial) (Rx) [*Adriamycin PFS* (sodium chloride 0.9%) [GENERIC (sodium chloride 0.9%)].
Canada—
   2 mg per mL (5- and 25-mL single-dose vials, and 200-mL multidose vial) (Rx) [*Adriamycin PFS* (sodium chloride 0.9%)].

**Packaging and storage**
Store between 2 and 8 °C (36 and 46 °F). Protect from light.

**Incompatibilities**
Doxorubicin should not be mixed with heparin, dexamethasone, fluorouracil, hydrocortisone sodium succinate, aminophylline, or cephalothin, since a precipitate may form.

**Caution**
Caution in handling the 100- or 200-mL (200- or 400-mg) multiple-dose vial is recommended to prevent confusion with the single-dose vial and possible inadvertent overdose. For example, the manufacturer recommends that the multiple-dose vial be stored in the original carton until the contents are used.

**Note**
Great care should be taken to prevent exposure of the skin to doxorubicin. The use of gloves is recommended. Any doxorubicin solution that comes in contact with the skin or mucosae should be washed off thoroughly with soap and water.

## DOXORUBICIN HYDROCHLORIDE FOR INJECTION USP

**Usual adult dose**
See *Doxorubicin Hydrochloride Injection USP*.

**Usual adult prescribing limits**
See *Doxorubicin Hydrochloride Injection USP*.

**Usual pediatric dose**
See *Doxorubicin Hydrochloride Injection USP*.

**Size(s) usually available**
U.S.—
   10 mg (single-dose vial) (Rx) [*Adriamycin RDF* (lactose 50 mg; methylparaben 1 mg); *Rubex* (lactose) [GENERIC (may contain lactose 50 mg)].
   20 mg (single-dose vial) (Rx) [*Adriamycin RDF* (lactose 100 mg; methylparaben 2 mg) [GENERIC (may contain lactose 100 mg)].
   50 mg (single-dose vial) (Rx) [*Adriamycin RDF* (lactose 250 mg; methylparaben 5 mg); *Rubex* (lactose 250 mg) [GENERIC (may contain lactose 250 mg)].
   100 mg (single-dose vial) (Rx) [*Rubex* (lactose 500 mg)].
   150 mg (multidose vial) (Rx) [*Adriamycin RDF* (lactose 750 mg; methylparaben 15 mg)].
Canada—
   10 mg (single-dose vial) (Rx) [*Adriamycin RDF* (lactose 50 mg; methylparaben 1 mg)].
   20 mg (single-dose vial) (Rx) [*Adriamycin RDF* (lactose 100 mg; methylparaben 2 mg)].
   50 mg (single-dose vial) (Rx) [*Adriamycin RDF* (lactose 250 mg; methylparaben 5 mg)].
   150 mg (multidose vial) (Rx) [*Adriamycin RDF* (lactose 750 mg; methylparaben 15 mg)].

**Packaging and storage**
Store below 40 °C (104 °F), preferably between 15 and 30 °C (59 and 86 °F), unless otherwise specified by the manufacturer. Protect from light.

**Preparation of dosage form**
Doxorubicin Hydrochloride for Injection USP is reconstituted for intravenous administration by adding 5 mL (10-mg vial), 10 mL (20-mg vial), 25 mL (50-mg vial), 50 mL (100-mg vial), or 75 mL (150-mg vial) of 0.9% sodium chloride injection to the vial and shaking to dissolve, producing a solution containing 2 mg of doxorubicin hydrochloride per mL. Use of bacteriostatic diluents is not recommended. An appropriate volume of air should be withdrawn from the vial during reconstitution to avoid excessive pressure buildup.

**Stability**
Reconstituted solutions of *Adriamycin RDF* are stable for 7 days at room temperature and under normal room light (100-foot candles) or 15 days between 2 and 8 °C (36 and 46 °F) when protected from sunlight. Unused solution from single-dose vials or unused solution from the multiple-dose vial remaining beyond the recommended storage time should be discarded.
Reconstituted solutions of *Rubex* or generic doxorubicin are stable for 24 hours at room temperature or 48 hours between 2 and 8 °C (36 and 46 °F). The solution should be protected from light and any unused solution should be discarded.

**Incompatibilities**
Doxorubicin should not be mixed with heparin, dexamethasone, fluorouracil, hydrocortisone sodium succinate, aminophylline, or cephalothin, since a precipitate may form.

**Note**
Great care should be taken to prevent inhalation of particles of doxorubicin hydrochloride and exposure of the skin to it. The use of gloves is recommended. Any doxorubicin powder or solution that comes in contact with the skin or mucosae should be washed off thoroughly with soap and water.

[1]Not included in Canadian product labeling.

Revised: 09/02/97
Interim revision: 06/17/98

# DOXORUBICIN, LIPOSOMAL   Systemic

VA CLASSIFICATION (Primary): AN200
Commonly used brand name(s): *Caelyx*; *Doxil*.
Note: For a listing of dosage forms and brand names by country availability, see *Dosage Forms* section(s).

## Category
Antineoplastic.

## Indications

**Accepted**
Note: Bracketed information in the *Indications* section refers to uses that are not included in U.S. product labeling.

Kaposi's sarcoma (KS), acquired immunodeficiency syndrome (AIDS)–associated (treatment)—Liposomal doxorubicin is indicated for treatment of patients with AIDS-associated KS disease that has progressed in spite of prior combination chemotherapy or patients who are intolerant of such therapy.
Note: The treatment of AIDS-associated KS is dependent on the extent and severity of the KS and the patient's clinical condition. For patients with minimal disease, local treatments such as excision, radiotherapy, or intralesional chemotherapy may be adequate. However, for those with severe cutaneous or systemic disease, systemic chemotherapy may be required. Patients with severe debilitation due to their general condition are best served by optimal palliative care.

[Carcinoma, ovarian][1]—Liposomal doxorubicin is indicated for treatment of refractory ovarian carcinoma.

[1]Not included in Canadian product labeling.

## Pharmacology/Pharmacokinetics

**Physicochemical characteristics**
Source—Doxorubicin is isolated from *Streptomyces peucetius* var. *caesius*. Liposomal doxorubicin is doxorubicin encapsulated in long-circulating liposomes. Liposomes are microscopic vesicles, composed of a phospholipid bilayer, that are capable of encapsulating active drugs. Liposomal doxorubicin is supplied as a sterile, translucent, red liposomal dispersion.
Molecular weight—579.99 (as hydrochloride).

**Mechanism of action/Effect**
Doxorubicin is an anthracycline cytostatic antibiotic with activity against a variety of malignancies including Kaposi's sarcoma (KS). Liposomal doxorubicin has been shown to inhibit the growth of KS cells both *in vitro* and *in vivo*. KS spindle cell cultures are more sensitive to lipo-

somal doxorubicin than are cultures of normal monocytes or normal endothelial or smooth muscle cells.

Tumor cell DNA fragmentation induced by doxorubicin is a result of topoisomerase II inhibition, which occurs when doxorubicin intercalates between DNA strands. The antitumor activity and toxicity of doxorubicin may also relate to the formation of intracellular oxygen free radicals, which are produced by reduction of the doxorubicin molecule. In addition, liposomal doxorubicin induces expression of monocyte chemoattractant protein-1, which results in intralesional recruitment of phagocytic cells in patients with KS.

The mechanism by which liposome encapsulation apparently enhances doxorubicin accumulation in lesions of acquired immunodeficiency syndrome (AIDS)–associated KS is not fully understood. However, polyethylene glycol (PEG)–containing liposomes of the same size and exhibiting approximately the same rate of plasma clearance as those used to encapsulate the doxorubicin, but containing entrapped colloidal gold designed to serve as a marker for following liposome distribution by light and electron microscopy, have been shown to enter solid colon tumors implanted in mice and KS-like lesions in human immunodeficiency virus (HIV)–transgenic mice.

Extravasation of liposomes also may occur by passage of the particles through endothelial cell gaps, which are reported to be present in certain solid tumors and which are known to be present in KS-like lesions. These processes may contribute to the enhanced accumulation of doxorubicin in lesions of AIDS-associated KS after administration of PEG-liposomal doxorubicin.

Once within the tumor, the active ingredient, doxorubicin, is presumably available to be released locally as the liposomes degrade and become permeable *in situ*.

**Distribution**
Limited to vascular fluid.
Vol$_D$—Steady-state: 2.7 to 2.8 liters per square meter of body surface area for doses of 20 and 10 mg per square meter of body surface area (mg/m$^2$), respectively.
Note: During circulation, at least 90% of liposomal doxorubicin remains encapsulated. This circulation is represented by a large area under the plasma concentration–time curve (AUC) of 277 and 590 mcg per mL (mcg/mL) per hour for doses of 10 and 20 mg/m$^2$, respectively.

**Protein binding**
Protein binding of liposomal doxorubicin has not been determined; however, the active ingredient, doxorubicin, binds extensively to tissues (70%).

**Biotransformation**
The major metabolite of standard doxorubicin is doxorubicinol; however, after administration of liposomal doxorubicin, neither doxorubicinol nor other metabolites were detectable in plasma. Metabolites of doxorubicin, including doxorubicinol and the sulfate and glucuronide conjugates of the 7-deoxyaglycones, were detected in small quantities in the urine.
The presence of small quantities of metabolites in urine, but not in plasma, indicates that liposomal doxorubicin probably undergoes metabolism similar to that of the standard formulation, but the rate of metabolite production is slower than the rate of metabolite elimination.

**Half-life**
First phase—4.7 and 5.2 hours for doses of 10 and 20 mg/m$^2$, respectively.
Second phase—52.3 and 55 hours for doses of 10 and 20 mg/m$^2$, respectively.

**Peak serum concentration**
4.1 and 8.3 mcg/mL for doses of 10 and 20 mg/m$^2$, respectively.

**Elimination**
Renal—Total plasma clearance of liposomal doxorubicin is slower than total plasma clearance of standard doxorubicin, with a rate of 0.041 and 0.056 liters per hour per square meter of body surface area (L/h/m$^2$) for doses of 20 and 10 mg/m$^2$, respectively.
Renal elimination of PEG-liposomal doxorubicin is slower than elimination of the standard doxorubicin; 5.5% of an injected dose of liposomal doxorubicin was recovered in urine after 72 hours, compared with 11% of an injected dose of standard doxorubicin after only 24 hours.

## Precautions to Consider

**Cross-sensitivity and/or related problems**
Patients hypersensitive to other doxorubicin formulations may be hypersensitive to liposomal doxorubicin also.

**Carcinogenicity/Mutagenicity**
Studies to evaluate the carcinogenic potential of liposomal doxorubicin injection have not been performed; however, the active ingredient, doxorubicin, is carcinogenic and mutagenic in experimental models. The liposome component of liposomal doxorubicin demonstrated no mutagenic effects in the Ames test, mouse lymphoma assay, an *in vitro* chromosomal aberration assay, and an *in vivo* mammalian micronucleus assay.

**Pregnancy/Reproduction**
Fertility—Adequate and well-controlled studies in humans have not been done. However, fertility studies in mice have shown that liposomal doxorubicin causes ovarian and testicular degeneration at five times the recommended human dose. Studies in dogs have shown that liposomal doxorubicin causes atrophy of the seminiferous tubules and diminished spermatogenesis at a dose equivalent to the recommended human dose. Studies in rats have shown that liposomal doxorubicin causes testicular degeneration at 7.7% of the recommended human dose.
Pregnancy—Adequate and well-controlled studies in humans have not been done. However, use is not recommended during pregnancy. Women of childbearing age should be advised to avoid pregnancy during treatment.
In general, use of a contraceptive method is recommended during cytotoxic drug therapy.
FDA Pregnancy Category D.

**Breast-feeding**
It is not known whether liposomal doxorubicin is distributed into breast milk. However, breast-feeding is not recommended while liposomal doxorubicin is being administered because of the potential risk of adverse reactions in the infant.

**Pediatrics**
Appropriate studies on the relationship of age to the effects of liposomal doxorubicin have not been performed in the pediatric population. Safety and efficacy have not been established. However, cardiotoxicity may occur frequently with the active ingredient, doxorubicin, in children up to 2 years of age.

**Geriatrics**
No information is available on the relationship of age to the effects of liposomal doxorubicin in geriatric patients. However, the active ingredient, doxorubicin, may increase the risk of cardiotoxicity in patients 70 years of age or older.

**Dental**
The leukopenic and thrombocytopenic effects of liposomal doxorubicin may result in an increased incidence of certain microbial infections of the mouth, delayed healing, and gingival bleeding. If leukopenia or thrombocytopenia occurs, dental work should be deferred until blood counts have returned to normal. Patients should be instructed in proper oral hygiene, including caution in use of regular toothbrushes, dental floss, and toothpicks.

**Drug interactions and/or related problems**
The following drug interactions and/or related problems have been selected on the basis of their potential clinical significance (possible mechanism in parentheses where appropriate)—not necessarily inclusive (» = major clinical significance):
Note: Combinations containing any of the following medications, depending on the amount present, may also interact with this medication.

» Anthracenedione antineoplastic agents, prior use of or
» Daunorubicin, prior use of or
» Doxorubicin, prior use of or
» Other anthracycline antineoplastics, prior use of
(use of liposomal doxorubicin in a patient who previously has received anthracenedione antineoplastic agents, daunorubicin, doxorubicin, or other anthracycline antineoplastics increases the risk of cardiotoxicity; dosage adjustment is necessary)

Blood dyscrasia–causing medications (see *Appendix II*)
(leukopenic and/or thrombocytopenic effects of liposomal doxorubicin may be increased with concurrent or recent therapy if these medications cause the same effects; dosage adjustment of liposomal doxorubicin, if necessary, should be based on blood counts)

» Bone marrow depressants, other (see *Appendix II*)
(additive bone marrow depression, including severe dermatitis and/or mucositis, may occur; dosage reduction may be required when two or more bone marrow depressants are used concurrently or consecutively)

Cyclophosphamide or
Dactinomycin or
Mitomycin or
Radiation therapy to mediastinal area
(concurrent use may result in increased cardiotoxicity)
(concurrent use of cyclophosphamide with liposomal doxorubicin may potentiate cyclophosphamide-induced hemorrhagic cystitis)

Hepatotoxic medications (see *Appendix II*)
(concurrent use may increase the risk of toxicity; for example, high-dose methotrexate may impair liver function and increase toxicity of subsequently administered liposomal doxorubicin)

Vaccines, killed virus
(because normal defense mechanisms may be suppressed by liposomal doxorubicin therapy, the patient's antibody response to the vaccine may be decreased. The interval between discontinuation of medications that cause immunosuppression and restoration of the patient's ability to respond to the vaccine depends on the intensity and type of immunosuppression-causing medication used, the underlying disease, and other factors; estimates vary from 3 months to 1 year)

» Vaccines, live virus
(because normal defense mechanisms may be suppressed by liposomal doxorubicin therapy, concurrent use with a live virus vaccine may potentiate the replication of the vaccine virus, may increase the side/adverse effects of the vaccine virus, and/or may decrease the patient's antibody response to the vaccine; immunization of these patients should be undertaken only with extreme caution after careful review of the patient's hematologic status and only with the knowledge and consent of the physician managing the liposomal doxorubicin therapy. The interval between discontinuation of medications that cause immunosuppression and restoration of the patient's ability to respond to the vaccine depends on the intensity and type of immunosuppression-causing medication used, the underlying disease, and other factors; estimates vary from 3 months to 1 year. Patients with leukemia in remission should not receive live virus vaccine until at least 3 months after their last chemotherapy. In addition, immunization with oral poliovirus vaccine should be postponed in persons in close contact with the patient, especially family members)

### Laboratory value alterations
The following have been selected on the basis of their potential clinical significance (possible effect in parentheses where appropriate)—not necessarily inclusive (» = major clinical significance):

With diagnostic test results
» Cardiac function tests
(echocardiography and radionuclide scans may be altered)

With physiology/laboratory test values
Alanine aminotransferase (ALT [SGPT]), serum
Alkaline phosphatase, serum or
Aspartate aminotransferase (AST [SGOT]), serum
(values may be increased)

Bilirubin, serum
(concentrations may be increased)

Blood urea nitrogen (BUN) or
Creatinine, serum
(values rarely may be increased)

Calcium, serum
(concentrations may be decreased)

Glucose, blood
(concentrations may be increased)

» Hemoglobin/hematocrit or
» Leukocyte counts or
» Platelet counts
(may be decreased)

Prothrombin time
(may be prolonged)

### Medical considerations/Contraindications
The medical considerations/contraindications included have been selected on the basis of their potential clinical significance (reasons given in parentheses where appropriate)—not necessarily inclusive (» = major clinical significance).

*Risk-benefit should be considered when the following medical problems exist:*

» Bone marrow depression
» Cardiovascular disease, history of
(may increase risk for cardiotoxicity)
» Chickenpox, existing or recent (including recent exposure) or
» Herpes zoster
(risk of severe generalized disease)
» Heart disease
(cardiotoxicity may occur at lower cumulative doses)

» Hepatic function impairment
(slowed excretion may occur. Reduction in dosage is recommended; one half of the normal dose is recommended in patients with serum bilirubin concentrations of 1.2 to 3 mg per 100 mL; one quarter of the normal dose is recommended in patients with serum bilirubin concentrations of greater than 3 mg per 100 mL)
» Sensitivity to doxorubicin or to liposomal components
» Tumor cell infiltration of the bone marrow
» Caution should be used also in patients with inadequate bone marrow reserves due to previous cytotoxic drug or radiation therapy.

### Patient monitoring
The following may be especially important in patient monitoring (other tests may be warranted in some patients, depending on condition; » = major clinical significance):

Alanine aminotransferase (ALT [SGPT]) values, serum and
Alkaline phosphatase values, serum and
Aspartate aminotransferase (AST [SGOT]) values, serum and
Bilirubin concentrations, serum
(recommended prior to initiation of therapy and at periodic intervals during therapy)

» Echocardiography and
Electrocardiogram (ECG) studies and
Radionuclide angiography determination of ejection fraction
(recommended prior to initiation of therapy and at periodic intervals during therapy)

» Hematocrit or hemoglobin and
» Leukocyte count, total and, if appropriate, differential and
» Platelet count
(determinations recommended prior to initiation of therapy and at periodic intervals during therapy)

## Side/Adverse Effects
Note: Clinical studies of liposomal doxorubicin to treat Kaposi's sarcoma (KS) were performed only in patients with acquired immunodeficiency syndrome (AIDS). Assessment of tolerability of liposomal doxorubicin is therefore complicated by underlying immune suppression and morbidity commonly present in these patients. Although liposomal doxorubicin was generally well tolerated, there was a strong likelihood that liposomal doxorubicin–related adverse effects would occur in the majority of the patients. In one study, 76% of patients reported at least one adverse effect that was probably or possibly related to liposomal doxorubicin and 30% of patients reported at least one severe adverse effect thought to be related to liposomal doxorubicin. However, the most common reason for termination of liposomal doxorubicin therapy in these studies was death from AIDS-related complications.

The following side/adverse effects have been selected on the basis of their potential clinical significance (possible signs and symptoms in parentheses where appropriate)—not necessarily inclusive:

### Those indicating need for medical attention
Incidence more frequent
*Anemia* (unusual tiredness or weakness); *asthenia* (loss of strength and energy); *infusion reactions* (chills; facial swelling; headache; low blood pressure; shortness of breath); *neutropenia* (fever and sore throat)—usually asymptomatic; *stomatitis* (sores in mouth and on lips); *thrombocytopenia* (black, tarry stools; unusual bleeding or bruising; blood in urine or stools; pinpoint red spots on skin)—usually asymptomatic

Note: Some patients may experience *infusion reactions* during the initial few minutes of the first infusion of liposomal doxorubicin. *Infusion reactions* will resolve upon cessation of infusion. However, these reactions often do not prevent further treatment with liposomal doxorubicin. Patients who do not experience *infusion reactions* during the first cycle of liposomal doxorubicin therapy are unlikely to react to subsequent cycles.

*Neutropenia* is the most common treatment-related side effect. In one study, 35% of enrolled patients had one or more episodes of grade 3 or 4 *neutropenia*. *Neutropenia* is manageable with the use of colony-stimulating factors. However, pre-existing immune system compromise complicates assessment of *neutropenia* and infectious events in patients with AIDS.

Incidence less frequent
*Allergic reaction* (chills; fever; skin rash or itching); *cardiotoxicity* (fast or irregular heartbeat; shortness of breath; swelling of the feet and lower legs); *dyspnea* (troubled breathing); *pain at injection site; palmar-plantar erythrodysesthesia* (reddening of skin; scaling of skin on hands

and feet; swelling of skin; ulceration of skin); **pneumonia** (cough; fever; shortness of breath; troubled breathing; wheezing); **postirradiation erythema, recall** (darkening or redness of skin); **tachycardia** (fast or irregular heartbeat)

  Note: Few data are available on the *cardiotoxicity* of liposomal doxorubicin. Although left ventricular failure has been reported in patients who received a high cumulative liposomal doxorubicin dose, some evidence suggests that the incidence and severity of these effects are lower than after similar doses of standard doxorubicin.

  *Palmar-plantar erythrodysesthesia*, characterized by ulceration, erythema, and desquamation on the hands and feet with pain and inflammation, occurs in some patients, most commonly after 6 to 8 weeks of treatment. At recommended dosages of liposomal doxorubicin, the incidence of this syndrome is less than 5%. Although reactions may occasionally be severe and debilitating, they are more often mild, and most patients with the syndrome do not require dosage reduction or prolonged treatment delay. However, in severe cases, *palmar-plantar erythrodysesthesia* can be managed by withholding treatment until its resolution and by resuming therapy with longer intervals between doses.

Incidence rare
  **Diabetes mellitus or hyperglycemia** (blurred vision; flushed, dry skin; frequent urination; fruit-like breath odor; unusual thirst); **jaundice** (yellowing of eyes and skin); **optic neuritis** (blurred vision; eye pain; loss of vision)

**Those indicating need for medical attention only if they continue or are bothersome**
Incidence more frequent
  **Diarrhea; nausea; vomiting**
Incidence less frequent
  **Back pain; constipation; dizziness; dysphagia** (difficulty swallowing); **headache**

**Those not indicating need for medical attention**
Incidence more frequent
  **Alopecia** (loss of hair)

**Those indicating the need for medical attention if they occur after medication is discontinued**
  **Cardiotoxicity** (fast or irregular heartbeat; shortness of breath; swelling of feet and lower legs)

## Overdose

For specific information on the agents used in the management of liposomal doxorubicin overdose, see:
- *Filgrastim* in *Colony Stimulating Factors (Systemic)* monograph; and/or
- *Sargramostim* in *Colony Stimulating Factors (Systemic)* monograph.

For more information on the management of overdose, **contact a Poison Control Center** (see *Poison Control Center Listing*).

**Clinical effects of overdose**
The following effects have been selected on the basis of their potential clinical significance (possible signs and symptoms in parentheses where appropriate)—not necessarily inclusive:

Acute
  **Mucositis** (sores in mouth and on lips); **neutropenia** (cough or hoarseness; fever or chills; lower back or side pain; painful or difficult urination)—usually asymptomatic; **thrombocytopenia** (black, tarry stools; unusual bleeding or bruising; blood in urine or stools; pinpoint red spots on skin)—usually asymptomatic

**Treatment of overdose**
Treatment of leukopenia includes antibiotic therapy and administration of colony stimulating factors (filgrastim [rG-CSF] or sargramostim [rGM-CSF]).
Treatment of thrombocytopenia includes hospitalization of the patient and platelet transfusions.

## Patient Consultation

As an aid to patient consultation, refer to *Advice for the Patient, Doxorubicin, Liposomal (Systemic)*.
In providing consultation, consider emphasizing the following selected information (» = major clinical significance):

**Before using this medication**
» Conditions affecting use, especially:
   Sensitivity to doxorubicin or liposomal component
   Pregnancy—Use is not recommended; women of childbearing age should be advised to avoid pregnancy during treatment
   Breast-feeding—Use is not recommended because of the potential for serious adverse effects in nursing infants
   Use in children—Cardiotoxicity in children younger than 2 years old may occur frequently
   Use in the elderly—Based on studies with the active ingredient, cardiotoxicity may be more frequent in patients 70 years of age and older
   Other medications, especially anthracenedione antineoplastic agents, daunorubicin, doxorubicin, live virus vaccines, other anthracycline antineoplastics, other bone marrow depressants, or previous cytotoxic drug or radiation therapy
   Other medical problems, especially bone marrow depression; cardiovascular disease, history of; chickenpox; heart disease; hepatic function impairment; herpes zoster; or tumor cell infiltration of bone marrow

**Proper use of this medication**
  Caution in taking combination therapy; taking each medication at the right time
  Importance of ample fluid intake and subsequent increase in urine output to aid in excretion of uric acid
  Frequency of nausea and vomiting; importance of continuing medication despite stomach upset
» Proper dosing

**Precautions while using this medication**
» Importance of close monitoring by the physician
» Avoiding immunizations unless approved by the physician; other persons in patient's household should avoid immunizations with oral poliovirus vaccine; avoiding persons who have taken oral poliovirus vaccine, or wearing a protective mask that covers nose and mouth
*Caution if bone marrow depression occurs*
» Avoiding exposure to persons with infections, especially during periods of low blood counts; checking with physician immediately if fever or chills, cough or hoarseness, lower back or side pain, or painful or difficult urination occurs
» Checking with physician immediately if unusual bleeding or bruising; black, tarry stools; blood in urine or stools; or pinpoint red spots on skin occur
  Caution in use of regular toothbrush, dental floss, or toothpick; physician, dentist, or nurse may suggest alternatives; checking with physician before having dental work done
  Not touching eyes or inside of nose unless hands washed immediately before
  Using caution to avoid accidental cuts with use of sharp objects such as safety razor or fingernail or toenail cutters
  Avoiding contact sports or other situations where bruising or injury could occur
» Telling doctor or nurse right away about redness, pain, or swelling at injection site

**Side/adverse effects**
  May cause adverse effects such as blood problems, loss of hair, and heart problems
  Signs of potential side effects, especially anemia; asthenia; infusion reaction; neutropenia; stomatitis; thrombocytopenia; allergic reaction; cardiotoxicity; dyspnea; pain at injection site; palmar-plantar erythrodysesthesia; pneumonia; postirradiation erythema, recall; tachycardia; diabetes mellitus or hyperglycemia; jaundice; and optic neuritis
  Physician or nurse can help in dealing with side effects
  Reddish urine for 1 to 2 days after administration may be alarming to patient although medically insignificant
  Possibility of hair loss; normal hair growth should resume after treatment has ended

## General Dosing Information

Patients receiving liposomal doxorubicin should be under the supervision of a physician experienced in cancer chemotherapy.

In patients with acquired immunodeficiency syndrome (AIDS)–associated Kaposi's sarcoma (KS) it is not known whether the combination of liposomal doxorubicin with other antineoplastic agents will improve response rates or quality of life (QOL) compared with currently used combination regimens or liposomal doxorubicin monotherapy. However, because tumor cells are heterogeneous and the development of tumor resistance to a single antineoplastic agent is probable, combinations of cancer chemotherapy agents generally are preferred to monotherapy. Nevertheless, liposomal doxorubicin is one of the most active single agents studied so far in patients with AIDS-associated KS. Furthermore, liposomal doxorubicin 20 mg per square meter of body surface area (mg/m$^2$) administered at 2- or 3-week intervals seems to be more efficacious than the best available combination regimens.

The recommended dose of liposomal doxorubicin for patients with AIDS-associated KS is 20 mg/m² administered intravenously over a period of 30 minutes at 3-week intervals. However, in several studies, liposomal doxorubicin was administered at 2-week intervals. Doses as high as 40 mg/m² and treatment intervals of 1 week have been evaluated in patients with KS, but offer no clear advantages over 20 mg/m² administered every 2 or 3 weeks.

Liposomal doxorubicin should be used with caution in patients who have previously received complete cumulative doses of other anthracycline or anthracenedione agents.

Unlike extravasation of standard doxorubicin, which may result in severe local inflammation and tissue damage, extravasation of liposomal doxorubicin was associated with only transient, mild irritation at the infusion site. However, liposomal doxorubicin should be considered an irritant and precautions should be taken to avoid extravasation. If extravasation of liposomal doxorubicin occurs during intravenous administration, as indicated by local burning or stinging (may also be painless), the infusion should be stopped immediately, and resumed, completing the dose, in another vein. Application of ice packs to the site of extravasation for 30 minutes may be necessary to relieve symptoms.

Patients who develop thrombocytopenia may require platelet transfusions.

Patients who develop leukopenia should be observed carefully for signs of infection. Antibiotic support may be required. Use of colony stimulating factors may be necessary.

Acute infusion-related hypersensitivity reactions can occur in some patients during the first infusion of liposomal doxorubicin, usually within the first few minutes after the start of the infusion. These acute reactions do not appear to occur with subsequent doses of liposomal doxorubicin in patients who do not react to the first cycle. Reactions generally resolve within 1 day once the infusion is terminated. Slowing the infusion rate can sometimes eliminate this problem. Most patients who react to liposomal doxorubicin are able to tolerate further infusions without complication.

The pharmacokinetics of liposomal doxorubicin have not been studied in patients with hepatic impairment. However, standard doxorubicin is known to be eliminated in large part by the liver. Therefore, dosage of liposomal doxorubicin should be reduced for patients with impaired hepatic function. A dose reduction of 50% is recommended if serum bilirubin concentrations are 1.2 to 3 mg per deciliter (mg/dL). A dose reduction of 75% is recommended if serum bilirubin concentrations are > 3 mg/dL.

Dosage adjustment or discontinuation of therapy may be necessary for patients who experience stomatitis, bone marrow depression, or palmar-plantar erythrodysesthesia.

### Safety considerations for handling this medication
There is limited but increasing evidence and concern that personnel involved in preparation and administration of parenteral antineoplastic agents may be at some risk because of the potential mutagenicity, teratogenicity, and/or carcinogenicity of these agents, although the actual risk is unknown. USP advisory panels recommend cautious handling both in preparation and disposal of antineoplastic agents. Precautions that have been suggested include:
- Use of a biological containment cabinet during reconstitution and dilution of parenteral medications and wearing of disposable surgical gloves and masks.
- Use of proper technique to prevent contamination of the medication, work area, and operator during transfer between containers (including proper training of personnel in this technique).
- Cautious and proper disposal of needles, syringes, vials, ampuls, and unused medication.

A number of medical centers have developed detailed guidelines for handling of antineoplastic agents.

## Parenteral Dosage Forms

Note: Bracketed uses in the *Dosage Forms* section refer to categories of use and/or indications that are not included in U.S. product labeling.

## DOXORUBICIN, LIPOSOMAL INJECTION

### Usual adult dose
Kaposi's sarcoma (KS), acquired immunodeficiency syndrome (AIDS)–associated—
  Intravenous infusion (over thirty minutes), 20 mg per square meter of body surface area, repeated every three weeks, for as long as patient responds satisfactorily and tolerates treatment.

Note: Although AIDS-associated KS may respond to treatment with single or multiagent chemotherapy, disease recurrence is common because the underlying immunodeficiency is unremitting. Thus, multiple courses of therapy may be required to control the disease. This repeated use of cytotoxic chemotherapy in patients with AIDS can cause significant morbidity.

[Carcinoma, ovarian][1]—
  Intravenous infusion (over one to two hours), 40 to 50 mg per square meter of body surface area, repeated every four weeks, for as long as patient responds satisfactorily and tolerates treatment.

### Usual pediatric dose
Safety and efficacy have not been established.

### Size(s) usually available
U.S.—
  2 mg per mL (single-dose vial) (Rx) [*Doxil* (ammonium sulfate 2 mg; histidine; sucrose)].
Canada—
  2 mg per mL (single-dose vial) (Rx) [*Caelyx* (ammonium sulfate 2 mg; histidine; sucrose)].

### Packaging and storage
Store between 2 and 8 °C (36 and 46 °F). Do not freeze for longer than 1 month.

### Preparation of dosage form
Liposomal doxorubicin (up to a maximum of 90 mg) must be diluted in 250 mL of 5% dextrose injection for administration by intravenous infusion.

### Stability
Diluted liposomal doxorubicin is stable for 24 hours when stored between 2 and 8 °C (36 and 46 °F). Undiluted liposomal doxorubicin contains no preservatives or bacteriostatic agents. Aseptic techniques should be observed when handling liposomal doxorubicin.

Do not freeze for longer than 1 month. Long-term freezing may harm the liposomal component.

### Incompatibilities
Liposomal doxorubicin should be diluted only in 5% dextrose injection. Liposomal doxorubicin should not be mixed with other medications, other diluents, or bacteriostatic agents. Mixing liposomal doxorubicin with any other diluent may cause precipitation.

### Caution
Do not use if a precipitate is present.

### Note
Liposomal doxorubicin is a red, translucent dispersion. In-line filters should not be used because liposomal doxorubicin is not a clear solution.

Great care should be taken to prevent exposure of the skin to liposomal doxorubicin. The use of gloves is recommended. Any liposomal doxorubicin solution that comes into contact with the skin or mucosa should be washed off thoroughly with soap and water.

[1]Not included in Canadian product labeling.

Developed: 06/30/98
Interim revision: 08/04/98

---

# DOXYCYCLINE—See *Tetracyclines (Systemic)*

---

# DOXYLAMINE—See *Antihistamines (Systemic)*

---

# DRONABINOL  Systemic

VA CLASSIFICATION (Primary/Secondary): GA700/GA900
Note: Controlled substance classification—
  U.S.: Schedule II.
  Canada: N.

Commonly used brand name(s): *Marinol*.

Another commonly used name is delta-9-tetrahydrocannabinol (THC).

Note: For a listing of dosage forms and brand names by country availability, see *Dosage Forms* section(s).

## Category
Antiemetic; appetite stimulant.

## Indications

**Accepted**

Nausea and vomiting, cancer chemotherapy–induced (prophylaxis)—Dronabinol is indicated in selected patients for the prevention of nausea and vomiting associated with emetogenic cancer chemotherapy when other antiemetic medications are not effective.

Anorexia, AIDS-associated (treatment)—Dronabinol is indicated for the treatment of anorexia associated with weight loss in patients with acquired immunodeficiency syndrome (AIDS). Tachyphylaxis and tolerance to some effects of dronabinol develop with chronic use; unlike cardiovascular and subjective adverse CNS effects, the appetite stimulant effects of dronabinol have been sustained for up to 5 months in AIDS patients receiving doses ranging from 2.5 to 20 mg per day.

## Pharmacology/Pharmacokinetics

**Physicochemical characteristics**
Chemical group—A cannabinoid.
Molecular weight—314.47.
pKa—10.6.

**Mechanism of action/Effect**
The exact mechanism of action of dronabinol is not known. Cannabinoid receptors in neural tissues may mediate the effects of dronabinol and other cannabinoids. Animal studies with other cannabinoids suggest that dronabinol's antiemetic effects may be due to inhibition of the vomiting control mechanism in the medulla oblongata.

**Other actions/effects**
Central sympathomimetic activity may result in tachycardia and/or conjunctival injection. Dose-related reversible effects on appetite, mood, cognition, memory, and perception also occur, subject to great interpatient variability.

**Absorption**
Although dronabinol is 90 to 95% absorbed after administration of single oral doses, only 10 to 20% reaches the systemic circulation, due to first-pass hepatic metabolism and high lipid solubility.

**Distribution**
Apparent volume of distribution is approximately 10 liters per kilogram (L/kg).
Distributed into breast milk.

**Protein binding**
Very high (97%).

**Biotransformation**
Extensive first-pass hepatic metabolism, primarily by microsomal hydroxylation, yields both active and inactive metabolites. Dronabinol and its principal active metabolite, 11-OH-delta-9-THC, are present in approximately equal concentrations in plasma.

**Half-life**
Elimination—
  Alpha phase: 4 hours.
  Terminal (beta) phase: 25 to 36 hours.

**Time to peak concentration**
2 to 4 hours.

**Duration of action**
Psychoactive effects—4 to 6 hours.
Appetite stimulant effects—24 hours or longer.

**Elimination**
Primarily fecal; approximately 50% of an oral dose appears in the feces and 10 to 15% in the urine (either as unchanged drug or as metabolite), within 72 hours.

## Precautions to Consider

**Cross-sensitivity and/or related problems**
Patients sensitive to other marijuana products or sesame oil may be sensitive to this preparation also.

**Carcinogenicity**
Studies to evaluate the carcinogenic potential of dronabinol have not been performed.

**Mutagenicity**
Dronabinol was not shown to be mutagenic in an Ames test.

**Pregnancy/Reproduction**
Fertility—In a long-term study in rats at doses 0.3 to 1.5 times the maximum recommended human dose (MRHD) in cancer patients or 2 to 10 times the MRHD in AIDS patients, a decrease in seminal fluid volume, as well as reduced ventral prostate, seminal vesicle, and epididymal weights were reported. Decreases in spermatogenesis, number of developing germ cells, and number of Leydig cells in the testes were also observed. However, sperm count, mating success, and testosterone levels were not affected. The significance of these animal findings for use in humans is not known.

Pregnancy—Adequate and well-controlled studies in humans have not been done.

Reproduction studies in mice (at doses 0.2 to 5 times the MRHD in cancer patients and 1 to 30 times the MRHD in AIDS patients) and in rats (at doses 0.8 to 3 times the MRHD in cancer patients and 5 to 20 times the MRHD in AIDS patients) have revealed no evidence of teratogenicity. However, dose-dependent effects of dronabinol, including decreased maternal weight gain and number of viable pups, and increased fetal mortality and early resorptions were observed.

FDA Pregnancy Category C.

**Breast-feeding**
Use is not recommended since dronabinol is distributed into and concentrated in breast milk and is absorbed by the nursing infant.

**Pediatrics**
No information is available on whether the risk of dronabinol-induced adverse effects is increased in children. However, because of this medication's psychoactive effects and potential for dependence, it should be used with caution, after less toxic alternatives have been considered and found ineffective. Recommended doses should not be exceeded, and children should be carefully monitored during therapy.

**Geriatrics**
Studies performed in a limited number of patients up to 82 years of age have not demonstrated geriatrics-specific problems that would limit the usefulness of dronabinol in the elderly. However, because of this medication's psychoactive effects and potential for creating dependency, therapy could be more troublesome in the elderly and should be used with caution, after less toxic alternatives have been considered and found ineffective. Recommended doses should not be exceeded, and the elderly patient should be carefully monitored during therapy.

**Drug interactions and/or related problems**
The following drug interactions and/or related problems have been selected on the basis of their potential clinical significance (possible mechanism in parentheses where appropriate)—not necessarily inclusive (» = major clinical significance):

Note: Combinations containing any of the following medications, depending on the amount present, may also interact with this medication.

Alcohol or
» Central nervous system (CNS) depression–producing medications, other (See *Appendix II*)
  (concurrent use may potentiate the CNS depressant effects of either these medications or dronabinol)

Apomorphine
  (prior administration of dronabinol may decrease the emetic response to apomorphine; also, concurrent use may potentiate the CNS depressant effects of either apomorphine or dronabinol)

**Medical considerations/Contraindications**
The medical considerations/contraindications included have been selected on the basis of their potential clinical significance (reasons given in parentheses where appropriate)—not necessarily inclusive (» = major clinical significance).

*Risk-benefit should be considered when the following medical problems exist:*

Cardiac disorders
  (dronabinol may cause cardiac effects including occasional hypotension, hypertension, syncope, and tachycardia)

Drug abuse or dependence, history of, including acute alcoholism
  (increased risk of dronabinol abuse and dependence)

Hypertension
  (increase in sympathomimetic activity may exacerbate condition)

Manic or depressive states or
Schizophrenia
  (symptoms may be exacerbated)

Sensitivity to dronabinol or sesame oil

**Patient monitoring**
The following may be especially important in patient monitoring (other tests may be warranted in some patients, depending on condition; » = major clinical significance):

Blood pressure determinations and
Cardiac function monitoring
(recommended for early detection of tachycardia and changes in blood pressure, especially in patients with hypertension or cardiac disease)

## Side/Adverse Effects

Note: Following abrupt withdrawal of dronabinol, an abstinence syndrome manifested by irritability, insomnia, and restlessness was observed within 12 hours in volunteers receiving dosages of 210 mg per day for 12 to 16 consecutive days; approximately 24 hours later, the withdrawal syndrome intensified with such symptoms as hot flashes, sweating, rhinorrhea, loose stools, hiccups, and anorexia. Withdrawal symptoms dissipated gradually over the next 48 hours. Electroencephalographic changes consistent with the hyperexcitation effects of drug withdrawal were recorded in patients after abrupt discontinuation.

Sleep disturbances, which continued for several weeks after discontinuation of high-dose dronabinol therapy, have been reported.

Although chronic abuse of cannabis has been associated with decreases in motivation, cognition, judgment, and perception, no such decrements in psychological, social, or neurological status have been associated with the administration of dronabinol for therapeutic purposes. In an open-label study in patients with AIDS who received dronabinol for up to 5 months, no abuse, diversion, or systematic change in personality or social functioning was observed, even in those patients with a history of drug abuse.

The following side/adverse effects have been selected on the basis of their potential clinical significance (possible signs and symptoms in parentheses where appropriate)—not necessarily inclusive:

**Those indicating need for medical attention**
Incidence less frequent
*Fast or pounding heartbeat; psychotomimetic effects* (changes in mood; confusion, including delusions and feelings of depersonalization or unreality; hallucinations; mental depression; nervousness or anxiety)

Note: The above side/adverse effects may also be symptoms of overdose.
An initial tachycardia may be followed by normal sinus rhythm and then bradycardia. These effects may disappear when tolerance develops after continued use.

**Those indicating need for medical attention only if they continue or are bothersome**
Incidence more frequent
*Clumsiness or unsteadiness; dizziness; drowsiness; nausea; trouble thinking; vomiting*
Incidence less frequent or rare
*Blurred vision or any changes in vision; dryness of mouth; orthostatic hypotension* (feeling faint or lightheaded; unusual tiredness or weakness); *restlessness*

## Overdose

For specific information on the agents used in the management of dronabinol overdose, see:
- Diazepam in *Benzodiazepines (Systemic)* monograph.

For more information on the management of overdose or unintentional ingestion, **contact a Poison Control Center** (see *Poison Control Center Listing*).

**Clinical effects of overdose**
The following effects have been selected on the basis of their potential clinical significance (possible signs and symptoms in parentheses where appropriate)—not necessarily inclusive:

*Mild intoxication*
*Heightened sensory awareness* (change in your sense of smell, taste, sight, sound, or touch)); *altered time perception* (change in how fast you think time is passing); *reddened conjunctiva* (redness of eyes)

*Moderate intoxication*
*Memory impairment* (being forgetful); *urinary retention* (problems in urinating); *reduced bowel motility* (constipation)

*Severe intoxication*
*Slurred speech*

**Treatment of overdose**
Overdose may occur either with therapeutic doses or with higher, nontherapeutic doses. Recommended treatment includes:
To decrease absorption—Gut decontamination, if ingestion is recent.

Specific treatment—Treatment of hypertension or hypotension, if necessary. Hypotension usually responds to Trendelenburg position and administration of IV fluids. Pressors are rarely required. Administration of benzodiazepines (5 to 10 mg of diazepam orally) may be used to treat extreme agitation.

Monitoring—Observation of patient in a quiet environment. Continuous blood pressure monitoring. Cardiac monitoring.

Supportive care—Supportive therapy. Patients in whom intentional overdose is confirmed or suspected should be referred for psychiatric consultation.

## Patient Consultation

As an aid to patient consultation, refer to *Advice for the Patient, Dronabinol (Systemic)*.

In providing consultation, consider emphasizing the following selected information (» = major clinical significance):

**Before using this medication**
» Conditions affecting use, especially:
Sensitivity to marijuana products or sesame oil
Pregnancy—No studies in humans; increased risk of fetal mortality and resorptions in animal studies with doses many times the usual human dose
Breast-feeding—Not recommended; distributed into breast milk
Use in children—Caution recommended because of psychoactive effects and potential for dependence
Use in the elderly—Caution recommended because of psychoactive effects and potential for dependence
Other medications, especially CNS depressants

**Proper use of this medication**
» Importance of not taking more medication than the amount prescribed because of danger of overdose
» Proper dosing
Missed dose: Taking as soon as possible; not taking if almost time for next dose; not doubling doses
» Proper storage

**Precautions while using this medication**
» Avoiding use of alcohol or other CNS depressants during therapy
» Caution if dizziness, drowsiness, lightheadedness, or false sense of well-being occurs
» Caution when getting up suddenly from a lying or sitting position
» Suspected overdose: Getting emergency help at once

**Side/adverse effects**
Signs of potential side effects, especially psychotomimetic effects and tachycardia

## General Dosing Information

Because of the potential for abuse and risk of diversion, the amount of dronabinol dispensed should be limited to the amount necessary for the period between clinic visits.

Patients should remain under the supervision of a responsible adult during initial use of dronabinol and following dosage adjustments. Also, patients taking dronabinol should be advised of possible changes in mood and other adverse behavioral effects of the medication, so that occurrence of such effects will not be alarming.

Psychological and physical dependence may occur with high doses or chronic administration of dronabinol; an abstinence syndrome may be precipitated when dronabinol is discontinued. However, this is very unlikely to occur with therapeutic doses and short-term use of dronabinol.

## Oral Dosage Forms

### DRONABINOL CAPSULES USP

**Usual adult and adolescent dose**
Antiemetic—
Oral, 5 mg per square meter of body surface one to three hours prior to the administration of chemotherapy, then every two to four hours after chemotherapy, for a total of four to six doses a day.

Note: The dose may be increased by increments of 2.5 mg per square meter of body surface if initial dose is ineffective and side effects are not significant.

Appetite stimulant—
Oral, initially 2.5 mg two times a day, before lunch and supper. Patients unable to tolerate this dose may be given 2.5 mg a day, administered as a single dose in the evening or at bedtime. The dose may be increased, if clinically indicated and in the absence of significant adverse effects, to a maximum of 20 mg a day; however, the inci-

dence of psychiatric symptoms increases significantly at maximum doses.

**Usual adult prescribing limits**
Antiemetic—
  Up to 15 mg per square meter of body surface per dose.
Appetite stimulant—
  20 mg a day.

**Usual pediatric dose**
See *Usual adult and adolescent dose.*

**Usual geriatric dose**
See *Usual adult and adolescent dose.*

**Strength(s) usually available**
U.S.—
  2.5 mg (Rx) [*Marinol* (sesame oil)].
  5 mg (Rx) [*Marinol* (sesame oil)].
  10 mg (Rx) [*Marinol* (sesame oil)].

Canada—
  2.5 mg (Rx) [*Marinol*].
  5 mg (Rx) [*Marinol*].

**Packaging and storage**
Store between 8 and 15 °C (46 and 59 °F), in a well-closed container, unless otherwise specified by manufacturer. Protect from freezing.

**Auxiliary labeling**
• Refrigerate.
• May cause drowsiness.
• Avoid alcoholic beverages.
• May be habit-forming.

**Note**
Controlled substance in the U.S.

Revised: 06/07/93

---

# DROPERIDOL  Systemic

VA CLASSIFICATION (Primary/Secondary): CN206/GA605; CN709
Commonly used brand name(s): *Inapsine.*
Note: For a listing of dosage forms and brand names by country availability, see *Dosage Forms* section(s).

## Category
Anesthesia, adjunct; antiemetic; antipsychotic.

## Indications
Note: Bracketed information in the *Indications* section refers to uses that are not included in U.S. product labeling.

### General considerations
Most of the adult patients included in published clinical trials of droperidol for prophylaxis of postoperative nausea and vomiting were women. Many of the trials involved gynecologic surgery. In these trials, droperidol was superior to placebo and usually equal to ondansetron in preventing postoperative nausea and vomiting. High-dose droperidol (i.e., 2.5 mg) was found to be superior to ondansetron (8 mg) in preventing postoperative nausea and vomiting in one trial; however, the patients receiving high-dose droperidol experienced increased sedation and delayed arousal compared to those receiving ondansetron. The degree to which these findings can be generalized to other types of surgery and male patients is not clear.

Most published trials in pediatric patients administered droperidol for prophylaxis of postoperative nausea and vomiting were placebo-controlled trials in strabismus surgery. Although droperidol was more effective than placebo, these studies did not establish the role of droperidol as compared to other antiemetic agents. In one trial in pediatric patients undergoing tonsillectomy, ondansetron was more effective than droperidol in preventing postoperative nausea and vomiting.

Although droperidol is not approved by the FDA to control severe agitation and combativeness, it can be used for this indication. Compared to haloperidol, droperidol is more sedating and controls agitation more quickly. Some, but not all, USP medical experts do not regard droperidol as first-line therapy for this indication.

Although droperidol is approved for use as an adjunctive agent in anesthesia, some USP medical experts do not regard droperidol as a first-line choice for use in anesthesia. When droperidol is used as an adjunctive agent in anesthesia, USP medical experts recommend lower doses than those indicated in the drug labeling.

### Accepted
Anesthesia, general, adjunct or
Anesthesia, local, adjunct—Droperidol is indicated for use in anesthesia as premedication and for adjunctive use in the induction and maintenance of general and regional anesthesia. Droperidol combined with an opioid analgesic induces neuroleptanalgesia to produce tranquility and decrease anxiety and pain.

Nausea and vomiting (prophylaxis)—Droperidol is indicated for the prevention of postoperative nausea and vomiting.

Droperidol is effective in controlling postoperative nausea and vomiting in children undergoing strabismus repair.

Droperidol has been used as part of a regimen to control nausea and vomiting associated with emetogenic chemotherapy; however, droperidol is considered to be only moderately effective in preventing chemotherapy-associated nausea and vomiting.

Sedation, conscious—Droperidol is indicated to produce sedation without loss of consciousness in patients undergoing various diagnostic procedures.

[*Psychotic disorder (treatment)*][1]—Droperidol is indicated in the treatment of acute psychotic episodes manifested by severe agitation and combativeness (Evidence rating: I). In a comparative study with haloperidol, intramuscular administration of 5 mg of droperidol provided more rapid control of symptoms than an equal dose of haloperidol, without an increase in adverse effects.

### Unaccepted
Droperidol has been used in the treatment of Meniere's disease, but it has been replaced by safer and more effective agents.

[1]Not included in Canadian product labeling.

## Pharmacology/Pharmacokinetics

### Physicochemical characteristics
Chemical group—A butyrophenone neuroleptic, chemically related to haloperidol.
Molecular weight—379.44.
pH—Saturated solution at ambient temperature: 7.
Droperidol injection has lactic acid added to the formulation to adjust the pH to 3 to 3.8.
pKa—7.64.
Solubility—Practically insoluble in water; slightly soluble in methanol and ethanol.
Partition coefficient—The log-partition coefficient (n-octanol/aqueous buffer at pH 9.9) is 3.58.

### Mechanism of action/Effect
The mechanism of action of droperidol is not known. It has been theorized that droperidol may bind postsynaptic gamma-aminobutyric acid (GABA) receptors. Binding of GABA receptors in the chemoreceptor trigger zone (CTZ) may be the mechanism by which droperidol produces an antiemetic effect. Droperidol may block dopaminergic receptors in the caudate nucleus and in the nucleus accumbens.

### Other actions/effects
Droperidol selectively blocks postsynaptic alpha-adrenergic receptors. This action may cause vasodilation and hypotension.
Droperidol causes a small, but statistically significant, prolongation of the QT interval.

### Absorption
Completely absorbed after intramuscular administration.

### Distribution
Volume of distribution at steady state (Vol$_{DSS}$)—
  Adults:
    1.5 L per kg of body weight (L/kg).
  Children:
    0.58 L/kg.

### Biotransformation
Extensively metabolized.

### Half-life
Distribution—
  Droperidol has biphasic distribution. The rapid distribution phase is 1.4 ± 0.5 minutes and the slower distribution phase is 14.3 ± 6.5 minutes.

Elimination—
 Adults: 134 ± 13 minutes; may be increased in geriatric patients.
 Children: 101.5 ± 26.4 minutes.

**Onset of action**
3 to 10 minutes.

**Time to peak effect**
Within 30 minutes of administration.

**Duration of action**
The duration of the sedative effects is 2 to 4 hours, although alteration of alertness may persist for up to 12 hours.

**Elimination**
Renal—
 About 75% of intramuscularly administered droperidol is excreted in the urine; only 1% is excreted unchanged.
Biliary/fecal—
 22% of intramuscularly administered droperidol is excreted in the feces; the high fraction of droperidol excreted in the feces suggests biliary excretion.

## Precautions to Consider

**Cross-sensitivity and/or related problems**
Patients sensitive to other butyrophenones may be sensitive to droperidol also.

**Carcinogenicity**
Carcinogenicity studies have not been done with droperidol.

**Mutagenicity**
The micronucleus test in female rats revealed no mutagenicity after single doses of up to 160 mg per kg of body weight.

**Pregnancy/Reproduction**
Pregnancy—Droperidol has been used in pregnant patients to manage hyperemesis gravidarum. Compared to the control group, the mean birth weight and the incidence of premature birth were not different in the neonates born to droperidol-treated mothers. A similar number of congenital anomalies occurred in the two groups.
FDA Pregnancy Category C.
Labor and delivery—Droperidol has been used in patients undergoing cesarean section. Respiratory depression in the neonates has not been reported.

**Breast-feeding**
Droperidol is distributed into breast milk. Although problems in humans have not been documented, the manufacturer recommends breast-feeding be avoided in patients using droperidol.

**Pediatrics**
Although patients under 2 years of age have been included in some clinical trials, no information is available on the relationship of age to the effects of droperidol in these pediatric patients; safety and efficacy have not been established.
The comparative incidence of extrapyramidal effects from droperidol in pediatric patients as compared to adult patients is not known. However, pediatric patients are more likely than adult patients to experience extrapyramidal reactions after receiving haloperidol. It is expected that pediatric patients may be more likely than adult patients to experience extrapyramidal effects from droperidol also. Of the extrapyramidal effects, acute dystonic effects are more likely in pediatric patients.

**Geriatrics**
Geriatric patients may be more sensitive to the sedating effects of droperidol; in addition, geriatric patients may be more likely to experience hypotension.

**Drug interactions and/or related problems**
The following drug interactions and/or related problems have been selected on the basis of their potential clinical significance (possible mechanism in parentheses where appropriate)—not necessarily inclusive (» = major clinical significance):

Note: Combinations containing any of the following medications, depending on the amount present, may also interact with this medication.
 Anesthetics, parenteral-local
  (peripheral vasodilation and hypotension due to sympathetic blockade may occur)
 Bromocriptine or
 Levodopa
  (dopamine agonists may be inhibited by droperidol)

Central nervous system (CNS) depression–producing medications (see *Appendix II*), including medications commonly used for anesthesia and analgesia
 (additive CNS depression may occur; lower doses may be needed)
Epinephrine
 (droperidol may antagonize the pressor effects of epinephrine, and may trigger a hypotensive episode)
Extrapyramidal reaction–causing medications, other (see *Appendix II*)
 (may increase the frequency and severity of extrapyramidal effects)
Hypotension-producing medications (see *Appendix II*)
 (orthostatic hypotension may occur; hypotension is especially likely if droperidol is used concurrently with drugs causing vasodilation)
Propofol
 (droperidol may compete with propofol for binding sites in the chemoreceptor trigger zone; concurrent use of propofol and droperidol to control nausea and vomiting is less effective than using propofol alone)

**Laboratory value alterations**
The following have been selected on the basis of their potential clinical significance (possible effect in parentheses where appropriate)—not necessarily inclusive (» = major clinical significance):

With physiology/laboratory test values
 Electrocardiogram
  (droperidol may cause prolongation of the QT interval)
 Prolactin, serum
  (droperidol causes dose-dependent increase in serum prolactin)

**Medical considerations/Contraindications**
The medical considerations/contraindications included have been selected on the basis of their potential clinical significance (reasons given in parentheses where appropriate)—not necessarily inclusive (» = major clinical significance).

*Except under special circumstances, this medication should not be used when the following medical problems exist:*
» Hypokalemia or
» Hypomagnesemia or
» QT interval prolongation, pre-existing
  (risk of arrhythmia, rarely including sudden death, may be increased)
» Hypersensitivity to droperidol
» Pheochromocytoma
  (hypertension and tachycardia may occur)

*Risk-benefit should be considered when the following medical problems exist:*
» Alcoholism, acute
  (risk of arrhythmia, rarely including sudden death, may be increased, especially with use of large doses of droperidol)
 Cardiovascular function impairment or
 Epilepsy or
 Mental depression, severe or
» Parkinsonism
  (may worsen condition)
 Hepatic function impairment
  (metabolism may be altered)
 Hypovolemia
  (risk of hypotension may be increased)

**Patient monitoring**
The following may be especially important in patient monitoring (other tests may be warranted in some patients, depending on condition; » = major clinical significance):

Blood pressure and
Body temperature and
Heart rate and
Respiratory and ventilatory status
 (routine monitoring of vital signs is recommended)
Electrocardiogram
 (recommended for patients receiving prolonged therapy with droperidol for agitation, and for patients with pre-existing heart rhythm abnormalities)
Motor functioning
 (recommended to monitor for extrapyramidal effects)

## Side/Adverse Effects

The following side/adverse effects have been selected on the basis of their potential clinical significance (possible signs and symptoms in parentheses where appropriate)—not necessarily inclusive:

**Those indicating need for medical attention**
Incidence less frequent
   *Akathisia* (restlessness)—extrapyramidal reaction; *anxiety*—extrapyramidal reaction; *hypertension* (high blood pressure)—asymptomatic
   Note: *Hypertension* has occurred following the use of droperidol combined with an opioid analgesic (e.g., fentanyl) and may be due to surgical stimulation during light anesthesia.
Incidence rare
   *Dystonia* (spasm of the muscles of the tongue, face, neck, and back)—extrapyramidal reaction; *hyperpyrexia* (fever)—may indicate neuroleptic malignant syndrome; *oculogyric crisis* (fixed upward position of eyeballs)—extrapyramidal reaction

**Those indicating need for medical attention only if they continue or are bothersome**
Incidence more frequent
   *Hypotension* (lightheadedness)—usually transient; *excessive sedation* (drowsiness); *tachycardia* (rapid heart rate)

**Those indicating possible extrapyramidal reaction and the need for medical attention if they occur after medication is discontinued**
   *Akathisia* (restlessness); *dystonia* (spasm of the muscles of the tongue, face, neck, and back); *oculogyric crisis* (fixed upward position of eyeballs)
   Note: *Dystonia* has been reported up to 30 hours after administration of a dose of droperidol.

## Overdose

For specific information on the agents used in the management of droperidol overdose, see:
- *Benztropine* in *Antidyskinetics (Systemic)* monograph;
- *Diphenhydramine* in *Antihistamines (Systemic)* monograph; and/or
- *Phenylephrine* in *Sympathomimetic Agents—Cardiovascular Use (Parenteral-Systemic)* monograph.

For more information on the management of overdose or unintentional ingestion, **contact a Poison Control Center** (see *Poison Control Center Listing*).

**Clinical effects of overdose**
The following effects have been selected on the basis of their potential clinical significance (possible signs and symptoms in parentheses where appropriate)—not necessarily inclusive:
Acute and/or chronic
   *Akathisia* (restlessness); *dystonia* (spasm of the muscles of the tongue, face, neck, and back); *hypotension* (dizziness); *prolongation of QT interval*—usually asymptomatic; *oculogyric crisis* (fixed upward position of eyeballs); *respiratory depression* (slowed breathing)
   Note: *Akathisia, dystonia,* and *oculogyric crisis* are effects that can occur with overdose of droperidol. However, these effects can also occur with usual therapeutic doses of droperidol.

**Treatment of overdose**
Discontinue droperidol.
Specific treatment—Extrapyramidal reactions (e.g., akathisia, dystonia, and oculogyric crisis) may be treated with anticholinergic agents such as benztropine or diphenhydramine.
Supportive care—A patent airway must be maintained, and respiration should be assisted or controlled if necessary. Oxygen should be administered. Blood pressure should be supported as needed. Phenylephrine may be needed to counteract the alpha-blocking effects of droperidol. In hypovolemic patients, administration of intravenous fluids may be required. Patients in whom intentional overdose is confirmed or suspected should be referred for psychiatric consultation.

## Patient Consultation

As an aid to patient consultation, refer to *Advice for the Patient, Droperidol (Systemic)*.
In providing consultation, consider emphasizing the following selected information (» = major clinical significance):

**Before using this medication**
» Conditions affecting use, especially:
   Hypersensitivity to droperidol
   Breast-feeding—Temporary discontinuation of breast-feeding is recommended in patients receiving droperidol, because droperidol is distributed into breast milk
   Use in children—Children may be more likely than adult patients to experience extrapyramidal effects
   Use in the elderly—Older patients may be more likely to experience drowsiness and hypotension
   Other medical problems, especially acute alcoholism, hypokalemia, hypomagnesemia, parkinsonism, pheochromocytoma or pre-existing QT interval prolongation

**Proper use of this medication**
» Proper dosing

**Precautions after receiving this medication**
   Not driving or operating machinery for 24 hours after receiving droperidol
   Not drinking alcohol or taking CNS depression–producing medications for about 24 hours after receiving droperidol

**Side/adverse effects**
   Signs of potential side effects, especially akathisia, anxiety, hypertension, dystonia, hyperpyrexia, and oculogyric crisis

## General Dosing Information

Geriatric, debilitated, or critically ill patients are more likely to experience excessive sedation and hypotension from the use of droperidol. It is recommended that the initial dose be lower in these patients. Subsequent doses may be titrated based on the response to the initial dose.

Droperidol should not be administered as the sole agent for anesthesia induction for surgery.

## Parenteral Dosage Forms

Note: Bracketed uses in the *Dosage Forms* section refer to categories of use and/or indications that are not included in U.S. product labeling.

### DROPERIDOL INJECTION USP

**Usual adult and adolescent dose**
Anesthesia, general, adjunct or
Anesthesia, local, adjunct—
   Premedication—
      Intramuscular, 2.5 to 5 mg thirty to sixty minutes before surgery.
   Induction—
      Intravenous, 1.25 mg per twenty to twenty-five pounds of body weight (0.1 to 0.14 mg [100 to 140 mcg] per kg of body weight).
   Maintenance—
      Intravenous, 1.25 to 2.5 mg. When droperidol is used as an adjunct to regional anesthesia, 2.5 to 5 mg may be administered intramuscularly or intravenously if additional sedation is required.
Nausea and vomiting, postoperative (prophylaxis)—
   Intravenous, 7 to 20 mcg per kg of body weight.
Sedation, conscious—
   Intramuscular, 1.25 to 5 mg thirty to sixty minutes prior to a diagnostic procedure.
[Psychotic disorder][1]—
   Intramuscular or intravenous, 2.5 to 5 mg for acute agitation. The dose should be based on the size of the patient and the degree of agitation.

**Usual pediatric dose**
Anesthesia, general, adjunct or
Anesthesia, local, adjunct—
   Premedication:
      Intramuscular or intravenous, 0.075 to 0.15 mg (75 to 150 mcg) per kg of body weight thirty to sixty minutes before surgery.
   Induction:
      Intravenous, 0.075 to 0.15 mg (75 to 150 mcg) per kg of body weight.
Nausea and vomiting, postoperative (prophylaxis)—
   Intramuscular or intravenous, 0.02 to 0.075 mg (20 to 75 mcg) per kg of body weight.

**Usual geriatric dose**
See *Usual adult and adolescent dose*. However, initial doses should be decreased for geriatric patients because geriatric patients are more likely to experience hypotension and excessive sedation after receiving droperidol.

**Strength(s) usually available**
U.S.—
   2.5 mg per mL (Rx) [*Inapsine* [GENERIC].
Note: The 10-mL multidose vials available generically contain 1.8 mg of methylparaben and 0.2 mg of propylparaben per mL.
Canada—
   2.5 mg per mL (Rx) [*Inapsine*].

**Packaging and storage**
Protect from light. Store between 15 and 30 °C (59 and 86 °F).

**Preparation of dosage form**
Droperidol may be diluted to a convenient volume with 5% dextrose injection, 0.9% sodium chloride injection, or lactated Ringer's injection.

---
[1]Not included in Canadian product labeling.

## Selected Bibliography

Desilva P, Darvish A, McDonald S, et al. The efficacy of prophylactic ondansetron, droperidol, perphenazine, and metoclopramide in the prevention of nausea and vomiting after major gynecologic surgery. Anesth Analg 1995; 81: 139-43.

Resnick M, Burton B. Droperidol vs. haloperidol in the initial management of acutely agitated patients. J Clin Psychiatry 1984; 45: 298-9.

Antrobus J, Abbott P, Carr C, et al. Midazolam–droperidol premedication for cardiac surgery. A comparison with papaveretum and hyoscine. Anaesthesia 1991; 46: 407-9.

Developed: 05/21/98

**DYCLONINE** — See Anesthetics (Mucosal-Local)

**DYPHYLLINE** — The Dyphylline (Systemic) monograph is not included in this published version of the USP DI database. Copies of the monograph are available on request from Micromedex, Inc. - Reprint Requests, 6200 S. Syracuse Way, Suite 300, Englewood, CO 80111; telephone (303) 486-6400; telefax (303) 486-6464; Email: USPDI@MDX.COM.

**ECHOTHIOPHATE**—See *Antiglaucoma Agents, Cholinergic, Long-acting (Ophthalmic)*

**ECONAZOLE**—See *Antifungals, Azole (Vaginal); Econazole (Topical)*

# ECONAZOLE Topical

VA CLASSIFICATION (Primary): DE102
Commonly used brand name(s): *Ecostatin; Spectazole*.
Note: For a listing of dosage forms and brand names by country availability, see *Dosage Forms* section(s).

## Category

Antifungal (topical).
Note: Econazole is a broad-spectrum antifungal, which has an antifungal spectrum similar to that of miconazole.

## Indications

Note: Bracketed information in the *Indications* section refers to uses that are not included in U.S. product labeling.

**Accepted**
Candidiasis, cutaneous (treatment)—Econazole is indicated as a primary agent in the topical treatment of cutaneous candidiasis (moniliasis) caused by *Candida (Monilia)* species.
Tinea corporis (treatment)
Tinea cruris (treatment) or
Tinea pedis (treatment)—Econazole is indicated as a primary agent in the topical treatment of tinea corporis (ringworm of the body), tinea cruris (ringworm of the groin; jock itch), or tinea pedis (ringworm of the foot; athlete's foot) caused by *Trichophyton rubrum*, *T. mentagrophytes*, *T. tonsurans*, *Microsporum canis*, *M. audouini*, *M. gypseum*, and *Epidermophyton floccosum (Acrothesium floccosum)*.
Tinea versicolor (treatment)—Econazole is indicated as a primary agent in the topical treatment of tinea versicolor (pityriasis versicolor; "sun fungus") caused by *Pityrosporon orbiculare (Malassezia furfur)*.
[Paronychia (treatment)][1]—Econazole is used in the topical treatment of paronychia caused by fungi.
[Tinea barbae (treatment)][1] or
[Tinea capitis (treatment)][1]—Econazole is used in combination with griseofulvin or systemic ketoconazole (for griseofulvin-resistant cases) in the treatment of tinea barbae and tinea capitis.
Not all species or strains of a particular organism may be susceptible to econazole.

[1]Not included in Canadian product labeling.

## Pharmacology/Pharmacokinetics

**Physicochemical characteristics**
Chemical group—Synthetic chlorinated imidazole derivative, structurally related to clotrimazole, ketoconazole, and miconazole.
Molecular weight—444.70.

**Mechanism of action/Effect**
Fungistatic; may be fungicidal, depending on concentration; inhibits biosynthesis of ergosterol or other sterols, damaging the fungal cell wall membrane and altering its permeability; as a result, loss of essential intracellular elements may occur; also inhibits biosynthesis of triglycerides and phospholipids by fungi; in addition, inhibits oxidative and peroxidative enzyme activity, resulting in intracellular buildup of toxic concentrations of hydrogen peroxide, which may contribute to deterioration of subcellular organelles and cellular necrosis. In *Candida albicans*, inhibits transformation of blastospores into invasive mycelial form.

**Other actions/effects**
Also has some activity against gram-positive bacteria.

**Absorption**
Minimal systemic absorption following topical application to normal skin.

**Stratum corneum concentration**
Far exceeded minimum inhibitory concentrations (MICs) for dermatophytes; inhibitory concentrations found in epidermis and as deep as middle region of dermis.

**Elimination**
Renal and fecal; < 1% of applied dose recovered in urine and feces.

## Precautions to Consider

**Carcinogenicity**
Long-term studies in animals have not been done.

**Pregnancy/Reproduction**
Fertility—Studies in rats have shown that econazole given orally causes prolonged gestation. However, studies in humans have not shown that econazole given intravaginally causes prolonged gestation or other adverse reproductive effects.
Pregnancy—Adequate and well-controlled studies in humans have not been done.
Segment I studies in rats have shown that econazole is fetotoxic or embryotoxic when given orally in doses 10 to 40 times the usual human dermal dose. Similar effects were seen in mice, rabbits, and/or rats in Segment II or Segment III studies when econazole was given orally in doses 80 or 40 times the usual human dermal dose, respectively. However, no teratogenic effects were seen in mice, rabbits, or rats when econazole was given orally.
FDA Pregnancy Category C.

**Breast-feeding**
It is not known whether econazole is distributed into human breast milk. However, problems in humans have not been documented. Econazole and/or its metabolites are distributed into the milk of rats following oral administration and were found in the nursing pups. Also, in lactating rats given large oral doses of econazole (40 or 80 times the usual human dermal dose), a decrease in the postpartum viability of pups and survival to weaning was seen.

**Pediatrics**
Appropriate studies on the relationship of age to the effects of econazole have not been performed in the pediatric population. However, pediatrics-specific problems that would limit the usefulness of this medicine in children are not expected.

**Geriatrics**
Appropriate studies on the relationship of age to the effects of econazole have not been performed in the geriatric population. However, geriatrics-specific problems that would limit the usefulness of this medicine in the elderly are not expected.

**Medical considerations/Contraindications**
The medical considerations/contraindications included have been selected on the basis of their potential clinical significance (reasons given in parentheses where appropriate)—not necessarily inclusive (» = major clinical significance).

*Risk-benefit should be considered when the following medical problem exists:*
Sensitivity to econazole

## Side/Adverse Effects

The following side/adverse effects have been selected on the basis of their potential clinical significance (possible signs and symptoms in parentheses where appropriate)—not necessarily inclusive:

**Those indicating need for medical attention**
Incidence less frequent
*Hypersensitivity* (burning, itching, stinging, redness, or other signs of irritation not present before therapy)

## Patient Consultation

As an aid to patient consultation, refer to *Advice for the Patient, Econazole (Topical)*.
In providing consultation, consider emphasizing the following selected information (» = major clinical significance):

**Before using this medication**
» Conditions affecting use, especially:
    Pregnancy—Fetotoxic and embryotoxic reactions were seen in rats, mice, and rabbits given large oral doses
    Breast-feeding—Econazole was distributed into breast milk of rats given large oral doses

## Econazole (Topical)

**Proper use of this medication**
  Applying sufficient medication to cover affected and surrounding areas, and rubbing in gently
» Avoiding contact with the eyes
» Not applying occlusive dressing over this medication unless directed to do so by physician
» Compliance with full course of therapy; fungal infections may require prolonged therapy
» Proper dosing
  Missed dose: Applying as soon as possible; not applying if almost time for next dose
» Proper storage

**Precautions while using this medication**
  Checking with physician if no improvement within 2 weeks or more
» Using hygienic measures to help cure infection or to help prevent re-infection
*For tinea cruris*
  Avoiding underwear that is tight-fitting or made from synthetic materials; wearing loose-fitting cotton underwear instead
  Using a bland, absorbent powder or an antifungal powder on the skin; not using cream and powder concurrently
*For tinea pedis*
  Carefully drying feet, especially between toes, after bathing
  Avoiding socks made from wool or synthetic materials; wearing clean, cotton socks and changing them daily or more often if feet perspire excessively
  Wearing well-ventilated shoes or sandals
  Using a bland, absorbent powder or an antifungal powder between toes, on feet, and in socks and shoes liberally once or twice daily; not using cream and powder concurrently

**Side/adverse effects**
  Signs of potential side effects, especially hypersensitivity reactions

## General Dosing Information

Use of topical antifungals may lead to skin sensitization, resulting in hypersensitivity reactions with subsequent topical use of the medication.

To reduce the possibility of recurrence, *Candida* infections, tinea cruris, and tinea corporis should be treated for at least 2 weeks and tinea pedis should be treated for at least 1 month.

When this medication is used in the treatment of candidiasis, occlusive dressings should be avoided since they provide conditions that favor growth of yeast and release of its irritating endotoxin.

## Topical Dosage Forms

### ECONAZOLE NITRATE CREAM

**Usual adult and adolescent dose**
Candidiasis, cutaneous—
  Topical, to the skin, two times a day, morning and evening.
Tinea corporis; or
Tinea cruris; or
Tinea pedis; or
Tinea versicolor—
  Topical, to the skin, once a day.

**Usual pediatric dose**
See *Usual adult and adolescent dose*.

**Strength(s) usually available**
U.S.—
  1% (Rx) [*Spectazole*].
Canada—
  1% (Rx) [*Ecostatin*].

**Packaging and storage**
Store below 30 °C (86 °F), in a well-closed container, unless otherwise specified by manufacturer. Protect from freezing.

**Auxiliary labeling**
• For external use only.
• Continue medicine for full time of treatment.

Revised: 04/14/92
Interim revision: 06/06/94

---

# EDETATE CALCIUM DISODIUM   Systemic

INN:   Sodium calcium edetate
VA CLASSIFICATION (Primary/Secondary): AD300/DX900
Commonly used brand name(s): *Calcium Disodium Versenate*.
Other commonly used names are calcium EDTA, edathamil calcium disodium, and sodium calcium edetate.
Note:   For a listing of dosage forms and brand names by country availability, see *Dosage Forms* section(s).

## Category

Chelating agent; diagnostic aid, lead mobilization.

## Indications

Note:   Bracketed information in the *Indications* section refers to uses that are not included in U.S. product labeling.

**Accepted**
Toxicity, lead (treatment)—Edetate calcium disodium is indicated for the treatment of acute and chronic lead poisoning (plumbism) and lead encephalopathy.
Dimercaprol complements edetate calcium disodium by rapidly removing lead from red blood cells and by assisting in mobilizing lead from skeletal stores. When the combination is used, the rate of lead excretion is doubled, thus decreasing the mortality rate and likelihood of permanent neurologic deficits from lead poisoning.
Signs and symptoms of lead poisoning include anemia, gastrointestinal complaints (abdominal pain and vomiting), nephropathy, and encephalopathy. Symptoms of lead encephalopathy include headache and insomnia; persistent vomiting, sometimes projectile; visual disturbances; irritability, restlessness, delirium, hallucinations; ataxia; convulsions and coma; and characteristically high intracranial pressure. Recovery is slow and often incomplete, with residual neurologic deficit.
Edetate calcium disodium may be used as sole therapy when blood lead levels fall between 45 and 69 mcg per deciliter, unless serious symptoms such as encephalopathy are present. Clinical signs and symptoms suggesting lead poisoning that should be treated with the dimercaprol, edetate calcium disodium combination include the following:
• Patient is symptomatic (with or without encephalopathy).
• Blood lead concentrations are greater than or equal to 70 mcg per deciliter.

[Lead mobilization determination][1]—Edetate calcium disodium may be used as a diagnostic agent to identify patients who qualify for a full course of chelation therapy by determining the magnitude of lead stores in high-risk, asymptomatic children with mild to moderate increases in lead absorption (25 to 44 mcg of lead per deciliter of whole blood). However, use of the lead mobilization test is controversial because of variable results, difficulty in collecting urine from non–toilet-trained children, possible increase in brain lead levels, and risk of iron deficiency causing a negative mobilization result.

**Unaccepted**
To a lesser extent, cadmium, manganese, iron, copper, chromium, and nickel are also chelated, but the value of edetate calcium disodium in poisoning caused by these metals is questionable or unproven.
Edetate calcium disodium is *not* effective in arsenic, gold, or mercury poisoning.
Edetate calcium disodium is *not* effective in preventing or retarding the progression of atherosclerosis.

[1]Not included in Canadian product labeling.

## Pharmacology/Pharmacokinetics

**Physicochemical characteristics**
Molecular weight—374.27.

**Mechanism of action/Effect**
Edetate calcium disodium reduces blood concentrations and depot stores of lead. The calcium is replaced by divalent and trivalent metals, especially any available lead, to form stable, soluble complexes that are readily excreted. Edetate calcium disodium is saturated with calcium but can be administered intravenously in large quantities without causing any significant changes in serum or total body calcium concentrations.

**Other actions/effects**
Edetate calcium disodium greatly increases chelation and urinary excretion of zinc, but this action is considered clinically insignificant unless ther-

apy is continued for more than 5 days or zinc stores are low prior to treatment. Edetate calcium disodium has been found to chelate iron, copper, calcium, and manganese.

**Absorption**
Well absorbed after parenteral administration; poorly absorbed from the gastrointestinal tract. The oral route of administration is no longer used because of poor GI absorption. The absorption of any lead in the intestines may be increased upon oral administration of edetate calcium disodium because the lead chelate formed is more soluble than the lead itself. After absorption, the chelate dissociates and releases free lead ions, producing increased symptoms of lead toxicity.

**Distribution**
Extracellular fluid (90%); edetate calcium disodium does not penetrate erythrocytes and only slowly diffuses into the cerebrospinal fluid.

**Biotransformation**
No metabolism occurs; after parenteral administration, edetate calcium disodium is excreted in the urine either unchanged or as the metal chelates.

**Half-life**
Plasma—
  Intravenous administration: 20 to 60 minutes.
  Intramuscular administration: 1.5 hours.

**Elimination**
Renal, by glomerular filtration; 50% of the chelate that is formed appears in urine within the first hour after parenteral administration; 70% or more during first 4 hours; and 95% in 24 hours. Excretion is unaffected by urinary pH. Theoretically, one gram of edetate calcium disodium chelates 620 mg of lead, but only 3 to 5 mg of lead is excreted in the urine after parenteral administration of one gram to patients with symptoms of acute lead poisoning or with high concentrations of lead in soft tissues.

## Precautions to Consider

### Pregnancy/Reproduction
Pregnancy—Studies in humans have not been done. Risk-benefit must be considered during early pregnancy or in women of child-bearing potential.

One reproduction study in rats at doses up to 13 times the human dose revealed no evidence of impaired fertility or harm to the fetus. Another reproduction study performed in rats at doses up to 25 to 40 times the human dose revealed evidence of fetal malformations, which were prevented by simultaneous administration of zinc supplements.

FDA Pregnancy Category B.

### Breast-feeding
It is not known whether edetate calcium disodium is distributed into breast milk.

### Pediatrics
Because the intramuscular route is painful and there may be poor blood flow to muscle, the intravenous route is recommended for children. In cases of lead encephalopathy, fluid restriction may necessitate giving edetate calcium disodium intramuscularly. Children may require repeated courses of therapy if blood lead levels are greater than 45 mcg per deciliter.

The preferred treatment for children with lead encephalopathy is combined therapy with edetate calcium disodium and dimercaprol.

### Geriatrics
No information is available on the relationship of age to the effects of edetate calcium disodium in geriatric patients.

### Drug interactions and/or related problems
The following drug interactions and/or related problems have been selected on the basis of their potential clinical significance (possible mechanism in parentheses where appropriate)—not necessarily inclusive (» = major clinical significance):

Insulin
  (concurrent use will decrease the duration of action of zinc insulin preparations by chelation of zinc)

Zinc supplements
  (concurrent use may decrease the effectiveness of edetate calcium disodium and zinc supplements due to chelation; zinc supplement therapy should be withheld until edetate calcium disodium therapy is completed)

### Laboratory value alterations
The following have been selected on the basis of their potential clinical significance (possible effect in parentheses where appropriate)—not necessarily inclusive (» = major clinical significance):

With diagnostic test results
  Electrocardiogram (ECG) readings
    (inversion of T-wave may occur)

### Medical considerations/Contraindications
The medical considerations/contraindications included have been selected on the basis of their potential clinical significance (reasons given in parentheses where appropriate)—not necessarily inclusive (» = major clinical significance).

*Except under special circumstances, this medication should not be used when the following medical problems exist:*

» Anuria or
» Oliguria, severe
  (fatal lower nephron necrosis may result; if anuria occurs during therapy or is present before therapy, urine flow should be restored before starting edetate calcium disodium therapy)

*Risk-benefit should be considered when the following medical problems exist:*

» Dehydration
  (when acutely ill patients are dehydrated from vomiting and/or diarrhea, urine flow must be established before administering the first dose of edetate calcium disodium; once the flow is established, intravenous fluids must be restricted to basal water and electrolyte requirements)

Hypercalcemia
  (transitory hypercalcemia during treatment may exacerbate an existing condition)

» Renal function impairment
  (reduced glomerular filtration may delay the excretion of the chelate and increase the risk of nephrotoxicity)

### Patient monitoring
The following may be especially important in patient monitoring (other tests may be warranted in some patients, depending on condition; » = major clinical significance):

Blood urea nitrogen (BUN) concentrations and
Calcium concentrations, serum and
Creatinine concentrations, serum and
Hepatocellular enzymes and
Phosphorus concentrations, serum and
Urine output
  (determinations recommended prior to treatment and on the first, third, and fifth day of each course of therapy for evidence of renal function impairment)

Cardiac monitoring
  (may be recommended periodically to find irregularities of cardiac rhythm, especially if edetate calcium disodium is given intravenously)

Fluid intake
  (must be kept to a minimum if cerebral edema is present; volume of urine and flow must be adequate for elimination of lead chelate)

Urinalysis, routine
  (recommended daily during each course of therapy; since severe, acute lead poisoning and edetate calcium disodium may both produce the same signs of renal damage, urinalyses should be performed to determine if proteinuria or hematuria is improving or if evidence of renal tubular injury is worsening; edetate calcium disodium must be discontinued immediately if large renal epithelial cells or increasing numbers of red blood cells are present in urinary sediment, or if there is evidence of increased proteinuria)

## Side/Adverse Effects

The following side/adverse effects have been selected on the basis of their potential clinical significance (possible signs and symptoms in parentheses where appropriate)—not necessarily inclusive:

### Those indicating need for medical attention
Incidence more frequent
  **Systemic febrile reaction** (chills or sudden fever; fatigue; headache; increased thirst; loss of appetite; malaise); **histamine-like reaction** (sneezing; stuffy nose; watery eyes)—possibly occurring 4 to 8 hours after intravenous infusion; **low blood pressure; nausea or vomiting; renal damage or renal tubular necrosis** (cloudy urine); **thrombophlebitis** (pain or swelling at site of injection)

  Note: Febrile reaction has been observed in some patients 4 to 8 hours after infusion; it may accompany *histamine-like reaction*.

    *Renal damage* or *tubular necrosis* may occur when daily dose is excessive. Microscopic hematuria, proteinuria, or large renal epithelial cells may be observed in urine.

*Thrombophlebitis* may be a result of inadequate dilution of injection. Concentration of solution should not exceed 0.5%.

Incidence less frequent

**Transient anemia or bone marrow depression** (bleeding and bruising; sore throat and fever; unusual tiredness or weakness); *dermatitis* (cracking and dry, scaly skin, or sores in mouth and on lips); *hypercalcemia* (constipation; drowsiness; dry mouth; continuing headache; loss of appetite; metallic taste)

Note: *Dermatitis* lesions are similar to those caused by vitamin $B_6$ deficiency; results from prolonged administration at high doses and may be due to zinc depletion.

*Hypercalcemia* is usually transitory and accompanied by a significant increase in urinary excretion of calcium from endogenous sources. However, since recurring hypercalcemia may be causally related to renal tubular injury, discontinuation of edetate calcium disodium therapy is recommended when hypercalcemia occurs in susceptible patients.

Incidence rare

**Frequent or sudden urge to urinate; secondary gout** (severe pain in feet, knees, hands, elbows)—hyperuricemia may result from renal tubular toxicity

## General Dosing Information

**Warning:** The dosage schedule should be followed and the recommended daily dose must not be exceeded because of the toxic and potentially fatal effects of edetate calcium disodium.

Edetate calcium disodium is equally effective when administered intramuscularly or intravenously. However, the intravenous route is preferred because the intramuscular route is painful and children have poor blood flow to muscle.

In patients with lead encephalopathy or cerebral edema, intravenous infusion is preferred, but rapid infusion may be lethal because of a sudden increase in intracranial pressure. An excess of fluids must be avoided in such patients, and the intramuscular route should be used.

If edetate calcium disodium is given intramuscularly, pain at site of intramuscular injection may be reduced by mixing a 20% solution of edetate calcium disodium with procaine or lidocaine. A final procaine or lidocaine concentration of 5 mg per mL (0.5%) can be obtained by mixing 0.25 mL of a 10% lidocaine solution per 5 mL of edetate calcium disodium or 1 mL of 1% procaine or lidocaine solution per mL of edetate calcium disodium. Crystalline procaine may be used instead to maintain minimum fluid volume.

Urine flow should be established before the first dose of edetate calcium disodium is administered to acutely ill, dehydrated patients. When urine flow has been established, further intravenous fluids should be restricted to basal water and electrolyte requirements.

Each course of therapy should not exceed 5 to 7 days, with a drug-free interval of at least 2 days (preferably 2 weeks) between courses. This allows redistribution of lead from inaccessible storage sites, such as soft tissue or bone, and will result in a greater amount of lead available for elimination.

In cases of lead encephalopathy, children may require repeated courses of therapy if blood lead levels are greater than 45 mcg per deciliter.

Successful chelation therapy requires the administration of a sufficient molar excess of chelating agent over lead. Since the maximum safe dose of edetate calcium disodium alone may cause a shift of lead into the CNS, dimercaprol is combined with edetate calcium disodium. The preferred route of administration for edetate calcium disodium is intravenous and dimercaprol is given by deep intramuscular injection in divided doses every 4 hours for 5 days. If both drugs are given by intramuscular injection, then they must be given at separate sites. Dimercaprol is given alone for the first dose 4 hours before the combination is begun. Injection sites should be rotated. In asymptomatic or mildly symptomatic patients, dimercaprol may be discontinued after 48 hours, with edetate calcium disodium being continued for an additional 48 to 72 hours at reduced dosage.

Oral penicillamine is used after initial therapy with edetate calcium disodium or combined dimercaprol and edetate calcium disodium for long-term chelation therapy, especially if long-bone radiographs show lead lines. The oral chelating agent succimer has recently been approved for treatment of children with blood lead levels greater than 45 mcg per deciliter. Although use to date has been limited, toxicity appears to be less than with other agents.

### For lead mobilization test

Use of the lead mobilization test is controversial because of variable results, difficulty in collecting urine from non–toilet-trained children, possible increase in brain lead levels, and risk of iron deficiency causing a negative mobilization result.

Since the blood lead (BL) concentrations may not be a sensitive indicator of the body burden of lead in asymptomatic children with BL 25 to 44 mcg per dL, diagnostic tests may be performed as follows:

- Edetate calcium disodium is given intravenously at a dose of 15 mg per kg of body weight (mg/kg) (500 mg per square meter) in 5% dextrose over 1 hour; or edetate calcium disodium given intramuscularly at a dose of 15 mg/kg (500 mg per square meter) mixed with an equivalent amount of procaine so that the final concentration of procaine is 0.5%.
- An 8-hour urine sample, collected in lead-free equipment, is obtained.
- The test is considered positive for increased body burden of lead when the 8-hour urinary excretion of lead is greater than 0.6 mcg per mg of edetate calcium disodium administered.
- If the diagnostic mobilization test is positive, a five-day course of therapy is administered. The test may be repeated if another course of therapy is necessary.
- The upper limit for acceptable blood lead concentrations is 10 mcg per deciliter of whole blood. At 20 mcg per deciliter, medical evaluation should occur.
- In symptomatic patients or those with whole blood lead concentrations greater than or equal to 45 mcg per dL, appropriate chelation therapy should be given immediately without performing the mobilization test.

### For treatment of adverse effects

Recommended treatment consists of the following:

- Cessation of urine flow during therapy—Administration of edetate calcium disodium must be stopped to avoid excessively high tissue concentrations of the chelating agent.
- Sores in mouth and on lips—Subside when edetate calcium disodium is discontinued; replacement of zinc by supplementation may be advisable during drug-free interval between courses of therapy.

## Parenteral Dosage Forms

Note: Bracketed uses in the *Dosage Forms* section refer to categories of use and/or indications that are not included in U.S. product labeling.

### EDETATE CALCIUM DISODIUM INJECTION USP

#### Usual adult and adolescent dose

Lead toxicity—

Intravenous or intramuscular, in conjunction with dimercaprol, 30 to 50 mg of edetate calcium disodium per kg of body weight (1 to 1.5 grams per square meter of body surface area) per day in two divided doses twelve hours apart for three to five days.

Note: Patients with blood lead levels between 45 and 69 mcg per deciliter may be treated with edetate calcium disodium alone using the same dosage given above for use with dimercaprol.

A second course of treatment may be administered for up to five additional days after at least a two-day drug-free interval (preferably two weeks).

When serum creatinine is 2 mg per deciliter or less, the dosage is 1 gram a day for 5 days. If the serum creatinine is 2 to 3 mg per deciliter, the dosage is 500 mg a day.

For intravenous administration, the dilution must be infused slowly over a period of at least two hours for symptomatic patients and one hour for asymptomatic patients.

[Lead mobilization test][1]

Intravenous, 1 gram over 1 hour. The same dose can be mixed with procaine, so that the final concentration of procaine is 0.5%, and given intramuscularly.

#### Usual adult prescribing limits

The maximum dose is 2 grams a day.

#### Usual pediatric dose

Lead toxicity—

For blood lead levels greater than 70 mcg per deciliter or serious symptoms: Intravenous or intramuscular, in conjunction with dimercaprol, 1500 mg of edetate calcium disodium per square meter of body surface area a day, administered on a four-hour schedule for 5 days.

Note: Some clinicians prefer that edetate calcium disodium be given by continuous intravenous infusion. If given by intramuscular route, it must be given at a separate site from dimercaprol.

Children with blood lead levels between 45 and 69 mcg per deciliter may be treated with edetate calcium disodium alone, using a dose of 1000 mg of edetate calcium disodium per square meter of body surface area a day for 5 days.

A second course of treatment may be administered after a drug-free interval of at least two days.

Children with lead encephalopathy may require additional courses of therapy. Therapy should continue if blood lead levels are greater than 45 mcg per dL.

[Lead mobilization test][1]—
Intravenous, 15 mg per kg of body weight (500 mg per square meter of body surface area) up to a maximum dose of 1 gram over 1 hour. The same dose can be mixed with procaine, so that the final concentration of procaine is 0.5%, and given intramuscularly.

### Strength(s) usually available
U.S.—
200 mg per mL (Rx) [*Calcium Disodium Versenate*].
Canada—
200 mg per mL (Rx) [*Calcium Disodium Versenate*].

### Packaging and storage
Store below 40 °C (104 °F), preferably between 15 and 30 °C (59 and 86 °F), unless otherwise specified by manufacturer.

### Preparation of dosage form
Intravenous—Dilute 1 gram of edetate calcium disodium with 250 to 500 mL of 0.9% sodium chloride injection or 5% dextrose injection.

### Incompatibilities
Edetate calcium disodium injection is physically incompatible with 10% dextrose injection, 10% invert sugar, 10% invert sugar in sodium chloride injection, lactated Ringer's injection, Ringer's injection, one-sixth molar sodium lactate injection, and injectable preparations of amphotericin B and hydralazine hydrochloride.

### Additional information
Contains 5.3 mEq of sodium per gram of edetate calcium disodium.

[1]Not included in Canadian product labeling.

Revised: 07/06/92

**EDETATE DISODIUM**—The *Edetate Disodium (Ophthalmic)* monograph is not included in this published version of the USP DI database. Copies of the monograph are available on request from Micromedex, Inc. - Reprint Requests, 6200 S. Syracuse Way, Suite 300, Englewood, CO 80111; telephone (303) 486-6400; telefax (303) 486-6464; Email: USPDI@MDX.COM.

# EDETATE DISODIUM Systemic†

VA CLASSIFICATION (Primary): AD300

Commonly used brand name(s): *Disotate; Endrate*.

Other commonly used names are disodium EDTA, edathamil disodium, and sodium edetate.

Note: For a listing of dosage forms and brand names by country availability, see *Dosage Forms* section(s).

†Not commercially available in Canada; however, it is available by emergency drug release from the Health Protection Branch.

## Category
Chelating agent.

## Indications

### Accepted
Hypercalcemia (treatment)—Edetate disodium is indicated in selected patients for the emergency treatment of acute hypercalcemia, but is recommended only when the severity of the clinical condition (as when there has been a judgment of imminent death from hypercalcemic crisis) justifies the aggressive measures associated with this therapy. Other therapies should be started simultaneously so that treatment with edetate disodium will not exceed 48 hours. Some physicians recommend not using edetate disodium for hypercalcemia, especially when it is associated with metastatic bone disease, because of minimal and temporary beneficial effects and the great risk of renal damage.

Toxicity, digitalis glycoside (treatment)—Edetate disodium is indicated for the control of ventricular arrhythmias associated with digitalis toxicity. Although its onset of action is rapid, the short-term effects require that alternative therapy be undertaken quickly. Edetate disodium is rarely used to treat digitalis-induced ventricular arrhythmias since other more effective agents are available. Although edetate disodium may have been useful when other medications, such as potassium or phenytoin, were contraindicated or ineffective, or when controlling arrhythmias caused by digitalis poisoning in children who had ingested massive doses, it has now been replaced by digoxin immune fab as the first-line agent for treatment of life-threatening digitalis glycoside toxicity.

### Unaccepted
Edetate disodium is *not* indicated for the treatment of arteriosclerosis or atherosclerotic vascular disease involving coronary or peripheral vessels associated with advancing age, since it has not been proven effective and severe nephrotoxicity may occur.

Edetate disodium is *not* indicated for the treatment of lead poisoning because, unlike edetate calcium disodium, it causes hypocalcemia.

Edetate disodium is *not* indicated for the treatment of renal calculi by retrograde irrigation.

## Pharmacology/Pharmacokinetics

### Mechanism of action/Effect
Hypercalcemia—Edetate disodium forms soluble complexes with calcium in the blood, which are filtered by the glomeruli and not reabsorbed by the renal tubules. Chelation with calcium produces a lowering of serum calcium concentrations and a mobilization of extracirculatory calcium stores, especially from bone, during slow intravenous infusion. Theoretically, 1 gram of edetate disodium will chelate 120 mg of calcium. Hypocalcemic tetany, seizures, severe cardiac arrhythmias, and respiratory arrest may occur with the rapid decrease in serum calcium concentrations. However, the mobilization of calcium from bone may lessen the risk of hypocalcemia. Calcium ion concentrations in cerebrospinal fluid are not affected by edetate disodium.

Digitalis toxicity—Edetate disodium exerts a negative inotropic effect on the heart. The chronotropic and inotropic effects of digitalis glycosides on the ventricles of the heart are transiently antagonized by the hypocalcemia induced by edetate disodium.

### Other actions/effects
Edetate disodium also forms chelates with and increases urinary excretion of other polyvalent metals, such as magnesium, zinc, and other trace elements.

Although edetate disodium does not form a chelate with potassium, the serum concentration of potassium may be decreased and the urinary excretion of potassium increased.

### Biotransformation
None.

### Elimination
Rapidly excreted by the kidneys, principally as the calcium chelate; 95% of a dose appears in the urine within 24 hours; changes in urine flow and pH do not affect the rate of excretion of the chelate.

## Precautions to Consider

### Pregnancy/Reproduction
Pregnancy—Edetate disodium crosses the placenta. Adequate and well-controlled studies in humans have not been done.

Studies in rats have shown that edetate disodium causes impaired reproduction and fetal malformations. Since these effects were prevented by simultaneous supplementation of dietary zinc, it is believed that zinc deficiency may be the cause.

FDA Pregnancy Category C.

### Breast-feeding
Problems in humans have not been documented.

### Pediatrics
No information is available on the relationship of age to the effects of edetate disodium in pediatric patients.

### Geriatrics
No information is available on the relationship of age to the effects of edetate disodium in geriatric patients.

## Drug interactions and/or related problems
The following drug interactions and/or related problems have been selected on the basis of their potential clinical significance (possible mechanism in parentheses where appropriate)—not necessarily inclusive (» = major clinical significance):

» Digitalis glycosides
(sudden drop in serum calcium concentrations induced by edetate disodium may reverse effects of digitalis)

Insulin
(concurrent use may require adjustments in dosage of insulin due to decreased serum glucose and possible chelation of zinc in insulin)

## Laboratory value alterations
The following have been selected on the basis of their potential clinical significance (possible effect in parentheses where appropriate)—not necessarily inclusive (» = major clinical significance):

With diagnostic test results
Electrocardiograms (ECGs)
(changes such as sagging of the S-T segment, depression of the T wave, and elevation of the U wave may occur as a result of reduced serum potassium concentrations)

Calcium determinations, serum
(the oxalate method of determining serum calcium tends to give low readings in the presence of edetate disodium; sampling just before a subsequent dose will produce the least interference; acidifying the sample or using an alternate method may be necessary)

With physiology/laboratory test values
Alkaline phosphatase, serum
(concentration may be lowered because of hypomagnesemia induced by edetate disodium)

Glucose, serum
(treatment with edetate disodium may cause a lowering of blood sugar concentrations)

Glucose, urine
(concentration may be increased)

Magnesium, serum or
Potassium, serum
(concentration may be decreased)

## Medical considerations/Contraindications
The medical considerations/contraindications included have been selected on the basis of their potential clinical significance (reasons given in parentheses where appropriate)—not necessarily inclusive (» = major clinical significance):

*Except under special circumstances, this medication should not be used when the following medical problems exist:*

» Anuria or
» Renal function impairment
(excretion of edetate disodium may be delayed by reduced glomerular filtration, increasing the risk of nephrotoxicity)

» Hypocalcemia
(may be exacerbated)

*Risk-benefit should be considered when the following medical problems exist:*

Diabetes mellitus
(treatment with edetate disodium may reduce blood sugar concentrations and require adjustment of insulin dosage in diabetic patients)

» Heart disease
(myocardial contractility may be affected)

Hypokalemia
(edetate disodium may exacerbate hypokalemia and produce ECG changes)

Intracranial lesions or
» Seizure disorders, history of
(edetate disodium may induce seizures because of hypocalcemia)

Sensitivity to edetate disodium

Tuberculosis, active or with healed calcified lesions
(may be provoked)

## Patient monitoring
The following may be especially important in patient monitoring (other tests may be warranted in some patients, depending on condition; » = major clinical significance):

Blood pressure determinations
(recommended prior to and periodically during therapy)

Blood urea nitrogen (BUN) concentrations and
Creatinine concentrations, serum
(determinations recommended prior to and during therapy for evidence of renal function impairment)

Cardiac function studies, including ECG and
Electrolyte determinations, serum and urinary, especially potassium and magnesium
(recommended prior to administration of edetate disodium and periodically, as clinically indicated, during therapy, especially in patients with ventricular arrhythmias, limited cardiac reserve, congestive heart failure, or a history of seizure disorders or intracranial lesions; reduced serum potassium concentrations may produce ECG changes; serum magnesium determinations may be required during prolonged therapy)

Liver function tests
(recommended if there is any clinical evidence of liver function impairment during treatment)

Urinalysis
(recommended daily during treatment)

## Side/Adverse Effects
The following side/adverse effects have been selected on the basis of their potential clinical significance (possible signs and symptoms in parentheses where appropriate)—not necessarily inclusive:

**Those indicating need for medical attention**
Incidence more frequent
*Thrombophlebitis* (pain, burning, or swelling at site of injection)

Incidence less frequent
*Anemia* (unusual tiredness or weakness); *exfoliative dermatitis* (skin rash or other skin and mucous membrane lesions); *febrile reaction, systemic* (chills or sudden fever; fatigue; headache; malaise; muscle cramps; excessive thirst; weakness); *gout, secondary* (severe pain or inflammation in feet, knees, hands, or elbows)—hyperuricemia may result from renal tubular toxicity; *hypocalcemia* (convulsions; difficulty in breathing; irregular heartbeats; mood or mental changes; muscle spasms [tetany] in hands, arms, feet, legs, or face; numbness and tingling around the mouth, fingertips, or feet)—due to sudden decrease in serum calcium concentration caused by rapid intravenous infusion or high dose of edetate disodium; *hypokalemia or hypomagnesemia* (drowsiness; loss of appetite; muscle twitching or trembling; nausea or vomiting; unusual tiredness or weakness)—may be accompanied by hypocalcemia; *nephrotoxicity* (cloudy urine; frequent or sudden urge to urinate; large or small volume of urine; painful or difficult urination)

Note: Prolonged use may cause lesions similar to those seen with pyridoxine deficiency, such as cracking and dry scaly skin and sores in mouth and on lips, possibly due to zinc depletion.

*Nephrotoxicity* may be due to damage to the reticuloendothelial system with hemorrhagic tendencies, or may indicate possible renal tubular necrosis. Microscopic hematuria, proteinuria, and/or large renal epithelial cells in urine may be observed. Nephrotoxicity is usually associated with high doses of edetate disodium. Signs are often reversible within a few days after discontinuation of medication.

**Those indicating need for medical attention only if they continue or are bothersome**
Incidence more frequent
*Abdominal or stomach pain or cramps; diarrhea; hypotension, postural* (dizziness or lightheadedness)

Incidence less frequent
*Headache, without other symptoms of a febrile reaction*

## General Dosing Information
Because of its irritant effect on the tissues and the danger of hypocalcemia, edetate disodium must be diluted before infusion.

Dilute solution must be infused slowly over three hours or more, preferably four to six hours, and the cardiac reserve of the patient not exceeded. Rapid intravenous infusion or high serum concentrations of edetate disodium may cause a sudden drop in serum calcium concentration, resulting in hypocalcemic tetany, convulsions, severe cardiac arrhythmias, and death from respiratory arrest.

**For treatment of adverse effects**
Recommended treatment consists of the following:
• Hypocalcemia—A parenteral calcium salt, such as calcium gluconate, should be immediately available before administration of edetate disodium for calcium ion replacement. However, intravenous calcium should be administered with caution, especially in patients who are digitalized, since a reversal of digitalis effects may occur.

- Nephrotoxicity—Edetate disodium must be discontinued; maximum hydration compatible with patient's cardiovascular reserve may be necessary.
- Postural hypotension—Patient should remain in bed for a short time after infusion.

## Parenteral Dosage Forms

### EDETATE DISODIUM INJECTION USP

**Usual adult dose**
Hypercalcemia or
Digitalis toxicity—
 Intravenous, 50 mg per kg of body weight in twenty-four hours. The dosage may be repeated for four more consecutive daily doses followed by a two-day drug-free interval, with repeated courses, as necessary, up to fifteen doses.

**Usual adult prescribing limits**
3 grams in twenty-four hours.

**Usual pediatric dose**
Hypercalcemia or
Digitalis toxicity—
 Intravenous, 40 mg per kg of body weight in twenty-four hours.

Note: The pediatric dose may go as high as 70 mg per kg in twenty-four hours.

**Strength(s) usually available**
U.S.—
 150 mg per mL (Rx) [*Disotate; Endrate;* GENERIC].
Canada—
 Edetate disodium injection is not commercially available in Canada; however, it is available by emergency drug release from the Health Protection Branch.

**Packaging and storage**
Store below 40 °C (104 °F), preferably between 15 and 30 °C (59 and 86 °F), unless otherwise specified by manufacturer. Protect from freezing.

**Preparation of dosage form**
Adult use—The calculated dose is dissolved in 500 mL of 5% dextrose injection or sodium chloride injection.
Pediatric use—The calculated dose is dissolved in a sufficient volume of 5% dextrose injection or sodium chloride injection to make a final concentration of not more than 3% (30 mg per mL).

**Additional information**
Injection contains 5.4 mEq of sodium per gram of edetate disodium.

Revised: 02/20/92

---

# EDROPHONIUM  Systemic

VA CLASSIFICATION (Primary/Secondary): AU300/DX900; AD900
Commonly used brand name(s): *Enlon; Reversol; Tensilon.*
Note: For a listing of dosage forms and brand names by country availability, see *Dosage Forms* section(s).

## Category

Cholinergic (cholinesterase inhibitor); diagnostic aid (myasthenia gravis); antidote (to nondepolarizing neuromuscular block).
Note: Cholinergic (cholinesterase inhibitor) is the basic category; the other categories are specific categories of use.

## Indications

**Accepted**
Myasthenia gravis (diagnosis)—Edrophonium is indicated in the differential diagnosis of myasthenia gravis and as an adjunct in the evaluation of treatment requirements in the disease. It is also indicated for evaluating emergency treatment in myasthenic crisis. Edrophonium is not recommended for maintenance therapy in myasthenia gravis because of its short duration of action.
Neuromuscular blockade, nondepolarizing (treatment) and
Toxicity, curare (treatment)—Edrophonium is indicated to reverse the neuromuscular blockade produced by many nondepolarizing agents, including atracurium, gallamine, metocurine, mivacurium, pancuronium, rocuronium, tubocurarine, and vecuronium. Although edrophonium is frequently used to reverse moderate degrees of residual neuromuscular blockade, other cholinesterase inhibitors (such as neostigmine) may better antagonize profound levels of neuromuscular blockade and neuromuscular blockade induced by doxacurium and pipecuronium.
Edrophonium is not effective against depolarizing agents such as decamethonium and succinylcholine.
Also, edrophonium is indicated as an adjunct in the treatment of respiratory depression caused by overdosage of nondepolarizing neuromuscular blocking agents.

**Unaccepted**
Edrophonium has been used to terminate supraventricular tachycardia (SVT; paroxysmal atrial tachycardia) but has generally been replaced by other antiarrhythmic agents.

## Pharmacology/Pharmacokinetics

**Physicochemical characteristics**
Molecular weight—201.7.
Other characteristics—Edrophonium injection: pH between 5 and 5.8.

**Mechanism of action/Effect**
Cholinergic (cholinesterase inhibitor)—
 Inhibits destruction of acetylcholine by acetylcholinesterase, thereby facilitating transmission of impulses across the myoneural junction.

Diagnostic aid (myasthenia gravis): By prolonging the duration of action of acetylcholine at the motor end plate, edrophonium transiently increases muscle strength in patients with myasthenia gravis, whereas patients with other disorders develop either no increase in strength or even a slight weakness and possibly fasciculations.
Antidote (to nondepolarizing neuromuscular block): Since nondepolarizing neuromuscular blocking agents combine reversibly with the receptors, preventing access of acetylcholine, antagonism can be overcome by increasing the amount of agonist at the receptors; therefore, muscle paralysis induced by nondepolarizing neuromuscular blocking agents is reversed by edrophonium, which increases the concentration of acetylcholine at the receptors.

**Distribution**
The volume of distribution (Vol$_D$) of edrophonium is 1.1 ± 0.2 L per kg.

**Half-life**
Distribution—7 to 12 minutes.
Elimination—33 to 110 minutes.

**Onset of action**
Intramuscular—2 to 10 minutes.
Intravenous—Within 30 to 60 seconds. Onset of reversal of muscle relaxant–induced depression in twitch tension occurs within 3 minutes.

**Time to peak effect**
Following a 0.5 to 1 mg per kg of body weight (mg/kg) intravenous dose—Within 1.2 minutes.

**Duration of action**
In the diagnosis of myasthenia gravis—
 Intramuscular: 5 to 30 minutes.
 Intravenous: 5 to 10 minutes.
For reversal of neuromuscular blockade—
 Following a 0.5 to 1 mg per kg of body weight (mg/kg) intravenous dose: 70 minutes.

**Elimination**
Renal. The clearance of edrophonium is about 0.5 L per kg per hour.

## Precautions to Consider

**Cross-sensitivity and/or related problems**
Patients sensitive to sulfites may be sensitive to edrophonium because of the sulfite preservatives present.

**Pregnancy/Reproduction**
Pregnancy—Studies have not been done in humans.
Studies have not been done in animals.
FDA Pregnancy Category C.

**Breast-feeding**
It is not known whether edrophonium is distributed into breast milk. However, problems in humans have not been documented.

**Pediatrics**
A study performed in 4 infants and 12 children did not show any pediatrics-specific problems that would limit the usefulness of edrophonium for

neuromuscular blockade in children. Caution and careful monitoring are recommended.

### Geriatrics
Extensive studies on the relationship of age to the effects of edrophonium have not been performed in the geriatric population. However, in two studies comparing small numbers of patients 76 to 87 years of age with younger adults, the onset of action and the duration of antagonism of neuromuscular blockade by edrophonium in the older group were no different from those in younger patients.

### Drug interactions and/or related problems
The following drug interactions and/or related problems have been selected on the basis of their potential clinical significance (possible mechanism in parentheses where appropriate)—not necessarily inclusive (» = major clinical significance):

Cholinesterase inhibitors, other, including antimyasthenics, demecarium, echothiophate, and isoflurophate and possibly topical malathion in excessive quantities
(caution is recommended when administering edrophonium to patients with symptoms of myasthenic weakness who are also receiving these medications, since symptoms of cholinergic crisis [overdosage] may be similar to those occurring with myasthenic crisis [underdosage], and the patient's condition may be worsened by use of edrophonium)

Digitalis glycosides
(when used concurrently with edrophonium, the additive vagomimetic effects may cause excessive bradycardia)

Neuromuscular blocking agents
(phase I block of depolarizing neuromuscular blocking agents such as succinylcholine may be prolonged when these medications are used concurrently with edrophonium; however, if these blocking agents have been used over a prolonged period of time and the depolarization block has changed to a nondepolarization block, edrophonium may reverse the nondepolarization block)
(effects of many nondepolarizing neuromuscular blocking agents are antagonized by edrophonium, especially moderate degrees of residual neuromuscular blockade; profound levels of neuromuscular blockade may be better antagonized by other agents such as neostigmine)

### Medical considerations/Contraindications
The medical considerations/contraindications included have been selected on the basis of their potential clinical significance (reasons given in parentheses where appropriate)—not necessarily inclusive (» = major clinical significance).

*Except under special circumstances, this medication should not be used when the following medical problem exists:*
» Intestinal or urinary tract obstruction, mechanical

*Risk-benefit should be considered when the following medical problems exist:*
» Asthma, bronchial
(increase in bronchial secretions and other respiratory effects of edrophonium may aggravate condition)
Cardiac dysrhythmias such as bradycardia and atrioventricular (AV) block
(increased risk of cardiac arrhythmias)
Sensitivity to edrophonium

## Side/Adverse Effects
Note: Severe side/adverse effects occur rarely with usual doses of edrophonium. Any side effects that may occur with edrophonium are usually short-lived because of its short duration of action and are usually less severe than those that occur with neostigmine, pyridostigmine, or ambenonium.

The following side/adverse effects have been selected on the basis of their potential clinical significance (possible signs and symptoms in parentheses where appropriate)—not necessarily inclusive:

### Those indicating need for medical attention
Incidence rare
*Muscarinic effects* (shortness of breath, troubled breathing, wheezing or tightness in chest; slow heartbeat; unusual tiredness or weakness); *nicotinic effects* (muscle weakness, cramps, or twitching)
Note: Cholinergic reaction includes severe muscarinic side effects in addition to nicotinic effects.

### Those indicating need for medical attention only if they continue or are bothersome
Incidence less frequent or rare
*Muscarinic effects* (blurred vision; diarrhea; frequent urge to urinate; increased sweating; increased watering of eyes or mouth; increase in bronchial secretions; nausea or vomiting; stomach cramps or pain)

## Overdose
For specific information on the agents used in the management of edrophonium overdose, see:
• *Atropine* in *Anticholinergics/Antispasmodics (Systemic)* monograph; and/or
• *Pralidoxime (Systemic)* monograph.

For more information on the management of overdose or unintentional ingestion, **contact a Poison Control Center** (see *Poison Control Center Listing*).

### Clinical effects of overdose
The following effects have been selected on the basis of their potential clinical significance (possible signs and symptoms in parentheses where appropriate)—not necessarily inclusive:

Acute and/or chronic
*Muscarinic effects* (diarrhea; bradycardia; increased bronchial and salivary secretions; nausea and/or vomiting; sweating)

### Treatment of overdose
Discontinuation of edrophonium.

Specific treatment—Use of intravenous atropine or pralidoxime to control muscarinic effects. See package insert or *Atropine* in *Anticholinergics/Antispasmodics (Systemic)* or *Pralidoxime (Systemic)* monographs for specific dosing guidelines. However, use may be limited due to the short half-life of edrophonium.

May include treatment of seizures or shock as appropriate.

Monitoring—May include monitoring of cardiac function.

Supportive care—May include maintaining an open airway and possible suctioning of bronchial secretions; and use of assisted respiration.

## General Dosing Information
When edrophonium is used for testing, atropine injection should always be readily available to counteract severe cholinergic reactions, which may occur in hypersensitive individuals.

Atropine will prevent or relieve the muscarinic side effects, but is usually not required, except in patients older than 50 years of age, who should be given atropine before myasthenic testing to prevent bradycardia and hypotension.

Atropine may be administered to relieve the transient bradycardia that may occur with the use of edrophonium.

When used to reverse the effects of nondepolarizing neuromuscular blockade, edrophonium should not be administered prior to the nondepolarizing neuromuscular blocking agent but at the time the effect is needed.

When used as a test for the evaluation of treatment requirements in myasthenia gravis:
• In patients who require additional anticholinesterase medication, a transient increase in muscle strength without fasciculation or muscarinic side effects will occur (myasthenic response).
• In patients who have been overtreated with anticholinesterase agents, muscle strength is decreased, muscle fasciculations may occur, and severe muscarinic effects usually occur (cholinergic response).
• In patients being adequately treated with anticholinesterase agents, there is no change in muscle strength, muscle fasciculations may occur, and side effects, if any occur, are mild.

When used to differentiate myasthenic crisis from cholinergic crisis, edrophonium may temporarily increase muscle strength if treatment has been inadequate (myasthenic crisis), whereas in overtreatment (cholinergic crisis) the condition may worsen.

## Parenteral Dosage Forms

### EDROPHONIUM CHLORIDE INJECTION USP
#### Usual adult and adolescent dose
For evaluation of treatment requirements in myasthenia gravis—
Intravenous, 1 to 2 mg one hour after administration of anticholinesterase agent.
To differentiate cholinergic crisis from myasthenic crisis—
Intravenous, initially 1 mg, followed after one minute by an additional 1 mg if the initial dose does not further impair patient.
Diagnostic aid (myasthenia gravis)—
Intramuscular, 10 mg.

Note: If cholinergic reaction occurs, test should be repeated after thirty minutes using a dose of 2 mg, to rule out a false-negative reaction.

Intravenous, initially 2 mg administered within fifteen to thirty seconds, followed by 8 mg if no response after forty-five seconds.

Note: If cholinergic reaction occurs after initial dose of 2 mg, test should be discontinued and 400 mcg (0.4 mg) of atropine given intravenously. Test may be repeated after thirty to sixty minutes.

Reversal of nondepolarizing neuromuscular blockade—
Intravenous, 10 mg administered over a period of thirty to forty-five seconds, repeated as needed, up to a maximum total dose of 40 mg. Alternatively, doses of 0.5 to 1 mg of edrophonium per kg of body weight are used.

### Usual pediatric dose
Diagnostic aid (myasthenia gravis)—
Infants:
Intramuscular or subcutaneous, 500 mcg (0.5 mg) to 1 mg.
Intravenous, 500 mcg (0.5 mg).
Children up to 34 kg of body weight:
Intramuscular, 2 mg.
Intravenous, 1 mg initially; if no response within forty-five seconds, then 1 mg every thirty to forty-five seconds up to a total dose of 5 mg.
Children 34 kg of body weight and over:
Intramuscular, 5 mg.
Intravenous, 2 mg initially; if no response within forty-five seconds, then 1 mg every thirty to forty-five seconds up to a total dose of 10 mg.

### Usual geriatric dose
See *Usual adult and adolescent dose*.

Note: Patients older than 50 years of age should be given atropine before myasthenic testing to prevent bradycardia and hypotension.

### Strength(s) usually available
U.S.—
10 mg per mL (Rx) [*Enlon* (phenol 0.45%; sodium sulfite 0.2%; sodium citrate; citric acid); *Reversol* (phenol 0.45%; sodium sulfite 0.2%; sodium citrate; citric acid); *Tensilon* (sodium sulfite 0.2%; sodium citrate; citric acid—in 1-mL ampuls; or phenol 0.45%; sodium sulfite 0.2%; sodium citrate; citric acid—in 10-mL vials)].

Canada—
10 mg per mL (Rx) [*Enlon* (phenol 0.45%; sodium sulfite 0.2%; sodium citrate; citric acid); *Tensilon* (phenol 0.45%; sodium sulfite 0.2%; sodium citrate; citric acid; sodium < 1 mmol per mL)].

### Packaging and storage
Store below 40 °C (104 °F), preferably between 15 and 30 °C (59 and 86 °F), unless otherwise specified by manufacturer. Protect from freezing.

### Additional information
A combination of edrophonium and atropine (*Enlon-Plus*) is available in the U.S.

Revised: 1/21/98

---

# EDROPHONIUM AND ATROPINE Systemic†

BAN: Atropine sulfate—Atropine sulphate
VA CLASSIFICATION (Primary/Secondary): AU300/AD900
Commonly used brand name(s): *Enlon-Plus*.
Note: For a listing of dosage forms and brand names by country availability, see *Dosage Forms* section(s).

†Not commercially available in Canada.

## Category
Cholinergic (cholinesterase inhibitor); antidote (to nondepolarizing neuromuscular blockade).

## Indications
### Accepted
Neuromuscular blockade, nondepolarizing (treatment)—Edrophonium and atropine combination is indicated to reverse the neuromuscular blockade produced by many nondepolarizing agents, including atracurium, gallamine, metocurine, mivacurium, pancuronium, rocuronium, tubocurarine, and vecuronium.

Edrophonium is not effective against depolarizing agents such as decamethonium and succinylcholine.

Toxicity, curare (treatment adjunct)—Edrophonium and atropine combination is indicated as an adjunct in the treatment of respiratory depression caused by curare overdosage.

### Unaccepted
Edrophonium and atropine combination is not recommended for use in the differential diagnosis of myasthenia gravis.

## Pharmacology/Pharmacokinetics
### Physicochemical characteristics
Molecular weight—
Edrophonium chloride: 201.7.
Atropine sulfate: 694.85.
pH—Edrophonium chloride and atropine sulfate: 4.4 to 4.6.

### Mechanism of action/Effect
Edrophonium—Since nondepolarizing neuromuscular blocking agents combine reversibly with the receptors, preventing access of acetylcholine, antagonism can be overcome by increasing the amount of agonist at the receptors; therefore, muscle paralysis induced by nondepolarizing neuromuscular blocking agents is reversed by edrophonium, which increases the concentration of acetylcholine at the receptors.

Atropine—An accumulation of acetylcholine at the sites of muscarinic cholinergic transmission occurs at the parasympathetic postganglionic receptors of the autonomic nervous system, which may cause parasympathomimetic side effects, such as bradycardia, bronchoconstriction, or increased secretions. The anticholinergic activity of atropine counteracts these muscarinic side effects.

### Other actions/effects
A local and direct action on smooth muscle to reduce tone and motility of the gastrointestinal tract has been suggested to explain the apparent gastrointestinal antispasmodic effect of atropine.

### Distribution
$Vol_D$—
Edrophonium: $1.1 \pm 0.2$ L per kg of body weight (L/kg).
Atropine: $1.6 \pm 0.4$ L/kg.

### Protein binding
Atropine—Low (14%).

### Biotransformation
Atropine—Hepatic; primarily to tropine (30%).

### Half-life
Elimination—
Edrophonium: Approximately 108 minutes (range, 33 to 110 minutes).
Atropine: Approximately 180 minutes.

### Onset of action
Edrophonium—
Intramuscular: 2 to 10 minutes.
Intravenous: Within 30 to 60 seconds. Reversal of skeletal muscle relaxant–induced depression in twitch tension occurs within 3 minutes.

### Time to peak effect
Edrophonium—Following a 0.5- to 1-mg-per-kg-of-body-weight (mg/kg) intravenous dose: Within 1.2 minutes.
Atropine—Following a 0.02-mg/kg intravenous dose (effect on heart rate): 2 to 16 minutes.

### Duration of action
Edrophonium—Following a 0.5- to 1-mg/kg intravenous dose: 70 minutes.
Atropine—Following a 0.02-mg/kg dose (effect on heart rate): 170 minutes.

### Elimination
Edrophonium—Renal: 67% unchanged. The clearance of edrophonium is approximately 0.5 L/kg/hour.
Atropine—Renal: 57% unchanged. The clearance of atropine is approximately 0.4 L/kg/hour.

## Precautions to Consider
### Cross-sensitivity and/or related problems
Patients sensitive to edrophonium or atropine may be sensitive to the edrophonium and atropine combination.
Patients sensitive to sulfites may be sensitive to edrophonium and atropine combination because of the sulfite preservatives present.

**Carcinogenicity/Mutagenicity**
Studies evaluating the carcinogenic or mutagenic potential of edrophonium and atropine combination have not been done.

**Pregnancy/Reproduction**
Pregnancy—Adequate and well-controlled studies in humans have not been done.
Studies have not been done in animals.
*Atropine—*
  Atropine crosses the placenta. Well-controlled studies in humans have not been done. Intravenous administration of atropine during pregnancy or near term may produce tachycardia in the fetus. Studies in mice have not shown that atropine given in doses of 50 mg per kg of body weight (mg/kg) has adverse effects on the fetus.
*Edrophonium—*
  Studies in humans or animals have not been done.
FDA Pregnancy Category C.

**Breast-feeding**
It is not known whether edrophonium and atropine combination is distributed into breast milk. However, problems in humans have not been documented.
Atropine—
  Atropine is distributed into breast milk. Although amounts have not been quantified, the long-term use of atropine should be avoided during nursing since infants are usually very sensitive to the effects of anticholinergics.
Edrophonium—
  It is not known whether edrophonium is distributed into breast milk. However, problems in humans have not been documented.

**Pediatrics**
Limited information is available on the relationship of age to the effects of edrophonium and atropine combination in pediatric patients. Safety and efficacy have not been established.

**Geriatrics**
Extensive studies on the relationship of age to the effects of the edrophonium and atropine combination have not been done in the geriatric population. However, no geriatrics-specific problems have been documented.
Edrophonium—
  In two studies comparing small numbers of patients 76 to 87 years of age with younger adults, the onset of action and the duration of antagonism of neuromuscular blockade by edrophonium in the older group were no different than in younger patients.

**Drug interactions and/or related problems**
The following drug interactions and/or related problems have been selected on the basis of their potential clinical significance (possible mechanism in parentheses where appropriate)—not necessarily inclusive (» = major clinical significance):
Note: Combinations containing any of the following medications, depending on the amount present, may also interact with this medication.
  Anesthetics, inhalation, especially with the combination of an opioid analgesic and nitrous oxide or
» Beta-adrenergic blocking agents, systemic
    (concurrent use with edrophonium and atropine combination may increase the risk of excessive bradycardia; administration of atropine alone prior to the combination edrophonium and atropine is recommended; caution is also recommended when administering edrophonium and atropine combination in patients with cardiovascular disease who are receiving anesthesia with an opioid (narcotic) analgesic and nitrous oxide without a potent inhalational anesthetic)
  Digitalis glycosides
    (when used concurrently with edrophonium, the additive vagomimetic effects may cause excessive slowing of the heart rate)
  Cholinesterase inhibitors, other, including antimyasthenics, demecarium, echothiophate, and isoflurophate, and possibly topical malathion in excessive quantities
    (caution is recommended when administering edrophonium and atropine combination to patients with symptoms of myasthenic weakness who are also receiving these medications, since symptoms of cholinergic crisis [overdosage] may be similar to those occurring with myasthenic crisis [underdosage]; the patient's condition may be worsened by use of the edrophonium and atropine combination)
» Neuromuscular blocking agents
    (edrophonium and atropine combination should not be administered prior to the administration of any nondepolarizing muscle relaxant)
    (concurrent use of edrophonium and atropine combination with vecuronium may be associated with bradycardia and first-degree heart block, due to the lack of vagolytic activity of the skeletal muscle relaxant)

**Medical considerations/Contraindications**
The medical considerations/contraindications included have been selected on the basis of their potential clinical significance (reasons given in parentheses where appropriate)—not necessarily inclusive (» = major clinical significance).

*Except under special circumstances, this medication should not be used when the following medical problems exist:*
» Cardiac dysrhythmias, such as bradycardia and atrioventricular (AV) block
    (increased risk of arrhythmias; it is recommended that additional doses of atropine be available for immediate use to counteract severe cholinergic reactions that may occur)
  Sensitivity to edrophonium and atropine

*Risk-benefit should be considered when the following medical problems exist:*
» Asthma, bronchial
    (increase in bronchial secretions and other respiratory effects of edrophonium may aggravate the condition)
» Glaucoma, angle-closure
    (mydriatic effect resulting in increased intraocular pressure may precipitate an acute attack of angle-closure glaucoma)
» Intestinal or urinary tract obstruction, mechanical or
» Pyloric stenosis
    (may be aggravated)
  Lung disease, chronic, especially in debilitated patients
    (increase in bronchial secretions and other respiratory effects of edrophonium may aggravate the condition)
  Prostatic hypertrophy
    (urinary retention may be aggravated or precipitated)

## Side/Adverse Effects

The following side/adverse effects have been selected on the basis of their potential clinical significance (possible signs and symptoms in parentheses where appropriate)—not necessarily inclusive:

**Those indicating need for medical attention**
Incidence more frequent
  *Arrhythmias* (irregular heartbeat)
    Note: Of the patients in whom arrhythmias occurred, 85% experienced onset within 2 minutes; 74% of these patients no longer had any arrhythmias after 10 minutes. Arrhythmias related to increased vagal tone, bradycardia, or second- and third-degree heart block responded to treatment with 0.2 to 0.4 mg of intravenous atropine.
Incidence rare
  *Muscarinic effects* (shortness of breath, troubled breathing, wheezing, or tightness in chest; slow heartbeat; unusual tiredness or weakness); *nicotinic effects* (muscle weakness, cramps, or twitching)
    Note: Cholinergic reaction includes severe muscarinic side effects in addition to nicotinic effects.

**Those indicating need for medical attention only if they continue or are bothersome**
Incidence less frequent or rare
  *Dry skin*—dose-related; *muscarinic effects* (blurred vision; diarrhea; frequent urge to urinate; increased sweating; increased watering of eyes or mouth; increase in mucus in the lungs; nausea or vomiting; stomach cramps or pain); *restlessness with asthenia* (restlessness with muscle weakness); *skin rash*—dose-related; *speech disturbances* (changes in speech)

## Overdose

For specific information on the agents used in the management of edrophonium and atropine combination overdose, see:
  • *Atropine* in *Anticholinergics/Antispasmodics (Systemic)* monograph;
  • *Physostigmine (Systemic)* monograph; and/or
  • *Pralidoxime (Systemic)* monograph.

For more information on the management of overdose or unintentional ingestion, **contact a Poison Control Center** (see *Poison Control Center Listing*).

**Clinical effects of overdose**
The following effects have been selected on the basis of their potential clinical significance (possible signs and symptoms in parentheses where appropriate)—not necessarily inclusive:

Acute and/or chronic
*Edrophonium*
**Muscarinic effects** (diarrhea; bradycardia; increased bronchial and salivary secretions; nausea and/or vomiting; sweating)
*Atropine*
**Delirium; dryness of mouth; fever; tachycardia**

### Treatment of overdose
Specific treatment—

Use of atropine or pralidoxime for the treatment of muscarinic symptoms. See package insert or *Atropine* in *Anticholinergics/Antispasmodics (Systemic)* or *Pralidoxime (Systemic)* for specific dosing guidelines.

Physostigmine must be administered with caution to reverse anticholinergic symptoms. See package insert or *Physostigmine (Systemic)* monograph for specific dosing guidelines.

Treatment of seizures or shock as appropriate.

Monitoring—Monitoring cardiac function.

Supportive care—May include maintaining an open airway and possible suctioning of bronchial secretions.

## General Dosing Information

Atropine slows gastric emptying and gastrointestinal activity, which may interfere with the absorption of other medications.

It is recommended that atropine be immediately available to counteract severe cholinergic reactions that may occur in patients hypersensitive to edrophonium.

After administration of edrophonium and atropine combination, the patient's response should be carefully monitored and ventilation secured.

## Parenteral Dosage Forms

### EDROPHONIUM AND ATROPINE SULFATE INJECTION

**Usual adult dose**
Reversal of nondepolarizing neuromuscular blockade—
Intravenous, 0.05 to 0.1 mL per kg of body weight given slowly over forty-five seconds to one minute at a point of at least 5% recovery of twitch response to neuromuscular stimulation (95% block).

Note: The dosage delivered is 0.5 to 1 mg per kg of body weight of edrophonium and 0.007 to 0.014 mg per kg of body weight of atropine.

**Usual adult and prescribing limits**
Edrophonium—1 mg per kg of body weight per dose.

**Pediatric prescribing limits**
Safety and efficacy have not been established.

**Usual geriatric dose**
See *Usual adult dose*.

**Strength(s) usually available**
U.S.—
10 mg per mL of edrophonium chloride and 0.14 mg per mL of atropine sulfate (Rx) [*Enlon-Plus* (0.2% sodium sulfite; sodium citrate; citric acid—in 5-mL ampuls; 0.2% sodium sulfite; sodium citrate; citric acid; phenol 0.45%—in 15-mL ampuls)].
Canada—
Not commercially available.

**Packaging and storage**
Store below 40 ºC (104 ºF), preferably between 15 and 30 ºC (59 and 86 ºF), unless otherwise specified by manufacturer.

Protect from freezing.

Revised: 08/08/97

**EFLORNITHINE**—The *Eflornithine (Systemic)* monograph is not included in this published version of the USP DI database. Copies of the monograph are available on request from Micromedex, Inc. - Reprint Requests, 6200 S. Syracuse Way, Suite 300, Englewood, CO 80111; telephone (303) 486-6400; telefax (303) 486-6464; Email: USPDI@MDX.COM.

# EMEDASTINE Ophthalmic—INTRODUCTORY VERSION

VA CLASSIFICATION (Primary): OP801
Commonly used brand name(s): *Emadine*.
Note: For a listing of dosage forms and brand names by country availability, see *Dosage Forms* section(s).

## Category
Antihistamine ($H_1$-receptor), ophthalmic; antiallergic, ophthalmic.

## Indications

**Accepted**
Conjunctivitis, allergic (treatment)—Ophthalmic emedastine is indicated for temporary relief of the symptoms of allergic conjunctivitis.

## Pharmacology/Pharmacokinetics

**Physicochemical characteristics**
Molecular weight—Emedastine difumarate: 534.57.
pH—Approximately 7.4.

**Mechanism of action/Effect**
Emedastine is a relatively selective histamine $H_1$-receptor antagonist according to *in vitro* studies. Topical ocular administration of emedastine produces concentration-dependent inhibition of histamine-stimulated vascular permeability in the conjunctiva. Emedastine does not affect adrenergic, dopamine, or serotonin receptors.

**Absorption**
Ophthalmic use of emedastine usually does not produce measurable plasma concentrations. A study in normal volunteers (10 subjects) who were administered emedastine 0.05% ophthalmic solution in each eye twice a day for 16 days found that plasma concentrations were generally below the quantitative limit of the assay (less than 0.3 nanogram per mL). Samples in which emedastine was quantifiable contained plasma concentrations ranging from 0.3 to 0.49 nanogram per mL.

**Biotransformation**
Two primary metabolites, 5- and 6-hydroxyemedastine, are found in the urine as both free and conjugated forms. Minor metabolites include the 5'-oxoanalogs of 5- and 6-hydroxyemedastine and the *N*-oxide.

**Half-life**
Elimination—3 or 4 hours.

**Elimination**
Renal, approximately 44% of an oral dose over 24 hours (3.6% unchanged).

## Precautions to Consider

**Carcinogenicity**
No evidence of carcinogenicity was found in lifetime studies in mice and rats given dietary doses of emedastine that were more than 80,000 times and 26,000 times, respectively, the maximum recommended ocular human use level of 0.002 mg per kg of body weight (mg/kg) per day for a 50-kg adult.

**Mutagenicity**
Emedastine was not found to be mutagenic in *in vitro* tests, including a bacterial reverse mutation (Ames) test, a modification of the Ames test, a mammalian chromosome aberration test, a mammalian forward mutation test, and a mammalian DNA repair synthesis test, or in *in vivo* tests including a mammalian sister chromatid exchange test and a mouse micronucleus test.

**Pregnancy/Reproduction**
Fertility—Studies in rats given doses of emedastine that were 15,000 times the maximum recommended ocular human use level found no evidence of impairment of fertility or reproductive capacity.

Pregnancy—Adequate and well-controlled studies in humans have not been done.

Studies in rats and rabbits given doses of emedastine that were 15,000 times the maximum recommended ocular human use level found no evidence of teratogenicity, and the same dose produced no effect on perinatal or postnatal development in rats. However, studies in rats given doses of emedastine that were 70,000 times the maximum recommended ocular human use level found an increased incidence of external, visceral, and skeletal anomalies.

FDA Pregnancy Category B.

**Breast-feeding**
It is not known whether ophthalmic emedastine is absorbed in sufficient quantities to be distributed into human breast milk. However, emedas-

# Emedastine (Ophthalmic)—Introductory Version

tine has been detected in the milk of lactating rats following oral administration. Risk-benefit should be considered before use of ophthalmic emedastine during breast-feeding.

### Pediatrics
Appropriate studies on the relationship of age to the effects of ophthalmic emedastine have not been performed in children up to 3 years of age. Safety and efficacy have not been established.

### Geriatrics
No information is available on the relationship of age to the effects of ophthalmic emedastine in geriatric patients.

### Medical considerations/Contraindications
The medical considerations/contraindications included have been selected on the basis of their potential clinical significance (reasons given in parentheses where appropriate)—not necessarily inclusive (» = major clinical significance).

*Risk-benefit should be considered when the following medical problem exists:*
» Sensitivity to emedastine

## Side/Adverse Effects
The following side/adverse effects have been selected on the basis of their potential clinical significance (possible signs and symptoms in parentheses where appropriate)—not necessarily inclusive:

**Those indicating need for medical attention**
Incidence less frequent—Less than 5%
*Abnormal dreams; asthenia* (weakness); *corneal infiltrates or staining* (blurred vision or other change in vision); *keratitis* (eye redness, irritation, or pain); *tearing, discomfort, or other eye irritation not present before therapy or becoming worse during therapy*

**Those indicating need for medical attention only if they continue or are bothersome**
Incidence more frequent
*Headache*—11%
Incidence less frequent—Less than 5%
*Bad taste; burning or stinging of the eye; dermatitis* (skin rash or itching); *dry eye; foreign body sensation* (feeling of something in the eye); *hyperemia* (redness of eye); *pruritis* (itching); *rhinitis* (stuffy or runny nose); *sinusitis* (headache or runny nose)

## Patient Consultation
As an aid to patient consultation, refer to *Advice for the Patient, Emedastine (Ophthalmic)—Introductory Version.*

In providing consultation, consider emphasizing the following selected information (» = major clinical significance):

**Before using this medication**
» Conditions affecting use, especially:
   Sensitivity to emedastine
   Breast-feeding—Detected in the milk of lactating rats following oral administration of emedastine

**Proper use of this medication**
» Not wearing contact lenses if eyes are red; if eyes are not red, removing contact lenses prior to administration; waiting at least 10 minutes after administration before reinserting lenses
» Proper administration; not touching applicator tip to any surface; keeping container tightly closed

» Proper dosing
   Missed dose: Using as soon as possible; not using if almost time for next dose; using next dose at regularly scheduled time
» Proper storage

**Precautions while using this medication**
» Checking with physician if symptoms do not improve or if condition worsens

**Side/adverse effects**
   Signs of potential side effects, especially abnormal dreams; asthenia; corneal infiltrates or staining; keratitis; sinusitis; and tearing, discomfort, or other eye irritation not present before therapy or becoming worse during therapy

## General Dosing Information
Emedastine contains benzalkonium chloride, which may be absorbed by contact lenses. The manufacturer does not recommend use of contact lenses if eyes are red. If eyes are not red, contact lenses should be removed prior to administration of emedastine and may be reinserted 10 minutes after administration.

## Ophthalmic Dosage Forms

### EMEDASTINE DIFUMARATE OPHTHALMIC SOLUTION

Note: The dosing and strength of the dosage form available are expressed in terms of emedastine base.

**Usual adult and adolescent dose**
Allergic conjunctivitis—
   Topical, to the conjunctiva, 1 drop in each affected eye up to four times a day.

**Usual pediatric dose**
Allergic conjunctivitis—
   Children younger than 3 years of age: Safety and efficacy have not been established.
   Children 3 years of age and older: See *Usual adult and adolescent dose.*

**Strength(s) usually available**
U.S.—
   0.05% (Rx) [*Emadine* (benzalkonium chloride 0.01%; tromethamine; sodium chloride; hydroxypropyl methylcellulose; hydrochloric acid/sodium hydroxide; purified water)].

Note: Each mL contains 0.884 mg emedastine difumarate, which is equivalent to 0.5 mg emedastine base.

**Packaging and storage**
Store between 4 and 30 °C (39 and 86 °F).

**Auxiliary labeling**
• For the eye.

Developed: 08/14/98

---

**ENALAPRIL**—See *Angiotensin-converting Enzyme (ACE) Inhibitors (Systemic)*

---

# ENALAPRIL AND DILTIAZEM   Systemic—INTRODUCTORY VERSION

VA CLASSIFICATION (Primary): CV401
Commonly used brand name(s): *Teczem.*
Note: For a listing of dosage forms and brand names by country availability, see *Dosage Forms* section(s).

## Category
Antihypertensive.

## Indications

**Accepted**
Hypertension (treatment)—The combination of enalapril maleate and diltiazem malate is indicated for the treatment of hypertension. It is not indicated as initial treatment for hypertension.

## Pharmacology/Pharmacokinetics

**Physicochemical characteristics**
Molecular weight—Enalapril maleate: 492.53.
Diltiazem malate: 548.61.

**Mechanism of action/Effect**
Enalapril is the ethyl ester and prodrug of the long-acting angiotensin-converting enzyme (ACE) inhibitor, enalaprilat. ACE, a peptidyl dipeptidase, catalyzes the conversion of angiotensin I to the vasoconstrictor angiotensin II. Angiotensin II stimulates secretion of aldosterone from the adrenal cortex and inhibits the release of renin through a negative feedback mechanism. When ACE is inhibited, angiotensin II formation is reduced and the interruption of the negative feedback mechanism results in increased plasma renin concentrations. The reduction of angiotensin II formation also causes decreased aldosterone secretion and vasopressor activity. The decrease in aldosterone secretion leads to

a small increase in serum potassium. Suppression of the renin-angiotensin-aldosterone system is thought to be the primary mechanism through which ACE inhibitors lower blood pressure.

Diltiazem is a calcium channel blocking agent that inhibits the influx of calcium ions into cell membranes of vascular smooth muscle and cardiac muscle. The action of diltiazem on vascular smooth muscle results in a decrease in peripheral vascular resistance and a consequent reduction in blood pressure with a slight reduction in heart rate. Diltiazem also decreases conduction through the sinoatrial (SA) and atrioventricular (AV) nodes, produces small increases in the PR interval, and reduces the renal and peripheral effects of angiotensin II. Diltiazem also has a negative inotropic effect in isolated preparations.

When enalapril is given in combination with diltiazem, the antihypertensive effects are additive.

### Other actions/effects
ACE is also known as kininase II, an enzyme that degrades bradykinin. Enalapril may increase concentrations of bradykinin, producing a therapeutic vasodilating effect.

### Absorption
Enalapril—Extent of absorption, based on urinary recovery, is approximately 60% and is not influenced by food.

Diltiazem—Well absorbed from the gastrointestinal tract. Bioavailability of extended-release tablets is approximately 40%. The area under the plasma concentration–time curve (AUC) increases proportionally after multiple dosing. Postprandially, the mean AUC of diltiazem is approximately 16% higher than when given during fasting. Release of diltiazem from extended-release tablets is dependent on gastrointestinal transit times. Release of 70% or more of diltiazem requires transit times of 10 hours or greater; shorter transit times result in proportionally less diltiazem released.

### Protein binding
Diltiazem—High (70 to 80%); to alpha$_1$-acid glycoprotein and albumin.

### Biotransformation
Enalapril is hydrolyzed to enalaprilat, the active metabolite. No other metabolites of enalapril have been identified.

Diltiazem undergoes extensive first-pass metabolism. Biotransformation occurs by cytochrome P450 mixed function oxidase. Major metabolic pathways include deacetylation, *N*-demethylation, *O*-demethylation, and aromatic oxidation followed by conversion to glucuronide and sulfate conjugates. The major metabolites are *N*-desmethyldiltiazem (DMD) and desacetyldiltiazem (DAD), reaching respective plasma concentrations of 10% and 30% of those for diltiazem. Both metabolites are pharmacologically less active than diltiazem and are eliminated by biliary and urinary excretion. Other unidentified metabolites exist in higher concentrations than that of diltiazem and are more slowly eliminated than diltiazem. Less than 4% of the dose is excreted in urine as unchanged drug.

### Half-life
Elimination—
  Enalaprilat: Effective—11 hours. Effective half-life is prolonged when glomerular filtration rate is ≤ 30 mL per minute (mL/min).
  Diltiazem: Apparent—2 to 5 hours.

### Time to peak concentration
Enalapril—Approximately 1 hour.
Enalaprilat—3 to 4 hours. May be increased when glomerular filtration rate is ≤ 30 mL/min.
Diltiazem—Average range, 9 to 16 hours for the extended-release formulation.

### Elimination
Enalapril—
  Primarily renal.
Enalaprilat—
  Renal: 40%.
Diltiazem—
  Renal: Approximately 71%.
  Fecal: Approximately 16%.
In dialysis—
  Enalaprilat: Removable by hemodialysis at a rate of 62 mL/min. Removable by peritoneal dialysis from neonatal circulation.
  Diltiazem: Does not appear to be removable by peritoneal dialysis or hemodialysis.

## Precautions to Consider

### Cross-sensitivity and/or related problems
Patients hypersensitive to other angiotensin-converting enzyme (ACE) inhibitors may also be hypersensitive to enalapril.

### Carcinogenicity
No carcinogenicity tests have been performed with enalapril and diltiazem combination.

### Tumorigenicity
Tumorigenicity was not detected when enalapril was given to male and female rats for 106 weeks at daily doses of up to 90 mg per kg of body weight (mg/kg) or when given to male and female mice for 94 weeks at daily doses of up to 90 and 180 mg/kg, respectively. These doses represent 26 times, in rats and female mice, and 13 times, in male mice, the maximum recommended human daily dose (MRHDD), based on body surface area.

Tumorigenicity was not detected in either male and female rats or in male mice given oral daily doses of up to 100 mg/kg of diltiazem for up to 104 weeks in the rats or up to 92 weeks in the mice. These doses represent approximately one and two times for mice and rats, respectively, the maximum recommended human dose (MRHD) of 480 mg per day on a mg per square meter (mg/m$^2$) basis. An increase in the incidence of benign ovarian granulosa cell tumor occurred in female mice given doses of 100 mg/kg of diltiazem per day for 92 weeks. A similar effect was not apparent at daily doses as high as 200 mg/kg of diltiazem given for up to 78 weeks.

### Mutagenicity
Enalapril and diltiazem combination was not found to be mutagenic in the Ames microbial mutagen test with or without metabolic activation. The combination did not produce DNA single strand breaks in an *in vitro* alkaline elution assay in rat hepatocytes or chromosomal aberrations in an *in vivo* mouse bone marrow assay. Increases in chromosomal aberrations were seen, including endoreduplication (a form of polyploidy) in an *in vitro* cytogenetics assay of enalapril and diltiazem combination. These increases were similar to increases seen when diltiazem was given alone.

Enalapril and enalaprilat were not found to be mutagenic in the Ames microbial mutagen test with or without metabolic activation. Enalapril was not found to be genotoxic in the rec-assay, reverse mutation assay with *E. coli*, sister chromatid exchange with cultured mammalian cells, the micronucleus test with mice, or in an *in vivo* cytogenic study using mouse bone marrow.

Diltiazem was not found to be mutagenic *in vitro* in the Ames microbial mutagenicity test, in a study using Chinese hamster lung cells, or in the alkaline elution assay with rat hepatocytes. Diltiazem was also negative *in vivo* for chromosomal aberrations in mouse and Chinese hamster bone marrow, and for induction of micronuclei in Chinese hamster bone marrow. Diltiazem was positive *in vitro* for induction of chromosomal aberrations in Chinese hamster ovary cells at concentrations of approximately 500 times the human clinical plasma levels.

### Pregnancy/Reproduction
Fertility—Impairment of fertility was not found in studies in female rats given oral daily doses of 10 and 120 mg/kg of enalapril and diltiazem, respectively, or in male rats given oral daily doses of 8 and 96 mg/kg of enalapril and diltiazem, respectively. These doses represent 12 and 3 times, respectively for female rats, and 9 and 2.5 times, respectively for male rats, the MRHDD on a body surface area basis. In the fertility study in female rats given 10 and 120 mg/kg of enalapril and diltiazem, respectively, per day, a slight decrease in litter size due to preimplantation loss occurred. It is uncertain if this occurrence was related to treatment.

No adverse effects on reproductive performance were found in studies in male and female rats given up to 90 mg/kg of enalapril per day. This dose represents 26 times the MRHDD, based on body surface area.

Impaired fertility or reproductive performance was not observed in studies in rats given daily doses of up to 30 mg/kg of diltiazem. However, decreased reproductive performance (mating) was observed in male rats given doses of 100 mg/kg of diltiazem per day.

Pregnancy—ACE inhibitors can cause fetal and neonatal morbidity and mortality when administered to pregnant women during the second and third trimesters. Enalapril and diltiazem combination should be discontinued as soon as possible when pregnancy is detected unless no alternative therapy can be used. In the latter instance, serial ultrasound examinations should be performed to assess the intra-amniotic environment. Perinatal diagnostic tests, such as contraction-stress testing (CST), a nonstress test (NST), or biophysical profiling (BPP) may also be appropriate during the applicable week of pregnancy. If oligohydramnios is present, enalapril and diltiazem combination should be discontinued unless it is considered lifesaving for the mother. However, oligohydramnios may not appear until after the fetus has sustained irreversible damage.

Fetal exposure to ACE inhibitors during the second and third trimesters can cause hypotension, reversible or irreversible renal failure, anuria, neonatal skull hypoplasia, and death of the fetus or neonate. Maternal oligohydramnios, which may result from decreased fetal renal function, has been reported and associated with fetal limb contractures, craniofacial deformation, and hypoplastic lung development. Other adverse effects that have been reported are prematurity, intrauterine growth retardation, and patent ductus arteriosus, although how these effects are related to exposure to ACE inhibitors is not clear. ACE inhibitor exposure, when limited to the first trimester, does not appear to be associated with these adverse effects.

Infants who have been exposed *in utero* to ACE inhibitors should be observed closely for hypotension, oliguria, and hyperkalemia. Oliguria should be treated with support of blood pressure and renal perfusion. Dialysis or exchange transfusion may be necessary to reverse hypotension and/or substitute for disordered renal function. Removing enalapril from neonatal circulation by peritoneal dialysis has shown some clinical benefit. There is no experience with removing enalapril by exchange transfusion.

Teratogenic effects were not observed in pregnant rats and rabbits given enalapril in doses representing 57 and 12 times, respectively, the MRHDD based on body surface area.

Reproduction studies in mice given daily doses of ≥ 50 mg/kg of diltiazem, in rats given daily doses of ≥ 200 mg/kg of diltiazem, and in rabbits given daily doses of ≥ 35 mg/kg of diltiazem resulted in embryo and fetal mortality. These doses are similar to, or lower than, the MRHD, on a mg/m² basis, and have also been associated with skeletal (primarily vertebral) malformations in rabbits and mice. In a peri-postnatal study in pregnant rats, doses of diltiazem ≥ 30 mg/kg per day were associated with abnormalities of the retina and tongue in dead rat pups that were examined.

Studies of enalapril and diltiazem combination in mice and rats produced no developmental toxicity. The mice were given daily doses of up to 0.5 and 6 mg/kg of enalapril and diltiazem, respectively, representing approximately 3 and 0.9 times the MRHDD, based on body weight, and 0.29 and 0.079 times the MRHDD, based on body surface area. The rats were given daily doses of up to 5 and 60 mg/kg of enalapril and diltiazem, respectively, representing approximately 30 and 9 times the MRHDD based on body weight, and 5.7 and 1.6 times the MRHDD based on body surface area.

A study in rats showed a decrease in fetal weight, an increase in the incidence of fetuses with visceral anomalies, such as a thin diaphragm with protruding liver and dilated renal pelvis/ureter, and a decrease in pup survival. The rats were given a daily dose of 12.5 and 150 mg/kg of enalapril and diltiazem, respectively, representing 83 and 22 times the MRHD based on body weight and 14.3 and 4 times the MRHDD based on body surface area.

A study in mice resulted in an increase in postimplantation loss and a decrease in fetal weight. The mice were given a daily dose of 2.5 and 30 mg/kg of enalapril and diltiazem, respectively, representing 17 and 4.5 times the MRHDD based on body weight and 1.4 and 0.4 times the MRHDD based on body surface area.

FDA Pregnancy Category C (first trimester).

FDA Pregnancy Category D (second and third trimesters).

Labor—A study in rats given approximately 1.5 times, on a mg/m² basis, the daily recommended therapeutic dose of diltiazem immediately prior to, and throughout the period of parturition resulted in prolonged gestation and dystocia leading to pup death and/or stillbirths.

### Breast-feeding
Enalapril and enalaprilat are distributed into breast milk and are detected in trace amounts. Diltiazem is distributed into breast milk, reaching concentrations approximate to maternal serum concentrations. Breast-feeding is not recommended for mothers taking enalapril and diltiazem combination.

### Pediatrics
No information is available on the relationship of age to the effects of enalapril and diltiazem combination in pediatric patients. Safety and efficacy have not been established.

### Geriatrics
A study with oral and intravenous diltiazem in healthy subjects, ages ranging from 65 to 77 years, showed an increase in the mean area under the plasma concentration–time curve (AUC) of approximately 50% when compared with younger subjects, due to slower elimination in the elderly. However, bioavailability of diltiazem extended-release tablets is unaffected by patient age. In addition, elderly patients may experience greater sensitivity to the effects of enalapril and diltiazem combination compared with younger patients.

### Pharmacogenetics
Black patients have a smaller average response to enalapril when compared with nonblack patients. Black patients also may have a higher incidence of ACE inhibitor–associated angioedema.

Diltiazem has a greater antihypertensive effect in females than in males.

### Surgical
Patients receiving enalapril and diltiazem combination and undergoing major surgery or receiving anesthesia with agents that produce hypotension may experience excessive hypotension. If hypotension in these patients is thought to be the result of ACE inhibition, it can be corrected by volume expansion.

### Drug interactions and/or related problems
The following drug interactions and/or related problems have been selected on the basis of their potential clinical significance (possible mechanism in parentheses where appropriate)—not necessarily inclusive (» = major clinical significance):

Note: Combinations containing any of the following medications, depending on the amount present, may also interact with this medication.

Anesthetics
 (concurrent use with calcium channel blocking agents, such as diltiazem, may further depress cardiac contractility, conductivity, and automaticity; anesthetic-associated vascular dilation may be potentiated; anesthetics and calcium channel blocking agents should be titrated carefully when used concurrently)

» Beta-adrenergic blocking agents, including:
 Propranolol
  (concurrent use with diltiazem malate may result in additive effects to prolong AV conduction; concurrent use in patients with left ventricular dysfunction or cardiac conduction abnormalities may result in unpredictable effects; concurrent use of diltiazem hydrochloride and propranolol in five normal volunteers resulted in increased propranolol serum concentrations and an approximate 50% increase in propranolol bioavailability. *In vitro*, diltiazem appears to displace propranolol from its binding sites; a dosage adjustment of propranolol may be necessary)

Carbamazepine
 (concurrent use with diltiazem has resulted in increases in carbamazepine serum concentrations of 40 to 72%, resulting in toxicity in some cases)

Cimetidine
 (a study in six healthy volunteers given a 1-week course of 1200 mg of cimetidine per day and a single 60 mg dose of diltiazem resulted in a 58% increase in peak diltiazem concentrations ($C_{max}$) and a 53% increase in AUC; concurrent use with ranitidine has produced smaller increases. This effect may be the result of cimetidine-induced inhibition of hepatic cytochrome P450, the enzyme system responsible for the first-pass metabolism of diltiazem; careful monitoring and/or a diltiazem dosage adjustment may be necessary when initiating and discontinuing cimetidine)

Cyclosporine
 (during studies involving renal and cardiac transplant recipients, concurrent use with diltiazem resulted in the need to reduce the cyclosporine dose by 15 to 48% in order to maintain cyclosporine trough concentrations similar to those seen prior to the addition of diltiazem; cyclosporine concentrations should be monitored, especially when diltiazem is initiated, adjusted, or discontinued)

» Digitalis glycosides
 (there have been conflicting results regarding the effect of diltiazem on serum digoxin concentrations; a study in 24 healthy male subjects revealed an approximate 20% increase in digoxin concentrations. A separate study in 12 patients with coronary artery disease resulted in no increase in digoxin concentrations. It is recommended that digoxin serum concentrations be monitored when initiating, adjusting, and discontinuing therapy with diltiazem, in order to avoid possible over- or under-digitalization)

» Diuretics
 (concurrent use with ACE inhibitors may have additive hypotensive effects, especially with recently instituted diuretic therapy; the diuretic dosage may need to be reduced or discontinued or salt intake cautiously increased prior to initiation of ACE inhibitor therapy in patients at risk for excessive hypotension and who are able to tolerate these adjustments)

» Diuretics, potassium-sparing, such as:
 Amiloride
 Spironolactone
 Triamterene or
» Potassium-containing salt substitutes or
» Potassium supplements
  (concurrent use with ACE inhibitors may increase the risk of hyperkalemia; serum potassium concentrations should be monitored as appropriate)

Enzyme inducers, hepatic, cytochrome P450 (see *Appendix II*) or
Enzyme inhibitors, hepatic, cytochrome P450 (see *Appendix II*) or
Medications metabolized by cytochrome P450 hepatic enzyme
  (concurrent use with hepatic enzyme inducers or inhibitors may alter diltiazem metabolism and pharmacokinetics. Concurrent use with medications metabolized by cytochrome P450 may result in competitive inhibition of metabolism; a dosage adjustment of similarly metabolized medications may be necessary when initiating or discontinuing diltiazem, especially for drugs with a low therapeutic ratio and particularly in patients with renal and/or hepatic function impairment)

Lithium
  (concurrent ACE inhibitor use has resulted in increased serum lithium concentrations and symptoms of lithium toxicity; frequent monitoring of serum lithium concentrations is recommended)

**Laboratory value alterations**
The following have been selected on the basis of their potential clinical significance (possible effect in parentheses where appropriate)—not necessarily inclusive (» = major clinical significance):

With physiology/laboratory test values
  Blood urea nitrogen (BUN) and
  Creatinine, serum
    (minor and transient increases in serum creatinine concentrations may occur, especially in patients pretreated with a diuretic or in patients with renal function impairment or renal artery stenosis; a dosage reduction of enalapril or discontinuation of the diuretic may be necessary)

  Hematocrit and
  Hemoglobin
    (in clinical trials with enalapril and diltiazem in combination, small decreases in hematocrit and hemoglobin occurred occasionally, but were rarely of clinical importance unless another cause of anemia occurred concurrently; less than 0.1% of patients discontinued therapy due to anemia)

  Liver function tests, including:
  Alanine aminotransferase (ALT [SGPT]), and
  Alkaline phosphatase, serum and
  Aspartate aminotransferase (AST [SGOT]) and
  Bilirubin, serum and
  Lactate dehydrogenase (LDH), serum
    (in clinical studies with diltiazem, mild elevations of transaminases with and without concurrent elevations in alkaline phosphatase and bilirubin have occurred; increases may be transient and may resolve with continued treatment; rare reactions consistent with acute hepatic injury, such as significant increases in alkaline phosphatase, LDH, SGOT, and SGPT have occurred with diltiazem therapy. The reactions have occurred within 1 to 8 weeks after initiation of therapy and have been reversible after discontinuation of diltiazem)

  Potassium, serum
    (increases in concentrations occurred in approximately 1% of patients in clinical trials with enalapril; patients treated with enalapril for up to 48 weeks had mean increases in serum potassium of approximately 0.2 mEq per liter [mEq/L]; increases may be minor and reversible with continued therapy; hyperkalemia was a cause of discontinuation of therapy in 0.28% of patients treated with enalapril)

  Sodium, serum
    (decreases in concentrations may be minor and reversible upon discontinuation of enalapril and diltiazem combination)

**Medical considerations/Contraindications**
The medical considerations/contraindications included have been selected on the basis of their potential clinical significance (reasons given in parentheses where appropriate)—not necessarily inclusive (» = major clinical significance).

*Except under special circumstances, this medication should not be used when the following medical problems exist:*
» Angioedema related to previous ACE inhibitor therapy, history of
    (increased risk of angioedema with ACE inhibitor therapy)
» Atrioventricular (AV) block, 2nd- or 3rd-degree, except in patients with a functioning artificial ventricular pacemaker
    (increased risk of complete AV block with concurrent use of diltiazem)
» Hypersensitivity to enalapril or diltiazem
» Hypotension (systolic pressure less than 90 mm Hg)
    (increased risk of excessive hypotension)
» Myocardial infarction, acute, accompanied by pulmonary congestion, documented by radiography on hospital admission
    (condition may be exacerbated)
» Sick sinus syndrome, except in patients with a functioning artificial ventricular pacemaker
    (diltiazem prolongs sinus cycle length by as much as 50% in some patients with sick sinus syndrome; diltiazem may interfere with sinus node impulse generation and precipitate an abnormally slow heart rate)

*Risk-benefit should be considered when the following medical problems exist:*
Angioedema unrelated to ACE inhibitor therapy, history of
  (increased risk of angioedema with ACE inhibitor therapy)
Cerebrovascular disease
  (excessive lowering of blood pressure may result in cerebrovascular accident)
Collagen-vascular disease, such as systemic lupus erythematosus (SLE) or scleroderma
  (increased risk of developing neutropenia or agranulocytosis, especially if renal function is impaired)
» Congestive heart failure with preexisting impairment of ventricular function or
» Ventricular dysfunction or cardiac conduction abnormalities and concurrent use of beta-adrenergic blocking agents
  (diltiazem may cause further deterioration of ventricular function or have unpredictable effects)
Diabetes mellitus
  (increased risk of hyperkalemia with ACE inhibitor therapy)
Dialysis with high-flux membranes or
Low-density lipoprotein apheresis with dextran sulfate absorption
  (anaphylactoid reactions have been reported in patients undergoing these procedures while being treated with an ACE inhibitor)
Hepatic function impairment
  (a 1-year-long oral dose toxicity study in dogs given daily doses of diltiazem of 10 to 20 mg/kg showed sporadic and occasionally transient elevations of transaminase values; diltiazem should be used with caution in patients with hepatic function impairment)
Hypotension, as associated with:
» Congestive heart failure
  Dialysis, renal
  Diuresis, recent intensive
  Diuretic dose increase
  Diuretic therapy, high dose
  Sodium or volume depletion, severe
    (increased risk of excessive hypotension with ACE inhibitor therapy; may be associated with oliguria, progressive azotemia, acute renal failure, and/or death)
Hymenoptera venom desensitization treatment
  (life-threatening anaphylactoid reactions have been reported in two patients undergoing desensitizing treatment while receiving ACE inhibitors)
Ischemic heart disease
  (excessive lowering of blood pressure may result in a myocardial infarction)
» Renal artery stenosis, unilateral or bilateral or
» Renal function impairment
  (enalaprilat half-life, time to peak concentration, peak and trough concentrations, and time to steady state may increase with a glomerular filtration rate of ≤ 30 mL/min; increased risk of developing neutropenia or agranulocytosis; increased risk of hyperkalemia; in clinical trials, increases in blood urea nitrogen [BUN] and serum creatinine occurred in 20% of patients with renal function impairment and were reversible upon discontinuation of enalapril and/or the concurrently administered diuretic; renal function should be monitored during the first few weeks of therapy)

**Patient monitoring**
The following may be especially important in patient monitoring (other tests may be warranted in some patients, depending on condition; » = major clinical significance):

» Blood pressure measurements
  (periodic monitoring is necessary for titration of dose according to the patient's response)
Electrocardiogram (ECG) determinations and
Heart rate determinations
  (monitoring may be necessary because of diltiazem-associated PR interval prolongation and heart rate lowering effects)
Hepatic function determinations and
Renal function determinations
  (monitoring at regular intervals is recommended, especially in patients with hepatic or renal function impairment)

Leukocyte count determinations
  (periodic monitoring may be necessary for patients at risk for neutropenia or agranulocytosis, such as those with renal function impairment and/or a collagen-vascular disease)

Potassium, serum concentrations
  (monitoring may be necessary in patients at risk for hyperkalemia, such as those with renal insufficiency, with diabetes mellitus, or those concurrently taking potassium-sparing diuretics, potassium supplements, or potassium-containing salt substitutes)

## Side/Adverse Effects

Note: Small increases in the PR interval, and sometimes abnormal PR interval prolongation, have occurred in patients administered multiple oral doses of up to 540 mg of diltiazem hydrochloride per day. In a study of six normal volunteers given a single oral 300-mg dose of diltiazem hydrochloride, the average maximum PR interval prolongation that occurred was 14%. Atrioventricular (AV) block beyond 1st degree did not occur in these patients. Diltiazem causes a prolongation of AV node refractory periods without a significant prolongation of sinus node recovery time, except in patients with sick sinus syndrome. These effects rarely may cause abnormally slow heart rates, especially in patients with sick sinus syndrome or 2nd- or 3rd-degree AV block. A patient with Prinzmetal's angina developed periods of asystole (2 to 5 seconds) after being administered a single 60-mg dose of diltiazem.

The following side/adverse effects have been selected on the basis of their potential clinical significance (possible signs and symptoms in parentheses where appropriate)—not necessarily inclusive:

### Those indicating need for medical attention
Incidence less frequent
  *Bradycardia* (slow heartbeat); *edema, peripheral* (swelling of ankles, feet, and lower legs); *hypotension* (dizziness, lightheadedness, or fainting)
  Note: *Hypotension* may be anticipated with ACE inhibitor use in volume-depleted patients. Diltiazem therapy may occasionally result in symptomatic hypotension.

Incidence rare
  *Anemia, hemolytic* (bleeding gums, nosebleeds, or pale skin); *angioedema* (sudden trouble in swallowing or breathing; swelling of face, mouth, hands, or feet; hoarseness); *chest pain; hepatotoxicity* (yellow eyes or skin); *hyperkalemia* (confusion; irregular heartbeat; nervousness; numbness or tingling in hands, feet, or lips; shortness of breath or difficulty breathing; weakness or heaviness of legs)—incidence approximately 1% in patients treated with enalapril alone; *neutropenia or agranulocytosis* (chills; fever; sore throat)—occurs rarely in uncomplicated hypertension; occurs more frequently in patients with renal function impairment, especially if accompanied by a collagen-vascular disease; *thrombocytopenia* (unusual bleeding or bruising)
  Note: *Angioedema* is associated with angiotensin-converting enzyme (ACE) inhibitor therapy and may involve the face, extremities, lips, tongue, glottis, and larynx. Angioedema associated with laryngeal edema, resulting in airway obstruction, could be fatal. ACE inhibitor–associated angioedema may occur at any time during treatment and occurs at a higher rate in black patients than in nonblack patients.
  ACE inhibitor–associated *hepatotoxicity* occurs by a mechanism that is not understood, but is manifest as a syndrome of cholestatic jaundice, fulminant hepatic necrosis, and possibly death. Enalapril and diltiazem combination therapy should be discontinued in patients who develop jaundice or marked elevations of hepatic enzymes. Patients should receive appropriate medical follow-up. Rare reactions consistent with acute hepatic injury, such as significant increases in alkaline phosphatase, LDH, SGOT, and SGPT have occurred with diltiazem therapy. Reactions have occurred within 1 to 8 weeks after initiation of therapy and were reversible after discontinuation of diltiazem use.

### Those indicating need for medical attention only if they continue or are bothersome
Incidence less frequent
  *Abdominal pain; cough, dry and persistent; dizziness; fatigue* (unusual tiredness); *nausea; skin rash or other dermatologic reactions*
  Note: *Cough* has been reported with ACE inhibitors and is thought to be due to increased concentrations of bradykinin as a result of kininase II inhibition. In clinical trials of enalapril in combination with diltiazem, the incidence of cough was 3.4%.
  *Dermatologic reactions* may be transient and may disappear even with continued use of diltiazem. Skin eruptions progressing to erythema multiforme and/or exfoliative dermatitis also have been reported occasionally with diltiazem. If a dermatologic reaction persists, diltiazem use should be discontinued.

## Overdose
For specific information on the agents used in the management of enalapril and diltiazem combination overdose, see
  • *Atropine* in *Anticholinergics/Antispasmodics (Systemic)* monograph;
  • *Charcoal, Activated (Oral-Local)* monograph; and/or
  • *Dobutamine, Dopamine, Isoproterenol,* or *Norepinephrine,* in *Sympathomimetic Agents—Cardiovascular Use (Parenteral-Systemic)* monograph.

For more information on the management of overdose or unintentional ingestion, **contact a Poison Control Center** (see *Poison Control Center Listing*).

### Clinical effects of overdose
The following effects have been selected on the basis of their potential clinical significance (possible signs and symptoms in parentheses where appropriate)—not necessarily inclusive:

Acute and/or chronic
  *Bradycardia* (slow heartbeat); *cardiac failure; heart block; hypotension, severe* (dizziness; fainting; lightheadedness)

### Treatment of overdose
No information is available on the clinical effects of overdose with enalapril and diltiazem combination. No specific information is available on overdose with diltiazem malate in humans. However, several cases of overdosing with diltiazem hydrochloride in doses as high as 10.8 grams have been reported, with most patients recovering from the reported overdose. In the few fatal cases, multiple drug ingestions usually were involved. Because diltiazem is metabolized extensively, blood concentrations after a standard dose may vary over tenfold and, therefore, may not be a useful indicator in cases of overdose.

Treatment is symptomatic and supportive and may include ventilatory support and/or intravenous calcium, although the effectiveness of the latter in calcium channel blocking agent overdose may be questionable. Enalapril and diltiazem combination should be discontinued and the patient observed closely.

To decrease absorption—Induced emesis, gastric lavage, and/or activated charcoal.

For severe hypotension—Repletion of central fluid volume by placement of the patient in a supine or Trendelenburg position and/or infusion of normal saline. If necessary, vasopressors, such as norepinephrine or dopamine, may be used.

For bradycardia—Atropine. If there is no response to vagal blockade, isoproterenol may be cautiously administered.

For high-degree atrioventricular (AV) block—Treatment is the same as for bradycardia. Fixed high-degree AV block should be treated with cardiac pacing.

For cardiac failure—Inotropic agents, such as isoproterenol, dopamine, or dobutamine, and diuretics.

Supportive care—Patients in whom intentional overdose is confirmed or suspected should be referred for psychiatric consultation.

## Patient Consultation
As an aid to patient consultation, refer to *Advice for the Patient, Enalapril and Diltiazem (Systemic)—Introductory Version*.

In providing consultation, consider emphasizing the following selected information (» = major clinical significance):

### Before using this medication
» Conditions affecting use, especially:
  Hypersensitivity to enalapril, other angiotensin-converting enzyme (ACE) inibitors, or diltiazem
  Pregnancy—Enalapril can cause fetal and neonatal morbidity and mortality during the second and third trimesters; not recommended for use during pregnancy
  Breast-feeding—Enalapril, enalaprilat, and diltiazem are distributed into human breast milk; breast feeding is not recommended for mothers taking enalapril and diltiazem combination
  Use in the elderly—May be more sensitive to the effects of enalapril and diltiazem combination
  Pharmacogenetics—Black patients may have a lower than average response to enalapril and a higher incidence of ACE inhibitor–associated angioedema; diltiazem has a greater antihypertensive effect in females than in males
  Surgical—Anesthesia with hypotension-producing agents may cause excessive hypotension

- Other medications, especially beta-adrenergic blocking agents, including propranolol; digitalis glycosides; diuretics; potassium-containing salt substitutes; potassium supplements; and potassium-sparing diuretics, such as amiloride, spironolactone, and triamterene
- Other medical problems, especially acute myocardial infarction accompanied by pulmonary congestion, documented by radiography on hospital admission; congestive heart failure with preexisting impairment of ventricular function; history of angioedema related to previous ACE inhibitor therapy; hypotension (systolic pressure less than 90 mm Hg); hypotension associated with congestive heart failure; renal function impairment; 2nd- or 3rd-degree atrioventricular (AV) block, except in patients with a functioning artificial ventricular pacemaker; sick sinus syndrome, except in patients with a functioning artificial ventricular pacemaker; unilateral or bilateral renal artery stenosis; or ventricular dysfunction or cardiac conduction abnormalities and concurrent use of beta-adrenergic blocking agents

**Proper use of this medication**
» Compliance with therapy; taking medication at the same time each day to maintain the therapeutic effect
  Swallowing tablets whole without dividing, crushing, or chewing
» Proper dosing
  Missed dose: Taking as soon as possible; not taking if almost time for next scheduled dose; not doubling doses
» Proper storage

**Precautions while using this medication**
Regular visits to physician to check progress
Notifying physician immediately if pregnancy is suspected because of possibility of fetal or neonatal injury and/or death
Not taking other medications, especially potassium supplements or salt substitutes that contain potassium, without consulting the physician
Caution when driving or doing other things requiring alertness because of possible dizziness, lightheadedness, or fainting due to symptomatic hypotension
Notifying physician if lightheadedness or fainting occurs, especially during the first few days of therapy
Reporting any signs of infection (fever, sore throat, chills) to physician because of risk of neutropenia
Reporting any signs of facial or extremity swelling and difficulty in swallowing or breathing because of risk of angioedema
Checking with physician if severe nausea, vomiting, or diarrhea occurs and continues because of risk of dehydration, which may result in hypotension
Caution when exercising or during exposure to hot weather because of risk of dehydration, which may result in hypotension
Caution if any kind of surgery (including dental surgery) or emergency treatment is required

**Side/adverse effects**
Signs of potential side effects, especially bradycardia, peripheral edema, hypotension, hemolytic anemia, angioedema, chest pain, hepatotoxicity, hyperkalemia, neutropenia or agranulocytosis, and thrombocytopenia

## General Dosing Information

Therapy with enalapril and diltiazem combination should be used only after a patient has failed to achieve the desired antihypertensive effect with one or the other alone or the dose of one agent or the other as single therapy cannot be increased further because of dose-limiting side effects. For dosage ranges for the individual agents when given as single therapy, see
- *Enalapril* in *Angiotensin-converting Enzyme (ACE) Inhibitors (Systemic)* monograph; and/or
- *Diltiazem* in *Calcium Channel Blocking Agents (Systemic)* monograph.

When enalapril therapy is initiated in patients concurrently taking a diuretic, it is recommended that the patient be under medical supervision after the initial dose for at least 2 hours, and preferably an additional hour, until blood pressure has stabilized.

In some patients, the antihypertensive effects of enalapril when administered once a day, as single therapy, may diminish toward the end of the dosing interval.

For patients at risk for excessive hypotension or those with ischemic heart or cerebrovascular disease in whom an excessive fall in blood pressure could result in a myocardial infarction or cerebrovascular accident, enalapril (as single therapy) should be started under very close medical supervision and monitoring should be provided for the first 2 weeks of treatment and whenever the dose of enalapril and/or the diuretic is increased.

In patients with a creatinine clearance ≤ 30 mL per min (mL/min) (serum creatinine > 3 mg per dL [mg/dL]), the individual components should be titrated prior to the start of therapy with the combination.

Enalapril and diltiazem combination is contained in a nondeformable dosage form and should be used with caution when administered to patients with preexisting, pathologic or iatrogenic, severe gastrointestinal narrowing because of the risk of obstruction.

The diltiazem component of the combination is contained in a nonabsorbable tablet shell that slowly releases diltiazem for absorption. After release, the empty shell is eliminated from the body in the feces.

**For treatment of adverse effects**
Recommended treatment consists of the following:
- Treatment of symptomatic hypotension involves placing the patient in a supine position and, if needed, administering normal saline intravenously; reducing or discontinuing the dose of enalapril or diuretic may be necessary.
- For treatment of ACE inhibitor–associated angioedema with swelling confined to the face and lips—treatment, other than withdrawal of the medication, is usually not necessary, although antihistamines may relieve the symptoms.
- For treatment of ACE inhibitor–associated angioedema with swelling involving the tongue, glottis, or larynx, possibly causing airway obstruction—withdrawal of the medication and appropriate treatment, such as subcutaneous epinephrine or measures to ensure an open airway, should be initiated immediately. The patient should be monitored until full resolution of the symptoms.

## Oral Dosage Forms

### ENALAPRIL MALEATE AND DILTIAZEM MALATE EXTENDED-RELEASE TABLETS

**Usual adult dose**
Antihypertensive—
  For patients not receiving diuretics, Oral, 1 or 2 tablets a day as determined by the individual component doses.

**Usual adult prescribing limits**
10 mg of enalapril maleate and 360 mg of diltiazem malate (dosage expressed as diltiazem hydrochloride).

**Usual pediatric dose**
Antihypertensive—
  Safety and efficacy have not been established.

**Strength(s) usually available**
U.S.—
  5 mg enalapril maleate and 180 mg diltiazem malate (expressed as diltiazem hydrochloride) (Rx) [*Teczem* (film-coated)].

**Packaging and storage**
Store in a well-closed container at room temperature, preferably between 15 and 30 °C (59 and 86 °F). Protect from moisture.

**Auxiliary labeling**
- Do not take other medicines without your doctor's advice.
- Swallow tablets whole. Do not break or chew.

Developed: 11/12/97

# ENALAPRIL AND FELODIPINE   Systemic—INTRODUCTORY VERSION

VA CLASSIFICATION (Primary): CV401
Commonly used brand name(s): *Lexxel*.
Note: For a listing of dosage forms and brand names by country availability, see *Dosage Forms* section(s).

## Category
Antihypertensive.

# Indications
## Accepted
Hypertension (treatment)—The combination of enalapril maleate and felodipine is indicated for the treatment of hypertension. It is not indicated as initial treatment for hypertension.

# Pharmacology/Pharmacokinetics
## Physicochemical characteristics
Molecular weight—
  Enalapril maleate: 492.53.
  Felodipine: 384.26.

## Mechanism of action/Effect
Enalapril is the ethyl ester and prodrug of the long-acting angiotensin-converting enzyme (ACE) inhibitor, enalaprilat. ACE, a peptidyl dipeptidase, catalyzes the conversion of angiotensin I to the vasoconstrictor, angiotensin II. Angiotensin II stimulates secretion of aldosterone from the adrenal cortex and inhibits the release of renin through a negative feedback mechanism. When ACE is inhibited, angiotensin II formation is reduced, and the interruption of the negative feedback mechanism results in increased plasma renin concentrations. The reduction of angiotensin II formation leads to decreased aldosterone secretion and vasopressor activity. The decrease in aldosterone secretion produces a small increase in serum potassium. Suppression of the renin-angiotensin-aldosterone system is thought to be the primary mechanism through which ACE inhibitors lower blood pressure. In clinical studies, blood pressure reduction in patients with essential hypertension was accompanied by a reduction in peripheral arterial resistance, an increase in cardiac output, and little or no change in heart rate.

Felodipine is a dihydropyridine calcium channel blocking agent that inhibits the influx of calcium ions across the L-channels in cell membranes of vascular smooth muscle and cardiac muscle. Inhibition of the influx of calcium ions is selective, with a greater effect occurring in vascular smooth muscle cells than in cardiac muscle cells. Felodipine has an *in vitro* negative inotropic effect, which may be overcome *in vivo*. The direct action of felodipine on vascular smooth muscle reduces peripheral vascular resistance and blood pressure, producing a mild reflex increase in heart rate. Heart rate may increase by 5 to 10 beats per minute at steady-state.

When enalapril is given in combination with felodipine, the antihypertensive effects are additive.

## Other actions/effects
ACE is also known as kininase II, an enzyme that degrades bradykinin. Enalapril may increase concentrations of bradykinin, producing a therapeutic vasodilating effect.

## Absorption
Enalapril—The extent of absorption, estimated from the urinary recovery of enalapril, is approximately 60%. Bioavailability is slightly reduced when taken with food with a high fat content.

Felodipine—Undergoes almost complete absorption and extensive first-pass metabolism. Bioavailability of the extended-release form of felodipine is approximately 20%. When taken with food with a high fat content, the peak and trough concentrations of the isomers of felodipine are approximately doubled and halved, respectively, although the area under the plasma concentration–time curve (AUC$_{[0-48]}$) of felodipine is not changed. Bioavailability of felodipine is greater when it is taken with grapefruit juice than when it is taken with water or orange juice.

## Distribution
Felodipine—Apparent volume of distribution (Vol$_D$): 10 liters per kg (L/kg).
Felodipine crosses the blood-brain barrier, with a plasma-to-brain concentration ratio of approximately 20:1.

## Protein binding
Felodipine—Very high (Approximately 99%).

## Biotransformation
Enalapril is hydrolyzed to enalaprilat, the active metabolite. No other metabolites of enalapril have been identified.

Felodipine has six metabolites that have been identified and account for 23% of the oral dose. None of these metabolites has significant vasodilating activity.

## Half-life
Elimination—
  Enalaprilat: Effective—11 hours. Effective half-life is prolonged when glomerular filtration rate is ≤ 30 mL per minute (mL/min).
  Felodipine: Terminal—11 to 16 hours.

## Time to peak concentration
Enalapril—Approximately 1 hour.
Enalaprilat—Approximately 3 hours; may be increased when glomerular filtration rate is ≤ 30 mL/min.
Felodipine—3 to 6 hours.

## Elimination
Enalapril—
  Primarily renal.
Enalaprilat—
  Renal: 40%.
Felodipine—
  Renal: 70%.
  Fecal: 10%.
In dialysis—
  Enalaprilat: Removable by hemodialysis at a rate of 62 mL/min. Removable by peritoneal dialysis from neonatal circulation.
  Felodipine: Removal by hemodialysis has not been established.

# Precautions to Consider
## Cross-sensitivity and/or related problems
Patients hypersensitive to other angiotensin-converting enzyme (ACE) inhibitors may also be hypersensitive to enalapril.

## Carcinogenicity
No long-term carcinogenicity tests have been performed with enalapril and felodipine combination.

A 2-year study in rats given felodipine in daily dietary doses of 7.7, 23.1, or 69.3 mg per kg (mg/kg) of body weight resulted in a dose-related increase in the incidence of benign interstitial cell tumors of the testes (Leydig cell tumors) in the male rats. At these doses, felodipine has been shown to lower testicular testosterone and to produce a corresponding increase in serum luteinizing hormone in rats. A dose-related increase in the incidence of focal squamous cell hyperplasia in the esophageal groove of male and female rats also occurred in all dose groups. These doses represent up to 28 times the maximum recommended human dose (MRHD) on a mg per square meter of body surface area (mg/m$^2$) basis, assuming a 50-kg patient. The occurrence of Leydig cell tumors was not observed in a similar study in mice given doses of up to 138.6 mg/kg per day of felodipine. This dose represents 28 times the MRHD on a mg/m$^2$ basis, assuming a 50-kg patient.

No evidence of carcinogenicity was found in mice given daily dietary doses of up to 138.6 mg/kg of felodipine for up to 80 weeks in males and 99 weeks in females. This dose represents 28 times the MRHD on a mg/m$^2$ basis, assuming a 50-kg patient.

## Tumorigenicity
Tumorigenicity was not seen when enalapril was given to male and female rats for 106 weeks at doses of up to 90 mg/kg per day or to male and female mice for 94 weeks at doses of up to 90 and 180 mg/kg per day, respectively. In rats and female mice this dose represents 26 times the maximum recommended human daily dose (MRHDD) based on body surface area, and in male mice this dose represent 13 times the MRHDD based on body surface area.

## Mutagenicity
Enalapril and felodipine combination was not found to be mutagenic with or without metabolic activation *in vitro* in the Ames microbial mutation test, the V-79 mammalian cell forward mutation assay, the alkaline elution assay with rat hepatocytes, or the CHO mammalian cell cytogenetics assay, or in a separate *in vivo* mouse bone marrow cytogenetics assay.

Enalapril or enalaprilat was not found to be mutagenic in the Ames microbial mutagen test with or without metabolic activation. Enalapril was not found to be genotoxic in the rec-assay, reverse mutation assay with *Escherichia coli*, sister chromatid exchange with cultured mammalian cells, and the micronucleus test with mice, or in an *in vivo* cytogenic study using mouse bone marrow.

Felodipine was not found to be mutagenic *in vitro* in the Ames microbial mutagenicity test or in the mouse lymphoma forward mutation assay. Felodipine was not found to be clastogenic *in vitro* in a human lymphocyte chromosome aberration assay or *in vivo* in the mouse micronucleus test at oral doses of up to 2500 mg/kg. This dose represents 506 times the MRHD on a mg/m$^2$ basis, assuming a 50-kg patient.

## Pregnancy/Reproduction
Fertility—No effect on fertility was found in studies in male rats given doses of up to 6.9 and 9 mg/kg per day of enalapril and felodipine combination, respectively, or in female rats given doses of up to 17.3 mg/kg and 22.5 mg/kg per day of enalapril and felodipine combination, respectively.

No adverse effects on reproductive performance were found in studies in male and female rats given doses of enalapril of up to 90 mg/kg per day. This dose represents 26 times the MRHDD, based on body surface area.

No significant effect on reproductive performance was seen in a study in male and female rats given doses of 3.8, 9.6, or 26.9 mg/kg per day of felodipine.

Pregnancy—ACE inhibitors can cause fetal and neonatal morbidity and mortality when administered to pregnant women during the second and third trimesters. Enalapril and felodipine combination should be discontinued as soon as possible when pregnancy is detected, unless no alternative therapy can be used. In the latter instance, serial ultrasound examinations should be performed to assess the intra-amniotic environment. Perinatal diagnostic tests, such as contraction-stress testing (CST), a nonstress test (NST), or biophysical profiling (BPP) also may be appropriate during the applicable week of pregnancy. If oligohydramnios is present, enalapril and felodipine combination should be discontinued unless it is considered lifesaving for the mother. Oligohydramnios may not become apparent until after the fetus has sustained irreversible damage.

Fetal exposure to ACE inhibitors during the second and third trimesters can cause hypotension, reversible or irreversible renal failure, anuria, neonatal skull hypoplasia, and death in the fetus or neonate. Maternal oligohydramnios, which may result from decreased fetal renal function, has been reported and associated with fetal limb contractures, craniofacial deformation, and hypoplastic lung development. Other adverse effects that have been reported are prematurity, intrauterine growth retardation, and patent ductus arteriosus, although how these effects are related to exposure to ACE inhibitors is not clear. ACE inhibitor exposure, when limited to the first trimester, does not appear to be associated with these adverse effects.

Infants that have been exposed *in utero* to ACE inhibitors should be observed closely for hypotension, oliguria, and hyperkalemia. If oliguria develops, it should be treated with support of blood pressure and renal perfusion. Dialysis or exchange transfusion may be necessary to reverse hypotension and/or substitute for disordered renal function. Removal of enalapril from neonatal circulation by peritoneal dialysis has shown some clinical benefit. There is no clinical experience with removing enalapril by exchange transfusion.

Teratogenic effects were not observed in rats and rabbits given enalapril in doses representing 57 and 12 times, respectively, the MRHDD based on body surface area.

Adequate and well-controlled studies with felodipine in pregnant women have not been done. However, felodipine crosses the placenta, producing fetal plasma concentrations similar to maternal plasma concentrations. Felodipine may be hazardous if used during pregnancy or if the patient becomes pregnant during therapy because of the possible effects on the fetus, occurrence of digital anomalies of the infant, effects on labor and delivery, and effects on the mammary glands of pregnant females.

Studies in pregnant rabbits given doses of 0.46, 1.2, 2.3, and 4.6 mg/kg of felodipine per day, representing 0.4 to 4 times the MRHD on a mg/m$^2$ basis, assuming a 50-kg patient, revealed fetal digital anomalies that consisted of a reduced size and degree of ossification of the terminal phalanges. The frequency and severity of the changes appeared dose-related and were noted at the lowest dose. These changes were not observed in rats. In a teratology study in cynomolgus monkeys, the size of the terminal phalanges was not reduced, but an abnormal position of the distal phalanges occurred in about 40% of the fetuses.

Studies in pregnant rabbits given doses of 1.2 mg/kg or greater per day of felodipine, equivalent to the MRHD on a mg/m$^2$ basis, showed a significant enlargement of the mammary glands in excess of the normal enlargement. This effect was not observed in rats or monkeys and regressed during lactation in pregnant rabbits.

An increase in the incidence of fetuses with dilated renal pelvis/ureter occurred in rats given enalapril and felodipine combination of 1.9 and 2.5 mg/kg per day, respectively. This effect did not occur in the offspring postweaning.

An increase in the incidence of both early and late *in utero* deaths occurred in mice given doses of 23 and 30 mg/kg per day or greater of enalapril and felodipine combination, respectively. Transient and slight decreases in body weight gain in the first generation offspring occurred. However, no adverse effects regarding sexual maturation, behavioral development, fertility, or fecundity occurred in offspring.

Pregnant mice given 20.8 and 27 mg/kg per day of enalapril and felodipine, respectively, and pregnant rats given 17.3 mg/kg and 22.5 mg/kg per day of enalapril and felodipine, respectively, produced peak plasma concentration ($C_{max}$) and area under the plasma concentration–time curve (AUC) values of enalapril and/or enalaprilat 76 to 418-fold greater, and values of felodipine 151 to 433-fold greater than those expected in nonpregnant humans given the recommended dose.

FDA Pregnancy Category C (first trimester).
FDA Pregnancy Category D (second and third trimesters).

Labor—Studies in rats given 9.6 mg/kg and above of felodipine per day showed a prolongation of parturition with difficult labor and an increased incidence of fetal and early postnatal death. The 9.6 mg/kg per day dose represents four times the maximum human dose on a mg/m$^2$ basis, assuming a 50-kg patient.

### Breast-feeding
Enalapril and enalaprilat are distributed into breast milk. It is not known whether felodipine is distributed into breast milk. Studies in rats given enalapril and felodipine combination showed that felodipine appears in milk at a concentration almost tenfold that found in plasma. Because of the potential for serious adverse reactions from enalapril and felodipine in the infant, caution should be used in deciding to use the combination in a nursing mother.

### Pediatrics
No information is available on the relationship of age to the effects of enalapril and felodipine combination in pediatric patients. Safety and efficacy have not been established.

### Geriatrics
Plasma concentrations of felodipine may be increased in elderly patients. In clinical trials, the mean clearance in elderly hypertensive patients with a mean age of 74 years was 45% of that for volunteers with a mean age of 26 years. At steady state, the mean AUC for young patients was 39% of that for the elderly.

### Pharmacogenetics
Black patients have a lower than average response to enalapril in comparison with nonblack patients. Black patients may also have a higher incidence of ACE inhibitor–associated angioedema.

### Dental
Mild gingival enlargement has been reported. The incidence and severity of gingival enlargement may be decreased with good dental hygiene.

### Surgical
Patients receiving enalapril and felodipine combination and undergoing major surgery or during anesthesia with agents that produce hypotension may experience excessive hypotension. If hypotension in these patients is thought to be the result of ACE inhibition, it can be corrected by volume expansion.

### Drug interactions and/or related problems
The following drug interactions and/or related problems have been selected on the basis of their potential clinical significance (possible mechanism in parentheses where appropriate)—not necessarily inclusive (» = major clinical significance):

Note: Combinations containing any of the following medications, depending on the amount present, may also interact with this medication.

» Anticonvulsant therapy, long-term, with medications such as:
  Carbamazepine
  Phenytoin
  Phenobarbital
  (a study with patients on long-term anticonvulsant therapy receiving concurrent felodipine resulted in a considerably lower $C_{max}$ and a reduction of the mean AUC of felodipine to approximately 6% of that observed in healthy volunteers; this may be considered a clinically significant interaction and alternative antihypertensive therapy may be necessary)

Cimetidine
  (concurrent use may increase felodipine plasma concentration [$C_{max}$] and AUC by approximately 50%)

» Diuretics
  (concurrent use with ACE inhibitors may have additive hypotensive effects, especially with recently instituted diuretic therapy; the diuretic may need to be reduced or discontinued or salt intake cautiously increased prior to initiation of enalapril and felodipine combination therapy)

» Diuretics, potassium-sparing, such as:
  Amiloride
  Spironolactone
  Triamterene or
» Potassium-containing salt substitutes or
» Potassium supplements
  (concurrent use with ACE inhibitor therapy may increase the risk of hyperkalemia; serum potassium concentrations should be monitored as appropriate)

Grapefruit juice
  (the bioavailability of felodipine is greater when it is taken with grapefruit juice than when it is taken with water or orange juice)

Lithium
  (concurrent use with ACE inhibitors has resulted in increased serum lithium concentrations and symptoms of lithium toxicity; frequent monitoring of serum lithium concentrations is recommended)

Metoprolol
  (concurrent use may increase $C_{max}$ and AUC of felodipine by approximately 31% and 38%, respectively)

**Laboratory value alterations**
The following have been selected on the basis of their potential clinical significance (possible effect in parentheses where appropriate)—not necessarily inclusive (» = major clinical significance):

With physiology/laboratory test values
　Blood urea nitrogen (BUN) and
　Creatinine, serum
　　(minor and transient increases in serum creatinine concentrations may occur, especially in patients pretreated with a diuretic or in patients with renal function impairment or renal artery stenosis; a dosage reduction of enalapril or discontinuation of the diuretic may be necessary)
　Potassium, serum
　　(increases in concentrations may be minor and reversible)

**Medical considerations/Contraindications**
The medical considerations/contraindications included have been selected on the basis of their potential clinical significance (reasons given in parentheses where appropriate)—not necessarily inclusive (» = major clinical significance).

*Except under special circumstances, this medication should not be used when the following medical problems exist:*
» Angioedema related to previous ACE inhibitor therapy, history of
　　(increased risk of angioedema with ACE inhibitor therapy)
» Hypersensitivity to enalapril or felodipine

*Risk-benefit should be considered when the following medical problems exist:*
　Angioedema unrelated to ACE inhibitor therapy, history of
　　(increased risk of angioedema with ACE inhibitor therapy)
　Cerebrovascular disease
　　(excessive lowering of blood pressure may result in cerebrovascular accident)
　Collagen-vascular disease, such as systemic lupus erythematosus (SLE) or scleroderma
　　(increased risk of developing neutropenia or agranulocytosis, especially if renal function is impaired)
　Diabetes mellitus
　　(increased risk of hyperkalemia with ACE inhibitor therapy)
　Dialysis with high-flux membranes or
　Low-density lipoprotein apheresis with dextran sulfate absorption
　　(anaphylactoid reactions have been reported in patients undergoing these procedures while being treated with an ACE inhibitor)
　Hepatic function impairment
　　(plasma concentrations of felodipine may be elevated; in clinical trials, clearance of felodipine was reduced to about 60% of the clearance in normal young volunteers)
　Hypotension, as associated with:
» 　Congestive heart failure
　　Dialysis, renal
　　Diuresis, recent intensive
　　Diuretic dose increase
　　Diuretic therapy, high dose
　　Sodium or volume depletion, severe
　　　(increased risk of excessive hypotension with ACE inhibitor therapy; sometimes associated with oliguria, azotemia, acute renal failure, and/or death)
　Hymenoptera venom desensitization treatment
　　(life-threatening anaphylactoid reactions have been reported in two patients undergoing desensitizing treatment while receiving ACE inhibitors)
　Ischemic heart disease
　　(excessive lowering of blood pressure may result in a myocardial infarction)
» Renal artery stenosis, bilateral or unilateral or
» Renal function impairment
　　(enalaprilat half-life, time to peak concentration, peak and trough concentrations, and time to steady state may increase; increased risk of developing neutropenia or agranulocytosis; increased risk of hyperkalemia; increases in blood urea nitrogen [BUN] and serum creatinine may occur, especially in patients who are pretreated with a diuretic; renal function should be monitored during the first few weeks of therapy; a dosage adjustment or discontinuation of the diuretic may be necessary)

**Patient monitoring**
The following may be especially important in patient monitoring (other tests may be warranted in some patients, depending on condition; » = major clinical significance):

» Blood pressure measurements
　(periodic monitoring is necessary for titration of dose according to the patient's response)
　Renal function determinations
　　(monitoring may be necessary in patients with renal function impairment)
　Leukocyte count determinations
　　(periodic monitoring may be necessary for patients at risk for neutropenia or agranulocytosis, such as those with renal function impairment and/or a collagen-vascular disease)
　Potassium, serum concentrations
　　(monitoring may be necessary in patients at risk for hyperkalemia, such as those with renal insufficiency, diabetes mellitus, or those concurrently taking potassium-sparing diuretics, potassium supplements, or potassium-containing salt substitutes)

## Side/Adverse Effects

The following side/adverse effects have been selected on the basis of their potential clinical significance (possible signs and symptoms in parentheses where appropriate)—not necessarily inclusive:

**Those indicating need for medical attention**
Incidence less frequent
　*Edema, peripheral* (swelling of ankles, feet, and lower legs); *hypotension* (dizziness, lightheadedness, or fainting)
　Note: *Peripheral edema* is generally mild and usually occurs within 2 to 3 weeks of the initiation of therapy. In clinical trials, peripheral edema was the most common adverse effect, with an incidence that was age- and dose-dependent.
　　*Hypotension* and rarely syncope may be precipitated by felodipine and may lead to reflex tachycardia. In susceptible individuals, this may precipitate angina pectoris.
Incidence rare
　*Angioedema* (sudden trouble in swallowing or breathing; swelling of face, mouth, hands, or feet; hoarseness); *hepatotoxicity* (yellow eyes or skin); *hyperkalemia* (confusion; irregular heartbeat; nervousness; numbness or tingling in hands, feet, or lips; shortness of breath or difficulty in breathing; weakness or heaviness of legs)—incidence approximately 1% in patients treated with enalapril alone; *neutropenia or agranulocytosis* (chills; fever; sore throat)—occurs rarely in uncomplicated hypertension; occurs more frequently in patients with renal function impairment, especially if accompanied by a collagen-vascular disease; *thrombocytopenia* (unusual bleeding or bruising)
　Note: *Angioedema* is associated with angiotensin-converting enzyme (ACE) inhibitor therapy and may involve the face, extremities, lips, tongue, glottis, and larynx. Angioedema associated with laryngeal edema, resulting in airway obstruction, could be fatal. ACE inhibitor–associated angioedema may occur at any time during treatment and occurs at a higher rate in black patients than in nonblack patients.
　　ACE inhibitor–associated *hepatotoxicity* occurs by a mechanism that is not understood, but is manifest as a syndrome of cholestatic jaundice, fulminant hepatic necrosis, and may result in death. Enalapril and felodipine combination therapy should be discontinued in patients who develop jaundice or marked elevations of hepatic enzymes. Patients should receive appropriate medical follow-up.

**Those indicating need for medical attention only if they continue or are bothersome**
Incidence more frequent
　*Dizziness; headache*
Incidence less frequent
　*Cough, dry and persistent; fatigue* (unusual tiredness); *flushing; gingival enlargement* (gum swelling)
　Note: *Cough* has been reported with ACE inhibitors and is thought to be due to increased concentrations of bradykinin as a result of kininase II inhibition. In clinical trials of enalapril in combination with felodipine, the incidence of cough was 2.2%.

## Overdose

For specific information on the agents used in the management of enalapril and felodipine combination overdose, see
　• *Dopamine* and/or *Norepinephrine* in *Sympathomimetic Agents—Cardiovascular Use (Parenteral-Systemic)* monograph.

For more information on the management of overdose or unintentional ingestion, **contact a Poison Control Center** (see *Poison Control Center Listing*).

**Clinical effects of overdose**
The following effects have been selected on the basis of their potential clinical significance (possible signs and symptoms in parentheses where appropriate)—not necessarily inclusive:

Acute and/or chronic
*Hypotension, severe* (dizziness; fainting; lightheadedness); *tachycardia* (fast heartbeat)

**Treatment of overdose**
Treatment is symptomatic and supportive.

For severe hypotension—Repletion of central fluid volume by placing the patient in a supine or Trendelenburg position and/or infusion of normal saline. If necessary, vasopressors, such as norepinephrine or high-dose dopamine may be used.

Supportive care—Patients in whom intentional overdose is confirmed or suspected should be referred for psychiatric consultation.

## Patient Consultation

As an aid to patient consultation, refer to *Advice for the Patient, Enalapril and Felodipine (Systemic)—Introductory Version.*

In providing consultation, consider emphasizing the following selected information (» = major clinical significance):

**Before using this medication**
» Conditions affecting use, especially:
  Hypersensitivity to enalapril or felodipine
  Pregnancy—Can cause fetal and neonatal morbidity and mortality; not recommended for use during pregnancy
  Breast-feeding—Enalapril and enalaprilat are distributed into breast milk; potential for serious adverse reactions in the infant
  Pharmacogenetics—Black patients may have a lower than average response to enalapril and a higher incidence of ACE inhibitor–associated angioedema
  Dental—Mild gum swelling has been reported; good dental hygiene may decrease incidence and severity
  Surgical—Anesthesia with hypotension-producing agents may cause excessive hypotension
  Other medications, especially anticonvulsants such as carbamazepine, phenytoin, and phenobarbital; diuretics, potassium-containing salt substitutes, potassium-sparing diuretics, or potassium supplements
  Other medical problems, especially history of angioedema related to previous ACE inhibitor therapy, hypotension associated with congestive heart failure, renal artery stenosis, or renal function impairment

**Proper use of this medication**
» Compliance with therapy; taking medication at the same time each day to maintain the therapeutic effect
  Swallowing tablets whole without dividing, crushing, or chewing
  Importance of not taking tablets with grapefruit juice
» Proper dosing
  Missed dose: Taking as soon as possible; not taking if almost time for next scheduled dose; not doubling doses
» Proper storage

**Precautions while using this medication**
Regular visits to physician to check progress
Notifying physician immediately if pregnancy is suspected because of possibility of fetal or neonatal injury and/or death
Not taking other medications, especially potassium supplements or salt substitutes that contain potassium, without consulting physician
Caution when driving or doing other things requiring alertness because of possible dizziness, lightheadedness, or fainting due to symptomatic hypotension
Notifying physician if lightheadedness or fainting occurs, especially during the first few days of therapy
Reporting any signs of infection (fever, sore throat, chills) to physician because of risk of neutropenia
Reporting any signs of facial or extremity swelling and/or difficulty in swallowing or breathing because of risk of angioedema
Checking with physician if severe nausea, vomiting, or diarrhea occurs and continues because of risk of dehydration, which may result in hypotension
Caution when exercising or during exposure to hot weather because of risk of dehydration, which may result in hypotension
Caution if any kind of surgery (including dental surgery) or emergency treatment is required

**Side/adverse effects**
Signs of potential side effects, especially peripheral edema, hypotension, angioedema, hepatotoxicity, hyperkalemia, neutropenia or agranulocytosis, and thrombocytopenia

## General Dosing Information

Dosage must be adjusted to meet the individual requirements of each patient, on the basis of clinical response. The maximum reduction in blood pressure is generally achieved after 1 to 2 weeks during long-term dosing.

It is recommended that enalapril and felodipine combination therapy be used only after a patient has failed to achieve the desired antihypertensive effect with one or the other agent as single therapy. For dosage ranges for the individual agents when given as single therapy, see
• *Enalapril* in *Angiotensin-converting Enzyme Inhibitors (Systemic)* monograph; and/or
• *Felodipine* in *Calcium Channel Blocking Agents (Systemic)* monograph.

In patients who are elderly, have hepatic function impairment, or renal function impairment, individual components should be titrated prior to initiation of therapy with the combination. In patients with a creatinine clearance ≤ 30 mL per minute (mL/min) (serum creatinine > 3 mg per dL [mg/dL] or 265 micromole per L [micromole/L]), the recommended initial dose of enalapril is 2.5 mg. In elderly patients or those with hepatic function impairment, the recommended initial dose of felodipine is 2.5 mg.

For patients at risk for excessive hypotension, enalapril and felodipine combination therapy should be started under very close medical supervision and monitoring for the first 2 weeks of treatment and whenever the dose of enalapril and/or the diuretic (if concurrently administered) is increased.

When enalapril therapy is initiated in patients concurrently taking a diuretic, it is recommended that the patient be under medical supervision after the initial dose for at least 2 hours, and possibly an additional hour until blood pressure has stabilized.

In some patients treated with enalapril alone, administered once a day, the antihypertensive effect of enalapril may diminish toward the end of the dosing interval. An increase in dosage or twice-daily administration may be appropriate for these patients.

**For oral dosage forms only**

**Diet/Nutrition**
When enalapril and felodipine combination is taken with food, the peak concentration of felodipine is almost doubled, and the trough (24-hour) concentration is approximately halved.

The bioavailability of felodipine is greater when it is taken with grapefruit juice than when it is taken with water or orange juice.

**Bioequivalenence information**
The felodipine component of the combination has not been shown to be bioequivalent to available single-component extended-release felodipine tablets.

**For treatment of adverse effects**
Recommended treatment consists of the following:
• Treatment of symptomatic hypotension involves placing the patient in a supine position and, if needed, administering normal saline intravenously; reducing or discontinuing the dose of enalapril or diuretic (if concurrently administered) may be necessary.
• For treatment of ACE inhibitor–associated angioedema with swelling confined to the face and lips: treatment other than withdrawal of the medication is usually not necessary, although antihistamines may relieve the symptoms.
• For treatment of ACE inhibitor–associated angioedema with swelling involving the tongue, glottis, or larynx, possibly causing airway obstruction: withdrawal of the medication and appropriate treatment, such as subcutaneous epinephrine or measures to ensure an open airway, should be initiated immediately. The patient should be monitored until resolution of the symptoms is complete.

## Oral Dosage Forms

### ENALAPRIL MALEATE AND FELODIPINE TABLETS

**Usual adult dose**
Antihypertensive—
  Oral, initially 1 tablet daily. If blood pressure is not adequately controlled after one or two weeks, the dose may be increased to 2 tablets daily. If blood pressure is still not controlled, a thiazide diuretic may be added.

**Usual adult prescribing limits**
10 mg enalapril and 10 mg felodipine in combination.

**Usual pediatric dose**
Antihypertensive—
  Safety and efficacy have not been established.

**Enalapril and Felodipine (Systemic)—Introductory Version**

**Strength(s) usually available**
U.S.—
  5 mg enalapril and 5 mg felodipine extended-release (Rx) [*Lexxel* (film-coated)].

**Packaging and storage**
Store at 25 °C (77 °F), with brief exposures permitted between 15 and 30 °C (59 and 86 °F). Store and/or dispense in a tightly closed container and protect from moisture and light.

**Auxiliary labeling**
- Do not take other medicines without your doctor's advice.

Developed: 10/31/97

# ENCAINIDE   Systemic*†

VA CLASSIFICATION (Primary): CV300

Note: Although this product is no longer commercially available, the manufacturer is making it available to physicians who had patients well managed on encainide prior to market withdrawal.

For a listing of dosage forms and brand names by country availability, see *Dosage Forms* section(s).

*Not commercially available in the U.S.
†Not commercially available in Canada.

## Category
Antiarrhythmic.

## Indications
**Accepted**
Arrhythmias, ventricular (treatment)—Encainide is indicated for suppression of documented life-threatening ventricular arrhythmias, including sustained ventricular tachycardia.

**Unaccepted**
Use of encainide is no longer accepted for treatment of less severe arrhythmias such as nonsustained ventricular tachycardias or frequent premature ventricular contractions, even if patients are symptomatic, because of results of a trial that found increased mortality in patients with non-life-threatening arrhythmias treated with encainide compared to those treated with placebo.

## Pharmacology/Pharmacokinetics
**Physicochemical characteristics**
Molecular weight—388.94.

**Mechanism of action/Effect**
Decreases excitability, conduction velocity, and automaticity as a result of slowed atrial, atrioventricular (AV) nodal, His-Purkinje, and intraventricular conduction, and causes a slight but significant prolongation of refractory periods in these tissues. The greatest effect is on the His-Purkinje system. Decreases the rate of rise of the action potential without markedly affecting its duration. Electrophysiologic effects are greater in ischemic than in normal myocardial tissue. In the Vaughan Williams classification of antiarrhythmics, encainide is considered to be a class IC agent.

**Other actions/effects**
Very little negative inotropic effect.

**Absorption**
Nearly complete; slowed by food, but bioavailability is unchanged.

**Protein binding**
Encainide and O-demethylencainide (ODE)—High (75 to 85%).
3-Methoxy-O-demethylencainide (MODE)—Very high (92%).

**Biotransformation**
Hepatic. In over 90% of patients, rapidly and extensively metabolized to two active metabolites, ODE and MODE. In less than 10% of patients, more slowly metabolized (these patients also have a diminished ability to metabolize debrisoquin); little, if any, MODE and only small amounts of ODE are present in plasma.

**Half-life**
In normal metabolizers—
  Encainide: 1 to 2 hours.
  ODE: 3 to 4 hours.
  MODE: 6 to 12 hours.
In slow metabolizers—
  Encainide: 6 to 11 hours.

**Onset of action**
1 to 3 hours.

**Time to peak plasma concentration**
30 to 90 minutes.

**Time to steady-state plasma concentration**
Multiple doses—3 to 5 days.

**Elimination**
Renal/fecal (in slow metabolizers, more predominantly renal and mainly unchanged).

## Precautions to Consider

**Carcinogenicity**
Studies in rats and mice at oral doses of up to 30 mg per kg of body weight (mg/kg) per day and 135 mg/kg per day, respectively, found no evidence of carcinogenicity.

**Mutagenicity**
Bacterial and mammalian mutagenicity tests were negative.

**Pregnancy/Reproduction**
Fertility—Studies in male and female rats at oral doses of 28 mg/kg per day (approximately 13 times the average human dose) prior to mating found a reduction in fertility; doses up to 14 mg/kg per day did not reduce fertility.

Pregnancy—Adequate and well-controlled studies in humans have not been done.

Studies in rats and rabbits at doses of up to 13 and 9 times the average human dose, respectively, have not shown that encainide causes adverse effects in the fetus.

FDA Pregnancy Category B.

**Breast-feeding**
Encainide is distributed into the milk of laboratory animals and has been reported to be present in human milk. However, problems in humans have not been documented.

**Pediatrics**
Appropriate studies on the relationship of age to the effects of encainide have not been performed in the pediatric population. Safety and efficacy have not been established.

**Geriatrics**
Appropriate studies on the relationship of age to the effects of encainide have not been performed in the geriatric population. However, elderly patients are more likely to have age-related renal function impairment, which may require dosage reduction and increase in dosage intervals in patients receiving encainide.

**Drug interactions and/or related problems**
The following drug interactions and/or related problems have been selected on the basis of their potential clinical significance (possible mechanism in parentheses where appropriate)—not necessarily inclusive (» = major clinical significance):

Antiarrhythmics, other
  (concurrent use with encainide may result in increased cardiac effects)

Cimetidine
  (concurrent use of cimetidine increases plasma concentrations of encainide and its active metabolites; dosage reduction of encainide is recommended if concurrent use with cimetidine is necessary)

**Laboratory value alterations**
The following have been selected on the basis of their potential clinical significance (possible effect in parentheses where appropriate)—not necessarily inclusive (» = major clinical significance):

With physiology/laboratory test values
  Electrocardiogram (ECG) changes such as:
    QRS widening and
    PR prolongation
      (occur in most patients; dose-related)

  QT prolongation
    (may occur secondary to QRS widening)

Note: ECG changes produced by encainide do not necessarily indicate efficacy, toxicity, or overdose.

**Medical considerations/Contraindications**

The medical considerations/contraindications included have been selected on the basis of their potential clinical significance (reasons given in parentheses where appropriate)—not necessarily inclusive (» = major clinical significance).

*Except under special circumstances, this medication should not be used when the following medical problems exist:*

» Atrioventricular (AV) block, pre-existing second or third degree without pacemaker or
» Right bundle branch block associated with a left hemiblock (bifascicular block) without pacemaker
  (risk of complete heart block)

*Risk-benefit should be considered when the following medical problems exist:*

» Cardiogenic shock
  Cardiomyopathy or
  Congestive heart failure
    (encainide may exacerbate these conditions)
  Diabetes mellitus
    (encainide may in rare cases increase serum glucose levels, resulting in symptomatic hyperglycemia, especially in patients with pre-existing glucose intolerance; monitoring of serum glucose levels is recommended)
  Hepatic function impairment
    (reduced conversion to metabolites O-demethylencainide [ODE] and 3-methoxy-O-demethylencainide [MODE], but concentrations of metabolites are not significantly changed; no specific dosage adjustment recommendations can be made, but dosage should be increased cautiously)
  Hypokalemia or hyperkalemia
    (effects of encainide may be altered; any electrolyte imbalance should be corrected prior to beginning therapy with encainide)
  Myocardial infarction, history of, with associated left ventricular function impairment
    (increased risk of encainide-induced arrhythmias)
  Renal function impairment
    (reduced elimination; in patients with renal function impairment, the interval between dosage increments should be greater than 3 to 5 days, usually at least 7 days, and dosage reduction may be necessary)
  Sensitivity to encainide
» Sick sinus syndrome
    (sinus node recovery time prolonged; sinus bradycardia, sinus pause, or sinus arrest may occur)
  Caution is also recommended in patients with permanent pacemakers or temporary pacing electrodes because encainide may increase endocardial pacing thresholds and may suppress ventricular escape rhythms; use is not recommended in patients with existing poor thresholds or nonprogrammable pacemakers unless suitable pacing rescue is available.

**Patient monitoring**

The following may be especially important in patient monitoring (other tests may be warranted in some patients, depending on condition; » = major clinical significance):

» ECG
    (Holter monitoring or 24-hour ambulatory ECG recommended prior to initiation of therapy and at periodic intervals during therapy to help assess efficacy and detect possible proarrhythmic effects)
  Glucose
    (serum concentrations recommended, especially in diabetic patients)

## Side/Adverse Effects

Note: In the National Heart Lung and Blood Institute's Cardiac Arrhythmia Suppression Trial (CAST), encainide treatment was found to be associated with excessive mortality or increased nonfatal cardiac arrest rate as compared with placebo in patients with asymptomatic, non–life-threatening arrhythmias who had a recent myocardial infarction.

Adverse cardiac effects reported with encainide administration include new or exacerbated ventricular arrhythmias in about 10% of patients and, in 1% or less of patients, new or exacerbated congestive heart failure, second or third degree atrioventricular (AV) block, sinus bradycardia, sinus pause, or sinus arrest.

Incidence of cardiac and other effects is at least partially dose-related. Proarrhythmic effects are much more frequent at doses exceeding 200 mg per day.

Signs of overdose include excessive QRS widening and QT prolongation, AV dissociation, hypotension, and bradycardia; asystole may develop. Seizures have been reported. Deaths have occurred.

The following side/adverse effects have been selected on the basis of their potential clinical significance (possible signs and symptoms in parentheses where appropriate)—not necessarily inclusive:

**Those indicating need for medical attention**
Incidence more frequent
  *Chest pain; ventricular tachyarrhythmias* (fast or irregular heartbeat)
  Note: *Ventricular tachyarrhythmias* are dose-related and potentially fatal; incidence increased in patients with sustained ventricular tachycardia, cardiomyopathy, congestive heart failure, or history of myocardial infarction with associated left ventricular function impairment. Proarrhythmic effects usually occur during the first week of therapy.
Incidence rare
  *Central nervous system (CNS) effect* (trembling or shaking); *congestive heart failure* (shortness of breath; swelling of feet or lower legs)

**Those indicating need for medical attention only if they continue or are bothersome**
Incidence less frequent
  *CNS effects* (blurred or double vision; dizziness; headache; unusual tiredness or weakness); *nausea; pain in arms or legs; skin rash*

## Overdose

For more information on the management of overdose or unintentional ingestion, **contact a Poison Control Center** (see *Poison Control Center Listing*).

**Treatment of overdose**

Treatment is primarily supportive and symptomatic and includes immediate evacuation of the stomach (gastric lavage followed by activated charcoal) and cardiac monitoring

## Patient Consultation

As an aid to patient consultation, refer to *Advice for the Patient, Encainide (Systemic)*.

In providing consultation, consider emphasizing the following selected information (» = major clinical significance):

**Before using this medication**
» Conditions affecting use, especially:
    Sensitivity to encainide
    Pregnancy—Reduces fertility in rats
    Other medical problems, especially second or third degree atrioventricular (AV) block, right bundle branch block associated with a left hemiblock, cardiogenic shock, or sick sinus syndrome

**Proper use of this medication**
» Compliance with therapy; taking as directed even if feeling well
» Importance of not missing doses and taking at evenly spaced intervals
» Proper dosing
    Missed dose: Taking as soon as possible if remembered within 4 hours; not taking if remembered later; not doubling doses
» Proper storage

**Precautions while using this medication**
  Regular visits to physician to check progress
  Carrying medical identification card or bracelet
» Caution if any kind of surgery (including dental surgery) or emergency treatment is required
  Caution when driving or doing things requiring alertness because of possible dizziness

**Side/adverse effects**
  Signs of potential side effects, especially chest pain, ventricular tachyarrhythmias, congestive heart failure, and trembling or shaking

## General Dosing Information

Because of the long half-life of encainide's metabolites and the long half-life of encainide in slow metabolizers, dosage increments should be made no more frequently than every 3 to 5 days.

In general, it is recommended that previous antiarrhythmic therapy be withdrawn 2 to 4 plasma half-lives before initiation of encainide therapy.

In patients with pacemakers, it is recommended that the pacing threshold be determined prior to initiation of therapy, after one week of administration, and then at regular intervals.

# Encainide (Systemic)

## Oral Dosage Forms

### ENCAINIDE HYDROCHLORIDE CAPSULES

**Usual adult dose**
Antiarrhythmic—
  Oral, initially 25 mg every eight hours, the dosage being increased, if necessary, after three to five days to 35 mg every eight hours; may be further increased after an additional three to five days, if necessary, to 50 mg every eight hours.

Note: Patients well controlled by doses of 50 mg every eight hours or less may be changed to every-twelve-hour dosing if necessary to aid in compliance. No more than 75 mg should be taken in each dose.
  Occasional patients may require doses of 50 mg every six hours or, for life-threatening arrhythmias, 75 mg every six hours.
  In patients with severe renal function impairment (serum creatinine greater than 3.5 mg per deciliter or creatinine clearance less than 20 mL per minute), therapy should be initiated at a dose of 25 mg once a day. If necessary, dosage may be increased to 25 mg every twelve hours after at least seven days, followed by 25 mg every eight hours after an additional seven days (up to a maximum of 150 mg per day).

**Usual pediatric dose**
Safety and efficacy have not been established.

**Strength(s) usually available**
U.S.—
Note: Although this product is no longer commercially available, the manufacturer is making it available to physicians who had patients adequately maintained on encainide prior to market withdrawal.

Canada—
  Not commercially available.

**Packaging and storage**
Store below 30 °C (85 °F), in a well-closed container, unless otherwise specified by manufacturer.

## Selected Bibliography

Brogden RN, Todd PA. Encainide. A review of its pharmacological properties and therapeutic efficacy. Drugs 1987; 34: 519-38.
Chase SL, Sloskey GE. Encainide hydrochloride and flecainide acetate: two class 1c antiarrhythmic agents. Clin Pharm 1987 Nov; 6: 839-50.
Woosley RL, Wood AJJ, Roden DM. Encainide. New Engl J Med 1988 Apr 28; 318: 1107-15.

Revised: 06/08/93
Interim revision: 01/26/95

---

**ENFLURANE**—See *Anesthetics, Inhalation (Systemic)*

---

**ENOXACIN**—See *Fluoroquinolones (Systemic)*

---

# ENOXAPARIN  Systemic

VA CLASSIFICATION (Primary): BL111
Commonly used brand name(s): *Lovenox*.

Note: For a listing of dosage forms and brand names by country availability, see *Dosage Forms* section(s).

## Category

Antithrombotic.

Note: Enoxaparin is one of a group of substances known as low molecular weight heparins (LMWHs).

## Indications

Note: Bracketed information in the *Indications* section refers to uses that are not included in U.S. product labeling.

**General considerations**
The use of low molecular weight heparins (LMWHs) has several advantages compared to heparin. Improved bioavailability at low doses when administered subcutaneously, a longer plasma half-life, and a more predictable anticoagulant response allow for simpler dosing without laboratory monitoring. Studies in animals show that with doses of equivalent antithrombotic effect, LMWHs produce less bleeding than standard heparin. The clinical importance of this observation is uncertain, but may allow the use of higher anticoagulant doses of LMWHs, thereby improving efficacy without compromising safety. The potential advantage of reduced bleeding has been demonstrated in studies in patients receiving high doses for the treatment of venous thrombosis. However, in studies using prophylactic doses, no difference in bleeding has been demonstrated. This contrasting effect may be due to inappropriate dosage regimens in early studies, and the difficulty of measuring hemorrhagic tendencies in humans. LMWHs are associated with a lower incidence of heparin-induced thrombocytopenia, possibly due to reduced effects on platelet function and binding. These advantages must be weighed against the higher cost of the LMWHs, although the simpler dosing regimens used with LMWHs may allow home treatment in selected patients, thereby reducing overall costs and improving patient satisfaction.

**Accepted**
Thromboembolism, pulmonary (prophylaxis); and
Thrombosis, deep venous (prophylaxis)—Enoxaparin is indicated to prevent deep venous thrombosis (DVT) and to reduce the risk of pulmonary embolism following hip or knee replacement surgery. In addition, following hip replacement surgery, enoxaparin is indicated for extended prophylaxis following hospitalization.[1]

Enoxaparin is also indicated to prevent DVT and reduce the risk of pulmonary embolism in patients undergoing abdominal surgery who are at increased risk of thromboembolic complications. Patients at risk include patients who are over 40 years of age, obese, undergoing surgery under general anesthesia lasting longer than 30 minutes, or patients who have additional risk factors such as malignancy or a history of DVT or pulmonary embolism.

[Enoxaparin has been shown to be as effective as unfractionated heparin in preventing deep venous thrombosis and is indicated following general surgical procedures, including gynecological, urological and colorectal surgery, that leave the patient immobilized.]

Thrombosis, coronary arterial, acute (prophylaxis)[1]—Enoxaparin is indicated to prevent ischemic complications associated with unstable angina and non–Q-wave myocardial infarction, when concurrently administered with aspirin.

[1]Not included in Canadian product labeling.

## Pharmacology/Pharmacokinetics

**Physicochemical characteristics**
Source—Obtained by alkaline depolymerization of heparin benzyl ester derived from porcine intestinal mucosa.
Molecular weight—3500 to 5500 daltons (average 4500 daltons).
pH—5.5 to 7.5
Specific activity—Anti-factor Xa: 100 to 160 International Units (IU) per mg.
Anti-factor IIa: 20 to 40 IU per mg.

**Mechanism of action/Effect**
Enoxaparin, like unfractionated heparin, potentiates the actions of an endogenous inhibitor of blood coagulation, antithrombin III (heparin cofactor). Antithrombin III combines in a 1:1 molar ratio with activated serine proteases of the intrinsic and common coagulation pathways (primarily thrombin [factor IIa] and factor Xa, and, to a lesser extent, factors IXa, XIa, and XIIa) to form inactive complexes. Enoxaparin binds to antithrombin III, producing a conformational change in the cofactor molecule that results in significantly more rapid binding with and inactivation of the clotting factors than is achieved by the endogenous inhibitor alone.
Enoxaparin acts primarily by increasing antithrombin III–mediated inhibition of the formation and activity of factor Xa. This activity, in turn, reduces thrombin generation. These actions decrease thrombin-mediated events in coagulation, including the conversion of fibrinogen to fibrin, thereby inhibiting fibrin clot formation. Unlike unfractionated heparin, which has an anti-factor Xa (antithrombotic) to anti-factor IIa (anticoagulant) activity ratio of approximately 1 to 1, enoxaparin has

an anti-factor Xa to anti-factor IIa activity ratio of approximately 3 to 1. Enoxaparin's higher ratio of antithrombotic to anticoagulant activity is thought to result in an antithrombotic effect equivalent to that of unfractionated heparin with a lower risk of bleeding. However, it has not been consistently demonstrated that the risk of bleeding is lower with enoxaparin than with unfractionated heparin. Enoxaparin also decreases inhibition of platelet function and disrupts vascular permeability to a lesser extent than does unfractionated heparin.

**Other actions/effects**
Enoxaparin has been shown to increase the plasma concentration of nonesterified fatty acids, without affecting plasma cholesterol, triglycerides, or phospholipids.

**Absorption**
Absorbed rapidly and almost completely following subcutaneous injection, with approximately 90% bioavailability.

**Distribution**
The volume of distribution is between 5.2 and 9.3 L.

**Biotransformation**
Hepatic; weakly metabolized by desulfation and depolymerization.

**Half-life**
Elimination, based on anti-factor Xa activity—3 to 6 hours. May be prolonged in the presence of chronic, severe renal failure.

**Time to peak effect**
3 to 5 hours following subcutaneous injection.

**Duration of action**
Up to 24 hours following subcutaneous injection.

**Elimination**
Primarily renal. Total clearance is decreased in patients with chronic, severe renal failure.

## Precautions to Consider

### Cross-sensitivity and/or related problems
Patients with a history of allergies, especially those who are allergic to heparin, or to pork or pork products, may be allergic to this medication also.

### Carcinogenicity
The carcinogenic potential of enoxaparin has not been investigated.

### Mutagenicity
No mutagenicity was demonstrated *in vitro*, in the Ames test, mouse lymphoma cell forward mutation test, or human lymphocyte chromosomal aberration test; or *in vivo*, in the rat bone marrow chromosomal aberration test.

No disruption of chromosomes was demonstrated *in vitro*, in rat bone marrow cells, or *in vivo*, in human peripheral lymphocytes.

### Pregnancy/Reproduction
Pregnancy—Enoxaparin does not appear to cross the placenta. Adequate and well-controlled studies in humans have not been done.

No evidence of teratogenicity was found in studies in mice receiving 30 mg per kg of body weight per day or 211 mg per square meter of body surface area per day, or in rabbits receiving 410 mg per square meter of body surface area per day.

FDA Pregnancy Category B.

### Breast-feeding
It is not known whether enoxaparin is distributed into breast milk.

### Pediatrics
Appropriate studies on the relationship of age to the effects of enoxaparin have not been performed in the pediatric population. Safety and efficacy have not been established.

### Geriatrics
Elderly patients, especially females, may be more susceptible than other patients to bleeding during enoxaparin therapy. Also, the time to peak concentration and the half-life of enoxaparin may be prolonged in elderly patients. However, it is not necessary to modify the dose or the frequency of dosing.

### Drug interactions and/or related problems
The following drug interactions and/or related problems have been selected on the basis of their potential clinical significance (possible mechanism in parentheses where appropriate)—not necessarily inclusive (» = major clinical significance):

Note: Combinations containing any of the following medications, depending on the amount present, may also interact with this medication.

In addition to the interactions listed below, the possibility should be considered that multiple effects leading to further impairment of blood clotting and/or increased risk of bleeding may occur if enoxaparin is administered to a patient receiving any medication having a significant potential for causing hypoprothrombinemia, thrombocytopenia, or gastrointestinal ulceration or hemorrhage.

Anticoagulants, coumarin- or indandione-derivative
  (concurrent use may increase the risk of bleeding)

Anti-inflammatory drugs, nonsteroidal (NSAIDs) or
» Platelet aggregation inhibitors, other (see *Appendix II*), especially:
» Aspirin
» Sulfinpyrazone
» Ticlopidine
  (inhibition of platelet function by these agents may increase the risk of bleeding)
  (hypoprothrombinemia induced by large [antirheumatic] doses of aspirin, and the potential occurrence of gastrointestinal ulceration or hemorrhage during therapy with NSAIDs, aspirin, or sulfinpyrazone, also may increase the risk of bleeding in patients receiving enoxaparin)

Cefamandole or
Cefoperazone or
Cefotetan or
» Plicamycin or
» Valproic acid
  (these medications may cause hypoprothrombinemia; in addition, plicamycin or valproic acid may inhibit platelet aggregation; concurrent use with enoxaparin may increase the risk of hemorrhage and is not recommended)

» Thrombolytic agents, such as:
» Alteplase (tissue-type plasminogen activator, recombinant)
» Anistreplase (anisoylated plasminogen-streptokinase activator complex; APSAC)
» Streptokinase
» Urokinase
  (concurrent or sequential use with enoxaparin may increase the risk of bleeding complications)

### Laboratory value alterations
The following have been selected on the basis of their potential clinical significance (possible effect in parentheses where appropriate)—not necessarily inclusive (» = major clinical significance):

With physiology/laboratory test values
  Alanine aminotransferase (ALT [SGPT]) and
  Alkaline phosphatase and
  Aspartate aminotransferase (AST [SGOT])
    (serum values may be increased)

  Hemoglobin concentration and
  Hematocrit value and
  Red blood cell count
    (values may be decreased)

### Medical considerations/Contraindications
The medical considerations/contraindications included have been selected on the basis of their potential clinical significance (reasons given in parentheses where appropriate)—not necessarily inclusive (» = major clinical significance).

*Except under special circumstances, this medication should not be used when the following medical problems exist:*

» Abortion, threatened, or
» Aneurysm, cerebral or dissecting aorta, except in conjunction with corrective surgery, or
» Cerebrovascular hemorrhage, confirmed or suspected
  (increased risk of uncontrollable hemorrhage)
» Hemorrhage, active uncontrollable
» Hypertension, severe uncontrolled
  (increased risk of cerebral hemorrhage)
» Thrombocytopenia, severe, enoxaparin- or heparin-induced, within past several months
  (risk of recurrence, which may cause resistance to enoxaparin and new thromboembolic complications)

*Risk-benefit should be considered when the following medical problems exist:*

Any medical or dental procedure or condition in which the risk of bleeding or hemorrhage is present, such as:
» Anesthesia, epidural or spinal (risk of epidural or spinal hematoma, which can result in long-term or permanent paralysis; this risk is increased with the use of indwelling epidural catheters or by the concomitant use of medications that affect hemostasis, such as nonsteroidal anti-inflammatory drugs, platelet inhibitors, or other anti-

coagulants; the risk may also be increased by traumatic or repeated epidural or spinal puncture. See *General Dosing Information* for guidelines regarding the use of regional anesthesia in patients receiving perioperative enoxaparin.)
» Blood dyscrasias, hemorrhagic, especially thrombocytopenia, hemophilia, or von Willebrand disease; or other hemorrhagic tendency
» Childbirth, recent
  Diabetes, severe
» Endocarditis, acute or subacute bacterial
  Gastrointestinal ulceration, history of
  Intrauterine contraceptive device, use of
» Neurosurgery, recent or contemplated
» Ophthalmic surgery, recent or contemplated
» Pericarditis or pericardial effusion
  Radiation therapy, recent
  Renal function impairment, mild to moderate
» Renal function impairment, severe
» Retinopathy, diabetic or hemorrhagic
» Spinal puncture, recent
» Trauma, severe, especially to the central nervous system (CNS)
  Tuberculosis, active
» Ulceration or other lesions of the gastrointestinal, respiratory, or urinary tract, active
» Vasculitis, severe
» Wounds resulting in large open surfaces
  Hepatic function impairment, mild to moderate
» Hepatic function impairment, severe
  Hypertension, mild to moderate
    (increased risk of cerebral hemorrhage)
  Sensitivity to enoxaparin or to heparin

**Patient monitoring**
The following may be especially important in patient monitoring (other tests may be warranted in some patients, depending on condition; » = major clinical significance):
» Blood coagulation tests
    (although enoxaparin, in therapeutic doses, does not alter activated partial thromboplastin time [APTT], prothrombin time [PT], or thrombin time test values, these tests should be performed prior to therapy to establish a baseline or control value; also recommended to identify pre-existing coagulation defects and aid in determining whether the patient is a suitable candidate for treatment)
  Blood pressure measurement
  Hemoglobin concentration and
  Hematocrit value
    (recommended periodically during therapy; an unexplained fall in the blood pressure or hematocrit may signal occult bleeding; bleeding should be considered major if the hemoglobin concentration is decreased by more than 2 grams per deciliter [20 grams per liter], or if a transfusion of 2 or more units of blood is required)
» Neurologic status
    (monitor for signs and symptoms of neurologic impairment such as paresthesias, leg weakness, sensory loss, motor deficit, or bowel/bladder dysfunction indicating a potential epidural or spinal hematoma; if neurologic compromise is noted, urgent intervention is necessary, which includes radiographic confirmation and decompressive laminectomy; good or partial recovery is more likely if surgery is performed within 8 hours of the development of paraplegia)
» Platelet aggregation test
    (recommended prior to initiation of therapy in patients who have developed thrombocytopenia following administration of unfractionated heparin; if the result is negative, enoxaparin therapy may be instituted, with daily monitoring of the platelet count; however, if the result is positive, enoxaparin should not be given)
» Platelet count
    (recommended prior to initiation of therapy, then twice weekly for the duration of therapy to detect thrombocytopenia)
  Stool tests for occult blood loss
    (recommended periodically during therapy)

## Side/Adverse Effects
The following side/adverse effects have been selected on the basis of their potential clinical significance (possible signs and symptoms in parentheses where appropriate)—not necessarily inclusive:

**Those indicating need for medical attention**
Incidence less frequent
  *Bleeding complications, which may include blood in urine; bloody or black, tarry stools; bruising; coughing up blood; ecchymosis* (large, nonelevated blue or purplish patches in the skin); *hematoma* (collection of blood under the skin); *hypochromic anemia* (fatigue; headache; irritability; lightheadedness); *nosebleed; persistent bleeding or oozing from mucous membranes or surgical wound; shortness of breath; vomiting of blood or material that looks like coffee grounds; confusion; fever; peripheral edema* (swelling of ankles, feet, fingers); *thrombocytopenia, which may cause gangrene* (moderate to severe pain or numbness in the arms, legs, hands, feet); *organ infarction; pulmonary embolism* (chest discomfort; convulsions; dizziness or lightheadedness when getting up from a lying or sitting position; shortness of breath or fast breathing); *and stroke*—caused by excessive platelet aggregation
Incidence rare
  *Angioedema* (swelling of the face, genitalia, larynx [voice box], mouth, or tongue); *cardiovascular toxicity* (chest pain; dizziness or lightheadedness when getting up from a lying or sitting position; fast or irregular heartbeat; shortness of breath; sudden fainting); *epidural or spinal hematoma* (back pain; bowel/bladder dysfunction; leg weakness; numbness; paralysis; paresthesias)—back pain is not a typical presentation but some patients may experience this symptom; *skin rash or hives*
  Note: If an *epidural or spinal hematoma* is suspected, urgent intervention is necessary, which includes radiographic confirmation and decompressive laminectomy. Good or partial recovery is more likely if surgery is performed within 8 hours of the development of paraplegia.

**Those indicating need for medical attention only if they continue or are bothersome**
Incidence less frequent or rare
  *Increased menstrual bleeding; irritation, pain, or redness at injection site; nausea; vomiting*

## Overdose
For specific information on the agents used in the management of enoxaparin overdose, see the *Protamine (Systemic)* monograph.
For more information on the management of overdose or unintentional ingestion, **contact a Poison Control Center** (see *Poison Control Center Listing*).

**Clinical effects of overdose**
The following effects have been selected on the basis of their potential clinical significance (possible signs and symptoms in parentheses where appropriate)—not necessarily inclusive:

Acute
  **Bleeding complications**

**Treatment of overdose**
Specific treatment—Administration of protamine sulfate by slow intravenous injection. The dose of protamine sulfate should be equivalent, on a mg-per-mg basis, to the dose of enoxaparin. An equivalent dose of protamine sulfate will neutralize the anti-factor IIa (anticoagulant) activity of enoxaparin, but will only neutralize approximately 60% of its anti-factor Xa (antithrombotic) activity. However, studies in animals indicate that protamine sulfate stops microvascular bleeding produced by very high concentrations of enoxaparin.

## Patient Consultation
As an aid to patient consultation, refer to *Advice for the Patient, Enoxaparin (Systemic)*.
In providing consultation, consider emphasizing the following selected information (» = major clinical significance):

**Before using this medication**
» Conditions affecting use, especially:
    Sensitivity to enoxaparin or to heparin
    Other medications, especially platelet aggregation inhibitors, hypoprothrombinemia-inducing medications, and thrombolytic agents
    Other medical problems, especially threatened abortion; aneurysm; hemorrhage; hypertension; thrombocytopenia; hemorrhagic blood dyscrasias; recent childbirth; endocarditis; pericarditis or pericardial effusion; severe renal function impairment; diabetic or hemorrhagic retinopathy; spinal puncture, surgery, or other trauma; ulcers or other lesions of the gastrointestinal, respiratory, or urinary tract; severe vasculitis; wounds resulting in large open surfaces; and severe hepatic function impairment

**Proper use of this medication**
» Proper injection technique
» Safe handling and disposal of syringe

» Proper dosing
  Missed dose: Using as soon as possible; not using if almost time for next dose; not doubling doses
» Proper storage

**Precautions while using this medication**
» Need to inform all physicians and dentists that this medicine is being used
» Notifying physician immediately if signs and symptoms of bleeding or epidural/spinal hematoma occur

**Side/adverse effects**
Signs and symptoms of potential side effects, including bleeding complications, confusion, fever, peripheral edema, thrombocytopenia, angioedema, cardiovascular toxicity, epidural/spinal hematoma, and skin rash or hives

## General Dosing Information

Enoxaparin is administered by deep subcutaneous (intrafat) injection into the abdominal fat layer; injection sites should be rotated. Enoxaparin must not be administered intramuscularly or intravenously.

A controlled, comparative study found that in non-dialyzed patients with severe renal impairment (mean creatinine clearance 11.4 mL per minute), the total clearance of enoxaparin was 1.9 times slower and the apparent half-lives of absorption and elimination were 1.7 times longer than in healthy subjects. Dosage modifications are therefore recommended in patients with severe renal impairment who are not receiving hemodialysis. However, dosage modifications are not required in dialysis patients.

**Guidelines regarding the use of regional anesthesia in patients receiving perioperative enoxaparin**
Preoperative enoxaparin—A single-dose spinal anesthetic may be the safest neuraxial technique. Needle placement should occur at least 10 to 12 hours after the last dose of enoxaparin. Subsequent dosing should be delayed for at least 2 hours after needle placement. The presence of blood during needle placement may justify a delay in the start of postoperative prophylaxis.

Postoperative enoxaparin—Patients may safely undergo single-dose and continuous catheter techniques. With a continuous technique, the epidural catheter should be left indwelling overnight and removed the following day, with the first dose of enoxaparin given 2 hours after catheter removal. Using postoperative prophylaxis in the presence of an indwelling catheter must be done carefully and with close surveillance of the patient's neurologic status. An opioid and/or dilute local anesthetic solution is recommended in these patients to allow intermittent assessment of neurologic function.

The timing of catheter removal is extremely important. Removal should be delayed for at least 10 to 12 hours after a dose of enoxaparin. Subsequent dosing should not occur for at least 2 hours following catheter removal.

## Parenteral Dosage Forms

### ENOXAPARIN INJECTION

**Usual adult dose**
Thromboembolism, pulmonary (prophylaxis); and
Thrombosis, deep venous (prophylaxis)—
Hip or knee replacement surgery—
  Subcutaneously, 30 mg every twelve hours for an average of seven to ten days. The initial dose should be given twelve to twenty-four hours postoperatively.
  Alternatively, for hip replacement surgery, enoxaparin may be given subcutaneously, 40 mg once a day, with the initial dose given nine to fifteen hours prior to surgery. Following the initial phase of thromboprophylaxis for hip replacement surgery (either 30 mg every twelve hours or 40 mg once a day), continued prophylaxis at a dose of 40 mg once a day for three weeks is recommended.[1]
Abdominal, [and gynecological, urological, or colorectal] surgery—
  Subcutaneously, 40 mg once a day for an average of seven to ten days. The initial dose should be given two hours prior to surgery.
Thrombosis, coronary arterial, acute; associated with unstable angina or non–Q-wave myocardial infarction (prophylaxis)[1]—
  Subcutaneous, 1 mg per kg of body weight every twelve hours in conjunction with oral aspirin therapy (100 to 325 mg once a day). Treatment should be prescribed for a minimum of two days, and continued until the patient is clinically stable (usual duration is two to eight days).
  Note: To minimize the risk of bleeding following vascular instrumentation during the treatment of unstable angina, adhere precisely to the recommended dosing intervals. The vascular access sheath for instrumentation should remain in place for six to eight hours following a dose of enoxaparin. Following sheath removal, the next scheduled dose of enoxaparin should be given no sooner than six to eight hours later. The site of the procedure should be observed for signs of bleeding or hematoma formation.

**Usual pediatric dose**
Safety and efficacy have not been established.

**Usual geriatric dose**
See *Usual adult dose*.

**Strength(s) usually available**
U.S.—
  30 mg in 0.3 mL of Water for Injection (Rx) [*Lovenox* (in ampuls and single unit-dose syringes)].
  40 mg in 0.4 mL of Water for Injection (Rx) [*Lovenox* (in single unit-dose syringes)].
  60 mg in 0.6 mL of Water for Injection (Rx) [*Lovenox* (in single unit-dose syringes)].
  80 mg in 0.8 mL of Water for Injection (Rx) [*Lovenox* (in single unit-dose syringes)].
  100 mg in 1 mL of Water for Injection (Rx) [*Lovenox* (in single unit-dose syringes)].
Canada—
  30 mg in 0.3 mL of Water for Injection (Rx) [*Lovenox* (in single unit-dose syringes)].
  40 mg in 0.4 mL of Water for Injection (Rx) [*Lovenox* (in single unit-dose syringes)].
  300 mg in 3 mL (10 mg per 0.1 mL) of Water for Injection (Rx) [*Lovenox* (in multiple-dose vials; benzyl alcohol 1.5% m/v)].

**Packaging and storage**
Store between 15 and 25 °C (59 and 77 °F), unless otherwise specified by manufacturer. Protect from freezing.

**Stability**
Because the injection contains no preservative, each syringe should be used to administer a single dose only.

**Incompatibilities**
Enoxaparin should not be admixed with intravenous fluids or other medications.

**Additional information**
The 300-mg-per-3-mL multi-dose vial contains benzyl alcohol, which is not recommended for use in neonates. A fatal syndrome consisting of metabolic acidosis, central nervous system depression, respiratory problems, renal failure, hypotension, and possibly seizures and intracranial hemorrhage has been associated with the administration of benzyl alcohol to neonates.

[1] Not included in Canadian product labeling.

## Selected Bibliography

Buckley MM, Sorkin EM. Enoxaparin. A review of its pharmacology and clinical applications in the prevention and treatment of thromboembolic disorders. Drugs 1992; 44: 465-97.

Hirsh J, Levine MN. Low molecular weight heparin. Blood 1992; 79: 1-17.

Developed: 11/22/93
Interim revision: 07/28/98

---

**ENTERAL NUTRITION FORMULAS**—The *Enteral Nutrition Formulas (Systemic)* monograph is not included in this published version of the USP DI database. Copies of the monograph are available on request from Micromedex, Inc. - Reprint Requests, 6200 S. Syracuse Way, Suite 300, Englewood, CO 80111; telephone (303) 486-6400; telefax (303) 486-6464; Email: USPDI@MDX.COM.

---

**EPHEDRINE**—See *Bronchodilators, Adrenergic (Systemic)*; *Sympathomimetic Agents—Cardiovascular Use (Parenteral-Systemic)*.

---

**EPINEPHRINE**—See *Bronchodilators, Adrenergic (Inhalation-Local)*; *Bronchodilators, Adrenergic (Systemic)*; *Sympathomimetic Agents—Cardiovascular Use (Parenteral-Systemic)*.

# EPINEPHRINE Ophthalmic

This monograph includes information on the following: 1) Epinephrine; 2) Epinephryl Borate.

VA CLASSIFICATION (Primary/Secondary): OP114/OP900

Commonly used brand name(s): *Epifrin*[1]; *Epinal*[2]; *Eppy/N*[2]; *Glaucon*[1].

Note: For a listing of dosage forms and brand names by country availability, see *Dosage Forms* section(s).

## Category
Antiglaucoma agent (ophthalmic); Surgical aid, ophthalmic.

## Indications
Note: Bracketed information in the *Indications* section refers to uses that are not included in U.S. product labeling.

**Accepted**

Glaucoma, open-angle (treatment)—Ophthalmic epinephrine is indicated primarily in the treatment of open-angle (chronic simple) glaucoma, either alone or in combination with miotics, beta-blockers, hyperosmotic agents, or carbonic anhydrase inhibitors.

[Congestion, conjunctival, during surgery (treatment)][1]—Ophthalmic epinephrine is used in the treatment of conjunctival congestion during surgery.

[Glaucoma, secondary (treatment)][1]—Ophthalmic epinephrine is used in the treatment of secondary glaucoma.

**Unaccepted**

Epinephrine is not an effective mydriatic when used topically in the eye.

[1]Not included in Canadian product labeling.

## Pharmacology/Pharmacokinetics

**Physicochemical characteristics**

Molecular weight—
  Epinephrine: 183.21.
  Epinephryl borate: 209.01.

pH
  Epinephryl borate ophthalmic solution: 7.4.

**Mechanism of action/Effect**

Epinephrine is a direct-acting sympathomimetic amine.

Antiglaucoma agent (ophthalmic)—The mechanism by which epinephrine lowers intraocular pressure is not completely known, but appears to involve both a decrease in production of aqueous humor and an increase in aqueous outflow facility.

Surgical aid (antihemorrhagic; mydriatic)—Epinephrine acts on alpha-adrenergic receptors in the conjunctiva to produce vasoconstriction and hemostasis in bleeding from small vessels. It contracts the dilator muscle of the pupil by acting on alpha-adrenergic receptors, resulting in dilation of the pupil (mydriasis).

**Onset of action**

Reduction in intraocular pressure—Within 1 hour.
Vasoconstriction—Within 5 minutes.

**Time to peak effect**

Reduction in intraocular pressure—4 to 8 hours.

**Duration of action**

Reduction in intraocular pressure—Up to 24 hours.
Vasoconstriction—Less than 1 hour.

## Precautions to Consider

**Carcinogenicity/Tumorigenicity**

Studies have not been done in either animals or humans.

**Pregnancy/Reproduction**

Pregnancy—Ophthalmic epinephrine may be systemically absorbed.
Studies have not been done in humans.
Studies have not been done in animals.
FDA Pregnancy Category C.

**Breast-feeding**

It is not known whether epinephrine is distributed into breast milk; however, ophthalmic epinephrine may be systemically absorbed.

**Pediatrics**

Appropriate studies on the relationship of age to the effects of this medication have not been performed in the pediatric population. Safety and efficacy have not been established.

**Geriatrics**

Appropriate studies on the relationship of age to the effects of this medication have not been performed in the geriatric population. However, no geriatrics-specific problems have been documented to date.

**Dental**

Epinephrine is used in gingival retraction cords, and systemic absorption may occur, especially from application of topical cords to abraded surfaces. Concurrent systemic absorption of ophthalmic epinephrine will result in an additive effect.

**Drug interactions and/or related problems**

The following drug interactions and/or related problems have been selected on the basis of their potential clinical significance (possible mechanism in parentheses where appropriate)—not necessarily inclusive (» = major clinical significance):

Note: Combinations containing any of the following medications, depending on the amount present, may also interact with this medication.

Anesthetics, hydrocarbon inhalation, such as:
  Chloroform
  Cyclopropane
  Desflurane
  Enflurane
  Halothane
  Isoflurane
  Methoxyflurane
  Trichloroethylene
    (if significant systemic absorption of ophthalmic epinephrine occurs, concurrent use of cyclopropane, halothane, or possibly chloroform may increase the risk of severe ventricular arrhythmias because these anesthetics greatly sensitize the myocardium to the effects of sympathomimetics; therapy with ophthalmic epinephrine should be interrupted prior to general anesthesia in patients receiving these anesthetics)
    (enflurane, methoxyflurane, or especially trichloroethylene may cause some sensitization of the myocardium to the effects of sympathomimetics; caution is recommended during concurrent use with ophthalmic epinephrine)
    (desflurane and isoflurane do not significantly sensitize the myocardium to the ventricular arrhythmogenic effects of epinephrine)

Antidepressants, tricyclic or
Maprotiline or
Nomifensine
  (if significant systemic absorption of ophthalmic epinephrine occurs, concurrent use of these medications may potentiate the cardiovascular effects of epinephrine, possibly resulting in arrhythmias, hypertension, or tachycardia)

Beta-adrenergic blocking agents, ophthalmic
  (concurrent use of ophthalmic betaxolol, levobunolol, or timolol with ophthalmic epinephrine may provide a beneficial additive effect in lowering intraocular pressure)

Digitalis glycosides
  (if significant systemic absorption of ophthalmic epinephrine occurs, concurrent use of digitalis glycosides may increase the risk of cardiac arrhythmias; caution is recommended if concurrent use is necessary)

Monoamine oxidase (MAO) inhibitors, including furazolidone, procarbazine, and selegiline
  (if significant systemic absorption of ophthalmic epinephrine occurs, concurrent use of MAO inhibitors may result in exaggerated adrenergic effects; adjustment of the ophthalmic epinephrine dose is required when it is administered concurrently or within 21 days after administration of MAO inhibitors)

Sympathomimetics, systemic or local
  (if significant systemic absorption of ophthalmic epinephrine occurs, concurrent use of systemic sympathomimetics may result in additive toxic effects; in addition, local anesthetics with vasoconstrictors should be avoided or a minimal amount of the vasoconstrictor should be used with the local anesthetic)

**Medical considerations/Contraindications**

The medical considerations/contraindications included have been selected on the basis of their potential clinical significance (reasons given in parentheses where appropriate)—not necessarily inclusive (» = major clinical significance).

***Risk-benefit should be considered when the following medical problems exist:***

    Aphakia
        (epinephrine therapy may cause reversible macular edema)

    Asthma, bronchial

» Cardiovascular disease or
    Cerebral arteriosclerosis or
    Hypertension or
    Hyperthyroidism
        (if systemic absorption occurs, the vasoconstrictive action of epinephrine may make condition worse)

    Diabetes mellitus

» Glaucoma, angle-closure, or predisposition to
        (may precipitate an acute attack of angle-closure glaucoma)

    Sensitivity to epinephrine or sulfites

**Patient monitoring**

The following may be especially important in patient monitoring (other tests may be warranted in some patients, depending on condition; » = major clinical significance):

    Gonioscopy
        (recommended prior to initiating therapy)

    Intraocular pressure determinations
        (recommended at periodic intervals during therapy)

## Side/Adverse Effects

Note: Pigmentary deposits in the conjunctiva may occur after prolonged use of ophthalmic epinephrine; on rare occasions, deposits in the eyelids or cornea may also occur.

The following side/adverse effects have been selected on the basis of their potential clinical significance (possible signs and symptoms in parentheses where appropriate)—not necessarily inclusive:

**Those indicating need for medical attention**
Incidence less frequent
    ***Maculopathy in aphakic eyes*** (blurred or decreased vision); ***systemic absorption*** (fast, irregular, or pounding heartbeat; feeling faint; increased sweating; paleness; trembling; increased blood pressure)

**Those indicating need for medical attention only if they continue or are bothersome**
Incidence more frequent
    ***Headache or browache; stinging, burning, redness, or other eye irritation; watering of eyes***
Incidence less frequent
    ***Blurred vision or other vision change; eye pain or ache***

## Overdose

For specific information on the agents used in the management of ophthalmic epinephrine overdose, see:
• *Beta-adrenergic Blocking Agents (Systemic)* monograph.

For more information on the management of overdose or unintentional ingestion, **contact a Poison Control Center** (see *Poison Control Center Listing*).

**Treatment of overdose**
Systemic effects should be treated symptomatically; however, overdosage is not likely to occur due to the limited rate of absorption and rapid inactivation of epinephrine once it enters the bloodstream. If tachycardia occurs and persists, a beta-adrenergic blocker may be administered.

Overdosage in eyes should be treated by immediately flushing eyes with water or normal saline.

## Patient Consultation

As an aid to patient consultation, refer to *Advice for the Patient, Epinephrine (Ophthalmic)*.

In providing consultation, consider emphasizing the following selected information (» = major clinical significance):

**Before using this medication**
» Conditions affecting use, especially:
    Sensitivity to epinephrine or sulfites
    Other medical problems, especially cardiovascular disease, angle-closure glaucoma, or predisposition to angle-closure glaucoma

**Proper use of this medication**
» Importance of not using more medication than the amount prescribed
    Proper administration technique
    Preventing contamination: Not touching applicator tip to any surface; keeping container tightly closed
    Not using if medication becomes discolored or contains a precipitate

» Proper dosing
    Missed dose: Applying as soon as possible; if almost time for next dose, skipping missed dose and returning to regular dosing schedule; not doubling doses
» Proper storage

**Precautions while using this medication**
    Regular visits to physician to check eye pressure during therapy
» Blurred vision may occur for short time after application; not driving, using machines, or doing anything else that could be dangerous if unable to see well

**Side/adverse effects**
    Signs of potential side effects, especially maculopathy in aphakic eyes or signs of systemic absorption

## General Dosing Information

Although some manufacturers recommend a dose of 2 drops of an ophthalmic solution at appropriate intervals, the conjunctival sac will usually hold only 1 drop.

To avoid excessive systemic absorption, patient should press finger to the lacrimal sac during and for 1 or 2 minutes following instillation of medication.

Caution is recommended when epinephrine is used in aphakic eyes, since maculopathy may occur rarely, resulting in decreased visual acuity. In this event, medication should be promptly discontinued.

Although some manufacturers recommend that patients not wear soft contact lenses during treatment with ophthalmic epinephrine, USP medical experts do not believe this precaution is necessary unless the patient has corneal epithelial problems and the medication is to be used more often than once every 1 to 2 hours. No significant problems have been documented with ophthalmic solutions containing 0.03% or less of benzalkonium chloride as a preservative, and used as eye drops in patients with no significant corneal surface problems.

---

### EPINEPHRINE

## Ophthalmic Dosage Forms

**EPINEPHRINE OPHTHALMIC SOLUTION USP**

**Usual adult and adolescent dose**
Antiglaucoma agent (ophthalmic)—
    Topical, to the conjunctiva, 1 drop one or two times a day.

**Usual pediatric dose**
Safety and efficacy have not been established.

**Usual geriatric dose**
See *Usual adult and adolescent dose*.

**Strength(s) usually available**
U.S.—
    0.1% (Rx) [GENERIC].
    0.5% (Rx) [*Epifrin* (benzalkonium chloride; sodium metabisulfite)].
    1% (Rx) [*Epifrin* (benzalkonium chloride; sodium metabisulfite); *Glaucon* (benzalkonium chloride 0.01%; sodium metabisulfite)].
    2% (Rx) [*Epifrin* (benzalkonium chloride; sodium metabisulfite); *Glaucon* (benzalkonium chloride 0.01%; sodium metabisulfite)].
Canada—
    1% (Rx) [*Epifrin* (benzalkonium chloride 0.004%; sodium metabisulfite)].

**Packaging and storage**
Store below 40 °C (104 °F), preferably between 15 and 30 °C (59 and 86 °F), unless otherwise specified by manufacturer. Store in a tight, light-resistant container. Protect from freezing.

**Stability**
Do not use if solution is pinkish or brownish in color or contains a precipitate.

**Auxiliary labeling**
• For the eye.
• Keep container tightly closed.

---

### EPINEPHRYL BORATE

## Ophthalmic Dosage Forms

**EPINEPHRYL BORATE OPHTHALMIC SOLUTION USP**

**Usual adult and adolescent dose**
Antiglaucoma agent (ophthalmic)—
    Topical, to the conjunctiva, 1 drop one or two times a day.

## Epinephrine (Ophthalmic)

### Usual pediatric dose
Safety and efficacy have not been established.

### Usual geriatric dose
See *Usual adult and adolescent dose.*

### Strength(s) usually available
U.S.—
- 0.5% (base) (Rx) [*Epinal* (benzalkonium choloride 0.01%)].
- 1% (base) (Rx) [*Epinal* (benzalkonium chloride 0.01%); *Eppy/N* (benzalkonium chloride 0.01%)].
- 2% (base) (Rx) [*Eppy/N* (benzalkonium chloride 0.01%)].

Canada—
- Not commercially available.

### Packaging and storage
Store below 40 °C (104 °F), preferably between 15 and 30 °C (59 and 86 °F), unless otherwise specified by manufacturer. Store in a tight, light-resistant container. Protect from freezing.

### Stability
The color of this solution may vary from colorless to amber yellow. Do not use if solution is dark brown or contains a precipitate.

### Auxiliary labeling
- For the eye.
- Keep container tightly closed.

Revised: 11/28/94

---

**EPINEPHRYL BORATE**—See *Epinephrine (Ophthalmic)*

---

# EPOETIN  Systemic

VA CLASSIFICATION (Primary): BL400

Commonly used brand name(s): *Epogen; Eprex; Procrit.*

Other commonly used names are human erythropoietin, recombinant; EPO; and r-HuEPO.

Note: For a listing of dosage forms and brand names by country availability, see *Dosage Forms* section(s).

## Category
Antianemic.

## Indications
Note: Bracketed information in the *Indications* section refers to uses that are not included in U.S. product labeling.

### Accepted
Anemia associated with renal failure (treatment)—Epoetin is indicated for the treatment of anemia associated with chronic renal failure. It is used for patients who do not require dialysis as well as patients receiving dialysis (continuous peritoneal dialysis, high-flux short-time hemodialysis, or conventional hemodialysis). However, in patients not receiving dialysis, use of epoetin should be limited to individuals having hematocrit values below 30%.

Anemia, severe, associated with zidovudine therapy in human immunodeficiency virus (HIV)–infected patients (treatment)—Epoetin is indicated for the treatment of severe anemia associated with zidovudine therapy in HIV-infected patients. Epoetin is not indicated for the treatment of anemia in HIV-infected patients due to other factors.

Anemia associated with chemotherapy in cancer patients (treatment)—Epoetin is indicated for the treatment of anemia in patients with nonmyeloid malignancies in which the anemia is due to the effect of concomitantly administered chemotherapy.

Blood transfusions, allogeneic, in anemic surgery patients, reduction of—Epoetin is indicated for use in anemic patients (hemoglobin > 10 to ≤ 13 grams per dL) who are scheduled to undergo elective, noncardiac, nonvascular surgery, to reduce the need for allogeneic blood transfusions. It is indicated for patients who are at high risk for perioperative transfusions with significant, anticipated blood loss.

[Anemia associated with frequent blood donation (prophylaxis)]—Epoetin is indicated to prevent anemia in patients who donate blood and to increase the capacity for donation (for future autologous transfusion) prior to elective surgery. The medication has been found to be effective in females, patients with low packed-cell volumes due to anemia or small body size, and patients requiring donation of 4 units or more of blood.

[Anemia associated with malignancy (treatment)]—Epoetin is indicated for treatment of chronic anemia associated with neoplastic diseases.

[Anemia associated with myelodysplastic syndromes (treatment)[1]]—Epoetin is indicated for treatment of anemia associated with myelodysplastic syndromes in selected patients. (Evidence rating: IIID)

Note: Epoetin is not a substitute for blood transfusions, which may be required for the emergency treatment of severe anemia. However, with chronic use, epoetin reduces the need for repeated maintenance blood transfusions.

[1]Not included in Canadian product labeling.

## Pharmacology/Pharmacokinetics

### Physicochemical characteristics
Molecular weight—Epoetin alfa: About 30,400 daltons.

### Mechanism of action/Effect
Epoetin alfa is a glycoprotein, produced by recombinant DNA technology, that contains 165 amino acids in a sequence identical to that of endogenous human erythropoietin. Recombinant epoetin has the same biological activity as the endogenous hormone, which induces erythropoiesis by stimulating the division and differentiation of committed erythroid progenitor cells, including burst-forming units–erythroid, colony-forming units–erythroid, erythroblasts, and reticulocytes, in bone marrow. Erythropoietin also induces the release of reticulocytes from the bone marrow into the blood stream, where they mature into erythrocytes.

Endogenous erythropoietin is produced primarily in the kidney. The anemia associated with chronic renal failure is caused primarily by inadequate production of the hormone. Administration of epoetin corrects the erythropoietin deficiency in patients with chronic renal failure. Epoetin also stimulates red blood cell production in patients who do not have a documented erythropoietin deficiency, i.e., patients with normal or slightly elevated concentrations of endogenous erythropoietin. However, it may not be effective in patients who are anemic despite having significantly elevated concentrations of erythropoietin.

### Other actions/effects
The increase in hematocrit induced by epoetin may increase blood viscosity and peripheral vascular resistance, leading to a rise in blood pressure. The medication does not appear to have a direct pressor effect.

Epoetin may correct the bleeding tendency associated with chronic renal failure, which may be caused partially by red blood cell deficiency. However, the medication may also increase the thrombotic tendency in some patients.

Correction of anemia by epoetin may result in an improved feeling of well-being; increased appetite; relief of anemia-induced fatigue, tachycardia, headache, weakness, or angina pectoris; increased exercise tolerance and physical activity; and improved sleep, sexual function, and cognitive function.

Administration of epoetin alfa apparently does not induce antibody formation, because antibodies have not been detected in the blood of patients treated with the recombinant hormone for up to 12 months.

Endogenous erythropoietin production may be suppressed by chronic administration of recombinant epoetin.

### Half-life
Elimination—May average 4 to 13 hours following intravenous or subcutaneous administration. The elimination half-life is generally higher after the first few doses (> 7.5 hours) than after 2 or more weeks of treatment (6.2 hours after 7 doses; 4.6 hours after 24 doses).

### Onset of action
Increase in reticulocyte count (initial effect)—Within 7 to 10 days.

Increase in red cell count, hematocrit, hemoglobin—Clinically significant increases generally occur in 2 to 6 weeks. The rate and extent of the response are dependent on dosage and availability of iron stores. Over a 2-week period, administration of 50 Units per kg of body weight 3 times weekly increases the hematocrit by an average of 1.5 points, administration of 100 Units per kg of body weight 3 times weekly increases the hematocrit by an average of 2.5 points, and administration of 150 Units per kg of body weight 3 times weekly increases the hematocrit by an average of 3.5 points.

**Time to peak concentration**
Single intravenous dose—15 minutes.
Single subcutaneous dose—5 to 24 hours. Peak concentrations may be maintained for 12 to 16 hours, and detectable quantities are present for at least 24 hours, after administration.
Note: With repeated subcutaneous administration, peak concentrations are achieved and maintained over the same time periods as with single subcutaneous doses, but are substantially lower than those achieved by a single dose. However, the lower epoetin concentrations are sufficient for achieving, and even lower concentrations are sufficient for maintaining, the desired response.

**Time to peak effect**
Increase in hematocrit to target area—Dose dependent; usually within 2 months with administration of 100 or 150 Units per kg of body weight 3 times weekly.

**Duration of action**
The hematocrit may begin to decrease about 2 weeks after treatment has been discontinued.

## Precautions to Consider

**Carcinogenicity**
The carcinogenic potential of epoetin alfa has not been investigated.

**Mutagenicity**
Epoetin alfa does not induce bacterial gene mutation (Ames test), chromosomal aberrations in mammalian cells, micronuclei in mice, or gene mutation at the HGPRT locus. Also, examination of the bone marrow of patients receiving epoetin for up to 8 weeks has revealed no evidence of karyotypic abnormalities or alteration in the sister chromatid exchange rate.

**Pregnancy/Reproduction**
Fertility—Administration of 100 or 500 Units per kg of body weight intravenously to male and female rats showed a trend toward slightly increased fetal wastage, but the trend was not statistically significant.

Pregnancy—Adequate and well-controlled studies in humans have not been done. However, administration of 500 Units per kg of body weight to female rats caused decreases in weight gain, delays in the appearance of abdominal hair, delayed eyelid opening, delayed ossification, and decreases in the number of caudal vertebrae in first generation fetuses. Administration of up to 500 Units per kg of body weight to female rabbits from Day 6 to Day 18 of gestation produced no adverse effects.

FDA Pregnancy Category C.

**Breast-feeding**
It is not known whether epoetin alfa is excreted in human breast milk. However, in animal studies, administration of up to 500 Units per kg of body weight to female rats during lactation produced no adverse effects in the pups.

**Pediatrics**
No pediatrics-specific information is available for children up to 12 years of age.
Note: The multi-dose vials contain benzyl alcohol, which is not recommended for use in neonates.

**Geriatrics**
No published geriatrics-specific information is available.

**Drug interactions and/or related problems**
The following drug interactions and/or related problems have been selected on the basis of their potential clinical significance (possible mechanism in parentheses where appropriate)—not necessarily inclusive (» = major clinical significance):

Note: Combinations containing any of the following medications, depending on the amount present, may also interact with this medication.

Antihypertensive agents
(epoetin may increase blood pressure, possibly to hypertensive levels, especially when the hematocrit is rising rapidly; more intensive antihypertensive therapy [increase in dosage, administration of additional and/or more potent medications] may be required to control blood pressure)

Heparin
(an increase in heparin dosage may be required in patients receiving hemodialysis, because epoetin-induced increases in red blood cell volume may lead to blood clotting in the dialyzer and/or vascular access [arteriovenous shunt])

Iron supplements
(iron requirement may be increased as existing iron stores are used for erythropoiesis; some clinicians recommend supplementation for all patients who are not overloaded with iron because of frequent blood transfusions; in some patients, oral iron supplementation may be insufficient and intravenous iron dextran may be required)

**Laboratory value alterations**
The following have been selected on the basis of their potential clinical significance (possible effect in parentheses where appropriate)—not necessarily inclusive (» = major clinical significance):

With physiology/laboratory test values
Bleeding time
(may be decreased; also, the prolonged bleeding time associated with chronic renal failure in some patients may be corrected during epoetin treatment)

Blood pressure
(may be increased, possibly to hypertensive levels)

Blood urea nitrogen (BUN) and
Serum creatinine concentrations and
Serum phosphorus concentrations and
Serum potassium concentrations and
Serum sodium concentrations and
Serum uric acid concentrations
(may be increased; however, whether the increases reported in patients with chronic renal failure are caused by a direct effect of epoetin on the renal clearance of these substances or the efficacy of dialysis and/or by noncompliance with required dietary restrictions, which may occur with improvement of anemia increases the patient's appetite and feeling of well-being, has not been established)

Iron concentration and
Serum ferritin
(usually are decreased, unless the patient is receiving adequate iron supplementation, as iron stores are utilized for hemoglobin synthesis functional iron deficiency may occur and lead to a decrease or loss of epoetin efficacy)

**Medical considerations/Contraindications**
The medical considerations/contraindications included have been selected on the basis of their potential clinical significance (reasons given in parentheses where appropriate)—not necessarily inclusive (» = major clinical significance):

*Except under special circumstances, this medication should not be used when the following medical problems exist:*

» Hypersensitivity to human albumin or to mammalian cell–derived products
(risk of a serious allergic reaction to the albumin present in the commercial formulation or to the recombinant product itself)

» Hypertension, uncontrolled
(may be exacerbated, especially during the early phase of treatment or when the hematocrit is rising too rapidly [> 4 points within 2 weeks]; a few cases of hypertensive encephalopathy have occurred in patients with poorly controlled blood pressure during epoetin therapy; initiation of therapy should be delayed until blood pressure is adequately controlled)

*Risk-benefit should be considered when the following medical problems exist:*

Any condition that may decrease or delay the response to epoetin alfa, such as:
Aluminum intoxication
Folic acid deficiency
Hemolysis
Infection
Inflammation
Malignancy
Osteitis fibrosa cystica
Vitamin $B_{12}$ deficiency

Cardiovascular system abnormalities caused by hypertension or
» Hypertension, previous, controlled
(increased risk of hypertension, which may lead to hypertensive encephalopathy)

Hematologic disorders, such as:
Hypercoagulable disorders
Myelodysplastic syndromes
Sickle cell anemia or
Vascular disease
(caution and close monitoring are recommended because of an increased thrombotic tendency or other potential complications associated with increases in blood viscosity and peripheral vascular resistance that may occur as a result of epoetin-induced increases in hematocrit)

(the safety and efficacy of epoetin therapy in patients with hematologic disorders have not been determined; also, the presence of myelodysplastic disorders may slow or decrease the bone marrow response to the medication)

Seizure disorders, history of
(seizures not associated with hypertensive encephalopathy have been reported during epoetin therapy; although a causal association has not been established [in clinical studies, seizures occurred at the same rate in both epoetin-treated and placebo-treated patients with chronic renal failure], caution is recommended)

**Patient monitoring**
The following may be especially important in patient monitoring (other tests may be warranted in some patients, depending on condition; » = major clinical significance):

» Blood pressure determinations
(recommended at frequent intervals because epoetin may increase blood pressure, possibly to hypertensive levels; although the risk may be greatest in patients with pre-existing hypertension [even if optimally controlled at the time epoetin therapy is initiated], epoetin may also increase blood pressure in previously normotensive patients; control of blood pressure is essential because a few cases of hypertensive encephalopathy have occurred during epoetin therapy in patients with poorly controlled hypertension and because hypertension may be especially hazardous to patients with chronic renal failure, who are predisposed to cardiovascular complications including myocardial ischemia, myocardial infarction, heart failure, and/or stroke; initiation of or increase in antihypertensive therapy, reduction in dosage or temporary withdrawal of epoetin alfa, or even phlebotomy may be required to control hypertension)

Complete blood count and
Platelet count
(recommended periodically because increases in white blood cell and platelet counts have been reported, although the counts have generally remained within the normal range)

» Hematocrit
(determinations recommended prior to initiation of therapy, then twice weekly during therapy as a guide to efficacy and dosage; because a too-rapid rise in hematocrit may be associated with an increased risk of adverse effects, it is recommended that epoetin dosage be reduced if the hematocrit increases by more than 4 points in a 2-week period; after the hematocrit has been stabilized in the target range [30 to 36%], the frequency of monitoring may be decreased; however, after each dosage adjustment, determinations should be performed twice a week for at least 2 to 6 weeks, until the hematocrit has stabilized at the new level; also, to prevent adverse effects, therapy should be discontinued if the hematocrit exceeds 36%)

» Iron status, including:
Serum ferritin
Transferrin saturation
(determination recommended prior to initiation of therapy, because epoetin's efficacy is decreased when the available iron is insufficient to support erythropoiesis; serum ferritin should be at least 100 nanograms per mL, and transferrin saturation at least 20%, before therapy is initiated)
(monitoring recommended at regular intervals throughout therapy to determine whether iron supplementation should be initiated or increased, because incorporation of iron into hemoglobin may decrease iron stores to the point of functional iron deficiency, leading to a decrease or loss of epoetin efficacy)

Neurologic evaluation
(recommended periodically, especially during the first 90 days of therapy, to detect premonitory signs indicative of a risk of seizures; although a causal association between a rapid rise in hematocrit and seizures has not been established, it is recommended that epoetin dosage be reduced if the hematocrit increases by more than 4 points within 2 weeks)

» Renal function, including:
Blood urea nitrogen (BUN) and
Serum creatinine and
Serum phosphorous and
Serum potassium and
Serum sodium and
Serum uric acid
(close monitoring recommended in patients with renal function impairment to determine the need for initiating or increasing dialysis; however, whether the increases in concentrations of these substances that have been reported during epoetin therapy are caused by a direct effect of the hormone on renal function or the efficacy of dialysis and/or by noncompliance with dietary restrictions required by patients with chronic renal failure, which may occur when improvement of anemia produces increased appetite and feeling of well-being, has not been established)

## Side/Adverse Effects

Note: Some of the side effects listed below are known sequelae of chronic renal failure; therefore, a causal association with epoetin therapy has not always been established.

Menses have resumed during treatment in some female patients. Therefore, the risk of pregnancy should be evaluated and an appropriate method of contraception instituted if necessary.

The following side/adverse effects have been selected on the basis of their potential clinical significance (possible signs and symptoms in parentheses where appropriate)—not necessarily inclusive:

**Those indicating need for medical attention**
Incidence more frequent
*Chest pain*—incidence 7%; *edema* (swelling of face, fingers, ankles, feet, or lower legs; weight gain)—incidence 9%; *fast heartbeat; headache*—incidence 16%; may rarely indicate hypertensive encephalopathy; *increased blood pressure*—incidence 24%; may reach hypertensive levels and, rarely, lead to cerebral ischemia or to hypertensive encephalopathy (blurred vision or other change in vision, grand mal seizures, headache); *polycythemia*—may lead to hyperviscosity resulting in increased peripheral vascular resistance, hypertension, and thrombotic complications, e.g., clotting of arteriovenous (AV) shunts [incidence 6.8%] and/or dialyzer, and rarely, transient ischemic attacks or cerebrovascular accident [incidence 0.4%] or myocardial infarction [incidence 0.4%]

Incidence less frequent
*Seizures*—incidence 1.1% overall, but 2.5% during the first 90 days of treatment in patients receiving dialysis; *shortness of breath*

Incidence rare
*Skin rash or hives*

**Those indicating need for medical attention only if they continue or are bothersome**
Incidence more frequent
*Arthralgias* (bone pain)—incidence 11%; *asthenia* (muscle weakness, severe)—incidence 7%; *diarrhea*—incidence 8.5%; *nausea*—incidence 10.5%; *skin reaction at administration site*—incidence 7%; *tiredness*—incidence 9%; *vomiting*—incidence 8%

Incidence less frequent or rare
*Influenza-like syndrome, mild* (bone pain; muscle aches; chills; shivering; sweating)—may appear 1 to 2 hours after intravenous administration and persist for up to 12 hours

## Patient Consultation

As an aid to patient consultation, refer to *Advice for the Patient, Epoetin (Systemic)*.
In providing consultation, consider emphasizing the following selected information (» = major clinical significance):

**Before using this medication**
» Conditions affecting use, especially:
Other medical problems, especially hypertension and a history of hypersensitivity to albumin or to mammalian cell–derived products

**Proper use of this medication**
» Proper injection technique (if dispensed for home use)
» Proper dosing
Missed dose: Administering as soon as possible; not administering if almost time for next dose; not doubling doses
» Proper storage

**Precautions while receiving this medication**
Risk of seizures, especially during the first 90 days of treatment; avoiding activities that may be hazardous should a seizure occur
» Importance of keeping medical and dialysis appointments
» Importance of compliance with antihypertensive regimen (medications and diet), if prescribed, and dietary restrictions pertinent to patients with chronic renal failure
» Importance of compliance with iron or other vitamin supplementation

**Side/adverse effects**
Signs of potential side effects, especially chest pain, edema, fast heartbeat, headache, hypertension, seizures, shortness of breath, and skin rash or hives

## General Dosing Information
Epoetin alfa is administered intravenously or subcutaneously. In general, it is given intravenously to patients with an available intravenous access, i.e., patients receiving hemodialysis, and either intravenously or subcutaneously to other patients.

An increase in dosage may be required if aluminum intoxication, which is not uncommon in patients with chronic renal failure, is present.

### Diet/Nutrition
Failure to achieve an adequate response to the medication, or loss of efficacy during therapy, may indicate a lack of sufficient iron to support erythropoiesis. Iron supplementation should be initiated or increased as needed. Also, folic acid and/or vitamin $B_{12}$ deficiency may reduce or delay the response to the medication; supplementation with these nutrients may also be required.

Correction of anemia often results in increased appetite and a feeling of well-being, which, in turn, may lead to noncompliance with dietary restrictions (e.g., regulated protein, sodium, and potassium intake) that are necessary in patients with chronic renal failure. Noncompliance with such restrictions may require institution of, or an increase in, dialysis.

### For treatment of adverse effects
Recommended treatment consists of the following
- For clotting of arteriovenous (AV) shunt and/or dialyzer—Clotting complications should be managed according to the dialysis center's policy and procedures. AV shunts may be cleared by use of a syringe with heparinized saline solution. If this is unsuccessful, a thrombolytic agent (streptokinase or urokinase) may be used, after allowing the effects of prior anticoagulation to diminish. Increasing heparin dosage helps prevent recurrent clotting complications.
- For hypertension—Instituting or increasing administration of antihypertensive medications. In some patients, a decrease in dosage or temporary withdrawal of epoetin and/or phlebotomy may be needed.
- For polycythemia—Decreasing the dosage of, or temporarily suspending therapy with, epoetin. In some patients, phlebotomy may be needed.

## Parenteral Dosage Forms
### EPOETIN ALFA, RECOMBINANT, INJECTION
#### Usual adult and adolescent dose
Anemia associated with renal failure—
Initial: Intravenous or subcutaneous, 50 to 100 Units per kg of body weight three times a week. Dosage may be increased if, after eight weeks of therapy, the hematocrit has not increased by five to six points and is still below the desired range (30 to 36%). Adjustments in dosage are generally made in increments of 25 Units per kg of body weight.
Note: Some clinicians begin therapy with lower doses, e.g., 40 Units per kg of body weight three times a week.

An interval of at least four weeks should elapse between dosage adjustments, unless clinical circumstances dictate otherwise, because the response to a change in dosage may require two to six weeks.

Because of a possible risk of hypertensive and/or thrombotic complications, it is recommended that dosage be decreased if the hematocrit increases by more than four points in a two-week period.

Administration of epoetin should be discontinued temporarily if the hematocrit reaches or exceeds the maximum recommended level of 36%. When the hematocrit has returned to the desired range, therapy may be resumed using a dose that is 25 Units per kg of body weight lower than the previous dose.
Maintenance: Dosage should be decreased gradually, by 25 Units per kg of body weight at intervals of four weeks or more, to the lowest dose that will maintain the hematocrit at the desired level (30 to 36%).
Note: Although maintenance doses of up to 525 Units per kg of body weight three times a week have been administered, the maximum maintenance dose recommended by the manufacturer is 300 Units per kg of body weight three times a week.

Once-weekly subcutaneous administration of the entire week's dosage requirement may be sufficient to maintain some patients at the desired hematocrit range.
Anemia in zidovudine-treated HIV-infected patients—
Initial: Intravenous or subcutaneous, 100 Units per kg of body weight three times a week for eight weeks for patients with serum erythropoietin levels ≤ 500 milliUnits per mL and who are receiving a dose of zidovudine ≤ 4200 mg per week. Dosage may be increased if, after eight weeks of therapy, a satisfactory increase in hematocrit or reduction of transfusion requirements is not obtained. The dose can be increased by 50 to 100 Units per kg of body weight three times a week, with weekly monitoring of the hematocrit. Thereafter, the response should be evaluated every four to eight weeks, with the dose adjusted accordingly by 50 to 100 Units per kg of body weight three times a week. Patients who do not have a satisfactory response to a dose of 300 Units per kg of body weight three times a week are unlikely to respond to higher doses.
Note: Prior to beginning treatment with epoetin, it is recommended that the endogenous serum erythropoietin level be determined. Available evidence suggests that patients receiving zidovudine who have endogenous serum erythropoietin levels > 500 m-Units/mL are unlikely to respond to therapy with epoetin.
Maintenance: Dosage should be titrated to maintain the desired response and should be based on factors such as variations in zidovudine dose and the presence of intercurrent infectious or inflammatory episodes. Treatment should be discontinued if the hematocrit exceeds 40%. When the hematocrit drops to 36%, treatment may be resumed at a dose 25% less than the previous dose and then titrated accordingly.

Anemia in cancer patients on chemotherapy—
Initial: Subcutaneous, 150 Units per kg of body weight three times a week. If the initial dose causes a very rapid rise in hematocrit (i.e., an increase of more than four points in a two-week period), the dose should be reduced. Dosage may be increased if, after eight weeks of therapy, a satisfactory increase in hematocrit or reduction of transfusion requirements is not obtained. The dose can be increased up to 300 Units per kg of body weight three times a week. Patients who do not have a satisfactory response to a dose of 300 Units per kg of body weight three times a week are unlikely to respond to higher doses. Treatment should be discontinued if the hematocrit exceeds 40%. When the hematocrit drops to 36%, treatment may be resumed at a dose 25% less than the previous dose and then titrated accordingly.
Note: Treatment of patients with grossly elevated serum erythropoietin levels (e.g., > 200 mUnits/mL) is not recommended.
Reduction of allogeneic blood transfusion in anemic surgery patients—
Subcutaneous, 300 Units per kg of body weight per day for ten days prior to surgery, on the day of surgery, and for four days after surgery. Alternatively, subcutaneous, 600 Units per kg of body weight once a week, twenty-one, fourteen, and seven days prior to surgery, and on the day of surgery.
Note: Prior to treatment with epoetin, it should be established that the patient's hemoglobin is > 10 and ≤ 13 grams per deciliter.

#### Usual pediatric dose
Children up to 12 years of age—Dosage has not been established.

#### Strength(s) usually available
U.S.—
  In 1-mL single-dose vials
    2000 Units per mL (Rx) [*Epogen* (human albumin 2.5 mg); *Procrit* (human albumin 2.5 mg)].
    3000 Units per mL (Rx) [*Epogen* (human albumin 2.5 mg); *Procrit* (human albumin 2.5 mg)].
    4000 Units per mL (Rx) [*Epogen* (human albumin 2.5 mg); *Procrit* (human albumin 2.5 mg)].
    10,000 Units per mL (Rx) [*Epogen* (human albumin 2.5 mg); *Procrit* (human albumin 2.5 mg)].
  In multi-dose vials
    10,000 Units per mL in 2-mL vials (Rx) [*Epogen* (human albumin 2.5 mg; benzyl alcohol 1%); *Procrit* (human albumin 2.5 mg; benzyl alcohol 1%)].
    20,000 Units per mL in 1-mL vials (Rx) [*Epogen* (human albumin 2.5 mg; benzyl alcohol 1%); *Procrit* (human albumin 2.5 mg; benzyl alcohol 1%)].
Canada—
  In 1-mL single-dose vials
    2000 International Units (IU) per mL (Rx) [*Eprex* (human albumin 2.5 mg)].
    4000 IU per mL (Rx) [*Eprex* (human albumin 2.5 mg)].
    10,000 IU per mL (Rx) [*Eprex* (human albumin 2.5 mg)].
  In multi-dose vials
    20,000 IU per mL in 1-mL vials (Rx) [*Eprex* (human albumin 2.5 mg; benzyl alcohol 1%)].
  In single-dose, pre-filled syringes
    1000 IU per 0.5 mL (Rx) [*Eprex*].
    2000 IU per 0.5 mL (Rx) [*Eprex*].
    3000 IU per 0.3 mL (Rx) [*Eprex*].
    4000 IU per 0.4 mL (Rx) [*Eprex*].
    10,000 IU per mL (Rx) [*Eprex*].

## Epoetin (Systemic)

### Packaging and storage
Store at 2 to 8 °C (36 to 46 °F), unless otherwise specified by manufacturer. Protect from freezing.

### Stability
*Do not shake the vial of epoetin alfa, recombinant, injection.* Shaking may denature the glycoprotein and render it biologically inactive.

Because the single-dose injection contains no preservative, each vial should be used to administer one dose only. Any unused portion of the solution must be discarded.

The multi-dose vials should be discarded 21 days after initial entry.

### Incompatibilities
It is recommended that epoetin alfa, recombinant, not be admixed with other medications.

### Additional information
The multi-dose vials contain benzyl alcohol, which is not recommended for use in neonates. A fatal syndrome consisting of metabolic acidosis, central nervous system depression, respiratory problems, renal failure, hypotension, and possibly seizures and intracranial hemorrhage has been associated with the administration of benzyl alcohol to neonates.

### Selected Bibliography
Eschbach JW, Egrie JC, Downing MR, et al. Correction of the anemia of end-stage renal disease with recombinant human erythropoietin: results of a combined phase I and II clinical trial. N Engl J Med 1987; 316: 73-8.

Mohini R. Clinical efficacy of recombinant human erythropoietin in hemodialysis patients. Semin Nephrol 1989; 9 Suppl 1: 16-21.

Schwenk MH, Halstenson CE. Recombinant human erythropoietin. DICP 1989; 23: 528-36.

Revised: 06/30/98

---

# EPTIFIBATIDE  Systemic—INTRODUCTORY VERSION

VA CLASSIFICATION (Primary): BL117

Commonly used brand name(s): *Integrilin*.

Note: For a listing of dosage forms and brand names by country availability, see *Dosage Forms* section(s).

## Category
Platelet aggregation inhibitor.

## Indications

### Accepted
Thrombosis, acute coronary syndrome–related (prophylaxis)—Eptifibatide is indicated, usually as an adjunct to aspirin and heparin, for the prevention of acute cardiac ischemic complications in patients with acute coronary syndrome (unstable angina or non–Q-wave myocardial infarction). These patients are at high risk for myocardial infarction and sudden death due to progression of total coronary artery occlusion, whether managed medically or with percutaneous coronary intervention (PCI).

Note: Acute coronary syndrome is defined as prolonged ($\geq$ 10 minutes) symptoms of cardiac ischemia within the previous 24 hours associated with either ST-segment changes (elevation between 0.6 mm and 1 mm or depression > 0.5 mm), T-wave inversion (> 1 mm), or positive CK-MB. This definition includes "unstable angina" and "non–Q-wave myocardial infarction" but excludes myocardial infarction that is associated with Q waves or greater degrees of ST-segment elevation.

Thrombosis, percutaneous coronary intervention–related (prophylaxis)—Eptifibatide is indicated, usually as an adjunct to aspirin and heparin, for the prevention of acute cardiac ischemic complications in patients undergoing PCI.

Note: PCI usually involves balloon angioplasty, but may also consist of directional atherectomy, transluminal extraction catheter atherectomy, rotational ablation atherectomy, or excimer-laser angioplasty.

## Pharmacology/Pharmacokinetics

### Physicochemical characteristics
Source—Synthetic. Produced by solution-phase peptide synthesis, with purification by preparative reverse-phase liquid chomatography and lyophilization.

Molecular weight—831.96.

pH—Eptifibatide injection: 5.25.

### Mechanism of action/Effect
Eptifibatide inhibits platelet aggregation by reversibly binding to the platelet receptor glycoprotein (GP) IIb/IIIa of human platelets, thus preventing the binding of fibrinogen, von Willebrand factor, and other adhesive ligands. Inhibition of platelet aggregation occurs in a dose- and concentration-dependent manner.

### Protein binding
Low (about 25%).

### Biotransformation
No major metabolites have been detected in human plasma. Deamidated eptifibatide and other, more polar metabolites have been detected in urine.

### Half-life
Elimination—
Plasma: Approximately 2.5 hours.

### Onset of action
Immediate.

### Time to steady-state concentration
Within 4 to 6 hours.

### Elimination
Renal, 50% (the majority as eptifibatide, deamidated eptifibatide, and more polar metabolites).
In dialysis—
There are *in vitro* data that eptifibatide may be cleared from plasma by dialysis.

Note: Clearance in patients with coronary artery disease has been found to be 55 to 58 mL per kg of body weight per hour.

## Precautions to Consider

### Carcinogenicity
No long-term studies in animals have been done.

### Mutagenicity
Eptifibatide was not found to be mutagenic in the Ames test, the mouse lymphoma cell (L 5178Y, TK$^{+/-}$) forward mutation test, the human lymphocyte chromosome aberration test, or the mouse micronucleus test.

### Pregnancy/Reproduction
Fertility—In animal studies eptifibatide had no effect on fertility and reproductive performance of male and female rats at total daily doses of up to 72 mg per kg of body weight (mg/kg) per day (about four times the maximum recommended human daily dose [MRHD] on a body surface area basis) administered as a continuous infusion.

Pregnancy—Adequate and well-controlled studies in humans have not been done.

Studies in rats at total daily doses of up to 72 mg/kg per day (about four times the MRHD on a body surface area basis) and in rabbits at total daily doses of up to 36 mg/kg per day (about four times the MRHD on a body surface area basis) found no evidence of teratogenicity or fetal toxicity.

Risk-benefit should be considered before use of eptifibatide during pregnancy.

FDA Pregnancy Category B.

### Breast-feeding
It is not known whether eptifibatide is distributed into breast milk.

### Pediatrics
Safety and efficacy have not been studied.

### Geriatrics
Studies performed, which included elderly patients (age range up to 94 years, mean age 60 years) showed no apparent differences in efficacy between elderly patients and younger adults.

An increased frequency of bleeding complications was observed in elderly patients in clinical trials. In one clinical study, patients over 75 years of age had to weigh at least 50 kg to be enrolled because of concern about an increased risk of bleeding in this subgroup.

### Drug interactions and/or related problems
The following drug interactions and/or related problems have been selected on the basis of their potential clinical significance (possible mechanism

in parentheses where appropriate)—not necessarily inclusive (» = major clinical significance):

Note: Combinations containing any of the following medications, depending on the amount present, may also interact with this medication.

Anticoagulants, coumarin- or indandione-derivative or
Clopidogrel or
Dipyridamole or
Nonsteroidal anti-inflammatory drugs (NSAIDs) or
Thrombolytic agents or
Ticlopidine
(caution is recommended because of the increased risk of bleeding)

» Platelet aggregation inhibitors, other (especially inhibitors of platelet receptor glycoprotein IIb/IIIa)
(concurrent use with eptifibatide is not recommended because of potentially additive pharmacologic effects)

### Medical considerations/Contraindications

The medical considerations/contraindications included have been selected on the basis of their potential clinical significance (reasons given in parentheses where appropriate)—not necessarily inclusive (» = major clinical significance).

*Except under special circumstances, this medication should not be used when the following medical problems exist:*

» Bleeding, active (within the last 30 days) or
» Bleeding diathesis or
» Cerebrovascular accident (CVA) within the past 30 days or
» Hemorrhagic stroke, history of or
» Hypertension, severe, uncontrolled, i.e., > 200 mm Hg systolic or > 110 mm Hg diastolic or
» Surgery, major, recent (within 6 weeks) or
» Thrombocytopenia (< 100,000 per mm³)
(increased risk of bleeding with eptifibatide)

*Risk-benefit should be considered when the following medical problems exist:*

» Renal function impairment, severe or
» Renal failure with dependence on renal dialysis
(no dosage adjustment was necessary for mild to moderate renal function impairment, i.e., serum creatinine concentrations between 1 and 2 mg/dL [for the 180 microgram per kg of body weight (mcg/kg) bolus and the 2 mcg/kg per minute intravenous infusion] or between 2 and 4 mg/dL [for the 135 mcg/kg bolus and the 0.5 mcg/kg per minute intravenous infusion]; although studies in patients with more severe renal function impairment have not been done, caution is recommended because clearance of eptifibatide would be expected to be reduced)

» Sensitivity to eptifibatide

### Patient monitoring

The following may be especially important in patient monitoring (other tests may be warranted in some patients, depending on condition; » = major clinical significance):

» Activated clotting time (ACT)
(for patients undergoing percutaneous coronary intervention (PCI), ACT measurement is recommended prior to initiation of eptifibatide therapy and during PCI; it is recommended that ACT be maintained between 200 and 250 seconds during PCI)

» Activated partial thromboplastin time (aPTT) and
» Prothrombin time (PT)
(recommended prior to initiation of eptifibatide therapy to provide a baseline and detect pre-existing hemostatic abnormalities)
(it is recommended that the aPTT be maintained between 50 and 70 seconds during therapy unless PCI is to be performed)
(it is recommended that the aPTT be checked before removal of the arterial sheath; the sheath should not be removed unless the aPTT is less than 45 seconds)
(monitoring of aPTT can also minimize bleeding incidents in patients who are also receiving heparin)

» Creatinine concentrations, serum and
» Hematocrit or hemoglobin and
» Platelet count
(recommended prior to initiation of eptifibatide therapy to detect pre-existing hemostatic abnormalities)

## Side/Adverse Effects

The following side/adverse effects have been selected on the basis of their potential clinical significance (possible signs and symptoms in parentheses where appropriate)—not necessarily inclusive:

*Those indicating need for medical attention*
Incidence more frequent
  *Bleeding; hypotension*
  Note: *Bleeding* is the most common complication of eptifibatide therapy. In the clinical trials, *major bleeding* was defined as an intracranial hemorrhage or a decrease in hemoglobin greater than 5 grams per dL. *Minor bleeding* included spontaneous gross hematuria, spontaneous hematemesis, other observed blood loss with a hemoglobin decrease of more than 3 grams per dL, and other hemoglobin decreases that were greater than 4 grams per dL, but less than 5 grams per dL. The most common bleeding complications were related to cardiac revascularization (coronary artery bypass graft–related or femoral artery access site bleeding).

Incidence rare
  *Anaphylaxis; thrombocytopenia*

## Overdose

Although there have been incidents where patients received doses more than double those called for in the study protocol, or where patients were identified by the physician as having received an overdose, no incidents of intracranial bleeding or other major bleeding occurred.

For more information on the management of overdose or unintentional ingestion, **contact a Poison Control Center** (see *Poison Control Center Listing*).

## General Dosing Information

Because of the risk of bleeding, arterial and venous punctures, intramuscular injections, and use of urinary catheters, nasotracheal intubation, and nasogastric tubes should be minimized. Noncompressible sites, such as subclavian or jugular veins, should be avoided when obtaining intravenous access.

It is recommended that eptifibatide be discontinued prior to surgery in patients who undergo coronary artery bypass graft surgery (CABG).

It is recommended that eptifibatide and heparin therapy be discontinued, and appropriate monitoring and therapy initiated, if a confirmed platelet count of less than 100,000 per mm³ occurs.

**Care of femoral artery access site in patients undergoing percutaneous coronary intervention (PCI)**

After PCI, eptifibatide infusion should be continued for 20 to 24 hours. The femoral artery sheath may be removed during treatment with eptifibatide, but only after heparin has been discontinued and its effects largely reversed. Prior to removing the sheath, it is recommended that heparin be discontinued for 3 to 4 hours and that an activated partial thromboplastin time (aPTT) of < 45 seconds and/or an activated clotting time (ACT) of < 150 seconds be documented. In any case, both heparin and eptifibatide should be discontinued and sheath hemostasis should be achieved by standard compressive techniques at least 4 hours before hospital discharge.

## Parenteral Dosage Forms

### EPTIFIBATIDE INJECTION

**Usual adult dose**

Note: For dosing charts by patient weight, see the *Integrilin* package insert. Most patients in the clinical trials received concomitant aspirin and heparin. The doses of aspirin and heparin used in the studies are outlined in the *Integrilin* package insert.

Acute coronary syndrome—
  Initial—
    Intravenous (over one to two minutes), 180 micrograms (0.18 mg) per kg of body weight as soon as possible following diagnosis, immediately followed by—
  Maintenance—
    Intravenous infusion (continuous), 2 micrograms (0.002 mg) per kg of body weight per minute until hospital discharge or initiation of coronary artery bypass graft (CABG) surgery, for up to seventy-two hours.

Note: It is recommended that eptifibatide be discontinued prior to surgery in patients who undergo CABG.

If a patient is scheduled to undergo percutaneous coronary intervention (PCI) while receiving eptifibatide, consideration may be given to decreasing the infusion rate to 0.5 microgram per kg per minute at the time of the procedure, and the infusion should be continued for twenty to twenty-four hours following the procedure (allowing for up to ninety-six hours of therapy).

In one study, patients weighing more than 121 kg received a maximum bolus injection of 22.6 mg followed by a maximum infusion rate of 15 mg per hour.

Prophylaxis of percutaneous coronary intervention (PCI)–related thrombosis—
Initial—
Intravenous (over one to two minutes), 135 micrograms (0.135 mg) per kg of body weight immediately before initiation of PCI, immediately followed by—
Maintenance—
Intravenous infusion (continuous), 0.5 microgram (0.0005 mg) per kg of body weight per minute for twenty to twenty-four hours.
Note: Prophylaxis of PCI–related thrombosis is only indicated in patients *not* presenting with an acute coronary syndrome.
There has been little experience in patients weighing more than 143 kg.

**Usual pediatric dose**
Safety and efficacy have not been established.

**Strength(s) usually available**
U.S.—
2 mg per mL (10-mL bolus vial) (Rx) [*Integrilin* (for intravenous bolus administration; citric acid 5.25 mg per mL; sodium hydroxide)].
750 mcg (0.75 mg) per mL (100-mL infusion vial) (Rx) [*Integrilin* (for continous intravenous infusion; citric acid 5.25 mg per mL; sodium hydroxide)].

**Packaging and storage**
Store between 2 and 8 °C (36 and 46 °F). Protect from light.

**Preparation of dosage form**
The bolus dose of eptifibatide should be withdrawn from the 10-mL bolus vial into a syringe.
For administration by continuous intravenous infusion (via an intravenous infusion pump or via gravity), eptifibatide should be administered undiluted directly from the 100-mL infusion vial, which should be spiked with a vented infusion set. It is important that care be taken to center the spike within the circle on the vial stopper top.

**Incompatibilities**
Eptifibatide should not be administered in the same intravenous line as furosemide.
Eptifibatide may be administered in the same intravenous line as alteplase, atropine, dobutamine, heparin, lidocaine, meperidine, metoprolol, midazolam, morphine, nitroglycerin, or verapamil.
Eptifibatide may be administered in the same intravenous line as 0.9% sodium chloride injection or 0.9% sodium chloride in 5% dextrose injection. Either infusion solution may contain potassium chloride up to 60 millequivalents (mEq) per liter.
No incompatibilities have been observed with intravenous infusion sets, and no compatability studies have been performed with polyvinyl chloride (PVC) bags.

**Auxiliary labeling**
When dispensed, the 10-mL bolus vial should carry a label indicating that it is "FOR INTRAVENOUS BOLUS USE ONLY." When dispensed, the 100-mL infusion vial should carry a label indicating that it is "FOR CONTINUOUS INTRAVENOUS INFUSION."

**Caution**
*It is very important to use only the 100-mL infusion vial for administration by continuous intravenous infusion.*

Developed: 08/12/98
Interim revision: 08/21/98

---

**ERGOCALCIFEROL**—See *Vitamin D and Analogs (Systemic)*

---

# ERGOLOID MESYLATES  Systemic

VA CLASSIFICATION (Primary): CN900
Commonly used brand name(s): *Gerimal; Hydergine; Hydergine LC.*
Another commonly used name is dihydrogenated ergot alkaloids.
Note: For a listing of dosage forms and brand names by country availability, see *Dosage Forms* section(s).

## Category
Dementia symptoms treatment adjunct.

## Indications

**Accepted**
Dementia, early (treatment adjunct)—Ergoloid mesylates has been used to treat symptoms of an idiopathic decline in mental capacity (such as cognitive and interpersonal skills, mood, self-care, and apparent motivation) related to aging or to an underlying dementing condition such as primary progressive dementia, Alzheimer's dementia, or senile-onset multi-infarct dementia. Careful diagnosis is recommended prior to use to rule out other causes of the presenting symptoms.

The role of this medication in the therapy of dementia is controversial. A recent controlled study in patients with Alzheimer's disease found no advantage to the use of ergoloid mesylates as compared to placebo, and suggested that ergoloid mesylates may worsen scores on certain cognitive and behavioral rating scales. More study is needed to determine the risk-benefit profile of ergoloid mesylates in the treatment of dementia.

## Pharmacology/Pharmacokinetics

**Physicochemical characteristics**
Molecular weight—
Dihydroergocornine mesylate: 659.80.
Dihydroergocristine mesylate: 707.84.
Dihydro-alpha-ergocryptine mesylate: 673.82.
Dihydro-beta-ergocryptine mesylate: 673.82.

**Mechanism of action/Effect**
Not established with regard to indications. Ergoloid mesylates acts centrally to decrease vascular tone and slow the heart rate, and acts peripherally to block alpha-receptors. Another possible mechanism is the effect of ergoloid mesylates on neuronal cell metabolism, possibly resulting in improved oxygen uptake and improved cerebral metabolism, which in turn may normalize depressed neurotransmitter levels.

**Absorption**
Ergoloid mesylates is rapidly but incompletely (approximately 25%) absorbed from the gastrointestinal tract. Approximately 50% of an absorbed dose is removed by first-pass metabolism.

**Biotransformation**
Hepatic.

**Half-life**
2 to 5 hours.

**Onset of action**
Clinical improvement may not be apparent for 3 to 4 weeks or longer.

**Time to peak plasma concentration**
1 to 2 hours.

## Precautions to Consider

**Medical considerations/Contraindications**
The medical considerations/contraindications included have been selected on the basis of their potential clinical significance (reasons given in parentheses where appropriate)—not necessarily inclusive (» = major clinical significance).

*Risk-benefit should be considered when the following medical problems exist:*
» Bradycardia or
» Hypotension
(may be exacerbated)
Hepatic function impairment
(impaired elimination and possible toxicity)
» Psychosis, acute or chronic
(bradycardia reported; dopamine agonist activity may aggravate existing psychosis)
Sensitivity to ergoloid mesylates or other ergot alkaloids

**Patient monitoring**
The following may be especially important in patient monitoring (other tests may be warranted in some patients, depending on condition; » = major clinical significance):

Blood pressure and
Pulse count
(determinations recommended prior to initiation of therapy and at periodic intervals during therapy)

## Side/Adverse Effects

Note: At recommended dosage, side effects usually are rare. Incidence and severity of side effects tend to be related to dose and duration of treatment and are usually reversible after therapy is discontinued.

Ergot alkaloids have been reported to precipitate attacks of acute intermittent porphyria in susceptible patients.

The following side/adverse effects have been selected on the basis of their potential clinical significance (possible signs and symptoms in parentheses where appropriate)—not necessarily inclusive:

**Those indicating need for medical attention**
Incidence less frequent or rare
*Bradycardia* (drowsiness; slow heartbeat); *orthostatic hypotension* (dizziness or lightheadedness when getting up from a lying or sitting position); *skin rash*

**Those indicating need for medical attention only if they continue or are bothersome**
Incidence less frequent or rare
*Soreness under tongue*—with sublingual use
Incidence dose-related—possible symptoms of overdose
*Blurred vision; dizziness; fainting; flushing; headache; loss of appetite; nausea or vomiting; stomach cramps; stuffy nose*

## Patient Consultation

As an aid to patient consultation, refer to *Advice for the Patient, Ergoloid Mesylates (Systemic)*.

In providing consultation, consider emphasizing the following selected information (» = major clinical significance):

**Before using this medication**
» Conditions affecting use, especially:
Sensitivity to ergoloid mesylates
Other medical problems, especially bradycardia, hypotension, or acute or chronic psychosis

**Proper use of this medication**
» Importance of not using more or less medication than the amount prescribed
Proper administration of sublingual tablet: Dissolving tablet under tongue; not eating, drinking or smoking while tablet is dissolving
» Proper dosing
Missed dose: Not taking missed dose; not doubling doses; checking with physician if two or more doses in a row are missed
» Proper storage

**Precautions while using this medication**
Importance of regular monitoring by physician
» May require several weeks before clinical response is noted; checking with physician before discontinuing medication

**Side/adverse effects**
Signs of potential side effects, especially bradycardia, orthostatic hypotension, and skin rash

## General Dosing Information

Clinical improvement may not be apparent for 3 to 4 weeks or longer. Continued clinical evaluation of the patient during ergoloid mesylates therapy is required to determine whether there is any initial benefit of the medication and if the benefits continue with time.

If marked bradycardia or hypotension occurs, it is recommended that therapy with ergoloid mesylates be permanently withdrawn.

Ergoloid mesylates does not have the vasoconstrictor properties of the natural ergot alkaloids.

## Oral Dosage Forms

### ERGOLOID MESYLATES CAPSULES

**Usual adult dose**
Dementia symptoms treatment adjunct—
Oral, 1 to 2 mg three times a day.

**Strength(s) usually available**
U.S.—
1 mg (Rx) [*Hydergine LC* (methyl paraben; propyl paraben; sorbitol)].
Note: 0.333 mg each of dihydroergocornine mesylate, dihydroergocristine mesylate, and dihydroergocryptine mesylate, per capsule.
Canada—
Not commercially available.

**Packaging and storage**
Store below 30 °C (86 °F), preferably between 15 and 30 °C (59 and 86 °F), unless otherwise specified by manufacturer. Store in a tight container. Protect from light.

### ERGOLOID MESYLATES ORAL SOLUTION USP

**Usual adult dose**
See *Ergoloid Mesylates Capsules*.

**Strength(s) usually available**
U.S.—
1 mg per mL (Rx) [*Hydergine* (alcohol 28.5%; glycerin; propylene glycol; purified water)].
Note: 0.333 mg each of dihydroergocornine mesylate, dihydroergocristine mesylate, and dihydroergocryptine mesylate, per mL.
Canada—
Not commercially available.

**Packaging and storage**
Store below 30 °C (86 °F), preferably between 15 and 30 °C (59 and 86 °F), unless otherwise specified by manufacturer. Store in a tight, light-resistant container. Protect from freezing.

### ERGOLOID MESYLATES TABLETS USP

**Usual adult dose**
See *Ergoloid Mesylates Capsules*.

**Strength(s) usually available**
U.S.—
0.5 mg (Rx) [GENERIC].
1 mg (Rx) [*Gerimal*; *Hydergine* (lactose); GENERIC].
Canada—
1 mg (Rx) [*Hydergine* (scored)].
Note: An equal quantity of dihydroergocornine mesylate, dihydroergocristine mesylate, and dihydroergocryptine mesylate (that is, 0.167 or 0.333 mg of each) per tablet.

**Packaging and storage**
Store below 40 °C (104 °F), preferably between 15 and 30 °C (59 and 86 °F), unless otherwise specified by manufacturer. Store in a tight, light-resistant container.

## Sublingual Dosage Forms

### ERGOLOID MESYLATES TABLETS (SUBLINGUAL) USP

**Usual adult dose**
Dementia symptoms treatment adjunct—
Sublingual, 1 to 2 mg three times a day.

**Strength(s) usually available**
U.S.—
0.5 mg (Rx) [*Gerimal*; *Hydergine* (sucrose); GENERIC].
1 mg (Rx) [*Gerimal*; *Hydergine* (sucrose); GENERIC].
Note: An equal quantity of dihydroergocornine mesylate, dihydroergocristine mesylate, and dihydroergocryptine mesylate (that is 0.167 or 0.333 mg of each) per tablet.
Canada—
Not commercially available.

**Packaging and storage**
Store below 40 °C (104 °F), preferably between 15 and 30 °C (59 and 86 °F), unless otherwise specified by manufacturer. Store in a tight, light-resistant container.

**Auxiliary labeling**
• Dissolve under the tongue.
• Do not swallow tablets whole.

Revised: 04/16/93

**1360 Ergonovine (Systemic)**

# ERGONOVINE  Systemic

INN: Ergometrine
VA CLASSIFICATION (Primary/Secondary): GU600/GU900; DX900
Commonly used brand name(s): *Ergotrate; Ergotrate Maleate.*
Another commonly used name is ergometrine.
Note: For a listing of dosage forms and brand names by country availability, see *Dosage Forms* section(s).

## Category
Uterine stimulant; diagnostic aid (coronary vasospasm).

## Indications
Note: Bracketed information in the *Indications* section refers to uses that are not included in U.S. product labeling.

### Accepted
Hemorrhage, postpartum and postabortal (prophylaxis and treatment)—
  Ergonovine is indicated in the prevention or treatment of postpartum or postabortal uterine bleeding due to uterine atony or subinvolution. Its use is not recommended prior to delivery of the placenta since placental entrapment may occur.

[Abortion, incomplete (treatment)][1]—In cases of incomplete abortion, ergonovine may be used to hasten expulsion of uterine contents.

[Angina pectoris (diagnosis)][1]—Ergonovine is used as an aid in the diagnosis of variant angina pectoris. Use of ergonovine for this indication should only be undertaken by cardiologists experienced in this use. Careful monitoring is required, as myocardial infarction and death have been reported with the use of ergonovine during this procedure.

### Unaccepted
Ergonovine is not as effective in treatment of migraine as other ergot alkaloids and, therefore, its use for this indication is not recommended.

Ergonovine is not indicated for induction or augmentation of labor, to induce abortion, or in cases of threatened spontaneous abortion because of its propensity to produce nonphysiologic, tetanic contractions and its long duration of action.

Ergonovine has been used in the diagnosis of esophageal spasm. However, its use for this procedure is not generally recommended.

[1]Not included in Canadian product labeling.

## Pharmacology/Pharmacokinetics
### Physicochemical characteristics
Chemical group—Amine ergot alkaloid.
Molecular weight—441.48.

### Mechanism of action/Effect
Uterine stimulant—
  Ergonovine directly stimulates the uterine muscle to increase force and frequency of contractions. With usual doses, these contractions precede periods of relaxation; with larger doses, basal uterine tone is elevated and these relaxation periods will be decreased. Contraction of the uterine wall around bleeding vessels at the placental site produces hemostasis. Ergonovine also induces cervical contractions. The sensitivity of the uterus to the oxytocic effect is much greater toward the end of pregnancy. The oxytocic actions of ergonovine are greater than its vascular effects.
Vasoconstriction—
  Ergonovine, like other ergot alkaloids, produces arterial vasoconstriction by stimulation of alpha-adrenergic and serotonin receptors and inhibition of endothelial-derived relaxation factor release. It is a less potent vasoconstrictor than ergotamine.
Diagnostic aid (coronary vasospasm)—
  Ergonovine causes vasoconstriction of coronary arteries.

### Other actions/effects
Ergonovine has minor actions on the central nervous system (CNS). In the CNS, ergonovine is a partial agonist and partial antagonist at some serotonin and dopamine receptors. Ergonovine also possesses weak dopaminergic antagonist actions in certain blood vessels and partial agonist actions at serotonin receptors in umbilical and placental blood vessels. It does not possess significant alpha-adrenergic blocking activity.

### Absorption
Absorption is rapid and complete after oral or intramuscular administration.

### Biotransformation
Hepatic.

### Onset of action
Contraction of uterus, postpartum:
  Oral: 6 to 15 minutes.
  Intramuscular: 2 to 3 minutes.
  Intravenous: One minute or less.

### Time to peak concentration
60 to 90 minutes (plasma), after oral dosing.

### Duration of action
Contraction of uterus, postpartum—
  Oral: Approximately 3 hours.
  Intramuscular: Approximately 3 hours.
  Intravenous: 45 minutes (although rhythmic contractions may persist for up to 3 hours).

### Elimination
Renal excretion of metabolites.
Note: It is not known if use of forced diuresis, peritoneal dialysis, hemodialysis, or charcoal hemoperfusion will hasten the elimination of ergonovine, especially in overdose.

## Precautions to Consider
### Cross-sensitivity and/or related problems
Patients sensitive to other ergot derivatives may be sensitive to this medication also, although there is some degree of variation among ergot alkaloids in their ability to elicit oxytocic, CNS, or vasoconstrictive effects.

### Pregnancy/Reproduction
Fertility—Ergonovine has been shown to increase fallopian tube motility.

Pregnancy—Use of ergonovine is contraindicated during pregnancy. Tetanic contractions may result in decreased uterine blood flow and fetal distress.

Labor and delivery—High doses of ergonovine administered prior to delivery may cause uterine tetany and problems in the infant (hypoxia, intracranial hemorrhage). Ergonovine should *not* be administered prior to delivery of the placenta. Administration prior to delivery of the placenta may cause captivation of the placenta or missed diagnosis of a second infant, due to excessive uterine contraction.

### Breast-feeding
Problems in humans have not been documented. However, ergot alkaloids are excreted in breast milk. Although inhibition of lactation has not been reported for ergonovine, other ergot alkaloids inhibit lactation. Also, studies have shown that ergonovine interferes with the secretion of prolactin (to a lesser degree than bromocriptine) in the immediate postpartum period. This could result in delayed or diminished lactation with prolonged use.

Ergot alkaloids have the potential to cause chronic ergot poisoning in the infant if used in higher-than-recommended doses or if used for a longer period of time than is generally recommended.

### Pediatrics
Elimination of ergonovine may be prolonged in newborns. Neonates inadvertently administered ergonovine in overdose amounts have developed respiratory depression, cyanosis, seizures, decreased urine output, and severe peripheral vasoconstriction.

### Geriatrics
No information is available on the effects of ergonovine in geriatric patients.

### Drug interactions and/or related problems
The following drug interactions and/or related problems have been selected on the basis of their potential clinical significance (possible mechanism in parentheses where appropriate)—not necessarily inclusive (» = major clinical significance):

Note: Combinations containing any of the following medications, depending on the amount present, may also interact with this medication.

  Anesthetics, general, especially halothane
    (peripheral vasoconstriction may be potentiated by the concurrent use of general anesthetics)

    (concurrent use of halothane in concentrations greater than 1% may interfere with the oxytocic actions of ergonovine, resulting in severe uterine hemorrhage)

  Bromocriptine or
  Ergot alkaloids, other
    (the incidence of rare cases of hypertension, strokes, seizures, and

myocardial infarction associated with the postpartum use of bromocriptine may be increased with the use of ergot alkaloids)

Nicotine or
Smoking, tobacco
(nicotine absorption from heavy smoking may result in enhanced vasoconstriction)

Nitroglycerin or
Antianginal agents, other
(ergot alkaloids may induce coronary vasospasm, lowering the efficacy of nitroglycerin or other antianginal agents; increased doses of nitroglycerin or antianginal agents and/or use of intracoronary nitroglycerin may be necessary)

Vasoconstrictors, other, including those present in some local anesthetics or
Vasopressors
(concurrent use may result in enhanced vasoconstriction; dosage adjustments may be necessary)

(the pressor effect of sympathomimetic pressor amines may be potentiated, resulting in potentially severe hypertension, headache, and rupture of cerebral blood vessels; gangrene developed in a patient receiving both dopamine and ergonovine infusions)

**Laboratory value alterations**

The following have been selected on the basis of their potential clinical significance (possible effect in parentheses where appropriate)—not necessarily inclusive (» = major clinical significance):

With physiology/laboratory test values
Blood pressure or
Central venous pressure
(may be elevated due to peripheral vasoconstriction, primarily of postcapillary vessels; has sometimes been associated with preeclampsia, history of hypertension, intravenous administration of ergonovine, or concurrent use of local anesthetics containing vasoconstrictors; hypotension has also been reported)

Heart rate
(may be decreased due primarily to an increase in vagal tone, and possibly to decreased central sympathetic activity and direct depression of the myocardium)

Prolactin
(serum concentrations may be decreased during the postpartum period)

**Medical considerations/Contraindications**

The medical considerations/contraindications included have been selected on the basis of their potential clinical significance (reasons given in parentheses where appropriate)—not necessarily inclusive (» = major clinical significance).

*Except under special circumstances, this medication should not be used when the following medical problems exist:*

For all indications
» Angina pectoris, unstable or
» Myocardial infarction, recent
(vasospasm caused by ergonovine may precipitate angina or myocardial infarction)
» Cerebrovascular accident, history of or
» Transient ischemic attack, history of
(patients may be susceptible to recurrence due to increases in blood pressure)
» Hypertension, severe, or history of
(may be exacerbated)

For obstetric uses only
» Coronary artery disease
(patients may be more susceptible to angina or myocardial infarction caused by ergonovine-induced vasospasm)
» Eclampsia or
» Preeclampsia
(may be exacerbated; patients may be more likely to develop ergonovine-induced hypertension; headaches, severe cardiac arrhythmias, seizures, and cerebrovascular accidents have occurred)
» Occlusive peripheral vascular disease or
» Raynaud's phenomenon, severe
(may be exacerbated; a patient with Raynaud's phenomenon developed impalpable arterial pulses)

*Risk-benefit should be considered when the following medical problems exist:*

Allergy, hypersensitivity, or intolerance to ergonovine or other ergot alkaloids

» Cardiovascular disease or
» Coronary artery disease (in diagnosis of angina) or
» Mitral valve stenosis or
» Venoatrial shunts
(vasospasm caused by ergonovine may precipitate angina or myocardial infarction)
(in patients with pre-existing coronary artery disease, careful monitoring is critical during the diagnosis of angina because severe chest pain, myocardial ischemia, myocardial infarction, and death may occur more frequently and/or as a result of overdose)
» Hepatic function impairment
(impaired metabolism of ergonovine may result in ergot overdose)
Hypocalcemia
(oxytocic response to ergonovine may be reduced; cautious use of intravenous calcium gluconate may restore oxytocic response to ergonovine)
» Positive response to ergonovine testing, history of or
» Electrocardiograph abnormalities such as ST changes during exercise or episodes of chest pain or prolonged QT interval (atrioventricular block) during chest pain, rest, or activity
(ergonovine should not be used routinely in the diagnosis of variant angina in these patients because prolonged coronary vasoconstriction may precipitate angina, acute myocardial infarction, or heart failure)
» Renal function impairment
» Sepsis
(possible increased sensitivity to the effects of ergonovine)

**Patient monitoring**

The following may be especially important in patient monitoring (other tests may be warranted in some patients, depending on condition; » = major clinical significance):

*For obstetric uses*
Blood pressure determinations and
Pulse rate determinations and
Uterine response
(recommended at frequent intervals after parenteral therapy to monitor for adverse reactions; especially important with intravenous administration)

*For diagnosis of variant angina pectoris*
Blood pressure and
Electrocardiogram (ECG)
(recommended throughout procedure)

## Side/Adverse Effects

Note: Because the duration of therapy with ergonovine is generally short, many of the side effects seen with other ergot alkaloids do not occur.

The following side/adverse effects have been selected on the basis of their potential clinical significance (possible signs and symptoms in parentheses where appropriate)—not necessarily inclusive:

**Those indicating need for medical attention**
Incidence less frequent
*Bradycardia* (slow heartbeat); *coronary vasospasm* (chest pain)
Incidence rare
*Allergic reaction, including shock; cardiac arrest or ventricular arrhythmias, including fibrillation and tachycardia* (irregular heartbeat); *dyspnea* (unexplained shortness of breath); *hypertension, sudden and severe* (sudden, severe headache; blurred vision; seizures); *myocardial infarction* (crushing chest pain; unexplained shortness of breath)—has occurred with the use of ergot preparations in the postpartum period and with the use of ergonovine for the diagnosis of variant angina; *peripheral vasospasm* (itching of skin; pain in arms, legs, or lower back; pale or cold hands or feet; weakness in legs)—dose-related

**Those indicating need for medical attention only if they continue or are bothersome**
Incidence more frequent
*Nausea*—especially after intravenous use; *uterine cramping; vomiting*—especially after intravenous use

Note: *Uterine cramping* will occur to some degree in all patients and is indicative of efficacy. However, dosage reduction may be required in occasional patients with severe or intolerable uterine cramps.

Incidence less frequent
*Abdominal or stomach pain; diarrhea; dizziness; headache, mild and transient; nasal congestion; sweating; tinnitus* (ringing in the ears); *unpleasant taste*

## Overdose

For specific information on the agents used in the management of ergonovine overdose, see:
- *Charcoal, Activated (Oral-Local)* monograph;
- *Chlorpromazine* in *Phenothiazines (Systemic)* monograph;
- *Diazepam* in *Benzodiazepines (Systemic)* monograph;
- *Hydralazine (Systemic)* monograph;
- *Laxatives (Local)* monograph;
- *Nitroglycerin* in *Nitrates (Systemic)* monograph;
- *Nitroprusside (Systemic)* monograph;
- *Phentolamine (Systemic)* monograph;
- *Phenytoin* in *Anticonvulsants, Hydantoin (Systemic)* monograph; and/or
- *Tolazoline (Parenteral-Systemic)* monograph.

For more information on the management of overdose or unintentional ingestion, **contact a Poison Control Center** (see *Poison Control Center Listing*).

### Clinical effects of overdose

The following effects have been selected on the basis of their potential clinical significance (possible signs and symptoms in parentheses where appropriate)—not necessarily inclusive:

Acute
 *Angina* (chest pain); *bradycardia* (slow heartbeat); *confusion; drowsiness; fast, weak pulse; miosis* (small pupils); *peripheral vasoconstriction, severe* (cool, pale, or numb arms or legs; muscle pain; weak or absent arterial pulse in arms or legs; tingling, itching, and cool skin); *respiratory depression* (decreased breathing rate or trouble in breathing; bluish color of skin or inside of nose or mouth); *seizures; tachycardia* (fast heartbeat); *unconsciousness; unusual thirst; uterine tetany* (severe cramping of the uterus)

Chronic
 *Formication* (false feeling of insects crawling on the skin); *gangrene* (dry, shriveled appearance of skin on hands, lower legs, or feet); *hemiplegia* (paralysis of one side of the body); *thrombophlebitis* (pain and redness in an arm or leg)

 Note: *Chronic overdose symptoms* are unlikely with proper use since treatment is of short duration.

### Treatment of overdose

Immediate discontinuation of ergonovine. Since there is no specific antidote for the management of ergonovine overdose, treatment is primarily supportive and symptomatic and may include the following:

To decrease absorption—Gastrointestinal decontamination for oral overdose, preferably with multiple doses of activated charcoal and an appropriate cathartic. Gastric lavage may also be considered. It is not known if use of forced diuresis, peritoneal dialysis, hemodialysis, or charcoal hemoperfusion will hasten the elimination of ergonovine, especially in overdose.

Specific treatment—

Use of nitroglycerin for treatment of myocardial ischemia. Intracoronary nitroglycerin may be necessary.

Use of diazepam or phenytoin for treatment of seizures.

Use of sodium nitroprusside, tolazoline, or phentolamine for treatment of peripheral ischemia.

Use of sodium nitroprusside, chlorpromazine 15 mg, or hydralazine for treatment of severe hypertension.

Monitoring—Frequent monitoring of vital signs, arterial blood gases, and electrolytes. Monitoring of serum ergonovine levels is not predictive of the outcome of overdose. Electrocardiogram monitoring to assess cardiac function and perfusion.

Supportive care—May include maintaining an open airway and breathing, maintaining proper fluid and electrolyte balance, correcting hypertension, and controlling seizures. Patients in whom intentional overdose is known or suspected should be referred for psychiatric consultation.

## Patient Consultation

As an aid to patient consultation, refer to *Advice for the Patient, Ergonovine/Methylergonovine (Systemic)*.

In providing consultation, consider emphasizing the following selected information (» = major clinical significance):

### Before using this medication
» Conditions affecting use, especially:
   Allergies, hypersensitivity, or intolerance to ergonovine or other ergot alkaloids
   Pregnancy—Should not be administered prior to delivery or delivery of the placenta
   Breast-feeding—Ergot alkaloids are excreted in breast milk

Other medical problems, especially cardiac or vascular disease, hepatic function impairment, severe hypertension or history of hypertension, renal function impairment, and sepsis

### Proper use of this medication
» Importance of not using more medication or for longer than prescribed; risk of ergotism and gangrene with prolonged use
» Proper dosing
   Missed dose: Not taking at all; not doubling doses
» Proper storage

### Precautions while using this medication
Notifying physician if infection develops, since infection may cause increased sensitivity to medication

### Side/adverse effects
Signs of potential side effects, especially allergic reaction, coronary vasospasm or other cardiovascular complications, dyspnea, severe hypertension, or peripheral vasospasm

## General Dosing Information

Antiemetic medications such as prochlorperazine may be administered prior to use of ergonovine.

### For parenteral dosage forms only

Because the risk of severe adverse effects is increased with intravenous use of ergonovine, its use is recommended only for emergencies such as excessive uterine bleeding.

If intravenous use is warranted, administration must be done slowly, over a period of at least 1 minute. Some clinicians recommend dilution of the solution before administration.

In some patients who do not respond to ergonovine because of hypocalcemia, cautious intravenous administration of calcium gluconate (provided the patient is not receiving digitalis) may restore the oxytocic action.

## Oral Dosage Forms

### ERGONOVINE MALEATE TABLETS USP

**Usual adult and adolescent dose**
Uterine stimulant—
 Oral or sublingual, 200 to 400 mcg (0.2 to 0.4 mg) two to four times a day (every six to twelve hours) until the danger of uterine atony and hemorrhage has passed.

Note: Generally, a treatment course of 48 hours is sufficient. Oral or sublingual administration usually follows an initial parenteral dose.

**Strength(s) usually available**
U.S.—
 200 mcg (0.2 mg) (Rx) [*Ergotrate*].
Canada—
 200 mcg (0.2 mg) (Rx) [*Ergotrate Maleate*].

**Packaging and storage**
Store below 40 °C (104 °F), preferably between 15 and 30 °C (59 and 86 °F), unless otherwise specified by manufacturer. Store in a well-closed container.

## Parenteral Dosage Forms

Note: Bracketed uses in the *Dosage Forms* section refer to categories of use and/or indications that are not included in U.S. product labeling.

### ERGONOVINE MALEATE INJECTION USP

**Usual adult and adolescent dose**
Uterine stimulant—
 Intravenous, administered over at least one minute, or intramuscular, 200 mcg (0.2 mg), repeated in two to four hours if necessary, up to five doses.
[Angina pectoris (diagnosis)][1]—
 Intravenous, 50 mcg (0.05 mg), repeated every five minutes until chest pain occurs or a total dose of 400 mcg (0.4 mg) has been given.

**Strength(s) usually available**
U.S.—
 200 mcg (0.2 mg) per mL (Rx) [*Ergotrate*].
Canada—
 250 mcg (0.25 mg) per mL (Rx) [GENERIC].

**Packaging and storage**
Store below 8 °C (46 °F), preferably between 2 and 8 °C (36 and 46 °F), unless otherwise specified by manufacturer. Protect from light. Protect from freezing.

## Stability

Ergonovine maleate ampules may be stored at room temperature for up to 60 days. At any time, discolored solutions or solutions containing visible particles should not be used.

¹Not included in Canadian product labeling.

Revised: 06/07/93

**ERGOTAMINE**—See *Vascular Headache Suppressants, Ergot Derivative–containing (Systemic)*

# ERGOTAMINE, BELLADONNA ALKALOIDS, AND PHENOBARBITAL Systemic

VA CLASSIFICATION (Primary/Secondary): CN105/AU900

**NOTE:** The *Ergotamine, Belladonna Alkaloids, and Phenobarbital (Systemic)* monograph is maintained on the USP DI electronic data base. For a printed copy of the most recent revision of the complete monograph, contact Micromedex, Inc. - Reprint Requests, 6200 S. Syracuse Way, Suite 300, Englewood, CO 80111; telephone (303) 486-6400; telefax (303) 486-6464; Email: USPDI@MDX.COM.

For information on the specific components of this combination, see the USP DI monographs for *Anticholinergics/Antispasmodics (Systemic), Barbiturates (Systemic),* and *Vascular Headache Suppressants, Ergot Derivative-containing (Systemic).*

The information that follows is selectively abstracted from the complete monograph and is provided to facilitate drug use review and patient counseling.

Note: For a listing of dosage forms and brand names by country availability, see *Dosage Forms* section(s).

## Category

Vascular headache prophylactic; menopausal symptoms suppressant.

## Indications

**Accepted**

Headache, vascular (prophylaxis)—Ergotamine, belladonna alkaloids, and phenobarbital combination is used in the prevention of vascular (migraine or cluster) headaches.

Menopausal symptoms (treatment)—Ergotamine, belladonna alkaloids, and phenobarbital combination is indicated to ameliorate symptoms such as hot flushes, sweating, restlessness, and insomnia in menopausal women. It is usually used for women who are unable to take estrogens. However, unlike estrogen replacement therapy, the ergotamine, belladonna, and phenobarbital combination does not protect against postmenopausal osteoporosis.

The ergotamine, belladonna alkaloids, and phenobarbital combination has also been used for its autonomic effects in the treatment of various cardiovascular, gastrointestinal, and genitourinary disorders. However, it generally *has been replaced* by more specific agents for these uses.

## Patient Consultation

As an aid to patient consultation, refer to *Advice for the Patient, Ergotamine, Belladonna Alkaloids, and Phenobarbital (Systemic).*

In providing consultation, consider emphasizing the following selected information (» = major clinical significance):

**Before using this medication**
» Conditions affecting use, especially:
   Allergies to ergotamine, belladonna alkaloids, or barbiturates
   Pregnancy—Use is not recommended because of ergotamine's oxytocic activity; also, belladonna alkaloids and barbiturates cross placenta; phenobarbital may cause fetal abnormalities and neonatal hemorrhage
   Breast-feeding—Ergot alkaloids inhibit lactation; also, they are distributed into breast milk and may cause ergotism in the infant; belladonna alkaloids may also inhibit lactation; phenobarbital is distributed into breast milk and may cause CNS depression in the infant
   Use in children—Increased susceptibility to toxic effects of belladonna alkaloids; increased response to belladonna alkaloids in children with spastic paralysis or brain damage; also, risk of paradoxical phenobarbital-induced excitement in hypersensitive children
   Use in the elderly—Increased risk of hypothermia and other adverse effects associated with peripheral vasoconstriction; also, increased susceptibility to mental and other toxic effects of anticholinergics and barbiturates; danger of precipitating undiagnosed glaucoma; possible memory impairment
   Other medications, especially other anticholinergics, antacids, anticoagulants, antidiarrheals, carbamazepine, CNS depressants, corticosteroids or corticotropin, estrogen- and progestin-containing oral contraceptives, other ergot alkaloids, ketoconazole, monoamine oxidase (MAO) inhibitors, potassium chloride, and other vasoconstrictors (including those present in local anesthetic solutions)
   Other medical problems, especially angina pectoris, coronary artery disease, gastrointestinal obstructive disease, glaucoma, hepatic function impairment, hypertension, severe infection, peripheral vascular disease, pruritus, renal function impairment, urinary retention, and recent or contemplated angioplasty or vascular surgery

**Proper use of this medication**
» Importance of not using more medication than the amount prescribed; risk of ergotism with overdosage; habit-forming potential
   Proper administration of extended-release tablets: Swallowing whole without crushing, breaking, or chewing
» Proper dosing
   Missed dose: Not taking missed dose at all; not doubling doses
» Proper storage

**Precautions while using this medication**
» Checking with physician before discontinuing medication after prolonged use; gradual dosage reduction may be necessary to avoid the possibility of withdrawal symptoms
   Avoiding antacids and antidiarrheal medication within 1 hour of taking this medication
» Avoiding use of alcohol or other central nervous system (CNS) depressants; alcohol also aggravates headache
» Caution when driving or doing jobs requiring alertness because of possible dizziness, lightheadedness, or drowsiness
   Avoiding smoking, since nicotine constricts blood vessels
   Avoiding exposure to excessive cold, which may aggravate peripheral vasoconstriction
» Caution during exercise and hot weather; overheating may result in heat stroke
   Possible increased sensitivity of eyes to light
   Notifying physician if infection develops, since infection may cause increased sensitivity to medication
   Possible dryness of mouth, nose, and throat; using sugarless candy or gum, ice or saliva substitute for relief; checking with physician or dentist if dry mouth continues for more than 2 weeks

**Side/adverse effects**
Signs and symptoms of potential side effects, especially agranulocytosis, allergic reactions, edema, fast or slow heartbeat, gangrene, hepatitis, increased intraocular pressure, cerebral or peripheral ischemia, thrombocytopenia, and coronary or ocular vasospasm

## Oral Dosage Forms

### ERGOTAMINE TARTRATE, BELLADONNA ALKALOIDS, AND PHENOBARBITAL SODIUM TABLETS

**Usual adult dose**
Vascular headache prophylactic and
Menopausal symptoms suppressant—
   Oral, 1 tablet in the morning and at noon and 2 tablets at bedtime. In more resistant cases, therapy may begin with 6 tablets per day, the dosage being gradually reduced at weekly intervals to the lowest effective dose.

Note: Geriatric and debilitated patients may react to usual doses of barbiturates with excitement, confusion, or mental depression. Lower doses may be required in these patients.

**Usual adult prescribing limits**
Not to exceed 33 tablets per week.

**Usual pediatric dose**
Safety and efficacy have not been established.

**Strength(s) usually available**
U.S.—
  Not commercially available.
Canada—
  300 mcg (0.3 mg) of ergotamine tartrate, 100 mcg (0.1 mg) of belladonna alkaloids, and 20 mg of phenobarbital (Rx) [*Bellergal* (lactose; tartrazine)].

**Auxiliary labeling**
- May cause drowsiness.
- Avoid alcoholic beverages.

## ERGOTAMINE TARTRATE, BELLADONNA ALKALOIDS, AND PHENOBARBITAL SODIUM EXTENDED-RELEASE TABLETS

**Usual adult dose**
Vascular headache prophylactic and
Menopausal symptoms suppressant—
  Oral, 1 tablet in the morning and 1 tablet in the evening.

Note: Geriatric and debilitated patients may react to usual doses of barbiturates with excitement, confusion, or mental depression. Lower doses may be required in these patients.

**Usual pediatric dose**
Safety and efficacy have not been established.

**Strength(s) usually available**
U.S.—
  600 mcg (0.6 mg) of ergotamine tartrate, 200 mcg (0.2 mg) of belladonna alkaloids, and 40 mg of phenobarbital (Rx) [*Bellergal-S* (scored; lactose)].
Canada—
  600 mcg (0.6 mg) of ergotamine tartrate, 200 mcg (0.2 mg) of belladonna alkaloids, and 40 mg of phenobarbital (Rx) [*Bellergal Spacetabs* (scored; lactose; tartrazine)].

**Auxiliary labeling**
- May cause drowsiness.
- Avoid alcoholic beverages.
- Swallow whole.

Revised: 08/30/94

## ERYTHRITYL TETRANITRATE—See *Nitrates (Systemic)*

# ERYTHROMYCIN  Ophthalmic

VA CLASSIFICATION (Primary): OP201
Commonly used brand name(s): *Ilotycin*.
Note: For a listing of dosage forms and brand names by country availability, see *Dosage Forms* section(s).

## Category
Antibacterial (ophthalmic).

## Indications
Note: Bracketed information in the *Indications* section refers to uses that are not included in U.S. product labeling.

**Accepted**
Conjunctivitis, neonatal (prophylaxis)—Erythromycin is indicated in the topical prophylaxis of neonatal conjunctivitis caused by *Chlamydia trachomatis*.

Ocular infections (treatment)—Erythromycin is indicated in the topical treatment of superficial ocular infections of the conjunctiva and/or cornea caused by susceptible organisms.

Ophthalmia neonatorum (prophylaxis)—Erythromycin is indicated alone in the prophylaxis of ophthalmia neonatorum caused by *Neisseria gonorrhoeae* or *C. trachomatis*. However, in infants born to mothers who have clinically apparent gonorrhea, ophthalmic erythromycin is indicated concurrently with parenteral aqueous penicillin G.

[Blepharitis, bacterial (treatment)][1]
[Blepharoconjunctivitis (treatment)][1]
[Chlamydial infections (treatment)][1]
[Conjunctivitis, bacterial (treatment)][1]
[Keratitis, bacterial (treatment)][1]
[Keratoconjunctivitis, bacterial (treatment)][1]
[Meibomianitis (treatment)][1] or
[Trachoma (treatment)][1]—Erythromycin is used in the topical treatment of bacterial blepharitis, blepharoconjunctivitis, chlamydial infections, bacterial conjunctivitis, bacterial keratitis, bacterial keratoconjunctivitis, meibomianitis, and trachoma.

Not all species or strains of a particular organism may be susceptible to erythromycin.

[1] Not included in Canadian product labeling.

## Pharmacology/Pharmacokinetics

**Physicochemical characteristics**
Molecular weight—733.94.
Family—Macrolide group of antibiotics.

**Mechanism of action/Effect**
Erythromycin is a bacteriostatic macrolide antibiotic. However, it may be bactericidal in high concentrations or when used against highly susceptible organisms. It is thought to penetrate the bacterial cell membrane and to reversibly bind to the 50 S subunit of bacterial ribosomes or near the "P" or donor site so that binding of tRNA (transfer RNA) to the donor site is blocked. Translocation of peptides from the "A" or acceptor site to the "P" or donor site is prevented, and subsequent protein synthesis is inhibited.
Erythromycin is effective only against actively dividing organisms.

**Absorption**
Topical application of the ophthalmic ointment to the eye may result in absorption into the cornea and aqueous humor.

## Precautions to Consider

**Cross-sensitivity and/or related problems**
Patients intolerant of one erythromycin may be intolerant of other erythromycins also.

**Tumorigenicity**
Two-year studies of rats administered erythromycin orally showed no evidence of tumorigenicity.

**Mutagenicity**
Studies have not been done.

**Pregnancy/Reproduction**
Fertility—Studies of rats, mice, and rabbits given high doses of systemic erythromycin showed no evidence of impaired fertility

Pregnancy—Problems in humans have not been documented.
Studies of rats, mice, and rabbits given high doses of systemic erythromycin showed no evidence of harm to the fetus.

FDA Pregnancy Category B.

**Breast-feeding**
Problems in humans have not been documented.

**Pediatrics**
Appropriate studies on the relationship of age to the effects of this medicine have not been performed in the pediatric population. However, no pediatrics-specific problems have been documented to date.

**Geriatrics**
Appropriate studies on the relationship of age to the effects of this medicine have not been performed in the geriatric population. However, no geriatrics-specific problems have been documented to date.

**Medical considerations/Contraindications**
The medical considerations/contraindications included have been selected on the basis of their potential clinical significance (reasons given in parentheses where appropriate)—not necessarily inclusive (» = major clinical significance).

*Risk-benefit should be considered when the following medical problem exists:*

Intolerance to erythromycin or parabens

## Side/Adverse Effects

The following side/adverse effects have been selected on the basis of their potential clinical significance (possible signs and symptoms in parentheses where appropriate)—not necessarily inclusive:

**Those indicating need for medical attention**
Incidence rare
*Eye irritation not present before therapy*

## Patient Consultation

As an aid to patient consultation, refer to *Advice for the Patient, Erythromycin (Ophthalmic)*.

In providing consultation, consider emphasizing the following selected information (» = major clinical significance):

**Before using this medication**
» Conditions affecting use, especially:
  Allergy to this or any of the other erythromycins

**Proper use of this medication**
Proper administration technique for ophthalmic ointment
» Compliance with full course of therapy
» Proper dosing
  Missed dose: Applying as soon as possible; not applying if almost time for next dose
» Proper storage

**Precautions while using this medication**
Checking with physician if no improvement within a few days
Blurred vision after application of ophthalmic ointments

**Side/adverse effects**
Signs of potential side effects, especially eye irritation not present before therapy

## General Dosing Information

Use of topical antibacterials may lead to skin sensitization, resulting in hypersensitivity reactions with subsequent topical or systemic use of the medication.

In the prophylaxis of ophthalmia neonatorum, erythromycin ophthalmic ointment should not be flushed from the eye following administration. In addition, ophthalmic erythromycin is given concurrently with parenteral aqueous penicillin G in infants born to mothers who have clinically apparent gonorrhea.

## Ophthalmic Dosage Forms

### ERYTHROMYCIN OPHTHALMIC OINTMENT USP

**Usual adult and adolescent dose**
Ocular infections—
  Topical, to the conjunctiva, a thin strip (approximately 1 cm) of ointment up to six times a day, depending on the severity of the infection.

**Usual pediatric dose**
Conjunctivitis, neonatal or
Ophthalmia neonatorum—
  Topical, to each conjunctiva, a thin strip (approximately 0.5 to 1 cm) of ointment as a single dose following cesarean or vaginal delivery.
Ocular infections—
  See *Usual adult and adolescent dose*.

**Strength(s) usually available**
U.S.—
  0.5% (Rx) [*Ilotycin* (methylparaben, propylparaben); GENERIC].
Canada—
  0.5% (Rx) [*Ilotycin;* GENERIC].

**Packaging and storage**
Store below 40 °C (104 °F), preferably between 15 and 30 °C (59 and 86 °F), unless otherwise specified by manufacturer. Protect from freezing.

**Auxiliary labeling**
• For the eye.
• Continue medicine for full time of treatment.

Revised: 11/28/94

---

# ERYTHROMYCIN  Topical

VA CLASSIFICATION (Primary/Secondary): DE752/DE101
Commonly used brand name(s): *A/T/S; A/T/S; Akne-Mycin; ETS; Ery-Sol; EryDerm; Erycette; Erygel; Erymax; Sans-Acne; Staticin; T-Stat*.

Note: For a listing of dosage forms and brand names by country availability, see *Dosage Forms* section(s).

## Category

Antiacne agent (topical)—Erythromycin Ointment; Erythromycin Pledgets; Erythromycin Topical Gel; Erythromycin Topical Solution..
Antibacterial (topical)—Erythromycin Ointment.

## Indications

Note: Bracketed information in the *Indications* section refers to uses that are not included in U.S. product labeling.

**Accepted**
Acne vulgaris (treatment)—Topical erythromycin is indicated in the topical treatment of acne vulgaris. It may be effective in grades II and III acne, which are characterized by inflammatory lesions such as papules and pustules. Topical antibacterials are not generally considered to be as effective as systemic antibacterials in the treatment of acne, especially more severe inflammatory acne.
[Skin infections, bacterial, minor (prophylaxis)][1] or
[Skin infections, bacterial, minor (treatment)][1]—Erythromycin ointment is used in the topical prophylaxis and treatment of superficial pyogenic infections of the skin.

**Unaccepted**
Topical erythromycin is not effective in deep cystic lesions or in noninflammatory lesions.

[1]Not included in Canadian product labeling.

## Pharmacology/Pharmacokinetics

**Physicochemical characteristics**
Molecular weight—733.94.

**Mechanism of action/Effect**
Antiacne agent (topical)—Probably due to its antibacterial activity. Topical erythromycin is thought to suppress the growth of *Propionibacterium acnes (Corynebacterium acnes)*, an anaerobe found in sebaceous glands and follicles. *P. acnes* produces proteases, hyaluronidases, lipases, and chemotactic factors, all of which can produce inflammatory components or inflammation directly.

## Precautions to Consider

**Cross-sensitivity and/or related problems**
Patients sensitive to one erythromycin may be sensitive to other erythromycins also.

**Carcinogenicity**
*For erythromycin pledgets; erythromycin topical gel; erythromycin topical solution—*
  Long-term studies in animals have not been done to evaluate carcinogenicity.

**Mutagenicity**
*For erythromycin pledgets; erythromycin topical gel—*
  Long-term studies in animals have not been done to evaluate mutagenicity.
*For erythromycin topical solution—*
  Erythromycin topical solution has not been shown to be mutagenic in the Ames Salmonella/Microsome Plate Test.

**Pregnancy/Reproduction**
Pregnancy—
  *For erythromycin pledgets*:
    Fertility; pregnancy—
      Studies have not been done in humans or animals.
      FDA Pregnancy Category C.
  *For erythromycin topical gel; erythromycin topical solution*:
    Fertility; pregnancy—
      Erythromycin crosses the placenta, although fetal serum concentrations are generally low. Adequate and well-controlled studies in humans have not been done.
      Studies in rats, fed erythromycin base in amounts up to 0.25% of their diet prior to and during mating, during gestation, and through weaning, have not shown that erythromycin

causes adverse effects on the fetus. In addition, studies in rats and rabbits, given 1.5, 4, and 13 times the estimated human dose, have not shown that erythromycin causes impaired fertility or adverse effects on the fetus.
FDA Pregnancy Category B.

**Breast-feeding**
For erythromycin pledgets; erythromycin topical gel—
It is not known whether erythromycin, applied topically, is distributed into breast milk. Erythromycin, given systemically, is distributed into breast milk. However, problems in humans have not been documented.

**Pediatrics**
For erythromycin topical gel—
Appropriate studies on the relationship of age to the effects of this medicine have not been performed in the pediatric population.
For erythromycin topical solution—
Appropriate studies on the relationship of age to the effects of this medicine have not been performed in children up to 12 years of age.

**Geriatrics**
Appropriate studies on the relationship of age to the effects of this medicine have not been performed in the geriatric population. However, geriatrics-specific problems that would limit the usefulness of this medication in the elderly are not expected.

**Drug interactions and/or related problems**
The following drug interactions and/or related problems have been selected on the basis of their potential clinical significance (possible mechanism in parentheses where appropriate)—not necessarily inclusive (» = major clinical significance):

Note: Combinations containing any of the following medications, depending on the amount present, may also interact with this medication.

Abrasive or medicated soaps or cleansers or
Acne preparations or preparations containing a peeling agent, such as:
Benzoyl peroxide
Resorcinol
Salicylic acid
Sulfur
Tretinoin or
Alcohol-containing preparations, topical, such as:
After-shave lotions
Astringents
Perfumed toiletries
Shaving creams or lotions or
Cosmetics or soaps with a strong drying effect or
Isotretinoin or
Medicated cosmetics or "cover-ups"
(concurrent use with erythromycin pledgets, topical gel, or topical solution may cause a cumulative irritant or drying effect, especially with the application of peeling, desquamating, or abrasive agents, resulting in excessive irritation of the skin)

**Medical considerations/Contraindications**
The medical considerations/contraindications included have been selected on the basis of their potential clinical significance (reasons given in parentheses where appropriate)—not necessarily inclusive (» = major clinical significance).

*Risk-benefit should be considered when the following medical problem exists:*
Sensitivity to erythromycin

## Side/Adverse Effects
The following side/adverse effects have been selected on the basis of their potential clinical significance (possible signs and symptoms in parentheses where appropriate)—not necessarily inclusive:

**Those indicating need for medical attention only if they continue or are bothersome**
For ointment
*Incidence less frequent*
**Peeling; redness**
For pledgets, topical gel, and topical solution
*Incidence more frequent*
**Dry or scaly skin; irritation; itching; stinging or burning feeling**
*Incidence less frequent*
**Peeling; redness**

## Patient Consultation
As an aid to patient consultation, refer to *Advice for the Patient, Erythromycin (Topical)*.
In providing consultation, consider emphasizing the following selected information (» = major clinical significance):

**Before using this medication**
» Conditions affecting use, especially:
Sensitivity to erythromycins
Pregnancy—Erythromycin crosses the placenta
Breast-feeding—Erythromycin enters breast-milk

**Proper use of this medication**
Proper administration technique
» Compliance with full course of therapy, which may take months or longer
» Proper dosing
Missed dose: Applying as soon as possible; not applying if almost time for next dose
» Proper storage
For pledgets, topical gel, and topical solution
» Not using near heat or open flame or while smoking
Not using medication more often than prescribed
Avoiding too frequent washing of affected areas
» Importance of applying medication to entire affected area
» Not using in eyes, nose, mouth, or on other mucous membranes

**Precautions while using this medication**
Checking with physician if no improvement in acne within 3 to 4 weeks; may take up to 8 to 12 weeks before full therapeutic benefit is seen
For pledgets, topical gel, and topical solution
Waiting at least 1 hour before applying any other topical medication for acne
Possibility of stinging or burning after application
Checking with physician if treated skin becomes excessively dry
Proper use of cosmetics

## General Dosing Information

**For topical solution dosage form**
If the treated area(s) become uncomfortable because of excessive dryness or irritation, the dosage of erythromycin topical solution may be reduced to once a day or less often until the symptoms have subsided.

In the treatment of acne with erythromycin topical solution, noticeable improvement may be seen in 3 to 4 weeks. However, 8 to 12 weeks of treatment may be required before maximum benefit is seen.

## Topical Dosage Forms

### ERYTHROMYCIN OINTMENT USP
Note: The composition of *Akne-Mycin* available in the U.S. is different from that of *Akne-Mycin* available in Europe.

**Usual adult and adolescent dose**
Acne vulgaris—
Topical, to the skin, two times a day, morning and evening.

**Usual pediatric dose**
See *Usual adult and adolescent dose*.

**Strength(s) usually available**
U.S.—
2% (Rx) [*Akne-Mycin*].
Canada—
Not commercially available.

**Packaging and storage**
Store preferably between 15 and 30 °C (59 and 86 °F). Store in a collapsible tube or in another tight container. Protect from freezing.

**Auxiliary labeling**
• For external use only.
• Continue medication for full time of treatment.

### ERYTHROMYCIN PLEDGETS USP

**Usual adult and adolescent dose**
Acne vulgaris—
Topical, to the skin, two times a day.

**Usual pediatric dose**
See *Usual adult and adolescent dose*.

**Strength(s) usually available**
U.S.—
2% (Rx) [*Erycette* (alcohol 66%; propylene glycol); *T-Stat* (alcohol 71.2%; propylene glycol)].

Canada—
  Not commercially available.
Note: Supplied as foil-covered pledgets (swabs) saturated with 2% erythromycin topical solution.

**Packaging and storage**
Store below 40 °C (104 °F), preferably between 15 and 30 °C (59 and 86 °F), unless otherwise specified by manufacturer. Store in a tight container.

**Auxiliary labeling**
- For external use only.
- Continue medication for full time of treatment.
- Flammable—Keep from heat and flame.

## ERYTHROMYCIN TOPICAL GEL

**Usual adult and adolescent dose**
See *Erythromycin Ointment USP*.

**Usual pediatric dose**
Dosage has not been established.

**Strength(s) usually available**
U.S.—
  2% (Rx) [*A/T/S* (alcohol 92%); *Erygel* (alcohol 92%)].
Canada—
  Not commercially available.

**Packaging and storage**
Store below 40 °C (104 °F), preferably between 15 and 30 °C (59 and 86 °F), unless otherwise specified by manufacturer. Protect from freezing.

**Auxiliary labeling**
- For external use only.
- Continue medication for full time of treatment.
- Flammable—Keep from heat and flame.

## ERYTHROMYCIN TOPICAL SOLUTION USP

**Usual adult and adolescent dose**
See *Erythromycin Ointment USP*.

**Usual pediatric dose**
Infants and children up to 12 years of age—Dosage has not been established.
Children 12 years of age and over—See *Usual adult and adolescent dose*.

**Strength(s) usually available**
U.S.—
  1.5% (Rx) [*Staticin* (alcohol 55%; propylene glycol); GENERIC].
  2% (Rx) [*Akne-Mycin* (alcohol 66%; propylene glycol); *A/T/S* (alcohol 66%; propylene glycol); *EryDerm* (alcohol 77%; propylene glycol); *Erymax* (alcohol 66%; propylene glycol); *Ery-Sol*; *ETS* (alcohol 66%; propylene glycol); *T-Stat* (alcohol 71.2%; propylene glycol); GENERIC].
Canada—
  1.5% (Rx) [*Staticin* ( alcohol 55%)].
  2% (Rx) [*Sans-Acne* ( alcohol 44%)].

**Packaging and storage**
Store below 40 °C (104 °F), preferably between 15 and 30 °C (59 and 86 °F), unless otherwise specified by manufacturer. Store in a tight container.

**Auxiliary labeling**
- For external use only.
- Continue medication for full time of treatment.
- Keep container tightly closed.
- Flammable—Keep from heat and flame.

**Note**
Explain administration technique.

Revised: 06/23/92
Interim revision: 07/06/94

---

**ERYTHROMYCIN BASE**—See *Erythromycin (Ophthalmic)*; *Erythromycins (Systemic)*; *Erythromycin (Topical)*

---

# ERYTHROMYCIN AND BENZOYL PEROXIDE Topical

VA CLASSIFICATION (Primary): DE752

**NOTE:** The *Erythromycin and Benzoyl Peroxide (Topical)* monograph is maintained on the USP DI electronic data base. For a printed copy of the most recent revision of the complete monograph, contact Micromedex, Inc. - Reprint Requests, 6200 S. Syracuse Way, Suite 300, Englewood, CO 80111; telephone (303) 486-6400; telefax (303) 486-6464; Email: USPDI@MDX.COM.

For information on the specific components of this combination, see the *USP DI* monographs for *Benzoyl Peroxide (Topical)* and *Erythromycin (Topical)*.

The information that follows is selectively abstracted from the complete monograph and is provided to facilitate drug use review and patient counseling.

Note: For a listing of dosage forms and brand names by country availability, see *Dosage Forms* section(s).

## Category
Antiacne agent (topical).

## Indications
Note: Bracketed information in the *Indications* section refers to uses that are not included in U.S. product labeling.

**Accepted**
Acne vulgaris (treatment)—Erythromycin and benzoyl peroxide combination is indicated [as a primary agent] in the topical treatment of acne vulgaris. [It may be effective in grades II and III acne, which are characterized by inflammatory lesions such as papules and pustules.]

[Topical antibacterials are not generally considered to be as effective as systemic antibacterials in the treatment of acne, especially more severe inflammatory acne.]

**Unaccepted**
Topical erythromycin-containing preparations are not as effective in deep cystic lesions or in noninflammatory lesions.

## Patient Consultation
As an aid to patient consultation, refer to *Advice for the Patient, Erythromycin and Benzoyl Peroxide (Topical)*.
In providing consultation, consider emphasizing the following selected information (» = major clinical significance):

**Before using this medication**
» Conditions affecting use, especially:
  Sensitivity to erythromycins

**Proper use of this medication**
» Not applying medication to raw or irritated skin
  Before applying, thoroughly washing affected area(s), rinsing well, and patting dry; after washing or shaving, waiting 30 minutes before applying medication
  Avoiding too frequent washing of affected area(s)
*To use*
» Importance of not using more medication than the amount prescribed
  After washing affected area(s), applying medication with fingertips; however, washing medication off hands afterward
» Importance of applying medication to entire affected area
» Not using in or around eyes, nose, or mouth, or on other mucous membranes
  Not using medication after expiration date
» Compliance with full course of therapy, which may take months or longer
» Proper dosing
  Missed dose: Applying as soon as possible; not applying if almost time for next dose
» Proper storage

**Precautions while using this medication**
Checking with physician if no improvement in acne within 3 to 4 weeks; may take up to 8 to 12 weeks before full therapeutic benefit is seen
Waiting at least 1 hour after applying the first medication before applying the second topical medication for acne
Possibility of mild stinging or burning of the skin after application; checking with physician if irritation continues; using medication less frequently
Checking with physician if treated skin becomes excessively dry

» Medication may bleach hair or colored fabrics
  Using only "oil-free" cosmetics to avoid worsening acne

**Side/adverse effects**
Signs of potential side effects, especially allergic contact dermatitis, painful irritation of the skin, or skin rash

## Topical Dosage Forms

### ERYTHROMYCIN AND BENZOYL PEROXIDE TOPICAL GEL USP

**Usual adult and adolescent dose**
Acne vulgaris—
  Topical, to the affected area(s), two times a day, morning and evening; or as directed by physician.

**Usual pediatric dose**
Acne vulgaris—
  Infants and children up to 12 years of age: Dosage has not been established.
  Children 12 years of age and over: See *Usual adult and adolescent dose*.

**When reconstituted and mixed according to manufacturer's instructions**
U.S.—
  3% of erythromycin and 5% of benzoyl peroxide (Rx) [*Benzamycin* (alcohol 22%; fragrance)].
Note: Erythromycin and benzoyl peroxide topical gel is supplied in a package containing 20 grams of benzoyl peroxide gel and a plastic vial containing 800 mg of active erythromycin powder. After reconstitution and mixing, the combined weight is 23.3 grams.
Canada—
  Not commercially available.

**Preparation of dosage form**
Prior to dispensing
  Add 3 mL of ethyl alcohol (to the mark) to the vial containing the erythromycin powder.
  Shake the vial well to dissolve the erythromycin powder.
  Add the erythromycin-containing solution to the benzoyl peroxide gel. Stir the mixture until it is homogeneous in appearance (approximately 1 to 1½ minutes).

**Auxiliary labeling**
- Refrigerate.
- For external use only.
- Keep container tightly closed.
- Continue medication for full time of treatment.
- Beyond-use date.

Revised: 06/26/92
Interim revision: 07/06/94

---

**ERYTHROMYCIN ESTOLATE**—See *Erythromycins (Systemic)*

**ERYTHROMYCIN ETHYLSUCCINATE**—See *Erythromycins (Systemic)*

**ERYTHROMYCIN GLUCEPTATE**—See *Erythromycins (Systemic)*

**ERYTHROMYCIN LACTOBIONATE**—See *Erythromycins (Systemic)*

---

# ERYTHROMYCINS  Systemic

This monograph includes information on the following: 1) Erythromycin Base; 2) Erythromycin Estolate; 3) Erythromycin Ethylsuccinate; 4) Erythromycin Gluceptate; 5) Erythromycin Lactobionate; 6) Erythromycin Stearate

BAN: Erythromycin ethylsuccinate—Erythromycin ethyl succinate
VA CLASSIFICATION (Primary/Secondary):
  Erythromycin Base—AM200/DE751
  Erythromycin Estolate—AM200/DE751
  Erythromycin Ethylsuccinate—AM200/DE751
  Erythromycin Gluceptate—AM200
  Erythromycin Lactobionate—AM200
  Erythromycin Stearate—AM200/DE751

Commonly used brand name(s): *Apo-Erythro*[1]; *Apo-Erythro E-C*[1]; *Apo-Erythro-ES*[3]; *Apo-Erythro-S*[6]; *E-Base*[1]; *E-Mycin*[1]; *E.E.S.*[3]; *ERYC*[1]; *ERYC-250*[1]; *ERYC-333*[1]; *Ery-Tab*[1]; *EryPed*[3]; *Erybid*[1]; *Erythro*[3]; *Erythrocin*[5]; *Erythrocot*[6]; *Erythromid*[1]; *Ilosone*[2]; *Ilotycin*[1]; *My-E*[6]; *Novo-Rythro*[3]; *Novo-rythro*[2]; *Novo-rythro Encap*[1]; *PCE*[1]; *Wintrocin*[6].

Note: For a listing of dosage forms and brand names by country availability, see *Dosage Forms* section(s).

## Category

Antibacterial (systemic)—Erythromycin Base; Erythromycin Estolate; Erythromycin Ethylsuccinate; Erythromycin Gluceptate; Erythromycin Lactobionate; Erythromycin Stearate.
Antiacne agent—Erythromycin Base; Erythromycin Estolate; Erythromycin Ethylsuccinate; Erythromycin Stearate.
Bowel preparation (preoperative) adjunct—Erythromycin Base.

## Indications

Note: Bracketed information in the *Indications* section refers to uses that are not included in U.S. product labeling.

**General considerations**
Erythromycin is a broad-spectrum antibiotic with activity against gram-positive and gram-negative bacteria, and other infectious agents, including *Chlamydia trachomatis*, mycoplasmas (*Mycoplasma pneumoniae* and *Ureaplasma urealyticum*), and spirochetes (*Treponema pallidum* and *Borrelia* species).
Erythromycin has good activity against *Streptococcus pneumoniae*, *S. pyogenes* (group A beta-hemolytic streptococci), and *Staphylococcus aureus*. Resistant strains of both streptococci have been encountered, especially in populations recently exposed to erythromycin. The incidence of resistance to group A streptococci has ranged from 1 to 18% in small studies to up to 60% in a population that had been widely treated with erythromycin for respiratory infections. Most strains of *S. aureus* are currently sensitive to erythromycin. However, the incidence of resistance is increasing. Resistance may develop to erythromycin alone, or may be the result of cross-resistance to other macrolides.
Erythromycin also has good activity against certain gram-negative bacteria, including *Legionella pneumophila*, *Campylobacter jejuni*, and *Bordetella pertussis*, and somewhat lower activity against *Haemophilus influenzae*. There is activity against some gram-negative anaerobes, but most strains of *Bacteroides fragilis* are resistant. Enterobacteriaceae are usually resistant.

**Accepted**
Bowel preparation, preoperative—Enteric-coated erythromycin base is indicated concurrently with oral-local neomycin as part of an adjunctive regimen for the suppression of normal bacterial flora in the preoperative preparation of the bowel.

Bronchitis, bacterial exacerbations (treatment)
Otitis media, acute (treatment) or
Sinusitis (treatment)—Erythromycins are indicated in the treatment of bacterial exacerbations of bronchitis and in the treatment of sinusitis caused by susceptible organisms. Erythromycins are indicated concurrently with sulfonamides in the treatment of acute otitis media caused by susceptible organisms.

Chlamydial infections, endocervical and urethral (treatment)—Erythromycins are indicated in the treatment of endocervical and urethral chlamydial infections caused by *Chlamydia trachomatis*. Erythromycins are recommended for the treatment of chlamydia in pregnant women. However, erythromycin estolate is contraindicated in pregnancy because of drug-related hepatotoxicity.

Conjunctivitis, chlamydial (treatment) or
Pneumonia, chlamydial (treatment)—Erythromycins are indicated in the treatment of conjunctivitis in newborns and pneumonia in infants caused by *Chlamydia trachomatis*. The efficacy of erythromycin treatment for these uses is approximately 80%; a second course of therapy may be required.

Diphtheria (prophylaxis and treatment)—Erythromycins are indicated as an adjunct to antitoxin, to prevent establishment of chronic carriers and to eradicate the organsim in carriers of diphtheria caused by *Corynebacterium diphtheriae*.

Endocarditis, bacterial (prophylaxis)—Erythromycins are indicated in the prophylaxis of bacterial endocarditis in penicillin-allergic patients who have congenital heart disease, rheumatic or other acquired valvular heart disease, prosthetic heart valves, previous bacterial endocarditis, hypertrophic cardiomyopathy, mitral valve prolapse with valvular regurgitation, and who undergo certain dental or surgical procedures.

Erythrasma (treatment)—Erythromycins are indicated in the treatment of erythrasma caused by *Corynebacterium minutissimum*.

Gonorrhea, endocervical (treatment) or
Gonorrhea, urethral (treatment)—Erythromycins are indicated in the treatment of gonorrhea caused by *Neisseria gonorrhoeae*; cephalosporins and fluoroquinolones are recommended for first-line treatment.

Legionnaires' disease (treatment)—Erythromycins are indicated in the treatment of Legionnaires' disease caused by *Legionella pneumophila*.

Listeriosis (treatment)—Erythromycins are indicated in the treatment of listeriosis caused by *Listeria monocytogenes*.

Pertussis (treatment)—Erythromycins are indicated in the treatment of pertussis (whooping cough) caused by *Bordetella pertussis*.

Pharyngitis, streptococcal (treatment)—Erythromycins are indicated in the treatment of pharyngitis caused by *Streptococcus pyogenes* (group A beta-hemolytic streptococci) in patients allergic to penicillin.

Pneumonia, mycoplasmal (treatment) or
Pneumonia, pneumococcal (treatment)—Erythromycins are indicated in the treatment of pneumonia caused by *Mycoplasma pneumoniae* and *Streptococcus pneumoniae*.

Rheumatic fever (prophylaxis)—Erythromycins are indicated as an alternative to penicillin in the long-term prophylaxis of rheumatic fever.

Skin and soft tissue infections (treatment)—Erythromycins are indicated in the treatment of skin and soft tissue infections, including burn wound infections, caused by *S. pyogenes* (group A beta-hemolytic streptococci).

Syphilis (treatment)—Erythromycins are indicated in the treatment of syphilis caused by *Treponema pallidum* in penicillin-allergic patients. However, erythromycin is less effective than other recommended regimens, and its use in pregnancy has failed to prevent congenital syphilis.

Urethritis, nongonococcal (treatment)—Erythromycins are indicated in the treatment of nongonococcal urethritis caused by *Chlamydia trachomatis* and *Ureaplasma urealyticum*.

[Acne vulgaris (treatment)]—Oral erythromycins are used in the treatment of acne vulgaris.

[Actinomycosis (treatment)][1];
[Anthrax (treatment)][1];
[Chancroid (treatment)][1];
[Lymphogranuloma venereum (treatment)][1]; or
[Relapsing fever (treatment)][1]—Erythromycins are used in the treatment of actinomycosis, anthrax, chancroid, lymphogranuloma venereum, and relapsing fever caused by *Borrelia* species.

[Enteritis, *Campylobacter* (treatment)][1]—Erythromycins are used in the treatment of enteritis caused by *Campylobacter jejuni*. Erythromycin therapy shortened the excretion of *C. jejuni* in the feces, but had no effect on the clinical course of the disease.

[Gastroparesis (treatment)][1]—Erythromycins are used in the treatment of gastroparesis, including severe diabetic gastroparesis, gastroparesis associated with progressive systemic sclerosis, and postvagotomy gastroparesis. Intravenous erythromycin appears to be more effective than oral erythromycin at increasing gastric emptying.

[Lyme disease (treatment)][1]—Erythromycins are used in the treatment of early stage Lyme disease in patients who are allergic to penicillin and in children under 9 years of age; however, erythromycins may be less effective than amoxicillin or doxycycline, possibly due to erratic absorption.

Not all species or strains of a particular organism may be susceptible to erythromycins.

---

[1] Not included in Canadian product labeling.

## Pharmacology/Pharmacokinetics

### Physicochemical characteristics
Molecular weight—
　Erythromycin base: 733.94.
　Erythromycin estolate: 1056.39.
　Erythromycin ethylsuccinate: 862.06.
　Erythromycin gluceptate: 960.12.
　Erythromycin lactobionate: 1092.23.
　Erythromycin stearate: 1018.42.

### Mechanism of action/Effect
Antibacterial—Erythromycin is a bacteriostatic macrolide antibiotic. However, it may be bactericidal in high concentrations or when used against highly susceptible organisms. It is thought to penetrate the bacterial cell membrane and to reversibly bind to the 50 S subunit of bacterial ribosomes; it does not directly inhibit peptide formation, but rather inhibits the translocation of peptides from the acceptor site on the ribosome to the donor site, inhibiting subsequent protein synthesis. Erythromycin is effective only against actively dividing organisms.

Gastroparesis—Erythromycin is thought to bind to motilin receptors and to act as an agonist. Erythromycin administration accelerates gastric emptying by increasing the amplitude of antral contractions and improving antroduodenal coordination. The effect appears to be dose-related. In patients with diabetic gastroparesis, low intravenous doses (40 mg) induce phase 3 of the migrating motor complex in the antrum of the stomach; and higher doses (200 mg) elicit prolonged periods of strong antral contractions. Faster emptying from the proximal stomach contributes to more rapid gastric emptying.

### Absorption
Bioavailability varies between 30 and 65%, depending on the salt. Erythromycin film-coated tablets (base and stearate) are subject to gastric acid inactivation and are best absorbed on an empty stomach. However, enteric-coated erythromycin base and erythromycin estolate are acid-stable and may be taken without regard to meals, and erythromycin ethylsuccinate is better absorbed when taken with meals.

### Distribution
Widely distributed to most tissues and fluids, including middle ear exudate, prostatic fluid, and semen. Highest concentrations are found in the liver, bile, and spleen. Low concentrations are found in the cerebrospinal fluid (CSF); however, penetration into CSF increases with meningeal inflammation.

$Vol_D$—0.9 L per kg.

### Protein binding
High (70 to 90%).

### Biotransformation
Hepatic; > 90% is hepatically metabolized, partially to inactive metabolites; may accumulate in patients with severe hepatic disease.

Erythromycin estolate (lauryl sulfate salt of the propanoate ester)—Propanoate ester is partially hydrolyzed in the gastrointestinal tract, then hydrolyzed in the blood to produce 20 to 40% of the dose as base in the serum.

Erythromycin ethylsuccinate—Absorbed into the blood as the ethylsuccinate salt and hydrolyzed to erythromycin base in the gastrointestinal tract and in the blood to produce 56 to 69% of the dose as base in the serum. Also, despite the high rate of biotransformation of erythromycin ethylsuccinate to active base, the area-under-the-curve (AUC) of active base generated from the ethylsuccinate salt was 1.6 times lower than that generated from a comparable dose of erythromycin estolate.

Erythromycin stearate—Dissociated to erythromycin base in the duodenum.

### Half-life
Normal renal function—1.4 to 2 hours.
Anuric patients—Approximately 5 hours.

### Time to peak concentration
2 to 4 hours, depending on the specific product (see *Peak serum concentration*).

### Peak serum concentration
Erythromycin base—
　Delayed-release capsules: Single dose of 250 mg—1.1 to 1.7 mcg per mL (mcg/mL) at 3 hours.
　Delayed-release tablets: Single dose of 250 mg—Approximately 0.9 mcg/mL at 4 hours.
　Delayed-release tablets: Multiple doses of 250 mg—Approximately 2.8 mcg/mL at 2 hours.
Erythromycin estolate—
　Single dose of 250 mg: Approximately 0.8 to 1.2 mcg/mL at 2 to 4 hours.

Erythromycin ethylsuccinate—
    Single dose of 400 mg: Approximately 0.8 mcg/mL at 1 hour.
    Multiple doses (400 mg twice a day), fasting: Approximately 1.4 mcg/mL.
    Multiple doses (400 mg twice a day), with food: Approximately 3 mcg/mL.
Erythromycin gluceptate—
    Single dose of 200 mg: 3 to 4 mcg/mL.
Erythromycin lactobionate—
    Single dose of 500 mg: Approximately 10 mcg/mL.
Erythromycin stearate—
    Single dose of 250 mg: Approximately 0.8 mcg/mL at 3 hours.

**Elimination**
Biliary; primarily excreted into the bile.
Renal, by glomerular filtration; 2 to 5% excreted unchanged following oral administration; 12 to 15% excreted unchanged following intravenous administration.
Erythromycins are not removed by hemodialysis or peritoneal dialysis.

## Precautions to Consider

**Cross-sensitivity and/or related problems**
Patients intolerant of one erythromycin or other macrolides may be intolerant of other erythromycins also.

**Tumorigenicity/Mutagenicity**
Long-term (20 month) oral studies done in rats did not demonstrate erythromycin base to be tumorigenic. Mutagenicity studies have not been conducted.

**Pregnancy/Reproduction**
Fertility—Adequate and well-controlled studies in humans have not been done.
Studies in rats fed erythromycin base at concentrations up to 0.25% of their diet found no apparent effect on male or female fertility.
Pregnancy—Erythromycins cross the placenta, resulting in low fetal plasma concentrations (5 to 20% of maternal plasma concentrations). Erythromycin estolate has been associated with an increased risk of reversible, subclinical hepatotoxicity in approximately 10% of pregnant women; its use during pregnancy is not recommended. However, problems with other erythromycins have not been documented.
There was no evidence of teratogenicity or any other adverse effect on reproduction in female rats fed erythromycin base (up to 0.25% of their diet) prior to and during mating, during gestation, and through weaning of 2 successive litters.
FDA Pregnancy Category B.

**Breast-feeding**
Erythromycins are distributed into breast milk. However, problems in humans have not been documented.

**Pediatrics**
Studies performed to date have not demonstrated pediatrics-specific problems that would limit the usefulness of erythromycin in children.

**Geriatrics**
Studies performed to date have not demonstrated geriatrics-specific problems that would limit the usefulness of erythromycin in the elderly. However, elderly patients may be at increased risk of hearing loss if they also have decreased renal or hepatic function associated with aging and are receiving high doses of erythromycin.

**Dental**
Systemic erythromycins may lead to oral candidiasis in patients undergoing long-term therapy.

**Drug interactions and/or related problems**
The following drug interactions and/or related problems have been selected on the basis of their potential clinical significance (possible mechanism in parentheses where appropriate)—not necessarily inclusive (» = major clinical significance):

Note: Combinations containing any of the following medications, depending on the amount present, may also interact with this medication.

  Alcohol
    (concurrent use with intravenous erythromycin was found to increase the peak blood alcohol concentration by 40%; erythromycin is not known to affect alcohol metabolism directly, but is thought to be related to more rapid gastric emptying; less exposure to alcohol dehydrogenase in the gastric mucosa and slower small intestine transit time may also favor the increase of alcohol absorption; there may be less of an effect with oral erythromycin)

» Alfentanil
    (chronic preoperative or perioperative use of erythromycins, which are hepatic enzyme inhibitors, may decrease the plasma clearance and prolong the duration of action of alfentanil)

» Astemizole or
» Terfenadine
    (concurrent use of astemizole or terfenadine with erythromycins is contraindicated; concurrent use may increase the risk of cardiotoxicity, such as torsades de pointes and ventricular tachycardia, and death)

» Carbamazepine or
  Valproic acid
    (erythromycins may inhibit carbamazepine and valproic acid metabolism, resulting in increased anticonvulsant plasma concentrations and toxicity; it is recommended that erythromycins be used with caution if at all in patients receiving carbamazepine or valproic acid)

» Chloramphenicol or
» Lincomycins
    (erythromycins may displace these medications from, or prevent them from binding to, 50 S subunits of bacterial ribosomes, thus antagonizing the effects of chloramphenicol and lincomycins; concurrent use is not recommended)

» Cyclosporine
    (erythromycin has been reported to increase cyclosporine plasma concentrations and may increase the risk of nephrotoxicity)

  Digoxin
    (although no clinical cases of toxicity have been reported, concurrent use of oral antibiotics may increase serum digoxin concentrations in some individuals; in these individuals, alteration of the gut flora by antibiotics may diminish digoxin conversion to inactive metabolites, resulting in increased serum digoxin concentrations; although limited data are available, this interaction has been reported with oral use of erythromycins, neomycin, and tetracyclines)

  Ergotamine
    (erythromycin inhibits the metabolism of ergotamine and has been reported to increase the vasospasm associated with ergotamines)

» Hepatotoxic medications, other (see *Appendix II*)
    (concurrent use of other hepatotoxic medications with erythromycins may increase the potential for hepatotoxicity)

  Lovastatin
    (concurrent use of lovastatin with erythromycin may increase the risk of rhabdomyolysis, which typically occurs after the completion of erythromycin therapy; this is thought to be due to erythromycin's inhibition of lovastatin metabolism, which increases lovastatin serum concentrations; simultaneous administration of erythromycin and lovastatin should be used with caution)

  Midazolam or
  Triazolam
    (concurrent use with erythromycin may decrease the clearance of these medications, increasing the pharmacological effect of midazolam or triazolam)

  Ototoxic medications, other (see *Appendix II*)
    (concurrent use of other ototoxic medications with high-dose erythromycin in patients with renal function impairment may increase the potential for ototoxicity)

  Penicillins
    (since bacteriostatic drugs may interfere with the bactericidal effect of penicillins in the treatment of meningitis or in other situations where a rapid bactericidal effect is necessary, it is best to avoid concurrent therapy)

» Warfarin
    (use of erythromycins in patients receiving chronic warfarin therapy may result in excessive prolongation of prothrombin time and increased risk of hemorrhage, especially in elderly patients, because of possible decreased warfarin metabolism and clearance; warfarin dosage adjustments may be necessary during and after therapy with erythromycins, and prothrombin times should be monitored closely)

» Xanthines, such as:
  Aminophylline
  Caffeine
  Oxtriphylline
  Theophylline
    (concurrent use of the xanthines [except dyphylline] with erythromycins may decrease hepatic clearance of theophylline, resulting in increased serum theophylline concentrations and/or toxicity; this effect may be more likely to occur after 6 days of concurrent therapy because the magnitude of theophylline clearance reduction is proportional to the peak serum erythromycin concentrations; dosage

adjustment of the xanthines may be necessary during and after therapy with erythromycins)

**Laboratory value alterations**
The following have been selected on the basis of their potential clinical significance (possible effect in parentheses where appropriate)—not necessarily inclusive (» = major clinical significance):

With diagnostic test results
  Aspartate aminotransferase (AST [SGOT])
    (use of erythromycin may interfere with AST [SGOT] determinations if azonefast violet B or diphenylhydrazine colorimetric tests are used)
  Catecholamines, urinary
    (erythromycin may produce false elevations of urinary catecholamines because of interference with the fluorometric determination)

With physiology/laboratory test values
  Alanine aminotransferase (ALT [SGPT]) and
  Alkaline phosphatase and
  Aspartate aminotransferase (AST [SGOT]) and
  Bilirubin, serum
    (values may be increased by all erythromycins, but more commonly by erythromycin estolate)

**Medical considerations/Contraindications**
The medical considerations/contraindications included have been selected on the basis of their potential clinical significance (reasons given in parentheses where appropriate)—not necessarily inclusive (» = major clinical significance).

*Risk-benefit should be considered when the following medical problems exist:*
» Cardiac arrhythmias, history of, or QT prolongation
    (patients with a history of cardiac arrhythmias or QT prolongation may be at risk for arrhythmias or torsades de pointes while receiving high doses of erythromycins)
» Hepatic function impairment, especially with erythromycin estolate
    (erythromycins, especially erythromycin estolate, may be hepatotoxic on rare occasion)
  Hypersensitivity to erythromycins
  Loss of hearing
    (patients with a history of hearing loss may be at increased risk of further hearing loss, especially if the patient has renal or hepatic function impairment, is elderly, and is receiving high doses of erythromycin)

**Patient monitoring**
The following may be especially important in patient monitoring (other tests may be warranted in some patients, depending on condition; » = major clinical significance):

  Electrocardiogram
    (monitoring of QT interval recommended, especially in patients receiving high doses of parenteral erythromycin)
» Hepatic function determinations
    (may be required periodically if signs of hepatic dysfunction occur with any of the erythromycins; erythromycins should be discontinued promptly if signs of hepatic dysfunction occur)

## Side/Adverse Effects

Note: Hepatotoxicity has been associated, rarely, with all erythromycin salts, but more frequently with erythromycin estolate. Reports suggest that a hypersensitivity mechanism may be involved. Symptoms include malaise, nausea, vomiting, abdominal cramps, skin rash, and fever. Jaundice may or may not be present. Liver function tests often indicate cholestasis. Symptoms typically appear within a few days to 1 or 2 weeks after the start of continuous therapy, and are reversible when erythromycin is discontinued. However, hepatotoxicity reappears promptly on readministration to sensitive patients.

Hearing loss is more likely to occur with administration of high doses (≥ 4 grams per day) in patients with renal or hepatic disease and/or in elderly patients. It appears to be related to high peak plasma concentrations, usually exceeding 12 mcg per mL. Hearing loss is usually reversible, although irreversible deafness has occurred. It occurs from 36 hours to 8 days after treatment is started, and begins to recover within 1 to 14 days after erythromycin is discontinued.

The following side/adverse effects have been selected on the basis of their potential clinical significance (possible signs and symptoms in parentheses where appropriate)—not necessarily inclusive:

**Those indicating need for medical attention**
Incidence less frequent
  *Hepatotoxicity* (fever; nausea; skin rash; stomach pain, severe; unusual tiredness or weakness; yellow eyes or skin; vomiting); *hypersensitivity* (skin rash, redness, or itching)

Incidence less frequent—parenteral erythromycins only
  *Inflammation or phlebitis at the injection site*

Incidence rare
  *Cardiac toxicity, especially QT prolongation and torsades de pointes* (irregular or slow heart rate; recurrent fainting; sudden death); *loss of hearing, usually reversible; pancreatitis* (severe abdominal pain, nausea, and vomiting)

**Those indicating need for medical attention only if they continue or are bothersome**
Incidence more frequent
  *Gastrointestinal disturbances* (abdominal or stomach cramping and discomfort; diarrhea, nausea or vomiting)

Incidence less frequent
  *Oral candidiasis* (sore mouth or tongue; white patches in mouth and/or on tongue); *vaginal candidiasis* (vaginal itching and discharge)

## Overdose

For specific information on the agents used in the management of erythromycin overdose, see:
• *Epinephrine (Systemic)* monograph;
• *Corticosteroids (Inhalation-Local)* monograph; and/or
• *Antihistamines (Systemic)* monograph.

For more information on the management of overdose or unintentional ingestion, **contact a Poison Control Center** (see *Poison Control Center Listing*).

**Treatment of overdose**
Recommended treatment consists of the following:
To decrease absorption—Evacuating the stomach to eliminate unabsorbed drug.

Specific treatment—Administering epinephrine, corticosteroids, and antihistamines for allergic reactions.

Supportive care—Using supportive measures as needed. Patients in whom intentional overdose is known or suspected should be referred for psychiatric consultation.

## Patient Consultation

As an aid to patient consultation, refer to *Advice for the Patient, Erythromycins (Systemic)*.

In providing consultation, consider emphasizing the following selected information (» = major clinical significance):

**Before using this medication**
» Conditions affecting use, especially:
  Hypersensitivity to erythromycins or other macrolides
  Pregnancy—Erythromycins cross the placenta; erythromycin estolate has been associated with an increased risk of reversible, subclinical hepatotoxicity in pregnant women
  Breast-feeding—Erythromycins are distributed into breast milk
  Dental—Oral candidiasis may occur with long-term therapy
  Other medications, especially alfentanil, astemizole, carbamazepine, chloramphenicol, cyclosporine, other hepatotoxic medications, lincomycins, terfenadine, warfarin, and xanthines
  Other medical problems, especially a history of cardiac arrhythmias or QT prolongation or hepatic function impairment

**Proper use of this medication**
  Taking with a full glass of water, on an empty stomach; may be taken with food if stomach upset occurs
  Proper administration technique for oral liquids and/or pediatric drops, chewable tablets, delayed-release capsules and tablets
  Not using oral liquids and/or pediatric drops after expiration date
» Compliance with full course of therapy, especially in streptococcal infections
» Importance of not missing doses and taking at evenly spaced times

» Proper dosing
  Missed dose: Taking as soon as possible; not taking if almost time for next dose; not doubling dose
» Proper storage

**Precautions while using this medication**
Checking with physician if no improvement within a few days

**Side/adverse effects**
Signs of potential side effects, especially, hepatotoxicity, hypersensitivity, inflammation or phlebitis at the injection site, cardiac toxicity, loss of hearing, or pancreatitis

## General Dosing Information

Therapy should be continued for at least 10 days in group A beta-hemolytic streptococcal infections to help prevent the occurrence of acute rheumatic fever.

**For oral dosage forms only**
Doses greater than 1 gram per dose are not recommended with twice-a-day dosing.

Erythromycin film-coated tablets (base and stearate) are best absorbed on an empty stomach; however, if gastrointestinal irritation occurs, they may be taken with food. Enteric-coated erythromycin base and erythromycin estolate may be taken without regard to meals; and erythromycin ethylsuccinate is better absorbed when taken with meals.

---

### ERYTHROMYCIN BASE

## Oral Dosage Forms

Note: Bracketed uses in the *Dosage Forms* section refer to categories of use and/or indications that are not included in U.S. product labeling.

### ERYTHROMYCIN DELAYED-RELEASE CAPSULES USP

**Usual adult and adolescent dose**
Antibacterial—
  Oral, 250 mg (base) every six hours; 333 mg every eight hours; or 500 mg every twelve hours if twice-a-day dosage is desired.
Note: Acne vulgaris—Oral, 250 mg (base) every six hours; 333 mg every eight hours; or 500 mg every twelve hours for four weeks. This dose may be reduced to 333 to 500 mg once a day for a maintenance dose.
  Bowel preparation (preoperative) adjunct—Oral, 1 gram (base) administered at nineteen hours, eighteen hours, and nine hours (total of 3 grams) before the start of surgery.
  Chlamydial infections, endocervical and urethral—Oral, 333 mg (base) every eight hours, or 500 mg every six hours for seven days; or 250 mg every six hours for fourteen days. Erythromycin base may be used in pregnant women.
  [Chancroid][1]—Oral, 500 mg (base) every six hours for seven days.
  Endocarditis prophylaxis—Oral, 1 gram (base) two hours prior to the procedure, and 500 mg six hours after the initial dose.
  [Enteritis, *Campylobacter*][1]—Oral, 250 mg (base) four times a day for five days.
  [Gastroparesis][1]—Oral, 250 mg (base) taken thirty minutes before meals, three times a day.
  Legionnaires' disease—Oral, 500 mg (base) to 1 gram every six hours.
  [Lyme disease][1]—Oral, 250 mg (base) four times a day for ten to twenty-one days.
  [Lymphogranuloma venereum][1]—Oral, 500 mg (base) every six hours for twenty-one days.
  Pelvic inflammatory disease, caused by *Neisseria gonorrhoeae*—Oral, 250 mg (base) every six hours for seven days, after intravenous administration of erythromycin 500 mg every six hours for three days.
  [Relapsing fever][1]—Oral, 10 mg (base) per kg of body weight every six hours for ten days.
  Streptococcal prophylaxis—Continuous prophylaxis of streptococcal infections in patients with a history of rheumatic heart disease: Oral, 250 mg (base) every twelve hours.
  Syphilis, primary—Oral, 30 to 40 grams (base) over a ten- to fifteen-day period.
  Urethritis, nongonococcal, caused by *Ureaplasma urealyticum*—Oral, 500 mg (base) every six hours for seven days; or 250 mg every six hours for fourteen days.

**Usual adult prescribing limits**
Antibacterial—
  Up to 4 grams (base) a day.

**Usual pediatric dose**
Antibacterial—
  Oral, 7.5 to 12.5 mg (base) per kg of body weight every six hours; or 15 to 25 mg per kg of body weight every twelve hours.
  Severe infections, 15 to 25 mg (base) per kg of body weight every six hours.
Note: Chlamydial infections, endocervical and urethral—
      Children up to 45 kg of body weight: Oral, 10 mg (base) per kg of body weight every six hours for ten to fourteen days.
      Children 45 kg of body weight and over but less than 8 years of age: See *Usual adult and adolescent dose*.
  Conjunctivitis, chlamydial[1]—Oral, 12.5 mg (base) per kg of body weight every six hours for at least ten to fourteen days.
  Diphtheria—Oral, 10 to 12.5 mg (base) per kg of body weight every six hours for fourteen days.
  Endocarditis prophylaxis—Oral, 20 mg (base) per kg of body weight two hours prior to the procedure, and 10 mg per kg of body weight six hours after the initial dose.
  [Enteritis, *Campylobacter*][1]—Oral, 10 mg (base) per kg of body weight every six hours for five days.
  [Lyme disease][1]—Oral, 7.5 mg (base) per kg of body weight every six hours for ten to twenty-one days.
  Pertussis—Oral, 10 to 12.5 mg (base) per kg of body weight every six hours for fourteen days.
  Pneumonia, chlamydial[1]—Oral, 12.5 mg (base) per kg of body weight every six hours for two weeks.
  [Relapsing fever][1]—Oral, 10 mg (base) per kg of body weight every six hours for ten days.
  Streptococcal pharyngitis—Oral, 5 to 7.5 mg (base) per kg of body weight every six hours; or 10 to 15 mg per kg of body weight every twelve hours for at least ten days.

**Strength(s) usually available**
U.S.—
  250 mg (base) (Rx) [*ERYC*; GENERIC].
Canada—
  250 mg (base) (Rx) [*Apo-Erythro E-C; ERYC-250; Novo-rythro Encap*].
  333 mg (base) (Rx) [*Apo-Erythro E-C; ERYC-333*].

**Packaging and storage**
Store below 40 °C (104 °F), preferably between 15 and 30 °C (59 and 86 °F), unless otherwise specified by manufacturer. Store in a tight container.

**Auxiliary labeling**
• Continue medicine for full time of treatment.
• Swallow capsules whole.

**Note**
Erythromycin delayed-release capsules contain enteric-coated pellets. The entire contents of a capsule may be sprinkled on applesauce, jelly, or ice cream immediately prior to ingestion. Subdividing the contents of the capsule is not recommended.

### ERYTHROMYCIN TABLETS USP

**Usual adult and adolescent dose**
See *Erythromycin Delayed-release Capsules USP*.

**Usual adult prescribing limits**
See *Erythromycin Delayed-release Capsules USP*.

**Usual pediatric dose**
See *Erythromycin Delayed-release Capsules USP*.

**Strength(s) usually available**
U.S.—
  250 mg (base) (Rx) [GENERIC].
  500 mg (base) (Rx) [GENERIC].
Canada—
  250 mg (base) (Rx) [*Apo-Erythro; Erythromid*].

**Packaging and storage**
Store below 40 °C (104 °F), preferably between 15 and 30 °C (59 and 86 °F), unless otherwise specified by manufacturer. Store in a tight container.

**Auxiliary labeling**
• Continue medicine for full time of treatment.

### ERYTHROMYCIN DELAYED-RELEASE TABLETS USP

**Usual adult and adolescent dose**
See *Erythromycin Delayed-release Capsules USP*.

Note: Endocarditis prophylaxis—The manufacturer of E-Mycin recommends taking 1 gram three to four hours prior to the procedure because of the pharmacokinetics of their enteric-coated product.

**Usual adult prescribing limits**
See *Erythromycin Delayed-release Capsules USP*.

**Usual pediatric dose**
See *Erythromycin Delayed-release Capsules USP*.

Note: Endocarditis prophylaxis—The manufacturer of E-Mycin recommends taking 1 gram three to four hours prior to the procedure because of the pharmacokinetics of their enteric-coated product.

**Strength(s) usually available**
U.S.—
  250 mg (base) (Rx) [*E-Mycin; Ery-Tab; Ilotycin;* GENERIC].
  333 mg (base) (Rx) [*E-Base; E-Mycin; Ery-Tab; PCE;* GENERIC].
  500 mg (base) (Rx) [*E-Base; Ery-Tab; PCE*].
Canada—
  250 mg (base) (Rx) [*E-Mycin;* GENERIC].
  333 mg (base) (Rx) [*PCE*].
  500 mg (base) (Rx) [*Erybid*].

**Packaging and storage**
Store below 40 °C (104 °F), preferably between 15 and 30 °C (59 and 86 °F), unless otherwise specified by manufacturer. Store in a tight container.

**Auxiliary labeling**
• Continue medicine for full time of treatment.
• Swallow tablets whole.

---

[1]Not included in Canadian product labeling.

---

### ERYTHROMYCIN ESTOLATE

## Summary of Differences

Precautions:
  Pregnancy—Associated with increased risk of reversible, subclinical hepatotoxicity.
  Laboratory value alterations—Serum alkaline phosphatase, bilirubin, AST (SGOT), and ALT (SGPT) concentrations may be increased more frequently than with other erythromycins.
Side/adverse effects:
  May also cause cholestatic jaundice less frequently (rare with other erythromycins).

## Oral Dosage Forms

Note: Bracketed uses in the *Dosage Forms* section refer to categories of use and/or indications that are not included in U.S. product labeling.
  The dosing and strengths of the dosage forms available are expressed in terms of erythromycin base (not the estolate salt).

### ERYTHROMYCIN ESTOLATE CAPSULES USP

**Usual adult and adolescent dose**
Antibacterial—
  Oral, 250 mg (base) every six hours; or 500 mg every twelve hours if twice-a-day dosage is desired.

Note: Chlamydial infections, endocervical and urethral—Oral, 500 mg (base) every six hours for seven days; or 250 mg every six hours for fourteen days. Erythromycin estolate is not recommended for use in pregnant women.
  Endocarditis prophylaxis—Oral, 1 gram (base) two hours prior to the procedure, and 500 mg six hours after the initial dose.
  [Gastroparesis][1]—Oral, 250 mg (base) taken thirty minutes before meals, three times a day.
  Legionnaires' disease—Oral, 500 mg (base) to 1 gram every six hours.
  Streptococcal prophylaxis—Continuous prophylaxis of streptococcal infections in patients with a history of rheumatic heart disease: Oral, 250 mg (base) every twelve hours.
  Syphilis, primary—Oral, 20 to 30 grams (base) over a ten-day period.

**Usual adult prescribing limits**
Antibacterial—
  Up to 4 grams (base) daily.

**Usual pediatric dose**
Antibacterial—
  Oral, 7.5 to 12.5 mg (base) per kg of body weight every six hours; or 15 to 25 mg per kg of body weight every twelve hours.
  Severe infections, 15 to 25 mg (base) per kg of body weight every six hours.

Note: Conjunctivitis, chlamydial[1]—Oral, 12.5 mg (base) per kg of body weight every six hours for at least two weeks.
  Diphtheria—Oral, 10 to 12.5 mg (base) per kg of body weight every six hours for fourteen days.
  Endocarditis prophylaxis—Oral, 20 mg (base) per kg of body weight two hours prior to the procedure, and 10 mg per kg of body weight six hours after the initial dose.
  Pertussis—Oral, 10 to 12.5 mg (base) per kg of body weight every six hours for fourteen days.
  Pneumonia, chlamydial[1]—Oral, 12.5 mg (base) per kg of body weight every six hours for two weeks.
  Streptococcal pharyngitis—Oral, 5 to 7.5 mg (base) per kg of body weight every six hours; or 10 to 15 mg per kg of body weight every twelve hours for at least ten days.

**Strength(s) usually available**
U.S.—
  250 mg (base) (Rx) [*Ilosone;* GENERIC].
Canada—
  250 mg (base) (Rx) [*Ilosone; Novo-rythro*].

**Packaging and storage**
Store below 40 °C (104 °F), preferably between 15 and 30 °C (59 and 86 °F), unless otherwise specified by manufacturer. Store in a tight container.

**Auxiliary labeling**
• Continue medicine for full time of treatment.

### ERYTHROMYCIN ESTOLATE ORAL SUSPENSION USP

**Usual adult and adolescent dose**
See *Erythromycin Estolate Capsules USP*.

**Usual adult prescribing limits**
See *Erythromycin Estolate Capsules USP*.

**Usual pediatric dose**
See *Erythromycin Estolate Capsules USP*.

**Strength(s) usually available**
U.S.—
  125 mg (base) per 5 mL (Rx) [*Ilosone* (methylparaben; propylparaben); GENERIC].
  250 mg (base) per 5 mL (Rx) [*Ilosone* (methylparaben; propylparaben); GENERIC].
Canada—
  125 mg (base) per 5 mL (Rx) [*Ilosone; Novo-rythro*].
  250 mg (base) per 5 mL (Rx) [*Ilosone; Novo-rythro*].

**Packaging and storage**
Store between 2 and 8 °C (36 and 46 °F). Store in a tight container.

**Auxiliary labeling**
• Refrigerate.
• Shake well.
• Continue medicine for full time of treatment.
• Take by mouth only (pediatric drops).

**Note**
Explain administration technique for pediatric drops (100 mg per mL).
When dispensing, include a calibrated liquid-measuring device.

### ERYTHROMYCIN ESTOLATE TABLETS USP

**Usual adult and adolescent dose**
See *Erythromycin Estolate Capsules USP*.

**Usual adult prescribing limits**
See *Erythromycin Estolate Capsules USP*.

**Usual pediatric dose**
See *Erythromycin Estolate Capsules USP*.

**Strength(s) usually available**
U.S.—
  250 mg (base) (Rx) [GENERIC].
  500 mg (base) (Rx) [*Ilosone*].
Canada—
  500 mg (base) (Rx) [*Ilosone*].

**Packaging and storage**
Store below 40 °C (104 °F), preferably between 15 and 30 °C (59 and 86 °F), unless otherwise specified by manufacturer. Store in a tight container.

**Auxiliary labeling**
- Continue medicine for full time of treatment.

[1]Not included in Canadian product labeling.

---

### ERYTHROMYCIN ETHYLSUCCINATE

## Summary of Differences

1.6 grams of erythromycin ethylsuccinate produce approximately the same blood levels as 1 gram erythromycin base.

In pediatric patients, equivalent doses of erythromycin ethylsuccinate and erythromycin base produce comparable blood levels.

## Oral Dosage Forms

Note: Bracketed uses in the *Dosage Forms* section refer to categories of use and/or indications that are not included in U.S. product labeling.

The dosing and dosage forms available are expressed in terms of ethylsuccinate salt. 400 mg of erythromycin ethylsuccinate produces approximately the same blood levels as 250 mg erythromycin base.

### ERYTHROMYCIN ETHYLSUCCINATE ORAL SUSPENSION USP

**Usual adult and adolescent dose**
Antibacterial—
 Oral, 400 mg every six hours; or 800 mg every twelve hours if twice-a-day dosing is desired.
Note: Chlamydial infections, endocervical and urethral—Oral, 800 mg (base) every six hours for seven days, or 400 mg every six hours for fourteen days. Erythromycin ethylsuccinate may be used in pregnant women.
 Endocarditis prophylaxis—Oral, 1.6 grams two hours prior to the procedure, and 800 mg six hours after the initial dose.
 [Gastroparesis][1]—Oral, 400 mg taken thirty minutes before meals, three times a day.
 Legionnaires' disease—Oral, 400 mg to 1 gram every six hours.
 Streptococcal prophylaxis—Continuous prophylaxis of streptococcal infections in patients with a history of rheumatic heart disease: Oral, 400 mg every twelve hours.
 Syphilis, primary—Oral, 48 to 64 grams (base) over a ten- to fifteen-day period.
 Urethritis, nongonococcal, caused by *Ureaplasma urealyticum*—Oral, 800 mg every eight hours for seven days; or 400 mg every six hours for fourteen days.

**Usual adult prescribing limits**
Antibacterial—
 Up to 4 grams daily.

**Usual pediatric dose**
Antibacterial—
 Oral, 7.5 to 12.5 mg per kg of body weight every six hours; or 15 to 25 mg per kg of body weight every twelve hours.
 Severe infections, 15 to 25 mg per kg body weight every six hours.
Note: Conjunctivitis, chlamydial[1]—Oral, 12.5 mg (base) per kg of body weight every six hours for ten to fourteen days.
 Diphtheria—Oral, 10 to 12.5 mg (base) per kg of body weight every six hours for fourteen days.
 Endocarditis prophylaxis—Oral, 20 mg per kg of body weight two hours prior to the procedure, and 10 mg per kg of body weight six hours after the initial dose.
 [Enteritis, *Campylobacter*][1]—Oral, 10 mg (base) per kg of body weight every six hours for five days.
 Pertussis—Oral, 10 to 12.5 mg per kg of body weight every six hours for fourteen days.
 Pneumonia, chlamydial[1]—Oral, 12.5 mg (base) per kg of body weight every six hours for ten to fourteen days.

**Strength(s) usually available**
U.S.—
 200 mg per 5 mL (Rx) [*E.E.S.* (methylparaben; propylparaben); *Erythro*; GENERIC].
 400 mg per 5 mL (Rx) [*E.E.S.* (methylparaben; propylparaben); *Erythro*; GENERIC].
Canada—
 Not commercially available.

**Packaging and storage**
Store between 2 and 8 °C (36 and 46 °F). Store in a tight container.
Note: After dispensing, suspensions do not require refrigeration if used within 14 days. Some manufacturers recommend storage in light-resistant containers to prevent discoloration.

**Auxiliary labeling**
- Shake well.
- Continue medicine for full time of treatment.
- Beyond-use date.

**Note**
When dispensing, include a calibrated liquid-measuring device.

### ERYTHROMYCIN ETHYLSUCCINATE FOR ORAL SUSPENSION USP

**Usual adult and adolescent dose**
See *Erythromycin Ethylsuccinate Oral Suspension USP*.

**Usual adult prescribing limits**
See *Erythromycin Ethylsuccinate Oral Suspension USP*.

**Usual pediatric dose**
See *Erythromycin Ethylsuccinate Oral Suspension USP*.

**Strength(s) usually available**
U.S.—
 200 mg per 5 mL (when reconstituted according to manufacturer's instructions) (Rx) [*E.E.S.*; *EryPed*; GENERIC].
 400 mg per 5 mL (when reconstituted according to manufacturer's instructions) (Rx) [*EryPed*; GENERIC].
Canada—
 100 mg per 5 mL (when reconstituted according to manufacturer's instructions) (Rx) [*Novo-Rythro*].
 200 mg per 5 mL (when reconstituted according to manufacturer's instructions) (Rx) [*E.E.S.*; *Novo-Rythro*].
 400 mg per 5 mL (when reconstituted according to manufacturer's instructions) (Rx) [*E.E.S.*].

**Packaging and storage**
Prior to reconstitution, store below 40 °C (104 °F), preferably between 15 and 30 °C (59 and 86 °F), unless otherwise specified by manufacturer. Store in a tight container.
Note: After reconstitution, depending on manufacturer or specific product, suspensions do not require refrigeration if used within 14 days.

**Auxiliary labeling**
- Shake well.
- Continue medicine for full time of treatment.
- Beyond-use date.
- Take by mouth only (pediatric drops).

**Note**
Explain administration technique for pediatric drops.
When dispensing, include a calibrated liquid-measuring device.

### ERYTHROMYCIN ETHYLSUCCINATE TABLETS USP

**Usual adult and adolescent dose**
See *Erythromycin Ethylsuccinate Oral Suspension USP*.

**Usual adult prescribing limits**
See *Erythromycin Ethylsuccinate Oral Suspension USP*.

**Usual pediatric dose**
See *Erythromycin Ethylsuccinate Oral Suspension USP*.

**Strength(s) usually available**
U.S.—
 400 mg (Rx) [*E.E.S.*; GENERIC].
Canada—
 600 mg (Rx) [*Apo-Erythro-ES*; *E.E.S.*].

**Packaging and storage**
Store below 40 °C (104 °F), preferably between 15 and 30 °C (59 and 86 °F), unless otherwise specified by manufacturer. Store in a tight container.

**Auxiliary labeling**
- Continue medicine for full time of treatment.

### ERYTHROMYCIN ETHYLSUCCINATE TABLETS (CHEWABLE) USP

**Usual adult and adolescent dose**
See *Erythromycin Ethylsuccinate Oral Suspension USP*.

**Usual adult prescribing limits**
See *Erythromycin Ethylsuccinate Oral Suspension USP*.

**Usual pediatric dose**
See *Erythromycin Ethylsuccinate Oral Suspension USP*.

**Strength(s) usually available**
U.S.—
  200 mg (Rx) [*EryPed*].
  400 mg (Rx) [*Erythro*].
Canada—
  200 mg (Rx) [*E.E.S.* (scored); *EryPed*].

**Packaging and storage**
Store below 40 °C (104 °F), preferably between 15 and 30 °C (59 and 86 °F), unless otherwise specified by manufacturer. Store in a tight container.

**Auxiliary labeling**
- Chew or crush tablets before swallowing.
- Continue medicine for full time of treatment.

[1]Not included in Canadian product labeling.

---

## ERYTHROMYCIN GLUCEPTATE

## Summary of Differences
Category: Indicated only as an antibacterial.

## Parenteral Dosage Forms
Note: Bracketed uses in the *Dosage Forms* section refer to categories of use and/or indications that are not included in U.S. product labeling.
  The dosing and strengths of the dosage forms available are expressed in terms of erythromycin base (not the gluceptate salt).

### ERYTHROMYCIN GLUCEPTATE STERILE USP

**Usual adult and adolescent dose**
Antibacterial—
  Intravenous infusion, 250 to 500 mg (base) every six hours; or 3.75 to 5 mg per kg of body weight every six hours.
Note: [Gastroparesis][1]—Oral, 200 mg taken thirty minutes before meals, three times a day.
  Legionnaires' disease—Intravenous infusion, 1 gram (base) every six hours.
  Pelvic inflammatory disease, caused by *Neisseria gonorrhoeae*—Intravenous infusion, 500 mg (base) every six hours for three days, then oral administration of erythromycin 250 mg every six hours for seven days.

**Usual adult prescribing limits**
Up to 4 grams (base) daily.

**Usual pediatric dose**
Antibacterial—
  Intravenous infusion, 3.75 to 5 mg (base) per kg of body weight every six hours.
  Note: Diphtheria—Oral, 10 to 12.5 mg (base) per kg of body weight every six hours for fourteen days.

**Size(s) usually available**
U.S.—
  1 gram (base) (Rx) [*Ilotycin*].
Canada—
  500 mg (base) (Rx) [*Ilotycin*].
  1 gram (base) (Rx) [*Ilotycin*].

**Packaging and storage**
Prior to reconstitution, store below 40 °C (104 °F), preferably between 15 and 30 °C (59 and 86 °F), unless otherwise specified by manufacturer.

**Preparation of dosage form**
To prepare initial dilution, add at least 10 mL of sterile water for injection (without preservatives) to each 500-mg vial and at least 20 mL of diluent to each 1-gram vial.
After initial dilution, solution may be further diluted to a concentration of 1 gram per liter in 0.9% sodium chloride injection or 5% dextrose injection for slow, continuous infusion.

**Stability**
After reconstitution, initial dilutions (25 to 50 mg per mL) retain their potency for 7 days if refrigerated.

**Additional information**
Infusions with a pH below 5.5 tend to lose potency rapidly and should be administered completely within 4 hours after dilution.
If administration time is prolonged, infusions should be buffered to neutrality with a suitable buffer and administered completely within 24 hours after dilution.
If administered by intermittent infusion, dose may be diluted in 100 to 250 mL of 0.9% sodium chloride injection or 5% dextrose injection and administered slowly over a 20- to 60-minute period.

[1]Not included in Canadian product labeling.

---

## ERYTHROMYCIN LACTOBIONATE

## Summary of Differences
Category: Indicated only as an antibacterial.

## Parenteral Dosage Forms
Note: Bracketed uses in the *Dosage Forms* section refer to categories of use and/or indications that are not included in U.S. product labeling.
  The dosing and strengths of the dosage forms available are expressed in terms of erythromcyin base (not the lactobionate salt).

### ERYTHROMYCIN LACTOBIONATE FOR INJECTION USP

**Usual adult and adolescent dose**
Antibacterial—
  Intravenous infusion, 250 to 500 mg (base) every six hours; or 3.75 to 5 mg per kg of body weight every six hours.
Note: [Gastroparesis][1]—Oral, 200 mg administered thirty minutes before meals, three times a day.
  Legionnaires' disease—Intravenous infusion, 1 gram (base) every six hours.
  Pelvic inflammatory disease, caused by *Neisseria gonorrhoeae*—Intravenous infusion, 500 mg (base) every six hours for three days, then oral administration of erythromycin 250 mg every six hours for seven days.

**Usual adult prescribing limits**
Up to 4 grams (base) daily.

**Usual pediatric dose**
Antibacterial—
  Intravenous infusion, 3.75 to 5 mg (base) per kg of body weight every six hours. This product should be used with caution in neonates since it contains benzyl alcohol.
Note: Diphtheria—Oral, 10 to 12.5 mg (base) per kg of body weight every six hours for fourteen days.

**Size(s) usually available**
U.S.—
  500 mg (base) (Rx) [*Erythrocin* (may contain benzyl alcohol 90 mg per 500 mg vial); GENERIC].
  1 gram (base) (Rx) [*Erythrocin* (may contain benzyl alcohol 180 mg per 1 gram vial); GENERIC].
Canada—
  500 mg (base) (Rx) [*Erythrocin* (may contain benzyl alcohol 0.9% per vial)].
  1 gram (base) (Rx) [*Erythrocin* (may contain benzyl alcohol 0.9% per vial)].

**Packaging and storage**
Prior to reconstitution, store below 40 °C (104 °F), preferably between 15 and 30 °C (59 and 86 °F), unless otherwise specified by manufacturer.

**Preparation of dosage form**
To prepare initial dilution, add 10 mL of sterile water for injection (without preservatives) to each 500-mg vial and 20 mL of diluent to each 1-gram vial.
After initial dilution, solution may be further diluted to a concentration of 1 to 5 mg per mL in 0.9% sodium chloride injection, lactated Ringer's injection, or other electrolyte solutions (see manufacturer's package insert) for slow, continuous infusion. Dextrose-containing solutions may also be used if suitably buffered by adding 1 mL of 4% sodium bicarbonate per 100 mL of solution.
For reconstitution of piggyback infusion bottles, see manufacturer's labeling for instructions.
Caution: Use of diluents containing benzyl alcohol is not recommended for preparation of medications for use in neonates. A fatal toxic syndrome consisting of metabolic acidosis, CNS depression, respiratory problems, renal failure, hypotension, and possibly seizures and intracranial hemorrhages has been associated with this use.

# Erythromycins (Systemic)

**Stability**

After reconstitution, initial dilutions (50 mg per mL) retain their potency for 14 days if refrigerated, or for 24 hours at room temperature.

Infusions prepared in piggyback infusion bottles retain their potency for 8 hours at room temperature, for 24 hours if refrigerated, or for 30 days if frozen.

Infusions prepared in the ADD-vantage system should not be stored.

**Additional information**

Acidic infusions are unstable and lose potency rapidly. A pH of at least 5.5 is recommended for final dilutions, which should be administered completely within 8 hours after dilution.

If administered by intermittent infusion, dose may be diluted to a maximum concentration of 5 mg per mL with specified diluent and administered slowly over a 20- to 60-minute period.

[1]Not included in Canadian product labeling.

---

## ERYTHROMYCIN STEARATE

## Oral Dosage Forms

Note: Bracketed uses in the *Dosage Forms* section refer to categories of use and/or indications that are not included in U.S. product labeling.

The dosing and strengths of the dosage forms available are expressed in terms of erythromycin base (not the stearate salt).

### ERYTHROMYCIN STEARATE ORAL SUSPENSION

**Usual adult and adolescent dose**

Antibacterial—
Oral, 250 mg (base) every six hours; or 500 mg every twelve hours if twice a day dosage is desired.

Note: Chlamydial infections, endocervical and urethral—Oral, 500 mg (base) every six hours for seven days; or 250 mg every six hours for fourteen days. Erythromycin stearate may be used in pregnant women.

Endocarditis prophylaxis—Oral, 1 gram (base) two hours prior to the procedure, and 500 mg six hours after the initial dose.

Legionnaires' disease—Oral, 500 mg (base) to 1 gram every six hours.

Pelvic inflammatory disease, caused by *Neisseria gonorrhoeae*—Oral, 250 mg (base) every six hours for seven days, after intravenous administration of erythromycin 500 mg (base) every six hours for three days.

Streptococcal prophylaxis—Continuous prophylaxis of streptococcal infections in patients with a history of rheumatic heart disease: Oral, 250 mg (base) every twelve hours.

Syphilis, primary—Oral, 30 to 40 grams (base) over a ten- to fifteen-day period.

[Gastroparesis][1]—Oral, 150 to 250 mg (base) taken thirty minutes before meals, three times a day.

**Usual adult prescribing limits**

Antibacterial—
Up to 4 grams (base) daily.

**Usual pediatric dose**

Antibacterial—
Oral, 7.5 to 12.5 mg (base) per kg of body weight every six hours; or 15 to 25 mg per kg of body weight every twelve hours.

Severe infections, 15 to 25 mg (base) per kg of body weight every six hours.

Note: Conjunctivitis, chlamydial[1]—Oral, 12.5 mg (base) per kg of body weight every six hours for at least two weeks.

Endocarditis prophylaxis—Oral, 20 mg (base) per kg of body weight two hours prior to the procedure, and 10 mg per kg of body weight six hours after the initial dose.

Pertussis—Oral, 10 to 12.5 mg (base) per kg of body weight every six hours for fourteen days.

Pneumonia, chlamydial[1]—Oral, 12.5 mg (base) per kg of body weight every six hours for two weeks.

Streptococcal pharyngitis—Oral, 5 to 7.5 mg (base) per kg of body weight every six hours; or 10 to 15 mg per kg of body weight every twelve hours for at least ten days.

**Strength(s) usually available**

U.S.—
Not commercially available.

Canada—
125 mg per 5 mL (base) (Rx) [*Erythrocin* (parabens); *Novo-rythro*].
250 mg per 5 mL (base) (Rx) [*Erythrocin* (parabens); *Novo-rythro*].

**Packaging and storage**

Prior to reconstitution, store below 40 °C (104 °F), preferably between 15 and 30 °C (59 and 86 °F), unless otherwise specified by manufacturer. Store in a tight container.

**Auxiliary labeling**

- Refrigerate.
- Shake well.
- Continue medicine for full time of treatment.
- Beyond-use date.

**Note**

When dispensing, include a calibrated liquid-measuring device.

### ERYTHROMYCIN STEARATE TABLETS USP

**Usual adult and adolescent dose**

See *Erythromycin Stearate Oral Suspension*.

**Usual adult prescribing limits**

See *Erythromycin Stearate Oral Suspension*.

**Usual pediatric dose**

See *Erythromycin Stearate Oral Suspension*.

**Strength(s) usually available**

U.S.—
250 mg (base) (Rx) [*Erythrocin; Erythrocot; My-E; Wintrocin;* GENERIC].
500 mg (base) (Rx) [*Erythrocin;* GENERIC].

Canada—
250 mg (base) (Rx) [*Apo-Erythro-S; Erythrocin; Novo-rythro*].
500 mg (base) (Rx) [*Apo-Erythro-S; Erythrocin*].

**Packaging and storage**

Store below 40 °C (104 °F), preferably between 15 and 30 °C (59 and 86 °F), unless otherwise specified by manufacturer. Store in a tight container.

Note: Some manufacturers recommend storage in light-resistant containers to prevent discoloration.

**Auxiliary labeling**

- Continue medicine for full time of treatment.

[1]Not included in Canadian product labeling.

Revised: 07/22/94
Interim revision: 08/14/97

---

**ERYTHROMYCIN STEARATE**—See *Erythromycins (Systemic)*

---

# ERYTHROMYCIN AND SULFISOXAZOLE    Systemic

VA CLASSIFICATION (Primary): AM900

NOTE: The *Erythromycin and Sulfisoxazole (Systemic)* monograph is maintained on the USP DI electronic data base. For a printed copy of the most recent revision of the complete monograph, contact Micromedex, Inc. - Reprint Requests, 6200 S. Syracuse Way, Suite 300, Englewood, CO 80111; telephone (303) 486-6400; telefax (303) 486-6464; Email: USPDI@MDX.COM.

For information on the specific components of this combination, see the USP DI monographs for *Erythromycins (Systemic)* and *Sulfonamides (Systemic)*.

The information that follows is selectively abstracted from the complete monograph and is provided to facilitate drug use review and patient counseling.

Note: For a listing of dosage forms and brand names by country availability, see *Dosage Forms* section(s).

## Category
Antibacterial (systemic).

## Indications
Note: Bracketed information in the *Indications* section refers to uses that are not included in U.S. product labeling.

### Accepted
Otitis media, acute (treatment)—Erythromycin and sulfisoxazole combination is indicated in the treatment of acute otitis media caused by *Haemophilus influenzae*, [pneumococci, group A streptococci, and *Branhamella catarrhalis*] in children.

[Sinusitis (treatment)][1]—Erythromycin and sulfisoxazole combination is used in the treatment of acute sinusitis caused by *H. influenzae*, pneumococci, group A streptococci, and *B. catarrhalis* in children.

Not all species or strains of a particular organism may be susceptible to erythromycin and sulfisoxazole combination.

[1] Not included in Canadian product labeling.

## Patient Consultation
As an aid to patient consultation, refer to *Advice for the Patient, Erythromycin and Sulfisoxazole (Systemic)*.

In providing consultation, consider emphasizing the following selected information (» = major clinical significance):

### Before using this medication
» Conditions affecting use, especially:
  Allergy to erythromycins or sulfonamides; patients allergic to furosemide, thiazide diuretics, sulfonylureas, or carbonic anhydrase inhibitors may also be allergic to this medication
  Pregnancy—Erythromycin crosses the placenta; sulfisoxazole also crosses the placenta and should not be used at term because it may cause kernicterus in the infant; it has also been associated with cleft palates and skeletal defects in the offspring of mice and rats
  Breast-feeding—Erythromycins are distributed into breast milk in concentrations that may exceed maternal serum concentrations; sulfisoxazole is also distributed into breast-milk and is not recommended in nursing women since sulfonamides may cause kernicterus in nursing infants
  Use in children—Sulfonamides should not be used in children up to 2 months of age because they may cause kernicterus
  Dental—Systemic erythromycins may cause oral candidiasis; the leukopenic and thrombocytopenic effects of sulfonamides may result in an increased incidence of certain microbial infections, delayed healing, and gingival bleeding
  Other medications, especially alfentanil; coumarin- or indandione-derivative anticoagulants; hydantoin anticonvulsants; oral antidiabetic agents; carbamazepine; chloramphenicol; cyclosporine; other hemolytics; other hepatotoxic medications; lincomycins; methenamine; methotrexate; or xanthines, especially theophylline
  Other medical problems, especially blood dyscrasias, glucose-6-phosphate dehydrogenase (G6PD) deficiency, hepatic function impairment, porphyria, or renal function impairment

### Proper use of this medication
» Maintaining adequate fluid intake; taking with food
» Not giving to infants under 2 months of age
  Proper administration technique for oral liquids; not using after expiration date
» Compliance with full course of therapy
» Importance of not missing doses and taking at evenly spaced times
» Proper dosing
  Missed dose: Taking as soon as possible; not taking if almost time for next dose; not doubling dose
» Proper storage

### Precautions while using this medication
» Regular visits to physician to check blood counts, especially in long-term therapy
  Checking with physician if no improvement within a few days
» Possible photosensitivity reactions
  Using caution in use of regular toothbrushes, dental floss, and toothpicks; delaying dental work until blood counts have returned to normal; checking with physician or dentist concerning proper oral hygiene

### Side/adverse effects
Signs of potential side effects, especially blood dyscrasias, crystalluria, goiter, hematuria, hepatitis, hypersensitivity reactions, interstitial nephritis, Lyell's syndrome, Stevens-Johnson syndrome, thyroid function disturbance, and tubular necrosis

## Oral Dosage Forms

### ERYTHROMYCIN ETHYLSUCCINATE AND SULFISOXAZOLE ACETYL FOR ORAL SUSPENSION USP

**Usual adult and adolescent dose**
Use is not indicated in adults.

**Usual pediatric dose**
Antibacterial—
  Infants up to 2 months of age:
    Use is contraindicated since sulfonamides may cause kernicterus in neonates.
  Infants and children 2 months of age and over
    The dose can be calculated, based on either the equivalent of erythromycin or sulfisoxazole base, as follows:
      Oral, 12.5 mg (erythromycin) per kg of body weight every six hours for ten days; or
      Oral, 37.5 mg (sulfisoxazole) per kg of body weight every six hours for ten days.
  The following dosage schedule can also be used

| Body Weight | Dose (Every 6 hours) |
|---|---|
| Less than 8 kg (Less than 18 lb) | Adjust dosage by body weight |
| 8 kg (18 lb) | 1/2 teaspoonful (2.5 mL) |
| 16 kg (35 lb) | 1 teaspoonful (5 mL) |
| 24 kg (53 lb) | 1 1/2 teaspoonfuls (7.5 mL) |
| Over 45 kg (over 100 lb) | 2 teaspoonfuls (10 mL) |

Note: The maximum dose for children should not exceed 6 grams (sulfisoxazole) daily.

**Strength(s) usually available**
U.S.—
  200 mg of erythromycin and 600 mg of sulfisoxazole per 5 mL (when reconstituted according to manufacturer's instructions) (Rx) [*Eryzole; Pediazole; Sulfimycin;* GENERIC].
Canada—
  200 mg of erythromycin and 600 mg of sulfisoxazole per 5 mL (when reconstituted according to manufacturer's instructions) (Rx) [*Pediazole*].

**Auxiliary labeling**
- Refrigerate.
- Shake well.
- Take with water.
- Avoid too much sun or use of sunlamp.
- Continue medicine for full time of treatment.
- Beyond-use date.

Revised: 08/27/92
Interim revision: 03/18/94

---

# ESMOLOL Systemic†

VA CLASSIFICATION (Primary/Secondary): CV100/CV300
Commonly used brand name(s): *Brevibloc*.
Note: For a listing of dosage forms and brand names by country availability, see *Dosage Forms* section(s).

†Not commercially available in Canada.

## Category
Antiadrenergic; antiarrhythmic.

## Indications
Note: Bracketed information in the *Indications* section refers to uses that are not included in U.S. product labeling.

## Accepted

**Arrhythmias, cardiac (treatment)**—Esmolol is indicated for rapid and short-term control of ventricular rate in patients with atrial fibrillation or atrial flutter in perioperative, postoperative, or other emergency situations. It is also indicated in noncompensatory sinus tachycardia judged by the physician to need intervention. [Esmolol is used for control of heart rate in patients with myocardial ischemia.] It is not recommended for use in chronic situations where transfer to another agent is anticipated.

**Tachycardia, intraoperative and postoperative (treatment)**—Esmolol is indicated for the treatment of refractory tachycardia that occurs during surgery, on emergence from anesthesia, and in the postoperative period. It is recommended for use only when other treatable causes of tachycardia, such as bleeding or hypovolemia, have been ruled out.

**Hypertension, intraoperative and postoperative (treatment)**—Esmolol is indicated for the treatment of refractory hypertension that occurs during surgery, on emergence from anesthesia, and in the postoperative period. Esmolol is not considered to be a first-line agent and should be reserved for situations in which agents known to be effective in treating the etiology of the hypertension have failed. It is not recommended for use in patients with hypertension secondary to the vasoconstriction associated with hypothermia.

## Pharmacology/Pharmacokinetics

**Physicochemical characteristics**
Molecular weight—331.84.

**Mechanism of action/Effect**
Like other beta-blockers, esmolol blocks the agonistic effect of the sympathetic neurotransmitters by competing for receptor binding sites. Because it predominantly blocks the beta-1 receptors in cardiac tissue, it is said to be cardioselective. In general, so-called cardioselective beta-blockers are relatively cardioselective; at lower doses they block beta-1 receptors only but begin to block beta-2 receptors as the dose increases. At therapeutic dosages, esmolol does not have intrinsic sympathomimetic activity (ISA) or membrane-stabilizing (quinidine-like) activity.

Antiarrhythmic activity is due to blockade of adrenergic stimulation of cardiac pacemaker potentials. In the Vaughan Williams classification of antiarrhythmics, beta-blockers are considered to be class II agents.

**Protein binding**
Moderate (55%).

**Biotransformation**
Rapid hydrolysis by esterases in red blood cells to a free acid metabolite (with 1/1500 the activity of esmolol) and methanol.

**Half-life**
Esmolol—
  Distribution: Approximately 2 minutes.
  Elimination: Approximately 9 minutes.
Free acid metabolite—
  Approximately 3.7 hours (increased up to tenfold in renal failure).

**Time to steady-state blood concentration**
With loading dose—Within 5 minutes.
Without loading dose—Approximately 30 minutes.
Note: Use of a loading dose expedites achievement of constant plasma drug concentrations, but true steady-state occurs at 30 minutes, with or without a loading dose.

**Duration of action**
10 to 20 minutes after infusion is discontinued.

**Elimination**
Renal, almost entirely as metabolite.

## Precautions to Consider

**Carcinogenicity/Mutagenicity**
Studies have not been done in either animals or humans.

**Pregnancy/Reproduction**
Fertility—Studies have not been done in either animals or humans.

Pregnancy—Adequate and well-controlled studies in humans have not been done.
Studies in rats and rabbits at intravenous doses of up to 10 and 3 times the maximum human maintenance dose (MHMD), respectively, for 30 minutes daily showed no evidence of maternal toxicity, embryotoxicity, or teratogenicity. However, doses of approximately 30 and 8 times the MHMD in rats and rabbits, respectively, caused maternal toxicity, death, and increased fetal resorptions.

FDA Pregnancy Category C.

**Breast-feeding**
Although it is not known whether esmolol is distributed into human breast milk, problems have not been documented.

**Pediatrics**
Appropriate studies on the relationship of age to the effects of esmolol have not been performed in the pediatric population. However, limited experience with esmolol in the evaluation and management of pediatric tachyarrhythmias have not demonstrated pediatrics-specific problems that would limit the usefulness of esmolol in children.

**Geriatrics**
Although appropriate studies on the relationship of age to the effects of esmolol have not been performed in the geriatric population, the elderly may be less sensitive to some of the effects of beta-blockers. However, reduced metabolic and excretory capabilities in many elderly patients may lead to increased myocardial depression and require dosage reduction of beta-blockers. The net effect is uncertain; dosage adjustment should be based on clinical response.

**Drug interactions and/or related problems**
The following drug interactions and/or related problems have been selected on the basis of their potential clinical significance (possible mechanism in parentheses where appropriate)—not necessarily inclusive (» = major clinical significance):

Note: Combinations containing any of the following medications, depending on the amount present, may also interact with this medication.

Because of esmolol's short duration of action and the short periods of time over which it is used, many of the drug interactions associated with other beta-blockers do not apply.

» Antidiabetic agents, sulfonylurea or
» Insulin
  (esmolol may mask certain symptoms of developing hypoglycemia, such as increases in pulse rate and blood pressure)

Gallamine or
Metocurine or
Pancuronium or
Tubocurarine
  (esmolol may potentiate and prolong the action of nondepolarizing neuromuscular blocking agents when used concurrently; careful postoperative monitoring of the patient may be necessary following concurrent or sequential use, especially if there is a possibility of incomplete reversal of neuromuscular blockade)

Hypotension-producing medications, other (See *Appendix II*)
  (antihypertensive effects may be potentiated when these medications are used concurrently with esmolol; dosage adjustments should be based on blood pressure measurements)

» Monoamine oxidase (MAO) inhibitors, including furazolidone, procarbazine, and selegiline
  (possible significant hypertension may theoretically occur up to 14 days following discontinuation of the MAO inhibitor; although sufficient clinical reports are lacking, concurrent use with esmolol is not recommended)

Phenytoin
  (concurrent use of esmolol with intravenous phenytoin may produce additive cardiac depressant effects)

Reserpine
  (concurrent use with esmolol may result in additive and possibly excessive beta-adrenergic blockade; close observation is recommended since bradycardia and hypotension may occur)

» Sympathomimetics
  (concurrent use of esmolol with sympathomimetic amines having beta-adrenergic stimulant activity may result in mutual but short-lived inhibition of therapeutic effects)

» Xanthines, especially aminophylline or theophylline
  (concurrent use with esmolol may result in mutual inhibition of therapeutic effects; in addition, concurrent use of beta-blockers with the xanthines [except dyphylline] may decrease theophylline clearance, especially in patients with increased theophylline clearance induced by smoking; concurrent use requires careful monitoring)

**Medical considerations/Contraindications**
The medical considerations/contraindications included have been selected on the basis of their potential clinical significance (reasons given in parentheses where appropriate)—not necessarily inclusive (» = major clinical significance).

*Except under special circumstances, this medication should not be used when the following medical problems exist:*

- » Cardiac failure, overt or
- » Cardiogenic shock or
- » Heart block, 2nd- or 3rd-degree atrioventricular (AV) block or
- » Sinus bradycardia (heart rate less than 45 beats per minute)
    (risk of further myocardial depression; may be used with extreme caution in some patients with cardiac failure [e.g., high output failure associated with thyrotoxicosis])

*Risk-benefit should be considered when the following medical problems exist:*
- » Allergy, history of or
- » Asthma, bronchial or
- » Emphysema or nonallergenic bronchitis
    (esmolol may promote bronchospasm and block the bronchodilating effect of epinephrine; however, because esmolol is cardioselective and may be less likely to cause such effects than less cardioselective beta-blockers, it may be used with caution)
- » Congestive heart failure
    (risk of further depression of myocardial contractility)
- » Diabetes mellitus
    (all beta-blockers may mask tachycardia associated with hypoglycemia, but not dizziness and sweating)
  - Renal function impairment
  - Sensitivity to esmolol

**Patient monitoring**
The following may be especially important in patient monitoring (other tests may be warranted in some patients, depending on condition; » = major clinical significance):
- » Blood pressure and
- » Electrocardiogram (ECG) and
- » Heart rate
    (should be carefully monitored during intravenous administration)

## Side/Adverse Effects

The following side/adverse effects have been selected on the basis of their potential clinical significance (possible signs and symptoms in parentheses where appropriate)—not necessarily inclusive:

**Those indicating need for medical attention**
Incidence less frequent
  *Confusion; redness or swelling at place of injection; reduced peripheral circulation* (cold hands and feet)
Incidence rare
  *Bradycardia, especially less than 50 beats per minute; breathing difficulty and/or wheezing; chest pain; fainting; fever; mental depression*

**Those indicating need for medical attention only if they continue or are bothersome**
Incidence more frequent
  *Hypotension* (dizziness; sweating)—symptomatic in about 12% of patients, asymptomatic in about 25% of patients
  Note: *Hypotension* can occur at any dose, but is dose-related.
Incidence less frequent
  *Anxiety or nervousness; drowsiness or tiredness; flushing or pale skin; headache; nausea or vomiting*

## Overdose

For specific information on the agents used in the management of esmolol overdose, see:
- *Atropine* in *Anticholinergics/Antispasmodics (Systemic)* monograph;
- *Bronchodilators, Theophylline (Systemic)* monograph;
- *Glucagon (Systemic)* monograph;
- *Isoproterenol* in *Bronchodilators, Adrenergic (Systemic)* monograph;
- *Lidocaine (Systemic)* monograph; and/or
- *Sympathomimetic Agents—Cardiovascular Use (Parenteral-Systemic)* monograph.

For more information on the management of overdose or unintentional ingestion, **contact a Poison Control Center** (see *Poison Control Center Listing*).

**Clinical effects of overdose (in order of occurrence)**
The following effects have been selected on the basis of their potential clinical significance (possible signs and symptoms in parentheses where appropriate)—not necessarily inclusive:
  *Slow heartbeat; dizziness, severe, or fainting; drowsiness, severe; difficulty in breathing; bluish-colored fingernails or palms of hands; seizures*

**Treatment of overdose**
In most cases, symptoms of esmolol overdose disappear quickly after esmolol is withdrawn.

Specific treatment—
  Clinical reports are increasing for the successful use of glucagon to counteract the cardiovascular effects (bradycardia, hypotension) resulting from overdose with beta-blockers. An intravenous dose of 2 to 3 mg is administered over a period of 30 seconds and repeated if necessary, followed by an intravenous glucagon infusion at the rate of 5 mg per hour until the patient has been stabilized.
Supportive care—
  Bradycardia—Atropine sulfate may be administered intravenously to correct severe bradycardia if the patient is hypotensive. If vagal blockade is unresponsive, atropine may be repeated or intravenous isoproterenol or dobutamine may be given cautiously. Intravenous epinephrine or a transvenous pacemaker may be necessary.
  Premature ventricular contractions—Intravenous lidocaine or phenytoin (quinidine, procainamide, and disopyramide should be avoided since they may further depress myocardial function).
  Cardiac failure—Provision of oxygen. Digitalization of patient and/or administration of diuretic.
  Hypotension—Trendelenburg position and intravenous fluids (unless pulmonary edema is present). Intravenous administration of a vasopressor such as epinephrine, norepinephrine, dopamine, or dobutamine (some reports indicate epinephrine may be the agent of choice). Serial monitoring of blood pressure. Hypotension does not respond to beta-2 agonists. (See *Drug interactions and/or related problems* for precautions in use of sympathomimetic vasopressors.)
  Bronchospasm—Administration of a beta-2 agonist such as isoproterenol and/or a theophylline derivative.

## General Dosing Information

The 250-mg-per-mL strength of esmolol hydrochloride injection must be diluted before it is administered by intravenous infusion. Concentrations of greater than 10 mg of esmolol hydrochloride per mL may produce irritation. The 10-mg-per-mL strength may be given by direct infusion.

If a reaction occurs at the infusion site, the infusion should be stopped and resumed at another site. Use of butterfly needles for administration is not recommended.
  To convert to other antiarrhythmic therapy after control has been achieved with esmolol
  —30 minutes after administration of the first dose of the alternative agent, infusion rate of esmolol should be reduced by one-half, and
  —after the second dose of the alternative agent, if a satisfactory response is maintained for 1 hour, esmolol should be discontinued.

**For treatment of adverse effects**
Hypotension is usually reversed within 30 minutes after dosage reduction or withdrawal of esmolol.

Dosage reduction or withdrawal of esmolol is recommended at the first sign of congestive heart failure.

## Parenteral Dosage Forms

### ESMOLOL HYDROCHLORIDE INJECTION

**Usual adult dose**
Antiarrhythmic—
  Dosage is established by means of a series of loading and maintenance doses
    Loading: Intravenous infusion, 500 mcg (0.5 mg) per kg of body weight per minute for one minute, followed by
    Maintenance: Intravenous infusion, 50 mcg (0.05 mg) per kg of body weight per minute for four minutes.
  If an adequate response is observed at the end of five minutes, the infusion dosage should be maintained with periodic adjustments as needed.
  If an adequate response is not observed at the end of the five minutes, the sequence is repeated with an increment of 50 mcg (0.05 mg) per kg of body weight per minute in the maintenance dose
    Loading: Intravenous infusion, 500 mcg (0.5 mg) per kg of body weight per minute for one minute, followed by
    Maintenance: Intravenous infusion, 100 mcg (0.1 mg) per kg of body weight per minute for four minutes.
  The sequence is repeated until an adequate response is obtained, with an increment of 50 mcg (0.05 mg) per kg of body weight per minute in the maintenance dose at each step. As the desired end-point (defined by desired heart rate or undesirable decrease in blood pressure) is approached, the loading dose may be omitted and increments in the maintenance dose reduced to 25 mcg (0.025 mg) per kg of body weight per minute or less. If desired, the interval between titration steps may be increased from five to ten minutes. The established

maintenance dose usually does not exceed 200 mcg (0.2 mg) per kg of body weight per minute and can be given for up to forty-eight hours.
- Note: Because of the time required for titration, the above dosage regimen may not be optimal for intraoperative use.

Tachycardia, intraoperative or postoperative or
Hypertension, intraoperative or postoperative—
- Initial: Intravenous, 250 to 500 mcg (0.25 to 0.5 mg) per kg of body weight over one minute.
- Maintenance: Intravenous infusion, 50 mcg (0.05 mg) per kg of body weight per minute for four minutes.
- If an adequate response is not observed, the sequence may be repeated, with an increment of 50 mcg (0.05 mg) per kg of body weight per minute in the maintenance dose
- Initial: Intravenous, 250 to 500 mcg (0.25 to 0.5 mg) per kg of body weight over one minute.
- Maintenance: Intravenous infusion, 100 mcg (0.1 mg) per kg of body weight per minute for four minutes.

The sequence may be repeated up to four times if needed, with an increment of 50 mcg (0.05 mg) per kg of body weight per minute in the maintenance dose at each step.

### Usual adult prescribing limits
Maintenance—Up to 200 mcg (0.2 mg) per kg of body weight per minute (because of the risk of hypotension).

### Usual pediatric dose
Arrhythmias, supraventricular—
- Intravenous infusion, 50 mcg (0.05 mg) per kg of body weight per minute; dosage may be titrated upwards every ten minutes up to 300 mcg (0.3 mg) per kg of body weight per minute.

### Strength(s) usually available
U.S.—
- 10 mg per mL (100 mg per 10-mL single-dose vial) (Rx) [*Brevibloc*].
- Note: The 10-mg-per-mL strength is prediluted and may be used for the loading dose.
- 250 mg per mL (2500 mg per 10-mL ampul) (Rx) [*Brevibloc* (alcohol 25%)].
- Note: The 250-mg-per-mL strength must be diluted before use. It is not intended for direct intravenous injection.

Canada—
Not commercially available.

### Packaging and storage
Store below 40 °C (104 °F), preferably between 15 and 30 °C (59 and 86 °F), unless otherwise specified by manufacturer. Not adversely affected by freezing.

### Preparation of dosage form
Esmolol hydrochloride injection (250-mg-per-mL strength) is prepared for administration by intravenous infusion by aseptically removing 20 mL from a 500-mL bottle of intravenous fluid (5% dextrose injection, 5% dextrose in Ringer's injection, 5% dextrose and 0.45% sodium chloride injection, 5% dextrose and 0.9% sodium chloride injection, lactated Ringer's injection, 0.45% sodium chloride injection, or 0.9% sodium chloride injection) and then adding 5 grams of esmolol hydrochloride injection to the bottle, producing a solution containing 10 mg of esmolol hydrochloride per mL.

### Stability
Diluted solutions of esmolol hydrochloride are stable for at least 24 hours at room temperature.

### Incompatibilities
Not compatible with 5% sodium bicarbonate injection.

### Auxiliary labeling
For 250-mg-per-mL vial
- Must be diluted before administration.

### Caution
Confusion caused by two significantly different concentrations of esmolol has resulted in massive overdoses, including several deaths. The incidents occurred when the 250-mg-per-mL ampul, which requires dilution prior to administration, was given undiluted. The 250-mg-per-mL ampul of esmolol must be diluted before administration. Caution should be utilized when dispensing, using, and storing this medication.

## Selected Bibliography
Angaran DM, Schultz NJ, Tschida VH. Esmolol hydrochloride: an ultrashort-acting, beta-adrenergic blocking agent. Clin Pharm 1986 Apr; 5: 288-303.
Murthy VS, Frishman WH. Controlled beta-receptor blockade with esmolol and flestolol. Pharmacother 1988; 8(3): 168-82.
Covinsky JO. Esmolol: a novel cardioselective, titratable, intravenous beta-blocker with ultrashort half-life. DICP, Ann Pharmacother 1987; 21: 316-21.

Revised: 09/13/94
Interim revision: 04/19/96

---

**ESTAZOLAM**—See *Benzodiazepines (Systemic)*

---

**ESTRADIOL**—See *Estrogens (Systemic)*; *Estrogens (Vaginal)*

---

# ESTRAMUSTINE  Systemic

VA CLASSIFICATION (Primary): AN900
Commonly used brand name(s): *Emcyt*.
Note: For a listing of dosage forms and brand names by country availability, see *Dosage Forms* section(s).

## Category
Antineoplastic.

## Indications
### Accepted
Carcinoma, prostatic (treatment)—Estramustine is indicated for palliative treatment of metastatic, progressive, and/or [hormone-refractory][1] (Evidence rating: IA) carcinoma of the prostate gland.

[1]Not included in Canadian product labeling.

## Pharmacology/Pharmacokinetics
### Physicochemical characteristics
Molecular weight—Estramustine phosphate sodium: 582.36.

### Mechanism of action/Effect
Exact mechanism of antineoplastic action is unknown. Structurally, estramustine is a phosphorylated combination of estradiol and mechlorethamine (nitrogen mustard). However, estramustine has very weak alkylating activity and may be effective in some patients refractory to estrogen therapy. Therefore, its antineoplastic activity may be due to the estrogen component, a direct effect of estramustine or one of its metabolites, other antimitotic activity, or a combination of effects. Prolonged use elevates total plasma estradiol concentrations to within ranges similar to those produced in prostatic carcinoma patients given conventional estradiol therapy. Estrogenic effects (changes in circulating concentrations of steroids and pituitary hormones) are also similar to those produced by estradiol. A suppressive effect on the hypothalamic-hypophyseal-gonadal axis with a resultant reduction in serum testosterone concentrations may also be involved. Estramustine is highly localized in prostatic tissue because of binding to an estramustine-specific protein.

### Absorption
Well absorbed (up to 75%) from the gastrointestinal tract; impaired by milk, milk products, and other substances high in calcium.

### Biotransformation
Rapidly dephosphorylated during absorption into peripheral circulation, then estramustine is oxidized and hydrolyzed to estromustine, with low levels of estradiol and estrone, and to mechlorethamine; metabolism is by conjugation in the liver.

### Half-life
Multiphasic; 20 hours (terminal phase).

### Elimination
Biliary/fecal; renal (minor). The metabolites derived from estramustine phosphate are excreted at a slower rate than the native agent.

## Precautions to Consider

### Cross-sensitivity and/or related problems
Patients sensitive to estradiol or mechlorethamine may be sensitive to estramustine also.

### Carcinogenicity/Mutagenicity
Secondary malignancies are potential delayed effects of many antineoplastic agents, although it is not clear whether the effect is related to their mutagenic or immunosuppressive action. The effect of dose and duration of therapy is also unknown, although risk seems to increase with long-term use. Although information is limited, available data seem to indicate that the carcinogenic risk is greatest with the alkylating agents.

Studies with estramustine have not been done. Antimitotic agents have been associated with an increased risk of development of secondary carcinomas in humans. Long-term continuous administration of estrogens in some animals has been associated with an increased frequency of carcinomas of the breast and liver. Compounds structurally similar to estramustine are carcinogenic in mice.

Although estramustine was not found to be mutagenic in Ames tests, both estradiol and nitrogen mustard alone are mutagenic.

### Pregnancy/Reproduction
*Fertility*—Gonadal suppression, resulting in azoospermia, has been reported in patients taking estramustine. These effects appear to be related to dose and length of therapy and may be irreversible. On the other hand, patients impotent from previous therapy may regain potency when taking estramustine.

Antimitotic agents have been reported to cause alterations in sperm cells that could result in mutagenicity and teratogenicity.

*Pregnancy*—Because of the possibility of mutagenic effects, patients or their partners should be advised to use contraceptive measures.

### Geriatrics
Appropriate studies on the relationship of age to the effects of estramustine have not been performed in the geriatric population. However, elderly patients are more likely to have age-related renal function impairment and/or peripheral vascular disease, which may require caution in patients receiving estrogens.

### Drug interactions and/or related problems
The following drug interactions and/or related problems have been selected on the basis of their potential clinical significance (possible mechanism in parentheses where appropriate)—not necessarily inclusive (» = major clinical significance):

Note: Combinations containing any of the following medications, depending on the amount present, may also interact with this medication.

Calcium-containing medications or
Calcium supplements
 (calcium binds with estramustine in the gastrointestinal tract and forms an insoluble calcium phosphate salt, which is not absorbed; simultaneous administration should be avoided)

Corticosteroids, glucocorticoid
 (concurrent use with estrogens may alter the metabolism and protein binding of the glucocorticoids, leading to decreased clearance, increased elimination half-life, and increased therapeutic and toxic effects of the glucocorticoids; glucocorticoid dosage adjustment may be required during and following concurrent use)

Corticotropin (chronic therapeutic use)
 (concurrent use with estrogens may potentiate the anti-inflammatory effects of endogenous cortisol [adrenal secretion of endogenous cortisol is increased by corticotropin])

» Hepatotoxic medications (see *Appendix II*)
 (concurrent use of these medications with estrogens may increase the risk of hepatotoxicity)

» Smoking, tobacco
 (not recommended during estrogen therapy because of the increased risk of serious cardiovascular side effects, including cerebrovascular accident, transient ischemic attacks, thrombophlebitis, and pulmonary embolism; risk increases with increasing tobacco usage and with age)

Vaccines, killed virus
 (because normal defense mechanisms may be suppressed by estramustine therapy, the patient's antibody response to the vaccine may be decreased. The interval between discontinuation of medications that cause immunosuppression and restoration of the patient's ability to respond to the vaccine depends on the intensity and type of immunosuppression-causing medication used, the underlying disease, and other factors; estimates vary from 3 months to 1 year)

Vaccines, live virus
 (because normal defense mechanisms may be suppressed by estramustine therapy, concurrent use with a live virus vaccine may potentiate the replication of the vaccine virus, may increase the side/adverse effects of the vaccine virus, and/or may decrease the patient's antibody response to the vaccine; immunization of these patients should be undertaken only with extreme caution after careful review of the patient's hematologic status and only with the knowledge and consent of the physician managing the estramustine therapy. The interval between discontinuation of medications that cause immunosuppression and restoration of the patient's ability to respond to the vaccine depends on the intensity and type of immunosuppression-causing medication used, the underlying disease, and other factors; estimates vary from 3 months to 1 year. Immunization with oral poliovirus vaccine should be postponed in persons in close contact with the patient, especially family members)

### Laboratory value alterations
The following have been selected on the basis of their potential clinical significance (possible effect in parentheses where appropriate)—not necessarily inclusive (» = major clinical significance):

With diagnostic test results

» Metyrapone test
 (reduced response)

Norepinephrine-induced platelet aggregability
 (may be increased)

Sulfobromophthalein (BSP) test
 (increased BSP retention)

Thyroid function test
 (protein-bound thyroxine [$T_4$] is increased; serum free $T_4$ concentrations may be unchanged or decreased; triiodothyronine [$T_3$] serum resin uptake is decreased, because estrogens increase serum thyroid-binding globulin [TBG]; serum $T_3$ may be increased)

With physiology/laboratory test values
Alanine aminotransferase (AST [SGOT]) values, and
Bilirubin concentrations, serum and
Lactate dehydrogenase (LDH) values
 (may be increased)

Antithrombin 3 concentrations and
Folate concentrations, serum and
Pregnanediol excretion and
Pyridoxine concentrations
 (may be decreased)

Ceruloplasmin and
Cortisol and
Glucose and
Phospholipids and
Prolactin and
Prothrombin and clotting factors VII, VIII, IX, and X and
Sodium and
Triglycerides
 (serum concentrations may be increased)

Phosphate
 (serum concentrations may be decreased)

### Medical considerations/Contraindications
The medical considerations/contraindications included have been selected on the basis of their potential clinical significance (reasons given in parentheses where appropriate)—not necessarily inclusive (» = major clinical significance).

Note: Estramustine may be poorly metabolized in patients with impaired liver function and should be administered with caution in such patients. Estramustine also may influence the metabolism of calcium and phosphorus. Therefore, it should be used with caution in patients who have metabolic bone diseases that are associated with hypercalcemia and in patients with renal insufficiency.

*Except under special circumstances, this medication should not be used when the following medical problems exist:*

» Hypersensitivity to estramustine or
» Hypersensitivity to estradiol or
» Hypersensitivity to mechlorethamine
 (estramustine is a molecule combining estradiol and normechlorethamine by a carbamate link. It should not be used if the patient is known to be hypersensitive to either estradiol or nitrogen mustard)

» Thromboembolic disorders, active, including recent myocardial infarction or stroke or
» Thrombophlebitis, active
 (may be aggravated by estrogen component; an exception may be made when the actual tumor mass is the cause of the thromboembolic phenomenon)

*Risk-benefit should be considered when the following medical problems exist:*

Asthma or
Cardiac insufficiency or
Epilepsy or
Mental depression, or history of or
Migraine headaches or
Renal function impairment
(fluid retention sometimes caused by estrogen component may aggravate these conditions)
Bone disease, metabolic, associated with hypercalcemia or
Renal insufficiency
(estrogens influence metabolism of calcium and phosphorus)
Bone marrow depression, moderate to severe
Cerebrovascular disease or
Coronary artery disease or
» Thrombophlebitis, thrombosis, or thromboembolic disorders, history of, especially if associated with estrogen therapy
(risk of thromboembolic disorders caused by estrogens)
» Chickenpox, existing or recent (including recent exposure) or
» Herpes zoster
(risk of severe generalized disease)
Cholestatic jaundice, history of, including previous jaundice that occurred with estrogens or as a reaction to other medication
Diabetes mellitus
(glucose tolerance may be decreased)
Gallbladder disease, or history of, especially gallstones
Hepatic function impairment
(reduced metabolism and possible hepatotoxicity)
» Hypercalcemia associated with metastatic breast disease
» Peptic ulcer

**Patient monitoring**
The following are especially important in patient monitoring (other tests may be warranted in some patients, depending on condition (» = major clinical significance):

Acid phosphatase values, serum and/or
Alkaline phosphatase values, serum
(to assess response; elevated values should be reduced)
Blood counts, complete and
Platelet counts
(may be appropriate at periodic intervals, although leukopenia and thrombocytopenia are rare with estramustine)
Blood pressure and
Hepatic function
(determinations recommended at periodic intervals)
Calcium concentrations, serum and
Phosphate concentrations, serum
(recommended at periodic intervals, especially in patients with bone metastases)

## Side/Adverse Effects

The following side/adverse effects have been selected on the basis of their potential clinical significance (possible signs and symptoms in parentheses where appropriate)—not necessarily inclusive):

**Those indicating need for medical attention**
Incidence more frequent
*Sodium and fluid retention* (swelling of feet or lower legs)
Incidence rare
*Allergic reaction* (skin rash or fever); *anemia* (unusual tiredness or weakness); *leukopenia* (fever or chills; cough or hoarseness; lower back or side pain; painful or difficult urination)—usually asymptomatic; *thrombocytopenia* (unusual bleeding or bruising; black, tarry stools; blood in urine or stools; pinpoint red spots on skin)—usually asymptomatic; *thrombosis* (severe or sudden headaches; sudden loss of coordination; pains in chest, groin, or leg, especially calf of leg; sudden and unexplained shortness of breath; sudden slurred speech; sudden vision changes; weakness or numbness in arm or leg)

**Those indicating need for medical attention only if they continue or are bothersome**
Incidence more frequent
*Breast tenderness or enlargement*—incidence 20 to 50%; *decreased interest in sex*—occurs in most patients; *diarrhea*—incidence 20 to 50%; *nausea*—incidence 20 to 50%

Incidence less frequent
*Trouble in sleeping; vomiting*
Note: *Vomiting* is intolerable in approximately 8% of patients.

## Overdose

For more information on the management of overdose or unintentional ingestion, **contact a Poison Control Center** (see *Poison Control Center Listing*).

**Clinical effects of overdose**
There has been no documented experience with estramustine overdose. However, it is reasonable to expect that such episodes may produce pronounced manifestations of the known adverse reactions.

**Treatment of overdose**
Treatment of overdose is symptomatic and supportive.
To decrease absorption—Removal of gastric contents by gastric lavage.
Monitoring—Monitoring of hematologic and hepatic parameters for at least 6 weeks.

## Patient Consultation

As an aid to patient consultation, refer to *Advice for the Patient, Estramustine (Systemic)*.
In providing consultation, consider emphasizing the following selected information (» = major clinical significance):

**Before using this medication**
» Conditions affecting use, especially:
Hypersensitivity to estramustine, estradiol, or mechlorethamine
Pregnancy—It is recommended that patients or their partners use contraceptive measures
Other medications, especially hepatotoxic medications
Other medical problems, especially chickenpox, herpes zoster, hypercalcemia, peptic ulcer, active or history of thromboembolic disorders (including recent myocardial infarction or stroke), or active or history of thrombophlebitis

**Proper use of this medication**
» Importance of not taking more or less medication than the amount prescribed
For best results, taking 1 hour before or 2 hours after meals or milk or milk products
» Frequently causes nausea and sometimes causes vomiting; checking with physician before discontinuing medication
Checking with physician if vomiting occurs shortly after dose is taken
» Proper dosing
Missed dose: Not taking at all; not doubling doses
» Proper storage

**Precautions while using this medication**
» Importance of close monitoring by physician
» Avoiding immunizations unless approved by physician; other persons in patient's household should avoid immunizations with oral poliovirus vaccine; avoiding persons who have taken oral poliovirus vaccine or wearing a protective mask that covers nose and mouth

**Side/adverse effects**
Signs of potential side effects, especially sodium and fluid retention, allergic reaction, anemia, leukopenia, thrombocytopenia, and thrombosis

## General Dosing Information

Patients receiving estramustine should be under supervision of a physician experienced in cancer chemotherapy.

Patients should be treated for 30 to 90 days before the physician determines the possible benefits of continued therapy. Therapy should be continued as long as the response to estramustine is favorable. Some patients have been maintained on therapy for more than 3 years at doses ranging from 10 to 16 mg per kg of body weight (mg/kg) per day.

Nausea and vomiting sometimes responds to treatment with phenothiazines but may be severe enough to necessitate withdrawal of estramustine in some patients.

**Diet/Nutrition**
Patients should be instructed to take estramustine at least 1 hour before or 2 hours after meals. Estramustine should be swallowed with water. Milk, milk products, or calcium-rich foods or medications should not be taken simultaneously with estramustine.

## Oral Dosage Forms

### ESTRAMUSTINE PHOSPHATE SODIUM CAPSULES

**Usual adult dose**
Carcinoma, prostatic—
  Oral, 600 mg (base) per square meter of body surface area per day in three divided doses (one hour before or two hours after meals) or 14 mg per kg of body weight (range 10 to 16 mg per kg) per day in three or four divided doses (one hour before or two hours after meals).

**Strength(s) usually available**
U.S.—
  140 mg (base) (Rx) [*Emcyt*].
Canada—
  140 mg (base) (Rx) [*Emcyt*].

**Packaging and storage**
Store between 2 and 8 °C (36 and 46 °F), in a tight container, unless otherwise specified by the manufacturer. Protect from light.

**Auxiliary labeling**
- Take 1 hour before or 2 hours after meals.
- Avoid milk or milk products.

Revised: 09/29/97
Interim revision: 06/24/98

# ESTROGENS  Systemic

This monograph includes information on the following: 1) Conjugated Estrogens; 2) Diethylstilbestrol; 3) Esterified Estrogens; 4) Estradiol; 5) Estrone†; 6) Estropipate; 7) Ethinyl Estradiol.

INN:
  Diethylstilbestrol diphosphate—Fosfestrol

BAN:
  Diethylstilbestrol diphosphate—Fosfestrol
  Diethylstilbestrol—Stilboestrol
  Estradiol—Oestradiol
  Estrone—Oestrone

JAN:
  Diethylstilbestrol diphosphate—Fosfestrol

VA CLASSIFICATION (Primary/Secondary):
  Conjugated Estrogens—HS102/AN500; HS104; MS900
  Diethylstilbestrol—HS102/AN500; HS104; MS900
  Esterified Estrogens—HS102/AN500; MS900
  Estradiol—HS102/AN500; MS900
  Estrone—HS102/AN500
  Estropipate—HS102/MS900
  Ethinyl Estradiol—HS102/AN500; HS104; MS900

Commonly used brand name(s): *Alora*[4]; *Aquest*[5]; *C.E.S.*[1]; *Climara*[4]; *Clinagen LA 40*[4]; *Congest*[1]; *Delestrogen*[4]; *Depo-Estradiol*[4]; *Depogen*[4]; *Dioval 40*[4]; *Dioval XX*[4]; *Dura-Estrin*[4]; *Duragen-20*[4]; *E-Cypionate*[4]; *Estinyl*[7]; *Estra-L 40*[4]; *Estrace*[4]; *Estraderm*[4]; *Estragyn 5*[5]; *Estragyn LA 5*[4]; *Estratab*[3]; *Estro-A*[5]; *Estro-Cyp*[4]; *Estro-L.A.*[4]; *Estro-Span*[4]; *Estrofem*[4]; *Estrone '5'*[5]; *FemPatch*[4]; *Femogex*[4]; *Gynogen L.A. 20*[4]; *Gynogen L.A. 40*[4]; *Honvol*[2]; *Kestrone-5*[5]; *Menaval-20*[4]; *Menest*[3]; *Neo-Estrone*[3]; *Ogen*[6]; *Ogen .625*[6]; *Ogen 1.25*[6]; *Ogen 2.5*[6]; *Ortho-Est .625*[6]; *Ortho-Est 1.25*[6]; *Premarin*[1]; *Premarin Intravenous*[1]; *Stilbestrol*[2]; *Stilphostrol*[2]; *Valergen-10*[4]; *Valergen-20*[4]; *Valergen-40*[4]; *Vivelle*[4]; *Wehgen*[5]; *depGynogen*[4].

Other commonly used names are: DES [Diethylstilbestrol], Fosfestrol [Diethylstilbestrol diphosphate], Oestradiol [Estradiol], Oestrone [Estrone], Piperazine Estrone Sulfate [Estropipate], and Stilboestrol [Diethylstilbestrol].

Note: For a listing of dosage forms and brand names by country availability, see *Dosage Forms* section(s).

†Not commercially available in Canada.

## Category

Estrogen (systemic)—Conjugated Estrogens; Diethylstilbestrol; Esterified Estrogens; Estradiol; Estrone; Estropipate; Ethinyl Estradiol.
Antineoplastic—Conjugated Estrogens Tablets; Diethylstilbestrol; Esterified Estrogens; Estradiol; Estradiol Valerate; Estrone; Ethinyl Estradiol.
Osteoporosis prophylactic—Conjugated Estrogens Tablets; Esterified Estrogens; Estradiol Tablets; Estradiol Transdermal System; Estropipate.
Ovarian hormone therapy agent—Conjugated Estrogens Tablets; Esterified Estrogens; Estradiol Tablets; Estradiol Transdermal System; Estropipate.

## Indications

Note: Bracketed information in the *Indications* section refers to uses that are not included in U.S. product labeling.

**General considerations**
Estrogen deficiency in women without a uterus is best treated with unopposed estrogen therapy; combined estrogen-progestin therapy is not needed.

**Accepted**
Bleeding, uterine, hormonal imbalance–induced (treatment)—Conjugated estrogens for injection and estrone are indicated in the treatment of abnormal uterine bleeding associated with a hypoplastic or atrophic endometrium without organic pathology. Continuous treatment with estrogen without a progestin may cause abnormal uterine bleeding with or without organic pathology.

Carcinoma, breast (treatment)—Conjugated estrogens tablets, esterified estrogens[1], estradiol tablets[1], and ethinyl estradiol are indicated for palliative treatment of metastatic breast carcinoma in selected men and postmenopausal or oophorectomized women.

Carcinoma, prostatic (treatment)—Conjugated estrogens tablets, diethylstilbestrol, esterified estrogens[1], estradiol tablets[1], estradiol valerate, estrone, and ethinyl estradiol are indicated for treatment of advanced prostatic carcinoma.

Estrogen deficiency, due to ovariectomy (treatment) or
Hypogonadism, female (treatment) or
Ovarian failure, primary (treatment)—Conjugated estrogens tablets, esterified estrogens, estradiol tablets[1], matrix-[1] or reservoir-type estradiol transdermal system, estrone, estropipate[1], and ethinyl estradiol[1] are indicated to replace estrogen in the treatment of female hypogonadism, primary ovarian failure, or ovariectomy. Estradiol cypionate and estradiol valerate[1] are indicated to replace estrogen in the treatment of female hypogonadism. Estradiol valerate also is indicated for the treatment of estrogen deficiency resulting from an ovariectomy or primary ovarian failure.

Menopause, vasomotor symptoms of (treatment) or
Vaginitis, atrophic (treatment) or
Vulvar atrophy (treatment)—Conjugated estrogens tablets, esterified estrogens, estradiol tablets, matrix- or reservoir-type estradiol transdermal system, estradiol valerate, estrone, and estropipate are indicated to replace estrogen in the treatment of atrophic vaginitis, vulvar atrophy (also called kraurosis vulvae), and moderate to severe vasomotor symptoms associated with menopause. Also, estradiol cypionate and ethinyl estradiol are indicated for treatment of moderate to severe vasomotor symptoms of menopause.

Osteoporosis, postmenopausal (prophylaxis)—Conjugated estrogens tablets, esterified estrogens[1], estradiol tablets, [matrix-][1] or reservoir-type estradiol transdermal system, and estropipate[1] are indicated in postmenopausal women to retard bone loss and estrogen deficiency–induced osteoporosis. Replacing estrogen can reduce the rate of bone loss and fractures in postmenopausal women. Proper diet, calcium supplementation, and physical activity should also be encouraged along with estrogen replacement therapy.

[Osteoporosis, premenopausal, estrogen deficiency–induced (prophylaxis)][1]—Conjugated estrogens tablets, esterified estrogens, estradiol tablets, matrix- or reservoir-type estradiol transdermal systems, and estropipate also are used in premenopausal women who are estrogen-deficient to protect them against bone loss.

[Atherosclerotic disease (prophylaxis)][1]—Estrogens may be effective in the prevention of cardiovascular disease in postmenopausal women.

[Turner's syndrome (treatment)][1]—Ethinyl estradiol is used in the treatment of Turner's syndrome (gonadal dysgenesis).

**Acceptance not established**
Conjugated estrogens, diethylstilbestrol tablets, and ethinyl estradiol have been used as *emergency contraception* (also called interception, morning-after treatment, or postcoital contraception). However, the combination oral contraceptive containing ethinyl estradiol with either norgestrel or levonorgestrel is more commonly prescribed for this indication. Although the failure rate for postcoital contraception is higher (2%

versus 1%) for these oral estrogen-progestin contraceptives compared to these estrogens used alone, the oral contraceptives cause fewer and less severe side effects (such as nausea or vomiting) and have better patient compliance.

**Unaccepted**
The use of estrogens to reduce postpartum breast engorgement is not recommended. In many patients, postpartum breast engorgement is a benign, self-limited condition that may respond to breast support and mild analgesics, such as acetaminophen and ibuprofen. Evidence supporting the efficacy of estrogens for this indication is lacking. Therefore, the questionable benefits of administering the large doses of estrogens required for this indication are outweighed by the risk of increasing the incidence of puerperal thromboembolism.

Although a few studies show estrogens having some effect on brain neurotransmitters in improving memory and cognitive function, estrogens are not indicated or effective in treatment of clinical mental depression.

Estradiol valerate, ethinyl estradiol, and the matrix-type estradiol transdermal system are indicated to treat abnormal uterine bleeding due to a hormonal imbalance but are not recommended. These estrogens are considered obsolete for this use.

Although estradiol valerate and estrone are indicated for palliative treatment of breast carcinoma, both have a long duration of action, making discontinuation of the medication or management of hypercalcemia more difficult if hypercalcemia develops. These estrogens are not recommended. These estrogens are considered obsolete for this use.

[1]Not included in Canadian product labeling.

## Pharmacology/Pharmacokinetics

**Physicochemical characteristics**
Physical description
Two types of estradiol transdermal systems are available:
Drug-in-adhesive matrix on film (ethylene vinyl acetate and rubber) (matrix-type)—Three layers that include a polyester liner that must be removed before using, an adhesive matrix containing estradiol, and the back outermost layer, a flexible polyurethane protective film with epoxy resin.
Membrane-controlled drug reservoir (reservoir-type)—Five layers that include a protective liner to be removed before using, an adhesive layer, a membrane providing a slow release of estradiol, a drug reservoir containing the estradiol and alcohol gelled with hydroxypropyl cellulose, and the back outermost layer, a polyester protective film.
Patch size may differ for products among different manufacturers and among products of different strengths from the same manufacturer. Generally, the matrix-type transdermal system is smaller and thinner than the reservoir-type transdermal system.
Source—
Naturally occurring compounds include estradiol ($E_2$), conjugated estrogens (sodium estrone sulfate, sodium equilin sulfate, and others as found in equine urine), esterified estrogens (sodium sulfate esters of estrogenic substances, primarily estrone), and estrone ($E_1$).
Semisynthetic compounds include estradiol cypionate, estradiol valerate, estropipate, and ethinyl estradiol.
Synthetic compounds include diethylstilbestrol and diethylstilbestrol phosphate.
Molecular weight—
Diethylstilbestrol: 268.36.
Diethylstilbestrol diphosphate: 428.32.
Estradiol: 272.39.
Estradiol cypionate: 396.57.
Estradiol valerate: 356.51.
Estrone: 270.37.
Estropipate: 436.58.
Ethinyl estradiol: 296.41.

**Mechanism of action/Effect**
At the cellular level, estrogens increase the synthesis of DNA, RNA, and various proteins in target tissues. Pituitary mass is also increased. Estrogens reduce the release of gonadotropin-releasing hormone from the hypothalamus, leading to a reduction in release of follicle-stimulating hormone and luteinizing hormone from the pituitary.
For ovarian hormone therapy—
In healthy females, endogenous estrogens maintain genitourinary function and vasomotor stability. Replacing estrogens helps to alleviate or prevent symptoms caused by the decreased amounts of estrogens produced by the ovaries after natural or surgical menopause or other estrogen-deficiency states.

For prevention of postmenopausal osteoporosis—
During periods of estrogen deficiency, the rate of bone resorption by osteoclasts greatly exceeds the rate of bone formation by osteoblasts. Replacing estrogen prevents this accelerated bone loss by inhibiting bone resorption to a level where the near equilibrium between bone resorption and formation is restored. However, estrogens do not replace previously lost bone or significantly increase total bone mass.
For prostatic carcinoma—
Inhibition of pituitary secretion of luteinizing hormone and a possible minor, direct effect on the testis, resulting in decreased serum concentrations of testosterone.

**Distribution**
To most tissues, especially breast, uterine, vaginal, hypothalamic, and pituitary tissues; high affinity for adipose tissue.

**Protein binding**
Moderate to high (50 to 80% to albumin and sex hormone–binding globulin).

**Biotransformation**
Primarily hepatic; some metabolism also occurs in muscle, kidneys, and gonads. The metabolic sites for all synthetic estrogens have not been completely determined, although some seem to undergo hepatic change.

**Elimination**
Primarily renal excretion of metabolites, some fecal; undergo extensive enterohepatic recirculation. Prolonged in obese patients.

## Precautions to Consider

**Carcinogenicity**
Independent studies have shown an increased risk of endometrial cancer in postmenopausal women placed on unopposed (without a progestin) estrogen therapy for prolonged periods. The risk of endometrial cancer in estrogen users, which appears to depend on duration of treatment and dose, was 5 to 10 times greater than in nonusers. However, studies have shown that administration of a progestin for at least 10 to 14 days of an estrogen cycle is associated with a lower incidence of endometrial hyperplasia and endometrial carcinoma than an estrogen-only cycle. There is no risk of endometrial cancer in patients who have undergone hysterectomies and, therefore, no documented need for concurrent progestin therapy.

Whether the use of systemic estrogens increases the incidence of breast cancer in some postmenopausal women is unresolved. Some large studies reported an increase in the relative risk for development of breast cancer for women taking high doses of estrogen or using estrogens for a prolonged period of time, especially longer than 10 years. At present, however, the majority of data have not shown an increased risk of breast cancer in women who have ever used ovarian hormone therapy.

In certain animal species, long-term, continuous administration of estrogens increases the frequency of cancers of the breast, cervix, liver, pancreas, testis, uterus, and vagina.

Estrogens have been reported to be associated with carcinoma of the male breast. Males treated with estrogens should have regular breast examinations.

**Pregnancy/Reproduction**
Pregnancy—Estrogens are not recommended for use during pregnancy or during the immediate postpartum period. Studies suggest an association of congenital malformations with use of some estrogens during pregnancy.
Diethylstilbestrol: Daughters of women who took diethylstilbestrol (DES) during pregnancy have developed abnormalities of the reproductive tract and, in rare cases, cancer of the vagina and/or uterine cervix upon reaching childbearing age. In addition, sons of women who took DES during pregnancy have developed urogenital tract abnormalities. Patients who become pregnant while taking estrogens should be informed of the potential risks to the fetus.

FDA Pregnancy Category X.

**Breast-feeding**
Estrogens are distributed into breast milk. Use by breast-feeding women is not recommended with estrogen doses larger than those used in oral contraceptives.
Ethinyl estradiol—Traces of ethinyl estradiol are distributed into breast milk when estrogen is given in high doses as an antineoplastic agent. Also, use of oral contraceptives containing ethinyl estradiol during lactation has been associated with a decrease in milk production and in the milk protein and nitrogen content. However, the magnitude of these effects is small and probably of clinical significance only in malnourished mothers.

**Pediatrics**

Estrogens may accelerate epiphyseal closure. Therefore, estrogens should be used with caution in children and adolescents in whom bone growth is not complete.

**Geriatrics**

Studies performed to date have not demonstrated geriatrics-specific problems that would limit the usefulness of estrogens in the elderly.

**Dental**

Estrogens may predispose the patient to bleeding of the gingival tissues. In addition, gingival hyperplasia may occur during estrogen therapy, usually starting as gingivitis or gum inflammation. A strictly enforced program of teeth cleaning by a professional, combined with plaque control by the patient, will minimize growth rate and severity of gingival enlargement.

**Drug interactions and/or related problems**

The following drug interactions and/or related problems have been selected on the basis of their potential clinical significance (possible mechanism in parentheses where appropriate)—not necessarily inclusive (» = major clinical significance):

Note: Combinations containing any of the following medications, depending on the amount present, may also interact with this medication.

Bromocriptine
(estrogens may interfere with the effects of bromocriptine; dosage adjustment may be needed)

Calcium supplements
(concurrent use with estrogens may increase calcium absorption and exacerbate nephrolithiasis in susceptible individuals; this can be used to therapeutic advantage to increase bone mass)

Corticosteroids, glucocorticoid
(concurrent use with estrogens may alter the metabolism and protein binding of the glucocorticoids, leading to decreased clearance, increased elimination half-life, and increased therapeutic and toxic effects of the glucocorticoids; glucocorticoid dosage adjustment may be required during and following concurrent use)

Corticotropin (chronic therapeutic use)
(concurrent use with estrogens may potentiate the anti-inflammatory effects of endogenous cortisol induced by corticotropin)

» Cyclosporine
(estrogens have been reported to inhibit cyclosporine metabolism and thereby increase plasma concentrations of cyclosporine, possibly increasing the risk of hepatotoxicity and nephrotoxicity; concurrent use is recommended only with great caution and frequent monitoring of blood cyclosporine concentrations and liver and renal function)

» Hepatotoxic medications, especially dantrolene and isoniazid (see *Appendix II*)
(concurrent use of these medications with estrogens may increase the risk of hepatotoxicity and fatal hepatitis has occurred; risk may be further increased with use in females over 35 years of age, prolonged use, or use in patients with a history of liver disease)

Medications associated with pancreatitis, especially
Didanosine or
Lamividine or
Zalcitabine
(estrogens should be used with caution with medications that cause pancreatitis, especially if the patient has pre-existing risk factors such as high triglyceride concentrations; however, physiologic doses of estrogen would not be expected to induce pancreatitis)

» Protease inhibitors, such as ritonavir
(ritonavir has decreased the area under the plasma concentration–time curve [AUC] of ethinyl estradiol by 40%; similar effects may occur with other estrogens or with other protease inhibitors)

Smoking, tobacco
(data from studies on tobacco smoking and the use of high-dose estrogen oral contraceptives indicate that there is an increased risk of serious cardiovascular side effects, including cerebrovascular accident, transient ischemic attacks, thrombophlebitis, and pulmonary embolism; risk increases with increasing tobacco usage and with age, especially in women over 35 years of age; it is not known whether any elevation of risk occurs with tobacco smoking during the use of ovarian hormone therapy)

(metabolism of estrogens may also be increased by smoking, resulting in a decreased estrogenic effect)

Somatrem or
Somatropin
(in prepubertal patients, concurrent use of estrogens with somatrem or somatropin may accelerate epiphyseal maturation)

Tamoxifen
(concurrent use may interfere with therapeutic effect of tamoxifen)

**Laboratory value alterations**

The following have been selected on the basis of their potential clinical significance (possible effect in parentheses where appropriate)—not necessarily inclusive (» = major clinical significance):

With diagnostic test results
Biopsy
(pathologist should be notified of relevant specimens)

Fasting blood sugar (FBS) and
Glucose tolerance test
(may be altered by large doses of estrogens)

Metyrapone test
(reduced response)

Norepinephrine-induced platelet aggregability
(may be increased)

Thyroid function tests, such as
Thyroxine ($T_4$) determinations
Triiodothyronine ($T_3$) determinations
(values for the $T_3$ uptake test may be decreased because of an increase in thyroid-binding globulin [TBG]; free $T_3$, thyroxine [$T_4$], and thyroid-stimulating hormone [TSH] concentrations remain unaltered and patient remains euthyroid, even though the total thyroid hormone may be increased)

With physiology/laboratory test values
Antithrombin III, serum and
Cholesterol, total, serum and
Folate, serum and
Lipoproteins, low density (LDL), serum and
Pregnanediol, urine and
Pyridoxine, serum
(concentrations may be decreased; however, transdermal estradiol may have little effect on lowering LDL, total serum cholesterol, or serum antithrombin III concentrations)

Calcium
(increased serum concentrations, especially for immobilized patients or for patients with bone cancer or metastatic breast cancer)

Ceruloplasmin and
Clotting factors VII, VIII, IX, and X and
Cortisol and
Glucose—especially in diabetic or prediabetic patients taking larger doses of estrogens, and
Lipoproteins, high density (HDL) and
Phospholipids and
Prolactin and
Prothrombin and
Sodium and
Triglycerides
(serum concentrations may be increased. Transdermal estradiol may lower serum triglyceride concentrations and have little effect on increasing HDL or hepatic clotting factors)

Renin substrate
(may be increased by conjugated estrogens and ethinyl estradiol; this effect may also occur with other estrogens; however, transdermal estradiol does not affect renin substrate)

**Medical considerations/Contraindications**

The medical considerations/contraindications included have been selected on the basis of their potential clinical significance (reasons given in parentheses where appropriate)—not necessarily inclusive (» = major clinical significance).

*Except under special circumstances, this medication should not be used when the following medical problems exist:*

» Genital or uterine bleeding, abnormal and undiagnosed
(use of estrogens may delay diagnosis; on occurrence, estrogen should be discontinued awaiting clinical evaluation. Condition may worsen if cause of abnormal uterine bleeding is endometrial hyperplasia or uterine cancer)

» Neoplasia, estrogen-dependent, known or suspected
(possible promotion of tumor growth or estrogen may interfere with the action of antiestrogen treatment regimens; when these conditions are present, estrogen therapy usually is discontinued)

*For all indications, except for the treatment of breast cancer or prostatic cancer*
» Thrombophlebitis or thromboembolic disorders, active
(estrogens should be discontinued if thromboembolic events occur)

**Risk-benefit should be considered when the following medical problems exist:**
Endometriosis
(endometrial implants may be aggravated by use of estrogens)
Gallbladder disease, or history of, especially gallstones
(conflicting evidence exists as to whether an increased risk of recurrence or exacerbation occurs secondary to oral estrogen use)
Hepatic function impairment, severe, including
Jaundice, or history of, during pregnancy
Porphyria, hepatic—acute, intermittent, or variegate or
Hyperlipoproteinemia, familial or
Pancreatitis
(may cause these conditions to worsen or recur; estrogens given to achieve serum concentrations at the premenopausal level can rarely increase triglycerides to concentrations that result in pancreatitis, especially in patients with familial defects in lipoprotein metabolism. Metabolism of estrogens may be impaired with hepatic function impairment)
» Hypercalcemia associated with bone or metastatic breast cancer
(severe hypercalcemia may occur in patients with bone cancer or metastatic breast cancer who are treated with estrogens; estrogens may aggravate breast cancer–induced hypercalcemia through alterations in the metabolism of calcium and phosphorus; appropriate monitoring is recommended)
Leiomyoma, uterine
(may increase in size during estrogen therapy)
Sensitivity to estrogens
*For all indications, except for the treatment of breast cancer or prostatic cancer*
» Thrombophlebitis, thrombosis, or thromboembolic disorders, estrogen-induced, history of
(resumption of estrogen therapy may result in recurrence. Hypercoagulability information for postmenopausal women taking ovarian hormone therapy is not available. Estrogens can be used cautiously in women with predisposing risk factors and should be discontinued if thromboembolic events occur)
*For treatment of male breast cancer or prostatic cancer only (in addition to those conditions listed above)*
Cerebrovascular disease or
Coronary artery disease or
Thrombophlebitis, active or
Thromboembolic disorders
(the large doses of estrogens used in males to treat breast and prostatic cancer have been associated with an increased risk of myocardial infarction, pulmonary embolism, and thrombophlebitis)

**Patient monitoring**
The following may be especially important in patient monitoring (other tests may be warranted in some patients, depending on condition; » = major clinical significance):
Blood pressure determinations
(blood pressure elevations that generally occur within a short time after initiation of therapy are due to a reversible effect on the renin-angiotensin system and have only been documented during the use of conjugated estrogens and high-dose combination oral contraceptives; hypertension occurring during the treatment of gonadal dysgenesis also may be a result of worsening of the disease state itself, and may not necessarily be attributable to estrogen therapy)
Bone age determinations
(x-ray of hand and wrist recommended every 6 months for children and adolescents to determine rate of bone maturation and effects on epiphyseal centers)
Breast examinations
(should be performed routinely by patient and physician for early detection of possible breast cancer; teaching patient about periodic self-examination of breasts)
Endometrial biopsy
(should be considered periodically as necessary in patients with an intact uterus; patients with a uterus should be monitored for signs of endometrial cancer and malignancy should be ruled out in cases of persistent or abnormal vaginal bleeding; there is no risk of endometrial cancer in patients who have undergone a hysterectomy)
Hepatic function determinations
(recommended at regular intervals, especially during therapy in patients who have or are suspected of having hepatic disease)
Lipid profile determinations, serum
(recommended annually in women who are receiving ovarian hormone therapy, especially if taking a progestin)
Mammogram
(every 12 months, or as determined by physician)
(sensitivity or specificity of mammography testing is decreased with concurrent use of estrogens due to detection problems caused by estrogen-induced breast tissue growth, especially if the postmenopausal breast is fibrous. Ordering mammography during week of no hormonal use or after cessation of therapy may help in recognizing false-positive or false-negative mammograms)
Papanicolaou (Pap) test and
Physical examinations
(every year or more frequently when so determined by physician, with special attention being given to abdomen, breast, and pelvic organs)

## Side/Adverse Effects
The following side/adverse effects have been selected on the basis of their potential clinical significance (possible signs and symptoms in parentheses where appropriate)—not necessarily inclusive:

**Those indicating need for medical attention**
Incidence more frequent
*Breast pain or tenderness*—in females as well as in males treated for prostatic cancer; *enlargement of breasts*—in females; *gynecomastia* (increased breast size)—in males treated for prostatic cancer; *peripheral edema* (swelling of feet and lower legs; rapid weight gain)
Incidence less frequent or rare
*Amenorrhea* (stopping of menstrual bleeding); *breakthrough bleeding* (heavier vaginal bleeding between regular menses); *menorrhagia* (prolonged or heavier menses); *or spotting* (lighter vaginal bleeding between regular menses); *breast tumors* (breast lumps; discharge from breast); *gallbladder obstruction; hepatitis; or pancreatitis* (pains in stomach, side, or abdomen; yellow eyes or skin)
Note: If persistent or recurring abnormal vaginal bleeding occurs, malignancy should be ruled out. However, *withdrawal bleeding* will frequently occur in patients placed on cyclic estrogen therapy with a progestin who have not undergone hysterectomy. Any unusual uterine bleeding persisting longer than 3 to 6 months should be investigated. With continuous estrogen-progestin therapy, withdrawal bleeding is eliminated, endometrial atrophy and amenorrhea are produced in most patients after 2 to 3 months and, in the remaining patients, after 7 to 13 months. Amenorrhea is highly desired by many women and not considered by them to be a true adverse effect.

For treatment of male breast cancer or prostatic cancer only (in addition to those listed above)
*Thromboembolism or thrombus formation* (severe or sudden headache; sudden loss of coordination; pains in chest, groin, or leg, especially calf; sudden and unexplained shortness of breath; sudden slurred speech; sudden vision changes; weakness or numbness in arm or leg)
Note: The use of large doses of estrogens (5 mg a day) in males to treat breast and prostate cancer has been associated with an increased risk of *myocardial infarction, pulmonary embolism*, and *thrombophlebitis*.

**Those indicating need for medical attention only if they continue or are bothersome**
Incidence more frequent
*Abdominal cramping or bloating; anorexia* (loss of appetite); *nausea; skin irritation and redness*—with transdermal system
Incidence less frequent
*Diarrhea, mild; dizziness, mild; headaches, mild; intolerance to contact lenses; libido decrease*—in males; *libido increase*—in females; *migraine headaches; vomiting*—primarily of central origin; usually with high doses

## Patient Consultation
As an aid to patient consultation, refer to *Advice for the Patient, Estrogens (Systemic)*.
In providing consultation, consider emphasizing the following selected information (» = major clinical significance):

**Before using this medication**
» Conditions affecting use, especially:
Sensitivity to estrogens

Carcinogenicity—Increased risk of endometrial cancer for patients with intact uteri placed on unopposed estrogen therapy; decreased risk occurs when used with a progestin; male breast cancer has occurred in association with estrogen use; continuous, long-term estrogen use in animal studies increased frequency of cancers of the breast, cervix, and liver

Pregnancy—Use of some estrogens may be associated with congenital abnormalities. Physician should be informed immediately if pregnancy is suspected

Breast-feeding—Use is not recommended because estrogens are distributed into breast milk and may have unpredictable effects

Use in children—Use in children or growing adolescents may slow or stop growth

Other medications, especially cyclosporine; hepatotoxic medications; or protease inhibitors

Other medical problems, especially abnormal or undiagnosed genital or uterine bleeding; active thrombophlebitis or thromboembolic disorders; estrogen-dependent neoplasia; history of estrogen-induced thrombophlebitis, thrombosis, or thromboembolic disorders; or hypercalcemia associated with bone cancer or metastatic breast cancer

**Proper use of this medication**
» Reading patient package insert carefully
» Compliance with therapy
*For oral or parenteral dosage forms*
Taking with or immediately after food to reduce nausea
*For transdermal estradiol*
Washing and drying hands thoroughly before and after application
Applying to clean, dry, nonoily, hairless, intact area of skin on the lower abdomen, hips below the waistline, or buttocks; not applying over cuts or irritation. The manufacturer of the 0.025-mg matrix transdermal system recommends applying its patch to the buttocks only, rotating the application site from left buttock to right buttock every 7 days
» Not applying to breasts; not applying to waistline or other areas where tight clothes may rub disk loose
Pressing the disk firmly in place with palm for about 10 seconds; making sure there is good contact, especially around edges
Reapplying disk if it comes loose, or discarding and applying a new one
Applying each patch to different area of skin on lower abdomen, hips below waistline, or buttocks so at least 1 week elapses before the area is used again to help prevent skin irritation
» Proper dosing
Missed dose: Taking or using as soon as possible; not using if almost time for next dose; not doubling doses
» Proper storage

**Precautions while using this medication**
» Regular visits to physician every year, or more often, as determined by physician
Possibility of dental problems, such as tenderness, swelling, or bleeding of gums; brushing and flossing teeth, massaging gums, and having dentist clean teeth regularly; checking with dentist if there are questions about care of teeth or gums or if tenderness, swelling, or bleeding of gums is noticed
» Checking breast by self-examination regularly and having clinical examination and mammography as required by physician; reporting unusual breast lumps or discharge
» Understanding that menstrual bleeding may begin again but, with continuous therapy, will stop by 10 months
» Understanding that intermenstrual uterine bleeding will occur for the first 3 months; importance of not stopping medicine; checking with doctor immediately if uterine bleeding is unusual or continuous, missed period occurs, or pregnancy is suspected
If scheduled for laboratory tests, telling physician about taking estrogens; certain blood tests and tissue biopsies are affected

**Side/adverse effects**
Withdrawal bleeding will occur in many postmenopausal patients with an intact uterus who are placed on cyclic estrogen therapy with a progestin
Signs of potential side effects, especially breast pain or tenderness, enlargement of breasts in females, gynecomastia in males treated for prostatic cancer, peripheral edema, amenorrhea, breakthrough bleeding, menorrhagia, or spotting; breast tumors; gallbladder obstruction, hepatitis, or pancreatitis; for treatment of prostatic cancer and male breast cancer only—thromboembolism or thrombus formation

## General Dosing Information

It is recommended that the patient package insert be given to patients.

As a general rule, estrogen therapy should be administered at the lowest effective dosage. If prolonged therapy is necessary, the patient should be re-evaluated at least every year to determine the need for continued therapy.

With chronic administration of estrogens in patients with the uterus *in situ*, the concurrent use of a progestin for at least 10 to 14 days of the cycle should be considered. Administration of a progestin decreases the risk of occurrence of endometrial hyperplasia and endometrial carcinoma. There is no risk of endometrial hyperplasia or endometrial carcinoma in patients who do not have an intact uterus.

An estrogen may be administered for the entire period of estrogen deficiency. Estrogens may be administered on a cyclic or continuous regimen when used to treat estrogen deficiency states, for prevention of osteoporosis, and for prevention of atherosclerotic disease. Some patients are placed on a cyclic regimen consisting of 3 weeks of estrogen therapy, with a progestin concurrently administered (if indicated) for the first or last 10 to 14 days of the 3-week period. During the fourth and final week of the cycle, no medication is administered. Other physicians advocate the use of continuous estrogen dosing with continuous progestin administration.

Use of the continuous regimen for both conjugated estrogen and medroxyprogesterone is a good choice for women who do not want to resume menses. If spotting or uterine bleeding occurs during the first 6 months, a higher dose of progestin may be used for a short time until endometrial atrophy occurs.

**For ovarian hormone therapy**
Decisions to treat menopausal symptoms with hormones for a limited time (1 to 5 years) or to use hormones to prevent diseases in postmenopausal women for a longer period of time (10 to 20 years), or a lifetime, should be made separately.

Counseling asymptomatic postmenopausal women about the benefits and risks of using long-term ovarian hormone therapy to prevent osteoporosis and coronary heart disease and to increase life expectancy is complex. Risk estimates are based on observational studies; the true estimates for long-term risks and benefits await controlled clinical trials. Women should understand that the benefits and risks of preventive hormone therapy depend on their risk status, and that women at higher risk for developing osteoporosis or coronary heart disease can derive the greatest benefit.

For women with a uterus, adding a progestin to estrogen therapy may benefit postmenopausal women at risk for osteoporosis, slightly reduce estrogen's protective effect against coronary heart disease, and slightly increase the risk of breast cancer over that of nonusers.

**Diet/Nutrition**
Estrogen therapy with either the oral or parenteral dosage form may cause nausea, especially in the morning. Although this nausea is primarily of central origin, eating solid food often provides some relief.

**For parenteral dosage forms only**
Intramuscular injections should be administered slowly and deeply into a large muscle area such as the upper outer quadrant of the buttock.

Rapid intravenous injections may cause perineal or vaginal burning.

A dry syringe and needle of at least 21 gauge should be used for the oil-vehicle preparations.

**For estradiol transdermal dosage forms**
Patients who are currently taking oral estrogens should wait 1 week after withdrawal of oral estrogens before the transdermal dosage system is initiated.

Transdermal estradiol generally is administered on a continuous regimen, with repeating cycles of 3 weeks on and 1 week off. In women with an intact uterus, administration of a progestin for at least 10 to 14 days of each month is recommended. For women who have had a hysterectomy, transdermal estradiol may be given continuously or cyclically without adding a progestin to the therapeutic regimen.

The adhesive side of the transdermal system should be placed on a clean, dry area of the skin on the trunk of the body. The lower abdomen is the preferred site, although the patch may be applied to the buttocks or sides of hip below the waist instead. However, the manufacturer of the 0.025-mg matrix transdermal system recommends applying its patch to the buttock site only, rotating the site of application between left and right buttocks. None of the transdermal systems should be applied to the breasts or waistline. The area selected should not be oily or irritated and the skin should not be broken. The application site should be rotated, and no site should be reused until 1 week has passed.

## CONJUGATED ESTROGENS

## Oral Dosage Forms
### CONJUGATED ESTROGENS TABLETS USP
**Usual adult dose**
Atrophic vaginitis or
Menopausal (vasomotor) symptoms or
Vulvar atrophy—
  Oral, 300 mcg (0.3 mg) to 1.25 mg a day, cyclically or continuously.
  Note: May be used in conjunction with vaginal dosage forms.
Breast carcinoma (inoperable and progressing in selected men and postmenopausal women)—
  Oral, 10 mg three times a day for at least three months.
Estrogen deficiency, due to ovariectomy or
Primary ovarian failure—
  Oral, 1.25 mg a day, cyclically or continuously. For maintenance, adjust estrogen dose to lowest level that provides control.
Female hypogonadism—
  Oral, 2.5 to 7.5 mg a day, in divided doses, cyclically.
Osteoporosis, postmenopausal (prophylaxis)—
  Oral, 625 mcg (0.625 mg) a day, cyclically or continuously as appropriate.
Prostatic carcinoma (inoperable and progressing)—
  Oral, 1.25 to 2.5 mg three times a day.

**Strength(s) usually available**
U.S.—
  300 mcg (0.3 mg) (Rx) [*Premarin*].
  625 mcg (0.625 mg) (Rx) [*Premarin*].
  Note: Premarin 0.625 mg is available as either white or purple tablets.
  900 mcg (0.9 mg) (Rx) [*Premarin*].
  1.25 mg (Rx) [*Premarin*].
  2.5 mg (Rx) [*Premarin*].
Canada—
  300 mcg (0.3 mg) (Rx) [*C.E.S.; Congest; Premarin*].
  625 mcg (0.625 mg) (Rx) [*C.E.S.; Congest; Premarin* GENERIC].
  900 mcg (0.9 mg) (Rx) [*C.E.S.; Congest; Premarin*].
  1.25 mg (Rx) [*C.E.S.; Congest; Premarin* GENERIC].
  2.5 mg (Rx) [*C.E.S.; Congest; Premarin*].

**Packaging and storage**
Store below 40 °C (104 °F), preferably between 15 and 30 °C (59 and 86 °F), unless otherwise specified by manufacturer. Store in a well-closed container.

**Note**
Include mandatory patient package insert (PPI) when dispensing.

## Parenteral Dosage Forms
### CONJUGATED ESTROGENS FOR INJECTION
**Usual adult dose**
Uterine bleeding, hormonal imbalance–induced—
  Intramuscular or intravenous, 25 mg, repeated in six to twelve hours if needed.
  Note: Intravenous administration is preferred because of the more rapid response obtained. To reduce the possibility of a flushing reaction, the medication should be administered slowly.

**Size(s) usually available**
U.S.—
  25 mg (Rx) [*Premarin Intravenous* (benzyl alcohol 2%—diluent)].
Canada—
  25 mg (Rx) [*Premarin Intravenous*].

**Packaging and storage**
Prior to reconstitution, store between 2 and 8 °C (36 and 46 °F), unless otherwise specified by manufacturer.

**Preparation of dosage form**
With aseptic technique, at least 5 mL of air should be withdrawn from the container of dry powder. Then 5 mL of the sterile diluent provided should be added slowly against the side of the container. The vial should be agitated gently to dissolve the contents. Do not shake vigorously.

**Stability**
When stored between 2 and 8 °C (36 and 46 °F), the reconstituted solution retains potency for about 60 days. Do not use if solution has darkened or if a precipitate is present.

**Incompatibilities**
The prepared injection is compatible with normal saline, dextrose, and invert sugar solutions. It is *not* compatible with solutions having an acid pH, such as protein hydrolysate or ascorbic acid.

**Note**
Include mandatory patient package insert (PPI) if dispensed to patient.

## DIETHYLSTILBESTROL

## Oral Dosage Forms
### DIETHYLSTILBESTROL TABLETS USP
**Usual adult dose**
Prostatic carcinoma (inoperable and progressing)—
  Oral, 1 to 3 mg initially and increased as needed in advanced cases, with the dosage later reduced to 1 mg a day.
  Note: Doses used to treat prostatic carcinoma have been found to have a maximal effect in maintenance doses of up to 1 mg a day. Higher doses do not appreciably increase the therapeutic results, but may increase the risk of cardiovascular embolism.

**Strength(s) usually available**
U.S.—
  Not commercially available.
Canada—
  100 mcg (0.1 mg) (Rx) [*Stilbestrol*].
  500 mcg (0.5 mg) (Rx) [*Stilbestrol*].
  1 mg (Rx) [*Stilbestrol*].

**Packaging and storage**
Store below 40 °C (104 °F), preferably between 15 and 30 °C (59 and 86 °F), unless otherwise specified by manufacturer. Store in a well-closed container.

**Note**
Include patient package insert (PPI) when dispensing.

### DIETHYLSTILBESTROL DIPHOSPHATE TABLETS
**Usual adult dose**
Prostatic carcinoma (inoperable and progressing)—
  Oral, 50 to 166 mg three times a day; the dosage being increased gradually to 200 mg or more, three times a day as needed and tolerated.

**Usual adult prescribing limits**
Oral, 1 gram a day.

**Strength(s) usually available**
U.S.—
  50 mg (Rx) [*Stilphostrol* (scored)].
Canada—
  83 mg (diethylstilbestrol diphosphate sodium 100 mg) (Rx) [*Honvol* (scored)].

**Packaging and storage**
Store below 40 °C (104 °F), preferably between 15 and 30 °C (59 and 86 °F), in a well-closed container, unless otherwise specified by manufacturer.

**Note**
Include mandatory patient package insert (PPI) when dispensing.

## Parenteral Dosage Forms
### DIETHYLSTILBESTROL DIPHOSPHATE INJECTION USP
**Usual adult dose**
Prostatic carcinoma (inoperable and progressing)—
  Induction: Intravenous infusion, initially 500 mg in 250 mL of Sodium Chloride Injection USP or 5% Dextrose Injection USP administered at a rate of 1 mL per minute during the first ten to fifteen minutes; then the flow is adjusted to permit dose completion within one hour. The dosage is increased to 1 gram a day for the subsequent five or more days as needed for relief.
  Maintenance: Intravenous infusion, 250 to 500 mg in 250 mL of Sodium Chloride Injection USP or 5% Dextrose Injection USP administered one or two times a week at the same rate as during induction.

---

The system should be applied immediately after removal from the pouch and removal of the protective liner. It should not be stored unprotected. The system should be pressed firmly in place with the palm of the hand for about 10 seconds, making sure there is good contact, especially around the edges.

If a transdermal system loosens or falls off, it may be reapplied or a new system may be applied instead. In either case, the patient should continue with the original treatment schedule.

**Strength(s) usually available**
U.S.—
   50 mg per mL (Rx) [*Stilphostrol*].
Canada—
   50 mg per mL (diethylstilbestrol diphosphate sodium 60 mg) (Rx) [*Honvol*].

**Packaging and storage**
Store below 21 °C (70 °F), unless otherwise specified by manufacturer. Protect from freezing.

**Note**
Include mandatory patient package insert (PPI) if dispensed to patient.

---

### ESTERIFIED ESTROGENS

## Oral Dosage Forms
### ESTERIFIED ESTROGENS TABLETS USP

**Usual adult dose**
Atrophic vaginitis or
Vulvar atrophy—
   Oral, 300 mcg (0.3 mg) to 1.25 mg or more a day, cyclically or continuously as appropriate.
   Note: May be used in conjunction with vaginal dosage forms.
Breast carcinoma (inoperable and progressing in selected men and postmenopausal women)[1]—
   Oral, 10 mg three times a day for at least three months.
Estrogen deficiency, due to ovariectomy or
Primary ovarian failure—
   Oral, 1.25 mg a day, cyclically or continuously. For maintenance, adjust estrogen dose to lowest level that provides control.
Female hypogonadism—
   Oral, 2.5 to 7.5 mg a day, in divided doses, cyclically or continuously.
Menopausal (vasomotor) symptoms—
   Oral, 625 mcg (0.625 mg) to 1.25 mg a day, cyclically or continuously as appropriate.
Osteoporosis, postmenopausal (prophylaxis)[1]—
   Oral, 300 mcg (0.3 mg) to 1.25 mg a day, cyclically or continuously.
Prostatic carcinoma (inoperable and progressing)[1]—
   Oral, 1.25 to 2.5 mg three times a day.

**Strength(s) usually available**
U.S.—
   300 mcg (0.3 mg) (Rx) [*Estratab; Menest*].
   625 mcg (0.625 mg) (Rx) [*Estratab; Menest*].
   1.25 mg (Rx) [*Estratab; Menest*].
   2.5 mg (Rx) [*Estratab; Menest*].
Canada—
   300 mcg (0.3 mg) (Rx) [*Neo-Estrone*].
   625 mcg (0.625 mg) (Rx) [*Neo-Estrone*].
   1.25 mg (Rx) [*Neo-Estrone*].

**Packaging and storage**
Store below 40 °C (104 °F), preferably between 15 and 30 °C (59 and 86 °F), unless otherwise specified by manufacturer. Store in a well-closed container.

**Note**
Include mandatory patient package insert (PPI) when dispensing.

[1]Not included in Canadian product labeling.

---

### ESTRADIOL

## Oral Dosage Forms
### ESTRADIOL TABLETS USP

**Usual adult dose**
Atrophic vaginitis or
Estrogen deficiency, due to ovariectomy[1] or
Female hypogonadism[1] or
Menopausal (vasomotor) symptoms or
Primary ovarian failure[1] or
Vulvar atrophy—
   Oral, 500 mcg (0.5 mg) to 2 mg a day, cyclically or continuously as appropriate.
Breast carcinoma (inoperable and progressing in selected men and postmenopausal women)[1]—
   Oral, 10 mg three times a day for at least three months.
Prostatic carcinoma (inoperable and progressing)[1]—
   Oral, 1 to 2 mg three times a day.
Osteoporosis, postmenopausal (prophylaxis)—
   Oral, 0.5 mg (500 mcg) a day, cyclically (twenty-three days on and five days off per month).

**Strength(s) usually available**
U.S.—
   500 mcg (0.5 mg) (Rx) [*Estrace* (scored); GENERIC (scored)].
   1 mg (Rx) [*Estrace* (scored); GENERIC (scored)].
   2 mg (Rx) [*Estrace* (scored); GENERIC (scored)].
Canada—
   500 mcg (0.5 mg) (Rx) [*Estrace* (scored)].
   1 mg (Rx) [*Estrace* (scored)].
   2 mg (Rx) [*Estrace* (scored)].

**Packaging and storage**
Store below 40 °C (104 °F), preferably between 15 and 30 °C (59 and 86 °F), unless otherwise specified by manufacturer. Store in a tight, light-resistant container.

**Note**
Include mandatory patient package insert (PPI) when dispensing.

## Parenteral Dosage Forms
### ESTRADIOL CYPIONATE INJECTION USP

**Usual adult dose**
Female hypogonadism—
   Intramuscular, 1.5 to 2 mg administered at monthly intervals.
Menopausal (vasomotor) symptoms—
   Intramuscular, 1 to 5 mg once a week for three to four weeks, usually administered cyclically (three weeks on and one week off).

**Strength(s) usually available**
U.S.—
   5 mg per mL (Rx) [*depGynogen* (chlorobutanol; cottonseed oil); *Depo-Estradiol* (chlorobutanol 5.4 mg; cottonseed oil); *Depogen* (chlorobutanol; cottonseed oil); *Dura-Estrin* (chlorobutanol; cottonseed oil); *E-Cypionate; Estragyn LA 5; Estro-Cyp* (chlorobutanol; cottonseed oil); *Estrofem* (chlorobutanol; cottonseed oil); *Estro-L.A.;* GENERIC].
Canada—
   Not commercially available.

**Packaging and storage**
Store below 40 °C (104 °F), preferably between 15 and 30 °C (59 and 86 °F), in a light-resistant container, unless otherwise specified by manufacturer. Protect from freezing.

**Note**
Include mandatory patient package insert (PPI) if dispensed to patient.

### ESTRADIOL VALERATE INJECTION USP

**Usual adult dose**
Atrophic vaginitis or
Estrogen deficiency, due to ovariectomy or
Female hypogonadism[1] or
Menopausal (vasomotor) symptoms or
Primary ovarian failure or
Vulvar atrophy—
   Intramuscular, 10 to 20 mg repeated every four weeks as needed.
Prostatic carcinoma (inoperable and progressing)—
   Intramuscular, 30 mg every one or two weeks, the dose being adjusted as needed.

**Strength(s) usually available**
U.S.—
   10 mg per mL (Rx) [*Delestrogen* (chlorobutanol 5 mg; sesame oil); *Valergen-10* (chlorobutanol; sesame oil); GENERIC].
   20 mg per mL (Rx) [*Delestrogen* (benzyl alcohol; benzyl benzoate; castor oil); *Dioval XX* (benzyl alcohol; benzyl benzoate; castor oil); *Duragen-20* (benzyl alcohol; benzyl benzoate; castor oil); *Gynogen L.A. 20* (benzyl alcohol; benzyl benzoate; castor oil); *Menaval-20; Valergen-20* (benzyl alcohol; benzyl benzoate; castor oil); GENERIC].
   40 mg per mL (Rx) [*Clinagen LA 40; Delestrogen* (benzyl alcohol; benzyl benzoate; castor oil); *Dioval 40* (benzyl alcohol; benzyl benzoate; castor oil); *Estra-L 40* (benzyl alcohol; benzyl benzoate; castor oil); *Estro-Span; Gynogen L.A. 40* (benzyl alcohol; benzyl benzoate; castor oil); *Valergen-40* (benzyl alcohol; benzyl benzoate; castor oil); GENERIC].
Canada—
   10 mg per mL (Rx) [*Delestrogen* (chlorobutanol 0.5%; sesame oil)].
   20 mg per mL (Rx) [*Femogex* (chlorobutanol 0.5%)].

## Estrogens (Systemic)

**Packaging and storage**
Store below 40 °C (104 °F), preferably between 15 and 30 °C (59 and 86 °F), unless otherwise specified by manufacturer. Store in a light-resistant container. Protect from freezing.

**Note**
Include mandatory patient package insert (PPI) if dispensed to patient.

## Topical Dosage Forms

Note: Bracketed uses in the *Dosage Forms* section refer to categories of use and/or indications that are not included in U.S. product labeling.

### ESTRADIOL TRANSDERMAL SYSTEM (Matrix-type)

**Usual adult dose**
Atrophic vaginitis or
Estrogen deficiency, due to ovariectomy[1] or
Female hypogonadism[1] or
Menopausal (vasomotor) symptoms or
[Osteoporosis, postmenopausal (prophylaxis)][1] or
Primary ovarian failure[1] or
Vulvar atrophy—
   Topical, to the skin, one transdermal system delivering 25 mcg to 50 mcg a day is worn continuously and replaced, depending on the product, every seven days or every three or four days (two times a week) for three weeks of a four-week cycle. No patch is worn for the fourth week of the cycle, although estrogen treatment may be continued uninterrupted for appropriate patients. After the first thirty days, the dosage may be adjusted and then re-evaluated every three to six months for treatment continuance. If osteoporosis is established, a higher dose of 100 mcg may be used initially.

**Strength(s) usually available**
U.S.—
   Once–weekly transdermal system:
      25 mcg (0.025 mg) delivered per day (Rx) [*FemPatch*].
      50 mcg (0.05 mg) delivered per day (Rx) [*Climara*].
      100 mcg (0.1 mg) delivered per day (Rx) [*Climara*].
   Twice–weekly transdermal system:
      37.5 mcg (0.0375 mg) delivered per day (Rx) [*Vivelle*].
      50 mcg (0.05 mg) delivered per day (Rx) [*Alora; Vivelle*].
      75 mcg (0.075 mg) delivered per day (Rx) [*Alora; Vivelle*].
      100 mcg (0.1 mg) delivered per day (Rx) [*Alora; Vivelle*].
Canada—
   Twice–weekly transdermal system:
      37.5 mcg (0.0375 mg) delivered per day (Rx) [*Vivelle*].
      50 mcg (0.05 mg) delivered per day (Rx) [*Vivelle*].
      75 mcg (0.075 mg) delivered per day (Rx) [*Vivelle*].
      100 mcg (0.1 mg) delivered per day (Rx) [*Vivelle*].

**Packaging and storage**
Store below 30 °C (86 °F).

**Note**
Include mandatory patient package insert (PPI) when dispensing.

### ESTRADIOL TRANSDERMAL SYSTEM (Reservoir-type)

**Usual adult dose**
Atrophic vaginitis or
Estrogen deficiency, due to ovariectomy or
Female hypogonadism or
Menopausal (vasomotor) symptoms or
Osteoporosis, postmenopausal (prophylaxis) or
Primary ovarian failure or
Vulvar atrophy—
   Topical, to the skin, one 50-mcg transdermal system delivering 50 mcg a day, worn continuously and replaced every three or four days (two times a week) for three weeks of a four-week cycle. No patch is worn for the fourth week of the cycle, although estrogen treatment may be continued uninterrupted for appropriate patients. After the first thirty days, the dosage may be adjusted and then re-evaluated every three to six months for treatment continuance. If osteoporosis is established, a higher dose of 100 mcg may be used initially.

**Strength(s) usually available**
U.S.—
   Twice–weekly transdermal system:
      50 mcg (0.05 mg) delivered per day (Rx) [*Estraderm*].
      100 mcg (0.1 mg) delivered per day (Rx) [*Estraderm*].
Canada—
   Twice–weekly transdermal system:
      25 mcg (0.025 mg) delivered per day (Rx) [*Estraderm*].
      50 mcg (0.05 mg) delivered per day (Rx) [*Estraderm*].
      100 mcg (0.1 mg) delivered per day (Rx) [*Estraderm*].

**Packaging and storage**
Store below 30 °C (86 °F).

**Note**
Include mandatory patient package insert (PPI) when dispensing.

[1]Not included in Canadian product labeling.

---

## ESTRONE

## Parenteral Dosage Forms

### ESTRONE INJECTABLE SUSPENSION USP

**Usual adult dose**
Atrophic vaginitis or
Menopausal (vasomotor) symptoms or
Vulvar atrophy—
   Intramuscular, 100 to 500 mcg (0.1 to 0.5 mg) two or three times a week, cyclically or continuously as appropriate.
Estrogen deficiency, due to ovariectomy or
Female hypogonadism or
Primary ovarian failure—
   Intramuscular, 100 mcg (0.1 mg) to 1 mg a week, administered as a single dose or in divided doses, cyclically or continuously. A few patients may need doses of up to 2 mg a week.
Prostatic carcinoma (inoperable and progressing)—
   Intramuscular, 2 to 4 mg two or three times a week.
Uterine bleeding, abnormal (hormonal imbalance–induced)—
   Intramuscular, 2 to 5 mg a day for several days.

**Strength(s) usually available**
U.S.—
   2 mg estrone per mL (Rx) [*Aquest; Wehgen;* GENERIC].
   5 mg estrone per mL (Rx) [*Estragyn 5; Estro-A; Estrone '5'; Kestrone-5;* GENERIC].
Canada—
   Not commercially available.

**Packaging and storage**
Store below 40 °C (104 °F), preferably between 15 and 30 °C (59 and 86 °F), unless otherwise specified by manufacturer. Protect from freezing.

**Note**
Include mandatory patient package insert (PPI) if dispensed to patient.

---

## ESTROPIPATE

## Oral Dosage Forms

### ESTROPIPATE TABLETS USP

**Usual adult dose**
Atrophic vaginitis or
Menopausal (vasomotor) symptoms or
Vulvar atrophy—
   Oral, 750 mcg (0.75 mg) to 6 mg of estropipate a day, cyclically or continuously.
Estrogen deficiency, due to ovariectomy[1] or
Primary ovarian failure[1]—
   Oral, 1.5 to 9 mg of estropipate a day, cyclically or continuously. For maintenance, adjust dose to lowest level that provides control.
Female hypogonadism[1]—
   Oral, 1.5 to 9 mg of estropipate a day, cyclically or continuously.
Osteoporosis, postmenopausal (prophylaxis)[1]—
   Oral, 750 mcg (0.75 mg) a day for twenty-five days of a thirty-one-day cycle and continued cyclically.

**Strength(s) usually available**
U.S.—
   750 mcg (0.75 mg) estropipate—equivalent to 625 mcg (0.625 mg) sodium estrone sulfate (Rx) [*Ogen .625* (scored); *Ortho-Est .625;* GENERIC].
   1.5 mg estropipate—equivalent to 1.25 mg sodium estrone sulfate (Rx) [*Ogen 1.25* (scored); *Ortho-Est 1.25;* GENERIC].
   3 mg estropipate—equivalent to 2.5 mg sodium estrone sulfate (Rx) [*Ogen 2.5* (scored); GENERIC].
   6 mg estropipate—equivalent to 5 mg sodium estrone sulfate (Rx) [GENERIC (may be scored)].
Canada—
   750 mcg (0.75 mg) estropipate—equivalent to 625 mcg (0.625 mg) sodium estrone sulfate (Rx) [*Ogen* (scored)].
   1.5 mg estropipate—equivalent to 1.25 mg sodium estrone sulfate (Rx) [*Ogen* (scored)].

3 mg estropipate—equivalent to 2.5 mg sodium estrone sulfate (Rx) [*Ogen* (scored)].

Note: Estropipate previously was called piperazine estrone sulfate and the strengths were calculated as sodium estrone sulfate (0.625 mg, 1.25 mg, 2.5 mg, and 5 mg). Both strengths may appear on the manufacturer's labeling.

**Packaging and storage**
Store below 40 °C (104 °F), preferably between 15 and 30 °C (59 and 86 °F), unless otherwise specified by manufacturer. Store in a well-closed container.

**Note**
Include mandatory patient package insert (PPI) when dispensing.

[1]Not included in Canadian product labeling.

---

## ETHINYL ESTRADIOL

## Oral Dosage Forms

**ETHINYL ESTRADIOL TABLETS USP**

**Usual adult dose**
Breast carcinoma (inoperable and progressing in selected men and postmenopausal women)—
  Oral, 1 mg three times a day.
Estrogen deficiency, due to ovariectomy[1] or
Primary ovarian failure[1]—
  Oral, 50 mcg (0.05 mg) three times a day for a few weeks, then reduced to 50 mcg (0.05 mg) once a day, cyclically or continuously.
Female hypogonadism[1]—
  Oral, 50 mcg (0.05 mg) one to three times a day, cyclically or continuously, followed by a progestin during the last half of the menstrual cycle. This treatment cycle can be repeated for three to six months to establish a normal menses.
Menopausal (vasomotor) symptoms—
  Oral, 20 to 50 mcg (0.02 to 0.05 mg) a day, cyclically or continuously.
Prostatic carcinoma (inoperable and progressing)—
  Oral, 150 mcg (0.15 mg) to 3 mg a day.

**Strength(s) usually available**
U.S.—
  20 mcg (0.02 mg) (Rx) [*Estinyl*].
  50 mcg (0.05 mg) (Rx) [*Estinyl*].
  500 mcg (0.5 mg) (Rx) [*Estinyl* (scored)].
Canada—
  20 mcg (0.02 mg) (Rx) [*Estinyl*].
  50 mcg (0.05 mg) (Rx) [*Estinyl*].
  500 mcg (0.5 mg) (Rx) [*Estinyl* (scored)].

**Packaging and storage**
Store below 40 °C (104 °F), preferably between 15 and 30 °C (59 and 86 °F), unless otherwise specified by manufacturer. Store in a well-closed container.

**Note**
Include mandatory patient package insert (PPI) when dispensing.

[1]Not included in Canadian product labeling.

## Selected Bibliography
Baker VL. Alternatives to oral estrogen replacement: transdermal patches, percutaneous gels, vaginal creams and rings, implants, and other methods of delivery. Obstet Gynecol Clin North Am 1994 Jun; 21(2): 271-97.

Revised: 08/24/97
Interim revision: 2/26/98; 5/28/98

---

# ESTROGENS  Vaginal

This monograph includes information on the following: 1) Conjugated Estrogens; 2) Dienestrol; 3) Estradiol; 4) Estrone*; 5) Estropipate†
BAN:
  Dienestrol—Dienoestrol
  Estradiol—Oestradiol
  Estrone—Oestrone
VA CLASSIFICATION (Primary/Secondary): GU500/HS102
Commonly used brand name(s): *Estrace*[3]; *Estring*[3]; *Oestrilin*[4]; *Ogen*[5]; *Ortho Dienestrol*[2]; *Premarin*[1].

Other commonly used names are Dienoestrol [Dienestrol], Oestradiol [Estradiol], Oestrone [Estrone], and Piperazine Estrone Sulfate [Estropipate].

Note: For a listing of dosage forms and brand names by country availability, see *Dosage Forms* section(s).

*Not commercially available in U.S.
†Not commercially available in Canada.

## Category
Urogenital symptoms suppressant.

## Indications

**General considerations**
Vaginal estrogen doses that maintain the serum estradiol concentration in the postmenopausal range do not produce systemic effects of the hormone, such as suppression of *vasomotor symptoms of menopause* or protection against *cardiovascular disease* or *osteoporosis*, and they are not indicated for these uses. While sufficiently high serum estradiol concentrations can be produced from use of vaginal estrogens, use of oral or transdermal estrogen therapy may be preferred instead if systemic benefits are desired.
After menopause, serum estradiol concentrations are approximately 10 to 20 picograms per mL (pg/mL) (40 to 70 picomoles per L [pmol/L]) and serum estrone concentrations are approximately 30 to 70 pg/mL (110 to 260 pmol/L). If vaginal administration provides serum estrogen concentrations greater than these concentrations, systemic effects of estrogen should be considered and their potential side effects appropriately managed, such as adding a progestin to the treatment regimen to decrease estrogen-induced endometrial hyperplasia.
Women without a uterus are best treated with unopposed estrogen therapy; combined estrogen-progestin therapy is not needed.

**Accepted**
Urethritis, atrophic, postmenopausal (treatment)—Estradiol vaginal insert is indicated to treat atrophic urethritis in postmenopausal women who have symptoms of dysuria or urinary frequency, urgency, or incontinence.

Vaginitis, atrophic (treatment)—Conjugated estrogens, dienestrol, estradiol vaginal cream, [estradiol vaginal insert], and estropipate are indicated to treat symptoms of atrophic vaginitis due to estrogen deficiency that may include dyspareunia. Estradiol vaginal insert[1] and estrone are indicated to treat atrophic vaginitis in postmenopausal women only (also called senile vaginitis).

Vulvar atrophy—Conjugated estrogens, dienestrol, estradiol vaginal cream, [estradiol vaginal insert], estrone, and estropipate are indicated for treatment of symptomatic atrophic vulva due to estrogen deficiency, including kraurosis vulvae and pruritus vulvae.

**Unaccepted**
Although a few studies show that estrogens have some effect on neurotransmitters and may improve memory and cognitive function, estrogen is not indicated or effective in the treatment of clinical depression.

[1]Not included in Canadian product labeling.

## Pharmacology/Pharmacokinetics

**Physicochemical characteristics**
Source—
  Naturally occurring estrogens: Estradiol ($E_2$), estrone ($E_1$), and estriol ($E_3$) in humans.
  Conjugated estrogens are a mixture of estrogenic metabolites found in equine urine; the complete profile is not known. The primary estrogens, sodium estrone sulfate and sodium equilin sulfate, make up 79.5 to 88% of the total mixture. Other estrogens defined by USP as concomitant components are the sodium sulfated conjugates of 17-alpha-dihydroequilin, 17-alpha-estradiol, and 17-beta-dihydroequilin.
  Semi-synthetic estrogen: Estropipate (estrone sulfate piperazine compound).
  Synthetic nonsteroidal estrogen: Dienestrol.
Molecular weight—
  Dienestrol: 266.34.
  Estradiol: 272.39.
  Estrone: 270.37.
  Estropipate: 436.58.

## Mechanism of action/Effect

Estrogens—
Estrogens passively diffuse into target cells of responsive tissues, complex with the estrogen receptors, and enter the cell's nucleus to initiate or enhance gene transcription of protein synthesis after binding to DNA.

The magnitude of estrogen's effect and its influence upon different hormones depends on the endogenous estrogen concentration in the plasma, and the product formulation and type and dose of exogenous estrogen administered. A 2:1 ratio of serum estradiol to estrone normally found in premenopausal women can be achieved with intravaginal or transdermal use; this ratio is not achievable with oral use. Total estrogen serum concentrations is dose-dependent.

Urogenital symptoms suppressant—
After the menopause when ovarian follicles are absent, symptoms of estrogen deficiency begin when the serum estradiol concentration falls. Restoring the more potent estrogens, such as estradiol, or increasing the estrone concentration helps to lessen or stop symptoms of genital itching, vaginal dryness, dyspareunia, dysuria, urinary frequency, urgency, and urinary or stress incontinence. Clinical data show estrogens cause the vaginal and urethral environment to return to normal. As the vaginal pH falls below 5, normal flora recolonize, and the vaginal and urethral mucosa mature. The maturation of the mucosa is clinically apparent with the disappearance of parabasal cells and an increase in the number of intermediate and superficial epithelial cells.

Estrogens may act to increase the collagen content in the urethra and bladder base and cause growth of urethral epithelium. How intravaginal administration distributes estrogen to the urethral mucosa is not known, but it is likely due to an increased systemic concentration or is provided by local access to urogenital tissue through a venous plexus.

In most menopausal patients, vaginal estrogen doses that maintain the serum estradiol concentrations at postmenopausal levels produce mainly local vaginal effects without sufficiently stimulating the endometrium to resume menstrual-like cycles. For some patients, the dose may be sufficient to stimulate the endometrium; rarely, endometrial hyperplasia occurs. Also, at these low doses, vaginal estrogens do not significantly suppress the gonadotropins FSH or LH, lessen systemic menopausal symptoms, or diminish the rate of bone loss. Systemic effects must be considered and expected if serum estrogen concentrations increase beyond the postmenopausal range.

## Other actions/effects

Estrogens help develop and maintain the female reproductive system, urogenital tissue tone and elasticity, and secondary sex characteristics. Estrogens, acting with other hormones and cytokines, stimulate the growth and development of breast tissue and skeleton formation, and are integral to the physiology of puberty, menstruation, ovulatory cycles, and pregnancy.

## Absorption

Estrogens are well absorbed from the vagina, mucous membranes, subcutaneous fat, and gastrointestinal tract. Vaginal absorption is dependent on estrogen particle size, dose and type of estrogen, vehicle used, and status of the vaginal mucosa. Smaller-sized particles of estrogens (micronized) show rapid absorption while coarser particles absorb slowly over a longer period of time. Low doses of estrogen used several times a week or ultralow doses given continuously, such as with the estradiol vaginal insert, achieve mainly local effects, while daily vaginal dosing can produce high systemic concentrations and effects. Conjugated or sulfated estrogens and creams and suppositories provide longer effects. Atrophied mucosa exhibits more systemic absorption for 3 to 4 months until mucosa is revitalized by estrogens, after which less of the estrogen is absorbed systemically.

For conjugated estrogens—Conjugates of estrogens, largely estrone sulfate, are absorbed intravaginally but to a lesser extent than estradiol.

For estradiol vaginal insert: 8% (range 3 to 13%) of the daily release from the estradiol vaginal insert is absorbed systemically. After an initial 24-hour peak release of 50 mcg, 7.5 mcg is released every 24 hours for 90 days of continuous use. Maximum peak concentration is approximately 38% lower after 3 months, when the second vaginal insert is used and the vaginal mucosa is no longer atrophied.

## Protein binding

Moderate to high (50 to 80%); to sex hormone–binding globulin and albumin.

Vaginal conjugated estrogens, by delivering supraphysiologic doses to the liver, are capable of inducing the synthesis of proteins, such as sex hormone–binding globulin, and sulfating estrogens to create a drug reservoir of estrogen. Except for conjugated estrogens, vaginally administered estrogens in appropriate doses can deliver physiologic doses of estrogen to the liver that do not induce production of hepatic proteins.

## Biotransformation

Estrogens are metabolized primarily by hepatic and local target tissues such as skeletal muscles, the kidneys, and the gonads. Tissues dynamically metabolize and interconvert between estrogens—estrone and estradiol—as well as between their metabolites, such as unconjugated and conjugated estrogen sulfates, and unesterified and esterified estrogens. On a dose-to-dose basis, a higher ratio of estradiol to estrone serum concentrations can be achieved through use of vaginal or transdermal products as compared with oral products.

During hepatic metabolism estrogens are desulfated, resulfated, and oxidized to less active estrogens, to nonestrogenic substances that interact with catecholamine receptors in the CNS, and to conjugates of glucuronic acid that may be quickly eliminated.

Vaginal metabolism of estradiol is minimal; conjugated estrogens, however, are metabolized in the vaginal epithelia.

## Half-life

For estradiol—20 minutes.

## Time to peak concentration

For estradiol vaginal insert—Time to peak is 0.5 to 1 hour, declining to a constant release after 24 hours, reaching the steady-state serum concentration within 7 to 10 days.

## Duration of action

For estradiol vaginal insert—3 months.

## Elimination

Renal—Major route for excretion of acidic ionized conjugates, such as glucuronides and sulfates.

Fecal—Minimal; reabsorbed from intestines and recirculated through portal venous system.

## Precautions to Consider

Note: Vaginally administered estrogen attains serum estradiol concentrations that are about 25 to 40% of that reached by the same dose given orally. Risk of endometrial proliferation should be considered with use of vaginal estrogen, even if systemic effects are not produced. If the serum estrone and estradiol concentrations increase beyond the postmenopausal range, systemic effects of the hormones should be considered with vaginal use.

## Carcinogenicity

Risk of developing endometrial cancer for users of vaginal estrogens has not been determined, but is probably related to estrogen dose and duration of treatment. Developing endometrial cancer is less likely if the vaginal dose affects only the urogenital tissue, not the uterine lining, and is not greatly absorbed systemically. Low doses used intravaginally for prolonged periods of time may increase risk of endometrial hyperplasia and, although no cases have been reported, endometrial carcinoma.

The following data are based on use of oral estrogens. Estrogens may increase the incidence of breast cancer in some postmenopausal women. Long-term studies are still needed to fully characterize potential risk. The majority of data available do not seem to support a significant increase in risk for patients using physiologic doses. Patients using estrogen in either high doses or low doses for a prolonged period of time, especially longer than 10 years, potentially may have greater risk. Short-term use of estrogens for treatment of menopausal symptoms does not appear to increase risk, and no additional risk has been attributed to adding a progestin to the therapy. Regular breast examinations or mammography will help detect any developing problems.

When nonusers were compared with users of an oral estrogen-only cycle, no risk of endometrial hyperplasia was shown for the first year of use. When oral estrogens were taken for a prolonged period of time or at higher-than-physiologic doses, the risk increased 2 to 12 times. Furthermore, the risk can be increased as much as 24 times when oral estrogens are used for 5 years or longer. Although the magnitude of the risk decreases substantially within 6 months after unopposed oral estrogen therapy is discontinued, some risk can continue for 8 to 15 years. Studies show a lower incidence of endometrial hyperplasia and, potentially, endometrial cancer when patients take a progestin for a minimum period of 10 to 14 days a month along with an estrogen cycle.

In certain animal species, long-term, continuous administration of systemic estrogens increases the frequency of cancers of the breast, cervix, liver, pancreas, testes, uterus, and vagina. Results of animal studies may not apply to humans because of the general hormonal differences in sex steroids among species.

## Pregnancy/Reproduction

Pregnancy—Estrogens are not recommended for use during pregnancy. This recommendation is based on studies showing an association of congenital malformations with use of oral diethylstilbestrol (DES). Patients who become pregnant while taking estrogens should be informed of the potential risks to the fetus. Pregnancy occurs rarely in menopausal women because of the natural change in their hormonal milieu; on the rare chance of its occurrence, a fetus surviving to term is unlikely.

FDA Pregnancy Category X.

**Breast-feeding**
Estrogens are distributed into breast milk. Use of estrogens by breast-feeding women is not recommended.

**Geriatrics**
Studies performed to date have not demonstrated geriatrics-specific problems that would limit the usefulness of vaginal estrogens in the elderly.

**Laboratory value alterations**
The following have been selected on the basis of their potential clinical significance (possible effect in parentheses where appropriate)—not necessarily inclusive (» = major clinical significance):

With physiology/laboratory test values
 Plasma binding globulins, such as:
  Sex hormone–binding globulin (SHBG), serum
  Thyroxine-binding globulin (TBG), serum
 Renin substrate
  (conjugated estrogens elevate SHBG, TBG, and renin substrate, but not corticosteroid-binding globulin, when doses of 0.2 to 2 mg are given vaginally; other estrogens given vaginally in doses to maintain physiologic concentrations of estradiol in postmenopausal women do not show these effects)

**Medical considerations/Contraindications**
The medical considerations/contraindications included have been selected on the basis of their potential clinical significance (reasons given in parentheses where appropriate)—not necessarily inclusive (» = major clinical significance).

Note: If vaginal doses increase the serum estradiol concentrations beyond the postmenopausal range, consider the precautions for systemic estrogens.

*Except under special circumstances, this medication should not be used when the following medical problems exist:*
» Allergy to cream components, including parabens
» Neoplasia, estrogen-dependent, known or suspected
  (may promote tumor growth or interfere with the action of antiestrogen treatment regimens for any systemically absorbed dose. Carefully chosen patients with these conditions have used low vaginal doses for treating urogenital conditions; however, estrogen use in these patients is still considered to introduce an unknown risk)
» Genital or uterine bleeding, abnormal or undiagnosed
  (use of estrogens may delay diagnosis; on occurrence, estrogen should be discontinued until clinical evaluation is completed. Condition may worsen if cause of abnormal uterine bleeding is endometrial hyperplasia or endometrial cancer)

*Risk-benefit should be considered when the following medical problems exist:*
 Cervicitis or
 Vaginal infection or
 Vaginitis
  (use of vaginal estrogen may worsen these conditions or, for the estradiol vaginal insert, cause ulceration; on occurrence, discontinuing use of estrogen may not be necessary but the underlying irritation or infection should be treated as appropriate)
 Endometriosis or
 Leiomyomata, uterine
  (may be aggravated by use of estrogens)
 Hepatic function impairment, severe
  (systemic doses may worsen this condition)
  (severe hepatic function impairment can decrease estrogen metabolism, especially when using conjugated estrogens. Carefully chosen patients with severe hepatic function impairment have used low vaginal doses of estrogens for treating urogenital conditions. Locally or vaginally administered estradiol and estrone have less effect on the liver than conjugated estrogens)
 Thrombophlebitis or thromboembolic disorders, active
  (concurrent use of any estrogen is not recommended by many physicians until condition is resolved; although low doses of vaginal estrogens to treat urogenital conditions make the association for exacerbation of an active condition unlikely)
 Vaginal narrowing or
 Vaginal prolapse or
 Vaginal stenosis
  (use of the estradiol vaginal insert may cause abdominal or back pain, vaginal irritation or ulceration, urinary incontinence, or frequent device expulsion in some of these patients)

**Patient monitoring**
The following may be especially important in patient monitoring (other tests may be warranted in some patients, depending on condition; » = major clinical significance):

Breast examination and
Mammography and
Papanicolaou (Pap) test and
Physical examinations
 (recommended annually or more often as determined by physician, with emphasis on examining blood pressure, breasts, abdomen, and pelvic organs, including a Papanicolaou [Pap] test; regular self-examination to detect breast problems should be done by patient)
Endometrial biopsy
 (patients with a uterus should be monitored for signs of endometrial cancer, and malignancy should be ruled out in cases of persistent or recurring abnormal vaginal bleeding)

## Side/Adverse Effects

Note: The risk of any serious adverse effect is minimal for women using low doses of estrogen. Even women who have special risk factors successfully use estrogens.

Consider the side effects of systemic estrogens if serum estradiol concentrations increase beyond the postmenopausal range as shown by laboratory tests or evidence of patient complaints, especially complaints of uterine bleeding or breast tenderness. Risk of endometrial proliferation should be considered with use of vaginal estrogens, with or without systemic effects.

The following side/adverse effects have been selected on the basis of their potential clinical significance (possible signs and symptoms in parentheses where appropriate)—not necessarily inclusive:

**Those indicating need for medical attention**
Incidence less frequent
 *Breast pain or enlargement; headache; nausea; vulvovaginal candidiasis* (itching of the vagina or genitals; thick, white vaginal discharge without odor or with a mild odor)—estrogens usually prevent; *vulvovaginitis* (itching, stinging, or redness of the genital area)—estrogens usually prevent

Note: *Vulvovaginal candidiasis* or *vulvovaginitis* occur more frequently in untreated postmenopausal patients, but since they are reported in up to 13% of vaginal estrogen users, infection or irritation should be evaluated and treated. Although estrogen is used in treating vulvovaginal irritation, *vulvovaginitis* may be caused by other ingredients in the vaginal formulation.

*Breast pain*, *headache*, or *nausea* can indicate systemic absorption, and may require reduction of dose or frequency if systemic absorption is not desired.

Incidence rare
 *Uterine bleeding or spotting, unusual or unexpected; vaginal discomfort, pain, or ulceration due to a foreign object* (feeling of vaginal pressure; vaginal burning or pain)—with use of estradiol vaginal insert

Note: Any *unusual or unexpected uterine bleeding or spotting*, especially if persistent or recurrent, should be evaluated for endometrial hyperplasia or endometrial cancer. If workup is uneventful, then lowering patient's estrogen dose or frequency or adding a progestin for at least 10 to 14 days a month may be needed.

**Those indicating need for medical attention only if they continue or are bothersome**
Incidence less frequent
 *Abdominal or back pain; leukorrhea* (clear vaginal discharge)—usually indicates therapeutic effect

## Patient Consultation

As an aid to patient consultation, refer to *Advice for the Patient, Estrogens (Vaginal)*.

In providing consultation, consider emphasizing the following selected information (» = major clinical significance):

**Before using this medication**
» Conditions affecting use, especially:
 Allergy to cream components, such as parabens
 Carcinogenicity—For patients taking estrogens or progestins, risk of endometrial cancer for vaginal estrogen users is not fully understood or easily quantified, but thought to be less likely if doses are kept low enough to treat urogenital conditions locally; also, endometrial hyperplasia is less likely to occur

Pregnancy—Use of estrogens during pregnancy is not recommended because of reported congenital abnormalities caused by diethylstilbestrol (DES); although pregnancy is not usually a concern for perimenopausal patients, patient should inform physician immediately if pregnancy is suspected

Breast-feeding—Use is not recommended because estrogens are distributed into breast milk

Other medical problems, especially estrogen-dependent neoplasia (known or suspected) or genital or uterine bleeding (abnormal or undiagnosed)

**Proper use of this medication**

» Reading patient package insert (PPI) carefully
Washing hands immediately before and after vaginal administration; avoiding contact with eyes; washing it out of eyes with water if medication accidentally gets into eyes

» Understanding directions of use and that full therapeutic effect may take 3 or 4 months to appear; checking with physician for changes in dose and not using medication longer than prescribed

*Proper administration technique*
For cream dosage form—Understanding the markings on applicator and how to withdraw the proper dose
For cream and suppository dosage form—Following directions regarding the filling of the applicator with medication; understanding the insertion technique; and, depending on the applicator type supplied by the product's packaging, either discarding the disposable applicators after each use or, if reusable, cleaning and drying applicators thoroughly after each use
For estradiol vaginal insert—Knowing how to place, reposition, or remove the vaginal insert in the upper part of vagina, and how to dispose of the old vaginal insert safely, especially avoiding flushing it down the toilet

» Compliance with therapy
» Proper dosing
Missed dose:
For weekly dosing of suppository or cream—Using as soon as possible within 1 or 2 days; however, not using if almost time for next dose; not doubling doses
For daily dosing of suppository or cream—Using missed dose within 12 hours. Not using missed dose if almost time for next dose; not doubling doses

» Proper storage

**Precautions while using this medication**

» Regular annual visits to physician, or more often, as determined by physician
» Checking breasts by self-examination regularly and having clinical examination and mammography as required by physician; reporting unusual breast lumps or discharge
» Stopping medication immediately and checking with physician if pregnancy is suspected
If scheduled for laboratory tests, telling physician about estrogen use; certain blood tests and tissue biopsies are affected

*For all vaginal creams*
» Not using latex condoms for up to 72 hours after vaginal estrogen treatment because oils in the vaginal cream dosage form may weaken latex products
Using medication at bedtime to increase effectiveness; wearing sanitary napkin to protect clothing
Avoiding exposing male partner to estrogen vaginal cream through sexual intercourse; having sexual intercourse, when desired, prior to administering vaginal dose

*For estradiol vaginal insert*
Not needing to remove for sexual intercourse unless desired
Washing the vaginal insert before reinsertion when expelled or if taken out for sexual intercourse
Replacing with new vaginal insert after 3 months

**Side/adverse effects**
Signs of potential side effects, especially breast pain or enlargement; headache; nausea; vulvovaginal candidiasis; vulvovaginitis; unusual or unexpected uterine bleeding or spotting; vaginal discomfort, pain, or ulceration due to a foreign object (for estradiol vaginal insert)
Reporting to physician if vaginal use produces systemic estrogen side/adverse effects, such as uterine bleeding or breast tenderness; understanding that vaginal administration can produce systemic estrogen effects and, on their occurrence, may warrant a dosage reduction

## General Dosing Information

It is required that the patient package insert (PPI) be given to patients.
Generally, the lowest dose to control urogenital symptoms is used. The patient is often titrated over a 6-week period and re-evaluated at 3- to 6-month intervals to assess whether to continue her estrogen treatment or to make dosage or frequency adjustments.

Doses that maintain serum estradiol concentrations within the postmenopausal range will not cause endometrial stimulation or monthly uterine bleeding. While serum estradiol concentrations of 140 to 200 picomoles per liter (pmol/L) suppress vasomotor symptoms, these concentrations do not frequently occur when low maintenance doses of estrogen are applied or used vaginally 2 to 3 times a week. Concentrations below 70 pmol/L associated with atrophy of the endometrium are produced instead.

Postmenopausal patients should be counseled that they will not show an improved lipoprotein cholesterol profile or be protected against bone loss while their serum estradiol concentration remains in the postmenopausal range. Although sufficiently high serum estradiol concentrations can be produced from use of vaginal estrogens, use of oral, transdermal, or parenteral estrogen therapy may be preferred instead for these uses.

*For vaginal creams*
The cream vehicles for some vaginal estrogen products contain mineral oil or other lipid-based components that may adversely affect the performance of latex barrier devices, such as condoms, cervical caps, or diaphragms, to prevent pregnancy or sexually transmitted diseases.

Low doses given vaginally cause few systemic effects and, rarely, cause endometrial stimulation; concomitant progestin treatment for 10 to 14 days is recommended by some medical organizations for patients with a uterus and is especially important when uterine bleeding or systemic effects occur. Usually when 2 or 3 low maintenance doses a week are used intravaginally, cyclic treatment of 3 weeks on and 1 week off is sufficient to prevent endometrial proliferation without adding a progestin.

If oral estrogens are given for 10 to 14 days as a priming dose, then the initial dosage regimen for vaginal treatment is discontinued and the maintenance treatment regimen is initiated instead.

Patient counseling on withdrawing the proper dose into applicator is important, especially when transferring a patient to a different product. Applicator markings indicate the amount of cream in grams. Patients may confuse the dose (in mg) with the amount of cream to be applied (in grams).

*For vaginal cream or suppository*
To properly place vaginal cream or suppository, patient lies on back with knees drawn up and apart, gently inserting applicator into vagina, carefully releasing dose by pressing plunger downward to original position. Cleaning the applicator, if reusable, is accomplished by separating the plunger from the barrel and washing each separately with soap and water; never using boiling or hot water. Applicator unit is reassembled after each part dries thoroughly. A new disposable applicator can be used with each dose if one is contained in the packaging.

*For estradiol vaginal insert*
Systemic effects from a daily dose of 7.5 mcg of estradiol released over 24 hours are minimal, making concomitant progestin treatment unnecessary as use of the vaginal insert at this dose rarely causes endometrial stimulation. Use of the vaginal insert beyond ninety days does not result in an overdose, but rather an underdose, and increases the likelihood of vaginal infections or epithelial ulcers occurring due to lack of efficacy.

Insertion technique—Pinching or pressing the sides of the vaginal insert together, between forefinger and middle finger, into a smaller oval-shape allows placement into the upper third of the vagina, and can be managed by patient or physician. Patient can place vaginal insert while lying on her back with knees up or while standing with one foot raised on a chair. Although an exact placement in the vagina is not critical, any discomfort felt by the patient requires that the vaginal insert be moved higher by gently pushing the insert further into the vagina.

Removal technique—Removed by hooking a finger through the ring-shaped vaginal insert and gently pulling it out through the vagina.

Removal of the vaginal insert is not needed for sexual intercourse unless preferred by the patient; in one study, only 6 of approximately 182 postmenopausal patients (17%) removed the vaginal insert for sexual intercourse. Straining on defecation may cause the vaginal insert to move lower in the vagina or to be expelled accidentally from the vagina.

If the vaginal insert is removed by the patient or expelled accidentally, rinsing in lukewarm water is sufficient before replacing the vaginal insert back into the vagina.

## CONJUGATED ESTROGENS

### Summary of Differences
Indications: Atrophic vaginitis and vulvar atrophy.
Pharmacology/pharmacokinetics: Mixture of estrogenic metabolites, extracted from the urine of pregnant mares; highly sulfated. Vaginal conjugated estrogens provide longer duration of action and induce liver to increase proteins, such as SHBG, TBG, and renin substrate; metabolized by vaginal mucosa; absorbed slower than other estrogens.
Medical considerations/Contraindications—May exacerbate existing hepatic function impairment.

### Vaginal Dosage Forms
#### CONJUGATED ESTROGENS VAGINAL CREAM
**Usual adult dose**
Atrophic vaginitis or
Vulvar atrophy—
Intravaginal or topical, 0.3 to 1.25 mg of conjugated estrogens (one-half to two grams of cream) daily or as directed by physician based on the lowest dose needed for three weeks, with no medication used in the fourth week; the schedule being repeated each month.

**Usual geriatric dose**
See *Usual adult dose*.

**Strength(s) usually available**
U.S.—
625 mcg (0.625 mg) per gram (Rx) [*Premarin* (benzyl alcohol; cetyl esters wax; cetyl alcohol; glycerin; glyceryl monostearate; methyl stearate; mineral oil; propylene glycol monostearate; sodium lauryl sulfate; white wax)].
Canada—
625 mcg (0.625 mg) per gram (Rx) [*Premarin* (cetyl alcohol; phenylethyl alcohol)].

**Packaging and storage**
Store below 40 °C (104 °F), preferably between 15 and 30 °C (59 and 86 °F), unless otherwise specified by manufacturer.

**Auxiliary labeling**
• For vaginal use only.

**Note**
Include mandatory patient package insert (PPI) when dispensing.

**Additional information**
Canadian brand of *Premarin* is gluten-, paraben-, sugar-, sulfite-, and tartazine-free. Calibrated applicator measures in 0.5 gram increments up to 2 grams of cream.

## DIENESTROL

### Summary of Differences
Indications: Atrophic vaginitis and vulvar atrophy.
Pharmacology/pharmacokinetics: Source—Synthetic, nonsteroidal estrogen.

### Vaginal Dosage Forms
#### DIENESTROL CREAM USP
**Usual adult dose**
Atrophic vaginitis or
Vulvar atrophy—
Initial: Intravaginal, 0.5 mg (one applicatorful) one or two times a day for one or two weeks, the dose then being reduced to either 0.25 or 0.5 mg (one-half or one applicatorful) a day for an additional one or two weeks.
Maintenance: Intravaginal, 0.5 mg (one applicatorful) one to three times a week for three weeks with no medication used in the fourth week after vaginal mucosa is no longer atrophied; this schedule being repeated each month.

**Usual geriatric dose**
See *Usual adult dose*.

**Strength(s) usually available**
U.S.—
0.01% (Rx) [*Ortho Dienestrol* (benzoic acid; butylated hydroxyanisole; citric acid; glutamic acid; glycerin; glyceryl monostearate; peanut oil; sodium hydroxide; water)].
Canada—
0.01% (Rx) [*Ortho Dienestrol* (benzoic acid; butylated hydroxyanisole; citric acid; glutamic acid; glycerin; glyceryl monostearate; peanut oil; sodium hydroxide; water)].

**Packaging and storage**
Store below 40 °C (104 °F), preferably between 15 and 30 °C (59 and 86 °F), unless otherwise specified by manufacturer. Store in collapsible tubes or tight containers.

**Auxiliary labeling**
• For vaginal use only.

**Note**
Include mandatory patient package insert (PPI) when dispensing.

**Additional information**
Applicator is not calibrated.

## ESTRADIOL

### Summary of Differences
Indications: Atrophic vaginitis, vulvar atrophy, and atrophic postmenopausal urethritis.
Pharmacology/pharmacokinetics: Natural estrogen easily absorbed vaginally without metabolism by vaginal mucosa; does not induce hepatic protein synthesis.
Medical considerations/Contraindications—Does not exacerbate existing hepatic function impairment; vaginal insert is more likely to be expelled or cause problems for women with narrow vaginas, vaginal prolapse or vaginal stenosis; cream may exacerbate allergy to parabens.
Side/Adverse effects: Vaginal insert, as a foreign device, may cause vaginal discomfort, pain, or ulceration.

### Vaginal Dosage Forms
Note: Bracketed uses in the *Dosage Forms* section refer to categories of use or indications that are not included in U.S. product labeling.

#### ESTRADIOL VAGINAL CREAM USP
**Usual adult dose**
Atrophic vaginitis or
Vulvar atrophy—
Initial: Intravaginal, 200 to 400 mcg of estradiol (two to four grams of cream) daily for one or two weeks, the dosage then being gradually reduced to one-half the initial dosage for one or two weeks.
Maintenance: Intravaginal, 100 mcg of estradiol (one gram of cream) one to three times a week for three weeks with no medication used in the fourth week after vaginal mucosa is no longer atrophied; this schedule being repeated each month.

**Usual geriatric dose**
See *Usual adult dose*.

**Strength(s) usually available**
U.S.—
0.01% (Rx) [*Estrace* (2208 4000 CPS; edetate disodium; glyceryl monostearate; hydroxypropyl methylcellulose; methylparaben; propylene glycol; sodium lauryl sulfate; stearyl alcohol; tertiary-butylhydroquinone; water; white ceresin wax)].
Canada—
Not commercially available.

**Packaging and storage**
Store below 40 °C (104 °F), preferably between 15 and 30 °C (59 and 86 °F), unless otherwise specified by manufacturer. Store in collapsible tubes or tight containers.

**Auxiliary labeling**
• For vaginal use only.

**Note**
Include mandatory patient package insert (PPI) when dispensing.

**Additional information**
Calibrated applicator measures 1 to 4 grams of cream in increments of 1 gram.

#### ESTRADIOL VAGINAL INSERT
Note: Also called estradiol vaginal ring.

**Usual adult dose**
[Atrophic vaginitis] or
Urethritis, atrophic, postmenopausal or

[Vulvar atrophy, postmenopausal]—
   Intravaginal, 2 mg (one vaginal insert) releases 7.5 mcg from its ring-shape over twenty-four hours when worn continuously high in the upper third of the vagina and is replaced every ninety days.

**Usual geriatric dose**
See *Usual adult dose*.

**Strength(s) usually available**
U.S.—
   2 mg delivering 7.5 mcg per 24 hours (Rx) [*Estring* (barium sulfate in device; silicone polymers in device)].
Canada—
   2 mg delivering 7.5 mcg per 24 hours (Rx) [*Estring* (barium sulfate in device; silicone polymers in device)].

**Packaging and storage**
Store below 40 °C (104 °F), preferably between 15 and 30 °C (59 and 86 °F), unless otherwise specified by manufacturer.

**Auxiliary labeling**
• For vaginal use only.

**Note**
Include mandatory patient package insert (PPI) when dispensing.

---

## ESTRONE

## Summary of Differences
Indications: Atrophic vaginitis, postmenopausal, and vulvar atrophy.
Pharmacology/pharmacokinetics: Natural estrogen easily absorbed vaginally without metabolism by vaginal mucosa; does not induce hepatic proteins synthesis.
Medical considerations/Contraindications—Does not exacerbate existing hepatic function impairment; cream may exacerbate allergy to parabens.

## Vaginal Dosage Forms
### ESTRONE VAGINAL CREAM

**Usual adult dose**
Atrophic vaginitis, postmenopausal or
Vulvar atrophy—
   Intravaginal, 2 to 4 mg of estrone (two to four grams of cream) daily or as directed by physician based on the lowest dose needed.

**Usual geriatric dose**
See *Usual adult dose*.

**Strength(s) usually available**
U.S.—
   Not commercially available.
Canada—
   1 mg per gram (Rx) [*Oestrilin* (methylparaben; mineral oil; propylparaben)].

**Packaging and storage**
Store below 40 °C (104 °F), preferably between 15 and 30 °C (59 and 86 °F), in a well-closed container, unless otherwise specified by manufacturer.

**Auxiliary labeling**
• For vaginal use only.

**Note**
Include mandatory patient package insert (PPI) when dispensing.

**Additional information**
Calibrated applicator measures 1 to 4 grams of cream in increments of 1 gram.

### ESTRONE VAGINAL SUPPOSITORIES
Note: Also called cones.

**Usual adult dose**
Atrophic vaginitis, postmenopausal or
Vulvar atrophy—
   Intravaginal, 250 to 500 mcg daily or as directed by physician based on the lowest dose needed.

**Usual geriatric dose**
See *Usual adult dose*.

**Strength(s) usually available**
U.S.—
   Not commercially available.
Canada—
   250 mcg (Rx) [*Oestrilin* (gelatin; glycerin)].

**Packaging and storage**
Store below 40 °C (104 °F), preferably between 15 and 30 °C (59 and 86 °F), in a well-closed container, unless otherwise specified by manufacturer.

**Auxiliary labeling**
• For vaginal use only.

**Note**
Include mandatory patient package insert (PPI) when dispensing.

---

## ESTROPIPATE

## Summary of Differences
Indications: Atrophic vaginitis and vulvar atrophy.
Pharmacology/pharmacokinetics: Semi-synthetic estrogen.
Medical considerations/Contraindications—Cream may exacerbate allergy to parabens.

## Vaginal Dosage Forms
### ESTROPIPATE VAGINAL CREAM USP
Note: Formerly called piperazine estrone sulfate.

**Usual adult dose**
Atrophic vaginitis or
Vulvar atrophy—
   Intravaginal, 3 to 6 mg of estropipate (two to four grams of cream) daily for three weeks with no medication used the fourth week, the schedule being repeated each month.

**Usual geriatric dose**
See *Usual adult dose*.

**Strength(s) usually available**
U.S.—
   1.5 mg per gram (Rx) [*Ogen* (anhydrous lanolin; cetyl alcohol; cis-*N*-(3-chloroallyl) hexaminium chloride; citric acid; glycerin; glyceryl monostearate; higher fatty alcohols; methylparaben; mineral oil; piperazine hexahydrate; propylparaben; sodium biphosphate; water)].
Canada—
   Not commercially available.

**Packaging and storage**
Store below 40 °C (104 °F), preferably between 15 and 30 °C (59 and 86 °F), unless otherwise specified by manufacturer.

**Auxiliary labeling**
• For vaginal use only.

**Note**
Include mandatory patient package insert (PPI) when dispensing.

**Additional information**
Calibrated applicator measures 1 to 4 grams of cream in increments of 1 gram.

## Selected Bibliography
Baker VL. Alternatives to oral estrogen replacement. Transdermal patches, percutaneous gels, vaginal creams and rings, implants, and other methods of delivery. Obstet Gynecol Clin North Am 1994 Jun; 21(2): 271-97.

Revised: 08/20/97

---

**ESTROGENS, CONJUGATED**—See *Estrogens (Systemic)*; *Estrogens (Vaginal)*

---

**ESTROGENS, ESTERIFIED**—See *Estrogens (Systemic)*

# ESTROGENS AND PROGESTINS (ORAL CONTRACEPTIVES) Systemic

This monograph includes information on the following: 1) Desogestrel and Ethinyl Estradiol; 2) Ethynodiol Diacetate and Ethinyl Estradiol; 3) Levonorgestrel and Ethinyl Estradiol; 4) Norethindrone Acetate and Ethinyl Estradiol; 5) Norethindrone and Ethinyl Estradiol; 6) Norethindrone and Mestranol; 7) Norgestimate and Ethinyl Estradiol; 8) Norgestrel and Ethinyl Estradiol

Note: For information pertaining to the use of progestin-only contraceptives, see *Progestins (Systemic)*.

INN:
Ethinyl estradiol—Ethinylestradiol
Ethynodiol diacetate—Etynodiol
Norethindrone—Norethisterone

BAN:
Ethinyl estradiol—Ethinyloestradiol
Ethynodiol diacetate—Etynodiol
Norethindrone—Norethisterone

JAN:
Ethinyl estradiol—Ethinylestradiol
Ethynodiol diacetate—Etynodiol acetate
Norethindrone—Norethisterone

VA CLASSIFICATION (Primary/Secondary): HS104/HS109

Commonly used brand name(s): *Alesse*[3]; *Brevicon*[5]; *Brevicon 0.5/35*[5]; *Brevicon 1/35*[5]; *Cyclen*[7]; *Demulen 1/35*[2]; *Demulen 1/50*[2]; *Demulen 30*[2]; *Demulen 50*[2]; *Desogen*[1]; *Estrostep*[4]; *Estrostep Fe*[4]; *Genora 0.5/35*[5]; *Genora 1/35*[5]; *Genora 1/50*[6]; *Intercon 0.5/35*[5]; *Intercon 1/35*[5]; *Intercon 1/50*[6]; *Jenest*[5]; *Levlen*[3]; *Levlite*[3]; *Levora 0.15/30*[3]; *Lo/Ovral*[8]; *Loestrin 1.5/30*[4]; *Loestrin 1/20*[4]; *Loestrin Fe 1.5/30*[4]; *Loestrin Fe 1/20*[4]; *Marvelon*[1]; *Min-Ovral*[3]; *Minestrin 1/20*[4]; *Mircette*[1]; *ModiCon*[5]; *N.E.E. 1/35*[5]; *N.E.E. 1/50*[5]; *Necon 0.5/35*[5]; *Necon 1/35*[5]; *Necon 1/50*[6]; *Necon 10/11*[5]; *Nelova 10/11*[5]; *Nelova 0.5/35E*[5]; *Nelova 1/35E*[5]; *Nelova 1/50M*[6]; *Nordette*[3]; *Norethin 1/35E*[5]; *Norethin 1/50M*[6]; *Norinyl 1+35*[5]; *Norinyl 1+50*[6]; *Norinyl 1/50*[6]; *Ortho 0.5/35*[5]; *Ortho 1/35*[5]; *Ortho 10/11*[5]; *Ortho 7/7/7*[5]; *Ortho Tri-Cyclen*[7]; *Ortho-Cept*[1]; *Ortho-Cyclen*[7]; *Ortho-Novum 1/35*[5]; *Ortho-Novum 1/50*[6]; *Ortho-Novum 10/11*[5]; *Ortho-Novum 7/7/7*[5]; *Ovcon-35*[5]; *Ovcon-50*[5]; *Ovral*[8]; *Select 1/35*[5]; *Synphasic*[5]; *Tri-Cyclen*[7]; *Tri-Levlen*[3]; *Tri-Norinyl*[5]; *Triphasil*[3]; *Triquilar*[3]; *Trivora*[3]; *Zovia 1/35E*[2]; *Zovia 1/50E*[2].

Other commonly used names are Ethinylestradiol and Ethinyloestradiol [Ethinyl estradiol]; Ethynodiol, Etynodiol, and Etynodiol acetate [Ethynodiol diacetate]; and Norethindrone [Norethisterone].

Note: For a listing of dosage forms and brand names by country availability, see *Dosage Forms* section(s).

## Category

Contraceptive, systemic—Desogestrel and Ethinyl Estradiol; Ethynodiol Diacetate and Ethinyl Estradiol; Levonorgestrel and Ethinyl Estradiol; Norethindrone Acetate and Ethinyl Estradiol; Norethindrone and Ethinyl Estradiol; Norethindrone and Mestranol; Norgestimate and Ethinyl Estradiol; Norgestrel and Ethinyl Estradiol.

Antiacne agent, systemic—Norgestimate and Ethinyl Estradiol (Triphasic formulation only).

Antiendometriotic agent—Desogestrel and Ethinyl Estradiol; Ethynodiol Diacetate and Ethinyl Estradiol; Levonorgestrel and Ethinyl Estradiol; Norethindrone Acetate and Ethinyl Estradiol; Norethindrone and Ethinyl Estradiol; Norethindrone and Mestranol; Norgestimate and Ethinyl Estradiol; Norgestrel and Ethinyl Estradiol.

Contraceptive, postcoital (systemic)—Levonorgestrel and Ethinyl Estradiol; Norgestrel and Ethinyl Estradiol.

Estrogen-progestin—Desogestrel and Ethinyl Estradiol; Ethynodiol Diacetate and Ethinyl Estradiol; Levonorgestrel and Ethinyl Estradiol; Norethindrone Acetate and Ethinyl Estradiol; Norethindrone and Ethinyl Estradiol; Norethindrone and Mestranol; Norgestimate and Ethinyl Estradiol; Norgestrel and Ethinyl Estradiol.

Gonadotropin inhibitor, female, noncontraceptive use—Desogestrel and Ethinyl Estradiol; Ethynodiol Diacetate and Ethinyl Estradiol; Levonorgestrel and Ethinyl Estradiol; Norethindrone Acetate and Ethinyl Estradiol; Norethindrone and Ethinyl Estradiol; Norethindrone and Mestranol; Norgestimate and Ethinyl Estradiol; Norgestrel and Ethinyl Estradiol.

## Indications

Note: Bracketed information in the *Indications* section refers to uses that are not included in U.S. product labeling.

### Accepted

Pregnancy, prevention of—Combination estrogen-progestin oral contraceptives are indicated for the prevention of pregnancy. The lowest expected failure rate for women who use oral contraceptives consistently and correctly under clinical conditions is 0.1% in the first year of use; however, under nonclinical conditions the typical use is less perfect and typical failures may range from 0 to 6%. All regimens are considered equally effective for preventing pregnancy.

The following table presents the results of studies examining contraceptive failure rates calculated using the life-table method. The first column lists the contraceptive method used. The second column indicates the percentage of women experiencing an accidental pregnancy in the first year of use of a contraceptive method while using the method perfectly under clinical conditions. The range of failure rates in the clinical trials may be explained by interstudy variations in study design or patient population characteristics, such as motivation, fecundity, or socioeconomic factors (including education). The third column indicates contraceptive failure rates in the first year of contraceptive use under clinical conditions for typical couples who start using a method (not necessarily for the first time). Failure rates among adolescents may be higher due to poorer compliance than in other age groups.

| Method used | Failure rate range (over 12 months) in clinical studies (%) | Typical first year failure rate (%) |
|---|---|---|
| None | 78–94 | 85 |
| Spermicides* | 0.3–37 | 21 |
| Periodic abstinence[†] | 13–35 | 20 |
| Withdrawal | 7–22 | 19 |
| Cervical cap with spermicide | 6–27 | 18 |
| Diaphragm with spermicide | 2–23 | 18 |
| Condom without spermicide | 2–14 | 12 |
| IUD | | |
| Progesterone-releasing | 1.9–2 | 2 |
| Copper-T 200 | 3–3.6 | |
| Copper-T 200Ag[‡] | 0–1.2 | |
| Copper-T 220C[§] | 0.9–1.8 | |
| Copper-T 380A | 0.5–0.8 | 0.8 |
| Copper-T 380S | 0.9 | |
| Oral contraceptive | | 3 |
| Estrogen and progestin | 0–6 | |
| Progestin only | 1–10 | |
| Medroxyprogesterone injection (90-day) | 0–0.3 | 0.3 |
| Levonorgestrel (subdermal) | | |
| Six implants | 0–0.09 | 0.09 |
| Two rods | 0–0.2 | 0.3 |
| Sterilization | | |
| Female[#] | 0–8 | 0.4 |
| Male | 0–0.5 | 0.15 |

*Spermicides studied include creams, foams, gels, jellies, and suppositories.

[†]Methods studied include calendar, ovulation method, and symptothermal (cervical mucus method supplemented by basal body temperature post-ovulation).

[‡]Life-table method rate is unavailable for Copper-T 200Ag and the Pearl method rate at 12 months was reported; these methods at 12 months are considered comparable.

[§]Copper-T 220C is manufactured with copper sleeves instead of copper wire; often used as a control in clinical studies.

[#]Methods studied include culdotomy laparoscopy, minilaparotomy, electrocoagulation, laparotomy, tubal diathermy and/or use of rings or clips.

[Contraception, emergency postcoital (prophylaxis)][1]—A combination of levonorgestrel or norgestrel with ethinyl estradiol is used as emergency contraception (also called intraception, morning-after treatment, or postcoital contraception) for postcoital birth control, after pregnancy has been ruled out. The dosing method using high doses of estrogen-progestin hormones is commonly called the Yuzpe method. Using oral contraceptives for emergency postcoital contraception is preferable to using ethinyl estradiol alone because, although the failure rate is higher (2% versus 1%) with oral contraceptives, they cause fewer and less severe side effects to occur. Treatment is initiated within the first 72 hours, preferably within the first 12 hours, after unprotected intercourse.

Acne vulgaris(treatment)[1]—The triphasic formulation of norgestimate and ethinyl estradiol is indicated to treat moderate acne vulgaris in females

15 years of age or older who need contraception and whose acne is unresponsive to other antiacne therapy.

[Amenorrhea (treatment)] or
[Dysfunctional uterine bleeding (DUB) (treatment)] or
[Dysmenorrhea (treatment)] or
[Hypermenorrhea (treatment)]—[Norethindrone and mestranol tablets (dose of 1/50)] are indicated [and other estrogen-progestin combinations and doses are used][1] as a hormonal treatment for hypoestrogenic or hyperandrogenic conditions, which may present as menstrual cycle abnormalities or unusual uterine bleeding, such as amenorrhea, dysfunctional uterine bleeding, or hypermenorrhea. When treating amenorrhea and hypermenorrhea, the abnormality should be diagnosed first and then treated appropriately; oral contraceptives have limited use for treating conditions not caused by a hypoestrogenic or hyperandrogenic state. Patients who require contraception as well as relief from primary dysmenorrhea, may benefit from treatment with oral contraceptives. If contraception is not needed, prostaglandin-inhibiting medications, such as nonsteroidal anti-inflammatory drugs (NSAIDs), are used. If dysmenorrhea is not relieved by oral contraceptives or NSAIDs, endometriosis or another organic cause should be considered.

Endometriosis (prophylaxis and treatment)—[Norethindrone and mestranol tablets (dose of 1/50)] are indicated [and other estrogen-progestin combinations and doses are used][1] to reduce the size and growth of endometrial tissue.

[Hirsutism, female (treatment and treatment adjunct)][1] or
[Hyperandrogenism, ovarian (treatment and treatment adjunct)][1] or
[Polycystic ovary syndrome (treatment)][1]—When treating these conditions, the basic cause should be ascertained first, if possible, and treated accordingly. When contraception is needed as well, oral contraceptives are used to help suppress hypothalamic-pituitary function in luteinizing hormone–dependent hyperandrogenism in conditions such as polycystic ovary syndrome. Oral contraceptive treatment results in regularity of the menstrual cycle and lessening of hirsutism in these conditions.

**Acceptance not established**
Only limited data are available evaluating the use of oral contraceptives as adjunct agents to replace the estrogen component as *add-back therapy* when gonadotropin-releasing hormone agonists are used to suppress the hypothalamic-pituitary axis. Using oral contraceptives as the estrogen replacement may be especially useful in women needing contraception as well. By replacing estrogen, hypoestrogenic side effects caused by the gonadotropin-releasing hormone agonist, such as bone loss and the associated vasomotor symptoms, are reduced. Further studies are needed to evaluate the safety and efficacy of this use.

Oral contraceptives, which have been effective in dysmenorrhea, have been used to reduce premenstrual pain associated with the *premenstrual syndrome* in some patients, but generally oral contraceptives are not considered useful for this indication.

**Unaccepted**
Administration of oral contraceptives to induce withdrawal bleeding should not be used as a test for pregnancy.

Oral contraceptives should not be used during pregnancy for the treatment of threatened or habitual abortion.

[1] Not included in Canadian product labeling.

## Pharmacology/Pharmacokinetics

**Physicochemical characteristics**
Chemical group—
Estrogens—
  Ethinyl estradiol.
  Mestranol.
Progestins, 19-nortestosterone derivatives—
  Desogestrel.
  Ethynodiol diacetate.
  Levonorgestrel (levorotatory isomer).
  Norethindrone.
  Norethindrone acetate.
  Norgestimate.
  Norgestrel (racemic mixture).
Molecular weight—
  Desogestrel: 310.48.
  Ethinyl estradiol: 296.41.
  Ethynodiol diacetate: 384.52.
  Levonorgestrel: 312.45.
  Mestranol: 310.44.
  Norethindrone: 298.43.
  Norethindrone acetate: 340.47.
  Norgestimate: 369.51.
  Norgestrel: 312.45.

**Mechanism of action/Effect**
Estrogen-progestin—Estrogens increase the cellular synthesis of chromatin (DNA), RNA, and various proteins in responsive tissues, and progestins increase the synthesis of RNA by means of an interaction with DNA.

Contraceptive, systemic—The synergistic anti-ovulatory effect from the combined use of estrogen and progestin directly decreases the secretion of the gonadotropin-releasing hormone (GnRH) from the hypothalamus and is considered the main action. This negative feedback mechanism disrupts ovulation by interfering with the hypothalamus-pituitary-ovary axis and gonadotropin secretion from the pituitary. Specifically, the progestin component blunts or suppresses luteinizing hormone (LH) release and the LH surge, which is necessary for ovulation, and the estrogen component blunts or suppresses the follicle-stimulating hormone (FSH), which prevents the selection and maturation of the dominant follicle. Neither the estrogen nor the progestin hormone dose used in combination hormonal oral contraceptives alone would be able to suppress ovulation but together the estrogen and progestin hormones work synergistically to suppress ovulation successfully. Other contributing effects include delayed maturation of the endometrium, which prevents implantation of ova; and the development of viscous cervical mucus, which slows spermatic ingress. The effects on the endometrium and cervical mucus are considered the mechanisms of action for the estrogen-progestin oral contraceptives used for emergency contraception (intraception).

Antiendometriotic agent—Oral contraceptives can produce a pseudopregnant state (especially when used continuously) in which the uterine endometrium and ectopic endometriotic implants undergo decidual reaction, necrosis, and eventual atrophy. Sometimes endometriotic symptoms may increase before improvement is noted.

Gonadotropin inhibitor, female, noncontraceptive use—Suppressed ovarian steroidogenesis secondary to LH concentration reduction prevents ovarian cyst formation in functional ovarian cysts, corpus luteum cysts, or polycystic ovary syndrome. Although a decrease in occurrence of repetitively forming functional ovarian cysts is possible, treatment to either speed the resolution of existing ovarian cysts or to treat functional ovarian cysts secondary to ovulation induction has not been established. The likelihood of suppressing ovarian cyst formation is greatest with 50-mcg ethinyl estradiol–containing monophasic formulations but 35-mcg ethinyl estradiol–containing monophasic formulations are used effectively, also. Suppression is least likely with triphasic formulations. In addition to suppression of ovarian steroidogenesis, there is an increase in sex hormone–binding globulin, which binds testosterone and decreases the quantity of free hormone. This effectively reduces the androgenic symptoms of hirsutism, polycystic ovary syndrome, and hyperandrogenism. Desogestrel and norgestimate additionally improve acne or hirsutism conditions because of their high level of progestational effects and absence of androgenic effects. Other progestins having androgenic properties, such as levonorgestrel, norgestrel, or norethindrone, may or may not worsen acne or hirsutism, depending on the progestin-estrogen dose relationship.

**Other actions/effects**
The following noncontraceptive effects have been observed with the use of oral contraceptives: menstrual cycle regularity, fewer occurrences of iron-deficient anemia associated with heavy menses flow or pelvic inflammatory disease; and fewer ectopic pregnancies. Although low-dose oral contraceptives may have less effect, high-dose formulations (containing ≥ 50 mcg [0.05 mg] estrogen) used long-term have decreased the occurrence of benign breast disease, including fibroadenomas and fibrocystic breast disease. Also, oral contraceptives may protect against or delay development of benign or malignant endometrial and ovarian cancers, atherosclerosis, or rheumatoid arthritis (although some of these are still controversial).

Norgestrel and levonorgestrel have the most androgenic activity of all the progestins. Norethindrone and ethynodiol diacetate possess slight estrogenic activity, and norethindrone has some androgenic activity. Norgestimate and desogestrel have high progestational activity and are low in androgenicity.

**Absorption**
Both estrogen and progestin components are rapidly and well absorbed.
  Ethinyl estradiol or
  Mestranol—Relative bioavailability is 83% because these estrogens have both a first-pass effect and enterohepatic recirculation with similar blood concentrations achieved for both 50 mcg of mestranol-containing and 35 mcg of ethinyl estradiol–containing oral contraceptives.

  Desogestrel—Desogestrel is primarily absorbed in the intestine as its active metabolite, etonogestrel, but because of a significant first-pass effect, the relative bioavailability of etonogestrel is 84%.

  Ethynodiol diacetate or
  Norethindrone or

Norethindrone acetate—Ethynodiol diacetate and norethindrone acetate are completely hydrolyzed by intestinal tissue to norethindrone, which is then absorbed. All of these progestins are rapidly and well absorbed but because of a first-pass effect, 53% bioavailability results.

Levonorgestrel or
Norgestimate or
Norgestrel—Intestinal absorption within 2 hours; completely bioavailable because these progestins do not exhibit a first-pass effect.

### Distribution
Oral contraceptives are widely distributed.
Ethinyl estradiol—Distributed into the uterus (0.9%), blood (8.8%), adipose tissue (28.2%), and other tissues. Fifty mcg of ethinyl estradiol taken orally would yield a concentration of 10 nanograms/100 mL a day in breast milk, which is not considered clinically significant.
Desogestrel (with ethinyl estradiol administration)—Volume of distribution (Vol$_D$) is 143 ± 61 liters (L).
Norethindrone (with ethinyl estradiol)—Vol$_D$ is approximately 236 ± 60 L.

### Protein binding
Oral contraceptives differ in their ability to increase the concentration of sex hormone–binding globulin (SHBG) that is induced by estrogen because contraceptive progestins differ in their ability to suppress this estrogenic effect. Also, contraceptive progestins have different affinities for albumin and SHBG. Therefore, progestins binding to serum proteins differ relative to how the estrogen and the progestin together affect serum proteins. For instance, a progestin with greater affinity for albumin than SHBG but faced with greater serum concentration of SHBG induced by estrogen would result in greater binding of progestin to SHBG.
Ethinyl estradiol—High; specifically, ethinyl estradiol is 95% bound to albumin, but not to SHBG; ethinyl estradiol induces production of SHBG. Tissue-specific receptor proteins form complexes with estrogens in estrogen-responsive tissues.
Desogestrel (with ethinyl estradiol administration)—High; albumin (66 ± 12%), SHBG (31 ± 12%), unbound (2.5 ± 0.2%). Because desogestrel does not counteract the increase in SHBG caused by daily estrogen administration, nonlinear kinetics result; desogestrel binds to a threefold increase in SHBG, which is highest between the third and sixth months of treatment.
Levonorgestrel (with ethinyl estradiol administration)—High; proportion bound to albumin or SHBG varies by strength and phasic relationship of both levonorgestrel and estrogen. Specifically, 250 mcg levonorgestrel and 50 mcg ethinyl estradiol have decreased SHBG by 24%, 150 mcg levonorgestrel and 30 mcg ethinyl estradiol decreased SHBG by 10%, and triphasic formulations increased SHBG. Levonorgestrel's affinity for SHBG is greater than its affinity for albumin.
Norethindrone—Without use of estrogen, norethindrone binds 61% to albumin and 35.5% to SHBG while 3.5% is unbound. With use of ethinyl estradiol, an 80 to 100% increase in SHBG may be expected, which will increase the SHBG-bound proportion of norethindrone.

### Biotransformation
Desogestrel—In Phase I hydroxylation, desogestrel, a prodrug, is metabolized in the intestinal tract and by hepatic first-pass metabolism to the biologically active metabolite etonogestrel and several inactive metabolites. The metabolism is completed in Phase II, resulting in polar conjugated glucuronide and sulfate metabolites.
Ethinyl estradiol or
Mestranol—Exhibits Phase I and Phase II metabolism. Seventy percent of the prodrug, mestranol, converts to ethinyl estradiol by demethylation. Estrogen metabolites, mainly conjugates, are hydroxylated by enzymes of intestinal bacteria then reabsorbed via enterohepatic recirculation.
Ethynodiol diacetate or
Norethindrone or
Norethindrone acetate—Hydrolysis of ethynodiol diacetate and norethindrone acetate to norethindrone occurs mainly in the intestines, but also in the liver. Norethindrone is metabolized to sulfate (predominately in plasma) and glucuronide conjugates, which may prolong activity if active metabolites are discovered. Also, it is postulated that the aromatization of norethindrone to ethinyl estradiol by tissues such as the liver, ovaries, and placenta may be of clinical significance.
Levonorgestrel or
Norgestrel—Metabolism of the inactive isomer L-(d)-norgestrel differs considerably from metabolism of the active isomer L-(l)-norgestrel; the latter is sulfated more rapidly than is the inactive isomer.
Norgestimate—Considered an incomplete prodrug for levonorgestrel; has biological activity, but 85% of activity is thought to be due to norgestrel acetate and, to a much lesser extent, norgestrel. Metabolized to active metabolites, levonorgestrel and 17-deactyl norgestimate (has activity similar to norgestimate), as well as to other hydroxy compounds.

### Half-life
With ethinyl estradiol administration:
Desogestrel or
Levonorgestrel—Elimination, plasma: 8 to 13 hours.
Ethynodiol diacetate or
Norethindrone or
Norethindrone acetate—Elimination, plasma: 8 hours.
Norgestimate—Elimination, plasma: 30 to 71 hours for norgestimate; 17 to 30 hours for 17-deactyl norgestimate, a metabolite.
With desogestrel administration:
Ethinyl estradiol—Elimination, plasma: 26 hours.
With norgestimate administration:
Ethinyl estradiol—Elimination, plasma: 6 to 14 hours.

### Elimination
Desogestrel—
 Renal: 45%, of which 14 to 28% is unchanged, and 38 to 61% is excreted as glucuronide and 23 to 39% as sulfate conjugates.
 Fecal: Up to 30%.
Ethinyl estradiol or
Mestranol—
 Renal: 22 to 58%.
 Fecal: 30 to 53%.
 Biliary: 26 to 43%.
Ethynodiol diacetate or
Norethindrone acetate or
Norethindrone—
 Renal: 37 to 87%, of which 3% is unchanged, and 40% is excreted as glucuronide and 15% as sulfate conjugates.
 Fecal: Up to 40%.
Levonorgestrel or
Norgestrel—Renal, as inactive metabolites.
Norgestimate—
 Renal: 45 to 49%.
 Fecal: 16 to 49%.

## Precautions to Consider

### Carcinogenicity
Recent and current users of high-dose oral contraceptives (containing 50 mcg or more of estrogen) for at least 2 years have shown a progressive reduction of up to 40% in incidence of benign fibrocystic breast disease; it is unknown if low-dose oral contraceptives (containing less than 50 mcg of estrogen) have similar effects.

Use of oral contraceptives in women between 25 and 39 years of age does not increase the risk of developing breast cancer at 45 years of age or older. Whether oral contraceptives increase the risk of breast cancer in certain subgroups of women, such as women under 20 years of age using oral contraceptives for more than 4 years or women 46 to 54 years of age using oral contraceptives for more than 3 years, is unresolved. Some case-control studies have shown no association between oral contraceptive use and breast cancer in women under 20 years of age and a protective effect or no enhancement of risk in women 46 to 54 years of age. Because risk factors vary for women of different age groups, parity, environment, and age at first use, controlling for these and other confounding factors and establishing whether additional risk occurs is difficult. The magnitude of increased risk, if it exists at all, is considered very small, and does not warrant withholding the use of oral contraceptives in any subgroup of women (including those women having a family history of either breast cancer or benign breast disease, or women having a history of benign breast disease) or restricting use for young nulliparous women. Further analyses of risks associated with using low-dose oral contraceptives as compared to high-dose contraceptives and to characterize effects of duration of use are being evaluated.

If an oral contraceptive containing 50 mcg of estrogen is taken for at least 12 months, a 15-year protective effect against the development of endometrial cancer persists after the oral contraceptive treatment is discontinued. Similar effects for low-dose oral contraceptives are expected but an evaluation is needed.

High and low doses of monophasic oral contraceptives used continuously for at least 3 years have shown a protective effect against ovarian cancer, an effect that is fully developed in 6 years and may persist for at least 10 years; shorter-term use has not shown a protective effect. Similar short- and long-term effects are expected for low-dose bi- and triphasic oral contraceptives since they suppress ovulation, but further evaluation is needed.

Epidemiologic studies suggest that women taking oral contraceptives for 8 or more years have an increased risk of developing hepatocellular carcinoma as compared to women not taking oral contraceptives. However, these cancers are extremely rare and occur in less than one per million women using oral contraceptives long-term.

Risk for dysplasia and carcinoma of the cervix is increased with oral contraceptive use for more than 1 year. The risk of invasive cervical cancer could increase twofold after 5 years of use; the greatest risk is in women using oral contraceptives for longer than 10 years. A great portion of the risk is thought to be due to the number of sexual partners a woman has and the age at first coitus, a factor that may be different between users and never-users.

**Tumorigenicity**
Although benign and rare, liver cell adenomas, many of which regressed with the cessation of oral contraceptive use, have occurred in women using oral contraceptives for longer than 5 years. Liver cell adenomas should be suspected in patients having abdominal pain and tenderness, abdominal mass, or hypovolemic shock. These adenomas may rupture and may cause death through intra-abdominal hemorrhage.

**Mutagenicity**
It is generally believed that there is no increased risk of mutagenicity or teratogenicity, including any development of fetal sexual malformation, when oral contraceptives are inadvertently taken in early pregnancy. This information is based on a small number of case reports, and well-designed studies still are needed.

**Pregnancy/Reproduction**
Fertility—Delayed fertility has been shown to occur rarely in users of oral contraceptives, especially in nulliparous women. In one study, the rate of impaired fertility normalized by 48 and 72 months for two groups of nulliparous women (25 to 29 years of age and 30 to 34 years of age, respectively). Infertility rates have not been shown to increase.

Pregnancy—Studies have shown that combination oral contraceptives do not appear to increase the risk of birth defects when they are used before pregnancy. Studies have also shown that oral contraceptives, when taken inadvertently during early pregnancy, do not seem to have a teratogenic effect. However, oral contraceptives are not recommended for use during pregnancy and should be discontinued immediately if pregnancy is suspected.

Any patient who has missed two consecutive menstrual periods while taking oral contraceptives should discontinue their use; a nonhormonal contraceptive method should be used until pregnancy is ruled out. If the patient has not followed the dosing schedule, pregnancy should be ruled out after the first missed menstrual period.

When considering pregnancy, it is recommended that conception be delayed for 1 or 2 months after cessation of oral contraceptives or until after the first regular menses to accurately date the gestation period.

FDA Pregnancy Category X.

Postpartum or postabortion—Oral contraceptive use and the immediate postpartum period are both associated with an increased risk of thromboembolism occurrence. Therefore, to lessen any potential risk that may exist, oral contraceptives should be started no sooner than 2 weeks after delivery in women choosing to not breast-feed. Also, ovulation usually does not occur before this time and contraception is not needed. However, the chance of early ovulation is high following abortion but the risk of thromboembolic phenomena is not great. Therefore, some clinicians recommend that use of a low-dose oral contraceptive may begin immediately after a first-trimester or second-trimester abortion. Also, immediate use of an oral contraceptive is recommended following a second-trimester premature delivery or after a pregnancy of less than 12 weeks; however, for a pregnancy of 12 or more weeks, use of a low-dose oral contraceptive is recommended after 2 weeks.

**Breast-feeding**
Oral contraceptives are distributed into breast milk, and may diminish its quantity or quality or shorten the time of lactation, especially for those women who are only partially breast-feeding and have less physical stimulus for lactation. Use of oral contraceptives by nursing mothers in the early postpartum period is generally not recommended. When used by mothers who are exclusively breast-feeding, oral contraceptive therapy is recommended to begin after the third postpartum month or, if only partially or not breast-feeding, to begin in the third postpartum week. If contraception is needed prior to this, some clinicians begin low-dose oral contraceptives after lactation has been well-established.

**Adolescents**
One of the most accepted, frequently prescribed, and, when used regularly, effective contraceptive methods for adolescents is oral contraceptives. However, the pregnancy rate for adolescents using oral contraceptives is estimated at 6 to 12 per 100 woman years, which is higher than the pregnancy rate, 0.3 to 0.7 per 100 woman years, for all age groups of women.

Studies generally have shown that adolescents tend to be less compliant users of any type of contraceptive. Any psychosocial factors involved and discussion of preconceived thoughts on side effects, including weight gain, fluid retention, or breakthrough uterine bleeding, are important areas for patient counseling to help aid in this age group's compliance problem with using oral contraceptives.

**Dental**
Increased concentrations of progestins increase the normal oral flora growth rate, leading to an increase in inflammation of the gingival tissues and increased bleeding. A strictly enforced program of teeth cleaning by a professional, combined with plaque control by the patient, will minimize severity.

An increased incidence of local alveolar osteitis (dry socket) after dental extractions has been seen with the use of estrogen and progestin combination oral contraceptives. A direct correlation exists between the incidence of dry socket occurrence and increasing estrogen dose. Therefore, it is recommended that patients inform their dentist or oral surgeon that they are taking an estrogen and progestin contraceptive.

**Drug interactions and/or related problems**
The following drug interactions and/or related problems have been selected on the basis of their potential clinical significance (possible mechanism in parentheses where appropriate)—not necessarily inclusive (» = major clinical significance):

Note: Combinations containing any of the following medications, depending on the amount present, may also interact with this medication.

Amoxicillin or
Ampicillin or
Doxycycline or
Penicillin V or
Tetracycline
(there have been rare case reports of reduced oral contraceptive effectiveness in women taking amoxicillin, ampicillin, doxycycline, penicillin V, or tetracycline, resulting in unplanned pregnancy. This is thought to be due to a reduction in enterohepatic circulation of estrogens, which may cause a lower estrogen plasma concentration than expected. Although the association is very weak, patients, especially long-term users of antibiotic therapy, should be advised of this information and given the option of using an alternate or additional method of contraception while taking any of these antibiotics, especially if the duration of antibiotic therapy is greater than 2 weeks)

Anticoagulants, coumarin- or indandione-derivative
(concurrent use with oral contraceptives has modestly increased, and in some cases decreased, the effectiveness of anticoagulants; however, the mechanism is unknown and appropriate studies have not been done. Because estrogens increase hepatic synthesis of procoagulant factors and decrease antithrombin III, it is possible that adjustment of the anticoagulant dosage based on prothrombin time determinations may be needed)

Antidiabetic agents, sulfonylurea or
Insulin
(estrogen-containing oral contraceptives may cause glucose or insulin resistance in diabetic patients, resulting in a loss, probably slight, of metabolic control of plasma glucose concentration; unless the changes can be controlled with diet, this may necessitate an increased sulfonylurea or insulin dose and regular monitoring)

Benzodiazepines
(metabolism of those benzodiazepines, such as diazepam, alprazolam, and triazolam, that undergo oxidation may be inhibited, resulting in delayed elimination of diazepam and triazolam and an increased risk of adverse effects. Although the pharmacokinetics of alprazolam were not affected with long-term use, a study has shown a greater sensitivity to alprazolam and psychomotor impairment with single doses of alprazolam in long-term contraceptive users; pharmacokinetic factors were not believed to contribute to this effect. Metabolism of those benzodiazepines that undergo conjugation, such as oxazepam, lorazepam, and temazepam, is not impaired)

(reduction of oral contraceptive effectiveness has not been shown with concurrent use of benzodiazepines)

Caffeine
(oral contraceptives reduce or inhibit the hepatic metabolism of caffeine, thereby increasing the plasma concentration of caffeine up to 30 to 40%; patient may need to be counseled about the increased effects of caffeine if warranted)

Clofibrate
(concurrent use with oral contraceptives may lower the effectiveness of clofibrate)

» Corticosteroids, glucocorticoid
(concurrent use with estrogens may lower the metabolism of glucocorticoids, decrease the elimination of potent metabolites, decrease the protein binding of glucocorticoids, and increase the production of the protein-binding globulin, transcortin (also called cortisol-binding globulin. This leads to decreased clearance [approximately 30 to 50% for prednisolone] of the glucocorticoid free fraction, prolonged elimination half-life, and increased effects of the glucocorticoids; lower doses of the glucocorticoid are needed with concurrent use of estrogen-containing oral contraceptives)

» Cyclosporine
(a case report has shown that concurrent use with oral contraceptives increased the plasma concentration of cyclosporine, which may increase its effects; monitoring of plasma cyclosporine concentration and hepatic factors for toxicity, reducing cyclosporine dose, or changing to nonhormonal contraception may be required to minimize the risk of cyclosporine toxicity)

» Hepatic enzyme inducers (see *Appendix II*), especially:
Barbiturates
Carbamazepine
Griseofulvin
Phenytoin
Primidone
Rifabutin
Rifampin
(concurrent use of these medications with oral contraceptives may induce hepatic enzyme oral contraceptive metabolism, especially of the estrogen component, which could result in reduced contraceptive reliability and increased incidence of breakthrough bleeding. High interindividual variability in hepatic enzyme induction exists. Patients should be advised to use a high-dose estrogen-containing contraceptive if oral contraceptives are used, or an alternative or additional method of contraception during use of any of these medications, especially if breakthrough bleeding occurs)

(additionally, phenobarbital and phenytoin have been shown to increase sex hormone–binding globulin [SHBG], which may lower the amount of free progestin available for biological action and contribute to the lowered effectiveness of the oral contraceptive)

» Hepatotoxic medications, especially troleandomycin (see *Appendix II*)
(the estrogen component of oral contraceptives increases hepatic blood flow and size of the liver with increased vesiculation of the smooth and rough endoplasmic reticulum, which results in altered hepatic metabolism. It is possible that concurrent use of these medications with estrogens may increase the risk of hepatotoxicity; more frequent monitoring of hepatic function is needed)

» Ritonavir
(area under the plasma concentration–time curve [AUC] of estrogen is decreased by 40% during use of ritonavir; the estrogen dose of the oral contraceptive should be increased or an alternative form of birth control used with concurrent use of ritonavir)

» Smoking, tobacco
(polycyclic hydrocarbons in cigarette smoke are potent inducers of certain hepatic cytochrome P450 isoenzymes; the consequences of this effect on metabolism have not been fully explored but may influence the associated risks of using oral contraceptives and smoking concurrently. Although some studies showed inhibition of metabolism of a metabolite of ethinyl estradiol, smoking did not affect the metabolism of ethinyl estradiol)

(oral contraceptives are not recommended with heavy tobacco use because of an increased risk of serious cardiovascular side effects, including cerebrovascular accident, transient ischemic attacks, thrombophlebitis, and pulmonary embolism. Risk increases with increased tobacco usage and with age, especially in women over 35 years of age. The mechanisms for these outcomes are still being explored. Some clinicians have used low-dose estrogen oral contraceptives in women who are light smokers or who use a nicotine patch)

Tamoxifen
(concurrent use with estrogens may interfere with the antiestrogenic therapeutic effect of tamoxifen)

» Theophylline
(although theophylline reduced the apparent clearance of ethinyl estradiol 30 to 35% in oral contraceptive users, clinical significance was not noted because of the wide interindividual variability in metabolism of the estrogen; however, reduction of the total plasma clearance of theophylline by 25 to 35% by oral contraceptives was considered clinically significant. These effects result in an increase in both the theophylline and ethinyl estradiol plasma concentration; a lower dose of the theophylline may be needed)

Tricyclic antidepressants
(inhibition of imipramine oxidation by oral contraceptives results in higher plasma concentrations of imipramine; imipramine dose may need to be adjusted)

(estrogen has facilitated the development of neuroleptic antipsychotic or tricyclic antidepressant medication–associated movement disorders, such as akathisia, but not tardive dyskinesia. It is not known if the low doses of estrogen used in oral contraceptives are also implicated in akathisia)

(rare cases of chorea have developed in women with chorea gravidarum using oral contraceptives, but oral contraceptives do not appear to create any additional risk in women not predisposed to develop chorea)

» Troglitazone
(troglitazone may induce drug metabolism by cytochrome P450 isoenzyme CYP3A4; ethinyl estradiol and norethindrone are substrates for this isoenzyme; therefore, caution is recommended when they are used concurrently with troglitazone)

(concurrent use may decrease the plasma concentrations of ethinyl estradiol and norethindrone by approximately 30%, resulting in a loss of efficacy)

**Laboratory value alterations**
The following have been selected on the basis of their potential clinical significance (possible effect in parentheses where appropriate)—not necessarily inclusive (» = major clinical significance):

With diagnostic test results
Aldosterone, serum or
Aldosterone, urine or
Renin, plasma
(the estrogen component decreases the plasma concentration of plasma renin but increases plasma renin activity; oral contraceptives should be discontinued at least 2 weeks, and preferably 4 weeks, before testing plasma renin activity)

Antipyrine test
(lower values result because oral contraceptives significantly reduce antipyrine metabolism, particularly the oxidative mechanism)

Corticotropin-releasing hormone stimulation test or
Metyrapone test
(corticotropin plasma levels were reduced approximately 25% overall in a study of women using triphasic oral contraceptives who had been given a morning corticotropin-releasing hormone [CRH] stimulation test; normal basal levels were unchanged. Reduced response also has been noted for the metyrapone test with other oral contraceptives)

Dexamethasone suppression test
(oral contraceptive users had a significantly higher plasma cortisol level pre- and post-dexamethasone testing; this effect caused by estrogen may persist for up to 1 month after oral contraceptive treatment ends)

Glucose tolerance test, oral
(significantly higher 2-hour oral glucose tolerance test results)

Norepinephrine-induced platelet aggregability
(may be increased)

*Thyroid function tests*
Thyroxine ($T_4$) determinations
(estrogen-induced thyroid-binding globulin elevates the amount of $T_4$ that is protein bound; this effect reverses in about 2 months after discontinuation of oral contraceptives; serum free $T_4$ concentrations are unchanged. Specifically, triphasic oral contraceptives containing 30 mcg of ethinyl estradiol have increased thyroid-binding globulin by about 20% and elevated total $T_4$ by 40%)

Triiodothyronine ($T_3$) determinations
(free $T_3$ and reverse $T_3$ are unchanged, but $T_3$ resin uptake is decreased because estrogens increase serum thyroid-binding globulin [TBG]; total $T_3$ radioimmunoassay [RIA] values are increased but proportionately less than total $T_4$ values)

With physiology/laboratory test values
Albumin or
Alkaline phosphatase
(levels were decreased in women taking norethindrone-ethinyl estradiol 1/35 throughout the 1-year treatment period in one study; these effects were not seen in the same study among women taking levonorgestrel-ethinyl estradiol 0.15/30)

Androstenedione or
Ceruloplasmin, serum or
Dehydroepiandrosterone sulfate (DHEA-S) or
Pregnenolone or
Sex hormone–binding globulin (SHBG), serum or
Testosterone or
Thyroid-binding globulin or
Transferrin or cortisol-binding globulin, serum
   (oral contraceptives increase protein synthesis of SHBG, thyroid-binding globulin, transferrin, and ceruloplasmin. The serum concentrations of total sex steroids, copper, and cortisol may also increase. The free thyroid concentration is unchanged, and thyroid function is unaltered. Response of the free non–protein-bound component may be variable)

   (oral contraceptives' net effect on SHBG is the result of the opposing actions of the estrogen and progestin. A dose-related response to progestins of greater androgenicity, such as norgestrel, has a greater suppressive effect on the estrogen-induced increases of SHBG than do those with low androgenic effect, such as desogestrel or norgestimate, which have little suppressive effect on estrogen-induced SHBG levels and can result in a three- to fourfold increase in SHBG. However, further elevations of SHBG, above some level that remains undetermined, do not appear to result in any further decrease in free testosterone. For instance, one study showed that an elevation of SHBG by 92% and 175% decreased free testosterone similarly [by 35%]. Ethinyl estradiol and norethindrone 1/35 and 1/50 increased SHBG levels by 183 to 390%; ethinyl estradiol and norgestrel increased SHBG by 12%. Testosterone levels are further changed by those progestins that have greater affinity for SHBG, such as levonorgestrel-containing oral contraceptives, that can displace testosterone from its SHBG binding site)

   (also, norgestrel-, ethynodiol diacetate–, and norethindrone-containing oral contraceptives reduce circulating DHEA-S by 28%, androstenedione by 47%, and testosterone by 40%, including the precursor, pregnenolone, by causing a decrease in corticotropin stimulation or by direct effect on hepatic enzyme inhibition. The complexity of these factors causes a variable clinical effect among individuals taking oral contraceptives)

Antithrombin III
   (may be decreased by most oral contraceptives, which contributes to decreased anticoagulant or increased fibrinolytic activity of oral contraceptives. A study showed that desogestrel increased fibrinolytic activity less than did a triphasic formulation of levonorgestrel but that there was significantly more activity in users of desogestrel than in nonusers. Although the increase in activity was generally within normal laboratory ranges, extreme values among individuals may need to be taken into consideration. Specifically, users of a triphasic formulation of levonorgestrel and ethinyl estradiol showed a slight increase in antithrombin III concentration at 12 weeks, followed by a decrease until the end of the 48-week study. In the same study, users of desogestrel and ethinyl estradiol showed a decreased concentration of antithrombin III at 24 weeks that returned to the normal range at 48 weeks)

Apolipoprotein $A_1$, $A_2$, or B or
Cholesterol, total or
Triglycerides
   (in general, the net effect on lipoproteins is the result of the opposing actions of the estrogen and progestin and depends on the ratio between the two hormones. The estrogen component increases triglyceride, very low density lipoproteins (VLDL), and total cholesterol concentrations and decreases low density lipoproteins (LDL). The progestin component, if androgenic, decreases high density lipoproteins (HDL) and increases LDL. The low concentrations of the androgenic progestins in oral contraceptives have slight effect, which is of clinical significance only for some predisposed individuals. Sometimes, older women with higher serum concentrations of cholesterol may experience a reduction caused by a lowering of the serum LDL concentrations. Triglycerides are increased by all oral contraceptives because of the predominant estrogen effects. The increase in total cholesterol caused by desogestrel- and norgestimate-containing oral contraceptives is considered favorable because it is the net result of the increase in $HDL_3$-C (an estrogen effect) without an increase in $HDL_2$-C concentrations. The increase in $HDL_2$-C caused by other low-dose oral contraceptives is considered an androgenic effect of some of the 19–nortestosterone-derived progestins)

*For monophasics*
   (users of ethynodiol diacetate-ethinyl estradiol 1/35 showed the greatest increase in apolipoprotein $A_1$ and levonorgestrel-ethinyl estradiol 0.15/30 showed the smallest increase. Users of ethinyl estradiol-norgestrel have shown significant decrease in apolipoproteins $A_1$ and $A_2$)

   (in one study, norethindrone-ethinyl estradiol 1/35 increased triglycerides to levels that continued throughout a 1-year treatment period while levonorgestrel-ethinyl estradiol 0.15/30 caused no change in triglyceride levels over a 1-year treatment period. Total cholesterol levels were slightly decreased for norethindrone-ethinyl estradiol 1/35 but returned toward baseline within the 1-year treatment period. Levonorgestrel-ethinyl estradiol 0.15/30 slightly reduced total cholesterol levels at 3-month and 1-year treatment periods)

*For triphasics*
   (in a study comparing users of triphasic formulations with nonusers, levonorgestrel-ethinyl estradiol [7/7/7- and 9/5/7-day regimens] and norethindrone-ethinyl estradiol produced significant increases in plasma triglyceride [28 to 52%] and plasma apolipoprotein B levels [20 to 23%] in each treatment group at 6 months compared with levels in nonusers. In the contraceptive users, total plasma cholesterol concentrations increased 3 to 11% and plasma apolipoprotein $A_1$ concentrations increased 5 to 12%. The increases in the concentrations shown in a 12-month study remained within an acceptable clinical range. Another study of oral triphasics showed a significant decrease in total cholesterol in users during the first week of use, an effect associated with a decrease in LDL; the total serum cholesterol returned to baseline over the next 3 weeks)

Aspartate aminotransferase (AST [SGOT]), serum or
Bilirubin, total, serum or
Urobilinogen, urine
   (these values are decreased with oral contraceptives containing 50 mcg of ethinyl estradiol; the incidence of abnormal liver test values is lower for oral contraceptives containing 35 mcg of ethinyl estradiol or 50 mcg of mestranol. Total bilirubin, urinary urobilinogen, and serum AST were significantly decreased at 3 months for norethindrone-ethinyl estradiol 1/35, but returned to baseline at 12 months. Users of levonorgestrel-ethinyl estradiol 0.15/30 showed only slightly decreased concentrations that were not considered clinically significant)

Clotting factors VII, VIII, IX, and X or
Prothrombin time or
Thromboplastin time, partial
   (oral contraceptives shorten partial thromboplastin and prothrombin time, but these results are neither consistent nor do they occur in all individuals. Activation of the segments of the intrinsic and extrinsic system of coagulation by oral contraceptives enhances, depending on the factor, either the fibrinolysis or procoagulation or affects both. If baseline values were increased, the increase was within normal laboratory ranges in most cases, and did not consistently alter bleeding or clotting times)

Cortisol, serum or urine
   (the net effect of oral contraceptives on serum cortisol is the result of the opposing actions of the estrogen and progestin and depends on the ratio between the two hormones. Progestins, such as norethindrone, having glucocorticoid effects decrease corticotropin release and adrenal cortisol production. Estrogens augment corticotropin release by downregulating pituitary glucocorticoid receptors and increase adrenal cortisol responsiveness to corticotropin stimulation. This results in an increase in serum cortisol concentrations and a decrease in urinary cortisol clearance)

Glucose, plasma or serum or
Insulin
   (reduced glucose tolerance and elevated fasting insulin and C-peptide values can occur with use of low-dose oral contraceptives during the first 12 months of use, returning to normal between 12 and 24 months of continued use. These changes from baseline were considered not to be of clinical significance in most prospective studies of low-dose oral contraceptives, as many values were still within the normal range. Levonorgestrel- or norgestrel-containing combinations caused the greatest insulin resistance, followed by combinations of desogestrel and low-dose norethindrone oral contraceptives. Levonorgestrel significantly increased second-phase pancreatic insulin production while desogestrel and norgestimate did not)

Growth hormone
   (physiologic levels may increase during the first year)

High density lipoproteins (HDL), serum
   (low-dose oral contraceptives show no change or a decrease in value of HDL; the estrogen component increases HDL and the progestin component, if androgenic, lowers HDL. If the progestin is nonan-

drogenic, HDL is not influenced. In studies clinically comparing oral contraceptives, formulations containing levonorgestrel and norgestrel had a greater adverse effect on lipids than did less androgenic formulations such as those containing ethynodiol diacetate, norethindrone, or norethindrone acetate. However, if levonorgestrel or norgestrel is given in low doses or if the total dose given is limited, such as in biphasic or triphasic formulations, these potent androgenic progestins exhibit only mild lipid changes similar to those of less potent androgenic progestins given in monophasic formulations. Nonandrogenic formulations, such as desogestrel and norgestimate, had little effect on lipid profile)

Low density lipoproteins (LDL), serum or
Very low density lipoproteins (VLDL), serum
  (low-dose oral contraceptives show no change or an increase in value of LDL; the estrogen component decreases LDL and the progestin component, if androgenic, raises LDL. If the progestin is nonandrogenic, LDL is not influenced. In clinical studies comparing oral contraceptives, formulations containing levonorgestrel and norgestrel had a greater adverse effect on lipids than did less androgenic formulations, such as those containing ethynodiol diacetate, norethindrone, or norethindrone acetate. However, if levonorgestrel or norgestrel is given in low doses or if the total dose given is limited, such as in biphasic or triphasic formulations, these potent androgenic progestins exhibit only mild lipid changes similar to those of less potent androgenic progestins given in monophasic formulations. Nonandrogenic formulations, such as desogestrel and norgestimate, had little effect)

Oxytocin, serum
  (mean basal oxytocin levels were higher in women on oral contraceptives)

Plasminogen activity
  (activity is increased above normal laboratory reference values)

## Medical considerations/Contraindications

The medical considerations/contraindications included have been selected on the basis of their potential clinical significance (reasons given in parentheses where appropriate)—not necessarily inclusive (» = major clinical significance).

*Except under special circumstances, this medication should not be used when the following medical problems exist:*

» Carcinoma, breast, known or suspected or
» Carcinoma, endometrium or
» Neoplasia, estrogen-dependent, known or suspected
  (may worsen conditions; estrogen-containing oral contraceptives should be discontinued and nonhormonal contraceptives initiated, although sometimes progestin-only contraceptives are used for selected patients)
» Cardiac insufficiency
  (oral contraceptives should not be used in patients with marginal cardiac reserve; fluid retention sometimes caused by estrogens may aggravate this condition)
» Cerebrovascular disease, active or history of or
» Coronary artery disease, active or history of
  (the estrogen component of oral contraceptives has a protective effect against atherosclerosis. Any association with risk in these conditions has been related to thrombosis or interference with cholesterol-lipoprotein profile, such as with levonorgestrel, a progestin, in doses greater than 150 to 250 mcg for those individuals predisposed to thrombosis. No correlation has been seen between coronary artery disease and use of low-dose oral contraceptives, including those formulated with levonorgestrel, in these women or in women who are not predisposed to these conditions. Oral contraceptives should be discontinued or strictly avoided if any cardiovascular or cerebrovascular accidents occur; users should switch to nonhormonal contraception. If oral contraceptives are used in women at risk, special monitoring may be required)
  (the progestins norgestimate and desogestrel have minimal negative impact and may improve the cholesterol-lipoprotein profile, which is thought to additionally protect against cardiovascular disease along with the estrogen component of oral contraceptives)
» Hepatic disease, cholestatic, active or
» Hepatic tumors, benign or malignant, or history of
  (metabolism of estrogens may be impaired; also, estrogens may worsen the condition. Oral contraceptives should be discontinued and nonhormonal contraception initiated; for those women with active hepatic disease, oral contraceptive use may be resumed after liver function tests return to normal)

» Thrombophlebitis, thrombosis, or thromboembolic disorders, active or history of
  (oral contraceptives are not recommended for women with predisposing factors, especially those who smoke tobacco or who have an underlying abnormality of the coagulation system, that place them at special risk for thrombosis. Although hormones can increase thrombin formation, the coagulation effect is offset by an increase in fibrolytic activity. Some women with coagulation disorders may successfully use oral contraceptives as evaluated by the physician if only a slight risk for a thrombogenic condition exists. Problems generally have not been associated with the low doses of hormones used for contraception for women not at risk for these conditions)
» Uterine bleeding, abnormal or undiagnosed
  (malignancy should be ruled out in cases of persistent or recurring abnormal uterine bleeding; use of a progestin-containing oral contraceptive may delay diagnosis by masking underlying conditions, including cancer)

*Risk-benefit should be considered when the following medical problems exist:*

Breast cancer, strong family history of or
Breast disease, benign
  (although studies have failed to conclusively prove that use of oral contraceptives causes any excess risk for developing breast disease in these women, caution and more frequent monitoring for potential problems may be warranted)

Chorea gravidarum
  (oral contraceptives do not cause chorea gravidarum but rarely they have aggravated pre-existing conditions)

Diabetes mellitus
  (use of oral contraceptives may slightly decrease glucose tolerance, slightly increase insulin release in patients with Type 2 diabetes mellitus, or produce a mild adverse effect on the cholesterol-lipoprotein profile. Depending on the oral contraceptive used, a change in the dose of the antidiabetic agent or more frequent monitoring for plasma glucose or lipid profile may be needed. If adverse metabolic effects cannot be controlled, the oral contraceptive should be discontinued)
  (norethindrone-, ethynodiol diacetate-, norgestimate-, and desogestrel-containing oral contraceptives affect carbohydrate metabolism less than do levonorgestrel- or norgestrel-containing oral contraceptives; many clinicians recommend low-dose oral contraceptives, such as the triphasic oral contraceptives, for patients with diabetes mellitus)
  (use of oral contraceptives in patients with Type 1 diabetes mellitus who are 35 years of age or older or in any patient having diabetes mellitus complications is generally not recommended because of the potential increased risk of thrombosis. Healthy patients up to 35 years of age who have diabetes mellitus have minimal risk for adverse effects from oral contraceptive use and usually do not need an adjustment in their insulin dose. They may require more frequent monitoring of the cholesterol-lipoprotein profile and serum glucose concentration)

Epilepsy
  (oral contraceptives can be used effectively with this condition but their use may affect the pharmacokinetics of certain antiepileptic medications; dose changes for both medications and special monitoring may be needed)

Gallbladder disease, or history of, especially gallstones
  (estrogens may alter the composition of gallbladder bile and can cause a rise in cholesterol saturation that may moderately accelerate the development of gallstones during the first 2 years of use in predisposed individuals. The overall risk is low and thought to be of minimal clinical importance; however, cautious use of oral contraceptives is recommended with known gallbladder disease)

» Hepatic function impairment
  (metabolism of estrogens may be impaired, resulting in a worsening of the condition; therefore, oral contraceptives should be discontinued and nonhormonal contraception initiated with active disease; oral contraceptive use may be resumed after liver function tests return to normal. Oral contraceptives are not thought to aggravate cirrhosis or exacerbate previous hepatitis)

Hypertension
  (low-dose monophasic oral contraceptives have been shown to raise blood pressure in some normotensive women considered to be at high risk [although these women cannot be easily identified] or further raise blood pressure in hypertensive women. Use of low-dose multiphasic contraceptives may be an appropriate choice for these women)

Immobilization, extended or
Surgery, major
(although controversial, many guidelines suggest that concurrent oral contraceptive usage increases the risk of postoperative thromboembolism in predisposed women, especially for smokers of tobacco or for those women with a history of thromboembolism. When possible or if appropriate, oral contraceptives should be discontinued at least 4 weeks before and for 2 weeks after an extended period of immobilization or scheduled major elective surgery. If not possible, prophylactic low-dose heparin therapy should be considered prior to surgery)

Jaundice, obstructive or history of during pregnancy
(estrogens may increase risk of recurrence but low-dose contraceptives have not done so consistently; risk is higher shortly after hormone exposure; increased monitoring may be needed)

Mental depression, or history of
(may be aggravated; however, low-dose contraceptives are considered to have minimal effect on mental depression; the oral contraceptive should be discontinued if significant depression occurs, especially in women with a history of depression)

Migraine headaches
(since migraine headaches have been associated with an increased risk of stroke, discontinuation of oral contraceptives may be warranted if migraine headaches are recurring, persistent, or more severe with use of oral contraceptives, especially for those individuals predisposed to thrombosis)

**Patient monitoring**

The following may be especially important in patient monitoring (other tests may be warranted in some patients, depending on condition; » = major clinical significance):

Blood pressure determinations and
Hepatic function determinations and
Papanicolaou (Pap) test and
Physical examinations
(recommended as determined by physician—generally every 12 months for healthy women with no risk factors but every 6 months if needed when such risk factors exist, although breast and pelvic examinations are needed only annually. New oral contraceptive users should be reassessed at 3 months. Special attention should be given to breast, liver, and pelvic area in the physical exam and patients should be encouraged to self-examine breasts monthly)
(special attention to rule out malignancy should be given to patients complaining of persistent or recurring uterine bleeding)

Glucose, serum and
Lipid profile, serum and
Lipoprotein profile, serum
(routine assessment is needed only for women at special risk, including women 35 years of age or older, women who have personal or strong family histories of heart disease, diabetes mellitus, or hypertension, or whose personal history includes gestational diabetes mellitus, xanthomatosis, or obesity)

*For perimenopausal women using oral contraceptives*
Gonadotropin determination
(FSH levels should be measured annually to determine when menopause occurs)

## Side/Adverse Effects

Note: The risk of any serious adverse effect is minimal for healthy women using low-dose oral contraceptives. Some women who are at special risk have successfully used low-dose oral contraceptives, although in others the use of oral contraceptives rarely will increase the incidence of life-threatening effects, such as benign hepatic adenomas, hepatocellular carcinoma, or thromboembolism or thromboembolic events such as deep vein thrombosis, cerebral or coronary ischemia and/or infarction, pulmonary embolism, or stroke. Pre-existing risk factors for these events include genetic predisposition (i.e., antiestrogen antibodies, activated protein C or antithrombin deficiencies or resistance, or genetic thrombotic disorder), hypertension, hyperlipidemia, obesity, diabetes, or smoking of cigarettes.

Low-dose oral contraceptives are recommended for most women throughout their reproductive years without need for discontinuance. Mortality rates in oral contraceptive users are lower than those that are associated with childbirth. This is true even for smokers 35 years and older and nonsmokers 40 years and older.

There is no evidence of an etiological relationship between oral contraceptive use and pituitary prolactinoma; however, the appearance of galactorrhea while on oral contraceptives merits investigation.

The following side/adverse effects have been selected on the basis of their potential clinical significance (possible signs and symptoms in parentheses where appropriate)—not necessarily inclusive:

**Those indicating need for immediate medical attention**
Incidence rare
*Thromboembolism or thrombosis* (abdominal pain, sudden, severe, or continuing; coughing up blood; headache, severe or sudden; loss of coordination, sudden; pains in chest, groin, or leg, especially calf of leg; shortness of breath, sudden, unexplained; slurring of speech, sudden; vision changes, sudden; weakness, numbness, or pain in arm or leg, unexplained)—mainly exhibited in women having predisposing or pre-existing conditions, especially for those who smoke tobacco, but the event may be idiopathic

**Those indicating need for medical attention**
Incidence more frequent, especially during the first 3 months of oral contraceptive use
*Changes in the menstrual bleeding pattern or intermenstrual bleeding, such as amenorrhea* (complete stoppage of menstrual bleeding over several months); *absence of withdrawal bleeding* (occasional stoppage of menses over nonconsecutive months); *breakthrough bleeding* (vaginal bleeding between regular menstrual periods, which may require the use of a pad or a tampon); *metrorrhagia* (prolonged bleeding); *scanty menses* (very light menstrual bleeding); *or spotting* (light vaginal bleeding between regular menstrual periods)

Note: Malignancy should be ruled out as the cause if persistent or recurring abnormal *uterine bleeding* occurs.

Up to 46% of women using oral contraceptives experience *changes in the intermenstrual uterine bleeding pattern*. These problems become less frequent with duration of use; women who use high-dose oral contraceptives or who are changing formulations have fewer uterine bleeding problems than do women who are new users. *Breakthrough bleeding* occurs in 6 to 12% of women; some may require a change to a higher formulation with progestin or a change to a monophasic oral contraceptive after 3 months. Intervention with therapeutic doses of estrogen and/or progestin may be necessary if breakthrough bleeding is heavy or further prolonged.

For women experiencing *changes in the menstrual bleeding pattern*, 6 to 12%, 6 to 10%, and less than 1% of women will experience *spotting*, *scanty menses*, or *metrorrhagia*, respectively. Up to 12% of women using norethindrone-containing oral contraceptives and less than 2% of women using desogestrel-, norgestimate-, or levonorgestrel-containing oral contraceptives will experience an *absence of withdrawal bleeding*. Early or mid-cycle spotting or absence of withdrawal bleeding may be seen with use of low doses of monophasic contraceptives and may not be an unexpected side effect but is a major reason for discontinuance. A change to a different formulation with a greater estrogen:progestin ratio or less progestin, such as multiphasic formulations, or temporary supplementation with an estrogen, may improve these adverse effects. Failure of oral contraceptives to induce *withdrawal uterine bleeding* may be caused by insufficient estrogen activity to induce endometrial development. A change to a different formulation with increased estrogen:progestin ratio may improve this effect.

Incidence less frequent
*Glucose tolerance, mildly reduced* (faintness; nausea; skin paleness; sweating)—usually for women with predisposing conditions; *headaches or migraines, worsening or increased frequency of*—21%; *hypertension, worsening or exacerbation; vaginal candidiasis or vaginitis, sporadic or recurrent* (vaginal discharge, thick, white, or curd-like, or vaginal itching or other irritation)—10 to 16%

Note: Several studies have confirmed that 15 to 18% of oral contraceptive users will experience an increase, but not a clinically significant elevation, in blood pressure. Another study has observed that 4% of contraceptive users will develop *hypertension*, especially when either a history of hypertension in pregnancy or a family history of hypertension exists. Severe or *malignant hypertension* has been rarely seen.

Although one large cross-sectional study has shown a 43 to 61% increase in the area under the plasma concentration–time curve for glucose, past or current use of oral contraceptives does not increase risk for developing Type 2 diabetes mellitus; the increase is considered transitory and reversible with discontinuation. Oral contraceptive formulations vary in the degree to which they cause *reduced glucose tolerance*, which is usually mild, and may be of clinical importance only for a subset of women at particular risk. In separate studies, norgestimate- and desogestrel-containing oral contraceptives showed minimal impact on glucose tolerance.

Frequency and severity of *headaches or migraines* are reduced in some patients using oral contraceptives, but can be increased in others if they experience fluid retention. If headaches or migraines worsen considerably, discontinuation of oral contraceptives should be considered since this may be a prodomal symptom of stroke.

Withdrawal of oral contraceptives does not seem to affect the frequency of *recurrent vaginal candidiasis or vaginitis;* the increased risk may depend on other factors, such as lifestyle.

Incidence rare

**Breast tumors** (lumps in breast)—primarily in women having a predisposing or pre-existing condition; **hepatic focal nodular hyperplasia, hepatitis, or hepatocellular carcinoma** (pains in stomach, side, or abdomen, or yellow eyes or skin)—primarily in women having a predisposing or pre-existing condition, especially those who smoke tobacco; **hepatic cell adenomas, benign** (swelling, pain, or tenderness in upper abdominal area); **mental depression, slight worsening**—in pre-existing conditions

Note: Association of increased incidence of *breast tumors* is controversial. One study of women 20 to 34 years of age who were long-term oral contraceptive users (10 or more years of use) or recent users (within 5 years of breast cancer diagnosis) found only 1 more case of invasive breast cancer per year among oral contraceptive users than in nonusers for every 100,000 women. It still has not been determined whether the risk of breast cancer increases for early users under 20 years of age or for long-term users.

Although very rare, *hepatic cell adenomas* should be considered in patients having abdominal pain and tenderness, abdominal mass, or hypovolemic shock; one third of patients are asymptomatic at diagnosis. Studies of developing countries that have a high incidence of primary liver cancer have not associated oral contraceptives with an increased risk; however, Western countries, with a low incidence of hepatic carcinoma, have shown a fivefold increase in incidence that persisted for 10 years or more in long-term (5 to 10 years) users of oral contraceptives after stopping treatment. Studies in the U.S., also a country with low incidence of hepatic carcinoma, have not confirmed this finding. Whether hepatic cell adenomas are premalignant is disputed. On occurrence, discontinuing the oral contraceptives is necessary and may result in spontaneous regression of the adenoma.

*Mental depression* has improved for many women with pre-existing conditions; otherwise, no effect with oral contraceptive use usually is noted but severe depression should be reported to and treatment continuance evaluated by a physician.

**Those indicating need for medical attention only if they continue or are bothersome**

Incidence more frequent

**Abdominal cramping or bloating; acne**—usually less frequent after the first 3 months of use; **breast pain, tenderness, or swelling**—8.5 to 25%; **dizziness**—10 to 14%; **nausea or vomiting**—6 to 12%; **sodium and fluid retention** (swelling of ankles and feet); **unusual tiredness or weakness**

Note: When compared with those patients using levonorgestrel, norgestrel, or norethindrone, patients using oral contraceptives containing desogestrel or norgestimate showed improvement in their condition of *acne. Nausea, vomiting, breast tenderness,* and *sodium and fluid retention* diminish after the first 2 or 3 months of oral contraceptive use.

Incidence less frequent

**Gain or loss of body or facial hair; increased skin sensitivity to sun; libido changes** (increase or decrease of interest in sexual intercourse); **melasma** (brown, blotchy spots on exposed skin); **weight gain or loss**—1%

Note: *Melasma* usually is temporary but can be permanent. Women having dark complexions, having a history of melasma during pregnancy, or having prolonged exposure to sunlight are most susceptible to developing melasma.

## Overdose

Serious adverse effects generally do not occur with an acute overdosage. When children have accidentally ingested a large amount of an oral contraceptive, more serious adverse effects also did not result. Withdrawal bleeding has occasionally occurred in young girls and does not require treatment.

For more information on the management of overdose or unintentional ingestion, **contact a Poison Control Center** (see *Poison Control Center Listing*).

**Clinical effects of overdose**

The following effects have been selected on the basis of their potential clinical significance (possible signs and symptoms in parentheses where appropriate)—not necessarily inclusive:

*Irregular bleeding cycle; nausea or vomiting*—occurring in less than 10% of patients; *withdrawal bleeding*

**Treatment of overdose**

Specific treatment—Nausea or vomiting is treated for symptomatic relief.

Supportive care—Patients in whom intentional overdose is known or suspected should be referred for psychiatric consultation.

## Patient Consultation

As an aid to patient consultation, refer to *Advice for the Patient, Estrogens and Progestins Oral Contraceptives (Systemic)*.

Consider advising the patient on the following (» = major clinical significance):

**Before using this medication**

» Conditions affecting use, especially:
  Sensitivity to estrogens or progestins
  Pregnancy—Not recommended for use during pregnancy
  Breast-feeding—Oral contraceptives are distributed into breast milk
  Use in adolescents—Careful counseling may be required to increase compliance
  Dental—May increase possibility of bleeding of gingival tissues, gingival hyperplasia, or local alveolar osteitis (dry socket)
  Other medications, especially corticosteroids, cyclosporine, hepatic enzyme inducers, hepatotoxic medications (especially troleandomycin), ritonavir, theophylline, tobacco smoking, or troglitazone
  Other medical problems, especially carcinoma of the breast (known or suspected); carcinoma of the endometrium; cardiac insufficiency; cerebrovascular disease—especially if patient smokes cigarettes (active or history of); coronary artery disease; estrogen-dependent neoplasia (known or suspected); hepatic disease, cholestatic (active); hepatic function impairment; hepatic tumors, benign or malignant (active or history of); thrombophlebitis, thrombosis, or thromboembolic disorders (active or history of); or uterine bleeding (abnormal or undiagnosed)

**Proper use of this medication**

» Reading patient package insert carefully
  Taking with or immediately after food to reduce nausea
  Using an additional method of birth control for the first 7 days; some clinicians may recommend that an additional method of birth control be used during the first cycle of oral contraceptive use
» Compliance with therapy; taking medication at the same time each day, at 24-hour intervals
  Keeping an extra 1-month supply available when possible
  Taking tablets in proper (color-coded) sequence
» Proper dosing
  Missed doses for the monophasic, biphasic, or triphasic cycle
    Missing the first tablet of a new cycle—Taking as soon as possible; if not remembered until next day, taking two tablets; continuing on regular dosing schedule and using another birth control method for 7 days after the last missed dose
    Missing 1 day—Taking as soon as possible; if not remembered until next day, taking 2 tablets; continuing on regular dosing schedule
    Missing 2 days in a row in the first or second week—Taking two tablets a day for next 2 days, then continuing on regular dosing schedule; using additional method of birth control for remainder of cycle
    Missing 2 days in a row in the third week or
    Missing 3 days in a row—
      Using Day-1 start: Discarding remaining doses for current cycle; beginning a new cycle following the recommended dosing schedule and using a second method of birth control, additionally, for 7 days after the last missed dose; contacting health care professional if two menstrual periods are missed
      Using Sunday start: Continuing on regular dosing schedule for current cycle until Sunday; on Sunday, throwing out remaining doses for current cycle and beginning a new cycle; using an additional method of birth control for 7 days after the last missed dose; contacting health care professional if two menstrual periods are missed

Missing any of the last seven tablets of a twenty-eight–day cycle is not important, but beginning new cycle on time is essential
» Proper storage

**Precautions while using this medication**
» Regular visits to physician at least every 6 to 12 months to check progress
» Caution if medical or dental surgery or emergency treatment is required—increased risk of thrombotic complications
» Using an additional method of birth control during each cycle in which the following medications are used: ampicillin, hepatic enzyme inducers, penicillin V, ritonavir, tetracyclines, or troglitazone
What to expect and do if vaginal bleeding occurs
What to expect and do if a menstrual period is missed; contacting health professional if two menstrual periods are missed
Possibility of dental problems, such as tenderness, swelling, or bleeding of gums; brushing and flossing teeth, massaging gums, and having dentist clean teeth regularly; checking with dentist if there are questions about care of teeth or gums or if tenderness, swelling, or bleeding of gums is noticed
Possibility of photosensitivity
» Stopping medication immediately and checking with physician if pregnancy is suspected
If scheduled for laboratory tests, telling physician if taking birth control pills; certain blood tests may be affected by oral contraceptives
Not refilling an old prescription for oral contraceptives without having a physical examination by physician, especially after a pregnancy

**Side/adverse effects**
Signs of potential side effects, especially thromboembolism or thrombosis; changes in the menstrual bleeding pattern or intermenstrual bleeding; headaches or migraines; hypertension, worsening; mildly reduced glucose tolerance (usually for predisposed individuals); vaginal candidiasis or vaginitis; breast tumors (usually for predisposed individuals); hepatic focal nodular hyperplasia, hepatitis, or hepatocellular carcinoma; hepatic cell adenomas, benign; slight worsening of mental depression
Cigarette smoking combined with oral contraceptive use causes increased risk of serious thromboembolic or hepatic side effects, especially for heavy smokers or women over age 35

## General Dosing Information

The doses of estrogens and progestins used for contraception are much greater than those doses of estrogens and progestins used for hormone replacement therapy. Perimenopausal women should be tested for serum FSH levels annually for accurate dating of menopause; oral contraceptives should be discontinued and hormone replacement therapy started if or when appropriate.

Low doses of estrogen (doses containing 35 mcg or less of ethinyl estradiol or 50 mcg mestranol) are preferred to higher doses (equal to 50 mcg of ethinyl estradiol). Many side effects are related to the dominance of either the estrogen or progestin present in the preparation. By changing to preparations of differing component ratios, side effects can often be lessened or eliminated. In some instances low-dose estrogen formulations are not acceptable and the high-dose estrogen formulations should be used, such as when the effectiveness of oral contraceptives is compromised because of increased hepatic metabolism. This may occur when some anticonvulsant medications are used concurrently. All effects of long-term use of the lower-dose oral contraceptives have not been determined. Most long-term studies performed have been in patients using higher doses of estrogens and progestins than are used commonly at present.

Thirty-five mcg of ethinyl estradiol and 50 mcg of mestranol are considered to have equal therapeutic potency as the estrogen component for contraception. Norgestrel (d,l-norgestrel) is a racemic mixture of dextro- and levonorgestrel and has one-half the potency of levonorgestrel on a weight basis. Dextronorgestrel can be considered an inactive isomer.

The multiphasic formulations were developed to supply the lowest possible total hormone dose over a treatment cycle. Monophasic, biphasic, and triphasic regimens are considered equally effective for preventing pregnancy and choice may be unique to an individual's lifestyle, health risks, or other factors. The success of an oral contraceptive is also highly dependent on proper selection of the formulation for an individual, according to her menstrual cycle regularity, her ability to be compliant, and her tolerance for side effects. When possible, the lowest dose of hormones should be used to achieve these goals.
• The *monophasic regimen* provides constant doses of estrogen and progestin in 21 days.
• The *biphasic regimen* provides two different dose ratios of two phases of the estrogen:progestin in 21 days and includes a constant estrogen dose throughout the cycle with a progestin dose increase either at the 7th or the 10th day, depending on the product.
• The *triphasic regimen* provides four different dose ratios of three phases of estrogen:progestin in 21 days and includes:
—Variable doses of estrogen and progestin changing after the 6th and 10th days.
—A constant progestin dose throughout the cycle plus an increase in the estrogen dose after the 5th and 7th days.
—A constant estrogen dose throughout the cycle plus an increase in the progestin dose for only 9 days (8th through the 16th day).
—A constant estrogen dose throughout the cycle with an increase in the progestin dose every 7 days.

**For routine contraception**
To begin taking oral contraceptives, the first tablet is taken either on Day 1 (first day of menstrual bleeding) of the menstrual cycle or the first Sunday following the start of menses. Dosage schedules are arranged on a 21- or 28-day cycle to correspond with the 28 days of the menstrual cycle. The 21-day regimens provide 21 active tablets containing estrogen and progestin hormone therapy. The 28-day cycle adds 7 inactive (nonhormonal) tablets to the 21-day regimen for either 7 days of placebo tablets for ease of daily counting or 7 days of iron (ferrous fumarate) companion tablets to supplement the diet. To help the patient to comply with this schedule, most manufacturers integrate the schedule into a non-childproof dispensing container, which should be utilized whenever possible. Tablets containing different strengths of hormones are colored differently to help the patient differentiate between the tablet strengths; this is especially helpful for biphasic and triphasic formulations. Also, the active and inactive tablets are different colors. Patients should be informed of the necessity of taking different colored tablets in the proper sequence and not mixing tablets of different colors indiscriminately. Also, even if the hormone formulation is the same for two products of different manufacturers, tablet colors do not always correspond.

Maximum contraceptive effect is obtained by taking doses at 24-hour intervals and beginning the new regimen on time; this enhances patient compliance, also. When initiating oral contraceptive treatment, many clinicians instruct patients to use a nonhormonal backup method for 7 days if contraceptive therapy is started within the first 5 days of the menstrual cycle. Other clinicians counsel patients to use a nonhormonal backup method of contraception for the first month. Contraceptive effectiveness is continued when transferring patients between oral contraceptive formulations when initiated at the beginning of the menstrual cycle, with minimal side effects. Breakthrough bleeding or spotting may recur for several months when an oral contraceptive is started, but is usually less for those patients transferred between formulations than for initial users.

A periodic pill-free *rest period* is not recommended, since it appears to provide no therapeutic advantage and does not enhance the resumption of ovulatory cycles after cessation of oral contraceptive therapy. Such intervals may result in noncompliance with the substituted contraceptive and unwanted pregnancies.

**For emergency postcoital contraception**
Therapy is initiated as soon as possible or up to 72 hours after intercourse; repeated courses in a single cycle are not recommended as efficacy may be compromised.

The use of norgestrel or levonorgestrel and ethinyl estradiol tablets as a postcoital contraceptive (the *morning-after pill*) has been employed primarily in emergency situations, such as when possible contraceptive method failure is realized early or when any unprotected sexual intercourse is of concern to the patient. Effectiveness depends on the time interval between coitus and administration of the medication. A pregnancy test should be performed prior to administering medication. A patient requesting treatment should be fully informed of the risks involved, such as potential increased risk of blood clot formation because of the higher dosage of hormone required, although treatment is of short duration. Also, nausea and vomiting may result, increasing the possibility of contraceptive failure because of the difficulty of maintaining compliance.

**For patients with endometriosis**
Oral contraceptives can be given continuously or cyclically for 6 to 9 months to aid in ectopic implant atrophy. Low-dose estrogen preparations containing a high progestational progestin, such as desogestrel, are probably best for this. Endometriotic symptoms may increase before improvement is noted by patient.

**For patients with hirsutisim**
Treatment with oral contraceptives for 6 months to 1 year may be required before effects are apparent. Although hormones suppress new hair growth, normal androgen levels maintain hair that is already present.

### Diet/Nutrition
Should be taken with food or milk to lessen gastrointestinal irritation if it occurs or tablets may be taken at bedtime.

---
## *DESOGESTREL AND ETHINYL ESTRADIOL*
---

## Summary of Differences

Pharmacology/pharmacokinetics—Desogestrel is a prodrug that is metabolized to a more active form, etonogestrel. Exhibits first-pass effect. Highly progestational and does not counteract the estrogen increase in sex hormone–binding globulin (SHBG) levels; highly bound to SHBG and albumin; low androgenicity.

Laboratory value alterations—Little effect on lipoproteins.

Medical considerations/contraindications—Desogestrel plus ethinyl estradiol increases glucose tolerance but does not affect 2-hour insulin release; has less effect on carbohydrate metabolism compared with other oral contraceptives.

Side/adverse effects—Absence of withdrawal menstrual bleeding is low; improves pre-existing acne.

## Oral Dosage Forms

Note: Bracketed uses in the *Dosage Forms* section refer to categories of use and/or indications that are not included in U.S. product labeling.

### DESOGESTREL AND ETHINYL ESTRADIOL TABLETS

**Usual adult and adolescent dose**
Contraceptive, systemic or
Estrogen-progestin or
[Antiendometriotic agent][1] or
[Gonadotropin inhibitor, female, noncontraceptive use][1]—
 Twenty-one–day cycle: Oral, 1 tablet a day for twenty-one days commencing on Day 1 of the menstrual cycle or on the first Sunday after the menstrual cycle begins; the next round of treatment is begun on the eighth day after the last tablet of the previous cycle has been taken.
 Twenty-eight–day cycle: Oral, 1 tablet a day for twenty-eight days commencing on Day 1 of the menstrual cycle, or on the first Sunday after the menstrual cycle begins; the next round of treatment is begun on the day after the last tablet of the previous cycle has been taken.

Note: With a Sunday start schedule, the patient should take her first tablet on the first Sunday after the onset of menstruation. If the patient's period begins on a Sunday, she should take her first tablet that same day.
 With a Day-1 start schedule, the patient should take her first tablet on Day 1 of the menstrual cycle.
 The last seven tablets of the twenty-eight–day cycle contain no hormones. These seven companion tablets are a different color from those containing hormones.
 Oral contraceptives may be given continuously or cyclically for endometriosis.

**Strength(s) usually available**
U.S.—
 Monophasic formulation:
  150 mcg (0.15 mg) of desogestrel and 30 mcg (0.03 mg) of ethinyl estradiol (Rx) [*Desogen*; *Ortho-Cept*].
Canada—
 Monophasic formulation:
  150 mcg (0.15 mg) of desogestrel and 30 mcg (0.03 mg) of ethinyl estradiol (Rx) [*Marvelon*; *Ortho-Cept*].

Note: *Marvelon* and *Ortho-Cept* are available in twenty-one– or twenty-eight–day cycles. The twenty-eight–day cycle includes an additional seven days of placebo tablets.

**Packaging and storage**
Store below 40 °C (104 °F), preferably between 15 and 30 °C (59 and 86 °F), unless otherwise specified by manufacturer. Store in a well-closed container.

**Auxiliary labeling**
• Take with food.
• Avoid too much sun or use of sunlamp.

**Note**
 Include mandatory patient package inserts (PPIs) (the brief summary of patient labeling and the detailed patient labeling) when dispensing.
 Caution first-time users to use an additional form of birth control as directed by their physicians until maximum contraceptive protection begins.

### DESOGESTREL AND ETHINYL ESTRADIOL TABLETS AND ETHINYL ESTRADIOL TABLETS USP

**Usual adult and adolescent dose**
Contraceptive, systemic or
Estrogen-progestin or
[Antiendometriotic agent][1] or
[Gonadotropin inhibitor, female, noncontraceptive use][1]—
 See *Desogestrel and Ethinyl Estradiol Tablets*.

**Strength(s) usually available**
U.S.—
 Monophasic formulation:
  150 mcg (0.15 mg) of desogestrel and 20 mcg ethinyl estradiol (0.02 mg) (Rx) [*Mircette*].
Canada—
 Not commercially available in Canada.

Note: Available in twenty-eight–day cycles. The twenty-eight–day cycle includes an additional seven days of tablets containing two placebo tablets for the first two days, then five tablets of 10 mcg (0.10 mg) of ethinyl estradiol. Similar to placebo tablets, the last seven days of a this twenty-eight–day cycle need not be taken, even though it contains a low-dose of estrogen; contraceptive efficacy is not dependent on the low doses of estrogen given Days 24 through 28.

**Packaging and storage**
Store below 40 °C (104 °F), preferably between 15 and 30 °C (59 and 86 °F), unless otherwise specified by manufacturer. Store in a well-closed container.

**Auxiliary labeling**
• Take with food.
• Avoid too much sun or use of sunlamp.

**Note**
 Include mandatory patient package inserts (PPIs) (the brief summary of patient labeling and the detailed patient labeling) when dispensing.
 Caution first-time users to use an additional form of birth control as directed by their physicians until maximum contraceptive protection begins.

---
[1]Not included in Canadian product labeling.

---
## *ETHYNODIOL DIACETATE AND ETHINYL ESTRADIOL*
---

## Summary of Differences

Pharmacology/pharmacokinetics—Ethynodiol diacetate hydrolyzed to norethindrone; aromatization by tissues may be clinically significant. Greater affinity for albumin but significant SHBG binding occurs because of estrogen-induced SHBG levels. Exhibits first-pass effect. Slightly estrogenic.

Laboratory value alterations—Triglycerides increase; shows the greatest increase in apolipoprotein A$_1$ of all contraceptives.

Dosage forms—High estrogen dose formulation available.

## Oral Dosage Forms

Note: Bracketed uses in the *Dosage Forms* section refer to categories of use and/or indications that are not included in U.S. product labeling.

### ETHYNODIOL DIACETATE AND ETHINYL ESTRADIOL TABLETS USP

**Usual adult and adolescent dose**
Contraceptive, systemic or
Estrogen-progestin or
[Antiendometriotic agent][1] or
[Gonadotropin inhibitor, female, noncontraceptive use][1]—
 Twenty-one–day cycle: Oral, 1 tablet a day for twenty-one days commencing on Day 1 of the menstrual cycle or on the first Sunday after the menstrual cycle begins; the next round of treatment is begun on the eighth day after the last tablet of the previous cycle has been taken.
 Twenty-eight–day cycle: Oral, 1 tablet a day for twenty-eight days commencing on Day 1 of the menstrual cycle, or on the first Sunday after the menstrual cycle begins; the next round of treatment is begun on the day after the last tablet of the previous cycle has been taken.

Note: With a Sunday start schedule, the patient should take her first tablet on the first Sunday after the onset of menstruation. If the patient's period begins on a Sunday, she should take her first tablet that same day.

With a Day-1 start schedule, the patient should take her first tablet on Day 1 of the menstrual cycle.

The last seven tablets of the twenty-eight–day cycle contain no hormones. These seven companion tablets are of a different color from those containing hormones.

Oral contraceptives may be given continuously or cyclically for endometriosis.

**Strength(s) usually available**
U.S.—
  Monophasic formulation:
    1 mg of ethynodiol diacetate and 35 mcg (0.035 mg) of ethinyl estradiol (Rx) [*Demulen 1/35; Zovia 1/35E*].
    1 mg of ethynodiol diacetate and 50 mcg (0.05 mg) of ethinyl estradiol (Rx) [*Demulen 1/50; Zovia 1/50E*].
Canada—
  Monophasic formulation:
    1 mg of ethynodiol diacetate and 50 mcg (0.05 mg) of ethinyl estradiol (Rx) [*Demulen 50*].
    2 mg of ethynodiol diacetate and 30 mcg (0.03 mg) of ethinyl estradiol (Rx) [*Demulen 30*].
Note: Available in twenty-one- or twenty-eight–day cycles. The twenty-eight–day cycle includes an additional seven days of placebo tablets.

**Packaging and storage**
Store below 40 °C (104 °F), preferably between 15 and 30 °C (59 and 86 °F), unless otherwise specified by manufacturer. Store in a well-closed container.

**Auxiliary labeling**
• Take with food.
• Avoid too much sun or use of sunlamp.

**Note**
Include mandatory patient package inserts (PPIs) (the brief summary of patient labeling and the detailed patient labeling) when dispensing.
Caution first-time users to use additional form of birth control as directed by their physicians until maximum contraceptive protection begins.

---

[1]Not included in Canadian product labeling.

---

### LEVONORGESTREL AND ETHINYL ESTRADIOL

## Summary of Differences

Indications—Also used for emergency postcoital contraception.
Pharmacology/pharmacokinetics—Levonorgestrel is the active enantiomer of norgestrel. Proportion bound to SHBG depends on both estrogen and levonorgestrel dose; suppresses estrogen-induced increase of SHBG levels except when the triphasic formulation is used, which slightly increases SHBG levels. No first-pass effect. One of the most androgenic progestins; androgenic effects depend on both progestin and estrogen dose.
Laboratory value alterations—No change in triglycerides over 1 year; may slightly decrease or increase total cholesterol; negatively affected lipoprotein—increases LDL and lowers HDL; increases apolipoprotein A$_1$ the least of all contraceptives; can increase free testosterone by displacing it from SHBG.
Dosage forms—High estrogen dose formulation available.

## Oral Dosage Forms

Note: Bracketed uses in the *Dosage Forms* section refer to categories of use and/or indications that are not included in U.S. product labeling.

### LEVONORGESTREL AND ETHINYL ESTRADIOL TABLETS USP

**Usual adult and adolescent dose**
Contraceptive, systemic or
Estrogen-progestin or
[Antiendometriotic agent][1] or
[Gonadotropin inhibitor, female, noncontraceptive use][1]—
  Twenty-one–day cycle: Oral, 1 tablet a day for twenty-one days commencing on Day 1 of the menstrual cycle or on the first Sunday after the menstrual cycle begins; the next round of treatment is begun on the eighth day after the last tablet of the previous cycle has been taken.
  Twenty-eight–day cycle: Oral, 1 tablet a day for twenty-eight days commencing on Day 1 of the menstrual cycle, or on the first Sunday after the menstrual cycle begins; the next round of treatment is begun on the day after the last tablet of the previous cycle has been taken.

Note: With a Sunday start schedule, the patient should take her first tablet on the first Sunday after the onset of menstruation. If the patient's period begins on a Sunday, she should take her first tablet that same day.

With a Day-1 start schedule, the patient should take her first tablet on Day 1 of the menstrual cycle.

The last seven tablets of the twenty-eight–day cycle contain no hormones. These seven companion tablets are a different color from those containing hormones.

Oral contraceptives may be given continuously or cyclically for endometriosis.

[Contraceptive, postcoital, systemic][1]—
  Four tablets (150 mcg levonorgestrel and 30 mcg of ethinyl estradiol per tablet) taken as soon as possible after unprotected coitus, preferably within twelve hours but not longer than seventy-two hours later. Then, four more tablets are taken twelve hours after the first dose.

Note: Monophasic or only phase-three tablets of the triphasic oral contraceptives contain sufficient hormone doses for postcoital emergency contraception use.

**Strength(s) usually available**
U.S.—
  Monophasic formulation:
    100 mcg (0.1 mg) of levonorgestrel and 20 mcg (0.02 mg) of ethinyl estradiol (Rx) [*Alesse; Levlite*].
    150 mcg (0.15 mg) of levonorgestrel and 30 mcg (0.03 mg) of ethinyl estradiol (Rx) [*Levlen; Levora 0.15/30; Nordette*].
  Triphasic formulation:
    **Phase one (six days)**—50 mcg (0.05 mg) of levonorgestrel and 30 mcg (0.03 mg) of ethinyl estradiol. **Phase two (five days)**—75 mcg (0.075 mg) of levonorgestrel and 40 mcg (0.04 mg) of ethinyl estradiol. **Phase three (ten days)**—125 mcg (0.125 mg) of levonorgestrel and 30 mcg (0.03 mg) of ethinyl estradiol. (Rx) [*Tri-Levlen; Triphasil; Trivora*].
Canada—
  Monophasic formulation:
    150 mcg (0.15 mg) of levonorgestrel and 30 mcg (0.03 mg) of ethinyl estradiol (Rx) [*Min-Ovral*].
  Triphasic formulation:
    **Phase one (six days)**—50 mcg (0.05 mg) of levonorgestrel and 30 mcg (0.03 mg) of ethinyl estradiol. **Phase two (five days)**—75 mcg (0.075 mg) of levonorgestrel and 40 mcg (0.04 mg) of ethinyl estradiol. **Phase three (ten days)**—125 mcg (0.125 mg) of levonorgestrel and 30 mcg (0.03 mg) of ethinyl estradiol. (Rx) [*Triphasil; Triquilar*].
Note: Available in twenty-one- or twenty-eight–day cycles. The twenty-eight–day cycle includes an additional seven days of placebo tablets.

**Packaging and storage**
Store below 40 °C (104 °F), preferably between 15 and 30 °C (59 and 86 °F), unless otherwise specified by manufacturer. Store in a well-closed container.

**Auxiliary labeling**
• Take with food.
• Avoid too much sun or use of sunlamp.

**Note**
Include mandatory patient package inserts (PPIs) (the brief summary of patient labeling and the detailed patient labeling) when dispensing.
Explain sequence of administration of triphasic cycle formula when dispensing, especially for twenty-eight–day cycle (colored tablet sequence).
Caution first-time users to use an additional form of birth control as directed by their physicians until maximum contraceptive protection begins.

---

[1]Not included in Canadian product labeling.

---

### NORETHINDRONE ACETATE AND ETHINYL ESTRADIOL

## Summary of Differences

Pharmacology/pharmacokinetics—Proportion bound to SHBG depends on both estrogen and norethindrone dose; does not suppress estrogen-induced increase in SHBG levels. Norethindrone acetate metabolized to norethindrone, which exhibits no first-pass effect. Androgenic effect depends on both progestin and estrogen dose; androgenic effects less than those of levonorgestrel or norgestrel; possesses slight estrogenic activity.

Laboratory value alterations—Slightly increases total cholesterol; negatively affects lipoproteins—increases LDL and lowers HDL; increases apolipoprotein $A_1$.

Dosage forms—High estrogen dose formulation available.

## Oral Dosage Forms

Note: Bracketed uses in the *Dosage Forms* section refer to categories of use and/or indications that are not included in U.S. product labeling.

### NORETHINDRONE ACETATE AND ETHINYL ESTRADIOL TABLETS USP

**Usual adult and adolescent dose**
Contraceptive, systemic or
Estrogen-progestin or
[Antiendometriotic agent][1] or
[Gonadotropin inhibitor, female, noncontraceptive use][1]—
    Twenty-one–day cycle: Oral, 1 tablet a day for twenty-one days commencing on Day 1 of the menstrual cycle or on the first Sunday after the menstrual cycle begins; the next round of treatment is begun on the eighth day after the last tablet of the previous cycle has been taken.
    Twenty-eight–day cycle: Oral, 1 tablet a day for twenty-eight days commencing on Day 1 of the menstrual cycle, or on the first Sunday after the menstrual cycle begins; the next round of treatment is begun on the day after the last tablet of the previous cycle has been taken.

Note: With a Sunday start schedule, the patient should take her first tablet on the first Sunday after the onset of menstruation. If the patient's period begins on a Sunday, she should take her first tablet that same day.

With a Day-1 start schedule, the patient should take her first tablet on Day 1 of the menstrual cycle.

The last seven tablets of the twenty-eight–day cycle contain no hormones. These seven companion tablets are a different color from those containing hormones.

Oral contraceptives may be given continuously or cyclically for endometriosis.

**Strength(s) usually available**
U.S.—
  Monophasic formulation:
    1 mg of norethindrone acetate and 20 mcg (0.02 mg) of ethinyl estradiol (Rx) [*Loestrin 1/20*].
    1.5 mg of norethindrone acetate and 30 mcg (0.03 mg) of ethinyl estradiol (Rx) [*Loestrin 1.5/30*].
  Triphasic formulation:
    **Phase one (five days)**—1 mg of norethindrone acetate and 20 mcg (0.02 mg) of ethinyl estradiol. **Phase two (seven days)**—1 mg of norethindrone acetate and 30 mcg (0.03 mg) of ethinyl estradiol. **Phase three (nine days)**—1 mg of norethindrone acetate and 35 mcg (0.035 mg) of ethinyl estradiol. (Rx) [*Estrostep*].
Canada—
  Monophasic formulation:
    1 mg of norethindrone acetate and 20 mcg (0.02 mg) of ethinyl estradiol (Rx) [*Minestrin 1/20*].
    1.5 mg of norethindrone acetate and 30 mcg (0.03 mg) of ethinyl estradiol (Rx) [*Loestrin 1.5/30*].

Note: Available in twenty-one– or twenty-eight–day cycles. The twenty-eight–day cycle includes an additional seven days of placebo tablets.

**Packaging and storage**
Store below 40 °C (104 °F), preferably between 15 and 30 °C (59 and 86 °F), unless otherwise specified by manufacturer. Store in a well-closed container.

**Auxiliary labeling**
• Take with food.
• Avoid too much sun or use of sunlamp.

**Note**
Include mandatory patient package inserts (PPIs) (the brief summary of patient labeling and the detailed patient labeling) when dispensing.
Caution first-time users to use an additional form of birth control as directed by their physicians until maximum contraceptive protection begins.

[1]Not included in Canadian product labeling.

### NORETHINDRONE ACETATE AND ETHINYL ESTRADIOL TABLETS USP
### FERROUS FUMARATE TABLETS USP

**Usual adult and adolescent dose**
Contraceptive, systemic or
Estrogen-progestin or
[Antiendometriotic agent][1] or
[Gonadotropin inhibitor, female, noncontraceptive use][1]—
    See *Norethindrone Acetate and Ethinyl Estradiol Tablets USP*.

**Strength(s) usually available**
U.S.—
  Monophasic formulation:
    1 mg of norethindrone acetate and 20 mcg (0.02 mg) of ethinyl estradiol (Rx) [*Loestrin Fe 1/20*].
    1.5 mg of norethindrone acetate and 30 mcg (0.03 mg) of ethinyl estradiol (Rx) [*Loestrin Fe 1.5/30*].
  Triphasic formulation:
    **Phase one (five days)**—1 mg of norethindrone acetate and 20 mcg (0.02 mg) of ethinyl estradiol. **Phase two (seven days)**—1 mg of norethindrone acetate and 30 mcg (0.03 mg) of ethinyl estradiol. **Phase three (nine days)**—1 mg of norethindrone acetate and 35 mcg (0.035 mg) of ethinyl estradiol. (Rx) [*Estrostep Fe*].
Canada—
  Not commercially available in Canada.

Note: Available in twenty-eight–day cycles. The twenty-eight–day cycle includes an additional seven days of tablets containing 75 mg ferrous fumarate each.

**Packaging and storage**
Store below 40 °C (104 °F), preferably between 15 and 30 °C (59 and 86 °F), unless otherwise specified by manufacturer. Store in a well-closed container.

**Auxiliary labeling**
• Take with food.
• Avoid too much sun or use of sunlamp.

**Note**
Include mandatory patient package inserts (PPIs) (the brief summary of patient labeling and the detailed patient labeling) when dispensing.
Caution first-time users to use an additional form of birth control as directed by their physicians until maximum contraceptive protection begins.

[1]Not included in Canadian product labeling.

---

### NORETHINDRONE AND ETHINYL ESTRADIOL

## Summary of Differences

Pharmacology/pharmacokinetics—Proportion bound to SHBG depends on both estrogen and norethindrone dose; does not suppress estrogen-induced increase in SHBG levels. Norethindrone exhibits no first-pass effect; less androgenic than levonorgestrel or norgestrel; its androgenic effect depends on both progestin and estrogen doses; slight estrogenic activity.

Laboratory value alterations—Triglycerides increase as with all oral contraceptives; slightly increases total cholesterol; negatively affects lipoproteins—increases LDL and lowers HDL; increases apolipoprotein $A_1$.

Dosage forms—High estrogen dose formulation available.

## Oral Dosage Forms

Note: Bracketed uses in the *Dosage Forms* section refer to categories of use and/or indications that are not included in U.S. product labeling.

### NORETHINDRONE AND ETHINYL ESTRADIOL TABLETS USP

**Usual adult and adolescent dose**
Contraceptive, systemic or
Estrogen-progestin or
[Antiendometriotic agent][1] or
[Gonadotropin inhibitor, female, noncontraceptive use][1]—
    Twenty-one–day cycle: Oral, 1 tablet a day for twenty-one days commencing on Day 1 of the menstrual cycle or on the first Sunday after the menstrual cycle begins; the next round of treatment is begun on the eighth day after the last tablet of the previous cycle has been taken.
    Twenty-eight–day cycle: Oral, 1 tablet a day for twenty-eight days commencing on Day 1 of the menstrual cycle, or on the first Sunday after the menstrual cycle begins; the next round of treatment is be-

gun on the day after the last tablet of the previous cycle has been taken.

Note: With a Sunday start schedule, the patient should take her first tablet on the first Sunday after the onset of menstruation. If the patient's period begins on a Sunday, she should take her first tablet that same day.

With a Day-1 start schedule, the patient should take her first tablet on Day 1 of the menstrual cycle.

The last seven tablets of the twenty-eight–day cycle contain no hormones. These seven companion tablets are a different color from those containing hormones.

Oral contraceptives may be given continuously or cyclically for endometriosis.

### Strength(s) usually available

U.S.—
- Monophasic formulation:
    - 400 mcg (0.4 mg) of norethindrone and 35 mcg (0.035 mg) of ethinyl estradiol (Rx) [*Ovcon-35*].
    - 500 mcg (0.5 mg) of norethindrone and 35 mcg (0.035 mg) of ethinyl estradiol (Rx) [*Brevicon; Genora 0.5/35; Intercon 0.5/35; ModiCon; Necon 0.5/35; Nelova 0.5/35E*].
    - 1 mg of norethindrone and 35 mcg (0.035 mg) of ethinyl estradiol (Rx) [*Genora 1/35; Intercon 1/35; Necon 1/35; N.E.E. 1/35; Nelova 1/35E; Norethin 1/35E; Norinyl 1+35; Ortho-Novum 1/35*].
    - 1 mg of norethindrone and 50 mcg (0.05 mg) of ethinyl estradiol (Rx) [*N.E.E. 1/50; Ovcon-50*].
- Biphasic formulation, Option one:
    - **Phase one (ten days)**—500 mcg (0.5 mg) of norethindrone and 35 mcg (0.035 mg) of ethinyl estradiol. **Phase two (eleven days)**—1 mg of norethindrone and 35 mcg (0.035 mg) of ethinyl estradiol. (Rx) [*Necon 10/11; Nelova 10/11; Ortho-Novum 10/11*].
- Biphasic formulation, Option two:
    - **Phase one (seven days)**—500 mcg (0.5 mg) of norethindrone and 35 mcg (0.035 mg) of ethinyl estradiol. **Phase two (fourteen days)**—1 mg norethindrone and 35 mcg (0.035 mg) of ethinyl estradiol. (Rx) [*Jenest*].
- Triphasic formulation, Option one:
    - **Phase one (seven days)**—500 mcg (0.5 mg) of norethindrone and 35 mcg (0.035 mg) of ethinyl estradiol. **Phase two (nine days)**—1 mg of norethindrone and 35 mcg (0.035 mg) of ethinyl estradiol. **Phase three (five days)**—500 mcg (0.5 mg) of norethindrone and 35 mcg (0.035 mg) of ethinyl estradiol. (Rx) [*Tri-Norinyl*].
- Triphasic formulation, Option two:
    - **Phase one (seven days)**—500 mcg (0.5 mg) of norethindrone and 35 mcg (0.035 mg) of ethinyl estradiol. **Phase two (seven days)**—750 mcg (0.75 mg) of norethindrone and 35 mcg (0.035 mg) of ethinyl estradiol. **Phase three (seven days)**—1 mg of norethindrone and 35 mcg (0.035 mg) of ethinyl estradiol. (Rx) [*Ortho-Novum 7/7/7*].

Canada—
- Monophasic formulation:
    - 500 mcg (0.5 mg) of norethindrone and 35 mcg (0.035 mg) of ethinyl estradiol (Rx) [*Brevicon 0.5/35; Ortho 0.5/35*].
    - 1 mg of norethindrone and 35 mcg (0.035 mg) of ethinyl estradiol (Rx) [*Brevicon 1/35; Ortho 1/35; Select 1/35 (povidone)*].
- Biphasic formulation:
    - **Phase one (ten days)**—500 mcg (0.5 mg) of norethindrone and 35 mcg (0.035 mg) of ethinyl estradiol. **Phase two (eleven days)**—1 mg of norethindrone and 35 mcg (0.035 mg) of ethinyl estradiol. (Rx) [*Ortho 10/11; Synphasic*].
- Triphasic formulation:
    - **Phase one (seven days)**—500 mcg (0.5 mg) of norethindrone and 35 mcg (0.035 mg) of ethinyl estradiol. **Phase two (seven days)**—750 mcg (0.75 mg) of norethindrone and 35 mcg (0.035 mg) of ethinyl estradiol. **Phase three (seven days)**—1 mg of norethindrone and 35 mcg (0.035 mg) of ethinyl estradiol. (Rx) [*Ortho 7/7/7*].

Note: Most products are available in twenty-one– or twenty-eight–day cycles. The twenty-eight–day cycle includes an additional seven days of placebo tablets.

### Packaging and storage

Store below 40 °C (104 °F), preferably between 15 and 30 °C (59 and 86 °F), unless otherwise specified by manufacturer. Store in a well-closed container.

### Auxiliary labeling

- Take with food.
- Avoid too much sun or use of sunlamp.

### Note

Include mandatory patient package inserts (PPIs) (the brief summary of patient labeling and the detailed patient labeling) when dispensing. Explain sequence of administration of biphasic or triphasic cycle formula when dispensing, especially for twenty-eight–day cycle (colored tablet sequence).

Caution first-time users to use an additional form of birth control as directed by their physicians until maximum contraceptive protection begins.

---

[1]Not included in Canadian product labeling.

---

## NORETHINDRONE AND MESTRANOL

## Summary of Differences

Pharmacology/pharmacokinetics—Proportion bound to SHBG depends on both estrogen and norethindrone dose; does not suppress estrogen-induced increase in SHBG levels. Norethindrone exhibits no first-pass effect. Mestranol is a prodrug metabolized to ethinyl estradiol at about 83% conversion rate; high first-pass effect and enterohepatic recirculation. Norethindrone is less androgenic than levonorgestrel or norgestrel; its androgenic effect depends on both progestin and estrogen doses; slight estrogenic activity.

Laboratory value alterations—Triglycerides increase as with all oral contraceptives; slightly increases total cholesterol; negatively affects lipoproteins—increases LDL and lowers HDL; increases apolipoprotein A$_1$.

Dosage forms—High estrogen dose formulation available.

## Oral Dosage Forms

Note: Bracketed uses in the *Dosage Forms* section refer to categories of use and/or indications that are not included in U.S. product labeling.

### NORETHINDRONE AND MESTRANOL TABLETS USP

**Usual adult and adolescent dose**

Contraceptive, systemic or
Estrogen-progestin or
[Antiendometriotic agent] or
[Gonadotropin inhibitor, female, noncontraceptive use][1]—

Twenty-one–day cycle: Oral, 1 tablet a day for twenty-one days commencing on Day 1 of the menstrual cycle or on the first Sunday after the menstrual cycle begins; the next round of treatment is begun on the eighth day after the last tablet of the previous cycle has been taken.

Twenty-eight–day cycle: Oral, 1 tablet a day for twenty-eight days commencing on Day 1 of the menstrual cycle, or on the first Sunday after the menstrual cycle begins; the next round of treatment is begun on the day after the last tablet of the previous cycle has been taken.

Note: With a Sunday start schedule, the patient should take her first tablet on the first Sunday after the onset of menstruation. If the patient's period begins on a Sunday, she should take her first tablet that same day.

With a Day-1 start schedule, the patient should take her first tablet on Day 1 of the menstrual cycle.

The last seven tablets of the twenty-eight–day cycle contain no hormones. These seven companion tablets are a different color from those containing hormones.

Oral contraceptives may be given continuously or cyclically for endometriosis.

### Strength(s) usually available

U.S.—
- Monophasic formulation:
    - 1 mg of norethindrone and 50 mcg (0.05 mg) of mestranol (Rx) [*Genora 1/50; Intercon 1/50; Necon 1/50; Nelova 1/50M; Norethin 1/50M; Norinyl 1+50; Ortho-Novum 1/50*].

Canada—
- Monophasic formulation:
    - 1 mg of norethindrone and 50 mcg (0.05 mg) of mestranol (Rx) [*Norinyl 1/50; Ortho-Novum 1/50*].

Note: Most products are available in twenty-one– or twenty-eight–day cycles. The twenty-eight–day cycle includes an additional seven days of placebo tablets.

### Packaging and storage

Store below 40 °C (104 °F), preferably between 15 and 30 °C (59 and 86 °F), unless otherwise specified by manufacturer. Store in a well-closed container.

### Auxiliary labeling
- Take with food.
- Avoid too much sun or use of sunlamp.

### Note
Include mandatory patient package inserts (PPIs) (the brief summary of patient labeling and the detailed patient labeling) when dispensing. Caution first-time users to use an additional form of birth control as directed by their physicians until maximum contraceptive protection begins.

---

[1]Not included in Canadian product labeling.

---

## NORGESTIMATE AND ETHINYL ESTRADIOL

## Summary of Differences
Pharmacology/pharmacokinetics—Norgestimate is an incomplete prodrug, which is metabolized to other active forms, such as levonorgestrel, norgestrel acetate, and norgestrel. No first-pass effect. Highly progestational; does not counteract the estrogen increase in SHBG levels—highly bound to SHBG and albumin; low androgenicity.

Laboratory value alterations—Triglycerides increase but little effect on lipoproteins.

Medical considerations/contraindications—Norgestimate plus ethinyl estradiol increase glucose tolerance; do not affect 2-hour insulin release; had one of the smallest effects on both areas of carbohydrate metabolism compared with other oral contraceptives.

Side/adverse effects—Absence of withdrawal menstrual bleed was low with norgestimate and ethinyl estradiol formulation; improves pre-existing acne.

## Oral Dosage Forms
Note: Bracketed uses in the *Dosage Forms* section refer to categories of use and/or indications that are not included in U.S. product labeling.

### NORGESTIMATE AND ETHINYL ESTRADIOL TABLETS

**Usual adult and adolescent dose**
Contraceptive, systemic or
Estrogen-progestin or
[Antiendometriotic agent][1] or
[Gonadotropin inhibitor, female, noncontraceptive use][1]—
Twenty-one–day cycle: Oral, 1 tablet a day for twenty-one days commencing on Day 1 of the menstrual cycle or on the first Sunday after the menstrual cycle begins; the next round of treatment is begun on the eighth day after the last tablet of the previous cycle has been taken.
Twenty-eight–day cycle: Oral, 1 tablet a day for twenty-eight days commencing on Day 1 of the menstrual cycle, or on the first Sunday after the menstrual cycle begins; the next round of treatment is begun on the day after the last tablet of the previous cycle has been taken.
Acne vulgaris, systemic[1]—
Twenty-one–day cycle (Triphasic formulation only):
For adults and adolescents 15 years of age and over—Oral, 1 tablet a day for twenty-one days commencing on Day 1 of the menstrual cycle or on the first Sunday after the menstrual cycle begins; the next round of treatment is begun on the eighth day after the last tablet of the previous cycle has been taken.
For adolescents up to 15 years of age—Safety and efficacy have not been established.
Twenty-eight–day cycle (Triphasic formulation only):
For adults and adolescents 15 years of age and over—Oral, 1 tablet a day for twenty-eight days commencing on Day 1 of the menstrual cycle, or on the first Sunday after the menstrual cycle begins; the next round of treatment is begun on the day after the last tablet of the previous cycle has been taken.
For adolescents up to 15 years of age—Safety and efficacy have not been established.

Note: With a Sunday start schedule, the patient should take her first tablet on the first Sunday after the onset of menstruation. If the patient's period begins on a Sunday, she should take her first tablet that same day.
With a Day-1 start schedule, the patient should take her first tablet on Day 1 of the menstrual cycle.
The last seven tablets of the twenty-eight–day cycle contain no hormones. These seven companion tablets are a different color from those containing hormones.
Oral contraceptives may be given continuously or cyclically for endometriosis.

**Strength(s) usually available**
U.S.—
Monophasic formulation:
250 mcg (0.25 mg) of norgestimate and 35 mcg (0.035 mg) of ethinyl estradiol (Rx) [*Ortho-Cyclen*].
Triphasic formulation:
**Phase one (seven days)**—180 mcg (0.18 mg) of norgestimate and 35 mcg (0.035 mg) of ethinyl estradiol. **Phase two (seven days)**—215 mcg (0.215 mg) of norgestimate and 35 mcg (0.035 mg) of ethinyl estradiol. **Phase three (seven days)**—250 mcg (0.25 mg) of norgestimate and 35 mcg (0.035 mg) of ethinyl estradiol. (Rx) [*Ortho Tri-Cyclen*].
Canada—
Monophasic formulation:
250 mcg (0.25 mg) of norgestimate and 35 mcg (0.035 mg) of ethinyl estradiol (Rx) [*Cyclen*].
Triphasic formulation:
**Phase one (seven days)**—180 mcg (0.18 mg) of norgestimate and 35 mcg (0.035 mg) of ethinyl estradiol. **Phase two (seven days)**—215 mcg (0.215 mg) of norgestimate and 35 mcg (0.035 mg) of ethinyl estradiol. **Phase three (seven days)**—250 mcg (0.25 mg) of norgestimate and 35 mcg (0.035 mg) of ethinyl estradiol. (Rx) [*Tri-Cyclen*].
Note: Available in twenty-one– or twenty-eight–day cycles. The twenty-eight–day cycle includes an additional seven days of placebo tablets.

**Packaging and storage**
Store below 40 °C (104 °F), preferably between 15 and 30 °C (59 and 86 °F), unless otherwise specified by manufacturer. Store in a well-closed container.

**Auxiliary labeling**
- Take with food.
- Avoid too much sun or use of sunlamp.

**Note**
Include mandatory patient package inserts (PPIs) (the brief summary of patient labeling and the detailed patient labeling) when dispensing.
Explain sequence of administration of biphasic or triphasic cycle formula when dispensing, especially for twenty-eight–day cycle (colored tablet sequence).
Caution first-time users to use an additional form of birth control as directed by their physicians until maximum contraceptive protection begins.

---

[1]Not included in Canadian product labeling.

---

## NORGESTREL AND ETHINYL ESTRADIOL

## Summary of Differences
Indications: Also used for emergency postcoital contraception.
Pharmacology/pharmacokinetics: Proportion bound to SHBG depends on both estrogen and norgestrel dose; suppressed estrogen-induced increase in SHBG levels in most contraceptive doses except for triphasic formulation which only slightly increased SHBG levels. No first-pass effect. Norgestrel is one of the most androgenic progestins; its androgenic effect depends on both progestin and estrogen doses.
Laboratory value alterations: No change of triglycerides over 1 year; may slightly decrease or increase total cholesterol; negatively affects lipoprotein—increases LDL and lowers HDL; increases apolipoprotein A$_1$ the least of all contraceptives; can increase free testosterone by displacing it from SHBG.
Dosage forms: High estrogen dose formulation available.

## Oral Dosage Forms
Note: Bracketed uses in the *Dosage Forms* section refer to categories of use and/or indications that are not included in U.S. product labeling.

### NORGESTREL AND ETHINYL ESTRADIOL TABLETS USP

**Usual adult and adolescent dose**
Contraceptive, systemic or
Estrogen-progestin or
[Antiendometriotic agent][1] or
[Gonadotropin inhibitor, female, noncontraceptive use][1]—
Twenty-one–day cycle: Oral, 1 tablet a day for twenty-one days commencing on Day 1 of the menstrual cycle or on the first Sunday after the menstrual cycle begins; the next round of treatment is begun on the eighth day after the last tablet of the previous cycle has been taken.

**1412  Estrogens and Progestins (Oral Contraceptives) (Systemic)**

Twenty-eight–day cycle: Oral, 1 tablet a day for twenty-eight days commencing on Day 1 of the menstrual cycle, or on the first Sunday after the menstrual cycle begins; the next round of treatment is begun on the day after the last tablet of the previous cycle has been taken.

Note: With a Sunday start schedule, the patient should take her first tablet on the first Sunday after the onset of menstruation. If the patient's period begins on a Sunday, she should take her first tablet that same day.

With a Day-1 start schedule, the patient should take her first tablet on Day 1 of the menstrual cycle.

The last seven tablets of the twenty-eight–day cycle contain no hormones. These seven companion tablets are a different color from those containing hormones.

Oral contraceptives may be given continuously or cyclically for endometriosis.

[Contraceptive, postcoital, systemic][1]—
Two tablets (500 mcg norgestrel and 50 mcg of ethinyl estradiol per tablet) or four tablets (300 mcg norgestrel and 30 mcg ethinyl estradiol per tablet) taken as soon as possible after unprotected coitus, preferably within twelve hours but not longer than seventy-two hours later. Then, repeat the dose twelve hours after the first dose.

**Strength(s) usually available**
U.S.—
Monophasic formulation:
300 mcg (0.3 mg) of norgestrel and 30 mcg (0.03 mg) of ethinyl estradiol (Rx) [*Lo/Ovral*].
500 mcg (0.5 mg) of norgestrel and 50 mcg (0.05 mg) of ethinyl estradiol (Rx) [*Ovral*].

Canada—
Monophasic formulation:
500 mcg (0.50 mg) of norgestrel and 50 mcg (0.05 mg) of ethinyl estradiol (Rx) [*Ovral*].

Note: Available in twenty-one– or twenty-eight–day cycles. The twenty-eight–day cycle includes an additional seven days of placebo tablets.

**Packaging and storage**
Store below 40 °C (104 °F), preferably between 15 and 30 °C (59 and 86 °F), unless otherwise specified by manufacturer. Store in a well-closed container.

**Auxiliary labeling**
• Take with food.
• Avoid too much sun or use of sunlamp.

**Note**
Include mandatory patient package inserts (PPIs) (the brief summary of patient labeling and the detailed patient labeling) when dispensing.
Caution first-time users to use an additional form of birth control as directed by their physicians until maximum contraceptive protection begins.

[1]Not included in Canadian product labeling.

## Selected Bibliography

**For norethindrone acetate and ethinyl estradiol**
Goldzieher JW. Pharmacokinetics and metabolism of ethynyl estrogens. In: Goldzieher JW, editor. Pharmacology of the contraceptive steroids. New York: Raven Press; 1994. p. 127-51.

**For norethindrone and ethinyl estradiol**
Godsland IF, Crook D, Simpson R, et al. The effects of different formulations of oral contraceptive agents on lipid and carbohydrate metabolism. N Engl J Med 1990 Nov 15; 323(20): 1375-81.

**For levonorgestrel and ethinyl estradiol**
Godsland IF, Walton C, Felton C, et al. Insulin resistance, secretion, and metabolism in users of oral contraceptives. J Clin Endocrinol Metab 1992; 74(1): 64-70.

**For ethynodiol diacetate and ethinyl estradiol**
Burkman RT, Robinson CJ, Kruszone-Moran DA, et al. Lipid and lipoprotein changes associated with oral contraceptive use: a randomized clinical trial. Obstet Gynecol 1988 Jan; 71(1): 33-8.

**For norgestrel and ethinyl estradiol**
Ayangade O, Akinyemi A. A comparative study of Norinyl 1/35 versus Lo-Ovral in Ile-Ife, Nigeria. Int J Gynaecol Obstet 1989; 30: 165-70.

**For norethindrone and mestranol**
Policar M. Clinical experience with multiphasic oral contraceptives. J Reprod Med 1986; 31(9): 939-45.

**General**
Fraser IS. Contraceptive choice for women with 'risk factors.' Drug Saf 1993 Apr; 8(4): 271-9.
Speroff L, DeCherney A, The Advisory Board for the New Progestins. Evaluation of a new generation of oral contraceptives. Obstet Gynecol 1993 Jun; 81(6): 1034-47.
World Health Organization. Oral contraceptives and neoplasia. WHO Technical Report Series 1992; 817: 1-45.

**For desogestrel and ethinyl estradiol**
Burkman RT, editor. Desogestrel: a progestin for the 1990s. Am J Obstet Gynecol 1993 May; 168(3 Pt 2): 1009-52.

**For norgestimate and ethinyl estradiol**
McGuire JL, Phillips A, Hahn DW, et al. Pharmacologic and pharmacokinetic characteristics of norgestimate and its metabolites. Am J Obstet Gynecol 1990; 163(6 Pt 2): 2127-31.

Revised: 07/29/98

---

**ESTRONE** — See *Estrogens (Systemic)*; *Estrogens (Vaginal)*

---

**ESTROPIPATE** — See *Estrogens (Systemic)*; *Estrogens (Vaginal)*

---

**ETHACRYNIC ACID** — See *Diuretics, Loop (Systemic)*

---

# ETHAMBUTOL  Systemic

VA CLASSIFICATION (Primary): AM500
Commonly used brand name(s): *Etibi*; *Myambutol*.
Note: For a listing of dosage forms and brand names by country availability, see *Dosage Forms* section(s).

## Category
Antibacterial (antimycobacterial).

## Indications
Note: Bracketed information in the *Indications* section refers to uses that are not included in U.S. product labeling.

**General considerations**
Tuberculosis is a highly infectious life-threatening bacterial disease with 8 million new cases and 3 million deaths reported worldwide each year to the World Health Organization (WHO). The vast majority of these cases are in developing countries; however, tuberculosis also has emerged as an important public health problem in the U.S. in recent years after the decline in number of cases observed between 1950 and 1980.

The resurgence of tuberculosis in the U.S. has been complicated by an increase in the proportion of patients with strains resistant to antituberculosis medications. Outbreaks of multidrug-resistant tuberculosis have been documented in hospitals and prisons. Drug-resistant tuberculosis, particularly that caused by strains resistant to isoniazid and rifampin, is much harder to treat and often is fatal. Among acquired immunodeficiency syndrome (AIDS) patients infected with tuberculosis bacilli resistant to both rifampin and isoniazid, a case-fatality rate of 91% has been reported. Recent investigations of outbreaks of multidrug-resistant tuberculosis have found an extraordinarily high case-fatality rate, with the median time to mortality being reached between 4 and 16 weeks. In almost all instances, these outbreaks have involved patients with severe immunosuppression by infection with the human immunodeficiency virus (HIV).

Acquired drug resistance develops during treatment for drug-sensitive tuberculosis with regimens that are poorly conceived or poorly complied with, allowing the emergence of naturally occurring drug-resistant mutations. Resistant organisms from affected patients may subsequently infect other people who have not been infected with *M. tuberculosis* previously, resulting in primary drug resistance.

Resistance to antituberculosis agents can develop not only in the strain that caused the initial disease, but also as a result of reinfection with a new strain of *M. tuberculosis* that is drug-resistant. Reinfection with a new multidrug-resistant *M. tuberculosis* strain can occur during therapy for the original infection or after completion of therapy. Most recent data suggest that outcomes can be improved if patients promptly begin therapy with two or more drugs that have *in vitro* activity against the multidrug-resistant isolate.

HIV infection is the strongest risk factor yet identified for the development of active tuberculosis disease in persons infected with tuberculosis. In addition, persons with HIV infection are at an increased risk of tuberculosis resulting either from newly acquired disease or from reactivation of latent infections. Tuberculosis is a major clinical manifestation of immunodeficiency induced by HIV. In hospital-based retrospective studies, high rates of tuberculosis have been found among patients with AIDS. In communities where tuberculosis and HIV infection are common, the prevalence of HIV seropositivity among patients with tuberculosis is greatly increasing.

WHO has estimated that 5.6 million people worldwide and 80,000 people in the U.S. are infected with both HIV and tuberculosis. Persons dually infected with *M. tuberculosis* and HIV have a high risk of developing clinically active tuberculosis. One study of HIV-positive drug users with positive tuberculin skin test results found a rate of the development of active tuberculosis to be 8 cases per 100 person-years (8% yearly) as compared with the 10% lifetime risk (1 to 3% risk within the first year after skin test conversion) in the general population.

Persons who are known to be HIV-infected and who are contacts of patients with infectious tuberculosis should be carefully evaluated for evidence of tuberculosis. If there are no findings suggestive of current tuberculosis, preventive therapy with isoniazid should be given. Because HIV-infected contacts are not managed in the same way as those who are not HIV-infected, HIV testing is recommended if there are known or suspected risk factors for their acquiring HIV infection.

According to investigators at the National Institute of Allergy and Infectious Diseases (NIAID), levels of HIV in the bloodstream increase 5- to 160-fold in HIV-infected persons who develop active tuberculosis. Clinical and epidemiologic observations have demonstrated that HIV-infected individuals have an estimated 113-times higher risk and AIDS patients have a 170-times higher risk as compared with uninfected persons. Furthermore, the problem of drug resistance may worsen as the HIV epidemic spreads. Immunosuppressed patients with HIV infection who subsequently become infected with *M. tuberculosis* have an extraordinarily high risk of developing active tuberculosis within a short period of time.

In addition to the convincing evidence that HIV infection increases the risk and worsens the course of tuberculosis, there is increasing clinical evidence that coinfection with *M. tuberculosis* accelerates progression of disease caused by HIV infection. Understanding the interaction of these two pathogens is clinically important, given the high prevalence of patients coinfected with HIV and *M. tuberculosis* in both the U.S. and Africa; it is estimated that by the year 2000 about 500,000 deaths per year will occur in coinfected patients worldwide.

Persons with a positive tuberculin skin test and HIV infection, and persons with a positive tuberculin skin test and at risk of acquiring HIV infection with unknown HIV status should be considered for tuberculosis preventive therapy regardless of age. One study showed that isoniazid prophylaxis in HIV-infected, tuberculin-positive individuals not only decreased the incidence of tuberculosis disease, but also delayed the progression to AIDS and death.

Twelve months of preventive therapy is recommended for adults and children with HIV infection and other conditions associated with immunosuppression. Persons with HIV infection should receive at least 6 months of preventive therapy. The American Academy of Pediatrics recommends that children receive 9 months of therapy.

Tuberculosis control programs should ensure that drug susceptibility tests are performed on all initial isolates of *M. tuberculosis* and the results are reported promptly to the primary care provider and the local health department. Tuberculosis control programs should monitor local drug resistance rates to assess the effectiveness of local tuberculosis control efforts and to determine the appropriateness of the currently recommended initial tuberculosis treatment regimen for the area.

Relapse of rifampin-resistant tuberculosis has been reported in HIV-infected patients. Reinfection with new strains of *M. tuberculosis* has also been reported in these patients. Rifampin-resistant tuberculosis is a serious threat because responses to therapy are more difficult to achieve and require long courses of treatment. Therefore, careful follow-up of HIV-infected patients with treated tuberculosis is essential.

Multidrug-resistant tuberculosis also has been transmitted to persons without HIV infection in health care facilities. Together with the lack of effective agents for second-line treatment and methods of prophylaxis, the transmission of multidrug-resistant strains of *M. tuberculosis* may create a substantial reservoir of latently infected people and the potential for clinical multidrug-resistant tuberculosis for many years to come.

Several studies have documented a high prevalence of extrapulmonary disease in HIV-infected patients with clinical tuberculosis disease, particularly in conjunction with pulmonary manifestations. Cutaneous miliary tuberculosis, also known as *tuberculosis cutis miliaris disseminata*, was in the past a rare condition in adults, with only 24 cases reported in nearly a century. However, since the first reported case of cutaneous miliary tuberculosis in 1990 in a patient with AIDS, five additional cases have been reported in HIV-infected patients. Its appearance can be quite nondescript; therefore, a high level of suspicion must be maintained, particularly for patients with CD4+ cell counts of < 200 per cubic millimeter, in order to diagnose the condition and initiate therapy appropriately.

### Accepted
Tuberculosis (treatment)—Ethambutol is indicated in combination with other antituberculosis medications in the treatment of all forms of tuberculosis, including tuberculous meningitis, caused by *Mycobacterium tuberculosis*.

[Mycobacterial infections, atypical (treatment)]—Ethambutol is used in the treatment of atypical mycobacterial infections, such as *Mycobacterium avium* complex (MAC).

No cross-resistance with other available antimycobacterial agents has been demonstrated.

Not all species or strains of a particular organism may be susceptible to ethambutol.

## Pharmacology/Pharmacokinetics

Note: Preliminary data suggest that patients coinfected with the human immunodeficiency virus (HIV) and mycobacteria (*Mycobacterium tuberculosis* or *M. avium*) have altered pharmacokinetic profiles for antimycobacterial agents. In particular, malabsorption of these agents appears to occur frequently, and could seriously affect the efficacy of treatment.

### Physicochemical characteristics
Molecular weight—277.24.

### Mechanism of action/Effect
Ethambutol is a synthetic, bacteriostatic antitubercular agent. Its mechanism of action is not fully known. It diffuses into mycobacteria and appears to suppress multiplication by interfering with RNA synthesis. It is effective only against mycobacteria that are actively dividing.

### Absorption
Rapidly absorbed (75 to 80%) from the gastrointestinal tract following oral administration.

### Distribution
Widely distributed to most tissues and body fluids except cerebrospinal fluid (CSF). CSF concentrations are 10 to 50% of the corresponding serum concentrations.
Erythrocytes—
  Equal to or double the plasma concentrations, which provide a depot effect for 24 hours.
  Distributed into breast milk.
CSF—
  Does not penetrate intact meninges, but 10 to 50% may penetrate the meninges of patients with tuberculous meningitis.
  $Vol_D$—1.6 liters per kg.

### Protein binding
Low (20 to 30%).

### Biotransformation
Hepatic; up to 15% metabolized to inactive metabolites.

### Half-life
Normal renal function—
  3 to 4 hours.
Impaired renal function—
  Up to 8 hours.

**Time to peak concentration**
2 to 4 hours.

**Peak serum concentration**
2 to 5 mcg per mL after a single oral dose of 25 mg per kg of body weight (mg/kg).

**Elimination**
Renal—
By glomerular filtration and tubular secretion; up to 80% excreted within 24 hours (at least 50% excreted unchanged and up to 15% as inactive metabolites).
Fecal—
20% excreted unchanged.
In dialysis—
Ethambutol is removed from the blood by hemodialysis and peritoneal dialysis.

## Precautions to Consider

### Pregnancy/Reproduction

Note: Tuberculosis in pregnancy should be managed in concert with an expert in the management of tuberculosis. Women who have only pulmonary tuberculosis are not likely to infect the fetus until after delivery, and congenital tuberculosis is extremely rare. *In utero* infections with tubercle bacilli, however, can occur after maternal bacillemia occurs at different stages in the course of tuberculosis. Miliary tuberculosis can seed the placenta and thereby gain access to the fetal circulation. In women with tuberculous endometritis, transmission of infection to the fetus can result from fetal aspiration of bacilli at the time of delivery. A third mode of transmission is through ingestion of infected amniotic fluid *in utero*.

If active disease is diagnosed during pregnancy, a 9-month regimen of isoniazid and rifampin, supplemented by an initial course of ethambutol if drug resistance is suspected, is recommended. Pyrazinamide usually is not given because of inadequate data regarding teratogenesis. Hence, a 9-month course of therapy is necessary for drug-susceptible disease. When isoniazid resistance is a possibility, isoniazid, ethambutol, and rifampin are recommended initially. One of these medications can be discontinued after 1 or 2 months, depending on results of susceptibility tests. If rifampin or isoniazid is discontinued, treatment is continued for a total of 18 months; if ethambutol is discontinued, treatment is continued for a total of 9 months. Prompt initiation of chemotherapy is mandatory to protect both the mother and fetus. If isoniazid or rifampin resistance is documented, an expert in the management of tuberculosis should be consulted.

Asymptomatic pregnant women with positive tuberculin skin tests and normal chest radiographs should receive preventive therapy with isoniazid for 9 months if they are HIV seropositive or have recently been in contact with an infectious person. For these individuals, preventive therapy should begin after the first trimester. In other circumstances in which none of these risk factors is present, although no harmful effects of isoniazid to the fetus have been observed, preventive therapy can be delayed until after delivery.

For all pregnant women receiving isoniazid, pyridoxine should be prescribed. Isoniazid, ethambutol, and rifampin appear to be relatively safe for the fetus. The benefit of ethambutol and rifampin for therapy of active disease in the mother outweighs the risk to the infant. Streptomycin and pyrazinamide should not be used unless they are essential to the control of the disease.

Pregnancy—Ethambutol crosses the placenta, resulting in fetal plasma concentrations that are approximately 30% of maternal plasma concentrations. However, problems in humans have not been documented.

Studies in mice given high doses of ethambutol have shown that this antimycobacterial causes a low incidence of cleft palate, exencephaly, and vertebral column abnormalities. In addition, studies in rats given high doses this medication have shown that ethambutol causes minor abnormalities of the cervical vertebrae. Studies in rabbits given high doses have shown that ethambutol may cause monophthalmia, limb reduction defects, hare lip, and cleft palate.

### Breast-feeding
Ethambutol is distributed into breast milk in concentrations approximating maternal serum concentrations. However, problems in humans have not been documented.

### Pediatrics

Note: If an infant is suspected of having congenital tuberculosis, a Mantoux tuberculin skin test, chest radiograph, lumbar puncture, and appropriate cultures should be performed promptly. Regardless of the skin test results, treatment of the infant should be initiated promptly with isoniazid, rifampin, pyrazinamide, and streptomycin or kanamycin. In addition, the mother should be evaluated for the presence of pulmonary or extrapulmonary (including uterine) tuberculosis. If the physical examination or chest radiograph support the diagnosis of tuberculosis, the patient should be treated with the same regimen as that used for tuberculous meningitis. The drug susceptibilities of the organism recovered from the mother and/or infant should be determined.

Possible isoniazid resistance should always be considered, particularly in children from population groups in which drug resistance is high, especially in foreign-born children from countries with a high prevalence of drug-resistant tuberculosis. For contacts who are likely to have been infected by an index case with isoniazid-resistant but rifampin-susceptible organisms, and in whom the consequences of the infection are likely to be severe (e.g., children up to 4 years of age), rifampin (10 mg per kg of body weight, maximum 600 mg, given daily in a single dose) should be given in addition to isoniazid (10 mg per kg, maximum 300 mg, given daily in a single dose) until susceptibility test results for the isolate from the index case are available. If the index case is known or proven to be excreting organisms resistant to isoniazid, then isoniazid should be discontinued and rifampin given for a total of 9 months. Isoniazid alone should be given if no proof of exposure to isoniazid-resistant organisms is found. Optimal therapy for children with tuberculosis infection caused by organisms resistant to isoniazid and rifampin is unknown. In deciding on therapy in this situation, consultation with an expert is advised.

Adjuvant treatment with corticosteroids in treating tuberculosis is controversial. Corticosteroids have been used for therapy in children with tuberculous meningitis to reduce vasculitis, inflammation, and, as a result, intracranial pressure. Data indicate that dexamethasone may lower mortality rates and lessen long-term neurologic impairment. The administration of corticosteroids should be considered in all children with tuberculous meningitis, and also may be considered in children with pleural and pericardial effusions (to hasten reabsorption of fluid), severe miliary disease (to mitigate alveolocapillary block), and endobronchial disease (to relieve obstruction and atelectasis). Corticosteroids should be given only when accompanied by appropriate antituberculosis therapy. Consultation with an expert in the treatment of tuberculosis should be obtained when corticosteroid therapy is considered.

Appropriate studies on the relationship of age to the effects of ethambutol have not been performed in children up to 13 years of age. Ethambutol is generally not recommended in children whose visual acuity cannot be monitored (younger than 6 years of age). However, ethambutol should be considered for all children with organisms resistant to other medications, and in whom susceptibility to ethambutol has been demonstrated or is likely.

### Geriatrics
No information is available on the relationship of age to the effects of ethambutol in geriatric patients. However, elderly patients are more likely to have an age-related decrease in renal function, which may require an adjustment of dosage in patients receiving ethambutol.

### Drug interactions and/or related problems
The following drug interactions and/or related problems have been selected on the basis of their potential clinical significance (possible mechanism in parentheses where appropriate)—not necessarily inclusive (» = major clinical significance):

Note: Combinations containing any of the following medications, depending on the amount present, may also interact with this medication.

Neurotoxic medications, other (see *Appendix II*)
(concurrent administration of ethambutol with other neurotoxic medications may increase the potential for neurotoxicity, such as optic and peripheral neuritis)

### Laboratory value alterations
The following have been selected on the basis of their potential clinical significance (possible effect in parentheses where appropriate)—not necessarily inclusive (» = major clinical significance):

With physiology/laboratory test values
Uric acid, serum
(concentrations may be increased)

### Medical considerations/Contraindications
The medical considerations/contraindications included have been selected on the basis of their potential clinical significance (reasons given in parentheses where appropriate)—not necessarily inclusive (» = major clinical significance).

*Risk-benefit should be considered when the following medical problems exist:*

Gouty arthritis, acute
(ethambutol may increase uric acid concentrations)

» Hypersensitivity to ethambutol

» Optic neuritis
(ethambutol may cause retrobulbar optic neuritis)

» Renal function impairment
(because ethambutol is excreted primarily through the kidneys, patients with renal function impairment may require a reduction in dosage)

**Patient monitoring**

The following may be especially important in patient monitoring (other tests may be warranted in some patients, depending on condition; » = major clinical significance):

Ophthalmologic examinations
(tests for visual fields and acuity and red-green discrimination may be required prior to and monthly during treatment, especially if treatment is prolonged or if dosage is greater than 15 mg per kg of body weight [mg/kg] daily)

Uric acid concentrations, serum
(may be required during treatment since elevated serum uric acid concentrations frequently occur, possibly precipitating acute gout)

## Side/Adverse Effects

Note: Retrobulbar optic neuritis is thought to be dose-related, occurring most frequently with daily doses of 25 mg per kg of body weight (mg/kg) and after 2 months of therapy; however, optic neuritis has occurred after only a few days of treatment. Most cases are reversible after several weeks or months. Visual changes may be unilateral or bilateral; therefore, each eye must be tested separately and both eyes tested together.

The following side/adverse effects have been selected on the basis of their potential clinical significance (possible signs and symptoms in parentheses where appropriate)—not necessarily inclusive:

**Those indicating need for medical attention**

Incidence less frequent
*Gouty arthritis, acute* (chills; pain and swelling of joints, especially big toe, ankle, or knee; tense, hot skin over affected joints)

Incidence rare
*Hypersensitivity* (skin rash; fever; joint pain); *peripheral neuritis* (numbness, tingling, burning pain, or weakness in hands or feet); *retrobulbar optic neuritis* (blurred vision, eye pain, red-green color blindness, or any loss of vision)

**Those indicating need for medical attention only if they continue or are bothersome**

Incidence less frequent
*Confusion; disorientation; gastrointestinal disturbances* (abdominal pain; loss of appetite; nausea and vomiting); *headache*

## Patient Consultation

As an aid to patient consultation, refer to *Advice for the Patient, Ethambutol (Systemic).*

In providing consultation, consider emphasizing the following selected information (» = major clinical significance):

**Before using this medication**

» Conditions affecting use, especially:

Pregnancy—Ethambutol crosses the placenta. However, problems in humans have not been documented

Breast-feeding—Ethambutol is distributed into breast milk

Use in children—Appropriate studies have not been done in children up to 13 years of age. Ethambutol is generally not recommended in children whose visual acuity cannot be monitored (younger than 6 years of age)

Other medical problems, especially optic neuritis and renal function impairment

**Proper use of this medication**

Taking with food if gastrointestinal irritation occurs

» Compliance with full course of therapy, which may take months or years

» Proper dosing
Missed dose: Taking as soon as possible; not taking if almost time for next dose; not doubling doses

» Proper storage

**Precautions while using this medication**

Checking with physician if no improvement within 2 or 3 weeks

» Regular visits to physician to check progress; need to report promptly to physician signs of optic neuritis and prodromal signs of peripheral neuritis; need for ophthalmologic examinations if signs of optic neuritis occur

» Caution if blurred vision or loss of vision occurs

**Side/adverse effects**

Signs of potential side effects, especially acute gouty arthritis, hypersensitivity, peripheral neuritis, or retrobulbar optic neuritis

## General Dosing Information

Ethambutol may be taken with food if gastrointestinal irritation occurs.

Since daily administration in divided doses may not result in therapeutic serum concentrations, ethambutol should be administered only in a single daily dose.

Since bacterial resistance may develop rapidly when ethambutol is administered alone, it should only be administered concurrently with other antituberculosis medications.

The duration of treatment with an antituberculosis regimen is at least 6 months, and may be continued for 2 years. Uncomplicated pulmonary tuberculosis is often successfully treated within 6 to 12 months. Several different treatment regimens are currently recommended.

The duration of antituberculosis therapy is based on the patient's clinical and radiographic responses, smear and culture results, and susceptibility studies of *Mycobacterium tuberculosis* isolates from the patient or the suspect source case. With directly observed therapy (DOT), clinical evaluation is an integral component of each visit for administration of medication. Careful monitoring of the clinical and bacteriologic responses to therapy on a monthly basis in sputum-positive patients is important.

If therapy is interrupted, the treatment schedule should be extended to a later completion date. Although guidelines cannot be provided for every situation, the following factors need to be considered in establishing a new date for completion:

• The length of interruption;

• The time during therapy (early or late) in which interruption occurred; and

• The patient's clinical, radiographic, and bacteriologic status before, during, and after interruption. Consultation with an expert is advised.

Therapy should be administered based on the following guidelines, published by the American Thoracic Society (ATS) and by the Centers for Disease Control and Prevention (CDC), and endorsed by the American Academy of Pediatrics (AAP).

• A 6-month regimen consisting of isoniazid, rifampin, and pyrazinamide given for 2 months followed by isoniazid and rifampin for 4 months is the preferred treatment for patients infected with fully susceptible organisms who adhere to the treatment course.

• Ethambutol (or streptomycin in children too young to be monitored for visual acuity) should be included in the initial regimen until the results of drug susceptibility studies are available, and unless there is little possibility of drug resistance (i.e., there is less than 4% primary resistance to isoniazid in the community, and the patient has had no previous treatment with antituberculosis medications, is not from a country with a high prevalence of drug resistance, and has no known exposure to a drug-resistant case).

• Alternatively, a 9-month regimen of isoniazid and rifampin is acceptable for persons who cannot or should not take pyrazinamide. Ethambutol (or streptomycin in children too young to be monitored for visual acuity) should also be included until the results of drug susceptibility studies are available, unless there is little possibility of drug resistance. If isoniazid resistance is demonstrated, rifampin and ethambutol should be continued for a minimum of 12 months.

• Consideration should be given to treating all patients with DOT. DOT programs have been demonstrated to increase adherence in patients receiving antituberculosis chemotherapy in both rural and urban settings.

• Multidrug-resistant tuberculosis (i.e., resistance to at least isoniazid and rifampin) presents difficult treatment problems. Treatment must be individualized and based on susceptibility studies. In such cases, consultation with an expert in tuberculosis is recommended.

• Children should be managed in essentially the same ways as adults, but doses of the medications must be adjusted appropriately and specific important differences between the management of adults and children addressed. However, optimal therapy of tuberculosis in children with HIV infection has not been established. The Committee on Infectious Diseases of the AAP recommends that therapy always should include at least three drugs initially, and should be continued for a minimum period of 9 months. Isoniazid, rifampin, and pyrazinamide with or without ethambutol or an aminoglycoside should be given for at least the first 2 months. A fourth drug may be needed for disseminated disease and whenever drug-resistant disease is suspected.

- Extrapulmonary tuberculosis should be managed according to the principles and with the drug regimens outlined for pulmonary tuberculosis, except in children who have miliary tuberculosis, bone/joint tuberculosis, or tuberculous meningitis. These children should receive a minimum of 12 months of therapy.
- A 4-month regimen of isoniazid and rifampin is acceptable therapy for adults who have active tuberculosis and who are sputum smear- and culture-negative, if there is little possibility of drug resistance.

Rifampin is an essential component of the currently recommended regimen for treating tuberculosis. This regimen is effective in treating HIV-infected patients with tuberculosis, and consists of isoniazid and rifampin for a minimum period of 6 months, plus pyrazinamide and either ethambutol or streptomycin for the first 2 months.

Because of the common association of tuberculosis with HIV infection, an increasing number of patients probably will be considered candidates for combined therapy with rifampin and protease inhibitors. Prompt initiation of appropriate pharmacologic therapy for patients with HIV infection who acquire tuberculosis is critical because tuberculosis may become rapidly fatal. The management of these patients is complex, requires an individualized approach, and should be undertaken only by or in consultation with an expert. In addition, all HIV-infected patients at risk for tuberculosis infection should be carefully evaluated and administered isoniazid preventive treatment if indicated, regardless of whether they are receiving protease inhibitor therapy.

For HIV-infected patients diagnosed with drug-susceptible tuberculosis and for whom protease inhibitor therapy is being considered but has not been initiated, the suggested management strategy is to complete tuberculosis treatment with a regimen containing rifampin before starting therapy with a protease inhibitor. The duration of antituberculosis regimen is at least 6 months, and therapy should be administered according to the guidelines developed by ATS and CDC, including the recommendation to carefully assess clinical and bacteriologic responses in patients coinfected with HIV and to prolong treatment if response is slow or suboptimal.

Health care or correctional institutions experiencing outbreaks of tuberculosis that are resistant to isoniazid and rifampin, or that are resuming therapy for a patient with a prior history of antitubercular therapy, may need to begin 5- or 6-drug regimens as initial therapy. These regimens should include the 4-drug regimen and at least 3 medications to which the suspected multidrug-resistant strain may be susceptible.

ATS, CDC, and AAP recommend preventive treatment of tuberculosis infection in the following patients:

- Preventive therapy with isoniazid given for 6 to 12 months is effective in decreasing the risk of future tuberculosis disease in adults and children with tuberculosis infection demonstrated by a positive tuberculin skin test reaction.
- Persons with a positive skin test and any of the following risk factors should be considered for preventive therapy regardless of age:
    — Persons with HIV infection.
    — Persons at risk for HIV infection with unknown HIV status.
    — Close contacts of sputum-positive persons with newly diagnosed infectious tuberculosis.
    — Newly infected persons (recent skin test convertors).
    — Persons with medical conditions reported to increase the risk of tuberculosis (i.e., diabetes mellitus, corticosteroid therapy and other immunosuppressive therapy, intravenous drug users, hematologic and reticuloendothelial malignancies, end-stage renal disease, and clinical conditions associated with rapid weight loss or chronic malnutrition).

In some circumstances, persons with negative skin tests should be considered for preventive therapy. These include children who are close contacts of infectious tuberculosis cases and anergic HIV-infected adults at increased risk of tuberculosis, tuberculin-positive adults with abnormal chest radiographs showing fibrotic lesions probably representing old healed tuberculosis, adults with silicosis, and persons who are known to be HIV-infected and who are contacts of patients with infectious tuberculosis.

- In the absence of any of the above risk factors, persons up to 35 years of age with a positive skin test who are in the following high-incidence groups should be also considered for preventive therapy:
    — Foreign-born persons from high-prevalence countries.
    — Medically underserved low-income persons from high-prevalence populations (especially blacks, Hispanics, and Native Americans).
    — Residents of facilities for long-term care (e.g., correctional institutions, nursing homes, and mental institutions).
- Twelve months of preventive therapy is recommended for adults and children with HIV infection and other conditions associated with immunosuppression. Persons without HIV infection should receive preventive therapy for at least 6 months.
- In persons younger than 35 years of age, routine monitoring for adverse effects of isoniazid should consist of a monthly symptom review. For persons 35 years of age and older, hepatic enzymes should be measured prior to starting isoniazid and monitored monthly throughout treatment, in addition to monthly symptom reviews.
- Persons who are presumed to be infected with isoniazid-resistant organisms should be treated with rifampin rather than with isoniazid.
- As with the treatment of active tuberculosis, the key to success of preventive treatment is patient adherence to the prescribed regimen. Although not evaluated in clinical studies, directly observed, twice-weekly preventive therapy may be appropriate for adults and children at risk, who cannot or will not reliably self-administer therapy.

Serum concentrations may be increased and half-life prolonged in patients with impaired renal function. Therefore, patients with impaired renal function may require a reduction in dose.

Most infants ≤ 12 months of age with tuberculosis are asymptomatic at the time of diagnosis, and the gastric aspirate cultures in these patients have a high yield for *M. tuberculosis*. When an infant is suspected of having tuberculosis, a thorough household investigation should be undertaken. A 6-month regimen of isoniazid and rifampin supplemented during the first 2 months by pyrazinamide has been found to be well-tolerated and effective in infants with pulmonary tuberculosis. Furthermore, twice-weekly DOT appears to be as effective as daily therapy, and is an essential alternative in patients for whom social issues prevent reliable daily therapy.

Physicians caring for children should be familiar with the clinical forms of the disease in infants to enable them to make an early diagnosis. Any child, especially one in a high-risk group or area, who has unexplained pneumonia, cervical adenitis, bone or joint infections, or aseptic meningitis should have a Mantoux tuberculin skin test performed, and a detailed epidemiologic history for tuberculosis should be obtained.

Management of a newborn infant whose mother, or other household contact, is suspected of having tuberculosis is based on individual considerations. If possible, separation of the mother, or contact, and infant should be minimized. The Committee on Infectious Diseases of the AAP offers the following recommendations in the management of the newborn infant whose mother, or any other household contact, has tuberculosis:

- *Mother, or any other household contact, with a positive tuberculin skin test reaction but no evidence of current disease:* Investigation of other members of the household or extended family to whom the infant may later be exposed is indicated. If no evidence of current disease is found in the mother or in members of the extended family, the infant should be tested with a Mantoux tuberculin skin test at 3 to 4 months of age. When the family members cannot be promptly tested, consideration should be given to administering isoniazid (10 mg per kg of body weight a day) to the infant until skin testing and other evaluation of the family members have excluded contact with a case of active tuberculosis. The infant does not need to be hospitalized during this time if adequate follow-up can be arranged, but adherence to medication administration should be closely monitored. The mother also should be considered for isoniazid therapy.
- *Mother with untreated (newly diagnosed) disease or disease that has been treated for 2 or more weeks and who is judged to be noncontagious at delivery:* Careful investigation of household members and extended family is mandatory. A chest radiograph and Mantoux tuberculin skin test should be performed on the infant at 3 to 4 months and at 6 months of age. Separation of the mother and infant is not necessary if adherence to treatment for the mother and infant is assured. The mother can breast-feed. The infant should receive isoniazid even if the tuberculin skin test and chest radiograph do not suggest clinical tuberculosis, since cell-mediated immunity of a degree sufficient to mount a significant reaction to tuberculin skin testing may develop as late as 6 months of age in an infant infected at birth. Isoniazid can be discontinued if the Mantoux skin test is negative at 3 to 4 months of age, the mother is adherent to treatment and has a satisfactory clinical response, and no other family members have infectious tuberculosis. The infant should be examined carefully at monthly intervals. If nonadherence is documented, the mother has an acid-fast bacillus (AFB)–posi-

tive sputum or smear, and supervision is impossible, the infant should be separated from the ill family member and Bacillus Calmette-Guérin (BCG) vaccine may be considered for the infant. However, the response to the vaccine in infants may be delayed and inadequate for prevention of tuberculosis.

• *Mother has current disease and is suspected of having been contagious at the time of delivery:* The mother and infant should be separated until the infant is receiving therapy or the mother is confirmed to be noncontagious. Otherwise, management is the same as when the disease is judged to be noncontagious to the infant at delivery.

• *Mother has hematogenously spread tuberculosis (e.g., meningitis, miliary disease, or bone involvement):* The infant should be evaluated for congenital tuberculosis. If clinical and radiographic findings do not support the diagnosis of congenital tuberculosis, the infant should be separated from the mother until she is judged to be noncontagious. The infant should be given isoniazid until 3 or 4 months of age, at which time the Mantoux skin test should be repeated. If the skin test is positive, isoniazid should be continued for a total of 12 months. If the skin test is negative and the chest radiograph is normal, isoniazid may be discontinued, depending on the status of the mother and whether there are other cases of infectious tuberculosis in the family. The infant should continue to be examined carefully at monthly intervals.

## Oral Dosage Forms

Note: Bracketed uses in the *Dosage Forms* section refer to categories of use and/or indications that are not included in U.S. product labeling.

### ETHAMBUTOL HYDROCHLORIDE TABLETS USP

**Usual adult and adolescent dose**
Tuberculosis—
  In combination with other antituberculosis medications: Oral, 15 to 25 mg per kg of body weight once a day; or 50 mg per kg of body weight, up to 2.5 grams, two times a week; or 25 to 30 mg per kg of body weight, up to 2.5 grams, three times a week.
  [Mycobacterial infections, atypical]—Oral, 15 to 25 mg per kg of body weight once a day.

**Usual adult prescribing limits**
Tuberculosis—
  2.5 grams daily.

**Usual pediatric dose**
Children up to 13 years of age—Dosage has not been established. However, ethambutol should be considered for all children with organisms resistant to other medications, and in whom susceptibility to ethambutol has been demonstrated or is likely. Ethambutol is generally not recommended in children whose visual acuity cannot be monitored (younger than 6 years of age).
Children 13 years of age and over—See *Usual adult and adolescent dose*.

**Strength(s) usually available**
U.S.—
  100 mg (Rx) [*Myambutol*].
  400 mg (Rx) [*Myambutol* (scored)].

Canada—
  100 mg (Rx) [*Etibi* (scored); *Myambutol*].
  400 mg (Rx) [*Etibi* (scored); *Myambutol* (scored)].

**Packaging and storage**
Store below 40 °C (104 °F), preferably between 15 and 30 °C (59 and 86 °F), unless otherwise specified by manufacturer. Store in a well-closed container.

**Auxiliary labeling**
• Continue medicine for full time of treatment.

## Selected Bibliography
The American Thoracic Society (ATS). Ad Hoc Committee on the Scientific Assembly on Microbology, Tuberculosis, and Pulmonary Infections. Treatment of tuberculosis and tuberculosis infection in adults and children. Clin Infect Dis 1995; 21: 9-27.

Revised: 08/29/97

---

**ETHANOLAMINE OLEATE**—The *Ethanolamine Oleate (Parenteral-Local)* monograph is not included in this published version of the USP DI database. Copies of the monograph are available on request from Micromedex, Inc. - Reprint Requests, 6200 S. Syracuse Way, Suite 300, Englewood, CO 80111; telephone (303) 486-6400; telefax (303) 486-6464; Email: USPDI@MDX.COM.

---

**ETHCHLORVYNOL**—The *Ethchlorvynol (Systemic)* monograph is not included in this published version of the USP DI database. Copies of the monograph are available on request from Micromedex, Inc. - Reprint Requests, 6200 S. Syracuse Way, Suite 300, Englewood, CO 80111; telephone (303) 486-6400; telefax (303) 486-6464; Email: USPDI@MDX.COM.

---

**ETHINAMATE**—The *Ethinamate (Systemic)* monograph is not included in this published version of the USP DI database. Copies of the monograph are available on request from Micromedex, Inc. - Reprint Requests, 6200 S. Syracuse Way, Suite 300, Englewood, CO 80111; telephone (303) 486-6400; telefax (303) 486-6464; Email: USPDI@MDX.COM.

---

**ETHINYL ESTRADIOL**—See *Estrogens (Systemic)*

---

# ETHIONAMIDE  Systemic†

VA CLASSIFICATION (Primary): AM500

Commonly used brand name(s): *Trecator-SC*.

Note: For a listing of dosage forms and brand names by country availability, see *Dosage Forms* section(s).

†Not commercially available in Canada.

## Category
Antibacterial (antimycobacterial; antileprosy agent).

## Indications
Note: Bracketed information in the *Indications* section refers to uses that are not included in U.S. product labeling.

**Accepted**
Tuberculosis (treatment)—Ethionamide is indicated in combination with other antituberculosis medications in the treatment of tuberculosis, including tuberculous meningitis, after failure with the primary medications (streptomycin, isoniazid, rifampin, and ethambutol) or when these cannot be used because of toxicity or development of resistant tubercle bacilli. Ethionamide is effective only against mycobacteria.

[Leprosy (treatment)]—Ethionamide is used in combination with other antileprosy agents in the treatment of Hansen's disease.

[Mycobacterial infections, atypical (treatment)]—Ethionamide is used in the treatment of atypical mycobacterial infections, such as *Mycobacterium avium* complex (MAC).

Not all species or strains of a particular organism may be susceptible to ethionamide.

## Pharmacology/Pharmacokinetics

**Physicochemical characteristics**
Molecular weight— 166.24.

**Mechanism of action/Effect**
Ethionamide's mechanism of action is not known, but it appears to inhibit peptide synthesis. Ethionamide is bacteriostatic against *Mycobacterium tuberculosis*.

**Absorption**
Rapidly absorbed from the gastrointestinal tract following oral administration. Bioavailability approximately 100%.

**Distribution**
Widely distributed to most tissues and fluids, including liver, kidneys, and spleen. Concentrations in various organs and cerebrospinal fluid (CSF) are approximately equal to plasma concentrations. Readily crosses the placenta, also.
Vol$_D$ = Approximately 2.8 L/kg.

**Protein binding**
Low (10%).

**Biotransformation**
Probably hepatic; metabolized to sulfoxide, which is active, and to inactive metabolites.

**Half-life**
Approximately 2 to 3 hours.

**Time to peak concentration**
Approximately 1.8 hours.

**Peak serum concentration**
Approximately 2.2 mcg/mL after a single oral 500-mg dose.

**Elimination**
Renal; 1% excreted unchanged; up to 5% excreted as active metabolite; the remainder excreted as inactive metabolites.

## Precautions to Consider

**Cross-sensitivity and/or related problems**
Patients sensitive to isoniazid, pyrazinamide, niacin (nicotinic acid), or other chemically related medications may be sensitive to this medication also.

**Pregnancy/Reproduction**
Pregnancy—Ethionamide crosses the placenta.
Ethionamide has been shown to be teratogenic in rabbits and rats given doses greater than the usual human dose.

**Breast-feeding**
It is not known whether ethionamide is distributed into breast milk. However, problems in humans have not been documented.

**Pediatrics**
Appropriate studies on the relationship of age to the effects of ethionamide have not been performed in the pediatric population. However, no pediatrics-specific problems have been documented to date.

**Geriatrics**
No information is available on the relationship of age to the effects of ethionamide in geriatric patients.

**Dental**
Ethionamide may cause a metallic taste and stomatitis (sore mouth).

**Drug interactions and/or related problems**
The following drug interactions and/or related problems have been selected on the basis of their potential clinical significance (possible mechanism in parentheses where appropriate)—not necessarily inclusive (» = major clinical significance):

Note: Combinations containing any of the following medications, depending on the amount present, may also interact with this medication.

» Cycloserine
(concurrent use may result in increased incidence of central nervous system [CNS] effects, especially seizures; dosage adjustments may be necessary and patients should be monitored closely for signs of CNS toxicity)

Neurotoxic medications, other (See *Appendix II*)
(concurrent administration of ethionamide with other neurotoxic medications may increase the potential for neurotoxicity, such as optic and peripheral neuritis)

**Laboratory value alterations**
The following have been selected on the basis of their potential clinical significance (possible effect in parentheses where appropriate)—not necessarily inclusive (» = major clinical significance):

With physiology/laboratory test values
Alanine aminotransferase (ALT [SGPT]) and
Aspartate aminotransferase (AST [SGOT])
(serum values may be increased)

**Medical considerations/Contraindications**
The medical considerations/contraindications included have been selected on the basis of their potential clinical significance (reasons given in parentheses where appropriate)—not necessarily inclusive (» = major clinical significance).

*Risk-benefit should be considered when the following medical problems exist:*
» Diabetes mellitus
(management of diabetes mellitus may be more difficult in patients taking ethionamide)
» Hepatic function impairment, severe
(may increase risk of hepatotoxicity)
» Hypersensitivity to ethionamide

**Patient monitoring**
The following may be especially important in patient monitoring (other tests may be warranted in some patients, depending on condition; » = major clinical significance):

Hepatic function determinations
(AST [SGOT] and ALT [SGPT] concentrations may increase during therapy; however, elevated serum enzyme values may not be predictive of clinical hepatitis and may return to normal despite continued treatment; patients with impaired hepatic function may require a reduction in dose)

Ophthalmologic examinations
(if loss of vision and other symptoms of optic neuritis occur during treatment, ophthalmologic examinations should be performed immediately and periodically thereafter)

## Side/Adverse Effects

Note: Peripheral neuritis may be alleviated by administering pyridoxine.

The following side/adverse effects have been selected on the basis of their potential clinical significance (possible signs and symptoms in parentheses where appropriate)—not necessarily inclusive:

**Those indicating need for medical attention**
Incidence less frequent
*Hepatitis or jaundice* (yellow eyes or skin); *peripheral neuritis* (clumsiness or unsteadiness; numbness, tingling, burning, or pain in hands and feet); *psychiatric disturbances* (mental depression, confusion, mood or other mental changes)

Incidence rare
*Goiter or hypothyroidism* (changes in menstrual periods; coldness; decreased sexual ability—males; dry, puffy skin; swelling of front part of neck; weight gain); *hypoglycemia* (difficulty in concentrating, faster heartbeat, increased hunger, nervousness, shakiness); *optic neuritis* (blurred vision or loss of vision, with or without eye pain); *skin rash*

**Those indicating need for medical attention only if they continue or are bothersome**
Incidence more frequent
*Gastrointestinal disturbances* (loss of appetite, metallic taste, nausea or vomiting, sore mouth); *orthostatic hypotension* (dizziness, especially when getting up from a lying or sitting position)

Incidence less frequent or rare
*gynecomastia* (enlargement of the breasts in males)

## Patient Consultation

As an aid to patient consultation, refer to *Advice for the Patient, Ethionamide (Systemic)*.
In providing consultation, consider emphasizing the following selected information (» = major clinical significance):

**Before using this medication**
» Conditions affecting use, especially:
Hypersensitivity to ethionamide
Pregnancy—Ethionamide crosses the placenta
Dental—Ethionamide may cause a metallic taste and stomatitis
Other medications, especially cycloserine
Other medical problems, especially diabetes mellitus or hepatic function impairment

**Proper use of this medication**
Taking with or after meals if gastrointestinal irritation occurs
» Compliance with full course of therapy, which may take months or years
» Taking pyridoxine concurrently to prevent or minimize signs of peripheral neuritis
» Proper dosing
Missed dose: Taking as soon as possible; not taking if almost time for next dose; not doubling doses
» Proper storage

### Precautions while using this medication
Checking with physician if no improvement within 2 or 3 weeks
» Regular visits to physician to check progress, as well as ophthalmologic examinations if signs of optic neuritis occur
» Caution if blurred vision or loss of vision occurs
» Need to report promptly to physician signs of optic neuritis and prodromal signs of peripheral neuritis

### Side/adverse effects
Signs of potential side effects, especially hepatitis or jaundice, peripheral neuritis, psychiatric disturbances, goiter or hypothyroidism, hypoglycemia, optic neuritis, and skin rash

## General Dosing Information
Ethionamide may be given with or after meals if gastrointestinal irritation occurs.

Ethionamide has been given as a single daily dose after the evening meal or at bedtime. Serum concentrations are higher and effectiveness may be greater than with divided doses. However, gastrointestinal irritation may also be increased.

Ethionamide has also been given rectally as suppositories, resulting in fewer side effects. However, serum concentrations may be inadequate.

Ethionamide should generally be given in the maximum daily dose that the patient can tolerate. However, approximately one-third of the patients taking ethionamide are unable to tolerate therapeutic doses and the dose must be reduced by ⅓ to ½ or the medication must be discontinued.

Since bacterial resistance may develop rapidly when ethionamide is administered alone in the treatment of tuberculosis, it should only be administered concurrently with other antituberculars.

Therapy may have to be continued for 1 to 2 years, and may even be required for up to several years or indefinitely, although in some patients shorter treatment regimens may be effective.

### For treatment of adverse effects
Recommended treatment consists of the following:
• Administration of pyridoxine concurrently with ethionamide to help prevent or minimize the symptoms of peripheral neuritis, especially in patients with prior isoniazid-induced peripheral neuritis.

## Oral Dosage Forms
Note: Bracketed uses in the *Dosage Forms* section refer to categories of use and/or indications that are not included in U.S. product labeling.

### ETHIONAMIDE TABLETS USP
**Usual adult and adolescent dose**
Tuberculosis; or
[Mycobacterial infections, atypical]—In combination with other antituberculosis medications: Oral, 250 mg every eight to twelve hours, as tolerated.

[Leprosy]—In combination with other antileprosy agents: Oral, 250 mg every eight to twelve hours.

**Usual adult prescribing limits**
Up to a maximum of 1 gram daily.

**Usual pediatric dose**
Tuberculosis—In combination with other antituberculosis medications: Oral, 4 to 5 mg per kg of body weight every eight hours, as tolerated.

Note: Some children have received up to 20 mg per kg of body weight per day. However, the maximum daily dose should not exceed 750 mg.

**Strength(s) usually available**
U.S.—
250 mg (Rx) [*Trecator-SC*].
Canada—
Not commercially available.

**Packaging and storage**
Store below 40 °C (104 °F), preferably between 15 and 30 °C (59 and 86 °F), unless otherwise specified by manufacturer. Store in a tight container.

**Auxiliary labeling**
• Continue medicine for full time of treatment.

Revised: 06/22/94

---

**ETHOPROPAZINE**—See *Antidyskinetics (Systemic)*

---

**ETHOTOIN**—See *Anticonvulsants, Hydantoin (Systemic)*

---

**ETHYLNOREPINEPHRINE**—See *Bronchodilators, Adrenergic (Systemic)*

---

**ETIDOCAINE**—See *Anesthetics (Parenteral-Local)*

---

# ETIDRONATE  Systemic

VA CLASSIFICATION (Primary/Secondary): HS303/HS302
Commonly used brand name(s): *Didronel*.
Another commonly used name is EHDP.
Note: For a listing of dosage forms and brand names by country availability, see *Dosage Forms* section(s).

## Category
Bone resorption inhibitor; antihypercalcemic.

## Indications
### Accepted
Paget's disease of bone (treatment)—Oral etidronate is indicated for the treatment of symptomatic Paget's disease (osteitis deformans), characterized by abnormal and accelerated bone turnover in one or more bones. Signs and symptoms may include bone pain, deformity, and/or fractures; increased concentrations of serum alkaline phosphatase and/or urinary hydroxyproline; neurologic disorders associated with skull lesions and vertebral deformities; and elevated cardiac output and other vascular disorders associated with increased vascularity of bones.

Although studies have not been done on etidronate's effects in *asymptomatic* Paget's disease, treatment may be considered for such patients if extensive involvement of the skull or vertebral column might lead to neurologic damage; if extensive involvement of weight-bearing bones threatens their integrity; or if juxta-articular involvement threatens the integrity of adjacent joints.

Ossification, heterotopic (prophylaxis and treatment)—Oral etidronate is indicated for the prevention and treatment of heterotopic ossification (myositis ossificans—circumscripta, progressiva, or traumatica; ectopic calcification; periarticular ossification; or paraosteoarthropathy) following total hip replacement or caused by spinal cord injury. Heterotopic ossification is characterized by metaplastic osteogenesis, and may be accompanied by localized inflammation and pain, and elevated skin temperature or redness. Also, loss of joint function or reduction in range of motion may occur when tissues near joints are involved.

Hypercalcemia, associated with neoplasms (treatment adjunct)—Parenteral etidronate is indicated as adjunctive therapy for the treatment of hypercalcemia of malignancy that is inadequately managed by dietary changes and/or oral hydration alone. It is used in conjunction with adequate saline hydration and with "high ceiling" or loop diuretics, such as bumetanide, ethacrynic acid, and furosemide. Limited clinical study results show that oral etidronate may be used in some patients after the last dose of etidronate infusion to maintain clinically acceptable serum calcium concentrations and to prolong normocalcemia.

### Unaccepted
Hypercalcemia caused by hyperparathyroidism, where increased tubular reabsorption of calcium may be a factor in the hypercalcemia, is refractory to parenteral etidronate.

# Etidronate (Systemic)

Note: Oral etidronate is presently being used experimentally in the U.S. to treat osteoporosis in adults. A small increase in bone mineral density has been noted. Some studies with continuous dosing of etidronate have found abnormal mineralization of osteoid and microfractures that might potentially result in increased susceptibility to fractures, especially nonvertebral fractures. Further studies are needed to determine the safety profile and dosing information.

## Pharmacology/Pharmacokinetics

**Physicochemical characteristics**
Molecular weight—249.99.

**Mechanism of action/Effect**
Although the exact mechanism is not completely understood, etidronate chemisorbs to calcium phosphate surfaces of calcium hydroxyapatite crystals and their amorphous precursors, and, *in vitro*, blocks the aggregation, growth, and mineralization of the crystals. A similar process is believed to be responsible *in vivo* for retarding the mineralization and growth of heterotopic ossification. This process may also be responsible for retarding bone resorption, and, secondarily, for retarding the accelerated rate of bone turnover in Paget's disease.

Paget's disease—Etidronate induces a reduction of bone resorption, which is accompanied by a reduction in the number of osteoclasts. Secondarily, coupled bone formation is reduced, which is associated with a reduction in the number of osteoblasts. New bone formed following the reduction in bone turnover is histologically more normal. Lamellar bone is formed, and the marrow becomes less vascular and fibrotic. Etidronate reduces serum alkaline phosphatase and urinary hydroxyproline concentrations, reduces radionuclide uptake at pagetic lesions, decreases elevated cardiac output by reducing bone vascularity, and reduces elevated skin temperature over pagetic lesions. The incidence of pagetic fractures may be reduced when etidronate is administered intermittently over a period of years.

Heterotopic ossification—Etidronate slows the progression of immature bone lesions, thus reducing the severity of the disease.

Hypercalcemia of malignancy—Bone resorption is increased in the presence of neoplastic tissue. Etidronate inhibits abnormal bone resorption and reduces the flow of calcium from the resorbing bone into the blood, effectively decreasing total and ionized serum calcium. When kidney function is adequate for the fluid load, hydration with saline increases urine output and the use of diuretics increases the rate of calcium excretion.

**Duration of therapeutic effect**
Paget's disease—Possibly up to a year or more after discontinuation of therapy.
Heterotopic ossification—Several months after discontinuation of therapy.
Hypercalcemia—Clinical studies indicate a median duration of normocalcemia of 11 days.

**Absorption**
Lower doses (5 mg per kg of body weight (mg/kg) a day)—1% (average).
Higher doses (10 to 20 mg per kg a day)—2.5 to 6% (average).

**Distribution**
Approximately half of absorbed dose is chemically adsorbed to bone, presumably upon hydroxyapatite crystals, in areas of elevated osteogenesis.

**Biotransformation**
None.

**Half-life**
Elimination—Approximately 50% of the absorbed/infused dose is eliminated from the body within 24 hours. The remainder is presumably chemisorbed to bone and slowly eliminated.
Plasma—5 to 7 hours.

**Onset of action**
Paget's disease—May be observed after 1 month of treatment; initially observed as a reduction in urinary hydroxyproline.
Hypercalcemia—Reductions in urinary calcium excretion, which accompany reductions in bone resorption, may become apparent after 24 hours.

**Time to peak effect**
Hypercalcemia—Decreases in serum calcium are maximal on the day following the third infusion, in most patients.

**Elimination**
Absorbed dose—50% excreted intact in the urine via the kidneys.
Unabsorbed dose—Intact in the feces.

## Precautions to Consider

**Carcinogenicity**
Long-term studies in rats have shown no evidence of carcinogenicity.

**Pregnancy/Reproduction**
Pregnancy—
  *For oral etidronate*—
    Adequate and well-controlled studies in humans have not been done.
    Studies in rats and rabbits administered oral doses up to 5 times the maximum human dose have shown no evidence of impaired fertility or harm to the fetus. However, studies in rats administered doses 22 times the maximum human dose of etidronate have shown a decrease in live fetuses.
    FDA Pregnancy Category B.
  *For parenteral etidronate*—
    Reproductive studies have not been done in either animals or humans. Rats administered large parenteral doses showed skeletal malformations, which were attributed to the pharmacologic action of the drug
    FDA Pregnancy Category C.

**Breast-feeding**
It is not known if etidronate is distributed into breast milk. However, problems in humans have not been documented.

**Pediatrics**
Appropriate studies have not been performed in the pediatric population. However, in children treated for heterotopic ossification or soft tissue calcifications at doses of 10 mg or more per kg of body weight a day for prolonged periods (approaching or exceeding a year), signs of a rachitic syndrome were infrequently reported. Epiphyseal radiologic changes associated with retarded mineralization of new osteoid and cartilage have been reversible upon discontinuation of etidronate.

**Geriatrics**
Appropriate studies have not been performed in the geriatric population. However, elderly patients may be more prone to overhydration when treated with parenteral etidronate in conjunction with hydration therapy. Careful monitoring of fluid and electrolyte status is recommended.

**Drug interactions and/or related problems**
The following drug interactions and/or related problems have been selected on the basis of their potential clinical significance (possible mechanism in parentheses where appropriate)—not necessarily inclusive (» = major clinical significance):

Note: Combinations containing any of the following medications, depending on the amount present, may also interact with this medication.

» Antacids containing calcium, magnesium, or aluminum or
» Foods containing large amounts of calcium, such as milk or other dairy products or
» Mineral supplements or other medications containing calcium, iron, magnesium, or aluminum
  (concurrent use may prevent absorption of oral etidronate; patients should be advised to avoid using within 2 hours of etidronate)

**Laboratory value alterations**
The following have been selected on the basis of their potential clinical significance (possible effect in parentheses where appropriate)—not necessarily inclusive (» = major clinical significance):

With diagnostic test results
  Technetium Tc 99m medronate or
  Technetium Tc 99m oxidronate or
  Technetium Tc 99m pyrophosphate
    (etidronate may theoretically interfere with bone uptake of these diagnostic agents; clinical significance is unknown)

**Medical considerations/Contraindications**
The medical considerations/contraindications included have been selected on the basis of their potential clinical significance (reasons given in parentheses where appropriate)—not necessarily inclusive (» = major clinical significance).

*Except under special circumstances, this medication should not be used when the following medical problem exists:*

For hypercalcemia
» Renal function impairment when serum creatinine is 5 mg per dL or greater
  (kidney function may be inadequate for the increased fluid load and the excretion of etidronate)

*Risk-benefit should be considered when the following medical problems exist:*

» Bone fractures, especially of long bones
  (mineralization of osteoid laid down during the bone accretion process may be retarded because of the inhibition of hydroxyapatite crystal growth; delay or interruption of etidronate treatment for

Paget's disease may be necessary until callus formation and calcification are evident)
» Cardiac failure
(overhydration should be avoided with use of parenteral etidronate in patients with cardiac failure)
» Enterocolitis
(risk of diarrhea is increased, particularly at higher doses)
Hyperphosphatemia
(high doses of oral etidronate may increase the tubular reabsorption of phosphate; occurs less frequently with parenteral therapy)
Hypocalcemia or
Hypovitaminosis D
(patients with restricted intake of calcium or vitamin D may be more sensitive to medications that affect calcium homeostasis)
» Renal function impairment when serum creatinine is 2.5 to 4.9 mg per dL
(excretion of etidronate may be reduced; reduction of dose may be necessary; in addition, renal function impairment may be exacerbated by etidronate infusion)
Sensitivity to etidronate

**Patient monitoring**
The following may be especially important in patient monitoring (other tests may be warranted in some patients, depending on condition; » = major clinical significance):

*For Paget's disease and hypercalcemia*
Renal function determinations, especially glomerular filtration rate (GFR) and/or blood urea nitrogen (BUN)
(recommended at periodic intervals during therapy; reduction in dosage in patients with impairment of renal function [GFR] should be considered and such patients closely monitored; occasional mild to moderate abnormalities in renal function [increases of serum creatinine >0.5 mg per dL and elevated BUN] may occur when etidronate infusion is given to patients with hypercalcemia; these increases are reversible or may remain stable without worsening after completion of the course of infusion)

*For Paget's disease only*
Pain relief, assessment of
(pain may be an indication of Paget's disease activity; however, in elderly patients, biochemical indices, periodically monitored during therapy, are more valuable)
» Serum alkaline phosphatase concentrations and
» Urine hydroxyproline concentrations
(determinations recommended every 3 to 6 months during therapy; decreases in urine hydroxyproline result from decreased collagen resorption following reduced osteoclastic activity and reduced bone resorption; decreases in alkaline phosphatase result from a secondary reduction in osteoblastic activity; reduction in both parameters are an indication of improvement; sustained decreases during drug-free period are evidence of remission; retreatment is started when biochemical indices re-elevate to 75% of pretreatment values or symptoms recur)
Serum phosphate concentrations
(determinations recommended prior to and 4 weeks after initiation of therapy; at higher doses [10 mg or more per kg of body weight per day], a rise of greater than 0.5 mg per deciliter over pretreatment is normal and without clinical consequence and is probably related to an alteration in renal tubular reabsorption of phosphate [normal values return within 2 to 4 weeks after discontinuation of etidronate]; a rise of 0.5 mg per deciliter or greater at lower doses [5 mg or less per kg of body weight per day] is uncommon and may indicate above average bioavailability; if such a rise is seen at the lower dose, the serum alkaline phosphatase and urinary hydroxyproline values should be examined for evidence that the drug is reducing bone turnover as expected; if there are no significant declines in these values, etidronate dosage should be reduced or the medication discontinued to avoid possible reduced mineralization of osteoid with no accompanying clinical benefit)

*For hypercalcemia only*
Serum albumin concentrations and
Serum calcium concentrations
(determinations recommended periodically during therapy; since serum proteins, especially albumin, may influence the ratio of free and bound calcium, corrected serum calcium values should be calculated by using an established algorithm; albumin-corrected serum calcium determinations may be useful when the signs and symptoms of hypercalcemia are inconsistent with unadjusted calcium values)

## Side/Adverse Effects

The following side/adverse effects have been selected on the basis of their potential clinical significance (possible signs and symptoms in parentheses where appropriate)—not necessarily inclusive:

**Those indicating need for medical attention**
Incidence more frequent
*Bone pain or tenderness, increased, continuing, or recurrent*—in patients with Paget's disease
Note: Usually occurs over the site of pagetic lesions, but sometimes occurs at previously asymptomatic sites, beginning within 4 to 6 weeks of initiation of therapy; more common with doses of 5 mg per kg of body weight (mg/kg) or greater for more than six months. Pain may persist in some patients, even with continued therapy; usually subsides days to months after etidronate is discontinued.

Incidence less frequent
*Osteomalacia* (bone fractures, especially of the femur)
Note: Usually occur in patients taking doses higher than 20 mg/kg or continuous administration of etidronate for longer than 6 months. Microfractures may be due to decreased strength of active pagetic bone or may be caused by a mineralization defect accompanying etidronate therapy.

Incidence rare
*Allergic reaction, specifically; angioedema* (swelling of the extremities, face, lips, tongue, glottis, and/or larynx); *skin rash or itching; urticaria* (hives)

**Those indicating need for medical attention only if they continue or are bothersome**
Incidence more frequent—at higher doses
*Diarrhea; nausea*

Incidence less frequent—with parenteral dosage form
*Loss of taste or metallic or altered taste*

## Patient Consultation

As an aid to patient consultation, refer to *Advice for the Patient, Etidronate (Systemic)*.
In providing consultation, consider emphasizing the following selected information (» = major clinical significance):

**Before using this medication**
» Conditions affecting use, especially:
Sensitivity to etidronate
Use in children—Children given adult dosages for nearly a year or more were reported to have signs of a rachitic syndrome that were reversible upon discontinuation of etidronate
Use in the elderly—Elderly patients may be more prone to overhydration when treated with parenteral etidronate in conjunction with hydration therapy
Other medications, especially antacids or mineral supplements
Other medical problems, especially renal function impairment, bone fractures, cardiac failure, or enterocolitis

**Proper use of this medication**
» Taking with water on an empty stomach, at least 2 hours before or after food (upon arising, midmorning, or at bedtime)
» Compliance with therapy; not taking more or less medication or for longer period of time than prescribed
Checking with physician before discontinuing medication; may require 1 to 3 months for symptomatic improvement
» Maintaining a well-balanced diet with adequate intake of calcium and vitamin D; not taking within 2 hours of milk or milk products, antacids, mineral supplements, or other medicines high in calcium, magnesium, iron, or aluminum
» Proper dosing
Missed dose: Taking as soon as possible; not taking if almost time for next dose; not doubling doses
» Proper storage

**Precautions while using this medication**
» Regular visits to physician to check progress even if between treatments
Checking with physician if nausea or diarrhea occurs and continues; dosage adjustment may be necessary
» Checking with physician if bone pain appears or worsens during treatment

**Side/adverse effects**
Signs of potential side effects, especially increased or continuing bone pain, fractures, or allergic reaction

# Etidronate (Systemic)

## General Dosing Information
See also *Patient monitoring*.

### For Paget's disease
Symptomatic improvement as evidence of therapeutic response may not be seen for 1 to 3 months; dosage should not be prematurely increased or discontinued during that time.

Although etidronate is usually taken as a single dose, divided doses may be preferred if diarrhea or nausea occurs.

In patients with Paget's disease, retreatment should be initiated only after a medication-free period of at least 3 months and only if there is evidence of active disease or if the biochemical indices have become re-elevated to 75% of pretreatment values or symptoms recur.

Analgesics may be required at any time if patient experiences bone pain.

In many patients with Paget's disease, the disease process may be suppressed for a year or more after discontinuing therapy.

Etidronate therapy in patients with total hip replacement does not promote loosening of the prosthesis or impede trochanteric reattachment.

The dosage of etidronate should be reduced when there is a decrease in the glomerular filtration rate

### For hypercalcemia
Retreatment with parenteral etidronate for more than 3 days and the safety and effectiveness of more than 2 courses of therapy have not been studied.

The daily dose must be diluted in at least 250 mL of normal saline solution or 5% dextrose injection. More of the diluent may be used, if convenient. The diluted dose should be administered over a period of at least 2 hours.

Limited clinical studies suggest that oral administration of etidronate in some patients may be started on the day following the last dose of parenteral therapy. If serum calcium levels remain normal, treatment may be extended for up to 90 days. Normocalcemia may be defined as serum calcium concentrations usually within 8.5 to 10.5 mg per dL.

### Diet/Nutrition
Etidronate should be taken with water on an empty stomach, at least 2 hours before or after food (e.g., upon arising, midmorning, or at bedtime) for maximum absorption.

A well-balanced diet with adequate intake of calcium and vitamin D should be maintained.

Foods containing large amounts of calcium, such as milk or other dairy products, mineral supplements, or other medicines high in calcium, magnesium, iron, or aluminum, may prevent absorption of etidronate and should not be taken within 2 hours of etidronate.

## Oral Dosage Forms

### ETIDRONATE DISODIUM TABLETS USP

**Usual adult dose**
Paget's disease of bone—
Oral, initially 5 mg per kg of body weight a day, usually as a single dose, for a period of time not to exceed six months; or 6 to 10 mg per kg of body weight a day, for a period of time not to exceed six months; or 11 to 20 mg per kg of body weight a day, for no longer than three months.

Note: Doses above 5 mg per kg of body weight are recommended only when lower doses are ineffective or there is an overriding requirement for suppression of increased bone turnover or when a more prompt reduction of elevated cardiac output is required.

The retreatment dose after a drug-free period remains the same as the initial dose for most patients.

Heterotopic ossification—
Patients with total hip replacement: Oral, 20 mg per kg of body weight a day for one month prior to and for three months after surgery.

Patients with spinal cord injury: Oral, initially 20 mg per kg of body weight a day for two weeks, beginning as soon as medically feasible after injury and preferably before evidence of heterotopic ossification, the dosage then being decreased to 10 mg per kg of body weight a day for an additional ten weeks.

Hypercalcemia—
Maintenance: Oral, 20 mg per kg of body weight a day for thirty days, up to a maximum of ninety days.

**Usual adult prescribing limits**
20 mg per kg of body weight a day.

**Usual pediatric dose**
Dosage has not been established.

**Strength(s) usually available**
U.S.—
200 mg (Rx) [*Didronel*].
400 mg (Rx) [*Didronel* (scored)].
Canada—
200 mg (Rx) [*Didronel*].

**Packaging and storage**
Store below 40 °C (104 °F), preferably between 15 and 30 °C (59 and 86 °F), unless otherwise specified by manufacturer. Store in a tight container.

**Auxiliary labeling**
- Take on an empty stomach.
- Do not take with milk or antacids.

## Parenteral Dosage Forms

### ETIDRONATE DISODIUM INJECTION

Note: Etidronate disodium injection is not commercially available in Canada.

**Usual adult dose**
Hypercalcemia—
Intravenous infusion, initially 7.5 mg per kg of body weight per day, administered over a period of at least two hours, for three consecutive days.

Note: Some patients may be treated for up to seven days, but the risk of hypocalcemia is increased after three days.

The retreatment dose after a seven-day drug-free interval remains the same as the initial dose for most patients.

**Usual pediatric dose**
Dosage has not been established.

**Strength(s) usually available**
U.S.—
50 mg per mL (Rx) [*Didronel*].

**Packaging and storage**
Store below 40 °C (104 °F), preferably between 15 and 30 °C (59 and 86 °F), unless otherwise specified by manufacturer. Protect from freezing.

**Preparation of dosage form**
Dilute the daily dose in at least 250 mL of 0.9% sodium chloride injection or 5% dextrose injection.

**Stability**
Diluted solution may be stored at controlled room temperature for at least 48 hours without loss of drug.

Revised: 08/05/97

---

**ETODOLAC**—See *Anti-inflammatory Drugs, Nonsteroidal (Systemic)*

---

# ETOMIDATE  Systemic†

VA CLASSIFICATION (Primary/Secondary): CN203/CN206;
Commonly used brand name(s): *Amidate*.
Note: For a listing of dosage forms and brand names by country availability, see *Dosage Forms* section(s).

†Not commercially available in Canada.

## Category
Anesthetic, general; anesthesia adjunct.

## Indications
Note: Bracketed information in the *Indications* section refers to uses that are not included in U.S. product labeling.

### Accepted

Anesthesia, general or

Anesthesia, general, adjunct—Etomidate is indicated for the induction of general anesthesia. It is also indicated to supplement low-potency anesthetics, such as nitrous oxide and oxygen, during maintenance of anesthesia for short operative procedures such as dilation and curettage or cervical conization.

Etomidate may be especially useful in patients with compromised cardiopulmonary function because of its minimal cardiovascular and respiratory depressant effects and lack of histamine release at usual doses.

Etomidate is a sedative-hypnotic, which has no analgesic action.

## Pharmacology/Pharmacokinetics

### Physicochemical characteristics
Molecular weight—244.29.

### Mechanism of action/Effect
Etomidate is a short-acting hypnotic, which appears to have gamma-aminobutyric acid (GABA)–like effects. Unlike the barbiturates, etomidate reduces subcortical inhibition at the onset of hypnosis while inducing neocortical sleep. Studies in animals suggest that a part of the action of etomidate consists of a depression of the activity and reactivity of the brain stem reticular formation.

### Other actions/effects
Etomidate does not cause significant cardiovascular or respiratory depression, but may cause a brief period of apnea. Also, it does not appear to elevate plasma histamine or cause histamine release when administered in recommended dosage. The decrease in cerebral blood flow produced by etomidate is approximately the same as that produced by thiopental and methohexital; this reduction appears to be uniform in the absence of intracranial tumors. Etomidate slightly lowers intracranial pressure and preliminary data suggest that it usually causes a moderate decrease in intraocular pressure. Also, etomidate (at induction doses of 0.3 mg per kg of body weight [mg/kg]) has been reported to reduce plasma cortisol concentrations; this effect persists for 6 to 8 hours and appears to be unresponsive to adrenocorticotropic hormone (ACTH).

### Protein binding
High (76%), primarily to serum albumin.

### Biotransformation
Hepatic; rapidly metabolized by ester hydrolysis to inactive metabolites.

### Half-life
About 75 minutes.

### Onset of action
Rapid, usually within 1 minute.

### Plasma concentration
Minimal hypnotic plasma concentrations of unchanged drug are equal to or higher than 0.23 mcg per mL; they decrease rapidly for up to 30 minutes following injection and more slowly thereafter.

### Duration of action
Dose dependent, but usually 3 to 5 minutes with an average dose of 0.3 mg/kg; may be prolonged by a sedative premedication or by repeated injections of etomidate.

### Time to recovery
As rapid as, or slightly faster than, immediate recovery after similar use of thiopental. The immediate recovery period will usually be shortened in adults by intravenous administration of approximately 0.1 mg of fentanyl 1 or 2 minutes before induction of anesthesia, possibly because less etomidate is generally required.

### Elimination
Renal; approximately 75% of a dose excreted in the urine the first day after injection. The major inactive acid metabolite accounts for approximately 80% of the urinary excretion.

## Precautions to Consider

### Carcinogenicity/Mutagenicity
Studies have not been done.

### Pregnancy/Reproduction
Fertility—Reproduction studies showed no impairment of fertility in male and female rats when etomidate was administered prior to pregnancy at 0.31, 1.25, and 5 mg per kg of body weight (mg/kg) (approximately 1, 4, and 16 times the human dose, respectively).

Pregnancy—Studies in humans have not been done. However, studies in animals have shown that etomidate causes an embryocidal effect in rats when given in doses 1 and 4 times the human dose; decreases pup survival in rats at doses of 0.3 and 5 mg per kg (approximately 1 and 16 times the human dose) and in rabbits at doses of 1.5 and 4.5 mg per kg (approximately 5 and 15 times the human dose); slightly increases the incidence of stillborn fetuses in rats at doses of 0.3 and 1.25 mg per kg (approximately 1 and 4 times the human dose); and causes maternal toxicity with deaths in 6 out of 20 rats at a dose of 5 mg per kg (approximately 16 times the human dose) and in 6 out of 20 rabbits at a dose of 4.5 mg per kg (approximately 15 times the human dose). However, studies in animals have not shown that etomidate causes teratogenic effects.

FDA Pregnancy Category C.

Labor and delivery—Use of etomidate is not recommended since data are insufficient to support its use in obstetrics, including cesarean section deliveries.

### Breast-feeding
It is not known whether etomidate is distributed into breast milk. However, problems in humans have not been documented.

### Pediatrics
Appropriate studies with etomidate have not been performed in children up to 10 years of age. Safety and efficacy have not been established.

### Geriatrics
Elderly patients are more sensitive to the effects of etomidate than are younger patients. In addition, geriatric patients are more likely to have age-related hepatic function impairment, which may require reduction of dosage in patients receiving etomidate.

### Drug interactions and/or related problems
The following drug interactions and/or related problems have been selected on the basis of their potential clinical significance (possible mechanism in parentheses where appropriate)—not necessarily inclusive (» = major clinical significance):

Note: Combinations containing any of the following medications, depending on the amount present, may also interact with this medication.

» Alcohol or
» Central nervous system (CNS) depression–producing medications, other (See *Appendix II*)
(concurrent use may increase the CNS depressant effects of either these medications or etomidate; dosage adjustment of etomidate may be necessary)

Hypotension-producing medications, other (See *Appendix II*)
(concurrent use may potentiate the hypotensive effect of etomidate; dosage adjustments may be necessary)

(caution is advised during titration of calcium channel blocker dosage for those patients taking medication, such as etomidate, known to promote hypotension, since the combination may result in excessive hypotension)

(concurrent use of diazoxide with etomidate may result in an additive hypotensive effect, which may be severe; dosage adjustments may be necessary, and patient should be continuously observed for excessive fall in blood pressure for several hours after concurrent use)

(concurrent use of mecamylamine or trimethaphan with etomidate may potentiate the hypotensive response, with increased risk of severe hypotension, shock, and cardiovascular collapse during surgery)

Ketamine
(concurrent use of ketamine, especially in high doses or when rapidly administered, with etomidate may increase the risk of hypotension and/or respiratory depression)

### Medical considerations/Contraindications
The medical considerations/Contraindications included have been selected on the basis of their potential clinical significance (reasons given in parentheses where appropriate)—not necessarily inclusive (» = major clinical significance).

***Risk-benefit should be considered when the following medical problems exist:***

Immunosuppression or
Sepsis or
Transplantation
(potential effects on adrenal function)

Sensitivity to etomidate

## Side/Adverse Effects

Note: Etomidate can block the adrenal gland's production of cortisol and other steroid hormones, possibly resulting in temporary adrenal gland failure. This may cause abnormal salt and water balance, low-

## Etomidate (Systemic)

ered blood pressure, and, ultimately, shock. Postoperative or critically ill patients may require adrenocorticoid supplementation.

Etomidate may cause brief periods of apnea.

The following side/adverse effects have been selected on the basis of their potential clinical significance (possible signs and symptoms in parentheses where appropriate)—not necessarily inclusive:

**Those indicating need for medical attention**
Incidence more frequent
*Nausea and/or vomiting*
Note: Incidence of postoperative *nausea* and *vomiting* more frequent than with thiopental when etomidate is used for both induction and maintenance of anesthesia in short procedures or when analgesia is insufficient.

Incidence less frequent or rare
*Fast or slow breathing; increase or decrease in blood pressure; irregular or fast or slow heartbeat*

**Those indicating need for medical attention only if they continue or are bothersome**
Incidence more frequent—less frequent when fentanyl is given immediately before induction
*Involuntary muscle movements, temporary*—observed incidence 32%; reported incidence 22.7 to 63%; *pain, temporary, at injection site*—observed incidence 20%; reported incidence 1.2 to 42%
Note: May last for less than 1 minute; self-limiting without residual effects; appear to be more frequent with occurrence of venous pain on injection.

Bilateral movements are possibly a manifestation of disinhibition of cortical activity; unilateral movements sometimes resemble localized response to stimuli such as venous pain on injection.

*Pain at injection site* occurs immediately and appears to be less frequent when larger, more proximal arm veins are used.

Incidence less frequent or rare
*Hiccups*

## Overdose

For more information on the management of overdose or unintentional ingestion, **contact a Poison Control Center** (see *Poison Control Center Listing*).

**Treatment of overdose**
Recommended treatment for suspected or apparent overdosage of etomidate includes the following:

Discontinuation of medication.

Supportive care—Supportive measures such as establishing and maintaining a patent airway (intubating, if necessary) and administering oxygen with assisted ventilation, if necessary. Patients in whom intentional overdose is known or suspected should be referred for psychiatric consultation.

## Patient Consultation

As an aid to patient consultation, refer to *Advice for the Patient, Anesthetics, General (Systemic)*.

In providing consultation, consider emphasizing the following selected information (» = major clinical significance):

**Before using this medicine**
» Conditions affecting use, especially:
Sensitivity to etomidate
Pregnancy—Studies in animals have shown etomidate to cause embryocidal effects in rats, decrease pup survival in rats, slightly increase incidence of stillborn fetuses in rats, and cause maternal toxicity in rats and rabbits
Labor and delivery—Use of etomidate is not recommended since data are insufficient to support its use in obstetrics
Other medications, especially alcohol or other CNS depression–producing medications

**Proper use of this medication**
Proper dosing

**Precautions after receiving this medication**
» Possibility of psychomotor impairment following use of anesthetics; using caution in driving or performing other tasks requiring alertness and coordination for about 24 hours following anesthesia
» Avoiding use of alcohol or other CNS depressants within 24 hours following anesthesia except as directed by physician or dentist

**Side/adverse effects**
Signs of potential side effects, especially fast or slow breathing; increase or decrease in blood pressure; irregular, fast, or slow heartbeat; and nausea and/or vomiting

## General Dosing Information

Etomidate injection is for intravenous administration only. It is not intended for administration by prolonged infusion because of potential prolonged suppression of endogenous cortisol and aldosterone production.

Although clinical experience and animal studies have shown that inadvertent intra-arterial injection of etomidate usually will not cause necrosis of tissue, intra-arterial injection of etomidate is not recommended.

**Intravenous etomidate should be administered only by individuals trained in the administration of general anesthetics and in the management of complications encountered during general anesthesia.**

Dosage of etomidate must be individualized for each patient.

Etomidate injection is compatible with commonly administered preanesthetics, which may be used as indicated.

Immediately before anesthesia induction with etomidate, narcotic analgesics (e.g., fentanyl) may be administered to provide analgesia and to minimize pain on injection and involuntary muscle movements. Diazepam also may be used to reduce the incidence and magnitude of involuntary muscle movements.

Concurrent use of etomidate with neuromuscular blocking agents does not significantly alter the usual dosage requirements of these agents when used for endotracheal intubation or other procedures shortly after induction of anesthesia.

## Parenteral Dosage Forms

### ETOMIDATE INJECTION

Note: Etomidate injection is not commercially available in Canada.

**Usual adult and adolescent dose**
Anesthesia, general (induction of anesthesia)—
Dosage must be individualized by physician; however, as a general guideline: Intravenous, 300 mcg (0.3 mg) (range, 200 to 600 mcg [0.2 to 0.6 mg]) per kg of body weight, administered over a period of thirty to sixty seconds.
Note: Smaller increments of etomidate may be administered during short operative procedures to supplement low-potency anesthetics, such as nitrous oxide and oxygen. Although the dosage is usually much smaller than the initial induction dose, it must be individualized.

**Usual pediatric dose**
Anesthesia, general (induction of anesthesia)—
Children up to 10 years of age: Safety and efficacy have not been established.
Children 10 years of age and over—See *Usual adult and adolescent dose*.

**Usual geriatric dose**
See *Usual adult and adolescent dose*.

**Strength(s) usually available**
U.S.—
2 mg per mL (Rx) [*Amidate* (propylene glycol 35% v/v)].

**Packaging and storage**
Store below 40 °C (104 °F), preferably between 15 and 30 °C (59 and 86 °F), unless otherwise specified by manufacturer. Protect from freezing.

**Stability**
Any unused portion should be discarded.

Revised: 06/26/90
Interim revision: 08/10/94

---

# ETOPOSIDE   Systemic

VA CLASSIFICATION (Primary): AN900
Commonly used brand name(s): *Etopophos*; *Toposar*; *VePesid*.
Another commonly used name is VP-16.

Note: For a listing of dosage forms and brand names by country availability, see *Dosage Forms* section(s).

## Category
Antineoplastic.

## Indications
Note: Bracketed information in the *Indications* section refers to uses that are not included in U.S. product labeling.

### Accepted
Carcinoma, testicular (treatment)—Etoposide injection is indicated, in combination with other antineoplastics, for treatment of testicular tumors.

Carcinoma, lung, small cell (treatment)—Etoposide is indicated in combination with other agents as first line treatment of small cell lung carcinoma.

[Lymphomas, Hodgkin's (treatment)][1]
[Lymphomas, non-Hodgkin's (treatment)] or
[Leukemia, acute nonlymphocytic (treatment)][1]—Etoposide also is indicated, alone and in combination with other agents, for treatment of Hodgkin's and non-Hodgkin's lymphomas and acute nonlymphocytic (myelocytic) leukemia.

[Ewing's sarcoma (treatment)][1] or
[Kaposi's sarcoma, autoimmune deficiency syndrome (AIDS)–associated (treatment)][1]—Etoposide is indicated for treatment of Ewing's sarcoma and AIDS-associated Kaposi's sarcoma.

[Carcinoma, adrenocortical (treatment)][1]
[Carcinoma, gastric (treatment)][1]
[Hepatoblastoma (treatment)][1]
[Leukemia, acute lymphocytic (treatment)][1]
[Lymphomas, cutaneous T-cell (treatment)][1]
[Multiple myeloma (treatment)][1]
[Neuroblastoma (treatment)][1]
[Sarcomas, soft tissue (treatment)][1]
[Tumors, brain, primary (treatment)][1] or
[Tumors, trophoblastic, gestational (treatment)][1]—Etoposide is indicated, alone or in combination with other agents, for treatment of adrenocortical carcinoma, gastric carcinoma, hepatoblastoma, acute lymphocytic leukemia, cutaneous T-cell lymphomas, multiple myeloma, neuroblastoma, soft tissue sarcomas, primary brain tumors, and gestational trophoblastic tumors.

[Carcinoma, lung, non–small cell (treatment)][1]—Etoposide is indicated, alone or in combination with other agents, for treatment of non–small cell lung carcinoma.

[Carcinoma, endometrial (treatment)][1]—Etoposide is considered reasonable medical therapy at some point in the management of endometrial carcinoma (Evidence rating: IIID).

[Retinoblastoma (treatment)][1]
[Thymoma (treatment)][1] or
[Wilms' tumor (treatment)][1]—Etoposide is considered reasonable medical therapy at some point in the management of retinoblastoma (Evidence rating: IIID), thymoma (Evidence rating: IIID), and Wilms' tumor (Evidence rating: IIID).

[Osteosarcoma (treatment)][1]—Etoposide is considered reasonable medical therapy at some point in the management of osteosarcoma (Evidence rating: IIID).

[1]Not included in Canadian product labeling.

## Pharmacology/Pharmacokinetics

### Physicochemical characteristics
Molecular weight—Etoposide: 588.57.
Etoposide phosphate: 668.55.
Other characteristics—Etoposide: Lipophilic.

### Mechanism of action/Effect
The exact mechanism of etoposide's antineoplastic effect is unknown. Etoposide is a topoisomerase II inhibitor. It seems to act at the premitotic stage of cell division to inhibit DNA synthesis; it is cell cycle–dependent and phase-specific, with maximum effect on the S and $G_2$ phases of cell division.

### Absorption
Variable, dose-dependent oral bioavailability; absorption decreases as the dose of etoposide increases; mean 50% (range, 25 to 75%).

### Distribution
Low and variable into cerebrospinal fluid (CSF). Concentrations are higher in normal lung than in lung metastases, and are similar in primary tumors and normal tissues of the myometrium.

### Protein binding
Very high (97%) *in vitro*. Etoposide binding ratio correlates directly with serum albumin in normal individuals and cancer patients. The unbound fraction has been found to correlate significantly with bilirubin in a group of cancer patients. Phenylbutazone, sodium salicylate, and aspirin displaced protein-bound etoposide *in vitro*.

### Biotransformation
Hepatic.

### Half-life
Terminal (biphasic)—7 hours (range, 3 to 12).

### Elimination
Renal—44 to 60% (67% of that unchanged).
Fecal—Up to 16% (as unchanged drug and metabolites).
Biliary—6% or less.

## Precautions to Consider

### Carcinogenicity
Secondary malignancies are potential delayed effects of many antineoplastic agents, although it is not clear whether the effect is related to their mutagenic or immunosuppressive action. The effect of dose and duration of therapy is also unknown, although risk seems to increase with long-term use. Although information is limited, available data seem to indicate that the carcinogenic risk is greatest with the alkylating agents.

Acute leukemia (onset 2 to 3 years) has been reported in patients treated with topoisomerase II inhibitors such as etoposide.

### Mutagenicity
Etoposide is mutagenic and genotoxic in mammalian cells. Etoposide caused aberrations in chromosome number and structure in embryonic murine cells and human hematopoietic cells, gene mutations in Chinese hamster ovary cells, and DNA damage by strand breakage and DNA-protein cross-links in mouse leukemia cells; it also caused a dose-related increase in sister chromatid exchanges in Chinese hamster ovary cells and was mutagenic in the Ames test.

### Pregnancy/Reproduction
Fertility—Gonadal suppression, resulting in amenorrhea or azoospermia, may occur in patients receiving antineoplastic therapy, especially with the alkylating agents. In general, these effects appear to be related to dose and length of therapy and may be irreversible. Prediction of the degree of testicular or ovarian function impairment is complicated by the common use of combinations of several antineoplastics, which makes it difficult to assess the effects of individual agents.

Pregnancy—Adequate and well-controlled studies in humans have not been done.

First trimester: It is usually recommended that use of antineoplastics, especially combination chemotherapy, be avoided whenever possible, especially during the first trimester. Although information is limited because of the relatively few instances of antineoplastic administration during pregnancy, the mutagenic, teratogenic, and carcinogenic potential of these medications must be considered.

Other hazards to the fetus include adverse reactions seen in adults.

In general, use of a contraceptive is recommended during cytotoxic drug therapy.

Etoposide has been shown to be teratogenic and embryotoxic in mice and rats. Dose-related maternal toxicity, embryotoxicity, and teratogenicity (major skeletal abnormalities, exencephaly, encephalocele, and anophthalmia) have been reported with intravenous administration of 0.4 mg of etoposide per kg of body weight per day (mg/kg per day) (one twentieth of the recommended clinical dose based on body surface area) to rats during organogenesis; doses of 1.2 and 3.6 mg/kg per day (one seventh and one half of the recommended clinical dose, respectively, based on body surface area) caused 90% and 100% embryonic resorptions, respectively. Embryotoxicity and teratogenicity (cranial abnormalities, major skeletal abnormalities) also have been reported in mice following intraperitoneal administration of 1 mg/kg (one sixteenth of the recommended clinical dose based on body surface area) on day 6, 7, or 8 of gestation; intraperitoneal administration of 1.5 mg/kg (one tenth of the recommended clinical dose based on body surface area) on day 7 of gestation caused an increase in the incidences of intrauterine fetal death, fetal malformations, and decreased fetal weights. Risk-benefit must be carefully considered when this medication is required in life-threatening situations or in serious diseases for which other medications cannot be used or are ineffective.

FDA Pregnancy Category D.

### Breast-feeding
Etoposide is distributed into breast milk. Breast-feeding is not recommended during chemotherapy because of the risks to the infant (adverse effects, mutagenicity, carcinogenicity).

## Pediatrics
Appropriate studies on the relationship of age to the effects of etoposide have not been performed in the pediatric population. However, use of higher-than-recommended dosages of etoposide has been associated with a higher incidence of anaphylactic reactions in the pediatric population.

## Geriatrics
No information is available on the relationship of age to the effects of etoposide in geriatric patients. However, elderly patients are more likely to have age-related renal function impairment, which may require adjustment of dosage in patients receiving etoposide.

## Dental
The bone marrow depressant effects of etoposide may result in an increased incidence of microbial infection, delayed healing, and gingival bleeding. Dental work, whenever possible, should be completed prior to initiation of therapy or deferred until blood counts have returned to normal. Patients should be instructed in proper oral hygiene during treatment, including caution in use of regular toothbrushes, dental floss, and toothpicks.

Etoposide may also cause stomatitis which may be associated with considerable discomfort.

## Drug interactions and/or related problems
The following drug interactions and/or related problems have been selected on the basis of their potential clinical significance (possible mechanism in parentheses where appropriate)—not necessarily inclusive (» = major clinical significance):

Note: Combinations containing any of the following medications, depending on the amount present, may also interact with this medication.

Blood dyscrasia–causing medications (see *Appendix II*)
(leukopenic and/or thrombocytopenic effects of etoposide may be increased with concurrent or recent therapy if these medications cause the same effects; dosage adjustment of etoposide, if necessary, should be based on blood counts)

» Bone marrow depressants, other (see *Appendix II*) or
Radiation therapy
(additive bone marrow depression may occur; dosage reduction may be required when two or more bone marrow depressants, including radiation, are used concurrently or consecutively)

Vaccines, killed virus
(because normal defense mechanisms may be suppressed by etoposide therapy, the patient's antibody response to the vaccine may be decreased. The interval between discontinuation of medications that cause immunosuppression and restoration of the patient's ability to respond to the vaccine depends on the intensity and type of immunosuppression-causing medication used, the underlying disease, and other factors; estimates vary from 3 months to 1 year)

» Vaccines, live virus
(because normal defense mechanisms may be suppressed by etoposide therapy, concurrent use with a live virus vaccine may potentiate the replication of the vaccine virus, may increase the side/adverse effects of the vaccine virus, and/or may decrease the patient's antibody response to the vaccine; immunization of these patients should be undertaken only with extreme caution after careful review of the patient's hematologic status and only with the knowledge and consent of the physician managing the etoposide therapy. The interval between discontinuation of medications that cause immunosuppression and restoration of the patient's ability to respond to the vaccine depends on the intensity and type of immunosuppression-causing medication used, the underlying disease, and other factors; estimates vary from 3 months to 1 year. Patients with leukemia in remission should not receive live virus vaccine until at least 3 months after their last chemotherapy. In addition, immunization with oral poliovirus vaccine should be postponed in persons in close contact with the patient, especially family members)

## Medical considerations/Contraindications
The medical considerations/contraindications included have been selected on the basis of their potential clinical significance (reasons given in parentheses where appropriate)—not necessarily inclusive (» = major clinical significance).

***Risk-benefit should be considered when the following medical problems exist:***

» Bone marrow depression
» Chickenpox, existing or recent (including recent exposure) or
» Herpes zoster
(risk of severe generalized disease)

Hepatic function impairment
(reduced clearance)

» Infection
Renal function impairment
(reduced elimination; lower dosage may be necessary)
Sensitivity to etoposide

» Caution should be used also in patients who have had previous cytotoxic drug therapy or radiation therapy.

## Patient monitoring
The following are especially important in patient monitoring (other tests may be warranted in some patients, depending on condition; » = major clinical significance):

» Examination of patient's mouth for ulceration
(recommended prior to each dose)

» Hematocrit or hemoglobin and
» Leukocyte count, total and, if appropriate, differential and
» Platelet count
(determinations recommended prior to initiation of therapy and at periodic intervals during therapy; frequency varies according to clinical state, agent, dose, and other agents being used concurrently)

Albumin, serum
(low concentrations may be associated with increased risk of etoposide-related toxicities)

# Side/Adverse Effects
Note: Many "side effects" of antineoplastic therapy are unavoidable and represent the medication's pharmacologic action. Some of these (for example, leukopenia and thrombocytopenia) are actually used as parameters to aid in individual dosage titration.

Hypotension may occur temporarily if etoposide is administered by intravenous infusion over a period of less than 30 minutes.

Use of higher-than-recommended doses has been associated with hepatic toxicity and metabolic acidosis.

The following side/adverse effects have been selected on the basis of their potential clinical significance (possible signs and symptoms in parentheses where appropriate)—not necessarily inclusive:

## Those indicating need for medical attention
Incidence more frequent
*Anemia* (unusual tiredness or weakness); *leukopenia* (fever or chills; cough or hoarseness; lower back or side pain; painful or difficult urination)—usually asymptomatic; *thrombocytopenia* (unusual bleeding or bruising; black, tarry stools; blood in urine or stools; pinpoint red spots on skin)—usually asymptomatic

Note: With *leukopenia*, the nadir of the granulocyte count occurs 7 to 14 days after administration, and recovery is usually complete by the 20th day; cumulative myelosuppression has not been reported.

With *thrombocytopenia*, the nadir of the platelet count occurs 9 to 16 days after administration, and recovery is usually complete by the 20th day; cumulative myelosuppression has not been reported.

Incidence less frequent
*Stomatitis* (sores in mouth or on lips)

Incidence rare
*Anaphylaxis* (fast heartbeat; fever or chills; shortness of breath or wheezing; back pain; cough; loss of consciousness; sweating; swelling of face or tongue; tightness in throat); *chemical phlebitis* (pain at site of injection); *neurotoxicity* (difficulty in walking; numbness or tingling in fingers and toes; weakness); *skin rash or itching*

Note: Anaphylaxis also is associated with hypotension; hypertension and flushing also have been reported; blood pressure usually returns to normal within a few hours after the intravenous infusion is discontinued. An apparent hypersensitivity-associated apnea has been reported rarely. Use of higher-than-recommended dosages of etoposide has been associated with a higher rate of anaphylaxis in pediatric patients. Rarely, anaphylaxis may be fatal.

At investigational doses, a generalized pruritic erythematous maculopapular *rash*, consistent with perivasculitis, has been reported.

## Those indicating need for medical attention only if they continue or are bothersome
Incidence more frequent
*Loss of appetite; nausea and vomiting*

Incidence less frequent
*Central nervous system (CNS) toxicity* (unusual tiredness); *diarrhea*

### Those not indicating need for medical attention
Incidence more frequent
> *Alopecia* (loss of hair)
>> Note: *Alopecia* sometimes progresses to total baldness; it is reversible.

## Patient Consultation

As an aid to patient consultation, refer to *Advice for the Patient, Etoposide (Systemic)*.

In providing consultation, consider emphasizing the following selected information (» = major clinical significance):

### Before using this medication
» Conditions affecting use, especially:
> Sensitivity to etoposide
> Pregnancy—Use not recommended because of mutagenic, teratogenic, and carcinogenic potential; advisability of using contraception; telling physician immediately if pregnancy is suspected
> Breast-feeding—Not recommended because of risk of serious side effects
> Use in children—Severe allergic reactions can occur if children receive higher than recommended doses
> Other medications, especially other bone marrow depressants or previous cytotoxic drug or radiation therapy
> Other medical problems, especially chickenpox, herpes zoster, or infection

### Proper use of this medication
» Importance of not taking more or less medication than the amount prescribed
> Caution in taking combination therapy; taking each medication at the right time
> Frequency of nausea, vomiting, and loss of appetite; importance of continuing medication despite stomach upset
> Checking with physician if vomiting occurs shortly after oral dose is taken

» Proper dosing
> Missed dose: Not taking at all; not doubling doses

» Proper storage

### Precautions while using this medication
» Importance of close monitoring by physician
» Avoiding immunizations unless approved by physician; other persons in patient's household should avoid immunizations with oral poliovirus vaccine; avoiding persons who have taken oral poliovirus vaccine or wearing a protective mask that covers nose and mouth

*Caution if bone marrow depression occurs*
» Avoiding exposure to persons with infections, especially during periods of low blood counts; checking with physician immediately if fever or chills, cough or hoarseness, lower back or side pain, or painful or difficult urination occurs
» Checking with physician immediately if unusual bleeding or bruising; black, tarry stools; blood in urine or stools; or pinpoint red spots on skin occur
> Caution in use of regular toothbrush, dental floss, or toothpick; physician, dentist, or nurse may suggest alternatives; checking with physician before having dental work done
> Not touching eyes or inside of nose unless hands are washed immediately before
> Using caution to avoid accidental cuts with use of sharp objects such as safety razor or fingernail or toenail cutters
> Avoiding contact sports or other situations where bruising or injury could occur

### Side/adverse effects
> Importance of discussing possible effects, including cancer, with physician
> Signs of potential side effects, especially anemia, leukopenia, thrombocytopenia, stomatitis, anaphylaxis, chemical phlebitis, neurotoxicity, and skin rash or itching
> Physician or nurse can help in dealing with side effects
> Possibility of hair loss; normal hair growth should resume after treatment has ended

## General Dosing Information

Patients receiving etoposide should be under supervision of a physician experienced in cancer chemotherapy.

A variety of dosage schedules of etoposide, alone or in combination with other antitumor agents, are used. The prescriber may consult the medical literature as well as the manufacturer's literature in choosing a specific dosage.

Dosage must be adjusted to meet the individual requirements of each patient, based on clinical response and appearance or severity of toxicity.

Frequency and duration of nausea and vomiting may be reduced in some patients by administration of antiemetics prior to dosing.

Special precautions are recommended in patients who develop thrombocytopenia as a result of administration of etoposide. These may include extreme care in performing invasive procedures; regular inspection of intravenous sites, skin (including perirectal area), and mucous membrane surfaces for signs of bleeding or bruising; limiting frequency of venipuncture and avoiding intramuscular injections; testing urine, emesis, stool, and secretions for occult blood; care in use of regular toothbrushes, dental floss, toothpicks, safety razors, and fingernail and toenail cutters; avoiding constipation; and using caution to prevent falls and other injuries. Such patients should avoid alcohol and aspirin intake because of the risk of gastrointestinal bleeding. Platelet transfusions may be required.

Patients who develop leukopenia should be observed carefully for signs of infection. Antibiotic support may be required. In neutropenic patients who develop fever, broad-spectrum antibiotic coverage should be initiated empirically, pending bacterial cultures and appropriate diagnostic tests.

It is recommended that the dosage of etoposide be reduced in patients with renal function impairment. A dose reduction of 25% is recommended if creatinine clearance is 15 to 50 mL per minute.

### For parenteral dosage form only
It is recommended that etoposide injection be diluted prior to use, and that it be administered by slow intravenous infusion over a period of 30 to 60 minutes to prevent hypotension. Etoposide should not be administered by rapid intravenous injection or any other route.

Etoposide phosphate may be administered intravenously over 5 to 210 minutes.

### Safety considerations for handling this medication
There is limited but increasing evidence and concern that personnel involved in preparation and administration of parenteral antineoplastics may be at some risk because of the potential mutagenicity, teratogenicity, and/or carcinogenicity of these agents, although the actual risk is unknown. USP advisory panels recommend cautious handling both in preparation and disposal of antineoplastic agents. Precautions that have been suggested include:
- Use of a biological containment cabinet during reconstitution and dilution of parenteral medications and wearing of disposable surgical gloves and masks.
- Use of proper technique to prevent contamination of the medication, work area, and operator during transfer between containers (including proper training of personnel in this technique).
- Cautious and proper disposal of needles, syringes, vials, ampuls, and unused medication.

A number of medical centers have developed detailed guidelines for handling of antineoplastic agents.

### Combination chemotherapy
Etoposide may be used in combination with other agents in various regimens. As a result, incidence and/or severity of side effects may be altered and different dosages (usually reduced) may be used. For example, etoposide is part of the following chemotherapeutic combinations (some commonly used acronyms are in parentheses):
—etoposide, cyclophosphamide, doxorubicin, and vincristine (CAVE).
—cyclophosphamide, doxorubicin, and etoposide (CAE).
—cisplatin, bleomycin, and etoposide (BEP).
—cisplatin and etoposide (EP).

For specific dosages and schedules, consult the literature. For information regarding each agent, consult the individual monograph.

### For treatment of adverse effects
Hypotension may be treated by stopping the infusion, administering fluids and other supportive treatment, then resuming the infusion at a slower rate.

Anaphylaxis should be treated by stopping the infusion and administering pressor agents, corticosteroids, antihistamines, or volume expanders as necessary.

## Oral Dosage Forms

### ETOPOSIDE CAPSULES USP
Note: The dosing and strengths of the dosage forms available are expressed in terms of etoposide base (not the phosphate salt).

#### Usual adult dose
Small cell lung carcinoma—
> Oral, 70 mg (base) per square meter of body surface area (rounded to the nearest 50 mg) per day for four days to 100 mg per square meter of body surface area (rounded to the nearest 50 mg) per day for five days, repeated every three to four weeks.

## Usual pediatric dose
Dosage has not been established.

## Strength(s) usually available
U.S.—
  50 mg (base) (Rx) [VePesid].
Canada—
  50 mg (base) (Rx) [VePesid].

## Packaging and storage
Store between 2 and 8 °C (36 and 46 °F), in a tight container. Protect from freezing.

# Parenteral Dosage Forms

Note: Bracketed uses in the *Dosage Forms* section refer to categories of use and/or indications that are not included in U.S. product labeling.

## ETOPOSIDE INJECTION

### Usual adult dose
Testicular carcinoma—
  Intravenous infusion, 50 to 100 mg (base) per square meter of body surface area per day on days 1 through 5 to 100 mg per square meter of body surface area on days 1, 3, and 5 of a regimen that is repeated every three to four weeks.
Small cell lung carcinoma—
  Intravenous infusion, 35 mg (base) per square meter of body surface area per day for four days to 50 mg per square meter of body surface area per day for five days, repeated every three to four weeks.
[Lymphomas, Hodgkin's][1] or
[Lymphomas, non-Hodgkin's][1] or
[Lymphomas, cutaneous T-cell][1] or
[Leukemia, acute nonlymphocytic][1] or
[Leukemia, acute lymphocytic][1] or
[Multiple myeloma][1] or
[Ewing's sarcoma][1] or
[Kaposi's sarcoma, autoimmune deficiency syndrome (AIDS)–associated][1] or
[Sarcomas, soft tissue][1] or
[Osteosarcoma][1] or
[Carcinoma, adrenocortical][1] or
[Carcinoma, gastric][1] or
[Carcinoma, lung, non–small cell][1] or
[Carcinoma, endometrial][1] or
[Hepatoblastoma][1] or
[Neuroblastoma][1] or
[Retinoblastoma ][1] or
[Thymoma][1] or
[Wilms' tumor][1] or
[Tumors, brain, primary][1] or
[Tumors, trophoblastic, gestational][1]—
  Consult medical literature and manufacturer's literature for specific dosage.

### Usual pediatric dose
Dosage has not been established.

### Strength(s) usually available
U.S.—
  20 mg (base) per mL (Rx) [VePesid (citric acid 2 mg per mL; benzyl alcohol 30 mg per mL; polysorbate 80/tween 80, 80 mg per mL; polyethylene glycol 300, 650 mg per mL; alcohol 30.5% v/v); Toposar (citric acid 2 mg per mL; benzyl alcohol 30 mg per mL; polysorbate 80/tween 80, 80 mg per mL; polyethylene glycol 300, 650 mg per mL; alcohol 30.5% v/v); GENERIC].
Canada—
  20 mg (base) per mL (Rx) [VePesid (benzyl alcohol 30 mg per mL; citric acid; polyethylene glycol 300; polysorbate 80; ethanol; GENERIC].

### Packaging and storage
Store below 40 °C (104 °F), preferably between 15 and 30 °C (59 and 86 °F), unless otherwise specified by the manufacturer. Protect from freezing.

### Preparation of dosage form
Etoposide injection may be diluted for administration by intravenous infusion in either 5% dextrose injection or 0.9% sodium chloride injection to produce a solution containing 200 to 400 mcg (0.2 to 0.4 mg) of etoposide per mL (precipitation may occur with concentrations greater than 400 mcg per mL).

Cracking and leaking of plastic containers made of ABS (a polymer composed of acrylonitrile, butadiene, and styrene) has been reported when used with undiluted (but not diluted) etoposide injection.

### Caution—
- Use of products containing benzyl alcohol is generally not recommended for preparation of medications for use in neonates. A fatal toxic syndrome consisting of metabolic acidosis, CNS depression, respiratory problems, renal failure, hypotension, and possibly seizures and intracranial hemorrhages has been associated with this use.
- Use of products containing polysorbate 80 is generally not recommended for preparation of medications for use in premature infants. A life-threatening syndrome consisting of hepatic and renal failure, pulmonary deterioration, thrombocytopenia, and ascites has been associated with this use.

### Stability
When diluted as recommended, 0.2 and 0.4 mg per mL solutions are stable for 96 and 24 hours, respectively, at 25 °C (77 °F) under normal room fluorescent light in glass or plastic containers.

## ETOPOSIDE PHOSPHATE FOR INJECTION

Note: The dosage and strength of the available dosage form are expressed in terms of etoposide base (not the phosphate salt).

### Usual adult dose
Testicular carcinoma—
  Intravenous infusion, 50 to 100 mg (base) per square meter of body surface area per day on days 1 through 5 to 100 mg per square meter of body surface area on days 1, 3, and 5 of a regimen that is repeated every three to four weeks.
Small cell lung carcinoma—
  Intravenous infusion, 35 mg (base) per square meter of body surface area per day for four days to 50 mg per square meter of body surface area per day for five days, repeated every three to four weeks.
[Lymphomas, Hodgkin's][1] or
[Lymphomas, non-Hodgkin's][1] or
[Lymphomas, cutaneous T-cell][1] or
[Leukemia, acute nonlymphocytic][1] or
[Leukemia, acute lymphocytic][1] or
[Multiple myeloma][1] or
[Ewing's sarcoma][1] or
[Kaposi's sarcoma, autoimmune deficiency syndrome (AIDS)–associated][1] or
[Sarcomas, soft tissue][1] or
[Osteosarcoma][1] or
[Carcinoma, adrenocortical][1] or
[Carcinoma, gastric][1] or
[Carcinoma, lung, non–small cell][1] or
[Carcinoma, endometrial][1] or
[Hepatoblastoma][1] or
[Neuroblastoma][1] or
[Retinoblastoma ][1] or
[Thymoma][1] or
[Wilms' tumor][1] or
[Tumors, brain, primary][1] or
[Tumors, trophoblastic, gestational][1]—
  Consult medical literature and manufacturer's literature for specific dosage.

### Usual pediatric dose
Dosage has not been established.

### Strength(s) usually available
U.S.—
  100 mg (base) (Rx) [Etopophos (sodium citrate 32.7 mg; dextran 40, 300 mg)].
Canada—
  Not commercially available.

### Packaging and storage
Store between 2 and 8 °C (36 and 46 °F), unless otherwise specified by the manufacturer.

### Preparation of dosage form
Etoposide phosphate for injection is reconstituted for intravenous use by the addition of 5 or 10 mL of either sterile water for injection, 5% dextrose injection, 0.9% sodium chloride injection, bacteriostatic water for injection with benzyl alcohol, or bacteriostatic sodium chloride for injection with benzyl alcohol, producing a solution containing 20 mg or 10 mg etoposide per mL (22.7 mg or 11.4 mg etoposide phosphate per mL), respectively. Following reconstitution, etoposide phosphate may be administered without further dilution, or it may be further diluted with 5% dextrose injection or 0.9% sodium chloride injection to a final concentration as low as 0.1 mg etoposide per mL.

**Stability**
When diluted as recommended, etoposide phosphate solution is stable for 24 hours at controlled room temperature (20 to 25 °C [68 to 77 °F]) or in a refrigerator (2 to 8 °C [36 to 46 °F]).

**Caution**
Use of products containing benzyl alcohol is generally not recommended for preparation of medications for use in neonates. A fatal toxic syndrome consisting of metabolic acidosis, CNS depression, respiratory problems, renal failure, hypotension, and possibly seizures and intracranial hemorrhages has been associated with this use.

[1]Not included in Canadian product labeling.

Revised: 06/24/98

# FACTOR IX  Systemic

BAN: Factor IX Fraction
VA CLASSIFICATION (Primary): BL116
Commonly used brand name(s): *AlphaNine SD; Bebulin VH; BeneFix; Immunine VH; Konÿne 80; Mononine; Profilnine SD; Proplex T.*
Other commonly used names are Christmas factor, plasma thromboplastin component (PTC), and prothrombin complex concentrate (PCC).
Note: For a listing of dosage forms and brand names by country availability, see *Dosage Forms* section(s).

## Category
Antihemorrhagic.

## Indications
Note: Some of the indications for factor IX formulations vary among different brand name products because of differences in composition. Some brand name products contain clinically useful quantities of clotting factors other than factor IX; other brand name products contain only factor IX, or factor IX with clinically insignificant quantities of other clotting factors.

### Accepted
Hemophilia B, hemorrhagic complications of (prophylaxis and treatment)—Factor IX is indicated for the control and prevention of bleeding in patients with hemophilia B (Christmas disease).

Hemorrhagic complications in hemophilic patients with factor VIII inhibitors (prophylaxis and treatment)—Factor IX complex concentrates may be indicated for the control and prevention of bleeding in patients with hemophilia A (classical hemophilia) who have developed inhibitor antibodies to, and therefore will not respond to treatment with, factor VIII.

Hemorrhagic complications of factor VII deficiency (prophylaxis and treatment)—*Proplex T* is indicated for the replacement of factor VII for the control and prevention of bleeding in patients lacking this clotting factor.

Hemorrhage, anticoagulant-induced (treatment)—Factor IX complex concentrates may be indicated to reverse life-threatening hemorrhage induced by coumarin- and indandione-derivative anticoagulants.

## Pharmacology/Pharmacokinetics

### Physicochemical characteristics
Source—Factor IX products are sterile, dried concentrates derived from pooled human plasma or produced by recombinant DNA technology. One type of factor IX product, which is also called prothrombin complex concentrate (PCC), may contain clinically useful quantities of vitamin K–dependent clotting factors II, VII, and X in addition to factor IX. PCCs also may contain other proteins, including proteins C and S; high molecular weight kininogen; and small quantities of activated clotting factors II, VII, IX, or X.

A second type of factor IX product, which is called coagulation factor IX, is purified of extraneous plasma proteins, including clotting factors II, VII, and X, by affinity chromatography (*AlphaNine SD*, *BeneFix*) or by immunoaffinity chromatography utilizing murine monoclonal antibodies to factor IX (*Mononine*). Products of this type contain clinically useful quantities of factor IX only.

Molecular weight—Factor IX: 55,000 to 71,000.

### Mechanism of action/Effect
Hemorrhagic complications of Hemophilia B—Factor IX is a vitamin K–dependent clotting factor synthesized in the liver. It is part of the intrinsic pathway of blood coagulation. Factor IX is converted to its activated form, factor IXa, by factor XIa in the presence of calcium ions. Factor IXa, in combination with activated factor VIII, calcium ions, and phospholipids, converts factor X to its activated form, factor Xa, resulting ultimately in the conversion of prothrombin to thrombin, and the formation of a fibrin clot. Hemophilia B is an inherited, X chromosome–linked disorder in which there is a deficiency of factor IX. Hemophilia B is classified as mild, moderate, or severe when plasma factor IX concentrations are more than 5%, 1 to 5%, or less than 1% of normal, respectively. The average normal plasma activity of factor IX is designated as 60 to 100%, and a plasma factor IX concentration of 25 to 40% of normal is required for hemostasis. The administration of factor IX products temporarily replaces the deficient clotting factor to correct or prevent bleeding episodes.

Hemorrhagic complications in hemophilic patients with factor VIII inhibitors—The exact mechanism of action is unclear. However, the clotting factors present in the prothrombin complex concentrates are believed to bypass the factor VIII inhibitors and directly activate factor X. *In vitro* experiments suggest the possibility of a factor Xa-like substance; or a complex of factor VIII coagulant antigen (FVIIIC:Ag), factor IXa, and phospholipid as the active principle, which is only minimally inhibited by an inhibitor.

Hemorrhagic complications of factor VII deficiency—Factor VII is part of the extrinsic pathway of blood coagulation. It is activated to factor VIIa by factor Xa. Factor VIIa, in combination with tissue factor, activates factors IX and X. The administration of the factor VII present in factor IX complex replaces the deficient clotting factor to correct or prevent bleeding episodes.

Anticoagulant-induced hemorrhage—Coumarin- and indandione-derivative anticoagulants act indirectly in the liver by inhibiting the vitamin K–mediated gamma-carboxylation of precursor proteins, thus preventing the activation of clotting factors II, VII, IX, and X. The administration of factor IX complex concentrates containing additional vitamin K–dependent clotting factors increases the plasma concentration of these clotting factors to overcome the effect of the anticoagulant.

### Half-life
Factor IX—
  Distribution: 3 to 6 hours.
  Elimination: 17 to 32 hours.

### Time to peak effect
10 to 30 minutes after intravenous administration.

## Precautions to Consider

### Pregnancy/Reproduction
Pregnancy—Studies have not been done in humans.
Studies have not been done in animals.
FDA Pregnancy Category C.

### Breast-feeding
It is not known whether the proteins present in factor IX products are distributed into breast milk. However, distribution into breast milk would be highly unlikely because of the large size of the protein molecules.

### Pediatrics
Premature infants and neonates may be at increased risk of developing thrombotic complications following the administration of factor IX products.

### Geriatrics
Appropriate studies performed to date have not demonstrated geriatrics-specific problems that would limit the usefulness of factor IX products in the elderly.

### Dental
Antifibrinolytic agents, such as aminocaproic acid and tranexamic acid, are used commonly in conjunction with clotting factor replacement to control excessive bleeding in hemophilic patients undergoing tooth extractions, or who have other oral bleeding. Care should be taken, however, as systemic use of antifibrinolytic agents may potentiate the thrombogenic effects of the concentrate, particularly factor IX complex. Using the antifibrinolytic agent as an oral rinse, or delaying its use for 8 to 12 hours after administration of the concentrate, may minimize this complication.

### Surgical
Factor IX concentrates should be used cautiously in patients undergoing surgical procedures, as the risk of thrombotic complications is increased in these patients who receive large, repeated doses of factor IX complex, or who have significant hepatic dysfunction.

### Drug interactions and/or related problems
The following drug interactions and/or related problems have been selected on the basis of their potential clinical significance (possible mechanism in parentheses where appropriate)—not necessarily inclusive (» = major clinical significance):

Note: Combinations containing any of the following medications, depending on the amount present, may also interact with this medication.

Aminocaproic acid or
Tranexamic acid
  (although these antifibrinolytic agents are used commonly in conjunction with clotting factor replacement to control and prevent excessive bleeding in hemophilic patients undergoing tooth extractions or who have other oral bleeding, systemic use with factor IX products (particularly factor IX complex) may increase the risk of thrombotic complications; this may be less of a problem with the

use of coagulation factor IX; using the antifibrinolytic agent as an oral rinse, or delaying its use for 8 to 12 hours following injection of factor IX products, may minimize this complication)

### Medical considerations/Contraindications
The medical considerations/contraindications included have been selected on the basis of their potential clinical significance (reasons given in parentheses where appropriate)—not necessarily inclusive (» = major clinical significance).

*Except under special circumstances, this medication should not be used when the following medical problems exist:*
» Disseminated intravascular coagulation (DIC) or
» Hyperfibrinolytic states or
» Thromboembolism, predisposition to or history of
  (risk of thrombotic complications)

*Risk-benefit should be considered when the following medical problems exist:*
Crush injuries or
Hepatic function impairment, severe or
Surgery, recent
  (increased risk of disseminated intravascular coagulation, fibrinolysis, or thrombosis)
Sensitivity to factor IX
Sensitivity to hamster protein
  (risk of allergic reaction to protein, which is present in recombinant product, *BeneFix*)
Sensitivity to mouse protein
  (risk of allergic reaction to protein, which is present in monoclonal antibody–derived product, *Mononine*)

### Patient monitoring
The following may be especially important in patient monitoring (other tests may be warranted in some patients, depending on condition; » = major clinical significance):

Activated partial thromboplastin time (APTT) tests
Plasma fibrinogen determinations
Platelet count and
Prothrombin time (PT) tests
  (recommended daily during therapy to detect disseminated intravascular coagulation [DIC]; prolonged APTT and PT test results in combination with a reduced fibrinogen concentration and thrombocytopenia are highly suggestive of DIC; additional laboratory findings that further corroborate the diagnosis of DIC include prolonged thrombin time, an increase in plasma D-dimer and fibrinogen degradation products, and a decrease in plasma clotting factors)
Factor IX plasma, determinations
  (recommended daily during therapy to assure that adequate factor IX concentrations have been achieved and are maintained)

## Side/Adverse Effects
Note: To reduce the risk of *transmission of viruses* by blood and blood components, potential blood donors are screened, and donor blood is tested and must be found negative for antibodies to human immunodeficiency virus (HIV), hepatitis B core antigen, hepatitis C (non-A, non-B) virus, and for hepatitis B surface antigen. The concentration of alanine aminotransferase (ALT) also must be within normal limits. However, these precautions are not totally effective in eliminating viral infectivity. To further reduce the risk, factor IX products are treated utilizing one or more methods of viral inactivation. Some of the methods employed include dry heating, vapor heating, heating in solvent suspension, use of solvent detergent, immunoaffinity chromatography, and ultrafiltration. These processes substantially decrease the risk of transmission of lipid-enveloped viruses such as HIV, hepatitis B, and hepatitis C (non-A, non-B). However, nonlipid-enveloped viruses, including human parvovirus B19 and hepatitis A, are potentially resistant to some of these measures and can still be transmitted. Also, unknown viruses and prions, such as the agent that causes Creutzfeldt-Jakob disease (CJD), may not be eliminated by current inactivation and purification methods and could be transmitted. There is no evidence, however, of CJD transmission through any transfused blood component, and it remains only a theoretical concern.

Approximately 1 to 4% of patients treated with factor IX products develop *inhibitors*, or antibodies, which neutralize the procoagulant activity of factor IX. Patients with inhibitor antibodies to factor IX may be treated with increased quantities of factor IX, which complex with and thereby inactivate the antibodies, or with an anti-inhibitor coagulant complex, which directly activates factor X. However, the success of either of these treatment options is variable. Recombinant activated factors VII and X are currently undergoing clinical trials to assess safety and efficacy in the treatment of patients with factor IX inhibitor antibodies.

The following side/adverse effects have been selected on the basis of their potential clinical significance (possible signs and symptoms in parentheses where appropriate)—not necessarily inclusive:

**Those indicating need for medical attention**
Incidence more frequent
  *Disseminated intravascular coagulation* (cyanosis [bluish coloring], especially of the hands and feet; ecchymoses at injection sites [large, nonelevated blue or purplish patches in the skin]; excessive sweating; persistent bleeding or oozing from puncture sites or mucous membranes [bowel, mouth, nose, or urinary bladder]); *myocardial infarction* (anxiety; cold sweating; increased heart rate; nausea or vomiting; severe pain or pressure in the chest and/or the neck, back, or left arm; shortness of breath); *pulmonary embolism* (chest discomfort; convulsions; dizziness or lightheadedness when getting up from a lying or sitting position; shortness of breath or fast breathing); *thrombosis or thromboembolism* (pains in chest, groin, or legs [especially calves]; severe, sudden headache; sudden and unexplained shortness of breath, slurred speech, vision changes, and/or weakness or numbness in arm or legs; sudden loss of coordination)—depending on site of thrombus formation or embolization

Note: The nonactivated clotting factors II, VII, and X; activated clotting factors II, VII, IX, and X; and coagulant-active phospholipids present in prothrombin complex concentrates (factor IX complex) are thought to be largely responsible for the *thrombotic complications* described. Intravascular thrombosis has occurred most frequently in patients who received large, repeated doses of factor IX complex while undergoing surgery, and may be more common in patients with underlying liver disease. These complications are less likely to occur after the administration of purified coagulation factor IX products *AlphaNine SD*, *BeneFix*, *Immunine VH*, or *Mononine*.

Incidence less frequent
  *Anaphylaxis or other allergic reaction* (changes in facial skin color; fast or irregular breathing; puffiness or swelling of the eyelids or around the eyes; shortness of breath, troubled breathing, tightness in chest, and/or wheezing; skin rash, hives, and/or itching)—may include anaphylactic shock with sudden, severe decrease in blood pressure and collapse; *injection reaction* (burning or stinging at injection site; changes in blood pressure or pulse rate; chills; drowsiness; fever; flushing [redness of face]; headache; nausea or vomiting; shortness of breath)—occurs with too rapid an injection rate

Note: An *allergic reaction* to mouse protein (incidence rare) may occur after the administration of the monoclonal antibody–derived product, *Mononine*.

## Patient Consultation
As an aid to patient consultation, refer to *Advice for the Patient, Factor IX (Systemic)*.
In providing consultation, consider emphasizing the following selected information (» = major clinical significance):

### Before using this medication
» Conditions affecting use, especially:
  Sensitivity to factor IX or to hamster or mouse protein
  Use in children—Thrombotic complications are more likely to occur in premature infants and neonates, who are usually more sensitive than adults to the effects of factor IX
  Other medical problems, especially disseminated intravascular coagulation, hyperfibrinolytic states, or predisposition to or history of thromboembolism

### Proper use of this medication
» Proper preparation of medication: bringing dry concentrate and diluent to room temperature before reconstitution; when reconstituting, directing stream of diluent against side of vial of concentrate to prevent foaming; gently swirling vial to dissolve contents; not shaking vigorously
» Administering within 3 hours of reconstitution
» Use of plastic disposable syringe and filter needle; safe handling and disposal of syringe and needle
» Proper dosing
Missed dose: Contacting physician immediately for instructions
» Proper storage

## Precautions while using this medication

Need for patients newly diagnosed with hemophilia to receive hepatitis A and hepatitis B vaccines

» Notifying physician if medication seems less effective than usual; this may indicate the development of antibodies to factor IX

» Need to carry identification stating condition

## Side/adverse effects

Signs and symptoms of potential adverse effects, including disseminated intravascular coagulation, myocardial infarction, pulmonary embolism, thrombosis or thromboembolism, and allergic reaction to factor IX or mouse protein

# General Dosing Information

## Choice of product

Because of the risk of thrombotic complications with the use of factor IX complex concentrates, use of a coagulation factor IX product should be strongly considered in the following situations: for surgery, for treatment of crush injuries, for treatment of large intramuscular hemorrhages for which several days of replacement therapy will be required, in persons with severe hepatocellular dysfunction, in neonates, and in persons who have a history of thrombotic complications associated with the use of factor IX complex.

Some clinicians recommend the use of heparin with factor IX complex, either administered to the patient directly (5000 USP Units subcutaneously every eight hours) or added to the concentrate (5 to 10 USP Units per mL), as a way to prevent thrombotic complications.

Factor IX products are recommended for intravenous use only.

Factor IX products should be administered via plastic disposable syringes because the proteins present tend to adhere to the ground-glass surface of all-glass syringes.

Factor IX products should be filtered before administration.

Factor IX may be administered as a continuous intravenous infusion via a minipump or syringe pump for severe, life-threatening bleeding, or following surgery.

Long-term prophylactic therapy for severe hemophilia, in which factor replacement is given several times a week to maintain the factor level above 1%, has been used extensively in Europe. The goal is to convert severe hemophilia to a mild or moderate form of the disease to prevent spontaneous bleeding and preserve joint function.

Antifibrinolytic therapy is useful adjunctive therapy in hemophilic patients with oral or mucous membrane bleeding, particularly that which occurs during dental and oral surgery. It prevents or controls bleeding, thus reducing the need for replacement therapy. Aminocaproic acid may be given orally or intravenously at a dose of 75 mg per kg of body weight (up to 6 grams) immediately after surgery, then every six hours for seven to ten days. Or, tranexamic acid may be given as a single dose of 25 mg per kg of body weight orally or 10 mg per kg of body weight intravenously two hours before surgery, followed, after surgery, by 25 mg per kg of body weight orally every six to eight hours for seven to ten days. When antifibrinolytic agents are used in this manner, a single coagulation factor IX infusion of 60 International Units per kg of body weight prior to surgery is often enough for normal hemostasis. These agents can also be given as an oral rinse (5 mL of aminocaproic acid syrup, or 10 mL of a 5% tranexamic acid solution four times a day for seven to ten days).

# Parenteral Dosage Forms

## FACTOR IX COMPLEX USP

Note: Each vial of factor IX concentrate is labeled with the factor IX activity expressed in International Units (IU) per vial. This potency assignment is referenced to the World Health Organization International Standard. One IU of factor IX activity per kg of body weight is approximately equal to the factor IX activity in 1 mL of fresh plasma and increases the plasma concentration of factor IX by 1%. The specific factor IX activity of the prothrombin complex concentrates ranges from 0.7 to 3 IU per mg of total protein. Although the dose of factor IX should be individualized for each patient based on body weight, type of hemorrhage, and desired plasma factor IX concentration, the following formula may be used as a guide in determining dosage:

Dose factor IX (IU) = Body weight (kg) × Desired factor IX increase (% of normal) × 1 IU/kg

*Bebulin VH* may be administered at a rate ≤ 2 mL per minute, *Konÿne 80* at a rate of 100 IU per minute, *Profilnine SD* at a rate ≤ 10 mL per minute, and *Proplex T* at a rate between 2 and 3 mL per minute. However, the rate at which factor IX complex is administered should be guided by the comfort of the patient.

## Usual adult and adolescent dose

Hemophilia B—
Prophylaxis of spontaneous hemorrhage—
Intravenous, 25 to 40 IU per kg of body weight, administered twice a week, maintaining the trough factor level above 1% between doses.

Treatment of hemorrhage—
Schedules for administration of clotting factor concentrates are based on the severity of the bleeding diathesis. Currently, there is no consensus among practitioners regarding the optimal dose of factor replacement therapy for the treatment of the various types of bleeding, and the optimal therapeutic level for control of such bleeding remains debatable. The doses in *Table 1* should be considered only as a guideline, since recommendations may vary from one hemophilia center to another. Doses and duration of treatment may be adjusted according to the patient's condition.

Table 1. General Factor Replacement Guidelines for the Treatment of Bleeding in Hemophilia

| Indication | Initial minimum desired factor level (%) | Factor IX dose* (IU/kg) | Duration (days) |
|---|---|---|---|
| Severe epistaxis | 20–30 | 20–30 | 1–2 |
| Oral mucosal bleeding† | 20–30 | 20–30 | 1–2 |
| Hemarthrosis | 30–50 | 30–50 | 1–2 |
| Hematoma | 30–50 | 30–50 | 1–2 |
| Persistent hematuria‡ | 30–50 | 30–50 | 1–2 |
| Gastrointestinal bleeding | 30–50 | 30–50 | at least 1–2 days after bleeding stops |
| Retroperitoneal bleeding | 30–50 | 30–50 | at least 3 |
| Trauma without signs of bleeding | 40–50 | 40–50 | 2–3 |
| Tongue/retropharyngeal bleeding† | 40–50 | 40–50 | 3–4 |
| Trauma with bleeding§ | 100 | 100 | 10–14 |
| Intracranial bleeding§ | 100 | 100 | 10–14 |

*Dosing intervals are based on a half-life for Factor IX of 18 to 24 hours (1 to 2 doses/day). Maintenance doses of one half the initial dose may be given at these intervals. The frequency depends on the severity of bleeding, with more frequent dosing for serious bleeding.

†In addition to antifibrinolytics.

‡Painless spontaneous hematuria usually requires no treatment. Increased oral or intravenous fluids are necessary to maintain renal output.

§Continuous factor infusion may be administered. Following the initial loading dose, a continuous infusion at a dose of 3 IU/kg per hour is given. Subsequent doses are adjusted according to the plasma factor levels.

Control of perisurgical hemostasis—
Dental and oral surgery—Intravenous, 60 IU per kg of body weight prior to surgery. A single dose is often sufficient for normal hemostasis when an antifibrinolytic agent, such as aminocaproic acid or tranexamic acid, is used as adjunctive treatment. Care should be taken, however, as systemic use of antifibrinolytic agents may potentiate the thrombogenic effects of the concentrate. Using the antifibrinolytic agent as an oral rinse, or delaying its use for 8 to 12 hours after administration of the concentrate, may minimize this complication. This may be less of a problem with the use of coagulation factor IX.

Other surgery—Intravenous, 50 to 60 IU per kg of body weight, or a quantity sufficient to raise the plasma factor IX concentration to 50 to 60% of normal, administered one hour prior to surgery. Subsequent doses equal to half the initial dose are given every twelve to twenty-four hours to maintain that plasma level for the first few days after surgery. The dose can then be tapered to maintain a plasma factor level > 30% for the following one to two weeks. Major orthopedic surgery may require several weeks of replacement therapy. However, because of the increased risk of thrombotic complications with the use of factor IX complex in surgical patients, the use of coagulation factor IX is preferred.

Hemophilia A—
Prevention and control of bleeding in patients with inhibitors to factor VIII—
Intravenous, 75 IU per kg of body weight. The dose may be repeated after six or twelve hours, if necessary.

Factor VII deficiency—
  Control of perisurgical hemostasis—
    *Proplex T*—Intravenous, a quantity sufficient to raise the plasma factor VII concentration to 25% of normal administered prior to the procedure, with repeat doses every four to six hours after the procedure, as needed, for at least seven days. To estimate the dose of factor IX complex required to treat factor VII deficiency, the following formula may be used:
    Dose factor IX complex (IU) = Body weight (kg) × Desired factor VII increase (% of normal) × 0.5 IU/kg
Anticoagulant-induced hemorrhage—
  Intravenous, 1500 IU, administered with vitamin $K_1$ if needed in severe cases.

### Usual pediatric dose
See *Usual adult and adolescent dose*.

### Size(s) usually available
U.S.—
  400 to 1200 IU of factor IX, as specified on the label, with sterile water for injection provided as diluent (Rx) [*Bebulin VH* (heparin ≤ 0.15 IU per IU of factor IX; diluent 20 mL)].
  450 to 1000 IU of factor IX, as specified on the label, with sterile water for injection provided as diluent (Rx) [*Proplex T* (heparin ≤ 1.5 USP units per mL; diluent 30 mL)].
  500 IU of factor IX with sterile water for injection provided as diluent (Rx) [*Konyne 80* (diluent 20 mL); *Profilnine SD* (diluent 5 mL)].
  1000 IU of factor IX, with sterile water for injection provided as diluent (Rx) [*Konyne 80* (diluent 40 mL); *Profilnine SD* (diluent 10 mL)].
  1500 IU of factor IX, with sterile water for injection provided as diluent (Rx) [*Profilnine SD* (diluent 10 mL)].
Canada—
  400 to 1200 IU of factor IX, as specified on the label, with sterile water for injection provided as diluent (Rx) [*Bebulin VH* (heparin ≤ 0.15 IU per IU of factor IX; diluent 20 mL)].
Note: The products listed also contain factors II, VII, and X. The quantities may be specified on the individual product labels.

### Packaging and storage
The dry concentrates are stored preferably between 2 and 8 °C (36 and 46 °F). However, *Konyne 80* may be stored at room temperatures not exceeding 25 °C (77 °F) for up to 1 month, and *Profilnine SD* may be stored at room temperatures not exceeding 30 °C (86 °F) for up to 3 months. The solution should not be refrigerated after reconstitution. The diluent should be protected from freezing.

### Preparation of dosage form
The diluent and dry concentrate should be brought to room temperature prior to reconstitution. The solution should be gently swirled, not shaken, until all of the concentrate is dissolved. Reconstitution generally requires 5 to 10 minutes. The reconstituted solution should be approximately at room temperature at the time of administration.

Note: Heparin may be added to prothrombin complex concentrates at a concentration of 5 to 10 USP units per mL of reconstituted product. The addition of heparin has been shown, in some cases, to reduce the likelihood of development of thrombotic complications.

### Stability
Administration should begin within 3 hours after reconstitution. Partially used vials should be discarded.

### Incompatibilities
It is recommended that factor IX complex, after reconstitution with the provided diluent, be administered through a separate line, by itself, and without mixing with other intravenous fluids or medications.

## COAGULATION FACTOR IX (HUMAN)

Note: Each vial of factor IX concentrate is labeled with the factor IX activity expressed in International Units (IU) per vial. This potency assignment is referenced to the World Health Organization International Standard. One IU of factor IX activity per kg of body weight is approximately equal to the factor IX activity in 1 mL of fresh plasma, and increases the plasma concentration of factor IX by 1%. The specific factor IX activities of coagulation factor IX products *AlphaNine SD* and *Mononine* are ≥ 50 IU per mg of total protein and 180 to 200 IU per mg of total protein, respectively. Although the dose of factor IX should be individualized for each patient based on body weight, type of hemorrhage, and desired plasma factor IX concentration, the following formula may be used as a guide in determining dosage:

Dose factor IX (IU) = Body weight (kg) × Desired factor IX increase (% of normal) × 1 IU/kg

*AlphaNine SD* may be administered at a rate not exceeding 10 mL per minute, and *Mononine* and *Immunine VH* at a rate of 2 mL per minute. However, the rate at which coagulation factor IX is administered should be guided by the comfort of the patient.

### Usual adult and adolescent dose
Hemophilia B—
  Prophylaxis of spontaneous hemorrhage—
    See *Factor IX Complex USP*.
  Treatment of hemorrhage—
    See *Factor IX Complex USP*.
  Control of perisurgical hemostasis—
    Dental and oral surgery— See *Factor IX Complex USP*.
    Other surgery—Intravenous, 100 IU per kg of body weight, or a quantity sufficient to raise the plasma factor IX concentration to 100% of normal, administered one hour prior to surgery. Subsequent doses equal to half the initial dose are given every twelve to twenty-four hours to maintain that plasma level for the first few days after surgery. As an alternative to the intermittent dosing of replacement factor, continuous infusion of factor IX may be given following surgery at a dose of 3 IU per kg of body weight per hour via a minipump or syringe pump. The dose can then be tapered to maintain a plasma factor level > 30% for the following one to two weeks. Major orthopedic surgery may require several weeks of replacement therapy.

### Usual pediatric dose
See *Usual adult and adolescent dose*.

### Size(s) usually available
U.S.—
  250 IU, with sterile water for injection provided as diluent (Rx) [*Mononine* (factors II, VII, and X ≤ 0.0025 units per unit of factor IX; sodium chloride 66 mmol; mouse protein ≤ 50 nanograms per 100 units of factor IX; diluent 2.5 mL)].
  500 IU, with sterile water for injection provided as diluent (Rx) [*AlphaNine SD* (factors II and VII < 5 units per 100 IU of factor IX; factor X < 20 units per IU of factor IX; heparin ≤ 0.04 USP units per IU of factor IX; dextrose ≤ 1 mg per IU of factor IX; diluent 10 mL); *Mononine* (factors II, VII, and X ≤ 0.0025 units per unit of factor IX; sodium chloride 66 mmol; mouse protein ≤ 50 nanograms per 100 units of factor IX; diluent 5 mL)].
  1000 IU, with sterile water for injection provided as diluent (Rx) [*AlphaNine SD* (factors II and VII < 5 units per 100 IU of factor IX; factor X < 20 units per IU of factor IX; heparin ≤ 0.04 USP units per IU of factor IX; dextrose ≤ 1 mg per IU of factor IX; diluent 10 mL); *Mononine* (factors II, VII, and X ≤ 0.0025 units per unit of factor IX; sodium chloride 66 mmol; mouse protein ≤ 50 nanograms per 100 units of factor IX; diluent 10 mL)].
  1250 IU, with sterile water for injection provided as diluent (Rx) [*AlphaNine SD* (factors II and VII < 5 units per 100 IU of factor IX; factor X < 20 units per IU of factor IX; dextrose ≤ 1 mg per IU of factor IX; diluent 10 mL)].
  1500 IU, with sterile water for injection provided as diluent (Rx) [*AlphaNine SD* (factors II and VII < 5 units per 100 IU of factor IX; factor X < 20 units per IU of factor IX; dextrose ≤ 1 mg per IU of factor IX; diluent 10 mL)].
Canada—
  160 to 240 IU, with sterile water for injection provided as diluent (Rx) [*Immunine VH* (heparin < 0.1 IU per mL; factors II, VII, and X < 0.02 IU per IU of factor IX)].
  500 IU, with sterile water for injection provided as diluent (Rx) [*AlphaNine SD* (factors II and VII < 5 units per 100 IU of factor IX; factor X < 20 units per IU of factor IX; dextrose ≤ 1 mg per IU of factor IX; diluent 10 mL)].
  480 to 720 IU, with sterile water for injection provided as diluent (Rx) [*Immunine VH* (heparin < 0.1 IU per mL; factors II, VII, and X < 0.02 IU per IU of factor IX)].
  1000 IU, with sterile water for injection provided as diluent (Rx) [*AlphaNine SD* (factors II and VII < 5 units per 100 IU of factor IX; factor X < 20 units per IU of factor IX; dextrose ≤ 1 mg per IU of factor IX; diluent 10 mL)].
  960 to 1440 IU, with sterile water for injection provided as diluent (Rx) [*Immunine VH* (heparin < 0.1 IU per mL; factors II, VII, and X < 0.02 IU per IU of factor IX)].
  1250 IU, with sterile water for injection provided as diluent (Rx) [*AlphaNine SD* (factors II and VII < 5 units per 100 IU of factor IX; factor X < 20 units per IU of factor IX; dextrose ≤ 1 mg per IU of factor IX; diluent 10 mL)].
  1500 IU, with sterile water for injection provided as diluent (Rx) [*AlphaNine SD* (factors II and VII < 5 units per 100 IU of factor IX; factor X < 20 units per IU of factor IX; dextrose ≤ 1 mg per IU of factor IX; diluent 10 mL)].

## Factor IX (Systemic)

**Packaging and storage**
The dry concentrates preferably are stored between 2 and 8 °C (36 and 46 °F). However, *Mononine* may be stored at room temperatures not exceeding 30 °C (86 °F) for up to 1 month. The diluent should be protected from freezing.

**Preparation of dosage form**
The diluent and dry concentrate should be brought to room temperature prior to reconstitution. The reconstituted solution should be gently swirled, not shaken, until all of the concentrate is dissolved. Reconstitution generally requires 1 to 5 minutes. The reconstituted solution should be approximately at room temperature at the time of administration.

**Stability**
Administration should begin within 3 hours after reconstitution. Partially used vials should be discarded.

**Incompatibilities**
It is recommended that coagulation factor IX, after reconstitution with the provided diluent, be administered through a separate line, by itself, and without mixing with other intravenous fluids or medications.

### COAGULATION FACTOR IX (RECOMBINANT)

Note: Each vial of factor IX concentrate is labeled with the factor IX activity expressed in International Units (IU) per vial. This potency assignment is referenced to the World Health Organization International Standard. One IU of factor IX activity per kg of body weight is approximately equal to the factor IX activity in 1 mL of fresh plasma. The specific activity of *BeneFix* is ≥ 200 IU per mg of total protein. Although the dose of factor IX should be individualized for each patient based on body weight, type of hemorrhage, and desired plasma factor IX concentration, recombinant factor IX may require higher doses than those used for plasma-derived factor IX to attain the desired factor IX level. Patients switching from plasma-derived factor IX to recombinant factor IX may be started at the same dose previously used for plasma-derived factor IX and titrated upward as needed, or the dose may be based on the following formula:

Dose factor IX (IU) = Body weight (kg) × Desired factor IX increase (% of normal) × 1.2 IU/kg

**Usual adult and adolescent dose**
Hemophilia B—
  Prophylaxis of spontaneous hemorrhage—
    See *Factor IX Complex USP*.
  Treatment of hemorrhage—
    See *Factor IX Complex USP*.
  Control of perisurgical hemostasis—
    See *Coagulation Factor IX (Human)*.

**Usual pediatric dose**
See *Usual adult and adolescent dose*.

**Size(s) usually available**
U.S.—
  250 IU, with sterile water for injection provided as diluent (Rx) [*BeneFix*].
  500 IU, with sterile water for injection provided as diluent (Rx) [*BeneFix*].
  1000 IU, with sterile water for injection provided as diluent (Rx) [*BeneFix*].
Canada—
  250 IU, with sterile water for injection provided as diluent (Rx) [*BeneFix*].
  500 IU, with sterile water for injection provided as diluent (Rx) [*BeneFix*].
  1000 IU, with sterile water for injection provided as diluent (Rx) [*BeneFix*].

**Packaging and storage**
The dry concentrate preferably is stored between 2 and 8 °C (36 and 46 °F). However, *BeneFix* may be stored at room temperatures not exceeding 25 °C (77 °F) for up to 6 months. The diluent should be protected from freezing.

**Preparation of dosage form**
The diluent and dry concentrate should be brought to room temperature prior to reconstitution. The reconstituted solution should be gently swirled, not shaken, until all of the concentrate is dissolved. The reconstituted solution should be approximately at room temperature at the time of administration.

**Stability**
Administration should begin within 3 hours after reconstitution. Partially used vials should be discarded.

### Selected Bibliography

Thompson AR. Factor IX concentrates for clinical use. Semin Thromb Hemost 1993; 19: 25-36.

Lusher JM. Considerations for current and future management of haemophilia and its complications. Haemophilia 1995; 1: 2-10.

Revised: 08/15/97

---

# FAMCICLOVIR Systemic

VA CLASSIFICATION (Primary): AM802

Commonly used brand name(s): *Famvir*.

Note: For a listing of dosage forms and brand names by country availability, see *Dosage Forms* section(s).

## Category

Antiviral (systemic).

## Indications

### Accepted

Herpes genitalis, recurrent episodes (suppression[1] or treatment)—Famciclovir is indicated in the suppression or treatment of recurrent episodes of genital herpes. Treatment of recurrent episodes is most effective when started within 6 hours of the onset of symptoms or lesions.

Herpes zoster (treatment)—Famciclovir is indicated in the treatment of herpes zoster infections (shingles) caused by varicella-zoster virus (VZV). Famciclovir has been found to decrease the duration of postherpetic neuralgia (defined as pain at or following healing) when compared to placebo (55 to 62 days versus 128 days, respectively). Famciclovir has also been found to be equivalent to acyclovir in decreasing the duration of acute pain. Therapy is most effective when started within 48 hours of the onset of rash.

### Unaccepted

The efficacy of famciclovir has not been established in the treatment of immunocompromised patients, nor for the treatment of initial episodes of genital herpes infection, ophthalmic zoster, or disseminated zoster.

[1]Not included in Canadian product labeling.

## Pharmacology/Pharmacokinetics

### Physicochemical characteristics
Molecular weight—321.3.

### Mechanism of action/Effect

Famciclovir is a pro-drug; it is the diacetyl 6-deoxy analog of the active antiviral compound, penciclovir. Penciclovir is phosphorylated by viral thymidine kinase to penciclovir monophosphate, which is then converted to penciclovir triphosphate by cellular kinases. Penciclovir inhibits herpes viral DNA synthesis, and, therefore, replication. Penciclovir does not inhibit DNA synthesis in uninfected cells because it is phosphorylated only in herpes-infected cells.

Penciclovir has antiviral activity against herpes simplex virus type 1 (HSV-1), HSV-2, varicella-zoster virus (VZV), and Epstein-Barr virus. *In vitro* studies have shown that penciclovir triphosphate has greater intracellular stability in HSV-2–infected cells than does acyclovir triphosphate. Also, unlike acyclovir, the antiviral activity of penciclovir persists in the absence of extracellular drug.

### Absorption

Famciclovir is absorbed in the upper intestine and rapidly converted in the intestinal wall to the active compound, penciclovir. The bioavailability of penciclovir after oral administration of famciclovir is approximately 77%.

Famciclovir may be taken without regard to meals; although a decrease in the time to peak serum concentration and peak serum concentration of penciclovir was seen when famciclovir was taken with food or after a meal, there was no decrease in the extent of systemic availability.

### Distribution

The steady-state volume of distribution of penciclovir is approximately 1 liter per kilogram (L/kg).

**Protein binding**
Low (20 to 25%).

**Biotransformation**
Famciclovir is deacetylated, and then oxidized to form the active agent, penciclovir. Little or no famciclovir is detected in the plasma or urine. Inactive metabolites include 6-deoxypenciclovir, monoacetylated penciclovir, and monoacetylated 6-deoxypenciclovir, all of which account for ≤ 1.5% of the dose.

**Half-life**
Normal renal function—
2.1 to 3 hours.
Severe renal failure (creatinine clearance < 30 mL/min [0.33 mL/sec])—
10 to 13 hours.
Intracellular half-life of penciclovir triphosphate—
In HSV-1–infected cells—Approximately 10 hours.
In HSV-2–infected cells—Approximately 20 hours.
In VZV-infected cells—Approximately 7 hours.

**Time to peak plasma concentration**
0.7 to 0.9 hours.

**Peak plasma concentration**
3.3 to 4.2 mcg/mL [10.3 to 13.1 micromoles/L] after a single oral dose (fasting) of 500 mg.

**Elimination**
Renal (glomerular filtration and tubular secretion); 60 to 65% of an oral dose is recovered as penciclovir in the urine; 27% in the feces over 72 hours.
In dialysis—It is not known if hemodialysis removes penciclovir from the blood.

## Precautions to Consider

### Carcinogenicity
Dietary carcinogenicity studies of famciclovir were conducted in rats and mice at the doses listed below for approximately 1.5 years. A significant increase in the incidence of mammary adenocarcinoma was seen in female rats receiving 600 mg per kg (mg/kg) per day (1.5 times the human systemic exposure at 500 mg three times a day, based on the area under the plasma concentration–time curve [AUC] for penciclovir). Marginal increases in the incidence of subcutaneous tissue fibrosarcomas or squamous cell carcinomas of the skin were seen in female rats and male mice dosed at 600 mg/kg per day (0.4 times the human exposure, based on AUC for penciclovir). There was no increase in tumor incidence reported in male rats treated with doses of up to 240 mg/kg per day (0.9 times the human AUC), or in female mice treated with doses of up to 600 mg/kg per day (0.4 times the human AUC).

### Mutagenicity
Famciclovir and penciclovir were negative in *in vitro* tests for gene mutations in bacteria (*S. typhimurium* and *E. coli*) and unscheduled DNA synthesis in mammalian HeLa 83 cells. Famciclovir was also negative in the L5178Y mouse lymphoma assay, the *in vivo* mouse micronucleus test, and rat dominant lethal study. Famciclovir induced increases in polyploidy in human lymphocytes *in vitro* in the absence of chromosomal damage.
Penciclovir was positive in the L5178Y mouse lymphoma assay for gene mutation/chromosomal aberrations, with and without metabolic activation. In human lymphocytes, penciclovir caused chromosomal aberrations in the absence of metabolic activation. Penciclovir caused an increased incidence of micronuclei in mouse bone marrow *in vivo* when administered intravenously at doses highly toxic to bone marrow, but not when administered orally.

### Pregnancy/Reproduction
Fertility—Testicular toxicity was observed in rats, mice, and dogs following repeated administration of famciclovir or penciclovir. Testicular changes included atrophy of the seminiferous tubules, reduction in sperm count, and/or increased incidence of sperm with abnormal morphology or reduced motility. The degree of toxicity was related to dose and duration of exposure. In male rats, decreased fertility was observed after 10 weeks of dosing at 500 mg/kg per day (1.9 times the human AUC). Testicular toxicity was observed following chronic administration to mice (104 weeks) and dogs (26 weeks) at doses of 600 mg/kg per day (0.4 times the human AUC) and 150 mg/kg per day (1.07 times the human AUC), respectively.
Famciclovir had no effect on general reproductive performance or fertility in female rats at doses up to 1000 mg/kg per day (3.6 times the human AUC).
Pregnancy—No adequate and well-controlled studies have been done in pregnant women.
No adverse effects were observed on embryo-fetal development in rats and rabbits given oral famciclovir at doses of up to 1000 mg/kg per day (approximately 3.6 and 1.8 times the human exposure based on AUC, respectively), and intravenous doses of 360 mg/kg per day in rats (2 times the human exposure based on body surface area [BSA]) and 120 mg/kg per day in rabbits (1.5 times the human exposure based on BSA). Also, no adverse effects were observed after intravenous administration of penciclovir to rats given 80 mg/kg per day (0.4 times the human exposure based on BSA), and rabbits given 60 mg/kg per day (0.7 times the human exposure based on BSA).

FDA Pregnancy Category B.

### Breast-feeding
Following oral administration of famciclovir, it is not known whether penciclovir is distributed into breast milk.
However, it has been found to pass into the milk of lactating rats at concentrations higher than those seen in the plasma. Also, because of the tumorigenicity seen in rats, it is recommended that either breast-feeding or administration of famciclovir to the mother be discontinued.

### Pediatrics
Safety and efficacy have not been established in children up to 18 years of age.

### Geriatrics
Studies performed to date have not demonstrated geriatric-specific problems that would limit the usefulness of famciclovir in the elderly. However, elderly patients are more likely to have an age-related decrease in renal function, which may require an adjustment of famciclovir dosage or of dosing interval.

### Drug interactions and/or related problems
The following drug interactions and/or related problems have been selected on the basis of their potential clinical significance (possible mechanism in parentheses where appropriate)—not necessarily inclusive (» = major clinical significance):

Note: Combinations containing any of the following medications, depending on the amount present, may also interact with this medication.

Probenecid
(probenecid may compete with penciclovir for active tubular secretion, resulting in increased plasma concentrations of penciclovir)

### Medical considerations/Contraindications
The medical considerations/contraindications included have been selected on the basis of their potential clinical significance (reasons given in parentheses where appropriate)—not necessarily inclusive (» = major clinical significance).

*Risk-benefit should be considered when the following medical problem exists:*

» Renal function impairment
(because penciclovir is renally excreted, patients with renal function impairment may be at increased risk of toxicity; patients with a creatinine clearance of < 60 mL/min [1 mL/sec] require a reduction in dose)

## Side/Adverse Effects
Note: No serious side effects have been noted to date with the administration of famciclovir.

**Those indicating need for medical attention only if they continue or are bothersome**
Incidence more frequent
*Headache*
Incidence less frequent
*Dizziness; fatigue* (unusual tiredness or weakness); *gastrointestinal disturbances* (diarrhea; nausea; vomiting)

## Patient Consultation
As an aid to patient consultation, refer to *Advice for the Patient, Famciclovir (Systemic)*.
In providing consultation, consider emphasizing the following selected information (» = major clinical significance):

**Before using this medication**
» Conditions affecting use, especially:
Breast-feeding—Because of the potential for tumorigenicity seen in rats, it is recommended that either breast-feeding or the use of famciclovir be discontinued
Use in children—Safety and efficacy have not been established in children up to 18 years of age
Other medical problems, especially renal function impairment

# Famciclovir (Systemic)

**Proper use of this medication**
Initiating use of famciclovir for herpes zoster at the earliest sign or symptom; it is most effective when started within 48 hours of the onset of rash
Initiating use of famciclovir for treatment of recurrent episodes of genital herpes at the earliest sign or symptom; it is most effective when started within 6 hours of the onset of symptoms or lesions
Famciclovir may be taken with meals
» Compliance with full course of therapy; not using more often or for longer than prescribed
» Proper dosing
Missed dose: Taking as soon as possible; not taking if almost time for next dose; not doubling doses
» Proper storage

**Precautions while using this medication**
Checking with physician if no improvement within a few days
Keeping affected areas as clean and dry as possible; wearing loose-fitting clothing to avoid irritation of lesions

## General Dosing Information

Therapy should be initiated as soon as possible following the onset of signs and symptoms of varicella-zoster infection. Treatment was started within 72 hours of the onset of rash in clinical studies; however, famciclovir was found to be more useful if started within 48 hours.

For treatment of recurrent episodes of herpes genitalis, therapy should be initiated as soon as possible following the onset of signs and symptoms. Treatment was started within 6 hours of the onset of symptoms or lesions in clinical studies.

In clinical trials, the effect of famciclovir on the resolution of rash was most pronounced in patients over 50 years of age.

Famciclovir tablets may be taken with meals since absorption has not been shown to be significantly affected by food.

## Oral Dosage Forms

### FAMCICLOVIR TABLETS

**Usual adult dose**
Genital herpes, recurrent episodes (suppression)[1]—
  Oral, 250 mg two times a day for up to one year.
Genital herpes, recurrent episodes (treatment)—
  Oral, 125 mg two times a day for five days.
Herpes zoster (treatment)—
  Oral, 500 mg every eight hours for seven days.
Note: Adults with impaired renal function may require a change in dosing as follows:

| Indication | Creatinine clearance (mL/min)/(mL/sec) | Dosing regimen |
|---|---|---|
| Herpes zoster | ≥ 60/1 | 500 mg every 8 hours |
|  | 40–59/0.67–0.98 | 500 mg every 12 hours |
|  | 20–39/0.33–0.65 | 500 mg every 24 hours |
|  | < 20/0.33 | 250 mg every 48 hours |
| Treatment of recurrent genital herpes | ≥ 40/0.67 | 125 mg every 12 hours |
|  | 20–39/0.33–0.65 | 125 mg every 24 hours |
|  | < 20/0.33 | 125 mg every 48 hours |

| Indication | Creatinine clearance (mL/min)/(mL/sec) | Dosing regimen |
|---|---|---|
| Suppression of recurrent genital herpes | ≥ 40/0.67 | 250 mg every 12 hours |
|  | 20–39/0.33–0.65 | 125 mg every 12 hours |
|  | < 20/0.33 | 125 mg every 24 hours |
| Hemodialysis patients | The recommended dose is 250 mg (herpes zoster) or 125 mg (treatment or suppression of recurrent genital herpes) administered after each dialysis session. | |

**Usual pediatric dose**
Safety and efficacy have not been established for patients up to 18 years of age.

**Strength(s) usually available**
U.S.—
  125 mg (Rx) [*Famvir* (lactose)].
  250 mg (Rx) [*Famvir* (lactose)].
  500 mg (Rx) [*Famvir* (lactose)].
Canada—
  125 mg (Rx) [*Famvir* (lactose)].
  250 mg (Rx) [*Famvir* (lactose)].
  500 mg (Rx) [*Famvir* (lactose)].

**Packaging and storage**
Store between 15 and 25 °C (59 and 77 °F), in a tight container, unless otherwise specified by manufacturer.

**Auxiliary labeling**
• Continue medicine for full time of treatment.

[1] Not included in Canadian product labeling.

Developed: 11/28/94
Interim revision: 01/28/98

---

**FAMOTIDINE**—See *Histamine H₂-receptor Antagonists (Systemic)*

---

**FAT EMULSIONS**—The *Fat Emulsions (Systemic)* monograph is not included in this published version of the USP DI database. Copies of the monograph are available on request from Micromedex, Inc. - Reprint Requests, 6200 S. Syracuse Way, Suite 300, Englewood, CO 80111; telephone (303) 486-6400; telefax (303) 486-6464; Email: USPDI@MDX.COM.

---

**FECAL OCCULT BLOOD TEST KITS**—The *Fecal Occult Blood Test Kits* monograph is not included in this published version of the USP DI database. Copies of the monograph are available on request from Micromedex, Inc. - Reprint Requests, 6200 S. Syracuse Way, Suite 300, Englewood, CO 80111; telephone (303) 486-6400; telefax (303) 486-6464; Email: USPDI@MDX.COM.

---

# FELBAMATE  Systemic†

VA CLASSIFICATION (Primary): CN400
Commonly used brand name(s): *Felbatol*.
Another commonly used name is FBM.
Note: For a listing of dosage forms and brand names by country availability, see *Dosage Forms* section(s).

†Not commercially available in Canada.

## Category
Anticonvulsant.

## Indications

**Accepted**
Epilepsy (treatment)—Felbamate is indicated as monotherapy or as an adjunct to other anticonvulsants for the treatment of partial seizures with

or without generalization in adults with severe epilepsy that has not responded to other treatment.

Epilepsy, Lennox-Gastaut syndrome (treatment adjunct)—Felbamate is indicated as adjunctive therapy in the treatment of partial and generalized seizures associated with Lennox-Gastaut syndrome in children who have not responded to other treatment.

## Pharmacology/Pharmacokinetics

**Physicochemical characteristics**
Chemical group—Dicarbamate. Structurally similar to meprobamate.
Molecular weight—238.24.

**Mechanism of action/Effect**
*In vitro* receptor binding studies suggest that felbamate may be an antagonist at the strychnine-insensitive glycine-recognition site of the N-methyl-D-aspartate (NMDA) receptor-ionophore complex. Antagonism of the NMDA receptor glycine binding site may block the effects of the excitatory amino acids and suppress seizure activity. Animal studies indicate that felbamate may increase the seizure threshold and may decrease seizure spread.

**Other actions/effects**
Animal studies have shown felbamate to induce the cytochrome P-450 enzyme system to some extent. In clinical studies, however, felbamate has acted as an enzyme inhibitor, possibly through competitive inhibition. In rat studies, felbamate has been shown to possess some neuroprotective activity against hypoxic-ischemic damage, probably through interaction with the strychnine-insensitive glycine receptor, at plasma concentrations achieved during clinical use; the relevance to humans is unknown.

**Absorption**
Complete (90%). Absorption is unaffected by food, and both tablet and suspension dosage forms exhibit similar kinetics.

**Distribution**
Felbamate enters the central nervous system (CNS), with a brain/plasma coefficient of approximately 0.9. The apparent volume of distribution ($Vol_D$) ranged from 0.73 to 0.85 L per kg of body weight (L/kg) in single and multiple dose studies. Felbamate is distributed into breast milk.

**Protein binding**
Low (20-36%).

**Biotransformation**
Hepatic, probably by the cytochrome P-450 system; primarily by hydroxylation and conjugation to metabolites that are neither pharmacologically active nor neurotoxic.

**Half-life**
Elimination—13 to 23 hours.

**Time to peak concentration**
1 to 6 hours.

**Therapeutic serum concentration**
The therapeutic concentration range for felbamate has yet to be established. Plasma concentrations in 21 patients receiving monotherapy with 3600 mg of felbamate per day ranged from 23.7 to 136.6 mcg per mL (mcg/mL) (99.5 to 573.7 micromoles per L [micromoles/L]), with a mean of 78.8 mcg/mL (329.3 micromoles/L).

**Elimination**
Renal—About 90% of an orally administered radioactive dose of felbamate was recovered in the urine, 40 to 50% of which was recovered unchanged.
Fecal—Less than 5% of an orally administered radioactive dose of felbamate was recovered in the feces.

## Precautions to Consider

**Cross-sensitivity and/or related problems**
Patients sensitive to other carbamate derivatives (for example, carbromal, carisoprodol, meprobamate, mebutamate, or tybamate) may also be sensitive to felbamate. Felbamate should be used cautiously in patients who have demonstrated hypersensitivity reactions to other carbamate derivatives.

**Carcinogenicity/Tumorigenicity**
In lifetime carcinogenicity studies, rats and mice received dosages of felbamate that resulted in steady state plasma concentrations less than or equal to those of humans receiving 3600 mg per day. The mice and the female rats showed a significant increase in hepatic cell adenomas, the mice showed a significant increase in hepatic hypertrophy, and the male rats showed a significant increase in benign interstitial cell tumors of the testes. The significance to humans is unknown.

As a result of the manufacturing process of felbamate, small amounts of two known animal carcinogens, ethyl carbamate (urethane) and methyl carbamate, may be present in the final dosage forms. The amounts present in felbamate used in lifetime carcinogenic studies were inadequate to cause tumors in rats and mice. A patient receiving 3600 mg per day of felbamate could be exposed to up to 0.72 mcg of urethane and 1800 mcg of methyl carbamate per day. These amounts are 1/10,000 and 1/1,600, respectively, of the dose levels shown to be carcinogenic in rodents, on a mg per square meter of body surface area ($mg/m^2$) basis.

**Mutagenicity**
No evidence of mutagenesis was revealed in microbial and mammalian cell assays.

**Pregnancy/Reproduction**
Fertility—No effect on male or female fertility was seen in rats at oral doses up to 3 times the human maximum daily dose on a $mg/m^2$ basis.
Pregnancy—Studies in humans have not been done.
Felbamate crosses the placenta in rats. Incidence of malformation in offspring was not increased in rats at doses up to 3 times, or in rabbits at doses less than 2 times, the human maximum daily dose on a $mg/m^2$ basis. However, rat pup weight was decreased, and pup mortality during lactation was increased. The cause of these deaths is unknown. No effect was seen in rats given 1.5 times the human maximum daily dose of felbamate on a $mg/m^2$ basis.
FDA Pregnancy Category C.
Labor and delivery—The effect of felbamate on labor and delivery is not known.

**Breast-feeding**
Felbamate is distributed into breast milk. However, the effect on the nursing infant is unknown.

**Pediatrics**
Felbamate has been associated with several deaths due to aplastic anemia and acute liver failure. It is not known whether children are at increased risk for developing these adverse effects. However, children may be less able than adults to articulate symptoms should these effects occur. Felbamate should be used in children only if other medications have failed to control seizures.

**Geriatrics**
Although appropriate studies on the relationship of age to the effects of felbamate have not been performed in the geriatric population, no geriatrics-specific problems have been documented to date. However, elderly patients are more likely to have age-related renal function impairment and other concomitant diseases, and to use other medications, which may require more cautious dosing of felbamate.

**Drug interactions and/or related problems**
The following drug interactions and/or related problems have been selected on the basis of their potential clinical significance (possible mechanism in parentheses where appropriate)—not necessarily inclusive (» = major clinical significance):

Note: Possible interactions with hepatic enzyme inducers, hepatic enzyme inhibitors, and medications that are metabolized by the hepatic P-450 enzyme system, other than those listed below, have not been studied, but the possibility of a significant interaction should be considered and the patient should be carefully monitored during and following concurrent use.

» Carbamazepine
(enzyme induction by carbamazepine may lead to decreased felbamate plasma concentrations; increased felbamate plasma concentrations may occur when carbamazepine dosage is reduced or carbamazepine is discontinued; concurrent use may also decrease carbamazepine plasma concentrations by about 20 to 30% and may increase the plasma concentrations of carbamazepine-10,11-epoxide, an active metabolite of carbamazepine, by about 60%, leading to an increase in adverse effects; carbamazepine dosage should be reduced by 20 to 33% when felbamate therapy is initiated, and plasma concentrations of carbamazepine should be monitored, with further dosage adjustments made as clinically necessary)

Methsuximide
(felbamate may increase plasma concentrations of N-desmethyl-methsuximide, an active metabolite of methsuximide, leading to increased adverse effects; methsuximide dosage should be reduced by 20 to 33% when felbamate therapy is initiated, with further dosage adjustments made as clinically necessary)

Phenobarbital
(felbamate may increase phenobarbital plasma concentrations, leading to increased adverse effects; phenobarbital dosage should be reduced by 20 to 33% when felbamate therapy is initiated, and

plasma phenobarbital concentrations should be monitored, with further dosage adjustments made as clinically necessary)

» Phenytoin
(enzyme induction by phenytoin may lead to decreased felbamate plasma concentrations during concurrent use; increased felbamate plasma concentrations may occur when phenytoin dosage is reduced or phenytoin is discontinued; since both felbamate and phenytoin are hydroxylated by the cytochrome P-450 system, possible competitive inhibition of phenytoin metabolism may result in phenytoin plasma concentrations being increased by 20 to 40%, leading to increased adverse effects; phenytoin dosage should be reduced by 20 to 33% when felbamate therapy is initiated, and plasma concentrations of phenytoin should be monitored, with further dosage adjustments made as necessary to maintain therapeutic plasma concentrations and limit adverse effects)

» Valproic acid
(felbamate may increase valproic acid plasma concentrations by approximately 20 to 40%, leading to increased adverse effects; valproic acid dosage should be reduced by 20 to 33% when felbamate therapy is initiated, and plasma concentrations of valproic acid should be monitored, with further dosage adjustments made as clinically necessary)

### Medical considerations/Contraindications
The medical considerations/contraindications included have been selected on the basis of their potential clinical significance (reasons given in parentheses where appropriate)—not necessarily inclusive (» = major clinical significance).

*Except under special circumstances, this medication should not be used when the following medical problems exist:*

» Blood disorders characterized by serious abnormalities in blood count, platelets, or serum iron or
» Bone marrow depression, or history of or
» Hepatic function impairment or history of
(condition may be exacerbated)

*Risk-benefit should be considered when the following medical problems exist:*

» Hematologic reactions to other medications, history of
(patients may be especially at risk for felbamate-induced bone marrow depression)
» Sensitivity to felbamate or other carbamate derivatives

### Patient monitoring
The following may be especially important in patient monitoring (other tests may be warranted in some patients, depending on condition; » = major clinical significance):

Note: Monitoring may not detect aplastic anemia or liver failure before serious illness has developed; however, early detection of these life-threatening adverse effects may facilitate optimal treatment.

» Hepatic function determinations
(ALT [SGPT], AST [SGOT], and serum bilirubin determinations are recommended prior to initiation of felbamate treatment, and regularly thereafter. Felbamate should be discontinued immediately if any indication of liver injury develops)
» Blood counts, complete (CBCs), including platelet and possibly reticulocyte counts and
» Iron concentrations, serum
(determinations recommended prior to initiation of therapy as a baseline. Patients who develop low or decreased white blood cell or platelet counts during the course of treatment should be monitored closely and felbamate discontinued if there is any evidence of significant bone marrow depression)

## Side/Adverse Effects

Note: There have been reports of deaths due to both aplastic anemia and acute liver failure associated with felbamate use. However, causal relationships have not been definitively established. Appropriate monitoring, including complete blood cell counts, determinations of serum iron concentrations, and liver function tests, should be conducted.

In clinical trials, the frequency of adverse effects was much lower during felbamate monotherapy than during polytherapy with other anticonvulsant medications. The adverse effects seen most frequently during felbamate monotherapy were anorexia, headache, insomnia, and weight loss.

The following side/adverse effects have been selected on the basis of their potential clinical significance (possible signs and symptoms in parentheses where appropriate)—not necessarily inclusive:

### Those indicating need for medical attention
Incidence more frequent
*Fever; gait abnormality* (walking in unusual manner); *purpura* (purple or red spots on skin)
Incidence less frequent
*CNS toxicity, specifically agitation, aggression or other mood or mental changes, ataxia* (clumsiness or unsteadiness); *or tremor* (trembling or shaking); *skin rash*
Incidence rare
*Anaphylactoid reaction* (nasal congestion; shortness of breath or troubled breathing; skin rash, hives or itching; swelling of face); *blood dyscrasias, including agranulocytosis* (chills; fever; sore throat; general feeling of tiredness or weakness); *aplastic anemia* (shortness of breath, troubled breathing, wheezing, or tightness in chest; sores, ulcers, or white spots on lips or in mouth; swollen or painful glands; unusual bleeding or bruising); *leukopenia* (chills; fever; sore throat); *pancytopenia* (nosebleeds or other unusual bleeding or bruising); *thrombocytopenia* (unusual bleeding or bruising; black, tarry stools; blood in urine or stools; pinpoint red spots on skin); *or qualitative platelet disorder* (unusual bruising or bleeding; black or tarry stools); *bone marrow depression* (chills; fever; sore throat; unusual bleeding or bruising); *liver failure, acute* (continuing headache; continuing stomach pain; continuing vomiting; dark-colored urine; general feeling of tiredness or weakness; light-colored stools; yellow eyes or skin); *lymphadenopathy* (swollen lymph nodes); *photosensitivity* (sensitivity of skin to sunlight); *psychosis* (severe mood or mental changes); *Stevens-Johnson syndrome* (skin rash or itching; sores or white spots on lips or in mouth; sore throat; fever; chills; muscle cramps; pain; weakness; chest pain)

Note: *Thrombocytopenia* is usually asymptomatic; rarely, symptoms are present.

### Those indicating need for medical attention only if they continue or are bothersome
Incidence more frequent
*Dizziness; gastrointestinal effects, specifically abdominal pain* (stomach pain); *anorexia* (loss of appetite); *constipation; dyspepsia* (indigestion); *nausea or vomiting; headache; insomnia* (trouble in sleeping); *taste perversion* (change in sense of taste)
Incidence less frequent
*Anxiety; diarrhea; drowsiness; nervousness; rhinitis* (runny nose); *upper respiratory tract infection* (coughing; ear congestion or pain; fever; head congestion; nasal congestion; runny nose; sneezing; sore throat); *vision abnormalities, including blurred vision and diplopia* (double vision); *weight loss*

## Overdose
For information on the management of overdose or unintentional ingestion, **contact a Poison Control Center** (see *Poison Control Center Listing*).

### Clinical effects of overdose
Experience with felbamate overdose is limited. One patient who ingested 12 grams of felbamate over 12 hours experienced mild gastric distress and a resting heart rate of 100 beats per minute.

### Treatment of overdose
There is no specific antidote for felbamate overdose. Recommended treatment includes:

To decrease absorption—Emesis or gastric lavage.

Supportive care—Patients in whom intentional overdose is confirmed or suspected should be referred for psychiatric consultation.

## Patient Consultation
As an aid to patient consultation, refer to *Advice for the Patient, Felbamate (Systemic)*.

In providing consultation, consider emphasizing the following selected information (» = major clinical significance):

### Before using this medication
» Conditions affecting use, especially:
Sensitivity to felbamate or to other carbamate derivatives
Pregnancy—Crosses the placenta in rats. Animal studies using up to 3 times the maximum human dose in mg/m$^2$ have shown decreased rat pup weight and decreased survival; clinical significance is unknown
Breast-feeding—Distributed into breast milk
Use in children—Children may be unable to articulate symptoms of aplastic anemia or acute liver failure; use only if other medications have failed to control seizures
Other medications, especially carbamazepine, phenytoin, and valproic acid
Other medical problems, especially blood disorders, bone marrow depression, or hepatic function impairment

**Proper use of this medication**
» Compliance with therapy; not taking more or less medicine than prescribed
Proper administration for liquid dosage form: Shaking well; using an accurate measuring device, such as a specially marked measuring spoon, a plastic syringe, or a small graduated cup
» Proper dosing
Missed dose: Taking as soon as possible; if almost time for next dose, skipping missed dose and going back to regular dosing schedule; not doubling doses
» Proper storage

**Precautions while using this medication**
» Regular visits to physician to check progress of therapy and to monitor for severe adverse effects
» Not discontinuing felbamate abruptly; consulting physician about gradually reducing dosage
» Possible dizziness, drowsiness, impairment of judgment, thinking, or motor skills; caution when driving or doing jobs requiring alertness

**Side/adverse effects**
Fever; gait abnormality; purpura; CNS toxicity, specifically agitation, aggression, or other mood or mental changes, ataxia, tremor; skin rash; anaphylactoid reaction; blood dyscrasias, including agranulocytosis, aplastic anemia, leukopenia, pancytopenia, thrombocytopenia, qualitative platelet disorder; bone marrow depression; liver failure, acute; lymphadenopathy; photosensitivity; psychosis; Stevens-Johnson syndrome

## General Dosing Information

Most adverse effects that emerge when adding felbamate to an anticonvulsant regimen resolve as dosages of concomitant anticonvulsant medications are reduced.

Adverse gastrointestinal effects may be reduced by taking felbamate after meals. If nausea persists, felbamate dosage may be decreased until tolerance to the gastrointestinal effects develops.

Neither felbamate nor other anticonvulsant medications should be suddenly discontinued because of the possibility of increased seizure frequency. The dosage should be reduced gradually when an anticonvulsant medication is being withdrawn.

**For treatment of adverse effects**
Treatment of bone marrow depression includes the following:
• Discontinuing felbamate therapy.
• Daily CBC, platelet and reticulocyte counts.
• Performing a bone marrow aspiration and trephine biopsy immediately and repeating with sufficient frequency to monitor recovery.
• Considering other studies that may be helpful, including white cell and platelet antibodies; [59]Fe—ferrokinetic studies; peripheral blood cell typing; cytogenic studies on marrow and peripheral blood; bone marrow culture studies for colony-forming units; hemoglobin electrophoresis for A[2] and F hemoglobin; and serum folic acid and B$_{12}$ concentrations. If aplastic anemia develops, specialized consultation should be sought for appropriate monitoring and treatment.

## Oral Dosage Forms

### FELBAMATE ORAL SUSPENSION

**Usual adult and adolescent dose**
Anticonvulsant—
Oral, initially 1200 mg per day, usually divided into three or four doses, the dosage being gradually increased over several weeks based on clinical response.

**Usual adult and adolescent prescribing limits**
3600 mg per day.

**Usual pediatric dose**
Anticonvulsant—
Children 2 to 14 years of age: Oral, initially 15 mg per kg of body weight per day, usually divided into three or four doses, the dosage being gradually increased over a few weeks based on clinical response.

**Usual pediatric prescribing limits**
Children 2 to 14 years of age—45 mg per kg per day or 3600 mg per day, whichever is less.

**Strength(s) usually available**
U.S.—
600 mg per 5 mL (Rx) [*Felbatol* (sorbitol; glycerin; microcrystalline cellulose; carboxymethylcellulose sodium; simethicone; polysorbate 80; methylparaben; saccharin sodium; propylparaben; FD&C Yellow No. 6; FD&C Red No. 40; flavorings; purified water)].
Canada—
Not commercially available.

**Packaging and storage**
Store below 40 °C (104 °F), preferably between 15 and 30 °C (59 and 86 °F), in a tight container, unless otherwise specified by manufacturer.

**Auxiliary labeling**
• Shake well before using.
• May cause dizziness or drowsiness.

**Additional information**
Use a specially marked measuring spoon, a plastic syringe, or a small marked measuring cup to measure each dose accurately.

### FELBAMATE TABLETS

**Usual adult and adolescent dose**
See *Felbamate Oral Suspension*.

**Usual adult and adolescent prescribing limits**
See *Felbamate Oral Suspension*.

**Usual pediatric dose**
See *Felbamate Oral Suspension*.

**Usual pediatric prescribing limits**
See *Felbamate Oral Suspension*.

**Strength(s) usually available**
U.S.—
400 mg (Rx) [*Felbatol* (scored; starch; microcrystalline cellulose; croscarmellose sodium; lactose; magnef rm stearate; FD&C Yellow No. 6; D&C Yellow No. 10)].
600 mg (Rx) [*Felbatol* (scored; starch; microcrystalline cellulose; croscarmellose sodium; lactose; magnesium stearate; FD&C Yellow No. 6; D&C Yellow No. 10; FD&C Red No. 40)].
Canada—
Not commercially available.

**Packaging and storage**
Store below 40 °C (104 °F), preferably between 15 and 30 °C (59 and 86 °F), in a tight container, away from moisture, unless otherwise specified by manufacturer.

**Auxiliary labeling**
• May cause dizziness or drowsiness.

## Selected Bibliography

Palmer KJ, McTavish D. Felbamate: A review of its pharmacodynamic and pharmacokinetic properties, and therapeutic efficacy in epilepsy. Drugs 1993; 45(6): 1041-65.
Graves NM. Felbamate. Ann Pharmacother 1993 Sep; 27: 1073-81.

Developed: 08/30/94
Interim revision: 10/06/94; 03/28/95

---

**FELODIPINE**—See *Calcium Channel Blocking Agents (Systemic)*

---

**FENFLURAMINE**—See *Appetite Suppressants (Systemic)*

---

# FENOFIBRATE  Systemic—INTRODUCTORY VERSION

VA CLASSIFICATION (Primary): CV603
Commonly used brand name(s): *Tricor*.
Note: For a listing of dosage forms and brand names by country availability, see *Dosage Forms* section(s).

## Category

Antihyperlipidemic.

# Indications

## Accepted

**Hyperlipidemia (treatment)**—Fenofibrate is indicated as an adjunct to diet for the treatment of adult patients with very high serum triglyceride concentrations (types IV and V hyperlipidemia) who have not responded adequately to diet and who are at risk of pancreatitis. A risk of pancreatitis is associated with a serum triglyceride concentration of over 2000 mg per dL and increases in very low–density lipoprotein (VLDL) cholesterol, as well as with fasting chylomicron (type V hyperlipidemia) concentrations. A total serum or plasma triglyceride concentration below 1000 mg per dL is not associated with a risk of pancreatitis. Fenofibrate therapy may be considered for those subjects with triglyceride concentrations between 1000 and 2000 mg per dL who have a history of pancreatitis or of recurrent abdominal pain typical of pancreatitis. Fenofibrate has not been adequately studied to decrease the risk of pancreatitis in patients with a type IV lipoprotein pattern, with triglyceride concentrations below 1000 mg per dL, who (through dietary indiscretion or alcohol consumption) convert to a type V lipoprotein pattern with large triglyceride concentrations accompanied by fasting chylomicronemia.

For additional information on initial therapeutic guidelines related to the treatment of hyperlipidemia, see *Appendix III*.

The effect of fenofibrate on coronary heart disease morbidity and mortality and noncardiovascular mortality has not been established. Because fenofibrate has chemical, pharmacologic, and clinical similarities to the other fibrate drugs, clofibrate and gemfibrozil, the adverse findings in four large randomized, placebo-controlled clinical studies with these drugs may also apply to fenofibrate. In one clofibrate study, there was no difference in mortality between the clofibrate-treated subjects and the placebo-treated subjects, but twice as many clofibrate-treated subjects developed cholelithiasis and cholecystitis requiring surgery. Another clofibrate study resulted in a 44% higher age-adjusted total mortality in the clofibrate-treated group than in a comparable placebo-treated group. The higher mortality rate was attributed to a 33% increase in noncardiovascular causes, including malignancy, postcholecystectomy complications, and pancreatitis. A third study with gemfibrozil resulted in a 22% higher total mortality, primarily due to a higher cancer mortality, in the gemfibrozil-treated group, while cancers (excluding basal cell carcinoma) were diagnosed in 2.5% of patients in both gemfibrozil- and placebo-treated patients. In a fourth study with gemfibrozil, cardiac deaths tended to be higher and gallbladder surgery and appendectomy were more frequent in the gemfibrozil-treated group than in the placebo-treated group.

## Unaccepted

Fenofibrate is not indicated for the treatment of either primary or secondary hyperlipoproteinemia as a form of prevention to reduce the risk of developing coronary heart disease.

# Pharmacology/Pharmacokinetics

## Physicochemical characteristics

Molecular weight—360.83.

## Mechanism of action/Effect

Fenofibrate is a lipid-regulating agent that has chemical, pharmacologic, and clinical similarities to the other fibrate drugs, clofibrate and gemfibrozil. Although the exact mechanism of action of fenofibrate is not completely understood, fenofibric acid, the active metabolite of fenofibrate, is thought to lower plasma triglyceride concentrations by inhibiting triglyceride synthesis (resulting in a lower level of very low-density lipoproteins [VLDL] released into the circulation) and by stimulating the catabolism of triglyceride-rich lipoproteins (i.e., VLDL). In clinical trials, patients with hypertriglyceridemia and normal cholesterolemia, with or without hyperchylomicronemia (type IV or V hyperlipidemia), treated with doses of 201 mg of fenofibrate per day had decreases in VLDL triglycerides and VLDL cholesterol. Treatment of patients with type IV hyperlipoproteinemia and elevated triglyceride concentrations often results in an increase in low-density lipoprotein (LDL) cholesterol.

## Other actions/effects

Fenofibrate reduces serum uric acid concentrations in hyperuricemic and normal individuals by increasing the urinary excretion of uric acid.

## Absorption

Fenofibrate is well absorbed from the gastrointestinal tract. Absorption of the micronized form of fenofibrate is increased by approximately 35% when administered with food, as compared with that in the fasting state.

## Distribution

Volume of distribution (Vol$_D$)—30 L.

## Protein binding

Very high (approximately 99% in normal and hyperlipidemic individuals).

## Biotransformation

Fenofibrate undergoes rapid metabolism by esterase hydrolysis and is converted to the active metabolite, fenofibric acid. Fenofibric acid undergoes conjugation with glucuronic acid and is excreted in urine. A small amount of fenofibric acid undergoes reduction at the carbonyl moiety, resulting in a benzhydrol metabolite which is then conjugated with glucuronic acid and excreted in urine.

## Half-life

Elimination—
  20 hours.

## Time to peak concentration

6 to 8 hours.

## Elimination

Renal—60%, primarily as fenofibric acid and fenofibric acid glucuronide.
Fecal—25%.
  *In dialysis*—
    Hemodialysis is not expected to remove fenofibrate significantly because of its extensive binding to plasma proteins.

# Precautions to Consider

## Cross-sensitivity and/or related problems

Fenofibrate has chemical, pharmacological, and clinical similarities to the other fibrate agents, clofibrate and gemfibrozil.

## Carcinogenicity

A 24-month study in rats, given fenofibrate doses of 10, 45, and 200 mg per kg of body weight (mg/kg), resulted in a significant increase in the incidence of liver carcinomas in both male and female rats given the 200-mg/kg dose. These doses represent 0.3, 1, and 6 times the maximum recommended human dose (MRHD) of fenofibrate, respectively, on a mg per square meter of body surface area (mg/m$^2$) basis. A significant increase in pancreatic carcinomas occurred in male rats given the 45- and 200-mg/kg doses of fenofibrate and increases in pancreatic adenomas and benign testicular interstitial cell tumors occurred in male rats given the 200-mg/kg fenofibrate dose. In a second 24-month study in a different strain of rats given fenofibrate in doses of 10 mg/kg and 60 mg/kg, significant increases in the incidence of pancreatic acinar adenomas occurred in both sexes and increases in interstitial cell tumors of the testes occurred in rats given the 60-mg/kg dose of fenofibrate. These doses represent 0.3 and 2 times the MRHD of fenofibrate, respectively, on a mg/m$^2$ basis.

A comparative carcinogenicity study was done in rats comparing three drugs: fenofibrate, given in doses of 10 mg/kg and 70 mg/kg or 0.3 and 1.6 times the MRHD of fenofibrate on a mg/m$^2$ basis; clofibrate, given in doses of 400 mg/kg or 1.6 times the MRHD of clofibrate on a mg/m$^2$ basis; and gemfibrozil, given in doses of 250 mg/kg or 1.7 times the MRHD of gemfibrozil on a mg/m$^2$ basis. An increased incidence of pancreatic acinar adenomas was observed in male and female rats given fenofibrate. An increase in hepatocellular carcinoma and pancreatic acinar adenomas occurred in male rats, and hepatic neoplastic nodules occurred in female rats given clofibrate; hepatic neoplastic nodules were increased in male and female rats given gemfibrozil, while an increase in testicular interstitial cell tumors occurred in male rats given all three drugs.

In a 21-month study in mice given fenofibrate in doses of 10, 45, and 200 mg/kg, significant increases in liver carcinoma occurred in both male and female mice given the 200-mg/kg dose of fenofibrate. These doses represent approximately 0.2, 0.7, and 3 times the MRHD of fenofibrate on a mg/m$^2$ basis, respectively. In a second 18-month study in mice given the same doses of fenofibrate, a significant increase in liver carcinoma in male mice and liver adenoma in female mice occurred when they were given the 200-mg/kg dose of fenofibrate.

Peroxisomal proliferation, as determined by electron microscopy studies, has occurred following administration of fenofibrate to rats. An adequate study to test for peroxisome proliferation in humans has not been done, but a comparison of liver biopsies before and after treatment of human subjects with other members of the fibrate class of medications has revealed changes in peroxisome morphology and numbers after treatment.

## Mutagenicity

Fenofibrate was not found to be mutagenic in the Ames test and mouse lymphoma, chromosomal aberration, and unscheduled DNA synthesis tests.

## Pregnancy/Reproduction

Pregnancy—Adequate and well-controlled studies in pregnant women have not been done. Fenofibrate should be used during pregnancy only if the potential benefit justifies the potential risk to the fetus. Fenofibrate has been shown to be embryocidal and teratogenic in rats given 7 to 10 times the MRHD of fenofibrate on a mg/m² basis, and embryocidal in rabbits given 9 times the MRHD of fenofibrate on a mg/m² basis.

A study in female rats given 9 times the MRHD of fenofibrate before and throughout gestation resulted in a delay of delivery in 100% of dams, a 60% increase in post implantation loss, a decrease in litter size, a decrease in birth weight, a 40% survival of pups at birth, a 4% survival of pups as neonates, a 0% survival of pups to weaning, and an increased occurrence of spina bifida. A study in female rats given 10 times the MRHD of fenofibrate on days 6 through 15 of gestation resulted in an increase in gross, visceral, and skeletal findings in fetuses, manifested as a domed head, hunched shoulders, a rounded body, an abnormal chest, kyphosis, stunted fetuses, elongated sternal ribs, malformed sternebrae, extra foramen in palatine, misshapen vertebrae, and supernumerary ribs.

A study in female rats given 7 times the MRHD of fenofibrate from day 15 of gestation through weaning resulted in a delay in delivery, a 40% decrease in live births, a 75% decrease in neonatal survival, and decreases in pup weight at birth, as well as on days 4 and 21 post partum. A study of fenofibrate in female rabbits resulted in abortions in 10% of dams given 9 times and 25% of dams given 18 times the MRHD of fenofibrate, and death of 7% of fetuses given 18 times the MRHD of fenofibrate.

FDA Pregnancy Category C.

**Breast-feeding**
Because of the potential for tumorigenicity as seen in animal studies, fenofibrate should not be used in women who are breast-feeding. A decision should be made whether to discontinue nursing or to discontinue fenofibrate.

**Pediatrics**
No information is available on the relationship of age to the effects of fenofibrate in pediatric patients. Safety and efficacy have not been established.

**Geriatrics**
Clearance of fenofibric acid following a single oral dose of fenofibrate in elderly volunteers, ages 77 through 87 years, was 1.2 L per hour (L/hr), compared to 1.1 L/hr in younger adults, indicating that a similar dosage regimen can be used in the elderly without resulting in an increase in accumulation of fenofibrate or its metabolites.

**Pharmacogenetics**
Fenofibrate is not metabolized by enzymes known for exhibiting interethnic variability, therefore, interethnic pharmacokinetic differences are not expected. Pharmacokinetic differences have not been observed between male and female individuals administered fenofibrate.

**Drug interactions and/or related problems**
The following drug interactions and/or related problems have been selected on the basis of their potential clinical significance (possible mechanism in parentheses where appropriate)—not necessarily inclusive (» = major clinical significance):

Note: Combinations containing any of the following medications, depending on the amount present, may also interact with this medication.

» Anticoagulants, oral
(concurrent use with fenofibrate may potentiate coumarin-type anticoagulant prolongation of prothrombin time; the dosage of the anticoagulant should be reduced to maintain the prothrombin time at the desired level in order to prevent bleeding complications)

Bile acid sequestrants, such as:
Cholestyramine or
Colestipol
(concurrent use with these agents may bind fenofibrate; in order to avoid interfering with the absorption of fenofibrate, it should be taken at least 1 hour before or 4 to 6 hours after taking a bile acid binding agent)

» Cyclosporine
(because fenofibrate is primarily eliminated by renal excretion and cyclosporine when used alone is potentially nephrotoxic, causing decreases in creatinine clearance and increases in serum creatinine concentrations, concurrent use of these agents may potentiate renal function deterioration; concurrent use of fenofibrate with immunosuppressants and other potentially nephrotoxic agents should be carefully considered, and the lowest effective dose should be used)

» HMG-CoA reductase inhibitors, such as:
Lovastatin or
Pravastatin or
Simvastatin
(although no data exists on the concurrent use of these agents with fenofibrate, concurrent use of gemfibrozil, another fibrate agent, with lovastatin has been associated with rhabdomyolysis, significantly increased creatine kinase [CK] concentrations, and myoglobinuria, resulting in a high percentage of acute renal failure cases; because the potential benefits of combined therapy do not outweigh the risks of severe myopathy, rhabdomyolysis, and acute renal failure, and because the use of fibrates alone, including fenofibrate, may occasionally be associated with myositis, myopathy, or rhabdomyolysis, their concurrent use with HMG-CoA reductase inhibitors is not recommended)

**Laboratory value alterations**
The following have been selected on the basis of their potential clinical significance (possible effect in parentheses where appropriate)—not necessarily inclusive (» = major clinical significance):

With physiology/laboratory test values
Creatine kinase (CK), serum
(myopathy should be considered in patients with marked elevations of CK concentrations accompanied by diffuse myalgias, muscle tenderness or weakness)

Hematocrit and
Hemoglobin concentrations and
Leukocyte counts
(mild to moderate decreases in hemoglobin and hematocrit concentrations, and leukocyte counts have occurred; however, these values stabilize with continued use of fenofibrate)

Aspartate aminotransferase (AST [SGOT]), serum and/or
Alanine aminotransferase (ALT [SGPT]), serum
(in an 8-week dose-ranging study, increases in serum transaminase values to at least 3 times the upper limit of normal occurred in 13% of patients receiving fenofibrate in doses equivalent to 134 or 201 mg of fenofibrate per day and occurred in 0% of patients receiving doses equivalent to 33.5 or 67 mg per day, or placebo; in two U.S. placebo-controlled studies, serum transaminase values increased to > 3 times the upper limit of normal in 8 to 10% of patients taking fenofibrate in doses equivalent to 201 mg of fenofibrate per day; in controlled multiple-dose trials lasting 3 to 24 weeks, increases in serum transaminase values to > 3 times the upper limit of normal occurred in 28 of 442 patients [6.3%] taking fenofibrate in doses equivalent to 134 or 201 mg per day; in the latter trial, in the patients whose serum transaminase values were followed, values usually returned to normal limits either with continued treatment or after discontinuation of treatment; however, values remained above normal limits in 2 of the 28 patients [7.1%] at the end of follow-up of treatment)

Uric acid, serum
(concentrations may be decreased; fenofibrate reduces serum uric acid concentrations in hyperuricemic and normal individuals by increasing the urinary excretion of uric acid)

**Medical considerations/Contraindications**
The medical considerations/contraindications included have been selected on the basis of their potential clinical significance (reasons given in parentheses where appropriate)—not necessarily inclusive (» = major clinical significance).

*Except under special circumstances, this medication should not be used when the following medical problems exist:*

» Gallbladder disease, pre-existing
(use of fibrate agents, such as fenofibrate, has been associated with cholelithiasis and, therefore, is contraindicated in patients with pre-existing gallbladder disease)

» Hepatic function impairment, including primary biliary cirrhosis and unexplained persistent liver function abnormality
(use of fenofibrate has been associated with hepatotoxicity, which may further aggravate these conditions)

» Hypersensitivity to fenofibrate

» Renal function impairment, severe
(the rate of clearance of fenofibric acid may be significantly reduced in patients with severe renal function impairment [creatinine clearance < 50 mL per minute (mL/min)], resulting in the medication's accumulation during chronic dosing; use of fibrate agents, such as fenofibrate, has been associated with rhabdomyolysis in patients with impaired renal function)

*Risk-benefit should be considered when the following medical problem exists:*

Renal function impairment, moderate
(in patients having moderate renal function impairment [creatinine clearance of 50 to 90 mL/min], clearance and volume of distribution of fenofibric acid are increased when compared to healthy adults [2.1 L/hr and 95 L versus 1.1 L/hr and 30 L, respectively]; however,

no modification of dosage is required in patients having moderate renal function impairment; use of fibrate agents, such as fenofibrate, has been associated with rhabdomyolysis in patients with impaired renal function)

**Patient monitoring**

The following may be especially important in patient monitoring (other tests may be warranted in some patients, depending on condition; » = major clinical significance):

Creatine kinase (CK), serum
(CK concentrations should be monitored in patients with symptoms of unexplained muscle pain, tenderness, or weakness, particularly if accompanied by malaise or fever; if marked CK concentrations occur, fenofibrate therapy should be discontinued)

Hematocrit
Hemoglobin concentrations and
Leukocyte counts
(periodic monitoring of blood counts are recommended during the first 12 months of fenofibrate therapy)

» Hepatic function determinations, such as:
Alanine aminotransferase (ALT [SGPT]), serum and
Aspartate aminotransferase (AST [SGOT]), serum
(regular periodic monitoring should be performed for the duration of fenofibrate therapy; fenofibrate should be discontinued if serum transaminase values of > 3 times the upper limit of normal persist)

» Lipid concentrations, serum
(periodic monitoring should be done during initiation of therapy in order to establish the lowest effective dose of fenofibrate; fenofibrate should be discontinued in patients who do not have an adequate response after 2 months of treatment with the maximum recommended dose [201 mg per day])

## Side/Adverse Effects

The following side/adverse effects have been selected on the basis of their potential clinical significance (possible signs and symptoms in parentheses where appropriate)—not necessarily inclusive:

**Those indicating need for medical attention**
Incidence less frequent
*Influenza syndrome* (chills, fever, muscle aches and pains, or nausea and/or vomiting); *infections; pruritus* (generalized itching); *skin rash and/or urticaria* (hives)

Note: In clinical trials, *skin rash* was the most frequent side effect, requiring discontinuation of fenofibrate treatment in 2% of patients. Acute hypersensitivity reactions, including severe skin rashes requiring patient hospitalization and treatment with steroids, have occurred very rarely during treatment with fenofibrate. *Urticaria* was seen in 1.25% versus 0% and rash in 2.82% versus 1.23% of fenofibrate-treated and placebo-treated patients, respectively, in controlled trials.

Incidence rare
*Agranulocytosis* (chills; fever; sore throat); *alveolitis, allergic* (cough; shortness of breath or troubled breathing); *cholecystitis* (abdominal pain, vague; indigestion, chronic; nausea); *cholelithiasis* (abdominal fullness, gaseous; abdominal pain, recurrent; fever; yellow eyes or skin); *eczema; hepatotoxicity* (abdominal fullness; dark urine; fever; general ill feeling; generalized itching; loss of appetite; unusual fatigue; yellow eyes or skin); *musculoskeletal symptoms, such as myalgia* (muscle pain); *myasthenia* (muscle weakness); *myositis* (inflammation or swelling of skeletal muscle); *and/or rhabdomyolysis* (fever; muscle cramps, pain, stiffness, or weakness; unusual tiredness); *pancreatitis* (abdominal pain and distention; fever; nausea; vomiting); *thrombocytopenia* (unusual bleeding or bruising)

Note: Rare cases of *agranulocytosis* and *thrombocytopenia* have been reported during postmarketing surveillance outside of the U.S.

Fenofibrate, like clofibrate and gemfibrozil, may increase cholesterol excretion into the bile, leading to *cholelithiasis*. A gallstone prevalence sub-study of a placebo-controlled trial with gemfibrozil revealed a trend toward a greater prevalence of gallstones in gemfibrozil-treated patients. If cholelithiasis is suspected, gallbladder studies should be performed and fenofibrate should be discontinued if gallstones are found.

*Hepatotoxicity* associated with fenofibrate therapy appears to be dose-related. Hepatocellular, chronic active, and cholestatic hepatitis have been reported after weeks to several years of exposure to fenofibrate. Rarely, cirrhosis has been reported in association with chronic active hepatitis.

Treatment with fibrate agents, such as fenofibrate, may occasionally be associated with *myositis*. Rhabdomyolysis has also been associated rarely with this class of agents, usually in patients with impaired renal function. Degradation of muscle occurs in rhabdomyolysis, resulting in the release of myoglobin into the urine, which can lead to acute renal failure. *Myopathy* and/or rhabdomyolysis should be considered in any patient with diffuse *myalgias*, muscle tenderness or weakness, and/or marked elevations of creatine kinase (CK) in serum. Patients receiving fenofibrate and complaining of muscle pain, tenderness, or weakness, especially if accompanied by malaise or fever, should have a prompt medical evaluation for myopathy, including serum CK determinations. If myopathy or myositis is suspected or diagnosed, or if serum CK concentrations are significantly elevated, fenofibrate therapy should be discontinued.

*Pancreatitis* has been reported in patients taking fenofibrate, gemfibrozil, and clofibrate and may be associated with a failure in fenofibrate efficacy or a blockage of the common bile duct by biliary tract stone or sludge formation.

**Those indicating need for medical attention only if they continue or are bothersome**
Incidence less frequent
*Dizziness; eye irritation; gastrointestinal symptoms, such as belching; constipation; flatulence* (gas); *libido, decreased; photosensitivity* (increased sensitivity of the skin to sunlight); *rhinitis* (stuffy nose)

## Overdose

For more information on the management of overdose or unintentional ingestion, **contact a Poison Control Center** (see *Poison Control Center Listing*).

**Treatment of overdose**

Treatment should be symptomatic and supportive.

Specific treatment—Hemodialysis should not be considered in the treatment of fenofibrate overdosage because fenofibrate is extensively bound to plasma proteins.

Supportive care—Patients in whom intentional overdose is confirmed or suspected should be referred for psychiatric consultation.

## Patient Consultation

As an aid to patient consultation, refer to *Advice for the Patient, Fenofibrate (Systemic)—Introductory Version*.

In providing consultation, consider emphasizing the following selected information (» = major clinical significance):

**Before using this medication**
» Conditions affecting use, especially:
Hypersensitivity to fenofibrate
Carcinogenicity—Liver carcinomas and pancreatic acinar adenomas have occurred in rats given long-term, high doses of fenofibrate
Pregnancy—Not recommended during pregnancy unless potential benefit outweighs the risk
Breast-feeding—Not recommended in women who are breast-feeding
Other medications, especially oral anticoagulants, cyclosporine, or HMG-CoA reductase inhibitors
Other medical problems, especially pre-existing gallbladder disease; hepatic function impairment, including primary biliary cirrhosis and unexplained persistent liver function abnormality; or severe renal function impairment

**Proper use of this medication**
» Compliance with therapy; taking medication at the same time each day to maintain the therapeutic effect; not taking more or less medication than the amount prescribed
» Compliance with prescribed diet during treatment
Taking medication with a meal to increase its bioavailability
» Proper dosing
Missed dose: Taking as soon as possible; not taking if almost time for next dose; not doubling doses
» Proper storage

**Precautions while using this medication**
» Regular visits to physician to check progress
» Notifying physician immediately if unexplained muscle pain, tenderness, or weakness occurs, especially if accompanied by unusual tiredness or fever
Notifying physician if pregnancy is suspected
Reporting any signs of infection (fever, sore throat, chills) to physician because of risk of agranulocytosis

### Side/adverse effects
Signs of potential side effects, especially influenza-like syndrome; infections; pruritus; skin rash and/or urticaria; agranulocytosis; allergic alveolitis; cholecystitis; cholelithiasis; eczema; hepatotoxicity; musculoskeletal symptoms, such as myalgia, myasthenia, myositis, and/or rhabdomyolysis; pancreatitis; and thrombocytopenia

### General Dosing Information
Prior to any drug therapy, an attempt should be made to treat hyperlipidemia with nondrug methods, such as dietary therapy specific for the type of lipoprotein abnormality, reduction of excess body weight, reduction of excess alcohol intake, and physical exercise. Secondary causes of hyperlipidemia, such as hypothyroidism or diabetes mellitus, should be ruled out or adequately treated. Treatment with estrogens, thiazide diuretics, and beta-adrenergic blocking agents may contribute to increases in plasma triglyceride levels, especially in individuals with familial hypertriglyceridemia. In such cases, the medication should be changed or discontinued if it is considered medically appropriate to do so. The use of lipid-lowering agents should be considered only when satisfactory results have not been obtained from using nondrug methods.

### Diet/Nutrition
Patients should be placed on an appropriate triglyceride-lowering diet before receiving fenofibrate and should continue this diet during treatment with fenofibrate.

Fenofibrate should be given with a meal to optimize the bioavailability of the medication.

### Oral Dosage Forms

#### FENOFIBRATE CAPSULES (MICRONIZED)

**Usual adult dose**
Antihyperlipidemic—
Oral, initially, 67 mg per day, depending on the physician's assessment of the patient's risk for pancreatitis. Dosage should be individualized according to patient response, and should be increased sequentially, if necessary, following repeat serum triglyceride estimations at 4- to 8-week intervals. Fenofibrate should be discontinued in patients who do not have an adequate response after two months of treatment with the maximum recommended dose (201 mg per day).

In patients with impaired renal function, treatment should be initiated at a dose of 67 mg per day and increased only after the effects of fenofibrate on renal function and triglyceride concentrations have been evaluated.

**Usual adult prescribing limits**
201 mg per day.

**Usual pediatric dose**
Safety and efficacy have not been established.

**Usual geriatric dose**
Antihyperlipidemic—
Oral, initially, 67 mg per day. See *Usual adult dose*.

**Strength(s) usually available**
U.S.—
67 mg (Rx) [*Tricor* (lactose; pregelatinized starch; sodium lauryl sulfate; crospovidone; magnesium stearate)].

**Packaging and storage**
Store at controlled room temperature, between 15 and 30 °C (59 and 86 °F). Protect from moisture.

**Auxiliary labeling**
• Take with a meal.

---

Developed: 05/18/98

---

# FENOLDOPAM Systemic—INTRODUCTORY VERSION

VA CLASSIFICATION (Primary/Secondary): CV402/CV500
Commonly used brand name(s): *Corlopam*.
Note: For a listing of dosage forms and brand names by country availability, see *Dosage Forms* section(s).

## Category
Antihypertensive.

## Indications

### Accepted
Hypertension (treatment)—Fenoldopam is indicated for the in-hospital, short-term (up to 48 hours) management of severe hypertension (including malignant hypertension with deteriorating end-organ function) when rapid, but quickly reversible, emergency reduction of blood pressure is clinically indicated. Transition to orally administered antihypertensive therapy can begin at any time after blood pressure is stable during infusion of fenoldopam.

## Pharmacology/Pharmacokinetics

**Physicochemical characteristics**
Molecular weight—401.87.

**Mechanism of action/Effect**
Fenoldopam is a rapid-acting vasodilator with agonist effects on dopamine $D_1$-like receptors, and only moderate affinity for the $alpha_2$-adrenergic receptors. Fenoldopam is a racemic mixture, with the R-isomer having an approximate 250-fold higher affinity for $D_1$-like receptors than the S-isomer. Fenoldopam has no agonist effect on presynaptic $D_2$-like dopamine receptors or on alpha- or beta-adrenergic receptors, and does not appear to affect angiotensin-converting enzyme activity. In animals, fenoldopam dilates coronary, renal, mesenteric, and peripheral arteries, although vasodilation is not equal in all vascular beds. In normal and hypertensive patients, fenoldopam appears to dilate renal efferent and afferent arterioles, thereby increasing renal blood flow; however, a beneficial clinical effect on renal fuction in patients with heart failure or hepatic or severe renal disease has not been demonstrated.

**Other actions/effects**
Fenoldopam may increase norepinephrine plasma concentrations.

**Distribution**
Steady-state plasma concentrations of intravenous fenoldopam are proportional to the infusion rates when fenoldopam is administered at a constant infusion rate ranging from 0.01 to 1.6 mcg per kg of body weight (mcg/kg) per minute. In rats, approximately 0.005% of a fenoldopam dose crosses the blood-brain barrier.

**Biotransformation**
Metabolism of fenoldopam is by conjugation and does not involve cytochrome P450 enzymes. Methylation, glucuronidation, and sulfation are the main routes of conjugation. The resulting metabolites are considered to be inactive. Approximately 4% of a fenoldopam dose is eliminated as unchanged drug.

**Half-life**
Elimination—
Approximately 5 minutes in patients with mild to moderate hypertension.

**Elimination**
Renal—Approximately 90%.
Fecal—Approximately 10%.
In dialysis—
In patients with end-stage renal disease, continuous ambulatory peritoneal dialysis does not affect the clearance of fenoldopam. It is not known if fenoldopam is removable by hemodialysis.

## Precautions to Consider

### Carcinogenicity
No increase in the incidence of neoplasms was found in a 2-year study in mice given daily oral fenoldopam doses of 12.5, 25, or 50 mg per kg of body weight (mg/kg) for the first 208 days of the study and then given oral daily fenoldopam doses of 25 mg/kg for the remainder of study. An increased incidence and degree of severity of a fibro-osseous lesion of the sternum occurred in female mice in the highest-dose group. A higher incidence and degree of severity of chronic nephritis occurred in female mice in the middle- and upper-dose groups. These pathologic findings did not occur in male mice treated with fenoldopam.

In rats, no increase in the incidence or type of neoplasms was found in a 2-year study that used daily oral fenoldopam doses of 5, 10, or 20 mg/kg for the first 371 days of the study and then increased the doses of the mid- and high-dose groups to daily fenoldopam doses of 15 or 25 mg/kg, respectively, thereafter. A higher incidence of hyperplasia of collecting duct epithelium at the tip of the renal papilla occurred in rats in the mid- and high-dose groups.

**Mutagenicity**
Mutagenicity was not detected in the *in vitro* Ames test or Chinese hamster ovary (CHO) cell assay. Fenoldopam was associated with statistically significant and dose-dependent increases in chromosomal aberrations and in the proportion of aberrant metaphases in the *in vitro* chromosomal aberration assay with CHO cells. However, chromosomal damage was not seen in the *in vivo* mice micronucleus or bone marrow assays.

**Pregnancy/Reproduction**
Fertility—Impairment of fertility or reproduction performance was not found in fertility and general reproduction performance studies in male and female rats given oral daily doses of fenoldopam of 12.5, 37.5, or 75 mg/kg.

Pregnancy—Adequate and well-controlled studies in pregnant women have not been done. No evidence of impaired fertility or harm to the fetus was found in reproduction studies in rats and rabbits given daily oral fenoldopam doses of 12.5 to 200 mg/kg and 6.25 to 25 mg/kg, respectively. However, maternal toxicity occurred at the highest doses tested. Because animal reproduction studies are not always predictive of human response, fenoldopam should be used in pregnant patients only if absolutely necessary.

FDA Pregnancy Category B.

**Breast-feeding**
It is not known whether fenoldopam is distributed into breast milk. However, fenoldopam is distributed into the milk of lactating rats. Caution should be used when fenoldopam is administered to a nursing woman.

**Pediatrics**
No information is available on the relationship of age to the effects of fenoldopam in pediatric patients. Safety and efficacy have not been established.

**Geriatrics**
The pharmacokinetics of fenoldopam are unaffected by patient age.

**Drug interactions and/or related problems**
The following drug interactions and/or related problems have been selected on the basis of their potential clinical significance (possible mechanism in parentheses where appropriate)—not necessarily inclusive (» = major clinical significance):

Note: Combinations containing any of the following medications, depending on the amount present, may also interact with this medication.

» Beta-adrenergic blocking agents
  (concurrent use with fenoldopam has not been studied in hypertensive patients and is not recommended; unexpected hypotension may result from beta-adrenergic blocking agent inhibition of the reflex response [tachycardia] to fenoldopam)

Alpha-adrenergic blocking agents or
Angiotensin-converting enzyme (ACE) inhibitors or
Calcium channel blocking agents or
Diuretics, loop or
Diuretics, thiazide
  (there is limited experience in the concurrent use of these agents with fenoldopam)

**Laboratory value alterations**
The following have been selected on the basis of their potential clinical significance (possible effect in parentheses where appropriate)—not necessarily inclusive (» = major clinical significance):

With physiology/laboratory test values
Electrolytes, serum, especially
Potassium, serum
  (decreases in serum potassium to concentrations below 3 mEq per liter [mEq/L] have occurred after less than 6 hours of fenoldopam administration; it is not known if hypokalemia results from a pressure natriuresis with enhanced potassium-sodium exchange or as a direct effect of the drug)

**Medical considerations/Contraindications**
The medical considerations/contraindications included have been selected on the basis of their potential clinical significance (reasons given in parentheses where appropriate)—not necessarily inclusive (» = major clinical significance).

*Risk-benefit should be considered when the following medical problems exist:*

Glaucoma, open-angle or
Hypertension, ocular (mean baseline intraocular pressure of 29.2 mm Hg with a range of 22 to 33 mm Hg)
  (in 12 patients with open-angle glaucoma or ocular hypertension, infusion of fenoldopam in escalating doses ranging from 0.05 to 0.5 mcg per kg of body weight [mcg/kg] per minute over a 3.5-hour period resulted in a dose-dependent increase in intraocular pressure [IOP]; the maximum mean increase in intraocular pressure that occurred was 6.5 mm Hg [range −2 to +8.5 mm Hg, corrected for placebo effect]; the IOP returned to baseline within 2 hours after discontinuation of fenoldopam; fenoldopam should be administered with caution in these patients)

Cerebral infarction or hemorrhage, acute
  (because fenoldopam may cause hypotension, close monitoring during fenoldopam administration is necessary in these patients)

Sensitivity to fenoldopam
Sensitivity to sulfites
  (fenoldopam injection contains sodium metabisulfite, which may cause allergic- or anaphylactic-type reactions and life-threatening or less severe asthmatic episodes in individuals who are sensitive to sulfites; sensitivity to sulfites is more common in asthmatic patients than in nonasthmatic patients)

**Patient monitoring**
The following may be especially important in patient monitoring (other tests may be warranted in some patients, depending on condition; » = major clinical significance):

Electrolytes, serum, especially
Potassium, serum
  (monitoring at 6-hour intervals is recommended; decreases in serum potassium to concentrations below 3 mEq/L have occurred after less than 6 hours of fenoldopam administration)

» Heart rate determinations
» Blood pressure determinations
  (monitoring at frequent intervals, such as every 15 minutes, is recommended)

Note: Intra-arterial blood pressure monitoring was not used in clinical trials in emergency hypertension

## Side/Adverse Effects

Note: ST-T wave abnormalities, primarily T-wave inversion, have occurred with administration of fenoldopam.

Arterial lesions characterized by medial necrosis and hemorrhage have occurred in renal and splanchnic arteries of rats given a continuous intravenous infusion of fenoldopam in doses of 1 to 100 mcg per kg of body weight (mcg/kg) per minute for 24 hours. The lesions are morphologically identical to those observed in rats given intravenous infusions of dopamine, and have a dose-related incidence. The occurrence of these lesions may involve activation of $D_1$-like dopaminergic receptors. Lesions have not been seen in dogs given continuous intravenous infusion of fenoldopam in doses of up to 100 mcg/kg per minute for 24 hours, or in dogs given the same dose for 6 hours daily for 24 days. No evidence of similar lesions have been observed in humans.

A higher incidence of polyarteritis nodosa occurred in rats given oral daily doses of fenoldopam of 10 to 15 mg per kg (mg/kg) or 20 to 25 mg/kg for 24 months. These lesions were not seen in rats given oral daily doses of fenoldopam of 5 mg/kg for 24 months or in mice given oral daily doses of fenoldopam of up to 50 mg/kg for 24 months.

The following side/adverse effects have been selected on the basis of their potential clinical significance (possible signs and symptoms in parentheses where appropriate)—not necessarily inclusive:

**Those indicating need for medical attention**
Incidence more frequent
  *Hypotension* (lightheadedness or fainting); *tachycardia* (fast heartbeat)

Note: In clinical studies in patients with severe hypertension and end-organ damage, 3% of patients withdrew because of excessive *hypotension*.

*Tachycardia* is dose-related and could lead to ischemic cardiac events or worsened heart failure in certain individuals, although these events have not been observed. Tachycardia is more prevalent with infusion rates above 0.1 mcg/kg per minute and decreases over time, but remains significant at higher fenoldopam doses.

Incidence less frequent
  *Vomiting*

## Those indicating need for medical attention only if they continue or are bothersome

*Incidence more frequent*
  *Flushing* (sudden reddening of the face, neck, and occasionally, upper chest); *headache; nausea*

*Incidence less frequent*
  *Abdominal pain and/or sensation of fullness; back pain; constipation; diarrhea; dizziness; insomnia; nasal congestion; nervousness and/or anxiety; sweating*

## Overdose

For more information on the management of overdose or unintentional ingestion, **contact a Poison Control Center** (see *Poison Control Center Listing*).

### Clinical effects of overdose
The following effects have been selected on the basis of their potential clinical significance (possible signs and symptoms in parentheses where appropriate)—not necessarily inclusive:

Acute and/or chronic
  **Hypotension, severe**

### Treatment of overdose
Fenoldopam should be discontinued and treatment should be symptomatic and supportive.

## General Dosing Information

Fenoldopam should be administered by continuous intravenous infusion using a calibrated mechanical infusion pump that can deliver the desired infusion rate accurately and reliably. *A bolus dose should not be used.* Hypotension and rapid decreases of blood pressure should be avoided.

### For treatment of adverse effects
Recommended treatment consists of the following:
- Hypokalemia may be treated with either oral or intravenous potassium supplementation.

## Parenteral Dosage Forms

### FENOLDOPAM MESYLATE INJECTION

Note: Fenoldopam infusion can be discontinued abruptly or tapered gradually prior to discontinuation. Orally administered antihypertensive agents can be added during fenoldopam infusion or following its discontinuation.

### Usual adult dose
Hypertension (treatment)—
  The optimal magnitude and rate of blood pressure reduction in acutely hypertensive patients have not been determined precisely. In clinical studies, doses ranging from 0.01 to 1.6 mcg per kg per minute have been used. Doses below 0.1 mcg per kg per minute have very limited effects and may be only minimally useful. In general, as the initial dose increases, blood pressure reduction is greater and more rapid. Lower initial doses, such as 0.03 to 0.1 mcg per kg per minute, titrated slowly, have been associated with less reflex tachycardia than have higher initial doses ($\geq$ 0.3 mcg per kg per minute). Most of the effect of a given infusion rate is attained within 15 minutes. The initial dose should be titrated upward or downward, no more frequently than every 15 minutes (and less frequently as goal blood pressure is approached), to achieve the desired therapeutic effect. The recommended increments for titration are 0.05 to 0.1 mcg per kg per minute. Blood pressure and heart rate should be monitored at frequent intervals, e.g., every 15 minutes.

  For initial doses of fenoldopam used in clinical trials to produce a desired magnitude and rate of blood pressure reduction in a given clinical situation, see prescriber information.

  The drug dose rate must be individualized according to the patient's body weight and according to the desired rapidity and extent of pharmacodynamic effect. The following table provides the calculated infusion volume in mL per minute (mL/min) for a range of drug doses and body weights.

Infusion rates (mL/min) to achieve a given drug dose rate (mcg/kg/min)

| Body weight (kg) | 0.025 mcg/kg/min | 0.05 mcg/kg/min | 0.1 mcg/kg/min | 0.2 mcg/kg/min | 0.3 mcg/kg/min |
|---|---|---|---|---|---|
| | Recommended infusion rate (mL/min) ||||| 
| 40 | 0.025 | 0.05 | 0.1 | 0.2 | 0.3 |
| 50 | 0.031 | 0.06 | 0.13 | 0.25 | 0.38 |
| 60 | 0.038 | 0.08 | 0.15 | 0.3 | 0.45 |
| 70 | 0.044 | 0.09 | 0.18 | 0.35 | 0.53 |
| 80 | 0.05 | 0.1 | 0.2 | 0.4 | 0.6 |
| 90 | 0.056 | 0.11 | 0.23 | 0.45 | 0.68 |
| 100 | 0.063 | 0.13 | 0.25 | 0.5 | 0.75 |
| 110 | 0.069 | 0.14 | 0.28 | 0.55 | 0.83 |
| 120 | 0.075 | 0.15 | 0.3 | 0.6 | 0.9 |
| 130 | 0.081 | 0.16 | 0.33 | 0.65 | 0.98 |
| 140 | 0.088 | 0.18 | 0.35 | 0.7 | 1.05 |
| 150 | 0.094 | 0.19 | 0.38 | 0.75 | 1.13 |

### Usual adult prescribing limits
1.6 mcg per kg per minute. Fenoldopam infusion has been administered to patients for as long as 48 hours.

### Usual pediatric dose
Safety and efficacy have not been established.

### Strength(s) usually available
U.S.—
  10 mg per mL (Rx) [*Corlopam* (citric acid; propylene glycol; sodium citrate dihydrate; sodium metabisulfite)].

### Packaging and storage
Store between 2 and 30 °C (36 and 86 °F).

### Preparation of dosage form
The contents of ampuls must be diluted before infusion. Each ampul is for single use only. Concentrated fenoldopam must be diluted in 0.9% Sodium Chloride Injection USP or 5% Dextrose Injection USP using the following dilution schedule:

Preparation of infusion solution

| Volume of concentrate (amount of drug) | Added to volume of 0.9% Sodium Chloride Injection USP or 5% Dextrose Injection USP | To make a final concentration of |
|---|---|---|
| 4 mL (40 mg) | 1000 mL | 40 mcg/mL |
| 2 mL (20 mg) | 500 mL | 40 mcg/mL |
| 1 mL (10 mg) | 250 mL | 40 mcg/mL |

### Stability
The diluted solution is stable under normal ambient light and temperature conditions for at least 24 hours. Diluted solution that is not used within 24 hours of preparation should be discarded. Parenteral products should be inspected visually. If particulate matter or cloudiness is observed, the drug should be discarded.

### Additional information
Fenoldopam injection contains sodium metabisulfite, which may cause allergic- or anaphylactic-type reactions and life-threatening or less severe asthmatic episodes in individuals who are sensitive to sulfites. Sensitivity to sulfites is more common in asthmatic patients than in nonasthmatic patients.

Developed: 03/10/98

---

**FENOPROFEN**—See *Anti-inflammatory Drugs, Nonsteroidal (Systemic)*.

---

**FENOTEROL**—See *Bronchodilators, Adrenergic (Inhalation-Local); Bronchodilators, Adrenergic (Systemic)*.

---

**FENTANYL**—See *Fentanyl Derivatives (Systemic); Fentanyl (Transdermal-Systemic)*.

# FENTANYL  Transdermal-Systemic

VA CLASSIFICATION (Primary): CN101
Note: Controlled substance classification—
  U.S.—II.
  Canada—N.
Commonly used brand name(s): *Duragesic*.
Note: For a listing of dosage forms and brand names by country availability, see *Dosage Forms* section(s).

## Category
Analgesic.

## Indications
Note: **Transdermal fentanyl should be prescribed, and its use monitored, only by persons knowledgeable in the continuous administration of potent opioid analgesics, in the care of patients requiring such treatment, and in the detection and management of hypoventilation** .

Use of this formulation requires that the advantages of providing a continuous, prolonged analgesic effect via a noninvasive, non-oral route of administration outweigh the disadvantage of being unable to adjust dosage rapidly should analgesic requirements change or adverse effects occur.

### Accepted
Pain, chronic (treatment)—Transdermal fentanyl is indicated to relieve chronic pain that requires continuous treatment with a potent opioid analgesic. Most patients will need supplemental administration of an analgesic with a rapid onset and a short duration of action for pain relief during the interval between application of the first transdermal system and the onset of effective analgesia (24 hours or longer) and for relief of breakthrough pain.

### Unaccepted
**Transdermal fentanyl is not recommended for treatment of acute pain (including postoperative pain).** Use of this formulation for postoperative pain may cause severe hypoventilation; a few fatalities have been reported. Also, clinical trials have shown that application of transdermal fentanyl 2 hours prior to anesthesia does not eliminate the need for postoperative administration of a rapidly acting analgesic, especially in the first 12 to 24 hours after surgery. However, transdermal fentanyl need not be discontinued perioperatively if a patient being treated for chronic pain requires surgery.

This formulation is **not** recommended for treatment of mild or intermittent pain that can be managed with less potent analgesics or with as-needed administration of short- or intermediate-acting opioid analgesics.

## Pharmacology/Pharmacokinetics

### Physicochemical characteristics
Source—Synthetic.
Chemical group—Phenylpiperidine derivative; chemically related to meperidine.
Molecular weight—336.5.
pKa—8.4.
*n*-Octanol:water partition coefficient—860:1.
Note: Physicochemical characteristics that facilitate percutaneous absorption of a medication include high lipid solubility (as indicated by a high *n*-octanol:water partition coefficient) and relatively low molecular weight (< 1000 daltons). Lipophilic opioid analgesics such as fentanyl are well absorbed through intact skin; hydrophilic opioid analgesics (e.g., morphine, codeine, and hydromorphone) are not.

### Mechanism of action/Effect
Opioid analgesics such as fentanyl bind with stereospecific receptors at many sites within the central nervous system (CNS) to alter processes affecting both the perception of and emotional response to pain. Although the precise sites and mechanisms of action have not been fully determined, alterations in the release of various neurotransmitters from afferent nerves sensitive to painful stimuli may be partially responsible for the analgesic effects.

Multiple subtypes of opioid receptors, each mediating various therapeutic and/or side effects of opioid analgesics, have been identified. The actions of an opioid analgesic may therefore depend on whether it acts as a full agonist or a partial agonist or is inactive at each type of receptor. Fentanyl probably produces its effects predominantly via agonist actions at the mu receptor.

On a weight basis, fentanyl is considerably more potent than morphine. Transdermal administration of fentanyl at a delivery rate of 100 mcg per hour (mcg/hr) is therapeutically equivalent to intramuscular administration of 60 mg of morphine, chronic oral administration of 180 mg of morphine, or intermittent oral administration of 360 mg of morphine per day in 6 divided doses administered at 4-hour intervals. This high potency permits a therapeutic dose to be applied to a relatively small skin area.

### Other actions/effects
Fentanyl, like other opioid analgesics, may cause respiratory depression (characterized by decreases in respiratory rate, tidal volume, minute ventilation, and ventilatory response to carbon dioxide), increased biliary tone, increased smooth muscle tone in the urinary tract, decreased gastrointestinal motility, euphoria, miosis, hypotension, and bradycardia. However, unlike many other opioid analgesics, fentanyl does not cause clinically significant histamine release with therapeutic doses (as determined by intravenous administration of single doses of up to 50 mcg per kg of body weight [mcg/kg]).

### Absorption
Following application of a transdermal system, some fentanyl is released relatively rapidly from the adhesive layer of the system. Most of the fentanyl is located in a reservoir layer within the system, from which it is released gradually at a rate controlled by a restrictive copolymer membrane located between the reservoir and adhesive layers. A very small quantity of alcohol present in the formulation enhances passage of the medication through both the rate-limiting restrictive membrane and the skin. Less than 0.2 mL of alcohol is released from a transdermal system. The rate at which fentanyl is delivered to the skin may vary across the 72-hour application time. The labeled strength of a transdermal system represents the average quantity of fentanyl delivered to the systemic circulation per hour across intact skin.

Absorption of fentanyl after application of a transdermal system is initially slow because a depot of fentanyl, from which the medication is subsequently absorbed into the systemic circulation, must first form in the upper skin layers. Absorption is subject to intra- as well as interindividual variability. The rate and/or extent of absorption may be altered by the temperature, state of hydration, and integrity of the skin at the application site. Also, absorption may depend on blood flow in the area of application, which may increase or decrease with the patient's level of activity. Despite these variables, the average quantity of fentanyl absorbed per hour into the systemic circulation of an individual patient is sufficiently consistent to permit dosage titration over extended periods of time.

Approximately 92% of the fentanyl contained in a transdermal system is absorbed into the systemic circulation over 72 hours (calculated value). In a multiple-dose study, absorption from the fifth consecutive transdermal system to be applied and kept in place for 72 hours was 47% complete after 24 hours, 88% complete after 48 hours, and 94% complete after 72 hours.

Absorption of fentanyl from the depot in the skin continues after removal of the transdermal system. When application sites are rotated, continued absorption prevents plasma concentrations from decreasing to subtherapeutic values while another depot is forming below the new application site. Failure to rotate application sites may lead to more rapid absorption and higher fentanyl concentrations, which may increase the risk of toxicity.

### Distribution
Fentanyl is distributed to and accumulates in adipose tissue and skeletal muscle. The medication is slowly released from these tissues to the systemic circulation. Fentanyl readily crosses the blood/brain barrier. Alterations in pH may affect the medication's distribution between CNS tissues and plasma.

Volume of distribution (determined with intravenous administration to surgical patients)—6 (range, approximately 3 to 8) L per kg of body weight.

### Protein binding
High (79 to 87%), primarily to albumin and lipoproteins; dependent on plasma pH.

### Biotransformation
Primarily hepatic, mostly via N-dealkylation to norfentanyl and other inactive metabolites. Fentanyl is not metabolized in the skin.

### Half-life
Elimination—Transdermal—
  Single application—17 (range, 13 to 22) hours
  Multiple applications—21.9±8.9 hours, determined after 5 consecutive 72-hour applications.

Note: The prolonged elimination half-life with transdermal administration (relative to that with intravenous administration—about 3.6 hours) is due to prolonged continued absorption from the skin depot below the transdermal system.

Values may be greatly prolonged in geriatric patients. In a single-dose study the mean value for patients 78 to 88 years of age was 43.1±23.4 hours.

The half-life of transdermal fentanyl has not been assessed in patients with renal or hepatic function impairment.

### Onset of action
Very slow (12 to 24 hours in most studies) because of delayed absorption following application of an initial transdermal dose.

### Time to peak concentration
Single 72-hour application—Generally between 24 and 72 hours.

Multiple applications—Concentrations continue to increase during the first few 72-hour applications.

### Peak serum concentration
Serum concentrations achieved with transdermal fentanyl have been studied primarily in clinical trials that investigated whether the formulation might be useful for postoperative pain control. In general, the studies found fentanyl concentrations to be proportional to the transdermal delivery rate in mcg per hour, subject to substantial interpatient variability, and significantly higher in geriatric patients than in younger adults. The concentrations produced were similar to those measured during continuous intravenous infusion of fentanyl at the same rate of administration, but took considerably longer to achieve. In many studies, measurable quantities of fentanyl were not present in serum within the first 2 hours after application of an initial transdermal system. Specific values determined during short-term use in postoperative patients are not likely to be relevant to prolonged use of this medication in chronic pain patients.

### Steady-state concentrations
A multiple-dose study in which pharmacokinetics of fentanyl were assessed during 5 consecutive 72-hour applications of a system designed to deliver 100 mcg per hour reported mean trough concentrations of 0.91±0.55 nanograms/mL (0.0027±0.0016 micromoles/L) prior to, and mean maximum concentrations of 2.6±1.3 nanograms/mL (0.0077±0.0039 micromoles/L) during, application of the fifth dose. Steady-state concentrations are subject to substantial interpatient variability because of individual differences in skin permeability and clearance of fentanyl. Although several sequential 72-hour applications may be required to achieve steady-state, measurement of trough concentrations prior to application of each dose in the multiple-dose study suggested that steady-state concentrations are approached by the second dose.

### Therapeutic concentrations
Generally 0.2 to 1.2 nanograms/mL (0.0006 to 0.0036 micromoles/L) in patients who are not tolerant to opioid analgesics. Required concentrations increase with the degree of tolerance to opioid analgesics. Fentanyl requirements are highly subject to intrapatient variability and dependent on the intensity of pain.

Effective concentrations were reached between 1.2 and 37.3 hours after application of a transdermal system in various postoperative pain studies. In 1 of these studies, concentrations decreased to subtherapeutic values between 2.3 and > 24.9 hours (mean, 16.1±7.1 hours) after the system was removed.

### Duration of action
Individual transdermal systems are designed to release fentanyl over 72 hours. Analgesic effects may persist for several hours after a system is removed because of continued absorption. This provides relatively constant analgesia during the time required for an effective quantity of fentanyl to be absorbed from the next dose.

### Elimination
Studies with intravenously administered fentanyl have shown that approximately 75% of a dose is eliminated in the urine (10% as unchanged fentanyl and the remainder as metabolites) and another 9% in the feces, mostly as metabolites. These studies also indicated that clearance rates are more variable and prolonged in patients with hepatic or renal function impairment than in patients with normal hepatic and renal function. Clearance rates for transdermally administered fentanyl have not been published.

## Precautions to Consider

### Cross-sensitivity and/or related problems
Patients hypersensitive to alfentanil or sufentanil may be hypersensitive to fentanyl also.

### Carcinogenicity
Long-term studies with fentanyl have not been done.

### Mutagenicity
No evidence of mutagenicity was demonstrated in the Ames test, primary rat hepatocyte unscheduled DNA synthesis assay, BALB/c-3T3 transformation test, and the human lymphocyte and CHO chromosomal aberration *in vitro* assays. In the mouse lymphoma assay, fentanyl concentrations more than 2000 times greater than those occurring with chronic systemic use were mutagenic only in the presence of metabolic activation.

### Pregnancy/Reproduction
Fertility—Intravenous administration of 0.3 times the human dose of fentanyl for 12 days impaired fertility in rats.

Pregnancy—Adequate and well-controlled studies with transdermal fentanyl have not been done in pregnant women. Chronic use of other opioids by pregnant women has caused physical dependence in the fetus, leading to withdrawal symptoms (convulsions, irritability, excessive crying, tremors, hyperactive reflexes, fever, vomiting, diarrhea, sneezing, and yawning) in the neonate. Also, use of opioid analgesics shortly before or during labor may cause respiratory depression in the neonate.

Studies in rats have not shown that fentanyl is teratogenic.

FDA Pregnancy Category C.

Labor and delivery—Use of transdermal fentanyl to provide analgesia during labor and delivery is not recommended.

### Breast-feeding
Fentanyl is distributed into human breast milk. Nursing infants may ingest quantities of fentanyl sufficient to produce adverse effects typical of potent opioid analgesics, including sedation, respiratory depression, and physical dependence when the mother is receiving chronic, high-dose treatment. Use of transdermal fentanyl by nursing women is therefore not recommended.

### Pediatrics
No information is available on the relationship of age to the effects of transdermal fentanyl in pediatric patients. Safety and efficacy have not been established. Administration to children younger than 12 years of age is not recommended except in an authorized investigational research setting.

### Adolescents
No information is available on the relationship of age to the effects of transdermal fentanyl in adolescents up to 18 years of age. Safety and efficacy have not been established. Administration to patients younger than 18 years of age who weigh less than 50 kg is not recommended except in an authorized investigational research setting.

### Geriatrics
No information is available on the relationship of age to the effects of transdermal fentanyl in geriatric patients with chronic pain. However, it is known that geriatric patients are generally more susceptible to the effects, especially the respiratory depressant effects, of opioid analgesics. Short-term pharmacokinetic studies with transdermal fentanyl have shown that the elimination half-life and serum concentrations are significantly higher in elderly individuals than in younger people. Also, in a study that utilized an investigational 24-hour transdermal system with a delivery rate of 50 mcg per hour, the systems were removed earlier than anticipated from all of the elderly subjects (planned application time 24 hours; mean time of removal 11.7 ± 4.9 hours), but none of the younger individuals, because of adverse effects. Caution and careful attention to dosage are recommended, especially if the patient is not tolerant to opioid analgesics.

### Drug interactions and/or related problems
The following drug interactions and/or related problems have been selected on the basis of their potential clinical significance (possible mechanism in parentheses where appropriate)—not necessarily inclusive (» = major clinical significance):

Note: Combinations containing any of the following medications, depending on the amount present, may also interact with this medication.

» Alcohol or
» CNS depression–producing medications, other (See *Appendix II*) (concurrent or sequential use with fentanyl may result in increased CNS depressant, respiratory depressant, and hypotensive effects; caution and careful titration of the dose of each agent are recommended)

(concurrent use of fentanyl with other CNS depressants that may cause habituation may increase the risk of habituation)

Anticholinergics or other medications with anticholinergic activity (See *Appendix II*)
(concurrent use with fentanyl may result in increased risk of severe constipation, which may lead to paralytic ileus, and/or urinary retention)

Antidiarrheals, antiperistaltic, such as:
Difenoxin and atropine
Diphenoxylate and atropine
Loperamide
Opium tincture
Paregoric
(repeated administration of any of these antidiarrheals with fentanyl, especially during chronic, high-dose fentanyl therapy, may increase the risk of severe constipation and CNS depression)

Antihypertensives, especially ganglionic blockers such as guanadrel, guanethidine, and mecamylamine or
Diuretics or
Hypotension-producing medications, other (see *Appendix II*)
(hypotensive effects of these medications may be potentiated when they are used concurrently with fentanyl; patients should be monitored for excessive fall in blood pressure)
(concurrent use of a beta-adrenergic blocking agent with fentanyl may also increase the risk of bradycardia)

Hydroxyzine
(concurrent use with fentanyl may result in increased analgesia as well as increased CNS depressant and hypotensive effects)

Metoclopramide
(fentanyl may antagonize the effects of metoclopramide on gastrointestinal motility)

Monoamine oxidase (MAO) inhibitors, including furazolidone, procarbazine, and selegiline
(caution is recommended when any opioid analgesic is given to patients who have received an MAO inhibitor within 14 days because administration of meperidine to patients receiving MAO inhibitors has caused unpredictable, severe, and sometimes fatal reactions, including immediate excitation, sweating, rigidity, and severe hypertension, or, in some patients, hypotension, severe respiratory depression, coma, seizures, hyperpyrexia, and vascular collapse; although a few reports indicated that intravenous injections of fentanyl did not cause adverse reactions when administered perioperatively to patients receiving MAO inhibitor therapy, administration of an intravenous test dose of fentanyl [to detect any possible interaction] may be advisable prior to initiation of transdermal therapy because the effects of transdermal fentanyl cannot be terminated rapidly)

Naloxone
(antagonizes the analgesic, CNS, and respiratory depressant effects of opioid analgesics; however, because naloxone may precipitate withdrawal symptoms in physically dependent patients, dosage of naloxone should be carefully titrated when it is used to treat opioid overdosage in dependent patients; also, because absorption of fentanyl from the depot that forms in the skin layers below the transdermal system continues after the system has been removed, prolonged infusion or repeated administration of naloxone may be required)

» Naltrexone
(fentanyl will be ineffective if administered to a patient receiving naltrexone, which blocks the therapeutic effects of opioid analgesics; administration of increased doses of an opioid analgesic to override naltrexone blockade of opioid receptors may result in increased and prolonged respiratory depression and/or circulatory collapse and is not recommended)
(administration of naltrexone to a patient who is physically dependent on fentanyl will precipitate withdrawal symptoms; symptoms may appear within 5 minutes of naltrexone administration, persist for up to 48 hours, and be very difficult to reverse)

Neuromuscular blocking agents and possibly other medications having some neuromuscular blocking activity
(respiratory suppressant effects of neuromuscular blockade may be additive to the central respiratory depressant effects of opioid analgesics; increased or prolonged respiratory depression [apnea] may occur but is of minor clinical significance if the patient is being ventilated mechanically; however, caution and careful monitoring of the patient are recommended during and following concurrent or sequential use, especially if there is a possibility of incomplete reversal of neuromuscular blockade)

» Opioid analgesics, other
(although most patients require supplemental administration of an analgesic with a rapid onset of action for pain relief during the interval between application of the first transdermal system and the onset of effective analgesia [24 hours or longer] and for relief of breakthrough pain, the risk of additive CNS and/or respiratory depression or other adverse effects must be considered, especially in patients who are not tolerant to opioid analgesics; use of long-acting opioid analgesics [or extended-release dosage forms of short-acting opioids] in conjunction with transdermal fentanyl may be especially hazardous and is not recommended)
(in addition to their potential for causing additive effects when used concurrently with fentanyl, opioids having partial mu-receptor activity [e.g., buprenorphine and dezocine] and some opioids having mixed agonist/antagonist activity [i.e., nalbuphine and pentazocine] have the potential to antagonize fentanyl's therapeutic and adverse effects; whether additive or antagonistic effects occur may depend on the dose of each medication as well as on the order in which the medications are given and the extent to which physical dependence has developed; administration of a partial mu-receptor agonist prior to an initial dose of fentanyl may reduce the therapeutic response to fentanyl, whereas administration of a partial mu-receptor agonist, nalbuphine, or pentazocine to a patient who is receiving fentanyl may antagonize fentanyl's effects to the extent of precipitating withdrawal symptoms in physically dependent patients)

**Laboratory value alterations**
The following have been selected on the basis of their potential clinical significance (possible effect in parentheses where appropriate)—not necessarily inclusive (» = major clinical significance):

With diagnostic test results
Gastric emptying studies
(opioid analgesics may delay gastric emptying, thereby invalidating test results)

Hepatobiliary imaging using a technetium Tc 99m–labeled iminodiacetic acid derivative
(delivery of the radiopharmaceutical to the small bowel may be slowed because of fentanyl-induced constriction of the sphincter of Oddi and increased biliary-tract pressure; these actions result in delayed visualization, which may be falsely interpreted as indicating obstruction of the common bile duct)

With physiology/laboratory test values
Amylase, plasma and
Lipase, plasma
(enzyme values may be increased because fentanyl can cause contractions of the sphincter of Oddi and increased biliary tract pressure; the diagnostic utility of determinations of these enzymes may be compromised during, and for a time following discontinuation of, transdermal fentanyl therapy)

Cerebrospinal fluid pressure
(fentanyl may increase cerebrospinal fluid pressure; effect is secondary to respiratory depression–induced carbon dioxide retention)

**Medical considerations/Contraindications**
The medical considerations/contraindications included have been selected on the basis of their potential clinical significance (reasons given in parentheses where appropriate)—not necessarily inclusive (» = major clinical significance).

*Except under special circumstances, this medication should not be used when the following medical problems exist:*

» Diarrhea associated with pseudomembranous colitis caused by cephalosporins, lincomycins (possibly including topical clindamycin), or penicillins or

» Diarrhea caused by poisoning, until toxic material has been eliminated from the gastrointestinal tract
(opioid analgesics may slow elimination of toxic material, thereby worsening and/or prolonging the diarrhea)

» Respiratory depression, acute
(may be exacerbated)

*Risk-benefit should be considered when the following medical problems exist:*

Abdominal conditions, acute
(diagnosis or clinical course may be obscured)

Allergic reaction to fentanyl, alfentanil, or sufentanil, or to the adhesives in the transdermal system
(risk of hypersensitivity reaction)

» Asthma, acute attack or
» Respiratory impairment or disease, chronic
    (opioids may decrease respiratory drive and increase airway resistance in patients with these conditions)
Bradyarrhythmias
    (may be exacerbated)
Drug abuse or dependence, current or history of, including alcoholism or
Emotional instability or
Suicidal ideation or attempts
    (patient predisposition to drug abuse; possibility of adverse effects if patient uses nonprescribed CNS depressants concurrently with fentanyl)
    (although this medication should not be withheld from known opioid addicts who require treatment for chronic pain, caution is recommended; addicts treated with fentanyl transdermal systems have been reported to increase the rate of fentanyl release by disrupting the restrictive membrane and to remove fentanyl from the reservoir for rapid administration by other routes)
Fever
    (temperature-dependent changes in fentanyl release from the transdermal system and increased skin permeability may result in a 33% increase in fentanyl plasma concentrations in patients with a fever of 40 °C [102 °F]; patients who develop a fever while a system is in place should be monitored for adverse effects and fentanyl dosage adjusted and/or treatment instituted as needed)
Gallbladder disease or gallstones
    (fentanyl may cause biliary contraction and increased biliary tract pressure; biliary colic may be exacerbated rather than relieved)
Gastrointestinal tract surgery, current or recent
    (alteration of gastrointestinal motility by fentanyl may be undesirable)
Head injury or
Increased intracranial pressure, pre-existing or
Intracranial lesions
    (risk of respiratory depression and further elevation of cerebrospinal fluid pressure, which may lead to complications such as impaired consciousness, is increased; also, opioid analgesics may cause sedation and pupillary changes that may obscure the clinical course of patients with head injury)
Hepatic function impairment or
Renal function impairment
    (potential for reduced clearance of fentanyl, leading to higher plasma concentrations; pharmacokinetic studies on which recommendations regarding use of transdermal fentanyl could be based have not been done in patients with these conditions)
    (fluid retention associated with renal function impairment may be exacerbated because fentanyl may also cause urinary retention)
Hypothyroidism
    (risk of respiratory depression and prolonged CNS depression is greatly increased)
» Inflammatory bowel disease, severe
    (risk of toxic megacolon, especially with prolonged use of fentanyl)
Prostatic hypertrophy or obstruction or
Urethral stricture or
Urinary tract surgery, current or recent
    (patient predisposition to urinary retention)
Caution is also recommended in administration to elderly or very ill or debilitated patients, who may be more sensitive to the effects, especially the respiratory depressant effects, of opioid analgesics.

**Patient monitoring**
The following may be especially important in patient monitoring (other tests may be warranted in some patients, depending on condition; » = major clinical significance):
Blood pressure and
Heart rate and
» Respiratory rate and
» Sedation, degree of
    (should be monitored at periodic intervals, especially at the beginning of therapy and after increases in dosage; if the system is removed because of adverse effects, monitoring should continue for at least 12 hours because absorption of fentanyl continues, and serum concentrations decrease slowly, after the system is removed)

## Side/Adverse Effects
Note: The frequencies of the adverse effects reported below were obtained in clinical studies in 510 patients (153 cancer patients, 56% of whom received treatment lasting from 30 days to more than a year, and 357 surgical patients who received the medication for 1 to 3 days), almost all of whom received supplemental doses of other opioid analgesics. The relative contribution of fentanyl, other opioid analgesic(s), the patient's underlying condition, and/or various surgical procedures to the occurrence of specific symptoms has not been established.

The risk of hypoventilation and of CNS adverse effects in opioid-naive individuals is increased when serum concentrations of fentanyl reach 2 nanograms per mL (nanograms/mL) (0.006 micromoles/liter [micromoles/L]) and more than 3 nanograms/mL (0.009 micromoles/L), respectively. The concentration at which toxicity occurs increases with increasing tolerance to the opioid analgesic.

In addition to the side/adverse effects listed below, a case of toxic delirium has been reported in an elderly patient receiving 125 mcg per hour of transdermal fentanyl together with other CNS depressants.

Physical dependence, with or without psychological dependence, may occur with chronic administration of fentanyl; an abstinence syndrome may occur when the medication is discontinued abruptly.

The following side/adverse effects have been selected on the basis of their potential clinical significance (possible signs and symptoms in parentheses where appropriate)—not necessarily inclusive:

**Those indicating need for medical attention**
Incidence more frequent (3 to 10%)
   *Apnea; CNS depression; difficult breathing; hypoventilation*—respiratory rate < 8 breaths per minute, pCO$_2$ > 55 mm Hg; *hallucinations* (seeing, hearing, or feeling things that are not there); *urinary retention* (decreased frequency of urination; decrease in urine volume)
Note: The risk of *hypoventilation* is higher in nontolerant women than in men, in patients weighing less than 63 kg, in patients with pre-existing respiratory function impairment, and in patients receiving doses of 75 mcg per hour or higher.

Incidence less frequent (1 to 3%)
   *Chest pain; CNS effects* (abnormal thinking; difficulty in speaking; fainting; problems with coordination or gait); *paranoia* (delusions of persecution, mistrust, suspiciousness, and/or combativeness)—frequency of CNS effects and paranoia symptoms is 1 to 3% in clinical studies; *irregular heartbeat; localized skin reaction* (redness, swelling, and/or bumps on the skin, with or without itching, at place of application); *spitting blood*
Note: *Fainting* occurs more frequently in ambulatory than in recumbent patients and may be associated with postural hypotension. Localized reactions to the transdermal system are probably caused by the adhesive rather than by fentanyl. These reactions have been characterized as mild, transient (generally disappearing within 6 to 24 hours after removal of the transdermal system), and more typical of local irritation and occlusion than of allergic contact dermatitis. Generalized skin reactions also may occur; at least 1 case of diffuse, nonpruritic macular papules has been attributed to transdermal fentanyl therapy.

Incidence rare (less than 1%)
   *Abdominal distention* (swelling of abdominal area); *amblyopia* (any change in vision); *bladder pain; bradycardia* (slow heartbeat); *cessation of urination; CNS toxicity* (inability to speak; depersonalization; stupor); *dermatitis, exfoliative* (fever with or without chills; red, thickened, orscaly skin; swollen and/or painful glands; unexplained bruising); *fluid-filled blisters; frequent urge to urinate; respiratory problems, including asthma* (noisy breathing; shortness of breath; troubled breathing; tightness in chest; wheezing)

**Those indicating need for medical attention only if they continue or are bothersome**
Incidence more frequent (each symptom 3% or higher)
   *CNS effects* (anxiety; confusion; dizziness; drowsiness; false sense of well-being; nervousness; weakness); *gastrointestinal effects* (abdominal pain; constipation; diarrhea; indigestion; loss of appetite); *headache; itching of skin; nausea; sweating; vomiting*
Note: *Nausea* and *vomiting* are more likely to occur in ambulatory than in recumbent patients. These effects may be induced by a direct effect on the chemoreceptor trigger zone in the CNS.

Incidence less frequent (1 to 3%)
   *Agitation* (feeling anxious and restless); *bloated feeling or gas; feeling of crawling, tingling, or burning of the skin; memory loss; unusual dreams*

# 1450  Fentanyl (Transdermal-Systemic)

Those indicating possible withdrawal and the need for medical attention if they occur after medication is discontinued
   *Body aches; diarrhea; fast heartbeat; fever, runny nose, or sneezing; gooseflesh; increased sweating; increased yawning; loss of appetite; nausea or vomiting; nervousness, restlessness, or irritability; shivering or trembling; stomach cramps; trouble in sleeping; unusually large pupils; weakness*

## Overdose

For specific information on the agents used in the management of fentanyl overdose, see:
- *Atropine* in *Anticholinergics/Antispasmodics (Systemic)* monograph; and/or
- *Naloxone (Systemic)* monograph.

For more information on the management of overdose or unintentional ingestion, **contact a Poison Control Center** (see *Poison Control Listing*).

### Clinical effects of overdose
The following effects have been selected on the basis of their potential clinical significance (possible signs and symptoms in parentheses where appropriate)—not necessarily inclusive:

Acute and chronic
   *Cold, clammy skin; confusion; convulsions; severe dizziness, drowsiness, nervousness, restlessness, or weakness; low blood pressure; pinpoint pupils of eyes; slow heartbeat; slow or troubled breathing; unconsciousness*

### Treatment of overdose
General measures—Removing the transdermal system (if symptoms are judged sufficiently severe to warrant removal) and monitoring the patient, keeping in mind that fentanyl absorption continues and plasma concentrations decline slowly after the system has been removed. Prolonged monitoring may be needed.

Specific treatment—

For hypoventilation:
   Verbal stimulation or waking the patient (if bradypnea occurs during sleep) may be sufficient to increase the respiratory rate and provide adequate ventilation.
   Use of the opioid antagonist naloxone if necessary. However, usual doses of naloxone may reverse analgesia and precipitate withdrawal in opioid-dependent patients. Since naloxone's duration of action is considerably shorter than that of transdermal fentanyl, administration via continuous intravenous infusion at a rate titrated to the needs of the individual patient may be necessary.

For bradycardia: Use of atropine.

For hypotension: Use of intravenous fluids and/or vasopressors and using other supportive measures as needed.

Supportive care—May include establishing adequate respiratory exchange through provision of a patent airway and institution of assisted or controlled respiration.

## Patient Consultation

As an aid to patient consultation, refer to *Advice for the Patient, Fentanyl (Transdermal-Systemic)*.

In providing consultation, consider emphasizing the following selected information (» = major clinical significance):

### Before using this medication
» Conditions affecting use, especially:
   Sensitivity to fentanyl, alfentanil, or sufentanil
   Pregnancy—Opioids cross the placenta; use by pregnant women may cause physical dependence in the fetus and withdrawal symptoms and/or respiratory depression in the neonate
   Breast-feeding—Fentanyl is distributed into breast milk; opioid effects including sedation, respiratory depression, and physical dependence may occur in the infant if the mother is receiving chronic, high-dose therapy
   Use in the elderly—Geriatric patients are more susceptible to the effects of opioids, especially respiratory depression
   Other medications, especially alcohol or other CNS depressants (including other opioid analgesics) and naltrexone
   Other medical problems, especially asthma or other acute or chronic respiratory problems, diarrhea caused by poisoning or antibiotic therapy, and severe inflammatory bowel disease

### Proper use of this medication
» Reading patient instructions carefully before using
» Proper application technique
   Keeping medication in sealed pouch until ready to apply
   Using caution in handling; not touching adhesive surface with the hand; washing area with clear water if medication does touch the skin in an unintended location
   Using care not to damage (puncture or tear) the surface of the transdermal system
   Applying to clean, dry skin area of upper arm or torso that is free of oil, hair, scars, cuts, burns, or irritation; avoiding areas that have been irradiated
   Clipping, not shaving, hair at application site, if necessary
   If cleansing site prior to application, using only clear water (not soaps, lotions, or cleansers that contain oils, alcohol, or other agents) and allowing area to dry completely prior to application
   Removing liner from adhesive layer, then pressing system in place with palm of hand for about 30 seconds; making sure that good contact is achieved, especially around the edges
   If dose requires applying 2 or more systems, keeping them far enough apart so that the edges do not touch or overlap
   Washing hands with clear water after applying or handling transdermal system
   Removing system after 3 days; applying next system, if treatment is being continued, at new site, preferably on opposite side of the body; not reusing a site for at least 3 days
   Disposing of used or unneeded systems by folding in half with adhesive layer inside the fold, then flushing down the toilet
» Not using more transdermal fentanyl than directed, even if medication appears ineffective; onset of action may require 24 hours or longer and several dosage adjustments may be required to achieve maximum effectiveness
» Taking "rescue" doses of short-acting opioid for first few days after initiation of therapy and for breakthrough pain, but not using more than prescribed because of danger of overdose
» Proper dosing
   Missed dose: Applying as soon as possible
» Proper storage

### Precautions while using this medication
Regular consultations with health care professional during long-term therapy
» Checking with health care professional before increasing dose of transdermal fentanyl and/or "rescue" medication if treatment becomes less effective
» Avoiding use of alcoholic beverages or other CNS depressants during therapy, unless prescribed or otherwise approved by physician
» Caution if dizziness, drowsiness, lightheadedness, or false sense of well-being occurs; checking with health care professional if severe drowsiness persists for more than a few days
» Getting up slowly from a lying or sitting position; lying down for a while may provide relief if patient becomes dizzy, lightheaded, or faint
Caution that nausea or vomiting may occur, especially during first several days of treatment, and may be relieved by lying down; checking with health care professional if severe, since an antiemetic may be needed
» Compliance with regimen for preventing severe constipation, if prescribed
» Avoiding external sources of heat (e.g., heating pad, sunlamps, heated water beds, electric blankets, sunbathing, prolonged baths or showers in hot water) and checking with health care professional if fever occurs; absorption of fentanyl may be accelerated
» Informing physician or dentist of use of medication if any kind of surgery (including dental surgery) or emergency treatment is required
System may be worn while bathing, showering, or swimming, but should not be rubbed vigorously because it may become loose or detached; discarding system and applying a new one in an alternate, dry location if this occurs
» Not discontinuing medication abruptly after prolonged use; checking with physician instead, since gradual withdrawal may be needed to minimize risk of precipitating abstinence syndrome
» Suspected overdose: Getting emergency help at once

### Side/adverse effects
Getting emergency help if symptoms of overdose occur, i.e., very slow (fewer than 8 breaths per minute) or troubled breathing, extreme drowsiness, convulsions, low blood pressure, or slow heartbeat
Other potential side effects, especially hallucinations or other CNS effects, urinary retention, chest pain, irregular heartbeat, localized skin reactions, skin rash or blisters, spitting blood, abdominal distention, amblyopia, bladder pain, bradycardia, exfoliative dermatitis, and urinary frequency

## General Dosing Information

Transdermal fentanyl may cause respiratory depression, especially in elderly, very ill, or debilitated patients and patients with pre-existing respiratory problems. Lower doses may be required for these patients, at least initially. However, elderly patients may also be more sensitive to the analgesic effects of opioid analgesics, and lower doses may be sufficient to provide effective analgesia.

Dosage must be individualized. Pre-existing tolerance to opioid analgesics is the primary factor to be considered in determining the appropriate initial dose of transdermal fentanyl. The rate at which tolerance develops varies widely among individuals. For patients who have been receiving chronic therapy with another opioid analgesic, initial dosage of transdermal fentanyl should be based on the patient's daily opioid requirement.

The transdermal system should be kept in the protective packaging until it is used. It should be applied to a dry, flat, nonirritated, non-irradiated skin surface of the upper arm or torso. If necessary, hair at the application site may be clipped (but not shaved) prior to application. Also, if the site is cleansed prior to application, clear water should be used; soaps, oils, lotions, alcohol, or other agents that may irritate the skin or change its characteristics should be avoided. The system should be pressed firmly in place with the palm of the hand for about 30 seconds, making sure that contact is complete, especially around the edges.

Because of the delayed onset of action after initial application of a fentanyl transdermal system, the adequacy of analgesia cannot be evaluated for 24 hours. A short-acting opioid analgesic must be administered as needed to relieve pain. If necessary, a higher dose may be applied for the second 72 hours, based on the quantity of supplemental opioid required during the second or third day of the first 72-hour application. Subsequent increases in dosage, if needed, should be made at 6-day intervals, with "rescue" doses continuing to be administered as needed until maximum analgesia has been attained. Some patients may require "rescue" dosing with a short-acting opioid analgesic for breakthrough pain throughout transdermal fentanyl therapy.

The fentanyl transdermal system should be removed after 72 hours. If treatment is being continued, a new system should be applied at a new site after the prior one has been removed.

Concurrent administration of a nonopioid analgesic (such as aspirin or other salicylates, other nonsteroidal anti-inflammatory drugs, or acetaminophen) with opioid analgesics provides additive analgesia and may permit lower doses of the opioid analgesic to be utilized.

The overall treatment regimen for chronic pain patients who are receiving long-term opioid analgesic therapy includes management of common side effects such as sedation, nausea and vomiting, and constipation. An antiemetic may be needed, especially during the first few weeks of therapy. Also, measures to prevent constipation and decrease the risk of intestinal obstruction may be needed, such as administration of a laxative (a bowel stimulant and/or a stool softener), a high fluid intake, and an increase in dietary fiber. Appropriate medications and dosages must be determined according to the physical condition and the needs of the individual patient.

Increases in the dosage of transdermal fentanyl and/or "rescue" medications may be required as tolerance to the medication develops or increases and/or the intensity of pain increases. Tolerance to the respiratory depressant effects of an opioid analgesic develops concurrently with tolerance to its analgesic effects. Careful adjustment of dosage as required to provide adequate analgesia is not likely to increase the risk of respiratory depression. However, a reduction in dose may be needed to prevent respiratory depression, which may occur even at a previously well-tolerated opioid dose, if the intensity of pain decreases because of changes in the patient's condition or institution of other pain-relieving treatments.

Psychological and physical dependence may occur with chronic administration of an opioid analgesic; an abstinence syndrome may occur when the medication is discontinued. However, physical dependence in patients receiving prolonged therapy for severe chronic pain rarely leads to true addiction, i.e., a desire to continue taking the medication (for its euphoric effect) after it is no longer required for pain relief. **Fear of causing addiction should not result in failure to provide adequate pain relief,** although caution is advised if patient predisposition toward drug abuse is known or strongly suspected. Reducing the dose gradually prior to discontinuation may minimize the development of withdrawal symptoms following prolonged use.

If a patient is being changed from transdermal fentanyl to another opioid analgesic, the transdermal system should be removed and the new analgesic administered in a low dose that may be gradually increased according to the patient's report of pain until adequate analgesia is achieved. The fact that fentanyl concentrations decrease very slowly after removal of the system must be considered when selecting a starting dose of the new agent. Also, the oral morphine–to–transdermal fentanyl conversion ratios recommended by the manufacturer for determining initial doses of transdermal fentanyl for opioid-tolerant patients are very conservative. Using the reverse of these ratios to calculate an appropriate dose of a subsequently administered opioid could result in an overdose and is not recommended.

### Safety considerations for handling this medication

The transdermal system is supplied in sealed systems that pose little risk of exposure to health care personnel. If any of the gel in the reservoir should contact the skin, the area should be flushed with copious quantities of water. Soap, alcohol, or other solvents may enhance penetration of fentanyl through the skin and should not be used.

## Transdermal Dosage Forms

### FENTANYL TRANSDERMAL SYSTEM

Note: The doses and strengths of the fentanyl transdermal system are expressed in terms of the delivery rate in mcg per hour.

### Usual adult dose

Analgesic—
 For chronic pain: Transdermal, the appropriate number of transdermal systems to be applied and kept in place for seventy-two hours.
 For patients who are not opioid-tolerant—Not more than one transdermal system rated to deliver 25 mcg (0.025 mg) per hour, initially. Dosage may be increased gradually as needed and tolerated until an adequate response has been attained.
 For opioid-tolerant patients—Initially, a quantity of fentanyl (in mcg per hour) equivalent to the patient's current twenty-four-hour oral morphine requirement, as follows:

| Fentanyl (mcg/hr) | Morphine* (mg/24 hr) |
|---|---|
| | Oral |
| 25 | 45–134 |
| 50 | 135–224 |
| 75 | 225–314 |
| 100 | 315–404 |
| 125 | 405–494 |
| 150 | 495–584 |
| 175 | 585–674 |
| 200 | 675–764 |
| 225 | 765–854 |
| 250 | 855–944 |
| 275 | 945–1034 |
| 300 | 1035–1124 |

*A 10-mg intramuscular (IM) dose of morphine is therapeutically equivalent to 30 mg of chronically administered oral morphine or 60 mg of intermittently administered oral morphine. For patients who are receiving opioid analgesics other than morphine, the patient's twenty-four-hour opioid requirement should be determined, then converted to the equianalgesic oral morphine dose. The following quantities are equivalent to 30 mg of chronically administered oral morphine or 60 mg of intermittently administered oral morphine:

 For buprenorphine—300 mcg (0.3 mg) IM.
 For butorphanol—2 mg IM.
 For codeine—200 mg orally; 130 mg IM.
 For dezocine—10 mg IM.
 For heroin—60 mg orally; 5 mg IM.
 For hydromorphone—7.5 mg orally; 1.5 mg IM.
 For levorphanol—4 mg orally; 2 mg IM.
 For meperidine—300 mg orally; 75 mg IM.
 For methadone—20 mg orally; 10 mg IM.
 For nalbuphine—10 mg IM.
 For oxycodone—30 mg orally.
 For oxymorphone—1 mg IM; 10 mg rectally.
 For pentazocine—180 mg orally; 60 mg IM.

Note: The oral morphine-to-transdermal fentanyl conversion ratios listed above are conservative; the need for an increase in dose should be anticipated. The second dose of transdermal fentanyl may be increased by 25 mcg per hour for each 90 mg per day of supplemental oral morphine (or equivalent dosage of other opioid analgesics) required during the second or third day of the first application. Six days may be required to reach equilibrium after each increase in dose; therefore, the higher dose should be worn for seventy-two-hour applications before further increases are made. If necessary, more than one transdermal system may be applied at a time.

A few patients may need replacement of the transdermal system(s) every forty-eight hours. Before the interval between applications is decreased, an attempt should be made to maintain the seventy-two-hour interval.

**Usual pediatric dose**
Children up to 18 years of age—Safety and efficacy have not been established.

**Usual geriatric dose**
See *Usual adult dose*

Note: It is recommended that initial dosage not exceed 25 mcg (0.025 mg) per hour unless the patient has been receiving chronic therapy with more than 135 mg per day of oral morphine or an equivalent dose of another opioid analgesic.

**Strength(s) usually available**
U.S.—
  25 mcg (0.025 mg) per hour (a total of 2.5 mg of fentanyl per 10 square centimeters [cm$^2$]) (Rx) [*Duragesic* (alcohol 0.1 mL)].
  50 mcg (0.05 mg) per hour (a total of 5 mg of fentanyl per 20 cm$^2$) (Rx) [*Duragesic* (alcohol 0.2 mL)].
  75 mcg (0.075 mg) per hour (a total of 7.5 mg of fentanyl per 30 cm$^2$) (Rx) [*Duragesic* (alcohol 0.3 mL)].
  100 mcg (0.1 mg) per hour (a total of 10 mg of fentanyl per 40 cm$^2$) (Rx) [*Duragesic* (alcohol 0.4 mL)].
Canada—
  25 mcg (0.025 mg) per hour (a total of 2.5 mg of fentanyl per 10 cm$^2$) (Rx) [*Duragesic* (alcohol 0.1 mL)].
  50 mcg (0.05 mg) per hour (a total of 5 mg of fentanyl per 20 cm$^2$) (Rx) [*Duragesic* (alcohol 0.2 mL)].
  75 mcg (0.075 mg) per hour (a total of 7.5 mg of fentanyl per 30 cm$^2$) (Rx) [*Duragesic* (alcohol 0.3 mL)].
  100 mcg (0.1 mg) per hour (a total of 10 mg of fentanyl per 40 cm$^2$) (Rx) [*Duragesic* (alcohol 0.4 mL)].

**Packaging and storage**
Store below 30 °C (59 °F), unless otherwise specified by manufacturer.

**Auxiliary labeling**
- May cause drowsiness.
- Avoid alcoholic beverages.
- May be habit-forming.

## Selected Bibliography
Calis KA, Kohler DR, Corso DM. Transdermally administered fentanyl for pain management. Clin Pharm 1992; 11: 22-36.
Yee LY, Lopez JR. Transdermal fentanyl. Ann Pharmacother 1992; 26: 1393-9.
Payne R. Transdermal fentanyl: Suggested recommendations for clinical use. J Pain Symptom Manage 1992; 7 No 3 (suppl): S40-S44.

Developed: 07/27/94

# FENTANYL DERIVATIVES   Systemic

This monograph includes information on the following: 1) Alfentanil; 2) Fentanyl; 3) Sufentanil.

VA CLASSIFICATION (Primary/Secondary): CN101/CN205

Note: Controlled substance classification—
  U.S.—II.
  Canada—N.

Commonly used brand name(s): *Alfenta*[1]; *Sublimaze*[2]; *Sufenta*[3].

Note: For a listing of dosage forms and brand names by country availability, see *Dosage Forms* section(s).

## Category
Anesthesia adjunct (opioid analgesic)—Alfentanil, Fentanyl, Sufentanil.
Analgesic—Fentanyl.

## Indications
Note: Bracketed information in the *Indications* section refers to uses that are not included in U.S. product labeling.

**Accepted**
Anesthesia, general [or local][1] adjunct—Fentanyl and its derivatives are indicated as opioid analgesic supplements to general anesthesia. During surgery, they are often used in conjunction with other agents, such as a combination of an ultrashort-acting barbiturate, a neuromuscular blocking agent, and an inhalation anesthetic (usually nitrous oxide), for the maintenance of "balanced" anesthesia.
  Fentanyl and its derivatives are also indicated as primary agents for the induction of anesthesia in patients undergoing general surgery.
  Fentanyl and sufentanil are also indicated as primary agents for the maintenance of anesthesia in selected patients undergoing major surgery. In these cases, they are administered in high doses with 100% oxygen or nitrous oxide plus oxygen and a neuromuscular blocking agent.
  Fentanyl [and sufentanil][1] are indicated to provide neuroleptanalgesia (in conjunction with a neuroleptic agent such as droperidol) or neuroleptanesthesia (in conjunction with a neuroleptic agent and nitrous oxide).
  Fentanyl [and sufentanil][1] are indicated to supplement regional or local anesthesia.
  Fentanyl is approved by U.S. and Canadian regulatory agencies for use as presurgical medication. However, because of its short duration of action (following administration of single analgesic doses), fentanyl may be less desirable than longer acting opioid analgesics for this purpose.
Pain, postoperative (treatment)—Fentanyl is also approved by U.S. and Canadian regulatory agencies for prevention or relief of pain in the immediate postoperative period; however, longer acting opioid analgesics are more commonly used in this situation.

**Unaccepted**
Alfentanil has also been investigated for use as the primary agent, administered in conjunction with 100% oxygen and a neuromuscular blocking agent, for the maintenance of anesthesia in selected patients undergoing cardiovascular surgery. Preliminary information indicates that the patient must be heavily premedicated and that continuous intravenous infusion of extremely high doses is required. Further study is needed to determine efficacy and appropriate dosage for such use.

[1] Not included in Canadian product labeling.

## Pharmacology/Pharmacokinetics

**Physicochemical characteristics**
Molecular weight—
  Alfentanil hydrochloride: 452.98.
  Fentanyl citrate: 528.60.
  Sufentanil citrate: 578.68.
pKa—
  Alfentanil: 6.5.
  Fentanyl: 8.43.
  Sufentanil: 8.01.
Partition coefficient (octanol:water; pH 7.4)—
  Alfentanil hydrochloride: 130
  Fentanyl citrate: 816
  Sufentanil citrate: 1727

**Mechanism of action/Effect**
Low to moderate doses of fentanyl and its derivatives produce analgesia. During surgery, analgesic actions provide dose-related protection against hemodynamic responses to surgical stress; however, patient responsiveness to the pharmacodynamic actions of these medications is highly variable. Although high doses of these medications produce loss of consciousness, the ability of opioid analgesics (when used alone) to induce a true anesthetic state has been questioned.
  Opioid analgesics bind with stereospecific receptors at many sites within the central nervous system (CNS) to alter processes affecting both the perception of and emotional response to pain. Although the precise sites and mechanisms of action have not been fully determined, alterations in the release of various neurotransmitters from afferent nerves sensitive to painful stimuli may be partially responsible for the analgesic effects.
  It has been proposed that there are multiple subtypes of opioid receptors, each mediating various therapeutic and/or side effects of opioid drugs. The actions of an opioid analgesic may therefore depend upon whether it acts as a full agonist or a partial agonist or is inactive at each type of receptor. Fentanyl and its derivatives probably produce their effects via agonist actions at the mu receptor.

**Other actions/effects**
Fentanyl and its derivatives may produce signs and symptoms common to opioid analgesics including respiratory depression (characterized by decreases in respiratory rate, tidal volume, minute ventilation, and ventilatory response to carbon dioxide), ureteral spasm, biliary spasm, decreased gastrointestinal motility, euphoria, miosis, hypotension, and

bradycardia. However, unlike many other opioid analgesics, fentanyl and its derivatives have not been shown to cause histamine release (in doses used clinically).

Fentanyl and its derivatives, especially in moderate or high doses, may induce skeletal muscle rigidity.

Fentanyl and its derivatives may produce a dose-related decrease in certain hormonal responses during surgery, such as increased blood concentrations of circulating growth hormone, catecholamines, cortisol, antidiuretic hormone, and prolactin. However, alfentanil's effects on endocrine responses to surgical stimulation have not been fully evaluated. Also, in patients undergoing coronary bypass surgery, these agents may not suppress such endocrine responses, especially increased catecholamine concentrations, during the period of cardiopulmonary bypass.

### Volume of distribution

Alfentanil—Usually 0.6 to 1.0 liter per kg of body weight but subject to interpatient variability; values ranging from 0.23 to 2.47 liters per kg of body weight have been reported. The volume of distribution may be increased during aortocoronary bypass or decreased in children, but is not altered by obesity or hepatic function impairment. However, the distribution volume of total alfentanil (but not of the unbound [free] fraction) may be increased in patients with renal failure.

Fentanyl—Usually 4 liters per kg of body weight, although values ranging from 3.1 to 7.8 liters per kg of body weight have been reported.

Sufentanil—1.08 to 2.78 liters per kg of body weight.

Note: Fentanyl and its derivatives readily cross the blood/brain barrier; however, because of alfentanil's lower degree of lipophilicity (and therefore lower degree of tissue binding) and its lower pKa, alfentanil reaches receptors in the brain significantly more rapidly than fentanyl.

Fentanyl and sufentanil are rapidly distributed to body tissues. The relatively poor blood flow to fatty tissues limits the rate of the medications' accumulation in these tissues. However, accumulation in body fat, as well as in other tissues, may occur with large or multiple doses or prolonged administration. Clearance of either of these agents from tissues may result in therapeutic blood concentrations being maintained following discontinuation of administration, leading to a prolonged duration of action.

Alfentanil is also rapidly distributed to body tissues. Although accumulation of alfentanil may occur with prolonged continuous infusion or with repeated administration of single doses and may lead to a prolonged duration of action, alfentanil's accumulation in body tissues is significantly less than that of fentanyl or sufentanil. Therefore, alfentanil's duration of action is less likely than that of fentanyl or sufentanil to be substantially prolonged by clearance from body tissues.

### Protein binding

Alfentanil—About 92%; primarily to glycoproteins (especially alpha-1-acidglycoprotein [AAG]). Although independent of alfentanil plasma concentration or plasma pH, alfentanil protein binding is subject to interpatient variability and may be decreased in patients with alcoholic hepatic cirrhosis or renal failure and during cardiopulmonary bypass.

Fentanyl—80 to 89%, primarily to albumin and lipoproteins; dependent on plasma pH.

Sufentanil—92.5%, primarily to AAG; independent of sufentanil plasma concentration but highly dependent on plasma pH.

### Biotransformation

Hepatic; sufentanil may also undergo some metabolism in the small intestine. The rate of metabolism is dependent on total dosage, hepatic function, and factors affecting hepatic blood flow (possibly including certain surgical manipulations or, to a much lesser extent, concurrent use of a potent inhalation anesthetic). The rate of fentanyl or sufentanil metabolism is also dependent on the rate of their release from various body tissues. The rate of alfentanil metabolism is decreased in geriatric patients, obese patients, and patients with hepatic function impairment. In addition, genetic polymorphism has been suspected as a cause of unusually slow alfentanil metabolism in a few patients.

### Half-life

Alfentanil—
 Triphasic (with a dose of 50 or 125 mcg per kg of body weight):
  Distribution—0.4 to 3.1 minutes.
  Redistribution—4.6 to 21.6 minutes.
  Elimination—Generally 1 to 2.1 hours, although values well outside this range have been reported. The elimination half-life is not altered in patients with renal failure but may be decreased in children. Also, the elimination half-life is highly dependent on factors affecting the rate of metabolism. Increased values have been reported in patients with reduced hepatic function (up to 4.9 hours in asymptomatic patients with abnormal liver function test values and up to 5.8 hours in patients with active hepatic [alcoholic] cirrhosis), geriatric patients (about 2.3 hours), and obese patients (about 3 hours).

Fentanyl—
 Triphasic (with a dose of 6.4 mcg per kg of body weight):
  Distribution—1.7 minutes.
  Redistribution—13 minutes.
  Elimination—3.6 hours; may be greatly prolonged during and following cardiopulmonary bypass and in geriatric patients. One study showed an average elimination half-life of 15.75 hours following administration of 10 mcg per kg of body weight to patients 60 years of age or older.

Sufentanil—
 Triphasic (with a dose of 5 mcg per kg of body weight):
  Distribution—1.4 minutes.
  Redistribution—18 minutes.
  Elimination—2.7 hours; may be greatly prolonged during and following cardiopulmonary bypass.

### Onset of action

Alfentanil—
 Analgesic effects (anesthesia adjunct doses):
  Within 1 minute.
 Time to loss of consciousness (induction doses):
  Dependent on rate of administration; generally within 1 to 2 minutes.

Fentanyl—
 Analgesic effects (anesthesia adjunct doses):
  Intramuscular—7 to 15 minutes.
  Intravenous—1 to 2 minutes.
 Time to loss of consciousness (induction doses):
  Dependent on rate of administration; 4 to 5 minutes when administered intravenously at a rate of 400 mcg per minute.

Sufentanil—
 Analgesic effects (anesthesia adjunct doses):
  Within 1 minute.
 Time to loss of consciousness (induction doses):
  Dependent on rate of administration; 1 to 1.6 minutes when administered intravenously at a rate of 300 mcg per minute.

Note: The time to loss of consciousness with induction doses of these medications may be substantially decreased by premedication with a benzodiazepine.

### Therapeutic plasma concentration

Requirements are highly subject to interpatient variability and dependent on the intensity of the surgical stimulus. With alfentanil, it has been shown that the highest plasma concentrations are required near the beginning of surgery (with intubation requiring higher concentrations than incision) and the lowest toward the end of surgery (i.e., 227 during skin closure). Studies of therapeutic plasma concentrations of fentanyl or sufentanil required for different types of surgery, or at different times during a surgical procedure, have not been done.

For use of alfentanil as a supplement to inhalation (nitrous oxide/oxygen) anesthesia—
 For superficial surgery: 100 to >300 nanograms per mL.
 For intra-abdominal surgery: 310 to >400 nanograms per mL.

### Time to peak effect

Alfentanil—
 Single analgesic dose of up to 500 mcg:
  Within 1.5 to 2 minutes (for both analgesia and respiratory depression).

Fentanyl—
 Analgesic effects:
  Intramuscular—20 to 30 minutes.
  Intravenous—3 to 5 minutes.
 Respiratory depressant effects:
  5 to 15 minutes following administration of a single intravenous dose.

### Duration of action

Alfentanil—
 Analgesic effects (single dose of up to 500 mcg):
  5 to 10 minutes.
 Time to awakening (when used as a supplement to nitrous oxide/oxygen anesthesia):
  Usually within 10 minutes following the end of surgery when administered either as single injections or as a variable-rate infusion that is discontinued approximately 15 minutes before the end of surgery.

Note: Alfentanil's duration of action may be decreased in children.

Fentanyl—
  Analgesic effects (anesthesia adjunct doses):
    Intramuscular—1 to 2 hours.
    Intravenous—0.5 to 1 hour (single dose of up to 100 mcg).
  Time to awakening (high doses):
    0.7 to 3.5 hours following an average total dose of 122 mcg per kg of body weight.
Sufentanil—
  Analgesic effects (anesthesia adjunct doses):
    5 minutes.
  Time to awakening (high doses):
    0.7 to 2.9 hours following an average total dose of 12.9 mcg per kg of body weight.

Note: The duration of action of fentanyl and its derivatives is dose-dependent. The effects of a low to moderate single dose of any of these medications are terminated rapidly because of redistribution.

With high or multiple doses or prolonged administration of fentanyl or sufentanil, the duration of action is prolonged because substantial plasma concentrations of these agents may be maintained during their clearance from tissue storage sites (although accumulation of sufentanil is less than that of fentanyl). Accumulation of alfentanil resulting in a prolonged duration of action may occur with prolonged continuous infusion or, to a lesser extent, with repeated administration of single injections during lengthy surgical procedures. However, because accumulation of alfentanil in body tissues is significantly less extensive than that of fentanyl or sufentanil, alfentanil's duration of action after multiple doses or prolonged continuous infusion is more highly dependent on total body clearance than on redistribution and subsequent removal from tissue storage sites. Therefore, alfentanil's duration of action may be affected to a greater extent than that of fentanyl or sufentanil by factors that tend to decrease the rate of metabolism (See *Biotransformation*).

When fentanyl or sufentanil is administered in high doses as the primary agent for maintenance of anesthesia, respiratory depression requiring continued mechanical ventilation may persist for many hours after the patient awakens.

**Elimination**
Alfentanil—Hepatic; only 0.2% of a dose is excreted in the urine as unchanged alfentanil. Inactive metabolites are also excreted in the urine. Approximately 81% of a dose is excreted within 24 hours.
Fentanyl—Primarily hepatic; 10 to 25% of a dose may be excreted in the urine as unchanged fentanyl. About 70% of a dose is excreted within 4 days.
Sufentanil—Via metabolism; about 2% of a dose is excreted in the urine as unchanged sufentanil. About 80% of a dose is excreted within 24 hours.

## Precautions to Consider

### Cross-sensitivity and/or related problems
Patients hypersensitive to fentanyl may be hypersensitive to the chemically related alfentanil or sufentanil also, and vice versa.

### Carcinogenicity
Long-term animal studies of the carcinogenic potential of alfentanil have not been done.

### Mutagenicity
For alfentanil—No evidence of mutagenicity was demonstrated in the Ames *Salmonella* metabolic activating test. Also, no mutagenicity was demonstrated in the micronucleus test in female rats or the dominant lethal assay in female and male mice with single intravenous doses up to 20 mg per kg of body weight (mg/kg) (approximately 40 times the upper recommended human dose).

For sufentanil—Sufentanil has not been shown to have mutagenic potential in the micronucleus test in female rats (with single intravenous doses up to 80 mcg per kg) or in the Ames test.

### Pregnancy/Reproduction
Pregnancy—
  *First trimester*
    For alfentanil:
      Although adequate and well-controlled studies in humans have not been done, one study demonstrated that alfentanil readily crosses the placenta. Studies in rats and rabbits have not shown that alfentanil is teratogenic. However, embryocidal effects (possibly related to maternal toxicity) occurred following administration of 2.5 times the upper recommended human dose for 10 to more than 30 days.
    FDA Pregnancy Category C.

    For fentanyl:
      Although studies on the teratogenic potential of fentanyl have not been done in either animals or humans, one study showed that fentanyl crosses the placenta when it is administered to the mother prior to cesarean section.
    FDA Pregnancy Category C.
    For sufentanil:
      Although adequate and well-controlled studies in humans have not been done, studies in rats and rabbits have not shown that sufentanil is teratogenic. However, embryocidal effects (possibly related to maternal toxicity, decreased food consumption, and anoxia) occurred in rats and rabbits following administration of up to 2.5 times the upper human dose for 10 to more than 30 days.
    FDA Pregnancy Category C.

Labor and delivery—The safety of fentanyl derivatives in obstetrics has not been established. However, in one study, drowsiness (but no other adverse effect) was observed in 4-hour-old neonates after administration of fentanyl to the mother prior to cesarean section. This effect was associated with a concentration of 0.8 nanograms (or more) of fentanyl per mL of cord blood. Drowsiness was not present 24 hours after birth.

### Breast-feeding
Problems in humans have not been documented.
*For alfentanil—*
  In one study, 0.88 nanograms of alfentanil per mL was measured in colostrum 4 hours following maternal administration of 60 mcg per kg of body weight. Measurable concentrations were not present 28 hours following administration.
*For sufentanil—*
  It is not known whether sufentanil is excreted in breast milk.

### Pediatrics
Neonates may be more susceptible to the effects, especially the respiratory depressant effects, of opioid analgesics. Caution is recommended if fentanyl is used as presurgical or postsurgical medication in these patients.

Neonates have been found to have low concentrations of alpha-1-acidglycoprotein, leading to a reduced protein-binding capacity for alfentanil and an increase in the quantity of the medication available to receptor sites. However, one study has demonstrated an increased alfentanil dosage requirement in neonates.

The elimination half-life and duration of action of alfentanil may be decreased in pediatric patients. More frequent administration of supplemental doses than is usually needed by adults may be required.

### Geriatrics
Geriatric patients may be more susceptible to the effects, especially the respiratory depressant effects, of opioid analgesics. Also, elderly patients are more likely to have age-related renal function impairment, which may require caution in patients receiving alfentanil (because of decreased protein-binding, which increases the effects of alfentanil by increasing its concentration at receptor sites) or fentanyl (because excretion of fentanyl may be slowed). Lower initial and supplemental doses, a slower infusion rate, and/or a longer interval between doses than are usually recommended for younger adults may be required for these patients. However, geriatric patients may also be more sensitive to the therapeutic effects of opioid analgesics so that lower doses may be sufficient. In one study, possible increased brain sensitivity to alfentanil was demonstrated in geriatric patients (compared with healthy young adults) as shown by a 40% reduction in the dose required to produce delta waves in the electroencephalogram (EEG).

Many studies have indicated that clearance of opioid analgesics is significantly reduced in geriatric patients. Specifically, studies have shown that alfentanil clearance is reduced by approximately 30% (leading to a prolonged elimination half-life) in patients older than 65 years of age, and that the elimination half-life of fentanyl may be greatly prolonged (in one study, to 15.75 hours) because of reduced clearance in patients 60 years of age and older. Reduced clearance may lead to a risk of delayed postoperative recovery.

### Drug interactions and/or related problems
The following drug interactions and/or related problems have been selected on the basis of their potential clinical significance (possible mechanism in parentheses where appropriate)—not necessarily inclusive (» = major clinical significance):

Note: Combinations containing any of the following medications, depending on the amount present, may also interact with this medication.

Anesthetics, peridural conduction or
Anesthetics, spinal
(alterations in respiration caused by high levels of spinal or peridural blockade may be additive to fentanyl derivative–induced alterations in respiratory rate and alveolar ventilation; also, the vagal effects of fentanyl derivatives may be more pronounced in patients with high levels of spinal or epidural anesthesia, possibly leading to bradycardia and/or hypotension)

Antihypertensives or
Diuretics or
Hypotension-producing medications, other (See *Appendix II*)
(hypotensive effects of these medications may be potentiated when they are used concurrently with a fentanyl derivative; patients should be monitored for excessive fall in blood pressure during and following concurrent use)

» Benzodiazepines
(premedication with a benzodiazepine such as diazepam, lorazepam, or midazolam may decrease the dose of a fentanyl derivative required for induction of anesthesia and decrease the time to loss of consciousness with induction doses; also, administration of a benzodiazepine prior to or during surgery may decrease the risk of patient recall of surgical events postoperatively; however, these potential benefits must be weighed against the potential risks of concurrent use, such as an increased risk of severe hypotension associated with decreases in systemic vascular resistance, increased risk of respiratory depression, and delayed recovery time, especially when the benzodiazepine is administered intravenously)

Beta-adrenergic blocking agents
(preoperative chronic use of systemic beta-adrenergic blocking agents may decrease the frequency and/or severity of hypertensive responses to surgery, especially during sternotomy and sternal spread in cardiac or coronary artery surgery; however, chronic preoperative use of systemic beta-adrenergic blocking agents or ophthalmic beta-adrenergic blocking agents [especially levobunolol or timolol] may also increase the risk of initial bradycardia following induction doses of a fentanyl derivative)

» Buprenorphine and other partial mu-receptor agonists
(use of buprenorphine as presurgical medication prior to opioid analgesic–assisted anesthesia should be undertaken with caution because this partial mu-receptor agonist has high affinity for, and dissociates slowly from, the mu receptor and may therefore decrease the therapeutic effects of subsequently administered mu-receptor agonist)
(buprenorphine and other partial mu-receptor agonists have the potential to reverse respiratory depressant effects induced by high doses of other opioid analgesics [while providing adequate postoperative analgesia] or to cause additive respiratory depression, hypotension, and/or CNS depression if administered in conjunction with low doses of other opioids; although the effects of buprenorphine administered following alfentanil- or sufentanil-assisted anesthesia have not been determined, in one study, administration of 0.3 or 0.45 mg of buprenorphine intramuscularly every 6 hours following opioid-assisted anesthesia with total doses of 0.2 or 0.3 mg of fentanyl caused a higher incidence of hypotension, respiratory depression, and CNS depression than equianalgesic doses [10 or 15 mg] of morphine intramuscularly every 6 hours)

» CNS depression–producing medications, other, including those commonly used as preanesthetic medication or for induction, supplementation, or maintenance of anesthesia (See *Appendix II*)
(concurrent use with a fentanyl derivative may result in increased CNS depressant, respiratory depressant, and hypotensive effects; caution is recommended and the dosage of each agent should be carefully titrated)
(it is recommended that initial dosage of other opioid agonist analgesics used during recovery from fentanyl- or sufentanil-assisted anesthesia be decreased to as low as one-fourth to one-third of the usual recommended dose)
(dosage requirements of volatile inhalation anesthetics may be decreased by 30 to 50% for the first hour of maintenance following administration of anesthetic induction doses of alfentanil)

» Hepatic enzyme inhibitors (See *Appendix II*)
(chronic preoperative administration or perioperative use of hepatic enzyme inhibitors may decrease plasma clearance and prolong the duration of action of alfentanil)

Monoamine oxidase (MAO) inhibitors, including furazolidone, pargyline, and procarbazine
(caution is recommended when using a fentanyl derivative in patients who have received an MAO inhibitor within 14 days because concurrent use of MAO inhibitors with meperidine has resulted in unpredictable, severe, and sometimes fatal reactions, including immediate excitation, sweating, rigidity, and severe hypertension, or, in some patients, hypotension, severe respiratory depression, coma, seizures, hyperpyrexia, and vascular collapse; the risk of a significant reaction with fentanyl-derivative opioid analgesics has been questioned because a few reports indicate that fentanyl caused no adverse reactions when administered to patients receiving MAO inhibitor therapy; however, administration of a small test dose of a fentanyl derivative [to detect any possible interaction] may be advisable until the relative risk of concurrent use has been better defined)

Nalbuphine or
Pentazocine
(these opioid agonist/antagonist analgesics may partially antagonize the analgesic, respiratory depressant, and CNS depressant effects of fentanyl derivatives; however, because of their agonist activity, concurrent use of these agents also has the potential to produce additive CNS, respiratory, and hypotensive effects; the extent to which antagonistic or additive effects will predominate may depend upon dosage of the fentanyl derivative, with antagonism being more likely with low to moderate doses)

Naloxone
(naloxone antagonizes the analgesic, hypotensive, CNS, and respiratory depressant effects of fentanyl derivatives; dosage of the antagonist should be carefully titrated when used to reverse the effects of opioid analgesics used during surgery in order to achieve the desired effect without interfering with control of postoperative pain or inducing other adverse effects)
(naloxone also reverses skeletal muscle rigidity induced by fentanyl derivatives)

» Naltrexone
(usual doses of opioid analgesics will be ineffective if administered to a patient receiving naltrexone, which blocks the therapeutic effects of opioid analgesics; if possible, alternative [nonopioid] medications should be used prior to, during, and following surgery, because administration of increased doses of opioids to override naltrexone blockade of opioid receptors may result in increased and more prolonged respiratory depression and/or circulatory collapse; naltrexone should be discontinued several days prior to elective surgery if administration of an opioid is unavoidable)

Neuromuscular blocking agents
(concurrent use with high doses of sufentanil may reduce the initial dosage requirements for a nondepolarizing neuromuscular blocking agent; it is recommended that a peripheral nerve stimulator be used to determine dosage)
(concurrent use of a neuromuscular blocking agent prevents or reverses muscle rigidity induced by fentanyl derivatives)
(a neuromuscular blocking agent having vagolytic activity such as pancuronium or gallamine may decrease the risk of fentanyl derivative–induced bradycardia or hypotension, especially in patients receiving chronic therapy with beta-adrenergic blocking agents and/or vasodilators for treatment of coronary artery disease; however, concurrent use may also increase the risk of tachycardia or hypertension in some patients)
(a nonvagolytic neuromuscular blocking agent such as succinylcholine will not decrease the risk of bradycardia or hypotension induced by a fentanyl derivative; however, in some patients, especially those with compromised cardiac function and/or those receiving a beta-adrenergic blocking agent preoperatively, concurrent use may increase the incidence and/or severity of these effects)
(respiratory depressant effects of neuromuscular blocking agents may be additive to respiratory depressant effects of fentanyl derivatives; although increased or prolonged respiratory depression or paralysis [apnea] may occur, clinical significance is minimal while the patient is being mechanically ventilated; however, patients should be carefully monitored during and following concurrent use, especially if there is a possibility of incomplete reversal of neuromuscular blockade postoperatively)

Nitrous oxide
(in addition to the increased CNS depressant, respiratory depressant, and hypotensive effects that may occur when a fentanyl derivative is used concurrently with any CNS depressant, concurrent use of nitrous oxide with high doses of these agents may decrease mean arterial pressure, heart rate, and cardiac output; these effects may be more pronounced in patients with poor left ventricular function)

Phenothiazines
(in addition to the increased CNS depressant, respiratory depressant, and hypotensive effects that may occur when a phenothiazine is

used concurrently with an opioid analgesic, some phenothiazines increase, while others decrease, the effects of opioid analgesic supplements to anesthesia; however, the effect of various phenothiazines on fentanyl derivative–assisted anesthesia has not been determined)

**Laboratory value alterations**
The following have been selected on the basis of their potential clinical significance (possible effect in parentheses where appropriate)—not necessarily inclusive (» = major clinical significance):

With diagnostic test results
  Gastric emptying studies
    (opioid analgesics may delay gastric emptying, thereby invalidating test results)
  Hepatobiliary imaging using technetium Tc 99m disofenin
    (delivery of technetium Tc 99m disofenin to the small bowel may be prevented because of opioid analgesic–induced constriction of the sphincter of Oddi and increased biliary tract pressure; these actions result in delayed visualization and thus resemble obstruction of the common bile duct; contraction of the sphincter of Oddi has been demonstrated with alfentanil and fentanyl and, although not yet documented, should be considered a possibility with sufentanil also)
  Plasma amylase determinations and
  Plasma lipase determinations
    (activity of these enzymes may be increased because alfentanil and fentanyl can cause contractions of the sphincter of Oddi and increased biliary tract pressure; the possibility should be considered that the diagnostic utility of determinations of these enzymes may be compromised for up to 24 hours after fentanyl administration or for several hours after alfentanil administration; although documentation is not yet available, the possibility exists that similar effects may occur with sufentanil)

With physiology/laboratory test values
  Cerebrospinal fluid pressure
    (opioid analgesics may increase cerebrospinal fluid pressure; effect is secondary to respiratory depression–induced carbon dioxide retention)

**Medical considerations/Contraindications**
The medical considerations/contraindications included have been selected on the basis of their potential clinical significance (reasons given in parentheses where appropriate)—not necessarily inclusive (» = major clinical significance).

*Risk-benefit should be considered when the following medical problems exist:*

For all indications
  Allergic reaction to fentanyl or its derivatives, history of
  Cardiac bradyarrhythmias
    (may be induced or exacerbated)
  Cardiac conditions leading to compromised cardiac reserve
    (increased risk of severe bradycardia and/or undesirably large decreases in mean blood pressure, especially following rapid administration of induction doses of a fentanyl derivative)
  Head injury or
  Increased intracranial pressure, pre-existing or
  Intracranial lesions
    (risk of respiratory depression and further elevation of cerebrospinal fluid pressure is increased; also, opioid analgesic–induced sedation and pupillary changes may obscure clinical course of head injury)
» Hepatic function impairment or cirrhosis
    (studies have demonstrated that alfentanil clearance rate is reduced, leading to increased elimination half-life and prolonged duration of action; although clearance of fentanyl or sufentanil may not be altered as greatly as that of alfentanil, caution is advised)
    (alfentanil's effects may also be increased because of decreased protein-binding leading to increased concentration of medication at receptor sites; a reduction of alfentanil dosage may be required)
  Hypothyroidism
    (risk of respiratory depression and prolonged CNS depression is greatly increased; a reduction in dosage of the fentanyl derivative may be required)
  Renal function impairment
    (elimination of fentanyl [up to 25% of a dose is excreted unchanged in the urine] may be slowed)
    (alfentanil's effects may be increased because of decreased protein-binding leading to increased concentration of medication at receptor sites; however, alfentanil's clearance rate and duration of action are not affected)

  Respiratory impairment or pulmonary disease, pre-existing
    (opioid analgesics may further decrease respiratory drive and increase airway resistance; although clinical significance is minimal if the patient is being mechanically ventilated during surgery, respiratory support may be required with doses that usually permit spontaneous breathing)
  Caution is also advised in elderly, very ill, or debilitated patients, who may be more sensitive to the effects, especially the respiratory depressant effects, of opioid analgesics.

*For use of a fentanyl derivative for indications other than as a component of anesthesia*
  Abdominal conditions, acute
    (diagnosis or clinical course may be obscured)
  Gallbladder disease or gallstones
    (opioid analgesics may cause biliary tract spasm)
  Gastrointestinal tract surgery
    (opioid analgesics may decrease gastrointestinal motility)
  Prostatic hypertrophy or obstruction or
  Urethral stricture or
  Urinary tract surgery
    (opioid analgesics may cause urinary retention)
» Respiratory impairment or pulmonary disease, pre-existing
    (opioid analgesics may further decrease respiratory drive and increase airway resistance)
» Caution is also advised in elderly, very ill, or very young patients, who may be more sensitive to the effects, especially the respiratory depressant effects, of opioid analgesics.

**Patient monitoring**
The following may be especially important in patient monitoring (other tests may be warranted in some patients, depending on condition; » = major clinical significance):

  Monitoring of vital signs, especially blood pressure and respiratory status
    (required during and following administration; prolonged postoperative surveillance may be necessary following high or multiple doses or prolonged administration because of the risk of prolonged respiratory depression, especially after use of fentanyl or sufentanil; also, following high or multiple doses or prolonged administration of alfentanil or fentanyl, respiratory depression, respiratory arrest, bradycardia, asystole, arrhythmias, and hypotension have occurred or recurred following initial recovery)

## Side/Adverse Effects

Note: *Fentanyl derivatives may cause rigidity in muscles of respiration in the chest and pharynx, which may lead to difficulty in establishing pulmonary ventilation.* Rigidity may occur more rapidly with alfentanil than with fentanyl or sufentanil. In addition, alfentanil may cause rigidity of abdominal muscles; flexion of the fingers, wrists, and elbows; extension of the toes, ankles, knees, and hips; contraction of neck muscles; immobility of the head; and/or clenching of the jaw. These effects are dose-dependent and must be anticipated with anesthetic induction doses. Abnormal eye movements (i.e., disconjugate gaze) have also been reported during induction with alfentanil. Chest wall rigidity has also been reported during emergence from fentanyl- or sufentanil-assisted anesthesia.

Delayed respiratory depression, respiratory arrest, bradycardia, asystole, arrhythmias, and hypotension have been reported to occur or recur following initial recovery from alfentanil- or fentanyl-assisted anesthesia and should be considered a possibility following sufentanil-assisted anesthesia also.

Like other opioid analgesics, fentanyl derivatives may cause physical dependence following prolonged use. It has been proposed that adverse effects (such as tachycardia, hypertension, hyperpnea, hyperalgesia, nausea, and vomiting) occurring (rarely) after naloxone is administered for reversal of opioid effects following lengthy surgical procedures may be manifestations of an induced abstinence syndrome in acutely dependent individuals. However, other symptoms more commonly associated with an opioid withdrawal syndrome have not been reported following perisurgical use.

In addition to the side effects listed below, hypertension, tachycardia, and skeletal muscle movements (not related to onset of rigidity) may occur during surgery. These effects may be indicative of a failure to suppress autonomic responses to surgical stimulation rather than a direct effect of the medication. The incidence and severity of these effects are lower with sufentanil than with alfentanil or fentanyl.

Although not all of the side/adverse effects listed below have been reported with all of the fentanyl derivatives, they have been reported with at least one of these medications and/or encountered during administration of other opioid analgesics. Therefore, they should be considered potential side effects of any of the fentanyl derivatives.

The following side/adverse effects have been selected on the basis of their potential clinical significance (possible signs and symptoms in parentheses where appropriate)—not necessarily inclusive:

**Those indicating need for medical attention**

*Bradycardia; hypotension*—most likely to occur shortly after administration; blood pressure may return to preadministration values with surgical stimulation; *respiratory depression, intra- or postoperative*—may progress to apnea

Incidence less frequent
*Cardiac arrhythmia*—incidence 2% with alfentanil or fentanyl; <1% with sufentanil; *confusion, postoperative*—rare with alfentanil

Incidence rare
*Bronchospasm, allergic*—not caused by histamine release; *circulatory depression*—may lead to cardiac arrest; *convulsions*—reported with fentanyl and sufentanil only; *dermatitis, allergic* (skin rash [fentanyl], hives [alfentanil, fentanyl], and/or itching [alfentanil, fentanyl, sufentanil]); *dysesthesia, opioid analgesic-induced* (itching, especially of the face); *laryngospasm*—may be a form of rigidity; *mental depression, postoperative; paradoxical CNS excitation or delirium*

**Those common to opioid analgesics (but not necessarily reported specifically with fentanyl derivatives) and indicating need for medical attention only if they continue or are bothersome**

Incidence more frequent
*Drowsiness, postoperative*—less frequent with alfentanil; *nausea or vomiting*—lower incidence reported with sufentanil than with alfentanil or fentanyl but highly variable; may depend on the specific surgical procedure performed, e.g., especially likely following gynecologic surgery

Incidence less frequent or rare
*Biliary spasm; blurred or double vision or other changes in vision; chills; CNS depression or hypotension, orthostatic* (dizziness, lightheadedness, feeling faint, unusual tiredness or weakness); *constipation; ureteral spasm* (decreased or difficult urination)

## Overdose

For specific information on the agents used in the management of an overdose, see:
- *Atropine* in *Anticholinergics/Antispasmodics (Systemic)* monograph;
- *Naloxone (Systemic)* monograph; and/or
- *Neuromuscular Blocking Agents (Systemic)* monograph; and/or
- *Sympathomimetic Agents—Cardiovascular Use (Parenteral-Systemic)* monograph.

For more information on the management of overdose or unintentional ingestion, **contact a Poison Control Center** (see *Poison Control Center Listing*).

**Clinical effects of overdose**

The following effects have been selected on the basis of their potential clinical significance (possible signs and symptoms in parentheses where appropriate)—not necessarily inclusive:

Acute
*Bradycardia; circulatory depression; cold, clammy skin; dizziness, severe; drowsiness, severe; hypotension; nervousness or restlessness, severe; pinpoint pupils of eyes; respiratory depression; weakness, severe*

**Treatment of overdose**

Specific treatment—
For bradycardia—Administering atropine. Alternatively, if a neuromuscular blocking agent is being used, administration of a neuromuscular blocking agent with vagolytic activity, such as pancuronium or gallamine, may antagonize fentanyl derivative-induced bradycardia.

For respiratory depression—During surgery, respiratory depression may be managed via endotracheal intubation and assisted or controlled respiration. If respiratory depression persists following surgery, prolonged mechanical ventilation may be required. Also, intravenous administration of the opioid antagonist naloxone may be required. Dosage of naloxone should be carefully titrated to achieve the desired effect without interfering with control of postoperative pain or causing other adverse effects; hypertension and tachycardia, sometimes resulting in left ventricular failure and pulmonary edema, have occurred following naloxone administration in these circumstances (especially in cardiac patients). Initial doses as small as 0.5 mcg (0.0005 mg) of naloxone per kg of body weight have been recommended. Because the duration of respiratory depression may exceed the duration of action of a single intravenous dose of the antagonist, continued monitoring of the patient is mandatory so that additional antagonist may be administered as necessary. Continuous intravenous infusion of naloxone may provide continuing control of undesirable opioid effects.

For hypotension—Administration of appropriate parenteral fluid therapy is recommended. Repositioning of the patient to improve venous return to the heart should be considered when surgical conditions permit. If necessary, a vasopressor (during or following surgery) and/or naloxone (postoperatively only) may be administered.

For muscle rigidity—Administering a neuromuscular blocking agent and assisting respiration via controlled ventilation with oxygen. Alternatively, if muscle rigidity should occur upon emergence, naloxone may be administered.

Supportive care—
Other supportive measures should also be employed as needed. Patients in whom intentional overdose is confirmed or suspected should be referred for psychiatric consultation.

## Patient Consultation

As an aid to patient consultation, refer to *Advice for the Patient, Narcotic Analgesics—For Surgery and Obstetrics (Systemic)*.

In providing consultation, consider emphasizing the following selected information (» = major clinical significance):

**Before receiving this medication**
» Conditions affecting use, especially:
    Allergic reaction to fentanyl or its derivatives
    Pregnancy—Alfentanil and fentanyl cross the placenta
    Breast-feeding—Fentanyl is excreted in breast milk
    Use in children—Increased sensitivity to the effects of opioid analgesics in neonates
    Use in the elderly—Increased sensitivity to the effects of opioid analgesics
    Any other medications, including "street" drugs
    Other medical problems, especially hepatic function impairment or cirrhosis and pulmonary disease

**Precautions after receiving this medication**

*To be followed for about 24 hours after receiving this medication as part of an outpatient regimen*
» Caution if dizziness, drowsiness, lightheadedness, or blurred vision occurs
» Avoiding use of alcohol or other CNS depressants unless specifically prescribed or otherwise approved by physician or dentist

**Side/adverse effects**
Signs and symptoms of potential side effects, especially postoperative CNS depression and allergic dermatitis

## General Dosing Information

Fentanyl derivatives should be administered only by personnel experienced in the use of intravenous anesthetics and in the management of the respiratory effects of opioid analgesics.

*An opioid antagonist, resuscitative medications, intubation equipment, and oxygen should be readily available during and following administration of a fentanyl derivative. Careful monitoring of the patient's respiratory status is necessary during and following surgery.* These medications suppress respiration, especially in elderly, very ill, or debilitated patients and those with respiratory problems. Postoperative respiratory depression may be prolonged or may recur following initial recovery, especially following use of moderate or high doses. Following administration of fentanyl or sufentanil, respiratory depression requiring mechanical ventilation may be greatly prolonged. Alfentanil-induced respiratory depression is of shorter duration than that induced by fentanyl or sufentanil. The peak respiratory depressant effect of fentanyl occurs 5 to 15 minutes following administration of a single intravenous dose and may persist longer than the analgesic effect.

Sufentanil is approximately 5 to 7 times more potent than fentanyl on a mcg-to-mcg (and mL-to-mL) basis. 100 mcg of fentanyl or 13 to 20 mcg of sufentanil produce analgesic effects equivalent to 10 mg of morphine. Alfentanil has been reported to be 3 to 10 times less potent than fentanyl on a mcg-to-mcg basis (as determined by dosage requirements). However, because of alfentanil's considerably smaller volume of distribution, much higher plasma concentrations are achieved with alfentanil than with equal doses of fentanyl; studies comparing plasma concentrations of fentanyl or alfentanil required to produce similar effects have indicated that fentanyl may be up to 75 times more potent than alfentanil. Also, interpatient variability in responsiveness to these medications and/or differences in analytic methodology may have contributed to the difficulty in determining relative potency.

## Fentanyl Derivatives (Systemic)

The usual adult and pediatric doses stated below are intended as a guideline only. Dosage must be individualized on the basis of the age, weight, body size, and physical status of the patient; underlying pathology; other medications used concurrently, especially the type of anesthesia to be used; type and anticipated duration of the surgical procedure involved; and patient response. Also, for obese patients (more than 20% above ideal body weight), the dosage of alfentanil or sufentanil should be determined on the basis of lean body weight.

It is recommended that initial dosage be reduced in elderly or debilitated patients. The effects of the initial dose should be considered in determining supplemental doses. Lower doses may also be required in patients with chronic hepatic disease (especially for alfentanil) or hypothyroidism.

Fentanyl derivatives may cause rigidity of chest and abdominal muscles, which may interfere with pulmonary ventilation. Alfentanil may also cause rigidity in other muscles. The risk of muscle rigidity may be reduced if intravenous injections are administered slowly. A neuromuscular blocking agent compatible with the patient's condition may be administered prophylactically to prevent muscle rigidity or to induce muscle relaxation after rigidity occurs. Rigidity has also been reported upon emergence from fentanyl- or sufentanil-assisted anesthesia and should be considered a possibility upon emergence from alfentanil-assisted anesthesia.

It is recommended that intravenous injections of fentanyl or sufentanil be given slowly over a period of at least 1 to 2 minutes, especially if high doses are being administered. It is recommended that induction doses of alfentanil also be given slowly. Although the manufacturer's prescribing information recommends that induction doses of alfentanil be administered over a period of approximately 3 minutes, many investigators have administered induction doses within 90 seconds. Slow intravenous administration of these medications may reduce the incidence and/or severity of rigidity, bradycardia, and hypotension. Also, rapid intravenous administration of other opioid analgesics has caused anaphylactoid reactions, severe respiratory depression, hypotension, peripheral circulatory collapse, and cardiac arrest.

Premedication with a benzodiazepine may reduce induction dose requirements and decrease the time to loss of consciousness. In addition, administration of a benzodiazepine or other amnestic agent may help to prevent patient recall of intrasurgical events postoperatively. Patient recall of intrasurgical events despite the absence of autonomic or hormonal responses indicative of light or inadequate anesthesia has been reported following use of high-dose fentanyl with 100% oxygen and, although not reported to date, should be considered a possibility following use of high-dose sufentanil with 100% oxygen or following administration of alfentanil also. However, the fact that concurrent use of a benzodiazepine with a fentanyl derivative may increase the risk of hypotension, respiratory depression, or delayed recovery must be kept in mind. Alternatively, detection of signs of inadequate anesthesia may be facilitated if the neuromuscular blocking agent being used is administered in doses titrated to avoid complete paralysis.

Fentanyl derivatives, even in very high doses, may fail to suppress autonomic responses to surgical stimulation. Tachycardia and hypertension may occur and are more likely to respond rapidly to additional doses of alfentanil or sufentanil than to additional fentanyl. However, administration of a suitable antihypertensive agent may be required in some patients. In patients undergoing cardiac surgery, administration of a beta-adrenergic blocking agent with the presurgical medication (or continuation of previously instituted therapy with a beta-adrenergic blocking agent up to the time of surgery) may reduce or prevent these responses.

Tolerance to the effects of fentanyl or sufentanil may occur with repeated dosing; in addition, patients who have become tolerant to other opioid analgesics may be at least partially cross-tolerant to the effects of a fentanyl derivative also.

Like other opioid analgesics, fentanyl derivatives may cause physical dependence following prolonged use. Rarely, symptoms possibly indicating a type of withdrawal syndrome (e.g., tachycardia, hypertension, hyperpnea, hyperalgesia, nausea, and vomiting) may occur following administration of naloxone (especially in high doses) for reversal of opioid effects postoperatively. However, other symptoms commonly associated with an opioid withdrawal syndrome do not occur.

### For treatment of adverse effects
Recommended treatment may include:
- For hypotension—Administration of appropriate parenteral fluid therapy is recommended. Repositioning of the patient to improve venous return to the heart should be considered when surgical conditions permit. If necessary, a vasopressor (during or following surgery) and/or naloxone (postoperatively only) may be administered.
- For muscle rigidity—Administering a neuromuscular blocking agent and assisting respiration via controlled ventilation with oxygen. Alternatively, if muscle rigidity should occur upon emergence, naloxone may be administered.

Other supportive measures should also be employed as needed.

---

## ALFENTANIL

### Summary of Differences
Indications: See *Indications*.
Pharmacology/pharmacokinetics: See *Pharmacology/Pharmacokinetics*.
Pediatrics: Duration of action may be reduced in children.
Drug interactions and/or related problems: Hepatic enzyme inhibitors may prolong duration of action.
Side/adverse effects: See *Side/Adverse Effects*.

### Additional Dosing Information
See also *General Dosing Information*.

The anesthetic $ED_{90}$ in unpremedicated patients (induction dose required to attenuate or abolish the response to placement of a nasopharyngeal airway in 90% of the patients) is approximately 169 to 182 mcg per kg of body weight (using a rapid induction); however, values ranging from 137 to 383 mcg per kg of body weight have been reported.

An initial loading dose of alfentanil is required to achieve therapeutic plasma concentrations rapidly. Administration of the induction or loading dose may be followed by continuous intravenous infusion of the medication and/or administration of supplemental single injections as required. Continuous intravenous infusion, with the rate of infusion adjusted according to the observed clinical effect, may reduce the total maintenance dosage requirement, decrease the risk of postoperative respiratory depression, and speed recovery time, and may be the preferred method of administration. If necessary, small single doses may be administered in addition to or instead of increasing the infusion rate as required to prevent or abolish responses to surgical stimuli or other signs of light or inadequate anesthesia.

Because alfentanil requirements are lowest near the end of surgery, it is recommended that the maintenance infusion be discontinued 10 to 20 minutes before the end of surgery. If further administration of alfentanil is required after the infusion is discontinued, single injections of 7 to 15 mcg per kg of body weight may be given.

Because of alfentanil's short duration of action, postoperative pain requiring treatment may occur relatively early in the recovery period.

### Parenteral Dosage Forms
#### ALFENTANIL HYDROCHLORIDE INJECTION
**Usual adult dose**
Anesthesia adjunct (opioid analgesic)—
  Induction of anesthesia (for procedures lasting 45 minutes or longer):
    Intravenous, 130 to 245 mcg (0.13 to 0.245 mg) (base) per kg of body weight. Induction with alfentanil may be followed by administration of an inhalation anesthetic (with the required concentration of inhalation anesthetic generally being reduced by 30 to 50% during the first hour of maintenance) or by further administration of alfentanil in maintenance doses.
  Maintenance of anesthesia (in conjunction with nitrous oxide and oxygen):
    Procedures lasting up to 30 minutes—Intravenous, 8 to 20 mcg (0.008 to 0.02 mg) (base) per kg of body weight as an initial loading dose, followed by administration of single doses of 3 to 5 mcg (0.003 to 0.005 mg) per kg of body weight as required or by continuous infusion at a rate of 0.5 to 1 mcg (0.0005 to 0.001 mg) per kg of body weight per minute.
    Procedures lasting longer than 30 minutes—Intravenous, 20 to 75 mcg (0.02 to 0.075 mg) (base) per kg of body weight as an initial loading dose (if an agent other than alfentanil has been used for induction), followed by continuous infusion at a rate of 0.5 to 4 mcg (0.0005 to 0.004 mg) per kg of body weight per minute and/or by single injections of 5 to 15 mcg (0.005 to 0.015 mg) per kg of body weight as required. Following induction with alfentanil, infusion rate requirements may be reduced by 30 to 50% during the first hour of maintenance.
    Note: For maintenance of anesthesia, continuous infusions of alfentanil are generally administered at an average rate of 0.5 to 1.5 mcg (0.0005 to 0.0015 mg) (base) per kg of body weight per minute. However, a variable rate of infusion is recommended, with the rate being increased in response to signs of light or inadequate anesthesia or decreased when

signs of light or inadequate anesthesia have been absent for a suitable period of time.

**Usual pediatric dose**
Anesthesia adjunct (opioid analgesic) for maintenance of anesthesia—Intravenous, 30 to 50 mcg (0.03 to 0.05 mg) (base) per kg of body weight as an initial loading dose, followed by supplemental single doses of 10 to 15 mcg (0.01 to 0.015 mg) per kg of body weight as required, or by continuous infusion at a rate of 0.5 to 1.5 mcg (0.0005 to 0.0015 mg) per kg of body weight per minute.

Note: Alfentanil half-life and duration of action are decreased in children as compared with adults; therefore, more frequent supplemental dosing may be required.

**Strength(s) usually available**
U.S.—
  Without preservative: 500 mcg (0.5 mg) (base) per mL (Rx) [*Alfenta*].
Canada—
  Without preservative: 500 mcg (0.5 mg) (base) per mL (Rx) [*Alfenta*].

**Packaging and storage**
Store between 15 and 30 °C (59 and 86 °F), protected from light, unless otherwise specified by manufacturer. Protect from freezing.

**Preparation of dosage form**
Alfentanil hydrochloride injection may be diluted with 0.9% sodium chloride injection, 5% dextrose and sodium chloride injection (0.9% sodium chloride), 5% dextrose injection, or lactated Ringer's injection to a convenient concentration. As an example, 20 mL of alfentanil hydrochloride injection may be added to 230 mL of diluent to provide a solution containing 40 mcg (0.04 mg) of alfentanil per mL.

**Stability**
Alfentanil hydrochloride injection is stable when diluted to a concentration of 25 to 80 mcg of alfentanil base per mL using any of the solutions listed in *Preparation of dosage form* above.

**Note**
Controlled substance in the U.S., Canada, and the U.K.

---

## FENTANYL

## Summary of Differences
Indications: See *Indications*.
Pharmacology/pharmacokinetics: See *Pharmacology/Pharmacokinetics*.
Pediatrics: Neonates may be more susceptible to respiratory depressant effects, especially if used as presurgical or postsurgical medication.
Side/adverse effects: See *Side/Adverse Effects*.

## Additional Dosing Information
See also *General Dosing Information*.
A reduction in dosage may be required in very young patients receiving fentanyl as presurgical or postsurgical medication.

## Parenteral Dosage Forms
### FENTANYL CITRATE INJECTION USP

**Usual adult dose**
Anesthesia, general, adjunct—
  For minor surgery:
    Intravenous, 2 mcg (0.002 mg) (base) per kg of body weight.
  For major surgery:
    Moderate dose—Intravenous, 2 to 20 mcg (0.002 to 0.02 mg) (base) per kg of body weight.
    High dose (for open-heart surgery or complicated neurological or orthopedic procedures requiring prolonged anesthesia and abolition of stress response)—Intravenous, 20 to 50 mcg (0.02 to 0.05 mg) (base) per kg of body weight.
  Note: The total moderate or high dosage recommended during major surgery may be given as a single dose or in divided doses. The quantity of fentanyl given as an initial loading dose and as subsequent maintenance doses must be individualized, depending upon the anesthetic regimen being used, the type and anticipated duration of the surgical procedure involved, and the occurrence of signs of surgical stress or lightening of anesthesia during surgery. Although fentanyl may be administered intramuscularly during surgery, it is usually administered intravenously.
Anesthesia, local, adjunct—
  Intravenous, 0.7 to 1.4 mcg (0.0007 to 0.0014 mg) (base) per kg of body weight.

Anesthesia, as primary agent in major surgery—
  Intravenous, 50 to 100 mcg (0.05 to 0.1 mg) (base) per kg of body weight, to be administered with 100% oxygen or oxygen plus nitrous oxide and a neuromuscular blocking agent.
  Note: Up to 150 mcg (0.15 mg) (base) per kg of body weight may be required in some patients.
    In order to provide both immediate and sustained effects throughout a prolonged surgical procedure, administration of an initial loading dose of fentanyl simultaneously with or followed by continuous intravenous infusion is recommended.
Presurgical medication—
  Intramuscular, 0.7 to 1.4 mcg (0.0007 to 0.0014 mg) (base) per kg of body weight thirty to sixty minutes prior to surgery.
Postoperative (in recovery room period)—
  Intramuscular, 0.7 to 1.4 mcg (0.0007 to 0.0014 mg) (base) per kg of body weight; may be repeated in one or two hours as needed.

**Usual pediatric dose**
Anesthesia, as primary agent in major surgery—
  Children up to 2 years of age: Dosage has not been established.
  Children 2 to 12 years of age: Intravenous, 2 to 3 mcg (0.002 to 0.003 mg) (base) per kg of body weight.

**Strength(s) usually available**
U.S.—
  Without preservative: 50 mcg (0.05 mg) (base) per mL (Rx) [*Sublimaze*; GENERIC].
Canada—
  Without preservative: 50 mcg (0.05 mg) (base) per mL (Rx) [*Sublimaze*].

**Packaging and storage**
Store below 40 °C (104 °F), preferably between 15 and 30 °C (59 and 86 °F), unless otherwise specified by manufacturer. Protect from light. Protect from freezing.

**Note**
Controlled substance in the U.S., Canada, and the U.K.

---

## SUFENTANIL

## Summary of Differences
Indications: See *Indications*.
Pharmacology/pharmacokinetics: See *Pharmacology/Pharmacokinetics*.
Drug interactions and/or related problems: See *interaction with neuromuscular blocking agents* for information that may not apply to alfentanil or fentanyl.
Side/adverse effects: See *Side/Adverse Effects*.

## Parenteral Dosage Forms
### SUFENTANIL CITRATE INJECTION USP

**Usual adult dose**
Anesthesia, general, adjunct—
  Low dose: Intravenous, 0.5 to 1 mcg (0.0005 to 0.001 mg) (base) per kg of body weight initially. Supplemental doses of 10 to 25 mcg (0.01 to 0.025 mg) may be administered as needed.
  Moderate dose (for major surgical procedures requiring some attenuation of sympathetic response to surgical stimuli): Intravenous, 2 to 8 mcg (0.002 to 0.008 mg) (base) per kg of body weight initially. Supplemental doses of 10 to 50 mcg (0.01 to 0.05 mg) may be administered as needed.
  Note: When administered with nitrous oxide and oxygen for procedures lasting up to 8 hours, total doses of 1 mcg (0.001 mg) per kg of body weight per hour, or less, are recommended.
Anesthesia, as primary agent in major surgery—
  Intravenous, 8 to 30 mcg (0.008 to 0.03 mg) (base) per kg of body weight initially, administered with 100% oxygen. Supplemental doses of 25 to 50 mcg (0.025 to 0.05 mg) may be administered as needed.
  Note: In order to provide both immediate and sustained effects throughout a prolonged surgical procedure, administration of an initial loading dose of sufentanil simultaneously with or followed by continuous intravenous infusion is recommended.

**Usual pediatric dose**
Anesthesia, as primary agent in cardiovascular surgery—
  Initial: Intravenous, 10 to 25 mcg (0.01 to 0.025 mg) (base) per kg of body weight, administered with 100% oxygen.
  Maintenance: Intravenous, up to 25 to 50 mcg (0.025 to 0.05 mg) (base).

**Strength(s) usually available**
U.S.—
Without preservative: 50 mcg (0.05 mg) (base) per mL (Rx) [*Sufenta*; GENERIC].
Canada—
Without preservative: 50 mcg (0.05 mg) (base) per mL (Rx) [*Sufenta*].

**Packaging and storage**
Store below 40 °C (104 °F), preferably between 15 and 30 °C (59 and 86 °F), protected from light, unless otherwise specified by manufacturer. Protect from freezing.

**Note**
Controlled substance in both the U.S. and Canada.

Revised: 06/19/90
Interim revision: 07/26/96

---

# FERROUS CITRATE FE 59  Systemic*

VA CLASSIFICATION (Primary): DX201

Note: For a listing of dosage forms and brand names by country availability, see *Dosage Forms* section(s).

*Not commercially available in U.S.

## Category
Diagnostic aid (iron metabolism; iron absorption).

## Indications
**Accepted**
Anemia (diagnosis) and
Iron metabolism studies—Ferrous citrate Fe 59 is indicated, by intravenous administration, to determine various parameters of the kinetics of iron metabolism, including plasma iron clearance, plasma iron turnover rate, and the utilization of iron in new red blood cells. The values of serum iron obtained from these studies provide diagnostic information in patients with anemias. Ferrous citrate Fe 59 is also useful to assess the role of the spleen in red blood cell production and destruction, and thus to help determine the advisability of splenectomy. Also, organ uptake measurements are used to measure the sites of red cell production (or lack thereof) in extramedullary erythropoiesis in myeloproliferative disorders.

Iron absorption studies—Ferrous citrate Fe 59 is indicated, by oral administration, to measure the absorption of iron from the intestine.

## Physical Properties
**Nuclear Data**

| Radionu-clide (half-life) | Decay constant | Mode of decay | Principal emissions (meV) | Mean number of emissions/ disintegration |
|---|---|---|---|---|
| Fe 59 (44.6 days) | 0.000649 hr⁻¹ | Beta emission | Beta-2 (mean 0.081) | 0.45 |
| | | | Beta-3 (mean 0.149) | 0.53 |
| | | | Gamma-2 (0.192) | 0.03 |
| | | | Gamma-5 (1.099) | 0.56 |
| | | | Gamma-6 (1.292) | 0.43 |

## Pharmacology/Pharmacokinetics
**Mechanism of action/Effect**
Iron from ferrous citrate is bound to plasma protein (transferrin) and carried to the blood-forming organs where it is utilized to form hemoglobin or is deposited in the reticuloendothelial cells of the liver and spleen. The amount of radioactive iron absorbed, transported, stored, utilized, and excreted can then be measured by the periodic collection of blood specimens and external counting.

**Protein binding**
Very high.

**Half-life**
Plasma iron clearance (biological)—
Normal: 1 to 2 hours.
Polycythemia, iron deficiency anemia, chronic blood loss, and hemolytic anemia: < 1 hour.
Hypoplastic anemia, myelofibrosis, and hemachromatosis: > 2 hours.

Note: Transferrin-bound radioactive iron concentration in plasma decreases as radioactive iron accumulates in the bone marrow. Rate of disappearance reflects erythropoiesis.

**Radiation dosimetry**

| Mode of administration | Target organ | Estimated absorbed radiation dose* | |
|---|---|---|---|
| | | mGy/MBq | rad/mCi |
| Intravenous | Spleen | 55 | 200 |
| | Heart wall | 24 | 90 |
| | Liver | 12 | 44 |
| | Red marrow | 12 | 43 |
| | Kidneys | 8.6 | 32 |
| | Ovaries | 6.4 | 24 |
| | Testes | 5.3 | 20 |
| | Total body | 6.4 | 24 |

*In normal subjects.

**Elimination**
No significant physiological system of excretion exists for iron. Very slowly excreted, mostly in feces; remainder excreted within cells shed by skin and gastrointestinal mucosa.

## Precautions to Consider
**Pregnancy/Reproduction**
Pregnancy—The possibility of pregnancy should be assessed in women of child-bearing potential. Clinical situations exist where the benefit to the patient and fetus derived from radiopharmaceutical use outweighs the risks from radiation exposure to the fetus. In these situations, the physician should use discretion and reduce the radiopharmaceutical dose to the lowest possible amount.

**Breast-feeding**
Ferrous citrate Fe 59 is excreted in breast milk. Because of the potential risk of radiation exposure to the infant, temporary discontinuation of nursing is recommended for a length of time that may be assessed by measuring the activity of breast milk and estimating the radiation exposure to the infant.

**Pediatrics**
There have been no specific studies evaluating safety and efficacy of ferrous citrate Fe 59 in children. When this radiopharmaceutical is used in children, the diagnostic benefit should be judged to outweigh the potential risk of radiation.

**Geriatrics**
Appropriate studies on the relationship of age to the effects of ferrous citrate Fe 159 have not been performed in the geriatric population. However, no geriatrics-specific problems have been documented to date.

**Diagnostic interference**
The following have been selected on the basis of their potential clinical significance (possible effect in parentheses where appropriate)—not necessarily inclusive (» = major clinical significance):

With results of *this* test
Foods
(absorption of oral ferrous citrate Fe 59 may be decreased by presence of food in the stomach; overnight fasting is recommended prior to its administration for iron absorption studies)

## Side/Adverse Effects
At present, there are no known side/adverse effects associated with the use of ferrous citrate Fe 59.

USP DI

## Patient Consultation
As an aid to patient consultation, refer to *Advice for the Patient, Radiopharmaceuticals (Diagnostic)*.
In providing consultation, consider emphasizing the following selected information (» = major clinical significance):

**Description of use**
Action in the body: Utilization by body of radioactive iron same as dietary iron
Collection of blood specimen allows measurement of iron
Small amounts of radioactivity used in diagnosis; radiation received is low and considered safe

**Before having this test**
» Conditions affecting use, especially:
Pregnancy—Risk of radiation exposure to fetus
Breast-feeding—Excreted in breast milk; temporary discontinuation of nursing recommended because of risk of radiation exposure to infant
Use in children—Risk of radiation exposure

**Preparation for this test**
Special preparatory instructions may be given; patient should inquire in advance

**Precautions after having this test**
No special precautions

## General Dosing Information
Radiopharmaceuticals are to be administered only by or under the supervision of physicians who have had extensive training in the safe use and handling of radionuclides and who are licensed by the Nuclear Regulatory Commission (NRC) or the appropriate Agreement State agency or, outside the U.S., the appropriate authority.
Overnight fasting is recommended prior to the oral administration of ferrous citrate Fe 59 for iron absorption studies.

**Safety considerations for handling this radiopharmaceutical**
Improper handling of this radiopharmaceutical may cause radioactive contamination. Guidelines for handling radioactive material have been prepared by scientific, professional, state, federal, and international bodies and are available to the specially qualified and authorized users who have access to radiopharmaceuticals.

## Parenteral Dosage Forms

**FERROUS CITRATE Fe 59 INJECTION USP**

**Usual adult and adolescent administered activity**
Diagnostic aid—
Intravenous or oral, 0.185 to 0.555 megabecquerel (5 to 15 microcuries).

**Usual pediatric administered activity**
Diagnostic aid—
Dosage must be individualized by physician.

**Usual geriatric administered activity**
See *Usual adult and adolescent administered activity*.

**Strength(s) usually available**
U.S.—
Not commercially available.
Canada—
0.185 to 3.7 megabecquerels (5 to 100 microcuries) per mL, having a specific activity ranging from 0.185 to 1.11 megabecquerels (5 to 30 microcuries) per microgram of iron, at time of calibration (Rx) [GENERIC].

**Packaging and storage**
Store below 40 °C (104 °F), preferably between 15 and 30 °C (59 and 86 °F), unless otherwise specified by manufacturer.

**Note**
Caution—Radioactive material.

Revised: 06/23/92
Interim revision: 08/02/94

---

**FERROUS FUMARATE**—See *Iron Supplements (Systemic)*

---

**FERROUS GLUCONATE**—See *Iron Supplements (Systemic)*

---

**FERROUS SULFATE**—See *Iron Supplements (Systemic)*

---

**FERUMOXIDES**—The *Ferumoxides (Systemic)* monograph is not included in this published version of the USP DI database. Copies of the monograph are available on request from Micromedex, Inc. - Reprint Requests, 6200 S. Syracuse Way, Suite 300, Englewood, CO 80111; telephone (303) 486-6400; telefax (303) 486-6464; Email: USPDI@MDX.COM.

# FEXOFENADINE Systemic—INTRODUCTORY VERSION

VA CLASSIFICATION (Primary): AH102
Commonly used brand name(s): *Allegra*.
Note: For a listing of dosage forms and brand names by country availability, see *Dosage Forms* section(s).

## Category
Antihistaminic ($H_1$-receptor).

## Indications

**Accepted**
Rhinitis, seasonal allergic (treatment)—Fexofenadine is indicated to relieve symptoms that are associated with seasonal allergic rhinitis, such as sneezing; rhinorrhea; itchy eyes, nose, and throat; and red, watery eyes.

## Pharmacology/Pharmacokinetics

**Physicochemical characteristics**
Chemical group—Metabolite of terfenadine.
Molecular weight—538.13.

**Mechanism of action/Effect**
Fexofenadine is an antihistamine with selective peripheral $H_1$-receptor antagonist activity. It inhibits antigen-induced bronchospasm in sensitized guinea pigs and histamine release from peritoneal mast cells in rats.

**Absorption**
Rapid following oral administration.

**Distribution**
Tissue distribution studies in rats using radiolabeled fexofenadine show that it does not cross the blood-brain barrier.

**Protein binding**
60 to 70% bound primarily to albumin and alpha$_1$-glycoprotein.

**Biotransformation**
About 5% of the total dose is metabolized; approximately 0.5 to 1.5% by hepatic metabolism and 3.5% by intestinal microflora.

**Half-life**
Elimination: 14.4 hours in healthy subjects; in patients with mild renal impairment (creatinine clearance of 41 to 80 mL per minute) and severe renal impairment (creatinine clearance of 11 to 40 mL per minute), the mean elimination half-life was 59% and 72% longer, respectively, than in healthy subjects. In patients on dialysis, half-life was 31% longer than in healthy subjects.

**Onset of action**
Within 1 hour, as determined by a reduction in rhinitis symptoms following administration of a single 60-mg dose to patients exposed to ragweed pollen and by human histamine skin wheal and flare studies following administration of single and twice-daily doses of 20 and 40 mg of fexofenadine.

### Time to peak effect
2 to 3 hours, as determined by human histamine skin wheal and flare studies following administration of single and twice-daily doses of 20 and 40 mg of fexofenadine.

### Duration of action
Effect evident 12 hours after administration, as determined by clinical studies in patients with seasonal allergic rhinitis given a single 60-mg dose, and by human histamine skin wheal and flare studies in patients given single and twice-daily doses of 20 and 40 mg of fexofenadine.

Note: Tolerance to the antihistamine effect of fexofenadine was not demonstrated following 28 days of dosing.

### Elimination
Approximately 80% and 11% of a radioactive fexofenadine dose is excreted in the feces and urine, respectively.

## Precautions to Consider

### Carcinogenicity
Fexofenadine showed no carcinogenic potential in 18- and 24-month studies in mice and rats given oral terfenadine doses of 50 and 150 mg per kg of body weight (mg/kg) per day, respectively. These doses resulted in area under the plasma concentration–time curve (AUC) values for fexofenadine of up to four times the human therapeutic value based on the recommended dosage.

### Mutagenicity
Fexofenadine was not mutagenic in *in vitro* bacterial or animal studies and *in vivo* animal studies.

### Pregnancy/Reproduction
Fertility—Dose-related reductions in implants and increases in postimplantation losses were seen in rats given oral doses of terfenadine ≥ 150 mg/kg. These doses resulted in AUC values for fexofenadine of up to three times the human therapeutic value based on the recommended dosage.

Pregnancy—Adequate and well-controlled studies in humans have not been done.

Fexofenadine was not teratogenic in studies in which rats or rabbits were given oral doses of terfenadine of up to 300 mg/kg per day. These doses resulted in AUC values for fexofenadine of up to 4 and 37 times the human therapeutic value based on the recommended dosage, respectively.

In rats given oral doses of terfenadine ≥ 150 mg/kg, dose-related decreases in pup weight and survival were observed. These doses resulted in AUC values for fexofenadine of three or more times the human therapeutic value based on the recommended dosage, respectively.

FDA Pregnancy Category C.

### Breast-feeding
It is not known whether fexofenadine is distributed into breast milk.

### Pediatrics
In clinical trials, 205 children 12 to 16 years of age have been safely treated with fexofenadine for up to 2 weeks; adverse effects were similar to those occurring in patients older than 16 years. However, the safety and efficacy of fexofenadine in children up to 12 years of age has not been established.

### Geriatrics
In patients 65 years of age and older, peak plasma concentrations of fexofenadine were 99% greater than those in healthy subjects younger than 65 years of age. Mean elimination half-lives were similar in the two groups. Adverse effects were similar to those occurring in patients up to 60 years of age.

### Drug interactions and/or related problems
The following drug interactions and/or related problems have been selected on the basis of their potential clinical significance (possible mechanism in parentheses where appropriate)—not necessarily inclusive (» = major clinical significance):

Note: Combinations containing any of the following medications, depending on the amount present, may also interact with this medication.

Erythromycin or
Ketoconazole
(concurrent administration with fexofenadine has been found to increase plasma fexofenadine concentrations; however, no differences in adverse effects or increased $QT_c$ intervals were seen)

### Medical considerations/Contraindications
The medical considerations/contraindications included have been selected on the basis of their potential clinical significance (reasons given in parentheses where appropriate)—not necessarily inclusive (» = major clinical significance).

*Risk-benefit should be considered when the following medical problems exist:*

» Renal function impairment
(based upon increases in the half-life of fexofenadine, once-daily administration is recommended initially in patients with impaired renal function)
Hypersensitivity to fexofenadine

## Side/Adverse Effects
The following side/adverse effects have been selected on the basis of their potential clinical significance (possible signs and symptoms in parentheses where appropriate)—not necessarily inclusive:

**Those indicating need for medical attention only if they continue or are bothersome**
Incidence less frequent—(≤ 2.5% but more common with fexofenadine than with placebo)
*Drowsiness; dysmenorrhea* (painful menstrual bleeding); *dyspepsia* (stomach upset); *fatigue* (unusual feeling of tiredness)

## Patient Consultation
As an aid to patient consultation, refer to *Advice for the Patient, Fexofenadine (Systemic)—Introductory Version*.

In providing consultation, consider emphasizing the following selected information (» = major clinical significance):

### Before using this medication
» Conditions affecting use, especially:
Hypersensitivity to fexofenadine
Other medical problems, especially renal function impairment

### Proper use of this medication
» Proper dosing
Missed dose
If used regularly—using as soon as possible; using any remaining doses for that day at regularly spaced intervals; not doubling doses
» Proper storage

### Side/adverse effects
Signs of potential side effects, especially drowsiness, dysmenorrhea, dyspepsia, and fatigue

## Oral Dosage Forms

### FEXOFENADINE HYDROCHLORIDE CAPSULES

#### Usual adult and adolescent dose
Antihistaminic ($H_1$-receptor)—
Oral, 60 mg two times a day.

Note: For patients with decreased renal function, an initial dose of 60 mg once a day is recommended.

#### Usual adult and adolescent prescribing limits
60 mg two times a day.

#### Usual pediatric dose
Antihistaminic ($H_1$-receptor)—
Children up to 12 years of age: Safety and efficacy have not been determined.
Children 12 years of age and older: See *Usual adult and adolescent dose*.

#### Usual geriatric dose
Antihistaminic ($H_1$-receptor)—
See *Usual adult and adolescent dose*.

#### Strength(s) usually available
U.S.—
60 mg (Rx) [*Allegra*].

#### Packaging and storage
Store at controlled room temperature, between 20 and 25 °C (68 and 77 °F). Protect from moisture.

Developed: 12/04/96
Interim revision: 08/12/98

# FEXOFENADINE AND PSEUDOEPHEDRINE Systemic—INTRODUCTORY VERSION

VA CLASSIFICATION (Primary): RE501

Commonly used brand name(s): *Allegra-D*.

Note: For a listing of dosage forms and brand names by country availability, see *Dosage Forms* section(s).

## Category
Antihistaminic ($H_1$-receptor)–decongestant.

## Indications

**Accepted**

Rhinitis, seasonal allergic (treatment)—Fexofenadine and pseudoephedrine combination is indicated for symptomatic relief of seasonal allergic rhinitis (including sneezing; rhinorrhea; itchy nose, palate, and/or throat; itchy, watery, red eyes; and nasal congestion) in adults and children 12 years of age and older when both antihistaminic and decongestant effects are desired.

## Pharmacology/Pharmacokinetics

**Physicochemical characteristics**

Chemical group—
  Fexofenadine hydrochloride—Piperidine derivative. Fexofenadine is the major active metabolite of terfenadine.
Molecular weight—
  Fexofenadine hydrochloride—538.13.
  Pseudoephedrine hydrochloride—201.7.
Solubility—
  Fexofenadine hydrochloride—Freely soluble in methanol and ethanol, slightly soluble in chloroform and water, and insoluble in hexane.
  Pseudoephedrine hydrochloride—Very soluble in water, freely soluble in alcohol, and sparingly soluble in chloroform.

**Mechanism of action/Effect**

Fexofenadine—
  A selective peripheral $H_1$-receptor antagonist that has been found to inhibit antigen-induced bronchospasm in sensitized guinea pigs and histamine release from peritoneal mast cells in rats.
Pseudoephedrine—
  A sympathomimetic amine that has a decongestant effect on the nasal mucosa. Its peripheral effects are similar to those of ephedrine and its central effects are similar to, but less intense than, those of amphetamines.

**Other actions/effects**

Fexofenadine:
  Animal studies have not found that fexofenadine has anticholinergic or $alpha_1$-adrenergic receptor activity, and no sedative or other central nervous system (CNS) effects have been observed.
  Pseudoephedrine has the potential for excitatory side effects, but has little or no pressor effect in normotensive adults.

**Absorption**

Bioavailability of fexofenadine and pseudoephedrine from the combination formulation is similar to that observed with administration as single agents. Coadministration with a high-fat meal has been found to decrease peak fexofenadine plasma concentrations and area under the curve (AUC) by 46% and 42%, respectively, and to delay the time to peak plasma concentration by 50%. The rate and extent of pseudoephedrine absorption have not been found to be affected by food.
Fexofenadine:
  Rapidly absorbed in combination form with pseudoephedrine. Absolute bioavailability has not been established.

**Distribution**

Fexofenadine has not been found to cross the blood-brain barrier.

**Protein binding**

Fexofenadine—
  Moderate (60 to 70%), primarily to albumin and $alpha_1$-acid glycoprotein.

**Biotransformation**

Fexofenadine—
  Hepatic; approximately 5% of the total dose is metabolized.
Pseudoephedrine—
  Hepatic, 25 to 45%.

**Half-life**

Elimination—
  Fexofenadine:
    Mean, 14.4 hours following administration to steady-state as a single agent to healthy volunteers.
  Pseudoephedrine:
    Mean, 4 to 6 hours, depending on urine pH (elimination half-life is reduced at a pH less than 6 and increased at a pH above 8).

**Onset of action**

Fexofenadine (antihistaminic effect):
  1 hour.

**Time to peak concentration**

Plasma—
  Fexofenadine:
    2 hours following single or multiple doses.
  Pseudoephedrine:
    6 hours following a single dose; 5 hours following multiple doses to steady-state.

**Peak plasma concentration**

Fexofenadine—
  191 nanograms per mL following administration of a single dose of the combination of 60 mg of fexofenadine hydrochloride and 120 mg of pseudoephedrine hydrochloride; 225 nanograms per mL following multiple dose administration to steady-state.
  Peak plasma concentrations have been found to be increased by 87% and mean elimination half-life increased by 59% in patients with mild renal function impairment (creatinine clearance 41 to 80 mL per minute [mL/min]), compared with those in normal volunteers. In patients with severe renal function impairment (creatinine clearance 11 to 40 mL/min), peak plasma concentrations were increased by 111% and mean elimination half-life increased by 72%. In patients on dialysis (creatinine clearance 10 mL/min or less), peak plasma concentrations and half-life were increased by 82% and 31%, respectively.
Pseudoephedrine—
  206 nanograms per mL following administration of a single dose of the combination of 60 mg of fexofenadine hydrochloride and 120 mg of pseudoephedrine hydrochloride; 411 nanograms per mL following multiple dose administration to steady-state.

**Time to peak effect**

Fexofenadine (antihistaminic effect)—
  2 to 3 hours.

**Duration of action**

Fexofenadine (antihistaminic effect)—
  At least 12 hours.

**Elimination**

Fexofenadine—
  Fecal, 80%. Because absolute bioavailability has not been established, it is not known if this component is unabsorbed drug or the result of biliary excretion.
  Renal, 11%.
Pseudoephedrine—
  Renal, 55 to 75% unchanged.
In dialysis—
  Fexofenadine is not effectively removed by hemodialysis. It is not known whether pseudoephedrine is removable by hemodialysis.

Note: Fexofenadine exhibits linear pharmacokinetics for oral doses of up to 120 mg administered twice a day.

## Precautions to Consider

**Cross-sensitivity and/or related problems**

Patients sensitive to other adrenergic agents may also be sensitive to pseudoephedrine.

**Carcinogenicity**

No animal or *in vitro* studies with the combination of fexofenadine and pseudoephedrine have been done.

Studies in mice and rats at oral daily doses of terfenadine of up to 150 mg per kg of body weight (mg/kg) (producing adequate fexofenadine exposure [area under the curve (AUC)], or up to three times the human AUC at the maximum recommended daily oral dose in adults) for 18 and 24 months, respectively, found no evidence of carcinogenicity.

Studies in rats and mice with ephedrine sulfate (an agent structurally related to and with similar pharmacologic properties as pseudoephedrine) at oral doses of up to 10 and 27 mg/kg, respectively (approximately one third and one half, respectively, the maximum recommended daily oral dose of pseudoephedrine hydrochloride in adults on a mg per square meter of body surface area basis) found no evidence of carcinogenicity.

**Mutagenicity**
Fexofenadine was not found to be mutagenic in *in vitro* (bacterial reverse mutation, CHO/HGPRT forward mutation, and rat lymphocyte chromosomal aberration assays) or *in vivo* (mouse bone marrow micronucleus assay) tests.

**Pregnancy/Reproduction**
Fertility—Studies in rats given oral doses of terfenadine of up to 300 mg/kg showed no effect on male or female fertility. However, a reduction in implants was observed at an oral dose of 150 mg/kg per day, and both a reduction in implants and postimplantation losses were reported at 300 mg/kg. (Oral doses of 150 and 300 mg/kg of terfenadine produced fexofenadine AUC values of approximately three and four times, respectively, the human AUC at the maximum recommended daily oral dose in adults.)

Pregnancy—Adequate and well-controlled studies in humans have not been done.

Studies in rats and rabbits given oral doses of terfenadine of up to 300 mg/kg (producing fexofenadine AUC values in rats and rabbits of approximately 4 and 30 times, respectively, the human AUC at the maximum recommended daily oral dose in adults) found no evidence of teratogenicity. However, studies in rats given an oral combination of terfenadine and pseudoephedrine at a dose of 150/300 mg/kg found reduced fetal weight and delayed ossification with a finding of wavy ribs. (The terfenadine dose produced a fexofenadine AUC value of approximately three times the human AUC at the maximum recommended daily oral dose in adults. The dose of pseudoephedrine was approximately 10 times the maximum recommended daily oral dose in adults on a mg per square meter of body surface area basis.)

Dose-related decreases in pup weight gain and survival occurred in rats at oral doses of 150 mg/kg of terfenadine (producing fexofenadine AUC values of approximately three times the human AUC at the maximum recommended daily oral dose in adults). Studies in rabbits given an oral combination of terfenadine and pseudoephedrine at a dose of 100/200 mg/kg found reduced fetal weight. (By extrapolation, the terfenadine dose produced a fexofenadine AUC value of approximately 10 times the human AUC at the maximum recommended daily oral dose in adults and the dose of pseudoephedrine was approximately 15 times the maximum recommended daily oral dose in adults on a mg per square meter of body surface area basis.)

Risk-benefit should be considered before using this medication during pregnancy.

FDA Pregnancy Category C.

**Breast-feeding**
It is not known whether fexofenadine is distributed into breast milk. Pseudoephedrine is distributed into breast milk in concentrations that are consistently higher than those in plasma (approximately two to three times higher in breast milk than the plasma AUC); the fraction of pseudoephedrine distributed into breast milk is estimated to be 0.4 to 0.7%. Risk-benefit should be considered before use of the combination medication in women who are breast-feeding.

**Pediatrics**
Safety and efficacy of fexofenadine and pseudoephedrine in children younger than 12 years of age have not been established.

**Geriatrics**
Appropriate studies on the relationship of age to the effects of fexofenadine and pseudoephedrine have not been performed in the geriatric population. However, peak plasma concentrations of fexofenadine have been observed to be 99% greater in patients 65 years of age and older, compared with those in younger subjects; no differences in elimination half-life were observed. Elderly patients are more likely to have adverse reactions to sympathomimetic amines. In general, cautious dosing is recommended for the elderly (beginning at the low end of the dosage range), keeping in mind the possibility that they may have decreased hepatic, renal, or cardiac function along with other concomitant diseases or use of other medications. Elderly patients are more likely to have age-related renal function impairment, which requires adjustment of dosage.

**Drug interactions and/or related problems**
The following drug interactions and/or related problems have been selected on the basis of their potential clinical significance (possible mechanism in parentheses where appropriate)—not necessarily inclusive (» = major clinical significance):

Note: Combinations containing any of the following medications, depending on the amount present, may also interact with this medication.

Antihypertensives that interfere with sympathomimetic activity, such as:
  Mecamylamine
  Methyldopa
  Reserpine
    (concurrent administration with pseudoephedrine may lead to reduced antihypertensive effects)
Digitalis glycosides
    (concurrent administration with pseudoephedrine can result in increased ectopic pacemaker activity)
Erythromycin or
Ketoconazole
    (concurrent administration with fexofenadine has been found to increase plasma fexofenadine concentrations; however, no differences in adverse effects or increased QTc intervals were seen)
» Monoamine oxidase (MAO) inhibitors, including furazolidone, procarbazine, and selegiline
    (pseudoephedrine should not be administered during or within 14 days following administration of MAO inhibitors)
Sympathomimetics, other
    (concurrent use may increase the cardiovascular effects of either the other sympathomimetics or pseudoephedrine and the potential for side effects)

**Medical considerations/Contraindications**
The medical considerations/contraindications included have been selected on the basis of their potential clinical significance (reasons given in parentheses where appropriate)—not necessarily inclusive (» = major clinical significance).

*Risk-benefit should be considered when the following medical problems exist:*
  Sensitivity to fexofenadine or pseudoephedrine or other sympathomimetics
*For pseudoephedrine*
» Coronary artery disease, severe or
» Hypertension, severe
    (condition may be exacerbated due to drug-induced cardiovascular effects)
  Diabetes mellitus
    (may lead to increased blood glucose concentrations)
» Glaucoma, narrow-angle or
  Increased intraocular pressure
    (condition may be exacerbated)
  Hyperthyroidism
    (symptoms may be exacerbated)
  Ischemic heart disease
    (condition may be exacerbated due to drug-induced cardiovascular effects)
  Prostatic hypertrophy
    (urinary retention may be precipitated)
» Renal function impairment
    (based upon the increases in bioavailability and half-life of fexofenadine and pseudoephedrine, once-daily administration is recommended initially in patients with impaired renal function)
» Urinary retention
    (condition may be exacerbated)

## Side/Adverse Effects

Note: Pseudoephedrine alone may cause mild CNS stimulation in hypersensitive patients, including nervousness, excitability, restlessness, dizziness, weakness, or insomnia. Other effects include headache, drowsiness, tachycardia, palpitation, pressor activity, and cardiac arrhythmias. Dizziness and insomnia may be manifestations of patient idiosyncrasy to adrenergic agents; other manifestations may include weakness, tremor, or cardiac arrhythmias.

Possible adverse effects of sympathomimetic amines include CNS stimulation with convulsions or cardiovascular collapse and accompanying hypotension. Sympathomimetic medications have been associated with fear, anxiety, tremor, hallucinations, seizures, pallor, respiratory difficulty, dysuria, and cardiovascular collapse.

The following side/adverse effects have been selected on the basis of their potential clinical significance (possible signs and symptoms in parentheses where appropriate)—not necessarily inclusive:

**Those indicating need for medical attention**
Incidence more frequent
  *Insomnia* (trouble in sleeping)

Incidence less frequent
*Dizziness; nervousness; palpitations* (irregular heartbeat); *upper respiratory infection* (cough; sore throat)

**Those indicating need for medical attention only if they continue or are bothersome**
Incidence more frequent
*Headache; nausea*
Incidence less frequent
*Abdominal or stomach pain; agitation; anxiety; back pain; dry mouth; dyspepsia* (heartburn); *sore throat*

## Overdose
For more information on the management of overdose or unintentional ingestion, **contact a Poison Control Center** (see *Poison Control Center Listing*).

### Clinical effects of overdose
No specific experience with combination fexofenadine/pseudoephedrine has been reported.
Large doses of sympathomimetics may cause giddiness, headache, nausea, vomiting, sweating, thirst, tachycardia, precordial pain, palpitations, difficulty in micturition, muscular weakness and tenseness, anxiety, restlessness, and insomnia. A toxic psychosis with delusions and hallucinations is common. Some patients may develop cardiac arrhythmias, circulatory collapse, convulsions, coma, and respiratory failure.

### Treatment of overdose
Standard measures to remove unabsorbed medication may be considered.
Hemodialysis does not effectively remove fexofenadine from blood (up to 1.7% removed); it is not known whether hemodialysis removes pseudoephedrine.
Supportive care—Symptomatic and supportive treatment is recommended. Patients in whom intentional overdose is confirmed or suspected should be referred for psychiatric consultation.

## Patient Consultation
As an aid to patient consultation, refer to *Advice for the Patient, Fexofenadine and Pseudoephedrine (Systemic)—Introductory Version*.
In providing consultation, consider emphasizing the following selected information (》 = major clinical significance):

### Before using this medication
》 Conditions affecting use, especially:
Sensitivity to fexofenadine or pseudoephedrine
Pregnancy—In animal studies, terfenadine and pseudoephedrine caused reduced weight and delayed ossification in the offspring
Breast-feeding—Pseudoephedrine is distributed into breast milk; risk-benefit should be considered
Use in the elderly—Older patients may be more sensitive to some of the effects of pseudoephedrine; and age-related decreases in hepatic, renal, or cardiac function are a possibility and may require a dosage reduction
Other medications, especially monoamine oxidase (MAO) inhibitors
Other medical problems, especially severe coronary artery disease, severe hypertension, narrow-angle glaucoma, renal function impairment and urinary retention

### Proper use of this medication
Swallowing tablet whole; not breaking or chewing tablet
Taking medication on an empty stomach

》 Proper dosing
Missed dose: Taking as soon as remembered; not taking if almost time for next dose; not doubling doses
Importance of not taking more than the prescribed dose or more frequently than recommended
》 Proper storage

### Side/adverse effects
Signs of potential side effects, especially dizziness, insomnia, nervousness, palpitations, or upper respiratory infection

## General Dosing Information
It is recommended by the manufacturer that patients stop taking the medication and check with their physician if dizziness, insomnia, or nervousness occurs.

### Diet/Nutrition
It is recommended by the manufacturer that the administration of fexofenadine/pseudoephedrine extended-release tablets with food be avoided.

## Oral Dosage Forms

### FEXOFENADINE HYDROCHLORIDE AND PSEUDOEPHEDRINE HYDROCHLORIDE EXTENDED-RELEASE TABLETS

**Usual adult and adolescent dose**
Antihistaminic-decongestant—
Oral, 1 tablet twice a day.
Note: In patients with reduced renal function, a starting dose of 1 tablet once a day is recommended.

**Usual pediatric dose**
Antihistaminic-decongestant—
Children younger than 12 years of age:
Safety and efficacy have not been established
Children 12 years of age and over:
See *Usual adult and adolescent dose*.

**Strength(s) usually available**
U.S.—
60 mg fexofenadine hydrochloride and 120 mg pseudoephedrine hydrochloride (Rx) [*Allegra-D*].
Note: The fexofenadine hydrochloride is in immediate-release form and the pseudoephedrine is in extended-release form controlled by an insoluable wax matrix.

**Packaging and storage**
Store between 20 and 25 °C (68 and 77 °F).

**Auxiliary labeling**
- Take on an empty stomach.
- Swallow tablets whole.

Developed: 08/12/98

---

**FILGRASTIM**—See *Colony Stimulating Factors (Systemic)*

---

# FINASTERIDE Systemic

VA CLASSIFICATION (Primary/Secondary): GU700/DE890
Commonly used brand name(s): *Propecia; Proscar*.
Note: For a listing of dosage forms and brand names by country availability, see *Dosage Forms* section(s).

## Category
Benign prostatic hyperplasia therapy agent; hair growth stimulant, alopecia androgenetica (systemic).

## Indications
**Accepted**
Note: SEE THE *PREGNANCY/REPRODUCTION* SECTION OF *PRECAUTIONS TO CONSIDER* FOR RESTRICTIONS ON THE USE OF FINASTERIDE. WOMEN OF CHILDBEARING POTENTIAL SHOULD NOT USE OR HANDLE CRUSHED FINASTERIDE TABLETS BECAUSE OF A POTENTIAL RISK TO A MALE FETUS.

Benign prostatic hyperplasia (treatment)—Finasteride is indicated for the treatment of symptomatic benign prostatic hyperplasia (BPH).

Approximately 60% of patients receiving finasteride experience increases of > 10% in urinary flow and 30% experience improvement in symptoms of BPH. Finasteride has been shown to reduce prostatic volume by an average of 27% in most treated patients.

One study comparing finasteride to terazosin for the treatment of BPH found that finasteride alone was no more effective than placebo, and that finasteride and terazosin given together were no more effective than terazosin alone. However, the patients receiving finasteride had, on average, smaller-volume prostates; a recent meta-analysis has determined that finasteride therapy is most useful in patients with large-volume prostates. Further studies are needed to assess the role of finasteride in the treatment of BPH.

The long-term effects of finasteride on reducing the incidences of surgery, acute urinary obstruction, or other complications of BPH have not been determined.

Because finasteride causes only slight improvement in symptoms, it is probably less useful in patients with severe symptoms than in patients with mild to moderate symptoms.

Prior to initiation of finasteride therapy, infection, prostate cancer, stricture disease, hypotonic bladder, or other neurogenic disorders that might mimic BPH should be ruled out.

Alopecia androgenetica (treatment)—Finasteride is indicated for the treatment of alopecia androgenetica (also known as male-pattern baldness) in men only. Safety and efficacy were demonstrated in men between the ages of 18 to 41 with mild to moderate hair loss of the vertex and anterior or midscalp area.

### Acceptance not established
Finasteride has been used for the treatment of hirsutism; however, because of potential risk to male fetuses, it should be used with caution, if at all, in women of childbearing years.

Finasteride has been used to treat prostate cancer; however, data are limited and results from ongoing trials are needed to define its role in this condition.

Efficacy of finasteride in the treatment of bitemporal hair recession has not been established.

### Unaccepted
Finasteride is not useful in patients with obstructive uropathy accompanied by urinary retention.

## Pharmacology/Pharmacokinetics

### Physicochemical characteristics
Source—Synthetic.
Chemical group—A 4-azasteroid compound.
Molecular weight—372.55.

### Mechanism of action/Effect
Finasteride competitively and specifically inhibits 5-alpha-reductase, a type 2 isoenzyme that metabolizes testosterone to dihydrotestosterone (DHT) in the prostate gland, liver, and skin. Finasteride has no affinity for the androgen receptors and does not appear to affect the hypothalamic-pituitary-testicular axis.

Benign prostatic hyperplasia—Development of the prostate gland is dependent on DHT, which is a potent androgen. After administration of finasteride, 5-alpha–reduced steroid metabolites in blood and urine are decreased; serum DHT is reduced by approximately 70% with daily dosing. Concentrations of both DHT and prostate-specific antigen (PSA) are decreased in prostatic tissue, whereas intraprostatic testosterone concentrations are significantly increased.

Alopecia androgenetica—The scalps of men with alopecia androgenetica contain miniaturized hair follicles and increased amounts of DHT compared with the scalps of men with normal hair growth. Scalp and serum DHT concentrations decrease after administration of finasteride, thus disrupting the development of male-pattern balding. It is not known why a decrease in scalp and serum DHT disrupts the development of male-pattern balding.

### Absorption
Finasteride is rapidly absorbed from the gastrointestinal tract. Mean bioavailability of a 5-mg tablet was 63% (range 34 to 108%) in a study in healthy male subjects. Mean bioavailability of a 1-mg tablet was 65% (range 26 to 70%) in a study in healthy male subjects. Bioavailability is not affected by food intake.

### Distribution
Finasteride crosses the blood-brain barrier. It also is distributed into semen; however, the amount of finasteride in the semen of patients receiving 5 mg per day has no effect on circulating DHT concentrations in adults.

### Protein binding
Plasma—Very high (90%).

### Biotransformation
Hepatic. The major metabolite isolated from urine is the monocarboxylic acid metabolite; the t-butyl side chain monohydroxylated metabolite has been isolated from plasma. These metabolites have no more than 20% of the 5-alpha-reductase inhibiting activity of finasteride.

### Half-life
Mean 6 hours (range 3 to 16 hours) following a single 5-mg dose in healthy male subjects 45 to 60 years of age; approximately 8 hours in subjects 70 years of age or older.

### Time to peak concentration
Plasma—Ranged from 1.8 to 2.8 hours after administration of single doses of 5, 10, 20, 50, and 100 mg of finasteride and 1 to 2 hours after administration of multiple doses of 1 mg per day.

### Peak serum concentration
Plasma—Ranged from 38.1 ± 7 to 835.5 ± 199.2 micrograms per L (mcg/L) after administration of single doses of 5, 10, 20, 50, and 100 mg of finasteride and 9.2 nanograms per mL (range 4.9 to 13.7 nanograms per mL) after administration of multiple doses of 1 mg per day. Slow accumulation occurs with multiple dosing; in one study, mean plasma concentrations were approximately 50% higher after 17 days of treatment than after the first dose, and mean trough concentrations in another study after 1 year were even higher. In one study, the mean area under the plasma concentration–time curve (AUC) (0 to 24 hours) after 17 days of administration was 15% higher in subjects 70 years of age or older.

### Time to peak effect
Reduction in serum DHT concentration—8 hours after the first dose.

### Duration of action
Single dose—Reduction in serum DHT concentration: 24 hours.
Multiple doses—DHT concentrations return to pretreatment levels within approximately 2 weeks after withdrawal of daily therapy. The prostate returns to pretreatment size in about 3 months.

### Elimination
Fecal, 57% (range 51 to 64%), as metabolites; renal, 39% (range 32 to 46%), as metabolites. In renal function impairment, urinary excretion of metabolites is decreased, but fecal excretion of metabolites is increased; therefore, no dosage adjustment is necessary.
In dialysis—Unknown.

## Precautions to Consider

### Carcinogenicity
A 19-month study in CD-1 mice at a dose of 250 mg per kg of body weight (mg/kg) per day (228 times the human exposure of 5 mg and 1824 times the human exposure of 1 mg) found a statistically significant increase in incidence of testicular Leydig cell adenomas. An increase in the incidence of Leydig cell hyperplasia was observed in mice at a dose of 25 mg/kg per day (23 times the human exposure of 5 mg and 184 times the human exposure of 1 mg, estimated) and in rats at a dose ≥ 40 mg/kg per day (39 times the human exposure of 5 mg and 312 times the human exposure of 1 mg). A positive correlation between the proliferative changes in the Leydig cells and an increase in serum luteinizing hormone (LH) concentrations (two- to threefold higher than control) has been demonstrated in both rodent species treated with high doses of finasteride. No drug-related Leydig cell changes were seen in either rats or dogs treated for 1 year at doses of 20 mg/kg per day and 45 mg/kg per day (30 and 350 times, respectively, the human exposure of 5 mg and 240 and 2800 times, respectively, the human exposure of 1 mg) or in mice treated for 19 months at a dose of 2.5 mg/kg per day (2.3 times the human exposure of 5 mg and 18.4 times the human exposure of 1 mg, estimated).

### Tumorigenicity
A 24-month study in Sprague-Dawley rats at doses up to 160 mg/kg per day in males and 320 mg/kg per day in females (producing 111 and 274 times, respectively, the systemic exposure observed in humans receiving the recommended human dose of 5 mg per day and 888 and 2192 times, respectively, the systemic exposure observed in humans receiving the recommended human dose of 1 mg per day) found no evidence of tumorigenicity.

### Mutagenicity
No evidence of mutagenicity was found in an in vitro bacterial mutagenesis assay, a mammalian cell mutagenesis assay, or an in vitro alkaline elution assay. In an in vitro chromosome aberration assay, when Chinese hamster ovary cells were treated with high concentrations (450 to 550 micromoles, corresponding to 4000 to 5000 times the peak plasma concentrations in humans given a total dose of 5 mg and 18,000 to 22,000 times the peak plasma concentration in humans given a total dose of 1 mg) of finasteride, there was a slight increase in chromosome aberrations. In addition, the concentrations (450 to 550 micromoles) used in in vitro studies are not achievable in a biological system. In an in vivo chromosome aberration assay in mice, no treatment-related increase in chromosome aberration was observed at the maximum tolerated finasteride dose of 250 mg/kg per day (228 times the human exposure of 5 mg and 1824 times the human exposure of 1 mg) as determined in the carcinogenicity studies.

## Pregnancy/Reproduction

Fertility—Volume of ejaculate may be decreased in some patients during therapy, but the decrease does not appear to interfere with normal sexual function.

No effect on fertility, sperm count, or ejaculation volume was found in sexually mature male rabbits treated with finasteride at doses of 80 mg/kg per day (543 times the human exposure of 5 mg and 4344 times the human exposure of 1 mg) for up to 12 weeks. No effects on fertility were found in sexually mature male rats treated with 80 mg/kg per day (61 times the human exposure of 5 mg and 488 times the human exposure of 1 mg) for 6 or 12 weeks. However, when treatment in male rats was continued for up to 24 or 30 weeks, there was an apparent decrease in fertility and fecundity and an associated significant decrease in the weights of the seminal vesicles and prostate, all of which were reversible within 6 weeks of withdrawal of finasteride. No drug-related effect on testes or on mating performance has been seen in rats or rabbits. The decrease in fertility in rats is secondary to an effect on accessory sex organs (prostate and seminal vesicles) that results in failure to form a seminal plug, which is essential for normal fertility in rats, but is not relevant in humans.

Pregnancy—Finasteride is not indicated for use in women.

Because of the ability of 5-alpha-reductase inhibitors to inhibit conversion of testosterone to dihydrotestosterone (DHT), finasteride administration to a pregnant woman may cause abnormalities of the external genitalia of a male fetus.

Because of the potential risk to a male fetus, a woman who is pregnant or who may become pregnant should not handle crushed finasteride tablets.

Administration of finasteride to pregnant rats at doses ranging from 100 mcg per kg of body weight (mcg/kg) per day to 100 mg/kg per day (approximately 1 to 1000 times the recommended human dose of 5 mg and 5 to 5000 times the recommended human dose of 1 mg) produced dose-dependent development of hypospadias in 3.6 to 100% of male offspring. Pregnant rats given doses ≥ 30 mcg/kg per day (≥ three tenths of the recommended human dose of 5 mg and ≥ 1.5 times the recommended human dose of 1 mg) produced male offspring with decreased prostatic and seminal vesicular weights, delayed preputial separation, and transient nipple development; doses of ≥ 3 mcg/kg per day (≥ 3% of the recommended human dose of 5 mg and one fifth of the recommended human dose of 1 mg) produced decreased anogenital distance. All of these changes are expected pharmacologic effects of 5-alpha-reductase inhibitors and are similar to those reported in male infants with a genetic deficiency of 5-alpha-reductase. The critical period during which these effects can be induced in male rats has been defined as days 16 to 17 of gestation. No abnormalities were observed in female offspring exposed *in utero* to any dose of finasteride.

In reproduction studies using male rats treated with finasteride doses of 80 mg/kg per day (61 times the human exposure of 5 mg and 488 times the human exposure of 1 mg) and untreated female rats, no developmental abnormalities were observed in first filial generation (F$_1$) male or female offspring. Administration of 3 mg/kg per day (30 times the recommended human dose of 5 mg and 150 times the recommended human dose of 1 mg) during the late gestation and lactation period resulted in slightly decreased fertility in F$_1$ male offspring; no effects were seen in female offspring. In rabbit fetuses exposed to finasteride *in utero* from days 6 to 18 of gestation at doses up to 100 mg/kg per day (1000 times the recommended human dose of 5 mg and 5000 times the recommended human dose of 1 mg), no evidence of malformations was observed; however, effects on male genitalia would not be expected since the rabbits were not exposed during the critical period of urogenital system development.

FDA Pregnancy Category X.

## Breast-feeding

Finasteride is not indicated for use in women. It is not known whether finasteride is distributed into breast milk.

## Pediatrics

Finasteride is not indicated for use in children. No information is available on the relationship of age to the effects of finasteride in pediatric patients.

## Geriatrics

The elimination rate of finasteride is decreased in the elderly (70 years of age or older); however, no dosage adjustment is necessary.

## Laboratory value alterations

The following have been selected on the basis of their potential clinical significance (possible effect in parentheses where appropriate)—not necessarily inclusive (» = major clinical significance):

With diagnostic test results
  Prostate-specific antigen (PSA)
    (serum concentrations are decreased by finasteride, even in the presence of prostatic cancer; the effect on usefulness of PSA determinations for prostatic cancer detection is unknown)

With physiology/laboratory test values
  Dihydrotestosterone (DHT)
    (serum and prostatic concentrations are rapidly reduced)
  Follicle-stimulating hormone (FSH) and
  Luteinizing hormone (LH) and
  Testosterone
    (median circulating serum concentrations are increased by 10% but remain within the physiologic range; testosterone concentrations in prostatic tissue increase by up to tenfold)

## Medical considerations/Contraindications

The medical considerations/contraindications included have been selected on the basis of their potential clinical significance (reasons given in parentheses where appropriate)—not necessarily inclusive (» = major clinical significance).

*Risk-benefit should be considered when the following medical problems exist:*

Hepatic function impairment
  (metabolism of finasteride may be reduced)
Large residual urinary volume or
Reduced urinary flow
  (because of possible presence of obstructive uropathy, patients with these conditions may not be candidates for finasteride therapy)
» Sensitivity to finasteride or to any component of the medication

## Patient monitoring

The following may be especially important in patient monitoring (other tests may be warranted in some patients, depending on condition; » = major clinical significance):

*For benign prostatic hyperplasia*
» Digital rectal examination
  (recommended prior to initiation of therapy and at periodic intervals during therapy, to detect possible prostate cancer)

## Side/Adverse Effects

The following side/adverse effects have been selected on the basis of their potential clinical significance (possible signs and symptoms in parentheses where appropriate)—not necessarily inclusive:

### Those indicating need for medical attention

### Incidence less frequent

*Gynecomastia* (breast enlargement and tenderness); **hypersensitivity reaction** (skin rash; swelling of lips)

Note: *Gynecomastia* has been reported to develop from 14 days to 2.5 years after initiation of 5-mg finasteride therapy. Discontinuation of therapy has led to a partial or complete remission in most cases; however, a small percentage of patients have required mastectomy. In addition, gynecomastia has led to primary intraductal breast carcinoma in at least two patients receiving finasteride therapy. Cause and effect are not known at this time. In clinical trials, gynecomastia and *hypersensitivity reaction* events in patients receiving 1 mg of finasteride therapy were not different from subjects receiving placebo.

### Those indicating need for medical attention only if they continue or are bothersome

Incidence less frequent or rare (< 4%)

*Abdominal pain; back pain; decreased libido; decreased volume of ejaculate; diarrhea; dizziness; headache; impotence*

Note: *Decreased libido, decreased volume of ejaculate,* and *impotence* usually resolve with continued treatment in over 60% of patients who report these side effects.

## Patient Consultation

As an aid to patient consultation, refer to *Advice for the Patient, Finasteride (Systemic)*.

In providing consultation, consider emphasizing the following selected information (» = major clinical significance):

### Before using this medication
» Conditions affecting use, especially:
  Sensitivity to finasteride or any component of the medication

  Carcinogenicity—Increased incidence of testicular tumors in mice and rats receiving very high doses

## Finasteride (Systemic)

Pregnancy—Pregnant women should not use or handle crushed tablets because of potential risk of abnormal external genitalia development in male fetuses

Breast-feeding—Not indicated for use in breast-feeding women

### Proper use of this medication
Tablets may be crushed; however, pregnant women should not handle crushed tablets

*For benign prostatic hyperplasia (BPH)*
Getting into the habit of taking at same time each day to help increase compliance
» Does not cure, but helps control BPH; taking for at least 6 months for full effect; possible need for lifelong therapy; checking with physician before discontinuing medication
All patients with BPH should avoid drinking fluids, especially coffee or alcohol, in the evening, to reduce nocturia

*For male-pattern balding*
Taking for at least 3 months to see effect; improvement lasts only as long as treatment continues; new hair will be lost within one year of stopping treatment
» Proper dosing
Missed dose: Taking as soon as possible; not taking if almost time for next dose; not doubling doses
» Proper storage

### Precautions while using this medication
» Women who are or who may become pregnant should not handle crushed tablets

### Side/adverse effects
Signs of potential side effects, especially gynecomastia (more likely with 5 mg dose), hypersensitivity reaction (more likely with 5 mg dose), decreased libido, decreased volume of ejaculate, and impotence

## General Dosing Information

### Diet/Nutrition
Finasteride may be taken with or without food.

## Oral Dosage Forms

### FINASTERIDE TABLETS

**Usual adult dose**
Benign prostatic hyperplasia—
   Oral, 5 mg once a day.
Note: At least six to twelve months of therapy may be required to assess clinical response.
Alopecia androgenetica—
   Oral, 1 mg once a day.
Note: Three months of therapy may be required to assess response as a hair growth stimulant. Discontinuation of finasteride treatment leads to reversal of effects within one year.

**Usual geriatric dose**
See *Usual adult dose*.

**Strength(s) usually available**
U.S.—
   1 mg (Rx) [*Propecia* (lactose)].
   5 mg (Rx) [*Proscar* (lactose)].
Canada—
   5 mg (Rx) [*Proscar*].

**Packaging and storage**
Store below 30 °C (86 °F), unless otherwise specified by the manufacturer. Store in a tight container. Protect from light.

## Selected Bibliography
Drugs for the treatment of benign prostatic hypertrophy: efficacy and safety criteria. Proceedings of meeting of the Endocrinology and Metabolic Drugs Advisory Committee, Center for Drug Evaluation and Research, Food and Drug Administration; 1992 Feb 3-4: Bethesda, MD.

Revised: 04/27/98

---

# FLAVOXATE  Systemic

VA CLASSIFICATION (Primary): GU201
Commonly used brand name(s): *Urispas*.
Note: For a listing of dosage forms and brand names by country availability, see *Dosage Forms* section(s).

## Category
Antispasmodic (urinary tract).

## Indications

**Accepted**
Urologic disorders, symptoms of (treatment); and
Irritative voiding, symptoms of (treatment)—Flavoxate is indicated for the symptomatic relief, but not the definitive treatment, of dysuria, urgency, nocturia, suprapubic pain, and frequency and incontinence associated with cystitis, prostatitis, urethritis, urethrocystitis, or urethrotrigonitis.

## Pharmacology/Pharmacokinetics

**Physicochemical characteristics**
Molecular weight—427.93.

**Mechanism of action/Effect**
Exerts direct antispasmodic (relaxant) effect on smooth muscle, mainly of the urinary tract.

**Other actions/effects**
Also has weak antihistaminic, local anesthetic, and analgesic action. With high doses, flavoxate has weak anticholinergic properties.

**Absorption**
Well absorbed from gastrointestinal tract.

**Elimination**
Renal (10 to 30% eliminated within 6 hours).

## Precautions to Consider

### Pregnancy/Reproduction
Pregnancy—Adequate and well-controlled studies in humans have not been done.

Reproduction studies in rats and rabbits at doses up to 34 times the recommended human dose have not shown that flavoxate causes impaired fertility or adverse effects on the fetus.

FDA Pregnancy Category B.

### Breast-feeding
Problems in humans have not been documented.

### Pediatrics
Appropriate studies on the relationship of age to the effects of flavoxate have not been performed in the pediatric population.

### Geriatrics
Confusion is more likely to occur in geriatric patients taking flavoxate.

### Dental
Prolonged use or use of large doses of flavoxate may decrease or inhibit salivary flow, thus contributing to the development of caries, periodontal disease, oral candidiasis, and discomfort.

### Medical considerations/Contraindications
The medical considerations/contraindications included have been selected on the basis of their potential clinical significance (reasons given in parentheses where appropriate)—not necessarily inclusive (» = major clinical significance).

*Risk-benefit should be considered when the following medical problems exist:*
» Gastrointestinal tract obstructive disease as in achalasia and pyloroduodenal stenosis
   (decrease in motility and tone may occur, resulting in obstruction and gastric retention)
   Glaucoma, angle-closure
   (mydriatic effect of flavoxate resulting in increased intraocular pressure may precipitate an acute attack of angle-closure glaucoma )
» Hemorrhage, gastrointestinal
   (may exacerbate condition)
» Paralytic ileus
   (may result in obstruction)
   Sensitivity to flavoxate

» Uropathy, obstructive, such as bladder neck obstruction due to prostatic hypertrophy
(urinary retention may be precipitated)

### Side/Adverse Effects

Note: Although weak, flavoxate's anticholinergic action should be taken into consideration when it is given to patients where the environmental temperature is high, since there is risk of a rapid increase in body temperature because of suppression of sweat gland activity.

The following side/adverse effects have been selected on the basis of their potential clinical significance (possible signs and symptoms in parentheses where appropriate)—not necessarily inclusive:

**Those indicating need for medical attention**
Incidence rare
*Confusion*—especially in the elderly; *hypersensitivity* (skin rash or hives); *increased intraocular pressure* (eye pain); *leukopenia* (sore throat and fever)

**Those indicating need for medical attention only if they continue or are bothersome**
Incidence more frequent
*Drowsiness; dryness of mouth and throat*

Incidence less frequent or rare
*Constipation*—more frequent with doses of 800 mg or above; *difficult urination; difficulty concentrating; difficulty in eye accommodation* (blurred vision); *dizziness; fast heartbeat; headache; increased sweating; mydriatic effect* (increased sensitivity of eyes to light); *nausea or vomiting; nervousness; stomach pain*

### Overdose

For specific information on the agents used in the management of flavoxate overdose, see:
*Thiopental* in *Anesthetics, Barbiturate (Systemic)* monograph;
*Benzodiazepines (Systemic)* monograph;
*Charcoal, Activated (Oral-Local)* monograph;
*Chloral Hydrate (Systemic)* monograph

For more information on the management of overdose or unintentional ingestion, **contact a Poison Control Center** (see *Poison Control Center Listing*).

**Clinical effects of overdose**
The following effects have been selected on the basis of their potential clinical significance (possible signs and symptoms in parenthesis where appropriate)—not necessarily inclusive:

*Anticholinergic effects* (clumsiness or unsteadiness; severe dizziness; severe drowsiness; fever; flushing or redness of face; hallucinations; shortness of breath or troubled breathing; unusual excitement; nervousness; restlessness; or irritability)

**Treatment of overdose**
Recommended treatment for overdose with flavoxate includes:
• To decrease absorption—Emesis or gastric lavage with 4% tannic acid solution or administration of an aqueous slurry of activated charcoal.
• Specific treatment—Administration of small doses of short-acting barbiturate (100 mg thiopental sodium) or benzodiazepines, or rectal infusion of 100 to 200 mL of a 2% solution of chloral hydrate, to control excitement. Artificial respiration with oxygen if needed for respiratory depression. Adequate hydration. Symptomatic treatment as necessary.
• Supportive care—Patients in whom intentional overdose is known or suspected should be referred for psychiatric consultation.

### Patient Consultation

As an aid to patient consultation, refer to *Advice for the Patient, Flavoxate (Systemic)*.

In providing consultation, consider emphasizing the following selected information (» = major clinical significance):

**Before using this medication**
» Conditions affecting use, especially:
Sensitivity to flavoxate
Use in the elderly—Confusion more likely
Dental—Possible development of dental problems because of decreased salivary flow
Other medical problems, especially gastrointestinal hemorrhage, paralytic ileus, or obstruction in gastrointestinal or urinary tract

**Proper use of this medication**
Taking medication on an empty stomach with water, or with food or milk to reduce gastric irritation
» Importance of not taking more medication than the amount prescribed
» Proper dosing
Missed dose: Taking as soon as possible; if almost time for next dose, not taking at all; not doubling doses
» Proper storage

**Precautions while using this medication**
Possible increased sensitivity of eyes to light
» Caution if drowsiness or blurred vision occurs
» Caution during exercise or hot weather; overheating may result in heat stroke
Possible dryness of mouth and throat; using sugarless gum or candy, ice, or saliva substitute for relief; checking with physician or dentist if dry mouth continues for more than 2 weeks

**Side/adverse effects**
Signs of potential side effects, especially hypersensitivity, confusion, increased intraocular pressure, and leukopenia

### General Dosing Information

Flavoxate may be taken on an empty stomach with water; however, if gastric irritation occurs it may be taken with food or milk.

If urinary tract infection is present, appropriate antibacterial therapy should be administered.

### Oral Dosage Forms

#### FLAVOXATE HYDROCHLORIDE TABLETS

**Usual adult and adolescent dose**
Urologic disorders or
Irritative voiding—
Oral, 100 to 200 mg three or four times a day, the dosage being adjusted as needed and tolerated.

**Usual pediatric dose**
Dosage has not been established.

**Usual geriatric dose**
See *Usual adult and adolescent dose*.

**Strength(s) usually available**
U.S.—
100 mg (Rx) [*Urispas*].
Canada—
200 mg (Rx) [*Urispas*].

**Packaging and storage**
Store below 40 °C (104 °F), preferably between 15 and 30 °C (59 and 86 °F), unless otherwise specified by manufacturer.

**Auxiliary labeling**
• May cause drowsiness or blurred vision.

Revised: 01/18/93

---

# FLECAINIDE Systemic

VA CLASSIFICATION (Primary): CV300
Commonly used brand name(s): *Tambocor*.
Note: For a listing of dosage forms and brand names by country availability, see *Dosage Forms* section(s).

### Category
Antiarrhythmic.

### Indications

**Accepted**
Arrhythmias, supraventricular (prophylaxis)[1]—In patients without structural heart disease, flecainide is indicated for the prevention of paroxysmal supraventricular tachycardias, including atrioventricular nodal reentrant tachycardia, atrioventricular reentrant tachycardia, and other supraventricular tachycardias of unspecified mechanism associated with disabling symptoms. It is also indicated for the prevention of paroxysmal atrial fibrillation/flutter associated with disabling symptoms in patients without structural heart disease.

**Arrhythmias, ventricular (prophylaxis and treatment)**—Flecainide is indicated for the prevention and suppression of documented life-threatening ventricular arrhythmias, such as sustained ventricular tachycardia.

### Unaccepted
Use of flecainide is no longer accepted for treatment of less severe arrhythmias such as nonsustained ventricular tachycardias or frequent premature ventricular contractions, even if patients are symptomatic, because of results of a trial that found increased mortality in patients with non–life-threatening arrhythmias treated with flecainide.

Flecainide is not accepted for use in the treatment of chronic atrial fibrillation because of the increased risk for development of ventricular arrhythmias such as ventricular tachycardia and ventricular fibrillation.

---

[1]Not included in Canadian product labeling.

## Pharmacology/Pharmacokinetics

### Physicochemical characteristics
Molecular weight—474.40.
pKa—9.3.

### Mechanism of action/Effect
Decreases excitability, conduction velocity, and automaticity as a result of slowed atrial, atrioventricular (AV) nodal, His-Purkinje, and intraventricular conduction, and causes a slight but significant prolongation of refractory periods in these tissues. The greatest effect is on the His-Purkinje system. Decreases the rate of rise of the action potential without affecting its duration. In the Vaughan Williams classification of antiarrhythmics, flecainide is considered to be a class IC agent.

### Other actions/effects
Mild to moderate negative inotropic effect; local anesthetic activity.

### Absorption
Nearly complete; not affected by food or antacids.

### Protein binding
Moderate (40%).

### Biotransformation
Hepatic.

### Half-life
Elimination—Approximately 20 hours (range, 12 to 27 hours); increased with renal or hepatic function impairment or congestive heart failure. In addition, elimination is slowed significantly in those rare conditions where urinary pH is 8 or higher (e.g., renal tubular acidosis, strict vegetarian diet).

### Time to peak plasma concentration
Single dose—Approximately 3 hours (range, 1 to 6 hours).

### Time to steady-state plasma concentration
Multiple doses—3 to 5 days.

### Therapeutic trough plasma concentration
0.2 to 1.0 mcg per mL.

### Elimination
Renal—Approximately 30% (range, 10 to 50%) unchanged.
Fecal—5%.
In dialysis—Hemodialysis removes only about 1% of a dose as unchanged drug.

## Precautions to Consider

### Cross-sensitivity and/or related problems
Patients sensitive to other amide-type anesthetics may rarely be sensitive to flecainide also. Cross-sensitivity with procainamide or quinidine has not been reported.

### Carcinogenicity
Studies with flecainide in rats and mice at doses up to 8 times the usual human dose found no evidence of carcinogenicity.

### Mutagenicity
Mutagenicity studies (Ames test, mouse lymphoma, *in vivo* cytogenetics) found no evidence of mutagenicity.

### Pregnancy/Reproduction
Fertility—A reproduction study in male and female rats given flecainide in doses up to 50 mg per kg of body weight (mg/kg) per day (7 times the usual human dose) did not reveal fertility impairment.

Pregnancy—Adequate and well-controlled studies in humans have not been done.
Studies in New Zealand White rabbits given doses of 30 and 35 mg/kg per day revealed teratogenic and embryotoxic effects. Teratogenic effects did not occur in Dutch Belted rabbits at the same dose or in rats and mice given doses up to 50 and 80 mg/kg per day, respectively. However, delayed sternebral and vertebral ossification was seen at the high dose in rats.

FDA Pregnancy Category C.

### Breast-feeding
Flecainide is distributed into human breast milk in concentrations as high as 4 times the corresponding plasma concentrations. The potential dose to a nursing infant, assuming a maternal plasma concentration of 1 mcg per mL (mcg/mL) and infant ingestion of 700 mL of breast milk over 24 hours, would be less than 3 mg.

### Pediatrics
Appropriate studies on the relationship of age to the effects of flecainide have not been performed in the pediatric population. Safety and efficacy have not been established.

### Geriatrics
The half-life of flecainide may be somewhat prolonged in the elderly, although dosage adjustment is usually not necessary. In addition, incidence of proarrhythmic effects may be increased in the elderly, who are more likely to have underlying cardiac function impairment. Elderly patients are also more likely to have age-related renal function impairment, which may require caution in patients receiving flecainide.

### Drug interactions and/or related problems
The following drug interactions and/or related problems have been selected on the basis of their potential clinical significance (possible mechanism in parentheses where appropriate)—not necessarily inclusive (» = major clinical significance):

Note: Combinations containing any of the following medications, depending on the amount present, may also interact with this medication.

Acidifiers, urinary
(by decreasing urine pH, may increase elimination of flecainide; dosage adjustment of flecainide may be necessary)

Alkalizers, urinary
(by increasing urine pH, may decrease elimination of flecainide; dosage adjustment of flecainide may be necessary)

» Antiarrhythmics, other
(concurrent use with flecainide may produce additive cardiac effects; irreversible ventricular tachycardia/fibrillation has been reported in patients with hypotensive ventricular tachycardia)

(concurrent use of amiodarone with flecainide has resulted in a two-fold or greater increase in plasma flecainide concentrations; it is recommended that the usual dose of flecainide be reduced by 50% and plasma flecainide concentrations monitored carefully during concurrent use)

Beta-adrenergic blocking agents
(concurrent use with flecainide may result in additive negative inotropic effects; in addition, concurrent use of propranolol with flecainide has resulted in increased plasma concentrations of both, but less depression of heart rate than occurs with propranolol alone)

Bone marrow depressants (See *Appendix II*)
(although problems have not been reported, concurrent use with flecainide may increase the risk of leukopenia and thrombocytopenia)

Digoxin
(concurrent use with flecainide has resulted in transiently increased plasma digoxin concentrations; no adverse effects have been reported)

### Laboratory value alterations
The following have been selected on the basis of their potential clinical significance (possible effect in parentheses where appropriate)—not necessarily inclusive (» = major clinical significance):

With physiology/laboratory test values
Electrocardiogram (ECG) changes such as:
QRS widening and
PR prolongation and
QT prolongation secondary to QRS widening
(occur in most patients)

Note: ECG changes produced by flecainide do not necessarily indicate efficacy, toxicity, or overdose.

### Medical considerations/Contraindications
The medical considerations/contraindications included have been selected on the basis of their potential clinical significance (reasons given in parentheses where appropriate)—not necessarily inclusive (» = major clinical significance).

*Except under special circumstances, this medication should not be used when the following medical problems exist:*
» Atrioventricular (AV) block, pre-existing second or third degree without pacemaker or
» Right bundle branch block associated with a left hemiblock (bifascicular block) without pacemaker
 (risk of complete heart block)

*Risk-benefit should be considered when the following medical problems exist:*
» Cardiogenic shock
 (negative inotropic effect of flecainide; increased risk of flecainide-induced arrhythmias)
 Congestive heart failure
 (may be aggravated as a result of small negative inotropic effect; elimination may be delayed; increased risk of flecainide-induced arrhythmias; dosage reduction may be necessary)
» Hepatic function impairment
 (elimination may be significantly slowed; the interval between dosage increments should be greater than 4 days, and dosage reduction may be necessary; dosage adjustments should be made on the basis of plasma flecainide determinations)
 Hypokalemia or hyperkalemia
 (effects of flecainide may be altered; pre-existing hypokalemia or hyperkalemia should be corrected before administration of flecainide)
 Myocardial infarction, history of, with associated left ventricular function impairment
 (increased risk of flecainide-induced arrhythmias)
 Renal function impairment
 (reduced elimination; the interval between dosage increments should be greater than 4 days, and dosage reduction may be necessary; dosage adjustments should be made on the basis of plasma flecainide determinations)
 Sensitivity to flecainide
» Sick sinus syndrome
 (flecainide prolongs sinus node recovery time; may cause sinus bradycardia, sinus pause, or sinus arrest)
 Caution is also recommended in patients with permanent pacemakers or temporary pacing electrodes because flecainide increases endocardial pacing thresholds and may suppress ventricular escape rhythms; use is not recommended in patients with existing high thresholds or nonprogrammable pacemakers unless suitable pacing rescue is available. In patients with pacemakers, it is recommended that the pacing threshold be determined prior to initiation of therapy, after one week of administration, and then at regular intervals.

**Patient monitoring**
The following may be especially important in patient monitoring (other tests may be warranted in some patients, depending on condition; » = major clinical significance):
 Blood counts
 (recommended at periodic intervals to detect bone marrow depression)
» ECG
 (Holter monitoring or 24-hour ambulatory ECG recommended prior to initiation of therapy and at periodic intervals during therapy to assess efficacy and detect possible proarrhythmic effects)
 Plasma flecainide determinations, trough
 (recommended at frequent intervals to aid in dosage adjustment in patients with severe renal or hepatic disease; may also be useful in patients with congestive heart failure or moderate renal disease)

## Side/Adverse Effects

Note: In the National Heart Lung and Blood Institute's Cardiac Arrhythmias Suppression Trial (CAST), flecainide treatment was found to be associated with excessive mortality or increased nonfatal cardiac arrest rate as compared with placebo in patients with asymptomatic, non–life-threatening arrhythmias who had a recent myocardial infarction.

Adverse cardiac effects reported with flecainide administration include new or exacerbated ventricular or supraventricular arrhythmias, new or exacerbated congestive heart failure, second or third degree atrioventricular (AV) block, and rarely, sinus bradycardia, sinus pause, or sinus arrest.

Incidence of cardiac and other effects is at least partially dose-related and is increased at plasma flecainide concentrations greater than 0.7 to 1.0 mcg per mL.

The following side/adverse effects have been selected on the basis of their potential clinical significance (possible signs and symptoms in parentheses where appropriate)—not necessarily inclusive:

**Those indicating need for medical attention**
Incidence less frequent
 *Arrhythmias, including new or worsened ventricular tachyarrhythmias, increased frequency of premature ventricular contractions, or new supraventricular arrhythmias* (irregular heartbeat); *chest pain; congestive heart failure* (shortness of breath; swelling of feet or lower legs); *trembling or shaking*
 Note: *Arrhythmias* are dose-related and potentially fatal; incidence increased in patients with congestive heart failure or history of myocardial infarction with associated left ventricular function impairment.
Incidence rare
 *Hepatic function impairment* (yellow eyes or skin)

**Those indicating need for medical attention only if they continue or are bothersome**
Incidence more frequent
 *Blurred vision or seeing spots; dizziness or lightheadedness*
Incidence less frequent
 *Anxiety or mental depression; constipation; headache; nausea or vomiting; skin rash; stomach pain or loss of appetite; unusual tiredness or weakness*

## Overdose

For specific information on the agents used in the management of flecainide overdose, see:
 • *Dobutamine, Dopamine,* or *Isoproterenol* in *Sympathomimetic Agents–Cardiovascular Use (Parenteral-Systemic)* monograph.

For more information on the management of overdose or unintentional ingestion, **contact a Poison Control Center** (see *Poison Control Center Listing*).

**Treatment of overdose**
To decrease absorption—Treatment should begin with immediate evacuation of the stomach.
Specific treatment—Treatment is primarily supportive and symptomatic and may include oxygen, mechanical respiratory assistance, circulatory assistance (e.g., intra-aortic balloon pumping), transvenous conduction pacing, administration of inotropic agents (dopamine, dobutamine, or isoproterenol), cardioversion defibrillation if sustained ventricular tachycardia attributable to flecainide's effects occurs, and if the sustained ventricular tachycardia has caused or may lead to hemodynamic decomposition and/or ventricular fibrillation.
Supportive care—Patients in whom intentional overdose is confirmed or suspected should be referred for psychiatric consultation.

## Patient Consultation

As an aid to patient consultation, refer to *Advice for the Patient, Flecainide (Systemic)*.
In providing consultation, consider emphasizing the following selected information (» = major clinical significance):

**Before using this medication**
» Conditions affecting use, especially:
 Sensitivity to flecainide or amide-type anesthetics
 Pregnancy—Teratogenic in rabbits
 Use in the elderly—Increased duration of action; increased risk of proarrhythmic effects
 Other medications, especially other antiarrhythmics
 Other medical problems, especially hepatic function impairment

**Proper use of this medication**
» Compliance with therapy; taking as directed even if feeling well
» Importance of not missing doses and taking at evenly spaced intervals
» Proper dosing
 Missed dose: Taking as soon as possible if remembered within 6 hours; not taking if remembered later; not doubling doses
» Proper storage

**Precautions while using this medication**
 Regular visits to physician to check progress
 Carrying medical identification card or bracelet
» Caution if any kind of surgery (including dental surgery) or emergency treatment is required
» Caution when driving or doing things requiring alertness because of possible dizziness
 Checking with physician before discontinuing medication; gradual dosage reduction may be necessary

## Flecainide (Systemic)

### Side/adverse effects
Signs of potential side effects, especially arrhythmias, chest pain, congestive heart failure, trembling or shaking, and hepatic function impairment

### General Dosing Information
Previous antiarrhythmic therapy should be withdrawn 2 to 4 half-lives before initiation of flecainide therapy (except lidocaine, which can be used for interim control).

Occasionally, patients intolerant to or not adequately controlled by every-twelve-hour dosing may be dosed at eight-hour intervals.

Because of flecainide's long half-life, dosage increments should be made no more frequently than every 4 days.

It is recommended that treatment be initiated in the hospital because of the increased risk of proarrhythmic effects associated with flecainide administration.

It is recommended that flecainide therapy be withdrawn if bone marrow depression occurs.

### For treatment of adverse effects
Digitalis or diuretic therapy may be useful in patients with flecainide-induced or -aggravated congestive heart failure. Dosage reduction or withdrawal of flecainide may be necessary.

## Oral Dosage Forms

### FLECAINIDE ACETATE TABLETS

**Usual adult dose**
Paroxysmal supraventricular tachycardias or paroxysmal atrial fibrillation/flutter—
  Oral, 50 mg every twelve hours, the dosage being increased in increments of 50 mg two times a day every four days as needed and tolerated.
Sustained ventricular tachycardia—
  Initial: Oral, 100 mg every twelve hours, the dosage being increased in increments of 50 mg two times a day every four days as needed and tolerated.
Note: In patients with severe renal function impairment (creatinine clearance of 35 mL per minute per 1.73 square meters of body surface or less), an initial dose of 100 mg once a day or 50 mg every twelve hours is recommended, and dosage should be adjusted on the basis of frequent plasma concentration determinations. In patients with less severe renal function impairment, an initial dose of 100 mg every twelve hours may be used; plasma concentration determinations may be useful in dosage adjustment.
  Maintenance: Oral, up to 150 mg every twelve hours.

**Usual adult prescribing limits**
Paroxysmal supraventricular arrhythmias—Up to 300 mg per day.
Sustained ventricular tachycardia—Up to 400 mg per day.

**Usual pediatric dose**
Safety and efficacy have not been established.

**Strength(s) usually available**
U.S.—
  50 mg (Rx) [*Tambocor;* GENERIC].
  100 mg (Rx) [*Tambocor* (scored); GENERIC].
  150 mg (Rx) [*Tambocor* (scored); GENERIC].
Canada—
  50 mg (Rx) [*Tambocor* (scored)].
  100 mg (Rx) [*Tambocor* (scored)].

**Packaging and storage**
Store below 40 °C (104 °F), preferably between 15 and 30 °C (59 and 86 °F), unless otherwise specified by manufacturer. Store in a tight container. Protect from light.

### Selected Bibliography
Nappi JM, Anderson JL. Flecainide: a new prototype antiarrhythmic agent. Pharmacother 1985; 5: 209-21.
A symposium. Flecainide. Am J Cardiol 1988 Aug 25; 62: 1D-66D.
Roden DM, Woosley AL. Flecainide. N Engl J Med 1986 Jul 3; 315: 36-41.

Revised: 09/24/92
Interim revision: 04/29/94; 08/19/97

---

**FLOCTAFENINE**—See *Anti-inflammatory Drugs, Nonsteroidal (Systemic)*

---

# FLOXURIDINE  Systemic†

VA CLASSIFICATION (Primary): AN300
Commonly used brand name(s): *FUDR*.
Note: For a listing of dosage forms and brand names by country availability, see *Dosage Forms* section(s).

†Not commercially available in Canada.

## Category
Antineoplastic.

## Indications
Note: Bracketed information in the *Indications* section refers to uses that are not included in U.S. product labeling.

**Accepted**
Carcinoma, colorectal (treatment)
Carcinoma, hepatic (treatment)
[Carcinoma, ovarian, epithelial (treatment)] or
[Carcinoma, renal (treatment)]—Floxuridine, given by continuous regional intra-arterial infusion, is indicated for palliative management of colorectal carcinoma metastatic to the liver that has not responded to other treatment. Floxuridine is most useful when the disease has not extended beyond an area capable of infusion via a single artery.
Floxuridine also is indicated for carcinoma of the ovary and kidney not responsive to other antimetabolites.

## Pharmacology/Pharmacokinetics

**Physicochemical characteristics**
Molecular weight—246.20.

**Mechanism of action/Effect**
Floxuridine is an antimetabolite of the pyrimidine analog type. Floxuridine is considered to be cell cycle–specific for the S-phase of cell division. Activity occurs as the result of activation in the tissues, and includes inhibition of DNA and, as a result of action of the fluorouracil metabolite, RNA synthesis.

**Distribution**
Some crosses the blood-brain barrier; active metabolites are localized intracellularly.

**Biotransformation**
Hepatic and in tissues, extensive, to the monophosphate derivative and fluorouracil; after continuous intra-arterial infusion, conversion to the monophosphate derivative is enhanced; largely converted to fluorouracil after rapid intravenous or intra-arterial injection.

**Elimination**
Respiratory (as carbon dioxide), about 60%.
Renal, 10 to 13% (as unchanged drug and metabolites).

## Precautions to Consider

**Carcinogenicity**
Secondary malignancies are potential delayed effects of many antineoplastic agents, although it is not clear whether the effect is related to their mutagenic or immunosuppressive action. The effect of dose and duration of therapy is also unknown, although risk seems to increase with long-term use. Although information is limited, available data seem to indicate that the carcinogenic risk is greatest with the alkylating agents. Studies with floxuridine have not been done.
Antimetabolites have been shown to be carcinogenic in animals and may be associated with an increased risk of development of secondary carcinomas in humans, although the risk appears to be less than with alkylating agents.

**Mutagenicity**
Floxuridine produces oncogenic transformation of fibroblasts in cultured C3H/10T1/2 mouse embryo cells.
Floxuridine is mutagenic in human leukocytes *in vitro* and in the *Drosophila* test system.

## Pregnancy/Reproduction

Fertility—Gonadal suppression, resulting in amenorrhea or azoospermia, may occur in patients taking antineoplastic therapy, especially with the alkylating agents. In general, these effects appear to be related to dose and length of therapy and may be irreversible. Prediction of the degree of testicular or ovarian function impairment is complicated by the common use of combinations of several antineoplastics, which makes it difficult to assess the effects of individual agents.

Studies with floxuridine have not been done. However, fluorouracil, which is a metabolite of floxuridine, has significant effects on fertility in animals.

Pregnancy—Adequate and well-controlled studies in humans have not been done.

First trimester: It is usually recommended that use of antineoplastics, especially combination chemotherapy, be avoided whenever possible, especially during the first trimester. Although information is limited because of the relatively few instances of antineoplastic administration during pregnancy, the mutagenic, teratogenic, and carcinogenic potential of these medications must be considered.

Other hazards to the fetus include adverse reactions seen in adults.

In general, use of a contraceptive is recommended during cytotoxic drug therapy.

Floxuridine is teratogenic in chick embryos, mice (at doses of 2.5 to 100 mg per kg of body weight [mg/kg]), and rats (at doses of 75 to 150 mg/kg); doses were 3.2 to 125 times, respectively, the recommended human therapeutic dose. Malformations included cleft palates, skeletal defects, and deformed appendages, paws, and tails.

FDA Pregnancy Category D.

## Breast-feeding

It is not known whether floxuridine is distributed into breast milk. Although very little information is available regarding distribution of antineoplastic agents into breast milk, breast-feeding is not recommended during chemotherapy, because of the risks to the infant (adverse effects, mutagenicity, carcinogenicity).

## Pediatrics

No information is available on the relationship of age to the effects of floxuridine in pediatric patients.

## Geriatrics

Although appropriate studies on the relationship of age to the effects of floxuridine have not been performed in the geriatric population, geriatrics-specific problems are not expected to limit the usefulness of this medication in the elderly. However, elderly patients are more likely to have age-related renal function impairment, which may require reduction of dosage in patients receiving floxuridine.

## Dental

The bone marrow depressant effects of floxuridine may result in an increased incidence of microbial infection, delayed healing, and gingival bleeding. Dental work, whenever possible, should be completed prior to initiation of therapy or deferred until blood counts have returned to normal. Patients should be instructed in proper oral hygiene during treatment, including caution in use of regular toothbrushes, dental floss, and toothpicks.

Floxuridine also commonly causes stomatitis, which may be associated with considerable discomfort.

## Drug interactions and/or related problems

The following drug interactions and/or related problems have been selected on the basis of their potential clinical significance (possible mechanism in parentheses where appropriate)—not necessarily inclusive (» = major clinical significance):

Blood dyscrasia–causing medications (see *Appendix II*)
(leukopenic and/or thrombocytopenic effects of floxuridine may be increased with concurrent or recent therapy if these medications cause the same effects; dosage adjustment of floxuridine, if necessary, should be based on blood counts)

» Bone marrow depressants, other (see *Appendix II*) or
Radiation therapy
(additive bone marrow depression may occur; dosage reduction may be required when two or more bone marrow depressants, including radiation, are used concurrently or consecutively)

Vaccines, killed virus
(because normal defense mechanisms may be suppressed by floxuridine therapy, the patient's antibody response to the vaccine may be decreased. The interval between discontinuation of medications that cause immunosuppression and restoration of the patient's ability to respond to the vaccine depends on the intensity and type of immunosuppression-causing medication used, the underlying disease, and other factors; estimates vary from 3 months to 1 year)

» Vaccines, live virus
(because normal defense mechanisms may be suppressed by floxuridine therapy, concurrent use with a live virus vaccine may potentiate the replication of the vaccine virus, may increase the side/adverse effects of the vaccine virus, and/or may decrease the patient's antibody response to the vaccine; immunization of these patients should be undertaken only with extreme caution after careful review of the patient's hematologic status and only with the knowledge and consent of the physician managing the floxuridine therapy. The interval between discontinuation of medications that cause immunosuppression and restoration of the patient's ability to respond to the vaccine depends on the intensity and type of immunosuppression-causing medication used, the underlying disease, and other factors; estimates vary from 3 months to 1 year. Immunization with oral poliovirus vaccine should also be postponed in persons in close contact with the patient, especially family members)

## Laboratory value alterations

The following have been selected on the basis of their potential clinical significance (possible effect in parentheses where appropriate)—not necessarily inclusive (» = major clinical significance):

With physiology/laboratory test values
Alanine aminotransferase (ALT [SGPT]) and
Alkaline phosphatase and
Aspartate aminotransferase (AST [SGOT]) and
Lactate dehydrogenase (LDH)
(serum values may be increased; possible chemical hepatitis or biliary sclerosis)

Bilirubin, serum
(concentrations may be increased)

## Medical considerations/Contraindications

The medical considerations/contraindications included have been selected on the basis of their potential clinical significance (reasons given in parentheses where appropriate)—not necessarily inclusive (» = major clinical significance).

*Risk-benefit should be considered when the following medical problems exist:*

» Bone marrow depression
» Chickenpox, existing or recent (including recent exposure) or
» Herpes zoster
   (risk of severe generalized disease)
» Hepatic function impairment
   (reduced biotransformation; lower dosage is recommended)
» Hepatitis, history of
   (increased risk of chemical hepatitis)
» Infection
» Renal function impairment
   (reduced elimination; lower dosage is recommended)
   Sensitivity to floxuridine
» Extreme caution should be used also in patients who have had previous cytotoxic drug therapy with alkylating agents or high-dose pelvic radiation therapy; a lower dosage is recommended.

## Patient monitoring

The following are especially important in patient monitoring (other tests may be warranted in some patients, depending on condition; » = major clinical significance):

Alanine aminotransferase (ALT [SGPT]) values, serum and
Aspartate aminotransferase (AST [SGOT]) values, serum and
Bilirubin concentrations, serum and
Lactate dehydrogenase (LDH) values, serum
(recommended prior to initiation of therapy and at periodic intervals during therapy; frequency varies according to clinical state, agent, dose, and other agents being used concurrently)

» Examination of patient's mouth for ulceration
   (recommended before administration of each dose)
» Hematocrit or hemoglobin and
» Leukocyte count, total and, if appropriate, differential and
» Platelet count
   (determinations recommended prior to initiation of therapy and at periodic intervals during therapy; frequency varies according to clinical state, agent, dose, and other agents being used concurrently)

## Side/Adverse Effects

Note: Many "side effects" of antineoplastic therapy are unavoidable and represent the medication's pharmacologic action. Some of these (for example, leukopenia and thrombocytopenia) are actually used as parameters to aid in individual dosage titration.

Floxuridine is a highly toxic medication and serious toxic effects frequently occur. When floxuridine is administered intra-arterially, local reactions are more prominent than systemic reactions.

Because floxuridine is converted to fluorouracil, there is a possibility that some side/adverse effects associated with fluorouracil may also occur.

Adverse effects associated with prolonged use of an arterial catheter include arterial ischemia, thrombosis, bleeding at the catheter site, blocked catheters, leakage at the site, embolism, fibromyositis, infection at the catheter site, abscesses, thrombophlebitis, and perforation of the duodenum or stomach.

Floxuridine administered via hepatic artery infusion may cause a chemical hepatitis, characterized by elevated hepatic enzymes and nausea and vomiting. However, elevated hepatic enzymes may also be a sign of biliary sclerosis.

The following side/adverse effects have been selected on the basis of their potential clinical significance (possible signs and symptoms in parentheses where appropriate)—not necessarily inclusive:

**Those indicating need for medical attention**
Incidence more frequent
*Aphthous stomatitis* (sores in mouth and on lips); *enteritis* (diarrhea; stomach pain or cramps)
Incidence less frequent
*Displaced hepatic artery catheter* (heartburn; black tarry stools); *esophagopharyngitis* (heartburn); *gastrointestinal ulceration or gastritis* (black tarry stools); *glossitis* (swelling or soreness of tongue); *nausea and vomiting; scaling or redness of hands or feet*—with prolonged infusion therapy
Incidence rare
*Anemia* (unusual tiredness or weakness); *hepatotoxicity or intra- and extrahepatic biliary sclerosis or acalculus cholecystitis* (yellow eyes or skin); *leukopenia or infection* (fever or chills; cough or hoarseness; lower back or side pain; painful or difficult urination)—usually asymptomatic; *thrombocytopenia* (unusual bleeding or bruising; black, tarry stools; blood in urine or stools; pinpoint red spots on skin)—usually asymptomatic; *trouble in walking*

**Those indicating need for medical attention only if they continue or are bothersome**
Incidence less frequent or rare
*Loss of appetite; skin rash or itching*

**Those not indicating need for medical attention**
Incidence less frequent or rare
*Thinning of hair*

## Patient Consultation

As an aid to patient consultation, refer to *Advice for the Patient, Floxuridine (Systemic)*.

In providing consultation, consider emphasizing the following selected information (» = major clinical significance):

**Before using this medication**
» Conditions affecting use, especially:
 Sensitivity to floxuridine
 Pregnancy—Use not recommended because of mutagenic, teratogenic, and carcinogenic potential; advisability of using contraception; telling physician immediately if pregnancy is suspected
 Breast-feeding—Not recommended because of risk of serious side effects
 Other medications, especially other bone marrow depressants or previous cytotoxic drug or radiation therapy
 Other medical problems, especially chickenpox, herpes zoster, hepatic function impairment, history of hepatitis, infection, or renal function impairment

**Proper use of this medication**
» Telling physician about nausea and vomiting, especially with stomach pain
» Proper dosing

**Precautions while using this medication**
» Importance of close monitoring by physician
» Avoiding immunizations unless approved by physician; other persons in patient's household should avoid immunizations with oral poliovirus vaccine; avoiding persons who have taken oral poliovirus vaccine or wearing a protective mask that covers nose and mouth

**Side/adverse effects**
May cause adverse effects such as blood problems, inflammation of gastrointestinal tract, chemical hepatitis, and cancer; importance of discussing possible effects with physician

Signs of potential side effects, especially aphthous stomatitis, enteritis, displaced hepatic artery catheter, esophagopharyngitis, gastrointestinal ulceration, gastritis, glossitis, nausea and vomiting, scaling or redness of hands or feet, anemia, hepatotoxicity, intra- and extrahepatic biliary sclerosis, acalculus cholecystitis, leukopenia, infection, thrombocytopenia, and trouble in walking
Physician or nurse can help in dealing with side effects
Possibility of thinning of hair; normal hair growth should return after treatment has ended

## General Dosing Information

Patients receiving floxuridine should be under supervision of a physician experienced in antimetabolite chemotherapy and the technique of intra-arterial infusion.

Floxuridine is recommended mainly for intra-arterial use. Use of an appropriate infusion pump is recommended to ensure a uniform rate of infusion. In selected patients, a portable or implantable pump may be used.

Therapy with floxuridine is continued as long as a response occurs, which may vary from 1 week to several months (with appropriate rest periods). However, floxuridine is an extremely toxic medication; therapy should be discontinued promptly at the first sign of:
 Diarrhea (five or more loose stools daily)
 Esophagopharyngitis
 Gastrointestinal ulceration and bleeding
 Hemorrhage from any site
 Leukopenia (particularly granulocytopenia), marked
 Myocardial ischemia
 Stomatitis
 Thrombocytopenia, marked
 Vomiting, intractable

Therapy may be reinitiated at a lower dosage when side effects have subsided. Floxuridine should be withdrawn if signs of obstructive jaundice occur and reinstituted only after careful evaluation of the patient.

Special precautions are recommended in patients who develop thrombocytopenia as a result of administration of floxuridine. These may include extreme care in performing invasive procedures; regular inspection of intravenous sites, skin (including perirectal area), and mucous membrane surfaces for signs of bleeding or bruising; limiting frequency of venipuncture and avoiding intramuscular injections; testing urine, emesis, stool, and secretions for occult blood; care in use of regular toothbrushes, dental floss, toothpicks, safety razors, and fingernail and toenail cutters; avoiding constipation; and using caution to prevent falls and other injuries. Such patients should avoid alcohol and aspirin intake because of the risk of gastrointestinal bleeding. Platelet transfusions may be required.

Patients who develop leukopenia should be observed carefully for signs of infection. Antibiotic support may be required. In neutropenic patients who develop fever, broad-spectrum antibiotic coverage should be initiated empirically, pending bacterial cultures and appropriate diagnostic tests.

**Safety considerations for handling this medication**
There is limited but increasing evidence and concern that personnel involved in preparation and administration of parenteral antineoplastics may be at some risk because of the potential mutagenicity, teratogenicity, and/or carcinogenicity of these agents, although the actual risk is unknown. USP advisory panels recommend cautious handling both in preparation and disposal of antineoplastic agents. Precautions that have been suggested include:
• Use of a biological containment cabinet during reconstitution and dilution of parenteral medications and wearing of disposable surgical gloves and masks.
• Use of proper technique to prevent contamination of the medication, work area, and operator during transfer between containers (including proper training of personnel in this technique).
• Cautious and proper disposal of needles, syringes, vials, ampuls, and unused medication.

A number of medical centers have developed detailed guidelines for handling of antineoplastic agents.

## Parenteral Dosage Forms

### FLOXURIDINE STERILE USP

**Usual adult dose**
Carcinoma, colorectal or
Carcinoma, hepatic—
 Intra-arterial, 100 to 600 mcg (0.1 to 0.6 mg) per kg of body weight per day continuously over twenty-four hours, continued until tox-

icity or a response occurs, usually for fourteen to twenty-one days, with a rest period of two weeks between courses.

**Usual pediatric dose**
Safety and efficacy have not been established.

**Size(s) usually available**
U.S.—
500 mg (Rx) [*FUDR*; GENERIC].
Canada—
Not commercially available.

**Packaging and storage**
Store below 40 °C (104 °F), preferably between 15 and 30 °C (59 and 86 °F), unless otherwise specified by manufacturer. Protect from light.

**Preparation of dosage form**
Sterile Floxuridine USP is reconstituted for use by adding 5 mL of sterile water for injection to the vial; may be further diluted in 5% dextrose injection or 0.9% sodium chloride injection for administration by infusion.

**Stability**
Reconstituted solutions of floxuridine are stable at 2 to 8 °C (36 to 46 °F) for not more than 2 weeks.

Revised: 07/26/94
Interim revision: 09/30/97

---

**FLUCLOXACILLIN**—See *Penicillins (Systemic)*

---

**FLUCONAZOLE**—See *Antifungals, Azole (Systemic)*

---

**FLUCYTOSINE**—The *Flucytosine (Systemic)* monograph is not included in this published version of the USP DI database. Copies of the monograph are available on request from Micromedex, Inc. - Reprint Requests, 6200 S. Syracuse Way, Suite 300, Englewood, CO 80111; telephone (303) 486-6400; telefax (303) 486-6464; Email: USPDI@MDX.COM.

---

# FLUDARABINE Systemic

VA CLASSIFICATION (Primary): AN300
Commonly used brand name(s): *Fludara*.

Note: For a listing of dosage forms and brand names by country availability, see *Dosage Forms* section(s).

## Category
Antineoplastic.

## Indications

**Accepted**
Leukemia, chronic lymphocytic (treatment)—Fludarabine is indicated for treatment of patients with B-cell chronic lymphocytic leukemia (CLL) who have not responded to or whose disease has progressed during treatment with at least one standard alkylating agent–containing regimen.

[Lymphomas, non-Hodgkin's (treatment)][1]—Fludarabine is indicated for treatment of non-Hodgkin's lymphomas.

[1]Not included in Canadian product labeling.

## Pharmacology/Pharmacokinetics

**Physicochemical characteristics**
Chemical group—Fludarabine is a fluorinated adenine analog (a fluorinated nucleotide analog of vidarabine [Ara-A], which differs from vidarabine in that it is resistant to deactivation by adenosine deaminase).
Molecular weight—365.22.

**Mechanism of action/Effect**
Fludarabine is a purine antimetabolite. Activity occurs as the result of activation to 2-fluoro-ara-ATP and includes inhibition of DNA synthesis (primarily in the S-phase of cell division) by inhibition of ribonucleotide reductase and the DNA polymerases. It is also postulated that fludarabine interferes with RNA by decreased incorporation of uridine and leucine into RNA and protein, respectively. Fludarabine is also active against non-proliferating cells.

**Other actions/effects**
Fludarabine appears to have immunosuppressant activity by inhibiting lymphocytes.

**Biotransformation**
Rapidly dephosphorylated in serum to 2-fluoro-ara-A (9-beta-D-arabinofuranosyl-2-fluoroadenine) within minutes after intravenous infusion, then phosphorylated intracellularly by deoxycytidine kinase to the active triphosphate, 2-fluoro-ara-ATP, the principal active metabolite.

**Half-life**
2-Fluoro-ara-A—Triphasic: Terminal—Approximately 10 hours.

**Onset of action**
In two studies, the median time to response was 7 weeks (range, 1 to 68 weeks) and 21 weeks (range, 1 to 53 weeks).

**Elimination**
2-Fluoro-ara-A—Renal, approximately 23% unchanged.

## Precautions to Consider

**Carcinogenicity**
Secondary malignancies are potential delayed effects of many antineoplastic agents, although it is not clear whether the effect is related to their mutagenic or immunosuppressive action. The effect of dose and duration of therapy is also unknown, although risk seems to increase with long-term use. Although information is limited, available data seem to indicate that the carcinogenic risk is greatest with the alkylating agents.
Antimetabolites have been shown to be carcinogenic in animals and may be associated with an increased risk of development of secondary carcinomas in humans, although the risk appears to be less than with alkylating agents.
Studies with fludarabine in animals have not been done.

**Mutagenicity**
Fludarabine was not found to be mutagenic in several strains of *Salmonella typhimurium*, including TA-98, TA-100, TA-1535, and TA-1537. It was also nonmutagenic to Chinese hamster ovary (CHO) cells at the hypoxanthine-guanine-phosphoribosyltransferase (HGPRT) locus under both activated and nonactivated metabolic conditions. However, chromosomal aberrations were observed in an *in vitro* assay using CHO cells under metabolically activated conditions. It was also determined to cause increased sister chromatid exchanges in an *in vitro* sister chromatid exchange (SCE) assay under both metabolically activated and non-activated conditions.

**Pregnancy/Reproduction**
Fertility—Gonadal suppression, resulting in amenorrhea or azoospermia, may occur in patients taking antineoplastic therapy, especially with the alkylating agents. In general, these effects appear to be related to dose and length of therapy and may be irreversible. Prediction of the degree of testicular or ovarian function impairment is complicated by the common use of combinations of several antineoplastics, which makes it difficult to assess the effects of individual agents.
Dose-related adverse effects on the male reproductive system have been demonstrated in mice, rats, and dogs; effects consisted of a decrease in mean testicular weights in mice and rats with a trend toward decreased testicular weights in dogs, and degeneration and necrosis of spermatogenic epithelium of the testes in mice, rats, and dogs.

Pregnancy—Adequate and well-controlled studies in women have not been done.
First trimester: It is usually recommended that use of antineoplastics, especially combination chemotherapy, be avoided whenever possible, especially during the first trimester. Although information is limited because of the relatively few instances of antineoplastic administration during pregnancy, the mutagenic, teratogenic, and carcinogenic potential of these medications must be considered.
Other hazards to the fetus include adverse reactions seen in adults.
In general, use of a contraceptive is recommended during cytotoxic drug therapy.

Studies in rats at intravenous doses of 0, 1, 10, or 30 mg per kg of body weight (mg/kg) per day on days 6 to 15 of gestation found an increased incidence of skeletal malformations. Studies in rabbits at doses of 5 and 8 mg/kg per day found dose-related teratogenic effects (external deformities and skeletal malformations).

FDA Pregnancy Category D.

**Breast-feeding**
Although very little information is available regarding distribution of antineoplastic agents into breast milk, breast-feeding is not recommended during chemotherapy because of the potential risks to the infant (adverse effects, mutagenicity, carcinogenicity). It is not known whether fludarabine is distributed into breast milk.

**Pediatrics**
No information is available on the relationship of age to the effects of fludarabine in pediatric patients. Safety and efficacy have not been established.

**Geriatrics**
Although appropriate studies on the relationship of age to the effects of fludarabine have not been performed in the geriatric population, clinical trials have included elderly patients and geriatrics-specific problems that would limit the usefulness of this medication in the elderly are not expected. However, elderly patients are more likely to have age-related renal function impairment, which may require reduction of dosage in patients receiving fludarabine.

**Dental**
The bone marrow depressant effects of fludarabine may result in an increased incidence of microbial infection, delayed healing, and gingival bleeding. Dental work, whenever possible, should be completed prior to initiation of therapy or deferred until blood counts have returned to normal. Patients should be instructed in proper oral hygiene during treatment, including caution in use of regular toothbrushes, dental floss, and toothpicks.

Fludarabine also sometimes causes stomatitis associated with considerable discomfort.

**Drug interactions and/or related problems**
The following drug interactions and/or related problems have been selected on the basis of their potential clinical significance (possible mechanism in parentheses where appropriate)—not necessarily inclusive (» = major clinical significance):

Note: Combinations containing any of the following medications, depending on the amount present, may also interact with this medication.

Allopurinol or
Colchicine or
» Probenecid or
» Sulfinpyrazone
(fludarabine may raise the concentration of blood uric acid as part of a tumor lysis syndrome; dosage adjustment of antigout agents may be necessary to control hyperuricemia and gout; allopurinol may be preferred to prevent or reverse fludarabine-induced hyperuricemia because of risk of uric acid nephropathy with uricosuric antigout agents)

Blood dyscrasia–causing medications (see *Appendix II*)
(leukopenic and/or thrombocytopenic effects of fludarabine may be increased with concurrent or recent therapy if these medications cause the same effects; dosage adjustment of fludarabine, if necessary, should be based on blood counts)

» Bone marrow depressants, other (see *Appendix II*) or
Radiation therapy
(additive bone marrow depression may occur; dosage reduction may be required when two or more bone marrow depressants, including radiation, are used concurrently or consecutively)

» Pentostatin
(concurrent use with fludarabine is not recommended because of a possible increased risk of fatal pulmonary toxicity)

Vaccines, killed virus
(because normal defense mechanisms may be suppressed by fludarabine therapy, the patient's antibody response to the vaccine may be decreased. The interval between discontinuation of medications that cause immunosuppression and restoration of the patient's ability to respond to the vaccine depends on the intensity and type of immunosuppression-causing medication used, the underlying disease, and other factors; estimates vary from 3 months to 1 year)

» Vaccines, live virus
(because normal defense mechanisms may be suppressed by fludarabine therapy, concurrent use with a live virus vaccine may potentiate the replication of the vaccine virus, may increase the side/adverse effects of the vaccine virus, and/or may decrease the patient's antibody response to the vaccine; immunization of these patients should be undertaken only with extreme caution after careful review of the patient's hematologic status and only with the knowledge and consent of the physician managing the fludarabine therapy. The interval between discontinuation of medications that cause immunosuppression and restoration of the patient's ability to respond to the vaccine depends on the intensity and type of immunosuppression-causing medication used, the underlying disease, and other factors; estimates vary from 3 months to 1 year. Patients with leukemia in remission should not receive live virus vaccine until at least 3 months after their last chemotherapy. In addition, immunization with oral poliovirus vaccine should be postponed in persons in close contact with the patient, especially family members)

**Laboratory value alterations**
The following have been selected on the basis of their potential clinical significance (possible effect in parentheses where appropriate)—not necessarily inclusive (» = major clinical significance):

With physiology/laboratory test values
Alkaline phosphatase and
Aspartate aminotransferase (AST [SGOT])
(serum values may rarely be increased)

Uric acid concentrations in blood and urine
(may be increased as part of a tumor lysis syndrome in patients with large tumor burdens)

**Medical considerations/Contraindications**
The medical considerations/contraindications included have been selected on the basis of their potential clinical significance (reasons given in parentheses where appropriate)—not necessarily inclusive (» = major clinical significance).

*Risk-benefit should be considered when the following medical problems exist:*

» Bone marrow depression
(lower dosage may be necessary)
» Chickenpox, existing or recent (including recent exposure) or
» Herpes zoster
(risk of severe generalized disease)
Gout, history of or
Urate renal stones, history of
(risk of hyperuricemia as part of a tumor lysis syndrome in patients with large tumor burdens)
» Infection
» Renal function impairment
(reduced elimination; dosage adjustment may be necessary)
» Sensitivity to fludarabine
» Caution should be used also in patients who have had previous cytotoxic drug therapy or radiation therapy.

**Patient monitoring**
The following are especially important in patient monitoring (other tests may be warranted in some patients, depending on condition; » = major clinical significance):

» Hematocrit or hemoglobin and
» Leukocyte count, total and, if appropriate, differential and
» Platelet count
(determinations recommended prior to initiation of therapy and at periodic intervals during therapy; frequency varies according to clinical state, agent, dose, and other agents being used concurrently)

Uric acid concentrations, serum
(recommended prior to initiation of therapy and at periodic intervals during therapy in patients with large tumor burdens, because of the risk of tumor lysis syndrome; frequency varies according to clinical state, agent, dose, and other agents being used concurrently)

# Side/Adverse Effects

Note: Many "side effects" of antineoplastic therapy are unavoidable and represent the medication's pharmacologic action. Some of these (for example, leukopenia and thrombocytopenia) are actually used as parameters to aid in individual dosage titration.

Dose-related bone marrow depression occurs in the majority of patients treated with fludarabine and may be severe and cumulative. Bone marrow fibrosis occurred in one patient.

High single doses (above 75 mg per square meter of body surface area) have been associated with severe, delayed, irreversible, and potentially fatal toxicity, including central nervous system (CNS) toxicity (cortical blindness, incontinence, seizure, continued deterioration of mental status, coma). Most patients experiencing neurotoxicity were found to have progressive CNS demyelination; leukoencephalopathy involving the subcortical white matter, optic nerves, and optic tract was found. High doses are also associated with severe thrombocytopenia and neutropenia.

The following side/adverse effects have been selected on the basis of their potential clinical significance (possible signs and symptoms in parentheses where appropriate)—not necessarily inclusive:

**Those indicating need for medical attention**
Incidence more frequent
*Anemia*—usually asymptomatic; **leukopenia or infection** (fever or chills; cough or hoarseness; lower back or side pain; painful or difficult urination)—usually asymptomatic; **pain; pneumonia** (cough; fever; shortness of breath); **thrombocytopenia** (unusual bleeding or bruising; black, tarry stools; blood in urine or stools; pinpoint red spots on skin)—usually asymptomatic

Note: In *leukopenia*, the median time to nadir of granulocyte counts in a phase I study in solid tumor patients was 13 days (range, 3 to 25 days). Cumulative and severe myelosuppression may occur.

*Infection* may be caused by opportunistic organisms including herpes zoster, cytomegalovirus, *Pneumocystis carinii*, and *Candida*, among others. In a study in patients with chronic lymphocytic leukemia (CLL), immunodeficiency in the form of a marked and prolonged decrease in CD4+ and CD8+ T cells, associated with delayed severe infection, was reported after two courses of fludarabine in all 17 patients.

In *thrombocytopenia*, the median time to nadir of platelet counts in a phase I study in solid tumor patients was 16 days (range, 2 to 32 days). Cumulative and severe myelosuppression may occur.

Incidence less frequent
*Edema* (swelling of feet or lower legs); **neurologic effects, including agitation or confusion; blurred vision; loss of hearing; peripheral neuropathy** (numbness or tingling in fingers, toes, or face); **or weakness; stomatitis or mucositis** (sores in mouth and on lips)

Incidence rare
**Delayed severe neurologic effects** (blindness; coma); **hemolytic anemia** (unusual tiredness or weakness); **hemorrhagic cystitis** (blood in urine; painful urination); **pulmonary edema or diffuse interstitial hypersensitivity pneumonitis** (cough; fever; shortness of breath); **tumor lysis syndrome, including hyperuricemia; hyperphosphatemia; hypocalcemia; metabolic acidosis; hyperkalemia; hematuria; urate crystalluria; renal failure** (blood in urine, lower back or side pain)

Note: Death may also occur as a result of *delayed neurologic effects*. This syndrome is rare in patients receiving fludarabine for chronic lymphocytic leukemia. However, it occurred commonly in patients treated for acute leukemia with high doses of fludarabine (approximately 4 times greater than the recommended dose); symptoms occurred 21 to 60 days following the last dose.

*Hemolytic anemia* has been reported after one or more cycles of fludarabine in patients with or without a history of autoimmune hemolytic anemia or a positive Coombs' test. Hospitalization and transfusion have been necessary in severe cases and a fatality has occurred.

*Tumor lysis syndrome* has been reported in chronic lymphocytic leukemia patients with large tumor burdens.

**Those indicating need for medical attention only if they continue or are bothersome**
Incidence more frequent
*Diarrhea; nausea or vomiting; skin rash; unusual tiredness*

Incidence less frequent
*Aching muscles; headache; loss of appetite; malaise* (general feeling of discomfort or illness)

**Those not indicating need for medical attention**
Incidence less frequent or rare
*Loss of hair*

## Overdose
For more information on the management of overdose or unintentional ingestion, **contact a Poison Control Center** (see *Poison Control Center Listing*).

**Treatment of overdose**
Treatment consists of withdrawal of fludarabine and supportive therapy.

## Patient Consultation
As an aid to patient consultation, refer to *Advice for the Patient, Fludarabine (Systemic)*.
In providing consultation, consider emphasizing the following selected information (» = major clinical significance):

**Before using this medication**
» Conditions affecting use, especially:
Sensitivity to fludarabine
Pregnancy—Use not recommended because of mutagenic, teratogenic, and carcinogenic potential; advisability of using contraception; telling physician immediately if pregnancy is suspected
Breast-feeding—Not recommended because of risk of serious side effects
Other medications, especially probenecid, sulfinpyrazone, other bone marrow depressants, or other cytotoxic drug or radiation therapy
Other medical problems, especially chickenpox, herpes zoster, renal function impairment, or infection

**Proper use of this medication**
Possibility of nausea and vomiting; importance of continuing medication despite stomach upset
» Proper dosing

**Precautions while using this medication**
» Importance of close monitoring by the physician
» Avoiding immunizations unless approved by physician; other persons in patient's household should avoid immunizations with oral poliovirus vaccine; avoiding persons who have taken oral poliovirus vaccine or wearing a protective mask that covers nose and mouth

*Caution if bone marrow depression occurs*
» Avoiding exposure to persons with infections, especially during periods of low blood counts; checking with physician immediately if fever or chills, cough or hoarseness, lower back or side pain, or painful or difficult urination occurs
» Checking with physician immediately if unusual bleeding or bruising; black, tarry stools; blood in urine or stools; or pinpoint red spots on skin occur
Caution in use of regular toothbrush, dental floss, or toothpick; physician, dentist, or nurse may suggest alternatives; checking with physician before having dental work done
Not touching eyes or inside of nose unless hands are washed immediately before
Using caution to avoid accidental cuts with use of sharp objects such as safety razor or fingernail or toenail cutters
Avoiding contact sports or other situations where bruising or injury could occur

**Side/adverse effects**
May cause adverse effects such as blood problems; importance of discussing possible effects with physician
Signs of potential side effects, especially leukopenia, infection, pneumonia, pain, thrombocytopenia, edema, neurologic effects, stomatitis, pulmonary edema, pneumonitis, and tumor lysis syndrome
Physician or nurse can help in dealing with side effects
Possibility of hair loss; normal hair growth should return after treatment has ended

## General Dosing Information
Patients receiving fludarabine should be under supervision of a physician experienced in cancer chemotherapy.

A variety of dosage schedules and regimens of fludarabine, alone or in combination with other antitumor agents, are used. The prescriber may consult the medical literature as well as the manufacturer's literature in choosing a specific dosage.

Dosage must be adjusted to meet the individual requirements of each patient, on the basis of clinical response and degree of bone marrow depression.

If neurotoxicity occurs, consideration should be given to delaying or discontinuing fludarabine.

Development of uric acid nephropathy in patients with leukemia or lymphoma may be prevented by adequate oral hydration and, in some cases, administration of allopurinol. Alkalinization of urine may be necessary if serum uric acid concentrations are elevated.

Special precautions are recommended in patients who develop thrombocytopenia as a result of administration of fludarabine. These may include extreme care in performing invasive procedures; regular inspection of intravenous sites, skin (including perirectal area), and mucous membrane surfaces for signs of bleeding or bruising; limiting frequency of venipuncture and avoiding intramuscular injections; testing urine, emesis, stool, and secretions for occult blood; care in use of regular

## Fludarabine (Systemic)

toothbrushes, dental floss, toothpicks, safety razors, and fingernail and toenail cutters; avoiding constipation; and using caution to prevent falls and other injuries. Such patients should avoid alcohol and aspirin intake because of the risk of gastrointestinal bleeding. Platelet transfusions may be required.

Patients who develop leukopenia should be observed carefully for signs of infection. Antibiotic support may be required. In neutropenic patients who develop fever, broad-spectrum antibiotic coverage should be initiated empirically, pending bacterial cultures and appropriate diagnostic tests.

**Safety considerations for handling of medication**
There is limited but increasing evidence and concern that personnel involved in preparation and administration of parenteral antineoplastics may be at some risk because of the potential mutagenicity, teratogenicity, and/or carcinogenicity of these agents, although the actual risk is unknown. USP advisory panels recommend cautious handling both in preparation and disposal of antineoplastic agents. Precautions that have been suggested include:
- Use of a biological containment cabinet during reconstitution and dilution of parenteral medications and wearing of disposable surgical gloves and masks.
- Use of proper technique to prevent contamination of the medication, work area, and operator during transfer between containers (including proper training of personnel in this technique).
- Cautious and proper disposal of needles, syringes, vials, ampuls, and unused medication.

A number of medical centers have developed detailed guidelines for handling of antineoplastic agents.

The manufacturer recommends use of latex gloves and safety glasses during handling and preparation of fludarabine to avoid exposure in case of breakage of the vial or other accidental spillage. If the solution contacts the skin or mucous membranes, they should be washed thoroughly with soap and water; eyes should be rinsed thoroughly with plain water. Exposure by inhalation or by direct contact of the skin or mucous membranes should be avoided.

## Parenteral Dosage Forms

### FLUDARABINE PHOSPHATE FOR INJECTION

**Usual adult dose**
Chronic lymphocytic leukemia—
  Intravenous (over approximately thirty minutes), 25 mg per square meter of body surface area per day for five consecutive days. Each five-day course of treatment should begin every twenty-eight days.
- Note: Dosage may be decreased or delayed based on evidence of hematologic or nonhematologic toxicity.

**Usual pediatric dose**
Safety and efficacy have not been established.

**Size(s) usually available**
U.S.—
  50 mg (Rx) [*Fludara* (mannitol 50 mg; sodium hydroxide)].
Canada—
  50 mg (Rx) [*Fludara* (mannitol 50 mg; sodium hydroxide)].

**Packaging and storage**
Store between 2 and 8 °C (36 and 46 °F), unless otherwise specified by manufacturer.

**Preparation of dosage form**
Fludarabine phosphate for injection is prepared for intravenous use by aseptically adding 2 mL of sterile water for injection to the 50-mg vial, producing a solution containing 25 mg of fludarabine phosphate per mL (the solid cake should fully dissolve within 15 seconds).

Fludarabine phosphate solutions may be further diluted in 100 or 125 mL of 5% dextrose injection or 0.9% sodium chloride injection for administration by intravenous infusion.

**Stability**
Reconstituted solutions contain no preservative and should be used within 8 hours of reconstitution.

## Selected Bibliography

Hood MA, Finley RS. Fludarabine: a review. DICP Ann Pharmacother 1991 May; 25: 518-24.

Chun HG, Leyland-Jones B, Cheson BD. Fludarabine phosphate: a synthetic purine antimetabolite with significant activity against lymphoid malignancies. J Clin Oncol 1991 Jan; 9: 175-88.

Revised: 08/02/94
Interim revision: 09/30/97

---

# FLUDEOXYGLUCOSE F 18   Systemic*†

VA CLASSIFICATION (Primary): DX201
Note: For a listing of dosage forms and brand names by country availability, see *Dosage Forms* section(s).

*Not commercially available in the U.S.
†Not commercially available in Canada.

## Category
Diagnostic aid, radioactive (brain disorders; cardiac disease; neoplastic disease).

## Indications
Note: Because fludeoxyglucose F 18 (FDG) is commercially available only on a limited basis in the U.S. and Canada, the bracketed information and the use of the superscript 1 in this monograph reflect the lack of labeled (approved) indications for this product.

**Accepted**
[Brain imaging, positron emission tomographic][1]—Positron emission tomography (PET) using FDG is used in studies of cerebral glucose metabolism in various physiological and pathological states. FDG-PET is currently used for the following diagnostic studies:

Seizures (diagnosis)[1]—FDG-PET is indicated for the identification of regions of abnormal glucose metabolism associated with foci of epileptic seizures. FDG-PET is used in patients with partial complex seizures who do not respond adequately to medication, in order to establish the site of the epileptogenic focus, when temporal lobectomy or focal resection is being considered. In interictal FDG-PET scans of patients with partial seizures, regions of focal or lateralized hypometabolism have been shown to correlate with the site of epileptogenic lesions. PET can complement electroencephalographic (EEG) studies in the preoperative evaluation of patients with partial seizures, making invasive depth electrode studies unnecessary in about 50% of the cases. In intractable childhood seizures, FDG-PET is used to identify site(s) for surgical resection, from focal resections to hemispherectomies. In large area resections, FDG-PET is also used to assess functional status of uninvolved areas of the brain before and after surgery. It provides a direct means of predicting postsurgical developmental response.

[Tumors, brain (diagnosis)][1]—FDG-PET is used to locate and differentiate primary brain tumors. It is helpful in staging the extent of malignant growth. It also provides indications of prognosis, as well as an ongoing means of assessing therapeutic response. Also, in patients with cerebral tumors who have undergone radiation therapy, FDG-PET is the primary means, other than biopsy, available to differentiate tumor recurrence from radiation necrosis and edema.

[Depression, mental (diagnosis)][1]—FDG-PET can be used to differentiate unipolar from bipolar depression, as well as to differentiate chronic depression (pseudodementia) from Alzheimer's.

[Behavior-metabolism relationship studies][1]—FDG-PET is used in behavior-metabolism relationship studies, since differences in regional rates of glucose metabolism are associated with different behavioral tasks. It can be used to test for normal function or deficits in motor, visual, sensory, memory, and cognitive functions in the brain.

[Dementia, Alzheimer-type (diagnosis)][1]—FDG-PET is used to examine glucose metabolism in dementia. Regional alterations, particularly in the temporal-parietal cortex, provide means of detecting early- to late-stage Alzheimer's, and provide differential diagnosis from confounding conditions, such as multi-infarct dementia, pseudodementia, thyroid disease, normal-pressure hydrocephalus, as well as normal aging.

[Stroke (diagnosis)][1]—FDG-PET can be used to determine the degree and extent of injury in acute and chronic stages. Also, the technique provides criteria for reversible injury and provides a means of establishing proper selection and evaluation of therapy.

[Cardiac imaging, positron emission tomographic][1]—FDG-PET is currently used for the following diagnostic studies:

[Ischemia, myocardial (diagnosis)][1]—FDG-PET is used to evaluate the extent and degree of regional alterations in myocardial metabolism associated with acute and chronic ischemia. These data are used to distinguish viable, but functionally impaired, ischemic myocardium from nonviable (infarcted) myocardium and are critical in deciding between angioplasty or surgical bypass versus a more conservative medical treatment. The technique is also useful for follow-up studies to determine therapeutic outcome.

[Cardiac wall-motion abnormalities assessment][1]—PET using ammonia N 13 ($^{13}NH_3$) or rubidium Rb 82 ($^{82}Rb$) to assess the distribution of blood flow in conjunction with FDG-PET to estimate myocardial metabolic viability in dysfunctional myocardial segments serves to predict, preoperatively, the presence of reversible regional wall-motion abnormalities, which is helpful in the selection of patients in whom revascularization may lead to improved ventricular function.

[Cardiac bypass surgery assessment][1]—FDG-PET is used in conjunction with $^{13}NH_3$-PET or $^{82}Rb$-PET before and after aortocoronary bypass surgery to help evaluate the effect of surgery on myocardial glucose metabolism. Also, graft patency can be established with postoperative images.

[Percutaneous transluminal coronary angioplasty assessment][1]—FDG-PET is used in conjunction with $^{13}NH_3$-PET or $^{82}Rb$-PET, before and after percutaneous transluminal coronary angioplasty, to evaluate the infarcted areas and assess the recovery of myocardial blood flow and metabolism in the ischemic myocardium.

[Whole-body imaging, positron emission tomographic][1]—FDG-PET currently is used in whole-body imaging of cancer patients for the following diagnostic studies:

[Carcinoma, breast (diagnosis)][1]—FDG-PET is used as an adjunct to mammography in the diagnosis of primary breast carcinoma, especially in patients with unclear, unpalpable lesions. In patients with breast carcinoma, FDG-PET is useful to help determine the extent of the disease at initial diagnosis. Also, it is useful for staging and for monitoring the effectiveness of therapy. FDG-PET is particularly useful to help localize lesions in patients with radiodense breasts, implants, or potential lobular carcinomas, which are poorly visualized on mammography. Also, FDG-PET may be effective in distinguishing malignant from benign processes in patients with suspected recurrence or in postoperative cases in which scar tissue may be present. In studies done to monitor the effects of preoperative chemotherapy in patients with locally advanced breast cancer, FDG-PET has demonstrated better sensitivity for primary tumor and better specificity for nodal metastasis than ultrasonography (US).

[Carcinoma, colorectal (diagnosis)][1]—FDG-PET is used for the detection of recurrent colorectal carcinoma. Also, FDG-PET assists with staging of patients with advanced disease, distinguishing recurrent disease from scar, and monitoring the response to therapy.

[Carcinoma, hepatic (diagnosis)][1]—FDG-PET is used to detect and characterize liver tumors and to monitor liver tumor therapy.

[Carcinoma, lung (diagnosis)][1]—FDG-PET is used for differentiating benign from malignant solitary pulmonary nodules, staging mediastinal or distant metastases at initial diagnosis, re-staging for recurrence, and for monitoring the effectiveness of therapy. In patients with a solitary pulmonary nodule that is smaller than 3 centimeters, in whom biopsy would be a medical risk or the risk of malignancy is considered low based on medical history or other radiographic findings, FDG-PET is recommended prior to biopsy and/or surgery, to differentiate benign from malignant processes. Also, FDG-PET is being used in the staging of non–small-cell lung cancer (NSCLC) and in the detection of distant metastases from NSCLC.

[Carcinoma, ovarian (diagnosis)][1]—FDG-PET is used for the detection and staging of ovarian carcinoma, including detection of residual or recurrent tumors, and in the follow-up of patients undergoing therapy. In assessing response to therapy, FDG-PET is particularly useful in ascertaining the presence of residual disease in those cases with normal anatomic imaging studies in which there is a rising CA-125 tumor marker. In patients with advanced ovarian disease, FDG-PET may be useful in the evaluation of suspected extraperitoneal disease.

[Carcinoma, pancreatic (diagnosis)][1]—FDG-PET is used for the detection and staging of pancreatic carcinoma, including detection of metastatic disease in the preoperative evaluation of patients. In patients with suspected pancreatic tumors, FDG-PET has accurately differentiated malignant neoplasm from benign diseases, such as chronic pancreatitis, mucinous cyst adenoma, and pseudocyst. FDG-PET should be used in cases identified by computerized tomography (CT) or US as suspicious for pancreatic tumor, and as follow-up examination in cases of nondiagnostic endoscopic retrograde cholangiopancreatography (ERCP) test results.

[Carcinoma, thyroid (diagnosis)][1]—FDG-PET is used in imaging of metastases of advanced thyroid carcinoma. FDG-PET may reveal less differentiated metastases that do not accumulate I 131. Also, FDG-PET may be useful for confirmation of complete remission after treatment with radioiodine. The utility of FDG-PET in the preoperative diagnosis of thyroid malignancy and in the differentiation of benign from malignant lesions is limited by the fact that FDG uptake has been shown to occur within the normal thyroid gland as well as in malignant thyroid tumors.

[Lymphoma (diagnosis)][1]—FDG-PET is used for the detection and staging of Hodgkin's or non-Hodgkin's lymphoma (especially high-grade malignancy) and its recurrence. Also, FDG-PET is used to monitor response to therapy. In patients with the acquired immunodeficiency syndrome (AIDS), FDG-PET is used to provide accurate differentiation of primary central nervous system (CNS) lymphoma from non-neoplastic lesions such as toxoplasmosis.

[Melanoma, malignant (diagnosis)][1]—FDG-PET is used for the detection of malignant melanoma and nodal metastases. Also, FDG-PET is used to monitor response to therapy.

[Musculoskeletal, carcinoma (diagnosis)][1]—FDG-PET is used for the detection of both primary and recurrent or residual musculoskeletal malignancies. When used for the detection of recurrent musculoskeletal tumors, FDG-PET has demonstrated a higher specificity than serial magnetic resonance imaging (MRI) and/or CT in distinguishing postoperative scar tissue from tumors. Also, FDG-PET is used to monitor response to therapy.

[Tumors, head and neck (diagnosis)][1]—FDG-PET is used for the detection of primary head and neck tumors. In patients previously treated for head and neck carcinoma, in whom postoperative and postradiation edema or scarring may mimic tumor recurrence, FDG-PET is useful in the differentiation of actual tumor recurrence from scar tissue. Since FDG uptake is decreased in patients with complete or partial response to radiation therapy, FDG-PET serves as a marker for the effectiveness of treatment in head and neck tumors. Also, FDG-PET is useful for identifying lymph node involvement in head and neck carcinoma.

[1]Not included in Canadian product labeling.

## Physical Properties

### Nuclear Data

| Radionuclide (half-life) | Decay constant | Mode of decay | Principal photon emissions (keV) | Mean number of photons/ disintegration |
|---|---|---|---|---|
| F 18 (110 min) | 0.0063 min$^{-1}$ | Positron decay | Gamma* (511) | 1.94 |

*The 2 gamma rays emitted in opposite directions at the moment of positron annihilation are used for imaging purposes. Detection devices usually used are positron emission tomography (PET) units; however, conventional planar scintillation cameras have also been used for some studies.

## Pharmacology/Pharmacokinetics

### Physicochemical characteristics
Molecular weight—182.

### Mechanism of action/Effect
FDG is transported from blood to tissues in a manner similar to glucose and competes with glucose for hexokinase phosphorylation to FDG-6-phosphate. However, since FDG-6-phosphate is not a substrate for subsequent glycolytic pathways and has a very low membrane permeability, the FDG becomes trapped in tissue in proportion to the rate of glycolysis or glucose utilization of that tissue.

Brain imaging; and

Neoplastic disease (diagnosis)—The rate of anaerobic glycolysis in tumors increases with higher degree of malignancy. It is believed that increased FDG uptake is caused by a shift in energy metabolism within malignant tumors from high yield oxidative pathways to inefficient anaerobic glycolysis, resulting in an increase in glucose utilization for a given energy demand. Accumulation of FDG in malignant tissue not only helps to locate and differentiate tumors, but can also be used to help distinguish recurrent malignant cerebral tumors from foci of radiation necrosis and edema, since glucose uptake takes place in tumors and in normal brain tissue, while active uptake is absent in an area of necrosis and reduced in edema.

Ischemia, myocardial (diagnosis)—The amount of FDG-6-phosphate accumulated in myocardial tissue is proportional to the tissue's rate of glucose consumption. Significant glucose consumption and uptake of FDG occurs in ischemic tissue because in severe oxygen-deprived states the primary source of energy for the myocardium shifts from fatty acids to anaerobic glucose metabolism.

**Distribution**
FDG accumulates mainly in the heart and brain because of the high glycolytic rate of these tissues; it also accumulates throughout the body in proportion to glucose metabolism. FDG also has been shown to accumulate in bone tumors and in primary and metastatic carcinomas throughout the body. Accumulation of FDG in tumors may be related to the degree of tumor differentiation, the number of viable cancer cells present in the tumor, and possibly, the tumor proliferation rate.

**Protein binding**
Minimal.

**Biotransformation**
FDG is phosphorylated to FDG-6-phosphate by hexokinase, with no further metabolism taking place throughout the remainder of the study.

**Half-life**
75% of the administered activity of FDG is retained with an effective half-life of 1.83 hours; 19% has an effective half-life of 0.26 hour; and the remaining 6% has an effective half-life of 1.53 hours.

**Time to peak concentration**
Approximately 30 minutes to peak tissue concentration.

**Time to peak diagnostic effect**
For most studies high tumor-to-background ratio has been obtained 30 to 45 minutes after injection of FDG. In one study, optimal differentiation of benign and malignant lesions was obtained when imaging of focal pulmonary abnormalities was done at 50 minutes after FDG administration.

**Radiation dosimetry**

| Organ | Estimated absorbed radiation dose*† |  |
|---|---|---|
|  | mGy/MBq | mrad/mCi |
| Bladder wall | 0.17 | 629 |
| Heart | 0.065 | 240 |
| Brain | 0.026 | 96 |
| Kidneys | 0.021 | 77 |
| Uterus | 0.02 | 74 |
| Ovaries | 0.015 | 55 |
| Testes | 0.015 | 55 |
| Adrenals | 0.014 | 51 |
| Small intestine | 0.013 | 48 |
| Liver | 0.012 | 44 |
| Pancreas | 0.012 | 44 |
| Spleen | 0.012 | 44 |
| Red marrow | 0.011 | 41 |
| Lungs | 0.011 | 41 |
| Thyroid | 0.0097 | 36 |
| Other tissue | 0.011 | 41 |

Effective dose: 0.027mSv/MBq (0.1 rem/mCi)

*For adults; intravenous injection.
†Data based on the International Commission on Radiological Protection (ICRP) Publication 53—Radiation Dose to Patients from Radiopharmaceuticals.

**Elimination**
Renal (approximately 20% of administered activity excreted within the first 2 hours).

## Precautions to Consider

**Pregnancy/Reproduction**
Pregnancy—The possibility of pregnancy should be assessed in women of child-bearing potential. Clinical situations exist where the benefit to the patient and fetus, based on information derived from radiopharmaceutical use, outweighs the risks from fetal exposure to radiation. In this situation, the physician should use discretion and reduce the administered activity to the lowest practical amount.

**Breast-feeding**
It is not known whether FDG is distributed into breast milk; however, it is expected that some will be present. Temporary discontinuation of nursing for a period of 12 to 24 hours is considered adequate.

**Pediatrics**
Although FDG is used in children, there have been no specific studies evaluating safety and efficacy.

**Geriatrics**
Diagnostic studies performed to date have not demonstrated geriatrics-specific problems that would limit the usefulness of FDG in the elderly.
In one study, older subjects (mean age, 66 years) demonstrated significantly lower cerebral metabolic rates than did the younger subjects (mean age, 27 years) in anterior, middle, and posterior temporal neocortex and in mesial temporal cortex. The largest differences occurred in anterior temporal cortex. These findings may indicate either decreases in regional cerebral metabolic rates for glucose that occur with normal aging, or may be early signs of cognitive dysfunction associated with age-related disorders.

**Drug interactions and/or related problems**
See *Diagnostic interference*.

**Diagnostic interference**
The following have been selected on the basis of their potential clinical significance (possible effect in parentheses where appropriate)—not necessarily inclusive (» = major clinical significance):
With results of *cardiac and whole-body imaging*
*Due to other medications*
  Dopamine and
  Insulin
    (concurrent intravenous administration of these medications with FDG may alter myocardial extraction of FDG; insulin may decrease FDG uptake in tumor cells)
With results of *cardiac imaging*
*Due to medical problems or conditions*
  Diabetes mellitus
    (patients with diabetes mellitus may require normalization of plasma glucose levels and insulin therapy for optimal myocardial image quality)

## Side/Adverse Effects

There are no known side/adverse effects associated with the use of FDG.

## Patient Consultation

As an aid to patient consultation, refer to *Advice for the Patient, Radiopharmaceuticals (Diagnostic)*.
In providing consultation, consider emphasizing the following selected information (» = major clinical significance):

**Description of use**
  Action in the body: Concentration of radioactivity in brain, heart, and other sites of high glucose utilization (e.g., certain tumors) allows images to be obtained
  Small amounts of radioactivity used in diagnosis; radiation received is low and considered safe

**Before having this test**
» Conditions affecting use, especially:
    Pregnancy—Risk to fetus from radiation exposure as opposed to benefit derived from use should be considered
    Breast-feeding—Not known if distributed into breast milk; temporary discontinuation of nursing recommended because of risk of radiation exposure to infant

**Preparation for this test**
  Special preparatory instructions may be given; patient should inquire in advance

**Precautions after having this test**
No special precautions

## General Dosing Information

Radiopharmaceuticals are to be administered only by or under the supervision of physicians who have had extensive training in the safe use and handling of radioactive materials and who are authorized by the appropriate Federal or State regulatory agency, if required, or, outside the U.S., the appropriate authority.

**For brain imaging**
Fasting for about 4 to 6 hours prior to the examination is sometimes recommended to increase the amount of FDG delivered to the brain.
To minimize the influence of external stimulation on the brain uptake of FDG, prior to the injection of FDG and for 30 minutes thereafter, the patient should be kept lying or sitting still in a quiet room.
Imaging is usually performed 30 minutes after administration of FDG.

**For cardiac imaging**
Optimal cardiac FDG-PET (e.g., better image quality) may be obtained if patients are in a glucose-loaded state rather than in the fasting state. Under fasting conditions with normal plasma levels of nonesterified fatty acids, only the ischemic areas of the myocardium use glucose preferentially, and thus, only these areas will accumulate FDG. This

renders an image in which the myocardial outline is not well seen, making it difficult to locate the ischemic area.

**For whole-body imaging**
Glucose and FDG compete for the same cell membrane receptors; thus, elevated glucose levels will cause a decrease in cellular FDG uptake. For this reason, fasting for several hours prior to the examination is recommended to increase the relative uptake of FDG by the tumor.

**Safety considerations for handling this radiopharmaceutical**
Guidelines for the receipt, storage, handling, dispensing, and disposal of radioactive materials are available from scientific, professional, state, federal, and international bodies. Handling of this radiopharmaceutical should be limited to those individuals who are appropriately qualified and authorized.

## Parenteral Dosage Forms

Note: Because fludeoxyglucose F 18 (FDG) is commercially available only on a limited basis in the U.S. and Canada, the bracketed information and the use of the superscript 1 in this monograph reflect the lack of labeled (approved) indications for this product.

### FLUDEOXYGLUCOSE F 18 INJECTION USP

**Usual adult and adolescent administered activity**
[Brain imaging][1]
[Cardiac imaging][1] or
[Whole-body imaging][1]—
   Intravenous, 370 megabecquerels (10 millicuries).

**Usual pediatric administered activity**
[Brain imaging][1]
[Cardiac imaging][1] or
[Whole-body imaging][1]—
   Intravenous, up to 5.3 megabecquerels (0.14 millicuries) per kg of body weight.

**Usual geriatric administered activity**
See *Usual adult and adolescent administered activity*.

**Strength(s) usually available**
U.S.—
   Prepared on-site at various clinical facilities or available from some nuclear pharmacies.
Canada—
   Prepared on-site at various clinical facilities or available from some nuclear pharmacies.

**Packaging and storage**
Store below 40 °C (104 °F), preferably between 15 and 30 °C (59 and 86 °F). Protect from freezing.

**Note**
Caution—Radioactive material.

[1]Not included in Canadian product labeling.

## Selected Bibliography

Chan SY, Brunken RC, Buxton DB. Cardiac positron emission tomography: the foundations and clinical applications. J Thorac Imaging 1990; 5(3): 9-19.
Conti PS, Lilien DL, Hawley K, et al. PET and F18–FDG in oncology: a clinical update. Nucl Med Biol 1996; 23: 717-35.
Jamieson D, Alavi A, Jolles P, et al. Positron emission tomography in the investigation of central nervous system disorders. Radiol Clin North Am 1988; 26(5): 1075-88.

Revised: 01/14/98

---

# FLUDROCORTISONE Systemic

VA CLASSIFICATION (Primary/Secondary): HS052/CV900; DX900
Commonly used brand name(s): *Florinef*.

Note: For a listing of dosage forms and brand names by country availability, see *Dosage Forms* section(s).

## Category

Corticosteroid (mineralocorticoid); antihypotensive (idiopathic orthostatic); diagnostic aid (renal tubular acidosis).

## Indications

Note: Bracketed information in the *Indications* section refers to uses that are not included in U.S. product labeling.

**Accepted**
Adrenocortical insufficiency, chronic primary (treatment) or
Adrenocortical insufficiency, chronic secondary (treatment)—Fludrocortisone is indicated as partial replacement therapy in the treatment of adrenocortical insufficiency.

Adrenogenital syndrome, congenital (treatment)—Fludrocortisone is indicated in salt-losing forms of adrenogenital syndrome.

[Hypotension, idiopathic orthostatic (treatment)][1]—Fludrocortisone is used in conjunction with increased sodium intake in the treatment of idiopathic orthostatic hypotension.

[Acidosis, in renal tubular disorders (diagnosis and treatment)][1]—Fludrocortisone is used in the treatment of Type IV renal tubular acidosis associated with hyporeninemic hypoaldosteronism. Fludrocortisone is also used as an aid in diagnosing the cause of the condition. Effectiveness of fludrocortisone therapy indicates that the condition is caused by hyporeninemic hypoaldosteronism rather than by renal tubular transport dysfunction.

[1]Not included in Canadian product labeling.

## Pharmacology/Pharmacokinetics

**Physicochemical characteristics**
Molecular weight—422.49.

**Mechanism of action/Effect**
Fludrocortisone acetate is an adrenal cortical steroid that has very high levels of mineralocorticoid activity and moderate levels of glucocorticoid activity. However, it is used only for its mineralocorticoid effects.

Mineralocorticoids act on the distal tubules to increase potassium excretion, hydrogen ion excretion, and sodium reabsorption and subsequent water retention. Cation transport in other secretory cells is similarly affected; excretion of water and electrolytes by the large intestine and by salivary and sweat glands is also altered, but to a lesser extent.

At the cellular level, corticosteroids diffuse across cell membranes and complex with specific cytoplasmic receptors. These complexes then enter the cell nucleus, bind to DNA (chromatin), and stimulate transcription of mRNA (messenger RNA) and subsequent protein synthesis of various enzymes thought to be ultimately responsible for the physiological effects of these hormones.

**Protein binding**
High.

**Biotransformation**
Hepatic, renal.

**Half-life**
≥3.5 hours (plasma); 18–36 hours (biological).

**Duration of action**
1–2 days.

**Elimination**
Renal, mostly as inactive metabolites.

## Precautions to Consider

**Carcinogenicity/Mutagenicity**
Adequate animal studies have not been conducted on the carcinogenicity or mutagenicity of fludrocortisone.

**Pregnancy/Reproduction**
Pregnancy—Studies on use of fludrocortisone during pregnancy have not been done in humans.
Infants born to mothers who have received substantial doses of corticosteroids during pregnancy should be closely observed for signs of hypoadrenalism.
Studies on use of fludrocortisone during pregnancy have not been done in animals.
FDA Pregnancy Category C.

**Breast-feeding**
Problems in humans have not been documented. However, corticosteroids are distributed into breast milk and may cause unwanted effects in the infant such as growth suppression and inhibition of endogenous steroid production.

## Fludrocortisone (Systemic)

**Pediatrics**
Although adequate and well-controlled studies have not been done in the pediatric population, corticosteroids may cause unwanted effects in children and growing adolescents, such as growth suppression and inhibition of endogenous steroid production.

**Geriatrics**
Appropriate studies have not been performed in the geriatric population. One published report described the use of fludrocortisone in the treatment of severe hyponatremia that occurred following head injury in 3 geriatric patients in whom syndrome of inappropriate antidiuretic hormone (SIADH) had been ruled out as the cause of the hyponatremia. Doses ranged from 0.1 to 0.4 mg of fludrocortisone per day.

**Drug interactions and/or related problems**
The following drug interactions and/or related problems have been selected on the basis of their potential clinical significance (possible mechanism in parentheses where appropriate)—not necessarily inclusive (» = major clinical significance):

Note: Combinations containing any of the following medications, depending on the amount present, may also interact with this medication.

» Digitalis glycosides
(risk of cardiac arrhythmias or digitalis toxicity associated with hypokalemia may be increased; serum potassium concentrations and cardiac function should be monitored; potassium supplements may be required)

» Hepatic enzyme inducers (See *Appendix II*)
(phenytoin and rifampin have been reported to increase 6-beta-hydroxylation of fludrocortisone, via induction of P-450 liver enzymes; fludrocortisone dosage increase may be required)

» Hypokalemia-causing medications (See *Appendix II*)
(risk of severe hypokalemia due to other hypokalemia-causing medications may be increased; monitoring of serum potassium concentrations and cardiac function and potassium supplementation may be required)

Lithium
(in one published case report, lithium antagonized the mineralocorticoid effects of fludrocortisone; increased fludrocortisone dose and dietary sodium supplementation were required during concurrent use)

» Sodium-containing medications or foods
(concurrent use with fludrocortisone in the treatment of Type IV renal tubular acidosis may result in hypernatremia, edema, and potentially severe increases in blood pressure; adjustment of sodium intake may be required)

**Laboratory value alterations**
The following have been selected on the basis of their potential clinical significance (possible effect in parentheses where appropriate)—not necessarily inclusive (» = major clinical significance):

With physiology/laboratory test values
Blood pressure
(may be increased)
Hematocrit percentage
(may be decreased due to increased blood volume)
Potassium
(serum concentration may be decreased due to increased potassium excretion)
Sodium
(serum concentration may be increased due to sodium retention)

**Medical considerations/Contraindications**
The medical considerations/contraindications included have been selected on the basis of their potential clinical significance (reasons given in parentheses where appropriate)—not necessarily inclusive (» = major clinical significance).

*Risk-benefit should be considered when the following medical problems exist:*

» Cardiac disease or
» Congestive heart failure or
» Hypertension or
Peripheral edema or
» Renal function impairment, except when fludrocortisone is used to treat Type IV renal tubular acidosis
(sodium- and fluid-retaining effects detrimental to these patients)
Glomerulonephritis, acute
Hepatic function impairment or
Hypothyroidism
(clearance of fludrocortisone may be decreased)
Hyperthyroidism
(clearance of fludrocortisone may be increased)
Nephritis, chronic
Osteoporosis
(may be exacerbated by increased calcium excretion)
Sensitivity to fludrocortisone

**Patient monitoring**
The following may be especially important in patient monitoring (other tests may be warranted in some patients, depending on condition; » = major clinical significance):

Blood pressure determinations and
Serum electrolyte concentrations
(recommended at onset of therapy and at periodic intervals during prolonged therapy)

## Side/Adverse Effects

The following side/adverse effects have been selected on the basis of their potential clinical significance (possible signs and symptoms in parentheses where appropriate)—not necessarily inclusive:

**Those indicating need for medical attention**
Incidence less frequent or rare
**Anaphylaxis, generalized** (cough; difficulty swallowing; hives; redness and itching of skin; redness of conjunctivae; shortness of breath; swelling of nasal membranes, face, and eyelids); **congestive heart failure** (cough; dilated neck veins; extreme fatigue; irregular breathing; irregular heartbeat); **dizziness; headache, severe or continuing; hypokalemic syndrome** (irregular heartbeat; loss of appetite; muscle cramps or pain; nausea; severe weakness of extremities and trunk; vomiting); **peripheral edema** (rapid weight gain; swelling of feet or lower legs)

## Patient Consultation

As an aid to patient consultation, refer to *Advice for the Patient, Fludrocortisone (Systemic)*.

In providing consultation, consider emphasizing the following selected information (» = major clinical significance):

**Before using this medication**
» Conditions affecting use, especially:
Sensitivity to fludrocortisone
Pregnancy—Infants born to mothers who received substantial doses of corticosteroids during pregnancy require close observation for signs of hypoadrenalism
Use in children and growing adolescents—May cause growth suppression and inhibition of endogenous steroid production
Other medications, especially hypokalemia-causing medications, digitalis glycosides, hepatic enzyme inducers, or sodium-containing medications or food
Other medical problems, especially cardiac disease, congestive heart failure, hypertension, or renal function impairment

**Proper use of this medication**
» Importance of not taking more medication than the amount prescribed
Missed dose: Taking as soon as possible; not taking if almost time for next dose; not doubling doses
» Proper dosing
» Proper storage

**Precautions while using this medication**
» Regular visits to physician to check progress duringtherapy
Carrying medical identification card during long-term therapy

**Side/adverse effects**
Signs of potential side effects, especially generalized anaphylaxis, congestive heart failure, dizziness, severe headache, hypokalemic syndrome, or peripheral edema

## General Dosing Information

When used in the treatment of adrenocortical insufficiency or salt-losing forms of adrenogenital syndrome, fludrocortisone should be administered with appropriate glucocorticoid therapy such as 10 to 30 mg of hydrocortisone per day or 10 to 37.5 mg of cortisone per day. Sodium supplementation may also be necessary.

In the treatment of Type IV renal tubular acidosis, concurrent use of a diuretic may be necessary to decrease the risk of sodium and fluid retention, especially in patients with hypertension, congestive heart failure, or renal function impairment.

## Oral Dosage Forms

Note: Bracketed uses in the *Dosage Forms* section refer to categories of use and/or indications that are not included in U.S. product labeling.

## FLUDROCORTISONE ACETATE TABLETS USP

**Usual adult and adolescent dose**
Adrenocortical insufficiency, chronic—
 Oral, 100 mcg (0.1 mg) per day.
  Note: Dose should be reduced to 50 mcg (0.05 mg) per day if transient hypertension occurs. Dosages of 100 mcg (0.1 mg) three times a week to 200 mcg (0.2 mg) once a day have been employed.
Adrenogenital syndrome, congenital—
 Oral, 100 to 200 mcg (0.1 to 0.2 mg) per day.
[Antihypotensive, idiopathic orthostatic][1]—
 Oral, 50 to 200 mcg (0.05 to 0.2 mg) per day.

**Usual pediatric dose**
Oral, 50 to 100 mcg (0.05 to 0.1 mg) per day.

**Strength(s) usually available**
U.S.—
 100 mcg (0.1 mg) (Rx) [*Florinef* (scored; lactose)].
Canada—
 100 mcg (0.1 mg) (Rx) [*Florinef* (scored; lactose)].

**Packaging and storage**
Store below 40 °C (104 °F), preferably between 15 and 30 °C (59 and 86 °F), unless otherwise specified by manufacturer. Store in a well-closed container.

[1] Not included in Canadian product labeling.

Revised: 06/15/93

---

# FLUMAZENIL  Systemic

VA CLASSIFICATION (Primary/Secondary): AD700/CN303
Commonly used brand name(s): *Anexate*; *Romazicon*.
Note: For a listing of dosage forms and brand names by country availability, see *Dosage Forms* section(s).

## Category
Benzodiazepine antagonist.

## Indications

**General considerations**
**Administering flumazenil to reverse the effects of benzodiazepines does not eliminate the need for monitoring and evaluating the patient and instituting needed interventions**, e.g., establishing an airway, assisting ventilation, and supporting circulation. Although flumazenil partially reverses benzodiazepine-induced hypoventilation, it should not be relied upon to provide complete or sustained reversal of hypoventilation, especially if the patient has also received an opioid analgesic. Also, resedation may occur after initial recovery, although most patients remain more alert than they were before flumazenil administration.

Before flumazenil is administered, the advantages of reversing benzodiazepine-induced sedation should be weighed against the possible disadvantages, especially in high-risk patients. The risks of antagonizing the anticonvulsant effects of benzodiazepines and/or of precipitating a withdrawal syndrome in physically dependent patients must be considered because seizures may result.

**Accepted**
Sedation, benzodiazepine-induced, reversal—Flumazenil is indicated for partial or complete reversal of post-procedure residual sedation resulting from use of benzodiazepines for induction and/or maintenance of anesthesia, conscious sedation, or deep sedation. The benefits of reversing post-procedure residual sedation are more apparent in patients who are heavily sedated at the time of administration than in patients who are only mildly or moderately sedated. Flumazenil facilitates patient management most significantly during the first hour following administration. After 1 hour, significant spontaneous recovery is also apparent in patients who have not received the medication. Flumazenil has been shown to speed recovery of patients who have received benzodiazepines concurrently with opioid analgesics, inhalation anesthetics, or local, regional, spinal, or topical anesthetics. However, its efficacy may be decreased when multiple anesthetic agents have been used or sedating medications are required post-procedure.

Flumazenil is indicated to reverse the effects of benzodiazepines used to sedate critical care patients.

Toxicity, benzodiazepine (treatment)—Flumazenil is indicated for the management of benzodiazepine overdose. However, if the patient has been intubated flumazenil may be unnecessary and may complicate patient management by causing agitation. In addition to reversing central nervous system (CNS) depression, flumazenil has been reported to reverse benzodiazepine-induced hypotension and bradycardia unresponsive to administration of intravenous fluids, atropine, and dopamine. Flumazenil is most effective in intoxications caused by a benzodiazepine alone, although resedation occurs frequently. Flumazenil may also be at least partially effective in treating mixed overdoses, but its efficacy depends on the extent to which a benzodiazepine contributes to the intoxication, especially if significant quantities of other sedating medications have been used concurrently. Flumazenil is not a substitute for other measures that may be necessary, but in some clinical trials its use decreased the need for interventions such as gastric lavage, urinary catheterization, and diagnostic tests.

**Extreme caution is recommended if flumazenil is considered for treating mixed overdoses in which medications with potential seizurogenic and/or arrhythmogenic activity or unidentified medications may have been taken.** Reversal of the protective effect of the benzodiazepine in such cases has resulted in seizures and/or arrhythmias, usually in mixed overdoses with tricyclic antidepressants. Some emergency care physicians recommend that flumazenil not be used until after a diagnostic electrocardiogram and/or quantitative analytical testing has ruled out severe cyclic (tricyclic or tetracyclic) antidepressant overdosage.

Note: Flumazenil does not reverse benzodiazepine-induced amnesia for events occurring prior to administration of the antagonist (retrograde amnesia). Although flumazenil may partially reverse amnesia for events occurring after it is given (anterograde amnesia), its effects on memory are less complete, less consistent, and of shorter duration than its effects on sedation. Also, although flumazenil may reverse post-procedure psychomotor deficits associated with benzodiazepine administration, normal levels of performance may not be achieved.

**Acceptance not established**
Flumazenil has been used to reverse benzodiazepine-maintained anesthesia intraoperatively during spinal surgery, to arouse the patient temporarily for assessment of sensory and motor function. Assessments could be performed within 1 or 2 minutes after administration of flumazenil. Postoperatively, the patients did not recall having been aroused. However, flumazenil has been used for this purpose in relatively few patients; more experience is needed before the risks and benefits of this procedure can be determined.

**Unaccepted**
Flumazenil should not be administered in mixed overdoses if signs of severe cyclic (tricyclic or tetracyclic) antidepressant toxicity are present. Instead, respiration and circulation should be supported until signs of cyclic antidepressant toxicity have abated.

Use of flumazenil for the treatment of benzodiazepine dependence is not recommended. Efficacy has not been established.

Because of the unacceptably high risk of adverse effects, flumazenil should not be used to determine whether dependence on sedating benzodiazepines has occurred in critical care patients.

Flumazenil is not recommended for treatment of hepatic encephalopathy. Although intravenously administered flumazenil has produced partial improvement of neurologic status in some patients, the beneficial effect was not sustained, and several patients became worse after treatment was discontinued. One patient who received twice-daily administration of oral flumazenil in an attempt to prevent return of symptoms experienced a psychotic reaction that began 48 hours after treatment was started and resolved within 12 hours after the medication was discontinued.

## Pharmacology/Pharmacokinetics

**Physicochemical characteristics**
Chemical group—Flumazenil is a 1,4-imidazobenzodiazepine derivative. It is structurally related to benzodiazepine agonists.
Molecular weight—303.29.
pKa—1.78.
Octanol:buffer partition coefficient—14.1

**Mechanism of action/Effect**
Flumazenil selectively antagonizes or attenuates the effects of benzodiazepines in the CNS by competitively inhibiting their actions at the benzodiazepine binding site of the gamma aminobutyric acid (GABA)–

benzodiazepine receptor complex. Flumazenil does not antagonize the effects of CNS-active substances that act via other receptors. Also, flumazenil does not alter the pharmacokinetics of benzodiazepines.

The extent to which flumazenil reverses the effects of a benzodiazepine depends on the dose and plasma concentration of both medications and on the effect being assessed. Flumazenil reverses some components of benzodiazepine-induced hypoventilation, leading to at least partial improvement in respiratory function. One study showed that midazolam's effect on respiration results primarily (but not exclusively) from a reduction in tidal volume, and that flumazenil completely reverses this effect. However, several studies have shown that flumazenil may not affect other measures of respiratory function, especially measures that are independent of patient effort or wakefulness. Also, amnesia is antagonized less consistently and less completely than psychomotor deficits, which may be reversed less completely than sedation.

### Other actions/effects
Animal studies have shown that flumazenil may have some weak agonist or inverse agonist activity when given in high doses. However, therapeutic doses of flumazenil have not produced clinically significant effects other than antagonism of administered benzodiazepines in humans.

### Distribution
Flumazenil is rapidly distributed into the brain. Concentrations are highest in the cerebral cortex (which contains the largest number of benzodiazepine receptors), intermediate in the inferior temporal lobe and cerebellum, and lowest in white matter.

Volume of distribution (Vol$_D$)—
Initially, 0.5 L per kg of body weight (L/kg). After redistribution, the apparent Vol$_D$ is approximately 1 L/kg (range, 0.77 to 1.6 L/kg). One study in children 5 to 9 years of age also reported a mean Vol$_D$ at steady-state of 1 ± 0.2 L/kg. These values are not altered in patients with moderately impaired hepatic function, but are increased by approximately 37% in patients with severe hepatic function impairment.

### Protein binding
Moderate (approximately 50%, of which 66% is bound to albumin). Protein binding is reduced in patients with hepatic cirrhosis; in one study, the free fraction was increased from 55% in controls to 64 and 79% in patients with moderate and severe hepatic function impairment, respectively.

### Biotransformation
Hepatic; rapid and extensive. Clearance is dependent on hepatic blood flow.

### Half-life
In plasma—
Distribution: 7 to 15 minutes.
Elimination: Approximately 54 minutes (range, 41 to 79 minutes) in adults. One study in children 5 to 9 years of age reported a mean elimination half-life of 35.3 ± 13.8 minutes. Prolonged to about 1.3 hours and 2.5 hours in patients with moderate and severe hepatic function impairment, respectively, but not affected by renal function impairment or by hemodialysis beginning 1 hour after flumazenil administration.
In brain—
Elimination: 20 to 30 minutes.

### Onset of action
Approximately 1 to 2 minutes.

### Time to peak concentration
In the CNS—Approximately 1 to 3 minutes.

### Peak serum concentration
1-mg dose, infused over 5 minutes—24 (range, 11 to 43) nanograms per mL (nanograms/mL) (0.08 [range, 0.036 to 0.14] micromoles/L); substantially higher in patients with moderate, stable, alcoholic cirrhosis. The concentration in the brain may be higher than the simultaneous plasma concentration.

### Therapeutic serum concentration
Dependent on the benzodiazepine being reversed and its concentration. In patients receiving usual sedating doses of benzodiazepines, partial reversal generally occurs at flumazenil concentrations of 3 to 6 nanograms/mL (0.01 to 0.02 micromoles/L) and complete reversal usually occurs at concentrations of 12 to 28 nanograms/mL (0.036 to 0.09 micromoles/L). These concentrations are generally produced by doses of 100 to 200 mcg (0.1 to 0.2 mg) and 400 mcg (0.4 mg) to 1 mg, respectively.

### Time to peak effect
6 to 10 minutes after completion of the injection.

### Duration of action
Dependent on the doses and concentrations of the benzodiazepine being antagonized and of flumazenil. In various clinical trials that assessed flumazenil's ability to reverse post-procedure residual sedation, the level of alertness achieved was maintained during the 3-hour observation period in 60 to 95% of the responders. Although up to 40% of the patients experienced partial resedation, most retained an adequate level of alertness. Up to 3% of the patients experienced clinically significant resedation, generally 1 to 2 hours after flumazenil administration. In a study that assessed flumazenil's ability to reverse much larger quantities (i.e., overdoses) of various benzodiazepines, resedation occurred in > 60% of the patients, generally 60 to 90 minutes after flumazenil administration.

### Elimination
Renal—90 to 95% of a dose, primarily as metabolites (following hepatic metabolism). In adults, < 1% of a dose is eliminated in the urine as unchanged flumazenil. However, in a study in children 5 to 9 years of age, 5.8 to 13.8% of a dose was eliminated in the urine as unchanged flumazenil.

Biliary/fecal—In adults: 5 to 10% of a dose.

Note: About 70% of a dose is excreted within 2 hours, and 86% of a dose is excreted within 4 hours, after administration. Elimination is complete within 72 hours.

Plasma clearance in healthy adult subjects ranges from 0.7 to 1.3 (mean, 1) L per hour per kg of body weight(L/hr/kg). Values in pediatric patients undergoing minor surgery are similar; a study in a small number of children 5 to 9 years of age reported a mean clearance rate of 1.2 L/hr/kg.

Ingestion of food during an infusion has been shown to increase flumazenil clearance by 50%, probably by increasing hepatic blood flow. The clinical significance of this effect is not known. Clearance rates may be increased by approximately 25% in patients with chronic stable renal failure (with or without dialysis), but are not affected by hemodialysis beginning 1 hour after administration of flumazenil or by advanced age. However, clearance rates are decreased to approximately 40 to 60% of normal values in patients with moderate hepatic function impairment and to 25% of normal values in patients with severely impaired hepatic function.

## Precautions to Consider

### Carcinogenicity
Studies have not been done.

### Mutagenicity
Flumazenil was not mutagenic in the Ames test (performed with 5 different test strains), assays in *S. cerevisiae* D7 and Chinese hamster cells, blastogenesis assays in peripheral human lymphocytes *in vitro*, and in a mouse micronucleus assay *in vivo*. Cytotoxic concentrations of flumazenil caused a slight increase in unscheduled DNA synthesis in rat hepatocyte culture, but no increase in DNA repair occurred in male mouse germ cells in an *in vivo* assay.

### Pregnancy/Reproduction
Fertility—Flumazenil did not impair fertility in male or female rats given oral doses of 125 mg per kg of body weight (mg/kg) per day. This dose is considered, on the basis of area under the concentration-time curve (AUC) comparisons, to represent 120 times the human exposure provided by the maximum recommended intravenous dose of 5 mg.

Pregnancy—Adequate and well-controlled studies in humans have not been done. However, after administration to a pregnant woman who took an overdose of diazepam, flumazenil (300 mcg [0.3 mg] intravenously) reversed tachycardia and occasional decelerations in the fetus as well as antagonizing sedation in the woman. Fetal cardiac abnormalities and maternal drowsiness recurred about 15 hours later and responded to a second dose of flumazenil.

Studies in rats given up to 150 mg/kg per day orally from Day 6 to Day 15 of gestation and in rabbits given up to 150 mg/kg per day orally from Day 6 to Day 18 of gestation (120 to 600 times the human exposure from an intravenous dose of 5 mg, based on AUC comparisons) found no evidence of teratogenicity. Embryocidal effects (higher rates of pre-implantation and post-implantation losses) occurred in rabbits given 50 mg/kg (200 times the human exposure to a 5-mg intravenous dose) but did not occur in rabbits given 15 mg/kg (60 times the human exposure to a 5-mg intravenous dose). Also, decreased survival during lactation, increased liver weight at weaning, delayed incisor eruption, and delayed ear opening (and, consequently, delayed appearance of the auditory startle response) were observed in offspring of rats given 125 mg/kg per day (120 times the human exposure to a 5-mg intravenous dose), but not in offspring of rats given 5 or 25 mg/kg per day (up to 24 times the human exposure to a 5-mg intravenous dose).

FDA Pregnancy Category C.

Labor and delivery—The safety of administering flumazenil to reverse the effects of benzodiazepines used during labor and delivery has not been established.

**Breast-feeding**
It is not known whether flumazenil is distributed into breast milk.

**Pediatrics**
Flumazenil has been administered to a limited number of pediatric patients up to 14 years of age, including a neonate with apnea (born at 38 weeks' gestation) who had been exposed to diazepam *in utero* during the last 3 weeks of pregnancy as well as children receiving the medication for reversal of benzodiazepine sedation or for treatment of benzodiazepine overdose. Although appropriate dosage has not been established, preliminary data indicate that the pharmacokinetics and pharmacodynamics of flumazenil in children (in doses ranging between 10 and 100 mcg/kg) are similar to those in adults, and that pediatrics-specific problems that would limit use of flumazenil in children are not expected.

**Geriatrics**
Flumazenil was found to be safe and effective in geriatric patients in clinical trials, which included patients up to 91 years of age. Other studies have shown that the pharmacokinetics of flumazenil are not altered, and no adjustment of dosage is needed, in geriatric patients. However, particularly careful monitoring of the patient may be needed because benzodiazepine-induced sedation tends to be deeper and more prolonged in geriatric patients than in younger adults.

**Drug interactions and/or related problems**
The following drug interactions and/or related problems have been selected on the basis of their potential clinical significance (possible mechanism in parentheses where appropriate)—not necessarily inclusive (» = major clinical significance):

Note:  Combinations containing any of the following medications, depending on the amount present, may also interact with this medication.

Benzodiazepines, chronic use of
(the risk of precipitating withdrawal symptoms and of other adverse effects, including those associated with reversal of the therapeutic effects of a benzodiazepine, is increased when flumazenil is administered to patients taking a benzodiazepine chronically)

Seizurogenic medications, especially:
» Cyclic (tricyclic or tetracyclic) antidepressants
(high risk of seizures, especially in a mixed overdose with a seizurogenic medication and a benzodiazepine, because flumazenil reverses the anticonvulsant, as well as the sedative, effects of benzodiazepines)

**Medical considerations/Contraindications**
The medical considerations/contraindications included have been selected on the basis of their potential clinical significance (reasons given in parentheses where appropriate)—not necessarily inclusive (» = major clinical significance).

*Risk-benefit should be considered when the following medical problems exist:*

Anxiety, chronic or episodic, history of or
Anxiety, existing or
Panic disorder
(reversal of benzodiazepines may cause anxiety and has precipitated panic attacks in susceptible patients; caution and careful titration of dosage to clinical response are recommended, especially in patients with cardiac disease)

Cardiac disease, especially with increased left ventricular end-diastolic pressure
(although studies in patients with cardiac disease undergoing cardiac catheterization or surgery have not shown that administration of flumazenil produces significant alterations in cardiac function or evidence of ischemia, caution is recommended if the patient has displayed significant pre-procedure nervousness because stress and/or anxiety associated with abrupt reversal of benzodiazepines has led to increased blood pressure in some patients, especially after cardiac surgery; also, flumazenil has increased left ventricular end-diastolic pressure in some patients with coronary artery disease who received the medication to reverse benzodiazepine-induced sedation after cardiac catheterization; although the increases generally represented a return to presedation values, caution is recommended in patients with pre-existing increases in left ventricular end-diastolic pressure)

Drug abuse or history of, especially:
» Benzodiazepine abuse or chronic use
(risk of precipitating withdrawal symptoms, including seizures, since the patient may be dependent on benzodiazepines; also, flumazenil administration may complicate treatment for withdrawal from alcohol, barbiturates, and sedatives to which cross-tolerance may exist)

» Head injury, severe
(flumazenil may induce seizures and/or alter cerebral blood flow in patients with head injury; flumazenil has increased intracranial pressure significantly in patients with severe head injuries when intracranial pressure was not well controlled [but not when intracranial pressure was adequately controlled]; it should therefore be used with caution, if at all, in cases of severe head injury with known or suspected increases in intracranial pressure or poor intracranial compliance)

Hepatic function impairment
(clearance of flumazenil is decreased to 40 to 60% of normal in patients with mild to moderate hepatic function impairment, and to 25% of normal in patients with severely impaired hepatic function; although no alteration of initial dosage is necessary, a reduction in the size or frequency of subsequent doses may be needed)

» Hypersensitivity to benzodiazepines or to flumazenil

» Seizure disorders, especially if treated with benzodiazepines
(high risk of precipitating seizures)

**Patient monitoring**
The following may be especially important in patient monitoring (other tests may be warranted in some patients, depending on condition; » = major clinical significance):

» Electrocardiographic determinations
(may be advisable to detect QRS prolongation, a possible sign of cyclic [tricyclic or tetracyclic] antidepressant toxicity, prior to flumazenil administration in overdose situations, especially when mixed overdosage with a cyclic antidepressant is suspected)

» Oxygenation, determined via pulse oximetry
(monitoring for an adequate period of time, depending on the dose and duration of action of the benzodiazepine being antagonized, is essential following flumazenil administration because benzodiazepine-induced hypoventilation may not be completely antagonized or may recur; it cannot be assumed that residual respiratory depression is not present in an alert patient; ventilatory assistance and/or supplemental oxygen may be required)

» Patient alertness
(monitoring for at least 1 to 2 hours following flumazenil administration is essential, although more prolonged monitoring may be needed, depending on the dose and the duration of action of the benzodiazepine being antagonized and whether other CNS depressants have been or are being given; resedation requiring additional treatment may occur, especially after initial reversal of the effects of large quantities of a benzodiazepine or of a benzodiazepine with a long elimination half-life or active metabolites; patients who do not show signs of resedation within 2 hours after post-procedure administration of 1 mg of flumazenil are not likely to experience severe resedation at a later time; however, resedation may occur 3 to 5 hours or longer [15 hours, in 1 reported case] after reversal of an overdose)

» Vital signs
(monitoring of blood pressure, heart rate, and respiratory rate is recommended so that supplemental treatment can be instituted as required)

## Side/Adverse Effects

Note:  Flumazenil caused no serious adverse effects when administered in large intravenous doses to volunteers who had not received a benzodiazepine agonist. Many side/adverse effects are caused by abrupt reversal of the effects of benzodiazepines.

Reversal of the effects of benzodiazepines in physically dependent patients may precipitate a withdrawal syndrome with symptoms ranging from anxiety, headache, and/or emotional lability to seizures, depending on the degree of dependence. Other possible signs and symptoms of benzodiazepine withdrawal include hypertension, dizziness, involuntary movements, irritability, muscle tension, palpitations, panic, paresthesias, perceptual disturbances, sweating, tachycardia, and tinnitus. The risk of precipitating a withdrawal syndrome is increased with flumazenil doses higher than 1 mg and/or rapid administration. Severe symptoms, especially seizures, may be more likely to occur in patients who have been receiving long-term benzodiazepine therapy, especially for seizure disorders. However, benzodiazepine dependence resulting in an increased risk of seizures or other withdrawal symptoms may develop after relatively short exposure (3 to 5 days) when a benzodiazepine is used to provide continuous sedation in critical care patients.

In addition to the side/adverse effects reported below, arrhythmias including atrial, nodal, and ventricular extrasystoles, bradycardia, and tachycardia; hypertension; and chest pain have been reported (frequencies of occurrence less than 1%). Arrhythmias have been reported mostly in mixed overdoses with potentially arrhythmogenic medications, including chloral hydrate and tricyclic antidepressants. Also, complete heart block occurred in a patient who overdosed on temazepam, atenolol, and nifedipine. It has been proposed that arrhythmias may occur in association with hypoxic seizures after other medications taken together with a benzodiazepine in an overdose have sensitized the myocardium to such complications.

The following side/adverse effects have been selected on the basis of their potential clinical significance (possible signs and symptoms in parentheses where appropriate)—not necessarily inclusive:

**Those indicating need for medical attention**
Incidence more frequent (3 to 9%)
*Agitation* (anxiety; dry mouth; dyspnea; hyperventilation; insomnia; nervousness; palpitations; tremor); **headache**
Incidence less frequent (1 to 3%)
*Emotional lability* (crying; depersonalization; dysphoria; euphoria; mental depression; paranoia); **hypertension; resedation, severe; skin rash**

Note: *Anxiety* and *emotional lability*, in addition to being symptoms of benzodiazepine withdrawal, may reflect reversal of the anxiolytic effects for which a benzodiazepine may have been prescribed.

Overall *resedation* rates of 3 to 9% and 10 to 15% were reported in clinical studies in which flumazenil was used to reverse conscious sedation and deep sedation or anesthesia, respectively, although substantially higher rates of partial resedation have been reported in individual studies. Resedation severe enough to be considered clinically significant occurred less frequently. Resedation may occur in 40 to > 60% of patients being treated for an overdose. The risk of resedation in critical care patients receiving flumazenil for reversal of prolonged sedation is also high. Clinically significant resedation is more likely to occur when large or repeated doses of a benzodiazepine have been administered, especially during a long procedure during which multiple anesthetics have been used, after initial reversal of a long-acting benzodiazepine, and in overdose situations.

Incidence rare (less than 1%)
***Convulsions without other signs or symptoms of withdrawal; hallucinations; hives or itching of skin***

Note: The risk of *convulsions* is increased in benzodiazepine-dependent patients, in patients with seizure disorders (especially if a benzodiazepine is being used for long-term treatment or for control of a convulsive episode), in patients treated for a mixed overdose with a cyclic (tricyclic or tetracyclic) antidepressant or other potentially seizurogenic medication, and in patients who are undergoing withdrawal from nonbenzodiazepine sedative-hypnotic agents.

**Those indicating need for medical attention only if they continue or are bothersome**
Incidence more frequent (3 to 11%, unless otherwise specified)
*Blurred vision or other vision disturbance; dizziness, possibly with ataxia and/or vertigo; drowsiness, residual or re-emergent*—incidence up to 40 to 60%; *nausea; pain at injection site; vomiting*
Incidence less frequent (1 to 3%) or rare (less than 1%)
*Fatigue, possibly with asthenia and malaise; flushing or hot flashes; hearing disturbances; thrombophlebitis at injection site*

## General Dosing Information

**Flumazenil administration is not a substitute for interventions such as establishing an airway, assisting ventilation, and supporting circulation.** Equipment and medications needed to institute such measures should be available for immediate use.

Equipment required for patient management, such as endotracheal tubes and intravenous access lines, should be securely in place before flumazenil is given. Some patients become confused and agitated when aroused, and may attempt to remove them.

**Preparation for managing seizures should be made prior to flumazenil administration,** especially when flumazenil is used to reverse long-term or high-dose use of a benzodiazepine for sedation in critical care patients or to treat a mixed overdose in which a potentially seizurogenic medication may have been ingested.

Flumazenil is to be administered intravenously. To minimize injection pain, it should be injected into a large vein through a freely flowing intravenous infusion. Extravasation may result in local irritation and should be avoided.

To allow control over the rate and degree of reversal while avoiding complications associated with too-rapid awakening or other adverse effects, it is recommended that flumazenil be administered as a series of small injections rather than as a single dose.

Dosage must be individualized according to the needs of the patient and clinical circumstances. Doses higher than the minimally effective dose are tolerated well by most patients, but administration of more flumazenil than is necessary increases the risk of adverse effects resulting from reversal of a benzodiazepine's therapeutic effects and may complicate the management of physically dependent patients.

The effects of a neuromuscular blocking agent, if used during surgery or for facilitating assisted ventilation in an intensive care patient, should be reversed completely before flumazenil is administered. Neuromuscular blocking agents should not be used without adequate sedation because the respiratory paralysis they induce is highly distressing to aware patients.

Post-procedure analgesic requirements are not increased in patients who have received flumazenil, but awake patients may report pain, and require earlier treatment, than patients who have not received the reversal agent.

Because psychomotor and memory deficits may persist after sedation has been completely reversed, patients receiving flumazenil following an outpatient procedure should be advised not to resume normal activities for at least 18 to 24 hours after discharge. Also, post-procedure instructions should be given to the patient in writing or given to a responsible caretaker.

### For treatment of adverse effects
Recommended treatment consists of the following
- For convulsions—Benzodiazepines are usually recommended for treatment of convulsions, but higher than usual doses may be needed after flumazenil has been administered. Therefore, the risk of substantial resedation after the effects of flumazenil have subsided must be considered. Administration of a barbiturate or phenytoin instead of a benzodiazepine should be considered.
- For CNS effects possibly associated with benzodiazepine withdrawal, e.g., anxiety and emotional lability—Signs and symptoms are usually mild and short-lived and may not require treatment. If severe, continuing symptoms occur, administration of a barbiturate, benzodiazepine, or other sedative may be required.

## Parenteral Dosage Forms

### FLUMAZENIL INJECTION

**Usual adult dose**
Benzodiazepine antagonist—
  Reversal of benzodiazepine-induced sedation—
    Intravenous, 200 mcg (0.2 mg), administered over fifteen seconds, initially. If the desired response has not been attained after forty-five seconds to one minute, additional 200-mcg (0.2-mg) doses may be administered over fifteen seconds at one-minute intervals, up to a maximum cumulative dose of 1 mg. Most patients require 600 mcg (0.6 mg) to 1 mg.
    If resedation occurs, additional flumazenil may be administered at a rate of 200 mcg (0.2 mg) per minute, up to a total cumulative dose of 1 mg. This dose may be repeated at twenty-minute intervals, up to a maximum of 3 mg in a one-hour period.
  Treatment of benzodiazepine overdose—
    Intravenous, 200 mcg (0.2 mg), administered over thirty seconds, initially. If the desired response has not been obtained after thirty seconds to one minute, 300 mcg (0.3 mg) may be administered over thirty seconds. If necessary, additional doses of 500 mcg (0.5 mg) may be administered over thirty seconds at one-minute intervals, up to a maximum cumulative dose of 3 mg. Most patients respond to a cumulative dose of 1 to 3 mg. Higher doses do not reliably produce additional benefit, but patients who have responded partially to 3 mg may obtain additional benefit from a total dose of 4 or 5 mg; occasional patients have required as much as 8 mg to achieve full reversal. If no response is attained after a cumulative dose of 5 mg, it can be assumed that a benzodiazepine was not responsible for the overdose and that further administration of flumazenil is not likely to be helpful. If resedation occurs, additional doses of up to a total of 1 mg of flumazenil may be administered at a rate of 500 mcg (0.5

mg) per minute. This dose may be repeated at twenty-minute intervals, up to a maximum of 3 mg in a one-hour period. Alternatively, flumazenil may be administered as an intravenous infusion at a rate adjusted to provide the desired level of arousal, generally 100 to 400 mcg (0.1 to 0.4 mg) per hour.

Note: Dosage should be titrated to produce the desired degree of arousal. Complete reversal may not be needed or desirable in certain circumstances.

For patients who may be tolerant to or dependent on benzodiazepines, a slower rate of administration (100 mcg [0.1 mg] per minute) and lower total doses may be required to minimize the risk of adverse effects.

The recommended one-minute interval between doses may not be sufficiently long for high-risk patients.

No adjustment of initial dosage is required for patients with significant hepatic function impairment, but a reduction in the size and/or frequency of subsequent doses is recommended.

To prevent resedation after initial reversal, up to 1 mg of flumazenil may be administered intravenously at a rate of 200 mcg (0.2 mg) per minute thirty minutes and possibly sixty minutes later.

**Usual adult prescribing limits**
For reversal of benzodiazepine-induced sedation—
  Not more than 1 mg at any one time or 3 mg per hour.

**Usual pediatric dose**
Dosage has not been established. However, the medication is being administered intravenously to pediatric patients in doses ranging from 10 mcg (0.01 mg) per kg of body weight (for reversing sedation) to 100 mcg (0.1 mg) per kg of body weight (for life-threatening overdose), up to a maximum cumulative dose of 1 mg. Some investigators have also administered flumazenil by intravenous infusion at a rate of 5 to 10 mcg (0.005 to 0.01 mg) per kg of body weight per hour.

**Usual geriatric dose**
See *Usual adult dose*.

**Strength(s) usually available**
U.S.—
  100 mcg (0.1 mg) per mL (Rx) [*Romazicon* (methylparaben 1.8 mg per mL; propylparaben 0.2 mg per mL; sodium chloride 0.9%; edetate disodium 0.01%; acetic acid 0.01%)].
Canada—
  100 mcg (0.1 mg) per mL (Rx) [*Anexate* (edetate disodium 0.1 mg per mL; sodium chloride; glacial acetic acid; sodium hydroxide)].

**Packaging and storage**
Store between 15 and 30 °C (59 and 86 °F), unless otherwise specified by manufacturer.

**Preparation of dosage form**
Flumazenil injection may be diluted with 5% dextrose injection, 0.9% sodium chloride injection, 0.45% sodium chloride and 2.5% dextrose injection, or lactated Ringer's injection.

**Stability**
Infusion solutions prepared with 5% dextrose injection, 0.9% sodium chloride injection, or 0.45% sodium chloride and 2.5% dextrose injection are stable for up to 24 hours at room temperature. Flumazenil injections that have been drawn into a syringe or mixed with intravenous infusion solutions should be discarded after 24 hours.

One study has shown that stability of 20 mcg per mL (mcg/mL) of flumazenil in 5% dextrose injection is maintained for 12 hours at 23 °C (73 to 74 °F) when admixed with 3.2 mcg/mL of dopamine hydrochloride and for 24 hours when admixed with 2 mg per mL (mg/mL) of aminophylline, 2 mg/mL of dobutamine, 2.4 mg/mL of cimetidine, 0.08 mg/mL of famotidine, 50 USP Units per mL of heparin sodium, 4 mg/mL of lidocaine hydrochloride, 4 mg/mL of procainamide hydrochloride, or 0.3 mg/mL of ranitidine. Whether flumazenil affected the stability of the other medications was not determined.

**Selected Bibliography**
Brogden RN, Goa KL. Flumazenil. A reappraisal of its pharmacological properties and therapeutic efficacy as a benzodiazepine antagonist. Drugs 1991; 42: 1061-89.
Ghouri AF, Ruiz MAR, White PF. Effect of flumazenil on recovery after midazolam and propofol sedation. Anesthesiology 1994; 81: 333-9.
Miller RD, supplemental section editor. U.S. clinical trials of flumazenil, a benzodiazepine antagonist. Clin Ther 1992; 14: 860-995.

Developed: 02/28/95

# FLUMETHASONE—See *Corticosteroids (Topical)*

# FLUNARIZINE—See *Calcium Channel Blocking Agents (Systemic)*

# FLUNISOLIDE—See *Corticosteroids (Inhalation-Local); Corticosteroids (Nasal)*

# FLUOCINOLONE—See *Corticosteroids (Topical)*

# FLUOCINONIDE—See *Corticosteroids (Topical)*

# FLUOROMETHOLONE—See *Corticosteroids (Ophthalmic)*

# FLUOROQUINOLONES Systemic

This monograph includes information on the following: 1) Ciprofloxacin; 2) Enoxacin†; 3) Lomefloxacin†; 4) Norfloxacin; 5) Ofloxacin.
VA CLASSIFICATION (Primary): AM402
Commonly used brand name(s): *Cipro*[1]; *Cipro I.V.*[1]; *Floxin*[5]; *Floxin I.V.*[5]; *Maxaquin*[3]; *Noroxin*[4]; *Penetrex*[2].

Note: For a listing of dosage forms and brand names by country availability, see *Dosage Forms* section(s).

†Not commercially available in Canada.

## Category
Antibacterial (systemic).

## Indications
Note: Bracketed information in the *Indications* section refers to uses that are not included in U.S. product labeling.

**General considerations**
Fluoroquinolones are broad-spectrum anti-infectives, active against a wide range of aerobic gram-positive and gram-negative organisms. They are active *in vitro* against most Enterobacteriaceae, including *Citrobacter diversus, Citrobacter freundii,* and *Citrobacter koseri; Enterobacter aerogenes* and *Enterobacter cloacae; Escherichia coli; Klebsiella oxytoca, Klebsiella ozaenae,* and *Klebsiella pneumoniae; Morganella morganii; Proteus mirabilis* and *Proteus vulgaris; Providencia alcalifaciens, Providencia rettgeri,* and *Providencia stuartii; Salmonella enteritidis* and *Salmonella typhi; Shigella boydii, Shigella dysenteriae, Shigella flexneri,* and *Shigella sonnei; Vibrio cholerae, Vibrio parahaemolyticus,* and *Vibrio vulnificus;* and *Yersinia enterocolitica.* All of the fluoroquinolones also have good *in vitro* activity against penicillin-resistant strains of *Neisseria gonorrhoeae,* beta-lactamase–producing strains of *Haemophilus influenzae* and *Moraxella (Branhamella) catarrhalis,* and some gram-negative bacilli that are resistant to other antimicrobial agents. Ciprofloxacin is the most active fluoroquinolone against *Pseudomonas aeruginosa.* It is not generally effective against most strains of *Burkholderia (Pseudomonas) cepacia* or some strains of *Stenotrophomonas (Pseudomonas) maltophilia.* Ofloxacin's potency against *P. aeruginosa* is similar to that of norfloxacin, and greater than that of enoxacin or lomefloxacin.

Fluoroquinolones also have good *in vitro* activity against *Staphylococcus saprophyticus, Staphylococcus epidermidis,* and *Staphylococcus aureus,* including some methicillin-resistant (MRSA) strains. However, most methicillin-resistant strains are also resistant to fluoroquinolones. Any bacteria that are resistant to one fluoroquinolone also may be resistant to another. Streptococci, including *Streptococcus pneumoniae*, *Streptococcus pyogenes*, and *Enterococcus faecalis*, are all moderately susceptible to ofloxacin and ciprofloxacin *in vitro*. Resistant strains of these species are often seen. The $MIC_{90}$ values for these species, especially *E. faecalis*, are often equal to or greater than the susceptible breakpoint for these two antimicrobials. Therapeutic failures have been reported in patients taking ciprofloxacin for the treatment of pneumococcal pneumonia.

Ciprofloxacin and ofloxacin have been found to have good *in vitro* activity against *Chlamydia trachomatis*, *Mycoplasma hominis*, *Mycoplasma pneumoniae*, and *Legionella pneumophila*. These two fluoroquinolones have moderate activity *in vitro* against *Mycobacterium tuberculosis*, but neither antimicrobial is indicated for tuberculosis. The susceptibility of *Mycobacterium avium-intracellulare*, however, is only fair to poor, and inhibition requires significantly higher drug concentrations.

The emergence of bacterial resistance to fluoroquinolones, and of cross-resistance within this class of antimicrobial agents, has become a significant clinical concern. Decreased susceptibility among Enterobacteriaceae, including *E. coli*, *K. pneumoniae*, and *Salmonella*, has been reported worldwide. Strains of *N. gonorrhoeae* with low-level resistance to fluoroquinolones have been isolated; strains with high-level resistance to ciprofloxacin have been documented, and treatment failures have been reported. Resistance also has been documented for *H. influenzae* in patients with cystic fibrosis, and for *S. epidermidis* in several cases of nosocomial infections. Use of fluoroquinolones in poultry may be at least partially responsible for the emergence of fluoroquinolone resistance in *Salmonella* and *Campylobacter*. Mechanisms underlying fluoroquinolone resistance may include plasmid transfer, chromosomal mutations in DNA gyrase (*gyrA*) or topoisomerase IV (*parC*), and/or antibiotic efflux mediated by outer membrane proteins. Extensive and continuous use of fluoroquinolones, and antimicrobials in general, encourages the multiplication and spread of resistant bacterial strains; therefore, the World Health Organization recommends that prescribing practices for antimicrobial agents should be modified to reflect this growing concern.

**Accepted**
Bone and joint infections (treatment)—Ciprofloxacin is indicated in the treatment of bone and joint infections caused by susceptible organisms.

Bronchitis, bacterial exacerbations (treatment)—Ciprofloxacin, lomefloxacin[1], and ofloxacin are indicated in the treatment of bacterial exacerbations of chronic bronchitis caused by susceptible organisms.

Chlamydial infections, endocervical and urethral (treatment)—Ofloxacin is indicated in the treatment of endocervical and urethral infections caused by *C. trachomatis*.

Gastroenteritis, bacterial (treatment)—Ciprofloxacin and [norfloxacin][1] are indicated in the treatment of bacterial gastroenteritis, including traveler's diarrhea and infectious diarrhea, caused by susceptible organisms.

Gonorrhea, endocervical and urethral (treatment)—Ciprofloxacin, enoxacin[1], norfloxacin, and ofloxacin are indicated in the treatment of endocervical and urethral infections caused by *N. gonorrhoeae*.

Intra-abdominal infections (treatment)—Ciprofloxacin, in combination with metronidazole, is indicated in the treatment of complicated intra-abdominal infections caused by *Bacteroides fragilis*, *E. coli*, *K. pneumoniae*, *P. mirabilis*, or *P. aeruginosa*.

Neutropenia, febrile, empiric therapy (treatment)[1]—Parenteral ciprofloxacin, in combination with piperacillin, is indicated for empiric therapy in patients with febrile neutropenia.

Pelvic inflammatory disease (treatment)—Ofloxacin is indicated in the treatment of pelvic inflammatory disease, including severe infection, caused by *C. trachomatis* and/or *N. gonorrhoeae*.

If anaerobic microorganisms are suspected of contributing to the infection, appropriate therapy for anaerobic pathogens should also be administered.

Pneumonia, bacterial (treatment)—Ciprofloxacin and ofloxacin are indicated in the treatment of pneumonia caused by susceptible organisms.

Caution should be used in treating streptococcal and pneumococcal pneumonia with fluoroquinolones. Although they have been effective in limited trials, treatment failures have been reported; fluoroquinolones should not be considered the drug of first choice in the treatment of presumed or confirmed pneumococcal pneumonia.

Prostatitis, bacterial (treatment)—Ciprofloxacin, norfloxacin[1], and ofloxacin are indicated in the treatment of bacterial prostatitis caused by susceptible organisms.

Sinusitis, acute (treatment)[1]—Oral ciprofloxacin is indicated in the treatment of acute sinusitis caused by *H. influenzae*, *M. catarrhalis*, or *S. pneumoniae*.

Skin and soft tissue infections (treatment)—Ciprofloxacin and ofloxacin are indicated in the treatment of skin and soft tissue infections caused by susceptible organisms.

Typhoid fever (treatment)—Oral ciprofloxacin is indicated in the treatment of typhoid fever caused by susceptible strains of *S. typhi*.

Urinary tract infections, bacterial (prophylaxis)[1]—Lomefloxacin is indicated preoperatively for the prophylaxis of urinary tract infections in patients undergoing transurethral surgical procedures.

Urinary tract infections, bacterial (treatment)—Ciprofloxacin, enoxacin[1], lomefloxacin[1], norfloxacin, and ofloxacin are indicated in the treatment of complicated and uncomplicated urinary tract infections, including cystitis, caused by susceptible organisms.

[Chancroid (treatment)][1]—Ciprofloxacin and enoxacin are indicated in the treatment of chancroid caused by *Haemophilus ducreyi*.

[Meningococcal carriers (treatment)]—Oral ciprofloxacin is indicated in the treatment of asymptomatic carriers of *Neisseria meningitidis* for the elimination of meningococci from the nasopharynx.

[Septicemia, bacterial (treatment)]—Parenteral ciprofloxacin is indicated in the treatment of septicemia caused by *E. coli* or *S. typhi*.

Not all species or strains of a particular organism may be susceptible to a particular fluoroquinolone.

**Unaccepted**
Fluoroquinolones have not been shown to be effective in the treatment of syphilis and have poor activity against most anaerobic bacteria (including *Bacteroides fragilis* and *Clostridium difficile*).

---

[1]Not included in Canadian product labeling.

## Pharmacology/Pharmacokinetics

See *Table 1*, page 1496, and *Table 2*, page 1496.

**Physicochemical characteristics**
Molecular weight—
  Ciprofloxacin: 331.35.
  Ciprofloxacin hydrochloride: 385.82.
  Enoxacin: 320.33.
  Lomefloxacin: 351.36.
  Lomefloxacin hydrochloride: 387.82.
  Norfloxacin: 319.34.
  Ofloxacin: 361.38.

**Mechanism of action/Effect**
Bactericidal; fluoroquinolones act intracellularly by inhibiting topoisomerase II (DNA gyrase) and/or topoisomerase IV. Topoisomerases are essential bacterial enzymes that are critical catalysts in the duplication, transcription, and repair of bacterial DNA.

**Distribution**
Fluoroquinolones are widely distributed to most body fluids and tissues; high concentrations are attained in the kidneys, gallbladder, liver, lungs, gynecologic tissue, prostatic tissue, phagocytic cells, urine, sputum, and bile. Ciprofloxacin is also distributed to skin, fat, muscle, bone, and cartilage. The skin, fascia, and subcutaneous fat concentrations of ofloxacin are less than 50% of those found in the serum.

Ciprofloxacin and ofloxacin have been found to penetrate into the cerebrospinal fluid (CSF). CSF concentrations of ciprofloxacin reach 10% of the peak serum concentration with noninflamed meninges, and 14 to 37% with inflamed meninges. Ofloxacin penetrates into the CSF in the presence and the absence of meningeal inflammation (range, 14 to 60%). This ability of these agents has resulted in their bactericidal CSF titers ranging from inadequate to high, depending on the microorganism and its sensitivity to these antibiotics.

## Precautions to Consider

**Cross-sensitivity and/or related problems**
Patients allergic to one fluoroquinolone or other chemically related quinolone derivatives (e.g., cinoxacin, nalidixic acid) may be allergic to other fluoroquinolones also.

**Carcinogenicity/Tumorigenicity**
*Ciprofloxacin*—Long-term carcinogenicity studies (up to 2 years) in rats and mice with oral ciprofloxacin have shown no evidence that ciprofloxacin had any carcinogenic or tumorigenic effects.

*Enoxacin and ofloxacin*—Long-term studies to determine the carcinogenic potential of enoxacin or ofloxacin in animals have not been conducted.

*Lomefloxacin*—One study lasting up to 52 weeks showed that 92% of hairless (Skh-1) mice that were exposed to UVA light for 3.5 hours, five times every two weeks, and that had received lomefloxacin concurrently developed skin tumors within 16 weeks. These tumors were well-differentiated squamous cell carcinomas of the skin that were nonmetastatic and endophytic in character. Two thirds of these squamous cell carcinomas contained large keratinous inclusion masses and were thought to arise from the vestigial hair follicles in these hairless animals. In this study, mice treated with lomefloxacin alone did not develop skin or systemic tumors. The clinical significance of these findings to humans is not known.

*Norfloxacin*—Studies lasting up to 96 weeks in rats given doses of eight to nine times the usual human dose have shown that norfloxacin causes no increase in neoplastic changes, compared with controls.

**Mutagenicity**

*Ciprofloxacin*—*In vitro* mutagenicity studies have shown both positive and negative results. Negative results were obtained in the *Salmonella*/microsome test, *Escherichia coli* DNA repair test, Chinese hamster V79 cell HGPRT test, Syrian hamster embryo cell transformation assay, *Saccharomyces cerevisiae* point mutation assay, and the *S. cerevisiae* mitotic crossover and gene conversion assay. Positive results were obtained in the mouse lymphoma cell forward mutation assay and the rat hepatocyte DNA repair assay. Although positive results were obtained in two of eight *in vitro* studies, negative results were obtained in the *in vivo* rat hepatocyte DNA repair assay, micronucleus test in mice, and the dominant lethal test in mice.

*Enoxacin*—Enoxacin did not induce point mutations in bacterial cells or mitotic gene conversion in yeast cells, with or without metabolic activation. Enoxacin did not induce sister chromatid exchanges or structural chromosomal aberrations in mammalian cells *in vitro*, with or without metabolic activation. Also, it did not induce chromosomal aberrations in mice. There was a minimal, dose-related, statistically significant increase in micronuclei at high doses of enoxacin in mice; however, the significance of these findings, in the absence of effects in other test systems, is not established.

*Lomefloxacin*—One *in vitro* mutagenicity test (CHO/HGPRT assay) was weakly positive at concentrations of 226 mcg per mL (mcg/mL) and higher, and negative at concentrations of less than 226 mcg/mL. Mutagenicity tests were negative in two other *in vitro* tests (chromosomal aberrations in Chinese hamster ovary cells and in human lymphocytes). Two *in vivo* mouse micronucleus mutagenicity tests were also negative.

*Norfloxacin*—Studies in mice have shown that norfloxacin causes no mutagenic effects in the dominant lethal test. Studies in hamsters and rats given doses of 30 to 60 times the usual human dose have shown that norfloxacin causes no chromosomal aberrations. The Ames test, studies in Chinese hamster fibroblasts, and the V79 mammalian cell assay have shown that norfloxacin causes no mutagenic activity *in vitro*.

*Ofloxacin*—Ofloxacin was not found to be mutagenic in the Ames test, *in vitro* and *in vivo* cytogenetic assay, sister chromatid exchange (Chinese hamster and human cell lines), unscheduled DNA repair test using human fibroblasts, mouse micronucleus assay, or dominant lethal assays. However, ofloxacin was mutagenic in the unscheduled DNA repair test using rat hepatocytes and in the mouse lymphoma assay.

**Pregnancy/Reproduction**

Fertility—
 *Ciprofloxacin*—
  Adequate and well-controlled studies in humans have not been done. Studies in rats and mice given doses of up to six times the usual daily human dose have not shown that ciprofloxacin causes adverse effects on fertility.
 *Enoxacin*—
  No consistent effects on fertility and reproductive parameters were noted in female rats given oral doses of up to 1000 mg per kg of body weight (mg/kg) of enoxacin. Decreased spermatogenesis and subsequent impaired fertility were noted in male rats given oral doses of 1000 mg/kg.
 *Lomefloxacin*—
  The fertility of male and female rats was not affected when lomefloxacin was administered at oral doses of up to eight times the recommended human dose on a mg per square meter of body surface area (mg/m²) basis, or 34 times the recommended human dose on a mg/kg basis.
 *Norfloxacin*—
  Studies in male and female mice given oral doses of up to 30 times the usual human dose have not shown that norfloxacin causes adverse effects on fertility.

Pregnancy—
 *Ciprofloxacin*—
  Ciprofloxacin crosses the placenta. Adequate and well-controlled studies in humans have not been done. However, since ciprofloxacin has been shown to cause arthropathy in immature animals, its use is not recommended during pregnancy.
  Studies in rats and mice given doses of up to six times the usual daily human dose have not shown that ciprofloxacin causes adverse effects on the fetus. Studies in rabbits given oral doses of 30 and 100 mg/kg have shown that ciprofloxacin causes gastrointestinal disturbances, resulting in maternal weight loss and an increased incidence of abortion. However, these studies have not shown that ciprofloxacin is teratogenic at either dose. Studies using intravenous doses of up to 20 mg/kg have not shown that ciprofloxacin causes maternal toxicity, embryotoxicity, or teratogenic effects.
  FDA Pregnancy Category C.
 *Enoxacin*—
  Adequate and well-controlled studies in humans have not been done. Since enoxacin has been shown to cause arthropathy in immature animals, its use is not recommended during pregnancy.
  Rats and mice given oral enoxacin have shown no evidence of teratogenic potential. Intravenous infusion of enoxacin into pregnant rabbits at doses of 10 to 50 mg/kg caused dose-related maternal toxicity (venous irritation, weight loss, and reduced food intake). At 50 mg/kg, there were increased incidences of postimplantation loss and stunted fetuses. The incidence of fetal malformations also was significantly increased at this dose in the presence of overt maternal and fetal toxicity.
  FDA Pregnancy Category C.
 *Lomefloxacin*—
  Adequate and well-controlled studies in humans have not been done. Since lomefloxacin has been shown to cause arthropathy in immature animals, its use is not recommended during pregnancy.
  Reproduction studies done in rats given oral doses of up to 34 times the recommended human dose on a mg/kg basis reported no harm to the fetus. An increased incidence of fetal loss in monkeys has been observed at approximately 6 to 12 times the recommended human dose on a mg/kg basis. No teratogenicity has been observed in rats and monkeys at doses of up to 16 times the recommended human dose. In rabbits, maternal toxicity and associated fetotoxicity, decreased placental weight, and variations of the coccygeal vertebrae occurred at doses two times the recommended human dose on a mg/m² basis.
  FDA Pregnancy Category C.
 *Norfloxacin*—
  Adequate and well-controlled studies in humans have not been done. The umbilical cord serum concentration ranges from undetectable to 0.5 mg per mL (mg/mL) and the amniotic fluid concentration ranges from undetectable to 0.92 mg/mL following the administration of a single 200-mg dose of norfloxacin. Since norfloxacin has been shown to cause arthropathy in immature animals, its use is not recommended during pregnancy.
  Studies in monkeys given doses of 10 times the maximum recommended human dose (MRHD) (800 mg daily) have shown that norfloxacin causes embryonic loss. Peak plasma concentrations were two to three times those seen in humans. Studies in cynomolgus monkeys given doses of 150 mg/kg per day or more have shown that norfloxacin is embryocidal and causes slight maternal toxicity (vomiting and anorexia) as well. However, studies in rats, rabbits, mice, and monkeys given doses of 6 to 50 times the usual human dose have not shown that norfloxacin is teratogenic.
  FDA Pregnancy Category C.
 *Ofloxacin*—
  Ofloxacin crosses the placenta. In one small study, umbilical cord serum concentrations reached 80 to 90% of maternal serum concentrations after mothers received 200-mg doses. Ofloxacin was also detected in the amniotic fluid from more than 50% of the mothers. Another small study found that ofloxacin concentrated in the amniotic fluid, reaching up to 35 to 257% of the simultaneous maternal serum concentration. Adequate and well-controlled studies in humans have not been done. However, since ofloxacin and other quinolones have been shown to cause arthropathy in immature animals, its use is not recommended during pregnancy.
  Studies in rats and rabbits given doses of up to 810 and 160 mg/kg per day, respectively, have not shown ofloxacin to be teratogenic. Studies in rats given doses of up to 360 mg/kg per day showed no adverse effect on late fetal development, labor, delivery, lactation, neonatal viability, or growth of the newborn. Doses equivalent to 50 and 10 times the MRHD were fetotoxic in rats (decreased fetal body weight) and rabbits (increased fetal mortality), respectively. Rats given 810 mg/kg per day, greater than 10 times the MRHD, were reported to have minor skeletal variations.
  FDA Pregnancy Category C.

## Breast-feeding

Ciprofloxacin and ofloxacin are known to be distributed into human breast milk. The concentration of ofloxacin in breast milk was similar to that found in plasma. One small study found that ofloxacin was highly concentrated in breast milk, reaching 98% of the simultaneous maternal serum level within 2 hours of administration. It is not known whether enoxacin, lomefloxacin, or norfloxacin is distributed into breast milk. Norfloxacin was not detected in breast milk following its administration in low (200-mg) doses to nursing mothers. However, other quinolone derivatives are distributed into human breast milk. Fluoroquinolones have been shown to cause permanent lesions of the cartilage of weight-bearing joints, as well as other signs of arthropathy, in immature animals. Therefore, if an alternative antibiotic cannot be prescribed and a fluoroquinolone must be administered, breast-feeding is not recommended.

## Pediatrics

*For all fluoroquinolones—*

Fluoroquinolones are not recommended for use in infants and children. Patients up to 18 years of age have not been included in clinical trials because fluoroquinolones caused lameness in immature dogs due to permanent lesions of the cartilage of weight-bearing joints. These medications and other related quinolones have been reported to cause arthropathy in immature animals of various species.

Fluoroquinolones have been used in infants and children with serious infections that have not responded to other therapeutic regimens, or infections caused by multiple organisms resistant to other antibiotics, without reported damage to cartilage tissue. However, there have been case reports of arthropathy that was thought to be due to ciprofloxacin developing in children with pseudomonal pneumonias associated with cystic fibrosis. The arthropathy completely resolved soon after the medication was discontinued.

## Adolescents

*For all fluoroquinolones—*

Fluoroquinolones are not recommended for use in adolescents. Patients up to 18 years of age have not been included in clinical trials because fluoroquinolones caused lameness in immature dogs due to permanent lesions of the cartilage of weight-bearing joints. These medications and other related quinolones have been reported to cause arthropathy in immature animals of various species.

Fluoroquinolones have been used in children and adolescents with serious infections that have not responded to other therapeutic regimens, or infections caused by multiple organisms resistant to other antibiotics, without reported damage to cartilage tissue. However, there have been case reports of arthropathy that was thought to be due to ciprofloxacin developing in children with pseudomonal pneumonias associated with cystic fibrosis. The arthropathy completely resolved soon after the medication was discontinued.

## Geriatrics

*For all fluoroquinolones—*

Studies performed to date have not demonstrated geriatrics-specific problems that would limit the usefulness of fluoroquinolones in the elderly. However, elderly patients are more likely to have an age-related decrease in renal function, which may require an adjustment of dosage in patients receiving any of these medications.

## Drug interactions and/or related problems

The following drug interactions and/or related problems have been selected on the basis of their potential clinical significance (possible mechanism in parentheses where appropriate)—not necessarily inclusive (» = major clinical significance):

Note: Combinations containing any of the following medications, depending on the amount present, may also interact with this medication.

Alkalizers, urinary, such as:
  Carbonic anhydrase inhibitors
  Citrates
  Sodium bicarbonate
    (urinary alkalizers may reduce the solubility of ciprofloxacin or norfloxacin in the urine; patients should be observed for signs of crystalluria and nephrotoxicity, although the incidence is rare)

» Aminophylline or
» Oxtriphylline or
» Theophylline
    (concurrent use of aminophylline, oxtriphylline, or theophylline with ciprofloxacin or enoxacin significantly reduces the hepatic metabolism and clearance of theophylline, probably by competitive inhibition at its binding sites within the cytochrome P450 enzyme system; this may result in a prolonged theophylline elimination half-life, increased serum concentration, and increased risk of theophylline-related toxicity; enoxacin has the greatest effect on theophylline clearance and it is recommended that the dose of theophylline be decreased by 50%; ciprofloxacin may also increase the risk of toxicity, especially in patients with theophylline concentrations at the upper end of the therapeutic range; serum theophylline concentrations should be monitored and dosage adjustments may be required; norfloxacin and ofloxacin have a minor effect on theophylline clearance; one study with ofloxacin found an increase of approximately 10% in the theophylline serum concentration; however, other studies have found that ofloxacin has a negligible effect on theophylline metabolism; theophylline dosage adjustment is usually not necessary in patients receiving norfloxacin or ofloxacin; theophylline clearance has not been found to be significantly altered by lomefloxacin)

» Antacids, aluminum-, calcium-, and/or magnesium-containing or
» Ferrous sulfate or
  Laxatives, magnesium-containing or
» Sucralfate or
  Zinc
    (antacids, ferrous sulfate, zinc, or sucralfate may reduce the absorption of fluoroquinolones by chelation, resulting in lower serum and urine concentrations; therefore, concurrent use is not recommended; because the bioavailability of enoxacin is decreased the most by concurrent administration of these medications, it is recommended that enoxacin be taken at least 2 hours before or 8 hours after any of these medications; ciprofloxacin should be taken at least 2 hours before or 6 hours after any of these medications; lomefloxacin should be taken at least 2 hours before or 4 hours after any of these medications; and norfloxacin or ofloxacin should be taken at least 2 hours before or after any of these medications)

Anticonvulsants, hydantoin, especially:
» Phenytoin
    (concurrent administration of ciprofloxacin with phenytoin has resulted in a 34 to 80% decrease in the plasma concentration of phenytoin; caution should be used when administering quinolones, especially ciprofloxacin, to patients stabilized on phenytoin; careful monitoring of phenytoin dosage after discontinuation of quinolones is highly recommended)

Antidiabetic agents, sulfonylurea, especially:
  Glyburide or
  Insulin
    (concurrent use of ciprofloxacin with glyburide has, on rare occasions, resulted in hypoglycemia; also, hyperglycemia and hypoglycemia have been reported in patients taking quinolone antibiotics and antidiabetic agents concurrently; since the mechanism is not understood, similar effects with other sulfonylurea antidiabetic agents should be considered when these medications are used with fluoroquinolones)

Anti-inflammatory drugs, nonsteroidal (NSAIDs)
    (fluoroquinolones, particularly enoxacin and norfloxacin, are competitive inhibitors of gamma-aminobutyric acid receptor binding, and some NSAIDs have been shown to enhance this effect; seizures have been reported in patients taking enoxacin and fenbufen concurrently; concurrent administration of NSAIDs with quinolone antibiotics may increase the risks of central nervous system [CNS] stimulation and convulsions)

Bismuth
    (the bioavailability of enoxacin is decreased by approximately 25% when bismuth subsalicylate is administered concurrently or within 60 minutes of enoxacin administration; concurrent administration of these medications is not recommended)

» Caffeine
    (concurrent use of caffeine with enoxacin has been found to decrease the hepatic metabolism of caffeine, resulting in a dose-related increase in the half-life of caffeine of up to five times normal; ciprofloxacin and, to a lesser extent, norfloxacin also reduce the hepatic metabolism and clearance of caffeine, increasing its half-life and the risk of caffeine-related CNS stimulation; lomefloxacin and ofloxacin do not produce any significant change in caffeine metabolism)

Cyclosporine
    (concurrent use with ciprofloxacin or norfloxacin has been reported to elevate serum creatinine and serum cyclosporine concentrations; other studies have not found ciprofloxacin or enoxacin to alter the pharmacokinetics of cyclosporine; cyclosporine concentrations should be monitored, and dosage adjustments may be required)

» Didanosine
    (concurrent use of didanosine with ciprofloxacin has been shown to reduce the absorption of ciprofloxacin due to chelation of ciprofloxacin by the aluminum and magnesium buffers in didanosine;

didanosine should not be administered concurrently with any fluoroquinolone)

Digoxin
(enoxacin may raise serum digoxin concentrations in some patients; digoxin serum concentrations should be monitored)

Probenecid
(concurrent use of probenecid decreases the renal tubular secretion of fluoroquinolones, resulting in decreased urinary excretion of the fluoroquinolone, prolonged elimination half-life, and increased risk of toxicity; this interaction is more significant with ofloxacin, which is excreted largely unchanged in the urine, and of less clinical significance with fluoroquinolones that have larger nonrenal elimination, such as ciprofloxacin and enoxacin)

» Warfarin
(concurrent use of warfarin with ciprofloxacin or norfloxacin has been reported to increase the anticoagulant effect of warfarin, increasing the chance of bleeding; other studies have not found fluoroquinolones to alter the prothrombin time [PT] significantly; enoxacin decreases the clearance of R-warfarin, the less active isomer of racemic warfarin, but not the active S-isomer; changes in clotting time have not been observed when enoxacin and warfarin are administered concurrently; the PT of patients receiving warfarin and fluoroquinolones concurrently should be monitored carefully)

**Laboratory value alterations**
The following have been selected on the basis of their potential clinical significance (possible effect in parentheses where appropriate)—not necessarily inclusive (» = major clinical significance):

With physiology/laboratory test values
Alanine aminotransferase (ALT [SGPT]) and
Alkaline phosphatase and
Aspartate aminotransferase (AST [SGOT]) and
Lactate dehydrogenase (LDH)
(serum values may be increased)

**Medical considerations/Contraindications**
The medical considerations/contraindications included have been selected on the basis of their potential clinical significance (reasons given in parentheses where appropriate)—not necessarily inclusive (» = major clinical significance).

*Except under special circumstances, this medication should not be used when the following medical problem exists:*
» Previous allergic reaction to fluoroquinolones or other chemically related quinolone derivatives

*Risk-benefit should be considered when the following medical problems exist:*
CNS disorders, including cerebral arteriosclerosis or epilepsy
(fluoroquinolones may cause CNS stimulation or toxicity)
Hepatic function impairment
(patients with severe hepatic function impairment, such as cirrhosis with ascites, may have decreased clearance of ofloxacin, resulting in an increase in peak serum concentration and elimination half-life; patients with *both* hepatic and renal function impairment may require a reduction in the dosage of ciprofloxacin; cirrhosis has not been found to decrease the nonrenal clearance of lomefloxacin)
» Renal function impairment
(fluoroquinolones are primarily excreted renally; it is recommended that a reduced dose be administered to patients with impaired renal function)

## Side/Adverse Effects

Note: The relative insolubility of ciprofloxacin and norfloxacin at an alkaline pH has resulted in crystalluria, usually when the urinary pH exceeds 7. Because normal urinary pH is acidic, approximately 5 to 6, crystalluria is very unlikely to occur unless the patient's urine has become alkalinized.

Seizures have been reported very rarely with ciprofloxacin therapy; however, the patients who did have seizures either had a previous seizure history, were alcoholic, or were taking ciprofloxacin concurrently with theophylline.

Achilles tendinitis and tendon rupture have been reported in patients receiving fluoroquinolones. The ruptures occurred 2 to 42 days after the start of therapy. These injuries may require surgical repair or result in prolonged disability. It is recommended that fluoroquinolone treatment be discontinued at the first sign of tendon pain or inflammation, and that patients refrain from exercising until the diagnosis of tendinitis has been excluded.

The following side/adverse effects have been selected on the basis of their potential clinical significance (possible signs and symptoms in parentheses where appropriate)—not necessarily inclusive:

**Those indicating need for medical attention**
Incidence rare
***CNS stimulation*** (acute psychosis; agitation; confusion; hallucinations; tremors); ***hepatotoxicity*** (dark or amber urine; loss of appetite; pale stools; stomach pain; unusual tiredness or weakness; yellow eyes or skin); ***hypersensitivity reactions*** (skin rash, itching, or redness; Stevens-Johnson syndrome; shortness of breath; swelling of face or neck; vasculitis); ***interstitial nephritis*** (bloody or cloudy urine; fever; skin rash; swelling of feet or lower legs); ***phlebitis*** (pain at site of injection)—for intravenous ciprofloxacin and ofloxacin; ***pseudomembranous colitis*** (abdominal or stomach cramps and pain, severe; abdominal tenderness; diarrhea, watery and severe, which may also be bloody; fever); ***tendinitis or tendon rupture*** (pain in calves, radiating to heels; swelling of calves or lower legs)

**Those indicating need for medical attention only if they continue or are bothersome**
Incidence more frequent
***CNS toxicity*** (dizziness or lightheadedness; headache; nervousness; drowsiness; insomnia); ***gastrointestinal reactions*** (abdominal or stomach pain or discomfort, mild; diarrhea, mild; nausea or vomiting)

Incidence less frequent or rare
***Photosensitivity*** (increased sensitivity of skin to sunlight)—more common with lomefloxacin

## Overdose

For more information on the management of overdose or unintentional ingestion, **contact a Poison Control Center** (see *Poison Control Center Listing*).

**Treatment of overdose**
Since there is no specific antidote for overdose of fluoroquinolone antibiotics, treatment should be symptomatic and supportive and may include the following:
To decrease absorption—Induction of emesis or use of gastric lavage to empty the stomach.
Specific treatment—Maintenance of adequate hydration.
Supportive care—Supportive therapy. Patients in whom intentional overdose is confirmed or suspected should be referred for psychiatric consultation.

## Patient Consultation

As an aid to patient consultation, refer to *Advice for the Patient, Fluoroquinolones (Systemic)*.

In providing consultation, consider emphasizing the following selected information (» = major clinical significance):

**Before using this medication**
» Conditions affecting use, especially:
Allergies to fluoroquinolones or other quinolone derivatives
Pregnancy—Fluoroquinolones are not recommended for use during pregnancy because they have been shown to cause arthropathy in immature animals
Breast-feeding—Not recommended since fluoroquinolones have been shown to cause arthropathy in immature animals
Use in children—Use of fluoroquinolones is not recommended in infants and children since these medications have been shown to cause arthropathy in immature animals
Use in adolescents—Use of fluoroquinolones is not recommended in adolescents since these medications have been shown to cause arthropathy in immature animals
Other medications, especially aluminum-, calcium-, and/or magnesium-containing antacids, aminophylline, caffeine-containing products, didanosine, ferrous sulfate, oxtriphylline, phenytoin, sucralfate, theophylline, or warfarin
Other medical problems, especially allergy to quinolones and renal function impairment

**Proper use of this medication**
» Not giving to infants, children, adolescents, or pregnant women; fluoroquinolones have been shown to cause arthropathy in immature animals
» Taking with full glass (240 mL) of water; maintaining adequate fluid intake
» For enoxacin or norfloxacin—taking on an empty stomach
» For ciprofloxacin, lomefloxacin, or ofloxacin—taking with meals or on an empty stomach
» Compliance with full course of therapy

- » Importance of not missing doses and taking at evenly spaced times
- » Proper dosing
  Missed dose: Taking as soon as possible; not taking if almost time for next dose; not doubling doses
- » Proper storage

**Precautions while using this medication**
Checking with physician if no improvement of symptoms within a few days
- » Avoiding concurrent use of antacids or sucralfate and fluoroquinolones; taking antacids or sucralfate at least 6 hours before or 2 hours after administration of ciprofloxacin, 2 hours before or after administration of norfloxacin or ofloxacin, 4 hours before or 2 hours after administration of lomefloxacin, and 8 hours before or 2 hours after administration of enoxacin
- » Possible photosensitivity reactions
- » Caution if dizziness, lightheadedness, or drowsiness occurs

**Side/adverse effects**
Signs of potential side effects, especially CNS stimulation, hepatotoxicity, hypersensitivity reactions, interstitial nephritis, phlebitis, pseudomembranous colitis, and tendinitis or tendon rupture

## General Dosing Information

Patients with impaired renal function may require a reduction in dosage based on creatinine clearance. Creatinine clearance (in mL per minute) may be calculated as follows:

Adult males—Creatinine clearance = [(140 − age) × (ideal body weight in kg)]/[72 × serum creatinine (in milligrams per dL)]

Adult females—Creatinine clearance = [(140 − age) × (ideal body weight in kg)]/[72 × serum creatinine (in milligrams per dL)] × 0.85

Creatinine clearance may also be calculated in SI units (as mL per second) as follows:

Adult males—Creatinine clearance = [(140 − age) × (ideal body weight in kg)]/[50 × serum creatinine (in micromoles per L)]

Adult females—Creatinine clearance = [(140 − age) × (ideal body weight in kg)]/[50 × serum creatinine (in micromoles per L)] × 0.85

### CIPROFLOXACIN

## Additional Dosing Information

**Diet/Nutrition**
The presence of food in the stomach may delay the rate of absorption of oral ciprofloxacin; however, the overall absorption is not affected. Therefore, ciprofloxacin may be taken with meals or on an empty stomach. Ciprofloxacin should be taken with a full glass (240 mL) of water.

Parenteral ciprofloxacin should be administered by intravenous infusion over a period of at least 60 minutes to minimize patient discomfort and reduce the risk of venous irritation.

Crystalluria has been reported, especially in patients with alkaline urine (pH 7 or above). Therefore, alkalinization of the urine should be avoided. Although crystalluria has been reported only rarely in humans, fluid intake should be sufficient to maintain urine output of at least 1200 to 1500 mL per day in adults.

**Bioequivalenence information**
The oral suspension and tablet dosage forms of ciprofloxacin are bioequivalent.

## Oral Dosage Forms

Note: Bracketed uses in the *Dosage Forms* section refer to categories of use and/or indications that are not included in U.S. product labeling. The dosing and strengths of the dosage forms available are expressed in terms of ciprofloxacin base.

### CIPROFLOXACIN FOR ORAL SUSPENSION

**Usual adult dose**
Bone and joint infections—
  Mild or moderate: Oral, 500 mg (base) every twelve hours for at least four to six weeks.
  Severe or complicated: Oral, 750 mg (base) every twelve hours for at least four to six weeks.
Diarrhea, bacterial—
  Mild to severe: Oral, 500 mg (base) every twelve hours for five to seven days.
Gonorrhea, endocervical and urethral—
  Oral, 250 mg (base) as a single dose.
Intra-abdominal infections[1]—
  Oral, 500 mg (base) every twelve hours for seven to fourteen days, in combination with oral metronidazole.
[Meningococcal carriers]—
  Oral, 750 mg (base) as a single dose.
Prostatitis—
  Mild or moderate: Oral, 500 mg (base) every twelve hours for twenty-eight days.
Sinusitis, mild or moderate[1] or
Typhoid fever—
  Oral, 500 mg (base) every twelve hours for ten days.
Skin and soft tissue infections—
  Mild or moderate: Oral, 500 mg (base) every twelve hours for seven to fourteen days.
  Severe or complicated: Oral, 750 mg (base) every twelve hours for seven to fourteen days.
Urinary tract infections—
  Acute uncomplicated: Oral, 100 mg (base) every twelve hours for three days.
  Mild or moderate: Oral, 250 mg (base) every twelve hours for seven to fourteen days.
  Severe or complicated: Oral, 500 mg (base) every twelve hours for seven to fourteen days.

Note: Adults with impaired renal function may require a reduction in dose as follows:

| Creatinine clearance (mL/min)/(mL/sec) | Dose (base) |
| --- | --- |
| > 50/0.83 | See *Usual adult dose* |
| 30–50/0.5–0.83 | 250–500 mg every 12 hours |
| 5–29/0.08–0.48 | 250–500 mg every 18 hours |
| Hemodialysis or Peritoneal dialysis patients | 250–500 mg every 24 hours after dialysis |

In patients with severe infection and severe renal function impairment, a unit dose of 750 mg may be administered at the intervals noted above; however, these patients should be monitored carefully and serum concentrations of ciprofloxacin should be measured periodically.

**Usual adult prescribing limits**
1.5 grams (base) daily.

**Usual pediatric dose**
Children up to 18 years of age—Use is not recommended in infants, children, or adolescents since ciprofloxacin causes arthropathy in immature animals. However, ciprofloxacin has been given to children at doses of 10 to 20 mg (base) per kg of body weight every twelve hours when alternative therapy could not be used.

**Usual geriatric dose**
See *Usual adult dose*.

**Strength(s) usually available**
U.S.—
  250 mg (base) per 5 mL (5%) (Rx) [*Cipro* (sucrose)].
  500 mg (base) per 5 mL (10%) (Rx) [*Cipro* (sucrose)].
Canada—
  Not commercially available.

**Packaging and storage**
Prior to reconstitution, store below 25 °C (77 °F). Protect from freezing.
After reconstitution, store below 30 °C (86 °F). Protect from freezing.

**Preparation of dosage form**
To prepare the oral suspension, the small bottle containing the microcapsules should be emptied into the large bottle containing the diluent. **Water should not be added to the suspension.** The large bottle should be closed and shaken vigorously for about 15 seconds.

**Stability**
The suspension is stable for 14 days when stored in a refrigerator or at room temperature (below 30 °C [86 °F]).

**Auxiliary labeling**
- Shake well before use.
- Take with a full glass of water.
- May cause dizziness or lightheadedness.
- Continue medicine for full time of treatment.
- Avoid too much sun or use of sunlamp.
- Do not take antacids or iron preparations within 4 hours of this medicine.

### CIPROFLOXACIN TABLETS USP

**Usual adult dose**
See *Ciprofloxacin for Oral Suspension*.

**Usual adult prescribing limits**
See *Ciprofloxacin for Oral Suspension*.

**Usual pediatric dose**
See *Ciprofloxacin for Oral Suspension*.

## Usual geriatric dose
See *Ciprofloxacin for Oral Suspension*.

## Strength(s) usually available
U.S.—
- 100 mg (base) (Rx) [*Cipro*].
- 250 mg (base) (Rx) [*Cipro*].
- 500 mg (base) (Rx) [*Cipro*].
- 750 mg (base) (Rx) [*Cipro*].

Canada—
- 100 mg (base) (Rx) [*Cipro*].
- 250 mg (base) (Rx) [*Cipro*].
- 500 mg (base) (Rx) [*Cipro*].
- 750 mg (base) (Rx) [*Cipro*].

## Packaging and storage
Store below 30 °C (86 °F) in a well-closed container.

## Auxiliary labeling
- Take with a full glass of water.
- May cause dizziness or lightheadedness.
- Continue medicine for full time of treatment.
- Avoid too much sun or use of sunlamp.
- Do not take antacids or iron preparations within 4 hours of this medicine.

# Parenteral Dosage Forms

Note: Bracketed uses in the *Dosage Forms* section refer to categories of use and/or indications that are not included in U.S. product labeling.

## CIPROFLOXACIN INJECTION USP

### Usual adult dose
Bone and joint infections or
Pneumonia, bacterial, gram-negative or
Skin and soft tissue infections—
- Mild or moderate: Intravenous infusion, 400 mg every twelve hours.
- Severe or complicated: Intravenous infusion, 400 mg every eight hours.

Intra-abdominal infections—
- Intravenous infusion, 400 mg every twelve hours, in combination with parenteral metronidazole.

Neutropenia, febrile, empiric therapy[1]—
- Severe: Intravenous infusion, 400 mg every eight hours, in combination with piperacillin 50 mg per kg of body weight every four hours (up to 24 grams per day), for seven to fourteen days.

Pneumonia, nosocomial—
- Mild to severe: Intravenous infusion, 400 mg every eight hours.

[Septicemia]—
- Intravenous infusion, 400 mg every twelve hours.

Urinary tract infections—
- Mild or moderate: Intravenous infusion, 200 mg every twelve hours.
- Severe or complicated: Intravenous infusion, 400 mg every twelve hours.

Note: Adults with impaired renal function may require a reduction in dose as follows:

| Creatinine clearance (mL/min)/(mL/sec) | Dose (base) |
| --- | --- |
| ≥ 30/0.5 | See *Usual adult dose* |
| 5–29/0.08–0.48 | 200–400 mg every 18 to 24 hours |

### Usual pediatric dose
Children up to 18 years of age—Use is not recommended in infants, children, or adolescents since ciprofloxacin causes arthropathy in animals. However, ciprofloxacin has been given to children at doses of 10 to 20 mg (base) per kg of body weight every twelve hours when alternative therapy could not be used.

### Usual geriatric dose
See *Usual adult dose*.

### Strength(s) usually available
U.S.—
- 200 mg per 20 mL (Rx) [*Cipro I.V.* (in sterile water for injection; requires dilution prior to administration)].
- 200 mg per 100 mL (Rx) [*Cipro I.V.* (in 5% dextrose injection; premixed)].
- 400 mg per 40 mL (Rx) [*Cipro I.V.* (in sterile water for injection; requires dilution prior to administration)].
- 400 mg per 200 mL (Rx) [*Cipro I.V.* (in 5% dextrose injection; premixed)].
- 1200 mg per 120 mL (Rx) [*Cipro I.V.* (in sterile water for injection; requires dilution prior to administration)].

Canada—
- 200 mg per 20 mL (Rx) [*Cipro I.V.* (in sterile water for injection; requires dilution prior to administration)].
- 400 mg per 40 mL (Rx) [*Cipro I.V.* (in sterile water for injection; requires dilution prior to administration)].

## Packaging and storage
Store in a cool place (between 8 and 15 °C [46 and 59 °F]) or at controlled room temperature (between 20 and 25 °C [68 and 77 °F]), unless otherwise specified by manufacturer. Protect from light and freezing.

## Preparation of dosage form
To prepare a solution for intravenous infusion, the concentrate in sterile water for injection should be withdrawn aseptically from the vial and diluted to a final concentration of 1 to 2 mg per mL with a suitable intravenous solution (see manufacturer's package insert). *Solutions that come from the manufacturer in 5% dextrose injection should not be diluted prior to intravenous infusion.* The resulting solution should be infused over a period of at least 60 minutes by direct infusion or through a Y-type intravenous infusion set. It is recommended that administration of any other solutions be discontinued during infusion of ciprofloxacin.

## Stability
When diluted with appropriate intravenous fluids (see manufacturer's package insert) to concentrations from 0.5 to 2 mg per mL, solutions retain their potency for up to 14 days when refrigerated or stored at room temperature.

## Incompatibilities
Ciprofloxacin is incompatible with aminophylline, amoxicillin, cefepime, clindamycin, dexamethasone, floxacillin, furosemide, heparin, and phenytoin.

If ciprofloxacin is to be given concurrently with another medication, each medication should be administered separately according to the recommended dosage and route of administration for each medication.

[1]Not included in Canadian product labeling.

---

## ENOXACIN

# Summary of Differences
Precautions: Drug interactions—Enoxacin has the greatest effect in decreasing the clearance of caffeine and theophylline, increasing the risk of toxicity for these medications.

# Additional Dosing Information

## Diet/Nutrition
The effect of food on the absorption of enoxacin tablets has not been studied; it is recommended that enoxacin be taken at least 1 hour before or 2 hours after a meal; however, decreased gastric acidity has been shown to decrease the bioavailability of enoxacin.

# Oral Dosage Forms

## ENOXACIN TABLETS

### Usual adult dose
Gonorrhea[1]—
- Oral, 400 mg as a single dose.

Urinary tract infections[1]—
- Complicated: Oral, 400 mg every twelve hours for fourteen days.
- Uncomplicated: Oral, 200 mg every twelve hours for seven days.

Note: Adults with impaired renal function may require a reduction in dose as follows:

| Creatinine clearance (mL/min)/(mL/sec) | Dose |
| --- | --- |
| > 30/0.5 | See *Usual adult dose* |
| ≤ 30/0.5 | 50% of the recommended dose every 12 hours |

### Usual pediatric dose
Children up to 18 years of age—Use is not recommended in infants, children, or adolescents since enoxacin causes arthropathy in immature animals.

### Usual geriatric dose
See *Usual adult dose*.

### Strength(s) usually available
U.S.—
- 200 mg (Rx) [*Penetrex*].
- 400 mg (Rx) [*Penetrex*].

Canada—
- Not commercially available.

**Packaging and storage**
Store below 40 °C (104 °F), preferably between 15 and 30 °C (59 and 86 °F), in a tight container.

**Auxiliary labeling**
- Take with a full glass of water.
- May cause dizziness, lightheadedness, or drowsiness.
- Continue medicine for full time of treatment.

---

[1]Not included in Canadian product labeling.

---

## LOMEFLOXACIN

### Summary of Differences

Pharmacology/pharmacokinetics: Longer half-life; may be dosed once a day.
Precautions: Drug interactions—Does not significantly interfere with the clearance of caffeine and theophylline.
Side/adverse effects: More likely to cause phototoxicity.

### Additional Dosing Information

**Diet/Nutrition**
When lomefloxacin was administered with food, the extent of absorption was only slightly decreased. Lomefloxacin may be taken with or without food.

### Oral Dosage Forms

Note: The dosing and strength of the dosage form available are expressed in terms of lomefloxacin base.

**LOMEFLOXACIN TABLETS**

**Usual adult dose**
Bronchitis, bacterial exacerbations[1]—
  Oral, 400 mg (base) once a day for ten days.
Urinary tract infections, prophylaxis[1]—
  Transrectal biopsy patients: Oral, 400 mg (base) as a single dose one to six hours prior to the start of surgery.
  Transurethral surgical patients: Oral, 400 mg (base) as a single dose two to six hours prior to the start of surgery.
Urinary tract infections, treatment[1]—
  Complicated: Oral, 400 mg (base) once a day for fourteen days.
  Uncomplicated, due to *Escherichia coli*: Oral, 400 mg (base) once a day for three days.
  Uncomplicated, due to *Klebsiella pneumoniae*, *Proteus mirabilis*, or *Staphylococcus saprophyticus*: Oral, 400 mg (base) once a day for ten days.

Note: Adults with impaired renal function may require a reduction in dose as follows:

| Creatinine clearance (mL/min)/(mL/sec) | Dose (base) |
|---|---|
| > 40/0.67 | See *Usual adult dose* |
| ≤ 40/0.67 or Hemodialysis | 400 mg for first dose, then 200 mg once a day |

**Usual pediatric dose**
Children up to 18 years of age—Use is not recommended in infants, children, and adolescents since lomefloxacin causes arthropathy in immature animals.

**Usual geriatric dose**
See *Usual adult dose*.

**Strength(s) usually available**
U.S.—
  400 mg (base) (Rx) [*Maxaquin* (scored; lactose)].
Canada—
  Not commerically available.

**Packaging and storage**
Store below 40 °C (104 °F), preferably between 15 and 30 °C (59 and 86 °F), in a tight container.

**Auxiliary labeling**
- Take with a full glass of water.
- May cause dizziness, lightheadedness, or drowsiness.
- Continue medicine for full time of treatment.

---

[1]Not included in Canadian product labeling.

---

## NORFLOXACIN

### Additional Dosing Information

**Diet/Nutrition**
The presence of food in the stomach may slightly decrease or delay absorption of norfloxacin. Therefore, norfloxacin should preferably be taken with a full glass (240 mL) of water on an empty stomach (either 1 hour before or 2 hours after meals or milk ingestion).
In studies with volunteers, crystalluria has been reported, especially with high doses (1200 or 1600 mg) and alkaline urine (pH 7 or above). Although crystalluria has not been reported with usual adult doses (400 mg twice a day), fluid intake should be sufficient to maintain urine output of at least 1200 to 1500 mL per day in adults.

### Oral Dosage Forms

Note: Bracketed uses in the *Dosage Forms* section refer to categories of use and/or indications that are not included in U.S. product labeling.

**NORFLOXACIN TABLETS USP**

**Usual adult dose**
[Gastroenteritis, bacterial][1]—
  Oral, 400 mg every eight to twelve hours for five days.
Gonorrhea—
  Oral, 800 mg as a single dose.
Prostatitis, acute or chronic[1]—
  Oral, 400 mg every twelve hours for twenty-eight days.
Urinary tract infections—
  Uncomplicated, due to *Escherichia coli*, *Klebsiella pneumoniae*, or *Proteus mirabilis*: Oral, 400 mg every twelve hours for three days.
  Uncomplicated, due to other indicated organisms: Oral, 400 mg every twelve hours for seven to ten days.

Note: Adults with impaired renal function may require a reduction in dose as follows:

| Creatinine clearance (mL/min)/(mL/sec) | Dose |
|---|---|
| > 30/0.5 | See *Usual adult dose* |
| ≤ 30/0.5 | 400 mg once a day |

**Usual adult prescribing limits**
1.2 grams per day for [gastroenteritis][1].
800 mg per day for all other indications.

**Usual pediatric dose**
Children up to 18 years of age—Use is not recommended in infants, children, or adolescents since norfloxacin causes arthropathy in immature animals.

**Usual geriatric dose**
See *Usual adult dose*.

**Strength(s) usually available**
U.S.—
  400 mg (Rx) [*Noroxin*].
Canada—
  400 mg (Rx) [*Noroxin*].

**Packaging and storage**
Store below 40 °C (104 °F), preferably between 15 and 30 °C (59 and 86 °F), in a tight container.

**Auxiliary labeling**
- Take with a full glass of water.
- Take on empty stomach.
- May cause dizziness, lightheadedness, or drowsiness.
- Continue medicine for full time of treatment.

---

[1]Not included in Canadian product labeling.

---

## OFLOXACIN

### Summary of Differences

Precautions: Drug interactions—Has a minor effect on the metabolism of theophylline.
General dosing information: Unlike intravenous ciprofloxacin, the dose of intravenous ofloxacin does not need to be changed from the oral dose.

## Additional Dosing Information

### Diet/Nutrition
Food has minor influence on the absorption of ofloxacin, causing only a slight decrease in the peak serum concentration and the area under the serum concentration–time curve (AUC). Therefore, ofloxacin may be taken with or without food.

Ofloxacin injection should only be administered by slow intravenous infusion over 60 minutes. Rapid or bolus injection may result in hypotension.

## Oral Dosage Forms

### OFLOXACIN TABLETS

#### Usual adult dose
Bronchitis, bacterial exacerbations or
Pneumonia, community-acquired or
Skin and soft tissue infections, uncomplicated—
    Oral, 400 mg every twelve hours for ten days.
Chlamydial infections, endocervical or urethral, with or without concurrent gonorrhea—
    Oral, 300 mg every twelve hours for seven days.
Gonorrhea, uncomplicated—
    Oral, 400 mg as a single dose.
Pelvic inflammatory disease, acute—
    Oral, 400 mg every twelve hours for ten to fourteen days.
Prostatitis—
    Oral, 300 mg every twelve hours for six weeks.
Urinary tract infections—
    Complicated: Oral, 200 mg every twelve hours for ten days.
    Cystitis, due to *Escherichia coli* or *Klebsiella pneumoniae*: Oral, 200 mg every twelve hours for three days.
    Cystitis, due to other indicated organisms: Oral, 200 mg every twelve hours for seven days.

Note: Adults with impaired renal function may require a reduction in dose as follows:

| Creatinine clearance (mL/min)/(mL/sec) | Dose (% of Usual adult dose) | Dosing interval (hr) |
|---|---|---|
| > 50/0.83 | 100 | 12 |
| 20–50/0.33–0.83 | 100 | 24 |
| < 20/0.33 | 50 | 24 |

#### Usual adult prescribing limits
400 mg per day for patients with severe hepatic function impairment (e.g., cirrhosis with or without ascites).

#### Usual pediatric dose
Children up to 18 years of age—Use is not recommended in infants, children, or adolescents since ofloxacin and other quinolones have been shown to cause arthropathy in immature animals.

#### Usual geriatric dose
See *Usual adult dose*.

#### Strength(s) usually available
U.S.—
    200 mg (Rx) [*Floxin* (lactose)].
    300 mg (Rx) [*Floxin* (lactose)].
    400 mg (Rx) [*Floxin* (lactose)].
Canada—
    200 mg (Rx) [*Floxin* (lactose)].
    300 mg (Rx) [*Floxin* (lactose)].
    400 mg (Rx) [*Floxin* (lactose)].

#### Packaging and storage
Store below 30 °C (86 °F). Store in a well-closed container.

#### Auxiliary labeling
- Take with a full glass of water.
- Continue medicine for full time of treatment.
- Do not take antacids, or zinc or iron preparations, within 2 hours of taking this medicine.

## Parenteral Dosage Forms

### OFLOXACIN IN DEXTROSE INJECTION

#### Usual adult dose
Bronchitis, bacterial exacerbations or
Pneumonia, community-acquired or
Skin and soft tissue infections, uncomplicated—
    Intravenous infusion, 400 mg, administered over a period of sixty minutes, every twelve hours for ten days.
Chlamydial infections, endocervical or urethral, with or without concurrent gonorrhea—
    Intravenous infusion, 300 mg, administered over a period of sixty minutes, every twelve hours for seven days.
Gonorrhea, uncomplicated—
    Intravenous infusion, 400 mg, administered over a period of sixty minutes, as a single dose.
Pelvic inflammatory disease, acute—
    Intravenous infusion, 400 mg, administered over a period of sixty minutes, every twelve hours for ten to fourteen days.
Prostatitis—
    Intravenous infusion, 300 mg, administered over a period of sixty minutes, every twelve hours for six weeks.
Urinary tract infections—
    Complicated: Intravenous infusion, 200 mg, administered over a period of sixty minutes, every twelve hours for ten days.
    Cystitis, due to *Escherichia coli* or *Klebsiella pneumoniae*: Intravenous infusion, 200 mg, administered over a period of sixty minutes, every twelve hours for three days.
    Cystitis, due to other indicated organisms: Intravenous infusion, 200 mg, administered over a period of sixty minutes, every twelve hours for seven days.

Note: Adults with renal function impairment may require a reduction in dose. See *Ofloxacin Tablets*.

#### Usual adult prescribing limits
See *Ofloxacin Tablets*.

#### Usual pediatric dose
Children up to 18 years of age—Use is not recommended in infants, children, or adolescents since ofloxacin and other quinolones have been shown to cause arthropathy in immature animals.

#### Usual geriatric dose
See *Usual adult dose*.

#### Strength(s) usually available
U.S.—
    200 mg per 50 mL (Rx) [*Floxin I.V.* (in 5% dextrose injection)].
    400 mg per 100 mL (Rx) [*Floxin I.V.* (in 5% dextrose injection)].
Canada—
    Not commercially available.

#### Packaging and storage
Store below 30 °C (86 °F). Protect from freezing and light.

#### Preparation of dosage form
Premixed ofloxacin in dextrose injection in flexible containers requires no further dilution prior to administration (see manufacturer's labeling for instructions). Since these injections contain no preservatives or bacteriostatic agent, they should be used promptly after opening; unused portions should be discarded.

Do not use the flexible containers in series connections. This may result in air embolism due to residual air being drawn from the primary container before administration of the fluid from the secondary container is complete.

#### Stability
Thaw frozen solutions at room temperature or in a refrigerator. Do not force thaw by microwave irradiation or immersion in water baths. Do not refreeze after initial thawing.

Ofloxacin in dextrose injection contains no preservatives or bacteriostatic agent. Do not use if injection is discolored or contains a precipitate.

#### Incompatibilities
Because only limited data are available on the compatibility of ofloxacin in dextrose injection with other intravenous substances, additives or other medications, including cefepime, should not be added to the preparation or infused simultaneously through the same intravenous line.

### OFLOXACIN INJECTION

#### Usual adult dose
See *Ofloxacin in Dextrose Injection*.

#### Usual adult prescribing limits
See *Ofloxacin in Dextrose Injection*.

#### Usual pediatric dose
See *Ofloxacin in Dextrose Injection*.

#### Usual geriatric dose
See *Ofloxacin in Dextrose Injection*.

#### Strength(s) usually available
U.S.—
    400 mg per 10 mL (Rx) [*Floxin I.V.* (in sterile water for injection; requires dilution prior to administration)].
Canada—
    Not commercially available.

### Packaging and storage
Store below 30 °C (86 °F). Protect from freezing and light.

### Preparation of dosage form
Ofloxacin in sterile water for injection requires dilution prior to administration. To prepare a solution at a concentration of 4 mg per mL for intravenous administration, add the volume of appropriate diluent (see manufacturer's package insert) as indicated below:

| Dose | Volume of ofloxacin concentrate to withdraw from vial | Volume of diluent to add |
|---|---|---|
| 200 mg | 5 mL | 45 mL |
| 300 mg | 7.5 mL | 67.5 mL |
| 400 mg | 10 mL | 90 mL |

The diluted solution should be administered only by intravenous infusion over a period of at least 60 minutes. Since these injections contain no preservatives or bacteriostatic agent, they should be used promptly after opening; unused portions should be discarded.

### Stability
When diluted to a concentration between 0.4 and 4 mg/mL, ofloxacin injection is stable for 72 hours when stored at or below 24 °C (75 °F) or for 14 days when refrigerated at 5 °C (41 °F) in glass bottles or plastic intravenous containers. Solutions that are diluted and frozen are stable for 6 months when stored at −20 °C (−4 °F). Once thawed, the solution is stable for up to 14 days when refrigerated (2 to 8 °C [36 to 46 °F]).

Thaw frozen solutions at room temperature or in a refrigerator. Do not force thaw by microwave irradiation or immersion in water baths. Do not refreeze after initial thawing.

Ofloxacin injection contains no preservatives or bacteriostatic agent. Do not use if injection is discolored or contains a precipitate.

### Incompatibilities
Because only limited data are available on the compatibility of ofloxacin injection with other substances, additives or other medications, including cefepime, should not be added to the preparation or infused simultaneously through the same intravenous line.

Revised: 07/07/98

### Table 1. Pharmacology/Pharmacokinetics

| Drug | Bioavailability (%) | Half-life (hr) Normal renal function | Half-life (hr) Impaired renal function | Time to peak serum concentration (hr) | Peak serum concentration after dose mcg/mL | Peak serum concentration after dose Dose (mg) | Peak urine concentration after dose mcg/mL | Peak urine concentration after dose Dose (mg) |
|---|---|---|---|---|---|---|---|---|
| Ciprofloxacin Oral | 70–80* | 4† | 6–8 | 1–2 | 1.2–1.4 / 2.4–4.3 / 3.4–4.3 / 5.4 | 250 / 500 / 750 / 1000 | >200 | 250 |
| IV | | 5–6 | | End of infusion | 2.1 / 4.6 | 200 / 400 | >200 | 200 |
| Enoxacin Oral | 90 | 3–6 | 9–10 | 1–3 | 0.9 / 2 | 200 / 400 | | |
| Lomefloxacin Oral | 95–98 | | 21–45 | 1.5 | 0.8 / 1.4 / 3–5.2 | 100 / 200 / 400 | >300 | 400 |
| Norfloxacin Oral | 30–70* | 3–4 | 6–9 | 1–2 | 1.4–1.6 / 2.5 | 400 / 800 | 98–200 | 400 |
| Ofloxacin Oral | 95–100 | 4.7–7‡ | 15–60§ | 1–2 | 1.5–2.6 / 4.6–5 | 200 / 400 | | |
| IV | | | | End of infusion | 2.3–2.7 / 5.5–7.2 | 200 / 400 | | |

*Absorption delayed in presence of food, although overall absorption not substantially affected.
†Half-life of ciprofloxacin slightly prolonged in elderly patients (approximately 6 hours).
‡Half-life of ofloxacin slightly prolonged in elderly patients (approximately 6 to 8.5 hours).
§Half-life of ofloxacin also prolonged in patients who have cirrhosis with ascites (approximately 7.3 to 19.5 hours).

### Table 2. Pharmacology/Pharmacokinetics*

| Drug | Protein binding (%) | Renal excretion (% unchanged/hrs) | Metabolism (%) | Biliary excretion (%) | Vol_D (liter/kg) | Removal by dialysis HD (%) | Removal by dialysis PD (%) |
|---|---|---|---|---|---|---|---|
| Ciprofloxacin | 20–40 | | 20 | | 2 | <10 | <10 |
| Oral | | 40–50/24 | | 20–35 | | | |
| IV | | 50–70/24 | | 15 | | | |
| Enoxacin | 40† | 40–60/48 | 20 | 18 | 1.6 | <5 | |
| Lomefloxacin | 10 | 60–80/48 | 5 | 10 | 1.8–2.5 | <3 | <3 |
| Norfloxacin | 10–15 | 26–40/24–48 | 20 | 28–30 | 3.2 | <10 | |
| Ofloxacin | 20–25 | 70–90/36 | 3 | 4–8 | 0.9–1.8 | 10–30 | 2–10 |

*Abbreviations: Vol_D = volume of distribution; HD = hemodialysis; PD = peritoneal dialysis; NS = not significant.
†Approximately 14% of enoxacin is bound to plasma proteins in patients with impaired renal function.

# FLUOROURACIL Systemic

VA CLASSIFICATION (Primary): AN300
Commonly used brand name(s): *Adrucil*.
Another commonly used name is 5-FU.

Note: For a listing of dosage forms and brand names by country availability, see *Dosage Forms* section(s).

## Category
Antineoplastic.

## Indications

Note: Bracketed information in the *Indications* section refers to uses that are not included in U.S. product labeling.

### Accepted
Carcinoma, colorectal (treatment)
Carcinoma, breast (treatment)
Carcinoma, gastric (treatment) or
Carcinoma, pancreatic (treatment)—Fluorouracil is indicated for palliative treatment of carcinoma of the colon, rectum, breast, stomach, and pancreas in patients considered to be incurable by surgery or other means.
[Carcinoma, bladder (treatment)]
[Carcinoma, prostatic (treatment)]
[Carcinoma, ovarian, epithelial (treatment)]
[Carcinoma, cervical (treatment)][1]
[Carcinoma, endometrial (treatment)][1]
[Carcinoma, anal (treatment)]
[Carcinoma, esophageal (treatment)]
[Carcinoma, skin (treatment)]
[Hepatoblastoma (treatment)]
[Carcinoma, hepatocellular, primary (treatment)][1] or
[Carcinoma, head and neck (treatment)]—Fluorouracil is also indicated for treatment of bladder carcinoma, prostatic carcinoma, epithelial ovarian carcinoma, cervical carcinoma, endometrial carcinoma, anal carcinoma, esophageal carcinoma, metastatic tumors of skin carcinoma, and hepatoblastoma, and is used by intra-arterial injection for treatment of hepatic tumors and head and neck tumors.
[Carcinoma, adrenocortical (treatment)][1]
[Carcinoma, vulvar (treatment)][1]
[Carcinoma, penile (treatment)][1] or
[Carcinoid tumors (treatment)][1]—Fluorouracil, in combination therapy, is reasonable medical therapy at some point in the management of adrenocortical carcinoma (Evidence rating: IIID), vulvar carcinoma (Evidence rating: IIID), penile carcinoma (Evidence rating: IIID), and carcinoid tumors (gastrointestinal and neuroendocrine tumors) (Evidence rating: IA).

Note: Although fluorouracil has been used for treatment of malignant pleural effusions, the USP Division of Information Development Hematology-Oncology Advisory Panel believes there is insufficient evidence to support the effectiveness of fluorouracil in the treatment of malignant pleural effusions.

[1]Not included in Canadian product labeling.

## Pharmacology/Pharmacokinetics

### Physicochemical characteristics
Molecular weight—130.08.

### Mechanism of action/Effect
Fluorouracil is an antimetabolite of the pyrimidine analog type. Fluorouracil is considered to be cell cycle–specific for the S phase of cell division. Activity results from its conversion to an active metabolite in the tissues, and includes inhibition of DNA and RNA synthesis.

### Distribution
Distributes into tumors, intestinal mucosa, bone marrow, liver, and other tissues; crosses the blood-brain barrier.

### Biotransformation
Rapidly, via a complex metabolic pathway in the tissues to produce an active metabolite, floxuridine monophosphate. Catabolic degradation occurs in the liver.

### Half-life
Intravenous—
  Approximately 16 minutes.

### Elimination
Primary route—Respiratory (approximately 90% as carbon dioxide).
Secondary route—Renal (approximately 7 to 20% unchanged; 90% of this in the first hour).

## Precautions to Consider

### Carcinogenicity
Secondary malignancies are potential delayed effects of many antineoplastic agents, although it is not clear whether the effect is related to their mutagenic or immunosuppressive action. The effect of dose and duration of therapy is also unknown, although risk seems to increase with long-term use.

Antimetabolites have been shown to be carcinogenic in animals and may be associated with an increased risk of development of secondary carcinomas in humans, although the risk appears to be less than with alkylating agents.

Long-term carcinogenicity studies in animals have not been done. However, studies in rats at oral doses of 0.01, 0.3, 1, or 3 mg per rat 5 days a week for 52 weeks, followed by a 6-month observation period, found no evidence of carcinogenicity. In addition, studies in male rats at intravenous doses of 33 mg per kg of body weight (mg/kg) once a week for 52 weeks, followed by observation for the rest of their lifetimes, found no evidence of carcinogenicity. Incidence of lung adenomas was unchanged in female mice given 1 mg of fluorouracil intravenously once a week for 16 weeks.

### Mutagenicity
Very high levels of fluorouracil produce oncogenic changes in cultured C3H/10T1/2 mouse embryo cells. In addition, fluorouracil has been found to be mutagenic in several strains of *Salmonella typhimurium*, including TA 1535, TA 1537, and TA 1538, and in *Saccharomyces cerevisiae*, but not in *Salmonella typhimurium* strains TA 92, TA 98, and TA 100. A positive effect was also observed in the micronucleus test on bone marrow cells of the mouse, and very high concentrations of fluorouracil produced chromosomal breaks in hamster fibroblasts *in vitro*.

### Pregnancy/Reproduction
Fertility—Gonadal suppression, resulting in amenorrhea or azoospermia, may occur in patients taking antineoplastic therapy, especially with the alkylating agents. In general, these effects appear to be related to the dose and duration of therapy and may be irreversible. Prediction of the degree of testicular or ovarian function impairment is complicated by the common use of combinations of several antineoplastics, which makes it difficult to assess the effects of individual agents.

In male rats given intraperitoneal doses of 125 or 250 mg/kg, fluorouracil induced chromosomal aberrations and changes in chromosomal organization of spermatogonia. In addition, inhibition of spermatogonial differentiation by fluorouracil resulted in transient infertility. However, fluorouracil did not produce any abnormalities at doses of up to 80 mg/kg per day in a strain of mouse that is sensitive to the induction of sperm head abnormalities after exposure to a range of chemical mutagens and carcinogens.

In female rats given intraperitoneal doses of 25 or 50 mg/kg per week for 3 weeks during the pre-ovulatory phase of oogenesis, fluorouracil significantly reduced the incidence of fertile matings, delayed the development of pre- and post-implantation embryos, increased the incidence of pre-implantation lethality, and induced chromosomal anomalies in these embryos. A limited study in rabbits with single doses of 25 mg/kg or five daily doses of 5 mg/kg found no effect on ovulation, no apparent effect on implantation, and only a limited effect in producing zygote destruction.

Pregnancy—Adequate and well-controlled studies in humans have not been done.
*First trimester*—
  It is usually recommended that use of antineoplastics, especially combination chemotherapy, be avoided whenever possible, especially during the first trimester. Although information is limited because of the relatively few instances of antineoplastic administration during pregnancy, the mutagenic, teratogenic, and carcinogenic potential of these medications must be considered.
  One case of multiple congenital anomalies has been reported with fluorouracil administration in the first trimester.
  Other hazards to the fetus include adverse reactions seen in adults.
  In general, use of a contraceptive is recommended during cytotoxic drug therapy.

*Teratogenic effects—*
Fluorouracil has been reported to be teratogenic in mice given single intraperitoneal doses of 10 to 40 mg/kg on days 10 and 12 of gestation, in rats given 12 to 37 mg/kg intraperitoneally between days 9 and 12 of gestation, and in hamsters given 3 to 9 mg intramuscularly between days 8 and 11 of gestation; these dosages, which are one to three times the maximum recommended human dose (MRHD), produced malformations including cleft palates, skeletal defects, and deformed appendages, paws, and tails. Teratogenicity did not occur in monkeys given divided doses of 40 mg/kg between days 20 and 24 of gestation.

*Nonteratogenic effects—*
Studies of effects of fluorouracil on perinatal and postnatal development in animals have not been done. However, in rats fluorouracil crosses the placenta and enters into fetal circulation, and use has resulted in increased resorptions and embryo deaths. Abortion occurred in all pregnant monkeys given doses of fluorouracil higher than 40 mg/kg.

FDA Pregnancy Category D.

**Breast-feeding**
It is not known whether fluorouracil is distributed into breast milk. Although very little information is available regarding distribution of antineoplastic agents into breast milk, breast-feeding is not recommended during chemotherapy because of the risks to the infant (adverse effects, mutagenicity, carcinogenicity).

**Pediatrics**
Appropriate studies on the relationship of age to the effects of fluorouracil have not been performed in the pediatric population. However, pediatrics-specific problems that would limit the usefulness of this medication in children are not expected.

**Geriatrics**
Although appropriate studies on the relationship of age to the effects of fluorouracil have not been performed in the geriatric population, geriatrics-specific problems are not expected to limit the usefulness of this medication in the elderly. However, elderly patients are more likely to have age-related renal function impairment, which may require reduction of dosage in patients receiving fluorouracil.

**Dental**
The bone marrow depressant effects of fluorouracil may result in an increased incidence of microbial infection, delayed healing, and gingival bleeding. Dental work, whenever possible, should be completed prior to initiation of therapy or deferred until blood counts have returned to normal. Patients should be instructed in proper oral hygiene during treatment, including caution in use of regular toothbrushes, dental floss, and toothpicks.

Fluorouracil also commonly causes ulcerative stomatitis, which may be associated with considerable discomfort.

**Drug interactions and/or related problems**
The following drug interactions and/or related problems have been selected on the basis of their potential clinical significance (possible mechanism in parentheses where appropriate)—not necessarily inclusive (» = major clinical significance):

Blood dyscrasia–causing medications (see *Appendix II*)
(leukopenic and/or thrombocytopenic effects of fluorouracil may be increased with concurrent or recent therapy if these medications cause the same effects; dosage adjustment of fluorouracil, if necessary, should be based on blood counts)

» Bone marrow depressants, other (see *Appendix II*) or
Radiation therapy
(additive bone marrow depression may occur; dosage reduction may be required when two or more bone marrow depressants, including radiation, are used concurrently or consecutively)

Leucovorin
(concurrent use may increase the therapeutic and toxic effects of fluorouracil; although the two medications may be used together for therapeutic advantage, dosage adjustment may be necessary)

Vaccines, killed virus
(because normal defense mechanisms may be suppressed by fluorouracil therapy, the patient's antibody response to the vaccine may be decreased. The interval between discontinuation of medications that cause immunosuppression and restoration of the patient's ability to respond to the vaccine depends on the intensity and type of immunosuppression-causing medication used, the underlying disease, and other factors; estimates vary from 3 months to 1 year)

» Vaccines, live virus
(because normal defense mechanisms may be suppressed by fluorouracil therapy, concurrent use with a live virus vaccine may potentiate the replication of the vaccine virus, may increase the side/adverse effects of the vaccine virus, and/or may decrease the patient's antibody response to the vaccine; immunization of these patients should be undertaken only with extreme caution after careful review of the patient's hematologic status and only with the knowledge and consent of the physician managing the fluorouracil therapy. The interval between discontinuation of medications that cause immunosuppression and restoration of the patient's ability to respond to the vaccine depends on the intensity and type of immunosuppression-causing medication used, the underlying disease, and other factors; estimates vary from 3 months to 1 year. Immunization with oral poliovirus vaccine should also be postponed in persons in close contact with the patient, especially family members)

Anticoagulants, coumarin-derivative, such as warfarin
(concurrent use may increase the anticoagulant effect; adjustment of anticoagulant dosage based on frequent prothrombin-time determinations is recommended)

**Laboratory value alterations**
The following have been selected on the basis of their potential clinical significance (possible effect in parentheses where appropriate)—not necessarily inclusive (» = major clinical significance):

With physiology/laboratory test values
Albumin, plasma
(may be decreased because of drug-induced protein malabsorption)

**Medical considerations/Contraindications**
The medical considerations/contraindications included have been selected on the basis of their potential clinical significance (reasons given in parentheses where appropriate)—not necessarily inclusive (» = major clinical significance).

*This medication should be used with extreme caution when the following medical problems exist:*

» Bone marrow depression
» Chickenpox, existing or recent (including recent exposure) or
» Herpes zoster
(risk of severe generalized disease)
» Hepatic function impairment
(reduced biotransformation; lower dosage is recommended)
» Infection
» Renal function impairment
(reduced elimination; lower dosage is recommended)
» Sensitivity to fluorouracil
» Tumor cell infiltration of bone marrow
» Extreme caution should be used also in patients who have had previous cytotoxic drug therapy with alkylating agents or high-dose pelvic radiation therapy; a lower dosage is recommended.

**Patient monitoring**
The following are especially important in patient monitoring (other tests may be warranted in some patients, depending on condition; » = major clinical significance):

Alanine aminotransferase (ALT [SGPT]) values and
Aspartate aminotransferase (AST [SGOT]) values and
Bilirubin concentrations, serum and
Lactate dehydrogenase (LDH) values
(recommended prior to initiation of therapy and at periodic intervals during therapy; frequency varies according to clinical state, agent, dose, and other agents being used concurrently)

» Examination of patient's mouth for ulceration
(recommended before administration of each dose)

» Hematocrit or hemoglobin and
» Leukocyte count, total and, if appropriate, differential and
» Platelet count
(determinations recommended prior to initiation of therapy and at periodic intervals during therapy; frequency varies according to clinical state, agent, dose, and other agents being used concurrently)

## Side/Adverse Effects

Note: Many "side effects" of antineoplastic therapy are unavoidable and represent the medication's pharmacologic action. Some of these (for example, leukopenia and thrombocytopenia) are actually used as parameters to aid in individual dosage titration.

Adverse effects associated with prolonged use of an arterial catheter include arterial ischemia, thrombosis, bleeding at the catheter site, blocked catheters, leakage at the site, embolism, fibromyositis, infection at the catheter site, abscesses, and thrombophlebitis.

The following side/adverse effects have been selected on the basis of their potential clinical significance (possible signs and symptoms in parentheses where appropriate)—not necessarily inclusive:

**Those indicating need for medical attention**
Incidence more frequent
*Diarrhea; esophagopharyngitis* (heartburn); *leukopenia or infection* (fever or chills; cough or hoarseness; lower back or side pain; painful or difficult urination)—usually asymptomatic; *ulcerative stomatitis* (sores in mouth and on lips)

Note: *Esophagopharyngitis* may lead to sloughing and ulceration.

*Leukopenia* usually occurs by 9 to 14 days after each course of treatment; the nadir of leukocyte count occurs about 9 to 14 days after the first day of a course of therapy (uncommonly, as long as 20 days) and usually recovers by about 30 days. Severity of bone marrow depression varies and determines subsequent dosage of fluorouracil.

Incidence less frequent
*Gastrointestinal ulceration* (black, tarry stools; severe nausea and vomiting; stomach cramps); *thrombocytopenia* (unusual bleeding or bruising; black, tarry stools; blood in urine or stools; pinpoint red spots on skin)—usually asymptomatic

Incidence rare
*Cerebellar syndrome, acute* (trouble with balance); *myocardial ischemia* (chest pain; shortness of breath); *palmar-plantar erythrodysesthesia syndrome* (tingling of hands and feet, followed by pain, redness, and swelling); *pneumopathy* (cough; shortness of breath)

Note: *Myocardial ischemia* may occur several hours after a dose; it usually develops after the second or later doses.

The *palmar-plantar erythrodysesthesia syndrome* is also known as hand-foot syndrome. It begins with tingling of hands and feet and may progress over the next few days to pain when holding objects or walking. Symmetrical swelling and erythema of palms and soles, with tenderness of the distal phalanges, occurs, possibly accompanied by desquamation. Symptoms gradually resolve over 5 to 7 days following withdrawal of fluorouracil. The syndrome may also be treatable with oral pyridoxine.

**Those indicating need for medical attention only if they continue or are bothersome**
Incidence more frequent
*Dermatitis* (skin rash and itching, usually on extremities and less frequently on trunk); *loss of appetite; nausea and vomiting; weakness*

Note: *Gastrointestinal distress* usually occurs on about the fourth day of therapy and subsides 2 or 3 days after the medication is stopped. *Weakness* usually occurs immediately and persists for 12 to 36 hours after administration.

Incidence less frequent
*Dry skin and fissuring*

**Those not indicating need for medical attention**
Incidence more frequent
*Alopecia* (loss of hair)

**Those indicating the need for medical attention if they occur after medication is discontinued**
Bone marrow depression (black, tarry stools; blood in urine or stools; cough or hoarseness; fever or chills; lower back or side pain; painful or difficult urination; pinpoint red spots on skin; unusual bleeding or bruising)

## Patient Consultation
As an aid to patient consultation, refer to *Advice for the Patient, Fluorouracil (Systemic)*.

In providing consultation, consider emphasizing the following selected information (» = major clinical significance):

**Before using this medication**
» Conditions affecting use, especially:
Sensitivity to fluorouracil
Pregnancy—Use not recommended because of mutagenic, teratogenic, and carcinogenic potential; advisability of using contraception; telling physician immediately if pregnancy is suspected
Breast-feeding—Not recommended because of risk of serious side effects
Other medications, especially other bone marrow depressants or previous cytotoxic drug or radiation therapy
Other medical problems, especially chickenpox, herpes zoster, hepatic function impairment, infection, or renal function impairment

**Proper use of this medication**
Caution with combination therapy; taking each medication at the right time
Frequency of nausea and vomiting; importance of continuing medication despite stomach upset

» Proper dosing

**Precautions while using this medication**
» Importance of close monitoring by the physician
» Avoiding immunizations unless approved by physician; other persons in patient's household should avoid immunizations with oral poliovirus vaccine; avoiding persons who have taken oral poliovirus vaccine or wearing a protective mask that covers nose and mouth

*Caution if bone marrow depression occurs*
» Avoiding exposure to persons with infections, especially during periods of low blood counts; checking with physician immediately if fever or chills, cough or hoarseness, lower back or side pain, or painful or difficult urination occurs
» Checking with physician immediately if unusual bleeding or bruising; black, tarry stools; blood in urine or stools; or pinpoint red spots on skin occur
Caution in use of regular toothbrush, dental floss, or toothpick; physician, dentist, or nurse may suggest alternatives; checking with physician before having dental work done
Not touching eyes or inside of nose unless hands are washed immediately before
Using caution to avoid accidental cuts with use of sharp objects such as safety razor or fingernail or toenail cutters
Avoiding contact sports or other situations where bruising or injury could occur

**Side/adverse effects**
May cause adverse effects such as blood problems and cancer; importance of discussing possible effects with physician
Signs of potential side effects, especially diarrhea, esophagopharyngitis, leukopenia, infection, ulcerative stomatitis, gastrointestinal ulceration, thrombocytopenia, acute cerebellar syndrome, myocardial ischemia, palmar-plantar erythrodysesthesia, and pneumopathy
Physician or nurse can help in dealing with side effects
Possibility of hair loss; normal hair growth should return after treatment has ended

## General Dosing Information
Patients receiving fluorouracil should be under supervision of a physician experienced in antimetabolite chemotherapy and should be hospitalized at least during the first course of treatment.

Dosage subsequent to the initial dose should be adjusted to meet the individual requirements of each patient, based on the patient's hematologic response to the previous dose. An additional course of fluorouracil should be given only after toxic effects from the first course have subsided.

Fluorouracil is recommended for parenteral use only. Fluorouracil should not be administered intrathecally because of neurotoxicity.

Administration of fluorouracil by slow intravenous infusion over 2 to 24 hours appears to reduce the toxicity, although rapid injections (over 1 to 2 minutes) may be more effective.

When fluorouracil is given intra-arterially, use of an appropriate infusion pump is recommended to ensure a uniform rate of infusion. In selected patients, a portable pump may be used.

Fluorouracil is an extremely toxic medication; therapy should be discontinued promptly at the first sign of:
Diarrhea
Esophagopharyngitis
Gastrointestinal ulceration and bleeding
Hemorrhage from any site
Leukopenia, marked, or rapidly falling leukocyte (particularly granulocyte) count
Stomatitis
Thrombocytopenia
Vomiting, intractable

Therapy may be reinitiated at a lower dose when side effects have subsided.

Special precautions are recommended in patients who develop thrombocytopenia as a result of administration of fluorouracil. These may include extreme care in performing invasive procedures; regular inspection of intravenous sites, skin (including perirectal area), and mucous membrane surfaces for signs of bleeding or bruising; limiting frequency of venipuncture and avoiding intramuscular injections; testing urine, emesis, stool, secretions for occult blood; care in use of regular toothbrushes, dental floss, toothpicks, safety razors, and fingernail and toenail cutters; avoiding constipation; and using caution to prevent falls and other injuries. Such patients should avoid alcohol and aspirin intake because of the risk of gastrointestinal bleeding. Platelet transfusions may be required.

Patients who develop leukopenia should be observed carefully for signs of infection. Antibiotic support may be required. In neutropenic patients who develop fever, broad-spectrum antibiotic coverage should be initiated empirically, pending bacterial cultures and appropriate diagnostic tests.

**Safety considerations for handling this medication**
There is limited but increasing evidence and concern that personnel involved in the preparation and administration of parenteral antineoplastics may be at some risk because of the potential mutagenicity, teratogenicity, and/or carcinogenicity of these agents, although the actual risk is unknown. USP advisory panels recommend cautious handling both in preparation and disposal of antineoplastic agents. Precautions that have been suggested include:
- Use of a biological containment cabinet during reconstitution and dilution of parenteral medications and wearing of disposable surgical gloves and masks.
- Use of proper technique to prevent contamination of the medication, work area, and operator during transfer between containers (including proper training of personnel in this technique).
- Cautious and proper disposal of needles, syringes, vials, ampuls, and unused medication.

A number of medical centers have developed detailed guidelines for handling of antineoplastic agents.

**Combination chemotherapy**
Fluorouracil may be used in combination with other agents in various regimens. As a result, incidence and/or severity of side effects may be altered and different dosages (usually reduced) may be used. For example, fluorouracil is part of the following chemotherapeutic combinations (some commonly used acronyms are in parentheses):
—cyclophosphamide, doxorubicin, and fluorouracil (CAF).
—cyclophosphamide, methotrexate, and fluorouracil (CMF).
—cyclophosphamide, methotrexate, fluorouracil, vincristine, and prednisone (CMFVP).
—fluorouracil, doxorubicin, and cyclophosphamide (FAC).
—fluorouracil, doxorubicin, and mitomycin (FAM).
—fluorouracil and leucovorin.

For specific dosages and schedules, consult the literature. For information regarding each agent, consult the individual monographs.

**For treatment of side/adverse effects**
The palmar-plantar erythrodysesthesia syndrome may be treated with oral pyridoxine in a dose of 100 to 150 mg per day.

## Parenteral Dosage Forms

Note: Bracketed uses in the *Dosage Forms* section refer to categories of use and/or indications that are not included in U.S. product labeling.

### FLUOROURACIL INJECTION USP

**Usual adult and adolescent dose**
Carcinoma, colorectal or
Carcinoma, breast or
Carcinoma, gastric or
Carcinoma, pancreatic or
[Carcinoma, bladder] or
[Carcinoma, prostatic] or
[Carcinoma, ovarian, epithelial]—
   Initial—
      Intravenous, 7 to 12 mg per kg of body weight per day for four days, then after three days if no toxicity has occurred, 7 to 10 mg per kg of body weight every three or four days, for a total course of two weeks or
      Intravenous, 12 mg per kg of body weight per day for four days, then after one day if no toxicity has occurred, 6 mg per kg of body weight every other day for four or five doses, for a total course of twelve days.
   Note: Poor-risk patients should receive a dose of 3 to 6 mg per kg of body weight per day for three days, then after one day if no toxicity has occurred, 3 mg per kg of body weight every other day for three doses.
   Maintenance—
      Intravenous, 7 to 12 mg per kg of body weight every seven to ten days or
      Intravenous, 300 to 500 mg per square meter of body surface area per day for four or five days, repeated monthly.
Note: Although dosages are based on the patient's actual weight, use of estimated lean body mass (dry weight) is recommended in obese patients or those with weight gain due to edema, ascites, or other abnormal fluid retention.

Fluorouracil has also been administered in a regimen containing no loading dose, at an intravenous dose of 15 mg per kg of body weight or 500 to 600 mg per square meter of body surface area once a week.
[Carcinoma, cervical][1] or
[Carcinoma, endometrial][1] or
[Carcinoma, anal] or
[Carcinoma, esophageal] or
[Carcinoma, skin] or
[Hepatoblastoma] or
[Carcinoma, hepatocellular, primary][1] or
[Carcinoma, head and neck] or
[Carcinoma, adrenocortical][1] or
[Carcinoma, vulvar][1] or
[Carcinoma, penile][1] or
[Carcinoid tumors][1]—
   Consult medical literature or manufacturer's literature for specific dosage.

**Usual adult prescribing limits**
800 mg daily (400 mg daily in poor-risk patients).

**Usual pediatric dose**
See *Usual adult and adolescent dose*.

**Strength(s) usually available**
U.S.—
   50 mg per mL (10-mL vials) (Rx) [*Adrucil*; GENERIC].
Canada—
   50 mg per mL (10- and 50-mL vials) (Rx) [*Adrucil* [GENERIC].

**Packaging and storage**
Store below 40 °C (104 °F), preferably between 15 and 30 °C (59 and 86 °F), unless otherwise specified by the manufacturer. Protect from light. Protect from freezing.

**Preparation of dosage form**
Fluorouracil Injection USP may be mixed with 5% dextrose injection or 0.9% sodium chloride injection for administration by intravenous infusion.

Note: The 50-mL vial is intended for intravenous admixture service use only. Entry into the vial should be made with a sterile dispensing device or transfer set that will accept a syringe hub; use of a syringe and needle is not recommended because of the risk of leakage and microbial and particulate contamination. Proper aseptic technique, under a laminar flow hood, should be used. Any unused portion should be discarded within 8 hours.

**Stability**
Although Fluorouracil Injection USP may discolor slightly during storage, potency and safety are not adversely affected. If a precipitate forms because of exposure to low temperatures, redissolve the medication by heating to 60 °C (140 °F) and shaking vigorously, then allow to cool to body temperature before using.

---

[1]Not included in Canadian product labeling.

Revised: 06/24/98

---

# FLUOROURACIL   Topical

VA CLASSIFICATION (Primary): DE600
Commonly used brand name(s): *Efudex*; *Fluoroplex*.
Another commonly used name is 5-FU.
Note: For a listing of dosage forms and brand names by country availability, see *Dosage Forms* section(s).

## Category
Antineoplastic, topical.

## Indications
Note: Bracketed information in the *Indications* section refers to uses that are not included in U.S. product labeling.

**Accepted**
Actinic keratoses, multiple (treatment)
[Actinic cheilitis (treatment)][1]
[Leukoplakia, mucosal (treatment)][1]
[Radiodermatitis (treatment)][1]
[Bowen's disease (treatment)][1] or

[Erythroplasia of Queyrat (treatment)][1]—Topical fluorouracil is indicated for treatment of precancerous skin conditions including multiple actinic (solar) keratoses, actinic cheilitis, mucosal leukoplakia, radiodermatitis, Bowen's disease, and erythroplasia of Queyrat.

Carcinoma, skin (treatment)—Topical fluorouracil is indicated for treatment of superficial basal cell carcinomas (multiple lesions or difficult access sites), although conventional treatment is preferred whenever possible.

Note: The diagnosis should be established prior to treatment, since topical fluorouacil has not been proven effective in other types of basal cell carcinomas. Surgery is preferred with isolated, easily accessible basal cell carcinomas, since success with such lesions is almost 100%. The success rate with fluorouracil cream and solution is approximately 93%.

---

[1]Not included in Canadian product labeling.

## Pharmacology/Pharmacokinetics

**Physicochemical characteristics**
Molecular weight—130.08.
pKa—8 and 13.

**Mechanism of action/Effect**
There is evidence that the metabolism of fluorouracil via the anabolic pathway blocks the methylation reaction of deoxyuridylic acid to thymidylic acid. In this manner fluorouracil interferes with the synthesis of DNA and, to a lesser extent, inhibits the formation of RNA. Since DNA and RNA are essential for cell division and growth, the effect of fluorouracil may be to create a thymine deficiency, which provokes unbalanced growth and death of the cell. The effects of DNA and RNA deprivation are most marked on cells that grow more rapidly and take up fluorouracil at a more rapid rate.

**Absorption**
Systemic absorption studies of topically applied fluorouracil have been performed on patients with actinic keratoses using tracer amounts of carbon-labeled fluorouracil added to a 5% preparation. All patients had been receiving nonlabeled fluorouracil until the peak of the inflammatory reaction occurred (2 to 3 weeks), ensuring that the time of maximum absorption was used for measurement. One gram of labeled preparation was applied to the entire face and neck and left in place for 12 hours. At the end of 3 days, urine samples were collected. The total recovery ranged between 0.48% and 0.94% with an average of 0.76%, indicating that approximately 5.98% of the topical dose was absorbed systemically. If applied twice daily, this would indicate systemic absorption of topical fluorouracil to be in the range of 5 to 6 mg per daily dose of 100 mg.

**Distribution**
In one clinical study, negligible amounts of labeled material were found in the plasma after 3 days of treatment with topically applied carbon-labeled fluorouracil.

**Onset of action**
2 to 3 days. A treatment period of 2 to 6 weeks is usually required to reach the erosion and necrosis stage, or up to 12 weeks in some patients with superficial basal cell carcinomas. Complete healing may not occur until 1 to 2 months after therapy is stopped.

## Precautions to Consider

**Carcinogenicity**
Studies have not been done. However, morphological transformation of cells was produced by fluorouracil in three *in vitro* cell transformation assays. In one of these assays, a metabolite of fluorouracil produced morphological transformation, and injection of the transformed cells into immunosuppressed syngeneic mice produced malignant tumors.

**Mutagenicity**
Parenteral administration of fluorouracil in humans at cumulative doses of 240 mg to 1 gram has produced an increase in numerical and structural chromosome aberrations in peripheral blood lymphocytes. Fluorouracil is mutagenic in yeast cells, *Bacillus subtilis*, and *Drosophila* assays. It produced chromosome damage in an *in vitro* hamster fibroblast assay at concentrations of 1 and 2 mcg per liter and increased micronuclei formation in the bone marrow of mice at intraperitoneal doses within the human therapeutic dose range of 12 to 15 mg per kg of body weight (mg/kg) per day. Results of the dominant lethal mutation assay performed in mice were negative.

**Pregnancy/Reproduction**
Fertility—Parenteral fluorouracil impairs fertility in rats. In mice, single-dose intravenous and intraperitoneal injections of fluorouracil killed differentiated spermatogonia and spermatocytes at a dose of 500 mg/kg and produced abnormalities in spermatids at a dose of 50 mg/kg.

Pregnancy—Adequate and well-controlled studies with either the topical or the parenteral forms of fluorouracil have not been done in humans. However, topical fluorouracil may cause fetal harm when administered to a pregnant woman. One case of birth defect, cleft lip and palate, has been reported in the newborn of a patient using topical fluorouracil as recommended. One case of birth defect, ventricular septal defect, and some cases of miscarriage have been reported when topical fluorouracil was applied to mucous membrane areas. Multiple birth defects were reported in the fetus of a patient treated with intravenous fluorouracil.

Studies with topical fluorouracil have not been done in animals. Fluorouracil administered parenterally has been shown to be teratogenic in mice, rats, and hamsters when given at doses equivalent to the usual human intravenous dose. However, the amount of fluorouracil absorbed systemically after topical administration to actinic keratoses is minimal.

FDA Pregnancy Category X.

**Breast-feeding**
It is not known whether topical fluorouracil is distributed into breast milk. However, there is some systemic absorption of fluorouracil after topical administration. Therefore, because of the potential for serious adverse reactions in nursing infants, a decision should be made whether to discontinue nursing or to discontinue use of topical fluorouracil, taking into account the importance of topical fluorouracil treatment to the mother.

**Pediatrics**
Appropriate studies on the relationship of age to the effects of topical fluorouracil have not been performed in the pediatric population. Safety and efficacy have not been established.

**Geriatrics**
Appropriate studies on the relationship of age to the effects of topical fluorouracil have not been performed in the geriatric population. However, geriatrics-specific problems that would limit the usefulness of this medication in elderly patients are not expected.

**Laboratory value alterations**
The following have been selected on the basis of their potential clinical significance (possible effect in parentheses where appropriate)—not necessarily inclusive (» = major clinical significance):

With physiology/laboratory test values
   Eosinophilia and
   Leukocytosis and
   Thrombocytopenia and
   Toxic granulation
     (may occur)

**Medical considerations/Contraindications**
The medical considerations/contraindications included have been selected on the basis of their potential clinical significance (reasons given in parentheses where appropriate)—not necessarily inclusive (» = major clinical significance).

*Risk-benefit should be considered when the following medical problems exist:*

Hemorrhagic ulcerated tissues
   (significant systemic absorption and toxicity may occur)
Pre-existing dermatoses, especially chloasma and rosacea
   (may be accentuated by the inflammatory response to fluorouracil)
» Sensitivity to fluorouracil

**Patient monitoring**
The following may be especially important in patient monitoring (other tests may be warranted in some patients, depending on condition; » = major clinical significance):

Biopsy
   (recommended to confirm diagnosis if actinic (solar) keratoses do not respond or if they recur after treatment, and to confirm cure of superficial basal cell carcinomas)

## Side/Adverse Effects

The following side/adverse effects have been selected on the basis of their potential clinical significance (possible signs and symptoms in parentheses where appropriate)—not necessarily inclusive:

**Those indicating need for medical attention**
Incidence more frequent
   *Inflammatory response or allergic reaction* (redness and swelling of normal skin)
   Note: A delayed *hypersensitivity* reaction may occur. Patch testing for hypersensitivity may be inconclusive.

## Fluorouracil (Topical)

**Those indicating need for medical attention only if they continue or are bothersome**
Incidence more frequent
  *Burning feeling at site of application; contact dermatitis* (skin rash); *increased sensitivity of skin to sunlight; itching; oozing; soreness or tenderness of skin*
Incidence less frequent or rare
  *Darkening of skin; scaling; watery eyes*

## Patient Consultation

As an aid to patient consultation, refer to *Advice for the Patient, Fluorouracil (Topical)*.

In providing consultation, consider emphasizing the following selected information (» = major clinical significance):

**Before using this medication**
» Conditions affecting use, especially:
    Sensitivity to fluorouracil
    Pregnancy—Use not recommended because of teratogenic potential; some systemic absorption occurs
    Breast-feeding—Not recommended because of risk of serious side effects; some systemic systemic absorption occurs

**Proper use of this medication**
» Compliance with therapy; applying enough medication to cover affected areas
   Washing area to be treated with soap and water and drying thoroughly; using cotton-tipped applicator or fingertips to apply
» Washing hands immediately after application if fingertips are used
   Possible unsightly and uncomfortable reaction during therapy and for several weeks after therapy is completed; possible temporary pink, smooth spot left during healing; checking with physician before discontinuing medication
» Proper dosing
   Missed dose: Applying as soon as remembered; not applying if not remembered within a few hours; checking with physician if more than one dose is missed
» Proper storage

**Precautions while using this medication**
» Importance of close monitoring by physician
» Caution in applying medication; avoiding eyes, nose, and mouth
» Possible photosensitivity reactions during therapy and for 1 or 2 months after therapy is completed; avoiding sun; using protective clothing and sun block product; avoiding use of sunlamp, tanning bed, or tanning booth

**Side/adverse effects**
   Signs of potential side effects, especially inflammatory response or allergic reaction

## General Dosing Information

Patients using topical fluorouracil should be under supervision of a physician experienced in use of the medication.

Patients should be forewarned that the reaction in the treated areas may be unsightly during therapy and, usually, following cessation of therapy. Patients should be instructed to avoid exposure to ultraviolet rays during and immediately following treatment with topical fluorouracil because the intensity of the reaction may be increased. If topical fluorouracil is applied with the fingers, the hands should be washed immediately afterward. Topical fluorouracil should not be applied on the eyelids or directly into the eyes, nose, or mouth, because irritation may occur.

When topical fluorouracil is applied to a lesion, a response occurs in the following sequence: erythema, usually followed by vesiculation, desquamation, erosion, and epithelialization.

Fluorouracil cream or solution should be applied twice daily on actinic or solar keratoses in an amount sufficient to cover the lesions. Medication should be continued until the inflammatory response reaches the erosion stage, at which time use of topical fluorouracil should be terminated. The usual duration of therapy is from 2 to 4 weeks. Complete healing of the lesions may not be evident for 1 to 2 months following cessation of topical fluorouracil therapy.

In superficial basal cell carcinomas, only the 5% strength is recommended. Fluorouracil cream or solution should be applied twice daily in an amount sufficient to cover the lesions. Treatment should be continued for at least 3 to 6 weeks. Therapy may be required for as long as 10 to 12 weeks before the lesions are obliterated. As in any neoplastic condition, the patient should be followed for a reasonable period of time to determine if a cure has been obtained.

Occlusion of the skin with consequent hydration has been shown to increase percutaneous penetration of several topical preparations. Therefore, if any occlusive dressing is used in treatment of basal cell carcinoma, there may be an increase in the severity of inflammatory reactions in the adjacent normal skin. A porous gauze dressing may be applied for cosmetic reasons without an increase in reaction.

It is recommended that treatment with fluorouracil be discontinued if an excessive inflammatory response occurs on normal skin.

## Topical Dosage Forms

### FLUOROURACIL CREAM USP

**Usual adult dose**
Actinic (solar keratoses)—
   Topical, to the skin, as a 1% cream once or twice a day in a sufficient amount to cover the lesions. Usually the 1% strength is effective on the head, neck, and chest; 2 to 5% may be needed on the hands.
Superficial basal cell carcinomas—
   Topical, to the skin, as a 5% cream twice a day in a sufficient amount to cover the lesions, for at least three to six weeks, and possibly up to twelve weeks.

**Usual pediatric dose**
Safety and efficacy have not been established.

**Strength(s) usually available**
U.S.—
   1% (Rx) [*Fluoroplex* (benzyl alcohol)].
   5% (Rx) [*Efudex* (methylparaben; propylparaben)].
Canada—
   1% (Rx) [*Fluoroplex* (benzyl alcohol)].
   5% (Rx) [*Efudex*].

**Packaging and storage**
Store below 40 °C (104 °F), preferably between 15 and 30 °C (59 and 86 °F), unless otherwise specified by the manufacturer. Store in a tight container.

**Auxiliary labeling**
• For the skin.
• Continue medicine for full course of treatment.
• Avoid overexposure to sun.

### FLUOROURACIL TOPICAL SOLUTION USP

**Usual adult dose**
Actinic (solar keratoses)—
   Topical, to the skin, as a 1 or 2% solution once or twice a day in a sufficient amount to cover the lesions. Usually the 1% strength is effective on the head, neck, and chest; 2 to 5% may be needed on the hands.
Superficial basal cell carcinomas—
   Topical, to the skin, as a 5% solution twice a day in a sufficient amount to cover the lesions, for at least three to six weeks, and possibly up to twelve weeks.

**Usual pediatric dose**
Safety and efficacy have not been established.

**Strength(s) usually available**
U.S.—
   1% (Rx) [*Fluoroplex*].
   2% (Rx) [*Efudex* (methylparaben; propylparaben)].
   5% (Rx) [*Efudex* (methylparaben; propylparaben)].
Canada—
   1% (Rx) [*Fluoroplex*].

**Packaging and storage**
Store between 15 and 30 °C (59 and 86 °F), unless otherwise specified by manufacturer. Store in a tight container. Protect from freezing.

**Auxiliary labeling**
• For the skin.
• Continue medicine for full course of treatment.
• Avoid overexposure to sun.

Revised: 09/30/97

# FLUOXETINE Systemic

VA CLASSIFICATION (Primary/Secondary): CN603/CN900
Commonly used brand name(s): *Prozac*.
Note: For a listing of dosage forms and brand names by country availability, see *Dosage Forms* section(s).

## Category

Antidepressant; antiobsessional agent; antibulimic agent.

## Indications

### Accepted

Depressive disorder, major (treatment)—Fluoxetine is indicated for the treatment of major depressive disorder. Treatment of acute depressive episodes typically requires 6 to 12 months of antidepressant therapy. Patients with recurrent or chronic depression may require long-term treatment. Fluoxetine has shown effective maintenance of antidepressant response for up to 50 weeks of treatment in a placebo-controlled trial.

Obsessive-compulsive disorder (treatment)—Fluoxetine is indicated for the treatment of obsessions and compulsions in patients with obsessive-compulsive disorder.

Bulimia nervosa (treatment)—Fluoxetine is indicated for the treatment of binge-eating and vomiting behaviors in patients with moderate to severe bulimia nervosa.

[Premenstrual dysphoric disorder (treatment)][1]—Fluoxetine is used to relieve the symptoms of premenstrual dysphoric disorder (PMDD). PMDD was formerly known as late luteal phase dysphoric disorder (LLPDD) and is distinguishable from the cyclic changes in mood commonly known as premenstrual syndrome (PMS) by its greater severity of symptoms. (Evidence rating: B-1)

[1] Not included in Canadian product labeling.

## Pharmacology/Pharmacokinetics

### Physicochemical characteristics

Chemical group—Cyclic, propylamine-derivative. Chemically unrelated to tricyclic or tetracyclic antidepressants. Fluoxetine is a 50:50 racemic mixture of R- and S-fluoxetine.
Molecular weight—Fluoxetine: 309.33.
  Fluoxetine hydrochloride: 345.79.
Solubility—14 mg per mL water.

### Mechanism of action/Effect

The antidepressant, antiobsessional, and antibulimic effects of fluoxetine are thought to be related to its effects on serotonergic neurotransmission. Fluoxetine is a potent and selective inhibitor of serotonin (5-HT) uptake, but not of norepinephrine or dopamine uptake, in the central nervous system (CNS). In depressed patients who had received 40 to 60 mg per day of fluoxetine for 6 weeks, the cerebrospinal fluid concentrations of the metabolites of 5-HT (5-HIAA), dopamine (HVA), and norepinephrine (HMPG) were reduced by 46%, 14%, and 18%, respectively. Because uptake inactivates serotonin by removing it from the synaptic cleft, uptake inhibition by fluoxetine enhances serotonergic function. As a consequence, the $5-HT_1$ receptors are desensitized or downregulated after long-term fluoxetine administration. Fluoxetine does not interact directly with postsynaptic serotonin receptors, muscarinic-cholinergic receptors, histaminergic receptors, or alpha-adrenergic receptors. Fluoxetine does not appear to cause downregulation of postsynaptic beta-adrenergic receptors or a decrease in beta-adrenergic–stimulated cyclic adenosine monophosphate (cAMP) generation as do older antidepressant medications.

### Other actions/effects

Fluoxetine may exhibit an acute anorectic effect and could potentially cause weight loss proportional to the degree of initial obesity as measured by the body mass index (BMI).

Fluoxetine and norfluoxetine inhibit the isoenzyme cytochrome P450 2D6 (CYP2D6) potently, and, to a lesser extent, CYP3A. Fluoxetine is a moderately potent inhibitor of CYP2C9 and CYP2C19.

Fluoxetine blocks the uptake of 5-HT into human platelets as well as into neurons.

### Absorption

Well absorbed with a small first-pass effect. Food does not affect the extent of absorption, although the rate may be slightly decreased.

### Distribution

Fluoxetine has a large volume of distribution. In eight patients being treated with fluoxetine for major depression or obsessive-compulsive disorder, the mean ratio of brain concentration to plasma concentration of fluoxetine plus its metabolites was 2.6.

### Protein binding

High (94.5%).

### Biotransformation

Metabolized by demethylation in the liver to the active metabolite, norfluoxetine, and other unidentified metabolites. *In vivo* studies indicate that cytochrome P450 2D6 (CYP2D6) is involved in fluoxetine metabolism. An *in vitro* study indicates that CYP2C9 and, to a lesser extent, CYP3A may also be involved in fluoxetine metabolism.

The active metabolite of fluoxetine, norfluoxetine, exists as a racemic mixture. The selective serotonin reuptake inhibition activity of S-norfluoxetine is comparable to that of fluoxetine. R-norfluoxetine is significantly less potent than the parent compound.

### Half-life

Elimination—
  Fluoxetine: 1 to 3 days after a single dose, and 4 to 6 days with long-term administration.
  Norfluoxetine: 4 to 16 days after single dose or long-term administration.
  After long-term or high-dose use, it may take 1 to 2 months for the active moieties to be eliminated from the body. In four patients who had received 80 mg of fluoxetine per day for 52 ± 8 weeks, the elimination half-lives of fluoxetine and norfluoxetine were found to be 8 days and 19.3 days, respectively. This extended elimination time may have reflected the increased plasma concentrations achieved with high dosing, since fluoxetine displays nonlinear pharmacokinetics, as well as the extensive distribution of fluoxetine in the body.

### Onset of action

Depression—Effects have been seen in 1 to 3 weeks; however, response may require 4 to 6 weeks to occur.
Obsessive-compulsive disorder—Full effectiveness may not occur for 5 or more weeks.
Bulimia nervosa—Significant improvement has been seen in 1 week; however, response may require 4 to 6 weeks to occur.

### Time to peak concentration

6 to 8 hours after a single oral dose of 40 mg.

### Time to steady-state concentration

Approximately 4 weeks for fluoxetine and norfluoxetine.

### Peak serum concentration

Single dose (40 mg)—
  Fluoxetine: 15 to 55 nanograms per mL. Fluoxetine exhibits nonlinear pharmacokinetics; higher doses lead to disproportionately higher plasma concentrations.
Multiple dose (40 mg a day for 30 days)—
  Fluoxetine: 91 to 302 nanograms per mL. After multiple dosing, plasma fluoxetine concentrations are higher than predicted by single-dose kinetics.
  Norfluoxetine: 72 to 258 nanograms per mL. Norfluoxetine appears to have linear kinetics.

### Elimination

Renal—
  80% excreted in the urine (11.6% fluoxetine, 7.4% fluoxetine glucuronide, 6.8% norfluoxetine, 8.2% norfluoxetine glucuronide, > 20% hippuric acid, 46% other). Renal function impairment does not alter fluoxetine or norfluoxetine pharmacokinetics; however, effects on other metabolites are unknown.
Biliary—
  Approximately 15% in the feces.
In dialysis—
  Not dialyzable because of high protein binding and large volume of distribution.

## Precautions to Consider

### Carcinogenicity

Two-year studies in rats and mice given dietary fluoxetine in doses equivalent to 1.2 and 0.7 times, respectively, the maximum recommended human dose (MRHD) on a mg per square meter of body surface area (mg/m²) basis showed no evidence of carcinogenicity.

### Mutagenicity
Fluoxetine and norfluoxetine have shown no genotoxic effects in the bacterial mutation assay, DNA repair assay in cultured rat hepatocytes, mouse lymphoma assay, or *in vivo* sister chromatid exchange assay in Chinese hamster bone marrow cells.

### Pregnancy/Reproduction
Fertility—No evidence of adverse effects on fertility was seen in rats given fluoxetine doses of 0.9 to 1.5 times the MRHD on a mg/m$^2$ basis.

Pregnancy—A study comparing birth outcomes between women who took fluoxetine only during the first and second trimesters of pregnancy and women who took fluoxetine during the third trimester of pregnancy found an increased risk of premature delivery and poor neonatal adaptation, including respiratory difficulties, cyanosis on feeding, and jitteriness, in the neonates who had been exposed during the third trimester. In addition, the number of neonates exhibiting more than three minor anomalies was greater among neonates who had been exposed to fluoxetine during the first trimester than among neonates with no *in utero* exposure to fluoxetine. However, a previous analysis of birth outcomes among women taking various antidepressant medications during pregnancy, including 96 women taking fluoxetine, either as monotherapy or in combination with other medications, found the rates of adverse pregnancy outcome to be within the normal limits. Also, an analysis of the manufacturer's registry of fluoxetine-exposed pregnancies, which comprised 123 pregnancies at the time of analysis, found the rates of adverse outcome to be within the normal limits, as did a prospective study comparing pregnancy outcomes of 128 women who took fluoxetine during the first trimester with pregnancy outcomes of 128 age-matched controls who took medications known to be nonteratogenic during the first trimester. A study of preschoolers and young children revealed no differences in global intelligence, language development, or behavioral development between a group of 55 preschoolers and young children with *in utero* fluoxetine exposure, either during the first trimester or throughout gestation, and a group of 84 preschoolers and young children with no fluoxetine exposure.

Petechiae and a cephalohematoma, in addition to jitteriness and hypertonia, were reported in a newborn whose mother was receiving 60 mg per day of fluoxetine to treat obsessive-compulsive disorder. However, at a 5-month follow-up, the infant was normal. Serum fluoxetine and norfluoxetine concentrations on the infant's second day of life were 129 and 227 nanograms per mL, respectively.

No evidence of teratogenicity was found in studies in rats and rabbits receiving fluoxetine doses that were 1.5 and 3.6 times, respectively, the MRHD on a mg/m$^2$ basis. However, an increase in stillbirths and pup deaths during the first postpartum week was seen in rats given 1.5 times the MRHD on a mg/m$^2$ basis during gestation or 0.9 times the MRHD on a mg/m$^2$ basis during gestation and lactation.

FDA Pregnancy Category C.

Labor and delivery—The effect of fluoxetine on labor and delivery is not known.

### Breast-feeding
Fluoxetine is distributed into breast milk. In a study of 10 mothers and 11 nursing infants ranging in age from 20 to 747 days, the concentration of fluoxetine in breast milk was found to be linearly correlated with maternal fluoxetine dose and, in most cases, to peak within 6 hours after the dose was taken. Infant exposure to fluoxetine plus norfluoxetine was estimated using mean fluoxetine and norfluoxetine milk concentrations and an assumed milk intake of one liter per day. The estimated infant exposure was 10.8% (range 6.3 to 13.9%) of the maternal fluoxetine dose in mg per kg of body weight (mg/kg). Mothers in this study reported no adverse effects in the infants. However, in one case report, vomiting, watery stools, crying, and sleep disorders were reported in the 6-week-old infant of a nursing mother taking 20 mg of fluoxetine a day; these symptoms remitted when breast-feeding was interrupted and recurred when the infant was rechallenged with breast milk. Total drug exposure will be affected by the maturity of the metabolic and excretory systems of the infant, with very young infants having lower drug clearance and higher exposure. Use of fluoxetine in nursing mothers is not recommended. However, the risks and benefits to both the mother and the infant must be considered in each case.

### Pediatrics
Fluoxetine has been studied for a variety of indications in over 300 patients 7 to 18 years of age. Most of the studies were open trials; almost all of the studies had 40 or fewer subjects; and results were variable. However, one randomized, double-blind, placebo-controlled study in 96 children 7 to 17 years of age (48 receiving 20 mg per day of fluoxetine and 48 receiving placebo), who were diagnosed with major depressive disorder, found fluoxetine to be superior to placebo in relieving depressive symptoms. The difference between the two groups became statistically significant after 5 weeks of treatment. Response in children 7 through 12 years of age did not differ from response in adolescents 13 through 17 years of age, nor was there a difference in response between males and females. Although the available information is insufficient to establish the efficacy of fluoxetine in children, it does provide some evidence of effectiveness of fluoxetine in the treatment of depression and obsessive-compulsive disorder.

Children may be more sensitive than adults to the behavioral adverse effects of fluoxetine, including mania or hypomania, social inhibition, irritability, restlessness, and insomnia.

### Geriatrics
No geriatric-specific problems have been documented in studies done to date that included elderly patients.

### Pharmacogenetics
Approximately 2 to 10% of the adult population has a reduced ability to metabolize substrates of cytochrome P450 2D6 (CYP2D6). In these patients, the rate of S-fluoxetine metabolism is decreased, leading to higher plasma concentrations of S-fluoxetine and lower plasma concentrations of S-norfluoxetine than are seen in normal metabolizers. However, the metabolism of R-fluoxetine appears to be unaffected. The sum concentration of the four active moieties is not significantly different between patients with reduced CYP2D6 activity and patients with normal CYP2D6 activity.

### Drug interactions and/or related problems
The following drug interactions and/or related problems have been selected on the basis of their potential clinical significance (possible mechanism in parentheses where appropriate)—not necessarily inclusive (» = major clinical significance):

Note: Because fluoxetine is a potent inhibitor of cytochrome P450 2D6 (CYP2D6) there is a potential for interaction with medications that are metabolized by this enzyme, other than those listed below, such as flecainide, metoprolol, risperidone, and vinblastine. A reduction in the dosage of medications that are metabolized by CYP2D6 may be needed when they are used concurrently with fluoxetine or within 5 weeks of discontinuing fluoxetine.

Fluoxetine also inhibits CYP3A, CYP2C9, and CYP2C19. Possible interactions with medications that are metabolized by these isoenzymes, other than those listed below, such as nifedipine (CYP3A), diclofenac (CYP2C9), and omeprazole (CYP2C19), should be considered.

Combinations containing any of the following medications, depending on the amount present, may also interact with this medication.

Alcohol
(although fluoxetine has not been shown to alter alcohol metabolism and does not appear to potentiate cognitive or psychomotor effects of alcohol in healthy subjects, concomitant use is not recommended)

» Alprazolam or
Diazepam
(concurrent use with fluoxetine may prolong the half-lives of these medications; decreased psychomotor performance has been reported with concurrent use of alprazolam but not with concurrent use of diazepam)

» Antidepressants, tricyclic (TCAs)
(plasma concentrations of the TCAs and/or their active metabolites may be increased twofold to tenfold when they are used with or within 3 or more weeks after discontinuation of fluoxetine; although beneficial effects of the combination have been reported, there have been reports of serious adverse effects, including seizures and death; if these medications are to be administered concurrently or if TCA therapy is to be initiated shortly after the discontinuation of fluoxetine, the initial TCA dosage should be reduced and TCA plasma concentrations should be monitored)

» Astemizole
(because of the possibility that fluoxetine may inhibit the metabolism of astemizole, leading to increased blood levels and risk of cardiac arrhythmias, including *torsades de pointes*, concurrent use is not recommended)

Carbamazepine
(although small drug interaction studies have yielded conflicting results regarding the effect of fluoxetine on the plasma concentrations of carbamazepine and its metabolite, carbamazepine-10,11-epoxide, there have been reports of increased anticonvulsant concentrations and toxicity after the initiation of fluoxetine treatment in patients stabilized on carbamazepine)

Cyproheptadine
(may reverse the therapeutic effects of fluoxetine)

Electroconvulsive therapy
  (prolonged seizures have been reported in patients on concomitant fluoxetine therapy)
Clozapine or
Haloperidol or
Loxapine or
Molindone or
Phenothiazines or
Pimozide or
Thioxanthenes
  (caution in concurrent use of other CNS-active medications with fluoxetine is recommended because of a potentially increased risk of side effects)
  (elevated concentrations of clozapine, fluphenazine, and haloperidol have been reported in patients receiving concomitant fluoxetine)
  (cases of bradycardia and mental status changes have been reported with concurrent pimozide and fluoxetine use)
» Highly protein-bound medications, especially:
  Anticoagulants
  Digitalis or digitoxin
    (caution in concurrent use with fluoxetine is recommended because of possible displacement of either medication from protein-binding sites, leading to increased plasma concentrations of the free [unbound] medications and increased risk of adverse effects)
    (increased international normalized ratio [INR] measurements and increased bleeding have been reported when warfarin and fluoxetine were used concurrently; the mechanism of this interaction is unknown; careful coagulation monitoring is recommended when treatment with fluoxetine is initiated or discontinued)
  Lithium
    (both increased and decreased lithium concentrations, as well as some cases of lithium toxicity, have been reported with concomitant fluoxetine use; close monitoring of lithium concentrations is recommended)
  Maprotiline or
  Trazodone
    (plasma concentrations of these medications may be doubled when fluoxetine is used concurrently)
» Moclobemide
    (because of the potentially fatal effects of concomitant use of fluoxetine and nonselective, irreversible monoamine oxidase [MAO] inhibitors, and the increased risk of development of the serotonin syndrome with concomitant use of fluoxetine and the selective, reversible, MAO type A inhibitor moclobemide, concurrent use is not recommended; a wash-out period of 7 days is advised between discontinuing moclobemide and initiating fluoxetine therapy, and a wash-out period of 5 weeks [approximately 5 half-lives of norfluoxetine] is advised between discontinuing fluoxetine and initiating moclobemide therapy)
» Monoamine oxidase (MAO) inhibitors, including furazolidone, procarbazine, and selegiline
    (concurrent use of fluoxetine with MAO inhibitors may result in confusion, agitation, restlessness, gastrointestinal symptoms, hyperpyretic episodes, severe convulsions, hypertensive crises, the serotonin syndrome, or death. Concurrent use is **contraindicated**, and at least 14 days should elapse between discontinuation of an MAO inhibitor and initiation of fluoxetine. However, because of the long half-lives of fluoxetine and its active metabolite, at least 5 weeks [approximately 5 half-lives of norfluoxetine] should elapse between discontinuation of fluoxetine and initiation of therapy with an MAO inhibitor. Deaths following the initiation of an MAO inhibitor shortly after stopping fluoxetine administration have been reported)
» Phenytoin
    (elevated plasma phenytoin concentrations resulting in symptoms of toxicity have been reported when fluoxetine was used concurrently with phenytoin; caution and close monitoring are suggested)
» Serotonergics or other medications or substances with serotonergic activity (see *Appendix II*)
    (increased risk of developing the serotonin syndrome, a rare but potentially fatal hyperserotonergic state; symptoms typically occur shortly [hours to days] after the addition of a serotonergic agent to a regimen that includes serotonin-enhancing drugs or an increase in dosage of a serotonergic agent; symptoms include agitation, diaphoresis, diarrhea, fever, hyperreflexia, incoordination, mental status changes [confusion, hypomania], myoclonus, shivering, or tremor)
    (use of tramadol with fluoxetine increases the risk of having seizures)
    (there have been reports of agitation, restlessness, and gastrointestinal distress occurring with concurrent use of tryptophan and fluoxetine)

**Medical considerations/Contraindications**
The medical considerations/contraindications included have been selected on the basis of their potential clinical significance (reasons given in parentheses where appropriate)—not necessarily inclusive (» = major clinical significance).

*Risk-benefit should be considered when the following medical problems exist:*
Diabetes mellitus
  (glycemic control may be altered due to improved peripheral and hepatic insulin action occurring with fluoxetine use)
» Hepatic function impairment
  (metabolism of fluoxetine is delayed; lower doses or less frequent dosing is recommended in patients with liver disease)
Neurological impairment, including developmental delay or
Seizures, history of
  (risk of seizures may be increased)
Parkinson's disease
  (exacerbation has been reported)
Renal function impairment
  (metabolites that are excreted renally may accumulate; however, routine dosage adjustments are not required)
Sensitivity to fluoxetine
Weight loss
  (although weight loss occurring with fluoxetine use in bulimia trials averaged 0.45 kg [about 1 pound], significant weight loss may be an undesirable effect of fluoxetine use in some patients)

**Patient monitoring**
The following may be especially important in patient monitoring (other tests may be warranted in some patients, depending on condition; » = major clinical significance):
Careful supervision of patients with suicidal tendencies
  (recommended especially during early treatment phase prior to peak effectiveness of fluoxetine; prescribing the smallest amount of medication necessary for good patient management is recommended to prevent overdosing)
Electrolytes, serum
  (recommended in bulimic patients prior to initiation of fluoxetine treatment since electrolyte disturbances, which can occur due to vomiting, may lower the seizure threshold or may cause cardiac conduction abnormalities)
Weight
  (recommended in bulimic patients periodically during treatment because of anorexia associated with fluoxetine use)

## Side/Adverse Effects
The following side/adverse effects have been selected on the basis of their potential clinical significance (possible signs and symptoms in parentheses where appropriate)—not necessarily inclusive:

**Those indicating need for medical attention**
Incidence more frequent
  *Akathisia* (inability to sit still; restlessness); *sexual dysfunction, including abnormal ejaculation; anorgasmia; decreased libido; genital anesthesia (rare); or impotence* (decreased sexual drive or ability); *skin rash, hives, or itching*
  Note: *Skin rash, hives, or itching* has been associated with systemic signs or symptoms, including arthralgia, carpal tunnel syndrome, edema, fever, leukocytosis, lymphadenopathy, mild transaminase elevations, proteinuria, and respiratory distress. Some patients have experienced syndromes resembling serum sickness. Rarely, systemic events involving the lung, kidney, or liver have developed in patients with skin rash. Deaths have occurred. However, most patients with fluoxetine-associated skin rash recovered with discontinuation of fluoxetine and/or with treatment with steroids or antihistamines. Fluoxetine should be discontinued if the patient develops skin rash or other allergic symptomatology for which no alternate etiology can be identified.
Incidence less frequent
  *Chills or fever; joint or muscle pain*
Incidence rare
  *Abnormal bleeding* (purple or red spots on skin); *breast enlargement or pain; dyspnea* (trouble in breathing); *galactorrhea* (unusual secretion of milk)—in females; *hypoglycemia* (anxiety; chills; cold sweats;

confusion; cool pale skin; difficulty in concentration; drowsiness; excessive hunger; fast heartbeat; headache; nervousness; shakiness; unsteady walk; unusual tiredness or weakness); *hyponatremia* (confusion; drowsiness; dryness of mouth; increased thirst; lack of energy; seizures)—especially in geriatric or volume-depleted patients; *mania or hypomania* (talking, feeling, and acting with excitement and activity that cannot be controlled); *movement disorders* (unusual or incomplete body or facial movements); *palpitation* (fast or irregular heartbeat); *seizures; serotonin syndrome* (diarrhea; fever; increased sweating; mood or behavior changes; overactive reflexes; racing heartbeat; restlessness; shivering or shaking)

- Note: *Dyspnea* may indicate a rare pulmonary event involving an inflammatory process and/or fibrosis.

  *Hyponatremia* results from the syndrome of inappropriate antidiuretic hormone (SIADH).

  *Movement disorders* are more likely to occur in patients with risk factors, such as pre-existing movement disorders or co-medication with drugs associated with movement disorders.

  The *serotonin syndrome* is most likely to occur shortly (hours to days) after a dosage increase or the addition of another serotonergic agent to the patient's regimen and may include cardiac arrhythmias, coma, disseminated intravascular coagulation, hypertension or hypotension, renal failure, respiratory failure, seizures, or severe hyperthermia. Although the serotonin syndrome has not been reported in patients receiving fluoxetine monotherapy, it has been reported in patients receiving monotherapy with other selective serotonin reuptake inhibitors and the possibility of occurrence with fluoxetine monotherapy exists.

**Those indicating need for medical attention only if they continue or are bothersome**
Incidence more frequent
  *Anxiety or nervousness; anorexia* (decreased appetite); *asthenia* (tiredness or weakness); *diarrhea; drowsiness; headache; increased sweating; insomnia* (trouble in sleeping); *nausea; tremor* (trembling or shaking)

Incidence less frequent or rare
  *Abnormal dreams; alopecia* (hair loss); *changes in vision; chest pain; dizziness or lightheadedness; frequent urination; gastrointestinal effects, including change in sense of taste; constipation; dryness of mouth; increased appetite; stomach cramps, gas, or pain; vomiting; weight gain; or weight loss; menstrual pain; photosensitivity* (increased sensitivity of skin to sunlight); *vasodilation* (feeling of warmth or heat; flushing or redness of skin, especially on face and neck); *yawning*

**Those indicating the need for medical attention if they occur after medication is discontinued**
  *Agitation; anxiety; dizziness; fatigue* (unusual tiredness or weakness); *headache; malaise* (general feeling of discomfort or illness); *nausea; sweating; vertigo* (feeling that body or surroundings are turning)

- Note: *Dizziness* and *vertigo* have been reported to occur in short bursts of a few seconds each.

  Discontinuation symptoms have been reported less frequently with fluoxetine than with other selective serotonin reuptake inhibitors, probably due to the long half-lives of fluoxetine and its active metabolite, norfluoxetine. The symptoms may begin up to 3½ weeks after discontinuation of fluoxetine and may require several weeks to resolve.

## Overdose

For specific information on the agents used in the management of fluoxetine overdose, see:
- *Charcoal, Activated (Oral-Local)* monograph; and/or
- *Diazepam* in *Benzodiazepines (Systemic)* monograph.

For more information on the management of overdose or unintentional ingestion, **contact a Poison Control Center** (see *Poison Control Center Listing*).

**Clinical effects of overdose**
The following effects have been selected on the basis of their potential clinical significance (possible signs and symptoms in parentheses where appropriate)—not necessarily inclusive:

- Note: Patients who take an overdose of fluoxetine only, with no other substances, may remain asymptomatic.

  *Agitation and restlessness; drowsiness; hypomania* (talking, feeling, and acting with excitement and activity that cannot be controlled); *nausea and vomiting; seizures; tachycardia* (fast heartbeat); *tremor* (trembling or shaking)

**Treatment of overdose**
There is no specific antidote for fluoxetine overdose. Treatment is essentially symptomatic and supportive.

To decrease absorption—Administering activated charcoal with sorbitol.

Specific treatment—Administering an anticonvulsant such as diazepam, if necessary, for seizure control.

Monitoring—Monitoring cardiovascular function (ECG).

Supportive care—Maintaining respiratory function. Maintaining body temperature. Patients in whom intentional overdose is confirmed or suspected should be referred for psychiatric consultation.

- Note: Dialysis, forced diuresis, hemoperfusion or exchange transfusions are unlikely to be of benefit due to the large volume of distribution and high degree of protein binding of fluoxetine.

  If a tricyclic antidepressant has been coingested, the tricyclic toxicity may be prolonged due to inhibition of metabolism by fluoxetine.

## Patient Consultation

As an aid to patient consultation, refer to *Advice for the Patient, Fluoxetine (Systemic)*.

In providing consultation, consider emphasizing the following selected information (» = major clinical significance):

**Before using this medication**
» Conditions affecting use, especially:
    Sensitivity to fluoxetine
    Pregnancy—Respiratory difficulties, cyanosis on feeding, jitteriness, hypertonia, petechiae, and cephalohematoma reported in newborns exposed during the third trimester; no effects seen in preschoolers and young children with *in utero* exposure; increased stillbirths and pup deaths in animal studies using doses approximating human doses
    Breast-feeding—Not recommended; vomiting, watery stools, crying, and sleep disturbance were reported in one infant; in several other infants, no problems were reported
    Contraindicated medications—Monoamine oxidase (MAO) inhibitors
    Other medications, especially alprazolam; astemizole; highly protein-bound medications such as anticoagulants, digitalis, or digitoxin; moclobemide; phenytoin; serotonergics or other medications or substances with serotonergic activity; or tricyclic antidepressants
    Other medical problems, especially hepatic function impairment

**Proper use of this medication**
» Compliance with therapy; not taking more or less medicine than prescribed
    May be taken with food to lessen possible stomach upset
» May require 4 weeks or longer of therapy to obtain antidepressant effects; may require 5 weeks or longer to obtain full antiobsessional effects; antibulimic effects may be seen after 1 week of therapy but may require 4 weeks or longer to occur
» Proper dosing
    Missed dose: Skipping the missed dose and continuing on regular schedule with next dose; not doubling doses
» Proper storage

**Precautions while using this medication**
    Regular visits to physician to check progress of therapy
» Not taking fluoxetine within 2 weeks of discontinuing an MAO inhibitor; not taking an MAO inhibitor for at least 5 weeks after discontinuing fluoxetine
    Avoiding use of alcoholic beverages
» Stopping fluoxetine and checking with physician as soon as possible if skin rash or hives occurs
    For diabetic patients: possible change in blood sugar levels; discussing with physician
» Possible drowsiness, impairment of judgment, thinking, or motor skills; caution when driving or doing jobs requiring alertness

**Side/adverse effects**
    Signs of potential side effects, especially akathisia; sexual dysfunction; skin rash, hives, or itching; chills or fever; joint or muscle pain; abnormal bleeding; breast enlargement or pain; dyspnea; galactorrhea, in females; hypoglycemia; hyponatremia; mania or hypomania; movement disorders; seizures; or serotonin syndrome

## General Dosing Information

Because of the long elimination half-lives of fluoxetine and norfluoxetine, dosing changes are not reflected in plasma for several weeks. This must be taken into consideration when titrating to a final dose.

Potentially suicidal patients, particularly those who may use alcohol excessively, should not have access to large quantities of this medication since these patients may continue to exhibit suicidal tendencies until significant improvement occurs. Some clinicians recommend that the patient be supplied with the least amount of medication necessary for satisfactory patient management.

Because of the long elimination half-lives of fluoxetine and norfluoxetine, tapering of the dosage prior to discontinuation generally is not necessary.

### Diet/Nutrition
Fluoxetine may be taken with food to lessen possible stomach upset.

### Bioequivalence information
Fluoxetine hydrochloride oral capsules and oral solution are bioequivalent.

### For treatment of adverse effects
Akathisia—Fluoxetine dosage reduction, addition of propranolol, or both may lessen or eliminate akathisia.

Discontinuation symptoms—Although tapering fluoxetine when discontinuing therapy generally is not required, patients who experience distressing symptoms upon discontinuation may benefit from reinstitution of fluoxetine followed by a gradual tapering of the dosage.

Serotonin syndrome—Serotonergic medications should be discontinued. Treatment is essentially symptomatic and supportive. The nonspecific serotonergic receptor antagonists cyproheptadine and methysergide have been reported to be of some use in shortening the duration of the syndrome.

Skin rash or hives—Fluoxetine should be discontinued on appearance of skin rash or hives. Treatment with antihistamines and/or steroids may be necessary.

## Oral Dosage Forms

Note: Bracketed uses in the *Dosage Forms* section refer to categories of use and/or indications that are not included in U.S. product labeling.

The available dosage forms contain fluoxetine hydrochloride, but dosage and strength are expressed in terms of fluoxetine base.

### FLUOXETINE CAPSULES USP

**Usual adult dose**
Antidepressant or
Antiobsessional agent or
[Premenstrual dysphoric disorder][1]—
  Oral, initially 20 mg (base) a day as a single morning dose. The dose may be increased as needed and tolerated at intervals of four to eight weeks.

Note: Some clinicians begin fluoxetine therapy with a single morning dose of 5 to 10 mg (base).
The manufacturer states that, in the treatment of depression or obsessive-compulsive disorder, doses over 20 mg (base) a day may be taken as a single morning dose or in two divided doses, in the morning and at noon.

Antibulimic agent—
  Oral, the target dose is 60 mg (base) a day as a single morning dose. Patients may need to be titrated up to this dose over several days.

Note: For all indications, patients with hepatic function impairment should receive a lower dosage or less frequent dosing. Also, for elderly patients and patients who have concurrent illness or who are taking multiple medications, a lower dosage or less frequent dosing should be considered. For patients with renal function impairment, dosage adjustments are not routinely required.

**Usual adult prescribing limits**
80 mg (base) a day.

**Usual pediatric dose**
Safety and efficacy have not been established.

**Usual geriatric dose**
See *Usual adult dose*.

Note: Dosage for elderly patients is often initiated at 10 mg (base) a day and usually does not exceed 60 mg (base) a day.

**Strength(s) usually available**
U.S.—
  10 mg (base) (Rx) [*Prozac* (FD&C Blue No.1; gelatin; iron oxide; silicon; starch; titanium dioxide)].
  20 mg (base) (Rx) [*Prozac* (FD&C Blue No.1; gelatin; iron oxide; silicon; starch; titanium dioxide)].
Canada—
  10 mg (base) (Rx) [*Prozac* (benzyl alcohol; carboxymethylcellulose sodium; edetate calcium disodium; FD&C Blue No. 1; gelatin; iron oxide black; iron oxide yellow; methylparaben; silicone; sodium lauryl sulfate; sodium propionate; starch; titanium dioxide)].
  20 mg (base) (Rx) [*Prozac* (benzyl alcohol; carboxymethylcellulose sodium; edetate calcium disodium; FD&C Blue No. 1; gelatin; iron oxide yellow; methylparaben; silicone; sodium lauryl sulfate; sodium propionate; starch; titanium dioxide)].

**Packaging and storage**
Store below 40 °C (104 °F), preferably between 15 and 30 °C (59 and 86 °F), unless otherwise specified by manufacturer. Store in a tight, light-resistant container.

**Auxiliary labeling**
• May cause drowsiness.
• Avoid alcoholic beverages.

### FLUOXETINE HYDROCHLORIDE ORAL SOLUTION

**Usual adult dose**
See *Fluoxetine Capsules USP*.

**Usual adult prescribing limits**
See *Fluoxetine Capsules USP*.

**Usual pediatric dose**
See *Fluoxetine Capsules USP*.

**Usual geriatric dose**
See *Fluoxetine Capsules USP*.

**Strength(s) usually available**
U.S.—
  20 mg (base) per 5 mL (Rx) [*Prozac* (alcohol 0.23%; benzoic acid; flavoring agent; glycerin; purified water; sucrose)].
Canada—
  20 mg (base) per 5 mL (Rx) [*Prozac* (benzoic acid; glycerin; mint flavor; purified water; sucrose)].

**Packaging and storage**
Store below 40 °C (104 °F), preferably between 15 and 30 °C (59 and 86 °F), in a tight, light-resistant container, unless otherwise specified by manufacturer. Protect from freezing.

**Stability**
Fluoxetine oral solution has been shown to be stable for up to 8 weeks at temperatures of 5 and 30 °C (41 and 86 °F) when diluted to strengths of 1 mg/mL or 2 mg/mL with deionized water, Simple Syrup British Pharmacopeia, Syrup NF, Aromatic Elixir NF, or grape-cranberry drink.

**Auxiliary labeling**
• May cause drowsiness.
• Avoid alcoholic beverages.

**Additional information**
The oral solution is mint-flavored.

[1] Not included in Canadian product labeling.

Revised: 08/07/98

---

# FLUOXYMESTERONE — See *Androgens (Systemic)*

---

# FLUPENTHIXOL — See *Thioxanthenes (Systemic)*

---

# FLUPHENAZINE — See *Phenothiazines (Systemic)*

---

# FLURANDRENOLIDE — See *Corticosteroids (Topical)*

---

# FLURAZEPAM — See *Benzodiazepines (Systemic)*

---

# FLURBIPROFEN — See *Anti-inflammatory Drugs, Nonsteroidal (Ophthalmic)*; *Anti-inflammatory Drugs, Nonsteroidal (Systemic)*

**FLUTAMIDE**—See *Antiandrogens, Nonsteroidal (Systemic)*

**FLUTICASONE**—See *Corticosteroids (Topical)*

# FLUTICASONE Inhalation-Local—INTRODUCTORY VERSION

VA CLASSIFICATION (Primary/Secondary): RE101/RE109
Commonly used brand name(s): *Flovent; Flovent Rotadisk*.
Note: For a listing of dosage forms and brand names by country availability, see *Dosage Forms* section(s).

## Category
Anti-inflammatory (inhalation); antiasthmatic.

## Indications

**Accepted**

*Asthma, chronic (treatment)*—Fluticasone is indicated as maintenance treatment in chronic asthma to improve lung function and reduce asthma symptoms. Use of fluticasone in patients who require oral corticosteroid therapy may allow the reduction or elimination of oral corticosteroids over time.

**Unaccepted**

Fluticasone is not indicated in the primary treatment of status asthmaticus or other acute asthma symptoms where intensive measures, such as rapid bronchodilation, are required.

## Pharmacology/Pharmacokinetics

**Physicochemical characteristics**
Source—Synthetic.
Molecular weight—Fluticasone propionate: 500.58.

**Mechanism of action/Effect**
Fluticasone acts as a human glucocorticoid receptor agonist with an affinity for the receptor that is 18 times greater than that of dexamethasone, almost twice that of beclomethasone-17-monopropionate, and over three times that of budesonide.

Studies have demonstrated that the clinical effectiveness of inhaled fluticasone is due to its direct local effect rather than an indirect effect through systemic absorption.

The anti-inflammatory actions of fluticasone may contribute to its efficacy in asthma; however, its precise mechanisms are unknown. Glucocorticoids have been shown to inhibit mast cells, eosinophils, basophils, lymphocytes, macrophages, and neutrophils. Glucocorticoids also inhibit production or secretion of cell mediators such as histamine, cytokines, and eicosanoids.

**Absorption**
*Inhalation aerosol*—Systemic bioavailability averages approximately 30% of the dose delivered from the actuator.
*Powder for inhalation*—Systemic bioavailability averages about 13.5% of the nominal dose.
*Oral*—Studies using radiolabeled and nonradiolabeled drug have demonstrated that the systemic bioavailability is less than 1%, primarily due to incomplete absorption and presystemic metabolism in the intestine and liver.

**Distribution**
The average volume of distribution (Vol$_D$) is 4.2 liters per kilogram of body weight (L/kg).

**Protein binding**
Plasma proteins—Very high (91%). Fluticasone is weakly and reversibly bound to erythrocytes. It is not significantly bound to transcortin.

**Biotransformation**
The total clearance of fluticasone is high, with renal clearance accounting for less than 0.02%. In humans, one circulating metabolite, formed through the cytochrome P450 3A4 pathway, is detectable; *in vitro* studies using human lung cytosol show that this metabolite has significantly less affinity for the glucocorticoid receptor than does the parent drug.

**Half-life**
After intravenous administration—7.8 hours.

**Onset of action**
Improvement following inhalation can occur within 24 hours.

**Peak plasma concentration**
*Inhalation aerosol*—Ranges from 0.1 to 1 nanogram per mL following an 880-microgram (mcg) dose.
*Powder for inhalation*—Ranges from 0.1 to 1 nanogram per mL following a 1000-mcg dose.

**Time to peak effect**
Maximum benefit may not be achieved for 1 to 2 weeks or longer after starting treatment.

**Duration of action**
Asthma stability persists for several days after withdrawal of corticosteroids.

**Elimination**
Fecal, as parent drug and metabolites.
Renal, less than 5% as metabolites.

## Precautions to Consider

**Carcinogenicity/Tumorigenicity**
Fluticasone showed no tumorigenic potential in a 78-week study in mice given oral doses of up to approximately 2 and 10 times the maximum human recommended daily inhalation dose on a mcg per square meter of body surface area (mcg/m$^2$) basis in adults and children, respectively, and in a 104-week study in rats given inhalation doses of up to approximately one fourth the maximum human recommended daily inhalation dose in adults and comparable to the maximum recommended human daily dose in children, on a mcg/m$^2$ basis.

**Mutagenicity**
Fluticasone was not mutagenic at high oral or subcutaneous doses in *in vitro* tests in prokaryotic or eukaryotic cells or in human peripheral lymphocytes or in an *in vivo* mouse micronucleus test. Fluticasone did not delay erythroblast division in bone marrow *in vitro*.

**Pregnancy/Reproduction**
*Fertility*—No evidence of impairment of fertility was seen in male and female rats given fluticasone subcutaneously in doses of up to 50 mcg per kg of body weight (approximately one fourth or one fifth the maximum human daily inhalation dose of the inhalation aerosol or powder for inhalation, respectively, on a mcg/m$^2$ basis). However, prostate weight was significantly reduced at a subcutaneous dose of 50 mcg/kg.

*Pregnancy*—Adequate and well-controlled studies in humans have not been done.

*Inhalation aerosol*—Less than 0.008% of a dose crosses the placenta following oral administration of fluticasone to rats and rabbits in doses approximately one half and three times the maximum human daily inhalation dose, respectively, on a mcg/m$^2$ basis. Studies in mice given fluticasone subcutaneously in doses approximately one half and one half the maximum human daily inhalation on a mcg/m$^2$ basis showed fetal toxicity characteristic of potent glucocorticoids, including embryonic growth retardation, omphalocele, cleft palate, and retarded cranial ossification. In rabbits, fetal weight reduction and cleft palate were observed following subcutaneous doses of approximately one twenty-fifth of the maximum human daily inhalation dose on a mcg/m$^2$ basis. However, following oral administration of fluticasone to rabbits in doses approximately three times the maximum human daily inhalation dose on a mcg/m$^2$ basis, no maternal effects or increased incidence of external, visceral, or skeletal fetal defects were shown.

*Powder for inhalation*—Studies in mice and rats at subcutaneous doses of 45 and 100 mcg/kg, respectively (approximately one tenth and one third, respectively, the maximum recommended daily inhalation dose in adults on a mcg/m$^2$ basis) found fetal toxicity characteristic of potent corticosteroid compounds, including embryonic growth retardation, omphalocele, cleft palate, and retarded cranial ossification. Studies in rabbits at subcutaneous doses of 4 mcg/kg (approximately one thirtieth the maximum recommended daily inhalation dose in adults on a mcg/m$^2$ basis) found fetal weight reduction and cleft palate. However, no teratogenic effects were reported at oral doses of up to 300 mcg/kg (approximately twice the maximum recommended daily inhalation dose in adults on a mcg/m$^2$ basis); in addition, no fluticasone propionate was detected in the plasma in this study, consistent with the established low bioavailability following oral administration. Fluticasone propionate crosses the placenta following oral administration of 100 mcg/kg to rats or 300 mcg/kg to rabbits (approximately one third and two times, respectively, the maximum recommended daily inhalation dose in adults on a mcg/m$^2$ basis).

Experience suggests that rodents are more susceptible to the teratogenic effects of pharmacologic doses of oral glucocorticoids than are humans. Additionally, because production of glucocorticoid increases naturally during pregnancy, most women will require a lower exogenous glucocorticoid dose and many may not need glucocorticoid treatment during pregnancy.

FDA Pregnancy Category C.

**Breast-feeding**

It is not known whether fluticasone is distributed into human breast milk. However, subcutaneous administration of radiolabeled fluticasone to lactating rats, in doses of approximately one twentieth the maximum human daily inhalation aerosol dose (one twenty fifth of the dose of the powder for inhalation) in adults on a mcg/m$^2$ basis, resulted in measurable radioactivity in milk.

**Pediatrics**

Clinical trials conducted with the inhalation aerosol in 137 patients between the ages of 12 and 16 years and with the powder for inhalation in 264 patients between 4 and 11 years of age have not demonstrated pediatrics-specific problems that would limit the usefulness of fluticasone in this age group. Safety and efficacy of the inhalation aerosol in children younger than 12 years of age, or of the powder for inhalation in children younger than 4 years of age, have not been established.

Plasma concentrations of fluticasone after an inhaled dose of 100 mcg were higher in children 4 to 11 years of age (median 58.7 picograms per mL) than in adults (median 39.5 picograms per mL).

Extended use of oral corticosteroids in children and adolescents has been shown to cause a reduction in growth velocity. A 52-week placebo-controlled study using fluticasone powder for inhalation at doses of 50 and 100 mcg twice a day in 325 patients between 4 and 11 years of age found a slight decrease in growth rate, although the clinical significance is uncertain. Therefore, close monitoring of the growth of children and adolescents taking corticosteroids, as well as use of the lowest effective dose, is recommended. In addition, patients using fluticasone may be more susceptible to infection; therefore, exposure to chickenpox or measles should be avoided.

**Geriatrics**

Studies performed with the inhalation aerosol in 574 patients and with the powder for inhalation in 173 patients 65 years of age and older have not demonstrated geriatrics-specific problems that would limit the usefulness of fluticasone in the elderly.

**Surgical**

Because of the possibility of systemic absorption of inhaled corticosteroids, postoperative patients treated with these drugs should be observed carefully for evidence of inadequate adrenal response.

**Critical/Emergency care**

Because of the possibility of systemic absorption of inhaled corticosteroids, patients treated with these drugs should be observed carefully during periods of stress for evidence of inadequate adrenal response.

**Drug interactions and/or related problems**

The following drug interactions and/or related problems have been selected on the basis of their potential clinical significance (possible mechanism in parentheses where appropriate)—not necessarily inclusive (» = major clinical significance):

Note: Combinations containing any of the following medications, depending on the amount present, may also interact with this medication.

Cytochrome P450 3A4 isoenzyme inhibitors, other
(may cause increased plasma concentrations of fluticasone or reductions in plasma cortisol area under the curve [AUC])

Ketoconazole
(concurrent use with fluticasone propionate powder for inhalation has been reported to lead to increased plasma fluticasone concentrations, decreased plasma cortisol AUC, and no effect on urinary excretion of cortisol; this effect may be related to inhibition, by ketoconazole, of cytochrome P450 3A4 isoenzyme system, which is involved in metabolism of fluticasone)

**Laboratory value alterations**

The following have been selected on the basis of their potential clinical significance (possible effect in parentheses where appropriate)—not necessarily inclusive (» = major clinical significance):

With physiology/laboratory test values
Hypothalamic-pituitary-adrenal (HPA) axis function as assessed by short cosyntropin test
(may occasionally be decreased with high doses)

**Medical considerations/Contraindications**

The medical considerations/contraindications included have been selected on the basis of their potential clinical significance (reasons given in parentheses where appropriate)—not necessarily inclusive (» = major clinical significance).

*Except under special circumstances, this medication should not be used when the following medical problems exist:*

» Herpes simplex, ocular or
» Infections, systemic, bacterial, fungal, parasitic, or viral, untreated
(possible increased risk of severe, uncontrollable infections)
Sensitivity to fluticasone
» Tuberculosis, pulmonary, active or quiescent
(may be exacerbated or reactivated)

**Patient monitoring**

The following may be especially important in patient monitoring (other tests may be warranted in some patients, depending on condition; » = major clinical significance):

» Growth and development in children and adolescents
(careful observation is recommended periodically during prolonged therapy with inhaled corticosteroids)

## Side/Adverse Effects

Note: Rarely, systemic corticosteroid effects such as hypercorticism and adrenal suppression may occur, especially with the use of higher doses.

The following side/adverse effects have been selected on the basis of their potential clinical significance (possible signs and symptoms in parentheses where appropriate)—not necessarily inclusive:

**Those indicating need for medical attention**
Incidence rare
*Aggression; angioedema* (swelling of face, lips, or eyelids); *bronchitis* (cough; shortness of breath); *bronchospasm, paradoxical or hypersensitivity-induced* (shortness of breath; tightness in chest; troubled breathing; wheezing); *cushingoid features* (increased fat deposits on face, neck, and trunk); *depression; glaucoma; increased intraocular pressure; or cataracts* (blurred vision); *growth velocity reduction in children or adolescents; hyperglycemia* (blurred vision; dry mouth or skin; increased hunger, thirst, or urination; weight loss); *hypersensitivity reaction, immediate or delayed, such as skin rash; or urticaria* (hives)

**Those indicating need for medical attention only if they continue or are bothersome**
Incidence more frequent—> 3%
*Dysphonia* (hoarseness or other voice changes); *fatigue* (unusual tiredness); *headache; influenza; insomnia* (trouble in sleeping); *malaise* (general feeling of illness); *muscle soreness; nasal problems, such as nasal congestion* (stuffy nose); *rhinitis* (runny or stuffy nose); *pain in nasal sinuses; or sinusitis* (headache); *nausea; oropharyngeal candidiasis* (creamy white, curd-like patches in mouth or throat; pain when eating or swallowing); *pharyngitis* (sore throat); *upper respiratory infections*

Incidence less frequent or rare
*Agitation; contusions or ecchymoses* (bruising); *pruritis* (itching); *restlessness; weight gain*

## Overdose

**Clinical effects of overdose**

The following effects have been selected on the basis of their potential clinical significance (possible signs and symptoms in parentheses where appropriate)—not necessarily inclusive:

Chronic
*Hypercorticism*

**Treatment of overdose**

The fluticasone dose should be reduced gradually, consistent with accepted procedures for reducing systemic corticosteroids and for management of the patient's asthma symptoms.

## Patient Consultation

As an aid to patient consultation, refer to *Advice for the Patient, Fluticasone (Inhalation-Local)—Introductory Version.*

In providing consultation, consider emphasizing the following selected information (» = major clinical significance):

**Before using this medication**

» Conditions affecting use, especially:
Hypersensitivity to fluticasone propionate
Use in children—Chronic use may result in decreased growth velocity; monitoring of growth and development is important; exposure to chickenpox or measles should be avoided

Other medical problems, especially active or quiescent pulmonary tuberculosis, herpes simplex infection of the eye, or untreated systemic bacterial, fungal, parasitic, or viral infections

**Proper use of this medication**
» Not using to relieve acute asthma attacks; continuing use of fluticasone even if using other medications for asthma attack
» Importance of not using more than the amount prescribed
» Compliance with therapy by using every day in regularly spaced doses Rinsing mouth with water after each dose; not swallowing rinse water
» Reading patient instructions carefully; checking frequently with health care professional for proper use of inhaler
» Proper dosing
Missed dose: Using as soon as possible; using any remaining doses for that day at regularly spaced intervals; not doubling doses
» Proper storage
*For inhalation aerosol*
Testing inhaler before using first time
Proper administration technique
Proper cleaning procedure for inhaler
*For powder for inhalation*
Proper loading technique for inhaler
Proper administration technique
Proper cleaning procedure for inhaler

**Precautions while using this medication**
» Checking with physician in the following circumstances:
Periods of potential stress
A severe asthma attack occurs
Asthma symptoms do not improve or condition worsens
Exposure to chickenpox or measles occurs
Carrying medical identification stating that supplemental systemic corticosteroid therapy may be required in emergency situations, periods of unusual stress, or acute asthma attack
» Caution if any kind of surgery or emergency treatment is required; informing health care professional that inhalation corticosteroid is being used

**Side/adverse effects**
Signs of potential side effects, especially aggression, angioedema, bronchitis, paradoxical or hypersensitivity-induced bronchospasm, cushingoid features, depression, glaucoma, increased intraocular pressure, cataracts, growth velocity reduction in children or adolescents, hyperglycemia, or immediate or delayed hypersensitivity reactions

## General Dosing Information

Caution is recommended when patients are transferred from systemic corticosteroids to inhaled fluticasone because deaths due to adrenal insufficiency have occurred in asthmatic patients during and after transfer from systemic corticosteroids to less systemically available inhaled corticosteroids. After withdrawal from systemic corticosteroids, several months are required for recovery of hypothalamic-pituitary-adrenal (HPA) function. Patients who have been maintained on the equivalent of 20 mg or more of prednisone per day (or its equivalent) may be most susceptible, particularly when their systemic corticosteroids have been almost completely withdrawn. During this period of HPA suppression, patients may exhibit signs and symptoms of adrenal insufficiency when exposed to trauma, surgery, infection (particularly gastroenteritis), or other conditions associated with severe electrolyte loss. In recommended doses, fluticasone by inhalation may control asthma symptoms during these episodes but supplies lower-than-normal physiological amounts of glucocorticoid systemically and does not provide the mineralocorticoid activity necessary for coping with these emergencies. During periods of stress or if a severe asthma attack occurs, patients who have been withdrawn from systemic corticosteroids should be instructed to immediately resume oral corticosteroids in large doses and to contact their physician for further instructions. These patients should also be instructed to carry a warning card indicating that they may need systemic corticosteroids during periods of stress or if a severe asthma attack occurs.

After at least 1 week of fluticasone inhalation therapy, the dose of oral corticosteroid should be tapered slowly. The daily prednisone dose should be reduced no faster than by 2.5 mg per day on a weekly basis. Reduction of the prednisone dose should be done only when lung function, asthma symptoms, and as-needed beta-adrenergic bronchodilator use are better than or comparable to that seen before starting the prednisone dose reduction. Careful monitoring of lung function forced expiratory volume (FEV) or a.m. peak expiratory flow rate (PEFR), beta-adrenergic agonist use, and asthma symptoms is recommended during withdrawal of oral corticosteroids. In addition, patients should be observed for signs of adrenal insufficiency, such as fatigue, hypotension, lassitude, nausea, vomiting, or weakness.

Transfer of patients from systemic corticosteroid therapy to fluticasone propionate by inhalation may unmask conditions previously suppressed by the systemic corticosteroid therapy, such as rhinitis, conjunctivitis, eczema, and arthritis. During withdrawal from oral corticosteroids, some patients may experience symptoms of systemically active corticosteroid withdrawal, such as joint and/or muscular pain, lassitude, and depression, despite maintenance or even improvement of respiratory function.

If bronchospasm, with an immediate increase in wheezing, occurs after dosing, it should be treated immediately with a fast-acting inhaled bronchodilator. It is recommended that treatment with inhaled fluticasone be discontinued and alternative therapy instituted.

Patients who are on medications that suppress the immune system are more susceptible to infections; therefore, children or adults using fluticasone who have not had diseases such as chickenpox or measles should avoid exposure. If the patient is exposed to chickenpox, prophylaxis with varicella zoster immune globulin (VZIG) may be indicated. If the patient is exposed to measles, prophylaxis with intramuscular pooled immune globulin (IG) may be indicated. If chickenpox develops, treatment with antiviral agents may be considered.

After asthma stability has been achieved with the initial dose of fluticasone, titration to the lowest effective dose is desirable to reduce the possibility of side effects. For patients who do not respond adequately to the initial dose after 2 weeks, higher doses may provide better asthma control.

If symptoms of hypercorticism or adrenal suppression occur, the dosage of fluticasone should be reduced slowly.

**For treatment of adverse effects**
Recommended treatment consists of the following:
- Appropriate local or systemic antifungal therapy should be given to treat localized infections of *Candida albicans* while fluticasone therapy is continued. Interruption of fluticasone therapy is required rarely.

## Inhalation Dosage Forms

### FLUTICASONE PROPIONATE INHALATION AEROSOL

**Usual adult and adolescent dose**
Asthma, chronic (treatment)—
Previous asthma therapy consisting of bronchodilators alone: Oral inhalation, 88 to 440 mcg two times a day.
Previous asthma therapy including inhaled corticosteroids: Oral inhalation, 88 to 440 mcg two times a day. Initial doses above 88 mcg two times a day may be considered for patients with inadequate asthma control or those who have required inhaled corticosteroids in the higher dosing range for that medication.
Previous asthma therapy including systemic corticosteroids: Oral inhalation, 880 mcg two times a day. After at least one week of therapy, slow reduction of the oral corticosteroid dosage may be considered.

**Usual adult and adolescent prescribing limits**
1660 mcg per day for patients previously taking oral corticosteroids.
880 mcg per day for patients previously using inhaled corticosteroids or bronchodilators alone.

**Usual pediatric dose**
Asthma, chronic (treatment)—
Children younger than 12 years of age: Safety and efficacy have not been established.
Children 12 years of age and older: See *Usual adult and adolescent dose*.

**Usual geriatric dose**
See *Usual adult and adolescent dose*.

**Strength(s) usually available**
U.S.—
44 mcg per metered spray (Rx) [*Flovent* (chlorofluorocarbons)].
110 mcg per metered spray (Rx) [*Flovent* (chlorofluorocarbons)].
220 mcg per metered spray (Rx) [*Flovent* (chlorofluorocarbons)].
Note: Each strength is available as a 13-gram canister that provides 120 metered sprays. Additionally, the 44-mcg strength is available as a 7.9-gram canister that provides 60 metered sprays.

**Packaging and storage**
Store between 2 and 30 °C (36 and 86 °F). Store canister with nozzle end down. Protect from freezing and direct sunlight.

**Auxiliary labeling**
- Shake well before using.

**Note**
Include patient instructions when dispensing.
Demonstrate administration technique.

**Additional information**
This product contains trichlorofluoromethane and dichlorodifluoromethane, substances that harm public health and the environment by destroying ozone in the upper atmosphere.

### FLUTICASONE PROPIONATE POWDER FOR INHALATION

**Usual adult and adolescent dose**
Asthma, chronic (treatment)—
  Previous asthma therapy consisting of bronchodilators alone: Oral inhalation, 100 mcg two times a day.
  Previous asthma therapy including inhaled corticosteroids: Oral inhalation, 100 to 250 mcg two times a day. Initial doses above 100 mcg two times a day may be considered for patients with inadequate asthma control or those who have required inhaled corticosteroids in the higher dosing range.
  Previous asthma therapy including systemic corticosteroids: Oral inhalation, 1000 mcg two times a day. After at least one week of therapy, slow reduction of the oral corticosteroid dosage may be considered.

**Usual adult and adolescent prescribing limits**
2000 mcg per day for patients previously taking oral corticosteroids.
1000 mcg per day for patients previously using inhaled corticosteroids or bronchodilators alone.
Note: The 2000-mcg-per-day limit recommendation is based on clinical data from a study using fluticasone inhalation aerosol; no dosing limit studies have been done with the powder for inhalation.

**Usual pediatric dose**
Asthma, chronic (treatment)—
  Children older than 11 years of age: See *Usual adult and adolescent dose*.
  Children 4 to 11 years of age:
    Previous asthma therapy consisting of bronchodilators alone—Oral inhalation, 50 mcg two times a day.
    Previous asthma therapy including inhaled corticosteroids—Oral inhalation, 50 mcg two times a day.
  Children younger than 4 years of age: Safety and efficacy have not been established.

**Usual pediatric prescribing limits**
Children 4 to 11 years of age—200 mcg per day.

**Usual geriatric dose**
See *Usual adult and adolescent dose*.

**Strength(s) usually available**
U.S.—
  50 mcg per disk (delivering 44 mcg) (Rx) [*Flovent Rotadisk* (lactose)].
  100 mcg per disk (delivering 88 mcg) (Rx) [*Flovent Rotadisk* (lactose)].
  250 mcg per disk (delivering 220 mcg) (Rx) [*Flovent Rotadisk* (lactose)].
Note: This product is supplied with 15 disks and one inhaler device per carton. The disks are in a white plastic tube that is protected from moisture by a foil pouch. Each circular disk comes in a double-foil pack containing four blisters of the medication.

**Packaging and storage**
Store between 20 and 25 °C (68 and 77 °F). Protect from moisture.

**Note**
Include patient instructions when dispensing.
Demonstrate administration technique.

Developed: 10/16/96
Interim revision: 08/12/98

---

# FLUTICASONE Nasal—INTRODUCTORY VERSION

VA CLASSIFICATION (Primary): NT201
Commonly used brand name(s): *Flonase*.
Note: For a listing of dosage forms and brand names by country availability, see *Dosage Forms* section(s).

## Category
Anti-inflammatory (steroidal), nasal; corticosteroid (nasal).

## Indications

**Accepted**
Rhinitis, perennial allergic (treatment)
Rhinitis, seasonal allergic (treatment)—Fluticasone is indicated in the treatment of perennial allergic rhinitis and seasonal allergic rhinitis.

**Acceptance not established**
Fluticasone is not indicated in the treatment of *nonallergic rhinitis*, since efficacy has not been adequately demonstrated in patients with this condition.

## Pharmacology/Pharmacokinetics

**Physicochemical characteristics**
Molecular weight—500.6.

**Mechanism of action/Effect**
The precise mechanism by which corticosteroids affect allergic rhinitis symptoms is not known. Corticosteroids have been shown to have a wide range of effects on multiple cell types (e.g., mast cells, eosinophils, neutrophils, macrophages, and lymphocytes) and mediators (e.g., histamine, eicosanoids, leukotrienes, and cytokines) involved in inflammation.

**Absorption**
Nasal fluticasone propionate has an absolute bioavailability averaging less than 2%. After nasal application for 3 weeks in patients with allergic rhinitis, fluticasone propionate plasma levels were above the level of detection (50 picograms per mL) only when the recommended dose (200 mcg per day) was exceeded and then only in occasional samples. In addition, absorption is low and bioavailability negligible following oral administration of fluticasone propionate.

**Protein binding**
Approximately 90%, to human plasma proteins following intravenous administration. Fluticasone propionate is weakly and reversibly bound to erythrocytes and freely equilibrates between erythrocytes and plasma. It is not significantly bound to human transcortin.

**Biotransformation**
Hepatic to a 17-beta-carboxylic acid derivative, which has negligible pharmacological activity in animal studies.

**Half-life**
Following intravenous administration, fluticasone propionate has an elimination half-life of approximately 3 hours.

**Onset of action**
Fluticasone, like other corticosteroids, does not have an immediate effect on allergic symptoms. In some patients, a decrease in nasal symptoms has been noted 12 hours after initial treatment.

**Time to peak effect**
Maximum benefit may not be reached for several days.

**Duration of action**
When treatment is discontinued, symptoms may not return for several days.

**Elimination**
Less than 5% of an oral dose is excreted in the urine as metabolites; the remainder is excreted in the feces as the parent drug and metabolites.

## Precautions to Consider

**Tumorigenicity**
There was no evidence of tumorigenicity in mice given fluticasone orally in doses of up to 1 mg per kg of body weight (mg/kg) for 78 weeks or in rats receiving inhalation doses of up to 57 mcg per kg of body weight (mcg/kg) for 104 weeks.

**Mutagenicity**
Fluticasone did not induce gene mutation in prokaryotic or eukaryotic cells *in vitro*. No significant clastogenic effect was seen in cultured human peripheral lymphocytes *in vitro* or in the mouse micronucleus test administered at high doses by the oral or subcutaneous routes. In addition, fluticasone did not delay erythroblast division in bone marrow.

**Pregnancy/Reproduction**
Fertility—There was no evidence of impairment of fertility in male and female rats given fluticasone in subcutaneous doses of up to 50 mcg/kg. However, prostate weight was significantly reduced.

Pregnancy—Studies have not been done in humans.
Animals given subcutaneous doses: Studies in mice and rats given doses of 45 and 100 mcg/kg, respectively, (approximately equivalent to and 4 times, respectively, the maximum recommended daily [MRD] intra-

nasal dose in adult humans on a mcg-per-square-meter [mcg/m$^2$] basis) have shown that fluticasone causes fetal toxicity characteristic of potent corticosteroids, including embryonic growth retardation, omphalocele, cleft palate, and retarded cranial ossification. Studies in rabbits given doses of 4 mcg/kg (approximately one-third the MRD intranasal dose in adult humans on a mcg/m$^2$ basis) have shown that fluticasone causes fetal weight reduction and cleft palate.

Animals given oral doses: In rats and rabbits, fluticasone crossed the placenta following oral administration of 100 and 300 mcg/kg, respectively (approximately 4 and 25 times, respectively, the MRD intranasal dose in adult humans on a mcg/m$^2$ basis). In addition, studies in rabbits given doses of 300 mcg/kg (approximately 25 times the MRD intranasal dose in adult humans on a mcg/m$^2$ basis) have not shown any maternal effects or increased incidence of external, visceral, or skeletal fetal defects.

FDA Pregnancy Category C.

### Breast-feeding
It is not known whether nasal fluticasone is distributed into human breast milk. However, systemic corticosteroids are distributed into human breast milk. In addition, studies in lactating rats given subcutaneous doses of 10 mcg/kg of fluticasone showed that fluticasone is distributed into animal milk.

### Pediatrics
For children up to 4 years of age—Safety and efficacy have not been established.

For children 4 years of age and older—With extended use, oral, and possibly intranasal, corticosteroids have been shown to have the potential to cause growth suppression in children and adolescents. If significant systemic absorption of nasal corticosteroids occurs in pediatric or adolescent patients, adrenal suppression and growth suppression may result. Prolonged or high-dose therapy with these medications requires careful attention to dosage and close monitoring of growth and development.

### Geriatrics
Appropriate studies on the relationship of age to the effects of nasal fluticasone have not been performed in the geriatric population. However, clinical trials included a limited number of older patients and the adverse reactions reported were similar to those of younger adults; therefore, geriatrics-specific problems that would limit the usefulness of the medication in the elderly are not expected.

### Medical considerations/Contraindications
The medical considerations/contraindications included have been selected on the basis of their potential clinical significance (reasons given in parentheses where appropriate)—not necessarily inclusive (» = major clinical significance).

*Except under special circumstances, this medication should not be used when the following medical problems exist:*
» Intolerance to corticosteroids
» Sensitivity to any ingredient in the product, such as benzalkonium chloride, dextrose, or phenylethyl alcohol

*Risk-benefit should be considered when the following medical problems exist:*
  Glaucoma
    (rare cases of glaucoma have been reported following use of nasal corticosteroids, including nasal fluticasone)
» Infections, fungal, bacterial, or systemic viral
    (corticosteroids may mask the infection; in addition, some infections, such as chickenpox or measles, may have a more serious course in patients on immunosuppressant doses of corticosteroids)
  Nasal septal ulcers, recent or
  Nasal surgery, recent or
  Nasal trauma, recent
    (corticosteroids inhibit wound healing)
» Ocular herpes simplex
    (corticosteroids may mask the infection)
» Tuberculosis, latent or active, of respiratory tract
    (corticosteroids may mask or activate the infection)

### Patient monitoring
The following may be especially important in patient monitoring (other tests may be warranted in some patients, depending on condition; » = major clinical significance):
  Adrenal function assessment
    (assessment of hypothalamic-pituitary-adrenal (HPA) axis function may be advisable at periodic intervals in patients receiving long-term nasal corticosteroid therapy; this is especially important in children and adolescents)
  Otolaryngologic examination
    (should be performed in patients on long-term therapy [several months or longer] to monitor nasal mucosa and nasal passages for infection, nasal septal perforation, nasal membrane ulceration, or other histologic changes)

## Side/Adverse Effects
Note: The risk of systemic effects is minimal with usual doses of nasal fluticasone. Rare cases of cataracts, glaucoma, and increased intraocular pressure have been reported following use of intranasal corticosteroids, including fluticasone.

Systemic effects including hypothalamic-pituitary-adrenal (HPA) axis suppression may occur with greater-than-recommended doses of nasal fluticasone. Use of greater-than-recommended doses is not recommended. If a patient is particularly sensitive or has recently used systemic corticosteroids prior to using nasal corticosteroids, the patient may also be predisposed to hypercorticism.

The following side/adverse effects have been selected on the basis of their potential clinical significance (possible signs and symptoms in parentheses where appropriate)—not necessarily inclusive:

### Those indicating need for medical attention
Incidence more common
  *Epistaxis* (bloody mucus; unexplained nosebleeds); *headache; pharyngitis* (sore throat)
Incidence less frequent
  *Bronchitis* (cough); *dizziness; nasal septal excoriation* (bloody mucus; unexplained nosebleeds); *nausea or vomiting; rhinorrhea* (runny nose); *sinusitis* (headache; runny or stuffy nose); *ulceration of nasal mucosa* (sores inside nose); *urticaria* (hives)
Incidence rare
  *Contact dermatitis* (skin rash); *hypersensitivity reaction, immediate* (hives; rash; shortness of breath or troubled breathing; swelling of eyelids, face, or lips); *nasal or pharyngeal candidiasis* (white patches inside nose or throat); *nasal septal perforation* (bloody mucus; unexplained nosebleeds); *wheezing*

### Those indicating need for medical attention only if they continue or are bothersome
Incidence more frequent
  *Burning, dryness, or other irritation inside the nose*
Incidence less frequent
  *Bad taste in mouth; nasal congestion* (stuffy nose); *sneezing; xerostomia* (dryness of mouth)

## Overdose
For more information on the management of overdose or unintentional ingestion, **contact a Poison Control Center** (see *Poison Control Center Listing*).

### Treatment of overdose
For acute overdose—Adverse effects due to acute overdose are unlikely with the small quantities of corticosteroid contained in each bottle.

For chronic overdose—If symptoms of chronic overdose occur, nasal corticosteroids should be discontinued slowly.

## Patient Consultation
As an aid to patient consultation, refer to *Advice for the Patient, Fluticasone (Nasal)—Introductory Version*.

In providing consultation, consider emphasizing the following selected information (» = major clinical significance):

### Before using this medication
» Conditions affecting use, especially:
  Intolerance to corticosteroids
  Sensitivity to any ingredient in the product, such as benzalkonium chloride, dextrose, or phenylethyl alcohol
  Pregnancy—Subcutaneous doses of fluticasone in mice, rats, and rabbits have shown fetal toxicity; oral doses in rabbits have not shown any fetal or maternal toxicity; studies in rats and rabbits have shown that fluticasone crosses the placenta
  Breast-feeding—Studies in rats showed that subcutaneous fluticasone is distributed into animal milk
  Use in children—Importance of monitoring growth and development with prolonged or high-dose therapy
  Other medical problems, especially fungal, bacterial, or systemic viral infections; latent or active tuberculosis of respiratory tract; or ocular herpes simplex

### Proper use of this medication
» Proper administration technique; reading patient directions carefully before use
  Clearing nasal passages before use; aiming spray toward inner corner of eye
» Compliance with therapy
» Importance of not using more medication than the amount prescribed, because of potential enhanced absorption and increased severity of side effects
» Proper dosing
  Missed dose: Using as soon as possible; skipping missed dose if almost time for next dose; not doubling doses
» Proper storage

### Precautions while using this medication
Regular visits to physician to check progress during prolonged therapy
» Checking with physician if:
  —signs of infection of nose, throat, or sinuses occur
  —no improvement within 3 weeks
  —condition becomes worse

### Side/adverse effects
Signs of potential side effects, especially epistaxis, headache, pharyngitis, bronchitis, dizziness, nasal septal excoriation, nausea or vomiting, rhinorrhea, sinusitis, ulceration of nasal mucosa, urticaria, contact dermatitis, immediate hypersensitivity reaction, nasal or pharyngeal candidiasis, nasal septal perforation, ocular hypertension, or wheezing

## General Dosing Information
Regular use of nasal fluticasone is required to obtain full therapeutic benefit.

Fluticasone propionate nasal suspension dosage form contains no fluorocarbon propellants.

The dosage of other corticosteroids being administered concurrently by other routes of administration, including oral inhalation, should be taken into account when determining the usual adult prescribing limits of nasal corticosteroids.

Caution is recommended if a nasal corticosteroid, such as fluticasone, is added to an alternate-day regimen of a systemic corticosteroid, since that may increase the likelihood of hypothalamic-pituitary-adrenal (HPA) axis suppression.

Caution is recommended if a systemic corticosteroid is replaced with a nasal corticosteroid, such as fluticasone, since adrenal insufficiency may occur. In addition, some patients may experience symptoms of withdrawal, such as joint or muscular pain, lassitude, or depression. It is recommended that patients previously treated for prolonged periods with systemic corticosteroids and transferred to nasal corticosteroids be carefully monitored for acute adrenal insufficiency in response to stress.

## Nasal Dosage Forms

### FLUTICASONE PROPIONATE NASAL SUSPENSION
**Usual adult dose**
Rhinitis, perennial allergic (treatment) or
Rhinitis, seasonal allergic (treatment)—
  Initial: Nasal, 200 mcg (0.2 mg) a day, administered as 2 metered sprays in each nostril once a day or 1 metered spray in each nostril two times a day. Each metered spray delivers 50 mcg (0.05 mg).
  Maintenance: Nasal, 100 mcg (0.1 mg) a day, administered as 1 metered spray in each nostril once a day. Each metered spray delivers 50 mcg (0.05 mg). It may be possible to switch to the maintenance dosage as early as 4 to 7 days after initial treatment is started.

**Usual adult prescribing limits**
Nasal, 200 mcg (0.2 mg) per day.

**Usual pediatric dose**
Rhinitis, perennial allergic (treatment) or
Rhinitis, seasonal allergic (treatment)—
  Infants and children up to 4 years of age: Safety and efficacy have not been established.
  Children 4 years of age and older (including adolescents): Nasal, 100 mcg (0.1 mg) a day, administered as 1 metered spray in each nostril once a day. Each metered spray delivers 50 mcg (0.05 mg).
Note: Children and adolescents not adequately responding to 100 mcg (0.1 mg) a day may use 200 mcg (0.2 mg) a day, administered as 2 metered sprays in each nostril once a day or 1 metered spray in each nostril two times a day. Once adequate control is achieved, the dosage should be decreased to 100 mcg (0.1 mg) once a day.

**Usual pediatric prescribing limits**
Nasal, 200 mcg (0.2 mg) per day.

**Strength(s) usually available**
U.S.—
  50 mcg (0.05 mg) per metered spray (0.05%) (Rx) [*Flonase* (benzalkonium chloride; dextrose; microcrystalline cellulose; microcrystalline carboxymethylcellulose sodium; phenylethyl alcohol; polysorbate 80)].

**Packaging and storage**
Store between 4 and 30 °C (39 and 86 °F), unless otherwise specified by manufacturer. Protect from freezing.

**Auxiliary labeling**
• For the nose.
• Shake gently before use.

**Note**
Explain administration technique.

Developed: 06/25/95
Interim revision: 11/14/97; 08/11/98

---

# FLUVASTATIN—See *HMG-CoA Reductase Inhibitors (Systemic)*

---

# FLUVOXAMINE Systemic

VA CLASSIFICATION (Primary/Secondary): CN900/CN603
Commonly used brand name(s): *Luvox*.
Note: For a listing of dosage forms and brand names by country availability, see *Dosage Forms* section(s).

## Category
Antiobsessional agent; antidepressant.

## Indications
Note: Bracketed information in the *Indications* section refers to uses that are not included in U.S. product labeling.

**Accepted**
Obsessive-compulsive disorder (treatment)—Fluvoxamine is used to relieve symptoms of obsessive-compulsive disorder (OCD) in children[1] and adults. The effectiveness of using fluvoxamine for longer than 10 weeks has not been evaluated in placebo-controlled trials.

[Depressive disorder, major (treatment)]—Fluvoxamine is used to relieve symptoms of depressive illness. The effectiveness of using fluvoxamine for longer than 10 weeks has not been evaluated in placebo-controlled trials. However, treatment of acute depressive episodes typically requires 6 to 12 months of antidepressant therapy. Patients with recurrent or chronic depression may require long-term treatment.

[1]Not included in Canadian product labeling.

## Pharmacology/Pharmacokinetics

**Physicochemical characteristics**
Chemical group—2-aminoethyl oxime ethers of aralkylketones. Fluvoxamine is chemically unrelated to other selective serotonin reuptake inhibitors (SSRIs) or clomipramine.
Molecular weight—Fluvoxamine base: 318.3.
  Fluvoxamine maleate: 434.41.
Solubility—Fluvoxamine maleate is sparingly soluble in water and freely soluble in ethanol.

## Mechanism of action/Effect
The mechanism of action of fluvoxamine as an antiobsessional agent and as an antidepressant is presumed to be linked to its specific serotonin (5-hydroxytryptamine [5-HT]) reuptake inhibition in brain neurons. Fluvoxamine potently and specifically inhibits presynaptic neuronal reuptake of 5-HT by blocking the membrane pump mechanism for neuronal 5-HT reuptake, thereby facilitating serotonergic transmission and decreasing 5-HT turnover. Noradrenergic and dopaminergic functioning is generally unaffected by fluvoxamine. *In vitro* studies have shown fluvoxamine to possess no significant affinity for histaminergic, alpha-adrenergic, beta-adrenergic, muscarinic, dopaminergic, 5-HT$_1$, or 5-HT$_2$ receptors.

## Other actions/effects
Fluvoxamine inhibits serotonin (5-HT) uptake by platelets as well as by neurons.

Fluvoxamine is a potent inhibitor of cytochrome P450 1A2 (CYP1A2). *In vitro* studies have also shown fluvoxamine to inhibit CYP3A4 and CYP2C9, and to weakly inhibit CYP2D6.

## Absorption
Fluvoxamine is well absorbed, but bioavailability is about 50%, probably due to first-pass metabolism. Absorption is nonlinear over a dosage range of 100 to 300 mg per day, and higher doses of fluvoxamine lead to higher plasma concentrations than predicted by lower dose kinetics. Food does not significantly affect oral bioavailability.

## Distribution
The mean apparent volume of distribution for fluvoxamine is approximately 25 liters per kg of body weight (L/kg), reflecting the lipophilic nature of fluvoxamine and suggesting extensive tissue distribution. Fluvoxamine is distributed into breast milk.

## Protein binding
High (approximately 77%), primarily to albumin.

## Biotransformation
Fluvoxamine is extensively metabolized in the liver, primarily by oxidative demethylation and oxidative deamination. The specific cytochrome P450 isoenzymes involved in fluvoxamine metabolism have yet to be completely identified. However, a study comparing fluvoxamine kinetics in poor and extensive metabolizers of CYP2D6 substrates indicates that the CYP2D6 isoenzyme is involved in fluvoxamine metabolism. Nine metabolites have been identified, none of which shows significant pharmacologic activity.

## Half-life
Elimination—
15 to 20 hours; may be slightly increased after multiple dosing.

## Onset of action
Antiobsessional agent—3 to 10 weeks.
Antidepressant—2 to 3 weeks.

## Time to peak concentration
About 3 to 8 hours with a single dose or at steady-state.

## Time to steady-state concentration
Steady-state plasma concentrations of fluvoxamine are attained in about 10 days of multiple dosing.

## Steady-state plasma concentrations
At steady state, fluvoxamine demonstrates nonlinear pharmacokinetics over a dosage range of 50 to 150 mg twice a day, and plasma concentrations after multiple dosing are greater than those predicted by single-dose kinetics. In 30 healthy volunteers, maximum steady-state plasma fluvoxamine maleate concentrations reached 88, 283, and 546 nanograms/mL (0.203, 0.651, and 1.26 micromoles/L) following dosing regimens of 100, 200, and 300 mg per day, respectively. A correlation between plasma fluvoxamine concentration and efficacy has not been demonstrated.

In one kinetics study, mean maximum plasma concentrations were 40% higher in elderly patients (66 to 73 years of age) than in younger subjects (19 to 35 years of age).

## Elimination
Renal; 94% within 71 hours following a single oral dose of 5 mg of fluvoxamine maleate, about 3% as unchanged drug. A comparison of mean minimum plasma concentrations at 4 and 6 weeks of treatment in 13 patients with renal function impairment (creatinine clearance of 5 to 45 mL per minute) receiving 50 mg of fluvoxamine two times per day showed comparable values, indicating no accumulation of medication.

# Precautions to Consider

## Carcinogenicity/Mutagenicity
There was no evidence of carcinogenicity or mutagenicity in animal or *in vitro* studies with fluvoxamine.

## Pregnancy/Reproduction
Fertility—Fertility studies in male and female rats that received up to two times the maximum recommended human dose (MRHD) of fluvoxamine on a mg per square meter of body surface area (mg/m$^2$) basis showed no effect on mating performance, duration of gestation, or pregnancy rate.

Pregnancy—Adequate and well-controlled studies have not been done in humans.

In teratology studies conducted in rats and rabbits receiving daily oral fluvoxamine doses approximately two times the MRHD on a mg/m$^2$ basis, no fetal malformations were seen. In other reproductive studies in which pregnant rats were dosed through weaning, there was an increase in pup mortality at birth at doses greater than or equal to two times the MRHD on a mg/m$^2$ basis, and decreases in postnatal pup survival at all doses tested (0.1 through 4 times the MRHD on a mg/m$^2$ basis). While the results of a cross-fostering study implied that at least some of these results probably occurred secondarily to maternal toxicity, a direct drug effect on the fetuses or pups could not be ruled out.

FDA Pregnancy Category C.

Labor and delivery—The effect of fluvoxamine on labor and delivery in humans is unknown.

## Breast-feeding
Fluvoxamine is distributed into breast milk, but does not appear to accumulate in breast milk. In one woman receiving fluvoxamine at a dosage of 100 mg two times a day, plasma and breast milk fluvoxamine base concentrations were 0.31 mg per L (mg/L; 0.97 micromole/L) and 0.09 mg/L (0.28 micromole/L), respectively, 4.75 hours after a 100-mg dose.

## Pediatrics
Appropriate studies performed to date have not demonstrated pediatrics-specific problems that would limit the usefulness of fluvoxamine in children.

Because decreased appetite and weight loss are associated with fluvoxamine use, monitoring of weight and growth parameters is recommended in children receiving long-term treatment with fluvoxamine.

## Geriatrics
No differences in safety or efficacy were seen between elderly and younger subjects in studies that included geriatric patients. However, fluvoxamine clearance is reduced by about 50% in elderly patients, and elderly patients may be less tolerant of adverse effects. A reduced initial fluvoxamine dosage and slower dosage titration may be appropriate in elderly patients.

## Pharmacogenetics
About 2 to 10% of the adult population are poor metabolizers of CYP2D6 substrates. A study comparing fluvoxamine single-dose kinetics in poor and extensive metabolizers found the mean maximum plasma concentration, the area under the plasma concentration–time curve (AUC), and the elimination half-life of fluvoxamine to be 52%, 200%, and 62% higher, respectively, in the poor metabolizers. This indicates that fluvoxamine is metabolized, at least in part, by the CYP2D6 isoenzyme.

## Drug interactions and/or related problems
The following drug interactions and/or related problems have been selected on the basis of their potential clinical significance (possible mechanism in parentheses where appropriate)—not necessarily inclusive (» = major clinical significance):

Note: Fluvoxamine is a potent inhibitor of cytochrome P450 1A2 (CYP1A2). *In vitro* studies have also shown fluvoxamine to inhibit CYP3A4 and CYP2C9, and to weakly inhibit CYP2D6. Interactions with medications other than those listed below that are metabolized by these enzymes, particularly medications having a narrow therapeutic window such as phenytoin, should be considered. If fluvoxamine is coadministered with a drug that is eliminated via oxidative metabolism and that has a narrow therapeutic window, plasma concentrations and/or pharmacodynamic effects of the latter drug should be monitored closely.

CYP2D6 appears to be involved in fluvoxamine metabolism. Therefore, interactions with medications that inhibit this isoenzyme, such as quinidine, should also be considered.

Combinations containing any of the following medications, depending on the amount present, may also interact with this medication.

Alcohol
(although studies indicate that there is no significant pharmacokinetic or pharmacodynamic interaction between fluvoxamine and alcohol, concomitant use is not recommended)

» Antidepressants, tricyclic (TCAs)
(coadministration of fluvoxamine with amitriptyline, clomipramine, or imipramine has resulted in significantly increased plasma con-

centrations of the TCAs; a reduced TCA dosage and monitoring of TCA plasma concentrations should be considered)

Antipsychotics of the butyrophenone type, including haloperidol
(concurrent administration has resulted in significantly increased serum concentrations of the antipsychotic or of two- to tenfold increases in fluvoxamine serum concentration)

» Astemizole or
» Cisapride or
» Terfenadine
(astemizole, cisapride, and terfenadine are metabolized via the cytochrome P450 3A4 [CYP3A4] isoenzyme; *in vitro* studies show that fluvoxamine is an inhibitor of this isoenzyme and, therefore, could block metabolism of these agents; other agents that block metabolism of astemizole, cisapride, or terfenadine via this isoenzyme have caused increased concentrations of these drugs, resulting in potentially fatal QT prolongation and *torsades de pointes*; coadministration of astemizole, cisapride, or terfenadine with fluvoxamine is **contraindicated**)

» Benzodiazepines that are metabolized by hepatic oxidation, such as
Alprazolam or
Bromazepam or
Diazepam or
Midazolam or
Triazolam
(fluvoxamine is likely to reduce the clearance of these benzodiazepines; concurrent use has been shown to reduce the clearance of alprazolam, bromazepam, diazepam, and the active metabolite of diazepam, *N*-desmethyldiazepam, by 50% or more, and to impair psychomotor performance and memory; when alprazolam is to be used with fluvoxamine, the initial alprazolam dosage should be reduced by at least 50%; it is recommended that diazepam not be used concurrently with fluvoxamine because of the probability of accumulation of diazepam and its active metabolite; benzodiazepines such as lorazepam, oxazepam, and temazepam, which are metabolized by glucuronidation, are unlikely to be affected by fluvoxamine)

» Beta-adrenergic blocking agents that are metabolized hepatically, such as
Metoprolol or
Propranolol
(coadministration of fluvoxamine with propranolol in healthy volunteers resulted in mean minimum propranolol plasma concentrations increasing fivefold; potentiation of propranolol-induced heart rate reduction and exercise diastolic pressure reduction were seen in this study; similarly, cases of bradycardia, hypotension, and orthostatic hypotension have been reported with the coadministration of fluvoxamine with metoprolol; if concurrent use is undertaken, reductions in initial beta-blocking agent dosage and cautious titration are recommended; the beta-adrenergic blocking agent atenolol undergoes minimal hepatic metabolism and effects on atenolol plasma concentrations have not been reported)

Caffeine or
» Theophylline
(clearance of caffeine and theophylline are decreased, probably due to inhibition of cytochrome P450 1A2 [CYP1A2] by fluvoxamine; symptoms of theophylline toxicity, including arrhythmias, headache, tiredness, tremor, or vomiting have been reported with concurrent use of theophylline and fluvoxamine; if theophylline is coadministered with fluvoxamine, the theophylline dosage should be reduced to one third of the usual daily maintenance dosage, and theophylline plasma concentrations should be monitored)

Carbamazepine
(elevated carbamazepine plasma concentrations and symptoms of toxicity have been reported following coadministration with fluvoxamine, although one small study found no change in plasma concentrations of carbamazepine or its active metabolite, carbamazepine-10,11-epoxide)

» Clozapine
(coadministration of clozapine with fluvoxamine has resulted in threefold and greater elevations of serum concentrations of clozapine and clinical symptoms of toxicity; patients receiving the combination should be closely monitored)

Diltiazem
(concurrent administration of diltiazem with fluvoxamine has resulted in bradycardia)

Methadone
(significantly increased methadone plasma concentration-to-dose ratios have been reported when fluvoxamine was added to the regimens of patients on methadone maintenance; symptoms of opioid intoxication were reported in one patient; one case of opioid withdrawal symptoms was reported when fluvoxamine was discontinued; fluvoxamine treatment should be initiated and discontinued with caution in patients receiving methadone)

» Monoamine oxidase (MAO) inhibitors, including furazolidone, procarbazine, and selegiline
(serious and sometimes fatal reactions have occurred in patients receiving another serotonin reuptake inhibitor with an MAO inhibitor; reactions have included hyperthermia, rigidity, myoclonus, autonomic instability with rapid fluctuation of vital signs, and mental status changes including extreme agitation progressing to delirium and coma; some cases presented with features resembling neuroleptic malignant syndrome [NMS]; concurrent use of an MAO inhibitor and fluvoxamine is **contraindicated**; at least 14 days should elapse between the discontinuation of one medication and the initiation of the other)

» Serotonergics or other medications or substances with serotonergic activity (see *Appendix II*)
(increased risk of developing the serotonin syndrome, a rare but potentially fatal hyperserotonergic state which may occur in patients receiving serotonergic medications such as fluvoxamine, usually in combination; symptoms typically occur shortly [hours to days] after the addition of a serotonergic agent to a regimen that includes other serotonin-enhancing drugs or after an increase in dosage of a serotonergic agent; symptoms include agitation, diaphoresis, diarrhea, fever, hyperreflexia, incoordination, mental status changes [confusion, hypomania], myoclonus, shivering, or tremor)

(concurrent use of lithium and fluvoxamine has resulted in seizures as well as a case resembling the serotonin syndrome, which included hyperreflexia, tremor, and decreased coordination; the combination of these agents should be administered with caution)

(severe vomiting has been reported with the combined use of tryptophan and fluvoxamine)

Smoking tobacco
(bioavailability of fluvoxamine is significantly decreased in smokers as compared with nonsmokers, possibly due to induction of metabolism of fluvoxamine)

» Warfarin
(fluvoxamine administered concomitantly with warfarin for 2 weeks resulted in warfarin plasma concentration increases of up to 98% and prolonged prothrombin times; patients receiving both medications should have their prothrombin times monitored and anticoagulant doses adjusted accordingly)

**Medical considerations/Contraindications**
The medical considerations/contraindications included have been selected on the basis of their potential clinical significance (reasons given in parentheses where appropriate)—not necessarily inclusive (» = major clinical significance).

*Risk-benefit should be considered when the following medical problems exist:*

Drug abuse or dependence, or history of
(patients with a history of drug abuse should be observed closely for signs of misuse or abuse, as with any new central nervous system [CNS] agent)

» Hepatic function impairment
(fluvoxamine elimination half-life is increased; initial fluvoxamine dosage should be reduced, and titration should proceed slowly; an increased dosing interval may be considered)

Mania or hypomania, history of
(condition may be re-activated)

Neurological impairment, including developmental delay or
» Seizure disorders, history of
(risk of seizures may be increased; if seizures occur, fluvoxamine should be discontinued)

Sensitivity to fluvoxamine maleate

**Patient monitoring**
The following may be especially important in patient monitoring (other tests may be warranted in some patients, depending on condition; » = major clinical significance):

Careful supervision of patients with suicidal tendencies
(recommended especially during early treatment phase before peak effectiveness of fluvoxamine is achieved; prescribing the least amount of medication necessary for good patient management is recommended to decrease risk of overdose)

Monitoring of growth parameters and weight in children
(recommended during long-term treatment because of anorexia and weight loss associated with fluvoxamine use)

## Side/Adverse Effects

The following side/adverse effects have been selected on the basis of their potential clinical significance (possible signs and symptoms in parentheses where appropriate)—not necessarily inclusive:

**Those indicating need for medical attention**
Incidence more frequent
*Sexual dysfunction, including abnormal ejaculation; anorgasmia; decreased libido; delayed orgasm; or impotence* (change in sexual performance or desire)

Incidence less frequent
*Behavior, mood, or mental changes, including agitation; anxiety; apathy; confusion; disinhibition; hallucinations (rare); malaise; mania or hypomania; nervousness; panic attack (rare); or psychotic reaction; dyspnea* (trouble in breathing); *myoclonus* (twitching); *urinary retention* (trouble in urinating)

Incidence rare
*Abnormal bleeding* (nose bleed; unusual bruising); *blurred vision; extrapyramidal effects, including akinesia or hypokinesia* (absence of or decrease in body movements); *ataxia* (clumsiness or unsteadiness); *dyskinesia* (unusual or incomplete body movements); *or dystonia* (unusual or sudden body or facial movements; inability to move eyes); *hyperkinesia* (increase in body movements); *menstrual changes; seizures; serotonin syndrome* (agitation; confusion; diarrhea; fever; overactive reflexes; poor coordination; restlessness; shivering; sweating; talking or acting with excitement you cannot control; trembling or shaking; twitching)—usually following an increase in dosage; *skin rash; syndrome of inappropriate antidiuretic hormone (SIADH)* (difficult urination; irritability; muscle twitching; weakness); *toxic epidermal necrolysis* (redness, tenderness, itching, burning or peeling of skin; red or irritated eyes; sore throat, fever, and chills); *unusual lactation* (unusual secretion of milk)—in females

Note: Cardiac arrhythmias, coma, disseminated intravascular coagulation, hyper- or hypotension, renal failure, respiratory failure, seizures, and severe hyperthermia have been reported effects of the *serotonin syndrome*.

**Those indicating need for medical attention only if they continue or are bothersome**
Incidence more frequent
*Asthenia or fatigue* (unusual tiredness or weakness); *constipation; dizziness; drowsiness; headache; insomnia* (trouble in sleeping); *nausea; vomiting*

Incidence less frequent
*Abdominal pain; anorexia* (decreased appetite); *diarrhea; dryness of mouth; dyspepsia* (heartburn); *increased sweating; palpitation* (feeling of fast or irregular heartbeat); *tachycardia* (fast heartbeat); *taste perversion* (change in sense of taste); *tremor* (trembling or shaking); *unusual weight gain or loss; urinary frequency; vertigo* (feeling of constant movement of self or surroundings)

Incidence rare
*Abnormal dreaming; flatulence* (gas); *polydypsia* (increased thirst); *yawning*

**Those indicating the need for medical attention if they occur after medication is discontinued**
*Confusion; decreased energy; dizziness; headache; irritability; nausea; problems with memory; weakness*

Note: Discontinuation symptoms usually start 24 to 72 hours after discontinuing fluvoxamine, and continue for 7 to 14 days.

## Overdose

For specific information on the agents used in the management of fluvoxamine overdose, see *Charcoal, Activated (Oral-Local)* monograph.

For more information on the management of overdose or unintentional ingestion, **contact a Poison Control Center** (see *Poison Control Center Listing*).

**Clinical effects of overdose**

Note: Overdose with fluvoxamine alone has resulted in death. However, patients have recovered completely from overdoses of 9000 to 10,000 mg.

The clinical effects of fluvoxamine overdose may be similar to side effects seen at therapeutic doses, but may be more severe or several may occur together.

The following effects have been selected on the basis of their potential clinical significance (possible signs and symptoms in parentheses where appropriate)—not necessarily inclusive:

Acute
Most commonly observed effects
*Diarrhea; dizziness; drowsiness; nausea; vomiting*
Other notable signs and symptoms
*Bradycardia* (slow heartbeat); *coma; dryness of mouth; electrocardiogram (ECG) abnormalities; hypotension* (low blood pressure); *liver function abnormalities; mydriasis* (large pupils); *myoclonus* (twitching); *seizures; tachycardia* (fast heartbeat); *tremor* (trembling or shaking); *urinary retention* (trouble in urinating)
Symptoms that may be secondary to vomiting or loss of consciousness
*Aspiration pneumonitis; hypokalemia; respiratory difficulties*

**Treatment of overdose**
There is no specific antidote for fluvoxamine. Treatment is essentially symptomatic and supportive.

To decrease absorption—The stomach should be emptied as soon as possible by emesis or gastric lavage. The administration of activated charcoal may be useful up to 24 hours post-ingestion, since absorption may be delayed in overdose.

Monitoring—Electrocardiogram (ECG) and vital signs monitoring is necessary. Because of prolonged absorption, monitoring should be continued for at least 48 hours.

Supportive care—Adequate airway, oxygenation, and ventilation must be maintained. Patients in whom intentional overdose is confirmed or suspected should be referred for psychiatric consultation.

Note: Dialysis and forced diuresisare not likely to be of benefit because of the large volume of distribution of fluvoxamine.
In managing overdose, the possibility of multiple drug involvement should be considered.

## Patient Consultation

As an aid to patient consultation, refer to *Advice for the Patient, Fluvoxamine (Systemic)*.

In providing consultation, consider emphasizing the following selected information (» = major clinical significance):

**Before using this medication**
» Conditions affecting use, especially:
    Sensitivity to fluvoxamine maleate
    Breast-feeding—Fluvoxamine is distributed into breast milk
    Use in children—Growth and weight monitoring is recommended during long-term treatment
    Use in the elderly—Clearance is reduced; elderly may be more sensitive to adverse effects
    Contraindicated medications—Astemizole, cisapride, monoamine oxidase (MAO) inhibitors, terfenadine
    Other medications, especially benzodiazepines that are metabolized by hepatic oxidation, beta-adrenergic blocking agents that are metabolized hepatically, clozapine, other serotonergics or medications or substances with serotonergic activity, theophylline, tricyclic antidepressants, or warfarin
    Other medical problems, especially hepatic function impairment or history of seizure disorders

**Proper use of this medication**
» Compliance with therapy; not taking more or less medicine than prescribed
    Taking with or without food, on a full or empty stomach.
» May require several weeks of therapy to obtain therapeutic effects
» Proper dosing
    Missed dose: If taking once a day, taking the missed dose as soon as possible if remembered the same day; continuing on regular schedule with next dose; not doubling doses
    If taking two times a day, skipping the missed dose and continuing on regular schedule with next dose; not doubling doses
» Proper storage

**Precautions while using this medication**
» Regular visits to physician to check progress of therapy
» Not taking astemizole, cisapride, or terfenadine while taking fluvoxamine
» Not taking fluvoxamine or an MAO inhibitor within 14 days of each other
    Avoiding use of alcoholic beverages
» Notifying physician as soon as possible if skin rash, hives, or other sign of allergic reaction occurs
» Possible drowsiness, impairment of thinking, vision, or motor skills; caution when driving or doing jobs requiring alertness, clear vision, or good muscle control
    Checking with physician before discontinuing medication; gradual dosage reduction may be required to avoid discontinuation symptoms

### Side/adverse effects
Sexual dysfunction; behavior, mood, or mental changes; dyspnea; myoclonus; urinary retention; abnormal bleeding; blurred vision; extrapyramidal effects; menstrual changes; seizures; serotonin syndrome; skin rash; syndrome of inappropriate antidiuretic hormone; toxic epidermal necrolysis; unusual lactation (in females)

## General Dosing Information
Although the long-term efficacy of fluvoxamine has not been documented in clinical trials, obsessive-compulsive disorder and depression may be frequently recurring or chronic conditions and it is reasonable to consider continuing drug therapy in a responding patient. The patient should be maintained on the lowest effective dosage, and be reassessed periodically to determine the need for continued therapy.

If obsessive-compulsive symptoms do not improve within 10 to 12 weeks, treatment with fluvoxamine should be reconsidered.

Potentially suicidal patients, particularly those who use alcohol excessively, should not have access to large quantities of this medication. Some clinicians recommend that the patient be supplied with the least amount of medication necessary for satisfactory patient management.

Skin rash, hives, or any other sign of allergic reaction should be reported to the physician as soon as possible.

Discontinuation of fluvoxamine treatment should be achieved by a gradual reduction in dosage to reduce the occurrence of discontinuation symptoms. A reduction rate of 50 mg per day every 5 to 7 days has been proposed.

### Diet/Nutrition
Fluvoxamine may be taken with or without food, on a full or empty stomach.

### For treatment of adverse effects
Serotonin syndrome—Treatment is essentially symptomatic and supportive. The nonspecific serotonergic receptor antagonists cyproheptadine and methysergide have been reported to be of some use in shortening the duration of the serotonin syndrome.

## Oral Dosage Forms
Note: Bracketed uses in the Dosage Forms section refer to categories of use and/or indications that are not included in U.S. product labeling.

### FLUVOXAMINE MALEATE TABLETS
**Usual adult dose**
Antiobsessional agent or
[Antidepressant]—
Oral, initially 50 mg in a single dose at bedtime. The dosage may be increased as needed and tolerated in increments of 50 mg a day at intervals of four to seven days. If the daily dosage exceeds 100 mg, it should be taken in two divided doses. If the doses are not equal, the larger dose should be taken at bedtime.

Note: In patients with hepatic function impairment, initial fluvoxamine dosage should be reduced, and titration should proceed slowly; an increased dosing interval may be considered.

Some clinicians recommend an initial dosage of 25 mg once a day in all adult patients to reduce the incidence of adverse effects.

**Usual adult prescribing limits**
300 mg per day.

**Usual pediatric dose**
Antiobsessional agent[1]—
Children younger than 8 years of age: Safety and efficacy have not been established.
Children 8 to 17 years of age: Oral, initially 25 mg in a single dose at bedtime. The dosage may be increased as needed and tolerated in increments of 25 mg a day at intervals of four to seven days. If the daily dosage exceeds 50 mg, it should be administered in two divided doses. If the doses are not equal, the larger dose should be administered at bedtime.

**Usual pediatric prescribing limits**
Antiobsessional agent—
Children 8 to 17 years of age: 200 mg a day.

**Usual geriatric dose**
See *Usual adult dose*.

Note: In elderly patients, modifications of the initial dosage and subsequent titration may be appropriate. Some clinicians recommend an initial dosage of 25 mg once a day and a maximum dosage of 100 mg two times a day for elderly patients.

**Strength(s) usually available**
U.S.—
25 mg (Rx) [*Luvox* (carnauba wax; hydroxypropyl methylcellulose; mannitol; polyethylene glycol; polysorbate 80; pregelatinized potato starch; silicon dioxide; sodium stearyl fumarate; corn starch; titanium dioxide)].
50 mg (Rx) [*Luvox* (scored; carnauba wax; hydroxypropyl methylcellulose; mannitol; polyethylene glycol; polysorbate 80; pregelatinized potato starch; silicon dioxide; sodium stearyl fumarate; corn starch; synthetic iron oxides; titanium dioxide)].
100 mg (Rx) [*Luvox* (scored; carnauba wax; hydroxypropyl methylcellulose; mannitol; polyethylene glycol; polysorbate 80; pregelatinized potato starch; silicon dioxide; sodium stearyl fumarate; corn starch; synthetic iron oxides; titanium dioxide)].
Canada—
50 mg (Rx) [*Luvox* (scored)].
100 mg (Rx) [*Luvox* (scored)].

**Packaging and storage**
Store at controlled room temperature, between 15 and 30 °C(59 and 86 °F), in a tight container, unless otherwise specified by manufacturer. Protect from humidity.

**Auxiliary labeling**
- Avoid alcoholic beverages.
- May cause drowsiness.

**Note**
Dispense in tight container.

[1]Not included in Canadian product labeling.

## Selected Bibliography
Claassen V, Davies, JE, Hertting G, et al. Fluvoxamine, a specific 5-hydroxytryptamine uptake inhibitor. Br J Pharmacol 1977; 60: 505-16.
Wilde MI, Plosker GL, Benfield P. Fluvoxamine: an updated review of its pharmacology, and therapeutic use in depressive illness. Drugs 1993; 46(5): 895-924.

Developed: 04/16/98
Interim revision: 08/07/98

---

# FOLIC ACID  Systemic

VA CLASSIFICATION (Primary): VT102
Commonly used brand name(s): *Apo-Folic*; *Folvite*; *Novo-Folacid*.
Another commonly used name is Vitamin B$_9$.
Note: For a listing of dosage forms and brand names by country availability, see *Dosage Forms* section(s).

## Category
Nutritional supplement (vitamin); diagnostic aid (folate deficiency).
Note: Folic acid (vitamin B$_9$) is a water-soluble vitamin.

## Indications
Note: Bracketed information in the *Indications* section refers to uses that are not included in U.S. product labeling.

**Accepted**
Folic acid deficiency (prophylaxis and treatment)—Folic acid is indicated for prevention and treatment of folic acid deficiency states. Folic acid deficiency may occur as a result of inadequate nutrition or intestinal malabsorption but does not occur in healthy individuals receiving an adequate balanced diet. Simple nutritional deficiency of individual B vitamins is rare since dietary inadequacy usually results in multiple deficiencies. For prophylaxis of folic acid deficiency, dietary improvement, rather than supplementation, is advisable. For treatment of folic acid deficiency, supplementation is preferred.

Folic acid should not be given until the diagnosis of pernicious anemia has been ruled out, since it corrects the hematologic manifestations and masks pernicious anemia while allowing neurologic damage to progress.

Deficiency of folic acid may lead to megaloblastic and macrocytic anemias and glossitis.

Recommended intakes may be increased and/or supplementation may be necessary in the following persons or conditions (based on documented folic acid deficiency):
Alcoholism
Anemia, hemolytic
Fever, chronic
Gastrectomy
Hemodialysis, chronic
Infants—low-birthweight, breast-fed, or those receiving unfortified formulas such as evaporated milk or goat's milk
Intestinal diseases—celiac disease, tropical sprue, persistent diarrhea
Malabsorption syndromes associated with hepatic-biliary disease—hepatic function impairment, alcoholism with cirrhosis
Stress, prolonged

Some unusual diets (e.g., reducing diets that drastically restrict food selection) may not supply minimum daily requirements of folic acid. Supplementation is necessary in patients receiving total parenteral nutrition (TPN) or undergoing rapid weight loss or in those with malnutrition, because of inadequate dietary intake.

Recommended intakes for all vitamins and most minerals are increased during pregnancy. Many physicians recommend that pregnant women receive multivitamin and mineral supplements, especially those pregnant women who do not consume an adequate diet and those in high-risk categories (i.e., women carrying more than one fetus, heavy cigarette smokers, and alcohol and drug abusers). Taking excessive amounts of a multivitamin and mineral supplement may be harmful to the mother and/or fetus and should be avoided.

Some studies have found that folic acid supplementation alone or in combination with other vitamins given before conception and during early pregnancy may reduce the incidence of neural tube defects in infants.

Recommended intakes for all vitamins and most minerals are increased during breast-feeding.

Recommended intakes may be increased by the following medications: Analgesics (long-term use), anticonvulsants, epoetin, estrogens, sulfasalazine

[Folate deficiency (diagnosis)][1]—Folic acid is being used in the diagnosis of folate deficiency.

**Unaccepted**
Folic acid has not been proven effective for prevention of mental disorders or in the treatment of normocytic, refractory, or aplastic anemias.

[1]Not included in Canadian product labeling.

## Pharmacology/Pharmacokinetics

### Physicochemical characteristics
Molecular weight—441.41.

### Mechanism of action/Effect
Folic acid, after conversion to tetrahydrofolic acid, is necessary for normal erythropoiesis, synthesis of purine and thymidylates, metabolism of amino acids such as glycine and methionine, and the metabolism of histidine.

### Absorption
Commercially available folic acid is almost completely absorbed from the gastrointestinal tract (mostly in the upper duodenum), even in the presence of malabsorption due to tropical sprue. However, absorption of food folates is impaired in malabsorption syndromes.

### Protein binding
Extensive (to plasma proteins).

### Storage
Hepatic (large proportion).

### Biotransformation
Hepatic. Folic acid is converted (in the presence of ascorbic acid) in the liver and plasma to its metabolically active form (tetrahydrofolic acid) by dihydrofolate reductase.

### Peak serum concentration
30 to 60 minutes.

### Elimination
Renal (almost entirely as metabolites). Excess beyond daily needs is excreted, largely unchanged, in urine.
In dialysis—Folic acid is removed by hemodialysis; therefore, dialysis patients should receive increased amounts (100 to 300% of USRDA [United States Recommended Daily Allowances]).

## Precautions to Consider

### Pregnancy/Reproduction
Pregnancy—Problems in humans have not been documented with intake of normal daily recommended amounts. Folic acid crosses the placenta. However, adequate and well-controlled studies in humans have not shown that folic acid causes adverse effects on the fetus.
Some studies have found that folic acid supplementation alone or in combination with other vitamins given before conception and during early pregnancy may reduce the incidence of neural tube defects in infants.
FDA Pregnancy Category A.

### Breast-feeding
Folic acid is distributed into breast milk. However, problems in humans have not been documented with intake of normal daily recommended amounts.

### Pediatrics
Problems in pediatrics have not been documented with intake of normal daily recommended amounts.
Folic acid injection that contains benzyl alcohol as a preservative should not be used in newborn and immature infants. The use of benzyl alcohol in neonates has been associated with a fatal toxic syndrome consisting of metabolic acidosis and CNS, respiratory, circulatory, and renal function impairment.

### Geriatrics
Problems in geriatrics have not been documented with intake of normal daily recommended amounts.

### Drug interactions and/or related problems
The following drug interactions and/or related problems have been selected on the basis of their potential clinical significance (possible mechanism in parentheses where appropriate)—not necessarily inclusive (» = major clinical significance):

Note: Combinations containing any of the following medications, depending on the amount present, may also interact with this medication.

Analgesics, long-term use or
Anticonvulsants, hydantoin or
Carbamazepine or
Estrogens or
Oral contraceptives
(requirements for folic acid may be increased in patients receiving these medications)
(concurrent use with folic acid may decrease the effects of hydantoin anticonvulsants by antagonism of their central nervous system [CNS] effects; an increase in hydantoin dosage may be necessary for patients who receive folic acid supplementation)

Antacids, aluminum- or magnesium-containing
(prolonged use of aluminum- and/or magnesium-containing antacids may decrease folic acid absorption by lowering the pH of the small intestine; patients should be advised to take antacids at least 2 hours after folic acid)

Antibiotics
(may interfere with the microbiologic method of assay for serum and erythrocyte folic acid concentrations and cause falsely low results)

Cholestyramine
(concurrent use with folic acid may interfere with absorption of folic acid; folic acid supplementation taken at least 1 hour before or 4 to 6 hours after cholestyramine is recommended in patients receiving cholestyramine for prolonged periods)

Methotrexate or
Pyrimethamine or
Triamterene or
Trimethoprim
(act as folate antagonists by inhibiting dihydrofolate reductase; most significant with high doses and/or prolonged use; leucovorin calcium must be used instead of folic acid in patients receiving these medications)

Sulfonamides, including sulfasalazine
(inhibit absorption of folate; folic acid requirements may be increased in patients receiving sulfasalazine)

Zinc supplements
(some studies have found that folate may decrease the absorption of zinc, but not in the presence of excessive zinc; other studies have found no inhibition)

### Laboratory value alterations
The following have been selected on the basis of their potential clinical significance (possible effect in parentheses where appropriate)—not necessarily inclusive (» = major clinical significance):

With physiology/laboratory test values
    Vitamin B$_{12}$ concentrations in blood
        (may be reduced by large and continuous doses of folic acid)

### Medical considerations/Contraindications
The medical considerations/contraindications included have been selected on the basis of their potential clinical significance (reasons given in parentheses where appropriate)—not necessarily inclusive (» = major clinical significance).

*Risk-benefit should be considered when the following medical problems exist:*

» Pernicious anemia
    (folic acid will correct hematologic abnormalities but neurologic problems will progress irreversibly; doses of folic acid greater than 0.4 mg per day are not recommended until pernicious anemia has been ruled out, except during pregnancy and lactation)

Sensitivity to folic acid

## Side/Adverse Effects
Note: No side effects other than an allergic reaction have been reported with folic acid administration, even at doses of up to 10 times the recommended dietary allowances (RDA) for 1 month.

The following side/adverse effects have been selected on the basis of their potential clinical significance (possible signs and symptoms in parentheses where appropriate)—not necessarily inclusive:

**Those indicating need for medical attention**
Incidence rare
    *Allergic reaction, specifically; bronchospasm* (shortness of breath; troubled breathing; tightness of chest; wheezing); *erythema* (reddened skin); *fever; skin rash or itching*

## Patient Consultation
As an aid to patient consultation, refer to *Advice for the Patient, Folic Acid (Vitamin B$_9$) (Systemic)*.

In providing consultation, consider emphasizing the following selected information (» = major clinical significance):

**Description of use**
    Description should include function in the body, signs of deficiency, and unproven uses

**Importance of diet**
    Importance of proper nutrition; supplement may be needed because of inadequate dietary intake
    Food sources of folic acid; effects of processing
    Not using vitamins as substitute for balanced diet
    Recommended daily intake for folic acid

**Before using this dietary supplement**
» Conditions affecting use, especially:
    Other medical problems, especially pernicious anemia

**Proper use of this dietary supplement**
» Proper dosing
    Missed dose: No cause for concern because of length of time necessary for depletion; remembering to take as directed
» Proper storage

**Side/adverse effects**
    Signs of potential side effects, especially allergic reaction

## General Dosing Information
Because of the infrequency of single B vitamin deficiencies, combinations are commonly administered. Many commercial combinations of B vitamins are available.

**For parenteral dosage forms only**
In most cases, parenteral administration is indicated only when oral administration is not acceptable (for example, in nausea, vomiting, preoperative and postoperative conditions) or possible (for example, in malabsorption syndromes or following gastric resection).

**Diet/Nutrition**
Recommended dietary intakes for folic acid are defined differently worldwide.

For U.S.—
    The Recommended Dietary Allowances (RDAs) for vitamins and minerals are determined by the Food and Nutrition Board of the National Research Council and are intended to provide adequate nutrition in most healthy persons under usual environmental stresses. In addition, a different designation may be used by the FDA for food and dietary supplement labeling purposes, as with Daily Value (DV). DVs replace the previous labeling terminology United States Recommended Daily Allowances (USRDAs).

For Canada—
    Recommended Nutrient Intakes (RNIs) for vitamins, minerals, and protein are determined by Health and Welfare Canada and provide recommended amounts of a specific nutrient while minimizing the risk of chronic diseases.

Daily recommended intakes for folic acid are generally defined as follows:

| Persons | U.S. (mcg) | Canada (mcg) |
|---|---|---|
| Infants and children | | |
|   Birth to 3 years of age | 25–50 | 50–80 |
|   4 to 6 years of age | 75 | 90 |
|   7 to 10 years of age | 100 | 125–180 |
| Adolescent and adult males | 150–200 | 150–220 |
| Adolescent and adult females | 150–180 | 145–190 |
| Pregnant females | 400 | 445–475 |
| Breast-feeding females | 260–280 | 245–275 |

These are usually provided by adequate diets.
Best dietary sources of folic acid include vegetables, especially green vegetables; potatoes; cereal and cereal products; fruits; and organ meats (liver, kidney). Heat destroys folic acid (50 to 90%) in foods.

## Oral Dosage Forms
Note: Bracketed uses in the *Dosage Forms* section refer to categories of use and/or indications that are not included in U.S. product labeling.

### FOLIC ACID TABLETS USP
**Usual adult and adolescent dose**
Deficiency (prophylaxis)—
    Oral, amount based on normal daily recommended intakes:

| Persons | U.S. (mcg) | Canada (mcg) |
|---|---|---|
| Adolescent and adult males | 150–200 | 150–220 |
| Adolescent and adult females | 150–180 | 145–190 |
| Pregnant females | 400 | 445–475 |
| Breast-feeding females | 260–280 | 245–275 |

Deficiency (treatment)—
    Treatment dose is individualized by prescriber based on severity of deficiency.

[Diagnostic aid (folate deficiency)][1]—
    Oral, 100 to 200 mcg (0.1 to 0.2 mg) a day for ten days plus low dietary folic acid and vitamin B$_{12}$.

**Usual pediatric dose**
Deficiency (prophylaxis)—
    Oral, amount based on normal daily recommended intakes:

| Persons | U.S. (mcg) | Canada (mcg) |
|---|---|---|
| Infants and children | | |
|   Birth to 3 years of age | 25–50 | 50–80 |
|   4 to 6 years of age | 75 | 90 |
|   7 to 10 years of age | 100 | 125–180 |

Deficiency (treatment)—
    Treatment dose is individualized by prescriber based on severity of deficiency.

**Strength(s) usually available**
U.S.—
    100 mcg (Rx) [GENERIC].
    400 mcg (Rx) [GENERIC].
    800 mcg (Rx) [GENERIC].
    1 mg (Rx) [*Folvite*; GENERIC].
Canada—
    5 mg (Rx) [*Apo-Folic* (scored); *Folvite* (scored); *Novo-Folacid*; GENERIC].

Note: Some strengths of these folic acid preparations may exceed the dosage range recommended by USP DI Advisory Panels based on the amount necessary to meet normal nutritional needs.

**Packaging and storage**
Store below 40 °C (104 °F), preferably between 15 and 30 °C (59 and 86 °F), unless otherwise specified by manufacturer. Store in a well-closed container.

## Parenteral Dosage Forms

Note: Bracketed uses in the *Dosage Forms* section refer to categories of use and/or indications that are not included in U.S. product labeling.

### FOLIC ACID INJECTION USP

**Usual adult and adolescent dose**
Deficiency (prophylaxis)—
  Intravenous infusion, as part of total parenteral nutrition solutions, the specific amount determined by individual patient need.
Deficiency (treatment)—
  Intramuscular, intravenous, or deep subcutaneous: 250 mcg (0.25 mg) to 1 mg a day until a hematologic response occurs.
[Diagnostic aid (folate deficiency)][1]—
  Intramuscular, 100 to 200 mcg (0.1 to 0.2 mg) a day for ten days plus low dietary folic acid and vitamin $B_{12}$.

**Usual pediatric dose**
See *Usual adult and adolescent dose*.

Note: Folic acid injection that contains benzyl alcohol as a preservative should not be used in newborn and immature infants. The use of benzyl alcohol in neonates has been associated with a fatal toxic syndrome consisting of metabolic acidosis and CNS, respiratory, circulatory, and renal function impairment.

**Strength(s) usually available**
U.S.—
  5 mg (base) per mL (Rx) [*Folvite* (benzyl alcohol 1.5%); GENERIC].
  10 mg per mL (Rx) [GENERIC].
Canada—
  5 mg (base) per mL (Rx) [*Folvite*].

**Packaging and storage**
Store below 40 °C (104 °F), preferably between 15 and 30 °C (59 and 86 °F), unless otherwise specified by manufacturer. Protect from light. Protect from freezing.

[1]Not included in Canadian product labeling.

Revised: 05/20/92
Interim revision: 08/17/94; 05/01/95

---

# FOLLITROPIN ALFA  Systemic—INTRODUCTORY VERSION

VA CLASSIFICATION (Primary): HS106
Commonly used brand name(s): *Gonal-F*.
Note: For a listing of dosage forms and brand names by country availability, see *Dosage Forms* section(s).

## Category
Gonadotropin; infertility therapy agent.

## Indications

**General considerations**
Special attention should be given to the underlying cause of female infertility in both female and male partners before follitropin alfa treatment is initiated.

**Accepted**
Infertility, female (treatment)—Follitropin alfa is indicated in the treatment of female infertility to stimulate ovarian follicular development in patients with ovulatory dysfunction not due to primary ovarian failure, such as anovulation or oligo-ovulation. Follitropin alfa replaces physiologic concentrations of follicle-stimulating hormone (FSH). It is used in conjunction with a properly timed injection of human chorionic gonadotropin (hCG) when the patient produces no ovulatory surge of endogenous luteinizing hormone (LH). In studies of patients using follitropin alfa for no more than three cycles for ovulation induction, the cumulative ovulation rate of 81% produced a cumulative pregnancy rate of 37%, which resulted in 63% single births, 14% multiple births, and 23% of pregnancies not reaching term.

Reproductive technologies, assisted—Follitropin alfa is indicated to stimulate the development of multiple oocytes in ovulatory patients enrolled in an assisted reproductive technology (ART) program, such as embryo transfer (ET) or *in vitro* fertilization (IVF). In some studies, patients were pretreated with a gonadotropin-releasing hormone agonist (GnRHa) to down-regulate the pituitary in order to reduce FSH and LH activity, giving control of hypothalamic-pituitary axis function and timing of exogenous gonadotropins (follitropin alfa and hCG) administration to the investigator or clinician. Follitropin alfa is used in conjunction with a properly timed injection of hCG when the patient produces no ovulatory surge of endogenous LH. In studies of patients undergoing ART, pregnancy outcome may be influenced by several factors, such as number of oocytes being inseminated, fertilization rate of oocytes, and number of embryos transferred *in utero* in a single treatment cycle. Many variables that will be different among patients and/or treatment protocols influence these results.

## Pharmacology/Pharmacokinetics

**Physicochemical characteristics**
Source—Follitropin alfa is derived from genetically modified Chinese hamster ovary (CHO) cells cultured in bioreactors. It is then purified to a consistent follicle-stimulating hormone (FSH) isoform profile by means of immunochromatography.
Chemical group—The primary and tertiary structures of follitropin alfa are identical to that of human FSH.
Molecular weight—10,205.88 for the alpha subunit of 92 amino acids; 12,485.34 for the beta subunit of 111 amino acids.
Other characteristics—Follitropin alfa may contain up to 15% of oxidized follitropin alfa.

**Mechanism of action/Effect**
Infertility, female or reproductive technologies, assisted—Follitropin alfa replaces deficient or abnormal FSH serum concentrations in patients experiencing ovulatory function impairment. Specifically, follitropin alfa, a recombinant FSH, stimulates follicle recruitment and follicular growth and maturation. Follitropin alfa's ability to increase serum concentrations of inhibin, estradiol, and total ovarian follicular volume varies widely among individuals. The rise in the serum inhibin concentration is an early indicator of follicular development; its concentration declines quickly after follitropin alfa treatment is discontinued. Total growth of ovarian follicles lags behind increasing FSH serum concentrations, and ovarian follicular growth continues to increase for a time with declining FSH serum concentrations. Maximum ovarian follicular volume correlates better with inhibin or estradiol serum concentrations than it does with FSH serum concentrations. Anovulatory patients who need luteinizing hormone (LH) activity at mid-cycle receive an injection of human chorionic gonadotropin (hCG) to stimulate ovulation and to continue follicular maturation. Follitropin alfa is not useful for patients experiencing infertility due to primary ovarian failure.

Before consecutive administration of gonadotropins as single agents to increase recruitment of multiple follicles, some assisted reproductive technology protocols include pretreatment with a gonadotropin-releasing hormone agonist (GnRHa) to suppress the pituitary release of gonadotropins. Once the pituitary is suppressed, the patient's physiologic concentrations of gonadotropins are then replaced.

**Absorption**
Absorption of follitropin alfa is slower than its elimination, and the pharmacokinetics are considered to be dependent on the absorption rate.

**Distribution**
Human tissue or organ distribution of subcutaneous follitropin alfa administration has not been determined.

**Biotransformation**
Biotransformation has not been studied in humans.

**Half-life**
Distribution—Intravenous: 2 to 5 hours.

**Elimination**
Renal, 12.5% of total clearance.

## Precautions to Consider

**Cross-sensitivity and/or related problems**
Patients hypersensitive to follicle-stimulating hormone (FSH) preparations may be hypersensitive to follitropin alfa also.

**Carcinogenicity**
Long-term studies have not been done in animals to evaluate the carcinogenic potential of follitropin alfa.

**Mutagenicity**
Follitropin alfa was not found to be mutagenic in a series of tests, including the bacterial and mammalian cell mutation tests, a chromosomal aberration test, and a micronucleus test.

### Pregnancy/Reproduction
Use of follitropin alfa in treatment of infertility or as an adjunct with assisted reproduction technologies is associated with a high incidence of multiple gestations and multiple births. This may increase the risk of neonatal prematurity, as well as other complications associated with multiple gestations.

Fertility—Follitropin alfa is used before a natural or artificial luteinizing hormone (LH) surge to develop and recruit follicles in humans.

Impaired fertility has been reported in rats given 40 international units per kg (IU/kg) or more of body weight once a day for extended periods.

Pregnancy—Use of follitropin alfa during pregnancy is unnecessary and not recommended. Ovarian hyperstimulation syndrome (OHSS), which may be induced by follitropin alfa therapy, is more common, more severe, and protracted in patients who conceive.

FDA Pregnancy Category X.

### Breast-feeding
It is not known whether follitropin alfa is distributed into breast milk.

### Medical considerations/Contraindications
The medical considerations/contraindications included have been selected on the basis of their potential clinical significance (reasons given in parentheses where appropriate)—not necessarily inclusive (» = major clinical significance).

*Risk-benefit should be considered when the following medical problems exist:*
» Abnormal uterine or genital bleeding, undiagnosed
 (may delay diagnosis of endocrinopathy, such as endometrial hyperplasia or hormone-dependent carcinoma; inducing fertility and pregnancy may not be advisable for such patients)
» Adrenal function impairment, uncontrolled or
» Thyroid function impairment, uncontrolled or
» Tumors, intracranial or sex hormone–dependent
 (increasing estrogen concentrations may make these conditions worse)
 Asthma
 (may be exacerbated)
 Hypersensitivity to FSH preparations
» Ovarian cyst or enlargement, undetermined cause
 (increased risk of further enlargement)
» Primary ovarian failure
 (follitropin alfa is ineffective in patients with primary ovarian failure)

### Patient monitoring
The following may be especially important in patient monitoring (other tests may be warranted in some patients, depending on condition; » = major clinical significance):

*For female patients*
Note: Patients should be examined for ovarian hyperstimulation syndrome (OHSS) every other day during treatment with follitropin alfa and for 14 days posttreatment.
 Daily basal body temperature and/or
 Progesterone, serum
 (measurement of serum progesterone concentrations can be made prior to follitropin alfa therapy to confirm anovulation. An increase in serum progesterone concentrations or a rise in basal body temperature can confirm ovulation)
» Estradiol, serum and/or
» Ultrasonography of ovaries and uterus
 (ultrasonography and monitoring of serum estradiol concentrations can be used to monitor follicular development, predict timing for human chorionic gonadotropin [hCG] administration, detect ovarian enlargement, and aid in minimizing risk of OHSS and multiple gestation)
 (ultrasonography of the ovaries can determine approximate time of ovulation by viewing fluid in the cul-de-sac, ovarian stigmata, collapsed follicle, or secretory endometrium. Ultrasonography is especially useful for evaluating the number of developing follicles, which is not predictable from serum estrogen concentration data)
 Pregnancy test
 (pregnancy can be confirmed by testing for serum hCG)

*For male partners*
 Sperm count and determinations of sperm motility and
 Testosterone, serum
 (baseline measurement of sperm count and activity in male partners is recommended to evaluate success of follitropin alfa treatment in females. If semen analysis is abnormal, serum testosterone concentration in the male partner may be measured)

## Side/Adverse Effects
Note: Serious pulmonary and vascular complications have been reported in patients who have received gonadotropins. Arterial thromboembolism has been reported both in association with and separate from ovarian hyperstimulation syndrome (OHSS) in patients who have received follitropin alfa. Complications resulting from thromboembolism have included venous thrombophlebitis, pulmonary embolism, pulmonary infarction, stroke, arterial occlusion necessitating limb amputation, and, in rare cases, death. Serious pulmonary complications that have occurred include atelectasis, acute respiratory distress syndrome, and, rarely, death.

The following side/adverse effects have been selected on the basis of their potential clinical significance (possible signs and symptoms in parentheses where appropriate)—not necessarily inclusive:

### Those indicating need for medical attention
Incidence more frequent
 *For patients treated for female infertility or patients pretreated with a gonadotropin-releasing hormone agonist (GnRHa) undergoing artificial reproductive technologies (ART)*
  **Abdominal or pelvic pain**—9 to 10%; *diarrhea*—8%; *flatulence* (passing of gas)—4 to 7%; *influenza-like or cold symptoms, including sinusitis; pharyngitis; and upper respiratory tract infection* (body aches or pain; coughing; fever; headache; loss of voice; runny nose; unusual tiredness or weakness)—4 to 12%; *intermenstrual bleeding* (uterine bleeding between menstrual periods)—4 to 9%; *nausea*—5 to 14%; *ovarian enlargement, mild and uncomplicated* (abdominal bloating; abdominal pain)—20%, usually regresses after 2 to 3 weeks

 *For patients treated for female infertility*
  **Acne**—4%; *breast pain or tenderness*—4%; *emotional lability* (mood swings)—5%; *ovarian cysts* (abdominal or pelvic pain; mild bloating)—15.3%; *ovarian hyperstimulation syndrome (OHSS)* (abdominal pain, severe; nausea; rapid weight gain; vomiting)—7%

Note: When comparing follitropin alfa to urofollitropin in one study of 454 patients treated for ovulation induction, 15% of patients using follitropin alfa and 29% of patients using urofollitropin developed *ovarian cysts*. Conversely, 7% of patients using follitropin alfa developed *ovarian hyperstimulation syndrome (OHSS)* while 4% of patients using urofollitropin developed OHSS; 0.8% of all patients were considered to have severe cases. Ovarian cysts and OHSS did not occur in two studies of 237 patients enrolled in an ART program who were pretreated with gonadotropin-releasing hormone agonists to down-regulate the pituitary before follitropin alfa or urofollitropin treatment was initiated.

Incidence less frequent
 *For patients treated for female infertility or patients pretreated with a GnRHa undergoing ART—1 to 3%*
  **Dizziness**; *dysmenorrhea* (painful menstrual periods); *leukorrhea* (white vaginal discharge); *redness, pain, or swelling at injection site*; *somnolence* (sleepiness); *vaginal hemorrhage* (heavy nonmenstrual vaginal bleeding)

 *For patients treated for female infertility—1 to 3%*
  **Dyspepsia** (stomach discomfort); *hypotension* (dizziness; lightheadedness; fainting); *lesion on cervix*; *migraine*; *nervousness*

 *For patients pretreated with a GnRHa undergoing ART—1 to 2%*
  **Anorexia** (loss of appetite); *chest pain or palpitations* (fast, racing heartbeat); *pruritus* (itching of skin); *unusual thirst*

### Those indicating possible need for medical attention if they occur after medication is discontinued
 *OHSS* (abdominal pain, severe; nausea; rapid weight gain; vomiting)—usually within seven to ten days after treatment discontinuation

## Patient Consultation
As an aid to patient consultation, refer to *Advice for the Patient, Follitropin Alfa (Systemic)*.

In providing consultation, consider emphasizing the following selected information (» = major clinical significance):

### Before using this medication
» Conditions affecting use, especially:
 Hypersensitivity to follicle-stimulating hormone (FSH) preparations
 Pregnancy—Use during pregnancy is not needed or recommended; increased risk of multiple gestations and their associated complications and protracted ovarian hyperstimulation syndrome (OHSS) in patients who conceive

Other medical problems, especially abnormal uterine or genital bleeding, undiagnosed; adrenal function impairment, uncontrolled; intracranial or sex hormone–dependent tumors; ovarian cyst or enlargement, undetermined cause; primary ovarian failure; or thyroid function impairment, uncontrolled

**Proper use of this medication**
» Carefully reading patient instructions provided
*For those patients self-administering the medication*
    Proper preparation of medication; using proper technique to prevent contamination of the medication, work area, and patient during transfer between containers
    Proper administration; using proper needle and syringe
    Knowing proper dose to use and not using more than prescribed
    Carefully selecting and rotating injection sites as directed by physician
    Disposing of needles, syringes, ampuls, and unused medication properly
    Alerting physician when last dose of follitropin alfa is given and knowing that another drug called human chorionic gonadotropin may be required as a single injection 24 hours after the last dose of follitropin alfa
» Proper dosing
    Missed dose: Calling physician for advice; do not double doses
» Proper storage

**Precautions while using this medication**
» Understanding the duration of treatment and the importance of required frequent monitoring by physician during treatment and for at least 2 weeks after follitropin alfa treatment is stopped
» Importance of following physician's instructions for recording basal body temperature, if requested, and timing of intercourse
    Understanding that dizziness can occur with use of follitropin alfa and may impair driving, using machines, or other dangerous tasks

**Side/adverse effects**
Signs of potential side effects, especially:
    For patients treated for female infertility or patients pretreated with a GnRHa undergoing ART—Abdominal or pelvic pain; diarrhea; flatulence; influenza-like or cold symptoms, including sinusitis, pharnygitis, and upper respiratory tract infection; intermenstrual bleeding; nausea; ovarian enlargement, mild and uncomplicated; dizziness; dysmenorrhea; leukorrhea; redness, pain, or swelling at injection site; somnolence; or vaginal hemorrhage
    For patients treated for female infertility—Acne; breast pain or tenderness; emotional lability; ovarian cysts; ovarian hyperstimulation syndrome; dyspepsia; hypotension; lesion on cervix; migraine; or nervousness
    For patients pretreated with a GnRHa undergoing ART—Anorexia; chest pain or palpitations; pruritus; or unusual thirst

## General Dosing Information

Patients receiving follitropin alfa should be under the supervision of a physician experienced in the treatment of gynecologic or endocrinologic disorders and willing to devote considerable time to case-management.

Dosage varies considerably and must be adjusted to meet the individual requirements of each patient on the basis of clinical response.

If the ovaries are abnormally enlarged on the last day of follitropin alfa treatment, human chorionic gonadotropin (hCG) should not be administered to minimize risk of ovarian hyperstimulation syndrome (OHSS). OHSS develops rapidly (between 24 and 72 hours) and is distinct from uncomplicated ovarian enlargement. Patients should be monitored for 2 weeks after treatment ends, since the risk of OHSS reaches its maximal potential at 7 to 10 days post-treatment.

Patients self-injecting follitropin alfa should be given the patient information sheet and instructed on how to prepare the medication and injection site, administer the medication, and safely discard used items. Injection sites should be rotated and medication administered to upper thigh or at waistline.

**For patients treated for ovulation induction**
Conception should be attempted daily beginning within 24 hours of administration of hCG until ovulation is thought to have occurred.

If ovulation does not occur after any cycle of therapy, the therapeutic regimen employed should be re-evaluated. After three to six cycles of nonovulatory menses, the appropriateness of continuing the use of follitropin alfa for ovulation induction should be reconsidered.

**Bioequivalenence information**
According to physicochemical tests and assays, the primary and tertiary structures of follitropin alfa, follitropin beta, and human follicle-stimulating hormone (FSH) are indistinguishable from one another. These hormones are similar to human menopausal urine-derived follicle-stimulating hormone (urofollitropin) but without urinary protein for the non-purified dosage form, and to menotropins without the urinary protein or luteinizing hormone (LH) components.

**Safety considerations for handling this medication**
Precautions include:
• Use of proper technique to prevent contamination of the medication, work area, and operator during transfer between containers, including proper training in this technique for those patients self-administering the medication
• Cautious and proper disposal of needles, syringes, vials, ampuls, and unused medication.

**For treatment of adverse effects**
Recommended treatment for OHSS consists of the following:
• Stopping treatment with follitropin alfa (or hCG).
• Hospitalizing patients with severe OHSS; less severe cases may spontaneously resolve at onset of menses.
• Managing electrolyte and fluid imbalances.

## Parenteral Dosage Forms

### FOLLITROPIN ALFA FOR INJECTION

**Usual adult dose**
Infertility, female—
    Subcutaneous, 75 international units (IU) a day, usually for fourteen days, then the dose is increased by 37.5 IU at weekly intervals if clinically indicated after measurement of the serum estradiol concentration and follicular development. Total dose should not routinely exceed 300 IU a day. Total length of treatment should not exceed thirty-five days, unless serum estradiol indicates imminent follicular development. Treatment should be discontinued if the ovaries become abnormally enlarged or abdominal pain occurs; at this time the patient should be advised not to have sexual intercourse. To complete follicular development and to induce ovulation in the absence of a luteinizing hormone (LH) surge, human chorionic gonadotropin (hCG) is administered one day after the last dose of follitropin alfa treatment, unless the serum estradiol concentration exceeds 2000 picograms per mL.
Reproductive technologies, assisted—
    Subcutaneous, 150 international units (IU) once a day, beginning cycle Day 2 or Day 3 until follicles are developed sufficiently. Dose adjustment can be considered after the first five days of treatment, and then adjusted every three to five days thereafter; dose should be adjusted by no more than 75 to 150 IU per day for each adjustment interval. For most patients, treatment should not exceed ten days. Doses greater than 450 IU a day are not recommended. For patients with suppressed endogenous gonadotropins, treatment may begin at 225 IU once a day. To complete follicular development in all patients not experiencing an LH surge, hCG is administered one day after the last dose of follitropin alfa treatment.

**Size(s) usually available**
U.S.—
    75 International Units (Rx) [*Gonal-F* (inactive dibasic sodium phosphate 1.11 mg; monobasic sodium phosphate monohydrate 0.45 mg; sucrose 30 mg)].
    150 International Units (Rx) [*Gonal-F* (inactive dibasic sodium phosphate 1.11 mg; monobasic sodium phosphate monohydrate 0.45 mg; sucrose 30 mg)].

**Packaging and storage**
Store between 2 and 25 °C (36 and 77 °F). Protect from light.

**Preparation of dosage form**
Using standard aseptic technique, follitropin alfa is reconstituted by adding 0.5 to 1 mL of Sterile Water for Injection USP to each ampul. A total concentration of 225 IU per 0.5 mL should not be exceeded.

**Stability**
The solution should be used immediately after reconstitution and any unused material discarded. The solution should not be used if it is cloudy or discolored.

**Auxiliary labeling**
• Protect from light.

**Note**
Include patient package information when dispensing.

Developed: 1/26/98

# FOLLITROPIN BETA  Systemic—INTRODUCTORY VERSION

VA CLASSIFICATION (Primary): HS106
Commonly used brand name(s): *Follistim*.
Note: For a listing of dosage forms and brand names by country availability, see *Dosage Forms* section(s).

## Category
Gonadotropin; infertility therapy agent.

## Indications

### General considerations
Special attention should be given to the underlying cause of female infertility in both female and male partners before follitropin beta treatment is initiated.

### Accepted
Infertility, female (treatment)—Follitropin beta is indicated in the treatment of female infertility to stimulate ovarian follicular development in patients with ovulatory dysfunction not due to primary ovarian failure, such as anovulation or oligo-ovulation. Follitropin beta replaces physiologic concentrations of follicle-stimulating hormone (FSH). It is used in conjunction with a properly timed injection of human chorionic gonadotropin (hCG) when the patient produces no ovulatory surge of endogenous luteinizing hormone (LH). In studies of patients unresponsive to clomiphene using follitropin beta for no more than three cycles for ovulation induction, the cumulative ovulation rate of 85% produced a cumulative pregnancy rate of 23%, which resulted in 63% single births, 6% multiple births, and 31% of pregnancies not reaching term.

Reproductive technologies, assisted—Follitropin beta is indicated to stimulate the development of multiple oocytes in ovulatory patients enrolled in an assisted reproductive technology (ART) program, such as embryo transfer (ET) or *in vitro* fertilization (IVF). In some studies, patients were pretreated with a gonadotropin-releasing hormone agonist (GnRHa) to down-regulate the pituitary in order to reduce FSH and LH activity, giving control of hypothalamic-pituitary axis function and timing of exogenous gonadotropins (follitropin beta and hCG) administration to the investigator or clinician. Follitropin beta is used in conjunction with a properly timed injection of hCG when the patient produces no ovulatory surge of endogenous LH. In studies of patients undergoing ART, pregnancy outcome may be influenced by several factors, such as number of oocytes being inseminated, fertilization rate of oocytes, and number of embryos transferred *in utero* in a single treatment cycle. Many variables that will be different among patients and/or treatment protocols influence these results.

## Pharmacology/Pharmacokinetics

### Physicochemical characteristics
Source—Follitropin beta is derived from a product produced from genetically modified Chinese hamster ovary (CHO) cells. Afterwards, it is purified to a consistent follicle-stimulating hormone (FSH) isoform profile.
Chemical group—The primary and tertiary structures of follitropin beta are identical to that of human FSH.
Molecular weight—10,205.88 for the alpha subunit of 92 amino acids; 12,485.34 for the beta subunit of 111 amino acids.
Other characteristics—Follitropin beta may contain up to 20% oxidized follitropin beta.

### Mechanism of action/Effect
Infertility, female, or reproductive technologies, assisted—Follitropin beta replaces deficient or abnormal FSH serum concentrations in patients experiencing ovulatory function impairment. Specifically, follitropin beta, a recombinant FSH, stimulates follicle recruitment and follicular growth and maturation. Follitropin beta's ability to increase serum concentrations of inhibin, estradiol, and total ovarian follicular volume varies widely among individuals. The rise in the serum inhibin concentration is an early indicator of follicular development; its concentration declines quickly after follitropin beta treatment is discontinued. Total growth of ovarian follicles lags behind increasing FSH serum concentrations, and ovarian follicular growth continues to increase for a time with declining FSH serum concentrations. Maximum ovarian follicular volume correlates better with inhibin or estradiol serum concentrations than it does with FSH serum concentrations. Anovulatory patients who need luteinizing hormone (LH) activity at mid-cycle receive an injection of human chorionic gonadotropin (hCG) to stimulate ovulation and to continue follicular maturation. Follitropin beta is not useful for patients experiencing infertility due to primary ovarian failure.

Before consecutive administration of gonadotropins as single agents to increase recruitment of multiple follicles, some assisted reproductive technology protocols include pretreatment with a gonadotropin-releasing hormone agonist (GnRHa) to suppress the pituitary release of gonadotropins. Once the pituitary is suppressed, the patient's physiologic concentrations of gonadotropins are replaced.

### Absorption
The area under the plasma concentration–time curve (AUC) for the subcutaneous and intramuscular routes for administering follitropin beta are considered equivalent; however, the peak plasma concentration ($C_{max}$) differs.

### Half-life
Elimination—
The mean half-lives for 7-day treatment for the following doses of follitropin beta given intramuscularly once a day are:
75 international units (IU)—26.9 hours ± 7.8 hours.
150 IU—30.1 hours ± 6.2 hours.
225 IU—28.9 hours ± 6.5 hours.
The mean half-life for a single dose of 300 IU of follitropin beta given intramuscularly is 43.9 ± 14.1 hours.

### Peak serum concentration
A 7-day treatment of 75 IU, 150 IU, and 225 IU of follitropin beta given once a day to pituitary-suppressed females produced the following mean peak serum concentrations ($C_{max}$):
75 IU—Intramuscular, 4.7 ± 1.5 IU per liter (IU/L). Subcutaneous, 4.3 ± 0.6 IU/L.
150 IU—Intramuscular, 9.5 ± 2.6 IU/L. Subcutaneous—8.5 ± 0.6 IU/L.
225 IU—Intramuscular, 11.3 ± 1.8 IU/L. Subcutaneous—13.9 ± 1.8 IU/L.
A single dose of 300 IU of follitropin beta given intramuscularly to healthy, gonadotropin-deficient females produced a $C_{max}$ of 4.3 ± 1.7 IU/L.

## Precautions to Consider

### Cross-sensitivity and/or related problems
Patients hypersensitive to follicle-stimulating hormone (FSH) preparations may be hypersensitive to follitropin beta also.

### Carcinogenicity
Long-term studies have not been done in animals to evaluate the carcinogenic potential of follitropin beta.

### Mutagenicity
Follitropin beta was not found to be mutagenic in the Ames test and an *in vitro* chromosomal aberration test using human lymphocytes.

### Pregnancy/Reproduction
Use of follitropin beta in treatment of infertility or as an adjunct with assisted reproduction technologies is associated with a high incidence of multiple gestations and multiple births. This may increase the risk of neonatal prematurity, as well as other complications associated with multiple gestations.
Fertility—Follitropin beta is used before a natural or an artificial luteinizing hormone (LH) surge to develop and recruit follicles in humans.
Pregnancy—Follitropin beta is not needed or recommended for use during pregnancy. Ovarian hyperstimulation syndrome (OHSS), which may be induced by follitropin beta therapy, is more common, more severe, and protracted in patients who conceive.
FDA Pregnancy Category X.

### Breast-feeding
It is not known whether follitropin beta is distributed into breast milk.

### Pharmacogenetics
Although drug clearance was comparable between groups of European women and Japanese women, the Japanese women absorbed more of a single 300 IU dose of follitropin beta given intramuscularly based on their lower body weight.

### Medical considerations/Contraindications
The medical considerations/contraindications included have been selected on the basis of their potential clinical significance (reasons given in parentheses where appropriate)—not necessarily inclusive (» = major clinical significance).

*Risk-benefit should be considered when the following medical problems exist:*
» Abnormal uterine or genital bleeding, undiagnosed
(may delay diagnosis of endocrinopathology, such as endometrial

- Adrenal function impairment, uncontrolled or
- Thyroid function impairment, uncontrolled or
- Tumors, intracranial or sex hormone–dependent
    (increasing estrogen concentrations may make these conditions worse)
  Asthma
    (may be exacerbated)
  Hypersensitivity to FSH preparations
- Ovarian cyst or enlargement, undetermined cause
    (increased risk of further enlargement)
- Primary ovarian failure
    (follitropin beta is ineffective in patients with primary ovarian failure)

**Patient monitoring**
The following may be especially important in patient monitoring (other tests may be warranted in some patients, depending on condition; » = major clinical significance):

*For female patients*
Note: Patients should be examined for ovarian hyperstimulation syndrome (OHSS) every other day during treatment with follitropin beta and for 14 days posttreatment.
  Daily basal body temperature and/or
  Progesterone, serum
    (measurement of serum progesterone concentrations can be made prior to follitropin beta therapy to confirm anovulation. An increase in serum progesterone concentrations or a rise in basal body temperature can confirm ovulation)
- Estradiol, serum and/or
  Examination, cervical secretions or vaginal cytology and
- Ultrasonography of ovaries and/or uterus
    (ultrasonography and monitoring of serum estradiol concentrations can be used to monitor follicular development, predict time of human chorionic gonadotropin [hCG] administration, detect ovarian enlargement, and aid in minimizing risk of OHSS and multiple gestation)
    (ultrasonography of the ovaries and endometrial lining can help confirm if ovulation occurs by viewing fluid in the cul-de-sac, ovarian stigmata, collapsed follicle, or secretory endometrium. Ultrasonography is especially helpful for evaluating the number of follicles, which is not predictable from serum estrogen concentration data)
    (when evaluating follicular development, estrogenic changes of vaginal cytology or changes in volume or appearance of cervical mucus may be assessed as an adjunct to direct measurement of serum estradiol concentrations or viewing of the ovaries or endometrial lining by ultrasonography)
  Pregnancy test
    (pregnancy can be confirmed by testing for serum hCG)

*For male partners*
  Sperm count and determinations of sperm motility and
  Testosterone, serum
    (baseline measurement of sperm count and activity in male partners is recommended to evaluate success of follitropin beta treatment in females. If semen analysis is abnormal, serum testosterone concentration in the male partner may be measured)

## Side/Adverse Effects

Note: Serious pulmonary and vascular complications and arterial thromboembolism have been reported both in association with and separate from ovarian hyperstimulation syndrome in patients who have received gonadotropins. Complications resulting from thromboembolism have included venous thrombophlebitis, pulmonary embolism, pulmonary infarction, stroke, arterial occlusion necessitating limb amputation, and, in rare cases, death. Serious pulmonary complications that have occurred include atelectasis, acute respiratory distress syndrome, and, rarely, death.

The following side/adverse effects have been selected on the basis of their potential clinical significance (possible signs and symptoms in parentheses where appropriate)—not necessarily inclusive:

**Those indicating need for medical attention**
Incidence more frequent
    *For patients treated for female infertility or patients pretreated with a gonadotropin-releasing hormone agonist (GnRHa) undergoing assisted reproductive technology (ART)*
        **Ovarian hyperstimulation syndrome (OHSS)** (abdominal pain, severe; nausea; rapid weight gain; vomiting)—7.6% for treatment of female infertility and 5.2% for ART

Incidence less frequent
    *For patients treated for female infertility or patients pretreated with a GnRHa undergoing ART*
        **Abdominal pain**—2.5 to 2.9%
    *For patients treated for female infertility*
        **Ovarian cyst**—2.9%
    *For patients pretreated with a GnRHa undergoing ART*
        **Redness, pain, or swelling at site of injection**—1.7%

**Those indicating need for medical attention only if they continue or are bothersome**
    *Breast tenderness; dermatological symptoms, such as dry skin; hair loss; hives; and skin rash; dizziness; dyspnea* (difficulty in breathing); *influenza-like symptoms, such as body aches or pain; chills; fever; headache; nausea; unusual tiredness; tachycardia* (fast, racing heart); *tachypnea* (quick, shallow breathing)

Note: The above side/adverse effects have not been reported in patients specifically receiving follitropin beta but have been reported for patients receiving gonadotropins and may potentially occur for follitropin beta.

**Those indicating possible development of OHSS and/or the need for medical attention if they occur after medication is discontinued**
    *OHSS* (abdominal pain, severe; nausea; rapid weight gain; vomiting)—usually occurring within 7 to 10 days after treatment discontinuation

## Patient Consultation

As an aid to patient consultation, refer to *Advice for the Patient, Follitropin Beta (Systemic)*.
In providing consultation, consider emphasizing the following selected information (» = major clinical significance):

**Before using this medication**
- Conditions affecting use, especially:
    Hypersensitivity to follicle-stimulating hormone (FSH) preparations
    Pregnancy—Use during pregnancy is not needed or recommended; increased risk of multiple gestations and their associated complications and protracted ovarian hyperstimulation syndrome (OHSS) in patients who conceive
    Other medical problems, especially abnormal uterine or genital bleeding, undiagnosed; adrenal function impairment, uncontrolled; intracranial or sex hormone–dependent tumors; ovarian cyst or enlargement, undetermined cause; primary ovarian failure; or thyroid function impairment, uncontrolled

**Proper use of this medication**
  Carefully reading patient instructions provided
*For patients self-administering the medication*
  Proper preparation of medication; using proper technique to prevent contamination of the medication, work area, and patient during transfer between containers
  Proper administration; using proper needle and syringe
  Knowing proper dose to use and not using more than prescribed
  Carefully selecting and rotating injection sites as directed by physician
  Disposing of needles, syringes, vials, and unused medication properly
  Alerting physician when last dose of follitropin beta is given and knowing that another drug called human chorionic gonadotropin may be required as a single injection 24 hours after the last dose of follitropin beta
- Proper dosing
  Missed dose: Calling physician for advice; do not double doses
- Proper storage

**Precautions while using this medication**
- Understanding the duration of treatment and the importance of being monitored every other day by physician during treatment and for at least 2 weeks after treatment stops
- Importance of following physician's instructions for recording basal body temperature, if requested, and timing of intercourse
- If abdominal pain occurs, discontinuing treatment of follitropin beta, notifying physician, not having injection of hCG, and avoiding sexual intercourse
  Understanding that dizziness can occur with use of follitropin beta and may impair driving, using machines, or other dangerous tasks

**Side/adverse effects**
  Signs of potential side effects, especially:
    For patients treated for female infertility or patients pretreated with a GnRHa undergoing ART—Ovarian hyperstimulation syndrome; abdominal pain
    For patients treated for female infertility—Ovarian cyst
    For patients pretreated with a GnRHa undergoing ART—Redness, pain, or swelling at site of injection

## General Dosing Information

Patients receiving follitropin beta should be under the supervision of a physician experienced in the treatment of gynecologic or endocrine disorders. Patient and physician should be willing to devote considerable time to case-management.

Dosage varies considerably and must be adjusted to meet the individual requirements of each patient, on the basis of clinical response.

If the ovaries are abnormally enlarged on the last day of follitropin beta treatment, hCG should not be administered to minimize risk of ovarian hyperstimulation syndrome (OHSS). OHSS develops rapidly (between 24 and 72 hours) and is distinct from uncomplicated ovarian enlargement. Patients should be monitored every other day for 2 weeks after treatment ends, since the risk of OHSS reaches its maximal potential at 7 to 10 days posttreatment.

Patients self-injecting follitropin beta should be given the patient information sheet and instructed on how to prepare the medication and injection site, administer the medication, and safely discard used items. Injection sites should be rotated and medication administered subcutaneously to upper thigh or at waistline or administered intramuscularly to the upper outer quadrant of the buttocks.

### For patients treated for ovulation induction

Conception should be attempted daily beginning within 24 hours of administration of hCG until ovulation is thought to have occurred.

If ovulation does not occur after any cycle of therapy, the therapeutic regimen employed should be re-evaluated. After three to six cycles of nonovulatory menses, the appropriateness of continuing the use of follitropin beta for ovulation induction should be reconsidered.

### Bioequivalenence information

According to physicochemical tests and assays, the primary and tertiary structures of follitropin alfa, follitropin beta, and human follicle-stimulating hormone (FSH) are indistinguishable from one another, but alfa and beta forms are based on different international reference standards. These hormones are similar to formulations of human menopausal urine-derived follicle-stimulating hormone (urofollitropin), but without urinary protein for the nonpurified dosage form. Also, follitropin beta's action is similar to that of menotropins, but follitropin beta does not contain the urinary protein or luteinizing hormone (LH) components.

### Safety considerations for handling this medication

Precautions include:
- Use of proper technique to prevent contamination of the medication, work area, and operator during transfer between containers, including proper training in this technique for patients self-administering the medication.
- Cautious and proper disposal of needles, syringes, vials, ampuls, and unused medication.

### For treatment of adverse effects

**Ovarian enlargement, ovarian cyst formation, or ovarian hyperstimulation syndrome (OHSS)—**
- Discontinuing therapy until ovarian size has returned to baseline. Human chorionic gonadotropin should also be withheld for that cycle.
- Prohibiting intercourse until ovarian size has returned to baseline to prevent cyst rupture.
- Reducing dosage of follitropin beta in next course of therapy.
- Most cases of ovarian enlargement, ovarian cyst formation, or OHSS will spontaneously resolve when menses begins. In selected cases, hospitalization of the patient and bed rest may be necessary.
- Limiting performance of pelvic examinations since they may result in rupture of ovarian cysts and hemoperitoneum.
- When treating OHSS, the general purpose of therapy is to prevent hemoconcentration and minimize risk of thromboembolism and renal injury.

  —*Acute phase of OHSS*: The electrolyte imbalance should be corrected cautiously while an acceptable intravascular volume is maintained; in the acute phase, intravascular volume deficit cannot be completely corrected without increasing third space fluid volume.
  - Specific treatment:
    —Avoiding diuretic use since it reduces intravascular volume further.
    —Administering intravenous fluids, electrolytes, and Albumin Human USP as needed to maintain adequate urine output and to avoid hemoconcentration.
    —Administering analgesics as needed.
  - Monitoring:
    —Monitoring fluid intake and output, body weight, hematocrit, serum and urine electrolytes, urine specific gravity, blood urea nitrogen (BUN) and creatinine, total protein with albumin:globulin ratio, coagulation studies, and abdominal girth daily or as often as required.
    —Monitoring serum potassium concentrations and electrocardiogram for development of hyperkalemia.
  - Supportive care:
    —Removing ascitic, pleural, or pericardial fluid *only* if it is imperative for relief of symptoms such as respiratory distress or cardiac tamponade; to do so may increase risk of injury to the ovary.
    —In patients who require surgery to control bleeding from ovarian cyst rupture, employing surgical measures that also maximally conserve ovarian tissue.

  —*Intermediate phase of OHSS*: Once patient is stabilized, minimize third spacing of fluids.
  - Specific treatment:
    —Avoiding diuretic use.
    —Restricting or cautiously replacing potassium, sodium, and fluids as required, based on monitoring of serum electrolyte concentrations.

  —*Resolution phase of OHSS*: In this phase, the third space fluid shifts to the intravascular compartment, resulting in decreased hematocrit value and increased urinary output.
  - Monitoring: Peripheral and/or pulmonary edema may result if mobilized third space fluid volume exceeds renal output.
  - Specific treatment: Administering diuretics when required to manage pulmonary edema.

## Parenteral Dosage Forms

### FOLLITROPIN BETA FOR INJECTION

**Usual adult dose**

Infertility, female—
  Subcutaneous or intramuscular, 75 international units (IU) once a day, for up to fourteen days. Then the dose is increased by 37.5 IU at weekly intervals if clinically indicated after measurement of the serum estradiol concentration and follicular development. Total daily dose should not routinely exceed 300 IU. Treatment should be discontinued if the ovaries become abnormally enlarged or abdominal pain occurs, and the patient should be advised to avoid sexual intercourse.

  To complete follicular development and to induce ovulation in the absence of a luteinizing hormone (LH) surge, human chorionic gonadotropin (hCG) is administered one day after the last dose of follitropin beta treatment. Human chorionic gonadotropin should not be injected if the ovaries are abnormally enlarged or the ovarian response is inappropriate, as shown by serum estradiol concentrations or ultrasonography.

Reproductive technologies, assisted—
  Subcutaneous or intramuscular, 150 to 225 international units (IU) once a day, beginning cycle Day 2 or Day 3 for the first four days of treatment. Dose may then be adjusted according to an individual's ovarian response; daily maintenance doses of 75 to 300 IU for six to twelve days are usually sufficient. About 10% of patients who do not respond may need higher doses of 375 to 600 IU.

  After a sufficient number of follicles are produced, hCG is administered one day after the last dose of follitropin beta treatment to complete follicular development in all patients not experiencing an LH surge, unless the ovaries are abnormally enlarged. Egg retrieval is attempted thirty-four to thirty-six hours later.

**Size(s) usually available**

U.S.—
  75 International Units (Rx) [*Follistim* (polysorbate 20; sucrose 25 mg; sodium citrate dihydrate 7.35 mg)].

**Packaging and storage**

Store between 2 and 25 °C (36 and 77 °F). Protect from light.

**Preparation of dosage form**

Using standard aseptic technique, follitropin beta is reconstituted by adding 1 mL of 0.45% Sodium Chloride Injection USP to a vial of follitropin beta to make 75 IU per mL. The vial should be swirled slowly, not shaken. For larger doses, the contents of the first vial can be used as the diluent for subsequent vials; up to four vials can be used to make a solution of 300 IU per mL. After reconstitution, the solution should be checked to determine that it is thoroughly mixed, clear, and free of particles before combining the contents of the next vial of follitropin beta.

**Stability**

The solution should be used immediately after reconstitution and any unused material discarded. The solution should not be used if it is cloudy or discolored.

# FOMEPIZOLE  Systemic—INTRODUCTORY VERSION

VA CLASSIFICATION (Primary): AD900
Commonly used brand name(s): *Antizol*.
Other commonly used names are 4-methylpyrazole and 4-MP.
Note: For a listing of dosage forms and brand names by country availability, see *Dosage Forms* section(s).

## Category
Antidote (to ethylene glycol poisoning).

## Indications
**Accepted**
Toxicity, ethylene glycol (treatment)—Fomepizole is indicated for use as an antidote in confirmed or suspected ethylene glycol (antifreeze) poisoning.

## Pharmacology/Pharmacokinetics
**Physicochemical characteristics**
Molecular weight—82.1.
Solubility—Soluble in water; very soluble in ethanol, diethyl ether, and chloroform.

**Mechanism of action/Effect**
Fomepizole is a competitive inhibitor of alcohol dehydrogenase, the enzyme that catalyzes the initial steps in the metabolism of ethylene glycol to glycoaldehyde. Glycoaldehyde then undergoes further oxidation to glycolate, glyoxylate, and oxalate. It is glycolate and oxalate that are primarily responsible for the metabolic acidosis and renal damage that are seen in ethylene glycol poisoning.

**Distribution**
Distributes rapidly into total body water. The volume of distribution is between 0.6 and 1.02 L per kg.

**Biotransformation**
Hepatic; the primary metabolite is 4-carboxypyrazole (approximately 80 to 85% of an administered dose). Other metabolites include 4-hydroxymethylpyrazole and the *N*-glucuronide conjugates of 4-carboxypyrazole and 4-hydroxymethylpyrazole.
Following multiple doses, fomepizole rapidly induces its own metabolism via the cytochrome P450 mixed-function oxidase system.

**Half-life**
Varies with dose and, therefore, has not been calculated.

**Time to peak concentration**
1 to 2 hours following single oral doses of 7 to 50 mg per kg of body weight to healthy volunteers.

**Therapeutic concentration**
8.2 to 24.6 mg (100 to 300 micromoles) per mL.

**Elimination**
In healthy volunteers, 1 to 3.5% of an administered dose was excreted unchanged in the urine. The metabolites also are excreted unchanged in the urine.
In dialysis—
  Fomepizole is dialyzable.

## Precautions to Consider

**Carcinogenicity**
Long-term animal studies to evaluate the carcinogenic potential of fomepizole have not been performed.

**Mutagenicity**
Fomepizole was found to be mutagenic in Ames tests utilizing *Escherichia coli* and *Salmonella typhimurium* test strains.

**Pregnancy/Reproduction**
Fertility—An 8% decrease in testicular mass was found in rats administered fomepizole at a dose of 110 mg per kg of body weight (approximately 0.6 time the human maximum daily exposure based on body surface area) for 40 to 42 days.

Pregnancy—Studies have not been done in humans.
Studies have not been done in animals.
FDA Pregnancy Category C.

**Breast-feeding**
It is not known whether fomepizole is distributed into breast milk.

**Pediatrics**
Appropriate studies on the relationship of age to the effects of fomepizole have not been performed in the pediatric population. Safety and efficacy have not been established.

**Geriatrics**
Although appropriate studies on the relationship of age to the effects of fomepizole have not been performed in the geriatric population, geriatrics-specific problems are not expected to limit the usefulness of fomepizole in the elderly. However, elderly patients are more likely to have renal function impairment, which may require adjustment of dosage in patients receiving fomepizole because its metabolites are excreted by the kidneys.

**Drug interactions and/or related problems**
The following drug interactions and/or related problems have been selected on the basis of their potential clinical significance (possible mechanism in parentheses where appropriate)—not necessarily inclusive (» = major clinical significance):

Note: Combinations containing any of the following medications, depending on the amount present, may also interact with this medication.

Ethanol
  (concurrent use can reduce the rate of elimination of fomepizole by 50% and the rate of elimination of ethanol by 40%)

**Laboratory value alterations**
The following have been selected on the basis of their potential clinical significance (possible effect in parentheses where appropriate)—not necessarily inclusive (» = major clinical significance):

With physiology/laboratory test values
  Cholesterol, serum and
  Triglycerides, serum
    (concentrations may be increased; however, no adverse clinical effects have been seen)
  Transaminase values
    (transient increases have been seen with repeated dosing)
  White blood count (WBC)
    (eosinophilia has been seen with repeated dosing)

**Medical considerations/Contraindications**
The medical considerations/contraindications included have been selected on the basis of their potential clinical significance (reasons given in parentheses where appropriate)—not necessarily inclusive (» = major clinical significance).

*Risk-benefit should be considered when the following medical problem exists:*
  Sensitivity to fomepizole or other pyrazoles

**Patient monitoring**
The following may be especially important in patient monitoring (other tests may be warranted in some patients, depending on condition; » = major clinical significance):

» Blood gases, arterial and
» Blood urea nitrogen (BUN) and
» Creatinine, serum and
» Electrolytes, serum and
» Urinalysis
    (frequent monitoring recommended to determine therapeutic efficacy of fomepizole)
» Electrocardiogram (ECG)
    (recommended because the acidosis and electrolyte imbalance caused by ethylene glycol poisoning can affect the cardiovascular system)
Electroencephalogram (EEG)
    (recommended in patients who are comatose)

- » Ethylene glycol concentrations, plasma and urine and
- » Oxylate crystals, urinary
    (frequent monitoring recommended to assess the status of ethylene glycol and metabolite clearance)
  Transaminase values
    (recommended because transient increases have been seen with repeated dosing)
  White blood count (WBC)
    (recommended because eosinophilia has been seen with repeated dosing)

## Side/Adverse Effects

The following side/adverse effects have been selected on the basis of their potential clinical significance (possible signs and symptoms in parentheses where appropriate)—not necessarily inclusive:

### Those indicating need for medical attention
Incidence less frequent or rare—incidence 6% or less
  *Allergic reaction* (skin rash); *bradycardia* (slow heartbeat); *hypotension* (dizziness or lightheadedness); *injection site reaction; nystagmus* (uncontrolled back-and-forth and/or rolling eye movements); *phlebosclerosis* (pain or tenderness over affected vein); *seizures; tachycardia* (fast heartbeat)

### Those indicating need for medical attention only if they continue or are bothersome
Incidence more frequent
  *Dizziness*—incidence 7%; *headache*—incidence 12%; *nausea*—incidence 11%
Incidence less frequent or rare—incidence 6% or less
  *Abdominal pain; anorexia* (loss of appetite); *blurred vision; change in sense of smell; decreased environmental awareness; diarrhea; feeling of drunkenness; fever; heartburn; hiccups; lightheadedness; metallic or unpleasant taste; pharyngitis* (sore throat); *sleepiness; slurred speech; vertigo* (dizziness; sensation of spinning); *vomiting*

## Overdose

For more information on the management of overdose or unintentional ingestion, **contact a Poison Control Center** (see *Poison Control Center Listing*).

### Clinical effects of overdose
Note: Clinical effects of overdose were seen in healthy volunteers given fomepizole at doses of 50 to 100 mg per kg of body weight (mg/kg) (three to six times the recommended dose). Plasma concentrations were 23.8 to 42.6 mg (290 to 520 micromoles) per liter.
The following effects are dose-dependent and have been selected on the basis of their potential clinical significance (possible signs and symptoms in parentheses where appropriate)—not necessarily inclusive:
  *Dizziness; nausea; vertigo* (dizziness; sensation of spinning)

### Treatment of overdose
To enhance elimination—Hemodialysis.

Supportive care—Patients in whom intentional overdose is confirmed or suspected should be referred for psychiatric consultation.

## General Dosing Information

Initiation of therapy with fomepizole should not be delayed if ethylene glycol concentrations are not readily available. Therapy should be started as soon as ethylene glycol poisoning is suspected based upon patient history and anion gap metabolic acidosis, increased osmolar gap, or presence of oxylate crystals in the urine. However, if ethylene glycol concentrations are available and are greater than 20 mg per dL, fomepizole therapy also should be initiated.

In addition to antidotal therapy, gastric lavage may be indicated if performed soon after ingestion or in patients who are comatose or at risk for seizures. A patent airway and support of ventilation should be maintained as there is a potential for central nervous system (CNS) and respiratory depression. Sodium bicarbonate should be administered to correct metabolic acidosis. Intravenous fluids may be needed to correct electrolyte imbalance and maintain adequate urine output. However, if renal failure develops, it may be necessary to discontinue administration of fluids to prevent fluid overload. Intravenous calcium should be administered to patients experiencing tetany and seizures, which often are caused by hypocalcemia, but should not be used to treat hypocalcemia itself because, when given under these circumstances, intravenous calcium may increase precipitation of calcium oxalate crystals in the tissues. Pyridoxine and thiamine may be administered to prevent the metabolism of glyoxylate to oxalate. However, data that support the efficacy of pyridoxine for this use are minimal. Hemodialysis should be considered in patients with high ethylene glycol concentrations (greater than or equal to 50 mg per dL), significant metabolic acidosis, or renal failure.

Fomepizole must be administered by intravenous infusion. Venous irritation and phlebosclerosis have occurred when fomepizole was administered undiluted or by bolus injection.

## Parenteral Dosage Forms

### FOMEPIZOLE INJECTION

**Usual adult dose**
Ethylene glycol toxicity—
  Intravenous infusion, initially 15 mg per kg of body weight, followed by 10 mg per kg of body weight every twelve hours for four doses, then 15 mg per kg of body weight every twelve hours until ethylene glycol concentration decreases to less than 20 mg per dL.
Note: Each dose of fomepizole should be administered over thirty minutes.
  Because fomepizole is dialyzable, the frequency of dosing should be increased to every four hours during hemodialysis.
  A regimen for dosing during hemodialysis is as follows:
    Dose at the beginning of hemodialysis—
      If less than six hours since the last dose: Do not administer dose.
      If six or more hours since last dose: Administer next scheduled dose.
    Dose during hemodialysis—
      Administer every four hours.
    Dose at time hemodialysis is completed—
      If less than one hour between last dose and end of hemodialysis: Do not administer dose.
      If one to three hours between last dose and end of hemodialysis: Administer one half of next scheduled dose.
      If more than three hours between last dose and end of hemodialysis: Administer next scheduled dose.
    Maintenance dose once hemodialysis has been completed—
      Administer next scheduled dose twelve hours from last dose administered.

**Usual pediatric dose**
Safety and efficacy have not been established.

**Strength(s) usually available**
U.S.—
  1 gram per mL (Rx) [*Antizol*].

**Packaging and storage**
Store between 20 and 25 °C (68 and 77 °F).

**Preparation of dosage form**
Fomepizole should be admixed with at least 100 mL of 0.9% sodium chloride injection or 5% dextrose injection.

**Stability**
Fomepizole solidifies at temperatures less than 25 °C (77 °F). If this occurs, the contents of the vial may be liquefied by holding the vial under warm running water or by holding it in the hand. Solidification does not affect the efficacy, safety, or stability of fomepizole.

Following dilution with 0.9% sodium chloride injection or 5% dextrose injection, fomepizole is stable for at least 48 hours when refrigerated or stored at room temperature. However, the manufacturer recommends that it be used within 24 hours.

**Caution**
Fomepizole must be diluted before use.

Developed: 05/14/98

1528    Foscarnet (Systemic)

# FOSCARNET   Systemic†

VA CLASSIFICATION (Primary): AM802
Commonly used brand name(s): *Foscavir*.
Other commonly used names are PFA, phosphonoformic acid, and trisodium phosphonoformate.
Note: For a listing of dosage forms and brand names by country availability, see *Dosage Forms* section(s).

†Not commercially available in Canada.

## Category
Antiviral (systemic).

## Indications
Note: Bracketed information in the *Indications* section refers to uses that are not included in U.S. product labeling.

**Accepted**

Cytomegalovirus retinitis (treatment)—Foscarnet is indicated in the treatment of cytomegalovirus (CMV) retinitis in patients with acquired immunodeficiency syndrome (AIDS).

[Cytomegalovirus disease (treatment)]—Foscarnet is used in the treatment of severe, life-threatening CMV disease, including CMV pneumonia, CMV gastrointestinal disease, and disseminated CMV infections, in immunocompromised patients.

[Herpes simplex (treatment)]—Foscarnet is used in the treatment of acyclovir-resistant mucocutaneous herpes simplex virus (HSV-1 and HSV-2) infections in human immunodeficiency virus (HIV)-infected patients.

[Varicella-zoster (treatment)]—Foscarnet is used in the treatment of acyclovir-resistant varicella-zoster virus infection in HIV-infected patients.

**Unaccepted**

Foscarnet is not active against bacteria or mycoplasma.

## Pharmacology/Pharmacokinetics

**Physicochemical characteristics**
Molecular weight—Foscarnet sodium hexahydrate: 300.1.

**Mechanism of action/Effect**
Virostatic. Foscarnet inhibits viral replication by noncompetitively blocking the pyrophosphate binding site of viral DNA polymerase, preventing cleavage of pyrophosphate from deoxynucleoside triphosphate and elongation of the viral DNA chain. Unlike acyclovir and ganciclovir, foscarnet does not require viral thymidine kinase for activation. Viral replication resumes after foscarnet is discontinued.

**Other actions/effects**
*In vitro* studies show that foscarnet inhibits the viral replication of all known herpes viruses—herpes simplex virus (HSV-1 and HSV-2), varicella-zoster, Epstein-Barr virus, human herpes virus 6 (HHV-6), and cytomegalovirus. It has also been found to noncompetitively inhibit human immunodeficiency virus (HIV) reverse transcriptase and hepatitis B virus DNA polymerase. However, the use of foscarnet in clinical practice for many of these viral infections has not been fully evaluated.

Foscarnet is also a specific competitive inhibitor of the sodium-phosphate cotransport by renal cortical brush border membrane vesicles. The inhibition is dose-dependent and specific for phosphate, which may decrease the tubular reabsorption and thus increase renal excretion of phosphate.

**Absorption**
Foscarnet is poorly absorbed after oral administration; bioavailability ranges from 12 to 22%.

**Distribution**
Foscarnet is sequestered into bone and cartilage; however, the extent to which this occurs is not known. Cerebrospinal fluid (CSF) concentration was approximately 43% (13 to 68%) of plasma concentration in HIV-infected patients receiving a continuous intravenous infusion; other CSF-to-plasma ratios have been 35 to 103%; variable penetration may be due to disease-related defects in the blood-brain barrier.
$Vol_D$—0.3 to 0.7 L per kg.

**Protein binding**
14 to 17%.

**Biotransformation**
Not metabolized.

**Half-life**
Normal renal function—
 Distribution: 0.4 to 1.4 hours.
 Elimination: 3.3 to 6.8 hours.
 Terminal: 18 to 88 hours.
Renal function impairment—
 Prolonged.

**Time to peak concentration**
End of infusion.

**Peak serum concentration**
Approximately 575 micromoles per L on both days 1 and 14 or 15 after administration of 57 (on day 1) and 47 mg (on days 14 or 15) per kg of body weight (mg/kg), infused over 1 hour, every 8 hours.

**Elimination**
Renal; approximately 80 to 87% excreted unchanged in the urine; in one study, glomerular filtration accounted for 44% of total renal excretion, and net tubular secretion accounted for 56%. Tubular reabsorption may also occur. Apparent extrarenal clearance reflects the uptake of foscarnet into bone matrix.

Dialysis—Foscarnet is cleared through hemodialysis; clearance is approximately 80 mL per minute.

## Precautions to Consider

**Carcinogenicity**
No evidence of carcinogenicity was found in rats and mice given oral doses of 500 mg per kg of body weight (mg/kg) per day and 250 mg/kg per day, respectively, resulting in plasma concentrations equal to one-third and one-fifth of those in humans as measured by area under the plasma concentration time curve (AUC).

**Mutagenicity**
Foscarnet was found to be genotoxic in the BALB/3T3 *in vitro* transformation assay at concentrations greater than 0.5 mcg per mL; there was also an increased frequency of chromosome aberrations in the sister chromatid exchange assay at 1000 mcg per mL. Foscarnet caused an increase in micronucleated polychromatic erythrocytes *in vivo* in mice at doses (350 mg/kg) that produced exposures (AUC) comparable to those anticipated clinically.

**Pregnancy/Reproduction**
Fertility—Foscarnet did not adversely affect the fertility and general reproductive performance of rats; however, because of the doses used, these studies do not adequately define the potential for fertility impairment at human doses.

Pregnancy—It is not known whether foscarnet crosses the placenta. Studies in humans have not been done.

A slight increase ($< 5\%$) in the number of skeletal anomalies compared with controls was seen in female rats given daily subcutaneous doses of up to 75 mg/kg administered prior to and during mating, during gestation, and 21 days postpartum. An increase in the frequency of skeletal anomalies/variations was found in rats and rabbits given daily subcutaneous doses of up to 75 mg/kg and 150 mg/kg, respectively. On the basis of estimated drug exposure (AUC), these doses were approximately one-eighth (rat) and one-third (rabbit) the estimated maximal daily human exposure. These studies are inadequate to define the potential teratogenicity at levels to which women will be exposed.

FDA Pregnancy Category C.

**Breast-feeding**
It is not known whether foscarnet is distributed into human breast milk. However, in lactating rats administered 75 mg/kg, foscarnet was distributed into milk at concentrations 3 times higher than peak maternal blood concentrations.

**Pediatrics**
No information is available on the relationship of age to the effects of foscarnet in pediatric patients. Safety and efficacy have not been established. Post mortem data show that foscarnet is deposited in the bones of human adults; 40% of an intravenous dose is also deposited in the teeth and bones of young and growing animals; therefore, it is likely that foscarnet also will deposit in developing bone in children.

**Geriatrics**
No information is available on the relationship of age to the effects of foscarnet in geriatric patients. However, elderly patients are more likely to have age-related renal function impairment, which may require adjustment of dosage or dosing interval in patients receiving foscarnet.

**Drug interactions and/or related problems**
The following drug interactions and/or related problems have been selected on the basis of their potential clinical significance (possible mechanism in parentheses where appropriate)—not necessarily inclusive (» = major clinical significance):

Note: Combinations containing any of the following medications, depending on the amount present, may also interact with this medication.

» Nephrotoxic medications, other (See *Appendix II*)
(concurrent use of foscarnet with other nephrotoxic drugs, such as aminoglycosides or amphotericin B, may increase the risk of renal toxicity)

» Pentamidine
(concurrent use of foscarnet with intravenous pentamidine may result in severe but reversible hypocalcemia, hypomagnesemia, and nephrotoxicity)

Zidovudine
(concurrent use of foscarnet with zidovudine may produce an additive effect, increasing the risk of anemia; however, there is no evidence of increased myelosuppression when these 2 drugs are used concurrently)

**Laboratory value alterations**
The following have been selected on the basis of their potential clinical significance (possible effect in parentheses where appropriate)—not necessarily inclusive (» = major clinical significance):

With physiology/laboratory test values
Alanine aminotransferase (ALT [SGPT]) and
Alkaline phosphatase and
Aspartate aminotransferase (AST [SGOT]) and
Bilirubin, serum
(values may be increased)

» Calcium, ionized, serum and
» Calcium, total, serum and
» Phosphate, serum
(concentrations of phosphate may be increased or decreased; concentrations of total calcium may be decreased; although the total calcium concentration may also appear normal, the level of ionized calcium may be decreased and result in symptomatic hypocalcemia)

» Creatinine, serum
(concentration may be increased)

» Magnesium, serum
(concentration may be decreased)

Potassium, serum
(concentration may be decreased)

**Medical considerations/Contraindications**
The medical considerations/contraindications included have been selected on the basis of their potential clinical significance (reasons given in parentheses where appropriate)—not necessarily inclusive (» = major clinical significance).

*Risk-benefit should be considered when the following medical problems exist:*

Anemia
(foscarnet may cause a decrease in hemoglobin concentration, worsening pre-existing anemia)

» Dehydration
(to help avoid renal toxicity, patients must be well hydrated both before and during treatment with foscarnet)

Hypersensitivity to foscarnet

» Renal function impairment
(because foscarnet is nephrotoxic and is excreted through the kidneys, patients with renal function impairment must receive a reduction in dosage or dosing interval)

**Patient monitoring**
The following may be especially important in patient monitoring (other tests may be warranted in some patients, depending on condition; » = major clinical significance):

» Calcium, ionized and total, serum and
» Magnesium, serum and
» Phosphate, serum and
Potassium, serum
(should be monitored 2 to 3 times a week during induction, and once a week during maintenance therapy; total serum calcium levels may appear normal in some patients; however, ionized calcium levels may be decreased, resulting in symptoms of hypocalcemia, such as perioral tingling, numbness in the extremities and paresthesias; there is an inverse linear relationship between the plasma foscarnet concentration and ionized calcium, not seen with total calcium concentrations; this is thought to be due to foscarnet complexing with ionized calcium; if abnormal neurologic or cardiac events occur, ionized calcium levels ideally should be measured at the end of the foscarnet infusion)

(decreases in magnesium and potassium, and an increase and decrease in calcium and phosphate have been observed; this may be a result of foscarnet replacing phosphate in the bone or of foscarnet inhibiting the tubular reabsorption of phosphate)

Complete blood counts (CBCs)
(foscarnet may cause a decrease in serum hemoglobin concentrations, resulting in anemia; there have also been rare reports of thrombocytopenia and leukopenia)

» Ophthalmologic examinations
(ophthalmologic examinations should be performed at the start of treatment, at the conclusion of induction, and every 4 weeks during maintenance; since foscarnet is virostatic and not a cure for cytomegalovirus [CMV] retinitis, progression of retinitis is expected to eventually occur during or following foscarnet treatment; examinations during maintenance therapy should be more frequent if there is residual disease activity [whitening of lesion borders] or if lesions are close to the macula or optic nerve head; in selected cases, examinations could be less frequent if lesions are completely inactive and located only in the peripheral retina)

» Renal function tests
(blood urea nitrogen and serum creatinine concentrations should be monitored at least 2 to 3 times a week during induction, and at least once a week during maintenance therapy since foscarnet is nephrotoxic and patients with renal function impairment will require an adjustment in dosage or discontinuation of the drug)

## Side/Adverse Effects

Note: Renal function impairment is the major dose-limiting side effect of foscarnet therapy. Acute tubular necrosis is the most common type of nephrotoxicity; however, nephrogenic diabetes insipidus and foscarnet crystal formation in the glomerular capillary lumen have also been described. Hydration with 0.5 to 1 liter of 0.9% sodium chloride per dose, throughout the course of foscarnet treatment, has been found to lessen the nephrotoxic effects.

The following side/adverse effects have been selected on the basis of their potential clinical significance (possible signs and symptoms in parentheses where appropriate)—not necessarily inclusive:

**Those indicating need for medical attention**
Incidence more frequent
*Nephrotoxicity* (decreased urination, or increased thirst and urination)

Incidence less frequent
*Anemia* (unusual tiredness and weakness); **granulocytopenia or leukopenia** (fever, chills, or sore throat); **neurotoxicity** (muscle twitching; tremor; seizures; tingling sensation around mouth; pain or numbness in hands or feet); **phlebitis** (pain at site of injection)

Note: *Anemia* was reported in 33% of 189 patients in the 5 controlled U.S. clinical trials. Only 1 patient required discontinuation of drug.

*Granulocytopenia or leukopenia* was reported in 17% of 189 patients in the 5 controlled U.S. clinical trials. Only 2 patients required discontinuation of drug.

*Neurotoxicity* may be related to drug-induced alterations in serum minerals and electrolytes, especially a decrease in ionized calcium concentrations.

Incidence rare
***Sores or ulcers of the mouth or throat, penis, or vulva***

**Those indicating need for medical attention only if they continue or are bothersome**
Incidence more frequent
*Gastrointestinal disturbances* (abdominal pain; anorexia; nausea and vomiting); **neurotoxicity** (anxiety; confusion; dizziness; fatigue; headache)

## Patient Consultation

As an aid to patient consultation, refer to *Advice for the Patient, Foscarnet (Systemic)*.

In providing consultation, consider emphasizing the following selected information (» = major clinical significance):

**Before using this medication**
» Conditions affecting use, especially:
Hypersensitivity to foscarnet
Other medications, especially other nephrotoxic medications or pentamidine
Other medical problems, especially dehydration or renal function impairment

## Proper use of this medication
» Importance of receiving medication for full course of therapy and on a regular schedule
» Maintaining adequate fluid intake
  Washing genitals after urination to decrease risk of genital ulceration
» Proper dosing

## Precautions while using this medication
» Regular visits to ophthalmologist to examine eyes since progression of retinitis and visual loss may occur during foscarnet therapy

### Side/adverse effects
Signs of potential side effects, especially nephrotoxicity, anemia, granulocytopenia, leukopenia, neurotoxicity, phlebitis, and sores or ulcers of the mouth or throat, penis, or vulva

## General Dosing Information

Foscarnet must be administered at a constant rate by an infusion pump and must not be administered by rapid intravenous injection. Rapid administration may result in excessive plasma levels of foscarnet and increased risk of acute hypocalcemia or other toxicity. Doses of 60 mg per kg of body weight (mg/kg) or less may be infused over 1 hour; higher doses should be infused over at least a 2-hour period. The recommended dosage, frequency, or infusion rate should not be exceeded.

Patients must be adequately hydrated during treatment to avoid nephrotoxicity.

Foscarnet may be administered undiluted (24 mg/mL) but only through a central venous line. When a peripheral vein is used, the solution must be diluted to 12 mg/mL (1:1) with 5% dextrose in water or 0.9% sodium chloride for injection prior to administration to avoid local irritation of peripheral veins.

Intravitreal administration of foscarnet has been used in patients with a history of intolerance to acyclovir and advanced renal function impairment. Intravitreal doses of 1200 to 2400 mcg of undiluted foscarnet (0.05 mL) were injected into the eye 6 times at 72-hour intervals, followed by a single, weekly maintenance injection. Intravitreal administration has resulted in improvement of patients' visual acuity and appeared to be well tolerated. The elimination half-life of foscarnet from the vitreous fluid was estimated to be approximately 32 hours, and the intravitreal concentration was calculated to remain above the mean 50% inhibition level for cytomegalovirus for approximately 41 hours after a single injection.

## Parenteral Dosage Forms

Note: Bracketed uses in the *Dosage Forms* section refer to categories of use and/or indications that are not included in U.S. product labeling.

### FOSCARNET SODIUM INJECTION

**Usual adult and adolescent dose**
Cytomegalovirus (CMV) retinitis—
  Induction—
    Intravenous infusion, 60 mg per kg of body weight, administered over at least 1 hour with an infusion pump, every eight hours for fourteen to twenty-one days, depending on the clinical response.

Note: Induction doses of 90 and 100 mg per kg of body weight every twelve hours also have been used; dosing twice a day was found to be as effective as the three-times-a-day dosing, and was more convenient.

Adults with impaired renal function require a reduction in dose as follows:

| Creatinine clearance (mL/min/kg)/ (mL/sec/kg) | Equivalent to 60 mg/kg dose every 8 hours |
| --- | --- |
| ≥1.6/0.027 | 60 |
| 1.5/0.025 | 57 |
| 1.4/0.023 | 53 |
| 1.3/0.022 | 49 |
| 1.2/0.020 | 46 |
| 1.1/0.018 | 42 |
| 1.0/0.017 | 39 |
| 0.9/0.015 | 35 |
| 0.8/0.013 | 32 |
| 0.7/0.012 | 28 |
| 0.6/0.010 | 25 |
| 0.5/0.008 | 21 |
| 0.4/0.007 | 18 |

Maintenance—
  Intravenous infusion, 90 to 120 mg per kg of body weight, administered over 2 hours with an infusion pump, once a day.

Note: It is recommended that most patients be started on maintenance treatment with a dose of 90 mg per kg of body weight per day since the superiority of 120 mg per kg of body weight per day has not been established in controlled trials, and higher plasma levels may lead to increased toxicity. Treatment with 120 mg per kg of body weight per day may be considered if early reinduction is required because of retinitis progression. Patients who show excellent tolerance to foscarnet may benefit from a maintenance dose of 120 mg per kg of body weight per day early in their treatment.

If CMV retinitis progresses during maintenance therapy, patients should be retreated with the induction regimen.

Adults with impaired renal function receiving a 90 mg per kg of body weight maintenance dose require a reduction in dose as follows:

| Creatinine clearance (mL/min/kg)/ (mL/sec/kg) | Equivalent to 90 mg/kg dose every 24 hours |
| --- | --- |
| ≥1.4/0.023 | 90 |
| 1.2–1.4/0.020–0.023 | 78 |
| 1.0–1.2/0.017–0.020 | 75 |
| 0.8–1.0/0.013–0.017 | 71 |
| 0.6–0.8/0.010–0.013 | 63 |
| 0.4–0.6/0.007–0.010 | 57 |

Adults with impaired renal function receiving a 120 mg per kg of body weight maintenance dose require a reduction in dose as follows:

| Creatinine clearance (mL/min/kg)/ (mL/sec/kg) | Equivalent to 120 mg/kg dose every 24 hours |
| --- | --- |
| ≥1.4/0.023 | 120 |
| 1.2–1.4/0.020–0.023 | 104 |
| 1.0–1.2/0.017–0.020 | 100 |
| 0.8–1.0/0.013–0.017 | 94 |
| 0.6–0.8/0.010–0.013 | 84 |
| 0.4–0.6/0.007–0.010 | 76 |

[Herpes simplex (treatment)] and
[Varicella-zoster (treatment)]—
  Intravenous infusion, 40 mg per kg of body weight, administered over at least 1 hour with an infusion pump, every eight hours for fourteen to twenty-one days, depending on the clinical response. The dose should be adjusted if the calculated creatinine clearance is less than 1.6 mL per kg of body weight.

**Usual pediatric dose**
See *Usual adult and adolescent dose*.

**Strength(s) usually available**
U.S.—
  6000 mg in 250 mL (Rx) [*Foscavir*].
  12,000 mg in 500 mL (Rx) [*Foscavir*].
Canada—
  Not commercially available.

**Packaging and storage**
Store below 40 °C (104 °F), preferably between 15 and 30 °C (59 and 86 °F), unless otherwise specified by manufacturer. Do not freeze. Refrigeration of stock or diluted solutions may result in crystallization of drug.

**Preparation of dosage form**
Undiluted foscarnet (24 mg per mL) can only be administered through a central line due to its potential for causing venous irritation.

For peripheral administration, dilute stock solution of foscarnet with an equal amount (1:1) of 5% dextrose injection or 0.9% sodium chloride injection, for a final concentration of 12 mg per mL. After calculation of the dose, based on body weight, it is advisable to remove and discard any excess foscarnet from the bottle before starting the infusion, to avoid accidental overdosage.

**Stability**
Undiluted foscarnet is stable for 24 months at 25 °C.
Because foscarnet contains no preservatives, diluted foscarnet should be discarded after 24 hours.
Foscarnet must not be frozen because precipitation is likely to occur. Any drug that has been frozen must be discarded.

**Incompatibilities**
Foscarnet must not be mixed with anything other than 5% dextrose injection or 0.9% sodium chloride injection. It is incompatible with 30% dextrose injection, lactated Ringer's solution, or any solution containing calcium.
Foscarnet has been found to precipitate immediately with acyclovir, amphotericin B, ganciclovir, pentamidine isethionate, trimethoprim-sulfamethoxazole, trimetrexate, and vancomycin. Delayed precipitation was observed when foscarnet was combined with dobutamine hydrochloride, droperidol, and haloperidol. Gas production was observed

when foscarnet was combined with diazepam, digoxin, lorazepam, midazolam, and promethazine hydrochloride. Cloudiness and/or color change was observed when foscarnet was combined with diphenhydramine hydrochloride, leucovorin calcium, and prochlorperazine.

## Selected Bibliography

Minor JR, Baltz JK. Foscarnet sodium. DICP, Ann Pharmacother 1991; 25: 41-7.

Chrisp P, Clissold SP. Foscarnet. Drugs 1991; 41(1): 104-29.

Revised: 07/22/94

# FOSFOMYCIN Systemic—INTRODUCTORY VERSION

VA CLASSIFICATION (Primary): AM900
Commonly used brand name(s): *Monurol*.
Note: For a listing of dosage forms and brand names by country availability, see *Dosage Forms* section(s).

## Category

Antibacterial (systemic).

## Indications

### General considerations

Fosfomycin is active against most strains of *Enterococcus faecalis* and *Escherichia coli*. Fosfomycin also exhibits *in vitro* minimum inhibitory concentrations of 64 micrograms per mL or less against most strains of *Citrobacter diversus*, *Citrobacter freundii*, *Enterobacter aerogenes*, *Enterococcus faecium*, *Klebsiella oxytoca*, *Klebsiella pneumoniae*, *Proteus mirabilis*, *Proteus vulgaris*, and *Serratia marcescens*.

There is generally no cross-resistance between fosfomycin and other classes of antibacterial agents, such as beta-lactams and aminoglycosides.

### Accepted

Urinary tract infections, uncomplicated (treatment)—Fosfomycin is indicated in the treatment of uncomplicated urinary tract infections and acute cystitis, caused by *E. coli* or *E. faecalis*, in women.

### Unaccepted

Fosfomycin is not indicated for the treatment of perinephric abscess or pyelonephritis.

## Pharmacology/Pharmacokinetics

### Physicochemical characteristics

Chemical group—Phosphonic acid derivative.
Molecular weight—Fosfomycin tromethamine: 259.2.

### Mechanism of action/Effect

Fosfomycin inactivates enolpyruvyl transferase, which irreversibly blocks the condensation of uridine diphosphate-*N*-acetylglucosamine with phospho*enol*pyruvate, and inhibits bacterial cell wall synthesis. Fosfomycin also decreases the adherence of bacteria to epithelial cells of the urinary tract.

### Absorption

Fosfomycin tromethamine is rapidly absorbed following oral administration and converted to fosfomycin. Oral bioavailability under fasting conditions is 37%. When given with food, oral bioavailability is reduced to 30%.

### Distribution

Fosfomycin is distributed to the bladder wall, kidneys, prostate, and seminal vesicles.

Vol$_D$—Mean steady-state following oral administration, 136.1 ± 44.1 L.

### Protein binding

Fosfomycin is not bound to plasma proteins.

### Biotransformation

Fosfomycin tromethamine is converted to the free acid fosfomycin.

### Half-life

Elimination—Mean, 5.7 ± 2.8 hours.
The elimination half-life is 40 hours in anuric patients undergoing hemodialysis.

### Onset of action

2 to 3 days.

### Elimination

With normal renal function—
  Fecal: 18% of a 3-gram fosfomycin dose is eliminated.
  Renal: 38% of a 3-gram fosfomycin dose is eliminated.
  Fosfomycin tromethamine is excreted as fosfomycin.
With renal function impairment—Fosfomycin recovery in urine decreases from 32% to 11%.

## Precautions to Consider

### Carcinogenicity

Long-term carcinogenicity studies in animals have not been done.

### Mutagenicity

Fosfomycin was not found to be mutagenic or genotoxic *in vitro* in the Ames test, in cultured human lymphocytes, or in Chinese hamster V79 cells, or *in vivo* in the mouse micronucleus assay.

### Pregnancy/Reproduction

Fertility—Fertility and reproductive performance of male and female rats were not affected.

Pregnancy—Adequate and well-controlled studies in humans have not been done. However, fosfomycin has been shown to cross the placenta. Studies in pregnant rabbits at dosages of 1000 mg per kg of body weight per day (approximately 9 and 2.7 times the human dose based on body weight and body surface area, respectively) showed fetotoxicity and maternal toxicity.

FDA Pregnancy Category B.

### Breast-feeding

It is not known whether fosfomycin is distributed into breast milk.

### Pediatrics

Safety and efficacy have not been established in children up to 12 years of age.

### Geriatrics

The bacteriologic effectiveness and safety profiles for women older than 65 years of age did not show clinically significant differences, as compared with those for women 65 years of age and younger.

### Drug interactions and/or related problems

The following drug interactions and/or related problems have been selected on the basis of their potential clinical significance (possible mechanism in parentheses where appropriate)—not necessarily inclusive (» = major clinical significance):

Note: Cimetidine does not affect the pharmacokinetics of fosfomycin.

Combinations containing the following medication, depending on the amount present, may also interact with this medication.

Metoclopramide
  (concurrent use of metoclopramide increases gastrointestinal motility and lowers the serum concentration and urinary excretion of fosfomycin; other medications that increase gastrointestinal motility may have the same effect)

### Laboratory value alterations

The following have been selected on the basis of their potential clinical significance (possible effect in parentheses where appropriate)—not necessarily inclusive (» = major clinical significance):

With physiology/laboratory test values
  Alanine aminotransferase (ALT [SGPT]) and
  Alkaline phosphatase and
  Aspartate aminotransferase (AST [SGOT])
    (serum values may be increased)

  Bilirubin, serum
    (concentration may be increased)

  Eosinophil count
    (may be increased)

  Hematocrit and
  Hemoglobin
    (concentrations may be decreased)

  Leukocyte count and
  Platelet count
    (may be increased or decreased)

### Medical considerations/Contraindications

The medical considerations/contraindications included have been selected on the basis of their potential clinical significance (reasons given in

## 1532 Fosfomycin (Systemic)—Introductory Version

parentheses where appropriate)—not necessarily inclusive (» = major clinical significance).

*Risk-benefit should be considered when the following medical problems exist:*
- » Sensitivity to fosfomycin
- » Renal function impairment
    (clearance of fosfomycin may be decreased)

**Patient monitoring**
The following may be especially important in patient monitoring (other tests may be warranted in some patients, depending on condition; » = major clinical significance):
- » Urine culture and susceptibility testing
    (recommended before and after completion of treatment)

### Side/Adverse Effects

Note: Use of more than one dose to treat a single episode of acute cystitis may increase the incidence of adverse effects.

The following side/adverse effects have been selected on the basis of their potential clinical significance (possible signs and symptoms in parentheses where appropriate)—not necessarily inclusive:

**Those indicating need for medical attention**
Incidence more frequent
  *Vaginitis* (vaginal discharge and pain)—7.6%

**Those indicating need for medical attention only if they continue or are bothersome**
Incidence more frequent
  *Diarrhea*—10.4%; *headache*—10.3%; *nausea*—5.2%
Incidence less frequent
  *Abdominal pain*—2.2%; *asthenia* (weakness)—1.7%; *back pain*—3%; *dizziness*—2.3%; *dysmenorrhea* (painful menstruation)—2.6%; *dyspepsia* (heartburn; indigestion)—1.8%; *pain, nonlocalized*—2.2%; *pharyngitis* (sore throat)—2.5%; *rhinitis* (runny or stuffy nose)—4.5%; *skin rash*—1.4%

### Overdose

For more information on the management of overdose or unintentional ingestion, **contact a Poison Control Center** (see *Poison Control Center Listing*).

**Clinical effects of overdose**
No cases of overdose in humans have been reported.

**Treatment of overdose**
Supportive care—Patient should receive symptomatic and supportive therapy. Patients in whom intentional overdose is confirmed or suspected should be referred for psychiatric consultation.

### Patient Consultation

As an aid to patient consultation, refer to *Advice for the Patient, Fosfomycin (Systemic)—Introductory Version*.
In providing consultation, consider emphasizing the following selected information (» = major clinical significance):

**Before using this medication**
- » Conditions affecting use, especially:
    Sensitivity to fosfomycin
    Pregnancy—Fosfomycin crosses the placenta
    Other medical problems, especially renal function impairment

**Proper use of this medication**
- » Not taking medication in its dry form; taking immediately after dissolving in water
    Taking with or without food
- » Proper dosing
- » Proper storage

**Precautions while using this medication**
- » Checking with physician if there is no improvement in symptoms within 2 to 3 days

**Side/adverse effects**
Signs of potential side effects, especially vaginitis

### Oral Dosage Forms

#### FOSFOMYCIN TROMETHAMINE FOR ORAL SOLUTION

Note: The dosing and strength of the dosage form available are expressed in terms of the fosfomycin free acid (not the tromethamine salt).

**Usual adult dose**
Urinary tract infections, uncomplicated—
  Oral, 3 grams (free acid) as a single dose.

**Usual adult prescribing limits**
3 grams (free acid) per episode of acute cystitis.

**Usual pediatric dose**
Children up to 12 years of age—
  Safety and efficacy have not been established.

**Usual geriatric dose**
See *Usual adult dose*.

**Strength(s) usually available**
U.S.—
  3 grams (free acid) per packet (Rx) [*Monurol* (saccharin; sucrose)].
Note: The single-dose packet contains 5.63 grams of fosfomycin tromethamine, equivalent to 3 grams of fosfomycin free acid.

**Packaging and storage**
Store between 15 and 30 °C (59 and 86 °F).

**Preparation of dosage form**
Empty entire contents of a single-dose packet into 3 or 4 ounces of water and stir until dissolved. Do not use hot water.

**Stability**
After reconstitution, fosfomycin solution should be taken immediately.

**Auxiliary labeling**
- Dissolve in water before taking.

Developed: 10/20/97
Interim revision: 07/28/98

---

**FOSINOPRIL**—See *Angiotensin-converting Enzyme (ACE) Inhibitors (Systemic)*

---

**FOSPHENYTOIN**—See *Anticonvulsants, Hydantoin (Systemic)*

---

# FRUCTOSE, DEXTROSE, AND PHOSPHORIC ACID   Oral-Local

VA CLASSIFICATION (Primary): GA605
Commonly used brand name(s): *Emetrol*.
Note: For a listing of dosage forms and brand names by country availability, see *Dosage Forms* section(s).

## Category
Antiemetic.

## Indications

**Accepted**
Fructose, dextrose, and phosphoric acid oral solution is used for the symptomatic relief of nausea and vomiting. However, to date, there is insufficient evidence to establish effectiveness (FDA Category III).

## Pharmacology/Pharmacokinetics

**Physicochemical characteristics**
Molecular weight—Fructose: 180.16.
  Dextrose: 198.17.
  Phosphoric acid: 98.0.

**Mechanism of action/Effect**
Exact mechanism has not been determined. Appears to have a direct local action on the wall of the gastrointestinal tract that reduces smooth muscle contraction and delays gastric emptying time through the high osmotic pressure exerted by the solution of simple sugars. Phosphoric acid is added to adjust pH to between 1.5 and 1.6.

**Absorption**
Fructose—Slowly absorbed from gastrointestinal tract.
Dextrose—Rapidly absorbed from gastrointestinal tract.

**Biotransformation**
Fructose—Hepatic, by phosphorylation; partly converted to liver glycogen and glucose.
Dextrose—Hepatic; metabolized to carbon dioxide and water.

## Precautions to Consider

**Pregnancy/Reproduction**
Pregnancy—Studies have not been done in humans.
Studies have not been done in animals.

**Breast-feeding**
Problems in humans have not been documented.

**Pediatrics**
In infants and children up to 3 years of age with vomiting, caution is recommended because of the risk of fluid and electrolyte loss; these patients should be referred to a physician.

**Geriatrics**
In geriatric patients with vomiting, caution is recommended because of the risk of fluid and electrolyte loss; these patients should be referred to a physician.

**Laboratory value alterations**
The following have been selected on the basis of their potential clinical significance (possible effect in parentheses where appropriate)—not necessarily inclusive (» = major clinical significance):

With physiology/laboratory test values
   Glucose
     (blood concentrations may be elevated)

**Medical considerations/Contraindications**
The medical considerations/contraindications included have been selected on the basis of their potential clinical significance (reasons given in parentheses where appropriate)—not necessarily inclusive (» = major clinical significance).

*Except under special circumstances, this medication should not be used when the following medical problems exist:*
» Appendicitis, symptoms of or
» Inflamed bowel, symptoms of
   (proper diagnosis required or severe condition may develop)
» Fructose intolerance, hereditary
   (severe side effects may occur)

*Risk-benefit should be considered when the following medical problems exist:*
» Diabetes mellitus
   (condition may be aggravated because of solution's high carbohydrate content)
   Intolerance to dextrose or phosphoric acid

## Side/Adverse Effects

The following side/adverse effects have been selected on the basis of their potential clinical significance (possible signs and symptoms in parentheses where appropriate)—not necessarily inclusive:

**Those indicating need for medical attention**
Incidence rare
   *Fructose intolerance* (fainting; swelling of face, arms, and legs; unusual bleeding; vomiting; weight loss; yellow eyes or skin)

**Those indicating need for medical attention only if they continue or are bothersome**
Incidence less frequent—more frequent with large doses
   *Diarrhea; stomach or abdominal pain*

## Patient Consultation

As an aid to patient consultation, refer to *Advice for the Patient, Fructose, Dextrose, and Phosphoric Acid (Oral)*.
In providing consultation, consider emphasizing the following selected information (» = major clinical significance):

**Before using this medication**
» Conditions affecting use, especially:
   Intolerance to fructose, dextrose, or phosphoric acid
   Use in children—Risk of fluid and electrolyte loss due to vomiting
   Use in the elderly—Risk of fluid and electrolyte loss due to vomiting
   Other medical problems, especially diabetes mellitus, symptoms of appendicitis, or inflamed bowel

**Proper use of this medication**
   Following physician's or manufacturer's instructions
   Not diluting or taking fluids before or after dose
» Proper dosing
» Proper storage

**Precautions while using this medication**
» Checking with physician if symptoms do not improve or become worse
» Not taking if symptoms of appendicitis or inflamed bowel are present; checking with physician for proper diagnosis

**Side/adverse effects**
   Signs of potential side effects, especially fructose intolerance

## General Dosing Information

The fructose, dextrose, and phosphoric acid oral solution should not be diluted. Also, oral fluids should not be taken immediately before or for at least 15 minutes after the dose.

## Oral Dosage Forms

### FRUCTOSE, DEXTROSE, AND PHOSPHORIC ACID ORAL SOLUTION

**Usual adult and adolescent dose**
Antiemetic—Oral, 15 to 30 mL. Dose may be repeated every fifteen minutes until distress subsides, but should not be taken for more than one hour (five doses) without consulting a physician.

Note: For morning sickness, dose should be taken on arising and repeated every three hours as needed.

**Usual pediatric dose**
Antiemetic—
   Children up to 3 years of age: Use is not recommended.
   Children over 3 years of age: Oral, 5 to 10 mL. Dose may be repeated every fifteen minutes until distress subsides, but should not be taken for more than one hour (five doses) without consulting a physician.

**Usual geriatric dose**
See *Usual adult and adolescent dose*.

**Strength(s) usually available**
U.S.—
   1.87 grams of fructose, 1.87 grams of dextrose, and 21.5 mg of phosphoric acid, per 5 mL (OTC) [*Emetrol*].
Canada—
   1.87 grams of fructose, 1.87 grams of dextrose, and 21.5 mg of phosphoric acid, per 5 mL (OTC) [*Emetrol*].

**Packaging and storage**
Store below 40 °C (104 °F), preferably between 15 and 30 °C (59 and 86 °F), in a well-closed container, unless otherwise specified by manufacturer. Protect from freezing.

Revised: 05/12/93

---

# FURAZOLIDONE    Oral-Local†

VA CLASSIFICATION (Primary/Secondary): AM600/AP109
Commonly used brand name(s): *Furoxone; Furoxone Liquid*.
Note: For a listing of dosage forms and brand names by country availability, see *Dosage Forms* section(s).

†Not commercially available in Canada.

## Category

Antibacterial (oral-local); antiprotozoal.
Note: Furazolidone is a broad-spectrum anti-infective that is effective against most gastrointestinal tract pathogens.

# Furazolidone (Oral-Local)

## Indications

### Accepted

Cholera (treatment)—Furazolidone is indicated as a secondary agent in the treatment of cholera caused by *Vibrio cholerae* (*V. comma*).

Diarrhea, bacterial (treatment)—Furazolidone is indicated as a secondary agent in the treatment of bacterial diarrhea caused by susceptible organisms. Furazolidone is active *in vitro* against *Campylobacter jejuni*, *Enterobacter aerogenes*, *Escherichia coli*, *Proteus* species, *Salmonella* species, *Shigella* species, and staphylococci. However, clinical studies on the effectiveness of furazolidone in some types of bacterial diarrhea have been inconclusive or conflicting.

Giardiasis (treatment)—Furazolidone is indicated as a secondary agent in the treatment of giardiasis caused by *Giardia lamblia*.

Not all species or strains of a particular organism may be susceptible to furazolidone.

## Pharmacology/Pharmacokinetics

### Physicochemical characteristics

Molecular weight—225.16.

### Mechanism of action/Effect

Microbicidal. Furazolidone interferes with several bacterial enzyme systems. It neither significantly alters normal bowel flora nor results in fungal overgrowth.

### Other actions/effects

Furazolidone also acts as a monoamine oxidase inhibitor (MAOI). MAOIs prevent the inactivation of tyramine by hepatic and gastrointestinal monoamine oxidase. Tyramine in the bloodstream releases norepinephrine from the sympathetic nerve terminals and produces a sudden increase in blood pressure.

### Absorption

Radiolabeled drug studies indicate that furazolidone is well absorbed following oral administration.

### Distribution

Limited pharmacokinetic information is available in humans; however, recent data have reported that variable plasma concentrations were measured in subjects given therapeutic doses. One study of 8 meningitis patients showed that cerebral spinal fluid (CSF) concentrations reached levels comparable to serum concentrations. Also, significant concentrations have been measured in the bile of rats.

### Biotransformation

Furazolidone is rapidly and extensively metabolized; the primary metabolic pathway identified begins with nitro-reduction to the aminofuran derivative.

### Elimination

Radiolabeled drug studies showed that more than 65% of an oral dose was recovered in the urine of humans and animals. Also found in feces.

## Precautions to Consider

### Cross-sensitivity and/or related problems

Patients hypersensitive to other nitrofurans may be hypersensitive to this medication also.

### Carcinogenicity/Tumorigenicity

Several studies in rodents, given chronic, high-dose furazolidone orally, have shown that this medication is tumorigenic. Furazolidone has been shown to cause mammary neoplasia in two strains of rats. In addition, furazolidone has been shown to cause pulmonary tumors in mice.

### Pregnancy/Reproduction

Pregnancy—Studies in humans have not been done. However, teratogenic effects on the human fetus or newborn infants have not been reported. Studies in animals have not shown that furazolidone, given in doses far exceeding recommended human doses for long periods of time, causes adverse effects on the fetus.

### Breast-feeding

It is not known whether furazolidone is distributed into breast milk. However, breast-feeding is not recommended in nursing infants up to 1 month of age because of the possibility of hemolytic anemia due to glutathione instability in the early neonatal period.

### Pediatrics

Use of furazolidone is not recommended in infants up to 1 month of age because of the possibility of hemolytic anemia due to immature enzyme systems (glutathione instability) in the early neonatal period.

### Geriatrics

No information is available on the relationship of age to the effects of furazolidone in geriatric patients.

### Drug interactions and/or related problems

The following drug interactions and/or related problems have been selected on the basis of their potential clinical significance (possible mechanism in parentheses where appropriate)—not necessarily inclusive (» = major clinical significance):

Note: Combinations containing any of the following medications, depending on the amount present, may also interact with this medication.

» Alcohol
 (concurrent use of alcohol with furazolidone may rarely result in a disulfiram-like reaction, characterized by facial flushing, difficult breathing, slight fever, and tightness of the chest; these effects usually subside spontaneously within 24 hours with no lasting ill effects; patients should be advised not to drink alcoholic beverages while taking furazolidone and for 4 days after discontinuing it)

» Antidepressants, tricyclic or
» Monoamine oxidase (MAO) inhibitors, other or
» Sympathomimetics, direct- or indirect-acting, such as amphetamines, ephedrine, or phenylephrine or
» Tyramine- or other high pressor amine–containing foods and beverages, such as aged cheese; beer; reduced-alcohol and alcohol-free beer and wine; red and white wine; sherry; liqueurs; yeast or protein extracts; fava or broad bean pods; smoked or pickled meat, poultry, or fish; fermented sausage (bologna, pepperoni, salami, summer sausage) or other fermented meat; and any overripe fruit
 (concurrent use of these medications, foods, and beverages with furazolidone may theoretically precipitate sudden and severe hypertensive reactions due to furazolidone's MAO inhibitory properties; a dose of 400 mg daily for 5 days was required to experimentally enhance tyramine and amphetamine sensitivity by 2- to 3-fold; this dose does not usually cause an undue risk of hypertensive crises in adults due to MAO inhibition, and no clinical reports of this interaction have been reported; however, if furazolidone is given in larger-than-recommended doses or for more than 5 days, there may be an increased risk of hypertensive crises due to accumulation of monoamine oxidase)

 (because of furazolidone's MAO inhibitory properties, dietary restrictions must be continued for at least 2 weeks after the medication is discontinued; other tyramine- or high pressor amine–containing foods, such as yogurt, sour cream, cream cheese, cottage cheese, chocolate, and soy sauce, if eaten when fresh and in moderation, are considered unlikely to cause serious problems)

### Medical considerations/Contraindications

The medical considerations/contraindications included have been selected on the basis of their potential clinical significance (reasons given in parentheses where appropriate)—not necessarily inclusive (» = major clinical significance).

*Risk-benefit should be considered when the following medical problems exist:*

Glucose-6-phosphate dehydrogenase (G6PD) deficiency
 (mild, reversible, hemolytic anemia may occur in G6PD-deficient patients; it is recommended that furazolidone be discontinued if hemolytic anemia occurs in patients with G6PD deficiency)

Hypersensitivity to furazolidone or other nitrofurans

### Patient monitoring

The following may be especially important in patient monitoring (other tests may be warranted in some patients, depending on condition; » = major clinical significance):

Glucose-6-phosphate dehydrogenase (G6PD) determinations
 (recommended prior to treatment in Caucasians of Mediterranean and Near Eastern origin, Orientals, and blacks; if a deficiency is found, furazolidone should be given with caution since hemolytic effects may be exacerbated in these patients; dosage adjustments and/or discontinuation of the medication may be required)

*For giardiasis*
» Stool examinations
 (3 stool examinations, taken several days apart, beginning 3 to 4 weeks following treatment are recommended if symptoms persist; however, in some successfully treated patients, the lactose intolerance brought on by infection may persist for a period of some weeks or months, mimicking the symptoms of giardiasis; in cases of treatment failure, alternate medications may be used)

## Side/Adverse Effects

Note: Furazolidone may cause mild, reversible hemolytic anemia in G6PD-deficient patients. Furazolidone should be discontinued if hemolytic anemia occurs in these patients.

The following side/adverse effects have been selected on the basis of their potential clinical significance (possible signs and symptoms in parentheses where appropriate)—not necessarily inclusive:

**Those indicating need for medical attention**
Incidence rare
*Hypersensitivity reactions* (fever; itching; joint pain; skin rash or redness)—incidence approximately 0.6%; *leukopenia* (sore throat and fever)—incidence approximately 0.2%

**Those indicating need for medical attention only if they continue or are bothersome**
Incidence less frequent
*Gastrointestinal disturbances* (abdominal pain, diarrhea, nausea, or vomiting); *headache*

**Those not indicating need for medical attention**
Incidence more frequent
*Dark yellow to brown discoloration of urine*

## Patient Consultation

As an aid to patient consultation, refer to *Advice for the Patient, Furazolidone (Oral)*.
In providing consultation, consider emphasizing the following selected information (» = major clinical significance):

**Before using this medication**
» Conditions affecting use, especially:
Sensitivity to furazolidone or other nitrofurans
Breast-feeding—Not recommended in infants up to 1 month of age because of possibility of hemolytic anemia
Use in children—Not recommended in infants up to 1 month of age because of possibility of hemolytic anemia
Other medications, especially direct-acting and indirect-acting sympathomimetics, other MAO inhibitors, or tricyclic antidepressants

**Proper use of this medication**
» Not giving to infants up to 1 month of age; may cause hemolytic anemia
May be taken with food to reduce gastrointestinal irritation
Proper administration technique for oral suspension: Using a specially marked measuring spoon or other device
» Compliance with full course of therapy
» Proper dosing
Missed dose: Taking as soon as possible; not taking if almost time for next dose; not doubling doses
» Proper storage

**Precautions while using this medication**
Regular visits to physician to check progress
Checking with physician if no improvement within a week
» Avoiding alcoholic beverages or other alcohol-containing preparations while taking, and for 4 days after discontinuing, furazolidone
» Avoiding tyramine- and other high pressor amine–containing foods and beverages, OTC appetite suppressants, cough and cold medications, and other medications unless prescribed by physician; also avoiding these products for at least 2 weeks after discontinuing furazolidone; asking health care professional to provide list of products that may or may not cause serious problems with furazolidone

**Side/adverse effects**
Signs of potential side effects, especially hypersensitivity reactions and leukopenia
Dark yellow to brown discoloration of urine may be alarming to patient, although medically insignificant

## General Dosing Information

Furazolidone has been used as adjunctive therapy with other antibacterial agents or bismuth salts with no problems reported.

**Diet/Nutrition**
Gastrointestinal intolerance may be decreased if furazolidone is taken with food or if the dose is reduced.
After discontinuation of furazolidone, the MAO inhibiting effects may persist for at least 2 weeks. During this time, food, beverage, and medication precautions must be observed by patients receiving larger-than-recommended doses or prolonged therapy (See *Drug interactions and/or related problems*).

**For treatment of adverse effects**
Recommended treatment consists of the following
• Administering direct-acting vasopressor agents (e.g., norepinephrine) to counteract hypotensive episodes. Avoiding indirect-acting vasopressor agents.
• Administering phentolamine or parenteral chlorpromazine to counteract hypertensive crises.

## Oral Dosage Forms

### FURAZOLIDONE ORAL SUSPENSION USP

**Usual adult and adolescent dose**
Cholera or
Diarrhea, bacterial—
Oral, 100 mg four times a day for five to seven days.
Note: Some medical experts recommend shorter courses of treatment (e.g., two to five days) for the above-listed infections.
Giardiasis—
Oral, 100 mg four times a day for seven to ten days.

**Usual pediatric dose**
Cholera or
Diarrhea, bacterial—
Infants up to 1 month of age: Use is not recommended because of the possibility of hemolytic anemia due to immature enzyme systems (glutathione instability) in these infants.
Infants and children 1 month of age and over: Oral, 1.25 mg per kg of body weight four times a day for five to seven days.
Giardiasis—
Infants up to 1 month of age: Use is not recommended because of the possibility of hemolytic anemia due to immature enzyme systems (glutathione instability) in these infants.
Infants and children 1 month of age and over: Oral, 1.25 to 2 mg per kg of body weight four times a day for seven to ten days.
Note: The maximum dose for children should not exceed 8.8 mg per kg of body weight daily because of the possibility of nausea or vomiting.

**Strength(s) usually available**
U.S.—
50 mg per 15 mL (Rx) [*Furoxone Liquid* (methylparaben; propylparaben)].
Canada—
Not commercially available.

**Packaging and storage**
Store below 40 °C (104 °F) in a tight, light-resistant container. Protect from freezing.

**Auxiliary labeling**
• Shake well.
• Avoid alcoholic beverages.
• Continue medication for full time of treatment.
• May discolor urine.

### FURAZOLIDONE TABLETS USP

**Usual adult and adolescent dose**
See *Furazolidone Oral Suspension USP*.

**Usual pediatric dose**
See *Furazolidone Oral Suspension USP*.

**Strength(s) usually available**
U.S.—
100 mg (Rx) [*Furoxone* (scored; sucrose)].
Canada—
Not commercially available.

**Packaging and storage**
Store below 40 °C (104 °F) in a tight, light-resistant container.

**Preparation of dosage form**
*For patients who cannot take oral solids*—Furazolidone tablets may be crushed and given in a teaspoonful of corn syrup.

**Auxiliary labeling**
• Avoid alcoholic beverages.
• Continue medication for full time of treatment.
• May discolor urine.

## Selected Bibliography

Strickland GT, editor. Hunter's tropical medicine. 6th ed. Philadelphia: W. B. Saunders Company, 1984: 279-82, 305-12.
Rabbani GH, Butler T, Shahrier M, et al. Efficacy of a single dose of furazolidone for treatment of cholera in children. Antimicrob Agents Chemother 1991; 35(9): 1864-7.

Revised: 08/11/95

---

# FUROSEMIDE—See *Diuretics, Loop (Systemic)*

# GABAPENTIN Systemic

VA CLASSIFICATION (Primary): CN400
Commonly used brand name(s): *Neurontin*.
Another commonly used name is GBP
Note: For a listing of dosage forms and brand names by country availability, see *Dosage Forms* section(s).

## Category
Anticonvulsant.

## Indications

**Accepted**

Epilepsy (treatment adjunct)—Gabapentin is indicated as an adjunct to other anticonvulsant medications in the treatment of partial seizures with or without secondary generalization in adults and adolescents over 12 years of age with epilepsy.

## Pharmacology/Pharmacokinetics

**Physicochemical characteristics**

Chemical group—Cyclohexane-acetic acid derivative. Structural analog to gamma-aminobutyric acid (GABA).
Molecular weight—171.24.
pKa—3.68 and 10.70.

**Mechanism of action/Effect**

The mechanism of action is unknown. Gabapentin does not interact with GABA receptors, is not metabolized to a GABA agonist or to GABA, and does not inhibit GABA uptake or degradation. In rats, gabapentin interacts with a novel binding site on cortical neurons that may be associated with the L-system amino acid transporter of brain cell membranes.

**Absorption**

Rapid. Gabapentin is absorbed in part by the L-amino acid transport system, which is a saturable transport system, and as the dose increases, bioavailability decreases. Bioavailability ranges from approximately 60% for a 300 mg dose, to approximately 35% for a 1600 mg dose. Therefore, as the total daily dosage is increased, it may be necessary to divide the total dosage into smaller doses given more frequently. Absorption is unaffected by food.

**Distribution**

Volume of distribution ($Vol_D$) is approximately 50 to 60 L Gabapentin penetrates the blood-brain barrier, yielding cerebrospinal fluid (CSF) concentrations approximately equal to 20% of corresponding steady state plasma trough concentrations in patients with epilepsy. Brain tissue concentrations in one patient undergoing temporal lobectomy were approximately 80% of corresponding plasma concentrations.

**Protein binding**

Very low (<5%).

**Biotransformation**

Gabapentin is not metabolized.

**Half-life**

Elimination—
  Normal renal function: 5 to 7 hours.
  In hemodialysis: In 11 anuric patients, a single 400 mg oral dose of gabapentin had an elimination half-life of 132 hours on days when patients did not receive dialysis, and 3.8 hours during dialysis.

**Time to peak concentration**

2 to 4 hours.

**Therapeutic serum concentration**

The therapeutic concentration range for gabapentin is not well defined. However, in one study it was noted that seizure frequency decreased significantly only in patients with gabapentin serum concentrations >2 mg/L (11.7 micromoles/L). After receiving gabapentin 400 mg three times per day for one week, patients maintained on phenytoin had minimum gabapentin plasma concentrations of 2 to 4.8 mg/L (11.7 to 28 micromoles/L) and maximum gabapentin plasma concentrations of 3.6 to 8.6 mg/L (21 to 50.2 micromoles/L). Titration of dosage is based on clinical response.

**Elimination**

Renal—Entire absorbed dose, as unchanged drug. Gabapentin clearance is directly proportional to creatinine clearance.
In dialysis—Gabapentin can be removed from plasma by hemodialysis.

## Precautions to Consider

**Carcinogenicity/Tumorigenicity**

In 2 year carcinogenicity studies, a statistically significant increase in the incidence of pancreatic acinar cell adenomas and carcinomas was found in male rats receiving doses of gabapentin that produced plasma concentrations 10 times higher than those seen in humans receiving 3600 mg per day. Tumors were noninvasive, did not metastasize, did not affect survival, and did not occur in female rats or in mice. The significance to humans is unknown.

**Mutagenicity**

No evidence of mutagenicity was found in appropriate *in vitro* and *in vivo* testing.

**Pregnancy/Reproduction**

Fertility—No adverse effect on fertility was seen in rats given up to 5 times an equivalent human dose of 3600 mg on a mg per square meter of body surface area (mg/m$^2$) basis.

Pregnancy—Gabapentin should be used during pregnancy only if the benefit justifies the potential risk to the fetus.
Studies have not been done in humans.
Mice given 1 to 4 times an equivalent human dose of 3600 mg on a mg/m$^2$ basis produced offspring with delayed ossification of several bones in the skull, vertebrae, and limbs. Rats given approximately 1 to 5 times an equivalent human dose of 3600 mg on a mg/m$^2$ basis produced offspring with an increased incidence of hydroureter and hydronephrosis. In rabbits given < ¼ to 8 times an equivalent human dose of 3600 mg on a mg/m$^2$ basis an increased incidence of postimplantation fetal loss occurred.

FDA Pregnancy Category C.

**Breast-feeding**

It is not known whether gabapentin is distributed into breast milk.

**Pediatrics**

No information is available on the relationship of age to the effects of gabapentin in children up to 12 years of age. Safety and efficacy have not been established.

**Adolescents**

Appropriate studies on the relationship of age to the effects of gabapentin have not been performed in the adolescent population. However, clinical trials that included a limited number of patients aged 12 to 18 years revealed no adolescence-specific problems.

**Geriatrics**

Plasma clearance of gabapentin is reduced in the elderly, probably due to age-related renal function decline. Dosage reduction based on creatinine clearance is recommended. Further dosage adjustments should be based on clinical response.

**Drug interactions and/or related problems**

The following drug interactions and/or related problems have been selected on the basis of their potential clinical significance (possible mechanism in parentheses where appropriate)—not necessarily inclusive (» = major clinical significance):

Note: Combinations containing any of the following medications, depending on the amount present, may also interact with this medication.

Alcohol or
Central nervous system (CNS) depression–producing medications, other (See *Appendix II*)
(increased CNS depression may occur)

Antacids, especially aluminum- and magnesium-containing
(antacid taken with or within 2 hours after gabapentin reduces gabapentin's bioavailability by 20%; gabapentin should be taken at least 2 hours after antacid)

**Laboratory value alterations**

The following have been selected on the basis of their potential clinical significance (possible effect in parentheses where appropriate)—not necessarily inclusive (» = major clinical significance):

With diagnostic test results
Dipstick tests for urinary protein (e.g., Ames N-Multistix SG, Chemstrip 3)
(gabapentin causes a false positive result; the sulfosalicylic acid precipitation procedure should be used to detect urinary protein in patients taking gabapentin)

With physiology/laboratory test values
　　White blood cell counts
　　　(may be decreased)

**Medical considerations/Contraindications**
The medical considerations/contraindications included have been selected on the basis of their potential clinical significance (reasons given in parentheses where appropriate)—not necessarily inclusive (» = major clinical significance).

*Risk-benefit should be considered when the following medical problems exist:*
» Renal function impairment
　　(elimination may be prolonged in patients not receiving hemodialysis, and shortened in patients during hemodialysis; dosage adjustment based on creatinine clearance is recommended)
　Sensitivity to gabapentin

## Side/Adverse Effects
The following side/adverse effects have been selected on the basis of their potential clinical significance (possible signs and symptoms in parentheses where appropriate)—not necessarily inclusive:

**Those indicating need for medical attention**
Incidence more frequent
　*Ataxia* (clumsiness or unsteadiness); *nystagmus* (continuous, uncontrolled back and forth and/or rolling eye movements)
Incidence less frequent
　*Amnesia* (loss of memory); *depression, irritability, or other mood or mental changes*
Incidence rare
　*Leukopenia* (usually asymptomatic; rarely, fever or chills; cough or hoarseness; lower back or side pain; painful or difficult urination)

**Those indicating need for medical attention only if they continue or are bothersome**
Incidence more frequent
　*Dizziness; drowsiness; fatigue* (unusual tiredness or weakness); *myalgia* (muscle ache or pain); *peripheral edema* (swelling of hands, feet, or lower legs); *tremor* (trembling or shaking); *vision abnormalities, including blurred vision and diplopia* (double vision)
Incidence less frequent or rare
　*Asthenia* (weakness or loss of strength); *dryness of mouth or throat; dysarthria* (slurred speech); *frequent urination; gastrointestinal effects, including diarrhea dyspepsia* (indigestion); *nausea and vomiting; headache; hypotension* (low blood pressure); *insomnia* (trouble in sleeping); *rhinitis* (runny nose); *tinnitus* (noise in ears); *trouble in thinking; weight gain*

## Overdose
For more information on the management of overdose or unintentional ingestion, **contact a Poison Control Center** (see *Poison Control Center Listing*).

**Clinical effects of overdose**
The following effects have been selected on the basis of their potential clinical significance (possible signs and symptoms in parentheses where appropriate)—not necessarily inclusive:
　*Diarrhea, severe; diplopia* (double vision); *dizziness, severe; drowsiness, severe; dysarthria, severe* (slurred speech); *lethargy* (sluggishness)

**Treatment of overdose**
Note: There is no specific antidote for gabapentin overdose.
　　Specific treatment—Hemodialysis (may be indicated by clinical state or in patients with significant renal impairment)
　　Supportive care—Patients in whom intentional overdose is confirmed or suspected should be referred for psychiatric consultation.

## Patient Consultation
As an aid to patient consultation, refer to *Advice for the Patient, Gabapentin (Systemic)*.
In providing consultation, consider emphasizing the following selected information (» = major clinical significance):

**Before using this medication**
» Conditions affecting use, especially:
　　Sensitivity to gabapentin
　　Use in the elderly—Elderly patients may excrete gabapentin more slowly; dosage reduction based on creatinine clearance, and dosage adjustment based on clinical response are recommended
　　Other medications, especially antacids
　　Other medical problems, especially renal function impairment

**Proper use of this medication**
» Compliance with therapy; not taking more or less medicine than prescribed; not missing any doses
» Importance of not exceeding 12 hour interval between any 2 doses while on 3 times a day dosing schedule
» Importance of dissolving each dose as needed when a liquid dosage form is required; not dissolving any doses to save for later use
　Missed dose: Taking as soon as possible; if less than 2 hours until next dose, taking missed dose immediately and taking next dose 1 to 2 hours later, then resuming regular dosing schedule; not doubling doses
» Proper storage

**Precautions while using this medication**
» Importance of regular visits to physician to check progress of therapy
　Discussing alcohol use or use of other CNS depressants with physician
» Possible blurred or double vision, dizziness, drowsiness, impairment of thinking or motor skills; caution when driving or doing jobs requiring alertness
　Possible false positive results with dipstick tests for urinary protein; using the sulfosalicylic acid precipitation procedure to determine presence of urinary protein
» Not discontinuing gabapentin abruptly; consulting physician about gradually reducing dosage

**Side/adverse effects**
　Ataxia; nystagmus; amnesia; depression, irritability, or other mood or mental changes; leukopenia

## General Dosing Information
Gabapentin dosage is titrated to clinical effect, not to plasma concentration.
Adverse effects are generally mild to moderate in severity, and tend to diminish with continued use of gabapentin.
Anticonvulsant medications should not be discontinued abruptly because of the possibility of increased seizure frequency. If gabapentin is to be discontinued, or if another anticonvulsant medication is to be added to the patient's therapy, the change should be made gradually, over a minimum period of one week, to avoid loss of seizure control.

## Oral Dosage Forms

### GABAPENTIN CAPSULES
**Usual adult and adolescent dose**
Anticonvulsant—
　Oral, 300 mg on the first day, 600 mg divided into two doses on the second day, 900 mg divided into three doses on the third day. The dosage may be gradually increased based on clinical response. Dosages of 900 to 1800 mg per day are effective for most patients. However, dosages as high as 2400 to 3600 mg per day have been well tolerated.
Note: Taking the initial dose at bedtime will minimize adverse effects.
　　Dosage may be increased more slowly to avoid CNS adverse effects.
　　When taking gabapentin three times a day, the maximum time between doses should not exceed twelve hours.
　　For patients with renal function impairment: See *Usual geriatric dose*
　　For patients undergoing hemodialysis: Oral, 300 to 400 mg initially for patients who have never received gabapentin, then 200 to 300 mg following each four hours of hemodialysis.

**Usual adult and adolescent prescribing limits**
Up to 3600 mg per day.

**Usual pediatric dose**
Anticonvulsant—
　Children up to 12 years of age: Safety and efficacy have not been established.
　Children 12 years of age and over: See *Usual adult and adolescent dose*.

# Gabapentin (Systemic)

**Usual geriatric dose**
Anticonvulsant—
   Oral, initial dosage recommendations, based on creatinine clearance, are as follows. Dosage adjustments may be made based on clinical response.

| Creatinine Clearance (mL per minute) | Total Daily Dose (mg per day) | Dosage Regimen (mg) |
|---|---|---|
| >60 | 1200 | 400 three times a day |
| 30 to 60 | 600 | 300 two times a day |
| 15 to 30 | 300 | 300 once a day |
| <15 | 150 | 300 once every other day |

**Strength(s) usually available**
U.S.—
   100 mg (Rx) [*Neurontin* (lactose; corn starch; talc; gelatin; titanium dioxide; FD&C Blue No.2)].
   300 mg (Rx) [*Neurontin* (lactose; corn starch; talc; gelatin; titanium dioxide; yellow iron oxide; FD&C Blue No.2)].
   400 mg (Rx) [*Neurontin* (lactose; corn starch; talc; gelatin; red iron oxide; titanium dioxide; yellow iron oxide; FD&C Blue No.2)].
Canada—
   100 mg (Rx) [*Neurontin* (lactose; corn starch; talc)].
   300 mg (Rx) [*Neurontin* (lactose; corn starch; talc)].
   400 mg (Rx) [*Neurontin* (lactose; corn starch; talc)].
   Note: Capsule shells may contain gelatin, titanium dioxide, silicon dioxide, sodium lauryl sulfate, yellow iron oxide, red iron oxide, and FD&C Blue No. 2.

**Packaging and storage**
Store below 40 °C (104 °F), preferably between 15 and 30 °C (59 and 86 °F), in a well closed container, unless otherwise specified by manufacturer.

**Preparation of dosage form**
For patients who cannot take oral solids—Individual doses may be dissolved in juice or sprinkled over soft foods, such as applesauce, immediately before use. However, gabapentin solutions degrade over time and should be taken immediately after preparation.

**Auxiliary labeling**
- May cause blurred vision.
- May cause dizziness.
- May cause drowsiness. Alcohol may intensify this effect.

**Selected Bibliography**
Goa KL, Sorkin EM. Gabapentin: A review of its pharmacological properties and clinical potential in epilepsy. Drugs 1993; 46(3): 409-27.

Developed: 02/28/95

---

**GADODIAMIDE**—The *Gadodiamide (Systemic)* monograph is not included in this published version of the USP DI database. Copies of the monograph are available on request from Micromedex, Inc. - Reprint Requests, 6200 S. Syracuse Way, Suite 300, Englewood, CO 80111; telephone (303) 486-6400; telefax (303) 486-6464; Email: USPDI@MDX.COM.

---

**GADOPENTETATE**—The *Gadopentetate (Systemic)* monograph is not included in this published version of the USP DI database. Copies of the monograph are available on request from Micromedex, Inc. - Reprint Requests, 6200 S. Syracuse Way, Suite 300, Englewood, CO 80111; telephone (303) 486-6400; telefax (303) 486-6464; Email: USPDI@MDX.COM.

---

**GADOTERIDOL**—The *Gadoteridol (Systemic)* monograph is not included in this published version of the USP DI database. Copies of the monograph are available on request from Micromedex, Inc. - Reprint Requests, 6200 S. Syracuse Way, Suite 300, Englewood, CO 80111; telephone (303) 486-6400; telefax (303) 486-6464; Email: USPDI@MDX.COM.

---

**GALLAMINE**—See *Neuromuscular Blocking Agents (Systemic)*

---

# GALLIUM CITRATE GA 67   Systemic

VA CLASSIFICATION (Primary): DX201
Commonly used brand name(s): *Neoscan*.
Note:   For a listing of dosage forms and brand names by country availability, see *Dosage Forms* section(s).

## Category
Diagnostic aid, radioactive (neoplastic disease; focal inflammatory lesions).

## Indications
Note:   Bracketed information in the *Indications* section refers to uses that are not included in U.S. product labeling.

**Accepted**
Neoplastic disease (diagnosis)—Gallium citrate Ga 67 is indicated to demonstrate the presence and extent of lymphoma, bronchogenic carcinoma, [acute myelocytic leukemia], [chronic myelocytic leukemia], [hepatoma], and [bone sarcoma]. May also be useful in the detection of [epithelial, head, and neck carcinoma]; [malignant melanoma]; [malignant fibrous histiocytoma]; and [testicular tumors].

Inflammatory lesions, focal (diagnosis)—Gallium citrate Ga 67 is indicated for the localization of focal inflammatory lesions, such as abscess, osteomyelitis, pneumonia, pyelonephritis, and granulomatous diseases (sarcoidosis). May also be useful in the detection of active tuberculosis; and for assessing the activity of the inflammatory process in certain interstitial pulmonary diseases, including sarcoidosis and fibrosing alveolitis.

In combination with thallous chloride Tl 201 imaging, gallium citrate Ga 67 imaging may be useful in the diagnosis of myocardial sarcoidosis and in predicting the response to corticosteroid therapy.

[Immunodeficiency syndrome, acquired, related disorders of (diagnosis)][1]—Gallium citrate Ga 67 is useful in the diagnosis and monitoring of *Pneumocystis carinii* pneumonia, tuberculosis, and other infections in acquired immunodeficiency syndrome (AIDS) patients.

[Fever, unknown origin, source of (diagnosis)][1]—Gallium citrate Ga 67 is useful as a diagnostic screening test in cases of prolonged fever, when physical examination, laboratory tests, and other imaging studies have failed to disclose the source of the fever.

In the absence of pre-existing symptoms, a positive uptake of gallium citrate Ga 67 justifies additional testing for potential disease.

[1]Not included in Canadian product labeling.

## Physical Properties
**Nuclear Data**

| Radionuclide (half-life) | Decay constant | Mode of decay | Principal photon emissions (keV) | Mean number of emissions/ disintegration (≥0.01) |
|---|---|---|---|---|
| Ga 67 (78.26 hr) | 0.00886 hr-1 | Electron capture | Gamma-3 (93.3) | 0.37 |
| | | | Gamma-4 (184.6) | 0.20 |
| | | | Gamma-5 (300.2) | 0.17 |

## Pharmacology/Pharmacokinetics
**Mechanism of action/Effect**
Diagnosis of neoplastic disease and
Diagnosis of inflammatory lesions—The exact mechanism of action is unknown, but gallium citrate Ga 67 has been found to concentrate in

certain viable primary and metastatic tumors as well as focal sites of inflammation. Studies of Ga 67 accumulation in acute inflammatory lesions suggest that a number of factors are involved in the accumulation and retention of Ga 67 at the site of inflammation. Adequate blood supply is essential for delivery of Ga 67 to the lesion. Ga 67, mainly in the form of transferrin-Ga-67 complex, is delivered to the lesion through capillaries with increased permeability. Some Ga 67 is taken up by the leukocytes and bacteria, if present at the site of inflammation.

### Distribution
Rapidly distributed throughout body; concentrating first in tumors and sites of infection, and renal cortex. Maximum concentration shifts to bone (including marrow) and lymph nodes after the first day, and to liver and spleen after the first week.

### Protein binding
High (mainly to plasma transferrin; to a lesser extent to albumins and globulins).

### Half-life
Biological—Approximately 2 to 3 weeks.

### Radiation dosimetry

| Estimated absorbed radiation dose* |||
| --- | --- | --- |
| Organ | mGy/MBq | rad/mCi |
| Bone surfaces | 0.59 | 2.18 |
| Intestine wall (lower) | 0.20 | 0.74 |
| Red marrow | 0.19 | 0.70 |
| Spleen | 0.15 | 0.55 |
| Adrenals | 0.14 | 0.52 |
| Liver | 0.12 | 0.44 |
| Intestine wall (upper) | 0.12 | 0.44 |
| Kidneys | 0.11 | 0.41 |
| Pancreas | 0.083 | 0.31 |
| Ovaries | 0.082 | 0.30 |
| Bladder wall | 0.081 | 0.30 |
| Uterus | 0.079 | 0.29 |
| Stomach wall | 0.072 | 0.27 |
| Lungs | 0.065 | 0.24 |
| Breast | 0.062 | 0.23 |
| Small intestine | 0.059 | 0.22 |
| Testes | 0.057 | 0.21 |
| Thyroid | 0.056 | 0.21 |
| Other tissue | 0.063 | 0.23 |
| Effective dose: 0.12 mSv/MBq (0.44 rem/mCi) |||

*For adults; intravenous injection.

### Elimination
Slow—
Primary:
Renal (26% of the administered dose of which 10 to 15% is eliminated within 24 hours).
Secondary:
Fecal (10% within the first week). Fecal excretion becomes primary route of excretion after the first 24 hours.
Note: Bowel radioactivity may interfere with the interpretation of abdominal scans. To cleanse the bowel prior to imaging, laxatives and/or enemas are recommended on the day of gallium citrate Ga 67 administration and/or subsequent days prior to imaging. Imaging is usually done 48 to 72 hours after administration of the radiotracer.

## Precautions to Consider

### Carcinogenicity/Mutagenicity
Long-term animal studies to evaluate carcinogenic or mutagenic potential of gallium citrate Ga 67 have not been performed.

### Pregnancy/Reproduction
Pregnancy—Gallium citrate Ga 67 crosses the placenta. Adequate and well-controlled studies have not been done in humans.
The possibility of pregnancy should be assessed in women of child-bearing potential. Clinical situations exist where the benefit to the patient and fetus, based on information derived from radiopharmaceutical use, outweighs the risks from fetal exposure to radiation. In these situations, the physician should use discretion and reduce the radiopharmaceutical dose to the lowest possible amount.
Studies have not been done in animals.
FDA Pregnancy Category C.

### Breast-feeding
Gallium citrate Ga 67 is excreted in breast milk. It has been recommended that nursing be resumed, after administration of a radiopharmaceutical, when the infant's ingested effective dose equivalent (EDE) is below 1 mSv (100 mrem). A method to calculate the EDE has been proposed based on the effective half-life of the radionuclide, the activity administered to the mother, the fraction of administered activity ingested by the infant, and the total body effective dose equivalent to the newborn infant per unit of activity ingested. According to this method, it has been estimated that, for gallium citrate Ga 67, the time to reduce the EDE to the infant to below 1 mSv (100 mrem) is approximately 3 weeks after administration to the mother. Because of the difficulty of maintaining the maternal milk supply for such an extended period of time, complete cessation of nursing is usually recommended.

### Pediatrics
There have been no specific studies evaluating safety and efficacy of gallium citrate Ga 67 in children. When this radiopharmaceutical is used in children, the diagnostic benefit should be judged to outweigh the potential risk of radiation.
Caution is recommended when using preparations that contain benzyl alcohol as preservative in neonates, particularly infants born prematurely.

### Geriatrics
Appropriate studies on the relationship of age to the effects of gallium citrate Ga 67 have not been performed in the geriatric population. However, no geriatrics-specific problems have been documented to date.

### Drug interactions and/or related problems
See *Diagnostic interference*.

### Diagnostic interference
The following have been selected on the basis of their potential clinical significance (possible effect in parentheses where appropriate)—not necessarily inclusive (» = major clinical significance):

With results of *this* test
*Due to other medications*
Antineoplastics, which cause an elevation of serum iron, such as:
Cytarabine
Fluorouracil
Methotrexate or
Iron
(concurrent use may result in more unbound Ga 67, thus increasing renal excretion and bone uptake of Ga 67, possibly by elevating serum iron, which in turn may displace Ga 67 from plasma protein-binding sites; tumor or abscess localization of gallium citrate Ga 67 is decreased)
Calcium gluconate, parenteral
(soft tissue accumulation of gallium citrate Ga 67 may occur as a result of extravasated calcium gluconate)
COPP chemotherapy
(thymic uptake of gallium citrate Ga 67 may occur during or after cyclophosphamide-vincristine-procarbazine-prednisone [COPP] chemotherapy)
Corticosteroids, glucocorticoid
(concurrent use may decrease gallium citrate Ga 67 uptake by brain tumor or abscess because of reduced peritumor edema caused by the steroid)
(thymic uptake of gallium citrate Ga 67 may occur with concurrent use of prednisone)
Gallium nitrate
(gallium nitrate competes with gallium citrate Ga 67 for plasma protein binding sites, resulting in reduced tumor or abscess uptake and increased skeletal uptake, increased renal excretion, and reduced liver uptake of gallium citrate Ga 67)
Iron dextran
(abscess-to-muscle ratio may be increased when iron dextran is given 24 hours after the injection of gallium citrate Ga 67, but may be decreased if given before or concurrently with it; this effect is probably due to a displacement of Ga 67 from plasma protein–binding sites by the iron, which results in increased elimination of the radiopharmaceutical)
Mechlorethamine or
Vincristine
(concurrent use may decrease whole body retention and increase bone deposition and urinary excretion of gallium citrate Ga 67)

*Due to medical problems or conditions*
Cardiotoxicity, doxorubicin-induced
(doxorubicin-induced cardiotoxicity may enhance myocardial uptake of gallium citrate Ga 67)
Gynecomastia or hyperprolactinemia, diethylstilbestrol-, imipramine-, metoclopramide-, oral contraceptive-, phenothiazine-, or reserpine-induced
(possible localization of gallium citrate Ga 67 in breast [females and males])

## 1540  Gallium Citrate Ga 67 (Systemic)

Lymphadenopathy, phenytoin-induced
(false positive images that resemble true lymphoma may occur since phenytoin has been associated with the development of local or generalized lymphadenopathy; condition should be differentiated from other types of lymph node pathology and the patient observed for an extended period of time)

Nephritis, drug-induced
(interstitial nephritis induced by drugs [e.g., allopurinol, cephalosporins, erythromycin, furosemide, gold compounds, nonsteroidal anti-inflammatory drugs, pentamidine, phenobarbital, rifampin, sulfonamides, thiazide diuretics] may result in kidney uptake of gallium citrate Ga 67 that resembles that observed with other inflammatory kidney disease and possibly may be mistaken for glomerulonephritis, pyelonephritis, or the nephrotoxic syndrome)

Pseudomembranous colitis, antibiotic-induced
(inflammation of the colon induced by antibiotics or other drugs may result in colonic uptake of gallium citrate Ga 67 that resembles that observed with other inflammatory bowel diseases)

Pulmonary disease, amiodarone-, bleomycin-, busulfan-, combination chemotherapeutic agent-, or nitrofurantoin-induced
(pulmonary interstitial pneumonitis and/or fibrosis induced by therapy with these medications may result in diffuse pulmonary localization of gallium citrate Ga 67 that resembles that observed with other diffuse pulmonary diseases not related to drug therapy)

**Medical considerations/Contraindications**
The medical considerations/contraindications included have been selected on the basis of their potential clinical significance (reasons given in parentheses where appropriate)—not necessarily inclusive (» = major clinical significance).
See also *Diagnostic interference*.

*Risk-benefit must be considered when the following medical problem exists:*
Sensitivity to the radiopharmaceutical preparation

## Side/Adverse Effects
The following side/adverse effects have been selected on the basis of their potential clinical significance (possible signs and symptoms in parentheses where appropriate)—not necessarily inclusive:

**Those indicating need for medical attention**
Incidence rare
*Fast heartbeat; nausea or vomiting; skin rash, hives, or itching*

## Patient Consultation
As an aid to patient consultation, refer to *Advice for the Patient, Radiopharmaceuticals (Diagnostic)*.
In providing consultation, consider emphasizing the following selected information (» = major clinical significance):

**Description of use**
Action in the body: Concentration of radioactivity in certain tumors and sites of inflammation allows images to be obtained
Small amounts of radioactivity used in diagnosis; radiation received is low and considered safe

**Before having this test**
» Conditions affecting use, especially:
Sensitivity to the radiopharmaceutical preparation
Pregnancy—Crosses the placenta; risk to fetus from radiation exposure as opposed to benefit derived from use should be considered
Breast-feeding—Excreted in breast milk; cessation of nursing recommended because of risk to infant from radiation exposure
Use in children—Risk from radiation exposure as opposed to benefit derived from use should be considered

**Preparation for this test**
Special preparatory instructions may apply; laxatives or enemas may be prescribed

**Precautions after having this test**
No special precautions

**Side/adverse effects**
Signs of potential side effects, especially fast heartbeat; nausea or vomiting; or skin rash, hives, or itching

## General Dosing Information
Radiopharmaceuticals are to be administered only by or under the supervision of physicians who have had extensive training in the safe use and handling of radioactive materials and who are authorized by the appropriate Federal or State agency, if required or, outside the U.S., the appropriate authority.

Gallium citrate Ga 67 is to be administered intravenously only.

Imaging is usually done 48 to 72 hours after administration of the radiotracer.

Abnormal gallium citrate Ga 67 concentration usually implies the existence of underlying pathology, but further diagnostic studies may be required to distinguish benign from malignant lesions.

To cleanse the bowel of radioactive material and minimize the possibility of false-positive test results, laxatives and/or enemas may be given daily until final images are obtained.

**Safety considerations for handling this radiopharmaceutical**
Improper handling of this radiopharmaceutical may cause radioactive contamination. Guidelines for handling radioactive material have been prepared by scientific, professional, state, federal, and international bodies and are available to the specially qualified and authorized users who have access to radiopharmaceuticals.

## Parenteral Dosage Forms
### GALLIUM CITRATE Ga 67 INJECTION USP
**Usual adult and adolescent administered activity**
Diagnostic aid, radioactive (neoplastic); and
Diagnostic aid, radioactive (focal inflammatory lesions)—
Intravenous, 74 to 185 megabecquerels (2 to 5 millicuries).
Note: In patients with known tumors, doses of 370 megabecquerels (10 millicuries) are used, to facilitate tomography (SPECT) and delayed imaging (>96 hours).

**Usual pediatric administered activity**
Dosage must be individualized by physician.

**Usual geriatric administered activity**
See *Usual adult and adolescent administered activity*.

**Strength(s) usually available**
U.S.—
74 megabecquerels (2 millicuries) ± 10% of gallium Ga 67 per mL at time of calibration (Rx) [*Neoscan;* GENERIC].
Canada—
As per labeling of supplier [GENERIC].

**Packaging and storage**
Store below 40 °C (104 °F), preferably between 15 and 30 °C (59 and 86 °F), unless otherwise specified by manufacturer. Protect from freezing.

**Note**
Caution—Radioactive material.

## Selected Bibliography
Tsan M. Mechanism of gallium 67 accumulation in inflammatory lesions. J Nucl Med 1985; 26: 88-92.
McNeil BJ, Sanders R, Alderson PO, et al. A prospective study of computed tomography, ultrasound, and gallium imaging in patients with fever. Radiology 1981; 139: 647-53.
Ganz WI, Serafini AN. The diagnostic role of nuclear medicine in the acquired immunodeficiency syndrome. J Nucl Med 1989; 30: 1935-45.

Revised: 10/21/92
Interim revision: 08/02/94

# GALLIUM NITRATE  Systemic†

VA CLASSIFICATION (Primary): HS309
Commonly used brand name(s): *Ganite*.
Note: For a listing of dosage forms and brand names by country availability, see *Dosage Forms* section(s).

†Not commercially available in Canada.

## Category
Antihypercalcemic.

## Indications

### Accepted
**Hypercalcemia, associated with neoplasms (treatment)**—Gallium nitrate is indicated in the treatment of hypercalcemia of malignancy that is inadequately managed by oral hydration alone. It is used with saline hydration and may be used with diuretics.

### Acceptance not established
Gallium nitrate has been used to treat moderate to severe symptoms of Paget's disease of bone (osteitis deformans), characterized by abnormal and accelerated bone metabolism in one or more bones. However, data are limited and further study is required to define the role of gallium nitrate in this condition.

## Pharmacology/Pharmacokinetics

### Physicochemical characteristics
Source—Gallium nitrate is a hydrated nitrate salt of the group IIIa element gallium.
Molecular weight—417.87.

### Mechanism of action/Effect
*In vivo* studies indicate that gallium nitrate preferentially accumulates in metabolically active areas of high bone turnover, where it reversibly inhibits osteoclast-mediated bone resorption.
Hypercalcemia of malignancy—Bone resorption is increased in the presence of neoplastic tissue. Gallium nitrate inhibits abnormal bone resorption and reduces the flow of calcium from the resorbing bone into the blood, effectively decreasing total and ionized serum calcium. When kidney function is adequate for the fluid load, hydration with saline increases urine output and the use of diuretics increases the rate of calcium excretion.

### Distribution
$Vol_D$—1.27 liters per kg of body weight (L/kg).

### Biotransformation
None.

### Half-life
Alpha—1 hour.
Beta—24 hours, but lengthens to 72 to 115 hours with prolonged intravenous infusion.

### Duration of action
Studies have reported a median duration of 6 to 8 days (range, 0 to 15+ days).

### Elimination
Renal.

## Precautions to Consider

### Carcinogenicity
Long-term carcinogenicity studies have not been performed in animals.

### Mutagenicity
Gallium nitrate has not been found to be mutagenic in standard tests such as Ames and chromosomal aberration studies on human lymphocytes.

### Pregnancy/Reproduction
Pregnancy—Studies have not been done in humans.
Studies have not been done in animals.
FDA Pregnancy Category C.

### Breast-feeding
It is not known whether gallium nitrate is distributed into breast milk. It is recommended that mothers taking gallium nitrate not breast-feed because of potentially serious adverse effects in nursing infants.

### Pediatrics
No information is available on the relationship of age to the effects of gallium nitrate in pediatric patients. Safety and efficacy have not been established.

### Geriatrics
Although appropriate studies on the relationship of age to the effects of gallium nitrate have not been performed in the geriatric population, no geriatrics-specific problems have been documented to date. However, elderly patients are more likely to have age-related renal function impairment, which may require caution in patients receiving gallium nitrate.

### Drug interactions and/or related problems
The following drug interactions and/or related problems have been selected on the basis of their potential clinical significance (possible mechanism in parentheses where appropriate)—not necessarily inclusive (» = major clinical significance):

» Nephrotoxic medications, other (See *Appendix II*)
(the possibility of additive toxicity should be considered if these medications are used concurrently with gallium nitrate)

### Laboratory value alterations
The following have been selected on the basis of their potential clinical significance (possible effect in parentheses where appropriate)—not necessarily inclusive (» = major clinical significance):

With diagnostic test results
Gallium citrate Ga 67 scintigraphy for tumor or abscess localization (gallium nitrate competes with gallium citrate Ga 67 for plasma protein binding sites, resulting in reduced tumor or abscess uptake and increased skeletal uptake, increased renal excretion, and reduced liver uptake of gallium citrate Ga 67)

### Medical considerations/Contraindications
The medical considerations/contraindications included have been selected on the basis of their potential clinical significance (reasons given in parentheses where appropriate)—not necessarily inclusive (» = major clinical significance).

*Except under special circumstances, this medication should not be used when the following medical problem exists:*
» Renal function impairment when serum creatinine is greater than 2.5 mg per deciliter (mg/dL)
(condition may be exacerbated)

*Risk-benefit should be considered when the following medical problem exists:*
» Renal function impairment when serum creatinine is 2 to 2.5 mg/dL
(frequent monitoring of patient's renal status is recommended; gallium nitrate treatment should be discontinued if serum creatinine exceeds 2.5 mg/dL)

### Patient monitoring
The following may be especially important in patient monitoring (other tests may be warranted in some patients, depending on condition; » = major clinical significance):

Albumin concentrations, serum and
Calcium concentrations, serum and
Phosphorus concentrations, serum
(serum calcium should be monitored daily, serum phosphorus two times a week, and serum albumin before and after each course of therapy; serum proteins, especially albumin, may influence the ratio of free and bound calcium; corrected serum calcium values should be calculated by using an established algorithm; albumin-corrected serum calcium determinations may be useful when the signs and symptoms of hypercalcemia are inconsistent with unadjusted calcium values)

» Renal function determinations, especially serum creatinine and blood urea nitrogen (BUN)
(recommended daily to every 2 to 3 days during therapy; treatment should be discontinued if serum creatinine is greater than 2.5 mg per dL)

## Side/Adverse Effects

The following side/adverse effects have been selected on the basis of their potential clinical significance (possible signs and symptoms in parentheses where appropriate)—not necessarily inclusive:

Note: Decreased serum bicarbonate, possibly secondary to mild respiratory alkalosis, has been reported. It has been asymptomatic and has not required specific treatment.

### Those indicating need for medical attention
Incidence more frequent
*Hypophosphatemia* (bone pain; loss of appetite; muscle weakness); *nephrotoxicity* (blood in urine; greatly increased or decreased frequency of urination or amount of urine; increased thirst; loss of appetite; nausea; vomiting)

Incidence less frequent
*Hypocalcemia* (abdominal cramps; confusion; muscle spasms)

Incidence rare
*Anemia* (unusual tiredness or weakness)—with doses of up to 1400 mg per square meter of body surface area

### Those indicating need for medical attention only if they continue or are bothersome
Incidence more frequent
*Diarrhea; metallic taste; nausea; vomiting*

# Gallium Nitrate (Systemic)

## Patient Consultation
As an aid to patient consultation, refer to *Advice for the Patient, Gallium Nitrate (Systemic)*.

In providing consultation, consider emphasizing the following selected information (» = major clinical significance):

**Before using this medication**
» Conditions affecting use, especially:
  Breast-feeding—Not known if distributed into breast milk; may cause potentially serious adverse effects in nursing infants
  Other medications, especially nephrotoxic medications
  Other medical problems, especially renal function impairment

**Proper use of this medication**
» Proper dosing
» Proper storage

**Precautions while using this medication**
  Importance of close monitoring by physician

**Side/adverse effects**
  Signs of potential adverse effects, especially hypophosphatemia, nephrotoxicity, hypocalcemia, and anemia

## General Dosing Information
The daily dose is usually diluted in 1000 mL of 0.9% sodium chloride injection or 5% dextrose injection. The diluted dose should be administered over a period of twenty-four hours. The solution can also be delivered undiluted via a metered ambulatory infusion pump.

During acute therapy for hypercalcemia, patients should maintain a urinary output of at least 2000 mL per day to decrease the chance of nephrotoxicity.

## Parenteral Dosage Forms

### GALLIUM NITRATE INJECTION

**Usual adult and adolescent dose**
Hypercalcemia (treatment)—
  Intravenous infusion, 100 to 200 mg per square meter of body surface area per day, administered over a period of twenty-four hours, for five days.

Note: If serum calcium concentrations decrease to normal in less than five days, treatment should be discontinued.
  Some clinicians recommend that therapy be repeated, if needed, after a waiting period of two to four weeks.

**Usual pediatric dose**
Safety and efficacy have not been established.

**Usual geriatric dose**
Safety and efficacy have not been established.

**Strength(s) usually available**
U.S.—
  25 mg per mL (Rx) [*Ganite*].
Canada—
  Gallium nitrate is not commercially available in Canada; however, it is available by emergency drug release from the Health Protection Branch.

**Packaging and storage**
Store below 40 °C (104 °F), preferably between 15 and 30 °C (59 and 86 °F), unless otherwise specified by manufacturer.

**Preparation of dosage form**
The daily dose is usually diluted in 1000 mL of 0.9% sodium chloride injection or 5% dextrose injection.

**Stability**
Diluted solution may be stored at controlled room temperature for 48 hours and under refrigeration for 7 days without loss of potency.

Revised: 08/05/97

---

# GANCICLOVIR  Implantation-Ophthalmic—INTRODUCTORY VERSION

VA CLASSIFICATION (Primary): OP900
Commonly used brand name(s): *Vitrasert*.
Note: For a listing of dosage forms and brand names by country availability, see *Dosage Forms* section(s).

## Category
Antiviral (ophthalmic).

## Indications

**Accepted**
Cytomegalovirus retinitis (treatment)—Ganciclovir intravitreal implant is indicated for the treatment of cytomegalovirus (CMV) retinitis in patients with acquired immunodeficiency syndrome (AIDS). However, ganciclovir therapy is not a cure for CMV retinitis, and progression will occur after all of the medication has been released from the implant.

The intravitreal implant provides localized treatment only and will not have any effect on extraocular CMV infection.

Note: Viral resistance to ganciclovir has been demonstrated *in vitro* using CMV isolates from patients receiving the medication intravenously. The possibility of viral resistance should be considered if a poor clinical response occurs.

## Pharmacology/Pharmacokinetics

**Physicochemical characteristics**
Molecular weight—255.23.
Solubility—In water at 25 °C: 4.3 mg per mL (mg/mL).

**Mechanism of action/Effect**
Ganciclovir inhibits virus replication.

**Duration of action**
The intravitreal implant is designed to release ganciclovir over a period of 5 to 8 months. In one clinical trial, the median time to progression of CMV retinitis after insertion of the implant was 210 days. With the comparison treatment (recommended induction and maintenance doses of intravenous ganciclovir), the median time to progression of CMV retinitis was 120 days.

## Precautions to Consider

**Cross-sensitivity and/or related problems**
Patients hypersensitive to acyclovir may be hypersensitive to ganciclovir also.

**Carcinogenicity/Tumorigenicity**
Ganciclovir is carcinogenic and tumorigenic in animals and should be considered a potential carcinogen in humans. Mice given oral doses of 20 mg per kg of body weight (mg/kg) per day showed slightly increased incidences of tumors in the preputial and harderian glands in males, forestomach in males and females, and liver in females. Mice given oral doses of 1000 mg/kg per day showed increased incidences of tumors of the preputial gland in males, forestomach in males and females, and reproductive tissues and liver in females. Except for histiocytic sarcoma of the liver, ganciclovir-induced tumors were of vascular or epithelial origin.

**Mutagenicity**
Ganciclovir was mutagenic in mouse lymphoma cells at concentrations between 50 and 500 micrograms per mL (mcg/mL) and caused DNA damage in human lymphocytes at concentrations between 250 and 2000 mcg/mL. Ganciclovir was clastogenic in the mouse micronucleus assay after intravenous administration of 150 and 500 mg/kg (2.8 and 10 times, respectively, the human exposure after intravenous administration based on the area under the concentration–time curve [AUC]), but not after intravenous administration of 50 mg/kg (exposure approximately equivalent to the human exposure after intravenous administration based on the AUC). However, no mutagenicity was found in the Ames *Salmonella* assay with ganciclovir concentrations of 500 to 5000 mcg/mL.

**Pregnancy/Reproduction**
Fertility—Systemic ganciclovir causes adverse effects on fertility in animals and may impair fertility in humans. Decreases in mating behavior and fertility occurred in female mice given intravenous doses of 90 mg/kg per day, and fetal resorptions occurred in at least 85% of rabbits and

mice given 60 mg/kg per day and 108 mg/kg per day, respectively. Also, decreases in sperm production and fertility occurred in male mice and dogs given oral or intravenous doses ranging from 0.2 to 10 mg/kg per day.

Pregnancy—Adequate and well-controlled studies with the intravitreous implant have not been done in humans.

Animal studies have shown systemic ganciclovir to be embryotoxic and teratogenic. In rabbits, ganciclovir administration resulted in maternal toxicity, fetal growth retardation, and teratogenic changes including cleft palate, anophthalmia or microphthalmia, aplastic kidney and pancreas, hydrocephaly, and brachygnathia. In mice, ganciclovir caused maternal and fetal toxicity. Also, intravenous administration of 90 mg/kg per day to female mice prior to mating, during gestation, and during lactation caused hypoplasia of the testes and seminal vesicles in month-old male offspring, and pathologic changes in the forestomach (non-glandular mucosa) of the mothers.

FDA Pregnancy Category C.

**Breast-feeding**

It is not known whether ganciclovir is distributed into human breast milk. However, because of the carcinogenicity, teratogenicity, and other adverse effects seen in animal studies, it is recommended that breast-feeding be discontinued if the mother receives a ganciclovir intravitreal implant.

**Pediatrics**

Appropriate studies on the relationship of age to the effects of ganciclovir intravitreal implants have not been done in children younger than 9 years of age. Safety and efficacy have not been established.

**Geriatrics**

No information is available on the relationship of age to the effects of ganciclovir intravitreal implants in geriatric patients.

**Medical considerations/Contraindications**

The medical considerations/contraindications included have been selected on the basis of their potential clinical significance (reasons given in parentheses where appropriate)—not necessarily inclusive (» = major clinical significance).

*Except under special circumstances, this medication should not be used when the following medical problems exist:*

» Any condition in which intraocular surgery is contraindicated, such as:
    Infection, external
    Thrombocytopenia, severe
» Hypersensitivity to ganciclovir or acyclovir, history of

**Patient monitoring**

The following may be especially important in patient monitoring (other tests may be warranted in some patients, depending on condition; » = major clinical significance):

» Ophthalmologic examinations, postoperative
    (recommended periodically to detect possible postoperative complications and to detect a progression of cytomegalovirus [CMV] retinitis in cases of drug resistance or after the medication is depleted from the implant)

## Side/Adverse Effects

Note: Side effects reported in conjunction with insertion of a ganciclovir intravitreous implant are probably due to the surgical procedure, rather than to the medication.

In addition to the side/adverse effects listed below, there is a risk of postoperative infection.

A decrease in visual acuity occurs in the implanted eye immediately after surgery in almost all patients. This effect is temporary and lasts approximately 2 to 4 weeks. This decrease in visual acuity is most likely a result of the surgical implant procedure itself.

The following side/adverse effects have been selected on the basis of their potential clinical significance (possible signs and symptoms in parentheses where appropriate)—not necessarily inclusive:

**Those indicating need for medical attention**

Incidence more frequent—10 to 20% within the first 2 months after surgery
*Hemorrhage, vitreous* (seeing floating spots before the eyes); *retinal detachment* (seeing flashes or sparks of light, seeing floating spots before the eyes, or a veil or curtain appearing across part of vision); *visual acuity loss of three or more lines* (decrease in vision, severe)

Incidence less frequent—1 to 5% within the first 2 months after surgery
*Cataract formation or lens opacities; increased intraocular pressure; macular abnormalities; or optic disk or nerve changes* (decreased vision or other change in vision); *hyphema* (red or bloodshot eye); *uveitis* (eye pain, tearing, sensitivity of eye to light, redness of eye, or blurred vision or other change in vision)

Incidence rare—less than 1% within the first 2 months after surgery
*Angle closure glaucoma with anterior chamber shallowing* (eye pain and blurred vision); *chemosis* (swelling of the membrane covering the white part of the eye); *choroidal folds; corneal dellen; keratopathy; phthisis bulbi; retinal hole or tear; synechia; or vitreous detachment or traction* (decreased vision or other change in vision); *choroiditis; endophthalmitis; or other severe postoperative inflammation* (eye pain, tearing, sensitivity of eye to light, redness of eye, or blurred vision or other change in vision); *gliosis* (decreased vision or other change in vision); *hypotony* (decreased vision or other change in vision); *pellet extrusion from scleral wound* (eye irritation or pain, eye redness, or tearing)

**Those indicating need for medical attention only if they continue or are bothersome**

Incidence more frequent
*Visual acuity loss, immediate and temporary* (decrease in vision lasting approximately 2 to 4 weeks)—in nearly all patients; most likely a result of the surgical implant procedure itself

Incidence rare—less than 1% within the first 2 months after surgery
*Hemorrhage, nonvitreous* (red or bloodshot eye); *sclerosis*

## Patient Consultation

As an aid to patient consultation, refer to *Advice for the Patient, Ganciclovir (Implantation-Ophthalmic)—Introductory Version.*

In providing consultation, consider emphasizing the following selected information (» = major clinical significance):

**Description of use**

» Describing the surgical procedure for inserting the implant
» Discussing with the patient the possible risks of the surgical procedure, including intraocular infection or inflammation, detachment of the retina, and formation of a cataract in the natural crystalline lens

**Before receiving this intravitreal implant**

» Conditions affecting use, especially:
    Sensitivity to ganciclovir or acyclovir

    Carcinogenicity/tumorigenicity—Ganciclovir is carcinogenic and tumorigenic in animals; ganciclovir should be considered a potential carcinogen in humans

    Mutagenicity—Mutagenicity has been demonstrated in various tests

    Pregnancy—The risk of adverse effects with the intravitreal implant has not been established; however, systemic ganciclovir is embryotoxic and teratogenic in animals

    Breast-feeding—Breast-feeding should be discontinued if an intravitreal implant is inserted because carcinogenicity and other adverse effects have been demonstrated in animals

    Use in children—Safety and efficacy in children up to 9 years of age have not been established

    Other medical problems, especially any condition in which intraocular surgery is contraindicated, such as external infection or severe thrombocytopenia

**Precautions after receiving this intravitreal implant**

» Importance of regular ophthalmologic examinations to check for possible postoperative complications and to check for a progression of cytomegalovirus (CMV) retinitis in cases of drug resistance or after the medication is depleted from the implant
» Decrease in visual acuity in the implanted eye is to be expected for the first 2 to 4 weeks after surgery; checking with physician if other vision changes occur or if the decrease in visual acuity worsens, continues for more than 4 weeks, or recurs after improving, since this may indicate postoperative complications

**Side/adverse effects**

Signs of potential postoperative complications, especially hemorrhage, vitreous; retinal detachment; visual acuity loss of three or more lines; cataract formation or lens opacities; increased intraocular pressure; macular abnormalities, or optic disk or nerve changes; hyphema; uveitis; angle closure glaucoma with anterior chamber shallowing; chemosis; choroidal folds, corneal dellen, keratopathy, phthisis bulbi, retinal hole or tear, synechia, or vitreous detachment or traction; choroiditis, endophthalmitis, or other severe postoperative inflammation; gliosis; hypotony; and pellet extrusion from scleral wound

## General Dosing Information

The ganciclovir intravitreal implant should be inserted only by a surgeon who previously has observed or assisted with the procedure. Aseptic technique should be maintained prior to and during the procedure.

The ganciclovir intravitreal implant has been sterilized by an ethylene oxide–freon mixture (a substance that may harm public health and the environment by destroying ozone in the upper atmosphere). **The implant should not be resterilized.**

To avoid damaging the polymer coatings, which could result in an increased rate of ganciclovir release from the implant, the product should be handled only by the suture tab.

### Safety considerations for handling this medication
Because ganciclovir shares some of the properties of antitumor agents (e.g., carcinogenicity, mutagenicity), consideration should be given to handling and disposing of the implant according to guidelines issued for antineoplastics.

## Ophthalmic Dosage Forms

### GANCICLOVIR IMPLANTS (INTRAVITREAL)

#### Usual adult and adolescent dose
Cytomegalovirus retinitis—
   Intravitreal, one implant inserted surgically into the affected eye. The implant may be removed and replaced when evidence of progression of retinitis indicates that the medication has been depleted from the implant.

Note: The product is designed to release ganciclovir over a period of five to eight months.

#### Usual pediatric dose
Cytomegalovirus retinitis—
   Children up to 9 years of age:
      Safety and efficacy have not been established.
   Children 9 years of age and older:
      See *Usual adult and adolescent dose*.

#### Strength(s) usually available
U.S.—
   4.5 mg (Rx) [*Vitrasert* (magnesium stearate 0.25%; polyvinyl alcohol polymer; ethylene vinyl acetate polymer)].

#### Packaging and storage
Store between 15 and 30 °C (59 and 86 °F), unless otherwise directed by manufacturer. Protect from freezing and from excessive heat and light.

Developed: 10/14/97
Interim revision: 08/12/98

# GANCICLOVIR  Systemic

VA CLASSIFICATION (Primary): AM809

Commonly used brand name(s): *Cytovene; Cytovene-IV*.

Another commonly used name is DHPG

Note: For a listing of dosage forms and brand names by country availability, see *Dosage Forms* section(s).

## Category
Antiviral (systemic).

## Indications
Note: Bracketed information in the *Indications* section refers to uses that are not included in U.S. product labeling.

### Accepted
Cytomegalovirus retinitis (treatment)—Parenteral ganciclovir is indicated for induction and maintenance in the treatment of cytomegalovirus (CMV) retinitis in immunocompromised patients, including patients with acquired immunodeficiency syndrome (AIDS). Oral ganciclovir is indicated only for the maintenance of CMV retinitis in patients who have had a complete resolution of active retinitis after an induction course of parenteral ganciclovir; however, oral ganciclovir has been associated with a shorter time to CMV retinitis progression. [Intravitreal administration of ganciclovir has also been used in patients who have been unresponsive to intravenous ganciclovir, or in whom serious myelosuppression has precluded the continuation of intravenous therapy.].

Cytomegalovirus disease (prophylaxis)[1]—Parenteral ganciclovir is indicated for the prophylaxis of CMV disease in transplant patients who are at risk for the disease.

[Cytomegalovirus disease (treatment)][1]—Parenteral ganciclovir is used in the treatment of severe CMV disease, including CMV pneumonia, CMV gastrointestinal disease, and disseminated CMV infections, in immunocompromised patients.

[Polyradiculopathy (treatment)][1]—Parenteral ganciclovir is used in the treatment of polyradiculopathy caused by CMV in patients with AIDS.

Resistance to ganciclovir has been reported. One paper described CMV disease refractory to ganciclovir therapy due to infections with a resistant virus, a susceptible virus that became resistant, and an infection first by a susceptible strain, and later by a genetically distinct, resistant one. The primary mechanism of resistance to ganciclovir is the decreased ability to form the active triphosphate moiety. Recurrence may be more frequent in patients treated with ganciclovir for prolonged periods, (> 3 to 6 months).

[1]Not included in Canadian product labeling.

## Pharmacology/Pharmacokinetics

### Physicochemical characteristics
High pH (11).
Molecular weight—Ganciclovir: 255.23.
Ganciclovir sodium: 277.22.

### Mechanism of action/Effect
Ganciclovir is a prodrug that is structurally similar to acyclovir. Its antiviral activity results from its intracellular conversion to the triphosphate form. In cytomegalovirus (CMV)-infected cells, ganciclovir is thought to be rapidly phosphorylated to the monophosphate form by a CMV-encoded enzyme, then subsequently converted to the diphosphate and triphosphate forms by cellular kinases. Ganciclovir is phosphorylated much more rapidly in infected cells; however, uninfected cells can also produce low levels of ganciclovir-triphosphate. Ganciclovir-triphosphate competitively inhibits DNA polymerase by acting as a substrate and becoming incorporated into the DNA. This inhibits DNA synthesis by suppressing DNA chain elongation. The drug inhibits viral DNA polymerases more effectively than it does cellular polymerase. Chain elongation resumes when ganciclovir is removed.

### Absorption
Ganciclovir is poorly absorbed after oral administration; bioavailability under fasting conditions is approximately 5%, and when administered with food, 6 to 9%.

### Distribution
Ganciclovir is widely distributed to all tissues and crosses the placenta; however, there is no marked accumulation in any one type of tissue. Penetration into the cerebral spinal fluid averaged 38% in one study, and ranged from 7 to 67% in others. Ganciclovir also appears to have good intraocular penetration. In one patient, the subretinal fluid ganciclovir concentration was 7.2 micromoles per L with a corresponding plasma concentration of 8.2 micromoles per L 5.5 hours after a dose of 5 mg per kg of body weight (mg/kg), and 2.58 micromoles per L with a corresponding plasma concentration of 1.3 micromoles per L 8 hours after a subsequent dose of 5 mg/kg.

Vol$_D$ (steady state)—Adults and neonates: Approximately 0.74 L per kg.

### Protein binding
Low (1 to 2%).

### Biotransformation
Little to no metabolism.

### Half-life
Serum—
   Intravenous:
      Adults—Normal renal function: 2.5 to 3.6 hours (average, 2.9 hours).
      Adults—Renal function impairment: 9 to 30 hours (creatinine clearance of 20 to 50 mL per minute [0.33 to 0.83 mL per second]).
      Neonates—Approximately 2.4 hours.
   Oral:
      Normal renal function—3.1 to 5.5 hours.
      Renal function impairment—15.7 to 18.2 hours (creatinine clearance of 10 to 50 mL per minute [0.17 to 0.83 mL per second]).
Vitreous fluid—
   Approximately 13 hours.

### Time to peak concentration
Intravenous—
   End of infusion (approximately 1 hour).
Oral—
   Fasting: Approximately 1.8 hours.
   With food: Approximately 3 hours.

**Peak concentrations**
Intravenous—
  Adults: 5 mg/kg over 1 hour—8.3 to 9 mcg/mL.
  Neonates: 4 and 6 mg/kg over 1 hour—Approximately 5.5 and 7 mcg/mL, respectively.
Oral—
  3 grams per day: 1 to 1.2 mcg/mL.
Intravitreal injection—
  1000 mcg administered in 5 divided doses over 15 days: 16.2 mcg/mL; ganciclovir was not detected in plasma.

**Elimination**
Renal; almost 100% excreted unchanged in the urine by glomerular filtration and tubular secretion.
In dialysis—Plasma ganciclovir concentrations are reduced by approximately 50% after a single, 4-hour hemodialysis.

## Precautions to Consider

**Cross-sensitivity and/or related problems**
Patients hypersensitive to acyclovir may also be hypersensitive to ganciclovir because of the chemical similarity of the 2 medications.

**Carcinogenicity/Tumorigenicity**
Ganciclovir is carcinogenic in animals and should be considered a potential carcinogen in humans. Ganciclovir was carcinogenic in the mouse at oral doses of 20 and 1000 mg/kg per day (approximately 0.1 and 1.4 times, respectively, the mean drug exposure in humans following the recommended intravenous dose of 5 mg/kg, based on the area under the concentration-time curve [AUC]) comparisons. Mice given oral doses of 20 mg per kg of body weight (mg/kg) per day showed a slightly increased incidence of tumors in the preputial and harderian glands in males, forestomach in males and females, and liver in females. Studies in mice given oral doses of 1000 mg/kg per day showed an increased incidence of tumors of the forestomach in males and females, preputial gland in males, and reproductive tissues and liver in females. All ganciclovir-induced tumors were of epithelial or vascular origin, except for histiocytic sarcoma of the liver. No carcinogenic effect occurred at a dose of 1 mg/kg per day.

**Mutagenicity**
Ganciclovir was mutagenic in mouse lymphoma cells at concentrations between 50 and 500 mcg/mL, and caused chromosomal damage *in vitro* in human lymphocytes at concentrations between 250 and 2000 mcg/mL. Parenteral ganciclovir was also clastogenic in the mouse micronucleus assay at doses of 150 and 500 mg/kg (2.8 to 10 times the human exposure based on area under the concentration-time curve [AUC] of a single intravenous dose of 5 mg/kg), but not at a dose of 50 mg/kg (exposure approximately comparable to the human dose based on AUC). Ganciclovir was not mutagenic in the Ames Salmonella assay at concentrations of 500 to 5000 mcg/mL.

**Pregnancy/Reproduction**
Fertility—Although data in humans have not been obtained, temporary or permanent suppression of fertility in women and spermatogenesis in men may occur.
In female mice, ganciclovir caused decreased mating behavior, decreased fertility, and increased death *in utero* at doses approximately 1.7 times the recommended human dose (based on the AUC of a single intravenous dose of 5 mg/kg). Ganciclovir was also found to cause decreased fertility in male mice, and hypospermatogenesis in mice and dogs following daily oral or intravenous administration of doses ranging from 0.2 to 10 mg/kg. Inhibition of spermatogenesis and subsequent infertility was reversible at lower doses and irreversible at higher doses in animals. Systemic drug exposure (as measured by AUC) at the lowest dose showing toxicity in each species ranged from 0.03 to 0.1 times the AUC of the recommended human intravenous dose.
Pregnancy—Adequate and well-controlled studies in humans have not been done. However, ganciclovir has been found to cross the placenta. Due to the high toxicity and mutagenic and teratogenic potential of ganciclovir, use during pregnancy should be avoided whenever possible. Women of childbearing age should use effective contraception. Men should use barrier contraception during, and for at least 90 days following, treatment with ganciclovir.
Ganciclovir was found to be carcinogenic in animals and teratogenic in rabbits, causing cleft palate, anophthalmia/microphthalmia, aplastic organs (kidneys and pancreas), hydrocephaly, bradygnathia, and fetal growth retardation. It also was found to be embryotoxic in mice, and to cause death in utero and maternal toxicity in both rabbits and mice. Fetal resorptions occurred in at least 85% of rabbits and mice administered 60 mg/kg per day and 108 mg/kg per day (2 times the human exposure based on AUC comparisons), respectively. Daily intravenous doses of 90 mg/kg administered to female mice prior to mating, during gestation, and during lactation caused hypoplasia of the testes and seminal vesicles in the month-old male offspring, as well as pathologic changes in the nonglandular region of the stomach. The drug exposure in mice as estimated by the AUC was approximately 1.7 times the human AUC.
FDA Pregnancy Category C.

**Breast-feeding**
It is not known whether ganciclovir is distributed into breast milk; however, it is likely that some drug will accumulate because of its pharmacokinetic properties. Because of the potential for serious adverse effects in nursing infants, breast-feeding should be stopped during ganciclovir therapy. Ganciclovir has caused irreversible toxicity in nursing animal pups.

**Pediatrics**
There is little information currently available on the use of ganciclovir in children, especially those up to the age of 12. At this time, the side effects seen in children appear to be similar to those seen in adults, especially granulocytopenia (17%) and thrombocytopenia (10%). However, the probability of long-term carcinogenicity and reproductive toxicity seen in animal studies should also be considered.

**Geriatrics**
No information is available on the relationship of age to the effects of ganciclovir in geriatric patients. However, elderly patients are more likely to have an age-related decrease in renal function, which may require an adjustment of dosage or dosing interval in patients receiving ganciclovir.

**Dental**
The neutropenic and thrombocytopenic effects of ganciclovir may result in an increased incidence of microbial infection, delayed healing, and gingival bleeding. Patients should be instructed in proper oral hygiene, including caution in use of regular toothbrushes, dental floss, and toothpicks.

**Drug interactions and/or related problems**
The following drug interactions and/or related problems have been selected on the basis of their potential clinical significance (possible mechanism in parentheses where appropriate)—not necessarily inclusive (» = major clinical significance):

Note: Combinations containing any of the following medications, depending on the amount present, may also interact with this medication.

Blood dyscrasia–causing medications (See *Appendix II*) or
» Bone marrow depressants, other (See *Appendix II*) or
Radiation therapy
  (concurrent use with ganciclovir may increase the bone marrow–depressant effects of these medications and radiation therapy)

Didanosine
  (concurrent and sequential [2 hours apart] administration of didanosine with ganciclovir results in a significant increase in the steady-state area under the concentration-time curve [AUC] of didanosine [range, 72 to 111%]; when didanosine was administered 2 hours before oral ganciclovir, the steady-state AUC of ganciclovir was decreased by approximately 21%; there was no significant change in renal clearance of either medication)

Imipenem and cilastatin combination
  (generalized seizures have been reported in patients receiving ganciclovir and imipenem and cilastatin combination concurrently)

» Nephrotoxic medications (See *Appendix II*)
  (concurrent use with ganciclovir may increase serum creatinine; concurrent use with nephrotoxic medications, such as cyclosporine or amphotericin B, may increase the chance of renal function impairment; this may also decrease elimination of ganciclovir and increase the risk of toxicity)

Probenecid
  (concurrent use with probenecid increases the AUC of ganciclovir by approximately 53% and decreases its renal clearance by approximately 22%; concurrent use of ganciclovir with probenecid, or other medications that inhibit renal tubular secretion, may reduce the renal clearance of ganciclovir and lead to toxicity)

» Zidovudine
  (concurrent use of ganciclovir with zidovudine has been associated with severe hematologic toxicity in some patients, even when the zidovudine dose was reduced to 300 mg per day; concurrent use increases the AUC of zidovudine by approximately 14 to 19%; *in vitro* studies found concurrent use of these 2 drugs to be synergistically cytotoxic; concurrent administration should be used with caution)

### Laboratory value alterations
The following have been selected on the basis of their potential clinical significance (possible effect in parentheses where appropriate)—not necessarily inclusive (» = major clinical significance):

With physiology/laboratory test values
Alanine aminotransferase (ALT [SGPT]), serum and
Alkaline phosphatase, serum and
Aspartate aminotransferase (AST [SGOT]), serum and
Bilirubin, serum
(values may be increased)
Blood urea nitrogen (BUN) or
Creatinine, serum
(values may be increased)

### Medical considerations/Contraindications
The medical considerations/contraindications included have been selected on the basis of their potential clinical significance (reasons given in parentheses where appropriate)—not necessarily inclusive (» = major clinical significance).

***Risk-benefit should be considered when the following medical problems exist:***

» Absolute neutrophil count (ANC) <500 cells/mm³ or platelet count <25,000 cells/mm³

» Hypersensitivity to acyclovir or ganciclovir

» Renal function impairment
(because ganciclovir is excreted through the kidneys, the dose of ganciclovir should be reduced or the dosing interval increased in patients with renal function impairment)

### Patient monitoring
The following may be especially important in patient monitoring (other tests may be warranted in some patients, depending on condition; » = major clinical significance):

» Complete blood counts (CBCs) and
» Platelet counts
(because ganciclovir may cause granulocytopenia and thrombocytopenia, neutrophil and platelet counts should be monitored prior to treatment, every 2 days during induction therapy, then at least weekly thereafter. Neutrophil and platelet counts should be performed daily in patients undergoing hemodialysis, patients with neutrophil counts less than 1000 cells/mm³ at the beginning of treatment, and those in whom use of ganciclovir or other nucleoside analogs previously resulted in leukopenia. When severe neutropenia [absolute neutrophil count < 500 cells/mm³] or severe thrombocytopenia [platelet count < 25,000 cells/mm³] occurs, discontinuation of ganciclovir may be necessary; however, a small number of patients have been successfully treated with concurrent use of sargramostim [GM-CSF; granulocyte-macrophage colony stimulating factor] or filgrastin [G-CSF; granulocyte colony stimulating factor])

Liver function tests
(liver function tests, including serum ALT [SGPT] and AST [SGOT] values, and serum bilirubin concentration, should be monitored periodically since elevations, usually reversible, have occurred during ganciclovir therapy)

» Renal function determinations
(blood urea nitrogen and serum creatinine determinations should be monitored at least every 2 weeks since patients with renal function impairment will require an adjustment in dosage or dosage interval)

*For treatment of cytomegalovirus [CMV] retinitis, in addition to the above*
» Ophthalmologic examinations
(ophthalmologic examinations should be performed weekly during induction and every 4 weeks during maintenance since ganciclovir is not a cure for cytomegalovirus [CMV] retinitis, and progression of retinitis may occur during or following ganciclovir treatment; however, the frequency of examinations may vary, depending on the extent of disease, activity, and proximity to the macula and optic disc)

## Side/Adverse Effects
The following side/adverse effects have been selected on the basis of their potential clinical significance (possible signs and symptoms in parentheses where appropriate)—not necessarily inclusive:

### Those indicating need for medical attention
Incidence more frequent
*For intravenous and oral administration*
**Granulocytopenia** (sore throat and fever); ***thrombocytopenia*** (unusual bleeding or bruising)

Note: *Granulocytopenia* is usually reversible, with an overall incidence of approximately 40%; the incidence of dose-limiting toxicity is <20%.
*Thrombocytopenia* is also usually reversible, with an overall incidence of approximately 20%; the incidence of dose-limiting toxicity is 5 to 10%.

Incidence less frequent
*For intravenous and oral administration*
**Anemia** (unusual tiredness and weakness); **central nervous system (CNS) effects** (mood or other mental changes; nervousness; tremor); **hypersensitivity** (fever; skin rash); **phlebitis** (pain at site of injection)

*For intravitreal administration*
**Bacterial endophthalmitis; conjunctival scarring, mild; foreign body sensation; retinal detachment; scleral induration; or subconjunctival hemorrhage** (decreased vision or any change in vision)

### Those indicating need for medical attention only if they continue or are bothersome
Incidence less frequent
**Gastrointestinal disturbances** (abdominal pain; loss of appetite; nausea and vomiting)

## Patient Consultation
As an aid to patient consultation, refer to *Advice for the Patient, Ganciclovir (Systemic)*.

In providing consultation, consider emphasizing the following selected information (» = major clinical significance):

### Before using this medication
» Conditions affecting use, especially:
Hypersensitivity to acyclovir or ganciclovir
Pregnancy—Use of ganciclovir during pregnancy should be avoided whenever possible. Ganciclovir crosses the placenta and has been found to be carcinogenic and teratogenic in animals. Use of effective contraception by men and women who are undergoing treatment and in men for 90 days following treatment is recommended
Breast-feeding—Because of ganciclovir's potential for severe toxicity, breast-feeding should be stopped during therapy
Use in children—There is little information currently available on the use of ganciclovir in children, especially those up to the age of 12; long-term carcinogenicity and reproductive toxicity due to ganciclovir use in children is unknown
Dental—The neutropenic and thrombocytopenic effects of ganciclovir may result in an increased incidence of microbial infection, delayed healing, and gingival bleeding
Other medications, especially other bone marrow depressants, nephrotoxic medications, or zidovudine
Other medical problems, especially renal function impairment, an absolute neutrophil count (ANC) <500 cells/mm³, or platelet count <25,000 cells/mm³

### Proper use of this medication
» Taking ganciclovir capsules with food
» Importance of receiving medication for full course of therapy and on a regular schedule
» Proper dosing

### Precautions while using this medication
*To reduce the risk of bleeding during periods of low blood counts:*
» Checking with physician immediately if getting an infection or fever or chills
» Checking with physician immediately if unusual bleeding or bruising; black, tarry stools; blood in urine or stools; or pinpoint red spots on skin occur
Using caution in use of regular toothbrushes, dental floss, and toothpicks; physician, dentist, or nurse may suggest alternative methods for cleaning teeth and gums; checking with physician before having dental work done
Using caution to avoid accidental cuts with use of sharp objects such as a safety razor or fingernail or toenail cutters
» Using contraception since ganciclovir has mutagenic and teratogenic potential; women should use effective contraception during treatment, and men should use barrier contraception during and for at least 90 days following treatment
» Regular visits to physician to check blood counts
» *For CMV retinitis*—Regular visits to ophthalmologist to examine eyes since progression of retinitis and visual loss may occur during ganciclovir therapy

### Side/adverse effects
Signs of potential side effects, especially granulocytopenia, thrombocytopenia, anemia, CNS effects, hypersensitivity, and phlebitis when ganciclovir is administered intravenously or orally; and bacterial endophthalmitis, mild conjunctival scarring, foreign body sensation, retinal detachment, scleral induration, and subconjunctival hemorrhage when it is administered intravitreally

## General Dosing Information
Ganciclovir is not a cure for cytomegalovirus infections. Maintenance therapy is almost always necessary in AIDS patients to prevent relapse, which is very common once the medication has been withdrawn.

Monitoring of serum ganciclovir concentrations has not been shown to be useful for ensuring efficacy or avoiding toxicity.

Ganciclovir sodium should be administered by intravenous infusion only. Intramuscular or subcutaneous injection will result in severe tissue irritation due to ganciclovir's high pH (11).

Intravenous infusions of ganciclovir should be administered at a constant rate *over at least a 1-hour period*, and patients must be adequately hydrated, to avoid increased toxicity. The recommended dosage, frequency, and infusion rate should not be exceeded.

Severe neutropenia or thrombocytopenia (absolute neutrophil count [ANC] <500 cells/mm$^3$ or platelet count <25,000 cells/mm$^3$) requires an interruption in therapy until there is evidence of bone marrow recovery (ANC ≥750 cells/mm$^3$); however, a small number of patients have been successfully treated with concurrent use of sargramostim (GM-CSF; granulocyte-macrophage colony stimulating factor).

Ganciclovir capsules should be taken with food for maximum absorption.

The dose of ganciclovir must be decreased in patients with renal function impairment.

Patients undergoing hemodialysis should not receive a dose in excess of 1.25 mg per kg of body weight (mg/kg) every 24 hours. On dialysis days, the dose of ganciclovir should be administered after hemodialysis has been performed since dialysis will reduce plasma ganciclovir concentrations by approximately 50%.

Ganciclovir capsules are indicated as an alternative to intravenous ganciclovir for maintenance therapy of CMV retinitis in immunocompromised patients, including those with AIDS. Oral ganciclovir should be used in patients in whom retinitis is stable and quiescent following appropriate induction therapy and for whom the risk of more rapid progression is balanced by the benefit associated with avoiding long-term daily intravenous infusions, usually requiring indwelling intravenous catheters.

Intravitreal administration of ganciclovir has been used in patients who have been unresponsive to intravenous ganciclovir, or in whom serious myelosuppression has precluded the continuation of intravenous therapy. Intravitreal doses of 200 micrograms have resulted in improvement or stabilization of retinitis, and have been well tolerated. In one report describing a patient who received 28 intravitreal injections, plasma concentrations after intravitreal injections showed no significant systemic absorption. The elimination half-life of ganciclovir from the vitreous fluid was estimated to be 13.3 hours, and the intravitreal concentration remained above the ID$_{50}$ of cytomegalovirus for approximately 62 hours after a single injection.

### Safety considerations for handling this medication
Caution should be exercised in the handling and preparation of ganciclovir. Because ganciclovir shares some properties of anti-tumor agents (i.e., carcinogenicity and mutagenicity), it should be handled and disposed of according to guidelines issued for cytotoxic drugs. Ganciclovir solution is alkaline (pH 11). Avoid inhalation, ingestion, or direct contact of ganciclovir with the skin or mucous membranes. If contact does occur, wash area thoroughly with soap and water; rinse eyes thoroughly with plain water. Ganciclovir capsules should not be opened or crushed.

## Oral Dosage Forms
### GANCICLOVIR CAPSULES
#### Usual adult and adolescent dose
Cytomegalovirus retinitis—
   Induction: Ganciclovir capsules should not be used for induction therapy. See *Sterile Ganciclovir Sodium*
   Maintenance: Oral, 1000 mg three times a day with food, or 500 mg six times a day every three hours with food, during waking hours.
   Note: For maintenance, patients with impaired renal function may require a reduction in dose as follows:

| Creatinine Clearance (mL/min)/(mL/sec) | Dose |
|---|---|
| ≥70/1.17 | See *Usual adult and adolescent dose* |
| 50–69/0.83–1.15 | 1500 mg once a day, or 500 mg three times a day |
| 25–49/0.42–0.82 | 1000 mg once a day, or 500 mg twice a day |
| 10–24/0.17–0.40 | 500 mg once a day |
| <10/0.17 | 500 mg three times a week, following hemodialysis |

#### Usual pediatric dose
Dosage has not been established.

#### Strength(s) usually available
U.S.—
   250 mg (Rx) [*Cytovene*].
Canada—
   Not commercially available.

#### Packaging and storage
Store below 40 °C (104 °F), preferably between 15 and 30 °C (59 and 86 °F), unless otherwise specified by manufacturer.

#### Auxiliary labeling
- Continue medicine for full time of treatment.

#### Note
Ganciclovir capsules should not be opened or crushed.

## Parenteral Dosage Forms
### STERILE GANCICLOVIR SODIUM
#### Usual adult and adolescent dose
Cytomegalovirus retinitis (treatment)—
   Induction—
      Intravenous infusion, 5 mg per kg of body weight, administered over at least one hour, every twelve hours for fourteen to twenty-one days.
   Note: Doses of 7.5 to 15 mg per kg of body weight per day divided into two or three doses have been used, and treatment has been continued for longer than twenty-one days; if retinitis does not show significant improvement, the possibility of viral resistance should be considered.
   Intravitreal injection, 200 mcg two times a week for three weeks.
   Note: For induction, patients with impaired renal function may require a reduction in dose as follows:

| Creatinine Clearance (mL/min)/(mL/sec) | Dose |
|---|---|
| ≥70/1.17 | See *Usual adult and adolescent dose* |
| 50–69/0.83–1.15 | 2.5 mg per kg every twelve hours |
| 25–49/0.42–0.82 | 2.5 mg per kg every twenty-four hours |
| 10–24/0.17–0.40 | 1.25 mg per kg every twenty-four hours |
| <10 | 1.25 mg per kg three times a week, following hemodialysis |

Maintenance—
   Intravenous infusion, 5 mg per kg of body weight a day, administered over at least one hour, once a day for seven days per week; or 6 mg per kg of body weight, administered over at least one hour, once a day for five days of the week.
   Note: If CMV retinitis progresses during maintenance therapy, patients should be retreated with the twice-a-day induction regimen.
   Intravitreal injection, 200 mcg once a week.
   Note: For maintenance, patients with impaired renal function may require a reduction in dose as follows:

| Creatinine Clearance (mL/min)/(mL/sec) | Dose |
|---|---|
| ≥70/1.17 | See *Usual adult and adolescent dose* |
| 50–69/0.83–1.15 | 2.5 mg per kg every twelve hours |
| 25–49/0.42–0.82 | 1.25 mg per kg every twenty-four hours |

## Ganciclovir (Systemic)

| Creatinine Clearance (mL/min)/(mL/sec) | Dose |
|---|---|
| ≥70/1.17 | See *Usual adult and adolescent dose* |
| 10–24/0.17–0.40 | 0.625 mg per kg every twenty-four hours |
| <10 | 0.625 mg per kg three times a week, following hemodialysis |

Cytomegalovirus disease (prophylaxis)—
  Intravenous infusion, 5 mg per kg of body weight, administered over at least one hour, every twelve hours for seven to fourteen days; then 5 mg per kg of body weight, administered over at least one hour, once a day for seven days of the week, or 6 mg per kg of body weight, administered over at least one hour, once a day for five days of the week.

**Usual pediatric dose**
Dosage has not been established. However, induction doses of 7.5 to 10 mg per kg of body weight divided into two or three doses, and maintenance doses of 2.5 to 5 mg per kg of body weight a day have been used in children.

**Strength(s) usually available**
U.S.—
  500 mg (Rx) [*Cytovene-IV* (sodium 46 mg)].
Canada—
  500 mg (Rx) [*Cytovene*].

**Packaging and storage**
Store below 40 °C (104 °F), preferably between 15 and 30 °C (59 and 86 °F), unless otherwise specified by manufacturer.

**Preparation of dosage form**
To prepare initial dilution for intravenous infusion, 10 mL of sterile water for injection (without parabens) should be added to each 500-mg vial to provide 50 mg per mL. To ensure complete dissolution, the vial should be shaken until solution is clear. The resulting solution should be further diluted, usually with 100 mL of 0.9% sodium chloride injection, 5% dextrose injection, Ringer's injection, or lactated Ringer's injection. Final concentrations of 10 mg per mL or less are recommended.

Note:  Caution should be exercised in the handling and preparation of ganciclovir. Because ganciclovir shares some properties of anti-tumor agents (i.e., carcinogenicity and mutagenicity), it should be handled and disposed of according to guidelines issued for cytotoxic drugs. Ganciclovir solution is alkaline (pH 11). Avoid inhalation, ingestion, or direct contact of ganciclovir with the skin or mucous membranes. If contact does occur, wash area thoroughly with soap and water; rinse eyes thoroughly with plain water.

**Stability**
The manufacturer states that after reconstitution, solutions at concentrations of 50 mg per mL retain their potency for 12 hours at room temperature. Refrigeration is not recommended. After further dilution for intravenous infusion, it is recommended that solutions be used within 24 hours since nonbacteriostatic infusion solutions must be used; refrigerate the diluted solution; do not freeze.
However, studies have found that ganciclovir, when diluted to concentrations of 1, 5, and 10 mg per mL in 5% dextrose injection and 0.9% sodium chloride injection, was stable when assayed at 28 and 35 days. These solutions were refrigerated in polyvinyl chloride (PVC) bags and syringes. Ganciclovir was also stable when 5 and 10 mg per mL solutions were frozen in PVC bags for 28 days.

**Incompatibilities**
Parabens are incompatible with ganciclovir sodium and may cause precipitation.

## Selected Bibliography
Markham A, Faulds D. Ganciclovir. An update of its therapeutic use in cytomegalovirus infections. Drugs 1994; 48(3): 455-84.

Revised: 08/08/95

---

# GEMCITABINE  Systemic

VA CLASSIFICATION (Primary): AN300
Commonly used brand name(s): *Gemzar*.
Note:  For a listing of dosage forms and brand names by country availability, see *Dosage Forms* section(s).

## Category
Antineoplastic.

## Indications
Note:  Bracketed information in the *Indications* section refers to uses that are not included in U.S. product labeling.

**Accepted**
Carcinoma, pancreatic (treatment)—Gemcitabine is indicated as first-line therapy for locally advanced (nonresectable Stage II or III) or metastatic (Stage IV) adenocarcinoma of the pancreas. It is also indicated as second-line therapy for patients who have previously been treated with fluorouracil. Treatment with gemcitabine is primarily palliative.

[Carcinoma, lung, non−small cell (treatment)]—Gemcitabine is indicated for palliative treatment of locally advanced or metastatic non−small cell lung carcinoma.

[Carcinoma, bladder][1]—Gemcitabine is indicated for treatment of metastatic bladder (urothelial) carcinoma, based on response rates (both complete and partial responses) achieved in clinical trials.

---
[1] Not included in Canadian product labeling.

## Pharmacology/Pharmacokinetics

**Physicochemical characteristics**
Chemical group—Gemcitabine is a nucleoside(deoxycytidine) analog.
Molecular weight—Gemcitabine hydrochloride: 299.66.
pH—2.7 to 3.3 (after reconstitution).
pKa—3.6.
Solubility—Practically insoluble in ethanol and polar organic solvents; soluble in water.

**Mechanism of action/Effect**
Gemcitabine is an antimetabolite of the pyrimidine analog type. Gemcitabine is cell cycle−specific for the S phase and for the $G_1$/S phase boundary of cell division. Activity occurs as a result of intracellular conversion to two active metabolites, gemcitabine diphosphate and gemcitabine triphosphate. Gemcitabine diphosphate inhibits the enzyme responsible for catalyzing synthesis of deoxynucleoside triphosphates required for DNA synthesis, and gemcitabine triphosphate competes with endogenous deoxynucleoside triphosphates for incorporation into DNA. The gemcitabine diphosphate−induced reduction in intracellular concentrations of deoxynucleoside triphosphates results in increased incorporation of gemcitabine triphosphate into DNA and, consequently, in inhibition of DNA synthesis. DNA polymerase epsilon is unable to remove the incorporated gemcitabine triphosphate and repair the DNA strands.

**Other actions/effects**
Gemcitabine is a potent radiation sensitizer. In *in vitro* studies, it produced significant radiosensitization even in lower-than-cytotoxic concentrations.

**Distribution**
The volume of distribution is significantly affected by the duration of the gemcitabine infusion and the gender of the patient.
  Short infusion (< 70 minutes)—50 liters per square meter of body surface area ($L/m^2$), indicating that gemcitabine is not distributed extensively into tissues.
  Long infusion (70 to 285 minutes)—370 $L/m^2$, indicating slow equilibration within the tissue compartment.

**Protein binding**
Very low (< 10%).

**Biotransformation**
Gemcitabine undergoes intracellular metabolism, via nucleoside kinases, to produce two active metabolites (gemcitabine diphosphate and gemcitabine triphosphate) and also undergoes deamination to an inactive uracil metabolite.

### Half-life
Gemcitabine—Elimination:
Short infusions (< 70 minutes)—
Females:
29 years of age—49 minutes.
45 years of age—57 minutes.
65 years of age—73 minutes.
79 years of age—94 minutes.
Males:
29 years of age—42 minutes.
45 years of age—48 minutes.
65 years of age—61 minutes.
79 years of age—79 minutes.
Long infusions (70 to 285 minutes)—245 to 638 minutes, depending on age and gender.
Gemcitabine triphosphate metabolite—Terminal (from peripheral blood mononuclear cells): 1.7 to 19.4 hours.

### Elimination
Renal—92 to 98% of a single dose of radiolabeled gemcitabine (1000 mg per square meter of body surface area, given over 30 minutes to five patients) was recovered within 1 week, primarily as the inactive uracil metabolite (approximately 89% of the excreted dose) and secondarily as unchanged gemcitabine (less than 10% of the excreted dose).
Clearance is affected by age and gender as follows:
Females—
29 years of age: 69.4 liters per hour per square meter of body surface area (L/hr/m$^2$).
45 years of age: 57 L/hr/m$^2$.
65 years of age: 41.5 L/hr/m$^2$.
79 years of age: 30.7 L/hr/m$^2$.
Males—
29 years of age: 92.2 L/hr/m$^2$.
45 years of age: 75.7 L/hr/m$^2$.
65 years of age: 55.1 L/hr/m$^2$.
79 years of age: 40.7 L/hr/m$^2$.

## Precautions to Consider

### Carcinogenicity
Secondary malignancies are potential delayed effects of many antineoplastic agents, although it is not clear whether the effect is related to their mutagenic or immunosuppressive action. The effect of dose and duration of therapy is also unknown, although risk seems to increase with long-term use. The risk of secondary malignancies developing after gemcitabine therapy is not known.
Long-term animal studies to evaluate the carcinogenic potential of gemcitabine have not been done.

### Mutagenicity
Gemcitabine was mutagenic in *in vitro* (mouse lymphoma assay) and *in vivo* (mouse micronucleus assay) mammalian test systems. However, it was not mutagenic in the Ames test, *in vivo* sister chromatid exchange, or in *in vitro* (chromosomal aberration assays and unscheduled DNA synthesis) test systems.

### Pregnancy/Reproduction
Fertility—Intraperitoneal administration to male mice of 0.5 mg per kg of body weight (mg/kg) per day (0.14% of the recommended human dose on a mg per square meter of body surface area [mg/m$^2$] basis) resulted in moderate to severe hypospermatogenesis, decreased fertility, and decreased implantations. The hypospermatogenesis was reversible. Gemcitabine did not impair fertility, but caused maternal toxicity in female mice given doses of 1.5 mg/kg per day (0.5% of the recommended human dose on a mg/m$^2$ basis).
Pregnancy—Studies in humans have not been done.
It is usually recommended that use of antineoplastics, especially combination chemotherapy, be avoided whenever possible, especially during the first trimester. Although information is limited because of the relatively few instances of antineoplastic administration during pregnancy, the mutagenic, teratogenic, and carcinogenic potential of these medications must be considered.
Other potential hazards to the fetus include adverse reactions seen in adults. In general, use of a contraceptive is recommended during therapy with cytotoxic medications.
Gemcitabine caused fetal malformations (fusion of the pulmonary artery and absence of the gall bladder) in rabbits given 0.1 mg/kg per day (0.17% of the recommended human dose on a mg/m$^2$ basis). The medication was embryotoxic (causing decreased fetal viability, reduced live litter sizes, and delayed development), and teratogenic (causing cleft palate and incomplete ossification) in mice given 1.5 mg/kg per day (0.5% of the recommended human dose on a mg/m$^2$ basis). In mice, embryolethality or fetotoxicity occurred with intravenous doses as low as 0.25 mg/kg per day (0.08% of the recommended human dose on a mg/m$^2$ basis).
FDA Pregnancy Category D.

### Breast-feeding
Although very little information is available regarding distribution of antineoplastic agents into breast milk, breast-feeding is not recommended while gemcitabine is being administered, because of the risks to the infant (adverse effects, mutagenicity, carcinogenicity). It is not known whether gemcitabine or its metabolites are distributed into breast milk.

### Pediatrics
Appropriate studies on the relationship of age to the effects of gemcitabine have not been performed in the pediatric population. Safety and efficacy have not been established.

### Geriatrics
Appropriate studies performed to date have not demonstrated geriatrics-specific problems that would limit the usefulness of gemcitabine in the elderly. Although some pharmacokinetic parameters are altered in geriatric patients (increased elimination half-life and decreased clearance), no adjustment of the initial dose is recommended for patients older than 65 years of age. However, the risk of hematologic toxicity requiring reduction, delay, or omission of subsequent doses is higher in geriatric patients than in younger adults. Specifically, Grade 3 or 4 thrombocytopenia is more likely to occur in geriatric men and women and Grade 3 or 4 neutropenia is more likely to occur in geriatric women. Nonhematologic toxicities did not occur more frequently in patients older than 65 years of age than in younger adults.

### Dental
The bone marrow depressant effects of gemcitabine may result in an increased incidence of microbial infection, delayed healing, and gingival bleeding. Dental work, whenever possible, should be completed prior to initiation of therapy or deferred until blood counts have returned to normal. Patients should be instructed in proper oral hygiene during treatment, including caution in use of regular toothbrushes, dental floss, and toothpicks.
Gemcitabine causes stomatitis, usually mild, in a minority of patients (incidence 11% or lower in various clinical trials).

### Drug interactions and/or related problems
The following drug interactions and/or related problems have been selected on the basis of their potential clinical significance (possible mechanism in parentheses where appropriate)—not necessarily inclusive (» = major clinical significance):

Blood dyscrasia–causing medications (see *Appendix II*)
(leukopenic and/or thrombocytopenic effects of gemcitabine may be increased with concurrent or recent therapy if these medications cause the same effects; dosage adjustment of gemcitabine, if necessary, should be based on blood counts)

» Bone marrow depressants, other (see *Appendix II*) or
» Radiation therapy
(additive bone marrow depression may occur; dosage reduction may be required when two or more bone marrow depressants, including radiation, are used concurrently or consecutively)

(gemcitabine is a potent radiosensitizer; depending on the site being irradiated, concurrent use of gemcitabine may cause severe, life-threatening esophagitis or pneumonitis; in one study, gemcitabine with radiation therapy caused severe stomatitis or pharyngeal damage requiring patients to be fed via feeding tube for as long as 10 to 12 months, even when gemcitabine was given in doses as low as 300 mg per square meter of body surface area [25% or less of the usual adult dose])

» Immunosuppressants, other, such as:
Azathioprine
Chlorambucil
Corticosteroids, glucocorticoid
Cyclophosphamide
Cyclosporine
Mercaptopurine
Muromonab CD-3
Tacrolimus
(concurrent use with gemcitabine may increase the risk of infection)

Vaccines, killed virus
(because normal defense mechanisms may be suppressed by gemcitabine therapy, the patient's antibody response to the vaccine may be decreased. The interval between discontinuation of medications that cause immunosuppression and restoration of the patient's ability to respond to the vaccine depends on the intensity and type of immunosuppression-causing medication used, the underlying disease, and other factors; estimates vary from 3 months to 1 year)

» Vaccines, live virus
(because normal defense mechanisms may be suppressed by gemcitabine therapy, concurrent use with a live virus vaccine may potentiate the replication of the vaccine virus, may increase the side/adverse effects of the vaccine virus, and/or may decrease the patient's antibody response to the vaccine; immunization of these patients should be undertaken only with extreme caution, after careful review of the patient's hematologic status, and only with the knowledge and consent of the physician managing the gemcitabine therapy. The interval between discontinuation of medications that cause immunosuppression and restoration of the patient's ability to respond to the vaccine depends on the intensity and type of immunosuppression-causing medication used, the underlying disease, and other factors; estimates vary from 3 months to 1 year. In addition, immunization with oral poliovirus vaccine should be postponed in persons in close contact with the patient, especially family members)

**Laboratory value alterations**
The following have been selected on the basis of their potential clinical significance (possible effect in parentheses where appropriate)—not necessarily inclusive (» = major clinical significance):

With physiology/laboratory test values
  Alanine aminotransferase (ALT [SGPT]) and
  Alkaline phosphatase and
  Aspartate aminotransferase (AST [SGOT]) and
  Bilirubin concentrations, serum
    (values may be increased; in clinical trials, Grade 3 or 4 increases in ALT, alkaline phosphatase, AST, and bilirubin occurred in 10%, 9%, 8%, and 3% of all patients and in 11%, 20%, 17%, and 8% of pancreatic cancer patients, respectively. However, continuation of gemcitabine therapy despite these elevations produced no evidence of increasing hepatotoxicity)
  Blood urea nitrogen (BUN) and
  Creatinine, serum
    (concentrations may be increased)
» Hemoglobin/hematocrit and
» Leukocyte count and
» Platelet count
    (may be decreased)

**Medical considerations/Contraindications**
The medical considerations/contraindications included have been selected on the basis of their potential clinical significance (reasons given in parentheses where appropriate)—not necessarily inclusive (» = major clinical significance).

*Risk-benefit should be considered when the following medical problems exist:*
» Bone marrow depression
    (will be exacerbated; reduction, delay, or omission of a gemcitabine dose may be necessary)
» Chickenpox, existing or recent (including recent exposure) or
» Herpes zoster
    (risk of severe generalized disease)
  Hepatic function impairment, severe or
  Renal function impairment
    (caution is recommended; gemcitabine has not been studied in patients with these medical problems)
    (caution and careful monitoring of patients with renal function impairment are also recommended because hemolytic-uremic syndrome has been reported in a few patients during or immediately following gemcitabine therapy)
» Hypersensitivity to gemcitabine
» Infection
    (gemcitabine may decrease the patient's ability to fight an infection)
» Caution should be used also in patients who have had previous cytotoxic chemotherapy or radiation therapy

**Patient monitoring**
The following may be especially important in patient monitoring (other tests may be warranted in some patients, depending on condition; » = major clinical significance):

  Alanine aminotransferase (ALT [SGPT]) and
  Alkaline phosphatase and
  Aspartate aminotransferase (AST [SGOT]) and
  Bilirubin, serum and
  Blood urea nitrogen (BUN) and
  Creatinine concentrations, serum
    (determinations recommended prior to initiation of gemcitabine therapy and at appropriate intervals during therapy)

» Hemoglobin concentration and
» Leukocyte count, total and, if appropriate, differential and
» Platelet count
    (determinations recommended prior to each course of gemcitabine therapy; reduction, delay, or omission of a dose may be required, depending on cell counts)

## Side/Adverse Effects

Note: Many "side effects" of antineoplastic therapy are unavoidable and represent the medication's pharmacologic action. Some of these (for example, leukopenia and thrombocytopenia) are actually used as parameters to aid in individual dosage titration.

The following side/adverse effects have been selected on the basis of their potential clinical significance (possible signs and symptoms in parentheses where appropriate)—not necessarily inclusive:

**Those indicating need for medical attention**
Incidence more frequent
  *Anemia* (unusual tiredness or weakness); *dyspnea* (shortness of breath)—may be due to underlying disease; *edema* (swelling of fingers, feet, or lower legs); *fever*—may occur in the absence of infection, usually in conjunction with other flu-like symptoms; *hematuria* (blood in urine); *leukopenia or neutropenia*—usually asymptomatic; *proteinuria* (cloudy urine); *skin rash, with or without itching; thrombocytopenia* (unusual bleeding or bruising; black, tarry stools; blood in urine or stools; pinpoint red spots on skin)—usually asymptomatic; symptoms occur less frequently

Note: Bone marrow suppression (*anemia, leukopenia,* and *thrombocytopenia*) is the dose-limiting adverse effect.
  *Edema* is usually peripheral, but rarely may become generalized.
  Typically, gemcitabine-induced *skin rashes* are mild to moderate in severity and consist of macular or finely granular maculopapular eruptions on the trunk and extremities.

Incidence less frequent
  *Bronchospasm* (shortness of breath, troubled breathing, tightness in chest, and/or wheezing); *cardiovascular effects, including arrhythmia* (fast or irregular heartbeat); *cerebrovascular accident* (headache, sudden and severe; slurred speech or inability to speak; weakness in arm and/or leg on one side of the body, sudden and severe); *hypertension* (high blood pressure); *or myocardial infarction* (pain in chest, arm, or back; pressure or squeezing in chest); *febrile neutropenia or other infection* (fever or chills; cough or hoarseness; lower back or side pain; painful or difficult urination); *hemorrhage*

Note: In clinical trials, *cardiovascular effects* occurred mostly in patients with a prior history of cardiovascular disease, and *hemorrhage* occurred mostly in patients with pancreatic carcinoma.
  Severe infections associated with *leukopenia* or *neutropenia* occurred in approximately 1% of patients in clinical studies.

Incidence rare
  *Anaphylactoid reaction* (change in facial skin color; shortness of breath, troubled breathing, tightness in chest, and/or wheezing; skin rash, hives, and/or itching; swelling or puffiness of the face, especially the eyelids or area around the eyes); *heart failure* (coughing; noisy, rattling, or troubled breathing); *hemolytic-uremic syndrome* (black, tarry stools; blood in urine or stools; fever; increased or decreased urination; pinpoint red spots on skin; swelling of face, fingers, feet, or lower legs; unusual bleeding or bruising; unusual tiredness or weakness; yellow eyes or skin); *lung toxicity, parenchymal, or pneumonitis* (coughing; shortness of breath); *pulmonary edema* (coughing; noisy, rattling, or troubled breathing)

Note: In clinical trials, *hemolytic-uremic syndrome* occurred in 6 of 2429 patients. Four cases occurred during gemcitabine treatment and two shortly after treatment had ended. This complication may result in irreversible renal failure requiring dialysis.
  *Heart failure* and *pulmonary edema* have been reported in patients being treated for lung carcinoma.

**Those indicating need for medical attention only if they continue or are bothersome**
Incidence more frequent
  *Constipation; diarrhea; flu-like syndrome* (chills; cough; fever; general feeling of illness; headache; loss of appetite; muscle pain; runny nose; sweating; trouble in sleeping; weakness); *nausea and vomiting*

Note: Weakness, while often occurring as part of a *flu-like syndrome*, may also occur as an isolated symptom.
  *Nausea and vomiting* are usually mild to moderate in severity, but may be severe in up to 15% of patients.

Incidence less frequent
> ***Irritation, pain, or redness at injection site***—if extravasation occurs; ***paresthesia*** (numbness or tingling of hands or feet); ***somnolence*** (drowsiness, severe); ***stomatitis*** (sores, ulcers, or white spots on lips and in mouth)

> Note: Gemcitabine is not a vesicant. Extravasation has not caused injection site necrosis.
>> *Paresthesia* is usually mild; however, severe paresthesia may occur rarely.

**Those not indicating need for medical attention**
Incidence more frequent
> *Alopecia* (loss of hair)—usually minimal

> Note: Complete hair loss, which was reversible after discontinuation of treatment, occurred in less than 0.5% of patients in clinical trials.

## Overdose

For more information on the management of overdose, **contact a Poison Control Center** (see *Poison Control Center Listing*).

**Clinical effects of overdose**
The following effects have been selected on the basis of their potential clinical significance (possible signs and symptoms in parentheses where appropriate)—not necessarily inclusive:

Acute and chronic
> ***Bone marrow suppression, including anemia*** (unusual tiredness or weakness); ***leukopenia or neutropenia, possibly with infection*** (chills; cough or hoarseness; lower back or side pain; painful or difficult urination); ***and thrombocytopenia*** (unusual bleeding or bruising; black, tarry stools; blood in urine or stools; pinpoint red spots on skin); ***paresthesia*** (numbness or tingling of hands or feet); **skin rash, severe**

**Treatment of overdose**
There is no specific antidote to gemcitabine.

The patient's blood count should be monitored and supportive therapy given, as needed. Severe bone marrow depression may require transfusion of needed blood components. Patients who develop leukopenia should be observed carefully for signs of infection. Antibiotic support may be required. In neutropenic patients who develop fever, broad-spectrum antibiotic coverage should be initiated empirically, pending bacterial cultures and appropriate diagnostic tests.

## Patient Consultation

As an aid to patient consultation, refer to *Advice for the Patient, Gemcitabine (Systemic)*.

In providing consultation, consider emphasizing the following selected information (» = major clinical significance):

**Before using this medication**
» Conditions affecting use, especially:
  Hypersensitivity to gemcitabine
  Pregnancy—Use not recommended because of mutagenic, teratogenic, embryotoxic, and fetotoxic potential; advisability of using contraception; telling physician immediately if pregnancy is suspected
  Breast-feeding—Not recommended because of risk of serious adverse effects
  Use in the elderly—Seriously low blood counts are more likely to occur in older patients
  Other medications, especially other bone marrow depressants, other immunosuppressants, or other cytotoxic medication or radiation therapy
  Other medical problems, especially chickenpox or recent exposure, herpes zoster, infection, or previous cytotoxic medication or radiation therapy

**Proper use of this medication**
Frequency of flu-like syndrome or nausea and vomiting; importance of continuing medication despite stomach upset or otherwise feeling ill
» Proper dosing

**Precautions while using this medication**
» Importance of close monitoring by the physician; periodic blood tests required to monitor blood counts
» Avoiding immunizations unless approved by physician; other persons in patient's household should avoid immunizations with oral poliovirus vaccine; avoiding persons who have taken oral poliovirus vaccine or wearing a protective mask that covers nose and mouth
» Checking with physician immediately if dyspnea develops or worsens during treatment

*Caution if bone marrow depression occurs*
» Avoiding exposure to persons with bacterial infections, especially during periods of low blood counts; checking with physician immediately if fever or chills, cough or hoarseness, lower back or side pain, or painful or difficult urination occur
» Checking with physician immediately if unusual bleeding or bruising; black, tarry stools; blood in urine or stools; or pinpoint red spots on skin occur
  Caution in use of regular toothbrush, dental floss, or toothpick; physician, dentist, or nurse may suggest alternatives; checking with physician before having dental work done
  Not touching eyes or inside of nose unless hands are washed immediately before
  Using caution to avoid accidental cuts with use of sharp objects such as safety razor or fingernail or toenail cutters
  Avoiding contact sports or other situations where bruising or injury could occur

**Side/adverse effects**
May cause adverse effects such as blood problems; importance of discussing possible effects with physician
Signs of potential side effects, especially anemia; dyspnea; edema; fever; hematuria; proteinuria; skin rash; thrombocytopenia; bronchospasm; cardiovascular effects; febrile neutropenia or other infection; hemorrhage; anaphylactoid reaction; hemolytic-uremic syndrome; and lung toxicity or pneumonitis
Physician or nurse can help in dealing with side effects
Possibility that some adverse effects may occur after treatment has ended; notifying physician if symptoms of serious adverse effects noted
Possibility of hair loss; normal hair growth should return after treatment has ended

## General Dosing Information

Patients receiving gemcitabine should be under the supervision of a physician experienced in cancer chemotherapy.

Gemcitabine is to be administered only by intravenous infusion.

Adverse effects associated with gemcitabine therapy may occur more frequently and be more severe if gemcitabine is administered more frequently than once weekly or infused over a time period longer than 60 minutes.

If gemcitabine-induced pneumonitis is confirmed or suspected, treatment should be discontinued permanently.

Special precautions are recommended in patients who develop thrombocytopenia as a result of administration of gemcitabine. These may include extreme care in performing invasive procedures; regular inspection of intravenous sites, skin (including perirectal area), and mucous membrane surfaces for signs of bleeding or bruising; limiting frequency of venipuncture and avoiding intramuscular injections; testing urine, emesis, stool, and secretions for occult blood; care in use of regular toothbrushes, dental floss, toothpicks, safety razors, and fingernail and toenail cutters; avoiding constipation; and using caution to prevent falls and other injuries. Such patients should avoid alcohol and aspirin intake because of the risk of gastrointestinal bleeding. Platelet transfusions may be required.

Patients who develop leukopenia should be observed carefully for signs of infection. Antibiotic support may be required. In neutropenic patients who develop fever, broad-spectrum antibiotic coverage should be initiated empirically, pending bacterial cultures and appropriate diagnostic tests.

**Safety considerations for handling this medication**
There is limited but increasing evidence and concern that personnel involved in preparation and administration of parenteral antineoplastics may be at some risk because of the potential mutagenicity, teratogenicity, and/or carcinogenicity of these agents, although the actual risk is unknown. USP advisory panels recommend cautious handling both in preparation and disposal of antineoplastic agents. Precautions that have been suggested include:
• Use of a biological containment cabinet during reconstitution and dilution of parenteral medications and wearing of disposable surgical gloves and masks.
• Use of proper technique to prevent contamination of the medication, work area, and operator during transfer between containers (including proper training of personnel in this technique).
• Cautious and proper disposal of needles, syringes, vials, ampuls, and unused medication.

A number of medical centers have developed detailed guidelines for handling of antineoplastic agents.

# Gemcitabine (Systemic)

Direct contact of skin or mucosa with gemcitabine requires immediate washing with soap and water or thoroughly flushing with water, respectively.

## Parenteral Dosage Forms

Note: Bracketed uses in the *Dosage Forms* section refer to categories of use and/or indications that are not included in U.S. product labeling.

### GEMCITABINE FOR INJECTION

**Usual adult dose**
Pancreatic carcinoma—
  Intravenous infusion (over thirty minutes), 1000 mg per square meter of body surface area, once a week for up to seven weeks (depending on toxicity experienced by the patient), followed by a one-week rest. Each subsequent cycle of therapy consists of administering the medication once a week for three weeks followed by a one-week rest.

[Non–small cell lung carcinoma]—
  Intravenous infusion (over thirty minutes), 1000 mg per square meter of body surface area, once a week for three weeks, followed by a one-week rest.

[Bladder carcinoma][1]—
  Intravenous infusion (over thirty minutes), 1000 to 1200 mg per square meter of body surface area, once a week for three weeks, followed by a one-week rest.

Note: The development of neutropenia and thrombocytopenia may require an adjustment of gemcitabine dosage. If the absolute granulocyte and platelet counts measured prior to each dose are—
  500 to 999 × $10^6$ cells per liter and 50,000 to 99,000 × $10^6$ cells per liter, respectively: The dosage of gemcitabine should be decreased to 75% of the full dose. However, some oncologists recommend that, because treatment for pancreatic carcinoma and lung carcinoma is primarily palliative, gemcitabine should be withheld until cell counts recover, then resumed at the lower dose level.
  Less than 500 × $10^6$ cells per liter and 50,000 × $10^6$ cells per liter, respectively: Gemcitabine should be withheld until cell counts recover.

If one complete cycle of therapy (seven weeks or three weeks) at the recommended initial dose is well tolerated (i.e., the granulocyte count nadir remains higher than 1500 × $10^6$ cells per liter, the platelet count nadir exceeds 100,000 × $10^6$ cells per liter, and nonhematologic toxicities are no more severe than Grade 1), the dose of gemcitabine for the next cycle may be increased by 25% (e.g., from 1000 to 1250 mg per square meter of body surface area). If the medication remains well tolerated during a complete cycle at this higher dose (i.e., toxicities remain within the specified parameters), the dose may be increased a second time (e.g., from 1250 to 1500 mg per square meter of body surface area).

**Usual pediatric dose**
Safety and efficacy have not been established.

**Usual geriatric dose**
See *Usual adult dose*.

**Size(s) usually available**
U.S.—
  200 mg (single-dose vial) (Rx) [*Gemzar* (mannitol 200 mg; sodium acetate 12.5 mg)].
  1 gram (single-dose vial) (Rx) [*Gemzar* (mannitol 1 gram; sodium acetate 62.5 mg)].
Canada—
  200 mg (single-dose vial) (Rx) [*Gemzar* (mannitol 200 mg; sodium acetate 12.5 mg)].
  1 gram (single-dose vial) (Rx) [*Gemzar* (mannitol 1 gram; sodium acetate 62.5 mg)].

**Packaging and storage**
Store between 20 and 25 °C (68 and 77 °F), unless otherwise specified by manufacturer.

**Preparation of dosage form**
Gemcitabine for injection is reconstituted for intravenous use by adding 5 or 25 mL of 0.9% sodium chloride injection (without preservative) to the 200-mg or 1-gram vial, respectively, producing a clear, colorless to light straw-colored solution containing 38 mg of gemcitabine per mL. Incomplete dissolution may occur if gemcitabine is reconstituted to a concentration greater than 40 mg per mL. The resulting solution may be further diluted with 0.9% sodium chloride injection, if necessary, to a concentration as low as 0.1 mg per mL.

**Stability**
After reconstitution, gemcitabine injections are stable for 24 hours at controlled room temperature (20 to 25 °C [68 to 77 °F]).
Unused portions of gemcitabine injection should be discarded.
Reconstituted gemcitabine should not be refrigerated because of the possibility of crystal formation.

**Auxiliary labeling**
• Do not refrigerate.

### Selected Bibliography

Gatzemeier U, Shepherd FA, Le Chavalier T, et al. Activity of gemcitabine in patients with non-small cell lung cancer: a multicentre, extended phase II study. Eur J Cancer 1996; 32A: 243-8.

Abratt RP, Bezwada WR, Falkson G, et al. Efficacy and safety profile of gemcitabine in non–small-cell lung cancer: a phase II study. J Clin Oncol 1994; 12: 1535-40.

Developed: 08/21/97
Interim revision: 03/24/98

---

# GEMFIBROZIL Systemic

VA CLASSIFICATION (Primary): CV603

Commonly used brand name(s): *Apo-Gemfibrozil*; *Gen-Fibro*; *Lopid*; *Novo-Gemfibrozil*; *Nu-Gemfibrozil*.

Note: For a listing of dosage forms and brand names by country availability, see *Dosage Forms* section(s).

## Category

Antihyperlipidemic.

## Indications

**Accepted**

Hyperlipidemia (treatment)—Gemfibrozil is indicated in the treatment of hyperlipidemia and to reduce the risk of coronary heart disease *only* in those patients with type IIb hyperlipidemia without history of or symptoms of existing coronary heart disease, who have not responded to diet, exercise, weight loss, or other pharmacologic therapy (bile acid sequestrants and niacin) alone *and* who have the triad of low high density lipoprotein (HDL) cholesterol levels, elevated low density lipoprotein (LDL) cholesterol levels, and elevated triglycerides.

Gemfibrozil is also recommended for use in patients with severe primary hyperlipidemia (types IV and V hyperlipidemia) and a significant risk of coronary artery disease, abdominal pain typical of pancreatitis, or pancreatitis, who have not responded to diet or other measures alone. Its use is limited in type III hyperlipidemia because of its limited effect on cholesterol concentrations. It is not useful in the treatment of type I hyperlipidemia.

Gemfibrozil is not indicated for treatment of patients with type IIa hyperlipidemia or patients with low HDL cholesterol as their only lipid abnormality because the potential benefits do not outweigh the risks.

Caution and close observation are recommended in patients with high triglyceride concentrations, since in some of these patients treatment with gemfibrozil is associated with significant increases in low density lipoprotein (LDL)-cholesterol concentrations.

For additional information on initial therapeutic guidelines related to the treatment of hyperlipidemia, see *Appendix III*.

Gemfibrozil is not recommended for community-wide prevention of ischemic heart disease.

Studies have suggested that control of elevated cholesterol and triglycerides may not lessen the danger of cardiovascular disease and mortality, although incidence of nonfatal myocardial infarctions may be decreased.

## Pharmacology/Pharmacokinetics

**Physicochemical characteristics**
Molecular weight—250.34.

**Mechanism of action/Effect**
Gemfibrozil reduces plasma triglyceride (very low–density lipoprotein [VLDL]) concentrations and increases high-density lipoprotein (HDL)

concentrations. Although gemfibrozil may slightly reduce total and low-density lipoprotein (LDL) cholesterol concentrations, use of gemfibrozil in patients with elevated triglycerides associated with type IV hyperlipidemia often results in significant increases in LDL; LDL concentrations are not significantly affected by gemfibrozil in patients with Type IIb hyperlipidemia (although HDL is significantly increased). The mechanism of this action is not completely understood but may involve inhibition of peripheral lipolysis; reduced hepatic extraction of free fatty acids, which reduces hepatic triglyceride production; inhibition of synthesis and increased clearance of VLDL carrier, apolipoprotein B, which also reduces VLDL production; and, according to animal studies, reduced incorporation of long-chain fatty acids into newly formed triglycerides, accelerated turnover and removal of cholesterol from the liver (stimulates incorporation of cholesterol precursors into liver sterols), and increased excretion of cholesterol in the feces.

**Absorption**
Well absorbed from gastrointestinal tract.

**Biotransformation**
Hepatic.

**Half-life**
Single dose—1.5 hours.
Multiple doses—1.3 hours.

**Onset of action**
Reduction of plasma VLDL concentrations—2 to 5 days.

**Time to peak concentration**
1 to 2 hours.

**Time to peak effect**
Reduction of plasma VLDL concentrations—4 weeks (major effect; further decreases occur over several months).

**Elimination**
Renal (70%; largely unchanged)/fecal (6%).

## Precautions to Consider

### Carcinogenicity/Tumorigenicity
During long term follow-up of patients in the Helsinki Heart Study, there was a trend toward an increased incidence of basal cell carcinomas and deaths attributed to cancer in the group of patients originally randomized to gemfibrozil. However, these data did not reach statistical significance.

Long-term studies in male rats have shown gemfibrozil to have a tumorigenic effect. Studies in rats given gemfibrozil for prolonged periods found an increased incidence of benign and malignant hepatic tumors in male and female rats, as well as benign testicular (Leydig cell) tumors in male rats, at doses of 1 and 10 times the human dose.

### Pregnancy/Reproduction
Fertility—Studies in male rats given gemfibrozil at doses 0.6 to 2 times the human dose (based on surface area) for 10 weeks revealed a dose-related decrease in fertility.

Pregnancy—Studies in humans have not been done.
Studies in female rats given gemfibrozil at 0.6 to 2 times the human dose (based on surface area) before and throughout gestation resulted in a dose-related decrease in conception rate and an increase in skeletal variations, including anophthalmia. At the high dose level an increase in stillbirths and reduction in pup weight during lactation were observed. In addition, similar doses given to female rats from gestation day 15 through weaning resulted in decreased birth weights and pup growth suppression during lactation.

Gemfibrozil, given at doses 1 to 3 times the human dose (based on surface area) to female rabbits during organogenesis, caused decreased litter sizes and, at the high dose, an increased incidence of parietal bone variations.

FDA Pregnancy Category C.

### Breast-feeding
It is not known whether gemfibrozil is excreted in breast milk. Problems in humans have not been documented; however, any decision regarding breast-feeding during therapy should take into account that gemfibrozil has a tumorigenic effect in rats.

### Pediatrics
Appropriate studies on the relationship of age to the effects of gemfibrozil have not been performed in the pediatric population. However, use in children under 2 years of age is not recommended since cholesterol is required for normal development.

### Geriatrics
No information is available on the relationship of age to the effects of gemfibrozil in geriatric patients. However, elderly patients are more likely to have age-related renal function impairment, which may require reduction of dosage in patients receiving gemfibrozil.

### Drug interactions and/or related problems
The following drug interactions and/or related problems have been selected on the basis of their potential clinical significance (possible mechanism in parentheses where appropriate)—not necessarily inclusive (» = major clinical significance):

» Anticoagulants, coumarin- or indandione-derivative
(concurrent use with gemfibrozil may significantly increase the anticoagulant effect of these medications; adjustment of anticoagulant dosage based on frequent prothrombin-time determinations is recommended)

Chenodiol or
Ursodiol
(effect may be decreased when chenodiol or ursodiol is used concurrently with gemfibrozil, which tends to increase cholesterol saturation of bile)

» Lovastatin
(concurrent use with gemfibrozil may be associated with an increased risk of rhabdomyolysis, significant increases in creatine kinase [CK] concentrations, and myoglobinuria that leads to acute renal failure; may be seen as early as 3 weeks or as late as several months after initiation of combined therapy; monitoring of CK has not been shown to prevent severe myopathy or renal damage)

### Laboratory value alterations
The following have been selected on the basis of their potential clinical significance (possible effect in parentheses where appropriate)—not necessarily inclusive (» = major clinical significance):

With physiology/laboratory test values
Alanine aminotransferase (ALT [SGPT]), serum and
Alkaline phosphatase, serum and
Aspartate aminotransferase (AST [SGOT]), serum and
Bilirubin, serum and
Creatine kinase (CK), plasma and
Lactate dehydrogenase (LDH), serum
(concentrations may be increased, indicating liver function abnormalities)

Hematocrit and
Hemoglobin concentrations and
Leukocyte counts
(may be mildly decreased, but usually stabilize with continued administration)

Potassium
(serum concentrations may be decreased)

### Medical considerations/Contraindications
The medical considerations/contraindications included have been selected on the basis of their potential clinical significance (reasons given in parentheses where appropriate)—not necessarily inclusive (» = major clinical significance).

*Except under special circumstances, this medication should not be used when the following medical problem exists:*

» Primary biliary cirrhosis
(use of gemfibrozil may further raise the cholesterol)

*Risk-benefit should be considered when the following medical problems exist:*

Gallbladder disease or
Gallstones
(increased risk of biliary complications, including possible formation of gallstones)

» Hepatic function impairment
(reduced biotransformation; reduced dosage is recommended)

» Renal function impairment, severe
(reduced clearance leads to increased incidence of side effects; reduced dosage is recommended)
(gemfibrozil may worsen pre-existing renal insufficiency)

Sensitivity to gemfibrozil

### Patient monitoring
The following may be especially important in patient monitoring (other tests may be warranted in some patients, depending on condition; » = major clinical significance):

Blood counts, complete and
Cholesterol, serum and
Liver function tests and
Triglycerides, serum
(determinations recommended prior to initiation of therapy and at periodic intervals during therapy)

## Side/Adverse Effects

Note: Because of the chemical, pharmacologic, and clinical similarity of gemfibrozil to clofibrate, the possibility of similar long-term effects should be kept in mind. Studies with clofibrate have associated long-term use of the medication with an increased incidence of deaths from noncardiovascular causes and have also found a greatly increased incidence of cholelithiasis and cholecystitis requiring surgery in clofibrate users (see *Clofibrate [Systemic]*). In addition, studies have suggested that control of elevated cholesterol and triglycerides may not lessen the danger of cardiovascular disease and mortality, although incidence of nonfatal myocardial infarctions may be decreased.

Subcapsular bilateral cataracts and unilateral cataracts have been reported in 10% and 6.3%, respectively, of male rats given 10 times the human dose.

The following side/adverse effects have been selected on the basis of their potential clinical significance (possible signs and symptoms in parentheses where appropriate)—not necessarily inclusive:

**Those indicating need for immediate medical attention**
Incidence rare
*Anemia or leukopenia* (cough or hoarseness; fever or chills; lower back or side pain; painful or difficult urination); *gallstones* (severe stomach pain with nausea and vomiting); *myositis* (muscle pain, unusual tiredness or weakness)

Note: Gemfibrozil may increase cholesterol secretion into the bile.

**Those indicating need for medical attention only if they continue or are bothersome**
Incidence more frequent
*Stomach pain, gas, or heartburn*
Incidence less frequent
*Diarrhea; nausea or vomiting; skin rash; unusual tiredness*

## Patient Consultation

As an aid to patient consultation, refer to *Advice for the Patient, Gemfibrozil (Systemic)*.

In providing consultation, consider emphasizing the following selected information (» = major clinical significance):

**Before using this medication**
Potential serious toxicity because of similarity to clofibrate
» Diet as preferred therapy
» Conditions affecting use, especially:
  Sensitivity to gemfibrozil
  Pregnancy—High doses in animals cause birth defects and an increase in fetal deaths
  Breast-feeding—High doses associated with increased incidence of tumors in rats; consider when deciding whether to breast-feed
  Use in children—Not recommended in children under 2 years of age since cholesterol is required for normal development
  Other medications, especially lovastatin or oral anticoagulants
  Other medical problems, especially primary biliary cirrhosis, hepatic function impairment, or severe renal function impairment

**Proper use of this medication**
» Importance of not taking more or less medication than the amount prescribed
  Taking 30 minutes before morning and evening meal
» Compliance with prescribed diet
» Proper dosing
  Missed dose: Taking as soon as possible; not taking if almost time for next dose; not doubling doses
» Proper storage

**Precautions while using this medication**
» Importance of close monitoring by physician
» Checking with physician before discontinuing medication; blood lipid concentrations may increase significantly

**Side/adverse effects**
Signs of potential side effects, especially gallstones, leukopenia, anemia, and myositis

## General Dosing Information

If response is inadequate after 3 months of treatment, gemfibrozil therapy should be withdrawn.

When gemfibrozil is discontinued, an appropriate hypolipidemic diet and monitoring of serum lipids are recommended until the patient stabilizes, since a rise in serum triglyceride and cholesterol concentrations to the original base may occur.

If results of hepatic function tests rise significantly or show significant abnormalities, it is recommended that gemfibrozil therapy be withdrawn and not resumed; laboratory abnormalities are usually reversible.

If gallstones are found, gemfibrozil therapy should be withdrawn.

If patients receiving gemfibrozil experience muscle pain or weakness, evaluation for myositis (including serum CK determinations) is recommended. It is recommended that gemfibrozil be withdrawn if myositis is suspected or diagnosed.

**Diet/Nutrition**
Gemfibrozil should be taken 30 minutes before the morning and evening meals.

## Oral Dosage Forms

### GEMFIBROZIL CAPSULES USP

**Usual adult dose**
Antihyperlipidemic—
  Oral, 1.2 grams a day in two divided doses thirty minutes before the morning and evening meals.

**Usual pediatric dose**
Dosage has not been established.

**Strength(s) usually available**
U.S.—
  Not commercially available.
Canada—
  300 mg (Rx) [*Lopid; Apo-Gemfibrozil; Gen-Fibro; Nu-Gemfibrozil;* GENERIC].

**Packaging and storage**
Store below 30 °C (86 °F), unless otherwise specified by manufacturer. Store in a tight container.

### GEMFIBROZIL TABLETS

**Usual adult dose**
Antihyperlipidemic—
  Oral, 1.2 grams a day in two divided doses thirty minutes before the morning and evening meals.

**Usual pediatric dose**
Dosage has not been established.

**Strength(s) usually available**
U.S.—
  600 mg (Rx) [*Lopid* (scored; methylparaben; propylparaben); GENERIC].
Canada—
  600 mg (Rx) [*Lopid; Apo-Gemfibrozil; Gen-Fibro; Novo-Gemfibrozil; Nu-Gemfibrozil;* GENERIC].

**Packaging and storage**
Store below 30 °C (86 °F), unless otherwise specified by manufacturer. Store in a tight container.

## Selected Bibliography

National Cholesterol Education Program. Second Report of the Expert Panel on Detection, Evaluation, and Treatment of High Blood Cholesterol in Adults (Adult Treatment Panel II). Circulation 1994; 89(3): 1329-445.

Knodel LC, Talbert RL. Adverse effects of hypolipidaemic drugs. Med Toxicol 1987; 2: 10-32.

Frick MH, Elo O, Haapa K, et al. Helsinki Heart Study: Primary-prevention trial with gemfibrozil in middle-aged men with dyslipidemia. N Engl J Med 1987; 317: 1237-45.

Revised: 05/24/93
Interim revision: 06/28/95; 08/12/98

---

**GENTAMICIN**—See *Aminoglycosides (Systemic); Gentamicin (Ophthalmic); Gentamicin (Otic); Gentamicin (Topical)*

# GENTAMICIN Ophthalmic

VA CLASSIFICATION (Primary): OP201

Commonly used brand name(s): *Alcomicin; Garamycin; Genoptic Liquifilm; Genoptic S.O.P.; Gentacidin; Gentafair; Gentak; Gentrasul; Ocu-Mycin; Spectro-Genta.*

Another commonly used name is gentamycin.

Note: For a listing of dosage forms and brand names by country availability, see *Dosage Forms* section(s).

## Category

Antibacterial (ophthalmic).

## Indications

**Accepted**
Blepharitis, bacterial (treatment)
Blepharoconjunctivitis (treatment)
Conjunctivitis, bacterial (treatment)
Dacryocystitis (treatment)
Keratitis, bacterial (treatment)
Keratoconjunctivitis, bacterial (treatment) or
Meibomianitis (treatment)—Ophthalmic gentamicin is indicated in the treatment of blepharitis, blepharoconjunctivitis, conjunctivitis, dacryocystitis, keratitis, keratoconjunctivitis, and acute meibomianitis caused by coagulase-negative and coagulase-positive staphylococci, *Pseudomonas aeruginosa,* indole-positive and indole-negative *Proteus* species, *Escherichia coli, Klebsiella pneumoniae, Hemophilus influenzae, H. aegyptius, Enterobacter aerogenes (Aerobacter aerogenes), Moraxella lacunata* (Morax-Axenfeld bacillus), and *Neisseria* species, including *N. gonorrhoeae.*

Note: Not all species or strains of a particular organism may be susceptible to gentamicin.

## Pharmacology/Pharmacokinetics

**Physicochemical characteristics**
Chemical group—Aminoglycosides.
pH—Gentamicin sulfate ophthalmic solution is buffered to pH of approximately 7.

**Mechanism of action/Effect**
Aminoglycoside; actively transported across the bacterial cell membrane, binds to a specific receptor protein on the 30 S subunit of bacterial ribosomes, and interferes with an initiation complex between mRNA (messenger RNA) and the 30 S subunit, inhibiting protein synthesis. DNA may be misread, thus producing nonfunctional proteins; polyribosomes are split apart and are unable to synthesize protein.

Note: Aminoglycosides are bactericidal, while most other antibiotics that interfere with protein synthesis are bacteriostatic.

**Absorption**
May be absorbed in minute quantities following topical application to the eye.

## Precautions to Consider

**Cross-sensitivity and/or related problems**
Patients sensitive to one aminoglycoside may be sensitive to other aminoglycosides also.

**Pregnancy/Reproduction**
Problems in humans have not been documented.

**Breast-feeding**
Problems in humans have not been documented.

**Pediatrics**
Appropriate studies on the relationship of age to the effects of this medicine have not been performed in the pediatric population. However, no pediatrics-specific problems have been documented to date.

**Geriatrics**
Appropriate studies on the relationship of age to the effects of this medicine have not been performed in the geriatric population. However, no geriatrics-specific problems have been documented to date.

**Medical considerations/Contraindications**
The medical considerations/contraindications included have been selected on the basis of their potential clinical significance (reasons given in parentheses where appropriate)—not necessarily inclusive (» = major clinical significance).

*Risk-benefit should be considered when the following medical problem exists:*
Sensitivity to gentamicin

## Side/Adverse Effects

The following side/adverse effects have been selected on the basis of their potential clinical significance (possible signs and symptoms in parentheses where appropriate)—not necessarily inclusive:

**Those indicating need for medical attention**
Incidence less frequent
*Hypersensitivity* (itching, redness, swelling, or other sign of irritation not present before therapy)

**Those indicating need for medical attention only if they continue or are bothersome**
Incidence less frequent
*Burning or stinging*

**Those not indicating need for medical attention**
For ophthalmic ointment dosage form only
*Blurred vision*

## Patient Consultation

As an aid to patient consultation, refer to *Advice for the Patient, Gentamicin (Ophthalmic).*

In providing consultation, consider emphasizing the following selected information (» = major clinical significance):

**Before using this medication**
» Conditions affecting use, especially:
Sensitivity to gentamicin or to any related antibiotic, such as amikacin, kanamycin, neomycin, netilmicin, streptomycin, or tobramycin

**Proper use of this medication**
Proper administration technique
» Compliance with full course of therapy
» Proper dosing
Missed dose: Applying as soon as possible; not applying if almost time for next dose
» Proper storage

**Precautions while using this medication**
Checking with physician if no improvement within a few days

**Side/adverse effects**
Blurred vision may occur for a few minutes after application of ophthalmic ointments
Signs of potential side effects, especially hypersensitivity

## General Dosing Information

Gentamicin sulfate ophthalmic solution is not for subconjunctival injection or for direct injection into the anterior chamber of the eye.

Although some manufacturers recommend a dose of 2 drops of an ophthalmic solution at appropriate intervals, the conjunctival sac will usually hold only 1 drop.

At night the ophthalmic ointment may be used as an adjunct to the ophthalmic solution to provide prolonged contact with the medication.

In infections of the tear sacs (dacryocystitis), often occurring in children with nonpatent tear passages, hot compresses and gentle massage of the area over the tear duct may be useful adjuncts to treatment with the ophthalmic solution.

## Ophthalmic Dosage Forms

### GENTAMICIN SULFATE OPHTHALMIC OINTMENT USP

**Usual adult and adolescent dose**
Antibacterial (ophthalmic)—
Topical, to the conjunctiva, a thin strip (approximately 1 cm) of ointment every eight to twelve hours.

**Usual pediatric dose**
See *Usual adult and adolescent dose.*

**Strength(s) usually available**
U.S.—
5 mg of gentamicin sulfate, equivalent to 3 mg of gentamicin base, per gram (Rx) [*Garamycin* (methylparaben; propylparaben); *Genoptic S.O.P.* (methylparaben; propylparaben); *Gentacidin; Gentafair* (may contain methylparaben; may contain propylparaben); *Gentak*

# Gentamicin (Ophthalmic)

(methylparaben; propylparaben); *Gentrasul* (methylparaben 0.05%; propylparaben 0.01%); *Ocu-Mycin* [GENERIC (may contain methylparaben; may contain propylparaben)].

Canada—
5 mg of gentamicin sulfate, equivalent to 3 mg of gentamicin base, per gram (Rx) [*Garamycin* (methylparaben; propylparaben); *Gentrasul*].

### Packaging and storage
Store below 40 °C (104 °F). Store in a collapsible ophthalmic ointment tube. Protect from freezing.

### Auxiliary labeling
- For the eye.
- Continue medicine for full time of treatment.

## GENTAMICIN SULFATE OPHTHALMIC SOLUTION USP

### Usual adult and adolescent dose
Antibacterial (ophthalmic)—
Mild to moderate infections: Topical, to the conjunctiva, 1 drop every four hours.
Severe infections: Topical, to the conjunctiva, 1 drop every hour.

### Usual pediatric dose
See *Usual adult and adolescent dose*.

### Strength(s) usually available
U.S.—
5 mg of gentamicin sulfate, equivalent to 3 mg of gentamicin base, per mL (Rx) [*Garamycin* (benzalkonium chloride); *Genoptic Liquifilm* (polyvinyl alcohol 1.4%; benzalkonium chloride); *Gentacidin* (benzalkonium chloride); *Gentafair* (may contain benzalkonium chloride); *Gentak* (benzalkonium chloride 0.01%); *Gentrasul* (benzalkonium chloride 0.01%); *Ocu-Mycin*; *Spectro-Genta* [GENERIC (may contain benzalkonium chloride)].

Canada—
5 mg of gentamicin sulfate, equivalent to 3 mg of gentamicin base, per mL (Rx) [*Alcomicin* (benzalkonium chloride 0.01%); *Garamycin* (benzalkonium chloride); *Gentrasul*].

### Packaging and storage
Store below 40 °C (104 °F). Store in a tight container. Protect from freezing.

### Auxiliary labeling
- For the eye.
- Continue medicine for full time of treatment.

### Note
Dispense in original unopened container.

Revised: 6/23/92
Interim revision: 8/30/93

---

# GENTAMICIN Otic*

VA CLASSIFICATION (Primary): OT101
Commonly used brand name(s): *Garamycin Otic Solution*.

Note: For a listing of dosage forms and brand names by country availability, see *Dosage Forms* section(s).

*Not commercially available in U.S.

## Category
Antibacterial (otic).

## Indications
### Accepted
Mastoidectomy cavity infections (treatment) or
Otitis media, chronic suppurative (treatment) or
Otitis media, subacute purulent (treatment) or
Otitis, external (treatment) —Gentamicin otic preparations are used in the treatment of mastoidectomy cavity infections, chronic suppurative otitis media, subacute purulent otitis media with tympanic membrane perforation, or external otitis.

Note: Not all species or strains of a particular organism may be susceptible to gentamicin.

## Pharmacology/Pharmacokinetics
### Physicochemical characteristics
Chemical group—Aminoglycosides.

### Mechanism of action/Effect
Aminoglycoside; actively transported across the bacterial cell membrane, binds to a specific receptor protein on the 30 S subunit of bacterial ribosomes, and interferes with an initiation complex between mRNA (messenger RNA) and the 30 S subunit, inhibiting protein synthesis. DNA may be misread, thus producing nonfunctional proteins; polyribosomes are split apart and are unable to synthesize protein.

Note: Aminoglycosides are bactericidal, while most other antibiotics that interfere with protein synthesis are bacteriostatic.

### Absorption
May be absorbed in minute quantities following topical application to the ear, especially if the eardrum is perforated or if tissue damage is present.

## Precautions to Consider

### Cross-sensitivity and/or related problems
Patients sensitive to one aminoglycoside may be sensitive to other aminoglycosides also.

### Pregnancy/Reproduction
Problems in humans have not been documented.

### Breast-feeding
It is not known whether otic gentamicin is excreted in breast milk. However, problems in humans have not been documented.

### Pediatrics
Appropriate studies on the relationship of age to the effects of this medicine have not been performed in the pediatric population. However, no pediatrics-specific problems have been documented to date.

### Geriatrics
Appropriate studies on the relationship of age to the effects of this medicine have not been performed in the geriatric population. However, no geriatrics-specific problems have been documented to date.

### Medical considerations/Contraindications
The medical considerations/contraindications included have been selected on the basis of their potential clinical significance (reasons given in parentheses where appropriate)—not necessarily inclusive (» = major clinical significance).

*Risk-benefit should be considered when the following medical problems exist:*
Perforated eardrum
Sensitivity to aminoglycosides

## Side/Adverse Effects
The following side/adverse effects have been selected on the basis of their potential clinical significance (possible signs and symptoms in parentheses where appropriate)—not necessarily inclusive:

### Those indicating need for medical attention
Incidence less frequent
*Hypersensitivity* (itching, redness, swelling, or other sign of irritation not present before therapy)

### Those indicating need for medical attention only if they continue or are bothersome
Incidence less frequent
*Burning or stinging*

## Patient Consultation
As an aid to patient consultation, refer to *Advice for the Patient, Gentamicin (Otic)*.

In providing consultation, consider emphasizing the following selected information (» = major clinical significance):

### Before using this medication
» Conditions affecting use, especially:
Sensitivity to aminoglycosides

### Proper use of this medication
Proper administration technique
» Compliance with full course of therapy

» Proper dosing
  Missed dose: Applying as soon as possible; not applying if almost time for next dose
» Proper storage
**Precautions while using this medication**
  Checking with physician if no improvement within a few days
**Side/adverse effects**
  Signs of potential side effects, especially hypersensitivity

## Otic Dosage Forms

### GENTAMICIN SULFATE OTIC SOLUTION

**Usual adult and adolescent dose**
Topical, to the ear canal, 3 or 4 drops three times a day.

**Usual pediatric dose**
See *Usual adult and adolescent dose*.

**Strength(s) usually available**
U.S.—
  Not commercially available. Gentamicin sulfate ophthalmic solution is being used for otic application.

Canada—
  0.3% (base) (Rx) [*Garamycin Otic Solution*].
Note: Each mL of solution contains 5 mg of gentamicin sulfate, equivalent to 3 mg of gentamicin base.

**Packaging and storage**
Store below 40 °C (104 °F), preferably between 15 and 30 °C (59 and 86 °F), unless otherwise specified by manufacturer. Store in a tight container. Protect from freezing.

**Auxiliary labeling**
• For the ear.
• Continue medicine for full time of treatment.

**Note**
Dispense in original unopened container.

Revised: 08/12/92
Interim revision: 04/11/94

---

# GENTAMICIN  Topical

VA CLASSIFICATION (Primary): DE101
Commonly used brand name(s): *G-Myticin; Garamycin; Gentamar*.
Note: For a listing of dosage forms and brand names by country availability, see *Dosage Forms* section(s).

## Category
Antibacterial (topical).

## Indications
Note: Bracketed information in the *Indications* section refers to uses that are not included in U.S. product labeling.

**Accepted**
Folliculitis (treatment)
Furunculosis (treatment)
Paronychia (treatment) or
Skin infections, bacterial, other minor (treatment)—Topical gentamicin is indicated in the topical treatment of folliculitis, furunculosis, paronychia, and other minor bacterial skin infections (including infected insect bites, infected minor burns, infected contact dermatitis, infectious eczematoid dermatitis, infected seborrheic dermatitis, infected excoriation, infected lacerations, infected skin abscesses and cysts, infected skin ulcers, infected stasis ulcers, infected stings, bacterial superinfections of minor fungal and viral infections, sycosis barbae, and minor surgical wounds) caused by staphylococci, streptococci, *Proteus vulgaris*, *Escherichia coli*, *Pseudomonas aeruginosa*, and *Enterobacter aerogenes* (*Aerobacter aerogenes*).

[Skin infections, bacterial, minor (prophylaxis)][1] or
[Ulcer, dermal (treatment)]—Topical gentamicin is used in the prophylaxis of minor bacterial skin infections and in the treatment of dermal ulcer.

Not all species or strains of a particular organism may be susceptible to gentamicin.

**Unaccepted**
Indiscriminate use of topical gentamicin may lead to the emergence of aminoglycoside-resistant organisms. Therefore, use in immunocompromised or other high-risk patients is not recommended.
Gentamicin is not effective against anaerobes, fungi, or viruses.

[1]Not included in Canadian product labeling.

## Pharmacology/Pharmacokinetics

**Physicochemical characteristics**
Chemical group—Aminoglycosides.

**Mechanism of action/Effect**
Aminoglycoside; actively transported across the bacterial cell membrane, binds to a specific receptor protein on the 30 S subunit of bacterial ribosomes, and interferes with an initiation complex between mRNA (messenger RNA) and the 30 S subunit, inhibiting protein synthesis. DNA may be misread, thus producing nonfunctional proteins; polyribosomes are split apart and are unable to synthesize protein.

Note: Aminoglycosides are bactericidal, while most other antibiotics that interfere with protein synthesis are bacteriostatic.

**Absorption**
Although not absorbed through intact skin, topical gentamicin is readily absorbed from large denuded, burned, or granulating areas. Greater and more rapid absorption occurs with gentamicin cream than with the ointment.

## Precautions to Consider

**Cross-sensitivity and/or related problems**
Patients sensitive to one aminoglycoside may be sensitive to other aminoglycosides also. However, patients who are sensitive to neomycin have been treated with gentamicin without apparent adverse effects.

**Pregnancy/Reproduction**
Problems in humans have not been documented.

**Breast-feeding**
It is not known whether topical gentamicin is distributed into breast milk. However, problems in humans have not been documented.

**Pediatrics**
Appropriate studies on the relationship of age to the effects of this medicine have not been performed in infants and children up to 1 year of age. In children over 1 year of age, appropriate studies performed to date have not demonstrated pediatrics-specific problems that would limit the usefulness of this medicine.

**Geriatrics**
Appropriate studies on the relationship of age to the effects of this medicine have not been performed in the geriatric population. However, no geriatrics-specific problems have been documented to date.

**Medical considerations/Contraindications**
The medical considerations/contraindications included have been selected on the basis of their potential clinical significance (reasons given in parentheses where appropriate)—not necessarily inclusive (» = major clinical significance).

*Risk-benefit should be considered when the following medical problem exists:*
  Sensitivity to topical gentamicin

## Side/Adverse Effects
The following side/adverse effects have been selected on the basis of their potential clinical significance (possible signs and symptoms in parentheses where appropriate)—not necessarily inclusive:

**Those indicating need for medical attention**
Incidence less frequent
  *Hypersensitivity* (itching, redness, swelling, or other sign of irritation not present before therapy)

## Patient Consultation
As an aid to patient consultation, refer to *Advice for the Patient, Gentamicin (Topical)*.
In providing consultation, consider emphasizing the following selected information (» = major clinical significance):

## Gentamicin (Topical)

### Before using this medication
» Conditions affecting use, especially:
   Sensitivity to aminoglycosides

### Proper use of this medication
Before applying, washing affected area with soap and water and drying thoroughly; applying small amount and rubbing in gently
After applying, covering with gauze dressing if desired
» Compliance with full course of therapy
» Proper dosing
   Missed dose: Applying as soon as possible; not applying if almost time for next dose
» Proper storage

### Precautions while using this medication
Checking with physician if no improvement within 1 week

### Side/adverse effects
Signs of potential side effects, especially hypersensitivity

## General Dosing Information
The treated area(s) may be covered with a gauze dressing if desired.

Serum concentrations up to 4 mcg per mL or more have been reported following topical administration. Nephrotoxicity and moderate to severe ototoxicity may occur, especially if renal function is impaired and systemic nephrotoxic and/or ototoxic drugs are given concurrently.

Use of topical antibacterials may lead to skin sensitization, resulting in hypersensitivity reactions with subsequent topical or systemic use of the medication.

## Topical Dosage Forms

### GENTAMICIN SULFATE CREAM USP

#### Usual adult and adolescent dose
Antibacterial—
  Topical, to the skin, three or four times a day.

#### Usual pediatric dose
Antibacterial—
  Infants and children over 1 year of age: See *Usual adult and adolescent dose*.

#### Strength(s) usually available
U.S.—
  0.1% (base) (Rx) [*Garamycin* (butylparaben 0.4%; methylparaben 0.1%); *Gentamar*; *G-Myticin*; GENERIC].
Canada—
  0.1% (base) (Rx) [*Garamycin* (chlororesol 0.1%)].

Note: Each gram of cream contains 1.7 mg of gentamicin sulfate, equivalent to 1 mg of gentamicin base.

#### Packaging and storage
Store below 40 °C (104 °F). Store in a collapsible tube or other tight container. Protect from freezing.

#### Auxiliary labeling
- For external use only.
- Continue medication for full time of treatment.

#### Note
Gentamicin sulfate cream is water-washable and may be useful in treating wet, oozing primary infections and greasy, secondary infections of the skin, such as pustular acne or infected seborrheic dermatitis.

### GENTAMICIN SULFATE OINTMENT USP

#### Usual adult and adolescent dose
See *Gentamicin Sulfate Cream USP*.

#### Usual pediatric dose
See *Gentamicin Sulfate Cream USP*.

#### Strength(s) usually available
U.S.—
  0.1% (base) (Rx) [*Garamycin* (methylparaben 0.05%; propylparaben 0.01%); *Gentamar*; *G-Myticin*; GENERIC].
Canada—
  0.1% (base) (Rx) [*Garamycin* (methylparaben 0.05%; propylparaben 0.01%)].

Note: Each gram of ointment contains 1.7 mg of gentamicin sulfate, equivalent to 1 mg of gentamicin base.

#### Packaging and storage
Store below 40 °C (104 °F). Store in a collapsible tube or other tight container. Protect from freezing.

#### Auxiliary labeling
- For external use only.
- Continue medication for full time of treatment.

#### Note
Gentamicin sulfate ointment helps retain moisture and may be useful in treating infections of dry, eczematous, or psoriatic skin.

Revised: 06/23/92
Interim revision: 06/08/94

---

**GENTIAN VIOLET**—The *Gentian Violet (Topical)* monograph is not included in this published version of the USP DI database. Copies of the monograph are available on request from Micromedex, Inc. - Reprint Requests, 6200 S. Syracuse Way, Suite 300, Englewood, CO 80111; telephone (303) 486-6400; telefax (303) 486-6464; Email: USPDI@MDX.COM.

**GENTIAN VIOLET**—The *Gentian Violet (Vaginal)* monograph is not included in this published version of the USP DI database. Copies of the monograph are available on request from Micromedex, Inc. - Reprint Requests, 6200 S. Syracuse Way, Suite 300, Englewood, CO 80111; telephone (303) 486-6400; telefax (303) 486-6464; Email: USPDI@MDX.COM.

---

# GLATIRAMER ACETATE   Systemic—INTRODUCTORY VERSION

VA CLASSIFICATION (Primary): IM900; CN900
Commonly used brand name(s): *Copaxone*.
Another commonly used name is copolymer-1.
Note: For a listing of dosage forms and brand names by country availability, see *Dosage Forms* section(s).

## Category
Multiple sclerosis (MS) therapy agent.

## Indications

### General considerations
Because glatiramer acetate can modify immune response, consideration must be given to the possibility that it may interfere with useful immune function. Theoretically, for example, it could interfere with the recognition of foreign antigens in a manner that would undermine the body's defenses against infections and tumor surveillance. There is no evidence of this, although no systematic evaluation of this risk has been conducted.

Because glatiramer acetate is an antigenic material, its use possibly could induce unwanted host responses. There is no evidence that this occurs in humans, although no systematic evaluation of this risk has been conducted. Studies in rats and monkeys, however, have suggested that immune complexes are deposited in the renal glomeruli. Furthermore, in a controlled trial of 125 patients with relapsing-remitting multiple sclerosis who received 20 mg of glatiramer acetate subcutaneously every day for 2 years, serum IgG levels reached approximately three times the baseline values in 80% of patients within 3 to 6 months of initiation of treatment. These values decreased to about 50% greater than baseline during the remainder of treatment.

Although treatment with glatiramer acetate is intended to minimize the autoimmune response to myelin, the possibility remains that continued alteration of cellular immunity due to long-term treatment may result in untoward effects.

### Accepted
Multiple sclerosis (treatment)—Glatiramer acetate is indicated for reduction of the frequency of relapses in patients with relapsing-remitting multiple sclerosis.

## Pharmacology/Pharmacokinetics

### Physicochemical characteristics
Chemical group—Glatiramer acetate is composed of the acetate salts of synthetic polypeptides, containing four naturally occurring amino acids: L-glutamic acid, L-alanine, L-tyrosine, and L-lysine, with an average molar fraction of 0.141, 0.427, 0.095, and 0.338, respectively.

Molecular weight—The average molecular weight of glatiramer acetate is 4700 to 11,000 daltons.

### Mechanism of action/Effect
The mechanism of action is unknown. However, glatiramer acetate is believed to modify immune processes that are thought to be responsible for the pathogenesis of multiple sclerosis (MS). Glatiramer acetate reduces the incidence and severity of experimentally induced allergic encephalomyelitis; this condition can be induced in several animal species through immunization against myelin-containing material derived from the central nervous system (CNS), and often is used as an experimental animal model of MS.

The ability of glatiramer acetate to modify immune functions raises concerns regarding its potential to alter naturally occurring immune responses. Results of a limited battery of tests designed to evaluate this risk were negative; however, the possibility cannot be absolutely excluded.

### Pharmacokinetics
Pharmacokinetic studies have not been performed in humans. Partly on the basis of animal studies, a substantial fraction of subcutaneously injected glatiramer acetate is assumed to be hydrolyzed locally. Some fraction of the injected material is presumed to enter the lymphatic circulation, enabling it to reach regional lymph nodes, and some may enter the systemic circulation intact.

## Precautions to Consider

### Carcinogenicity
Studies to assess the carcinogenic potential of glatiramer acetate in mice and rats are in progress.

### Mutagenicity
Glatiramer acetate was not mutagenic in four strains of *Salmonella typhimurium* and two strains of *Escherichia coli* (Ames test) or in the *in vitro* mouse lymphoma assay in L5178Y cells. Glatiramer acetate was found to be clastogenic in two separate *in vitro* chromosomal aberration assays in cultured human lymphocytes; it was not clastogenic in an *in vivo* mouse bone marrow micronucleus assay.

### Pregnancy/Reproduction
Fertility—In a multigeneration reproduction and fertility study in rats, glatiramer acetate at subcutaneous doses of up to 36 mg per kg of body weight (mg/kg) (18 times the recommended human daily dose) had no adverse effects on reproductive parameters.

Pregnancy—Adequate and well-controlled studies in humans have not been done.

In reproduction studies in rats and rabbits receiving subcutaneous doses of glatiramer acetate up to 37.5 mg/kg during the period of organogenesis, no adverse effects on embryo/fetal development occurred. In a prenatal and postnatal study in which rats received subcutaneous glatiramer acetate doses of up to 36 mg/kg from day 15 of pregnancy through lactation, no significant effects on delivery or on offspring growth and development were observed.

FDA Pregnancy Category B.

### Breast-feeding
It is not known whether glatiramer acetate is distributed into human milk.

### Pediatrics
Safety and efficacy have not been established in patients younger than 18 years of age.

### Geriatrics
Glatiramer acetate has not been studied specifically in elderly patients.

### Drug interactions and/or related problems
Note: Interactions between glatiramer acetate and other medications have not been fully evaluated. Results from clinical trials do not suggest any significant interactions of glatiramer acetate with other therapies commonly used in multiple sclerosis patients, including concurrent use of corticosteroids for up to 28 days. Glatiramer acetate has not been evaluated formally in combination with interferon beta; however, ten patients who switched from therapy with interferon beta to glatiramer acetate have not reported any serious or unexpected adverse events thought to be related to treatment.

### Medical considerations/Contraindications
The medical considerations/contraindications included have been selected on the basis of their potential clinical significance (reasons given in parentheses where appropriate)—not necessarily inclusive (» = major clinical significance).

*Risk-benefit should be considered when the following medical problem exists:*

Sensitivity to glatiramer acetate or mannitol

## Side/Adverse Effects

Note: Approximately 10% of patients exposed to glatiramer acetate in premarketing studies experienced a constellation of symptoms immediately after injection. Symptoms included flushing, chest pain, palpitations, anxiety, dyspnea, constriction of the throat, and urticaria. These symptoms were invariably transient and self-limited and did not require specific treatment. In general, these symptoms appear several months after the initiation of therapy, although they may occur earlier in the course of treatment, and a patient may experience one or several episodes of these symptoms. It is not certain if this constellation of symptoms represents a specific syndrome. Whether these episodes are mediated by an immunologic or nonimmunologic mechanism, or whether several similar episodes seen in a particular patient have identical mechanisms is not known.

Approximately 26% of patients receiving glatiramer acetate in the premarketing multicenter controlled trial experienced at least one episode of transient chest pain, as compared with 10% of the patients receiving placebo. Some, but not all, of these episodes occurred in the context of the immediate postinjection reaction. Chest pain usually lasted only a few minutes, was often unassociated with other symptoms, and appeared to have no important sequelae. Electrocardiogram (ECG) monitoring was not performed during these episodes. Chest pain episodes usually began at least 1 month after initiation of treatment, and some patients experienced more than one episode. The pathogenesis of this symptom is unknown.

The following side/adverse effects have been selected on the basis of their potential clinical significance (possible signs and symptoms in parentheses where appropriate)—not necessarily inclusive:

**Those indicating need for medical attention**
Incidence more frequent
*Anxiety; arthralgia* (joint pain); *chest pain; dyspnea* (troubled breathing); *facial edema* (swelling or puffiness of face); *hypertonia* (excessive muscle tone); *injection-site reactions; including hemorrhage* (bleeding); *induration* (hard lump); *inflammation; pain; pruritus* (itching); *redness; urticaria* (hives or welts); *lymphadenopathy* (swollen lymph glands); *neck pain; palpitations* (irregular or pounding heartbeat); *vaginal moniliasis* (vaginal yeast infection); *vasodilatation* (flushing)

Incidence less frequent
*Agitation; bronchitis* (tightness in chest or wheezing); *chills; confusion; ecchymosis* (purple spots under the skin); *edema* (bloating or swelling); *flu-like syndrome* (chills; fever; muscle aches); *infection; laryngismus* (spasm of throat); *migraine; pain; peripheral edema* (swelling of fingers, arms, feet, or legs); *skin nodules* (small lumps under the skin); *skin rash; syncope* (fainting); *urinary urgency* (strong urge to urinate); *urticaria* (hives)

Incidence rare
*Anorexia* (loss of appetite); *back pain; diarrhea; dysmenorrhea or other menstrual changes; ear pain; hematuria* (blood in urine); *hypertension* (high blood pressure); *hyperventilation* (fast breathing); *impotence* (decreased sexual ability); *nystagmus* (continuous, uncontrolled back-and-forth and/or rolling eye movements); *oral moniliasis* (irritation of mouth and tongue [thrush] ); *speech problems; suspicious Papanicolaou test; tachycardia* (fast or racing heartbeat); *vertigo* (sensation of motion, usually whirling, either of oneself or of one's surroundings); *vision problems*

**Those indicating need for medical attention only if they continue or are bothersome**
Incidence more frequent
*Asthenia* (unusual tiredness or weakness); *nausea; sweating, increased; tremor* (trembling); *vomiting*

Incidence less frequent
*Rhinitis* (runny nose); *weight gain*

## Overdose
For information on the management of overdose or unintentional ingestion, **contact a Poison Control Center** (see *Poison Control Center Listing*).

## Patient Consultation

In providing consultation, consider emphasizing the following selected information (» = major clinical significance)

**Before using this medication**
- » Conditions affecting use, especially:
    Sensitivity to glatiramer acetate or mannitol

**Proper use of this medication**
- » Receiving instructions in self-injection techniques to assure safe administration
- » Carefully reading patient instructions contained in package
- » Importance of using medication exactly as directed
- » Not discontinuing medication without checking with physician
- » Proper dosing
    Missed dose: Using as soon as remembered; not using if not remembered until next day; not doubling doses
- » Proper storage

**Side/adverse effects**
Signs of potential side effects, especially anxiety, arthralgia, chest pain, dyspnea, facial edema, hypertonia, injection-site reactions, lymphadenopathy, neck pain, palpitations, vaginal moniliasis, vasodilatation, agitation, bronchitis, chills, confusion, ecchymosis, edema, flu-like syndrome, infection, laryngismus, migraine, pain, peripheral edema, skin nodules, skin rash, syncope, urinary urgency, urticaria, anorexia, back pain, diarrhea, dysmenorrhea or other menstrual changes, ear pain, hematuria, hypertension, hyperventilation, impotence, nystagmus, oral moniliasis, speech problems, suspicious Papanicolaou test, tachycardia, vertigo, and vision problems

## General Dosing Information

Patients should be instructed in self-injection techniques to assure safe administration.

Patients should be instructed not to change the dose or dosing schedule and not to discontinue the medication without consulting physician.

## Parenteral Dosage Forms

### GLATIRAMER ACETATE FOR INJECTION

**Usual adult dose**
Relapsing-remitting multiple sclerosis—
    Subcutaneously, 20 mg a day.

**Usual pediatric dose**
Safety and efficacy in patients up to 18 years of age have not been established.

**Strength(s) usually available**
U.S.—
    20 mg (Rx) [*Copaxone* (diluent—Sterile Water for Injection; Mannitol USP)].

**Packaging and storage**
Vials containing glatiramer acetate should be stored between 2 and 8 °C (36 and 46 °F) and protected from light. If refrigeration is not available, vials containing glatiramer acetate may be stored between 15 and 30 °C (59 and 86 °F) for up to one week. Vials containing diluent should be stored between 15 and 30 °C (59 and 86 °F).

**Preparation of dosage form**
The contents of the diluent vial are transferred into the lyophilized glatiramer acetate vial using aseptic technique. The vial is gently swirled and allowed to stand at room temperature until the solid material is completely dissolved; this occurs in about 5 minutes. If particulate matter remains, glatiramer acetate should not be used, and the vial should be discarded.

After reconstitution, the solution should be withdrawn into a sterile syringe fitted with a new 27-gauge needle and injected subcutaneously.

**Stability**
Glatiramer acetate contains no preservatives and should be used immediately after reconstitution or must be discarded.

**Auxiliary labeling**
- Store glatiramer acetate vials in refrigerator.

**Additional information**
The manufacturer has established a program entitled Shared Solutions™ to provide support to any patient with multiple sclerosis; the program is accessible with a toll-free telephone number.

Developed: 11/12/97

---

# GLIMEPIRIDE Systemic—INTRODUCTORY VERSION

VA CLASSIFICATION (Primary): HS502

Commonly used brand name(s): *Amaryl*.

Note: For a listing of dosage forms and brand names by country availability, see *Dosage Forms* section(s).

## Category

Antidiabetic agent.

## Indications

**Accepted**

Diabetes, type 2 (treatment)—Glimepiride is indicated as adjunctive therapy to diet and exercise to lower blood glucose in patients with type 2 diabetes (previously referred to as non–insulin-dependent diabetes mellitus [NIDDM]) whose hyperglycemia cannot be controlled by diet and exercise alone. An attempt to control diabetes through changes in diet and level of physical activity is usually first-line management before beginning pharmacologic treatment.

Glimepiride also is indicated for use in combination with insulin to lower blood glucose in patients with type 2 diabetes whose hyperglycemia cannot be controlled by diet and exercise in conjunction with an oral hypoglycemic agent. However, combined use of glimepiride and insulin may increase the potential for hypoglycemia.

## Pharmacology/Pharmacokinetics

**Physicochemical characteristics**
Chemical group—Sulfonylurea.
Molecular weight—490.62.

**Mechanism of action/Effect**
Antidiabetic agent—Glimepiride lowers blood glucose in patients with type 2 diabetes by stimulating the release of insulin from functioning pancreatic beta cells. Glimepiride also produces an increase in the sensitivity of peripheral tissues to insulin via an extrapancreatic mechanism.

**Absorption**
Following oral administration, glimepiride is 100% absorbed from the gastrointestinal tract.

Following oral administration with meals to normal volunteers, the mean peak drug concentration ($C_{max}$) and area under the plasma concentration–time curve (AUC) were slightly decreased (8% and 9%, respectively), and the mean time to reach $C_{max}$ ($T_{max}$) was slightly increased (12%).

**Distribution**
Following intravenous administration to normal volunteers, the volume of distribution was 8.8 L (113 mL per kg of body weight) and the total body clearance was 47.8 mL per minute.

**Protein binding**
Very high (99.5%).

**Biotransformation**
Following either an intravenous or oral dose, glimepiride is completely metabolized by oxidative biotransformation to a major metabolite, cyclohexyl hydroxymethyl derivative (M1), via the hepatic cytochrome P450 II C9 subsystem. M1 is further metabolized to the carboxyl derivative (M2) by one or several cytosolic enzymes. M1, but not M2, possessed approximately one third of the pharmacologic activity of its parent in an animal model. However, whether the glucose-lowering effect of M1 is clinically significant is not clear.

**Half-life**
Approximately 5.3 hours following a single oral dose when administered to normal volunteers; and approximately 5 and 9.2 hours following single and multiple doses, respectively, when administered to patients with type 2 diabetes.

**Time to peak concentration**
2 to 3 hours.

**Time to peak effect**
2 to 3 hours.

**Elimination**
Renal, approximately 60% of an oral dose, primarily as M1 and M2 metabolites (80 to 90%), within 7 days. Fecal, approximately 40% of an oral dose, primarily as M1 and M2 metabolites (70%).

No significant biliary excretion of glimepiride or its M1 metabolite has been observed following intravenous administration.

# Precautions to Consider

### Carcinogenicity
In a 30-month study in rats, glimepiride at doses approximately 340 times the maximum recommended human dose based on surface area showed no evidence of carcinogenic potential.

### Tumorigenicity
In a 24-month study in mice, glimepiride at doses greater than 35 times the maximum recommended human dose based on surface area showed a dose-related increase in the incidence of benign pancreatic adenoma formation. This increase is believed to be the result of chronic pancreatic stimulation.

### Mutagenicity
No evidence of mutagenicity was found in a series of *in vitro* and *in vivo* studies, including the Ames test, somatic cell mutation, chromosomal aberration, unscheduled DNA synthesis, and mouse micronucleus test.

### Pregnancy/Reproduction
Fertility—Glimepiride had no effect on the fertility of male mice and male and female rats administered doses greater than 1700 times and approximately 4000 times, respectively, the maximum recommended human dose based on surface area.

Pregnancy—Studies have not been done in humans.

Based on the results of animal studies, glimepiride is not recommended for use during pregnancy. Use of insulin during pregnancy allows for the maintenance of blood glucose concentrations that are as close to normal as possible. Abnormal blood glucose concentrations have been associated with a higher incidence of congenital abnormalities.

No evidence of teratogenicity was found in rats following oral administration of glimepiride at doses approximately 4000 times the maximum recommended human dose based on surface area, or in rabbits following administration of glimepiride at doses approximately 60 times the maximum recommended human dose based on surface area. However, glimepiride has been associated with intrauterine death in rats administered doses 50 times the human dose based on surface area, and in rabbits administered doses 0.1 time the human dose based on surface area. This fetotoxicity, observed only at doses inducing maternal hypoglycemia, has been similarly noted with other sulfonylureas and is believed to be directly related to the hypoglycemic action of glimepiride.

FDA Pregnancy Category C.

Delivery—Severe hypoglycemia lasting 4 to 10 days has been reported in neonates born to mothers who were receiving a sulfonylurea at the time of delivery. This effect has been observed more frequently with the use of sulfonylureas with prolonged half-lives.

### Breast-feeding
It is not known whether glimepiride is distributed into human breast milk. However, some sulfonylureas are distributed into human breast milk.

In reproduction studies, significant concentrations of glimepiride were observed in the milk of rats and in the serum of their pups. In some studies, pups of rats exposed to high concentrations of glimepiride during pregnancy developed skeletal abnormalities after nursing. These abnormalities included shortening, thickening, and bending of the humerus during the postnatal period.

Because of its potential to cause hypoglycemia in nursing infants, and because of its effect on nursing animals, glimepiride is not recommended for use by nursing mothers.

### Pediatrics
Appropriate studies on the relationship of age to the effects of glimepiride have not been performed in the pediatric population. Safety and efficacy have not been established.

### Geriatrics
No significant pharmacokinetic differences were apparent in patients with type 2 diabetes older than 65 years of age when compared with patients younger than 65 years of age taking glimepiride. However, the mean area under the plasma concentration–time curve (AUC) at steady state for the older patients was about 13% lower than that for the younger patients. Also, the mean weight-adjusted clearance for the older patients was about 11% higher than that for the younger patients.

Hypoglycemia may be difficult to recognize in elderly patients. In addition, elderly patients are more likely to have age-related renal function impairment, which may cause increased sensitivity to the glucose-lowering effect of glimepiride. Therapy should be initiated with the minimum dose of glimepiride in these patients.

### Pharmacogenetics
Pharmacogenetic studies to determine the effects of glimepiride in different races have not been performed. However, in placebo-controlled studies, the antihyperglycemic effect of glimepiride in patients with type 2 diabetes was comparable in blacks, Hispanics, and whites.

### Drug interactions and/or related problems
The following drug interactions and/or related problems have been selected on the basis of their potential clinical significance (possible mechanism in parentheses where appropriate)—not necessarily inclusive (» = major clinical significance):

Note: Combinations containing any of the following medications, depending on the amount present, may also interact with this medication.

Highly protein-bound medications, such as:
Anti-inflammatory drugs, nonsteroidal (NSAIDs)
Anticoagulants, coumarin-derivative
Chloramphenicol
Monoamine oxidase (MAO) inhibitors
Probenecid
Salicylates
Sulfonamides
(these medications enhance the hypoglycemic effects of sulfonylureas when given concurrently; patients should be observed closely for symptoms of hypoglycemia or loss of glycemic control when glimepiride is added to or withdrawn from a regimen containing these medications)

Hyperglycemia-causing agents, such as:
Corticosteroids
Diuretics, especially thiazide diuretics
Estrogens
Isoniazid
Niacin
Oral contraceptives
Phenothiazines
Phenytoin
Sympathomimetic agents
Thyroid hormones
(these medications may cause loss of glycemic control; patients should be observed closely for symptoms of hypoglycemia or loss of glycemic control when glimepiride is added to or withdrawn from a regimen containing these medications)

Miconazole
(severe hypoglycemia has been reported shortly after concurrent use of some sulfonylureas with miconazole)

» Sympatholytics, such as beta-adrenergic blocking agents
(sympatholytics may blunt some of the symptoms of developing hypoglycemia, making detection of this condition more difficult)

### Laboratory value alterations
The following have been selected on the basis of their potential clinical significance (possible effect in parentheses where appropriate)—not necessarily inclusive (» = major clinical significance):

With physiology/laboratory test values
Transaminases, serum
(elevations have been reported)

### Medical considerations/Contraindications
The medical considerations/contraindications included have been selected on the basis of their potential clinical significance (reasons given in parentheses where appropriate)—not necessarily inclusive (» = major clinical significance).

*Except under special circumstances, this medication should not be used when the following medical problem exists:*

» Diabetic ketoacidosis, with or without coma
(this condition should be treated with insulin)

*Risk-benefit should be considered when the following medical problems exist:*

Adrenal insufficiency or
Debilitated physical condition or
Hepatic function impairment or
Malnutrition or
Pituitary insufficiency or
» Renal function impairment
(these conditions may cause increased sensitivity to the glucose-lowering effect of glimepiride; therapy with glimepiride should be initiated at the minimum recommended dose in these patients)

Fever, high or
Infection or
Surgery or
Trauma
(these conditions may cause loss of glycemic control; temporary therapy in combination with insulin or with insulin alone may be necessary)
Hypersensitivity to glimepiride

**Patient monitoring**
The following may be especially important in patient monitoring (other tests may be warranted in some patients, depending on condition; » = major clinical significance):

» Blood glucose determinations
(periodic monitoring recommended to determine therapeutic efficacy)
(daily monitoring of capillary blood glucose recommended in stable diabetics using combination insulin-glimepiride therapy)

» Glycosylated hemoglobin (hemoglobin $A_{1c}$) determinations
(monitoring recommended every 3 to 6 months to assess long-term glycemic control)

## Side/Adverse Effects

Note: It has been suggested, based on a study conducted by the University Group Diabetes Program (UGDP), that certain sulfonylurea antidiabetic agents increase cardiovascular mortality in diabetic patients, a population that already has a greater risk of cardiovascular disease and mortality when blood glucose is not controlled. Despite questions regarding the interpretation of the results and the adequacy of the experimental design, the findings of the UGDP study provide an adequate basis for caution, especially for certain high risk patients with coronary artery disease, congestive heart failure, or angina pectoris. The patient should be informed of the potential risks and advantages of sulfonylurea antidiabetic agents and of alternative modes of therapy.

The following side/adverse effects have been selected on the basis of their potential clinical significance (possible signs and symptoms in parentheses where appropriate)—not necessarily inclusive:

**Those indicating need for medical attention**
Incidence less frequent
*Hypoglycemia* (anxiety; behavior change similar to drunkenness; blurred vision; cold sweats; coma; confusion; cool pale skin; difficulty in concentrating; drowsiness; excessive hunger; fast heartbeat; headache; nausea; nervousness; nightmares; restless sleep; seizures; shakiness; slurred speech; unusual tiredness or weakness)—incidence 0.9 to 1.7%

Note: *Hypoglycemia* is more likely to occur when caloric intake is deficient, following ingestion of alcohol, following intense or prolonged exercise, or when more than one glucose-lowering medication is used.

Incidence rare
*Allergic skin reactions* (erythema; morbilliform or maculopapular eruptions; pruritus; urticaria); *blurred vision and/or changes in accommodation* (difficulty in focusing eyes); *hyponatremia* (depression; dizziness; headache; lethargy; nausea; swelling or puffiness of face, ankles, or hands with occasional progression to seizures, coma, or stupor)

Note: *Allergic skin reactions* may be transient and may disappear despite continued use of glimepiride. However, if skin reactions persist, use of glimepiride should be discontinued.

*Blurred vision and/or changes in accommodation* may be more pronounced when therapy with glimepiride is initiated and are thought to be caused by changes in blood glucose concentration.

**Those indicating need for medical attention only if they continue or are bothersome**
Incidence less frequent or rare
*Diarrhea; dizziness; gastrointestinal pain; headache; nausea; unusual tiredness or weakness; vomiting*

## Overdose

For more information on the management of overdose or unintentional ingestion, **contact a Poison Control Center** (see *Poison Control Center Listing*).

**Clinical effects of overdose**
The following effects have been selected on the basis of their potential clinical significance (possible signs and symptoms in parentheses where appropriate)—not necessarily inclusive:

*Hypoglycemia* (anxiety; behavior change similar to drunkenness; blurred vision; cold sweats; coma; confusion; cool pale skin; difficulty in concentrating; drowsiness; excessive hunger; fast heartbeat; headache; nausea; nervousness; nightmares; restless sleep; seizures; shakiness; slurred speech; unusual tiredness or weakness)

**Treatment of overdose**
Specific treatment—
Mild hypoglycemia without neurologic symptoms or loss of consciousness should be treated with immediate ingestion of glucose and adjustments to medication dosage and/or meal patterns.
Severe hypoglycemia including coma, seizures, or other neurologic impairment requires immediate emergency medical assistance. The patient should immediately be given an intravenous injection of a 50% glucose solution followed by a continuous infusion of a 10% glucose solution to maintain a blood glucose concentration of 100 mg per dL.
Monitoring—
Patients with severe hypoglycemia should be monitored for at least 24 to 48 hours.

## Patient Consultation

As an aid to patient consultation, refer to *Advice for the Patient, Glimepiride (Systemic)—Introductory Version*.
In providing consultation, consider emphasizing the following selected information (» = major clinical significance):

**Before using this medication**
» Conditions affecting use, especially:
Hypersensitivity to glimepiride
Pregnancy—Based on results of animal studies, glimepiride is not recommended for use during pregnancy; use of insulin during pregnancy allows for maintenance of blood glucose concentrations as close to normal as possible
Breast-feeding—May be distributed into human breast milk; not recommended because of potential for causing hypoglycemia in nursing infants
Use in the elderly—Hypoglycemia may be difficult to recognize in elderly patients
Other medications, especially sympatholytics
Other medical problems, especially diabetic ketoacidosis with or without coma and renal function impairment

**Proper use of this medication**
» Importance of adherence to recommended regimens for diet, exercise, and glucose monitoring
» Taking medication with breakfast or first main meal
» Proper dosing
» Proper storage

**Precautions while using this medication**
» Regular visits to physician to check progress
» *Carefully following special instructions of health care team*
Discussing use of alcohol
Not taking other medications unless discussed with physician
Getting counseling for family members to help them assist the patient with diabetes; also, special counseling for pregnancy planning and contraception
Making travel plans to include preparedness for diabetic emergencies and keeping meal times near the usual times with changing time zones
» Preparing for and understanding what to do in case of emergency; carrying medical history and current medication list and wearing medical identification
» Recognizing what brings on symptoms of hypoglycemia, such as using other antidiabetic medications; delaying or missing a meal or snack; exercising more than usual; drinking significant amounts of alcohol; illness, including vomiting or diarrhea
» Recognizing symptoms of hypoglycemia: anxiety; behavior change similar to drunkenness; blurred vision; cold sweats; confusion; cool, pale skin; difficulty in concentrating; drowsiness; excessive hunger; fast heartbeat; headache; nausea; nervousness; nightmares; restless sleep; shakiness; slurred speech; and unusual tiredness and weakness
» Knowing what to do if symptoms of hypoglycemia occur, such as eating glucose tablets or gel, corn syrup, honey, or sugar cubes; drinking fruit juice, nondiet soft drink, or sugar dissolved in water; or getting emergency medical assistance if symptoms are severe
» Recognizing what brings on symptoms of hyperglycemia, such as not taking enough or skipping a dose of antidiabetic medication, overeating or not following meal plan, having a fever or infection, exercising less than usual

» Recognizing symptoms of hyperglycemia and ketoacidosis: blurred vision; drowsiness; dry mouth; flushed, dry skin; fruit-like breath odor; increased urination (frequency and volume); ketones in urine; loss of appetite; stomachache, nausea, or vomiting; tiredness; troubled breathing (rapid and deep); unconsciousness; unusual thirst
» Knowing what to do if symptoms of hyperglycemia occur, such as checking blood glucose and contacting a member of the health care team

**Side/adverse effects**
Signs of potential side effects, especially hypoglycemia, allergic skin reactions, blurred vision and/or changes in accommodation, or hyponatremia

## General Dosing Information

Temporary use of glimepiride may be warranted during periods of loss of glycemic control in patients usually well-controlled with diet and exercise.

Secondary failure of oral antidiabetic therapy may occur in certain patients. This may be due to increasing severity of diabetes or to diminished responsiveness to the medication. Secondary failure may be treated by using insulin in combination with glimepiride. The fasting glucose concentration for instituting combination therapy is 150 mg per dL in plasma or serum. Periodic adjustments in insulin dosage may be necessary as guided by glucose and glycosylated hemoglobin concentrations. Combination insulin-glimepiride therapy may increase the potential for development of hypoglycemia.

When patients are transferred to glimepiride from another oral antidiabetic agent (with the exception of chlorpropamide), no transition period is required. When transferring patients from chlorpropamide, caution should be exercised during the first 1 to 2 weeks because of the prolonged retention of chlorpropamide in the body.

## Oral Dosage Forms

### GLIMEPIRIDE TABLETS

**Usual adult dose**
Antidiabetic—
Monotherapy—
Initial—Oral, 1 to 2 mg once a day with breakfast or the first main meal.
Maintenance—Oral, 1 to 4 mg once a day. After reaching a dose of 2 mg, increases in dosage should be made in increments of up to 2 mg every one to two weeks based on blood glucose response.
Note: Patients with renal function impairment should receive an initial dose of 1 mg once a day.
Combination therapy with insulin—
Oral, 8 mg once a day with breakfast or the first main meal.

**Usual adult prescribing limits**
8 mg once a day.

**Usual pediatric dose**
Safety and efficacy have not been established.

**Usual geriatric dose**
See *Usual adult dose*.
Note: Geriatric patients should receive an initial dose of 1 mg once a day.

**Strength(s) usually available**
U.S.—
1 mg (Rx) [*Amaryl* (scored; lactose [hydrous]; sodium starch glycolate; povidone; microcrystalline cellulose; magnesium stearate)].
2 mg (Rx) [*Amaryl* (scored; lactose [hydrous]; sodium starch glycolate; povidone; microcrystalline cellulose; magnesium stearate)].
4 mg (Rx) [*Amaryl* (scored; lactose [hydrous]; sodium starch glycolate; povidone; microcrystalline cellulose; magnesium stearate)].

**Packaging and storage**
Store between 15 and 30 °C (59 and 86 °F) in a well-closed container.

Revised: 08/04/98

---

**GLICLAZIDE**—See *Antidiabetic Agents, Sulfonylurea (Systemic)*

---

**GLIPIZIDE**—See *Antidiabetic Agents, Sulfonylurea (Systemic)*

---

# GLUCAGON  Systemic

VA CLASSIFICATION (Primary/Secondary): HS508/AD900; DX900; GA801
Commonly used brand name(s): *Glucagon Emergency Kit*.
Note: For a listing of dosage forms and brand names by country availability, see *Dosage Forms* section(s).

## Category

Antihypoglycemic; diagnostic aid adjunct (antispasmodic); antispasmodic; antidote (to beta-adrenergic blocking agents; to calcium channel blocking agents).

## Indications

Note: Bracketed information in the *Indications* section refers to uses that are not included in U.S. product labeling.

**Accepted**

Hypoglycemia (treatment)—Glucagon is indicated in the correction of severe hypoglycemic conditions. Glucagon is helpful in hypoglycemia only if liver glycogen is available. Glucagon and glucose may be used together without decreasing the effects of either. When glucagon is used for patients in a very deep state of coma (such as Stage IV or Stage V of Himwich), intravenous glucose is given in addition to glucagon for a more immediate response.

Radiography, gastrointestinal, adjunct—Glucagon is indicated in barium radiographic examinations to produce hypotonicity and relaxation of the esophagus, stomach, duodenum, small bowel, and colon. Glucagon is administered to provide relaxation of smooth musculature, and to decrease peristalsis thereby reducing patient discomfort, slowing emptying, and improving the examination quality.

[Abdominal imaging, digital angiographic, adjunct][1] or
[Abdominal imaging, computed tomographic, adjunct][1] or
[Abdominal imaging, magnetic resonance, adjunct][1] or
[Pelvic imaging, magnetic resonance, adjunct][1]—Glucagon is being used to inhibit bowel peristalsis in abdominal digital vascular imaging, abdominal and pelvic magnetic resonance imaging, and in abdominal CT scanning to prevent motion-related artifact.

[Bleeding, gastrointestinal (diagnosis adjunct)][1]—Glucagon may be beneficial as an adjuvant to Tc 99m–labeled red blood cells in the scintigraphic diagnosis of small bowel hemorrhage.

[Hysterosalpingography, adjunct][1]—Glucagon is used rarely by some clinicians to eliminate possible spasm of the fallopian tubes during hysterosalpingography in those patients whose fallopian tubes are not visualized during examination.

[Toxicity, beta-adrenergic blocking agent (treatment)][1]—Glucagon administered in large intravenous doses is used to treat the cardiotoxic effects, specifically bradycardia and hypotension, in overdoses of beta-adrenergic blocking agents. Glucagon may be used with isoproterenol or dobutamine. Supplemental potassium may be necessary for treated patients since glucagon tends to reduce serum potassium.

[Toxicity, calcium channel blocking agent (treatment)][1]—Glucagon may be of use in treating myocardial depression due to calcium channel blocking agents in those patients in whom conventional therapies have been ineffective.

[Esophageal obstruction, foreign body (treatment)][1]—Glucagon is used in the treatment of lower esophageal obstruction due to foreign bodies, including food boluses.

**Unaccepted**

Glucagon is of little or no help in the treatment of hypoglycemia in conditions where hepatic glycogen stores are depleted, such as starvation, adrenal insufficiency, or chronic hypoglycemia.

Glucagon should not be used to treat birth asphyxia or hypoglycemia in premature infants or in infants who have had intrauterine growth retardation.

Glucagon has been used as an aid in the diagnosis of insulinoma and pheochromocytoma; however, USP advisory panels do not generally recommend this use because of questions about safety.

[1]Not included in Canadian product labeling.

## Pharmacology/Pharmacokinetics

### Physicochemical characteristics
Source—Beef or porcine pancreas.
Chemical group—Glucagon is a single-chain polypeptide containing 29 amino acid residues. Chemically unrelated to insulin. One USP Unit of glucagon is equivalent to 1 International Unit of glucagon and also to about 1 mg of glucagon.
Molecular weight—3482.78.

### Mechanism of action/Effect
Promotes hepatic glycogenolysis and gluconeogenesis. Stimulates adenylate cyclase to produce increased cyclic-AMP, which is involved in a series of enzymatic activities. The resultant effects are increased concentrations of plasma glucose, a relaxant effect on smooth musculature, and an inotropic myocardial effect. Hepatic stores of glycogen are necessary for glucagon to elicit an antihypoglycemic effect.

### Biotransformation
Primarily hepatic and renal through enzymatic proteolysis.

### Half-life
10 minutes (plasma).

### Onset of action
Hyperglycemic action—
    Intravenous: 5 to 20 minutes.
    Intramuscular—15 minutes.
    Subcutaneous—30 to 45 minutes.
Smooth muscle relaxation—
    Intravenous:
        0.25 to 2 USP Units—45 seconds.
    Intramuscular:
        1 USP Unit—8 to 10 minutes.
        2 USP Units—4 to 7 minutes.

### Duration of action
Hyperglycemic action—
    90 minutes.
Smooth muscle relaxation—
    Intravenous:
        0.25 to 0.5 USP Units—9 to 17 minutes.
        2 USP Units—22 to 25 minutes.
    Intramuscular:
        1 USP Unit—12 to 27 minutes.
        2 USP Units—21 to 32 minutes.

## Precautions to Consider

### Cross-sensitivity and/or related problems
Patients who are allergic to beef or porcine proteins may be allergic to glucagon, since glucagon is either of beef or porcine origin.

### Carcinogenicity/Mutagenicity
No studies have been done on carcinogenicity or mutagenicity.

### Pregnancy/Reproduction
Fertility—Studies in rats have not shown that glucagon causes impaired fertility.
Pregnancy—Adequate and well-controlled studies in humans have not been done.
Studies in rats have not shown that glucagon causes adverse effects on the fetus.
FDA Pregnancy Category B.

### Breast-feeding
Problems in humans have not been documented. It is not known whether glucagon is distributed into breast milk. However, because glucagon is inactivated by gastric acid, problems are unlikely. Also, glucagon has a short half-life and is usually used for a short duration.

### Pediatrics
Appropriate studies performed to date have not demonstrated pediatrics-specific problems that would limit the usefulness of glucagon in children.

### Geriatrics
Appropriate studies on the relationship of age to the effects of glucagon have not been performed in the geriatric population. However, geriatrics-specific problems that would limit the usefulness of this medication in the elderly are not expected.

### Drug interactions and/or related problems
The following drug interactions and/or related problems have been selected on the basis of their potential clinical significance (possible mechanism in parentheses where appropriate)—not necessarily inclusive (» = major clinical significance):

Anticoagulants, coumarin- or indandione-derivative
    (concurrent use with glucagon may potentiate the anticoagulant effects; enhanced anticoagulant activity has been reported with unusually high doses such as 25 mg or more per day for 2 or more days)

### Laboratory value alterations
The following have been selected on the basis of their potential clinical significance (possible effect in parentheses where appropriate)—not necessarily inclusive (» = major clinical significance):

With physiology/laboratory test values
    Potassium
        (serum concentrations may be decreased with use of large doses)

### Medical considerations/Contraindications
The medical considerations/contraindications included have been selected on the basis of their potential clinical significance (reasons given in parentheses where appropriate)—not necessarily inclusive (» = major clinical significance).

*Risk-benefit should be considered when the following medical problems exist:*

Allergy to beef or porcine proteins, history of
» Diabetes mellitus
    (risk of hyperglycemia when glucagon is used as a diagnostic adjunct; however, glucagon is commonly used by diabetic patients to treat hypoglycemia resulting from overdose of oral antidiabetic agents or insulin)
» Insulinoma, or history of
    (may paradoxically decrease blood glucose concentrations)
» Pheochromocytoma
    (may cause hypertension due to stimulation of the release of catecholamines)
Sensitivity to glucagon

## Side/Adverse Effects
The following side/adverse effects have been selected on the basis of their potential clinical significance (possible signs and symptoms in parentheses where appropriate)—not necessarily inclusive:

### Those indicating need for medical attention
Incidence less frequent
    *Allergic reaction* (dizziness; lightheadedness; skin rash; trouble in breathing)

### Those indicating need for medical attention only if they continue or are bothersome
*Nausea or vomiting*—incidence is generally dependent upon dose and (with intravenous use) the rate of injection; these effects may be diminished by slower intravenous administration

## Overdose
For specific information on the agents used in the management of glucagon overdose, see *Potassium Supplements (Systemic)* monograph.
For more information on the management of overdose or unintentional ingestion, **contact a Poison Control Center** (see *Poison Control Center Listing*).

### Clinical effects of overdose (in order of usual occurrence)
The following effects have been selected on the basis of their potential clinical significance (possible signs and symptoms in parentheses where appropriate)—not necessarily inclusive:

*Continuing nausea; continuing vomiting; hypokalemic syndrome* (severe weakness of extremities and trunk; loss of appetite; nausea; vomiting; irregular heartbeat; muscle cramps or pain)

### Treatment of overdose
Due to the short half-life of glucagon, treatment of glucagon overdose is primarily symptomatic and supportive.
Specific treatment—Treating hypokalemia with potassium supplementation as required.
Monitoring—Monitoring of serum electrolytes, especially potassium; monitoring blood glucose concentrations and blood pressure.
Supportive care—Replacing fluids as necessary, due to excessive nausea and vomiting. Patients in whom intentional overdose is confirmed or suspected should be referred for psychiatric consultation.

## Patient Consultation
As an aid to patient consultation, refer to *Advice for the Patient, Glucagon (Systemic)*.
In providing consultation, consider emphasizing the following selected information (» = major clinical significance):

### Before using this medication
» Conditions affecting use, especially:
 Sensitivity to glucagon
 Other medical problems, especially diabetes mellitus (for diagnostic procedures only), insulinoma or history of, or pheochromocytoma

### Proper use of this medication
» Using medication only as directed by physician; need to explain use to family or friend; reviewing use on a regular basis
» Reading directions in glucagon kit before medication is actually needed; knowing how to reconstitute and inject properly
» Knowing which type of syringe to use; keeping sterile syringe and needles always readily available; knowing how to use syringe supplied with some kits
 May be reconstituted when emergency occurs or ahead of time, but must be used within 48 hours of reconstitution
» Not keeping after expiration date on vial; checking date regularly; replacing medication before it expires
» Proper dosing
» *Proper storage*
 Storing unmixed medication at room temperature
 Storing mixed solution in refrigerator for no longer than 48 hours and protecting from freezing

### Precautions while using this medication
» Importance of knowing symptoms of hypoglycemia: mild abdominal or stomach pain; anxious feeling; continuing chills; cold sweats; confusion; convulsions; cool, pale skin; difficulty in concentrating; drowsiness; fast heartbeat; continuing headache; excessive hunger; continuing nausea or vomiting; nervousness; shakiness; unconsciousness; unsteady walk; vision changes; unusual tiredness or weakness
» Importance of eating some form of sugar (glucose tablets or gel; fruit juice; corn syrup; honey; nondiet soft drinks; sugar cubes or table sugar dissolved in water) if symptoms of hypoglycemia occur
» *Steps to be taken after glucagon is injected for hypoglycemia in unconscious patient:*
» After injection, turning patient on one side to avoid choking if emesis occurs
 Contacting an emergency medical service and physician
 Monitoring blood glucose concentrations throughout episode, treatment, and for 3 to 4 hours after patient becomes conscious
 If patient not conscious in 5 minutes (intravenous use) or 15 minutes (intramuscular use), giving second dose; simultaneously, getting emergency help
 When patient conscious enough to swallow, initially giving some form of sugar to take orally then having patient eat crackers and cheese or half a sandwich or drink a glass of milk to prevent hypoglycemia from recurring before the next scheduled meal or snack
 If nausea and vomiting prevent a patient from swallowing some form of sugar for an hour after injection, getting medical assistance
» Importance of keeping physician informed of hypoglycemic episodes and use of glucagon
» Replacing supply of glucagon as soon as possible

### Side/adverse effects
Signs of potential side effects, especially allergic reaction

## General Dosing Information

### For use as an antihypoglycemic
For ambulatory-care use of glucagon kits that do not supply the user with a syringe, USP medical advisory panelists generally recommend that a standard 1-mL insulin syringe be used for injection. Using an insulin syringe will ensure availability when needed and reduce the potential for confusion or improper injection. However, the injection should be made at a 90-degree angle rather than the standard subcutaneous approach. Although the standard insulin syringe will not generally allow for a true intramuscular injection, the deeper injection may provide for a more rapid response time than would the subcutaneous route. A different syringe may be considered if the user is able to make such an injection in an appropriate manner and/or if the insulin syringe being used will not hold the appropriate amount of glucagon solution required.

A rapid blood glucose test should be performed to confirm that the patient has low blood sugar. Emergency medical assistance should also be obtained as soon as possible. Blood glucose should also be monitored throughout the hypoglycemic episode, treatment period, and for 3 to 4 hours after the patient regains consciousness.

Patient response usually occurs 5 minutes following intravenous administration or 15 minutes following intramuscular administration. Dose may be repeated if no response is evident within this time. Medical care will be needed if response is not obtained following a second glucagon dose; intravenous glucose will be required if the patient fails to respond to glucagon.

After the patient is sufficiently alert and oriented, oral supplemental sugar (glucose or sucrose) must be given to prevent secondary hypoglycemia. Patients with insulin-dependent diabetes (type I) do not have as great a response in blood glucose levels as do the non-insulin-dependent (type II), stable diabetic patients. Therefore, it is especially important that supplemental carbohydrates be given as soon as possible to patients with type I diabetes. Emergency room evaluation and/or hospital admission should be considered for all patients experiencing a hypoglycemic episode from oral antidiabetic agents (especially chlorpropamide), since hypoglycemia may recur after blood glucose concentrations are normalized.

If nausea and vomiting result from glucagon administration and the patient is unable to ingest some form of sugar for 1 hour, medical assistance should be obtained immediately. Severe hypoglycemia may rapidly recur under these circumstances.

## Parenteral Dosage Forms

Note: Bracketed uses in the *Dosage Forms* section refer to categories of use and/or indications that are not included in U.S. product labeling.

### GLUCAGON FOR INJECTION USP

**Usual adult and adolescent dose**
Antihypoglycemic—
 Intramuscular, intravenous, or subcutaneous, 0.5 to 1 mg (0.5 to 1 USP Unit), repeated in twenty minutes if necessary.
Diagnostic aid—Radiography, gastrointestinal or
[Abdominal imaging, computed tomographic or magnetic resonance][1] or
[Pelvic imaging, computed tomographic or magnetic resonance][1] or
[Hysterosalpingography]—
 Intravenous, 0.25 to 1 mg (0.25 to 1 USP Unit).
 Note: Doses in the upper range and/or intramuscular dosing may be preferred by some clinicians to achieve hypotonicity during the prolonged scan times associated with magnetic resonance imaging. The duration of action of glucagon is longer with intramuscular dosing.
[Antidote (to beta-adrenergic blocking agents)][1]—
 Intravenous, initially, 50 to 150 mcg (0.05 to 0.15 USP Unit) per kg of body weight over one minute, to be followed by a 1 to 5 mg-per-hour infusion.
[Antidote (to calcium channel blocking agents)][1]—
 Intravenous, initially 2 mg (2 USP Units). Maintenance dosing is then titrated according to patient response.
[Antispasmodic (esophageal obstruction due to foreign body)][1]—
 Intravenous, 0.5 to 2 mg (0.5 to 2 USP Units), repeated in ten to twenty minutes if necessary.

**Usual pediatric dose**
Antihypoglycemic—
 Intramuscular, intravenous, or subcutaneous, 25 mcg (0.025 USP Unit) per kg of body weight, up to a maximum dose of 1 mg (1 USP Unit), repeated in twenty minutes if necessary.

**Size(s) usually available**
U.S.—
 1 mg (1 USP Unit) (Rx) [*Glucagon Emergency Kit* (phenol 0.2%, in diluent) [GENERIC (Lilly—phenol 0.2%, in diluent)].
 10 mg (10 USP Units) (Rx) [GENERIC (Lilly—phenol 0.2%, in diluent)].
Canada—
 1 mg (1 USP Unit) (Rx) [*Glucagon Emergency Kit* (phenol 0.2%, in diluent) [GENERIC (Lilly—phenol 0.2%, in diluent)].

**Packaging and storage**
Prior to reconstitution, store between 15 and 30 °C (59 and 86 °F), unless otherwise specified by manufacturer.

**Preparation of dosage form**
Check expiration dating.
See patient instruction sheet in glucagon package.
Use the diluent provided in the package for doses of 2 USP Units (2 mg) or less. When more than 2 USP Units (2 mg) are needed, sterile water for injection should be used, rather than the diluent provided, to minimize the possibility of thrombophlebitis, central nervous system toxicity, or myocardial depression, which may be caused by the phenol preservative in the manufacturer-supplied diluent.

**Stability**
When stored between 2 and 8 °C (36 and 46 °F) and reconstituted with diluent provided, the reconstituted solution retains potency for 48 hours.
Solutions prepared with sterile water for injection should be used immediately.

## Glucagon (Systemic)

**Incompatibilities**
Glucagon may precipitate from saline solution and solutions having a pH of 3 to 9.5.

**Auxiliary labeling**
- Refrigerate after reconstituting.
- After reconstituting, discard after 48 hours.

**Note**
Make sure patient has syringe and needles or understands use of syringe supplied with kit.
Check patient's understanding of preparing and administering medication.
Make sure patient routinely checks expiration date of medication.

[1]Not included in Canadian product labeling.

Revised: 01/13/93

---

**GLUTETHIMIDE**—The *Glutethimide (Systemic)* monograph is not included in this published version of the USP DI database. Copies of the monograph are available on request from Micromedex, Inc. - Reprint Requests, 6200 S. Syracuse Way, Suite 300, Englewood, CO 80111; telephone (303) 486-6400; telefax (303) 486-6464; Email: USPDI@MDX.COM.

---

**GLYBURIDE**—See *Antidiabetic Agents, Sulfonylurea (Systemic)*

---

**GLYCERIN**—See *Glycerin (Systemic)*; *Laxatives (Local)*

---

**GLYCERIN**—The *Glycerin (Systemic)* monograph is not included in this published version of the USP DI database. Copies of the monograph are available on request from Micromedex, Inc. - Reprint Requests, 6200 S. Syracuse Way, Suite 300, Englewood, CO 80111; telephone (303) 486-6400; telefax (303) 486-6464; Email: USPDI@MDX.COM.

---

**GLYCOPYRROLATE**—See *Anticholinergics/Antispasmodics (Systemic)*

---

# GOLD COMPOUNDS Systemic

This monograph includes information on the following: 1) Auranofin; 2) Aurothioglucose; 3) Gold Sodium Thiomalate.

INN: Gold Sodium Thiomalate—Sodium Aurothiomalate

VA CLASSIFICATION (Primary): MS109

Commonly used brand name(s): *Myochrysine*[3]; *Ridaura*[1]; *Solganal*[2].

A commonly used name for gold sodium thiomalate is sodium aurothiomalate.

Note: For a listing of dosage forms and brand names by country availability, see *Dosage Forms* section(s).

## Category
Antirheumatic (disease-modifying).

## Indications
Note: Bracketed information in the *Indications* section refers to uses that are not included in U.S. product labeling.

**Accepted**
Arthritis, rheumatoid (treatment) or
Arthritis, juvenile (treatment)—Auranofin is indicated in the treatment of adult rheumatoid arthritis and is used in the treatment of [juvenile arthritis][1] Aurothioglucose and gold sodium thiomalate are indicated in the treatment of adult or juvenile rheumatoid arthritis. These agents are usually used for treating patients who show evidence of continued or additional disease activity despite conservative therapy, e.g., with salicylates (especially aspirin) or other nonsteroidal anti-inflammatory agents, glucocorticoids, etc. Gold compounds may induce remission or suppression of rheumatoid arthritis. In chronic advanced rheumatoid arthritis, they may prevent further damage to affected joints; however, they do not reverse existing damage.

[Arthritis, psoriatic (treatment)][1] or
[Felty's syndrome (treatment)][1]—Gold compounds are used in the treatment of these rheumatic conditions.

[1]Not included in Canadian product labeling.

## Pharmacology/Pharmacokinetics

**Physicochemical characteristics**
Molecular weight—
  Auranofin: 678.48.
  Aurothioglucose: 392.18.
  Gold sodium thiomalate: 758.16.

**Mechanism of action/Effect**
The predominant clinical effect of the gold compounds appears to be suppression of the synovitis of the active stage of rheumatoid disease. The precise mechanism of anti-inflammatory effect is unknown, but it has been suggested that these agents alter cellular mechanisms by inhibiting sulfhydryl systems. Other proposed mechanisms for gold compounds' effects in patients with rheumatoid arthritis include alteration or inhibition of various enzyme systems, suppression of the phagocytic activity of macrophages and polymorphonuclear leukocytes, alteration of immune response, and alteration of collagen biosynthesis. *In vitro*, the gold compounds have been shown to inhibit prostaglandin synthesis.

**Absorption**
Approximately 25% of the gold in a dose of auranofin is absorbed from the gastrointestinal tract.

**Protein binding**
Auranofin—Moderate. In blood, approximately 60% of the gold is bound to plasma proteins; the remainder is present in red blood cells.
Aurothioglucose and
Gold sodium thiomalate—Very high; to plasma proteins only.

**Biotransformation**
Auranofin—Metabolized so rapidly that the intact molecule has not been detected in blood.
Aurothioglucose and
Gold sodium thiomalate—The metabolic fate is unknown, but it is believed that these compounds are not broken down to elemental gold.

**Half-life**
Elimination—
  Oral (determined [as gold] after reaching steady-state blood concentrations):
    Blood—21 to 31 days; average 26 days.
    Tissue (body)—42 to 128 days; average 80 days.
  Parenteral:
    Dependent on dose and duration of therapy.

**Onset of action**
Oral—Usually 3 to 4 months but up to 6 months in some patients.
Parenteral—At least 6 to 8 weeks.

**Time to steady-state blood concentration**
Auranofin (measured as blood gold concentration)—3 months.

**Steady-state blood concentration**
Auranofin—Blood gold concentrations of about 68 mcg per mL are achieved with administration of 6 mg per day.

**Elimination**
Oral—60% of the absorbed gold (15% of the administered dose) is excreted in the urine; the remainder of the dose is excreted in the feces.
Parenteral—60 to 90% renal, very slowly; 10 to 40% fecal, mostly via biliary secretion.

## Precautions to Consider

**Cross-sensitivity and/or related problems**
Patients sensitive to gold or other heavy metals may be sensitive to this medication also.
Patients sensitive to sesame products may also be sensitive to the sesame oil vehicle of parenteral aurothioglucose.
Patients intolerant of parabens may be intolerant of parenteral aurothioglucose, which may contain propylparaben, also.

### Carcinogenicity/Tumorigenicity
For auranofin—Renal tubular cell karyomegaly and cytomegaly, renal adenoma, and malignant renal epithelial tumors have been reported in rats receiving 1 and 2.5 mg per kg of body weight (mg/kg) per day (8 and 21 times the usual human dose, respectively) for 24 months. In another study, renal tubular epithelial tumors occurred in rats receiving 23 mg/kg per day (192 times the human dose) for 12 months. In a third study, no tumorigenicity was demonstrated in mice receiving 1, 3, or 9 mg/kg per day (8, 24, and 72 times the human dose, respectively) for 18 months.

For aurothioglucose and gold sodium thiomalate—Renal adenoma and adenocarcinoma have been reported in rats with prolonged administration of frequent, high doses of parenteral gold compounds (2 mg per kg weekly for 45 weeks followed by 6 mg per kg daily for 47 weeks in one study; 3 mg per kg or 6 mg per kg daily for up to 2 years in a second study). The adenomas were similar to those produced in rats by chronic administration of other heavy metals such as lead or nickel. Renal adenoma has not been reported in humans receiving these medications therapeutically.

### Mutagenicity
High concentrations (313 to 700 nanograms per mL) of auranofin increased the frequency of mutations in the mouse lymphoma forward mutation assay in the presence of a rat liver microsomal preparation. No mutagenic activity was observed in the Ames (salmonella) test, the forward and reverse mutation inducement assay with *Saccharomyces*, the *in vitro* transformation of BALB/T3 cell mouse assay, or the dominant lethal assay.

### Pregnancy/Reproduction
Fertility—Studies in rats have shown that auranofin decreases litter size, probably because of maternal toxicity, when given in doses of 5 mg/kg per day (42 times the human dose) but not when given in doses of 2.5 mg/kg per day (21 times the human dose).

Pregnancy—For auranofin: Well-controlled and adequate studies in humans have not been done. However, studies in rabbits have shown that auranofin increases the incidence of resorptions and abortions, decreases fetal weight, and causes congenital abnormalities, mainly abdominal defects such as gastroschisis and umbilical hernia, when administered in doses of 0.5, 3, or 6 mg/kg per day (up to 50 times the usual human dose). Other studies in animals have shown that auranofin increases the incidence of resorptions and decreases fetal weight in rats receiving 5 mg/kg per day (42 times the human dose), probably because of maternal toxicity, but not in those receiving 2.5 mg/kg per day (21 times the human dose). Studies in mice receiving 5 mg/kg per day (42 times the human dose) showed no teratogenic effects

FDA Pregnancy Category C.

For aurothioglucose and gold sodium thiomalate: Studies in humans have not been done. However, studies in animals have shown parenteral gold compounds to cause hydrocephalus and microphthalmia in rats (at a dose of 25 mg per kg per day from Day 6 through Day 15 of gestation); and gastroschisis; umbilical hernia; anomalies of the brain, heart, lung, and skeleton; microphthalmia; and limb defects in rabbits (at a dose of 20 to 45 mg per kg per day from Day 6 through Day 18 of gestation)

FDA Pregnancy Category C.

### Breast-feeding
Problems in humans have not been documented. However, use by nursing mothers is not recommended because of the potential for serious adverse effects in the infant. Parenterally administered gold is excreted in human breast milk and has been detected in the blood of a nursing infant. It is not known whether auranofin is excreted in human breast milk, but gold has been detected in the milk of lactating rats and mice following auranofin administration.

### Pediatrics
For auranofin—Although appropriate studies have not been done in the pediatric population, auranofin is being used in the treatment of juvenile arthritis.

For aurothioglucose and gold sodium thiomalate—Studies performed to date have not demonstrated pediatrics-specific problems that would limit the usefulness of these medications in children.

### Geriatrics
Studies performed to date have not demonstrated geriatrics-specific problems that would limit the usefulness of these medications in the elderly. However, elderly patients are more likely to have age-related renal function impairment, which may require caution in patients receiving gold compounds.

### Dental
The leukopenic and/or thrombocytopenic effects of gold compounds may result in an increased incidence of microbial infection, delayed healing, and gingival bleeding. If leukopenia or thrombocytopenia occurs, dental work should be deferred until blood counts have returned to normal and patients should be instructed in proper oral hygiene, including caution in use of regular toothbrushes, dental floss, and toothpicks.

Gold compounds may cause glossitis, gingivitis, or stomatitis.

### Drug interactions and/or related problems
The following drug interactions and/or related problems have been selected on the basis of their potential clinical significance (possible mechanism in parentheses where appropriate)—not necessarily inclusive (» = major clinical significance):

Bone marrow depressants (See *Appendix II*) or
Dermatitis-causing medications, other or
Hepatotoxic medications, other (See *Appendix II*) or
Nephrotoxic medications, other (See *Appendix II*)
 (the possibility of additive toxicity should be considered if these medications are used concurrently with gold compounds)

» Penicillamine
 (concurrent use of penicillamine with gold compounds may be especially likely to increase the risk of serious hematologic and/or renal adverse effects; concurrent use is not recommended)

### Laboratory value alterations
The following have been selected on the basis of their potential clinical significance (possible effect in parentheses where appropriate)—not necessarily inclusive (» = major clinical significance):

With physiology/laboratory test values
 Hematocrit and
 Hemoglobin concentration and
 Platelet count and
 White blood cell count
  (may be decreased)

 Liver function tests
  (abnormalities may occur)

 Urine protein concentrations
  (may be increased)

### Medical considerations/Contraindications
The medical considerations/contraindications included have been selected on the basis of their potential clinical significance (reasons given in parentheses where appropriate)—not necessarily inclusive (» = major clinical significance).

*Except under special circumstances, this medication should not be used when the following medical problems exist:*

» Serious adverse effects associated with previous gold therapy, such as bone marrow aplasia or other severe hematologic disorders, exfoliative dermatitis, necrotizing enterocolitis, or pulmonary fibrosis, history of
 (high risk of recurrence)

*Risk-benefit should be considered when the following medical problems exist:*

» Blood dyscrasias or a history of agranulocytosis or hemorrhagic diathesis

 Blood dyscrasias, such as granulocytopenia or anemia caused by drug sensitivity, history of

 Colitis—especially for auranofin

» Debilitation, severe

 Inadequate or compromised cerebral or cardiovascular circulation

 Renal disease, or history of

» Sensitivity to any of the gold compounds, history of

» Sjögren's syndrome in rheumatoid arthritis

 Skin rash

» Systemic lupus erythematosus

» Urticaria or eczema

### Patient monitoring
The following may be especially important in patient monitoring (other tests may be warranted in some patients, depending on condition; » = major clinical significance):

Hepatic function tests and
Renal function tests
 (recommended prior to initiation of auranofin therapy and at appropriate intervals during therapy)

Platelet counts and
Total white blood cell counts and
Urinalyses, especially urinary protein determination
 (recommended prior to therapy; urinalysis or urinary protein determination recommended prior to each injection and blood and platelet counts [or platelet estimations] recommended before every sec-

ond injection; also, blood and platelet counts and urinalysis recommended at least monthly during auranofin administration)

## Side/Adverse Effects
See *Table 1*, page 1569.

## Patient Consultation
As an aid to patient consultation, refer to *Advice for the Patient, Gold Compounds (Systemic)*.

In providing consultation, consider emphasizing the following selected information (» = major clinical significance):

### Before using this medication
» Conditions affecting use, especially:
  Sensitivity to gold, other heavy metals, or sesame products
  Pregnancy—Studies in humans have not been done, but gold compounds have caused teratogenic and fetotoxic effects in animal studies
  Breast-feeding—Use is not recommended because of potential adverse effects in the nursing infant; aurothioglucose and gold sodium thiomalate are excreted in human breast milk; it is not known whether auranofin is excreted in human breast milk
  Dental—Risk of adverse effects such as infection, delayed healing, and gingival bleeding associated with blood dyscrasias, as well as gold compound–induced gingivitis, glossitis, and/or stomatitis
  Other medications, especially penicillamine
  Other medical problems, especially serious adverse effects to prior gold therapy, blood dyscrasias (especially hemorrhagic or caused by sensitivity to a medication), severe debilitation, Sjögren's syndrome, systemic lupus erythematosus, eczema, or urticaria

### Proper use of this medication
Compliance with therapy; symptomatic relief may not occur until after three to six months of continuous use
» Proper dosing
*For auranofin (oral dosage form) only*
» Not taking more medication than amount prescribed
  Missed dose: If dosing schedule is
    Once a day: Taking as soon as possible; not taking if not remembered until next day; not doubling doses
    More than once a day: Taking as soon as possible; not taking if almost time for next dose; not doubling doses
» Proper storage

### Precautions while using this medication
Possibility of phototoxicity
*For oral dosage form only*
Regular visits to physician to check progress during therapy; blood and urine tests may be required to detect possible adverse effects
*For parenteral dosage forms only*
Possibility of nitritoid reactions immediately following injection
Possibility of joint pain occurring for 1 or 2 days after injection

### Side/adverse effects
Signs and symptoms of potential side effects, especially allergic reactions, blood dyscrasias, central nervous system or neurologic effects, cutaneous or dermatologic effects, difficulty in swallowing, fever, ulcerative enterocolitis, gastrointestinal bleeding, hepatotoxicity, mucous membrane reactions, ocular effects, pulmonary effects, and renal effects
Possibility of side effects occurring up to many months after discontinuation of medication

## General Dosing Information
Concurrent therapy with salicylates or other nonsteroidal anti-inflammatory drugs or glucocorticoids is necessary, especially during the first few months of gold therapy, to provide symptomatic relief.

Following mild adverse reactions, therapy should be discontinued temporarily. After the reactions have cleared, therapy may be resumed using a reduced dosage schedule.

Therapy should not be reinstituted after severe or idiosyncratic reactions.

### For treatment of adverse effects
Recommended treatment may include
• Discontinuing the medication promptly.
• Administering appropriate therapy, such as topical adrenocorticoids, soothing lotions, or local anesthetics, for relief of mild to moderately severe skin or mucous membrane reactions.
• Administering systemic glucocorticoids (i.e., 10 to 40 mg of prednisone daily in divided doses) for severe or generalized dermatitis or stomatitis.
• Administering high doses of glucocorticoids (i.e., 40 to 100 mg of prednisone daily in divided doses) if required for severe pulmonary or other complications. If symptoms do not improve with high-dose glucocorticoid treatment, or if significant glucocorticoid-induced adverse effects develop, use of a chelating agent such as dimercaprol (BAL) to enhance gold excretion may be considered. However, the efficacy of BAL has not been established. Also, caution in use of BAL is recommended because of its toxicity.
• Administering other supportive treatment as required for specific complications.

---

### AURANOFIN

## Summary of Differences
Pharmacology/pharmacokinetics:
  Protein-binding—Less extensive than with parenteral gold formulations.
  Onset of action—Usually 3 to 4 months, but up to 6 months in some patients.
Precautions:
  Patient monitoring—
    Hepatic and renal function tests also recommended.
Side/adverse effects:
  Nitritoid reactions and temporary joint pain that sometimes occur following injections have not been reported.
  Lower incidence of mucous membrane reactions (other than stomatitis) than with injectible gold formulations.
  Higher incidence of gastrointestinal irritation (e.g., cramping, indigestion, constipation, diarrhea, nausea) than with injectible gold products.

## Additional Dosing Information
See also *General Dosing Information*.

Diarrhea occurring during auranofin therapy may respond to a reduction in dosage.

## Oral Dosage Forms
### AURANOFIN CAPSULES
**Usual adult dose**
Oral, 6 mg once a day or 3 mg twice a day.

Note: Initiation of therapy with doses higher than 6 mg per day is associated with an increased incidence of diarrhea and is not recommended.

If an adequate response has not been achieved after six months, the daily dose may be increased to 9 mg, administered in three divided doses. If an adequate response has not been achieved after three months of treatment at the higher dose, therapy should be discontinued.

**Usual adult prescribing limits**
9 mg per day.

**Usual pediatric dose**
Dosage has not been established.

**Strength(s) usually available**
U.S.—
  3 mg (Rx) [*Ridaura* (lactose)].
Canada—
  3 mg (Rx) [*Ridaura* (lactose)].

**Packaging and storage**
Store below 40 °C (104 °F), preferably between 15 and 30 °C (59 and 86 °F), unless otherwise specified by manufacturer.

---

### AUROTHIOGLUCOSE

## Summary of Differences
Pharmacology/pharmacokinetics:
  Protein-binding—More extensive than with auranofin.
  Onset of action—Usually 6 to 8 weeks.
Side/adverse effects:
  May cause nitritoid reactions and temporary joint pain after an injection.
  Higher incidence of mucous membrane reactions (other than stomatitis) than with auranofin.

Lower incidence of gastrointestinal irritation (e.g., cramping, indigestion, constipation, diarrhea, nausea) than with auranofin.

## Additional Dosing Information
See also *General Dosing Information*.

Aurothioglucose is for intramuscular injection only. Injections should be administered deeply into the upper outer quadrant of the gluteal region, using an 18-gauge, 1½-inch (2-inch for obese patients) needle.

Before withdrawing the dose, the vial should be thoroughly shaken to obtain a uniform suspension.

The needle and syringe used to withdraw the dose from the vial must be dry.

To facilitate withdrawing the suspension from the vial, the vial may be heated by immersing in warm water.

## Parenteral Dosage Forms
### STERILE AUROTHIOGLUCOSE SUSPENSION USP
**Usual adult and adolescent dose**
Initial—
  Intramuscular, 10 mg the first week, 25 mg the second and third weeks, then 25 to 50 mg once a week until a total dose of 800 mg to 1 gram has been given.
Maintenance—
  Intramuscular, 25 to 50 mg every two weeks for two to twenty weeks, then 25 to 50 mg every three to four weeks.

**Usual adult prescribing limits**
Up to 50 mg per week.

**Usual pediatric dose**
Children up to 6 years of age—Dosage has not been established.
Children 6 to 12 years of age—Intramuscular, 2.5 mg the first week, 6.25 mg the second and third weeks, then 12.5 mg every week until a total dose of 200 to 250 mg has been given; thereafter, 6.25 to 12.5 mg every three to four weeks.

**Strength(s) usually available**
U.S.—
  50 mg per mL (Rx) [*Solganal* (propylparaben)].

**Packaging and storage**
Store below 40 °C (104 °F), preferably between 15 and 30 °C (59 and 86 °F), unless otherwise specified by manufacturer. Protect from light. Protect from freezing.

**Auxiliary labeling**
• Shake well.

---

## GOLD SODIUM THIOMALATE

## Summary of Differences
Pharmacology/pharmacokinetics:
  Protein-binding—More extensive than with auranofin.
  Onset of action—Usually 6 to 8 weeks.

Side/adverse effects:
  May cause nitritoid reactions and temporary joint pain after an injection.
  Higher incidence of mucous membrane reactions (other than stomatitis) than with auranofin.
  Lower incidence of gastrointestinal irritation (e.g., cramping, indigestion, constipation, diarrhea, nausea) than with auranofin.

## Additional Dosing Information
See also *General Dosing Information*.

Gold sodium thiomalate should be administered only by intramuscular injection, preferably intraglutteally.

To reinstitute therapy following mild adverse reactions, an initial dose of 5 mg is given. If the medication is well tolerated, the dose may be increased in 5- to 10-mg increments at weekly to monthly intervals until a dose of 25 to 50 mg is reached.

Maintenance treatment at intervals of 1 to 3 weeks may be required for some patients.

## Parenteral Dosage Forms
### GOLD SODIUM THIOMALATE INJECTION USP
**Usual adult and adolescent dose**
Initial—
  Intramuscular, 10 mg the first week, 25 mg the second week, then 25 to 50 mg once a week until the desired therapeutic response is obtained or until toxicity occurs, up to a total dose of 1 gram.
Maintenance—
  Intramuscular, 25 to 50 mg every two weeks for two to twenty weeks, then 25 to 50 mg every three or four weeks.

**Usual pediatric dose**
Intramuscular, 10 mg the first week, then 1 mg per kg of body weight, not to exceed 50 mg per dose. See *Usual adult and adolescent dose* for recommended spacing of doses.

**Strength(s) usually available**
U.S.—
  10 mg per mL (Rx) [GENERIC].
  25 mg per mL (Rx) [*Myochrysine* (benzyl alcohol); GENERIC].
  50 mg per mL (Rx) [*Myochrysine* (benzyl alcohol); GENERIC].
Canada—
  10 mg per mL (Rx) [*Myochrysine*].
  25 mg per mL (Rx) [*Myochrysine*].
  50 mg per mL (Rx) [*Myochrysine*].

**Packaging and storage**
Store below 40 °C (104 °F), preferably between 15 and 30 °C (59 and 86 °F), unless otherwise specified by manufacturer. Protect from light. Protect from freezing.

**Stability**
Do not use if solution has darkened to more than a pale yellow.

---

Revised: June 1990
Interim revision: 08/22/94

---

## Table 1. Side/Adverse Effects*

| The following side/adverse effects have been selected on the basis of their potential clinical significance (possible signs and symptoms in parentheses where appropriate)—not necessarily inclusive: | Legend: I=Auranofin; II=Aurothioglucose; III=Gold Sodium Thiomalate | | |
|---|---|---|---|
| | I | II | III |
| **Medical attention needed** | | | |
| *Allergic reactions* | | | |
| **Anaphylactic shock** (changes in facial skin color; skin rash, hives, and/or itching; fast or irregular breathing; puffiness or swelling of the eyelids or around the eyes; shortness of breath, troubled breathing, tightness in chest, and/or wheezing; sudden, severe decrease in blood pressure and collapse) | U | R | R |
| **Angioedema** without other signs and symptoms of nitritoid or allergic reaction (large hive-like swellings on face, eyelids, mouth, lips, and/or tongue) | R | U | U |

*Differences in frequency of occurrence may reflect either lack of clinical-use data or actual pharmacologic distinctions among agents (although their pharmacologic similarity suggests that side effects occurring with one may occur with the others).
  For auranofin: M=3–9%; L=1–3%; R=<1%; U=unknown; unless otherwise specified.
  For aurothioglucose and gold sodium thiomalate (actual percentages not available): M=more frequent; F=less frequent; R=rare; U=unknown.
†Has not been reported with auranofin.
‡May occur during therapy or up to several months after cessation of therapy.
§If severe, may indicate overdose (parenteral dosage forms only).

## Table 1. Side/Adverse Effects* *(continued)*

| | Legend:<br>**I** = Auranofin<br>**II** = Aurothioglucose<br>**III** = Gold Sodium Thiomalate | | |
|---|:---:|:---:|:---:|
| The following side/adverse effects have been selected on the basis of their potential clinical significance (possible signs and symptoms in parentheses where appropriate)—not necessarily inclusive: | **I** | **II** | **III** |
| *Nitritoid or allergic reaction, severe* (difficulty in breathing or swallowing; fainting; slow heartbeat; large hive-like swellings on face, eyelids, mouth, lips, and/or tongue; thickening of tongue)—may occur up to 10 minutes after injection | † | R | R |
| *Central nervous system (CNS)/Neurologic effects* | | | |
|     Confusion | U | U | R |
|     Convulsions | U | U | R |
|     Encephalitis | U | R | U |
|     Electroencephalographic (EEG) abnormalities | U | R | U |
|     *Guillain-Barre syndrome* (tingling, numbness, and weakness in arms, trunk, or face; problems with muscle coordination) | U | U | R |
|     Hallucinations | U | U | R |
|     *Neuropathy, peripheral* (numbness, tingling, pain, or weakness in hands or feet)‡ | R | R | R |
| *Cutaneous/dermatologic effects* | | | |
|     *Dermatitis, allergic*‡ | | | |
|       (hives) | L | U | U |
|       (itching)—may occur first and indicate an impending cutaneous reaction | M (17%) | M | M |
|       (skin rash)—both papular and vesicular dermatitis have been reported with aurothioglucose; in some patients, skin rash may indicate toxicity rather than an allergic reaction; also, skin rash may be caused or aggravated by exposure to sunlight | M (24%) | M | M |
|     *Dermatitis, exfoliative* (fever with or without chills; red, thickened, or scaly skin; swollen and/or painful glands; unusual bruising)—may lead to alopecia and shedding of nails | U | R | R |
|     *Hair loss without symptoms of exfoliative dermatitis* | L | U | U |
|     *Reddened skin* | U | M | U |
| *Difficulty in swallowing* without other symptoms of nitritoid or allergic reaction | R | U | U |
| *Fever* | U | R | R |
| *Gastrointestinal effects* | | | |
|     *Enterocolitis, ulcerative* (abdominal pain, cramping, or burning, severe; bloody or black tarry stools; vomiting of blood or material that looks like coffee grounds; nausea, heartburn, and/or indigestion, severe and continuing) | R | R | R |
|     *Gastrointestinal bleeding* without other signs and symptoms of ulcerative enterocolitis (bloody or black tarry stools)—occult blood in the stool has also been reported with auranofin | R | U | U |
| *Hematologic effects*—may occur individually or in combination | | | |
|     *Agranulocytosis* (sore throat and fever with or without chills; sores, ulcers, or white spots on lips or in mouth) | R | R | R |
|     *Anemia* (unusual tiredness or weakness)‡ | R | U | U |
|     *Anemia, aplastic [anemia, hypoplastic; pancytopenia; red cell aplasia]* (shortness of breath, troubled breathing, tightness in chest, and/or wheezing; sores, ulcers, or white spots on lips or in mouth; swollen and/or painful glands; unusual bleeding or bruising; unusual tiredness or weakness)‡ | R | R | R |
|     *Eosinophilia* | L | R | R |
|     *Leukopenia [neutropenia]* (usually asymptomatic; rarely, fever or chills, cough or hoarseness, lower back or side pain, painful or difficult urination)‡ | L | R | U |
|     *Thrombocytopenia with or without purpura* (usually asymptomatic; rarely, unusual bleeding or bruising; black, tarry stools; blood in urine or stools; pinpoint red spots on skin)‡ | L | R | R |
| *Hepatotoxicity* (dark urine, pale stools, and/or yellow eyes or skin)—cholestatic hepatitis and toxic hepatitis have both been reported‡ | R | R | R |
| *Mucous membrane reactions* | | | |
|     *Gingivitis* (redness, soreness, swelling, or bleeding of gums)‡ | R | M | M |
|     *Glossitis* (irritation or soreness of tongue)‡ | L | M | M |
|     *Metallic taste*—may indicate impending gingivitis, glossitis, or stomatitis‡ | R | M | M |
|     *Pharyngitis, tracheitis, or upper respiratory tract inflammation* (irritation of nose, throat, and/or upper chest area, possibly with hoarseness and/or coughing) | U | R | U |
|     *Stomatitis*‡ (ulcers, sores, or white spots in mouth or throat)—indicative of toxicity | M (13%) | M | M |
|     *Vaginitis* (irritation of vagina) | U | R | U |
| *Ocular effects* | | | |
|     *Conjunctivitis* (redness, itching, or tearing of eyes; feeling of something in the eye)‡ | M | R | R |
|     *Corneal ulcers* | U | R | R |
|     *Iritis* (eye pain, tearing, decreased vision) | U | R | R |

## Table 1. Side/Adverse Effects* (continued)

Legend:
I = Auranofin
II = Aurothioglucose
III = Gold Sodium Thiomalate

The following side/adverse effects have been selected on the basis of their potential clinical significance (possible signs and symptoms in parentheses where appropriate)—not necessarily inclusive:

| | I | II | III |
|---|---|---|---|
| **Pulmonary effects** (coughing, shortness of breath) | | | |
|   *Bronchitis [gold bronchitis],* or | U | R | R |
|   *Fibrosis, pulmonary*‡, or | U | R | R |
|   *Pneumonitis*‡, *interstitial* | R | R | R |
| **Renal effects**‡ | | | |
|   *Glomerulitis* (pain in lower back or abdomen; bloody urine; difficulty in breathing; decreased urination; swelling of face and/or legs) | U | R | R |
|   *Hematuria* without other signs or symptoms of renal toxicity (bloody urine)—may be detected microscopically before bleeding is visually apparent | L | R | R |
|   *Nephrotic syndrome* (swelling of face, fingers, ankles, lower legs, and/or feet; cloudy urine) | U | R | R |
|   *Proteinuria* without other signs or symptoms of renal toxicity (cloudy urine) | M | L | L |
| **Medical attention needed only if continuing or bothersome** | | | |
| *Allergic reaction* | | | |
|   *Nitritoid or allergic reaction, mild* (dizziness, feeling faint, flushing or redness of face, increased sweating, nausea with or without vomiting, weakness)—may occur immediately after injection | † | R | R |
| **Gastrointestinal effects** | | | |
|   *Abdominal or stomach cramps or pain, mild to moderate*‡ | M (14%) | R | R |
|   *Bloated feeling, gas, or indigestion, mild to moderate* | M | U | U |
|   *Constipation* | L | U | U |
|   *Decrease or loss of appetite* | M | R | R |
|   *Diarrhea or loose stools*‡ | M (47%) | R§ | R§ |
|   *Loss of or other change in taste sense* | L | U | U |
|   *Nausea with or without vomiting, mild to moderate* | M (10%) | R§ | R§ |
| *Joint pain*—may occur for 1 or 2 days after injection | — | L | L |

*Differences in frequency of occurrence may reflect either lack of clinical-use data or actual pharmacologic distinctions among agents (although their pharmacologic similarity suggests that side effects occurring with one may occur with the others).
  For auranofin: M=3–9%; L=1–3%; R=<1%; U=unknown; unless otherwise specified.
  For aurothioglucose and gold sodium thiomalate (actual percentages not available): M=more frequent; F=less frequent; R=rare; U=unknown.
†Has not been reported with auranofin.
‡May occur during therapy or up to several months after cessation of therapy.
§If severe, may indicate overdose (parenteral dosage forms only).

## GOLD SODIUM THIOMALATE—See *Gold Compounds (Systemic)*

# GONADORELIN Systemic

JAN: Gonadorelin acetate—Gonadorelin diacetate
VA CLASSIFICATION (Primary/Secondary): HS900/DX900
Commonly used brand name(s): *Factrel; Lutrepulse; Relisorm.*

Other commonly used names are luteinizing hormone–releasing hormone (LHRH), luteinizing hormone–releasing factor dihydrochloride (for gonadorelin hydrochloride), luteinizing hormone–releasing factor diacetate tetrahydrate (for gonadorelin acetate), and luteinizing hormone–/follicle-stimulating hormone–releasing hormone (LH/FSH–RH).

Note: For a listing of dosage forms and brand names by country availability, see *Dosage Forms* section(s).

## Category

Gonadotropin-releasing hormone; diagnostic aid (hypothalamic-pituitary-gonadal axis function); infertility therapy agent.

## Indications

Note: Bracketed information in the *Indications* section refers to uses that are not included in U.S. product labeling.

**Accepted**

Hypogonadism (diagnosis)—Gonadorelin as a single dose (gonadorelin test) is indicated for evaluation of the functional capacity and response of gonadotropes in the anterior pituitary in postpubertal patients who are suspected of having gonadotropin deficiency, whether due to hypothalamic function impairment alone or in combination with anterior pituitary function failure. The gonadorelin test can confirm, with other laboratory and clinical tests, the diagnosis of hypogonadotropic hypogonadism in adult males and females. The single-dose test is also indicated for evaluation of residual gonadotropic function of the pituitary in patients following removal of a pituitary tumor by surgery, irradiation, or their combination. In long-standing gonadotropin-releasing hormone (GnRH) deficiency, a single dose will not stimulate the pituitary. However, repetitive dosing can prime the pituitary and increase the gonadotropins luteinizing hormone and follicle-stimulating hormone.

A single-dose or series of gonadorelin tests will confirm the presence of functional pituitary gonadotropes, but it can not differentiate pituitary disorders from hypothalamic disorders or measure pituitary gonadotropic reserve. A single dose of gonadorelin will not stimulate a gonadal steroid response large enough or reproducible enough to test gonadal steroidogenic potential. Also, single-dose gonadorelin administration is not capable of stimulating prepubertal gonadotropes in children or adolescents when the hypothalamic-pituitary-gonadal axis is relatively inactive.

Amenorrhea, primary hypothalamic (treatment) or
Infertility, female, due to primary hypothalamic hypogonadism (treatment) or
[Infertility, male, due to primary hypothalamic hypogonadism (treatment)][1] or
[Puberty, delayed (treatment)][1]—Gonadorelin acetate administered through an infusion pump set for pulsatile or intermittent dosing is indicated for induction of ovulation in females who experience hypogonadotropic amenorrhea or infertility due to hypogonadotropic hypogonadism. It may be used alone or in conjunction with other agents, such as chorionic gonadotropin, as a separate injection. Intermittent administration of gonadorelin, which is postulated to simulate normal release of gonadotropin-releasing hormone from the hypothalamus, may be useful in males experiencing infertility due to hypothalamic hypogonadism and in children experiencing delayed puberty resulting from hypothalamic impairment.

---

[1]Not included in Canadian product labeling.

## Pharmacology/Pharmacokinetics

**Physicochemical characteristics**
Source—Gonadorelin is synthetic gonadotropin-releasing hormone (GnRH).
Molecular weight—Base: 1182.33.

**Mechanism of action/Effect**
Like naturally occurring gonadotropin-releasing hormone (GnRH), gonadorelin primarily stimulates the synthesis and release of luteinizing hormone (LH) from the anterior pituitary gland. Follicle-stimulating hormone (FSH) production and release is also increased by gonadorelin, but to a lesser degree. In prepubertal females and some gonadal function disorders, the FSH response may be greater than the LH response.

For the treatment of amenorrhea, delayed puberty, and infertility—
Administration of gonadorelin is used to simulate the physiologic release of GnRH from the hypothalamus in treatment of delayed puberty, treatment of infertility caused by hypogonadotropic hypogonadism, and induction of ovulation in those women with hypothalamic amenorrhea. This results in increased levels of pituitary gonadotropins LH and FSH, which subsequently stimulate the gonads to produce reproductive steroids.

For diagnosis of hypogonadism—
After intravenous or subcutaneous administration of a single dose of gonadorelin, quantitation of the LH response to gonadorelin allows for detection of hypothalamic or pituitary dysfunction. It is recommended that a series of seven blood samples be drawn to evaluate the LH response to gonadorelin. A response is considered subnormal if three or more LH values fall below the 10th percentile curve established in the clinical studies for patients with normal LH responses using gonadorelin. The incidence of patients with hypogonadism who showed subnormal responses in the clinical studies when they were tested with a single dose of gonadorelin included:
- Postpubertal panhypopituitarism—100%.
- Prader-Willi syndrome—100%.
- Prepubertal panhypopituitarism—95%.
- Sheehan's syndrome—84%.
- Kallmann's syndrome—77%; response may increase with repetitive dosing.

**Biotransformation**
Rapid metabolism to various biologically inactive peptide fragments.

**Half-life**
Initial, 2 to 10 minutes; terminal, 10 to 40 minutes.

**Duration of action**
3 to 5 hours.

**Elimination**
Renal excretion of inactive metabolites.

## Precautions to Consider

**Pregnancy/Reproduction**
Fertility—High doses admininistered repeatedly in humans may lead to luteolysis and inhibition of spermatogenesis.

Pregnancy—Studies in pregnant humans show that gonadorelin did not cause adverse effects in the fetus when it was used in the first trimester. Intermittent pulse dosing of gonadorelin used for 2 weeks after conception helps to establish the corpus luteum, and then it is discontinued. Multiple follicle development, multiple gestations, and spontaneous termination of pregnancy have been reported. Multiple gestations occurred in 12% of 89 patients using intermittent pulse dosing (10 sets of twins, one set of triplets).

In animal studies, gonadorelin did not cause adverse effects in the fetuses of mice, rats, and rabbits.
FDA Pregnancy Category B.

**Breast-feeding**
It is not known whether gonadorelin is distributed into breast milk. Problems in humans have not been documented.

**Pediatrics**
Appropriate studies on the relationship of age to the effects of gonadorelin as a diagnostic test have not been performed in children up to 12 years of age. Safety and efficacy have not been established. Children would not be sensitive to single doses of gonadorelin until after the onset of puberty.
Newborn infants are very sensitive to the effects of GnRH (peak responsiveness is at 1 to 3 months of age). Responsiveness declines dramatically until puberty (except for FSH in prepubertal females). However, there are no medically accepted indications for the use of gonadorelin in newborn infants.

**Adolescents**
Appropriate diagnostic studies performed to date using the single-dose gonadorelin test have not demonstrated specific problems in postpubertal adolescents that would limit the usefulness of gonadorelin in this age group. Safety and efficacy for use of gonadorelin in an intermittent pulse dosing schedule have not been established for adolescents up to 18 years of age. Use of gonadotropin-releasing hormone analogs in multiple doses or intermittent pulse dose schedules for the treatment of delayed puberty have been successful.

**Drug interactions and/or related problems**
The following drug interactions and/or related problems have been selected on the basis of their potential clinical significance (possible mechanism in parentheses where appropriate)—not necessarily inclusive (» = major clinical significance):
See also *Laboratory value alterations*.
» Infertility therapy agents, other, including clomiphene
(gonadorelin should not be used for ovulation induction concurrently with other infertility therapy agents because of the rare risk of causing ovarian hyperstimulation)

**Laboratory value alterations**
The following have been selected on the basis of their potential clinical significance (possible effect in parentheses where appropriate)—not necessarily inclusive (» = major clinical significance):
With results of *this* test
*Due to other medications*
Androgens or
Estrogens or
Glucocorticoids or
Progestins
(may alter results of the gonadorelin test by affecting pituitary secretion of gonadotropins through feedback mechanism)
Contraceptives, estrogen and progestin oral or
Digoxin
(may suppress serum gonadotropin concentrations)
Dopaminergic blocking agents, including metoclopramide
Phenothiazines
(may blunt the response to gonadorelin by increasing serum prolactin concentrations)
Levodopa or
Spironolactone
(may elevate serum gonadotropin concentrations)

With physiology/laboratory test values
Estradiol in females
(serum concentrations may initially decrease within the first 90 minutes after gonadorelin administration, then increase, reaching a peak at 6 hours and returning to normal by 18 hours)
Testosterone in males
(serum concentrations may increase transiently)

**Medical considerations/Contraindications**
The medical considerations/contraindications included have been selected on the basis of their potential clinical significance (reasons given in parentheses where appropriate)—not necessarily inclusive (» = major clinical significance).

*Risk-benefit should be considered when the following medical problems exist:*
» Adenoma, gonadotropin-releasing hormone
(pituitary apoplexy and sudden blindness occurred in one patient receiving a single dose of a gonadotropin-releasing hormone analog; this may occur also with gonadorelin)

Allergy to gonadorelin
» Any condition that may be worsened by reproductive hormones, such as hormone-dependent tumor
(the increase of estrogen and progestins in women or androgens in men that results from multiple doses of gonadorelin may exacerbate any condition dependent on reproductive hormones)

**Patient monitoring**
The following may be especially important in patient monitoring (other tests may be warranted in some patients, depending on condition; » = major clinical significance):

Catheter site inspection and
Physical examination and
Progesterone concentration, serum, at mid-luteal phase and
Ultrasound examination of ovaries
(monitoring of patient for asepsis may be accomplished by regular inspection of the catheter site; monitoring of patient for ovulation by measuring ovarian follicle size and mid-luteal serum progesterone concentration, physical examination, especially of the pelvic area, and ultrasound examination of the ovaries for baseline measurements and on the seventh and fourteenth days of gonadorelin pulse therapy)

Luteinizing hormone (LH)
(measurement of serum concentrations recommended at timed intervals before and after gonadorelin administration for diagnostic procedures. The LH peak occurs approximately 30 minutes after injection; however, the time to peak response and the peak LH concentrations vary significantly in the control population and measurements will depend on each laboratory's standards and the different assay methods used for the age-group tested. It is recommended that seven venous blood samples be taken—at baseline and at 15, 30, 45, 60, and 120 minutes after administration. Two samples should be averaged for the baseline value and should be taken at least 15 to 20 minutes apart. A response is considered subnormal if three or more blood LH concentrations fall below the 10th percentile curve established in the clinical studies for patients with normal LH responses using gonadorelin)

## Side/Adverse Effects

The following side/adverse effects have been selected on the basis of their potential clinical significance (possible signs and symptoms in parentheses where appropriate)—not necessarily inclusive:

**Those indicating need for medical attention**
*Anaphylaxis, generalized* (difficulty in breathing; hardening of skin at injection site; hives; persistent flushing; rapid heartbeat)—following multiple doses; *infection; mild phlebitis; or hematoma, local* (itching, pain, redness, or swelling at place of injection)—following single or multiple doses; *skin rash, generalized or local*—following multiple doses

**Those indicating need for medical attention only if they continue or are bothersome**
Incidence rare
*For single dose injection only*
*Abdominal or stomach discomfort; flushing, transient; headaches; lightheadedness; nausea*

## Patient Consultation

As an aid to patient consultation, refer to *Advice for the Patient, Gonadorelin (Systemic)*.
In providing consultation, consider emphasizing the following selected information (» = major clinical significance):

**Before using this medication**
» Conditions affecting use, especially:
Allergy to gonadorelin
Pregnancy—Gonadorelin has not caused adverse effects in the fetus when used in the first trimester; multiple births occur
Other medications, especially infertility therapy agents, such as clomiphene
Other medical problems, especially gonadotropin-releasing hormone adenoma (for single or multiple doses of gonadorelin) or any condition that may be worsened by reproductive hormones, such as a hormone-dependent tumor (for multiple dose gonadorelin)

**Proper use of this medication**
Test procedure: Blood samples taken; injection given; several blood samples taken again; measurement of luteinizing hormone in blood
» Understanding the directions for use if using the pump for gonadorelin at home

» For brand name *Lutrepulse*: Proper care of catheter site and pump, including warning signals for pump malfunction and proper placement of tubing on body
» Proper dosing
Proper storage

**Precautions while using this medication**
*For brand name Lutrepulse*
» Importance of close and frequent monitoring by physician during use of the pump
» If desiring pregnancy, importance of following physician's instructions for timing of sexual intercourse to become pregnant and to reduce the chances of multiple gestations
» Telling physician immediately if pregnancy is suspected

**Side/adverse effects**
Signs of potential side effects, especially anaphylaxis (following multiple dosing); generalized or local skin rash (following multiple dosing); infection, mild phlebitis, or hematoma, local (following single or multiple dosing)

## General Dosing Information

**For single-dose use (diagnostic)**
Results of the gonadorelin test should be interpreted by someone familiar with hypothalamic-pituitary-gonadal physiology and the clinical status of the patient. For accurate interpretation of the test, the controls for the assay being used should be established and relayed to physician. If the results are blunted or borderline, the gonadorelin test should be repeated.

To determine the baseline luteinizing hormone (LH) concentration, the LH concentrations of two samples of venous blood drawn at least 15 to 20 minutes apart are averaged.

Following gonadorelin administration, venous blood samples are drawn at regular intervals (for example, at 15, 30, 45, 60, and 120 minutes after administration) and analyzed for serum LH concentration.

Depending on the laboratory and assay method used, normal baseline serum LH concentrations may vary. Even though the LH response is greatest in females when gonadorelin is given during the luteal phase, the gonadorelin test is given to females during the follicular phase, if that can be established, since females respond the same as males during this phase.

In menopausal and postmenopausal females, baseline LH concentrations are elevated and the maximum LH increases are exaggerated compared to premenopausal concentrations.

Basal LH and follicle-stimulating hormone (FSH) concentrations increase with age (over 50 years) in males; however, time to peak LH response after gonadorelin administration in older males is significantly delayed and may be diminished.

**For pulsatile dosing (brand name *Lutrepulse* only)**
Physicians prescribing intermittent pulsatile dosing with gonadorelin should be familiar with its use and with the clinical response to ovulation induction. Ovarian hyperstimulation is rare when using pulsatile dosing because of the body's natural negative feedback mechanism, but the physician should be aware of its symptoms (ascites, pleural effusion, hemoconcentration, rupture of a cyst, fluid or electrolyte imbalance, or sepsis). Hyperstimulation is more likely to occur if the patient is taking an ovulation induction agent, such as clomiphene, or has spontaneous changes in the endogenous gonadotropin-releasing hormone.

Pituitary hyperstimulation or multiple follicle development can be minimized by adhering to recommended dosing schedules. The possibility of a multiple pregnancy may be minimized by monitoring ovarian follicles by ultrasound examination at baseline and on the seventh and fourteenth days of therapy and by recommending proper timing of sexual intercourse to patient.

If a malfunction of the device occurs and all contents of its reservoir are released at full dose, no harmful effects are expected, since doses as high as 3000 mcg of gonadorelin have not caused adverse effects. However, patients should be monitored for multiple follicles, and temporary pituitary desensitization would be expected. Also, continuous, nonpulsatile exposure to gonadorelin acetate would temporarily reduce pituitary responsiveness.

Patients should be provided with oral and written instructions on proper use of the pump and proper care of the pump and catheter site to minimize the chance of pump malfunction and development of sepsis (inflammation, infection, mild phlebitis) or hematoma. The injection site should be monitored and the cannula and catheter site should be changed at 48-hour intervals.

Response to intermittent dosing usually occurs within 2 to 3 weeks after treatment initiation.

Eight milliliters of solution will supply 90-minute pulsatile doses for approximately 7 consecutive days. The pump can be set to deliver 25 or 50 microliters of solution, based on the dose selected, over a pulse period of 1 minute, and at a pulse frequency of 90 minutes.

A reconstituted 0.8 mg vial of gonadorelin acetate yields:
  2.5 mcg/25 microliters per 90-minute pulse.
  5 mcg/50 microliters per 90-minute pulse.

A reconstituted 3.2 mg vial of gonadorelin acetate yields:
  10 mcg/25 microliters per 90-minute pulse.
  20 mcg/50 microliters per 90-minute pulse.

## Parenteral Dosage Forms

Note: Dosage and strength of gonadorelin hydrochloride for injection is expressed in terms of gonadorelin base.

### GONADORELIN ACETATE FOR INJECTION

#### Usual adult and adolescent dose
Hypogonadism (diagnosis)—
  Intravenous or subcutaneous, 100 mcg (0.1 mg).
  Note: In females, gonadorelin should be administered within the early follicular phase of the menstrual cycle, if the phase can be determined.
Amenorrhea, primary hypothalamic or
Infertility, female, due to primary hypothalamic hypogonadism or
[Infertility, male, due to primary hypothalamic hypogonadism][1]—
  Adults: Intravenous or subcutaneous, 5 mcg every 90 minutes delivered by intravenous or subcutaneous pump, usually for twenty-one days. Doses between 1 and 20 mcg have been used clinically. Check the manufacturer's labeling for the doses the pump is capable of delivering. The pump should be set to deliver 25 or 50 microliters of solution, based on the dose selected, over a pulse period of one minute and at a pulse frequency of ninety minutes. Dose may be changed in a stepwise fashion if no results are seen after three doses while monitoring patient for an inappropriate response. When ovulation occurs, treatment should continue for two more weeks to maintain the corpus luteum.
  Adolescents up to 18 years of age: Safety and efficacy have not been established.

#### Usual pediatric dose
Hypogonadism (diagnosis)—
  Children 12 years of age and over: Intravenous or subcutaneous, 2 mcg per kilogram of body weight, not to exceed a single-dose of 100 mcg.
  Children up to 12 years of age: Safety and efficacy have not been established.
[Puberty, delayed][1]—
  Adolescents up to 18 years of age: Intravenous or subcutaneous, 5 mcg every 90 minutes delivered by intravenous or subcutaneous pump. Doses between 1 and 20 mcg have been used clinically. Check the manufacturer's labeling for the doses the pump is capable of delivering. The pump should be set to deliver 25 or 50 microliters of solution, based on the dose selected, over a pulse period of one minute and at a pulse frequency of ninety minutes. Dose may be changed in a stepwise fashion if appropriate.

#### Size(s) usually available
U.S.—
  Not commercially available.
Canada—
  For intermittent dosing
    0.8 mcg (Rx) [*Lutrepulse*].
    3.2 mcg (Rx) [*Lutrepulse*].
  For single-dose
    100 mcg (0.1 mg) (Rx) [*Relisorm* (mannitol 5 mg)].
    500 mcg (0.5 mg) (Rx) [*Relisorm* (mannitol 500 mg)].

#### Packaging and storage
Store unreconstituted gonadorelin for injection and diluent below 40 °C (104 °F), preferably between 15 and 30 °C (59 and 86 °F), unless otherwise specified by manufacturer.

#### Preparation of dosage form
For brand name *Lutrepulse*—Using standard aseptic technique, add provided diluent (8 mL of Sodium Chloride Injection USP containing hydrochloric acid) to the 0.8-mg vial to make 5 mcg of gonadorelin in 50 microliters or to the 3.2-mg vial to make 20 mcg of gonadorelin in 50 microliters.
For brand name *Relisorm*—Using standard aseptic technique, add provided diluent.
  100-mcg vial: Add 1 mL of Sodium Chloride Injection USP.
  500-mcg vial: Add 5 mL of Bacteriostatic Sodium Chloride Injection USP.

#### Stability
Reconstituted solutions should be clear and colorless. Do not use if precipitate has formed or solution is discolored in appearance.
For brand name *Lutrepulse*—Reconstituted gonadorelin acetate for injection should be made immediately before use and placed within the pump's plastic reservoir.
For brand name *Relisorm*—Reconstituted 100 mcg gonadorelin acetate for injection should be made immediately before use. Unused reconstituted 500 mcg gonadorelin acetate for injection can be stored in the refrigerator for up to 14 days.

#### Note
*Lutrepulse* for injection is intended for use in *Lutrepulse* pumps that are included in the kits. Injection may be intravenously or subcutaneously administered, depending on the kit used, *Lutrepulse IV Kit* or *Lutrepulse SC Kit*. The injection volumes and concentrations are specific to the type of pump to achieve proper dosing. Eight milliliters of solution will supply 90-minute pulsatile doses for approximately 7 consecutive days.

### GONADORELIN HYDROCHLORIDE FOR INJECTION

#### Usual adult and adolescent dose
Hypogonadism (diagnosis)—
  Intravenous or subcutaneous, 100 mcg (0.1 mg) (base).
  Note: In females, gonadorelin should be administered within the early follicular phase of the menstrual cycle, if that can be determined.

#### Usual pediatric dose
Hypogonadism (diagnosis)—
  Children 12 years of age and over: Intravenous or subcutaneous, 2 mcg per kilogram of body weight, not to exceed a single dose of 100 mcg (base).
  Children up to 12 years of age: Safety and efficacy have not been established.

#### Size(s) usually available
U.S.—
  For single-dose
    100 mcg (0.1 mg) (base) (Rx) [*Factrel* (diluent—benzyl alcohol 2%; lactose 100 mg)].
    500 mcg (0.5 mg) (base) (Rx) [*Factrel* (diluent—benzyl alcohol 2%; lactose 100 mg)].
Canada—
  For single-dose
    100 mcg (0.1 mg) (base) (Rx) [*Factrel* (diluent—benzyl alcohol 2%; lactose 100 mg)].
    500 mcg (0.5 mg) (base) (Rx) [*Factrel* (diluent—benzyl alcohol 2%; lactose 100 mg)].

#### Packaging and storage
Store below 40 °C (104 °F), preferably between 15 and 30 °C (59 and 86 °F), unless otherwise specified by manufacturer.

#### Preparation of dosage form
Using standard aseptic technique, add 1 mL of diluent provided to the 100-mcg vial or 2 mL of diluent to the 500-mcg vial. The solution should be made immediately before use. Unused reconstituted solution and diluent should be discarded.

#### Stability
Reconstituted gonadorelin injection should be stored at room temperature and used within 24 hours.

[1]Not included in Canadian product labeling.

## Selected Bibliography
Goodpasture JC, Rosenfield RL, Ehrman DA. In: Polan ML, Henzl MR. Infertility and reproductive medicine: Clinics of North America. The clinical use of GnRH superactive analogs. Philadelphia: W.B. Saunders; 1993. p. 129-45.

Revised: 06/29/98

# GOSERELIN Systemic

VA CLASSIFICATION (Primary/Secondary): HS900/AN500

Commonly used brand name(s): *Zoladex; Zoladex 3-Month; Zoladex LA.*

Note: For a listing of dosage forms and brand names by country availability, see *Dosage Forms* section(s).

## Category

Gonadotropin-releasing hormone analog; antiendometriotic agent; antineoplastic; gonadotropin inhibitor.

## Indications

Note: Bracketed information in the *Indications* section refers to uses that are not included in U.S. product labeling.

### Accepted

Carcinoma, breast (treatment)[1]—Goserelin, as the 3.6-mg implant, is indicated for the palliative treatment of advanced breast carcinoma in pre- and perimenopausal females. The 10.8-mg implant should not be used for this indication because it has not been shown to suppress serum estradiol reliably.

Carcinoma, prostatic (treatment)—Goserelin is indicated for the palliative treatment of advanced prostatic carcinoma, especially as an alternative to orchiectomy or estrogen administration.

[Endometrial thinning]—Goserelin, as the 3.6-mg implant, is indicated as an endometrial thinning agent prior to endometrial ablation.

Endometriosis (treatment)—Goserelin, as the 3.6-mg implant, is indicated for the management of endometriosis, including treatment of pelvic pain and reduction in the size and number of lesions. The 10.8-mg implant should not be used for this indication because it has not been shown to suppress serum estradiol reliably.

---

[1]Not included in Canadian product labeling.

## Pharmacology/Pharmacokinetics

### Physicochemical characteristics

Physical description—Goserelin acetate, dispersed in a matrix of D,L-lactic and glycolic acids copolymer, is available in a biodegradable and biocompatible, sterile, white- to cream-colored cylinder.

3.6-mg implant: Contains 13.3 to 14.3 mg of copolymer per dose with less than 2.5% acetic acid and up to 12% goserelin-related substances.

10.8-mg implant: Contains 12.82 to 14.76 mg of copolymer per dose with less than 2% acetic acid and up to 10% goserelin-related substances.

Molecular weight—Goserelin: 1269.44.
Goserelin acetate: 1328.
pKa—Goserelin: 6.2.

### Mechanism of action/Effect

Goserelin is a synthetic gonadotropin-releasing hormone analog (GnRHa). Like naturally occurring luteinizing hormone–releasing hormone (LH-RH) that is produced by the hypothalamus, initial or intermittent administration of goserelin stimulates release of gonadotropins, luteinizing hormone (LH) and follicle-stimulating hormone (FSH), from the anterior pituitary. Long-term, sustained use of goserelin is associated with an early phase of increased LH and FSH levels, followed by their suppression.

Prostatic carcinoma—

In males, the release of LH and FSH results in a transient increase in testosterone concentrations. However, continuous daily administration of goserelin in the treatment of prostatic carcinoma suppresses secretion of LH and FSH, with a resultant fall in testosterone concentrations and a pharmacologic castration within 2 to 4 weeks following initial administration.

Endometriosis; breast carcinoma; endometrial thinning—

In females, the release of LH and FSH results in a transient increase in estradiol concentrations. However, continuous daily administration of goserelin suppresses secretion of LH and FSH, with a resultant reduction in ovarian size and function, reduction in the size of the uterus and mammary glands, and regression of sex hormone–responsive tumors. Estradiol and progesterone concentrations are suppressed to postmenopausal levels within 2 to 4 weeks following initial administration. In consequence of suppression of ovarian function, both normal and ectopic endometrial tissues become inactive and atrophic. As a result, amenorrhea usually occurs within 4 to 8 weeks of treatment initiation.

### Absorption

Slower during the first 8 days after injection of the 3.6-mg implant than during the remainder of the 28-day dosing period.

### Distribution

Following subcutaneous administration of 250 mcg of an aqueous solution of goserelin, the apparent volume of distribution was 44.1 and 20.3 L for males and females, respectively.

### Protein binding

Low (27.3%).

### Biotransformation

Via hydrolysis of the C-terminal amino acids.

### Half-life

Following subcutaneous administration of 250 mcg of an aqueous solution of goserelin—

Males with normal renal function (creatinine clearance > 70 mL per minute [mL/min]): 4.2 hours.

Males with renal function impairment (creatinine clearance < 20 mL/min): 12.1 hours.

Females: 2.3 hours.

Although half-life is increased in patients with renal function impairment, dosage adjustment is not required.

### Onset of action

Transient increases in testosterone and estradiol concentrations occur within the first week of therapy. A decline in testosterone to castrate level and in estradiol to postmenopausal level occurs within 2 to 4 weeks.

### Time to peak concentration

3.6-mg implant:
Males: 12 to 15 days.
Females: 8 to 22 days.
10.8-mg implant:
Males: 2 hours.

### Peak plasma concentration

3.6-mg implant—
Males: 2.84 ± 1.81 nanograms per mL (nanograms/mL).
Females 1.46 ± 0.82 nanograms/mL.
10.8-mg implant—
Males: 8 nanograms/mL.

### Duration of action

Suppression of testosterone concentrations to castrate levels and suppression of estradiol concentrations to postmenopausal levels persist for the duration of therapy.

### Elimination

Following subcutaneous administration of the aqueous solution—
Hepatic: < 10%.
Renal: > 90% (20% unchanged).

## Precautions to Consider

### Cross-sensitivity and/or related problems

Patients sensitive to gonadorelin (synthetic gonadotropin-releasing hormone [GnRH]) or to gonadotropin-releasing hormone analogs (GnRHa), such as buserelin, histrelin, leuprolide, and nafarelin, may be sensitive to goserelin also.

### Carcinogenicity

Extensive experience with GnRHa, including with goserelin in humans, has shown no evidence of pituitary tumors in humans.

A 1-year study in male rats given daily subcutaneous doses of 80 and 150 mcg per kg of body weight (mcg/kg) and in female rats given daily subcutaneous doses of 50 and 100 mcg/kg (three to nine times the recommended human dose on a mg per square meter of body surface area [mg/m$^2$] basis) every 4 weeks found an increased incidence of pituitary adenomas. Similar doses given to male rats over a period of 72 weeks and to female rats over a period of 101 weeks also resulted in an increased incidence of pituitary adenomas. Relevance of these data to humans has not been established; animal data suggest that the effects on the pituitary are a species-specific response.

A 2-year study in mice given daily subcutaneous doses of up to 2400 mcg/kg (approximately 70 times the recommended human dose on a mg/m$^2$ basis) every 3 weeks found an increased incidence of histiocytic sarcoma of the vertebral column and femur.

### Mutagenicity

Mutagenicity tests using bacterial and mammalian systems for point mutations and cytogenetic effects were negative.

**Pregnancy/Reproduction**

Fertility—Suppression of estrogen and testosterone secretion results in impairment of fertility in males and females and is consistent with the expected gonadal suppression action of goserelin. Menses should resume within 8 weeks after discontinuation of therapy. Of 500 patients treated for endometriosis for 6 months and followed for 1 year, 100 patients (20%) became pregnant. Of 177 patients thought to be infertile, 53 patients (30%) conceived.

Studies in male rats found that goserelin produced changes consistent with gonadal suppression as a result of its endocrine action, including decreased weight and atrophic histological changes in the testes, epididymis, seminal vesicle, and prostate gland with complete suppression of spermatogenesis. In female rats, suppression of ovarian function resulted in decreased size and weight of the ovaries and secondary sex organs. Also, follicular development was arrested at the antral stage and the corpora lutea were reduced in size and number. Except for the testes, almost complete histologic reversal of these changes occurred several weeks after the end of dosing. In male and female dogs, suppression of fertility was fully reversible after continuous administration of goserelin at 20 to 40 times the recommended daily human dose (on a mg/m$^2$ basis) for 1 year.

Pregnancy—Goserelin is not recommended for use during pregnancy. Goserelin can cause serious adverse effects in the fetus. The pre-existence of a pregnancy should be ruled out prior to its use. When used every 28 days, goserelin usually inhibits ovulation and stops menstruation. However, contraception cannot be ensured. A nonhormonal contraceptive method should be used by all premenopausal females during and for 12 weeks following goserelin therapy.

Goserelin crosses the placenta of rats and rabbits following subcutaneous doses of 50 and 1000 mcg/kg, respectively. Dose-related increases in pregnancy loss and embryotoxicity and fetotoxicity were seen in rats and rabbits at doses equivalent to one tenth and two times the maximum recommended daily human dose, respectively, on a mg/m$^2$ basis. A decrease in fetal and pup survival also was seen in a reproduction study in rats.

FDA Pregnancy Category D (for treatment of advanced breast carcinoma).
FDA Pregnancy Category X (for treatment of endometriosis).

**Breast-feeding**

Goserelin is distributed into the milk of lactating rats. It is not known whether goserelin is distributed into human breast milk. However, goserelin is not recommended for use by nursing mothers.

**Pediatrics**

Appropriate studies on the relationship of age to the effects of goserelin have not been performed in pediatric patients up to 18 years of age. Safety and efficacy have not been established.

**Geriatrics**

Appropriate studies on the relationship of age to the effects of goserelin have not been performed in the geriatric population. However, clinical trials were conducted mainly in older patients and geriatrics-specific problems that would limit the usefulness of this medication in the elderly are not expected.

**Laboratory value alterations**

The following have been selected on the basis of their potential clinical significance (possible effect in parentheses where appropriate)—not necessarily inclusive (» = major clinical significance):

With diagnostic test results
» Pituitary gonadotropic function testing and
» Gonadal function testing
(therapeutic doses of goserelin suppress the pituitary-gonadal hormone regulatory system; baseline values usually are restored within 8 to 12 weeks after treatment is discontinued)

With physiology/laboratory test values
Acid phosphatase
(values may increase early in treatment of prostatic carcinoma but usually decrease to or near baseline by the fourth week; may decrease to below baseline levels if elevated values were present before treatment)

Alanine aminotransferase (ALT [SGPT]) and
Aspartate aminotransferase (AST [SGOT])
(increased serum values have been reported in females)

» Bone mineral density
(bone mineral density usually decreases, more substantially in females than in males, with losses being greater in females with osteoporotic risk factors; may be irreversible)

Calcium, serum
(concentrations may be increased, usually in patients with bone metastases)

Estradiol, serum
(concentrations may increase early in treatment of females with breast cancer, become suppressed within 3 weeks of treatment, and remain suppressed throughout treatment)

High-density lipoprotein (HDL) cholesterol and
Low-density lipoprotein (LDL) cholesterol and
Total cholesterol and
Triglycerides
(concentrations may be increased)

Testosterone, serum
(concentrations usually are increased in males during the first week of therapy, become suppressed within 3 weeks of treatment, and remain suppressed throughout treatment)

**Medical considerations/Contraindications**

The medical considerations/contraindications included have been selected on the basis of their potential clinical significance (reasons given in parentheses where appropriate)—not necessarily inclusive (» = major clinical significance).

*Risk-benefit should be considered when the following medical problems exist:*

Sensitivity to gonadorelin (synthetic gonadotropin-releasing hormone [GnRH]) or to gonadotropin-releasing hormone analogs (GnRHa), such as buserelin, goserelin, histrelin, leuprolide, and nafarelin
For endometrial thinning or treatment of endometriosis
Conditions causing decrease in bone density or
Osteoporosis, or history of, or family history of
(hypoestrogenism-induced loss of bone mineral density may occur in females treated with goserelin and may be irreversible; major risk factors include chronic alcohol and/or tobacco abuse, family history of severe osteoporosis, and chronic use of medications, such as anticonvulsants or corticosteroids, that decrease bone mineral density; goserelin should be used with caution in these patients)
» Uterine bleeding, abnormal, undiagnosed
(use of goserelin may delay diagnosis)
*For treatment of prostatic carcinoma*
» Urinary tract obstruction or history of
(existing urinary obstruction should be treated before beginning treatment with goserelin; for patients with a history of urinary tract obstruction, there is an increased incidence of a disease flare during initial goserelin treatment because of the initial increase in serum testosterone concentrations; close monitoring is recommended during the first month of treatment and catheterization may be needed on its occurrence)
» Vertebral metastases
(risk of spinal cord compression and neurologic problems, including paralysis, as a result of a disease flare during first few weeks of goserelin treatment; close monitoring is recommended during the first month of treatment)

**Patient monitoring**

The following may be especially important in patient monitoring (other tests may be warranted in some patients, depending on condition; » = major clinical significance):

Bone density assessment
(recommended as needed to monitor response in patients during long-term use of goserelin, including treatment of endometriosis for longer than 6 months)
*For endometrial thinning or treatment of endometriosis*
Pregnancy test
(recommended for females of reproductive potential if treatment is not started during menstruation, if irregular menstrual cycles exist, or if a scheduled dose is delayed)
*For treatment of prostatic carcinoma*
Acid phosphatase, plasma prostatic or serum or
Prostate-specific antigen (PSA) concentrations, serum and
Testosterone concentrations, serum
(recommended at periodic intervals to monitor response in patients with prostatic carcinoma)
Bone scans
(recommended as needed to monitor response in patients at risk for vertebral metastases)
Imaging studies
(intravenous pyelogram, computerized tomography [CT] scan, and/or ultrasonography may be used to diagnose or assess obstructive uropathy in patients at risk for obstructive uropathy, especially useful during the first week of therapy)

## Side/Adverse Effects

Note: Many of the side/adverse effects of goserelin are related to hypoestrogenism in females and hypotestosteronism in males. The reversibility of clinical hypogonadism produced by goserelin has not been established for long-term use.

There is a risk of increased loss of vertebral trabecular bone density during treatment for endometriosis or breast cancer; some of this loss may be irreversible. However, the loss usually is small when treatment is limited to 6 months for endometriosis, except in patients with existing risk factors (e.g., history of osteoporosis). Decreased bone density also has been reported in males who have had an orchiectomy or who have been treated with a gonadotropin-releasing hormone analog (GnRHa).

The following side/adverse effects have been selected on the basis of their potential clinical significance (possible signs and symptoms in parentheses where appropriate)—not necessarily inclusive:

**Those indicating need for medical attention**
Incidence less frequent—> 5%
   *In females and males*
      **Cardiac arrhythmias or palpitations** (fast or irregular heartbeat)
Incidence rare— < 5%
   *In females and males*
      **Anaphylaxis** (changes in facial skin color; fast or irregular breathing; puffiness or swelling of the eyelids or around the eyes; shortness of breath, troubled breathing, tightness in chest, and/or wheezing; skin rash, hives, and/or itching; sudden, severe decrease in blood pressure and collapse); **bone, muscle, or joint pain, continuing**; **paresthesias** (numbness or tingling of hands or feet); **syncope** (fainting)
   *In females only*
      **Androgenic effects** (deepening of voice; increased hair growth); **personality or behavioral changes** (anxiety; mental depression; mood changes; nervousness)
   *In males only*
      **Angina or myocardial infarction** (pains in chest); **pulmonary embolism** (sudden shortness of breath); **thrombophlebitis** (pains in groin or legs, especially calves of legs)

**Those indicating need for medical attention only if they continue or are bothersome**
Incidence more frequent— > 50%
   *In females and males*
      **Hot flashes** (sudden sweating and feelings of warmth)
   *In females only*
      **Amenorrhea** (stopping of menstrual periods); **or spotting** (light, irregular vaginal bleeding)
Incidence less frequent—5 to 13%
   *In females and males*
      **Blurred vision; decreased libido** (decreased interest in sexual intercourse); **dizziness; edema** (swelling of feet or lower legs); **headache; injection site reaction** (burning, itching, redness, or swelling at place of injection); **nausea or vomiting; swelling or increased tenderness of breasts; trouble in sleeping; weight gain**
   *In females only*
      **Endometriotic disease flare, transient** (pelvic pain); **vaginitis** (burning, dryness, or itching of vagina)
   Note: An *endometriotic disease flare*, with a transient increase in symptoms (pelvic pain, dysmenorrhea, dyspareunia, pelvic tenderness, induration), may occur shortly after initiation of therapy for endometriosis as a result of the temporary increase in serum estradiol.
   *In males only*
      **Constipation; decreased size of testicles; impotence** (inability to have or keep an erection); **prostatic carcinoma disease flare, transient** (bone pain)
   Note: A *prostatic carcinoma disease flare*, with a transient, sometimes severe, increase in bone or tumor pain, may occur shortly after initiation of therapy for prostatic carcinoma, usually is associated with the increase in serum testosterone, and usually subsides with continued goserelin treatment. Analgesics may be required during this time. Other signs and symptoms of prostatic carcinoma, including difficult urination and spinal compression, also may worsen transiently. In addition, worsening of neurologic signs and symptoms in patients with vertebral metastases may result in temporary weakness and paresthesias of the lower extremities; paralysis, with or without fatal complications, is possible.

## Patient Consultation

As an aid to patient consultation, refer to *Advice for the Patient, Goserelin (Systemic)*.

In providing consultation, consider emphasizing the following selected information (» = major clinical significance):

### Before using this medication
» Conditions affecting use, especially:
   Sensitivity to gonadorelin (synthetic gonadotropin-releasing hormone [GnRH]) or to gonadotropin-releasing hormone analogs (GnRHa), such as buserelin, goserelin, histrelin, leuprolide, or nafarelin
   Pregnancy—Not recommended for use during pregnancy; pregnancy should be ruled out prior to use of goserelin; nonhormonal contraceptive should be used during and for 12 weeks following therapy
   Breast-feeding—Not recommended for use by nursing mothers
   Other medical problems, especially undiagnosed, abnormal uterine bleeding (for endometrial thinning or endometriosis); urinary tract obstruction or history of (for prostatic carcinoma); or vertebral metastases (for prostatic carcinoma)

### Proper use of this medication
» Importance of continuing medication despite side effects
» Proper dosing
   Missed dose: Receiving as soon as possible

### Precautions while using this medication
» Importance of close monitoring by the physician
» Notifying physician if regular menstruation continues following regular use of goserelin or if regular menstrual periods do not begin again within 2 to 3 months after discontinuing medication; however, missing one or more successive doses may cause breakthrough menstrual bleeding
   For women of reproductive potential, using a nonhormonal contraceptive while being treated with goserelin

### Side/adverse effects
Signs of potential side effects, especially cardiac arrhythmias or palpitations; anaphylaxis; bone, muscle, or joint pain; paresthesias; syncope; androgenic effects (for females only); personality or behavioral changes (for females only); angina or myocardial infarction (for males only); pulmonary embolism (for males only); or thrombophlebitis (for males only)

## General Dosing Information

Patients receiving goserelin should be under supervision of a physician experienced in its use. Administration of goserelin should be carried out, using sterile technique, under supervision of a physician.

If the implant needs to be removed for any reason, it can be located by ultrasound.

Dosage adjustment is not needed for patients with hepatic or renal function impairment.

### For endometrial thinning
When used as an endometrial thinning agent, goserelin may cause an increase in cervical resistance. Therefore, care should be taken when dilating the cervix.

### For treatment of endometriosis
It is recommended that therapy begin with the first day of the menstrual cycle after pregnancy has been ruled out.

Development of amenorrhea is usually evidence of a clinical response, although spotting or bleeding from the atrophic endometrium can still occur.

Therapy should continue uninterrupted for 6 months. Re-treatment is not recommended. However, if re-treatment is contemplated, bone density should be assessed prior to beginning treatment, to verify that values are in the normal range.

### For treatment of prostatic carcinoma
A 10.8-mg, 3-month implant of goserelin suppresses testosterone levels equivalent to a 3.6-mg implant inserted every 28 days.

### For treatment of side/adverse effects
Recommended treatment:
   Bone pain—Mild oral analgesics with rest or, if severe, parenteral narcotics. Bone pain usually subsides after 2 weeks.
   Urinary obstruction, worsening of, in treatment of prostatic carcinoma—Catheterization if needed. Urinary obstruction usually resolves after the first week of goserelin therapy.

## Parenteral Dosage Forms

Note: Bracketed uses in the *Dosage Forms* section refer to categories of use and/or indications that are not included in U.S. product labeling.

The available dosage form contains goserelin acetate, but dosage and strength are expressed in terms of the base.

### GOSERELIN ACETATE IMPLANTS

**Usual adult dose**
Breast carcinoma[1]—
    Subcutaneous (into upper abdominal wall), 3.6 mg (base) every twenty-eight days.
Prostatic carcinoma—
    Subcutaneous (into upper abdominal wall), 3.6 mg (base) every twenty-eight days or 10.8 mg every twelve weeks.
[Endometrial thinning]—
    Subcutaneous (into upper abdominal wall), 3.6 mg (base) every twenty-eight days for two doses. The second dose should be given between zero and two weeks prior to endometrial ablation.
Endometriosis—
    Subcutaneous (into upper abdominal wall), 3.6 mg (base) every twenty-eight days for six months.
Note: Safety of goserelin when used for this indication for re-treatment or for periods greater than six months has not been established.

**Usual pediatric dose**
Carcinoma, breast or
Carcinoma, prostate or
[Endometrial thinning]—
    Children up to 18 years of age—Safety and efficacy have not been established.

Endometriosis—
    Children up to 18 years of age—Safety has not been established.

**Size(s) usually available**
U.S.—
    1-month formulation
        3.6 mg (base) (preloaded in a special single-use syringe) (Rx) [*Zoladex*].
    3-month formulation
        10.8 mg (base) (preloaded in a special single-use syringe) (Rx) [*Zoladex 3-Month*].
Canada—
    1-month formulation
        3.6 mg (base) (preloaded in a special single-use syringe) (Rx) [*Zoladex*].
    3-month formulation
        10.8 mg (base) (preloaded in a special single-use syringe) (Rx) [*Zoladex LA*].

**Packaging and storage**
Store below 25 °C (77 °F), unless otherwise specified by manufacturer. Protect from light. Protect from moisture.

---

[1]Not included in Canadian product labeling.

Revised: 07/02/98

---

# GRANISETRON   Systemic

VA CLASSIFICATION (Primary): GA605

Commonly used brand name(s): *Kytril*.

Note: For a listing of dosage forms and brand names by country availability, see *Dosage Forms* section(s).

## Category
Antiemetic.

## Indications

Note: Bracketed information in the *Indications* section refers to uses that are not included in U.S. product labeling.

**Accepted**
Nausea and vomiting, cancer chemotherapy–induced (prophylaxis)—
    Granisetron is indicated for the prevention of nausea and vomiting associated with initial and repeat courses of moderately or severely emetogenic cancer chemotherapy, including high-dose cisplatin.

    Studies have found intravenous granisetron to be as effective as high-dose metoclopramide plus dexamethasone, and superior to dexamethasone plus chlorpromazine or prochlorperazine in preventing nausea and vomiting induced by high-dose cisplatin, and by moderately emetogenic chemotherapy, respectively, during the acute phase lasting 24 hours after the start of chemotherapy. However, the dose of granisetron used in many of these studies was higher than the dose that is currently recommended. Unlike metoclopramide, granisetron has no dopamine receptor antagonist activity and thus does not induce extrapyramidal side effects.

[Nausea and vomiting, cancer radiotherapy–induced (prophylaxis)][1]—
    Granisetron injection may be used to prevent the nausea and vomiting associated with total body or upper hemibody irradiation in patients undergoing bone marrow transplantation.

---

[1]Not included in Canadian product labeling.

## Pharmacology/Pharmacokinetics

**Physicochemical characteristics**
Molecular weight—348.9.
pH—4.7 to 7.3

**Mechanism of action/Effect**
Antiemetic—Granisetron is a potent, selective antagonist of 5-hydroxytryptamine (serotonin) subtype 3 ($5-HT_3$) receptors. $5-HT_3$ receptors are present peripherally on vagal nerve terminals and centrally in the area postrema of the brain. Cytotoxic drugs and radiation damage gastrointestinal mucosa, causing the release of serotonin from the enterochromaffin cells of the gastrointestinal tract. Stimulation of $5-HT_3$ receptors causes transmission of sensory signals to the vomiting center via vagal afferent fibers to induce vomiting. By binding to $5-HT_3$ receptors, granisetron blocks vomiting mediated by serotonin release.

Granisetron has little or no affinity for other serotonin receptors, including $5-HT_1$, $5-HT_{1A}$, $5-HT_{1B/C}$, or $5-HT_2$; for $alpha_1$-, $alpha_2$-, or beta-adrenoreceptors; for dopamine $D_2$ receptors; for histamine $H_1$ receptors; for benzodiazepine receptors; for picrotoxin receptors; or for opioid receptors. In most human studies, granisetron has had little effect on blood pressure, heart rate, or electrocardiogram (ECG). Other studies have found no effect on plasma prolactin or aldosterone concentrations.

**Other actions/effects**
Granisetron, administered in single or multiple oral doses to volunteers, reduced colonic transit time, perhaps by antagonizing the effects of serotonin on the cholinergic neurons of the colon. However, a single intravenous infusion (of 50 or 200 micrograms of granisetron per kg of body weight [mcg/kg]) administered to volunteers showed no effect on oro-cecal transit time.

**Distribution**
The volume of distribution in cancer patients following a 5-minute infusion of 40 mcg/kg was 2 to 3 L/kg. The volume of distribution in healthy volunteers following administration of a single 1-mg oral dose of granisetron was 3.94 L/kg. Granisetron distributes freely between plasma and erythrocytes.

**Protein binding**
Moderate (65%).

**Biotransformation**
Hepatic; undergoes *N*-demethylation and aromatic ring oxidation followed by conjugation. Animal studies suggest that some of the metabolites may have $5-HT_3$ receptor antagonist activity.

**Half-life**
Intravenous—The elimination half-life in healthy volunteers following a single intravenous dose of 40 mcg/kg has been reported as 4 to 5 hours. The elimination half-life in cancer patients following a single intravenous dose of 40 mcg/kg has been reported as 9 to 12 hours. However, there is wide intrapatient and interpatient variability.
Oral—The elimination half-life in healthy volunteers following a single 1-mg dose has been reported as 6.23 hours.

**Peak plasma concentration**
Intravenous—Following a 5-minute infusion of 40 mcg of granisetron per kg of body weight, a mean peak plasma concentration of 63.8 nanograms per mL (nanograms/mL) was reported in adult cancer patients, and a mean value of 42.8 nanograms/mL was reported in healthy volunteers. Following a 3-minute infusion of 40 mcg of granisetron per kg

of body weight to healthy volunteers, a mean peak plasma concentration of 64.3 nanograms/mL was reported in subjects 21 to 42 years of age, and a mean value of 57 nanograms/mL was reported in subjects 65 to 81 years of age.

Oral—Following an oral dose of 1 mg of granisetron twice a day for 7 days, a mean peak plasma concentration of 5.99 nanograms/mL (range, 0.63 to 30.9 nanograms/mL) was reported in adult cancer patients. Following a single oral dose of 1 mg, a mean value of 3.63 nanograms/mL (range, 0.27 to 9.14 nanograms/mL) was reported in healthy volunteers. When healthy volunteers received a single oral 10-mg dose of granisetron with food, the area under the plasma concentration–time curve (AUC) was decreased by 5% and the peak plasma concentration was increased by 30%.

### Elimination
Predominantly hepatic. In healthy volunteers, approximately 8 to 15% of an intravenous dose, and 11% of an oral dose, of granisetron is recovered unchanged in the urine. The remainder of the dose is excreted as metabolites, 48 to 49% in the urine and 34 to 38% in the feces.

## Precautions to Consider

### Cross-sensitivity and/or related problems
Patients sensitive to ondansetron may also be sensitive to dolasetron and granisetron.

### Carcinogenicity/Tumorigenicity
In a 2-year study in rats, granisetron—given orally in doses corresponding to 20 and 101 times the recommended human oral dose (81 and 405 times the recommended human intravenous dose, respectively)—produced a statistically significant increase in the incidence of hepatocellular carcinomas and adenomas in males and females. In a 1-year study in rats, granisetron given orally in a dose corresponding to 405 times the recommended human oral dose (1622 times the recommended human intravenous dose) produced hepatocellular adenomas in males and females.

### Mutagenicity
Granisetron was not mutagenic in the *in vitro* Ames test and mouse lymphoma cell forward mutation assay, the *in vivo* mouse micronucleus test, and *in vitro* and *ex vivo* rat hepatocyte unscheduled DNA synthesis (UDS) assays. However, granisetron produced a significant increase in UDS in HeLa cells *in vitro* and a significantly increased incidence of cells with polyploidy in an *in vitro* human lymphocyte chromosomal aberration test.

### Pregnancy/Reproduction
Fertility—Granisetron was found to have no effect on the fertility and reproductive performance of male or female rats when given subcutaneously a dose corresponding to 97 times the recommended human intravenous dose (405 times the recommended human oral dose).

Pregnancy—Adequate and well-controlled studies have not been done in humans.

Studies in pregnant rats and rabbits given intravenous doses corresponding to 146 and 96 times the recommended human intravenous dose (507 and 255 times the recommended human oral dose), respectively, have not shown that granisetron causes adverse effects in the fetus.

FDA Pregnancy Category B.

### Breast-feeding
It is not known whether granisetron is distributed into breast milk.

### Pediatrics
Intravenous—Appropriate studies performed to date have not demonstrated pediatrics-specific problems that would limit the use of intravenous granisetron in children 2 years of age and older. Safety and efficacy in children up to 2 years of age have not been established.

Oral—Appropriate studies on the relationship of age to the effects of oral granisetron have not been performed in the pediatric population. Safety and efficacy have not been established.

### Geriatrics
Studies performed in patients 65 years of age or older have not demonstrated geriatrics-specific problems that would limit the usefulness of granisetron in the elderly.

### Drug interactions and/or related problems
The following drug interactions and/or related problems have been selected on the basis of their potential clinical significance (possible mechanism in parentheses where appropriate)—not necessarily inclusive (» = major clinical significance):

Note: Combinations containing any of the following medications, depending on the amount present, may also interact with this medication.

Enzyme inducers, hepatic, cytochrome P450 (see *Appendix II*) or
Enzyme inhibitors, hepatic, various (see *Appendix II*)
  (because granisetron is metabolized by hepatic cytochrome P450 3A enzymes, inducers or inhibitors of this enzyme may alter granisetron's clearance and half-life)

### Laboratory value alterations
The following have been selected on the basis of their potential clinical significance (possible effect in parentheses where appropriate)—not necessarily inclusive (» = major clinical significance):

With physiology/laboratory test values
  Alanine aminotransferase (ALT [SGPT]), serum and
  Aspartate aminotransferase (AST [SGOT]), serum
    (values may be increased)

### Medical considerations/Contraindications
The medical considerations/contraindications included have been selected on the basis of their potential clinical significance (reasons given in parentheses where appropriate)—not necessarily inclusive (» = major clinical significance).

*Risk-benefit should be considered when the following medical problem exists:*

» Sensitivity to granisetron, dolasetron, or ondansetron

## Side/Adverse Effects

The following side/adverse effects have been selected on the basis of their potential clinical significance (possible signs and symptoms in parentheses where appropriate)—not necessarily inclusive:

### Those indicating need for medical attention
Incidence less frequent
  *Fever*

Incidence rare
  *Arrhythmias* (irregular heartbeat); **chest pain; fainting; hypersensitivity reaction** (shortness of breath; skin rash, hives, and itching)

Note: *Alopecia, anemia, anorexia, leukopenia,* and *thrombocytopenia* have also been reported. However, it is not clear whether these effects were caused by granisetron or by the chemotherapy.

### Those indicating need for medical attention only if they continue or are bothersome
Incidence more frequent
  *Abdominal pain; constipation; diarrhea; headache; unusual tiredness or weakness*

Incidence less frequent
  *Agitation; dizziness; drowsiness; dyspepsia* (heartburn; indigestion; sour stomach); *insomnia* (trouble in sleeping); *unusual taste in mouth*

## Patient Consultation

As an aid to patient consultation, refer to *Advice for the Patient, Granisetron (Systemic)*.

In providing consultation, consider emphasizing the following selected information (» = major clinical significance):

### Before receiving this medication
» Conditions affecting use, especially:
    Sensitivity to granisetron

### Proper use of this medication
» Proper dosing

### Precautions while receiving this medication
Consulting physician if severe nausea and vomiting occur after administration of chemotherapy

### Side/adverse effects
Signs of potential side effects, especially fever, arrhythmias, chest pain, fainting, and hypersensitivity reaction

## Oral Dosage Forms

Note: The dosing and strength of the dosage form available are expressed in terms of granisetron base (not the hydrochloride salt).

### GRANISETRON HYDROCHLORIDE TABLETS

**Usual adult and adolescent dose**
Nausea and vomiting, cancer chemotherapy–induced, prophylaxis—
  Oral, 2 mg (base) given up to one hour before chemotherapy. Alternatively, 1 mg (base) administered up to one hour prior to chemotherapy, then 1 mg administered twelve hours after the initial dose.

Note: Dosage adjustment is not required in the elderly, or in patients with hepatic or renal function impairment.

**Usual pediatric dose**
Dosage has not been established.

# Granisetron (Systemic)

**Usual geriatric dose**
See *Usual adult and adolescent dose*.

**Strength(s) usually available**
U.S.—
- 1 mg (base) (Rx) [*Kytril* (hydroxypropyl methylcellulose; lactose; magnesium stearate; microcrystalline cellulose; polyethylene glycol; polysorbate 80; sodium starch glycolate; titanium dioxide)].

Canada—
- 1 mg (base) (Rx) [*Kytril* (hydroxypropyl methylcellulose; lactose; magnesium stearate; microcrystalline cellulose; polyethylene glycol; polysorbate 80; sodium starch glycolate; titanium dioxide)].

**Packaging and storage**
Store between 15 and 30 °C (59 and 86 °F), unless otherwise specified by manufacturer. Protect from light.

## Parenteral Dosage Forms

Note: Bracketed uses in the *Dosage Forms* section refer to categories of use and/or indications that are not included in U.S. product labeling.

The dosing and strength of the dosage form available are expressed in terms of granisetron base (not the hydrochloride salt).

### GRANISETRON HYDROCHLORIDE INJECTION

**Usual adult and adolescent dose**
Nausea and vomiting, cancer chemotherapy–induced, prophylaxis; or
[Nausea and vomiting, cancer radiotherapy–induced, prophylaxis][1]—
Intravenous, 10 mcg (base) per kg of body weight, administered within thirty minutes before initiation of emetogenic chemotherapy or radiotherapy. The dose may be administered undiluted over thirty seconds, or diluted with 5% dextrose injection or 0.9% sodium chloride injection and infused over five minutes. (See *Preparation of dosage form*.)

Note: Dosage adjustment is not required in the elderly, or in patients with hepatic or renal function impairment.

**Usual pediatric dose**
Children up to 2 years of age—Dosage has not been established.
Children 2 years of age and older—See *Usual adult and adolescent dose*.

**Usual geriatric dose**
See *Usual adult and adolescent dose*.

**Strength(s) usually available**
U.S.—
- 1 mg (base) per mL (Rx) [*Kytril* (sodium chloride 9 mg; citric acid 2 mg—in multi-dose vial; benzyl alcohol 10 mg—in multi-dose vial)].

Canada—
- 1 mg (base) per mL (Rx) [*Kytril* (sodium chloride 9 mg)].

**Packaging and storage**
Store between 2 and 30 °C (36 and 86 °F), unless otherwise specified by manufacturer. Do not freeze. Protect from light.

**Preparation of dosage form**
Granisetron may be diluted with 5% dextrose injection or 0.9% sodium chloride injection to a total volume of 20 to 50 mL.

**Stability**
Intravenous infusions of granisetron retain their potency for 24 hours at room temperature under normal lighting after dilution with 5% dextrose injection or 0.9% sodium chloride injection.

**Incompatibilities**
The chemical stability of granisetron with the following medications injected into Y-sites of administration sets has been verified:

| Medication | Concentration |
| --- | --- |
| Cyclophosphamide | 2 mg/mL |
| Cytarabine | 2 mg/mL |
| Dacarbazine | 1.7 mg/mL |
| Dexamethasone | 0.24 mg/mL |
| Doxorubicin | 0.2 mg/mL |
| Fluorouracil | 2 mg/mL |
| Furosemide | 0.4 mg/mL |
| Ifosfamide | 4 mg/mL |
| Magnesium sulfate | 4 grams/250 mL |
| Methotrexate | 12.5 mg/mL |
| Potassium chloride | 40 mEq/L |

Additionally, granisetron admixed with dexamethasone and mannitol is stable for 24 hours. However, no data are available on the compatibility of granisetron injection with other substances; therefore, other medications should not be added to the preparation or infused simultaneously through the same intravenous line.

**Caution**
Granisetron dosage is expressed in terms of mcg; however, the vial concentration is identified in terms of mg per mL.
Granisetron hydrochloride injection that contains benzyl alcohol as a preservative must not be used in newborns and immature infants. The use of benzyl alcohol in neonates has been associated with a fatal toxic syndrome consisting of metabolic acidosis and central nervous system (CNS), respiratory, circulatory, and renal function impairment.

[1] Not included in Canadian product labeling.

### Selected Bibliography

Joss RA, Dott CS, on behalf of the Granisetron Study Group. Clinical studies with granisetron, a new 5-HT$_3$ receptor antagonist for the treatment of cancer chemotherapy–induced emesis. Eur J Cancer 1993; 29A(1 Suppl): S22-S29.

Plosker GL, Goa KL. Granisetron. A review of its pharmacological properties and therapeutic use as an antiemetic. Drugs 1991; 42: 805-24.

Developed: 12/16/94
Revised: 06/23/98

---

# GREPAFLOXACIN Systemic—INTRODUCTORY VERSION

VA CLASSIFICATION (Primary): AM402
Note: For a listing of dosage forms and brand names by country availability, see *Dosage Forms* section(s).

## Category
Antibacterial (systemic).

## Indications

**General considerations**
Grepafloxacin is a fluoroquinolone antibiotic with *in vitro* activity against a wide variety of microorganisms. Grepafloxacin has been shown to be active *in vitro* and in clinical infections against most strains of *Chlamydia trachomatis*, *Haemophilus influenzae*, *Moraxella catarrhalis*, *Mycoplasma pneumoniae*, *Neisseria gonorrhoeae*, and penicillin-susceptible strains of *Streptococcus pneumoniae*. *In vitro* tests demonstrate that grepafloxacin has reduced activity against some gram-positive microorganisms when combined with rifampin.

Resistance to grepafloxacin *in vitro* occurs infrequently. In clinical trials, grepafloxacin-resistant mutants were observed rarely during the treatment of infections caused by susceptible isolates. When resistance did occur, it was usually in *Pseudomonas* species isolates. Although cross-resistance has been observed between grepafloxacin and some other fluoroquinolones, some organisms resistant to other quinolones remain susceptible to grepafloxacin.

**Accepted**
Bronchitis, bacterial exacerbations (treatment)—Grepafloxacin is indicated in the treatment of acute bacterial exacerbations of chronic bronchitis caused by *H. influenzae*, *M. catarrhalis*, or *S. pneumoniae*.

Cervicitis, nongonococcal (treatment) or
Urethritis, nongonococcal (treatment)—Grepafloxacin is indicated in the treatment of nongonococcal cervicitis or urethritis caused by *C. trachomatis*.

Gonorrhea, endocervical, uncomplicated (treatment)
Gonorrhea, rectal, uncomplicated, in females (treatment) or
Gonorrhea, urethral, uncomplicated (treatment)—Grepafloxacin is indicated in males for the treatment of uncomplicated urethral gonorrhea or in females for the treatment of uncomplicated endocervical or rectal gonorrhea caused by *N. gonorrhoeae*.

Pneumonia, bacterial (treatment)—Grepafloxacin is indicated in the treatment of community-acquired pneumonia caused by *H. influenzae*, *M. catarrhalis*, *M. pneumoniae*, or *S. pneumoniae*.

## Pharmacology/Pharmacokinetics

**Physicochemical characteristics**
Chemical group—Fluoroquinolone.
Molecular weight—422.88.

### Mechanism of action/Effect
Grepafloxacin inhibits the bacterial enzymes topoisomerase II (DNA gyrase) and topoisomerase IV, which are essential for duplication, transcription, and repair of bacterial DNA.

### Absorption
Rapid and extensive. The absolute bioavailability is approximately 70%.

### Distribution
$Vol_D$—5.07 ± 0.95 L per kg, following an oral dose of 400 mg.

### Protein binding
Moderate (approximately 50%).

### Biotransformation
The major metabolite is a glucuronide conjugate; minor metabolites include sulfate conjugates and oxidative metabolites. The oxidative metabolites are formed mainly by the cytochrome P450 enzyme CYP1A2, while the cytochrome P450 enzyme CYP3A4 plays a minor role. The nonconjugated metabolites have little antimicrobial activity compared with the parent drug, and the conjugated metabolites have no antimicrobial activity.

### Half-life
Elimination (at steady state)—15.7 ± 4.2 hours.

### Time to peak concentration
2 to 3 hours.

### Peak plasma concentration
In healthy adult males, after a single dose of—
  400 mg: 1.11 ± 0.34 mcg per mL.
  600 mg: 1.58 ± 0.37 mcg per mL.
In healthy adult males, at steady state, following 7 days of dosing with a single daily dose of—
  400 mg: 1.35 ± 0.25 mcg per mL.
  600 mg: 2.25 ± 0.48 mcg per mL.

Note: The peak plasma concentration in females is approximately 30 to 50% higher than that in males, a difference that appears to be due primarily to differences in body weight. Total clearance, renal clearance, and half-life are similar between males and females. No gender-specific dosage adjustments are necessary.

### Elimination
Primarily through hepatic metabolism and biliary excretion.
Fecal—Approximately 50% of an oral dose of 400 mg is recovered over 7 days; 27% of the dose is recovered unchanged; 1.83 to 3.91% of the dose is recovered as metabolites.
Renal—Approximately 38% of an oral dose of 400 mg is recovered over 7 days; 6% of the dose is recovered unchanged; 0.08 to 5.57% of the dose is recovered as metabolites.

## Precautions to Consider

### Cross-sensitivity and/or related problems
Patients allergic to one fluoroquinolone or other chemically related quinolone derivatives (e.g., cinoxacin, nalidixic acid) may be allergic to grepafloxacin also.

### Carcinogenicity
Long-term studies to determine the carcinogenic potential of grepafloxacin have not been performed.

### Mutagenicity
Grepafloxacin was not mutagenic in the Ames test, the forward gene mutation assay, the mouse micronucleus assay, or the unscheduled DNA repair test using rat hepatocytes. However, grepafloxacin was mutagenic in a bacterial DNA repair test and in an *in vitro* chromosome aberration test.

### Pregnancy/Reproduction
Fertility—Parenteral grepafloxacin produced no medication-related changes in the estrous cycle of female rats, or in the copulation behavior or fertility of male or female rats.

Pregnancy—Adequate and well-controlled studies in humans have not been done. Grepafloxacin should be used in pregnancy only if the potential benefit to the mother outweighs the potential risk to the fetus.

Administration of oral or parenteral grepafloxacin to rats did not result in embryo lethality or teratogenicity. There were no medication-related effects on maintenance of pregnancy, parturition, implantation of females, ovulation, or nursing; or on fetal viability, body weight, or morphology. However, decreases in placental weight and in the number of ossified sacrococcygeal vertebrae were observed in rats given 2.4 times the maximum recommended human dose (MRHD) on a mg per square meter of body surface area ($mg/m^2$) basis (15 times the MRHD on a mg per kg of body weight [mg/kg] basis); these effects were associated with maternal toxicity (demonstrated by decreased body weight and food consumption). No effect was observed in rats given 420 $mg/m^2$, which is equivalent to the recommended human dose.

Administration of grepafloxacin to rabbits did not result in embryo lethality or teratogenicity. However, fetal body weight was decreased, and there was a tendency for a decrease in placental weight for rabbits given doses of 60 mg/kg. Maternal toxicity was demonstrated by abortion in rabbits given doses of 40 mg/kg or higher.

In a perinatal/postnatal study in rats, death and prolongation of delivery time were observed at doses of 2.4 times the MRHD on a $mg/m^2$ basis (15 times the MRHD on a mg/kg basis). There were no medication-related effects on delivery index, lactation, or offspring.

FDA Pregnancy Category C.

### Breast-feeding
Grepafloxacin is distributed into breast milk. Fluoroquinolones have been shown to cause permanent lesions of the cartilage of weight-bearing joints, as well as other signs of arthropathy, in immature animals. Because of the potential for serious adverse effects in nursing infants, a decision should be made to discontinue breast-feeding or discontinue administration of grepafloxacin.

### Pediatrics
Safety and efficacy have not been established for pediatric patients. Use is not recommended because fluoroquinolones have been shown to cause arthropathy in immature animals.

### Adolescents
Safety and efficacy have not been established for patients less than 18 years of age. Use is not recommended because fluoroquinolones have been shown to cause arthropathy in immature animals.

### Geriatrics
Studies performed in approximately 343 elderly patients 65 years of age or older have not demonstrated geriatrics-specific problems that would limit the usefulness of grepafloxacin in the elderly.

### Drug interactions and/or related problems
The following drug interactions and/or related problems have been selected on the basis of their potential clinical significance (possible mechanism in parentheses where appropriate)—not necessarily inclusive (» = major clinical significance):

Note: Combinations containing any of the following medications, depending on the amount present, may also interact with this medication.

» Amiodarone or
» Antidepressants, tricyclic or
» Astemizole or
» Bepridil or
» Cisapride or
» Erythromycin or
» Pentamidine or
» Phenothiazines or
» Procainamide or
» Quinidine or
» Sotalol or
» Terfenadine or
» Other medications reported to prolong the QTc interval
  (prolongation of the QTc interval was observed in healthy volunteers receiving grepafloxacin; concurrent administration of these agents with grepafloxacin may potentiate the risk of cardiac arrhythmias, including torsades de pointes; grepafloxacin is **contraindicated** in patients being treated concurrently with medications known to produce an increase in the QTc interval and/or torsades de pointes, unless appropriate cardiac monitoring can be assured [i.e., hospital patients])

Antacids, aluminum-, calcium-, and/or magnesium-containing or
Iron supplements or
Sucralfate or
Zinc supplements
  (concurrent use of antacids, iron or zinc supplements, or sucralfate with grepafloxacin may chelate metal cations and interfere with the absorption of grepafloxacin; these agents should not be taken within 4 hours before or 4 hours after taking grepafloxacin)

» Antidiabetic agents
  (disturbances of blood glucose concentrations, including hyperglycemia and hypoglycemia, have been reported with concurrent use of antidiabetic agents and quinolones other than grepafloxacin; careful monitoring of blood glucose concentrations is recommended when these medications are used concurrently)

» Anti-inflammatory drugs, nonsteroidal (NSAIDs)
  (concurrent administration of NSAIDs with quinolone antibiotics may increase the risks of central nervous system [CNS] stimulation and convulsions)

Methylxanthines, such as:
» Caffeine or
  Theobromine or
» Theophylline or
  Other medications metabolized by the cytochrome P450 enzyme system
    (grepafloxacin may inhibit the metabolism of caffeine or theobromine, enhancing the effects of caffeine or theobromine)
    (grepafloxacin is a competitive inhibitor of the metabolism of theophylline; serum theophylline concentrations may increase when grepafloxacin is administered to patients receiving theophylline therapy; when initiating a multi-day course of grepafloxacin therapy in a patient maintained on theophylline, the theophylline maintenance dose should be halved for the period of concurrent use with grepafloxacin; serum theophylline concentrations should be monitored to guide further dosage adjustments)
    (grepafloxacin is metabolized primarily by the cytochrome P450 enzyme system; this may result in impaired metabolism of other medications that are also metabolized via this system; however, studies have not been done to evaluate these interactions)
  Warfarin
    (some quinolones have been reported to enhance the effects of warfarin or its derivatives; although no significant change in clotting time was observed when grepafloxacin was administered concurrently to patients receiving warfarin, it is recommended that prothrombin time [PT] or other suitable anticoagulation test be monitored closely)

**Medical considerations/Contraindications**
The medical considerations/Contraindications included have been selected on the basis of their potential clinical significance (reasons given in parentheses where appropriate)—not necessarily inclusive (» = major clinical significance).

*Except under special circumstances, this medication should not be used when the following medical problems exist:*
» Hepatic function failure
    (grepafloxacin is **contraindicated** in patients with hepatic function failure because it is metabolized primarily by the liver)
» Hypersensitivity to grepafloxacin or other quinolone antibiotics
» Proarrhythmias
    (grepafloxacin is not recommended for use in patients with ongoing proarrhythmic conditions, including atrial fibrillation, congestive heart failure, hypokalemia, myocardial infarction, and significant bradycardia)
» QTc-interval prolongation
    (prolongation of the QTc interval has been observed in healthy volunteers receiving grepafloxacin; therefore, grepafloxacin is **contraindicated** in patients with known QTc-interval prolongation)

*Risk-benefit should be considered when the following medical problems exist:*
  CNS disorders, including:
» Cerebral arteriosclerosis, severe or
» Epilepsy or
» Other factors that predispose to seizures
    (convulsions, increased intracranial pressure, and toxic psychosis have been reported in patients receiving quinolones; quinolones may also cause CNS stimulation, which may lead to confusion, hallucinations, lightheadedness, restlessness, or tremors; therefore, grepafloxacin should be used with caution in patients with confirmed or suspected CNS disorders)

**Patient monitoring**
The following may be especially important in patient monitoring (other tests may be warranted in some patients, depending on condition; » = major clinical significance):

  Blood glucose determinations
    (disturbances of blood glucose concentrations, including hyperglycemia and hypoglycemia, have been reported with concurrent administration of antidiabetic agents and quinolones other than grepafloxacin; careful monitoring of blood glucose concentrations is recommended for patients with diabetes mellitus who are taking antidiabetic agents and grepafloxacin concurrently)
» Electrocardiogram (ECG)
    (patients who are being treated concurrently with grepafloxacin and medications known to produce an increase in the QTc interval and/or torsades de pointes should receive appropriate cardiac monitoring)

  Prothrombin time (PT)
    (the PT of patients concurrently receiving grepafloxacin and warfarin should be monitored closely)
  Syphilis testing
    (the efficacy of grepafloxacin for treatment of syphilis is not known; antimicrobial agents used in high doses for short periods of time to treat gonorrhea may mask or delay the symptoms of incubating syphilis; it is recommended that all patients with gonorrhea have a serologic test for syphilis at the time of diagnosis, and that patients treated with grepafloxacin have a follow-up test for syphilis 3 months after treatment for gonorrhea)

## Side/Adverse Effects
Note: Adverse events during clinical trials were generally transient, mild to moderate in severity, and required no treatment. However, prolongation of the QTc interval was observed in healthy male and female volunteers receiving grepafloxacin.

The following side/adverse effects have been selected on the basis of their potential clinical significance (possible signs and symptoms in parentheses where appropriate)—not necessarily inclusive:

**Those indicating need for medical attention**
Incidence more frequent
  *QTc-interval prolongation* (irregular or slow heart rate; recurrent fainting)
Incidence rare
  *Central nervous system (CNS) stimulation* (acute psychosis; confusion; hallucinations; restlessness; seizures; tremors); *hypersensitivity reactions* (difficulty in breathing or swallowing; rapid heartbeat; skin itching, rash, or redness; shortness of breath; swelling of face, throat, or tongue); *pseudomembranous colitis* (abdominal or stomach cramps and pain; abdominal tenderness; diarrhea, watery and severe, which may also be bloody; fever); *tendinitis or tendon rupture* (pain in calves, radiating to heels; swelling of calves or lower legs)

**Those indicating need for medical attention only if they continue or are bothersome**
Incidence more frequent
  *Change in sense of taste; diarrhea, mild; dizziness or lightheadedness; headache; nausea or vomiting; vaginitis* (vaginal pain and discharge)
Incidence less frequent
  *Photosensitivity* (increased sensitivity of skin to sunlight)

**Those indicating possible pseudomembranous colitis and the need for medical attention if they occur after medication is discontinued**
  *Abdominal or stomach cramps and pain; abdominal tenderness; diarrhea, watery and severe, which may also be bloody; fever*

## Overdose
For more information on the management of overdose or unintentional ingestion, **contact a Poison Control Center** (see *Poison Control Center Listing*).

**Treatment of overdose**
To decrease absorption—The stomach should be emptied by gastric lavage or by inducing vomiting.

To enhance elimination—It is not known whether grepafloxacin is efficiently removed by hemodialysis or peritoneal dialysis.

Monitoring—Electrocardiogram (ECG) monitoring is recommended due to the possibility of prolongation of the QTc interval and other cardiac complications, including arrhythmias.

Supportive care—Patients in whom intentional overdose is confirmed or suspected should be referred for psychiatric consultation.

## Patient Consultation
In providing consultation, consider emphasizing the following selected information (» = major clinical significance):

**Before using this medication**
» Conditions affecting use, especially:
  Hypersensitivity to grepafloxacin or other quinolone antibiotics
  Pregnancy—Use is recommended only if the potential benefit to the mother outweighs the potential risk to the fetus
  Breast-feeding—Grepafloxacin is distributed into breast milk
  Use in children—Use is not recommended because fluoroquinolones have been shown to cause arthropathy in immature animals
  Use in adolescents—Use is not recommended in adolescents less than 18 years of age because fluoroquinolones have been shown to cause arthropathy in immature animals
  Contraindicated medications—Amiodarone, astemizole, bepridil, cisapride, erythromycin, pentamidine, phenothiazines, procain-

amide, quinidine, sotalol, terfenadine, tricyclic antidepressants, or other medications reported to prolong the QTc interval

Other medications, especially antidiabetic agents, caffeine, nonsteroidal anti-inflammatory drugs (NSAIDs), and theophylline

Other medical problems, especially CNS disorders, including epilepsy, severe cerebral arteriosclerosis, and other factors predisposing to seizures; hepatic function failure; proarrhythmias; and QTc-interval prolongation

**Proper use of this medication**
» Not giving to infants, children, or adolescents
» Compliance with full course of therapy
» Taking with full glass (8 ounces) of water; maintaining adequate fluid intake
» Proper dosing
  Missed dose: Taking as soon as possible if remembered the same day; if dose is missed on one day, not doubling dose the following day
» Proper storage

**Precautions while using this medication**
Checking with physician if no improvement within a few days
» Not taking antacids, iron- or zinc-containing vitamins or supplements, or sucralfate within 4 hours before or 4 hours after taking grepafloxacin
» Possible photosensitivity reactions
» Caution if dizziness or lightheadedness occurs

**Side/adverse effects**
Signs of potential side effects, especially QTc-interval prolongation, CNS stimulation, hypersensitivity reactions, pseudomembranous colitis, and tendinitis or tendon rupture

## General Dosing Information
Dosage adjustment is not required in patients with renal function impairment.

### Diet/Nutrition
Grepafloxacin may be taken either with food or on an empty stomach.

Antacids, iron- or zinc-containing vitamins or supplements, or sucralfate should not be taken within 4 hours before or 4 hours after taking grepafloxacin.

## Oral Dosage Forms

### GREPAFLOXACIN HYDROCHLORIDE TABLETS

Note: The dosing and strength of the dosage form available are expressed in terms of grepafloxacin base, not the hydrochloride salt.

**Usual adult dose**
Bronchitis, bacterial exacerbations—
  Oral, 400 or 600 mg (base) once a day for ten days.
Cervicitis, nongonococcal or
Urethritis, nongonococcal—
  Oral, 400 mg (base) once a day for seven days.
Gonorrhea, uncomplicated—
  Oral, 400 mg (base) as a single dose.
Pneumonia, community-acquired—
  Oral, 600 mg (base) once a day for ten days.

**Usual pediatric dose**
Children up to 18 years of age—Safety and efficacy have not been established. Use is not recommended.

**Usual geriatric dose**
See *Usual adult dose*.

**Strength(s) usually available**
U.S.—
  200 mg (base) (Rx) [*Raxar*].

**Packaging and storage**
Store at room temperature (20 to 25 °C [68 to 77 °F]).

Developed: 02/09/98

---

# GRISEOFULVIN  Systemic

VA CLASSIFICATION (Primary): AM700

Commonly used brand name(s): *Fulvicin P/G; Fulvicin U/F; Fulvicin-U/F; Grifulvin V; Gris-PEG; Grisactin; Grisactin Ultra; Grisovin-FP*.

Note: For a listing of dosage forms and brand names by country availability, see *Dosage Forms* section(s).

## Category
Antifungal (systemic).

## Indications

**Accepted**
Tinea barbae (treatment)
Tinea capitis (treatment)
Tinea corporis (treatment)
Tinea cruris (treatment)
Tinea pedis (treatment) or
Tinea unguium—Griseofulvin is indicated in the treatment of tinea barbae, tinea capitis, tinea corporis, tinea cruris, tinea pedis, and tinea unguium (onychomycosis) caused by *Trichophyton rubrum, T. tonsurans, T. mentagrophytes, T. interdigitale, T. verrucosum, T. megninii, T. gallinae, T. schoenleinii, Microsporum audouinii, M. canis, M. gypseum,* and *Epidermophyton floccosum*.

Not all species or strains of a particular organism may be susceptible to griseofulvin. In addition, griseofulvin may not be effective because of poor absorption or inadequate tissue concentrations of griseofulvin.

**Unaccepted**
Griseofulvin is not indicated in the treatment of minor or trivial infections that will respond to topical antifungals alone.

Griseofulvin is not effective in the treatment of bacterial infections, candidiasis, histoplasmosis, actinomycosis, sporotrichosis, chromoblastomycosis, coccidioidomycosis, North American blastomycosis, cryptococcosis, tinea versicolor, or nocardiosis.

## Pharmacology/Pharmacokinetics

**Physicochemical characteristics**
Molecular weight—352.77.

**Mechanism of action/Effect**
Fungistatic; griseofulvin inhibits fungal cell mitosis by causing disruption of the mitotic spindle structure, thereby arresting the metaphase of cell division. It is deposited in varying concentrations in the keratin precursor cells of skin, hair, and nails, rendering the keratin resistant to fungal invasion. As the infected keratin is shed, it is replaced with healthy tissue.

**Absorption**
Microsize—Variable, ranging from 25 to 70% of an oral dose.
Ultramicrosize—Almost completely absorbed.
Absorption is significantly enhanced by administration with or after a fatty meal.

**Distribution**
Griseofulvin is deposited in varying concentrations in the keratin layer of the skin, hair, and nails. It can be detected in the stratum corneum of the skin within a few hours following administration. Only a very small fraction of an oral dose is distributed in the body fluids and tissues.

**Biotransformation**
Hepatic; major metabolites are 6-methyl-griseofulvin and its glucuronide conjugate.

**Half-life**
Approximately 24 hours.

**Time to peak serum concentration**
Approximately 4 hours following administration of a single dose of 250 mg of ultramicrosize griseofulvin or 500 mg of microsize griseofulvin.

**Elimination**
Renal. Less than 1% of a dose is excreted as unchanged drug in the urine. Approximately 36% of griseofulvin is excreted unchanged in the feces.

## Precautions to Consider

**Cross-sensitivity and/or related problems**
Since griseofulvin is derived from a species of *Penicillium*, it is theoretically possible that patients intolerant of penicillins or penicillamine may be intolerant of griseofulvin also. However, cross-sensitivity between griseofulvin and penicillins or penicillamine has not been clinically substantiated. In addition, penicillin-sensitive patients have received griseofulvin without difficulty.

## Carcinogenicity/Tumorigenicity/Mutagenicity

Griseofulvin has been shown to cause hepatomas in several strains of mice, particularly males, that were chronically fed griseofulvin at levels ranging from 0.5% to 2.5% of their diet. Smaller particle-size griseofulvin resulted in an enhanced tumorigenic effect. Griseofulvin, given subcutaneously in relatively small doses once a week during the first 3 weeks of life, has also been shown to cause hepatomas in mice.

Griseofulvin has been shown to cause thyroid tumors, mostly adenomas but also some carcinomas, in male rats that were fed griseofulvin at levels of 0.2%, 1%, and 2% of their diet. Thyroid tumors were also reported in female rats that were fed the two higher dosage levels of griseofulvin.

Studies in other animal species have not shown that griseofulvin is tumorigenic, however.

Griseofulvin has been shown to have a colchicine-like effect on mitosis and to be cocarcinogenic with methylcholanthrene in cutaneous tumor induction studies in laboratory animals.

## Pregnancy/Reproduction

Fertility—Griseofulvin has been shown to suppress spermatogenesis in rats, although this has not been confirmed in humans.

Pregnancy—Griseofulvin crosses the placenta. Conjoined twins have been reported rarely in patients taking griseofulvin during the first trimester of pregnancy. Therefore, this medication is not recommended for use during pregnancy.

Studies in rats have shown that griseofulvin is embryotoxic and teratogenic. In addition, studies in dogs have shown that griseofulvin may cause adverse effects in pups.

## Breast-feeding

It is not known whether griseofulvin is excreted in breast milk. However, problems in humans have not been documented.

## Pediatrics

Appropriate studies on the relationship of age to the effects of griseofulvin have not been performed in children up to 2 years of age.

## Geriatrics

Appropriate studies on the relationship of age to the effects of griseofulvin have not been performed in the geriatric population. However, no geriatrics-specific problems have been documented to date.

## Dental

Griseofulvin may cause oral thrush (soreness or irritation of mouth or tongue).

## Drug interactions and/or related problems

The following drug interactions and/or related problems have been selected on the basis of their potential clinical significance (possible mechanism in parentheses where appropriate)—not necessarily inclusive (» = major clinical significance):

Note: Combinations containing any of the following medications, depending on the amount present, may also interact with this medication.

Alcohol
(effects may be potentiated when alcohol is used concurrently with griseofulvin; also, concurrent use with griseofulvin may result in tachycardia, diaphoresis, and flushing)

» Anticoagulants, coumarin- or indandione-derivative
(anticoagulant effects may be decreased when these agents are used concurrently with griseofulvin; decrease is thought to be due to accelerated metabolism of anticoagulants secondary to stimulation of hepatic microsomal enzyme activity; prothrombin time should be monitored until a stable level is maintained; dosage adjustments may be necessary during and after griseofulvin therapy)

Barbiturates or
Primidone
(antifungal effects of griseofulvin may be decreased when it is used concurrently with primidone or barbiturates, especially phenobarbital, because of impaired absorption, resulting in decreased serum concentrations; although the effect of decreased serum concentrations on therapeutic response has not been established, concurrent use is preferably avoided)

» Contraceptives, estrogen-containing, oral
(concurrent long-term use of griseofulvin may decrease the effectiveness of oral contraceptives, possibly because of stimulation of hepatic microsomal enzyme activity, resulting in decreased serum estrogen concentrations; this may lead to intermenstrual bleeding, amenorrhea, or unplanned pregnancies; patients should be advised to use an alternate or additional method of contraception while taking griseofulvin concurrently with estrogen-containing oral contraceptives and for 1 month after stopping griseofulvin)

## Medical considerations/Contraindications

The medical considerations/contraindications included have been selected on the basis of their potential clinical significance (reasons given in parentheses where appropriate)—not necessarily inclusive (» = major clinical significance).

*Risk-benefit should be considered when the following medical problems exist:*

» Hepatic dysfunction
(griseofulvin may on rare occasion be hepatotoxic)

Hypersensitivity to griseofulvin

Lupus erythematosus or lupus-like syndromes
(griseofulvin may precipitate or exacerbate lupus)

» Porphyria
(griseofulvin may precipitate porphyria attacks)

## Patient monitoring

The following may be especially important in patient monitoring (other tests may be warranted in some patients, depending on condition; » = major clinical significance):

Complete blood count (CBC) and
Creatinine concentration, serum and
Hepatic function determinations
(recommended at periodic intervals during therapy)

Urinalysis
(recommended at periodic intervals during therapy since proteinuria has been rarely reported)

# Side/Adverse Effects

The following side/adverse effects have been selected on the basis of their potential clinical significance (possible signs and symptoms in parentheses where appropriate)—not necessarily inclusive:

## Those indicating need for medical attention

Incidence less frequent
*Confusion; hypersensitivity* (skin rash, hives, or itching); *oral thrush* (soreness or irritation of mouth or tongue); *photosensitivity* (increased sensitivity of skin to sunlight)

Incidence rare—more frequent with prolonged use and/or high doses
*Granulocytopenia or leukopenia* (sore throat and fever); *hepatitis* (yellow eyes or skin); *peripheral neuritis* (numbness, tingling, pain, or weakness in hands or feet)

## Those indicating need for medical attention only if they continue or are bothersome

Incidence more frequent
*Headache*

Incidence less frequent
*Dizziness; gastrointestinal reactions* (diarrhea; nausea or vomiting; stomach pain); *insomnia* (trouble in sleeping); *unusual tiredness*

# Patient Consultation

As an aid to patient consultation, refer to *Advice for the Patient, Griseofulvin (Systemic)*.

In providing consultation, consider emphasizing the following selected information (» = major clinical significance):

## Before using this medication

» Conditions affecting use, especially:
Hypersensitivity to griseofulvin; theoretic cross-sensitivity with penicillin, however, penicillin-sensitive patients have received griseofulvin without difficulty
Pregnancy—Griseofulvin crosses the placenta; use is not recommended during pregnancy since griseofulvin has been shown to be embryotoxic and teratogenic in rats
Dental—Griseofulvin may cause oral thrush
Other medications, especially coumarin- or indandione-derivative anticoagulants or estrogen-containing oral contraceptives
Other medical problems, especially hepatic dysfunction or porphyria

## Proper use of this medication

» Taking with or after meals, especially fatty ones, to minimize gastrointestinal irritation and to increase absorption; checking with physician if on low-fat diet
Proper administration technique for oral suspension
» Compliance with full course of therapy
» Proper dosing
Missed dose: Taking as soon as possible; not taking if almost time for next dose; not doubling doses
» Proper storage

**Precautions while using this medication**
  Regular visits to physician to check progress during therapy
» Use of an alternate or additional means of contraception if taking estrogen-containing oral contraceptives concurrently and for 1 month after stopping griseofulvin
  Caution in drinking alcoholic beverages during griseofulvin therapy
» Caution if dizziness occurs
» Possible photosensitivity reactions

**Side/adverse effects**
  Signs of potential side effects, especially confusion, hypersensitivity, photosensitivity, oral thrush, granulocytopenia, leukopenia, and peripheral neuritis

## General Dosing Information

An oral dose of 250 to 330 mg of ultramicrosize griseofulvin produces serum concentrations equal to 500 mg of microsize griseofulvin.

Griseofulvin should be administered with or after meals (preferably meals high in fat content) to minimize possible gastrointestinal irritation and to increase absorption.

To help prevent relapse, therapy should be continued until the infecting organism is completely eradicated as determined by clinical or laboratory examination. Representative treatment periods are: tinea capitis, 8 to 10 weeks; tinea corporis, 2 to 4 weeks; tinea pedis, 4 to 8 weeks; onychomycosis, at least 4 months for fingernails and at least 6 months for toenails. However, recurrence rates in the treatment of onychomycosis of the toenails are very high.

Concurrent use of an appropriate topical agent is usually required, particularly in the treatment of tinea pedis, since both yeasts and bacteria as well as fungi may be involved in some forms of athlete's foot. Also, griseofulvin is not effective against bacterial or monilial infections. In addition, concurrent use with a topical antifungal agent may reduce the likelihood of relapse.

## Oral Dosage Forms

### GRISEOFULVIN CAPSULES (MICROSIZE) USP

**Usual adult and adolescent dose**
Antifungal—
  Onychomycosis; or
  Tinea pedis: Oral, 500 mg every twelve hours.
  Tinea capitis
  Tinea corporis or
  Tinea cruris: Oral, 250 mg every twelve hours; or 500 mg once a day.

**Usual pediatric dose**
Antifungal—
  Oral, 5 mg per kg of body weight or 150 mg per square meter of body surface every twelve hours; or 10 mg per kg of body weight or 300 mg per square meter of body surface once a day; or for
  Children 14 to 23 kg: Oral, 62.5 to 125 mg every twelve hours; or 125 to 250 mg once a day.
  Children 23 kg and over: Oral, 125 to 250 mg every twelve hours; or 250 to 500 mg once a day.

**Strength(s) usually available**
U.S.—
  250 mg (Rx) [*Grisactin*].
Canada—
  Not commercially available.

**Packaging and storage**
Store below 40 °C (104 °F), preferably between 15 and 30 °C (59 and 86 °F), unless otherwise specified by manufacturer. Store in a tight container.

**Auxiliary labeling**
• May cause dizziness.
• Avoid alcoholic beverages.
• Avoid too much sun or use of sunlamp.
• Continue medicine for full time of treatment.
• Take with or after meals or milk.

### GRISEOFULVIN ORAL SUSPENSION (MICROSIZE) USP

**Usual adult and adolescent dose**
See *Griseofulvin Capsules USP (Microsize)*.

**Usual pediatric dose**
See *Griseofulvin Capsules USP (Microsize)*.

**Strength(s) usually available**
U.S.—
  125 mg per 5 mL (Rx) [*Grifulvin V* (alcohol 0.008%; methylparaben; propylparaben)].

Canada—
  Not commercially available.

**Packaging and storage**
Store below 40 °C (104 °F), preferably between 15 and 30 °C (59 and 86 °F), unless otherwise specified by manufacturer. Store in a tight container. Protect from freezing.

**Auxiliary labeling**
• Shake well.
• May cause dizziness.
• Avoid alcoholic beverages.
• Avoid too much sun or use of sunlamp.
• Continue medicine for full time of treatment.
• Take with or after meals or milk.

**Note**
When dispensing, include a calibrated liquid-measuring device.

### GRISEOFULVIN TABLETS (MICROSIZE) USP

**Usual adult and adolescent dose**
See *Griseofulvin Capsules USP (Microsize)*.

**Usual pediatric dose**
See *Griseofulvin Capsules USP (Microsize)*.

**Strength(s) usually available**
U.S.—
  250 mg (Rx) [*Fulvicin-U/F* (scored); *Grifulvin V* (scored)].
  500 mg (Rx) [*Fulvicin-U/F* (scored); *Grifulvin V* (scored); *Grisactin*].
Canada—
  125 mg (Rx) [*Fulvicin U/F* (scored); *Grisovin-FP*].
  250 mg (Rx) [*Fulvicin U/F* (scored); *Grisovin-FP*].
  500 mg (Rx) [*Fulvicin U/F* (scored); *Grisovin-FP*].

**Packaging and storage**
Store below 40 °C (104 °F), preferably between 15 and 30 °C (59 and 86 °F), unless otherwise specified by manufacturer. Store in a tight container.

**Auxiliary labeling**
• May cause dizziness.
• Avoid alcoholic beverages.
• Avoid too much sun or use of sunlamp.
• Continue medicine for full time of treatment.
• Take with or after meals or milk.

### ULTRAMICROSIZE GRISEOFULVIN TABLETS USP

**Usual adult and adolescent dose**
Antifungal—
  Onychomycosis or
  Tinea pedis: Oral, 250 to 375 mg every twelve hours.
  Tinea capitis
  Tinea corporis or
  Tinea cruris: Oral, 125 to 187.5 mg every twelve hours; or 250 to 375 mg once a day.

**Usual pediatric dose**
Antifungal—
  Oral, 2.75 to 3.65 mg per kg of body weight every twelve hours; or 5.5 to 7.3 mg per kg of body weight once a day; or for
  Children 14 to 23 kg: Oral, 31.25 to 82.5 mg every twelve hours; or 62.5 to 165 mg once a day.
  Children 23 kg and over: Oral, 62.5 to 165 mg every twelve hours; or 125 to 330 mg once a day.
Note: Infants and children up to 2 years of age—Dosage has not been established.

**Strength(s) usually available**
U.S.—
  100 mg (Rx) [GENERIC].
  125 mg (Rx) [*Fulvicin P/G* (scored); *Gris-PEG* (scored; methylparaben)].
  165 mg (Rx) [*Fulvicin P/G* (scored); GENERIC].
  250 mg (Rx) [*Fulvicin P/G* (scored); *Grisactin Ultra* (scored); *Gris-PEG* (scored; methylparaben)].
  330 mg (Rx) [*Fulvicin P/G* (scored); *Grisactin Ultra* (scored); GENERIC].
Canada—
  165 mg (Rx) [*Fulvicin P/G*].
  330 mg (Rx) [*Fulvicin P/G*].

**Packaging and storage**
Store below 40 °C (104 °F), preferably between 15 and 30 °C (59 and 86 °F), unless otherwise specified by manufacturer. Store in a well-closed container.

# GROWTH HORMONE  Systemic

This monograph includes information on the following: 1) Somatrem; 2) Somatropin, Recombinant.

VA CLASSIFICATION (Primary): HS701

Commonly used brand name(s): *Humatrope*[2]; *Nutropin*[2]; *Protropin*[1].

Other commonly used names are GH and human growth hormone (hGH)

Note: For a listing of dosage forms and brand names by country availability, see *Dosage Forms* section(s).

## Category
Growth hormone.

## Indications
Note: Bracketed information in the *Indications* section refers to uses that are not included in U.S. product labeling.

**Accepted**

Growth failure (treatment)—Somatrem and recombinant somatropin are indicated for long-term treatment of growth failure in children caused by pituitary growth hormone (GH) deficiency (pituitary dwarfism), including GH deficiency caused by cranial irradiation. Failure to grow must be documented by a subnormal growth rate, and GH deficiency is usually identified by a lack of response to 2 standard pharmacologic stimuli that would normally provoke the release of somatropin or evidence of impaired spontaneous secretion or bioactivity of endogenous GH.

Human growth hormone is ineffective in patients with closed epiphyses; use in patients with epiphyseal maturation of greater than 15 to 16 years in males or 14 to 15 years in females is not generally recommended, although therapy may be useful in some older patients if epiphyses have not closed.

[Human growth hormone is also being used to treat growth failure associated with Turner's syndrome.]

There are currently insufficient data to establish the efficacy and the long-term safety of the use of human growth hormone in treating idiopathic short stature.

**Unaccepted**

The use of human growth hormone in older males to change body composition (e.g., to decrease adiposity and to prevent decline in muscle mass) is not recommended.

## Pharmacology/Pharmacokinetics

**Physicochemical characteristics**

Source—
  Somatrem: Biosynthetic. A single polypeptide chain of 192 amino acids, one more (methionine) than naturally occurring human growth hormone, produced by a recombinant DNA process in *Escherichia coli*.
  Somatropin, recombinant: Biosynthetic, produced by a recombinant DNA process in *Escherichia coli*; same amino acid sequence as naturally occurring human growth hormone. A single polypeptide chain of 191 amino acids.

Chemical name—
  Somatrem: Somatotropin (human), *N*-L-methionyl-.
  Somatropin, recombinant: Somatotropin (human).

**Mechanism of action/Effect**

Human growth hormone is an anterior pituitary hormone. Most anabolic actions are thought to be mediated by insulin-like growth factor-I (IGF-I, which has also been known as somatomedin-C), synthesized in the liver and other tissues in response to growth hormone stimulation.

Stimulates linear growth by affecting cartilaginous growth areas of long bones. Also stimulates growth by increasing the number and size of skeletal muscle cells, influencing the size of organs, and increasing red cell mass through erythropoietin stimulation.

Influences metabolism of carbohydrates by decreasing insulin sensitivity and possibly by affecting glucose transport; of fats by causing mobilization of fatty acids; of minerals by causing the retention of phosphorus, sodium, and potassium through promotion of cellular growth; and of proteins by increasing protein synthesis, which results in nitrogen retention.

**Biotransformation**
Hepatic, approximately 90%.

**Half-life**
Intravenous injection—Approximately 20 to 30 minutes (elimination).
Intramuscular or subcutaneous injection—Serum concentrations decline with a half-life of approximately 3 to 5 hours, reflecting continued release of the hormone from the injection site.

**Duration of action:**
Approximately 12 to 48 hours.

**Elimination**
Biliary (approximately 0.1% of a dose as unchanged drug).

## Precautions to Consider

**Carcinogenicity/Mutagenicity**

Carcinogenicity and mutagenicity testing has not been performed in animals or humans. Mutagenicity testing *in vitro* with recombinant somatropin did not reveal any mutagenic effects.

Anecdotal cases of acute and chronic leukemia have been reported in patients treated with human growth hormone, at an incidence slightly higher than that expected in the overall population. However, the exact relationship to human growth hormone therapy is unknown. Leukemia has also been reported in hypopituitary patients who have not been treated with growth hormone.

**Drug interactions and/or related problems**

The following drug interactions and/or related problems have been selected on the basis of their potential clinical significance (possible mechanism in parentheses where appropriate)—not necessarily inclusive (» = major clinical significance):

Note: Combinations containing any of the following medications, depending on the amount present, may also interact with this medication.

Anabolic steroids or
Androgens or
Estrogens or
Thyroid hormones
  (concurrent use of excessive doses of these hormones may accelerate epiphyseal closure, although supplemental use of these hormones may be necessary in patients with those deficiencies, to maintain the growth response to human growth hormone)

» Corticosteroids, glucocorticoid or
» Corticotropin (ACTH), especially with chronic therapeutic use
  (inhibition of the growth response to human growth hormone may occur with chronic therapeutic use of corticotropin or with daily oral doses [per square meter of body surface] in excess of:
    Betamethasone: 300 to 450 mcg)
    Cortisone: 12.5 to 18.8 mg)
    Dexamethasone: 250 to 500 mcg)
    Hydrocortisone: 10 to 15 mg)
    Methylprednisolone: 2 to 3 mg)
    Paramethasone: 1 to 1.5 mg)
    Prednisolone: 2.5 to 3.75 mg)
    Prednisone: 2.5 to 3.75 mg)
    Triamcinolone: 2 to 3 mg)

Maximum parenteral corticosteroid doses are approximately one-half maximum oral doses. In general, it is recommended that these doses not be exceeded during human growth hormone therapy and if larger doses are required, administration of human growth hormone should be postponed, except for brief administration of stress dosages during acute febrile illness or other acute stress; however, there is great interindividual variation. Also, concurrent use with corticotropin is not recommended; of the others, hydrocortisone or cortisone is usually preferred, except in extenuating circumstances)

**Laboratory value alterations**
The following have been selected on the basis of their potential clinical significance (possible effect in parentheses where appropriate)—not necessarily inclusive (» = major clinical significance):

With physiology/laboratory test values
  Glucose tolerance
    (may be reduced by high doses)
  Inorganic phosphate
    (serum concentrations may be increased to normal during treatment with growth hormone as a result of metabolic activity associated with bone growth as well as increased tubular reabsorption of phosphate by the kidney)
  Nonesterified fatty acids
    (plasma concentrations may be increased as a result of lipid mobilization from body fat stores)
  Thyroid function
    (serum thyroxine [T$_4$] concentration, radioactive iodine uptake [RAIU], and thyroxine-binding capacity may be slightly decreased; asymptomatic hypothyroidism usually occurs in less than 5%, but possibly up to 10 to 20%, of patients with hypopituitarism)

**Medical considerations/Contraindications**
The medical considerations/contraindications included have been selected on the basis of their potential clinical significance (reasons given in parentheses where appropriate)—not necessarily inclusive (» = major clinical significance).

*Risk-benefit should be considered when the following medical problems exist:*
  Hypothyroidism, untreated
    (interferes with growth response to human growth hormone; prior and/or concurrent thyroid hormone replacement therapy is recommended)
  Malignancy, especially intracranial tumor, actively growing within the previous 12 months
    (human growth hormone should not be used if there is evidence of progression or recurrent growth of an underlying tumor; antitumor therapy and a reasonable period of observation should be complete before growth hormone therapy is initiated)
  Sensitivity to the growth hormone product prescribed

**Patient monitoring**
The following may be especially important in patient monitoring (other tests may be warranted in some patients, depending on condition; » = major clinical significance):
  Antibodies to growth hormone, serologic evaluation for
    (in some cases, where growth rate falls during therapy and all other sources of growth inhibition have been ruled out, serologic evaluation for the presence of antibodies to growth hormone may be performed, with emphasis on binding capacity; antibodies to somatrem may be formed in the first 3 to 6 months of treatment, but only rarely cause failure to respond to therapy; antibodies to recombinant somatropin have been detected in patients treated for 6 months or more; relative incidence of antibody formation is difficult to compare because different assays have been used; however, growth inhibition appears to be correlated more with high binding capacity than with titer, and differences in antibody formation have demonstrated minimal clinical significance to date)
  Bone age determinations
    (recommended annually during therapy, especially in pubertal patients on concurrent androgen, estrogen, or thyroid replacement therapy since concurrent use may accelerate epiphyseal maturation)
  Examinations to monitor intracranial lesion
    (recommended at frequent intervals in patients with growth hormone deficiency secondary to an intracranial lesion)
  Growth rate determinations from stadiometer measurements
    (recommended every 3 to 6 months during therapy; if the growth rate does not exceed the pretreatment growth rate by at least 2 cm per year, the patient should be checked for noncompliance or the presence of antibodies or other medical problems such as hypothyroidism or malnutrition)
  Thyroid function determinations
    (recommended at regular intervals during therapy to detect hypothyroidism that develops during treatment; untreated hypothyroidism interferes with response to human growth hormone)

## Side/Adverse Effects

Note: Prolonged use of excessive doses of human growth hormone in patients who are not growth hormone deficient may theoretically cause acromegalic features (face, hands, feet), and other problems associated with acromegaly, including organ enlargement, diabetes mellitus, atherosclerosis, hypertension, and nerve entrapment syndrome (carpal tunnel syndrome).

The following side/adverse effects have been selected on the basis of their potential clinical significance (possible signs and symptoms in parentheses where appropriate)—not necessarily inclusive:

**Those indicating need for medical attention**
Incidence rare
  *Allergic reaction* (skin rash or itching); **pain and swelling at site of injection; slipped capital femoral epiphysis** (limp; pain in hip or knee)

  Note: *Slipped femoral epiphyses* may also occur in growth hormone–deficient children not treated with growth hormone.

## Patient Consultation

As an aid to patient consultation, refer to *Advice for the Patient, Growth Hormone (Systemic)*.
In providing consultation, consider emphasizing the following selected information (» = major clinical significance):

**Before using this medication**
» Conditions affecting use, especially:
    Sensitivity to growth hormone
    Other medications, especially corticosteroids or corticotropin (ACTH)

**Proper use of this medication**
» Proper dosing

**Precautions while using this medication**
» Importance of regular visits to physician

**Side/adverse effects**
  Signs of potential side effects, especially allergic reaction, and pain and swelling at site of injection

## General Dosing Information

Patients receiving human growth hormone should be under the supervision of a physician trained in the use of and familiar with growth hormone therapy.

The dosage and schedule of administration must be individualized for each patient.

The dosage of human growth hormone may be increased above the recommended dosage in older children with hypopituitarism, especially those who have open epiphyses.

Generally, after 2 or more years of treatment, growth rate will decrease, if therapy is continued. Attenuation of growth may be spontaneous. However, if this occurs, the patient should be checked for poor compliance with therapy, other medical problems (such as malnutrition or hypothyroidism), or the presence of antibodies. An increased dose of human growth hormone may be effective. In some patients, low doses of androgens or estrogens may be given concomitantly to restore the response, as long as epiphyseal maturation of 11 years or greater is present.

Human growth hormone therapy should be continued as long as the patient is responsive, until the patient reaches a mature adult height or until epiphyses close.

---

### SOMATREM

## Parenteral Dosage Forms

### SOMATREM FOR INJECTION

Note: The specific activity of growth hormone is defined as International Units (IU) per mg of protein. In October 1994, a new standard was developed that changed the conversion amount from 2.6 IU per mg of growth hormone to 3 IU per mg of growth hormone. This change did not affect the milligram-per-kg dosing or the quantity (mg) of growth hormone per vial. The only change was the increase of IUs per mg.

**Usual pediatric dose**
Growth hormone—
  Intramuscular or subcutaneous, up to 0.3 mg (0.9 International Unit [IU]) per kg of body weight a week with dosing and dosing regimen individualized according to the patient's needs. It is recommended by the manufacturer that this dose be divided into the appropriate dose for daily injection (six or seven times per week). The subcutaneous route of administration is preferred to the intramuscular route.

**Growth Hormone (Systemic)**

Note: If the growth rate does not exceed the pretreatment growth rate by at least 2 cm per year, the patient should be checked for noncompliance or the presence of antibodies or other medical problems such as hypothyroidism or malnutrition. If increasing the dose is not effective, treatment should be discontinued and the patient re-evaluated.

**Size(s) usually available**
U.S.—
- 5 mg (approximately 15 IU) per vial (Rx) [*Protropin* (diluent—benzyl alcohol)].
- 10 mg (approximately 30 IU) per vial (Rx) [*Protropin* (diluent—benzyl alcohol)].

Canada—
- 5 mg (approximately 15 IU) per vial (Rx) [*Protropin* (diluent—benzyl alcohol)].
- 10 mg (approximately 30 IU) per vial (Rx) [*Protropin* (diluent—benzyl alcohol)].

**Packaging and storage**
Prior to and following reconstitution, store between 2 and 8 °C (36 and 46 °F). Protect the reconstituted solution and diluent from freezing.

**Preparation of dosage form**
Using standard aseptic technique, add 1 to 5 mL of Bacteriostatic Water for Injection USP (benzyl alcohol preserved only) to a 5-mg vial or 1 to 10 mL to a 10-mg vial. Swirl gently to dissolve. The vial should not be shaken. Cloudy solution should not be used.

If somatrem is to be administered to a neonate, Water for Injection should be used for reconstitution; benzyl alcohol used as a preservative has been associated with toxicity in neonates. Each vial should then be used only for one dose and any unused portion discarded.

**Stability**
When prepared with the diluent provided by the manufacturer, reconstituted solutions should be stored in the refrigerator and used within 14 days. If water for injection is used for reconstitution, each vial should be used only for one dose and any unused portion discarded. If these procedures are not followed, sterility of the solution cannot be assured.

---

### SOMATROPIN, RECOMBINANT

## Parenteral Dosage Forms

**SOMATROPIN, RECOMBINANT, FOR INJECTION**

Note: The specific activity of growth hormone is defined as International Units (IU) per mg of protein. In October 1994, a new standard was developed that changed the conversion amount from 2.6 IU per mg of growth hormone to 3 IU per mg of growth hormone. This change did not affect the milligram-per-kg dosing or the quantity (mg) of growth hormone per vial. The only change was the increase of IUs per mg.

**Usual pediatric dose**
Growth hormone—
Intramuscular or subcutaneous, 0.18 to 0.3 mg (0.54 to 0.9 International Unit [IU]) per kg of body weight a week with dosing and dosing regimen individualized according to the patient's needs. This can be divided into the appropriate dose for daily injection (six or seven times per week) or, as an alternative, divided and injected three times a week (every other day). The subcutaneous route of administration is preferred to the intramuscular route.

Note: If the growth rate does not exceed the pretreatment growth rate by at least 2 cm per year, the patient should be checked for noncompliance or the presence of antibodies or other medical problems such as hypothyroidism or malnutrition. If increasing the dose is not effective, treatment should be discontinued and the patient re-evaluated.

**Size(s) usually available**
U.S.—
- 5 mg (approximately 15 IU) per vial (Rx) [*Humatrope* (diluent—m-cresol; glycerin); *Nutropin* (diluent—benzyl alcohol)].
- 10 mg (approximately 30 IU) per vial (Rx) [*Nutropin* (diluent—benzyl alcohol)].

Canada—
- 2 mg (approximately 6 IU) per vial (Rx) [*Humatrope* (diluent—m-cresol; glycerin)].
- 5 mg (approximately 15 IU) per vial (Rx) [*Humatrope* (diluent—m-cresol; glycerin)].

**Packaging and storage**
Prior to and following reconstitution, store between 2 and 8 °C (36 and 46 °F). Protect the reconstituted solution and diluent from freezing.

**Preparation of dosage form**
Some brands of *Humatrope* are packaged in a system with the diluent and somatropin in the same vial, with a rubber stopper separating each component. The product can be reconstituted by depressing the stopper, which allows the two components to mix.

For products that package the diluent and somatropin in separate vials, using standard aseptic technique the following amount of diluent should be added:
- For *Humatrope*—1.5 to 5 mL of the diluent provided by the manufacturer is added to a 2-mg or 5-mg vial.
- For *Nutropin*—1 to 10 mL of the diluent provided by the manufacturer or Bacteriostatic Water for Injection USP (benzyl alcohol preserved only) is added to a 5-mg or 10-mg vial.
- To mix the diluent with the somatropin, the diluent must be injected while aimed against the glass wall of the vial, then swirled gently to dissolve the contents of the vial. The vial should not be shaken. Cloudy solutions or those containing particulate matter should not be used.

If somatropin is to be administered to a neonate, Water for Injection should be used for reconstitution; benzyl alcohol used as a preservative has been associated with toxicity in neonates. Each vial should then be used only for one dose and any unused portion discarded.

**Stability**
Somatropin is stable for up to 14 days if stored in the refrigerator following reconstitution with the diluent provided by the manufacturer. If sterile water for injection is used for reconstitution, each vial should be refrigerated and used within 24 hours.

## Selected Bibliography

Frasier SD, Lippe BM. The rational use of growth hormone during childhood [review]. J Clin Endocrinol Metab 1990; 71(2): 269-73.

Laron Z, Butenandt O. Optimum use of growth hormone in children [review]. Drugs 1991; 42(1): 1-8.

Revised: 11/18/92
Interim revision: 06/30/94; 08/15/95

---

# GUAIFENESIN  Systemic

VA CLASSIFICATION (Primary): RE302

Commonly used brand name(s): *Anti-Tuss; Balminil Expectorant; Benylin-E; Breonesin; Calmylin Expectorant; Diabetic Tussin EX; Fenesin; GG-CEN; Gee-Gee; Genatuss; Glycotuss; Glytuss; Guiatuss; Halotussin; Humibid L.A; Humibid Sprinkle; Hytuss; Hytuss-2X; Naldecon Senior EX; Organidin NR; Pneumomist; Resyl; Robitussin; Scot-tussin Expectorant; Sinumist-SR; Touro EX; Uni-tussin.*

Another commonly used name is glyceryl guaiacolate.

Note: For a listing of dosage forms and brand names by country availability, see *Dosage Forms* section(s).

## Category

Expectorant.

## Indications

**Accepted**

Cough (treatment)—Guaifenesin is indicated as an expectorant in the temporary symptomatic management of cough due to minor upper respiratory infections and related conditions, such as sinusitis, pharyngitis, and bronchitis, when these conditions are complicated by viscous mucus and congestion. However, because supporting data are very limited, there is some controversy about its effectiveness.

## Pharmacology/Pharmacokinetics

**Physicochemical characteristics**
Molecular weight—198.22.

**Mechanism of action/Effect**
Guaifenesin is thought to act as an expectorant by increasing the volume and reducing the viscosity of secretions in the trachea and bronchi.

Thus, it may increase the efficiency of the cough reflex and facilitate removal of the secretions; however, objective evidence for this is limited and conflicting.

**Absorption**
Readily absorbed from gastrointestinal tract.

**Elimination**
Renal, as inactive metabolites.

## Precautions to Consider

### Carcinogenicity/Tumorigenicity/Mutagenicity
Studies to determine the carcinogenicity, tumorigenicity, or mutagenicity of guaifenesin in animals have not been conducted.

### Pregnancy/Reproduction
Pregnancy—Although adequate and well-controlled studies in pregnant women have not been done, the Collaborative Perinatal Project monitored 197 mother-child pairs exposed to guaifenesin during the first trimester. An increased occurrence of inguinal hernias was found in the neonates. However, congenital defects were not strongly associated with guaifenesin use during pregnancy in 2 large groups of mother-child pairs.

Studies have not been done in animals.

FDA Pregnancy Category C.

### Breast-feeding
It is not known whether guaifenesin is distributed into breast milk. However, problems in humans have not been documented.

### Pediatrics
Appropriate studies on the relationship of age to the effects of guaifenesin have not been performed in the pediatric population. However, no pediatrics-specific problems have been documented to date.

Caution is recommended in children up to 12 years of age with persistent or chronic cough, such as occurs with asthma, or if the cough is accompanied by excessive phlegm (mucus). The condition of these children may need a physician's evaluation before guaifenesin is administered.

Guaifenesin should not be given to children younger than 2 years of age unless recommended by a physician.

### Geriatrics
Appropriate studies on the relationship of age to the effects of guaifenesin have not been performed in the geriatric population. However, no geriatrics-specific problems have been documented to date.

### Laboratory value alterations
The following have been selected on the basis of their potential clinical significance (possible effect in parentheses where appropriate)—not necessarily inclusive (» = major clinical significance):

With diagnostic test results
5-hydroxyindoleacetic acid (5-HIAA), urine
(urinary determinations may be falsely increased when nitrosonaphthol reagent is used because of color interference by guaifenesin metabolites; guaifenesin should be discontinued 48 hours before collection of urine for this test)

Vanillylmandelic acid (VMA), urine
(guaifenesin or its metabolites may cause color interference with urinary determinations and may falsely elevate VMA test for catechols; guaifenesin should be discontinued 48 hours before collection of urine for this test)

### Medical considerations/Contraindications
The medical considerations/contraindications included have been selected on the basis of their potential clinical significance (reasons given in parentheses where appropriate)—not necessarily inclusive (» = major clinical significance).

*Risk-benefit should be considered when the following medical problem exists:*
Sensitivity to guaifenesin

## Side/Adverse Effects

The following side/adverse effects have been selected on the basis of their potential clinical significance (possible signs and symptoms in parentheses where appropriate)—not necessarily inclusive:

**Those indicating need for medical attention only if they continue or are bothersome**
Less frequent or rare
*Diarrhea; dizziness; headache; nausea or vomiting; skin rash; stomach pain; urticaria* (hives)

## Patient Consultation

As an aid to patient consultation, refer to *Advice for the Patient, Guaifenesin (Systemic).*

In providing consultation, consider emphasizing the following selected information (» = major clinical significance):

### Before using this medication
» Conditions affecting use, especially:
Sensitivity to guaifenesin
Pregnancy—Increased incidence of inguinal hernias in the babies of one group of women taking guaifenesin during pregnancy; however, this did not occur in other groups
Use in children—For self-medication, caution if cough is persistent or occurs with excessive phlegm; not administering to children younger than 2 years of age unless directed by a physician

### Proper use of this medication
*Proper administration*
Importance of maintaining adequate fluid intake
» For extended-release dosage forms
Swallowing capsules whole or opening capsules and sprinkling contents on soft food, then swallowing without crushing or chewing
Not breaking (unless scored for breakage), crushing, or chewing tablets; swallowing tablet whole
» Proper dosing
Missed dose (if on a scheduled dosing regimen): Taking as soon as possible; not taking if almost time for next dose; not doubling doses
» Proper storage

### Precautions while using this medication
Checking with physician if cough persists after medication has been used for 7 days or if fever, skin rash, continuing headache, or sore throat is present with cough

## General Dosing Information

Before prescribing or recommending medication to suppress or modify cough, it is important that the underlying cause of the cough be assessed.

For self-medication, guaifenesin should not be taken for chronic cough unless directed by a physician.

Patient should be advised to maintain adequate hydration.

## Oral Dosage Forms

### GUAIFENESIN CAPSULES USP

**Usual adult and adolescent dose**
Expectorant—
Oral, 200 to 400 mg every four hours, not to exceed 2400 mg a day.

**Usual pediatric dose**
Expectorant—
Children 2 to 6 years of age: The liquid or extended-release capsule dosage forms may be preferable for children in this age group.
Children 6 to 12 years of age: Oral, 100 to 200 mg every four hours, not to exceed 1200 mg a day.

**Usual geriatric dose**
See *Usual adult and adolescent dose.*

**Strength(s) usually available**
U.S.—
200 mg (OTC) [*Breonesin; GG-CEN; Hytuss-2X*].
Canada—
Not commercially available.

**Packaging and storage**
Store below 40 °C (104 °F), preferably between 15 and 30 °C (59 and 86 °F), unless otherwise specified by manufacturer. Store in a tight container.

### GUAIFENESIN EXTENDED-RELEASE CAPSULES

**Usual adult and adolescent dose**
Expectorant—
Oral, 600 to 1200 mg every twelve hours, not to exceed 2400 mg a day.

**Usual pediatric dose**
Expectorant—
Children 2 to 6 years of age: Oral, 300 mg every twelve hours, not to exceed 600 mg a day.
Note: The liquid dosage forms may be preferable for children 2 to 6 years of age, who cannot always be relied upon to swallow the contents of the capsule without chewing.
Children 6 to 12 years of age: Oral, 600 mg every twelve hours, not to exceed 1200 mg a day.

## 1590 Guaifenesin (Systemic)

**Usual geriatric dose**
See *Usual adult and adolescent dose.*

**Strength(s) usually available**
U.S.—
　300 mg (Rx) [*Humibid Sprinkle*].
Canada—
　Not commercially available.

**Packaging and storage**
Store between 15 and 30 °C (59 and 86 °F), unless otherwise specified by manufacturer. Store in a tight container.

**Additional information**
Extended-release capsules may be swallowed whole or opened and the contents sprinkled on soft food immediately prior to ingestion, then swallowed without crushing or chewing. Capsule contents should not be subdivided.

### GUAIFENESIN ORAL SOLUTION

**Usual adult and adolescent dose**
See *Guaifenesin Capsules USP.*

**Usual pediatric dose**
Expectorant—
　Children 6 months to 2 years of age—Dosage must be individualized by physician. A commonly used regimen is 25 to 50 mg every four hours, not to exceed 300 mg a day.
　Children 2 to 6 years of age—Oral, 50 to 100 mg every four hours, not to exceed 600 mg a day.
　Children 6 to 12 years to age—See *Guaifenesin Capsules USP.*

**Usual geriatric dose**
See *Usual adult and adolescent dose.*

**Strength(s) usually available**
U.S.—
　100 mg per 5 mL (OTC) [*Diabetic Tussin EX* (alcohol free; sugar free); *Scot-tussin Expectorant* (alcohol 3.5%; sugar free)].
　100 mg per 5 mL (Rx) [*Organidin NR* (sorbitol; alcohol free)].
　200 mg per 5 mL (OTC) [*Naldecon Senior EX* (alcohol free; sugar free)].
Canada—
　Not commercially available.

**Packaging and storage**
Store below 40 °C (104 °F), preferably between 15 and 30 °C (59 and 86 °F), unless otherwise specified by manufacturer. Store in a tight container. Protect from freezing.

### GUAIFENESIN SYRUP USP

**Usual adult and adolescent dose**
See *Guaifenesin Capsules USP.*

**Usual pediatric dose**
See *Guaifenesin Oral Solution.*

**Usual geriatric dose**
See *Usual adult and adolescent dose.*

**Strength(s) usually available**
U.S.—
　100 mg per 5 mL (OTC) [*Anti-Tuss* (alcohol 3.5%); *Genatuss* (alcohol 3.5%); *Guiatuss; Halotussin* (alcohol 3.5%); *Robitussin* (alcohol 3.5%); *Uni-tussin* (alcohol 3.5%); GENERIC].
Canada—
　100 mg per 5 mL (OTC) [*Balminil Expectorant; Benylin-E* (alcohol 5%); *Calmylin Expectorant* (sorbitol; alcohol free); *Robitussin* (alcohol 3.5%)].

**Packaging and storage**
Store below 40 °C (104 °F), preferably between 15 and 30 °C (59 and 86 °F), unless otherwise specified by manufacturer. Store in a tight container. Protect from freezing.

### GUAIFENESIN TABLETS USP

**Usual adult and adolescent dose**
See *Guaifenesin Capsules USP.*

**Usual pediatric dose**
See *Guaifenesin Capsules USP.*

**Usual geriatric dose**
See *Usual adult and adolescent dose.*

**Strength(s) usually available**
U.S.—
　100 mg (OTC) [*Glycotuss; Hytuss* (scored; sugar free)].
　200 mg (OTC) [*Gee-Gee; Glytuss*].
　200 mg (Rx) [*Organidin NR* (scored)].
Canada—
　100 mg (OTC) [*Resyl*].

**Packaging and storage**
Store below 40 °C (104 °F), preferably between 15 and 30 °C (59 and 86 °F), unless otherwise specified by manufacturer. Store in a tight container.

### GUAIFENESIN EXTENDED-RELEASE TABLETS

**Usual adult and adolescent dose**
See *Guaifenesin Extended-release Capsules.*

**Usual pediatric dose**
See *Guaifenesin Extended-release Capsules.*

**Strength(s) usually available**
U.S.—
　600 mg (Rx) [*Fenesin* (scored); *Humibid L.A* (scored); *Pneumomist* (scored); *Sinumist-SR* (scored); *Touro EX* (scored); GENERIC].
Canada—
　Not commercially available.

**Packaging and storage**
Store between 15 and 30 °C (59 and 86 °F), unless otherwise specified by manufacturer. Store in a tight container.

## Selected Bibliography

Irwin RS, Curley FJ, Bennett FM. Appropriate use of antitussives and protussives. Drugs 1993; 46(1): 80-91.

Revised: 08/04/95

---

# GUANABENZ  Systemic†

VA CLASSIFICATION (Primary): CV409

Commonly used brand name(s): *Wytensin.*

Note:　For a listing of dosage forms and brand names by country availability, see *Dosage Forms* section(s).

　†Not commercially available in Canada.

## Category
Antihypertensive.

## Indications

**Accepted**
Hypertension (treatment)—Guanabenz is indicated for treatment of hypertension. Because it usually does not cause postural hypotension, guanabenz may be useful as a substitute for other central adrenergic blockers in patients who cannot tolerate these agents because of severe orthostatic hypotension.

## Pharmacology/Pharmacokinetics

**Physicochemical characteristics**
Molecular weight—Guanabenz acetate: 291.14.

**Mechanism of action/Effect**
Guanabenz is a centrally acting alpha-2 adrenergic agonist. The antihypertensive effect is thought to be due to central alpha-adrenergic stimulation, which results in a decreased sympathetic outflow to the heart, kidneys, and peripheral vasculature; decreased systolic and diastolic blood pressure; and slight slowing of pulse rate. Chronic administration of guanabenz also causes a decrease in peripheral vascular resistance.

**Absorption**
Approximately 75% absorbed from gastrointestinal tract; however, bioavailability is very low because of extensive first-pass metabolism.

**Protein binding**
Very high (90%).

**Biotransformation**
Hepatic.

**Half-life**
Average, 6 hours.
**Onset of action**
Within 60 minutes (after a single dose).
**Time to peak plasma concentration**
2 to 5 hours.
**Time to peak effect**
2 to 4 hours.
**Duration of action**
12 hours (after a single dose).
**Elimination**
Renal (less than 1% unchanged); fecal, about 16%.

## Precautions to Consider

### Carcinogenicity
Studies in rats at doses up to 10 times the maximum recommended human dose have not shown that guanabenz causes carcinogenic effects.

### Mutagenicity
Dose-related increases in the number of mutants occurred in one (TA 1537) of five *Salmonella typhimurium* strains in the Ames test at doses of 200 to 500 mcg per plate or 30 to 50 mcg per mL in suspension. No mutagenic activity was seen in other assays.

### Pregnancy/Reproduction
Fertility—Guanabenz has been found to impair fertility in both male and female rats given high doses (9.6 mg per kg of body weight [mg/kg]).

Pregnancy—Studies have not been done in humans.

Animal studies suggest that guanabenz crosses the placenta. Studies in mice have shown that guanabenz at doses of 3 to 6 times the maximum recommended human dose of 1 mg/kg causes an increase in skeletal abnormalities; these did not occur in rabbits or rats. Other studies have found increased fetal loss in rats and rabbits given 14 to 20 mg/kg. Slightly decreased live-birth indexes, decreased fetal survival rate, and decreased pup body weight occurred in rats given 6.4 to 9.6 mg/kg.

FDA Pregnancy Category C.

### Breast-feeding
It is not known whether guanabenz is distributed into breast milk. However, problems in humans have not been documented.

### Pediatrics
Appropriate studies on the relationship of age to the effects of guanabenz have not been performed in the pediatric population. Safety and efficacy have not been established.

### Geriatrics
Although appropriate studies on the relationship of age to the effects of guanabenz have not been performed in the geriatric population, no geriatrics-specific problems have been documented to date. However, elderly patients are more likely to have age-related renal function impairment, which may require caution in patients receiving guanabenz. In addition, elderly patients may be more sensitive to the hypotensive and sedative effects of guanabenz.

### Dental
Use of guanabenz may decrease or inhibit salivary flow, thus contributing to the development of caries, periodontal disease, oral candidiasis, and discomfort.

### Drug interactions and/or related problems
The following drug interactions and/or related problems have been selected on the basis of their potential clinical significance (possible mechanism in parentheses where appropriate)—not necessarily inclusive (» = major clinical significance):

Note: Combinations containing any of the following medications, depending on the amount present, may also interact with this medication.

Alcohol or
Central nervous system (CNS) depression-producing medications (See *Appendix II*)
(concurrent use may enhance the CNS depressant effects of either these medications or guanabenz)

Anti-inflammatory drugs, nonsteroidal (NSAIDs), especially indomethacin
(concurrent use may reduce antihypertensive effects of guanabenz; indomethacin, and possibly other NSAIDs, may antagonize the antihypertensive effect by inhibiting renal prostaglandin synthesis and/or by causing sodium and fluid retention; the patient should be carefully monitored to confirm that the desired effect is being obtained)

Beta-adrenergic blocking agents, ophthalmic
(if significant systemic absorption of ophthalmic beta-adrenergic blocking agents occurs, concurrent use may increase the hypotensive effect of guanabenz)

» Beta-adrenergic blocking agents, systemic or
Hypotension-producing medications, other (See *Appendix II*)
(antihypertensive effects may be potentiated when these medications are used concurrently with guanabenz; although some antihypertensive and/or diuretic combinations are frequently used for therapeutic advantage, dosage adjustments may be necessary during concurrent use)

(when therapy is discontinued in patients receiving a systemic beta-adrenergic blocking agent and guanabenz concurrently, the beta-adrenergic blocking agent should be gradually discontinued in order to avoid beta-adrenergic blocking agent–withdrawal hypertensive crisis; blood pressure control may also be impaired when the two are combined)

Sympathomimetics
(concurrent use may reduce the antihypertensive effects of guanabenz; the patient should be carefully monitored to confirm that the desired effect is being obtained)

### Laboratory value alterations
The following have been selected on the basis of their potential clinical significance (possible effect in parentheses where appropriate)—not necessarily inclusive (» = major clinical significance):

With physiology/laboratory test values
Cholesterol and total triglyceride
(serum values may be reduced with chronic administration)

### Medical considerations/Contraindications
The medical considerations/contraindications included have been selected on the basis of their potential clinical significance (reasons given in parentheses where appropriate)—not necessarily inclusive (» = major clinical significance).

*Risk-benefit should be considered when the following medical problems exist:*

Cerebrovascular disease or
Coronary insufficiency or
Myocardial infarction, recent
(may be aggravated by reduced blood pressure)

Hepatic function impairment
(plasma concentrations of guanabenz may increase; careful monitoring of blood pressure during dosage titration is recommended)

Renal function impairment
(half-life of guanabenz is increased and clearance is decreased; careful monitoring of blood pressure during dosage titration is recommended)

Sensitivity to guanabenz

### Patient monitoring
The following may be especially important in patient monitoring (other tests may be warranted in some patients, depending on condition; » = major clinical significance):

» Blood pressure measurements
(recommended at periodic intervals in patients being treated for hypertension; selected patients may be trained to perform blood pressure measurements at home and report the results at regular physician visits)

## Side/Adverse Effects

The following side/adverse effects have been selected on the basis of their potential clinical significance (possible signs and symptoms in parentheses where appropriate)—not necessarily inclusive:

**Those indicating need for medical attention only if they continue or are bothersome**
Incidence more frequent
*Dizziness; drowsiness; dryness of mouth; weakness*

Note: Incidence of *drowsiness* is dose-related and usually declines with continued administration.

Incidence less frequent or rare
*Decreased sexual ability; headache; nausea*

**Those indicating possible withdrawal and the need for medical attention if they occur after medication is abruptly discontinued**
*Anxiety or tenseness; chest pain; fast or irregular heartbeat; headache; increased salivation; increase in sweating; nausea or vomiting;*

*nervousness or restlessness; shaking or trembling of hands or fingers; stomach cramps; trouble in sleeping*

Note: The above are symptoms of sympathetic overactivity; elevation of blood pressure above baseline levels occurs rarely. The risk appears to be increased in patients receiving doses of greater than 32 mg of guanabenz per day.

## Overdose

For specific information on the agents used in the management of guanabenz overdose, see:
- *Atropine* in *Anticholinergics/Antispasmodics (Systemic)* monograph;
- *Charcoal (Oral-Local)* monograph; and/or
- *Dopamine* in *Sympathomimetic Agents—Cardiovascular Use (Systemic)* monograph.

For more information on the management of overdose or unintentional ingestion, **contact a Poison Control Center** (see *Poison Control Center Listing*).

### Clinical effects of overdose
The following effects have been selected on the basis of their potential clinical significance (possible signs and symptoms in parentheses where appropriate)—not necessarily inclusive:

*Bradycardia* (slow heartbeat); *hypotension* (dizziness, severe); *irritability; lethargy* (unusual tiredness or weakness); *miosis* (pinpoint pupils); *somnolence*

### Treatment of overdose
To decrease absorption—
Gastric lavage and administration of activated charcoal.
Specific treatment—
Treatment is mainly supportive. Maintaining adequate airway and fluid balance is recommended.
For bradycardia: Atropine has been used successfully.
For hypotension: Vasopressor agents, such as dopamine, have been used successfully.
Monitoring—
Carefully monitor vital signs and fluid balance.
Supportive care—
Patients in whom intentional overdose is known or suspected should be referred for psychiatric evaluation.

## Patient Consultation

As an aid to patient consultation, refer to *Advice for the Patient, Guanabenz (Systemic)*.

In providing consultation, consider emphasizing the following selected information (» = major clinical significance):

### Before using this medication
» Conditions affecting use, especially:
Sensitivity to guanabenz
Pregnancy—High doses in animals cause decreased fertility, birth defects, and fetal death
Use in the elderly—Increased sensitivity to hypotensive and sedative effects
Dental—May decrease or inhibit salivary flow
Other medications, especially systemic beta-adrenergic blocking agents

### Proper use of this medication
Possible need for control of weight and diet, especially sodium intake
» Patient may not experience symptoms of hypertension; importance of taking medication even if feeling well
» Does not cure but helps control hypertension; possible need for lifelong therapy; serious consequences of untreated hypertension
Compliance with therapy; taking medication at the same time(s) each day to maintain the therapeutic effect
» Proper dosing
Missed dose: Taking as soon as possible; not taking if almost time for next dose; checking with physician if two or more doses in a row are missed; possible unpleasant effects if stopped abruptly
» Proper storage

### Precautions while using this medication
Making regular visits to physician to check progress
Checking with physician before discontinuing medication; possible need for gradual dosage reduction
Caution if any kind of surgery (including dental surgery) or emergency treatment is required
» Not taking other medications, especially nonprescription sympathomimetics, unless discussed with physician
» Caution in taking alcohol or other CNS depressants
» Caution when driving or doing things requiring alertness because of possible dizziness or drowsiness
Possible dryness of mouth; using sugarless candy or gum, ice, or saliva substitute for relief; checking with physician or dentist if dry mouth continues for more than 2 weeks

### Side/adverse effects
Signs of potential side effects, especially signs and symptoms of overdose or withdrawal reaction

## General Dosing Information

It is recommended that the last daily dose be taken at bedtime to ensure overnight control of blood pressure and reduce daytime drowsiness.

Recent evidence suggests that withdrawal of antihypertensive therapy prior to surgery is not necessary, but that the anesthesiologist must be aware of such therapy.

The possibility of withdrawal syndrome should be kept in mind if guanabenz is discontinued abruptly, since rebound hypertension occurs rarely.

## Oral Dosage Forms

### GUANABENZ ACETATE TABLETS USP

**Usual adult dose**
Antihypertensive—
Oral, 4 mg two times a day initially, the dosage being increased if necessary in increments of 4 to 8 mg per day every one to two weeks up to the minimum effective dose.

Note: Geriatric patients may be more sensitive to the effects of the usual adult dose.

**Usual adult prescribing limits**
32 mg per day.

**Usual pediatric dose**
Safety and efficacy have not been established.

**Strength(s) usually available**
U.S.—
4 mg (Rx) [*Wytensin* (lactose)].
8 mg (Rx) [*Wytensin* (lactose)].
Canada—
Not commercially available.

**Packaging and storage**
Store below 40 °C (104 °F), preferably between 15 and 30 °C (59 and 86 °F), unless otherwise specified by manufacturer. Store in a tight, light-resistant container.

**Auxiliary labeling**
- Do not take other medicines without your doctor's advice.
- May cause dizziness.
- May cause drowsiness.

## Selected Bibliography

The fifth report of the Joint National Committee on Detection, Evaluation, and Treatment of High Blood Pressure (JNC V). Arch Intern Med 1993; 153(2): 154-83.

Revised: 07/22/96
Interim revision: 08/19/98

---

# GUANADREL Systemic†

VA CLASSIFICATION (Primary): CV409
Commonly used brand name(s): *Hylorel*.
Note: For a listing of dosage forms and brand names by country availability, see *Dosage Forms* section(s).

†Not commercially available in Canada.

## Category

Antihypertensive.

# Indications

### Accepted
Hypertension (treatment)—Guanadrel is indicated in the treatment of hypertension.

# Pharmacology/Pharmacokinetics

### Physicochemical characteristics
Molecular weight—524.63.

### Mechanism of action/Effect
Guanadrel is a postganglionic adrenergic blocking agent. Uptake of guanadrel and storage in sympathetic neurons occurs via the norepinephrine pump; guanadrel slowly displaces norepinephrine from its storage in nerve endings and thereby blocks the release of norepinephrine normally produced by nerve stimulation. The reduction in neurotransmitter release in response to sympathetic nerve stimulation, as a result of catecholamine depletion, leads to reduced arteriolar vasoconstriction, especially the reflex increase in sympathetic tone that occurs with a change in position.

### Absorption
Rapidly and well absorbed from gastrointestinal tract.

### Protein binding
Low (approximately 20%).

### Biotransformation
Hepatic.

### Half-life
Approximately 10 hours, with wide interindividual variability; may be prolonged up to 19.2 hours in the presence of renal function impairment.

### Onset of action
2 hours (after a single dose).

### Time to peak concentration
1.5 to 2 hours.

### Time to peak effect
4 to 6 hours (after a single dose).

### Duration of action
Average—9 hours (range 4 to 14 hours) after a single dose.

### Elimination
Renal, 85% (about 40% unchanged).

# Precautions to Consider

### Carcinogenicity
Two-year studies in mice found no carcinogenic effect of guanadrel. In a 2-year study in rats, an increased incidence of benign testicular interstitial cell tumors was observed at doses of 100 mg per kg of body weight (mg/kg) per day and 400 mg/kg per day. However, the significance of these findings is not known since these spontaneous tumors are common in aged rats.

### Mutagenicity
*Salmonella* testing (Ames test) showed no evidence of mutagenicity.

### Pregnancy/Reproduction
Fertility—Suppressed libido and reduced fertility were observed in male and female rats at a dose of 100 mg/kg per day (12 times the maximum human dose in a 50-kg person). Suppressed libido was evident to a lesser extent at a dose of 30 mg/kg per day.

Pregnancy—Studies in humans have not been done.

Studies in rats and rabbits at doses up to 12 times the maximum recommended human dose have not shown that guanadrel causes adverse effects in the fetus.

FDA Pregnancy Category B.

### Breast-feeding
It is not known whether guanadrel is distributed into breast milk. However, problems in humans have not been documented.

### Pediatrics
Appropriate studies on the relationship of age to the effects of guanadrel have not been performed in the pediatric population. Safety and efficacy have not been established.

### Geriatrics
Appropriate studies on the relationship of age to the effects of guanadrel have not been performed in the geriatric population. However, the elderly may be more sensitive to the hypotensive effects of guanadrel.

### Drug interactions and/or related problems
The following drug interactions and/or related problems have been selected on the basis of their potential clinical significance (possible mechanism in parentheses where appropriate)—not necessarily inclusive (» = major clinical significance):

Note: Because of the similarity of guanadrel's actions to those of guanethidine, some of the following potential interactions are stated for cautionary reference.

Combinations containing any of the following medications, depending on the amount present, may also interact with this medication.

Alcohol or
Barbiturates or
Opioid (narcotic) analgesics
   (concurrent use with guanadrel will produce additive orthostatic hypotensive effects)

Alpha-adrenergic blocking agents or
Other medications with alpha-adrenergic blocking action, such as:
   Dihydroergotamine
   Ergoloid mesylates
   Ergotamine
   Haloperidol
   Loxapine
   Phenothiazines
   Thioxanthenes or

Beta-adrenergic blocking agents or
Rauwolfia alkaloids
   (concurrent use with guanadrel may cause an increased incidence of orthostatic hypotension or bradycardia)

Amphetamines or
» Antidepressants, tricyclic or
Appetite suppressants, with the exception of fenfluramine or
Cyclobenzaprine or
Haloperidol or
» Loxapine or
Maprotiline or
Methylphenidate or
Phenothiazines, especially chlorpromazine or
» Thioxanthenes or
» Trimeprazine
   (concurrent use may decrease the hypotensive effects of guanadrel because of its displacement from and inhibition of uptake by adrenergic neurons; caution is recommended when these medications are discontinued, especially if discontinued abruptly, because effects of guanadrel might be suddenly increased)

Anticholinergics, especially atropine and related compounds
   (concurrent use with guanadrel may antagonize the inhibitory action of these medications on gastric acid secretion)

Anti-inflammatory drugs, nonsteroidal (NSAIDs), especially indomethacin
   (antihypertensive effects of guanadrel may be reduced when it is used concurrently with these agents; indomethacin, and possibly other NSAIDs, may antagonize the antihypertensive effect by inhibiting renal prostaglandin synthesis and/or by causing sodium and fluid retention; the patient should be carefully monitored to confirm that the desired effect is being obtained)

Fenfluramine
   (concurrent use with guanadrel may produce additive hypotensive effects, and may result in postural hypotension; dosage adjustments of the antihypertensive may be necessary)

Hypotension-producing medications, other (See *Appendix II*)
   (antihypertensive effects may be potentiated when these medications are used concurrently with guanadrel; although some antihypertensive and/or diuretic combinations are frequently used for therapeutic advantage, dosage adjustments may be necessary during concurrent use)

» Monoamine oxidase (MAO) inhibitors, including furazolidone, procarbazine, and selegiline
   (concurrent use with guanadrel may result in moderate to severe hypertension due to release of catecholamines; withdrawal of MAO inhibitors at least 1 week prior to initiation of guanadrel therapy is recommended)

Sympathomimetic agents, such as:
   Cocaine or
   Dobutamine or
   Dopamine or
   Ephedrine or
   Epinephrine or
»   Metaraminol or
   Methoxamine or
   Norepinephrine or

Phenylephrine or
Phenylpropanolamine
   (concurrent use of any sympathomimetics with guanadrel may reduce the antihypertensive effects of guanadrel; the patient should be carefully monitored to confirm that the desired effect is being obtained)
   (in addition to possibly decreasing the hypotensive effects of guanadrel, concurrent use of cocaine, dobutamine, dopamine, ephedrine, epinephrine, metaraminol, methoxamine, norepinephrine, phenylephrine, or phenylpropanolamine with guanadrel may potentiate the pressor effect of these medications, as a result of inhibition of sympathomimetic uptake by adrenergic neurons, possibly resulting in hypertension and cardiac arrhythmias)
   (concurrent use of ephedrine or phenylpropanolamine with guanadrel may decrease the hypotensive effects of guanadrel because of its displacement from and inhibition of uptake by adrenergic neurons)
   (concurrent use of metaraminol with guanadrel may cause a hypertensive crisis. When metaraminol is used within 5 days after discontinuation of guanadrel, a hypertensive potential may remain)
   (concurrent use of phenylephrine ophthalmic solution with guanadrel may increase the pupillary response)

**Medical considerations/Contraindications**
The medical considerations/contraindications included have been selected on the basis of their potential clinical significance (reasons given in parentheses where appropriate)—not necessarily inclusive (» = major clinical significance).

*Risk-benefit should be considered when the following medical problems exist:*

Asthma, history of
   (may be aggravated because of hypersensitivity to catecholamine depletion)
Cerebrovascular insufficiency or
Coronary insufficiency or
Myocardial infarction, recent
   (ischemia may be aggravated as a result of reduced blood pressure)
» Congestive heart failure, frank, not due to hypertension
   (may be aggravated by fluid retention; in addition, guanadrel may directly depress the myocardium)
Diarrhea
   (may be aggravated)
Fever
   (dosage requirements may be reduced)
Peptic ulcer, history of
   (may be aggravated by relative increase in parasympathetic tone)
» Pheochromocytoma
   (release of catecholamines and increased sensitivity to circulating norepinephrine may exacerbate symptoms)
Sensitivity to guanadrel
Sinus bradycardia
   (may be aggravated)

**Patient monitoring**
The following may be especially important in patient monitoring (other tests may be warranted in some patients, depending on condition; » = major clinical significance):

» Blood pressure measurements
   (recommended at periodic intervals in patients being treated for hypertension; selected patients may be trained to perform blood pressure measurements at home and report the results at regular physician visits)

## Side/Adverse Effects

Note: Side/adverse effects are largely due to selective sympathetic blockade and unopposed parasympathetic activity.
   Side/adverse effects are usually reduced after the first 8 weeks of therapy.

The following side/adverse effects have been selected on the basis of their potential clinical significance (possible signs and symptoms in parentheses where appropriate)—not necessarily inclusive:

**Those indicating need for medical attention**
Incidence more frequent
   *Edema, peripheral* (swelling of feet or lower legs)
Incidence less frequent or rare
   *Angina* (chest pain); *dyspnea* (shortness of breath)

**Those indicating need for medical attention only if they continue or are bothersome**
Incidence more frequent
   *Difficulty in ejaculating; drowsiness; fatigue* (unusual tiredness or weakness); *orthostatic hypotension* (dizziness, lightheadedness, or fainting, especially when getting up from a lying or sitting position); *weight gain or loss, excessive*
   Note: Morning *orthostatic hypotension* is less frequent with guanadrel than with guanethidine.
Incidence less frequent or rare
   *Diarrhea or increase in bowel movements; dryness of mouth; headache; muscle pain or tremors; nocturia* (nighttime urination)
   Note: *Diarrhea* is more commonly reported with guanethidine than with guanadrel.

## Overdose

For specific information on the agents used in the management of guanadrel overdose, see *Phenylephrine* in *Sympathomimetic Agents—Cardiovascular Use (Parenteral-Systemic)* monograph.

For more information on the management of overdose or unintentional ingestion, **contact a Poison Control Center** (see *Poison Control Center Listing*).

**Clinical effects of overdose**
The following effects have been selected on the basis of their potential clinical significance (possible signs and symptoms in parentheses where appropriate)—not necessarily inclusive:

   *Orthostatic hypotension, marked* (marked dizziness, blurred vision, or syncope when getting up from a lying or sitting position)

**Treatment of overdose**
For excessive hypotension—A vasoconstrictor, such as phenylephrine, may be necessary, keeping in mind that patients may be extra sensitive to these agents; symptomatic and supportive.

## Patient Consultation

As an aid to patient consultation, refer to *Advice for the Patient, Guanadrel (Systemic)*.

In providing consultation, consider emphasizing the following selected information (» = major clinical significance):

**Before using this medication**
» Conditions affecting use, especially:
   Sensitivity to guanadrel
   Use in the elderly—Increased sensitivity to hypotensive effects
   Other medications, especially loxapine, MAO inhibitors, thioxanthenes, tricyclic antidepressants, or trimeprazine
   Other medical problems, especially congestive heart failure or pheochromocytoma

**Proper use of this medication**
Importance of diet; possible need for sodium restriction and/or weight reduction
» Patients may not experience symptoms of hypertension; importance of taking medication even if feeling well
» Does not cure, but helps control hypertension; possible need for lifelong therapy; checking with physician before discontinuing medication; serious consequences of untreated hypertension
Compliance with therapy; taking medication at the same times each day to maintain the therapeutic effect
» Proper dosing
Missed dose: Taking as soon as possible; not taking if almost time for next dose; not doubling doses
» Proper storage

**Precautions while using this medication**
Making regular visits to physician to check progress
» Caution when getting up suddenly from a lying or sitting position, especially in the morning
» Caution in using alcohol, while standing for long periods or exercising, and during hot weather because of enhanced orthostatic hypotensive effects
» Not taking other medications, especially nonprescription sympathomimetics, unless discussed with physician
Caution if any kind of surgery (including dental surgery) or emergency treatment is required
Reporting fever to physician; dosage adjustment may be required

**Side/adverse effects**
Signs of potential side effects, especially peripheral edema, angina, and dyspnea

### General Dosing Information
Because of wide variation in response to guanadrel, dosage must be adjusted to meet the requirements of each patient on the basis of clinical response.

The hypotensive effect of guanadrel is especially pronounced when the patient is standing. If feasible, blood pressure readings should be taken in the supine position, after standing for 10 minutes, and immediately after exercise. Dosage increases should be made only if there has been no decrease in the standing blood pressure from previous levels.

Hospitalized patients should not be discharged until the effect of guanadrel on their standing blood pressure has been determined.

With continuing use, apparent tolerance to the antihypertensive effects of guanadrel may develop as a result of fluid retention and expanded plasma volume. Concurrent administration of a diuretic is recommended.

Recent evidence suggests that withdrawal of antihypertensive therapy prior to surgery is not necessary, but that the anesthesiologist must be aware of such therapy.

Dosage reduction is indicated if the patient has:
- Excessive orthostatic fall in pressure
- Normal supine pressure
- Severe diarrhea

### Oral Dosage Forms

#### GUANADREL SULFATE TABLETS USP

**Usual adult dose**
Antihypertensive—
Initial: Oral, 5 mg two times a day, the dosage being increased at weekly or monthly intervals as necessary to control blood pressure.
Maintenance: Oral, 20 to 75 mg per day in two to four divided doses.

Note: Geriatric patients may be more sensitive to the effects of the usual adult dose.

**Usual pediatric dose**
Safety and efficacy not been established.

**Strength(s) usually available**
U.S.—
 10 mg (Rx) [*Hylorel* (scored; lactose)].
Canada—
 Not commercially available.

**Packaging and storage**
Store below 40 °C (104 °F), preferably between 15 and 30 °C (59 and 86 °F), unless otherwise specified by manufacturer. Store in a tight, light-resistant container.

**Auxiliary labeling**
- Avoid alcoholic beverages.
- Do not take other medicines without your doctor's advice.

**Note**
Check refill frequency to determine compliance in hypertensive patients.

### Selected Bibliography
The fifth report of the Joint National Committee on Detection, Evaluation, and Treatment of High Blood Pressure (JNC V). Arch Intern Med 1993; 153(2): 154-83.

Finnerty FA, Brogden RN. Guanadrel. A review of its pharmacodynamic and pharmacokinetic properties and therapeutic use in hypertension. Drugs 1985 Jul; 30: 22-31.

Palmer JD, Nugent CA. Guanadrel sulfate: a postganglionic sympathetic inhibitor for the treatment of mild to moderate hypertension. Pharmacotherapy 1983; 3(4): 220-9.

Revised: 01/03/96
Interim revision: 08/19/98

# GUANETHIDINE  Systemic

VA CLASSIFICATION (Primary): CV409

Commonly used brand name(s): *Apo-Guanethidine; Ismelin.*

Note: For a listing of dosage forms and brand names by country availability, see *Dosage Forms* section(s).

### Category
Antihypertensive.

### Indications

**Accepted**
Hypertension (treatment)—Guanethidine is indicated in the treatment of moderate to severe hypertension.

Guanethidine is also indicated in the treatment of renal hypertension, including that secondary to pyelonephritis, renal amyloidosis, and renal artery stenosis.

### Pharmacology/Pharmacokinetics

**Physicochemical characteristics**
Molecular weight—296.38.
pKa—9 and 12.

**Mechanism of action/Effect**
Guanethidine is a postganglionic adrenergic blocking agent. Uptake of guanethidine and storage in sympathetic neurons occur via the norepinephrine pump. Guanethidine slowly displaces norepinephrine from its storage in nerve endings and thereby blocks the release of norepinephrine normally produced by nerve stimulation. Catecholamine depletion leads to reduced arteriolar vasoconstriction, especially the reflex increase in sympathetic tone that occurs with a change in position.

**Absorption**
With chronic oral administration, absorption of guanethidine is highly variable among patients; between 3 and 30% of an oral dose is absorbed.

**Biotransformation**
Hepatic, to 3 metabolites that are pharmacologically less active than guanethidine.

**Half-life**
Following chronic oral administration, the initial phase of elimination with a half-life of 1.5 days is followed by a second phase of elimination with a half-life of 4 to 8 days.

**Time to peak effect**
Single dose—The peak effect occurs within 8 hours after a single dose.
Multiple doses—The full therapeutic effects may not be noticed until 1 to 3 weeks after initiation of therapy.

**Duration of action**
Multiple doses—Blood pressure returns gradually to pretreatment levels within 1 to 3 weeks after withdrawal.

**Elimination**
Renal, 25 to 50% unchanged.

### Precautions to Consider

**Carcinogenicity/Mutagenicity**
Studies have not been done.

**Pregnancy/Reproduction**
Fertility—Reversible inhibition of ejaculation has been reported in men taking guanethidine.

Guanethidine given to rats and rabbits, subcutaneously or intraperitoneally, for several weeks at doses of 5 or 10 mg per kg of body weight (mg/kg) per day has been shown to inhibit sperm passage and result in accumulation of sperm debris. However, recovery of ejaculatory function and fertility has been shown in rats given guanethidine intramuscularly for 8 weeks at a dose of 25 mg/kg per day.

Pregnancy—Studies have not been done in humans.
Studies have not been done in animals.
FDA Pregnancy Category C.

**Breast-feeding**
Small quantities of guanethidine are distributed into breast milk. However, problems in humans have not been documented.

**Pediatrics**
Appropriate studies on the relationship of age to the effects of guanethidine have not been performed in the pediatric population. However, pediatrics-specific problems that would limit the usefulness of this medication in children are not expected.

## Geriatrics
Although appropriate studies on the relationship of age to the effects of guanethidine have not been performed in the geriatric population, the elderly may be more sensitive to the hypotensive effects. In addition, elderly patients are more likely to have age-related renal function impairment, which may require caution in patients receiving guanethidine.

## Drug interactions and/or related problems
The following drug interactions and/or related problems have been selected on the basis of their potential clinical significance (possible mechanism in parentheses where appropriate)—not necessarily inclusive (» = major clinical significance):

Note: Combinations containing any of the following medications, depending on the amount present, may also interact with this medication.

Alcohol or
Barbiturates or
Methotrimeprazine or
Opioid (narcotic) analgesics
   (concurrent use with guanethidine will contribute to additive orthostatic hypotensive effects)

Alpha-adrenergic blocking agents or
Other medications with alpha-adrenergic blocking action, such as:
   Dihydroergotamine
   Ergoloid mesylates
   Ergotamine
   Haloperidol
   Loxapine
   Phenothiazines
   Thioxanthenes or
Beta-adrenergic blocking agents or
Rauwolfia alkaloids
   (concurrent use with guanethidine may cause an increased incidence of orthostatic hypotension or bradycardia)

Amphetamines or
» Antidepressants, tricyclic or
Appetite suppressants, with the exception of fenfluramine or
Cyclobenzaprine or
Haloperidol or
» Loxapine or
Maprotiline or
Methylphenidate or
Phenothiazines, especially chlorpromazine or
» Thioxanthenes or
» Trimeprazine
   (concurrent use may decrease the hypotensive effects of guanethidine because of its displacement from and inhibition of uptake by adrenergic neurons)
   (however, up to 150 mg of doxepin a day can be given without antagonizing the antihypertensive effect of guanethidine)

Anticholinergics, especially atropine and related compounds
   (concurrent use with guanethidine may antagonize the inhibitory action of these medications on gastric acid secretion)

» Antidiabetic agents, sulfonylurea or
Insulin
   (concurrent use with guanethidine may enhance the hypoglycemic effect, in part through displacement of sulfonylurea antidiabetic agents from serum proteins; dosage adjustments may be necessary)

Anti-inflammatory drugs, nonsteroidal (NSAIDs), especially indomethacin
   (antihypertensive effects of guanethidine may be reduced when it is used concurrently with these agents; indomethacin, and possibly other NSAIDs, may antagonize the antihypertensive effect by inhibiting renal prostaglandin synthesis and/or by causing sodium and fluid retention; the patient should be carefully monitored to confirm that the desired effect is being obtained)

Fenfluramine
   (concurrent use with guanethidine may produce additive hypotensive effects, and may result in postural hypotension; dosage adjustments of the antihypertensive may be necessary)

Hypotension-producing medications, other (See *Appendix II*) or
» Minoxidil
   (antihypertensive effects may be potentiated when these medications are used concurrently with guanethidine; although some antihypertensive and/or diuretic combinations are frequently used for therapeutic advantage, when used concurrently dosage adjustments may be necessary; concurrent use with minoxidil is not recommended)

» Monoamine oxidase (MAO) inhibitors, including furazolidone, procarbazine, and selegiline
   (concurrent use with guanethidine may result in moderate to severe hypertension due to release of catecholamines; withdrawal of MAO inhibitors at least 1 week prior to initiation of guanethidine therapy is recommended)

Sympathomimetic agents, such as:
   Cocaine
   Dobutamine
   Dopamine
   Ephedrine
   Epinephrine
» Metaraminol
   Methoxamine
   Norepinephrine
   Phenylephrine
   Phenylpropanolamine
   (antihypertensive effects of guanethidine may be reduced when it is used concurrently with any sympathomimetics; the patient should be carefully monitored to confirm that the desired effect is being obtained)
   (in addition to possibly decreasing the hypotensive effects of guanethidine, concurrent use of cocaine, dobutamine, dopamine, epinephrine, metaraminol, methoxamine, norepinephrine, or phenylephrine may potentiate the pressor effect of these medications as a result of inhibition of sympathomimetic uptake by adrenergic neurons, possibly resulting in hypertension and cardiac arrhythmias)
   (concurrent use of ephedrine or phenylpropanolamine with guanethidine may decrease the hypotensive effects of guanethidine because of its displacement from and inhibition of uptake by adrenergic neurons)
   (concurrent use of metaraminol with guanethidine may cause a hypertensive crisis. When metaraminol is used within 5 days of discontinuation of guanethidine, a hypertensive potential may remain)
   (concurrent use of phenylephrine ophthalmic solution with guanethidine may increase the pupillary response)

## Medical considerations/Contraindications
The medical considerations/contraindications included have been selected on the basis of their potential clinical significance (reasons given in parentheses where appropriate)—not necessarily inclusive (» = major clinical significance).

***Risk-benefit should be considered when the following medical problems exist:***

Asthma, history of
   (may be aggravated because of hypersensitivity to catecholamine depletion)

Cerebrovascular insufficiency or
Coronary insufficiency or
Myocardial infarction, recent
   (ischemia may be aggravated as a result of reduced blood pressure)

» Congestive heart failure, frank, not due to hypertension or
» Congestive heart failure, severe
   (may be aggravated by fluid retention; in addition, guanethidine may interfere with the compensatory response of the adrenergic system in these patients)

Diabetes mellitus
   (guanethidine may enhance effects of hypoglycemic medications)

Diarrhea or
Sinus bradycardia
   (may be aggravated)

Fever
   (dosage requirements may be reduced)

Hepatic function impairment
   (reduced metabolism and excessive accumulation of guanethidine may occur; lower doses may be required)

Peptic ulcer, history of
   (may be aggravated by relative increase in parasympathetic tone)

» Pheochromocytoma
   (release of catecholamines may exacerbate symptoms)

Renal function impairment
   (guanethidine further reduces glomerular filtration rate and renal plasma flow; may produce transient urinary retention; severe orthostatic hypotension may occur because of excessive accumulation)

Sensitivity to guanethidine

**Patient monitoring**

The following may be especially important in patient monitoring (other tests may be warranted in some patients, depending on condition; » = major clinical significance):

» Blood pressure measurements
(recommended at periodic intervals in patients being treated for hypertension; selected patients may be trained to perform blood pressure measurements at home and report the results at regular physician visits)

## Side/Adverse Effects

Note: Side effects are largely due to selective sympathetic blockade and unopposed parasympathetic activity.

The following side/adverse effects have been selected on the basis of their potential clinical significance (possible signs and symptoms in parentheses where appropriate)—not necessarily inclusive:

**Those indicating need for medical attention**
Incidence more frequent
   *Edema, peripheral* (swelling of feet or lower legs)
Incidence less frequent or rare
   *Angina* (chest pain); *edema, pulmonary* (shortness of breath)

**Those indicating need for medical attention only if they continue or are bothersome**
Incidence more frequent
   *Bradycardia* (slow heartbeat); *diarrhea or increase in bowel movements; difficulty in ejaculating; nasal congestion* (stuffy nose); *orthostatic hypotension* (dizziness, lightheadedness, or fainting, especially when getting up from a lying or sitting position); *unusual tiredness or weakness*
   Note: *Orthostatic hypotension* may be most marked in the morning possibly due to an early morning reduction in vascular volume or by an inhibitory effect of guanethidine on the diurnal rhythm of catecholamine excretion. Hot weather, alcohol, or exercise may accentuate this effect.
Incidence less frequent or rare
   *Blurred vision; drooping eyelids; dryness of mouth; headache; loss of hair on scalp; muscle pain or tremors; nausea or vomiting; nocturia* (nighttime urination); *skin rash*

## Overdose

For specific information on the agents used in the management of guanethidine overdose, see:
• *Atropine (Systemic)* monograph;
• *Charcoal, Activated (Oral-Local)* monograph; and/or
• *Laxatives (Local)* monograph.

For more information on the management of overdose or unintentional ingestion, **contact a Poison Control Center** (see *Poison Control Center Listing*).

**Clinical effects of overdose**
The following effects have been selected on the basis of their potential clinical significance (possible signs and symptoms in parentheses where appropriate)—not necessarily inclusive:
   *Bradycardia; diarrhea; nausea; orthostatic hypotension; shock*

**Treatment of overdose**
To decrease absorption—
   Gastric lavage. If conditions permit, activated charcoal and laxatives may be administered.
Specific treatment—
   For sinus bradycardia: Atropine should be administered.
   For diarrhea: If severe and persistent, anticholinergic agents may be administered to reduce intestinal hypermotility. Hydration and electrolyte balance should be maintained.
Monitoring—
   Cardiovascular and renal function should be monitored for several days.
Supportive care—
   For previously normotensive patients: Restoring blood pressure and heart rate to normal by keeping patient in supine position. Normal homeostatic control usually returns over a 72-hour period.
   For previously hypertensive patients: Supporting vital functions and controlling cardiac irregularities that might present. Keeping patient in supine position. Use of vasopressors, if necessary, with extreme caution since guanethidine may increase the responsiveness to these agents, potentially resulting in a rise in blood pressure and cardiac arrhythmias.

## Patient Consultation

As an aid to patient consultation, refer to *Advice for the Patient, Guanethidine (Systemic)*.

In providing consultation, consider emphasizing the following selected information (» = major clinical significance):

**Before using this medication**
» Conditions affecting use, especially:
   Sensitivity to guanethidine
   Breast-feeding—Small quantities distributed into breast milk
   Use in the elderly—Increased sensitivity to hypotensive effects
   Other medications, especially loxapine, MAO inhibitors, minoxidil, sulfonylurea antidiabetic agents, thioxanthenes, tricyclic antidepressants, or trimeprazine
   Other medical problems, especially congestive heart failure or pheochromocytoma
   Fertility—Reversible inhibition of ejaculation

**Proper use of this medication**
Possible need for control of weight and diet, especially sodium intake
» Patient may not experience symptoms of hypertension; importance of taking medication even if feeling well
» Does not cure, but helps control hypertension; possible need for lifelong therapy; checking with physician before discontinuing medication; serious consequences of untreated hypertension
   Compliance with therapy; taking medication at the same time each day to maintain the therapeutic effect
» Proper dosing
   Missed dose: Taking as soon as possible; not taking if almost time for next dose; not doubling doses
» Proper storage

**Precautions while using this medication**
Making regular visits to physician to check progress
» Caution when getting up suddenly from a lying or sitting position, especially in the morning
» Caution in using alcohol, while standing for long periods or exercising, and during hot weather because of enhanced orthostatic hypotensive effects
» Not taking other medications, especially nonprescription sympathomimetics, unless discussed with physician
   Caution if any kind of surgery (including dental surgery) or emergency treatment is required
   Reporting fever to physician; dosage adjustment may be required
   Male patients: Guanethidine may interfere with ejaculation

**Side/adverse effects**
Signs of potential side effects, especially peripheral and pulmonary edema and angina

## General Dosing Information

Because of wide individual variation in response to guanethidine, dosage must be adjusted to meet the requirements of each patient on the basis of clinical response.

Because of its long half-life, the effects of guanethidine are cumulative over long periods. Initial doses should be small with gradual increases being made if necessary. Unless the patient is hospitalized, dosage increases should not be made more often than every 5 to 7 days.

The hypotensive effect of guanethidine is especially pronounced when the patient is standing. If feasible, blood pressure readings should be taken in the supine position, after standing for 10 minutes, and immediately after exercise. Dosage increases should be made only if there has been no decrease in the standing blood pressure from previous levels.

Hospitalized patients should not be discharged until the effect of guanethidine on their standing blood pressure has been determined.

With continuing use, apparent tolerance to the antihypertensive effects of guanethidine may develop as a result of fluid retention and expanded plasma volume. Concurrent administration of a diuretic is recommended.

Recent evidence suggests that withdrawal of antihypertensive therapy prior to surgery is not necessary, but that the anesthesiologist must be aware of such therapy.
   Dosage reduction is indicated if the patient has:
   • Excessive orthostatic fall in pressure
   • Normal supine pressure
   • Severe diarrhea

## Oral Dosage Forms

### GUANETHIDINE MONOSULFATE TABLETS USP

**Usual adult dose**
Antihypertensive—
Ambulatory patients—
  Initial—Oral, 10 or 12.5 mg once a day, the daily dosage being increased by 10 or 12.5 mg at five- to seven-day intervals if necessary for control of blood pressure.
  Maintenance—Oral, 25 to 50 mg once a day.
Hospitalized patients—
  Initial—Oral, 25 to 50 mg once a day, the daily dosage being increased by 25 to 50 mg at daily or every-other-day intervals if necessary for control of blood pressure.
Note: Geriatric patients may be more sensitive to the effects of the usual adult dose.

**Usual pediatric dose**
Antihypertensive—
  Oral, 200 mcg (0.2 mg) per kg of body weight or 6 mg per square meter of body surface area once a day, the daily dosage being increased by 200 mcg (0.2 mg) per kg of body weight or 6 mg per square meter of body surface area at seven- to ten-day intervals if necessary for control of blood pressure.

**Strength(s) usually available**
U.S.—
  10 mg (Rx) [*Ismelin* (scored; lactose) [GENERIC (may be scored; may contain lactose)].
  25 mg (Rx) [*Ismelin* (scored; lactose) [GENERIC (may be scored; may contain lactose)].
Canada—
  10 mg (Rx) [*Apo-Guanethidine* (scored); *Ismelin* (scored)].
  25 mg (Rx) [*Apo-Guanethidine* (scored); *Ismelin* (scored)].

**Packaging and storage**
Store below 40 °C (104 °F), preferably between 15 and 30 °C (59 and 86 °F), unless otherwise specified by manufacturer. Store in a well-closed container.

**Auxiliary labeling**
- Avoid alcoholic beverages.
- Do not take other medicines without your doctor's advice.

**Note**
Check refill frequency to determine compliance in hypertensive patients.

### Selected Bibliography
The fifth report of the Joint National Committee on Detection, Evaluation, and Treatment of High Blood Pressure (JNC V). Arch Intern Med 1993; 153(2): 154-83.

Revised: 01/03/96
Interim revision: 08/18/98

---

# GUANFACINE  Systemic†

VA CLASSIFICATION (Primary): CV409
Commonly used brand name(s): *Tenex*.
Note: For a listing of dosage forms and brand names by country availability, see *Dosage Forms* section(s).

†Not commercially available in Canada.

## Category
Antihypertensive.

## Indications

**Accepted**
Hypertension (treatment)—Guanfacine is indicated, usually in combination with a thiazide diuretic, in the treatment of hypertension.

## Pharmacology/Pharmacokinetics

**Physicochemical characteristics**
Molecular weight— 282.56.

**Mechanism of action/Effect**
Thought to be due to central $alpha_2$-adrenergic stimulation, which results in a decreased sympathetic outflow to the heart, kidneys, and peripheral vasculature; decreased systolic and diastolic blood pressure; and slightly decreased heart rate.

**Other actions/effects**
Growth hormone secretion stimulated by single doses (no effect with long-term use).

**Absorption**
Rapid and complete; bioavailability approximately 80%.

**Protein binding**
Moderate (70%; 50% to erythrocytes).

**Biotransformation**
Hepatic.

**Half-life**
Approximately 17 hours (range, 10–30 hours); 13 to 14 hours in younger patients.

**Onset of action**
Multiple doses—Within 1 week.

**Time to peak plasma concentration**
1 to 4 hours (average, 2.6 hours).

**Time to peak effect**
Single dose—8 to 12 hours.
Multiple doses—1 to 3 months.

**Duration of action**
Single dose—24 hours.

**Elimination**
Renal, approximately 40% unchanged.
In dialysis—Not significantly removed by dialysis (2.4%).

## Precautions to Consider

**Carcinogenicity**
Studies in mice for 78 weeks at doses greater than 150 times the maximum recommended human dose and in rats for 102 weeks at doses greater than 100 times the maximum recommended human dose found no evidence of carcinogenicity.

**Mutagenicity**
Mutagenicity studies were negative.

**Pregnancy/Reproduction**
Fertility—Studies in male and female rats found no adverse effects on fertility.
Pregnancy—Adequate and well-controlled studies in humans have not been done.
Studies in rats and rabbits at doses 70 and 20 times the maximum recommended human dose, respectively, have not shown that guanfacine causes adverse effects in the fetus. Studies with doses of 100 and 200 times the maximum recommended human dose in rabbits and rats respectively, showed maternal toxicity and reduced fetal survival. Guanfacine crosses the placenta in rats.
FDA Pregnancy Category B.

**Breast-feeding**
It is not known whether guanfacine is distributed into human breast milk. However, problems have not been documented. Guanfacine is distributed into the milk of lactating rats.

**Pediatrics**
Appropriate studies on the relationship of age to the effects of guanfacine have not been performed in the pediatric population. Safety and efficacy have not been established.

**Geriatrics**
Appropriate studies on the relationship of age to the effects of guanfacine have not been performed in the geriatric population. However, the elderly may be more sensitive to the hypotensive and sedative effects.

**Dental**
Use of guanfacine may decrease or inhibit salivary flow, thus contributing to the development of caries, periodontal disease, oral candidiasis, and discomfort.

# HAEMOPHILUS B CONJUGATE VACCINE   Systemic

This monograph includes information on the following: 1) Haemophilus b conjugate vaccine (HbOC—diptheria CRM197 protein conjugate); 2) Haemophilus b conjugate vaccine (PRP-D—diphtheria toxoid conjugate); 3) Haemophilus b conjugate vaccine (PRP-OMP—meningococcal protein conjugate); 4) Haemophilus b conjugate vaccine (PRP-T—tetanus protein conjugate)

Note: It is recommended that, whenever possible, persons with indications for haemophilus b (Hib) vaccine be immunized with this newer, more immunogenic conjugate vaccine instead of with the polysaccharide vaccine. This is especially important for children 2 months to 24 months of age. See *Haemophilus b Polysaccharide Vaccine (Systemic)* for information on the polysaccharide vaccine.

This vaccine is not an immunizing agent against diphtheria, meningococcal disease, or tetanus.

VA CLASSIFICATION (Primary): IM100

Commonly used brand name(s): *Act-Hib*[4]; *Hibtiter*; *Pedvaxhib*[3]; *Prohibit*[2].

Other commonly used names for HbOC are oligo-CRM and PRP-HbOC.

Note: For a listing of dosage forms and brand names by country availability, see *Dosage Forms* section(s).

## Category
Immunizing agent (active).

## Indications

### Accepted
*Haemophilus influenzae* type b disease (prophylaxis)—Haemophilus b conjugate vaccine is indicated for routine immunization of all children 2 to 59 months of age against diseases caused by *Haemophilus influenzae* type b (Hib).

Note: *Act-Hib* (PRP-T), *Hibtiter* (HbOC), and *Pedvaxhib* (PRP-OMP) are licensed for use in infants and children 2 months of age and older.

*Prohibit* (PRP-D) is licensed for use in children 15 months of age and older (U.S.) and in children 18 months of age and older (Canada).

There are no efficacy data available on the use of Hib vaccine for children 5 years of age and older and adults. Moreover, healthy adults and children 5 and older are not at risk for invasive Hib disease. However, studies suggest that patients in this age group who have chronic conditions associated with an increased risk of Hib disease, such as sickle cell disease, leukemia, splenectomy, or HIV infection, demonstrate good immune responses when immunized with Hib vaccine and may benefit from such immunization. Persons infected with human immunodeficiency virus (HIV) may receive this vaccine whether they are asymptomatic or symptomatic.

The following children should be included:
- Children attending day-care facilities.
- Children in residential institutions, such as orphanages.
- Children with chronic illnesses associated with increased risk of Hib disease. These illnesses include asplenia, sickle cell disease, antibody deficiency syndromes, immunosuppression, and Hodgkin's disease. Children scheduled to undergo immunosuppressive therapy, including that for Hodgkin's disease, should receive the conjugate vaccine at least 10 to 14 days prior to the therapy's initiation. The interval between discontinuation of therapy that causes immunosuppression and the restoration of the patient's ability to respond to an active immunizing agent depends on the intensity and type of immunosuppressive therapy used, the underlying disease, and other factors; estimates vary from 3 months to 1 year. Children with immunodeficiency syndromes secondary to deficient synthesis of immunoglobulins (e.g., agammaglobulinemia) probably will not benefit from immunization with the conjugate vaccine. Instead, passive immunity should be considered in these children.
- Infants and children under 24 months of age who have already had invasive Hib disease. Many infants and children under 24 months of age do not develop an adequate immune response to Hib disease and may contract the disease again if they are not immunized. The vaccine series can be initiated, or continued, at the time of discharge from the hospital. Children 24 months of age or older who contract Hib disease do not need to be immunized, since most children in this age group will develop protective levels of antibody from their illnesses.
- Children with asymptomatic or symptomatic human immunodeficiency virus (HIV) infection. Immunization is recommended even though immunization may be less effective than it would be for immunocompetent children.
- Children of certain racial groups, such as American Indian and Alaskan Eskimo. These racial groups appear to be at increased risk of Hib disease.
- Children of low socioeconomic status. Low socioeconomic status is often associated with crowded living conditions, which increase a child's risk of contact with Hib-infected persons.
- Children who have been previously immunized with the polysaccharide vaccine. Children previously immunized before 24 months of age should be reimmunized with the conjugate vaccine. Reimmunization should take place at least 2 months after the polysaccharide immunization. Children previously immunized at 24 months of age or older do not need to be reimmunized.

Even though they may be protected from invasive disease themselves, household, nursery, and day-care contacts, both adults and children, exposed to children with Hib disease may become asymptomatic carriers of Hib organisms and may infect unimmunized contacts. Therefore, the Immunization Practices Advisory Committee (ACIP) recommends that all contacts (whether immunized or unimmunized) of children with Hib disease receive rifampin chemoprophylaxis with the precautions that apply to the medication. Immunization of unimmunized contacts should not be used to prevent Hib disease in these contacts, because of the time required to generate an immunologic response. In addition, routinely immunizing health-care and day-care workers who may come into close contact with children with invasive Hib disease is not necessary, because healthy adults are not at risk for invasive Hib disease.

### Unaccepted
This vaccine should not be used as an immunizing agent against diphtheria, tetanus, or meningococcal disease, even though there will be some increase in serum diphtheria or tetanus antitoxin levels or antibody levels to the outer membrane protein complex (OMPC) of *Neisseria meningitidis*, respectively, following immunization. No changes in the schedule for administration of diphtheria or tetanus toxoid or meningococcal vaccine are necessitated by the administration of this vaccine.

The conjugate vaccine protects against only *Haemophilus influenzae* type b (Hib). Protection against other strains of *H. influenzae*, such as nonencapsulated strains associated with recurrent upper respiratory disease (including otitis media and sinusitis) should not be anticipated following administration of this vaccine.

## Pharmacology/Pharmacokinetics

### Physicochemical characteristics
Source—
Purified capsular polysaccharide, a polymer of ribose, ribitol, and phosphate (PRP), from the bacterium *Haemophilus influenzae* type b (Hib). It has been conjugated in one of the following ways:
- For the diphtheria toxoid conjugate—The polysaccharide has been conjugated to the diphtheria toxoid via a 6-carbon linker molecule
- For the diphtheria CRM$_{197}$ protein conjugate—The oligosaccharide has been derived from the polysaccharide and has been bound directly to CRM$_{197}$ (a nontoxic variant of diphtheria toxin) by reductive amination
- For the meningococcal protein conjugate—The polysaccharide has been covalently bound to an outer membrane protein complex (OMPC) of the B11 strain of *Neisseria meningitidis* serogroup B
- For the tetanus protein conjugate—The polysaccharide has been covalently bound to tetanus toxoid protein

### Mechanism of action/Effect
*Haemophilus influenzae* type b (Hib) bacteria are surrounded by polysaccharide capsules, which make these bacteria resistant to attack by white blood cells. However, human blood serum contains antibodies that render the bacteria vulnerable to attack. The vaccine, which is derived from the purified polysaccharide from Hib cells, stimulates production of anticapsular antibodies and provides active immunity to the *Haemophilus influenzae* type b bacteria.

Whereas the nonconjugated polysaccharide vaccine predominantly stimulates B-cells to produce antibodies (known as being T-cell independent), haemophilus b conjugate vaccine stimulates T-cells also. The additional stimulation of T-cells (known as being T-cell dependent) is particularly important in young children to ensure an adequate and persistent antibody response. Stimulation of T-cells also results in an anamnestic response to future doses of the conjugate or nonconjugate vaccine and to future natural exposure to *Haemophilus influenzae* type b, resulting in elevated antibody levels.

## Protective effect
The exact protective level of anti-Haemophilus b polysaccharide antibody has not been established; however, 0.15 mcg per mL is considered by many experts to be protective, and 1 mcg per mL in post-immunization sera is considered indicative of long-term protection.

Antibody response to the vaccine is age related in children, with the immune response improving with increasing age.

Some differences in immunogenicity may exist among the different conjugates of haemophilus b conjugate vaccine; however, further studies are needed to confirm these differences and to evaluate their clinical relevance.

Haemophilus b conjugate vaccine is significantly more immunogenic than the nonconjugated polysaccharide vaccine.

## Time to protective effect
Approximately 1 to 2 weeks for onset of a detectable antibody response to the vaccine.

## Duration of protective effect
The duration of immunity of the conjugate vaccine is unknown.

# Precautions to Consider

## Cross-sensitivity and/or related problems
Patients sensitive to haemophilus b polysaccharide vaccine may be sensitive to the conjugate vaccine also.

Patients sensitive to diphtheria toxoid, meningococcal vaccine, or tetanus toxoid protein may be sensitive to the conjugate vaccines available in the U.S. and Canada. These vaccines contain either diphtheria toxoid, a nontoxic variant of diphtheria toxin, an outer membrane protein complex (OMPC) of *Neisseria meningitidis*, or tetanus toxoid protein.

## Carcinogenicity/Mutagenicity
The conjugate vaccine has not been evaluated for its carcinogenic or mutagenic potential.

## Pregnancy/Reproduction
Pregnancy—Studies have not been done in humans or animals.

FDA Pregnancy Category C.

## Breast-feeding
Problems in humans have not been documented.

## Pediatrics
Immunization is not recommended for children less than 2 months of age, since the safety and efficacy of the conjugate vaccine have not been established in this age group.

## Geriatrics
Appropriate studies on the relationship of age to the effects of Hib vaccine have not been performed in the geriatric population. However, no geriatrics-specific problems have been documented to date.

## Drug interactions and/or related problems
The following drug interactions and/or related problems have been selected on the basis of their potential clinical significance (possible mechanism in parentheses where appropriate)—not necessarily inclusive (» = major clinical significance):

Note: Combinations containing any of the following medications, depending on the amount present, may also interact with this medication.

Immunosuppressive agents or
Radiation therapy
(because normal defense mechanisms are suppressed by immunosuppressive agents or radiation treatment, the patient's antibody response to the conjugate vaccine may be decreased. If possible, children who are to undergo therapy with agents that cause immunosuppression, including treatment for Hodgkin's disease, should receive the vaccine at least 10 days, and preferably more than 14 days, before receiving the immunosuppressive agent; otherwise, it may be preferable to postpone the immunization until after the immunosuppressive therapy is completed. The interval between discontinuation of therapy that causes immunosuppression and the restoration of the patient's ability to respond to an active immunizing agent depends on the intensity and type of immunosuppressive therapy used, the underlying disease, and other factors; estimates vary from 3 months to 1 year. The precaution does not apply to corticosteroids used as replacement therapy, for short-term [less than 2 weeks] systemic therapy, or by other routes of administration that do not cause immunosuppression)

## Laboratory value alterations
The following have been selected on the basis of their potential clinical significance (possible effect in parentheses where appropriate)—not necessarily inclusive (» = major clinical significance):

With diagnostic test results
Antigen detection tests
(there is a possibility that the conjugate vaccine may interfere with interpretation of antigen detection tests, such as latex agglutination and countercurrent immunoelectrophoresis, that are used for diagnosis of systemic Hib disease. PRP [a polymer of ribose, ribitol, and phosphate] derived from haemophilus b meningococcal protein conjugate vaccine may be detected in the urine of some persons for up to 7 days following immunization)

## Medical considerations/Contraindications
The medical considerations/contraindications included have been selected on the basis of their potential clinical significance (reasons given in parentheses where appropriate)—not necessarily inclusive (» = major clinical significance).

*Except under special circumstances, this medication should not be used when the following medical problems exist:*

» Illness, acute or febrile
(administration of the conjugate vaccine should be postponed to avoid confusing the symptoms of the illness with the side effects of the vaccine; minor illnesses, such as mild upper respiratory infections, do not preclude administration of the vaccine)

*Risk-benefit should be considered when the following medical problem exists:*

Sensitivity to haemophilus b conjugate vaccine

## Side/Adverse Effects
Note: Side effects generally are minor and last 48 hours or less; in addition, no serious systemic reactions have been observed.

In one person, thrombocytopenia was temporally noted; however, no causative relationship was established.

There are no significant differences in the frequency or types of side effects between haemophilus b polysaccharide vaccine and haemophilus b conjugate vaccine.

The following side/adverse effects have been selected on the basis of their potential clinical significance (possible signs and symptoms in parentheses where appropriate)—not necessarily inclusive:

### Those indicating need for medical attention
Incidence rare
*Anaphylactic reaction* (difficulty in breathing or swallowing; hives; itching, especially of soles or palms; reddening of skin, especially around ears; swelling of eyes, face, or inside of nose; unusual tiredness or weakness, sudden and severe); *convulsions*

### Those indicating need for medical attention only if they continue or are bothersome
Incidence more frequent
*Anorexia* (loss of appetite); *erythema at injection site* (redness); *fever up to 39 °C (102.2 °F)* (usually resolves within 48 hours); *irritability; lethargy* (lack of interest; reduced physical activity); *tenderness at injection site*

Incidence less frequent
*Diarrhea; fever over 39 °C (over 102.2 °F)* (usually resolves within 48 hours); *induration* (hard lump); *swelling, or warm feeling at injection site; skin rash; urticaria* (hives); *vomiting*

# Patient Consultation
As an aid to patient consultation, refer to *Advice for the Patient, Haemophilus b Conjugate Vaccine (Systemic)*.

In providing consultation, consider emphasizing the following selected information (» = major clinical significance):

## Before receiving this vaccine
» Conditions affecting use, especially:
Sensitivity to haemophilus b conjugate vaccine, haemophilus b polysaccharide vaccine, diphtheria toxoid, meningococcal vaccine, or tetanus toxoid
Use in children—Not recommended for use in children up to 2 months of age
Other medical problems, especially fever or serious illness

## Proper use of this vaccine
» Proper dosing

## Side/adverse effects
Signs of potential side effects, especially anaphylactic reaction or convulsions

## General Dosing Information

When sterilizing syringes before vaccination, care should be taken to avoid use of preservatives, antiseptics, detergents, and disinfectants, since the conjugate vaccine may be inactivated by these substances. Disposable syringes and needles are recommended.

The conjugate vaccine is for intramuscular administration only. It should not be administered intravenously.

This vaccine should not be used as an immunizing agent against diphtheria, meningococcal meningitis, or tetanus, even though there may be some slight increase in serum antitoxin or antibody levels following immunization. No changes in the schedule for administration of diphtheria or tetanus toxoid or meningococcal vaccine are necessitated by the administration of this vaccine.

Polysaccharide vaccines, including haemophilus b conjugate vaccine, may be administered concurrently with the vaccines listed below, using separate syringes for the parenterals, and the precautions that apply to each immunizing agent. If DTP, MMR, and IPV are administered concurrently with Hib conjugate vaccine, any 2 of the vaccines may be administered in the same deltoid, and any of these vaccines may be administered in the thigh. If any of the other vaccines listed below is to be administered concurrently with Hib conjugate vaccine, each parenteral vaccine should be administered at a separate body site.
- Polysaccharide vaccines, other, such as meningococcal polysaccharide vaccine or pneumococcal polyvalent vaccine.
- Influenza vaccine, whole or split virus.
- Diphtheria toxoid, tetanus toxoid, and/or pertussis vaccine.
- Live virus vaccines, such as measles, mumps, and/or rubella vaccines.
- Poliovirus vaccines (oral [OPV], inactivated [IPV], or enhanced-potency inactivated [enhanced-potency IPV]).
- Hepatitis B recombinant or plasma-derived vaccine.
- Immune globulin and disease-specific immune globulins.
- Inactivated vaccines, except cholera, typhoid (parenteral), and plague. It is recommended that cholera, typhoid (parenteral), and plague vaccines be administered on separate occasions because there are no data available on the concurrent administration of haemophilus b conjugate vaccine and these vaccines and because of these vaccines' propensity for causing side/adverse effects.

The first conjugate vaccine was licensed for use in the U.S. in December 1987. Persons immunized against Hib disease before that date can be presumed to have received the polysaccharide vaccine.

**For treatment of adverse effects**
Recommended treatment includes:
- For mild hypersensitivity reaction—Administering antihistamines, and, if necessary, glucocorticoids.
- For severe hypersensitivity or anaphylactic reaction—Administering epinephrine. Antihistamines or glucocorticoids may also be administered as required.

---

### HAEMOPHILUS B CONJUGATE VACCINE (HbOC—DIPTHERIA CRM$_{197}$ PROTEIN CONJUGATE)

## Parenteral Dosage Forms

### HAEMOPHILUS B CONJUGATE VACCINE INJECTION
(HbOC—diphtheria CRM$_{197}$ protein conjugate)

**Usual adult and adolescent dose**
Active immunizing agent—
Use is not recommended in these age groups, except for patients with certain chronic conditions associated with an increased risk of Hib disease.

**Usual pediatric dose**
Active immunizing agent—
Intramuscular, 0.5 mL, into the outer aspect of the upper arm (deltoid) or into the lateral mid thigh (vastus lateralis), according to the following dosage schedules:
In the U.S.—
Infants:
First dose—At 2 months of age.
Note: The vaccine series may be initiated as early as 6 weeks of age.
Second dose—At 4 months of age.
Third dose—At 6 months of age.
Booster—At 15 months of age.
Children up to 59 months of age who did not follow the above schedule:
Age 2 to 6 months of age at first dose—Three doses, two months apart, then a booster dose at 15 months of age or as soon as possible thereafter, but not less than two months after previous dose.
Age 7 to 11 months of age at first dose—Two doses, two months apart, then a booster dose at 15 months of age or as soon as possible thereafter, but not less than two months after previous dose.
Age 12 to 14 months of age at first dose—One dose, then a booster dose at 15 months of age or as soon as possible thereafter, but not less than two months after previous dose.
Age 15 to 59 months of age at first dose—One dose.
Note: An interval as short as 1 month between doses is acceptable, but is not optimal.
Any of the other conjugate vaccines may be used for the booster dose; however, there are no data demonstrating that a booster response will occur if one of these other vaccines is used. Ideally, the same conjugate vaccine should be used throughout the vaccination series, including the booster.
Children 5 years of age and older—
Use is not recommended, except for patients with certain chronic conditions associated with an increased risk of Hib disease.
In Canada—
Infants:
First dose—At 2 months of age.
Note: The vaccine series may be initiated as early as 6 weeks of age.
Second dose—At 4 months of age.
Third dose—At 6 months of age.
Booster—At 15 to 18 months of age.
Children up to 59 months of age who did not follow the above schedule:
Age 2 to 6 months of age at first dose—Three doses, two months apart, then a booster dose at 15 to 18 months of age or as soon as possible thereafter, but not less than two months after previous dose.
Age 7 to 11 months of age at first dose—Two doses, two months apart, then a booster dose at 15 to 18 months of age or as soon as possible thereafter, but not less than two months after previous dose.
Age 12 to 17 months of age at first dose—One dose, then a booster dose at 15 to 18 months of age or as soon as possible thereafter, but not less than two months after previous dose.
Age 18 to 59 months of age at first dose—One dose.
Note: An interval as short as 1 month between doses is acceptable, but is not optimal.
Any of the other conjugate vaccines may be used for the booster dose; however, there are no data demonstrating that a booster response will occur if one of these other vaccines is used. Ideally, the same conjugate vaccine should be used throughout the vaccination series, including the booster.
Children 5 years of age and older:
Use is not recommended.
Note: Children 5 years of age and older with certain chronic conditions associated with an increased risk of Hib disease may profit from Hib immunization.

**Strength(s) usually available**
U.S.—
10 mcg (0.01 mg) of purified haemophilus b saccharide and approximately 25 mcg (0.025 mg) of CRM$_{197}$ protein, a nontoxic variant of diphtheria toxin, per 0.5 mL dose (Rx) [*Hibtiter* (in multidose vials—thimerosal 1:10,000)].
Canada—
10 mcg (0.01 mg) of purified haemophilus b saccharide and approximately 25 mcg (0.025 mg) of CRM$_{197}$ protein, a nontoxic variant of diphtheria toxin, per 0.5 mL dose (Rx) [*Hibtiter*].

**Packaging and storage**
Store between 2 and 8 °C (35 and 46 °F), unless otherwise specified by manufacturer. Do not freeze.

## HAEMOPHILUS B CONJUGATE VACCINE (PRP-D—DIPHTHERIA TOXOID CONJUGATE)

### Parenteral Dosage Forms

**HAEMOPHILUS B CONJUGATE VACCINE INJECTION (PRP-D—diphtheria toxoid conjugate)**

**Usual adult and adolescent dose**
Active immunizing agent—
 Use is not recommended in these age groups, except for patients with certain chronic conditions associated with an increased risk of Hib disease.

**Usual pediatric dose**
Active immunizing agent—
 Intramuscular, 0.5 mL, into the outer aspect of the upper arm (deltoid) or into the lateral mid thigh (vastus lateralis), according to the following dosage schedules:
 In the U.S.—
  Infants and children up to 15 months of age: Use is not recommended.
  Children 15 to 59 months of age who were not previously immunized: One dose.
  Children 5 years of age and older: Use is not recommended, except for patients with certain chronic conditions associated with an increased risk of Hib disease.
 In Canada—
  Infants and children up to 18 months of age: Use is not recommended.
  Children 18 to 60 months of age who were not previously immunized: One dose.
  Children 5 years of age and older: Use is not recommended, except for patients with certain chronic conditions associated with an increased risk of Hib disease.

**Strength(s) usually available**
U.S.—
 25 mcg (0.025 mg) of purified haemophilus b capsular polysaccharide and 18 mcg (0.018 mg) of diphtheria toxoid protein, per 0.5 mL dose (Rx) [*Prohibit* (thimerosal 1:10,000)].
Canada—
 25 mcg (0.025 mg) of purified haemophilus b capsular polysaccharide and 18 mcg (0.018 mg) of diphtheria toxoid protein, per 0.5 mL dose (Rx) [*Prohibit* (thimerosal 1:10,000)].

**Packaging and storage**
Store between 2 and 8 °C (35 and 46 °F), unless otherwise specified by manufacturer. Do not freeze.

## HAEMOPHILUS B CONJUGATE VACCINE (PRP-OMP—MENINGOCOCCAL PROTEIN CONJUGATE)

### Parenteral Dosage Forms

**HAEMOPHILUS B CONJUGATE VACCINE INJECTION (PRP-OMP—meningococcal protein conjugate)**

**Usual adult and adolescent dose**
Active immunizing agent—
 Use is not recommended in these age groups, except for patients with certain chronic conditions associated with an increased risk of Hib disease.

**Usual pediatric dose**
Active immunizing agent—
 Intramuscular, 0.5 mL, into the outer aspect of the upper arm (deltoid) or into the lateral mid thigh (vastus lateralis), according to the following dosage schedules:
 In the U.S.—
  Infants:
   First dose—At 2 months of age.
   Note: the vaccine series may be initiated as early as 6 weeks of age.
   Second dose—At 4 months of age.
   Booster—At 12 months of age.
  Children up to 59 months of age who did not follow the above schedule:
   Age 2 to 6 months of age at first dose—Two doses, two months apart, then a booster dose at 12 months of age or as soon as possible thereafter, but not less than two months after previous dose.
   Age 7 to 11 months of age at first dose—Two doses, two months apart, then a booster dose at 15 months of age or as soon as possible thereafter, but not less than two months after previous dose.
   Age 12 to 14 months of age at first dose—One dose, then a booster dose at 15 months of age or as soon as possible thereafter, but not less than two months after previous dose.
   Age 15 to 59 months of age at first dose—One dose.
   Note: The U.S. manufacturer's labeling gives the age ranges and dosages as: 2 to 10 months of age at first dose—2 doses, 2 months apart, with a booster at 12 to 15 months; 11 to 14 months of age at first dose—2 doses, 2 months apart; 15 to 71 months of age at first dose—1 dose. These recommendations differ somewhat from those of the Immunization Practices Advisory Committee (ACIP) that are used above.
    An interval as short as 1 month between doses is acceptable, but is not optimal.
    Any of the other conjugate vaccines may be used for the 15-month booster dose; however, there are no data demonstrating that a booster response will occur if one of these other vaccines is used. Ideally, the same conjugate vaccine should be used throughout the vaccination series, including the booster.
  Children 5 years of age and older:
   Use is not recommended, except for patients with certain chronic conditions associated with an increased risk of Hib disease.
 In Canada—
  Infants:
   First dose—At 2 months of age.
   Note: The vaccine series may be initiated as early as 6 weeks of age.
   Second dose—At 4 months of age.
   Booster—At 12 months of age.
  Children up to 59 months of age who did not follow the above schedule:
   Age 2 to 6 months of age at first dose—Two doses, two months apart, then a booster dose at 12 months of age or as soon as possible thereafter, but not less than two months after previous dose.
   Age 7 to 11 months of age at first dose—Two doses, two months apart, then a booster dose at 15 months of age or as soon as possible thereafter, but not less than two months after previous dose.
   Age to 12 to 17 months of age at first dose—One dose, then a booster dose at 18 months of age or as soon as possible thereafter, but not less than two months after previous dose.
   Age 18 to 59 months of age at first dose—One dose.
   Note: An interval as short as 1 month between doses is acceptable, but is not optimal.
    Any of the other conjugate vaccines may be used for the 15- or 18-month booster dose; however, there are no data demonstrating that a booster response will occur if one of these other vaccines is used. Ideally, the same conjugate vaccine should be used throughout the vaccination series, including the booster.
  Children 5 years of age and older:
   Use is not recommended.
   Note: Children 5 years of age and older with certain chronic conditions associated with an increased risk of Hib disease may profit from Hib immunization.

**Strength(s) usually available**
U.S.—
 15 mcg (0.015 mg) of purified haemophilus b capsular polysaccharide and 250 mcg (0.25 mg) of an outer membrane protein complex (OMPC) of the B11 strain of *Neisseria meningitidis* serogroup B, per 0.5 mL dose (Rx) [*Pedvaxhib* (in lyophilized product—lactose 2 mg; in diluent—aluminum 225 mcg as aluminum hydroxide; thimerosal 1:20,000)].
Canada—
 15 mcg (0.015 mg) of purified haemophilus b capsular polysaccharide and 250 mcg (0.25 mg) of an outer membrane protein complex (OMPC) of the B11 strain of *Neisseria meningitidis* serogroup B, per 0.5 mL dose (Rx) [*Pedvaxhib* (in lyophilized product—lactose

2 mg; in diluent—aluminum 225 mcg as aluminum hydroxide; thimerosal 1:20,000)].

**Packaging and storage**
Store between 2 and 8 °C (35 and 45 °F), unless otherwise specified by manufacturer. Do not freeze reconstituted vaccine or aluminum hydroxide diluent.

**Preparation of dosage form**
*Pedvaxhib* should be reconstituted only with the aluminum hydroxide diluent that is supplied. The diluent should be agitated prior to its withdrawal. The vaccine should be agitated at the time of reconstitution, prior to withdrawal of the vaccine dose into the syringe, and prior to injection.

**Stability**
*Pedvaxhib* should be used as soon as possible after reconstitution. Reconstituted vaccine should be stored between 2 and 8 °C (35 and 46 °F) and discarded if not used within 24 hours.

**Auxiliary labeling**
- Shake gently before use.

---

## HAEMOPHILUS B CONJUGATE VACCINE (PRP-T—TETANUS PROTEIN CONJUGATE)

## Parenteral Dosage Forms

### HAEMOPHILUS B CONJUGATE VACCINE INJECTION (PRP-T—tetanus protein conjugate)

**Usual adult and adolescent dose**
Active immunizing agent—
Use is not recommended in these age groups, except for patients with certain chronic conditions associated with an increased risk of Hib disease.

**Usual pediatric dose**
Active immunizing agent—
Intramuscular, 0.5 mL, into the outer aspect of the upper arm (deltoid) or into the lateral mid thigh (vastus lateralis), according to the following dosage schedules:
In the U.S.—
　Infants:
　　First dose—At 2 months of age.
　　Note: The vaccine series may be initiated as early as 6 weeks of age.
　　Second dose—At 4 months of age.
　　Third dose—At 6 months of age.
　　Booster—At 15 months of age.
　Children up to 59 months of age who did not follow the above schedule:
　　Age 2 to 6 months of age at first dose—Three doses, two months apart, then a booster dose at 15 months of age or as soon as possible thereafter, but not less than two months after previous dose.
　　Age 7 to 11 months of age at first dose—Two doses, two months apart, then a booster dose at 15 months of age or as soon as possible thereafter, but not less than two months after previous dose.
　　Age 12 to 14 months of age at first dose—One dose, then a booster dose at 15 months of age or as soon as possible thereafter, but not less than two months after previous dose.
　　Age 15 to 59 months of age at first dose—One dose.
　　Note: An interval as short as 1 month between doses is acceptable, but is not optimal.
　　　Any of the other conjugate vaccines may be used for the booster dose; however, there are no data demonstrating that a booster response will occur if one of these other vaccines is used. Ideally, the same conjugate vaccine should be used throughout the vaccination series, including the booster.
　Children 5 years of age and older:
　　Use is not recommended, except for patients with certain chronic conditions associated with an increased risk of Hib disease.
In Canada—
　Infants:
　　First dose—At 2 months of age.
　　Note: The vaccine series may be initiated as early as 6 weeks of age.
　　Second dose—At 4 months of age.
　　Third dose—At 6 months of age.
　　Booster—At 18 months of age.
　Children up to 59 months of age who did not follow the above schedule:
　　Age 3 to 6 months of age at first dose—Three doses, two months apart, then a booster dose at 18 months of age or as soon as possible thereafter, but not less than two months after previous dose.
　　Age 7 to 11 months of age at first dose—Two doses, two months apart, then a booster dose at 18 months of age or as soon as possible thereafter, but not less than two months after previous dose.
　　Age 12 to 14 months of age at first dose—One dose, then a booster dose at 18 months of age or as soon as possible thereafter, but not less than two months after previous dose.
　　Age 15 to 59 months of age at first dose—One dose.
　　Note: An interval as short as 1 month between doses is acceptable, but is not optimal.
　　　The booster dose may be given as early as 15 months of age or as soon as possible thereafter, but not less than two months after previous dose.
　　　Any of the other conjugate vaccines may be used for the booster dose; however, there are no data demonstrating that a booster response will occur if one of these other vaccines is used. Ideally, the same conjugate vaccine should be used throughout the vaccination series, including the booster.
　Children 5 years of age and older
　　Use is not recommended, except for patients with certain chronic conditions associated with an increased risk of Hib disease.

**Strength(s) usually available**
U.S.—
　10 mcg (0.01 mg) of purified haemophilus b capsular polysaccharide and 20 mcg (0.02 mg) of tetanus protein, per 0.5 mL dose (Rx) [*Act-Hib*].
Canada—
　10 mcg (0.01 mg) of purified haemophilus b capsular polysaccharide and 20 mcg (0.02 mg) of tetanus protein, per 0.5 mL dose (Rx) [*Act-Hib*].

**Packaging and storage**
Store between 2 and 8 °C (35 and 46 °F), unless otherwise specified by manufacturer. Do not freeze the reconstituted vaccine.

**Preparation of dosage form**
*Act-Hib* should be reconstituted only with the 0.4% saline diluent that is supplied. The vaccine should be shaken gently until a clear, colorless solution results. (In Canada, *Act-Hib* may be reconstituted also with the Connaught-Canada brand of DTP vaccine.)

**Stability**
*Act-Hib* should be discarded if it is not used immediately after reconstitution.

## Selected Bibliography

Centers for Disease Control. ACIP update: prevention of Haemophilus influenzae type b disease. MMWR 1988 Jan 22; 37: 13-6.
Berkowitz CD, et al. Safety and immunogenicity of Haemophilus influenzae type b polysaccharide and polysaccharide diphtheria toxoid conjugate vaccines in children 15 to 24 months of age. J Pediatr 1987 Apr: 509-14.
Weinberg GA, Granoff DM. Polysaccharide-protein conjugate vaccines for the prevention of Haemophilus influenzae type b disease. J Pediatr 1988 Oct; 113(4): 621-31.
Centers for Disease Control. Haemophilus b conjugate vaccines for prevention of Haemophilus influenzae type b disease among infants and children two months of age and older: recommendation of the Immunization Practices Advisory Committee (ACIP). MMWR 1991 Jan 11: 40 (RR-1).
Centers for Disease Control. Update on adult immunization: recommendations of the Immunization Practices Advisory Committee (ACIP). MMWR 1991 Nov 15: 40 (RR-12).

Revised: 06/21/93
Interim revision: 03/29/94

# HAEMOPHILUS B CONJUGATE VACCINE (HBOC—DIPHTHERIA CRM₁₉₇ PROTEIN CONJUGATE)—See *Haemophilus b Conjugate Vaccine (Systemic)*

# HAEMOPHILUS B CONJUGATE VACCINE (PRP-D—DIPHTHERIA TOXOID CONJUGATE)—See *Haemophilus b Conjugate Vaccine (Systemic)*

# HAEMOPHILUS B CONJUGATE VACCINE (PRP-OMP—MENINGOCOCCAL PROTEIN CONJUGATE)—See *Haemophilus b Conjugate Vaccine (Systemic)*

# HAEMOPHILUS B CONJUGATE VACCINE (PRP-T—TETANUS PROTEIN CONJUGATE)—See *Haemophilus b Conjugate Vaccine (Systemic)*

# HAEMOPHILUS B POLYSACCHARIDE VACCINE   Systemic*†

VA CLASSIFICATION (Primary): IM100

Note:   This monograph applies only to the polysaccharide vaccine.
    It is recommended that, whenever possible, children with indications for haemophilus b vaccine be immunized with the more immunogenic conjugate vaccine instead of with this polysaccharide vaccine. This is especially important for children under 24 months of age. See *Haemophilus b Conjugate Vaccine (Systemic)* for information on the conjugate vaccine.

Commonly used names are: Haemophilus influenzae type b polysaccharide vaccine; HbPV; Hib CPS; Hib polysaccharide vaccine; and PRP.

Note:   For a listing of dosage forms and brand names by country availability, see *Dosage Forms* section(s).

*Not commercially available in the U.S.
†Not commercially available in Canada.

## Category
Immunizing agent (active).

## Indications

### Accepted
*Haemophilus influenzae* type b disease (prophylaxis)—Haemophilus b polysaccharide vaccine is indicated for routine immunization of children 24 months to 5 years of age (i.e., up to the 5th birthday) against diseases caused by *Haemophilus influenzae* type b (Hib). Although the polysaccharide vaccine was licensed for use up to the 6th birthday, pediatric experts recommend that the vaccine be used only up to the 5th birthday.

In addition, immunization with haemophilus b polysaccharide vaccine should be considered for children 18 to 24 months of age, especially those in known high-risk groups, only if the more immunogenic conjugate vaccine is not available. These groups include:
• Children attending day-care facilities.
• Children in residential institutions, such as orphanages.
• Children with chronic illnesses associated with increased risk of Hib disease. These illnesses include asplenia, sickle cell disease, antibody deficiency syndromes, immunosuppression, and Hodgkin's disease. Children scheduled to undergo immunosuppressive therapy, including that for Hodgkin's disease, should receive the polysaccharide vaccine at least 10 to 14 days prior to the initiation of therapy. The interval between discontinuation of immunosuppressive therapy and the restoration of the patient's ability to respond to an active immunizing agent depends on the intensity and type of immunosuppression-causing therapy, the underlying disease, and other factors; estimates vary from 3 months to 1 year. Children with immunodeficiency syndromes secondary to deficient synthesis of immunoglobulins (e.g., agammaglobulinemia) probably will not benefit from immunization with the polysaccharide vaccine. Instead, passive immunity should be maintained in these children.
• Children under 24 months of age who have already had invasive Hib disease. Most children under 24 months of age do not develop an immune response to Hib disease and may contract the disease again if they are not immunized. The vaccine should be administered to these children no sooner than 2 months following Hib disease and not until they have reached 24 months of age. Children 24 months of age or older who contract Hib disease do not need to be immunized, since most children in this age group will develop protective levels of antibody from their illnesses.
• Children with asymptomatic or symptomatic human immunodeficiency virus (HIV) infection. Immunization is recommended even though immunization of symptomatic children may be less effective than it would be for immunocompetent children.
• Children of certain racial groups, such as American Indian and Alaskan Eskimo. These racial groups appear to be at increased risk of Hib disease.
• Children of low socioeconomic status. Low socioeconomic status is often associated with crowded living conditions, which increase a child's risk of contact with Hib-infected persons.

Even though they may be protected from invasive disease themselves, household, nursery, and day-care contacts, both adults and children, exposed to children with Hib disease may become asymptomatic carriers of Hib organisms and may infect unimmunized contacts. There is an increased risk of invasive Hib disease among unimmunized household contacts less than 4 years of age; in addition, unimmunized nursery and day-care contacts may also be at increased risk, especially if they are younger than 2 years of age. In households where there is at least one contact younger than 48 months of age, it is recommended that all household contacts, both adults and children, receive rifampin chemoprophylaxis, regardless of the immunization status of any of the contacts. For nursery and day-care contacts where the facility provides for children less than 2 years of age for at least 25 hours per week, rifampin chemoprophylaxis is recommended for all contacts, both adults and children, regardless of the immunization status of any of the contacts. For nursery and day-care facilities where all contacts are more than 2 years of age, rifampin chemoprophylaxis is not necessary.

Since satisfactory response to the polysaccharide vaccine is not consistent among children 18 to 24 months of age, most authorities believe that these children should be reimmunized. The optimal timing of this second dose is not known; however, it appears that reimmunization of these children should occur at or after 24 months of age, with 2 to 18 months having elapsed between the first immunization and the second one. Previous immunization does not affect the immune response or adverse reaction to a subsequent dose of the vaccine.

### Unaccepted
Because the polysaccharide vaccine protects against only *Haemophilus influenzae* type b (Hib), protection against other strains of *H. influenzae*, such as nonencapsulated strains associated with recurrent upper respiratory disease (including otitis media and sinusitis), should not be anticipated following administration of this vaccine.

## Pharmacology/Pharmacokinetics

### Physicochemical characteristics
Source—Purified capsular polysaccharide, a polymer of ribose, ribitol, and phosphate (PRP), from the bacterium *Haemophilus influenzae* type b (Hib).

### Mechanism of action/Effect
*Haemophilus influenzae* type b (Hib) bacteria are surrounded by polysaccharide capsules, which make the bacteria resistant to attack by white blood cells. However, human blood serum contains antibodies, which render the bacteria vulnerable to attack. The vaccine, which is composed of the purified polysaccharide from Hib bacterial cells, stimulates production of anticapsular antibodies and provides active immunity to the *Haemophilus influenzae* type b bacteria represented by the polysaccharide in the vaccine.

Haemophilus b polysaccharide vaccine, unlike the conjugate vaccine, predominantly stimulates B-cells to produce antibodies. This is known as being T-cell independent and is characteristic of polysaccharide vaccines. The initial stimulation of T-cells followed by stimulation of B cells (known as a T-cell response) is particularly important in young children to ensure adequate and persisting antibody production. Stimulation of T-cells also results in an anamnestic response to future doses of the vaccine and future natural exposure to *Haemophilus influenzae* type b. The poor T-cell response stimulated by the polysaccharide vaccine is thought to be one reason why the polysaccharide vaccine is not adequately immunogenic in children up to 18 months of age and may not be fully immunogenic in children 18 to 24 months of age. In addition, lack of initial T-cell stimulation probably is the reason that repeat doses of the polysaccharide vaccine do not boost the antibody response consistently.

**Protective efficacy**

The exact protective level of anti-Haemophilus b polysaccharide antibody has not been established; however, 0.15 mcg/mL is considered by many experts to be protective, and 1 mcg/mL in post-immunization sera is considered indicative of long-term protection.

Antibody response to the vaccine is age related in children. Children up to 18 months of age develop very little immunologic response to the vaccine. Children 18 to 24 months of age have inconsistent and less than optimal response to the vaccine. Children over 24 months of age have a high rate of seroconversion. Antibody response continues to improve until it reaches adult levels in children approximately 6 years of age.

**Time to protective efficacy**

Approximately 1 week for onset of an antibody response to the vaccine; approximately 3 weeks for attainment of the protective level of 1 mcg per mL, which is considered indicative of long-term protection.

**Duration of protective effect**

The duration of immunity after a single dose of the polysaccharide vaccine has not been completely described. However, it may be less than the duration of immunity following administration of the conjugate vaccine, which is expected to be at least 1.5 to 3 years.

Duration of antibody response is age related in children. In one study of children 15 to 24 months of age, an antibody concentration of 1 mcg per mL, which is considered indicative of long-term protection, was reached in less than 30% of children.

## Precautions to Consider

**Cross-sensitivity and/or related problems**

Patients sensitive to haemophilus b conjugate vaccine may be sensitive to the polysaccharide vaccine also.

**Pediatrics**

For children up to 18 months of age—Immunization is not recommended, since children in this age group will not have an adequate antibody response to the polysaccharide vaccine.

For children 18 to 24 months of age—Immunization is recommended for children in this age group, especially those in known high risk groups. However, the efficacy of the polysaccharide vaccine in these children appears to be less than in children 24 months of age or older, and some of these children will not have an adequate antibody response to the polysaccharide vaccine. It is recommended that, whenever possible, the more immunogenic conjugate vaccine be used instead of the polysaccharide vaccine.

**Drug interactions and/or related problems**

The following drug interactions and/or related problems have been selected on the basis of their potential clinical significance (possible mechanism in parentheses where appropriate)—not necessarily inclusive (» = major clinical significance):

Note: Combinations containing any of the following medications, depending on the amount present, may also interact with this medication.

Immunosuppressive agents or
Radiation therapy
(because immunosuppressive agents and radiation therapy suppress normal defense mechanisms, the patient's antibody response to the polysaccharide vaccine may be decreased. If possible, children who are to undergo therapy with agents that cause immunosuppression, including that for Hodgkin's disease, should receive the vaccine at least 10 days, and preferably more than 14 days, prior to receiving the immunosuppression-causing agent; otherwise, it may be preferable to postpone the immunization until after the immunosuppression-causing therapy is completed. The interval between discontinuation of therapy that causes immunosuppression and the restoration of the patient's ability to respond to an active immunizing agent depends on the intensity and type of immunosuppression-causing therapy, the underlying disease, and other factors; estimates vary from 3 months to 1 year. The precaution does not apply to corticosteroids used as replacement therapy, for short-term [less than 2 weeks] systemic therapy, or by other routes of administration that do not cause immunosuppression)

**Laboratory value alterations**

The following have been selected on the basis of their potential clinical significance (possible effect in parentheses where appropriate)—not necessarily inclusive (» = major clinical significance):

With diagnostic test results
Antigen detection tests
(the polysaccharide vaccine may interfere with interpretation of antigen detection tests, such as latex agglutination and countercurrent immunoelectrophoresis, that are used for diagnosis of systemic Hib disease. Antigenuria from administration of the haemophilus b polysaccharide vaccine can produce positive urinary latex agglutination tests for up to 11 days after immunization)

**Medical considerations/Contraindications**

The medical considerations/contraindications included have been selected on the basis of their potential clinical significance (reasons given in parentheses where appropriate)—not necessarily inclusive (» = major clinical significance).

*Except under special circumstances, this medication should not be used when the following medical problem exists:*

» Illness, acute or febrile
(administration of the polysaccharide vaccine should be postponed to avoid confusing the symptoms of the illness with the side effects of the vaccine; minor illnesses, such as mild upper respiratory infections, do not preclude administration of the vaccine)

*Risk-benefit should be considered when the following medical problem exists:*

Sensitivity to haemophilus b polysaccharide vaccine

## Side/Adverse Effects

Note: Side effects generally are minor, occur within 24 hours, and last 24 hours or less.
There are no significant differences in the frequency or types of side effects between haemophilus b polysaccharide vaccine and haemophilus b conjugate vaccine.

The following side/adverse effects have been selected on the basis of their potential clinical significance (possible signs and symptoms in parentheses where appropriate)—not necessarily inclusive:

**Those indicating need for medical attention**

Incidence rare
*Anaphylactic reaction* (difficulty in breathing or swallowing; hives; itching, especially of soles or palms; reddening of skin, especially around ears; swelling of eyes, face, or inside of nose; unusual tiredness or weakness, sudden and severe); *convulsions*

**Those indicating need for medical attention only if they continue or are bothersome**

Incidence more frequent
*Anorexia* (lack of appetite); *diarrhea; erythema at injection site* (redness at place of injection); *fever up to 39 °C (102.2 °F)*—usually resolves within 48 hours; *irritability; lethargy* (lack of interest; reduced physical activity); *tenderness at injection site*

Incidence less frequent or rare
*Fever over 39 °C (over 102.2 °F)*—usually resolves within 48 hours; *induration at injection site* (hard lump at place of injection); *serum sickness–like reaction* (itching; skin rash; swelling of face; arthralgia; joint pain); *sleep disturbance* (trouble in sleeping); *swelling at injection site; vomiting*

## Patient Consultation

As an aid to patient consultation, refer to *Advice for the Patient, Haemophilus b Polysaccharide Vaccine (Systemic)*.

In providing consultation, consider emphasizing the following selected information (» = major clinical significance):

**Before receiving this vaccine**

» Conditions affecting use, especially:
Sensitivity to haemophilus b polysaccharide vaccine or haemophilus b conjugate vaccine
Use in children—Not recommended for use in children up to 18 months of age
Other medical problems, especially fever or serious illness

**Proper use of this vaccine**

» Proper dosing

**Side/adverse effects**

Signs of potential side effects, especially anaphylactic reaction or convulsions

## General Dosing Information

When sterilizing syringes and skin before vaccination, care should be taken to avoid use of preservatives, antiseptics, detergents, and disinfectants, since the polysaccharide vaccine may be inactivated by these substances.

The polysaccharide vaccine is for intramuscular or subcutaneous administration. It should not be administered intradermally or intravenously.

To prevent inactivation of the vaccine, it is recommended that only the diluent provided by the manufacturer be used for vaccine reconstitution.

Persons infected with human immunodeficiency virus (HIV) may receive this vaccine whether they have asymptomatic or symptomatic HIV infection.

Polysaccharide vaccines, including haemophilus b polysaccharide vaccine, may be administered concurrently with the following, using separate body sites, separate syringes, and the precautions that apply to each immunizing agent:
- Polysaccharide vaccines, other, such as meningococcal polysaccharide vaccine or pneumococcal polyvalent vaccine.
- Influenza vaccine, whole or split virus.
- Diphtheria toxoid, tetanus toxoid, and/or pertussis vaccine.
- Live virus vaccines, such as measles, mumps, and/or rubella vaccines.
- Poliovirus vaccines (oral [OPV], inactivated [IPV], or enhanced-potency inactivated [enhanced-potency IPV]).
- Hepatitis B recombinant or plasma-derived vaccine.
- Immune globulin and disease-specific immune globulins.
- Inactivated vaccines, except cholera, typhoid, and plague. It is recommended that cholera, typhoid, and plague vaccines be administered on separate occasions because there are no data available on the concurrent administration of haemophilus b polysaccharide vaccine and these vaccines and because of these vaccines' propensity to cause side/adverse effects.

Parents should be informed that the polysaccharide vaccine is not as effective in children 18 to 24 months of age as it is in older children and that reimmunization may be necessary.

Most authorities believe that children immunized between 18 and 24 months of age should be reimmunized. The optimal timing of this second dose is not known; however, it appears that reimmunization of these children should occur at or after 24 months of age, with 2 to 18 months having elapsed between the first immunization and the second one. Previous immunization does not affect the immune response or adverse reaction to a subsequent dose of the vaccine.

### For treatment of adverse effects

Recommended treatment consists of the following—
For children
- If anaphylaxis occurs, 0.01 mg of epinephrine per kg of body weight or 0.3 mg of epinephrine per square meter of body surface, up to a maximum of 0.5 mg per dose, may be administered subcutaneously, the dose being repeated every fifteen minutes for two doses, then administered every four hours as needed.
- If anaphylactic shock occurs, 0.01 mg of epinephrine per kg of body weight, up to a maximum of 0.3 mg, may be administered intramuscularly or subcutaneously, the dose being repeated every five minutes if necessary. If there is an inadequate response to the intramuscular or subcutaneous dosage, 0.01 mg of epinephrine per kg of body weight may be administered intravenously every five to fifteen minutes as needed.

## Parenteral Dosage Forms

### HAEMOPHILUS B POLYSACCHARIDE VACCINE (FOR INJECTION)

**Usual adult and adolescent dose**
Use is not recommended.

**Usual pediatric dose**
Children up to 18 months of age—Use is not recommended.
Children 18 to 24 months of age (especially if they are in known high risk groups) and
Children 24 months to 5 years of age (i.e., up to the 5th birthday)—Intramuscular or subcutaneous, 0.5 mL, into the outer aspect of the upper arm (deltoid) or into the lateral mid thigh (vastus lateralis).

Note: Since satisfactory response to the polysaccharide vaccine is not consistent among children 18 to 24 months of age, most authorities believe that these children should be reimmunized. The optimal timing of this second dose is not known; however, it appears that reimmunization of these children should occur at or after 24 months of age with 2 to 18 months having elapsed between the first immunization and the second one. Previous immunization does not affect the immune response or adverse reaction to a subsequent dose of the vaccine.

**Strength(s) usually available**
U.S.—
Not commercially available.
Canada—
Not commercially available.

**Packaging and storage**
Store lyophilized and reconstituted polysaccharide vaccine and diluent between 2 to 8 °C (35 to 46 °F), unless otherwise specified by manufacturer. Do not freeze.

**Preparation of dosage form**
The appropriate measured amount of the sterile diluent supplied by the manufacturer should be injected into the vial of lyophilized polysaccharide vaccine and then the vial should be gently shaken to dissolve the contents; the lyophilized vaccine dissolves rapidly. The reconstituted solution is clear and colorless.

**Stability**
The reconstituted polysaccharide vaccine should be administered as soon as possible; discard unused reconstituted vaccine after 8 hours.
The date and time of reconstitution should be recorded on the label of the vaccine vial.

## Selected Bibliography

Centers for Disease Control and Prevention. ACIP: Polysaccharide vaccine for prevention of haemophilus influenzae type b disease. MMWR 1985 Apr 19: 201-5.
Preblud, et al. Progress in haemophilus type b polysaccharide vaccine use in the United States. Pediatrics 1988 Jan; 81(1): 166-8.
Centers for Disease Control and Prevention. ACIP Update: Prevention of haemophilus influenzae type b disease. MMWR 1986 Mar 21: 170-80.

Revised: 06/21/93
Interim revision: 03/29/94

---

**HALAZEPAM**—See *Benzodiazepines (Systemic)*

---

**HALCINONIDE**—See *Corticosteroids (Topical)*

---

**HALOBETASOL**—See *Corticosteroids (Topical)*

---

# HALOFANTRINE   Systemic*†

VA CLASSIFICATION (Primary): AP101
Commonly used brand name(s): *Halfan*.

Note: For a listing of dosage forms and brand names by country availability, see *Dosage Forms* section(s).

*Not commercially available in the U.S.
†Not commercially available in Canada.

## Category
Antimalarial.

## Indications

Note: Because halofantrine is not commercially available in the U.S or Canada, the bracketed information and the use of the superscript 1 in this monograph reflect the lack of labeled (approved) indications for this medication.

## Accepted

[Malaria (treatment)][1]—Halofantrine is indicated as alternative treatment for acute malaria (single or mixed infections) caused by chloroquine-resistant or multi-drug resistant strains of *Plasmodium falciparum* or *P. vivax*. Limited data indicate favorable results with the use of halofantrine in the treatment of malaria caused by *Plasmodium ovale* and *Plasmodium malariae*. Halofantrine does not exert any effect on the exoerythrocytic (intrahepatic) stage of *Plasmodium ovale* or *Plasmodium vivax* infection; therefore, subsequent treatment with an 8-aminoquinoline derivative such as primaquine is recommended to eliminate the hepatic forms and thus effect a cure.

## Unaccepted

Halofantrine is not recommended for use as a causal or suppressive prophylactic medication against malaria. Indiscriminate use of halofantrine should be avoided to prevent or minimize the emergence of resistance to the drug by some strains of *Plasmodium falciparum*. A recent study on the large scale use of halofantrine in the Congo confirmed the existence of a high frequency and degree of resistance of *Plasmodium falciparum* to halofantrine. Use of halofantrine should be restricted to those individuals with suspected chloroquine, or multi-drug resistant malaria.

[1]Not included in Canadian product labeling.

## Pharmacology/Pharmacokinetics

### Physicochemical characteristics
Molecular weight—536.89.

### Mechanism of action/Effect
Blood schizontocidal; halofantrine acts on the erythrocytic stage of the life cycle (trophozoites and schizonts) of the parasite.

Although the mechanism of action is still uncertain, it is believed that halofantrine forms complexes with ferriprotoporphyrin IX, which is formed during digestion of hemoglobin by plasmodia. The resulting toxic complex damages cell membranes, thereby causing lysis and death of the schizont.

Halofantrine also may act by inhibiting the proton pump, which is believed to be present at the host-parasite interface in the intraerythrocytic stage of the parasite's life cycle. Halofantrine is not effective against exoerythrocytic or hepatic schizonts and hypnozoites, or against the sporozoites, merozoites, or gametocytic stages of the life cycle of the *Plasmodium* species studied.

### Absorption
Following oral administration—Slow with wide intra- and intersubject variability, which may be attributed to poor drug solubility in water (<0.01%), notably at high pH; food enhances the rate and extent of absorption, especially food with high fat content, which increases absorption approximately 6-fold.

### Distribution
Large volume of distribution both in healthy volunteers and in patients with malaria; animal studies have shown that halofantrine is widely distributed in the tissues, with drug-related material persisting for at least 72 hours.

### Biotransformation
Metabolized primarily to N-desbutyl halofantrine, the desbutyl derivative of halofantrine; animal studies have shown that at peak concentrations, N-desbutyl halofantrine may represent 20 to 30% of all halofantrine-related material.

### Half-life
Highly variable for both halofantrine and its principal metabolite, N-desbutyl halofantrine.
Mean half-life in healthy volunteers—
  Halofantrine: Approximately 1 to 2 days.
  N-desbutyl halofantrine: Approximately 3 to 5 days.
Mean half-life in patients with malaria—
  Halofantrine: Approximately 4 to 5 days.
  N-desbutyl halofantrine: Approximately 4 to 5 days.

### Time to peak concentration
Oral doses of 250 to 2000 mg:
  Halofantrine: Approximately 6 hours.
  N-desbutyl halofantrine: Approximately 10 to 18 hours (range 6 to 32 hours).

### Peak serum concentration
Variable.
  Following three 500-mg oral doses—
    Halofantrine: Averages 1134 nanograms per mL.
    N-desbutyl halofantrine: Averages about one-half the concentration of halofantrine.

### Elimination
Eliminated mainly in the feces as unchanged drug.

## Precautions to Consider

### Mutagenicity
Halofantrine has not been shown to be mutagenic either in animals or in *in vitro* tests utilizing the following assay techniques: Ames test, HGPRT gene mutation assay, CHO chromosome aberration test, mouse micronucleus test, and dominant lethal assays in rats. There were no adverse effects observed at the proposed clinical doses in the animal tests.

### Pregnancy/Reproduction
Fertility—Studies in male rats given halofantrine hydrochloride at doses of 15 to 30 mg per kg of body weight (mg/kg) per day for 16 weeks have not shown that halofantrine causes adverse effects on fertility.

Pregnancy—Adequate and well-controlled studies in humans have not been done. Halofantrine is not recommended for use in pregnancy since it has been found to be embryotoxic in animals.

Studies in animals have shown that halofantrine is not teratogenic at doses below 45 mg/kg of body weight per day (halofantrine base) in rats and 120 mg/kg per day (halofantrine base) in rabbits. However, halofantrine base was found to be embryotoxic at doses of 30 mg/kg per day in rats and 60 mg/kg per day in rabbits. In addition to the increased frequency of post-implantation embryonic death, reduced fetal body weight was observed at doses in excess of 15 mg/kg given for 5 days.

### Breast-feeding
Halofantrine may be distributed into breast milk. Animal studies have shown that halofantrine is distributed into milk in quantities sufficient to cause a reduced rate of weight gain, growth, and survival of the nursing offspring. In rats, these dose-related decreases were observed in pups exposed to the milk of dams receiving halofantrine at a dose of 50 mg/kg per day. However, no adverse effect was seen at a dose of 25 mg/kg per day.

### Pediatrics
Appropriate studies on the relationship of age to the effects of halofantrine have not been performed in the pediatric population. However, no pediatrics-specific problems have been documented to date.

### Geriatrics
Appropriate studies on the relationship of age to the effects of halofantrine have not been performed in the geriatric population. However, no geriatrics-specific problems have been documented to date.

### Drug interactions and/or related problems
The following drug interactions and/or related problems have been selected on the basis of their potential clinical significance (possible mechanism in parentheses where appropriate)—not necessarily inclusive (» = major clinical significance):

Note: Combinations containing any of the following medications, depending on the amount present, may also interact with this medication.

» Mefloquine
  (recent or concomitant treatment with mefloquine further prolongs the QT interval and may potentiate the risk of adverse cardiac effects)

### Laboratory value alterations
The following have been selected on the basis of their potential clinical significance (possible effect in parentheses where appropriate)—not necessarily inclusive (» = major clinical significance):

With physiology/laboratory test values
  Alanine aminotransferase (ALT [SGPT]), serum, and
  Aspartate aminotransferase (AST [SGOT]), serum
    (values may be transiently increased; however, their relation to medication is not clear since such enzymic changes are also commonly seen in acute malaria; values return to normal usually within 1 week after treatment)

  Electrocardiogram (ECG) changes, such as prolongation of QT interval (occur at both the recommended therapeutic and higher doses)

### Medical considerations/Contraindications
The medical considerations/contraindications included have been selected on the basis of their potential clinical significance (reasons given in parentheses where appropriate)—not necessarily inclusive (» = major clinical significance).

*Except under special circumstances, this medication should not be used when the following medical problem exists:*

» Known congenital QT prolongation, or family history of
  (risk of arrhythmia)

*Risk-benefit should be considered when the following medical problems exist:*

» Atrioventricular (AV) conduction disorders or
» Syncope, unexplained, or
» Thiamine deficiency or
» Ventricular dysrhythmias
    (these conditions prolong the QT interval which may cause an increased risk of arrhythmia)
   Cerebral malaria and other complicated malarial conditions
    (caution is required since there is no experience with the use of halofantrine in these conditions)
   Hypersensitivity to halofantrine

**Patient monitoring**

The following may be especially important in patient monitoring (other tests may be warranted in some patients, depending on condition; » = major clinical significance):

   Electrocardiogram (ECG)
    (may be advisable to check arrhythmia)

## Side/Adverse Effects

Note: Side/adverse effects of halofantrine may be difficult to distinguish from the symptoms of acute malarial infection, since most of these side effects also occur in clinical malaria.

The following side/adverse effects have been selected on the basis of their potential clinical significance (possible signs and symptoms in parentheses where appropriate)—not necessarily inclusive:

**Those indicating need for medical attention**
Incidence rare
   *Acute intravascular hemolysis* (anxiety; chest or lower back pain; fast heartbeat; flushing; nausea; rapid breathing; restlessness; scanty and black urine); *cardiovascular toxicity, specifically prolonged QT interval* (fast and irregular heartbeat)

**Those indicating need for medical attention only if they continue or are bothersome**
Incidence less frequent
   *Gastrointestinal disturbances* (abdominal pain, diarrhea, nausea, and vomiting); *hypersensitivity* (skin itching or rash)

## Overdose

For more information on the management of overdose or unintentional ingestion, **contact a Poison Control Center** (See *Poison Control Center Listing*).

**Treatment of overdose**
Recommended treatment consists of the following:
   To decrease absorption—
     Immediate induction of emesis and/or gastric lavage may be performed.
   Specific treatment—
     Symptomatic treatment may be given.
   Monitoring—
     ECG monitoring should be done.
   Supportive care—
     Supportive measures such as maintaining an open airway, respiration, and circulation may be administered. Patients in whom intentional overdose is known or suspected should be referred for psychiatric consultation.

## Patient Consultation

As an aid to patient consultation, refer to *Advice for the Patient, Halofantrine (Systemic)*.
In providing consultation, consider emphasizing the following selected information (» = major clinical significance):

**Before using this medication**
» Conditions affecting use, especially:
   Hypersensitivity to halofantrine
   Pregnancy—Not recommended for use in pregnancy because of its embryotoxic effects in animals
   Breast-feeding—May be distributed into breast milk, resulting in reduced rate of weight gain, growth, and survival of nursing offspring as shown in animals; breast-feeding is not recommended while the patient is taking halofantrine
   Other medications, especially mefloquine
   Other medical problems, especially, atrioventricular conduction disorders, prolonged QT interval, thiamine deficiency, unexplained syncope, or ventricular dysrhythmias

**Proper use of this medication**
» Taking on an empty stomach due to cardiotoxicity
» Compliance with full course of therapy
» Repeating treatment after 1 week
» Proper dosing
   Missed dose: Taking as soon as possible; not taking if almost time for next dose; not doubling doses
» Proper storage

**Precautions while using this medication**
   Regular visits to physician to check progress
   Checking with physician if symptoms persist or if no improvement occurs after the full course of treatment
*Self-protection measures against mosquitoes to help prevent infection or reinfection:*
   Avoiding exposure to mosquitoes, especially at peak feeding times (between dusk and dawn)
   Wearing suitable clothing (long-sleeved shirt and long trousers) to protect arms and legs when mosquitoes are out
   Applying insect repellant (containing diethylmetatoluamide [DEET]) sparingly to exposed skin
   Sleeping in screened or air-conditioned room
   Using bed netting impregnated with repellant or permethrin
   Using mosquito coils or sprays

**Side/adverse effects**
   Signs of potential side effects, especially acute intravascular hemolysis and cardiovascular toxicity

## General Dosing Information

Halofantrine has been shown to prolong QT interval at the recommended therapeutic dose. Higher than recommended doses or recent or concomitant treatment with mefloquine further prolongs the QT interval.

Because of the variability of absorption of halofantrine within individuals, oral halofantrine should be given in three doses over a 12-hour period every six hours to ensure adequate blood concentration. Due to its cardiotoxic effects, it is recommended that halofantrine be taken on an empty stomach, because food enhances its absorption.

Since halofantrine does not exert any effect on the exoerythrocytic or intrahepatic stage of *Plasmodium ovale* or *P. vivax*, subsequent treatment with an 8-aminoquinoline derivative such as primaquine is recommended to eliminate the hepatic forms of these parasites.

A second course of treatment with halofantrine is recommended one week after the first course to prevent recrudescence.

## Oral Dosage Forms

Note: Bracketed uses in the *Dosage Forms* section refer to categories of use and/or indications that are not included in U.S. product labeling.

### HALOFANTRINE HYDROCHLORIDE ORAL SUSPENSION

**Usual adult and adolescent dose**
[Malaria][1]—
   Oral, 500 mg taken on an empty stomach every six hours three times a day for one day. Treatment should be repeated after one week.

**Usual pediatric dose**
[Malaria)][1]—
   Children weighing less than 40 kg: Oral, 8 mg per kg of body weight taken on an empty stomach every six hours three times a day for one day. Treatment should be repeated after one week. The following doses also have been given—
   Children 1 to 2 years of age (10 to 12 kg of body weight): Oral, 100 mg taken on an empty stomach every six hours three times a day for one day. Treatment should be repeated after one week.
   Children 2 to 5 years of age (13 to 18 kg of body weight): Oral, 150 mg taken on an empty stomach every six hours three times a day for one day. Treatment should be repeated after one week.
   Children 5 to 8 years of age (19 to 25 kg of body weight): Oral, 200 mg taken on an empty stomach every six hours three times a day for one day. Treatment should be repeated after one week.
   Children 8 to 10 years of age (26 to 31 kg of body weight): Oral, 250 mg taken on an empty stomach every six hours three times a day for one day. Treatment should be repeated after one week.
   Children 10 to 12 years of age (32 to 40 kg of body weight): Oral, 300 mg taken on an empty stomach every six hours three times a day for one day. Treatment should be repeated after one week.
   Children 12 years of age and over (over 40 kg of body weight): See *Usual adult and adolescent dose*.

**Strength(s) usually available**
U.S.—
   Not commercially available.

Canada—
   Not commercially available.
Other (United Kingdom)—
   100 mg (93 mg base) per 5 mL (Rx) [*Halfan*].

**Packaging and storage**
Store below 40 °C (104 °F), preferably between 15 and 30 °C (59 and 86 °F), in a well-closed light-resistant container, unless otherwise specified by manufacturer. Protect from freezing.

**Auxiliary labeling**
• Shake well.

### HALOFANTRINE HYDROCHLORIDE TABLETS

**Usual adult and adolescent dose**
See *Halofantrine Hydrochoride Oral Suspension*.

**Usual pediatric dose**
[Malaria][1]—
   Children weighing less than 40 kg: Oral, 8 mg per kg of body weight taken on an empty stomach every six hours three times a day for one day. Treatment should be repeated after one week. The following doses also have been given
   Children up to 23 kg of body weight: Dosage has not been established.
   Children 23 to 31 kg of body weight: Oral, 250 mg taken on an empty stomach every six hours three times a day for one day. Treatment should be repeated after one week.
   Children 32 to 37 kg of body weight: Oral, 375 mg taken on an empty stomach every six hours three times a day for one day. Treatment should be repeated after one week.
   Children 37 kg of body weight and over: See *Usual adult and adolescent dose*.

**Strength(s) usually available**
U.S.—
   Not commercially available.
Canada—
   Not commercially available.
Other (United Kingdom)—
   250 mg (233 mg base) (Rx) [*Halfan*].

**Packaging and storage**
Store below 40 °C (104 °F), preferably between 15 and 30 °C (59 and 86 °F), in a well-closed container. Protect from light.

[1]Not included in Canadian product labeling.

### Selected Bibliography
Bryson HM, Goa KL. Halofantrine: a review of its antimalarial activity, pharmacokinetic properties and therapeutic potential. Drugs 1992; 43(2): 236-58.
Weinke T, Loscher T, Fleischer K, Kretschmer H, Pohle HD, Kohler B, et al. The efficacy of halofantrine in the treatment of acute malaria in nonimmune travelers. Am J Trop Med Hyg 1992; 47(1): 1-5.
Shanks GD, Watt G, Edstein MD, Webster HK, Suriyamongkol V, Watanasook C, et al. Halofantrine for the treatment of mefloquine chemoprophylaxis failures in Plasmodium falciparum infections. Am J Trop Med Hyg 1991; 45(4): 488-91.

Revised: 8/27/93

# HALOPERIDOL Systemic

VA CLASSIFICATION (Primary/Secondary): CN709/CN900; GA605
Commonly used brand name(s): *Apo-Haloperidol; Haldol; Haldol Decanoate; Haldol LA; Novo-Peridol; PMS Haloperidol; Peridol*.

Note: For a listing of dosage forms and brand names by country availability, see *Dosage Forms* section(s).

### Category
Antipsychotic; antidyskinetic (Gilles de la Tourette's syndrome; Huntington's chorea); antiemetic.

### Indications
Note: Bracketed information in the *Indications* section refers to uses that are not included in U.S. product labeling.

**Accepted**
Psychotic disorders (treatment)—Haloperidol is indicated for the management of the manifestations of acute and chronic psychotic disorders including schizophrenia, manic states, and drug-induced psychoses, such as steroid psychosis. It may also be useful in the management of aggressive and agitated patients, including patients with organic mental syndrome or mental retardation. Haloperidol decanoate, a long-acting parenteral form, is intended for maintenance use in the management of patients requiring prolonged parenteral therapy, as in chronic schizophrenia.

Behavior problems, severe (treatment)—Haloperidol is effective in the treatment of children with severe behavior problems of apparently unprovoked, combative, explosive hyperexcitability. It is also effective in the *short-term* treatment of hyperactivity in children who show excessive motor activity with accompanying conduct disorders such as aggressiveness, impulsiveness, easy frustration, short attention span, and/or rapid mood fluctuations. In these two groups of children, haloperidol should be tried only in patients who fail to respond to psychotherapy or other non-neuroleptic medication.

Gilles de la Tourette's syndrome (treatment)—Haloperidol is used to control tics and vocalizations of Tourette's syndrome in children and adults.

[Autism, infantile (treatment)][1]—Haloperidol has been used to reduce abnormal behaviors, such as withdrawal, stereotypy, abnormal object relationships, fidgetiness, hyperactivity, negativism, angry affect, and labile affect, and may improve learning, in some patients with autism.

[Chorea, Huntington's (treatment)][1]—Because of its strong extrapyramidal effects, haloperidol is used to reduce disabling choreiform movements in Huntington's disease.

[Nausea and vomiting, cancer chemotherapy–induced (prophylaxis and treatment)][1]—Haloperidol is used as a second-line agent to control nausea and vomiting associated with antineoplastic therapy and surgery.

[1]Not included in Canadian product labeling.

### Pharmacology/Pharmacokinetics

Note: Pharmacological effects of haloperidol are similar to the effects of piperazine-derivative phenothiazines, which include acetophenazine, fluphenazine, perphenazine, prochlorperazine, and trifluoperazine.

**Physicochemical characteristics**
Chemical group—A butyrophenone derivative.
Molecular weight—
   Haloperidol: 375.87.
   Haloperidol decanoate: 530.12.
Other characteristics—
   Haloperidol oral solution: pH 2.75–3.75.
   Haloperidol injection: pH 3.0–3.8.

**Mechanism of action/Effect**
Although the complex mechanism of the therapeutic effect is not clearly established, haloperidol is known to produce a selective effect on the central nervous system (CNS) by competitive blockade of postsynaptic dopamine ($D_2$) receptors in the mesolimbic dopaminergic system and an increased turnover of brain dopamine to produce its tranquilizing effects. With subchronic therapy, depolarization blockade, or diminished firing rate of the dopamine neuron (decreased release) along with $D_2$ postsynaptic blockade results in the antipsychotic action.
The long-acting decanoate form acts as a pro-drug, slowly and steadily releasing haloperidol from the vehicle.

**Other actions/effects**
Blockade of dopamine receptors in the nigrostriatal dopamine pathway produces extrapyramidal motor reactions; blockade of dopamine receptors in the tuberoinfundibular system decreases growth hormone release and increases prolactin release by the pituitary. There is also some blockade of alpha-adrenergic receptors of the autonomic system.

**Absorption**
Oral—60%.

**Distribution**
The volume of distribution of haloperidol at steady state ($Vd_{SS}$) is 18 L per kg.

**Protein binding**
Very high (92%).

**Biotransformation**
Hepatic; extensive.

### Half-life
Haloperidol, Elimination—
Oral: 24 hours (range, 12 to 37 hours).
Intramuscular: 21 hours (range, 17 to 25 hours).
Intravenous: 14 hours (range, 10 to 19 hours).
Haloperidol decanoate, Elimination—
Approximately 3 weeks (single or multiple doses).

### Time to peak plasma concentration
Oral—3 to 6 hours.
Intramuscular—10 to 20 minutes.
Long-acting intramuscular—3 to 9 days, although variable. May occur on first day in some patients, notably the elderly.

### Therapeutic plasma concentration
4 to 20 nanograms per mL (0.01 to 0.05 micromoles per L).

### Elimination
Renal—
   About 40% of a single oral dose is excreted in the urine within 5 days, 1% of which is unchanged drug. A mean clearance value of 12 mL per kg per minute has been reported.
Biliary—
   15% of an oral dose is excreted in the feces by biliary elimination.

## Precautions to Consider

### Carcinogenicity/Tumorigenicity
Neuroleptic drugs (including haloperidol) elevate prolactin concentrations; the elevation persists during chronic administration. Tissue culture experiments indicate that approximately one third of human breast cancers are prolactin dependent *in vitro*, a factor of potential importance if the prescription of these drugs is contemplated in a patient with a previously detected breast cancer. Although disturbances such as galactorrhea, amenorrhea, gynecomastia, and impotence have been reported, the clinical significance of elevated serum prolactin concentrations is unknown for most patients. An increase in mammary neoplasms has been found in rodents after chronic administration of neuroleptic drugs. However, neither clinical studies nor epidemiologic studies conducted to date have shown an association between chronic administration of these drugs and mammary tumorigenesis; the available evidence is considered too limited to be conclusive at this time.

### Mutagenicity
Haloperidol decanoate—No mutagenic potential was found in the Ames *Salmonella* microsomal activation assay.

### Pregnancy/Reproduction
Fertility—Animal reproduction studies have shown decreased fertility with doses 2 to 20 times the usual maximum human dose of haloperidol.
Pregnancy—
   *For haloperidol*—
      Adequate studies in humans have not been done. However, there have been some reports of limb malformations with maternal use of haloperidol along with other drugs of suspected teratogenicity during the first trimester.
      Some rodent studies have shown an increase in incidence of fetal resorption, delayed delivery, and neonatal death with doses 2 to 20 times the usual maximum human dose of haloperidol. Cleft palate has been observed in a study with mice given 15 times the human dose of haloperidol.
   *For haloperidol decanoate*—
      Adequate studies in humans have not been done.
      Studies in rats given up to three times the usual maximum human dose showed an increase in incidence of fetal resorption, fetal mortality, and neonatal mortality.
   FDA Pregnancy Category C.

### Breast-feeding
Haloperidol is distributed into breast milk. Animal studies have shown that haloperidol is distributed into milk in quantities sufficient to cause sedation and motor function impairment in the nursing offspring. Breast-feeding during haloperidol therapy is not recommended.

### Pediatrics
Haloperidol is not recommended for use in children up to 3 years of age. Children are highly susceptible to the extrapyramidal side effects, especially dystonias, of haloperidol.

### Geriatrics
Geriatric patients tend to develop higher plasma concentrations of haloperidol because of changes in distribution due to decreases in lean body mass, total body water, and albumin, and often an increase in total body fat composition. These patients usually require lower initial dosage and a more gradual titration of dose.

Elderly patients appear to be more prone to orthostatic hypotension and exhibit an increased sensitivity to the anticholinergic and sedative effects of haloperidol. In addition, they are more prone to develop extrapyramidal side effects, such as tardive dyskinesia and parkinsonism. The symptoms of tardive dyskinesia are persistent, difficult to control, and, in some patients, appear to be irreversible. The symptoms may be masked during long-term treatment, but may appear if haloperidol is discontinued. There is no known effective treatment. Careful observation during haloperidol therapy for early signs of tardive dyskinesia and reduction of dosage or discontinuation of medication may prevent a more severe manifestation of the syndrome.

It has been suggested that elderly patients receive half the usual adult dose. Patients with organic mental syndrome or acute confusional states should initially receive one-third to one-half the usual adult dose, with the dose being increased no more frequently than every 2 or 3 days, and preferably at intervals of 7 to 10 days. A periodic attempt should be made to discontinue medication as soon as the patient improves.

### Dental
The peripheral anticholinergic effects of haloperidol may decrease or inhibit salivary flow, especially in middle-aged or elderly patients, thus contributing to the development of caries, periodontal disease, oral candidiasis, and discomfort.

Extrapyramidal reactions induced by haloperidol will result in increased motor activity of the head, face, and neck. Occlusal adjustments, bite registrations, and treatment for bruxism may be made less reliable.

The leukopenic and thrombocytopenic effects of haloperidol may result in an increased incidence of microbial infection, delayed healing, and gingival bleeding. If leukopenia or thrombocytopenia occurs, dental work should be deferred until blood counts have returned to normal. Patients should be instructed in proper oral hygiene, including caution in use of regular toothbrushes, dental floss, and toothpicks.

### Drug interactions and/or related problems
The following drug interactions and/or related problems have been selected on the basis of their potential clinical significance (possible mechanism in parentheses where appropriate)—not necessarily inclusive (» = major clinical significance):

Note: Combinations containing any of the following medications, depending on the amount present, may also interact with this medication.

» Alcohol or
» CNS depression–producing medications, other (see *Appendix II*)
   (concurrent use with haloperidol may result in increased CNS and respiratory depression and increased hypotensive effects)
   (concurrent use with haloperidol may potentiate alcohol intoxication)

Amphetamines
   (concurrent use may decrease stimulant effects of amphetamines due to alpha-adrenergic blockade by haloperidol; also, the antipsychotic effects of haloperidol may be reduced when amphetamines and haloperidol are used concurrently)

Anticholinergics or other medications with anticholinergic activity (see *Appendix II*) or
Antidyskinetic agents or
Antihistamines
   (concurrent use with haloperidol may intensify anticholinergic side effects, especially those of confusion, hallucinations, nightmares, and increased intraocular pressure, because of secondary anticholinergic effects of haloperidol; also, patients should be advised to report occurrence of gastrointestinal problems since paralytic ileus may occur with concurrent therapy; in addition, antipsychotic effectiveness of haloperidol may be decreased because of reduced gastrointestinal absorption; dosage adjustments may be necessary)

Anticoagulants, coumarin- or indandione-derivative
   (concurrent use with haloperidol may either increase or decrease anticoagulant activity; although the clinical significance has not been determined, caution is recommended )

Anticonvulsants, including barbiturates
   (concurrent use with haloperidol may cause a change in the pattern and/or frequency of epileptiform seizures; dosage adjustments of anticonvulsants may be necessary; serum concentrations of haloperidol may be significantly reduced)

Antidepressants, tricyclic or
Maprotiline or
Monoamine oxidase (MAO) inhibitors, including furazolidone, procarbazine, or selegiline or

Trazodone
(concurrent use with haloperidol may prolong and intensify the sedative and anticholinergic effects of either these medications or haloperidol)

Bromocriptine
(concurrent use with haloperidol may increase serum prolactin concentrations and interfere with effects of bromocriptine; dosage adjustment of bromocriptine may be necessary)

Bupropion
(concurrent use of bupropion with haloperidol may lower the seizure threshold and increase the risk of major motor seizures)

Diazoxide
(concurrent use antagonizes the inhibition of insulin release by diazoxide)

Dopamine
(concurrent use may antagonize peripheral vasoconstriction produced by high doses of dopamine because of the alpha-adrenergic blocking action of haloperidol)

Ephedrine
(concurrent use may decrease the pressor response to ephedrine)

» Epinephrine
(concurrent use may block the alpha-adrenergic effects of epinephrine, possibly resulting in severe hypotension and tachycardia)

» Extrapyramidal reaction–causing medications, other (see *Appendix II*)
(concurrent use with haloperidol may increase the severity and frequency of extrapyramidal effects)

Fluoxetine
(caution in concurrent use of fluoxetine with haloperidol is recommended because of a potentially increased risk of CNS side effects, particularly extrapyramidal reactions)

Guanadrel or
Guanethidine
(concurrent use with haloperidol may decrease the hypotensive effects of these agents because of displacement from and inhibition of uptake into alpha-adrenergic neurons)

» Levodopa or
Pergolide
(concurrent use may decrease the therapeutic effects of these agents because of blockade of dopamine receptors by haloperidol)

» Lithium
(lithium is frequently used concurrently with haloperidol during the first week or two of treatment for acute manic episodes; lithium alone may be adequate thereafter, although some patients may continue to need both; however, concurrent use with haloperidol has been associated with irreversible neurological toxicity and brain damage, especially in patients with organic mental syndrome or other CNS impairment, although this interaction has been reported only with high doses; extrapyramidal symptoms may be increased by haloperidol's enhancement of dopamine blockade; patients should be monitored closely during concurrent use; dosage adjustments or discontinuation of treatment may be necessary)

(admixture of the liquid forms of lithium and haloperidol may result in precipitation of free haloperidol)

Metaraminol
(concurrent use with haloperidol usually decreases, but does not reverse or completely block, the pressor response to metaraminol, because of the alpha-adrenergic blocking action of haloperidol)

Methoxamine
(prior administration of haloperidol may decrease the pressor effect and duration of action of methoxamine because of the alpha-adrenergic blocking action of haloperidol)

Methyldopa
(concurrent use with haloperidol may cause unwanted mental effects such as disorientation and slowed or difficult thought processes)

Phenylephrine
(prior administration of haloperidol may decrease the pressor response to phenylephrine because of the alpha-adrenergic blocking action of haloperidol)

**Laboratory value alterations**
The following have been selected on the basis of their potential clinical significance (possible effect in parentheses where appropriate)—not necessarily inclusive (» = major clinical significance):

With diagnostic test results
ECG
(prolongation of the Q-T interval and changes compatible with configuration of *torsades de pointes* may occur)

**Medical considerations/Contraindications**
The medical considerations/contraindications included have been selected on the basis of their potential clinical significance (reasons given in parentheses where appropriate)—not necessarily inclusive (» = major clinical significance).

*Except under special circumstances, this medication should not be used when the following medical problem exists:*

» CNS depression, toxic, drug-induced, severe
(may be potentiated)

*Risk-benefit should be considered when the following medical problems exist:*

Alcoholism, active
(CNS depression may be potentiated; risk of heat stroke may be increased)

» Cardiovascular disease, severe, especially angina
(transient hypotension and anginal pain may be provoked)

» Epilepsy
(seizure threshold may be lowered)

Glaucoma or predisposition to
(may be potentiated because of secondary anticholinergic effects of haloperidol)

Hepatic function impairment
(metabolism may be altered)

Hyperthyroidism or thyrotoxicosis
(severe neurotoxicity such as rigidity and inability to walk or talk may result)

» Parkinson's disease
(may be potentiated)

Pulmonary insufficiency, such as asthma, emphysema, or acute pulmonary infections
(potentiation of breathing impairment may possibly lead to "silent pneumonias")

Renal function impairment
(excretion may be altered; more applicable to higher dosage since renal clearance of unchanged drug is relatively low)

» Sensitivity to haloperidol
(patients with known allergies or with a history of allergic reactions to other medications may also be sensitive to haloperidol)

» Urinary retention
(may be potentiated)

**Patient monitoring**
The following may be especially important in patient monitoring (other tests may be warranted in some patients, depending on condition; » = major clinical significance):

Blood cell counts and differential in patients with sore throat and fever or infections
(may be required during high-dose or prolonged therapy when symptoms of infection develop; if significant cellular depression occurs, medication should be discontinued and appropriate therapy initiated; rechallenge in recovered patients will usually cause a recurrence of agranulocytosis)

Careful observation for early signs of dehydration, such as lethargy and decreased sensation of thirst
(recommended at periodic intervals, especially in elderly or debilitated persons, for prevention of bronchopneumonia)

Careful observation for early symptoms of tardive dyskinesia
(recommended at periodic intervals, especially in the elderly and patients on high or extended maintenance dosage; since there is no known effective treatment if syndrome should develop, haloperidol should be discontinued, if clinically feasible, at earliest signs, usually fine, worm-like movements of the tongue, to stop further development)

Careful observation for early symptoms of tardive dystonia
(recommended at periodic intervals; since there is no known effective treatment if syndrome should develop, haloperidol should be discontinued, if clinically feasible, at the earliest signs)

Careful observation for signs of overdose or insufficient dosing with haloperidol decanoate
(recommended during initial dosing adjustments; since haloperidol decanoate slowly increases to steady state plasma concentration over 2 to 4 months, accumulation to excessive levels may occur; if psychotic symptoms reappear before next dose, therapy can be supplemented with short-acting forms of haloperidol)

Hepatic function determinations
(may be required at periodic intervals during high-dose or prolonged therapy or if jaundice or grippe-like symptoms occur, to detect liver function impairment)

## Side/Adverse Effects

Note: A few cases of sudden and unexpected death have been reported in patients who were receiving haloperidol therapy. However, there is no definite evidence that haloperidol is a causative factor.

Children are highly susceptible to extrapyramidal effects.

Geriatric and debilitated patients are more prone to develop extrapyramidal side effects and orthostatic hypotension and usually require a lower initial dosage and a more gradual titration of dose.

The following side/adverse effects have been selected on the basis of their potential clinical significance (possible signs and symptoms in parentheses where appropriate)—not necessarily inclusive:

### Those indicating need for medical attention
Incidence more frequent
*Akathisia* (restlessness or need to keep moving); *dystonic extrapyramidal effects* (muscle spasms of face, neck, and back; tic-like or twitching movements; twisting movements of body; inability to move eyes; weakness of arms and legs); *parkinsonian extrapyramidal effects* (difficulty in speaking or swallowing; loss of balance control; mask-like face; shuffling walk; stiffness of arms or legs; trembling and shaking of hands and fingers)

Note: *Akathisia* may appear within first 6 hours after dose; often indistinguishable from psychotic agitation; differentiation with benztropine may improve haloperidol-induced akathisia but not psychotic agitation.

*Dystonic extrapyramidal effects* appear most often in children and young adults and early in treatment; may subside within 24 to 48 hours after drug has been discontinued.

*Parkinsonian extrapyramidal effects* are more frequent in the elderly; symptoms may be seen in the first few days of treatment or after prolonged treatment, and can recur after even a single dose.

Incidence less frequent
*Allergic reaction* (red and raised, or acne-like skin rash); *anticholinergic effects* (difficult urination; hallucinations); *CNS effect* (hallucinations); *decreased thirst, or unusual tiredness or weakness; orthostatic hypotension* (dizziness, lightheadedness, or fainting); *persistent tardive dyskinesia* (lip smacking or puckering; puffing of cheeks; rapid or worm-like movements of tongue; uncontrolled chewing movements; uncontrolled movements of the arms and legs)

Note: *Decreased thirst* or *unusual tiredness or weakness* may precede dehydration, hemoconcentration, reduced pulmonary ventilation, and bronchopneumonia; occur most often in elderly or debilitated patients.

*Tardive dyskinesia* is more frequent in elderly patients, women, and patients with brain damage; initially dose related, but may increase with long-term treatment and total cumulative dose; may persist after discontinuation of haloperidol.

Incidence rare
*Agranulocytosis* (sore throat and fever; unusual bleeding or bruising); *heat stroke* (hot, dry skin; inability to sweat; muscle weakness; confusion); *obstructive jaundice* (yellow eyes or skin); *neuroleptic malignant syndrome (NMS)* (difficult or unusually fast breathing; fast heartbeat or irregular pulse; high fever; high or low [irregular] blood pressure; increased sweating; loss of bladder control; severe muscle stiffness; seizures; unusual tiredness or weakness; unusually pale skin); *tardive dystonia* (increased blinking or spasms of eyelid; unusual facial expressions or body positions; uncontrolled twisting movements of neck, trunk, arms, or legs)

Note: *Heat stroke,* caused by haloperidol-induced suppression of central and peripheral temperature regulation in the hypothalamus, may occur during environmental conditions of high heat and high humidity. The effectiveness of sweating as a cooling mechanism may be reduced by humid conditions and by the anticholinergic effects of haloperidol, used alone or in combination with other anticholinergic medications such as nonprescription cold medications or antihistamines. Adequate interior temperature control (air conditioning) must be maintained for institutionalized patients during hot weather because of the increased risk of heat stroke and NMS. Patients should be advised to avoid exertion, stay in cool areas, and avoid dehydration and other anticholinergic medications.

*NMS* may occur at any time during neuroleptic therapy, but is more commonly seen soon after start of therapy, or after patient has switched from one neuroleptic to another, during combined therapy with another psychotropic medication, or after a dosage increase. Along with the overt signs of skeletal muscle rigidity, hyperthermia, autonomic dysfunction, and altered consciousness, differential diagnosis may reveal leukocytosis (9500 to 26,000 cells per cubic millimeter), elevated liver function test values, and elevated creatine kinase (CK).

### Those indicating need for medical attention only if they continue or are bothersome
Incidence more frequent
*Blurred vision; changes in menstrual period; constipation; dryness of mouth; swelling or soreness in breasts in females; unusual secretion of milk; weight gain*

Incidence less frequent
*Decreased sexual ability; drowsiness; increased sensitivity of skin to sun; nausea or vomiting*

### Those indicating the need for medical attention if they occur after the medication is discontinued
*Withdrawal emergent dyskinesia* (trembling of fingers and hands; uncontrolled, repetitive movements of mouth, tongue, and jaw)—more frequent in elderly patients, women, and patients with brain damage

## Overdose

For specific information on the agents used in the management of haloperidol overdose, see:
- *Albumin Human (Systemic)* monograph;
- *Benztropine* in *Antidyskinetics (Systemic)* monograph;
- *Charcoal, Activated (Oral-Local)* monograph;
- *Diphenhydramine* in *Antihistamines (Systemic)* monograph; and/or
- *Norepinephrine* in *Sympathomimetic Agents—Cardiovascular Use (Parenteral-Systemic)* monograph.

For more information on the management of overdose or unintentional ingestion, **contact a Poison Control Center** (see *Poison Control Center Listing*).

### Clinical effects of overdose
In general, symptoms of overdose may be an exaggeration of adverse effects. Patient would appear comatose with respiratory depression and hypotension severe enough to produce a shock-like state.

The following effects have been selected on the basis of their potential clinical significance (possible signs and symptoms in parentheses where appropriate)—not necessarily inclusive:

*Severe breathing difficulty; dizziness; severe drowsiness or comatose state; severe muscle trembling, jerking, stiffness, or uncontrolled movements; severe tiredness or weakness*

### Treatment of overdose
Treatment is essentially symptomatic and supportive.
To decrease absorption—
Inducing emesis or initiating gastric lavage, immediately followed by administration of activated charcoal.
Specific treatment—
Counteracting hypotension and circulatory collapse by use of intravenous fluids, plasma, or concentrated albumin, and vasopressor agents such as norepinephrine. Epinephrine should *not* be used since it may cause paradoxical hypotension.
Administering benztropine or diphenhydramine to manage severe extrapyramidal reactions.
Monitoring—
Monitoring ECG for signs of Q-T prolongation or *torsades de pointes.* Severe arrhythmias should be treated with appropriate antiarrhythmic measures.
Supportive care—
Establishing a patent airway.
Mechanically assisting respiration, if necessary.
Patients in whom intentional overdose is known or suspected should be referred for psychiatric consultation.

Note: Dialysis is not effective in removing excessive systemic haloperidol.

## Patient Consultation

As an aid to patient consultation, refer to *Advice for the Patient, Haloperidol (Systemic)*.

In providing consultation, consider emphasizing the following selected information (» = major clinical significance):

### Before using this medication
» Conditions affecting use, especially:
Sensitivity to haloperidol
Pregnancy—Reports of limb malformations after maternal use of haloperidol with other drugs of suspected teratogenicity during first trimester; animal reproduction studies have shown a de-

crease in fertility, increased incidence of fetal resorption, delayed delivery, and neonatal death with very high doses
Breast-feeding—Distributed into breast milk; animal studies have shown sedation, impaired motor function in nursing offspring; not recommended for use during breast-feeding
Use in children—Children are more prone to extrapyramidal symptoms, especially dystonias
Use in the elderly—Elderly patients are more likely to develop extrapyramidal, anticholinergic, hypotensive, and sedative effects; reduced dosage recommended
Dental—Haloperidol-induced blood dyscrasias may result in infections, delayed healing, and bleeding; dry mouth may cause caries, candidiasis, periodontal disease, and discomfort; increased motor activity of face, head, and neck may interfere with some dental procedures
Other medications, especially alcohol, other CNS depression–producing medications, epinephrine, other extrapyramidal reaction–producing medications, levodopa, or lithium
Other medical problems, especially severe cardiovascular disease, severe CNS depression, Parkinson's disease, allergies, epilepsy, or urinary retention

**Proper use of this medication**
Taking with food or milk to reduce gastrointestinal irritation
Proper administration of oral liquid form:
  Using special dropper
  Mixing with water or a beverage such as orange juice, apple juice, tomato juice, or cola; not mixing with tea or coffee
» Importance of not taking more or less medication than the amount prescribed
» Compliance with therapy; may require several weeks of therapy to obtain desired effects
» Proper dosing
  Missed dose: Taking as soon as possible; taking any remaining doses for that day at regularly spaced intervals; not doubling doses
» Proper storage

**Precautions while using this medication**
Regular visits to physician to check progress of therapy
» Checking with physician before discontinuing medication; gradual dosage reduction may be needed
» Avoiding use of alcoholic beverages or other CNS depressants during therapy
» Possible drowsiness or dizziness; caution when driving, using machinery, or doing things requiring alertness
Possible dizziness or lightheadedness: caution when getting up suddenly from a lying or sitting position
» Possible heat stroke: caution during exercise, hot baths, or hot weather
Avoiding the use of over-the-counter medications for colds or allergies, to prevent increased anticholinergic effects and risk of heat stroke
» Caution if any kind of surgery, dental treatment, or emergency treatment is required; telling physician or dentist in charge about taking haloperidol because of possible drug interactions or blood dyscrasias
Possible skin photosensitivity; avoiding unprotected exposure to sun; using protective clothing; using a sun block product that includes protection against both UVA-caused photosensitivity reactions and UVB-caused sunburn reactions; avoiding use of sunlamp, tanning bed, or tanning booth
Possible dryness of mouth; using sugarless gum or candy, ice, or saliva substitute for relief; checking with physician or dentist if dry mouth continues for more than 2 weeks
If taking liquid form, avoiding contact with skin (to prevent contact dermatitis)
Observing precautions for up to 6 weeks with long-acting parenteral form

**Side/adverse effects**
» Stopping medication and notifying physician immediately if symptoms of neuroleptic malignant syndrome (NMS) appear
Extrapyramidal effects are more likely to occur in children, the elderly, and debilitated patients
Notifying physician as soon as possible if early symptoms of tardive dyskinesia appear
Possibility of withdrawal symptoms
Signs of potential side effects, especially akathisia, dystonias, parkinsonism, allergic reaction, anticholinergic effects, CNS effect, decreased thirst, unusual tiredness or weakness, orthostatic hypotension, tardive dyskinesia or dystonia, blood dyscrasias, heat stroke, obstructive jaundice, and neuroleptic malignant syndrome (NMS)

## General Dosing Information
See also *Patient monitoring*.

Dosage must be individualized by titration from the lower dose range. After a favorable response is noted (usually within 3 weeks), the proper maintenance dosage should be determined by gradually decreasing to the lowest level of therapeutic dosage that will maintain an adequate clinical response.

The antiemetic effect of haloperidol may mask signs of drug toxicity or may obscure diagnosis of conditions in which the primary symptom is nausea.

When extended therapy is discontinued, a gradual reduction in haloperidol dosage over several weeks is recommended, since abrupt withdrawal may cause some patients on high or long-term dosage to experience withdrawal-emergent neurological symptoms.

Avoid skin contact with haloperidol oral solution; contact dermatitis has been reported.

**For oral dosage forms only**
Because undiluted haloperidol concentrated oral solution may irritate mucous membranes, the dose should be diluted with water or beverages having a pH less than 4 (such as orange juice, apple juice, tomato juice, or cola). The dilution should be prepared immediately prior to administration to prevent precipitation. If mixed with coffee, tea, or lithium citrate syrup, free haloperidol will precipitate.

**For long-acting dosage form only**
Patients being considered for haloperidol decanoate therapy should be first converted to oral haloperidol from any other neuroleptic they may have been taking to prevent unexpected adverse sensitivity to haloperidol.

Variations in patient response may require adjustments of dose and dosing intervals. Each patient must be carefully supervised to determine the optimal dosing interval and lowest effective dose, depending on patient's response, age, physical condition, symptoms, severity of illness, and drug history.

Effects of the extended-action injectable form may last up to 6 weeks in some patients. The side effects information and precautions apply during this period of time.

**Diet/Nutrition**
Haloperidol tablets may be taken with food or a full glass (240 mL) of water or milk if necessary to lessen gastrointestinal irritation.

To prevent mucosal irritation, haloperidol oral solution should be diluted in water or beverages such as orange juice, apple juice, tomato juice, or cola immediately prior to administration.

**For treatment of adverse effects**
Neuroleptic malignant syndrome (NMS)
  Treatment is essentially symptomatic and supportive and includes the following
  • *Discontinuing haloperidol immediately*. Neuroleptic malignant syndrome after injection of long-acting haloperidol decanoate may be difficult to treat because of this dosage form's long half-life.
  • Hyperthermia—Administering antipyretics (aspirin or acetaminophen); using cooling blanket.
  • Dehydration—Restoring fluids and electrolytes.
  • Cardiovascular instability—Monitoring blood pressure and cardiac rhythm closely.
  • Hypoxia—Administering oxygen; considering airway insertion and assisted ventilation.
  • Muscle rigidity—Dantrolene sodium may be administered (100 to 300 mg per day in divided doses; 1.25 to 1.5 mg per kg of body weight, intravenously). Bromocriptine (5 to 7.5 mg every eight hours) has been used to reverse hyperpyrexia and muscle rigidity.

Parkinsonism, severe—
  Many authorities advise that the only appropriate treatment of extrapyramidal symptoms is reduction of the antipsychotic dosage, if possible. Oral antidyskinetic agents such as trihexyphenidyl, 2 mg three times per day, or benztropine, may be effective in treating more severe parkinsonism and acute motor restlessness but are used sparingly, and then usually for no longer than 3 months. Extrapyramidal symptoms may reappear if both haloperidol and the antidyskinetic agent are discontinued simultaneously. The antidyskinetic agent may have to be continued after haloperidol is discontinued because of different excretion rates. Milder effects may be treated by adjusting dosage.

Akathisia—
  May be treated with antiparkinsonian medications, or with propranolol (30 to 120 mg per day), nadolol (40 mg per day), pindolol (5 to 60 mg per day), lorazepam (1 or 2 mg two or three times a day), or diazepam (2 mg two or three times a day).

Dystonia—
Acute dystonic postures or oculogyric crisis may be relieved by parenteral administration of benztropine (2 mg intramuscularly); or diphenhydramine (50 mg intramuscularly); or diazepam (5 to 7.5 mg intravenously), to be followed by oral antidyskinetic medication for one or two days to prevent recurrent dystonic episodes. Dosage adjustments of haloperidol may control these effects, and discontinuation of haloperidol may reverse severe symptoms in weeks to months.

Tardive dyskinesia or tardive dystonia—
No known effective treatment. Dosage of haloperidol should be lowered or medication discontinued, if clinically feasible, at earliest signs of tardive dyskinesia or tardive dystonia, to prevent possible irreversible effects.

## Oral Dosage Forms

Note: Bracketed uses in the *Dosage Forms* section refer to categories of use and/or indications that are not included in U.S. product labeling.

### HALOPERIDOL ORAL SOLUTION USP

**Usual adult and adolescent dose**
Antipsychotic; antidyskinetic—
Oral, 500 mcg (0.5 mg) to 5 mg two or three times a day initially, the dosage being gradually adjusted as needed and tolerated.

**Usual adult prescribing limits**
100 mg a day.

**Usual pediatric dose**
Psychotic disorders—
Children younger than 3 years of age: Safety and efficacy have not been established.
Children 3 to 12 years of age or 15 to 40 kg of body weight: Oral, initially 50 mcg (0.05 mg) per kg of body weight a day (in two or three divided doses), the daily dose being increased as needed and tolerated by 500-mcg (0.5 mg) increments at five- to seven-day intervals up to a total of 150 mcg (0.150 mg) per kg of body weight a day.

Nonpsychotic behavior disorders and Tourette's syndrome—
Children younger than 3 years of age: Safety and efficacy have not been established.
Children 3 to 12 years of age or 15 to 40 kg of body weight: Oral, initially 50 mcg (0.05 mg) per kg of body weight a day (in two or three divided doses), the daily dose being increased as needed and tolerated by 500-mcg (0.5 mg) increments at five- to seven-day intervals up to a total of 75 mcg (0.075 mg) per kg of body weight a day. Alternatively, some clinicians recommend that, in the treatment of Tourette's syndrome, the initial daily dose be administered at bedtime to avoid daytime sedation.

[Infantile autism][1]—
Children younger than 3 years of age: Safety and efficacy have not been established.
Children 3 to 12 years of age or 15 to 40 kg of body weight: Oral, 25 mcg (0.025 mg) per kg of body weight a day, up to 50 mcg (0.05 mg) per kg of body weight a day.

Note: There is little evidence that pediatric dosages exceeding 6 mg a day produce additional improvement in behavior or in tics.

**Usual geriatric dose**
Oral, 500 mcg (0.5 mg) to 2 mg two or three times a day, the dosage being increased gradually as needed and tolerated.

Note: The dose for debilitated patients is the same as the geriatric dose.

**Strength(s) usually available**
U.S.—
2 mg per mL (Rx) [*Haldol* (methylparaben); GENERIC].
Canada—
2 mg per mL (Rx) [*Apo-Haloperidol; Novo-Peridol; Peridol; PMS Haloperidol;* GENERIC].

**Packaging and storage**
Store below 40 °C (104 °F), preferably between 15 and 30 °C (59 and 86 °F), unless otherwise specified by manufacturer. Store in a tight, light-resistant container. Protect from freezing.

**Incompatibilities**
Insoluble precipitate of haloperidol is formed when mixed with coffee, tea or lithium citrate syrup.

**Auxiliary labeling**
• May cause drowsiness.
• Avoid alcoholic beverages.

**Note**
Avoid skin contact with liquid forms of this medication; contact dermatitis has been reported.

Each dose must be diluted in water or a beverage such as orange juice, apple juice, tomato juice, or cola, immediately prior to administration. Provide patient with specially marked dosage dropper and explain use if necessary.

### HALOPERIDOL TABLETS USP

**Usual adult and adolescent dose**
See *Haloperidol Oral Solution USP*.

**Usual adult prescribing limits**
See *Haloperidol Oral Solution USP*.

**Usual pediatric dose**
See *Haloperidol Oral Solution USP*.

**Usual geriatric dose**
See *Haloperidol Oral Solution USP*.

**Strength(s) usually available**
U.S.—
500 mcg (0.5 mg) (Rx) [*Haldol;* GENERIC].
1 mg (Rx) [*Haldol* (tartrazine); GENERIC].
2 mg (Rx) [*Haldol;* GENERIC].
5 mg (Rx) [*Haldol* (tartrazine); GENERIC].
10 mg (Rx) [*Haldol* (tartrazine); GENERIC].
20 mg (Rx) [*Haldol;* GENERIC].
Canada—
500 mcg (0.5 mg) (Rx) [*Apo-Haloperidol; Haldol; Novo-Peridol; Peridol* (scored); GENERIC].
1 mg (Rx) [*Apo-Haloperidol; Haldol* (tartrazine); *Novo-Peridol; Peridol* (scored); GENERIC].
2 mg (Rx) [*Apo-Haloperidol; Haldol* (metabisulfite); *Novo-Peridol; Peridol* (scored); GENERIC].
5 mg (Rx) [*Apo-Haloperidol; Haldol* (tartrazine); *Novo-Peridol; Peridol* (scored); GENERIC].
10 mg (Rx) [*Apo-Haloperidol; Haldol* (tartrazine); *Novo-Peridol; Peridol* (scored); GENERIC].
20 mg (Rx) [*Haldol* (metabisulfite); *Novo-Peridol;* GENERIC].

**Packaging and storage**
Store below 40 °C (104 °F), preferably between 15 and 30 °C (59 and 86 °F), unless otherwise specified by manufacturer. Store in a tight, light-resistant container.

**Auxiliary labeling**
• May cause drowsiness.
• Avoid alcoholic beverages.

## Parenteral Dosage Forms

### HALOPERIDOL INJECTION USP

**Usual adult and adolescent dose**
Acute psychosis—
Intramuscular, 2 to 5 mg initially, the dosage being repeated at one-hour intervals if necessary, or at four- to eight-hour intervals if symptoms are satisfactorily controlled.

Note: For the rapid control of acute psychosis or delirium, haloperidol has also been administered intravenously, in doses of 0.5 to 50 mg at a rate of 5 mg per minute, the dose being repeated as needed at 30-minute intervals. Alternatively, the dose of haloperidol can be diluted in 30 to 50 mL of compatible intravenous fluid and administered over 30 minutes.

**Usual adult prescribing limits**
Intramuscular: 100 mg daily.

**Usual pediatric dose**
Safety and efficacy have not been established.

**Strength(s) usually available**
U.S.—
5 mg per mL (Rx) [*Haldol* (methylparaben 1.8 mg; propylparaben 0.2 mg; lactic acid); GENERIC].
Canada—
5 mg per mL (Rx) [*Haldol* (methylparaben 1.8 mg; propylparaben 0.2 mg; lactic acid); GENERIC].

**Packaging and storage**
Store below 40 °C (104 °F), preferably between 15 and 30 °C (59 and 86 °F), unless otherwise specified by manufacturer. Protect from light. Protect from freezing.

**Incompatibilities**
Haloperidol injection may be precipitated by phenytoin or heparin.

### HALOPERIDOL DECANOATE INJECTION

Note: The dosing of haloperidol decanoate injection is expressed in terms of haloperidol base (not the decanoate).

**Usual adult and adolescent dose**
Chronic psychosis—
Intramuscular, initially 10 to 15 times the previous daily oral dose of haloperidol, up to a maximum initial dose of 100 mg (base), at monthly intervals, the dosing interval and dose being adjusted as needed and tolerated.

Note: Administration is by deep intramuscular injection into gluteal region using Z-track technique. A 2-inch long, 21-gauge needle is recommended.

The maximum volume per injection site should not exceed 3 mL.

**Usual adult prescribing limits**
300 mg (base) per month.
Note: Monthly doses as high as 900 mg (base) have been reported.

**Usual pediatric dose**
Safety and efficacy have not been established.

**Strength(s) usually available**
U.S.—
50 mg (base) (70.52 mg of haloperidol decanoate) per mL (Rx) [*Haldol Decanoate* (benzyl alcohol 1.2%; sesame oil) GENERIC].
100 mg (base) (141.04 mg of haloperidol decanoate) per mL (Rx) [*Haldol Decanoate* (benzyl alcohol 1.2%; sesame oil) GENERIC].
Canada—
50 mg (base) (70.52 mg of haloperidol decanoate) per mL (Rx) [*Haldol LA* (benzyl alcohol 15 mg/mL)].
100 mg (base) (141.04 mg of haloperidol decanoate) per mL (Rx) [*Haldol LA* (benzyl alcohol 15 mg/mL)].

**Packaging and storage**
Store below 40 °C (104 °F), preferably between 15 and 30 °C (59 and 86 °F), unless otherwise specified by manufacturer. Protect from light. Protect from freezing. Do not refrigerate.

**Note**
Not to be administered intravenously.

[1]Not included in Canadian product labeling.

Revised: 03/19/93
Interim revision: 08/04/95; 08/11/98

---

**HALOPROGIN**—The *Haloprogin (Topical)* monograph is not included in this published version of the USP DI database. Copies of the monograph are available on request from Micromedex, Inc. - Reprint Requests, 6200 S. Syracuse Way, Suite 300, Englewood, CO 80111; telephone (303) 486-6400; telefax (303) 486-6464; Email: USPDI@MDX.COM.

---

**HALOTHANE**—See *Anesthetics, Inhalation (Systemic)*

---

# HEPARIN Systemic

VA CLASSIFICATION (Primary): BL110
Commonly used brand name(s): *Calcilean; Calciparine; Hepalean; Heparin Leo; Liquaemin.*

Note: For a listing of dosage forms and brand names by country availability, see *Dosage Forms* section(s).

## Category
Anticoagulant.

## Indications
Note: Bracketed information in the *Indications* section refers to uses that are not included in U.S. product labeling.

Note: Some of the indications for heparin therapy are identical to those for thrombolytic (alteplase [tissue-type plasminogen activator, recombinant], anistreplase [anisoylated plasminogen-streptokinase activator complex, APSAC], streptokinase, or urokinase) or coumarin- or indandione-derivative anticoagulant therapy. However, thrombolytic agents are used primarily to lyse obstructive thrombi and restore blood flow in a recently occluded blood vessel, whereas anticoagulants are used primarily to prevent thrombus formation and extension of existing thrombi. For treatment of acute deep venous thrombosis and acute pulmonary embolism, a thrombolytic agent may be the treatment of choice in selected patients. However, the selection of thrombolytic therapy or anticoagulant therapy as opposed to other forms of treatment, including vascular surgery, must be based on determination of the severity of thrombotic disease and assessment of patient condition and history.

Heparin is the anticoagulant of choice when an immediate effect is required. When long-term anticoagulant therapy is required, a coumarin or indandione derivative is usually administered as a follow-up to heparin therapy. However, in some patients (especially pregnant women) long-term anticoagulation with heparin may be desirable.

### Accepted
Thrombosis, deep venous (prophylaxis and treatment) and
Thromboembolism, pulmonary (prophylaxis and treatment)—Heparin is indicated using a full-dose regimen in the treatment of patients with recent thrombosis or thrombophlebitis of the deep veins to prevent extension and embolization of the thrombus and to reduce the risk of pulmonary embolism or recurrent thrombus formation. In acute pulmonary embolism, full-dose heparin is indicated to decrease the risk of extension, recurrence, or death.

Heparin is also indicated using a low-dose regimen to prevent the development of venous thrombosis and pulmonary embolism following major abdominal or thoracic surgery in high-risk patients, such as patients with a history of thromboembolism and patients requiring prolonged immobilization following surgery, especially if they are 40 years of age or older. Low-dose heparin may be ineffective for this purpose in some patients, especially following hip surgery. Many clinicians question the validity of data showing the efficacy and safety of low-dose heparin prophylaxis.

[Low-dose heparin prophylaxis is also used to prevent thrombus formation in selected immobilized medical patients who are not at risk of hemorrhage.]

Heparin is also administered using an adjusted-dose regimen for prophylaxis against thromboembolic complications when low-dose heparin may not be effective, e.g., for general abdominal or thoracic surgery in very high-risk patients, high-risk orthopedic procedures such as elective hip surgery or knee reconstruction, and [the second half of the third trimester in pregnant women with a history of venous thrombosis or pulmonary embolism][1].

Adjusted-dose subcutaneous heparin is also recommended when long-term anticoagulation is required and use of a coumarin- or indandione-derivative anticoagulant is contraindicated or inadvisable (e.g., during pregnancy). In addition, after the dosage of heparin has been stabilized (i.e., the desired level of anticoagulation has been achieved and maintained for a 2-week period without additional dosage adjustment), further anticoagulant monitoring and dosage adjustment are not needed (except during pregnancy, when heparin requirements increase with the patient's blood volume as pregnancy progresses). Therefore, this regimen can be utilized for the long-term treatment of nonpregnant patients when anticoagulant therapy cannot be monitored on a regular basis.

Thromboembolism (prophylaxis)—Heparin is indicated prior to and during attempted cardioversion or surgery to prevent systemic thromboembolism that may occur in patients with chronic atrial fibrillation, especially those with rheumatic mitral stenosis, congestive heart failure, left atrial enlargement, or cardiomyopathy.

Heparin is indicated as adjunctive therapy in acute myocardial infarction to reduce the risk of thromboembolic complications, especially in high-risk patients such as those with shock, congestive heart failure, prolonged arrhythmias (especially atrial fibrillation), previous myocardial infarction, or history of venous thrombosis or pulmonary embolism. Also, heparin may be administered to help prevent reocclusion following thrombolytic therapy in patients with acute myocardial infarction.

[Heparin is also used to prevent catheter-induced thromboembolism during coronary angiography and percutaneous transluminal angioplasty.][1]

Blood clotting (prophylaxis)—Heparin is indicated to prevent blood clotting during extracorporeal circulation in cardiac surgery and dialysis procedures.

Heparin is indicated to prevent blood clotting during and following arterial surgery. It is administered systemically or by local intra-arterial injection.

Heparin is indicated to prevent blood clotting during blood transfusions and in blood sampling for laboratory purposes. However, heparinized blood should not be used for isoagglutinin, complement, or erythrocyte fragility tests, or for platelet counts. In addition, leukocyte counts should be performed within 2 hours after heparin is added to the blood sample.

Heparin is also available as a lock flush solution, which is not intended for anticoagulant therapy. This solution is used to maintain the patency of an indwelling intravascular device.

Coagulation, disseminated intravascular (treatment)—Although heparin is indicated as a temporary measure in the treatment of disseminated intravascular coagulation, especially if there is clinical evidence of intravascular thrombosis, its use in this condition is controversial. The underlying cause of the condition must be determined and treated.

Thromboembolism, arterial (treatment)—Heparin is indicated as adjunctive therapy for peripheral arterial embolism. It may prevent further thrombus formation when surgery must be delayed.

Thrombosis, cerebral (prophylaxis)—Heparin is indicated to decrease the risk of cerebral thrombosis and death in patients with progressive stroke (stroke-in-evolution).

[Thromboembolism, cerebral, recurrence (prophylaxis)][1]—Heparin is also used in the treatment of patients with recent cerebral embolism to decrease the risk of recurrence and death; however, this use is controversial. Although administration of an anticoagulant too soon after a cerebral embolism may increase the risk of cerebral hemorrhage, recent studies have indicated that the risk of early recurrence may be greater than the risk of anticoagulant therapy. It is recommended that heparin therapy be initiated only if the patient is not hypertensive and a computerized tomography (CT) scan performed 24 hours or longer following the onset of the stroke shows no evidence of hemorrhagic transformation. If severe hypertension is present, or the embolic stroke is large, there is a risk of late hemorrhagic transformation and anticoagulant therapy should be delayed for several days. If hemorrhagic transformation is documented, anticoagulant therapy should be postponed for at least 8 to 10 days. Long-term anticoagulation is recommended.

### Unaccepted
Prophylactic use of heparin (low-dose or full-dose) is not recommended for patients with bleeding disorders; patients having neurosurgery, ophthalmic surgery, or spinal anesthesia; or patients who are receiving a coumarin- or indandione-derivative anticoagulant or a platelet active agent.

[Heparin has also been used to reduce the risk of thrombosis and/or occlusion of the aortocoronary bypass following coronary bypass surgery; however, its efficacy has not been established and this use is controversial. Also, platelet aggregation inhibitors, especially aspirin, are more commonly used for this indication.]

---

[1] Not included in Canadian product labeling.

## Pharmacology/Pharmacokinetics

### Mechanism of action/Effect
Heparin acts indirectly at multiple sites in both the intrinsic and extrinsic blood clotting systems to potentiate the inhibitory action of antithrombin III (heparin cofactor) on several activated coagulation factors, including thrombin (factor IIa) and factors IXa, Xa, XIa, and XIIa, by forming a complex with and inducing a conformational change in the antithrombin III molecule. Inhibition of activated factor Xa interferes with thrombin generation and thereby inhibits the various actions of thrombin in coagulation. Heparin also accelerates the formation of an antithrombin III–thrombin complex, thereby inactivating thrombin and preventing the conversion of fibrinogen to fibrin; these actions prevent extension of existing thrombi. Larger doses of heparin are required to inactivate thrombin than are required to inhibit thrombin formation. Heparin also prevents formation of a stable fibrin clot by inhibiting the activation of the fibrin stabilizing factor by thrombin. Heparin has no fibrinolytic activity.

Full-dose heparin prolongs partial thromboplastin time, thrombin time, whole blood clotting time, and activated clotting time (ACT).

### Other actions/effects
Heparin reduces the concentration of triglycerides in plasma by releasing the enzyme lipoprotein lipase from tissues and stabilizing the enzyme. The resultant hydrolysis of triglycerides leads to increased blood concentrations of free fatty acids.

### Protein binding
Very high; primarily to low-density lipoproteins; also bound to globulins and to fibrinogen.

### Biotransformation
Hepatic; however, the primary route of removal from the circulation is uptake by the reticuloendothelial system.

### Half-life
1 to 6 hours (average 1.5 hours); dose and route dependent and subject to inter- and intrapatient variation. May be increased above the average in patients with renal failure, hepatic function impairment, or obesity. May be decreased in patients with pulmonary embolism, infections, or malignancy.

### Onset of action
Direct intravenous injection—Immediate.

Intravenous infusion—Immediate when infusion is preceded by the recommended intravenous loading dose. If no loading dose is given, the onset of action may depend upon the rate of infusion.

Subcutaneous—Generally within 20 to 60 minutes but subject to interpatient variability.

### Elimination
Renal, usually as metabolites. However, after intravenous administration of high doses, up to 50% of a dose may be excreted unchanged.

In dialysis—Not removed via hemodialysis.

## Precautions to Consider

### Cross-sensitivity and/or related problems
Patients with a history of allergies, especially those who are allergic to swine, beef, or other animal proteins, may be allergic to this medication also (depending on heparin source).

### Pregnancy/Reproduction
Pregnancy—Heparin does not cross the placenta and is the anticoagulant of choice for use during pregnancy because it does not affect blood clotting mechanisms in the fetus. Although heparin has not been reported to cause birth defects, use during pregnancy has been reported to increase the risk of stillbirth or prematurity. However, the underlying condition, rather than heparin itself, may have been responsible. Also, the reported incidence (13 to 22%) of these complications is lower than that reported with coumarin-derivative anticoagulants (31%). In addition, caution is recommended when heparin is used during the last trimester of pregnancy or during the postpartum period because of the increased risk of maternal bleeding.

Especially careful monitoring of the patient and attention to dosage are recommended during pregnancy. Heparin requirements increase, because of expansion of the patient's blood volume, as pregnancy progresses. Readjustment of heparin dosage may be needed following delivery.

FDA Pregnancy Category C.

### Breast-feeding
Heparin is not distributed into breast milk. However, administration to lactating women has rarely been reported to cause rapid (within 2 to 4 weeks) development of severe osteoporosis and vertebral collapse.

### Pediatrics
Appropriate studies performed to date have not demonstrated pediatrics-specific problems that would limit the usefulness of heparin in children. However, heparin injections that contain benzyl alcohol should not be administered to premature neonates because the preservative has been associated with a fatal "gasping syndrome" in these patients.

### Geriatrics
Patients 60 years of age or older, especially females, may be more susceptible to hemorrhaging during heparin therapy. Also, elderly patients are more likely to have age-related renal function impairment, which may increase the risk of bleeding in patients receiving anticoagulants.

### Dental
Bleeding from gingival tissue may be a symptom of heparin overdose.

Heparin therapy increases the risk of localized hemorrhage during and following oral surgical procedures. Consultation with the prescribing physician may be advisable prior to oral surgery, to determine whether a temporary dosage reduction or withdrawal of heparin therapy is feasible. Also, local measures to minimize bleeding should be used at the time of surgery.

### Drug interactions and/or related problems
The following drug interactions and/or related problems have been selected on the basis of their potential clinical significance (possible mechanism in parentheses where appropriate)—not necessarily inclusive (» = major clinical significance):

Note: Combinations containing any of the following medications, depending on the amount present, may also interact with this medication.

Interactions listed below may not apply to short-term use of heparin followed by protamine reversal, as in cardiovascular surgery.

In addition to the documented interactions listed below, the possibility should be considered that multiple effects leading to further impairment of blood clotting and/or increased risk of bleeding may occur if heparin is administered to a patient receiving any medication having a significant potential for causing hypoprothrombinemia, thrombocytopenia, or gastrointestinal ulceration or hemorrhage.

Acid citrate dextrose (ACD)–converted blood—blood collected in heparin and later converted to ACD blood
(heparin anticoagulant activity lasts for up to 22 days after conversion to ACD blood when refrigerated; use of ACD blood in heparin-treated patients may increase the risk of hemorrhage)

Adrenocorticoids, glucocorticoid or
Corticotropin, especially chronic therapeutic use or
Ethacrynic acid or
Salicylates, nonacetylated
(the potential occurrence of gastrointestinal ulceration or hemorrhage during therapy with these medications may cause increased risk of bleeding in patients receiving anticoagulant therapy)

(large [antirheumatic] doses of salicylates may cause hypoprothrombinemia, which may increase the risk of bleeding in patients receiving anticoagulant therapy)

Anticoagulants, coumarin- or indandione-derivative
(although these medications are commonly used concurrently with heparin, the fact that concurrent use may lead to a severe deficiency of vitamin K–dependent procoagulant factors, leading to increased risk of bleeding, must be considered)

(heparin may prolong the prothrombin time used for dosage adjustments of these agents)

Antihistamines or
Digitalis glycosides or
Nicotine or
Tetracyclines
(these medications may partially counteract the anticoagulant effect of heparin; heparin dosage adjustment may be required during and following concurrent use)

Anti-inflammatory drugs, nonsteroidal (NSAIDs) or
» Platelet aggregation inhibitors, other, (See *Appendix II*) especially:
» Aspirin
» Sulfinpyrazone
(inhibition of platelet function by these agents may lead to hemorrhage because it impairs a hemostatic mechanism on which heparin-treated patients depend to prevent bleeding)

(hypoprothrombinemia induced by large [antirheumatic] doses of aspirin, and the potential occurrence of gastrointestinal ulceration or hemorrhage during therapy with NSAIDs, aspirin, or sulfinpyrazone, may also cause increased risk of bleeding in patients receiving heparin therapy)

» Cefamandole or
» Cefoperazone or
» Cefotetan or
» Plicamycin or
» Valproic acid
(these medications may cause hypoprothrombinemia; in addition, plicamycin or valproic acid may inhibit platelet aggregation; concurrent use with heparin may increase the risk of hemorrhage and is not recommended)

Chloroquine or
Hydroxychloroquine
(these agents may cause thrombocytopenia, which may increase the risk of hemorrhage because heparin-treated patients depend on platelet aggregation to prevent bleeding)

» Methimazole or
» Propylthiouracil
(these medications may cause hypoprothrombinemia, which may enhance the anticoagulant effect of heparin and increase the risk of bleeding)

Nitroglycerin, intravenous
(the anticoagulant effect of heparin may be decreased in patients receiving nitroglycerin via intravenous infusion; adjustment of heparin dosage may be required to maintain the desired degree of anticoagulation during and following administration of a nitroglycerin infusion)

» Probenecid
(probenecid may increase and prolong the anticoagulant effect of heparin)

» Thrombolytic agents, such as:
» Alteplase (tissue-type plasminogen activator, recombinant)

» Anistreplase (anisoylated plasminogen-streptokinase activator complex; APSAC)
» Streptokinase
» Urokinase
(concurrent or sequential use with heparin increases the risk of bleeding complications; although heparin is sometimes given before, and is usually given to decrease the risk of reocclusion following, thrombolytic therapy, caution and especially careful monitoring of the patient are recommended)

**Diagnostic interference**
The following have been selected on the basis of their potential clinical significance (possible effect in parentheses where appropriate)—not necessarily inclusive (» = major clinical significance):

With diagnostic test results
Blood pool imaging studies
(heparin may impair blood pool images by decreasing the radiolabeling of red blood cells with sodium pertechnetate Tc 99m)

$^{125}$I-fibrinogen uptake test
(some reports have indicated that heparin may cause false-negative test results in patients with actively forming or established venous thrombosis)

Platelet scintigraphy using indium In 111 oxyquinoline
(although studies of the effect of heparin on In 111–labeled platelet accumulation on venous thrombi have yielded contradictory results, the possibility should be considered that false negative test results may occur in heparin-treated patients)

Prothrombin-time test, one-stage
(may be prolonged; single intravenous injections or subcutaneous injection of full therapeutic doses of heparin may prolong the prothrombin time considerably because of the high concentrations of heparin in the blood, whereas usual prophylactic [low] doses of heparin given subcutaneously or full therapeutic doses given by continuous intravenous infusion usually do not increase the prothrombin time by more than a few seconds; to minimize problems, draw blood for the prothrombin time test just prior to, or at least 5 hours after, a single intravenous dose or 12 to 24 hours following subcutaneous injection of a full therapeutic dose)

Radionuclide imaging using technetium Tc 99m sulfur colloid
(heparin may reduce the quantity of technetium Tc 99m sulfur colloid reaching the site being studied by causing the radiotracer to accumulate in the lung, probably by increasing the number of free intravascular macrophages, which may migrate to, and phagocytize colloidal particles in, the pulmonary capillary bed)

Skeletal imaging, radionuclide
(subcutaneously administered heparin calcium may cause extraosseus accumulation of technetium Tc 99m medronate, technetium Tc 99m oxidronate, or technetium Tc 99m pyrophosphate, thereby interfering with the bone scan, if injected near the site to be studied; the interference involves precipitation of calcium, which may occur if the tissue concentration of calcium exceeds its solubility limits, and therefore does not occur with subcutaneously administered heparin sodium)

Thyroid function tests
(increases in serum thyroxine concentrations may occur, depending on the test method used; also, resin $T_3$ uptake may be increased)

With physiology/laboratory test values
Plasma free fatty acid concentration
(may be increased)

Plasma triglyceride concentration
(may be decreased)

Serum alanine aminotransferase (ALT [SGPT]) activity and
Serum aspartate aminotransferase (AST [SGOT]) activity
(may be increased during, and for a time following, heparin therapy; the usefulness of determinations of these enzymes in the differential diagnosis of myocardial infarction, pulmonary embolism, or liver disease may therefore be decreased)

Serum cholesterol concentration
(may be decreased with doses of 15,000 to 20,000 USP Units of heparin)

**Medical considerations/Contraindications**
The medical considerations/contraindications included have been selected on the basis of their potential clinical significance (reasons given in parentheses where appropriate)—not necessarily inclusive (» = major clinical significance).

*Except under special circumstances, this medication should not be used when the following medical problems exist:*
- » Abortion, threatened or
- » Aneurysm, cerebral or dissecting aorta, except in conjunction with corrective surgery or
- » Cerebrovascular hemorrhage, confirmed or suspected
  (increased risk of uncontrollable hemorrhage)
- » Hemorrhage, active uncontrollable, except in disseminated intravascular coagulation
- » Hypertension, severe uncontrolled
  (increased risk of cerebral hemorrhage)
- » Thrombocytopenia, severe, heparin-induced, within past several months
  (risk of recurrence, which may cause resistance to heparin and new thromboembolic complications)

*Risk-benefit should be considered when the following medical problems exist:*
  Allergic reaction to heparin, history of
  Allergy or asthma, history of
  (increased risk of allergic reactions because heparin is derived from animal tissue)
  Any medical or dental procedure or condition in which the risk of bleeding or hemorrhage is present, such as:
- » Anesthesia, regional or lumbar block
- » Blood dyscrasias, hemorrhagic, especially thrombocytopenia or hemophilia; or other hemorrhagic tendency
- » Childbirth, recent
  Diabetes, severe
- » Endocarditis, subacute bacterial
  Gastrointestinal ulceration, history of
  Intrauterine contraceptive device, use of
- » Neurosurgery, recent or contemplated
- » Ophthalmic surgery, recent or contemplated
- » Pericarditis or pericardial effusion
  Radiation therapy, recent
  Renal function impairment, mild to moderate
- » Renal function impairment, severe
- » Spinal puncture, recent
- » Surgery, major, or wounds resulting in large open surfaces
- » Trauma, severe, especially to the central nervous system (CNS)
  Tuberculosis, active
- » Ulceration or other lesions of the gastrointestinal, respiratory, or urinary tract, active
- » Vasculitis, severe
  Hepatic function impairment, mild to moderate
  Hepatic function impairment, severe
  Hypertension, mild to moderate
  (increased risk of cerebral hemorrhage)
- » Caution in use is also recommended for lactating women, who may develop severe osteoporosis after only 2 to 4 weeks of heparin therapy, and geriatric patients, who may be at increased risk of heparin-induced hemorrhage.

**Patient monitoring**
The following may be especially important in patient monitoring (other tests may be warranted in some patients, depending on condition; » = major clinical significance):
- » Blood coagulation tests
  (except in rare acute or emergency situations, should be performed prior to full-dose therapy to establish a baseline or control value; also, recommended prior to initiation of low-dose prophylaxis to identify pre-existing coagulation defects and aid in determining whether the patient is a suitable candidate for such treatment)
- » Blood coagulation tests, heparin-specific, such as:
  Activated clotting time (ACT) test or
  Partial thromboplastin time (PTT) tests
  (must be performed at periodic intervals during full-dose therapy as a guide to dosage, efficacy, and safety)
  (PTT tests are used to establish dosage requirements during the initial phase of adjusted-dose therapy; they are also required at periodic intervals throughout adjusted-dose therapy, as a guide to dosage and efficacy, if the patient is pregnant)
  Hematocrit determinations and
  Stool tests for occult blood loss
  (should be performed at regular intervals during full-dose therapy)
- » Platelet counts
  (recommended prior to initiation of therapy and at intervals of every 2 to 3 days during full-dose, adjusted-dose, or low-dose therapy to detect thrombocytopenia)

## Side/Adverse Effects

Note: The occurrence of hemorrhage (especially in the gastrointestinal tract) during heparin therapy, especially if blood coagulation tests are within the therapeutic range, may indicate the presence of an underlying occult lesion such as a tumor or ulcer.

Two forms of reversible thrombocytopenia related to heparin therapy have been identified, either of which may occur in up to 30% of patients receiving the medication. A mild form may occur on the second to fourth day of heparin therapy and may improve despite continuing heparin usage. This condition is characterized by a moderate decrease in platelet count and by the absence of thrombotic or hemorrhagic complications; it may occur more frequently with bovine lung heparin than with porcine mucosal heparin. A severe form of thrombocytopenia, associated with the development of heparin-dependent antiplatelet antibodies resulting in greatly increased platelet aggregation, has also been reported. This condition usually occurs after the eighth day of therapy, although it has occurred within as little as 2 days in some patients, and is characterized by reduction of platelet count to as low as 5000 per cu. mm. and by increased resistance to heparin therapy. Continued use of heparin may lead to the "white clot syndrome", i.e., the formation of new thrombi composed primarily of fibrin platelet aggregates, which may cause thrombotic complications including organ infarction, skin necrosis, gangrene of the extremities, pulmonary embolism, and stroke. Rarely, hemorrhage may occur. This severe form of thrombocytopenia is independent of the source of heparin, dosage, or route of administration; however, patients who have recently received a prior course of heparin therapy may be at greater risk of developing this complication. Heparin should be discontinued immediately if severe thrombocytopenia occurs or is suspected. Severe thrombocytopenia may recur if heparin is administered to the patient within several months following the development of this complication.

Adrenal hemorrhage resulting in acute adrenal insufficiency has been reported to occur rarely during anticoagulant therapy. Diagnosis may be difficult because the initial symptoms (abdominal pain, apprehension, diarrhea, dizziness or fainting, headache, loss of appetite, nausea or vomiting, and weakness) are nonspecific and variable. If acute adrenal insufficiency is suspected, anticoagulant therapy must be discontinued and high-dose adrenocorticoid therapy (preferably with hydrocortisone, since other glucocorticoids do not provide sufficient sodium retention) instituted immediately. Delay of treatment while laboratory confirmation of the diagnosis is awaited may prove fatal to the patient. It has been proposed that abdominal computerized axial tomographic (CAT) scanning may be of use in diagnosing this condition more rapidly.

Heparin may suppress aldosterone synthesis. Rarely, with prolonged use, inhibition of renal function, hyperkalemia, and metabolic acidosis may result.

The following side/adverse effects have been selected on the basis of their potential clinical significance (possible signs and symptoms in parentheses where appropriate)—not necessarily inclusive:

### Those indicating need for medical attention
Incidence less frequent or rare
  *Allergic reaction* (fever with or without chills; runny nose; headache; nausea with or without vomiting; shortness of breath, troubled breathing, wheezing, or tightness in chest; skin rash, itching, or hives; tearing of eyes); *anaphylactoid reaction, possibly including anaphylactic shock* (changes in facial skin color; skin rash, hives, and/or itching; fast or irregular breathing; puffiness or swelling of the eyelids or around the eyes; shortness of breath, troubled breathing, tightness in chest, and/or wheezing; sudden, severe decrease in blood pressure and collapse); *chest pain; frequent or persistent erection; itching and burning feeling, especially on the plantar site of the feet; pain, coldness, and blue color of skin of arms or legs; peripheral neuropathy* (numbness or tingling in hands or feet).

Note: Signs and symptoms suggestive of *ischemia* may occur in one or more limbs approximately 6 to 10 days following initiation of therapy. If heparin therapy is continued, progression of the reaction may lead to cyanosis, tachypnea, and headache. Protamine sulfate will not reverse these effects, which in the past have been attributed to an allergic vasospastic reaction. Whether these effects are actually identical to complications associated with heparin-induced thrombocytopenia has not been determined.

### Signs and symptoms of hemorrhage indicating need for medical attention
Early signs of hemorrhage
> *Bleeding from gums when brushing teeth; heavy bleeding or oozing from cuts or wounds; unexplained bruising or purplish areas on skin; unexplained nosebleeds; unusually heavy or unexpected menstrual bleeding*
>> Note: *Unexplained bleeding or bruising* may also indicate thrombocytopenia.

Signs and symptoms of internal bleeding—incidence 5 to 15%
> *Abdominal pain or swelling; back pain or backaches; blood in urine; bloody or black, tarry stools; constipation caused by hemorrhage-induced paralytic ileus or intestinal obstruction; coughing up blood; dizziness; headaches, severe or continuing; joint pain, stiffness, or swelling; vomiting of blood or material that looks like coffee grounds*

### Those occurring during long-term (6 months or longer) therapy and indicating need for medical attention
> *Osteoporosis* (back or rib pain; decrease in height); *unusual hair loss*

### Those occurring at site of administration and indicating need for medical attention
Incidence less frequent or rare with deep subcutaneous injections
> *Hematoma* (collection of blood under skin [blood blister]); *histamine-like reaction; hives, localized; irritation, pain, redness, or ulceration; necrosis, cutaneous* (peeling or sloughing of skin)—several cases of tissue necrosis, possibly associated with cutaneous hemorrhage, have also been reported following intravenous administration

## Overdose
For specific information on the agents used in the management of heparin overdose, see the *Protamine (Systemic)* monograph.

For more information on the management of overdose, **contact a Poison Control Center** (see *Poison Control Center Listing*).

### Clinical effects of overdose
The following effects have been selected on the basis of their potential clinical significance (possible signs and symptoms in parentheses where appropriate)—not necessarily inclusive:

Early signs of excessive anticoagulation
> *Bleeding from gums when brushing teeth; heavy bleeding or oozing from cuts or wounds; unexplained bruising or purplish areas on skin; unexplained nosebleeds; unusually heavy or unexpected menstrual bleeding*
>> Note: *Unexplained bleeding or bruising* may also indicate thrombocytopenia.

Signs and symptoms of internal bleeding
> *Abdominal pain or swelling; back pain or backaches; blood in urine; bloody or black, tarry stools; constipation caused by hemorrhage-induced paralytic ileus or intestinal obstruction; coughing up blood; dizziness; headaches, severe or continuing; joint pain, stiffness, or swelling; vomiting of blood or material that looks like coffee grounds*

### Treatment of overdose
For mild effects of heparin overdose, withdrawal of heparin therapy may be sufficient.

Specific treatment—
> For more severe overdose, administration of the heparin antagonist protamine is required. One milligram of protamine sulfate will neutralize approximately 100 USP Units of heparin. However, heparin blood concentrations decrease rapidly following intravenous administration; 30 minutes after intravenous administration of heparin, half as much protamine sulfate may be sufficient to neutralize the remaining heparin. In most cases, it is recommended that protamine sulfate be administered intravenously, slowly (over a one- to three-minute period), and in doses not exceeding 50 mg in any ten-minute period. It is strongly recommended that blood coagulation tests be used to determine optimum protamine dosage, especially when neutralizing large doses of heparin given during cardiac or arterial surgery.

> Because absorption of heparin may be prolonged following subcutaneous administration, it has been recommended that protamine (when used to neutralize heparin administered via that route) be administered as an initial loading dose of 25 to 50 mg that is followed by continuous intravenous infusion (over a period of 8 to 16 hours) of the remainder of the calculated dose. It is recommended that blood coagulation tests and/or direct titration of a sample of the patient's blood with protamine be used as a guide to protamine dosage.

> When protamine is used to neutralize large doses of heparin, such as those used during cardiopulmonary bypass surgery, a rebound of heparin activity resulting in hemorrhage may occur despite initial complete neutralization of heparin. Prolonged monitoring of the patient is necessary; additional protamine should be administered as determined by coagulation test results. Also, it is recommended that no more than 100 mg of protamine sulfate be administered over a short period of time (2 hours) unless accurate titrations or other tests indicate that larger doses are required.

> For severe hemorrhaging, transfusion of whole blood or plasma may also be required. This may dilute, but will not neutralize the effects of, heparin.

## Patient Consultation
As an aid to patient consultation, refer to *Advice for the Patient, Heparin (Systemic)*.

In providing consultation, consider emphasizing the following selected information (» = major clinical significance):

### Before using this medication
» Conditions affecting use, especially:
> Allergies, especially to heparin or to swine, beef, or other animal proteins
> Pregnancy—Although heparin does not cross the placenta and is not likely to adversely affect the fetus or neonate, there is a risk of maternal bleeding
> Breast-feeding—Although heparin is not distributed into breast milk and poses no danger to the infant, severe osteoporosis and vertebral collapse may develop rapidly in lactating women
> Use in the elderly—Increased risk of hemorrhage, especially in elderly females
> Other medications, especially platelet aggregation inhibitors, hypoprothrombinemia-inducing medications, and probenecid
> Other medical problems, especially hypertension; hemorrhagic blood dyscrasias; recent childbirth, spinal puncture, surgery, or other trauma; endocarditis; hepatic function impairment; renal function impairment; ulcers or other lesions of the gastrointestinal, respiratory, or urinary tract; and history of heparin-induced thrombocytopenia

### Proper use of this medication
» Proper administration of injections at home (if applicable)
» Importance of strict compliance with dosage measurement and dosage schedule to achieve maximum effectiveness and to lessen chance of bleeding
» Regular visits to physician and regular blood coagulation tests to check progress during therapy
» Proper dosing
> Missed dose: Using as soon as possible; not using if almost time for next dose; not doubling doses; keeping record of doses taken to avoid mistakes; keeping record of missed doses to give physician
» Proper storage—if dispensed to patient

### Precautions while using this medication
» Not taking aspirin while using this medication; checking all medications for aspirin content; not taking ibuprofen or other platelet-active medications (unless prescribed by physician) while using heparin
» Need to inform all physicians and dentists that this medication is being used

Need to carry identification stating that medication is being used
Avoiding activities that may lead to injuries
Using care in brushing teeth and shaving

### Side/adverse effects
Signs of potential side effects, especially allergic reactions, including anaphylaxis and anaphylactic shock; bleeding, including internal bleeding; chest pain; pain, coldness, or blue color of skin of arms or legs; peripheral neuropathy; skin necrosis; and local reactions at the injection site
Notifying physician immediately if signs and symptoms of bleeding are evident

## General Dosing Information
Full-dose heparin is administered by deep subcutaneous (intrafat) injection, direct intravenous injection, or intravenous infusion. Heparin should not be administered by intramuscular injection because of the increased incidence of hematomas, irritation, and pain at the injection site. Low-dose heparin is generally administered by deep subcutaneous injection.

The deep subcutaneous (intrafat) injections should be made deep into fatty tissue such as above the iliac crest or into the abdominal fat layer, and the sites should be rotated to prevent formation of hematomas. Aspiration of blood should not be attempted, and the needle should not be moved while the solution is being injected. Other measures recommended to reduce the risk of tissue trauma during subcutaneous injections include use of a small needle, use of a concentrated heparin solution to minimize the injection volume, and injection of the solution into a 2 to 2.5 cm (1 to 2 inch) area of fat which is grasped and held away from deeper tissues. The injection sites should not be massaged before or after the injections; however, application of pressure over the injection sites for up to two minutes following each injection has been recommended.

For intravenous administration, many clinicians prefer continuous intravenous infusion because several studies have indicated that a more constant degree of anticoagulation may be achieved with lower total daily dosages and that the incidence of bleeding complications may be decreased. However, other clinicians prefer intermittent intravenous administration. Use of an indwelling, rubber-capped needle (heparin-lock) has been recommended for intermittent intravenous therapy. Use of a constant infusion pump or mechanical syringe pump has been recommended for administration of the continuous intravenous infusion, to control the flow rate and infusion volume. **It is recommended that other medications not be added to infusion solutions containing heparin**, even if compatibility has been established, because changes in the infusion rate that may be needed to adjust heparin dosage will also affect the delivery rate of other medications present in the solution.

When heparin is administered using a full-dose regimen, the dosage must be individualized and adjusted according to the results of periodic coagulation tests. *Full-dose heparin therapy is contraindicated whenever suitable blood coagulation tests cannot be performed at the required intervals.* However, the effect of low-dose heparin usually does not require monitoring if the patient has normal pretreatment coagulation parameters. During the first day of treatment, a coagulation test is usually performed prior to each injection (if given via an intermittent dosage schedule). When the medication is given by continuous intravenous infusion, the test is usually performed 1½ to 2 hours after the infusion is started, then every 4 hours during the early stages of treatment. However, the frequency of testing must be adjusted to the needs of the individual patient. Coagulation tests should be performed at least once daily for the duration of therapy; however, increased monitoring may be necessary in patients who may be more sensitive to the effects of heparin, such as elderly patients or those with hypertension, renal function impairment, or hepatic function impairment.

When heparin is administered using an adjusted-dose regimen, dosage must be established according to the results of daily coagulation tests. When no dosage adjustments have been needed for two weeks, further monitoring at regular frequent intervals may be unnecessary for most patients. However, pregnant women should be monitored throughout therapy because their dosage requirements increase as pregnancy progresses.

The standard tests used for measuring heparin's general effect on clotting include the Lee-White whole blood clotting time, the whole blood activated partial thromboplastin time (WBAPTT), the activated partial thromboplastin time (APTT), and the activated clotting time (ACT). Other tests may be used in some cases. The Lee-White whole blood clotting time has been reported to be less reproducible than other tests and has largely been replaced by partial thromboplastin time tests. If the Lee-White whole blood clotting time is used to monitor therapy, the clotting time should be elevated to 2½ to 3 times the control value in minutes. The generally accepted value for the APTT is 1½ to 2½ times the control value in seconds. However, the specific reagent used must be considered when evaluating APTT test results because the various reagents used in the APTT test vary widely in their sensitivity to heparin. The generally accepted value for the ACT test is 2 to 3 times the control value in seconds. The ACT has been recommended as being particularly useful during extracorporeal circulation because it can be performed at the bedside; however, one study has indicated that the ACT may be ineffective for monitoring heparin dosage and protamine neutralization during cardiopulmonary bypass procedures in which hypothermia has been induced. Hypothermia may also interfere with the results of other coagulation tests. It is recommended that a single laboratory be employed for each patient, and that the laboratory understand the test will be used to monitor heparin therapy.

Because heparin is derived from animal tissue, it is recommended that patients with a history of allergies or asthma be given a test dose of 1000 USP Units before therapy is initiated.

Postsurgical patients and those with active thromboembolic disease (especially pulmonary embolism or myocardial infarction), infections with thrombosing tendency, malignancy, or a fever may be resistant to the effects of heparin and may require larger doses than other patients. Resistance to the effects of heparin also occurs in patients with familial antithrombin III deficiency. However, this type of resistance cannot always be overcome by increasing the dosage of heparin; a coumarin- or indandione-derivative anticoagulant is indicated for such patients. Also, local antithrombin III depletion resulting in loss of heparin effect may occur when heparin is administered intraperitoneally during peritoneal dialysis procedures.

If clinical evidence of thromboembolism occurs in a patient receiving low-dose heparin prophylaxis, full therapeutic doses of an anticoagulant should be administered. However, before full therapeutic doses of heparin are given, the possibility that the thrombosis may be due to the severe form of heparin-induced thrombocytopenia must be ruled out.

Heparin may be administered prior to or following thrombolytic therapy with alteplase (tissue-type plasminogen activator, recombinant), streptokinase, or urokinase. However, heparin should be discontinued and the patient's TT or APTT should be less than twice the control value prior to initiation of intravenous thrombolytic therapy. Also, following thrombolytic therapy, the patient's TT or APTT should return to less than twice the control value prior to administration of heparin.

When anticoagulant therapy is initiated with heparin and continued with a coumarin or indandione derivative, it is recommended that both agents be given concurrently until prothrombin time determinations indicate an adequate response to the coumarin or indandione derivative. The fact that early changes in prothrombin time may reflect initial depletion of factor VII rather than peak antithrombogenic activity must be kept in mind. Some clinicians recommend continuation of heparin therapy for several days after prothrombin time determinations have shown a reduction of activity to ensure that peak antithrombogenic activity has been reached.

Intramuscular injection of other medications is not recommended in patients receiving heparin because hematomas and bleeding into adjacent areas may occur.

A concentration of 400 to 600 USP Units of heparin per 100 mL of whole blood is usually used to prevent clotting during blood transfusion; a concentration of 70 to 150 USP Units of heparin per 10 to 20 mL of whole blood is usually used to prevent clotting in blood used for laboratory sampling. Consult manufacturers' prescribing information for specific directions. For use of heparin lock-flush solution in maintaining the patency of an indwelling venipuncture device, consult manufacturers' prescribing information. For use of heparin to prevent clotting during extracorporeal dialysis procedures, consult the equipment manufacturers' operating directions.

## Parenteral Dosage Forms

Note: The following doses are given in USP Heparin Units. The strengths of heparin preparations available in the U.S. are labeled in USP Heparin Units per mL. The strengths of heparin preparations available in Canada may be labeled in USP Units or in International Units (IU) per mL. The strengths of heparin preparations available in many other countries, including the U.K., are labeled only in IU per mL. *USP Heparin Units are not identical to IU.* The relative potency between USP Units and IU may vary, depending upon the test method and specific reagents used to measure heparin activity. Also, a new International Standard for Heparin (used to calibrate potency in IU) was adopted in 1983. Therefore, equivalence in USP Units of dosages in clinical studies using heparin preparations labeled in IU may be difficult to determine.

Consult current labeling for specific dosage recommendations for heparin preparations labeled in IU.

At one time, 1 mg of heparin sodium was equivalent to 100 USP Units. However, this is no longer the case because of increased purification.

### HEPARIN CALCIUM INJECTION USP

#### Usual adult dose
Full-dose (therapeutic) regimen—
Subcutaneous, deep (intrafat), 10,000 to 20,000 USP Units initially, then 8000 to 10,000 USP Units every eight hours or 15,000 to 20,000 USP Units every twelve hours, or as determined by coagulation test results. This dosage schedule is usually preceded by a loading dose of 5000 USP Units administered by intravenous injection.

Intravenous, 10,000 USP Units initially, then 5000 to 10,000 USP Units every four to six hours or 100 USP Units per kg of body weight every four hours, or as determined by coagulation test results. The dose may be administered undiluted or diluted with 50 to 100 mL of 0.9% sodium chloride injection.

Intravenous infusion, 20,000 to 40,000 USP Units in 1000 mL of 0.9% sodium chloride injection, administered over a twenty-four-hour period. This dosage schedule is usually preceded by a loading dose of 35 to 70 USP Units per kg of body weight or 5000 USP Units, administered by intravenous injection. The infusion is often administered at a rate of 1000 USP Units per hour; however, dosage must be adjusted as determined by coagulation test results.

Note: Recommendations for specific indications include:
Heart and blood vessel surgery—Intravenous, initially not less than 150 USP Units per kg of body weight. Doses of 300 USP Units per

kg of body weight are often used for procedures expected to last less than 60 minutes and doses of 400 USP units per kg of body weight are often used for procedures expected to last longer than 60 minutes. It is recommended that subsequent doses be based on coagulation test results.

Disseminated intravascular coagulation—Intravenous, 50 to 100 USP Units per kg of body weight every four hours, administered by continuous infusion or as a single injection. The medication should be discontinued if no improvement occurs within 4 to 8 hours.

Adjusted-dose regimen—
Subcutaneous, deep (intrafat), an established dose to be injected every twelve hours. The required dose is determined by adjusting heparin dosage until the midinterval (six hours after an injection) activated partial thromboplastin time (APTT) is maintained at one and one-half times the control value.

Low-dose (prophylactic) regimen—
Subcutaneous, deep (intrafat), 5000 USP Units two hours before surgery and every eight to twelve hours thereafter for seven days or until the patient is fully ambulatory, whichever is longer.

**Usual pediatric dose**
Intravenous, 50 USP Units per kg of body weight initially, then 50 to 100 USP Units per kg of body weight every four hours, or as determined by coagulation test results.

Intravenous infusion, 50 USP Units per kg of body weight as a loading dose initially, then 100 USP Units per kg of body weight added and absorbed every four hours or 20,000 USP Units per square meter of body surface every twenty-four hours, or as determined by coagulation test results.

Note: Recommendations for specific indications include:

Disseminated intravascular coagulation—Intravenous, 25 to 50 USP Units per kg of body weight every four hours, administered by continuous infusion or as a single injection. The medication should be discontinued if no improvement occurs within 4 to 8 hours.

Heart and blood vessel surgery—Intravenous, initially not less than 150 USP Units per kg of body weight. Doses of 300 USP Units per kg of body weight are often used for procedures expected to last less than 60 minutes. It is recommended that subsequent doses be based on coagulation test results.

**Strength(s) usually available**
U.S.—
Derived from porcine intestinal mucosa
25,000 USP Units per mL (Rx) [*Calciparine* (in single unit-dose containers providing 5000 USP Units per 0.2 mL; 12,500 USP Units per 0.5 mL; and 20,000 USP Units per 0.8 mL)].

Canada—
Derived from porcine intestinal mucosa
25,000 International Units (IU) per mL (Rx) [*Calcilean* (in single unit-dose containers providing 20,000 IU per 0.8 mL); *Calciparine* (in single unit-dose containers providing 5000 IU per 0.2 mL; 12,500 IU per 0.5 mL; and 20,000 IU per 0.8 mL)].

**Packaging and storage**
Store below 40 °C (104 °F), preferably between 15 and 30 °C (59 and 86 °F), unless otherwise specified by manufacturer. Protect from freezing.

**Stability**
Do not use if the solution is discolored or contains a precipitate. Some studies have indicated that loss of heparin activity may occur if heparin is diluted with 5% dextrose injection and the diluted solution is not used within 24 hours, or if diluted solutions of heparin in any diluent are stored in glass containers.

**Incompatibilities**
Heparin is strongly acidic and is incompatible with many solutions containing medications, although no loss of activity occurs when the agents are given via separate administration sites. Also, heparin may be incompatible with solutions containing a phosphate buffer, sodium carbonate, or sodium oxalate. It is recommended that heparin not be mixed, or administered through the same intravenous line, with other medications unless compatibility has first been established. In addition, heparin may be inactivated when used in conjunction with an artificial kidney because of an influx of calcium, magnesium, and acetate ions from the dialysate.

**Note**
When preparing the label, indicate that heparin calcium is of porcine mucosal origin.

## HEPARIN SODIUM INJECTION USP

**Usual adult dose**
Full-dose (therapeutic) regimen—
Subcutaneous, deep (intrafat), 10,000 to 20,000 USP Units initially, then 8000 to 10,000 USP Units every eight hours or 15,000 to 20,000 USP Units every twelve hours, or as determined by coagulation test results. This dosage schedule is usually preceded by a loading dose of 5000 USP Units administered by intravenous injection.

Intravenous, 10,000 USP Units initially, then 5000 to 10,000 USP Units every four to six hours or 100 USP Units per kg of body weight every four hours, or as determined by coagulation test results. The dose may be administered undiluted or diluted with 50 to 100 mL of 0.9% sodium chloride injection.

Intravenous infusion, 20,000 to 40,000 USP Units in 1000 mL of 0.9% sodium chloride injection, administered over a twenty-four-hour period. This dosage schedule is usually preceded by a loading dose of 35 to 70 USP Units per kg of body weight or 5000 USP Units, administered by intravenous injection. The infusion is often administered at a rate of 1000 USP Units per hour; however, dosage must be adjusted as determined by coagulation test results.

Note: Recommendations for specific indications include:

Heart and blood vessel surgery—Intravenous, initially not less than 150 USP Units per kg of body weight. Doses of 300 USP Units per kg of body weight are often used for procedures expected to last less than 60 minutes and doses of 400 USP units per kg of body weight are often used for procedures expected to last longer than 60 minutes. It is recommended that subsequent doses be based on coagulation test results.

Disseminated intravascular coagulation—Intravenous, 50 to 100 USP Units per kg of body weight every four hours, administered by continuous infusion or as a single injection. The medication should be discontinued if no improvement occurs within 4 to 8 hours.

Adjusted-dose regimen—
Subcutaneous, deep (intrafat), an established dose to be injected every twelve hours. The required dose is determined by adjusting heparin dosage until the midinterval (six hours after an injection) activated partial thromboplastin time (APTT) is maintained at one and one-half times the control value.

Low-dose (prophylactic) regimen—
Subcutaneous, deep (intrafat), 5000 USP Units two hours before surgery and every eight to twelve hours thereafter for seven days or until the patient is fully ambulatory, whichever is longer.

**Usual pediatric dose**
Intravenous, 50 USP Units per kg of body weight initially, then 50 to 100 USP Units per kg of body weight every four hours, or as determined by coagulation test results.

Intravenous infusion, 50 USP Units per kg of body weight as a loading dose initially, then 100 USP Units per kg of body weight added and absorbed every four hours or 20,000 USP Units per square meter of body surface every twenty-four hours, or as determined by coagulation test results.

Note: Recommendations for specific indications include:

Disseminated intravascular coagulation—Intravenous, 25 to 50 USP Units per kg of body weight every four hours, administered by continuous infusion or as a single injection. The medication should be discontinued if no improvement occurs within 4 to 8 hours.

Heart and blood vessel surgery—Intravenous, initially not less than 150 USP Units per kg of body weight. Doses of 300 USP Units per kg of body weight are often used for procedures expected to last less than 60 minutes. It is recommended that subsequent doses be based on coagulation test results.

**Strength(s) usually available**
U.S.—
Derived from beef lung: With preservative
1000 USP Units per mL (Rx) [GENERIC].
5000 USP Units per mL (Rx) [GENERIC].
10,000 USP Units per mL (Rx) [GENERIC].
20,000 USP Units per mL (Rx) [GENERIC].
Derived from beef lung: Without preservative
1000 USP Units per mL (Rx) [GENERIC].
5000 USP Units per mL (Rx) [GENERIC].
Derived from porcine intestinal mucosa: With preservative
1000 USP Units per mL (Rx) [*Liquaemin* (benzyl alcohol); GENERIC].
2500 USP Units per mL (Rx) [GENERIC].

5000 USP Units per mL (Rx) [*Liquaemin* (benzyl alcohol); GENERIC].
7500 USP Units per mL (Rx) [GENERIC].
10,000 USP Units per mL (Rx) [*Liquaemin* (benzyl alcohol); GENERIC].
15,000 USP Units per mL (Rx) [GENERIC].
20,000 USP Units per mL (Rx) [*Liquaemin* (benzyl alcohol); GENERIC].
25,000 USP Units per mL (Rx) [GENERIC].
40,000 USP Units per mL (Rx) [*Liquaemin* (benzyl alcohol); GENERIC].

Derived from porcine intestinal mucosa: Without preservative
1000 USP Units per mL (Rx) [*Liquaemin;* GENERIC].
5000 USP Units per mL (Rx) [*Liquaemin;* GENERIC].

Note: Single unit-dose containers may also provide the quantities of heparin sodium listed above in volumes other than 1 mL.

Canada—
Derived from porcine intestinal mucosa: With preservative
1000 International Units (IU) per mL (Rx) [*Heparin Leo* (chlorobutanol)].
1000 USP Units per mL (Rx) [*Hepalean* (benzyl alcohol); [GENERIC]].
10,000 IU per mL (Rx) [*Heparin Leo* (chlorobutanol)].
10,000 USP Units per mL (Rx) [*Hepalean* (benzyl alcohol); [GENERIC]].
25,000 IU per mL (Rx) [*Heparin Leo* (in 2-mL containers; chlorobutanol)].
25,000 USP Units per mL (Rx) [*Hepalean* (in single-dose containers providing 5000 USP Units in 0.2 mL and in 2-mL containers; benzyl alcohol)].

Derived from porcine intestinal mucosa: Without preservative
1000 IU per mL (Rx) [*Heparin Leo*].
1000 USP Units per mL (Rx) [*Hepalean*].
10,000 IU per mL (Rx) [*Heparin Leo*].
25,000 IU per mL (Rx) [*Heparin Leo* (in single-dose containers providing 5000 IU in 0.2 mL)].

**Packaging and storage**
Store below 40 °C (104 °F), preferably between 15 and 30 °C (59 and 86 °F), unless otherwise specified by manufacturer. Protect from freezing.

**Stability**
Do not use if the solution is discolored or contains a precipitate. Some studies have indicated that loss of heparin activity may occur if heparin is diluted with 5% dextrose injection and the diluted solution is not used within 24 hours, or if diluted solutions of heparin in any diluent are stored in glass containers.

**Incompatibilities**
Heparin is strongly acidic and is incompatible with many solutions containing medications, although no loss of activity occurs when the agents are given via separate administration sites. Also, heparin may be incompatible with solutions containing a phosphate buffer, sodium carbonate, or sodium oxalate. It is recommended that heparin not be mixed, or administered through the same intravenous line, with other medications unless compatibility has first been established. In addition, heparin may be inactivated when used in conjunction with an artificial kidney because of an influx of calcium, magnesium, and acetate ions from the dialysate.

**Note**
When preparing the label, indicate the organ and species from which the heparin is derived.

**Additional information**
Heparin sodium injections that contain benzyl alcohol should not be administered to premature neonates because the preservative has been associated with a fatal "gasping syndrome" in these patients.

## HEPARIN SODIUM IN DEXTROSE INJECTION

**Usual adult dose**
Intravenous infusion, 20,000 to 40,000 USP Units, administered over a twenty-four-hour period. This dosage schedule is usually preceded by a loading dose of 35 to 70 USP Units per kg of body weight or 5000 USP Units, administered by intravenous injection. The infusion is often administered at a rate of 1000 USP Units per hour; however, dosage must be adjusted as determined by coagulation test results.

**Usual pediatric dose**
Intravenous infusion, 50 USP Units per kg of body weight as a loading dose initially, then 100 USP Units per kg of body weight added and absorbed every four hours or 20,000 USP Units per square meter of body surface every twenty-four hours, or as determined by coagulation test results.

**Strength(s) usually available**
U.S.—
Derived from porcine intestinal mucosa
20 USP Units per mL (10,000 USP Units per 500 mL), with 5% of dextrose (Rx) [GENERIC].
40 USP Units per mL (20,000 USP Units per 500 mL), with 5% of dextrose (Rx) [GENERIC].
50 USP Units per mL (12,500 USP Units per 250 mL and 25,000 USP Units per 500 mL), with 5% of dextrose (Rx) [GENERIC].
100 USP Units per mL (10,000 USP Units per 100 mL and 25,000 USP Units per 250 mL), with 5% of dextrose (Rx) [GENERIC].

Canada—
Derived from porcine intestinal mucosa
40 USP Units per mL (20,000 USP Units per 500 mL), with 5% of dextrose (Rx) [[GENERIC]].

**Packaging and storage**
Store below 40 °C (104 °F), preferably between 15 and 30 °C (59 and 86 °F), unless otherwise specified by manufacturer. Protect from freezing.

**Incompatibilities**
Heparin is strongly acidic and is incompatible with many solutions containing medications, although no loss of activity occurs when the agents are given via separate administration sites. Also, heparin may be incompatible with solutions containing a phosphate buffer, sodium carbonate, or sodium oxalate. It is recommended that heparin not be mixed, or administered through the same intravenous line, with other medications unless compatibility has first been established.

## HEPARIN SODIUM IN SODIUM CHLORIDE INJECTION

**Usual adult dose**
Intravenous infusion, 20,000 to 40,000 USP Units, administered over a twenty-four-hour period. This dosage schedule is usually preceded by a loading dose of 35 to 70 USP Units per kg of body weight or 5000 USP Units, administered by intravenous injection. The infusion is often administered at a rate of l000 USP Units per hour; however, dosage must be adjusted as determined by coagulation test results.

**Usual pediatric dose**
Intravenous infusion, 50 USP Units per kg of body weight as a loading dose initially, then 100 USP Units per kg of body weight added and absorbed every four hours or 20,000 USP Units per square meter of body surface every twenty-four hours, or as determined by coagulation test results.

**Strength(s) usually available**
U.S.—
Derived from porcine intestinal mucosa
2 USP Units per mL (1000 USP Units per 500 mL and 2000 USP Units per 1000 mL), with 0.9% of sodium chloride (Rx) [GENERIC].
50 USP Units per mL (12,500 USP Units per 250 mL and 25,000 USP Units per 500 mL), with 0.45% of sodium chloride (Rx) [GENERIC].
100 USP Units per mL (25,000 USP Units per 250 mL), with 0.45% of sodium chloride (Rx) [GENERIC].

Canada—
Derived from porcine intestinal mucosa
2 USP Units per mL (1000 USP Units per 500 mL and 2000 USP Units per 1000 mL), with 0.9% of sodium chloride (Rx) [[GENERIC]].
5 USP Units per mL (5000 USP Units per 1000 mL), with 0.9% of sodium chloride (Rx) [[GENERIC]].

**Packaging and storage**
Store below 40 °C (104 °F), preferably between 15 and 30 °C (59 and 86 °F), unless otherwise specified by manufacturer. Protect from freezing.

**Incompatibilities**
Heparin is strongly acidic and is incompatible with many solutions containing medications, although no loss of activity occurs when the agents are given via separate administration sites. Also, heparin may be incompatible with solutions containing a phosphate buffer, sodium carbonate, or sodium oxalate. It is recommended that heparin not be mixed, or administered through the same intravenous line, with other medications unless compatibility has first been established.

Revised: August 1990
Interim revision: 08/23/94

# HEPATITIS A VACCINE INACTIVATED  Systemic

VA CLASSIFICATION (Primary): IM100

Note: This monograph is specific for the inactivated whole virus vaccine derived from hepatitis A virus (HAV) and grown in human diploid cell (MRC-5) culture.

Commonly used brand name(s): *Havrix; Vaqta*.

Note: For a listing of dosage forms and brand names by country availability, see *Dosage Forms* section(s).

Note: All cases of suspected or confirmed side/adverse effects following the administration of hepatitis A vaccine inactivated should be reported to the U.S. Department of Health and Human Services' Vaccine Adverse Events Reporting System (VAERS).

## Category

Immunizing agent (active).

## Indications

### General considerations

Hepatitis A virus (HAV), previously known as the infectious hepatitis virus, is acquired by ingesting uncooked or undercooked seafood from polluted water, swimming in polluted water, and by person-to-person spread. Food and water are the leading sources of HAV transmission because of the relative stability of the virus itself, poor sanitation in large areas of the world, and abundant HAV shedding in feces.

Travelers to HAV-endemic areas should avoid eating uncooked or undercooked food, especially fruits and vegetables contaminated by polluted water or human fecal fertilizer, and shellfish taken from polluted waters, and should peel fruits themselves. Travelers also should avoid drinking polluted water and the ice and drinks made from it, and should avoid swimming or bathing in polluted fresh or ocean water.

General improvement in hygiene, especially in water supplies and sewage disposal, in many industrialized and industrializing countries has resulted in a falling level of natural immunity to the disease. This in turn has led to a substantial rise in the proportion of persons with no protective antibodies, which places them at risk for HAV infection. It has been shown that seronegative travelers and military personnel visiting regions where HAV is endemic are at higher risk of hepatitis A. This higher risk has also been demonstrated in seronegative health care workers and day-care center staff.

In developing countries, HAV infection in children is frequent and typically mild, leading to the formation of antibodies and immunity. In such areas, there is at present little need for hepatitis A vaccine. However, in certain industrialized countries that have a higher level of sanitation, immunity is not acquired during childhood, and hepatitis A typically occurs in adults. Tourism is one of the largest businesses in many developing countries where hepatitis A is endemic, and susceptible travelers are at high risk of acquiring infection.

Many travel medicine experts estimate that the morbidity from HAV among international travelers is much higher than that from other vaccine-preventable infections. HAV infection accounts for 20 to 25% of clinically apparent acute hepatitis cases worldwide. In the U.S., 20 to 30% of all documented cases of acute viral hepatitis are due to HAV. Therefore, travelers to areas in which there is a recognized risk of exposure to HAV should take the necessary precautions. Risk is greatest for travelers to countries of Africa, Asia (except Japan), parts of the Caribbean, Central and South America, eastern Europe, the Mediterranean basin, the Middle East, and Mexico. For travelers to these areas of the world, risk of infection increases with duration of travel, and will be highest in those who live in or visit rural areas, travel through back country areas, or frequently eat or drink in settings of poor sanitation.

### Accepted

Hepatitis A (prophylaxis)—Hepatitis A vaccine inactivated is indicated for preexposure immunization against disease caused by hepatitis A virus (HAV) in persons 2 years of age or older.

Unless otherwise contraindicated, hepatitis A vaccine inactivated is indicated in persons 2 years of age or older who are at increased risk of infection by HAV and for any person wishing to obtain immunity. Examples of groups identified as being at increased risk of infection include:
- International travelers. Persons from areas of low endemicity who travel to areas of intermediate or high endemicity are at risk for acquiring hepatitis A. These areas include, but are not limited to, Africa, Asia (except Japan), parts of the Caribbean, Central and South America, eastern Europe, the Mediterranean basin, the Middle East, and Mexico. Current advisories from the Centers for Disease Control and Prevention (CDC) should be consulted for information about specific locales. Immunization should be considered for persons traveling to areas where hepatitis A is highly endemic, for travel of long duration, and for those who travel repeatedly. Primary immunization with hepatitis A vaccine inactivated should be completed at least 2 weeks prior to expected exposure to HAV. Travelers to Australia, Canada, Japan, New Zealand, the U.S., and western Europe do not have a significantly increased risk of hepatitis A and, therefore, vaccination is not warranted.
- Military personnel identified as being at increased risk. Prevention of hepatitis A in military personnel is essential. This is especially important for military personnel from developed countries who are deployed in areas where hepatitis A is common, particularly during conflicts. Immunization should be considered for military personnel traveling to areas of higher endemicity for hepatitis A.
- People living in or relocating to areas of higher HAV endemicity.
- Populations that experience cyclic hepatitis A epidemics, such as Alaskan Eskimos and Native Americans. Hepatitis A is endemic in Native Americans; infection rates approach 100 cases per 100,000 people. In Alaskan Eskimos, large HAV epidemics occur every 10 to 12 years, resulting in thousands of cases of clinical illness and a few deaths. Studies have shown the effectiveness of the hepatitis A vaccine in Alaskan Eskimos. Consideration should be given to vaccination of these groups of people.
- Persons engaging in high-risk sexual activity, such as sexually active homosexual and bisexual males. Extensive hepatitis A outbreaks among homosexual men have been recognized in urban areas of the U.S., England, and Australia. Therefore, sexually active homosexual and bisexual men should be considered for vaccination with hepatitis A vaccine.
- Users of illicit injectable drugs. Within the past decade, hepatitis A outbreaks have been reported with increasing frequency among users of illicit injectable drugs, both in the U.S. and Europe. As these individuals may have underlying liver disease due to chronic infection with other hepatotropic viruses, they may be at higher risk for severe complications from hepatitis A. Consideration should be given to vaccination of these individuals.
- Residents of a community experiencing an outbreak of hepatitis A.
- Certain institutional workers, such as caretakers for the developmentally disabled.
- Employees of child day-care centers. Outbreaks have been recognized among children and employees in day-care centers, and in some instances these outbreaks may be the source of larger community epidemics. Outbreaks have been recognized predominantly in centers with children who are not toilet-trained, and where clinical disease occurs in staff, parents, and older siblings of day-care center children. The use of immune globulin (IG) has been well documented to control outbreaks of disease in these settings. Although use of hepatitis A vaccine has not yet been studied in the day-care center setting, the available data from efficacy studies suggest that the vaccine may be able to replace IG in control of day-care center outbreaks.
- Laboratory workers who handle live HAV.
- Handlers of primate animals that may be harboring HAV. Since viral hepatitis was recognized among primates caretakers, consideration should be given to vaccination of handlers of primate animals that may be harboring HAV.
- Patients with hemophilia. Outbreaks of HAV infection in patients with hemophilia receiving solvent detergent–treated factor concentrates have been reported primarily in Europe. However, in the U.S., three cases of HAV infection were reported in the mid-1990s in patients with hemophilia who received factor VIII concentrate from a single lot from one manufacturer. Available seroprevalence data in the U.S. from patients with hemophilia do not allow accurate determination of risk. Nevertheless, patients with hemophilia, especially those receiving solvent detergent–treated factor concentrates, may benefit from protection against HAV infection and should be considered for immunization. Preimmunization testing for anti-HAV antibody may be cost-effective because seroprevalence rates among persons with hemophilia may be higher.
- Food handlers. Food-borne outbreaks usually are associated with contamination of uncooked food during preparation by a food handler who is infected with HAV. The most effective means to prevent these outbreaks is by careful hygienic practices during food preparation. Little information is available concerning seroprevalence rates of HAV antibody in food handlers compared with that in the general population. Therefore, routine hepatitis A vaccination is not indicated in this population. However, economic, medicolegal, and public relations implications of a food-borne HAV outbreak from a commercial establishment may indicate that use of hepatitis A vaccine inactivated should be

considered in some circumstances. Factors to consider in this decision include the nature of the food (e.g., materials for salads) as well as the demographic characteristics, the average duration of employment, and the number of food handlers.
- Persons with chronic liver disease, including those with alcoholic cirrhosis, chronic hepatitis B, chronic hepatitis C, autoimmune hepatitis, and primary biliary cirrhosis. Since clinical hepatitis A may be more severe in persons with chronic liver disease due to hepatitis viruses or other etiologies, vaccination of these persons should be considered. Although few data exist about the immunogenicity and protective efficacy of hepatitis A vaccine inactivated in persons with chronic liver disease, no reason exists to suspect that the hepatitis A vaccine inactivated would aggravate the chronic condition.

### Unaccepted
Hepatitis A vaccine inactivated will not give protection from hepatitis caused by infectious agents other than HAV.

## Pharmacology/Pharmacokinetics

### Physicochemical characteristics
Source—Hepatitis A vaccine inactivated is a sterile suspension for intramuscular injection. The vaccine is a whole virus vaccine derived from hepatitis A virus (HAV), grown in human diploid cell (MRC-5) culture, and inactivated with formalin. The vaccine contains HAV antigen adsorbed onto aluminum provided as aluminum hydroxide.

### Protective effect
Clinical studies in animals and humans have shown that hepatitis A vaccine inactivated is safe and highly immunogenic. Immunogenicity studies have shown that 70 to 90% of persons develop antibodies to HAV (anti-HAV) following a single dose, and nearly 100% of persons develop antibodies following two doses of vaccine. The presence of anti-HAV confers protection against hepatitis A infection. However, the lowest titer needed to confer protection has not been determined. Antibody levels obtained after a single dose of vaccine are often higher than those obtained after a single dose of IG, and substantial levels of anti-HAV neutralizing antibody are present in the majority of recipients of a complete immunization series. One immunogenicity study has suggested that simultaneous administration of large doses of immune globulin (IG) with the first vaccine dose may lower the active antibody response. However, the lowering of antibody titer levels does not appear great enough to have an impact on the protective effect of the vaccine.

### Time to protective effect
After receiving the initial dose of hepatitis A vaccine, persons are considered protected in 4 weeks. For long-term protection, a second dose is needed 6 to 12 months later. For persons who will travel to high-risk areas in < 4 weeks after the initial vaccine dose, IG (0.02 mL per kg of body weight) should be administered simultaneously with the first dose of vaccine but at different injection sites.

### Duration of protective effect
The duration of protection after vaccination is unknown. However, antibody decay studies suggest that measurable antibody will persist for many years. Continued observation of immunized persons will be required to determine the need for later booster doses of vaccine.

## Precautions to Consider

### Pregnancy/Reproduction
Pregnancy—Adequate and well-controlled studies have not been done in humans. However, hepatitis A vaccine inactivated, if indicated, should be given to pregnant women. Although data on the safety of hepatitis A vaccine inactivated for the developing fetus are not available, no risk would be expected because the vaccine contains inactivated, purified viral proteins. In contrast, infection with the hepatitis A virus (HAV) in a pregnant woman can result in severe disease in the mother.
Studies have not been done in animals.
FDA Pregnancy Category C.

### Breast-feeding
It is not known whether hepatitis A vaccine inactivated is distributed into breast milk. However, problems in humans have not been documented.

### Pediatrics
Children have the highest age-specific incidence of hepatitis A and are likely to play a role in its spread. Hepatitis A vaccine inactivated is well tolerated and highly immunogenic and effective in children 2 years of age and older. In a double-blind, controlled study in the U.S. involving 1037 children, aged 2 to 16 years, who were randomly assigned to receive either one intramuscular injection of inactivated hepatitis A vaccine or placebo, 25 cases of clinical hepatitis A occurred in the control group while none were noted in the vaccinated group, establishing a protective efficacy of 100%. A similar study performed in Thailand showed similar results. Safety and efficacy of hepatitis A vaccine inactivated in infants and children younger than 2 years of age have not been established, and use is not recommended.

### Geriatrics
No information is available on the relationship of age to the effects of hepatitis A vaccine inactivated in geriatric patients.

### Drug interactions and/or related problems
The following drug interactions and/or related problems have been selected on the basis of their potential clinical significance (possible mechanism in parentheses where appropriate)—not necessarily inclusive (» = major clinical significance):

Note: Combinations containing any of the following medications, depending on the amount present, may also interact with this medication.

Immunosuppressive agents or
Radiation therapy
(because normal defense mechanisms are suppressed, the patient's antibody response to hepatitis A vaccine inactivated may be decreased)

### Laboratory value alterations
The following have been selected on the basis of their potential clinical significance (possible effect in parentheses where appropriate)—not necessarily inclusive (» = major clinical significance):

With physiology/laboratory test values
Alanine aminotransferase (ALT [SGPT]) and
Alkaline phosphatase and
Aspartate aminotransferase (AST [SGOT])
(serum values may be increased)

### Medical considerations/Contraindications
The medical considerations/contraindications included have been selected on the basis of their potential clinical significance (reasons given in parentheses where appropriate)—not necessarily inclusive (» = major clinical significance).

*Risk-benefit should be considered when the following medical problem exists:*
» Hypersensitivity to hepatitis A vaccine inactivated
(there have been rare reports of anaphylaxis/anaphylactoid reactions following the use of hepatitis A vaccine inactivated in some countries; therefore, persons experiencing hypersensitivity reactions after a dose of hepatitis A vaccine inactivated should not receive further doses of the vaccine.)

## Side/Adverse Effects

Note: Cases of convulsions, dizziness, encephalopathy, Guillain-Barré syndrome, multiple sclerosis, myelitis, neuropathy, and paresthesia have been reported following administration of hepatitis A vaccine inactivated. However, no causal relationship has been established.
Angioedema, dyspnea, erythema multiforme, hepatitis, hyperhidrosis, jaundice, lymphadenopathy, and syncope have been reported since market introduction of the vaccine, but the relationship to the vaccine is unclear.

The following side/adverse effects have been selected on the basis of their potential clinical significance (possible signs and symptoms in parentheses where appropriate)—not necessarily inclusive:

### Those indicating need for medical attention
Incidence rare
*Anaphylactic reaction* (difficulty in breathing or swallowing; hives; itching, especially of soles or palms; reddening of skin, especially around ears; swelling of eyes, face, or inside of nose; unusual tiredness or weakness, sudden and severe)

### Those indicating need for medical attention only if they continue or are bothersome
Incidence more frequent
*Soreness at injection site*—incidence 21 to 56%
Note: Local reactions are common but generally mild. Although rare, since market introduction of the vaccine, localized edema has also been reported following administration of the vaccine.

Incidence less frequent
*Anorexia* (lack of appetite); *fever ≥ 37.7 °C (100 °F); headache; malaise* (general feeling of discomfort or illness); *nausea; tenderness or warmth at injection site*

Incidence rare
*Arthralgia, arthritis, or myalgia* (aches or pain in joints or muscles); *diarrhea or stomach cramps or pain; lymphadenopathy* (swelling of glands in armpits or neck); *pruritus* (itching); *urticaria* (welts); *vomiting*

## Patient Consultation

As an aid to patient consultation, refer to *Advice for the Patient, Hepatitis A Vaccine Inactivated (Systemic)*.

In providing consultation, consider emphasizing the following selected information (» = major clinical significance):

**Before using this medication**
» Conditions affecting use, especially:
    Hypersensitivity to hepatitis A vaccine inactivated
    Use in children—Use is not recommended in infants and children younger than 2 years of age

**Proper use of this medication**
» Proper dosing

**Side/adverse effects**
Signs of potential side effects, especially anaphylactic reaction

## General Dosing Information

Appropriate precautions should be taken prior to vaccine injection to prevent allergic or other unwanted reactions. Precautions should include a review of the patient's history regarding possible sensitivity and the ready availability of epinephrine 1:1000 and other appropriate agents used for control of immediate allergic reactions.

Hepatitis A vaccine inactivated is administered by *intramuscular* injection. It should not be injected intravenously, intradermally, or subcutaneously.

The deltoid muscle (outer aspect of the upper arm) is the recommended site for the immunization of adults and older children. The vaccine should not be administered in the gluteal region since administration at this site may result in suboptimal response.

Vaccination of an immune person is not contraindicated and does not increase the risk of adverse effects. Prevaccination serologic testing may be indicated for adult travelers who probably have had prior hepatitis A virus (HAV) infection, if the cost of testing is less than the cost of vaccination and if testing will not interfere with completion of the vaccine series. Such persons may include those older than 40 years of age and those born in areas of the world having a high endemicity of HAV infection. Postvaccination testing for serologic response is not indicated.

The Advisory Committee on Immunization Practices (ACIP) offers the following recommendations for the use of inactivated hepatitis A vaccine among international travelers:
- All susceptible persons traveling to or working in countries with intermediate or high HAV endemicity (countries other than Australia, Canada, Japan, New Zealand, the U.S., and countries in Scandinavia and western Europe) should be vaccinated or receive immune globulin (IG) before departure. Hepatitis A vaccine at the age-appropriate dose is preferred for persons who plan to travel repeatedly to, or reside for long periods in, these high-risk areas. IG is recommended for travelers younger than 2 years of age.
- After receiving the initial dose of hepatitis A vaccine, persons are considered protected in 4 weeks. For long-term protection, a second dose is needed 6 to 12 months later. For persons who will travel to high-risk areas in less than 4 weeks after the initial vaccine dose, IG (0.02 mL per kg of body weight) should be administered simultaneously with the first dose of vaccine but at a different injection site.
- Persons who are allergic to a vaccine component or otherwise elect not to receive the vaccine should receive a single dose of IG (0.02 mL per kg of body weight), which provides effective protection against hepatitis A for up to 3 months. IG should be administered at 0.06 mL per kg of body weight and must be repeated if travel is longer than 5 months.

Hepatitis A vaccine inactivated can be administered simultaneously with other vaccines and toxoids, including cholera, diphtheria, hepatitis B, Japanese encephalitis, rabies, tetanus, oral typhoid, and yellow fever, without affecting immunogenicity or increasing the frequency of adverse effects. However, during simultaneous administration, the vaccines should be given at separate injection sites. Hepatitis A and hepatitis B vaccines induce a similar immune response when given either separately or concomitantly.

When IG is given concurrently with the first dose of vaccine, the proportion of persons who develop protective levels of anti-HAV antibody is not affected, but antibody concentrations are lower. Because the final concentrations of anti-HAV antibody are substantially higher than those considered to be protective, this reduced immunogenicity is not expected to be clinically important.

Hepatitis A vaccine inactivated should replace IG for use in preexposure prophylaxis against HAV. On the other hand, hepatitis A vaccine inactivated has little to offer after a person has been exposed to HAV, because the need for protection is immediate and exposure is almost always limited to a brief period. Thus, when hepatitis A is recognized in a patient, close family member, or household contact, IG should be given for prophylaxis, optimally within two weeks after exposure.

Hepatitis A vaccine inactivated does not enhance disease progression in human immunodeficiency virus (HIV)–infected persons and can be administered safely to persons who are HIV-positive.

### For treatment of adverse effects

Recommended treatment consists of the following:
- For mild hypersensitivity reaction—Administering antihistamines, and, if necessary, corticosteroids. In mild anaphylaxis, antihistamines or subcutaneous epinephrine may be all that is necessary if the condition is progressing slowly and is not life-threatening, regardless of the organ or system affected. Under these circumstances the risks associated with intravenous epinephrine administration outweigh the benefits.
- For severe hypersensitivity or anaphylactic reaction—Administering epinephrine. Antihistamines or corticosteroids may also be administered as required. Epinephrine is the treatment of choice for severe hypersensitivity or anaphylactic reaction. If the patient's condition is not stable, epinephrine should be infused. Norepinephrine may be preferable if there is no bronchospasm. For bronchospasm, epinephrine should be given with corticosteroids. Other bronchodilators, such as intravenous aminophylline or albuterol by nebulization, also should be considered.

## Parenteral Dosage Forms

### HEPATITIS A VACCINE INACTIVATED INJECTION

**Usual adult dose**
Hepatitis A (prophylaxis)—
    Intramuscular, a single dose of 1440 enzyme linked immunosorbent assay (ELISA) Units (*Havrix*) or 50 Units (*Vaqta*).

Note: A booster dose is recommended six months after the first dose of (*Vaqta*), or six to twelve months after the first dose of (*Havrix*).

**Usual pediatric dose**
Hepatitis A (prophylaxis)—
    Children 2 to 18 years of age—Intramuscular, a single dose of 720 enzyme linked immunosorbent assay (ELISA) Units or two doses of 360 enzyme linked immunosorbent assay (ELISA) Units given one month apart (*Havrix*—U.S. and Canada).
    Children 2 to 17 years of age—Intramuscular, a single dose of 25 Units (*Vaqta*—U.S.).
    Children younger than 2 years of age—Use is not recommended.

Note: A booster dose is recommended six months after the first dose of (*Vaqta*—U.S.), or six to twelve months after the first dose of (*Havrix*—U.S. and Canada).

**Strength(s) usually available**
U.S.—
    1440 enzyme linked immunosorbent assay (ELISA) units viral antigen, adsorbed on 0.5 mg of aluminum hydroxide in each 1-mL adult dose (Rx) [*Havrix* (formalin approximately 0.1 mg)].
    360 enzyme linked immunosorbent assay (ELISA) units viral antigen, adsorbed on 0.25 mg of aluminum hydroxide in each 0.5-mL pediatric dose (Rx) [*Havrix* (formalin approximately 0.05 mg)].
    720 enzyme linked immunosorbent assay (ELISA) units viral antigen, adsorbed on 0.25 mg of aluminum hydroxide in each 0.5-mL pediatric dose (Rx) [*Havrix* (formalin approximately 0.05 mg)].
    50 units viral antigen, adsorbed on 0.45 mg of aluminum hydroxide in each 1-mL adult dose (Rx) [*Vaqta* (formaldehyde approximately 0.8 mcg)].
    25 units viral antigen, adsorbed on 0.225 mg of aluminum hydroxide in each 0.5-mL pediatric dose (Rx) [*Vaqta* (formaldehyde approximately 0.4 mcg)].
Canada—
    1440 enzyme linked immunosorbent assay (ELISA) units viral antigen, adsorbed on 0.5 mg of aluminum hydroxide in each 1-mL adult dose (Rx) [*Havrix* (formalin approximately 0.1 mg)].
    360 enzyme linked immunosorbent assay (ELISA) units viral antigen, adsorbed on 0.25 mg of aluminum hydroxide in each 0.5-mL pediatric dose (Rx) [*Havrix* (formalin approximately 0.05 mg)].
    50 units viral antigen, adsorbed on 0.45 mg of aluminum hydroxide in each 1-mL adult dose (Rx) [*Vaqta* (formaldehyde approximately 0.8 mcg)].
    25 units viral antigen, adsorbed on 0.225 mg of aluminum hydroxide in each 0.5-mL pediatric dose (Rx) [*Vaqta* (formaldehyde approximately 0.4 mcg)].

**Packaging and storage**
Store between 2 and 8 °C (36 and 46 °F), unless otherwise specified by the manufacturer. Protect from freezing.

## Preparation of dosage form
The vaccine should be used as supplied, and should not be diluted. The vial should be shaken well immediately before withdrawal of the dose. In addition, thorough agitation at the time of administration is necessary to maintain suspension of the vaccine. After agitation, the vaccine is a slightly opaque, white suspension. The vaccine should be discarded if the suspension does not appear homogenous.

## Stability
Storage below the recommended temperature may reduce potency. Freezing destroys potency, and the vaccine should be discarded if freezing occurs.

## Auxiliary labeling
- Do not freeze; discard if freezing occurs.
- Shake well.

## Selected Bibliography
Centers for Disease Control. Recommendations of the Advisory Committee on Immunization Practices (ACIP): prevention of hepatitis A through active or passive immunization. MMWR Morb Mortal Wkly Rep 1996; 45(15): 1-30.

American Academy of Pediatrics. Hepatitis A. In: Peter G, editor. 1997 Red Book: report of the Committee on Infectious Diseases. 24th ed. Elk Grove Village, IL: American Academy of Pediatrics; 1997. p. 237-46.

Developed: 02/06/97
Interim revision: 07/31/98

# HEPATITIS B VACCINE RECOMBINANT  Systemic

VA CLASSIFICATION (Primary): IM100

Note: This monograph is specific to the recombinant DNA hepatitis B vaccine derived from the surface antigen of hepatitis B virus (HBsAg) and produced in yeast (*Saccharomyces cerevisiae*) cells.

Commonly used brand name(s): *Engerix-B*; *Recombivax HB*; *Recombivax HB Dialysis Formulation*.

Another commonly used name is HB vaccine.

Note: For a listing of dosage forms and brand names by country availability, see *Dosage Forms* section(s).

## Category
Immunizing agent (active).

## Indications

### General considerations
Hepatitis B virus (HBV) (previously known as the serum hepatitis virus) infection is a major cause of acute and chronic hepatitis, cirrhosis, and primary hepatocellular carcinoma worldwide. It is estimated that more than 200 million persons are chronically infected with HBV worldwide, and up to 80% of new liver cancer cases each year are attributable to HBV infection.

Viral hepatitis is the second most reported disease in the U.S., with hepatitis B accounting for about 45% of cases. HBV infection is a significant cause of morbidity and mortality in the U.S., and there are approximately 200,000 to 300,000 new cases of hepatitis B infection each year. Among infected persons, approximately 4000 to 5000 die each year of HBV-induced chronic liver disease or hepatocellular carcinoma. It is estimated that more than 1 million Americans have chronic HBV infection. In the U.S., most persons infected with HBV acquire the infection during adolescence or young adulthood. HBV is transmitted primarily through sexual contact, intravenous drug use, regular household contact with a chronically infected person, or occupational exposure. However, for approximately one third of persons who have acute hepatitis B, the source of infection is unknown.

Because of lifestyle, occupation, or ethnicity, certain groups have a much higher risk of hepatitis B infection than the general population. These groups include health care workers, those undergoing dialysis, persons from areas in which HBV infection is endemic, homosexual men, heterosexual persons with multiple sex partners, intravenous drug users, household contacts of HBV carriers, children of carrier mothers, and clients and staff of programs for the developmentally disabled.

In pregnancy, HBV is thought to be transmitted primarily at the time of delivery. Vertical transmission is an effective route for neonatal infection, and 10 to 85% of infants born to hepatitis B surface antigen (HBsAg)–positive mothers will become infected, depending on the hepatitis B e antigen (HBeAg) status of the mother. Morbidity and mortality rates are significant higher among infected infants than in the general newborn population, with 90% having chronic infection, and 25% of this population ultimately dying of complications of liver disease. However, 90% of infections can be prevented if HBsAg–positive mothers are identified, and their offspring are treated promptly after delivery with hepatitis B immune globulin and hepatitis B vaccine.

The Centers for Disease Control and Prevention (CDC) and the American College of Obstetricians and Gynecologists recommend adding HBsAg to routine early prenatal tests and notifying the pediatrician as soon as possible as to the HBV status of the mother so the newborn can be given HBV vaccination and hepatitis B immune globulin as appropriate.

After a person has been exposed to HBV, appropriate immunoprophylactic treatment can effectively prevent infection. The mainstay of postexposure immunoprophylaxis is hepatitis B vaccine, but in some settings the addition of hepatitis B immune globulin will provide some increase in protection.

Coinfection with HBV and human immunodeficiency virus (HIV) is common in the U.S. The two viruses are transmitted through similar routes, including sexual contact, sharing of infected needles, and exposure to infected blood products. In one study, the prevalence of HBV markers in patients with acquired immune deficiency syndrome (AIDS) was reported to be as high as 89%. These patients are at high risk of developing a chronic carrier state, viremia, and chronic hepatitis. At present, no medication therapy can reliably treat patients with chronic HBV infection. Theoretically, early identification and vaccination of high-risk groups against HBV before they acquire HIV infection should produce the best response to the vaccine. However, this strategy has not been successful, and coinfection continues to be a significant cause of morbidity and mortality in these patients.

### Accepted
Hepatitis B virus infection (prophylaxis)—Hepatitis B recombinant vaccine is indicated for immunization of persons of all ages against infection caused by all subtypes of hepatitis B virus. The dialysis formulation of hepatitis B recombinant vaccine is indicated for immunization of adult predialysis and dialysis patients.

Hepatitis B recombinant vaccine is also recommended in conjunction with hepatitis B immune globulin (HBIG) for postexposure prophylaxis.

Unless otherwise contraindicated, hepatitis B recombinant vaccine is recommended for all infants (whether at high or low risk), adolescents, and persons of all ages who live in areas of high prevalence of hepatitis B infection or who are, or will be, at increased risk of infection from hepatitis B virus. The Committee on Infectious Diseases of the American Academy of Pediatrics, the Advisory Committee on Immunization Practices of the Centers for Disease Control and Prevention, and the American Academy of Family Physicians recommend that all adolescents who have not previously received three doses of hepatitis B vaccine should initiate or complete the series at the 11- to 12-year-old visit to the physician.

Examples of groups identified as being at increased risk of infection include:

- Newborn infants, including those born to HBsAg-positive mothers whether or not the infants are HBeAg-positive. The routine hepatitis B vaccination series should begin at birth for all infants. Infants of HBsAg-positive mothers should receive the first dose of vaccine along with immunoprophylaxis with hepatitis B immune globulin.
- Health care personnel. HBV infection is a major infectious occupational hazard for healthcare and public safety workers. The risk of acquiring HBV infection from occupational exposure is dependent on the frequency of percutaneous and permucosal exposures to blood or blood products. Risk is often the highest during the professional training period of medical personnel. Therefore, immunization should be completed during training in the schools of medicine, dentistry, nursing, laboratory technology, and other allied health professions before workers have their first occupational contact with human blood.
- Employees in medical facilities, such as paramedical personnel and custodial staff, who may be exposed to the virus via blood, blood products, or other patient specimens.
- Patients and staff of institutions or residential settings for the developmentally disabled. Staff who work closely with patients, and the patients themselves, should be immunized. The risk in institutional en-

vironments is associated not only with blood exposure, but also with bites and contact with skin lesions and other infective secretions.
- Staff of nonresidential day-care programs for the developmentally disabled, such as schools and sheltered workshops. Staff who have clients who are HBV carriers are at a risk of HBV infection comparable to that of health care workers. Although the risk of HBV infection to other clients appears to be lower than the risk to staff, immunization of clients is recommended if a client who is an HBV carrier is aggressive or has special medical problems that increase the risk of others exposure to his or her blood or serous secretions.
- Sexually active homosexual and bisexual males, including those with human immunodeficiency virus (HIV) infection. Sexually active homosexual and bisexual males should be immunized regardless of their age or the duration of their homosexual practices. Males should be immunized as soon as possible after their homosexual activity begins or if they anticipate initiating homosexual activity.
- Sexually active heterosexual persons with multiple sexual partners. Heterosexual persons with multiple sexual partners are at increased risk of HBV infection; the risk increases with the number of sexual partners. Immunization is recommended for prostitutes, persons with a history of multiple sexual partners in the last 6 months, and persons who have recently or repeatedly acquired other sexually transmitted diseases.
- Hemodialysis patients. Although seroconversion rates and antibody to hepatitis B surface antigen (anti-HBs) titers are lower after vaccination in hemodialysis patients than in healthy persons, for the patients who do respond, hepatitis B recombinant vaccine will protect them from HBV infection and reduce the need for frequent serologic screening.
- Patients with renal disease. Some studies have shown higher seroconversion rates and antibody titers after vaccination for patients with uremia who were immunized before they required dialysis. Therefore, it is recommended that patients be immunized early in the course of renal disease.
- Users of illicit injection drugs. Injection drug abusers should be immunized as soon as possible after drug abuse begins.
- Patients with clotting disorders who receive clotting factor concentrates. These patients are at increased risk of HBV infection and should be immunized at the time that their specific clotting disorder is identified. Preimmunization testing for HBsAg may be cost-effective in patients who have already received multiple infusions of these blood products.
- Household and sexual contacts of HBV carriers. Household contacts of HBV carriers are at high risk, and their sexual contacts appear to be at the greatest risk, of HBV infection.
- Persons accepting orphans or adoptees from countries of high or intermediate HBV endemicity. The children should be tested for HBsAg. If the children are found to be positive, the adopting family members should be immunized.
- Populations with high endemicity of HBV infection, such as Alaskan Eskimos, Pacific Islanders, Haitian and Indochinese immigrants, and refugees from HBV-endemic areas.
- Inmates of long-term correctional facilities.
- International travelers. Immunization should be considered for travelers who plan to reside abroad for more than 6 months and will have close contact with the local population in areas with high levels of endemic HBV. Immunization also should be considered for short-term travelers who are likely to have sexual contact with, or contact with blood from, members of the local population in endemic areas.
- Military personnel identified as being at increased risk.
- Morticians and embalmers.
- Police and fire department personnel. Paramedical or other personnel who render first aid or medical assistance may be exposed to the hepatitis B virus.

Hepatitis D virus infection (prophylaxis)—Since hepatitis D infection (caused by the delta hepatitis virus) can occur only in the presence of hepatitis B infection, it can be expected that hepatitis D infection will be prevented by immunization with hepatitis B recombinant vaccine.

### Unaccepted
Because this vaccine protects only against infection with subtypes of hepatitis B virus (and indirectly against infection with hepatitis D virus), immunization with hepatitis B recombinant vaccine is not an indication for, and will not provide protection against, hepatitis caused by other hepatitis viruses or by other viruses known to infect the liver.

## Pharmacology/Pharmacokinetics

### Physicochemical characteristics
Hepatitis B recombinant vaccines are produced from *Saccharomyces cerevisiae*, into which a plasmid containing the gene for the hepatitis B surface antigen (HBsAg) has been inserted. Purified HBsAg is obtained by lysis of the yeast cells and separation of the HBsAg from the yeast components. These vaccines contain more than 95% HBsAg protein. Yeast-derived protein constitutes no more than 5% of the final product. Hepatitis B recombinant vaccines are adsorbed with aluminum hydroxide (0.5 mg per mL). No substances of human origin are used in their manufacture.

### Protective effect
Well-designed clinical trials have demonstrated the efficacy of hepatitis B recombinant vaccines. Immunization reduced the incidence of hepatitis B by 90 to 95% in cohorts of homosexual men and of health care workers frequently exposed to blood. Protection is evident within weeks after the first two doses of vaccine in adults and, in large prospective studies, is correlated with anti-HBs titers above 10 milliInternational Units per milliliter (mIU/mL). Pre-exposure vaccination produces protective levels of antibody in 95 to 100% of infants after three doses, in 80 to 95% after two doses, and in 20 to 50% after one dose. For infants born to HBsAg-positive mothers, the average efficacy of postexposure prophylaxis with hepatitis B recombinant vaccine and hepatitis B immune globulin is 95%; vaccination alone and the combined regimen have similar efficacy.

Studies have revealed that the percentage of infants who develop protective levels ($\geq$ 10 mIU/mL) of antibody to HBsAg (anti-HBs) and the final anti-HBs concentrations may be lower in premature infants given the hepatitis B recombinant vaccines beginning at birth than if the initial dose is delayed until they are older or weigh more than 2000 grams. In one study, the response rates for premature infants who received their first doses of hepatitis B recombinant vaccine at a weight of either 1000 to 1999 grams or 2000 grams or more were 79% and 91% respectively; the response rate was 100% for full-term infants. The second dose was given 1 month later, and the third dose was given approximately 5 months after the first dose.

In a study of premature Thai infants with gestational ages of 28 to 32 weeks, 11 of 14 (78%) developed protective levels of anti-HBs after receiving three 10-mcg doses of hepatitis B recombinant vaccine; doses were given at birth, 1 month of age, and 6 months of age. Eleven of 11 infants with gestational ages of 33 to 37 weeks developed protective levels. The overall response rate for premature infants was 22 of 25 (88%).

A third study in Italy revealed that 37 of 37 premature infants (< 37 weeks' gestation) developed anti-HBs levels of 10 mIU/mL or greater after receiving 10-mcg doses of hepatitis B recombinant vaccine at birth, 1 month of age, and 3 months of age; or at birth, 1 month of age, and 6 months of age. Lower gestational age but not lower birth weight was associated with lower final antibody concentrations.

As is seen with other vaccines, serologic response of human immunodeficiency virus (HIV)-infected patients to both plasma-derived and recombinant HBV vaccines have been suboptimal. Protective antibody responses after three doses of hepatitis B recombinant vaccine were achieved in 28% of 32 HIV-infected patients, as compared with 88% of 75 HIV-negative individuals. An additional dose given 9 months after the last of three doses led to only one additional HIV-infected patient achieving protective level. The CD4+ cell count was significantly higher in responders than in nonresponders. In addition, nonresponders were significantly more likely to progress to HIV-related diseases within 24 months than were responders.

In one study, hepatitis B recombinant vaccine was administered to 16 HIV-positive and 68 HIV-negative patients. One month after the last vaccine of the series, low or no antibody response had occurred in 44% of the HIV-positive group as compared with only 9% in the HIV-negative group.

### Duration of protective effect
Long-term protection (6 to 13 years) from hepatitis B virus (HBV) infection has been shown in approximately 3700 immunized persons from populations that continue to be exposed to HBV. Vaccine-induced antibody levels may decline with age. Loss of antibody has occurred in one third of adults and 15% of infants and children. Asymptomatic infections have been identified in approximately 3% of these individuals, and HBsAg-positive infections in less than 0.5%, but not all infections were chronic. Protection against HBV infection persists even when antibody titers subsequently decline; therefore, booster doses are not necessary.

In contrast, a lower proportion (50 to 60%) of vaccinated hemodialysis patients develops a protective antibody response. Booster doses are necessary to maintain protection against hepatitis B infection when antibody titers decline below protective levels. However, more than 50% of hemodialysis patients can be protected from hepatitis B infection by vaccination, and maintaining immunity among these patients will reduce the frequency and cost of serologic screening.

## Precautions to Consider

### Cross-sensitivity and/or related problems
Patients sensitive to the plasma-derived hepatitis B vaccine may be sensitive to the recombinant hepatitis B vaccine also.

## Pregnancy/Reproduction

*Pregnancy*—Adequate and well-controlled studies have not been done in humans. However, risk from vaccination is largely theoretical; there is no convincing evidence of risk from vaccinating pregnant women. Hepatitis B recombinant vaccine is recommended for pregnant women at risk of hepatitis B infection. All pregnant women should be tested for the presence of hepatitis B virus surface antigen (HBsAg), and those infected with hepatitis B virus (HBV) should be monitored carefully to ensure that the infant receives hepatitis B immune globulin and begins the hepatitis B vaccine series shortly after birth.

Studies have not been done in animals.

FDA Pregnancy Category C.

## Breast-feeding

It is not known whether the vaccine is distributed into breast milk. However, the vaccine does not affect the safety of breast-feeding for mothers or infants. Breast-feeding does not adversely affect immunization, and is not a contraindication for vaccination. Breast-fed infants should be vaccinated according to the routine, recommended schedule.

## Pediatrics

Note: Because infants born to HBsAg-negative women are not at immediate risk of exposure to HBV, the first dose of vaccine can be deferred. Infants born to HBsAg-positive women, however, are at immediate risk of contracting HBV infection. Immunization, together with a dose of hepatitis B immune globulin, should be given at birth and these infants should be tested for anti-HBs antibody. Infants born to mothers who have not been screened should receive the first dose of hepatitis B vaccine at birth using the dose of vaccine recommended for infants born to HBsAg-positive mothers. Subsequent management of these infants is dependent on the results of the serologic screening of the mother.

Hepatitis B recombinant vaccine has been shown to be well tolerated and highly immunogenic in infants and children of all ages. Neonates also respond well, and maternally transferred antibodies do not interfere with the active immune response to the vaccine.

No published pediatrics-specific information is available for the dialysis formulation of hepatitis B recombinant vaccine. Safety and efficacy have not been established.

Although long-term carriage of HBV in children is usually asymptomatic, it may lead to chronic hepatitis, liver cirrhosis, and hepatocellular carcinoma in later life. Many studies have demonstrated the efficacy of hepatitis B vaccine in reducing long-term carriage in neonates at high risk. The World Health Organization (WHO) has endorsed the inclusion of hepatitis B vaccine in routine childhood immunization programs, especially in areas where hepatitis B is endemic. Studies suggest that universal hepatitis B vaccination of infants in the first year of life is effective in the improvement of the endemic status of the infection.

Premature infants born to HBsAg-positive mothers should receive immunoprophylaxis with hepatitis B recombinant vaccine and hepatitis B immune globulin, beginning at birth. For premature infants of HBsAg-negative mothers, the optimal timing of hepatitis B vaccination has not been determined. Some studies suggest that decreased seroconversion rates may occur in some premature infants with low birthweight (i.e., less than 2000 grams) following administration of hepatitis B recombinant vaccine at birth. Such low-birthweight premature infants born to HBsAg-negative mothers should receive the hepatitis B vaccine series at discharge from the nursery, if the infant weighs at least 2000 grams, or at 2 months of age along with diphtheria, tetanus, and pertussis vaccine; oral poliovirus vaccine; and haemophilus b conjugate vaccine.

## Adolescents

Studies have shown that hepatitis B recombinant vaccine is highly immunogenic in adolescents and young adults when administered in varying three-dose schedules. Routine vaccination of adolescents 11 to 12 years of age who have not been vaccinated previously is an effective strategy for rapidly lowering the incidence of HBV infection and its transmission in the U.S. Studies performed in Canada, and Italy indicated that universal vaccination of this age group can be highly acceptable and efficient. An adolescent's visit to a physician at 11 to 12 years of age gives the provider an opportunity to initiate protection against HBV before the adolescent begins high-risk behaviors. Unvaccinated adolescents older than 12 years of age who are at increased risk for HBV infection also should be vaccinated.

## Geriatrics

Studies have shown that the adult response to hepatitis B recombinant vaccine is inversely related to age: more than 90% response in young adults, 70% in persons 50 to 59 years of age, and 50 to 70% in persons 60 years of age and over. Other geriatrics-specific problems that would limit the usefulness of this medication in the elderly are not expected.

## Drug interactions and/or related problems

The following drug interactions and/or related problems have been selected on the basis of their potential clinical significance (possible mechanism in parentheses where appropriate)—not necessarily inclusive (» = major clinical significance):

Note: Combinations containing any of the following medications, depending on the amount present, may also interact with this medication.

Immunosuppressive agents or
Radiation therapy
(because normal defense mechanisms are suppressed, the patient's antibody response to hepatitis B recombinant vaccine may be decreased. Larger vaccine doses [2 to 4 times the normal adult dose] or an increased number of doses [4 doses] may be required to induce protective levels of antibody in immunocompromised persons)

## Laboratory value alterations

The following have been selected on the basis of their potential clinical significance (possible effect in parentheses where appropriate)—not necessarily inclusive (» = major clinical significance):

With physiology/laboratory test values
Erythrocyte sedimentation (SED) rate
(may be increased)

## Medical considerations/Contraindications

The medical considerations/contraindications included have been selected on the basis of their potential clinical significance (reasons given in parentheses where appropriate)—not necessarily inclusive (» = major clinical significance).

*Except under special circumstances, this medication should not be used when the following medical problem exists:*

» Previous hypersensitivity reaction to hepatitis B recombinant vaccine (rare cases of anaphylaxis [1 per 600,000 vaccine doses administered] among vaccine recipients has been reported to the Vaccine Adverse Events Reporting System [VAERS]; although none of the persons who developed anaphylaxis died, this adverse event can be fatal; in addition, hepatitis B vaccine can, in rare instances, cause a life-threatening hypersensitivity reaction in some persons; therefore, subsequent vaccination with hepatitis B vaccine is contraindicated for persons who previously had anaphylactic responses to a dose of this vaccine)

*Risk-benefit should be considered when the following medical problems exist:*

Allergy to yeast
(hepatitis B recombinant vaccine is produced using yeast; a maximum of 1 or 5%, depending on the manufacturer, of yeast-derived protein may be present in the final vaccine; although there have not been any proven allergic reactions to the yeast, the possibility exists that they may occur)

Cardiopulmonary status, severely compromised
(a febrile or systemic reaction to the vaccine could pose a significant risk to persons with this condition)

Illness, moderate or severe, with or without fever
(administration of the vaccine should be delayed, except when withholding the vaccine entails a greater risk to the patient than a possible superimposed reaction to the vaccine)

Immune deficiency conditions
(antibody response to hepatitis B recombinant vaccine may be decreased; larger vaccine doses [2 to 4 times the normal adult dose] or an increased number of doses [4 doses] may be required to induce protective levels of antibody in immunocompromised persons)

# Side/Adverse Effects

Note: In the U.S., an estimated 2.5 million adults received one or more doses of hepatitis B recombinant vaccine between 1986 and 1990, and available data concerning these vaccinees do not indicate an association between receipt of hepatitis B recombinant vaccine and Guillain-Barré syndrome (GBS). Moreover, large-scale hepatitis B immunization programs for infants in Alaska, New Zealand, and Taiwan have not established an association between vaccination and the occurrence of GBS. However, systematic surveillance for adverse reactions in these populations has been limited, and only a minimal number of children have received the recombinant vaccine. Any presumed risk for adverse events that could be causally associated with hepatitis B vaccination must be balanced against the expected risk for hepatitis B virus (HBV)-related liver disease. Currently, an estimated 2000 to 5000 persons in each U.S. birth cohort will die as a result of HBV–related liver disease because of the 5% lifetime risk for HBV infection.

Agitation, conjunctivitis, constipation, erythrocyte sedimentation rate increase, hepatic enzyme elevation, herpes zoster, hypesthesia, irritability, keratitis, migraine, myelitis, petechiae, radiculopathy, somnolence, Stevens-Johnson syndrome, syncope, tachycardia, thrombocytopenia, tinnitus, and visual disturbances also have been reported in temporal association with administration of hepatitis B recombinant vaccine, but their relationship to the vaccine is unclear.

The following side/adverse effects have been selected on the basis of their potential clinical significance (possible signs and symptoms in parentheses where appropriate)—not necessarily inclusive:

**Those indicating need for medical attention**
Incidence rare
   *Anaphylactic reaction* (difficulty in breathing or swallowing; hives; itching, especially of feet or hands; reddening of skin, especially around ears; swelling of eyes, face, or inside of nose; unusual tiredness or weakness, sudden and severe); *neuropathy* (muscle weakness or numbness or tingling of limbs); *optic neuritis* (blurred vision or other vision changes); *serum sickness–like reaction* (aches or pain in joints, fever, or skin rash or welts)—may occur days or weeks following administration of the vaccine

**Those indicating need for medical attention only if they continue or are bothersome**
Incidence more frequent
   *Soreness at injection site*—20 to 30%
Incidence less frequent (1 to 10% frequency)
   *Fatigue* (unusual tiredness or weakness); *fever of 37.7 °C (100 °F) or over; headache; induration* (hard lump); *erythema* (redness); *swelling; pain; pruritus* (itching); *ecchymosis* (purple spot); *tenderness; or warmth at injection site; vertigo* (dizziness)
Incidence rare (less than 1% frequency)
   *Anorexia* (lack of appetite); *or decreased appetite; arthralgia, arthritis, or myalgia* (aches or pain in joints or muscles); *back pain; chills; diarrhea or abdominal cramps or pain* (stomach cramps or pain); *flushing* (sudden redness of skin); *hypotension* (unusual tiredness or weakness); *increased sweating; influenza-like symptoms or upper respiratory tract illness* (headache, sore throat, runny nose, or fever); *insomnia or sleep disturbance* (trouble in sleeping); *lymphadenopathy* (swelling of glands in armpit or neck); *malaise* (general feeling of discomfort or illness); *nausea or vomiting; nodule at injection site* (lump at place of injection)—probably from the aluminum content of the vaccine and may persist for a few weeks; *pruritus* (itching); *skin rash; or urticaria* (welts); *stiffness or pain in neck or shoulder*

## Patient Consultation

As an aid to patient consultation, refer to *Advice for the Patient, Hepatitis B Vaccine Recombinant (Systemic)*.

In providing consultation, consider emphasizing the following selected information (» = major clinical significance):

**Before receiving this vaccine**
» Conditions affecting use, especially:
   Hypersensitivity to plasma-derived hepatitis B vaccine or recombinant hepatitis B vaccine or allergy to yeast
   Use in the elderly—Compared with younger adults, persons over 50 years of age may be less likely to develop a protective antibody level following immunization with hepatitis B recombinant vaccine

**Proper use of this vaccine**
» Proper dosing

**Side/adverse effects**
Signs of potential side effects, especially anaphylactic reaction, neuropathy, optic neuritis, or serum sickness–like reaction

## General Dosing Information

Although systemic reactions to hepatitis B recombinant vaccine are rare, anaphylaxis among vaccine recipients has been reported to the Vaccine Adverse Events Reporting System (VAERS). Therefore, appropriate precautions should be taken prior to hepatitis B recombinant vaccine injection to prevent allergic or any other unwanted reactions. Precautions should include review of the patient's history regarding possible sensitivity and the ready availability of 1:1000 epinephrine injection and other appropriate agents used for control of immediate allergic reactions.

Only persons who have not been infected with hepatitis B virus (HBV) previously need to be immunized with hepatitis B recombinant vaccine. Therefore, as a cost-effective measure, testing for prior HBV infection should be considered for adults in groups having a high prevalence of HBV infection (e.g., users of injection drugs, homosexual men, and household contacts of HBV carriers). If the group to be tested is also expected to have a high prevalence of carriers, it may be preferable to test for antibody to hepatitis B core antigen (anti-HBc), since this test identifies previously infected persons, both carriers and noncarriers. If the group to be tested is not expected to have a high rate of carriers, the test for antibody to hepatitis B surface antigen (anti-HBs) will be adequate, since this test identifies previously infected persons, except for carriers.

There is no harm but also no proven benefit in immunizing those already infected with HBV. Recent claims of a therapeutic response in carriers of hepatitis B surface antigen (HBsAg) have not been confirmed.

Although the dosages are different for the products of different manufacturers, the resulting immunogenicity of each is comparable. An immunization schedule started with one manufacturer's vaccine and dose may be completed with the other manufacturer's vaccine and dose. However, in the dialysis setting, the two vaccines should not be used interchangeably.

Because of the long incubation period of HBV, unrecognized infection may be present at the time of immunization; the vaccine may not prevent hepatitis B in already-infected patients.

Passively acquired antibody, whether acquired by administration of immune globulins or via the transplacental route, will not interfere with active immunization with hepatitis B recombinant vaccine. In addition, there is no interference with the induction of protective antibodies elicited by hepatitis B recombinant vaccine when hepatitis B immune globulin (HBIG) is administered at the same time at different body sites.

The Committee on Infectious Diseases of the American Academy of Pediatrics, the Advisory Committee on Immunization Practices of the Centers for Disease Control and Prevention, and the American Academy of Family Physicians offer the following recommendations for the use of hepatitis B recombinant vaccine among infants, children, and adolescents:

• Infants born to HBsAg-negative mothers should receive 2.5 mcg *Recombivax HB* or 10 mcg *Engerix-B*. A second dose should be administered 1 or more months after the first dose.
• Infants born to HBsAg-positive mothers should receive 0.5 mL HBIG within 12 hours of birth, and either 5 mcg *Recombivax HB* or 10 mcg *Engerix-B* at a separate injection site. A second dose should be administered at 1 to 2 months of age and a third dose at 6 months of age.
• Infants born to mothers whose HBsAg status is unknown should receive either 5 mcg *Recombivax HB* or 10 mcg *Engerix-B* within 12 hours of birth. A second dose should be administered at 1 month of age and a third dose at 6 months of age.
• Adolescents who have not previously received three doses of hepatitis B vaccine should initiate or complete the series at the 11- to 12-year-old visit to the physician. A second dose should be administered at least 1 month after the first dose, and a third dose should be administered at least 4 months after the first dose, and at least 2 months after the second dose.

If within 7 days after delivery, a mother of unknown HBsAg status is found to be HBsAg positive, the infant should receive HBIG immediately. In addition, immunization with the appropriate dosage of hepatitis B recombinant vaccine should be initiated or continued. If hepatitis B recombinant vaccine and HBIG are administered at the same time, they should be administered in the anterolateral aspects of opposite thighs. If a mother of unknown HBsAg status is found not to be HBsAg-positive, the infant should complete the immunization series with the appropriate dosage of hepatitis B recombinant vaccine.

For known or presumed exposure to the hepatitis B virus, HBIG should be administered according to its directions as soon as possible after exposure and within 24 hours if possible. (HBIG's value if given later than 7 days after exposure is unclear; in addition, the period after sexual exposure to HBV during which HBIG is effective is unknown, but extrapolation from other data suggests that this period does not exceed 14 days.) In addition, hepatitis B recombinant vaccine should be administered at a separate body site, using one of the following dosage schedules and the dosage that applies to it:
• If using *Recombivax HB*—At the same time as HBIG or within 7 days after exposure, then 1 month and 6 months after the first dose, for a total of three doses.
• If using *Engerix-B*—
   —At the same time as HBIG or within 7 days after exposure, then 1 month and 6 months after the first dose, for a total of three doses.
   —Alternatively, at the same time as HBIG or within 7 days after exposure, then 1 month, 2 months, and 12 months after the first dose, for a total of four doses.

If the exposed person has begun, but not completed, immunization with hepatitis B recombinant vaccine, HBIG should be given as usual, and immunization with the vaccine should be completed as scheduled.

For travelers: Ideally, immunization with hepatitis B recombinant vaccine should begin at least 6 months before travel to allow completion of the full three-dose vaccine series (given at 0, 1, and 6 months). However, if there is less time available before travel than a full 6 months, the first three doses of an alternative four-dose schedule (given at 0, 1, 2, and 12 months) may provide earlier protection during travel if the doses can be administered before travel begins.

Although the alternative four-dose schedule (given at 0, 1, 2, and 12 months)(*Engerix-B*) provides a more rapid induction of immunity, there is no clear evidence that this schedule provides greater long-term protection than the standard three-dose schedule (given at 0, 1, and 6 months).

Vaccine doses administered at longer-than-recommended intervals (recommended intervals being 0, 1, and 6 months) provide equally satisfactory protection. However, optimal protection is not conferred until after the third dose. If the vaccine series is interrupted after the first dose, the second dose should be given as soon as possible, followed by the third dose 3 to 5 months later. Persons who receive the third dose later than 6 months after the initial dose should be given the third dose as soon as is practical. In healthy persons it is not considered necessary to perform postvaccination testing to ensure an adequate antibody response, in either of the above situations.

When sterilizing syringes and skin before vaccination, care should be taken to avoid contact of the vaccine with preservatives, antiseptics, detergents, and disinfectants, since the vaccine virus particles may be easily denatured by these substances.

The hepatitis B recombinant vaccine should be administered by intramuscular (IM) injection. The needle should be of sufficient length and bore to reach the muscle mass itself and to prevent vaccine from seeping into subcutaneous tissue. For adults, the suggested needle length is 1½ inches. For children, a 20- or 22-gauge needle 1 to 1¼ inches long is recommended. For small infants, a 25-gauge needle 5/8 inch long may be adequate. However, for persons at risk of hemorrhage following IM injections, the vaccine may be administered subcutaneously, although the subsequent antibody titer may be lower and there may be an increased risk of local reactions. The vaccine should not be administered intravenously or intradermally.

The deltoid muscle (outer aspect of the upper arm) is the recommended site for the immunization of adults and older children. For infants and young children, the anterolateral aspect of the thigh muscle is the recommended site. The vaccine should not be administered in the gluteal region (buttock), because the immunogenicity of the vaccine is substantially lowered.

The 40 mcg/mL strength (*Recombivax HB Dialysis Formulation*) is given in a three-dose regimen, with a total of three doses required. The 20 mcg/mL strength (*Engerix-B*) requires either one 2-mL injection or two separate 1-mL injections during a four-dose regimen for a total of either four or eight injections.

Larger vaccine doses (2 to 4 times the normal adult dose) or an increased number of doses (4 doses) may be necessary for immunocompromised persons (such as those on immunosuppressive medications or with human immunodeficiency virus [HIV] infection). However, although persons with HIV infection have an impaired response to hepatitis B recombinant vaccine, the immunogenicity of higher doses of the vaccine in these persons is unknown, and specific recommendations on dosage are not available.

Although postimmunization testing for serologic response and immunity is not routinely recommended, it is recommended for the following:
- Persons whose subsequent management depends on knowledge of their immune status, such as dialysis patients, medical staff, and infants born to HBsAg-positive mothers.
- Persons in whom a less-than-optimal response may be anticipated, such as those who were administered the vaccine in the buttock or subcutaneously, persons over 50 years of age, and persons with HIV infection or other immune deficiencies.
- Persons at occupational risk who may have HBV exposures necessitating postexposure prophylaxis.

Postimmunization testing should be done 1 to 6 months after completion of the immunization series to provide definitive information on the response to the vaccine.

Reimmunization of persons who did not originally respond to the primary series produces adequate antibody response in 15 to 25% after 1 additional dose and in 30 to 50% after 3 additional doses, when the original immunization was administered in the deltoid muscle. Data suggest that in more than 75% of persons who did not adequately respond to a primary vaccine series given in the buttock, reimmunization in the arm induces adequate antibody response.

In adult predialysis and dialysis patients, hepatitis B recombinant vaccine–induced protection is less complete and may persist only as long as antibody levels remain at or above 10 milliInternational Units (mIU) per mL. The need for additional doses of the vaccine should be assessed by annual antibody testing. It is recommended that additional doses of 40 mcg of hepatitis B recombinant vaccine be given when antibody levels decline to below 10 mIU per mL.

Hepatitis B recombinant vaccine, an inactivated product, can be administered concurrently with the following, using separate body sites (in infants, selecting separate sites in the same anterolateral aspect of the thigh muscle is preferable to administering hepatitis B recombinant vaccine in the buttock or deltoid muscle), separate syringes (for parenterals), and the precautions that apply to each immunizing agent:
- Polysaccharide vaccines, such as haemophilus b conjugate vaccine, haemophilus b polysaccharide vaccine, meningococcal polysaccharide vaccine, or pneumococcal polyvalent vaccine.
- Influenza virus vaccine, whole or split virus.
- Diphtheria toxoid, tetanus toxoid, and/or pertussis (whole cell or acellular) vaccine.
- Live virus vaccines, such as measles, mumps, and/or rubella vaccines.
- Poliovirus vaccines (oral [OPV], inactivated [IPV], or enhanced-potency inactivated [enhanced-potency IPV]).
- Immune globulin and disease-specific immune globulins.
- Inactivated vaccines, other, except cholera, typhoid (parenteral), and plague. It is recommended that cholera, typhoid (parenteral), and plague vaccines be administered on separate occasions because of these vaccines' propensity to cause side/adverse effects.

### For treatment of adverse effects
Recommended treatment includes:
- For mild hypersensitivity reaction—Administering antihistamines, and, if necessary, corticosteroids. In mild anaphylaxis, antihistamines or subcutaneous epinephrine may be all that is necessary if the condition is progressing slowly and is not life-threatening, regardless of the organ or system affected. Under these circumstances the risks associated with intravenous epinephrine administration outweigh the benefits.
- For severe hypersensitivity or anaphylactic reaction—Administering epinephrine. Antihistamines or corticosteroids may also be administered as required. Epinephrine is the treatment of choice for severe hypersensitivity or anaphylactic reaction. If the patient's condition is not stable, epinephrine should be infused. Norepinephrine may be preferable if there is no bronchospasm. For bronchospasm, epinephrine should be given with corticosteroids. Other bronchodilators, such as intravenous aminophylline or albuterol by nebulization, also should be considered.

## Parenteral Dosage Forms

### STERILE HEPATITIS B VACCINE RECOMBINANT SUSPENSION

#### Usual adult and adolescent dose
Immunizing agent (active)—
- Adolescents 11 to 19 years of age: Intramuscular, into the deltoid muscle, 5 mcg (*Recombivax HB*—U.S. and Canada), or 10 mcg (*Recombivax HB*—Canada), or 20 mcg (*Engerix-B*—U.S. and Canada), at initial visit, then one month and six months after the first dose, for a total of three doses.
- Adults 19 years of age and older: Intramuscular, into the deltoid muscle, 10 mcg (*Recombivax HB*—U.S. and Canada) or 20 mcg (*Engerix-B*—U.S. and Canada), at initial visit, then one month and six months after the first dose, for a total of three doses.
- Adult predialysis and dialysis patients—Intramuscular, into the deltoid muscle, 40 mcg (*Recombivax HB Dialysis Formulation*—U.S. and Canada), at initial visit, then one month and six months after the first dose, for a total of three doses;

Or

40 mcg (*Engerix-B*—U.S. and Canada), at initial visit, then one month, two months, and six months after the first dose, for a total of four doses. The 20 mcg/mL strength (*Engerix-B*) requires either one 2-mL injection or two separate 1-mL injections during a four-dose regimen for a total of either four or eight injections.

#### Usual pediatric dose
Immunizing agent (active)—
- Neonates born to hepatitis B surface antigen (HBsAg)-positive mothers: Intramuscular, into the anterolateral aspect of the thigh—5 mcg (*Recombivax HB*—U.S. and Canada), 10 mcg (*Engerix-B*—U.S. and Canada), within twelve hours after birth (preferably) or within seven days after birth, then one month and six months after the first dose, for a total of three doses;

Or

10 mcg (*Engerix-B*—U.S. and Canada), within twelve hours after birth (preferably) or within seven days after birth, then one

month, two months, and twelve months after the first dose, for a total of four doses.

Neonates born to mothers of unknown HBsAg status: Intramuscular, into the anterolateral aspect of the thigh: 5 mcg (*Recombivax HB*—U.S.), 10 mcg (*Engerix-B*—U.S. and Canada), within twelve hours after birth (preferably) or within seven days after birth, then:

Infants of mothers subsequently determined to be HBsAg-positive:
- 5 mcg (*Recombivax HB*—U.S.), 10 mcg (*Engerix-B*—U.S. and Canada), one month and six months after the first dose, for a total of three doses;

Or
- 10 mcg (*Engerix-B*—U.S. and Canada), one month, two months, and twelve months after the first dose, for a total of four doses.

Infants of mothers subsequently determined to be HBsAg-negative:
- 2.5 mcg (*Recombivax HB*—U.S.), 10 mcg (*Engerix-B*—U.S. and Canada), one month and six months after the first dose, for a total of three doses.

Neonates born to HBsAg-negative mothers or

Infants and children up to 11 years of age: Intramuscular, into the anterolateral aspect of the thigh for neonates, infants, and young children and into the deltoid muscle for older children, 2.5 mcg (*Recombivax HB*—U.S. and Canada), 10 mcg (*Engerix-B*—U.S. and Canada), at initial visit, then one month and six months after the first dose, for a total of three doses.

Note: Physicians have a great deal of flexibility in scheduling the three-dose immunization series for full-term infants born to HBsAg-negative mothers. The recommended schedule is to give the first dose during the neonatal period or by two months of age, the second dose one to two months later, and the third dose at six to eighteen months of age. The vaccines, however, are highly immunogenic when given according to other schedules. Although the highest titers of anti-HBs are achieved when the last two doses of vaccine are spaced four months apart or longer, schedules with two-month intervals between doses have been shown to produce high rates of seroconversion. Some pediatricians have adopted other three-dose schedules in order to minimize the number of simultaneous injections. Schedules with intervals of up to ten months between the second and the third doses have been shown to be highly effective. Intervals longer than two months between the first two doses or more than one year between the second and the third dose have not been evaluated in controlled trials. The American Academy of Pediatrics currently recommends that children of all ages for whom a longer time than recommended has elapsed between doses of hepatitis B vaccine can complete the series without repeating a dose or starting the series over.

**Strength(s) usually available**

U.S.—
- 2.5 mcg (0.0025 mg) of hepatitis B surface antigen (HBsAg) protein per 0.5 mL (Rx) [*Recombivax HB* (0.25 mg aluminum as aluminum hydroxide; thimerosal 1:20,000)].
- 5 mcg (0.005 mg) of HBsAg protein per 0.5 mL (Rx) [*Recombivax HB* (0.25 mg aluminum as aluminum hydroxide; thimerosal 1:20,000)].
- 10 mcg (0.01 mg) of HBsAg protein per mL (Rx) [*Recombivax HB* (0.5 mg aluminum as aluminum hydroxide; thimerosal 1:20,000)].
- 10 mcg (0.01 mg) of HBsAg protein per 0.5 mL (Rx) [*Engerix-B* (0.25 mg aluminum as aluminum hydroxide; thimerosal 1:20,000)].
- 20 mcg (0.02 mg) of HBsAg protein per mL (Rx) [*Engerix-B* (0.5 mg aluminum as aluminum hydroxide; thimerosal 1:20,000)].
- 40 mcg (0.04 mg) of HBsAg protein per mL (Rx) [*Recombivax HB Dialysis Formulation* (0.5 mg aluminum as aluminum hydroxide; thimerosal 1:20,000)].

Canada—
- 5 mcg (0.005 mg) of HBsAg protein per 0.5 mL (Rx) [*Recombivax HB* (alum adjuvant; thimerosal 1:20,000)].
- 10 mcg (0.01 mg) of HBsAg protein per mL (Rx) [*Recombivax HB* (alum adjuvant; thimerosal 1:20,000)].
- 10 mcg (0.01 mg) of HBsAg protein per mL (Rx) [*Engerix-B* (0.25 mg aluminum as aluminum hydroxide; thimerosal 1:20,000)].
- 20 mcg (0.02 mg) of HBsAg protein per mL (Rx) [*Engerix-B* (0.5 mg aluminum as aluminum hydroxide; thimerosal 1:20,000)].
- 40 mcg (0.04 mg) of HBsAg protein per mL (Rx) [*Recombivax HB Dialysis Formulation* (thimerosal 1:20,000)].

**Packaging and storage**

Store between 2 and 8 °C (36 and 46 °F), unless otherwise specified by manufacturer. Protect from freezing.

**Preparation of dosage form**

The vaccine should be used as supplied, and should not be diluted. The vial should be shaken well immediately before withdrawal of the dose. In addition, thorough agitation at the time of administration is necessary to maintain suspension of the vaccine. After agitation, the vaccine is a slightly opaque, white suspension.

**Stability**

Storage above or below the recommended temperature may reduce potency. Freezing destroys potency, and the vaccine should be discarded if freezing occurs.

**Auxiliary labeling**
- Do not freeze; discard if freezing occurs.
- Shake well.

Revised: 06/20/97

---

**HISTAMINE**—The *Histamine (Systemic)* monograph is not included in this published version of the USP DI database. Copies of the monograph are available on request from Micromedex, Inc. - Reprint Requests, 6200 S. Syracuse Way, Suite 300, Englewood, CO 80111; telephone (303) 486-6400; telefax (303) 486-6464; Email: USPDI@MDX.COM.

---

# HISTAMINE H$_2$-RECEPTOR ANTAGONISTS  Systemic

This monograph includes information on the following: 1) Cimetidine; 2) Famotidine; 3) Nizatidine; 4) Ranitidine.

VA CLASSIFICATION (Primary/Secondary):
Cimetidine—GA301/DE890
Famotidine—GA301
Nizatidine—GA301
Ranitidine—GA301

Commonly used brand name(s): *Acid Control*[2]; *Act*[2]; *Apo-Cimetidine*[1]; *Apo-Famotidine*[2]; *Apo-Nizatidine*[3]; *Apo-Ranitidine*[4]; *Axid*[3]; *Axid AR*[3]; *Dyspep HB*[2]; *Gen-Cimetidine*[1]; *Gen-Famotidine*[2]; *Gen-Ranitidine*[4]; *Mylanta-AR*[2]; *Novo-Cimetine*[1]; *Novo-Famotidine*[2]; *Novo-Ranitidine*[4]; *Nu-Cimet*[1]; *Nu-Famotidine*[2]; *Nu-Ranit*[4]; *PMS-Cimetidine*[1]; *Pepcid*[2]; *Pepcid AC*[2]; *Pepcid I.V.*[2]; *Peptol*[1]; *Tagamet*[1]; *Tagamet HB*[1]; *Tagamet HB 200*[1]; *Ulcidine*[2]; *Ulcidine-HB*[2]; *Zantac*[4]; *Zantac 150 GELdose*[4]; *Zantac 300 GELdose*[4]; *Zantac 75*[4]; *Zantac EFFERdose Granules*[4]; *Zantac EFFERdose Tablets*[4]; *Zantac-C*[4].

Note: For a listing of dosage forms and brand names by country availability, see *Dosage Forms* section(s).

## Category

Histamine H$_2$-receptor antagonist—All drugs in this monograph are used as histamine H$_2$-receptor antagonists.

Antiulcer agent—All drugs in this monograph are used as antiulcer agents.
Gastric acid secretion inhibitor—All drugs in this monograph are used as gastric acid secretion inhibitors.
Urticaria therapy adjunct—Cimetidine.

## Indications

Note: Bracketed information in the *Indications* section refers to uses that are not included in U.S. product labeling.

**Accepted**

Ulcer, duodenal (prophylaxis and treatment)—Histamine H$_2$-receptor antagonists are indicated in the short-term treatment of active duodenal ulcer. They are also indicated (at reduced dosage) in the prevention of duodenal ulcer recurrence in selected patients.

Ulcer, gastric (treatment)—Cimetidine, famotidine, nizatidine, and ranitidine are indicated in the short-term treatment of active benign gastric ulcer.

Ulcer, gastric (prophylaxis)—Cimetidine and ranitidine are indicated (at reduced dosage) in the prevention of gastric ulcer recurrence after the healing of acute ulcers.

Heartburn, acid indigestion, and sour stomach associated with hyperacidity (prophylaxis and treatment)—Nonprescription strengths of the histamine H$_2$-receptor antagonists cimetidine, famotidine, and ranitidine are indicated for relief of symptoms associated with hyperacidity, including heartburn, acid indigestion, and sour stomach. Nonprescription strengths of cimetidine, famotidine, nizatidine, and ranitidine are also indicated in prevention of hyperacidity symptoms brought on by the consumption of food or beverages.

Hypersecretory conditions, gastric (treatment)
Zollinger-Ellison syndrome (treatment)
Mastocytosis, systemic (treatment) or
Adenoma, multiple endocrine (treatment)—Cimetidine, famotidine, [nizatidine][1], and ranitidine are indicated in the treatment of pathological gastric hypersecretion associated with Zollinger-Ellison syndrome (alone or as part of multiple endocrine neoplasia Type-1), systemic mastocytosis, and multiple endocrine adenoma.

Reflux, gastroesophageal (treatment)—Cimetidine, famotidine, nizatidine[1], and ranitidine are indicated in the treatment of acute gastroesophageal reflux disease, which may or may not cause erosive or ulcerative esophagitis.

[Pancreatic insufficiency (treatment adjunct)][1]—Cimetidine is used to enhance pancreatic enzyme replacement by reducing peptic acid deactivation and to enhance the efficacy of orally administered pancreatic enzymes in patients with pancreatic insufficiency by reducing the secretion of hydrochloric acid. However, the efficacy of cimetidine in acute pancreatitis has not been established, and some studies have demonstrated that cimetidine may increase and prolong hyperamylasemia.

Bleeding, upper gastrointestinal (treatment)—Cimetidine, [famotidine][1], and [ranitidine] are used to treat upper gastrointestinal bleeding secondary to gastric ulcer, duodenal ulcer, or hemorrhagic gastritis.

Stress-related mucosal damage (prophylaxis and treatment)—[Parenteral ranitidine] is used to prevent and treat and parenteral cimetidine is indicated to prevent and used to treat upper gastrointestinal, stress-induced ulceration and bleeding, especially in intensive care patients. However, the efficacy of histamine H$_2$-receptor antagonists in treating hemorrhage in critically ill patients has not been established.

[Pneumonitis, aspiration (prophylaxis)]—Cimetidine, ranitidine, and famotidine are also used before anesthesia induction for the prophylaxis of aspiration pneumonitis.

Arthritis, rheumatoid (treatment adjunct)—[Cimetidine] and [ranitidine][1] are used for the relief of gastrointestinal symptoms associated with the use of nonsteroidal anti-inflammatory drugs in the treatment of rheumatoid arthritis.

[Urticaria, acute (treatment adjunct)][1]—Cimetidine is used in combination with an antihistamine to treat acute urticaria.

---
[1]Not included in Canadian product labeling.

## Pharmacology/Pharmacokinetics
See *Table 1*, page 1643 and *Table 2*, page 1643.

### Physicochemical characteristics
Molecular weight—
　Cimetidine: 252.34.
　Famotidine: 337.43.
　Nizatidine: 331.45.
　Ranitidine: 350.87.
pKa—
　Cimetidine: 7.09.
　Cimetidine hydrochloride: 7.11.
　Ranitidine: 8.2 and 2.7.

### Mechanism of action/Effect
H$_2$-receptor antagonists inhibit basal and nocturnal gastric acid secretion by competitive inhibition of the action of histamine at the histamine H$_2$-receptors of the parietal cells. They also inhibit gastric acid secretion stimulated by food, betazole, pentagastrin, caffeine, insulin, and physiological vagal reflex.

Urticaria therapy adjunct—Cimetidine blocks H$_2$-receptors, which in part are responsible for the inflammatory response, in the cutaneous blood vessels of humans.

### Other actions/effects
Cimetidine—Inhibits hepatic cytochrome P-450 and P-448 mixed function oxidase (microsomal enzyme) systems; antagonizes dihydrotestosterone (antiandrogenic action); produces transient and clinically insignificant increases in prolactin concentrations (with intravenous bolus administration only). May enhance gastromucosal defense and healing in acid-related disorders, particularly stress-induced ulceration and bleeding, by increasing production of gastric mucus, content of mucus glycoprotein, mucosal secretion of bicarbonate, gastric mucosal blood flow, endogenous mucosal prostaglandin synthesis, and rate of epithelial cell renewal.

Famotidine—Weak inhibitor of hepatic cytochrome P-450 mixed function oxidase system.

Nizatidine—Weak inhibitor of hepatic cytochrome P-450 mixed function oxidase system.

Ranitidine—Weak inhibitor of hepatic cytochrome P-450 mixed function oxidase system; produces small, transient, and clinically insignificant increases in serum prolactin concentrations (reported with intravenous bolus administration of 100 mg or more).

### Distribution
All H$_2$-receptor antagonists are distributed in breast milk and cerebrospinal fluid.

### Onset of action
Famotidine—Oral: 1 hour.

## Precautions to Consider

### Cross-sensitivity and/or related problems
Patients sensitive to one of the histamine H$_2$-receptor antagonists may be sensitive to the other histamine H$_2$-receptor antagonists also.

### Carcinogenicity/Mutagenicity/Tumorigenicity
It is not known whether the histamine H$_2$-receptor antagonists are carcinogenic or mutagenic in humans.
　For cimetidine—Long-term toxicity studies in rats have shown a significantly higher incidence of benign Leydig cell tumors in cimetidine-treated groups than in controls at doses approximately 8 to 48 times the recommended human dose.
　For famotidine—Studies in rats and mice with oral doses approximately 2500 times the recommended human dose showed no evidence of carcinogenicity. Studies in mice with a micronucleus test and a chromosomal aberration test showed no evidence of mutagenicity.
　For nizatidine—Studies in rats and mice with oral doses many times the recommended human dose showed no evidence of carcinogenicity.
　For ranitidine—Long-term studies in mice and rats with doses up to 2 grams per kg of body weight have not shown ranitidine to be carcinogenic.

### Pregnancy/Reproduction
Fertility—For cimetidine: There has been no evidence of impaired mating performance or fertility at doses 40 times the human dose in rats, rabbits, and mice.
For famotidine: Studies in rats and rabbits with oral doses of up to 2000 and 500 mg per kg of body weight (mg/kg) per day, respectively, have not shown that famotidine impairs fertility.
For nizatidine: Studies in rats and rabbits with oral doses up to 300 and 55 times the human dose, respectively, have not shown that nizatidine impairs fertility.
For ranitidine: Studies in rats and rabbits at doses up to 160 times the human dose have not shown that ranitidine impairs fertility.

Pregnancy—
　*For cimetidine—*
　　Adequate and well-controlled studies in humans have not been done.
　　Animal studies have shown that cimetidine crosses the placenta. Also, a study in rats exposed to cimetidine during intrauterine life and the immediate neonatal period showed a hypoandrogenization in adult life with decreased weights of androgen-dependent tissues and decreased concentrations of testosterone.
　　FDA Pregnancy Category B.
　*For famotidine—*
　　Famotidine crosses the placenta. Adequate and well-controlled studies in humans have not been done.
　　Studies in rats and rabbits with oral doses of up to 2000 and 500 mg/kg per day, respectively, have not shown that famotidine has adverse effects on the fetus.
　　FDA Pregnancy Category B.
　*For nizatidine—*
　　Nizatidine crosses the placenta. Adequate and well-controlled studies in humans have not been done.
　　Rabbits treated with a dose equivalent to 300 times the human dose had abortions, a decreased number of live fetuses, and depressed fetal weights.
　　FDA Pregnancy Category B.
　*For ranitidine—*
　　Ranitidine crosses the placenta. Adequate and well-controlled studies in humans have not been done.
　　Studies in rats and rabbits at doses up to 160 times the human dose have not shown that ranitidine causes adverse effects on the fetus.
　　FDA Pregnancy Category B.

**Breast-feeding**

Problems in humans have not been documented; however, cimetidine, famotidine, nizatidine, and ranitidine are distributed into breast milk and could possibly suppress gastric acidity, inhibit drug metabolism, and cause central nervous system (CNS) stimulation in the nursing infant. It has been found that very high acute and chronic milk/plasma ratios occur with the use of cimetidine; therefore, the Committee on Drugs of the American Academy of Pediatrics has recommended that cimetidine not be taken by mothers while they are breast-feeding. Although, at present, data for ranitidine are insufficient, it appears that high milk/plasma ratios may also occur with ingestion of ranitidine.

**Pediatrics**

For cimetidine, famotidine, and ranitidine—Studies performed to date have not demonstrated pediatrics-specific problems that would limit the usefulness of cimetidine, famotidine, and ranitidine in children for short-term (6 to 8 weeks) use. Cimetidine, famotidine, and ranitidine have been used for long-term treatment of chronic gastroesophageal reflux disease in children; however, cimetidine-induced cerebral toxicity and reported cimetidine effects on the hormonal system in adults may be of concern with long-term use in children.

For nizatidine—Appropriate studies have not been performed in children up to 16 years of age.

**Geriatrics**

For cimetidine, famotidine, and ranitidine—Although appropriate studies on the relationship of age to the effects of these medicines have not been performed in the geriatric population, no geriatrics-specific problems have been documented to date. However, confusion is more likely to occur in elderly patients with impaired hepatic or renal function.

For nizatidine—Studies performed to date have not demonstrated geriatrics-specific problems that would limit the usefulness of nizatidine in the elderly.

**Drug interactions and/or related problems**

The following drug interactions and/or related problems have been selected on the basis of their potential clinical significance (possible mechanism in parentheses where appropriate)—not necessarily inclusive (» = major clinical significance):

Note: Only specific interactions between histamine $H_2$-receptor antagonists and other medications have been identified in this monograph. However, histamine $H_2$-receptor antagonists, by increasing gastric pH, have the potential to affect the bioavailability of those medications and dosage forms (e.g., enteric-coated) whose absorption is pH-dependent. Also, histamine $H_2$-receptor antagonists may prevent the degradation of acid-labile drugs.

In addition, because of cimetidine's documented ability to inhibit hepatic microsomal drug metabolism, elimination of other medications that require hepatic metabolism via the cytochrome (P-450) system or that are highly extracted by the liver, may be decreased during concurrent use with cimetidine. This same possibility should be kept in mind for ranitidine, although ranitidine's ability to inhibit hepatic microsomal drug metabolism is significantly less than that for cimetidine. To date, there is no evidence that famotidine or nizatidine binds to cytochrome P-450 to a significant extent, and interactions with medications metabolized by this system have not been reported; however, clinical experience with famotidine and nizatidine is very limited.

Combinations containing any of the following medications, depending on the amount present, may also interact with this medication.

*For all histamine $H_2$-receptor antagonists*

Antacids
(concurrent use with histamine $H_2$-receptor antagonists in the treatment of peptic ulcer may be indicated for the relief of pain; however, simultaneous administration of antacids of medium to high potency [80 mmol to 150 mmol HCl] is not recommended since absorption of histamine $H_2$-receptor antagonists may be decreased; patients should be advised not to take any antacids within one-half to one hour of histamine $H_2$-receptor antagonists)

Bone marrow depressants (see *Appendix II*)
(concurrent use with $H_2$-receptor antagonists may increase the risk of neutropenia or other blood dyscrasias)

» Itraconazole or
» Ketoconazole
(histamine $H_2$-receptor antagonists may increase gastrointestinal pH; concurrent administration with histamine $H_2$-receptor antagonists may result in a marked reduction in absorption of itraconazole or ketoconazole; patients should be advised to take histamine $H_2$-receptor antagonists at least 2 hours after itraconazole or ketoconazole)

Sucralfate
(although a decrease in absorption is only reported in the literature for cimetidine and ranitidine, concurrent use with sucralfate may decrease the absorption of any $H_2$-receptor antagonist; patients should be advised to take an $H_2$-receptor antagonist 2 hours before sucralfate)

*For cimetidine*

Alcohol
(some studies in humans have found increased blood alcohol levels when oral cimetidine was given in conjunction with alcohol; the clinical significance of this effect has not been documented)

» Anticoagulants, coumarin- or indandione-derivative or
» Antidepressants, tricyclic or
Benzodiazepines, especially chlordiazepoxide, diazepam, and midazolam or
Glipizide or
Glyburide or
» Metoprolol or
Metronidazole or
» Phenytoin or
» Propranolol or
» Xanthines, such as:
Aminophylline
Caffeine
Oxtriphylline
Theophylline
(inhibition of the cytochrome P-450 enzyme system by cimetidine may cause a decrease in the hepatic metabolism of these medications, which may result in delayed elimination and increased blood concentrations, when these medications are used concurrently with cimetidine)

(monitoring of blood concentrations, or prothrombin time for anticoagulants, as a guide to dosage is recommended since dosage adjustment of these medications may be necessary during and after cimetidine therapy to prevent bleeding due to anticoagulant potentiation)

(concurrent use of phenytoin with cimetidine may increase the risk of ataxia due to increased blood concentrations of phenytoin)

(concurrent use of metoprolol or propranolol with cimetidine may require monitoring of blood pressure)

Calcium channel blocking agents
(concurrent use with cimetidine may result in accumulation of the calcium channel blocking agent as a result of inhibition of first-pass metabolism; caution and careful titration of the calcium channel blocking agent dose is recommended on initiation of therapy in patients receiving cimetidine)

Cyclosporine
(although this effect is rare, cimetidine has been reported to increase plasma concentrations of cyclosporine and may increase the risk of nephrotoxicity)

Lidocaine
(concurrent administration of lidocaine with cimetidine may result in reduced hepatic clearance of lidocaine, possibly resulting in delayed elimination and increased blood concentrations; lower doses of lidocaine may be required)

Procainamide
(renal elimination of procainamide may be decreased due to competition between cimetidine and procainamide for active tubular secretion, resulting in increased blood concentration of procainamide)

Quinine
(concurrent use of quinine with cimetidine may reduce the clearance of quinine)

*For ranitidine*

Alcohol
(some studies in humans have found increased blood alcohol levels when oral ranitidine was given in conjunction with alcohol; the clinical significance of this effect has not been documented)

Glipizide or
Glyburide or
Metoprolol or
Midazolam or
Nifedipine or
Phenytoin or
Theophylline or
Warfarin
(ranitidine is a weak inhibitor of hepatic drug metabolism; isolated cases of drug interactions have been reported between ranitidine

and glipizide, glyburide, metoprolol, midazolam, nifedipine, phenytoin, theophylline, and warfarin)
(monitoring of blood concentrations or prothrombin time for anticoagulants as a guide to dosage is recommended since dosage adjustment of these medications may be necessary during and after ranitidine therapy to prevent bleeding due to anticoagulant potentiation)
(concurrent use of phenytoin with ranitidine may increase the risk of ataxia due to increased blood concentrations of phenytoin)
Procainamide
(renal elimination of procainamide may be decreased due to competition between ranitidine and procainamide for active tubular secretion, resulting in increased blood concentration of procainamide)

**Laboratory value alterations**
The following have been selected on the basis of their potential clinical significance (possible effect in parentheses where appropriate)—not necessarily inclusive (» = major clinical significance):
With diagnostic test results
*For all histamine H₂-receptor antagonists*
» Gastric acid secretion test
(histamine H₂-receptor antagonists may antagonize the effect of pentagastrin and histamine in the evaluation of gastric acid secretory function; administration of histamine H₂-receptor antagonists is not recommended during the 24 hours preceding the test)
Skin tests using allergen extracts
(histamine H₂-receptor antagonists may inhibit the cutaneous histamine response, thus producing false-negative results; it is recommended that histamine H₂-receptor antagonists be discontinued before the diagnostic use of immediate skin tests)
*For nizatidine only (in addition to those listed above for all histamine H₂-receptor antagonists)*
Urine urobilinogen test
(a false-positive reaction may be produced during nizatidine therapy)
*For ranitidine only (in addition to those listed above for all histamine H₂-receptor antagonists)*
Urine protein test
(a false-positive reaction may be produced during ranitidine therapy; testing with sulphosalicylic acid is recommended)
With physiology/laboratory test values
*For cimetidine*
Creatinine and
Transaminase
(serum values may be increased)
Parathyroid hormone
(concentrations may be decreased, especially when abnormally elevated as in primary hyperparathyroidism)
Prolactin
(serum concentrations may be increased after intravenous bolus administration)
*For famotidine*
Transaminase
(serum values may be increased)
*For nizatidine*
Alanine aminotransferase (ALT [SGPT]) and
Alkaline phosphatase and
Aspartate aminotransferase (AST [SGOT])
(serum values may be increased)
*For ranitidine*
Creatinine and
Gamma-glutamyl transpeptidase and
Transaminase
(serum values may be increased)

**Medical considerations/Contraindications**
The medical considerations/contraindications included have been selected on the basis of their potential clinical significance (reasons given in parentheses where appropriate)—not necessarily inclusive (» = major clinical significance).

***Risk-benefit should be considered when the following medical problems exist:***
Cirrhosis, with history of portal systemic encephalopathy or
Hepatic function impairment or
» Renal function impairment
(decreased hepatic or renal clearance of histamine H₂-receptor antagonists may result in increased plasma concentrations thus increasing the risk of side effects, especially CNS effects; dosage reduction of histamine H₂-receptor antagonists or longer intervals between doses are recommended with renal function impairment and may be necessary with hepatic function impairment)
Immunocompromised patients
(decreased gastric acidity may increase the possibility of a hyperinfection of strongyloidiasis)
Phenylketonuria (PKU)
(certain dosage forms of the Zantac brand of ranitidine contain phenylalanine)
Sensitivity to any of the histamine H₂-receptor antagonists

**Patient monitoring**
The following may be especially important in patient monitoring (other tests may be warranted in some patients, depending on condition; » = major clinical significance):
Cyanocobalamin (vitamin B₁₂) concentration determinations
(monitoring may be needed in long-term treatment of patients likely to have impaired secretion of intrinsic factor, such as those with severe fundic gastritis, to prevent malabsorption of cyanocobalamin)

## Side/Adverse Effects

See *Table 3*, page 1643.
Note: Rapid intravenous bolus administration (an infusion time of less than 5 minutes) of histamine H₂-receptor antagonists may cause significant, transient hypotension. Also, rare instances of cardiac arrhythmias have been reported with intravenous boluses of cimetidine and ranitidine.
Rare cases of hepatitis, with or without jaundice, have been reported in patients using histamine H₂-receptor antagonists; however, a direct association with the use of histamine H₂-receptor antagonists has not been established.

## Overdose

For specific information on the agents used in the management of overdose with histamine H₂-receptor antagonists, see:
• *Atropine* in *Anticholinergics/Antispasmodics (Systemic)* monograph;
• *Diazepam* in *Benzodiazepines (Systemic)* monograph; and/or
• *Lidocaine Hydrochloride (Systemic)* monograph.
For more information on the management of overdose or unintentional ingestion, **contact a Poison Control Center** (see *Poison Control Center Listing*).

**Clinical effects of overdose**
Experience with overdose in humans is limited. In animals, toxic doses of cimetidine have caused respiratory failure and tachycardia. Toxic doses of famotidine given intravenously to dogs caused emesis, restlessness, pallor of mucous membranes or redness of mouth and ears, hypotension, tachycardia, and collapse. Muscular tremors, vomiting, and rapid respiration have been reported with daily doses in excess of 225 mg of ranitidine per kg of body weight in animals.

**Treatment of overdose**
Since there is no specific antidote for overdose with histamine H₂-receptor antagonists, treatment is symptomatic and supportive with possible utilization of the following:
To decrease absorption—
Induction of emesis and/or use of gastric lavage.
Specific treatment—
For seizures—Treatment with intravenous diazepam.
For bradycardia—Treatment with atropine.
For ventricular arrhythmias—Treatment with lidocaine.
Monitoring—
Possible laboratory monitoring for adverse reactions.
Supportive care—
Patients in whom intentional overdose is confirmed or suspected should be referred for psychiatric consultation.

## Patient Consultation

As an aid to patient consultation, refer to *Advice for the Patient, Histamine H₂-receptor Antagonists (Systemic)*.
In providing consultation, consider emphasizing the following selected information (» = major clinical significance):

### Before using this medication
» Conditions affecting use, especially:
Sensitivity to any of the H₂-receptor antagonists
Pregnancy—All cross placenta
Breast-feeding—Cimetidine, famotidine, nizatidine, and ranitidine distributed into breast milk; nursing not recommended during cimetidine therapy, because of high concentration in breast milk

Use in the elderly—Confusion more likely with cimetidine, famotidine, and ranitidine in elderly patients with impaired hepatic or renal function

Other medications, especially itraconazole, ketoconazole (with all histamine $H_2$-receptor antagonists); anticoagulants, metoprolol, phenytoin, xanthines (with cimetidine and possibly ranitidine only); propranolol or tricyclic antidepressants (with cimetidine only)

Other medical problems, especially renal function impairment

**Proper use of this medication**

For patients taking nonprescription strengths: not taking maximum daily dose continuously for more than 2 weeks unless directed by physician; seeing physician promptly if having trouble swallowing or persistent abdominal pain

Dosing schedule for patients taking prescription strengths:
1 dose a day—Taking at bedtime
2 doses a day—Taking in the morning and at bedtime
Several doses a day—Taking with meals and at bedtime

For patients taking famotidine chewable tablets, chewing the tablet well before swallowing

For patients taking ranitidine effervcescent granules or tablets, removing foil wrapping and dissolving dose in 6 to 8 ounces of water before drinking

Taking antacids for relief of ulcer pain; not taking within one-half to one hour of histamine $H_2$-receptor antagonists

» Compliance with full course of therapy
» Proper dosing
Missed dose: Taking as soon as possible; not taking if almost time for next dose; not doubling doses
» Proper storage

**Precautions while using this medication**

Possible interference with gastric acid secretion tests or skin tests using allergens; need to inform physician of use of medication

Avoiding use of foods, drinks, or other medication that may cause gastrointestinal irritation

Discontinuing smoking or at least avoiding smoking after last dose of day

Avoiding alcoholic beverages

Checking with physician if condition does not improve or worsens

**Side/adverse effects**

Signs of possible side effects, especially allergic reaction, bradycardia or tachycardia, bronchospasm, confusion, fever, and neutropenia or other blood dyscrasias

## General Dosing Information

Use of histamine $H_2$-receptor antagonists in the treatment of duodenal ulcer rarely continues beyond 8 weeks, since no long-term, carefully monitored studies have been done with these medications. Also, most patients taking histamine $H_2$-receptor antagonists heal within 6 to 8 weeks.

Although the symptoms of duodenal ulcers may subside within 1 or 2 weeks after initiation of therapy, therapy should be continued for at least 4 to 6 weeks, unless healing has been documented by endoscopic examination or x-rays.

Histamine $H_2$-receptor antagonists may be used, in reduced doses, to prevent ulcer recurrence. However, until consequences of very long term use are fully determined, such use should be limited to patients likely to need surgical treatment, patients with concomitant illnesses in whom surgery would constitute a greater-than-usual risk, and patients with recurrent ulcers.

Initial titration of doses and subsequent dosage adjustment of histamine $H_2$-receptor antagonists is recommended in the long-term treatment of pathological hypersecretory conditions (e.g., Zollinger-Ellison syndrome, systemic mastocytosis, multiple endocrine adenomas). Doses of cimetidine should generally not exceed 2.4 grams per day; however, doses up to 12 grams per day have been used. Up to 160 mg of famotidine every 6 hours and up to 6 grams of ranitidine per day have been administered to some patients with severe Zollinger-Ellison syndrome.

The efficacy of histamine $H_2$-receptor antagonists in inhibiting nocturnal gastric acid secretion may be decreased by cigarette smoking. Patients with peptic ulcer disease should discontinue smoking, or at least avoid smoking after their last dose of the day.

Dosage of histamine $H_2$-receptor antagonists may need to be increased in burn patients to achieve adequate control of gastric pH, because of enhanced clearance of histamine $H_2$-receptor antagonists in these patients. Individualization of dosage should be based on monitoring of gastric pH and/or plasma concentrations of histamine $H_2$-receptor antagonists since their clearance varies in proportion to burn size.

No dosage adjustment of histamine $H_2$-receptor antagonists is necessary for hemodialysis and peritoneal dialysis patients, since only small amounts of the medications are removed.

**For oral dosage forms only**

In the treatment of peptic ulcer and other hypersecretory conditions, optimal therapeutic effect is obtained when histamine $H_2$-receptor antagonists are taken with meals and at bedtime. By administering histamine $H_2$-receptor antagonists with meals, maximum serum concentrations and antisecretory effects are achieved when the stomach is no longer protected by the buffering capacity of the food. However, more recent information indicates that ulcer healing rates may be greatest with a bedtime-only dosage regimen.

If required, antacids of standard neutralizing capacity (e.g., 13 mEq per 15 mL) may be administered concurrently with histamine $H_2$-receptor antagonists for the relief of pain. However, spacing of doses one-half to one hour apart is recommended, especially with antacids of greater neutralizing capacity, since absorption of histamine $H_2$-receptor antagonists may be decreased.

**For parenteral dosage forms only**

Parenteral administration may be indicated in hospitalized patients with pathological hypersecretory disorders or intractable ulcers, or in patients who are unable to take oral medication.

Rapid intravenous bolus administration of cimetidine, famotidine, or ranitidine is not recommended because it may increase the risk of cardiac arrhythmias and hypotension.

**Diet/Nutrition**

Patients with phenylketonuria (PKU) should be informed that some dosage forms of the Zantac brand of ranitidine (EFFERdose Tablets and EFFERdose Granules) contain 16.84 mg of phenylalanine per 150 mg dose.

---

### CIMETIDINE

## Summary of Differences

Indications:
  Also used in treatment of pancreatic insufficiency and as a treatment adjunct in acute urticaria.
Pharmacology/pharmacokinetics:
  Other actions/effects—Inhibits hepatic cytochrome P-450 and P-448 mixed function oxidase (microsomal enzyme) systems; possesses antiandrogenic activity; increases prolactin concentration (with IV bolus injection); enhances gastromucosal defense and healing in stress-induced ulceration and bleeding.
Precautions:
  Drug interactions and/or related problems—May interact with alcohol, anticoagulants, tricyclic antidepressants, benzodiazepines, glipizide, glyburide, metoprolol, metronidazole, phenytoin, propranolol, xanthines, calcium channel blocking agents, cyclosporine, lidocaine, procainamide, sucralfate, quinine.
  Laboratory value alterations—May increase serum prolactin concentrations; may decrease parathyroid hormone concentrations.
Side/adverse effects:
  Constipation has not been reported. Bronchospasms have not been reported as a side/adverse effect with cimetidine.

## Oral Dosage Forms

Note: Bracketed uses in the *Dosage Forms* section refer to categories of use and/or indications that are not included in U.S. product labeling.

### CIMETIDINE TABLETS USP

**Usual adult and adolescent dose**

Duodenal ulcer—
  Treatment: Oral, 300 mg four times a day, with meals and at bedtime; 400 or 600 mg two times a day, in the morning and at bedtime; or 800 mg at bedtime.

  Note: A 1600-mg dose of cimetidine at bedtime has been found to produce a more rapid healing in some ulcer patients who have an endoscopically demonstrated ulcer larger than 1 cm and are also heavy smokers.

  Prophylaxis of recurrent duodenal ulcer: Oral, 300 mg two times a day, in the morning and at bedtime; or 400 mg at bedtime. Patients have been maintained on continued treatment with 400 mg at bedtime for periods of up to five years.

Gastric ulcer, benign, active—
  Oral, 300 mg four times a day, with meals and at bedtime; or 600 mg two times a day, in the morning and at bedtime; or 800 mg at bedtime.

**Heartburn, acid indigestion, and sour stomach—**
Treatment: Oral, 200 mg with water as symptoms occur; dose may be repeated once in twenty-four hours
Prophylaxis: Oral, 100 to 200 mg with water up to one hour before consuming food or beverages expected to cause symptoms

**Gastric hypersecretory conditions (e.g., Zollinger-Ellison syndrome, systemic mastocytosis, multiple endocrine adenomas)—**
Oral, 300 mg four times a day, with meals and at bedtime, the dosage being adjusted as needed, and therapy continued for as long as clinically indicated.

**Gastroesophageal reflux—**
Oral, 800 to 1600 mg per day in divided doses for 12 weeks.

**Upper gastrointestinal bleeding—**
Oral, 300 mg every six hours; or 600 mg two times a day, in the morning and at bedtime.

Note: For patients with impaired renal function—Oral, 300 mg every twelve hours, the dosage being increased to 300 mg every eight hours or more frequently, if necessary. Further reduction in dosage may be required if hepatic function impairment is also present.

### Usual adult prescribing limits
Up to 2.4 grams daily; however, doses up to 12 grams per day have been used in the treatment of pathological hypersecretory conditions.

### Usual pediatric dose
Duodenal ulcer; or
Gastric ulcer—
Oral, 20 to 40 mg per kg of body weight a day in divided doses four times a day, with meals and at bedtime.
Gastroesophageal reflux —
Oral, 40 to 80 mg per kg of body weight a day in divided doses four times a day.

Note: In certain circumstances, doses may be titrated based on gastric pH.
Clinical experience with the use of cimetidine in children up to 16 years of age is limited; risk-benefit must be considered.
In children with impaired renal function, dosage should be reduced to 10 to 15 mg per kg of body weight a day, and the dosing interval increased to eight hours.

### Usual geriatric dose
See *Usual adult and adolescent dose*.

### Strength(s) usually available
U.S.—
100 mg (OTC) [*Tagamet HB;* GENERIC].
200 mg (OTC) [*Tagamet HB 200;* GENERIC].
200 mg (Rx) [*Tagamet;* GENERIC].
300 mg (Rx) [*Tagamet;* GENERIC].
400 mg (Rx) [*Tagamet;* GENERIC].
800 mg (Rx) [*Tagamet;* GENERIC].
Canada—
100 mg (OTC) [*Apo-Cimetidine* (film-coated)].
200 mg (Rx) [*Apo-Cimetidine; Gen-Cimetidine* (film-coated); *Novo-Cimetine* (scored; film-coated); *Nu-Cimet* (film-coated); *Peptol; PMS-Cimetidine* (film-coated); *Tagamet* (film-coated); GENERIC].
300 mg (Rx) [*Apo-Cimetidine; Gen-Cimetidine* (film-coated); *Novo-Cimetine* (scored; film-coated); *Nu-Cimet* (film-coated); *Peptol; PMS-Cimetidine* (film-coated); *Tagamet* (film-coated); GENERIC].
400 mg (Rx) [*Apo-Cimetidine; Gen-Cimetidine* (film-coated); *Novo-Cimetine* (scored; film-coated); *Nu-Cimet* (film-coated); *Peptol; PMS-Cimetidine* (film-coated); *Tagamet* (film-coated); GENERIC].
600 mg (Rx) [*Apo-Cimetidine; Gen-Cimetidine* (film-coated); *Novo-Cimetine* (scored; film-coated); *Nu-Cimet* (film-coated); *Peptol; PMS-Cimetidine* (film-coated); *Tagamet* (film-coated); GENERIC].
800 mg (Rx) [*Apo-Cimetidine; Gen-Cimetidine* (film-coated); *Novo-Cimetine* (scored; film-coated); *Peptol; PMS-Cimetidine* (film-coated); GENERIC].

### Packaging and storage
Store between 15 and 30 °C (59 and 86 °F), in a tight, light-resistant container.

### Auxiliary labeling
• Continue medicine for full time of treatment.

### Note
Tablets have a characteristic odor, which does not represent any risk to the patient.

## CIMETIDINE HYDROCHLORIDE ORAL SOLUTION
Note: The dosing and strengths of the dosage forms available are expressed in terms of cimetidine base (not the hydrochloride salt).

### Usual adult and adolescent dose
See *Cimetidine Tablets USP*.

### Usual adult prescribing limits
See *Cimetidine Tablets USP*.

### Usual pediatric dose
See *Cimetidine Tablets USP*.

### Usual geriatric dose
See *Usual adult and adolescent dose*.

### Strength(s) usually available
U.S.—
300 mg (base) per 5 mL (Rx) [*Tagamet* (alcohol 2.8%); GENERIC].
Canada—
300 mg (base) per 5 mL (Rx) [*Tagamet* (alcohol 2.8%)].

### Packaging and storage
Store between 15 and 30 °C (59 and 86 °F), in a tight, light-resistant container, unless otherwise specified by manufacturer. Protect from freezing.

### Auxiliary labeling
• Continue medicine for full time of treatment.

# Parenteral Dosage Forms

Note: Bracketed uses in the *Dosage Forms* section refer to categories of use and/or indications that are not included in U.S. product labeling.

## CIMETIDINE HYDROCHLORIDE INJECTION
Note: The dosing and strengths of the dosage forms available are expressed in terms of cimetidine base (not the hydrochloride salt).

### Usual adult and adolescent dose
Duodenal ulcer or
Gastric ulcer or
Gastric hypersecretory conditions (e.g., Zollinger-Ellison syndrome, systemic mastocytosis, multiple endocrine adenomas) or
Upper gastrointestinal bleeding—
Intramuscular, 300 mg (base) every six to eight hours.
Intravenous, 300 mg (base) every six to eight hours, diluted with a compatible intravenous solution and administered over a period of not less than five minutes.
Intravenous infusion, 300 mg (base) every six to eight hours, diluted in a compatible intravenous solution and administered over a fifteen- to twenty-minute period.

Note: If necessary, increases in dosage should be made by more frequent administration of a 300 mg dose.

Continuous intravenous infusion, 37.5 (base) mg per hour (900 mg per day), diluted in a compatible intravenous solution. The infusion rate should be adjusted to individual patient requirements.

Note: For patients requiring a rapid elevation of gastric pH, a loading dose of 150 mg may be administered by intravenous infusion before continuous infusion is begun.

Prophylaxis of stress-related mucosal bleeding—
Continuous intravenous infusion, 50 mg (base) per hour, diluted in a compatible intravenous solution for up to 7 days.

Note: Patients with a creatinine clearance less than 30 mL per minute should receive 25 mg per hour.

[Prophylaxis of aspiration pneumonitis]—
Intramuscular, 300 mg (base) one hour before induction of anesthesia, and 300 mg (base) given intramuscularly or intravenously every four hours until patient responds to verbal commands.

[Urticaria therapy adjunct]—
Intravenous, 300 mg over 15 to 20 minutes.

Note: For patients with impaired renal function—Intravenous, 300 mg (base) every twelve hours, the dosage being increased to 300 mg every eight hours or more frequently, if necessary. Further reduction in dosage may be required if hepatic function impairment is also present.

### Usual adult prescribing limits
Up to 2.4 grams (base) daily.

### Usual pediatric dose
Duodenal ulcer or
Gastric ulcer—
Intramuscular, 5 to 10 mg (base) per kg of body weight every six to eight hours.
Intravenous, 5 to 10 mg (base) per kg of body weight every six to eight hours, diluted to a suitable volume with a compatible intravenous solution and administered over a period of not less than two minutes.
Intravenous infusion, 5 to 10 mg (base) per kg of body weight every six to eight hours, diluted to a suitable volume with a compatible

intravenous solution and administered over a fifteen- to twenty-minute period.

Note: In certain circumstances, doses may be titrated based on gastric pH.
Clinical experience with the use of cimetidine in children up to 16 years of age is limited; risk-benefit must be considered.
In children with impaired renal function, doses should be reduced and dosing interval increased.

**Usual geriatric dose**
See *Usual adult and adolescent dose*.

**Strength(s) usually available**
U.S.—
   300 mg (base) per 2 mL (Rx) [*Tagamet*; GENERIC].
   300 mg (base) per 50 mL (premixed) (Rx) [*Tagamet*].
Canada—
   300 mg (base) per 2 mL (Rx) [*Novo-Cimetine; Tagamet*].
   300 mg (base) per 50 mL (premixed) (Rx) [*Tagamet*].

**Packaging and storage**
Store between 15 and 30 °C (59 and 86 °F), unless otherwise specified by manufacturer. Protect from light. Protect from freezing.

**Preparation of dosage form**
Not for premixed dosage form
- For intravenous use, cimetidine hydrochloride injection must be diluted prior to use with a compatible intravenous solution, such as sodium chloride injection (0.9%).
- For intermittent intravenous infusion, cimetidine hydrochloride injection must be diluted prior to use in 50 mL of a compatible intravenous solution, such as dextrose injection (5%).

**Stability**
Diluted solutions of cimetidine hydrochloride injection are stable for 48 hours at room temperature.
Exposure to cold may lead to development of cloudiness. However, this is of no clinical significance, and solution clears on returning to room temperature.
Injection should not be used if discolored or if a precipitate is present.

---

## FAMOTIDINE

## Summary of Differences
Side/adverse effects: Loss of appetite, dryness of mouth or skin, ringing or buzzing in ears have been reported. A decrease in sexual ability has not been reported with famotidine.

## Oral Dosage Forms
Note: Bracketed uses in the *Dosage Forms* section refer to categories of use and/or indications that are not included in U.S. product labeling.

### FAMOTIDINE FOR ORAL SUSPENSION

**Usual adult and adolescent dose**
Duodenal ulcer—
   Treatment: Oral, 40 mg once a day at bedtime or 20 mg two times a day.
   Prophylaxis of recurrent duodenal ulcer: Oral, 20 mg at bedtime.
Gastric ulcer, benign, active—
   Treatment: Oral, 40 mg once a day at bedtime.
Gastric hypersecretory conditions (e.g., Zollinger-Ellison syndrome, systemic mastocytosis, multiple endocrine adenomas)—
   Oral, 20 mg every six hours, the dosage being adjusted as needed and therapy continued for as long as clinically indicated. Doses up to 160 mg every six hours have been administered to some patients with severe Zollinger-Ellison syndrome.
Gastroesophageal reflux—
   Oral, 20 mg two times a day for up to six weeks.
Note: The recommended oral dose for esophagitis due to gastroesophageal reflux disease is 20 to 40 mg two times a day for up to twelve weeks.
[Prophylaxis of aspiration pneumonitis]—
   Oral, 40 mg given either the night before or the morning of surgery.
Note: For patients with severely impaired renal function (creatinine clearance less than 10 mL per minute)—Oral, 20 mg at bedtime. Depending on patient's response, the dosing interval may have to be increased to thirty-six to forty-eight hours.

**Usual pediatric dose**
Gastroesophageal reflux disease—
   For children weighing more than 10 kg: Oral, 1 to 2 mg per kg of body weight a day, in two divided doses.
   For children weighing less than 10 kg: Oral, 1 to 2 mg per kg per day, in three divided doses.

Note: In certain circumstances, doses may be titrated based on gastric pH.

**Usual geriatric dose**
See *Usual adult and adolescent dose*.

**Strength(s) usually available**
U.S.—
   40 mg per 5 mL (Rx) [*Pepcid*].
Canada—
   Not commercially available.

**Packaging and storage**
Prior to constitution, store below 40 °C (104 °F), preferably between 15 and 30 °C (59 and 86 °F), unless otherwise specified by manufacturer.
After constitution, store below 30 °C (86 °F), unless otherwise specified by manufacturer. Protect from freezing.

**Preparation of dosage form**
At time of dispensing, slowly add 46 mL of purified water. Shake vigorously for 5 to 10 seconds immediately after adding the water and immediately before use.

**Stability**
Unused oral suspension of famotidine should be discarded after 30 days.

**Auxiliary labeling**
- Shake well.
- Continue medicine for full time of treatment.

### FAMOTIDINE TABLETS USP

**Usual adult and adolescent dose**
Duodenal ulcer—
   Treatment: Oral, 40 mg once a day at bedtime or 20 mg two times a day.
   Prophylaxis of recurrent duodenal ulcer: Oral, 20 mg at bedtime.
Gastric ulcer, benign, active—
   Treatment: Oral, 40 mg once a day at bedtime.
Heartburn, acid indigestion, and sour stomach—
   Treatment: Oral, 10 mg at onset of symptoms; dose may be repeated once in twenty-four hours
   Prophylaxis: Oral, 10 mg up to one hour before consuming food or beverages expected to cause symptoms
Gastric hypersecretory conditions (e.g., Zollinger-Ellison syndrome, systemic mastocytosis, multiple endocrine adenomas)—
   Oral, 20 mg every six hours, the dosage being adjusted as needed and therapy continued for as long as clinically indicated. Doses up to 160 mg every six hours have been administered to some patients with severe Zollinger-Ellison syndrome.
Gastroesophageal reflux—
   Oral, 20 mg two times a day for up to six weeks.
Note: The recommended oral dose for esophagitis due to gastroesophageal reflux disease is 20 to 40 mg two times a day for up to twelve weeks.
[Prophylaxis of aspiration pneumonitis]—
   Oral, 40 mg given either the night before or the morning of surgery.
Note: For patients with severely impaired renal function (creatinine clearance less than 10 mL per minute)—Oral, 20 mg at bedtime. Depending on patient's response, the dosing interval may have to be increased to thirty-six to forty-eight hours

**Usual pediatric dose**
See *Famotidine for Oral Suspension*.

**Usual geriatric dose**
See *Usual adult and adolescent dose*.

**Strength(s) usually available**
U.S.—
   10 mg (OTC) [*Mylanta-AR; Pepcid AC*].
   20 mg (Rx) [*Pepcid*].
   40 mg (Rx) [*Pepcid*].
Canada—
   10 mg (OTC) [*Acid Control* (film-coated); *Act* (film-coated); *Apo-Famotidine; Dyspep HB* (film-coated); *Gen-Famotidine; Pepcid AC* (film-coated); *Ulcidine-HB*].
   20 mg (Rx) [*Novo-Famotidine; Nu-Famotidine* (film-coated); *Pepcid; Ulcidine* (film-coated); GENERIC].
   40 mg (Rx) [*Novo-Famotidine; Nu-Famotidine* (film-coated); *Pepcid; Ulcidine* (film-coated); GENERIC].

**Packaging and storage**
Store below 40 °C (104 °F), preferably between 15 and 30 °C (59 and 86 °F), in a well-closed container, unless otherwise specified by manufacturer. Protect from light.

## Histamine H₂-receptor Antagonists (Systemic)

**Auxiliary labeling**
- Continue medicine for full time of treatment.

### FAMOTIDINE TABLETS (CHEWABLE)

**Usual adult and adolescent dose**
See *Famotidine Tablets USP*.

**Usual pediatric dose**
See *Famotidine for Oral Suspension*.

**Usual geriatric dose**
See *Famotidine Tablets USP*.

**Strength(s) usually available**
U.S.—
   Not commercially available.
Canada—
   10 mg (OTC) [*Pepcid AC*].

**Packaging and storage**
Store between 15 and 30 °C (59 and 86 °F), in a well-closed container, unless otherwise specified by manufacturer.

**Auxiliary labeling**
- Chew tablets well before swallowing.

## Parenteral Dosage Forms

Note: Bracketed uses in the *Dosage Forms* section refer to categories of use and/or indications that are not included in U.S. product labeling.

### FAMOTIDINE INJECTION

**Usual adult and adolescent dose**
Duodenal ulcer
Gastric ulcer, benign, active and
Gastric hypersecretory conditions (e.g., Zollinger-Ellison syndrome, systemic mastocytosis, multiple endocrine adenomas)—
   Intravenous, 20 mg every twelve hours, diluted with a compatible intravenous solution and administered over a period of not less than two minutes.
   Intravenous infusion, 20 mg every twelve hours, diluted with a compatible intravenous solution and administered over a fifteen- to thirty-minute period.
[Prophylaxis of aspiration pneumonitis]—
   Intramuscular, 20 mg given either the night before or the morning of surgery.

**Usual pediatric dose**
Dosage has not been established.

**Usual geriatric dose**
See *Usual adult and adolescent dose*.

**Strength(s) usually available**
U.S.—
   10 mg per mL (Rx) [*Pepcid I.V.*].
   20 mg per 50 mL (premixed) [*Pepcid*].
Canada—
   10 mg per mL (Rx) [*Pepcid I.V.* (benzyl alcohol 0.9%)].

**Packaging and storage**
Store between 2 and 8 °C (36 and 46 °F), unless otherwise specified by manufacturer. Protect from freezing.

**Preparation of dosage form**
For intravenous use, famotidine must be diluted prior to use with a compatible intravenous solution, such as sodium chloride injection (0.9%) to a total volume of either 5 or 10 mL.
For intravenous infusion, famotidine must be diluted prior to use in 100 mL of a compatible intravenous solution, such as dextrose injection (5%).
Caution—Famotidine products containing benzyl alcohol are not recommended for use in neonates (first 30 days of postnatal life). A fatal toxic syndrome consisting of metabolic acidosis, CNS depression, respiratory problems, renal failure, hypotension, and possibly seizures and intracranial hemorrhages has been associated with this use.

**Stability**
Diluted solutions of famotidine injection are stable for 48 hours at room temperature.
Injection should not be used if discolored or if a precipitate is present.

---

### NIZATIDINE

## Summary of Differences

Pharmacology/pharmacokinetics: Nizatidine is moderately protein bound, approximately 35%.

Precautions: Laboratory value alterations—Increases serum aspartate aminotransferase concentrations. May cause false-positive reaction with urine urobilinogen test.

Side/adverse effects: Agranulocytosis, diarrhea, joint or muscle pain, and loss of hair have not been reported with nizatidine. Increase in sweating has been reported.

## Oral Dosage Forms

### NIZATIDINE CAPSULES USP

**Usual adult and adolescent dose**
Duodenal ulcer—
   Treatment: Oral, 300 mg once a day at bedtime or 150 mg two times a day.
   Note:  For patients with impaired renal function:
      With creatinine clearance less than 20 mL per minute: Oral, 150 mg every other day.
      With creatinine clearance from 20 to 50 mL per minute: Oral, 150 mg every day.
Duodenal ulcer, recurrent—
   Prophylaxis: Oral, 150 mg once a day at bedtime.
   Note:  For patients with impaired renal function:
      With creatinine clearance less than 20 mL per minute: Oral, 150 mg every three days.
      With creatinine clearance from 20 to 50 mL per minute: Oral, 150 mg every other day.
Gastric ulcer, benign, active—
   Treatment: Oral, 300 mg once a day at bedtime or 150 mg two times a day.
Gastroesophageal reflux[1]—
   Oral, 150 mg two times a day.

**Usual pediatric dose**
Dosage has not been established.

**Usual geriatric dose**
See *Usual adult and adolescent dose*.

**Strength(s) usually available**
U.S.—
   150 mg (Rx) [*Axid*].
   300 mg (Rx) [*Axid*].
Canada—
   150 mg (Rx) [*Apo-Nizatidine*; *Axid*].
   300 mg (Rx) [*Apo-Nizatidine*; *Axid*].

**Packaging and storage**
Store between 15 and 30 °C (59 and 86 °F), in a well-closed container, unless otherwise specified by manufacturer.

**Auxiliary labeling**
- Continue medicine for full time of treatment.

### NIZATIDINE TABLETS

**Usual adult and adolescent dose**
Heartburn, acid indigestion, and sour stomach—
   Prophylaxis: Oral, 75 mg thirty to sixty minutes before consuming food or beverages expected to cause symptoms.

**Usual pediatric dose**
Dosage has not been established.

**Usual geriatric dose**
See *Usual adult and adolescent dose*.

U.S.—
   75 mg (OTC) [*Axid AR*].
Canada—
   Not commercially available.

**Packaging and storage**
Store between 20 and 25 °C (68 and 77 °F), in a well-closed container, unless otherwise specified by manufacturer. Protect from light.

[1]Not included in Canadian product labeling.

---

### RANITIDINE

## Summary of Differences

Pharmacology/pharmacokinetics:
   Other actions/effects:
      Weak inhibitor of P-450 mixed function oxidase (microsomal enzyme) system; produces small, transient increase in prolactin concentration (with IV bolus injection).

Precautions:
  Laboratory value alterations—May increase glutamyl transpeptidase. May cause false-positive reaction with urine protein test.
  Drug interactions and/or related problems—May interact with alcohol, antacids, glipizide, glyburide, metoprolol, midazolam, nifedipine, phenytoin, theophylline, warfarin, procainamide, sucralfate.
Side/adverse effects:
  Blurred vision has been reported.

## Oral Dosage Forms

Note: The dosing and strengths of the dosage forms available are expressed in terms of ranitidine base (not the hydrochloride salt).

### RANITIDINE HYDROCHORIDE CAPSULES

**Usual adult and adolescent dose**
Duodenal ulcer—
  Treatment: Oral, 150 mg two times a day or 300 mg at bedtime.
  Prophylaxis of recurrent duodenal ulcer: Oral, 150 mg at bedtime.
Gastric ulcer, benign, active—
  Treatment: Oral, 150 mg two times a day.
  Prophylaxis of recurrent gastric ulcer: Oral, 150 mg at bedtime.
Gastric hypersecretory conditions (e.g., Zollinger-Ellison syndrome, systemic mastocytosis, multiple endocrine adenomas)—
  Oral, 150 mg two times a day, the dosage being adjusted as needed and therapy continued as long as clinically indicated. Doses up to 6 grams per day have been used in severe cases.
Gastroesophageal reflux—
  Oral, 150 mg two times a day.
  Note: The recommended oral dose for erosive esophagitis is 150 mg four times a day.
Note: For patients with impaired renal function (creatinine clearance of less than 50 mL per minute)—Oral, 150 mg every twenty-four hours, the frequency of the dosage being increased to every twelve hours or more frequently, if necessary. Reductions in dosage may also be required if hepatic function impairment is present.

**Usual pediatric dose**
Duodenal ulcer or
Gastric ulcer—
  Oral, 2 to 4 mg per kg of body weight, two times a day up to a maximum dose of 300 mg per day.
Gastroesophageal reflux—
  Oral, 2 to 8 mg per kg of body weight per dose three times a day.
Note: In certain circumstances, doses may be titrated based on gastric pH.

**Usual geriatric dose**
See *Usual adult and adolescent dose*.

**Strength(s) usually available**
U.S.—
  150 mg (base) (Rx) [*Zantac 150 GELdose*; GENERIC].
  300 mg (base) (Rx) [*Zantac 300 GELdose*; GENERIC].
Canada—
  150 mg (base) (Rx) [*Zantac-C*].
  300 mg (base) (Rx) [*Zantac-C*].

**Packaging and storage**
Store between 2 and 25 °C (36 and 77 °F), unless otherwise specified by manufacturer. Store in a tight, light-resistant container.

**Auxiliary labeling**
• Continue medicine for full time of treatment.

### RANITIDINE HYDROCHORIDE EFFERVESCENT GRANULES

**Usual adult and adolescent dose**
See *Ranitidine Capsules*.

**Usual pediatric dose**
See *Ranitidine Capsules*.

**Usual geriatric dose**
See *Ranitidine Capsules*.

U.S.—
  150 mg (base) (Rx) [*Zantac EFFERdose Granules* (phenylalanine 16.84 mg)].
Canada—
  Not commercially available.

**Packaging and storage**
Store between 2 and 30 °C (36 and 86 °F), unless otherwise specified by manufacturer.

**Preparation of dosage form**
Dissolve each dose in 6 to 8 ounces (180 to 240 mL) of water before drinking.

**Auxiliary labeling**
• Continue medicine for full time of treatment.

### RANITIDINE HYDROCHLORIDE SYRUP USP

**Usual adult and adolescent dose**
See *Ranitidine Capsules*.

**Usual pediatric dose**
See *Ranitidine Capsules*.

**Usual geriatric dose**
See *Ranitidine Capsules*.

**Strength(s) usually available**
U.S.—
  150 mg (base) per 10 mL (Rx) [*Zantac* (alcohol 7.5%)].
Canada—
  75 mg (base) per 5 mL (Rx) [*Zantac* (alcohol 7.5%)].

**Packaging and storage**
Store between 4 and 25 °C (39 and 77 °F), in a tight, light-resistant container, unless otherwise specified by manufacturer. Protect from freezing.

**Auxiliary labeling**
• Continue medicine for full time of treatment.

### RANITIDINE HYDROCHLORIDE TABLETS USP

**Usual adult and adolescent dose**
Duodenal ulcer—
  Treatment: Oral, 150 mg two times a day or 300 mg at bedtime.
  Prophylaxis of recurrent duodenal ulcer: Oral, 150 mg at bedtime.
Gastric ulcer, benign, active—
  Treatment: Oral, 150 mg two times a day.
Heartburn, acid indigestion, and sour stomach—
  Treatment: Oral, 75 mg at onset of symptoms; dose may be repeated once in twenty-four hours.
  Prophylaxis: Oral, 75 mg thirty to sixty minutes before consuming food or beverages expected to cause symptoms.
Gastric hypersecretory conditions (e.g., Zollinger-Ellison syndrome, systemic mastocytosis, multiple endocrine adenomas)—
  Oral, 150 mg two times a day, the dosage being adjusted as needed and therapy continued as long as clinically indicated. Doses up to 6 grams per day have been used in severe cases.
Gastroesophageal reflux—
  Oral, 150 mg two times a day.
  Note: The recommended oral dose for erosive esophagitis is 150 mg four times a day.
Note: For patients with impaired renal function (creatinine clearance of less than 50 mL per minute)—Oral, 150 mg every twenty-four hours, the frequency of the dosage being increased to every twelve hours or more frequently, if necessary. Reductions in dosage may also be required if hepatic function impairment is present.

**Usual pediatric dose**
Duodenal ulcer or
Gastric ulcer—
  Oral, 2 to 4 mg per kg of body weight, two times a day up to a maximum dose of 300 mg per day.
Gastroesophageal reflux—
  Oral, 2 to 8 mg per kg of body weight per dose three times a day.
Note: In certain circumstances, doses may be titrated based on gastric pH.

**Usual geriatric dose**
See *Usual adult and adolescent dose*.

**Strength(s) usually available**
U.S.—
  75 mg (base) (OTC) [*Zantac 75* (film-coated)].
  150 mg (base) (Rx) [*Zantac* (film-coated); GENERIC].
  300 mg (base) (Rx) [*Zantac* (film-coated); GENERIC].
Canada—
  75 mg (base) (OTC) [*Zantac 75*].
  150 mg (base) (Rx) [*Apo-Ranitidine; Gen-Ranitidine; Novo-Ranitidine* (film-coated); *Nu-Ranit* (film-coated); *Zantac*].
  300 mg (base) (Rx) [*Apo-Ranitidine; Gen-Ranitidine; Novo-Ranitidine* (film-coated); *Nu-Ranit* (film-coated); *Zantac*].

**Packaging and storage**
Store between 15 and 30 °C (59 and 86 °F), unless otherwise specified by manufacturer. Store in a tight, light-resistant container.

**Auxiliary labeling**
• Continue medicine for full time of treatment.

## RANITIDINE HYDROCHORIDE EFFERVESCENT TABLETS

**Usual adult and adolescent dose**
See *Ranitidine Capsules*.

**Usual pediatric dose**
See *Ranitidine Capsules*.

**Usual geriatric dose**
See *Ranitidine Capsules*.

U.S.—
　150 mg (base) (Rx) [*Zantac EFFERdose Tablets* (phenylalanine 16.84 mg)].
Canada—
　Not commercially available.

**Packaging and storage**
Store between 2 and 30 °C (36 and 86 °F), unless otherwise specified by manufacturer.

**Preparation of dosage form**
Dissolve each dose in 6 to 8 ounces (180 to 240 mL) of water before drinking.

**Auxiliary labeling**
• Continue medicine for full time of treatment.

# Parenteral Dosage Forms

Note: Bracketed uses in the *Dosage Forms* section refer to categories of use and/or indications that are not included in U.S. product labeling. The dosing and strengths of the dosage forms available are expressed in terms of ranitidine base (not the hydrochloride salt).

## RANITIDINE HYDROCHORIDE INJECTION USP

**Usual adult and adolescent dose**
Duodenal ulcer
Gastric ulcer
Gastric hypersecretory conditions (e.g., Zollinger-Ellison syndrome, systemic mastocytosis, multiple endocrine adenomas) and
[Prophylaxis of stress-related mucosal bleeding]—
　Intramuscular, 50 mg every six to eight hours.
　Intravenous, 50 mg every six to eight hours, diluted to a total volume of 20 mL with a compatible intravenous solution and administered over a period of not less than five minutes.
　Intravenous infusion, 50 mg every six to eight hours, diluted in 100 mL of a compatible intravenous solution and administered over a fifteen- to twenty-minute period.
　Continuous intravenous infusion, 6.25 mg per hour, diluted in a compatible intravenous solution.

Note: For gastric hypersecretory conditions, the infusion should be started at 1 mg per kg of body weight per hour and increased by 0.5 mg per kg of body weight per hour increments (if gastric acid output is greater than 10 mEq per hour or patient is symptomatic), up to 2.5 mg per kg of body weight per hour.

[Prophylaxis of aspiration pneumonitis]—
　Intramuscular or slow intravenous injection, 50 mg administered forty-five to sixty minutes before induction of general anesthesia.

Note: For patients with impaired renal function (creatinine clearance of less than 50 mL per minute)—Intravenous, 50 mg every eighteen to twenty-four hours, the frequency of the dosage being increased to every twelve hours or more frequently, if necessary. Further reduction in dosage may be required if hepatic function impairment is also present.

**Usual adult prescribing limits**
Up to 400 mg a day.

**Usual pediatric dose**
Duodenal ulcer or
Gastric ulcer—
　Intravenous infusion, 2 to 4 mg per kilogram of body weight a day, diluted to a suitable volume with a compatible intravenous solution and administered over a fifteen- to twenty-minute period

Gastroesophageal reflux—
　Intravenous infusion, 2 to 8 mg per kg of body weight, diluted in a suitable volume with a compatible intravenous solution and administered over a fifteen- to twenty-minute period, three times a day.

Note: In certain circumstances, doses may be titrated based on gastric pH.

**Usual geriatric dose**
See *Usual adult and adolescent dose*.

**Strength(s) usually available**
U.S.—
　50 mg (base) per 2 mL (Rx) [*Zantac* (phenol 0.5%)].
Canada—
　50 mg (base) per 2 mL (Rx) [*Zantac*].

**Packaging and storage**
Store below 30 °C (86 °F), unless otherwise specified by manufacturer. Protect from light. Protect from freezing.

**Preparation of dosage form**
For 50 mg per 2 mL strength:
　For intravenous use, ranitidine injection must be diluted prior to use to a total volume of 20 mL with a compatible intravenous solution, such as sodium chloride injection (0.9%).
　For intermittent intravenous infusion, ranitidine injection must be diluted prior to use in 100 mL of a compatible intravenous solution, such as dextrose injection (5%).

**Stability**
Diluted solutions of ranitidine injection are stable for 48 hours at room temperature.
Injection should not be used if discolored or if a precipitate is present.
The bulk package of ranitidine should be discarded within twenty-four hours after it is opened.

## RANITIDINE HYDROCHLORIDE IN SODIUM CHLORIDE INJECTION

**Usual adult and adolescent dose**
See *Ranitidine Injection USP*

**Usual adult prescribing limits**
See *Ranitidine Injection USP*

**Usual pediatric dose**
See *Ranitidine Injection USP*

**Usual geriatric dose**
See *Ranitidine Injection USP*

U.S.—
　50 mg (base) per 50 mL (premixed), in 0.45% sodium chloride (Rx) [*Zantac*].
Canada—
　50 mg (base) per 50 mL (premixed), in 0.45% sodium chloride (Rx) [*Zantac*].

**Packaging and storage**
Store between 2 °C and 25 °C (36 °F and 77 °F). Protect from light. Protect from freezing.

Note: Brief exposure to temperatures up to 40 °C (104 °F) has not adversely affected the premixed product.

# Selected Bibliography

Feldman M, Burton M. Histamine$_2$-receptor antagonists standard therapy for acid-peptic diseases (first of two parts). N Engl J Med 1990; 323(24): 1672-80.

Feldman M, Burton M. Histamine$_2$-receptor antagonists standard therapy for acid-peptic diseases (second of two parts). N Engl J Med 1990; 323(25): 1749-55.

Revised: 08/15/97
Interim revision: 03/06/98; 08/14/98

## Table 1. Pharmacology/Pharmacokinetics

| Drug | Absorption* (% oral bioavailability) | Protein binding | Biotransformation | Half-life (elimination) With normal renal function (hr) | Half-life (elimination) With reduced creatinine clearance (mL/min: hr) |
|---|---|---|---|---|---|
| Cimetidine | Rapid (60–70) | Low (15–20%) | Hepatic (30–40% of oral dose) | Oral: 2.0 Parenteral: 1.6–2.1† | 20–50: 2.9 <20: 3.7 Anephric: 5 |
| Famotidine | Rapid; incomplete (40–45) | Low (15–20%) | Hepatic (minimal first pass metabolism) | Oral/Parenteral: 2.5–3.5 | <10: 20 or more |
| Nizatidine | Rapid (>90) | Moderate (35%) | Hepatic (minimal first pass metabolism) | Oral: 1–2 | Anephric: 3.5–11 |
| Ranitidine | Rapid (39–87) | Low (15%) | Hepatic | Oral: 2.5 Parenteral: 2–2.5 | Oral—20–30: 8–9 Parenteral—25–35: 4.8 |

*Rate of absorption, but not extent, is delayed by food. Younger patients usually have better absorption of cimetidine than elderly patients. Absorption of famotidine and nizatidine is slightly increased by food, while the absorption of ranitidine is not significantly affected by the presence of food.

†In burn patients with thermal injury ranging from 6 to 80% of the body surface, and with normal renal function, elimination half-life of cimetidine has been found to be significantly reduced.

## Table 2. Pharmacology/Pharmacokinetics

| Drug | Mean serum concentration resulting in 50% inhibition*(ng/mL) | Time to peak concentration after oral dose (hr) | Time to peak effect (hr) | Duration of action (hr) | Elimination† (% excreted unchanged) |
|---|---|---|---|---|---|
| Cimetidine | 500 | ¾–1½ | Oral: 1–2 | Nocturnal: 6–8 Basal: 4–5 | Primarily renal (48% of oral dose; 75% of parenteral dose)‡ |
| Famotidine | 13 | 1–3 | Oral: 1–3 Parenteral: ½ | Nocturnal and basal: 10–12 (oral and IV) | Primarily renal (30–35% of oral dose; 65–70% of parenteral dose) |
| Nizatidine | 295 | ½–3 | Oral: ½–3 | Nocturnal: Up to 12 Basal: Up to 8 | Primarily renal (60% of oral dose) |
| Ranitidine | 100 | 2–3 | Oral: 1–3 | Nocturnal: 13 Basal: 4 | Primarily renal (30% of oral dose; 70% of parenteral dose) |

*Refers to inhibition of pentagastrin-stimulated acid secretion.

†Trace amounts of H$_2$-receptor antagonists are removable by hemodialysis and peritoneal dialysis.

‡In burn patients with thermal injury ranging from 6 to 80% of the body surface, and with normal renal function, total clearance of cimetidine has been found to be significantly increased.

## Table 3. Side/Adverse Effects*

The following side/adverse effects have been selected on the basis of their potential clinical significance (possible signs and symptoms in parentheses where appropriate)—not necessarily inclusive:

Legend:
I=Cimetidine
II=Famotidine
III=Nizatidine
IV=Ranitidine

| | I | II | III | IV |
|---|---|---|---|---|
| **Medical attention needed** | | | | |
| *Agranulocytosis* (fever, sore throat, or unusual tiredness or weakness) | R§ | R§ | – | R§ |
| *Allergic reaction* (burning, redness, skin rash, or swelling) | ✔ | R | R | ✔ |

*Differences in frequency of occurrence may reflect either lack of clinical-use data or actual pharmacologic distinctions among agents (although their pharmacologic similarity suggests that side effects occurring with one may occur with the others). M = more frequent; L = less frequent; R = rare; – = not reported; ✔ = reported, but percentage of occurrence and/or direct relationship to therapy has not been established.

†More likely to occur in severely ill patients or in patients with impaired hepatic or renal function, particularly elderly patients. Reversible within 3 to 4 days following discontinuation of medication. This side effect may mimic alcohol withdrawal syndrome (delirium tremens) in patients treated for gastrointestinal complications of alcoholism.

‡Cardiac effects after intravenous bolus injection.

§Neutropenia or other blood dyscrasias are more likely to occur in patients with serious concomitant illnesses or in those who also received antimetabolites, alkylating agents, or other medications and/or treatment known to produce neutropenia. Appear to be reversible and tend to occur within the first 30 days of administration.

**Rare; more likely to occur in patients with Zollinger-Ellison syndrome receiving high doses (3 to 10 grams of cimetidine a day) for at least 1 year.

††Rare; more frequent (about 4%) with long-term therapy.

## Table 3. Side/Adverse Effects* *(continued)*

The following side/adverse effects have been selected on the basis of their potential clinical significance (possible signs and symptoms in parentheses where appropriate)—not necessarily inclusive:

Legend:
I=Cimetidine
II=Famotidine
III=Nizatidine
IV=Ranitidine

| | I | II | III | IV |
|---|---|---|---|---|
| *Bradycardia* (slow heartbeat) | R‡ | R | R | R |
| *Bronchospasm* (tightness in chest) | – | R | R | R |
| *Confusion* | R† | ✔ | R | R† |
| *Fever* | R | R | R | R |
| *Neutropenia* (sore throat and fever) | R§ | R§ | R§ | R§ |
| *Tachycardia* (fast, pounding, or irregular heartbeat) | R | R | R | R |
| *Thrombocytopenia* (unusual bleeding or bruising) | R§ | R§ | R§ | R§ |
| **Medical attention needed only if continuing or bothersome** | | | | |
| *Antiandrogenic effect* | | | | |
| (decreased sexual ability) | R** | – | ✔ | ✔ |
| (swelling of the breasts or breast soreness in females and males) | R†† | ✔ | ✔ | ✔ |
| *Blurred vision* | – | – | – | ✔ |
| *Constipation* | – | <2% | ✔ | <2% |
| *Decrease in sexual desire* | ✔ | ✔ | ✔ | ✔ |
| *Diarrhea* | <2% | <2% | – | <2% |
| *Dizziness* | <2% | <2% | ✔ | <2% |
| *Drowsiness* | <2% | ✔ | 2.4% | <2% |
| *Dryness of mouth or skin* | – | ✔ | – | – |
| *Headache* | <3.5% | <5% | ✔ | 2% |
| *Increased sweating* | – | – | 1% | – |
| *Joint or muscle pain* | ✔ | ✔ | – | ✔ |
| *Loss of appetite* | – | ✔ | – | – |
| *Loss of hair* | ✔ | ✔ | – | ✔ |
| *Nausea or vomiting* | <2% | ✔ | ✔ | <2% |
| *Ringing or buzzing in ears* | – | ✔ | – | – |
| *Skin rash* | <2% | ✔ | ✔ | <2% |

*Differences in frequency of occurrence may reflect either lack of clinical-use data or actual pharmacologic distinctions among agents (although their pharmacologic similarity suggests that side effects occurring with one may occur with the others). M = more frequent; L = less frequent; R = rare; – = not reported; ✔ = reported, but percentage of occurrence and/or direct relationship to therapy has not been established.

†More likely to occur in severely ill patients or in patients with impaired hepatic or renal function, particularly elderly patients. Reversible within 3 to 4 days following discontinuation of medication. This side effect may mimic alcohol withdrawal syndrome (delirium tremens) in patients treated for gastrointestinal complications of alcoholism.

‡Cardiac effects after intravenous bolus injection.

§Neutropenia or other blood dyscrasias are more likely to occur in patients with serious concomitant illnesses or in those who also received antimetabolites, alkylating agents, or other medications and/or treatment known to produce neutropenia. Appear to be reversible and tend to occur within the first 30 days of administration.

**Rare; more likely to occur in patients with Zollinger-Ellison syndrome receiving high doses (3 to 10 grams of cimetidine a day) for at least 1 year.

††Rare; more frequent (about 4%) with long-term therapy.

# HISTRELIN  Systemic—INTRODUCTORY VERSION

VA CLASSIFICATION (Primary): HS109

Commonly used brand name(s): *Supprelin*.

Note: For a listing of dosage forms and brand names by country availability, see *Dosage Forms* section(s).

## Category

Gonadotropin inhibitor; gonadotropin-releasing hormone analog.

## Indications

### Accepted

Puberty, central precocious (treatment)—Histrelin is indicated for the treatment of central precocious puberty (CPP) of either neurogenic or idiopathic origin in children of both genders. Children who have CPP usually develop secondary sexual characteristics at an earlier age than cohorts (up to 8 years of age in girls; up to 9.5 years of age in boys). They also show a significantly advanced bone age that can result in diminished adult height attainment. Before initiation of treatment with histrelin, diagnosis of CPP should be confirmed by measuring blood concentrations of total sex steroids, adrenal steroid, and human chorionic gonadotropin; testing stimulation response to gonadotropin-releasing hormone (GnRH or gonadorelin); assessing diagnostic imaging of the brain; and performing pelvic, adrenal, and testicular ultrasound examinations.

Before beginning treatment for CPP with histrelin, it is especially important to ascertain that the patient is willing to comply with the daily regimen of injections and frequent monitoring by the physician during the first 6 to 8 weeks of treatment to assure rapid suppression of gonadal-pituitary function.

## Pharmacology/Pharmacokinetics

**Physicochemical characteristics**

Chemical group—Histrelin acetate is a synthetic nonapeptide gonadotropin-releasing hormone analog (GnRHa) and is of greater potency than the endogenous gonadotropin–releasing hormone (GnRH).

Molecular weight—1323.53 (anhydrous free peptide).

pH—200 micrograms per mL (mcg/mL) of histrelin injection: 4.5 to 6.5 (unbuffered).

500 mcg/mL and 1000 mcg/mL of histrelin injection: 4.5 to 6 (unbuffered).

**Mechanism of action/Effect**

Like GnRH, initial or intermittent administration of histrelin acetate stimulates release of the gonadotropins, luteinizing hormone (LH), and follicle-stimulating hormone (FSH) from the pituitary gland, which in turn transiently increases the gonadal production of estradiol in females and testosterone in both sexes. However, with daily administration, histrelin continuously occupies the GnRH receptor, causing a reversible down-regulation of the GnRH receptors in the pituitary gland and desensitization of the pituitary gonadotropes. These inhibitory effects cause a significant and sustained decline in the production of LH and FSH. A decline in gonadotropin production and release causes a dramatic, reversible decrease in the synthesis of estradiol, progesterone, and testosterone by the ovaries or testes.

Gonadotropin inhibitor—When used regularly in boys and girls for treatment of central precocious puberty, histrelin suppresses LH response to gonadotropin-releasing hormone to prepubertal LH levels within 1 month of treatment. As a result, serum concentrations of the sex steroids estrogen and testosterone decrease. Consequently, secondary sexual development ceases or regresses in girls and boys. Also, linear growth velocity slows, improving the chance of attaining the predicted adult height.

**Onset of action**

For up to 3 weeks after histrelin therapy is initiated, an agonistic action occurs and manifestations of puberty worsen. However, within approximately 4 weeks of histrelin therapy, complete suppression of gonadal steroids occurs and manifestations of puberty lessen.

**Duration of action**

Control of the biochemical and physical manifestations of puberty continue as long as histrelin therapy continues.

## Precautions to Consider

**Carcinogenicity/Tumorigenicity**

Two-year carcinogenicity studies of histrelin given to rats in doses of 5, 25, or 150 micrograms per kg (mcg/kg) of body weight a day (up to fifteen times the human recommended dose [HRD]) resulted in a significant increase in pituitary adenomas, pancreatic islet cell adenomas in female rats, nondose–related testicular Leydig cell tumors (highest incidence in the group using the lowest dose), and stomach papillomas in male rats that were given high doses. Eighteen-month studies of histrelin given to mice in doses of 20, 200, or 2000 mcg/kg per day (up to two hundred times the HRD) resulted in a significant increase in mammary gland adenocarcinomas in all female mice and histiocytic sarcomas in female mice given the highest doses. Generally, tumorigenicity in rodents is particularly sensitive to hormonal stimulation.

**Mutagenicity**

Mutagenicity studies have not been done.

**Pregnancy/Reproduction**

Histrelin is expected to induce reversible anovulation and amenorrhea in most human female adults.

Fertility—Long-term, posttreatment follow-up studies of fertility in children treated for central precocious puberty (CPP) with histrelin have not been done. If an inadequate dose of histrelin is used or successive doses are missed, breakthrough bleeding or ovulation may occur.

Pregnancy—Histrelin should not be given during the course of pregnancy. It is not known how histrelin may affect an embryo if it is administered during pregnancy. The pre-existence of a pregnancy should be ruled out before beginning treatment. A nonhormonal contraceptive method should be used during histrelin therapy if conception is likely or possible.

Major fetal abnormalities, such as dystocia, unilateral hydroureter, and incomplete ossification, were observed in rats, but not in mice or rabbits, after administration of histrelin during gestation. An increase in fetal size occurred in rats and an increase in mortality occurred in rats and rabbits, but not in mice. An increase of fetal resorptions occurred in rats when they were given histrelin in doses of 1 to 15 mcg per kg [mcg/kg] of body weight per day (corresponding to 0.1 to 1.5 times the human dose [HRD]) on the 7th through 20th days of pregnancy. Early termination of the pregnancy and an increase in incidence of fetal death occurred when rabbits were given histrelin in doses of 20 to 80 mcg/kg per day (corresponding to two to eight times the HRD) on the 6th through 18th days of pregnancy. No adverse effects occurred in mice when they were given histrelin in doses 10 to 20 times the HRD on the 6th through the 15th days of pregnancy. The effects on animal fetal mortality were expected results of the changes in gonadal steroid levels induced by histrelin.

FDA Pregnancy Category X.

**Breast-feeding**

It is not known whether histrelin is distributed into breast milk. However, it is recommended that histrelin not be used by nursing mothers.

**Pediatrics**

Appropriate studies on the relationship of age to the effects of histrelin have not been performed in children up to 2 years of age. Safety and efficacy have not been established in children up to 2 years of age. Long-term, posttreatment follow-up studies of fertility in children treated for CPP with histrelin have not been done.

**Medical considerations/Contraindications**

The medical considerations/contraindications included have been selected on the basis of their potential clinical significance (reasons given in parentheses where appropriate)—not necessarily inclusive (» = major clinical significance).

*Risk-benefit should be considered when the following medical problems exist:*

Allergy to histrelin

Hypersensitivity to gonadotropin-releasing hormone or analogs or other ingredients in product formulation

**Patient monitoring**

The following may be especially important in patient monitoring (other tests may be warranted in some patients, depending on condition; » = major clinical significance):

Bone age velocity, bone density, and linear growth velocity determinations
(radiography of the left hand and wrist for bone density determination is recommended prior to initiation of histrelin therapy; during therapy, periodic measurement is suggested after 3 months and every 6 to 12 months to measure linear growth velocity; yearly bone age velocity determinations also are recommended during histrelin treatment)

Imaging studies
(adrenal and pelvic ultrasonography and magnetic resonance imaging or computerized axial tomography of the brain are recommended prior to initiation of histrelin therapy)

Dehydroepiandrosterone concentrations, serum and/or

Estradiol concentrations, serum and/or

Human chorionic gonadotropin concentrations, serum and/or

Hydroxyprogesterone concentrations, serum and/or

Luteinizing hormone concentrations, serum and/or

Prolactin concentrations, serum and/or

Testosterone concentrations, serum
(recommended prior to treatment initiation to establish prepubertal gonadotropin response. If gonadal-pituitary function suppression is not apparent within the first 3 months after therapy with histrelin is initiated and lack of patient compliance is ruled out, histrelin should be discontinued and the diagnosis of gonadotropin-independent sexual precocity should be reconsidered. Other possible causes of sexual precocity include adrenal hyperplasia and chorionic gonadotropin–secreting, intracranial, or testicular tumors)

Gonadotropin-releasing hormone (GnRH) stimulation test
(recommended prior to treatment initiation to establish present gonadotropin response initially and serial GnRH stimulation testing periodically during histrelin treatment as needed to confirm that the patient's pituitary response remains prepubertal)

## Side/Adverse Effects

Note: Some transient signs of puberty, including uterine bleeding, breast enlargement, vaginal secretions, moodiness, and enlarged testes, are expected and will occur in the first month with use of histrelin for treatment of central precocious puberty (CPP) until the hypothalamic-pituitary-gonadal axis becomes suppressed. Suppression usually occurs within the first 3 weeks of treatment.

Inadequate suppression of gonadal hormone secretion, whether due to poor patient compliance or improper dose or management, may have long-term consequences that could include a further compromise of adult stature. Also, it is possible that, in the rare occurrence that the hypothalamic-pituitary-gonadal axis fails to normalize after a patient discontinues histrelin treatment, hypogonadism could result.

The following side/adverse effects have been selected on the basis of their potential clinical significance (possible signs and symptoms in parentheses where appropriate)—not necessarily inclusive:

**Those indicating need for medical attention**
Incidence more frequent
*Headache*—incidence 22%; *leukorrhea* (white vaginal discharge)—incidence 6%; *skin rash*—incidence 7%; *skin reactions at injection site* (itching, redness, and swelling of skin at place of injection)—incidence 45%; *uterine bleeding* (vaginal bleeding)—incidence 22%, transient, occurring within first 3 weeks of therapy initiation

Incidence less frequent—1 to 3%
*Alopecia* (hair loss); *anaphylaxis or hypersensitivity reactions, including angioedema or generalized edema* (difficulty in swallowing; swelling of skin); *bronchospasm or dypsnea* (flushing; trouble in breathing); *cardiovascular collapse* (loss of consciousness); *hypotension* (lightheadedness); *and pruritus or urticaria* (itching or redness of skin); *anemia* (unusual tiredness or weakness); *anxiety; breast discharge, swelling, or pain; cardiovascular effects, including epistaxis* (bloody mucus or unexplained nosebleeds); *hypertension* (increased blood pressure); *migraine headaches*; *palpitations* and *tachycardia* (feeling of fast or irregular heartbeat); *chills; conduct disorder; convulsion; dizziness; dysuria, hematuria, or urinary tract infection* (blood in urine; lower back pain; pain or burning while urinating); *hot flashes* (feeling of warmth; sudden sweating); *infections of upper respiratory tract* (cough; sore throat); *or vagina* (brownish vaginal discharge with odor; irritation or itching of vaginal area); *keratoderma* (thickened patches of skin); *loss of appetite; mental depression; nervousness; otalgia* (earache); *pain in chest, joints, legs, or neck; pallor* (paleness of skin); *purpura* (red or purple spots on skin varying in size from pinpoint to large bruises); *tremor* (trembling or shaking); *visual disturbances, including abnormal pupillary function* (difficulty in seeing); *photophobia* (increased sensitivity of eyes to light); *or polyopia* (seeing two objects instead of just one)

**Those indicating need for medical attention only if they continue or are bothersome**
*Incidence more frequent—3 to 10%*
*Abdominal pain or cramping; diarrhea; nausea; vomiting*

Incidence less frequent—1 to 3%
*Constipation; increased appetite; increased thirst*

## Patient Consultation

As an aid to patient consultation, refer to *Advice for the Patient, Histrelin (Systemic)—Introductory Version*.

In providing consultation, consider emphasizing the following selected information (» = major clinical significance):

**Before using this medication**
» Conditions affecting use, especially:
  Hypersensitivity to gonadotropin-releasing hormone or its analogs or other ingredients in the product formulation
  Pregnancy—Use is not recommended because of potential problems occurring in the fetus; nonhormonal contraception should be used if a pregnancy is likely or possible
  Breast-feeding—Use is not recommended because of possible side effects
  Use in children—Use in children up to 2 years of age has not been established; long-term fertility studies have not been done in children who received histrelin for treatment of central precocious puberty

**Proper use of this medication**
» Carefully reading patient instructions provided
*For those patients receiving medication at home*
  Proper preparation of medication; using proper technique to prevent contamination of the medication, work area, and patient during administration
  Knowing how to prepare injection including removing package from refrigerator, allowing it to warm to room temperature, then removing vial from package just before administering
  Carefully selecting and rotating injection sites (upper arms, thighs, and abdomen) as directed by physician
  Understanding how to inject dose, discarding any unused medication after injection
  Knowing proper dose to use; knowing proper use of needle and syringe included in packaging
  Disposing of needles, syringes, ampules, and unused medication properly

» Not using more medication or using medication more frequent than directed
» Importance of compliance using injection each day at proper time
» Proper dosing
  Missed dose: Checking with your physician if you miss a dose of this medicine
» Proper storage

**Precautions while using this medication**
» Understanding the duration of treatment and the importance of required frequent monitoring by physician during treatment and after histrelin treatment is stopped
» Telling physician if signs of puberty do not stop within 6 to 8 weeks
» Understanding that dizziness can occur with use of histrelin and may impair using machines or other dangerous tasks; on occurrence, reporting these effects to physician

**Side/adverse effects**
Signs of potential side effects, especially headache; leukorrhea; skin rash; skin reactions at site of injection; uterine bleeding; alopecia; anaphylaxis or hypersensitivity reactions, including angioedema or generalized edema, bronchospasm or dyspnea, cardiovascular collapse, hypotension, and pruritus or urticaria; anemia; anxiety; breast swelling, pain, or discharge; cardiovascular effects including epistaxis, hypertension, palpitations, and tachycardia; chills; conduct disorder; convulsion; dizziness; dysuria or hematuria; hot flashes; infections of upper respiratory tract, urinary tract, or vagina; keratoderma; loss of appetite; mental depression; nervousness; otalgia; pain in chest, joints, legs, or neck; pallor; purpura; tremor; visual disturbances, including abnormal pupillary function, photophobia, or polyopia

Advising that transient signs of puberty will worsen during the first 3 weeks of histrelin treatment and may include uterine bleeding, breast enlargement, vaginal secretions, mood changes, and enlarged testes

Advising of long-term consequences, including compromised adult stature, that can occur because of poor control or compliance with therapy. If hypothalamic-pituitary-gonadal axis fails to normalize when puberty is desired and treatment is stopped, hypogonadism may result

## General Dosing Information

Those individuals using histrelin at home should be given the patient information sheet and instructed on medication and injection site preparation, medication administration, and safety precautions for used items. Place of daily injection should be rotated through different areas or body sites, including upper arms, thighs, and abdomen.

The patient and guardian should understand that lack of daily compliance may reactivate the pubertal process. The long-term results of noncompliance or therapy interruption are not known, but may include further compromise of adult stature attainment.

Histrelin should be discontinued when puberty is desired.

Following treatment discontinuation, progress of puberty should be documented and the patient monitored for fertility potential, reproductive function, and ultimate adult height. The patient and guardian should understand that hypogonadism may result if the hypothalamic-pituitary-gonadal axis fails to reactivate after histrelin is discontinued.

**Safety considerations for handling this medication**
Precautions include:
• Use of proper technique to prevent contamination of the medication, work area, and operator during transfer between containers, including proper training in this technique.
• Cautious and proper disposal of needles, syringes, vials, ampules, and unused medication.

## Parenteral Dosage Forms

### HISTRELIN ACETATE INJECTION

**Usual pediatric dose**
Puberty, central precocious—
  Children up to 2 years of age: Safety and efficacy have not been established.
  Children 2 years of age and older: Subcutaneous, 10 mcg per kilogram of body weight once a day at twenty-four-hour intervals; injection site should be varied with each dose.

**Strength(s) usually available**
U.S.—
  200 mcg/mL (120 mcg per 0.6 mL vial) (Rx) [*Supprelin* (mannitol 10%; sodium chloride 0.9%)].

*USP DI*

500 mcg/mL (300 mcg per 0.6 mL vial) (Rx) [*Supprelin* (mannitol 10%; sodium chloride 0.9%)].
1000 mcg/mL (600 mcg per 0.6 mL vial) (Rx) [*Supprelin* (mannitol 10%; sodium chloride 0.9%)].

Note: Packaging includes a 30-day supply of single-use vials containing 0.6 mL of premixed medication and 30 syringes with needles.

**Packaging and storage**
Store between 2 and 8 °C (36 and 46 °F). Protect from light.

**Stability**
Do not use if medication shows particulate matter or discoloration.

**Auxiliary labeling**
- May cause dizziness.
- Refrigerate.
- Do not freeze.

**Note**
Include patient information when dispensing.

**Additional information**
Remove from refrigerator and allow to warm to room temperature before injection.
Remove vial from packaging just before use.
Discard any unused medication after injection.

Developed: 04/27/98

# HMG-COA REDUCTASE INHIBITORS    Systemic

This monograph includes information on the following: 1) Fluvastatin†; 2) Lovastatin; 3) Pravastatin; 4) Simvastatin.

VA CLASSIFICATION (Primary): CV601

Commonly used brand name(s): *Lescol*[1]; *Mevacor*[2]; *Pravachol*[3]; *Zocor*[4].

Other commonly used names are: Epistatin [Simvastatin] Eptastatin [Pravastatin] Mevinolin [Lovastatin] Synvinolin [Simvastatin]

Note: For a listing of dosage forms and brand names by country availability, see *Dosage Forms* section(s).

†Not commercially available in Canada.

## Category
HMG-CoA reductase inhibitor; antihyperlipidemic.

## Indications
**Accepted**
Hyperlipidemia (treatment)—3-Hydroxy-3-methylglutaryl coenzyme A (HMG-CoA) reductase inhibitors are indicated as adjuncts to diet in the treatment of primary hypercholesterolemia (type IIa and IIb hyperlipoproteinemia) caused by elevated low-density lipoprotein (LDL) cholesterol concentrations in patients with a significant risk of coronary artery disease, who have not responded to diet or other measures alone. The HMG-CoA reductase inhibitors may also be useful for the reduction of elevated LDL cholesterol concentrations in patients with combined hypercholesterolemia and hypertriglyceridemia.

For additional information on initial therapeutic guidelines related to the treatment of hyperlipidemia, see *Appendix III*.

## Pharmacology/Pharmacokinetics
**Physicochemical characteristics**
Source—
   Fluvastatin: Synthetic.
   Lovastatin, pravastatin, simvastatin: Fungus-derived.
Molecular weight—
   Fluvastatin sodium: 433.45.
   Lovastatin: 404.55.
   Pravastatin sodium: 446.52.
   Simvastatin: 418.57.

**Mechanism of action/Effect**
The active beta-hydroxy acid form of the 3-hydroxy-3-methylglutaryl coenzyme A (HMG-CoA) reductase inhibitors competitively inhibits the enzyme HMG-CoA reductase. Fluvastatin and pravastatin are administered in the active (open acid) form, while lovastatin and simvastatin must be hydrolyzed to the beta-hydroxyacid in tissues.

Inhibition of HMG-CoA reductase prevents conversion of HMG-CoA to mevalonate, the rate-limiting step in cholesterol biosynthesis. The primary site of action of HMG-CoA reductase inhibitors is the liver. Inhibition of cholesterol synthesis in the liver leads to upregulation of LDL receptors and an increase in catabolism of LDL cholesterol. There may also be some reduction in LDL production as a result of inhibition of hepatic synthesis of very low-density lipoprotein (VLDL), the precursor of LDL. HMG-CoA reductase inhibitors reduce LDL cholesterol, VLDL cholesterol, and to a lesser extent, plasma triglyceride concentrations, and slightly increase high-density lipoprotein (HDL) concentrations.

**Absorption**
Fluvastatin—Rapidly and almost completely absorbed from the gastrointestinal tract (greater than 90%); bioavailability 19 to 29%.
Lovastatin—Reduced by approximately 30% when administered on an empty stomach rather than with food.
Pravastatin—Approximately 34%; bioavailability approximately 18%.

**Protein binding**
Fluvastatin—Very high (greater than 98%).
Lovastatin—Very high (greater than 95%).
Pravastatin—Moderate (50%).
Simvastatin—Very high (approximately 95%).

**Biotransformation**
Fluvastatin—Administered in active (open acid) form. Biotransformation by hydroxylation, N-dealkylation, and beta-oxidation; the major metabolic products present in plasma are pharmacologically inactive.
Lovastatin and simvastatin—By hydrolysis in tissues, to several metabolites, including a major active beta-hydroxy metabolite.
Pravastatin—Administered in active (open acid) form and converted to inactive metabolites and active metabolites with minimal activity.

**Half-life**
Fluvastatin—Approximately 1.2 hours (range, 0.5 to 3.1 hours).
Lovastatin—3 hours.
Pravastatin—1.3 to 2.7 hours.

**Time to peak concentration**
Fluvastatin—0.5 to 0.7 hour.
Lovastatin—2 to 4 hours.
Pravastatin—Approximately 1 hour.
Simvastatin—1.3 to 2.4 hours.

**Duration of action**
Lovastatin—After withdrawal of continuous therapy: 4 to 6 weeks.

**Elimination**
Fluvastatin—
   Fecal (biliary): 90%.
   Renal: 5%.
Lovastatin—
   Fecal (biliary and unabsorbed): 83%.
   Renal: 10%.
Pravastatin—
   Fecal (biliary and unabsorbed): 70%.
   Renal: 20%.
Simvastatin—
   Fecal (biliary and unabsorbed): 60%.
   Renal: 13%.

## Precautions to Consider
**Carcinogenicity**
*Fluvastatin*—A study in rats given fluvastatin in doses of 6, 9, and 18 to 24 mg per kg of body weight (mg/kg) per day (plasma drug concentrations of approximately 9, 13, and 26 to 35 times the mean human plasma drug concentration after a 40-mg dose) found a low incidence of forestomach squamous papillomas and one carcinoma of the forestomach at the 24 mg/kg dose. However, these results were thought to reflect prolonged hyperplasia induced by direct contact with fluvastatin sodium rather than a systemic drug effect. Similar results were found in mice studies. In addition, an increased incidence of thyroid follicular cell adenomas and carcinomas was found in male rats treated with the 18 to 24 mg/kg doses.
*Lovastatin*—Studies in male and female mice given lovastatin in doses of 500 mg/kg per day (a total plasma drug exposure [total HMG-CoA reductase inhibitory activity in extracted plasma] 3 to 4 times that of

humans given the highest recommended dose) for 21 months found an increased incidence of hepatocellular carcinomas and adenomas. In female mice, an increase in pulmonary adenomas was observed at approximately 4 times the human drug exposure. The incidence of papillomas in nonglandular mucosa of the stomach was also increased beginning at exposures 1 to 2 times that of humans; however, the human stomach contains only glandular mucosa. In rats given lovastatin for 24 months at drug exposures between 2 and 7 times human exposure at 80 mg per day, a positive dose–response relationship for hepatocellular carcinogenicity was observed in males.

*Pravastatin*—A study in rats given pravastatin doses producing serum drug concentrations 6 to 10 times higher than those in humans receiving 40 mg showed an increased incidence of hepatocellular carcinomas in male rats at the highest dose. Administration of pravastatin (producing plasma drug concentrations 0.5 to 5 times the human drug concentrations at 40 mg) in mice for 22 months resulted in an increased incidence of malignant lymphomas in females.

*Simvastatin*—A 72-week study in mice given simvastatin at doses producing serum concentrations 3, 15, and 33 times higher than the mean human plasma drug concentration after a 40-mg dose revealed increased incidences of liver adenomas, liver carcinomas, and lung adenomas in the middle- and high-dose groups. In addition, a higher incidence of Harderian gland (a gland of the eye in rodents) adenomas was observed in the high-dose group.

A 2-year study in rats exposed to simvastatin concentrations 45 times higher than those in humans given 40 mg revealed an increased incidence of thyroid follicular adenomas.

**Mutagenicity**
*Fluvastatin*—No evidence of mutagenicity was observed in *in vitro* studies with or without rat-liver activation, including microbial mutagen tests, unscheduled DNA synthesis in rat primary hepatocytes, and chromosomal aberration tests. Additionally, there was no evidence of mutagenicity in *in vivo* rat or mouse micronucleus tests.

*Lovastatin* and *simvastatin*—A microbial mutagen test using mutant strains of *Salmonella typhimurium* with or without rat or mouse liver metabolic activation found no evidence of mutagenicity. There was also no evidence of damage to genetic material in *in vitro* alkaline elution assays using rat or mouse hepatocytes, a V-79 mammalian cell forward mutation study, an *in vitro* chromosome aberration study in CHO cells, or an *in vivo* chromosomal aberration assay in mouse bone marrow.

*Pravastatin*—No evidence of mutagenicity was observed in *in vitro* tests with or without liver metabolic activation, including microbial mutagen tests, a chromosomal aberration test, a gene conversion assay, a dominant lethal test in mice, and a micronucleus test in mice.

**Pregnancy/Reproduction**
Fertility—*Fluvastatin*: No adverse effects on fertility or reproductive performance were observed in rats given fluvastatin sodium at doses of up to 6 mg/kg per day in females and 20 mg/kg per day in males.

*Lovastatin*: Testicular atrophy, decreased spermatogenesis, spermatocytic degeneration, and giant cell formation were seen in dogs given lovastatin starting at doses of 20 mg/kg per day. However, no adverse effects on fertility were observed in rats.

*Pravastatin*: No adverse effects on fertility or general reproductive performance were observed in rats given pravastatin at doses of up to 500 mg/kg per day.

*Simvastatin*: Decreased fertility was noted in rats given simvastatin for 34 weeks at 15 times the maximum human exposure level. However, this effect was not observed in another study in rats given simvastatin for 11 weeks at the same dosage level. Seminiferous tubule degeneration was observed in rats given simvastatin at a dose of 180 mg/kg per day (44 times the exposure level of humans given 40 mg per day). Testicular atrophy, decreased spermatogenesis, spermatocytic degeneration, and giant cell formation were observed in dogs given simvastatin at a dose of 10 mg/kg per day (7 times the human exposure level at a dose of 40 mg per day).

Pregnancy—HMG-CoA reductase inhibitors are not recommended for use during pregnancy or in women who plan to become pregnant in the near future.

Adequate and well-controlled studies in humans have not been done. However, because HMG-CoA reductase inhibitors interfere with biosynthesis of mevalonic acid, a cholesterol precursor that may have an essential function in DNA replication and, therefore, may be closely tied to fetal development (including synthesis of steroids and cell membranes), there is a possibility that fetal harm may be caused by administration of these medications during pregnancy. Vertebral anomalies, anal atresia, tracheo-esophageal fistula with esophageal atresia, and renal and radial dysplasias occurred in a neonate born to a mother who took lovastatin during the first trimester of pregnancy. However, a direct causal relationship has not been proven.

Use of birth control is recommended during use of these medications. If pregnancy occurs during HMG-CoA reductase inhibitor therapy, it is recommended that the HMG-CoA reductase inhibitor be discontinued for the duration of the pregnancy. Because of the long-term nature of antihyperlipidemic treatment, temporary suspension of therapy is not expected to be deleterious.

*Fluvastatin*—
No evidence of teratogenicity was found in rats or rabbits given doses of up to 36 mg/kg and 10 mg/kg per day, respectively. Administration of fluvastatin at 12 and 24 mg/kg per day to female rats during the third trimester resulted in maternal mortality at or near term and postpartum. Fetal and neonatal deaths were also observed. These results were confirmed by a second study.

FDA Pregnancy Category X.

*Lovastatin*—
Studies in mice and rats at doses producing plasma concentrations 40 (mouse fetus) and 80 (rat fetus) times the human exposure found an increased incidence of skeletal malformations. No changes occurred in rats or mice at multiples of 8 and 4 times, respectively, or in rabbits at exposures up to 3 times the highest tolerated human exposure.

FDA Pregnancy Category X.

*Pravastatin*—
Studies in rats and rabbits given pravastatin at doses of 1000 mg/kg per day (240 times the human exposure based on surface area) and 50 mg/kg per day (20 times the human exposure based on surface area), respectively, did not reveal teratogenic effects.

FDA Pregnancy Category X.

*Simvastatin*—
No teratogenic effects were observed in rats or rabbits given simvastatin at doses of 25 mg/kg per day (6 times the human exposure based on surface area) and 10 mg/kg per day (4 times the human exposure based on surface area), respectively.

FDA Pregnancy Category X.

**Breast-feeding**
Use of HMG-CoA reductase inhibitors while breast-feeding is not recommended, because of the potential for serious adverse effects in nursing infants.

*Fluvastatin*—
Fluvastatin is distributed into breast milk and is present in breast milk in a 2 to 1 ratio (milk to plasma).

*Lovastatin*—
It is not known whether lovastatin is distributed into human breast milk, but it is distributed into the milk of rats.

*Pravastatin*—
Trace amounts of pravastatin are distributed into human breast milk.

*Simvastatin*—
It is not known whether simvastatin is distributed into human breast milk.

**Pediatrics**
Appropriate studies on the relationship of age to the effects of HMG-CoA reductase inhibitors have not been performed in the pediatric population. Safety and efficacy have not been established.

Limited experience with use of lovastatin and simvastatin in children younger than 18 years of age seems to indicate that these medications are well tolerated and may be useful in severely hypercholesterolemic children who need medication therapy. However, the long-term safety of HMG-CoA reductase inhibitor use in children has not been studied. Use of these agents should be reserved for severe cases under the care of a lipid specialist. Caution is recommended in use of cholesterol-lowering agents in children younger than 10 years of age.

**Geriatrics**
Studies performed to date in a limited number of patients 65 years of age or older have not demonstrated geriatrics-specific problems that would limit the usefulness of HMG-CoA reductase inhibitors in the elderly.

**Drug interactions and/or related problems**
The following drug interactions and/or related problems have been selected on the basis of their potential clinical significance (possible mechanism in parentheses where appropriate)—not necessarily inclusive (» = major clinical significance):

Note: Combinations containing any of the following medications, depending on the amount present, may also interact with this medication.

Anticoagulants, coumarin- or indandione-derivative
(concurrent use with HMG-CoA reductase inhibitors may increase bleeding or prothrombin time; prothrombin time should be moni-

tored in patients taking HMG-CoA reductase inhibitors with anticoagulants)

Cholestyramine or
Colestipol
(concurrent use may decrease the bioavailability of HMG-CoA reductase inhibitors; therefore, when these agents are used with HMG-CoA reductase inhibitors for therapeutic advantage, it is recommended that the HMG-CoA reductase inhibitor be given 4 hours after cholestyramine or colestipol)

» Cyclosporine or
Erythromycin or
» Gemfibrozil or
Immunosuppressants or
» Niacin
(concurrent use with HMG-CoA reductase inhibitors may be associated with an increased risk of rhabdomyolysis and acute renal failure; although cases have been reported only with lovastatin, the potential also exists with other HMG-CoA reductase inhibitors; combined therapy of HMG-CoA reductase inhibitors with gemfibrozil, niacin, or immunosuppressants should include careful monitoring for symptoms of myopathy or rhabdomyolysis)

*For simvastatin (in addition to those listed above)*
Digoxin
(concurrent use with simvastatin may cause a slight elevation in serum digoxin concentrations)

**Laboratory value alterations**
The following have been selected on the basis of their potential clinical significance (possible effect in parentheses where appropriate)—not necessarily inclusive (» = major clinical significance):

With physiology/laboratory test values
Creatine kinase (CK) concentrations
(mild transient increases are common and may not be drug-related; drug-related marked increases, with myositis and possible renal failure, occur in about 0.5 to 1% of patients, although the incidence may be higher in organ transplant patients treated concurrently with immunosuppressants or gemfibrozil)

Transaminase, serum
(values may be increased, usually to less than 3 times the upper limit of normal; in slightly less than 1 to 2% of patients receiving HMG-CoA reductase inhibitors for at least 1 year, marked increases to more than 3 times the upper limit of normal have occurred)

**Medical considerations/Contraindications**
The medical considerations/contraindications included have been selected on the basis of their potential clinical significance (reasons given in parentheses where appropriate)—not necessarily inclusive (» = major clinical significance).

*Except under special circumstances, this medication should not be used when the following medical problem exists:*
» Hepatic disease, active
(condition may be exacerbated)

*Risk-benefit should be considered when the following medical problems exist:*
Alcoholism, active or in remission or
Hepatic disease, history of
(further increases in liver enzymes may occur)
» Organ transplant, with immunosuppressant therapy
(increased risk of rhabdomyolysis and renal failure)
Sensitivity to any HMG-CoA reductase inhibitor
» Serious conditions predisposing to the development of renal failure secondary to rhabdomyolysis, such as hypotension, severe acute infection, severe metabolic, endocrine, or electrolyte disorders, uncontrolled seizures, major surgery, or trauma
(increased risk of secondary renal failure if rhabdomyolysis occurs)

**Patient monitoring**
The following may be especially important in patient monitoring (other tests may be warranted in some patients, depending on condition; » = major clinical significance):
» Cholesterol, serum
(determinations recommended 4 weeks after initiation of therapy and at periodic intervals during therapy)
» Creatine kinase (CK), serum
(determinations recommended if patient develops muscle tenderness during therapy or during concurrent therapy with niacin or immunosuppressive medications)

» Liver function tests, including serum transaminase
(determinations recommended prior to initiation of therapy, every 6 weeks during the first 3 months of therapy, every 8 weeks during the remainder of the first year of therapy, and then at periodic intervals [approximately every 6 months])

## Side/Adverse Effects

Note: Recent data on patients receiving lovastatin do not reveal clinically significant differences between lovastatin and placebo in the incidence, type, or progression of lens opacities. To date, no increased incidence of lens opacities has been found with fluvastatin, pravastatin, or simvastatin.

Acute *pancreatitis* has been reported during clinical use with simvastatin and lovastatin. A causal relationship with the HMG-CoA reductase inhibitors has not been clearly established. However, onset of symptoms appears to occur within 3 months of initiation of therapy. Rapid regression of symptoms and laboratory anomalies has been observed upon discontinuation of the HMG-CoA reductase inhibitor. Patients should be advised to report immediately to physician acute onset of severe abdominal pain. Although reports of fluvastatin- or pravastatin-associated pancreatitis are lacking, patients taking these medications should also be properly advised, since the mechanism of the effect is poorly understood.

The following side/adverse effects have been selected on the basis of their potential clinical significance (possible signs and symptoms in parentheses where appropriate)—not necessarily inclusive:

**Those indicating need for medical attention**
Incidence less frequent or rare
*Myalgia, myositis, or rhabdomyolysis* (fever; muscle aches or cramps; unusual tiredness or weakness)
Note: *Rhabdomyolysis* may lead to renal failure. Incidence may be increased in patients treated with immunosuppressants, gemfibrozil, erythromycin, or niacin. Onset may occur weeks to months after initiation of treatment. Patients should be advised to report immediately to physician any unexplained muscle pain, tenderness, or weakness, especially if it is accompanied by malaise or fever.

**Those indicating need for medical attention only if they continue or are bothersome**
Incidence more frequent
*Constipation, diarrhea, gas, heartburn, or stomach pain; dizziness; headache; nausea; skin rash*
Incidence rare
*Impotence* (decreased sexual ability); *insomnia* (trouble in sleeping)

## Patient Consultation

As an aid to patient consultation, refer to *Advice for the Patient, HMG-CoA Reductase Inhibitors (Systemic)*.
In providing consultation, consider emphasizing the following selected information (» = major clinical significance):

**Before using this medication**
Diet as preferred therapy; importance of following prescribed diet
» Conditions affecting use, especially:
Sensitivity to any HMG-CoA reductase inhibitor
Pregnancy—Use not recommended in pregnancy or in women who plan to become pregnant in near future, because inhibited formation of cholesterol may impair fetal development; birth defects reported with lovastatin
Breast-feeding—Use not recommended, because of potentially serious adverse effects in nursing infants
Other medications, especially cyclosporine, gemfibrozil, or niacin
Other medical problems, especially, active hepatic disease; hypotension; major surgery; organ transplant with immunosuppressant therapy; severe infection; severe metabolic, endocrine, or electrolyte disorders; trauma; or uncontrolled seizures

**Proper use of this medication**
*For all HMG-CoA reductase inhibitors*
» Importance of not taking more or less medication than the amount prescribed
This medication does not cure the condition but instead helps control it
» Compliance with prescribed diet
» Proper dosing
Missed dose: Taking as soon as possible; not taking if almost time for next dose; not doubling doses
» Proper storage
*For lovastatin*
Taking with meals, since medication is more effective with food

## HMG-CoA Reductase Inhibitors (Systemic)

**Precautions while using this medication**
- Importance of close monitoring by physician
- Notifying physician immediately if pregnancy is suspected
- Checking with physician before discontinuing medications; blood lipid levels may increase significantly
- Caution if any kind of surgery (including dental surgery) or emergency treatment is required

**Side/adverse effects**
Signs of potential side effects, especially myalgia, myositis, or rhabdomyolysis

## General Dosing Information

If serum transaminase concentrations increase to 3 times the upper limit of normal, HMG-CoA reductase inhibitor therapy should be withdrawn.

If creatine kinase (CK) concentrations are markedly increased or myositis occurs, HMG-CoA reductase inhibitor therapy should be withdrawn.

**Diet/Nutrition**
Nonpharmacologic management (dietary and weight control) of hypercholesterolemia is recommended as an adjunct to all pharmacologic therapy.

---
### FLUVASTATIN
---

## Summary of Differences

Pharmacology/pharmacokinetics:
  Biotransformation—By hydroxylation, N-dealkylation, and beta-oxidation to inactive metabolites.
  Time to peak concentration—0.5 to 0.7 hour.

## Additional Dosing Information

Can be taken with meals or on an empty stomach.

## Oral Dosage Forms

Note: The dosing and strengths of the dosage forms available are expressed in terms of fluvastatin base (not the sodium salt).

### FLUVASTATIN SODIUM CAPSULES

**Usual adult and adolescent dose**
Antihyperlipidemic—
  Initial: Oral, 20 mg (base) once a day at bedtime, the dosage being adjusted at four-week intervals as needed and tolerated.
  Maintenance: Oral, 20 to 40 mg (base) once a day in the evening.
  Note: A 40-mg (base) daily dose may be split and taken two times a day.

**Usual pediatric dose**
Safety and efficacy have not been established.

**Strength(s) usually available**
U.S.—
  20 mg (base) (Rx) [*Lescol* (lactose)].
  40 mg (base) (Rx) [*Lescol* (lactose)].
Canada—
  Not commercially available.

**Packaging and storage**
Store below 30 °C (86 °F) in a tight container. Protect from light.

---
### LOVASTATIN
---

## Summary of Differences

Pharmacology/pharmacokinetics:
  Absorption—Reduced by one-third on empty stomach.
  Biotransformation—By hydrolysis to active metabolites.
  Time to peak concentration—2 to 4 hours.
  Duration of action—After withdrawal of continuous therapy: 4 to 6 weeks.

## Additional Dosing Information

Should be taken with meals to maximize absorption.

## Oral Dosage Forms

### LOVASTATIN TABLETS USP

**Usual adult and adolescent dose**
Antihyperlipidemic—
  Initial: Oral, 20 mg once a day with the evening meal, the dosage being adjusted at four-week intervals as needed and tolerated.
  Maintenance: Oral, 20 to 80 mg per day, as a single dose or in divided doses, with meals.
Note: For patients on concomitant immunosuppressive therapy, it is recommended that lovastatin therapy begin with 10 mg per day and not exceed 20 mg per day.
  For patients with severe renal function impairment (creatinine clearance less than 30 mL per min), doses above 20 mg per day should be carefully considered and dosage titration should proceed cautiously.

**Usual adult prescribing limits**
80 mg per day.

**Usual pediatric dose**
Safety and efficacy have not been established.

**Strength(s) usually available**
U.S.—
  10 mg (Rx) [*Mevacor* (lactose)].
  20 mg (Rx) [*Mevacor* (lactose)].
  40 mg (Rx) [*Mevacor* (lactose)].
Canada—
  20 mg (Rx) [*Mevacor* (lactose)].
  40 mg (Rx) [*Mevacor* (lactose)].

**Packaging and storage**
Store below 40 °C (104 °F), preferably between 15 and 30 °C (59 and 86 °F), in a tight, light-resistant container, unless otherwise specified by manufacturer.

**Auxiliary labeling**
- Take with meals.

---
### PRAVASTATIN
---

## Summary of Differences

Pharmacology/pharmacokinetics:
  Biotransformation—Administered in active form.
  Time to peak concentration—1 hour.

## Additional Dosing Information

Can be taken with meals or on an empty stomach.

## Oral Dosage Forms

### PRAVASTATIN SODIUM TABLETS

**Usual adult and adolescent dose**
Antihyperlipidemic—
  Initial:
    Oral, 10 to 20 mg once a day at bedtime, the dosage being adjusted at four-week intervals as needed and tolerated.
    Note: An initial dose of 10 mg once a day at bedtime is recommended in patients with significant renal function impairment or hepatic function impairment, and for the elderly.
  Maintenance:
    10 to 40 mg once a day at bedtime.
    Note: In the elderly, maintenance doses of 20 mg a day or less are usually effective.

**Usual pediatric dose**
Safety and efficacy have not been established.

**Strength(s) usually available**
U.S.—
  10 mg (Rx) [*Pravachol*].
  20 mg (Rx) [*Pravachol*].
  40 mg (Rx) [*Pravachol*].
Canada—
  10 mg (Rx) [*Pravachol*].
  20 mg (Rx) [*Pravachol*].

**Packaging and storage**
Store below 40 °C (104 °F), preferably between 15 and 30 °C (59 and 86 °F), in a well-closed container, unless otherwise specified by manufacturer.

---
### SIMVASTATIN
---

## Summary of Differences

Pharmacology/pharmacokinetics:
  Biotransformation—By hydrolysis to active metabolites.
  Time to peak concentration—1.3 to 2.4 hours.

Precautions:
Drug interactions and/or related problems—Elevation of serum digoxin.

## Additional Dosing Information
Can be taken with meals or on an empty stomach.

## Oral Dosage Forms
### SIMVASTATIN TABLETS
**Usual adult and adolescent dose**
Antihyperlipidemic—
Initial: Oral, 5 to 10 mg once a day in the evening, the dosage being adjusted at four-week intervals.
Maintenance: 5 to 40 mg once a day in the evening.

Note: For patients taking concurrent immunosuppressive medications, it is recommended that simvastatin therapy begin with 5 mg per day and not exceed 10 mg per day.

**Usual adult prescribing limits**
40 mg per day.

**Usual pediatric dose**
Safety and efficacy have not been established.

**Strength(s) usually available**
U.S.—
5 mg (Rx) [Zocor].
10 mg (Rx) [Zocor].
20 mg (Rx) [Zocor].
40 mg (Rx) [Zocor].
Canada—
5 mg (Rx) [Zocor].
10 mg (Rx) [Zocor].
20 mg (Rx) [Zocor].

**Packaging and storage**
Store below 40 °C (104 °F), preferably between 15 and 30 °C (59 and 86 °F), in a well-closed container, unless otherwise specified by manufacturer.

## Selected Bibliography
**General**
Grundy SM. HMG-CoA reductase inhibitors for treatment of hypercholesterolemia. N Engl J Med 1988 Jul 7; 319: 24-33.
**Fluvastatin**
Levy RI, Troendle AJ, Fattu JM. A quarter century of drug treatment of dyslipoproteinemia, with a focus on the new HMG-CoA reductase inhibitor fluvastatin. Circulation 1993; 87(Suppl III): III45-III53.
**Lovastatin**
Zeller FP, Uvodich KC. Lovastatin for hypercholesterolemia. Drug Intell Clin Pharm 1988 Jul/Aug; 2: 542-5.
**Pravastatin**
Jungnickel PW, Cantral KA, Maloley PA. Pravastatin: a new drug for the treatment of hypercholesterolemia. Clin Pharm 1992; 11: 677-89.
**Simvastatin**
Todd P, Goa K. Simvastatin: a review of its pharmacological properties and therapeutic potential in hypercholesterolaemia. Drugs 1990; 40(4): 583-607.

Revised: 03/06/95; 08/18/98

**HOMATROPINE**—See *Anticholinergics/Antispasmodics (Systemic)*; *Homatropine (Ophthalmic)*

# HOMATROPINE Ophthalmic

VA CLASSIFICATION (Primary): OP600
Commonly used brand name(s): *AK-Homatropine; I-Homatrine; Isopto Homatropine; Minims Homatropine; Spectro-Homatropine.*
Note: For a listing of dosage forms and brand names by country availability, see *Dosage Forms* section(s).

## Category
Cycloplegic; mydriatic.

## Indications
**Accepted**
Refraction, cycloplegic—Homatropine is indicated for measurement of refractive errors.
Uveitis (treatment)—Homatropine is indicated for pupil dilation and ciliary muscle relaxation, which are desirable in acute inflammatory conditions of the uveal tract.
Mydriasis, postoperative or
Mydriasis, preoperative—Homatropine may be indicated to produce mydriasis in some preoperative and postoperative conditions.
Lens opacities, axial—Homatropine is indicated as an optical aid in some cases of axial lens opacities.

## Pharmacology/Pharmacokinetics
**Mechanism of action/Effect**
Homatropine (a belladonna alkaloid) is an anticholinergic agent that blocks the responses of the sphincter muscle of the iris and the accommodative muscle of the ciliary body to stimulation by acetylcholine. Dilation of the pupil (mydriasis) and paralysis of accommodation (cycloplegia) result.

**Duration of action**
Moderately long-acting cycloplegic and mydriatic.
Has a shorter duration of action than atropine.
Residual cycloplegia and mydriasis may persist for 24 to 72 hours following instillation of medication.

## Precautions to Consider
**Cross-sensitivity and/or related problems**
Patients sensitive to any of the other belladonna alkaloids may be sensitive to homatropine also.

**Carcinogenicity**
No long-term studies in animals have been done.

**Pregnancy/Reproduction**
Pregnancy—Studies have not been done in humans; however, ophthalmic homatropine may be systemically absorbed.
Studies have not been done in animals.
FDA Pregnancy Category C.

**Breast-feeding**
It is not known whether homatropine is distributed into breast milk. Problems in humans have not been documented; however, ophthalmic homatropine may be systemically absorbed.

**Pediatrics**
An increased susceptibility to homatropine and similar drugs (such as atropine) has been reported in infants and young children and in children with blond hair, blue eyes, Down's syndrome, spastic paralysis, or brain damage; therefore, homatropine should be used with great caution in these patients.

**Geriatrics**
Geriatric patients are more susceptible to the effects of homatropine and similar drugs (such as atropine), thus increasing the potential for systemic side effects.

**Drug interactions and/or related problems**
The following drug interactions and/or related problems have been selected on the basis of their potential clinical significance (possible mechanism in parentheses where appropriate)—not necessarily inclusive (» = major clinical significance):

Note: Combinations containing any of the following medications, depending on the amount present, may also interact with this medication.

Anticholinergics or medications with anticholinergic activity, other (See *Appendix II*)
(if significant systemic absorption of ophthalmic homatropine occurs, concurrent use of other anticholinergics or medications with anticholinergic activity may result in potentiated anticholinergic effects)

Antiglaucoma agents, cholinergic, long-acting, ophthalmic
(concurrent use with homatropine may antagonize the antiglaucoma and miotic actions of ophthalmic long-acting cholinergic antiglaucoma agents, such as demecarium, echothiophate, and isoflurophate; concurrent use with homatropine may also antagonize the antiaccommodative convergence effects of these medications when they are used for the treatment of strabismus)

Antimyasthenics or
Potassium citrate or
Potassium supplements
(if significant systemic absorption of ophthalmic homatropine occurs, concurrent use may increase the chance of toxicity and/or side effects of these systemic medications because of the anticholinergic-induced slowing of gastrointestinal motility)

Carbachol or
Physostigmine or
Pilocarpine
(concurrent use with homatropine may interfere with the antiglaucoma action of carbachol, physostigmine, or pilocarpine. Also, concurrent use counteracts the mydriatic effect of homatropine; this counteraction may be used to therapeutic advantage)

CNS depression–producing medications (See *Appendix II*)
(if significant systemic absorption of ophthalmic homatropine occurs, concurrent use of medications having CNS effects, such as antiemetic agents, phenothiazines, or barbiturates, may result in opisthotonos, convulsions, coma, and extrapyramidal symptoms)

### Medical considerations/Contraindications

The medical considerations/contraindications included have been selected on the basis of their potential clinical significance (reasons given in parentheses where appropriate)—not necessarily inclusive (» = major clinical significance).

*Risk-benefit should be considered when the following medical problems exist:*

Brain damage, in children

Down's syndrome (mongolism), in children and adults

» Glaucoma, primary, or predisposition to angle closure

Keratoconus
(homatropine may produce fixed dilated pupil)

Sensitivity to homatropine

Spastic paralysis, in children

Synechiae between the iris and lens

## Side/Adverse Effects

Note: An increased susceptibility to homatropine and similar drugs (such as atropine) has been reported in infants, young children, children with blond hair or blue eyes, adults and children with Down's syndrome, children with brain damage or spastic paralysis, and the elderly. This susceptibility increases the potential for systemic side effects.

Prolonged use of homatropine may produce local irritation, resulting in follicular conjunctivitis, vascular congestion, edema, exudate, contact dermatitis, or an eczematoid dermatitis.

The following side/adverse effects have been selected on the basis of their potential clinical significance (possible signs and symptoms in parentheses where appropriate)—not necessarily inclusive:

### Those indicating need for medical attention

Symptoms of systemic absorption
*Clumsiness or unsteadiness; confusion or unusual behavior; dryness of skin; fever; flushing or redness of face; hallucinations; skin rash; slurred speech; swollen stomach in infants; tachycardia* (fast or irregular heartbeat); *unusual drowsiness; tiredness or weakness; xerostomia* (thirst or dryness of mouth)

### Those indicating need for medical attention only if they continue or are bothersome

*Blurred vision; eye irritation not present before therapy; increased sensitivity of eyes to light; swelling of the eyelids*

## Overdose

For specific information on the agents used in the management of ophthalmic homatropine overdose, see:
- *Atropine* in *Anticholinergics/Antispasmodics (Systemic)* monograph;
- *Diazepam* in *Benzodiazepines (Systemic)* monograph; and/or
- *Physostigmine (Systemic)* monograph.

For more information on the management of overdose or unintentional ingestion, **contact a Poison Control Center** (see *Poison Control Center Listing*).

### Treatment of overdose

For accidental ingestion, emesis or gastric lavage with 4% tannic acid solution is recommended.

For systemic effects, 0.2 to 1 mg (0.2 mg in children) physostigmine should be administered intravenously, as a dilution containing 1 mg in 5 mL of normal saline. The solution should be injected over a period of not less than 2 minutes. Dosage may be repeated every 5 minutes up to a total dose of 2 mg in children and 6 mg in adults in each 30-minute period.

Physostigmine is contraindicated in hypotensive reactions.

ECG monitoring is recommended during physostigmine administration.

Excitement may be controlled by diazepam or a short-acting barbiturate.

It is recommended that 1 mg of atropine be available for immediate injection if the physostigmine causes bradycardia, convulsion, or bronchoconstriction.

Supportive therapy may require oxygen and assisted respiration; cool water baths for fever, especially in children; and catheterization for urinary retention. In infants and small children, the body surface should be kept moist.

## Patient Consultation

As an aid to patient consultation, refer to *Advice for the Patient, Atropine/Homatropine/Scopolamine (Ophthalmic)*.

In providing consultation, consider emphasizing the following selected information (» = major clinical significance):

### Before using this medication

» Conditions affecting use, especially:

Sensitivity to atropine, homatropine, or scopolamine

Use in children—Infants and young children and children with blond hair or blue eyes may be especially sensitive to the effects of homatropine; this may increase the chance of side effects during treatment

Use in the elderly—Geriatric patients are more susceptible to the effects of homatropine and similar drugs (such as atropine), thus increasing the potential for systemic side effects

Other medical problems, especially primary glaucoma or predisposition to angle closure

### Proper use of this medication

Proper administration technique

Washing hands immediately after application to remove any medication that may be on them; if applying medication to infants or children, washing their hands immediately afterwards also, and not letting any medication get into their mouths; wiping off any medication that may have accidentally gotten on the infant or child, including his or her face and eyelids

Preventing contamination: Not touching applicator tip to any surface; keeping container tightly closed

» Importance of not using more medication than the amount prescribed

» Proper dosing

Missed dose: If dosing schedule is—

Once a day: Applying as soon as possible if remembered same day; if remembered later, skipping missed dose and going back to regular dosing schedule; not doubling doses

More than once a day: Applying as soon as possible; if almost time for next dose, skipping missed dose and going back to regular dosing schedule; not doubling doses

» Proper storage

### Precautions while using this medication

» Medication causes blurred vision and increased sensitivity of the eyes to light; checking with physician if these effects continue longer than 3 days after discontinuation of homatropine

### Side/adverse effects

Signs of potential side effects, especially symptoms of systemic absorption

## General Dosing Information

Although some manufacturers recommend a dose of 2 drops of an ophthalmic solution at appropriate intervals, the conjunctival sac will usually hold only 1 drop.

More frequent instillation or use of a stronger solution may be required to produce adequate cycloplegia in eyes with brown or hazel irides than in eyes with blue irides.

To avoid excessive systemic absorption, patient should press finger to the lacrimal sac during, and for 2 or 3 minutes following, instillation of the solution.

## Ophthalmic Dosage Forms

### HOMATROPINE HYDROBROMIDE OPHTHALMIC SOLUTION USP

**Usual adult and adolescent dose**
Cycloplegic refraction—
 Topical, to the conjunctiva, 1 drop of a 2 or 5% solution. May be repeated every five to ten minutes if needed for two or three doses immediately prior to refraction.
Uveitis—
 Topical, to the conjunctiva, 1 drop of a 2 or 5% solution two or three times a day. In some cases, a frequency of up to every 3 or 4 hours may be required.

**Usual pediatric dose**
Cycloplegic refraction—
 Topical, to the conjunctiva, 1 drop of a 2 to 5% solution every ten minutes for two or three doses immediately prior to refraction.
Uveitis—
 Topical, to the conjunctiva, 1 drop of a 2 to 5% solution two or three times a day.

**Strength(s) usually available**
U.S.—
 2% (Rx) [*Isopto Homatropine* (benzalkonium chloride 0.01%); *Spectro-Homatropine* (benzalkonium chloride 0.01%); GENERIC].
 5% (Rx) [*AK-Homatropine* (benzalkonium chloride 0.01%); *I-Homatrine; Isopto Homatropine* (benzethonium chloride 0.005%); *Spectro-Homatropine;* GENERIC].
Canada—
 2% (Rx) [*Isopto Homatropine* (benzalkonium chloride); *Minims Homatropine;* GENERIC].
 5% (Rx) [*Isopto Homatropine* (benzethonium chloride); GENERIC].

**Packaging and storage**
Store below 40 °C (104 °F), preferably between 15 and 30 °C (59 and 86 °F), unless otherwise specified by manufacturer. Store in a tight container. Protect from freezing.

**Auxiliary labeling**
• For the eye.
• Keep container tightly closed.

Revised: 06/21/94

---

# HYALURONATE SODIUM   Systemic—INTRODUCTORY VERSION

BAN: Hyaluronic acid.
VA CLASSIFICATION (Primary): MS900
Commonly used brand name(s): *Hyalgan.*
Note: For a listing of dosage forms and brand names by country availability, see *Dosage Forms* section(s).

## Category
Analgesic.

## Indications

**General considerations**
Hyaluronate sodium should not be used for osteoarthritis in joints other than the knee.

**Accepted**
Pain (treatment)—Hyaluronate sodium is indicated for the treatment of pain in osteoarthritis of the knee for patients who have failed to respond adequately to other therapy, such as nonpharmacological therapy and simple analgesics.

## Pharmacology/Pharmacokinetics

**Physicochemical characteristics**
Source—Obtained from rooster combs. Hyaluronic acid is a natural sugar of the glycosaminoglycan family that contains a long-chain polymer with repeating disaccharide units of Na-glucuronate-N-acetylglucosamine.
Molecular weight—500,000 to 730,000 daltons.
pH—6.8 to 7.5.

**Mechanism of action/Effect**
The exact mechanism of action is unknown.

## Precautions to Consider

**Cross-sensitivity and/or related problems**
Patients with known hypersensitivities to avian proteins, feathers, and egg products may be sensitive to hyaluronate sodium also.

**Pregnancy/Reproduction**
Fertility—No evidence of impairment of fertility was seen in rats and rabbits given hyaluronate sodium in doses of up to 1.43 mg per kg of body weight (mg/kg), approximately 11 times the maximum recommended human dose (MRHD), per treatment cycle.
Pregnancy—Adequate and well-controlled studies in humans have not been done.
No evidence of harm to the fetus was seen in rats and rabbits given hyaluronate sodium in doses of up to 1.43 mg/kg, approximately 11 times the MRHD, per treatment cycle.

**Breast-feeding**
It is not known whether hyaluronate sodium is distributed into breast milk. However, problems in humans have not been documented.

**Pediatrics**
No information is available on the relationship of age to the effects of hyaluronate sodium in pediatric patients. Safety and efficacy have not been established.

**Geriatrics**
No information is available on the relationship of age to the effects of hyaluronate sodium in geriatric patients.

**Medical considerations/Contraindications**
The medical considerations/contraindications included have been selected on the basis of their potential clinical significance (reasons given in parentheses where appropriate)—not necessarily inclusive (» = major clinical significance).

*Except under special circumstances, this medication should not be used when the following medical problems exist:*
» Skin disease or infection around the injection site
» Hypersensitivity to hyaluronate sodium

## Side/Adverse Effects

The following side/adverse effects have been selected on the basis of their potential clinical significance (possible signs and symptoms in parentheses where appropriate)—not necessarily inclusive:

**Those indicating need for medical attention**
Incidence less frequent
 *Allergic reaction* (fever; injection site reaction; skin rash, hives and/or itching); *anaphylactoid reaction* (bluish discoloration or flushing or redness of skin; coughing; difficulty in swallowing; dizziness or feeling faint, severe; skin rash; hives [may include giant urticaria and/or itching]; stuffy nose; swelling of eyelids, face, or lips; tightness in chest, troubled breathing, and/or wheezing)

**Those indicating need for medical attention only if they continue or are bothersome**
Incidence more frequent
 *Ecchymosis* (large, nonelevated blue or purplish patches in the skin); *gastrointestinal effects* (diarrhea; loss of appetite; nausea and/or vomiting; stomach pain); *headache; inflammation of the knee* (swelling of the knee); *pain at the injection site; pruritus* (itching of the skin)

## Patient Consultation

In providing consultation consider emphasizing the following selected information (» = major clinical significance):

**Before using this medication**
» Conditions affecting use, especially:
  Hypersensitivity to hyaluronate sodium, avian proteins, feathers, or egg products
  Other medical problems, especially skin disease or infection around the injection site

**Proper use of this medication**
» Reading patient instructions carefully
» Proper dosing

**Precautions while using this medication**
» Avoiding any strenuous activities or prolonged weight-bearing activities, such as jogging, heavy lifting, tennis, or standing on feet for a long time within 48 hours following the intra-articular injection with hyaluronate sodium

**Side/adverse effects**
Signs of potential side effects, especially anaphylactoid or allergic reaction

## General Dosing Information
Preparation for injection
- Prior to administration of hyaluronate sodium, it is recommended that subcutaneous lidocaine or a similar anesthetic be administered.
- A strict aseptic technique is recommended during administration of hyaluronate sodium. An aseptic technique should also be used to remove the tip cap from the syringe and needle.
- A 20-gauge needle should be used to administer hyaluronate sodium injection.
- If a joint effusion is present, it should be removed with a syringe before hyaluronate sodium is administered. However, a different syringe should be used to administer hyaluronate sodium.
- If treatment is bilateral, a separate 2-mL vial or prefilled syringe should be used for each knee.

Following the hyaluronate sodium injection, some patients who also have rheumatoid arthritis and gouty arthritis may experience transient increases in inflammation in the knee that is injected with hyaluronate sodium.

Safety and efficacy of repeated cycles of hyaluronate sodium have not been established.

## Parenteral Dosage Forms

### HYALURONATE SODIUM INJECTION
**Usual adult dose**
Pain—
Intra-articular, 20 mg once a week for a total of five injections.

Note: Injections should be given one week apart. Efficacy for the use of less than five injections has not been established.

**Usual adult prescribing limits**
20 mg once a week for a total of five injections.

Note: Safety and efficacy for repeat treatment cycles have not been established.

**Usual pediatric dose**
Safety and efficacy have not been established.

**Usual geriatric dose**
See *Usual adult dose*.

**Strength(s) usually available**
U.S.—
10 mg per mL (single-dose 2-mL vial or 2-mL prefilled syringe) (Rx) [*Hyalgan* (sodium chloride; monobasic sodium phosphate; dibasic sodium phosphate)].

**Packaging and storage**
Store below 25 °C (77 °F).
Protect from freezing and light.

**Stability**
Each vial or syringe should be used to administer a single dose only. Any unused portion of the solution must be discarded.

**Incompatibilities**
Hyaluronic acid may precipitate in the presence of quaternary salts; therefore, skin disinfectants with quaternary salts should not be used for skin preparation.

Developed: 11/05/97

# HYALURONATE SODIUM DERIVATIVE Systemic—INTRODUCTORY VERSION

VA CLASSIFICATION (Primary): MS900
Another commonly used name is hylan G-F 20.
Note: For a listing of dosage forms and brand names by country availability, see *Dosage Forms* section(s).

## Category
Analgesic.

## Indications

**Accepted**
Pain (treatment)—Hyaluronate sodium derivative is indicated for the treatment of pain in osteoarthritis of the knee for patients who have failed to respond adequately to other therapy, such as nonpharmacological therapy and simple analgesics.

## Pharmacology/Pharmacokinetics

**Physicochemical characteristics**
Source—Combination of hylan A and hylan B. Hylans are a derivative of hyaluronate sodium, which is obtained from chicken combs. Hyaluronate sodium is a natural sugar of the glycosaminoglycan family that contains a long-chain polymer with repeating disaccharide units of Na-glucuronate-*N*-acetylglucosamine.
Molecular weight—6,000,000.
pH—7.2.

**Mechanism of action/Effect**
The exact mechanism of action is unknown.

## Precautions to Consider

**Cross-sensitivity and/or related problems**
Patients with known hypersensitivities to hyaluronate sodium, avian proteins, feathers, and egg products may be sensitive to hyaluronate sodium derivative also.

**Pregnancy/Reproduction**
Pregnancy—Adequate and well-controlled studies in humans have not been done.

**Breast-feeding**
It is not known whether hyaluronate sodium derivative is distributed into breast milk. However, problems in humans have not been documented.

**Pediatrics**
No information is available on the relationship of age to the effects of hyaluronate sodium derivative in pediatric patients. Safety and efficacy have not been established.

**Geriatrics**
No information is available on the relationship of age to the effects of hyaluronate sodium derivative in geriatric patients. Safety and efficacy have not been established.

**Medical considerations/Contraindications**
The medical considerations/contraindications included have been selected on the basis of their potential clinical significance (reasons given in parentheses where appropriate)—not necessarily inclusive (» = major clinical significance).

*Except under special circumstances, this medication should not be used when the following medical problems exist:*
» Skin disease or infection around the injection site
» Hypersensitivity to hylans

## Side/Adverse Effects

The following side/adverse effects have been selected on the basis of their potential clinical significance (possible signs and symptoms in parentheses where appropriate)—not necessarily inclusive:

**Those indicating need for medical attention**
Incidence rare
*Hives; respiratory problems* (difficulty breathing; shortness of breath)

**Those indicating need for medical attention only if they continue or are bothersome**
Incidence more frequent
*Knee pain; pain at the injection site; swelling of the knee*
Incidence rare
*Calf cramps; dizziness; facial flushing with swelling of the lips; headache; infection of the joint; itching of the skin; muscle pain; nausea;*

*pain on one side of the body with anxiety, nausea, and tiredness; skin rash; tachycardia* (rapid heartbeat)

### Patient Consultation
As an aid to patient consultation, refer to *Advice for the Patient, Hyaluronate Sodium Derivative (Systemic)—Introductory version.*
In providing consultation, consider emphasizing the following selected information (» = major clinical significance):

**Before using this medication**
» Conditions affecting use, especially:
   Sensitivity to hyaluronate sodium derivative, hyaluronate sodium, other hylans, avian proteins, feathers, or egg products
   Other medical problems, especially skin disease, infection around the injection site, or knee joint infections

**Proper use of this medication**
» Proper dosing
» Proper storage

**Precautions while using this medication**
Avoiding any strenuous activities or prolonged weight-bearing activities, such as jogging, heavy lifting, tennis, or standing on feet for a long time within 48 hours following the intra-articular injection with hyaluronate sodium derivative

**Side/adverse effects**
Signs of potential side effects, especially hives or respiratory problems

### General Dosing Information
Preparation for injection
- A strict aseptic technique is recommended during administration of hyaluronate sodium derivative. An aseptic technique also should be used to remove the tip cap from the syringe and needle.
- An 18- to 22-gauge needle should be used to administer hyaluronate sodium derivative.
- If a joint effusion is present, it should be removed with a syringe before hyaluronate sodium derivative is administered. However, a different syringe should be used to administer hyaluronate sodium derivative.
- If treatment is bilateral, a separate 2-mL prefilled syringe should be used for each knee.

Do not inject sodium hyaluronate derivative extra-articularly or into the synovial tissues or cavity.
Intravascular injections may cause systemic adverse events.

### Parenteral Dosage Forms

#### HYALURONATE SODIUM DERIVATIVE INJECTION

**Usual adult dose**
Pain—
   Intra-articular, 16 mg once a week for a total of three injections.
   Note: Injections should be given one week apart.

**Usual adult prescribing limits**
16 mg once a week for a total of three injections.
Note: Safety and efficacy for repeat treatment cycles have not been established.

**Usual pediatric dose**
Safety and efficacy have not been established.

**Usual geriatric dose**
See *Usual adult dose.*

**Strength(s) usually available**
U.S.—
   16 mg (single-dose 2-mL prefilled syringe) (Rx) [*Synvisc* (sodium chloride; disodium hydrogen phosphate; sodium dihydrogen phosphate monohydrate)].

**Packaging and storage**
Store below 30 ºC (86 ºF). Protect from freezing.

**Stability**
Each prefilled syringe should be used to administer a single dose only. Any unused portion of the solution must be discarded.

**Incompatibilities**
Hyaluronate sodium derivative may precipitate in the presence of quaternary salts; therefore, skin disinfectants with quaternary salts should not be used for skin preparations.
Anesthetics or any other medications intra-articularly into the knee simultaneously with hyaluronate sodium derivative may dilute it and affect its safety and effectiveness.

Developed: 07/08/98
Interim revision: 08/11/98

---

# HYDRALAZINE  Systemic

VA CLASSIFICATION (Primary/Secondary): CV490/CV900
Commonly used brand name(s): *Apresoline; Novo-Hylazin.*
Note: For a listing of dosage forms and brand names by country availability, see *Dosage Forms* section(s).

## Category
Antihypertensive; vasodilator, congestive heart failure.

## Indications
Note: Bracketed information in the *Indications* section refers to uses that are not included in U.S. product labeling.

**Accepted**
Hypertension (treatment)—Hydralazine is indicated orally for the treatment of hypertension.
   For additional information on initial therapeutic guidelines related to the treatment of hypertension, see *Appendix III.*
   Hydralazine is indicated intravenously when oral therapy cannot be given or when there is an urgent need to lower blood pressure, such as in hypertensive crisis or pre-eclampsia or eclampsia.
[Congestive heart failure (treatment)][1]—Hydralazine may be used in combination with isosorbide dinitrate plus diuretics and digitalis in the treatment of congestive heart failure. Hydralazine and isosorbide dinitrate combination has been shown to improve 3-year mortality when compared to placebo. A more favorable effect on 2-year mortality was shown with an angiotensin-converting enzyme (ACE) inhibitor than with hydralazine and isosorbide dinitrate combination in a subsequent study. However, hydralazine plus isosorbide dinitrate still improved survival and exerted a more favorable effect on exercise performance and left ventricular ejection fraction than the ACE inhibitor. This combination may be considered in patients with left ventricular systolic dysfunction who cannot tolerate ACE inhibitors.

[1]Not included in Canadian product labeling.

## Pharmacology/Pharmacokinetics

**Physicochemical characteristics**
Molecular weight—Hydralazine hydrochloride: 196.64.
pKa—7.3.

**Mechanism of action/Effect**
Antihypertensive—The exact mechanism of antihypertensive action is not fully understood. The predominant effect of hydralazine is direct vasodilation of arterioles with little effect on veins, resulting in a decrease in peripheral resistance and an increase in heart rate, stroke volume, and cardiac output.
Vasodilator, congestive heart failure—Beneficial effects are due to increased cardiac output, decreased systemic resistance, and afterload reduction when hydralazine is used in combination with isosorbide dinitrate.

**Absorption**
Hydralazine is well absorbed (up to 90%) after oral administration, although plasma concentrations are considerably lower than after intramuscular or intravenous administration of the same dose because of first-pass metabolism. Oral bioavailability is approximately 50% (slow acetylators) or 30% (fast acetylators).

**Protein binding**
High (87%).

**Biotransformation**
Hydralazine undergoes extensive hepatic metabolism. Hydralazine is subject to polymorphic acetylation, although this does not appear to be the major metabolic pathway. Formation of hydrazone metabolites consti-

tutes the other important metabolic pathway. The active metabolites, hydralazine acetonide hydrazone and hydralazine pyruvate hydrazone, are equipotent with the parent, hydralazine.

**Half-life**
3 to 7 hours; prolonged in renal failure.
Some references state a difference in half-life between slow and fast acetylators, but there is generally thought to be little difference.
The half-life of antihypertensive action is much longer than the plasma half-life, possibly because hydralazine persists within muscular arterial walls.

**Onset of action**
Oral—45 minutes.
Intravenous—10 to 20 minutes.

**Time to peak concentration**
Oral—1 to 2 hours.

**Time to peak effect**
Intravenous—15 to 30 minutes.

**Duration of action**
Oral or intravenous—3 to 8 hours.

**Elimination**
Renal, 2 to 4% unchanged after oral administration and 11 to 14% unchanged after intravenous administration.

## Precautions to Consider

### Cross-sensitivity and/or related problems
Patients sensitive to tartrazine may be sensitive to the tablet dosage form also, since some tablets contain tartrazine.

### Carcinogenicity
In a 2-year carcinogenicity study of rats, hydralazine given at dose levels of 15, 30, and 60 mg per kg of body weight (mg/kg) per day (about 5 to 20 times the recommended human daily dose) produced a small, but statistically significant, increase in benign neoplastic nodules in male and female rats from the high-dose group and in female rats from the intermediate-dose group. Furthermore, benign interstitial cell tumors of the testes were significantly increased in male rats from the high-dose group.

### Tumorigenicity
A lifetime study in Swiss male and female albino mice given hydralazine continuously in their drinking water at a dose of about 250 mg/kg per day (approximately 80 times the maximum recommended human dose) revealed an increase in the incidence of lung tumors (adenomas and adenocarcinomas).

### Mutagenicity
Hydralazine was shown to be mutagenic in bacterial systems (gene mutation and DNA repair). Mutagenicity was also found in 1 of 2 rat and 1 rabbit hepatocyte *in vitro* DNA repair studies. However, *in vivo* and *in vitro* studies using mice lymphoma cells, germinal cells, and fibroblasts, Chinese hamster bone marrow cells, and human cell fibroblasts did not reveal any mutagenic potential for hydralazine.

### Pregnancy/Reproduction
Pregnancy—Hydralazine crosses the placenta. Studies in humans have not been done. However, thrombocytopenia, leukopenia, petechial bleeding, and hematomas have been reported in newborns whose mothers took hydralazine; symptoms resolved spontaneously in 1 to 3 weeks. Furthermore, there have been some reports of fetal distress following intravenous use of hydralazine to control maternal hypertension. The risk of fetal distress appears to be greater when vasodilation with hydralazine is undertaken without prior volume expansion. Preterm infants and growth-retarded infants appear to be particularly at risk.
Studies in mice given hydralazine at 20 to 30 times the maximum daily human dose of 200 to 300 mg revealed teratogenic effects. Furthermore, studies in rabbits indicate teratogenic effects at doses 10 to 15 times the maximum daily human dose. Teratogenic effects observed were cleft palate and malformations of facial and cranial bones. However, hydralazine was not shown to be teratogenic in rats.

FDA Pregnancy Category C.

### Breast-feeding
It is not known whether hydralazine is distributed into human milk.

### Pediatrics
Appropriate studies on the relationship of age to the effects of hydralazine have not been performed in the pediatric population. However, pediatrics-specific problems that would limit the usefulness of this medication in children are not expected.

### Geriatrics
Although appropriate studies on the relationship of age to the effects of hydralazine have not been performed in the geriatric population, geriatrics-specific problems are not expected to limit the usefulness of hydralazine in the elderly. However, elderly patients may be more sensitive to the hypotensive effects of hydralazine and are more likely to have age-related renal function impairment, both of which may require dosage reduction.

### Pharmacogenetics
All patients may be divided into two groups, slow and fast acetylators of hydralazine. Patients who are slow acetylators may be more prone to develop adverse effects (especially the systemic lupus erythematosus [SLE]–like syndrome) and may require lower-than-usual doses. Eskimo, Oriental, and American Indian populations have the lowest prevalence of slow acetylators, while Egyptian, Israeli, Scandanavian, other Caucasian, and black populations have the highest prevalence of slow acetylators.

### Drug interactions and/or related problems
The following drug interactions and/or related problems have been selected on the basis of their potential clinical significance (possible mechanism in parentheses where appropriate)—not necessarily inclusive (» = major clinical significance):

Note: Combinations containing any of the following medications, depending on the amount present, may also interact with this medication.

Anti-inflammatory drugs, nonsteroidal (NSAIDs), especially indomethacin
(may reduce antihypertensive effects of hydralazine; indomethacin, and possibly other NSAIDs, may antagonize the antihypertensive effect by inhibiting renal prostaglandin synthesis and/or by causing sodium and fluid retention; the patient should be carefully monitored to confirm that the desired effect is being obtained)

» Diazoxide or
Hypotension-producing medications, other (See *Appendix II*)
(antihypertensive effects may be potentiated when these medications are used concurrently with hydralazine; concurrent use of diazoxide or other potent parenteral antihypertensives with hydralazine may result in a severe, additive hypotensive effect; although some antihypertensive and/or diuretic combinations are frequently used for therapeutic advantage, dosage adjustments may be necessary during concurrent use)

(patients should be continuously observed for excessive fall in blood pressure for several hours after concurrent administration of diazoxide or other potent parenteral antihypertensives)

Estrogens
(estrogen-induced fluid retention may increase blood pressure)

Sympathomimetics
(may reduce antihypertensive effects of hydralazine; the patient should be carefully monitored to confirm that the desired effect is being obtained)

### Laboratory value alterations
The following have been selected on the basis of their potential clinical significance (possible effect in parentheses where appropriate)—not necessarily inclusive (» = major clinical significance):

With physiology/laboratory test values
Direct antiglobulin (Coombs') tests
(may produce positive results)

### Medical considerations/Contraindications
The medical considerations/contraindications included have been selected on the basis of their potential clinical significance (reasons given in parentheses where appropriate)—not necessarily inclusive (» = major clinical significance).

*Risk-benefit should be considered when the following medical problems exist:*

Aortic aneurysm or
» Aortic dissection, acute
(reflexive increase in heart rate, cardiac output, and shear stress associated with hydralazine may exacerbate condition)

Cerebrovascular disease or accident
(decreased blood pressure may increase cerebral ischemia)

Congestive heart failure
(use of hydralazine alone is not recommended, although it may improve cardiac performance in some patients with intractable left ventricular failure)

» Coronary artery disease
(myocardial stimulation and increased myocardial oxygen demands may cause or aggravate ischemia and angina and reportedly may precipitate myocardial infarction)

Renal function impairment, advanced
(accumulation of hydralazine may occur because of slower acetylation and reduced elimination, although incidence of toxic side effects is not increased; lower dosage may be required)
» Rheumatic heart disease, mitral valvular
(hydralazine may increase pulmonary artery pressure)
Sensitivity to hydralazine

Note: There is no substantial evidence that use of hydralazine in the treatment of hypertension in patients with systemic vasculitis or systemic lupus erythematosus exacerbates the underlying disease process.

**Patient monitoring**
The following may be especially important in patient monitoring (other tests may be warranted in some patients, depending on condition; » = major clinical significance):

Antinuclear antibody (ANA) titer determinations and
Complete blood counts and
Lupus erythematosus cell preparations
(may be indicated if patient develops arthralgia, fever, chest pain, continued malaise, or other unexplained symptoms)
» Blood pressure measurements
(recommended at periodic intervals in patients being treated for hypertension; selected patients may be trained to perform blood pressure measurements at home and report the results at regular physician visits)

## Side/Adverse Effects

Note: Side/adverse effects are rare at lower dosages and are generally reversible.
Hepatotoxicity has been reported in a few patients.

The following side/adverse effects have been selected on the basis of their potential clinical significance (possible signs and symptoms in parentheses where appropriate)—not necessarily inclusive:

**Those indicating need for medical attention**
Incidence less frequent
*Allergic reaction* (skin rash or itching); *angina pectoris* (chest pain); *cutaneous vasculitis* (blisters on skin); *lymphadenopathy* (swelling of lymph glands); *peripheral neuritis* (numbness, tingling, pain, or weakness in hands or feet); *sodium and water retention and edema* (swelling of feet or lower legs); *systemic lupus erythematosus (SLE)–like syndrome, including glomerulonephritis* (blisters on skin; chest pain; general feeling of discomfort, illness, or weakness; muscle pain; joint pain; skin rash or itching; sore throat and fever)

Note: The SLE-like syndrome is a pharmacologic rather than an allergic effect. Risk factors include high daily doses of hydralazine (greater than 200 mg per day), slow acetylator or HLA-DRw4 phenotype, and family history of autoimmune disease. It is rarely seen with doses lower than 200 mg per day. The most common symptoms associated with hydralazine-induced SLE-like syndrome involve the musculoskeletal system, including arthralgias, arthritis, and myalgias. Other symptoms may include malaise, fever, or skin changes. Renal or central nervous system involvement is rare. A positive antinuclear antibody (ANA) is evident in virtually all cases of hydralazine-induced SLE-like syndrome. However, approximately 30% of all patients receiving hydralazine develop a positive ANA within one year of continuous therapy. Therefore, an isolated positive ANA does not necessarily mean that hydralazine-induced SLE-like syndrome is present. The clinical manifestations of hydralazine-induced SLE-like syndrome resolve within days to weeks of medication withdrawal. Resolution of positive ANA usually takes several months.

Incidence rare
*Blood dyscrasias, including agranulocytosis, leukopenia, and purpura* (fever; general feeling of discomfort or illness; sore throat; weakness)

**Those indicating need for medical attention only if they continue or are bothersome**
Incidence more frequent
*Anorexia* (loss of appetite); *diarrhea; headache; nausea or vomiting; palpitations* (pounding heartbeat); *tachycardia* (fast heartbeat)

Note: In patients with severe heart failure, sympathetic tone is already high and there will be little or no change in heart rate.

Incidence less frequent
*Constipation; dyspnea* (shortness of breath); *hypotension* (dizziness or lightheadedness); *lacrimation* (watering eyes); *nasal congestion* (stuffy nose); *redness or flushing of face*

## Overdose

For specific information on the agents used in the management of hydralazine overdose, see:
• *Beta-adrenergic Blocking Agents (Systemic) monograph;*
• *Charcoal, Activated (Oral-Local) monograph; and/or*
• *Sympathomimetic Agents—Cardiovascular Use (Parenteral-Systemic) monograph.*

For more information on the management of overdose or unintentional ingestion, **contact a Poison Control Center** (see *Poison Control Center Listing*).

**Clinical effects of overdose**
The following effects have been selected on the basis of their potential clinical significance (possible signs and symptoms in parentheses where appropriate)—not necessarily inclusive:

*Headache; hypotension; myocardial infarction; myocardial ischemia* (chest pain); *skin flushing; shock; tachycardia* (fast heartbeat)

Note: Myocardial ischemia with marked ST segment depression has been reported.

**Treatment of overdose**
To decrease absorption—
Evacuation of gastric contents. If conditions permit, activated charcoal may be administered.
Specific treatment—
For shock: Plasma expanders. If a vasopressor is required, care should be taken not to precipitate or aggravate cardiac arrhythmia.
For tachycardia: Beta-adrenergic blocking agents.
Monitoring—
Fluid and electrolyte status and renal function should be monitored.
Supportive care—
Support of cardiovascular system is most important. Patients in whom intentional overdose is known or suspected should be referred for psychiatric consultation.

## Patient Consultation

As an aid to patient consultation, refer to *Advice for the Patient, Hydralazine (Systemic)*.
In providing consultation, consider emphasizing the following selected information (» = major clinical significance):

**Before using this medication**
» Conditions affecting use, especially:
Sensitivity to hydralazine
Pregnancy—Blood problems and fetal distress reported in infants of mothers who took hydralazine; causes birth defects in animals
Use in the elderly—Increased sensitivity to hypotensive effects
Other medications, especially diazoxide
Other medical problems, especially acute aortic dissection, coronary artery disease, or rheumatic heart disease

**Proper use of this medication**
Getting into the habit of taking at same times each day to help increase compliance
» Proper dosing
Missed dose: Taking as soon as possible; not taking if almost time for next dose; not doubling doses
» Proper storage
*For use as an antihypertensive*
Possible need for control of weight and diet, especially sodium intake
» Patient may not experience symptoms of hypertension; importance of taking medication even if feeling well
» Does not cure, but helps control hypertension; possible need for lifelong therapy; checking with physician before discontinuing medication; serious consequences of untreated hypertension

**Precautions while using this medication**
Regular visits to physician to check progress
» Caution when driving or doing things requiring alertness because of possible headache or dizziness
*For use as an antihypertensive*
» Not taking other medications, especially nonprescription sympathomimetics, unless discussed with physician

**Side/adverse effects**
Signs of potential side effects, especially allergic reaction, angina pectoris, cutaneous vasculitis, lymphadenopathy, peripheral neuritis, sodium and water retention, edema, SLE-like syndrome, and blood dyscrasias

## General Dosing Information

Apparent tolerance to the antihypertensive effects of hydralazine may develop with chronic administration, as a result of fluid retention and expanded plasma volume and reflex activation of the sympathetic nervous system, which increases heart rate and cardiac output. Concurrent administration of a diuretic may decrease this likelihood and will enhance the antihypertensive effects of hydralazine.

If combination therapy is indicated, individual titration is required to ensure the lowest possible therapeutic dose of each drug.

Incidence and severity of some of the side effects of hydralazine can be minimized if the dosage is increased slowly to its therapeutic level. In addition, some side effects (especially tachycardia, headache, and dizziness) may be less pronounced if beta-adrenergic blocking agents are administered concurrently.

Recent evidence suggests that withdrawal of antihypertensive therapy prior to surgery is not necessary, but that the anesthesiologist must be aware of such therapy.

Peripheral neuritis has been observed in some patients on hydralazine therapy. Evidence suggests that this may be due to an antipyridoxine effect. Discontinuation of hydralazine or continuation of hydralazine with supplemental vitamin $B_6$(pyridoxine)—100 to 200 mg per day—usually results in remission of the neuritis over a period of 4 to 6 weeks.

It is recommended that hydralazine therapy be discontinued if a systemic lupus erythematosus (SLE)-like syndrome occurs.

To avoid a sudden increase in blood pressure, patients on hydralazine who have shown a significant decrease in blood pressure should have the medication withdrawn gradually at cessation of therapy.

### For oral dosage forms
Food may enhance the bioavailability of hydralazine by reducing first-pass metabolism in the gastrointestinal wall. Consistent administration in relation to meals is recommended.

### For parenteral dosage forms
Most patients can be transferred to the oral dosage form of hydralazine within 24 to 48 hours after initiation of parenteral therapy.

## Oral Dosage Forms
Note: Bracketed uses in the *Dosage Forms* section refer to categories of use and/or indications that are not included in U.S. product labeling.

### HYDRALAZINE HYDROCHLORIDE TABLETS USP
**Usual adult dose**
Hypertension—
　Initial: Oral, 10 mg four times a day for the first two to four days, followed by 25 mg four times a day for the balance of the first week.
　Maintenance: Oral, 50 mg four times a day for the second and subsequent weeks; dosage should be adjusted to the lowest effective levels.
[Congestive heart failure][1]—
　Initial: Oral, 25 to 37.5 mg four times a day. This dose may be increased as tolerated.
　Maintenance: Oral, 75 mg four times a day; or 100 mg three times a day.

Note: Geriatric patients may be more sensitive to the effects of the usual adult dose.

**Usual adult prescribing limits**
Up to 300 mg daily (higher doses have been used in treatment of congestive heart failure).

**Usual pediatric dose**
Hypertension—
　Oral, 750 mcg (0.75 mg) per kg of body weight a day divided into four doses, the dosage being increased gradually over three to four weeks as needed, up to a maximum of 7.5 mg per kg of body weight or 200 mg a day.

**Strength(s) usually available**
U.S.—
　10 mg (Rx) [*Apresoline* (lactose); GENERIC].
　25 mg (Rx) [*Apresoline* (lactose); GENERIC].
　50 mg (Rx) [*Apresoline* (lactose); GENERIC].
　100 mg (Rx) [*Apresoline* (tartrazine; lactose); GENERIC].
Canada—
　10 mg (Rx) [*Apresoline* (scored; tartrazine)].
　25 mg (Rx) [*Apresoline* (lactose); *Novo-Hylazin*].
　50 mg (Rx) [*Apresoline* (lactose); *Novo-Hylazin*].

**Packaging and storage**
Store below 40 °C (104 °F), preferably between 15 and 30 °C (59 and 86 °F), unless otherwise specified by manufacturer. Store in a tight, light-resistant container.

**Auxiliary labeling**
- Do not take other medicines without your doctor's advice.

**Note**
Check refill frequency to determine compliance in hypertensive patients.

## Parenteral Dosage Forms

### HYDRALAZINE HYDROCHLORIDE INJECTION USP
**Usual adult dose**
Antihypertensive—
　Intramuscular or intravenous, 5 to 40 mg, repeated as needed.
　Pre-eclampsia or eclampsia: Intravenous, 5 mg every fifteen to twenty minutes. If a therapeutic response is not achieved after a total dose of 20 mg, another agent should be considered.

Note: Geriatric patients may be more sensitive to the effects of the usual adult dose.

**Usual pediatric dose**
Antihypertensive—
　Intramuscular or intravenous, 1.7 to 3.5 mg per kg of body weight a day, divided into four to six daily doses.

**Strength(s) usually available**
U.S.—
　20 mg per mL (Rx) [GENERIC].
Canada—
　Not commercially available.

Note: The brand name product is no longer commercially available in the U.S. or Canada. However, the manufacturer is making it available to physicians on an emergency basis.

**Packaging and storage**
Store below 40 °C (104 °F), preferably between 15 and 30 °C (59 and 86 °F), unless otherwise specified by manufacturer. Protect from freezing.

**Stability**
Hydralazine hydrochloride injection should be used immediately after the ampul is opened.

**Incompatibilities**
Hydralazine hydrochloride injection may undergo color changes when added to infusion fluids. It is recommended that hydralazine hydrochloride injection not be added to infusion solutions.

---
[1]Not included in Canadian product labeling.

## Selected Bibliography
Stratton MA. Drug-induced systemic lupus erythematosus. Clin Pharm 1985; 4: 657-63.

The fifth report of the Joint National Committee on Detection, Evaluation, and Treatment of High Blood Pressure (JNC V). Arch Intern Med 1993; 153(2): 154-83.

---
Revised: 08/22/96

---

# HYDRALAZINE AND HYDROCHLOROTHIAZIDE　Systemic

VA CLASSIFICATION (Primary): CV401

**NOTE:** The *Hydralazine and Hydrochlorothiazide (Systemic)* monograph is maintained on the USP DI electronic data base. For a printed copy of the most recent revision of the complete monograph, contact Micromedex, Inc. - Reprint Requests, 6200 S. Syracuse Way, Suite 300, Englewood, CO 80111; telephone (303) 486-6400; telefax (303) 486-6464; Email: USPDI@MDX.COM.

For information on the specific components of this combination, see the *USP DI* monographs for *Diuretics, Thiazide (Systemic)* and *Hydralazine (Systemic)*.

The information that follows is selectively abstracted from the complete monograph and is provided to facilitate drug use review and patient counseling.

Note: For a listing of dosage forms and brand names by country availability, see *Dosage Forms* section(s).

## Category
Antihypertensive.

## Indications
### Accepted
Hypertension (treatment)—Hydralazine and hydrochlorothiazide combination is indicated in the treatment of hypertension.

Fixed-dosage combinations are generally not recommended for initial therapy and are useful for subsequent therapy only when the proportion of the component agents corresponds to the dose of the individual agents, as determined by titration.

## Patient Consultation
As an aid to patient consultation, refer to *Advice for the Patient, Hydralazine and Hydrochlorothiazide (Systemic)*.

In providing consultation, consider emphasizing the following selected information (» = major clinical significance):

### Before using this medication
» Conditions affecting use, especially:
  Sensitivity to hydralazine, hydrochlorothiazide, sulfonamide-type medications, bumetanide, furosemide, or carbonic anhydrase inhibitors
  Pregnancy—Blood problems reported in infants of mothers who took hydralazine and birth defects found in animals; hydrochlorothiazide may cause jaundice, thrombocytopenia, hypokalemia in infant
  Breast-feeding—Hydrochlorothiazide is distributed into breast milk
  Use in the elderly—Increased sensitivity to hypotensive and electrolyte effects; increased risk of hydralazine-induced hypothermia
  Other medications, especially diazoxide, digitalis glycosides, lithium
  Other medical problems, especially coronary artery disease, rheumatic heart disease, anuria or severe renal function impairment, or infants with jaundice

### Proper use of this medication
Diuretic effects of the medication and timing of doses to minimize inconvenience of diuresis
Possible need for control of weight and diet, especially sodium intake
» Patient may not experience symptoms of hypertension; importance of taking medication even if feeling well
» Does not cure, but helps control hypertension; possible need for lifelong therapy; checking with physician before discontinuing medication; serious consequences of untreated hypertension
Compliance with therapy; taking medication at the same times each day to maintain the therapeutic effect
» Proper dosing
Missed dose: Taking as soon as possible; not taking if almost time for next dose; not doubling doses
» Proper storage

### Precautions while using this medication
Making regular visits to physician to check progress
» Not taking other medications, especially nonprescription sympathomimetics, unless discussed with physician
» Caution when driving or doing things requiring alertness because of possible headache or dizziness
» Caution when getting up suddenly from a lying or sitting position
» Caution in using alcohol, while standing for long periods or exercising, and during hot weather because of enhanced orthostatic hypotensive effects
» Possibility of hypokalemia; possible need for additional potassium in diet; not changing diet without first checking with physician
  To prevent dehydration, checking with physician if severe nausea, vomiting, or diarrhea occurs and continues
  Diabetics: May increase blood sugar levels
  Possible photosensitivity; avoiding unprotected exposure to sun; using protective clothing and sun block product; avoiding use of sunlamp, tanning bed, or tanning booth

### Side/adverse effects
Signs of potential side effects, especially electrolyte imbalance, agranulocytosis, allergic reaction, angina pectoris, cutaneous vasculitis, lymphadenopathy, peripheral neuritis, SLE-like syndrome, agranulocytosis, cholecystitis, pancreatitis, hepatic function impairment, hyperuricemia, gout, and thrombocytopenia

## Oral Dosage Forms

### HYDRALAZINE HYDROCHLORIDE AND HYDROCHLOROTHIAZIDE CAPSULES

**Usual adult dose**
Antihypertensive—
  Oral, 1 capsule two times a day, as determined by individual titration with the component agents.

Note: Geriatric patients may be more sensitive to the effects of the usual adult dose.

**Usual pediatric dose**
Antihypertensive—
  Oral, as determined by individual titration with the component agents.

**Strength(s) usually available**
U.S.—
  25 mg of hydralazine hydrochloride and 25 mg of hydrochlorothiazide (Rx) [*Apresazide* (sodium bisulfite); GENERIC].
  50 mg of hydralazine hydrochloride and 50 mg of hydrochlorothiazide (Rx) [*Apresazide* (sodium bisulfite); GENERIC].
Canada—
  Not commercially available.

**Auxiliary labeling**
• Do not take other medicines without your doctor's advice.

Revised: 08/24/92
Interim revision: 04/29/94; 08/13/98

---

**HYDROCHLOROTHIAZIDE**—See *Diuretics, Thiazide (Systemic)*

---

**HYDROCODONE**—See *Opioid (Narcotic) Analgesics (Systemic)*

---

# HYDROCODONE AND IBUPROFEN Systemic—INTRODUCTORY VERSION

VA CLASSIFICATION (Primary): CN900
Note: Controlled substance classification—
  U.S.—Schedule III
Note: For a listing of dosage forms and brand names by country availability, see *Dosage Forms* section(s).

## Category
Analgesic.

## Indications
### Accepted
Pain (treatment)—Hydrocodone and ibuprofen combination is indicated for the short-term (< 10 days) management of acute pain.

### Unaccepted
Hydrocodone and ibuprofen combination is not indicated for the treatment of osteoarthritis and rheumatoid arthritis.

## Pharmacology/Pharmacokinetics

**Physicochemical characteristics**
Molecular weight—Hydrocodone bitartrate: 494.5.
Ibuprofen: 206.29.

**Mechanism of action/Effect**
Hydrocodone—The exact mechanism of action of hydrocodone is unknown. Hydrocodone is an opioid analgesic. It has been proposed that opioid analgesics bind with specific opioid receptors at many sites in the central nervous system (CNS) to alter processes affecting pain sensation.
Ibuprofen—Ibuprofen is a nonsteroidal anti-inflammatory drug (NSAID) with anti-inflammatory, analgesic, and antipyretic therapeutic effects. The exact mechanism of action of ibuprofen has not been determined.

However, it has been proposed that ibuprofen, like other NSAIDs, inhibits the activity of the enzyme cyclo-oxygenase, resulting in a decreased formation of precursors of prostaglandins. The resulting decrease in prostaglandin synthesis may be responsible for the therapeutic effects of ibuprofen.

### Other actions/effects
Hydrocodone also has antitussive activity.

### Absorption
Rapid.

### Protein binding
Hydrocodone—The extent of hydrocodone protein binding in human plasma is not known. However, it is expected to fall in the low-to-moderate range (19 to 45%), similar to that of other opioid agents.
Ibuprofen—Very high (99%).

### Biotransformation
Hydrocodone—Hepatic. Extensively metabolized by N- and O-demethylation via hepatic cytochrome P450 enzymes (CYP2D6 and CYP3A4, respectively) and 6-keto reduction to hydroxy metabolites. The O-demethylation of hydrocodone forms the potent opioid analgesic hydromorphone that contributes to the total analgesic action of hydrocodone.
Ibuprofen—Hepatic. Ibuprofen is present as a racemate, which undergoes conversion in the plasma from an R-isomer to an S-isomer following absorption. These isomers are metabolized to two primary phenyl propionic acid metabolites, which appear in the plasma at lower concentration levels than the parent.

### Half-life
Hydrocodone—4.5 hours.
Ibuprofen—2.2 hours.

### Time to peak concentration
Hydrocodone—1.7 hours.
Ibuprofen—1.8 hours.

### Peak serum concentration
Hydrocodone—27 nanograms/mL.
Ibuprofen—30 mcg/mL.

### Elimination
Hydrocodone—Renal.
Ibuprofen—Renal, approximately 50 to 60% is excreted in the urine as metabolites (15% as unchanged drug and conjugate).

## Precautions to Consider

### Cross-sensitivity and/or related problems
Patients sensitive to ibuprofen, other nonsteroidal anti-inflammatory drugs (NSAIDs), hydrocodone, or one of the other opioid analgesics may be sensitive to hydrocodone and ibuprofen combination also.
Hydrocodone and ibuprofen combination may cause bronchoconstriction or anaphylaxis in aspirin-sensitive asthmatics, especially those with aspirin-induced nasal polyps, asthma, and other allergic reactions (the "aspirin triad").

### Carcinogenicity/Mutagenicity
Studies have not been done to evaluate the carcinogenic or mutagenic potential of hydrocodone and ibuprofen combination.

### Pregnancy/Reproduction
Fertility—Reproductive studies have not been done to determine the effect of hydrocodone and ibuprofen combination on fertility.
Pregnancy—Adequate and well-controlled trials in humans have not been done.
In rabbits receiving doses of hydrocodone and ibuprofen combination of up to 95 mg per kilogram of body weight (mg/kg) (approximately 5.72 times and 1.9 times the maximum recommended human dose [MRHD] on a mg/kg basis and mg/m² basis, respectively), an increase in major and minor fetal abnormalities was observed. However, no reproductive toxicity was observed in rats receiving doses of hydrocodone and ibuprofen combination of up to 166 mg/kg (approximately 10 times and 1.66 times the MRHD on a mg/kg basis and mg/m² basis, respectively).
The use of NSAIDs, such as ibuprofen, is not recommended in the last trimester due to the possible adverse effects on the fetus, such as premature closure of the ductus arteriosus. In addition, regular use of an opioid during pregnancy will cause physical dependence in the fetus, leading to withdrawal symptoms, such as convulsions, irritability, excessive crying, tremors, hyperactive reflexes, fever, vomiting, diarrhea, sneezing, and yawning in the neonate. The dose and duration of maternal use of opioids is not necessarily reflective of the intensity of the withdrawal symptoms in the neonate.

FDA Pregnancy Category C.
Labor and delivery—The use of hydrocodone and ibuprofen combination is not recommended during labor and delivery.

In rats receiving hydrocodone and ibuprofen combination, an increased incidence of dystocia and delayed parturition was observed.

### Breast-feeding
It is not known whether hydrocodone and ibuprofen combination is distributed into breast milk. However, use of hydrocodone and ibuprofen combination is not recommended in nursing mothers due to the potential adverse effects of the ibuprofen, a prostaglandin-inhibiting drug, on neonates.
Hydrocodone—It is not known whether hydrocodone is distributed into human breast milk.
Ibuprofen—In studies using a 1 mg/mL assay to determine the concentration of ibuprofen in nursing mothers, no measurable quantity of ibuprofen was detected.

### Pediatrics
No information is available on the relationship of age to the effects of hydrocodone and ibuprofen combination in pediatric patients. Safety and efficacy in children up to 16 years of age have not been established.

### Geriatrics
Studies performed to date have demonstrated an increase in the incidence of constipation in geriatric patients to be the only difference in the tolerability of hydrocodone and ibuprofen combination compared with younger adults. However, elderly patients may be more likely to be more sensitive to nonsteroidal anti-inflammatory drug–induced renal and gastrointestinal effects and opioid-induced respiratory depression. Therefore, caution and dosage adjustment are recommended in geriatric patients receiving hydrocodone and ibuprofen combination.

### Dental
Hydrocodone and ibuprofen combination may cause soreness of the oral mucosa. Also, hydrocodone and ibuprofen combination may decrease or inhibit salivary flow, thus contributing to the development of caries, periodontal disease, oral candidiasis, and discomfort.

### Drug interactions and/or related problems
The following drug interactions and/or related problems have been selected on the basis of their potential clinical significance (possible mechanism in parentheses where appropriate)—not necessarily inclusive (» = major clinical significance):

Note: Combinations containing any of the following medications, depending on the amount present, may also interact with this medication.

» Alcohol or
» Central nervous system (CNS) depression–producing medications, other (see *Appendix II*)
(concurrent use with hydrocodone and ibuprofen combination may result in increased CNS depressant effects; caution is recommended and dosage of one or both agents should be reduced)

» Angiotensin-converting enzyme (ACE) inhibitors
(concurrent use with hydrocodone and ibuprofen combination may reduce the effects of the ACE inhibitor; concurrent use may also result in an increased risk of renal failure)

Anticholinergics
(concurrent use with hydrocodone and ibuprofen combination may result in paralytic ileus)

» Anticoagulants, coumarin- or indandione-derivative
(concurrent use with hydrocodone and ibuprofen combination may increase the risk of gastrointestinal bleeding)

» Antidepressants, tricyclic (TCAs)
(concurrent use with hydrocodone and ibuprofen combination may result in increased adverse effects of hydrocodone or increased antidepressant effects of the TCAs)

Aspirin or
Corticosteroids, glucocorticoid or
Nonsteroidal anti-inflammatory drugs (NSAIDs)
(concurrent use is not recommended due to the increased risk of gastrointestinal effects, including ulceration and hemorrhage)

» Diuretics
(ibuprofen has been shown to reduce the effects of antihypertensive agents, possibly by inhibiting renal prostaglandin synthesis; increased monitoring of the response to the diuretic agent is recommended when it is used concurrently with hydrocodone and ibuprofen combination)
(concurrent use of diuretics with hydrocodone and ibuprofen also may increase the risk of renal failure secondary to a decrease in renal blood flow caused by the inhibition of the renal prostaglandin synthesis by ibuprofen)

» Lithium
(inhibition of renal prostaglandin activity by ibuprofen has been reported to result in an increase in the plasma concentration of lith-

ium and a decrease in its renal clearance; increased monitoring for lithium toxicity is recommended during concurrent use with hydrocodone and ibuprofen combination)

» Methotrexate
(ibuprofen may decrease renal elimination of methotrexate, thereby resulting in increased and prolonged methotrexate plasma concentration and an increased risk of toxicity; caution is recommended with the concurrent use of hydrocodone and ibuprofen combination and methotrexate)

» Monoamine oxidase (MAO) inhibitors, including furazolidone, pargyline, and procarbazine
(concurrent use with hydrocodone and ibuprofen combination may result in increased adverse effects of hydrocodone or of the antidepressant effects of the MAO inhibitor)

**Laboratory value alterations**
The following have been selected on the basis of their potential clinical significance (possible effect in parentheses where appropriate)—not necessarily inclusive (» = major clinical significance):

With physiology/laboratory test values
Bleeding time
(may be prolonged by ibuprofen because of suppressed platelet aggregation)
Hemoglobin
(values may be decreased)
Liver function tests, including
Alkaline phosphatase, serum and
Lactate dehydrogenase (LDH), serum and
Transaminases
(values may be increased; liver function test abnormalities may return to normal despite continued use; however, if significant abnormalities occur, clinical signs and symptoms consistent with liver disease develop, or systemic manifestations such as eosinophilia or skin rash occur, hydrocodone and ibuprofen combination should be discontinued; routine monitoring is recommended in patients with severe hepatic or renal function impairment)

**Medical considerations/Contraindications**
The medical considerations/contraindications included have been selected on the basis of their potential clinical significance (reasons given in parentheses where appropriate)—not necessarily inclusive (» = major clinical significance).

*Except under special circumstances, this medication should not be used when the following medical problems exist:*

» Allergic reaction, severe, such as anaphylaxis or angioedema, induced by aspirin, other NSAIDs, history of, or other opioids, history of or
» Nasal polyps associated with bronchospasm, aspirin-induced
(high risk of severe allergic reactions because of cross-sensitivity)
» Peptic ulcer disease, active
(may be exacerbated; increased risk of perforation and/or bleeding)
» Renal disease, severe
(adverse renal effects may be increased in the presence of pre-existing renal disease)
» Respiratory depression
(may be exacerbated, especially in patients sensitive to opioids)

*Risk-benefit should be considered when the following medical problems exist:*

Abdominal conditions, acute
(diagnosis or clinical course may be obscured)
Addison's disease or
Hepatic function impairment, severe or
Hypothyroidism or
Prostatic hypertrophy or
Urethral stricture
(increased risk of respiratory depression)
Allergic reaction, mild, induced by aspirin, other NSAIDs, or opioids, history of
(possibility of cross-sensitivity)
Anemia or
» Respiratory impairment or disease, including
Asthma, pre-existing
(may be exacerbated; caution is recommended)
» Coagulation or platelet function disorders
(increased risk of bleeding; caution is recommended)
Conditions predisposing to and/or exacerbated by fluid retention, such as:
Compromised cardiac function
Congestive heart disease
Hypertension
(ibuprofen has been reported to cause fluid retention and edema; therefore, hydrocodone and ibuprofen combination should be used with caution in patients with these conditions)
Conditions predisposing to gastrointestinal toxicity, such as:
Alcoholism, active
Peptic ulcer disease, active or history of
Tobacco use, or recent history of
(nonsteroidal anti-inflammatory drugs (NSAIDs) should be used with extreme caution in patients with peptic ulcer disease or gastrointestinal bleeding; dosage adjustment of NSAIDs is recommended to minimize potential risk of gastrointestinal bleeding)
Congestive heart failure or
Extracellular volume depletion or
Hepatic function impairment
(increased risk of renal failure; patients who are dehydrated should be rehydrated before receiving hydrocodone and ibuprofen combination)
Drug abuse or dependence, current or history of
(patient predisposition to drug abuse)
Head injury or
Increased intracranial pressure, pre-existing or
Intracranial lesions
(risk of respiratory depression and further elevation of cerebrospinal fluid pressure is increased; also, hydrocodone and ibuprofen combination may cause sedation and pupillary changes that may obscure clinical course of head injury)
» Renal function impairment
(increased risk of adverse renal effects and respiratory depressant effects; careful monitoring of the patient is recommended, especially for patients with severe renal function impairment)
(ibuprofen and its metabolites are excreted primarily via the kidneys; a reduction in dosage of hydrocodone and ibuprofen combination may be required to prevent accumulation)
Sensitivity to hydrocodone and ibuprofen combination
» Caution is also advised in administration to very elderly, very ill, debilitated, or postoperative patients, who may be more sensitive to the effects, especially the respiratory depressant effects, of hydrocodone and ibuprofen combination
» Caution is also recommended in geriatric patients, who may be more likely to develop adverse hepatic or renal effects with hydrocodone and ibuprofen combination and in whom gastrointestinal ulceration or bleeding is more likely to cause serious consequences

**Patient monitoring**
The following may be especially important in patient monitoring (other tests may be warranted in some patients, depending on condition; » = major clinical significance):

» Liver function tests or
» Renal function tests
(routine monitoring may be required during hydrocodone and ibuprofen combination therapy in patients with severe hepatic or renal function impairment)

## Side/Adverse Effects

Note: Physical dependence, with or without psychological dependence, and tolerance may occur with long-term administration of opioid analgesics. However, the manufacturer states that psychological dependence is not likely to develop with the short-term use of hydrocodone and ibuprofen combination.

The following side/adverse effects have been selected on the basis of their potential clinical significance (possible signs and symptoms in parentheses where appropriate)—not necessarily inclusive:

**Those indicating need for medical attention**
Incidence less frequent or rare
*Allergic reaction* (changes in facial skin color; skin rash, hives, and/or itching; fast or irregular breathing; puffiness or swelling of the eyelids or around the eyes; shortness of breath, troubled breathing, tightness in chest and/or wheezing); *arrythmia* (irregular heartbeat); *bronchitis* (congestion in chest; cough); *dyspnea* (shortness of breath); *fever; frequent urge to urinate; gastrointestinal effects, including esophagitis* (difficulty in swallowing); *gastritis* (burning feeling in chest or stomach; tenderness in the stomach area); *gastroenteritis* (diarrhea; nausea; stomach pain); *hypotension* (lightheadedness or dizziness); *melena* (bloody stools); *tachycardia* (increased heart rate); *tinnitus* (ringing or buzzing in the ears); *urinary incontinence* (loss of bladder control); *urinary retention* (inability to urinate)

Note: Meningitis has been reported to occur in patients taking ibuprofen. Signs and symptoms of meningitis, including severe headache, drowsiness, confusion, stiff neck and/or back, or general feeling of illness or nausea, may be related to the ibuprofen in the hydrocodone and ibuprofen combination.

**Those indicating need for medical attention only if they continue or are bothersome**
Incidence more frequent
*Anxiety; asthenia* (unusual tiredness or weakness); *constipation; dry mouth; edema* (swelling of feet or lower legs); *flatulence* (gas); *headache; increased sweating; insomnia* (trouble in sleeping); *nausea and vomiting; nervousness; palpitations* (pounding heart beat); *pruritus* (itching of the skin); *somnolence* (sleepiness)

Incidence less frequent or rare
*Anorexia* (decreased appetite); *central nervous system (CNS) effects, including confusion; dizziness; depression; euphoria* (unusual feeling of well-being); *irritability; mood or mental changes; paresthesias* (sensation of burning, warmth, heat, numbness, tightness, or tingling); *slurred speech; thinking abnormalities; tremor* (trembling or shaking of hands or feet); *dyspepsia* (stomach upset); *dysphagia* (difficulty swallowing); *impotence* (decrease in sexual ability); *increased thirst; mouth ulcers; pharyngitis* (pain or burning in throat); *rhinitis* (runny nose); *sinusitis* (runny nose; headache); *visual disturbances; weight loss, unexplained*

## Overdose

For specific information on the agents used in the management of hydrocodone and ibuprofen combination overdose, see:
- *Charcoal, Activated (Oral-Local)* monograph; and/or
- *Naloxone (Systemic)* monograph.

For more information on the management of overdose or unintentional ingestion, **contact a Poison Control Center** (see *Poison Control Center Listing*).

**Clinical effects of overdose**
The following effects have been selected on the basis of their potential clinical significance (possible signs and symptoms in parentheses where appropriate)—not necessarily inclusive:

Acute and/or chronic
Hydrocodone
*Cold, clammy skin; drowsiness, severe; slow heartbeat; slow or troubled breathing*
Ibuprofen
*Blurred vision; difficulty hearing or ringing or buzzing in ears; dizziness; headache; meningitis* (severe headache; drowsiness; confusion; stiff neck and/or back; general feeling of illness or nausea); *mood or mental changes; nausea and/or vomiting; skin rash; stomach pain, severe; swelling of the face, fingers, feet, or lower legs*

**Treatment of overdose**
To decrease absorption—Emptying the stomach via emesis or gastric lavage. However, if gastric lavage is performed more than an hour after ingestion, the effectiveness of recovering the drug decreases. Activated charcoal may also be used to reduce the absorption and reabsorption of ibuprofen.

To enhance elimination—Administering urinary alkalizers may increase ibuprofen excretion.

Dialysis is not likely to be of value because of ibuprofen's high degree of protein binding.

Specific treatment—Administering the opioid antagonist naloxone. See the package insert or the *Naloxone (Systemic)* monograph for specific dosing guidelines for this product.

Monitoring—Continuing to monitor the patient and administering additional naloxone as needed.

Supportive care—Establishing adequate respiratory exchange through provision of a patent airway and institution of assisted or controlled respiration. Administering supportive measures as needed. Patients in whom intentional overdose is confirmed or suspected should be referred for psychiatric consultation.

## Patient Consultation

As an aid to patient consultation, refer to *Advice for the Patient, Hydrocodone and Ibuprofen (Systemic)—Introductory Version*.

In providing consultation, consider emphasizing the following selected information (» = major clinical significance):

**Before using this medication**
» Conditions affecting use, especially:
   Sensitivity to hydrocodone or ibuprofen
   Allergies to aspirin or any other nonsteroidal anti-inflammatory drugs (NSAIDs), or other opioid analgesics

Pregnancy—Regular use of opioids by pregnant women may cause physical dependence in the fetus and withdrawal symptoms in the neonate; use of NSAIDs are not recommended during the last trimester of pregnancy due to the potential adverse effects on renal blood flow

Breast-feeding—Use of hydrocodone and ibuprofen combination is not recommended for nursing mothers due to the potential adverse effects of ibuprofen on the neonate

Use in the elderly—Increased risk of toxicity, especially respiratory depression and gastrointestinal effects

Other medications, especially alcohol or other central nervous system (CNS) depressants; angiotensin-converting enzyme (ACE) inhibitors; anticoagulants, coumarin- or indandione-derivative; diuretics; lithium; methotrexate; monoamine oxidase (MAO) inhibitors; and tricylic antidepressants

Other medical problems, especially allergic reaction; aspirin-induced nasal polyps associated with bronchospasm; coagulation disorders or platelet function disorders; peptic ulcer disease (active); renal disease (severe); renal function impairment; respiratory disease or impairment

**Proper use of this medication**
» Not taking more medication than prescribed
» Proper dosing
   Missed dose: Taking as soon as possible; not taking if almost time for next dose; not doubling doses
» Proper storage

**Precautions while using this medication**
» Avoiding use of alcoholic beverages or other CNS depressants during therapy, unless prescribed or otherwise approved by physician
» Caution if dizziness, drowsiness, lightheadedness, false sense of well-being occurs, or vision problems occur
» Caution when getting up from a lying or sitting position
   Need to inform physician or dentist of use of medication if any kind of surgery (including dental) or emergency treatment is required
   Possible dryness of mouth; using sugarless gum or candy, ice, or saliva substitute for relief; checking with dentist if dry mouth continues for more than 2 weeks

**Side/adverse effects**
Signs of potential side effects, especially allergic reaction; arrythmia; bronchitis; dyspnea; fever; frequent urge to urinate; gastrointestinal effects, including esophagitis; gastritis; gastroenteritis; hypotension; melena; tachycardia; tinnitus; urinary incontinence; urinary retention

## General Dosing Information

Hydrocodone and ibuprofen combination may suppress respiration, especially in very young, elderly, very ill, or debilitated patients and those with respiratory problems. Lower doses may be required for these patients. Elderly patients also may be more sensitive to the analgesic effect of this medication so that lower doses or an increased dosing interval may be sufficient to provide effective analgesia.

Dosage and dosing intervals should be individualized on the basis of the severity of pain, the condition of the patient, other medications given concurrently, and patient response.

Concurrent use of other analgesics provides additive analgesia and may permit lower doses of the hydrocodone and ibuprofen combination to be utilized.

Tolerance to many of the effects of hydrocodone and ibuprofen combination may develop with repeated administration.

Psychological and physical dependence may occur with repeated administration of opioid analgesics. However, the manufacturer states that physical dependence is not likely to develop with the short-term use of hydrocodone and ibuprofen combination.

A reduction of the dosage may be required to prevent accumulation of hydrocodone and ibuprofen and/or their metabolites in patients with renal function impairment.

## Oral Dosage Forms

### HYDROCODONE AND IBUPROFEN TABLETS

**Usual adult dose**
Analgesic—
   Oral, 1 tablet containing 7.5 mg of hydrocodone and 200 mg of ibuprofen every four to six hours as needed.

**Usual adult prescribing limits**
5 tablets containing 7.5 mg of hydrocodone and 200 mg of ibuprofen in twenty-four hours.

**Usual pediatric dose**
Safety and efficacy have not been established.

**Usual geriatric dose**
See *Usual adult dose.*

Note: Dosage adjustment may be required.

**Strength(s) usually available**
U.S.—
  7.5 mg of hydrocodone and 200 mg of ibuprofen (Rx) [*Vicoprofen* (colloidal silicon dioxide; corn starch; croscarmellose sodium; hydroxypropyl methylcellulose; magnesium stearate; microcrystalline cellulose; polyethylene glycol; polysorbate 80; titanium dioxide)].

**Packaging and storage**
Store at 20 to 25 °C (68 to 77 °F).

**Auxiliary labeling**
• May cause drowsiness.
• Avoid alcoholic beverages.
• May be habit-forming

**Note**
Controlled substance in the U.S.

Developed: 07/13/98

---

**HYDROCORTISONE**—See *Corticosteroids—Glucocorticoid Effects (Systemic); Corticosteroids (Ophthalmic); Corticosteroids (Otic); Corticosteroids (Topical)*

---

**HYDROFLUMETHIAZIDE**—See *Diuretics, Thiazide (Systemic)*

---

**HYDROMORPHONE**—See *Opioid (Narcotic) Analgesics (Systemic)*

---

**HYDROXOCOBALAMIN**—See *Vitamin B$_{12}$ (Systemic)*

---

# HYDROXYCHLOROQUINE Systemic

VA CLASSIFICATION (Primary/Secondary): AP101/MS109; TN900
Commonly used brand name(s): *Plaquenil.*
Note: For a listing of dosage forms and brand names by country availability, see *Dosage Forms* section(s).

## Category
Antiprotozoal; antirheumatic (disease-modifying); lupus erythematosus suppressant; antihypercalcemic; polymorphous light eruption suppressant; porphyria cutanea tarda suppressant.

## Indications
Note: Bracketed information in the *Indications* section refers to uses that are not included in U.S. product labeling.

**Accepted**
Malaria (prophylaxis and treatment)—Hydroxychloroquine is indicated in the suppressive treatment and the treatment of acute attacks of malaria caused by *Plasmodium vivax, P. malariae, P. ovale,* and susceptible strains of *P. falciparum.* The radical cure of *P. vivax* and *P. ovale* malaria requires the concurrent or subsequent administration of primaquine.

Arthritis, rheumatoid (treatment)—Hydroxychloroquine is indicated in the treatment of acute and chronic rheumatoid arthritis in patients who do not respond adequately to other less toxic antirheumatics. [It may be used in addition to nonsteroidal anti-inflammatory agents.]

Lupus erythematosus, discoid (treatment) or
Lupus erythematosus, systemic (treatment)—Hydroxychloroquine is indicated as a suppressant for chronic discoid and systemic lupus erythematosus.

[Arthritis, juvenile (treatment)][1]—Hydroxychloroquine is used in the treatment of juvenile arthritis.

[Hypercalcemia, sarcoid-associated (treatment)][1]—Hydroxychloroquine is used to reduce urinary calcium excretion and the levels of 1,25-dihydroxyvitamin D in the serum of sarcoid patients who are unable to take corticosteroids.

[Polymorphous light eruption (treatment)][1]—Hydroxychloroquine is used as a suppressant for polymorphous light eruption.

[Porphyria cutanea tarda (treatment)][1]—Hydroxychloroquine is used in the treatment of porphyria cutanea tarda.

[Urticaria, solar (treatment)][1] or
[Vasculitis, chronic cutaneous (treatment)][1]—Hydroxychloroquine is used in the treatment of solar urticaria and chronic cutaneous vasculitis unresponsive to other therapy.

Chloroquine-resistant strains of *P. falciparum*, originally seen only in Southeast Asia and South America, are now documented in all malarious areas except Central America west of the Canal Zone, the Middle East, and the Caribbean. Chloroquine is still the drug of choice for the treatment of susceptible strains of *P. falciparum* and the other 3 malarial species; however, chloroquine-resistant *P. vivax* has recently been reported.

**Unaccepted**
Hydroxychloroquine does not prevent relapses in patients with *P. vivax* or *P. ovale* malaria since it is not effective against exo-erythrocytic forms of the parasite. In these species, "hypnozoites," which remain dormant in the liver, are responsible for relapses.

[1]Not included in Canadian product labeling.

## Pharmacology/Pharmacokinetics
Note: Because hydroxychloroquine concentrates in the cellular fraction of blood, hydroxychloroquine concentrations measured in the blood are higher than those measured in the plasma.

**Physicochemical characteristics**
Molecular weight—433.95.

**Mechanism of action/Effect**
Antiprotozoal—Malaria: Unknown, but may be based on ability of hydroxychloroquine to bind to and alter the properties of DNA. Also has been found to be taken up into the acidic food vacuoles of the parasite in the erythrocyte. This increases the pH of the acid vesicles, interfering with vesicle functions and possibly inhibiting phospholipid metabolism. In suppressive treatment, hydroxychloroquine inhibits the erythrocytic stage of development of plasmodia. In acute attacks of malaria, it interrupts erythrocytic schizogony of the parasite. Its ability to concentrate in parasitized erythrocytes may account for their selective toxicity against the erythrocytic stages of plasmodial infection.

Antirheumatic—Hydroxychloroquine is thought to act as a mild immunosuppressant, inhibiting the production of rheumatoid factor and acute phase reactants. It also accumulates in white blood cells, stabilizing lysosomal membranes and inhibiting the activity of many enzymes, including collagenase and the proteases that cause cartilage breakdown.

**Absorption**
Variable rate of absorption; absorption half-life of 3.6 hours (range, 1.9 to 5.5 hours). Bioavailability is approximately 74%.

**Distribution**
Widely distributed in body tissues such as the eyes, kidneys, liver, and lungs where retention is prolonged. Concentrations are 2 to 5 times higher in erythrocytes than in plasma. Very low concentrations in intestinal wall. Crosses the placenta, also.

Apparent Vol$_D$=5,522 L (measured in blood); 44,257 L (measured in plasma).

**Protein binding**
Moderate (approximately 45%).

**Biotransformation**
Hepatic (partially), to active de-ethylated metabolites.

### Half-life
Terminal elimination half-life—
  In blood: Approximately 50 days.
  In plasma: Approximately 32 days.

### Time to peak concentration
Approximately 3.2 hours (range, 2 to 4.5 hours).

### Peak concentrations
Steady state concentration in whole blood (achieved at 6 months)—
  155 mg (base) daily: 948 nanograms per mL.
  310 mg (base) daily: 1895 nanograms per mL.

### Elimination
Renal; 23 to 25% of hydroxychloroquine excreted unchanged in the urine. Hydroxychloroquine is excreted very slowly; may persist in urine for months or years after medication is discontinued. Also excreted in bile.

Hemodialysis does not remove appreciable amounts of hydroxychloroquine from blood.

## Precautions to Consider

### Cross-sensitivity and/or related problems
Patients hypersensitive to chloroquine, a 4-aminoquinoline compound structurally similar to hydroxychloroquine, may also be hypersensitive to hydroxychloroquine.

### Pregnancy/Reproduction
Pregnancy—Hydroxychloroquine crosses the placenta. Use is not recommended during pregnancy except in the suppression or treatment of malaria or hepatic amebiasis since malaria poses greater potential danger to the mother and fetus (i.e., abortion and death) than prophylactic administration of hydroxychloroquine. Hydroxychloroquine, given in weekly chemoprophylactic doses, has not been shown to cause adverse effects on the fetus. However, risk-benefit must be considered since 4-aminoquinolines, given in therapeutic doses, have been shown to cause central nervous system (CNS) damage, including ototoxicity (auditory and vestibular); congenital deafness; retinal hemorrhages; and abnormal retinal pigmentation. In addition, hydroxychloroquine has been shown to accumulate selectively in melanin structures of fetal eyes. It may be retained in ocular tissues for up to 5 months after elimination from the blood.

### Breast-feeding
One case report found that a very small amount of hydroxychloroquine is distributed into breast milk; chloroquine is also distributed into breast milk. Although problems in humans have not been documented, risk-benefit must be considered since infants and children are especially sensitive to the effects of 4-aminoquinolines.

### Pediatrics
Infants and children are especially sensitive to the effects of hydroxychloroquine and chloroquine. Fatalities have been reported following the ingestion of as little as 750 mg to 1 gram of chloroquine; hydroxychloroquine is assumed to be equally toxic. Long-term therapy with hydroxychloroquine is not generally recommended in children. However, it has been used in juvenile arthritis for as long as 6 months with little or no toxicity.

### Geriatrics
No information is available on the relationship of age to the effects of hydroxychloroquine in geriatric patients.

### Drug interactions and/or related problems
The following drug interactions and/or related problems have been selected on the basis of their potential clinical significance (possible mechanism in parentheses where appropriate)—not necessarily inclusive (» = major clinical significance):

Note: Combinations containing any of the following medications, depending on the amount present, may also interact with this medication.

Penicillamine
  (concurrent use of penicillamine with hydroxychloroquine may increase penicillamine plasma concentrations, increasing the potential for serious hematologic and/or renal adverse reactions, as well as the possibility of severe skin reactions)

### Medical considerations/Contraindications
The medical considerations/contraindications included have been selected on the basis of their potential clinical significance (reasons given in parentheses where appropriate)—not necessarily inclusive (» = major clinical significance).

*Risk-benefit should be considered when the following medical problems exist:*

» Blood disorders, severe
  (hydroxychloroquine may cause blood dyscrasias, including agranulocytosis, aplastic anemia, neutropenia, or thrombocytopenia)

Gastrointestinal disorders, severe
  (hydroxychloroquine may cause gastrointestinal irritation)

Glucose-6-phosphate dehydrogenase (G6PD) deficiency
  (hydroxychloroquine may cause hemolytic anemia in G6PD-deficient patients, although this is unlikely when hydroxychloroquine is given in therapeutic doses)

» Hepatic function impairment
  (because hydroxychloroquine is metabolized in the liver, hepatic function impairment may increase blood concentrations of hydroxychloroquine, increasing the risk of side effects)

Hypersensitivity to hydroxychloroquine or chloroquine

» Neurological disorders, severe
  (hydroxychloroquine may cause neuromyopathy, ototoxicity, polyneuritis, or seizures)

Porphyria
  (hydroxychloroquine may cause exacerbation of porphyria)

Psoriasis
  (hydroxychloroquine may precipitate severe attacks of psoriasis)

» Retinal or visual field changes, presence of
  (hydroxychloroquine may cause corneal opacities, keratopathy, or retinopathy)

### Patient monitoring
The following may be especially important in patient monitoring (other tests may be warranted in some patients, depending on condition; » = major clinical significance):

» Complete blood counts (CBCs)
  (recommended periodically during prolonged daily therapy with hydroxychloroquine; if severe blood dyscrasias occur that are not attributable to the disease being treated, discontinuation of hydroxychloroquine should be considered)

» Neuromuscular examinations, including knee and ankle reflexes
  (recommended periodically during long-term therapy with hydroxychloroquine to detect muscle weakness; if muscle weakness occurs, hydroxychloroquine should be discontinued)

» Ophthalmologic examinations, including visual acuity, expert slitlamp, funduscopic, and visual field tests
  (recommended before and at least every 3 to 6 months during prolonged daily therapy since irreversible retinal damage has been reported with long-term or high-dosage therapy; serious ocular injury has been thought to be correlated with a total cumulative dose of greater than 100 grams (base) of chloroquine; however, a daily dose of greater than 310 mg (base), or 5 mg (base) per kg daily, of hydroxychloroquine may be a more important determinant; any retinal or visual abnormality that is not fully explainable by difficulties of accommodation or corneal opacities should be monitored following discontinuation of therapy, since retinal changes and visual disturbances may progress even after cessation of therapy)

## Side/Adverse Effects

Note: Side/adverse effects of hydroxychloroquine are usually dose-related. When hydroxychloroquine is used for the short-term treatment of malaria or other parasitic diseases, side/adverse effects are usually mild and reversible. However, following prolonged use and/or high-dose therapy such as in the treatment of rheumatoid arthritis, lupus erythematosus, or polymorphous light eruption, side/adverse effects may be serious and sometimes irreversible.

Irreversible retinal damage may be more likely to occur when the daily dosage equals or exceeds the equivalent of 310 mg (base), or 5 mg (base) per kg daily, of hydroxychloroquine.

The following side/adverse effects have been selected on the basis of their potential clinical significance (possible signs and symptoms in parentheses where appropriate)—not necessarily inclusive:

### Those indicating need for medical attention
Incidence less frequent
  *Ocular toxicity specifically corneal opacities* (blurred vision or any other change in vision); *keratopathy* (blurred vision or any other change in vision); *or retinopathy* (blurred vision or any other change in vision)

Incidence rare
  *Blood dyscrasias, specifically agranulocytosis* (sore throat and fever); *aplastic anemia* (fatigue; weakness); *neutropenia* (sore throat and fever); *or thrombocytopenia* (unusual bleeding or bruising); *emotional*

*changes or psychosis* (mood or other mental changes); *neuromyopathy* (increased muscle weakness); *ototoxicity* (any loss of hearing; ringing or buzzing in ears)—usually in patients with pre-existing auditory damage; *seizures*

**Those indicating need for medical attention only if they continue or are bothersome**
Incidence more frequent
*Ciliary muscle dysfunction* (difficulty in reading); *gastrointestinal irritation* (diarrhea; loss of appetite; nausea; stomach cramps or pain; vomiting); *headache; itching* (especially in black patients)—not an indication for discontinuation of therapy in black patients

Incidence less frequent
*Bleaching of hair or increased hair loss; blue-black discoloration of skin, fingernails, or inside of mouth; dizziness or lightheadedness; nervousness or restlessness; skin rash or itching*

**Those indicating possible retinal changes, visual disturbances and the need for medical attention if they occur or progress after medication is discontinued**
*Blurred vision or any other change in vision*

## Overdose

For specific information on the agents used in the management of hydroxychloroquine overdose, see:
- *Charcoal, Activated (Oral-Local)* monograph;
- *Diazepam* in *Benzodiazepines (Systemic)* monograph; and/or
- *Sympathomimetic Agents—Cardiovascular Use (Parenteral-Systemic)* monograph.

For more information on the management of overdose or unintentional ingestion, **contact a Poison Control Center** (see *Poison Control Center Listing*).

**Clinical effects of overdose**
After ingestion of an overdose of hydroxychloroquine, toxic symptoms may occur within 30 minutes. These include drowsiness, visual disturbances, cardiovascular collapse, and seizures, followed by sudden respiratory and cardiac arrest.

Doses of chloroquine phosphate as small as 0.75 to 1 gram in children, and 2.25 to 3 grams in adults, may be fatal. It is assumed that hydroxychloroquine is equally toxic.

The following effects have been selected on the basis of their potential clinical significance (possible signs and symptoms in parenthesis where appropriate)—not necessarily inclusive:

Acute
*Cardiovascular toxicities, specifically conduction disturbances or hypotension; neurotoxicity, specifically drowsiness; headache; hyperexcitability; seizures; or coma; respiratory and cardiac arrest; visual disturbances* (blurred vision)

**Treatment of overdose**
Since there is no specific antidote, treatment of hydroxychloroquine overdose should be symptomatic and supportive with possible utilization of the following:
To decrease absorption—
  Emptying stomach with gastric lavage.
  Administering activated charcoal with a cathartic. The dose of activated charcoal should be 5 to 10 times the estimated dose of the drug ingested.
To enhance elimination—
  Forcing diuresis and acidifying the urine, with ammonium chloride, for example, can help promote urinary excretion of 4-aminoquinolines. Adjusting the dose of the acidifying agent to maintain a urinary pH of 5.5 to 6.5. Monitoring of plasma potassium is recommended. Using with caution in patients with renal function impairment and/or metabolic acidosis.
Specific treatment—
  For seizures—Treating repetitive seizures or status epilepticus with intravenous diazepam (in 2.5 to 5 mg increments).
  For arrhythmias—Managing life-threatening ventricular arrhythmias or cardiac arrest appropriately, as per Advanced Cardiac Life Support guidelines.
  For hypotension and circulatory shock—Administering fluids at a sufficient rate to maintain urine output. Administering intravenous pressors and/or inotropic drugs, such as norepinephrine, dopamine, isoproterenol, or dobutamine, if required. One study found that administration of a high-dose diazepam infusion improved hemodynamic function, and epinephrine decreased the myocardial depressant and vasodilatory effects of chloroquine overdose. This may also apply to a hydroxychloroquine overdose.

Monitoring—
  Monitoring of plasma potassium is recommended.
Supportive care—
  Securing and maintaining a patent airway, administering oxygen, and instituting assisted or controlled respiration as required. In severe overdoses, early mechanical ventilation has been suggested to prevent hypoxemia. Patients in whom intentional overdose is known or suspected should be referred for psychiatric consultation.

## Patient Consultation

As an aid to patient consultation, refer to *Advice for the Patient, Hydroxychloroquine (Systemic)*.

In providing consultation, consider emphasizing the following selected information (» = major clinical significance):

**Before using this medication**
» Conditions affecting use, especially:
  Hypersensitivity to hydroxychloroquine or chloroquine
  Pregnancy—May cause toxicity to the fetus when given to mother in therapeutic doses; however, hydroxychloroquine has not been shown to cause adverse effects in the fetus when used as a prophylactic agent against malaria
  Use in children—Infants and children are especially sensitive to effects of hydroxychloroquine
  Other medical problems, especially impaired hepatic function, presence of retinal or visual field changes, severe blood disorders, or severe neurologic disorders

**Proper use of this medication**
» Taking with meals or milk to minimize possible gastrointestinal irritation
» Keeping medication out of reach of children; fatalities reported with as few as 3 or 4 tablets (250-mg strength) of chloroquine phosphate; hydroxychloroquine is assumed to be equally toxic
» Importance of not taking more medication than the amount prescribed
» Compliance with full course of therapy
» Importance of not missing doses and taking medication on regular schedule
» Proper dosing
  Missed dose: Taking as soon as possible; not taking if almost time for next dose; not doubling doses
» Proper storage
*For prevention of malaria*
  Starting medication 1 to 2 weeks before entering malarious area to ascertain patient response and allow time to substitute another medication if reactions occur
» Continuing medication while staying in area and for 4 to 6 weeks after leaving area; checking with physician immediately if fever develops while traveling or within 2 months after departure from endemic area
*For arthritis and lupus erythematosus*
  Importance of taking medication on regular schedule
  May require up to 6 months for full benefit
*For patients unable to swallow hydroxychloroquine tablets*
  Crushing tablets and putting each dose in capsules; contents of capsules may be mixed with jam, jelly, or jello

**Precautions while using this medication**
» Regular visits to physician to check for blood problems, muscle weakness, and ophthalmologic examinations during or after long-term therapy
  Checking with physician if no improvement within a few days (or a few weeks or months for arthritis)
» Caution if blurred vision, difficulty in reading, other change in vision, dizziness, or lightheadedness occurs
  Mosquito-control measures to reduce the chance of getting malaria:
    Sleeping under mosquito netting
    Wearing long-sleeved shirts or blouses and long trousers to protect arms and legs between dusk and dawn
    Applying mosquito repellent to uncovered areas of skin between dusk and dawn

**Side/adverse effects**
  Signs of potential side effects, especially ocular toxicity, blood dyscrasias, emotional or psychological changes, neuromyopathy, ototoxicity, and seizures

## General Dosing Information

Long-term and/or high-dosage therapy may cause irreversible retinal damage and/or neurosensorial deafness.

Hydroxychloroquine should be discontinued if any of the following problems occur: any abnormality in visual acuity, visual fields, retinal macular changes, or any visual symptoms; muscle weakness; or severe blood disorders.

Malaria-suppressive therapy should be started 1 to 2 weeks before the patient enters a malarious area and should be continued for 4 to 6 weeks after patient leaves the area. Starting the medication in advance will help to determine the patient's tolerance to the medication and allow time to substitute other antimalarials if the patient develops allergies to the medication or develops other adverse effects.

Hydroxychloroquine should be taken with meals or milk to minimize the possibility of gastrointestinal irritation.

Corticosteroids and/or nonsteroidal anti-inflammatory analgesics (including salicylates) may be given concurrently with hydroxychloroquine in the treatment of rheumatoid arthritis. These medications can usually be reduced gradually in dosage or discontinued after hydroxychloroquine has been given for several weeks.

When hydroxychloroquine is used in the treatment of rheumatoid arthritis, several months of therapy may be required for it to reach its maximum effectiveness. If improvement (such as reduced joint swelling and increased mobility) does not occur within 6 months, the medication should be discontinued.

## Oral Dosage Forms

Note: Bracketed uses in the *Dosage Forms* section refer to categories of use and/or indications that are not included in U.S. product labeling.

### HYDROXYCHLOROQUINE SULFATE TABLETS USP

**Usual adult and adolescent dose**
Malaria—
  Suppressive: Oral, 400 mg (310 mg base) once every seven days.
  Therapeutic: Oral, 800 mg (620 mg base) as a single dose; or 800 mg (620 mg base) initially, followed by 400 mg (310 mg base) in six to eight hours, and 400 mg (310 mg base) once a day on the second and third days.
Antirheumatic (disease-modifying)—
  Oral, up to 6.5 mg (5 mg base) per kg of lean body weight daily, with meals or a glass of milk.
  Note: In a small number of patients who experience side effects with the usual initial dose in the treatment of rheumatoid arthritis, a temporary reduction in the initial dose of hydroxychloroquine may be required. After five to ten days the dose may be gradually increased until the desired response is obtained.
  If relapse occurs after withdrawal of hydroxychloroquine, therapy may be resumed or continued on an intermittent schedule if there are no ocular contraindications.
Lupus erythematosus suppressant—
  Oral, up to 6.5 mg (5 mg base) per kg of lean body weight daily.
[Polymorphous light eruption suppressant][1]—
  Oral, 200 mg (155 mg base) two or three times a day.

**Usual pediatric dose**
Malaria—
  Suppressive: Oral, 6.4 mg (5 mg base) per kg of body weight, not to exceed the adult dose, once every seven days.
  Therapeutic: Oral, 32 mg (25 mg base) per kg of body weight administered over a period of three days as follows: 12.9 mg (10 mg base) per kg of body weight, not to exceed a single dose of 800 mg (620 mg base); then 6.4 mg (5 mg base) per kg of body weight, not to exceed a single dose of 400 mg (310 mg base), six, twenty-four, and forty-eight hours after the first dose.

Note: Children are especially sensitive to the effects of the 4-aminoquinolines.
  Long-term therapy with hydroxychloroquine is not recommended in children.

**Strength(s) usually available**
U.S.—
  200 mg (equivalent to 155 mg base) (Rx) [*Plaquenil*].
Canada—
  200 mg (equivalent to 155 mg base) (Rx) [*Plaquenil* (scored)].

**Packaging and storage**
Store below 40 °C (104 °F), preferably between 15 and 30 °C (59 and 86 °F), unless otherwise specified by manufacturer. Store in a well-closed container.

**Preparation of dosage form**
According to the manufacturer, the tablets may be crushed and each dose placed in a capsule. The contents of each compounded capsule may then be mixed with a teaspoonful of jam, jelly, or jello prior to administration. Preparation of hydroxychloroquine sulfate oral suspensions is not recommended.

**Auxiliary labeling**
• Continue medication for full time of treatment.
• Keep out of reach of children.
• Take with food or milk.
• May cause dizziness.

**Note**
Explain potential danger of accidental overdose in children.
Consider dispensing in unit-dose packaging in child-resistant containers ("double-barrier" packaging).

[1] Not included in Canadian product labeling.

Revised: 12/30/94

---

**HYDROXYPROGESTERONE**—See *Progestins (Systemic)*

---

**HYDROXYPROPYL CELLULOSE**—The *Hydroxypropyl Cellulose (Ophthalmic)* monograph is not included in this published version of the USP DI database. Copies of the monograph are available on request from Micromedex, Inc. - Reprint Requests, 6200 S. Syracuse Way, Suite 300, Englewood, CO 80111; telephone (303) 486-6400; telefax (303) 486-6464; Email: USPDI@MDX.COM.

---

**HYDROXYPROPYL METHYLCELLULOSE**—The *Hydroxypropyl Methylcellulose (Ophthalmic)* monograph is not included in this published version of the USP DI database. Copies of the monograph are available on request from Micromedex, Inc. - Reprint Requests, 6200 S. Syracuse Way, Suite 300, Englewood, CO 80111; telephone (303) 486-6400; telefax (303) 486-6464; Email: USPDI@MDX.COM.

---

# HYDROXYUREA    Systemic

VA CLASSIFICATION (Primary): AN300
Commonly used brand name(s): *Hydrea*.
Note: For a listing of dosage forms and brand names by country availability, see *Dosage Forms* section(s).

## Category
Antineoplastic.

## Indications
Note: Bracketed information in the *Indications* section refers to uses that are not included in U.S. product labeling.

**Accepted**
Carcinoma, ovarian, epithelial (treatment) or
[Carcinoma, cervical (treatment)][1]—Hydroxyurea is indicated for treatment of recurrent, metastatic, or inoperable epithelial carcinoma of the ovary and for treatment of cervical carcinoma.

Leukemia, chronic myelocytic (treatment)—Hydroxyurea is indicated for treatment of resistant chronic myelocytic leukemia.

[Thrombocytosis, essential (treatment)][1] or
[Polycythemia vera (treatment)][1]—Hydroxyurea is indicated for treatment of essential thrombocytosis and polycythemia vera.

[1] Not included in Canadian product labeling.

## Pharmacology/Pharmacokinetics

**Physicochemical characteristics**
Molecular weight—76.05.

**Mechanism of action/Effect**
Hydroxyurea is classified as an antimetabolite. Hydroxyurea is thought to be cell cycle–specific for the S phase of cell division. The exact mechanism of antineoplastic activity is unknown but is thought to involve interference with synthesis of DNA, with no effect on synthesis of RNA or protein.

**Absorption**
Well absorbed from the gastrointestinal tract.

**Distribution**
Crosses the blood-brain barrier.

**Biotransformation**
Hepatic.

**Half-life**
3 to 4 hours.

**Time to peak serum concentration**
2 hours.

**Elimination**
Renal—80% within 12 hours(50% unchanged).
Respiratory—As carbon dioxide.

## Precautions to Consider

**Cross-sensitivity and/or related problems**
Patients sensitive to tartrazine may be sensitive to the capsule dosage form available in Canada also, since the capsules may contain tartrazine.

**Carcinogenicity/Mutagenicity**
Secondary malignancies are potential delayed effects of many antineoplastic agents, although it is not clear whether the effect is related to their mutagenic or immunosuppressive action. The effect of dose and duration of therapy is also unknown, although risk seems to increase with long-term use. Although information is limited, available data seem to indicate that the carcinogenic risk is greatest with the alkylating agents.

Antimetabolites have been shown to be carcinogenic in animals and may be associated with an increased risk of development of secondary carcinomas in humans, although the risk appears to be less than with alkylating agents.

**Pregnancy/Reproduction**
Fertility—Gonadal suppression, resulting in amenorrhea or azoospermia, may occur in patients taking antineoplastic therapy, especially with the alkylating agents. In general, these effects appear to be related to dose and length of therapy and may be irreversible. Prediction of the degree of testicular or ovarian function impairment is complicated by the common use of combinations of several antineoplastics, which makes it difficult to assess the effects of individual agents. Hydroxyurea causes reversible germ cell toxicity.

Pregnancy—First trimester: It is usually recommended that use of antineoplastics, especially combination chemotherapy, be avoided whenever possible, especially during the first trimester. Although information is limited because of the relatively few instances of antineoplastic administration during pregnancy, the mutagenic, teratogenic, and carcinogenic potential of these medications must be considered.

Other hazards to the fetus include adverse reactions seen in adults.

In general, use of a contraceptive is recommended during cytotoxic drug therapy.

Hydroxyurea is teratogenic in animals.

**Breast-feeding**
Although very little information is available regarding distribution of antineoplastic agents into breast milk, breast-feeding is not recommended during chemotherapy because of the risks to the infant (adverse effects, mutagenicity, carcinogenicity).

**Pediatrics**
Although appropriate studies on the relationship of age to the effects of hydroxyurea have not been performed in the pediatric population, children may be more sensitive to the effects of hydroxyurea.

**Geriatrics**
Although appropriate studies on the relationship of age to the effects of hydroxyurea have not been performed in the geriatric population, the elderly may be more sensitive to effects of hydroxyurea. In addition, elderly patients are more likely to have age-related renal function impairment, which may require reduction of dosage in patients receiving hydroxyurea.

**Dental**
The bone marrow depressant effects of hydroxyurea may result in an increased incidence of microbial infection, delayed healing, and gingival bleeding. Dental work, whenever possible, should be completed prior to initiation of therapy or deferred until blood counts have returned to normal. Patients should be instructed in proper oral hygiene during treatment, including caution in use of regular toothbrushes, dental floss, and toothpicks.

Hydroxyurea may also cause stomatitis associated with considerable discomfort.

**Drug interactions and/or related problems**
The following drug interactions and/or related problems have been selected on the basis of their potential clinical significance (possible mechanism in parentheses where appropriate)—not necessarily inclusive (» = major clinical significance):

Allopurinol or
Colchicine or
» Probenecid or
» Sulfinpyrazone
   (hydroxyurea may raise the concentration of blood uric acid; dosage adjustment of antigout agents may be necessary to control hyperuricemia and gout; allopurinol may be preferred to prevent or reverse hydroxyurea-induced hyperuricemia because of risk of uric acid nephropathy with uricosuric antigout agents)

Blood dyscrasia–causing medications (see *Appendix II*)
   (leukopenic and/or thrombocytopenic effects of hydroxyurea may be increased with concurrent or recent therapy if these medications cause the same effects; dosage adjustment of hydroxyurea, if necessary, should be based on blood counts)

» Bone marrow depressants, other (see *Appendix II*) or
Radiation therapy
   (additive bone marrow depression may occur; dosage reduction may be required when two or more bone marrow depressants, including radiation, are used concurrently or consecutively)

Vaccines, killed virus
   (because normal defense mechanisms may be suppressed by hydroxyurea therapy, the patient's antibody response to the vaccine may be decreased. The interval between discontinuation of medications that cause immunosuppression and restoration of the patient's ability to respond to the vaccine depends on the intensity and type of immunosuppression-causing medications used, the underlying disease, and other factors; estimates vary from 3 months to 1 year)

» Vaccines, live virus
   (because normal defense mechanisms may be suppressed by hydroxyurea therapy, concurrent use with a live virus vaccine may potentiate the replication of the vaccine virus, may increase the side/adverse effects of the vaccine virus, and/or may decrease the patient's antibody response to the vaccine; immunization of these patients should be undertaken only with extreme caution after careful review of the patient's hematologic status and only with the knowledge and consent of the physician managing the hydroxyurea therapy. The interval between discontinuation of medications that cause immunosuppression and restoration of the patient's ability to respond to the vaccine depends on the intensity and type of immunosuppression-causing medications used, the underlying disease, and other factors; estimates vary from 3 months to 1 year. Patients with leukemia in remission should not receive live virus vaccine until at least 3 months after their last chemotherapy. Immunization with oral poliovirus vaccine should also be postponed in persons in close contact with the patient, especially family members)

**Laboratory value alterations**
The following have been selected on the basis of their potential clinical significance (possible effect in parentheses where appropriate)—not necessarily inclusive (» = major clinical significance):

With physiology/laboratory test values
   Blood urea nitrogen (BUN) and
   Creatinine, serum
      (concentrations may occasionally be temporarily increased as a result of impairment of renal tubular function)

   Uric acid, serum
      (concentrations may be increased)

**Medical considerations/Contraindications**
The medical considerations/contraindications included have been selected on the basis of their potential clinical significance (reasons given in parentheses where appropriate)—not necessarily inclusive (» = major clinical significance).

**1668  Hydroxyurea (Systemic)**

*Risk-benefit should be considered when the following medical problems exist:*
» Anemia
(if severe, must be corrected with whole blood replacement before initiation of hydroxyurea therapy)
» Bone marrow depression
» Chickenpox, existing or recent (including recent exposure) or
» Herpes zoster
(risk of severe generalized disease)
Gout, history of or
Urate renal stones, history of
(risk of hyperuricemia)
» Infection
» Renal function impairment
(reduced elimination; lower dosage is recommended)
Sensitivity to hydroxyurea
» Caution should be used in patients who have had previous cytotoxic drug therapy and radiation therapy.

**Patient monitoring**
The following may be especially important in patient monitoring (other tests may be warranted in some patients, depending on condition; » = major clinical significance):

Blood urea nitrogen (BUN) concentrations and
Creatinine concentrations, serum
(recommended prior to initiation of therapy and at periodic intervals during therapy; frequency varies according to clinical state, agent, dose, and other agents being used concurrently)
» Hematocrit or hemoglobin and
» Leukocyte count, total and, if appropriate, differential and
» Platelet count
(determinations recommended prior to initiation of therapy and at periodic intervals during therapy; frequency varies according to clinical state, agent, dose, and other agents being used concurrently)
Uric acid concentrations, serum
(recommended prior to initiation of therapy and at periodic intervals during therapy; frequency varies according to clinical state, agent, dose, and other agents being used concurrently)

## Side/Adverse Effects

Note: Many "side effects" of antineoplastic therapy are unavoidable and represent the medication's pharmacologic action. Some of these (for example, leukopenia and thrombocytopenia) are actually used as parameters to aid in individual dosage titration.
Administration of hydroxyurea to patients with severe renal function impairment may produce visual and auditory hallucinations and pronounced hematologic toxicity.
Skin changes resembling atrophic lichen planus, including atrophy, brittle nails, darkening or redness of skin, and skin ulcers, have been reported rarely in patients receiving prolonged (over several years) daily treatment with hydroxyurea.

The following side/adverse effects have been selected on the basis of their potential clinical significance (possible signs and symptoms in parentheses where appropriate)—not necessarily inclusive:

**Those indicating need for medical attention**
Incidence more frequent
*Anemia or erythrocytic abnormalities; leukopenia* (fever or chills; cough or hoarseness; lower back or side pain; painful or difficult urination)—usually asymptomatic
Note: Self-limiting *megaloblastic erythropoiesis* occurs commonly early in the course of therapy; morphologic changes resemble pernicious anemia, but are not related to vitamin $B_{12}$ or folic acid deficiency. Plasma iron clearance may be delayed and rate of iron utilization by erythrocytes reduced, but hydroxyurea does not appear to alter red blood cell survival time.
Onset of *leukopenia* occurs about 10 days after initiation of therapy.
Incidence less frequent
*Stomatitis* (sores in mouth and on lips); *thrombocytopenia* (unusual bleeding or bruising; black, tarry stools; blood in urine or stools; pinpoint red spots on skin)—usually asymptomatic
Incidence rare
*Hyperuricemia or uric acid nephropathy* (joint pain; lower back or side pain; swelling of feet or lower legs); *neurotoxicity or cerebral metastatic disease* (confusion; convulsions; dizziness; hallucinations; headache); *renal function impairment*

Note: *Hyperuricemia or uric acid nephropathy* occurs most commonly during initial treatment of patients with leukemia, as a result of rapid cell breakdown, which leads to elevated serum uric acid concentrations.

**Those indicating need for medical attention only if they continue or are bothersome**
Incidence more frequent—dose-related
*Diarrhea; drowsiness*—large doses; *loss of appetite; nausea or vomiting*
Incidence less frequent
*Constipation; exacerbation of postirradiation erythema* (redness of skin); *skin rash and itching*

**Those indicating the need for medical attention if they occur after medication is discontinued**
*Bone marrow depression* (black, tarry stools; blood in urine; cough or hoarseness; fever or chills; lower back or side pain; painful or difficult urination; pinpoint red spots on skin; unusual bleeding or bruising)

## Patient Consultation

As an aid to patient consultation, refer to *Advice for the Patient, Hydroxyurea (Systemic)*.
In providing consultation, consider emphasizing the following selected information (» = major clinical significance):

**Before using this medication**
» Conditions affecting use, especially:
Sensitivity to hydroxyurea
Pregnancy—Use not recommended because of mutagenic, teratogenic, and carcinogenic potential; advisability of using contraception; telling physician immediately if pregnancy is suspected
Breast-feeding—Not recommended because of risk of serious side effects
Use in children—Children may be more sensitive to effects
Use in the elderly—Elderly patients may be more sensitive to effects
Other medications, especially probenecid, sulfinpyrazone, other bone marrow depressants, or previous cytotoxic drug or radiation therapy
Other medical problems, especially chickenpox, herpes zoster, anemia, infection, or renal function impairment

**Proper use of this medication**
» Importance of not taking more or less medication than the amount prescribed
For patients who cannot swallow capsules: Contents of capsules may be emptied into glass of water and taken immediately; some inert material may not dissolve and may float on surface
Caution in taking combination chemotherapy; taking each medication at the right time
Importance of ample fluid intake and subsequent increase in urine output to aid in excretion of uric acid
» Frequency of nausea, vomiting, and diarrhea; importance of continuing medication despite stomach upset
Checking with physician if vomiting occurs shortly after dose is taken
» Proper dosing
Missed dose: Not taking at all; not doubling doses
» Proper storage

**Precautions while using this medication**
» Importance of close monitoring by the physician
» Avoiding immunizations unless approved by physician; other persons in patient's household should avoid immunizations with oral poliovirus vaccine; avoiding other persons who have taken oral poliovirus vaccine or wearing a protective mask that covers nose and mouth
*Caution if bone marrow depression occurs*
» Avoiding exposure to persons with infections, especially during period of low blood counts; checking with physician immediately if fever or chills, cough or hoarseness, lower back or side pain, or painful or difficult urination occurs
» Checking with physician immediately if unusual bleeding or bruising; black, tarry stools; blood in urine; or pinpoint red spots on skin occur
Caution in use of regular toothbrush, dental floss, or toothpick; physician, dentist, or nurse may suggest alternatives; checking with physician before having dental work done
Not touching eyes or inside of nose unless hands washed immediately before
Using caution to avoid accidental cuts with use of sharp objects such as safety razor or fingernail or toenail cutters
Avoiding contact sports or other situations where bruising or injury could occur

### Side/adverse effects
- May cause adverse effects such as blood problems and cancer; importance of discussing possible effects with physician
- Signs of potential side effects, especially anemia, leukopenia, stomatitis, thrombocytopenia, neurotoxicity, cerebral metastatic disease, hyperuricemia, and uric acid nephropathy
- Physician or nurse can help in dealing with side effects

## General Dosing Information

Patients receiving hydroxyurea should be under supervision of a physician experienced in antimetabolite chemotherapy.

Dosage must be adjusted to meet the individual requirements of each patient, based on clinical response and appearance or severity of toxicity.

Dosage reduction may be necessary in children and in the elderly, who may be more sensitive to effects of the drug.

If the patient is unable to swallow capsules, the contents of the capsule may be emptied into a glass of water (some inert material may float on the surface) and taken immediately.

Development of uric acid nephropathy in patients with leukemia or lymphoma may be prevented by adequate oral hydration and, in some cases, administration of allopurinol. Alkalinization of urine may be necessary if serum uric acid concentrations are elevated.

If there is no clinical response after 6 weeks of therapy, the medication should be discontinued; if a response occurs, the medication may be continued indefinitely.

Combination therapy with radiation may be associated with more frequent and severe side effects of the radiation, including gastric distress and inflammation of mucous membranes at the irradiated site. Severe reactions may require temporary withdrawal of hydroxyurea therapy.

It is recommended that hydroxyurea therapy be temporarily withdrawn if marked leukopenia (particularly granulocytopenia) or thrombocytopenia occurs. Therapy may be resumed if, after 3 days, the counts rise significantly towards normal values; counts usually return to normal within 10 to 30 days after discontinuation of hydroxyurea. If anemia occurs, it may be corrected with whole blood replacement, without interruption of hydroxyurea therapy.

Special precautions are recommended in patients who develop thrombocytopenia as a result of administration of hydroxyurea. These may include extreme care in performing invasive procedures; regular inspection of intravenous sites, skin (including perirectal area), and mucous membrane surfaces for signs of bleeding or bruising; limiting frequency of venipuncture and avoiding intramuscular injections; testing urine, emesis, stool, and secretions for occult blood; care in use of regular toothbrushes, dental floss, toothpicks, safety razors, and fingernail and toenail cutters; avoiding constipation; and using caution to prevent falls and other injuries. Such patients should avoid alcohol and any aspirin intake because of the risk of gastrointestinal bleeding. Platelet transfusions may be required.

Patients who develop leukopenia should be observed carefully for signs of infection. Antibiotic support may be required. In neutropenic patients who develop fever, broad-spectrum antibiotic coverage should be initiated empirically, pending bacterial cultures and appropriate diagnostic tests.

## Oral Dosage Forms

### HYDROXYUREA CAPSULES USP

**Usual adult dose**
Carcinoma, ovarian, epithelial—
   Oral, 60 to 80 mg per kg of body weight or 2000 to 3000 mg per square meter of body surface in a single dose every third day, alone or in combination with radiation therapy, or 20 to 30 mg per kg of body weight per day in a single dose.

Note: Administration of hydroxyurea should begin at least seven days prior to initiation of radiation therapy, and should be continued during radiation therapy and indefinitely afterwards.

Leukemia, chronic myelocytic, resistant—
   Oral, 20 to 30 mg per kg of body weight a day in a single dose or two divided daily doses.

Note: Although dosages are based on the patient's actual weight, use of estimated lean body mass (dry weight) is recommended in obese patients or those with abnormal fluid retention.

In general, use of intermittent dosage is associated with less risk of serious toxicity than continuous daily dosage.

**Usual pediatric dose**
Dosage has not been established.

**Strength(s) usually available**
U.S.—
   500 mg (Rx) [*Hydrea* (lactose); GENERIC].
Canada—
   500 mg (Rx) [*Hydrea* (tartrazine 3 mg)].

**Packaging and storage**
Store below 40 °C (104 °F), preferably between 15 and 30 °C (59 and 86 °F), unless otherwise specified by manufacturer. Store in a tight container.

**Auxiliary labeling**
- Keep container tightly closed.

Revised: 06/16/92
Interim revision: 06/21/94; 09/26/97

---

## HYDROXYZINE — See *Antihistamines (Systemic)*

---

## HYOSCYAMINE — See *Anticholinergics/Antispasmodics (Systemic)*

**IBUPROFEN**—See *Anti-inflammatory Drugs, Nonsteroidal (Systemic)*

# IBUTILIDE Systemic—INTRODUCTORY VERSION

VA CLASSIFICATION (Primary): CV300
Commonly used brand name(s): *Corvert*.
Note: For a listing of dosage forms and brand names by country availability, see *Dosage Forms* section(s).

## Category
Antiarrhythmic.

## Indications

**Accepted**

Arrhythmias, atrial (treatment)—Ibutilide is indicated for the rapid conversion of recent onset atrial fibrillation or atrial flutter to sinus rhythm.

## Pharmacology/Pharmacokinetics

**Physicochemical characteristics**
Molecular weight—442.62.

**Mechanism of action/Effect**
Ibutilide prolongs action potential duration in isolated adult cardiac myocytes and increases both the atrial and ventricular refractory periods *in vivo*. The mechanism of action may involve activation of a slow, inward, predominantly sodium current, or blockage of outward potassium currents. The result of these effects is a prolongation of atrial and ventricular action potential duration and refractory periods. In the Vaughan Williams classification of antiarrhythmics, ibutilide is considered to be a class III agent.

**Other actions/effects**
Ibutilide produces a mild slowing of the sinus rate and atrioventricular conduction. It produces a dose-related prolongation of the QT interval.

**Distribution**
Volume of distribution (Vol$_D$)—11 L per kg of body weight.

**Protein binding**
Moderate (40%).

**Biotransformation**
Of eight metabolites, formed primarily by omega oxidation followed by sequential beta oxidation of the heptyl side chain of ibutilide, the omega-hydroxy metabolite appears to be the only active metabolite. Plasma concentrations of the active metabolite are less than 10% of that of ibutilide.

**Half-life**
Elimination—Average, 6 hours (range, 2 to 12 hours).

**Time to peak effect**
30 to 90 minutes to convert to normal sinus rhythm.

**Elimination**
Renal—Approximately 82% (about 7% unchanged).
Fecal—Approximately 19%.

## Precautions to Consider

**Carcinogenicity**
Studies in animals have not been done to evaluate the carcinogenic potential of ibutilide.

**Mutagenicity**
Mutagenicity was not detected in the Ames test, mammalian cell forward gene mutation assay, unscheduled DNA synthesis assay, and mouse micronucleus assay.

**Pregnancy/Reproduction**
Fertility—No impairment of fertility was detected in a reproductive study in rats.
Pregnancy—Adequate and well-controlled studies in humans have not been done.
Reproduction studies in rats have shown orally administered ibutilide to be teratogenic and embryocidal.
FDA Pregnancy Category C.

**Breast-feeding**
It is not known whether ibutilide is distributed into breast milk. However, breast-feeding is not recommended.

**Pediatrics**
Appropriate studies on the relationship of age to the effects of ibutilide have not been performed in the pediatric population. Safety and efficacy have not been established.

**Geriatrics**
Use of ibutilide in patients with a mean age of 65 has not demonstrated geriatric-specific problems that would limit the usefulness of ibutilide in the elderly.

**Drug interactions and/or related problems**
The following drug interactions and/or related problems have been selected on the basis of their potential clinical significance (possible mechanism in parentheses where appropriate)—not necessarily inclusive (» = major clinical significance):

Note: Combinations containing any of the following medications, depending on the amount present, may also interact with this medication.

» Antiarrhythmics, other
(class Ia antiarrhythmic agents such as disopyramide, quinidine, and procainamide, and other class III antiarrhythmic agents, such as amiodarone and sotalol, should not be given concurrently or within 4 hours postinfusion of ibutilide because of their potential to prolong the refractory period)

» Medications causing QT interval prolongation, such as:
Antidepressants, tricyclic
Astemizole
Disopyramide
Maprotiline
Phenothiazines
Procainamide
Quinidine
Terfenadine
(concurrent use of these medications with ibutilide may increase the risk for proarrhythmia)

**Medical considerations/Contraindications**
The medical considerations/contraindications included have been selected on the basis of their potential clinical significance (reasons given in parentheses where appropriate)—not necessarily inclusive (» = major clinical significance).

*Except under special circumstances, this medication should not be used when the following medical problem exists:*

» Hypersensitivity to ibutilide

*Risk-benefit should be considered when the following medical problems exist:*

» Atrial fibrillation, chronic
(increased risk of recurrence after conversion to sinus rhythm)

» Congestive heart failure, history of
(increased risk of sustained polymorphic ventricular tachycardia)

» Hypokalemia or hypomagnesemia
(increased risk of proarrhythmia)

» Low left ventricular ejection fraction, history of
(increased risk of sustained polymorphic ventricular tachycardia)

» Ventricular tachycardia, polymorphic, history of
(increased risk of recurrence of polymorphic ventricular tachycardia)

**Patient monitoring**
The following may be especially important in patient monitoring (other tests may be warranted in some patients, depending on condition; » = major clinical significance):

» Electrocardiogram (ECG)
(continuous monitoring recommended during administration and for at least 4 hours following infusion or until QTc has returned to baseline; if any arrhythmic activity is noted, longer monitoring is required; patients with abnormal liver function should be monitored for more than the 4 hour period)

## Side/Adverse Effects

Note: Side/adverse effects involving the cardiovascular system have occurred at therapeutic plasma concentrations of ibutilide in approximately 25% of patients during phase II/III clinical trials. These include sustained (1.7%) and nonsustained (2.7%) polymorphic ventricular tachycardia.

The following side/adverse effects have been selected on the basis of their potential clinical significance (possible signs and symptoms in parentheses where appropriate)—not necessarily inclusive:

**Those indicating need for medical attention**
Incidence less frequent
*Cardiovascular effects, including atrioventricular block; bradycardia* (slow heartbeat); *bundle branch block; hypertension; hypotension* (dizziness or lightheadedness when getting up from a lying or sitting position; sudden fainting); *nonsustained monomorphic ventricular tachycardia; palpitation; QT segment prolongation; sustained and nonsustained polymorphic ventricular tachycardia; tachycardia; ventricular extrasystoles*
Incidence rare
*Cardiovascular effects, including congestive heart failure; idioventricular rhythm; nodal arrhythmia; supraventricular extrasystoles; renal failure; syncope* (fainting)

**Those indicating need for medical attention only if they continue or are bothersome**
Incidence less frequent
*Headache; nausea*

## Overdose

For more information on the management of overdose or unintentional ingestion, **contact a Poison Control Center** (see *Poison Control Center Listing*).

**Clinical effects of overdose**
The following effects have been selected on the basis of their potential clinical significance (possible signs and symptoms in parentheses where appropriate)—not necessarily inclusive:

Acute and chronic
*Atrioventricular (AV) block (third degree); increased prolongation of repolarization; increased ventricular ectopy; ventricular tachycardia, monomorphic; ventricular tachycardia, nonsustained polymorphic*

**Treatment of overdose**
Treatment is symptomatic and supportive.

## General Dosing Information

The continuous infusion of ibutilide should be stopped upon the termination of the presenting arrhythmia or in the event of sustained or nonsustained ventricular tachycardia or marked prolongation of QT or QTc.

The use of ibutilide necessitates continuous ECG monitoring for at least 4 hours following infusion or until QTc has returned to baseline. Detection of any arrhythmic activity requires longer monitoring. The availability of proper resuscitative cardiovascular equipment and emergency medication for the treatment of sustained ventricular tachycardia, including polymorphic ventricular tachycardia, is necessary.

## Parenteral Dosage Forms

### IBUTILIDE FUMARATE INJECTION

**Usual adult dose**
Antiarrhythmic—
Patients weighing less than 60 kg: Intravenous infusion, 0.01 mg per kg of body weight administered over a ten-minute period. Dose may be repeated ten minutes after the completion of the first infusion if the arrhythmia does not stop within ten minutes after the end of initial administration.
Patients weighing 60 kg or more: Intravenous infusion, 1 mg administered over a ten-minute period. Dose may be repeated ten minutes after the completion of the first infusion if the arrhythmia does not stop within ten minutes after the end of initial administration.

**Usual pediatric dose**
Safety and efficacy have not been established.

**Strength(s) usually available**
U.S.—
0.1 mg per mL (Rx) [*Corvert*].

**Packaging and storage**
Store between 20 and 25 °C (68 and 77 °F). Store vial in carton until ready to use.

**Preparation of dosage form**
Ibutilide may be administered undiluted or diluted. Ibutilide may be diluted in 50 mL of 0.9% sodium chloride injection or 5% dextrose injection. The contents of one 10-mL (0.1 mg per mL) vial of ibutilide may be added to a 50-mL infusion bag to form an admixture of approximately 0.017 mg per mL.

**Stability**
Ibutilide admixtures are stable for 24 hours at room temperature (15 to 30 °C [59 to 86 °F]), and for 48 hours at refrigerated temperatures (2 to 8 °C [36 to 46 °F]).

**Incompatibilities**
Only polyvinyl chloride plastic bags or polyolefin bags should be used for ibutilide admixtures.

Developed: 08/07/96

# IDARUBICIN Systemic

VA CLASSIFICATION (Primary): AN200
Commonly used brand name(s): *Idamycin*.
Note: For a listing of dosage forms and brand names by country availability, see *Dosage Forms* section(s).

## Category
Antineoplastic.

## Indications

**Accepted**
Leukemia, acute nonlymphocytic (treatment) or
[Leukemia, acute lymphocytic (treatment)]—Idarubicin is indicated for treatment of acute nonlymphocytic leukemia (including French-American-British [FAB] classifications M1 through M7) and acute lymphocytic leukemia.

## Pharmacology/Pharmacokinetics

**Physicochemical characteristics**
Source—Synthetic. Analog of daunorubicin.
Molecular weight—Idarubicin hydrochloride: 533.97.
Other characteristics—Lipophilic.

**Mechanism of action/Effect**
Idarubicin is an anthracycline glycoside; it is classified as an antibiotic but is not used as an antimicrobial agent. Its exact mechanism of antineoplastic activity is unknown; however, it intercalates DNA strands, inhibits DNA synthesis, interacts with RNA polymerases, and inhibits topoisomerase II (an enzyme that promotes DNA strand supercoiling).

**Distribution**
High volume of distribution (approximately 2225 liters). Concentrations of both idarubicin and its primary metabolite idarubicinol are 400- and 200-fold higher, respectively, in nucleated blood and bone marrow cells than in plasma. Data about whether idarubicin crosses the blood-brain barrier are conflicting.

**Protein binding**
Extensive tissue binding.
Plasma—
Idarubicin: Very high (97%).
Idarubicinol: Very high (94%).

**Biotransformation**
Rapidly and extensively, both hepatically and extrahepatically, to produce the primary metabolite, idarubicinol, which is equipotent with idarubicin.

**Half-life**
Idarubicin—
As a single agent: Average, 22 hours (range, 4 to 46 hours).
In combination with cytarabine: Average, 20 hours (range, 7 to 38 hours).
Idarubicinol—
> 45 hours.

**Time to peak concentration**
Cellular (nucleated cells of blood and bone marrow)—Within a few minutes after injection.

**Elimination**
Primarily biliary, as idarubicinol.
Renal elimination occurs to a lesser extent, as idarubicinol.
In dialysis—Studies have not been done. However, because of the multicompartmental behavior, along with the extensive extravascular distribution and tissue binding, it is unlikely that significant amounts of idarubicin would be removable by dialysis.

## Precautions to Consider

### Carcinogenicity/Mutagenicity
Secondary malignancies are potential delayed effects of many antineoplastic agents, although it is not clear whether the effect is related to their mutagenic or immunosuppressive action. The effect of dose and duration of therapy is also unknown, although the risk seems to increase with long-term use.

Long-term carcinogenicity studies have not been done. However, studies in experimental models (including bacterial systems, mammalian cells in culture, and female Sprague-Dawley rats) indicate that idarubicin has mutagenic and carcinogenic properties.

### Pregnancy/Reproduction
Fertility—Idarubicin caused testicular atrophy (with inhibition of spermiogenesis and sperm maturation, resulting in few or no mature sperm) in male dogs given idarubicin in doses of 1.8 mg per square meter of body surface area per day three times a week for 13 weeks. Effects were not readily reversible after an 8-week recovery period.

Pregnancy—Adequate and well-controlled studies in humans have not been done.
First trimester: It is usually recommended that use of antineoplastics, especially combination chemotherapy, be avoided whenever possible, especially during the first trimester. Although information is limited because of the relatively few instances of antineoplastic administration during pregnancy, the mutagenic, teratogenic, and carcinogenic potential of these medications must be considered. There is one report of fetal death following maternal exposure to idarubicin during the second trimester.

Other hazards to the fetus include adverse reactions seen in adults.

Studies in rats at a dose of 1.2 mg per square meter of body surface area per day (one tenth the human dose), which was nontoxic to dams, found idarubicin to be embryotoxic and teratogenic. Studies in rabbits at a dose of 2.4 mg per square meter of body surface area (two tenths the human dose), which was toxic to dams, found idarubicin to be embryotoxic but not teratogenic.

FDA Pregnancy Category D.
In general, use of contraception is recommended during cytotoxic drug therapy.

### Breast-feeding
It is not known whether idarubicin is distributed into breast milk. Although very little information is available regarding distribution of antineoplastic agents into breast milk, breast-feeding is not recommended during chemotherapy because of the potential risks to the infant (adverse effects, mutagenicity, carcinogenicity).

### Pediatrics
Appropriate studies on the relationship of age to the effects of idarubicin have not been performed in the pediatric population. In two small studies of the pharmacokinetics, conflicting results were obtained about a possible difference in clearance rate. Safety and efficacy have not been established.

### Geriatrics
Although appropriate studies on the relationship of age to the effects of idarubicin have not been performed in the geriatric population, cardiotoxicity may be more frequent in older persons (over 60 years of age). Caution should also be used in patients who have inadequate bone marrow reserves due to old age. In addition, elderly patients are more likely to have age-related renal function impairment, which when severe may require reduction of dosage in patients receiving idarubicin.

### Dental
The bone marrow depressant effects of idarubicin may result in an increased incidence of microbial infection, delayed healing, and gingival bleeding. Dental work, whenever possible, should be completed prior to initiation of therapy or deferred until blood counts have returned to normal. Patients should be instructed in proper oral hygiene during treatment, including caution in use of regular toothbrushes, dental floss, and toothpicks.

Idarubicin also commonly causes mucositis, which may be associated with considerable discomfort.

### Drug interactions and/or related problems
The following drug interactions and/or related problems have been selected on the basis of their potential clinical significance (possible mechanism in parentheses where appropriate)—not necessarily inclusive (» = major clinical significance):

Note: Combinations containing any of the following medications, depending on the amount present, may also interact with this medication.

Allopurinol or
Colchicine or
» Probenecid or
» Sulfinpyrazone
(idarubicin may raise the concentration of blood uric acid; dosage adjustment of antigout agents may be necessary to control hyperuricemia and gout; allopurinol may be preferred to prevent or reverse idarubicin-induced hyperuricemia because of risk of uric acid nephropathy with uricosuric antigout agents)

Blood dyscrasia–causing medications (see *Appendix II*)
(leukopenic and/or thrombocytopenic effects of idarubicin may be increased with concurrent or recent therapy if these medications cause the same effects; dosage adjustment of idarubicin, if necessary, should be based on blood counts)

» Bone marrow depressants, other (see *Appendix II*) or
Radiation therapy
(additive bone marrow depression may occur; dosage reduction may be required when two or more bone marrow depressants, including radiation, are used concurrently or consecutively)

Daunorubicin or
Doxorubicin
(use of idarubicin in a patient who has previously received daunorubicin or doxorubicin increases the risk of cardiotoxicity; in general, idarubicin should not be used in patients who have previously received complete cumulative doses of daunorubicin or doxorubicin)

Radiation therapy to mediastinal area
(concurrent use with idarubicin may result in increased cardiotoxicity)

Vaccines, killed virus
(because normal defense mechanisms may be suppressed by idarubicin therapy, the patient's antibody response to the vaccine may be decreased. The interval between discontinuation of medications that cause immunosuppression and restoration of the patient's ability to respond to the vaccine depends on the intensity and type of immunosuppression-causing medication used, the underlying disease, and other factors; estimates vary from 3 months to 1 year)

» Vaccines, live virus
(because normal defense mechanisms may be suppressed by idarubicin therapy, concurrent use with a live virus vaccine may potentiate the replication of the vaccine virus, may increase the side/adverse effects of the vaccine virus, and/or may decrease the patient's antibody response to the vaccine; immunization of these patients should be undertaken only with extreme caution after careful review of the patient's hematologic status and only with the knowledge and consent of the physician managing the idarubicin therapy. The interval between discontinuation of medications that cause immunosuppression and restoration of the patient's ability to respond to vaccines depends on the intensity and type of immunosuppression-causing medication used, the underlying disease, and other factors; estimates vary from 3 months to 1 year. Patients with leukemia in remission should not receive live virus vaccine until at least 3 months after their last chemotherapy. In addition, immunization with oral poliovirus vaccine should be postponed in persons in close contact with the patient, especially family members)

### Laboratory value alterations
The following have been selected on the basis of their potential clinical significance (possible effect in parentheses where appropriate)—not necessarily inclusive (» = major clinical significance):

With physiology/laboratory test values
Alanine aminotransferase (ALT [SGPT]), serum and
Alkaline phosphatase, serum and

Aspartate aminotransferase (AST [SGOT]), serum
    (values may be increased transiently)
Bilirubin, serum
    (concentrations may be increased transiently)
Electrocardiogram (ECG) changes, transient, including:
    Arrhythmias (atrial or ventricular premature beats, tachycardia)
    ST-T wave changes
    T-wave flattening
    T-wave inversion
        (may occur)
Left ventricular ejection fraction (LVEF)
    (decrease from pretreatment baseline values usually occurs with idarubicin-induced cardiomyopathy)
Uric acid concentrations in blood and urine
    (may be increased)

### Medical considerations/Contraindications
The medical considerations/contraindications included have been selected on the basis of their potential clinical significance (reasons given in parentheses where appropriate)—not necessarily inclusive (» = major clinical significance).

*Risk-benefit should be considered when the following medical problems exist:*

» Bone marrow depression
» Chickenpox, existing or recent (including recent exposure) or
» Herpes zoster
    (risk of severe generalized disease)
Gout, history of or
Urate renal stones, history of
    (risk of hyperuricemia)
» Heart disease
    (increased risk of cardiotoxicity)
» Hepatic function impairment
    (reduction in dosage is recommended; one half the normal dose is recommended in patients with serum bilirubin concentrations of 2.35 to 5 mg per 100 mL; administration of idarubicin is not recommended in patients with serum bilirubin concentrations of greater than 5 mg per 100 mL)
» Infection
    (should be controlled before initiation of idarubicin treatment)
Renal function impairment
    (dosage reduction should be considered in patients with a serum creatinine of greater than 2.5 mg per 100 mL)
Sensitivity to idarubicin
» Caution should be used also in patients with inadequate bone marrow reserves due to previous cytotoxic drug or radiation therapy

### Patient monitoring
Alanine aminotransferase (ALT [SGPT]) and
Alkaline phosphatase and
Aspartate aminotransferase (AST [SGOT]) and
Bilirubin, serum and
Lactate dehydrogenase (LDH), serum
    (determinations recommended prior to initiation of therapy and at periodic intervals during therapy to monitor hepatic function; frequency varies according to clinical state, agent, dose, and other agents being used concurrently)
Chest x-ray and
» Echocardiography and
Electrocardiogram (ECG) studies and
» Radionuclide angiography determination of ejection fraction
    (recommended prior to initiation of therapy and at periodic intervals during therapy)
Creatinine, serum
    (recommended prior to treatment and at periodic intervals during treatment to monitor renal function)
» Examination of patient's mouth for ulceration
    (recommended before administration of each dose)
» Hematocrit or hemoglobin and
» Platelet count and
» Leukocyte count, total and, if appropriate, differential
    (determinations recommended prior to initiation of therapy and at periodic intervals during therapy; frequency varies according to clinical state, agent, dose, and other agents being used concurrently)
Uric acid, serum
    (determinations recommended prior to initiation of therapy and at periodic intervals during therapy; frequency varies according to clinical state, agent, dose, and other agents being used concurrently)

## Side/Adverse Effects
Note: Many "side effects" of antineoplastic therapy are unavoidable and represent the medication's pharmacologic action. Some of these (for example, leukopenia and thrombocytopenia) are actually used as parameters to aid in individual dosage titration.

The following side/adverse effects have been selected on the basis of their potential clinical significance (possible signs and symptoms in parentheses where appropriate)—not necessarily inclusive:

### Those indicating need for medical attention
Incidence more frequent
    ***Leukopenia*** (fever or chills; cough or hoarseness; lower back or side pain; painful or difficult urination); ***mucositis*** (sores in mouth and on lips); ***thrombocytopenia*** (unusual bleeding or bruising; black, tarry stools; blood in urine or stools; pinpoint red spots on skin)
    Note: Severe *leukopenia* occurs in all patients; deaths due to infection have been reported. Nadir of leukocyte counts occurs 10 to 14 days after a dose; recovery usually occurs within 21 days after a dose.
    Severe *thrombocytopenia* occurs in all patients; deaths due to bleeding have been reported. Nadir of platelet counts occurs 10 to 14 days after a dose; recovery usually occurs within 21 days after a dose.
Incidence less frequent
    ***Cardiotoxicity, in the form of arrhythmias, congestive heart failure, or other cardiomyopathies*** (shortness of breath; swelling of feet and lower legs; fast or irregular heartbeat); ***hyperuricemia or uric acid nephropathy*** (joint pain, lower back or side pain); ***tissue necrosis caused by extravasation*** (pain at injection site)
    Note: Incidence of *cardiotoxicity* is more frequent in patients who have received previous chest irradiation or medications increasing cardiotoxicity and in patients with a history of cardiac disease or mediastinal radiation, and may be more frequent in the elderly. Cumulative cardiotoxicity has not been studied.
    *Extravasation* may occur with or without accompanying stinging or burning and even if blood returns well on aspiration of the infusion needle.
    *Hyperuricemia or uric acid nephropathy* occurs most commonly during initial treatment of patients with leukemias a result of rapid cell breakdown, which leads to elevated serum uric acid concentrations.
Incidence rare
    ***Enterocolitis, with perforation*** (severe stomach pain); ***skin rash or hives***

### Those indicating need for medical attention only if they continue or are bothersome
Incidence more frequent
    ***Diarrhea or stomach cramps; headache; nausea and vomiting***
    Note: *Nausea and vomiting* are usually mild.
Incidence less frequent
    ***Peripheral neuropathy*** (numbness or tingling of fingers, toes, or face); ***recall postirradiation erythema*** (darkening or redness of skin)
    Note: *Recall postirradiation erythema* occurs if patient has received previous radiation therapy.

### Those not indicating need for medical attention
Incidence more frequent
    ***Alopecia*** (loss of hair); ***reddish urine***
    Note: *Alopecia* occurs in most patients. Hair growth should return after treatment has ended.

### Those indicating the need for medical attention if they occur after medication is discontinued
    ***Cardiotoxicity*** (fast or irregular heartbeat; shortness of breath; swelling of feet and lower legs)

## Overdose
For more information on the management of overdose or unintentional ingestion, **contact a Poison Control Center** (see *Poison Control Center Listing*).

### Treatment of overdose
Treatment of overdose involves supportive care, including:
    Platelet transfusions and antibiotics for severe and prolonged myelosuppression.
    Symptomatic treatment of mucositis.

It is unlikely that dialysis would remove significant amounts of idarubicin or its metabolites.

## Patient Consultation

As an aid to patient consultation, refer to *Advice for the Patient, Idarubicin (Systemic)*.

In providing consultation, consider emphasizing the following selected information (» = major clinical significance):

### Before using this medication
» Conditions affecting use, especially:
   Sensitivity to idarubicin
   Pregnancy—Use not recommended because of mutagenic, teratogenic, and carcinogenic potential; advisability of using contraception; telling physician immediately if pregnancy is suspected
   Breast-feeding—Not recommended because of risk of serious side effects
   Use in the elderly—Cardiotoxicity may be more frequent in patients over 60 years of age
   Other medications, especially probenecid, sulfinpyrazone, other bone marrow depressants, or previous cytotoxic drug or radiation therapy
   Other medical problems, especially chickenpox, herpes zoster, heart disease, hepatic function impairment, or other infections

### Proper use of this medication
Caution in taking combination therapy; taking each medication at the right time
Importance of ample fluid intake and subsequent increase in urine output to aid in excretion of uric acid
Frequency of nausea and vomiting; importance of continuing medication despite stomach upset
» Proper dosing

### Precautions while using this medication
» Importance of close monitoring by the physician
» Avoiding immunizations unless approved by physician; other persons in patient's household should avoid immunizations with oral poliovirus vaccine; avoiding persons who have taken oral poliovirus vaccine or wearing a protective mask that covers nose and mouth

*Caution if bone marrow depression occurs*
» Avoiding exposure to persons with infections, especially during periods of low blood counts; checking with physician immediately if fever or chills, cough or hoarseness, lower back or side pain, or painful or difficult urination occurs
» Checking with physician immediately if unusual bleeding or bruising; black, tarry stools; blood in urine or stools; or pinpoint red spots on skin occur
Caution in use of regular toothbrush, dental floss, or toothpick; physician, dentist, or nurse may suggest alternatives; checking with physician before having dental work done
Not touching eyes or inside of nose unless hands washed immediately before
Using caution to avoid accidental cuts with use of sharp objects such as safety razor or fingernail or toenail cutters
Avoiding contact sports or other situations where bruising or injury could occur
» Possibility of local tissue injury and scarring if infiltration of intravenous solution occurs; telling doctor or nurse right away about redness, pain, or swelling at injection site

### Side/adverse effects
Importance of discussing possible effects, including cancer, with physician
Signs of potential side effects, especially leukopenia, mucositis, thrombocytopenia, cardiotoxicity, tissue necrosis caused by extravasation, hyperuricemia, uric acid nephropathy, enterocolitis, and skin rash or hives
Possibility of hair loss; growth should return after treatment has ended

## General Dosing Information

Patients receiving idarubicin should be under supervision of a physician experienced in cancer chemotherapy.

A variety of dosage schedules of idarubicin, alone or in combination with other antitumor agents, are used. The prescriber may consult the medical literature as well as the manufacturer's literature in choosing a specific dosage.

Dosage must be adjusted to meet the individual requirements of each patient, on the basis of clinical response and appearance or severity of toxicity.

The desired dose of idarubicin is withdrawn from the vial of reconstituted solution and then injected over 10 to 15 minutes into the tubing of a freely running intravenous infusion of 5% dextrose injection or 0.9% sodium chloride injection. The tubing should be attached to a butterfly needle or other suitable device and inserted preferably into a large vein.

Care must be taken to avoid extravasation during intravenous administration because of the risk of severe ulceration and necrosis.

If extravasation of idarubicin occurs during intravenous administration, possibly indicated by local burning or stinging (may also be painless), the injection and infusion should be stopped immediately and resumed, completing the dose, in another vein. Treatment of known or suspected subcutaneous extravasation may include intermittent ice packs (one-half hour immediately, then one-half hour four times a day for 3 days) over the area of extravasation and elevation of the affected extremity. Frequent examinations of the area, as well as an early plastic surgery consultation, are recommended if there is any sign of a local reaction such as pain, erythema, edema, or vesication. Early excision of the involved area should be considered if ulceration begins or there is severe persistent pain at the site.

Because it will cause local tissue necrosis, idarubicin must not be administered intramuscularly or subcutaneously.

Development of uric acid nephropathy in patients with leukemia may be prevented by adequate oral hydration and, in some cases, administration of allopurinol. Alkalinization of urine may be necessary if serum uric acid concentrations are elevated.

In patients who experience severe mucositis, a second course of idarubicin should be delayed until recovery has occurred and a dose reduction of 25% is recommended.

In acute leukemia, idarubicin may be administered despite the presence of thrombocytopenia and bleeding; stoppage of bleeding and increase in platelet count can occur during or after treatment. Platelet transfusions may be necessary.

Special precautions are recommended in patients who develop thrombocytopenia as a result of administration of idarubicin. The precautions may include extreme care in performing invasive procedures; regular inspection of intravenous sites, skin (including perirectal area), and mucous membrane surfaces for signs of bleeding or bruising; limiting frequency of venipuncture and avoiding intramuscular injections; testing urine, emesis, stool, and secretions for occult blood; care in use of regular toothbrushes, dental floss, toothpicks, safety razors, and fingernail and toenail cutters; avoiding constipation; and using measures to prevent falls and other injuries. Such patients should avoid alcohol and aspirin intake because of the risk of gastrointestinal bleeding. Platelet transfusions may be required.

Patients who develop leukopenia should be observed carefully for signs of infection. Antibiotic support may be required. In neutropenic patients who develop fever, broad-spectrum antibiotic coverage should be initiated empirically, pending bacterial cultures and appropriate diagnostic tests.

### Safety considerations for handling this medication
There is concern and limited evidence that personnel involved in preparation and administration of parenteral antineoplastics may be at some risk because of the potential mutagenicity, teratogenicity, and/or carcinogenicity of these agents, although the actual risk is unknown. USP advisory panels recommend cautious handling both in preparation and disposal of antineoplastic agents. Precautions that have been suggested include:
- Use of a biological containment cabinet during reconstitution and dilution of parenteral medications and wearing of disposable surgical gloves and masks.
- Use of proper technique to prevent contamination of the medication, work area, and operator during transfer between containers (including proper training of personnel in this technique).
- Cautious and proper disposal of needles, syringes, vials, ampuls, and unused medication.

A number of medical centers have developed detailed guidelines for handling of antineoplastic agents.

### Combination chemotherapy
Idarubicin may be used in combination with other agents in various regimens. As a result, incidence and/or severity of side effects may be altered and different dosages (usually reduced) may be used.

For specific dosages and schedules, consult the literature. For information regarding each agent, consult the individual monographs.

## Parenteral Dosage Forms

### IDARUBICIN HYDROCHLORIDE FOR INJECTION USP

#### Usual adult dose
Leukemia, acute nonlymphocytic—
   Intravenous, slow (over ten to fifteen minutes), 12 mg per square meter of body surface area per day for three days. This is given in combination with cytarabine in a dose of either 100 mg per square meter of body surface area per day by continuous intravenous infusion for

seven days or 25 mg per square meter of body surface area intravenously, followed by 200 mg per square meter of body surface area per day by continuous intravenous infusion for five days.

Note: A second course may be given to patients with unequivocal evidence of leukemia after the first course.

**Usual pediatric dose**
Safety and efficacy have not been established.

**Size(s) usually available**
U.S.—
  5 mg (Rx) [*Idamycin* (lactose 50 mg)].
  10 mg (Rx) [*Idamycin* (lactose 100 mg)].
Canada—
  5 mg (Rx) [*Idamycin* (lactose 50 mg)].
  10 mg (Rx) [*Idamycin* (lactose 100 mg)].

**Packaging and storage**
Store below 40 °C (104 °F), preferably between 15 and 30 °C (59 and 86 °F), unless otherwise specified by the manufacturer. Protect from light.

**Preparation of dosage form**
Idarubicin Hydrochloride for Injection USP is reconstituted for intravenous administration by adding 5 or 10 mL, respectively, of 0.9% sodium chloride injection to the 5- or 10-mg vial, producing a solution containing 1 mg of idarubicin hydrochloride per mL. Use of bacteriostatic diluents is not recommended. Care should be taken when the needle is inserted in the vial, whose contents are under negative pressure to minimize aerosol formation during reconstitution.

**Stability**
Reconstituted solutions of idarubicin are physically and chemically stable for 72 hours at room temperature or at least 168 hours (7 days) between 2 and 8 °C (36 and 46 °F) when protected from light.

**Incompatibilities**
Idarubicin should not be mixed with heparin, since a precipitate may form.

**Note**
Great care should be taken to prevent exposure of the skin to idarubicin. Any idarubicin powder or solution that comes into contact with the skin or mucosa should be washed off thoroughly with soap and water.

Revised: 06/18/93
Interim revision: 06/21/94; 09/29/97; 07/07/98

# IDOXURIDINE Ophthalmic

VA CLASSIFICATION (Primary): OP203
Commonly used brand name(s): *Herplex Liquifilm; Stoxil.*
Note: For a listing of dosage forms and brand names by country availability, see *Dosage Forms* section(s).

## Category
Antiviral (ophthalmic).

## Indications
Note: Bracketed information in the *Indications* section refers to uses that are not included in U.S. product labeling.

**Accepted**
Keratitis, herpes simplex virus (treatment) or
[Keratitis, vaccinia virus (treatment)][1]—Idoxuridine is indicated in the treatment of keratitis caused by herpes simplex virus (HSV) and [vaccinia virus].

[Keratoconjunctivitis, herpes simplex virus (treatment)][1]—Idoxuridine is used in the treatment of keratoconjunctivitis caused by herpes simplex virus (HSV).

**Unaccepted**
Idoxuridine has no effect on accumulated scarring, vascularization, or progressive loss of vision that may result from the infection. It also has no effect on corneal inflammation that may follow HSV keratitis when the virus is absent, nor on adenoviral keratoconjunctivitis.

[1]Not included in Canadian product labeling.

## Pharmacology/Pharmacokinetics

**Physicochemical characteristics**
Chemical group—Chemically related to thymidine.
Molecular weight—354.10.

**Mechanism of action/Effect**
Idoxuridine, which closely resembles thymidine, inhibits thymidylic phosphorylase and specific DNA polymerases, which are necessary for the incorporation of thymidine into viral DNA. Idoxuridine is incorporated in place of thymidine into viral DNA, resulting in faulty DNA and the inability to infect or destroy tissue or to reproduce. Idoxuridine is incorporated into mammalian DNA as well.

**Distribution**
Idoxuridine penetrates the cornea poorly and therefore is ineffective in the treatment of iritis or deep stromal infections.

**Biotransformation**
Idoxuridine is rapidly inactivated by deaminases or nucleotidases.

## Precautions to Consider

**Cross-sensitivity and/or related problems**
Patients sensitive to iodine or iodine-containing preparations may be sensitive to this medication also.

**Pregnancy/Reproduction**
Pregnancy—Idoxuridine crosses the placenta. Studies in humans have not been done.
Fetal malformations in rabbits (including exophthalmos and clubbing of forelegs) and chromosomal aberrations in mice have been reported.

**Breast-feeding**
It is not known whether idoxuridine is distributed into breast milk. However, problems in humans have not been documented.

**Pediatrics**
Appropriate studies on the relationship of age to the effects of this medicine have not been performed in the pediatric population. However, no pediatrics-specific problems have been documented to date.

**Geriatrics**
Appropriate studies on the relationship of age to the effects of this medicine have not been performed in the geriatric population. However, no geriatrics-specific problems have been documented to date.

**Drug interactions and/or related problems**
The following drug interactions and/or related problems have been selected on the basis of their potential clinical significance (possible mechanism in parentheses where appropriate)—not necessarily inclusive (» = major clinical significance):

Note: Combinations containing any of the following medications, depending on the amount present, may also interact with this medication.

» Boric acid
  (concurrent use of boric acid with idoxuridine formulations is not recommended; boric acid may interact with inactive ingredients in some idoxuridine formulations, resulting in precipitate formation; in addition, boric acid may interact with preservatives, especially higher concentrations of thimerosal, in other idoxuridine formulations, resulting in increased ocular toxicity)

**Medical considerations/Contraindications**
The medical considerations/contraindications included have been selected on the basis of their potential clinical significance (reasons given in parentheses where appropriate)—not necessarily inclusive (» = major clinical significance).

*Risk-benefit should be considered when the following medical problem exists:*
Sensitivity to idoxuridine

**Patient monitoring**
The following may be especially important in patient monitoring (other tests may be warranted in some patients, depending on condition; » = major clinical significance):

Ophthalmologic, including slit-lamp, examinations
  (may be required periodically during therapy)

## Side/Adverse Effects

The following side/adverse effects have been selected on the basis of their potential clinical significance (possible signs and symptoms in parentheses where appropriate)—not necessarily inclusive:

## Idoxuridine (Ophthalmic)

**Those indicating need for medical attention**
Incidence less frequent
*Hypersensitivity* (itching, redness, swelling, pain, or other sign of irritation not present before therapy); *increased sensitivity of eyes to light*
Incidence rare
*Corneal clouding* (blurring, dimming, or haziness of vision)

**Those indicating need for medical attention only if they continue or are bothersome**
Incidence less frequent
*Lacrimal punctal stenosis or occlusion* (excess flow of tears)

**Those not indicating need for medical attention**
For ophthalmic ointment dosage form only
*Blurred vision*

## Patient Consultation

As an aid to patient consultation, refer to *Advice for the Patient, Idoxuridine (Ophthalmic)*.
In providing consultation, consider emphasizing the following selected information (» = major clinical significance):

**Before using this medication**
» Conditions affecting use, especially:
   Sensitivity to idoxuridine or to iodine or iodine-containing preparations
   Pregnancy—Ophthalmic idoxuridine crosses the placenta and has been shown to cause protruding eyes and deformed forelegs in rabbits. However, the medication has not been shown to cause birth defects or other problems in humans
   Other medications, especially boric acid

**Proper use of this medication**
Proper administration technique for ophthalmic ointment and solution
» Not administering more frequently or for longer than ordered by physician
» Compliance with full course of therapy
» Proper dosing
Missed dose: Applying as soon as possible; not applying if almost time for next dose
» Proper storage

**Precautions while using this medication**
Regular visits to physician to check progress
Checking with physician if no improvement within a week
Possible photophobic reactions; wearing sunglasses and avoiding prolonged exposure to bright light

**Side/adverse effects**
Blurred vision may occur for a few minutes after application of ophthalmic ointments
Signs of potential side effects, especially hypersensitivity, increased sensitivity of eyes to light, or corneal clouding

## General Dosing Information

At night the ophthalmic ointment may be used as an adjunct to the ophthalmic solution to provide prolonged contact with the medication.

Although some manufacturers recommend a dose of 2 drops of an ophthalmic solution at appropriate intervals, the conjunctival sac will usually hold only 1 drop.

Idoxuridine may be administered concurrently with cycloplegics, antibiotics, or corticosteroids. Corticosteroids can accelerate the spread of viral infections and are usually contraindicated in superficial herpes simplex virus keratitis. However, steroids may be used concurrently with idoxuridine in the treatment of herpes simplex infections with stromal lesions, corneal edema, or iritis. Prolonged administration with corticosteroids may be required. Idoxuridine should be continued for a few days after the steroid has been discontinued.

Since idoxuridine inhibits the formation of DNA in the cornea, prolonged administration of idoxuridine alone may damage the corneal epithelium and prevent healing of the ulcers. Treatment should usually not be continued for more than 21 days total or for more than 3 to 5 days after healing is complete. However, chronic or particularly difficult infections may require up to 3 to 6 weeks of treatment. Too frequent administration may result in small punctate defects in the cornea.

Burning after application or failure to respond to treatment may suggest deterioration of the ophthalmic solution; replace with fresh solution.

Herpetic keratitis may recur if idoxuridine is discontinued before microscopic staining with fluorescein has cleared.

## Ophthalmic Dosage Forms

Note: Bracketed uses in the *Dosage Forms* section refer to categories of use and/or indications that are not included in U.S. product labeling.

### IDOXURIDINE OPHTHALMIC OINTMENT USP

**Usual adult and adolescent dose**
Keratitis, herpes simplex virus—
   Topical, to the conjunctiva, a thin strip (approximately 1 cm) of ointment every four hours (five times a day) during the day. The last dose may be administered at bedtime. Treatment should be continued until definite improvement occurs, as demonstrated by loss of staining with fluorescein.
[Keratitis, vaccinia virus][1] or
[Keratoconjunctivitis, herpes simplex virus][1]—
   Topical, to the conjunctiva, a thin strip (approximately 1 cm) of ointment five times a day.

**Usual adult prescribing limits**
Up to 8 times daily.

**Usual pediatric dose**
See *Usual adult and adolescent dose*.

**Strength(s) usually available**
U.S.—
   0.5% (Rx) [*Stoxil*].
Canada—
   0.5% (Rx) [*Stoxil*].

**Packaging and storage**
Store between 8 and 15 °C (46 and 59 °F). Store in a collapsible ophthalmic ointment tube.

Note: Some manufacturers indicate that the ointment does not require refrigeration.

**Stability**
Idoxuridine is rapidly inactivated by deaminases or nucleotidases.

**Auxiliary labeling**
• Store in a cool place. May be refrigerated.
• For the eye.
• Continue medicine for full time of treatment.
• Do not use more often or longer than ordered.

### IDOXURIDINE OPHTHALMIC SOLUTION USP

**Usual adult and adolescent dose**
Keratitis, herpes simplex virus—
   Topical, to the conjunctiva, 1 drop every hour during the day and every two hours during the night; or 1 drop every minute for five minutes with the dosage schedule repeated every four hours day and night. Treatment should be continued until definite improvement occurs, as demonstrated by loss of staining with fluorescein. Dose may then be reduced to 1 drop every two hours during the day and every four hours during the night.
[Keratitis, vaccinia virus][1] or
[Keratoconjunctivitis, herpes simplex virus][1] —
   Topical, to the conjunctiva, 1 drop every hour during the day and every two hours during the night.

**Usual pediatric dose**
See *Usual adult and adolescent dose*.

**Strength(s) usually available**
U.S.—
   0.1% (Rx) [*Herplex Liquifilm* (polyvinyl alcohol 1.4%; benzalkonium chloride); *Stoxil* (thimerosal 1:50,000)].
Canada—
   0.1% (Rx) [*Herplex Liquifilm* (polyvinyl alcohol 1.4%; benzalkonium chloride 0.004%); *Stoxil* (thimerosal 1:50,000)].

**Packaging and storage**
Store between 2 and 8 °C (36 and 46 °F). Store in a tight, light-resistant container.

**Stability**
Idoxuridine is rapidly inactivated by deaminases or nucleotidases. To ensure stability, the ophthalmic solution should not be mixed with other medications. Burning after application or failure to respond to treatment may suggest deterioration of the ophthalmic solution; replace with fresh solution.

**Auxiliary labeling**
• Refrigerate.
• For the eye.
• Continue medicine for full time of treatment.
• Do not use more often or longer than ordered.

**Note**
Dispense in original unopened container.

---

[1] Not included in Canadian product labeling.

Revised: 06/21/93

# IFOSFAMIDE Systemic

VA CLASSIFICATION (Primary): AN100
Commonly used brand name(s): *IFEX*.
Note: For a listing of dosage forms and brand names by country availability, see *Dosage Forms* section(s).

## Category
Antineoplastic.

## Indications
Note: Bracketed information in the *Indications* section refers to uses that are not included in U.S. product labeling.

**Accepted**

Tumors, germ cell, testicular (treatment)[1]—Ifosfamide is indicated, in combination with other antineoplastic agents and a prophylactic agent against hemorrhagic cystitis (such as mesna), for treatment of germ cell testicular tumors.

[Carcinoma, head and neck (treatment)][1]—Ifosfamide is indicated as reasonable medical therapy for treatment of head and neck carcinoma. (Evidence rating: IIID)

[Sarcomas, soft-tissue (treatment)]
[Ewing's sarcoma (treatment)][1]
[Lymphomas, Hodgkin's (treatment)][1] or
[Lymphomas, non-Hodgkin's (treatment)][1]—Ifosfamide is used for treatment of soft-tissue sarcomas, Ewing's sarcoma, and Hodgkin's and non-Hodgkin's lymphomas.

[Carcinoma, breast (treatment)][1]
[Carcinoma, cervical (treatment)]
[Carcinoma, lung, small cell (treatment)][1]
[Carcinoma, lung, non–small cell (treatment)][1]
[Carcinoma, ovarian epithelial (treatment)][1]
[Leukemia, acute lymphocytic (treatment)][1]
[Neuroblastoma (treatment)][1] or
[Osteosarcoma (treatment)][1]—Ifosfamide is indicated for treatment of breast carcinoma, cervical carcinoma, small cell lung carcinoma, non–small cell lung carcinoma, ovarian epithelial carcinoma, acute lymphocytic leukemia, neuroblastoma, and osteosarcoma.

[1]Not included in Canadian product labeling.

## Pharmacology/Pharmacokinetics

**Physicochemical characteristics**
Molecular weight—261.09.

**Mechanism of action/Effect**
Ifosfamide is classified as an alkylating agent of the nitrogen mustard type. After metabolic activation, active metabolites of ifosfamide alkylate or bind with many intracellular molecular structures, including nucleic acids. The cytotoxic action is primarily due to cross-linking of strands of DNA and RNA, as well as inhibition of protein synthesis.

**Distribution**
Active metabolites cross the blood-brain barrier to only a limited extent.

**Biotransformation**
Hepatic (including initial activation and subsequent degradation). Metabolic pathways appear to be saturated at high doses.

**Half-life**
At single doses of 3.8 to 5 grams per square meter of body surface area—Biphasic: Terminal—15 hours.
At doses of 1.6 to 2.4 grams per square meter of body surface area per day—Monophasic: 7 hours.

**Elimination**
Renal, 70 to 86%; 61% unchanged at single doses of 5 grams per square meter of body surface area. 12 to 18% unchanged at doses of 1.2 to 2.4 grams per square meter of body surface area.

## Precautions to Consider

**Carcinogenicity**
Secondary malignancies are potential delayed effects of many antineoplastic agents, although it is not clear whether the effect is related to their mutagenic or immunosuppressive action. The effects of dose and duration of therapy are also unknown, although risk seems to increase with long-term use. Although information is limited, available data seem to indicate that the carcinogenic risk is greatest with the alkylating agents.

Studies in rats have found ifosfamide to be carcinogenic, with female rats showing a significant incidence of leiomyosarcomas and mammary fibroadenomas.

**Mutagenicity**
Ifosfamide has been shown to be mutagenic in bacterial studies *in vitro* and mammalian cells *in vivo*. *In vivo*, ifosfamide has induced mutagenic effects in mice and *Drosophila melanogaster* germ cells, and has induced a significant increase in dominant lethal mutations in male mice as well as recessive sex-linked lethal mutations in *Drosophila*.

**Pregnancy/Reproduction**
Fertility—Gonadal suppression, resulting in amenorrhea or azoospermia, may occur in patients taking antineoplastic therapy, especially with the alkylating agents. In general, these effects appear to be related to dose and length of therapy and may be irreversible. Prediction of the degree of testicular or ovarian function impairment is complicated by the common use of combinations of several antineoplastics, which makes it difficult to assess the effects of individual agents.

Pregnancy—First trimester: It is usually recommended that use of antineoplastics, especially combination chemotherapy, be avoided whenever possible, especially during the first trimester. Although information is limited because of the relatively few instances of antineoplastic administration during pregnancy, the mutagenic, teratogenic, and carcinogenic potential of these medications must be considered.

Other hazards to the fetus include adverse reactions seen in adults.

In general, use of a contraceptive is recommended during cytotoxic drug therapy.

Studies in animals have shown that ifosfamide is teratogenic in mice, rats, and rabbits given 0.05 to 0.075 times the human dose.

FDA Pregnancy Category D.

**Breast-feeding**
Ifosfamide is distributed into breast milk. Breast-feeding is not recommended during chemotherapy because of the risks to the infant (adverse effects, mutagenicity, carcinogenicity).

**Pediatrics**
Appropriate studies on the relationship of age to the effects of ifosfamide have not been performed in the pediatric population. However, no pediatrics-specific problems have been documented to date.

**Geriatrics**
No information is available on the relationship of age to the effects of ifosfamide in geriatric patients. However, elderly patients are more likely to have age-related renal function impairment, which may require caution.

**Dental**
The bone marrow depressant effects of ifosfamide may result in an increased incidence of microbial infection, delayed healing, and gingival bleeding. Dental work, whenever possible, should be completed prior to initiation of therapy or deferred until blood counts have returned to normal. Patients should be instructed in proper oral hygiene during treatment, including caution in use of regular toothbrushes, dental floss, and toothpicks.

Ifosfamide may also rarely cause stomatitis associated with considerable discomfort.

**Drug interactions and/or related problems**
The following drug interactions and/or related problems have been selected on the basis of their potential clinical significance (possible mechanism in parentheses where appropriate)—not necessarily inclusive (» = major clinical significance):

Note: Combinations containing any of the following medications, depending on the amount present, may also interact with this medication.

Blood dyscrasia–causing medications (see *Appendix II*)
(leukopenic and/or thrombocytopenic effects of ifosfamide may be increased with concurrent or recent therapy if these medications cause the same effects; dosage adjustment of ifosfamide, if necessary, should be based on blood counts)

» Bone marrow depressants, other (see *Appendix II*) or
» Radiation therapy
(additive bone marrow depression may occur; dosage reduction may be required when two or more bone marrow depressants, including radiation, are used concurrently or consecutively)

Hepatic enzyme inducers (see *Appendix II*)
(these agents may induce microsomal metabolism to increase formation of alkylating metabolites of ifosfamide; although it is unknown whether activity of ifosfamide is increased, neurotoxicity may be increased; caution is recommended)

Nephrotoxic medications
(prior or concurrent use with ifosfamide may increase ifosfamide's nephrotoxic effects)

(previous use of large cumulative doses of cisplatin may increase the risk of central nervous system (CNS) toxicity with ifosfamide)

Vaccines, killed virus
(because normal defense mechanisms may be suppressed by ifosfamide therapy, the patient's antibody response to the vaccine may be decreased. The interval between discontinuation of medications that cause immunosuppression and restoration of the patient's ability to respond to the vaccine depends on the intensity and type of immunosuppression-causing medication used, the underlying disease, and other factors; estimates vary from 3 months to 1 year)

» Vaccines, live virus
(because normal defense mechanisms may be suppressed by ifosfamide therapy, concurrent use with a live virus vaccine may potentiate the replication of the vaccine virus, may increase the side/adverse effects of the vaccine virus, and/or may decrease the patient's antibody response to the vaccine; immunization of these patients should be undertaken only with extreme caution after careful review of the patient's hematologic status and only with the knowledge and consent of the physician managing the ifosfamide therapy. The interval between discontinuation of medications that cause immunosuppression and restoration of the patient's ability to respond to the vaccine depends on the intensity and type of immunosuppression-causing medication used, the underlying disease, and other factors; estimates vary from 3 months to 1 year. Patients with leukemia in remission should not receive live virus vaccine until at least 3 months after their last chemotherapy. In addition, immunization with oral poliovirus vaccine should be postponed in persons in close contact with the patient, especially family members)

**Laboratory value alterations**
The following have been selected on the basis of their potential clinical significance (possible effect in parentheses where appropriate)—not necessarily inclusive (» = major clinical significance):

With physiology/laboratory test values
Alanine aminotransferase (ALT [SGPT]) and
Aspartate aminotransferase (AST [SGOT]) and
Lactate dehydrogenase (LDH)
(serum values may be increased as a sign of hepatotoxicity)
Bilirubin
(serum concentrations may be increased as a sign of hepatotoxicity)
Blood urea nitrogen (BUN) or
Creatinine, serum
(concentrations may be increased transiently as a sign of renal toxicity)
Creatinine clearance
(may be decreased transiently as a sign of renal toxicity)

**Medical considerations/Contraindications**
The medical considerations/contraindications included have been selected on the basis of their potential clinical significance (reasons given in parentheses where appropriate)—not necessarily inclusive (» = major clinical significance).

*Risk-benefit should be considered when the following medical problems exist:*

» Bone marrow depression
» Chickenpox, existing or recent (including recent exposure) or
» Herpes zoster
(risk of severe generalized disease)
» Hepatic function impairment
(effect of ifosfamide may be reduced or enhanced because of its dependence on hepatic microsomal enzyme activation and degradation)
» Infection
» Renal function impairment
(reduced elimination; incidence of CNS toxicity and renal toxicity may be increased; dosage reduction may be necessary)
Sensitivity to ifosfamide
Tumor cell infiltration of bone marrow
(bone marrow depression)
» Caution should be used also in patients who have had previous cytotoxic drug therapy or radiation therapy.

**Patient monitoring**
The following are especially important in patient monitoring (other tests may be warranted in some patients, depending on condition; » = major clinical significance):

Alanine aminotransferase (ALT [SGPT]) values, serum and
Alkaline phosphatase values, serum and
Aspartate aminotransferase (AST [SGOT]) values, serum and
Lactate dehydrogenase (LDH) values, serum
(recommended prior to initiation of therapy and at periodic intervals during therapy; frequency varies according to clinical state, agent, dose, and other agents being used concurrently)

Bilirubin, concentrations, serum and
Blood urea nitrogen (BUN) concentrations and
Creatinine concentrations, serum
(recommended prior to initiation of therapy and at periodic intervals during therapy; frequency varies according to clinical state, agent, dose, and other agents being used concurrently)

» Examination of urine for microscopic hematuria
(recommended prior to each dose)
» Hematocrit or hemoglobin and
» Leukocyte count, total and, if appropriate, differential and
» Platelet count
(determinations recommended prior to initiation of therapy and at periodic intervals during therapy; frequency varies according to clinical state, agent, dose, and other agents being used concurrently)

Phosphate concentrations, serum and
Potassium concentrations, serum
(recommended at periodic intervals during therapy)

## Side/Adverse Effects

Note: Many "side effects" of antineoplastic therapy are unavoidable and represent the medication's pharmacologic action. Some of these (for example, leukopenia and thrombocytopenia) are actually used as parameters to aid in individual dosage titration.

The following side/adverse effects have been selected on the basis of their potential clinical significance (possible signs and symptoms in parentheses where appropriate)—not necessarily inclusive:

### Those indicating need for medical attention
Incidence more frequent—dose-related
***CNS effects or encephalopathy*** (agitation; confusion; hallucinations; unusual tiredness; less frequently, dizziness; rarely, seizures; coma); ***leukopenia; thrombocytopenia*** (rarely associated with unusual bleeding or bruising; black, tarry stools; blood in urine or stools; pinpoint red spots on skin); ***urotoxicity, including hemorrhagic cystitis; dysuria; urinary frequency*** (blood in urine; frequent urination; painful urination)

Note: *CNS effects and encephalopathy* do not appear to be dose-related. They may be associated with electroencephalogram (EEG) changes. Signs and symptoms usually resolve within 3 days after withdrawal of ifosfamide, but may persist longer. Fatalities have been reported.

*Leukopenia* is usually mild to moderate. Nadir of leukocyte count occurs within 7 to 14 days and counts usually recover by 21 days after a course.

With *thrombocytopenia*, nadir of platelet count occurs within 7 to 14 days and counts usually recover by 21 days after a course.

*Urotoxicity* may occur within a few hours or be delayed by several weeks; it is thought to be caused by a metabolite of ifosfamide (acrolein). Urotoxicity usually resolves a few days after withdrawal of ifosfamide, but may persist and may be fatal. Incidence is reduced by fractionation of dosage, adequate hydration, and administration of mesna.

Incidence less frequent
***Hepatotoxicity; infection, resulting from leukopenia*** (fever or chills; cough or hoarseness; lower back or side pain; painful or difficult urination); ***nephrotoxicity; phlebitis*** (redness, swelling, or pain at site of injection)

Note: *Hepatotoxicity* is usually asymptomatic and detected on laboratory tests.

*Nephrotoxicity* is usually asymptomatic with signs of tubular damage detected on laboratory tests. Metabolic acidosis as a manifestation of *nephrotoxicity* has been reported to occur frequently in patients receiving high doses of ifosfamide. Renal tubular acidosis, Fanconi syndrome, and renal rickets have been reported.

Incidence rare
> *Cardiotoxicity; polyneuropathy; pulmonary toxicity* (cough or shortness of breath); *stomatitis* (sores in mouth and on lips)

**Those indicating need for medical attention only if they continue or are bothersome**
Incidence more frequent
> *Nausea and vomiting*

Note: *Nausea and vomiting* are usually controlled by antiemetics.

**Those not indicating need for medical attention**
Incidence more frequent
> *Loss of hair*

**Those indicating the need for medical attention if they occur after medication is discontinued**
> *Hemorrhagic cystitis* (blood in urine)

## Patient Consultation

As an aid to patient consultation, refer to *Advice for the Patient, Ifosfamide (Systemic)*.

In providing consultation, consider emphasizing the following selected information (» = major clinical significance):

**Before using this medication**
» Conditions affecting use, especially:
 Sensitivity to ifosfamide
 Pregnancy—Use not recommended because of mutagenic, teratogenic, and carcinogenic potential; advisability of using contraception; telling physician immediately if pregnancy is suspected
 Breast-feeding—Not recommended because of risk of serious side effects
 Other medications, especially other bone marrow depressants, previous cytotoxic drug therapy or radiation therapy
 Other medical problems, especially chickenpox, herpes zoster, hepatic function impairment, infection, renal function impairment

**Proper use of this medication**
 Caution in taking combination therapy; taking each medication at the right time
 Importance of ample fluid intake and subsequent increase in urine output, as well as frequent voiding (including at least once during night), to prevent hemorrhagic cystitis and aid in excretion of uric acid; following physician instructions for recommended fluid intake; some patients may require up to 3000 mL (3 quarts) per day
 Probability of nausea and vomiting; importance of continuing medication despite stomach upset
» Proper dosing

**Precautions while using this medication**
» Importance of close monitoring by physician
» Avoiding immunizations unless approved by physician; other persons in patient's household should avoid immunizations with oral poliovirus vaccine; avoiding other persons who have taken oral poliovirus vaccine within the past several months or wearing a protective mask that covers nose and mouth

*Caution if bone marrow depression occurs*
» Avoiding exposure to persons with infections, especially during periods of low blood counts; checking with physician immediately if fever or chills, cough or hoarseness, lower back or side pain, or painful or difficult urination occurs
» Checking with physician immediately if unusual bleeding or bruising; black, tarry stools; blood in urine or stools; or pinpoint red spots on skin occur
 Caution in use of regular toothbrush, dental floss, or toothpick; physician, dentist, or nurse may suggest alternatives; checking with physician before having dental work done
 Not touching eyes or inside of nose unless hands washed immediately before
 Using caution to avoid accidental cuts with use of sharp objects such as safety razor or fingernail or toenail cutters
 Avoiding contact sports or other situations where bruising or injury might occur

**Side/adverse effects**
 May cause adverse effects such as blood problems; loss of hair; toxicity to lungs, heart, liver, or bladder; and cancer; importance of discussing possible effects with physician
 Signs of potential side effects, especially CNS effects, leukopenia, thrombocytopenia, urotoxicity, hepatotoxicity, infection, nephrotoxicity, phlebitis, cardiotoxicity, polyneuropathy, pulmonary toxicity, and stomatitis
 Physician or nurse can help in dealing with side effects
 Possibility of hair loss; normal hair growth should return after treatment has ended

## General Dosing Information

Patients receiving ifosfamide should be under supervision of a physician experienced in cancer chemotherapy.

A variety of dosage schedules and regimens of ifosfamide, alone or in combination with other antitumor agents, are used. The prescriber may consult the medical literature as well as the manufacturer's literature in choosing a specific dosage.

Dosage must be adjusted to meet the individual requirements of each patient, based on clinical response and appearance or severity of toxicity.

To reduce the risk of hemorrhagic cystitis, adequate hydration is recommended prior to ifosfamide treatment and for at least 72 hours following treatment to ensure ample urine output. Concurrent use of an agent to prevent hemorrhagic cystitis (such as mesna) is recommended. In addition, the patient should be encouraged to void frequently to prevent prolonged contact of irritating metabolites with bladder mucosa.

Development of mild bladder irritation (microscopic hematuria) may require adjustment of mesna dosage. Although concurrent use of mesna greatly reduces the risk, ifosfamide should be discontinued at the first sign of hemorrhagic cystitis. In severe cases, blood replacement may be necessary. Electrocautery diversion of urine flow, cryosurgery, and formaldehyde bladder instillations have been used. Resumption of therapy should be undertaken with caution since recurrence is common.

Each subsequent dose should be given only after microscopic hematuria, if present (defined as greater than 10 red blood cells per high power field), has resolved.

Ifosfamide therapy should be discontinued if severe CNS symptoms occur.

Special precautions are recommended in patients who develop thrombocytopenia as a result of administration of ifosfamide. These may include extreme care in performing invasive procedures; regular inspection of intravenous sites, skin (including perirectal area), and mucous membrane surfaces for signs of bleeding or bruising; limiting frequency of venipuncture and avoiding intramuscular injections; testing urine, emesis, stool, and secretions for occult blood; care in use of regular toothbrushes, dental floss, toothpicks, safety razors, and fingernail and toenail cutters; avoiding constipation; and using caution to prevent falls and other injuries. Such patients should avoid alcohol and any aspirin intake because of the risk of gastrointestinal bleeding. Platelet transfusions may be required.

Patients who develop leukopenia should be observed carefully for signs of infection. Antibiotic support may be required. In neutropenic patients who develop fever, broad-spectrum antibiotic coverage should be initiated empirically, pending bacterial cultures and appropriate diagnostic tests.

If marked leukopenia (particularly granulocytopenia) or thrombocytopenia occurs, ifosfamide therapy should be withdrawn until leukocyte and platelet counts return to satisfactory levels. Then therapy may be reinstituted, possibly at a lower dose.

**Safety considerations for handling this medication**

There is limited but increasing evidence and concern that personnel involved in preparation and administration of parenteral antineoplastics may be at some risk because of the potential mutagenicity, teratogenicity, and/or carcinogenicity of these agents, although the actual risk is unknown. USP advisory panels recommend cautious handling both in preparation and disposal of antineoplastic agents. Precautions that have been suggested include:
- Use of a biological containment cabinet during reconstitution and dilution of parenteral medications and wearing of disposable surgical gloves and masks.
- Use of proper technique to prevent contamination of the medication, work area, and operator during transfer between containers (including proper training of personnel in this technique).
- Cautious and proper disposal of needles, syringes, vials, ampuls, and unused medication.

A number of medical centers have developed detailed guidelines for handling of antineoplastic agents.

**Combination chemotherapy**

Ifosfamide may be used in combination with other agents in various regimens. As a result, incidence and/or severity of side effects may be altered and different dosages (usually reduced) may be used. For example, ifosfamide is part of the following chemotherapeutic combinations (some commonly used acronyms are in parentheses):
—etoposide, ifosfamide, and cisplatin (VIP).
—vinblastine, ifosfamide, and cisplatin (VeIP).

For specific dosages and schedules, consult the literature. For information regarding each agent, consult the individual monograph.

# Ifosfamide (Systemic)

## Parenteral Dosage Forms

Note: Bracketed uses in the *Dosage Forms* section refer to categories of use and/or indications that are not included in U.S. product labeling.

### STERILE IFOSFAMIDE USP

**Usual adult and adolescent dose**
Germ cell testicular tumors[1]—
    Intravenous infusion (over at least thirty minutes), 1.2 grams per square meter of body surface area per day for five consecutive days, the course being repeated every three weeks or after hematologic recovery.
    Note: Mesna is also administered during ifosfamide therapy to reduce hemorrhagic cystitis.
[Carcinoma, breast][1] or
[Carcinoma, cervical] or
[Carcinoma, head and neck][1] or
[Carcinoma, lung, non–small cell][1] or
[Carcinoma, lung, small cell][1] or
[Carcinoma, ovarian epithelial][1] or
[Ewing's sarcoma][1] or
[Leukemia, acute lymphocytic][1] or
[Lymphomas, Hodgkin's][1] or
[Lymphomas, non-Hodgkin's][1] or
[Neuroblastoma][1] or
[Osteosarcoma][1] or
[Sarcomas, soft-tissue]—
    Consult medical literature or manufacturer's literature for information on appropriate dosage.

**Usual pediatric dose**
Dosage has not been established.

**Size(s) usually available**
U.S.—
    1 gram (Rx) [*IFEX* (plus 1 gram vial of mesna)].
    3 grams (Rx) [*IFEX* (plus 1 gram vial of mesna)].

Canada—
    1 gram (Rx) [*IFEX*].
    2 grams (Rx) [*IFEX*].
    3 grams (Rx) [*IFEX*].

**Packaging and storage**
Store below 40 °C (104 °F), preferably between 15 and 30 °C (59 and 86 °F), unless otherwise specified by manufacturer.

**Preparation of dosage form**
May be prepared for parenteral use by adding 20, 40, or 60 mL of sterile water for injection or bacteriostatic water for injection (benzyl alcohol– or paraben-preserved) to the 1-gram, 2-gram, or 3-gram vial, respectively, and shaking to dissolve, to provide a solution containing 50 mg of ifosfamide per mL. The resulting solution may be added to 5% dextrose injection, 0.9% sodium chloride injection, lactated Ringer's injection, or sterile water for injection for administration by intravenous infusion. Use of intermediate concentrations or mixtures of excipients (e.g., 2.5% dextrose injection, 0.45% sodium chloride injection, 5% dextrose and 0.9% sodium chloride injection) is also acceptable.

Caution: Use of diluents containing benzyl alcohol is not recommended for preparation of medications for use in neonates. A fatal toxic syndrome consisting of metabolic acidosis, CNS depression, respiratory problems, renal failure, hypotension, and possibly seizures and intracranial hemorrhages has been associated with this use.

**Stability**
Reconstituted or diluted solutions of ifosfamide are stable for up to 24 hours in a refrigerator (2 to 8 °C [36 to 46 °F]).

**Note**
Because ifosfamide for injection contains no preservative, caution in preparing and storing solutions is required to ensure sterility.
Ifosfamide and mesna may be mixed in the same infusion.

---

[1]Not included in Canadian product labeling.

Revised: 06/30/98

---

# IMIGLUCERASE Systemic

VA CLASSIFICATION (Primary): HS451
Commonly used brand name(s): *Cerezyme*.
Note: For a listing of dosage forms and brand names by country availability, see *Dosage Forms* section(s).

## Category
Enzyme (glucocerebrosidase) replenisher.

## Indications

**Accepted**
Gaucher's disease, (treatment)—Imiglucerase is indicated as enzyme replacement therapy in Type I Gaucher's disease, in which glucocerebrosidase is deficient, resulting in an accumulation of glycolipids in the spleen, liver, and bone marrow. Clinical manifestations requiring treatment include moderate to severe anemia, thrombocytopenia with bleeding tendency, bone disease, and/or significant hepatomegaly or splenomegaly.

## Pharmacology/Pharmacokinetics

**Mechanism of action/Effect**
Imiglucerase catalyzes the hydrolysis of the glycolipid, glucocerebroside, to glucose and ceramide as part of the normal degradation pathway for membrane lipids.

**Distribution**
Vol$_D$—0.09 to 0.15 L per kg of body weight.

**Half-life**
Elimination—3.6 to 10.4 minutes.

**Time to peak effect**
During one-hour intravenous infusions of four doses (7.5, 15, 30, 60 Units per kg of body weight) steady-state enzymatic activity was achieved by 30 minutes.

## Precautions to Consider

**Cross-sensitivity and/or related problems**
Patients sensitive to alglucerase may be sensitive to imiglucerase also.

**Carcinogenicity/Mutagenicity**
Carcinogenicity and mutagenicity studies have not been performed in either animals or humans.

**Pregnancy/Reproduction**
Pregnancy—Studies have not been done in humans.
Studies have not been done in animals.
FDA Pregnancy Category C.

**Breast-feeding**
It is not known whether imiglucerase is distributed into breast milk.

**Pediatrics**
Appropriate studies on the relationship of age to the effects of imiglucerase have not been performed in the pediatric population. However, pediatrics-specific problems that would limit the usefulness of this medication in children are not expected.

**Geriatrics**
No information is available on the relationship of age to the effects of imiglucerase in geriatric patients.

**Medical considerations/Contraindications**
The medical considerations/contraindications included have been selected on the basis of their potential clinical significance (reasons given in parentheses where appropriate)—not necessarily inclusive (» = major clinical significance).

*Except under special circumstances, this medication should not be used when the following medical problem exists:*
» Sensitivity to alglucerase or imiglucerase

**Patient monitoring**
The following may be especially important in patient monitoring (other tests may be warranted in some patients, depending on condition; » = major clinical significance):

Acid phosphatase, serum or
Angiotensin-converting enzymes, serum
(determinations recommended every 2 to 3 months by some clinicians; values should decrease with imiglucerase treatment)
Alanine aminotransferase (ALT [SGPT]) and
Aspartate aminotransferase (AST [SGOT])
(some clinicians recommend monitoring every 6 to 12 months; values should decrease during imiglucerase therapy)
Bilirubin concentrations, serum and
Calcium, serum and
Creatinine, serum and
Electrolyte concentrations, serum and
Phosphorus, serum
(some clinicians recommend monitoring every 6 to 12 months)
Hemoglobin and
Platelet count
(recommended monthly to assess effectiveness of imiglucerase therapy; if hemoglobin falls below 7 grams/dL [70 grams/L] and platelet count is under 50,000, monitoring at 2-week intervals may be recommended; both values should increase with treatment)
Liver volume and
Spleen volume
(recommended every 6 months to assess effectiveness of therapy; liver and spleen should decrease in volume with imiglucerase treatment)
Magnetic resonance imaging (MRI) of long bones
(some clinicians recommend monitoring every 1 to 2 years; skeletal response should improve with imiglucerase therapy)

## Side/Adverse Effects

The following side/adverse effects have been selected on the basis of their potential clinical significance (possible signs and symptoms in parentheses where appropriate)—not necessarily inclusive:

**Those indicating need for medical attention only if they continue or are bothersome**
Incidence less frequent
*Abdominal discomfort; decrease in blood pressure; decrease in urinary frequency; dizziness; headache; nausea; pruritus* (itching); *rash*

Note: Decrease in blood pressure, nausea, pruritus, and rash may be due to antibody formation, which occurs in approximately 10 to 16% of patients receiving imiglucerase. Antibody levels decrease in most patients with continuous therapy.

## Patient Consultation

As an aid to patient consultation, refer to *Advice for the Patient, Imiglucerase (Systemic)*.
In providing consultation, consider emphasizing the following selected information (» = major clinical significance):

**Before using this medication**
» Conditions affecting use, especially:
Sensitivity to alglucerase or imiglucerase

**Proper use of this medication**
Helps control and reverse problems caused by Gaucher's disease; possible need for lifelong therapy; serious consequences of untreated Gaucher's disease
» Proper dosing

**Precautions while using this medication**
Importance of monitoring by the physician

## Parenteral Dosage Forms

### IMIGLUCERASE INJECTION

**Usual adult and adolescent dose**
Enzyme replenisher—
Intravenous infusion, 15 to 60 Units per kg of body weight administered over one to two hours. The usual frequency of infusion is once every two weeks, but disease severity and patient convenience may dictate administration several times a week to once every two weeks. Dosage can be lowered depending on patient response. Dosage may be lowered at 6-month intervals, while monitoring response parameters.

**Usual pediatric dose**
See *Usual adult and adolescent dose*.

**Strength(s) usually available**
U.S.—
200 Units per vial (Rx) [*Cerezyme*].
Canada—
200 Units per vial (Rx) [*Cerezyme*].

**Packaging and storage**
Store at 2 to 8 °C (36 to 46 °F).

**Preparation of dosage form**
On the day of use, the vial is reconstituted with 5.1 mL of Sterile Water for Injection USP to give a volume of 5.3 mL. Then, 5 mL is withdrawn from the vial and diluted with 0.9% Sodium Chloride Injection USP to a final volume of 100 to 200 mL.

**Stability**
Imiglucerase does not contain a preservative. The product information for imiglucerase states that when diluted to 50 mL and stored at 2 to 8 °C (36 to 46 °F), the reconstituted product is stable for up to 24 hours.

Developed: 06/16/95
Interim revision: 08/13/98

---

# IMIPENEM AND CILASTATIN  Systemic

VA CLASSIFICATION (Primary): AM119
Commonly used brand name(s): *Primaxin; Primaxin IM; Primaxin IV*.
Note: For a listing of dosage forms and brand names by country availability, see *Dosage Forms* section(s).

## Category

Antibacterial (systemic).

## Indications

### General considerations

Imipenem is the first of a class of beta-lactam antibiotics called carbapenems. It has a very wide spectrum of activity *in vitro*, including most gram-positive and gram-negative aerobic and anaerobic bacteria. It is also stable in the presence of bacterial beta-lactamases. Imipenem is administered with an equal amount of cilastatin, a renal dehydropeptidase inhibitor that blocks the renal metabolism of imipenem and increases its urinary recovery. Cilastatin has no antibacterial activity or effect on beta-lactamases, and does not potentiate or antagonize the effects of imipenem.

Imipenem has excellent *in vitro* activity against aerobic gram-positive organisms, including most strains of staphylococci, streptococci, and some enterococci. Exceptions to this include *Enterococcus faecium*, which is usually resistant, and an increasing number of strains of methicillin-resistant *Staphylococcus aureus* and coagulase-negative staphylococci.

Imipenem also has excellent *in vitro* activity against most species of Enterbacteriaceae, including *Escherichia coli*, *Klebsiella* species, *Citrobacter* sp., *Morganella morganii*, and *Enterobacter* sp. It is slightly less potent *in vitro* against *Serratia marcescens*, *Proteus mirabilis*, indole-positive *Proteus* sp., and *Providencia stuartii*. Most strains of *Pseudomonas aeruginosa* are susceptible; however, increasing resistance has been seen in patients receiving imipenem who have advanced, refractory infections. Many strains of *Ps. cepacia* and virtually all strains of *Xanthamonas maltophilia* are resistant.

Most anaerobic species are inhibited by imipenem, including *Bacteroides* sp., *Fusobacterium* sp., and *Clostridium* sp. However, *C. difficile* is only moderately susceptible. Other susceptible organisms *in vitro* include *Campylobacter* sp., *Haemophilus influenzae*, *Neisseria gonorrhoeae*, including penicillinase-producing strains, *Yersinia enterocolitica*, *Nocardia asteroides*, and *Legionella* sp. *Chlamydia trachomatis* is resistant to imipenem.

### Accepted

Bone and joint infections (treatment)—Intravenous imipenem and cilastatin combination is indicated in the treatment of bone and joint infections caused by susceptible organisms.

Endocarditis, bacterial (treatment)—Intravenous imipenem and cilastatin combination is indicated in the treatment of bacterial endocarditis caused by susceptible organisms.

**Intra-abdominal infections (treatment)**—Intravenous and intramuscular imipenem and cilastatin combination is indicated in the treatment of intra-abdominal infections caused by susceptible organisms.

**Pelvic infections, female (treatment)**—Intravenous and intramuscular imipenem and cilastatin combination is indicated in the treatment of female pelvic infections caused by susceptible organisms.

**Pneumonia, bacterial (treatment)**—Intravenous and intramuscular imipenem and cilastatin combination is indicated in the treatment of bacterial pneumonia caused by susceptible organisms.

**Septicemia, bacterial (treatment)**—Intravenous imipenem and cilastatin combination is indicated in the treatment of bacterial septicemia caused by susceptible organisms.

**Skin and soft tissue infections (treatment)**—Intravenous and intramuscular imipenem and cilastatin combination is indicated in the treatment of skin and soft tissue infections caused by susceptible organisms.

**Urinary tract infections, bacterial (treatment)**—Intravenous imipenem and cilastatin combination is indicated in the treatment of bacterial urinary tract infections caused by susceptible organisms.

## Pharmacology/Pharmacokinetics

**Physicochemical characteristics**
Molecular weight—
  Imipenem: 317.36.
  Cilastatin sodium: 380.43.
pKa at 25 °C (77 °F)
  Imipenem—
    $pKa_1$—3.2
    $pKa_2$—9.9
  Cilastatin sodium (with aqueous sodium hydroxide)—
    $pKa_1$—2.0
    $pKa_2$—4.4
    $pKa_3$—9.2

**Mechanism of action/Effect**
Imipenem—Bactericidal; binds to penicillin-binding proteins (PBP) 1A, 1B, 2, 4, 5, and 6 of *E. coli* and to PBP 1A, 1B, 2, 4, and 5 of *Ps. aeruginosa*; this results in inhibition of bacterial cell wall synthesis; imipenem apparently has greatest affinity for PBP 1A, 1B, and 2, and the least affinity for PBP 3; imipenem's ability to bind to bacterial PBP 2 causes development of small spheres or ellipsoids without formation of filaments commonly seen with penicillins and cephalosporins, ultimately resulting in lysis and death; its lethal effect may also be related to binding to PBP 1A and 1B as well; imipenem is highly resistant to degradation by bacterial beta-lactamases and may demonstrate a "post-antibiotic" effect in some bacteria.

Cilastatin—A competitive, reversible, highly specific inhibitor of the renal dipeptidase, dehydropeptidase I (DHP I); cilastatin blocks tubular secretion of imipenem by competitive exclusion at its transport site, thereby preventing the renal metabolism of imipenem and resulting in significantly improved urinary recovery of imipenem; cilastatin may also prevent proximal renal tubular necrosis that occurs when imipenem is used alone; cilastatin does not inhibit bacterial beta-lactamases and has no intrinsic antibacterial activity.

**Absorption**
Bioavailability
  Intramuscular:
    Imipenem—95%.
    Cilastatin—75%.

**Distribution**
Imipenem rapidly and widely distributed to most tissues and fluids; distributed to sputum, pleural fluid, peritoneal fluid, interstitial fluid, bile, aqueous humor, reproductive organs, and bone; highest concentrations found in pleural fluid, interstitial fluid, peritoneal fluid, and reproductive organs; low concentrations have been detected in the cerebrospinal fluid (CSF).
  $Vol_D$—
    Neonates: 0.4 to 0.5 L/kg.
    Children (2 to 12 years old): Approximately 0.7 L/kg.
    Adults: 0.23 to 0.31 L/kg.

**Protein binding**
Imipenem—Low (20%).
Cilastatin—Moderate (40%).

**Biotransformation**
Imipenem—Renal; when given alone, imipenem is metabolized in the kidneys by hydrolysis of the beta-lactam ring caused by the renal dipeptidase, dehydropeptidase I (DHP I), resulting in low urinary concentrations; DHP I is an enzyme located on the brush border of the proximal renal tubular epithelium; DHP I acts only after imipenem has been cleared from the plasma by glomerular filtration or tubular secretion ("post-excretory" metabolism); metabolism occurs only in the tubular cell or glomerular filtrate; virtually all of the secreted fraction and approximately 75% of the filtered fraction are metabolized (a total of 60 to 95%).

Cilastatin—Metabolized to *N*-acetyl conjugate.

**Half-life**
Adults—
  Intravenous:
    Normal renal function—
      Imipenem: Approximately 1 hour.
      Cilastatin: Approximately 1 hour.
    Impaired renal function—
      Imipenem: 2.9 to 4.0 hours.
      Cilastatin: 13.3 to 17.1 hours.
  Intramuscular:
    Normal renal function—
      Imipenem: 2 to 3 hours.
Neonates—
  Intravenous:
    Imipenem—1.7 to 2.4 hours.
    Cilastatin—3.8 to 8.4 hours.
Children (2 to 12 years of age)—
  Intravenous: 1 to 1.2 hours.

**Time to peak concentration**
Intramuscular:
  Imipenem: Within 2 hours.
  Cilastatin: Within 1 hour.

**Peak serum concentration**
Imipenem—
  Intravenous: Approximately 14 to 24, 21 to 58, and 41 to 83 mcg per mL following a dose of 250 mg, 500 mg, and 1 gram, respectively, over 20 minutes.
  Intramuscular: Approximately 10 and 12 mcg per mL following a dose of 500 mg and 750 mg, respectively.
Cilastatin—
  Intravenous: Approximately 15 to 25, 31 to 49, and 56 to 80 mcg per mL following a dose of 250 mg, 500 mg, and 1 gram, respectively, over 20 minutes.
  Intramuscular: Approximately 24 and 33 mcg per mL following a dose of 500 mg and 750 mg, respectively.

**Urine concentration**
Imipenem—
  >10 mcg per mL up to 8 hours following a 500 mg intravenous dose.
  >10 mcg per mL for 12 hours following a 500 mg and 750 mg intramuscular dose.

**Elimination**
Imipenem alone—
  Renal; approximately 5 to 40% excreted in urine by both glomerular filtration and tubular secretion.
Cilastatin alone—
  Renal; approximately 70 to 78% excreted in urine within 10 hours, by both glomerular filtration and tubular secretion.
  Dialysis: Substantial amounts (approximately 40 to 82%) rapidly cleared from the blood by hemodialysis.
Imipenem with cilastatin—
  Renal; approximately 70 to 76% excreted in urine within 10 hours, by both glomerular filtration and active tubular secretion (approximately two-thirds of that amount by glomerular filtration and one-third by tubular secretion); no further urinary excretion detectable.
  Nonrenal; approximately 20 to 25% excreted by unknown nonrenal mechanism, possibly including up to 1 to 2% excreted via the bile in the feces.
  Dialysis: Substantial amounts (approximately 73 to 90%) rapidly cleared from the blood by hemodialysis. A 3-hour session of intermittent hemofiltration has removed approximately 75% of a given dose.

## Precautions to Consider

**Cross-sensitivity and/or related problems**
Patients allergic to other beta-lactam antibacterials (e.g., penicillins, cephalosporins) may be allergic to imipenem also.
Although imipenem has been administered without incident to some patients with rash-type penicillin allergy, caution is recommended when imipenem is administered to patients with a history of penicillin anaphylaxis because of cross-reactivity.

**Carcinogenicity/Mutagenicity**
Gene toxicity studies such as the V79 mammalian cell mutation assay, Ames test, unscheduled DNA synthesis assay, and *in vivo* mouse cy-

togenicity test have shown no evidence of genetic damage with imipenem and cilastatin combination.

**Pregnancy/Reproduction**
Pregnancy—Studies in humans have not been done.
Studies in mice, rats, and rabbits given doses ranging from the usual human dose up to 33 times the usual human dose have not shown that imipenem, cilastatin, or the combination causes adverse effects on the fetus. Studies in pregnant cynomolgus monkeys given intravenous bolus doses of 40 mg per kg of body weight (mg/kg) per day or 160 mg/kg per day subcutaneously resulted in maternal toxicity, including emesis, inappetence, weight loss, diarrhea, abortion, and death. No significant toxicity was observed when non-pregnant cynomolgus monkeys were given subcutaneous doses of up to 180 mg/kg per day. When doses of 100 mg/kg per day were administered to pregnant cynomolgus monkeys at an intravenous infusion rate which mimics human clinical use, there was minimal maternal intolerance (occasional emesis), no maternal deaths, no teratogenicity, but an increase in embryonic loss relative to the control groups.
FDA Pregnancy Category C.

**Breast-feeding**
It is not known whether imipenem or cilastatin is distributed into breast milk. However, problems in humans have not been documented.

**Pediatrics**
The half-life of imipenem in neonates is longer (1.7 to 2.4 hours) than that in adults with normal renal function (approximately 1 hour). The half-life in older pediatric patients (2 to 12 years of age) is 1 to 1.2 hours. The half-life of cilastatin in neonates is longer (3.8 to 8.4 hours) than that in adults with normal renal function (approximately 1 hour).
Appropriate studies have not been performed in children up to 12 years of age.

**Geriatrics**
No information is available on the relationship of age to the effects of imipenem and cilastatin combination in geriatric patients. However, elderly patients are more likely to have an age-related decrease in renal function, which may require a reduction of dosage in patients receiving imipenem and cilastatin.

**Dental**
Imipenem and cilastatin may cause glossitis (inflammation of the tongue), tongue papillar hypertrophy, and increased salivation.

**Drug interactions and/or related problems**
The following drug interactions and/or related problems have been selected on the basis of their potential clinical significance (possible mechanism in parentheses where appropriate)—not necessarily inclusive (» = major clinical significance):
Note: Combinations containing any of the following medications, depending on the amount present, may also interact with this medication.
Probenecid
(since concurrent use of probenecid results in only minimal increases in the serum concentrations and half-life of imipenem, concurrent use is not recommended where higher imipenem serum concentrations may be desirable)

**Laboratory value alterations**
The following have been selected on the basis of their potential clinical significance (possible effect in parentheses where appropriate)—not necessarily inclusive (» = major clinical significance):
With diagnostic test results
Positive direct antiglobulin (Coombs') tests
(may occur during therapy)

With physiology/laboratory test values
» Alanine aminotransferase (ALT [SGPT]), serum and
» Alkaline phosphatase, serum and
» Aspartate aminotransferase (AST [SGOT]), serum and
Lactate dehydrogenase (LDH), serum
(values may be transiently increased)
Bilirubin, serum and
Blood urea nitrogen (BUN) concentrations and
Creatinine, serum
(concentrations may be transiently increased)
Hematocrit (HCT) and
Hemoglobin (Hb) concentrations
(may be decreased)

**Medical considerations/Contraindications**
The medical considerations/contraindications included have been selected on the basis of their potential clinical significance (reasons given in parentheses where appropriate)—not necessarily inclusive (» = major clinical significance).

*Risk-benefit should be considered when the following medical problems exist:*
» Allergy to imipenem, cilastatin, or other beta-lactams (penicillin, cephalosporins)
» Central nervous system (CNS) disorders (e.g., brain lesions or history of seizures)
(seizures are more likely to occur in patients receiving higher doses of imipenem, or in patients with CNS lesions, a history of seizure disorders, or renal function impairment)
» Renal function impairment
(because imipenem and cilastatin are primarily excreted through the kidneys, this medicine must be administered in a reduced dosage to patients with impaired renal function)

## Side/Adverse Effects

Note: The following side/adverse effects of imipenem and cilastatin combination are similar in nature and incidence to those of other beta-lactam antibacterials. However, the incidence of seizures is higher than that seen with other beta-lactam antibiotics; it is reported to be 1.5 to 2%. The risk of seizures increases in patients receiving more than 2 grams of imipenem per day, those with a pre-existing seizure disorder, and patients with decreased renal function.

The following side/adverse effects have been selected on the basis of their potential clinical significance (possible signs and symptoms in parentheses where appropriate)—not necessarily inclusive:

**Those indicating need for medical attention**
Incidence more frequent
*Allergic reactions* (fever; hives; itching; skin rash; wheezing); *CNS toxicity* (confusion; dizziness; seizures; tremors); *thrombophlebitis* (pain at site of injection)
Incidence less frequent
*Infusion rate reaction* (dizziness; nausea and vomiting; sweating; unusual tiredness or weakness)—occurs with too rapid an infusion rate
Incidence rare
*Pseudomembranous colitis* (abdominal or stomach cramps and pain, severe; diarrhea, watery and severe, which may also be bloody; fever)

**Those indicating need for medical attention only if they continue or are bothersome**
Incidence more frequent
*Gastrointestinal disturbances* (diarrhea; nausea and vomiting)

**Those indicating the need for medical attention if they occur after medication is discontinued**
*Pseudomembranous colitis* (severe abdominal or stomach cramps and pain; watery and severe diarrhea, which may also be bloody; fever)

## Patient Consultation

As an aid to patient consultation, refer to *Advice for the Patient, Imipenem and Cilastatin (Systemic)*.
In providing consultation, consider emphasizing the following selected information (» = major clinical significance):

**Before using this medication**
» Conditions affecting use, especially:
Allergy to imipenem or cilastatin; patients allergic to other beta-lactams may also be allergic to imipenem
Dental—Imipenem and cilastatin may cause glossitis, tongue papillar hypertrophy, and increased salivation
Other medical problems, especially CNS disorders or renal function impairment

**Proper use of this medication**
» Importance of receiving medication for full course of therapy and on regular schedule
» Proper dosing

**Precautions while using this medication**
» Continuing anticonvulsant therapy in patients with a history of seizures
» For severe diarrhea, checking with physician before taking any antidiarrheals; for mild diarrhea, taking kaolin- or attapulgite-containing, but not other, antidiarrheals; checking with physician or pharmacist if mild diarrhea continues or worsens

**Side/adverse effects**
Signs of potential side effects, especially allergic reactions, CNS toxicity, infusion rate reaction, pseudomembranous colitis, and thrombophlebitis

## General Dosing Information

Intravenous doses of 250 or 500 mg of imipenem should be given over a 20- to 30-minute period in adults. Doses of 1 gram should be given over a 40- to 60-minute period. In pediatric patients, imipenem may be administered over a 20- to 30-minute period.

Intramuscular imipenem and cilastatin combination should be administered by deep IM injection into a large muscle mass, such as the gluteal muscles or lateral part of the thigh.

In patients receiving more than 2 grams of imipenem per day, there is an increased risk of seizures.

If a dose of this medication is missed, give it as soon as possible. However, if it is almost time for the next dose, skip the missed dose and go back to the regular dosing schedule. Do not double doses.

### For treatment of adverse effects

Anticonvulsants should be continued in the treatment of patients receiving imipenem and cilastatin combination who have known seizure disorders. In patients who develop symptoms of CNS toxicity (e.g., focal tremors, myoclonus, or seizures) during treatment with imipenem, anticonvulsant therapy (e.g., phenytoin or benzodiazepines) should be initiated, and the dosage of imipenem should be reduced or the drug should be discontinued.

If an allergic reaction to imipenem and cilastatin combination occurs, the drug should be discontinued. Severe hypersensitivity reactions may require the administration of epinephrine or other emergency measures.

Some patients may develop nausea, vomiting, hypotension, dizziness, or sweating during administration of imipenem and cilastatin combination, especially after rapid infusion. If these symptoms develop, the rate of infusion should be slowed. If this is not effective, it may be necessary to discontinue the drug.

*For antibiotic-associated pseudomembranous colitis (AAPMC)—*
   Some patients may develop AAPMC, caused by *Clostridium difficile* toxin, during or following administration of imipenem. Mild cases may respond to discontinuation of the drug alone. Moderate to severe cases may require fluid, electrolyte, and protein replacement.
   In cases not responding to the above measures or in more severe cases, oral metronidazole, oral bacitracin, or oral vancomycin may be used. Oral vancomycin is effective in doses of 125 to 500 mg every 6 hours for 5 to 10 days. The dose of metronidazole is 250 to 500 mg every 8 hours for 5 to 10 days. Recurrences may be treated with a second course of these medications.
   Cholestyramine and colestipol resins have been shown to bind *C. difficile* toxin *in vitro*. If cholestyramine or colestipol resin is administered in conjunction with oral vancomycin, the medications should be administered several hours apart since the resins have been shown to bind oral vancomycin also.
   In addition, AAPMC may result in severe watery diarrhea which may occur during therapy or up to several weeks after therapy is discontinued. If diarrhea occurs, administration of antiperistaltic antidiarrheals is not recommended since they may delay the removal of toxins from the colon, thereby prolonging and/or worsening the diarrhea.

## Parenteral Dosage Forms

### IMIPENEM AND CILASTATIN FOR INJECTION USP

#### Usual adult and adolescent dose
Antibacterial—
   Intravenous infusion, based on anhydrous imipenem content:
   Mild infections—250 to 500 mg every six hours.
   Moderate infections—500 mg every six to eight hours to 1 gram every eight hours.
   Severe, life-threatening infections—500 mg every six hours to 1 gram every six to eight hours.
   Note: Lower doses are used in the treatment of infections caused by gram-positive organisms, anaerobes, and highly susceptible gram-negative organisms. Infections caused by other gram-negative organisms require higher doses.
      Uncomplicated urinary tract infections: 250 mg every six hours.
      Complicated urinary tract infections: 500 mg every six hours.
      Adults with impaired renal function may require a reduction in dose as given below. Doses are based on an average body weight of 70 kg. Patients weighing less than 70 kg should receive a proportional reduction in dosage.

| Creatinine Clearance (mL/min/1.73 M²)/ (mL/sec) | Dose |
|---|---|
| >70/1.17 | See *Usual adult and adolescent dose* |
| 30–70/0.50–1.17 | 500 mg every 6 to 8 hours |
| 20–30/0.33–0.50 | 500 mg every 8 to 12 hours |
| 0–20/0–0.33 | 250 to 500 mg every 12 hours |
| Hemodialysis patients | Supplemental dose after hemodialysis, unless next dose scheduled within 4 hours |

#### Usual adult prescribing limits
Up to a maximum of 50 mg (imipenem) per kg of body weight or 4 grams daily, whichever is lower.

#### Usual pediatric dose
Antibacterial—
   Infants and children up to 12 years of age: Dosage has not been established.
   Children 12 years of age and older: See *Usual adult and adolescent dose*.

#### Size(s) usually available
U.S.—
   250 mg (anhydrous imipenem) and 250 mg (cilastatin) (Rx) [*Primaxin IV*].
   500 mg (anhydrous imipenem) and 500 mg (cilastatin) (Rx) [*Primaxin IV*].
Canada—
   250 mg (anhydrous imipenem) and 250 mg (cilastatin) (Rx) [*Primaxin*].
   500 mg (anhydrous imipenem) and 500 mg (cilastatin) (Rx) [*Primaxin*].

#### Packaging and storage
Prior to reconstitution, store below 30 °C (86 °F), unless otherwise specified by manufacturer.

#### Preparation of dosage form
To prepare initial dilution for intravenous infusion, add approximately 10 mL of diluent (see manufacturer's package insert) to each 250- or 500-mg vial (13-mL) and shake well. The resulting suspension should be transferred to not less than 100 mL of suitable intravenous fluids. Do not administer the initially prepared suspension intravenously. Add an additional 10 mL of diluent to each previously reconstituted vial and shake well. Transfer the remaining contents of the vial to the infusion container. Shake the resulting mixture well until clear. Do not administer a cloudy solution.

For reconstitution of piggyback infusion bottles (120-mL), add 100 mL of diluent (see manufacturer's package insert) to each 250- or 500-mg infusion bottle. Shake the resulting mixture well until clear. Do not administer a cloudy solution.

#### Stability
After reconstitution with sterile water for injection, solutions retain their potency for 8 hours at room temperature or for 48 hours if refrigerated at 4 °C (39 °F).

After reconstitution with 0.9% sodium chloride injection, solutions retain their potency for 10 hours at room temperature or for 48 hours if refrigerated at 4 °C (39 °F).

After reconstitution with other diluents, solutions retain their potency for 4 hours at room temperature or for 24 hours if refrigerated at 4 °C (39 °F).

Solutions of imipenem and cilastatin combination should not be frozen.

Solutions may vary from colorless to yellow in color; color changes within this range do not affect potency. Imipenem and cilastatin combination may become slightly discolored under strong ultraviolet (UV) light.

#### Incompatibilities
Extemporaneous admixtures of beta-lactam antibacterials and aminoglycosides may result in substantial mutual inactivation. If they are administered concurrently, they should be administered in separate sites. Do not mix them in the same intravenous bag or bottle.

### IMIPENEM AND CILASTATIN FOR INJECTABLE SUSPENSION USP

#### Usual adult and adolescent dose
Antibacterial—
   Intramuscular, mild to moderate infections:
   Female pelvic infections and
   Pneumonia and
   Skin and soft tissue infections—500 to 750 mg every twelve hours.
   Intra-abdominal infections—750 mg every twelve hours.

USP DI    Imipenem and Cilastatin (Systemic)  1685

Note: Safety and efficacy have not been studied in patients with a creatinine clearance of less than 20 mL/min.

**Usual adult prescribing limits**
Up to 1500 mg daily.

**Usual pediatric dose**
Antibacterial—
  Infants and children up to 12 years of age: Dosage has not been established.
  Children 12 years of age and older: See *Usual adult and adolescent dose.*

**Size(s) usually available**
U.S.—
  500 mg (anhydrous imipenem) and 500 mg (cilastatin) (Rx) [*Primaxin IM*].
  750 mg (anhydrous imipenem) and 750 mg (cilastatin) (Rx) [*Primaxin IM*].
Canada—
  Not commercially available.

**Packaging and storage**
Prior to reconstitution, store below 30 °C (86 °F), unless otherwise specified by manufacturer.

**Preparation of dosage form**
To prepare initial dilution for intramuscular use, add 2 mL of 1% lidocaine injection (without epinephrine) to each 500-mg vial, or 3 mL of 1% lidocaine injection (without epinephrine) to each 750-mg vial.

**Stability**
After reconstitution with 1% lidocaine injection, the suspension should be used within one hour.
Suspensions are white to light tan in color; variations of color within this range do not affect the potency.

**Incompatibilities**
Intramuscular imipenem and cilastatin combination should not be mixed with or physically added to other antibiotics. However, it may be administered concomitantly, but at separate sites, with other antibiotics.

Revised: 09/08/92
Interim revision: 04/01/94; 01/11/95; 06/20/95

**IMIPRAMINE**—See *Antidepressants, Tricyclic (Systemic)*

# IMIQUIMOD   Topical—INTRODUCTORY VERSION

VA CLASSIFICATION (Primary): IM700
Commonly used brand name(s): *Aldara.*
Note: For a listing of dosage forms and brand names by country availability, see *Dosage Forms* section(s).

## Category
Biological response modifier.

## Indications

**Accepted**
Condyloma acuminatum (treatment)—Imiquimod is indicated for the treatment of external genital and perianal warts (condyloma acuminatum). Imiquimod is not a cure and new warts may develop during treatment; effect of imiquimod on transmission of genital warts is not known.

**Unaccepted**
Imiquimod has not been evaluated for the treatment of urethral, intravaginal, cervical, rectal, or anal human papilloma viral disease and is not recommended for these uses.

## Pharmacology/Pharmacokinetics

**Physicochemical characteristics**
Molecular weight—240.31.

**Mechanism of action/Effect**
The mechanism of action is not known. Imiquimod does not have direct antiviral activity. Studies of mice show that imiquimod may induce cytokines, including interferon-alpha, in mouse skin; clinical significance or relevance of this finding to humans is not known. Imiquimod potentially can exacerbate inflammatory conditions of the skin.
In one clinical trial that had a 4 to 6 ratio of females to males, 50% of patients, approximately 75% of females and 33% of males, experienced complete wart clearance after using imiquimod for 10 weeks (median, range 4 to 16 weeks). Of the remaining 50% of patients, 33% still had genital warts at 16 weeks and 17% withdrew from the clinical trial. Of those who had complete wart clearance at 10 weeks and could be followed for 12 additional weeks, 23% of patients remained wart-free.

**Absorption**
Percutaneous absorption is minimal for a median wart area of 69 square millimeters (mm$^2$) (range, 8 to 5525 mm$^2$).

## Precautions to Consider

**Carcinogenicity**
Rodent carcinogenicity data are not available.

**Mutagenicity**
Imiquimod was not found to be mutagenic in a series of tests, including the Ames, mouse lymphoma, Chinese hamster ovary (CHO) chromosome aberration, human lymphocyte chromosome aberration, SHE cell transformation, rat and hamster bone marrow cytogenetics, and mouse dominant lethal test.

**Pregnancy/Reproduction**
Fertility—Daily oral administration of imiquimod to rats at eight times the human recommended (topical) daily dose, based on mg per square meter of body surface area, produced no impairment of fertility.
Pregnancy—Adequate and well-controlled studies in humans have not been done. Problems in humans have not been documented.
Researchers studied imiquimod's effect on reproduction in rats and rabbits. Maternotoxicity, but not teratogenicity, as shown by reduced pup weights and delayed ossification, occurred in studies of female rats given doses 28 times the recommended human dose (based on mg per square meter of body surface area). In developmental studies, no adverse effects appeared in the offspring of pregnant rats who received eight times the recommended human dose.
FDA Pregnancy Category B.

**Breast-feeding**
It is not known whether topical imiquimod is distributed into breast milk. Problems in humans have not been documented.

**Pediatrics**
No information is available on the relationship of age to the effects of imiquimod in pediatric patients. Safety and efficacy have not been established in patients up to 18 years of age.

**Geriatrics**
No information is available on the relationship of age to the effects of topical imiquimod in geriatric patients.

**Medical considerations/Contraindications**
The medical considerations/contraindications included have been selected on the basis of their potential clinical significance (reasons given in parentheses where appropriate)—not necessarily inclusive (» = major clinical significance).

*Except under special circumstances, this medication should not be used when the following medical problems exist:*
»  Dermatitis, genital or
»  Surgery, genital, recent
    (may exacerbate inflammatory conditions of skin; imiquimod is not recommended for application to areas that have recently involved surgery until genital skin has healed)

*Risk-benefit should be considered when the following medical problem exists:*
Sensitivity to imiquimod

## Side/Adverse Effects
The following side/adverse effects have been selected on the basis of their potential clinical significance (possible signs and symptoms in parentheses where appropriate)—not necessarily inclusive:

**Those indicating need for medical attention**
Incidence more frequent
  *Erosion or excoriation of skin* (self-induced skin lesion, such as a scratch)—30%, at site of application; *fungal infection, including tinea cruris* (itching in genital or other skin areas; scaling)—11% in females, 2% in males; *scabbing*—4 to 13%, at site of application; *ulceration or*

## Imiquimod (Topical)—Introductory Version (continued)

*vesicles on skin* (blisters; open sores on skin)—3 to 5%, at site of application

Incidence less frequent
*Erythema, severe* (redness of skin)—4%, at site of application

Signs and symptoms of systemic effects
*Influenza-like symptoms* (diarrhea; fatigue; fever; headache; muscle pain)

**Those indicating need for medical attention only if they continue or are bothersome**

Incidence more frequent
*Burning or stinging of skin, mild*—26%, at remote site and at site of application; *edema of skin* (swelling of skin)—12 to 17%, at site of application; *erythema, mild* (redness of skin)—54 to 61%, at site of application; *flaking of skin, mild*—18 to 25%, at site of application; *pain, soreness, or tenderness of skin, mild*—8%, at remote site and at site of application; *pruritus, mild* (itching of skin)—32%, at remote site and at site of application; *rash*—at site of application

Incidence less frequent
*Hypopigmentation* (lightening of normal skin color)—at site of application

### Patient Consultation

As an aid to patient consultation, refer to *Advice for the Patient, Imiquimod (Topical)—Introductory version*.

In providing consultation, consider emphasizing the following selected information (» = major clinical significance):

**Before using this medication**
» Conditions affecting use, especially:
    Sensitivity to imiquimod
    Other medical problems, especially genital dermatitis or recent genital surgery

**Proper use of this medication**
» Not using occlusive dressing, such as bandages; if covering is needed, only using nonocclusive material, such as cotton gauze or cotton underclothes

*Proper administration*
» Importance of washing hands before and after administration to help avoid translocation of cream. Avoiding contact with eyes
» Understanding amount to use and avoiding excessive administration
    Allowing medication to remain on skin for 6 to 10 hours; removing medication by thoroughly washing area with soap and water
    Discarding any unused cream from the single-dose packet
» Proper dosing
    Missed dose: Applying as soon as possible, then returning to normal dosing schedule
» Proper storage

**Precautions while using this medication**
» Reporting severe local skin reactions and rare systemic reactions to physician
» Delaying next dose for several days when experiencing any discomfort or if severe reaction occurs
» Avoiding genital, oral, or anal sexual contact while the cream is on the skin; washing cream off before engaging in sexual activities. Also, oils in the cream may weaken latex contraceptive devices, such as cervical caps, condoms, and diaphragms
» Avoiding use of other topical medications on the same treatment area, unless recommended by physician
» Not sharing medication with others

**Side/adverse effects**
Erosion or excoriation of skin (at site of application); fungal infection, including tinea cruris; scabbing (at site of application); ulceration or vesicles (at site of application); erythema, severe (at site of application)

Signs or symptoms of systemic effects—Influenza-like symptoms, including myalgia

### General Dosing Information

Occlusive dressings, such as bandages, should be avoided. If covering is needed, patient should use nonocclusive material, such as cotton gauze or cotton underclothes.

It is important for patients to avoid transferring cream to uninvolved skin sites or to their partners during sexual contact and not to share medication with others. Patient should wash hands before and after administration to help avoid translocation of cream, especially to eyes, and should wash the treatment area thoroughly with mild soap and water before engaging in sexual activities. Also, oils in the cream can weaken latex contraceptive devices, such as cervical caps, condoms, and diaphragms, and reduce their efficacy.

Patient should understand correct amount of imiquimod to use and avoid excessive administration, discarding the unused portion in the single-dose packets. When experiencing any discomfort or if severe reaction occurs, patient should delay next dose for several days, and report severe local skin reactions and rare systemic reactions to physician.

**For treatment of adverse effects**
Recommended treatment consists of the following:
• Discontinuing medication or decreasing frequency of dosing as needed.
• Using nonocclusive dressing, such as gauze, or cotton underclothes to help manage skin reactions.

### Topical Dosage Forms

#### IMIQUIMOD CREAM

**Usual adult dose**
Condyloma acuminatum—
    Topical, to the wart, once every other day (three times a week) during waking hours as a thin film, rubbing in well, leaving on skin for six to ten hours, then removing medication by washing with mild soap and water. Treatment is continued until wart is gone or for up to sixteen weeks.

Note: Each single-use packet containing 250 mg of cream is sufficient to cover a wart area of up to 20 square centimeters; excessive application should be avoided.

**Usual pediatric dose**
Up to 18 years of age—Safety and efficacy have not been established.

**Usual geriatric dose**
See *Usual adult dose*.

**Strength(s) usually available**
U.S.—
    5% (Rx) [*Aldara* (benzyl alcohol; cetyl alcohol; glycerin; isostearic acid; methylparaben; propylparaben; purified water; stearyl alcohol; xanthan gum)].

**Packaging and storage**
Store below 30 °C (86 °F), preferably between 15 and 30 °C (59 and 86 °F). Protect from freezing.

**Auxiliary labeling**
• For external use only.

Developed: 11/13/97
Interim revision: 06/30/98

---

# IMMUNE GLOBULIN INTRAVENOUS (HUMAN)   Systemic

VA CLASSIFICATION (Primary/Secondary): IM500/AM900; BL900; CV900; XX000

Commonly used brand name(s): *Gamimune N; Gammagard; Gammar-IV; Iveegam; Polygam; Sandoglobulin; Venoglobulin-I*.

Other commonly used names are IGIV and IVIG.

Note: For a listing of dosage forms and brand names by country availability, see *Dosage Forms* section(s).

### Category

Immunizing agent (passive); platelet count stimulator (systemic); anti-Kawasaki disease (systemic); antibacterial (systemic); antiviral (systemic); antipolyneuropathy agent.

### Indications

Note: Bracketed information in the *Indications* section refers to uses that are not included in U.S. product labeling.

**Accepted**
Immunodeficiency, primary (treatment)—Immune globulin intravenous (IGIV) is indicated for the treatment of patients with primary immu-

nodeficiency syndromes, such as congenital agammaglobulinemia (x-linked agammaglobulinemia), hypogammaglobulinemia, common variable immunodeficiency, x-linked immunodeficiency with hyperimmunoglobulin M (IgM), severe combined immunodeficiency, and Wiskott-Aldrich syndrome, to replace or boost immunoglobulin G (IgG).

Although IGIV may be of benefit in severe combined immunodeficiency, the cellular immunodeficit in this disease will not be corrected.

IGIV may be the preferred form of immune globulin for treatment of patients who have bleeding disorders for which an intramuscular injection of immune globulin is not recommended, patients who need an immediate increase in intravascular immunoglobulin concentrations, or patients who have limited muscle mass.

Thrombocytopenic purpura, idiopathic (treatment)—IGIV is indicated for the treatment of idiopathic thrombocytopenic purpura (ITP) when a rapid rise in the platelet count is required, such as prior to surgery, to control excessive bleeding, or to defer or avoid splenectomy. Not all patients will respond however, and, if the rise does occur, it may be transient. This treatment should not be considered curative, although remissions have occurred.

[Kawasaki disease (treatment adjunct)][1]—IGIV along with aspirin is considered to be a standard treatment for Kawasaki disease to prevent the development of coronary artery abnormalities, such as dilation, aneurysm, or ectasia, which in turn could lead to myocardial infarction.

Leukemia, chronic lymphocytic (treatment adjunct)[1]—IGIV is indicated for the prevention of recurrent bacterial infections in patients with hypogammaglobulinemia associated with B-cell chronic lymphocytic leukemia (CLL).

[Immunodepression, iatrogenically induced or disease-associated (treatment or treatment adjunct)][1]—IGIV is used, either alone or in conjunction with appropriate anti-infective therapy, to prevent or modify acute bacterial or viral infections (e.g., cytomegalovirus infections) in patients with iatrogenically induced or disease-associated immunodepression who are undergoing major surgery, such as bone marrow or cardiac transplants, or who have hematologic malignancies, extensive burns, or collagen-vascular diseases.

[Immunodeficiency syndrome, acquired, (AIDS) (treatment)][1] or [Immunodeficiency syndrome–related complex, acquired, (ARC) (treatment)][1]—IGIV is used to control or prevent infections and improve immunologic conditions in infants and children who are immunosuppressed in association with AIDS or ARC.

[Neonates, high-risk, preterm, low-birthweight, infections in (prophylaxis and treatment adjunct)][1]—IGIV is used for the prophylaxis of, and as a treatment adjunct in, infections in some high-risk, preterm, low-birthweight neonates. Controlled studies to assess its efficacy in the prevention of infection are ongoing. Until these studies are completed, IGIV is not recommended as a standard prophylactic agent in low-birthweight infants. In addition, since trials have yielded mixed results, IGIV is not recommended for routine use as adjunctive therapy in neonatal infections.

[Polyneuropathies, chronic inflammatory demyelinating (treatment)][1]—IGIV is used in the treatment of chronic inflammatory demyelinating polyneuropathies. IGIV is used either alone or following therapeutic plasma exchange to prolong its effect. IGIV is considered easier to use than repeated therapeutic plasma exchange and to have fewer complications than long-term glucocorticoid therapy.

[1]Not included in Canadian product labeling.

## Pharmacology/Pharmacokinetics

### Physicochemical characteristics
Other characteristics—
The pH of the reconstituted solution of the lyophilized product is approximately 6.8
The pH of the sterile solution is 4.0 to 4.5

### Mechanism of action/Effect
Immune globulin intravenous (IGIV) is a sterile, highly purified preparation of intact, unmodified immunoglobulin (IgG). The immunoglobulin is isolated from large pools of human plasma. All IgG antibody activities present in the donor population are conserved. The distribution of IgG subclasses corresponds to that in normal human plasma.
Immunodeficiency—
  IGIV is used to provide passive immunity against infection by increasing a person's antibody titer and antigen-antibody reaction potential.
  IGIV supplies a broad spectrum of IgG antibodies against bacterial, viral, parasitic, and mycoplasmal antigens. These antibodies have retained full biological function for the prevention or attenuation of a wide variety of infectious diseases, including the abilities to promote opsonization, fix complement, and neutralize microbes and their toxins.
Idiopathic thrombocytopenic purpura (ITP)—
  IGIV is used to induce a rapid increase in platelet counts in patients with ITP. The mechanism by which this occurs is not fully understood. In addition, it is not possible to predict which patients with ITP will respond to this therapy, although the increase in platelet counts seems to be greater in children than in adults.
Kawasaki disease—
  IGIV has been shown to have a striking anti-inflammatory effect in Kawasaki disease. Reductions in fever, neutrophil counts, and acute phase reactants usually occur within a day or so of initiation of IGIV treatment. The mechanism by which this occurs is not known.

### Distribution
100% in the serum immediately following intravenous administration. During the first week, the distribution equilibrates to approximately 60% in the serum and approximately 40% in the extravascular space.

### Time to peak concentration
Essentially 100% of a dose of IGIV is immediately available in the patient's circulation. A relatively rapid fall in serum IgG level that occurs in the first week following IGIV administration is to be expected.

### Time to peak effect
Immediately following intravenous administration.

### Duration of action
ITP—The rise in platelets most often lasts from several days to several weeks. Rarely, the rise in platelets may last up to 1 year or longer.

## Precautions to Consider

### Cross-sensitivity and/or related problems
Patients allergic to other immune globulins, either intramuscular or intravenous, may be allergic to immune globulin intravenous (IGIV) also.

### Pregnancy/Reproduction
Fertility—It is not known whether IGIV affects fertility.

Pregnancy—IGIV crosses the placenta. IGIV should be administered to pregnant women only if clearly needed.

Past experience with immune globulin intramuscular has shown no adverse effect on the fetus; however, it is not known whether IGIV can cause harm to the fetus. Although studies specific for pregnancy have not been done in humans, other studies on the use of IGIV during pregnancy for treatment of disease have not shown IGIV to cause harm to the fetus.

Studies have not been done in animals.

FDA Pregnancy Category C.

### Breast-feeding
It is not known whether IGIV is distributed into breast milk. However, problems in humans have not been documented.

### Pediatrics
Appropriate studies on the relationship of age to the effects of IGIV have not been performed in the pediatric population. However, administration of high doses of IGIV to children with idiopathic thrombocytopenic purpura did not cause any pediatrics-specific problems.

### Geriatrics
Appropriate studies on the relationship of age to the effects of IGIV have not been performed in the geriatric population. However, no geriatrics-specific problems have been documented to date.

### Drug interactions and/or related problems
The following drug interactions and/or related problems have been selected on the basis of their potential clinical significance (possible mechanism in parentheses where appropriate)—not necessarily inclusive (» = major clinical significance):
Live virus vaccines
  (antibodies contained in IGIV may interfere with the body's immune response to certain live virus vaccines; live virus vaccines, such as measles, mumps, and rubella, should be administered at least 14 days prior to, or at least 3 months after, administration of IGIV; however, there appears to be no interference between IGIV and oral polio vaccine [OPV], yellow fever vaccine, or diphtheria and tetanus toxoids and pertussis vaccine adsorbed [DTP])

### Medical considerations/Contraindications
The medical considerations/contraindications included have been selected on the basis of their potential clinical significance (reasons given in parentheses where appropriate)—not necessarily inclusive (» = major clinical significance).

# 1688  Immune Globulin Intravenous (Human) (Systemic)

*Except under special circumstances, this medication should not be used when the following medical problems exist:*

» Allergic reaction to IGIV
» Immunoglobulin A (IgA) deficiencies, selective, in patients who have known antibody to IgA
(small amounts of IgA may be present in IGIV and may cause a severe allergic reaction in patients with antibody to IgA; IgA-sensitive patients may be more tolerant of *Gammagard* or *Polygam* brands of IGIV, since they are very low in IgA [not more than 10 mcg per mL])

*Risk-benefit should be considered when the following medical problems exist:*

Acid-base compensatory mechanisms, limited or compromised
(because of its pH [4.0 to 4.5], the effect of the additional acid load of *Gamimune N* brand of IGIV should be considered when it is administered to patients with limited or compromised acid-base compensatory mechanisms)

Agammaglobulinemia or
Hypogammaglobulinemia, extreme
(patients who have never received immune globulin substitution therapy or who were last treated more than 8 weeks ago may be at risk, if administered IGIV by rapid infusion, of developing inflammatory reactions, which may lead to shock)

» Cardiac function impairment in seriously ill patients
(these patients may be at increased risk of vasomotor or cardiac complications, such as elevated blood pressure and cardiac failure)

Sensitivity to maltose or sucrose
(these ingredients may be present in some IGIV products)

**Patient monitoring**

The following may be especially important in patient monitoring (other tests may be warranted in some patients, depending on condition; » = major clinical significance):

Vital signs
(patients with agammaglobulinemia or severe hypogammaglobulinemia who have never received immune globulin substitution therapy or who were last treated more than 8 weeks ago may be at risk, if administered IGIV by rapid infusion, of developing inflammatory reactions, which may lead to shock; the patient's vital signs should be monitored continuously and the patient should be carefully observed throughout the infusion)

## Side/Adverse Effects

Note: Occasionally, immune globulin intravenous (IGIV) has caused a precipitous fall in blood pressure and signs of anaphylaxis. These reactions generally become evident within 30 to 60 minutes after the initiation of the infusion, and include fever, chills, nausea and vomiting, flushing, chest tightness, dizziness, sweating, and hypotension. Patients with agammaglobulinemia or extreme hypogammaglobulinemia who have never received immune globulin substitution therapy or who were last treated more than 8 weeks ago may be at increased risk of developing these reactions.

It appears that most side effects of IGIV are related to the rate of infusion, and may be relieved by decreasing the rate or temporarily stopping the infusion.

Backache, chills, flushing, headache, hypotension, myalgia, nausea, or pyrexia usually begins within 1 hour of the start of the infusion with IGIV. Symptoms usually subside within 30 minutes. Headache also may occur 3 to 24 hours after administration of IGIV.

IGIV appears to be safe with respect to the transmission of hepatitis B virus. Potential blood donors are screened, and studies have shown no evidence of the transmission of hepatitis B virus to patients who receive IGIV.

IGIV appears to be safe with respect to the transmission of the human immunodeficiency virus (HIV). Potential blood donors are screened for HIV. In addition, even when the donor plasma is deliberately spiked with HIV, tests of the final IGIV product do not show HIV in large enough quantities to be infective.

The following side/adverse effects have been selected on the basis of their potential clinical significance (possible signs and symptoms in parentheses where appropriate)—not necessarily inclusive:

**Those indicating need for medical attention**
Incidence more frequent
*Dyspnea* (troubled breathing); *tachycardia* (fast or pounding heartbeat)

Incidence less frequent
*Burning sensation in head; cyanosis* (bluish coloring of lips or nailbeds); *faintness or lightheadedness; fatigue* (unusual tiredness or weakness); *wheezing*

**Those indicating need for medical attention only if they continue or are bothersome**
Incidence more frequent
*Back ache or pain; headache; joint pain; malaise* (general feeling of discomfort or illness); *myalgia* (muscle pain)

Incidence less frequent
*Chest, back, or hip pain; erythema* (redness); *rash; or pain at injection site; leg cramps; urticaria* (hives)

## Overdose

For more information on the management of overdose or unintentional ingestion, **contact a Poison Control Center** (see *Poison Control Center Listing*).

**Clinical effects of overdose**
Symptoms of overdose apparently may be caused by too-rapid infusion.
The following effects have been selected on the basis of their potential clinical significance (possible signs and symptoms in parentheses where appropriate)—not necessarily inclusive:

Acute
*Chest tightness; chills; diaphoresis* (sweating); *dizziness; flushing* (redness of face); *hypotension* (unusual tiredness or weakness)—may become severe; *nausea; pyrexia* (fever); *vomiting*

## Patient Consultation

As an aid to patient consultation, refer to *Advice for the Patient, Immune Globulin Intravenous (Human) (Systemic)*.

In providing consultation, consider emphasizing the following selected information (» = major clinical significance):

**Before using this medication**
» Conditions affecting use, especially:
Sensitivity to intramuscular or intravenous immune globulins
Other medical problems, especially allergic reaction to IGIV, selective IgA deficiencies, or cardiac function impairment in seriously ill patients

**Proper use of this medication**
» Proper dosing

**Side/adverse effects**
Signs of potential side effects, especially dyspnea, tachycardia, burning sensation in head, cyanosis, faintness or lightheadedness, fatigue, and wheezing

## General Dosing Information

Since there is individual patient variation in the half-life of immune globulin intravenous (IGIV), the frequency of administration of IGIV should be based on both the patient's immune globulin half-life and the dose of IGIV administered.

It is suggested that a patient's trough serum IgG concentration 4 weeks after a treatment be maintained at 400 to 500 mg per deciliter, which is a value close to the lower limit of the normal range. Although IGIV is usually administered every 4 weeks, the interval should be adjusted depending on the trough serum IgG concentration and the patient's clinical condition.

IGIV is recommended for intravenous administration only. The intramuscular and subcutaneous routes have not been evaluated for this medication and are not recommended.

The infusion of IGIV should be at approximately room temperature for administration.

Diluents are product-specific. Only the specific diluent indicated by each manufacturer should be used for its particular product.

**For treatment of adverse effects**
Recommended treatment includes
• For mild hypersensitivity reaction—Administering antihistamines and, if necessary, glucocorticoids.
• For severe hypersensitivity or anaphylactic reaction—Administering epinephrine. Antihistamines and/or glucocorticoids may also be administered as required.

## Parenteral Dosage Forms

Note: Bracketed uses in the *Dosage Forms* section refer to categories of use and/or indications that are not included in U.S. product labeling.

## IMMUNE GLOBULIN INTRAVENOUS (HUMAN) INJECTION

**Usual adult and adolescent dose**
Immunodeficiency—
> Intravenous, 100 to 200 mg (2 to 4 mL) per kg of body weight once a month. If the patient's response is felt to be inadequate, the frequency of dosing may be increased to two times a month, or the dose may be increased to 400 mg (8 mL) per kg of body weight once a month.
>
> Note: For immunodeficiency, the National Institutes of Health (NIH) 1990 consensus panel for IGIV states that dose ranges of 200 to 800 mg per kg of body weight per month have been effective.

Idiopathic thrombocytopenic purpura (ITP)—
> Intravenous, 400 mg per kg of body weight per day for five consecutive days. If the patient's response to this five-day treatment period is inadequate, an additional 400 mg per kg of body weight may be administered as a single maintenance dose, repeated intermittently as needed.
>
> Note: For ITP, the NIH 1990 consensus panel for IGIV states that doses of either 400 mg per kg of body weight per day for two to five days or 1 gram per kg of body weight per day for one or two days have been effective. Administration every ten to twenty-one days is usually required to maintain adequate platelet counts.

[Kawasaki disease][1]—
> Intravenous, 400 mg per kg of body weight a day for four days; alternatively, a single dose of 2 grams per kg of body weight may be administered.
>
> Note: For *Gamimune N*, the rate of infusion of the undiluted medication should be 0.01 to 0.02 mL per kg of body weight per minute for thirty minutes. If the patient does not experience any discomfort, the rate may be gradually increased up to a maximum of 0.08 mL per kg of body weight per minute.

**Usual pediatric dose**
See *Usual adult and adolescent dose*.

**Size(s) usually available**
U.S.—
> 500 mg protein in 10 mL solution (Rx) [*Gamimune N* (maltose 9 to 11%)].
> 2.5 grams protein in 50 mL solution (Rx) [*Gamimune N* (maltose 9 to 11%)].
> 5 grams protein in 100 mL solution (Rx) [*Gamimune N* (maltose 9 to 11%)].
> 12.5 grams protein in 250 mL solution (Rx) [*Gamimune N* (maltose 9 to 11%)].

Canada—
> 500 mg protein in 10 mL solution (Rx) [*Gamimune N* (maltose 9 to 11%)].
> 2.5 grams protein in 50 mL solution (Rx) [*Gamimune N* (maltose 9 to 11%)].
> 5 grams protein in 100 mL solution (Rx) [*Gamimune N* (maltose 9 to 11%)].
> 10 grams protein in 200 mL solution (Rx) [*Gamimune N* (maltose 9 to 11%)].
> 12.5 grams protein in 250 mL solution (Rx) [*Gamimune N* (maltose 9 to 11%)].
> 25 grams protein in 500 mL solution (Rx) [*Gamimune N* (maltose 9 to 11%)].

Note: Each mL contains approximately 50 mg of protein of which not less than 98% is gamma globulin (IgG). Not less than 90% of the IgG is monomer. Also present are traces of immune globulin A (IgA) and immune globulin M (IgM).

**Packaging and storage**
Store at 2 to 8 °C (35 to 45 °F), unless otherwise specified by manufacturer. Protect from freezing.
The Canadian product may be stored also at temperatures not exceeding 25 °C (77 °F) for 30 days, after which it must be discarded.

**Preparation of dosage form**
The medication may be diluted only with 5% dextrose in water.

**Stability**
A solution that has been frozen should be discarded.
The contents of any vial that has been entered should be used promptly. The solution should not be used if it is not clear and colorless. Partially used vials should be discarded.

**Incompatibilities**
Incompatibilities have not been evaluated. It is recommended that IGIV be administered through a separate line, by itself, and without mixing with other intravenous fluids (with the exception of 5% dextrose in water for this particular product) or medications.

## IMMUNE GLOBULIN INTRAVENOUS HUMAN FOR INJECTION

**Usual adult and adolescent dose**
Immunodeficiency—
> *Gammagard* or *Polygam:* Intravenous, initially, 200 to 400 mg per kg of body weight once a month. Thereafter, monthly doses of at least 100 mg per kg of body weight may be adequate.
>
> *Gammar-IV:* Intravenous, 100 to 200 mg per kg of body weight every three to four weeks. Initially, a loading dose of at least 200 mg per kg of body weight at more frequent intervals than every three weeks may be used.
>
> *Iveegam:* Intravenous, 200 mg per kg of body weight once a month. If the patient's response is inadequate, the frequency of dosing may be increased, or the dose may be increased up to 800 mg per kg of body weight once a month.
>
> *Sandoglobulin:* Intravenous, 200 mg per kg of body weight once a month. If the patient's response is inadequate, the frequency of dosing may be increased, or the dose may be increased to 300 mg per kg of body weight once a month.
>
> *Venoglobulin-I:* Intravenous, 200 mg per kg of body weight once a month. If the patient's response is inadequate, the frequency of dosing may be increased, or the dose may be increased to 300 to 400 mg per kg of body weight once a month.
>
> Note: For immunodeficiency, the NIH 1990 consensus panel for IGIV states that dose ranges of 200 to 800 mg per kg of body weight per month have been effective.

Idiopathic thrombocytopenic purpura (ITP)—
> *Gammagard* or *Polygam:* Intravenous, 1 gram per kg of body weight as a single dose. If the patient's response is inadequate, 1 gram per kg of body weight may be administered on alternate days for up to three doses.
>
> *Sandoglobulin:* Intravenous, 400 mg per kg of body weight per day for two to five consecutive days. If the patient's response is inadequate, 400 mg per kg of body weight may be administered as a single maintenance dose once every several weeks. In some patients, it may be necessary to increase the maintenance dose up to 800 mg or 1 gram per kg of body weight.
>
> *Venoglobulin-I:* Intravenous, initially, up to 2 grams per kg of body weight per day for two to seven consecutive days. If the patient's response is inadequate, up to 2 grams per kg of body weight may be administered as a single maintenance dose every two weeks or more frequently as needed.
>
> Note: For ITP, the NIH 1990 consensus panel for IGIV states that doses of either 400 mg per kg of body weight per day for two to five days or 1 gram per kg of body weight per day for one or two days have been effective. Administration every ten to twenty-one days is usually required to maintain adequate platelet counts.

Bacterial infections secondary to B-cell chronic lymphocytic leukemia (CLL)[1]—
> *Gammagard* or *Polygam:* Intravenous, 400 mg per kg of body weight once every three to four weeks.

[Kawasaki disease][1]—
> Intravenous, 400 mg per kg of body weight a day for four days; alternatively, a single dose of 2 grams per kg of body weight may be administered.

Note: *Gammagard* or *Polygam*—Initially, the 50-mg-per-mL solution should be administered at a rate of approximately 0.008 mL per kg of body weight per minute (0.5 mL per kg of body weight per hour). If the patient does not experience any discomfort, the rate may be gradually increased up to a maximum of approximately 0.066 mL per kg of body weight per minute (4 mL per kg of body weight per hour).

*Gammar-IV*—Initially, the 50-mg-per-mL solution should be administered at a rate of 0.01 mL per kg of body weight per minute (0.6 mL per kg of body weight per hour) for fifteen to thirty minutes. The rate may then be increased to 0.02 mL per kg of body weight per minute (1.2 mL per kg of body weight per hour). If the patient does not experience any discomfort, the rate may be gradually increased to 0.03 to 0.06 mL per kg of body weight per minute (1.8 to 3.6 mL per kg of body weight per hour).

*Iveegam*—The usual rate of administration for the 5% solution is 1 mL per minute up to a maximum of 2 mL per minute. In order to prevent adverse reactions, some previously untreated patients with severe immunodeficiency have had treatment initiated with lower doses that have been diluted with saline or 5% dextrose. The dosage was then gradually increased.

*Sandoglobulin*—Previously untreated patients with agammaglobulinemia or hypogammaglobulinemia should have their first infusion administered as a 3% solution. Initially the flow rate should be 10 to 20 drops (0.5 to 1 mL) per minute. After 15 to 30 minutes, the rate of infusion may be increased to 30 to 50 drops (1.5 to 2.5 mL) per minute. After the initial bottle of 3% solution is infused, and if the patient shows good tolerance, subsequent infusions may be administered at a higher concentration. Such increases should be made gradually, allowing fifteen to thirty minutes before each increment.

*Venoglobulin-I*—Initially, the 50-mg-per-mL solution should be administered at a rate of 0.01 to 0.02 mL per kg of body weight per minute (0.6 to 1.2 mL per kg of body weight per hour) for thirty minutes. If the patient does not experience any discomfort, the rate may be gradually increased to 0.04 mL per kg of body weight per minute (2.4 mL per kg of body weight per hour). If the patient tolerates the higher infusion rate, subsequent infusions may be administered at this higher rate.

**Usual pediatric dose**
See *Usual adult and adolescent dose*.

**Size(s) usually available**
U.S.—
- 0.5 gram with 10 mL sterile water for injection as diluent (Rx) [*Gammagard* (sodium chloride 0.15 M; glucose 20 mg per mL; polyethylene glycol 2 mg per mL; glycine 0.3 M; human albumin 3 mg per mL); *Iveegam* (glucose 50 mg per mL; sodium chloride 3 mg per mL; polyethylene glycol < 0.5 gram per dL); *Polygam* (sodium chloride 0.15 M; glucose 20 mg per mL; polyethylene glycol 2 mg per mL; glycine 0.3 M; human albumin 3 mg per mL); *Venoglobulin-I* (D-mannitol 20 mg per mL; human albumin 10 mg per mL; sodium chloride 5 mg per mL; polyethylene glycol ≤ 6 mg per mL)].
- 1 gram with 20 mL sterile water for injection as diluent (Rx) [*Gammar-IV* (human albumin 3%; sucrose 5%; sodium chloride 0.5%; citric acid; sodium carbonate); *Iveegam* (glucose 50 mg per mL; sodium chloride 3 mg per mL; polyethylene glycol < 0.5 gram per dL)].
- 1 gram with 33 mL sodium chloride injection as diluent (Rx) [*Sandoglobulin*].
- 2.5 grams with 50 mL sterile water for injection as diluent (Rx) [*Gammagard* (sodium chloride 0.15 M; glucose 20 mg per mL; polyethylene glycol 2 mg per mL; glycine 0.3 M; human albumin 3 mg per mL); *Gammar-IV* (human albumin 3%; sucrose 5%; sodium chloride 0.5%; citric acid; sodium carbonate); *Iveegam* (glucose 50 mg per mL; sodium chloride 3 mg per mL; polyethylene glycol < 0.5 gram per dL); *Polygam* (sodium chloride 0.15 M; glucose 20 mg per mL; polyethylene glycol 2 mg per mL; glycine 0.3 M; human albumin 3 mg per mL)].
- 2.5 grams with or without 50 mL sterile water for injection as diluent (Rx) [*Venoglobulin-I* (D-mannitol 20 mg per mL; human albumin 10 mg per mL; sodium chloride 5 mg per mL; polyethylene glycol ≤ 6 mg per mL)].
- 3 grams with or without 100 mL sodium chloride injection as diluent (Rx) [*Sandoglobulin*].
- 5 grams with 100 mL sterile water for injection as diluent (Rx) [*Gammagard* (sodium chloride 0.15 M; glucose 20 mg per mL; polyethylene glycol 2 mg per mL; glycine 0.3 M; human albumin 3 mg per mL); *Gammar-IV* (human albumin 3%; sucrose 5%; sodium chloride 0.5%; citric acid; sodium carbonate); *Iveegam* (glucose 50 mg per mL; sodium chloride 3 mg per mL; polyethylene glycol < 0.5 gram per dL); *Polygam* (sodium chloride 0.15 M; glucose 20 mg per mL; polyethylene glycol 2 mg per mL; glycine 0.3 M; human albumin 3 mg per mL)].
- 5 grams with or without 100 mL sterile water for injection as diluent (Rx) [*Venoglobulin-I* (D-mannitol 20 mg per mL; human albumin 10 mg per mL; sodium chloride 5 mg per mL; polyethylene glycol ≤ 6 mg per mL)].
- 6 grams with or without 200 mL sodium chloride injection as diluent (Rx) [*Sandoglobulin*].
- 10 grams with 200 mL sterile water for injection as diluent (Rx) [*Gammagard* (sodium chloride 0.15 M; glucose 20 mg per mL; polyethylene glycol 2 mg per mL; glycine 0.3 M; human albumin 3 mg per mL); *Polygam* (sodium chloride 0.15 M; glucose 20 mg per mL; polyethylene glycol 2 mg per mL; glycine 0.3 M; human albumin 3 mg per mL)].

Note: When reconstituted according to directions, *Gammagard*, *Gammar-IV*, *Polygam*, and *Venoglobulin-I* contain approximately 50 mg of protein per mL, of which at least 90% is gamma globulin (IgG); *Iveegam* contains a 5% protein solution, which yields 50 mg ± 5 mg per mL of IgG; and *Sandoglobulin* contains either approximately 30 mg or 60 mg of protein per mL, of which at least 96% is IgG.

Also present are traces of IgA and IgM.

*Sandoglobulin* can be reconstituted with sterile water, 5% dextrose, or 0.9% saline to make solutions with protein concentrations of 3 to 12%.

Canada—
- 0.5 gram with 10 mL sterile water for injection as diluent (Rx) [*Iveegam* (glucose 50 mg ± 5 mg per mL; sodium chloride 3 mg ± 1 mg per mL)].
- 1 gram with 20 mL sterile water for injection as diluent (Rx) [*Iveegam* (glucose 50 mg ± 5 mg per mL; sodium chloride 3 mg ± 1 mg per mL)].
- 2.5 grams with 50 mL sterile water for injection as diluent (Rx) [*Iveegam* (glucose 50 mg ± 5 mg per mL; sodium chloride 3 mg ± 1 mg per mL)].
- 5 grams with 100 mL sterile water for injection as diluent (Rx) [*Iveegam* (glucose 50 mg ± 5 mg per mL; sodium chloride 3 mg ± 1 mg per mL)].
- 7.5 grams with 150 mL sterile water for injection as diluent (Rx) [*Iveegam* (glucose 50 mg ± 5 mg per mL; sodium chloride 3 mg ± 1 mg per mL)].
- 10 grams with 200 mL sterile water for injection as diluent (Rx) [*Iveegam* (glucose 50 mg ± 5 mg per mL; sodium chloride 3 mg ± 1 mg per mL)].

Note: When reconstituted according to directions, *Iveegam* contains 55 mg ± 5 mg of protein per mL, of which 50 mg ± 5 mg per mL is gamma globulin (IgG).

May also contain traces of IgA and IgM.

**Packaging and storage**
Store at temperatures not exceeding 25 °C (77 °F), unless otherwise specified by manufacturer. Protect the diluent from freezing.

**Preparation of dosage form**
The diluent and lyophilized product should be brought to room temperature prior to reconstitution. When the diluent is added, dissolution usually occurs within a few minutes, although in rare cases, or when the product and/or diluent are cold, dissolution may take up to 20 minutes. The reconstituted solution should not be shaken, since excessive shaking will cause foaming. Reconstituted solution should be at approximately room temperature at the time of administration.

**Stability**
Only the specific diluent that the product's manufacturer indicates for that particular product should be used. The solution should not be used if it is not clear and colorless to slightly straw colored, or if there is particulate matter present. Administration should begin promptly after reconstitution, or within 2 or 3 hours, according to the individual manufacturer's instructions. Partially used vials should be discarded.

**Incompatibilities**
Incompatibilities have not been evaluated. It is recommended that IGIV be administered through a separate line, by itself, and without mixing with other intravenous fluids (with the exception of the product's specified diluent) or medications. However, for *Iveegam*-Canada, if lower immune globulin concentrations are desired, the reconstituted 5% solution can be diluted using isotonic saline, isotonic glucose, or isotonic levulose solutions.

---

[1]Not included in Canadian product labeling.

## Selected Bibliography

Buckley RH, Schiff RI. The use of intravenous immune globulin in immunodeficiency diseases. N Engl J Med 1991 July 11; 325(2): 110-17.

Intravenous immunoglobulin: prevention and treatment of disease. NIH Consens Dev Conf Consens Statement 1990 May 21-23; 8(5).

ASHP Commission on Therapeutics. ASHP therapeutic guidelines for intravenous immune globulin. Clin Pharm 1992 Feb; 11: 117-36.

---

Revised: 06/21/93
Interim revision: 02/23/94

# INDAPAMIDE Systemic

VA CLASSIFICATION (Primary/Secondary): CV701/CV490
Commonly used brand name(s): *Lozide; Lozol.*
Note: For a listing of dosage forms and brand names by country availability, see *Dosage Forms* section(s).

## Category
Antihypertensive; diuretic.

## Indications
**Accepted**
Hypertension (treatment)—Indapamide is indicated, alone or in combination with other agents, for treatment of hypertension. Indapamide is effective in treating hypertension in patients with renal function impairment, although its diuretic effect is reduced.

For additional information on initial therapeutic guidelines related to the treatment of hypertension, see *Appendix III*.

Edema (treatment)—Indapamide is indicated for treatment of salt and fluid retention associated with congestive heart failure.

## Pharmacology/Pharmacokinetics
**Physicochemical characteristics**
Molecular weight—365.83.
pKa—8.8.

**Mechanism of action/Effect**
Antihypertensive—Not clearly understood, but may involve both renal and extrarenal effects. The diuretic effect (reduction of extracellular fluid and blood volume) probably contributes only minimally since indapamide decreases blood pressure at a dose well below the effective diuretic dose. The antihypertensive effect is thought to be the result of reduction in peripheral vascular resistance.
Diuretic—Indapamide inhibits reabsorption of water and electrolytes, primarily as a result of action on the cortical diluting segment of the distal tubule.

**Protein binding**
High (71 to 79%), to plasma proteins. Also bound to elastin in vascular smooth muscle.

**Biotransformation**
Hepatic (extensive).

**Half-life**
In whole blood—Approximately 14 hours.
Terminal half-life of excretion of total radioactivity ($^{14}C$-labeled indapamide)—26 hours.

**Onset of action**
Antihypertensive—Multiple dose: 1 to 2 weeks.

**Time to peak concentration**
Within 2 hours.

**Peak serum concentration**
Approximately 260 nanograms per mL after oral administration of 5 mg.

**Time to peak effect**
Antihypertensive—
  Single dose: Approximately 24 hours.
  Multiple doses: 8 to 12 weeks.

**Duration of action**
Antihypertensive—Multiple doses: Up to 8 weeks.

**Elimination**
Renal—60 to 70% (5 to 7% unchanged).
Fecal—20 to 23%.

## Precautions to Consider

**Cross-sensitivity and/or related problems**
Patients sensitive to other sulfonamide-type medications may be sensitive to indapamide also.

**Carcinogenicity/Tumorigenicity**
Studies in rats and mice found no evidence of carcinogenicity or tumorigenicity.

**Pregnancy/Reproduction**
Fertility—Studies in animals have not shown that indapamide causes adverse effects on the fetus at up to 6250 times the therapeutic human dose.

Pregnancy—Adequate and well-controlled studies in humans have not been done. However, pregnant women should be advised to contact physician before taking this medication, since routine use of diuretics during normal pregnancy is inappropriate and exposes mother and fetus to unnecessary hazard.
Studies in animals have not shown that indapamide causes adverse effects on the fetus at up to 6250 times the therapeutic human dose.
FDA Pregnancy Category B.

**Breast-feeding**
It is not known whether indapamide is excreted in breast milk. However, problems in humans have not been documented.

**Pediatrics**
Appropriate studies on the relationship of age to the effects of indapamide have not been performed in the pediatric population. Safety and efficacy have not been established.

**Geriatrics**
Although appropriate studies on the relationship of age to the effects of indapamide have not been performed in the geriatric population, the elderly may be more sensitive to the hypotensive and electrolyte effects. In addition, elderly patients are more likely to have age-related renal function impairment, which may require caution in patients receiving indapamide.

**Drug interactions and/or related problems**
The following drug interactions and/or related problems have been selected on the basis of their potential clinical significance (possible mechanism in parentheses where appropriate)—not necessarily inclusive (» = major clinical significance):

Note: Combinations containing any of the following medications, depending on the amount present, may also interact with this medication.

Amiodarone
  (concurrent use of indapamide with amiodarone may lead to an increased risk of arrhythmias associated with hypokalemia)

Anticoagulants, coumarin- or indandione-derivative
  (effects may be decreased when these medications are used concurrently with indapamide, as a result of reduction of plasma volume leading to concentration of procoagulant factors in the blood; in addition, diuretic-induced improvement of hepatic congestion may lead to improved hepatic function resulting in increased procoagulant factor synthesis; dosage adjustments may be necessary)

» Digitalis glycosides
  (concurrent use with indapamide may enhance the possibility of digitalis toxicity associated with hypokalemia)

Hypotension-producing medications, other (See *Appendix II*)
  (antihypertensive and/or diuretic effects may be increased when these medications are used concurrently with indapamide; although some antihypertensive and/or diuretic combinations are used frequently for therapeutic advantage, dosage adjustment may be necessary during concurrent use)

» Lithium
  (concurrent use with indapamide is not recommended, as it may provoke lithium toxicity because of reduced renal clearance; in addition, lithium has nephrotoxic effects)

Neuromuscular blocking agents, nondepolarizing
  (indapamide may induce hypokalemia, which may enhance the blockade of nondepolarizing neuromuscular blocking agents; serum potassium determinations may be necessary prior to administration of nondepolarizing neuromuscular blocking agents; careful postoperative monitoring of the patient may be necessary following concurrent or sequential use, especially if there is a possibility of incomplete reversal of neuromuscular blockade)

Sympathomimetics
  (antihypertensive effects of indapamide may be reduced when it is used concurrently with sympathomimetics; the patient should be carefully monitored to confirm that the desired effect is being obtained)

  (indapamide may decrease arterial responsiveness to norepinephrine, but does not usually significantly interfere with its clinical effects)

**Laboratory value alterations**
The following have been selected on the basis of their potential clinical significance (possible effect in parentheses where appropriate)—not necessarily inclusive (» = major clinical significance):

With physiology/laboratory test values
    Calcium and
    Protein-bound iodine (PBI)
        (serum concentrations may be slightly decreased)
    Plasma renin activity (PRA)
        (may be increased)
    Potassium and
    Sodium
        (serum concentrations may be decreased but usually remain within normal limits)
    Uric acid
        (serum concentrations may be increased but usually remain within normal limits)

**Medical considerations/Contraindications**
The medical considerations/contraindications included have been selected on the basis of their potential clinical significance (reasons given in parentheses where appropriate)—not necessarily inclusive (» = major clinical significance).

*Risk-benefit should be considered when the following medical problems exist:*
» Anuria or severe renal function impairment
    (diuretic effect reduced; may precipitate azotemia)
  Diabetes mellitus
    (possible impaired glucose tolerance)
  Gout, history of or
  Hyperuricemia
    (serum uric acid concentrations may be elevated)
  Hepatic function impairment
    (risk of dehydration, which may precipitate hepatic coma and death)
  Sensitivity to indapamide or other sulfonamide-type medications
  Sympathectomy
    (antihypertensive effects may be enhanced)

**Patient monitoring**
The following may be especially important in patient monitoring (other tests may be warranted in some patients, depending on condition; » = major clinical significance):

  Blood glucose concentration and
  Blood urea nitrogen (BUN) concentration and
  Uric acid concentration, serum
    (determinations recommended prior to initiation of therapy and at periodic intervals during therapy)
» Blood pressure measurements
    (recommended at periodic intervals in patients being treated for hypertension; selected patients may be trained to perform blood pressure measurements at home and report the results at regular physician visits)
  Electrolyte concentrations, serum
    (determinations recommended at periodic intervals for patients on long-term therapy, especially if they are also taking cardiac glycosides or systemic steroids, or when severe cirrhosis is present)

## Side/Adverse Effects

The following side/adverse effects have been selected on the basis of their potential clinical significance (possible signs and symptoms in parentheses where appropriate)—not necessarily inclusive:

**Those indicating need for medical attention**
Incidence rare
    *Allergic reaction* (skin rash, itching, or hives); *electrolyte imbalance, specifically hyponatremia, hypochloremic alkalosis, or hypokalemia* (dryness of mouth; increased thirst; irregular heartbeat; mood or mental changes; muscle cramps or pain; nausea or vomiting; unusual tiredness or weakness; weak pulse)
    Note: *Electrolyte imbalance* is dose-related (*hypokalemia* occurs fairly frequently) but is not usually symptomatic.

**Those indicating need for medical attention only if they continue or are bothersome**
Incidence less frequent or rare
    *Anorexia* (loss of appetite); *diarrhea; headache; orthostatic hypotension as a result of volume depletion* (dizziness or lightheadedness, especially when getting up from a lying or sitting position); *trouble in sleeping; stomach upset*

## Overdose

For more information on the management of overdose or unintentional ingestion, **contact a Poison Control Center** (see *Poison Control Center Listing*).

**Treatment of overdose**
Indapamide overdose should be treated by immediate evacuation of the stomach followed by supportive, symptomatic treatment and monitoring of serum electrolyte concentrations and renal function.

## Patient Consultation

As an aid to patient consultation, refer to *Advice for the Patient, Indapamide (Systemic)*.
In providing consultation, consider emphasizing the following selected information (» = major clinical significance):

**Before using this medication**
» Conditions affecting use, especially:
    Sensitivity to indapamide or other sulfonamide-type medications
    Pregnancy—Routine use not recommended
    Use in the elderly—Increased sensitivity to hypotensive and electrolyte effects
    Other medications, especially digitalis glycosides or lithium
    Other medical problems, especially anuria or severe renal function impairment

**Proper use of this medication**
    Diuretic effects of the medication and timing of doses to minimize inconvenience of diuresis
    Getting into habit of taking at same time each day to help increase compliance
» Proper dosing
    Missed dose: Taking as soon as possible; not taking if almost time for next dose; not doubling doses
» Proper storage
*For use as an antihypertensive*
    Possible need for control of weight and diet, especially sodium intake
» Patients may not experience symptoms of hypertension; importance of taking medication even if feeling well
» Does not cure but helps control hypertension; possible need for lifelong therapy; checking with physician before discontinuing therapy; serious consequences of untreated hypertension

**Precautions while using this medication**
    Regular visits to physician to check progress
» Possibility of hypokalemia; possible need for additional potassium in diet; not changing diet without first checking with physician
    To prevent dehydration, checking with physician if severe nausea, vomiting, or diarrhea occurs and continues
*For use as an antihypertensive*
» Not taking other medications, especially nonprescription sympathomimetics, unless discussed with physician

**Side/adverse effects**
    Signs of potential side effects, especially allergic reaction and electrolyte imbalance

## General Dosing Information

The lowest effective dosage should be utilized to minimize potential electrolyte imbalance.

When used to promote diuresis, a single daily dose is preferably taken on arising in order to minimize the effect of increased frequency of urination on sleep. Intermittent dosage schedules (drug-free days) may reduce the possibility of electrolyte imbalance or hyperuricemia resulting from therapy.

Concurrent administration of potassium supplements or potassium-sparing diuretics may be indicated in patients considered to be at higher risk for developing hypokalemia. Caution in administering potassium supplements is recommended, however, since loss of potassium is not clinically significant in most patients, and supplementation leads to a risk of development of hyperkalemia.

Recent evidence suggests that withdrawal of antihypertensive therapy prior to surgery is not necessary, but that the anesthesiologist must be aware of such therapy.

## Oral Dosage Forms

### INDAPAMIDE TABLETS

**Usual adult dose**
Diuretic—
    Oral, 2.5 mg once a day, adjusted according to response after one (for edema) to four (for hypertension) weeks up to 5 mg once a day.

Note: Geriatric patients may be more sensitive to the effects of the usual adult dose.

**Usual pediatric dose**
Safety and efficacy have not been established.

**Strength(s) usually available**
U.S.—
  2.5 mg (Rx) [*Lozol* (lactose)].
Canada—
  2.5 mg (Rx) [*Lozide*].

**Packaging and storage**
Store below 40 °C (104 °F), preferably between 15 and 30 °C (59 and 86 °F), in a well-closed container, unless otherwise specified by manufacturer. Protect from light.

**Note**
Check refill frequency to determine compliance in hypertensive patients.

**Selected Bibliography**
Thomas JR. A review of 10 years of experience with indapamide as an antihypertensive agent. Hypertension 1985; 7 (Suppl 2): II–152–II–156.
The fifth report of the Joint National Committee on Detection, Evaluation, and Treatment of High Blood Pressure (JNC V). Arch Intern Med 1993; 153(2): 154-83.

Revised: 01/20/93

# INDINAVIR Systemic—INTRODUCTORY VERSION

VA CLASSIFICATION (Primary): AM803
Commonly used brand name(s): *Crixivan*.
Note: For a listing of dosage forms and brand names by country availability, see *Dosage Forms* section(s).

## Category
Antiviral (systemic).

## Indications

**General considerations**
Human immunodeficiency virus (HIV) isolates with reduced susceptibility to indinavir have been recovered from some patients treated with this medication. Resistance correlated with the accumulation of mutations that resulted in the expression of amino acid substitutions at eleven residue positions in the viral protease.

Cross-resistance between indinavir and reverse transcriptase inhibitors is thought to be unlikely because they affect different enzyme targets. However, cross-resistance was observed between indinavir and ritonavir, another protease inhibitor. Varying degrees of resistance have been noted between indinavir and other protease inhibitors.

**Accepted**
Human immunodeficiency virus (HIV) infection (treatment) or
Immunodeficiency syndrome, acquired (AIDS) (treatment)—Indinavir is indicated in combination with the nucleoside analogs or as monotherapy for the treatment of HIV infection or AIDS.

## Pharmacology/Pharmacokinetics

**Physicochemical characteristics**
Molecular weight—Indinavir sulfate: 711.88.

**Mechanism of action/Effect**
Indinavir binds to the protease active site and inhibits the activity of human immunodeficiency virus (HIV) protease, an enzyme required for the proteolytic cleavage of viral polyprotein precursors into individual functional proteins found in infectious HIV. This inhibition prevents cleavage of viral polyproteins and results in the formation of immature noninfectious viral particles.

**Absorption**
Rapidly absorbed when taken on an empty stomach. Administration of indinavir with a meal high in calories, fat, and protein resulted in an 84% reduction in peak plasma concentration ($C_{max}$) and a 77% reduction in area under the plasma concentration–time curve (AUC). Administration with a lighter meal resulted in little or no change in $C_{max}$ or AUC.

**Protein binding**
Moderate (60%).

**Biotransformation**
Hepatic; seven metabolites have been identified. One is a glucuronide conjugate and six are oxidative metabolites; cytochrome P450 3A4 (CYP3A4) has been found to be the major enzyme responsible for formation of the oxidative metabolites.

**Half-life**
Approximately 1.8 hours.

**Time to peak concentration**
Approximately 0.8 hour after administration in the fasted state.

**Elimination**
Fecal—Approximately 83% of an administered radioactive dose was recovered in the feces. Radioactivity due to the parent medication in the feces was approximately 19%.
Renal—Approximately 19% of an administered radioactive dose was recovered in the urine. Radioactivity due to the parent medication in the urine was approximately 9%.
In dialysis—It is not known whether indinavir is dialyzable by peritoneal or hemodialysis.

## Precautions to Consider

**Carcinogenicity**
Long-term carcinogenicity studies in rats and mice have not been completed.

**Mutagenicity**
There has been no evidence of mutagenicity or genotoxicity in *in vitro* microbial mutagenesis (Ames) tests, *in vitro* alkaline elution assays for DNA breakage, *in vitro* and *in vivo* chromosomal aberration studies, and *in vitro* mammalian cell mutagenesis assays.

**Pregnancy/Reproduction**
Fertility—There were no effects on mating, fertility, or embryo survival in female rats and no effects on mating performance seen in male rats at doses providing systemic exposure comparable to or slightly higher than that attained with the clinical dose. Also, there were no effects observed on fertility or fecundity of untreated females mated with treated males.

Pregnancy—Adequate and well-controlled studies have not been done in humans. Hyperbilirubinemia has occurred during treatment with indinavir; it is unknown whether administration to the mother in the perinatal period will exacerbate physiologic hyperbilirubinemia in neonates.

No evidence of teratogenicity was found in developmental toxicity studies performed in rats and rabbits administered doses comparable to or slightly greater than those administered to humans. In rats, there were treatment-related increases over controls in the incidence of supernumerary ribs at exposures at or below those in humans, and of cervical ribs at exposures comparable to or slightly greater than those in humans. There were no external, visceral, or skeletal changes observed in rabbits. In rats and rabbits, there were no treatment-related effects on embryonic/fetal survival or fetal weights. Since fetal exposure was low in rabbits, a developmental toxicity study in dogs is in progress.

FDA Pregnancy Category C.

**Breast-feeding**
It is not known whether indinavir is distributed into human breast milk; however, there exists the potential for adverse effects in nursing infants. Nursing mothers are advised to discontinue breast-feeding if they are receiving indinavir.

Indinavir is distributed into the milk of lactating rats.

**Pediatrics**
No information is available on the relationship of age to the effects of indinavir in pediatric patients. Safety and efficacy have not been established.

**Geriatrics**
No information is available on the relationship of age to the effects of indinavir in geriatric patients.

**Drug interactions and/or related problems**
The following drug interactions and/or related problems have been selected on the basis of their potential clinical significance (possible mechanism

in parentheses where appropriate)—not necessarily inclusive (» = major clinical significance):

Note: Combinations containing any of the following medications, depending on the amount present, may also interact with this medication.

- » Astemizole or
- » Cisapride or
- » Midazolam or
- » Terfenadine or
- » Triazolam

    (studies have not been done with the cytochrome P450 CYP3A4 substrates astemizole, cisapride, midazolam, terfenadine, and triazolam; because competition for CYP3A4 by indinavir could result in inhibition of the metabolism of these medications and elevated plasma concentrations, there is a potential for serious and/or life-threatening side effects; concurrent use of indinavir with any of these medications is not recommended)

  Cimetidine
    (concurrent administration does not affect the area under the plasma concentration-time curve [AUC] of indinavir)

  Clarithromycin
    (concurrent use results in a 29% increase in the AUC of indinavir and a 53% increase in the AUC of clarithromycin; dosing modification is not required)

  Contraceptives, estrogen-containing, oral
    (concurrent use of indinavir with an estrogen-containing oral contraceptive [*Ortho-Novum 1/35®*] results in a 24% increase in the AUC of ethinyl estradiol and a 26% increase in the AUC of norethindrone; dosing modification is not required)

- » Didanosine
    (if indinavir and didanosine are both part of a treatment regimen, they should be administered at least 1 hour apart on an empty stomach; a normal acidic pH may be necessary for the optimal absorption of indinavir, and didanosine requires a buffer to increase the pH so that acid does not rapidly degrade didanosine)

  Fluconazole
    (concurrent use results in a 19% decrease in the AUC of indinavir and no change in the AUC of fluconazole; dosing modification is not required)

  Grapefruit juice
    (administration of a single 400-mg dose of indinavir with grapefruit juice results in a 26% decrease in the AUC of indinavir; dosing modification is not required)

  Isoniazid
    (concurrent administration results in a 13% increase in the AUC of isoniazid and no change in the AUC of indinavir; dosing modification is not required)

- » Ketoconazole
    (concurrent use results in a 68% increase in the AUC of indinavir; a dosage reduction of indinavir to 600 mg every 8 hours is recommended when coadministered with ketoconazole)

  Lamivudine or
  Zidovudine
    (concurrent administration of zidovudine and indinavir results in a 13% increase in the AUC of indinavir and a 17% increase in the AUC of zidovudine; administration of indinavir with zidovudine and lamivudine results in no change in the AUC of indinavir, a 36% increase in AUC of zidovudine and a 6% decrease in AUC of lamivudine; dosing modification is not required)

  Quinidine
    (administration of a single 400-mg dose of indinavir with 200 mg of quinidine sulfate results in a 10% decrease in the AUC of indinavir; dosing modification is not required)

- » Rifabutin
    (concurrent use results in a 32% increase in the AUC of indinavir and a 204% increase in the AUC of rifabutin; dosage reduction of rifabutin to 400 mg every 8 hours is necessary when it is coadministered with indinavir)

- » Rifampin
    (because rifampin is a potent inducer of CYP3A4, which could significantly decrease the plasma concentration of indinavir, concurrent use with indinavir is not recommended)

  Sulfamethoxazole and trimethoprim combination
    (concurrent administration results in no change in the AUC of indinavir and sulfamethoxazole, and a 19% increase in the AUC of trimethoprim; dosing modification is not required)

  Stavudine
    (concurrent administration results in no change in the AUC of indinavir and a 25% increase in the AUC of stavudine; dosing modification is not required)

**Laboratory value alterations**
The following have been selected on the basis of their potential clinical significance (possible effect in parentheses where appropriate)—not necessarily inclusive (» = major clinical significance):

With physiology/laboratory test values
  Alanine aminotransferase (ALT [SGPT]), serum and
  Amylase, serum and
  Aspartate aminotransferase (AST [SGOT]), serum
    (values may be increased)

- » Bilirubin, total serum
    (asymptomatic hyperbilirubinemia [total bilirubin ≥ 2.5 mg per dL], reported primarily as elevated indirect bilirubin, has occurred in approximately 10% of patients treated with indinavir; this was associated with elevations in ALT or AST in less than 1% of patients; it also occurred more frequently at doses > 2.4 grams per day)

  Glucose, plasma
    (concentrations may be increased)

**Medical considerations/Contraindications**
The medical considerations/contraindications included have been selected on the basis of their potential clinical significance (reasons given in parentheses where appropriate)—not necessarily inclusive (» = major clinical significance).

*Except under special circumstances, this medication should not be used when the following medical problem exists:*

- » Hypersensitivity to indinavir

*Risk-benefit should be considered when the following medical problems exist:*

  Hemophilia
    (spontaneous bleeding has been reported in patients with hemophilia types A and B who are being treated with protease inhibitors; a causal relationship has not been established)

- » Hepatic function impairment
    (it is recommended that the dosage of indinavir be lowered to 600 mg every 8 hours in patients with mild to moderate hepatic function impairment due to cirrhosis)

**Patient monitoring**
The following may be especially important in patient monitoring (other tests may be warranted in some patients, depending on condition; » = major clinical significance):

- » Blood glucose determinations
    (recommended to closely monitor patient's plasma glucose concentrations; development of hyperglycemia or diabetes may be associated with the use of protease inhibitors)

## Side/Adverse Effects

Note: Nephrolithiasis (kidney stones) was reported in approximately 4% of patients treated with indinavir. It was not usually associated with renal function impairment and resolved with hydration and temporary interruption of therapy. Nephrolithiasis was more likely to occur at doses > 2.4 grams per day.

The following side/adverse effects have been selected on the basis of their potential clinical significance (possible signs and symptoms in parentheses where appropriate)—not necessarily inclusive:

**Those indicating need for medical attention**
Incidence more frequent
  *Kidney stones* (blood in urine; sharp back pain just below ribs)
Incidence rare
  *Diabetes or hyperglycemia* (dry or itchy skin; fatigue; hunger, increased; thirst, increased; unexplained weight loss; urination, increased); *ketoacidosis* (confusion; dehydration; mouth odor, fruity; nausea; vomiting; weight loss)

**Those indicating need for medical attention only if they continue or are bothersome**
Incidence more frequent
  *Asthenia* (generalized weakness); *gastrointestinal disturbances* (abdominal or stomach pain; diarrhea; nausea; vomiting); *headache; insomnia* (difficulty in sleeping); *taste perversion* (change in sense of taste)

Incidence less frequent
  *Dizziness; somnolence* (sleepiness)

## Overdose

There are no reports of indinavir overdose in humans. Single oral and intraperitoneal doses of indinavir up to 20 times the human dose in rats and 10 times the human dose in mice did not result in any deaths.

For more information on the management of overdose or unintentional ingestion, **contact a Poison Control Center** (see *Poison Control Center Listing*).

## Patient Consultation

As an aid to patient consultation, refer to *Advice for the Patient, Indinavir (Systemic)—Introductory Version.*

In providing consultation, consider emphasizing the following selected information (» = major clinical significance)

### Before using this medication
» Conditions affecting use, especially:
   Hypersensitivity to indinavir
   Pregnancy—Hyperbilirubinemia has occurred during treatment with indinavir; it is unknown whether administration to the mother in the perinatal period will exacerbate physiologic hyperbilirubinemia in the neonate
   Breast-feeding—Indinavir is distributed into the milk of lactating rats; it is not known if indinavir is distributed into human breast milk; therefore, breast-feeding should be discontinued
   Other medications, especially astemizole, cisapride, didanosine, ketoconazole, midazolam, rifabutin, rifampin, terfenadine, or triazolam
   Other medical problems, especially hepatic function impairment

### Proper use of this medication
» Importance of taking indinavir with water 1 hour before or 2 hours after a meal; indinavir may also be taken with other liquids (skim milk, juice, coffee, or tea) or with a light meal (dry toast with jelly, juice, and coffee with skim milk and sugar, or corn flakes, skim milk and sugar)
» Importance of drinking at least 1.5 liters (approximately 48 ounces) of liquids over each 24-hour period
» Importance of not taking more medication than prescribed; importance of not discontinuing indinavir without checking with physician
» Compliance with full course of therapy
» Importance of not missing doses and of taking at evenly spaced times
   Not sharing medication with others
» Proper dosing
   Missed dose: Taking as soon as possible; not taking if almost time for next dose; not doubling doses
» Proper storage; indinavir capsules are sensitive to moisture; indinavir should be stored and used in the original container and the desiccant should remain in the bottle

### Precautions while using this medication
» Because indinavir may interact with other medications, not taking any other medications (prescription or nonprescription) without first consulting your physician

» Regular visits to physician for blood tests and monitoring of blood glucose concentrations

### Side/adverse effects
Signs of potential side effects, especially kidney stones, diabetes or hyperglycemia, and ketoacidosis

## General Dosing Information

The recommended dose of indinavir is 800 mg every eight hours, whether it is used alone or in combination with other antiretroviral agents.

To help prevent kidney stones, it is recommended that patients drink at least 1.5 liters (approximately 48 ounces) of liquids over each 24-hour period. Patients who experience kidney stones may require temporary interruption of therapy (e.g., 1 to 3 days) during the acute episode or discontinuation of therapy.

Patients with mild to moderate hepatic function impairment due to cirrhosis require a dosage reduction to 600 mg every eight hours.

### Diet/Nutrition
Administration of a single 400-mg dose of indinavir with grapefruit juice results in a 26% decrease in the area under the plasma concentration–time curve (AUC) of indinavir; dosing modification is not required.

## Oral Dosage Forms

Note: The dosing and strengths of the dosage form available are expressed in terms of indinavir base (not the sulfate salt).

### INDINAVIR SULFATE CAPSULES

#### Usual adult dose
Antiviral—
   Oral, 800 mg (base) every eight hours used alone or in combination with other antiretroviral agents.

#### Usual pediatric dose
Safety and efficacy have not been established.

#### Strength(s) usually available
U.S.—
   200 mg (base) (Rx) [*Crixivan* (lactose)].
   400 mg (base) (Rx) [*Crixivan* (lactose)].

#### Packaging and storage
Store at room temperature, preferably between 15 and 30 °C (59 and 86 °F). Store in a tight container. Protect from moisture.

#### Auxiliary labeling
• Take on an empty stomach.
• Continue medicine for full time of treatment.
• Do not take other medications without physician's advice.

Developed: 01/27/97
Revised: 09/11/97

---

# INDIUM In 111 OXYQUINOLINE Systemic†

VA CLASSIFICATION (Primary): DX201
Note: For a listing of dosage forms and brand names by country availability, see *Dosage Forms* section(s).

†Not commercially available in Canada.

## Category

Diagnostic aid, radioactive (inflammatory lesions; thrombosis).

## Indications

Note: Bracketed information in the *Indications* section refers to uses that are not included in U.S. product labeling.

### Accepted
Leukocytes, labeling of:
   Indium In 111 oxyquinoline is indicated for the labeling of autologous leukocytes. Indium In 111–labeled leukocytes are used for the following diagnostic studies:

Inflammatory lesions (diagnosis)—To locate inflammatory lesions such as abscesses. Indium In 111–labeled leukocytes are commonly used for the diagnosis of intra-abdominal abscesses, which may occur as complications of surgery, injuries, or inflammatory diseases of the gastrointestinal tract. Also, since labeled leukocytes localize in the inflamed gut mucosa, they are useful for demonstrating the presence, distribution, and extent of inflammatory bowel disease, including Crohn's disease and ulcerative colitis. In addition, labeled leukocytes are useful for demonstrating infections of prosthetic vascular grafts, and pyelonephritis and cystitis. Labeled leukocytes serve to evaluate acute and chronic osteomyelitis and are effective in demonstrating or excluding infection of orthopedic prostheses. The pattern of pulmonary uptake (diffuse vs. focal) of indium In 111–labeled leukocytes is used to rule out pulmonary or pleural infection, especially when chest x-rays are abnormal.

Indium In 111–labeled leukocyte scans have become useful as an adjunct to other diagnostic procedures in the detection of gastrointestinal and central nervous system (CNS) infections, such as focal encephalitis, cryptococcal meningitis, and cytomegalovirus encephalitis, in acquired immunodeficiency syndrome (AIDS) patients.

Ultrasound or computed tomography may be the preferred method for anatomical delineation of the infectious process when the location of the abscess is fairly well known. Indium In 111 oxyquinoline–labeled leukocyte imaging is recommended when neither of those methods has been successful or when the results have been ambiguous.

[Platelets, labeling of]:
Indium In 111 oxyquinoline is used for the labeling of autologous platelets to be used for the following studies:

[Platelet survival studies]—For the evaluation of platelet kinetics in patients with thrombocytopenia of uncertain etiology (where accelerated platelet destruction may be a contributory mechanism).

[Thrombosis, cardiac (diagnosis)]; and

[Thrombosis, arterial and deep venous (diagnosis)]—For the scintigraphic localization of cardiac thrombi and arterial or deep venous thrombosis.

## Physical Properties
### Nuclear data

| Radionuclide (half-life) | Mode of decay | Principal photon emissions (keV) | Mean number of emissions/ disintegration |
| --- | --- | --- | --- |
| In 111 (2.83 days) | Electron capture | Gamma (171.3) Gamma (245.3) | 0.90 0.94 |

## Pharmacology/Pharmacokinetics
### Mechanism of action/Effect
Labeling of leukocytes—
When incubated with leukocytes, which have been isolated from whole blood, the indium-oxyquinoline complex, being lipid-soluble, penetrates the cell membrane of the leukocytes. Within the cell the radioactive indium dissociates from oxyquinoline and becomes firmly attached to cytoplasmic components, while the nonradioactive oxyquinoline is released by the cell.

Diagnosis of inflammatory lesions: The radioactive autologous leukocytes are subsequently reinjected to permit the detection of inflammatory lesions based on the normal physiological accumulation of leukocytes at such sites.

Labeling of platelets—
Diagnosis of thrombosis: The radiolabeled autologous platelets, when reinjected, deposit at sites of vascular endothelium injury as a normal hemostatic response. This permits detection of thrombi.

### Distribution
Indium In 111–labeled leukocytes—
Distribution of labeled leukocytes is dependent on the predominance of the cell types labeled and their condition.

Leukocytes tend to concentrate at sites of inflammation (50 to 75% of circulating cells). However, there is an initial accumulation of radioactivity in the lungs, half of which is cleared in 15 minutes and the remainder slowly (by 4 hours after injection there is no notable radioactivity in normal lungs). Twenty-five to 50% of the radioactivity is subsequently distributed in spleen, liver, and bone marrow. Cells with lowered viability give high levels of activity in the liver, while a preparation with higher viability but contaminated with red cells and lymphocytes results in high levels of radioactivity in the spleen.

Radioactivity in liver and spleen reaches a plateau at 2 to 48 hours after injection with no significant clearance observed at 72 hours.

Indium In 111–labeled platelets—
Some of the labeled platelets are rapidly taken up in the spleen and liver (about 30 and 10% of the injected dose, respectively). The remaining cells (60%) are cleared from the blood with a half-time of 4 to 5 days, and are distributed in red bone marrow, liver, spleen, and other tissues (about 25, 20, 5, and 10% of the injected dose, respectively).

### Half-life
Biological—
Clearance of indium In 111–labeled leukocytes from whole blood: 5 to 10 hours.
Clearance of indium In 111–labeled platelets from whole blood: 7 to 10 days.

### Time to radioactivity visualization
Images of indium In 111–labeled leukocyte (or platelet) localization at inflammatory sites may be obtained as early as 4 hours after injection, but optimal images are obtained at 18 to 24 hours following administration.

### Radiation dosimetry

| | Estimated absorbed radiation dose* | | | |
| --- | --- | --- | --- | --- |
| Organ | Indium-labeled leukocytes† | | Indium-labeled platelets | |
| | mGy/ MBq | rad/ mCi | mGy/ MBq | rad/ mCi |
| Spleen | 5.5 | 20.35 | 7.5 | 27.75 |
| Liver | 0.71 | 2.63 | 0.73 | 2.70 |
| Red marrow | 0.69 | 2.55 | 0.36 | 1.33 |
| Pancreas | 0.52 | 1.92 | 0.66 | 2.44 |
| Bone surfaces | 0.35 | 1.30 | 0.23 | 0.85 |
| Kidneys | 0.33 | 1.22 | 0.41 | 1.52 |
| Adrenals | 0.31 | 1.15 | 0.37 | 1.37 |
| Stomach wall | 0.28 | 1.04 | 0.35 | 1.30 |
| Heart | 0.17 | 0.63 | 0.39 | 1.44 |
| Small intestine | 0.16 | 0.59 | 0.14 | 0.52 |
| Large intestine (upper) | 0.16 | 0.59 | 0.14 | 0.52 |
| Lungs | 0.16 | 0.59 | 0.28 | 1.04 |
| Large intestine (lower) | 0.13 | 0.48 | 0.097 | 0.36 |
| Ovaries | 0.12 | 0.44 | 0.098 | 0.36 |
| Uterus | 0.12 | 0.44 | 0.095 | 0.35 |
| Breast | 0.090 | 0.33 | 0.10 | 0.37 |
| Bladder wall | 0.072 | 0.27 | 0.066 | 0.24 |
| Thyroid | 0.061 | 0.23 | 0.081 | 0.30 |
| Testes | 0.045 | 0.17 | 0.043 | 0.16 |
| Other tissue | 0.11 | 0.41 | 0.12 | 0.44 |

| Radionuclide and impurities | Effective dose* | | | |
| --- | --- | --- | --- | --- |
| | Indium-labeled leukocytes | | Indium-labeled platelets | |
| | mSv/ MBq | rem/ mCi | mSv/ MBq | rem/ mCi |
| In 111 | 0.59 | 2.18 | 0.70 | 2.59 |
| In 114m‡ | 69 | 255 | 83 | 307 |

*For adults. Data based on the International Commission on Radiological Protection (ICRP) Publication 53—Radiation Dose to Patients from Radiopharmaceuticals.

†The actual leukocyte suspension used for labeling may also contain erythrocytes and thrombocytes, which become labeled at the same time. There may also be some unbound activity. Radiation contributions from these other fractions of activity have to be considered.

‡Impurity. Radionuclidic impurity at calibration time is not greater then 0.037 MBq (1 microcurie) of indium In 114m per 37 MBq (1 millicurie) of indium In 111.

### Elimination
Renal and fecal. Negligible amount (less than 1%) of the injected dose eliminated in 24 hours.

## Precautions to Consider
### Carcinogenicity
Although earlier studies suggested oxyquinoline might have a carcinogenic potential, recent studies have not shown a carcinogenic effect in rats or mice given oxyquinoline in feed at concentrations of 1500 or 3000 parts per million for 103 weeks. In any case, the carcinogenic potential of oxyquinoline is of no real concern since the oxyquinoline that is released from the cell following radiolabeling is probably removed from the preparation by subsequent cell washings.

### Pregnancy/Reproduction
Pregnancy—The possibility of pregnancy should be assessed in women of child-bearing potential. Clinical situations exist where the benefit to the patient and fetus, from information derived from radiopharmaceutical use, outweighs the risks from fetal exposure to radiation. In these situations, the physician should use discretion and reduce the radiopharmaceutical dose to the lowest possible amount.

For indium In 111 oxyquinoline–labeled leukocytes—
Indium In 111 (injected as chloride) crosses the placenta. Studies have not been done in humans with indium In 111 oxyquinoline–labeled leukocytes.
Studies have not been done in animals.
FDA Pregnancy Category C.

### Breast-feeding
Indium In 111 is excreted in breast milk in small concentrations (0.09 Bq/mL per megabecquerel [0.09 nCi/mL per millicurie] injected). Because of the potential risk to the infant from radiation exposure, temporary discontinuation of nursing is recommended for a short period of time (e.g., 24 hours), at the end of which milk should be expressed and discarded.

### Pediatrics
Although indium In 111–labeled leukocytes (and platelets) are used in children, there have been no specific studies evaluating safety and efficacy of indium In 111 oxyquinoline in pediatric patients. When this radiopharmaceutical is used in children, the diagnostic benefit should be judged to outweigh the potential risk of radiation.

### Geriatrics
Appropriate studies on the relationship of age to the effects of indium In 111–labeled leukocytes (or platelets) have not been performed in the geriatric population. However, no geriatrics-specific problems have been documented to date.

### Drug interactions and/or related problems
See *Diagnostic interference*.

### Diagnostic interference
The following have been selected on the basis of their potential clinical significance (possible effect in parentheses where appropriate)—not necessarily inclusive (» = major clinical significance):

With results of *indium In 111–labeled leukocyte* studies

Cell clumping
(clumping of cells in final preparation may produce false positive results, especially if images are taken early after injection [approximately 4 hours] because of focal accumulation of radioactivity in lungs)

Contamination by red blood cells or platelets
(red blood cells or platelets in final preparation may produce cardiac blood pool activity)

Plasma contamination
(plasma contamination may impair labeling efficiency of leukocytes since transferrin in plasma competes for indium In 111 oxyquinoline)

*Due to other medications*

Antibiotics, long-term therapy, or
Corticosteroids or
Hyperalimentation or
Lidocaine, with higher-than-therapeutic concentrations or
Procainamide, with higher-than-therapeutic concentrations
(may produce false negative results because of decreased chemotaxis)

*Due to medical problems or conditions*

Aspiration or
Atelectasis or
Congestive heart failure or
Cystic fibrosis or
Embolism, pulmonary or
Metastases or
Post-cardiopulmonary resuscitation or
Post-radiation therapy or
Pulmonary hemorrhage or
Respiratory distress syndrome, adult or
Uremia or
Vasculitis or
Wegener's granulomatosis
(may produce diffuse pulmonary uptake of indium In 111–labeled leukocytes)

Gastrointestinal bleeding
(may produce false positive images because of localization in bowel)

Hematomas
(may produce false positive images)

Infection, chronic
(may produce false negative images)

Leukopenia
(may decrease leukocyte labeling efficiency because of small number of available leukocytes; the use of donor cells may be considered in leukopenic patients)

Pneumonitis or
Respiratory infections, upper
(swallowed purulent sputum may cause false positive images)

*Due to other diagnostic tests*

Gallium citrate Ga 67 scan, previous
(background Ga 67 activity may preclude In 111–leukocyte study for at least 1 month)

With results of *indium In 111–labeled platelet* studies

Contamination by red blood cells
(red blood cells in final preparation may produce cardiac blood pool activity)

*Due to other medications*

Heparin
(although studies of the effect of heparin on In 111–labeled platelet accumulation on venous thrombi have yielded contradictory results, the possibility should be considered that false negative test results may occur in heparin-treated patients)

*Due to medical problems or conditions*

Hematoma
(false positive images may result because of accumulation of indium In 111–labeled platelets at sites of bleeding [e.g., due to venipuncture])

### Medical considerations/Contraindications
The medical considerations/contraindications included have been selected on the basis of their potential clinical significance (reasons given in parentheses where appropriate)—not necessarily inclusive (» = major clinical significance).
See also *Diagnostic interference*.

**Risk-benefit should be considered when the following medical problem exists:**

Sensitivity to the radiopharmaceutical preparation

## Side/Adverse Effects
The following side/adverse effects have been selected on the basis of their potential clinical significance (possible signs and symptoms in parentheses where appropriate)—not necessarily inclusive:

**Those indicating need for medical attention**
Incidence less frequent or rare
*Allergic reaction* (skin rash, hives, or itching); *pyrogenic reaction from indium In 111–labeled leukocytes (or platelets)* (fever)—may also be clinical sign of abscess

## Patient Consultation
As an aid to patient consultation, refer to *Advice for the Patient, Radiopharmaceuticals (Diagnostic)*.
In providing consultation, consider emphasizing the following selected information (» = major clinical significance):

### Description of use
Action in the body: Concentration of radioactivity at sites of infection or thrombosis allows images to be obtained

Small amounts of radioactivity used in diagnosis; radiation received is low and considered safe

### Before having this test
» Conditions affecting use, especially:
Pregnancy—Indium In 111 (administered as chloride) crosses the placenta; risk to fetus from radiation exposure as opposed to benefit derived from use should be considered

Breast-feeding—Small concentration of radioactivity excreted in breast milk; temporary discontinuation of nursing recommended because of risk to infant from radiation exposure

Use in children—Risk from radiation exposure as opposed to benefit derived from use should be considered

### Preparation for this test
Special preparatory instructions may apply; patient should inquire in advance

### Precautions after having this test
No special precautions

### Side/adverse effects
Signs of potential side effects, especially pyrogenic and allergic reactions

## General Dosing Information
Radiopharmaceuticals are to be administered only by or under the supervision of physicians who have had extensive training in the safe use and handling of radioactive materials and who are authorized by the appropriate Federal or State agency, if required, or, outside the U.S., the appropriate authority.

# Indium In 111 Oxyquinoline (Systemic)

Indium In 111 oxyquinoline solution is *not* administered directly. It is intended only for use in the preparation of indium In 111–labeled leukocytes (or platelets).

The manufacturer's package insert or other appropriate literature should be consulted for the specific method of labeling leukocytes and for optimal times when imaging should be performed.

### Safety considerations for handling this radiopharmaceutical
Improper handling of this radiopharmaceutical may cause radioactive contamination. Guidelines for handling radioactive material have been prepared by scientific, professional, state, federal, and international bodies and are available to the specially qualified and authorized users who have access to radiopharmaceuticals.

## Parenteral Dosage Forms

Note: Bracketed uses in the *Dosage Forms* section refer to categories of use and/or indications that are not included in U.S. product labeling.

### INDIUM In 111 OXYQUINOLINE SOLUTION USP

**Usual adult and adolescent administered activity**
Diagnosis of inflammatory lesions—
   Intravenous, 7.4 to 18.5 megabecquerels (200 to 500 microcuries) of indium In 111 oxyquinoline–labeled leukocytes.
[Platelet survival studies]—
   Intravenous, 0.74 to 18.5 megabecquerels (20 to 500 microcuries) of indium In 111 oxyquinoline–labeled platelets.
[Diagnosis of thrombosis]—
   Intravenous, 18.5 megabecquerels (500 microcuries) of indium In 111 oxyquinoline–labeled platelets.

**Usual pediatric administered activity**
Dosage has not been established.

Note: In the diagnosis of acute inflammatory conditions, in children and adolescents, dosages of 0.26 to 0.30 megabecquerel (7 to 8 microcuries) of indium In 111 oxyquinoline–labeled leukocytes per kg of body weight have been used. However, in most clinical studies a total dosage of 1.8 to 3.7 megabecquerels (50 to 100 microcuries) is recommended for optimal imaging quality.

**Usual geriatric administered activity**
See *Usual adult and adolescent administered activity*.

**Strength(s) usually available**
U.S.—
   37 megabecquerels (1 millicurie) per mL at calibration date (Rx) [GENERIC].
Note: Indium In 111 oxyquinoline solution is *not* administered directly. It is intended only for use in the preparation of indium In 111 oxyquinoline–labeled leukocytes (or platelets).
Canada—
   Not commercially available.

**Packaging and storage**
Store between 15 and 25 °C (59 and 77 °F), unless otherwise specified by manufacturer.

Note: The labeled leukocytes may be stored between 15 and 30 °C (59 and 86 °F), for up to 3 hours.

**Stability**
Do not use if cell clumping is observed in final preparation.
Indium In 111 oxyquinoline solution should be used for labeling within 5 days after the calibration date.
Indium In 111 oxyquinoline–labeled leukocytes should preferably be administered within 1 hour of labeling. Administration of labeled leukocytes beyond 3 hours after preparation is not recommended since chemotaxis of granulocytes deteriorates during storage, causing false negative images.

**Note**
Caution—Radioactive material.

## Selected Bibliography

Gerzof SG, Oates ME. Imaging techniques for infections in the surgical patient. Surg Clin North Am 1988; 68(1): 147-65.
Loken MK, Clay ME, Carpenter RT, et al. Clinical use of indium-111 labeled blood products. Clinical Nucl Med 1985; 10(12): 902-11.
Datz FL. Physiologic imaging of radiolabeled leukocytes. Am J Physiol Imaging 1987; 2(4): 196-207.
Datz FL. Radiolabeled leukocytes and platelets. Invest Radiol 1986; 21(3): 191-200.
Intenzo CM, Desai AG, Thakur ML, et al. Comparison of leukocytes labeled with indium 111-2-mercaptopyridine-N-oxide and indium 111 oxine for abscess detection. J Nucl Med 1987; 28(4): 438-41.

Revised: 01/18/93
Interim revision: 08/02/94

---

# INDIUM In 111 PENTETATE   Systemic†

VA CLASSIFICATION (Primary): DX201
Commonly used brand name(s): *Indium DTPA In 111*.
Note: For a listing of dosage forms and brand names by country availability, see *Dosage Forms* section(s).

†Not commercially available in Canada.

## Category
Diagnostic aid, radioactive (cerebrospinal fluid flow disorders).

## Indications

### Accepted
Cisternography, radionuclide—Indium In 111 pentetate ($^{111}$In-DTPA) is indicated as an imaging agent in cisternography to study the flow of cerebrospinal fluid (CSF) in the brain, to diagnose abnormalities in CSF circulation, to assess and help localize the site of CSF leakage, and to test the patency of or localize blocks in CSF shunts.

Also, cisternography with $^{111}$In-DTPA is used in the diagnosis and classification of hydrocephalus, especially normal pressure hydrocephalus, and in the evaluation of obstructive hydrocephalus.

$^{111}$In-DTPA cisternography is useful to detect, localize, and quantify CSF rhinorrhea, especially when the CSF leaks are small, intermittent, or questionable.

In preterm infants with hydrocephalus, lumbar cisternography using $^{111}$In-DTPA helps to evaluate CSF dynamics and the patency of the cerebral ventricular system.

## Physical Properties

### Nuclear data

| Radionuclide (half-life) | Mode of decay | Principal photon emissions (keV) | Mean number of emissions/ disintegration |
|---|---|---|---|
| In 111 (2.83 days) | Electron capture | Gamma (171.3) | 0.90 |
| | | Gamma (245.4) | 0.94 |

## Pharmacology/Pharmacokinetics

### Mechanism of action/Effect
The use of indium In 111 pentetate ($^{111}$In-DTPA) in radionuclide cisternography is based on its distribution. When administered intrathecally, this agent diffuses to the basal, sylvian, and cerebral cisterns and subarachnoid space around the convexity of the brain; it is then absorbed via the subarachnoid granulations into the bloodstream. Since this transit can be followed by means of external imaging, any deviations from the normal pattern can be detected. Significant abnormalities may be manifest as delayed or non-appearance of the agent in the subarachnoid space around the convexity of the brain or as reflux of the agent into the cerebral ventricles. The site of CSF leakage may be identified by an abnormal collection of activity. When $^{111}$In-DTPA is used to test the patency of CSF shunts (e.g., ventriculoperitoneal), absent or markedly diminished accumulation in and transit through the shunt tubing is an indication of obstruction.

### Distribution
Diffuses to the basal, sylvian, and cerebral cisterns and subarachnoid space around the convexity of the brain, and is subsequently absorbed into the bloodstream.

### Time to radioactivity visualization
Basal cisterns—2 to 4 hours.
Subarachnoid space around the convexity of the brain—24 hours (in patients with no significant abnormalities).

### Radiation dosimetry

| Organ | Estimated absorbed radiation dose* | | | |
|---|---|---|---|---|
| | Lumbar injection | | Cisternal injection | |
| | mGy/MBq | rad/mCi | mGy/MBq | rad/mCi |
| Spinal cord | 0.95 | 3.51 | 0.57 | 2.10 |
| Red marrow | 0.24 | 0.88 | 0.14 | 0.52 |
| Bladder wall | 0.20 | 0.74 | 0.18 | 0.67 |
| Adrenals | 0.16 | 0.59 | 0.065 | 0.24 |
| Bone surfaces | 0.072 | 0.27 | 0.076 | 0.28 |
| Small intestine | 0.060 | 0.22 | 0.023 | 0.085 |
| Large intestine (upper) | 0.047 | 0.17 | 0.019 | 0.070 |
| Uterus | 0.044 | 0.16 | 0.029 | 0.11 |
| Spleen | 0.040 | 0.15 | 0.019 | 0.070 |
| Stomach wall | 0.040 | 0.15 | 0.027 | 0.10 |
| Ovaries | 0.039 | 0.14 | 0.020 | 0.074 |
| Liver | 0.036 | 0.13 | 0.017 | 0.063 |
| Lungs | 0.033 | 0.12 | 0.022 | 0.081 |
| Large intestine (lower) | 0.024 | 0.089 | 0.015 | 0.056 |
| Thyroid | 0.021 | 0.078 | 0.039 | 0.14 |
| Testes | 0.011 | 0.040 | 0.0085 | 0.031 |
| Breast | 0.010 | 0.037 | 0.0096 | 0.035 |
| Other tissue | 0.027 | 0.10 | 0.017 | 0.063 |

| Radionuclide and impurities | Effective dose* | | | |
|---|---|---|---|---|
| | Lumbar injection | | Cisternal injection | |
| | mSv/MBq | rem/mCi | mSv/MBq | rem/mCi |
| In 111 | 0.14 | 0.52 | 0.12 | 0.44 |
| In 114m † | 1.8 | 6.67 | 2.1 | 7.78 |

*For adults. Data based on the International Commission on Radiological Protection (ICRP) Publication 53—Radiation dose to patients from radiopharmaceuticals.

†Impurity. Radionuclidic purity at calibration time is at least 99.88% with less than 0.06% indium In 114m and 0.06% zinc Zn 65. The concentration of each radionuclidic contaminant changes with time.

### Elimination
Renal; about 65% of the injected activity eliminated within 24 hours in normal subjects.

## Precautions to Consider

### Carcinogenicity/Mutagenicity
Long-term animal studies to evaluate carcinogenic or mutagenic potential of indium In 111 pentetate ([111]In-DTPA) have not been performed.

### Pregnancy/Reproduction
Pregnancy—Indium In 111 crosses the placenta. However, studies have not been done in humans with [111]In-DTPA.

The possibility of pregnancy should be assessed in women of child-bearing potential. Clinical situations exist where the benefit to the patient and fetus, based on information derived from radiopharmaceutical use, outweighs the risks from fetal exposure to radiation. In these situations, the physician should use discretion and reduce the radiopharmaceutical dose to the lowest possible amount.

Studies have not been done in animals.

FDA Pregnancy Category C.

### Breast-feeding
It is not known whether indium In 111 is distributed into breast milk. Because of the potential risk to the infant from radiation exposure, temporary discontinuation of nursing is recommended for a length of time that may be assessed by measuring the activity of breast milk and estimating the radiation exposure to the infant.

### Pediatrics
Although [111]In-DTPA is used in children, there have been no specific studies evaluating safety and efficacy of [111]In-DTPA in pediatric patients. When this radiopharmaceutical is used in children, the diagnostic benefit should be judged to outweigh the potential risk of radiation.

### Geriatrics
Appropriate studies on the relationship of age to the effects of [111]In-DTPA have not been performed in the geriatric population. However, no geriatrics-specific problems have been documented to date.

### Drug interactions and/or related problems
The following drug interactions and/or related problems have been selected on the basis of their potential clinical significance (possible mechanism in parentheses where appropriate)—not necessarily inclusive (» = major clinical significance):

Note: Combinations containing any of the following medications, depending on the amount present, may also interfere with the diagnostic imaging.

Acetazolamide
(inhibition of carbonic anhydrase by acetazolamide may decrease the rate of cerebrospinal fluid [CSF] production by the choroid plexus, thus altering CSF kinetics; may result in a false-positive cisternogram)

### Medical considerations/Contraindications
The medical considerations/contraindications included have been selected on the basis of their potential clinical significance (reasons given in parentheses where appropriate)—not necessarily inclusive (» = major clinical significance).

*Risk-benefit should be considered when the following medical problems exist:*
Renal function impairment, severe
(elimination of the agent may be delayed or impaired)
Sensitivity to the radiopharmaceutical preparation

## Side/Adverse Effects
The following side/adverse effects have been selected on the basis of their potential clinical significance (possible signs and symptoms in parentheses where appropriate)—not necessarily inclusive:

**Those indicating need for medical attention**
Incidence rare
*Aseptic meningitis* (severe drowsiness; fever; severe headache; continuing loss of appetite; nausea; vomiting)

## Patient Consultation
As an aid to patient consultation, refer to *Advice for the Patient, Radiopharmaceuticals (Diagnostic).*

In providing consultation, consider emphasizing the following selected information (» = major clinical significance):

### Description of use
Action in the body: Distribution mimics that of cerebrospinal fluid
Transit of agent may be visualized by external imaging
Small amounts of radioactivity used in diagnosis; radiation received is low and considered safe

### Before having this test
» Conditions affecting use, especially:
Sensitivity to the radiopharmaceutical preparation
Pregnancy—[111]In-DTPA may cross placenta; risk to fetus from radiation exposure as opposed to benefit derived from use should be considered
Breast-feeding—Not known if distributed into breast milk; temporary discontinuation of nursing recommended because of risk to infant from radiation exposure
Use in children—Risk from radiation exposure as opposed to benefit derived from use should be considered

### Preparation for this test
Special preparatory instructions may be given; patient should inquire in advance

### Side/adverse effects
Signs of potential side effects, especially aseptic meningitis

## General Dosing Information
Radiopharmaceuticals are to be administered only by or under the supervision of physicians who have had extensive training in the safe use and handling of radioactive materials and who are authorized by the the appropriate Federal or State agency, if required, or, outside the U.S., the appropriate authority.

### Safety considerations for handling this radiopharmaceutical
Improper handling of this radiopharmaceutical may cause radioactive contamination. Guidelines for handling radioactive material have been pre-

## Parenteral Dosage Forms

### INDIUM In 111 PENTETATE INJECTION USP

**Usual adult and adolescent administered activity**
Cisternography—
  Intrathecal, 18.5 megabecquerels (500 microcuries).

**Usual pediatric administered activity**
Dosage must be individualized by physician.

**Usual geriatric administered activity**
See *Usual adult and adolescent administered activity.*

**Strength(s) usually available**
U.S.—
  37 megabecquerels (1 millicurie) per mL (total activity, 55.5 megabecquerels [1.5 millicuries] per single-dose vial) at calibration time (Rx) [*Indium DTPA In 111*].
Canada—
  Not commercially available.

**Packaging and storage**
Store between 5 and 30 °C (41 and 86 °F), unless otherwise specified by manufacturer.

**Stability**
Do not use if contents are turbid.
Injection should be administered within 7 days after the calibration date.
Discard after single use.

**Note**
Caution—Radioactive material.

### Selected Bibliography

Wolbers JG, van Halderen P, van Lingen A, et al. Quantitative radioisotope cisternography for the investigation of CSF circulation in the posterior fossa and basal cisterns—a preliminary report. Neurosurgery 1986; 9(1–2): 125-8.

Maeda T, Ishida H, Matsuda H, et al. The utility of radionuclide myelography and cisternography in the progress of cerebrospinal fluid leaks. Eur J Nucl Med 1984; 9(9): 416-8.

Revised: 04/30/96

---

# INDIUM IN 111 PENTETREOTIDE Systemic†

VA CLASSIFICATION (Primary): DX201

Commonly used brand name(s): *OctreoScan.*

Note: For a listing of dosage forms and brand names by country availability, see *Dosage Forms* section(s).

†Not commercially available in Canada.

## Category
Diagnostic aid, radioactive (neuroendocrine tumors).

## Indications

**Accepted**

Neuroendocrine tumors (diagnosis)—Indium In 111 pentetreotide is indicated for the scintigraphic localization of primary and metastatic neuroendocrine tumors bearing somatostatin receptors, mainly growth hormone–secreting pituitary tumors, endocrine pancreatic tumors, carcinoids, other neuroendocrine tumors with typical amine precursor uptake and decarboxylation (APUD) characteristics (e.g., paragangliomas, medullary thyroid carcinomas, some pheochromocytomas, and small cell lung carcinomas), neuroblastomas, brain tumors (e.g., meningiomas and glial tumors, especially astrocytomas), Merkel cell tumors, lymphomas, and certain breast carcinomas.

A drawback of indium In 111 pentetreotide for the localization of pheochromocytomas in the adrenal gland is its relatively high accumulation in the kidneys; therefore, I 123 or I 131 iobenguane ($^{123}$I- or $^{131}$I-mIBG) may be preferable for this use. However, indium In 111 pentetreotide and $^{123}$I- or $^{131}$I-mIBG appear to be similar and complementary, providing comparable information in many patients; each provides superior results in some patients.

## Physical Properties

**Nuclear Data**

| Radionuclide (half-life) | Mode of decay | Principal photon emissions (keV) | Mean number of emissions/ disintegration |
|---|---|---|---|
| In 111 (2.83 days) | Electron capture | Gamma (171.3) | 0.90 |
| | | Gamma (245.4) | 0.94 |

## Pharmacology/Pharmacokinetics

**Mechanism of action/Effect**

Pentetreotide, a diethylenetriaminepentaacetic (DTPA) conjugate of octreotide (an analog of somatostatin), binds to somatostatin receptors on cell surfaces throughout the body. Tumors containing a high density of somatostatin receptors concentrate indium In 111-labeled pentetreotide. After clearance of blood activity, visualization of somatostatin receptor-positive tissue is achieved with scintigraphic imaging techniques.

**Distribution**

Within one hour of intravenous administration, indium In 111 pentetreotide is distributed from plasma to extravascular tissues and localizes in tumors as a function of the density of somatostatin receptors. Also, it localizes in the normal pituitary gland, thyroid gland, liver, spleen, urinary bladder, and to a lesser extent, in the bowel. Hepatic and biliary accumulation is 2% of the administered activity 4 hours after injection.

**Time to radioactivity visualization**
Optimal diagnostic images (planar and SPECT)—24 hours.

Note: Early scintigraphic demonstration of carcinoid liver metastases has been observed at 30 minutes, of meningiomas at 2 hours, and of small cell lung carcinomas at 4 hours postinjection of indium In 111 pentetreotide.

Repeat scintigraphy may be indicated at 48 hours when the 24-hour scintigram shows accumulation of radioactivity in the abdomen, which can represent normal bowel elimination of the indium In 111 pentetreotide.

**Radiation dosimetry**

| | Estimated absorbed radiation dose* | |
|---|---|---|
| Organ | mGy/MBq | rad/mCi |
| Spleen | 0.66 | 2.46 |
| Kidneys | 0.49 | 1.80 |
| Bladder wall | 0.27 | 1.01 |
| Liver | 0.11 | 0.41 |
| Large intestine (lower) | 0.07 | 0.26 |
| Adrenals | 0.068 | 0.25 |
| Thyroid | 0.067 | 0.25 |
| Uterus | 0.057 | 0.21 |
| Large intestine (upper) | 0.052 | 0.19 |
| Stomach wall | 0.052 | 0.19 |
| Ovaries | 0.044 | 0.16 |
| Small intestine | 0.043 | 0.16 |
| Red marrow | 0.031 | 0.12 |
| Testes | 0.026 | 0.097 |

Effective dose: 0.12 mSv/MBq (0.43 rem/mCi)†

*For adults; intravenous injection. Includes correction for maximum 0.1% indium In 114m contaminant, at calibration. Assumes 4.8 hour voiding interval. Data based on calculations by Oak Ridge Associated Universities, Radiopharmaceutical Internal Dose Information Center.

†Data estimated according to International Commission on Radiological Protection (ICRP) Publication 53—Radiation dose to patients from radiopharmaceuticals.

**Elimination**

Primarily renal. Fifty percent of the administered activity is excreted within 6 hours of injection, 85% within the first 24 hours, and over 90% by 2 days. During the first 4 hours after injection, indium In 111 pentetreotide appears predominantly in intact form (peptide-bound radioactivity) in the urine.

Less than 2% of the administered activity is found in the feces within 3 days after injection.

It is not known whether indium In 111 pentetreotide can be removed by dialysis.

## Precautions to Consider

### Carcinogenicity
Long-term animal studies to evaluate carcinogenic potential of indium In 111 pentetreotide have not been performed.

### Mutagenicity
No evidence of mutagenicity was found in an *in vitro* mouse lymphoma forward mutation assay and an *in vivo* mouse micronucleus assay.

### Pregnancy/Reproduction
Pregnancy—Indium In 111 administered as indium chloride crosses the placenta. Studies have not been done with indium In 111 pentetreotide in humans.

The possibility of pregnancy should be assessed in women of child-bearing potential. Clinical situations exist in which the benefit to the patient and fetus, based on information derived from radiopharmaceutical use, outweighs the risks from fetal exposure to radiation. In these situations, the physician should use discretion and reduce the radiopharmaceutical dose to the lowest possible amount.

Studies have not been done in animals.

FDA Pregnancy Category C.

### Breast-feeding
It is not known whether indium In 111 pentetreotide is distributed into breast milk. Because of the potential risk to the infant from radiation exposure, temporary discontinuation of nursing is recommended for a length of time that may be assessed by measuring the activity of breast milk and estimating the radiation exposure to the infant.

### Pediatrics
There have been no specific studies evaluating the safety and efficacy of indium In 111 pentetreotide in pediatric patients. When this radiopharmaceutical is used in children, the diagnostic benefit should be judged to outweigh the potential risk of radiation.

### Geriatrics
Diagnostic studies performed to date using indium In 111 pentetreotide have not demonstrated geriatrics-specific problems that would limit its usefulness in the elderly.

### Diagnostic interference
The following have been selected on the basis of their potential clinical significance (possible effect in parentheses where appropriate)—not necessarily inclusive (» = major clinical significance):

With results of *this* test
*Due to other medications*
Bleomycin
(may cause local pulmonary accumulation of indium In 111 pentetreotide)
Octreotide acetate
(concurrent administration of indium In 111 pentetreotide to patients receiving therapeutic doses of octreotide acetate may decrease the accumulation of radioactivity in the tumor; octreotide withdrawal for at least 12 hours is recommended)
Total parenteral nutrition (TPN) solutions
(administration of indium In 111 pentetreotide in TPN admixtures or into TPN intravenous lines may cause the formation of a complex glycosyl octreotide conjugate)
*Due to medical problems or conditions*
Cold/influenza
(may cause accumulation of radioactivity in the nasal region and lung hili)
Insulinomas
(administration of octreotide has produced severe hypoglycemia in patients with insulinomas; since pentetreotide is an analog of octreotide, an intravenous solution containing glucose should be administered before and during administration of indium In 111 pentetreotide to minimize the possibility of hypoglycemia)
Irradiation of lung, external
(may cause local pulmonary accumulation of indium In 111 pentetreotide)
Surgery, recent
(possible accumulation of radioactivity at sites of recent surgery)

### Medical considerations/Contraindications
The medical considerations/contraindications included have been selected on the basis of their potential clinical significance (reasons given in parentheses where appropriate)—not necessarily inclusive (» = major clinical significance).

*Risk-benefit should be considered when the following medical problems exist:*
Renal function impairment
(excretion of indium In 111 pentetreotide may be decreased)
Sensitivity to the radiopharmaceutical preparation

## Side/Adverse Effects

The following side/adverse effects have been selected on the basis of their potential clinical significance (possible signs and symptoms in parentheses where appropriate)—not necessarily inclusive:

**Those indicating need for medical attention only if they continue or are bothersome**
Incidence less frequent or rare (less than 1%)
*Dizziness; fever; flushing of skin; headache; hypotension* (dizziness or lightheadedness); *increased sweating; joint pain; nausea; unusual weakness*

## Patient Consultation

As an aid to patient consultation, refer to *Advice for the Patient, Radiopharmaceuticals (Diagnostic)*.

In providing consultation, consider emphasizing the following selected information (» = major clinical significance):

### Description of use
Action in the body: Localization at sites of tumor spread or growth
Tumor sites may be visualized by external imaging
Small amounts of radioactivity used in diagnosis; radiation received is relatively low and considered safe

### Before having this test
» Conditions affecting use, especially:
Sensitivity to the radiopharmaceutical preparation
Pregnancy—Indium In 111 as indium chloride crosses placenta; risk to fetus from radiation exposure as opposed to benefit derived from use should be considered
Breast-feeding—Not known if distributed into breast milk; temporary discontinuation of nursing recommended because of risk to infant from radiation exposure
Use in children—Risk of radiation exposure as opposed to benefit derived from use should be considered

### Preparation for this test
Special preparatory instructions may be given; patient should inquire in advance
Adequate intake of fluids before and after administration of indium In 111 pentetreotide; voiding as often as possible for 24 hours after administration to promote urine flow and to minimize radiation to bladder
Possible administration of a laxative before imaging, to minimize imaging interference due to radioactivity localization in stool

## General Dosing Information

Radiopharmaceuticals are to be administered only by or under the supervision of physicians who have had extensive training in the safe use and handling of radioactive materials and who are authorized by the appropriate Federal or State agency, if required, or, outside the U.S., the appropriate authority.

Adequate hydration of the patient is recommended before and after administration of indium In 111 pentetreotide to promote urinary flow and blood pool clearance. Also, urination is recommended as often as possible for 24 hours after examination to promote urine flow, thereby minimizing radiation to the bladder.

Laxative administration prior to initial or follow-up images may be considered to minimize radioactivity, which may interfere with image interpretation, in bowel, due to excretion of radiopharmaceutical into stool.

### Safety considerations for handling this radiopharmaceutical
Improper handling of this radiopharmaceutical may cause radioactive contamination. Guidelines for handling radioactive material have been prepared by scientific, professional, state, federal, and international bodies and are available to the specially qualified and authorized users who have access to radiopharmaceuticals.

## Parenteral Dosage Forms

### INDIUM In 111 PENTETREOTIDE INJECTION

**Usual adult and adolescent administered activity**
For diagnosis of neuroendocrine tumors—
  For planar imaging: Intravenous, 111 megabecquerels (3 millicuries).
  For SPECT imaging: Intravenous, 222 megabecquerels (6 millicuries).

**Usual pediatric administered activity**
Safety and efficacy have not been established.

**Usual geriatric administered activity**
See *Usual adult and adolescent administered activity*.

**Strength(s) usually available**
U.S.—
  10 micrograms of pentetreotide (DTPA-octreotide), 2 mg of gentisic acid, 4.9 mg of trisodium citrate (anhydrous), 0.37 mg of citric acid (anhydrous), and 10 mg of inositol, per 10-mL reaction vial; and in a separate 10-mL vial, 111 megabecquerels (3 millicuries) per mL of indium In 111 chloride sterile solution (Rx) [*OctreoScan*].
Canada—
  Not commercially available.

**Packaging and storage**
Before radiolabeling, store between 2 and 8 °C (36 and 46 °F), unless otherwise specified by manufacturer.

Note: After radiolabeling, injection should be stored at or below 25 °C (77 °F) and administered within 6 hours.

**Preparation of dosage form**
To prepare injection, the sterile, pyrogen-free indium In 111 chloride solution is combined with the contents of the reaction vial. See manufacturer's package insert for complete instructions.
Immediately before injection, the indium In 111 pentetreotide solution may be diluted with 0.9% sodium chloride injection to a maximum volume of 3 mL.

**Stability**
Injection should be administered within 6 hours after radiolabeling.

**Note**
Caution—Radioactive material.

## Selected Bibliography

Krenning EP, Kwekkeboom DJ, Bakker WH, et al. Somatostatin receptor scintigraphy with [$^{111}$In-DTPA-D-Phe$^1$]- and [$^{123}$I-Tyr$^3$]-octreotide: the Rotterdam experience with more than 1000 patients. Eur J Nucl Med 1993; 20(8): 716-31.

Developed: 01/24/95

---

# INDIUM In 111 SATUMOMAB PENDETIDE  Systemic†

VA CLASSIFICATION (Primary): DX201

Commonly used brand name(s): *OncoScint CR/OV*.

Note: For a listing of dosage forms and brand names by country availability, see *Dosage Forms* section(s).

†Not commercially available in Canada.

## Category

Diagnostic aid, radioactive (extrahepatic malignant disease).

## Indications

**Accepted**

Extrahepatic malignant disease (diagnosis)—Indium In 111 satumomab pendetide is indicated for use in immunoscintigraphy in patients with known colorectal or ovarian cancer. Indium In 111 satumomab pendetide helps determine the extent and location of extrahepatic foci of disease, and can be helpful in the preoperative determination of the resectability of malignant lesions in these patients. It helps clarify equivocal results of, and serves to complement, other diagnostic evaluations.

Indium In 111 satumomab pendetide immunoscintigraphy, when combined with computed tomography (CT) scans results and carcinoembryonic antigen (CEA) or serum tumor marker levels, provides complementary information useful in the presurgical evaluation of colorectal or ovarian cancer patients.

**Unaccepted**
Not indicated as a screening test for ovarian or colorectal cancer.

## Physical Properties

**Nuclear data**

| Radionuclide (half-life) | Mode of decay | Principal photon emissions (keV) | Mean number of emissions/ disintegration |
| --- | --- | --- | --- |
| In 111 (2.83 days) | Electron capture | Gamma (171.3) | 0.90 |
|  |  | Gamma (245.4) | 0.94 |

## Pharmacology/Pharmacokinetics

**Mechanism of action/Effect**
The murine monoclonal antibody of the immunoglobulin subclass IgG$_1$, satumomab (MAb B72.3), localizes or binds specifically to a tumor-associated glycoprotein (TAG-72), a cell surface antigen expressed at high levels on nearly all colorectal and ovarian adenocarcinomas. The monoclonal antibody B72.3 is site-specifically labeled with indium In 111 chloride using the linker-chelator, glycyl-tyrosyl-(N,epsilon-diethylenetriaminepentaacetic acid)-lysine or GYK-DTPA. The resultant radiolabeled monoclonal antibody conjugate, $^{111}$In satumomab pendetide (CYT-103), retains the immunoreactivity of the unconjugated monoclonal antibody. Following intravenous administration, the indium In 111–labeled satumomab pendetide travels through the bloodstream until it encounters tumors bearing the TAG-72 antigen. The distribution of radioactivity is recorded by imaging.

**Distribution**
Following intravenous administration, indium In 111 satumomab pendetide localizes rapidly in colorectal adenocarcinomas and common epithelial ovarian carcinomas. In *in vitro* immunohistologic studies indium In 111 satumomab pendetide has been reported to be reactive with the majority of breast, non–small cell lung, pancreatic, gastric, and esophageal carcinomas. Some non-antigen-dependent localization occurs, probably secondary to catabolism, in normal liver, spleen, and bone marrow. In some individuals, some radioactivity may localize in the bowel, blood pool, kidneys, urinary bladder, male genitalia, and breast nipples in women.

**Half-life**
Elimination—56±14 hours (mean±SD).

**Time to radioactivity visualization**
Optimal diagnostic images—48 to 72 hours.

Note: Variability occurs; diagnostic images have been obtained as early as 24 hours and as late as 120 hours after administration of the radiopharmaceutical. Delayed imaging allows clearance of the radiopharmaceutical from the cardiac and vascular pool, which improves image contrast.

### Radiation dosimetry

| Organ | Estimated absorbed radiation dose* | |
|---|---|---|
|  | mGy/MBq | rad/mCi |
| Spleen | 0.86 | 3.2 |
| Liver | 0.81 | 3.0 |
| Red marrow | 0.65 | 2.41 |
| Kidney | 0.52 | 1.93 |
| Lungs | 0.26 | 0.96 |
| Adrenal | 0.24 | 0.89 |
| Pancreas | 0.20 | 0.74 |
| Bone | 0.18 | 0.67 |
| Heart wall | 0.17 | 0.63 |
| Stomach wall | 0.17 | 0.63 |
| Large intestine wall (upper) | 0.17 | 0.63 |
| Small intestine | 0.16 | 0.59 |
| Ovaries | 0.16 | 0.59 |
| Bladder | 0.15 | 0.56 |
| Uterus | 0.15 | 0.56 |
| Large intestine wall (lower) | 0.14 | 0.52 |
| Other tissues | 0.12 | 0.44 |
| Skin | 0.09 | 0.33 |
| Thyroid | 0.08 | 0.30 |
| Testes | 0.08 | 0.30 |
| Total body | 0.15 | 0.55 |

Effective dose: 0.32 mSv/MBq (1.2 rem/mCi)

*For adults; intravenous injection. Includes absorbed radiation doses from both the indium In 111 and the indium In 114 contaminant. The maximum permissible level (0.16% at expiration time) of indium In 114 was used for dose estimates.

**Elimination**
Renal (10% of the administered activity excreted within 72 hours).
Note: The radioligand is excreted in the urine as a small molecular weight entity, which indicates that the indium In 111 has become catabolized from the immunoglobulin molecule.

## Precautions to Consider

**Cross-sensitivity and/or related problems**
Patients sensitive to murine antibody–based products may be sensitive to indium In 111 satumomab pendetide also.

**Carcinogenicity/Mutagenicity**
Long-term animal studies to evaluate carcinogenic or mutagenic potential of indium In 111 satumomab pendetide have not been performed.

**Pregnancy/Reproduction**
Pregnancy—Indium In 111 crosses the placenta. Studies have not been done with indium In 111 satumomab pendetide in humans.
The possibility of pregnancy should be assessed in women of child-bearing potential. Clinical situations exist where the benefit to the patient and fetus, based on information derived from radiopharmaceutical use, outweighs the risks from fetal exposure to radiation. In these situations, the physician should use discretion and reduce the radiopharmaceutical dose to the lowest possible amount.
Studies have not been done in animals.
FDA Pregnancy Category C.

**Breast-feeding**
In some women, indium In 111 satumomab pendetide has been found to localize in breast nipples. Because of the potential risk to the infant from radiation exposure, temporary discontinuation of nursing is recommended.

**Pediatrics**
There have been no specific studies evaluating the safety and efficacy of indium In 111 satumomab pendetide in pediatric patients. When this radiopharmaceutical is used in children, the diagnostic benefit should be judged to outweigh the potential risk of radiation.

**Geriatrics**
Diagnostic studies performed to date using indium In 111 satumomab pendetide have not demonstrated geriatrics-specific problems that would limit the usefulness of indium In 111 satumomab pendetide in the elderly.

**Laboratory value alterations**
The following have been selected on the basis of their potential clinical significance (possible effect in parentheses where appropriate)—not necessarily inclusive (» = major clinical significance):

With *other* diagnostic test results
Immunoassays, including carcinoembryonic antigen (CEA) and serum tumor marker (CA 125)
(human anti-murine antibodies [HAMAs] production may be induced by the administration of indium In 111 satumomab pendetide; HAMAs in serum may cause falsely elevated values of *in vitro* immunoassays; interference may persist for months; use of non-murine immunoassays, or HAMAs removal by adsorption, blocking, or heat inactivation is recommended to avoid interference)

**Diagnostic interference**
The following have been selected on the basis of their potential clinical significance (possible effect in parentheses where appropriate)—not necessarily inclusive (» = major clinical significance):

With results of *this* test
*Due to other medications*
Murine antibody–based products
(previous administration of murine antibody–based products, including this agent, may induce human anti-murine antibodies [HAMAs], which may alter the clearance and tissue biodistribution of indium In 111 satumomab pendetide; however, more studies are needed to establish the effects of circulating HAMAs on monoclonal antibody–based products)

*Due to medical problems or conditions*
Aneurysms, abdominal or
Bowel adhesions, postoperative or
Colostomy or
Inflammatory lesions, local or
Joint disease, degenerative or
Ovarian tumors, benign
(localization of indium In 111 satumomab pendetide may occur at these sites)

**Medical considerations/Contraindications**
The medical considerations/contraindications included have been selected on the basis of their potential clinical significance (reasons given in parentheses where appropriate)—not necessarily inclusive (» = major clinical significance):

*Risk-benefit should be considered when the following medical problem exists:*
Sensitivity to murine antibody–based products or to the radiopharmaceutical preparation

## Side/Adverse Effects

The following side/adverse effects have been selected on the basis of their potential clinical significance (possible signs and symptoms in parentheses where appropriate)—not necessarily inclusive:

**Those indicating need for medical attention**
Incidence less frequent
*Fever*

Incidence rare
*Allergic reaction, including anaphylaxis; chest pain; confusion; hypertension; hypotension; hypothermia; skin rash*

**Those indicating need for medical attention only if they continue or are bothersome**
Incidence less frequent or rare
*Chills; diarrhea; dizziness; flushing of skin; headache; joint pain; nausea; nervousness*

## Patient Consultation

As an aid to patient consultation, refer to *Advice for the Patient, Radiopharmaceuticals (Diagnostic)*.
In providing consultation, consider emphasizing the following selected information (» = major clinical significance):

**Description of use**
Action in the body: Localization at sites of tumor spread or growth
Tumor sites may be visualized by external imaging
Small amounts of radioactivity used in diagnosis; radiation received is low and considered safe

**Before having this test**
» Conditions affecting use, especially:
Sensitivity to murine antibody–based products or to the radiopharmaceutical preparation
Pregnancy—Indium In 111 crosses placenta; risk to fetus from radiation exposure as opposed to benefit derived from use should be considered

Breast-feeding—Indium In 111 satumomab pendetide may be distributed into breast milk; temporary discontinuation of nursing recommended because of risk to infant from radiation exposure

Use in children—Risk of radiation exposure as opposed to benefit derived from use should be considered

**Preparation for this test**

Special preparatory instructions may be given; patient should inquire in advance

Administration of a laxative, before imaging, to minimize imaging interference due to radioactivity localization in stool

**Side/adverse effects**

Signs of potential side effects, especially allergic reactions including anaphylaxis, fever, chest pain, confusion, hypertension, hypotension, hypothermia, skin rash

## General Dosing Information

Radiopharmaceuticals are to be administered only by or under the supervision of physicians who have had extensive training in the safe use and handling of radioactive materials and who are authorized by the Nuclear Regulatory Commission (NRC) or the appropriate Agreement State agency, if required, or, outside the U.S., the appropriate authority.

Laxative administration prior to initial or follow-up images is recommended to minimize radioactivity in bowel, which is due to uptake of isotope in stool and which may interfere with image interpretation.

**Safety considerations for handling this radiopharmaceutical**

Improper handling of this radiopharmaceutical may cause radioactive contamination. Guidelines for handling radioactive material have been prepared by scientific, professional, state, federal, and international bodies and are available to the specially qualified and authorized users who have access to radiopharmaceuticals.

**For treatment of adverse effects**

Epinephrine, antihistamines, and corticosteroid agents should be available during the administration of indium In 111 satumomab pendetide because of the possibility of allergic reactions.

## Parenteral Dosage Forms

### INDIUM In 111 SATUMOMAB PENDETIDE INJECTION

**Usual adult and adolescent administered activity**

For diagnosis of extrahepatic disease—Intravenous, 1 mg of satumomab pendetide radiolabeled with 185 megabecquerels (5 millicuries) of indium In 111 chloride, administered over a period of five minutes.

**Usual pediatric administered activity**

Safety and efficacy have not been established.

**Usual geriatric administered activity**

See *Usual adult and adolescent administered activity*.

**Strength(s) usually available**

U.S.—

1 mg of satumomab pendetide per 2 mL-single-dose vial of sodium phosphate–buffered saline solution (Rx) [*OncoScint CR/OV*].

Canada—

Not commercially available.

**Packaging and storage**

Before radiolabeling, store between 2 and 8 °C (36 and 46 °F), unless otherwise specified by manufacturer.

Note: Product should be brought to room temperature before radiolabeling.

After radiolabeling, injection may be kept at room temperature, up to 8 hours, until administration.

**Preparation of dosage form**

To prepare injection, a sterile, pyrogen-free indium In 111 chloride solution is used. Isoptope solution must be buffered with sodium acetate before adding to the satumomab pendetide solution. See manufacturer's package insert for instructions.

**Stability**

Injection should be administered within 8 hours after radiolabeling.

**Note**

Caution—Radioactive material.

## Selected Bibliography

Doerr RJ, Abdel-Nabi HH, Krag D, et al. Radiolabeled antibody imaging in the management of colorectal cancer. Ann Surg 1991; 214(2): 118-24.

Harwood SJ, Carroll RG, Webster WB, et al. Human biodistribution of $^{111}$In-labeled B72.3 monoclonal antibody. Cancer Res 1990;(Suppl) 50: 932S-936S.

Revised: 06/14/93
Interim revision: 08/02/94

---

**INDOMETHACIN**—See *Anti-inflammatory Drugs, Nonsteroidal (Ophthalmic)*; *Anti-inflammatory Drugs, Nonsteroidal (Systemic)*; *Indomethacin—For Patent Ductus Arteriosus (Systemic)*

---

# INDOMETHACIN—For Patent Ductus Arteriosus  Systemic

INN: Indometacin

VA CLASSIFICATION (Primary/Secondary):
Oral—MS102/MS400; CN850; CN105; CV900
Parenteral—CV900

Note: For information pertaining to use of indomethacin for other indications, see *Anti-inflammatory Drugs, Nonsteroidal (Systemic)*.

Commonly used brand name(s): *Apo-Indomethacin; Indameth; Indocid; Indocid PDA; Indocin; Indocin I.V; Novomethacin*.

Another commonly used name is indometacin.

Note: For a listing of dosage forms and brand names by country availability, see *Dosage Forms* section(s).

## Category

Ductus arteriosus, patent, closure adjunct.

## Indications

Note: Bracketed information in the *Indications* section refers to uses that are not included in U.S. product labeling.

### Accepted

Ductus arteriosus, patent (treatment)—Intravenous indomethacin sodium is indicated to induce pharmacologic closure of a hemodynamically significant patent ductus arteriosus (PDA) in premature infants weighing 500 to 1750 grams. Evidence of a hemodynamically significant PDA (such as respiratory distress, continuous murmur, hyperactive precordium, enlarged heart, congestion in the lungs, and associated constitutional symptoms) should be present prior to therapy. In the U.S., indomethacin is FDA-approved for administration only if these signs and symptoms persist after 48 hours of conservative treatment, such as fluid restriction, diuretics, and respiratory support. [However, some neonatologists recommend that indomethacin therapy be instituted as soon as possible after identification of the PDA, especially if echocardiography shows the presence of a significant left-to-right shunt and/or the infant is being mechanically ventilated.][1]

Some investigators have not found successful closure to be associated with birth weight or postnatal age. However, others have reported the medication's efficacy to be decreased in infants > 2 weeks of age (possibly because metabolism and/or clearance of indomethacin increases with neonatal age) and in infants weighing < 1000 grams (possibly because of insufficient muscular development in the ductal wall). Reopening of the ductus may occur following initial closure; although reclosure may occur spontaneously or in response to additional indomethacin, some infants may require surgery to achieve permanent closure.

[Indomethacin has also been administered orally (via a nasogastric tube) or rectally, as a suspension prepared from capsule contents, for this purpose.][1] However, intravenous administration is preferred because it produces more predictable indomethacin serum concentrations, leading to a higher closure rate (> 80%), than oral or rectal administration. Also, intravenous administration produces fewer gastrointestinal adverse effects than oral indomethacin.

[Indomethacin is not specifically approved by U.S. or Canadian regulatory agencies for administration to premature neonates without substantial evidence of a hemodynamically significant PDA. However, preliminary evidence suggests that administration at the first sign of a murmur (but no other symptoms) may prevent development of a symptomatic PDA in infants weighing < 1000 grams. These infants may be at greater risk of developing a symptomatic PDA than those with a murmur (but no other symptoms) weighing > 1000 grams.][1]

[1] Not included in Canadian product labeling.

## Pharmacology/Pharmacokinetics

### Physicochemical characteristics
Molecular weight—Indomethacin: 357.79.
Indomethacin sodium (trihydrate): 433.80.
pKa—4.5.

### Mechanism of action/Effect
Indomethacin inhibits the activity of the enzyme cyclo-oxygenase to decrease the formation of precursors of prostaglandins and thromboxanes from arachidonic acid. Inhibition of prostaglandin synthesis (and the consequent reduction of prostaglandin activity) permits constriction of the patent ductus arteriosus, which may be due to excessive production, and/or increased sensitivity of the premature ductus to the dilating effects, of prostaglandins of the E series.

### Other actions/effects
Indomethacin reversibly inhibits platelet aggregation. However, its antiplatelet effect, unlike that of aspirin, is reversible.

### Absorption
When administered via nasogastric tube—Poor and incomplete, possibly because of indomethacin's insolubility and/or abnormalities in gastric function (gastric acid secretion, gastric motility, etc.) or pH in premature neonates with a patent ductus arteriosus.

### Protein binding
Has not been determined in the premature neonate. Very high (99%), to albumin, in adults.

### Biotransformation
Hepatic; the rate of metabolism increases with neonatal age.

### Half-life
Greatly prolonged as compared with that reported in adults; varies inversely with postnatal age and weight. The prolonged half-life may reflect extensive and/or repeated enterohepatic circulation and re-entry into plasma.
Infants <7 days of age—3 to 60 hours; average 20 hours.
Infants >7 days of age—4 to 38 hours; average 12 hours.
Infants <1000 grams—9 to 60 hours; average 21 hours.
Infants >1000 grams—2 to 52 hours; average 15 hours.

### Peak serum concentration
Subject to wide individual variation when administered by any route but especially following oral administration.

### Elimination
Renal and biliary excretion of metabolites and of unchanged indomethacin. In adults, 10 to 20% of a dose is excreted in the urine as unchanged indomethacin; the quantity excreted unchanged in the premature neonate has not been determined.
In dialysis—Indomethacin is not dialyzable.

## Precautions to Consider

### Drug interactions and/or related problems
The following drug interactions and/or related problems have been selected on the basis of their potential clinical significance (possible mechanism in parentheses where appropriate)—not necessarily inclusive (» = major clinical significance):

Note: In addition to the interactions listed below, the possibility should be considered that additive or multiple effects leading to impaired blood clotting and/or increased risk of bleeding may occur if indomethacin is used concurrently with any medication having a significant potential for causing hypoprothrombinemia, thrombocytopenia, or gastrointestinal ulceration or hemorrhage.

» Aminoglycosides or
» Digitalis glycosides
(indomethacin may decrease renal clearance of aminoglycosides or digitalis glycosides, leading to increased plasma concentrations, elimination half-lives, and risk of aminoglycoside or digitalis toxicity; digitalis is not recommended for administration to a premature infant with an "isolated" patent ductus arteriosus; however, if digitalis administration should be required by an individual patient, it is recommended that digitalis dosage be reduced by 50% when indomethacin therapy is initiated and that further digitalis dose adjustment be based on monitoring of electrocardiogram (ECG) and digitalis concentration; dosage adjustment of aminoglycosides may also be required, based on evidence of toxicity and/or measurement of plasma concentration)

Nephrotoxic medications, other (See *Appendix II*)
(concurrent use with indomethacin may increase the risk and/or severity of adverse renal effects)

### Laboratory value alterations
The following have been selected on the basis of their potential clinical significance (possible effect in parentheses where appropriate)—not necessarily inclusive (» = major clinical significance):

With diagnostic test results
Urinary 5-hydroxyindoleacetic acid (5-HIAA) determinations
(false 5-HIAA concentration values may be measured via the Goldenberg modification of Undenfriend's method because indomethacin metabolites are structurally similar to 5-HIAA)

With physiology/laboratory test values
Bleeding time
(may be prolonged because of suppressed platelet aggregation; effects in the premature neonate may persist for several days after the medication is discontinued)

Blood glucose concentration
(may be decreased or, less frequently, increased)

Blood urea nitrogen (BUN) concentration and
Creatinine concentration, serum and
Glucose concentration, urine and
Potassium concentration, serum and
Protein (including albumin) concentrations, urine
(may be increased because indomethacin decreases glomerular filtration rate)

Chloride concentration, urine and
Creatinine clearance and
Free water clearance and
Glomerular filtration rate and
Osmolality, urine and
Potassium concentration, urine and
Sodium concentration, urine and
Sodium concentration, serum and
Urine volume
(may be decreased)

Note: Indomethacin may decrease both sodium and water excretion; however, water retention may exceed that of sodium so that the net effect is a reduction of serum sodium concentration (dilutional hyponatremia).

Leukocyte count and
Platelet count
(may be decreased)

Liver function tests, especially transaminase (AST [SGOT]; ALT [SGPT]) activity
(values may be increased; if significant abnormalities occur, clinical signs and symptoms consistent with liver disease develop, or systemic manifestations such as eosinophilia or rash occur, indomethacin should be discontinued)

Plasma renin activity (PRA)
(may be decreased; also, indomethacin may block the increase in PRA usually produced by bumetanide, furosemide, or indapamide)

### Medical considerations/Contraindications
The medical considerations/contraindications included have been selected on the basis of their potential clinical significance (reasons given in parentheses where appropriate)—not necessarily inclusive (» = major clinical significance).

*Except under special circumstances, this medication should not be used when the following medical problems exist:*

» Bleeding, active, especially intracranial or gastrointestinal or
» Coagulation defects
(increased risk of severe hemorrhage because indomethacin inhibits platelet aggregation and may cause gastrointestinal bleeding)

» Enterocolitis, necrotizing, proven or suspected
(may be exacerbated)

» Heart disease, congenital, such as:
Coarctation of the aorta, severe
Pulmonary atresia
Tetralogy of Fallot, severe or

» Lesions, severely obstructive, left-sided, other
(patency of the ductus arteriosus may be required to provide satisfactory pulmonary or systemic blood flow; indomethacin should not be administered until the safety of inducing closure has been determined)

» Infection, untreated, confirmed or suspected
    (symptoms of progression may be masked; also, sepsis may predispose the patient to renal insufficiency and increase the risk of renal impairment or failure; in addition, an unexpectedly high rate of treatment failure has been reported following indomethacin administration to infants with sepsis)

Jaundice, severe
    (in patients with severe jaundice, indomethacin may cause displacement of bilirubin and increased risk of kernicterus, and should be used with caution)

» Renal function impairment, severe, as determined by serum creatinine concentration higher than 1.2 to 1.4 mg per dL (106-124 micromols/L) or other appropriate tests
    (may be exacerbated)

*Risk-benefit should be considered when the following medical problems exist:*

Conditions predisposing to renal insufficiency, such as:
    Congestive heart failure
    Extracellular volume depletion
    Hepatic function impairment
        (increased risk of renal function impairment, including acute renal failure)

» Thrombocytopenia
    (increased risk of severe hemorrhage because indomethacin inhibits platelet aggregation and may cause gastrointestinal bleeding; although platelets may be administered if necessary, indomethacin should be used only when the risk of surgery outweighs the risk of administering blood products)

**Patient monitoring**

The following may be especially important in patient monitoring (other tests may be warranted in some patients, depending on condition; » = major clinical significance):

Electrolyte concentrations, serum and
Renal function tests
    (monitoring recommended during and following indomethacin administration; if renal function impairment occurs [as shown by a serum creatinine concentration greater than 1.2 to 1.4 mg per dL (106-124 micromols/L) or other appropriate tests], therapy should be suspended until adequate renal function has been restored)

## Side/Adverse Effects

The following side/adverse effects have been selected on the basis of their potential clinical significance (possible signs and symptoms in parentheses where appropriate)—not necessarily inclusive:

**Those indicating need for medical attention**
Incidence more frequent
    *Gastrointestinal problems; renal function impairment*

Note: *Renal function impairment* (incidence >40%) is characterized by decreases in urine volume; free water clearance; urine osmolality; glomerular filtration rate; creatinine clearance; and excretion of sodium, potassium, and chloride. Corresponding increases in blood urea nitrogen (BUN), blood creatinine, and serum potassium occur. Water retention may be greater than sodium retention, leading to dilutional hyponatremia.

*Gastrointestinal problems* reported include bleeding (incidence 3 to 9%), vomiting, abdominal distention, ileus, and gastric perforation (incidences 1 to 3%). These effects have been reported more frequently with oral (via a nasogastric tube) than with intravenous administration.

Incidence less frequent
    *Bleeding problems; hypoglycemia*

Note: *Bleeding problems* reported (in addition to gastrointestinal bleeding) include pulmonary hemorrhage, disseminated intravascular coagulopathy, microscopic hematuria, and oozing at needle puncture sites.

*Intracranial hemorrhage, necrotizing enterocolitis, and retrolental fibroplasia* have also been reported; however, the incidence in indomethacin-treated infants is not greater than that reported in other premature infants, who are known to be at risk for these complications.

Incidence rare
    *Acidosis; alkalosis; apnea; bradycardia; exacerbation of pre-existing pulmonary infection*

## General Dosing Information

Sterile indomethacin sodium is to be administered intravenously only, over a 5- to 10-second period. Extravasation must be avoided because the solution is irritating to tissues.

Restriction of fluid intake (recommended for treatment of premature neonates with a patent ductus arteriosus) should be continued during indomethacin treatment.

Administration of 1 mg per kg of body weight (mg/kg) of furosemide immediately following indomethacin has been reported to prevent or reduce indomethacin-induced adverse renal effects without interfering with ductus arteriosus closure. However, furosemide administration is not a generally accepted measure for achieving this purpose. If a significant decrease in renal function occurs following a dose of indomethacin as indicated by a serum creatinine concentration greater than 1.2 to 1.4 mg per dL (106-124 micromols/L) or other appropriate tests, additional doses should be withheld until urine volume increases to normal levels (i.e., > 1 mL per kg of body weight per hour) and/or laboratory studies indicate return of normal renal function.

The medication should be discontinued if any severe adverse reaction, especially hepatic function impairment or disease, occurs.

If significant constriction or closure of the ductus arteriosus does not occur following 2 courses (3 doses per course) of indomethacin therapy, surgery may be required.

Reopening of the ductus arteriosus may occur following initial closure. Although spontaneous reclosure has occurred in many patients, additional indomethacin or surgery may be required.

**For treatment of adverse effects or overdose**
Recommended treatment may include:
- Discontinuing or temporarily suspending administration.
- Monitoring the patient and treating observed symptoms. The possibility must be considered that gastrointestinal ulceration or hemorrhage may not occur until several days after administration.

Hemodialysis is not effective in removing indomethacin from the circulation.

## Oral Dosage Forms

Note: Bracketed uses in the *Dosage Forms* section refer to categories of use and/or indications that are not included in U.S. product labeling.

### INDOMETHACIN CAPSULES USP

**Usual pediatric dose**
[Patent ductus arteriosus closure adjunct][1]—
    Infants up to 48 hours of age at time of first dose:
        Oral, via nasogastric tube, 200 mcg (0.2 mg) of anhydrous indomethacin per kg of body weight initially. If necessary, one or two additional doses of 100 mcg (0.1 mg) of anhydrous indomethacin per kg of body weight may be given at twelve- to twenty-four-hour intervals.
    Infants 2 to 7 days of age at time of first dose:
        Oral, via nasogastric tube, 200 mcg (0.2 mg) of anhydrous indomethacin per kg of body weight initially. If necessary, one or two additional doses of 200 mcg (0.2 mg) of anhydrous indomethacin per kg of body weight may be given at twelve- to twenty-four-hour intervals.
    Infants over 7 days of age at time of first dose:
        Oral, via nasogastric tube, 200 mcg (0.2 mg) of anhydrous indomethacin per kg of body weight initially. If necessary, one or two additional doses of 250 mcg (0.25 mg) of anhydrous indomethacin per kg of body weight may be given at twelve- to twenty-four-hour intervals.

Note: Some investigators have used initial doses of 300 mcg (0.3 mg) per kg of body weight.

The recommended dose may also be administered rectally (as a suspension prepared from capsule contents); however, intravenous administration is preferred if available.

**Strength(s) usually available**
U.S.—
    25 mg (Rx) [*Indameth; Indocin;* GENERIC].
    50 mg (Rx) [*Indameth; Indocin;* GENERIC].
Canada—
    25 mg (Rx) [*Apo-Indomethacin; Indocid; Novomethacin*].
    50 mg (Rx) [*Apo-Indomethacin; Indocid; Novomethacin*].

**Packaging and storage**
Store below 40 °C (104 °F), preferably between 15 and 30 °C (59 and 86 °F). Store in a well-closed container.

## Parenteral Dosage Forms

### INDOMETHACIN SODIUM STERILE

**Usual pediatric dose**
Patent ductus arteriosus closure adjunct—
  Infants up to 48 hours of age at time of first dose:
    Intravenous, 200 mcg (0.2 mg) of anhydrous indomethacin per kg of body weight initially. If necessary, one or two additional doses of 100 mcg (0.1 mg) of anhydrous indomethacin per kg of body weight may be given at twelve- to twenty-four-hour intervals.
  Infants 2 to 7 days of age at time of first dose:
    Intravenous, 200 mcg (0.2 mg) of anhydrous indomethacin per kg of body weight initially. If necessary, one or two additional doses of 200 mcg (0.2 mg) of anhydrous indomethacin per kg of body weight may be given at twelve- to twenty-four-hour intervals.
  Infants over 7 days of age at time of first dose:
    Intravenous, 200 mcg (0.2 mg) of anhydrous indomethacin per kg of body weight initially. If necessary, one or two additional doses of 250 mcg (0.25 mg) of anhydrous indomethacin per kg of body weight may be given at twelve- to twenty-four-hour intervals.
Note: Some investigators have used initial doses of 300 mcg (0.3 mg) of anhydrous indomethacin per kg of body weight.

**Size(s) usually available**
U.S.—
  1 mg (anhydrous indomethacin) (Rx) [*Indocin I.V*].
Canada—
  1 mg (anhydrous indomethacin) (Rx) [*Indocid PDA*].

**Packaging and storage**
Store below 30 °C (86 °F), unless otherwise directed by manufacturer. Protect from light.

**Preparation of dosage form**
Add 1 or 2 mL of preservative-free 0.9% sodium chloride injection or preservative-free sterile water for injection to the contents of the vial. A solution prepared using 1 mL of diluent contains 100 mcg (0.1 mg) of anhydrous indomethacin per 0.1 mL; a solution prepared using 2 mL of diluent contains 50 mcg (0.05 mg) of anhydrous indomethacin per 0.1 mL.

**Stability**
Sterile indomethacin sodium contains no preservatives. Therefore, the medication should be reconstituted immediately prior to use and any unused solution should be discarded.

**Incompatibilities**
Sterile indomethacin sodium contains no buffering agents. Further dilution of the reconstituted solution with intravenous infusion solutions is not recommended because free indomethacin may be precipitated if the pH of the solution is < 6.

---

[1]Not included in Canadian product labeling.

Revised: 03/10/93

---

**INFANT FORMULAS**—The *Infant Formulas (Systemic)* monograph is not included in this published version of the USP DI database. Copies of the monograph are available on request from Micromedex, Inc. - Reprint Requests, 6200 S. Syracuse Way, Suite 300, Englewood, CO 80111; telephone (303) 486-6400; telefax (303) 486-6464; Email: USPDI@MDX.COM.

---

# INFLUENZA VIRUS VACCINE   Systemic

VA CLASSIFICATION (Primary): IM100

Note: This monograph refers to the current (1998–99 season) inactivated whole-virus influenza vaccine prepared from the intact, purified virus particles; the subvirion influenza vaccine prepared by the additional step of disrupting the lipid-containing membrane of the virus; and purified surface-antigen influenza vaccine.

Based on the detected antigenic changes in the circulating strains of influenza viruses in the U.S. and worldwide, the U.S. Food and Drug Administration's Vaccines and Related Biological Products Advisory Committee (VRBPAC) and the World Health Organization (WHO) recommended that the 1998–99 trivalent influenza virus vaccine contain A/Beijing/262/95–like (H1N1), A/Sydney/5/97–like (H3N2), and B/Beijing/184/93–like viruses. For the B/Beijing/184/93–like antigen, U.S. manufacturers will use the antigenically equivalent strain B/Harbin/07/94 because of its better growth properties.

However, as in previous years, the specific viruses used in vaccine manufacturing in each country must be approved by the national control authorities.

Commonly used brand name(s): *FluShield; Fluviral; Fluviral S/F; Fluvirin; Fluzone*.

Another commonly used name is flu vaccine.

Note: For a listing of dosage forms and brand names by country availability, see *Dosage Forms* section(s).

## Category
Immunizing agent (active).

## Indications

**General considerations**
Influenza A viruses are classified into subtypes on the basis of their two surface antigens: hemagglutinin (H) and neuraminidase (N). Three subtypes of hemagglutinin (H1, H2, and H3) and two types of neuraminidase (N1 and N2) are recognized among influenza A viruses that have caused widespread human disease. Immunity to these antigens, especially to the hemagglutinin, reduces the likelihood of infection and lessens the severity of disease if infection occurs.

Infection with a virus of one subtype confers little or no protection against viruses of other subtypes. Furthermore, over time, antigenic variation (antigenic drift) within a subtype may be so marked that infection or vaccination with one strain may not induce immunity to distantly related strains of the same subtype.

Although influenza B viruses have shown more antigenic stability than influenza A viruses, antigenic variations do occur in influenza B viruses. For these reasons, major epidemics of respiratory disease caused by new variants of influenza continue to occur. The antigenic characteristics of circulating strains provide the basis for selecting the virus strains included in each year's vaccine.

Typical influenza illness is characterized by abrupt onset of fever, myalgia, sore throat, and nonproductive cough. Unlike other common respiratory illnesses, influenza can cause severe malaise lasting for several days. More severe illness can result if either primary influenza develops into viral pneumonia or if secondary bacterial pneumonia occurs. During influenza epidemics, high attack rates of acute illness result in increased numbers of visits to physicians' offices, walk-in clinics, and emergency rooms, and increased hospitalizations for management of lower respiratory tract complications.

Elderly persons and persons with underlying chronic health problems are at increased risk for complications of influenza. If they become ill with influenza, such members of high-risk groups are more likely than the general population to require hospitalization. During major epidemics, hospitalization rates for persons at high risk may increase twofold to fivefold, depending on the age group. Previously healthy children and younger adults may also require hospitalization for influenza-related complications, but the relative increase in their hospitalization rates is less than for persons who belong to high-risk groups.

An increase in mortality further indicates the impact of influenza epidemics. Increased mortality results not only from influenza and pneumonia, but also from cardiopulmonary and other chronic diseases that can be exacerbated by influenza. More than 90% of the deaths attributed to pneumonia and influenza occur among persons ≥ 65 years of age.

Because the proportion of elderly persons in the U.S. population is increasing, and because age and its associated chronic diseases are risk factors for severe influenza illness, the number of deaths attributed to influenza can be expected to increase unless control measures are implemented more vigorously. In addition, the number of persons < 65 years of age at increased risk for influenza-related complications is increasing. Better survival rates for organ-transplant recipients, the success of neonatal intensive-care units, and better management of diseases such as cystic fibrosis and acquired immunodeficiency syndrome (AIDS) contribute to a growing population of younger persons at high risk.

More than 8 million children and adolescents in the U.S., including 2.2 million persons 10 to 18 years of age who have asthma, have at least one medical condition that places them at high risk for complications associated with influenza. Such children and adolescents should be vaccinated annually against influenza; currently, however, few actually receive the vaccine.

Adolescents who meet any of the following criteria should be vaccinated against influenza:
- Adolescents who have chronic disorders of the pulmonary system (including those who have asthma) or the cardiovascular system.
- Adolescents who reside in long-term facilities.
- Adolescents who have required regular medical follow-up or hospitalization during the preceding year because of chronic metabolic disease (including those who have diabetes mellitus), renal dysfunction, hemoglobinopathy, or immunosuppression (including those who have immunosuppression caused by medication).
- Adolescents who receive long-term aspirin therapy and, therefore, may be at risk for contracting Reye's syndrome after an influenza infection.

In addition, adolescents who have close contact with persons who meet any of these conditions or with persons ≥ 65 years of age should be administered influenza virus vaccine annually, to reduce the likelihood of their acquiring influenza infection.

In the U.S., influenza virus vaccine campaigns are targeted at approximately 32 million persons ≥ 65 years of age, and 27 to 31 million persons < 65 years of age who are at high risk for influenza-associated complications. National health objectives for the year 2000 include vaccination of at least 60% of persons at risk for severe influenza-related illnesses. Influenza virus vaccination levels among persons ≥ 65 years of age improved substantially from 1989 (33%) to 1993 (52%); however, vaccination levels among persons < 65 years of age at high risk are estimated to be < 30%.

Successful vaccination programs have combined education for health care workers, publicity and education targeted at potential recipients, a plan for identifying persons at high risk (usually by medical record review), and efforts to remove administrative and financial barriers that prevent persons from receiving the vaccine. Persons for whom influenza virus vaccine is recommended can be identified and vaccinated in the following settings:
- Outpatient clinics and physicians' offices. Staff in physicians' offices, clinics, health maintenance organizations, and employee health clinics should be instructed to identify and label the medical records of patients who should receive vaccination. Vaccination should be offered during visits beginning in September and lasting throughout the influenza season. The offer of vaccination and its receipt or refusal should be documented in the medical records. Patients in high-risk groups who do not have regularly scheduled visits during the fall should be reminded by mail or telephone of the need for vaccination. If possible, arrangements should be made to provide vaccination with minimal waiting time and at the lowest possible cost.
- Facilities providing episodic or acute care. Health care providers in these settings (e.g., emergency rooms and walk-in clinics) should be familiar with influenza virus vaccine recommendations. They should offer vaccination to persons in high-risk groups or should provide written information giving the reason for this vaccination, the locations where it is available, and the health care personnel to contact. Written information should be available in language(s) appropriate for the population served by the facility.
- Nursing homes and other residential long-term care facilities. Vaccination should be routinely provided to all residents of long-term care facilities with the concurrence of the attending physicians rather than by obtaining individual vaccination orders for each patient. Consent for vaccination should be obtained from the resident or a family member at the time of admission to the facility, and all residents should be vaccinated at one time, immediately preceding the influenza season. Residents admitted during the winter months after completion of the vaccination program should be vaccinated when they are admitted.
- Acute care hospitals. All persons ≥ 65 years of age and younger persons (including children) with high-risk conditions who are hospitalized at any time from September through March should be offered and strongly encouraged to receive the influenza virus vaccine before they are discharged. Household members and others with whom they will have contact also should receive written information about the need for influenza virus vaccination, and where it is available.
- Outpatient facilities providing continuing care to patients at high risk. All patients should be offered vaccination before the beginning of the influenza season. Patients admitted to such programs (e.g., hemodialysis centers, hospital specialty care clinics, and outpatient rehabilitation programs) during the winter months after the earlier vaccination program has been conducted should be vaccinated at the time of admission. Household members and others with whom they will have contact also should receive written information about the need for influenza virus vaccination, and where it is available.
- Visiting nurses and others providing home care to persons at high risk. Nursing care plans should identify patients in high-risk groups, and vaccination should be provided in the home if necessary. Caregivers and other persons in the household (including children) should be referred for vaccination.
- Facilities providing services to persons ≥ 65 years of age. In these facilities (e.g., retirement communities and recreation centers), all unvaccinated residents/attendees should be offered vaccination on site before the influenza season begins. Education/publicity programs should also be provided; these programs should emphasize the need for influenza virus vaccination and provide specific information on the vaccination programs, their schedules, and locations.
- Clinics and other settings providing health care for travelers. Indications for influenza virus vaccination should be reviewed before travel, and vaccination should be offered, if appropriate.
- Health care workers. Administrators of all health care facilities should arrange for influenza vaccination to be offered to all personnel before the influenza season begins. Personnel should be provided with appropriate educational materials, and should be strongly encouraged to receive the vaccine. Particular emphasis should be placed on vaccination of persons who care for members of high risk groups (e.g., staff of intensive care units [including neonatal intensive care units], staff of medical/surgical units, and employees of nursing homes and long-term care facilities). Using a mobile cart to carry the vaccine doses to hospital wards or other work sites and making the vaccine available during night and weekend work shifts can enhance compliance, as can a follow-up campaign early in the course of a community outbreak.

An alternative strategy for controlling influenza type A infection among high-risk patients is the use of the antiviral agents amantadine and rimantadine, especially for chronically ill, institutionalized, or severely debilitated persons who have been or may be exposed to influenza type A during an outbreak. Amantadine and rimantadine are equally effective in the prevention and treatment of influenza type A infections.

**Accepted**

Influenza (prophylaxis)—Influenza virus vaccine is indicated for any person ≥ 6 months of age who, because of age or underlying medical condition, is at increased risk of complications of influenza, including:
- Targeted high-risk children. Yearly immunization is recommended for children 6 months of age and older with one or more specific risk factors. Data are insufficient regarding the potential severity of influenza in several of these groups of children; however, based on available data and knowledge of the pathophysiology of these disorders, children with the following risk factors warrant immunization:
  —Those with asthma and other chronic pulmonary diseases. Influenza vaccination can be given safely and effectively to children with asthma regardless of asthma symptoms or concurrent prednisone therapy. Vaccination of all patients with moderate to severe asthma who visit clinics or emergency departments would improve the overall vaccination rate significantly.
  —Those with hemodynamically significant cardiac disease.
  —Those undergoing immunosuppressive therapy.
  —Those with sickle-cell anemia and other hemoglobinopathies.
- Other high-risk children. Children who are potentially at increased risk for complicated influenza illness and who may benefit from influenza immunization are those with one or more of the following conditions:
  —Human immunodeficiency virus (HIV) infection.
  —Diabetes mellitus.
  —Chronic metabolic diseases.
  —Recipients of long-term aspirin therapy, such as children with rheumatoid arthritis or Kawasaki disease, who may have an increased risk of developing Reye's syndrome.
  —Influenza virus vaccination also may be considered for children who are marginally immunocompromised as a result of any underlying condition, since even uncomplicated influenza can have adverse effects on the course of an underlying illness.
- Adults at increased risk for influenza-related complications:
  —Persons ≥ 65 years of age.
  —Residents of nursing homes and other long-term care facilities that house persons of any age with chronic medical conditions.
  —Those with chronic disorders of the pulmonary or cardiovascular systems.
  —Those who have required regular medical follow-up or hospitalization during the preceding year because of chronic metabolic diseases (including diabetes mellitus), renal dysfunction, hemoglobi-

nopathies, or immunosuppression (including immunosuppression caused by medications).
— Women who will be in the second or third trimester of pregnancy during the influenza season.

- Persons who can transmit influenza to others who are at high risk. Persons who are clinically or subclinically infected with influenza and who care for or live with members of high-risk groups can transmit influenza virus to them. Some persons at high risk (e.g., the elderly, transplant recipients, and persons with AIDS) can have a low antibody response to influenza vaccine. Efforts to protect these members of high-risk groups against influenza may be improved by reducing the likelihood of influenza virus exposure from their caregivers. Immunization of adults who are in close contact with children at high risk may be an important means of protecting these children, especially for infants < 6 months of age for whom vaccination is not recommended. Immunization of pregnant women may be beneficial to the neonates, as well, since transplacentally acquired antibody appears to protect neonates from infection with influenza A virus. Therefore, the following groups should be immunized:
— Physicians, nurses, and other personnel in both hospital and outpatient settings.
— Employees of nursing homes and long-term care facilities who have contact with patients or residents.
— Providers of home care to persons at high risk (e.g., visiting nurses and volunteer workers).
— Household contacts of persons at high risk, including children, siblings, and primary caretakers of children at high risk. HIV-infected children who are members of households with adults at high risk also should be immunized.

- General population. Physicians should administer influenza virus vaccine to any person who wishes to reduce the likelihood of becoming ill with influenza. Persons who provide essential community services should be considered for vaccination, to minimize disruption of essential activities during influenza outbreaks. Vaccination should be considered for groups of individuals whose close contact with each other facilitates rapid transmission of the virus infection resulting in disruption of routine activities. Examples are students in colleges, schools, and other institutions of learning, particularly those who reside in dormitories or who are members of athletic teams, and those living in residential institutions.

- Persons infected with HIV. Limited information exists regarding the frequency and severity of influenza illness among HIV-infected persons, but reports suggest that symptoms may be prolonged and the risk for complications increased for some HIV-infected persons. Influenza vaccine has produced protective antibody titers against influenza in vaccinated HIV-infected persons who have minimal AIDS-related symptoms and high CD4+ T-lymphocyte cell counts. In patients who have advanced HIV infection–related disease and low CD4+ T-lymphocyte cell counts, however, influenza virus vaccine may not induce protective antibody titers; furthermore, a second dose of vaccine does not improve the immune response for these persons. Recent studies have examined the effect of influenza vaccination on replication of HIV type 1 (HIV-1). Although some studies have demonstrated a transient (i.e., 2- to 4-week) increase in replication of HIV-1 in the plasma or peripheral blood mononuclear cells of HIV-1–infected persons after vaccine administration, other studies using similar laboratory techniques have not indicated any substantial increase in replication. Decline in CD4+ T-lymphocyte cell counts and progression of clinical HIV infection–related disease have not been demonstrated among HIV-infected persons who receive influenza virus vaccine. Since influenza can result in serious illness and complications, and because influenza virus vaccination may result in protective antibody titers, vaccination will benefit many HIV-infected patients.

- International travelers. The risk of exposure to influenza during foreign travel varies, depending on the season and destination. In the tropics, influenza outbreaks can occur throughout the year; in the southern hemisphere, most outbreaks occur between April and September. Because of the short incubation period for influenza, exposure to the virus during travel can result in clinical illness that begins while traveling, which could be an inconvenience or a potential danger, especially for persons at increased risk for complications. Persons preparing to travel to the tropics at any time of the year or to the southern hemisphere from April through September should review their influenza vaccination histories. If they were not vaccinated during the previous fall or winter, they should consider receiving influenza vaccination before travel.

## Pharmacology/Pharmacokinetics

### Physicochemical characteristics

Source—Each year's influenza vaccine contains three virus strains (usually two type A strains and one type B strain) representing the influenza viruses that are likely to circulate in the U.S. in the upcoming winter. The vaccine is made from highly purified, egg-grown viruses that have been made noninfectious (inactivated). Whole-virus, subvirion, and purified-surface-antigen preparations are available.

In collaboration with the World Health Organization (WHO), its international network of collaborating laboratories, and state and local health departments, the Centers for Disease Control and Prevention (CDC) conducts surveillance to monitor influenza activity and detect antigenic changes in the circulating strains of influenza viruses.

### Mechanism of action/Effect

Humoral defenses against influenza infection are mainly conferred by serum and local immune globulin G (IgG) and immune globulin A (IgA) antibodies to the surface glycoproteins, hemagglutinin (H) and neuraminidase (N). Anti-H antibodies inhibit the attachment of the influenza virus to target cell membrane receptors and thus neutralize viral infectivity. Depending on their concentration, these antibodies can either provide complete protection from the acquisition of infection or prevent the development of serious illness. Protection studies have indicated that an anti-H antibody titer of ≥ 40 is the protection threshold beyond which serious illness is unlikely to develop.

### Protective effect

Most vaccinated children and young adults develop high titers of postvaccination hemagglutinin-inhibition (HI) antibody. These antibodies protect the individual against illness caused by strains similar to those in the vaccine. Elderly persons and persons with certain chronic diseases may develop lower postvaccination antibody titers than healthy young adults and thus may remain susceptible to influenza-related upper respiratory tract infection. However, even if such persons develop influenza illness despite vaccination, the vaccine can be effective in preventing lower respiratory tract involvement or other complications, thereby reducing the risks of hospitalization and death.

The effectiveness of influenza vaccine in preventing or attenuating illness varies, depending primarily on the age and immunocompetence of the vaccine recipient and the degree of similarity between the virus strains included in the vaccine and those that circulate during the influenza season. When there is a good match between the vaccine and circulating viruses, influenza virus vaccine has been shown to prevent illness in approximately 70% of healthy persons < 65 years of age. In these circumstances, studies have also indicated that the effectiveness of influenza virus vaccine in preventing hospitalization for pneumonia and influenza among elderly persons living in settings other than nursing homes or similar long-term care facilities ranges from 30 to 70%.

Among elderly persons residing in nursing homes, influenza virus vaccine is very effective in preventing severe illness, secondary complications, and death. Studies in this population have indicated that the vaccine can be 50 to 60% effective in preventing hospitalization and pneumonia, and 80% effective in preventing death, even though the vaccine's efficacy in preventing influenza illness may only be in the range of 30 to 40% among the frail elderly. Achieving a high rate of vaccination among nursing home residents can reduce the spread of infection in a facility, thus preventing disease through herd immunity.

### Duration of protective effect

Since the antigenic properties of influenza virus surface antigens frequently change, the vaccine-induced protective immunity is short-lived. For this reason, health authorities recommend annual revaccination of persons at risk, using influenza virus vaccines containing the expected epidemic strains for the next season.

## Precautions to Consider

### Pregnancy/Reproduction

Pregnancy—Influenza-associated excess mortality among pregnant women has not been documented except during the pandemics of 1918–19 and 1957–58. However, because death-certificate data often do not indicate whether a woman was pregnant at the time of death, studies conducted during interpandemic periods may underestimate the impact of influenza in this population. Case reports and limited studies suggest that pregnancy may increase the risk of serious medical complications of influenza, as a result of increases in heart rate, increases in stroke volume and oxygen consumption, decreases in lung capacity, and changes in immunologic functions. A recent study of the impact of influenza during 17 interpandemic influenza seasons documented that the relative risk of hospitalization for selected cardiorespiratory conditions among pregnant women increased from 1.4 during weeks 14 to 20 of gestation to 4.7 during weeks 37 to 42, as compared with rates among women who were 1 to 6 months postpartum. Women in their third trimesters of pregnancy were hospitalized at a rate comparable to that of nonpregnant women with high-risk medical conditions for whom influenza virus vaccine has traditionally been recommended. Using data from this study, it was estimated that an average of 1 to 2 hospitalizations among pregnant women could be prevented for every 1000 pregnant women immunized.

On the basis of these and other data suggesting that influenza infection may cause increased morbidity in women during the second and third trimesters of pregnancy, the Advisory Committee on Immunization Practices (ACIP) of the Centers for Disease Control and Prevention (CDC) recommends that women who will be beyond the first trimester of pregnancy (14 weeks of gestation) during the influenza season be vaccinated. Pregnant women who have medical conditions that increase the risk of complications from influenza should be vaccinated before the influenza season, regardless of the stage of pregnancy. Studies of influenza immunization of more than 2000 pregnant women have demonstrated no adverse fetal effects associated with influenza virus vaccine; however, more data are needed. Because influenza virus vaccine is not a live virus vaccine and major systemic reactions are rare, many experts consider influenza vaccination safe during any stage of pregnancy. However, because spontaneous abortion is common in the first trimester and unnecessary exposures have traditionally been avoided during this time, some experts prefer influenza vaccination during the second trimester to avoid coincidental association of the vaccine with early pregnancy loss.

Studies have not been done in animals.

FDA Pregnancy Category C.

**Breast-feeding**

Influenza vaccine does not affect the safety of breast-feeding for mothers or infants. Breast-feeding does not adversely affect the immune response and is not a contraindication for vaccination.

**Pediatrics**

In immunosuppressed children receiving chemotherapy, influenza immunization with a new vaccine antigen results in a sufficient immune response in only a minority of children. The optimal time to immunize children with malignancies who still must undergo chemotherapy is 3 to 4 weeks after chemotherapy has been discontinued and the peripheral granulocyte and lymphocyte counts are greater than 1000 per cubic millimeter. Children who are no longer receiving chemotherapy generally have high rates of seroconversion.

The immune response and safety of influenza vaccine in children with hemodynamically unstable cardiac disease (another large group of children potentially at high risk for complications of influenza) are comparable to those in healthy children.

The effect of corticosteroid therapy on influenza vaccine immunogenicity is unknown. Since a high dose of corticosteroids (i.e., a dose equivalent to either 2 mg per kg of body weight or a total of 20 mg per day of prednisone) may impair antibody responses, particularly in unvaccinated or previously uninfected persons, vaccination may be deferred temporarily during high-dose corticosteroid therapy, provided deferral does not compromise the likelihood of immunization before the start of the influenza season. Corticosteroid therapy should not unnecessarily delay the administration of influenza vaccine, particularly in children with asthma who require intermittent or maintenance corticosteroid therapy.

Infants younger than 6 months of age with high-risk conditions, especially those with compromised cardiopulmonary function may have the same or greater risk from influenza complications as of older children. However, no information is available about the reactivity, immunogenicity, or the efficacy of the influenza vaccine in infants during the first 6 months of life. In addition, the effect of influenza antigens in an inactivated vaccine on the infant's future immune response to influenza is unknown. Therefore, alternative methods of protection for young infants should be considered.

Children and young adults with cystic fibrosis (CF) will benefit from annual influenza vaccination. In a 10-year observational study with a cohort design of 38 children and young adults with CF, serum hemagglutinin-inhibition (HI) antibody titers were determined at the time of vaccination, and 4 weeks later each year in the fall before the influenza epidemic. While the prevaccination and postvaccination geometric mean serum HI antibody titers varied from year to year, no upward or downward trend was evident over the 10-year period. In addition, the majority of vaccinees had a presumably protective postvaccination serum HI titer ≥ 1:40 each year for all three vaccine strains.

In children with little previous experience with influenza, two doses of vaccine, administered 1 month apart, are necessary to produce a satisfactory antibody response. Children previously primed with a related strain of influenza virus by infection or vaccination almost uniformly exhibit a brisk antibody response to one dose of the vaccine.

Only the subviron or purified surface-antigen vaccines, i.e., those termed "split-virus" vaccines, should be used for children younger than 12 years of age.

**Geriatrics**

Although influenza vaccine reportedly provides 65 to 85% protection against influenza illness in young, healthy adults, studies of its effectiveness in high-risk groups, such as the elderly, have yielded inconsistent results. In observational studies of high-risk patients, respiratory illness during influenza epidemics occurred often, despite vaccination. A review of studies of influenza vaccination in nursing homes disclosed that the median protective effect in 16 outbreaks of influenza A was 26%, and it was only 19% in seven studies of influenza B outbreaks. Among noninstitutionalized elderly persons, the number of medical care visits for upper respiratory illnesses during two influenza outbreaks was the same for those who had received influenza vaccine and those who had not.

Despite the apparent ineffectiveness of influenza vaccination in preventing respiratory infection, other nonrandomized studies have shown that it reduces serious complications and mortality due to influenza in the elderly or chronically ill. In nursing homes, for example, significant reductions in pneumonia and mortality among vaccinees were documented during influenza A outbreaks.

Among noninstitutionalized elderly persons, compelling evidence for the effectiveness of influenza vaccine comes from retrospective studies of more than 10,000 elderly members of a prepaid health plan during four influenza epidemics from 1968 to 1981. Hospitalizations and deaths from influenza and pneumonia among elderly vaccinees with chronic illnesses were reduced by more than 70% during two of these outbreaks. Healthy elderly persons who received the vaccine also had fewer hospitalizations and deaths than their unvaccinated counterparts, although the differences were not statistically significant. During a third epidemic in which there was pronounced antigenic drift, a statistically insignificant trend toward protection against hospitalization and death among vaccine recipients was observed. Antigenic shift to a subtype different from that in the vaccine occurred during the fourth epidemic studied, and no protection from vaccination was observed. More recently, several case-control studies during the influenza seasons from 1989 to 1992 showed that influenza vaccination was 31 to 45% effective in preventing hospitalizations for pneumonia.

**Drug interactions and/or related problems**

The following drug interactions and/or related problems have been selected on the basis of their potential clinical significance (possible mechanism in parentheses where appropriate)—not necessarily inclusive (» = major clinical significance):

Note: Combinations containing any of the following medications, depending on the amount present, may also interact with this medication.

Aminophylline or
Carbamazepine or
Phenobarbital or
Phenytoin or
Theophylline preparations or
Warfarin sodium
(influenza virus vaccine is listed in some references among the therapeutic agents that may increase theophylline levels or the anticoagulant effects of warfarin. Such warnings are apparently based on a report that influenza vaccination depresses hepatic cytochrome P450 activity and on case reports of complications or altered pharmacologic characteristics in vaccinated patients taking these medications. More recent studies have failed to show a significant impact of influenza virus vaccine on the laboratory or clinical effects of warfarin or theophylline, and patients taking these medications can be vaccinated safely without special precautions or monitoring)

Immunosuppressive agents or
Radiation therapy
(since normal defense mechanisms are suppressed, the patient's antibody response to influenza virus vaccine may be decreased. The precaution does not apply to corticosteroids used as replacement therapy, for short-term [less than 2 weeks] systemic therapy, or by other routes of administration that do not cause immunosuppression)

**Laboratory value alterations**

The following have been selected on the basis of their potential clinical significance (possible effect in parentheses where appropriate)—not necessarily inclusive (» = major clinical significance):

Human immunodeficiency virus (HIV), serum and
Hepatitis C virus (HCV), serum
(it was reported that patients who receive influenza virus vaccine may develop false-positive results of enzyme-linked immunosorbent assays for HIV and HCV. Such false-positive test results are uncommon, probably occurring in less than 2% of vaccine recipients; results usually revert to negative within several months. There is no evidence that recipients of influenza virus vaccine are at increased risk of acquiring HIV or HCV infection. However, physi-

**Medical considerations/Contraindications**
The medical considerations/contraindications included have been selected on the basis of their potential clinical significance (reasons given in parentheses where appropriate)—not necessarily inclusive (» = major clinical significance).

*Except under special circumstances, this medication should not be used when the following medical problems exist:*
» Febrile illness, severe
(to avoid confusing the manifestations of illness with possible side/adverse effects of vaccine)
» Respiratory disease, acute
(influenza virus vaccine should not be administered until the acute symptoms of the patient's illness have abated, since the symptoms of the condition may be confused with the possible side effects of the vaccine)

*Risk-benefit should be considered when the following medical problems exist:*
» Allergy to eggs
(immediate, presumably allergic, reactions [e.g., hives, angioedema, allergic asthma, and systemic anaphylaxis] occur rarely after influenza vaccination. These reactions probably result from hypersensitivity to some vaccine component; the majority of reactions are most likely related to residual egg protein in the vaccine)
(although current influenza vaccines contain only a small quantity of egg protein, this protein can induce immediate hypersensitivity reactions among persons who have severe egg allergy. Persons who have developed hives, have had swelling of the lips or tongue, or have experienced acute respiratory distress or collapse after eating eggs should consult a physician for appropriate evaluation to determine if influenza virus vaccine should be administered)
(persons with documented immunoglobulin E [IgE]-mediated hypersensitivity to eggs, including those who have had occupational asthma or other allergic responses due to exposure to egg protein, may also be at increased risk of reactions from influenza vaccine, and similar consultation with a physician should be considered. The protocol for influenza virus vaccination developed by Murphy and Strunk may be considered for patients who have egg allergies and other medical conditions that place them at increased risk for influenza-associated complications)
Guillain-Barré syndrome (GBS), history of
(the likelihood of coincidentally developing GBS after influenza virus vaccination is expected to be greater among persons with a history of GBS than among persons with no history of this syndrome; whether influenza virus vaccination might be causally associated with the risk of recurrence is not known; although it would seem prudent to avoid subsequent influenza virus vaccination of a person known to have developed GBS within 6 weeks of a previous influenza virus vaccination, for most persons with a history of GBS who are at high risk for severe complications from influenza, the established benefits of influenza virus vaccination justify their yearly immunization)
Neurologic disorders, active
(influenza vaccine should not be administered to a patient with an active neurologic disorder; the vaccine should be considered only after the disease process has been stabilized)
Sensitivity to influenza virus vaccine
Sensitivity to thimerosal, sodium bisulfite, gentamicin sulfate, streptomycin sulfate, or other aminoglycosides
(hypersensitivity reactions to any vaccine component can occur; although exposure to vaccines containing thimerosal can lead to induction of hypersensitivity, most patients do not develop reactions to thimerosal when administered as a component of vaccines, even when patch or intradermal tests for thimerosal indicate hypersensitivity; when reported, hypersensitivity to thimerosal usually has consisted of local, delayed-type hypersensitivity reactions)

## Side/Adverse Effects

Note: Because influenza vaccine contains only noninfectious viruses, it cannot cause influenza. Respiratory disease after vaccination represents coincidental illness unrelated to influenza vaccination.

Unlike the 1976 swine influenza vaccine, subsequent vaccines prepared from other viral strains have not been clearly associated with an increased frequency of Guillain-Barré syndrome (GBS). However, a precise estimate of risk is difficult to determine for a rare condition such as GBS, which has an annual background incidence of only one to two cases per 100,000 in the adult population. Among persons who received the swine influenza vaccine, the rate of GBS that exceeded the background rate was slightly less than one case per 100,000 vaccinations.

An investigation of GBS cases in 1990–91 indicated no overall increase in frequency of GBS among persons who were administered influenza vaccine; a slight increase in GBS cases among vaccinated persons may have occurred in the age group of 18 to 64 years, but not among persons ≥ 65 years of age. In contrast to the swine influenza vaccine, the epidemiologic features of the possible associations of the 1990–91 vaccine and GBS were not as convincing. The rate of GBS cases after vaccination that was passively reported to the Vaccine Adverse Event Reporting System (VAERS) during 1993–94 was estimated to be approximately twice the average rate reported during other seasons (i.e., 1990–91, 1991–92, 1992–93, and 1994–5). The data currently available are not sufficient to determine whether this represents an actual risk. However, even if GBS were a true side effect, the very low estimated risk for GBS is less than that of severe influenza prevented by vaccination.

Whereas the incidence of GBS in the general population is very low, persons with a history of GBS have a substantially greater likelihood of subsequently developing GBS than persons without such a history. Thus, the likelihood of coincidentally developing GBS after influenza vaccination is expected to be greater among persons with a history of GBS than among persons with no history of this syndrome. Whether influenza vaccination is causally associated with the risk for recurrence is not known. Although it would seem prudent to avoid a subsequent influenza vaccination in a person known to have developed GBS within 6 weeks of a previous influenza vaccination, for most persons with a history of GBS who are at high risk of severe complications from influenza, the established benefits of influenza virus vaccination justify their yearly immunization.

The following side/adverse effects have been selected on the basis of their potential clinical significance (possible signs and symptoms in parentheses where appropriate)—not necessarily inclusive:

**Those indicating need for medical attention**
Incidence rare
*Anaphylactic reaction, most likely to residual egg protein in the influenza virus vaccine* (difficulty in breathing or swallowing; hives; itching, especially of feet or hands; reddening of skin, especially around ears; swelling of eyes, face, or inside of nose; unusual tiredness or weakness, sudden and severe)

**Those indicating need for medical attention only if they continue or are bothersome**
Incidence more frequent
*Tenderness, redness, or induration at the site of injection, lasting 1 or 2 days* (tenderness, redness, or hard lump at place of injection)—incidence approximately 30%
Incidence less frequent
*Fever, malaise, myalgia, and headache starting 6 to 12 hours after administration and persisting 1 or 2 days* (aches or pains in muscles; general feeling of discomfort or illness)—most often affecting children and adults who have had no previous exposure to the influenza virus antigens in the vaccine

Note: Recent placebo-controlled trials suggest that in elderly persons and healthy young adults, split-virus influenza vaccine is not associated with higher rates of systemic symptoms (e.g., *fever, malaise, myalgia, and headache*) when compared with placebo injections.

## Patient Consultation

As an aid to patient consultation, refer to *Advice for the Patient, Influenza Virus Vaccine (Systemic).*
In providing consultation, consider emphasizing the following selected information (» = major clinical significance):

**Before using this medication**
» Conditions affecting use, especially:
Sensitivity to influenza virus vaccine or allergy to eggs, sodium bisulfite, thimerosal, gentamicin sulfate, streptomycin sulfate, or other aminoglycosides
Use in children—Use is not recommended for infants up to 6 months of age; for children 6 months to 12 years of age, only the split-virus vaccines (split, subvirion, or purified-surface-antigen type) should be used; if two doses are needed, they should be spaced 4 weeks apart

Use in the elderly—Influenza vaccine may be less effective in elderly persons; however, vaccine may be still effective in preventing other complications of influenza in these persons

Other medical problems, especially severe febrile illness, acute respiratory disease, or allergy to eggs

**Proper use of this medication**
» Proper dosing

**Side/adverse effects**
Signs of potential side effects, especially anaphylactic reaction

## General Dosing Information

Appropriate precautions should be taken prior to vaccine injection to prevent allergic or any other unwanted reactions. This should include a review of the patient's history regarding possible sensitivity, and the ready availability of epinephrine 1:1000 and other appropriate agents (e.g., antihistamines) used to control immediate allergic reactions.

Inactivated influenza virus vaccine should not be administered to persons known to have anaphylactic hypersensitivity to eggs or to other components of the influenza vaccine without first consulting a physician. Use of an antiviral agent (i.e., amantadine or rimantadine) instead of influenza virus vaccine is an option for prevention of influenza A in such persons. However, persons who have a history of anaphylactic hypersensitivity to vaccine components but who are also at high risk of complications of influenza can benefit from the vaccine after appropriate allergy evaluation and desensitization procedures.

Children with severe chronic asthma at risk for adverse reactions to influenza virus vaccine should be identified, and appropriate steps should be taken to assure their proper immunization. With the protocol of administering increasing doses of the influenza virus vaccine in small increments, individuals with hypersensitivity to egg proteins can be safely and effectively immunized. Therefore, the following desensitization protocol for influenza virus vaccination developed by Murphy and Strunk may be considered for patients who have egg allergies and other medical conditions that place them at increased risk of influenza-associated complications.

Desensitization of the patient should be carried out by serial injections of diluted and undiluted influenza virus vaccine as indicated below at intervals of 15 minutes for a total cumulative dose of 0.5 mL undiluted influenza virus vaccine.

Schedules for desensitization:
- 0.05 mL of 1:100 dilution intramuscularly.
- 0.05 mL of 1:10 dilution intramuscularly.
- 0.05 mL of undiluted vaccine intramuscularly.
- 0.1 mL of undiluted vaccine intramuscularly.
- 0.15 mL of undiluted vaccine intramuscularly.
- 0.2 mL of undiluted vaccine intramuscularly.

Because of their decreased potential for causing febrile reactions, only split-virus vaccines should be used for children younger than 13 years of age. They may be labeled as split, subvirion, or purified-surface-antigen type vaccine. Immunogenicity and side effects of split- and whole-virus vaccines are similar among adults when vaccines are administered at the recommended dosage.

Elderly patients may develop lower antibody titers after immunization than healthy young adults and, therefore, may remain susceptible to influenza infection of the upper respiratory tract. Nonetheless, influenza virus vaccine may still be effective in preventing lower respiratory tract involvement or other complications of influenza.

During recent decades, data on influenza virus vaccine immunogenicity and side effects have been obtained for intramuscularly administered vaccine. Because recent influenza vaccines have not been adequately evaluated when administered by other routes, the intramuscular route is recommended. Adults and older children should be vaccinated in the deltoid muscle and infants and young children in the anterolateral aspect of the thigh.

Beginning each September, when vaccine for the upcoming influenza season becomes available, persons at high risk who are seen by health care providers for routine care or as a result of hospitalization should be offered influenza virus vaccine. Opportunities to vaccinate persons at high risk of complications of influenza should not be missed.

The optimal time for organized vaccination campaigns for persons in high-risk groups is usually the period from October through mid-November. This period has been extended to include the first 2 weeks in October. In the U.S., influenza activity generally peaks between late December and early March. High levels of influenza activity infrequently occur in the contiguous 48 states before December. Administering the vaccine too far in advance of the influenza season should be avoided in facilities such as nursing homes, because antibody levels might begin to decline within a few months of vaccination. Vaccination programs can be undertaken as soon as the current vaccine is available, if regional influenza activity is expected to begin earlier than December.

Children younger than 9 years of age who have not been vaccinated previously should receive two doses of vaccine at least 1 month apart, to maximize the likelihood of a satisfactory antibody response to all three vaccine antigens. The second dose should preferably be administered before December. Vaccine should be offered to both children and adults prior to, and even after, influenza activity is documented in a community.

The target groups for influenza and pneumococcal vaccination overlap considerably. For persons at high risk who have not been previously vaccinated with pneumococcal vaccine, health care providers should strongly consider administering both pneumococcal and influenza virus vaccines concurrently. Both vaccines can be administered at the same time at different body sites without increasing potential side effects. However, influenza virus vaccine is administered each year, whereas the pneumococcal vaccine is not. Children at high risk of influenza-related complications can receive influenza virus vaccine at the same time they receive other routine vaccinations, including pertussis vaccine (as DTP or as DTaP). Because influenza virus vaccine can cause fever when administered to young children, DTaP (which is less frequently associated with fever and other adverse reactions) is preferable.

**For treatment of adverse effects**
Recommended treatment includes:
- For mild hypersensitivity reaction—Administering antihistamines and, if necessary, corticosteroids. In mild anaphylaxis, antihistamines or subcutaneous epinephrine may be all that is necessary if the condition is progressing slowly and is not life-threatening, regardless of the organ or system affected. Under these circumstances, the risks associated with intravenous epinephrine administration outweigh the benefits.
- For severe hypersensitivity or anaphylactic reaction—Administering epinephrine. Antihistamines and/or corticosteroids also may be administered as required. Epinephrine is the treatment of choice for severe hypersensitivity or anaphylactic reaction. If the patient's condition is not stable, epinephrine may be infused. Norepinephrine may be preferable if there is no bronchospasm. For bronchospasm, epinephrine should be given with corticosteroids. Other bronchodilators, such as intravenous aminophylline or albuterol by nebulization, also should be considered.

## Parenteral Dosage Forms

### INFLUENZA VIRUS VACCINE (Injection—Split virus [purified-surface-antigen type]) USP

**Usual adult and adolescent dose**
Influenza prophylaxis—
Adults and children 12 years of age and older: Intramuscular, 0.5 mL as a single dose.

**Usual pediatric dose**
Influenza prophylaxis—
Infants up to 6 months of age: Use is not recommended.
Infants 6 to 35 months of age: Two doses of 0.25 mL each, 4 weeks apart.
Children 3 to 8 years of age: Intramuscular, 0.5 mL of the split-virus vaccine. Two doses of 0.5 mL each, 4 weeks apart, are recommended for maximum protection in persons under 9 years of age who have not been previously vaccinated.
Children 8 to 12 years of age: Intramuscular, 0.5 mL as a single dose of the split-virus vaccine.

**Usual geriatric dose**
See *Usual adult and adolescent dose*.

**Strength(s) usually available**
U.S.—
Each 0.5-mL dose contains the proportions, and not less than the microgram amounts, of hemagglutinin antigens (mcg HA) representative of the specific components recommended for the present year's vaccine (Rx) [*Fluvirin* (thimerosal 0.01%)].
Canada—
Not commercially available.

**Packaging and storage**
Store between 2 and 8 °C (36 and 46 °F), unless otherwise specified by manufacturer. Do not freeze.

**Stability**
Potency is destroyed by freezing; vaccine that has been frozen should not be used.

**Auxiliary labeling**
- Shake well.
- Do not freeze.

## INFLUENZA VIRUS VACCINE (Injection—Split virus [split or subvirion type]) USP

**Usual adult and adolescent dose**
Influenza prophylaxis—
  Adults and children 12 years of age and older: Intramuscular, 0.5 mL as a single dose.

**Usual pediatric dose**
Influenza prophylaxis—
  Infants up to 6 months of age: Use is not recommended.
  Infants 6 to 35 months of age: Intramuscular, 0.25 mL of the split-virus vaccine. Dose should be repeated in four or more weeks if the patient has not been previously vaccinated.
  Children 3 to 8 years of age: Intramuscular, 0.5 mL of the split-virus vaccine. Two doses of 0.5 mL each, 4 weeks apart, are recommended for maximum protection in children under 8 years of age who have not been previously vaccinated.
  Children 8 to 12 years of age: Intramuscular, 0.5 mL as a single dose of the split-virus vaccine.

**Usual geriatric dose**
See *Usual adult and adolescent dose*.

**Strength(s) usually available**
U.S.—
  Each 0.5-mL dose contains the proportions, and not less than the microgram amounts, of hemagglutinin antigens (mcg HA) representative of the specific components recommended for the present year's vaccine (Rx) [*FluShield* (1:10,000 thimerosal; gentamicin sulfate); *Fluzone* (1:10,000 thimerosal) [GENERIC (may contain gentamicin sulfate; 1:10,000 thimerosal)].
Canada—
  Each 0.5-mL dose contains the proportions, and not less than the microgram amounts, of hemagglutinin antigens (mcg HA) representative of the specific components recommended for the present year's vaccine (Rx) [*Fluviral S/F* (thimerosal 0.01%); *Fluzone* (thimerosal)].

Note: Gentamicin sulfate, streptomycin sulfate, neomycin, polymyxin, and/or sodium bisulfite may be used in the production of influenza virus vaccine. By current assay procedures, concentrations of these products are not detectable in the final vaccine; however, even in trace amounts they may be able to cause hypersensitivity reactions in susceptible persons.

**Packaging and storage**
Store between 2 and 8 °C (36 and 46 °F), unless otherwise specified by the manufacturer. Do not freeze.

**Stability**
Potency is destroyed by freezing; vaccine that has been frozen should not be used.

**Auxiliary labeling**
  • Shake well.
  • Do not freeze.

## INFLUENZA VIRUS VACCINE (Injection—Whole virus) USP

**Usual adult and adolescent dose**
Influenza prophylaxis—
  Adults and children 13 years of age and older: Intramuscular, 0.5 mL as a single dose.

**Usual pediatric dose**
Influenza prophylaxis—
  Use is not recommended in children up to 12 years of age.

Note: Only split-virus influenza vaccines (split, subvirion, or purified-surface-antigen type) should be used for children up to 12 years of age because of the vaccines' lower potential for causing febrile adverse reactions when compared to the whole-virus influenza vaccine. None of the influenza virus vaccines is recommended for infants up to 6 months of age.

**Usual geriatric dose**
See *Usual adult and adolescent dose*.

**Strength(s) usually available**
U.S.—
  Each 0.5-mL dose contains the proportions, and not less than the microgram amounts, of hemagglutinin antigens (mcg HA) representative of the specific components recommended for the present year's vaccine (Rx) [*Fluzone* (1:10,000 thimerosal)].
Canada—
  Each 0.5-mL dose contains the proportions, and not less than the microgram amounts, of hemagglutinin antigens (mcg HA) representative of the specific components recommended for the present year's vaccine (Rx) [*Fluviral* (thimerosal 0.01%); *Fluzone* (thimerosal)].

**Packaging and storage**
Store between 2 and 8 °C (35 and 46 °F), unless otherwise specified by manufacturer. Do not freeze.

**Stability**
Potency is destroyed by freezing; vaccine that has been frozen should not be used.

**Auxiliary labeling**
  • Shake well.
  • Do not freeze.

### Selected Bibliography
Centers for Disease Control and Prevention (CDC). Prevention and control of influenza: recommendations of the Advisory Committee on Immunization Practices (ACIP). MMWR Morb Mortal Wkly Rep 1997; 46(RR-9): 1-25.

Revised: 07/25/97
Interim revision: 08/12/98

# INSULIN  Systemic

This monograph includes information on the following: 1) Buffered Insulin Human; 2) Extended Insulin Zinc*; 3) Extended Insulin Zinc, Human; 4) Insulin; 5) Insulin Human; 6) Insulin Zinc; 7) Insulin Zinc, Human; 8) Isophane Insulin; 9) Isophane Insulin, Human; 10) Isophane Insulin, Human, and Insulin Human; 11) Prompt Insulin Zinc*.

INN:
  Extended Insulin Zinc Suspension—Insulin Zinc Suspension (Crystalline)
  Insulin Human Injection—Insulin (Human)
  Insulin Zinc Suspension—Insulin Zinc Suspension, Compound
  Prompt Insulin Zinc Suspension—Insulin Zinc Suspension (Amorphous)

BAN:
  Extended Insulin Zinc Suspension—Insulin Zinc Suspension (Crystalline)
  Insulin Human Injection—Insulin (Human)
  Insulin Zinc Suspension—Insulin Zinc
  Isophane Insulin Suspension—Isophane Insulin
  Prompt Insulin Zinc Suspension—Insulin Zinc Suspension (Amorphous)

JAN:
  Extended Insulin Zinc Suspension—Crystalline Insulin Zinc Injection (Aqueous Suspension)
  Insulin Human Injection—Insulin Human (Biosynthesis) and Insulin Human (Synthesis)
  Isophane Insulin Suspension—Isophane Insulin Injection (Aqueous Suspension)
  Insulin Zinc Suspension—Insulin Zinc Injection (Aqueous Suspension) and Insulin Zinc Purified Porcine (Suspension)
  Prompt Insulin Zinc Suspension—Amorphous Insulin Zinc Injection (Aqueous Solution)

VA CLASSIFICATION (Primary/Secondary): HS501/GA900; DX900

Commonly used brand name(s): *Humulin 10/90*[10]; *Humulin 20/80*[10]; *Humulin 30/70*[10]; *Humulin 40/60*[10]; *Humulin 50/50*[10]; *Humulin 70/30*[10]; *Humulin L*[7]; *Humulin N*[9]; *Humulin R*[5]; *Humulin U Ultralente*[3]; *Humulin-L*[7]; *Humulin-N*[9]; *Humulin-R*[5]; *Humulin-U*[3]; *Insulin-Toronto*[4]; *Lente Iletin*[6]; *Lente Iletin I*[6]; *Lente Iletin II*[6]; *Lente Insulin*[6]; *Lente L*[6]; *NPH Iletin*[8]; *NPH Iletin I*[8]; *NPH Iletin II*[8]; *NPH Insulin*[8]; *NPH-N*[8]; *Novolin 70/30*[10]; *Novolin 70/30 PenFill*[10]; *Novolin 70/30 Prefilled*[10]; *Novolin L*[7]; *Novolin N*[9]; *Novolin N PenFill*[9]; *Novolin N Prefilled*[9]; *Novolin R*[5]; *Novolin R PenFill*[5]; *Novolin R Prefilled*[5]; *Novolin ge 10/90 Penfill*[10]; *Novolin ge 20/80 Penfill*[10]; *Novolin ge 30/70*[10]; *Novolin ge 30/70 Penfill*[10]; *Novolin ge 40/60 Penfill*[10]; *Novolin ge 50/50 Penfill*[10]; *Novolin ge Lente*[7]; *Novolin ge NPH*[9]; *Novolin ge NPH Penfill*[9]; *Novolin ge Toronto*[5]; *Novolin ge Toronto Penfill*[5]; *Novolin ge Ultralente*[3]; *Regular (Concentrated) Iletin II, U-500*[4]; *Regular Iletin*[4];

*Regular Iletin I*[4]; *Regular Iletin II*[4]; *Regular Insulin*[4]; *Semilente Insulin*[11]; *Ultralente Insulin*[2]; *Velosulin BR*[1]; *Velosulin Human*[1].

Other commonly used names are: Lente insulin [Insulin Zinc] NPH insulin [Isophane Insulin] Regular insulin [Insulin] Semilente insulin [Prompt Insulin Zinc] Ultralente insulin [Extended Insulin Zinc]

Note: For a listing of dosage forms and brand names by country availability, see *Dosage Forms* section(s).

*Not commercially available in U.S.

## Category

Antidiabetic agent; diagnostic aid (pituitary growth hormone reserve).

## Indications

Note: Bracketed information in the *Indications* section refers to uses that are not included in U.S. product labeling.

### Accepted

Diabetes mellitus (treatment), including

Diabetes mellitus, insulin-dependent (IDDM)—Insulin is indicated in the treatment of insulin-dependent diabetes mellitus (Type I diabetes; previously called ketosis-prone, brittle, or juvenile-onset diabetes), which occurs in individuals who produce little or no endogenous insulin. One of two regimens (conventional or intensive therapy) is commonly used to treat this condition. The intensive regimen provides more rigid control of blood glucose than the conventional regimen does, but requires more frequent monitoring and more frequent dosage adjustment, and, unless insulin is administered via an insulin pump, a larger number of injections.

Diabetes mellitus, non–insulin-dependent (NIDDM)—Insulin is indicated in the treatment of certain patients with NIDDM (Type II diabetes; previously known as adult-onset diabetes, maturity-onset diabetes, ketosis-resistant diabetes, or stable diabetes), which occurs in individuals who produce or secrete insufficient quantities of endogenous insulin or who have developed resistance to endogenous insulin. Insulin therapy in NIDDM is reserved for patients whose disease is not controlled by other measures (i.e., diet, exercise, oral antidiabetic agents) or who cannot tolerate oral antidiabetic agents.

Diabetes mellitus, gestational (GDM)

Diabetes mellitus, malnutrition-related or

Diabetes mellitus, other, associated with certain conditions or syndromes, such as:

Pancreatic disease (congenital absence of the pancreatic islets, transient diabetes of the newborn, functional immaturity of insulin secretion in the neonate, or cystic fibrosis)

Endocrine disease (endocrine overactivity due to Cushing's syndrome, hyperthyroidism, pheochromocytoma, somatostatinoma, or aldosteronoma; or endocrine underactivity due to hypoparathyroidism-hypocalcemia, type I isolated growth hormone deficiency, or multitropic pituitary deficiency) or

Genetic syndromes, including inborn errors of metabolism, (glycogen-storage disease type I or insulin-resistant syndromes, such as muscular dystrophies, late onset proximal myopathy, and Huntington's chorea)—Insulin is indicated for the treatment of GDM and for the treatment of diabetes mellitus associated with certain conditions and syndromes uncontrolled by other treatment measures (diet, exercise, and oral antidiabetic agents). Insulin requirements increase eventually during pregnancy for all diabetics. Need for additional exogenous insulin usually stops postpartum for GDM patients due to hormonal and metabolic changes; however, some GDM patients progress to NIDDM or IDDM within 5 to 10 years. Insulin is also used to treat diabetes induced by hormones, medications, or chemicals. Insulin has been added to total parenteral nutrition or glucose solutions in order to facilitate glucose utilization in patients with poor glucose tolerance.

Insulin is also used to treat acute complications associated with diabetes, such as ketoacidosis, significant acidosis, ketosis, hyperglycemic hyperosmolar nonketotic coma, or diabetic coma. Also, temporary insulin dosing for diabetics not using insulin or an increased insulin dose for IDDM or insulin-requiring NIDDM patients may be warranted when these patients are subjected to physical stress (i.e., pregnancy, fever, severe infection, severe burns, major surgery, or other severe trauma).

Combination use of insulin and oral antidiabetic agents in IDDM patients is controversial because many studies have indicated that oral antidiabetic agents are not effective in the treatment of these patients. Some NIDDM patients resistant to sulfonylureas alone may benefit from the combination of low-dose insulin and oral sulfonylurea agents for diabetes; however, resultant weight gain and effects of hyperinsulinemia should be considered. In addition, the combination of metformin and sulfonylurea agents has been used successfully before discontinuation of oral agents and initiation of insulin therapy.

Concentrated insulin (500 USP Insulin Units) is used only to treat insulin-resistant patients needing a high dose (over 200 USP units) of insulin.

[Growth hormone deficiency (diagnosis)][1]—Intravenous regular insulin is used to assess the capacity of the pituitary gland to release growth hormone. Reliable results may require that more than one test using regular insulin be performed or that one additional test be conducted, such as one using arginine. Also, information regarding release of corticotropin from the pituitary can be assessed. A physician experienced in the use of the insulin tolerance test should be present because of the risk of hypoglycemia.

[1]Not included in Canadian product labeling.

## Pharmacology/Pharmacokinetics

### Physicochemical characteristics

Source—

Bovine: Obtained from the pancreas of oxen; differs from human insulin by 2 amino acids at positions 8 and 10 on the A-chain and from porcine insulin by 1 amino acid at position 30 on the B-chain.

may contribute to an increase in peripheral vascular resistance through vascular hypertrophy.

| USP Insulin Type | Onset of action† (hrs) | Time to peak† (hrs) | Duration of action† (hrs) |
|---|---|---|---|
| Intravenous<br>　Insulin injection U-100<br>　　(regular insulin)<br>　　　mixed*, pork, purified pork,<br>　　　biosynthetic human<br>　　　semisynthetic human | 1/6–1/2 | 1/4–1/2 | 1/2–1 |
| Subcutaneous<br>　Insulin injection U-100<br>　　(regular insulin)<br>　　　mixed*, pork, purified pork,<br>　　　biosynthetic human<br>　　　semisynthetic human | 1/2–1 | 2–4 | 5–7 |
| Insulin injection U-500<br>　(regular insulin)<br>　　purified pork | | | 24‡ |
| Isophane insulin suspension<br>　U-100<br>　　(NPH insulin)<br>　　　mixed*, purified pork, biosynthetic human | 3–4 | 6–12 | 18–28 |
| Isophane insulin suspension<br>　(70%) and insulin injection<br>　(30%) U-100<br>　　biosynthetic human | 1/2 | 4–8 | 24 |
| Insulin zinc suspension U-100<br>　(lente insulin)<br>　　mixed*, purified pork, biosynthetic human | 1–3 | 8–12 | 18–28 |
| Extended insulin zinc<br>　suspension U-100<br>　　(ultralente)<br>　　　mixed*, biosynthetic human | 4–6 | 18–24 | 36 |
| Prompt insulin zinc suspension<br>　U-100<br>　　(semilente)<br>　　　mixed* | 1–3 | 2–8 | 12–16 |

*Mixed = Mixture of beef and pork insulins.
†Mean values; individual responses vary widely.
‡U-500 strength is absorbed slowly, resulting in a long duration of action.

**Absorption**
Rate of subcutaneous and intramuscular insulin absorption is highly variable (up to 50% inter- and intraindividual variability) and is dependent on many factors including insulin formulation, injection site, injection technique, and route of injection. The addition of protamine or zinc to insulin produces a crystallized insulin in suspension that has a longer absorption phase (and a longer duration of action) than dissolved insulin does and is dependent on enzymatic degradation of the suspension at the injection site for absorption. Absorption of regular insulin, when mixed with equal or greater quantities of zinc insulin, may be slowed if the mixture is not injected immediately after preparation. Mixing regular insulin with isophane insulin does not alter the rate of absorption of either. Studies have shown that the absorption rate of human insulins is no different from, or only slightly higher than, the rate for animal insulins. The speed of injection and temperature of insulin do not alter absorption; however, capillary surface area and exercise do affect the intramuscular blood flow and can alter absorption. Exercising the limb into which the insulin was injected within 30 to 40 minutes postinjection may increase insulin absorption (delay of exercise may be warranted). Although longer-acting insulins have less pronounced variability in absorption among injection sites, the absorption rate for 12 USP Units of regular insulin given subcutaneously declined per region as follows: abdominal (87 minutes), deltoid (141 minutes), gluteal (155 minutes), and femoral (164 minutes). Finally, insulin absorption is faster with intramuscular injection than with subcutaneous injection, and is slower with very high insulin concentrations or high dose volumes.

A subcutaneous depot of insulin forms slowly at the injection site when a continuous subcutaneous infusion insulin pump is used, resulting in less variation in insulin availability and a smaller depot than occurs with use of subcutaneous injections. When injection sites are rotated, continued absorption from the first depot usually prevents plasma concentrations from decreasing to subtherapeutic values while another depot is forming.

**Distribution**
Distributed into most cells.

**Biotransformation**
Insulin—Hepatic and renal.
Isophane or zinc insulins—Split into protamine or zinc and insulin by subcutaneous enzymes prior to absorption.

**Half-life**
Insulin—5 to 6 minutes; can be longer in some diabetics. Insulin antibodies, if present, bind to circulating plasma insulin and prolong its biologic half-life.

**Elimination**
Renal, 30 to 80%; unchanged insulin is reabsorbed.

## Precautions to Consider

### Cross-sensitivity and/or related problems
Patients intolerant of beef or pork insulins may use the alternative single-source insulin under the direction of their physician. Intolerance of beef insulin is more common than intolerance of pork insulin. Intolerance is often reduced by the use of purified pork insulin, biosynthetic human insulin, or semisynthetic human insulin.

Patients hypersensitive to protamine sulfate also may be hypersensitive to protamine-containing insulins. Patients who have become sensitized to protamine through administration of a protamine-containing insulin are at risk for severe anaphylactoid reactions if protamine sulfate is subsequently administered for reversal of heparin effect.

### Pregnancy/Reproduction
*Pregnancy*—Insulin does not cross the placenta. However, maternal glucose and maternal insulin antibodies do cross the placenta and can cause fetal hyperinsulinemia and related problems, such as large-for-gestational-age infants and macrosomnia, possibly resulting in a need for early induced or cesarean delivery. Furthermore, high blood glucose concentrations occurring during early pregnancy (5 to 8 weeks gestation) have been associated with a higher incidence of major congenital abnormalities and, later in pregnancy, increased perinatal morbidity and mortality.

Diabetic women must be educated about the necessity of maintaining strict metabolic control before conception and throughout pregnancy, especially during early pregnancy, to significantly decrease the risk of maternal mortality, congenital anomalies, and perinatal morbidity and mortality. A study reported that initial hemoglobin $A_{1c}$ (a measurement of blood glucose control for the preceding 3 months) concentrations of 10% or more, 8 to 9.9%, and below 8% produced infant malformation rates of 35%, 12.9%, and 4.8%, respectively; the malformation rate in infants born to nondiabetic mothers is approximately 2%. Use of insulin rather than oral antidiabetic agents for the treatment of NIDDM and GDM permits maintenance of blood glucose at concentrations as close to normal as possible. Insulin requirements in pregnant diabetic patients are often decreased during the first trimester. Requirements are usually increased in the last 2 trimesters of pregnancy in response to the anti-insulin hormone activity associated with increased concentrations of human placental estrogen, progesterone, chorionic gonadotropin, and prolactin; peripheral insulin resistance due to increasing levels of fatty acids and triglycerides; and increased degradation of insulin by the placenta.

*Postpartum*—Insulin requirements drop quickly after childbirth, and GDM patients usually no longer need insulin. Inadequately controlled maternal blood glucose late in pregnancy may cause increased insulin production in the fetus resulting in neonatal hypoglycemia. Treatment may be necessary until euglycemic control is established by the neonate.

### Breast-feeding
Insulin is not distributed into breast milk. Problems in humans have not been documented. The insulin requirement in lactating women is reduced because of hormonal changes; in patients with IDDM, insulin requirements during lactation may be up to 27% lower than the patients' pre-pregnancy requirements. Daily monitoring for several months is important until insulin needs stabilize or until insulin is no longer needed.

### Pediatrics
Insulin therapy in pediatric patients is similar to that in other age groups. However, strict intensive insulin therapy is not generally used for this age group because noncompliance may be a problem and because this regimen may be less beneficial before puberty while risks of hypoglycemia may be higher due to higher insulin sensitivity.

## Adolescents

Insulin therapy in adolescents is similar to that in other age groups. Appropriate use of intensive insulin therapy may be beneficial when used cautiously. Diabetic patients have a transient increase in insulin requirement (by approximately 20 to 50%) at puberty during the growth spurt only. Adolescent females usually require more insulin than do adolescent males because of increased insulin resistance; this is thought to be due, in part, to an increased secretion of growth hormone, but not to an increased secretion of sex hormones. Increased growth hormone secretion also may require alteration of the timing of insulin doses to overcome the prominent *dawn phenomenon* of hyperglycemia in diabetic adolescents of both sexes.

## Geriatrics

Insulin therapy in older patients is similar to that in other age groups. However, strict intensive insulin therapy is not generally used. Also, dehydration, which may mask early signs of hypoglycemia and permit development of more severe symptoms; vision problems, which may lead to inaccurate dosage measurement and/or glucose monitoring; shakiness, which may interfere with measurement and self-administration of a dose; and lack of compliance with prescribed diet commonly occur in the elderly and may interfere with control of diabetes. Instructions may be needed to help the patient monitor urine or blood glucose if visual problems are present or early symptoms of hypoglycemia are missing or delayed, a particular problem in this age group. Special devices are available to help administer the insulin dose when help with visual clarity or steadiness is needed.

## Drug interactions and/or related problems

The following drug interactions and/or related problems have been selected on the basis of their potential clinical significance (possible mechanism in parentheses where appropriate)—not necessarily inclusive (» = major clinical significance):

Note: Combinations containing any of the following medications, depending on the amount present, may also interact with this medication.

If the need exists to administer any medications that may affect metabolic or glycemic control of diabetes mellitus, blood glucose concentrations should be monitored by the patient or health care professional. This is particularly important when any medication is added to or removed from an established drug regimen. Subsequent adjustments in diet or insulin dosage or both may be necessary; these adjustments may differ depending on the severity of the diabetes mellitus and other factors.

» Alcohol
(consumption of moderate or large amounts of alcohol enhances insulin's hypoglycemic effect, increasing the risk of prolonged, severe hypoglycemia, especially under fasting conditions or when liver glycogen stores are low; small amounts of alcohol consumed with meals do not usually present problems)

Anabolic steroids, especially stanozolol, oxandrolone, and methandrostenolone or
Androgens
(increased tissue sensitivity to insulin and increased tissue resistance to glucagon may occur, resulting in hypoglycemia, especially when insulin resistance is present; a decrease in insulin dose may be required)

Antidiabetic agents, oral, sulfonylurea or
Carbonic anhydrase inhibitors, especially acetazolamide
(these medications chronically stimulate the pancreatic beta cell to release insulin and increase receptor and tissue sensitivity to insulin; although concurrent use of these medications with insulin may increase the hypoglycemic response, the effect may be unpredictable)

(sulfonylurea antidiabetic agents have been used concurrently with insulin in treating a select group of NIDDM patients whose condition is not well-controlled with either agent alone; however, the long-term benefit of this use has not been established; many studies have shown there is generally no additional benefit from using sulfonylurea antidiabetic agents for the treatment of IDDM patients)

Anti-inflammatory drugs, nonsteroidal (NSAIDs) or
Salicylates, large doses
(these medications inhibit synthesis of prostaglandin E [which inhibits endogenous insulin secretion], thereby increasing basal insulin secretion, the response to a glucose load, and the hypoglycemic effect of concurrently administered insulin; dosage adjustment of the NSAID or salicylate and/or insulin may be necessary, especially during and following chronic concurrent use)

» Beta-adrenergic blocking agents, including ophthalmics, if significant systemic absorption occurs
(beta-adrenergic blocking agents may inhibit insulin secretion, modify carbohydrate metabolism, and increase peripheral insulin resistance, leading to hyperglycemia; however, they may also cause hypoglycemia and block the normal catecholamine-mediated response to hypoglycemia [glycogenolysis and mobilization of glucose], thereby prolonging the time it takes to achieve euglycemia and increasing the risk of a severe hypoglycemic reaction. Selective beta$_1$-adrenergic blocking agents [such as acebutolol, atenolol, betaxolol, bisoprolol, and metoprolol] exhibit the above actions to a lesser extent; however, any of these agents can blunt some of the symptoms of developing hypoglycemia, such as increased heart rate or blood pressure [increased sweating may not be altered], making detection of this complication more difficult)

Chloroquine or
Quinidine or
Quinine
(concurrent use with insulin may increase the risk of hypoglycemia and increased blood insulin concentrations because of decreased insulin degradation)

» Corticosteroids
(these agents antagonize insulin's effects by stimulating release of catecholamines, causing hyperglycemia; corticosteroid-induced diabetes can occur in up to 14% of the patients taking systemic corticosteroids for several weeks or with prolonged use of topical corticosteroids, but this condition rarely produces acidosis or ketonuria even with high glucose concentrations; reversal of effects may take several weeks or months; changes in insulin dose may be necessary for diabetics during and following concurrent use)

Diuretics, loop or
Diuretics, thiazide
(concurrent use with insulin may increase the risk of hyperglycemia because the potassium-depleting effect of these diuretics may inhibit insulin secretion and decrease tissue sensitivity to insulin)

Guanethidine or
Monoamine oxidase (MAO) inhibitors, including furazolidone, procarbazine, and selegiline
(epinephrine release by these agents may cause hyperglycemia; however, chronic use results in hypoglycemia; the mechanism of the latter is unknown but may include stored catecholamine depletion and interference with the compensatory adrenergic response to a fall in blood glucose; a change in dose of insulin before, during, and after treatment with these agents may be necessary)

Hyperglycemia-causing agents, such as:
Calcium channel blockers
Clonidine
Danazol
Dextrothyroxine
Diazoxide, parenteral
Epinephrine
Estrogen
Estrogen-progestin–containing oral contraceptives
Glucagon
Growth hormone
Heparin
Histamine$_2$ receptor antagonists
Marijuana
Morphine
Nicotine
Phenytoin
Sulfinpyrazone
Thyroid hormones
(these medications may change metabolic control of glucose concentrations and, unless the changes can be controlled with diet, may necessitate an increase in the amount or a change in the timing of the insulin dose)

Hypoglycemia-causing agents, such as:
Angiotensin-converting enzyme inhibitors
Bromocriptine
Clofibrate
Ketoconazole
Lithium
Mebendazole
Pyridoxine
Sulfonamides
Theophylline
(these medications may change metabolic control of glucose concentrations and, unless the changes can be controlled with diet, may necessitate a decrease in the amount or a change in the timing of the insulin dose)

Octreotide
(octreotide can cause changes in the counterregulatory hormones secretion [insulin, glucagon, and growth hormone] and slow gastric

emptying and gastrointestinal contractility resulting in delayed meal absorption and mild transient hypo- or hyperglycemia in normal and diabetic patients; insulin therapy may need to be reduced in diabetic patients following the initiation of octreotide and monitored for adjustments during and after octreotide treatment)

» Pentamidine
(pentamidine has a toxic effect on pancreatic beta cells resulting in a biphasic effect on glucose concentration, i.e., initial insulin release and hypoglycemia followed by hypoinsulinemia and hyperglycemia with continued use of pentamidine; initially, insulin dose should be reduced, then the dose should be increased with continued use of pentamidine)

Tetracycline
(a delayed onset of increased tissue sensitivity to insulin may occur in diabetic patients; reaction has not appeared in individuals with normal glucose tolerance)

Tobacco, smoking
(may antagonize insulin effects by stimulating release of catecholamines, causing hyperglycemia; also, smoking reduces subcutaneous insulin absorption; dosage reduction of insulin may be necessary when an insulin-dependent diabetic patient suddenly stops smoking)

### Medical considerations/Contraindications

The medical considerations/contraindications included have been selected on the basis of their potential clinical significance (reasons given in parentheses where appropriate)—not necessarily inclusive (» = major clinical significance).

*Risk-benefit should be considered when the following medical problems exist:*

Note: The following medical problems may necessitate a change in insulin therapy and are not intended as contraindications.

» Diarrhea or
» Gastroparesis or
» Intestinal obstruction or
» Vomiting or
» Other conditions causing delayed food absorption or malabsorption
(vomiting or delayed stomach emptying may require a change in timing of the insulin dose to realign peak action to peak blood glucose concentrations)

Hepatic disease
(insulin requirements are complex, and an increase or decrease of dosage may be needed partly because of modifications in hepatic metabolism of insulin and alterations in hepatic and plasma glucose concentrations)

» Hyperglycemia-causing conditions, such as:
Female hormonal changes or
Fever, high or
Hyperadrenalism, not optimally controlled or
Infection, severe or
Psychological stress
(these conditions may increase blood glucose, increase or change the insulin requirement, and necessitate more frequent blood glucose monitoring)
(insulin requirements may be increased near or during a menstrual cycle and may return to normal after menstruation; also, a change to intravenous insulin administration may be needed during labor when close glucose control is needed)

Hyperthyroidism, not optimally controlled
(hyperthyroidism increases both the activity and the clearance of insulin, making glycemic control difficult until the patient is euthyroid)

» Hypoglycemia-causing conditions, such as:
Adrenal insufficiency, not optimally controlled or
Pituitary insufficiency, not optimally controlled
(these conditions, by reducing blood glucose concentrations, may decrease the insulin requirement and necessitate more frequent blood glucose monitoring)
(also, untreated or not optimally controlled adrenal or pituitary insufficiency may increase tissue sensitivity to insulin and reduce the patient's insulin requirement)

Renal disease
(insulin requirements are complex, and an increase or decrease of dosage may be needed due to modifications in renal clearance of insulin)

Surgery or
Trauma
(hypo- or hyperglycemia may occur depending on the surgery or trauma; a change to intravenous insulin administration may be needed when close glucose control is necessary)

### Patient monitoring

The following may be especially important in patient monitoring (other tests may be warranted in some patients, depending on condition; » = major clinical significance):

» Blood glucose determinations
(the concentration of blood or plasma glucose reflects the current degree of metabolic control and should be routinely monitored by the patient at home and by the physician [every 3 months and more often when patient is not stabilized] to confirm that blood glucose concentration is maintained within agreed upon targets by the selected diet and dosing regimen; particularly important during dosage adjustments. Self monitoring of blood glucose by patient may require testing at multiple times during the day for intensive insulin therapy or once to several times a week for conventional insulin therapy)

(caution in interpreting blood glucose concentrations is needed because normal whole blood glucose values are approximately 15% lower than plasma glucose values. Normal fasting whole blood glucose for adults of all ages is 65 to 95 mg/dL [3.6 to 5.3 mmol/L]. Normal fasting serum glucose is 70 to 105 mg/dL [3.9 to 5.8 mmol/L] for adults younger than 60 years of age and 80 to 115 mg/dL [4.4 to 6.4 mmol/L] for adults 60 years of age and older. For children, normal fasting serum glucose is less than 130 mg/dL [7.2 mmol/L] and fasting whole blood glucose is less than 115 mg/dL [5.6 mmol/L]. For pregnant diabetic women, normal fasting serum glucose is less than 105 mg/dL [5.8 mmol/L] and fasting whole blood glucose is less than 120 mg/dL [6.7 mmol/L]. Goals for intensive insulin therapy are to maintain fasting blood glucose between 60 and 120 mg/dL [3.3 and 6.7 mmol/L] and postprandial blood glucose at less than 180 mg/dL [10 mmol/L], while goals of conventional insulin therapy are based on the absence of symptoms of hyper- and hypoglycemia)

(capillary blood glucose measurement provides important information when done properly, but caution is warranted because of potential errors in technique and readings; it has been suggested that the values be relied upon only if the reported glucose concentration for stable diabetics is between 75 mg/dL and 325 mg/dL [4.12 mmol/L and 17.88 mmol/L, respectively])

Body weight determinations
(significant increase in body weight may require increase in insulin dosage)

Glucose, urine or
Ketones, urine
(if blood glucose concentrations exceed 200 mg/dL [11.1 mmol/L], it may be necessary to monitor urine for the presence of glucose and ketones; normalization of glucose in the urine generally lags quantitatively behind serum glucose concentrations; test methods are generally capable of detecting serum glucose concentrations greater than 180 mg/dL [10 mmol/L])

Glycosylated hemoglobin (hemoglobin $A_{1c}$) determinations
(hemoglobin $A_{1c}$ values [normal whole blood hemoglobin $A_{1c}$ is 4 to 6% of total hemoglobin; specific values are laboratory-dependent] reflect the metabolic control over the preceding 3 months, but assessment of this parameter does not eliminate the need for daily blood glucose monitoring. Hemoglobin $A_{1c}$ is falsely elevated in nonstabilized diabetics when the intermediate precursor is elevated [i.e., in alcoholism] and falsely lowered in conditions of shortened red blood cell lifespan [i.e., in anemia and acute or chronic blood loss] or in patients with hemoglobinopathies [i.e., sickle cell])

pH measurements, serum or
Potassium concentrations, serum
(determinations may be important if patient is hypoglycemic and ketoacidotic)

## Side/Adverse Effects

The following side/adverse effects have been selected on the basis of their potential clinical significance (possible signs and symptoms in parentheses where appropriate)—not necessarily inclusive:

### Those indicating need for medical attention

Incidence more frequent
*Hypoglycemia—mild, including nocturnal hypoglycemia* (anxiety; behavior change, similar to drunkenness; blurred vision; cold sweats; confusion; cool pale skin; difficulty in concentrating; drowsiness; excessive hunger; fast heartbeat; headache; nausea; nervousness; nightmares; restless sleep; shakiness; slurred speech; unusual tiredness or weakness); *hypoglycemia—severe* (convulsions or coma); *weight gain*

Note: The occurrence of a recent episode of *hypoglycemia* may lessen the symptoms of a second episode. In children and the elderly, *hypoglycemia* symptoms are variable and harder to identify. Furthermore, *nocturnal hypoglycemia* may be asymptomatic in 33% or more of affected patients. Also, rebound hyperglycemia may appear from ½ to 24 hours after moderate to severe hypoglycemia (Somogyi phenomenon).

Hypoglycemic episodes, including severe hypoglycemic coma, occur 3 times more frequently with intensive insulin therapy than with conventional therapy.

*Weight gain* of 120% above ideal weight (mean of 4.6 kg after 5 years of treatment) is experienced by 12.7 patients per 100 patient-years during intensive insulin therapy and by 9.3 patients per 100 patient-years during conventional insulin therapy.

Incidence rare
  *Edema* (swelling of face, fingers, feet, or ankles); *lipoatrophy at injection site* (depression of the skin at the injection site); *lipohypertrophy at injection site* (thickening of skin tissues at the injection site)
  Note: *Edema* due to sodium retention caused by insulin is reversible over several days to a week after euglycemic recovery from severe hyperglycemia or ketoacidosis.

  The risk of *lipohypertrophy* may be decreased by rotating injection sites; risk of *lipoatrophy* may be reduced by injecting insulin into the periphery of the atrophic site in order to restore subcutaneous adipose tissue.

# Patient Consultation

As an aid to patient consultation, refer to *Advice for the Patient, Insulin (Systemic)*.

In providing consultation, consider emphasizing the following selected information (» = major clinical significance):

**Before using this medication**
» Conditions affecting use, especially:
  Allergy or local skin sensitivity to insulins
  Pregnancy—Importance of controlling and monitoring blood glucose to meet changing needs for insulin during and after pregnancy and to prevent maternal and fetal problems, including fetal macrosomnia, anomalies, and hyperglycemia; alerting physician to plans before becoming pregnant when possible
  Breast-feeding—Insulin is not distributed into breast milk; however, the maternal requirement for insulin is less during breast-feeding because of hormonal changes; checking blood glucose every day for several months to help determine variable insulin dosing needs
  Use in children—Use in children is similar to use in other age groups. However, prepubertal children have increased risk of hypoglycemia because they have greater sensitivity to insulin than do pubertal children
  Use in adolescents—Use in adolescents is similar to use in other age groups. However, insulin needs increase by 20–50% at puberty and decrease afterwards; girls may need higher insulin doses than boys
  Use in the elderly—Risk of hypoglycemia is increased in elderly patients. Special counseling with emphasis on hydration, diet, and exercise may be necessary because of the greater risk of hypoglycemia in this age group. Special training and equipment are available to help overcome these problems
  Other medications, especially alcohol, beta-adrenergic blocking agents, corticosteroids, or pentamidine
  Other medical problems, especially adrenal insufficiency, pituitary insufficiency, or other conditions causing hypoglycemia, diarrhea, gastroparesis, intestinal obstruction, vomiting, or other conditions causing delayed food absorption; female hormonal changes, high fever, hyperadrenalism, psychological distress, severe infection, or other conditions causing hyperglycemia

**Proper use of this medication**
» Understanding what is meant by source of insulin (beef and pork, pork, mixed insulins, and human) and only buying insulin derived from the source and of the type and strength that are prescribed; otherwise, consulting physician
» Selecting syringe of proper units of measure for insulin capacity; syringe should be made to measure insulin in units to facilitate accurate dose measurement; a 3/10 cc syringe measures up to 30 USP Units, a ½ cc syringe measures up to 50 USP Units, and a 1 cc syringe measures up to 100 USP Units
  Carefully selecting and rotating injection sites, following physician's recommendations
» Proper preparation of medication
  Washing hands with soap and water
  Measuring 1 type of insulin per dose
  Measuring and mixing 2 types of insulin per dose
» Proper administration technique
*Using various injection devices*
» Carefully reading patient instruction sheet contained in insulin or device package
» Disposing of syringes by separating needle from syringe, capping or clipping needle, and disposing in puncture-resistant container
  Understanding how to use insulin in insulin devices, such as automatic injector, continuous subcutaneous insulin infusion pump, disposable and nondisposable syringes, insulin pen devices, and insulin spray injector
» Compliance with therapy, including alternative dosing for changes in diet and exercise or sick day management
» Proper dosing
» Proper storage

**Precautions while using this medication**
» Regular visits to physician to check progress, especially during the first few weeks of treatment
» Carefully following special instructions of health care team:
  Discussing use of alcohol
  Discussing plans to stop chronic smoking of tobacco
  Not taking other medications unless discussed with physician
  Getting counseling for family to help assist diabetic; also, special counseling for pregnancy planning and contraception
  Discussing travel arrangements, including transporting insulin and carrying medical history and extra supplies of insulin and syringes
» Preparing for and knowing what to do in case of an emergency by carrying medical history and current drug list, wearing medical identification, and keeping nonexpired glucagon kit and needles, quick acting sugar, and having extra needed medical supplies nearby
» Recognizing symptoms of hypoglycemia
» Recognizing what brings on symptoms of hypoglycemia, such as delaying or missing a meal, exercising more than usual, drinking significant amounts of alcohol, taking certain medicines, using too much insulin, sickness including vomiting or diarrhea
» Knowing what to do if symptoms of hypoglycemia occur, such as using glucagon, eating glucose tablets or gel, corn syrup, honey, or sugar cubes, or drinking fruit juice, nondiet soft drink, or dissolved sugar in water; also, eating small snack, such as cheese and crackers, milk, or half sandwich when scheduled meal is longer than 1 hour away; not eating foods high in fat, such as chocolate, since fat slows gastric emptying
» Recognizing symptoms of hyperglycemia and ketoacidosis:
  Blurred vision
  Drowsiness
  Dry mouth
  Flushed, dry skin
  Fruit-like breath odor
  Increased urination (frequency and volume)
  Ketones in urine
  Loss of appetite
  Somnolence (sleepiness)
  Stomachache, nausea, or vomiting
  Tiredness
  Troubled breathing (rapid and deep)
  Unconsciousness
  Unusual thirst
» Recognizing what brings on symptoms of hyperglycemia, such as fever or infection; not taking enough insulin; skipping an insulin dose; exercising less than usual; taking certain medicines; over-eating or not following meal plan
» Knowing what to do if symptoms of hyperglycemia occur, such as checking blood glucose and increasing the insulin dose (short term for supplementary or anticipatory doses) according to the individualized dosing schedule developed; contacting physician for more permanent dose changes; changing only 1 type of insulin dose (usually the first dose); anticipating how one change in an insulin dose affects other doses of the day; delaying a meal if blood glucose concentration exceeds 200 mg/dL (11.1 mmol/L); checking with physician when blood glucose concentration is above 240 mg/dL (13.3 mmol/L); not exercising when blood glucose concentration is above 240 mg/dL (13.3 mmol/L); or being hospitalized if ketoacidosis or coma occurs

**Side/adverse effects**
  Signs of potential side effects, especially mild hypoglycemia, including nocturnal; severe hypoglycemia; weight gain; edema; lipoatrophy or lipohypertrophy at injection site

## General Dosing Information

In the United States, the potency of insulin is expressed in terms of USP Insulin Units or USP Insulin Human Units. Bovine or porcine insulin contains not less than 26 USP Insulin Units per mg of insulin on the dried basis. Human insulin contains not less than 27.5 USP Insulin Human Units per mg of insulin on the dried basis. International Units cannot be compared directly to USP Units because the reference standards and the methodologies for manufacturing are different.

It is generally not recommended that patients whose diabetes is well-controlled with animal insulins automatically be switched to human insulins. Human insulins may not offer any significant advantage over the highly purified pork insulins, with the exception of reduced antibody levels, which may be a consideration for some patients, especially children, young adults, patients who are pregnant or considering pregnancy, patients with allergies, or patients using insulin intermittantly. Patients should be informed of the possible need for dosage adjustment during the first 1 to 2 weeks following a change in the source (bovine and porcine, porcine, or human) of their insulin products and advised not to make such a change without first consulting their physicians.

Transferring patients from oral hypoglycemic agents to insulin can be immediate, although blood glucose concentrations should be evaluated for several days following the change and the prolonged effects of chlorpropamide should be considered when determining the insulin dose.

The vial of insulin must not be shaken hard before being used. Frothing or bubble formation can cause an incorrect dose. Contents are mixed well by rolling the bottle slowly between the palms of the hands or by gently tipping the bottle over a few times. Insulin should not be used if it looks lumpy or grainy, or sticks to the bottle. Also, regular insulin should not be used if it becomes viscous or cloudy; only clear, colorless solutions should be used.

Dilution of insulin preparations generally should be avoided. However, some pediatric doses may be too small to measure accurately. If needed, diluting from U-100 to U-10 has been suggested to aid in accurate dosing for very small doses in pediatric patients. Such dilutions are stable for 2 months when stored at 4 °C (39 °F) or until the date of expiration of the insulin, whichever occurs first. Occasionally insulin must be diluted to avoid crystallization in the catheters when it is administered as a low-dose infusion via an insulin pump. In these rare cases, dilution should be performed aseptically in a laminar flow hood using diluents and mixing vials provided or recommended by the manufacturer. The differences in strength, dosage volume, and expiration date should be clearly labeled by the pharmacist and emphasized to the patient. If insulin needs to be diluted during an emergency and the diluents are not readily available, 0.9% sodium chloride injection without preservative may be used for dilution of small insulin doses. However, these solutions are not stable and should be used promptly. Stinging or burning at the site of injection may also occur due to the lower pH of these solutions.

Different types of insulin are sometimes mixed in the syringe in proportions ordered by the physician in order to achieve a more accurate matching of insulin availability to the patient's requirements in a single dose. If insulins are to be mixed, several factors should be considered:

- Each patient should always follow the same sequence of mixing the separate insulin preparations. As a general rule, regular insulin should be drawn first to avoid contamination and clouding of the vial of regular insulin by the other insulin. A mixture of regular insulin and another insulin will have a longer duration of action than does regular insulin alone.
- Insulin zinc, prompt insulin zinc, and extended insulin zinc may be mixed in any proportion without loss of the characteristics of the individual insulins. Such mixtures are stable for up to 18 months.
- Unbuffered regular insulin and isophane insulin may be mixed in any proportion in a syringe and stored upright if possible. The prefilled syringe can be used immediately, stored at room temperature and used within 14 days, or stored in a refrigerator for use within 3 weeks. Mixtures containing buffered regular insulin should be used immediately.
- Mixing unbuffered regular insulin and insulin zinc insulins (lente, semilente, and ultralente) is not recommended because the excess zinc in the insulin zinc insulin can form an extra zinc insulin complex with the regular insulin. This can lengthen the insulin's duration of action and give unpredictable clinical results. However, if these insulins are combined, it is recommended that the mixture be used immediately.
- Phosphate buffered regular insulin or isophane insulins should not be mixed with insulin zinc insulins. Zinc phosphate may precipitate from the mixture, which can shorten the expected duration of action and provide unpredictable clinical results.
- Phosphate buffered regular insulin should not be mixed with any other insulin when used in an external insulin infusion pump because of the potential problem of precipitation.

After receiving insulin at first diagnosis of IDDM, 20 to 30% of diabetics appear to normalize for a few weeks or months (called the honeymoon phase). Some clinicians continue insulin treatment in small doses of 0.2 to 0.5 USP Units per kg of body weight during this time.

Conventional and intensive insulin therapies are individualized insulin regimens that provide different levels of blood glucose control. Conventional therapy consists of 1 or 2 insulin injections a day and daily self-monitoring of urine or blood glucose, but not daily adjustments of insulin dose. Intensive insulin therapy provides tighter blood glucose control via administration of 3 or more injections a day or by use of an insulin pump. Also, adjustments of insulin dose according to the results of self-monitoring of blood glucose determinations are performed at least 4 times a day and before anticipated dietary intake and exercise. Close glucose control has been proven to delay the onset and slow the progression of diabetic retinopathy, nephropathy, and neuropathy. The dosage and the timing of administration of insulin can vary greatly and must therefore be determined for each individual patient by the attending physician. Matching the patient's specific insulin needs over a 24-hour period through the use of short-acting and longer-acting preparations may decrease long-term complications of diabetes mellitus.

If a pattern of metabolic noncontrol ensues (blood glucose concentrations changing for 3 days), the total daily insulin dose is usually adjusted by changing only 1 type of insulin and only 1 segment of the daily dose; the first preprandial dose is the one most commonly changed because it more prominently affects the other doses of the day.

Insulin requirements may change with diet or physical activity. Algorithms can be developed to aid a patient with supplemental or anticipatory insulin dosing needs based on the patient's sensitivity to insulin. Supplemental doses of regular insulin can be used to correct excessive preprandial blood glucose concentrations after the basic dose of insulin is established. Anticipatory insulin doses are based on anticipated dietary or physical activity changes. Patients should be cautioned against exercising if the blood glucose concentration exceeds 240 mg/dL (13.3 mmol/L), or when a condition exists that causes low glucagon stores, because of the increased risk of secondary hyperglycemia due to exercise.

Additional low doses of regular insulin (1 to 2 USP Units for each 30 to 40 mg/dL [1.7 to 2.2 mmol/L] incremental rise above the target blood glucose concentration) every 3 to 4 hours may be needed on sick days. Patients should be warned to inform the physician if the concentration remains above 240 mg/dL (13.3 mmol/L) after 3 supplementary insulin doses or if symptoms of ketoacidosis develop.

The patient should always use only one brand or type of syringe and should consult the physician before changing brands or syringe types. Among different brands or syringe types, the unmeasured volume between the needle point and the bottom calibration on the syringe barrel (called dead space) may differ enough to cause improper dosage.

The use of a disposable syringe and needle to administer more than one injection is controversial. Although USP medical advisory panels do not recommend this practice, it must be recognized that some patients reuse disposable syringes and needles because of economic constraints. Where this is occurring, it must be emphasized that the syringe and needle be used only for that particular patient, the needle should be wiped with alcohol, and the needle's cap replaced after each use. Also, the syringe and needle should be reused only for a limited number of injections. Disposable syringes and needles should not be reused on a continuing basis.

### For intravenous infusion

Regular insulin (Insulin Injection USP and Insulin Human Injection USP) in the 100-USP-Unit concentration is the only insulin type suitable for intravenous administration.

Insulin can be adsorbed to the surfaces of glass and plastic intravenous infusion containers (including PVC, ethylene vinyl acetate, and polyethylene). Adsorption is unpredictable and the clinical significance is uncertain. Recommendations for minimizing adsorption include adding 0.35% serum albumin human or approximately 5 mL of the patient's blood or using a syringe pump with a short cannula. For admixtures of insulin greater than 100 USP Units per 500 mL of intravenous solution, decant 50 mL of intravenous solution containing insulin through the administration apparatus and store for 30 minutes before using for optimal results. Afterwards, insulin dosage should be adjusted to meet patient's targeted blood glucose concentration. Regular insulin is compatible with dextrose in water, sodium chloride 0.9%, and combinations of these.

### For continuous subcutaneous insulin infusion pump
Generally, buffered regular insulin is used in insulin pumps, although unbuffered regular insulin has been used. The phosphate-buffered regular insulins are less likely to crystallize and block insulin pump catheters and are preferred over unbuffered regular insulin. Following insulin pump manufacturers' recommendations and suggested maintenance procedures is important to ensure optimal performance and to avoid problems, such as insulin adhesion or clogging. Consult individual manufacturer's package inserts.

When initiating a continuous subcutaneous insulin infusion with an insulin pump, a priming dose may be needed. Without an initial priming dose, the depot forms at a very slow rate. Pumps with a short pulse-rate interval have little superiority over pumps with a longer interval in relation to the depot formation. An additional priming dose is not necessary when the infusion site is changed. Absorption of insulin from the depot at the first site continues after discontinuation of the infusion, preventing insulin concentrations from decreasing to subtherapeutic values while another depot is forming at the new site.

### For treatment of adverse effects and/or overdose
Recommended treatment may include:
- For mild to moderate hypoglycemia—
  —Treating with immediate ingestion of a source of sugar, such as glucose gel, glucose tablets, fruit juice, corn syrup, non-diet soda, honey, sugar cubes, or table sugar dissolved in water. A frequently used source of sugar is a glassful of orange juice containing 2 or 3 teaspoonfuls of table sugar.
  —Documenting blood glucose and rechecking in 15 minutes.
  —Counseling patient to seek medical assistance promptly.
- For severe hypoglycemia or acute overdose, including coma—
  —Need for patient to obtain emergency medical assistance immediately.
  —Immediately treating with 50 mL of 50% dextrose given intravenously to stabilize, then administering a continuous infusion of 5 to 10% dextrose in water to maintain slight hyperglycemia (approximately 100 mg/dL blood glucose concentration) for up to 12 days. A nondiabetic adult usually exhibits a higher maximal hypoglycemic effect from insulin than does a diabetic adult. It is important to note that oral glucose cannot be relied upon to maintain euglycemia because 60% of an oral glucose dose is stored as hepatic glycogen with only 15% left for brain utilization and 15% for insulin-dependent tissues.
  —Glucagon, 1 to 2 mg intramuscular, is useful for fast onset of action to mobilize hepatic glucose stores but may be ineffective or variable in its effect if glycogen stores are depleted.
  —Monitoring vital signs, arterial blood gases, blood glucose, and serum electrolytes (especially calcium, potassium, and sodium) as required. Initially, blood glucose concentrations should be monitored as frequently as every 1 to 3 hours. Blood urea nitrogen and serum creatinine concentrations should also be obtained.
- Cerebral edema—Managed with mannitol and dexamethasone.
- Hypokalemia—Managed with potassium supplements.

Other supportive measures should also be employed as needed.

---

## BUFFERED INSULIN HUMAN

## Parenteral Dosage Forms
Note: Bracketed uses in the *Dosage Forms section* refer to categories of use and/or indications that are not included in U.S. product labeling.

### BUFFERED INSULIN HUMAN INJECTION
#### Usual adult and adolescent dose
Insulin-dependent diabetes mellitus (IDDM)—
  Initial:
    Subcutaneous or continuous subcutaneous insulin infusion, a total insulin dose, using one or more types of insulin, is 0.5 to 1.2 USP Insulin Human Units per kg of body weight a day in divided doses—taking body fat, blood glucose, and insulin sensitivity also under consideration. A few patients will require less than 0.5 USP Insulin Human Unit per kg of body weight a day. Dose titration to a targeted blood glucose goal is achieved over several days; a change in total daily insulin dose does not usually exceed 10% of the existing total daily insulin dose.
    When using a continuous subcutaneous insulin infusion pump, the basal insulin dose (usually forty to sixty percent of the total insulin daily dose) is divided into a dose that can be continuously infused subcutaneously over twenty-four hours. Also, a premeal injection (also, forty to sixty percent of total insulin dose) can be delivered preprogrammed or manually by the patient through the insulin pump.
    When using subcutaneous injections, regular human insulin is usually injected in low doses, e.g., less than 10 USP Insulin Human Units a dose.
    Both subcutaneous injections and premeal injections of regular human insulin using a continuous subcutaneous insulin infusion pump generally are given fifteen to thirty minutes before one or more meals and/or a bedtime snack.
  Maintenance:
    Subcutaneous or continuous subcutaneous insulin infusion, dosage must be determined by the physician, based on blood glucose concentrations.
Non–insulin-dependent diabetes mellitus (NIDDM)—
  Initial:
    Subcutaneous, a total insulin dose, using one or more types of insulin, may vary from 5 to 10 USP Insulin Human Units per day to 0.7 to 2.5 USP Insulin Human Units per kg of body weight a day in divided doses—taking body fat, blood glucose, and insulin sensitivity into consideration. Dose titration to a targeted blood glucose goal is achieved over several days with changes of no more than 2 to 6 USP Insulin Human Units a day in the existing total daily insulin dose; again, with consideration of body weight. Very insulin-resistant patients using large doses, 200 USP Insulin Human Units or greater, may need to use a concentrated regular insulin (U-500) instead. Regular human insulin is usually given in low doses, i.e., often less than 10 USP Insulin Human Units a dose, fifteen or thirty minutes before one or more meals and/or a bedtime snack.
  Maintenance:
    Subcutaneous, dosage must be determined by the physician, based on blood glucose concentrations.
Gestational diabetes mellitus—
  Subcutaneous, dosage must be determined by the physician, based on blood glucose concentrations and gestational duration.
Diabetes mellitus, other, associated with certain conditions or syndromes—
  Subcutaneous, dosage must be determined by the physician, based on body weight and blood glucose concentrations.
Note: For treatment of diabetic ketoacidosis, an optional loading dose of 0.15 USP Insulin Human Unit per kg of body weight is given intravenously, followed by 0.1 USP Insulin Human Unit per kg of body weight per hour by continuous infusion. The rate of insulin infusion should be decreased when the plasma glucose concentration reaches 300 mg per dL. Infusion of 5% dextrose injection should be started separately from the insulin infusion when plasma glucose concentration reaches 250 mg per dL. Thirty minutes before discontinuing the insulin infusion, an appropriate dose of insulin should be injected subcutaneously; intermediate-acting insulin has been recommended. Alternatively, a loading dose of 0.5 USP Insulin Human Unit per kg of body weight is injected intramuscularly, followed by 0.1 USP Insulin Human Unit per kg of body weight injected intramuscularly every hour until the blood glucose concentration reaches 300 mg per dL. Then to maintain blood glucose concentration at 250 mg per dL, 0.1 USP Insulin Human Unit per kg of body weight is injected intramuscularly every 2 hours as needed. With either type of insulin administration, capillary blood glucose monitoring should be followed at least hourly and the insulin dose adjusted accordingly.

Insulin requirements may change during illness or events causing psychological or physical stress. Dosage changes for patients receiving conventional therapy should be determined by the physician, based on each patient's needs and insulin sensitivity. Patients receiving intensive therapy may adjust individual doses to compensate for anticipated changes in diet or exercise but should consult a physician if the permitted adjustments are inadequate and/or glucose monitoring indicates the need for a permanent change in the daily dose.

Some patients experience a honeymoon phase after initial therapy and lose their requirement for insulin altogether or require much less for a limited period of time (several months to several years).

Adolescents during puberty may require an increase in their total daily insulin dose.

[Diagnostic aid (pituitary growth hormone reserve)][1]—
  Intravenous, 0.05 to 0.15 USP Insulin Human Unit per kg of body weight as a single rapid injection.

#### Usual pediatric dose
Antidiabetic—
  Subcutaneous, dosage must be determined by the physician, based on body weight and blood glucose concentrations.

**Strength(s) usually available**
U.S.—
　100 USP Insulin Human Units per mL (OTC) [*Velosulin BR* (semisynthetic, phosphate buffered)].
Canada—
　100 USP Insulin Human Units per mL (OTC) [*Velosulin Human* (semisynthetic, phosphate buffered)].

**Packaging and storage**
Store between 2 and 8 °C (36 and 46 °F). Protect from freezing.

**Stability**
Do not use if cloudy, discolored, or unusually viscous.

**Auxiliary labeling**
• Refrigerate.
• Do not freeze.

**Note**
Patients should be advised not to mix phosphate buffered insulin with zinc-containing insulins.

Also, patients should be advised not to mix with any other insulin when using a continuous subcutaneous external insulin pump.

Buffered insulin human is the preferred regular insulin for use in continuous subcutaneous infusion insulin pumps, but may also be injected subcutaneously or intramuscularly with an insulin syringe, or used intravenously. When this insulin is used in a continuous subcutaneous infusion insulin pump, the catheter tubing and the insulin in the reservoir must be changed every 48 hours or the manufacturer's recommendations followed for specific external insulin pumps.

[1]Not included in Canadian product labeling.

---

### EXTENDED INSULIN ZINC

## Parenteral Dosage Forms

**EXTENDED INSULIN ZINC SUSPENSION (ULTRALENTE INSULIN) USP**

**Usual adult and adolescent dose**
Insulin-dependent diabetes mellitus (IDDM)—
　Initial: Subcutaneous, a total insulin dose is 0.5 to 0.8 USP Insulin Unit per kg of body weight sometimes as a single dose, depending on insulin type, or 0.5 to 1.2 USP Insulin Units per kg of body weight per day in divided doses. Body fat, blood glucose, and insulin sensitivity should also be considered. This total daily dose of insulin may be provided by one or more types of insulin. A few patients will require less than 0.5 USP Insulin Unit per kg of body weight per day. Dose titration to a targeted blood glucose goal is achieved over several days; a change in total daily insulin dose does not usually exceed 10% of the existing total daily insulin dose. Extended insulin zinc is given once or twice a day thirty to sixty minutes before a meal and/or a bedtime snack.
　Maintenance: Subcutaneous, dosage must be determined by the physician, based on blood glucose concentrations.
Non–insulin-dependent diabetes mellitus (NIDDM)—
　Initial: Subcutaneous, a total insulin dose may vary from 5 to 10 USP Insulin Units per day to 0.7 to 2.5 USP Insulin Units per kg of body weight per day—taking body fat, blood glucose, and insulin sensitivity also under consideration. This total daily dose of insulin may be provided by one or more types of insulin and, depending on insulin type, may be given as a single dose or as divided doses. Dose titration to a targeted blood glucose goal is achieved over several days with changes from the existing total daily insulin dose of no more than 2 to 6 USP Insulin Units a day; again, body weight should be considered. Very insulin-resistant patients using large doses, 200 USP Insulin Units or greater, may need to use a concentrated regular insulin (U-500) instead. Extended insulin zinc is given once or twice a day thirty or sixty minutes before a meal and/or a bedtime snack.
　Maintenance: Subcutaneous, dosage must be determined by the physician, based on blood glucose concentrations.
Gestational diabetes mellitus—
　Subcutaneous, dosage must be determined by the physician, based on blood glucose concentrations and gestational duration.
Diabetes mellitus, other, associated with certain conditions or syndromes—
　Subcutaneous, dosage must be determined by the physician, based on body weight and blood glucose concentrations.
Note: Insulin requirements may change during illness or events causing psychological or physical stress. Dosage changes for patients receiving conventional therapy should be determined by the physician, based on each patient's needs and insulin sensitivity. Patients receiving intensive therapy may adjust individual doses to compensate for anticipated changes in diet or exercise but should consult a physician if the permitted adjustments are inadequate and/or glucose monitoring indicates the need for a permanent change in the daily dose.

Some patients experience a honeymoon phase after initial therapy and lose their requirement for insulin altogether or require much less for a limited period of time (several months to several years).

Adolescents during puberty may require an increase in their total daily insulin dose.

**Usual pediatric dose**
Antidiabetic—
　Subcutaneous, dosage must be determined by the physician, based on body weight and blood glucose concentrations.

**Strength(s) usually available**
U.S.—
　Not commercially available.
Canada—
　100 USP Insulin Units per mL (OTC) [*Ultralente Insulin* (beef and pork)].

**Packaging and storage**
Store between 2 and 8 °C (36 and 46 °F). Protect from freezing.

**Stability**
Do not use if precipitate has become clumped or granular in appearance.

**Auxiliary labeling**
• Shake gently.
• Refrigerate.
• Do not freeze.

**Note**
Extended insulin zinc suspension is sometimes mixed with other insulin types as directed by physician.

---

### EXTENDED INSULIN ZINC, HUMAN

## Parenteral Dosage Forms

**EXTENDED INSULIN ZINC, HUMAN, SUSPENSION**

**Usual adult and adolescent dose**
Insulin-dependent diabetes mellitus (IDDM)—
　Initial: Subcutaneous, a total insulin dose is 0.5 to 0.8 USP Insulin Human Unit per kg of body weight as a single dose, depending on insulin type, or 0.5 to 1.2 USP Insulin Human Units per kg of body weight per day in divided doses. Body fat, blood glucose, and insulin sensitivity should also be considered. This total daily dose of insulin may be provided by one or more types of insulin. A few patients will require less than 0.5 USP Insulin Human Unit per kg of body weight per day. Dose titration to a targeted blood glucose goal is achieved over several days; a change in total daily insulin dose does not usually exceed 10% of the existing total daily insulin dose. Human extended insulin zinc is given once or twice a day thirty to sixty minutes before a meal and/or a bedtime snack.
　Maintenance: Subcutaneous, dosage must be determined by the physician, based on blood glucose concentrations.
Non–insulin-dependent diabetes mellitus (NIDDM)—
　Initial: Subcutaneous, a total insulin dose may vary from 5 to 10 USP Insulin Human Units per day to 0.7 to 2.5 USP Human Insulin Units per kg of body weight per day—taking body fat, blood glucose, and insulin sensitivity also under consideration. This total daily dose of insulin may be provided by one or more types of insulin and, depending on insulin type, may be given as a single dose or as divided doses. Dose titration to a targeted blood glucose goal is achieved over several days with changes from the existing total daily insulin dose of no more than 2 to 6 USP Insulin Human Units a day; again, body weight should be considered. Very insulin-resistant patients using large doses, 200 USP Insulin Human Units or greater, may need to use a concentrated regular insulin (U-500) instead. Human extended insulin zinc is given once or twice a day thirty to sixty minutes before a meal and/or a bedtime snack.
　Maintenance: Subcutaneous, dosage must be determined by the physician, based on blood glucose concentrations.
Gestational diabetes mellitus—
　Subcutaneous, dosage must be determined by the physician, based on blood glucose concentrations and gestational duration.
Diabetes mellitus, other, associated with certain conditions or syndromes—
　Subcutaneous, dosage must be determined by the physician, based on body weight and blood glucose concentrations.

**1722 Insulin (Systemic)**

Note: Insulin requirements may change during illness or events causing psychological or physical stress. Dosage changes for patients receiving conventional therapy should be determined by the physician, based on each patient's needs and insulin sensitivity. Patients receiving intensive therapy may adjust individual doses to compensate for anticipated changes in diet or exercise but should consult a physician if the permitted adjustments are inadequate and/or glucose monitoring indicates the need for a permanent change in the daily dose.

Some patients experience a honeymoon phase after initial therapy and lose their requirement for insulin altogether or require much less for a limited period of time (several months to several years).

Adolescents during puberty may require an increase in their total daily insulin dose.

### Usual pediatric dose
Antidiabetic—
Subcutaneous, dosage must be determined by the physician, based on body weight and blood glucose concentrations.

### Strength(s) usually available
U.S.—
100 USP Insulin Human Units per mL (OTC) [*Humulin U Ultralente* (biosynthetic)].
Canada—
100 USP Insulin Human Units per mL (OTC) [*Humulin-U* (biosynthetic); *Novolin ge Ultralente* (biosynthetic)].

### Packaging and storage
Store between 2 and 8 °C (36 and 46 °F). Protect from freezing.

### Stability
Do not use if precipitate has become clumped or granular in appearance.

### Auxiliary labeling
- Shake gently.
- Refrigerate.
- Do not freeze.

---

## INSULIN

## Parenteral Dosage Forms

Note: Bracketed uses in the *Dosage Forms section* refer to categories of use and/or indications that are not included in U.S. product labeling.

### INSULIN INJECTION (REGULAR INSULIN, CRYSTALLINE ZINC INSULIN) USP

#### Usual adult and adolescent dose
Insulin-dependent diabetes mellitus (IDDM)—
Initial:
Subcutaneous or continuous subcutaneous insulin infusion, a total insulin dose, using one or more types of insulin, is 0.5 to 1.2 USP Insulin Units per kg of body weight a day in divided doses—taking body fat, blood glucose, and insulin sensitivity also under consideration. A few patients will require less than 0.5 USP Insulin Unit per kg of body weight a day. Dose titration to a targeted blood glucose goal is achieved over several days; a change in total daily insulin dose does not usually exceed 10% of the existing total daily insulin dose.

When using a continuous subcutaneous insulin infusion pump, the basal insulin dose (usually forty to sixty percent of the total insulin daily dose) is divided into a dose that can be continuously infused subcutaneously over twenty-four hours. Also, a premeal injection (also, forty to sixty percent of total insulin dose) can be delivered preprogrammed or manually by the patient through the insulin pump.

When using subcutaneous injections, regular insulin is usually injected in low doses, i.e., often less than 10 USP Insulin Units a dose.

Both subcutaneous injections and premeal injections using a continuous subcutaneous insulin infusion pump of regular insulin generally are given fifteen to thirty minutes before one or more meals and/or a bedtime snack.

Maintenance:
Subcutaneous or continuous subcutaneous insulin infusion, dosage must be determined by the physician, based on blood glucose concentrations.

Non–insulin-dependent diabetes mellitus (NIDDM)—
Initial:
Subcutaneous, a total insulin dose, using one or more types of insulin, may vary from 5 to 10 USP Insulin Units per day to 0.7 to 2.5 USP Insulin Units per kg of body weight a day in divided doses—taking body fat, blood glucose, and insulin sensitivity into consideration. Dose titration to a targeted blood glucose goal is achieved over several days with changes from the existing total daily insulin dose of no more than 2 to 6 USP Insulin Units a day; again, with consideration of body weight. Very insulin-resistant patients using large doses, 200 USP Insulin Units or greater, may need to use a concentrated regular insulin (U-500) instead. Regular insulin is usually given in low doses, i.e., often less than 10 USP Insulin Units a dose, fifteen to thirty minutes before one or more meals and/or a bedtime snack.

Maintenance:
Subcutaneous, dosage must be determined by the physician, based on blood glucose concentrations.

Gestational diabetes mellitus—
Subcutaneous, dosage must be determined by the physician, based on blood glucose concentrations and gestational duration.

Diabetes mellitus, other, associated with certain conditions or syndromes—
Subcutaneous, dosage must be determined by the physician, based on body weight and blood glucose concentrations.

Note: For treatment of diabetic ketoacidosis, an optional loading dose of 0.15 USP Insulin Unit per kg of body weight is given intravenously, followed by 0.1 USP Insulin Unit per kg of body weight per hour by continuous infusion. The rate of insulin infusion should be decreased when the plasma glucose concentration reaches 300 mg per dL. Infusion of 5% dextrose injection should be started separately from the insulin infusion when plasma glucose concentration reaches 250 mg per dL. Thirty minutes before discontinuing the insulin infusion, an appropriate dose of insulin should be injected subcutaneously; intermediate-acting insulin has been recommended. Alternatively, a loading dose of 0.5 USP Unit per kg of body weight is injected intramuscularly, followed by 0.1 USP Insulin Unit per kg of body weight injected intramuscularly every hour until the blood glucose concentration reaches 300 mg per dL. Then to maintain blood glucose concentration at 250 mg per dL, 0.1 USP Insulin Unit per kg of body weight is injected intramuscularly every 2 hours as needed. With either type of insulin administration, capillary blood glucose monitoring should be followed at least hourly and the insulin dose adjusted accordingly.

Insulin requirements may change during illness or events causing psychological or physical stress. Dosage changes for patients receiving conventional therapy should be determined by the physician, based on each patient's needs and insulin sensitivity. Patients receiving intensive therapy may adjust individual doses to compensate for anticipated changes in diet or exercise but should consult a physician if the permitted adjustments are inadequate and/or glucose monitoring indicates the need for a permanent change in the daily dose.

Some patients experience a honeymoon phase after initial therapy and lose their requirement for insulin altogether or require much less for a limited period of time (several months to several years).

Adolescents during puberty may require an increase in their total daily insulin dose.

[Diagnostic aid (pituitary growth hormone reserve)][1]—
Intravenous, 0.05 to 0.15 USP Insulin Unit per kg of body weight as a single rapid injection.

#### Usual pediatric dose
Antidiabetic—
Subcutaneous, dosage must be determined by the physician, based on body weight and blood glucose concentrations.

#### Strength(s) usually available
U.S.—
100 USP Insulin Units per mL (OTC) [*Regular Iletin I* (beef and pork); *Regular Iletin II* (purified pork); *Regular Insulin* (pork); *Regular Insulin* (purified pork)].
500 USP Insulin Units per mL (Rx) [*Regular (Concentrated) Iletin II, U-500* (purified pork)].
Canada—
100 USP Insulin Units per mL (OTC) [*Insulin-Toronto* (beef and pork); *Regular Iletin* (beef and pork); *Regular Iletin II* (pork)].

#### Packaging and storage
Store between 2 and 8 °C (36 and 46 °F). Protect from freezing.

#### Stability
Do not use if cloudy, discolored, or unusually viscous.

#### Auxiliary labeling
- Refrigerate.
- Do not freeze.

**Note**

The 500-Unit strength is available only with a prescription and is used only for the treatment of insulin-resistant diabetic patients.

Insulin Injection USP is sometimes mixed with other insulin types as directed by physician.

Patient should be advised not to mix with any other insulin when using a continuous subcutaneous external insulin pump.

Regular insulin can be used in continuous subcutaneous infusion insulin pumps but may also be injected subcutaneously or intramuscularly with an insulin syringe or used intravenously. Phosphate-buffered insulin is preferred over nonphosphate-buffered insulin in insulin pumps. When this insulin is used in a continuous subcutaneous infusion insulin pump, the catheter tubing and the insulin in the reservoir must be changed every 48 hours or the manufacturer's recommendations followed for specific external insulin pumps.

[1]Not included in Canadian product labeling.

---

## INSULIN HUMAN

## Parenteral Dosage Forms

Note: Bracketed uses in the *Dosage Forms section* refer to categories of use and/or indications that are not included in U.S. product labeling.

### INSULIN HUMAN INJECTION (REGULAR INSULIN HUMAN) USP

**Usual adult and adolescent dose**

Insulin-dependent diabetes mellitus (IDDM)—
  Initial:
    Subcutaneous or continuous subcutaneous insulin infusion, a total insulin dose, using one or more types of insulin, is 0.5 to 1.2 USP Insulin Human Units per kg of body weight a day in divided doses—taking body fat, blood glucose, and insulin sensitivity also under consideration. A few patients will require less than 0.5 USP Insulin Human Unit per kg of body weight a day. Dose titration to a targeted blood glucose goal is achieved over several days; a change in total daily insulin dose does not usually exceed 10% of the existing total daily insulin dose.
    When using a continuous subcutaneous insulin infusion pump, the basal insulin dose (usually forty to sixty percent of the total insulin daily dose) is divided into a dose that can be continuously infused subcutaneously over twenty-four hours. Also, a premeal injection (also, forty to sixty percent of total insulin dose) can be delivered preprogrammed or manually by the patient through the insulin pump.
    When using subcutaneous injections, regular human insulin is usually injected in low doses, i.e., often less than 10 USP Insulin Human Units a dose.
    Both subcutaneous injections and premeal injections of regular human insulin using a continuous subcutaneous insulin infusion pump generally are given fifteen to thirty minutes before one or more meals and/or a bedtime snack.
  Maintenance:
    Subcutaneous or continuous subcutaneous insulin infusion, dosage must be determined by the physician, based on blood glucose concentrations.
Non–insulin-dependent diabetes mellitus (NIDDM)—
  Initial:
    Subcutaneous, a total insulin dose, using one or more types of insulin, may vary from 5 to 10 USP Insulin Human Units per day to 0.7 to 2.5 USP Insulin Human Units per kg of body weight a day in divided doses—taking body fat, blood glucose, and insulin sensitivity into consideration. Dose titration to a targeted blood glucose goal is achieved over several days with changes from the existing total daily insulin dose of no more than 2 to 6 USP Insulin Human Units a day; again, with consideration of body weight. Very insulin-resistant patients using large doses, 200 USP Insulin Human Units or greater, may need to use a concentrated regular insulin (U-500) instead. Regular human insulin is usually given in low doses, i.e., often less than 10 USP Insulin Human Units a dose, fifteen to thirty minutes before one or more meals and/or a bedtime snack.
  Maintenance:
    Subcutaneous, dosage must be determined by the physician, based on blood glucose concentrations.
Gestational diabetes mellitus—
  Subcutaneous, dosage must be determined by the physician, based on blood glucose concentrations and gestational duration.
Diabetes mellitus, other, associated with certain conditions or syndromes—
  Subcutaneous, dosage must be determined by the physician, based on body weight and blood glucose concentrations.

Note: For treatment of diabetic ketoacidosis, an optional loading dose of 0.15 USP Insulin Human Unit per kg of body weight is given intravenously, followed by 0.1 USP Insulin Human Unit per kg of body weight per hour by continuous infusion. The rate of insulin infusion should be decreased when the plasma glucose concentration reaches 300 mg per dL. Infusion of 5% dextrose injection should be started separately from the insulin infusion when plasma glucose concentration reaches 250 mg per dL. Thirty minutes before discontinuing the insulin infusion, an appropriate dose of insulin should be injected subcutaneously; intermediate-acting insulin has been recommended. Alternatively, a loading dose of 0.5 USP Insulin Human Unit per kg of body weight is injected intramuscularly, followed by 0.1 USP Insulin Human Unit per kg of body weight injected intramuscularly every hour until the blood glucose concentration reaches 300 mg per dL. Then, to maintain blood glucose concentration at 250 mg per dL, 0.1 USP Insulin Human Unit per kg of body weight is injected intramuscularly every 2 hours as needed. With either type of insulin administration, capillary blood glucose monitoring should be followed at least hourly and the insulin dose adjusted accordingly.

Insulin requirements may change during illness or events causing psychological or physical stress. Dosage changes for patients receiving conventional therapy should be determined by the physician, based on each patient's needs and insulin sensitivity. Patients receiving intensive therapy may adjust individual doses to compensate for anticipated changes in diet or exercise but should consult a physician if the permitted adjustments are inadequate and/or glucose monitoring indicates the need for a permanent change in the daily dose.

Some patients experience a honeymoon phase after initial therapy and lose their requirement for insulin altogether or require much less for a limited period of time (several months to several years).

Adolescents during puberty may require an increase in their total daily insulin dose.

[Diagnostic aid (pituitary growth hormone reserve)][1]—
  Intravenous, 0.05 to 0.15 USP Insulin Human Unit per kg of body weight as a single rapid injection.

**Usual pediatric dose**
Antidiabetic—
  Subcutaneous, dosage must be determined by the physician, based on body weight and blood glucose concentrations.

**Strength(s) usually available**
U.S.—
  100 USP Insulin Human Units per mL (OTC) [*Humulin R* (biosynthetic); *Novolin R* (biosynthetic); *Novolin R PenFill* (biosynthetic); *Novolin R Prefilled* (biosynthetic), prefilled single use syringe contains 150 USP Units in 1.5 mL)].
Canada—
  100 USP Insulin Human Units per mL (OTC) [*Humulin-R* (biosynthetic); *Novolin ge Toronto* (biosynthetic); *Novolin ge Toronto PenFill* (biosynthetic)].

**Packaging and storage**
Store between 2 and 8 °C (36 and 46 °F). Protect from freezing.

**Stability**
Do not use if cloudy, discolored, or unusually viscous.

**Auxiliary labeling**
• Refrigerate.
• Do not freeze.

**Note**

Insulin Human Injection USP is sometimes mixed with other insulin types as directed by physician.

Patient should be advised not to mix with any other insulin when using a continuous subcutaneous infusion insulin pump.

Insulin human may be used in continuous subcutaneous infusion insulin pumps but may also be injected subcutaneously or intramuscularly with an insulin syringe, or used intravenously. Phosphate-buffered insulin is preferred over nonphosphate-buffered insulin in insulin pumps. When this insulin is used in a continuous subcutaneous infusion insulin pump, the catheter tubing and the insulin in the reservoir must be changed every 48 hours or the manufacturer's recommendations followed for specific external insulin pumps.

[1]Not included in Canadian product labeling.

## INSULIN ZINC

### Parenteral Dosage Forms
**INSULIN ZINC SUSPENSION (LENTE INSULIN) USP**

**Usual adult and adolescent dose**
Insulin-dependent diabetes mellitus (IDDM)—
  Initial: Subcutaneous, a total insulin dose is 0.5 to 0.8 USP Insulin Unit per kg of body weight as a single dose, depending on insulin type, or 0.5 to 1.2 USP Insulin Units per kg of body weight per day in divided doses. Body fat, blood glucose, and insulin sensitivity should also be considered. This total daily dose of insulin may be provided by one or more types of insulin. A few patients will require less than 0.5 USP Insulin Unit per kg of body weight per day. Dose titration to a targeted blood glucose goal is achieved over several days; a change in total daily insulin dose does not usually exceed 10% of the existing total daily insulin dose. Insulin zinc is given thirty minutes before a meal and/or a bedtime snack.
  Maintenance: Subcutaneous, dosage must be determined by the physician, based on blood glucose concentrations.
Non–insulin-dependent diabetes mellitus (NIDDM)—
  Initial: Subcutaneous, a total insulin dose may vary from 5 to 10 USP Insulin Units per day to 0.7 to 2.5 USP Insulin Units per kg of body weight per day—taking body fat, blood glucose, and insulin sensitivity also under consideration. This total daily dose of insulin may be provided by one or more types of insulin and, depending on insulin type, may be given as a single dose or as divided doses. Dose titration to a targeted blood glucose goal is achieved over several days with changes from the existing total daily insulin dose of no more than 2 to 6 USP Insulin Units a day; again, body weight should be considered. Very insulin-resistant patients using large doses, 200 USP Insulin Units or greater, may need to use a concentrated regular insulin (U-500) instead. Insulin zinc is given thirty minutes before a meal and/or a bedtime snack.
  Maintenance: Subcutaneous, dosage must be determined by the physician, based on blood glucose concentrations.
Gestational diabetes mellitus—
  Subcutaneous, dosage must be determined by the physician, based on blood glucose concentrations and gestational duration.
Diabetes mellitus, other, associated with certain conditions or syndromes—
  Subcutaneous, dosage must be determined by the physician, based on body weight and blood glucose concentrations.
Note: Insulin requirements may change during illness or events causing psychological or physical stress. Dosage changes for patients receiving conventional therapy should be determined by the physician, based on each patient's needs and insulin sensitivity. Patients receiving intensive therapy may adjust individual doses to compensate for anticipated changes in diet or exercise but should consult a physician if the permitted adjustments are inadequate and/or glucose monitoring indicates the need for a permanent change in the daily dose.
  Some patients experience a honeymoon phase after initial therapy and lose their requirement for insulin altogether or require much less for a limited period of time (several months to several years).
  Adolescents during puberty may require an increase in their total daily insulin dose.

**Usual pediatric dose**
Antidiabetic—
  Subcutaneous, dosage must be determined by the physician, based on body weight and blood glucose concentrations.

**Strength(s) usually available**
U.S.—
  100 USP Insulin Units per mL (OTC) [*Lente Iletin I* (beef and pork); *Lente Iletin II* (purified pork); *Lente L* (purified pork)].
Canada—
  100 USP Insulin Units per mL (OTC) [*Lente Iletin* (beef and pork); *Lente Iletin II* (pork); *Lente Insulin* (beef and pork)].

**Packaging and storage**
Store between 2 and 8 °C (36 and 46 °F). Protect from freezing.

**Stability**
Do not use if precipitate has become clumped or granular in appearance.

**Auxiliary labeling**
- Shake gently.
- Refrigerate.
- Do not freeze.

**Note**
Insulin zinc suspension is sometimes mixed with other insulin types as directed by physician.

## INSULIN ZINC, HUMAN

### Parenteral Dosage Forms
**INSULIN ZINC, HUMAN, SUSPENSION**

**Usual adult and adolescent dose**
Insulin-dependent diabetes mellitus (IDDM)—
  Initial: Subcutaneous, a total insulin dose is 0.5 to 0.8 USP Insulin Human Unit per kg of body weight as a single dose, depending on insulin type, or 0.5 to 1.2 USP Insulin Human Units per kg of body weight per day in divided doses. Body fat, blood glucose, and insulin sensitivity should also be considered. This total daily dose of insulin may be provided by one or more types of insulin. A few patients will require less than 0.5 USP Insulin Human Unit per kg of body weight per day. Dose titration to a targeted blood glucose goal is achieved over several days; a change in total daily insulin dose does not usually exceed 10% of the existing total daily insulin dose. Human insulin zinc is given thirty minutes before a meal and/or a bedtime snack.
  Maintenance: Subcutaneous, dosage must be determined by the physician, based on blood glucose concentrations.
Non–insulin-dependent diabetes mellitus (NIDDM)—
  Initial: Subcutaneous, a total insulin dose may vary from 5 to 10 USP Insulin Human Units per day to 0.7 to 2.5 USP Insulin Human Units per kg of body weight per day—taking body fat, blood glucose, and insulin sensitivity also under consideration. This total daily dose of insulin may be provided by one or more types of insulin and, depending on insulin type, may be given as a single dose or as divided doses. Dose titration to a targeted blood glucose goal is achieved over several days with changes from the existing total daily insulin dose of no more than 2 to 6 USP Insulin Human Units a day; again, body weight should be considered. Very insulin-resistant patients using large doses, 200 USP Insulin Human Units or greater, may need to use a concentrated regular insulin (U-500) instead. Human insulin zinc is given thirty minutes before a meal and/or a bedtime snack.
  Maintenance: Subcutaneous, dosage must be determined by the physician, based on blood glucose concentrations.
Gestational diabetes mellitus—
  Subcutaneous, dosage must be determined by the physician, based on blood glucose concentrations and gestational duration.
Diabetes mellitus, other, associated with certain conditions or syndromes—
  Subcutaneous, dosage must be determined by the physician, based on body weight and blood glucose concentrations.
Note: Insulin requirements may change during illness or events causing psychological or physical stress. Dosage changes for patients receiving conventional therapy should be determined by the physician, based on each patient's needs and insulin sensitivity. Patients receiving intensive therapy may adjust individual doses to compensate for anticipated changes in diet or exercise but should consult a physician if the permitted adjustments are inadequate and/or glucose monitoring indicates the need for a permanent change in the daily dose.
  Some patients experience a honeymoon phase after initial therapy and lose their requirement for insulin altogether or require much less for a limited period of time (several months to several years).
  Adolescents during puberty may require an increase in their total daily insulin dose.

**Usual pediatric dose**
Antidiabetic—
  Subcutaneous, dosage must be determined by the physician, based on body weight and blood glucose concentrations.

**Strength(s) usually available**
U.S.—
  100 USP Insulin Human Units per mL (OTC) [*Humulin L* (biosynthetic); *Novolin L* (biosynthetic)].
Canada—
  100 USP Insulin Human Units per mL (OTC) [*Humulin-L* (biosynthetic); *Novolin ge Lente* (biosynthetic)].

**Packaging and storage**
Store between 2 and 8 °C (36 and 46 °F). Protect from freezing.

**Stability**
Do not use if precipitate has become clumped or granular in appearance.

**Auxiliary labeling**
- Shake gently.
- Refrigerate.
- Do not freeze.

---

## ISOPHANE INSULIN

## Parenteral Dosage Forms
**ISOPHANE INSULIN SUSPENSION (NPH INSULIN) USP**

**Usual adult and adolescent dose**
Insulin-dependent diabetes mellitus (IDDM)—
  Initial: Subcutaneous, a total insulin dose is 0.5 to 0.8 USP Insulin Unit per kg of body weight as a single dose, depending on insulin type, or 0.5 to 1.2 USP Insulin Units per kg of body weight per day in divided doses. Body fat, blood glucose, and insulin sensitivity should also be considered. This total daily dose of insulin may be provided by one or more types of insulin. A few patients will require less than 0.5 USP Insulin Unit per kg of body weight per day. Dose titration to a targeted blood glucose goal is achieved over several days; a change in total daily insulin dose does not usually exceed 10% of the existing total daily insulin dose. Isophane insulin is given thirty to sixty minutes before a meal and/or a bedtime snack.
  Maintenance: Subcutaneous, dosage must be determined by the physician, based on blood glucose concentrations.
Non–insulin-dependent diabetes mellitus (NIDDM)—
  Initial: Subcutaneous, a total insulin dose may vary from 5 to 10 USP Insulin Units per day to 0.7 to 2.5 USP Insulin Units per kg of body weight per day—taking body fat, blood glucose, and insulin sensitivity also under consideration. This total daily dose of insulin may be provided by one or more types of insulin and, depending on insulin type, may be given as a single dose or as divided doses. Dose titration to a targeted blood glucose goal is achieved over several days with changes from the existing total daily insulin dose of no more than 2 to 6 USP Insulin Units a day; again, body weight should be considered. Very insulin-resistant patients using large doses, 200 USP Insulin Units or greater, may need to use a concentrated regular insulin (U-500) instead. Isophane insulin is given thirty to sixty minutes before a meal and/or a bedtime snack.
  Maintenance: Subcutaneous, dosage must be determined by the physician, based on blood glucose concentrations.
Gestational diabetes mellitus—
  Subcutaneous, dosage must be determined by the physician, based on blood glucose concentrations and gestational duration.
Diabetes mellitus, other, associated with certain conditions or syndromes—
  Subcutaneous, dosage must be determined by the physician, based on body weight and blood glucose concentrations.
Note: Insulin requirements may change during illness or events causing psychological or physical stress. Dosage changes for patients receiving conventional therapy should be determined by the physician, based on each patient's needs and insulin sensitivity. Patients receiving intensive therapy may adjust individual doses to compensate for anticipated changes in diet or exercise but should consult a physician if the permitted adjustments are inadequate and/or glucose monitoring indicates the need for a permanent change in the daily dose.
  Some patients experience a honeymoon phase after initial therapy and lose their requirement for insulin altogether or require much less for a limited period of time (several months to several years).
  Adolescents during puberty may require an increase in their total daily insulin dose.

**Usual pediatric dose**
Antidiabetic—
  Subcutaneous, dosage must be determined by the physician, based on body weight and blood glucose concentrations.

**Strength(s) usually available**
U.S.—
  100 USP Insulin Units per mL (OTC) [*NPH Iletin I* (beef and pork); *NPH Iletin II* (purified pork); *NPH-N* (purified pork)].
Canada—
  100 USP Insulin Units per mL (OTC) [*NPH Iletin* (beef and pork); *NPH Iletin II* (pork); *NPH Insulin* (beef and pork)].

**Packaging and storage**
Store between 2 and 8 °C (36 and 46 °F). Protect from freezing.

**Stability**
Do not use if precipitate has become clumped or granular in appearance or clings to sides of vial.

**Auxiliary labeling**
- Shake gently.
- Refrigerate.
- Do not freeze.

**Note**
Isophane insulin suspension is sometimes mixed with insulin injection as directed by physician.

---

## ISOPHANE INSULIN, HUMAN

## Parenteral Dosage Forms
**ISOPHANE INSULIN, HUMAN, SUSPENSION**

**Usual adult and adolescent dose**
Insulin-dependent diabetes mellitus (IDDM)—
  Initial: Subcutaneous, a total insulin dose is 0.5 to 0.8 USP Insulin Human Unit per kg of body weight as a single dose, depending on insulin type, or 0.5 to 1.2 USP Insulin Human Units per kg of body weight per day in divided doses. Body fat, blood glucose, and insulin sensitivity should also be considered. This total daily dose of insulin may be provided by one or more types of insulin. A few patients will require less than 0.5 USP Insulin Human Unit per kg of body weight per day. Dose titration to a targeted blood glucose goal is achieved over several days; a change in total daily insulin dose does not usually exceed 10% of the existing total daily insulin dose. Human isophane insulin is given thirty minutes before a meal and/or a bedtime snack.
  Maintenance: Subcutaneous, dosage must be determined by the physician, based on blood glucose concentrations.
Non–insulin-dependent diabetes mellitus (NIDDM)—
  Initial: Subcutaneous, a total insulin dose may vary from 5 to 10 USP Insulin Human Units per day to 0.7 to 2.5 USP Insulin Human Units per kg of body weight per day—taking body fat, blood glucose, and insulin sensitivity also under consideration. This total daily dose of insulin may be provided by one or more types of insulin and, depending on insulin type, may be given as a single dose or as divided doses. Dose titration to a targeted blood glucose goal is achieved over several days with changes from the existing total daily insulin dose of no more than 2 to 6 USP Insulin Human Units a day; again, body weight should be considered. Very insulin-resistant patients using large doses, 200 USP Insulin Human Units or greater, may need to use a concentrated regular insulin (U-500) instead. Human isophane insulin is given thirty minutes before a meal and/or a bedtime snack.
  Maintenance: Subcutaneous, dosage must be determined by the physician, based on blood glucose concentrations.
Gestational diabetes mellitus—
  Subcutaneous, dosage must be determined by the physician, based on blood glucose concentrations and gestational duration.
Diabetes mellitus, other, associated with certain conditions or syndromes—
  Subcutaneous, dosage must be determined by the physician, based on body weight and blood glucose concentrations.
Note: Insulin requirements may change during illness or events causing psychological or physical stress. Dosage changes for patients receiving conventional therapy should be determined by the physician, based on each patient's needs and insulin sensitivity. Patients receiving intensive therapy may adjust individual doses to compensate for anticipated changes in diet or exercise but should consult a physician if the permitted adjustments are inadequate and/or glucose monitoring indicates the need for a permanent change in the daily dose.
  Some patients experience a honeymoon phase after initial therapy and lose their requirement for insulin altogether or require much less for a limited period of time (several months to several years).
  Adolescents during puberty may require an increase in their total daily insulin dose.

**Usual pediatric dose**
Antidiabetic—
  Subcutaneous, dosage must be determined by the physician, based on body weight and blood glucose concentrations.

**Strength(s) usually available**
U.S.—
  100 USP Insulin Human Units per mL (OTC) [*Humulin N* (biosynthetic); *Novolin N* (biosynthetic); *Novolin N PenFill* (biosynthetic); *Novolin N Prefilled* (biosynthetic, prefilled single-use syringe contains 150 USP Insulin Human Units in 1.5 mL)].

Canada—
- 100 USP Insulin Human Units per mL (OTC) [*Humulin-N* (biosynthetic); *Novolin ge NPH* (biosynthetic); *Novolin ge NPH Penfill* (biosynthetic)].

**Packaging and storage**
Store between 2 and 8 °C (36 and 46 °F). Protect from freezing.

**Stability**
Do not use if precipitate has become clumped or granular in appearance or clings to sides of vial.

**Auxiliary labeling**
- Shake gently.
- Gently rotate prefilled syringe up and down before injection.
- Refrigerate.
- Do not freeze.

---

## ISOPHANE INSULIN, HUMAN AND INSULIN HUMAN

## Parenteral Dosage Forms

### ISOPHANE INSULIN, HUMAN, SUSPENSION AND INSULIN HUMAN INJECTION

**Usual adult and adolescent dose**
Insulin-dependent diabetes mellitus (IDDM)—
  Initial: Subcutaneous, a total insulin dose is 0.5 to 0.8 USP Insulin Human Unit per kg of body weight as a single dose, depending on insulin type, or 0.5 to 1.2 USP Insulin Human Units per kg of body weight per day in divided doses. Body fat, blood glucose, and insulin sensitivity should also be considered. This total daily dose of insulin may be provided by one or more types of insulin. A few patients will require less than 0.5 USP Insulin Human Unit per kg of body weight per day. Dose titration to a targeted blood glucose goal is achieved over several days; a change in total daily insulin dose does not usually exceed 10% of the existing total daily insulin dose. Human isophane insulin and human insulin is given fifteen or thirty minutes before a meal and/or a bedtime snack.
  Maintenance: Subcutaneous, dosage must be determined by the physician, based on blood glucose concentrations.
Non–insulin-dependent diabetes mellitus (NIDDM)—
  Initial: Subcutaneous, a total insulin dose may vary from 5 to 10 USP Insulin Human Units per day to 0.7 to 2.5 USP Insulin Human Units per kg of body weight per day—taking body fat, blood glucose, and insulin sensitivity also under consideration. This total daily dose of insulin may be provided by one or more types of insulin and, depending on insulin type, may be given as a single dose or as divided doses. Dose titration to a targeted blood glucose goal is achieved over several days with changes from the existing total daily insulin dose of no more than 2 to 6 USP Insulin Human Units a day; again, body weight should be considered. Very insulin-resistant patients using large doses, 200 USP Insulin Human Units or greater, may need to use a concentrated regular insulin (U-500) instead. Human isophane insulin and human insulin is given fifteen to thirty minutes before a meal and/or a bedtime snack.
  Maintenance: Subcutaneous, dosage must be determined by the physician, based on blood glucose concentrations.
Gestational diabetes mellitus—
  Subcutaneous, dosage must be determined by the physician, based on blood glucose concentrations and gestational duration.
Diabetes mellitus, other, associated with certain conditions or syndromes—
  Subcutaneous, dosage must be determined by the physician, based on body weight and blood glucose concentrations.
Note: Insulin requirements may change during illness or events causing psychological or physical stress. Dosage changes for patients receiving conventional therapy should be determined by the physician, based on each patient's needs and insulin sensitivity. Patients receiving intensive therapy may adjust individual doses to compensate for anticipated changes in diet or exercise but should consult a physician if the permitted adjustments are inadequate and/or glucose monitoring indicates the need for a permanent change in the daily dose.

  Some patients experience a honeymoon phase after initial therapy and lose their requirement for insulin altogether or require much less for a limited period of time (several months to several years).

  Adolescents during puberty may require an increase in their total daily insulin dose.

**Usual pediatric dose**
Antidiabetic—
  Subcutaneous, dosage must be determined by the physician, based on body weight and blood glucose concentrations.

**Strength(s) usually available**
U.S.—
- 100 USP Insulin Human Units per mL (50% isophane insulin, human, suspension and 50% insulin human injection) (OTC) [*Humulin 50/50* (biosynthetic)].
- 100 USP Insulin Human Units per mL (70% isophane insulin, human, suspension and 30% insulin human injection) (OTC) [*Humulin 70/30* (biosynthetic); *Novolin 70/30* (biosynthetic); *Novolin 70/30 PenFill* (biosynthetic); *Novolin 70/30 Prefilled* (biosynthetic, prefilled single-use syringe contains 150 USP Insulin Human Units in 1.5 mL)].

Canada—
- 100 USP Insulin Human Units per mL (10% insulin human injection and 90% isophane insulin, human) (OTC) [*Humulin 10/90* (biosynthetic); *Novolin ge 10/90 Penfill* (biosynthetic)].
- 100 USP Insulin Human Units per mL (20% insulin human injection and 80% isophane insulin, human) (OTC) [*Humulin 20/80* (biosynthetic); *Novolin ge 20/80 Penfill* (biosynthetic)].
- 100 USP Insulin Human Units per mL (30% insulin human injection and 70% isophane insulin, human) (OTC) [*Humulin 30/70* (biosynthetic); *Novolin ge 30/70* (biosynthetic); *Novolin ge 30/70 Penfill* (biosynthetic)].
- 100 USP Insulin Human Units per mL (40% insulin human injection and 60% isophane insulin, human) (OTC) [*Humulin 40/60* (biosynthetic); *Novolin ge 40/60 Penfill* (biosynthetic)].
- 100 USP Insulin Human Units per mL (50% insulin human injection and 50% isophane insulin, human) (OTC) [*Humulin 50/50* (biosynthetic); *Novolin ge 50/50 Penfill* (biosynthetic)].

**Packaging and storage**
Store between 2 and 8 °C (36 and 46 °F), unless otherwise specified by manufacturer. Protect from freezing.

**Stability**
Do not use if precipitate has become clumped or granular in appearance.

**Auxiliary labeling**
- Shake gently.
- Gently rotate prefilled syringe up and down before injection.
- Refrigerate.
- Do not freeze.

---

## PROMPT INSULIN ZINC

## Parenteral Dosage Forms

### PROMPT INSULIN ZINC SUSPENSION (SEMILENTE INSULIN) USP

**Usual adult and adolescent dose**
Insulin-dependent diabetes mellitus (IDDM)—
  Initial: Subcutaneous, a total insulin dose is 0.5 to 0.8 USP Insulin Unit per kg of body weight as a single dose, depending on insulin type, or 0.5 to 1.2 USP Insulin Units per kg of body weight per day in divided doses. Body fat, blood glucose, and insulin sensitivity should also be considered. This total daily dose of insulin may be provided by one or more types of insulin. A few patients will require less than 0.5 USP Insulin Unit per kg of body weight per day. Dose titration to a targeted blood glucose goal is achieved over several days; a change in total daily insulin dose does not usually exceed 10% of the existing total daily insulin dose. Prompt insulin zinc is given thirty to sixty minutes before a meal and/or a bedtime snack.
  Maintenance: Subcutaneous, dosage must be determined by the physician, based on blood glucose concentrations.
Non–insulin-dependent diabetes mellitus (NIDDM)—
  Initial: Subcutaneous, a total insulin dose may vary from 5 to 10 USP Insulin Units per day to 0.7 to 2.5 USP Insulin Units per kg of body weight per day—taking body fat, blood glucose, and insulin sensitivity also under consideration. This total daily dose of insulin may be provided by one or more types of insulin and, depending on insulin type, may be given as a single dose or as divided doses. Dose titration to a targeted blood glucose goal is achieved over several days with changes from the existing total daily insulin dose of no more than 2 to 6 USP Insulin Units a day; again, body weight should be considered. Very insulin-resistant patients using large doses, 200 USP Insulin Units or greater, may need to use a concentrated regular insulin (U-500) instead. Prompt insulin zinc is given thirty to sixty minutes before a meal and/or a bedtime snack.

USP DI

Maintenance: Subcutaneous, dosage must be determined by the physician, based on blood glucose concentrations.

Gestational diabetes mellitus—
Subcutaneous, dosage must be determined by the physician, based on blood glucose concentrations and gestational duration.

Diabetes mellitus, other, associated with certain conditions or syndromes—
Subcutaneous, dosage must be determined by the physician, based on body weight and blood glucose concentrations.

Note: Insulin requirements may change during illness or events causing psychological or physical stress. Dosage changes for patients receiving conventional therapy should be determined by the physician, based on each patient's needs and insulin sensitivity. Patients receiving intensive therapy may adjust individual doses to compensate for anticipated changes in diet or exercise but should consult a physician if the permitted adjustments are inadequate and/or glucose monitoring indicates the need for a permanent change in the daily dose.

Some patients experience a honeymoon phase after initial therapy and lose their requirement for insulin altogether or require much less for a limited period of time (several months to several years).

Adolescents during puberty may require an increase in their total daily insulin dose.

**Usual pediatric dose**
Antidiabetic—
Subcutaneous, dosage must be determined by the physician, based on body weight and blood glucose concentrations.

**Strength(s) usually available**
U.S.—
Not commercially available.
Canada—
100 USP Insulin Units per mL (OTC) [*Semilente Insulin* (beef and pork)].

**Packaging and storage**
Store between 2 and 8 °C (36 and 46 °F). Protect from freezing.

**Stability**
Do not use if precipitate has become clumped or granular in appearance.

**Auxiliary labeling**
• Shake gently.
• Refrigerate.
• Do not freeze.

**Note**
Prompt Insulin Zinc Suspension USP is sometimes mixed with other insulin types as directed by physician.

### Selected Bibliography
The Diabetes Control and Complications Trial Research Group. The effect of intensive treatment of diabetes on the development and progression of long-term complications in insulin-dependent diabetes mellitus. N Engl J Med 1993; 329(14): 977-86.

Koda-Kimble MA. Diabetes mellitus. In: Young LY, Koda-Kimble MA, editors. Applied therapeutics. The clinical use of drugs. 5th ed. Vancouver, WA: Applied Therapeutics, Inc., 1992: 72(1)-72(53).

Revised: 07/26/95

---

**INSULIN HUMAN**—See *Insulin (Systemic)*

---

**INSULIN HUMAN, BUFFERED**—See *Insulin (Systemic)*

---

# INSULIN LISPRO  Systemic—INTRODUCTORY VERSION

VA CLASSIFICATION (Primary): HS501
Commonly used brand name(s): *Humalog*.
Note: For a listing of dosage forms and brand names by country availability, see *Dosage Forms* section(s).

## Category
Antidiabetic agent.

## Indications
**Accepted**
Diabetes mellitus (treatment adjunct)—Insulin lispro is indicated in the treatment of diabetes mellitus for the control of hyperglycemia. Insulin lispro has a more rapid onset and shorter duration of action than regular human insulin and, therefore, should be used in a regimen that includes a longer acting insulin.

## Pharmacology/Pharmacokinetics
**Physicochemical characteristics**
Source—Analog of human insulin created by reversing amino acids at positions 28 (proline) and 29 (lysine) on the B-chain. Synthesized by recombinant DNA process involving genetically engineered *Escherichia coli*.
Molecular weight—5808.
pH—7 to 7.8.

**Mechanism of action/Effect**
Like other types of insulin, the primary activity of insulin lispro is to control the metabolism of glucose. Also, like other types of insulin, insulin lispro acts in muscle and other tissues (except the brain) to increase intracellular transport of glucose and amino acids, promote anabolism, and inhibit protein catabolism. In the liver, insulin lispro promotes conversion of glucose to glycogen or fat, and inhibits gluconeogenesis.

**Absorption**
The rate of absorption of insulin lispro demonstrates inter- and intraindividual variability and is dependent upon many factors, including the site of injection; temperature of, and blood flow to, the site; and exercise. Insulin lispro was absorbed at a consistently faster rate than regular human insulin in healthy male volunteers given 0.2 USP Insulin Human Units of regular human insulin or insulin lispro at abdominal, deltoid, or femoral sites. Following abdominal administration of insulin lispro, serum drug concentrations were higher and the duration of action slightly shorter than following deltoid or femoral administration.
Bioavailability ranges from 55 to 77% following doses of 0.1 to 0.2 USP Insulin Human Units per kg of body weight.

**Distribution**
The volume of distribution ranges from 0.26 to 0.36 L per kg.

**Biotransformation**
Studies have not been done in humans. However, studies in animals indicate that the metabolism of insulin lispro is identical to that of regular human insulin.

**Half-life**
Elimination—
Intravenous: 26 and 52 minutes following doses of 0.1 and 0.2 USP Insulin Human Units, respectively (identical to that of regular human insulin).
Subcutaneous: 1 hour (versus 1.5 hours for regular human insulin).

**Onset of action**
Studies in healthy volunteers and patients with diabetes have shown that insulin lispro has a more rapid onset of action than regular human insulin.

**Time to peak serum concentration**
30 to 90 minutes following subcutaneous doses ranging from 0.1 to 0.4 USP Insulin Human Units per kg of body weight to healthy volunteers. Similar results were seen in patients with type 1 diabetes.

**Time to peak effect**
Studies in healthy volunteers and patients with diabetes have shown that insulin lispro has an earlier time to peak effect than regular human insulin.

**Duration of action**
Studies in healthy volunteers and patients with diabetes have shown that insulin lispro has a shorter duration of action than regular human insulin.

## Precautions to Consider

**Cross-sensitivity and/or related problems**
Production of antibodies cross-reactive to human insulin and insulin lispro was observed in patients participating in large clinical trials. During the

12-month trials, the largest increase in antibody concentration to human insulin and insulin lispro was seen in patients new to insulin therapy.

**Carcinogenicity**
Long-term studies to evaluate the carcinogenic potential of insulin lispro have not been done in animals.

**Mutagenicity**
No evidence of mutagenicity was found in a series of *in vitro* and *in vivo* studies, including bacterial mutation tests, unscheduled DNA synthesis, mouse lymphoma assay, chromosomal aberration tests, and a micronucleus test.

**Pregnancy/Reproduction**
Fertility—No evidence of impaired fertility was found in animal studies.
Pregnancy—Studies have not been done in humans. However, women with diabetes must be educated about the necessity of maintaining glycemic control before conception and during pregnancy to improve fetal outcome. Insulin requirements often are decreased during the first trimester and increased during the second and third trimesters.
Studies in pregnant rats and rabbits given doses 4 and 0.3 times, respectively, the average human dose of 40 units per day based on body surface area have not shown that insulin lispro causes adverse effects in the fetus.
FDA Pregnancy Category B.

**Breast-feeding**
It is not known whether insulin lispro is distributed into breast milk. Women who are breast-feeding may require adjustments in their dosages of insulin lispro, in their meal plans, or in both.

**Pediatrics**
No information is available on the relationship of age to the effects of insulin lispro in pediatric patients younger than 12 years of age. Safety and efficacy have not been established.

**Geriatrics**
Appropriate studies on the relationship of age to the effects of insulin lispro have not been performed in the geriatric population. However, in clinical trial subgroup analyses based on age, no difference in postprandial glucose parameters between insulin lispro and regular human insulin was shown.

**Drug interactions and/or related problems**
The following drug interactions and/or related problems have been selected on the basis of their potential clinical significance (possible mechanism in parentheses where appropriate)—not necessarily inclusive (» = major clinical significance):

Note: Combinations containing any of the following medications, depending on the amount present, may also interact with this medication.

Antidiabetic agents, oral
  (concurrent use may necessitate a decrease in insulin lispro dosage)
Hyperglycemia-causing agents, such as:
  Corticosteroids
  Estrogens
  Isoniazid
  Niacin
  Oral contraceptives
  Phenothiazines
  Thyroid hormones
    (these medications may cause loss of glycemic control; insulin requirements may be increased)
Hypoglycemia-causing agents, such as:
  Alcohol
  Angiotensin-converting enzyme (ACE) inhibitors
  Monoamine oxidase (MAO) inhibitors, including furazolidone, procarbazine, and selegiline
  Octreotide
  Salicylates
  Sulfonamides
    (these medications may change metabolic control of glucose concentrations; insulin requirements may be decreased)
» Sympatholytics, such as beta-adrenergic blocking agents
    (sympatholytics may mask some of the symptoms of developing hypoglycemia, making detection of this condition more difficult)

**Medical considerations/Contraindications**
The medical considerations/contraindications included have been selected on the basis of their potential clinical significance (reasons given in parentheses where appropriate)—not necessarily inclusive (» = major clinical significance).

*Except under special circumstances, this medication should not be used when the following medical problem exists:*
» Hypoglycemia

*Risk-benefit should be considered when the following medical problems exist:*
» Diarrhea or
» Vomiting
    (may precipitate hypoglycemia; adjustment of insulin and/or insulin lispro dosage may be required)
» Fever or
» Infection
    (may precipitate hyperglycemia; adjustment of insulin and/or insulin lispro dosage may be required)
Hepatic function impairment or
Renal function impairment
    (studies have shown increased concentrations of circulating insulin in patients with hepatic or renal function impairment; careful glucose monitoring and adjustment of insulin lispro dosage may be necessary)
Hypersensitivity to insulin lispro
» Hypoglycemia-causing conditions, such as:
    Adrenal insufficiency
    Pituitary insufficiency

**Patient monitoring**
The following may be especially important in patient monitoring (other tests may be warranted in some patients, depending on condition; » = major clinical significance):

» Glucose concentrations, blood and/or urine
    (monitoring essential as a guide to therapeutic efficacy)
» Glycosylated hemoglobin (hemoglobin $A_{1c}$) determinations
    (periodic monitoring recommended to assess long-term glycemic control)

## Side/Adverse Effects

The following side/adverse effects have been selected on the basis of their potential clinical significance (possible signs and symptoms in parentheses where appropriate)—not necessarily inclusive:

**Those indicating need for medical attention**
Incidence more frequent
    *Hypoglycemia* (anxiety; behavior change similar to drunkenness; blurred vision; cold sweats; coma; confusion; depression; difficulty in concentrating; dizziness or lightheadedness; drowsiness; excessive hunger; fast heartbeat; headache; irritability or abnormal behavior; nervousness; nightmares; restless sleep; seizures; shakiness; slurred speech; tingling in the hands, feet, lips, or tongue)
    Note: In patients with type 1 diabetes, the risk of *nocturnal hypoglycemia* is less with insulin lispro than with regular human insulin.
Incidence less frequent or rare
    *Allergy, local* (itching, redness, or swelling at injection site); *allergy, systemic* (decrease in blood pressure; rapid pulse; shortness of breath; skin rash or itching over the entire body; sweating; wheezing)—may be life-threatening; *hypokalemia* (dryness of mouth; increased thirst; irregular heartbeat; mood or mental changes; muscle cramps or pain; nausea or vomiting; unusual tiredness or weakness; weak pulse); *lipoatrophy at injection site* (depression of the skin at injection site); *lipohypertrophy at injection site* (thickening of the skin at injection site)
    Note: *Local allergic reactions* are usually minor and resolve within a few days to a few weeks. In some cases, the reactions may be related to irritants in a skin cleansing agent or poor injection technique rather than to the medication.

## Overdose

For specific information on the agent used in the management of insulin lispro overdose, see the *Glucagon (Systemic)* monograph.
For more information on the management of overdose, **contact a Poison Control Center** (see *Poison Control Center Listing*).

**Clinical effects of overdose**
The following effects have been selected on the basis of their potential clinical significance (possible signs and symptoms in parentheses where appropriate)—not necessarily inclusive:

*Hypoglycemia* (anxiety; behavior change similar to drunkenness; blurred vision; cold sweats; coma; confusion; depression; difficulty in concentrating; dizziness or lightheadedness; drowsiness; excessive hunger; fast heartbeat; headache; irritability or abnormal behavior; nervousness; nightmares; restless sleep; seizures; shakiness; slurred speech; tingling in the hands, feet, lips, or tongue)

**Treatment of overdose**
Specific treatment—
Mild hypoglycemia without neurologic symptoms or loss of consciousness should be treated with immediate ingestion of glucose and adjustments to medication dosage and/or meal plan.
Severe hypoglycemia including coma, seizures, or other neurologic impairment requires immediate emergency medical assistance. The patient should immediately be given intramuscular or subcutaneous glucagon, or intravenous glucose, and observed because relapse may occur following apparent clinical recovery.

## Patient Consultation

As an aid to patient consultation, refer to *Advice for the Patient, Insulin Lispro (Systemic)—Introductory Version.*
In providing consultation, consider emphasizing the following selected information (» = major clinical significance):

**Before using this medication**
» Conditions affecting use, especially:
  Hypersensitivity to insulin lispro
  Pregnancy—Importance of maintaining glycemic control to improve fetal outcome; insulin requirements may change during pregnancy
  Breast-feeding—Women who are breast-feeding may require adjustments in their dosages of insulin lispro, in their meal plans, or in both
  Other medications, especially sympatholytics
  Other medical problems, especially adrenal insufficiency; diarrhea; fever; hypoglycemia; infection; pituitary insufficiency; or vomiting

**Proper use of this medication**
» Carefully reading patient instruction sheet contained in insulin lispro package and understanding:
  How to prepare the medication
  How to inject the medication
  How to dispose of syringes, needles, and injection devices
» Carefully selecting and rotating injection sites, following health care professional's recommendations
» Taking insulin lispro within 15 minutes before the meal when used as a mealtime insulin
» Adhering to recommended regimens for diet, exercise, and glucose monitoring
» Proper dosing
» Proper storage

**Precautions while using this medication**
» Regular visits to physician to check progress, especially during the first few weeks of treatment
» *Carefully following special instructions of health care team*
  Discussing use of alcohol
  Not taking other medications unless discussed with physician
  Getting counseling for family members to help the patient with diabetes; also, special counseling for pregnancy planning and contraception
  Discussing travel arrangements, including transporting insulin lispro, carrying medical history and extra supplies of insulin lispro and syringes or injection devices, and adjusting dosage if traveling across more than two time zones
» Preparing for and knowing what to do in case of an emergency by carrying medical history and current medication list, wearing medical identification, keeping extra needed medical supplies and quick-acting sugar, and having nonexpired glucagon kit and needles nearby
» Recognizing what brings on symptoms of hypoglycemia, such as using other antidiabetic medication; delaying or missing a meal or snack; exercising more than usual; drinking significant amounts of alcohol; or sickness, such as vomiting or diarrhea
» Recognizing symptoms of hypoglycemia: anxiety; behavior change similar to drunkenness; blurred vision; cold sweats; confusion; depression; difficulty in concentrating; dizziness or lightheadedness; drowsiness; excessive hunger; fast heartbeat; headache; irritability or abnormal behavior; nervousness; nightmares; restless sleep; shakiness; slurred speech; and tingling in the hands, feet, lips, or tongue
» Knowing what to do if symptoms of hypoglycemia occur, such as eating glucose tablets or gel, corn syrup, honey, or sugar cubes; drinking fruit juice, nondiet soft drink, or sugar dissolved in water; or injecting glucagon if symptoms are severe
» Recognizing what brings on symptoms of hyperglycemia, such as not taking enough or skipping a dose of insulin lispro or insulin; over-eating or not following meal plan; having a fever or infection; or exercising less than usual
» Recognizing symptoms of hyperglycemia and ketoacidosis: blurred vision; drowsiness; dry mouth; flushed, dry skin; fruit-like breath odor; increased urination (frequency and volume); ketones in urine; loss of appetite; stomachache, nausea, or vomiting; tiredness; troubled breathing (rapid and deep); unconsciousness; and unusual thirst
» Knowing what to do if symptoms of hyperglycemia occur, such as checking blood glucose and contacting a member of the health care team

**Side/adverse effects**
Signs of potential side effects, especially hypoglycemia, local allergy, systemic allergy, hypokalemia, and lipoatrophy or lipohypertrophy at injection site

## General Dosing Information

The glucose-lowering capability of one unit of insulin lispro is equal to that of one unit of regular human insulin.

Because of the short duration of action of insulin lispro, supplementation with a longer acting insulin may be required to maintain glycemic control.

Changes in insulin strength, type (e.g., analog, NPH, regular), source (beef and pork, human, pork), method of manufacture (naturally occurring, recombinant DNA process), or manufacturer should be made cautiously and only under medical supervision. A change in any of these parameters may require an adjustment of insulin dosage. Adjustment of insulin dosage also may be necessary following a change in meal plan or amount of exercise, or following an acute illness, emotional disturbance, or period of stress.

Different types of insulin are sometimes mixed in the same syringe to achieve a more accurate matching of insulin availability to the patient's requirements in a single dose. If insulin lispro is to be mixed, several factors should be considered:
• Physicochemical changes in the mixture may occur (immediately or over time), resulting in a physiological response to the mixture that differs from the response to the individual insulin preparations. A decrease in absorption rate, but not in total bioavailability, was seen when insulin lispro was mixed with human isophane insulin (NPH insulin), but not with human extended insulin zinc suspension (ultralente insulin).
• When insulin lispro is mixed with longer acting insulins, the mixture should be administered within 15 minutes before a meal.
• When it is mixed with a longer acting insulin, insulin lispro should be drawn into the syringe first to prevent clouding by the longer acting insulin. The mixture should be used immediately and should not be administered intravenously.
• The effects of mixing insulin lispro with insulins of animal source or other manufacturers have not been studied.

## Parenteral Dosage Forms

### INSULIN LISPRO INJECTION

**Usual adult and adolescent dose**
Antidiabetic agent—
Subcutaneous, dosage must be determined by the physician based on the patient's metabolic needs, eating habits, and other lifestyle variables.

Note: When used as a mealtime insulin, insulin lispro should be administered within fifteen minutes before the meal.

**Usual pediatric dose**
Safety and efficacy have not been established.

**Usual geriatric dose**
See *Usual adult and adolescent dose.*

**Strength(s) usually available**
U.S.—
100 USP Insulin Human Units per mL (Rx) [*Humalog* (glycerin 16 mg; dibasic sodium phosphate 1.88 mg; *m*-cresol 3.15 mg; zinc oxide content adjusted to provide 0.0197 mg zinc ion; phenol trace; water for injection)].

Note: Insulin lispro is available in 10-mL vials and 1.5-mL cartridges. The cartridges may be used with any of the following insulin delivery devices: Becton Dickinson and Company's *B-D® Pen* or Novo Nordisk's *NovoPen®*, *NovolinPen®*, or *NovoPen® 1.5*.

**Packaging and storage**
Store between 2 and 8 °C (36 and 46 °F). Protect from freezing. If refrigeration is not possible, insulin lispro may be stored unrefrigerated, at temperatures not exceeding 30 °C (86 °F) and protected from direct light, for up to 28 days.

1730  Insulin Lispro (Systemic)—Introductory Version

**Auxiliary labeling**
- Refrigerate.
- Do not freeze.

Revised: 08/04/98

**INSULIN ZINC**—See *Insulin (Systemic)*

**INSULIN ZINC, EXTENDED**—See *Insulin (Systemic)*

**INSULIN ZINC, EXTENDED, HUMAN**—See *Insulin (Systemic)*

**INSULIN ZINC, HUMAN**—See *Insulin (Systemic)*

**INSULIN ZINC, PROMPT**—See *Insulin (Systemic)*

**INTERFERON ALFA-2A, RECOMBINANT**—See *Interferons, Alpha (Systemic)*

**INTERFERON ALFA-2B, RECOMBINANT**—See *Interferons, Alpha (Systemic)*

# INTERFERON ALFACON-1   Systemic—INTRODUCTORY VERSION

VA CLASSIFICATION (Primary): IM700
Commonly used brand name(s): *Infergen*.
Note: For a listing of dosage forms and brand names by country availability, see *Dosage Forms* section(s).

## Category
Biological response modifier.

## Indications
**Accepted**
Hepatitis, chronic, active (treatment)—Recombinant interferon alfacon-1 is indicated in the treatment of chronic hepatitis C virus (HCV) infection associated with anti-HCV serum antibodies and/or HCV RNA, in patients 18 years of age or older who have compensated hepatic disease. In some of these patients, recombinant interferon alfacon-1 reduces serum alanine aminotransferase (ALT [SGPT]) concentrations to normal, reduces serum HCV RNA concentrations to undetectable levels (< 100 copies per mL), and improves liver histology.

Note: Other causes of hepatitis, such as viral hepatitis B or autoimmune hepatitis, should be ruled out prior to therapy with recombinant interferon alfacon-1.

## Pharmacology/Pharmacokinetics
Note: Pharmacokinetic data for interferon alfacon-1 are the results of studies in normal, healthy individuals. No pharmacokinetic studies have been conducted in patients with chronic hepatitis C infection.

**Physicochemical characteristics**
Source—Synthetic. A protein chain of 166 amino acids produced by a recombinant DNA process involving genetically engineered *Escherichia coli*. The amino acid sequence was derived by comparison of the sequences of several natural interferon alpha subtypes and assigning the most frequently observed amino acid in each corresponding position. Four additional amino acid changes were made to facilitate molecular construction. Interferon alfacon-1 differs from interferon alfa-2 at 20/166 amino acids (88% homology), and is 30% identical to interferon beta, which is closer than any natural alpha interferon subtype.

Following oxidation of recombinant interferon alfacon-1 to its native state, the purification procedure includes sequential passage over a series of chromatography columns.

Chemical group—Type-I interferon, related to naturally occurring alpha and beta interferons.
Molecular weight—19,434 daltons.
pH—7 ± 0.2.

**Mechanism of action/Effect**
In general, type-I interferons have antiviral, antiproliferative, and immunomodulatory activities, and regulate the expression of cell surface major histocompatibility antigens (HLA class I and class II) and cytokines. Activities of type-I interferons occur as a result of binding to a cell-surface receptor and stimulation of production of several gene products, including 2′5′ oligoadenylate synthetase (2′5′ OAS) and beta-2 microglobulin.

**Time to peak concentration**
2′5′ OAS—24 hours.
Beta-2 microglobulin—24 to 36 hours.
Plasma concentrations of interferon alfacon-1 itself after subcutaneous administration are undetectable by either ELISA or inhibition of viral cytopathic effect. However, analysis of the interferon-induced gene products (2′5′ OAS and beta-2 microglobulin) reveals a statistically significant, dose-related increase in the area under the plasma concentration–time curve (AUC) (p < 0.001 for all comparisons).

## Precautions to Consider
**Cross-sensitivity and/or related problems**
Patients sensitive to other *Escherichia coli*–derived products or to other alpha interferons may also be sensitive to interferon alfacon-1.

**Carcinogenicity**
Studies in humans or animals have not been done.

**Mutagenicity**
Interferon alfacon-1 was not found to be mutagenic in several *in vitro* assays, including the Ames bacterial mutagenicity test, or in an *in vivo* cytogenetic assay in human lymphocytes in the presence or the absence of metabolic activation.

**Pregnancy/Reproduction**
Fertility—Studies in male and female golden Syrian hamsters at subcutaneous doses as high as 100 mcg per kg of body weight (mcg/kg) given for 70 and 14 days before mating, respectively, and then through mating and to day 7 of pregnancy found no effect on reproductive performance or development of the offspring.

Pregnancy—Interferon alfacon-1 should not be used during pregnancy. If a woman becomes pregnant or plans to become pregnant while taking interferon alfacon-1, she should be informed of the potential hazards to the fetus. Males and females treated with interferon alfacon-1 should be advised to use effective contraception. Adequate and well-controlled studies in humans have not been done.

Studies in golden Syrian hamsters at 135 times the human dose and in cynomologus and rhesus monkeys at 9 to 81 times the human dose (based on body surface area) found embryolethal or abortifacient effects.

FDA Pregnancy Category C.

**Breast-feeding**
It is not known whether interferon alfacon-1 is distributed into breast milk.

**Pediatrics**
Safety and efficacy have not been established in patients up to 18 years of age. Use in pediatric patients is not recommended.

**Drug interactions and/or related problems**
The following drug interactions and/or related problems have been selected on the basis of their potential clinical significance (possible mechanism in parentheses where appropriate)—not necessarily inclusive (» = major clinical significance):

Note: Combinations containing any of the following medications, depending on the amount present, may also interact with this medication.

Blood dyscrasia–causing medications (see *Appendix II*) or
Bone marrow depressants, other (see *Appendix II*)
  (leukopenic and/or thrombocytopenic effects of interferon alfacon-1 may be increased)
Medications metabolized by the cytochrome P450 enzyme system
  (patients should be monitored closely for changes in concentrations of these medications during concurrent use with interferon alfacon-1)

**Laboratory value alterations**
The following have been selected on the basis of their potential clinical significance (possible effect in parentheses where appropriate)—not necessarily inclusive (» = major clinical significance):

With physiology/laboratory test values
  Hemoglobin and
  Hematocrit
    (concentrations may be decreased)
  Leukocyte counts (including neutrophils) and
  Platelet counts
    (counts may be decreased)
  Thyroid function tests
    (thyroxine [T₄] concentrations may be decreased and thyroid-stimulating hormone [TSH] concentrations may be increased, indicating possible hypothyroidism; thyroid supplements may be necessary in some patients)
  Triglycerides
    (serum concentrations may be increased to as much as three times pretreatment values; reversible upon withdrawal)

**Medical considerations/Contraindications**
The medical considerations/contraindications included have been selected on the basis of their potential clinical significance (reasons given in parentheses where appropriate)—not necessarily inclusive (» = major clinical significance).

*Except under special circumstances, this medication should not be used when the following medical problems exist:*
» Autoimmune hepatitis or
» Psychiatric disorders, severe, or history of
    (use is not recommended)

*Risk-benefit should be considered when the following medical problems exist:*
» Autoimmune disease, history of
    (caution is recommended because exacerbation of autoimmune disease has been reported with type-1 interferon therapy; use is not recommended in patients with autoimmune hepatitis)
» Bone marrow depression
    (interferon alfacon-1 may cause leukopenia, which may be severe, and/or thrombocytopenia)
» Cardiac disease
    (alpha interferons may cause hypertension, supraventricular arrhythmias, chest pain, and myocardial infarction)
» Endocrine disorders, history of
    (interferon alfacon-1 may cause hypothyroidism, sometimes requiring administration of thyroid supplements)
» Hepatic disease, decompensated
    (studies on the use of interferon alfacon-1 have not been done; use of interferon alfacon-1 is not recommended in patients with decompensated hepatic disease; if symptoms [ascites, coagulopathy, decreased serum albumin, jaundice] occur, interferon alfacon-1 therapy should be discontinued)
  Immunosuppression, such as:
    Transplantation
      (caution is recommended)
» Mental depression, history of
    (interferon alfacon-1 may cause mental depression, which may be severe and include suicidal thoughts or attempts)
» Sensitivity to interferon alfacon-1

**Patient monitoring**
The following may be especially important in patient monitoring (other tests may be warranted in some patients, depending on condition; » = major clinical significance):

» Absolute neutrophil count (ANC) and
» Platelet counts
    (counts should be monitored prior to initiation of therapy, 2 weeks after initiation of therapy, and at periodic intervals during the 24 weeks of therapy, at the discretion of the physician)
» Albumin and
» Bilirubin and
» Creatinine and
» Hemoglobin and
» Thyroid-stimulating hormone (TSH) and
» Thyroxine (T₄)
    (serum concentrations should be monitored prior to initiation of therapy, 2 weeks after initiation of therapy, and at periodic intervals during the 24 weeks of therapy, at the discretion of the physician)
  Blood pressure measurements
    (recommended at periodic intervals)
  Electrocardiogram (ECG)
    (recommended prior to initiation of therapy and at periodic intervals during therapy in patients with cardiac disease or advanced malignancy)
  Monitoring for signs and symptoms of anaphylaxis
    (recommended during and for at least 2 hours after administration)
  Neuropsychiatric monitoring
    (recommended especially in patients receiving high doses of alpha interferons)
  Triglycerides
    (serum concentrations should be monitored at periodic intervals during therapy)

## Side/Adverse Effects
Note: Development of positive binding antibodies has been reported; the titer of neutralizing antibodies has not been measured. The response rate (as measured by serum alanine aminotransferase [ALT (SGPT)]) in hepatitis C was similar in patients who developed binding antibodies to those who did not. The most frequently observed time to first antibody response was week 16 of interferon therapy.

The following side/adverse effects have been selected on the basis of their potential clinical significance (possible signs and symptoms in parentheses where appropriate)—not necessarily inclusive:

**Those indicating need for medical attention**
Incidence more frequent
  *Anxiety; hematologic effects* (leukopenia; thrombocytopenia); *injection erythema* (redness at site of injection); *neurotoxicity* (confusion; mental depression; nervousness; trouble in sleeping; trouble in thinking or concentrating)
Note: Depression may include suicidal ideation or suicide attempt. All patients should be monitored for evidence of depression. It is recommended that interferon alfacon-1 therapy be discontinued if severe mental depression, suicidal ideation, or other severe psychiatric disorders occur.

Incidence less frequent
  *Cardiovascular effects* (chest pain; irregular heartbeat); *hypoesthesia or paresthesia* (numbness or tingling of fingers, toes, or face)

Incidence rare
  *Abnormality or loss of vision; allergic reaction* (skin rash, hives, or itching); *hypothyroidism*—usually asymptomatic

**Those indicating need for medical attention only if they continue or are bothersome**
Incidence more frequent
  *Abdominal pain; anorexia* (decreased appetite); *coughing; diarrhea; dizziness; dyspepsia* (heartburn; indigestion); *flu-like syndrome* (aching muscles; fever and chills; headache; general feeling of discomfort or illness; pain in back or joints; unusual tiredness or weakness); *nausea or vomiting; pharyngitis* (sore throat)
Note: Although fever may be part of the flu-like syndrome caused by interferon alfacon-1, if persistent fever occurs other possible causes should be ruled out.

**Those not indicating need for medical attention**
Incidence less frequent
  *Alopecia* (hair loss)

## Overdose
For more information on the management of overdose or unintentional ingestion, **contact a Poison Control Center** (see *Poison Control Center Listing*).

**Clinical effects of overdose**
One patient enrolled in a phase I advanced malignancy clinical trial received 150 mcg interferon alfacon-1 (10 times the prescribed dosage) for 3 days. The patient experienced a mild increase in anorexia, chills, fever, and myalgia; increases in alanine aminotransferase (ALT [SGPT]), aspartate aminotransferase (AST [SGOT]), and lactate de-

**1732 Interferon Alfacon-1 (Systemic)—Introductory Version**

hydrogenase (LDH) were reported. These laboratory values returned to normal or to the patient's baseline values within 30 days.

### Treatment of overdose
Supportive care—Patients in whom intentional overdose is confirmed or suspected should be referred for psychiatric consultation.

## Patient Consultation
In providing consultation, consider emphasizing the following selected information (» = major clinical significance):

**Before using this medication**
» Conditions affecting use, especially:
   Sensitivity to interferon alfacon-1, other alpha interferons, or *Escherichia coli*-derived products
   Pregnancy—Use is not recommended; contraception is recommended for both males and females receiving interferon alfacon-1 therapy
   Use in children—Use is not recommended
   Other medical problems, especially a history of autoimmune disease, endocrine disorders, mental depression, or psychiatric disorders; autoimmune hepatitis; bone marrow depression; cardiac disease; or decompensated hepatic disease

**Proper use of this medication**
» Compliance with therapy
» Reading patient directions carefully with regard to:
   —Preparation of the injection
   —Use of disposable syringes
   —Proper administration technique
   —Stability of the injection
   Injecting at the same time each day
» Proper dosing
   Missed dose: Checking with physician if dose is missed by more than a few hours
» Proper storage

**Precautions while using this medication**
» Importance of close monitoring by the physician
» Not changing brands of interferon without consulting with physician because of differences in dosage
» Frequency of fever and flu-like symptoms
» Checking with physician immediately if signs of mental depression, especially suicidal thoughts, occur
» Checking with physician if blurred vision or loss of visual field occurs

**Side/adverse effects**
Signs of potential side effects, especially anxiety, hematologic effects, injection erythema, neurotoxicity, cardiovascular effects, hypoesthesia or paresthesia, abnormality or loss of vision, allergic reaction, or hypothyroidism
Possibility of some hair loss

## General Dosing Information
Patients receiving interferon alfacon-1 should be under the supervision of a physician experienced in immunomodulatory therapy.

If severe adverse effects occur, temporary withdrawal of interferon alfacon-1 is recommended. Dose reduction may be necessary if the adverse effect is intolerable. If the adverse effect does not become tolerable, the medication should be discontinued.

Dosage reduction may be necessary if leukopenia, especially granulocytopenia, is severe. If the absolute neutrophil count (ANC) decreases to less than $500 \times 10^6$ per liter, it is recommended that interferon alfacon-1 therapy be withheld.

It is recommended that interferon alfacon-1 therapy be withheld if platelet counts fall to less than $50 \times 10^9$ per liter.

If symptoms of hepatic decompensation (ascites, coagulopathy, decreased serum albumin, jaundice) occur, interferon alfacon-1 therapy should be discontinued.

If a hypersensitivity reaction (e.g., anaphylaxis, angioedema, bronchodilation, urticaria) occurs, it is recommended that interferon alfacon-1 therapy be discontinued immediately and appropriate medical treatment begun.

If the patient complains of any loss of visual acuity or disturbances in visual field, an eye examination should be performed to detect possible retinal hemorrhage, cotton wool spots, or retinal artery or vein obstruction.

## Parenteral Dosage Forms

### INTERFERON ALFACON-1 RECOMBINANT INJECTION

**Usual adult dose**
Hepatitis C, chronic, active—
   Subcutaneous, 9 mcg per dose three times per week, at intervals of at least forty-eight hours for twenty-four weeks.
   Note: Patients who relapse or do not respond, and who tolerated the initial dose, may be treated with 15 mcg per dose three times per week for six months.

   If a severe adverse effect occurs, interferon alfacon-1 should be withheld temporarily. If the adverse effect is intolerable, dose reduction to 7.5 mcg may be necessary. Further decreases in dose are possible, but may result in decreased efficacy. If the adverse effect does not become tolerable, the medication should be discontinued.

   In patients subsequently treated at a dose of 15 mcg, dose reductions in 3-mcg increments have been found to be necessary in 33% of patients.

**Usual pediatric dose**
Safety and efficacy have not been established in patients younger than 18 years of age. Use is not recommended.

**Strength(s) usually available**
U.S.—
   9 mcg per 0.3 mL (Rx) [*Infergen* (sodium chloride 5.9 mg per mL)].
   15 mcg per 0.5 mL (Rx) [*Infergen* (sodium chloride 5.9 mg per mL)].

**Packaging and storage**
Store between 2 and 8 °C (36 and 46 °F). Protect from freezing.
Note: Interferon alfacon-1 injection may be allowed to reach room temperature just prior to administration.

**Stability**
Any unused portion of the contents of a vial should be discarded.

**Note**
Do not shake.
Interferon alfacon-1 and interferon alfa-2a, -2b, -n1, and -n3 are not interchangeable.

Developed: 11/18/97

---

**INTERFERON ALFA-N1 (LNS)**—See *Interferons, Alpha (Systemic)*

---

**INTERFERON ALFA-N3**—See *Interferons, Alpha (Systemic)*

---

# INTERFERON, BETA-1A  Systemic—INTRODUCTORY VERSION

VA CLASSIFICATION (Primary): CN900; IM900
Commonly used brand name(s): *Avonex*.
Note: For a listing of dosage forms and brand names by country availability, see *Dosage Forms* section(s).

## Category
Multiple sclerosis (MS) therapy agent.

## Indications

**Accepted**
Multiple sclerosis (treatment)—Interferon beta-1a is indicated for treatment of relapsing forms of multiple sclerosis (MS) to slow the accumulation of physical disability and decrease the frequency of clinical exacerbations. The safety and efficacy in patients with chronic progressive MS have not been evaluated.

## Pharmacology/Pharmacokinetics

### Physicochemical characteristics

Source—Synthetic. Interferon beta-1a is a 166 amino acid glycoprotein produced by recombinant DNA techniques. It is produced by mammalian cells (Chinese hamster ovary cells) into which the human interferon beta gene has been introduced. The amino acid sequence is identical to that of human interferon beta.

Chemical group—Interferons are a family of naturally occurring proteins and glycoproteins produced by eukaryotic cells in response to viral infection and other biological inducers. Interferon beta, one member of this family, is produced by various cell types including fibroblasts and macrophages. Natural interferon beta and interferon beta-1a are glycosylated, with each containing a single N-linked complex carbohydrate moiety. Glycosylation of other proteins is known to affect their stability, activity, biodistribution, and half-life in blood. However, the effects of glycosylation of interferon beta on these properties have not been fully defined.

Molecular weight—Approximately 22,500 daltons.

pH—7.3 (reconstituted injection).

Note: Interferon beta-1a has a specific activity of approximately 200 million international units (IU) of antiviral activity per mcg. The unit measurement is derived using the World Health Organization (WHO) natural interferon beta standard, Second International Standard for Interferon, Human Fibroblast (Gb-23-902-531). The activity against other standards is not known.

### Mechanism of action/Effect

Interferons are cytokines that mediate antiviral, antiproliferative, and immunomodulatory activities in response to viral infection and other biological inducers. Three major classes have been identified: alpha, beta, and gamma. Interferons alpha and beta form the Type 1 class of interferons, and interferon gamma is a Type 2 interferon; these interferons have overlapping yet distinct biologic activities.

Interferon beta-1a exerts its biological effects by binding to specific receptors on the surface of human cells. This binding initiates a complex cascade of intracellular events that leads to the expression of numerous interferon-induced gene products and markers including 2′,5′-oligoadenylate synthetase, beta$_2$-microglobulin, and neopterin. The specific interferon-induced proteins and mechanisms by which interferon beta-1a exerts its effects in MS have not been fully defined.

Biological response markers (e.g., neopterin and beta$_2$-microglobulin) are induced by interferon beta-1a following parenteral doses of 15 to 75 mcg in both healthy subjects and treated patients. Concentrations of these markers increase within 12 hours of dosing, and remain elevated for at least 4 days. Peak biological response marker concentrations typically are observed 48 hours after dosing. The relationship of serum interferon beta-1a concentrations or of the concentrations of these induced biological response markers to the mechanisms by which interferon beta-1a exerts its effects in MS is unknown.

### Pharmacokinetics

Pharmacokinetic information on patients with multiple sclerosis (MS) has not been evaluated. Serum concentrations of interferon beta-1a, as measured by its antiviral activity, are only slightly above detectable limits following a 30 mcg intramuscular dose, but increase with higher doses. Pharmacokinetic and pharmacodynamic profiles in healthy subjects following doses of 30 to 75 mcg have been determined.

### Half-life

Elimination—
10 hours, following a 60-mcg dose administered intramuscularly.
8.6 hours, following a 60-mcg dose administered subcutaneously.

### Time to peak concentration

9.8 (range, 3 to 15) hours following a 60-mcg dose administered intramuscularly.

7.8 hours (range, 3 to 18 hours) following a 60-mcg dose administered subcutaneously.

Note: Serum concentrations of interferon beta-1a may be sustained after its intramuscular administration due to prolonged absorption from the injection site.

### Peak serum concentration

45 international units (IU) per mL following a 60-mcg dose administered intramuscularly.

30 IU per mL following a 60-mcg dose administered subcutaneously.

Systemic exposure, as determined by peak serum concentrations and area under the serum concentration–time curve (AUC) values, is greater following intramuscular than following subcutaneous administration.

## Precautions to Consider

### Carcinogenicity

No carcinogenicity data are available for interferon beta-1a in animals or humans.

### Mutagenicity

Interferon beta-1a was not mutagenic in the Ames bacterial test or in an *in vitro* cytogenetic assay in human lymphocytes in the presence and absence of metabolic activation; these assays are designed to detect agents that interact directly with and cause damage to cellular DNA. Interferon beta-1a is a glycosylated protein that does not directly bind to DNA.

### Pregnancy/Reproduction

Fertility—No studies have been conducted in healthy women or women with MS. It is not known if interferon beta-1a can affect human reproductive capacity.

Menstrual irregularities were observed in monkeys receiving interferon beta at a dose 100 times the recommended weekly human dose, based upon a body surface area comparison; anovulation and decreased serum progesterone concentrations also occurred transiently in some animals. These effects were reversible upon discontinuation of interferon beta treatment. Monkeys receiving interferon beta at a dose two times the recommended weekly human dose exhibited no changes in cycle duration or ovulation. In the placebo-controlled premarketing clinical trial, 6% of patients receiving placebo and 5% of patients receiving interferon beta-1a reported menstrual disorders. It is not known if, or for how long, menstrual irregularities will persist in women following treatment.

Pregnancy—Adequate and well-controlled studies have not been done in humans.

Studies in pregnant monkeys receiving 100 times the recommended weekly human dose, based on a body surface comparison, revealed no teratogenic or other adverse effects on fetal development; however, abortifacient activity was evident following administration of three to five doses. No abortifacient activity was seen in monkeys receiving two times the recommended weekly human dose, based on a body surface comparison. Although no teratogenic effects were demonstrated in these studies, it is not known if such effects would occur in humans. If a woman becomes pregnant or plans to become pregnant, it is recommended that interferon beta-1a therapy be discontinued due to potential risks to the fetus.

FDA Pregnancy Category C.

### Breast-feeding

It is not known whether interferon beta-1a is distributed into human breast milk. However, because of the potential for serious adverse reactions in nursing infants, discontinuation of interferon beta-1a or discontinuation of breast-feeding is recommended.

### Pediatrics

Appropriate studies on the relationship of age to the effects of interferon beta-1a have not been performed in children up to 18 years of age. Safety and efficacy have not been established.

### Geriatrics

No information is available on the relationship of age to the effects of interferon beta-1a in geriatric patients.

### Drug interactions and/or related problems

The following drug interactions and/or related problems have been selected on the basis of their potential clinical significance (possible mechanism in parentheses where appropriate)—not necessarily inclusive (» = major clinical significance):

Note: Studies designed to evaluate drug interactions with interferon beta-1a have not been conducted. However, treatment of exacerbations with corticosteroids or ACTH, and concomitant administration of antidepressants and/or oral contraceptives to some patients during the placebo-controlled premarketing clinical trial did not result in unexpected adverse effects.

Other interferons have been shown to reduce cytochrome P450 oxidase-mediated drug metabolism. Formal studies in humans have not been conducted, but hepatic microsomes isolated from interferon beta-1a–treated monkeys showed no influence on hepatic cytochrome P450 enzyme-mediated metabolic activity.

Combinations containing any of the following medications, depending on the amount present, may also interact with this medication.

» Myelosuppressive agents
(as with all interferon products, the potential for additive myelosuppressant effects exists)

### Laboratory value alterations

The following have been selected on the basis of their potential clinical significance (possible effect in parentheses where appropriate)—not necessarily inclusive (» = major clinical significance):

With physiology/laboratory test values
Aspartate aminotransferase (AST [SGOT]) values
(during the placebo-controlled premarketing clinical trial, 3% of patients receiving interferon beta-1a had values greater than or equal

to three times the upper limits of normal, as compared with 1% of the patients receiving placebo)

Eosinophil counts
(during the placebo-controlled premarketing clinical trial, 5% of patients receiving interferon beta-1a had counts ≥ 10%, as compared with 4% of patients receiving placebo)

Hematocrit
(during the placebo-controlled premarketing clinical trial, 3% of patients receiving interferon beta-1a had hematocrits ≤ 37% (males) and ≤ 32% (females), as compared with 1% of patients receiving placebo)

Serum neutralizing activity
(during the placebo-controlled premarketing clinical trial, 24% of patients treated with interferon beta-1a were found to have serum neutralizing activity at one or more time points tested; 15% of these patients tested positive for serum neutralizing activity at a level at which no placebo patient tested)

## Medical considerations/Contraindications

The medical considerations/contraindications included have been selected on the basis of their potential clinical significance (reasons given in parentheses where appropriate)—not necessarily inclusive (» = major clinical significance).

*Risk-benefit should be considered when the following medical problems exist:*

Cardiac disease, such as:
Angina
Arrhythmias
Congestive heart failure
(symptoms of influenza-like syndrome resulting from interferon beta-1a therapy may be stressful to patients with severe cardiac conditions)

» Depression, mental, especially with suicidal ideation
(condition may be exacerbated; patients should be monitored carefully; causal relationship to medication is not proven)

» Seizure disorder
(condition may be exacerbated, although causal relationship to medication is not proven)

Sensitivity to natural or recombinant interferon beta or human albumin

## Patient monitoring

The following may be especially important in patient monitoring (other tests may be warranted in some patients, depending on condition; » = major clinical significance):

Blood chemistry values, including liver function tests
(recommended at periodic intervals during treatment)
Platelet counts and
White blood cell counts, complete and differential
(recommended at periodic intervals during treatment)

## Side/Adverse Effects

The following side/adverse effects have been selected on the basis of their potential clinical significance (possible signs and symptoms in parentheses where appropriate)—not necessarily inclusive:

**Those indicating need for medical attention**
Incidence more frequent
*Anemia* (unusual bleeding or bruising; unusual tiredness or weakness); *asthenia* (unusual tiredness or weakness); *diarrhea; infection* (fever; chills); *influenza-like syndrome including arthralgia* (joint pain); *chills; fever; headache; and myalgia* (muscle aches); *nausea; pain*

Incidence less frequent
*Abdominal pain; ataxia* (clumsiness or unsteadiness); *chest pain; decreased hearing; dizziness; dyspnea* (troubled breathing); *hypersensitivity reaction* (coughing; difficulty in swallowing; hives or itching; swelling of face, lips, or eyelids; wheezing or difficulty in breathing); *injection-site reactions* (redness; swelling; tenderness); *mental depression, especially with suicidal ideation* (mood changes, especially with thoughts of suicide); *muscle spasms; nevi* (skin lesions); *ovarian cyst* (pelvic discomfort, aching, or heaviness); *seizures; speech problems; syncope* (fainting); *upper respiratory infection* (runny or stuffy nose; sneezing; sore throat); *urticaria* (hives or itching); *vaginitis* (pain or discharge from the vagina); *vasodilation* (flushing)

Incidence rare
*Anorexia* (loss of appetite); *herpes simplex* (painful cold sores or blisters on lips, nose, eyes, or genitals); *herpes zoster* (painful blisters on trunk of body)—also known as "shingles"; *malaise* (general feeling of discomfort or illness); *otitis media* (earache); *sinusitis* (headache; stuffy nose)

**Those indicating need for medical attention only if they continue or are bothersome**
Incidence more frequent
*Dyspepsia* (heartburn; acid indigestion; sour stomach)
Incidence less frequent
*Alopecia* (hair loss); *insomnia* (trouble in sleeping)

## Overdose

For information on the management of interferon beta-1a overdose, **contact a Poison Control Center** (see *Poison Control Center Listing*).

## Patient Consultation

In providing consultation, consider emphasizing the following selected information (» = major clinical significance):

**Before using this medication**
» Conditions affecting use, especially:
Sensitivity to natural or recombinant interferon beta or Albumin Human USP
Pregnancy—Potential abortifacient effects
Breast-feeding—Not recommended due to potential serious adverse effects in the nursing infant
Other medications, especially myelosuppressive agents
Other medical problems, especially mental depression with suicidal ideation, and seizure disorder

**Proper use of this medication**
» Proper administration: Importance of aseptic technique
Importance of training patient or caregiver in administration of intramuscular injections
Importance of proper disposal of syringes and needles
» Proper dosing
Missed dose: Using as soon as remembered; the next injection should be scheduled at least 48 hours later
» Proper storage

**Side/adverse effects**
Signs of potential side effects, especially anemia; asthenia; diarrhea; infection; influenza-like syndrome, including arthralgia, chills, fever, headache, and myalgia; nausea; pain; abdominal pain; ataxia; chest pain; decreased hearing; dizziness; dyspnea; hypersensitivity reaction; injection site reactions; mental depression, especially with suicidal ideation; muscle spasms; nevi; ovarian cyst; seizures; speech problems; syncope; upper respiratory infection; urticaria; vaginitis; vasodilation; anorexia; herpes simplex; herpes zoster; malaise; otitis media; and sinusitis

## General Dosing Information

If it is determined that interferon beta-1a can be used outside of the physician's office, the person who will be administering the injections should be instructed in proper aseptic technique for reconstitution and injection, and in proper disposal of syringes and needles. If the patient is to self-administer interferon beta-1a, the physical ability of that patient to self-inject intramuscularly should be assessed. The first injection should be performed under the supervision of a qualified health care professional.

**For treatment of adverse effects**
Recommended treatment consists of the following:
• Systemic acetaminophen may lessen the impact of influenza-like symptoms.

## Parenteral Dosage Forms

### INTERFERON BETA-1a FOR INJECTION

**Usual adult dose**
Relapsing forms of multiple sclerosis—
Intramuscular, 30 mcg once a week.

**Usual pediatric dose**
Safety and efficacy in children up to 18 years of age have not been established.

**Strength(s) usually available**
U.S.—
33 mcg (6.6 million International Units [IU]) (Rx) [*Avonex* (diluent: Sterile Water for Injection USP; Albumin Human USP 16.5 mg; Sodium Chloride USP 6.4 mg; Dibasic Sodium Phosphate USP 6.3 mg; Monobasic Sodium Phosphate USP 1.3 mg)].

**Packaging and storage**
Store between 2 and 8 °C (36 and 46 °F). Protect from freezing.
If refrigeration is not available, the vials may be stored at 25 °C (77 °F) for up to 30 days.

### Preparation of dosage form

The vials of drug and diluent should be allowed to come to room temperature before reconstitution. Using aseptic technique, 1.1 mL of the supplied diluent is transferred into the lyophilized interferon beta-1a vial. The vial should be swirled gently until the solid material is completely dissolved. If particulate matter remains or the reconstituted product is discolored, the vial should be discarded before use. Following reconstitution with the accompanying diluent, the resulting solution will contain 30 mcg of interferon beta-1a per mL.

After reconstitution, 1 mL of solution should be withdrawn into a sterile syringe to be injected intramuscularly.

### Stability

Interferon beta-1a contains no preservatives; after reconstitution, if not used immediately, it should be refrigerated and used within 6 hours.

### Auxiliary labeling

- Refrigerate.
- Do not freeze.

Developed: 12/19/97

---

# INTERFERON, BETA-1B   Systemic—INTRODUCTORY VERSION

VA CLASSIFICATION (Primary): CN900; IM900
Commonly used brand name(s): *Betaseron*.
Note: For a listing of dosage forms and brand names by country availability, see *Dosage Forms* section(s).

## Category

Multiple sclerosis (MS) therapy agent.

## Indications

### Accepted

Multiple sclerosis (treatment)—Interferon beta-1b is indicated for use in ambulatory patients with relapsing-remitting multiple sclerosis (MS) to reduce the frequency of clinical exacerbations. The safety and efficacy of interferon beta-1b in chronic-progressive MS have not been evaluated.

## Pharmacology/Pharmacokinetics

### Physicochemical characteristics

Source—Synthetic. Interferon beta-1b is a sterile lyophilized protein product produced by recombinant DNA techniques. It is manufactured by bacterial fermentation of a strain of *Escherichia coli* that bears a genetically engineered plasmid containing the gene for human interferon $beta_{ser17}$. The native gene was obtained from human fibroblasts and altered in a way that substitutes serine for the cysteine residue found at position 17. Interferon beta-1b is a highly purified protein with 165 amino acids; it does not include the carbohydrate side chains found in the natural material.

Chemical group—Interferons are a family of naturally occurring proteins. Three major classes have been identified: alfa, beta, and gamma. Interferon alfa, interferon beta-1b, and interferon gamma have overlapping yet distinct biologic activities; the activities of interferon beta-1b are species-restricted.

Molecular weight—Approximately 18,500 daltons.

### Mechanism of action/Effect

Interferon beta-1b has both antiviral and immunoregulatory properties. The mechanism by which it exerts its effects in multiple sclerosis (MS) are not clearly understood. It is known, however, that the biologic response-modifying properties of interferon beta-1b are mediated through its interactions with specific cell receptors found on the surface of human cells. Binding of interferon beta-1b to these receptors induces the expression of a number of interferon-induced gene products (e.g., 2',5'-oligoadenylate synthetase, protein kinase, and indoleamine 2, 3-dioxygenase) that are believed to be the mediators of this interferon's biological actions.

### Pharmacokinetics

Pharmacokinetic information on patients with multiple sclerosis (MS) receiving the recommended dose of interferon beta-1b is not available because serum concentrations following subcutaneous administration of ≤ 0.25 mg are low or undetectable. Healthy volunteers who received single or multiple daily subcutaneous doses of 0.5 mg generally had serum interferon beta-1b concentrations of less than 100 international units per mL (IU/mL). Pharmacokinetic parameters in non-MS patients following single and multiple intravenous doses of interferon beta-1b were comparable, and dosing three times a week for two weeks did not result in accumulation of interferon beta-1b in these patients.

### Absorption

Bioavailability was approximately 50%, based on a total dose of 0.5 mg given as two subcutaneous injections at different sites to healthy volunteers.

### Distribution

Mean steady-state volume of distribution ($Vol_D$) values ranged from 0.25 to 2.88 L per kg in healthy volunteers and non-MS patients who received single intravenous doses of up to 2 mg of interferon beta-1b.

### Half-life

Terminal elimination—
  Mean, 8 minutes to 4.3 hours in non-MS patients who received single intravenous doses of up to 2 mg of interferon beta-1b.

### Time to peak concentration

1 to 8 hours following subcutaneous administration of 0.5 mg to healthy volunteers.

### Peak serum concentration

Mean, 40 IU/mL following subcutaneous administration of 0.5 mg to healthy volunteers. Increases in serum concentrations were dose-proportional in non-MS patients receiving single intravenous doses of up to 2 mg of interferon beta-1b.

### Elimination

Mean serum clearance values ranged from 9.4 to 28.9 mL/minute·kg, and were independent of dose.

## Precautions to Consider

### Carcinogenicity

No carcinogenicity data in humans or animals are available. However, the effect of interferon beta-1b on the morphological transformation of the mammalian cell line BALBc-3T3 was studied to evaluate carcinogenic potential, and no significant increases in transformation frequency were noted.

### Mutagenicity

Interferon beta-1b was not mutagenic when assayed for genotoxicity in the Ames bacterial test in the presence or absence of metabolic activation.

### Pregnancy/Reproduction

Fertility—The effects of interferon beta-1b on normally cycling human females are not known. Studies on female rhesus monkeys showed no apparent adverse effects on the menstrual cycle or on associated hormonal profiles when interferon beta-1b was administered at doses of up to 32 times the recommended human dose (based on body surface area comparison) over three consecutive menstrual cycles.

Pregnancy—Adequate and well-controlled studies have not been done in humans. Spontaneous abortions were reported in four women who participated in the premarketing clinical trial.

Studies in female rhesus monkeys demonstrated a dose-related abortifacient activity when interferon beta-1b was administered at doses ranging from 2.8 to 40 times the recommended human dose based on body surface area comparison. It is not known if animal doses can be extrapolated to human doses. Interferon beta-1b administered to female rhesus monkeys on gestation days 20 to 70 did not cause teratogenic effects; it is not known if teratogenic effects would occur in humans.

FDA Pregnancy Category C.

### Breast-feeding

It is not known if interferon beta-1b is distributed into human milk; however, because of the potential for serious adverse reactions in nursing infants, risk-benefit must be considered.

### Pediatrics

Safety and efficacy in children up to 18 years of age have not been established.

### Geriatrics

The premarketing clinical trial of interferon beta-1b enrolled patients ranging from 18 to 50 years of age. No information is available on the effects of interferon beta-1b in geriatric patients.

### Drug interactions and/or related problems

Note: Studies designed to evaluate drug interactions with interferon beta-1b have not been conducted. However, ACTH or corticosteroids have been administered for periods of up to 28 days to treat relapses in patients receiving interferon beta-1b. The effect of alternate-day administration on drug metabolism in MS patients is unknown. Interferon beta-1b administered to three cancer patients over a dose range of 0.025 to 2.2 mg led to dose-dependent inhibition of antipyrine elimination.

### Laboratory value alterations

The following have been selected on the basis of their potential clinical significance (possible effect in parentheses where appropriate)—not necessarily inclusive (» = major clinical significance):

With physiology/laboratory test values
Alanine aminotransferase, serum (ALT [SGPT])
(values more than five times baseline occurred in 19% of patients receiving interferon beta-1b, as compared with 6% of patients receiving placebo in the premarketing clinical trial)
Aspartate aminotransferase, serum (AST [SGOT])
(values more than five times baseline occurred in 4% of patients receiving interferon beta-1b, as compared with 0% of patients receiving placebo in the premarketing clinical trial)
Bilirubin, total
(concentrations greater than 2.5 times the baseline occurred in 6% of patients receiving interferon beta-1b, as compared with 2% of patients receiving placebo in the premarketing clinical trial)
Glucose, blood
(concentrations of less than 55 mg/dL occurred in 15% of patients receiving interferon beta-1b, as compared with 13% of patients receiving placebo in the premarketing clinical trial)
Lymphocyte count
(counts less than 1500/mm$^3$ occurred in 82% of patients receiving interferon beta-1b, as compared with 67% of patients receiving placebo in the premarketing clinical trial)
Neutrophil count, absolute
(counts less than 1500/mm$^3$ occurred in 18% of patients receiving interferon beta-1b, as compared with 6% of patients receiving placebo in the premarketing clinical trial)
Protein, urine
(values greater than 1+ occurred in 5% of patients receiving interferon beta-1b, as compared with 3% of patients receiving placebo in the premarketing clinical trial)
White blood cell count
(counts less than 3000/mm$^3$ occurred in 16% of patients receiving interferon beta-1b, as compared with 5% of patients receiving placebo in the premarketing clinical trial)

### Medical considerations/Contraindications

The medical considerations/contraindications included have been selected on the basis of their potential clinical significance (reasons given in parentheses where appropriate)—not necessarily inclusive (» = major clinical significance).

*Risk-benefit should be considered when the following medical problems exist:*
» Depression, mental, especially with suicidal ideation
  (condition may be exacerbated; patients should be closely monitored)
Sensitivity to natural or recombinant interferon beta, Albumin Human USP, or dextrose

### Patient monitoring

The following may be especially important in patient monitoring (other tests may be warranted in some patients, depending on condition; » = major clinical significance):

» Blood chemistry values, including liver function tests and
» Hemoglobin and
» Platelet counts and
» White blood cell counts, complete and differential
  (recommended prior to initiation of therapy and at periodic intervals thereafter)

## Side/Adverse Effects

Note: In the premarketing clinical trial, one suicide and four attempted suicides were observed among 372 study patients during a 3-year period. All five of these cases were patients receiving interferon beta-1b; no attempted suicides occurred in study patients who were not receiving interferon beta-1b. Depression and suicide also have been reported in patients receiving interferon alfa, a related compound. Patients should be informed of these side effects and instructed to report symptoms of depression and suicidal ideation immediately to the prescribing physician. If depression occurs, the patient should be closely monitored, and discontinuation of interferon beta-1b should be considered.

Injection site necrosis (ISN) was reported in 5% of patients in premarketing clinical trials. Although typically occurring within the first 4 months of interferon beta-1b therapy, postmarketing surveillance reports ISN occurring over a year after initiation of therapy. ISN may occur at single or multiple injection sites; lesions are typically 3 cm or less in diameter, although larger areas have been reported. While necrosis has commonly extended only to subcutaneous fat, there are reports of necrosis extending to and including fascia overlying muscle. In some lesions, vasculitis has been reported. Debridement and, infrequently, skin grafting have been required for some lesions. Any infection of the necrotic site should be treated appropriately. Time to healing varies depending on the severity of the necrosis; in most cases, healing has been associated with scarring. In some patients, healing of necrotic skin lesions has occurred while interferon beta-1b therapy has continued. The decision to discontinue therapy following a single site of necrosis is dependent on the extent of necrosis. If patients continue using interferon beta-1b after ISN has occurred, injection into the affected area should be avoided until the site is fully healed. If multiple lesions have occurred, therapy should be discontinued until healing is complete. Patients should be instructed to contact the physician promptly if any break in the skin, which may be associated with blue-black discoloration, swelling, or drainage of fluid from the injection site, occurs.

Other injection site reactions, including redness, pain, swelling, and discoloration, occurred in 85% of patients at one or more times during the controlled MS trial. In general, these reactions were transient and did not require discontinuation of therapy, but the nature and severity of all reported reactions need to be carefully assessed.

The following side/adverse effects have been selected on the basis of their potential clinical significance (possible signs and symptoms in parentheses where appropriate)—not necessarily inclusive:

### Those indicating need for medical attention

Incidence more frequent
*Abdominal pain; headache or migraine; hypertension* (high blood pressure); *injection site reactions including hypersensitivity* (hives; itching; swelling); *inflammation* (redness; feeling of heat); *necrosis* (break in the skin, especially associated with blue-black discoloration, swelling, or drainage of fluid); *and pain; influenza-like syndrome; including chills; fever; increased sweating; malaise* (general feeling of discomfort or illness); *and myalgia* (muscle pain); *palpitations* (irregular or pounding heartbeat); *sinusitis* (headache; stuffy nose)

Incidence less frequent
*Abnormal vision* (any change in vision); *breast pain; cystitis* (bloody or cloudy urine; difficult, burning, or painful urination; frequent urge to urinate); *dyspnea* (troubled breathing); *lymphadenopathy* (swollen lymph glands); *pain; pelvic pain; peripheral vascular disorder* (cold hands and feet); *tachycardia* (fast or racing heartbeat); *weight gain, unusual*

Incidence rare
*Amnesia* (loss of memory); *breast neoplasm* (abnormal growth in breast); *confusion; conjunctivitis* (red, itching, or swollen eyes); *cyst* (abnormal growth filled with fluid or semisolid material); *edema, generalized* (bloating or swelling); *fibrocystic breast* (benign lumps in breast); *goiter* (dry, puffy skin; increased weight gain; swelling of front part of neck; changes in menstrual periods; decreased sexual ability in males; feeling cold); *hemorrhage* (bleeding problems); *hyperkinesia* (hyperactivity); *hypertonia* (increased muscle tone); *mental depression with suicidal ideation* (depression with thoughts of suicide); *seizure; speech disorder* (problems in speaking); *urinary urgency* (increased urge to urinate); *weight loss, unusual*

### Those indicating need for medical attention only if they continue or are bothersome

Incidence more frequent
*Asthenia* (unusual tiredness or weakness); *constipation; diarrhea; dizziness; dysmenorrhea or other menstrual disorders* (menstrual pain or other menstrual changes); *laryngitis*

Incidence less frequent
*Alopecia* (hair loss); *anxiety; nervousness; somnolence* (drowsiness); *vomiting*

## Overdose

For information on the management of overdose of interferon beta-1b, contact a **Poison Control Center** (see *Poison Control Center Listing*).

## Patient Consultation

In providing consultation, consider emphasizing the following selected information (» = major clinical significance)

### Before using this medication
» Conditions affecting use, especially:
    Sensitivity to interferon beta-1b, Albumin Human USP, or dextrose
    Pregnancy—Not recommended
    Breast-feeding—Possible need to avoid during interferon beta-1b therapy because of risk of serious adverse effects on infant
    Other medical problems, especially mental depression with suicidal ideation

### Proper use of this medication
» Proper administration:
    Importance of aseptic technique
    Choosing an appropriate injection site
    Importance of rotating injection sites
» Proper dosing
    Missed dose: Using as soon as remembered; the next injection should be scheduled about 48 hours later
» Proper storage

### Side/adverse effects
Signs of potential side effects, especially abdominal pain; headache or migraine; hypertension; injection site reactions including hypersensitivity, inflammation, necrosis, and pain; influenza-like syndrome including chills, fever, increased sweating, malaise, and myalgia; palpitations; sinusitis; abnormal vision; breast pain; cystitis; dyspnea; lymphadenopathy; pain; pelvic pain; peripheral vascular disorder; tachycardia; unusual weight gain; amnesia; breast neoplasm; confusion; conjunctivitis; cyst; edema, generalized; fibrocystic breast; goiter; hemorrhage; hyperkinesia; hypertonia; mental depression with suicidal ideation; seizure; speech disorder; urinary urgency; unusual weight loss

## General Dosing Information

Activity of interferon beta-1b is approximately 32 million international units (IU) per mg. The unit measurement is derived by comparing the antiviral activity of the product to the World Health Organization (WHO) reference standard of recombinant human interferon beta. Prior to 1993, a different analytical standard was used to determine potency; it assigned 54 million IU to 0.3 mg interferon beta-1b, as compared with the currently assigned potency of 9.6 million IU per 0.3 mg interferon beta-1b.

Patient understanding and use of aseptic self-injection techniques and procedures should be reevaluated periodically, particularly if injection site necrosis (ISN) has occurred.

Patient understanding of the importance of rotating areas of injection to minimize the likelihood of severe injection site reactions should be reinforced.

Taking interferon beta-1b at bedtime may help lessen the impact of influenza-like symptoms.

## Parenteral Dosage Forms

### INTERFERON BETA-1b FOR INJECTION

**Usual adult dose**
Relapsing-remitting multiple sclerosis—
    Subcutaneously, 0.25 mg every other day.

**Usual pediatric dose**
Safety and efficacy in patients up to 18 years of age have not been established.

**Strength(s) usually available**
U.S.—
    0.3 mg (Rx) [*Betaseron* (diluent: sodium chloride 0.54%; Albumin Human USP 15 mg; Dextrose USP 15 mg)].

**Packaging and storage**
Store between 2 and 8 °C (36 and 46 °F). Do not freeze.
If refrigeration is not possible, the drug and diluent should be kept as cool as possible (below 30 °C [86 °F]), stored away from heat and light, and used within 7 days.

**Preparation of dosage form**
Using aseptic technique, 1.2 mL of the supplied diluent should be transferred into the lyophilized interferon beta-1b vial. The vial should be swirled gently until the solid material is completely dissolved. If particulate matter remains or the reconstituted product is discolored, it should be discarded before use. Following reconstitution with the accompanying diluent, the resulting solution will contain 0.25 mg interferon beta-1b per mL.
After reconstitution, withdraw 1 mL of solution into a sterile syringe fitted with a new 27-gauge needle to be injected subcutaneously.

**Stability**
Interferon beta-1b contains no preservatives; after reconstitution, if not immediately used, it should be refrigerated and used within 3 hours.

**Auxiliary labeling**
- Refrigerate.
- Do not freeze.

Developed: 11/12/97

---

# INTERFERON, GAMMA  Systemic†

VA CLASSIFICATION (Primary/Secondary): IM700
Commonly used brand name(s): *Actimmune*.
Note: For a listing of dosage forms and brand names by country availability, see *Dosage Forms* section(s).

†Not commercially available in Canada.

## Category

Biological response modifier; immunomodulator.

## Indications

### Accepted
Chronic granulomatous disease (treatment)—Interferon gamma-1b, recombinant, is indicated for reducing the frequency and severity of serious infections associated with chronic granulomatous disease (CGD). Interferon gamma-1b appears to be effective in all genetic types of CGD.

## Pharmacology/Pharmacokinetics

Note: Pharmacokinetic studies have been conducted in healthy male subjects only.

### Physicochemical characteristics
Source—Synthetic. Structurally identical to naturally occurring human gamma interferon. A protein chain of 140 amino acids produced by a recombinant DNA process involving genetically engineered *Escherichia coli*. Purification procedure involves conventional column chromatography.
Chemical group—Related to naturally occurring gamma interferon. Interferons are produced and secreted by cells in response to viral infections or various synthetic and biologic stimuli; gamma interferon is produced mainly by T-lymphocytes.

### Mechanism of action/Effect
In general, interferons have antiviral, antiproliferative, and immunomodulatory activities.
Naturally occurring gamma interferon, which is secreted by antigen-stimulated T-lymphocytes (mainly CD4+ [helper] cells, plus CD8+ [suppressor] cells and natural killer [NK] cells), probably interacts with other lymphokines (cytokines) such as interleukin-2 in a complex immunoregulatory network. Gamma interferon induces activation of quiescent macrophages in blood monocytes to phagocytes, which have augmented antimicrobial and tumoricidal activity involving release of toxic oxygen metabolites. Macrophage activation is critical in the cellular immune response to intracellular and extracellular pathogens. Gamma interferon also enhances antibody-dependent cellular cytotoxicity and NK cell activity, histocompatibility class I and class II antigen expression, lymphocyte proliferation, and monocyte Fc receptor expression. Treatment with gamma interferon is associated with increased serum concentrations of beta-2 microglobulin and $H_2O_2$ secretion by peripheral blood monocytes, as well as a temporary increase in the T4/T8 cell ratio. Gamma interferon is also known as Type II interferon (based on interferon receptor types) and immune interferon.

In chronic granulomatous disease (CGD; an inherited disorder characterized by deficient phagocyte oxidative metabolism), gamma interferon enhances phagocytic function, resulting in an increase in superoxide anion production by granulocytes and monocytes; gamma interferon also enhances the oxygen-independent antimicrobial activity of monocytes from patients with classic X-linked CGD.

### Other actions/effects
May inhibit the hepatic microsomal cytochrome P450 system.

### Absorption
Intramuscular or subcutaneous—Slow; apparent fraction of dose absorbed is more than 89%.

### Biotransformation
Unknown.

### Half-life
Intramuscular—Mean: 2.9 hours
Intravenous—Mean: 38 minutes
Subcutaneous—Mean: 5.9 hours

### Time to peak plasma concentration
Intramuscular—4 hours.
Subcutaneous: 7 hours.

### Peak plasma concentration
After dose of 100 mcg per square meter of body surface—
  Intramuscular: 1.5 nanograms per mL.
  Subcutaneous: 0.6 nanograms per mL.

Note: Not related to blood monocyte activation capacity.

### Elimination
*In vitro* studies indicate that rabbit livers and kidneys are capable of clearing gamma interferon from perfusate; in nephrectomized mice and squirrel monkeys, clearance of gamma interferon from blood is reduced but elimination is not prevented.

## Precautions to Consider

### Cross-sensitivity and/or related problems
Patients sensitive to any *Escherichia coli* product may also be sensitive to gamma interferon.

### Carcinogenicity
Studies have not been done in either animals or humans.

### Mutagenicity
Results of Ames tests using five different tester strains of bacteria with and without metabolic activation showed no evidence of mutagenicity. No evidence of chromosomal damage was found in a micronucleus assay in bone marrow cells of mice following two intravenous doses of 20 mg per kg of body weight (mg/kg).

### Pregnancy/Reproduction
Fertility—In female cynomolgus monkeys, irregular menstrual cycles or absence of cyclicity occurred during treatment with daily subcutaneous doses of 150 mcg per kg of body weight (mcg/kg) (approximately 100 times the human dose), but not with doses of 3 or 30 mcg/kg.

Pregnancy—Adequate and well-controlled studies in humans have not been done.
Studies in primates at doses approximately 100 times the human dose found an increased incidence of abortions. No evidence of teratogenicity was found with intravenous doses of 2 to 100 times the human dose. Studies using recombinant murine gamma interferon in pregnant mice found increased incidences of uterine bleeding and abortifacient activity and decreased neonatal viability at maternally toxic doses; however, the clinical significance of this effect is unknown.

FDA Pregnancy Category C.

### Breast-feeding
It is not known whether gamma interferon is excreted in breast milk. However, because of the potential for serious adverse effects in nursing infants, avoidance of breast-feeding should be considered while gamma interferon is being administered.

### Pediatrics
Safety and efficacy in children less than 1 year of age have not been established. In one study, flu-like symptoms were twice as frequent in children 10 years of age or older as in those less than 10 years of age; the lowest incidence was in children 5 years of age or younger.

### Geriatrics
No information is available on the relationship of age to the effects of gamma interferon in geriatric patients.

### Drug interactions and/or related problems
The following drug interactions and/or related problems have been selected on the basis of their potential clinical significance (possible mechanism in parentheses where appropriate)—not necessarily inclusive (» = major clinical significance):

Note: Combinations containing any of the following medications, depending on the amount present, may also interact with this medication.

Blood dyscrasia–causing medications (See *Appendix II*)
  (leukopenic and/or thrombocytopenic effects of gamma interferon, although usually not significant except at high doses, may be increased with concurrent or recent therapy if these medications cause the same effects; dosage adjustment of gamma interferon, if necessary, should be based on blood counts)

Bone marrow depressants, other (See *Appendix II*) or
Radiation therapy
  (additive bone marrow depression may rarely occur; dosage reduction may be required when two or more bone marrow depressants, including radiation, are used concurrently or consecutively)

### Laboratory value alterations
The following have been selected on the basis of their potential clinical significance (possible effect in parentheses where appropriate)—not necessarily inclusive (» = major clinical significance):

With physiology/laboratory test values
  Alanine aminotransferase (ALT [SGPT]) and
  Alkaline phosphatase and
  Aspartate aminotransferase (AST [SGOT]) and
  Lactate dehydrogenase (LDH)
    (serum values may be slightly increased; dose related; reversible on withdrawal of gamma interferon)

Blood pressure
  (may be decreased)

Cortisol concentrations, plasma
  (may be increased; peak concentrations occur 2 to 4 hours after administration of gamma interferon)

Leukocyte counts (including neutrophils)
  (may be decreased; dose-related)

Platelet counts
  (may rarely be decreased)

Triglyceride concentrations, serum
  (may be increased; dose-related; resolve after treatment is withdrawn)

### Medical considerations/Contraindications
The medical considerations/contraindications included have been selected on the basis of their potential clinical significance (reasons given in parentheses where appropriate)—not necessarily inclusive (» = major clinical significance).

*Risk-benefit should be considered when the following medical problems exist:*

Bone marrow depression
  (may be exacerbated)
» Cardiac disease, including symptoms of ischemia, congestive heart failure, or arrhythmia
  (may be exacerbated as a result of the stress of the fever and chills that occur in patients receiving gamma interferon; no direct cardiotoxic effect of gamma interferon has been demonstrated)
» CNS function, compromised or
» Seizure disorders
  (risk of CNS side effects)
» Multiple sclerosis or
» Systemic lupus erythematosus
  (there is some evidence that these may be exacerbated; however, there is also some evidence of a helpful effect of gamma interferon)
» Sensitivity to gamma interferon or *Escherichia coli*–derived products
Caution should be used also in patients who have had previous cytotoxic drug therapy or radiation therapy.

### Patient monitoring
The following may be especially important in patient monitoring (other tests may be warranted in some patients, depending on condition; » = major clinical significance):

Alanine aminotransferase (ALT [SGPT]) values, serum and
Aspartate aminotransferase (AST [SGOT]) values, serum and
Bilirubin concentrations, serum and
Lactate dehydrogenase (LDH) values, serum
  (recommended prior to initiation of therapy and at periodic intervals during therapy)

» Leukocyte count, total and, if appropriate, differential and
» Platelet count
(determinations recommended prior to initiation of therapy and at periodic intervals during therapy)

## Side/Adverse Effects

Note: Most side/adverse effects, except the flu-like syndrome, are dose-related.

Development of neutralizing antibodies has not been reported with interferon gamma-1b, although it has been reported with interferon gamma-4a.

Neutropenia and elevation of hepatic enzymes may occur at doses of 100 mcg per square meter of body surface per day and may be dose-limiting at doses above 250 mcg per square meter of body surface per day; they resolve after treatment is withdrawn. Thrombocytopenia and proteinuria are also rare.

The following side/adverse effects have been selected on the basis of their potential clinical significance (possible signs and symptoms in parentheses where appropriate)—not necessarily inclusive:

**Those indicating need for medical attention**
Incidence more frequent
*Leukopenia* (usually asymptomatic; rarely, fever or chills; cough or hoarseness; lower back or side pain; painful or difficult urination)
Note: In *leukopenia*, neutrophil counts usually do not fall out of the normal range and usually recover within 2 to 5 days after a dose.

Incidence rare
*Hypotension* (not symptomatic); *neurotoxicity* (confusion, parkinsonian symptoms [loss of balance control, mask-like face, shuffling walk, stiffness of arms or legs, trembling and shaking of hands and fingers, trouble in speaking or swallowing], trouble in thinking or concentrating, trouble in walking); *thrombocytopenia* (usually asymptomatic; rarely, unusual bleeding or bruising; black, tarry stools; blood in urine or stools; pinpoint red spots on skin)
Note: *Neurotoxicity* is usually reversible after withdrawal.

**Those indicating need for medical attention only if they continue or are bothersome**
Incidence more frequent
*Diarrhea; flu-like syndrome* (aching muscles; fever and chills; general feeling of discomfort or illness; headache; less frequently, back pain; joint pain); *nausea or vomiting; skin rash; unusual tiredness*
Note: The *flu-like syndrome* occurs in most patients; it may decrease in severity with continued treatment. Severity is dose-related.

Incidence less frequent
*Dizziness; loss of appetite; weight loss*
Note: *Dizziness* is a CNS effect.

## Patient Consultation

As an aid to patient consultation, refer to *Advice for the Patient, Interferon, Gamma (Systemic)*.

In providing consultation, consider emphasizing the following selected information (» = major clinical significance):

### Before using this medication
» Conditions affecting use, especially:
Sensitivity to gamma interferon
Pregnancy—Abortifacient effects found in monkeys and mice
Breast-feeding—Possible need to avoid during gamma interferon therapy because of risk of serious adverse effects
Other medical problems, especially cardiac disease, compromised CNS function, multiple sclerosis, seizure disorders, and systemic lupus erythematosus

### Proper use of this medication
» Compliance with therapy
» Reading patient directions carefully with regard to:
Preparation of the injection
Use of disposable syringes
Proper administration technique
Stability of the injection
Importance of ample fluid intake to reduce risk of hypotension
Administration at bedtime to minimize flu-like symptoms
» Proper dosing
Missed dose: Skipping missed dose and going back to regular schedule; not doubling doses; checking with physician
» Proper storage

### Precautions while using this medication
» Importance of close monitoring by physician
» Frequency of fever and flu-like symptoms; possible need for acetaminophen before and after a dose is given

### Side/adverse effects
Signs of potential side effects, especially leukopenia, neurotoxicity, and thrombocytopenia

## General Dosing Information

Patients receiving gamma interferon should be under supervision of a physician experienced in immunomodulatory therapy.

The patient may be premedicated with acetaminophen at the time of gamma interferon dosing and the acetaminophen may be continued as needed to treat fever and headache.

If severe adverse effects occur, dosage reduction by 50% or temporary withdrawal of gamma interferon is recommended.

It is recommended that patients be well hydrated, especially during initial treatment with gamma interferon, to reduce the risk of hypotension associated with fluid depletion. Hypotension may require supportive treatment, including fluid replacement to maintain intravascular volume.

Patients who develop leukopenia should be observed carefully for signs of infection. Antibiotic support may be required. In neutropenic patients who develop fever, broad-spectrum antibiotic coverage should be initiated empirically, pending bacterial cultures and appropriate diagnostic tests. In some cases, it may be difficult to distinguish fever due to infection from fever associated with the flu-like syndrome.

Special precautions are recommended in patients who develop thrombocytopenia as a result of administration of gamma interferon. These may include extreme care in performing invasive procedures; regular inspection of intravenous sites, skin (including perirectal area), and mucous membrane surfaces for signs of bleeding or bruising; limiting frequency of venipuncture and avoiding intramuscular injections; testing urine, emesis, stool, and secretions for occult blood; care in use of regular toothbrushes, dental floss, toothpicks, safety razors, and fingernail and toenail cutters; avoiding constipation; and using caution to prevent falls and other injuries. Such patients should avoid alcohol and any aspirin intake because of the risk of gastrointestinal bleeding. Platelet transfusions may be required.

## Parenteral Dosage Forms

### INTERFERON GAMMA-1b, RECOMBINANT, INJECTION

**Usual pediatric dose**
Chronic granulomatous disease—
Body surface area greater than 0.5 square meter: Subcutaneous, 50 mcg (1.5 million Units) per square meter of body surface three times a week.
Body surface area less than or equal to 0.5 square meter: Subcutaneous, 1.5 mcg per kg of body weight three times a week.

Note: The optimum injection sites are the right and left deltoid and anterior thigh.

Either sterilized glass or plastic disposable syringes may be used for administration.

Safety and efficacy in children less than 1 year of age have not been established.

**Strength(s) usually available**
U.S.—
200 mcg per mL (100 mcg [3 million Units] per 0.5-mL vial) (Rx) [*Actimmune* (mannitol; sodium succinate; polysorbate 20)].
Canada—
Not commercially available.

**Packaging and storage**
Store between 2 and 8 °C (36 and 46 °F), unless otherwise specified by manufacturer. Protect from freezing.

**Stability**
Contains no preservative; any unused portion should be discarded. Vials left at room temperature for a total time exceeding 12 hours should be discarded.

### Note
Do not shake.

When dispensing for self-administration by the patient, make sure that patient instructions are included and that the patient understands how to prepare and administer the injection, including proper use of disposable syringes.

### Selected Bibliography

Ijzermans JNM, Marquet RL. Interferon-gamma: a review. Immunobiol 1989; 179: 456-73.

Murray HW. Interferon-gamma, the activated macrophage, and host defense against microbial challenge. Ann Intern Med 1988 Apr; 108: 595-608.

Revised: 06/04/92
Interim revision: 07/05/94

---

# INTERFERONS, ALPHA   Systemic

This monograph includes information on the following: 1) Interferon Alfa-2a, Recombinant; 2) Interferon Alfa-2b, Recombinant; 3) Interferon Alfa-n1(lns)*; 4) Interferon Alfa-n3†.

VA CLASSIFICATION (Primary/Secondary): IM700/AN900

Commonly used brand name(s): *Alferon N*[4]; *Intron A*[2]; *Roferon-A*[1]; *Wellferon*.

Note: For a listing of dosage forms and brand names by country availability, see *Dosage Forms* section(s).

*Not commercially available in U.S.
†Not commercially available in Canada.

## Category
Biological response modifier; antineoplastic.

## Indications
Note: Bracketed information in the *Indications* section refers to uses that are not included in U.S. product labeling.

### Accepted

Leukemia, hairy cell (treatment)—Recombinant interferon alfa-2a, recombinant interferon alfa-2b, and interferon alfa-n1 (lns) are indicated for treatment of hairy cell leukemia in splenectomized or nonsplenectomized patients. [Interferon alfa-n3] is also indicated for treatment of hairy cell leukemia.

Condyloma acuminatum (treatment)—Recombinant interferon alfa-2b[1], interferon alfa-n1 (lns), and interferon alfa-n3 are indicated by intralesional injection for treatment of refractory or recurrent external condyloma acuminatum (genital warts).

Hepatitis, chronic, active (treatment)—[Recombinant interferon alfa-2a][1], recombinant interferon alfa-2b, interferon alfa-n1 (lns)[1], and [interferon alfa-n3] are indicated for treatment of non-A, non-B/C hepatitis in patients 18 years of age or older with compensated liver disease who have a history of blood or blood product exposure and/or are HCV (hepatitis C virus) antibody positive. Safety and efficacy have not been established for treatment of patients with decompensated liver disease or for immune suppressed transplant recipients. Use is not recommended in patients with autoimmune hepatitis or a history of autoimmune disease.

Available data indicate that serum transaminase activity and markers of viral activity are reduced during alpha interferon treatment, although abnormalities may recur when treatment is withdrawn. Long-term effects of alpha interferon on development of chronic hepatitis are not established.

Hepatitis B, chronic (treatment)—Recombinant interferon alfa-2b[1] is indicated for treatment of chronic hepatitis B in patients 18 years of age or older with compensated liver disease and hepatitis B virus (HBV) replication. Patients must test positive for hepatitis B serum antigen for at least 6 months and have HBV replication with elevated serum alanine aminotransferase.

Kaposi's sarcoma, AIDS-associated (treatment)—Recombinant interferon alfa-2a and recombinant interferon alfa-2b are indicated for treatment of AIDS-associated Kaposi's sarcoma in selected patients 18 years of age and older. Interferon alfa-n1 (lns)[1] and [interferon alfa-n3] are also indicated for this indication.

Carcinoma, bladder (treatment)—Interferon alfa-n1 (lns)[1] and [interferon alfa-n3] are indicated for the treatment of superficial bladder carcinoma (intravesically).

Note: Recombinant interferon alfa-2a and recombinant interferon alfa-2b have been studied, in combination therapy, for intravesical use in the treatment of *bladder carcinoma* (Evidence rating: IIID,). Although some medical experts agree that these medications may be useful in the management of bladder carcinoma, others state there is not enough medical literature or clinical experience to consider the use of these alpha interferons for this indication outside of a clinical trial setting.

Carcinoma, renal (treatment) or
Leukemia, chronic myelocytic (treatment)—[Recombinant interferon alfa-2a], [recombinant interferon alfa-2b][1], interferon alfa-n1 (lns)[1], and [interferon alfa-n3] are indicated for the treatment of renal carcinoma and chronic myelocytic leukemia.

Papillomatosis, laryngeal (treatment)—[Recombinant interferon alfa-2b][1], interferon alfa-n1 (lns), and [interferon alfa-n3] are indicated for treatment of laryngeal papillomatosis, including juvenile laryngeal papilloma.

Lymphomas, non-Hodgkin's (treatment)
Malignant melanoma (treatment)
Multiple myeloma (treatment) or
Mycosis fungoides (treatment)—[Recombinant interferon alfa-2a][1], recombinant interferon alfa-2b[1], interferon alfa-n1 (lns)[1], and [interferon alfa-n3] are indicated for treatment of non-Hodgkin's lymphomas, especially follicular small cleaved cell lymphoma (nodular poorly differentiated types), malignant melanoma, multiple myeloma, and mycosis fungoides.

[Carcinoid tumors (treatment)][1]—Alpha interferons are indicated as reasonable medical therapy in the management of carcinoid tumors (Evidence rating: IID,).

[Carcinoma, ovarian, epithelial (treatment)][1] or
[Carcinoma, skin (treatment)]—Alpha interferons are indicated for treatment of epithelial ovarian (intraperitoneal administration) and skin (recombinant interferon alfa-2b) carcinomas.

[Polycythemia vera (treatment)][1]—Recombinant interferon alfa-2a and recombinant interferon alfa-2b are indicated as reasonable medical therapy at some point in the management of polycythemia vera (Evidence rating: IIID,). However, these medications are not recommended for first-line treatment.

[Thrombocytosis, essential (treatment)][1]—Alpha interferons are indicated for treatment of essential thrombocytosis.

Although efficacy of all alpha interferons for various indications appears to be similar, differences in relative efficacy for a particular indication may exist.

### Acceptance not established

Recombinant interferon alfa-2b, in combination therapy, has been studied for use in the treatment of *cervical carcinoma* (Evidence rating: IIID,). Some medical experts consider this agent to be reasonable medical therapy at some point in the management of advanced cervical carcinoma (although it is not recommended as first-line treatment). However, other experts state that there is not enough medical literature or clinical experience to consider the use of recombinant interferon alfa-2b for the treatment of cervical carcinoma outside of a clinical trial setting.

Recombinant interferon alfa-2a and recombinant interferon alfa-2b have been studied, in combination therapy, for use in the treatment of *esophageal carcinoma*(Evidence rating: IIID,). However, medical experts agree that, at this point in time, there is not enough medical literature or clinical experience to consider the use of these medications for the treatment of esophageal carcinoma outside of a clinical trial setting.

### Unaccepted

Recombinant interferon alfa-2a and recombinant interferon alfa-2b, in combination therapy, have been shown in several studies to be ineffective in the treatment of *colorectal carcinoma* (Evidence rating: IIC,). Their use is not recommended.

[1]Not included in Canadian product labeling.

## Pharmacology/Pharmacokinetics

### Physicochemical characteristics
Source—
- Interferon alfa-2a, recombinant: Synthetic. A protein chain of 165 amino acids produced by a recombinant DNA process involving genetically engineered *Escherichia coli*. Has a lysine group at position 23. Purification procedure includes affinity chromatography using a murine monoclonal antibody. Contains only a single alpha interferon subtype.
- Interferon alfa-2b, recombinant: Synthetic. A protein chain of 165 amino acids produced by a recombinant DNA process involving genetically engineered *Escherichia coli*. Has an arginine group at position 23. Purification is done by proprietary methods. Contains only a single alpha interferon subtype.
- Interferon alfa-n1 (lns): A highly purified blend of natural human alpha interferons, obtained from human lymphoblastoid cells following induction with Sendai virus. Is a mixture of natural alpha interferon subtypes, but in different proportions than in human leukocyte interferon.
- Interferon alfa-n3: A highly purified mixture of up to 14 natural human alpha interferon subtypes. A protein chain of approximately 166 amino acids. Manufactured from pooled units of human leukocytes that have been induced by incomplete infection with an avian virus (Sendai virus) to produce interferon alfa-n3. The manufacturing process includes immunoaffinity chromatography with a murine monoclonal antibody, acidification (pH 2) for 5 days at 4 °C, and gel filtration chromatography.

Chemical group—
- Interferon alfa-n1 and -n3: Naturally occurring alpha interferons.
- Interferon alfa-2a and -2b, recombinant: Related to naturally occurring alpha interferons.
- Interferons are produced and secreted by cells in response to viral infections or various synthetic and biologic inducers; alpha interferons are produced mainly by leukocytes.

### Mechanism of action/Effect
In general, interferons have antiviral, antiproliferative, and immunomodulatory activities. Antiviral and antiproliferative actions are thought to be related to alterations in synthesis of RNA, DNA, and cellular proteins, including oncogenes. The exact mechanism of antineoplastic activity is unknown, but may be related to any of these three actions.

Antiviral—Inhibit virus replication in virus-infected cells.

Antiproliferative—Suppress cell proliferation.

Immunomodulatory—Enhance phagocytic activity of macrophages and augment specific cytotoxicity of lymphocytes for target cells.

### Absorption
Intralesional—Plasma concentrations achieved are below detectable levels; however, systemic effects have been reported, indicating some systemic absorption.

Intramuscular and subcutaneous—Greater than 80%.

### Biotransformation
Renal, complete. Alpha interferons are totally filtered through the glomeruli and undergo rapid proteolytic degradation during tubular reabsorption.

### Half-life
Recombinant interferon alfa-2a—
- Intramuscular: 6 to 8 hours.
- Intravenous infusion: 3.7 to 8.5 (mean 5.1) hours.

Recombinant interferon alfa-2b—
- Intramuscular or subcutaneous: 2 to 3 hours.

Interferon alfa-n1—
- Intravenous infusion: About 8 hours.

Note: Accumulation may occur with daily intramuscular dosing.

### Onset of action
Hepatitis, chronic, active—Normalization of serum alanine aminotransferase (ALT) concentrations may occur as early as 2 weeks after initiation of treatment, although 6 months of treatment is usually recommended.

### Time to peak concentration
Recombinant interferon alfa-2a (single dose)—
- Intramuscular: 3.8 hours.
- Subcutaneous: 7.3 hours.

Recombinant interferon alfa-2b (single dose)—
- Intramuscular or subcutaneous: 3 to 12 hours.

### Time to peak effect
Condyloma acuminatum—4 to 8 weeks after initiation of treatment.

### Elimination
With systemic use—Renal; metabolites almost completely reabsorbed in renal tubules, with only negligible amounts of unchanged alpha interferon reappearing in systemic circulation.

## Precautions to Consider

### Cross-sensitivity and/or related problems
Patients sensitive to any alpha interferon may also be sensitive to any other alpha interferon.

Patients sensitive to mouse immunoglobulin may also be sensitive to recombinant interferon alfa-2a.

Patients sensitive to mouse immunoglobulin, egg protein, or neomycin may also be sensitive to interferon alfa-n3.

### Carcinogenicity
Studies have not been done in either animals or humans.

### Mutagenicity
Results of Ames tests and *in vitro* treatment of human lymphocyte cultures with recombinant alpha interferon at noncytotoxic concentrations showed no evidence of mutagenicity. However, both genotoxicity and protection from chromosomal abnormalities produced by gamma rays have been reported in association with human leukocyte interferon *in vitro*.

### Pregnancy/Reproduction
Fertility—In humans, alpha interferon has been shown to affect the menstrual cycle and decrease serum estradiol and progesterone concentrations in adult females.

In Macaca mulatta (rhesus) monkeys given high doses (e.g., in the case of interferon alfa-n3, 326 times the average intralesional dose [120 times the maximum recommended dose]) intramuscularly daily, recombinant alpha interferon has been shown to cause menstrual cycle changes; normal menstrual rhythm returned when alpha interferon was withdrawn.

For interferon alfa-2a, recombinant: Has been shown to cause reversible menstrual irregularities, including prolonged or shortened menstrual periods and erratic bleeding with anovulation, in Macaca mulatta (rhesus) monkeys given 5 million and 25 million Units per kg of body weight per day.

For interferon alfa-n3: No menstrual changes were reported in humans.

Pregnancy—Adequate and well-controlled studies in humans have not been done.

*For interferon alfa-2a, recombinant*—
Studies in Macaca mulatta (rhesus) monkeys at doses approximately 20 to 500 times the therapeutic human dose found a significant increase in abortifacient activity but no evidence of teratogenic activity.

FDA Pregnancy Category C.

*For interferon alfa-2b, recombinant*—
Studies in Macaca mulatta (rhesus) monkeys at doses of 90 and 180 times the intramuscular or subcutaneous dose of 2 million Units per square meter of body surface area found an abortifacient effect.

FDA Pregnancy Category C.

*For interferon alfa-n1 (lns)*—
Studies have not been done in animals.

*For interferon alfa-n3*—
Studies have not been done in animals.

FDA Pregnancy Category C.

### Breast-feeding
It is not known whether alpha interferon is distributed into breast milk; in mice, mouse interferons are distributed into milk. However, because of the potential for serious adverse effects in nursing infants, avoidance of breast-feeding should be considered while alpha interferon is being administered.

### Pediatrics
Appropriate studies on the relationship of age to the effects of alpha interferons have not been performed in the pediatric population.

### Adolescents
Alpha interferons have been shown to affect the menstrual cycle in animals and decrease serum estradiol and progesterone concentrations in human females. These effects should be kept in mind when considering alpha interferon treatment in adolescent females.

### Geriatrics
Although appropriate studies on the relationship of age to the effects of alpha interferons have not been performed in the geriatric population, neurotoxicity and cardiotoxicity may be more likely to occur in the elderly, who may have underlying central nervous system (CNS) and cardiac function impairment. In addition, elderly patients are more likely to have age-related renal function impairment, which may require caution in patients receiving alpha interferons.

### Dental
The bone marrow depressant effects of alpha interferons may result in an increased incidence of microbial infection, delayed healing, and gin-

gival bleeding. If leukopenia or thrombocytopenia occurs, dental work should be deferred until blood counts have returned to normal and patients should be instructed in proper oral hygiene, including caution in use of regular toothbrushes, dental floss, and toothpicks.

Interferon alfa-2a and alfa-2b may cause stomatitis and discomfort. Use of interferon alfa-2a or alfa-2b may decrease or inhibit salivary flow, thus contributing to the development of caries, periodontal disease, oral candidiasis, and discomfort.

### Drug interactions and/or related problems
The following drug interactions and/or related problems have been selected on the basis of their potential clinical significance (possible mechanism in parentheses where appropriate)—not necessarily inclusive (» = major clinical significance):

Note: Combinations containing any of the following medications, depending on the amount present, may also interact with this medication.

The following information applies to systemic use.

Alcohol or
CNS depression–producing medications (see *Appendix II*)
(concurrent use may enhance the CNS depressant effects of either these medications or alpha interferon)

Blood dyscrasia–causing medications (see *Appendix II*)
(leukopenic and/or thrombocytopenic effects of interferon may be increased with concurrent or recent therapy if these medications cause the same effects; dosage adjustment of alpha interferon, if necessary, should be based on blood counts)

Bone marrow depressants, other (see *Appendix II*) or
Radiation therapy
(additive bone marrow depression may occur; dosage reduction may be required when two or more bone marrow depressants, including radiation, are used concurrently or consecutively)

### Laboratory value alterations
The following have been selected on the basis of their potential clinical significance (possible effect in parentheses where appropriate)—not necessarily inclusive (» = major clinical significance):

With physiology/laboratory test values

Note: The following information applies to systemic use.

Alanine aminotransferase (ALT [SGPT]) and
Alkaline phosphatase and
Aspartate aminotransferase (AST [SGOT]) and
Lactate dehydrogenase
(serum values may be increased; dose-related; reversible on withdrawal of alpha interferon)

Blood pressure
(mild and transient increase may occur; hypotension is more likely and may occur during administration or up to 2 days after administration)

Hemoglobin concentrations and
Hematocrit
(may be decreased)

Leukocyte counts (including neutrophils) and
Platelet counts
(may be decreased; dose-related)

Prothrombin time (PT) and
Partial thromboplastin time (PTT)
(may be increased by recombinant interferon alfa-2b; dose-related)

### Medical considerations/Contraindications
The medical considerations/contraindications included have been selected on the basis of their potential clinical significance (reasons given in parentheses where appropriate)—not necessarily inclusive (» = major clinical significance).

*Risk-benefit should be considered when the following medical problems exist:*
» Autoimmune disease, history of
(caution is recommended because alpha interferon may increase the activity of the immune system and thereby worsen the condition; use for treatment of non-A, non-B/C hepatitis or hepatitis B is not recommended)

Bone marrow depression
(may be exacerbated)

» Cardiac disease, severe, including recent myocardial infarction or
» Diabetes mellitus prone to ketoacidosis or
» Pulmonary disease
(may be exacerbated as a result of the stress of the fever and chills that occur in most patients receiving alpha interferon)

(the risk of cardiotoxicity of alpha interferon may be increased in patients with a history of cardiac disease; myocardial infarction has been reported rarely)

» Chickenpox, existing or recent, including recent exposure or
» Herpes zoster
(risk of severe generalized disease)

» CNS function, compromised or
» Psychiatric conditions, severe, or history of or
» Seizure disorders
(risk of severe CNS side effects)

Hepatic disease, severe
(alpha interferons may elevate serum hepatic enzyme concentrations)

Herpes labialis, history of
(may be reactivated)

Renal disease, severe
(may be exacerbated by fever and dehydration caused by alpha interferon)

» Sensitivity to alpha interferon

Caution should be used also in patients who have had previous cytotoxic drug therapy or radiation therapy.

*For treatment of non-A, non-B/C hepatitis, or hepatitis B (in addition to the above)*
» Thyroid function impairment
(recombinant interferon alfa-2b has been reported to cause thyroid function abnormalities; serum thyroid-stimulating hormone [TSH] concentrations must be within normal limits before initiation of treatment)

*For recombinant interferon alfa-2b and interferon alfa-n3 only (in addition to the above)*
Coagulation disorders
(caution is recommended; recombinant interferon alfa-2b may prolong PT and PTT)

### Patient monitoring
The following may be especially important in patient monitoring (other tests may be warranted in some patients, depending on condition; » = major clinical significance):

Note: The following information applies to systemic use.

Alanine aminotransferase (ALT [SGPT]) values and
Aspartate aminotransferase (AST [SGOT]) values and
Bilirubin concentrations, serum and
Lactate dehydrogenase (LDH) values
(recommended prior to initiation of therapy and at periodic intervals during therapy)

Blood pressure measurements
(recommended at periodic intervals)

Electrocardiogram (ECG)
(recommended prior to initiation of therapy and at periodic intervals during therapy in patients with cardiac disease or advanced malignancy)

» Hematocrit or hemoglobin and
» Platelet count and
» Total and, if appropriate, differential leukocyte count
(determinations recommended prior to initiation of therapy and at periodic intervals during therapy)

Liver biopsy
(recommended prior to discontinuing alpha interferon treatment when hepatic enzyme values return to normal)

Neuropsychiatric monitoring
(recommended especially in patients receiving high doses of alpha interferon)

Thyroid-stimulating hormone (TSH) concentrations, serum
(recommended prior to initiation of treatment for non-A, non-B/C hepatitis, or hepatitis B and if symptoms of thyroid function impairment occur during treatment)

## Side/Adverse Effects
See *Table 1*, page 1746.

## Patient Consultation
As an aid to patient consultation, refer to *Advice for the Patient, Interferons, Alpha (Systemic)*.

In providing consultation, consider emphasizing the following selected information (» = major clinical significance):

### Before using this medication
» Conditions affecting use, especially:
    Sensitivity to alpha interferons
    Pregnancy—Abortifacient effects found in rhesus monkeys
    Breast-feeding—Possible need to avoid breast-feeding during alpha interferon therapy because of risk of serious adverse effects in the nursing infant
    Use in adolescents—Possible effects on menstrual cycle
    Use in the elderly—Risk of cardiotoxic and neurotoxic effects may be increased
    Other medical problems, especially history of autoimmune disease, severe cardiac disease, chickenpox, compromised CNS function, diabetes mellitus, herpes zoster, history of psychiatric disease, pulmonary disease, seizure disorders, and thyroid function impairment

### Proper use of this medication
» Compliance with therapy
» Reading patient directions carefully with regard to:
    —Preparation of the injection
    —Use of disposable syringes
    —Proper administration technique
    —Stability of the injection
    Importance of ample fluid intake to reduce risk of hypotension
    Administration at bedtime to minimize inconvenience of fatigue
» Proper dosing
    Missed dose: Skipping missed dose and going back to regular schedule; not doubling doses; checking with physician
» Proper storage

### Precautions while using this medication
» Importance of close monitoring by physician
» Not changing brands of interferon without consulting physician because of differences in dosage
» Caution in taking alcohol or other CNS depressants during therapy
» Caution when driving or doing anything else requiring alertness because of possible fatigue and dizziness
» Frequency of fever and flu-like symptoms; possible need for acetaminophen before and after a dose is given

*Caution if bone marrow depression occurs*
» Avoiding exposure to persons with bacterial infections, especially during periods of low blood counts; checking with physician immediately if fever or chills, cough or hoarseness, lower back or side pain, or painful or difficult urination occur
» Checking with physician immediately if unusual bleeding or bruising; black, tarry stools; blood in urine or stools; or pinpoint red spots on skin occur
    Caution in use of regular toothbrush, dental floss, or toothpick; physician, dentist, or nurse may suggest alternatives; checking with physician before having dental work done
    Not touching eyes or inside of nose unless hands washed immediately before
    Using caution to avoid accidental cuts with use of sharp objects such as safety razor or fingernail or toenail cutters
    Avoiding contact sports or other situations where bruising or injury could occur

### Side/adverse effects
Signs of potential side effects, especially cardiotoxicity, neurotoxicity, peripheral neuropathy, leukopenia, and thrombocytopenia
Possibility of minor hair loss; normal hair growth should return after treatment has ended

## General Dosing Information

Strengths and dosages of recombinant interferon alfa-2a and alfa-2b, interferon alfa-n1, and interferon alfa-n3 are expressed in terms of Units. Units are determined by comparison of the antiviral activity of the interferon with the activity of the international reference preparation of human leukocyte interferon established by the World Health Organization (WHO).

Patients receiving alpha interferon should be under supervision of a physician experienced in immunomodulatory and/or cancer chemotherapy.

It is recommended that the patient be premedicated with acetaminophen at the time of alpha interferon dosing and that the acetaminophen be continued as needed to treat fever and headache. Dosage reduction of alpha interferon may be necessary if headache persists.

Patients who develop leukopenia should be observed carefully for signs of infection. Antibiotic support may be required. In neutropenic patients who develop fever, broad-spectrum antibiotic coverage should be initiated empirically, pending bacterial cultures and appropriate diagnostic tests. In some cases, it may be difficult to distinguish fever due to infection from fever associated with the flu-like syndrome.

Special precautions are recommended in patients who develop thrombocytopenia as a result of administration of alpha interferons. These may include extreme care in performing invasive procedures; regular inspection of intravenous sites, skin (including perirectal area), and mucous membrane surfaces for signs of bleeding or bruising; limiting frequency of venipuncture and avoiding intramuscular injections; testing urine, emesis, stool, and secretions for occult blood; care in use of regular toothbrushes, dental floss, toothpicks, safety razors, and fingernail and toenail cutters; avoiding constipation; and using caution to prevent falls and other injuries. Such patients should avoid alcohol and any aspirin intake because of the risk of gastrointestinal bleeding. Platelet transfusions may be required.

### For systemic use
The subcutaneous route of administration is recommended for patients with thrombocytopenia or at risk for bleeding.

If severe adverse effects occur, dosage reduction by 50% or temporary withdrawal of alpha interferon is recommended.

It is recommended that patients be well hydrated, especially during initial treatment with alpha interferon, to reduce the risk of hypotension associated with fluid depletion. Hypotension may require supportive treatment, including fluid replacement to maintain intravascular volume.

---

### *INTERFERON ALFA-2a, RECOMBINANT*

## Summary of Differences
Pharmacology/pharmacokinetics:
    Source—Synthetic; produced by a recombinant DNA process. Purification procedure includes affinity chromatography using a murine monoclonal antibody. Single alpha interferon subtype.
    Half-life—
        Intramuscular: 6 to 8 hours.
        Intravenous infusion: 3.7 to 8.5 hours.
    Time to peak concentration (single dose)—
        Intramuscular: 3.8 hours.
        Subcutaneous: 7.3 hours.

## Parenteral Dosage Forms

### INTERFERON ALFA-2a, RECOMBINANT, INJECTION

**Usual adult dose**
Hairy cell leukemia—
    Induction: Intramuscular or subcutaneous, 3 million Units per day for sixteen to twenty-four weeks.
    Maintenance: Intramuscular or subcutaneous, 3 million Units three times per week.
Kaposi's sarcoma, AIDS-associated—
    Induction:
        Intramuscular or subcutaneous, 36 million Units (1 mL) per day for ten to twelve weeks, or
        Intramuscular or subcutaneous, 3 million Units per day on Days 1 to 3, 9 million Units per day on Days 4 to 6, and 18 million Units per day on Days 7 to 9, followed by 36 million Units (1 mL) per day for the remainder of the ten- to twelve-weeks induction period.
    Maintenance:
        Intramuscular or subcutaneous, 36 million Units (1 mL) three times per week.
Note: A variety of dosage schedules of interferon have been used for the unlabeled indications. Since these regimens are still largely investigational, the prescriber should consult the medical literature in choosing a specific dosage.

**Usual pediatric dose**
Dosage has not been established.

**Strength(s) usually available**
U.S.—
    3 million Units per mL (Rx) [*Roferon-A* (sodium chloride; albumin; phenol)].
    6 million Units per mL (18 million Units per vial) (Rx) [*Roferon-A* (sodium chloride; albumin; phenol)].
    10 million Units per mL (9 million Units per 0.9-mL vial) (Rx) [*Roferon-A* (sodium chloride; albumin; phenol)].
    36 million Units per mL (Rx) [*Roferon-A* (sodium chloride; albumin; phenol)].
    Note: The 10-million-Units-per-mL and 36-million-Units-per-mL strengths are for use for treatment of AIDS-associated Kaposi's sarcoma. They should *not* be used for treatment of hairy cell leukemia.

# Interferons, Alpha (Systemic)

Canada—
3 million Units per mL (Rx) [*Roferon-A* (sodium chloride; albumin; phenol)].
6 million Units per mL (Rx) [*Roferon-A* (phenol)].

**Packaging and storage**
Store between 2 and 8 °C (36 and 46 °F), unless otherwise specified by manufacturer. Protect from freezing.

**Note**
Do not shake.

When dispensing for self-administration by the patient, make sure that patient instructions are included and that the patient understands how to prepare and administer the injection, including proper use of disposable syringes.

Interferon alfa-2a, -2b, -n1, and -n3 are not interchangeable.

## INTERFERON ALFA-2a, RECOMBINANT, FOR INJECTION

**Usual adult dose**
Hairy cell leukemia—
 Induction: Intramuscular or subcutaneous, 3 million Units per day for sixteen to twenty-four weeks.
 Maintenance: Intramuscular or subcutaneous, 3 million Units three times per week.
Note: A variety of dosage schedules of interferon have been used for the unlabeled indications. Since these regimens are still largely investigational, the prescriber should consult the medical literature in choosing a specific dosage.

**Usual pediatric dose**
Dosage has not been established.

**Size(s) usually available**
U.S.—
 18 million Units (Rx) [*Roferon-A* (diluent contains sodium chloride, albumin, phenol)].
Canada—
 18 million Units (Rx) [*Roferon-A* (diluent contains sodium chloride, albumin, phenol)].

**Packaging and storage**
Store between 2 and 8 °C (36 and 46 °F), unless otherwise specified by manufacturer. Protect from freezing.

**Preparation of dosage form**
Interferon alfa-2a, recombinant, for injection is prepared for parenteral use by adding 3 mL of diluent (containing sodium chloride, albumin, and phenol) provided by the manufacturer and swirling gently to dissolve, producing a solution containing 6 million Units per mL.

**Stability**
Reconstituted solution of interferon alfa-2a, recombinant, for injection should be used within 30 days and stored between 2 and 8 °C (36 and 46 °F).

**Note**
When dispensing for self-administration by the patient, make sure that patient instructions are included and that the patient understands how to prepare and administer the injection, including proper use of disposable syringes.

Interferon alfa-2a, -2b, -n1, and -n3 are not interchangeable.

---

## INTERFERON ALFA-2b, RECOMBINANT

## Summary of Differences

Pharmacology/pharmacokinetics:
 Source—Synthetic; produced by a recombinant DNA process. Purification is done by proprietary methods. Single alpha interferon subtype.
 Half-life—Intramuscular or subcutaneous: 2 to 3 hours.
 Time to peak concentration—Intramuscular or subcutaneous: 3 to 12 hours.
Precautions:
 Laboratory value alterations—
  Nadir of leukocyte and platelet counts is at 3 to 5 days, with recovery within 3 to 5 days after withdrawal.
  Prothrombin time (PT) and partial thromboplastin time (PTT) may be increased.
 Medical considerations/contraindications—Caution in coagulation disorders.

## Parenteral Dosage Forms

### INTERFERON ALFA-2b, RECOMBINANT, FOR INJECTION

**Usual adult dose**
Hairy cell leukemia—
 Intramuscular or subcutaneous, 2 million Units per square meter of body surface area three times per week.
Condyloma acuminatum[1]—
 Intralesional, 1 million Units (using only the 10-million-Units-per-mL strength) per wart (up to five warts) three times a week on alternate days for three weeks. If response is not satisfactory twelve to sixteen weeks after the initial treatment course, a second course may be given. Patients with six to ten warts may be given a second (sequential) course of treatment at the same dose to treat up to five additional warts per course; for patients with more than ten warts, additional courses may be given as needed with up to five additional warts per course.
Kaposi's sarcoma, AIDS-associated—
 Intramuscular or subcutaneous, 30 million Units (using 50-million-Units-per-mL strength) per square meter of body surface area three times a week.
Hepatitis, chronic, active—
 Non-A, non-B/C hepatitis: Intramuscular or subcutaneous, 3 million Units three times per week. Patients who relapse may be re-treated with the same dose to which they had previously responded.
Hepatitis B, chronic[1]—
 Intramuscular or subcutaneous, 30 to 35 million Units per week, either as 5 million Units per day or 10 million Units three times per week, for sixteen weeks.
Malignant melanoma[1]—
 Induction: Intravenous infusion, 20 million Units per square meter of body surface area for five consecutive days per week for four weeks.
 Maintenance: Subcutaneous, 10 million Units per square meter of body surface area three times per week for forty-eight weeks.
Note: A variety of dosage schedules of interferon have been used for the unlabeled indications. Since these regimens are still largely investigational, the prescriber should consult the medical literature in choosing a specific dosage.

**Usual pediatric dose**
Safety and efficacy have not been established.

**Size(s) usually available**
U.S.—
 3 million Units (Rx) [*Intron A* (albumin)].
 5 million Units (Rx) [*Intron A* (albumin)].
 10 million Units (Rx) [*Intron A* (albumin)].
 18 million Units (Rx) [*Intron A* (albumin)].
 25 million Units (Rx) [*Intron A* (albumin)].
 50 million Units (Rx) [*Intron A* (albumin)].
Note: The 10-million-Unit size is the only one that should be used for treatment of condyloma acuminatum. Dilution of the other available sizes (3, 5, 18, 25, or 50 million Units) that would be required for intralesional use with the volume of diluent recommended for preparing an intralesional injection would produce a hypertonic solution.
 The 50-million-Unit size is a special formulation for use for treatment of AIDS-associated Kaposi's sarcoma or malignant melanoma. It should *not* be used for treatment of hairy cell leukemia or condyloma acuminatum.

Canada—
 3 million Units (Rx) [*Intron A* (albumin)].
 5 million Units (Rx) [*Intron A* (albumin)].
 10 million Units (Rx) [*Intron A* (albumin)].

**Packaging and storage**
Store between 2 and 8 °C (36 and 46 °F), unless otherwise specified by manufacturer.

**Preparation of dosage form**
Interferon alfa-2b, recombinant, for injection is prepared for parenteral use by adding the appropriate amount of diluent (in the U.S., bacteriostatic water for injection provided by the manufacturer; in Canada, either sterile water for injection or bacteriostatic water for injection) and agitating gently to dissolve, producing a clear, colorless to light yellow solution.

| Size (Units) | Diluent (mL) | Final concentration (Units/mL) |
|---|---|---|
| U.S.— | | |
| *For treatment of hairy cell leukemia* | | |
| 3 million | 1 | 3 million |
| 5 million | 1 | 5 million |
| 10 million | 2 | 5 million |
| 25 million | 5 | 5 million |
| *For treatment of condyloma acuminatum* | | |
| 10 million | 1 | 10 million |
| *For treatment of AIDS-associated Kaposi's sarcoma* | | |
| 50 million | 1 | 50 million |
| *For treatment of malignant melanoma (induction or maintenance phase)* | | |
| 3 million | 1 | 3 million |
| 5 million | 1 | 5 million |
| 10 million | 1 | 10 million |
| 18 million | 1 | 18 million |
| 25 million | 5 | 5 million |
| 50 million | 1 | 50 million |
| *For treatment of chronic hepatitis B* | | |
| 5 million | 1 | 5 million |
| 10 million | 1 | 10 million |
| *For treatment of chronic active non-A, non-B/C hepatitis* | | |
| 3 million | 1 | 3 million |
| Canada— | | |
| 3 million | 1 | 3 million |
| 5 million | 1 | 5 million |
| 10 million | 1 | 10 million |

**Stability**
Reconstituted solutions of interferon alfa-2b, recombinant, prepared with sterile water for injection are stable for 24 hours when stored between 2 and 8 °C (36 and 46 °F); solutions prepared with bacteriostatic water for injection are stable for 1 month when stored between 2 and 8 °C (36 and 46 °F).

**Note**
When dispensing for self-administration by the patient, make sure that patient instructions are included and that the patient understands how to prepare and administer the injection, including proper use of disposable syringes.

Interferon alfa-2a, -2b, -n1, and -n3 are not interchangeable.

[1]Not included in Canadian product labeling.

---

### INTERFERON ALFA-n1 (LNS)

## Summary of Differences
Pharmacology/pharmacokinetics:
  Source—Obtained from pooled units of human lymphoblastoid cells following induction with Sendai virus. Mixture of natural alpha interferon subtypes, but in different proportions than in human leukocyte interferon.
  Half-life—Intravenous infusion: About 8 hours.

## Parenteral Dosage Forms
### INTERFERON ALFA-n1 (LNS) INJECTION
**Usual adult dose**
Hairy cell leukemia—
  Induction: Intramuscular or subcutaneous, 3 million Units per day for sixteen to twenty-four weeks.
  Maintenance: Intramuscular or subcutaneous, 3 million Units three times per week.
Condyloma acuminatum—
  Intramuscular or subcutaneous, 1 to 3 million Units per square meter of body surface area five times a week for two weeks, followed by three times a week for four weeks. The same dose is then continued every other day or three times a week for one month.
Note: As an adjunct to laser surgery or cryosurgery, the dose is 1 million Units per square meter of body surface area intramuscularly or subcutaneously per day for seven days prior to and seven days following surgical resection of the lesions.

  A variety of dosage schedules of interferon have been used for the unlabeled indications. Since these regimens are still largely investigational, the prescriber should consult the medical literature in choosing a specific dosage.

**Usual pediatric dose**
Hairy cell leukemia or
Condyloma acuminatum—
  Dosage has not been established.
Juvenile laryngeal papillomatosis—
  For children older than 1 year of age:
    Body surface area less than 0.5 square meter—Intramuscular or subcutaneous, 1.5 million Units per day for twenty-eight days, followed by maintenance dosage three times a week for at least six months.
    Body surface area 0.5–1 square meter—Intramuscular or subcutaneous, 3 million Units per day for twenty-eight days, followed by maintenance dosage three times a week for at least six months.
    Body surface area greater than 1 square meter—Intramuscular or subcutaneous, 5 million Units per day for twenty-eight days, followed by maintenance dosage three times a week for at least six months.

**Size(s) usually available**
U.S.—
  Not commercially available.
Canada—
  3 million Units (Rx) [*Wellferon*].
  10 million Units (Rx) [*Wellferon*].

**Packaging and storage**
Store between 2 and 8 °C (36 and 46 °F), unless otherwise specified by manufacturer. Protect from light.

**Note**
Interferon alfa-2a, -2b, -n1, and -n3 are not interchangeable.

---

### INTERFERON ALFA-n3

## Summary of Differences
Pharmacology/pharmacokinetics:
  Source—Obtained from pooled units of human leukocytes that have been induced to produce interferon alfa-n3. Contains up to 14 natural alpha interferon subtypes. Human leukocyte interferon.
Precautions:
  Medical considerations/contraindications—Caution in coagulation disorders.

## Parenteral Dosage Forms
### INTERFERON ALFA-n3 INJECTION
**Usual adult dose**
Condyloma acuminatum—
  Intralesional (at the base of the wart, preferably using a 30 gauge needle), 250,000 Units two times a week for up to eight weeks.
Note: For large warts, it may be injected at several points around the periphery of the wart, using a total dose of 250,000 Units.

  Safety and efficacy of more than one 8-week course have not been established.

  A variety of dosage schedules of interferon have been used for the unlabeled indications. Since these regimens are still largely investigational, the prescriber should consult the medical literature in choosing a specific dosage.

**Usual adult prescribing limits**
2.5 million Units per treatment session.

**Usual pediatric dose**
Dosage has not been established.

**Strength(s) usually available**
U.S.—
  5 million Units per mL (Rx) [*Alferon N* (phenol 3.3 mg per mL; human albumin 1 mg per mL)].
Canada—
  Not commercially available.

**Packaging and storage**
Store between 2 and 8 °C (36 and 46 °F), unless otherwise specified by manufacturer. Protect from freezing.

**Note**
Do not shake.
Interferon alfa-2a, -2b, -n1, and -n3 are not interchangeable.

Revised: 06/25/98
Interim revision: 07/07/98

## Table 1. Side/Adverse Effects

Note: Most side/adverse effects, except the flu-like syndrome, are dose-related. They are usually mild to moderate at systemic doses less than 10 million Units per day; hematologic and hepatic toxicities tend to be more frequent with doses above 10 million Units, and cardiovascular and neurologic toxicities tend to be more frequent with doses above 30 million Units. However, patient sensitivity varies.

Reduced blood pressure occurs frequently with systemic use but is rarely symptomatic; hypotension may occur during administration or up to two days after therapy, and may require supportive therapy including fluid replacement to maintain intravascular volume; hypertension may occur but is usually mild and transient.

Development of neutralizing antibodies has been reported. Relationship of the presence of neutralizing antibodies to loss of antitumor effects is controversial; a possible correlation with titer of neutralizing antibodies has been suggested but not confirmed. Differences in frequency of antibody formation have been reported among alpha interferons but relative frequency has not been studied prospectively. Differences may be related to the differences in the sensitivity of tests used in antibody detection, as well as to disease state, dose, schedule, and route of administration.

| The following side/adverse effects have been selected on the basis of their potential clinical significance (possible signs and symptoms in parentheses where appropriate)—not necessarily inclusive:* | Hairy cell leukemia | Other malignancies | Condyloma acuminatum | Kaposi's sarcoma | Hepatitis |
|---|---|---|---|---|---|
| **Those indicating need for medical attention** | | | | | |
| ***Anemia*** (usually asymptomatic) | N/A | M | L | M | M |
| ***Cardiotoxicity*** (chest pain, irregular heartbeat) | R | R | U | R | R |
| Note: Arrhythmias are usually supraventricular. | | | | | |
| ***Hepatotoxicity*** (usually asymptomatic) | L | L | L | M | L |
| ***Hyperthyroidism or hypothyroidism*** (usually asymptomatic) | U | U | U | U | R |
| ***Leukopenia*** (usually asymptomatic; rarely, fever or chills, cough or hoarseness, lower back or side pain, painful or difficult urination) | N/A | M | M | M | M |
| ***Neurotoxicity*** (confusion, mental depression, nervousness, trouble in sleeping, trouble in thinking or concentrating | L | L | L | L | L |
| Note: Usually reversible after withdrawal; in some patients, especially the elderly or those treated with high doses, stupor, obtundation, and coma have occurred. | | | | | |
| ***Peripheral neuropathy*** (numbness or tingling of fingers, toes, or face) | L | L | L | L | R |
| ***Thrombocytopenia*** (usually asymptomatic; rarely, unusual bleeding or bruising; black, tarry stools; blood in urine or stools; pinpoint red spots on skin) | N/A | M | L | M | M |
| **Those indicating need for medical attention only if they continue or are bothersome** | | | | | |
| ***Blurred vision*** | L | L | L | L | L |
| ***Change in taste or metallic taste*** | M | M | R | M | R |
| ***Cold sores or stomatitis*** (sores in mouth and on lips) | L | L | R | R | R |
| ***Diarrhea*** | M | M | L | M | M |
| ***Dizziness*** | M | M | L | M | L |
| Note: Dizziness is a CNS effect. | | | | | |
| ***Dry mouth*** | M | M | R | M | L |
| ***Dry skin or itching*** | L | L | L | L | L |
| ***Flu-like syndrome*** (aching muscles, fever and chills, headache, general feeling of discomfort or illness; less frequently, joint pain, back pain) | M | M | M | M | M |
| Note: Occurs in most patients; most pronounced in first week of treatment and gradually reduced, as a result of tachyphylaxis, within 2 to 4 weeks with continued treatment. | | | | | |
| ***Increased sweating*** | L | L | L | L | L |
| ***Leg cramps*** | L | L | L | U | R |
| ***Loss of appetite*** | M | M | L | M | M |
| Note: Loss of appetite tends to become more prominent with continued treatment and may necessitate dosage reduction; usually resolves within 4 weeks after withdrawal of alpha interferon. | | | | | |
| ***Nausea or vomiting*** | M | M | M | M | M |
| Note: Nausea or vomiting usually resolves within 3 to 5 days after withdrawal of alpha interferon. | | | | | |
| ***Skin rash*** | M | M | L | M | L |
| ***Unusual tiredness*** | M | M | M | M | M |
| Note: Unusual tiredness tends to become more prominent with continued treatment and may necessitate dosage reduction; usually resolves several weeks after withdrawal of alpha interferon. | | | | | |
| ***Weight loss*** | R | R | R | L | R |
| **Those not indicating need for medical attention** | | | | | |
| ***Loss of hair, partial*** | L | L | U | M | M |
| Note: Hair growth returns promptly after withdrawal of alpha interferon. | | | | | |

*Differences in frequency of occurrence may reflect either lack of clinical-use data or actual pharmacologic distinctions among agents (although their pharmacologic similarity suggests that side effects occurring with one may occur with the others). M = more frequent; L = less frequent; R = rare; U = unknown; X = does not occur; N/A = not applicable.

**INULIN**—The *Inulin (Systemic)* monograph is not included in this published version of the USP DI database. Copies of the monograph are available on request from Micromedex, Inc. - Reprint Requests, 6200 S. Syracuse Way, Suite 300, Englewood, CO 80111; telephone (303) 486-6400; telefax (303) 486-6464; Email: USPDI@MDX.COM.

**IOBENGUANE I 123**—See *Iobenguane, Radioiodinated (Systemic—Diagnostic)*

**IOBENGUANE I 131**—See *Iobenguane, Radioiodinated (Systemic—Diagnostic)*

# IOBENGUANE, RADIOIODINATED  Systemic—Diagnostic†

VA CLASSIFICATION (Primary): DX201

A commonly used name for iobenguane is meta-iodobenzylguanidine or mIBG.

Note: For a listing of dosage forms and brand names by country availability, see *Dosage Forms* section(s).

†Not commercially available in Canada.

## Category
Diagnostic aid, radioactive (adrenomedullary disorders; neuroendocrine tumors).

## Indications
Note: Bracketed information in the *Indications* section refers to uses that are not included in U.S. product labeling. In addition, because iobenguane I 123 ($^{123}$I-mIBG) injection is not commercially available in the U.S. or Canada, the bracketed information and the use of the superscript 1 in this monograph reflect the lack of labeled (approved) indications for this product.

### Accepted
Tumors, adrenal medulla (diagnosis)[1]—[$^{123}$I]- and $^{131}$I-mIBG are used for diagnostic imaging of the adrenal medulla, for the evaluation and localization of intra- and extra-adrenal pheochromocytomas, paragangliomas, and neuroblastomas, as well as for localization of metastatic lesions from these tumors. [$^{123}$I]- and $^{131}$I-mIBG can also be used for confirmation of diagnosis of pheochromocytoma when catecholamine determination tests are unclear.

[Tumors, carcinoid (diagnosis)][1]—$^{123}$I- and $^{131}$I-mIBG scintigraphy are used as screening procedures for suspected carcinoid tumors, especially those of intestinal origin.

[Hyperplasia, adrenal medulla (diagnosis)][1]—$^{123}$I- and $^{131}$I-mIBG are used in the evaluation of the adrenal medulla for disorders such as medullary hyperplasia in patients at risk of developing medullary disease (e.g., multiple endocrine neoplasia [MEN type 2, MEN type 3]).

[Carcinoma, thyroid (diagnosis)][1]—$^{123}$I- and $^{131}$I-mIBG are used for diagnostic imaging of medullary thyroid carcinoma.

[1]Not included in Canadian product labeling.

## Physical Properties
### Nuclear data

| Radionuclide (half-life) | Decay constant | Mode of decay | Principal emissions (keV) | Mean number of emissions/ disintegration |
|---|---|---|---|---|
| I 123 (13.2 hr) | 0.0533 h$^{-1}$ | Electron capture | Gamma (159) | 0.83 |
| I 131 (8.08 days) | 0.00358 h$^{-1}$ | Beta | Beta (191.6) Gamma (364.5) | 0.90 0.81 |

## Pharmacology/Pharmacokinetics
### Mechanism of action/Effect
Iobenguane or meta-iodobenzylguanidine (mIBG) is a physiological analog of the guanidines, such as guanethidine and phenethylguanidine. In adrenergic nerves, guanidines are believed to share the same transport pathway as norepinephrine and to accumulate in, and displace norepinephrine from, intraneuronal storage granules. Similarly, $^{123}$I- and $^{131}$I-mIBG are concentrated in, stored in, and released from chromaffin granules. The retention of $^{123}$I- and $^{131}$I-mIBG in the adrenal medulla may be a result of their uptake in adrenergic neurons and subsequent sequestration into chromaffin storage granules. Due to their selective uptake mechanism, $^{123}$I- and $^{131}$I-mIBG allow specific detection and localization of neuroendocrine tumors and adrenal medullary hyperplasia. The gamma emissions given off by $^{123}$I- and $^{131}$I-mIBG allow detection of adrenergic tumors by scintigraphy.

Medullary thyroid carcinoma—Although the mechanism of $^{123}$I- and $^{131}$I-mIBG uptake by medullary thyroid carcinoma (MTC) is not completely understood, it has been found that MTC can produce catecholamines (epinephrine and norepinephrine). Therefore, $^{123}$I- and $^{131}$I-mIBG could be taken up and stored in catecholamine vesicles of MTC.

### Distribution
After intravenous administration, there is rapid uptake of mIBG mainly in the liver, and in lesser amounts in the lungs, heart, spleen, and salivary glands. Although the uptake in normal adrenal glands is very low, hyperplastic adrenals and tumors such as pheochromocytoma, neuroblastoma, and other tumors with neurosecretory granules have a relatively higher uptake.

Significant clearance of $^{131}$I-mIBG from the liver and the spleen occurs within 72 hours.

### Time to radioactivity visualization
$^{123}$I-mIBG—In adrenal medullary tumors: Initial images may be obtained 2 to 3 hours after injection. Images may also be obtained at 18 to 24 hours, and as late as 48 hours post injection. Most pheochromocytomas are visualized at 24 hours. However, due to the short half-life of $^{123}$I-mIBG, images may not be possible at times when background (e.g., liver) activity is low and imaging would be optimal.

$^{131}$I-mIBG—In adrenal medullary tumors: 48 hours. Early images at 24 hours after administration of $^{131}$I-mIBG are frequently positive in patients with pheochromocytoma. Decline in liver activity may permit optimal imaging at 48 or 72 hours.

### Radiation dosimetry

| Organ | I 123-mIBG mGy/MBq | I 123-mIBG rad/mCi | I 131-mIBG mGy/MBq | I 131-mIBG rad/mCi |
|---|---|---|---|---|
| Liver | 0.071 | 0.27 | 0.83 | 3.07 |
| Bladder wall | 0.070 | 0.30 | 0.59 | 2.18 |
| Spleen | 0.020 | 0.074 | 0.49 | 1.81 |
| Salivary glands | 0.017 | 0.063 | 0.23 | 0.85 |
| Lungs | 0.016 | 0.059 | 0.19 | 0.70 |
| Kidneys | 0.014 | 0.052 | 0.12 | 0.44 |
| Adrenals | 0.011 | 0.041 | 0.17 | 0.63 |
| Heart | 0.011 | 0.041 | 0.072 | 0.26 |
| Pancreas | 0.011 | 0.041 | 0.10 | 0.37 |
| Uterus | 0.011 | 0.041 | 0.080 | 0.29 |
| Red marrow | 0.0092 | 0.034 | 0.067 | 0.25 |
| Large intestine wall (upper) | 0.0089 | 0.033 | 0.080 | 0.29 |
| Small intestine | 0.0083 | 0.031 | 0.074 | 0.27 |
| Ovaries | 0.0080 | 0.030 | 0.066 | 0.24 |
| Stomach wall | 0.0078 | 0.029 | 0.077 | 0.28 |
| Large intestine wall (lower) | 0.0077 | 0.028 | 0.068 | 0.25 |
| Bone surfaces | 0.0076 | 0.028 | 0.061 | 0.23 |
| Breast | 0.0062 | 0.023 | 0.069 | 0.25 |
| Testes | 0.0054 | 0.020 | 0.059 | 0.22 |
| Thyroid (blocked)† | 0.0042 | 0.016 | 0.050 | 0.18 |
| Other tissue | 0.0065 | 0.024 | 0.062 | 0.23 |

| Radionuclide and impurities | Effective dose* | | | |
|---|---|---|---|---|
| | I 123-mIBG | | I 131-mIBG | |
| | mSv/MBq | rem/mCi | mSv/MBq | rem/mCi |
| I 123 | 0.018 | 0.067 | — | — |
| I 124 | 0.24 | 0.88 | — | — |
| I 125 | 0.049 | 0.18 | — | — |
| I 131 | — | — | 0.20 | 0.74 |

*For adults; intravenous injection. Data based on the International Commission on Radiological Protection (ICRP) Publication 53—Radiation dose to patients from radiopharmaceuticals.

†Thyroid dose listed assumes 0% thyroid uptake. However, uptakes ranging from 0.5 to 2% are more typical; consequently the absorbed radiation dose to the thyroid will be many times higher than listed.

**Elimination**
Renal; about 40 to 50% of the injected activity is eliminated within 24 hours and about 70 to 90% within 4 days (mainly as unchanged drug with small amounts of $^{123}$I- or $^{131}$I-m-iodohippuric acid [$^{123}$I- or $^{131}$I-mIHA], $^{123}$I or $^{131}$I iodide, and $^{123}$I- or $^{131}$I-m-iodobenzoic acid [$^{123}$I- or $^{131}$I-mIBA]).

## Precautions to Consider

### Pregnancy/Reproduction
Pregnancy—The possibility of pregnancy should be assessed in women of child-bearing potential. Clinical situations exist where the benefit to the patient and fetus, based on information derived from radiopharmaceutical use, outweighs the risks from fetal exposure to radiation. In these situations, the physician should use discretion and reduce the administered activity to the lowest possible amount.

### Breast-feeding
It is not known whether $^{123}$I- or $^{131}$I-mIBG is distributed into breast milk. However, this preparation may be contaminated with free radioiodide, which may be distributed into breast milk. It has been recommended that, after administration of a radiopharmaceutical, nursing be resumed only after the infant's ingested effective dose equivalent (EDE) is below 1 mSv (100 mrem). A method to calculate the EDE has been proposed based on the effective half-life of the radionuclide, the activity administered to the mother, the fraction of administered activity ingested by the infant, and the total body effective dose to the newborn infant per unit of activity ingested. According to this method, it has been estimated that, for sodium iodide I 131, the time to reduce the EDE to the infant to below 1 mSv (100 mrem) is approximately 10 weeks after administration of 40 megabecquerels (1.08 millicuries) to the mother. For sodium iodide I 123, the time period required is 3 days with administration of an uncontaminated preparation, 40 days with a preparation contaminated with I 124, and 340 days for a product contaminated with I 125. Because of the difficulty of maintaining the maternal milk supply for such an extended period of time, complete cessation of nursing is usually recommended for all radioiodines, except for uncontaminated I 123.

### Pediatrics
$^{123}$I- and $^{131}$I-mIBG are used in children. When $^{123}$I- or $^{131}$I-mIBG is used in children, the diagnostic benefit should be judged to outweigh the potential risk of radiation.

### Geriatrics
Diagnostic studies performed to date using $^{123}$I- or $^{131}$I-mIBG have not demonstrated geriatrics-specific problems that would limit the usefulness of either agent in the elderly.

### Drug interactions and/or related problems
The following drug interactions and/or related problems have been selected on the basis of their potential clinical significance (possible mechanism in parentheses where appropriate)—not necessarily inclusive (» = major clinical significance):

» Amphetamines or
» Antidepressants, tricyclic or
» Bretylium or
» Calcium channel blocking agents or
» Cocaine or
» Guanethidine or
» Haloperidol or
» Labetalol or
» Loxapine or
» Metaraminol or
» Phenothiazines or
» Reserpine or
» Sympathomimetics or
» Thiothixene
  (these medications may interfere with the uptake of $^{123}$I- or $^{131}$I-mIBG; although the ideal time to stop treatment with potential interacting medicines is 1 week prior to administration of $^{123}$I- or $^{131}$I-mIBG, the following withdrawal periods are usually recommended based on the individual half-life of each medication: 24 hours for bretylium, cocaine, and metaraminol; 48 hours for amphetamines, calcium channel blocking agents, guanethidine, haloperidol, loxapine, tricyclic antidepressants, phenothiazines, sympathomimetics, and thiothixene; 72 hours for labetalol and reserpine)

Phenoxybenzamine
  (although usual doses of phenoxybenzamine do not interfere with $^{123}$I- or $^{131}$I-mIBG uptake, when given in high doses necessary to control blood pressure in patients with pheochromocytomas or paragangliomas preparing for surgery, tumor uptake of $^{123}$I- or $^{131}$I-mIBG may be suppressed resulting in false-negative studies)

## Side/Adverse Effects
At present, there are no known side/adverse effects associated with the use of diagnostic dosages of $^{123}$I- or $^{131}$I-mIBG.

## Patient Consultation
As an aid to patient consultation, refer to *Advice for the Patient, Radiopharmaceuticals (Diagnostic)*.

In providing consultation, consider emphasizing the following selected information (» = major clinical significance):

### Description of use
Action in the body: Localization of $^{123}$I- or $^{131}$I-mIBG in adrenal medulla allows visualization of hyperactive adrenal medulla and neuroendocrine tumors

Small amounts of radioactivity used in diagnosis; radiation received is low and considered safe

### Before having this test
» Conditions affecting use, especially:
  Pregnancy—Risk to fetus from radiation exposure as opposed to benefit derived from study should be considered
  Breast-feeding—Not known if distributed into breast milk; however, free radioiodide, if present, may be distributed; cessation of nursing may be recommended to avoid any unnecessary absorbed radiation dose to the infant
  Use in children—Diagnostic benefit should be judged to outweigh potential risk of radiation
  Other medications, especially amphetamines, tricyclic antidepressants, bretylium, calcium channel blocking agents, cocaine, guanethidine, haloperidol, labetalol, loxapine, phenothiazines, reserpine, sympathomimetics, and thiothixene

### Preparation for this test
Special preparatory instructions may apply; patient should inquire in advance

Administration of potassium iodide or Lugol's solution one day before administration of $^{123}$I- or $^{131}$I-mIBG and for 6 days after administration to prevent or reduce thyroid uptake of radioiodide contaminant

## General Dosing Information
Radiopharmaceuticals are to be administered only by or under the supervision of physicians who have had extensive training in the safe use and handling of radioactive materials and who are authorized by the Nuclear Regulatory Commission (NRC) or the appropriate State agency, if required, or, outside the U.S., the appropriate authority.

To minimize uptake of radioactive iodine by the thyroid, potassium iodide (SSKI, 60 mg twice a day) or Lugol's solution (1 drop three times a day) may be used, beginning at least 24 hours before and continuing for 6 days after administration of $^{123}$I- or $^{131}$I-mIBG.

### Safety considerations for handling this radiopharmaceutical
Improper handling of this radiopharmaceutical may cause radioactive contamination. Guidelines for handling radioactive material have been prepared by scientific, professional, state, federal, and international bodies and are available to the specially qualified and authorized users who have access to radiopharmaceuticals.

## Parenteral Dosage Forms

Note: Bracketed information in the *Indications* section refers to uses that are not included in U.S. product labeling. In addition, because $^{123}$I-mIBG sulfate injection is not commercially available in the U.S. or Canada, the bracketed information and the use of the superscript 1 in the *Dosage Forms* section reflect the lack of labeled (approved) indications for this product.

The dosing and strengths of both the $^{123}$I- and $^{131}$I-mIBG dosage forms are expressed in terms of the sulfate salt of iobenguane.

### IOBENGUANE I 123 INJECTION USP

**Usual adult administered activity**
[Diagnosis of tumors][1] or
[Diagnosis of medullary disease][1]—
Intravenous, 370 megabecquerels (10 millicuries) of $^{123}$I-mIBG, with a specific activity of 740 megabecquerels to 1.3 gigabecquerels (20 to 35.6 millicuries) per mg (at time of calibration), administered over a period of fifteen to thirty seconds.

**Usual pediatric administered activity**
[Diagnosis of tumors][1] or
[Diagnosis of medullary disease][1]—
Children up to 18 years of age: Dosage must be individualized by physician.

**Usual geriatric administered activity**
See *Usual adult administered activity*.

**Strength(s) usually available**
U.S.—
Not commercially available. In most cases, may be obtained from the University of Michigan Nuclear Pharmacy (UMNP) by physicians who have filed their own Investigational New Drug Application (IND).
Canada—
Not commercially available. In most cases, may be obtained by physicians who have filed their own IND.

**Packaging and storage**
Store between −20 and −10 °C (−4 and −14 °F).

**Note**
Caution—Radioactive material.

### IOBENGUANE SULFATE I 131 INJECTION

**Usual adult administered activity**
Diagnosis of tumors[1] or
[Diagnosis of medullary disease][1]—
Intravenous, 18.5 to 37 megabecquerels (0.5 to 1 millicurie) of $^{131}$I-mIBG with a specific activity of 103.6 to 199 megabecquerels (2.8 to 5.38 millicuries) per mg (at time of calibration), administered over a period of fifteen seconds.

**Usual pediatric administered activity**
Diagnosis of tumors[1] or
[Diagnosis of medullary disease][1]—
Children up to 18 years of age: Dosage must be individualized by physician.
Note: In patients 1 year of age or older, the minimum dose necessary for a clinically acceptable study should not be less than 5 megabecquerels (0.135 millicuries).

**Usual geriatric administered activity**
See *Usual adult administered activity*.

**Strength(s) usually available**
U.S.—
85.1 megabecquerels (2.3 millicuries) per mL (Rx) [GENERIC].
Canada—
Not commercially available. In most cases, may be obtained by physicians who have filed their own IND.

**Packaging and storage**
Store between −20 and −10 °C (−4 and −14 °F), unless otherwise specified by manufacturer.

**Note**
Caution—Radioactive material.

[1]Not included in Canadian product labeling.

## Selected Bibliography

McEwan AJ, Shapiro B, Sisson JC, et al. Radio-iodobenzylguanidine for the scintigraphic location and therapy of adrenergic tumors. Semin Nucl Med 1985; 15(2): 132-53.

Solanki KK, Bomanji J, Moyes J, et al. A pharmacological guide to medicines which interfere with the biodistribution of radiolabelled meta-iodobenzylguanidine (MIBG). Nucl Med Commun 1992; 13: 513-21.

Revised: 05/05/93
Interim revision: 08/19/94; 04/25/95

---

# IOBENGUANE, RADIOIODINATED  Systemic—Therapeutic*†

VA CLASSIFICATION (Primary): AN600

A commonly used name for iobenguane is meta-iodobenzylguanidine or mIBG.

Note: For a listing of dosage forms and brand names by country availability, see *Dosage Forms* section(s).

*Not commercially available in the U.S.
†Not commercially available in Canada.

## Category

Antineoplastic.

## Indications

Note: Because I 131 iobenguane ($^{131}$I-mIBG) sulfate injection is not commercially available in the U.S. or Canada, the bracketed information and the use of the superscript 1 in this monograph reflect the lack of labeled (approved) indications for this product.

**Accepted**
[Carcinoid syndrome (treatment)][1] or
[Pheochromocytoma (treatment)][1]—$^{131}$I-mIBG is used in the treatment of pheochromocytoma and may be useful in other neuroendocrine tumors (e.g., carcinoid syndrome).

[Neuroblastoma (treatment)][1]—$^{131}$I-mIBG is used in the treatment of neuroblastomas unresponsive to conventional chemotherapy. Although complete remissions have been achieved in only a few cases, partial remissions have occurred in nearly half the reported cases in which $^{131}$I-mIBG has been used.

[1]Not included in Canadian product labeling.

## Physical Properties

### Nuclear data

| Radionuclide (half-life) | Decay constant | Mode of decay | Principal emissions (keV) | Mean number of emissions/ disintegration |
|---|---|---|---|---|
| I 131 (8.08 days) | 0.00358 h$^{-1}$ | Beta (90%) | Beta (191.6) Gamma (364.5) | 0.90 0.81 |

## Pharmacology/Pharmacokinetics

**Mechanism of action/Effect**
Iobenguane or meta-iodobenzylguanidine (mIBG) is a physiological analog of the guanidines, such as guanethidine and phenethylguanidine. In adrenergic nerves, guanidines are believed to share the same transport pathway as norepinephrine and to accumulate in, and displace norepinephrine from, intraneuronal storage granules. Similarly, $^{131}$I-mIBG is concentrated in, stored in, and released from chromaffin granules. The retention of $^{131}$I-mIBG in the adrenal medulla may be a result of its uptake in adrenergic neurons and subsequent sequestration into chromaffin storage granules. Due to its selective uptake mechanism, when $^{131}$I-mIBG is used at high levels of administered activity, the radionuclidic emissions can result in localized radiation therapy of tumor tissue.

**Distribution**
After intravenous administration, there is rapid uptake of mIBG mainly in the liver, and in lesser amounts in the lungs, heart, spleen, and salivary glands. Although the uptake in normal adrenal glands is very low, hyperplastic adrenals and tumors such as pheochromocytoma, neuroblastoma, and other tumors with neurosecretory granules have a relatively higher uptake.

## Onset of therapeutic action:
In malignant pheochromocytoma—Variable (after 1 to 8 doses).

## Radiation dosimetry

Estimated absorbed radiation dose*

| Organ | mGy/MBq | rad/mCi |
|---|---|---|
| Liver | 0.83 | 3.07 |
| Bladder wall | 0.59 | 2.18 |
| Spleen | 0.49 | 1.81 |
| Salivary glands | 0.23 | 0.85 |
| Lungs | 0.19 | 0.70 |
| Adrenals | 0.17 | 0.63 |
| Kidneys | 0.12 | 0.44 |
| Pancreas | 0.10 | 0.37 |
| Intestine wall (upper) | 0.080 | 0.29 |
| Uterus | 0.080 | 0.29 |
| Stomach wall | 0.077 | 0.28 |
| Small intestine | 0.074 | 0.27 |
| Heart | 0.072 | 0.26 |
| Breast | 0.069 | 0.25 |
| Intestine wall (lower) | 0.068 | 0.25 |
| Red marrow | 0.067 | 0.25 |
| Ovaries | 0.066 | 0.24 |
| Bone surface | 0.061 | 0.23 |
| Testes | 0.059 | 0.22 |
| Thyroid (blocked)† | 0.050 | 0.18 |
| Other tissue | 0.062 | 0.23 |

Effective dose: 0.20 mSv/MBq (0.74 rem/mCi)

*For adults; intravenous injection. Data based on the International Commission on Radiological Protection (ICRP) Publication 53—Radiation dose to patients from radiopharmaceuticals.

†Thyroid dose listed assumes 0% thyroid uptake. However, uptakes ranging from 0.5 to 2% are more typical; consequently the absorbed radiation dose to the thyroid will be many times higher than listed.

## Elimination
Renal; about 40 to 50% of the injected activity is eliminated within 24 hours and about 70 to 90% within 4 days (mainly as unchanged drug with small amounts of $^{131}$I-m-iodohippuric acid [$^{131}$I-mIHA], $^{131}$I iodide, and $^{131}$I-m-iodobenzoic acid [$^{131}$I-mIBA]).

# Precautions to Consider

## Pregnancy/Reproduction
Pregnancy—$^{131}$I-mIBG is not recommended for the treatment of disease during pregnancy.

To avoid the possibility of fetal exposure to radiation, in those circumstances where the patient's pregnancy status is uncertain a pregnancy test will help to prevent inadvertent administration of this preparation during pregnancy.

## Breast-feeding
It is not known whether $^{131}$I-mIBG is distributed into breast milk. However, this preparation may be contaminated with free radioiodide, which may be distributed into breast milk. In addition, free radioiodide will be produced during normal metabolism. In order to decrease the absorbed radiation dose to the breast and to avoid risk to the infant, complete cessation of nursing is recommended after $^{131}$I-mIBG is administered.

## Pediatrics
$^{131}$I-mIBG is used in children; however, the therapeutic benefit should be judged to outweigh the potential risk of radiation.

## Geriatrics
Treatment performed to date has not demonstrated geriatrics-specific problems that would limit the usefulness of $^{131}$I-mIBG in the elderly.

## Drug interactions and/or related problems
The following drug interactions and/or related problems have been selected on the basis of their potential clinical significance (possible mechanism in parentheses where appropriate)—not necessarily inclusive (» = major clinical significance):

» Amphetamines or
» Antidepressants, tricyclic or
» Bretylium or
» Calcium channel blocking agents or
» Cocaine or
» Guanethidine or
» Haloperidol or
» Labetalol or
» Loxapine or
» Metaraminol or
» Phenothiazines or
» Reserpine or
» Sympathomimetics or
» Thiothixene
(these medications may interfere with the uptake of $^{131}$I-mIBG; although the ideal amount of time to stop treatment with potential interacting medicines is 1 week prior to administration of $^{131}$I-mIBG, the following withdrawal periods are usually recommended based on the individual half-life of each medication: 24 hours for bretylium, cocaine, and metaraminol; 48 hours for amphetamines, calcium channel blocking agents, guanethidine, haloperidol, loxapine, tricyclic antidepressants, phenothiazines, sympathomimetics, and thiothixene; 72 hours for labetalol and reserpine)

Blood dyscrasia–causing medications (See *Appendix II*)
(leukopenic and/or thrombocytopenic effects of $^{131}$I-mIBG may be increased with concurrent or recent therapy with these medications)

Bone marrow depressants, other (See *Appendix II*)
(concurrent use of bone marrow depressants with $^{131}$I-mIBG may increase leukopenic and/or thrombocytopenic effects)

Chemotherapy and/or
Radiation therapy
(previous chemotherapy and/or radiotherapy may impair effectiveness of $^{131}$I-mIBG therapy)

## Laboratory value alterations
The following have been selected on the basis of their potential clinical significance (possible effect in parentheses where appropriate)—not necessarily inclusive (» = major clinical significance):

With physiology/laboratory test values
Alanine aminotransferase (ALT [SGPT], serum and
Aspartate aminotransferase (AST [SGOT]), serum
(concentrations may be increased)

Catecholamines, urinary
(concentration may be increased transiently)

# Side/Adverse Effects
The following side/adverse effects have been selected on the basis of their potential clinical significance (possible signs and symptoms in parentheses where appropriate)—not necessarily inclusive:

## Those indicating need for medical attention
Incidence rare
*Leukopenia and thrombocytopenia* (pale skin, sore throat and fever, unusual bleeding or bruising, unusual tiredness or weakness)

## Those indicating need for medical attention only if they continue or are bothersome
Incidence less frequent or rare
*Flushing of skin; nausea; slight and transient increase in blood pressure*

# Patient Consultation
As an aid to patient consultation, refer to *Advice for the Patient, Iobenguane, Radioiodinated (Therapeutic)*.

In providing consultation, consider emphasizing the following selected information (» = major clinical significance):

## Description of use
Action in the body: Localization of $^{131}$I-mIBG in adrenal medulla and neuroendocrine tumors; large doses are used therapeutically to damage or destroy tissue in management of adrenal carcinoma, pheochromocytomas, and other neuroendocrine tumors

## Before using this medication
» Conditions affecting use, especially:
Pregnancy—Use not recommended because of risk to fetus from radiation exposure
Breast-feeding—Not known if distributed into breast milk; however, free radioiodide, if present, may be distributed; cessation of nursing is recommended because of risk to infant from radiation exposure
Use in children—Benefit derived from treatment should be judged to outweigh potential risk of radiation
Other medications, especially amphetamines, tricyclic antidepressants, bretylium, calcium channel blocking agents, cocaine, guanethidine, haloperidol, labetalol, loxapine, phenothiazines, reserpine, sympathomimetics, and thiothixene

## Proper use of this medication
Special preparatory instructions may apply; patient should inquire in advance

Administration of potassium iodide or Lugol's solution to block thyroid uptake of radioiodide contaminants before and for several weeks after treatment

**Side/adverse effects**
Signs of potential side effects, especially leukopenia and thrombocytopenia

## General Dosing Information

Radiopharmaceuticals are to be administered only by or under the supervision of physicians who have had extensive training in the safe use and handling of radioactive materials and who are authorized by the Nuclear Regulatory Commission (NRC) or the appropriate Federal or Agreement State agency, if required, or, outside the U.S., the appropriate authority.

To minimize uptake of radioactive iodine by the thyroid, potassium iodide (SSKI, 60 mg twice a day) or Lugol's solution (1 drop three times a day) may be used, beginning at least 24 hours before and continuing for at least 4 weeks after therapy with $^{131}$I-mIBG.

When $^{131}$I-mIBG is used for the treatment of pheochromocytoma, concurrent use of an alpha-adrenergic blocking agent, such as phenoxybenzamine is recommended to control episodes of hypertension.

Following administration of $^{131}$I-mIBG the patient should be observed for possible reactions; competent personnel and emergency facilities should be available during this period.

**Safety considerations for handling this radiopharmaceutical**
Improper handling of this radiopharmaceutical may cause radioactive contamination. Guidelines for handling radioactive material have been prepared by scientific, professional, state, federal, and international bodies and are available to the specially qualified and authorized users who have access to radiopharmaceuticals.

## Parenteral Dosage Forms

Note: Because I 131 iobenguane ($^{131}$I-mIBG) sulfate injection is not commercially available in the U.S. or Canada, the bracketed information and the use of the superscript 1 in the *Dosage Forms* section reflect the lack of labeled (approved) indications for this product.

### I 131 IOBENGUANE SULFATE INJECTION

**Usual adult administered activity**
[Treatment of malignant pheochromocytoma][1]—
A safe and effective dosage has not been established. However, dosages in the range of 2.9 to 9.25 gigabecquerels (80 to 250 millicuries) of $^{131}$I-mIBG, with a specific activity of 103.6 to 199 megabecquerels (2.8 to 5.38 millicuries) per mg (at time of calibration), administered by slow intravenous infusion over a 20- to 30-second period every three to six months, have been used.

**Usual pediatric administered activity**
[Treatment of neuroblastoma][1]—
A safe and effective dosage has not been established for children up to 18 years of age. However, dosages in the range of 2.6 to 6.8 gigabecquerels (70 to 184 millicuries), administered in two fractions by slow (four to eight hours) intravenous infusion at two- to four-day intervals have been used.

Note: Dosages ranging from 1.3 to 8 gigabecquerels (35 to 215 millicuries) have also been used.

**Usual geriatric administered activity**
See *Usual adult administered activity*.

**Strength(s) usually available**
U.S.—
Not commercially available for therapeutic use. In most cases, may be obtained from the University of Michigan Nuclear Pharmacy (UMNP) by physicians who have filed their own Investigational New Drug Application (IND).
Canada—
Not commercially available. In most cases, may be obtained by physicians who have filed their own IND.

**Packaging and storage**
Store between 2 and 8 °C (35.6 and 46.4 °F), but preferably between −20 and −10 °C (−4 and −14 °F), unless otherwise specified by manufacturer.

**Note**
Caution—Radioactive material.

[1]Not included in Canadian product labeling.

## Selected Bibliography
McEwan AJ, Shapiro B, Sisson JC, et al. Radio-iodobenzylguanidine for the scintigraphic location and therapy of adrenergic tumors. Semin Nucl Med 1985; 15(2): 132-53.

Revised: 05/05/93
Interim revision: 08/02/94

---

**IOCETAMIC ACID**—See *Cholecystographic Agents, Oral (Systemic)*

---

**IODINATED I 125 ALBUMIN**—See *Radioiodinated Albumin (Systemic)*

---

**IODINATED I 131 ALBUMIN**—See *Radioiodinated Albumin (Systemic)*

---

**IODINE**—The *Iodine (Topical)* monograph is not included in this published version of the USP DI database. Copies of the monograph are available on request from Micromedex, Inc. - Reprint Requests, 6200 S. Syracuse Way, Suite 300, Englewood, CO 80111; telephone (303) 486-6400; telefax (303) 486-6464; Email: USPDI@MDX.COM.

---

# IODINE, STRONG   Systemic

VA CLASSIFICATION (Primary/Secondary): HS852/AD900; TN499
Another commonly used name is Lugol's solution.
Note: For a listing of dosage forms and brand names by country availability, see *Dosage Forms* section(s).

## Category
Antihyperthyroid agent; radiation protectant (thyroid gland); iodine replenisher.

## Indications
Note: Bracketed information in the *Indications* section refers to uses that are not included in U.S. product labeling.

**Accepted**
[Hyperthyroidism (treatment adjunct)][1]—Strong iodine is used as an adjunct in the treatment of hyperthyroidism.

[Radiation protection, thyroid gland][1]—Strong iodine is used as a radiation protectant (thyroid gland) prior to and following administration of radioactive isotopes of iodine or in radiation emergencies.

[Thyroid involution, preoperative (treatment adjunct)][1]—Strong iodine is used concurrently with an antithyroid agent to induce thyroid involution prior to thyroidectomy.

[Thyrotoxic crisis (treatment adjunct)][1]—Strong iodine is used as an adjunct in the treatment of thyrotoxic crisis.

[Iodine deficiency (treatment)]—Strong iodine is used in the treatment of iodine deficiency

[1]Not included in Canadian product labeling.

## Pharmacology/Pharmacokinetics

**Physicochemical characteristics**
Molecular weight—
Iodine: 126.90.
Potassium iodide: 166.00.

### Mechanism of action/Effect
Antihyperthyroid agent—In hyperthyroid patients, strong iodine produces rapid remission of symptoms by inhibiting the release of thyroid hormone into the circulation. The effects of strong iodine on the thyroid gland include reduction of vascularity, a firming of the glandular tissue, shrinkage of the size of individual cells, reaccumulation of colloid in the follicles, and increases in bound iodine. These actions may facilitate thyroidectomy when the medication is given prior to surgery.

Radiation protectant—Prior to and following administration of radioactive isotopes and in radiation emergencies, strong iodine protects the thyroid gland by blocking the thyroidal uptake of radioactive isotopes of iodine.

## Precautions to Consider

### Pregnancy/Reproduction
Iodides cross the placenta; use during pregnancy may result in abnormal thyroid function and/or goiter in the infant.

### Breast-feeding
Iodides are distributed into breast milk; use by nursing mothers may cause skin rash and thyroid suppression in the infant.

### Pediatrics
Iodides may cause skin rash and thyroid suppression in infants.

### Geriatrics
Appropriate studies on the relationship of age to the effects of strong iodine have not been performed in the geriatric population. However, geriatrics-specific problems that would limit the usefulness of this medication in the elderly are not expected.

### Dental
Strong iodine may cause salivary swelling or tenderness, burning of mouth or throat, metallic taste, soreness of teeth and gums, and unusual increase in salivation.

### Drug interactions and/or related problems
The following drug interactions and/or related problems have been selected on the basis of their potential clinical significance (possible mechanism in parentheses where appropriate)—not necessarily inclusive (» = major clinical significance):

Note: Combinations containing any of the following medications, depending on the amount present, may also interact with this medication.

» Antithyroid agents
(concurrent use of these medications with strong iodine may potentiate the hypothyroid and goitrogenic effects of antithyroid agents or strong iodine; baseline thyroid status should be determined at periodic intervals to detect changes in the thyroid-pituitary response)

Captopril or
Enalapril or
Lisinopril
(concurrent use of captopril, enalapril, or lisinopril with strong iodine may result in hyperkalemia; serum potassium concentrations should be monitored)

» Diuretics, potassium-sparing
(concurrent use with strong iodine may increase the effects of potassium, possibly resulting in hyperkalemia and cardiac arrhythmias or cardiac arrest; serum potassium concentrations should be monitored)

» Lithium
(concurrent use with strong iodine may potentiate the hypothyroid and goitrogenic effects of either medication; baseline thyroid status should be determined at periodic intervals to detect changes in the thyroid-pituitary response)

Sodium iodide I 131, therapeutic
(strong iodine solution may decrease thyroidal uptake of I 131)

### Laboratory value alterations
The following have been selected on the basis of their potential clinical significance (possible effect in parentheses where appropriate)—not necessarily inclusive (» = major clinical significance):

With diagnostic test results
Thyroid function studies and
Thyroid imaging, radionuclide and
Thyroid uptake tests
(strong iodine solution may decrease thyroidal uptake of I 131, I 123 and sodium pertechnetate Tc 99m)

### Medical considerations/Contraindications
The medical considerations/contraindications included have been selected on the basis of their potential clinical significance (reasons given in parentheses where appropriate)—not necessarily inclusive (» = major clinical significance).

*Risk benefit should be considered when the following medical problems exist:*
» Bronchitis, acute or
» Edema, pulmonary or
Tuberculosis, pulmonary
(may cause irritation and increase secretions)
» Hyperkalemia
(condition may be exacerbated)
Hyperthyroidism—for use other than thyroid inhibitor
(prolonged use of iodine may cause thyroid gland hyperplasia, thyroid adenoma, goiter, or hypothyroidism)
» Renal function impairment
(may cause excessive serum potassium concentrations)
Sensitivity to iodine or potassium iodide

### Patient monitoring
The following may be especially important in patient monitoring (other tests may be warranted in some patients, depending on condition; » = major clinical significance):

Potassium, serum, concentrations
(determinations recommended at periodic intervals during therapy in patients with renal function impairment)

## Side/Adverse Effects
The following side/adverse effects have been selected on the basis of their potential clinical significance (possible signs and symptoms in parentheses where appropriate)—not necessarily inclusive:

### Those indicating need for medical attention
Incidence less frequent
*Allergic reactions, specifically angioedema* (swelling of the arms, face, legs, lips, tongue, and/or throat); *arthralgia* (joint pain); *eosinophilia; swelling of lymph nodes; urticaria* (hives)

With prolonged use
*Iodism* (burning of mouth or throat; gastric irritation; increased watering of mouth; metallic taste; severe headache; soreness of teeth and gums; symptoms of head cold); *potassium toxicity* (confusion; irregular heartbeat; numbness, tingling, pain, or weakness in hands or feet; unusual tiredness; weakness or heaviness of legs)

### Those indicating need for medical attention only if they continue or are bothersome
Incidence less frequent
*Diarrhea; nausea or vomiting; stomach pain*

## Patient Consultation
As an aid to patient consultation, refer to *Advice for the Patient, Strong Iodine (Systemic)*

In providing consultation, consider emphasizing the following selected information (» = major clinical significance):

### Before using this medication
» Conditions affecting use, especially:
Sensitivity to iodine or potassium iodide
Pregnancy—May cause thyroid problems or goiter in the newborn infant
Breast-feeding—May cause skin rash and thyroid problems in nursing babies
Use in children—May cause skin rash and thyroid problems in infants
Other medications, especially antithyroid agents, potassium-sparing diuretics, or lithium
Other medical problems, especially bronchitis, hyperkalemia, or renal function impairment

### Proper use of this medication
» Taking after meals or with food or milk to minimize gastrointestinal irritation
Proper administration technique for oral liquids
» Taking medication by mouth even if dispensed in a dropper bottle
Not using if solution turns brownish yellow
Taking medication in a full glass (240 mL) of water or in fruit juice, milk, or broth to improve taste and lessen gastric upset; drinking full dose
If crystals form in solution, warming closed container in warm water and gently shaking container
» Proper dosing
Missed dose: Taking as soon as possible; not taking if almost time for next dose; not doubling doses

» Proper storage

*For use as a radiation protectant (thyroid gland)*
   Taking medication only upon instructions from state or local health authorities
» Taking medication daily for 10 days, unless otherwise instructed; not taking more medication or more often than instructed

**Precautions while using this medication**
Regular visits to physician to check progress during therapy
» Caution in patients on potassium-restricted diet

**Side/adverse effects**
» Signs of potential side effects, especially allergic reactions, iodism, or potassium toxicity

## General Dosing Information

The potassium content is 0.6 mEq (23.4 mg) per mL of strong iodine.

To protect against possible gastrointestinal injury, which has been associated with the oral ingestion of concentrated potassium salt preparations, and to improve the taste, it is recommended that the oral solution be administered in a full glass (240 mL) of water or in fruit juice, milk, or broth.

## Oral Dosage Forms

Note: Bracketed uses in the *Dosage Forms* section refer to categories of use and/or indications that are not included in U.S. product labeling.

### STRONG IODINE SOLUTION USP

**Usual adult and adolescent dose**
[Antihyperthyroid agent][1]—
   Oral, 1 mL three times a day, the first dose being given at least one hour after the initial dose of antithyroid agent.
[Thyroid involution, preoperative][1]—
   Prior to thyroidectomy: Oral, 3 to 5 drops (approximately 0.1 to 0.3 mL) three times a day for ten days before surgery, usually administered concurrently with an antithyroid agent.
[Radiation protectant (thyroid gland)][1]—
   Oral, 130 mg a day for ten days.
[Iodine replenisher]—
   Oral, 0.3 to 1 mL three or four times a day.

**Usual pediatric dose**
[Thyroid involution, preoperative][1]—
   See *Usual adult and adolescent dose*.
[Radiation protectant (thyroid gland)][1]—
   Oral, 65 mg per day for ten days.

**Strength(s) usually available**
U.S.—
   50 mg of iodine and 100 mg of potassium iodide per mL (Rx) [GENERIC].
Canada—
   50 mg of iodine and 100 mg of potassium iodide per mL (OTC) [GENERIC].

**Packaging and storage**
Store below 40 °C (104 °F), preferably between 15 and 30 °C (59 and 86 °F), unless otherwise specified by manufacturer. Store in a tight container. Protect from freezing.

**Stability**
Crystallization may occur under normal conditions of storage, especially if refrigerated; however, on warming and shaking, the crystals will redissolve.
Free iodine may be liberated by oxidation of the strong iodine, causing the solution to turn brownish yellow in color. If this occurs, the solution should be discarded.

**Auxiliary labeling**
• For oral use only.

[1] Not included in Canadian product labeling.

Revised: 04/15/92
Interim revision: 08/10/94

---

**IODIPAMIDE**—The *Iodipamide (Systemic)* monograph is not included in this published version of the USP DI database. Copies of the monograph are available on request from Micromedex, Inc. - Reprint Requests, 6200 S. Syracuse Way, Suite 300, Englewood, CO 80111; telephone (303) 486-6400; telefax (303) 486-6464; Email: USPDI@MDX.COM.

---

**IODIXANOL**—The *Iodixanol (Systemic)—Introductory Version* monograph is not included in this published version of the USP DI database. Copies of the monograph are available on request from Micromedex, Inc. - Reprint Requests, 6200 S. Syracuse Way, Suite 300, Englewood, CO 80111; telephone (303) 486-6400; telefax (303) 486-6464; Email: USPDI@MDX.COM.

---

# IODOHIPPURATE SODIUM I 123   Systemic*

VA CLASSIFICATION (Primary): DX201
Commonly used brand name(s): *Nephropure*.
Note: For a listing of dosage forms and brand names by country availability, see *Dosage Forms* section(s).

*Not commercially available in U.S.

## Category

Diagnostic aid, radioactive (renal disorders; urinary tract obstructions).

## Indications

**Accepted**

Renography—Iodohippurate sodium I 123 is indicated in renography to determine renal function, effective renal blood flow, and urinary tract obstruction.

Renal imaging, radionuclide—Iodohippurate sodium I 123 is indicated as a renal imaging agent to assess renal size, position, configuration, and function.

## Physical Properties

**Nuclear data**

| Radionuclide (half-life) | Mode of decay | Principal photon emissions (keV) | Mean number of emissions/disintegration |
|---|---|---|---|
| I 123 (13.2 hr) | Electron capture | Gamma (159) | 0.83 |

## Pharmacology/Pharmacokinetics

**Mechanism of action/Effect**
Based on its elimination by both tubular secretion and glomerular filtration, which can be monitored or observed by appropriate imaging or detection equipment.

**Half-life**
For iodohippurate sodium (biological)—Approximately 20 to 30 minutes.

**Time to peak concentration**
Kidneys—Approximately 3 to 6 minutes.

## Iodohippurate Sodium I 123 (Systemic)

**Radiation dosimetry**

| Organ | Estimated absorbed radiation dose*† | | | |
|---|---|---|---|---|
| | With normal kidney function | | With impaired kidney function | |
| | mGy/MBq | rad/mCi | mGy/MBq | rad/mCi |
| Bladder wall | 0.20 | 0.74 | 0.11 | 0.41 |
| Uterus | 0.17 | 0.63 | 0.013 | 0.048 |
| Large intestine (lower) | 0.0075 | 0.028 | 0.0078 | 0.029 |
| Ovaries | 0.0073 | 0.027 | 0.0079 | 0.029 |
| Kidneys | 0.0064 | 0.024 | 0.027 | 0.099 |
| Testes | 0.0046 | 0.017 | 0.0053 | 0.020 |
| Small intestine | 0.0032 | 0.012 | 0.0060 | 0.022 |
| Large intestine (upper) | 0.0025 | 0.0093 | 0.0056 | 0.021 |
| Red marrow | 0.0025 | 0.0093 | 0.0064 | 0.024 |
| Bone surfaces | 0.0013 | 0.0048 | 0.0051 | 0.019 |
| Adrenals | 0.00092 | 0.0034 | 0.0053 | 0.020 |
| Pancreas | 0.00089 | 0.0033 | 0.0051 | 0.019 |
| Spleen | 0.00082 | 0.0030 | 0.0049 | 0.018 |
| Stomach wall | 0.00079 | 0.0029 | 0.0044 | 0.016 |
| Liver | 0.00072 | 0.0027 | 0.0059 | 0.022 |
| Lungs | 0.00048 | 0.0018 | 0.0038 | 0.014 |
| Breast | 0.00044 | 0.0016 | 0.0034 | 0.013 |
| Thyroid | 0.00037 | 0.0014 | 0.0030 | 0.011 |
| Other tissue | 0.0022 | 0.0081 | 0.0045 | 0.017 |
| Effective dose | 0.015 mSv/MBq | 0.056 rem/mCi | 0.013 mSv/MBq | 0.048 rem/mCi |

*For adults; intravenous administration.
†Data based on the International Commission on Radiological Protection (ICRP) Publication 53—Radiation Dose to Patients from Radiopharmaceuticals.

**Elimination**
Renal, 50 to 75% within 25 minutes; 90 to 95% within 8 hours; primarily by tubular cell secretion, but also by glomerular filtration.
Iodide I 123 is excreted in breast milk, also.

## Precautions to Consider

**Carcinogenicity/Mutagenicity**
Long-term animal studies to evaluate carcinogenic or mutagenic potential of iodohippurate sodium I 123 have not been performed.

**Pregnancy/Reproduction**
Pregnancy—Studies have not been done in humans. Other radioiodines (e.g., iodide I 131) cross the placenta and may cause severe and irreversible hypothyroidism in the newborn and are not recommended for use during pregnancy.
The possibility of pregnancy should be assessed in women of child-bearing potential. Clinical situations exist where the benefit to the patient and fetus, based on information derived from radiopharmaceutical use, outweighs the risks from fetal exposure to radiation. In these situations, the physician should use discretion and reduce the radiopharmaceutical dose to the lowest possible amount.
Studies have not been done in animals.
FDA Pregnancy Category C.

**Breast-feeding**
Iodide I 123 is excreted in breast milk. Because of the potential risk to the infant from radiation exposure, temporary discontinuation of nursing is recommended for approximately 3 days.

**Pediatrics**
Although iodohippurate sodium I 123 is used in children, there have been no specific studies evaluating its safety and efficacy in pediatric patients. When this radiopharmaceutical is used in children, the diagnostic benefit should be judged to outweigh the potential risk of radiation.

**Geriatrics**
Appropriate studies on the relationship of age to the effects of iodohippurate sodium I 123 have not been performed in the geriatric population. However, no geriatrics-specific problems have been documented to date.

**Drug interactions and/or related problems**
See *Diagnostic interference*.

**Diagnostic interference**
The following have been selected on the basis of their potential clinical significance (possible effect in parentheses where appropriate)—not necessarily inclusive (» = major clinical significance):

With results of *this* test
  Due to other medications
    Probenecid
      (concurrent use may decrease kidney uptake of iodohippurate sodium I 123 due to a direct inhibition of the enzyme transport system in the proximal tubule by probenecid)
  Due to medical problems or conditions
    Dehydration
      (may prolong renal transit time of iodohippurate sodium I 123, thus increasing the time required to reach peak radioactivity level in kidney)
  Due to other diagnostic tests
    Retrograde pyelogram
      (may alter renogram curve; renogram should be performed before or at least 24 hours after this procedure)
With *other* diagnostic test results
  Thyroid function determinations and
  Thyroid imaging
    (Lugol's solution used prior to the administration of iodohippurate sodium I 123 may cause a decrease in radioactive iodine or pertechnetate ion uptake for several weeks)

**Medical considerations/Contraindications**
The medical considerations/contraindications included have been selected on the basis of their potential clinical significance (reasons given in parentheses where appropriate)—not necessarily inclusive (» = major clinical significance).
See also *Diagnostic interference*.

*Risk-benefit should be considered when the following medical problem exists:*
  Sensitivity to the radiopharmaceutical preparation

## Side/Adverse Effects

The following side/adverse effects have been selected on the basis of their potential clinical significance (possible signs and symptoms in parentheses where appropriate)—not necessarily inclusive:

**Those indicating need for medical attention**
Incidence rare
  *Allergic reaction* (skin rash, hives, or itching); *fainting; nausea or vomiting*

## Patient Consultation

As an aid to patient consultation, refer to *Advice for the Patient, Radiopharmaceuticals (Diagnostic)*.
In providing consultation, consider emphasizing the following selected information (» = major clinical significance):

**Description of use**
  Action in the body: Elimination by tubular cell secretion and glomerular filtration
  Appearance, concentration, and elimination of iodohippurate sodium I 123 in kidneys allows monitoring and visualization
  Small amounts of radioactivity used in diagnosis; radiation received is low and considered safe

**Before having this test**
» Conditions affecting use, especially:
    Sensitivity to the radiopharmaceutical preparation
    Pregnancy—Risk to fetus from radiation exposure as opposed to benefit derived from use should be considered; possibility of hypothyroidism in newborn
    Breast-feeding—Iodide I 123 excreted in breast milk; temporary discontinuation of nursing recommended because of risk to infant from radiation exposure
    Use in children—Risk from radiation exposure as opposed to benefit derived from use should be considered

**Preparation for this test**
  Special preparatory instructions may apply; patient should inquire in advance

**Precautions after having this test**
  Possible interference with future thyroid tests

**Side/adverse effects**
  Signs of potential side effects, especially allergic reaction, fainting, nausea or vomiting

## General Dosing Information

Radiopharmaceuticals are to be administered only by or under the supervision of physicians who have had extensive training in the safe use and handling of radioactive materials and who are authorized by the appropriate Federal or state agency, if required, or, outside the U.S., the appropriate authority.

To help minimize thyroidal uptake of free iodide I 123, a thyroid blocking agent such as a saturated solution of potassium iodide or potassium perchlorate should be given prior to administration of iodohippurate sodium I 123 and for several days afterwards.

To assure adequate urine flow, increased oral intake of fluids is recommended 1 hour prior to the diagnostic procedure, unless contraindicated because of the presence of edema or congestive heart failure.

Manufacturer's package insert or other appropriate literature should be consulted for optimal times when imaging should be performed. In general, imaging should be performed as close to time of calibration as possible since the quality of the image will degrade with time because of the increase in the proportion of radionuclidic contaminants (primarily I 124).

### Safety considerations for handling this radiopharmaceutical
Improper handling of this radiopharmaceutical may cause radioactive contamination. Guidelines for handling radioactive material have been prepared by scientific, professional, state, federal, and international bodies and are available to the specially qualified and authorized users who have access to radiopharmaceuticals.

## Parenteral Dosage Forms

### IODOHIPPURATE SODIUM I 123 INJECTION USP

**Usual adult and adolescent administered activity**
Renography—
  Intravenous, 3.7 to 14.8 megabecquerels (100 to 400 microcuries).
Renal imaging, radionuclide—
  Intravenous, 37 megabecquerels (1 millicurie).

**Usual pediatric administered activity**
Dosage must be individualized by physician.

**Usual geriatric administered activity**
See *Usual adult and adolescent administered activity*.

**Strength(s) usually available**
U.S.—
  Not commercially available.
Canada—
  37 megabecquerels (1 millicurie) of iodohippurate sodium I 123, at time of calibration, per vial (Rx) [*Nephropure*].
  74 megabecquerels (2 millicuries) of iodohippurate sodium I 123, at time of calibration, per vial (Rx) [*Nephropure*].

**Packaging and storage**
Store below 40 °C (104 °F), preferably between 15 and 30 °C (59 and 86 °F), unless otherwise specified by manufacturer. Protect from freezing.

**Note**
Caution—Radioactive material.

### Selected Bibliography
Eshima D, Fritzber AR, Taylor A Jr. Tc 99m renal tubular function agents: current status. Sem Nuc Med 1990; 20(1): 28-40.
Thrall JH, Koff SA, Keyes JW. Diuretic radionuclide renography and scintigraphy in the differential diagnosis of hydroureteronephrosis. Sem Nuc Med 1981; 11(2): 89-104.

Revised: 02/01/93
Interim revision: 08/02/94

---

# IODOHIPPURATE SODIUM I 131   Systemic

VA CLASSIFICATION (Primary): DX201
Commonly used brand name(s): *Hippuran*; *Hipputope*.
Note: For a listing of dosage forms and brand names by country availability, see *Dosage Forms* section(s).

## Category
Diagnostic aid, radioactive (renal disorders; urinary tract obstructions).

## Indications

**Accepted**
Renography—Iodohippurate sodium I 131 is indicated in renography to determine renal function, effective renal plasma flow, and urinary tract obstruction.
Renal imaging, radionuclide—Iodohippurate sodium I 131 is indicated as an imaging agent to assess renal size, position, configuration, and function.

## Physical Properties

**Nuclear Data**

| Radionuclide (half-life) | Mode of decay | Principal photon emissions (keV) | Mean number of emissions/ disintegration |
|---|---|---|---|
| I 131 (8.08 days) | Beta | Beta (191.6) Gamma (364.4) | 0.90 0.81 |

## Pharmacology/Pharmacokinetics

**Mechanism of action/Effect**
Based on its excretion by both tubular secretion and glomerular filtration, which can be observed by appropriate imaging or detection systems.

**Half-life**
For iodohippurate sodium (biological)—Approximately 20 to 30 minutes.

**Time to peak concentration**
Kidneys—Approximately 3 to 6 minutes.

**Radiation dosimetry**

| Organ | Estimated absorbed radiation dose*† |||||
|---|---|---|---|---|
| | With normal kidney function || With impaired kidney function ||
| | mGy/ MBq | rad/mCi | mGy/ MBq | rad/mCi |
| Bladder wall | 0.96 | 3.55 | 0.63 | 2.33 |
| Uterus | 0.35 | 1.30 | 0.039 | 0.14 |
| Kidneys | 0.30 | 1.11 | 0.15 | 0.56 |
| Large intestine (lower) | 0.17 | 0.63 | 0.027 | 0.099 |
| Ovaries | 0.17 | 0.63 | 0.026 | 0.096 |
| Testes | 0.12 | 0.44 | 0.022 | 0.081 |
| Small intestine | 0.0078 | 0.029 | 0.022 | 0.081 |
| Large intestine (upper) | 0.0069 | 0.026 | 0.021 | 0.078 |
| Red marrow | 0.0049 | 0.018 | 0.019 | 0.070 |
| Bone surfaces | 0.0030 | 0.011 | 0.017 | 0.063 |
| Adrenals | 0.0028 | 0.010 | 0.021 | 0.081 |
| Pancreas | 0.0026 | 0.0096 | 0.019 | 0.070 |
| Spleen | 0.0024 | 0.0089 | 0.019 | 0.070 |
| Stomach wall | 0.0025 | 0.0093 | 0.018 | 0.067 |
| Liver | 0.0023 | 0.0085 | 0.025 | 0.093 |
| Lungs | 0.0016 | 0.0059 | 0.015 | 0.056 |
| Thyroid | 0.0014 | 0.0052 | 0.014 | 0.052 |
| Other tissue | 0.0054 | 0.020 | 0.018 | 0.067 |
| Effective dose | 0.066 mSv/MBq | 0.24 rem/mCi | 0.065 mSv/MBq | 0.24 rem/mCi |

*For adults; intravenous administration.
†Data based on the International Commission on Radiological Protection (ICRP) Publication 53—Radiation dose to patients from radiopharmaceuticals.

**Elimination**
Renal, 50 to 75% within 25 minutes and 90 to 95% within 8 hours (primarily by tubular cell secretion [80%], but also by glomerular filtration [20%]). Iodide I 131 is eliminated in breast milk, also.

## Precautions to Consider

**Pregnancy/Reproduction**
Pregnancy—Studies have not been done in humans with iodohippurate sodium I 131. However, iodide I 131 crosses the placenta and may cause

severe and irreversible hypothyroidism in the newborn. Iodohippurate sodium I 131 is not recommended for use during pregnancy.

The possibility of pregnancy should be assessed in women of child-bearing potential. Clinical situations exist where the benefit to the patient and fetus, based on information derived from radiopharmaceutical use, outweighs the risks from fetal exposure to radiation. In these situations, the physician should use discretion and reduce the radiopharmaceutical dose to the lowest possible amount.

Studies have not been done in animals.

FDA Pregnancy Category C.

**Breast-feeding**
Iodide I 131 is excreted in breast milk. Because of the potential risk to the infant from radiation exposure, temporary discontinuation of nursing is recommended for approximately 5 days.

**Pediatrics**
Although iodohippurate sodium I 131 is used in children, there have been no specific studies evaluating its safety and efficacy in children. When this radiopharmaceutical is used in children, the diagnostic benefit should be judged to outweigh the potential risk of radiation.

**Geriatrics**
Appropriate studies on the relationship of age to the effects of iodohippurate sodium I 131 have not been performed in the geriatric population. However, no geriatrics-specific problems have been documented to date.

**Drug interactions and/or related problems**
See *Diagnostic interference*.

**Diagnostic interference**
The following have been selected on the basis of their potential clinical significance (possible effect in parentheses where appropriate)—not necessarily inclusive (» = major clinical significance):

With results of *this* test
*Due to other medications*
Probenecid
(concurrent use may decrease kidney uptake of iodohippurate sodium I 131 due to a direct inhibition of the enzyme transport system in the proximal tubule by probenecid)
*Due to medical problems or conditions*
Dehydration
(kidney uptake of iodohippurate sodium I 131 may be reduced and renal transit time may be prolonged)
*Due to other diagnostic tests*
Retrograde pyelogram
(may alter renogram curve; renogram should be performed before or at least 24 hours after this procedure)
With *other* diagnostic test results
Thyroid function determinations and
Thyroid imaging
(Lugol's solution used prior to the administration of iodohippurate sodium I 131 may cause a decrease in radioactive iodine or pertechnetate ion uptake for several weeks)

**Medical considerations/Contraindications**
The medical considerations/contraindications included have been selected on the basis of their potential clinical significance (reasons given in parentheses where appropriate)—not necessarily inclusive (» = major clinical significance).
See also *Diagnostic interference*.

***Risk-benefit should be considered when the following medical problem exists:***
Sensitivity to the radiopharmaceutical preparation

## Side/Adverse Effects

The following side/adverse effects have been selected on the basis of their potential clinical significance (possible signs and symptoms in parentheses where appropriate)—not necessarily inclusive:

**Those indicating need for medical attention**
Incidence rare—not clearly related to iodohippurate sodium I 131
*Fainting; nausea or vomiting*

## Patient Consultation

As an aid to patient consultation, refer to *Advice for the Patient, Radiopharmaceuticals (Diagnostic)*.
In providing consultation, consider emphasizing the following selected information (» = major clinical significance):

**Description of use**
Action in the body: Elimination by tubular cell secretion and glomerular filtration

Appearance, concentration, and elimination of iodohippurate sodium I 131 in kidneys allows monitoring and visualization
Small amounts of radioactivity used in diagnosis; radiation received is low and considered safe

**Before having this test**
» Conditions affecting use, especially:
Sensitivity to the radiopharmaceutical preparation
Pregnancy—Risk to fetus from radiation exposure as opposed to benefit derived from use should be considered; possibility of hypothyroidism in newborn
Breast-feeding—Iodide I 131 excreted in breast milk; temporary discontinuation of nursing recommended because of risk to infant from radiation exposure
Use in children—Risk from radiation exposure as opposed to benefit derived from use should be considered

**Preparation for this test**
Special preparatory instructions may apply; patient should inquire in advance

**Precautions after having this test**
Possible interference with future thyroid tests

**Side/adverse effects**
Signs of potential side effects, especially fainting, nausea, or vomiting

## General Dosing Information

Radiopharmaceuticals are to be administered only by or under the supervision of physicians who have had extensive training in the safe use and handling of radioactive materials and who are authorized by the Nuclear Regulatory Commission (NRC) or the appropriate Agreement State agency, if required, or, outside the U.S., the appropriate authority.

Approximately 25% of the free iodide content of iodohippurate sodium I 131 is taken up by the thyroid gland following intravenous administration. To help minimize thyroidal uptake of free iodide I 131, a thyroid blocking agent such as a saturated solution of potassium iodide or potassium perchlorate should be given prior to administration of iodohippurate sodium I 131 and for several days afterwards.

To assure adequate urine flow, increased oral intake of fluids is recommended 1 hour prior to the diagnostic procedure, unless contraindicated because of the presence of edema or congestive heart failure.

Iodohippurate Sodium I 131 Injection USP is not intended for intra-arterial use. Also, precautions should be taken to avoid extravasation during intravenous administration.

**Safety considerations for handling this radiopharmaceutical**
Improper handling of this radiopharmaceutical may cause radioactive contamination. Guidelines for handling radioactive material have been prepared by scientific, professional, state, federal, and international bodies and are available to the specially qualified and authorized users who have access to radiopharmaceuticals.

## Parenteral Dosage Forms

### IODOHIPPURATE SODIUM I 131 INJECTION USP

**Usual adult and adolescent administered activity**
Renography—
Intravenous, 0.0185 megabecquerel (0.5 microcurie) per kg of body weight.
Renal imaging, radionuclide—
Intravenous, 0.1 to 0.185 megabecquerel (3 to 5 microcuries) per kg of body weight.

**Usual pediatric administered activity**
Dosage must be individualized by physician.

**Usual geriatric administered activity**
See *Usual adult and adolescent administered activity*.

**Strength(s) usually available**
U.S.—
At time of calibration: Per multiple-dose vial—
37 megabecquerels (1 millicurie) (Rx) [*Hippuran; Hipputope;* GENERIC].
74 megabecquerels (2 millicuries) (Rx) [*Hipputope;* GENERIC].
Canada—
Various concentrations as per manufacturer's labeling (Rx) [GENERIC].

**Packaging and storage**
Store below 40 °C (104 °F), preferably between 15 and 30 °C (59 and 86 °F), unless otherwise specified by manufacturer. Protect from freezing.

**Note**
Caution—Radioactive material.

## Selected Bibliography

Eshima D, Fritzber AR, Taylor A Jr. Tc 99m renal tubular function agents: current status. Semin Nucl Med 1990; 20(1): 28-40.

Thrall JH, Koff SA, Keyes JW. Diuretic radionuclide renography and scintigraphy in the differential diagnosis of hydroureteronephrosis. Semin Nucl Med 1981; 11(2): 89-104.

Revised: 02/01/93
Interim revision: 08/02/94

**IODOQUINOL** — The *Iodoquinol (Oral-Local)* monograph is not included in this published version of the USP DI database. Copies of the monograph are available on request from Micromedex, Inc. - Reprint Requests, 6200 S. Syracuse Way, Suite 300, Englewood, CO 80111; telephone (303) 486-6400; telefax (303) 486-6464; Email: USPDI@MDX.COM.

# IOFETAMINE I 123    Systemic

VA CLASSIFICATION (Primary): DX201

Commonly used brand name(s): *Spectamine*.

Note: For a listing of dosage forms and brand names by country availability, see *Dosage Forms* section(s).

## Category

Diagnostic aid, radioactive (cerebrovascular disease).

## Indications

Note: Bracketed information in the *Indications* section refers to uses that are not included in U.S. product labeling.

### Accepted

Brain imaging, radionuclide—Iofetamine hydrochloride I 123 is indicated as a brain imaging agent in the localization and evaluation of nonlacunar stroke. It should be used within 96 hours of onset of focal neurological deficit.

[Seizures (diagnosis)][1]—Iofetamine hydrochloride I 123 is used in patients with partial complex seizures to establish the site of epileptogenic focus, which aids in the diagnosis and treatment of epilepsy.

[Dementia, Alzheimer-type (diagnosis)][1]—Iofetamine hydrochloride I 123 is used to study changes in regional cerebral blood flow in patients with senile dementia, which aids in the early diagnosis and classification of patients with senile dementia of the Alzheimer's type.

[1]Not included in Canadian product labeling.

## Physical Properties

### Nuclear Data

| Radionuclide (half-life) | Decay constant | Mode of decay | Principal emissions (keV) | Mean number of emissions/ disintegration |
|---|---|---|---|---|
| I 123 (13.2 h) | 0.0533 h$^{-1}$ | Electron capture | 159 | 0.83 |

## Pharmacology/Pharmacokinetics

### Physicochemical characteristics
Molecular weight—335.74.

### Mechanism of action/Effect
Iofetamine I 123, due to its high lipid solubility, passes through the blood-brain barrier and is distributed within the brain as a function of relative cerebral perfusion. Although the mechanism by which it localizes in the brain is not fully understood, it is assumed that much of its retention within the brain is probably due to binding by relatively nonspecific, high-capacity binding sites.

### Distribution
Rapidly distributed from the blood into body tissues. After 6 to 10 minutes, concentration in blood falls to about 3 to 8.5% of the administered dose; after 20 minutes, concentration falls to about 2.5%. Most of the injected dose is sequestered in the lung, from which it is rapidly released. Brain uptake increases progressively for 30 minutes and remains stable after that until 60 minutes after administration. During this phase, the lungs act as a reservoir to supply additional activity as it is lost from the brain. The ratio of concentration in gray to white matter varies with time, being 2.4 at 15 minutes, 2.2 at 1 hour, 1.8 at 4 hours, and 0.6 at 24 hours. The percentages remaining in the brain, liver, and lungs, respectively, at 1, 5, and 22 hours post-injection are: 5.7, 4.1, 2.1; 12.5, 14.1, 5.5; and 16.8, 10.6, 6.1.

### Protein binding
Low (<10%).

### Biotransformation
First-pass extraction primarily by the brain and liver. The two major metabolites are p-iodoamphetamine and p-iodobenzoic acid; p-iodoamphetamine is further metabolized to p-iodobenzoic acid.

### Half-life
Elimination—1.6±1.2 hours and 10.9±6.1 hours.

### Time to radioactivity visualization
10 minutes to 5 hours after administration of iofetamine I 123. However, since cerebral distribution of iofetamine I 123 changes over time, regional perfusion studies should be performed within 30 minutes after injection.

### Radiation dosimetry

| Organ | Estimated absorbed radiation dose* | |
|---|---|---|
|  | mGy/MBq | rad/mCi |
| Lungs | 0.12 | 0.44 |
| Liver | 0.11 | 0.41 |
| Bladder wall | 0.029 | 0.11 |
| Brain | 0.029 | 0.11 |
| Adrenals | 0.017 | 0.063 |
| Pancreas | 0.017 | 0.063 |
| Red marrow | 0.014 | 0.052 |
| Kidneys | 0.014 | 0.052 |
| Breast | 0.012 | 0.044 |
| Stomach wall | 0.012 | 0.044 |
| Bone surfaces | 0.011 | 0.041 |
| Spleen | 0.011 | 0.041 |
| Large intestine (upper) | 0.010 | 0.037 |
| Small intestine | 0.0087 | 0.032 |
| Uterus | 0.0082 | 0.030 |
| Ovaries | 0.0068 | 0.025 |
| Large intestine (lower) | 0.0064 | 0.024 |
| Thyroid | 0.0059 | 0.022 |
| Testes | 0.0045 | 0.017 |
| Other tissue | 0.0089 | 0.033 |

Effective dose: 0.032 mSv/MBq (0.12 rem/mCi)[†]

*For adults; intravenous injection.
[†]Effective dose of I 124 and I 125 impurities is 0.56 mSv/MBq (2.07 rem/mCi) and 0.094 mSv/MBq (0.027 rem/mCi), respectively.

### Elimination
Renal, as p-iodohippuric acid—About 20% of dose eliminated after 1 day; about 40% after 2 days; and about 48% after 3 days.

## Precautions to Consider

### Cross-sensitivity and/or related problems
Patients sensitive to sympathomimetics (for example, albuterol, amphetamines, ephedrine, epinephrine, isoproterenol, metaproterenol, norepinephrine, phenylephrine, phenylpropanolamine, terbutaline) may be sensitive to this imaging agent also because of iofetamine's amphetamine-like structure.

### Carcinogenicity/Mutagenicity
Long-term animal studies to evaluate carcinogenic or mutagenic potential of iofetamine I 123 have not been performed.

### Pregnancy/Reproduction
Pregnancy—Well-controlled studies have not been done in humans with iofetamine I 123. However, risk-benefit must be considered since other radioiodines (e.g., iodide I 131) cross the placenta and have caused severe and irreversible hypothyroidism in the fetus.

The possibility of pregnancy should be assessed in women of child-bearing potential. Clinical situations exist where the benefit to the patient and fetus from information derived from radiopharmaceutical use outweighs the risks from fetal exposure to radiation. In this situation, the physician should use discretion and reduce the radiopharmaceutical dose to the lowest possible amount.

Studies have not been done in animals.

FDA Pregnancy Category C.

**Breast-feeding**
Although it is currently unknown whether I 123 will appear in breast milk following intravenous administration of iofetamine I 123, it does appear when administered as sodium iodide I 123 and may reach concentrations equal to or greater than concentrations in maternal plasma. Because of the potential risk to the infant from radiation exposure, temporary discontinuation of nursing is recommended for a length of time that may be assessed by measuring the activity of breast milk and estimating the radiation exposure to the infant.

**Pediatrics**
Although iofetamine I 123 is used in children, there have been no specific studies evaluating its safety and efficacy in children. When this radiopharmaceutical is used in children, the diagnostic benefit should be judged to outweigh the potential risk of radiation.

**Geriatrics**
Appropriate studies on the relationship of age to the effects of iofetamine I 123 have not been performed in the geriatric population. However, no geriatric-specific problems have been documented to date.

**Drug interactions and/or related problems**
The following drug interactions and/or related problems have been selected on the basis of their potential clinical significance (possible mechanism in parentheses where appropriate)—not necessarily inclusive (» = major clinical significance):

See also *Diagnostic interference*.

Note: Combinations containing any of the following medications, depending on the amount present, may also interact with this medication.

» Monoamine oxidase (MAO) inhibitors, including furazolidone, procarbazine, and selegiline
  (concurrent use may precipitate hypertensive crisis; iofetamine I 123 should not be administered during or within 14 days following the administration of an MAO inhibitor)

**Diagnostic interference**
The following have been selected on the basis of their potential clinical significance (possible effect in parentheses where appropriate)—not necessarily inclusive (» = major clinical significance):

With results of *this* test
*Due to other medications*
  Sympathomimetics
    (sympathomimetics when used concurrently with iofetamine I 123 may alter its biodistribution, therefore, affecting the image quality and usefulness)

**Medical considerations/Contraindications**
The medical considerations/contraindications included have been selected on the basis of their potential clinical significance (reasons given in parentheses where appropriate)—not necessarily inclusive (» = major clinical significance).

*Risk-benefit should be considered when the following medical problems exist:*

Hypertension, history of
  (increased systolic blood pressure and dizziness with transient chest tightness may result [to date only one case has been reported in a patient with a history of hypertension])

Respiratory tract infection
  (hearing loss may occur [to date only one case has been reported of transient unilateral hearing loss that occurred several hours after the administration of iofetamine I 123])

## Side/Adverse Effects
As with any organic iodine–containing preparation, allergic reactions are possible.

## Patient Consultation
As an aid to patient consultation, refer to *Advice for the Patient, Radiopharmaceuticals (Diagnostic)*.

In providing consultation, consider emphasizing the following selected information (» = major clinical significance):

**Description of use**
  Action in the body: Distribution of radioactive iofetamine in brain tissues as a function of respective blood flow
  Retention of radioactivity in brain tissues allows visualization
  Small amount of radioactivity used in diagnosis; radiation received is low and considered safe

**Before having this test**
» Conditions affecting use, especially:
    Sensitivity to sympathomimetics
    Pregnancy—Risk to fetus from radiation exposure as opposed to benefit derived from use should be considered; possibility of hypothyroidism in fetus
    Breast-feeding—Risk to infant from radiation exposure
    Use in children—Risk from radiation exposure as opposed to benefit derived from use should be considered
    Other medications, especially MAO inhibitors

**Preparation for this test**
  Special preparatory instructions may be given; patient should inquire in advance

**Precautions after having this test**
  Increasing intake of fluids and voiding as often as possible after examination to minimize radiation exposure to bladder

**Side/adverse effects**
  Allergic reactions are possible

## General Dosing Information
Radiopharmaceuticals are to be administered only by or under the supervision of physicians who have had extensive training in the safe use and handling of radioactive materials and who are authorized by the appropriate Federal or Agreement State agency, if required or, outside the U.S., the appropriate authority.

To help minimize thyroidal uptake of free iodide I 123, a thyroid blocking agent such as a saturated solution of potassium iodide or potassium perchlorate should be given ½ to 1 hour prior to administration of iofetamine I 123.

Adequate hydration of the patient is recommended before and after examination to assure adequate urinary flow.

Urination is recommended as often as possible after the examination to reduce radiation exposure to the bladder.

Manufacturer's package insert or other appropriate literature should be consulted for optimal times when imaging should be performed.

**Safety considerations for handling this radiopharmaceutical**
Improper handling of this radiopharmaceutical may cause radioactive contamination. Guidelines for handling radioactive material have been prepared by scientific, professional, state, federal, and international bodies and are available to the specially qualified and authorized users who have access to radiopharmaceuticals.

## Parenteral Dosage Forms

### IOFETAMINE HYDROCHLORIDE I 123 INJECTION

**Usual adult and adolescent administered activity**
Brain imaging—
  Intravenous, 111 to 222 megabecquerels (3 to 6 millicuries).

**Usual pediatric administered activity**
Dosage has not been established.

**Strength(s) usually available**
U.S.—
  At calibration time
  37 megabecquerels (1 millicurie) of iofetamine hydrochloride I 123, per mL (Rx) [*Spectamine*].
Canada—
  At calibration time
  37 megabecquerels (1 millicurie) of iofetamine hydrochloride I 123, per mL (Rx) [*Spectamine*].

**Packaging and storage**
Store between 5 and 30 °C (41 and 86 °F). Protect from freezing.

**Stability**
Injection should be administered within 12 hours after calibration.

**Note**
Caution—Radioactive material.

## Selected Bibliography

Royal HD, Hill TC, Holman BL. Clinical brain imaging with Isopropyl-Iodoamphetamine and SPECT. Semin Nucl Med. 1985; 15(4): 357-76.

Johnson KA et al. Cerebral perfusion imaging in Alzheimer's disease. Use of single-photon emission computed tomography and iofetamine hydrochloride I 123. Arch Neurol Feb 1987; 44(2): 165-8.

Park CH et al. Iofetamine HCl I 123 Brain scanning in stroke: a comparison with transmission CT. Radiographics 1988; 8(2): 305-26.

Revised: 09/28/92
Interim revision: 08/02/94

---

**IOHEXOL**—The *Iohexol (Local)* monograph is not included in this published version of the USP DI database. Copies of the monograph are available on request from Micromedex, Inc. - Reprint Requests, 6200 S. Syracuse Way, Suite 300, Englewood, CO 80111; telephone (303) 486-6400; telefax (303) 486-6464; Email: USPDI@MDX.COM.

---

**IOHEXOL**—The *Iohexol (Systemic)* monograph is not included in this published version of the USP DI database. Copies of the monograph are available on request from Micromedex, Inc. - Reprint Requests, 6200 S. Syracuse Way, Suite 300, Englewood, CO 80111; telephone (303) 486-6400; telefax (303) 486-6464; Email: USPDI@MDX.COM.

---

**IOPAMIDOL**—The *Iopamidol (Systemic)* monograph is not included in this published version of the USP DI database. Copies of the monograph are available on request from Micromedex, Inc. - Reprint Requests, 6200 S. Syracuse Way, Suite 300, Englewood, CO 80111; telephone (303) 486-6400; telefax (303) 486-6464; Email: USPDI@MDX.COM.

---

**IOPANOIC ACID**—See *Cholecystographic Agents, Oral (Systemic)*

---

**IOPROMIDE**—The *Iopromide (Systemic)—Introductory Version* monograph is not included in this published version of the USP DI database. Copies of the monograph are available on request from Micromedex, Inc. - Reprint Requests, 6200 S. Syracuse Way, Suite 300, Englewood, CO 80111; telephone (303) 486-6400; telefax (303) 486-6464; Email: USPDI@MDX.COM.

---

**IOTHALAMATE**—The *Iothalamate (Local)* monograph is not included in this published version of the USP DI database. Copies of the monograph are available on request from Micromedex, Inc. - Reprint Requests, 6200 S. Syracuse Way, Suite 300, Englewood, CO 80111; telephone (303) 486-6400; telefax (303) 486-6464; Email: USPDI@MDX.COM.

---

**IOTHALAMATE**—The *Iothalamate (Systemic)* monograph is not included in this published version of the USP DI database. Copies of the monograph are available on request from Micromedex, Inc. - Reprint Requests, 6200 S. Syracuse Way, Suite 300, Englewood, CO 80111; telephone (303) 486-6400; telefax (303) 486-6464; Email: USPDI@MDX.COM.

---

**IOVERSOL**—The *Ioversol (Systemic)* monograph is not included in this published version of the USP DI database. Copies of the monograph are available on request from Micromedex, Inc. - Reprint Requests, 6200 S. Syracuse Way, Suite 300, Englewood, CO 80111; telephone (303) 486-6400; telefax (303) 486-6464; Email: USPDI@MDX.COM.

---

**IOXAGLATE**—The *Ioxaglate (Local)* monograph is not included in this published version of the USP DI database. Copies of the monograph are available on request from Micromedex, Inc. - Reprint Requests, 6200 S. Syracuse Way, Suite 300, Englewood, CO 80111; telephone (303) 486-6400; telefax (303) 486-6464; Email: USPDI@MDX.COM.

---

**IOXAGLATE**—The *Ioxaglate (Systemic)* monograph is not included in this published version of the USP DI database. Copies of the monograph are available on request from Micromedex, Inc. - Reprint Requests, 6200 S. Syracuse Way, Suite 300, Englewood, CO 80111; telephone (303) 486-6400; telefax (303) 486-6464; Email: USPDI@MDX.COM.

---

**IOXILAN**—The *Ioxilan (Systemic)—Introductory Version* monograph is not included in this published version of the USP DI database. Copies of the monograph are available on request from Micromedex, Inc. - Reprint Requests, 6200 S. Syracuse Way, Suite 300, Englewood, CO 80111; telephone (303) 486-6400; telefax (303) 486-6464; Email: USPDI@MDX.COM.

---

# IPECAC  Oral-Local

VA CLASSIFICATION (Primary): GA600

Note: For a listing of dosage forms and brand names by country availability, see *Dosage Forms* section(s).

## Category
Emetic.

## Indications

**Accepted**

Toxicity, nonspecific (treatment)—Ipecac syrup is indicated as an emetic for emergency use in the treatment of drug overdose and in some cases of poisoning. Ipecac should not be used if strychnine or corrosives such as alkalies (lye) or strong acids have been ingested. Use in strychnine poisoning may precipitate seizures, and use in corrosive poisoning may cause additional injury to the esophagus.

Also, ipecac should not be used in semiconscious or unconscious persons since there is an increased risk that the vomited material may enter the lungs and cause pneumonia.

In addition, ipecac is usually not used in patients who have ingested petroleum distillates such as kerosene, gasoline, coal oil, fuel oil, paint thinner, or cleaning fluid because of the high risk of pulmonary aspiration, possibly resulting in pneumonia; however, this is controversial. The benefits of ipecac may outweigh the risks of aspiration or toxic reactions from the petroleum distillate, depending on the amount ingested and the relative toxicity of the petroleum distillate or the chemical dissolved in it.

## Pharmacology/Pharmacokinetics

**Mechanism of action/Effect**

The actions of ipecac are mainly those of its major alkaloids, emetine and cephaeline. They act locally by irritating the gastric mucosa and centrally by stimulating the medullary chemoreceptor trigger zone to induce vomiting.

**Onset of action**
20 to 30 minutes.

**Duration of action**
20 to 25 minutes.

## Elimination
Emetine—Eliminated from body very slowly; may be detected in urine up to 60 days after ipecac use.

## Precautions to Consider

### Pregnancy/Reproduction
Pregnancy—Studies have not been done in humans.
Studies have not been done in animals.
FDA Pregnancy Category C.

### Breast-feeding
It is not known whether ipecac is distributed into breast milk. However, problems in humans have not been documented.

### Pediatrics
In children under 1 year of age, there is an increased risk of aspiration of vomitus. Medical advice and/or supervision on proper positioning to avoid aspiration is important in this age group.

### Geriatrics
Appropriate studies performed to date have not demonstrated geriatrics-specific problems that would limit the usefulness of ipecac in the elderly.

### Drug interactions and/or related problems
The following drug interactions and/or related problems have been selected on the basis of their potential clinical significance (possible mechanism in parentheses where appropriate)—not necessarily inclusive (» = major clinical significance):

Note: Combinations containing any of the following medications, depending on the amount present, may also interact with this medication.

Antiemetics
(prior ingestion of these medications may decrease the emetic response to ipecac)

Beverages, carbonated
(concurrent use with ipecac is not recommended since these beverages may cause distention of the stomach)

Charcoal, activated
(if both ipecac and activated charcoal are to be used in the treatment of poisoning, it is generally recommended that activated charcoal be administered only after vomiting has been induced and completed; however, in some clinical trials in which activated charcoal was administered pre-emesis 10 minutes after high doses of ipecac, the emetic properties of ipecac were not inhibited)

Milk or milk products
(concurrent use is not recommended since milk has been reported to decrease the effectiveness of ipecac)

### Medical considerations/Contraindications
The medical considerations/contraindications included have been selected on the basis of their potential clinical significance (reasons given in parentheses where appropriate)—not necessarily inclusive (» = major clinical significance).

*Except under special circumstances, this medication should not be used when the following medical problems exist:*
» Any condition in which there is an increased risk of aspiration of vomitus, such as:
» Decreased patient alertness or
» Depressed gag reflex or
» Seizures or history of or
» Shock or
» Unconsciousness
(risk of aspiration pneumonia)
» Ingestion of corrosive materials, such as alkalies (lye) or strong acids
(vomiting may cause additional injury to the esophagus)

*Risk-benefit should be considered when the following medical problems exist:*
Heart disease
(increased risk of tachycardia, hypotension, precordial chest pain, dyspnea, and electrocardiogram (ECG) abnormalities if ipecac is not vomited)
» Ingestion of petroleum distillates, such as kerosene, gasoline, coal oil, fuel oil, paint thinner, or cleaning fluid
(risk of aspiration pneumonia)
Strychnine poisoning
(increased risk of seizures)

## Side/Adverse Effects
Note: Toxic myopathy, cardiac toxicity, and several deaths have been reported as a result of the chronic use of ipecac among young women with anorexia nervosa, bulimia, and related eating disorders. These patients used ipecac as a means of inducing emesis to lose weight.

## Overdose
For more information on the management of overdose or unintentional ingestion, **contact a Poison Control Center** (see *Poison Control Center Listing*).

### Clinical effects of overdose
The following effects have been selected on the basis of their potential clinical significance (possible signs and symptoms in parentheses where appropriate)—not necessarily inclusive (may also be symptoms of chronic abuse):

*Diarrhea; fast or irregular heartbeat; nausea or vomiting, continuing more than 30 minutes; stomach cramps or pain; troubled breathing; unusual tiredness or weakness; weakness, aching, and stiffness of muscles, especially those of the neck, arms, and legs*

Note: *Cardiac and muscle disorders* are related to emetine toxicity.

## Patient Consultation
As an aid to patient consultation, refer to *Advice for the Patient, Ipecac (Oral)*.

In providing consultation, consider emphasizing the following selected information (» = major clinical significance):

### Before using this medication
» Calling physician, poison control center, or emergency room before taking medication
» Conditions affecting use, especially:
Use in children—Increased risk of aspiration of vomitus in children under 1 year of age
Other medical problems, especially any condition in which there is an increased risk of aspiration of vomitus, and ingestion of corrosive materials or petroleum distillates

### Proper use of this medication
» Importance of not taking more medication than recommended on the label or otherwise directed
» Not giving medication to semiconscious or unconscious persons
Importance of drinking water immediately after taking medication
» Avoiding concurrent use with milk or carbonated beverages
Getting medical attention immediately if vomiting does not occur within 20 minutes after second dose
» Taking activated charcoal only after vomiting has been induced by this medication and completed, if both are to be used
» Proper dosing
» Proper storage

### Side/adverse effects
Signs of potential side effects, especially cardiac and muscle disorders related to emetine toxicity (with chronic abuse)

## General Dosing Information
To increase the emetic action of ipecac, it is recommended that adults drink 1 full glass (240 mL) of water and children drink ½ to 1 full glass (120 to 240 mL) of water immediately after taking the ipecac syrup. In young and frightened children, water may be given before the ipecac syrup if necessary.

No more than 2 doses of ipecac syrup should be taken since ipecac can be cardiotoxic.

## Oral Dosage Forms

### IPECAC SYRUP USP

Note: *Ipecac Fluidextract* and *Ipecac Tincture* have been replaced by *Ipecac Syrup*, the preferred dosage form. *Ipecac Fluidextract* is 14 times more concentrated than *Ipecac Syrup*, and is not recommended for use because of its high potency and toxicity.

### Usual adult and adolescent dose
Emetic—
Oral, 15 to 30 mL, followed immediately by one full glass (240 mL) of water. Dose may be repeated after twenty to thirty minutes if emesis does not occur. If emesis does not occur after the second dose, gastric lavage should be performed.

### Usual pediatric dose
Emetic—
Children up to 6 months of age: Ipecac syrup should be administered only under the supervision of a physician.
Children 6 months to 1 year of age: Oral, 5 to 10 mL, preceded or followed by one-half to one full glass (120 to 240 mL) of water.
Children 1 to 12 years of age: Oral, 15 mL, preceded or followed by one-half to one full glass (120 to 240 mL) of water.

Note: Doses may be repeated after twenty to thirty minutes if emesis does not occur. If emesis does not occur after the second dose, gastric lavage should be performed.

For children 6 months to 1 year of age, professional advice on proper positioning to avoid aspiration of vomitus is important.

### Strength(s) usually available
U.S.—
 15 mL (OTC) [GENERIC].
 30 mL (OTC) [GENERIC].
Canada—
 15 mL (OTC) [GENERIC].
 30 mL (OTC) [GENERIC].

Note: Each mL of ipecac syrup contains 1.23 to 1.57 mg of the total ether-soluble alkaloids of ipecac.
Alcohol content ranges from 1 to 2%.

### Packaging and storage
Store preferably at a temperature below 25 °C (77 °F), in a tight container.

Note: Containers intended for sale to the public without prescription contain not more than 30 mL of ipecac syrup.

### Note
If ipecac syrup is to be used as an emetic for emergency use in poisoning, consider providing on the label the telephone number for physician, poison control center, or emergency room.

### Selected Bibliography
Manno BR, Manno JE. Toxicology of ipecac: a review. Clin Toxicol 1977; 10: 221-42.

Revised: 08/04/94

---

**IPODATE**—See *Cholecystographic Agents, Oral (Systemic)*

---

# IPRATROPIUM   Inhalation-Local

VA CLASSIFICATION (Primary): RE105
Commonly used brand name(s): *Apo-Ipravent; Atrovent; Kendral-Ipratropium*.

Note: For a listing of dosage forms and brand names by country availability, see *Dosage Forms* section(s).

## Category
Bronchodilator.

## Indications
Note: Bracketed information in the *Indications* section refers to uses that are not included in U.S. product labeling.

### Accepted
Bronchitis (treatment) or
Emphysema, pulmonary (treatment) or
Pulmonary disease, chronic obstructive, other (treatment)—Ipratropium is indicated for maintenance treatment of bronchospasm associated with chronic obstructive pulmonary disease, including chronic bronchitis and pulmonary emphysema. Regular use of ipratropium results in at least as great an increase in airflow as that with use of other bronchodilators and fewer adverse effects. If additional bronchodilation is needed in these patients, an adrenergic bronchodilator may be used as an adjunct to ipratropium.

[Ipratropium is indicated as an adjunct to adrenergic bronchodilators for treatment of acute exacerbations of chronic obstructive pulmonary disease.]

[Asthma (treatment adjunct)]—Ipratropium is used as an adjunct to anti-inflammatory therapy or bronchodilators to prevent[1] exacerbations of asthma in patients who respond poorly to therapy or as an alternative to other bronchodilators in patients who develop significant side effects with these medications.

Ipratropium is used as an adjunct to adrenergic bronchodilators for the treatment of acute exacerbations of asthma. It is not used alone because it has a relatively slower onset of action and time to peak effect as compared with adrenergic bronchodilators.

[1]Not included in Canadian product labeling.

## Pharmacology/Pharmacokinetics

### Physicochemical characteristics
Source—A synthetic quaternary ammonium compound, chemically related to atropine.
Molecular weight—430.38.
Other characteristics—Fairly stable in neutral solutions and in acid solutions; rapidly hydrolyzed in alkaline solutions

### Mechanism of action/Effect
The bronchodilation produced by ipratropium is primarily a local, site-specific effect rather than a systemic effect. Ipratropium appears to produce bronchodilation by competitive inhibition of cholinergic receptors on bronchial smooth muscle. This effect antagonizes the action of acetylcholine at its membrane-bound receptor site and thereby blocks the bronchoconstrictor action of vagal efferent impulses.

### Absorption
Systemic absorption is minimal following inhalation. Blood concentration and renal and fecal excretion studies have shown that ipratropium is poorly absorbed into the systemic circulation from both the surface of the lung and the gastrointestinal tract. At a dose of 14 times the recommended therapeutic inhalation dose, the peak plasma concentration is 0.06 nanograms/mL. Plasma concentrations after inhalation of usual doses are about 1000 times lower than equipotent oral or intravenous doses (15 and 0.15 mg, respectively).

### Distribution
Studies in rats have shown that ipratropium does not penetrate the blood-brain barrier.

### Biotransformation
Hepatic, for the small amount of ipratropium systemically absorbed; metabolites have little or no anticholinergic activity.

### Onset of action
Within 5 to 15 minutes.

### Time to peak effect
About 90 minutes (range, 1 to 2 hours).

### Duration of action
About 3 to 4 hours in the majority of patients, but up to 6 to 8 hours in some patients.

### Elimination
Primarily fecal; up to 90% of inhaled dose is swallowed and eliminated as unchanged drug. Absorbed portion of dose is excreted primarily in the urine.

## Precautions to Consider

### Cross-sensitivity and/or related problems
Patients sensitive to belladonna alkaloids may be sensitive to ipratropium also, since ipratropium is chemically related to atropine. Although rare, allergic reactions to ipratropium metered-dose inhaler have been reported; however, the causative component has not been identified. Therefore, patients allergic to soybean protein or other legumes, such as peanuts, may be allergic to soya lecithin contained in the metered-dose inhaler as a suspending agent.

### Carcinogenicity/Tumorigenicity
Two-year carcinogenicity studies in mice and rats have shown that ipratropium, at oral doses up to 1250 times the maximum recommended human daily dose, has no carcinogenic potential. Also, studies in mice and rats have shown that ipratropium, at oral doses up to 6 mg per kg of body weight (mg/kg), does not have a carcinogenic or tumorigenic effect.

# Ipratropium (Inhalation-Local)

**Mutagenicity**
Various studies in mice and hamsters have shown that ipratropium is not mutagenic.

**Pregnancy/Reproduction**
Fertility—Although studies in male and female rats have shown that ipratropium, at oral doses up to approximately 10,000 times the maximum recommended human daily dose, does not affect fertility, ipratropium has been shown to increase resorption and decrease conception rates when the medication was administered at doses above 18,000 times the maximum recommended human daily dose.

Pregnancy—Although adequate and well-controlled studies in humans have not been done, no increased risk of congenital malformation has been reported.

Reproduction studies with ipratropium in mice, rats, and rabbits given oral doses of 10, 100, and 125 mg per kg of body weight (mg/kg), respectively, and in rats and rabbits given inhalation doses of 1.5 and 1.8 mg/kg (or approximately 38 and 45 times the recommended human daily dose), respectively, have shown no evidence of teratogenic effects.

FDA Pregnancy Category B.

**Breast-feeding**
It is not known whether ipratropium is distributed into breast milk. However, problems in humans have not been documented. Although lipid-insoluble quaternary bases, such as ipratropium, are distributed into breast milk, it is unlikely that inhaled ipratropium would reach significant concentrations in maternal serum, and the concentration in breast milk would probably be undetectable.

**Pediatrics**
Appropriate studies performed to date have not demonstrated pediatrics-specific problems that would limit the usefulness of ipratropium in children.

**Geriatrics**
Studies performed to date on patients over 65 years of age have not demonstrated geriatrics-specific problems that would limit the usefulness of ipratropium inhalation in the elderly.

**Drug interactions and/or related problems**
The following drug interactions and/or related problems have been selected on the basis of their potential clinical significance (possible mechanism in parentheses where appropriate)—not necessarily inclusive (» = major clinical significance):

Note: Combinations containing any of the following medications, depending on the amount present, may also interact with this medication.

Anticholinergics, other, or other medications with anticholinergic activity (see *Appendix II*)
(concurrent use of other anticholinergics, including ophthalmic preparations, or other medications with anticholinergic action with ipratropium may result in additive effects)

Tacrine
(because tacrine is thought to act by increasing effective acetylcholine concentrations, concurrent use may decrease the effects of either ipratropium or tacrine)

**Medical considerations/Contraindications**
The medical considerations/contraindications included have been selected on the basis of their potential clinical significance (reasons given in parentheses where appropriate)—not necessarily inclusive (» = major clinical significance).

*Risk-benefit should be considered when the following medical problems exist:*

» Glaucoma, angle-closure
(an acute attack may be precipitated or condition may be exacerbated if ipratropium inhalation aerosol is sprayed directly into the eyes or if a poorly fitting face mask is used with nebulized ipratropium inhalation solution, alone or in combination with an adrenergic bronchodilator)

Sensitivity to ipratropium or belladonna alkaloids; also, allergy to soya lecithin, soybean protein, or other legumes such as peanuts for patients using the metered-dose inhaler

Urinary retention
(rarely, condition may be aggravated)

## Side/Adverse Effects

Note: Usual therapeutic doses of ipratropium generally do not cause systemic side/adverse effects because of the low blood concentrations achieved with the inhalation; however, the potential for systemic side/adverse effects exists.

Although rare, cases of precipitation or worsening of narrow-angle glaucoma and acute eye pain have been reported following use of ipratropium aerosol, and inhalation solution alone or in combination with an adrenergic bronchodilator, when the spray came into contact with the eyes.

Acute overdose of ipratropium by inhalation is unlikely since the medication is not well absorbed systemically.

The following side/adverse effects have been selected on the basis of their potential clinical significance (possible signs and symptoms in parentheses where appropriate)—not necessarily inclusive:

**Those indicating need for medical attention**
Incidence rare
*Bronchospasm, increased* (increased wheezing; tightness in chest; difficulty in breathing); *dermatitis, hypersensitivity-induced; angioedema* (swelling of face, lips, or eyelids); *skin rash; urticaria* (hives); *eye pain, acute; paralytic ileus* (continuing constipation; lower abdominal pain or distention)—especially in patients with cystic fibrosis

Note: *Increased bronchospasm* may be due to sensitivity to benzalkonium chloride and edetate disodium present in the multiple-dose container of inhalation solution.

**Those indicating need for medical attention only if they continue or are bothersome**
Incidence more frequent
*Cough; dryness of mouth; unpleasant taste*

Incidence rare
*Blurred vision or other changes in vision; burning eyes; dizziness; headache; nausea; nervousness; palpitations* (pounding heartbeat); *sweating; trembling; urinary retention* (difficult urination)

## Overdose

**Treatment of overdose**
Cholinesterase inhibitors may be used for serious anticholinergic toxicity.

## Patient Consultation

As an aid to patient consultation, refer to *Advice for the Patient, Ipratropium (Inhalation).*
In providing consultation, consider emphasizing the following selected information (» = major clinical significance):

**Before using this medication**
» Conditions affecting use, especially:
Sensitivity to ipratropium or belladonna alkaloids; also, allergy to soya lecithin, soybean protein, or peanuts for patients using metered-dose inhaler
Other medical problems, especially angle-closure glaucoma

**Proper use of this medication**
» Helps control symptoms of lung disease; inhalation solution used only with other bronchodilators when treating acute asthma attacks
» Importance of not using more medication than the amount prescribed
» Avoiding contact with the eyes; closing eyes if necessary when inhaling; if accidentally sprayed into the eyes or if nebulized solution escapes into the eyes, irritation or blurring of vision may occur; rinsing eyes with cool water if necessary
Reading patient instructions carefully before using
» If using regularly, importance of using every day at regularly spaced times.
» Proper dosing
Missed dose: If used regularly, using as soon as possible; using any remaining doses for that day at regularly spaced intervals
» Proper storage

*For inhalation aerosol dosage form*
Checking periodically with health care professional for proper use of inhaler to prevent improper technique and incorrect dosage
Testing or priming inhaler before using first time or first time in a while
Proper administration technique without spacer device
Proper administration technique with spacer device
Proper cleaning procedure for inhaler

*For inhalation solution dosage form*
Using only in nebulizer as instructed by physician
Preparing solution for nebulizer
Proper administration technique: Using in a power-operated nebulizer with an adequate flow rate and equipped with a face mask or mouthpiece

**Precautions while using this medication**
» Checking with physician immediately if symptoms do not improve within 30 minutes after using this medication or if condition becomes worse

*For patients using ipratropium inhalation solution*
» If also using cromolyn inhalation solution, not mixing cromolyn inhalation solution with ipratropium inhalation solution containing the preservative benzalkonium chloride for use in a nebulizer

**Side/adverse effects**
Signs of potential side effects, especially increased bronchospasm, hypersensitivity-induced dermatitis, acute eye pain, and paralytic ileus

## General Dosing Information

For nebulization of ipratropium bromide inhalation solution, a gas flow (oxygen or compressed air) of 6 to 10 liters per minute should be used. Nebulizers with either a face mask or mouthpiece have been used, although a mouthpiece may be preferable to a face mask because it reduces the risk of solution entering the eyes.

Patients should be advised to contact their physician immediately if they do not respond to the usual dose of ipratropium because this may be a sign of seriously worsening airflow obstruction or the development of concurrent illness requiring reassessment of therapy.

The contents of metered dose inhalers should generally not be floated in water to assess the contents since this method may not reliably predict the amount of medication remaining in the canister. A record should be kept of the number of inhalations used.

## Inhalation Dosage Forms

Note: Bracketed uses in the *Dosage Forms* section refers to indications that are not included in U.S. product labeling.

### IPRATROPIUM BROMIDE INHALATION AEROSOL

**Usual adult and adolescent dose**
Bronchitis (treatment)
Emphysema, pulmonary (treatment) or
Pulmonary disease, chronic obstructive, other (treatment)—
  Oral inhalation, 2 to 4 inhalations (36 to 72 mcg) three or four times a day. Some patients may require up to 6 to 8 inhalations (108 to 144 mcg) three times a day. For severe exacerbations, 6 to 8 inhalations may be administered, using a spacer device, every three to four hours.
[Asthma (treatment adjunct)][1]—
  Oral inhalation, 1 to 4 inhalations (18 to 72 mcg) four times a day as necessary.

**Usual pediatric dose**
[Asthma (treatment adjunct)][1]—
  Children up to 12 years of age: Oral inhalation, 1 to 2 inhalations (18 to 36 mcg) every six to eight hours as necessary.

**Strength(s) usually available**
U.S.—
  18 mcg per metered spray (Rx) [*Atrovent* (dichlorodifluoromethane; dichlorotetrafluoroethane; trichloromonofluoromethane; soya lecithin)].
Canada—
  20 mcg per metered spray (Rx) [*Atrovent* (dichlorodifluoromethane; dichlorotetrafluoroethane; trichloromonofluoromethane; soya lecithin)].
Note: In Canada, metered dose inhalers are labeled according to the amount of ipratropium delivered at the valve; in the U.S., metered dose inhalers are labeled according to the amount of ipratropium delivered at the mouthpiece or actuator. Therefore, 20 mcg of ipratropium delivered at the valve is equivalent to 18 mcg delivered at the mouthpiece.

**Packaging and storage**
Store between 15 and 30 °C (59 and 86 °F), unless otherwise specified by manufacturer.

**Auxiliary labeling**
• For oral inhalation only.
• Shake well before using.
• Store away from heat and direct sunlight.

**Note**
Include patient instructions when dispensing.
Demonstrate inhalation technique to patient when dispensing.

**Additional information**
Each canister contains medication for about 200 inhalations.

### IPRATROPIUM BROMIDE INHALATION SOLUTION

**Usual adult and adolescent dose**
Bronchitis (treatment)
Emphysema, pulmonary (treatment) or
Pulmonary disease, chronic obstructive, other (treatment)—
  Oral inhalation, 250 to 500 mcg (0.25 to 0.5 mg), diluted, if necessary; dose is administered via nebulization three or four times a day, every six to eight hours. For severe exacerbations of COPD, 500 mcg may be administered every four to eight hours.
[Asthma (treatment adjunct)][1]—
  Oral inhalation, 500 mcg (0.5 mg), diluted, if necessary; dose is administered via nebulization three or four times a day, every six to eight hours as necessary.

**Usual pediatric dose**
[Asthma (treatment adjunct)][1]—
  Children up to 5 years of age: Safety and efficacy have not been established.
  Children 5 to 12 years of age: Oral inhalation, 125 to 250 mcg (0.125 to 0.25 mg), diluted, if necessary, to three to five mL with preservative-free sterile sodium chloride inhalation solution 0.9%; dose is administered via nebulization every four to six hours as necessary.

**Strength(s) usually available**
U.S.—
  Single-dose vial
    0.02% (200 mcg per mL [2.5 mL]) (Rx) [*Atrovent*; GENERIC].
Canada—
  Single-dose vial
    0.0125% (125 mcg per mL [2 mL]) (Rx) [*Atrovent*].
    0.025% (250 mcg per mL [1 or 2 mL]) (Rx) [*Atrovent*].
  Multiple-dose vial
    0.025% (250 mcg per mL) (Rx) [*Apo-Ipravent* (benzalkonium chloride; EDTA-disodium); *Atrovent* (benzalkonium chloride; EDTA-disodium); *Kendral-Ipratropium*].

**Packaging and storage**
Prior to opening container, store between 15 and 30 °C (59 and 86 °F), unless otherwise specified by manufacturer. Protect from freezing. Protect from light.

**Preparation of dosage form**
Ipratropium inhalation solution can be diluted with preservative-free sterile 0.9% sodium chloride.

**Stability**
Solutions of ipratropium containing the preservative benzalkonium chloride may be diluted with preservative-free sterile sodium chloride inhalation solution 0.9%. The solution should be used within twenty-four hours from time of dilution when stored at room temperature and within forty-eight hours when stored in the refrigerator.
Preservative-free albuterol inhalation solution can be mixed in the nebulizer with ipratropium inhalation solution, if used within one hour.
Preservative-free ipratropium inhalation solution is recommended when combining ipratropium with cromolyn inhalation solution. This combination is compatible for up to one hour. Mixing ipratropium inhalation solution containing the preservative benzalkonium chloride with cromolyn in a nebulizer results in cloudiness of the solution, which is due to complexation between cromolyn sodium and benzalkonium chloride. No precipitation or significant decrease in the concentration of cromolyn or ipratropium occurs.

**Auxiliary labeling**
• For oral inhalation only.

**Note**
Include patient instructions for preparation of solution when dispensing.

---

[1]Not included in Canadian product labeling.

## Selected Bibliography

Gross NJ. Ipratropium bromide. N Engl J Med 1988; 319: 486-94.
Spector SL, Nicklas RA, editors. Practice parameters for the diagnosis and treatment of asthma. J Allergy Clin Immunol 1995; 96: 786-9.
American Thoracic Society. Standards for the diagnosis and care of patients with chronic obstructive pulmonary disease. Am J Respir Crit Care Med 1995; 152 Suppl: 77S-120S.

Revised: 06/21/96

# IPRATROPIUM Nasal*

VA CLASSIFICATION (Primary): NT900
Commonly used brand name(s): *Atrovent*.
Note: For a listing of dosage forms and brand names by country availability, see *Dosage Forms* section(s).

*Not commercially available in U.S.

## Category
Anticholinergic (nasal).

## Indications

**Accepted**
Rhinorrhea (treatment)—Ipratropium nasal aerosol is indicated for the symptomatic treatment of rhinorrhea associated with vasomotor rhinitis. Ipratropium nasal aerosol has not been shown to control rhinitis symptoms other than rhinorrea; it has little or no effect on sneezing, itching, or nasal congestion caused by vasodilation.

## Pharmacology/Pharmacokinetics

**Physicochemical characteristics**
Source—A synthetic quaternary ammonium compound, chemically related to atropine.

**Mechanism of action/Effect**
Ipratropium antagonizes the actions of acetylcholine at parasympathetic, postganglionic, effector-cell junctions by competing with acetylcholine for receptor sites. When administered intranasally, ipratropium has a localized parasympathetic blocking action, which reduces watery hypersecretion from mucosal glands in the nose.

**Absorption**
Systemic absorption from the nasal mucosa is rapid but minimal following nasal administration.

**Biotransformation**
Hepatic, for the small amount of nasal ipratropium systemically absorbed; metabolites have little or no anticholinergic activity.

**Half-life**
Elimination—About 3.5 hours (range, 1.5 to 4 hours).

**Onset of action**
Within 5 minutes.

**Time to peak effect**
1 to 4 hours.

**Duration of action**
About 4 to 8 hours.

**Elimination**
Absorbed portion of dose is excreted primarily in the urine; also excreted in the bile.

## Precautions to Consider

**Cross-sensitivity and/or related problems**
Patients sensitive to belladonna alkaloids may be sensitive to ipratropium also, since ipratropium is chemically related to atropine.

**Carcinogenicity/Tumorigenicity**
Studies of several weeks duration in mice and rats have shown that ipratropium, at oral doses of up to 6 mg/kg of body weight, does not have a carcinogenic or tumorigenic effect.

**Mutagenicity**
Although several studies have shown that ipratropium is not mutagenic, one study has shown a dose-related increase in the number of chromatoid gaps; however, the significance of this finding is not known.

**Pregnancy/Reproduction**
Fertility—A fertility study in rats given oral doses of 5, 50, and 500 mg of ipratropium per kg of body weight for 60 days before and during early gestation showed that fertility was delayed in 8 of 20 females; the conception rate was decreased in 75% of females given the 500 mg/kg dose.

Pregnancy—Adequate and well-controlled studies in humans have not been done.

Reproduction studies in mice, rats, and rabbits given ipratropium at oral doses of approximately 2, 10, and 20 mg/kg, and reproduction studies in rabbits given ipratropium at inhalation doses of 0.3, 0.9, and 1.8 mg/kg, have shown no evidence of embryotoxic or teratogenic effects.

**Breast-feeding**
It is not known whether ipratropium is distributed into breast milk. Problems in humans have not been documented.

**Pediatrics**
Appropriate studies on the relationship of age to the effects of ipratropium nasal aerosol have not been performed in children up to 12 years of age. However, no pediatrics-specific problems have been documented to date.

**Geriatrics**
No information is available on the relationship of age to the effects of ipratropium nasal aerosol in geriatric patients.

**Dental**
Higher doses and prolonged use of ipratropium nasal aerosol may decrease or inhibit salivary flow, thus contributing to the development of caries, periodontal disease, oral candidiasis, and discomfort.

**Drug interactions and/or related problems**
The following drug interactions and/or related problems have been selected on the basis of their potential clinical significance (possible mechanism in parentheses where appropriate)—not necessarily inclusive (» = major clinical significance):

Note: Combinations containing any of the following medications, depending on the amount present, may also interact with this medication.

Anticholinergics, other, or other medications with anticholinergic activity (See *Appendix II*)
(concurrent use of other anticholinergics, including ophthalmic preparations, or other medications with anticholinergic action with ipratropium nasal aerosol may result in additive effects)

**Medical considerations/Contraindications**
The medical considerations/contraindications included have been selected on the basis of their potential clinical significance (reasons given in parentheses where appropriate)—not necessarily inclusive (» = major clinical significance).

*Risk-benefit should be considered when the following medical problems exist:*

Glaucoma, angle-closure
(an acute attack may be precipitated or condition may be exacerbated if ipratropium nasal aerosol is sprayed directly into the eyes)
Sensitivity to ipratropium or belladonna alkaloids

## Side/Adverse Effects

Note: Usual therapeutic doses of ipratropium given intranasally generally do not cause systemic side/adverse effects because of the low blood concentrations achieved with nasal administration; however, the potential for systemic side/adverse effects exists.

In addition, acute overdose of ipratropium nasal aerosol is unlikely, since the medication is not well absorbed systemically.

The following side/adverse effects have been selected on the basis of their potential clinical significance (possible signs and symptoms in parentheses where appropriate)—not necessarily inclusive:

**Those indicating need for medical attention**
Incidence rare
*Blurred vision or other changes in vision; bronchospasm* (wheezing, tightness in chest, or difficulty in breathing); *difficult or painful urination; difficulty in swallowing; eye pain, severe; fast or irregular heartbeat; skin rash or hives; stomatitis* (sores in mouth and on lips); *swelling of tongue or lips*

**Those indicating need for medical attention only if they continue or are bothersome**
Incidence more frequent
*Dryness of nose or mouth; headache; irritation and crusting in nose*
Incidence less frequent or rare
*Bleeding or burning in nose; diarrhea or constipation; dryness of throat; nausea; nervousness; stomach pain; stuffy nose*

## Patient Consultation

As an aid to patient consultation, refer to *Advice for the Patient, Ipratropium (Nasal)*.
In providing consultation, consider emphasizing the following selected information (» = major clinical significance):

### Before using this medication
» Conditions affecting use, especially:
  Sensitivity to ipratropium or belladonna alkaloids

### Proper use of this medication
» Compliance with therapy; importance of not using more medication than the amount prescribed
» Avoiding contact with the eyes; if accidentally sprayed into the eyes, irritation or blurring of vision may occur; rinsing eyes with cool water if necessary
  Reading patient instructions carefully before using; clearing nasal passages before each use
  Checking with health care professional for proper use of aerosol spray device to prevent incorrect dosage
  Testing aerosol spray device before using first time
  Proper administration technique
  Proper cleaning procedure for aerosol spray device
» Proper dosing
  Missed dose: Using as soon as possible; not using if almost time for next dose; using any remaining doses for that day at regularly spaced intervals
» Proper storage

### Precautions while using this medication
» Checking with physician if symptoms do not improve within 1 or 2 weeks or if condition becomes worse
  Possible dryness of mouth or throat; using sugarless candy or gum, ice, or saliva substitute for relief; checking with physician or dentist if dryness of mouth continues for more than 2 weeks

### Side/adverse effects
Signs of potential side effects, especially severe eye pain, blurred vision or other changes in vision, bronchospasm, difficult or painful urination, difficulty in swallowing, fast or irregular heartbeat, skin rash or hives, stomatitis, and swelling of tongue or lips

## General Dosing Information
The smallest dose required to control symptoms should be used as a maintenance dose after the desired clinical response is achieved.

Prior to administration of ipratropium nasal aerosol, the nasal passages should be carefully cleared. During administration, patient should not breathe in so the medication will be deposited only on nasal mucosa. The patient may sniff gently, but not deeply inhale, to distribute the medication into the nose.

## Intranasal Dosage Form

### IPRATROPIUM BROMIDE NASAL AEROSOL

**Usual adult and adolescent dose**
Anticholinergic—
  Intranasal, 40 mcg (0.04 mg—2 metered sprays) into each nostril two times a day.
Note: The dosage frequency may be increased to three or four times a day as needed; however, administration should not be more frequent than every six hours.

**Usual adult prescribing limits**
320 mcg (0.32 mg—16 metered sprays) per twenty-four hours.

**Usual pediatric dose**
Children up to 12 years of age—Use is not recommended.

**Strength(s) usually available**
U.S.—
  Not commercially available.
Canada—
  20 mcg (0.02 mg) per metered spray (Rx) [*Atrovent* (dichlorodifluoromethane; dichlorotetrafluoroethane; trichloromonofluoromethane; soya lecithin)].

**Packaging and storage**
Store below 30 °C (86 °F), unless otherwise specified by manufacturer. Protect from freezing.

**Auxiliary labeling**
• For the nose.
• Shake well before using.
• Store away from heat and direct sunlight.

**Note**
Include patient instructions when dispensing.
Demonstrate nasal administration technique to patient.

**Additional information**
Each 10-mL canister contains medication for approximately 200 metered sprays.

### Selected Bibliography
Borts MR, Druce HM. The use of intranasal anticholinergic agents in the treatment of nonallergic perennial rhinitis. J Allergy Clin Immunol 1992; 90: 1065-70.
Meltzer EO. Intranasal anticholinergic therapy of rhinorrhea. J Allergy Clin Immunol 1992; 90: 1055-64.

Developed: 08/09/94

---

# IPRATROPIUM AND ALBUTEROL Inhalation-Local—INTRODUCTORY VERSION

INN: Albuterol—Salbutamol
BAN: Albuterol—Salbutamol
VA CLASSIFICATION (Primary): RE109
Commonly used brand name(s): *Combivent*.
Note: For a listing of dosage forms and brand names by country availability, see *Dosage Forms* section(s).

## Category
Bronchodilator.

## Indications

**Accepted**
Pulmonary disease, chronic obstructive (treatment)—Ipratropium and albuterol combination is indicated for the treatment of chronic obstructive pulmonary disease (COPD) in patients who are using an aerosol bronchodilator and who continue to have symptoms of bronchospasm that require treatment with a second bronchodilator.

## Pharmacology/Pharmacokinetics

**Physicochemical characteristics**
Source—
  Ipratropium: A synthetic quaternary ammonium compound, chemically related to atropine.

Molecular weight—
  Albuterol sulfate: 576.7.
  Ipratropium bromide: 430.4.

**Mechanism of action/Effect**
Ipratropium and albuterol combination reduces bronchospasm through both anticholinergic and sympathomimetic mechanisms. Simultaneous administration of both drugs produces a greater bronchodilator effect than when either drug is used alone at recommended dosages.
Albuterol—Albuterol is a sympathomimetic agent that has a relatively high degree of selectivity for beta$_2$-adrenergic receptors. Activation of these receptors on airway smooth muscle leads to the activation of the enzyme adenylyl cyclase and to an increase in the intracellular concentration of cyclic-3, 5-adenosine monophosphate (cAMP). Increased cAMP concentrations indirectly lower intracellular ionic calcium, which results in airway smooth muscle relaxation.
Ipratropium—Ipratropium is an anticholinergic agent that produces a local, site-specific effect rather than a systemic effect. It appears to produce bronchodilation by inhibition of cholinergic receptors on bronchial smooth muscle.

**Absorption**
Albuterol—Rapidly and completely absorbed, although whether primarily from pulmonary or from gastrointestinal site is unknown.
Ipratropium—Not readily absorbed into the systemic circulation either from the surface of the lung or from the gastrointestinal tract, as confirmed by blood concentration and renal excretion studies.

**Onset of action**
Ipratropium and albuterol combination—In clinical trials, the median time to onset of a 15% increase in forced expiratory volume in 1 second ($FEV_1$) was 15 minutes.

**Time to peak effect**
Ipratropium and albuterol combination—1 hour.

**Duration of action**
Ipratropium and albuterol combination—4 to 5 hours.

## Precautions to Consider

**Cross-sensitivity and/or related problems**
Patients allergic to soybean protein or other legumes, such as peanuts, may be allergic to the soya lecithin contained in the metered-dose inhaler.
Ipratropium—Patients sensitive to atropine or its derivatives may be sensitive to ipratropium.

**Carcinogenicity/Tumorigenicity**
Albuterol—A 2-year study in rats showed that albuterol, administered orally in doses of 20, 100, and 500 times the maximum recommended human inhalation dose, on a mg per square meter of body surface area ($mg/m^2$) basis, causes a dose-related increase in the incidence of benign leiomyomas of the mesovarium. This effect was blocked by the administration of propranolol in another study. An 18-month study in mice and a 99-week study in hamsters showed no evidence of tumorigenicity.
Ipratropium—Two-year studies in mice and rats have shown that ipratropium, at oral doses of up to 360 and 180 times, respectively, the maximum recommended human inhalation dose, on a $mg/m^2$ basis, has no carcinogenic potential.

**Mutagenicity**
Albuterol—*In vitro* studies with albuterol showed no evidence of tumorigenicity.
Ipratropium—Results of various *in vitro* mutagenicity studies were negative.

**Pregnancy/Reproduction**
Fertility—
Albuterol: Reproduction studies in rats given albuterol sulfate revealed no evidence of impaired fertility.
Ipratropium: Although studies in rats have shown that ipratropium, at oral doses of up to approximately 3000 times the maximum recommended human inhalation dose, on a $mg/m^2$ basis, does not affect fertility, ipratropium has been shown to increase fetal resorption and decrease conception rates when administered at doses above approximately 5400 times the maximum recommended human inhalation dose, on a $mg/m^2$ basis.
Pregnancy—
Albuterol: Adequate and well-controlled studies in humans have not been done.
Mice given albuterol subcutaneously at doses one-tenth of, comparable to, and 10 times the maximum recommended human daily inhalation dose on a $mg/m^2$ basis showed cleft palate formation in 0%, 4.5%, and 9.3% of fetuses, respectively. In rabbits given oral albuterol at doses approximately 1000 times the maximum recommended human daily inhalation dose on a $mg/m^2$ basis showed cranioschisis in 37% of fetuses.
Ipratropium: Adequate and well-controlled studies in humans have not been done.
Reproduction studies in mice, rats, and rabbits revealed no evidence of teratogenicity.
FDA Pregnancy Category C.
Labor—
Albuterol:
Beta-adrenergic agonists have been shown to decrease uterine contractions when administered systemically.

**Breast-feeding**
It is not known whether ipratropium or albuterol is distributed into breast milk. However, problems in humans have not been documented.

**Pediatrics**
No information is available on the relationship of age to the effects of the metered-dose inhalation dosage form of ipratropium and albuterol in pediatric patients. Safety and efficacy have not been established.

**Geriatrics**
Appropriate studies performed to date have not demonstrated geriatrics-specific problems that would limit the usefulness of ipratropium and albuterol combination in older adults.

**Drug interactions and/or related problems**
The following drug interactions and/or related problems have been selected on the basis of their potential clinical significance (possible mechanism in parentheses where appropriate)—not necessarily inclusive (» = major clinical significance):

Note: Combinations containing any of the following medications, depending on the amount present, may also interact with this medication.
Anticholinergics, other, or other medications with anticholinergic activity (see *Appendix II*)
(concurrent use of other medications with anticholinergic activity together with ipratropium may result in additive effects)
Beta-adrenergic blocking agents
(concurrent use with adrenergic bronchodilators may result in mutual inhibition of therapeutic effects)

**Laboratory value alterations**
The following have been selected on the basis of their potential clinical significance (possible effect in parentheses where appropriate)—not necessarily inclusive (» = major clinical significance):

With physiology/laboratory test values
Electrocardiogram
(flattened T waves, prolongation of the $QT_c$ interval, and ST segment depression have been reported with beta-adrenergic bronchodilators)
Potassium, serum
(beta-adrenergic bronchodilators may decrease serum potassium concentrations, especially when the recommended dose is exceeded)

**Medical considerations/Contraindications**
The medical considerations/contraindications included have been selected on the basis of their potential clinical significance (reasons given in parentheses where appropriate)—not necessarily inclusive (» = major clinical significance).

*Risk-benefit should be considered when the following medical problems exist:*
» Sensitivity to ipratropium, atropine, or albuterol
» Allergy to soya lecithin, soybean protein, or other legumes such as peanuts
For ipratropium
» Glaucoma, angle-closure
(an acute attack may be precipitated or condition may be exacerbated if ipratropium-containing inhalation aerosol is sprayed directly into the eyes)
Urinary retention
(rarely, condition may be aggravated)
For albuterol
Cardiac arrhythmias or
» Coronary insufficiency or
Hypertension
(although uncommon after administration of ipratropium and albuterol combination at recommended doses, albuterol can produce a clinically significant cardiovascular effect in some patients, as measured by pulse rate or blood pressure)

## Side/Adverse Effects

The following side/adverse effects have been selected on the basis of their potential clinical significance (possible signs and symptoms in parentheses where appropriate)—not necessarily inclusive:

**Those indicating need for medical attention**
Incidence rare
*Angioedema* (swelling of the face, lips, or eyelids); *bronchospasm, paradoxical or hypersensitivity-induced* (shortness of breath; wheezing); *chest discomfort or pain; irregular heartbeat; oropharyngeal edema* (swelling of the mouth or throat); *skin rash; tachycardia* (fast heartbeat); *urticaria* (hives)

**Those indicating need for medical attention only if they continue or are bothersome**
Incidence less frequent (2 to 6%)
*Coughing; headache; nausea*
Incidence rare
*Change in sense of taste; dizziness; dryness of mouth; nervousness; tremor*

## Patient Consultation

As an aid to patient consultation, refer to *Advice for the Patient, Ipratropium and Albuterol (Inhalation-Local)—Introductory Version*.
In providing consultation, consider emphasizing the following selected information (» = major clinical significance):

### Before using this medication
» Conditions affecting use, especially:
Sensitivity to ipratropium, atropine, or albuterol; allergy to soya lecithin, soybean protein, or other legumes such as peanuts
Other medical problems, especially angle-closure glaucoma or coronary insufficiency

### Proper use of this medication
Proper administration technique: reading patient instructions carefully before using
Performing three priming sprays before using first time or if not used for more than 24 hours
» Avoiding contact with eyes
» Importance of not using more medication than the recommended dose
» Proper dosing
Missed dose: Using as soon as possible; using any remaining doses for that day at regularly spaced intervals
» Proper storage

### Precautions while using this medication
» Checking with physician immediately if difficulty in breathing persists after using this medication or if condition becomes worse

### Side/adverse effects
Signs of potential side effects, especially angioedema, paradoxical or hypersensitivity-induced bronchospasm, chest discomfort or pain, irregular heartbeat, oropharyngeal edema, skin rash, tachycardia, and urticaria

## General Dosing Information
Three priming sprays should be performed before the metered-dose inhaler is used for the first time or when it has not been used in more than 24 hours.

## Inhalation Dosage Forms
Note: The strength of the dosage form available is expressed in terms of albuterol base.

### IPRATROPIUM BROMIDE AND ALBUTEROL SULFATE INHALATON AEROSOL

**Usual adult dose**
Pulmonary disease, chronic obstructive—
Oral inhalation, 2 inhalations four times a day and as required; however, the total number of inhalations should not exceed 12 inhalations in twenty-four hours.

**Usual adult prescribing limits**
12 inhalations in twenty-four hours.

**Usual pediatric dose**
Safety and efficacy have not been established.

**Usual geriatric dose**
See *Usual adult dose*.

**Strength(s) usually available**
U.S.—
18 mcg ipratropium bromide and 90 mcg albuterol (base) per metered spray (Rx) [*Combivent* (chlorofluorocarbons (CFCs))].

**Packaging and storage**
Store between 15 and 30 °C (59 and 86 °F); avoid excessive humidity.

**Auxiliary labeling**
• Shake well before using.
• For oral inhalation only.

**Note**
Include patient instructions when dispensing.

Developed: 06/17/97
Interim revision: 07/29/98

---

# IRBESARTAN  Systemic—INTRODUCTORY VERSION

VA CLASSIFICATION (Primary/Secondary): CV805/CV409
Note: For a listing of dosage forms and brand names by country availability, see *Dosage Forms* section(s).

## Category
Antihypertensive.

## Indications
**Accepted**
Hypertension (treatment)—Irbesartan is indicated for the treatment of hypertension. It may be used alone or in combination with other antihypertensive medications.

## Pharmacology/Pharmacokinetics

**Physicochemical characteristics**
Molecular weight—428.5.

**Mechanism of action/Effect**
Irbesartan is a nonpeptide angiotensin II antagonist that selectively blocks the binding of angiotensin II to the $AT_1$ receptor. In the renin-angiotensin system, angiotensin I is converted by angiotensin-converting enzyme (ACE) to form angiotensin II. Angiotensin II stimulates the adrenal cortex to synthesize and secrete aldosterone, which decreases the excretion of sodium and increases the excretion of potassium. Angiotensin II also acts as a vasoconstrictor in vascular smooth muscle. Irbesartan, by blocking the binding of angiotensin II to the $AT_1$ receptor, promotes vasodilation and decreases the effects of aldosterone. The negative feedback regulation of angiotensin II on renin secretion also is inhibited, but the resulting rise in plasma renin concentrations and consequent rise in angiotensin II plasma concentrations do not counteract the blood pressure–lowering effect that occurs.

**Absorption**
Rapid and complete; average absolute bioavailability ranges from 60 to 80%. Food does not affect the bioavailability of irbesartan.

**Distribution**
Volume of distribution ($Vol_D$)—53 to 93 liters. Irbesartan crosses the blood-brain barrier and placenta in low concentrations.

**Protein binding**
High (90%), primarily to albumin and alpha$_1$-acid glycoprotein.

**Biotransformation**
Irbesartan is metabolized by glucuronide conjugation and oxidation. Following oral or intravenous administration of radiolabeled irbesartan, more than 80% of the circulating plasma radioactivity is attributed to unchanged irbesartan. The primary metabolite is the inactive irbesartan glucuronide conjugate and accounts for approximately 6% of circulating metabolites. The remaining oxidative metabolites are considered to be inactive. *In vitro* studies indicate that irbesartan is oxidized primarily by the cytochrome P450 2C9 isoenzyme.

**Half-life**
Elimination—11 to 15 hours.

**Time to peak concentration**
1.5 to 2 hours.

**Elimination**
Renal—Approximately 20%.
Fecal (biliary)—Approximately 80%.
In dialysis—Irbesartan is not removable by hemodialysis.

## Precautions to Consider

**Carcinogenicity**
No evidence of carcinogenicity was found in a 2-year study in male rats given irbesartan in doses of up to 500 mg per kg of body weight (mg/kg) per day or in female rats given irbesartan in doses of up to 1000 mg/kg per day or in mice given irbesartan in doses of up to 1000 mg/kg per day. In male and female rats, a 500 mg/kg dose represents 3 and 11 times, respectively, the maximum recommended human daily dose (MRHDD) of 300 mg of irbesartan. In female rats, a 1000 mg/kg dose represents approximately 21 times the MRHDD of 300 mg of irbesartan. For male and female mice a 1000 mg/kg dose represents approximately 3 and 5 times, respectively, the MRHDD of 300 mg of irbesartan.

**Mutagenicity**
Irbesartan was not found to be mutagenic in the Ames microbial test, rat hepatocyte DNA repair test, or V79 mammalian-cell forward gene mu-

tation assay. Irbesartan was found to be negative for the induction of chromosomal aberrations in the *in vitro* human lymphocyte assay and in the *in vivo* mouse micronucleus study.

**Pregnancy/Reproduction**

Fertility—Irbesartan had no adverse effects on fertility or mating behavior of male or female rats given oral doses of ≤ 650 mg/kg per day. The 650 mg/kg dose of irbesartan represents approximately five times the MRHDD of 300 mg.

Pregnancy—Fetal exposure to drugs that act directly on the renin-angiotensin system during the second and third trimesters can cause hypotension, reversible or irreversible renal failure, anuria, neonatal skull hypoplasia, and death in the fetus or neonate. Irbesartan should be discontinued as soon as possible when pregnancy is detected, unless no alternative therapy can be used. If medication is continued, serial ultrasound examinations should be performed to assess the intra-amniotic environment. Perinatal diagnostic tests, such as contraction-stress testing (CST), a nonstress test (NST), or biophysical profiling (BPP) also may be appropriate during the applicable week of pregnancy.

Maternal oligohydramnios, which may result from decreased fetal renal function, has been reported, and is associated with fetal limb contractures, craniofacial deformation, and hypoplastic lung development. If oligohydramnios is observed, irbesartan should be discontinued unless it is considered lifesaving for the mother. Oligohydramnios may not appear until after the fetus has sustained irreversible damage. Other adverse effects that have been reported are prematurity, intrauterine growth retardation, and patent ductus arteriosus, although it is not clear how these effects are related to drug exposure. When limited to the first trimester, exposure to this medication does not appear to be associated with these adverse effects.

Infants exposed *in utero* to angiotensin II receptor antagonists should be observed closely for hypotension, oliguria, and hyperkalemia. Oliguria should be treated with support of blood pressure and renal perfusion. Dialysis or exchange transfusion may be necessary to reverse hypotension and/or substitute for disordered renal function.

Studies in pregnant rats given oral daily doses of 50, 180, and 650 mg/kg of irbesartan from day 0 to day 20 of gestation revealed increased incidences of renal pelvic cavitation, hydroureter, and/or absence of renal papilla in fetuses at doses ≥ 50 mg/kg (approximately equivalent to the MRHDD of 300 mg, based on a body surface area). Subcutaneous edema was observed in fetuses of rats given daily doses of ≥ 180 mg/kg. This dose represents approximately four times the maximum recommended human dose (MRHD) on a body surface area basis. Because these anomalies were not observed in rats given daily oral irbesartan doses of 50, 150, and 450 mg/kg limited to gestation days 6 through 15, they appear to reflect late gestational effects of irbesartan. In pregnant rabbits, oral daily doses of irbesartan of 30 mg/kg were associated with maternal mortality and abortion. In the surviving female rabbits given this dose (equivalent to approximately 1.5 times the MRHD on a body surface area basis), a slight increase in early resorptions and a corresponding decrease in live fetuses occurred. Irbesartan was found to cross the placental barrier in rats and rabbits. Radioactivity was present in the fetuses of rats and rabbits during late gestation following oral doses of radiolabeled irbesartan.

FDA Pregnancy Category C (first trimester).
FDA Pregnancy Category D (second and third trimesters).

**Breast-feeding**

It is not known whether irbesartan is distributed into breast milk, but irbesartan and/or its metabolite(s) is distributed into the milk of lactating rats at a low concentration. Because of the potential for adverse effects in the nursing infant, irbesartan should not be administered to nursing mothers.

**Pediatrics**

No information is available on the relationship of age to the effects of irbesartan in pediatric patients. Safety and efficacy have not been established in patients younger than 18 years of age. Infants exposed *in utero* to angiotensin II receptor antagonists should be observed closely for hypotension, oliguria, and hyperkalemia. Oliguria should be treated with support of blood pressure and renal perfusion. Dialysis or exchange transfusion may be necessary to reverse hypotension and/or substitute for disordered renal function. See *Pregnancy/Reproduction* section.

**Geriatrics**

In subjects 65 to 80 years of age, irbesartan elimination half-life is not significantly altered, but the area under the plasma concentration–time curve (AUC) and maximum plasma concentration ($C_{max}$) values may be greater by 20 to 50% than those in subjects 18 to 40 years of age. No dosage adjustment is necessary in the elderly. However, the elderly may experience greater sensitivity to the effects of irbesartan.

**Pharmacogenetics**

In female patients with hypertension, irbesartan plasma concentrations are increased by 11 to 44%; however, no gender-related dosage adjustment is necessary. In healthy black subjects, the AUC is 25% greater than in white patients. Black patients, usually a low-renin population, may experience a smaller reduction in blood pressure with irbesartan treatment than white patients.

**Drug interactions and/or related problems**

The following drug interactions and/or related problems have been selected on the basis of their potential clinical significance (possible mechanism in parentheses where appropriate)—not necessarily inclusive (» = major clinical significance):

Note: Combinations containing any of the following medications, depending on the amount present, may also interact with this medication.

» Diuretics
  (concurrent use with irbesartan may have additive hypotensive effects)

Medications that inhibit the cytochrome P450 2C9 isoenzyme or
Medications that are metabolized by cytochrome P450 2C9 (the isoenzyme responsible for irbesartan metabolism), such as
  Tolbutamide
  (*in vitro* studies show that irbesartan metabolism may be affected by medications that are metabolized by or inhibit the cytochrome P450 2C9 isoenzyme, although no clinically relevant interactions have been observed)

**Laboratory value alterations**

The following have been selected on the basis of their potential clinical significance (possible effect in parentheses where appropriate)—not necessarily inclusive (» = major clinical significance):

With physiology/laboratory test values
  Creatinine, serum and
  Blood urea nitrogen (BUN)
    (increases in serum creatinine or BUN concentrations have occurred in patients with unilateral or bilateral renal artery stenosis who were treated with angiotensin-converting enzyme (ACE) inhibitors, and a similar effect may occur with irbesartan treatment; minor increases in concentrations occurred in 0.7% of patients treated with irbesartan in clinical trials)

**Medical considerations/Contraindications**

The medical considerations/contraindications included have been selected on the basis of their potential clinical significance (reasons given in parentheses where appropriate)—not necessarily inclusive (» = major clinical significance).

*Except under special circumstances, this medication should not be used when the following medical problem exists:*

» Hypersensitivity to irbesartan

*Risk-benefit should be considered when the following medical problems exist:*

» Congestive heart failure, severe
  (therapy with angiotensin receptor antagonists in these patients, who may be especially susceptible to changes in the renin-angiotensin-aldosterone system, has been associated with oliguria, azotemia, acute renal failure, and/or death)

Dehydration
  (sodium or volume depletion, due to excessive perspiration, vomiting, diarrhea, prolonged diuretic therapy, dialysis, or dietary salt restriction)
  (a reduction in salt or fluid volume may increase the risk of symptomatic hypotension)

Renal artery stenosis, unilateral or bilateral or
Renal function impairment
  (increases in serum creatinine or BUN concentrations have occurred in patients with unilateral or bilateral renal artery stenosis who were treated with ACE inhibitors and a similar effect may occur with irbesartan treatment; therapy with angiotensin receptor–antagonists in patients susceptible to changes in the renin-angiotensin-aldosterone system, such as patients with severe congestive heart failure, has been associated with oliguria, progressive azotemia, acute renal failure, and/or death)

**Patient monitoring**

The following may be especially important in patient monitoring (other tests may be warranted in some patients, depending on condition; » = major clinical significance):

» Blood pressure measurements
  (periodic monitoring is necessary for titration of dose according to the patient's response)

## Side/Adverse Effects

The following side/adverse effects have been selected on the basis of their potential clinical significance (possible signs and symptoms in parentheses where appropriate)—not necessarily inclusive:

**Those indicating need for medical attention**
Incidence rare
> *Hypotension* (dizziness, lightheadedness, or fainting)—usually seen in volume- or salt-depleted patients receiving high doses of a diuretic
>> Note: *Hypotension* occurred in 0.4% of patients receiving irbesartan in clinical trials.

**Those indicating need for medical attention only if they continue or are bothersome**
Incidence less frequent
> *Anxiety and/or nervousness; diarrhea; dizziness; dyspepsia* (belching; heartburn; stomach discomfort); *fatigue* (unusual tiredness); *headache; musculoskeletal pain* (muscle or bone pain); *upper respiratory infection* (cold symptoms)

## Overdose

For more information on the management of overdose or unintentional ingestion, **contact a Poison Control Center** (see *Poison Control Center Listing*).

**Clinical effects of overdose**
The following effects have been selected on the basis of their potential clinical significance (possible signs and symptoms in parentheses where appropriate)—not necessarily inclusive:

Acute and/or chronic
> *Bradycardia* (slow heartbeat); *hypotension* (dizziness, lightheadedness, or fainting); *tachycardia* (fast heartbeat)

**Treatment of overdose**
Treatment should be symptomatic and supportive.

Supportive care—Patients in whom intentional overdose is confirmed or suspected should be referred for psychiatric consultation.

## Patient Consultation

As an aid to patient consultation, refer to *Advice for the Patient, Irbesartan (Systemic)—Introductory Version*.
In providing consultation, consider emphasizing the following selected information (» = major clinical significance):

**Before using this medication**
» Conditions affecting use, especially:
>> Hypersensitivity to irbesartan
>> Pregnancy—Fetal and neonatal hypotension, skull hypoplasia, renal failure, and death have been reported in humans; irbesartan should be discontinued as soon as possible when pregnancy is detected
>> Breast-feeding—Irbesartan is distributed into milk of lactating rats; use is not recommended in nursing mothers
>> Use in the elderly—Elderly patients may experience greater sensitivity to the effects of irbesartan
>> Other medications, especially diuretics
>> Other medical problems, especially severe congestive heart failure

**Proper use of this medication**
» Compliance with therapy; taking medication at the same time each day to maintain the therapeutic effect
» Proper dosing
> Missed dose: Taking as soon as possible; not taking if almost time for next scheduled dose; not doubling doses
» Proper storage

**Precautions while using this medication**
> Regular visits to physician to check progress
» Notifying physician immediately if pregnancy is suspected because of possibility of fetal or neonatal injury and/or death
> Not taking other medications without consulting the physician
» Caution when driving or doing other things requiring alertness because of possible dizziness
> Checking with physician if severe nausea, vomiting, or diarrhea occurs and continues because of risk of dehydration, which may result in hypotension
> Caution when exercising or during exposure to hot weather because of risk of dehydration, which may result in hypotension

**Side/adverse effects**
> Signs of potential side effects, especially hypotension

## General Dosing Information

Dosage must be adjusted, on the basis of clinical response to meet the individual requirements of each patient.

**Diet/Nutrition**
Irbesartan may be administered with or without food.

**For treatment of adverse effects**
Recommended treatment consists of the following:
• Treatment of symptomatic hypotension involves placing the patient in a supine position and, if needed, administering normal saline intravenously.

## Oral Dosage Forms

### IRBESARTAN TABLETS

**Usual adult dose**
Hypertension—
> Oral, initially 150 mg once a day. If blood pressure reduction is not adequate, the dosage may be increased to up to 300 mg once a day.
> If blood pressure is not controlled by irbesartan alone, a low dose of a diuretic, such as hydrochlorothiazide, may be added. Patients not adequately controlled by the maximum irbesartan dose of 300 mg once a day are unlikely to derive additional benefit from a higher dose or twice-daily dosing.
> In patients who are volume- and/or salt-depleted, such as those treated vigorously with diuretics or on hemodialysis, a lower initial dose of 75 mg of irbesartan is recommended.

**Usual adult prescribing limits**
300 mg.

**Usual pediatric dose**
Safety and efficacy have not been established in children younger than 18 years of age.

**Strength(s) usually available**
U.S.—
> 75 mg (Rx) [*Avapro*].
> 150 mg (Rx) [*Avapro*].
> 300 mg (Rx) [*Avapro*].

**Packaging and storage**
Store between 15 and 30 ºC (59 and 86 ºF).

**Auxiliary labeling**
• Do not take other medicines without your doctor's advice.

Developed: 01/05/98
Interim revision: 08/10/98

---

# IRINOTECAN    Systemic

VA CLASSIFICATION (Primary): AN900
Commonly used brand name(s): *Camptosar*.
Another commonly used name is CPT-11.
Note: For a listing of dosage forms and brand names by country availability, see *Dosage Forms* section(s).

## Category
Antineoplastic.

## Indications

**Accepted**
Carcinoma, colorectal (treatment)—Irinotecan is indicated for treatment of metastatic carcinoma of the colon or rectum that has progressed during or recurred following first-line chemotherapy with fluorouracil (5-FU).

## Pharmacology/Pharmacokinetics

**Physicochemical characteristics**
Source—Semisynthetic derivative of camptothecin, an alkaloid extracted from plants, e.g., *Camptotheca acuminata*.

**Molecular weight**—Irinotecan hydrochloride: 677.2.
**pH**—3.5.
**Solubility**—Slightly soluble in water and in organic solvents.

### Mechanism of action/Effect
Irinotecan and its active metabolite, SN-38, inhibit the action of topoisomerase I, an enzyme that produces reversible single-strand breaks in DNA during DNA replication. These single-strand breaks relieve torsional strain and allow DNA replication to proceed. Irinotecan and SN-38 bind to the topoisomerase I–DNA complex and prevent religation of the DNA strand, resulting in double-strand DNA breakage and cell death.

Note: Although SN-38 is approximately 2 to 2000 times more potent than the parent compound in various *in vitro* cytotoxicity assays, the precise contribution of the metabolite to the activity of irinotecan in humans is not known because its protein binding is significantly higher, and its area under the plasma concentration–time curve (AUC) is much lower, than those of irinotecan.

### Distribution
The volume of distribution (Vol$_D$) of the terminal elimination phase for irinotecan is 110 liters per square meter of body surface area.

### Protein binding
Irinotecan—Moderate (30 to 68%), primarily to albumin.
SN-38 metabolite—Very high (95%), primarily to albumin.

### Biotransformation
Primarily hepatic, via carboxylase-mediated cleavage of the carbamate bond. Conversion to the active metabolite (SN-38) is rapid. SN-38 undergoes conjugation to form a glucuronide metabolite, which is 50 to 100 times less active than SN-38.

Irinotecan and SN-38 both undergo reversible, pH-dependent conversion between their two forms, an active lactone and an inactive hydroxyacid. Whereas only the lactone form is present at an acidic pH, the hydroxyacid form predominates at physiologic pH.

### Half-life
Terminal—
Irinotecan: Mean, 5.8 hours (5.5 hours in patients younger than 65 years of age and 6 hours in older patients).
SN-38 metabolite: Mean, 10.4 hours.

### Time to peak concentration
SN-38 metabolite—Peak plasma concentrations occur within 1 hour after administration of a 90-minute infusion.

### Peak plasma concentration
Following a dose of 125 mg per square meter of body surface area (mg/m$^2$)—
Irinotecan: 1660 ± 797 nanograms per mL.
SN-38 metabolite: 26.3 ± 11.9 nanograms per mL.

Note: AUC values for 24 hours following a 125-mg/m$^2$ dose of irinotecan, administered as a 90-minute infusion, are 10,200 ± 3270 nanograms per mL per hour for irinotecan and 229 ± 108 nanograms per mL per hour for the SN-38 metabolite. Values in patients with hepatic metastases are somewhat higher. Also, dose-normalized values are 11% higher in patients 65 years of age or older than in younger patients.

### Elimination
Renal—11 to 20% of a dose as unchanged irinotecan; < 1% of a dose as SN-38; 1 to 3% of a dose as SN-38 glucuronide.
Combined biliary and renal—In two patients, 25% of a 100-mg/m$^2$ dose and 50% of a 300-mg/m$^2$ dose were excreted within 48 hours after intravenous administration.
Total systemic clearance of irinotecan—13.3 ± 6.01 liters per hour per square meter of body surface area after a 125-mg/m$^2$ dose.

Note: The effect of hepatic or renal function impairment on elimination of irinotecan and its metabolites has not been formally studied. However, because relatively small quantities of irinotecan are eliminated via renal excretion, it is unlikely that renal function impairment would have a major influence on the pharmacokinetics of irinotecan.

## Precautions to Consider

### Carcinogenicity
Secondary malignancies are potential delayed effects of many antineoplastic agents, although it is not clear whether the effect is related to their mutagenic or immunosuppressive action. The effect of dose and duration of therapy is also unknown, although the risk seems to increase with long-term use. There is some evidence linking therapy with topoisomerase I inhibitors, such as irinotecan, to the development of acute leukemias associated with specific chromosomal translocations.

Long-term carcinogenicity studies in animals have not been done with irinotecan. However, a significant dose-related trend for the development of uterine horn endometrial stromal polyps and endometrial stromal sarcomas was found in studies in rats given 2 mg per kg of body weight (mg/kg) or 25 mg/kg once weekly for 13 weeks, then allowed to recover for 91 weeks. The 25-mg/kg dose produced maximum plasma concentration (C$_{max}$) and area under the plasma concentration–time curve (AUC) values equivalent to seven times and 1.3 times, respectively, the values for irinotecan in humans receiving 125 mg per square meter of body surface area (mg/m$^2$).

### Mutagenicity
Irinotecan was clastogenic in *in vitro* (chromosome aberrations in Chinese hamster ovary cells) and *in vivo* (micronucleus test in mice) mammalian test systems. However, neither irinotecan nor its active metabolite, SN-38, was mutagenic in the Ames test.

### Pregnancy/Reproduction
Fertility—Irinotecan produced no significant effect on reproductive performance or fertility in rats and rabbits given up to 6 mg/kg per day. However, atrophy of male reproductive organs occurred in rodents given multiple daily intravenous doses of 20 mg/kg (producing C$_{max}$ values approximately five times, and AUC values approximately equal to, the values for irinotecan in humans receiving 125 mg/m$^2$), and in dogs given multiple daily intravenous doses of 0.4 mg/kg (producing C$_{max}$ and AUC values approximately 50% and 6.6%, respectively, of the values for irinotecan in humans receiving 125 mg/m$^2$).

Pregnancy—Adequate and well-controlled studies in humans have not been done.

It is usually recommended that use of antineoplastics, especially combination chemotherapy, be avoided whenever possible, especially during the first trimester. Although information is limited because of the relatively few instances of antineoplastic therapy during pregnancy, the mutagenic, teratogenic, and carcinogenic potential of these medications must be considered.

Other potential hazards to the fetus include adverse reactions seen in adults. In general, use of a contraceptive is recommended during therapy with cytotoxic medications.

Studies in rats have demonstrated that irinotecan crosses the placenta. Irinotecan was embryotoxic, causing increased postimplantation losses and decreased numbers of live fetuses, in rats and rabbits given 6 mg/kg per day (a dose that produced C$_{max}$ and AUC values in rats that are approximately two times and 0.2 times the respective values in humans receiving 125 mg/m$^2$. In rabbits, this dose is equivalent to approximately half of the recommended human dose on a mg/m$^2$ basis). Also, irinotecan was teratogenic, causing external, visceral, and skeletal abnormalities in rats given more than 1.2 mg/kg per day (producing C$_{max}$ and AUC values equivalent to two thirds and one fortieth the respective values in humans receiving 125 mg/m$^2$) and in rabbits administered 6 mg/kg per day (a dose equivalent to approximately half of the recommended human dose on a mg/m$^2$ basis).

FDA Pregnancy Category D.

### Breast-feeding
Although very little information is available regarding distribution of antineoplastic agents into breast milk, breast-feeding is not recommended while irinotecan is being administered because of the risks to the infant (adverse effects, mutagenicity, carcinogenicity). It is not known whether irinotecan is distributed into human breast milk.

Animal studies have shown that irinotecan is rapidly distributed into the milk of lactating rats. Four hours after administration, the concentration in milk was 65 times higher than the simultaneous plasma concentration, indicating that the medication accumulates in breast milk. Also, administration of 6 mg/kg per day of irinotecan to rat dams from the period following organogenesis through weaning caused lower female body weight and decreased learning ability in the offspring.

### Pediatrics
Appropriate studies on the relationship of age to the effects of irinotecan have not been performed in the pediatric population. Safety and efficacy have not been established.

### Geriatrics
Approximately 54% of the patients in clinical trials were 65 years of age or older. These studies showed that the risk of severe diarrhea (but not of severe neutropenia) is significantly increased in geriatric patients. Careful monitoring is recommended. Although some pharmacokinetic parameters are altered in the geriatric population (slight increases in terminal half-life and AUC), no adjustment of initial dosage on the basis of age is needed.

### Dental
The bone marrow depressant effects of irinotecan may result in an increased incidence of microbial infection, delayed healing, and gingival bleeding. Dental work, whenever possible, should be completed prior to initiation of therapy or deferred until blood counts have returned to normal. Patients should be instructed in proper oral hygiene during treat-

ment, including caution in use of regular toothbrushes, dental floss, and toothpicks.

Irinotecan may cause stomatitis, which is usually mild. In clinical trials, stomatitis occurred in 11.8%, and was severe (U.S. National Cancer Institute [NCI] grades 3 or 4) in 0.7% of the patients.

### Drug interactions and/or related problems

The following drug interactions and/or related problems have been selected on the basis of their potential clinical significance (possible mechanism in parentheses where appropriate)—not necessarily inclusive (» = major clinical significance):

Note: Combinations containing any of the following medications, depending on the amount present, may also interact with this medication.

Blood dyscrasia–causing medications (see *Appendix II*)
(the leukopenic and/or thrombocytopenic effects of irinotecan may be increased with concurrent or recent therapy if these medications cause the same effects; dosage adjustment of irinotecan, if necessary, should be based on blood cell counts)

» Bone marrow depressants, other (see *Appendix II*) or
» Radiation therapy, current or history of
(additive bone marrow depression may occur; dosage reduction may be required when two or more bone marrow depressants, including radiation, are used concurrently or consecutively. Studies have shown that the risk of severe irinotecan-induced myelosuppression is significantly higher in patients who have received previous radiation therapy of the pelvis or abdomen. Concurrent use of irinotecan with radiation therapy has not been adequately studied and is not recommended)

Dexamethasone
(prophylactic use of dexamethasone as an antiemetic prior to irinotecan administration may result in hyperglycemia, especially in patients with a history of diabetes or glucose intolerance, and may also increase the occurrence of lymphocytopenia)

» Diuretics
(careful monitoring during concurrent therapy with irinotecan is recommended because diuretics may increase the severity of dehydration associated with irinotecan-induced diarrhea or vomiting; withholding diuretic treatment during periods of active diarrhea or vomiting may be prudent)

» Immunosuppressants, other, such as:
Azathioprine
Chlorambucil
Corticosteroids, glucocorticoid
Cyclophosphamide
Cyclosporine
Mercaptopurine
Muromonab-CD3
Mycophenolate
Tacrolimus
(concurrent use with irinotecan may increase the risk of infection)

» Laxatives
(concurrent use with irinotecan may increase the risk of severe diarrhea and should be avoided)

Vaccines, killed virus
(because normal defense mechanisms may be suppressed by irinotecan therapy, the patient's antibody response to the vaccine may be decreased. The interval between discontinuation of medications that cause immunosuppression and restoration of the patient's ability to respond to the vaccine depends on the intensity and type of immunosuppression-causing medication used, the underlying disease, and other factors; estimates vary from 3 months to 1 year)

» Vaccines, live virus
(because normal defense mechanisms may be suppressed by irinotecan therapy, concurrent use with a live virus vaccine may potentiate the replication of the vaccine virus, may increase the side/adverse effects of the vaccine virus, and/or may decrease the patient's antibody response to the vaccine; immunization of these patients should be undertaken only with extreme caution after careful review of the patient's hematologic status and only with the knowledge and consent of the physician managing the irinotecan therapy. The interval between discontinuation of medications that cause immunosuppression and restoration of the patient's ability to respond to the vaccine depends on the intensity and type of immunosuppression-causing medication used, the underlying disease, and other factors; estimates vary from 3 months to 1 year. In addition, immunization with oral poliovirus vaccine should be postponed in persons in close contact with the patient, especially family members)

### Laboratory value alterations

The following have been selected on the basis of their potential clinical significance (possible effect in parentheses where appropriate)—not necessarily inclusive (» = major clinical significance):

With physiology/laboratory test values
Alkaline phosphatase, serum and
Aspartate aminotransferase (AST [SGOT]), serum
(values may be increased, especially in patients with hepatic metastases)

» Hemoglobin concentration and
» Leukocyte count and
Platelet count
(may be decreased; anemia, leukopenia, and neutropenia occurred in approximately 60%, 63%, and 54%, respectively, of the patients in clinical trials, but severe thrombocytopenia was uncommon)

### Medical considerations/Contraindications

The medical considerations/contraindications included have been selected on the basis of their potential clinical significance (reasons given in parentheses where appropriate)—not necessarily inclusive (» = major clinical significance).

***Risk-benefit should be considered when the following medical problems exist:***

» Bone marrow depression, pre-existing or treatment-related
(will be increased; delay, omission, and/or reduction of subsequent doses of irinotecan may be needed, depending on cell counts; a new course of irinotecan therapy should not be initiated until the granulocyte count has recovered to 1500 cells per cubic millimeter [cells/mm³] and the platelet count has recovered to 100,000 cells/mm³)

» Chickenpox, existing or recent (including recent exposure) or
» Herpes zoster
(risk of severe, generalized disease)

» Hepatic function impairment
(the risk of severe [U.S. National Cancer Institute (NCI) grade 3 or 4] neutropenia during the first course of irinotecan therapy may be substantially increased in patients with modest increases in serum bilirubin [concentrations between 1 and 2 mg/dL], and there is some evidence that patients with abnormal glucuronidation of bilirubin [e.g., patients with Gilbert's syndrome] may also be at relatively higher risk of irinotecan-induced myelosuppression. Studies have not been done in patients with more severe hepatic function impairment [serum bilirubin concentrations > 2 mg/dL or transaminase values > 3 times the upper limit of normal (ULN) in the absence of hepatic metastases, or transaminase values > 5 times the ULN in the presence of hepatic metastases]. A reduction in the initial dose of irinotecan should be considered)

» Infection, pre-existing
(recovery may be impaired)

Sensitivity to irinotecan

» Pulmonary disease or impairment
(a potentially life-threatening syndrome consisting of dyspnea, fever, and reticulonodular pattern on chest radiograph occurred in some patients with pre-existing lung tumors or nonmalignant pulmonary disease in early clinical trials [conducted in Japan]; although the extent to which irinotecan may have been responsible for this complication has not been established, caution is recommended)

» Caution should also be used in patients who have had previous cytotoxic drug therapy or radiation therapy. In addition, caution should be used in patients with poor performance status because of a higher risk of diarrhea and neutropenia.

### Patient monitoring

The following may be especially important in patient monitoring (other tests may be warranted in some patients, depending on condition; » = major clinical significance):

» Hemoglobin concentration and
» Leukocyte count, total and differential and
» Platelet count
(determinations recommended prior to each course of irinotecan therapy; delay, omission, and/or reduction of subsequent doses is recommended if significant hematologic toxicity is present [e.g., granulocyte count lower than 1500 cells/mm³ and/or platelet count lower than 100,000 cells/mm³])

## Side/Adverse Effects

Note: In addition to the side/adverse effects listed below, a potentially life-threatening syndrome consisting of dyspnea, fever, and a reti-

## 1772  Irinotecan (Systemic)

culonodular pattern on chest radiograph occurred in some patients in early clinical trials. Because this pulmonary syndrome appeared in patients with lung tumors or other pulmonary disease, the extent to which irinotecan may have contributed to this complication has not been established.

The following side/adverse effects have been selected on the basis of their potential clinical significance (possible signs and symptoms in parentheses where appropriate)—not necessarily inclusive:

### Those indicating need for medical attention
Incidence more frequent
>   *Anemia* (unusual tiredness or weakness, severe)—usually asymptomatic; *diarrhea, possibly preceded by abdominal cramping and/or sweating; dyspnea* (shortness of breath or troubled breathing)—may be associated with pulmonary metastases or other pre-existing lung disease; *fever; leukopenia*—usually asymptomatic; *neutropenia*—usually asymptomatic

>   Note: Phase I trials with irinotecan identified *diarrhea* as one of the medication's dose-limiting toxicities. Diarrhea may occur early (during or within 24 hours after administration of irinotecan) or late (more than 24 hours after administration of irinotecan; the median time to onset in clinical trials was 11 days), and may be severe. The early form of diarrhea is cholinergic in nature; it may be preceded by other symptoms of a cholinergic syndrome, including abdominal cramping and diaphoresis, and is usually short-lasting. In clinical trials, early diarrhea occurred in 50.7%, and was severe (U.S. National Cancer Institute [NCI] grade 3 or 4) in 7.9%, of the patients. The late form of diarrhea may be severe and prolonged enough to cause life-threatening dehydration and electrolyte disturbances. In clinical trials, late diarrhea occurred in 87.8%, and was severe (NCI grade 3 or 4) in 30.6%, of the patients. The median durations of late diarrhea of any grade and of NCI grade 3 or 4 were 3 days and 7 days, respectively. Ulceration of the colon, sometimes with bleeding, has also been reported during therapy.

>   *Neutropenia* is the other dose-limiting toxicity of irinotecan. Although neutropenia occurred in 53.9%, and was severe (NCI grade 3 or 4) in 26.3%, of the patients in clinical trials, the incidence of neutropenic fever (grade 4 neutropenia with grade 2 or higher fever) was relatively low (3%). However, deaths due to myelosuppression-related sepsis have been reported.

Incidence less frequent
>   *Abdominal enlargement* (swelling of abdominal or stomach area); *dehydration* (decreased urination; dizziness or lightheadedness, severe; dryness of mouth; fainting; increased thirst; wrinkled skin)—associated with severe diarrhea and/or vomiting; *edema* (swelling of face, fingers, feet or lower legs); *infection, minor, usually upper respiratory* (cough; hoarseness; runny or stuffy nose; sore throat); *neutropenic fever* (fever or chills; cough or hoarseness; lower back or side pain; painful or difficult urination; sore throat)

Incidence rare
>   *Thrombocytopenia* (unusual bleeding or bruising; black, tarry stools; blood in urine or stools; pinpoint red spots on skin)—usually asymptomatic

### Those indicating need for medical attention only if they continue or are bothersome
Incidence more frequent
>   *Abdominal cramps or pain; asthenia* (weakness); *constipation; decrease in or loss of appetite; nausea and vomiting; weight loss*

>   Note: *Nausea and vomiting* may occur early (within 24 hours after administration of irinotecan) or late (more than 24 hours after administration of irinotecan), and may be severe.

Incidence less frequent
>   *Bloated feeling or gas; headache; increased sweating; indigestion; rhinitis* (runny nose); *skin rash; stomatitis* (sores, ulcers, or white spots on lips or in mouth)

### Those not indicating need for medical attention
Incidence more frequent
>   *Alopecia* (loss of hair); *vasodilation* (flushing)

## Overdose
For specific information on the agents used in the management of irinotecan overdose, see the *Colony Stimulating Factors (Systemic)* monograph.
For more information on the management of overdose, **contact a Poison Control Center** (see *Poison Control Center Listing*).

### Clinical effects of overdose
The following effects have been selected on the basis of their potential clinical significance (possible signs and symptoms in parentheses where appropriate)—not necessarily inclusive:

Acute and chronic
>   *Diarrhea; leukopenia or neutropenia, including neutropenic fever* (fever or chills; cough or hoarseness; lower back or side pain; painful or difficult urination; sore throat)

>   Note: Single doses as high as 750 mg per square meter of body surface area (mg/m$^2$) have been given to some participants in clinical trials. The adverse effects were similar to, but more severe than, those that typically occur with usual doses of irinotecan.

>   In acute toxicity studies in animals, lethal single doses of irinotecan (111 mg per kg of body weight [mg/kg] in mice and 73 mg/kg in rats) produced cyanosis, tremors, respiratory distress, and convulsions prior to death.

### Treatment of overdose
It is recommended that the patient be hospitalized for close monitoring of vital functions and treatment of observed effects. Severe bone marrow depression may require transfusion of required blood components. A colony-stimulating factor may also be used to treat leukopenia or neutropenia. Febrile neutropenia should be treated empirically with broad-spectrum antibiotics, pending bacterial cultures and appropriate diagnostic tests.

Supportive care to prevent and treat dehydration associated with severe diarrhea is also recommended.

## Patient Consultation
As an aid to patient consultation, refer to *Advice for the Patient, Irinotecan (Systemic)*.
In providing consultation, consider emphasizing the following selected information (» = major clinical significance):

### Before using this medication
» Conditions affecting use, especially:
> Sensitivity to irinotecan
> Pregnancy—Use not recommended because of embryotoxic, teratogenic, and carcinogenic potential; advisability of using contraception; notifying physician immediately if pregnancy is suspected
> Breast-feeding—Not recommended because of risk of serious side effects
> Use in the elderly—Increased risk of severe diarrhea; close monitoring is recommended
> Other medications, especially other bone marrow depressants, diuretics, other immunosuppressants, laxatives, and radiation therapy or history of
> Other medical problems, especially ascites; chickenpox, current or recent (including recent exposure); herpes zoster; infection; pleural effusions; and pulmonary disease or impairment

### Proper use of this medication
» Frequency of nausea and vomiting; importance of continuing treatment despite stomach upset; physician or nurse can advise on methods of minimizing discomfort
» Proper dosing

### Precautions while using this medication
» Importance of close monitoring by the physician; need for periodic blood tests to check for asymptomatic side effects
» Avoiding immunizations unless approved by physician; other persons in patient's household should avoid immunizations with oral poliovirus vaccine; avoiding other persons who have taken oral poliovirus vaccine or wearing a protective mask that covers the nose and mouth

*Caution if diarrhea occurs*
» Notifying physician of occurrence immediately; informing physician if diarrhea is occurring within 24 hours after an infusion or was preceded by abdominal cramping or diaphoresis
» For late diarrhea (starting more than 24 hours after a dose): Starting treatment with loperamide as soon as an increased frequency or decreased consistency of bowel movement is noted, using a dosage regimen prescribed by physician or taking 4 mg initially, then 2 mg every 2 hours (or, at night, 4 mg every 4 hours), and continuing until free of diarrhea for 12 hours; not following maximum daily dosage recommendation for loperamide on nonprescription package labeling, which is insufficient for treating this complication
» Notifying physician if vomiting also occurs
» Ensuring adequate fluid replacement; ingesting the type and quantity of fluid recommended by physician

» Avoiding alcohol- or caffeine-containing beverages or medications, which can exacerbate fluid loss, and avoiding bran, raw fruits or vegetables, and fatty, fried, or spicy foods, which can aggravate diarrhea
» Notifying physician if signs and symptoms of dehydration (e.g., decreased urination, dizziness or lightheadedness, dryness of the mouth, fainting, increased thirst, wrinkled skin) occur

*Caution if bone marrow depression occurs*
» Avoiding exposure to persons with infections, especially during periods of low blood counts; checking with physician immediately if fever with or without chills, cough or hoarseness, lower back or side pain, or painful or difficult urination occurs
» Checking with physician immediately if unusual bleeding or bruising; black, tarry stools; blood in urine or stools; or pinpoint red spots on skin occur

Caution in use of regular toothbrush, dental floss, or toothpick; physician, dentist, or nurse may suggest alternatives; checking with physician before having dental work done

Not touching eyes or inside of nose unless hands washed immediately before

Using caution to avoid accidental cuts when using sharp objects, such as safety razor or fingernail or toenail cutters

Avoiding contact sports or other situations where bruising or injury could occur

**Side/adverse effects**
May cause asymptomatic adverse effects such as bone marrow depression; importance of discussing possible effects with physician
Signs of potential side effects, especially anemia, diarrhea with or without abdominal cramping and sweating, dyspnea, fever, abdominal enlargement, dehydration, edema, upper respiratory tract infection, neutropenic fever, and thrombocytopenia
Possibility of hair loss and of vasodilation

## General Dosing Information

It is recommended that irinotecan be administered to patients only under the supervision of a physician experienced in cancer chemotherapy. It is also recommended that equipment and medications necessary for treatment of complications be readily available.

Irinotecan is to be given only by intravenous infusion. Care must be taken to avoid extravasation, and the infusion site should be monitored for signs of inflammation.

To reduce nausea and vomiting associated with irinotecan administration, patients should be premedicated with antiemetic agents, starting at least 30 minutes before the irinotecan infusion. A commonly used prophylactic regimen consists of 10 mg of dexamethasone plus a 5-hydroxytryptamine (serotonin) subtype 3 (5-HT$_3$) receptor antagonist (e.g., ondansetron or granisetron). Another antiemetic, e.g., prochlorperazine, may also be made available to the patient for postinfusion treatment of nausea and vomiting, if necessary.

Prophylactic administration of loperamide, to decrease the occurrence or severity of late diarrhea, is not recommended.

If severe (U.S. National Cancer Institute [NCI] grade 3 or 4) diarrhea or other toxicity occurs, further treatment should be withheld until recovery occurs. A delay of 1 or 2 weeks is usually sufficient. Treatment may then be resumed at a lower dose. However, if recovery does not occur within 2 weeks, discontinuation of treatment should be considered.

Special precautions are recommended for patients who develop thrombocytopenia (platelet count lower than 50,000 cells per cubic millimeter) during treatment. These may include extreme care in performing invasive procedures; regular inspection of intravenous access sites, skin (including the perirectal area), and mucous membrane surfaces for signs of bleeding or bruising; testing urine, emesis, stool, and secretions for occult blood; care in use of regular toothbrushes, dental floss, toothpicks, safety razors, and fingernail and toenail cutters; avoiding constipation; and using caution to prevent falls and other injuries. Such patients should avoid alcohol and aspirin intake because of the risk of gastrointestinal bleeding.

Treatment with irinotecan may be continued as long as a response is achieved or the disease remains stable, provided that therapy is well tolerated.

**Safety considerations for handling this medication**
There is limited but increasing evidence and concern that personnel involved in the preparation and administration of parenteral antineoplastics may be at some risk because of the potential mutagenicity, teratogenicity, and/or carcinogenicity of these agents, although the actual risk is unknown. USP advisory panels recommend cautious handling both in preparation and disposal of antineoplastic agents. Precautions that have been suggested include:

- Use of a biological containment cabinet during reconstitution and dilution of parenteral medications and wearing of disposable surgical gloves and masks.
- Use of proper technique to prevent contamination of the medication, work area, and operator during transfer between containers (including proper training of personnel in this technique).
- Cautious and proper disposal of needles, syringes, vials, ampuls, and unused medication.

A number of medical centers have developed detailed guidelines for handling antineoplastic agents.

If irinotecan comes into contact with the skin, the skin should be washed immediately and thoroughly with soap and water. If the medication comes into contact with a mucous membrane, the area should be immediately and thoroughly flushed with water.

**For treatment of adverse effects**

Early diarrhea (occurring during, or within 24 hours following, an irinotecan infusion, sometimes preceded by abdominal cramping and/or diaphoresis)—0.25 to 1 mg of intravenous atropine, unless contraindicated.

Late diarrhea (occurring more than 24 hours postinfusion)—4 mg of loperamide immediately upon onset of increased frequency or decreased consistency of bowel movements, followed by 2 mg every 2 hours (at night, 4 mg every 4 hours) until diarrhea has been absent for at least 12 hours. Also, experience in a limited number of patients suggests that an alternative regimen consisting of 4 mg of loperamide every three hours plus 25 mg of diphenhydramine every six hours, starting immediately upon onset of increased frequency or decreased consistency of bowel movements, may decrease the occurrence of severe diarrhea significantly. Severe diarrhea also requires careful patient monitoring and fluid and electrolyte replacement as needed.

Leukopenia/neutropenia—Patients who develop leukopenia should be observed carefully for signs and symptoms of infection. Antibiotic support may be required. In neutropenic patients who develop fever, broad-spectrum antibiotic coverage should be initiated empirically, pending bacterial cultures and appropriate diagnostic tests. Use of a colony-stimulating factor may be considered. However, routine use of a colony-stimulating factor to prevent neutropenia during irinotecan treatment is not necessary.

Thrombocytopenia—Platelet transfusions may be required.

Extravasation-induced inflammation—Flushing the site with sterile water, then applying ice.

## Parenteral Dosage Forms

### IRINOTECAN HYDROCHLORIDE INJECTION

**Usual adult dose**
Carcinoma, colorectal—
Intravenous infusion (over ninety minutes), 125 mg per square meter of body surface area once a week for four weeks, followed by a rest period of two weeks. An alternate regimen of 240 to 350 mg per square meter of body surface area (infused over ninety minutes) every three weeks may also be considered.

Note: When the weekly dosage regimen is used, a lower initial dose of 100 mg per square meter of body surface area once a week should be considered for patients with a combined history of prior pelvic/abdominal irradiation and modestly elevated total serum bilirubin concentrations (1 to 2 mg/dL) because of the increased likelihood of first-course grade 3 or 4 neutropenia (graded according to U.S. National Cancer Institute [NCI] criteria). Although an appropriate initial dose has not been established for patients with pretreatment total serum bilirubin concentrations higher than 2 mg/dL, a starting dose that is even lower than 100 mg per square meter of body surface area should be considered.

When the weekly dosing regimen is used, dosage may be increased to up to 150 mg per square meter of body surface area or reduced to as low as 50 mg per square meter of body surface area, in increments of 25 or 50 mg per square meter of body surface area, according to individual patient tolerance. In general, dosage should be decreased by 25 mg per square meter of body surface area if an NCI grade 2 toxicity occurs, by 25 to 50 mg per square meter of body surface area if an NCI grade 3 toxicity occurs, and by 50 mg per square meter of body surface area if an NCI grade 4 toxicity occurs. After a grade 2 toxicity, if using the lower dose for the remainder of that course of therapy results in adequate recovery, the original dosage may be used for the next course of treatment. After a grade 3 or 4 toxicity, irinotecan should be withheld until recovery to at least the grade 2 level has taken place, after which the lower dose should be used (unless further reduction is needed) for the duration of therapy. Detailed recommendations are included in the

## Irinotecan (Systemic)

manufacturer's product labeling. For toxicities occurring with the every-three-week dosage regimen, subsequent doses may be delayed and/or decreased by increments of 50 mg per square meter of body surface area as necessary.

**Usual adult prescribing limits**
Per single weekly dose, 150 mg per square meter of body surface area.

**Usual pediatric dose**
Safety and efficacy have not been established.

**Usual geriatric dose**
See *Usual adult dose*.

**Size(s) usually available**
U.S.—
   20 mg per mL (40 mg per 2-mL and 100 mg per 5-mL single-use vials) (Rx) [*Camptosar* (sorbitol 45 mg; lactic acid 0.9 mg; hydrochloric acid or sodium hydroxide as needed to adjust pH)].
Canada—
   20 mg per mL (40 mg per 2-mL and 100 mg per 5-mL single-use vials) (Rx) [*Camptosar* (sorbitol 45 mg; lactic acid 0.9 mg; hydrochloric acid or sodium hydroxide as needed to adjust pH)].

**Packaging and storage**
Store between 15 and 30 °C (59 and 86 °F), protected from light and from freezing.

**Preparation of dosage form**
Irinotecan is prepared for administration by intravenous infusion by diluting the 20-mg-per-mL injection in 5% dextrose injection (preferred) or 0.9% sodium chloride injection to obtain a concentration of 0.12 to 1.1 mg per mL.

**Stability**
When diluted in 5% dextrose injection, irinotecan is stable for 48 hours if refrigerated at 2 to 8 °C (36 to 46 °F) and protected from light, or for up to 24 hours at room temperature (approximately 25 °C [77 °F]) in ambient fluorescent lighting. However, because irinotecan hydrochloride injection contains no antimicrobial preservative, the medication should preferably be used within 6 hours after dilution if kept at room temperature and within 24 hours after dilution if kept under refrigeration.

When diluted in 0.9% sodium chloride injection, irinotecan is stable for 24 hours at room temperature in ambient fluorescent lighting, but, because irinotecan hydrochloride injection contains no antimicrobial preservative, the medication should preferably be used within 6 hours after dilution. Dilutions in 0.9% sodium chloride injection should not be refrigerated because of the possibility of precipitate formation.

The 2-mL and 5-mL vials of irinotecan are intended for single use only; unused portions of the injection should be discarded.

**Incompatibilities**
It is recommended that other medications not be added to the irinotecan infusion.

**Auxiliary labeling**
• Must be diluted prior to administration.

### Selected Bibliography
Rothenberg ML, Eckardt JR, Kuhn JG, et al. Phase II trial of irinotecan in patients with progressive or rapidly recurrent colorectal cancer. J Clin Oncol 1996; 14: 1128-35.
Rougier P, Bugat R, Douillard JY, et al. Phase II study of irinotecan in the treatment of advanced colorectal cancer in chemotherapy-naive patients and patients pretreated with fluorouracil-based chemotherapy. J Clin Oncol 1997; 15: 251-60.

Developed: 06/26/98

---

**IRON DEXTRAN** — See *Iron Supplements (Systemic)*

**IRON-POLYSACCHARIDE** — See *Iron Supplements (Systemic)*

**IRON SORBITOL** — See *Iron Supplements (Systemic)*

---

# IRON SUPPLEMENTS   Systemic

This monograph includes information on the following: 1) Ferrous Fumarate; 2) Ferrous Gluconate; 3) Ferrous Sulfate; 4) Iron Dextran; 5) Iron-Polysaccharide†; 6) Iron Sorbitol*.

VA CLASSIFICATION (Primary): TN401

Commonly used brand name(s): *Apo-Ferrous Gluconate*[2]; *Apo-Ferrous Sulfate*[3]; *DexFerrum*[4]; *DexIron*[4]; *Femiron*[1]; *Feosol*[3]; *Feostat*[1]; *Feostat Drops*[1]; *Fer-In-Sol Capsules*[3]; *Fer-In-Sol Drops*[3]; *Fer-In-Sol Syrup*[3]; *Fer-Iron Drops*[3]; *Fer-gen-sol*[3]; *Feratab*[3]; *Fergon*[2]; *Fero-Grad*[3]; *Fero-Gradumet*[3]; *Ferospace*[3]; *Ferra-TD*[3]; *Ferralet*[2]; *Ferralet Slow Release*[2]; *Ferralyn Lanacaps*[3]; *Ferretts*[1]; *Fertinic*[2]; *Fumasorb*[1]; *Fumerin*[1]; *Hemocyte*[1]; *Hytinic*[5]; *InFeD*[4]; *Ircon*[1]; *Jectofer*[6]; *Mol-Iron*[3]; *Neo-Fer*[1]; *Nephro-Fer*[1]; *Niferex*[5]; *Niferex-150*[5]; *Novoferrogluc*[2]; *Novoferrosulfa*[3]; *Novofumar*[1]; *Nu-Iron*[5]; *Nu-Iron 150*[5]; *PMS-Ferrous Sulfate*[3]; *Palafer*[1]; *Simron*[2]; *Slow Fe*[3]; *Span-FF*[1].

Another commonly used name for dried ferrous sulfate is ferrous sulfate exsiccated.

Note:  For a listing of dosage forms and brand names by country availability, see *Dosage Forms* section(s).

*Not commercially available in U.S.
†Not commercially available in Canada.

## Category
Antianemic; nutritional supplement (mineral).

## Indications

**Accepted**

Iron deficiency anemia (prophylaxis and treatment)—Iron supplements are indicated in the prevention and treatment of iron deficiency anemia, which may result from inadequate diet, malabsorption, pregnancy, rapid growth during childhood, and/or blood loss.

Iron dextran and iron sorbitol are recommended for patients in whom iron deficiency has been determined, only after the cause has been corrected, if possible, and only when oral administration has been found unsatisfactory or impossible.

Note:  The cause of iron deficiency states should always be determined, as it may relate to a serious condition.

Deficiency of iron may lead to fatigue, shortness of breath, decreased physical performance, impaired learning in children and adults, altered body temperature, and altered immune function.

Requirements may be increased and/or supplementation may be necessary in the following persons or conditions (based on documented iron deficiency):
   Achlorhydria
   Blood loss, excessive
   Burns
   Gastrectomy
   Hemodialysis
   Hemorrhage
   Infants—full-term infants after 4 months of age and preterm infants after 2 months of age, especially those receiving breast milk or low-iron formulas
   Intestinal diseases—celiac, Crohn's, diarrhea, inflammatory bowel disease, malabsorption

In addition, individuals with conditions that cause chronic blood loss (e.g., peptic ulcer, hemorrhoids, hookworms) may be at risk for iron deficiency anemia.

Some unusual diets (e.g., reducing diets that drastically restrict food selection) may not supply minimum daily requirements of iron. Supplementation may be necessary in patients receiving total parenteral nutrition (TPN) or undergoing rapid weight loss or in those with malnutrition, because of inadequate dietary intake.

Recommended intakes for all vitamins and most minerals are increased during pregnancy. Many physicians recommend that pregnant women receive multivitamin and mineral supplements, especially those pregnant women who do not consume an adequate diet and those in high-risk categories (i.e., women carrying more than one fetus, heavy cigarette smokers, and alcohol and drug abusers). However, taking excessive amounts of multivitamin and mineral supplements may be harmful to the mother and/or fetus and should be avoided.

Recommended intakes for all vitamins and most minerals are increased during breast-feeding.

Recommended intakes may be increased by the following medications: Antacids, calcium supplements, epoetin, penicillamine, trientine, zinc supplements, and any medications that cause bleeding from the gastrointestinal tract.

## Pharmacology/Pharmacokinetics

**Physicochemical characteristics**
Molecular weight—
　Ferrous fumarate: 169.91.
　Ferrous gluconate: 482.18.
　Ferrous sulfate: 278.02.
　Ferrous sulfate, dried: 151.91.

**Mechanism of action/Effect**
Iron is an essential component in the physiological formation of hemoglobin, adequate amounts of which are necessary for effective erythropoiesis and the resultant oxygen transport capacity of the blood. A similar function is provided by iron in myoglobin production. Iron also serves as a cofactor of several essential enzymes, including cytochromes that are involved in electron transport. Iron is necessary for catecholamine metabolism and the proper functioning of neutrophils.

**Absorption**
Absorption is increased when iron stores are depleted or red blood cell production is increased. Conversely, high iron blood concentrations decrease absorption.
　Oral dosage forms—
　　When taken orally, in food or as a supplement, iron passes through the mucosal cells in the ferrous state and is bound with the protein transferrin.
　　Iron-deficient individuals: 10 to 30% is absorbed, the amount being approximately proportional to the degree of deficiency.
　　Non–iron-deficient individuals: Approximately 5 to 15% of ingested iron is absorbed.
　　Absorption occurs principally in the duodenum and proximal jejunum.
　　Absorption is most efficient when iron is ingested in its ferrous rather than its ferric form, on an empty stomach. Gastric acid increases absorption by maintaining ferric iron in a soluble form.
　　Twenty to 30% of heme iron is absorbed from the diet. Two to 10% of nonheme iron is absorbed from the diet, and its absorption is affected by other foods ingested. Ascorbic acid, as a supplement or in foods, reduces ferric salts to the ferrous form and thus enhances the absorption of nonheme iron. Meat and other animal tissues also enhance the absorption of nonheme iron. Certain foods and supplements, such as coffee, tea, milk, eggs, calcium, whole grains, and phosphorus, may inhibit nonheme iron absorption.
　Parenteral dosage forms—
　　Iron dextran: Iron dextran is absorbed from the injection site into the capillaries and lymphatic system. The majority of the intramuscular injection is absorbed within 72 hours. The remaining iron is absorbed in the following 3 to 4 weeks. Evidence of a therapeutic response is observed in a few days as an increase in reticulocyte count. The intravenous dose is available much more rapidly.
　　Iron sorbitol: Iron sorbitol is absorbed directly into the bloodstream as well as via the lymphatic system. Sixty-six percent of the intramuscular injection is absorbed within 3 hours.

**Distribution**
Oral dosage forms—Iron is transported in the body to bone marrow for red blood cell production in the iron-transferrin complex form.
Iron dextran—Iron dextran is removed from the plasma by cells of the reticuloendothelial system and dissociated into iron and dextran. The released iron is immediately bound to protein moieties to form hemosiderin or ferritin or, to a lesser extent, transferrin. The protein-bound iron eventually replenishes the depleted iron stores and is incorporated into hemoglobin.

**Protein binding**
Very high (90% or more).
Hemoglobin—High.
Myoglobin, enzymes, and transferrin—Low.
Ferritin and hemosiderin—Low.

**Storage**
Iron is stored as ferritin or hemosiderin, primarily in hepatocytes and in the reticuloendothelial system, with some storage in muscle.

**Half-life**
Ferrous sulfate—6 hours.
Iron dextran, intravenously administered—5 to more than 20 hours. However, half-life values do not represent clearance of iron from the body.

**Time to peak concentration**
Iron sorbitol—2 hours.

**Elimination**
No physiological system of elimination exists for iron, and it can accumulate in the body to toxic amounts; however, small amounts are lost daily in the shedding of skin, hair, and nails; and in feces, perspiration, breast milk (0.5 to 1 mg per day), menstrual blood, and urine.
　Average daily loss of iron for healthy adults is—
　　Males: 1 mg per day.
　　Postmenopausal females: 1 mg per day.
　　Healthy premenopausal adult females: 1.5 to 2 mg per day.
　Iron sorbitol—
　　30% of dose excreted in urine in 24 hours.

## Precautions to Consider

**Carcinogenicity/Tumorigenicity**
For iron dextran—Tumors at the injection site have been reported in humans who had previously received intramuscular injections of iron-carbohydrate complexes. However, the actual risk of such tumors is unknown because of the long latency period between injection and appearance of a tumor. Animal studies have shown the production of sarcoma in rodents injected repeatedly at the same site with large doses of iron-carbohydrate complexes. However, the rodent tumors were a different type than those reported in humans.
For iron sorbitol—There was no evidence of lymphatic obstruction or tumors at the injection site in mice receiving iron sorbitol subcutaneously at doses of 1 mg a week for seven months.

**Pregnancy/Reproduction**
Pregnancy—
*For ferrous fumarate, ferrous gluconate, ferrous sulfate, and iron-polysaccharide—*
　In the first trimester of pregnancy, adequate iron intake is usually obtained from a proper diet; however, in the second and third trimesters, when iron deficiency is more prevalent because of greatly increased requirements, iron supplements may be recommended. However, some clinicians prefer to evaluate the patient before giving routine iron supplementation.
　Studies in humans have not been done, and problems in humans have not been documented with intake of normal daily recommended amounts.
　Studies in animals have not been done.
*For iron dextran—*
　Iron dextran crosses the placenta. Studies in humans have not been done.
　Iron dextran has been shown to be teratogenic and embryocidal in mice, rats, rabbits, dogs, and monkeys when given in doses three times the maximum human dose.
　FDA Pregnancy Category C.
*For iron sorbitol—*
　Although no adequate and well-controlled studies have been done in humans, there have been a few reports of abortion after use of iron sorbitol in early pregnancy. Use is not recommended in the first 3 to 4 months of pregnancy.
　Studies in animals have not been done.

**Breast-feeding**
*For ferrous fumarate, ferrous gluconate, ferrous sulfate, and iron-polysaccharide—*
　Problems in humans have not been documented with intake of normal daily recommended amounts.
*For iron dextran—*
　Only traces of unmetabolized iron dextran are distributed into breast milk.

**Pediatrics**
The American Academy of Pediatrics recommends that iron supplementation (as iron-fortified formula or cereal or as iron-containing drops) be given to preterm infants after 2 months of age and to full-term infants after 4 months of age, whether breast or formula fed.
Problems in pediatrics have not been documented with intake of normal daily recommended amounts. Iron dextran is not normally given to infants under 4 months of age. There have been reports from other countries of increased gram-negative sepsis in neonates given iron dextran, probably due to *Escherichia coli*, after intramuscular injection.

## Geriatrics
Problems in geriatrics have not been documented with intake of normal daily recommended amounts. Some geriatric patients may require a larger than usual daily ingestion of bioavailable iron to correct an iron deficiency, because their ability to absorb iron has been diminished by reduced gastric secretions and achlorhydria.

## Drug interactions and/or related problems
The following drug interactions and/or related problems have been selected on the basis of their potential clinical significance (possible mechanism in parentheses where appropriate)—not necessarily inclusive (» = major clinical significance):

Note: Combinations containing any of the following, depending on the amount present, may also interact with this iron supplement.

» Acetohydroxamic acid
(iron, and possibly other heavy metals, when taken orally, are chelated by acetohydroxamic acid; this may result in reduced intestinal absorption of both acetohydroxamic acid and oral iron supplements; if iron therapy is indicated during treatment with acetohydroxamic acid, parenteral administration of iron is recommended)

Alcohol
(concurrent use with ferric iron for a prolonged period may result in toxicity since absorption and hepatic storage of iron are increased, especially if alcohol usage is high)

» Antacids or
Calcium supplements (calcium carbonate or phosphate) or
Coffee or
Eggs or
Foods or medications containing bicarbonates, carbonates, oxalates, or phosphates or
Milk or milk products or
Tea containing tannic acid or
Whole-grain breads and cereals (contain phytic acid) and dietary fiber
(concurrent use with iron maydecrease iron absorption because of the formation of less soluble or insoluble complexes; iron supplements should not be taken within 1 hour before or 2 hours after ingestion of any of the above)

Cimetidine
(the decrease in gastric acid caused by cimetidine may decrease the absorption of nonheme iron; concurrent use with iron supplements is not recommended; iron supplements should be taken at least 2 hours before or after cimetidine)

Deferoxamine, and possibly other chelating agents
(deferoxamine chelates iron and is used in the treatment of iron overdose and other iron overload conditions; iron may be necessary in patients receiving other chelating agents; however, it should be given at least 2 hours after the chelating agent)

» Dimercaprol
(concurrent administration of medicinal iron with dimercaprol results in the formation of a toxic complex; if iron deficiency is present, its treatment should be postponed until therapy with dimercaprol has been discontinued for at least 24 hours; severe iron deficiency anemia occurring during dimercaprol therapy should be managed with blood transfusion)

» Etidronate
(concurrent use may prevent absorption of oral etidronate; patients should be advised to avoid using iron supplements within 2 hours of etidronate)

» Fluoroquinolones
(iron may reduce absorption of fluoroquinolones by chelation, resulting in lower serum and urine concentrations of fluoroquinolones; fluoroquinolones should be taken at least 2 hours before or 2 hours after iron supplements)

Pancreatin or
Pancrelipase
(concurrent use of these medications with iron supplements may decrease iron absorption)

Penicillamine or
Trientine
(concurrent use with iron supplements may decrease the therapeutic effects of these medications; if necessary, iron may be administered in short courses, but a period of 2 hours should elapse between administration of penicillamine or trientine and iron)

» Tetracyclines, oral
(concurrent use with iron reduces absorbability and resultant therapeutic effects of oral tetracyclines; patients should be advised to take iron supplements 2 hours after tetracycline)

Zinc supplements, oral
(large doses of iron supplements have been found to inhibit the intestinal absorption of zinc; this may be a problem in individuals taking commercial multivitamin-mineral preparations or infant formulas that have a high iron-to-zinc ratio; however, most firms in the U.S. have reformulated their products; zinc supplements should be taken at least 2 hours after iron supplements)

## Laboratory value alterations
The following have been selected on the basis of their potential clinical significance (possible effect in parentheses where appropriate)—not necessarily inclusive (» = major clinical significance):

With diagnostic test results
*For all iron supplements*
Iron concentrations, serum
(caution in interpretation of serum iron values in blood samples drawn within 1 to 2 weeks of administration of large doses of iron dextran and within 4 hours of oral iron)

Orthotolidine test
(presence of iron may give false-positive results)

Technetium Tc 99m–labeled phosphates and phosphonates
(iron supplements may cause a decrease in bone uptake of technetium Tc 99m-labeled phosphates and phosphonates because of iron overload; bone scans with Tc 99m diphosphonate, taken 1 to 6 days after intramuscular iron dextran administration, may show dense areas of activity in the buttock, following the contour of the iliac crest)

Tumor and/or abscess imaging with Ga-67 gallium citrate
(iron supplements may cause a decrease in tumor and/or abscess uptake of Ga-67 gallium citrate due to competition for the same binding sites)

*For ferrous sulfate only (in addition to those laboratory value alterations listed above)*
Glucose oxidase tests
(presence of ferrous sulfate may give false-negative results)

With physiology/laboratory test values
Occult blood in stools
(may be obscured by black coloration of iron in stool)

Serum discoloration
(large doses of iron dextran have been reported to impart a brown color to serum in blood drawn 4 hours after intravenous administration)

## Medical considerations/Contraindications
The medical considerations/contraindications included have been selected on the basis of their potential clinical significance (reasons given in parentheses where appropriate)—not necessarily inclusive (» = major clinical significance).

*Except under special circumstances, this medication should not be used when the following medical problems exist:*

» Hemochromatosis or
» Hemosiderosis
(existing iron overload may be increased)

» Other anemic conditions, unless accompanied by iron deficiency (some conditions, such as hemolytic anemia or thalassemia, may cause excess storage of iron)

» Porphyria cutanea tarda
(may be caused by hepatic accumulation of iron, as in iron overload)

*Risk-benefit should be considered when the following medical problems exist:*

Alcoholism, active or in remission
(alcohol may increase absorption and hepatic storage of iron and increase iron toxicity)

Allergies or
Asthma
(increased risk of hypersensitivity reactions with parenteral administration)

Cardiovascular disease
(may be exacerbated by possible adverse reactions caused by administration of iron dextran)

Hepatitis or hepatic function impairment or
Kidney disease, acute, infectious
(may cause an accumulation of iron)

Intestinal tract inflammatory conditions, such as enteritis, colitis, diverticulitis, and ulcerative colitis or
Peptic ulcer
(may be exacerbated with oral iron dosage forms)

Rheumatoid arthritis
   (acute exacerbation of joint pain and swelling following intravenous administration of parenteral iron)
Sensitivity to iron
» Caution is recommended also in patients receiving repeated blood transfusions because the addition of high erythrocytic iron content may produce iron overload.

### Patient monitoring

The following may be especially important in patient monitoring (other tests may be warranted in some patients, depending on condition; » = major clinical significance):

Ferritin concentrations, serum and
Iron concentrations, serum
   (determinations are recommended when deemed necessary to recognize and prevent hemosiderosis and progressive accumulation of iron in patients with chronic renal failure, Hodgkin's disease, or rheumatoid arthritis, or in patients receiving large doses of iron dextran; patients on chronic renal dialysis may not show a valid correlation of serum iron ferritin with body iron stores while receiving iron dextran)

Hemoglobin and hematocrit determinations and
Reticulocyte counts
   (suggested at 3-week intervals for the first 2 months of therapy; recommended a few days after parenteral administration to determine therapeutic response; if there has not been at least a 1-gram-per-100-mL rise in hemoglobin within 2 weeks of initiation of iron dextran therapy, a review of the diagnosis of iron deficiency anemia may be necessary)

Total iron binding capacity (TIBC) or
Transferrin, percentage saturation of
   (some clinicians recommend monthly determinations during parenteral iron administration; however, while transferrin saturation may reflect a depletion of stored iron, it is less sensitive to changes in iron stores than serum ferritin; some clinicians recommend that TIBC and/or transferrin be monitored only in the case of suspected iron overload)

## Side/Adverse Effects

Note: Stools commonly become dark green or black when iron preparations are taken orally. This is caused by the presence of unabsorbed iron and is harmless. However, bleeding in the gastrointestinal tract may also cause black stools of a sticky consistency, often accompanied by other symptoms such as red streaks in the stool, cramping, soreness, or sharp pains in the stomach or abdominal region. Medical attention is needed for proper evaluation of the cause.

The parenteral administration of iron has resulted in anaphylactic reactions that, on rare occasions, have been fatal. Such reactions occur within the first several minutes of administration and have been characterized by sudden onset of respiratory difficulties and/or cardiovascular collapse. Therefore, epinephrine should be kept near the patient in case of emergency.

The following effects have been selected on the basis of their potential clinical significance (possible signs and symptoms in parentheses where appropriate)—not necessarily inclusive:

### Those indicating need for medical attention
Incidence more frequent
   *Oral use only*
      **Abdominal or stomach pain, cramping, or soreness**
   *Parenteral use only*
      **Allergic reaction** (skin rash or hives; trouble in breathing); **backache or muscle pain; chills; dizziness; fever with increased sweating; headache; metallic taste; nausea or vomiting; numbness, pain, or tingling of hands or feet; chest pain; hypotension** (dizziness or fainting); **fast heartbeat; flushing or redness of skin**—with excessive rate of intravenous administration; **pain and redness or sores at intramuscular injection site; redness at intravenous injection site**
      Note: Backache or muscle pain, chills, dizziness, fever with increased sweating, headache, metallic taste, nausea or vomiting, or numbness, pain, or tingling of hands or feet due to delayed reaction, with recommended doses; onset may be in 24 to 48 hours after administration and subsides in 3 to 7 days.

Incidence less frequent or rare
   *Oral use only*
      **Contact irritation** (chest or throat pain, especially when swallowing; stools containing fresh or digested blood)

Note: *Contact irritation* due to contact with ulcerous areas or high concentration of iron in one area resulting from improper release from dosage form or delayed passage of dosage form through alimentary tract.

### Those indicating need for medical attention only if they continue or are bothersome
Incidence more frequent
   *Oral use only*
      **Constipation; diarrhea; nausea; vomiting**
   *Parenteral use only*
      **Brown discoloration of skin**—usually fading within several weeks or months

Incidence less frequent
   *Oral use only*
      **Darkened urine** (iron sulfide formation following large doses); **heartburn; staining of teeth**—with liquid dosage forms

## Overdose

Note: Acute toxicity, with symptoms ranging from vomiting to coma, has been reported with ingestion of 200 to 250 mg per kg of body weight (mg/kg) of ferrous sulfate in adults and 20 mg/kg of elemental iron in children. There have been no reports of chronic iron toxicity in individuals who do not have genetic defects that increase iron absorption.

For specific information on the agents used in the management of iron overdose, see
   • *Deferoxamine (Systemic)* monograph;
   • *Ipecac (Oral-Local)* monograph; and/or
   • *Sodium Bicarbonate (Systemic)* monograph.

For more information on the management of overdose or unintentional ingestion, **contact a Poison Control Center** (see *Poison Control Center Listing*).

### Clinical effects of overdose

The following effects have been selected on the basis of their potential clinical significance (possible signs and symptoms in parentheses where appropriate)—not necessarily inclusive:

Acute effects
Early symptoms of acute iron toxicity
   Oral use only
      **Diarrhea, sometimes containing blood; fever; nausea, severe; stomach pain or cramping, sharp; vomiting, severe, sometimes containing blood**
      Note: Early symptoms may not be evident for up to 60 minutes or longer; if overdose is suspected, emergency room treatment should not be delayed for evidence of symptoms, but should begin immediately.

      Early signs may also include increased blood glucose and leukocytosis.

      A latency period lasting from 2 to about 48 hours after ingestion may occur between the 2 symptomatic phases. During this time, the patient may appear to improve clinically.

Late symptoms of acute iron toxicity
   Oral use only
      **Bluish-colored lips, fingernails, palms of hands; drowsiness; pale, clammy skin; seizures; unusual tiredness or weakness; weak and fast heartbeat**
      Note: Late signs may also include metabolic acidosis, hypotension, hypoglycemia, hepatic injury or failure, cardiovascular collapse, and gastrointestinal scarring.

### For treatment of acute overdose

**Overdose of ingested iron can be fatal, especially in small children. Immediate treatment is essential.** Serious poisoning may result in small children from ingestion of 3 or 4 ferrous sulfate tablets (200 mg of elemental iron).

Acute overdose of iron requires immediate medical treatment that should be completed as soon as possible following ingestion.

After one hour, excessive systemic absorption of iron and possible erosion of stomach and intestinal tissues complicate evacuative and supportive procedures.

Transport of patient to emergency room should not be delayed. If syrup of ipecac has been administered, emesis may require up to 30 minutes or even a repeat dose. However, patient transport must not wait for emetic effect.

Overdose symptoms may be delayed (10 to 60 minutes or longer) because of many intervening factors such as the iron salt taken, amount of food in stomach, and size of dose.

To decrease absorption—
Inducing emesis with syrup of ipecac or lavaging with sodium bicarbonate if patient is comatose or having convulsions may be used, depending on the patient's condition.

If intact radiopaque tablets are visualized on x-ray, repeating lavage may be necessary.

Monitoring—
Laboratory studies on heparinized blood should include serum iron, hemoglobin, hematocrit, electrolytes, blood gases and blood glucose, total iron-binding capacity (TIBC), complete blood count, blood type, and cross-match.

Serum iron determinations should be repeated. Serum drawn early (within 2 hours of ingestion) may have artificially high concentrations of iron. Peak serum concentrations are reached about 6 hours after ingestion. However, achievement of peak serum concentrations is delayed if the iron was in extended-release form, if the patient had a significant amount of food in his/her stomach, and if the dose of iron was large.

Specific treatment—
Fluid and electrolyte balance must be maintained. Acidosis may be corrected with intravenous sodium bicarbonate.

Antidote—Deferoxamine, administered slowly, intravenously or intramuscularly, is used in more severe iron toxicity, when symptoms are other than minimal vomiting or diarrhea. Deferoxamine chelates iron to form a red soluble ferric complex (ferrioxamine) that is excreted in the urine. Children with a history of ingesting > 40 mg of elemental iron per kg of body weight, or if serum iron determinations and TIBC are not available, should receive an intramuscular test dose of deferoxamine, regardless of symptoms. If the urine turns an orange-rose (vin rosé) color, deferoxamine should be continued intravenously. However, a negative test dose does not rule out iron toxicity, since false negative tests have been reported with deferoxamine. When results of serum iron determinations and TIBC are available, dosing should continue, if necessary.

Avoid deferoxamine in patients who have developed renal failure.

Dialysis is of no value in removing serum iron alone, but may be used to increase excretion of the iron-deferoxamine complex, and is indicated in the presence of anuria or oliguria.

Exchange transfusion may be successful.

Whole bowel irrigation is being used by some clinicians, but is not standard practice.

Supportive care—
Patient must be observed for a minimum of 24 hours after becoming asymptomatic. Delayed effects may include shock and severe gastrointestinal bleeding (24 to 48 hours), and gastrointestinal obstruction (weeks to months). Residual damage may be ruled out with liver and upper gastrointestinal studies.

Patients in whom intentional overdose is confirmed or suspected should be referred for psychiatric consultation.

## Patient Consultation

As an aid to patient consultation, refer to *Advice for the Patient, Iron Supplements (Systemic)*.

In providing consultation, consider emphasizing the following selected information (» = major clinical significance):

### Description of use
Description should include function in body, signs of deficiency, and conditions that may cause deficiency

### Importance of diet
Importance of proper nutrition; supplement may be needed because of inadequate dietary intake
Best dietary sources of iron
Recommended daily intake for iron

### Before using this dietary supplement
» Conditions affecting use, especially:
Sensitivity to iron
Other medications, especially acetohydroxamic acid, antacids, dimercaprol, etidronate, fluoroquinolones, or oral tetracyclines
Other medical problems, especially hemochromatosis, hemosiderosis, other anemic conditions, or prophyria cutanea tarda

### Proper use of this dietary supplement
» Proper dosing
Taking on empty stomach 1 hour before or 2 hours after meals; or with food to lessen possibility of stomach upset
Taking with water or fruit juice, a full glass (240 mL) for adults, ½ glass (120 mL) for children
Following health care professional's directions if dietary supplement was prescribed
Following manufacturer's package directions on nonprescription (OTC) iron

*For preventing, reducing, or removing iron stains on teeth*
Diluting liquid forms in water or fruit juice
Using drinking tube or straw
Placing dropper doses well back on tongue
Brushing teeth with baking soda or hydrogen peroxide 3%
Missed dose: Skipping missed dose; going back to regular schedule; not doubling doses
» Proper storage

### Precautions while using this dietary supplement
Taking iron supplements 1 hour before or 2 hours after eating dairy products, eggs, coffee, tea, whole-grain breads and cereals, antacids, or calcium supplements
Not taking iron supplements orally if receiving iron by injection
Avoiding regular use of large amounts of iron supplements several times daily for more than 6 months unless approved by health care professional
Extended-release dosage forms may not release iron properly; checking with health care professional if stools are not black during therapy
Keeping iron preparations out of the reach of children. Keeping syrup of ipecac readily available in case ordered for emergency
Keeping telephone numbers of poison control center, nearest hospital emergency room, and doctor readily available
» Suspected overdose: Immediately contacting physician, poison control center, or emergency room; following any instructions given on phone; not delaying emergency treatment; taking container of iron medicine to emergency room

### Side/adverse effects
Iron supplements cause black stools, which may be alarming to patient although medically insignificant; checking with physician if black stools occur with other symptoms of internal blood loss
Signs of potential side effects, especially abdominal pain or contact irritation in alimentary tract

## General Dosing Information

The elemental iron content of iron salts is as follows:

| Iron Salt | % Elemental Iron |
| --- | --- |
| Ferrous fumarate | Ferrous 33 |
| Ferrous gluconate | Ferrous 11.6 |
| Ferrous sulfate | Ferrous 20 |
| Ferrous sulfate, dried | Ferrous ≈30 |
| Iron dextran | Ferric* |
| Iron-polysaccharide | Ferric* |

*Variable, depending on product.

Noncompliance is a major factor in slow therapeutic results, especially in patients requiring prolonged treatment.

In healthy adult males, there are approximately 50 mg per kg of body weight (mg/kg) of iron and 14 to 18 grams of hemoglobin per 100 mL of whole blood.

In healthy adult females, there are approximately 35 mg/kg of iron and 12 to 16 grams of hemoglobin per 100 mL of whole blood.

The hemoglobin concentration of an iron-deficient patient usually reaches normal parameters after iron therapy of 1 or 2 months, but the plasma iron concentration often requires 3 to 6 months of therapy to reflect the normalization of body iron stores.

The American Academy of Pediatrics recommends that breast-fed preterm infants 2 months of age and older receive 2 to 3 mg/kg a day of elemental iron in the form of ferrous sulfate. Full-term infants 4 months of age and older should receive 1 mg/kg a day of elemental iron, preferably from iron-fortified formula or cereal.

Concurrent use of ascorbic acid with iron in proper ratio is thought to enhance iron absorption by maintaining ferrous salts in the reduced state and by reducing ferric salts to the more absorbable ferrous form; the suggested ratio is over 200 mg of ascorbic acid to 30 mg of elemental iron.

### Diet/Nutrition
Absorption of iron is most effective when the iron is ingested on an empty stomach; taking it with food will lessen absorption but will also lessen the chance of gastrointestinal irritation.

Taking iron supplements 1 hour before or 2 hours after eating dairy products, eggs, coffee, tea, or whole-grain breads and cereals will prevent the formation of less soluble or insoluble complexes, which decrease iron absorption.

Recommended dietary intakes for iron are defined differently worldwide.

For U.S.—
The Recommended Dietary Allowances (RDAs) for vitamins and minerals are determined by the Food and Nutrition Board of the National Research Council and are intended to provide adequate nutrition in most healthy persons under usual environmental stresses. In addition, a different designation may be used by the FDA for food and dietary supplement labeling purposes, such as Daily Value (DV). DVs replace the previous labeling terminology United States Recommended Daily Allowances (USRDAs).

For Canada—
Recommended Nutrient Intakes (RNIs) for vitamins, minerals, and protein are determined by Health and Welfare Canada and provide recommended amounts of a specific nutrient while minimizing the risk of chronic diseases.

Daily recommended intakes for elemental iron are generally defined as follows:

| Persons | U.S. (mg) | Canada (mg) |
|---|---|---|
| Infants and children | | |
| Birth to 3 years of age | 6–10 | 0.3–6 |
| 4 to 6 years of age | 10 | 8 |
| 7 to 10 years of age | 10 | 8–10 |
| Adolescent and adult males | 10 | 8–10 |
| Adolescent and adult females | 10–15 | 8–13 |
| Pregnant females | 30 | 17–22 |
| Breast-feeding females | 15 | 8–13 |

The best dietary source of iron is lean red meat. Chicken, turkey, and fish are less important sources of iron. Foods rich in vitamin C (e.g., citrus fruits and fresh vegetables) and heme iron–containing foods (such as found in meats) enhance nonheme iron absorption from cereals, beans, and other vegetables. Foods containing phytates, oxalates, fiber, and calcium may inhibit the absorption of nonheme iron. In food preparation, additional iron may be added through cooking in iron pots.

### For treatment of allergic reaction
Treatment may include the following:
- Administering epinephrine subcutaneously or intramuscularly. The usual adult dose for acute allergic (anaphylactic) reactions is 0.5 mL of a 1:1000 (1 mg/mL) solution (500 mcg of epinephrine base).
- Isoproterenol or similar beta-agonists may be required in patients taking beta-blockers because of an inadequate response to epinephrine.

---

### FERROUS FUMARATE

## Summary of Differences
General dosing information: Contains 33% elemental ferrous iron.

## Oral Dosage Forms

### FERROUS FUMARATE CAPSULES

**Usual adult and adolescent dose**
Deficiency (prophylaxis)—
Oral, amount based on normal daily recommended intakes of elemental iron:

| Persons | U.S. (mg) | Canada (mg) |
|---|---|---|
| Adolescent and adult males | 10 | 8–10 |
| Adolescent and adult females | 10–15 | 8–13 |
| Pregnant females | 30 | 17–22 |
| Breast-feeding females | 15 | 8–13 |

Deficiency (treatment)—
Treatment dose is individualized by prescriber based on severity of deficiency.

**Usual pediatric dose**
Dosage form is not recommended for use in children.

**Strength(s) usually available**
U.S.—
Not commercially available.
Canada—
300 mg (100 mg of elemental iron) (OTC) [*Neo-Fer; Palafer*].

Note: The strength of these iron preparations may exceed the dosage range recommended by USP DI Advisory Panels based on the amount necessary to meet normal nutritional needs.

**Packaging and storage**
Store below 40 °C (104 °F), preferably between 15 and 30 °C (59 and 86 °F), in a tight container, unless otherwise specified by manufacturer.

**Auxiliary labeling**
- Keep out of reach of children.

**Note**
Caution patients about toxic effects of accidental overdose, especially in children, and need for immediate medical aid.

### FERROUS FUMARATE EXTENDED-RELEASE CAPSULES

**Usual adult and adolescent dose**
See *Ferrous Fumarate Capsules*.

**Usual pediatric dose**
Dosage form is not recommended for use in children.

**Strength(s) usually available**
U.S.—
325 mg (106 mg of elemental iron) (OTC) [*Span-FF* (sucrose)].
Canada—
Not commercially available.

Note: The strength of this iron preparation may exceed the dosage range recommended by USP DI Advisory Panels based on the amount necessary to meet normal nutritional needs.

**Packaging and storage**
Store below 40 °C (104 °F), preferably between 15 and 30 °C (59 and 86 °F), in a well-closed container, unless otherwise specified by manufacturer.

**Auxiliary labeling**
- Swallow capsules whole.
- Keep out of reach of children.

**Note**
Caution patients about toxic effects of accidental overdose, especially in children, and need for immediate medical aid.

### FERROUS FUMARATE ORAL SOLUTION

**Usual adult and adolescent dose**
See *Ferrous Fumarate Capsules*.

**Usual pediatric dose**
Deficiency (prophylaxis)—
Oral, amount based on normal daily recommended intakes of elemental iron:

| Persons | U.S. (mg) | Canada (mg) |
|---|---|---|
| Infants and children | | |
| Birth to 3 years of age | 6–10 | 0.3–6 |
| 4 to 6 years of age | 10 | 8 |
| 7 to 10 years of age | 10 | 8–10 |

Deficiency (treatment)—
Treatment dose is individualized by prescriber based on severity of deficiency.

**Strength(s) usually available**
U.S.—
45 mg (15 mg of elemental iron) per 0.6 mL (OTC) [*Feostat Drops*].
Canada—
Not commercially available.

Note: The strength of this iron preparation may exceed the dosage range recommended by USP DI Advisory Panels based on the amount necessary to meet normal nutritional needs.

**Packaging and storage**
Store below 40 °C (104 °F), preferably between 15 and 30 °C (59 and 86 °F), in a tight container, unless otherwise specified by manufacturer. Protect from freezing.

**Auxiliary labeling**
- Protect from freezing.
- Keep out of reach of children.

**Note**
Explain dosage measurement; provide dropper or other dose-measuring device if indicated.

Explain dilution requirements.

Caution patients about toxic effects of overdose, especially in children, and need for immediate medical aid.

## FERROUS FUMARATE ORAL SUSPENSION

### Usual adult and adolescent dose
See *Ferrous Fumarate Capsules*.

### Usual pediatric dose
See *Ferrous Fumarate Oral Solution*.

### Strength(s) usually available
U.S.—
  100 mg (33 mg of elemental iron) per 5 mL (OTC) [*Feostat*].
Canada—
  300 mg (100 mg of elemental iron) per 5 mL (OTC) [*Palafer*].

Note: The strength of these iron preparations may exceed the dosage range recommended by USP DI Advisory Panels based on the amount necessary to meet normal nutritional needs.

### Packaging and storage
Store below 40 °C (104 °F), preferably between 15 and 30 °C (59 and 86 °F), in a tight container, unless otherwise specified by manufacturer. Protect from freezing.

### Auxiliary labeling
- Shake well before using.
- Protect from freezing.
- Keep out of reach of children.

### Note
Explain dosage measurement; provide dropper or other dose-measuring device if indicated.

Explain dilution requirements.

Caution patients about toxic effects of overdose, especially in children, and need for immediate medical aid.

## FERROUS FUMARATE TABLETS USP

### Usual adult and adolescent dose
See *Ferrous Fumarate Capsules*.

### Usual pediatric dose
See *Ferrous Fumarate Oral Solution*.

### Strength(s) usually available
U.S.—
  63 mg (20 mg of elemental iron) (OTC) [*Femiron*].
  195 mg (64 mg of elemental iron) (OTC) [*Fumerin*].
  200 mg (66 mg of elemental iron) (OTC) [*Fumasorb; Ircon*].
  300 mg (99 mg of elemental iron) (OTC) [GENERIC].
  325 mg (106 mg of elemental iron) (OTC) [*Ferretts; Hemocyte;* GENERIC].
  350 mg (115 mg of elemental iron) (OTC) [*Nephro-Fer*].
Canada—
  200 mg (66 mg of elemental iron) (OTC) [*Novofumar* (sucrose)].

Note: The strength of these iron preparations may exceed the dosage range recommended by USP DI Advisory Panels based on the amount necessary to meet normal nutritional needs.

### Packaging and storage
Store below 40 °C (104 °F), preferably between 15 and 30 °C (59 and 86 °F), unless otherwise specified by manufacturer. Store in a tight container.

### Auxiliary labeling
- Keep out of reach of children.

### Note
Caution patients about toxic effects of accidental overdose, especially in children, and need for immediate medical aid.

## FERROUS FUMARATE CHEWABLE TABLETS

### Usual adult and adolescent dose
See *Ferrous Fumarate Capsules*.

### Usual pediatric dose
See *Ferrous Fumarate Oral Solution*.

### Strength(s) usually available
U.S.—
  100 mg (33 mg of elemental iron) (OTC) [*Feostat*].
Canada—
  Not commercially available.

Note: The strength of this iron preparation may exceed the dosage range recommended by USP DI Advisory Panels based on the amount necessary to meet normal nutritional needs.

### Packaging and storage
Store below 40 °C (104 °F), preferably between 15 and 30 °C (59 and 86 °F), in a tight container, unless otherwise specified by manufacturer.

### Auxiliary labeling
- Chew well before swallowing.
- Keep out of reach of children.

### Note
Caution patients about toxic effects of accidental overdose, especially in children, and need for immediate medical aid.

---

## FERROUS GLUCONATE

## Summary of Differences
General dosing information: Contains 11.6% elemental ferrous iron.

## Oral Dosage Forms

### FERROUS GLUCONATE CAPSULES USP

#### Usual adult and adolescent dose
Deficiency (prophylaxis)—
  Oral, amount based on normal daily recommended intakes of elemental iron:

| Persons | U.S. (mg) | Canada (mg) |
|---|---|---|
| Adolescent and adult males | 10 | 8–10 |
| Adolescent and adult females | 10–15 | 8–13 |
| Pregnant females | 30 | 17–22 |
| Breast-feeding females | 15 | 8–13 |

Deficiency (treatment)—
  Treatment dose is individualized by prescriber based on severity of deficiency.

#### Usual pediatric dose
Deficiency (prophylaxis)—
  Oral, amount based on normal daily recommended intakes of elemental iron:

| Persons | U.S. (mg) | Canada (mg) |
|---|---|---|
| Infants and children | | |
| Birth to 3 years of age | 6–10 | 0.3–6 |
| 4 to 6 years of age | 10 | 8 |
| 7 to 10 years of age | 10 | 8–10 |

Deficiency (treatment)—
  Treatment dose is individualized by prescriber based on severity of deficiency.

#### Strength(s) usually available
U.S.—
  86 mg (10 mg of elemental iron) (OTC) [*Simron* (not USP)].
Canada—
  Not commercially available.

Note: The strength of this iron preparation may exceed the dosage range recommended by USP DI Advisory Panels based on the amount necessary to meet normal nutritional needs.

#### Packaging and storage
Store below 40 °C (104 °F), preferably between 15 and 30 °C (59 and 86 °F), unless otherwise specified by manufacturer. Store in a tight container.

#### Auxiliary labeling
- Keep out of reach of children.

#### Note
Caution patients about toxic effects of overdose, especially in children, and need for immediate medical aid.

### FERROUS GLUCONATE ELIXIR USP

#### Usual adult and adolescent dose
See *Ferrous Gluconate Capsules USP*.

#### Usual pediatric dose
See *Ferrous Gluconate Capsules USP*.

#### Strength(s) usually available
U.S.—
  300 mg (34 mg of elemental iron) per 5 mL (OTC) [*Fergon* (alcohol 7%); GENERIC].
Canada—
  Not commercially available.

Note: The strength of these iron preparations may exceed the dosage range recommended by USP DI Advisory Panels based on the amount necessary to meet normal nutritional needs.

**Packaging and storage**
Store below 40 °C (104 °F), preferably between 15 and 30 °C (59 and 86 °F), unless otherwise specified by manufacturer. Store in a tight, light-resistant container. Protect from freezing.

**Auxiliary labeling**
- Keep out of reach of children.

**Note**
Caution patients about toxic effects of overdose, especially in children, and need for immediate medical aid.

### FERROUS GLUCONATE SYRUP

**Usual adult and adolescent dose**
See *Ferrous Gluconate Capsules USP*.

**Usual pediatric dose**
See *Ferrous Gluconate Capsules USP*.

**Strength(s) usually available**
U.S.—
  Not commercially available.
Canada—
  300 mg (35 mg of elemental iron) per 5 mL (OTC) [*Fertinic*].

Note: The strength of this iron preparation may exceed the dosage range recommended by USP DI Advisory Panels based on the amount necessary to meet normal nutritional needs.

**Packaging and storage**
Store below 40 °C (104 °F), preferably between 15 and 30 °C (59 and 86 °F), in a tight container, unless otherwise specified by manufacturer. Protect from light. Protect from freezing.

**Auxiliary labeling**
- Keep out of reach of children.

**Note**
Caution patients about toxic effects of overdose, especially in children, and need for immediate medical aid.

### FERROUS GLUCONATE TABLETS USP

**Usual adult and adolescent dose**
See *Ferrous Gluconate Capsules USP*.

**Usual pediatric dose**
See *Ferrous Gluconate Capsules USP*.

**Strength(s) usually available**
U.S.—
  300 mg (34 mg of elemental iron) (OTC) [GENERIC].
  320 mg (37 mg of elemental iron) (OTC) [*Fergon* (not USP); *Ferralet*].
  325 mg (38 mg of elemental iron) (OTC) [GENERIC].
Canada—
  300 mg (35 mg of elemental iron) (OTC) [*Apo-Ferrous Gluconate; Fertinic; Novoferrogluc;* GENERIC].

Note: The strength of these iron preparations may exceed the dosage range recommended by USP DI Advisory Panels based on the amount necessary to meet normal nutritional needs.

**Packaging and storage**
Store below 40 °C (104 °F), preferably between 15 and 30 °C (59 and 86 °F), unless otherwise specified by manufacturer. Store in a tight container.

**Auxiliary labeling**
- Keep out of reach of children.

**Note**
Caution patients about toxic effects of overdose, especially in children, and need for immediate medical aid.

### FERROUS GLUCONATE EXTENDED-RELEASE TABLETS

**Usual adult and adolescent dose**
See *Ferrous Gluconate Capsules USP*.

**Usual pediatric dose**
Dosage form is not recommended for use in children.

**Strength(s) usually available**
U.S.—
  320 mg (37 mg of elemental iron) (OTC) [*Ferralet Slow Release*].
Canada—
  Not commercially available.

Note: The strength of this iron preparation may exceed the dosage range recommended by USP DI Advisory Panels based on the amount necessary to meet normal nutritional needs.

**Packaging and storage**
Store below 40 °C (104 °F), preferably between 15 and 30 °C (59 and 86 °F), unless otherwise specified by manufacturer.

**Auxiliary labeling**
- Keep out of reach of children.

**Note**
Caution patients about toxic effects of overdose, especially in children, and need for immediate medical aid.

---

### FERROUS SULFATE

## Summary of Differences

Precautions: Laboratory value alterations—Ferrous sulfate may give false-negative results for glucose oxidase tests.
General dosing information: Contains 20% of elemental ferrous iron (dried ferrous sulfate contains approximately 32% of elemental iron).

## Oral Dosage Forms

### FERROUS SULFATE CAPSULES

**Usual adult and adolescent dose**
Deficiency (prophylaxis)—
  Oral, amount based on normal daily recommended intakes of elemental iron:

| Persons | U.S. (mg) | Canada (mg) |
|---|---|---|
| Adolescent and adult males | 10 | 8–10 |
| Adolescent and adult females | 10–15 | 8–13 |
| Pregnant females | 30 | 17–22 |
| Breast-feeding females | 15 | 8–13 |

Deficiency (treatment)—
  Treatment dose is individualized by prescriber based on severity of deficiency.

**Usual pediatric dose**
Deficiency (prophylaxis)—
  Oral, amount based on normal daily recommended intakes of elemental iron:

| Persons | U.S. (mg) | Canada (mg) |
|---|---|---|
| Infants and children | | |
| Birth to 3 years of age | 6–10 | 0.3–6 |
| 4 to 6 years of age | 10 | 8 |
| 7 to 10 years of age | 10 | 8–10 |

Deficiency (treatment)—
  Treatment dose is individualized by prescriber based on severity of deficiency.

**Strength(s) usually available**
U.S.—
  250 mg (50 mg of elemental iron) (OTC) [*Ferospace;* GENERIC].
Canada—
  Not commercially available.

Note: The strength of these iron preparations may exceed the dosage range recommended by USP DI Advisory Panels based on the amount necessary to meet normal nutritional needs.

**Packaging and storage**
Store below 40 °C (104 °F), preferably between 15 and 30 °C (59 and 86 °F), in a tight container, unless otherwise specified by manufacturer.

**Auxiliary labeling**
- Keep out of reach of children.

**Note**
Caution patients about toxic effects of overdose, especially in children, and need for immediate medical aid.

### FERROUS SULFATE (DRIED) CAPSULES

**Usual adult and adolescent dose**
See *Ferrous Sulfate Capsules*.

**Usual pediatric dose**
See *Ferrous Sulfate Capsules*.

**Strength(s) usually available**
U.S.—
   190 mg, dried (60 mg of elemental iron) (OTC) [*Fer-In-Sol Capsules* (lecithin)].
Canada—
   Not commercially available.
Note: The strength of this iron preparation may exceed the dosage range recommended by USP DI Advisory Panels based on the amount necessary to meet normal nutritional needs.

**Packaging and storage**
Store below 40 °C (104 °F), preferably between 15 and 30 °C (59 and 86 °F), in a tight container, unless otherwise specified by manufacturer.

**Auxiliary labeling**
• Swallow capsules whole.
• Keep out of reach of children.

**Note**
Caution patients about toxic effects of overdose, especially in children, and need for immediate medical aid.

## FERROUS SULFATE (DRIED) EXTENDED-RELEASE CAPSULES

**Usual adult and adolescent dose**
See *Ferrous Sulfate Capsules*.

**Usual pediatric dose**
Dosage form is not recommended for use in children.

**Strength(s) usually available**
U.S.—
   150 mg (30 mg of elemental iron) (OTC) [GENERIC].
   159 mg (50 mg of elemental iron) (OTC) [*Feosol* (sucrose)].
   250 mg (50 mg of elemental iron) (OTC) [*Ferralyn Lanacaps; Ferra-TD;* GENERIC].
Canada—
   Not commercially available.
Note: The strength of these iron preparations may exceed the dosage range recommended by USP DI Advisory Panels based on the amount necessary to meet normal nutritional needs.

**Packaging and storage**
Store below 40 °C (104 °F), preferably between 15 and 30 °C (59 and 86 °F), in a well-closed container, unless otherwise specified by manufacturer.

**Auxiliary labeling**
• Swallow capsules whole.
• Keep out of reach of children.

**Note**
Caution patients about toxic effects of overdose, especially in children, and need for immediate medical aid.

## FERROUS SULFATE ELIXIR

**Usual adult and adolescent dose**
See *Ferrous Sulfate Capsules*.

**Usual pediatric dose**
See *Ferrous Sulfate Capsules*.

**Strength(s) usually available**
U.S.—
   220 mg (44 mg of elemental iron) per 5 mL (OTC) [*Feosol* (alcohol 5%); GENERIC].
Canada—
   Not commercially available.
Note: The strength of these iron preparations may exceed the dosage range recommended by USP DI Advisory Panels based on the amount necessary to meet normal nutritional needs.

**Packaging and storage**
Store below 40 °C (104 °F), preferably between 15 and 30 °C (59 and 86 °F), in a tight container, unless otherwise specified by manufacturer. Protect from freezing.

**Auxiliary labeling**
• Keep out of reach of children.

**Note**
Caution patients about toxic effects of overdose, especially in children, and need for immediate medical aid.

## FERROUS SULFATE ORAL SOLUTION USP

Note: The oral solution is sometimes known as concentrate, drops, or syrup.

**Usual adult and adolescent dose**
See *Ferrous Sulfate Capsules*.

**Usual pediatric dose**
See *Ferrous Sulfate Capsules*.

**Strength(s) usually available**
U.S.—
   75 mg (15 mg of elemental iron) per 0.6 mL (OTC) [*Fer-gen-sol* (alcohol 0.2%); *Fer-In-Sol Drops* (alcohol 0.2% v/v); GENERIC].
   90 mg (18 mg of elemental iron) per 5 mL (OTC) [*Fer-In-Sol Syrup* (alcohol 5%)].
   125 mg (25 mg of elemental iron) per mL (OTC) [*Fer-Iron Drops;* GENERIC].
   300 mg (60 mg elemental iron) per 5 mL [].
Canada—
   75 mg (15 mg of elemental iron) per 0.6 mL (OTC) [*Fer-In-Sol Drops* (alcohol 0.2%); *PMS-Ferrous Sulfate*].
   150 mg (30 mg of elemental iron) per 5 mL (OTC) [*Fer-In-Sol Syrup; PMS-Ferrous Sulfate*].
Note: The strength of these iron preparations may exceed the dosage range recommended by USP DI Advisory Panels based on the amount necessary to meet normal nutritional needs.

**Packaging and storage**
Store below 40 °C (104 °F), preferably between 15 and 30 °C (59 and 86 °F), unless otherwise specified by manufacturer. Store in a tight container. Protect from light. Protect from freezing.

**Auxiliary labeling**
• Keep out of reach of children.

**Note**
Caution patients about toxic effects of overdose, especially in children, and need for immediate medical aid.

## FERROUS SULFATE TABLETS USP

**Usual adult and adolescent dose**
See *Ferrous Sulfate Capsules*.

**Usual pediatric dose**
See *Ferrous Sulfate Capsules*.

**Strength(s) usually available**
U.S.—
   195 mg (39 mg of elemental iron) (OTC) [*Mol-Iron* (sucrose)].
   300 mg (60 mg of elemental iron) (OTC) [*Feratab;* GENERIC].
   325 mg (65 mg of elemental iron) (OTC) [GENERIC].
Canada—
   300 mg (60 mg of elemental iron) (OTC) [*Apo-Ferrous Sulfate; Novoferrosulfa; PMS-Ferrous Sulfate*].
Note: The strength of these iron preparations may exceed the dosage range recommended by USP DI Advisory Panels based on the amount necessary to meet normal nutritional needs.

**Packaging and storage**
Store below 40 °C (104 °F), preferably between 15 and 30 °C (59 and 86 °F), unless otherwise specified by manufacturer. Store in a tight container.

**Auxiliary labeling**
• Swallow tablets whole.
• Keep out of reach of children.

**Note**
Caution patients about toxic effects of overdose, especially in children, and need for immediate medical aid.

## FERROUS SULFATE TABLETS (DRIED) USP

**Usual adult and adolescent dose**
See *Ferrous Sulfate Capsules*.

**Usual pediatric dose**
See *Ferrous Sulfate Capsules*.

**Strength(s) usually available**
U.S.—
   200 mg, dried (65 mg of elemental iron) (OTC) [*Feosol* (glucose)].
Canada—
   Not commercially available.
Note: The strength of this iron preparation may exceed the dosage range recommended by USP DI Advisory Panels based on the amount necessary to meet normal nutritional needs.

**Packaging and storage**
Store below 40 °C (104 °F), preferably between 15 and 30 °C (59 and 86 °F), unless otherwise specified by manufacturer. Store in a tight container.

**Auxiliary labeling**
- Swallow tablets whole.
- Keep out of reach of children.

**Note**
Caution patients about toxic effects of overdose, especially in children, and need for immediate medical aid.

### FERROUS SULFATE ENTERIC-COATED TABLETS

**Usual adult and adolescent dose**
See *Ferrous Sulfate Capsules*.

**Usual pediatric dose**
Dosage form is not recommended for use in children.

**Strength(s) usually available**
U.S.—
 325 mg (approximately 65 mg of elemental iron) (OTC) [GENERIC].
Canada—
 300 mg (60 mg of elemental iron) (OTC) [*Apo-Ferrous Sulfate; Novoferrosulfa;* GENERIC].
Note: The strength of these iron preparations may exceed the dosage range recommended by USP DI Advisory Panels based on the amount necessary to meet normal nutritional needs.

**Packaging and storage**
Store below 40 °C (104 °F), preferably between 15 and 30 °C (59 and 86 °F), in a tight container, unless otherwise specified by manufacturer.

**Auxiliary labeling**
- Swallow tablets whole.
- Keep out of reach of children.

**Note**
Caution patients about toxic effects of overdose, especially in children, and need for immediate medical aid.

### FERROUS SULFATE EXTENDED-RELEASE TABLETS

**Usual adult and adolescent dose**
See *Ferrous Sulfate Capsules*.

**Usual pediatric dose**
Dosage form is not recommended for use in children.

**Strength(s) usually available**
U.S.—
 325 mg (65 mg elemental iron) (OTC) [GENERIC].
 525 mg (105 mg of elemental iron) (OTC) [*Fero-Gradumet*].
Canada—
 525 mg (105 mg of elemental iron) (OTC) [*Fero-Grad*].
Note: The strength of these iron preparations may exceed the dosage range recommended by USP DI Advisory Panels based on the amount necessary to meet normal nutritional needs.

**Packaging and storage**
Store below 40 °C (104 °F), preferably between 15 and 30 °C (59 and 86 °F), in a tight container, unless otherwise specified by manufacturer.

**Auxiliary labeling**
- Swallow tablets whole.
- Keep out of reach of children.

**Note**
Caution patients about toxic effects of overdose, especially in children, and need for immediate medical aid.

**Additional information**
Products utilize a plastic matrix that may appear intact in the stool.

### FERROUS SULFATE (DRIED) EXTENDED-RELEASE TABLETS

**Usual adult and adolescent dose**
See *Ferrous Sulfate Capsules*.

**Usual pediatric dose**
Dosage form is not recommended for use in children.

**Strength(s) usually available**
U.S.—
 160 mg, dried (50 mg of elemental iron) (OTC) [*Slow Fe* (lactose; wax matrix)].
Canada—
 160 mg, dried (50 mg of elemental iron) (OTC) [*Slow Fe* (lactose; wax matrix)].
Note: The strength of these iron preparations may exceed the dosage range recommended by USP DI Advisory Panels based on the amount necessary to meet normal nutritional needs.

**Packaging and storage**
Store below 40 °C (104 °F), preferably between 15 and 30 °C (59 and 86 °F), in a tight container, unless otherwise specified by manufacturer.

**Auxiliary labeling**
- Swallow tablets whole.
- Keep out of reach of children.

**Note**
Caution patients about toxic effects of overdose, especially in children, and need for immediate medical aid.

**Additional information**
Products utilize a porous wax matrix that may appear intact in the stool.

---

## *IRON DEXTRAN*

### Summary of Differences

General dosing information: Contains elemental ferric form of iron.

### Additional Dosing Information

Oral iron must be discontinued before the administration of parenteral iron.

Epinephrine should be immediately available during injection of iron dextran, especially in patients with allergies or asthma.

Overdose with iron dextran produces no acute toxicity. However, excessive doses beyond the amounts required for restoration of hemoglobin and replenishment of iron stores may result in hemosiderosis. Excess iron may also increase a patient's susceptibility to infection, especially *Yersinia enterocolitica*.

Factors contributing to the formula for determining dosages for patients with iron deficiency include:
 Blood volume—7.0% of body weight
 Normal hemoglobin (males and females)—
  15 kg (33 lb) or less: 12 grams/deciliter (dL)
  Over 15 kg (33 lb): 14.8 grams/dL
 Iron content of hemoglobin—0.34%
 Body weight

Serum ferritin peaks approximately 7 to 9 days after an intravenous dose of iron dextran, and returns to baseline after about 3 weeks.

*For intravenous injection*
 Iron dextran is administered undiluted and injected slowly at a rate not exceeding 1 mL per minute. However, some clinicians recommend that the calculated dose of iron dextran for the patient be added to 500 mL of dextrose 5% and infused over 4 to 5 hours, after a test infusion of 10 drops per minute for 10 minutes.
 The manufacturer does not recommend that iron dextran be mixed with other medications or added to parenteral nutrition solutions for intravenous infusion; however, iron dextran is added to total parenteral nutrition solutions in current medical practice. Iron dextran should not be added to total nutrient admixtures (TNA) because it has been reported to affect lipid emulsion stability.

For intramuscular injection
- Iron dextran should be injected only into the muscle mass of the upper outer quadrant of the buttock. It should *never* be injected into the arm or other exposed areas.
- Deep injection with a 2- to 3-inch, 19- or 20-gauge needle is recommended.
- If the patient is standing during administration of iron dextran, body weight should be on the leg opposite to the injection site.
- If the patient is lying down during administration of iron dextran, he/she should be in a lateral position with injection site uppermost.
- A Z-track technique (displacement of the skin laterally prior to injection) is recommended to avoid injection or leakage into subcutaneous tissue.

Test dose—An intramuscular or intravenous test dose of 25 mg (elemental iron) should be given to all patients before receiving their first therapeutic dose. Although anaphylactic reactions may be evident within the first few minutes after injection, one hour or longer should elapse before the initial therapeutic dose. The intramuscular test dose should be administered in the same injection site and by the same technique as the therapeutic dose.

If no adverse reactions are observed after the test dose, the daily dose of iron dextran may be given according to the following schedule until the total calculated amount has been reached:
 For infants up to 5 kg of body weight—25 mg (elemental iron)
 For children under 10 kg—50 mg (elemental iron)
 Other patients—100 mg (elemental iron)

## Parenteral Dosage Forms

### IRON DEXTRAN INJECTION USP

**Usual adult and adolescent dose**
Deficiency (treatment)—
To restore hemoglobin and replenish iron stores: Intravenous or intramuscular, the dosage being determined by the following dosage table:

| Patient Weight || Total Iron Dextran Requirement (mL)* <br> Based on Observed Hemoglobin (grams/dL) of: |||||||
|---|---|---|---|---|---|---|---|---|
| lb | kg | 3 | 4 | 5 | 6 | 7 | 8 | 9 | 10 |
| 11 | 5 | 3 | 3 | 3 | 3 | 2 | 2 | 2 | 2 |
| 22 | 10 | 7 | 6 | 6 | 5 | 5 | 4 | 4 | 3 |
| 33 | 15 | 10 | 9 | 9 | 8 | 7 | 7 | 6 | 5 |
| 44 | 20 | 16 | 15 | 14 | 13 | 12 | 11 | 10 | 9 |
| 55 | 25 | 20 | 18 | 17 | 16 | 15 | 14 | 13 | 12 |
| 66 | 30 | 23 | 22 | 21 | 19 | 18 | 17 | 15 | 14 |
| 77 | 35 | 27 | 26 | 24 | 23 | 21 | 20 | 18 | 17 |
| 88 | 40 | 31 | 29 | 28 | 26 | 24 | 22 | 21 | 19 |
| 99 | 45 | 35 | 33 | 31 | 29 | 27 | 25 | 23 | 21 |
| 110 | 50 | 39 | 37 | 35 | 32 | 30 | 28 | 26 | 24 |
| 121 | 55 | 43 | 41 | 38 | 36 | 33 | 31 | 28 | 26 |
| 132 | 60 | 47 | 44 | 42 | 39 | 36 | 34 | 31 | 28 |
| 143 | 65 | 51 | 48 | 45 | 42 | 39 | 36 | 34 | 31 |
| 154 | 70 | 55 | 52 | 49 | 45 | 42 | 39 | 36 | 33 |
| 165 | 75 | 59 | 55 | 52 | 49 | 45 | 42 | 39 | 35 |
| 176 | 80 | 63 | 59 | 55 | 52 | 48 | 45 | 41 | 38 |
| 187 | 85 | 66 | 63 | 59 | 55 | 51 | 48 | 44 | 40 |
| 198 | 90 | 70 | 66 | 62 | 58 | 54 | 50 | 46 | 42 |
| 209 | 95 | 74 | 70 | 66 | 62 | 57 | 53 | 49 | 45 |
| 220 | 100 | 78 | 74 | 69 | 65 | 60 | 56 | 52 | 47 |
| 231 | 105 | 82 | 77 | 73 | 68 | 63 | 59 | 54 | 50 |
| 242 | 110 | 86 | 81 | 76 | 71 | 67 | 62 | 57 | 52 |
| 253 | 115 | 90 | 85 | 80 | 75 | 70 | 64 | 59 | 54 |
| 264 | 120 | 94 | 88 | 83 | 78 | 73 | 67 | 62 | 57 |

*Dosage calculations based on a normal adult hemoglobin of 14.8 grams per dL for patients weighing more than 15 kg (33 pounds) and on hemoglobin of 12 grams/dL for patients weighing 15 kg (33 pounds) or less than or equal to 15 kg (33 pounds).

To calculate the total amount of iron dextran (mL) required to restore hemoglobin and to replenish iron stores in adults and children weighing over 15 kg (33 pounds), when LBW = lean body weight in kg and H = hemoglobin in grams/dL:
- Iron dextran (mL) = 0.0442 (Desired H − Observed H) × LBW + (0.26 × LBW)
- The dosage table above is *not* to be used for simple iron replacement from periodic blood loss in patients with hemorrhagic diatheses (familial telangiectasia; hemophilia; gastrointestinal bleeding) or patients on renal hemodialysis.

To replace the equivalent amount of iron represented in blood loss (based on the approximation that 1 mL of normocytic, normochromic red cells contains 1 mg of elemental iron)—Intramuscular or intravenous, the total iron requirement to be determined as follows:
- Replacement iron (mg) = Blood loss (mL) × hematocrit.
- To calculate dose in mL of iron dextran injection, divide result by 50.

**Usual pediatric dose**
Deficiency (treatment)—
To restore hemoglobin and replenish iron stores: Intravenous or intramuscular, the dosage being determined by the following dosage table:

| Patient Weight || Total Iron Dextran Requirement (mL)* <br> Based on Observed Hemoglobin (grams/dL) of: |||||||
|---|---|---|---|---|---|---|---|---|
| lb | kg | 3 | 4 | 5 | 6 | 7 | 8 | 9 | 10 |
| 11 | 5 | 3 | 3 | 3 | 3 | 2 | 2 | 2 | 2 |
| 22 | 10 | 7 | 6 | 6 | 5 | 5 | 4 | 4 | 3 |
| 33 | 15 | 10 | 9 | 9 | 8 | 7 | 7 | 6 | 5 |
| 44 | 20 | 16 | 15 | 14 | 13 | 12 | 11 | 10 | 9 |
| 55 | 25 | 20 | 18 | 17 | 16 | 15 | 14 | 13 | 12 |
| 66 | 30 | 23 | 22 | 21 | 19 | 18 | 17 | 15 | 14 |
| 77 | 35 | 27 | 26 | 24 | 23 | 21 | 20 | 18 | 17 |
| 88 | 40 | 31 | 29 | 28 | 26 | 24 | 22 | 21 | 19 |
| 99 | 45 | 35 | 33 | 31 | 29 | 27 | 25 | 23 | 21 |
| 110 | 50 | 39 | 37 | 35 | 32 | 30 | 28 | 26 | 24 |
| 121 | 55 | 43 | 41 | 38 | 36 | 33 | 31 | 28 | 26 |
| 132 | 60 | 47 | 44 | 42 | 39 | 36 | 34 | 31 | 28 |
| 143 | 65 | 51 | 48 | 45 | 42 | 39 | 36 | 34 | 31 |
| 154 | 70 | 55 | 52 | 49 | 45 | 42 | 39 | 36 | 33 |
| 165 | 75 | 59 | 55 | 52 | 49 | 45 | 42 | 39 | 35 |
| 176 | 80 | 63 | 59 | 55 | 52 | 48 | 45 | 41 | 38 |
| 187 | 85 | 66 | 63 | 59 | 55 | 51 | 48 | 44 | 40 |
| 198 | 90 | 70 | 66 | 62 | 58 | 54 | 50 | 46 | 42 |
| 209 | 95 | 74 | 70 | 66 | 62 | 57 | 53 | 49 | 45 |
| 220 | 100 | 78 | 74 | 69 | 65 | 60 | 56 | 52 | 47 |
| 231 | 105 | 82 | 77 | 73 | 68 | 63 | 59 | 54 | 50 |
| 242 | 110 | 86 | 81 | 76 | 71 | 67 | 62 | 57 | 52 |
| 253 | 115 | 90 | 85 | 80 | 75 | 70 | 64 | 59 | 54 |
| 264 | 120 | 94 | 88 | 83 | 78 | 73 | 67 | 62 | 57 |

*Dosage calculations based on a normal adult hemoglobin of 14.8 grams per dL for patients weighing more than 15 kg (33 pounds) and on hemoglobin of 12 grams/dL for patients weighing less than or equal to 15 kg.

Note: To calculate the total amount of iron dextran (mL) required to restore hemoglobin and to replenish iron stores in children weighing between 5 and 15 kg (11 and 33 pounds), when W = body weight in kg and H = hemoglobin in grams/dL:
- Iron dextran (mL) = 0.0442 (Desired H − Observed H) × W + (0.26 × W)
- The dosage table above is *not* to be used for simple iron replacement from periodic blood loss in patients with hemorrhagic diatheses (familial telangiectasia; hemophilia; gastrointestinal bleeding) or patients on renal hemodialysis.

**Strength(s) usually available**
U.S.—
50 mg (elemental ferric iron) per mL (Rx) [*DexFerrum; InFeD*].
Canada—
50 mg (elemental ferric iron) per mL (Rx) [*DexIron*].

**Packaging and storage**
Store below 40 °C (104 °F), preferably between 15 and 30 °C (59 and 86 °F), unless otherwise specified by manufacturer. Protect from freezing.

**Incompatibilities**
Addition of iron dextran to blood for transfusion is not recommended. Iron dextran has been reported to affect lipid emulsion stability in certain total nutrient admixture (TNA) formulations.

**Additional information**
Vehicle in iron dextran injection is 0.9% sodium chloride injection.

---

### IRON-POLYSACCHARIDE

## Summary of Differences
General dosing information: Contains elemental ferric form of iron.

## Additional Dosing Information
Strengths of products expressed in terms of elemental iron content only.

## Oral Dosage Forms

### IRON-POLYSACCHARIDE CAPSULES

**Usual adult and adolescent dose**
Deficiency (prophylaxis)—
Oral, amount based on normal daily recommended intakes of elemental iron:

| Persons | U.S. (mg) | Canada (mg) |
|---|---|---|
| Adolescent and adult males | 10 | 8–10 |
| Adolescent and adult females | 10–15 | 8–13 |
| Pregnant females | 30 | 17–22 |
| Breast-feeding females | 15 | 8–13 |

Deficiency (treatment)—
Treatment dose is individualized based on severity of deficiency.

**Usual pediatric dose**
Dosage form is not recommended for use in children.

**Strength(s) usually available**
U.S.—
  150 mg (elemental ferric iron) (OTC) [*Hytinic; Niferex-150; Nu-Iron 150*].
Canada—
  Not commercially available.
Note: The strength of these iron preparations may exceed the dosage range recommended by USP DI Advisory Panels based on the amount necessary to meet normal nutritional needs.

**Packaging and storage**
Store below 40 °C (104 °F), preferably between 15 and 30 °C (59 and 86 °F), unless otherwise specified by manufacturer. Store in a tight container.

**Auxiliary labeling**
• Keep out of reach of children.

**Note**
Caution patients about toxic effects of overdose, especially in children, and need for immediate medical aid.

### IRON-POLYSACCHARIDE ELIXIR

**Usual adult and adolescent dose**
See *Iron-Polysaccharide Capsules*.

**Usual pediatric dose**
Deficiency (prophylaxis)—
  Oral, amount based on normal daily recommended intakes of elemental iron:

| Persons | U.S. (mg) | Canada (mg) |
|---|---|---|
| Infants and children | | |
| Birth to 3 years of age | 6–10 | 0.3–6 |
| 4 to 6 years of age | 10 | 8 |
| 7 to 10 years of age | 10 | 8–10 |

Deficiency (treatment)—
  Treatment dose is individualized by prescriber based on severity of deficiency.

**Strength(s) usually available**
U.S.—
  100 mg (elemental ferric iron) per 5 mL (OTC) [*Niferex* (alcohol 10%); *Nu-Iron* (alcohol 10%)].
Canada—
  Not commercially available.
Note: The strength of these iron preparations may exceed the dosage range recommended by USP DI Advisory Panels based on the amount necessary to meet normal nutritional needs.

**Packaging and storage**
Store below 40 °C (104 °F), preferably between 15 and 30 °C (59 and 86 °F), unless otherwise specified by manufacturer. Store in a tight container. Protect from freezing.

**Auxiliary labeling**
• Keep out of reach of children.

**Note**
Caution patients about toxic effects of overdose, especially in children, and need for immediate medical aid.
When indicated by dosage, include a calibrated liquid-measuring device and explain use.

### IRON-POLYSACCHARIDE TABLETS

**Usual adult and adolescent dose**
See *Iron-Polysaccharide Capsules*.

**Usual pediatric dose**
See *Iron-Polysaccharide Elixir*.

**Strength(s) usually available**
U.S.—
  50 mg (elemental ferric iron) (OTC) [*Niferex*].
Canada—
  Not commercially available.
Note: The strength of this iron preparation may exceed the dosage range recommended by USP DI Advisory Panels based on the amount necessary to meet normal nutritional needs.

**Packaging and storage**
Store below 40 °C (104 °F), preferably between 15 and 30 °C (59 and 86 °F), unless otherwise specified by manufacturer. Store in a tight container.

**Auxiliary labeling**
• Keep out of reach of children.

**Note**
Caution patients about toxic effects of overdose, especially in children, and need for immediate medical aid.

### IRON SORBITOL

## Summary of Differences
General dosing information: Contains elemental ferric form of iron.

## Additional Dosing Information
Oral iron must be discontinued before the administration of parenteral iron.
*For intramuscular injection*
  • Iron sorbitol should be injected only into the muscle mass of the upper outer quadrant of the buttock. It should *never* be injected into the arm or other exposed areas.
  • Deep injection with a 2- to 3-inch, 19- or 20-gauge needle is recommended.
  • If the patient is standing during administration of iron sorbitol, body weight should be on the leg opposite to the injection site.
  • If the patient is lying down during administration of iron sorbitol, he/she should be in a lateral position with injection site uppermost.
  • A Z-track technique (displacement of the skin laterally prior to injection) is recommended to avoid injection or leakage into subcutaneous tissue.

## Parenteral Dosage Forms

### IRON SORBITOL INJECTION

**Usual adult and adolescent dose**
Deficiency (treatment)—
  To restore hemoglobin and replenish iron stores: Intramuscular, the daily dosage is determined based on 1.5 mg of elemental iron per kg of body weight. The calculated daily dose may be administered daily or every other day until hemoglobin values are normal.
  To increase hemoglobin by 1 gram per 100 mL: Intramuscular administration of 200 mg elemental iron for women and 250 mg for men is necessary. To replenish iron stores, an additional 250 to 1000 mg of elemental iron is needed.
  Note: Some clinicians recommend that iron sorbitol injection be given in divided doses of 50 mg per week because larger doses are painful to the patient.

**Usual adult prescribing limits**
100 mg per day.

**Usual pediatric dose**
Deficiency (treatment)—
  To restore hemoglobin and replenish iron stores: Intramuscular, the daily dosage is determined based on 1.5 mg of elemental iron per kg of body weight. The calculated daily dose may be administered daily or every other day until hemoglobin values are normal.
  Note: Some clinicians recommend that iron sorbitol injection be given in doses of 50 mg per week because larger doses are painful to the patient.

**Strength(s) usually available**
U.S.—
  Not commercially available.
Canada—
  50 mg (elemental ferric iron) per mL (Rx) [*Jectofer*].

**Packaging and storage**
Store below 40 °C (104 °F), preferably between 15 and 30 °C (59 and 86 °F), unless otherwise specified by manufacturer.

Revised: 04/16/92
Interim revision: 06/29/92; 06/19/95; 07/11/97

---

**ISOETHARINE**—See *Bronchodilators, Adrenergic (Inhalation-Local)*

---

**ISOFLURANE**—See *Anesthetics, Inhalation (Systemic)*

**ISOFLUROPHATE**—See *Antiglaucoma Agents, Cholinergic, Long-acting (Ophthalmic)*

# ISOMETHEPTENE, DICHLORALPHENAZONE, AND ACETAMINOPHEN Systemic

INN: Acetaminophen—Paracetamol
VA CLASSIFICATION (Primary/Secondary): CN103/CN105
Commonly used brand name(s): *Amidrine; I.D.A; Iso-Acetazone; Isocom; Midchlor; Midrin; Migquin; Migrapap; Migratine; Migrazone; Migrend; Migrex; Mitride.*

Note: For a listing of dosage forms and brand names by country availability, see *Dosage Forms* section(s).

## Category
Vascular headache suppressant (migraine).

Note: Some headache specialists question the validity of the term "vascular headache" because a correlation between dilatation of cerebral blood vessels and symptoms of migraine has not been demonstrated conclusively.

## Indications

**Accepted**

Headache, migraine (treatment) and

Headache, tension-type (treatment)—Isometheptene, dichloralphenazone, and acetaminophen combination is indicated to relieve occasional migraine headaches (with or without aura) and coexisting migraine and tension-type headaches ("mixed" headache syndrome). However, the U.S. FDA has classified this combination as being "possibly" effective in the treatment of migraine headaches. This classification requires the submission of adequate and well-controlled studies in order to provide substantial evidence of effectiveness.

Note: Some headache specialists question the value of this formulation in pure tension-type headaches. However, the distinction between vascular, tension-type, and "mixed" headaches is often difficult or uncertain, and the medication may relieve some headaches characterized as tension-type.

Because frequent use of headache-aborting medications by headache-prone individuals may lead to tolerance and dependence, this medication is not recommended for regular use by patients who experience frequent, especially daily, headaches.

To reduce analgesic use, underlying problems that may contribute to tension-type headaches, such as inflammation or structural abnormalities in the cervical or temporomandibular areas, should be identified and treated. In some patients, application of heat, muscle relaxants, and/or physical therapy may be helpful. Other medications having the potential to cause habituation (e.g., benzodiazepines used as muscle relaxants) should be used as infrequently as possible.

Chronic tension-type headaches and severe migraines that occur more frequently than twice a month may require additional prophylactic treatment to reduce the frequency, severity, and/or duration of the headaches. The prophylactic agents most commonly used for tension-type headaches are tricyclic antidepressants, especially amitriptyline, and/or beta-adrenergic blocking agents, especially propranolol. For migraines, beta-adrenergic blocking agents, calcium channel blocking agents, tricyclic antidepressants, monoamine oxidase inhibitors, methysergide, pizotyline (not commercially available in the U.S.), and sometimes cyproheptadine (especially in children) are used as prophylaxis. The combination of amitriptyline plus propranolol has been found superior to either agent used alone as prophylaxis against "mixed" headaches.

Identification and avoidance of precipitating factors is also important in the overall management of the patient with migraine headaches. Relaxation and/or biofeedback techniques may also be helpful in controlling some types of headache, and may reduce the need for medication.

## Pharmacology/Pharmacokinetics

**Physicochemical characteristics**
Molecular weight—
  Isometheptene mucate: 492.7.
  Dichloralphenazone: 519.04.
  Acetaminophen: 151.16.

**Mechanism of action/Effect**
Isometheptene—The mechanism of action has not been established. Isometheptene is an indirect-acting sympathomimetic agent with vasoconstricting activity. It has been proposed that constriction of cerebral blood vessels reduces the pulsation in cerebral arteries that may be responsible for the pain of migraine headaches. However, studies have not consistently shown a significant correlation between dilatation of cerebral blood vessels and pain or other symptoms of migraine headaches, or between a vasoconstrictive action and relief of migraine.

Dichloralphenazone—A complex of chloral hydrate and antipyrine (INN: phenazone). It is present in this formulation as a mild sedative and relaxant.

Acetaminophen—The mechanism of analgesic action has not been fully determined. Acetaminophen may act predominantly by inhibiting prostaglandin synthesis in the central nervous system (CNS) and, to a lesser extent, through a peripheral action by blocking pain-impulse generation. The peripheral action may also be due to inhibition of prostaglandin synthesis or to inhibition of the synthesis or actions of other substances that sensitize pain receptors to mechanical or chemical stimulation.

**Absorption**
Acetaminophen—Rapid and almost complete; may be decreased if taken following a high-carbohydrate meal.

**Distribution**
In breast milk—Acetaminophen: Peak concentrations of 10 to 15 mcg per mL (66.2 to 99.3 micromoles/L) have been measured 1 to 2 hours following maternal ingestion of a single 650-mg dose.

**Biotransformation**
Dichloralphenazone—Hydrolyzed to the active compounds chloral hydrate and antipyrine. Chloral hydrate is metabolized in the liver and erythrocytes to the active metabolite trichloroethanol, which may be further metabolized to inactive metabolites. It is also metabolized in the liver and kidneys to inactive metabolites.

Acetaminophen—Approximately 90 to 95% of a dose is metabolized in the liver, primarily by conjugation with glucuronic acid, sulfuric acid, and cysteine. An intermediate metabolite, which may accumulate in overdosage after the primary metabolic pathways become saturated, is hepatotoxic and possibly nephrotoxic.

**Half-life**
Acetaminophen—
  1 to 4 hours; does not change with renal failure but may be prolonged in acute overdosage, in some forms of hepatic disease, and in the elderly; may be somewhat shortened in children.
  In breast milk: 1.35 to 3.5 hours.

**Time to peak concentration**
Acetaminophen—0.5 to 2 hours.

**Peak plasma concentration**
Acetaminophen—5 to 20 mcg per mL (with doses up to 650 mg).

**Time to peak effect**
Acetaminophen—1 to 3 hours.

**Duration of action**
Acetaminophen—3 to 4 hours.

**Elimination**
Acetaminophen—Renal, as metabolites, primarily conjugates; 3% of a dose may be excreted unchanged.
  In dialysis:
    Hemodialysis: 120 mL per minute (for unmetabolized drug); metabolites are also cleared rapidly.
    Hemoperfusion: 200 mL per minute.
    Peritoneal dialysis: <10 mL per minute.

## Precautions to Consider

Note: The quantity of dichloralphenazone in this combination formulation does not provide full therapeutic doses of its active components chloral hydrate and antipyrine (phenazone). However, the possibility should be considered that precautions applying to chloral hydrate (see *Chloral Hydrate [Systemic]*) and to antipyrine may apply to ingestion of an overdose or to overuse of this combination medication.

**Cross-sensitivity and/or related problems**
Patients sensitive to aspirin are usually not sensitive to acetaminophen; however, acetaminophen has caused mild bronchospastic reactions in some aspirin-sensitive asthmatics (less than 5% of those tested).

**Pregnancy/Reproduction**
Fertility—Chronic toxicity studies in animals have shown that high doses of acetaminophen cause testicular atrophy and inhibition of spermatogenesis; the relevance of this finding to use in humans is not known.

Pregnancy—Acetaminophen crosses the placenta. However, problems in humans have not been documented.

**Breast-feeding**
Problems in humans have not been documented. Although peak concentrations of 10 to 15 mcg per mL (66.2 to 99.3 micromoles/L) of acetaminophen have been measured in breast milk 1 to 2 hours following maternal ingestion of a single 650-mg dose, neither acetaminophen nor its metabolites were detected in the urine of the nursing infants. The half-life in breast milk is 1.35 to 3.5 hours.

**Pediatrics**
No published information is available on the relationship of age to the effects of this combination medication in pediatric patients.

**Geriatrics**
No published information is available on the relationship of age to the effects of this combination medication in geriatric patients. Geriatric patients are more likely to have peripheral vascular disease, and are therefore more likely to be adversely affected by peripheral vasoconstriction, than are younger adults. However, isometheptene may be safer for elderly patients than the ergot derivatives used to abort acute vascular headaches. Also, elderly patients are more likely to have age-related renal function impairment, which may require caution in patients receiving acetaminophen and isometheptene.

**Drug interactions and/or related problems**
The following drug interactions and/or related problems have been selected on the basis of their potential clinical significance (possible mechanism in parentheses where appropriate)—not necessarily inclusive (» = major clinical significance):

Note: Combinations containing any of the following medications, depending on the amount present, may also interact with this medication.

Alcohol or
CNS depressants
(concurrent use with dichloralphenazone may cause additive sedation)

Alcohol, especially chronic abuse of or
Hepatic enzyme inducers (See *Appendix II*) or
Hepatotoxic medications, other (See *Appendix II*)
(risk of hepatotoxicity with single toxic doses of acetaminophen may be increased in alcoholics or in patients regularly taking other hepatotoxic medications or hepatic enzyme–inducing agents)

(chronic use of barbiturates [except butalbital] or primidone has been reported to decrease the therapeutic effects of acetaminophen, probably because of increased metabolism resulting from induction of hepatic microsomal enzyme activity; the possibility should be considered that similar effects may occur with other hepatic enzyme inducers)

» Monoamine oxidase (MAO) inhibitors
(concurrent use with an indirect-acting sympathomimetic such as isometheptene may cause sudden and severe hypertension and hyperpyrexia, which can reach crisis levels)

**Laboratory value alterations**
The following value have been selected on the basis of their potential clinical significance (possible effect in parentheses where appropriate)—not necessarily inclusive (» = major clinical significance):

With diagnostic test results
Glucose, blood, determinations
(acetaminophen may cause values to be falsely decreased when measured by the glucose oxidase/peroxidase method but probably not when measured by the hexokinase [glucose-6-phosphate dehydrogenase (G6PD)] method)

5-Hydroxyindoleacetic acid (5-HIAA), serum, determinations
(acetaminophen may cause false-positive results with qualitative screening tests using nitrosonaphthol reagent; the quantitative test is unaffected)

Pancreatic function test using bentiromide
(administration of acetaminophen prior to the bentiromide test will invalidate test results because acetaminophen is also metabolized to an arylamine and will thus increase the apparent quantity of para-aminobenzoic acid [PABA] recovered; it is recommended that acetaminophen be discontinued at least 3 days prior to administration of bentiromide)

Uric acid, serum, determinations
(acetaminophen may cause falsely increased values when the phosphotungstate uric acid test method is used)

With physiology/laboratory test values
Bilirubin, serum and
Lactate dehydrogenase (LDH), serum and
Prothrombin time and
Transaminase, serum
(values may be increased indicating acetaminophen-induced hepatotoxicity, especially in alcoholics, patients taking other hepatic enzyme inducers, or patients with pre-existing hepatic disease, when single toxic doses [> 8 to 10 grams] are taken)

**Medical considerations/Contraindications**
The medical considerations/contraindications included have been selected on the basis of their potential clinical significance (reasons given in parentheses where appropriate)—not necessarily inclusive (» = major clinical significance).

*Risk-benefit should be considered when the following medical problems exist:*

» Alcoholism, active or
» Hepatic function impairment or
» Viral hepatitis
(increased risk of acetaminophen-induced hepatotoxicity)

Any condition in which the vasoconstrictive or other sympathomimetic effects of isometheptene may be hazardous, such as:
Cardiovascular or cerebrovascular insufficiency, including recent myocardial infarction or stroke
» Glaucoma, not optimally controlled
» Hypertension, not optimally controlled
» Organic heart disease
Peripheral vascular disease
» Renal function impairment, severe

Sensitivity to acetaminophen or to isometheptene, history of

## Side/Adverse Effects

Note: The quantity of dichloralphenazone in this combination formulation does not provide full therapeutic doses of its active metabolites chloral hydrate and antipyrine (phenazone). However, the possibility should be considered that ingestion of an overdose or overuse of this combination medication may induce side effects characteristic of chloral hydrate (see *Chloral Hydrate [Systemic]*) and/or antipyrine.

The following side/adverse effects have been selected on the basis of their potential clinical significance (possible signs and symptoms in parentheses where appropriate)—not necessarily inclusive:

**Those indicating need for medical attention**
Incidence less frequent
*Anemia or methemoglobinemia* (unusual tiredness or weakness)
Incidence rare
*Agranulocytosis* (unexplained sore throat and fever); *anemia* (unusual tiredness or weakness); *dermatitis, allergic* (skin rash, hives, or itching); *hepatitis* (yellow eyes or skin); *thrombocytopenia* (usually asymptomatic; rarely, unusual bleeding or bruising; black, tarry stools; blood in urine or stools; pinpoint red spots on skin)

Symptoms of tolerance and/or dependence—with overuse
*Headaches*—more frequent, severe, and difficult to treat than previously

**Those indicating need for medical attention only if they continue or are bothersome**
Incidence more frequent
*Drowsiness*

Incidence less frequent or rare—dose-related
*Dizziness; fast or irregular heartbeat*

## Overdose

For specific information on the agents used in the management of isometheptene, dichloralphenazone, and acetaminophen overdose, see:
• *Acetylcysteine (Systemic)* monograph.

For more information on the management of overdose or unintentional ingestion, **contact a Poison Control Center** (see *Poison Control Center Listing*).

**Clinical effects of overdose**
The following effects have been selected on the basis of their potential clinical significance (possible signs and symptoms in parentheses where appropriate)—not necessarily inclusive:

Acute
   *Gastrointestinal upset* (diarrhea; loss of appetite; nausea or vomiting; stomach cramps or pain); *increased sweating*
   Note: Early signs and symptoms of acetaminophen overdose, i.e., *gastrointestinal upset* and *increased sweating* often do not occur. However, when they do occur, they usually appear within 6 to 14 hours after ingestion of an overdose and persist for about 24 hours.

Chronic
   *Hepatotoxicity* (pain, tenderness, and/or swelling in upper abdominal area)
   Note: The first indications of overdosage may be signs and symptoms of possible *liver damage* and abnormalities in liver function tests, which may not occur until 2 to 4 days after ingestion of the overdose. Maximal changes in liver function tests usually occur 3 to 5 days after ingestion of the overdose.
      Overt *hepatic disease or failure* may occur 4 to 6 days after ingestion of the overdose. *Hepatic encephalopathy* (with mental changes, confusion, agitation, or stupor), *convulsions, respiratory depression, coma, cerebral edema, coagulation defects, gastrointestinal bleeding, disseminated intravascular coagulation, hypoglycemia, metabolic acidosis, cardiac arrhythmias, and cardiovascular collapse* may occur.
      *Renal tubular necrosis* leading to *renal failure* (signs may include bloody or cloudy urine and sudden decrease in amount of urine) has also been reported in acetaminophen overdose, usually, but not exclusively, in conjunction with acetaminophen-induced *hepatotoxicity*.

**Treatment of overdose**
For acetaminophen—
   To decrease absorption—Emptying the stomach via induction of emesis or gastric lavage.
   Removing activated charcoal (if used) by gastric lavage may be advisable. Although activated charcoal is recommended in cases of mixed drug overdose, it may interfere with absorption of orally administered acetylcysteine (antidote used to protect against acetaminophen-induced hepatotoxicity) and decrease its efficacy.
   To enhance elimination—Instituting hemodialysis or hemoperfusion to remove acetaminophen from the circulation may be beneficial if acetylcysteine administration cannot be instituted within 24 hours following ingestion of a massive acetaminophen overdose. However, the efficacy of such treatment in preventing acetaminophen-induced hepatotoxicity is not known.
   Specific treatment—Use of acetylcysteine. *It is recommended that acetylcysteine administration be instituted as soon as possible after ingestion of an overdose has been reported,* without waiting for the results of plasma acetaminophen determinations or other laboratory tests. Acetylcysteine is most effective if treatment is started within 10 to 12 hours after ingestion of the overdose; however, it may be of some benefit if treatment is started within 24 hours. See the package insert or *Acetylcysteine (Systemic)* monograph for specific dosing guidelines for use of this product.
   Monitoring—Determining plasma acetaminophen concentration at least 4 hours following ingestion of the overdose. Determinations performed prior to this time are not reliable for assessing potential hepatotoxicity. Initial plasma concentrations above 150 mcg per mL (mcg/mL [993 micromoles/L]) at 4 hours, 100 mcg/mL (662 micromoles/L) at 6 hours, 70 mcg/mL (463.4 micromoles/L) at 8 hours, 50 mcg/mL (331 micromoles/L) at 10 hours, 20 mcg/mL (132.4 micromoles/L) at 15 hours, 8 mcg/mL (53 micromoles/L) at 20 hours, or 3.5 mcg/mL (23.2 micromoles/L) at 24 hours postingestion indicate possible hepatotoxicity and the need for completing the full course of acetylcysteine treatment. If the initial determination indicates a plasma concentration below those listed at the times indicated, cessation of acetylcysteine therapy can be considered. However, some clinicians advise that more than one determination should be performed to ascertain peak absorption and half-life of acetaminophen prior to considering discontinuation of acetylcysteine.
   Monitoring renal and cardiac function and administering appropriate therapy as required.
   Performing liver function tests (serum aspartate aminotransferase [AST; SGOT], serum alanine aminotransferase [ALT; SGPT], prothrombin time, and bilirubin) at 24-hour intervals for at least 96 hours postingestion if the plasma acetaminophen concentration indicates potential hepatotoxicity. If no abnormalities are detected within 96 hours, further determinations are not needed.
   Supportive care—May include maintaining fluid and electrolyte balance, correcting hypoglycemia, and administering vitamin K$_1$ (if prothrombin time ratio exceeds 1.5) and fresh frozen plasma or clotting factor concentrate (if prothrombin time ratio exceeds 3.0).

For dichloralphenazone—
   To decrease absorption—May include gastric lavage (endotracheal tube with inflated cuff should be in place to prevent aspiration of vomitus).
   To enhance elimination—Hemodialysis may be effective in promoting the clearance of the active metabolite trichloroethanol.
   Specific treatment—May include providing artificial respiration with oxygen.
   Monitoring—Continuous cardiac monitoring is important, especially in patients with predisposing cardiac disease.
   Supportive care— May include maintaining normal body temperature, maintaining appropriate fluid and electrolyte therapy and urinary output, and supporting respiration and circulation. Patients in whom intentional overdose is known or suspected should be referred for psychiatric consultation.

For isometheptene—
   To decrease absorption—Emptying the stomach by induction of emesis or gastric lavage.
   Monitoring—May include monitoring the patient, especially for signs and symptoms of excessive sympathetic stimulation or vasoconstriction, and treating observed symptoms as necessary.

## Patient Consultation

As an aid to patient consultation, refer to *Advice for the Patient, Isometheptene, Dichloralphenazone, and Acetaminophen (Systemic)*.
In providing consultation, consider emphasizing the following selected information (» = major clinical significance):

**Before using this medication**
» Conditions affecting use, especially:
   Allergic reaction to acetaminophen or to this combination medication, history of
   Pregnancy—Acetaminophen crosses the placenta
   Breast-feeding—Acetaminophen is excreted in breast milk
   Other medications, especially monoamine oxidase inhibitors
   Other medical problems, especially alcoholism (active), glaucoma, hypertension, heart disease, hepatic disease or viral hepatitis, and severe renal function impairment

**Proper use of this medication**
» Importance of not taking more medication than the amount prescribed; risk of tolerance and dependence with too frequent use; also, acetaminophen may cause liver damage with long-term use or greater than recommended doses
» Most effective when taken as soon as headache appears or at first sign of migraine attack (prodromal stage)
» Lying down in a quiet, dark room after taking initial dose
» Compliance with prophylactic therapy, if prescribed
   Proper dosing
» Proper storage

**Precautions while using this medication**
» Checking with physician if usual dose fails to relieve headaches, or if frequency and/or severity of headaches increases; possibility that tolerance to the medication has developed and/or withdrawal (rebound) or chronic, daily headaches are occurring
» Caution if other medications containing acetaminophen are used
» Caution when driving or doing jobs requiring alertness because of possible drowsiness or dizziness, especially if also taking a CNS depressant
» Avoiding use of alcohol, which increases the risk of liver toxicity with high doses of acetaminophen, especially in alcoholics; also, alcohol may aggravate or induce headache

**Side/adverse effects**
   Signs of potential side effects, especially allergic dermatitis, blood dyscrasias, hepatotoxicity, and methemoglobinemia

## General Dosing Information

Therapy is most effective when initiated at the first symptoms of a headache (during the prodrome, for migraine with aura).

After the first dose has been administered, it is recommended that the patient lie down and relax in a quiet, darkened room, because this contributes to relief of headaches.

In headache-prone individuals, frequent use of headache relievers may cause tolerance, leading to an increased dosage requirement, and to physical dependence, leading to both medication abuse and chronic (daily or near-daily) headaches. Patients who experience frequent headaches may also be dependent on a variety of other medications, including opioid analgesics, barbiturate-containing analgesic combinations, simple analgesics such as acetaminophen or aspirin, ergotamine, and antianxiety agents or sedatives.

Chronic headaches resulting from overmedication may be difficult to relieve, especially if the patient continues to take headache suppressants and/or analgesics. It is recommended that all such medications be discontinued. In-patient treatment may be necessary during detoxification. Naproxen, alone or together with amitriptyline, may reduce the severity of the headaches. Repetitive intravenous administration of dihydroergotamine (in conjunction with metoclopramide [to control dihydroergotamine-induced nausea and vomiting]) is recommended by some headache specialists to relieve chronic, intractable headaches associated with dependency on headache-aborting medications. Appropriate treatment for symptoms of withdrawal from other substances frequently used or abused by chronic headache patients may also be needed. In addition, appropriate prophylactic treatment should be initiated or adjusted to reduce the frequency and/or severity of future headaches.

## Oral Dosage Forms

### ISOMETHEPTENE MUCATE, DICHLORALPHENAZONE, AND ACETAMINOPHEN CAPSULES USP

**Usual adult dose**
Tension-type headache—
   Oral, 1 or 2 capsules every four hours as needed, up to 8 capsules a day.

Vascular headache suppressant (migraine)—
   Oral, 2 capsules at the start of the attack (during the prodrome, for migraine with aura), followed by 1 capsule every hour as needed, up to 5 capsules in twelve hours.

**Usual pediatric dose**
Dosage has not been established.

**Strength(s) usually available**
U.S.—
   65 mg of isometheptene mucate, 100 mg of dichloralphenazone, and 325 mg of acetaminophen (Rx) [*Amidrine; I.D.A; Iso-Acetazone; Isocom; Midchlor; Midrin; Migrapap; Migquin; Migratine; Migrazone; Migrend; Migrex; Mitride*].

**Packaging and storage**
Store below 40 °C (104 °F), preferably between 15 and 30 °C (59 and 86 °F). Store in a well-closed container.

### Selected Bibliography

Kunkel RS. Diagnosis and treatment of muscle contraction (tension-type) headaches. Med Clin N Amer 1991; 75: 595-603.
Anthony M. The treatment of migraine and other headaches. Curr Opin Neurol Neurosurg 1991; 4: 245-52.
Diamond S. Migraine headache. Med Clin N Amer 1991; 75: 545-66.

Revised: 08/18/92
Interim revision: 05/17/95

# ISONIAZID   Systemic

VA CLASSIFICATION (Primary): AM500
Commonly used brand name(s): *Isotamine; Laniazid; Nydrazid; PMS Isoniazid*.
Another commonly used name is INH.
Note:   For a listing of dosage forms and brand names by country availability, see *Dosage Forms* section(s).

## Category
Antibacterial (antimycobacterial).

## Indications

Note:   Bracketed information in the *Indications* section refers to uses that are not included in U.S. product labeling.

**General considerations**
Tuberculosis is a highly infectious life-threatening bacterial disease with 8 million new cases and 3 million deaths reported worldwide each year to the World Health Organization (WHO). The vast majority of these cases are in developing countries; however, tuberculosis also has emerged as an important public health problem in the U.S. in recent years after the decline in number of cases observed between 1950 and 1980.

The resurgence of tuberculosis in the U.S. has been complicated by an increase in the proportion of patients with strains resistant to antituberculosis medications. Outbreaks of multidrug-resistant tuberculosis have been documented in hospitals and prisons. Drug-resistant tuberculosis, particularly that caused by strains resistant to isoniazid and rifampin, is much harder to treat and often is fatal. Among acquired immunodeficiency syndrome (AIDS) patients infected with tuberculosis bacilli resistant to both rifampin and isoniazid, a case-fatality rate of 91% has been reported. Recent investigations of outbreaks of multidrug-resistant tuberculosis have found an extraordinarily high case-fatality rate, with the median time to mortality being reached between 4 and 16 weeks. In almost all instances, these outbreaks have involved patients with severe immunosuppression by infection with the human immunodeficiency virus (HIV).

Acquired drug resistance develops during treatment for drug-sensitive tuberculosis with regimens that are poorly conceived or poorly complied with, allowing the emergence of naturally occurring drug-resistant mutations. Resistant organisms from affected patients may subsequently infect other people who have not been infected with *M. tuberculosis* previously, resulting in primary drug resistance.

Resistance to antituberculosis agents can develop not only in the strain that caused the initial disease, but also as a result of reinfection with a new strain of *M. tuberculosis* that is drug-resistant. Reinfection with a new multidrug-resistant *M. tuberculosis* strain can occur during therapy for the original infection or after completion of therapy. Most recent data suggest that outcomes can be improved if patients promptly begin therapy with two or more drugs that have *in vitro* activity against the multidrug-resistant isolate.

HIV infection is the strongest risk factor yet identified for the development of active tuberculosis disease in persons infected with tuberculosis. In addition, persons with HIV infection are at an increased risk of tuberculosis resulting either from newly acquired disease or from reactivation of latent infections. Tuberculosis is a major clinical manifestation of immunodeficiency induced by HIV. In hospital-based retrospective studies, high rates of tuberculosis have been found among patients with AIDS. In communities where tuberculosis and HIV infection are common, the prevalence of HIV seropositivity among patients with tuberculosis is greatly increasing.

WHO has estimated that 5.6 million people worldwide and 80,000 people in the U.S. are infected with both HIV and tuberculosis. Persons dually infected with *M. tuberculosis* and HIV have a high risk of developing clinically active tuberculosis. One study of HIV-positive drug users with positive tuberculin skin test results found a rate of the development of active tuberculosis to be 8 cases per 100 person-years (8% yearly) as compared with the 10% lifetime risk (1 to 3% risk within the first year after skin test conversion) in the general population.

Persons who are known to be HIV-infected and who are contacts of patients with infectious tuberculosis should be carefully evaluated for evidence of tuberculosis. If there are no findings suggestive of current tuberculosis, preventive therapy with isoniazid should be given. Because HIV-infected contacts are not managed in the same way as those who are not HIV-infected, HIV testing is recommended if there are known or suspected risk factors for their acquiring of HIV infection.

According to investigators at the National Institute of Allergy and Infectious Diseases (NIAID), levels of HIV in the bloodstream increase 5-

to 160-fold in HIV-infected persons who develop active tuberculosis. Clinical and epidemiologic observations have demonstrated that HIV-infected individuals have an estimated 113-times higher risk and AIDS patients have a 170-times higher risk compared with uninfected persons. Furthermore, the problem of drug resistance may worsen as the HIV epidemic spreads. Immunosuppressed patients with HIV infection who subsequently become infected with *M. tuberculosis* have an extraordinarily high risk of developing active tuberculosis within a short period of time.

In addition to the convincing evidence that HIV infection increases the risk and worsens the course of tuberculosis, there is increasing clinical evidence that coinfection with *M. tuberculosis* accelerates progression of disease caused by HIV infection. Understanding the interaction of these two pathogens is clinically important, given the high prevalence of patients coinfected with HIV and *M. tuberculosis* in both the U.S. and Africa; it is estimated that by the year 2000 about 500,000 deaths per year will occur in coinfected patients worldwide.

Persons with a positive tuberculin skin test and HIV infection, and persons with a positive tuberculin skin test and at risk of acquiring HIV infection with unknown HIV status should be considered for tuberculosis preventive therapy regardless of age. One study showed that isoniazid prophylaxis in HIV-infected, tuberculin-positive individuals not only decreased the incidence of tuberculosis disease, but also delayed the progression to AIDS and death.

Twelve months of preventive therapy is recommended for adults and children with HIV infection and other conditions associated with immunosuppression. Persons with HIV infection should receive at least 6 months of preventive therapy. The American Academy of Pediatrics recommends that children receive 9 months of therapy.

Tuberculosis control programs should ensure that drug susceptibility tests are performed on all initial isolates of *M. tuberculosis* and the results are reported promptly to the primary care provider and the local health department. Tuberculosis control programs should monitor local drug resistance rates to assess the effectiveness of local tuberculosis control efforts and to determine the appropriateness of the currently recommended initial tuberculosis treatment regimen for the area.

Relapse of rifampin-resistant tuberculosis has been reported in HIV-infected patients. Reinfection with new strains of *M. tuberculosis* has also been reported in these patients. Rifampin-resistant tuberculosis is a serious threat because responses to therapy are more difficult to achieve and require long courses of treatment. Therefore, careful follow-up of HIV-infected patients with treated tuberculosis is essential.

Multidrug-resistant tuberculosis also has been transmitted to persons without HIV infection in health care facilities. Together with the lack of effective agents for second-line treatment and methods of prophylaxis, the transmission of multidrug-resistant strains of *M. tuberculosis* may create a substantial reservoir of latently infected people and the potential for clinical multidrug-resistant tuberculosis for many years to come.

Several studies have documented a high prevalence of extrapulmonary disease in HIV-infected patients with clinical tuberculosis disease, particularly in conjunction with pulmonary manifestations. Cutaneous miliary tuberculosis, also known as *tuberculosis cutis miliaris disseminata*, was in the past, a rare entity in adults, with only 24 cases reported in nearly a century. However, since the first reported case of cutaneous miliary tuberculosis in 1990 in a patient with AIDS, five additional cases have been reported in HIV-infected patients. Its appearance can be quite nondescript; therefore, a high level of suspicion must be maintained, particularly for patients with a CD4+ cell count of < 200 per cubic millimeter, in order to diagnose the condition and initiate therapy appropriately.

### Accepted

Tuberculosis (prophylaxis)—Isoniazid is indicated alone in the prophylaxis of all forms of tuberculosis in the following persons:
- Household members and other close contacts of patients with recently diagnosed tuberculosis who have a positive tuberculin skin test (PPD) of ≥ 5 mm; [tuberculin-negative children and adolescents who have been close contacts of infectious persons within the past 3 months are also candidates for preventative therapy until a repeat PPD is done 12 weeks after contact with the infectious source][1];
- [Human immunodeficiency virus (HIV)–infected persons of any age with a positive PPD of ≥ 5 mm or a past history of a positive PPD; also, persons with risk factors for HIV infection whose HIV status is unknown but who are suspected of having HIV infection][1];
- Positive PPD reactors of ≥ 5 mm with chest radiograph findings consistent with nonprogressive tuberculosis in whom there are neither positive bacteriologic findings nor a history of adequate chemotherapy for tuberculosis;
- [Children with a positive PPD of ≥ 5 mm who have an immunosuppressive condition, including HIV infection or immunosuppression due to corticosteroids][1];
- Adults with positive PPD reactions of ≥ 10 mm who are receiving immunosuppressives or prolonged therapy with corticosteroids, who have certain hematologic and reticuloendothelial diseases such as leukemia or Hodgkin's disease, who have diabetes mellitus or silicosis, or who have undergone gastrectomy;
- Children up to 4 years of age with a positive PPD of ≥ 10 mm who are at increased risk of dissemination because of their young age[1];
- [Children with a positive PPD of ≥ 10 mm who are at increased risk of dissemination because of medical risk factors other than immunosuppression due to corticosteroid therapy or HIV infection, such as Hodgkin's disease, lymphoma, diabetes mellitus, chronic renal failure, and malnutrition][1];
- [Positive PPD reactors with a PPD ≥ 10 mm among intravenous drug abusers (IVDA) known to be HIV-negative, alcoholics, or homeless persons of any age, and children frequently exposed to these persons][1];
- [Positive PPD reactions of ≥ 10 mm in foreign-born persons up to 35 years of age, or children whose parents are from high-prevalence areas, such as Asia, Africa, or Latin America][1];
- [Positive PPD reactions of ≥ 10 mm in residents of long-term care facilities, prisons, nursing homes, and mental institutions, and children frequently exposed to these persons][1];
- [Positive PPD reactions of ≥ 10 mm in medically underserved low-income populations, up to 35 years of age, including high-risk racial or ethnic minority populations, especially blacks, Hispanics, and Native Americans][1]; or
- Recent converters, as indicated by a PPD increase of ≥ 10 mm within 2 years for those up to 35 years of age, and a PPD increase of ≥ 15 mm for those 35 years of age and older; [also, children 4 years of age and older with a PPD of ≥ 15 mm without any risk factors][1].

Tuberculosis (treatment)—Isoniazid is indicated, in combination with other antituberculars, in the treatment of all forms of tuberculosis, including tuberculous meningitis.

Resistance to isoniazid is a rapidly increasing problem. The primary cause of drug-resistance to antitubercular medications is inadequate therapy due to patient noncompliance. To try to avoid this continuing trend, administration of four-drug directly observed therapy (DOT) is currently recommended. (See *General Dosing Information*.)

Not all species or strains of a particular organism may be susceptible to isoniazid.

### Unaccepted

Isoniazid is not recommended for use in the treatment of atypical mycobacterial infections, such as *Mycobacterium avium* complex (MAC), because isoniazid has weak activity against MAC compared to other antimycobacterial agents.

---

[1]Not included in Canadian product labeling.

## Pharmacology/Pharmacokinetics

Note: Preliminary data suggest that patients coinfected with human immunodeficiency virus (HIV) and mycobacteria (*Mycobacterium tuberculosis* or *M. avium*) have altered pharmacokinetic profiles for antimycobacterial agents. In particular, malabsorption of these agents appears to occur frequently, and could seriously affect the efficacy of treatment.

### Physicochemical characteristics
Molecular weight—137.14.

### Mechanism of action/Effect
Isoniazid (INH) is a synthetic, bactericidal antitubercular agent that is active against many mycobacteria, primarily those that are actively dividing. Its exact mechanism of action is not known, but it may relate to inhibition of mycolic acid synthesis and disruption of the cell wall in susceptible organisms.

### Absorption
Readily absorbed following oral administration; however, may undergo significant first pass metabolism. Absorption and bioavailability are reduced when isoniazid is administered with food.

### Distribution
Widely distributed to all fluids and tissues, including cerebrospinal fluid (CSF), pleural and ascitic fluids, skin, sputum, saliva, lungs, muscle, and caseous tissue. INH crosses the placenta and is distributed into breast milk.

Vol$_D$—0.57 to 0.76 L per kg.

### Protein binding
Very low (0 to 10%).

### Biotransformation
Hepatic; isoniazid is acetylated by *N*-acetyl transferase to *N*-acetylisoniazid; it is then biotransformed to isonicotinic acid and monoacetylhydrazine. Monoacetylhydrazine is associated with hepatotoxicity via formation of a reactive intermediate metabolite when *N*-hydroxylated by the cytochrome P450 mixed oxidase system. The rate of acetylation is genetically determined; slow acetylators are characterized by a relative lack of hepatic *N*-acetyltransferase.

### Half-life
Adults (including elderly patients)—
 Fast acetylators: 0.5 to 1.6 hours.
 Slow acetylators: 2 to 5 hours.
 Acute and chronic liver disease: May be prolonged (6.7 hours vs 3.2 hours in controls).
Children (age 1.5 to 15 years)—
 2.3 to 4.9 hours.
Neonates—
 7.8 and 19.8 hours in two newborns who received isoniazid transplacentally. The long half-life may be due to the limited acetylation capacity of neonates.

### Time to peak concentration
1 to 2 hours.

### Peak serum concentration
3 to 7 mcg per mL after a single 300-mg oral dose.

### Elimination
Renal; approximately 75–95% excreted by the kidneys within 24 hours, primarily as the inactive metabolites, *N*-acetylisoniazid and isonicotinic acid; of this amount, 93% of the isoniazid excreted in the urine may occur as the acetylated form in fast acetylators and 63% in slow acetylators, with the remainder, in both cases, occurring as the free or conjugated form.
Small amounts are excreted in feces.
In dialysis—
 Significant amounts of isoniazid are removed from the blood by hemodialysis. A single 5-hour hemodialysis period has removed up to 73% of the isoniazid in the blood.
 Peritoneal dialysis is of limited benefit.

## Precautions to Consider

### Cross-sensitivity and/or related problems
Patients hypersensitive to ethionamide, pyrazinamide, niacin (nicotinic acid), or other chemically related medications may be hypersensitive to this medication also.

### Carcinogenicity/Tumorigenicity
Isoniazid has been shown to cause pulmonary tumors in a number of strains of mice. However, isoniazid has not been shown to be carcinogenic or tumorigenic in humans.

### Pregnancy/Reproduction
Note: Tuberculosis in pregnancy should be managed in concert with an expert in the management of tuberculosis. Women who have only pulmonary tuberculosis are not likely to infect the fetus until after delivery, and congenital tuberculosis is extremely rare. *In utero* infections with tubercle bacilli, however, can occur after maternal bacillemia occurs at different stages in the course of tuberculosis. Miliary tuberculosis can seed the placenta and thereby gain access to the fetal circulation. In women with tuberculous endometritis, transmission of infection to the fetus can result from fetal aspiration of bacilli at the time of delivery. A third mode of transmission is through ingestion of infected amniotic fluid *in utero*.

If active disease is diagnosed during pregnancy, a 9-month regimen of isoniazid and rifampin, supplemented by an initial course of ethambutol if drug resistance is suspected, is recommended. Pyrazinamide usually is not given because of inadequate data regarding teratogenesis. Hence, a 9-month course of therapy is necessary for drug-susceptible disease. When isoniazid resistance is a possibility, isoniazid, ethambutol, and rifampin are recommended initially. One of these medications can be discontinued after 1 or 2 months, depending on results of susceptibility tests. If rifampin or isoniazid is discontinued, treatment is continued for a total of 18 months; if ethambutol is discontinued, treatment is continued for a total of 9 months. Prompt initiation of chemotherapy is mandatory to protect both the mother and fetus. If isoniazid or rifampin resistance is documented, an expert in the management of tuberculosis should be consulted.

Asymptomatic pregnant women with positive tuberculin skin tests and normal chest radiographs should receive preventive therapy with isoniazid for 9 months if they are HIV seropositive or have recently been in contact with an infectious person. For these individuals, preventive therapy should begin after the first trimester. In other circumstances in which none of these risk factors is present, although no harmful effects of isoniazid to the fetus have been observed, preventive therapy can be delayed until after delivery.

For all pregnant women receiving isoniazid, pyridoxine should be prescribed. Isoniazid, ethambutol, and rifampin appear to be relatively safe for the fetus. The benefit of ethambutol and rifampin for therapy of active disease in the mother outweighs the risk to the infant. Streptomycin and pyrazinamide should not be used unless they are essential to the control of the disease.

Pregnancy—Isoniazid crosses the placenta, resulting in fetal serum concentrations that may exceed maternal serum concentrations. However, problems in humans have not been documented.

Studies in rats and rabbits have shown that isoniazid may be embryocidal. However, isoniazid has not been shown to be teratogenic in mice, rats, or rabbits.

FDA Pregnancy Category C.

### Breast-feeding
Isoniazid is distributed into breast milk. An estimated 0.75 to 2.3% of the daily adult dose could be ingested by the nursing infant. Problems in nursing newborns have not been documented and breast-feeding should not be discouraged. However, because isoniazid concentrations are so low in breast milk, breast-feeding cannot be relied upon for adequate tuberculosis prophylaxis or therapy for nursing infants.

### Pediatrics
Note: If an infant is suspected of having congenital tuberculosis, a Mantoux tuberculin skin test, chest radiograph, lumbar puncture, and appropriate cultures should be performed promptly. Regardless of the skin test results, treatment of the infant should be initiated promptly with isoniazid, rifampin, pyrazinamide, and streptomycin or kanamycin. In addition, the mother should be evaluated for the presence of pulmonary or extrapulmonary (including uterine) tuberculosis. If the physical examination or chest radiograph support the diagnosis of tuberculosis, the patient should be treated with the same regimen as that used for tuberculous meningitis. The drug susceptibilities of the organism recovered from the mother and/or infant should be determined.

Possible isoniazid resistance should always be considered, particularly in children from population groups in which drug resistance is high, especially in foreign-born children from countries with a high prevalence of drug-resistant tuberculosis. For contacts who are likely to have been infected by an index case with isoniazid-resistant but rifampin-susceptible organisms, and in whom the consequences of the infection are likely to be severe (e.g., children up to 4 years of age), rifampin (10 mg per kg of body weight, maximum 600 mg, given daily in a single dose) should be given in addition to isoniazid (10 mg per kg, maximum 300 mg, given daily in a single dose) until susceptibility test results for the isolate from the index case are available. If the index case is known or proven to be excreting organisms resistant to isoniazid, then isoniazid should be discontinued and rifampin given for a total of 9 months. Isoniazid alone should be given if no proof of exposure to isoniazid-resistant organisms is found. Optimal therapy for children with tuberculosis infection caused by organisms resistant to isoniazid and rifampin is unknown. In deciding on therapy in this situation, consultation with an expert is advised.

Adjuvant treatment with corticosteroids in treating tuberculosis is controversial. Corticosteroids have been used for therapy in children with tuberculous meningitis to reduce vasculitis, inflammation, and, as a result, intracranial pressure. Data indicate that dexamethasone may lower mortality rates and lessen long-term neurologic impairment. The administration of corticosteroids should be considered in all children with tuberculous meningitis, and also may be considered in children with pleural and pericardial effusions (to hasten reabsorption of fluid), severe miliary disease (to mitigate alveolocapillary block), and endobronchial disease (to relieve obstruction and atelectasis). Corticosteroids should be given only when accompanied by appropriate antituberculosis therapy. Consultation with an expert in the treatment of tuberculosis should be obtained when corticosteroid therapy is considered.

Studies performed in children have not demonstrated pediatrics-specific problems that would limit the usefulness of isoniazid in children. However, newborn infants may have a limited acetylation capacity, prolonging the elimination half-life of isoniazid.

Children do not require routine hepatic function determinations unless they have pre-existing hepatic disease.

Pyridoxine supplementation is not usually required in children if dietary intake is adequate.

## Geriatrics
Appropriate studies on the relationship of age to the effects of isoniazid have not been performed in the geriatric population. However, patients over 50 years of age are more likely to develop hepatitis while receiving isoniazid than are patients in younger age groups.

## Pharmacogenetics
Patients can be divided into two groups: slow and rapid acetylators of isoniazid. Approximately 50% of blacks and Caucasians are slow acetylators; the majority of Eskimos and Asians are rapid acetylators. The rate of acetylation does not significantly alter the effectiveness of isoniazid. However, slow acetylation may lead to higher blood levels of isoniazid and thus, an increase in toxic reactions. Slow acetylators are characterized by a relative lack of hepatic N-acetyltransferase. Patients who are slow acetylators may be more prone to develop adverse effects, especially peripheral neuritis, and may require lower-than-usual doses. Rapid acetylators generally do not require higher doses, nor is isoniazid less effective in these patients.

## Drug interactions and/or related problems
The following drug interactions and/or related problems have been selected on the basis of their potential clinical significance (possible mechanism in parentheses where appropriate)—not necessarily inclusive (» = major clinical significance):

Note: Combinations containing any of the following medications, depending on the amount present, may also interact with this medication.

Acetaminophen
(concurrent use of acetaminophen with isoniazid may increase the potential for hepatotoxicity and, possibly, nephrotoxicity; isoniazid is thought to induce cytochrome P450, resulting in a greater proportion of acetaminophen being converted to toxic metabolite)

» Alcohol
(concurrent daily use of alcohol may result in increased incidence of isoniazid-induced hepatotoxicity and increased metabolism of isoniazid; dosage adjustments of isoniazid may be necessary; patients should be monitored closely for signs of hepatotoxicity and should be advised to restrict intake of alcoholic beverages)

» Alfentanil
(chronic preoperative or perioperative use of isoniazid, a hepatic enzyme inhibitor, may decrease the plasma clearance and prolong the duration of action of alfentanil)

Antacids, especially aluminum-containing
(antacids may delay and decrease absorption and serum concentrations of orally administered isoniazid; concurrent use should be avoided, or patients should be advised to take oral isoniazid at least 1 hour before aluminum-containing antacids)

Anticoagulants, coumarin- or indandione-derivative
(concurrent use with isoniazid may result in increased anticoagulant effect because of the inhibition of enzymatic metabolism of anticoagulants)

Benzodiazepines
(isoniazid may decrease the hepatic metabolism of benzodiazepines, such as diazepam, chlordiazepoxide, flurazepam, and prazepam, that are metabolized by phase I reactions [N-demethylation and hydroxylation]; it may also impair the oxidation of triazolam, increasing plasma benzodiazepine concentrations; isoniazid may decrease first-pass metabolism and elimination of midazolam in the liver, probably by competitive inhibition at the cytochrome P450 binding sites, increasing steady-state plasma concentrations of midazolam)

» Carbamazepine
(concurrent use with isoniazid increases serum carbamazepine levels and toxicity, probably through inhibition of carbamazepine metabolism; also, carbamazepine may induce microsomal metabolism of isoniazid, increasing formation of an INH-reactive intermediate metabolite, which may lead to hepatotoxicity)

Cheese, such as Swiss or Cheshire, or
Fish, such as tuna, skipjack, or Sardinella
(concurrent ingestion with isoniazid may result in redness or itching of the skin, hot feeling, rapid or pounding heartbeat, sweating, chills or clammy feeling, headache, or lightheadedness; this is thought to be due to the inhibition of plasma monoamine oxidase and diamine oxidase by isoniazid, interfering with the metabolism of histamine and tyramine found in fish and cheese)

Corticosteroids, glucocorticoid
(concurrent use of prednisolone, and probably other related corticosteroids, with isoniazid may increase hepatic metabolism and/or excretion of isoniazid, leading to decreased plasma concentrations and effectiveness of isoniazid, especially in patients who are rapid acetylators; isoniazid dosage adjustments may be required)

Cycloserine
(concurrent use may result in increased incidence of central nervous system [CNS] effects such as dizziness or drowsiness; dosage adjustments may be necessary and patients should be monitored closely for signs of CNS toxicity)

» Disulfiram
(concurrent use in alcoholics may result in increased incidence of CNS effects such as dizziness, incoordination, irritability, or insomnia; reduced dosage or discontinuation of disulfiram may be necessary)

Enflurane
(isoniazid may increase formation of the potentially nephrotoxic inorganic fluoride metabolite when used concurrently with enflurane)

» Hepatotoxic medications, other (see Appendix II)
(concurrent use of other hepatotoxic medications with isoniazid may increase the potential for hepatotoxicity and should be avoided)

» Ketoconazole
(concurrent use of ketoconazole with isoniazid has been reported to decrease serum concentrations of ketoconazole; isoniazid should be used with caution when given concurrently with ketoconazole)

Neurotoxic medications, other (see Appendix II)
(concurrent use of other neurotoxic medications with isoniazid may produce additive neurotoxicity)

» Phenytoin
(concurrent use with isoniazid inhibits the metabolism of phenytoin, resulting in increased phenytoin serum concentrations and toxicity; phenytoin dosage adjustments may be necessary during and after isoniazid therapy, especially in slow acetylators of isoniazid)

Pyridoxine
(isoniazid may cause peripheral neuritis by acting as a pyridoxine antagonist or increasing renal excretion of pyridoxine; requirements for pyridoxine may be increased in patients receiving isoniazid concurrently)

» Rifampin
(concurrent use of rifampin with isoniazid may increase the risk of hepatotoxicity, especially in patients with pre-existing hepatic impairment and/or in fast acetylators of isoniazid; patients receiving rifampin and isoniazid concurrently should be monitored closely for signs of hepatotoxicity during the first 3 months of therapy)

Theophylline
(concurrent use may reduce the metabolism of theophylline, increasing theophylline plasma concentrations)

## Laboratory value alterations
The following have been selected on the basis of their potential clinical significance (possible effect in parentheses where appropriate)—not necessarily inclusive (» = major clinical significance):

With diagnostic test results
Glucose, urine
(isoniazid may cause hyperglycemia with a secondary glycosuria, giving a positive response to copper sulfate tests; glucose enzymatic tests are not affected)

With physiology/laboratory test values
Alanine aminotransferase (ALT [SGPT]) and
Aspartate aminotransferase (AST [SGOT]) and
(values may be transiently and asymptomatically increased in approximately 10 to 20% of patients tested)

Bilirubin, serum
(concentrations may be transiently and asymptomatically increased in approximately 10 to 20% of patients tested)

## Medical considerations/Contraindications
The medical considerations/contraindications included have been selected on the basis of their potential clinical significance (reasons given in parentheses where appropriate)—not necessarily inclusive (» = major clinical significance).

### Risk-benefit should be considered when the following medical problems exist:

» Alcoholism, active or in remission, or
» Hepatic function impairment
(increased risk of hepatitis with daily consumption of alcohol or hepatic function impairment)

» Hypersensitivity to isoniazid, ethionamide, pyrazinamide, niacin (nicotinic acid), or other chemically related medications

Renal failure, severe
(there may be an increased risk of toxicity in patients who have severe renal failure [creatinine clearance < 10 mL/min])

Seizure disorders
(isoniazid may be neurotoxic and cause seizures)

**Patient monitoring**
The following may be especially important in patient monitoring (other tests may be warranted in some patients, depending on condition; » = major clinical significance):

Hepatic function determinations
(AST [SGOT], ALT [SGPT], and serum bilirubin determinations may be required prior to and monthly or more frequently during treatment; however, elevated serum enzyme values may not be predictive of clinical hepatitis and values may return to normal despite continued treatment; therefore, routine measurement of hepatic function is generally not recommended unless there is pre-existing hepatic disease; patients should be instructed to report promptly any prodromal symptoms of hepatitis; if signs and symptoms of hepatotoxicity occur, isoniazid should be promptly discontinued; if isoniazid therapy must be reinstituted, very small and gradually increasing doses should be used, and then only after signs and symptoms of hepatotoxicity have cleared; isoniazid should be withdrawn immediately if any further evidence of hepatotoxicity occurs)

» Ophthalmologic examinations
(if symptoms of optic neuritis occur in either adults or children during treatment, ophthalmologic examinations may be required immediately and periodically thereafter; ophthalmologic examinations are not recommended in asymptomatic patients)

## Side/Adverse Effects

Note: Isoniazid has been reported to cause severe, and sometimes fatal, age-related hepatitis. If signs and symptoms of hepatotoxicity occur, isoniazid should be discontinued promptly. The incidence of clinical hepatitis in young, healthy adults is 0.3%, but can increase to 2.6% for those who drink alcohol daily, have chronic liver disease, or are elderly.

Patients with advanced HIV disease have been reported to have an increased incidence of adverse reactions to antitubercular medications. This was not found in HIV-seropositive patients being treated for tuberculosis.

Pyridoxine deficiency is sometimes observed in adults receiving high doses of isoniazid and probably results from isoniazid's competetion with pyridoxal phosphate for the enzyme apotryptophanase.

Peripheral neuritis usually is preventable by administering 10 to 25 mg of pyridoxine per day. It is recommended for patients at risk of neuritis, including those over 65 years of age, pregnant women, patients with diabetes mellitus, chronic renal failure, alcoholism, malnutrition, and those taking anticonvulsant medications.

The following side/adverse effects have been selected on the basis of their potential clinical significance (possible signs and symptoms in parentheses where appropriate)—not necessarily inclusive:

**Those indicating need for medical attention**
Incidence more frequent
*Hepatitis* (dark urine, yellow eyes or skin); **hepatitis prodromal symptoms** (loss of appetite, nausea or vomiting, unusual tiredness or weakness); **peripheral neuritis** (clumsiness or unsteadiness; numbness, tingling, burning, or pain in hands and feet)

Incidence rare
*Blood dyscrasias* (fever and sore throat, unusual bleeding and bruising, unusual tiredness or weakness); **hypersensitivity** (fever, joint pain, skin rash); **neurotoxicity** (seizures, mental depression, mood or other mental changes); *optic neuritis* (blurred vision or loss of vision, with or without eye pain)

**Those indicating need for medical attention only if they continue or are bothersome**
Incidence more frequent
*Gastrointestinal disturbances* (diarrhea, nausea and vomiting, stomach pain)

Incidence not reported
*Local irritation at the site of intramuscular injections*

## Overdose

For specific information on the agents used in the management of isoniazid overdose, see
- *Pyridoxine (Systemic)* monograph;
- *Diazepam* in *Benzodiazepines (Systemic)* monograph; and/or
- *Thiopental* in *Barbiturates (Systemic)* monograph.

For more information on the management of overdose or unintentional ingestion, **contact a Poison Control Center** (see *Poison Control Center Listing*).

The information below applies to the clinical effects and treatment of isoniazid overdose.

**Clinical effects of isoniazid overdose**
The following effects have been selected on the basis of their potential clinical significance (possible signs and symptoms in parentheses where appropriate)—not necessarily inclusive:

Acute and chronic effects
*Gastrointestinal disturbances* (severe nausea and vomiting); **neurotoxicity** (dizziness; slurred speech; lethargy; disorientation; hyperreflexia; seizures; coma)

Note: Patients may be asymptomatic for 30 minutes to 2 hours after an acute overdose. Early symptoms include *nausea and vomiting, dizziness, slurred speech, lethargy, disorientation,* and *hyperreflexia. Seizures* usually occur within 1 to 3 hours after ingestion, and are often repetitive and refractory to treatment with usual anticonvulsants. Lactic acid accumulation produces an anion-gap metabolic acidosis within a few hours, which is often severe and refractory to treatment with sodium bicarbonate. Hyperglycemia, glycosuria, and ketonuria have also been reported.

**Treatment of isoniazid overdose**
To decrease absorption—
Because seizures may occur soon after ingestion, induction of emesis with ipecac is not recommended. Gastric lavage may be performed within 2 to 3 hours of ingestion, and activated charcoal and a cathartic may be administered if the patient's seizures are controlled and the airway protected.

Specific treatment—
Administering intravenous pyridoxine in a gram-for-gram dose, equivalent to the amount of isoniazid ingested; dose should be administered as a 5 or 10% solution in water for injection over 30 to 60 minutes. If the amount of isoniazid ingested is unknown, administering 5-gram doses of pyridoxine every 5 to 30 minutes until seizures stop or consciousness is regained.

Controlling seizures with diazepam, which acts synergistically with pyridoxine. Phenytoin should be used with caution, if at all, since isoniazid inhibits phenytoin metabolism. Thiopental has been effective in treating refractory seizures.

Carefully administering sodium bicarbonate if pyridoxine and diazepam do not control seizure activity. Use caution against overcorrection and watch for hypokalemia or hyperkalemia.

Supportive care—
Supportive measures such as establishing intravenous lines, hydration, correction of electrolyte imbalance, oxygenation, and support of ventilatory function are essential for maintaining the vital functions of the patient. Patients in whom intentional overdose is confirmed or suspected should be referred for psychiatric consultation.

## Patient Consultation

As an aid to patient consultation, refer to *Advice for the Patient, Isoniazid (Systemic)*.

In providing consultation, consider emphasizing the following selected information (» = major clinical significance):

**Before using this medication**
» Conditions affecting use, especially:
Hypersensitivity to isoniazid, ethionamide, pyrazinamide, niacin (nicotinic acid), or other chemically related medications
Pregnancy—Isoniazid crosses the placenta; fetal serum concentrations may exceed maternal serum concentrations
Breast-feeding—Isoniazid is distributed into breast milk
Use in children—Children may be less susceptible to pyridoxine deficiency and hepatotoxicity than adults, unless they have pre-existing hepatic disease; newborn infants may have prolonged elimination
Use in the elderly—Patients over the age of 50 have the highest incidence of hepatitis
Other medicines, especially daily alcohol use, alfentanil, carbamazepine, disulfiram, other hepatotoxic medications, ketoconazole, phenytoin, or rifampin
Other medical problems, especially alcoholism, active or in remission, or hepatic function impairment

**Proper use of this medication**
Taking this medication with food or antacids, but not within 1 hour of aluminum-containing antacids, if gastrointestinal irritation occurs (oral only)
Proper administration technique for oral liquids

- » Compliance with full course of therapy, which may take 6 months to 2 years
- » Taking pyridoxine concurrently to prevent or minimize symptoms of peripheral neuritis; not usually required in children if dietary intake is adequate
- » Proper dosing
  Missed dose: Taking as soon as possible; not taking if almost time for next dose; not doubling doses
- » Proper storage

**Precautions while using this medication**
- » Regular visits to physician to check progress, as well as ophthalmologic examinations if signs of optic neuritis occur in either adults or children
  Checking with physician if no improvement within 2 to 3 weeks
  Checking with physician if vascular reactions occur following concurrent ingestion of cheese or fish with isoniazid
- » Avoiding alcoholic beverages while taking this medication
- » Need to report to physician promptly prodromal signs of hepatitis or peripheral neuritis
- » Diabetics: False-positive reactions with copper sulfate urine glucose tests may occur

**Side/adverse effects**
  Hepatitis may be more likely to occur in patients over 50 years of age
  Signs of potential side effects, especially hepatitis, peripheral neuritis, blood dyscrasias, hypersensitivity, neurotoxicity, and optic neuritis

## General Dosing Information

All patients may be divided into two groups: slow and fast acetylators of isoniazid. Patients who are slow acetylators may be more prone to development of adverse effects, especially peripheral neuritis, and may require lower-than-usual doses. Fast acetylators do not generally require higher doses, nor is isoniazid less effective in these patients. Eskimo, Oriental, and American Indian populations have the lowest prevalence of slow acetylators, while Egyptian, Israeli, Scandinavian, other Caucasian, and black populations have the highest prevalence of slow acetylators.

The duration of treatment with an antituberculosis regimen is at least 6 months, and may be continued for 2 years. Uncomplicated pulmonary tuberculosis is often successfully treated within 6 to 12 months. Several different treatment regimens are currently recommended.

The duration of antituberculosis therapy is based on the patient's clinical and radiographic responses, smear and culture results, and susceptibility studies of *Mycobacterium tuberculosis* isolates from the patient or the suspect source case. With directly observed therapy (DOT), clinical evaluation is an integral component of each visit for administration of medication. Careful monitoring of the clinical and bacteriologic responses to therapy on a monthly basis in sputum-positive patients is important.

If therapy is interrupted, the treatment schedule should be extended to a later completion date. Although guidelines cannot be provided for every situation, the following factors need to be considered in establishing a new date for completion:
- The length of interruption;
- The time during therapy (early or late) in which interruption occurred; and
- The patient's clinical, radiographic, and bacteriologic status before, during, and after interruption. Consultation with an expert is advised.

Therapy should be administered based on the following guidelines, published by the American Thoracic Society (ATS) and by the Centers for Disease Control and Prevention (CDC), and endorsed by the American Academy of Pediatrics (AAP).
- A 6-month regimen consisting of isoniazid, rifampin, and pyrazinamide given for 2 months followed by isoniazid and rifampin for 4 months is the preferred treatment for patients infected with fully susceptible organisms who adhere to the treatment course.
- Ethambutol (or streptomycin in children too young to be monitored for visual acuity) should be included in the initial regimen until the results of drug susceptibility studies are available, and unless there is little possibility of drug resistance (i.e., there is less than 4% primary resistance to isoniazid in the community, and the patient has had no previous treatment with antituberculosis medications, is not from a country with a high prevalence of drug resistance, and has no known exposure to a drug-resistant case).
- Alternatively, a 9-month regimen of isoniazid and rifampin is acceptable for persons who cannot or should not take pyrazinamide. Ethambutol (or streptomycin in children too young to be monitored for visual acuity) should also be included until the results of drug susceptibility studies are available, unless there is little possibility of drug resistance. If isoniazid resistance is demonstrated, rifampin and ethambutol should be continued for a minimum of 12 months.
- Consideration should be given to treating all patients with DOT. DOT programs have been demonstrated to increase adherence in patients receiving antituberculosis chemotherapy in both rural and urban settings.
- Multidrug-resistant tuberculosis (i.e., resistance to at least isoniazid and rifampin) presents difficult treatment problems. Treatment must be individualized and based on susceptibility studies. In such cases, consultation with an expert in tuberculosis is recommended.
- Children should be managed in essentially the same ways as adults, but doses of the medications must be adjusted appropriately and specific important differences between the management of adults and children addressed. However, optimal therapy of tuberculosis in children with HIV infection has not been established. The Committee on Infectious Diseases of the AAP recommends that therapy always should include at least three drugs initially, and should be continued for a minimum period of 9 months. Isoniazid, rifampin, and pyrazinamide with or without ethambutol or an aminoglycoside should be given for at least the first 2 months. A fourth drug may be needed for disseminated disease and whenever drug-resistant disease is suspected.
- Extrapulmonary tuberculosis should be managed according to the principles and with the drug regimens outlined for pulmonary tuberculosis, except in children who have miliary tuberculosis, bone/joint tuberculosis, or tuberculous meningitis. These children should receive a minimum of 12 months of therapy.
- A 4-month regimen of isoniazid and rifampin is acceptable therapy for adults who have active tuberculosis and who are sputum smear– and culture–negative, if there is little possibility of drug resistance.

ATS, CDC, and AAP recommend preventive treatment of tuberculosis infection in the following patients:
- Preventive therapy with isoniazid given for 6 to 12 months is effective in decreasing the risk of future tuberculosis disease in adults and children with tuberculosis infection demonstrated by a positive tuberculin skin test reaction.
- Persons with a positive skin test and any of the following risk factors should be considered for preventive therapy regardless of age:
  —Persons with HIV infection.
  —Persons at risk for HIV infection with unknown HIV status.
  —Close contacts of sputum-positive persons with newly diagnosed infectious tuberculosis.
  —Newly infected persons (recent skin test convertors).
  —Persons with medical conditions reported to increase the risk of tuberculosis (i.e., diabetes mellitus, corticosteroid therapy and other immunosuppressive therapy, intravenous drug users, hematologic and reticuloendothelial malignancies, end-stage renal disease, and clinical conditions associated with rapid weight loss or chronic malnutrition).

In some circumstances, persons with negative skin tests should be considered for preventive therapy. These include children who are close contacts of infectious tuberculosis cases and anergic HIV-infected adults at increased risk of tuberculosis, tuberculin-positive adults with abnormal chest radiographs showing fibrotic lesions probably representing old healed tuberculosis, adults with silicosis, and persons who are known to be HIV-infected and who are contacts of patients with infectious tuberculosis.
- In the absence of any of the above risk factors, persons up to 35 years of age with a positive skin test who are in the following high-incidence groups should be also considered for preventive therapy:
  —Foreign-born persons from high-prevalence countries.
  —Medically underserved low-income persons from high-prevalence populations (especially blacks, Hispanics, and Native Americans).
  —Residents of facilities for long-term care (e.g., correctional institutions, nursing homes, and mental institutions).
- Twelve months of preventive therapy is recommended for adults and children with HIV infection and other conditions associated with immunosuppression. Persons without HIV infection should receive preventive therapy for at least 6 months.
- In persons younger than 35 years of age, routine monitoring for adverse effects of isoniazid should consist of a monthly symptom review. For persons 35 years of age and older, hepatic enzymes should be measured prior to starting isoniazid and monitored monthly throughout treatment, in addition to monthly symptom reviews.
- Persons who are presumed to be infected with isoniazid-resistant organisms should be treated with rifampin rather than with isoniazid.
- As with the treatment of active tuberculosis, the key to success of preventive treatment is patient adherence to the prescribed regimen. Although not evaluated in clinical studies, directly observed, twice-weekly preventive therapy may be appropriate for adults and children at risk, who cannot or will not reliably self-administer therapy.

The currently recommended regimen for treating tuberculosis is effective in treating HIV-infected patients with tuberculosis, and consists of isoniazid and rifampin for a minimum period of 6 months, plus pyrazinamide and either ethambutol or streptomycin for the first 2 months.

Because of the common association of tuberculosis with HIV infection, an increasing number of patients probably will be considered candidates for combined therapy with rifampin and protease inhibitors. Prompt initiation of appropriate pharmacologic therapy for patients with HIV infection who acquire tuberculosis is critical because tuberculosis may become rapidly fatal. The management of these patients is complex, requires an individualized approach, and should be undertaken only by or in consultation with an expert. In addition, all HIV-infected patients at risk for tuberculosis infection should be carefully evaluated and administered isoniazid preventive treatment if indicated, regardless of whether they are receiving protease inhibitor therapy.

For HIV-infected patients diagnosed with drug-susceptible tuberculosis and for whom protease inhibitor therapy is being considered but has not been initiated, the suggested management strategy is to complete tuberculosis treatment with a regimen containing rifampin before starting therapy with a protease inhibitor. The duration of the antituberculosis regimen is at least 6 months, and therapy should be administered according to the guidelines developed by ATS and CDC, including the recommendation to carefully assess clinical and bacteriologic response in patients coinfected with HIV and to prolong treatment if response is slow or suboptimal.

Most infants ≤ 12 months of age with tuberculosis are asymptomatic at the time of diagnosis, and the gastric aspirate cultures in these patients have a high yield for *M. tuberculosis*. When an infant is suspected of having tuberculosis, a thorough household investigation should be undertaken. A 6-month regimen of isoniazid and rifampin supplemented during the first 2 months by pyrazinamide has been found to be well-tolerated and effective in infants with pulmonary tuberculosis. Furthermore, twice-weekly DOT appears to be as effective as daily therapy, and is an essential alternative in patients for whom social issues prevent reliable daily therapy.

Physicians caring for children should be familiar with the clinical forms of the disease in infants to enable them to make an early diagnosis. Any child, especially one in a high-risk group or area, who has unexplained pneumonia, cervical adenitis, bone or joint infections, or aseptic meningitis should have a Mantoux tuberculin skin test performed, and a detailed epidemiologic history for tuberculosis should be obtained.

Management of a newborn infant whose mother, or other household contact, is suspected of having tuberculosis is based on individual considerations. If possible, separation of the mother, or contact, and infant should be minimized. The Committee on Infectious Diseases of the AAP offers the following recommendations in the management of the newborn infant whose mother, or any other household contact, has tuberculosis:

- *Mother, or any other household contact, with a positive tuberculin skin test reaction but no evidence of current disease:* Investigation of other members of the household or extended family to whom the infant may later be exposed is indicated. If no evidence of current disease is found in the mother or in members of the extended family, the infant should be tested with a Mantoux tuberculin skin test at 3 to 4 months of age. When the family members cannot be promptly tested, consideration should be given to administering isoniazid (10 mg per kg of body weight a day) to the infant until skin testing and other evaluation of the family members have excluded contact with a case of active tuberculosis. The infant does not need to be hospitalized during this time if adequate follow-up can be arranged, but adherence to medication administration should be closely monitored. The mother also should be considered for isoniazid therapy.
- *Mother with untreated (newly diagnosed) disease or disease that has been treated for 2 or more weeks and who is judged to be noncontagious at delivery:* Careful investigation of household members and extended family is mandatory. A chest radiograph and Mantoux tuberculin skin test should be performed on the infant at 3 to 4 months and at 6 months of age. Separation of the mother and infant is not necessary if adherence to treatment for the mother and infant is assured. The mother can breast-feed. The infant should receive isoniazid even if the tuberculin skin test and chest radiograph do not suggest clinical tuberculosis, since cell-mediated immunity of a degree sufficient to mount a significant reaction to tuberculin skin testing may develop as late as 6 months of age in an infant infected at birth. Isoniazid can be discontinued if the Mantoux skin test is negative at 3 to 4 months of age, the mother is adherent to treatment and has a satisfactory clinical response, and no other family members have infectious tuberculosis. The infant should be examined carefully at monthly intervals. If nonadherence is documented, the mother has an acid-fast bacillus (AFB)–positive sputum or smear, and supervision is impossible, the infant should be separated from the ill family member and Bacillus Calmette-Guérin (BCG) vaccine may be considered for the infant. However, the response to the vaccine in infants may be delayed and inadequate for prevention of tuberculosis.
- *Mother has current disease and is suspected of having been contagious at the time of delivery:* The mother and infant should be separated until the infant is receiving therapy or the mother is confirmed to be noncontagious. Otherwise, management is the same as when the disease is judged to be noncontagious to the infant at delivery.
- *Mother has hematogenously spread tuberculosis (e.g., meningitis, miliary disease, or bone involvement):* The infant should be evaluated for congenital tuberculosis. If clinical and radiographic findings do not support the diagnosis of congenital tuberculosis, the infant should be separated from the mother until she is judged to be noncontagious. The infant should be given isoniazid until 3 or 4 months of age, at which time the Mantoux skin test should be repeated. If the skin test is positive, isoniazid should be continued for a total of 12 months. If the skin test is negative and the chest radiograph is normal, isoniazid may be discontinued, depending on the status of the mother and whether there are other cases of infectious tuberculosis in the family. The infant should continue to be examined carefully at monthly intervals.

Health care or correctional institutions experiencing outbreaks of tuberculosis that are resistant to isoniazid and rifampin, or that are resuming therapy for a patient with a prior history of antitubercular therapy, may need to begin five- or six-drug regimens as initial therapy. These regimens should include the four-drug regimen and at least three medications to which the suspected multidrug-resistant strain may be susceptible.

Patients with impaired renal function do not generally require a reduction in dose if the plasma creatinine concentration is less than 6 mg per 100 mL. If renal impairment is more severe or if patients are slow acetylators, a reduction in dose and/or serum determinations may be required. Slow acetylators may require dosage adjustments to ensure isoniazid serum concentrations of less than 1 mcg per mL measured 24 hours after the preceding dose. In anuric patients, one-half the usual maintenance dose is recommended.

### For oral dosage forms only
Isoniazid may be taken with meals if gastrointestinal irritation occurs. Antacids may also be taken. However, isoniazid should be taken at least 1 hour before aluminum-containing antacids.

Oral absorption may be decreased if isoniazid is taken with food or antacids.

## Oral Dosage Forms

### ISONIAZID SYRUP USP

**Usual adult and adolescent dose**
Tuberculosis—
Prophylaxis: Oral, 300 mg once a day.
Treatment: In combination with other antituberculosis medications—Oral, 300 mg of isoniazid once a day for the entire treatment period; or 15 mg per kg of body weight, up to 900 mg, two or three times a week, as specified by the treatment regimen.

**Usual adult prescribing limits**
300 mg daily.

**Usual pediatric dose**
Tuberculosis—
Prophylaxis: Oral, 10 mg per kg of body weight, up to 300 mg, once a day.
Treatment: In combination with other antituberculosis medications—Oral, 10 to 20 mg of isoniazid per kg of body weight, up to 300 mg, once a day; or 20 to 40 mg per kg of body weight, up to 900 mg, two or three times a week, as specified by the treatment regimen.

**Strength(s) usually available**
U.S.—
  50 mg per 5 mL (Rx) [*Laniazid*; GENERIC].
Canada—
  50 mg per 5 mL (Rx) [*Isotamine*; *PMS Isoniazid*].

**Packaging and storage**
Store below 40 °C (104 °F), preferably between 15 and 30 °C (59 and 86 °F), unless otherwise specified by the manufacturer. Store in a tight, light-resistant container. Protect from freezing.

**Auxiliary labeling**
- Continue medicine for full time of treatment.
- Avoid alcoholic beverages.

**Note**
When dispensing, include a calibrated liquid-measuring device.

# ISONIAZID TABLETS USP

**Usual adult and adolescent dose**
See *Isoniazid Syrup USP*.

**Usual adult prescribing limits**
See *Isoniazid Syrup USP*.

**Usual pediatric dose**
See *Isoniazid Syrup USP*.

**Strength(s) usually available**
U.S.—
  50 mg (Rx) [*Laniazid;* GENERIC].
  100 mg (Rx) [*Laniazid;* GENERIC].
  300 mg (Rx) [*Laniazid;* GENERIC].
Canada—
  50 mg (Rx) [*PMS Isoniazid*].
  100 mg (Rx) [*PMS Isoniazid*].
  300 mg (Rx) [*PMS Isoniazid*].

**Packaging and storage**
Store below 40 °C (104 °F), preferably between 15 and 30 °C (59 and 86 °F), unless otherwise specified by the manufacturer. Store in a well-closed, light-resistant container.

**Auxiliary labeling**
• Continue medicine for full time of treatment.
• Avoid alcoholic beverages.

## Parenteral Dosage Forms

### ISONIAZID INJECTION USP

**Usual adult and adolescent dose**
Tuberculosis—
  Prophylaxis: Intramuscular, 300 mg once a day.
  Treatment: In combination with other antituberculosis medications—Intramuscular, 5 mg of isoniazid per kg of body weight, up to 300 mg, once a day for the entire treatment period; or 15 mg per kg of body weight, up to 900 mg, two or three times a week, as specified by the treatment regimen.

**Usual adult prescribing limits**
300 mg daily.

**Usual pediatric dose**
Tuberculosis—
  Prophylaxis: Intramuscular, 10 mg per kg of body weight, up to 300 mg, once a day.
  Treatment: In combination with other antituberculosis medications—Intramuscular, 10 to 20 mg of isoniazid per kg of body weight, up to 300 mg, once a day; or 20 to 40 mg per kg of body weight, up to 900 mg, two or three times a week, as specified by the treatment regimen.

**Strength(s) usually available**
U.S.—
  100 mg per mL (Rx) [*Nydrazid*].
Canada—
  Not commercially avrolable.

**Packaging and storage**
Store below 40 °C (104 °F), preferably between 15 and 30 °C (59 and 86 °F), unless otherwise specified by the manufacturer. Protect from light. Protect from freezing.
Note: Crystallization may occur at low temperatures. Upon warming to room temperature, the crystals will redissolve.

## Selected Bibliography

The American Thoracic Society (ATS). Ad Hoc Committee on the Scientific Assembly on Microbology, Tuberculosis, and Pulmonary Infections. Treatment of tuberculosis and tuberculosis infection in adults and children. Clin Infect Dis 1995; 21: 9-27.

Revised: 08/22/97

---

**ISONIAZID AND THIACETAZONE**—The *Isoniazid and Thiacetazone (Systemic)* monograph is not included in this published version of the USP DI database. Copies of the monograph are available on request from Micromedex, Inc. - Reprint Requests, 6200 S. Syracuse Way, Suite 300, Englewood, CO 80111; telephone (303) 486-6400; telefax (303) 486-6464; Email: USPDI@MDX.COM.

---

**ISOPHANE INSULIN**—See *Insulin (Systemic)*

---

**ISOPHANE INSULIN, HUMAN**—See *Insulin (Systemic)*

---

**ISOPHANE INSULIN, HUMAN, AND INSULIN HUMAN (SYSTEMIC)**—See *Insulin (Systemic)*

---

**ISOPROTERENOL**—See *Bronchodilators, Adrenergic (Inhalation-Local); Bronchodilators, Adrenergic (Systemic); Sympathomimetic Agents—Cardiovascular Use (Parenteral-Systemic)*

---

**ISOSORBIDE DINITRATE**—See *Nitrates (Systemic)*

---

**ISOSORBIDE MONONITRATE**—See *Nitrates (Systemic)*

---

# ISOTRETINOIN Systemic

VA CLASSIFICATION (Primary/Secondary): DE751/DE890
Commonly used brand name(s): *Accutane; Accutane Roche*.
Another commonly used name is 13-*cis*-retinoic acid.
Note: For a listing of dosage forms and brand names by country availability, see *Dosage Forms* section(s).

## Category
Antiacne agent (systemic); antirosacea agent (systemic); keratinization stabilizer (systemic).

## Indications
Note: Bracketed information in the *Indications* section refers to uses that are not included in U.S. product labeling.

**General considerations**
Note: FOR INFORMATION REGARDING PROBLEMS THAT HAVE OCCURRED DURING PREGNANCY SEE THE *PREGNANCY/REPRODUCTION* SECTION OF *PRECAUTIONS TO CONSIDER*.

Since **isotretinoin is a teratogen in pregnant females**, it should be prescribed only by physicians experienced in its use. Isotretinoin should not be used in females of childbearing potential, unless the patient is unresponsive to or intolerant of other treatments and can accept the strict measures to prevent pregnancy during treatment and for 1 month after treatment discontinuation.

FOR FEMALES OF CHILDBEARING POTENTIAL:
  Use of isotretinoin is contraindicated in females of childbearing potential, unless all of the following criteria have been met:
    • Patient shows severe, disfiguring, nodular acne or one of the other accepted indications.

- Patient is capable of complying with the mandatory contraceptive measures, even if she has a history of infertility. Two effective forms of contraception should be used at least 1 month before isotretinoin therapy begins, during therapy, and for 1 month following discontinuation of therapy. Contraceptive measures are not needed for patients who have had a hysterectomy or for those planning to abstain from sexual intercourse.
- Patient is not pregnant, as concluded from a negative pregnancy test. The pregnancy test should be performed after normal menstrual cycles are achieved and within 1 week prior to initiation of isotretinoin therapy. If isotretinoin therapy is initiated, it should begin within the same week as the pregnancy test, on Day 2 or Day 3 of the menstrual period.
- Patient receives both verbal and written warnings of the hazards associated with pregnancy during and following isotretinoin therapy and she acknowledges in writing her responsibility to avoid pregnancy.
- Patient understands treatment instructions and intends to follow them.

**For males and females**:

During treatment and 1 month after discontinuation of isotretinoin treatment, *patients should not donate blood* intended for transfusion purposes. Although the risk is small, a blood transfusion from such donors to pregnant women during their first trimester may expose the fetus to the medication.

**Accepted**

Acne vulgaris (treatment)—Isotretinoin is indicated in the treatment of severe, recalcitrant nodular acne, where severe is defined as numerous lesions of at least 5 millimeters in diameter that may be suppurative or hemorrhagic. [Isotretinoin is also indicated for severe, inflammatory acne and acne conglobata. Taking into consideration its potential adverse effects, isotretinoin may be considered in patients with moderately severe acne who are prone to scarring or dyspigmentation.] Because of its potential adverse effects, isotretinoin should be reserved for patients who are unresponsive to or intolerant of conventional therapy, including systemic antibiotics.

[Folliculitis, gram-negative (treatment)][1] or
[Rosacea, severe (treatment)][1]—Isotretinoin is used in the treatment of gram-negative folliculitis and severe rosacea.

[Hidradenitis suppurativa (treatment)][1]—Isotretinoin is used in the treatment of hidradenitis suppurativa and is more effective for less established conditions and for those mild in severity (less scarring). Complete suppression or prolonged remission is uncommon. Using isotretinoin as adjunctive therapy to intralesional steroids, systemic antibiotics, or local surgery has proved beneficial for some patients with hidradentitis suppurativa.

[Keratinization disorders][1], such as [Ichthyosis, lamellar][1], [Keratosis follicularis][1], [Palmoplantar keratoderma][1], [Pityriasis rubra pilaris][1]—Isotretinoin has been used for treatment of severe keratinization disorders, such as lamellar ichthyosis, keratosis follicularis (Darier's disease), palmoplantar keratoderma (keratosis palmaris et plantaris), and pityriasis rubra pilaris (PRP). Longer periods of isotretinoin therapy are usually required for keratinization disorders than for acne vulgaris, thus increasing the risk of side effects, including skeletal changes.

**Unaccepted**

Isotretinoin should not be used in the treatment of mild to moderate acne vulgaris that may be successfully controlled with topical acne medications and products or systemic antibiotics.

---

[1]Not included in Canadian product labeling.

## Pharmacology/Pharmacokinetics

**Physicochemical characteristics**
Chemical group—Vitamin A derivative (retinoid).
Molecular weight—300.44.
Chemical name—Retinoic acid, 13-*cis*-.

**Mechanism of action/Effect**
The exact mechanism of action for isotretinoin is not known. Although isotretinoin is produced naturally in the body as a retinoid, it does not bind directly to any of the two classes of nuclear retinoic acid receptors (RARs or RXRs) or their subclasses of receptors (alpha, beta, and gamma receptors). It does isomerize rapidly to all-*trans*-retinoic acid (tretinoin) and may metabolize to other compounds that act as a ligand for a retinoid receptor to alter gene expression and cause transcription or transrepression changes in protein synthesis. Other pathways outside of the retinoid receptor pathway may be responsible for the sebosuppressive action of isotretinoin.

Antiacne agent (systemic) and antirosacea agent (systemic)—The exact mechanism of action is not known. However, isotretinoin reduces sebaceous gland size and inhibits sebaceous gland activity, thereby decreasing sebum secretion. This action is probably responsible for the rapid initial clinical improvement in nodular acne. Isotretinoin also has been shown to decrease the number of *Propionibacterium acnes* organisms within the follicle. However, since isotretinoin has no effect on *P. acnes in vitro*, this action is probably a secondary effect due to decreased sebum secretion and the resulting decrease in nutrients and not a direct effect of isotretinoin. In addition, isotretinoin has been shown to have anti-keratinizing and anti-inflammatory actions. The exact role of these actions in clinical improvement of nodular acne is not known, especially with respect to prolonged remissions.

Hidradenitis suppurativa—If given early enough in the treatment of hidradenitis suppurativa, isotretinoin may prevent a potentially affected apocrine gland from being occluded by ductal hypercornification.

Keratinization stabilizer (systemic)—Isotretinoin is thought to interfere with the terminal differentiation of keratinocytes.

**Absorption**
Rapidly absorbed from the gastrointestinal tract; amount absorbed increases when isotretinoin is taken with food. Data suggest that isotretinoin and 4-oxo-isotretinoin may be reabsorbed from the bile.

**Distribution**
Radiolabeled doses administered to rats showed high concentrations of radioactivity in many tissues after 15 minutes, maximizing at 1 hour and declining to nondetectable concentrations in most tissues after 24 hours. Low radioactive concentrations in rats were still detectable in the liver, ureter, ovary, and adrenal and lacrimal glands after 7 days.

**Protein binding**
Very high (99.9%), almost exclusively to albumin.

**Biotransformation**
Metabolized in liver and possibly in the gut wall. The major identified metabolite in blood and urine is 4-oxo-isotretinoin; other identified metabolites are tretinoin and 4-oxo-tretinoin.

**Half-life**
Isotretinoin—
   10 to 20 hours, terminal half-life.
   90 hours, biologic half-life, following a radiolabeled 80-mg dose.
4-oxo-isotretinoin (major metabolite)—25 hours (range 17 to 50 hours), elimination half-life.

**Time to peak plasma concentration**
Isotretinoin—Approximately 3 hours, following an 80-mg dose.
4-oxo-isotretinoin—6 to 20 hours, following an 80-mg dose of isotretinoin.

**Peak plasma concentration**
Isotretinoin—98 to 535 nanograms per mL (mean, 256 nanograms per mL) in acne patients, following an 80-mg dose. Steady-state blood concentration for isotretinoin is 160 ± 19 nanograms per mL, following doses of 40 mg twice a day.
4-oxo-isotretinoin—87 to 399 nanograms per mL, following an 80-mg dose of isotretinoin. Steady-state blood concentration for 4-oxo-isotretinoin concentration exceeded that of isotretinoin after about 6 hours, following doses of 40 mg of isotretinoin twice a day.

**Elimination**
Biliary or feces—83%.
Renal—65%.

## Precautions to Consider

**Cross-sensitivity and/or related problems**
Patients sensitive to acitretin, tretinoin, or vitamin A derivatives may be sensitive to this medication also, since isotretinoin is related to both retinoic acid and retinol (vitamin A). Also, paraben-sensitive patients may be sensitive to isotretinoin capsules, since the gelatin capsule contains the preservatives methylparaben and propylparaben.

**Carcinogenicity/Tumorigenicity**
Studies in the Fischer 344 rat given isotretinoin doses of 8 or 32 mg per kg of body weight (mg/kg) per day for more than 18 months show an increased incidence of pheochromocytoma and, at the higher dose, adrenal medullary hyperplasia. However, pheochromocytoma is known to occur with a relatively high frequency in the particular species of rat tested. At doses of 8 and 32 mg/kg per day, rats show a decreased incidence of hepatic adenomas, hepatic angiomas, and leukemia.

**Mutagenicity**
Isotretinoin was not found to be mutagenic in a series of tests or assays, including the Ames test (for one of two laboratories), Chinese hamster cell assay, mouse micronucleus test, *S. cerevisiae* D7 assay, *in vitro* clastogenesis assay with human-derived lymphocytes, and unscheduled DNA synthesis assay. In one laboratory, isotretinoin produced a weakly

positive response for the Ames test when the test was conducted with metabolic activation.

**Pregnancy/Reproduction**
Fertility—Reproduction studies in male and female rats receiving isotretinoin in doses of 2, 8, or 32 mg/kg a day show no evidence of adverse effects on gonadal function, fertility, or conception rate. However, reproduction studies in male dogs receiving isotretinoin in doses of 20 or 60 mg/kg a day for approximately 30 weeks show incomplete testicular atrophy and microscopic evidence of depression of spermatogenesis. Studies in human males receiving isotretinoin for the treatment of nodular acne show no clinically significant changes in the number, motility, or morphology of spermatozoa in the ejaculate or in the production of ejaculate volume.

Pregnancy—**Isotretinoin is teratogenic in humans and is contraindicated during pregnancy.** Unless abstinence is the chosen method, it is recommended that the patient use two forms of effective contraception to prevent pregnancy, starting 1 month before initiation of treatment, during treatment, and for 1 month after discontinuation of treatment.

Although not every fetus exposed to isotretinoin has been affected, **the risk is high that an infant will have a deformity or abnormality if the pregnancy occurred while the mother was taking isotretinoin, even for a short period of time.** Whenever an unexpected pregnancy occurs during the time of teratogenic risk, the risk-benefit ratio of continuing the pregnancy must be considered. The risks include: 15% incidence of major malformations, 5% incidence of perinatal mortality, 16% incidence of premature birth, and 40% incidence of spontaneous abortion.

Major human fetal deformities or abnormalities associated with the use of isotretinoin include:
- Central nervous system (CNS) abnormalities, including hydrocephalus, microcephaly, and cranial nerve deficit;
- Eye abnormalities, including microphthalmia;
- Heart defects;
- Parathyroid deficiency;
- Skeletal or connective tissue abnormalities, including absence of terminal phalanges, alterations of the skull and cervical vertebra, and malformations of hip, ankle, and forearm; facial dysmorphia; cleft or high palate; low-set ears, micropinna, and small or absent external auditory canals; meningomyelocele; multiple synostoses; and syndactyly; and
- Thymus gland abnormality.

Cases of intelligence quotient scores lower than 85 have been reported with or without other CNS abnormalities.

One study of pregnant rats, who were given isotretinoin in doses of 5, 15, and 50 mg/kg a day on gestation days 7 through 15, produced no teratogenicity; in another study, isotretinoin was teratogenic in doses of 150 mg/kg a day. When rats were administered isotretinoin in doses of 5, 15, or 32 mg/kg a day on the 14th day of gestation through the 21st day of lactation, pup mortality increased, secondary to reduced maternal food intake.

In one study of pregnant New Zealand white rabbits given isotretinoin in doses of 1, 3, and 10 mg/kg of isotretinoin per day on the 7th through 18th days of gestation, no teratogenic or embryotoxic effects were seen at 1 and 3 mg/kg a day, but the 10 mg/kg dose caused nine of thirteen rabbits to abort and produced teratogenic effects in the remaining litters.

FDA Pregnancy Category X.

**Breast-feeding**
It is not known whether isotretinoin is distributed into breast milk. Isotretinoin is not recommended for use in women who are breast-feeding because of isotretinoin's potential to cause adverse effects in nursing infants.

**Pediatrics**
The long-term use of isotretinoin in children has not been studied. Although appropriate studies on the relationship of age to the effects of isotretinoin have not been performed in the pediatric population, many preteens have a high rate of clinical relapse for acne vulgaris. Prepubertal children may be more sensitive to some effects of isotretinoin. During clinical trials of disorders of keratinization that use higher doses of isotretinoin than that used for acne vulgaris, two children showed x-ray changes suggestive of premature epiphyseal closure.

**Adolescents**
Adolescents may have a high rate of clinical relapse for acne vulgaris.

**Geriatrics**
No information is available on the relationship of age to the effects of isotretinoin in geriatric patients.

**Dental**
Isotretinoin can increase or decrease saliva production. Continuing dryness of the mouth may increase the risk of dental disease, including tooth decay, gum disease, and fungal infection. Having regular dental checkups and using artificial saliva or dissolving sugarless candy or ice in the mouth may help to reduce the incidence of dental problems. Patient should check with a physician or dentist if dry mouth continues for more than 2 weeks.

**Drug interactions and/or related problems**
The following drug interactions and/or related problems have been selected on the basis of their potential clinical significance (possible mechanism in parentheses where appropriate)—not necessarily inclusive (» = major clinical significance):

Note: Combinations containing any of the following medications, depending on the amount present, may also interact with this medication.

Photosensitizing medications, other, such as sulfonamides, tetracyclines, or thiazide diuretics
(although isotretinoin is not phototoxic or photoallergic, it may increase the patient's sensitivity to sunlight or ultraviolet light for several months as the horny layer of skin thins; concurrent use of isotretinoin and these medications may increase susceptibility to sunburn)

Retinoids, other, systemic, such as:
» Acitretin
» Tretinoin, oral
Vitamin A and its derivatives, including vitamin supplements containing vitamin A or
Retinoids, topical, such as adapalene, tazarotene, and tretinoin
(concurrent use of retinoids or doses of vitamin A larger than the minimum recommended daily allowance (RDA) increase the risk of clinical symptoms resembling those of excessive vitamin A intake or toxicity, also called hypervitaminosis A)

» Tetracyclines, oral, including minocycline
(can increase intracranial pressure; concomitant use with isotretinoin is not recommended because of the combination's potential to exacerbate this effect)

**Laboratory value alterations**
The following have been selected on the basis of their potential clinical significance (possible effect in parentheses where appropriate)—not necessarily inclusive (» = major clinical significance):

With physiology/laboratory test values
Alanine aminotransferase (ALT [SGPT]), serum and
Alkaline phosphatase (ALP), serum and
Aspartate aminotransferase (AST [SGOT]), serum and
Gamma-glutamyltransferase (GGT), serum and
Lactate dehydrogenase (LDH), serum
(increases in concentrations have occurred in about 10 to 20% of patients; some of these concentrations returned to normal levels with dosage reduction or continued administration of isotretinoin; if normalization does not readily occur or if hepatitis is suspected, isotretinoin should be discontinued)

Blood, urine and
Creatine kinase (CK) concentration, serum and
Glucose concentration, fasting, plasma or serum and
Uric acid concentration, urine and
Urinalysis, protein
(increases have occurred in less than 10% of patients. Elevated CK concentrations have occurred in some patients engaging in vigorous physical activity)

High-density lipoprotein (HDL) concentration
(decreases in serum HDL concentrations have occurred in about 16% of patients; this effect is reversible upon discontinuation of medication)

Platelet counts, whole blood and
Sedimentation rate, erythrocyte (ESR), whole blood
(elevated sedimentation rates have been reported in about 40% of patients; increases in platelet counts have occurred in about 10 to 20% of patients)

Red blood cell indices, whole blood and
White blood cell count, whole blood
(decreases have occurred in about 10 to 20% of patients)

Triglyceride, plasma and
Cholesterol, total, serum
(elevated plasma triglyceride concentrations occur in about 25% of patients and are dose-related. Triglyceride concentrations greater than 500 mg/dL were experienced by 32 of 298 patients treated for all diagnoses and by 5 of 135 patients treated for nodular acne; elevation of serum triglycerides to concentrations in excess of 800 mg/dL occasionally has been associated with acute pancreatitis. A minimal increase in serum total cholesterol concentration has occurred in about 7% of patients; these effects are reversible upon discontinuation of medication)

### Medical considerations/Contraindications
The medical considerations/contraindications included have been selected on the basis of their potential clinical significance (reasons given in parentheses where appropriate)—not necessarily inclusive (» = major clinical significance).

*Risk-benefit should be considered when the following medical problems exist:*

Conditions predisposing to hypertriglyceridemia, such as
  High alcohol intake, or history of
  Hypertriglyceridemia, family history of
  Obesity
    (isotretinoin may increase plasma triglyceride concentrations and, to a lesser extent, total cholesterol and may decrease high density lipoprotein [HDL] cholesterol concentrations, possibly increasing the risk of cardiovascular disease for patients with these conditions who take isotretinoin over a long period of time)

Diabetes mellitus, or family history of
    (possible alteration in blood glucose concentrations; insulin requirements do not appear to be affected when isotretinoin is used for treatment of acne for several months. Isotretinoin may increase plasma triglyceride concentrations and decrease HDL cholesterol concentrations, possibly increasing the risk of cardiovascular disease for patients with diabetes mellitus who take isotretinoin over a long period of time)

Sensitivity to retinoids, vitamin A (also called retinol), or their derivatives

### Patient monitoring
The following may be especially important in patient monitoring (other tests may be warranted in some patients, depending on condition; » = major clinical significance):

Blood count, complete (CBC), whole blood
    (baseline determinations are recommended prior to therapy and may be repeated as needed after 4 to 6 weeks of therapy)

Glucose, fasting, plasma or serum and/or
Glucose, 2-hour postprandial, plasma or serum
    (recommended during therapy in patients known or suspected to have diabetes mellitus because some patients have experienced problems in controlling their blood glucose)

Lipid profile, serum
    (recommended under fasting conditions prior to therapy, then repeated at 1- or 2-week intervals until the lipid response to isotretinoin is established, which usually occurs within 4 weeks. After 1 month, the test is repeated only if there are significant increases in blood lipid concentrations, or if the patient has associated risk factors. Following consumption of alcohol, 36 hours should elapse before determining blood lipid concentrations)

Liver profile, serum
    (recommended prior to therapy and at 1- or 2-week intervals until the hepatic function response is established, or as determined by the physician. Testing is repeated only if there are liver function abnormalities at 1 month. Since transient abnormalities of liver function have been reported, special monitoring is warranted for patients with a history of liver disease and for those patients undergoing vigorous physical exercise)

Pregnancy testing
    (recommended within 1 week of treatment initiation, on a monthly basis thereafter during treatment, and 1 month after treatment discontinuation; testing serves to remind the patient of the importance of avoiding pregnancy. If pregnancy occurs, patient should be counseled on whether to continue the pregnancy)

## Side/Adverse Effects
Note: Most side/adverse reactions in nodular acne patients have been reversible upon discontinuation of therapy.

Studies in animals have shown that prolonged isotretinoin therapy increased the incidence of focal calcification; fibrosis and inflammation of the myocardium; calcification of coronary, pulmonary, and mesenteric arteries; and metastatic calcification of the gastric mucosa. Also, long bone fractures have been reported in rats given isotretinoin at a dosage of 32 mg per kg of body weight (mg/kg) per day for 15 weeks.

The following side/adverse effects have been selected on the basis of their potential clinical significance (possible signs and symptoms in parentheses where appropriate)—not necessarily inclusive:

### Those indicating need for medical attention
Incidence more frequent
  *Arthralgia* (bone or joint pain; difficulty in moving); **burning, redness, itching, or other signs of inflammation of eyes**—incidence about 40%; *cheilitis* (scaling, redness, burning, pain, or other signs of inflammation of lips)—incidence 90%; *epistaxis* (nosebleeds)—incidence of up to 80% in treatment of acne; *skin infection*—incidence about 5%; *skin rash*—incidence about 10%

Incidence rare
  **Bleeding or inflammation of gums; cataracts or corneal opacities** (blurred vision or other changes in vision); **decreased night vision** (decreased vision after sunset and before sunrise)—may occur suddenly, may continue after treatment discontinuation; *hepatitis* (yellow eyes or skin); **inflammatory bowel disease or regional ileitis** (rectal bleeding; severe abdominal or stomach pain; severe diarrhea); **mental depression; psychosis; or suicidal ideation** (attempts at suicide or thoughts of suicide; changes in behavior); *optic neuritis* (pain or tenderness of eyes); *pseudotumor cerebri* (blurred vision or other changes in vision; headache, severe or continuing; nausea; vomiting); **skeletal hyperostosis** (back pain; bone or joint pain; difficulty in moving; stiff, painful muscles)—generally with long-term treatment

Note: If symptoms of *inflammatory bowel disease*, *visual disturbances*, or signs or symptoms of *pseudotumor cerebri* occur, isotretinoin should be discontinued. Patients with signs or symptoms of pseudotumor cerebri should be referred to a neurologist for further diagnosis and care.

Although isotretinoin has caused *corneal opacities* and diffuse interstitial *skeletal hyperostosis* in patients treated for acne, these conditions occur more frequently when higher doses of isotretinoin are used in patients who are treated for keratinization disorders. A more extensive skeletal hyperostosis occurs in adults who use a mean dose of 2.24 mg of isotretinoin per kg of body weight a day. Premature closure of the epiphyses in children has occurred.

*Mental depression*, *psychosis*, or *suicidal ideation* is uncommon with isotretinoin treatment and is probably more prevalent in patients being treated for severe acne. The mechanism for these side/adverse effects is unknown. In many patients, mental depression subsided with discontinuation of isotretinoin and recurred when treatment was resumed. Any patient continuing to experience these effects after treatment discontinuation may need further evaluation.

### Those indicating need for medical attention only if they continue or are bothersome
Incidence more frequent
  *Delayed or exaggerated healing response* (crusting of skin); **difficulty in wearing contact lenses**—may continue after treatment discontinuation; *dryness of eyes*—may continue after treatment discontinuation; **dryness of mouth or nose**—incidence 80% in treatment of acne; **dryness or itching of skin**—incidence 80% in treatment of acne; **headache, mild**—incidence about 5%; **increased sensitivity of skin to sunlight**—incidence about 5%; **peeling of skin on palms of hands or soles of feet**—incidence about 5%; **stomach upset**—incidence about 5%; **thinning of hair**—incidence less than 10%, may continue after treatment discontinuation; **unusual tiredness**—incidence about 5%

## Overdose
For more information on the management of overdose or unintentional ingestion, **contact a Poison Control Center** (see *Poison Control Center Listing*).

### Clinical effects of overdose
The following effects have been selected on the basis of their potential clinical significance (possible signs and symptoms in parentheses where appropriate)—not necessarily inclusive:

Acute and/or chronic
  **Abdominal pain; dizziness; drowsiness; intracranial pressure, elevated** (headache, severe; nausea; vomiting); **irritability; itchy skin**

### Treatment of overdose
To decrease absorption—Evacuation of stomach should be considered within 2 hours of ingestion of acute overdose. Medication should be discontinued in patients with symptoms of overdose who were given therapeutic doses.

Monitoring—
• Monitor for increased intracranial pressure.
• Female patients of childbearing potential should have a pregnancy test at time of overdose and 1 month later; if positive, teratogenic risk and continuance of pregnancy should be discussed.

- Blood samples should be collected and isotretinoin and metabolite concentrations determined.

Supportive care—Female patients of childbearing potential need to use two effective contraceptive methods for 1 month after overdose or until isotretinoin and its metabolites are no longer measurable in the blood. Patients in whom intentional overdose is confirmed or suspected should be referred for psychiatric consultation.

## Patient Consultation

As an aid to patient consultation, refer to *Advice for the Patient, Isotretinoin (Systemic)*.

In providing consultation, consider emphasizing the following selected information (» = major clinical significance):

### Before using this medication
» Conditions affecting use, especially:
- Sensitivity to isotretinoin, acitretin, tretinoin, or vitamin A derivatives
- Pregnancy—Not taking isotretinoin during pregnancy because it causes birth defects in humans. In addition, not taking if there is a chance that pregnancy may occur during treatment or within 1 month following treatment. Not taking isotretinoin unless an effective form of contraception is used for at least 1 month before beginning treatment. Contraception must be continued during treatment and for 1 month after isotretinoin is stopped
- Breast-feeding—Although it is not known whether isotretinoin passes into the breast milk, medication is not recommended during breast-feeding because it may cause unwanted effects in nursing babies
- Use in children—Preadolescents may be more sensitive to the effects of isotretinoin and preadolescents and adolescents may experience high rates of relapse for acne vulgaris
- Other medications, especially retinoids, such as acitretin, tretinoin (oral); or tetracyclines (oral)

### Proper use of this medication
» Reading accompanying patient information before using this medication
» For women of reproductive potential—Special precautions are needed before beginning treatment to ensure that the patient is not pregnant, such as using an effective form of birth control for 1 month before initiating treatment, obtaining a negative pregnancy test after a normal menstrual period pattern has been established and within 1 week before initiating treatment, then starting medication on Day 2 or 3 of normal menses. Women of reproductive age or potential are required to use two forms of contraception during treatment, beginning at least 1 month before initiation of treatment with isotretinoin and continuing for 1 month after medication is discontinued
» Taking isotretinoin dose with food
» Importance of not taking more medication than the amount prescribed
» Proper dosing
Missed dose: Taking as soon as possible; not taking if almost time for next dose; not doubling doses
» Proper storage

### Precautions while using this medication
» Regular visits to physician to check progress during therapy
» Stopping medication immediately and checking with physician if pregnancy is suspected, since isotretinoin causes birth defects in humans
» Checking with physician if skin condition does not improve within 1 to 2 months, full improvement may take 5 to 6 months; expecting that skin irritation may occur or skin condition may worsen within the first several weeks of treatment but will lessen in severity with continued use
» Not donating blood to a blood bank during treatment or for 30 days after isotretinoin therapy has been completed to prevent possibility of a pregnant patient receiving the blood
» Understanding that vision impairment can occur, including sudden night vision impairment, photophobia, blurred vision, or dryness of eyes. Vision problems can make driving a car or operating machinery dangerous
Checking with physician anytime vision problems occur; wearing contact lenses may be uncomfortable
Understanding that dental problems can occur resulting from dryness of mouth and may increase dental disease, including tooth decay, gum disease, and fungus infections; regular dental appointments are needed and use of sugarless candy or saliva substitute or melting ice in mouth may be necessary to lessen dental problems
» Minimizing exposure of skin to wind, cold temperatures, and sunlight, including limiting exposure on cloudy days, to avoid sunburn, dryness, or irritation, especially during the first months of treatment.

Also, not using artificial sunlight or sunlamp, unless directed otherwise by physician
Using sunscreen preparations (minimum sun protection factor [SPF] of 15) and wearing protective clothing over exposed areas and UV-blocking sunglasses when sunlight exposure cannot be avoided; avoiding direct sunlight between 10 a.m. and 3 p.m.; checking with physician at any time skin becomes too dry or irritated; choosing proper skin products to reduce skin dryness or irritation
» Not using vitamin A or vitamin A–containing supplements in doses that exceed the minimum recommended daily allowances (RDA)
Patients with diabetes mellitus: Understanding that use of isotretinoin may alter blood glucose concentrations; insulin requirements do not appear to be affected when using isotretinoin for treatment of acne for several months

### Side/adverse effects
Signs of potential side effects, especially arthralgia; burning, redness, itching, or other signs of inflammation of eye; cheilitis; epistaxis; skin infection; or skin rash; bleeding or inflammation of gums; cataracts; corneal opacities; decreased night vision; hepatitis; inflammatory bowel disease; regional ileitis; mental depression, psychosis, or suicidal ideation; optic neuritis; pseudotumor cerebri; or skeletal hyperostosis

## General Dosing Information

Generally, the initial dose of isotretinoin should be individualized according to the patient's weight and the severity and location of the disease.

### Diet/Nutrition
Isotretinoin should be given with food.

### For use as an antiacne agent
Prescribing or dispensing a 30-day supply of isotretinoin may encourage communication to reinforce criteria for pregnancy prevention.

Isotretinoin doses of 0.5 and 1 mg per kilogram of body weight (mg/kg) a day provide initial clearing of nodular acne, but the need to re-treat the patient is less with the larger dose, providing that it can be tolerated by the patient. For best, long-lasting results and to lessen the chance of re-treatment, most physicians aim to achieve a cumulative isotretinoin dose of 100 to 150 mg/kg.

Higher doses of isotretinoin (i.e., up to 2 mg/kg per day) may be required in patients whose disease is very severe or is primarily located on the chest and back instead of on the face.

During the initial period of isotretinoin therapy, transient exacerbation of acne may occur. Severe flares sometimes occur. This usually can be prevented by starting with a lower initial dose for a short time, such as 0.5 mg/kg per day or less for 2 weeks.

Following 4 or more weeks of therapy, dosage adjustment should be based on response of the disease to isotretinoin and the occurrence of side effects.

Improvement in nodular acne may occur after 1 to 2 months, but marked improvement may require 4 to 5 months of therapy. Also, improvement may continue after discontinuation of isotretinoin use.

In most patients, a single course of therapy may result in complete and prolonged remission of severe nodular acne. However, if a second course of therapy is necessary, it should not be initiated for at least 8 weeks (possibly 16 to 20 weeks, depending on individual response) after completion of the first course. Improvement in the condition may continue following discontinuation of isotretinoin use.

## Oral Dosage Forms

Note: Bracketed uses in the *Dosage Forms* section refer to categories of use and/or indications that are not included in U.S. product labeling.

### ISOTRETINOIN CAPSULES

**Usual adult and adolescent dose**
Acne vulgaris—
Oral, 0.5 mg per kg of body weight a day for two to four weeks, then increased to 1 mg per kg of body weight per day for twelve to twenty weeks; the maximum recommended dose is 2 mg per kg of body weight per day.
[Folliculitis, gram-negative][1] or
[Rosacea, severe][1]—
Oral, 0.5 to 1 mg per kg of body weight per day in two divided doses.
[Hidradenitis suppurativa (treatment)][1]—
Oral, 1 mg per kg of body weight per day for four months. A lower dose of 0.5 to 1 mg per kg may be effective if isotretinoin is used as adjunctive therapy.
[Keratinization disorders][1]—
Oral, up to 4 mg per kg of body weight per day, the dosage depending on the specific disease and its severity, for up to four months. Lowest dose to achieve clinical effect should be used.

**Strength(s) usually available**
U.S.—
- 10 mg (Rx) [*Accutane* (edetate disodium; methylparaben; propylparaben)].
- 20 mg (Rx) [*Accutane* (edetate disodium; methylparaben; propylparaben)].
- 40 mg (Rx) [*Accutane* (edetate disodium; methylparaben; propylparaben)].

Canada—
- 10 mg (Rx) [*Accutane Roche* (methylparaben; propylparaben)].
- 40 mg (Rx) [*Accutane Roche* (methylparaben; propylparaben)].

**Packaging and storage**
Store between 15 and 30 °C (59 and 86 °F), in a tight, light-resistant container, unless otherwise specified by manufacturer.

**Auxiliary labeling**
- Do not take this medication if you become pregnant.
- Take with food.
- Avoid prolonged or excessive exposure to sunlight.
- May cause dizziness or blurred vision.
- This medication may impair your ability to drive or operate machinery. Use care until you become familar with its effects.

**Note**
Include patient directions when dispensing.
Counsel female patients about using two forms of birth control 1 month before starting treatment, during treatment, and for 1 month after discontinuing treatment.
Counsel male and female patients:
- Not to donate blood for transfusion during treatment and for at least 1 month after discontinuing treatment.
- Be aware that sudden night vision inadequacies can occur, which can be hazardous when operating a vehicle.

[1]Not included in Canadian product labeling.

## Selected Bibliography
Ruiz-Maldonado R, Tamayo L. Retinoids in keratinizing diseases and acne. Pediatr Clin North Am 1983 Aug; 30(4): 721-34.

Ward A, Brogden RN, Heel RC, et al. Isotretinoin: a review of its pharmacological properties and therapeutic efficacy in acne and other skin disorders. Drugs 1984 Jul; 28(1): 6-37.

Revised: 08/13/98

---

**ISOXUPRINE**—The *Isoxuprine (Systemic)* monograph is not included in this published version of the USP DI database. Copies of the monograph are available on request from Micromedex, Inc. - Reprint Requests, 6200 S. Syracuse Way, Suite 300, Englewood, CO 80111; telephone (303) 486-6400; telefax (303) 486-6464; Email: USPDI@MDX.COM.

---

**ISRADIPINE**—See *Calcium Channel Blocking Agents (Systemic)*

---

**ITRACONAZOLE**—See *Antifungals, Azole (Systemic)*

---

**IVERMECTIN**—The *Ivermectin (Systemic)* monograph is not included in this published version of the USP DI database. Copies of the monograph are available on request from Micromedex, Inc. - Reprint Requests, 6200 S. Syracuse Way, Suite 300, Englewood, CO 80111; telephone (303) 486-6400; telefax (303) 486-6464; Email: USPDI@MDX.COM.

---

**JAPANESE ENCEPHALITIS VIRUS VACCINE**—The *Japanese Encephalitis Virus Vaccine (Systemic)* monograph is not included in this published version of the USP DI database. Copies of the monograph are available on request from Micromedex, Inc. - Reprint Requests, 6200 S. Syracuse Way, Suite 300, Englewood, CO 80111; telephone (303) 486-6400; telefax (303) 486-6464; Email: USPDI@MDX.COM.

**KANAMYCIN**—See *Aminoglycosides (Systemic)*; *Kanamycin (Oral-Local)*

**KANAMYCIN**—The *Kanamycin (Oral-Local)* monograph is not included in this published version of the USP DI database. Copies of the monograph are available on request from Micromedex, Inc. - Reprint Requests, 6200 S. Syracuse Way, Suite 300, Englewood, CO 80111; telephone (303) 486-6400; telefax (303) 486-6464; Email: USPDI@MDX.COM.

# KAOLIN AND PECTIN   Oral-Local

VA CLASSIFICATION (Primary): GA208

Commonly used brand name(s): *Donnagel-MB*; *K-P*; *Kao-Spen*; *Kapectolin*.

Note: For a listing of dosage forms and brand names by country availability, see *Dosage Forms* section(s).

## Category
Antidiarrheal (adsorbent).

## Indications

Note: The efficacy of any antidiarrheal medication for treatment of most cases of nonspecific diarrhea is questionable, especially in children. **Preferred treatment for acute, nonspecific diarrhea consists of fluid and electrolyte replacement, nutritional therapy, and, if possible, elimination of the underlying cause of the diarrhea.**

**Accepted**
Diarrhea (treatment)—Kaolin and pectin may be indicated as an adjunct to rest, fluids, and an appropriate diet in the symptomatic treatment of mild to moderately acute diarrhea. Use is recommended in chronic diarrhea only as temporary symptomatic treatment until the etiology is determined. Kaolin and pectin combination should not be used if diarrhea is accompanied by fever or if there is blood or mucus in the stool.

## Pharmacology/Pharmacokinetics

**Mechanism of action/Effect**
Adsorbent and protectant. Kaolin is a natural hydrated aluminum silicate that is believed to adsorb large numbers of bacteria and toxins and reduce water loss. Pectin is a polyuronic polymer for which the mechanism of action is unknown. Pectin consists of purified carbohydrate extracted from citrus fruit or apple pomace. Studies have shown no decrease in stool frequency or fecal weight and water content with this combination even though stools appeared more formed.

**Absorption**
Not absorbed (up to 90% of pectin is decomposed in gastrointestinal tract).

## Precautions to Consider

**Pregnancy/Reproduction**
Pregnancy—Problems in humans have not been documented. Kaolin and pectin combination is poorly absorbed after oral administration.

**Breast-feeding**
Problems in humans have not been documented. Kaolin and pectin combination is poorly absorbed after oral administration.

**Pediatrics**
In infants and children up to 3 years of age with diarrhea, use is not recommended unless directed by a physician because of the risk of fluid and electrolyte loss. Oral rehydration therapy is recommended in children with diarrhea to prevent loss of fluids and electrolytes.

**Geriatrics**
In geriatric patients with diarrhea, caution is recommended because of the risk of fluid and electrolyte loss; these patients should be referred to a physician.

**Drug interactions and/or related problems**
The following drug interactions and/or related problems have been selected on the basis of their potential clinical significance (possible mechanism in parentheses where appropriate)—not necessarily inclusive (» = major clinical significance):

Note: Combinations containing any of the following medications, depending on the amount present, may also interact with this medication.

Anticholinergics or other medications with anticholinergic activity (See *Appendix II*), or

Antidyskinetics or
Digitalis glycosides or
Lincomycins or
Loxapine or
Phenothiazines or
Thioxanthenes
  (concurrent use with kaolin and pectin combination may impair absorption of these medications when it is administered orally, resulting in decreased therapeutic effectiveness; it is recommended that kaolin and pectin combination be administered not less than 2 hours before or 3 to 4 hours after oral lincomycins; patients receiving digitalis should be monitored closely for evidence of altered effect)

Oral medications, other
  (prolonged use of adsorbents may interfere with absorption of other oral agents administered concurrently; it is recommended that kaolin and pectin combination be administered at least 2 to 3 hours before or after other oral medications)

**Medical considerations/Contraindications**
The medical considerations/contraindications included have been selected on the basis of their potential clinical significance (reasons given in parentheses where appropriate)—not necessarily inclusive (» = major clinical significance).

*Risk-benefit should be considered when the following medical problems exist:*

» Dehydration
  (although adsorbent antidiarrheals may increase the consistency of feces and decrease the frequency of evacuation, they do not reduce the amount of fluid loss, but only mask its extent; rehydration therapy is essential if signs or symptoms of dehydration, such as dryness of mouth, excessive thirst, wrinkled skin, decreased urination, and dizziness or lightheadedness are present; fluid loss may have serious consequences, such as circulatory collapse and renal failure, especially in young children)

Diarrhea, parasite-associated, suspected
  (use of adsorbent antidiarrheals may make recognition of parasitic causes of diarrhea more difficult; if parasitic agents are suspected pathogens, appropriate stool analyses should be performed prior to therapy with adsorbents)

» Dysentery, acute, characterized by bloody stools and elevated temperature
  (sole treatment with adsorbent antidiarrheals may be inadequate; antibiotic therapy may be required)

## Side/Adverse Effects

The following side/adverse effects have been selected on the basis of their potential clinical significance (possible signs and symptoms in parentheses where appropriate)—not necessarily inclusive:

**Those indicating need for medical attention only if they continue or are bothersome**
Incidence dose-related
  *Constipation*—usually mild and transient, but may rarely lead to fecal impaction

## Patient Consultation

As an aid to patient consultation, refer to *Advice for the Patient, Kaolin and Pectin (Oral)*.

In providing consultation, consider emphasizing the following selected information (» = major clinical significance):

**Before using this medication**
» Conditions affecting use, especially:
    Use in children—Not using in infants and children up to 3 years of age unless prescribed by a physician because of risk of dehydration associated with diarrhea; oral rehydration therapy recommended in children with diarrhea

Use in the elderly—Risk of dehydration associated with diarrhea
Other medical problems, especially dehydration and acute dysentery

**Proper use of this medication**
» Not using if diarrhea is accompanied by fever or by blood or mucus in the stool; contacting physician
Taking after each loose bowel movement until diarrhea is controlled
» Importance of maintaining adequate hydration and proper diet
» Proper dosing
» Proper storage

**Precautions while using this medication**
» Checking with physician if diarrhea is not controlled within 48 hours and/or fever develops
Taking doses of other oral medications 2 to 3 hours before or after doses of kaolin and pectin combination

## Oral Dosage Forms

### KAOLIN AND PECTIN ORAL SUSPENSION

**Usual adult dose**
Antidiarrheal—
Oral, 60 to 120 mL after each loose bowel movement.

**Usual pediatric dose**
Antidiarrheal—
Children up to 3 years of age: Use is not recommended unless directed by a physician.
Children 3 to 6 years of age: Oral, 15 to 30 mL after each loose bowel movement.
Children 6 to 12 years of age: Oral, 30 to 60 mL after each loose bowel movement.
Children 12 years of age and over: Oral, 45 to 60 mL after each loose bowel movement.

Note: In general, dietary treatment of diarrhea in children is preferred whenever possible.

**Strength(s) usually available**
U.S.—
5.2 grams of kaolin and 260 mg of pectin per 30 mL (OTC) [*Kao-Spen; K-P*].
5.85 grams of kaolin and 130 mg of pectin per 30 mL (OTC) [*Kapectolin*; GENERIC].
Canada—
6 grams of kaolin and 143 mg of pectin per 30 mL (OTC) [*Donnagel-MB* (alcohol 3.8%)].

**Packaging and storage**
Store below 40 °C (104 °F), preferably between 15 and 30 °C (59 and 86 °F), in a well-closed container, unless otherwise specified by manufacturer. Protect from freezing.

**Auxiliary labeling**
• Shake well.

**Note**
Refer patients with recurrent or persistent diarrhea to a physician.

## Selected Bibliography
Brownlee HJ. Family practitioner's guide to patient self-treatment of acute diarrhea. Am J Med 1990; 88(6A Suppl): 27S-29S.

Revised: 08/04/94

# KAOLIN, PECTIN, AND BELLADONNA ALKALOIDS  Systemic

VA CLASSIFICATION (Primary): GA208

NOTE: The *Kaolin, Pectin, and Belladonna Alkaloids (Systemic)* monograph is maintained on the USP DI electronic data base. For a printed copy of the most recent revision of the complete monograph, contact Micromedex, Inc. - Reprint Requests, 6200 S. Syracuse Way, Suite 300, Englewood, CO 80111; telephone (303) 486-6400; telefax (303) 486-6464; Email: USPDI@MDX.COM.

For information on the specific components of this combination, see the USP DI monographs for *Anticholinergics/Antispasmodics (Systemic)* and *Kaolin and Pectin (Oral-Local)*.

The information that follows is selectively abstracted from the complete monograph and is provided to facilitate drug use review and patient counseling.

Note: For a listing of dosage forms and brand names by country availability, see *Dosage Forms* section(s).

## Category
Antidiarrheal (adsorbent).

## Indications
Note: The efficacy of any antidiarrheal medication for treatment of most cases of nonspecific diarrhea is questionable, especially in children. **Preferred treatment for acute, nonspecific diarrhea consists of fluid and electrolyte replacement, nutritional therapy, and, if possible, elimination of the underlying cause of the diarrhea.**

**Unaccepted**
The U.S. Food and Drug Administration (FDA) has banned the inclusion of belladonna alkaloids in antidiarrheal preparations because of lack of proof of their effectiveness. FDA has requested that manufacturers wishing to obtain the agency's approval for inclusion of these ingredients in their product provide FDA with evidence that the ingredients are safe and effective for their intended use. This medication has been replaced by equally or more effective, and safer, agents for the treatment of diarrhea.

## Patient Consultation
As an aid to patient consultation, refer to *Advice for the Patient, Kaolin, Pectin, and Belladonna Alkaloids (Systemic)*.
In providing consultation, consider emphasizing the following selected information (» = major clinical significance):

**Before using this medication**
» Conditions affecting use, especially:
Sensitivity to any of the belladonna alkaloids
Pregnancy—Belladonna alkaloids cross the placenta
Breast-feeding—Belladonna alkaloids are distributed into breast milk
Use in children—Not using in infants and children up to 6 years of age because use does not preclude, and may aggravate, risk of dehydration associated with diarrhea; oral rehydration therapy recommended in children with diarrhea; increased susceptibility to side/adverse effects of belladonna alkaloids
Use in the elderly—Risk of dehydration associated with diarrhea; increased sensitivity to effects of belladonna alkaloids
Dental—Possible development of dental problems because of decreased salivary flow
Other medications, especially CNS depressants, ketoconazole, MAO inhibitors, or potassium chloride
Other medical problems, especially acute dysentery, asthma or respiratory disease, dehydration, diarrhea caused by poisoning, glaucoma, hepatic and/or renal function impairment, prostatic hyperplasia or urinary retention, or severe colitis

**Proper use of this medication**
Taking with food or meals if gastric irritation occurs
» Importance of not taking more medication than the amount prescribed
Proper administration technique
» Importance of maintaining adequate hydration and proper diet
» Proper dosing
» Proper storage

**Precautions while using this medication**
» Consulting physician if diarrhea is not controlled within 48 hours and/or fever develops
Possible interference with laboratory values
» Avoiding use of alcohol or other CNS depressants
» Caution if drowsiness occurs
Possible increased sensitivity of eyes to light
» Caution during exercise and hot weather; overheating may result in heatstroke
Possible dryness of mouth, nose, and throat; using sugarless candy or gum, ice, or saliva substitute for relief; checking with physician or dentist if dry mouth continues for more than 2 weeks

**Side/adverse effects**
Signs of potential side effects, especially allergic reaction, CNS depression, hallucinations, increased intraocular pressure, paralytic ileus or toxic megacolon, or slow heartbeat

## Oral Dosage Forms

### KAOLIN, PECTIN, HYOSCYAMINE SULFATE, ATROPINE SULFATE, AND SCOPOLAMINE HYDROBROMIDE ORAL SUSPENSION

**Usual adult and adolescent dose**
Oral, 30 mL every three hours as needed to control diarrhea.

**Usual adult prescribing limits**
Four doses in twenty-four hours.

**Usual pediatric dose**
Children up to 6 years of age: Use is not recommended unless directed by a physician.
Children over 6 years of age: Oral, 5 to 10 mL every three hours as needed to control diarrhea, up to four doses in twenty-four hours.
Note: In general, oral rehydration therapy and dietary treatment of diarrhea in children are preferred whenever possible.

**Usual geriatric dose**
See *Usual adult and adolescent dose*.

Note: Geriatric patients may be more sensitive to the effects of the usual adult dose.

**Strength(s) usually available**
U.S.—
　Not commercially available.
Canada—
　6 grams of kaolin, 142.8 mg of pectin, 104 mcg (0.104 mg) of hyoscyamine sulfate, 19 mcg (0.019 mg) of atropine sulfate, and 7 mcg (0.007 mg) of scopolamine hydrobromide per 30 mL (Rx) [*Donnagel* (alcohol 3.8%; sodium <2.6 mg per 5 mL; sugar)].

**Auxiliary labeling**
- May cause drowsiness.
- Avoid alcoholic beverages.
- Do not take other medicines without your doctor's advice.
- Keep out of reach of children.
- Shake well before using.

Revised: 04/27/95

---

# KAOLIN, PECTIN, AND PAREGORIC　Systemic

**VA CLASSIFICATION (Primary):** GA208

**NOTE:** The *Kaolin, Pectin, and Paregoric (Systemic)* monograph is maintained on the USP DI electronic data base. For a printed copy of the most recent revision of the complete monograph, contact Micromedex, Inc. - Reprint Requests, 6200 S. Syracuse Way, Suite 300, Englewood, CO 80111; telephone (303) 486-6400; telefax (303) 486-6464; Email: USPDI@MDX.COM.

For information on the specific components of this combination, see the *USP DI* monographs for *Kaolin and Pectin (Oral-Local)* and *Paregoric (Systemic)*.

The information that follows is selectively abstracted from the complete monograph and is provided to facilitate drug use review and patient counseling.

Note: For a listing of dosage forms and brand names by country availability, see *Dosage Forms* section(s).

## Category
Antidiarrheal (adsorbent).

## Indications
Note: The efficacy of any antidiarrheal medication for treatment of most cases of nonspecific diarrhea is questionable, especially in children. **Preferred treatment for acute, nonspecific diarrhea consists of fluid and electrolyte replacement, nutritional therapy, and, if possible, elimination of the underlying cause of the diarrhea.**

**Unaccepted**
The U.S. Food and Drug Administration (FDA) has banned the inclusion of paregoric in antidiarrheal preparations because of lack of proof of its effectiveness. FDA has requested that manufacturers wishing to obtain the agency's approval for inclusion of this ingredient in their product provide FDA with evidence that the ingredient is safe and effective for its intended use. Paregoric-containing medications have been replaced by equally or more effective, and safer, agents for the treatment of diarrhea.

## Patient Consultation
As an aid to patient consultation, refer to *Advice for the Patient, Kaolin, Pectin, and Paregoric (Systemic)*.
In providing consultation, consider emphasizing the following selected information (» = major clinical significance):

**Before using this medication**
» Conditions affecting use, especially:
　Sensitivity to paregoric or other opiates
　Pregnancy—Opium alkaloids cross placenta; possible fetal dependence with regular use late in pregnancy
　Breast-feeding—Opium alkaloids distributed into breast milk
　Use in children—Not using in infants and children up to 2 years of age because of risk of dehydration associated with diarrhea; oral rehydration therapy recommended in children with diarrhea; increased sensitivity to opiate effects
　Use in the elderly—Risk of dehydration associated with diarrhea; increased sensitivity to opiate effects
　Other medications, especially antiperistaltic antidiarrheals, CNS depressants, naloxone, and naltrexone; spacing doses of other oral medications 2 to 3 hours before or after doses of kaolin and pectin–containing medication is recommended
　Other medical problems, especially acute dysentery, acute respiratory depression, asthma or respiratory disease, dehydration, diarrhea associated with *C. difficile* or caused by poisoning, and severe inflammatory bowel disease

**Proper use of this medication**
　Taking with food or meals if gastric irritation occurs
» Importance of not taking more medication than the amount prescribed because of habit-forming potential
　Using specially marked spoon or measuring device
» Importance of maintaining adequate hydration and proper diet
» Proper dosing
» Proper storage

**Precautions while using this medication**
» Consulting physician if diarrhea is not controlled within 48 hours and/or fever develops
» Caution if taking alcohol or other central nervous system (CNS) depressants
» Caution if drowsiness occurs

**Side/adverse effects**
　Signs of potential side effects, especially allergic reaction, histamine-release related effects, mental depression, and toxic megacolon

## Oral Dosage Forms

### KAOLIN, PECTIN, AND PAREGORIC ORAL SUSPENSION

**Usual adult and adolescent dose**
Antidiarrheal—Oral, 30 mL after each loose bowel movement.

**Usual adult prescribing limits**
Four doses within twelve hours.

**Usual pediatric dose**
Antidiarrheal—
　Children up to 2 years of age:
　　Use is not recommended.
　Children 2 years of age and over:
　　Children up to 4.5 kg of body weight—Dosage must be individualized by physician.
　　Children 4.5 to 9 kg of body weight—Oral, 2.5 mL after each loose bowel movement.
　　Children 9 to 13.5 kg of body weight—Oral, 5 mL after each loose bowel movement.
　　Children 13.5 kg of body weight and over—Oral, 5 to 10 mL after each loose bowel movement.
Note: No more than 4 doses should be administered within twelve hours.
　In general, oral rehydration therapy and dietary treatment of diarrhea in children are preferred whenever possible.

**Usual geriatric dose**
See *Usual adult and adolescent dose*.

Note: Geriatric patients may be more sensitive to the effects of the usual adult dose.

**Strength(s) usually available**
U.S.—
  Not commercially available.
Canada—
  6 grams of kaolin, 142.8 mg of pectin, and 6 mL of paregoric, per 30 mL (N) [*Donnagel-PG* (alcohol 5%; sodium <1 mmol per 5 mL)].

**Auxiliary labeling**
- May cause drowsiness.
- Avoid alcoholic beverages.
- Do not take other medicines without your doctor's advice.
- Keep out of reach of children.
- May be habit-forming.
- Shake well before using.

Revised: 04/26/95

# KETAMINE   Systemic

VA CLASSIFICATION (Primary/Secondary): CN203/CN206
Commonly used brand name(s): *Ketalar*; *Ketalar*; *Ketalar*.
Note:  For a listing of dosage forms and brand names by country availability, see *Dosage Forms* section(s).

## Category
Anesthetic (general).

## Indications
Note:  Bracketed information in the *Indications* section refers to uses that are not included in U.S. product labeling.

**Accepted**
Anesthesia, general—Ketamine is indicated to provide anesthesia for short diagnostic and surgical procedures that do not require skeletal muscle relaxation. It is also indicated to induce anesthesia prior to administration of other general anesthetics.

  [Ketamine is used to provide obstetrical anesthesia.][1]

Anesthesia, general, adjunct—Ketamine is indicated to supplement low-potency anesthetics such as nitrous oxide.

[Anesthesia, local, adjunct][1]—Ketamine is used as a supplement to local and regional anesthesia.

Caution is recommended when ketamine is considered for use in surgical procedures of the pharynx, larynx, or trachea because it increases salivary and tracheal-bronchial secretions and does not reliably suppress pharyngeal and laryngeal reflexes.

In subhypnotic doses, ketamine produces a dissociative state. The patient does not appear to be asleep and experiences a feeling of being dissociated from the environment.

[1] Not included in Canadian product labeling.

## Pharmacology/Pharmacokinetics

**Physicochemical characteristics**
Molecular weight—274.19.

**Mechanism of action/Effect**
The precise mechanism of action is unknown. Ketamine has been shown to block afferent impulses associated with the affective-emotional component of pain perception within the medial medullary reticular formation, to suppress spinal cord activity, and to interact with several central nervous system (CNS) transmitter systems.

**Absorption**
Rapid.

**Distribution**
Rapidly distributed into highly perfused tissues including the brain. Animal studies have shown ketamine to be highly concentrated in body fat, liver, and lung.

**Biotransformation**
Hepatic. However, termination of anesthetic effects may be caused by redistribution from the brain to other tissues.

**Half-life**
Distribution—Approximately 7 to 11 minutes.
Elimination—Approximately 2 to 3 hours.

**Time to induction of anesthesia**
Intravenous (following a dose of 1 to 2 mg per kg of body weight [mg/kg])—
  Sensation of dissociation: 15 seconds.
  Anesthesia: 30 seconds.
Intramuscular (following a dose of 5 to 10 mg/kg)—
  Anesthesia: 3 to 4 minutes.

**Duration of anesthesia**
Intravenous (following a dose of 2 mg/kg)—5 to 10 minutes.
Intramuscular (following a dose of 10 mg/kg)—12 to 25 minutes.

**Time to recovery**
Rapid.

**Elimination**
Renal, 90%; about 4% as unchanged ketamine.
Fecal, up to 5%.

## Precautions to Consider

**Pregnancy/Reproduction**
Studies in animals have not shown that ketamine causes birth defects; however, it crosses the placenta. Also, in one study in rats, ketamine produced histologic changes in the heart, liver, and kidneys of the offspring, including focal nuclear hypochromatosis, interfibrillary edema, parenchymal cell degeneration, proximal convoluted tubule degeneration, and diffuse hematopoietic cell infiltration. The degenerative effects were dependent on both dosage and duration of administration. Ketamine is used in low doses to provide obstetrical anesthesia. It has not been shown to cause adverse effects.

**Breast-feeding**
Problems in humans have not been documented.

**Pediatrics**
Appropriate studies performed to date have not demonstrated pediatrics-specific problems that would limit the usefulness of ketamine in children.

**Geriatrics**
Appropriate studies performed to date have not demonstrated geriatrics-specific problems that would limit the use of ketamine in the elderly.

**Drug interactions and/or related problems**
The following drug interactions and/or related problems have been selected on the basis of their potential clinical significance (possible mechanism in parentheses where appropriate)—not necessarily inclusive (» = major clinical significance):

Note:  Combinations containing any of the following medications, depending on the amount present, may also interact with this medication.

Anesthetics, halogenated hydrocarbon inhalation, such as:
  Enflurane
  Halothane
  Isoflurane
  Methoxyflurane
    (halogen hydrocarbon inhalation anesthetics may prolong the elimination half-life of ketamine; recovery from anesthesia may be prolonged following concurrent use)

Antihypertensives or
CNS depression–producing medications, including those commonly used as preanesthetic medication or for induction, supplementation, or maintenance of anesthesia (See *Appendix II*)
    (concurrent use with ketamine, especially high-dose or rapidly administered ketamine, may increase the risk of hypotension and/or respiratory depression)

Thyroid hormones
    (ketamine should be administered with caution to patients receiving thyroid hormones because of the increased risk of hypertension and tachycardia)

**Laboratory value alterations**
The following have been selected on the basis of their potential clinical significance (possible effect in parentheses where appropriate)—not necessarily inclusive (» = major clinical significance):

With physiology/laboratory test values
    Cerebrospinal fluid (CSF) pressure, or
    Intraocular pressure
        (may be increased)

### Medical considerations/Contraindications

The medical considerations/contraindications included have been selected on the basis of their potential clinical significance (reasons given in parentheses where appropriate)—not necessarily inclusive (» = major clinical significance).

*Except under special circumstances, this medication should not be used when the following medical problems exist:*

» Any condition in which a significant elevation of blood pressure would be hazardous, such as:
» Cardiovascular disease, severe
» Heart failure
» Hypertension, severe or poorly controlled
» Myocardial infarction, recent
» Stroke, history of
» Cerebral trauma
» Intracerebral mass or hemorrhage

*Risk-benefit should be considered when the following medical problems exist:*

    Alcohol abuse (or history of)
    Alcohol intoxication, acute
· Congestive heart failure or
    Hypertension, mild, uncomplicated or
    Myocardial ischemia or
    Tachyarrhythmias
        (may be exacerbated)
» Eye injury, open globe
» Increased cerebrospinal fluid (CSF) pressure
        (ketamine may further elevate CSF pressure)
» Increased intraocular pressure
        (ketamine may further elevate intraocular pressure)
» Psychiatric disorders such as schizophrenia or acute psychosis
    Sensitivity to ketamine
» Thyrotoxic states
        (increased risk of hypertension and tachycardia)

### Patient monitoring

The following may be especially important in patient monitoring (other tests may be warranted in some patients, depending on condition; » = major clinical significance):

    Cardiac function
        (monitoring throughout the procedure is recommended, especially in patients with congestive heart failure, hypertension, myocardial ischemia, or tachyarrhythmias)

## Side/Adverse Effects

The following side/adverse effects have been selected on the basis of their potential clinical significance (possible signs and symptoms in parentheses where appropriate)—not necessarily inclusive:

### Those indicating need for medical attention

Incidence more frequent
    *Increased blood pressure*—may reach hypertensive levels; *tachycardia; tonic and clonic muscle movements*—may resemble seizures; *tremor; vocalization*

Incidence less frequent
    *Bradycardia; hypotension; respiratory depression*—may lead to apnea; *vomiting*—following administration

Incidence rare
    *Cardiac arrhythmias; laryngospasm or other forms of airway obstruction*

### Those indicating need for medical attention only if they continue or are bothersome

Incidence more frequent in patients between 15 and 45 years of age; less frequent in other age groups
    *Emergence reaction* (alterations in mood or body image; delirium; dissociative or floating sensations); *vivid dreams or illusions; visual hallucinations*

    Note: Although *vivid dreams* and/or *hallucinations* usually disappear upon wakening, some patients may experience flashbacks several weeks postoperatively.

Incidence less frequent or rare
    *Double vision; loss of appetite; nausea with or without vomiting; nystagmus* (wandering or back-and-forth eye movements); *pain at injection site; reddened skin or skin rash*

## Patient Consultation

As an aid to patient consultation, refer to *Advice for the Patient, Anesthetics, General (Systemic).*

In providing consultation, consider emphasizing the following selected information (» = major clinical significance):

### Before receiving this medication

» Conditions affecting use, especially:
    Sensitivity to ketamine
    Pregnancy—Ketamine crosses the placenta
    Any other medication, including use of "street" drugs
    Other medical problems, especially cardiac or cardiovascular disease, glaucoma, hypertension, hyperthyroidism, psychiatric disorders, and stroke

### Proper use of this medication
    Proper dosing

### Precautions after receiving this medication

» Possibility of psychomotor impairment following anesthesia; using caution in driving or performing other tasks requiring alertness for about 24 hours postanesthesia
» Avoiding alcohol or other CNS depressants within 24 hours following anesthesia unless prescribed or otherwise approved by physician or dentist

### Side/adverse effects

Signs of potential delayed side effects, especially mood or mental changes, nightmares or unusual dreams, and blurred vision

## General Dosing Information

The usual adult dosages are intended as a guideline. Actual dosage must be individualized to meet the needs of each patient.

Ketamine may cause vomiting following administration. To prevent possible aspiration of vomitus, ketamine should be administered to the patient on an empty stomach.

Because ketamine increases salivary and tracheal-bronchial mucous gland secretions, use of atropine, scopolamine, or another drying agent is recommended prior to induction of anesthesia. The fact that atropine has been shown to increase the frequency of unpleasant dreams should be kept in mind.

Ketamine may be administered intramuscularly or intravenously. Intravenous administration produces anesthesia more rapidly than intramuscular administration.

Administration of an overdose, or administering ketamine at too rapid a rate, may produce respiratory depression, apnea, and hypertension. Intravenous ketamine should be administered over a period of 60 seconds unless a rapid-sequence induction technique is indicated.

Tolerance to the effects of ketamine has been reported following repeated administration.

A state of confusion (emergence delirium) may occur during recovery. Although it has been suggested that minimizing verbal, tactile, and visual stimulation during recovery may reduce the incidence of emergence reactions, the efficacy of such measures has not been documented. Administration of a benzodiazepine prior to or concurrently with ketamine, or just prior to termination of surgery, may decrease the incidence of emergence delirium.

### For treatment of adverse effects

Recommended treatment may include
    • For respiratory depression or apnea—Assisting respiration mechanically may be preferred over administration of analeptics.
    • For severe emergence reaction—Administering a short- or ultrashort-acting barbiturate.

## Parenteral Dosage Forms

Note: Bracketed uses in the *Dosage Forms* section refer to categories of use and/or indications that are not included in U.S. product labeling.

### KETAMINE HYDROCHLORIDE INJECTION USP

#### Usual adult and adolescent dose

Anesthetic (general)—
    Induction—
        Intravenous, 1 to 2 mg (base) per kg of body weight, administered as a single dose or by intravenous infusion at a rate of 500 mcg (0.5 mg) (base) per kg of body weight per minute; or
        Intramuscular, 5 to 10 mg (base) per kg of body weight.

Maintenance—
  Intravenous, 10 to 50 mcg (0.01 to 0.05 mg) (base) per kg of body weight by continuous infusion at a rate of 1 to 2 mg per minute.
  Note: Maintenance dosage must be adjusted as determined by the patient's anesthetic requirements and concurrent use of an additional anesthetic agent.
  Tonic-clonic movements that may appear during anesthesia are not indicative of the need for additional ketamine.
[Anesthesia, local, adjunct][1]—
  Intravenous, 5 to 30 mg (base), prior to administration of the local anesthetic. May be repeated if necessary.
[Sedation and analgesia][1]—
  Intravenous: 200 to 750 mcg (0.2 to 0.75 mg) (base) per kg of body weight administered over 2 to 3 minutes initially, followed by 5 to 20 mcg (0.005 to 0.02 mg) (base) per kg of body weight per minute as a continuous intravenous infusion.
  Intramuscular: 2 to 4 mg (base) per kg of body weight initially, followed by 5 to 20 mcg (0.005 to 0.02 mg) (base) per kg of body weight per minute as a continuous intravenous infusion.

**Usual adult prescribing limits**
Anesthesia, general, induction—
  Intravenous: Up to 4.5 mg (base) per kg of body weight.
  Intramuscular: Up to 13 mg (base) per kg of body weight.
[Anesthesia, local, adjunct][1]—
  Intravenous, up to 30 mg (base).

**Usual pediatric dose**
See *Usual adult and adolescent dose.*

**Usual geriatric dose**
See *Usual adult and adolescent dose.*

**Strength(s) usually available**
U.S.—
  10 mg (base) per mL (Rx) [*Ketalar* [GENERIC (benzethonium chloride)].
  50 mg (base) per mL (Rx) [*Ketalar* [GENERIC (benzethonium chloride)].
  100 mg (base) per mL (Rx) [*Ketalar* [GENERIC (benzethonium chloride)].
Canada—
  10 mg (base) per mL (Rx) [*Ketalar*].
  50 mg (base) per mL (Rx) [*Ketalar*].
U.K.—
  10 mg (base) per mL (Rx) [*Ketalar*].
  50 mg (base) per mL (Rx) [*Ketalar*].
  100 mg (base) per mL (Rx) [*Ketalar*].

**Packaging and storage**
Store below 40 °C (104 °F), preferably between 15 and 30 °C (59 and 86 °F), unless otherwise specified by manufacturer. Protect from light and heat. Protect from freezing.

**Preparation of dosage form**
For direct intravenous administration—The 100-mg-per-mL concentration of ketamine must be diluted with an equal volume of sterile water for injection, 0.9% sodium chloride injection, or 5% dextrose injection prior to injection.
For intravenous infusion—Add 10 mL of the 50-mg-per-mL concentration, or 5 mL of the 100-mg-per-mL concentration, of ketamine (base) to 500 mL of 5% dextrose injection or 0.9% sodium chloride injection and mix well. The resultant solution will contain 1 mg of ketamine (base) per mL. If fluid restriction is necessary, 250 mL of the diluent may be used to provide a solution containing 2 mg of ketamine (base) per mL.

**Incompatibilities**
Ketamine and barbiturates should not be injected from the same syringe because they will form a precipitate.
If diazepam is administered concurrently with ketamine, the two medications should be given separately. The two medications should not be mixed together in a syringe or added to the same intravenous infusion solution.

[1]Not included in Canadian product labeling.

Revised: 06/21/90
Interim revision: 08/23/94

---

**KETAZOLAM**—See *Benzodiazepines (Systemic)*

---

**KETOCONAZOLE**—See *Antifungals, Azole (Systemic)*

---

# KETOCONAZOLE Topical

VA CLASSIFICATION (Primary): DE102
Commonly used brand name(s): *Nizoral Cream; Nizoral Shampoo.*
Note: For a listing of dosage forms and brand names by country availability, see *Dosage Forms* section(s).

## Category
Antifungal (topical).

## Indications
Note: Bracketed information in the *Indications* section refers to uses that are not included in U.S. product labeling.

**Accepted**
Tinea corporis (treatment) or
Tinea cruris (treatment)—Ketoconazole cream is indicated as a primary agent in the topical treatment of tinea corporis (ringworm of the body) and tinea cruris (ringworm of the groin; jock itch) caused by *Trichophyton rubrum, T. mentagrophytes,* and *Epidermophyton floccosum (Acrothesium floccosum).*
Tinea pedis (treatment)—Ketoconazole cream is indicated as a primary agent in the topical treatment of tinea pedis (athlete's foot).
Pityriasis versicolor (treatment)—Ketoconazole cream is indicated as a primary agent in the topical treatment of pityriasis versicolor (tinea versicolor; "sun fungus") caused by *Malassezia furfur (Pityrosporon orbiculare).*
Candidiasis, cutaneous (treatment)[1]—Ketoconazole cream is indicated as a primary agent in the topical treatment of cutaneous candidiasis caused by *Candida* species.
Dermatitis, seborrheic (treatment)—Ketoconazole cream is indicated in the treatment of seborrheic dermatitis.
Dandruff (treatment)—Ketoconazole shampoo is indicated for the reduction of scaling due to dandruff.
[Paronychia (treatment)][1]
[Tinea barbae (treatment)][1] or
[Tinea capitis (treatment)][1]—Ketoconazole cream is used as a primary agent in the topical treatment of paronychia. Ketoconazole cream is used as a secondary agent in the topical treatment of tinea barbae and tinea capitis.

Not all species or strains of a particular organism may be susceptible to ketoconazole.

[1]Not included in Canadian product labeling.

## Pharmacology/Pharmacokinetics

**Physicochemical characteristics**
Chemical group—Imidazoles.
Molecular weight—531.44.

**Mechanism of action/Effect**
Fungistatic; may be fungicidal, depending on concentration; inhibits biosynthesis of ergosterol or other sterols, damaging the fungal cell membrane and altering its permeability; as a result, loss of essential intracellular elements may occur; also inhibits biosynthesis of triglycerides and phospholipids by fungi; in addition, inhibits oxidative and peroxidative enzyme activity, resulting in intracellular buildup of toxic concentrations of hydrogen peroxide, which may contribute to deterioration of subcellular organelles and cellular necrosis. In the treatment of *Candida albicans*, inhibits transformation of blastospores into invasive mycelial form.

## Ketoconazole (Topical)

**Absorption**
No systemic absorption detected at a sensitivity level of 5 nanograms per mL in the blood over a 72-hour period following a single topical application to the chest, back, and arms of normal volunteers.

## Precautions to Consider

**Cross-sensitivity and/or related problems**
Persons sensitive to miconazole or other imidazoles may be sensitive to ketoconazole also.

**Carcinogenicity**
A long-term feeding study in Swiss albino mice and Wistar rats has shown no evidence of carcinogenicity.

**Mutagenicity**
The dominant lethal mutation test in male and female mice, given single oral doses of ketoconazole as high as 80 mg per kg of body weight (mg/kg), has shown no mutations at any stage of germ cell development. The Ames *Salmonella* microsomal activator assay has also shown negative results.

**Pregnancy/Reproduction**
Pregnancy—Ketoconazole crosses the placenta. Adequate and well-controlled studies in humans have not been done.
Studies in rats, given oral doses of 80 mg/kg per day (10 times the maximum recommended human dose [MRHD]), have shown ketoconazole to be teratogenic, causing syndactyly and oligodactyly.
FDA Pregnancy Category C.

**Breast-feeding**
It is not known whether ketoconazole, applied topically on a regular basis, is absorbed systemically in sufficient amounts to be distributed into breast milk in detectable quantities. However, no systemic absorption was detected following a single application to the chest, back, and arms of healthy volunteers. Therefore, topical ketoconazole is unlikely to be distributed into breast milk in significant amounts or to cause adverse effects in the nursing infant.

**Pediatrics**
No information is available on the relationship of age to the effects of this medicine in pediatric patients. Safety and efficacy have not been established.

**Geriatrics**
No information is available on the relationship of age to the effects of this medicine in geriatric patients.

**Medical considerations/Contraindications**
The medical considerations/contraindications included have been selected on the basis of their potential clinical significance (reasons given in parentheses where appropriate)—not necessarily inclusive (» = major clinical significance).

*Risk-benefit should be considered when the following medical problem exists:*
Sensitivity to topical ketoconazole

## Side/Adverse Effects

The following side/adverse effects have been selected on the basis of their potential clinical significance (possible signs and symptoms in parentheses where appropriate)—not necessarily inclusive:

**Those indicating need for medical attention**
Incidence more frequent
*Itching, stinging, or irritation not present before therapy*

## Patient Consultation

As an aid to patient consultation, refer to *Advice for the Patient, Ketoconazole (Topical)*.
In providing consultation, consider emphasizing the following selected information (» = major clinical significance):

**Before using this medication**
» Conditions affecting use, especially:
　　Sensitivity to topical ketoconazole
　　Pregnancy—Ketoconazole crosses the placenta; studies in animals found ketoconazole to be teratogenic

**Proper use of this medication**
» Avoiding contact with the eyes
» Proper dosing
　　Missed dose: Applying as soon as possible; not applying if almost time for next dose
» Proper storage

*For the cream form*
　　Applying sufficient medication to cover affected and surrounding areas, and rubbing in gently
» Compliance with full course of therapy; fungal infections may require prolonged therapy

*For the shampoo form*
　　Wetting hair and scalp with water
　　Applying adequate shampoo for lather and massaging in for approximately 1 minute
　　Rinsing and repeating application
　　Leaving shampoo on an additional 3 minutes
　　Rinsing thoroughly and drying hair

**Precautions while using this medication**
*For the cream form*
　　Checking with physician if no improvement within 2 to 4 weeks
» Using hygienic measures to cure infection and prevent reinfection

*For tinea pedis*
　　Carefully drying feet, especially between toes, after bathing
　　Not wearing socks made from wool or synthetic materials; wearing clean, cotton socks and changing them daily or more often if feet perspire excessively
　　Wearing sandals or well-ventilated shoes
　　Using a bland, absorbent powder or an antifungal powder between toes, on feet, and in socks and shoes liberally once or twice daily; using the powder between administration times for the cream

*For tinea cruris*
　　Not wearing underwear that is tight-fitting or made from synthetic materials; wearing loose-fitting cotton underwear instead
　　Using a bland, absorbent powder or an antifungal powder on the skin between administration times for the cream

**Side/adverse effects**
　　Signs of potential side effects, especially itching, stinging, or irritation

## General Dosing Information

Prolonged use of topical ketoconazole may rarely lead to skin sensitization, resulting in hypersensitivity reactions with subsequent topical or systemic use of the medication.

**For cream dosage form**
To reduce the possibility of recurrence of infection, candida, tinea corporis, tinea cruris, and pityriasis versicolor should be treated for at least 2 weeks. Seborrheic dermatitis should be treated for at least 4 weeks or until clinical clearing. Tinea pedis should be treated for approximately 6 weeks.

## Topical Dosage Forms

Note: Bracketed uses in the *Dosage Forms* section refer to categories of use and/or indications that are not included in U.S. product labeling.

### KETOCONAZOLE CREAM

**Usual adult and adolescent dose**
Tinea corporis or
Tinea cruris or
Tinea pedis or
Pityriasis versicolor—
　　Topical, to the affected skin and surrounding areas, once a day.
Candidiasis, cutaneous—
　　Topical, to the affected skin and surrounding areas, once a day.
Seborrheic dermatitis—
　　Topical, to the affected skin and surrounding areas, two times a day.
[Paronychia][1] or
[Tinea barbae][1] or
[Tinea capitis][1]—
　　Topical, to the affected skin and surrounding areas, two or three times a day.

**Usual pediatric dose**
Safety and efficacy have not been established.

**Strength(s) usually available**
U.S.—
　　2% (Rx) [*Nizoral Cream* (stearyl alcohol; cetyl alcohol; sodium sulfite anhydrous)].
Canada—
　　2% (Rx) [*Nizoral Cream*].

**Packaging and storage**
Store below 30 °C (86 °F), in a well-closed container, unless otherwise specified by manufacturer. Protect from freezing.

USP DI

**Auxiliary labeling**
- For external use only.
- Continue medicine for full time of treatment.

### KETOCONAZOLE SHAMPOO

**Usual adult and adolescent dose**
Dandruff—
    Topical, as a shampoo, every four days for four weeks, then once every one or two weeks.

**Usual pediatric dose**
Safety and efficacy have not been established.

**Strength(s) usually available**
U.S.—
    2% (Rx) [*Nizoral Shampoo*].

Canada—
    2% (Rx) [*Nizoral Shampoo*].

[1]Not included in Canadian product labeling.

Revised: 06/21/93

**KETOPROFEN**—See *Anti-inflammatory Drugs, Nonsteroidal (Systemic)*

# KETOROLAC   Ophthalmic

VA CLASSIFICATION (Primary/Secondary): OP302/OP900
Commonly used brand name(s): *Acular*.
Note:  For a listing of dosage forms and brand names by country availability, see *Dosage Forms* section(s).

## Category
Anti-inflammatory, nonsteroidal (ophthalmic); antipruritic (ophthalmic).

## Indications
Note:  Bracketed information in the *Indications* section refers to uses that are not included in U.S. product labeling.

**Accepted**
Conjunctivitis, allergic (treatment)[1]—Ketorolac ophthalmic is indicated for the treatment of ocular itching caused by seasonal allergic conjunctivitis.

[Inflammation, ocular (prophylaxis and treatment)]—Ketorolac ophthalmic is indicated for the prophylaxis and treatment of postoperative ocular inflammation in patients undergoing cataract extraction with or without implantation of an intraocular lens.

[1]Not included in Canadian product labeling.

## Pharmacology/Pharmacokinetics

**Physicochemical characteristics**
Molecular weight—Ketorolac tromethamine: 376.41.
Osmolality—290 mOsmol per kg.
pKa—3.5.
pH—7.4.

**Mechanism of action/Effect**
Ketorolac is a nonsteroidal anti-inflammatory drug (NSAID) that is chemically related to indomethacin and tolmetin. Ocular administration of ketorolac reduces prostaglandin $E_2$ levels in aqueous humor, secondary to inhibition of prostaglandin biosynthesis.

**Other actions/effects**
Ketorolac ophthalmic has no significant effect on intraocular pressure.

**Absorption**
Negligible.

**Distribution**
Plasma—In a study where 26 subjects were administered 1 drop of 0.5% ketorolac ophthalmic solution in 1 eye 3 times a day for 21 days, 5 of 26 subjects had detectable (greater than 10 nanograms per mL) plasma levels of 11 to 22 nanograms per mL of ketorolac when they were tested 15 minutes after the first dose on day 10. When the subjects were tested on day 24, none had detectable plasma levels. In comparison, 10 mg of systemic ketorolac administered every 6 hours results in a steady state plasma level of approximately 960 nanograms per mL.

Aqueous humor—Eight of 9 patients administered 2 drops of 0.5% ketorolac ophthalmic solution in each eye 12 hours and 1 hour prior to cataract extraction had detectable (greater than or equal to 40 nanograms per mL) levels of 40 to 170 nanograms per mL (mean concentration 95 nanograms per mL) of ketorolac in the aqueous humor.

## Precautions to Consider

**Cross-sensitivity and/or related problems**
Patients sensitive to aspirin; phenylacetic acid derivatives, such as diclofenac; or other systemic or ophthalmic nonsteroidal anti-inflammatory drugs (NSAIDs) may be sensitive to ketorolac also.

**Tumorigenicity**
No evidence of tumorigenicity was found in an 18-month study in mice given oral doses of ketorolac equivalent to the parenteral maximum recommended human dose (MRHD) and a 24-month study in rats given oral doses of ketorolac equivalent to 2.5 times the parenteral MRHD.

**Mutagenicity**
Ketorolac was not mutagenic in the Ames test, the unscheduled DNA synthesis and repair test, and in forward mutation assays. In addition, ketorolac did not cause chromosome breakage in the *in vivo* mouse micronucleus assay. However, at 1590 mcg per mL and higher concentrations of ketorolac, there was an increased incidence of chromosomal aberrations in Chinese hamster ovarian cells.

**Pregnancy/Reproduction**
Fertility—Male and female rats given ketorolac at oral doses of 9 mg per kg of body weight (mg/kg) and 16 mg/kg, respectively, did not show impairment of fertility.

Pregnancy—Adequate and well-controlled studies in humans have not been done.

Studies in rabbits and rats given ketorolac at oral doses of 3.6 mg/kg a day and 10 mg/kg a day, respectively, during organogenesis did not show evidence of teratogenicity. However, rats given oral doses of 1.5 mg/kg after gestation day 17 had a higher pup mortality rate.

FDA Pregnancy Category C.

Labor—Rats given oral doses of 1.5 mg/kg of ketorolac after gestation day 17 developed dystocia.

**Breast-feeding**
Problems in humans have not been documented.

**Pediatrics**
Appropriate studies on the relationship of age to the effects of ophthalmic ketorolac have not been performed in the pediatric population. Safety and efficacy have not been established.

**Geriatrics**
Appropriate studies on the relationship of age to the effects of ophthalmic ketorolac have not been performed in the geriatric population. However, no geriatrics-specific problems have been documented to date.

**Drug interactions and/or related problems**
The following drug interactions and/or related problems have been selected on the basis of their potential clinical significance (possible mechanism in parentheses where appropriate)—not necessarily inclusive (» = major clinical significance):

Note:  Combinations containing any of the following medications, depending on the amount present, may also interact with this medication.

Any medication that may interfere with blood clotting or prolong bleeding time, such as:
  Anticoagulants, coumarin- or indandione-derivative, or
  Heparin or
  Platelet aggregation inhibitors
    (ophthalmic NSAIDs, such as ketorolac, may also increase the tendency to bleed; concurrent use may increase the risk of postoperative ocular bleeding)

**Medical considerations/Contraindications**
The medical considerations/contraindications included have been selected on the basis of their potential clinical significance (reasons given in parentheses where appropriate)—not necessarily inclusive (» = major clinical significance).

## Ketorolac (Ophthalmic)

*Risk-benefit should be considered when the following medical problems exist:*

Hemophilia or other bleeding problems or coagulation defects or
Prolonged bleeding time
   (increased risk of bleeding following ocular surgery)
Sensitivity to ophthalmic ketorolac

### Side/Adverse Effects

The following side/adverse effects have been selected on the basis of their potential clinical significance (possible signs and symptoms in parentheses where appropriate)—not necessarily inclusive:

**Those indicating need for medical attention**
Incidence less frequent or rare
   *Hypersensitivity* (itching, rash, redness, swelling, or other sign of irritation not present before therapy); *keratitis, superficial* (redness of the clear part of the eye); *ocular irritation* (itching, redness, tearing, or other sign of eye irritation not present before use of this medicine or becoming worse during use)

**Those indicating need for medical attention only if they continue or are bothersome**
Incidence more frequent
   *Stinging or burning upon instillation of medication*

### Patient Consultation

As an aid to patient consultation, refer to *Advice for the Patient, Ketorolac (Ophthalmic)*.
In providing consultation, consider emphasizing the following selected information (» = major clinical significance):

**Before using this medication**
» Conditions affecting use, especially:
   Sensitivity to ophthalmic or systemic ketorolac; aspirin; phenylacetic acid derivatives, such as diclofenac; or other systemic or ophthalmic nonsteroidal anti-inflammatory drugs (NSAIDs)

**Proper use of this medication**
Proper administration; using a second drop if necessary; not touching applicator tip to any surface; keeping container tightly closed
» Proper dosing
Missed dose: Using as soon as possible; not using if almost time for next dose; using next dose at regularly scheduled time; not doubling doses
» Proper storage

**Precautions while using this medication**
Checking with doctor if symptoms do not improve or if they become worse
Expecting stinging or burning of eye upon administration of medication

**Side/adverse effects**
Signs of potential side effects, especially hypersensitivity; keratitis, superficial; or ocular irritation

### General Dosing Information

The manufacturer recommends that patients not wear soft contact lenses during treatment with ketorolac ophthalmic solution. However, medical experts do not believe this precaution is necessary unless the patient has corneal epithelial problems and the medication is to be used more often than once every 1 to 2 hours. No significant problems have been documented with ophthalmic solutions that contain 0.03% or less of benzalkonium chloride as a preservative and are used as eye drops in patients with no significant corneal surface problems.

Ketorolac ophthalmic may be administered in conjunction with other ophthalmic medications, such as antibiotics, beta-adrenergic blocking agents, carbonic anhydrase inhibitors, cycloplegics, and mydriatics.

### Ophthalmic Dosage Forms

Note: Bracketed uses in the *Dosage Forms* section refer to categories of use and/or indications that are not included in U.S. product labeling.

#### KETOROLAC TROMETHAMINE OPHTHALMIC SOLUTION

**Usual adult and adolescent dose**
Conjunctivitis, allergic (treatment)[1]—
   Topical, to the conjunctiva, 1 drop in each eye four times a day.
[Inflammation, ocular (prophylaxis and treatment)]—
   Topical, to the conjunctiva, 1 drop in each eye every six to eight hours beginning twenty-four hours before surgery and continuing for three to four weeks.

**Usual pediatric dose**
Safety and efficacy have not been established.

**Strength(s) usually available**
U.S.—
   0.5% (Rx) [*Acular* (benzalkonium chloride 0.01%)].
Canada—
   0.5% (Rx) [*Acular* (benzalkonium chloride)].

**Packaging and storage**
Store between 15 and 30 °C (59 and 86 °F), unless otherwise specified by manufacturer. Protect from light.

**Auxiliary labeling**
• For the eye.

[1]Not included in Canadian product labeling.

### Selected Bibliography

Ketorolac for seasonal allergic conjunctivitis. Med Lett Drugs Ther 1993 Sep 17; 35(905): 88-9.

Tinkelman DG, Rupp G, Kaufman H, et al. Double-masked, paired-comparison clinical study of ketorolac tromethamine 0.5% ophthalmic solution compared with placebo eyedrops in the treatment of seasonal allergic conjunctivitis. Surv Ophthalmol 1993 Jul-Aug; 38 suppl: 133-40.

Ballas Z, Blumenthal M, Tinkelman DG, et al. Clinical evaluation of ketorolac tromethamine 0.5% ophthalmic solution for the treatment of seasonal allergic conjunctivitis. Surv Ophthalmol 1993 Jul-Aug; 38 suppl: 141-8.

Developed: 08/11/94
Interim revision: 08/12/98

---

# KETOROLAC Systemic

VA CLASSIFICATION (Primary): CN103
Commonly used brand name(s): *Toradol*.
Note: For a listing of dosage forms and brand names by country availability, see *Dosage Forms* section(s).

## Category
Analgesic.

## Indications

Note: Ketorolac, like other nonsteroidal anti-inflammatory drugs (NSAIDs), has antipyretic and anti-inflammatory, as well as analgesic actions. However, indications for specific NSAIDs may vary because of lack of specific testing and/or clinical-use data as well as the toxicity of the individual agent.

**Accepted**
Pain (treatment)—Ketorolac is indicated for the short-term management of moderately severe acute pain that would otherwise require treatment with an opioid analgesic. It is most commonly used to relieve postoperative pain. The oral dosage form is indicated only for continuation of therapy following initial parenteral administration. Because the risk of gastrointestinal bleeding and other severe adverse effects increases with the duration of treatment, **ketorolac should not be administered by any route or combination of routes for longer than 5 days**.

Before ketorolac is used perioperatively, its platelet aggregation–inhibiting activity, which increases the risk of bleeding, must be considered. Postoperative hematomas and other signs of wound bleeding have been reported in ketorolac-treated patients. Therefore, **ketorolac should not be given prior to major surgery to prevent postoperative pain; nor should it be administered intraoperatively when control of bleeding is critical**. Also, ketorolac lacks the sedative and anti-anxiety activity usually desired in a preoperative medication.

**Unaccepted**
Although ketorolac may be used for short-term (up to 5 days) treatment of moderately severe acute arthritic pain in patients who are not receiving chronic treatment with other NSAIDs, it is not recommended for the long-term treatment of chronic rheumatic disease.

Ketorolac is not recommended for treatment of mild pain or for long-term treatment of chronic pain.

Ketorolac is not recommended for obstetrical analgesia because its safety has not been studied adequately. Inhibition of prostaglandin synthesis by NSAIDs such as ketorolac may decrease uterine contractility, increase the risk of intrauterine bleeding, and/or cause premature constriction of the fetal ductus arteriosus.

## Pharmacology/Pharmacokinetics

### Physicochemical characteristics
Molecular weight—376.41.
pKa—3.5.

### Mechanism of action/Effect
Ketorolac is a nonsteroidal anti-inflammatory drug (NSAID) chemically related to indomethacin and tolmetin. Currently available NSAIDs inhibit the activity of the enzyme cyclo-oxygenase, leading to decreased formation of precursors of prostaglandins and thromboxanes from arachidonic acid. The resultant reduction in prostaglandin synthesis and activity may be at least partially responsible for many of the adverse, as well as the therapeutic, effects of these medications. Analgesia is probably produced via a peripheral action in which blockade of pain impulse generation results from decreased prostaglandin activity. However, inhibition of the synthesis or actions of other substances that sensitize pain receptors to mechanical or chemical stimulation may also contribute to the analgesic effect.

### Other actions/effects
Ketorolac has anti-inflammatory and antipyretic actions that, together with its analgesic effects, may mask the onset and/or progression of an infection.

Ketorolac inhibits platelet aggregation. This effect is reversible (unlike aspirin-induced platelet inhibition, which persists for the life of the exposed platelets). Recovery of platelet function usually occurs within 24 to 48 hours following discontinuation of ketorolac.

Like other NSAIDs, ketorolac may cause gastrointestinal ulceration and bleeding. These effects probably result from ketorolac-induced reduction of the synthesis and activity of prostaglandins that exert a protective effect on the gastrointestinal mucosa; they may occur after parenteral as well as after oral administration. However, when administered orally, this acidic medication probably also exerts a direct irritant or erosive effect on the mucosa.

Like other NSAIDs, ketorolac may cause renal toxicity (i.e., sodium and fluid retention, decreased renal perfusion, and decreased renal function), probably by inhibiting the synthesis and activity of renal prostaglandins, which are directly involved in the maintenance of renal hemodynamics and sodium and fluid balance. Renal prostaglandins are especially important in maintaining renal function in the presence of generalized vasoconstriction or volume depletion.

### Absorption
Intramuscular—Rapid and complete.

Oral—Rapid (more rapid than after intramuscular administration in some individuals) and complete. The rate, but not the extent, of absorption is decreased when the medication is taken with a high fat meal. Absorption is not altered by concurrent administration with an antacid.

### Distribution
The volume of distribution (Vol$_D$) of racemic ketorolac in patients with normal renal function is 0.15 to 0.33 L per kg of body weight. In patients with renal function impairment, the Vol$_D$ of the active S-enantiomer of ketorolac is twice as large as in individuals with normal renal function, and the Vol$_D$ of the inactive R-enantiomer is approximately 20% larger. Penetration of ketorolac across the blood-brain barrier is poor; concentrations in cerebrospinal fluid are 0.2%, or less, of those achieved in plasma.

In breast milk—Maximum concentrations of 7.3 nanograms per mL (0.019 micromoles/L) 2 hours after the first dose and 7.9 nanograms per mL (0.021 micromoles/L) 2 hours after the fifth dose were measured in the breast milk of women receiving 10 mg of ketorolac, orally, 4 times a day. However, in 40% of the subjects tested, the concentration in breast milk did not reach the lowest detection limit of 5 nanograms per mL (0.013 micromoles/L).

### Protein binding
Very high (> 99%).

### Biotransformation
Primarily hepatic. Less than 50% of a dose is metabolized. The major metabolites are a glucuronide conjugate, which may also be formed in the kidney, and p-hydroxy ketorolac. Neither metabolite has significant analgesic activity.

### Half-life
Terminal—
Individuals with normal renal function—
About 5.3 hours in healthy young adults (ranges, 3.5 to 9.2 hours after 30 mg intramuscularly, 4 to 7.2 hours after 30 mg intravenously, and 2.4 to 9.0 hours after 10 mg orally). Mean values are higher in healthy geriatric subjects, but remain within the same ranges reported for younger adults. Hepatic function impairment does not significantly prolong the half-life.
Patients with renal function impairment—
About 10.3 to 10.8 hours in patients with a serum creatinine of 1.9 to 5 mg per 100 mL (168 to 442 micromoles/L) (ranges, 5.9 to 19.2 hours after 30 mg intramuscularly and 3.4 to 18.9 hours after 10 mg orally). Values are even higher in patients receiving renal dialysis (13.6 [range, 8 to 39.1] hours after 30 mg intramuscularly).

Note: The above values apply to racemic ketorolac. In patients with normal renal function, terminal half-life values for the active S-enantiomer and the inactive R-enantiomer are approximately 2.5 hours and 5 hours, respectively.

### Onset of action
Dose-dependent; generally within 30 minutes to 1 hour.

### Time to peak plasma concentration
Intramuscular:
Single dose of up to 60 mg—30 to 60 minutes.
Intravenous:
Single 15-mg dose: 1.1 ± 0.7 minutes.
Single 30-mg dose: 2.9 ± 1.8 minutes.
Oral:
Single 10-mg dose—44 ± 34 minutes.

### Time to steady-state plasma concentration
Intramuscular or oral—About 24 hours, when the medication is administered at 6-hour intervals.

### Steady-state plasma concentration
With administration 4 times a day at 6-hour intervals
Intramuscular—
15 mg—Average, 0.94 ± 0.29 mcg/mL (2.5 ± 0.77 micromoles/L).
30 mg—Average, 1.88 ± 0.59 mcg/mL (5 ± 1.57 micromoles/L).
Intravenous—
15 mg—Average, 1.09 ± 0.3 mcg/mL (2.89 ± 0.8 micromoles/L).
30 mg—Average, 2.17 ± 0.59 mcg/mL (5.77 ± 1.57 micromoles/L).
Oral—
10 mg—Average, 0.59 ± 0.2 mcg/mL (1.57 ± 0.53 micromoles/L).

Note: Determination of minimum (trough) concentrations for each of the above routes of administration has shown that ketorolac concentrations do not decrease to subtherapeutic levels between doses.

### Peak plasma concentration
Following administration of a single dose

| Route* | Dose (mg) | Concentration mcg/mL | micromoles/L |
|---|---|---|---|
| IM | 15 | 1.14±0.32 | 3.03±0.85 |
|  | 30 | 2.42±0.68 | 6.44±1.81 |
|  | 60 | 4.5±1.27 | 11.97±3.38 |
| IV | 15 | 2.47±0.51 | 6.57±1.36 |
|  | 30 | 4.65±0.96 | 12.37±2.55 |
| PO | 10 | 0.87±0.22 | 2.31±0.58 |

*IM = intramuscular; IV = intravenous; PO = oral.

### Therapeutic plasma concentration
0.3 mcg/mL (0.8 micromoles/L), at steady-state.

### Time to peak effect
Intramuscular or intravenous—1 to 2 hours.
Oral—2 to 3 hours.

### Duration of action
Intramuscular—
6 hours or longer in approximately 50% of patients receiving a single 10-mg dose and in approximately 60% of patients receiving a single 30-mg dose in clinical studies.
Oral—
Approximately 4 hours in 75 to 80% of patients and 6 hours or longer in about 65% of patients receiving a single 10-mg dose in clinical studies.

## Elimination

91% renal; approximately 6% biliary/fecal. The active S-enantiomer is cleared approximately twice as rapidly as the inactive R-enantiomer. Average total clearance rates following administration of a single dose—

Healthy young adults:
Intramuscular, 30 mg—0.023 (range, 0.01 to 0.046) liters per hour per kg of body weight (L/hr/kg).
Intravenous, 30 mg—0.03 (range, 0.017 to 0.051) L/hr/kg.
Oral, 10 mg—0.025 (range, 0.013 to 0.05) L/hr/kg.

Elderly adults:
Intramuscular, 30 mg—0.019 (range, 0.013 to 0.034) L/hr/kg.
Oral, 10 mg—0.024 (range, 0.018 to 0.034) L/hr/kg.

Patients with hepatic function impairment:
Intramuscular, 30 mg—0.029 (range, 0.13 to 0.066) L/hr/kg.
Oral, 10 mg—0.033 (range, 0.019 to 0.051) L/hr/kg.

Patients with renal function impairment:
Serum creatinine 1.9 to 5 mg/100 mL (168 to 442 micromoles/L):
Intramuscular, 30 mg: 0.015 (range, 0.005 to 0.043) L/hr/kg.
Oral, 10 mg: 0.016 (range, 0.007 to 0.052) L/hr/kg.

Renal dialysis patients:
Intravenous, 30 mg: 0.016 (range, 0.003 to 0.036) L/hr/kg.

In dialysis—
Hemodialysis does not remove significant quantities of ketorolac from the body.

## Precautions to Consider

### Cross-sensitivity and/or related problems

Patients sensitive to aspirin or other nonsteroidal anti-inflammatory drugs (NSAIDs) may be sensitive to ketorolac also. Severe asthmatic and anaphylactoid reactions have occurred in such patients.

### Tumorigenicity

No evidence of tumorigenicity was found in an 18-month study in mice receiving up to 2 mg per kg of body weight (mg/kg) per day or a 24-month study in rats receiving up to 5 mg/kg per day orally. These doses are considered, on the basis of area under the concentration-time curve (AUC) comparisons, to be equivalent to 0.9 and 0.5 times, respectively, the human exposure resulting from intramuscular or intravenous administration of 30 mg 4 times a day.

### Mutagenicity

No evidence of mutagenicity was found in the Ames test, unscheduled DNA synthesis and repair, and forward mutation assays. Also, ketorolac did not cause chromosome breakage in the *in vivo* mouse micronucleus assay. However, in a concentration of 1590 mcg per mL (mcg/mL) (approximately 1000 times average human plasma concentrations), ketorolac increased the occurrence of chromosomal aberrations in Chinese hamster ovarian cells.

### Pregnancy/Reproduction

Fertility—No impairment of fertility was observed in male rats given 9 mg/kg per day or female rats given 16 mg/kg per day, orally (53.1 and 50 mg per square meter of body surface area [mg/m$^2$] per day). These doses are equivalent to 0.9 and 1.6 times, respectively, the human exposure resulting from intramuscular or intravenous administration of 30 mg 4 times a day, based on AUC comparisons.

Pregnancy—
*First trimester*—
Adequate and well-controlled studies have not been done in pregnant women.

No teratogenicity occurred in offspring of rabbits receiving oral doses of up to 3.6 mg/kg per day (42.35 mg/m$^2$ per day; equivalent to 0.37 times the human exposure resulting from intramuscular or intravenous administration of 30 mg 4 times a day, based on AUC comparisons) or rats receiving up to 10 mg/kg per day (59 mg/m$^2$ per day; equivalent to the human exposure, based on AUC comparisons).

*Second and third trimesters*—
Although studies in pregnant women have not been done with ketorolac, chronic use of any NSAID during the second half of pregnancy is not recommended because of possible adverse effects in the fetus, such as premature closure of the ductus arteriosus, which may lead to persistent pulmonary hypertension in the newborn. Such effects have been documented in animal studies with other NSAIDs.

Chronic administration of 1.5 mg/kg per day (8.8 mg/m$^2$ per day) of ketorolac to rats after Day 17 of gestation caused dystocia and higher pup mortality. This dose is equivalent to 0.14 times the human exposure resulting from intramuscular or intravenous administration of 30 mg 4 times a day, based on AUC comparisons. Higher doses (9 mg/kg or more per day, administered to rats from Day 15 of gestation) significantly increased the length of gestation, in addition to increasing the incidence of maternal deaths associated with dystocia and decreasing birth weights and survival rates in the offspring.

FDA Pregnancy Category C.

Labor and delivery—Although a few studies have investigated the use of ketorolac in obstetrics, it is not recommended for obstetrical preoperative medication or obstetrical analgesia. When administered during labor, ketorolac crosses the placenta and inhibits platelet aggregation in the neonate. Also, potential adverse effects on uterine contractility and the fetal ductus arteriosus, resulting in a risk of increased uterine bleeding and fetal circulatory disturbances, respectively, must be considered.

### Breast-feeding

Because of potential adverse effects in the nursing infant, use of ketorolac by nursing mothers is not recommended. Ketorolac is distributed into breast milk in small quantities. Maximum concentrations of 7.3 nanograms per mL (nanograms/mL) (0.019 micromoles/L) 2 hours after the first dose and 7.9 nanograms/mL (0.021 micromoles/L) 2 hours after the fifth dose were measured in the breast milk of women receiving 10 mg of ketorolac, orally, 4 times a day, although the concentration in breast milk failed to reach the lowest detection limit of 5 nanograms/mL (0.013 micromoles/L) in 40% of the subjects tested. Milk-to-plasma concentration ratios of 0.037 and 0.025 have been calculated after administration of a single dose and at steady-state, respectively.

### Pediatrics

No information is available on the relationship of age to the effects of ketorolac in pediatric patients. Safety and efficacy in patients younger than 16 years of age have not been established.

### Geriatrics

Studies have shown that clearance of ketorolac is reduced in healthy individuals 65 years of age or older, leading to significant prolongation of the elimination half-life. Also, geriatric patients are more likely to have age-related renal function impairment, which may further reduce ketorolac clearance and increase the risk of NSAID-induced renal or hepatic toxicity. The risk of gastrointestinal ulceration, bleeding, and perforation is higher in elderly patients receiving ketorolac than in younger adults. Also, ketorolac-induced gastrointestinal ulceration and/or bleeding is more likely to cause serious consequences, including fatalities, in geriatric patients. It is recommended that ketorolac be used with caution, in the lower of the recommended dosage regimens, and with careful monitoring of the patient.

### Drug interactions and/or related problems

The following drug interactions and/or related problems have been selected on the basis of their potential clinical significance (possible mechanism in parentheses where appropriate)—not necessarily inclusive (» = major clinical significance):

Note: Combinations containing any of the following medications, depending on the amount present, may also interact with this medication.

All of the interactions listed below have not been documented with ketorolac. However, they have been reported with other NSAIDs and should be considered potential precautions to the use of ketorolac also.

In addition to the interactions listed below, the possibility should be considered that additive or multiple effects leading to impaired blood clotting and/or increased risk of bleeding may occur if any NSAID is used concurrently with any medication having a significant potential for causing hypoprothrombinemia, thrombocytopenia, or gastrointestinal ulceration or hemorrhage.

Acetaminophen
(prolonged concurrent use of acetaminophen with an NSAID may increase the risk of adverse renal effects; it is recommended that patients be under close medical supervision while receiving such combined therapy)

Alcohol or
Corticosteroids, glucocorticoid or
Corticotropin (chronic therapeutic use) or
Potassium supplements
(concurrent use with an NSAID may increase the risk of gastrointestinal side effects, including ulceration or hemorrhage)

» Anticoagulants, coumarin- or indandione-derivative or
» Heparin or
» Thrombolytic agents, such as:
Alteplase
Anistreplase

Streptokinase
Urokinase
(ketorolac has not been shown to alter the pharmacokinetic or pharmacodynamic properties of warfarin or heparin; however, inhibition of platelet aggregation by ketorolac, and the potential occurrence of ketorolac-induced gastrointestinal ulceration or bleeding, may be hazardous to patients receiving anticoagulant or thrombolytic therapy; caution and careful monitoring of the patient are recommended, as there is evidence that administration of ketorolac to patients receiving an anticoagulant, possibly including low [prophylactic] doses of heparin [2500 to 5000 Units every 12 hours], increases the risk of bleeding and intramuscular hematoma formation)

Antihypertensives or
Diuretics
(increased monitoring of the response to any antihypertensive agent may be advisable when ketorolac is used concurrently because several other NSAIDs have been shown to reduce or reverse the effects of many antihypertensives, possibly by inhibiting renal prostaglandin synthesis and/or by causing sodium and fluid retention)

(NSAIDs may decrease the diuretic and natriuretic, as well as the antihypertensive, effects of diuretics, probably by inhibiting renal prostaglandin synthesis; ketorolac inhibited the diuretic effect of furosemide, decreasing sodium and urine output by about 20%, in a study in normovolemic healthy subjects)

(concurrent use of an NSAID and a diuretic may also increase the risk of renal failure secondary to a decrease in renal blood flow caused by inhibition of renal prostaglandin synthesis)

(concurrent use of ketorolac with an angiotensin-converting enzyme [ACE] inhibitor may also increase the risk of renal function impairment, especially in hypovolemic patients)

» Aspirin or other salicylates or
» Other NSAIDs
(concurrent use of aspirin or other NSAIDs with ketorolac is not recommended because of the potential for additive toxicity)

(concurrent use of ketorolac with antirheumatic doses of salicylates other than aspirin should be undertaken with caution and in reduced doses because therapeutic plasma concentrations of salicylate [30 mg per 100 mL (2.17 mmol per L)] decrease the protein binding of ketorolac sufficiently to potentially double the plasma concentration of free [unbound] ketorolac)

» Cefamandole or
» Cefoperazone or
» Cefotetan or
» Plicamycin or
» Valproic acid
(these medications may cause hypoprothrombinemia; in addition, plicamycin or valproic acid may inhibit platelet aggregation; concurrent use with an NSAID may increase the risk of bleeding because of additive interferences with blood clotting and/or the potential occurrence of gastrointestinal ulceration or hemorrhage during NSAID therapy)

Gold compounds
(although other NSAIDs are commonly used concurrently with gold compounds in the treatment of arthritis, the possibility should be considered that concurrent use of a gold compound with any NSAID, including ketorolac, may increase the risk of adverse renal effects)

» Lithium
(although the effect of ketorolac on lithium plasma concentration has not been studied, increases in lithium concentration have been reported during concomitant administration of ketorolac; increased monitoring of lithium plasma concentrations is recommended during and following concurrent use so that lithium dosage can be adjusted if necessary)

» Methotrexate
(the effect of ketorolac on methotrexate concentrations and/or toxicity has not been studied; however, administration of moderate- or high-dose methotrexate infusions to patients receiving other NSAIDs has resulted in severe, sometimes fatal, methotrexate toxicity, possibly because NSAIDs may reduce renal function, thereby decreasing methotrexate excretion; it is recommended that ketorolac not be administered for 24 hours prior to, and for at least 12 hours [or until the methotrexate plasma concentration has decreased to a nontoxic level] following, a high-dose methotrexate infusion)

(severe, sometimes fatal, methotrexate toxicity has also been reported with the relatively low to moderate doses of methotrexate used in the treatment of rheumatoid arthritis or psoriasis when an NSAID was given concurrently; it is recommended that concurrent use of ketorolac with low to moderate doses of methotrexate also be undertaken with caution, with methotrexate dosage being adjusted as determined by monitoring plasma methotrexate concentration and/or adequacy of the patient's renal function)

Nephrotoxic medications, other (See *Appendix II*)
(concurrent use with an NSAID may increase the risk and/or severity of adverse renal effects)

Platelet aggregation inhibitors, other (See *Appendix II*)
(concurrent use of any of these medications with an NSAID, including ketorolac, may increase the risk of bleeding because of additive inhibition of platelet aggregation as well as the potential occurrence of gastrointestinal ulceration or hemorrhage during NSAID therapy)

» Probenecid
(concurrent use with ketorolac is not recommended because probenecid decreases elimination of ketorolac, resulting in significantly increased ketorolac plasma concentrations [the area under the concentration-time curve (AUC) being increased about 3-fold, from 5.4 to 17.8 mcg per hour per mL] and half-life [which is more than doubled, to about 15 hours])

**Laboratory value alterations**
The following have been selected on the basis of their potential clinical significance (possible effect in parentheses where appropriate)—not necessarily inclusive (» = major clinical significance):

With physiology/laboratory test values
Bleeding time
(may be prolonged because ketorolac inhibits platelet aggregation; effects may persist for 24 to 48 hours after discontinuation of therapy)

Blood urea nitrogen (BUN) or
Creatinine, serum, or
Potassium, serum
(may be increased)

Liver function tests, especially serum transaminase activity
(although borderline elevations in test values may occur in up to 15% of patients receiving ketorolac, significant elevations [3 times the upper limit] of serum transaminases have occurred in fewer than 1%; ketorolac therapy should be discontinued if significant abnormalities occur)

**Medical considerations/Contraindications**
The medical considerations/contraindications included have been selected on the basis of their potential clinical significance (reasons given in parentheses where appropriate)—not necessarily inclusive (» = major clinical significance).

*Except under special circumstances, this medication should not be used when the following medical problems exist:*
» Cerebrovascular bleeding, suspected or confirmed or
» Hemophilia or other bleeding problems including coagulation or platelet function disorders
(increased risk of bleeding because ketorolac inhibits platelet aggregation and may also cause gastrointestinal ulceration or hemorrhage)

» Gastrointestinal bleeding, active, recent, or history of or
» Gastrointestinal perforation, recent or
» Peptic ulceration, ulcerative colitis, or other ulcerative gastrointestinal disease, active or history of
(increased risk of gastrointestinal ulceration, perforation, and/or hemorrhage)

» Nasal polyps associated with bronchospasm, aspirin-induced, or angioedema, anaphylaxis, or other severe allergic reaction induced by aspirin, ketorolac, or other NSAIDs, history of
(high risk of severe allergic reactions because of cross-sensitivity)

» Renal function impairment, severe
(increased risk of renal failure)

*Risk-benefit should be considered when the following medical problems exist:*
» Allergic reaction, mild, such as allergic rhinitis, urticaria, or skin rash, induced by aspirin, ketorolac, or other NSAIDs, history of
(possibility of cross-sensitivity)

Asthma
(may be exacerbated)

Cholestasis or
Hepatitis, active
(although other forms of hepatic function impairment apparently do not alter the clearance of ketorolac, studies to assess the possible

effect of cholestasis or active hepatitis on the pharmacokinetics of the medication have not been done)

Conditions predisposing to gastrointestinal toxicity, such as:
Alcoholism, active or
» Inflammatory bowel disease or
Tobacco use, or recent history of
(caution and close supervision are recommended for patients in whom there is a significant risk of gastrointestinal toxicity; misoprostol or sucralfate should be considered as prophylaxis for those at high risk)

Conditions predisposing to and/or exacerbated by fluid retention, such as:
Compromised cardiac function or
Congestive heart disease or
Edema, pre-existing or
Hypertension
(ketorolac may cause fluid retention and edema)

Congestive heart failure or
Diabetes mellitus or
Edema, pre-existing or
Hepatic function impairment or
» Hypovolemia or
Sepsis
(increased risk of renal failure; caution and monitoring of urine output, serum urea, and serum creatinine are advised; hypovolemia should be corrected before ketorolac therapy is initiated)

(hepatotoxicity, as indicated by significant abnormalities in liver function tests, is more likely to occur in patients with pre-existing hepatic function impairment)

» Renal function impairment, mild to moderate
(ketorolac and its metabolites are excreted primarily via the kidney, which may also be a site of ketorolac metabolism; a substantial reduction in ketorolac clearance, leading to significant prolongation of its half-life, has been demonstrated in patients with renal function impairment; a reduction in dosage is recommended for patients with moderate elevations of serum creatinine)

(caution and careful monitoring of the patient are also recommended because of possible patient predisposition toward development of NSAID-induced adverse renal effects, including acute renal failure)

Systemic lupus erythematosus (SLE)
(increased risk of renal function impairment)

## Side/Adverse Effects

Note: Ketorolac shares the risks associated with other nonsteroidal anti-inflammatory drugs (NSAIDs), including gastrointestinal and/or renal toxicity.

The risk of adverse effects increases with the duration of treatment as well as with the total daily dose of ketorolac. Also, side effects are more frequent when plasma concentrations of ketorolac exceed 5 mcg per mL (13.3 micromoles/L). In a long-term study in patients with chronic pain, oral administration of 10 mg 4 times a day of ketorolac caused more gastrointestinal toxicity than 650 mg 4 times a day of aspirin; the frequency of occurrence of gastrointestinal ulceration or bleeding was 0.69% after 3 months and 1.59% after 6 months in patients receiving ketorolac and 0% after 3 months and 0.73% after 6 months in patients receiving aspirin. An unusually large number of cases of upper gastrointestinal bleeding (20% of which were fatal) has been reported with ketorolac, mostly in elderly patients.

Studies have shown that there is also a substantial risk of gastrointestinal bleeding during short-term parenteral administration of ketorolac (a maximum of 20 doses, administered over 5 days), especially in patients older than 65 years of age and/or patients with a history of gastrointestinal perforation, ulcer, or bleeding (PUB). The following percentages of patients experienced clinically significant gastrointestinal bleeding in these studies:

| Patient | | Total dose/day (mg) | | | |
|---|---|---|---|---|---|
| Age (yr) | PUB History | ≤60 | >60–90 | >90–120 | >120 |
| <65 | No | 0.4% | 0.4% | 0.9% | 4.6% |
|  | Yes | 2.1% | 4.6% | 7.8% | 15.4% |
| ≥65 | No | 1.2% | 2.8% | 2.2% | 7.7% |
|  | Yes | 4.7% | 3.7% | 2.8% | 25% |

The following side/adverse effects have been selected on the basis of their potential clinical significance (possible signs and symptoms in parentheses where appropriate)—not necessarily inclusive:

**Those indicating need for medical attention**
Incidence more frequent (4%)
*Edema* (swelling of face, fingers, lower legs, ankles, and/or feet; unusual weight gain)
Incidence less frequent (1 to 3%)
*Hypertension* (high blood pressure); *purpura* (small, red spots on skin; bruising); *skin rash*—rarely including maculopapular rash, or itching; *stomatitis* (sores, ulcers, or white spots on lips or in mouth)
Incidence rare (< 1%)
*Anaphylaxis or anaphylactoid reaction* (changes in facial skin color; skin rash, hives, and/or itching; fast or irregular breathing; puffiness or swelling of the eyelids or around the eyes; shortness of breath, troubled breathing, tightness in chest, and/or wheezing); *anemia* (unusual tiredness or weakness); *aseptic meningitis* (fever; severe headache; drowsiness; confusion; stiff neck and/or back; general feeling of illness; nausea); *asthma, bronchospasm, or dyspnea* (shortness of breath, troubled breathing, tightness in chest, and/or wheezing); *bleeding from wound, postoperatively; bloody stools; blurred vision or other vision change; cholestatic jaundice* (dark urine; fever; itching; light-colored stools; pain, tenderness, and/or swelling in upper abdominal area; skin rash; swollen glands; yellow eyes or skin); *convulsions; edema of tongue; eosinophilia; exfoliative dermatitis* (fever with or without chills; red, thickened, or scaly skin; swollen and/or painful glands; unusual bruising); *fainting; fever; flank pain, with or without hematuria and/or azotemia* (pain in lower back and/or side; bloody or cloudy urine); *gastrointestinal, usually peptic, ulceration, possibly with perforation and/or bleeding* (abdominal pain, cramping, or burning, severe; bloody or black, tarry stools; vomiting of blood or material that looks like coffee grounds; nausea, heartburn, and/or indigestion, severe and continuing); *hallucinations; hearing loss; hemolytic uremic syndrome; hepatitis* (loss of appetite; nausea; vomiting; yellow eyes or skin; swelling in upper abdominal area); *hives; hyperactivity* (restlessness, severe); *hypotension* (low blood pressure); *increase in frequency of urination; increased urine volume; laryngeal edema* (shortness of breath or troubled breathing); *leukopenia* (rarely, fever or chills; cough or hoarseness; lower back or side pain; painful or difficult urination)—usually asymptomatic; *mental depression; nephritis* (bloody or cloudy urine; increased blood pressure; sudden decrease in amount of urine; swelling of face, fingers, feet, and/or lower legs; rapid weight gain); *nosebleeds; oliguria* (decrease in amount of urine); *pancreatitis, acute* (abdominal pain; fever with or without chills; swelling and/or tenderness in upper abdominal or stomach area); *psychosis* (mood changes; unusual behavior); *pulmonary edema* (difficult, fast, noisy breathing, sometimes with wheezing; blue lips and fingernails; pale skin; increased sweating); *rectal bleeding; renal failure, acute* (increased blood pressure; shortness of breath, troubled breathing, tightness in chest, and/or wheezing; sudden decrease in amount of urine; swelling of face, fingers, feet, and/or lower legs; continuing thirst; unusual tiredness or weakness; weight gain); *rhinitis* (runny nose); *Stevens-Johnson syndrome* (bleeding or crusting sores on lips; chest pain; fever with or without chills; muscle cramps or pain; skin rash; sores, ulcers, or white spots in mouth; sore throat); *thrombocytopenia* (rarely, unusual bleeding or bruising; black, tarry stools; blood in urine or stools; pinpoint red spots on skin)—usually asymptomatic; *tinnitus* (ringing or buzzing in ears); *toxic epidermal necrolysis [Lyell's syndrome]* (redness, tenderness, itching, burning, or peeling of skin; sore throat; fever with or without chills)

Note: *Hemolytic uremic syndrome* is characterized by hemolytic *anemia, renal failure, thrombocytopenia*, and *purpura*. These adverse effects may also occur independently of hemolytic uremic syndrome and are listed separately above.

**Those indicating need for medical attention only if they continue or are bothersome**
Incidence more frequent (> 3%)
*Abdominal pain*—[13%]; *bruising at injection site; diarrhea*—[7%]; *dizziness*—[7%]; *drowsiness*—[6%]; *headache*—[17%]; *indigestion*—[12%]; *nausea*—[12%]
Incidence less frequent (1 to 3%)
*Bloated feeling or gas; burning or pain at injection site; constipation; feeling of fullness in gastrointestinal tract; increased sweating; vomiting*

## Overdose

For specific information on the agents used in the management of ketorolac overdose, see:
• *Antacids (Oral-Local)* monograph;
• *Charcoal, Activated (Oral-Local)* monograph;
• *Histamine H$_2$-receptor Antagonists (Systemic)* monograph;
• *Misoprostol (Systemic)* monograph;

- *Omeprazole (Systemic)* monograph; and/or
- *Sucralfate (Oral-Local)* monograph.

For more information on the management of overdose or unintentional ingestion, **contact a Poison Control Center** (see *Poison Control Center Listing*).

Factors that are associated with an increased risk of ketorolac toxicity (in addition to total daily dosage and duration of treatment) include hypovolemia; renal insufficiency; a patient history of gastrointestinal perforation, ulceration, or bleeding; and patient age of 65 years or older.

### Clinical effects of overdose
The following effects have been selected on the basis of their potential clinical significance (possible signs and symptoms in parentheses where appropriate)—not necessarily inclusive:
***Abdominal pain; gastrointestinal ulceration and bleeding; metabolic acidosis***

### Treatment of overdose
To decrease absorption—

Administering activated charcoal (if the medication was ingested orally). The initial dose of charcoal may be followed by a cathartic, such as magnesium citrate, if the charcoal is not pre-mixed with sorbitol. Gastric lavage may also be performed.

Induction of emesis may also be helpful.

To enhance elimination—Hemodialysis does not remove significant quantities of ketorolac from the body.

Specific treatment—

For treatment of abdominal pain: Administering an antacid. See the product label or *Antacids (Oral-Local)* for specific dosing guidelines.

For treatment of gastrointestinal ulceration or bleeding: Discontinuing ketorolac therapy immediately. Depending on the site and severity of the ulcer, administering antacids, histamine H$_2$-receptor antagonists (cimetidine, famotidine, nizatidine, ranitidine), misoprostol, omeprazole, and/or sucralfate. See the package inserts or *Antacids (Oral-Local)*, *Histamine H$_2$-receptor Antagonists (Systemic)*, *Misoprostol (Systemic)*, *Omeprazole (Systemic)*, or *Sucralfate (Oral-Local)* for specific dosing guidelines for these products.

Supportive care—Supportive measures, such as establishing intravenous lines, hydration, administration of plasma volume expanders, and support of ventilatory function, should be instituted as needed. Patients in whom intentional overdose is confirmed or suspected should be referred for psychiatric consultation.

## Patient Consultation
As an aid to patient consultation, refer to *Advice for the Patient, Ketorolac (Systemic)*.

In providing consultation, consider emphasizing the following selected information (» = major clinical significance):

### Before using this medication
» Conditions affecting use, especially:

Sensitivity to ketorolac, aspirin, or any other nonsteroidal anti-inflammatory drug (NSAID)

Pregnancy—Crosses the placenta; use during second half of pregnancy may cause adverse effects on fetal or neonatal blood flow

Breast-feeding—Not recommended because of potential adverse effects in the infant; ketorolac is distributed into breast milk

Use in the elderly—Higher risk of gastrointestinal and/or renal toxicity, possibly because of reduced clearance in addition to increased sensitivity

Other medications, especially anticoagulants, aspirin or other salicylates, other NSAIDs, those cephalosporins that may adversely affect blood clotting, lithium, methotrexate, plicamycin, probenecid, and valproic acid

Other medical problems, especially bleeding (active, history of, or predisposition to), peptic ulcer or other ulcerative or inflammatory gastrointestinal tract disease (active or history of), and renal function impairment

### Proper use of this medication
Proper administration:

*For oral dosage form*

Taking with food (a meal or snack) to reduce gastrointestinal irritation, or with an antacid

Taking with a full glass of water, then remaining in an upright position for at least 15 to 30 minutes, to reduce risk of esophageal irritation

*For injection*

Proper injection technique (if self-medicating at home)

» Not using more medication than prescribed or using for longer than 5 days

Not saving unused medication for the future, and not sharing it with others

» Proper dosing

Missed dose (scheduled dosing): Using as soon as possible; not using if almost time for next dose; not doubling doses

» Proper storage

### Precautions while using this medication
» Not using acetaminophen concurrently for more than a few days, and not using aspirin, other salicylates, or other NSAIDs concurrently, unless combination therapy prescribed and monitored by physician or dentist

» Caution if dizziness or drowsiness occurs; not driving, using machines, or doing anything else that requires alertness

### Side/adverse effects
Signs of potential side effects, especially edema; hypertension; purpura; skin rash or itching; stomatitis; anaphylaxis or anaphylactoid reaction; aseptic meningitis; asthma, bronchospasm, or dyspnea; anemia; aseptic meningitis; bloody stools; blurred vision or other vision change; cholestatic jaundice; convulsions; edema of tongue; exfoliative dermatitis; fainting; fever; flank pain; gastrointestinal ulceration or bleeding; hallucinations; hearing loss; hemolytic uremic syndrome; hepatitis; hives; hyperactivity; hypotension; increase in frequency or volume of urination; laryngeal edema; leukopenia; mental depression; nephritis; nosebleeds; oliguria; pancreatitis, acute; psychosis; pulmonary edema; rectal bleeding; renal failure; rhinitis; Stevens-Johnson syndrome; thrombocytopenia; tinnitus; or toxic epidermal necrolysis

## General Dosing Information
Ketorolac may be administered on a scheduled or on an as-needed basis, depending on the type and severity of pain.

Ketorolac may be administered intramuscularly, intravenously, or orally. An intravenous dose should be given over at least 15 seconds. An intramuscular injection should be given slowly, deep into the muscle. Ketorolac injection contains alcohol and should not be administered intrathecally or epidurally.

**Because of the risk of anaphylaxis or other severe allergic reactions, equipment and medications to treat these complications should be available for immediate use when the first dose of ketorolac is administered.**

Hypovolemia increases the risk of adverse renal effects and should be corrected before ketorolac therapy is instituted.

Ketorolac therapy should be initiated with parenteral administration, after which additional doses may be given parenterally or orally. However, **the duration of treatment by any route or combination of routes is not to exceed 5 days.** The patient should be transferred to another analgesic as quickly as possible.

Concurrent use of ketorolac with an opioid analgesic provides additive analgesia and may permit lower doses of both medications to be utilized. Breakthrough pain that occurs during ketorolac treatment may be treated with an opioid analgesic (unless contraindicated); **increasing the dose or the frequency of administration of ketorolac is not recommended.**

### For treatment of adverse effects
For abdominal pain—Administering an antacid. See the product label or *Antacids (Oral-Local)* for specific dosing guidelines for these products.

For gastrointestinal ulceration or bleeding—Discontinuing ketorolac therapy immediately. Depending on the site and severity of the ulcer, administering antacids, histamine H$_2$-receptor antagonists (cimetidine, famotidine, nizatidine, ranitidine), misoprostol, omeprazole, and/or sucralfate. See the package inserts or *Antacids (Oral-Local)*, *Histamine H$_2$-receptor Antagonists (Systemic)*, *Misoprostol (Systemic)*, *Omeprazole (Systemic)*, or *Sucralfate (Oral-Local)* for specific dosing guidelines for these products.

For severe hypersensitivity reactions (e.g., anaphylaxis or anaphylactoid reaction or laryngeal edema)—Depending on the nature and severity of the symptoms, administering epinephrine and corticosteroids, and, in some cases, antihistamines. See the package inserts or *Antihistamines (Systemic), Corticosteroids—Glucocorticoid Effects (Systemic),* or *Sympathomimetic Agents—Cardiovascular Use (Parenteral)* for specific dosing guidelines for individual agents.

For renal failure—Dialysis may be needed. However, dialysis is not likely to assist in removing ketorolac from the body after an overdose; decreased clearance and prolongation of half-life have been reported in patients receiving dialysis.

## Oral Dosage Forms

### KETOROLAC TROMETHAMINE TABLETS USP

**Usual adult dose**
Analgesic:—
   Oral, as a continuation of initial parenteral therapy
Patients 16 to 64 years of age who weigh at least 50 kg and have normal renal function—
   20 mg initially, followed by 10 mg up to four times a day at four- to six-hour intervals as needed.
Patients weighing less than 50 kg; and/or
Patients with renal function impairment—
   10 mg up to four times a day, at four- to six-hour intervals as needed.
Note: The recommended doses and frequency of administration should not be increased if pain relief is inadequate or breakthrough pain occurs between doses. Supplemental doses of opioid analgesic may be used, if not contraindicated, to provide additional analgesia.

**Usual adult prescribing limits**
Oral, 40 mg per day. The duration of treatment (parenteral followed by oral administration) is not to exceed five days.

**Usual pediatric dose**
Patients up to 16 years of age— Safety and efficacy have not been established.

**Usual geriatric dose**
Analgesic—
   Oral, as a continuation of initial parenteral therapy: 10 mg up to four times a day at four- to six-hour intervals as needed.
   Note: The recommended doses and frequency of administration should not be increased if pain relief is inadequate or breakthrough pain occurs between doses. Supplemental doses of opioid analgesic may be used, if not contraindicated, to provide additional analgesia.

**Usual geriatric prescribing limits**
Oral, 40 mg per day. The duration of treatment (parenteral followed by oral administration) is not to exceed five days.

**Strength(s) usually available**
U.S.—
   10 mg (Rx) [*Toradol* (lactose)].
Canada—
   10 mg (Rx) [*Toradol* (lactose)].

**Packaging and storage**
Store between 15 and 30 °C (59 and 86 °F), unless otherwise specified by manufacturer. Protect from light and excessive humidity.

## Parenteral Dosage Forms

### KETOROLAC TROMETHAMINE INJECTION USP

**Usual adult dose**
Analgesic—
Patients 16 to 64 years of age who weigh at least 50 kg and have normal renal function—
   Intramuscular, a single dose of 60 mg followed, if necessary, by oral ketorolac (See *Ketorolac Tromethamine Tablets USP*) or by other analgesic therapy, or
   Intramuscular, 30 mg every six hours, up to a maximum of twenty doses given over five days, or
   Intravenous, 30 mg as a single dose or as multiple doses administered every six hours, up to a maximum of twenty doses given over five days.
Patients weighing less than 50 kg; and/or
Patients with renal function impairment—
   Intramuscular, a single dose of 30 mg followed, if necessary, by oral ketorolac (See *Ketorolac Tromethamine Tablets USP*) or by other analgesic therapy, or
   Intramuscular, 15 mg every six hours, up to a maximum of twenty doses given over five days, or
   Intravenous, 15 mg as a single dose or as multiple doses administered every six hours, up to a maximum of twenty doses given over five days.
Note: The recommended doses and frequency of administration should not be increased if pain relief is inadequate or breakthrough pain occurs between doses. Supplemental doses of opioid analgesic may be used, if not contraindicated, to provide additional analgesia.

**Usual adult prescribing limits**
Patients 16 to 64 years of age who weigh at least 50 kg and have normal renal function—
   Intramuscular or intravenous, 120 mg per day. The duration of therapy is not to exceed five days.
Patients weighing less than 50 kg; and/or
Patients with renal function impairment—
   Intramuscular or intravenous, 60 mg per day. The duration of therapy is not to exceed five days.

**Usual pediatric dose**
Patients up to 16 years of age—Safety and efficacy have not been established.

**Usual geriatric dose**
Analgesic—
   Intramuscular, a single dose of 30 mg, followed, if necessary, by oral ketorolac (See *Ketorolac Tromethamine Tablets USP*) or by other analgesic therapy, or
   Intramuscular, 15 mg every six hours, up to a maximum of twenty doses administered over five days, or
   Intravenous, 15 mg as a single dose or as multiple doses administered every six hours, up to a maximum of twenty doses administered over five days.
Note: The recommended doses and frequency of administration should not be increased if pain relief is inadequate or breakthrough pain occurs between doses. Supplemental doses of opioid analgesic may be used, if not contraindicated, to provide additional analgesia.

**Usual geriatric prescribing limits**
Intramuscular or intravenous, 60 mg per day. The duration of therapy is not to exceed five days.

**Strength(s) usually available**
U.S.—
   1.5% (15 mg per mL) (Rx) [*Toradol* (alcohol 10%)].
   3% (30 mg per mL; 60 mg per 2 mL) (Rx) [*Toradol* (alcohol 10%)].
Canada—
   1% (10 mg per mL) (Rx) [*Toradol* (alcohol 10%)].
   1.5% (15 mg per mL) (Rx) [*Toradol* (alcohol 10%)].
   3% (30 mg per mL; 60 mg per 2 mL) (Rx) [*Toradol* (alcohol 10%)].
Note: The product containing 60 mg in 2 mL is not recommended for intravenous administration.

**Packaging and storage**
Store between 15 and 30 °C (59 and 86 °F), unless otherwise specified by manufacturer. Protect from light.

## Selected Bibliography

O'Hara DA, Fragen RJ, Kinzer M, Pemberton D. Ketorolac tromethamine as compared with morphine sulfate for treatment of postoperative pain. Clin Pharmacol Ther 1987 May; 41: 556-61.

Revised: 07/24/95

# KRYPTON Kr 81m  Systemic

VA CLASSIFICATION (Primary): DX201
Commonly used brand name(s): *Krypton Kr 81m Gas Generator*.
Note: For a listing of dosage forms and brand names by country availability, see *Dosage Forms* section(s).

## Category
Diagnostic aid, radioactive (pulmonary disease; pulmonary emboli).

## Indications
Note: Bracketed information in the *Indications* section refers to uses that are not included in U.S. product labeling.

**Accepted**
Pulmonary function studies—Krypton Kr 81m for inhalation is indicated in pulmonary ventilation studies to assess and evaluate regional pulmonary function in lung diseases.

[Embolism, pulmonary (diagnosis)]—Krypton Kr 81m is used to complement lung perfusion studies to detect pulmonary emboli.

## Physical Properties
### Nuclear Data

| Radionuclide (half-life) | Mode of decay | Principal photon emissions (keV) | Mean number of emissions/ disintegration |
|---|---|---|---|
| Kr 81m (13.1 seconds) | Isomeric transition | Gamma (191) | 0.66 |
| Kr 81* (2.1 × 10⁵ years) | | | |

*Decay product.

## Pharmacology/Pharmacokinetics
### Mechanism of action/Effect
Krypton Kr 81m diffuses easily, passing through cell membranes and exchanging freely between blood and tissue. It is distributed in the lungs in a manner similar to air, thus representing the regions of the lung that are aerated. The gamma photons of krypton Kr 81m can then be employed to obtain counts per minute per lung or region of the lung, or to display their distribution as a scan.

### Distribution
When inhaled, krypton Kr 81m enters the alveolar wall and passes to the pulmonary venous circulation via capillaries. Most of it that enters the circulation from a single breath returns to the lungs and is exhaled after a single pass through the peripheral circulation.

### Radiation dosimetry

| | Estimated absorbed radiation dose* | |
|---|---|---|
| Organ | mGy/MBq | mrad/mCi |
| Lungs | 0.00021 | 0.78 |
| Breast | 0.0000046 | 0.017 |
| Pancreas | 0.0000035 | 0.013 |
| Adrenals | 0.0000034 | 0.013 |
| Liver | 0.0000034 | 0.013 |
| Spleen | 0.0000031 | 0.011 |
| Stomach wall | 0.0000025 | 0.0093 |
| Red marrow | 0.0000021 | 0.0078 |
| Bone surfaces | 0.0000017 | 0.0063 |
| Kidneys | 0.0000012 | 0.0044 |
| Large intestine (upper) | 0.00000032 | 0.0012 |
| Small intestine | 0.00000027 | 0.0010 |
| Ovaries | 0.00000017 | 0.00063 |
| Large intestine (lower) | 0.00000014 | 0.00052 |
| Uterus | 0.00000013 | 0.00048 |
| Bladder wall | 0.000000068 | 0.00025 |
| Testes | 0.000000017 | 0.000063 |
| Other tissue | 0.0000018 | 0.0067 |

Effective dose: 0.000027 mSv/MBq (0.0001 rem/mCi)

*For adults; by continuous inhalation. Data based on the International Commission on Radiological Protection (ICRP) Publication 53—Radiation dose to patients from radiopharmaceuticals.

### Elimination
Eliminated via lungs.

## Precautions to Consider
### Carcinogenicity/Mutagenicity
Long-term animal studies to evaluate carcinogenic or mutagenic potential of krypton Kr 81m have not been performed.

### Pregnancy/Reproduction
Pregnancy—Studies have not been done in humans. The possibility of pregnancy should be assessed in women of child-bearing potential. Clinical situations exist where the benefit to the patient and fetus from information derived from radiopharmaceutical use outweighs the risks of fetal exposure to radiation. In these situations, the physician should use discretion and reduce the radiopharmaceutical dose to the lowest possible amount.

Studies have not been done in animals.

FDA Pregnancy Category C.

### Breast-feeding
It is not known whether krypton Kr 81m is distributed into breast milk. However, risk to the infant from radiation exposure is considered negligible because of the short half-life of krypton Kr 81m. Also, most of the amount that passes into the venous circulation returns to the lungs to be exhaled.

### Pediatrics
Because of the potential risk of radiation exposure, risk-benefit must be considered. Although krypton Kr 81m is used in children, there have been no specific studies evaluating its safety and efficacy in children. When this radiopharmaceutical is used in children, the diagnostic benefit should be judged to outweigh the potential risk of radiation.

### Geriatrics
Appropriate studies on the relationship of age to the effects of krypton Kr 81m have not been performed in the geriatric population. However, geriatrics-specific problems that would limit the usefulness of this radiopharmaceutical in the elderly are not expected.

## Side/Adverse Effects
At the present time, there are no known side/adverse effects associated with diagnostic doses of krypton Kr 81m.

## Patient Consultation
As an aid to patient consultation, refer to *Advice for the Patient, Radiopharmaceuticals (Diagnostic)*.

In providing consultation, consider emphasizing the following selected information (» = major clinical significance):

### Description of use
Action in the body: Accumulation of radioactivity in lungs during continuous breathing

Radioactivity retained in lungs during continuous breathing allows visualization

Small amounts of radioactivity used in diagnosis; radiation exposure is low and considered safe

### Before having this test
» Conditions affecting use, especially:
  Pregnancy—Risk to fetus from radiation exposure as opposed to benefit derived from use should be considered
  Breast-feeding—Not known if krypton Kr 81m is distributed into breast milk; however, based on the short half-life of krypton Kr 81m, discontinuation of nursing is not necessary
  Use in children—Risk from radiation exposure as opposed to benefit derived from use should be considered

### Preparation for this test
Special preparatory instructions may be given; patient should inquire in advance

### Precautions after having this test
No special precautions when used for diagnosis

## General Dosing Information
Radiopharmaceuticals are to be administered only by or under the supervision of physicians who have had extensive training in the safe use and handling of radioactive materials and who are authorized by the Nuclear Regulatory Commission (NRC) or the appropriate Federal or Agreement State agency, if required or, outside the U.S., the appropriate authority.

The manufacturer's package insert or other appropriate literature should be consulted for optimal times when imaging should be performed.

### Safety considerations for handling this radiopharmaceutical
Improper handling of this radiopharmaceutical may cause radioactive contamination. Guidelines for handling radioactive material have been prepared by scientific, professional, state, federal, and international bodies and are available to the specially qualified and authorized users who have access to radiopharmaceuticals.

## Inhalation Dosage Forms

### KRYPTON Kr 81m USP

#### Usual adult and adolescent administered activity
Pulmonary function studies—
  Inhalation (continuous), 37 to 370 megabecquerels (1 to 10 millicuries) of krypton Kr 81m, not to exceed 3.7 gigabecquerel-minutes (100 millicurie-minutes).

#### Usual pediatric administered activity
Dosage must be individualized by physician.

#### Usual geriatric administered activity
See *Usual adult and adolescent administered activity*.

## Krypton Kr 81m (Systemic)

**Strength(s) usually available**

U.S.—
  At calibration time
    As rubidium Rb 81, with an activity of 74 to 370 megabecquerels (2 to 10 millicuries) (Rx) [*Krypton Kr 81m Gas Generator*].

Canada—
  At calibration time
    As rubidium Rb 81, with an activity of 74 to 370 megabecquerels (2 to 10 millicuries) (Rx) [*Krypton Kr 81m Gas Generator*].

  Note: Thirty-seven megabecquerels (one millicurie) of rubidium Rb 81 yields 35.5 megabecquerels (0.96 millicurie) of krypton Kr 81m at equilibrium.

**Packaging and storage**
Store below 40 °C (104 °F), preferably between 15 and 30 °C (59 and 86 °F), unless otherwise specified by manufacturer.

**Stability**
Gas generator expires 12 hours after date and time of calibration.

**Note**
Caution—Radioactive material.

Revised: 04/30/96

**LABETALOL**—See *Beta-adrenergic Blocking Agents (Systemic)*

**LACTULOSE**—See *Laxatives (Local)*

# LAMIVUDINE Systemic

VA CLASSIFICATION (Primary): AM804
Commonly used brand name(s): *3TC; Epivir*.
Note: For a listing of dosage forms and brand names by country availability, see *Dosage Forms* section(s).

## Category
Antiviral (systemic).

## Indications
Note: Bracketed information in the *Indications* section refers to uses that are not included in U.S. product labeling.

**General considerations**
Lamivudine is the negative enantiomer of 2'-deoxy-3'-thiacytidine. Both the positive and negative enantiomers have *in vitro* activity against human immunodeficiency virus (HIV), but the negative enantiomer has greater activity and less toxicity. *In vitro* inhibition of DNA polymerase gamma, which is thought to be associated with peripheral neuropathy, is minimal.

Lamivudine has *in vitro* activity against HIV-1 and HIV-2, including zidovudine-resistant isolates, as well as hepatitis B virus. Lamivudine is indicated in combination with zidovudine for the treatment of HIV infection. Lamivudine and zidovudine have been found to act synergistically *in vitro*. This is thought to produce better efficacy than either medication alone. Resistance to lamivudine is associated with a mutation at codon 184 in HIV-1 reverse transcriptase; this can suppress the expression of pre-existing resistance to zidovudine in a number of different HIV isolates. Strains of HIV-1 resistant to both lamivudine and zidovudine have been isolated.

**Accepted**
Human immunodeficiency virus (HIV) infection (treatment) or
Immunodeficiency syndrome, acquired (AIDS) (treatment)—Lamivudine is indicated, in combination with zidovudine, in the treatment of HIV infection or AIDS when therapy is warranted based on clinical and/or immunological evidence of disease progression.

[Human immunodeficiency virus (HIV) infection, occupational exposure (prophylaxis)][1]—Lamivudine may be used prophylactically in health care workers at risk of acquiring HIV infection after occupational exposure to the virus. It is being used in combination with zidovudine and, in some cases, a protease inhibitor.

**Acceptance not established**
Lamivudine is being studied for the treatment of *chronic hepatitis B infection*. However, reactivation of hepatitis B virus infection has been reported after lamivudine therapy was discontinued.

[1]Not included in Canadian product labeling.

## Pharmacology/Pharmacokinetics

**Physicochemical characteristics**
Molecular weight—229.26.

**Mechanism of action/Effect**
Lamivudine is metabolized intracellularly to its active 5'-triphosphate metabolite, lamivudine triphosphate (L-TP), which inhibits human immunodeficiency virus (HIV) reverse transcription via viral DNA chain termination.

**Other actions/effects**
Lamivudine also potently inhibits the replication of hepatitis B virus by interfering with reverse transcriptase activity.

**Absorption**
Rapidly absorbed; bioavailability in adults and adolescents is 80 to 88% and in children is approximately 66 to 68%. Food delays the peak serum concentration and the time to peak serum concentration; however, there is no significant difference in bioavailability. Therefore, lamivudine may be administered with or without food.

**Distribution**
Lamivudine is widely distributed. Lamivudine crosses the blood-brain barrier and is distributed into the cerebrospinal fluid (CSF) to a limited extent. In children, CSF concentrations ranged from 10 to 17% of the corresponding, non-steady-state serum concentration. Lamivudine crosses the placenta in rats, rabbits, and humans.
Apparent Vol $_D$ =Approximately 1.3 liters per kg.

**Protein binding**
Low (36%).

**Biotransformation**
Trans-sulfoxide is the only known metabolite of lamivudine; serum concentrations of this metabolite have not been determined.

**Half-life**
Intracellular lamivudine triphosphate—
  11 to 15 hours.
Lamivudine (serum)—
  Adults: 2 to 11 hours.
  Children (4 months to 14 years of age): 1.7 to 2 hours.
Renal function impairment—
  Creatinine clearance, 10 to 40 mL per min (mL/min) (0.17 to 0.67 mL per sec [mL/sec])—Approximately 13.6 hours.
  Creatinine clearance, less than 10 mL/min (0.17 mL/sec)—Approximately 19.4 hours.

**Time to peak concentration**
With food:
  Approximately 3.2 hours.
Fasting:
  Approximately 1 hour.

**Peak serum concentration**
Adults and adolescents—
  2 mg per kg of body weight (mg/kg): 1.5 micrograms per mL (mcg/mL) (6.5 micromoles per liter).
Children—
  8 mg/kg: 1.1 mcg/mL (4.8 micromoles per liter).

**Elimination**
Renal; the majority of lamivudine is eliminated unchanged in the urine (68 to 71%); approximately 5.2% of the trans-sulfoxide metabolite is excreted in the urine within 12 hours. The renal clearance of lamivudine is greater than the glomerular filtration rate, implying active secretion into the renal tubules.
In dialysis—
  It is not known whether lamivudine is removed by peritoneal dialysis or hemodialysis.

## Precautions to Consider

**Carcinogenicity**
Long-term carcinogenicity studies in animals have not been completed.

**Mutagenicity**
Lamivudine was not active in a microbial mutagenicity screen or in an *in vitro* cell transformation assay. It showed weak *in vitro* mutagenic activity in a cytogenic assay using cultured human lymphocytes and in the mouse lymphoma assay. However, lamivudine showed no evidence of *in vivo* genotoxic activity in rats at oral doses of up to 2000 mg per kg of body weight (mg/kg), which is approximately 65 times the recommended human dose based on body surface area.

**Pregnancy/Reproduction**
Fertility—Rats given doses of lamivudine up to 130 times the usual adult dose based on body surface area revealed no evidence of impaired fertility.

Pregnancy—Adequate and well-controlled studies have not been done in humans. However, lamivudine has been found to cross the placenta in humans.

Lamivudine crosses the placenta in rats and rabbits. Studies have been done in rats and rabbits administered doses up to approximately 130 and 60 times the usual adult dose, respectively. Some evidence of embryolethality in rabbits, but not in rats, at doses similar to the usual adult dose or higher has been seen.
FDA Pregnancy Category C.

**Breast-feeding**
It is not known whether lamivudine is distributed into human breast milk. Lamivudine is distributed into the milk of lactating rats in concentrations that are slightly higher than those in the plasma.

## Pediatrics

In one study, pancreatitis was reported in 14 of 97 (14%) and paresthesias and peripheral neuropathies were seen in 13 of 97 (13%) of pediatric patients receiving lamivudine monotherapy. However, the patients who developed these complications had advanced HIV disease and a prior history of pancreatitis, most commonly associated with the use of didanosine. The combination of lamivudine and zidovudine should be used with caution in children with advanced HIV disease and/or a history of pancreatitis. In addition, an increase in serum transaminases (greater than 10 times the upper limits of normal) was observed in 3 of 89 (3%) of pediatric patients receiving lamivudine monotherapy.

The pharmacokinetics of lamivudine have not been studied in combination with zidovudine in children. Pharmacokinetic properties of lamivudine monotherapy were assessed in 57 children (ages 4.8 months to 16 years). The absolute bioavailability was 66 to 68%, which is less than the 86% seen in adults and adolescents. The mechanism for this diminished bioavailability in infants and children is unknown. The area under the serum concentration–time curve (AUC) was comparable for pediatric patients receiving a dose of 8 mg/kg per day and adults receiving a dose of 4 mg/kg per day.

## Geriatrics

No information is available on the relationship of age to the effects of lamivudine in geriatric patients. However, elderly patients are more likely to have age-related renal function impairment, which may require a dosage adjustment in patients receiving lamivudine.

Lamivudine pharmacokinetics have not been studied in patients over 65 years of age.

## Drug interactions and/or related problems

The following drug interactions and/or related problems have been selected on the basis of their potential clinical significance (possible mechanism in parentheses where appropriate)—not necessarily inclusive (» = major clinical significance):

Note: Combinations containing any of the following medications, depending on the amount present, may also interact with this medication.

Drugs associated with pancreatitis, such as alcohol, didanosine, intravenous pentamidine, sulfonamides, or zalcitabine
(pancreatitis was seen in 14% (14 of 97) of pediatric patients receiving lamivudine monotherapy; this population had advanced HIV disease and a history of pancreatitis; although no interactions have been documented to date, concurrent use of lamivudine with medications associated with the development of pancreatitis should be avoided or, if concurrent use is necessary, used with caution)

Drugs associated with peripheral neuropathy, such as dapsone, didanosine, isoniazid, stavudine, or zalcitabine
(paresthesias and peripheral neuropathy were seen in 13% (13 of 97) of pediatric patients with advanced HIV disease receiving lamivudine monotherapy; although no interactions have been documented to date, other medications associated with the development of neuropathy should be avoided or, if concurrent use is necessary, used with caution)

Indinavir
(concurrent administration of lamivudine 150 mg twice a day, indinavir 800 mg every eight hours, and zidovudine 200 mg every eight hours resulted in a 6% decrease in the AUC of lamivudine, no change in AUC of indinavir, and a 36% increase in the AUC of zidovudine; no adjustment in dose is necessary)

Sulfamethoxazole and trimethoprim combination
(in one small study, concurrent administration of sulfamethoxazole and trimethoprim combination resulted in a 44% increase in lamivudine AUC and a 30% decrease in lamivudine renal clearance; the pharmacokinetic properties of sulfamethoxazole and trimethoprim were not altered by concurrent administration of lamivudine; no adjustment in dose is necessary unless the patient has renal function impairment)

Zidovudine
(in one small study, concurrent administration of lamivudine resulted in a 39% increase in the peak plasma concentration of zidovudine; although statistically significant, this increase is not thought to be significant to patient safety; no significant changes were observed in the AUC or total clearance of lamivudine or zidovudine)

## Laboratory value alterations

The following have been selected on the basis of their potential clinical significance (possible effect in parentheses where appropriate)—not necessarily inclusive (» = major clinical significance):

With physiology/laboratory test values
Alanine aminotransferase (ALT [SGPT]) and
Aspartate aminotransferase (AST [SGOT])
(an increase in serum transaminases [greater than 10 times the upper limits of normal] was observed in 3 of 89 (3%) of pediatric patients receiving lamivudine monotherapy)

Amylase, serum
(values may be increased)

Hemoglobin concentration and
Neutrophil count
(values may be decreased)

## Medical considerations/Contraindications

The medical considerations/contraindications included have been selected on the basis of their potential clinical significance (reasons given in parentheses where appropriate)—not necessarily inclusive (» = major clinical significance).

*Risk-benefit should be considered when the following medical problems exist:*

Hypersensitivity to lamivudine

Pancreatitis, or history of
(pancreatitis occurred in 14% (14 of 97) of pediatric patients receiving lamivudine monotherapy; these patients had advanced HIV disease and a history of pancreatitis; pancreatitis has been reported rarely in adults; lamivudine should be used with extreme caution in patients who have pancreatitis or a history of pancreatitis)

Peripheral neuropathy, or history of
(peripheral neuropathy occurred in approximately 13% (13 of 97) of pediatric patients receiving lamivudine monotherapy; these patients had advanced HIV disease; it has also been reported rarely in adults; lamivudine should be used with caution in patients who have peripheral neuropathy or a history of peripheral neuropathy)

» Renal function impairment
(decreased renal function has been found to result in an increase in the peak plasma concentration and elimination half-life of lamivudine; dosage modification is recommended in patients with a creatinine clearance of < 50 mL/min [0.83 mL/sec])

## Patient monitoring

The following may be especially important in patient monitoring (other tests may be warranted in some patients, depending on condition; » = major clinical significance):

Alanine aminotransferase (ALT [SGPT]) and
Aspartate aminotransferase (AST [SGOT])
(an increase in serum transaminases [greater than 10 times the upper limits of normal] was observed in 3 of 89 (3%) of pediatric patients receiving lamivudine monotherapy)

» Amylase, serum, and
» Lipase, serum, and
Triglycerides, serum
(lamivudine administration has been associated with pancreatitis in approximately 14% of pediatric patients; patients should be monitored for laboratory changes consistent with pancreatitis, such as elevated amylase, lipase, and triglyceride concentrations)

» Blood urea nitrogen (BUN) and
» Creatinine, serum
(blood urea nitrogen and serum creatinine concentrations should be monitored in patients with renal function impairment; an adjustment in dosage or dosage interval may be required)

## Side/Adverse Effects

Note: Lamivudine is given in combination with zidovudine, and, in some cases, it may also be given with other antiretroviral agents. Some side effects, such as pancreatitis, peripheral neuropathy, and hematologic abnormalities, may be seen with other antiretroviral agents, such as zidovudine, and/or severe human immunodeficiency virus (HIV) disease; therefore, differentiation between the side effects of lamivudine and other medications or the complications of HIV disease may be difficult.

In one study, 14 of 97 pediatric patients (14%) being treated with lamivudine monotherapy developed pancreatitis; in a second pediatric study, 7 of 47 patients (15%) receiving lamivudine in combination therapy with other antiretroviral agents developed pancreatitis. Pancreatitis was most commonly seen in patients who had advanced HIV disease, as well as a prior history of pancreatitis, most commonly associated with the use of didanosine. The combination of lamivudine and zidovudine therapy should be used with caution in pediatric patients with a history of pancreatitis or other risk factors for pancreatitis. Pancreatitis was seen in only 3 of 656 adult patients (< 0.5%) who received lamivudine. Lamivudine should be discontinued immediately if any signs or symptoms of pancreatitis occur. In addition, an increase in serum transaminases (greater than 10 times the upper limits of normal) was observed in 3 of 89 (3%) of pediatric patients receiving lamivudine monotherapy.

Paresthesias and peripheral neuropathy were reported in 13% of pediatric patients and have been reported rarely in adults.

The following side/adverse effects have been selected on the basis of their potential clinical significance (possible signs and symptoms in parentheses where appropriate)—not necessarily inclusive:

**Those indicating need for medical attention**
Incidence more frequent
> *Pancreatitis* (nausea; vomiting; severe abdominal or stomach pain)—more frequent in children; *paresthesias and peripheral neuropathy* (tingling, burning, numbness, or pain in the hands, arms, feet, or legs)—more frequent in children

Incidence rare
> *Anemia* (unusual tiredness or weakness); *neutropenia* (fever, chills, or sore throat); *skin rash*

**Those indicating need for medical attention only if they continue or are bothersome**
Incidence less frequent
> *Cough; dizziness; fatigue* (unusual tiredness or weakness); *gastrointestinal distress* (abdominal or stomach pain; diarrhea; nausea; vomiting); *headache; insomnia* (trouble in sleeping)

Incidence rare
> *Hair loss*

## Overdose

There is no known antidote for lamivudine. There is one reported case in which an adult ingested 6 grams of lamivudine; no clinical signs and symptoms were noted and hematologic tests remained normal. It is not known whether lamivudine is removed by peritoneal dialysis or hemodialysis.

For more information on the management of overdose or unintentional ingestion, **contact a Poison Control Center** (see *Poison Control Center Listing*).

## Patient Consultation

As an aid to patient consultation, refer to *Advice for the Patient, Lamivudine (Systemic)*.

In providing consultation, consider emphasizing the following selected information (» = major clinical significance):

**Before using this medication**
» Conditions affecting use, especially:
  Hypersensitivity to lamivudine
  Pregnancy—Lamivudine has caused embryolethality in rabbits at doses similar to the usual adult dose or higher
  Use in children—Lamivudine monotherapy has resulted in the development of pancreatitis in 14% (14 of 97) of children with advanced HIV disease and a prior history of pancreatitis, and paresthesias and peripheral neuropathies in 13% (13 of 97) of pediatric patients with advanced HIV disease; in addition, an increase in serum transaminases (greater than 10 times the upper limits of normal) was observed in 3 of 89 (3%) of pediatric patients receiving lamivudine monotherapy; the absolute bioavailability is 66 to 68% in children, less than the 86% seen in adults and adolescents
  Other medical problems, especially renal function impairment

**Proper use of this medication**
» Importance of not taking more medication than prescribed; importance of not discontinuing lamivudine or zidovudine without checking with physician
» Compliance with full course of therapy
» Importance of not missing doses and of taking at evenly spaced times
  Proper administration technique for oral liquids
  Not sharing medication with others
» Proper dosing
  Missed dose: Taking as soon as possible; not taking if almost time for next dose; not doubling doses
» Proper storage

**Precautions while using this medication**
» Regular visits to physician for blood tests
» Importance of not taking other medications concurrently without checking with physician

**Side/adverse effects**
Signs of potential side effects, especially pancreatitis, paresthesias, peripheral neuropathy, anemia, neutropenia, or skin rash

## General Dosing Information

Lamivudine may be taken on a full or empty stomach.

Patients 16 years of age and older with renal function impairment require a reduction in dose as follows:

| Creatinine Clearance (mL/min)/(mL/sec) | Dose |
| --- | --- |
| ≥50/0.83 | 150 mg twice a day |
| 30–49/0.50–0.82 | 150 mg once a day |
| 15–29/0.25–0.48 | 150 mg first dose, then 100 mg once a day |
| 5–14/0.08–0.23 | 150 mg first dose, then 50 mg once a day |
| <5/<0.08 | 50 mg first dose, then 25 mg once a day |

## Oral Dosage Forms

Note: Bracketed uses in the *Dosage Forms* section refer to categories of use and/or indications that are not included in U.S. product labeling.

### LAMIVUDINE ORAL SOLUTION

**Usual adult and adolescent dose**
Human immunodeficiency virus (HIV) infection (treatment) or
Immunodeficiency syndrome, acquired (AIDS) (treatment)—
  Adults and adolescents weighing 50 kg (110 pounds) or more: Oral, 150 mg of lamivudine twice a day in combination with zidovudine 200 mg three times a day.
  Adults weighing less than 50 kg (110 pounds): Oral, 2 mg per kg of body weight of lamivudine twice a day in combination with zidovudine 200 mg three times a day.
[Human immunodeficiency virus (HIV) infection, occupational exposure (prophylaxis)][1]—
  Oral, 150 mg of lamivudine twice a day, in combination with zidovudine 200 mg three times a day, for four weeks. In certain cases, a protease inhibitor may also be added to the regimen.

**Usual pediatric dose**
Children 3 months to 12 years of age—Oral, 4 mg per kg of body weight of lamivudine, up to a 150-mg dose, twice a day in combination with 180 mg per square meter of body surface of zidovudine every six hours.

**Strength(s) usually available**
U.S.—
  10 mg per mL (Rx) [*Epivir* (ethanol 6% v/v; methylparaben; propylparaben; sucrose)].
Canada—
  10 mg per mL (Rx) [*3TC* (ethanol 6% v/v; methylparaben; propylparaben; sucrose)].

**Packaging and storage**
Store between 2 and 25 °C (36 and 77 °F) in a tight container.

**Auxiliary labeling**
• Continue medicine for full time of treatment.

**Note**
When dispensing, include a calibrated liquid-measuring device.

### LAMIVUDINE TABLETS

**Usual adult and adolescent dose**
See *Lamivudine Oral Solution*.

**Usual pediatric dose**
See *Lamivudine Oral Solution*.

**Strength(s) usually available**
U.S.—
  150 mg (Rx) [*Epivir*].
Canada—
  150 mg (Rx) [*3TC*].

**Packaging and storage**
Store between 2 and 30 °C (36 and 86 °F) in a tight container.

**Auxiliary labeling**
• Continue medicine for full time of treatment.

---

[1] Not included in Canadian product labeling.

Developed: 08/08/96

# LAMIVUDINE AND ZIDOVUDINE  Systemic—INTRODUCTORY VERSION

VA CLASSIFICATION (Primary): AM809
Commonly used brand name(s): *Combivir*.
Note: For a listing of dosage forms and brand names by country availability, see *Dosage Forms* section(s).

## Category
Antiviral (systemic).

## Indications

### General considerations
Lamivudine and zidovudine are nucleoside inhibitors of reverse transcriptase in human immunodeficiency virus (HIV). Monotherapy with lamivudine or combination therapy with lamivudine and zidovudine has resulted in HIV isolates that were phenotypically and genotypically resistant to lamivudine within 12 weeks. In some patients harboring zidovudine-resistant virus at baseline, phenotypic sensitivity to zidovudine was restored by 12 weeks of therapy with lamivudine and zidovudine. Combination therapy with lamivudine and zidovudine delayed the emergence of mutations conferring resistance to zidovudine.

HIV strains resistant to both lamivudine and zidovudine have been isolated from patients after prolonged therapy with lamivudine and zidovudine. Dual resistance requires the presence of multiple mutations, the most essential of which appears to be at codon 333. The incidence of dual resistance and the duration of combination therapy required before dual resistance develops are unknown.

Cross-resistance among certain reverse transcriptase inhibitors has been recognized. However, cross-resistance between lamivudine and zidovudine has not been reported. In some patients treated with lamivudine alone or in combination with zidovudine, HIV isolates have emerged with a mutation at codon 184, which confers resistance to lamivudine. In the presence of this mutation, cross-resistance to didanosine and zalcitabine has been seen in some patients; the clinical significance of this is unknown. In some patients treated with zidovudine plus didanosine or zalcitabine, HIV isolates that are resistant to multiple drugs, including lamivudine, have emerged. Multiple drug resistance has been observed in 2 of 39 patients receiving zidovudine and didanosine combination therapy for 2 years.

### Accepted
Human immunodeficiency virus (HIV) infection (treatment)—Lamivudine and zidovudine combination is indicated in the treatment of HIV infection.

## Pharmacology/Pharmacokinetics

### Physicochemical characteristics
Molecular weight—Lamivudine: 229.3.
Zidovudine: 267.2.

### Mechanism of action/Effect
Lamivudine and zidovudine are synthetic nucleoside analogs of cytidine and thymidine, respectively. Intracellularly, lamivudine and zidovudine are phosphorylated to their respective active metabolites, lamivudine triphosphate and zidovudine triphosphate. HIV reverse transcriptase utilizes these nucleotide analogs when transcribing viral RNA to DNA. Incorporation of lamivudine triphosphate and zidovudine triphosphate into the growing chain of viral DNA results in termination of reverse transcription and thus inhibition of HIV reverse transcriptase.

Lamivudine triphosphate is a weak inhibitor of mammalian DNA polymerases alpha and beta, and of mitochondrial DNA polymerase gamma. Zidovudine triphosphate is a weak inhibitor of mammalian DNA polymerase alpha and mitochondrial DNA polymerase gamma; it also has been reported to be incorporated into the DNA of cells in culture.

### Absorption
Lamivudine—Rapidly absorbed; oral bioavailability is 86 ± 16% (mean ± SD).
Zidovudine—Rapidly absorbed; oral bioavailability is 64 ± 10% (mean ± SD).

### Distribution
Lamivudine—$Vol_D$ is approximately 1.3 ± 0.4 L per kg.
Zidovudine—$Vol_D$ is approximately 1.6 ± 0.6 L per kg.

### Protein binding
Lamivudine—Low to moderate (< 36%).
Zidovudine—Low to moderate (< 38%).

### Biotransformation
Lamivudine—In humans, the only known metabolite is the trans-sulfoxide metabolite, which accounts for approximately 5% of an oral dose after 12 hours.
Zidovudine—The major metabolites are 3'-azido-3'-deoxy-5'-*O*-beta-D-glucopyranuronosylthymidine (GZDV) and 3'-amino-3'-deoxythymidine (AMT).

### Half-life
Elimination—
Lamivudine: 5 to 7 hours.
Zidovudine: 0.5 to 3 hours.

### Elimination
Lamivudine—Renal; approximately 70% of an intravenous dose is recovered unchanged in the urine.
Zidovudine—Primarily hepatic; following oral administration, unchanged zidovudine and GZDV account for 14% and 74% of the dose, respectively, recovered in the urine.

## Precautions to Consider

### Carcinogenicity/Tumorigenicity
Lamivudine:
Long-term carcinogenicity studies in mice and rats showed no evidence of carcinogenic potential at exposures of up to 10 and 58 times, respectively, those observed in humans at the recommended therapeutic dose.

Zidovudine:
In mice given 120 mg per kg of body weight (mg/kg) per day for 90 days then 40 mg/kg per day thereafter, seven vaginal neoplasms (five nonmetastasizing squamous cell carcinomas, one squamous cell papilloma, and one squamous polyp) occurred after 19 months of treatment. In mice given 60 mg/kg per day for 90 days then 30 mg/kg per day thereafter, one vaginal squamous cell papilloma occurred after 19 months of treatment. No vaginal tumors were found in mice given 30 mg/kg per day for 90 days then 20 mg/kg per day thereafter. No other medication-related tumors were observed in any of the male or female mice. At doses that produced tumors in mice, the estimated exposure of zidovudine (as measured by the area under the plasma concentration–time curve [AUC]) was approximately three times the estimated human exposure at the recommended therapeutic dose of 100 mg every 4 hours.

In rats given 600 mg/kg per day for 90 days, then 450 mg/kg per day until day 279, then 300 mg/kg per day thereafter, two nonmetastasizing vaginal squamous cell carcinomas occurred after 20 months of treatment; no vaginal tumors were found in rats given 80 or 220 mg/kg per day. No other medication-related tumors were observed in any of the male or female rats. At doses that produced tumors in rats, the estimated exposure of zidovudine (as measured by the AUC) was approximately 24 times the estimated human exposure at the recommended therapeutic dose.

Two transplacental carcinogenicity studies were conducted in mice. In the first study, pregnant mice were administered zidovudine at doses of 20 or 40 mg/kg per day from gestation day 10 through parturition and lactation with dosing continuing in offspring for 24 months postnatally. After 24 months, an increase in the incidence of vaginal tumors was noted in the offspring of mice receiving 40 mg/kg per day with no increase in the incidence of any other tumors in male or female offspring. In the second study, pregnant mice were administered zidovudine at maximum tolerated doses of 12.5 or 25 mg per day (approximately 1000 or 450 mg/kg of nonpregnant or term body weight, respectively) from days 12 through 18 of gestation. There was an increase in the number of tumors in the liver, lung, and female reproductive tracts in the offspring of mice receiving the higher dose of zidovudine.

### Mutagenicity
Lamivudine:
Lamivudine was mutagenic in the L5178Y/TK$^{+/-}$ mouse lymphoma assay and clastogenic in a cytogenetic assay using cultured human lymphocytes. Lamivudine was not mutagenic in a microbial mutagenicity screen, an *in vitro* cell transformation assay, the rat micronucleus test, a rat bone marrow cytogenetic assay, or the unscheduled DNA synthesis test in rat liver.

Zidovudine:
Zidovudine was mutagenic in the L5178Y/TK$^{+/-}$ mouse lymphoma assay, an *in vitro* cell transformation assay, and mouse and rat micronucleus tests after repeated doses, and clastogenic in a cytogenetic

assay using cultured human lymphocytes. Zidovudine was not mutagenic in rats given a single dose in a cytogenetic study.

**Pregnancy/Reproduction**
Fertility—
*Lamivudine*—At doses of up to 130 times the usual adult human dose (on a body surface area basis), lamivudine administered to male and female rats showed no evidence of impairing fertility and had no effect on the survival, growth, or development of offspring to weaning.

*Zidovudine*—At doses of up to seven times the usual adult human dose (on a body surface area basis), zidovudine administered to male and female rats had no effects on fertility.

Pregnancy—Adequate and well-controlled studies of lamivudine and zidovudine combination have not been done in humans. However, zidovudine has been shown to cross the placenta.

*Lamivudine*—Studies in rats and rabbits revealed no evidence of teratogenicity at doses of 130 and 60 times, respectively, the usual adult human dose (on a body surface area basis). Early embryo lethality was observed in rabbits at doses similar to those produced by the usual adult human dose and higher; embryo lethality was not observed in rats administered doses of up to 130 times the usual adult human dose. Lamivudine crosses the placenta in rats and rabbits.

*Zidovudine*—Studies in rats and rabbits revealed no evidence of teratogenicity at doses of up to 500 mg/kg per day. Zidovudine was embryotoxic or fetotoxic in rats given 150 or 450 mg/kg per day and in rabbits given 500 mg/kg per day. In rats, 3000 mg/kg per day (resulting in peak plasma concentrations of 350 times the peak human plasma concentration) caused marked maternal toxicity and an increase in the incidence of fetal malformations.

FDA Pregnancy Category C.

Note: To monitor maternal-fetal outcomes of pregnant women exposed to lamivudine and zidovudine combination and other antiretroviral agents, an Antiretroviral Pregnancy Registry has been established. Physicians are encouraged to register patients by calling (800) 722-9292, ext. 39437.

**Breast-feeding**
Zidovudine is distributed into breast milk; it is not known whether lamivudine is distributed into breast milk. **The Centers for Disease Control and Prevention recommend that HIV-infected mothers do not breast-feed their infants to avoid potential postnatal transmission of HIV.**

**Pediatrics**
Lamivudine and zidovudine combination should not be administered to children younger than 12 years of age because the fixed-dose combination product cannot be adjusted.

**Adolescents**
Lamivudine and zidovudine combination should not be administered to patients who weigh less than 50 kg because the fixed-dose combination product cannot be adjusted.

**Geriatrics**
The pharmacokinetics of lamivudine and zidovudine combination have not been studied in patients 65 years of age and older.

**Drug interactions and/or related problems**
The following drug interactions and/or related problems have been selected on the basis of their potential clinical significance (possible mechanism in parentheses where appropriate)—not necessarily inclusive (» = major clinical significance):

Note: No drug interaction studies have been conducted using lamivudine and zidovudine combination.

Combinations containing any of the following medications, depending on the amount present, may also interact with this medication.

Atovaquone or
Fluconazole or
Methadone or
Nelfinavir or
Probenicid or
Ritonavir or
Trimethoprim and sulfamethoxazole combination or
Valproic acid
(concurrent use of lamivudine with nelfinavir or trimethoprim and sulfamethoxazole combination increases the area under the plasma concentration–time curve [AUC] of lamivudine; no dosing modifications are necessary)

(concurrent use of zidovudine with atovaquone, fluconazole, methadone, probenecid, or valproic acid increases the AUC of zidovudine; concurrent use with nelfinavir or ritonavir decreases the AUC of zidovudine; no dosing modifications are necessary)

» Ganciclovir or
» Interferons, alpha or
» Bone marrow depressants, other (see *Appendix II*)
(concurrent use of bone marrow depressing agents with zidovudine may increase the hematologic toxicity of zidovudine; caution should be used when bone marrow depressants are administered concurrently with lamivudine and zidovudine combination)

» Lamivudine or
» Zidovudine
(lamivudine and zidovudine combination is a fixed-dose product; concurrent use of either lamivudine or zidovudine with the combination product is not recommended)

**Laboratory value alterations**
The following have been selected on the basis of their potential clinical significance (possible effect in parentheses where appropriate)—not necessarily inclusive (» = major clinical significance):

With physiology/laboratory test values
» Alanine aminotransferase (ALT [SGPT]) and
Amylase and
Aspartate aminotransferase (AST [SGOT])
(serum values may be increased)

Bilirubin
(serum concentrations may be increased)

» Hemoglobin
(concentration may be decreased)

» Neutrophils and
Platelets
(counts may be decreased)

**Medical considerations/Contraindications**
The medical considerations/contraindications included have been selected on the basis of their potential clinical significance (reasons given in parentheses where appropriate)—not necessarily inclusive (» = major clinical significance).

*Except under special circumstances, this medication should not be used when the following medical problems exist:*
» Hypersensitivity to lamivudine or zidovudine
» Renal function impairment
(reduction of the dosages of lamivudine and zidovudine is recommended for patients with renal function impairment; therefore, patients with creatinine clearance ≤ 50 mL per minute should not receive lamivudine and zidovudine combination)

*Risk-benefit should be considered when the following medical problems exist:*
» Bone marrow depression
(lamivudine and zidovudine combination should be used with caution in patients with bone marrow compromise evidenced by granulocyte count < 1000 cells per cubic millimeter or hemoglobin < 9.5 grams per deciliter)

» Hepatic function impairment or
» Hepatitis B virus infection
(caution should be used when administering lamivudine and zidovudine combination to patients with known risk factors for hepatic dysfunction; lamivudine and zidovudine combination therapy should be discontinued in patients who develop clinical or laboratory findings suggestive of lactic acidosis or hepatotoxicity)

(some patients with human immunodeficiency virus [HIV] infection who have chronic liver disease due to hepatitis B virus infection experienced clinical or laboratory evidence of recurrent hepatitis upon discontinuation of lamivudine; consequences may be more severe in patients with decompensated hepatic disease)

**Patient monitoring**
The following may be especially important in patient monitoring (other tests may be warranted in some patients, depending on condition; » = major clinical significance):

» Complete blood counts (CBCs)
(frequent blood counts are strongly recommended in patients with advanced HIV disease who are treated with lamivudine and zidovudine combination; periodic blood counts are recommended in HIV-infected patients and patients with asymptomatic or early HIV disease)

# Lamivudine and Zidovudine (Systemic)—Introductory Version

## Side/Adverse Effects

Lactic acidosis and severe hepatomegaly with steatosis, including fatal cases, have been reported with the use of antiretroviral nucleoside analogs alone or in combination, including lamivudine and zidovudine. A majority of these effects have occurred in women.

The following side/adverse effects have been selected on the basis of their potential clinical significance (possible signs and symptoms in parentheses where appropriate)—not necessarily inclusive:

**Those indicating need for medical attention**
Incidence more frequent
   *Anemia* (pale skin; unusual tiredness or weakness); *neutropenia* (chills; fever; sore throat)
Incidence less frequent
   *Hepatotoxicity* (abdominal pain, severe; fever; nausea; skin rash; unusual tiredness or weakness; vomiting; yellow eyes or skin)—more frequent in women; *myopathy or myositis* (muscle tenderness and weakness); *neuropathy* (burning, tingling, numbness or pain in the hands, arms, feet, or legs)
Incidence rare
   *Pancreatitis* (abdominal pain, severe; nausea; vomiting)

**Those indicating need for medical attention only if they continue or are bothersome**
Incidence more frequent
   *Headache; nausea*
Incidence less frequent
   *Abdominal pain; anorexia* (decreased appetite); *coughing; diarrhea; dizziness; insomnia* (trouble in sleeping); *skin rash*

## Overdose

For more information on the management of overdose or unintentional ingestion, **contact a Poison Control Center** (see *Poison Control Center Listing*).

**Clinical effects of overdose**
For lamivudine, one case of an adult ingesting 6 grams has been reported. There were no clinical signs or symptoms noted, and hematologic tests remained normal.
For zidovudine, acute overdoses in children and adults ingesting up to 50 grams have been reported. Nausea and vomiting were consistently noted among these cases. Other reported occurrences included confusion, dizziness, drowsiness, headache, lethargy, and one report of a grand mal seizure. Hematologic changes were transient, and all patients recovered.

**Treatment of overdose**
To enhance elimination—It is not known whether lamivudine can be removed by hemodialysis or peritoneal dialysis. Hemodialysis and peritoneal dialysis have a negligible effect on the removal of zidovudine. However, either process may be used to enhance the removal of the primary metabolite of zidovudine (GZDV).

Supportive care—Patients in whom intentional overdose is confirmed or suspected should be referred for psychiatric consultation.

## Patient Consultation

In providing consultation, consider emphasizing the following selected information (» = major clinical significance):

**Before using this medication**
» Conditions affecting use, especially:
   Hypersensitivity to lamivudine or zidovudine
   Pregnancy—Zidovudine crosses the placenta
   Breast-feeding—Zidovudine is distributed into breast milk; it is recommended that HIV-infected mothers do not breast-feed their infants to avoid potential postnatal transmission of HIV
   Use in children—Lamivudine and zidovudine combination is not recommended for use in children younger than 12 years of age
   Use in adolescents—Lamivudine and zidovudine combination is not recommended for use in patients who weigh less than 50 kg
   Other medications, especially alpha interferons, ganciclovir, lamivudine, other bone marrow depressants, or zidovudine
   Other medical problems, especially bone marrow depression, hepatic function impairment, hepatitis B virus infection, or renal function impairment

**Proper use of this medication**
» Importance of not taking more medication than prescribed; importance of not discontinuing medication without checking with physician
» Importance of not missing doses and of taking at evenly spaced times
   Not sharing medication with others
» Proper dosing
   Missed dose: Taking as soon as possible; not taking if almost time for next dose; not doubling doses
» Proper storage

**Precautions while using this medication**
» Regular visits to physician for blood tests
» Importance of not taking other medications concurrently without checking with physician

**Side/adverse effects**
Signs of potential side effects, especially anemia, neutropenia, hepatotoxicity, myopathy or myositis, neuropathy, and pancreatitis

## General Dosing Information

May be taken with or without food.

**Bioequivalenence information**
One lamivudine and zidovudine combination tablet is bioequivalent to 150 mg lamivudine and 300 mg zidovudine; given two times a day, this combination tablet is an alternative dosing regimen to lamivudine 150 mg two times a day plus zidovudine 600 mg per day in divided doses.

## Oral Dosage Forms

### LAMIVUDINE AND ZIDOVUDINE TABLETS

**Usual adult and adolescent dose**
Human immunodeficiency virus (HIV) infection—
   Adults and adolescents 50 kg of body weight and over: Oral, 150 mg of lamivudine and 300 mg of zidovudine two times a day.
   Adults and adolescents up to 50 kg of body weight: Use is not recommended.

**Usual pediatric dose**
Use is not recommended.

**Usual geriatric dose**
See *Usual adult and adolescent dose*.

**Strength(s) usually available**
U.S.—
   150 mg of lamivudine and 300 mg of zidovudine (Rx) [*Combivir*].

**Packaging and storage**
Store between 2 and 30 °C (36 and 86 °F).

Developed: 11/14/97

---

# LAMOTRIGINE   Systemic

VA CLASSIFICATION (Primary): CN400
Commonly used brand name(s): *Lamictal*.
Another commonly used name is LTG.
Note:  For a listing of dosage forms and brand names by country availability, see *Dosage Forms* section(s).

## Category

Anticonvulsant.

## Indications

**Accepted**
Epilepsy (treatment adjunct)—Lamotrigine is indicated as an adjunct to other anticonvulsant medications in the treatment of partial seizures in adults 16 years of age and older with epilepsy.

**Acceptance not established**
Additional data are required to confirm the safety and effectiveness of lamotrigine use in children, as monotherapy, in the treatment of *secondary generalized seizures*, in the treatment of *primary generalized seizures* including *absence seizures*, and in the treatment of *Lennox-Gastaut syndrome*.

Note:  Although lamotrigine is approved in some countries for use in children, as monotherapy, and in the treatment of both primary and secondary generalized seizures, the USP DI Advisory Panels believe that currently there is insufficient evidence to support the safety and effectiveness of lamotrigine for use in these indications.

## Pharmacology/Pharmacokinetics

### Physicochemical characteristics
Chemical group—Phenyltriazine. Structurally unrelated to existing anticonvulsant medications.
Molecular weight—256.09.
pKa—5.7.

### Mechanism of action/Effect
The exact mechanism of action is unknown. *In vitro* studies suggest that lamotrigine blocks voltage-sensitive sodium channels, thereby stabilizing neuronal membranes and inhibiting the presynaptic release of neurotransmitters, principally glutamate. Lamotrigine may also directly inhibit high-frequency sustained repetitive firing of sodium-dependent action potentials.

### Other actions/effects
Lamotrigine is a weak dihydrofolate reductase inhibitor *in vitro* and in animal studies. No effect on folate concentrations has been noted in clinical studies. However, complete inhibition of erythropoiesis occurred in one patient with heterozygous beta-thalassemia, possibly due to inhibition of dihydrofolate reductase by lamotrigine.

Animal studies have shown that lamotrigine binds to melanin-containing tissues, such as eye tissues and pigmented skin. The long-term effects of this binding are not known, but no effects have been seen in humans.

The 2-*N*-methyl metabolite of lamotrigine causes cardiac conduction disturbances in dogs in a dose-dependent manner. This metabolite is present in trace amounts in the urine of people taking lamotrigine, but the clinical significance of its presence is unknown.

### Absorption
Rapid. Bioavailability of lamotrigine is approximately 98% and is unaffected by food.

### Distribution
Volume of distribution (Vol$_D$) is approximately 1.2 liters per kg (L/kg). In a 10-year-old patient undergoing topectomy 4 hours post-dose, lamotrigine concentration in brain tissue was greater than unbound lamotrigine concentration in plasma. Lamotrigine is distributed into breast milk.

### Protein binding
Moderate (55%).

### Biotransformation
Hepatic glucuronic acid conjugation. Evidence of autoinduction has been seen in some studies but not in others. Further evaluation of possible lamotrigine autoinduction is needed. The 2-*N*-methyl metabolite of lamotrigine is present in trace amounts in the urine of people taking lamotrigine, but the clinical significance of its presence is unknown.

### Half-life
Elimination—
With no other medication: 25±10 hours.
With enzyme-inducing anticonvulsants only: 14±6 hours.
With valproic acid only: Approximately 59 hours.
With enzyme-inducing anticonvulsants and valproic acid: Approximately 28 hours.

### Time to peak concentration
1.4 to 4.8 hours. A second peak may be seen 4 to 6 hours after oral or intravenous administration; this peak may reflect enterohepatic recirculation.

### Therapeutic serum concentration
The therapeutic concentration range for lamotrigine has not been determined. Over a range of 50 to 400 mg given as a single dose, peak plasma concentrations increased linearly from 0.58 to 4.63 mg/L in healthy subjects. In 2 small studies of patients with epilepsy, plasma concentrations increased linearly with doses of 50 to 350 mg given 2 times a day. Titration of dosage is based on clinical response.

### Elimination
Renal—Approximately 73% (about 10% unchanged, 80 to 90% as glucuronide conjugates, less than 5% as other metabolites, and trace amounts as the 2-*N*-methyl metabolite).
Fecal—Approximately 2%.
In dialysis—In 6 patients, 17 ± 10% of the lamotrigine in the body was removed in 4 hours of hemodialysis.

## Precautions to Consider

### Carcinogenicity
In 2-year studies, at plasma concentrations equal to those seen in humans receiving 300 to 500 mg of lamotrigine a day, rats and mice showed no evidence of carcinogenicity.

### Mutagenicity
No evidence of mutagenicity was found in appropriate *in vitro* and *in vivo* testing.

### Pregnancy/Reproduction
Fertility—No adverse effect on fertility was seen in rats given up to 0.4 times an equivalent human dose of 500 mg per day (mg/day) on a mg per square meter of body surface area (mg/m$^2$) basis.

Pregnancy—Lamotrigine should be used during pregnancy only if the potential benefit justifies the potential risk to the fetus.
Folic acid supplementation should be considered for all women of childbearing potential who are taking lamotrigine.
Studies have not been done in humans.
Studies in rats and rabbits indicate that lamotrigine crosses the placenta, yielding placental and fetal concentrations comparable to concentrations in maternal plasma. No teratogenic effects were seen in animal studies employing up to 1.2 times an equivalent human dose of 500 mg per day on a mg/m$^2$ basis. However, rats receiving up to 0.5 times an equivalent human dose of 500 mg per day on a mg/m$^2$ basis produced offspring with decreased fetal folate concentrations, an effect known to be associated with teratogenicity in humans and animals. In addition, stillbirths and postnatal deaths were increased among offspring of rats receiving lamotrigine in doses less than half of an equivalent human dose of 500 mg per day on a mg/m$^2$ basis, probably due to *in utero* exposure to lamotrigine. The clinical significance of these effects is unknown.

FDA Pregnancy Category C.

Labor and delivery—The effect of lamotrigine on labor and delivery is not known.

### Breast-feeding
Lamotrigine is distributed into breast milk. However, the effects on the nursing infant are unknown.

### Pediatrics
Uncontrolled studies performed in a limited number of pediatric epilepsy patients 2 to 16 years of age have not demonstrated pediatrics-specific problems that would limit the usefulness of lamotrigine in children. Pharmacokinetic data from these studies indicate that lamotrigine elimination half-life may be shorter, and clearance may be more rapid, in children than in adults. However, data from controlled trials are still needed to establish safety and efficacy in children.

### Geriatrics
Appropriate studies on the relationship of age to the effects of lamotrigine have not been performed in the geriatric population. However, one single-dose pharmacokinetic study comparing 12 healthy volunteers 65 to 76 years of age and 12 healthy volunteers 26 to 38 years of age found that lamotrigine clearance was 37% lower, area under the concentration-time curve (AUC) was 55% higher, peak plasma concentration was 27% higher, and elimination half-life was 6 hours longer in the older group. In addition, elderly patients are more likely to have age-related renal function impairment, which may require dosage adjustment. It is recommended that elderly patients receive dosages at the low end of the normal range.

### Drug interactions and/or related problems
The following drug interactions and/or related problems have been selected on the basis of their potential clinical significance (possible mechanism in parentheses where appropriate)—not necessarily inclusive (» = major clinical significance):

Note: Combinations containing any of the following medications, depending on the amount present, may also interact with this medication.

Possible interactions between lamotrigine and hepatic enzyme inducers or inhibitors not listed below should be considered.

Acetaminophen
(half-life and area under the concentration-time curve of lamotrigine may be reduced slightly by chronic, high-dose acetaminophen use)

Alcohol or central nervous system (CNS) depression-producing medications, other (See *Appendix II*)
(lamotrigine may enhance the CNS depressant effects of these medications or alcohol)

» Carbamazepine or
» Phenobarbital or
» Phenytoin or

# Lamotrigine (Systemic)

- » Primidone
  (clearance of lamotrigine is increased; clearance may be expected to decrease when concomitant enzyme-inducing therapy is discontinued; initial lamotrigine dosage and rate of lamotrigine dosage escalation should be based on concomitant anticonvulsant therapy; monitoring of plasma concentrations of lamotrigine and other anticonvulsant medications should be considered, especially during dosage adjustments)

  (an increased incidence of CNS adverse effects, including ataxia, blurred vision, diplopia, dizziness, or increased excitation, may occur with concomitant carbamazepine use; reduction of dosage of either lamotrigine or carbamazepine may reduce these effects)

- Folate antagonists, other (See *Appendix II*)
  (lamotrigine inhibits dihydrofolate reductase, and should be used with caution with other folate antagonists)

- » Valproic acid
  (half-life and plasma concentrations of lamotrigine are increased, probably due to competition for hepatic glucuronidation; half-life and plasma concentrations may be expected to decrease when valproic acid is discontinued; initial lamotrigine dosage, and rate of lamotrigine dosage escalation, should be based on concomitant anticonvulsant therapy; monitoring of plasma concentrations of lamotrigine and valproic acid should be considered, especially during dosage adjustments)

  (disabling tremor and an increased incidence of rash, including severe rash, have occurred with concomitant valproic acid use)

  (there is some evidence that the combination of lamotrigine and valproic acid may improve seizure control in patients who are refractory to either agent used alone, but controlled studies have not been done)

## Medical considerations/Contraindications

The medical considerations/contraindications included have been selected on the basis of their potential clinical significance (reasons given in parentheses where appropriate)—not necessarily inclusive (» = major clinical significance).

*Except under special circumstances, this medication should not be used when the following medical problem exists:*

- » Hypersensitivity to lamotrigine

*Risk-benefit should be considered when the following medical problems exist:*

- Cardiac conduction abnormalities
  (in one clinical trial, minor electrocardiogram [ECG] changes were seen in some patients with normal cardiac function who were taking lamotrigine; there is no experience with lamotrigine treatment in patients with cardiac conduction disturbances)

- Hepatic function impairment
  (lamotrigine metabolism may be decreased)

- » Renal function impairment
  (large interindividual differences in lamotrigine plasma concentration were seen in uremic patients, and elimination half-life is prolonged in patients with significant renal function impairment; patients with renal function impairment may require reduced maintenance doses)

- » Thalassemia
  (erythropoiesis may be decreased significantly)

## Side/Adverse Effects

Note: Disseminated intravascular coagulation and multi-organ failure have occurred very rarely in patients taking lamotrigine. Most cases have been in association with other serious medical events, such as status epilepticus and overwhelming sepsis, and it is uncertain whether these effects were related to lamotrigine use.

An increased incidence of CNS adverse effects, including ataxia, blurred vision, diplopia, dizziness, or increased excitation, may occur with concomitant carbamazepine use; reduction of dosage of either lamotrigine or carbamazepine may reduce these effects.

Lamotrigine may be less sedating than other anticonvulsant medications.

The following side/adverse effects have been selected on the basis of their potential clinical significance (possible signs and symptoms in parentheses where appropriate)—not necessarily inclusive:

### Those indicating need for medical attention

Incidence more frequent
  *Ataxia* (clumsiness or unsteadiness); *skin rash; vision abnormalities, including blurred vision; and diplopia* (double vision)

Note: The incidence of *skin rash* is highly dependent upon the initial rate of lamotrigine dosage escalation. Higher incidence of *skin rash* is seen with concurrent valproic acid therapy, higher lamotrigine starting doses, or rapid lamotrigine dosage escalation. Rash is usually maculopapular and/or erythematous and occurs within the first 4 to 6 weeks of treatment. Rash usually resolves when lamotrigine is discontinued. A mild rash may subside even with continuation of lamotrigine therapy; however, close monitoring is essential. Some patients have been successfully rechallenged with lamotrigine after discontinuation due to mild rash. Rarely, more severe rashes with systemic involvement may occur. It is recommended that any patient who acutely develops any combination of unexplained rash, fever, flu-like symptoms, or worsening of seizure control should discontinue lamotrigine and should be closely monitored; monitoring should include determinations of hepatic and renal function, and clotting parameters.

Incidence less frequent
  *CNS toxicity, specifically anxiety; confusion; depression; irritability; or other mood or mental changes; increased seizures; or nystagmus* (continuous, uncontrolled back and forth and/or rolling eye movements)

Incidence rare
  *Angioedema* (trouble in breathing; swelling of face, mouth, hands, or feet); *blood dyscrasias, including anemia; eosinophilia; leukopenia; or thrombocytopenia* (fever and sore throat; unusual bleeding or bruising; unusual tiredness or weakness); *erythema multiforme, Stevens-Johnson syndrome, or toxic epidermal necrolysis* (blistering, peeling, or loosening of skin; muscle cramps, pain, or weakness; red or irritated eyes; skin rash or itching; sore throat, fever, and chills; sores, ulcers, or white spots in mouth or on lips); *fever; hypersensitivity syndrome* (dark-colored urine; fever; flu-like symptoms; skin rash; facial swelling; swollen lymph nodes; unusual tiredness or weakness; yellow eyes or skin); *petechia* (small red or purple spots on skin)

### Those indicating need for medical attention only if they continue or are bothersome

Incidence more frequent
  *CNS effects, specifically dizziness; drowsiness; or headache; gastrointestinal effects, specifically nausea; or vomiting*

Note: A higher incidence of *dizziness* is seen in females than in males.

Incidence less frequent or rare
  *Asthenia* (loss of strength); *dysarthria* (slurred speech); *dyspepsia* (indigestion); *insomnia* (trouble in sleeping); *rhinitis* (runny nose); *tremor* (trembling or shaking)

## Overdose

For specific information on the agents used in the management of lamotrigine overdose, see:
- *Charcoal, Activated (Oral-Local)* monograph.

For more information on the management of overdose or unintentional ingestion, **contact a Poison Control Center** (see *Poison Control Center Listing*).

### Clinical effects of overdose

The following effects have been selected on the basis of their potential clinical significance (possible signs and symptoms in parentheses where appropriate)—not necessarily inclusive:

Acute effects
  *CNS toxicity, specifically ataxia, severe* (clumsiness or unsteadiness); *coma; dizziness, severe; drowsiness, severe; dysarthria, severe* (slurred speech); *or nystagmus, severe* (continuous, uncontrolled back and forth and/or rolling eye movements); *dryness of mouth; electrocardiogram (ECG) changes, specifically prolonged QRS interval; increased heart rate*

Note: Experience with lamotrigine overdose is very limited. Overdoses with lamotrigine have ranged from 1350 to over 4000 milligrams. Some of these clinical effects have occurred in only one patient, and general applicability to lamotrigine overdose is unknown.

### Treatment of overdose

To decrease absorption—Emesis may be induced or gastric lavage may be performed, if indicated, with precautions taken to protect the airway, keeping in mind the rapid absorption of lamotrigine. Activated charcoal also may be administered. These procedures may need to be repeated several times. The use of a cathartic to accelerate elimination of charcoal and medication from the lower gastrointestinal tract should be considered.

To enhance elimination—Hemodialysis is of questionable efficacy. The extraction ratio of lamotrigine in 6 patients with renal failure was 17±10% in 4 hours of hemodialysis.

Specific treatment—There is no known antidote to lamotrigine overdose.

Monitoring—Patient should be observed closely, with frequent monitoring of vital signs. Close electrocardiogram (ECG) monitoring may be advisable in patients showing QRS interval prolongation.

Supportive care—General supportive care is the basis of lamotrigine overdose treatment. Patients in whom intentional overdose is confirmed or suspected should be referred for psychiatric consultation.

## Patient Consultation

As an aid to patient consultation, refer to *Advice for the Patient, Lamotrigine (Systemic)*.

In providing consultation, consider emphasizing the following selected information (» = major clinical significance):

### Before using this medication
» Conditions affecting use, especially:
  Hypersensitivity to lamotrigine
  Pregnancy—Crossed the placenta in animal studies; increased stillbirths and postnatal deaths among offspring of rats receiving less than maximum human dose
  Breast-feeding—Distributed into breast milk; effect on nursing infant is unknown
  Other medications, especially carbamazepine, phenobarbital, phenytoin, primidone, or valproic acid
  Other medical problems, especially renal function impairment or thalassemia

### Proper use of this medication
» Compliance with therapy; not taking more or less medicine than prescribed; not missing any doses
  Taking with or without food or on a full or empty stomach, as directed by physician
» Proper dosing
  Missed dose: Taking as soon as possible; if almost time for next dose, skipping missed dose and returning to regular dosing schedule; not doubling doses
» Proper storage

### Precautions while using this medication
» Regular visits to physician to check progress of therapy
  Discussing alcohol use and use of other CNS depressants with physician
» Possible blurred or double vision, dizziness, drowsiness, impairment of motor skills; caution when driving or doing jobs requiring alertness, coordination, or clear vision
» Immediately notifying physician if skin rash or increase in seizures occurs
» Not discontinuing lamotrigine abruptly; consulting physician about gradually reducing dosage

### Side/adverse effects
Signs of potential side effects, especially ataxia; skin rash; vision abnormalities; anxiety, confusion, depression, irritability, or other mood or mental changes; increased seizures; nystagmus; angioedema; blood dyscrasias; erythema multiforme, Stevens-Johnson syndrome, or toxic epidermal necrolysis; fever; hypersensitivity syndrome; or petechia

## General Dosing Information

Lamotrigine should be initiated at a low dose, and dosage escalation should proceed slowly, to minimize the occurrence of skin rash. The incidence of skin rash is highly dependent upon the initial rate of lamotrigine dosage escalation.

Physician should be notified immediately if an acute worsening of seizure control or a skin rash occurs.

Anticonvulsant medications should not be discontinued abruptly because of the possibility of increased seizures. Lamotrigine dosage may be decreased by 25 to 33% every 2 weeks. If more rapid discontinuation is required, the dosage should be tapered over at least 2 weeks, if possible, with the dose decreased by 50% each week.

## Oral Dosage Forms

### LAMOTRIGINE TABLETS

Note: Lamotrigine therapy should be initiated at a low dose, and dosage escalation should proceed slowly to minimize the occurrence of skin rash, including severe skin rash.

### Usual adult dose
Anticonvulsant—
  With enzyme-inducing anticonvulsants only: Oral, 50 mg once a day for two weeks, then 100 mg a day, divided into two doses, for two weeks. The dosage may be increased by 100 mg a day every week based on clinical response.
  With enzyme-inducing anticonvulsants and valproic acid: Oral, 25 mg once every other day for two weeks, then 25 mg once a day for two weeks. The dosage may be increased by 25 to 50 mg a day every one or two weeks based on clinical response.

Note: Lamotrigine dosing in patients receiving only valproic acid concurrently has not been firmly established. However, lamotrigine dosing identical to that used in patients receiving lamotrigine with valproic acid and enzyme-inducing anticonvulsants has been used in some patients and is the recommended dosing in the United Kingdom. Lamotrigine plasma concentrations in patients receiving only valproic acid concurrently may be up to two times those seen in patients who are also receiving enzyme-inducing anticonvulsants.

Lamotrigine is approved for use as monotherapy in some countries. Monotherapy dosage being used for patients over 12 years of age is 25 mg per day for the first two weeks then 50 mg per day for the second two weeks. The dosage may be increased, based on clinical response, up to 200 mg per day given in one dose or two divided doses.

### Usual adult prescribing limits
With enzyme-inducing anticonvulsants only—500 mg a day in two divided doses.
With enzyme-inducing anticonvulsants and valproic acid—200 mg a day in two divided doses.

### Usual pediatric dose
Safety and efficacy have not been established.

### Strength(s) usually available
U.S.—
  25 mg (Rx) [*Lamictal* (scored; lactose; magnesium stearate; microcrystalline cellulose; povidone; sodium starch glycolate)].
  100 mg (Rx) [*Lamictal* (scored; FD&C Yellow No. 6 Lake; lactose; magnesium stearate; microcrystalline cellulose; povidone; sodium starch glycolate)].
  150 mg (Rx) [*Lamictal* (scored; ferric oxide yellow; lactose; magnesium stearate; microcrystalline cellulose; povidone; sodium starch glycolate)].
  200 mg (Rx) [*Lamictal* (scored; FD&C Blue No. 2 Lake; lactose; magnesium stearate; microcrystalline cellulose; povidone; sodium starch glycolate)].
Canada—
  25 mg (Rx) [*Lamictal* (scored; cellulose; lactose; magnesium stearate; povidone; sodium starch glycolate)].
  50 mg (Rx) [*Lamictal* (scored; cellulose; ferric oxide red; lactose; magnesium stearate; povidone; sodium starch glycolate)].
  100 mg (Rx) [*Lamictal* (scored; cellulose; lactose; magnesium stearate; povidone; sodium starch glycolate; Sunset Yellow FCF Lake)].
  150 mg (Rx) [*Lamictal* (scored; cellulose; ferric oxide yellow; lactose; magnesium stearate; povidone; sodium starch glycolate)].
  200 mg (Rx) [*Lamictal* (scored; cellulose; Indigotine Lake; lactose; magnesium stearate; povidone; sodium starch glycolate)].
  250 mg (Rx) [*Lamictal* (scored; cellulose; lactose; magnesium stearate; povidone; sodium starch glycolate)].

### Packaging and storage
Store between 15 and 25 °C (59 and 77 °F), in a well-closed container, unless otherwise specified by manufacturer. Protect from light and moisture.

### Auxiliary labeling
- May cause blurred vision.
- May cause dizziness.
- May cause drowsiness. Alcohol may intensify this effect.

## Selected Bibliography

Gilman JT. Lamotrigine: An antiepileptic agent for the treatment of partial seizures. Ann Pharmacother 1995 Feb; 29: 144-51.

Burstein AH. Lamotrigine. Pharmacotherapy 1995; 15(2): 129-43.

Fitton A, Goa KL. Lamotrigine: An update of its pharmacology and therapeutic use in epilepsy. Drugs 1995; 50(4): 691-713.

Developed: 05/23/96

# LANSOPRAZOLE Systemic

VA CLASSIFICATION (Primary): GA304
Commonly used brand name(s): *Prevacid*.
Note: For a listing of dosage forms and brand names by country availability, see *Dosage Forms* section(s).

## Category
Gastric acid pump inhibitor; antiulcer agent.

## Indications

**Accepted**

Gastroesophageal reflux disease [GERD] (prophylaxis and treatment)—Lansoprazole is indicated for the short-term treatment of heartburn and other symptoms associated with gastroesophageal reflux disease (GERD). Lansoprazole is indicated for the short-term (up to 8 weeks) treatment for symptom relief and healing of all grades of erosive esophagitis (associated with GERD). Lansoprazole may be indicated for an additional 8 weeks of treatment in patients in whom healing has not occurred. If erosive esophagitis recurs, an additional course of lansoprazole treatment may be considered. Lansoprazole also is indicated to maintain healing of erosive esophagitis.

Ulcer, gastric (treatment)—Lansoprazole is indicated for short-term (up to 8 weeks) treatment in patients with active benign gastric ulcer.

Ulcer, duodenal (prophylaxis and treatment)—Lansoprazole is indicated for short-term (up to 4 weeks) treatment for symptom relief and healing in patients with active duodenal ulcer. Lansoprazole also is indicated to maintain healing of duodenal ulcers.

Ulcer, duodenal, *Helicobacter pylori*–associated (treatment)—Lansoprazole is indicated in combination with amoxicillin plus clarithromycin for the treatment of duodenal ulcer associated with *H. pylori* infection. Lansoprazole also is indicated in combination with amoxicillin in patients who are either allergic or intolerant to clarithromycin or in whom resistance to clarithromycin is known or suspected. Eradication of *H. pylori* has been shown to reduce the risk of ulcer recurrence.

Hypersecretory conditions, gastric (treatment)—Lansoprazole is indicated for the long-term treatment of pathological hypersecretory conditions, including Zollinger-Ellison syndrome.

## Pharmacology/Pharmacokinetics

Note: A wide range of intersubject variability has been observed in the pharmacokinetic parameters of lansoprazole.

**Physicochemical characteristics**

Note: Lansoprazole is chemically and pharmacologically related to omeprazole.
Chemical group—Substituted benzimidazole.
Molecular weight—369.37.
pKa—8.5.

**Mechanism of action/Effect**

Lansoprazole is a selective and irreversible proton pump inhibitor. In the acidic environment of the gastric parietal cell, lansoprazole is converted to active sulphenamide derivatives that bind to the sulfhydryl group of $(H^+, K^+)$-adenosine triphosphatase $[(H^+, K^+)$-ATPase], also known as the proton pump. $(H^+, K^+)$-ATPase catalyzes the final step in the gastric acid secretion pathway. Lansoprazole's inhibition of $(H^+, K^+)$-ATPase results in inhibition of both centrally and peripherally mediated gastric acid secretion. The inhibitory effect is dose-related. Lansoprazole inhibits both basal and stimulated gastric acid secretion regardless of the stimulus.

Following oral administration, lansoprazole significantly decreases basal acid output and significantly increases the mean gastric pH and percent of time the gastric pH remains above 3 and 4. It also significantly reduces meal-stimulated gastric acid output and secretion volume, as well as pentagastrin-stimulated acid output. In addition, lansoprazole inhibits the normal increases in secretion volume, acidity, and acid output induced by insulin.

Lansoprazole does not have anticholinergic or histamine $H_2$-receptor antagonist properties.

**Other actions/effects**

Due to the normal physiologic effects caused by the inhibition of gastric acid secretion, blood flow in the antrum, pylorus, and duodenal bulb is decreased by about 17%; however, mucosal blood flow in the fundus of the stomach is not significantly affected by lansoprazole. Gastric emptying of digestible solids following intake of lansoprazole is significantly slowed. Lansoprazole increases serum pepsinogen levels and decreases pepsin activity under basal conditions and in response to meal stimulation or insulin injection. As with other agents that elevate intragastric pH, lansoprazole may cause an increase in the number of nitrate-reducing bacteria and an elevation in the nitrate concentration of gastric secretions in patients with gastric ulcer; however, significantly elevated nitrosamine levels have not been reported to date, suggesting no risk of carcinogenesis by this mechanism.

Lansoprazole and its active metabolites have demonstrated antimicrobial activity *in vitro* against *Helicobacter pylori*, a gram-negative bacilli strongly associated with peptic ulcers. Lansoprazole may influence the mucosal immune response to *H. pylori*. Mucosal *H. pylori*–specific IgA response is significantly enhanced after short-term treatment with lansoprazole, strongly suggesting that the secretory immune system is actively involved in host defense against *H. pylori*, and that the efficacy of such a system at the gastric mucosal level is crucial for complete eradication of *H. pylori*. Although lansoprazole alone has a relatively low clearance effect on *H. pylori*, it may enhance the ability of other agents to eradicate the organism; lansoprazole's activity as an antisecretory agent may be the more important factor explaining its effectiveness.

Lansoprazole has the ability to inhibit the hepatic cytochrome P450 enzyme system.

**Absorption**

Since lansoprazole is acid-labile, it is administered as a capsule containing enteric-coated granules to prevent gastric decomposition and to increase bioavailability. Once lansoprazole has left the stomach, absorption is rapid and relatively complete, with absolute bioavailability over 80%. Bioavailability may be decreased if lansoprazole is administered within 30 minutes of food intake as compared to that of a fasting state. Absorption may be delayed in patients with hepatic cirrhosis.

**Distribution**

Distributed in tissue, particularly gastric parietal cells. Apparent oral volume of distribution following administration of 30 mg of lansoprazole is about 0.5 liters per kilogram (L/kg).

**Protein binding**

Very high (around 97%); protein binding remains constant over the concentration range of 0.05 to 5 mcg per mL. In patients with renal function impairment, protein binding may be decreased by 1 to 1.5%.

**Biotransformation**

Lansoprazole is extensively metabolized in the liver to two main excretory metabolites that are inactive. In the acidic environment of the gastric parietal cell, lansoprazole is converted to two active compounds that inhibit acid secretion by $(H+, K+)$-ATPase within the parietal cell canaliculus, but that are not present in the systemic circulation.

**Half-life**

Elimination—
 Normal renal function: Approximately 1.5 hours.
 Renal function impairment: Shortened elimination half-life.
 Elderly patients: 1.9 to 2.9 hours.
 Hepatic function impairment: 3.2 to 7.2 hours.

**Onset of action**

An increase in gastric pH is seen within 2 to 3 hours following a single 15-mg dose, 1 to 2 hours following a single 30-mg dose or a 15-mg multiple-dose regimen, and 1 hour following a 30-mg multiple-dose regimen.

**Time to peak concentration**

Approximately 1 to 2 hours. Time to peak concentration ($t_{max}$) is shorter when lansoprazole is administered in the morning as opposed to the evening.

**Peak serum concentration**

Mean peak serum concentrations ($C_{max}$) ranged from 0.75 to 1.15 milligrams per Liter (mg/L) following administration of a single oral 30-mg dose of lansoprazole to volunteers. Although there is no correlation with serum concentrations of lansoprazole per se, inhibition of gastric secretion appears to be dose-proportional. Serum concentrations after morning dosing may be increased by twofold or more as compared to evening dosing regimens. Both $C_{max}$ and the area under the plasma concentration–time curve (AUC) decrease by about 50% when lansoprazole is administered within 30 minutes of food intake as opposed to fasting conditions. The concentration of lansoprazole and its active metabolites within the gastric parietal cell is the main determining factor of antisecretory efficacy.

**Duration of action**

More than 24 hours. Following discontinuation of lansoprazole, gastric acid levels do not increase to half the basal output until 39 hours have elapsed. No rebound gastric acidity has been observed following discontinuation of lansoprazole. In patients with Zollinger-Ellison syndrome, the duration of action of lansoprazole is prolonged.

### Elimination
Renal—Approximately 14 to 25% of a dose of lansoprazole is excreted in the urine, as conjugated and unconjugated hydroxylated metabolites. Less than 1% of unchanged lansoprazole is detectable in the urine.

Biliary/fecal—Approximately two-thirds of a dose of lansoprazole is detected as metabolites in the feces.

In dialysis—Lansoprazole and its metabolites are not significantly dialyzed; no appreciable fraction is removed by hemodialysis.

Note: Elimination is prolonged in healthy elderly subjects, in adult and elderly patients with mild renal impairment, and in patients with severe liver disease.

## Precautions to Consider

### Carcinogenicity
In 2-year studies in rats receiving up to 40 times the recommended human dose, lansoprazole produced dose-related gastric enterochromaffin-like (ECL) cell hyperplasia and ECL cell carcinoids in both male and female rats. Lansoprazole also increased the incidence of intestinal metaplasia of the gastric epithelium, and produced dose-related increases in the incidence of testicular interstitial adenomas. In a 1-year toxicity study in rats receiving 13 times the recommended human dose, testicular interstitial cell adenoma also occurred in 1 of 30 rats. In a 2-year study in mice receiving up to 80 times the recommended human dose, lansoprazole produced an increased incidence of liver tumors (hepatocellular adenomas and carcinomas), a dose-related increase in the incidence of gastric ECL cell hyperplasia, and adenomas of the rete testis in males.

### Mutagenicity
Lansoprazole was not genotoxic in the Ames test, the *ex vivo* rat hepatocyte unscheduled DNA synthesis (UDS) test, the *in vivo* mouse micronucleus test, or the rat bone marrow cell chromosomal aberration test. It was positive in *in vitro* human lymphocyte chromosomal aberration assays.

### Pregnancy/Reproduction
Fertility—Reproduction studies in rats and rabbits have shown no evidence of impaired fertility.

Pregnancy—Adequate and well-controlled studies in humans have not been done.

Reproductive studies in rats and rabbits at doses 40 times the recommended human dose have not shown that lansoprazole causes adverse effects in the fetus.

FDA Pregnancy Category B.

### Breast-feeding
It is not known whether lansoprazole is distributed into breast milk. However, lansoprazole or its metabolites are distributed into the milk of rats. Because lansoprazole has been shown to cause tumorigenic effects in animals, a decision should be made as to whether nursing should be discontinued or the medication withdrawn, taking into account the importance of lansoprazole to the mother.

### Pediatrics
No information is available on the relationship of age to the effects of lansoprazole in pediatric patients up to 18 years of age. Safety and efficacy have not been established.

### Geriatrics
Studies in elderly patients indicate that the clearance of lansoprazole is decreased in the elderly, resulting in a 50 to 100% increase in the elimination half-life. Because the mean half-life in the elderly remains between 1.9 and 2.9 hours, repeated once-daily dosing does not result in accumulation of lansoprazole. However, subsequent doses higher than 30 mg a day should not be administered unless additional gastric acid suppression is necessary.

### Drug interactions and/or related problems
The following drug interactions and/or related problems have been selected on the basis of their potential clinical significance (possible mechanism in parentheses where appropriate)—not necessarily inclusive (» = major clinical significance):

Note: Only specific interactions between lansoprazole and other medications have been identified in this monograph. However, lansoprazole, by decreasing gastric pH, has the potential to affect the bioavailability of any medication whose absorption is pH-dependent. Also, lansoprazole may prevent the degradation of acid-labile drugs.

Possible interactions of lansoprazole with medications known to be metabolized by the hepatic cytochrome P450 enzyme system should be considered. To date, however, lansoprazole appears to interact minimally with other agents, and no clinically relevant interactions have been reported with antipyrine; diazepam; ibuprofen, indomethacin, or other nonsteroidal anti-inflammatory drugs (NSAIDs); oral contraceptives; phenytoin; prednisone or prednisolone; propranolol; or warfarin.

Combinations containing any of the following medications, depending on the amount present, may also interact with this medication.

Ampicillin esters or
Digoxin or
Iron salts or
Ketoconazole
 (lansoprazole causes prolonged inhibition of gastric acid secretion, and thereby may interfere with the absorption of these medications and others for which bioavailability is determined by gastric pH)

Cyanocobalamin
 (lansoprazole appears to produce a dose-dependent decrease in the absorption of cyanocobalamin; this may be due to lansoprazole-induced hypochlorhydria or achlorhydria)

» Sucralfate
 (lansoprazole absorption is delayed and bioavailability is decreased; lansoprazole should be taken at least 30 minutes prior to sucralfate)

Theophylline
 (minor increases in the clearance of theophylline may occur, but the interaction is unlikely to be clinically significant; however, some patients may require adjustment of theophylline dosage when initiating or stopping lansoprazole therapy to maintain clinically effective concentrations of theophylline)

### Laboratory value alterations
The following have been selected on the basis of their potential clinical significance (possible effect in parentheses where appropriate)—not necessarily inclusive (» = major clinical significance):

Note: Although abnormalities in test values reported to date have generally not been of substantial clinical significance, the following have been selected on the basis of their *potential* clinical significance.

With physiology/laboratory test values
Alanine aminotransferase (ALT [SGPT]) and
Alkaline phosphatase and
Aspartate aminotransferase (AST [SGOT]) and
Bilirubin and
Gamma-glutamyltransferase (GGT) and
Globulins and
Lactate dehydrogenase (LDH)
 (serum values may be increased)

Albumin/globulin (AG) ratio
 (may be abnormal)

Cholesterol and
Electrolytes
 (serum concentrations may be increased or decreased)

Creatinine, serum and
Glucocorticoids and
Triglycerides, serum and
Uric acid
 (concentrations may be increased)

Gastrin, serum
 (concentrations may be increased; median fasting gastrin concentrations may increase 50 to 100% from baseline but remain in the normal range following treatment with lansoprazole at doses of 15 to 60 mg; observations in over 2100 patients showed that elevations reached a plateau after 2 months of therapy and returned to baseline after treatment was discontinued)

Hematocrit and
Hemoglobin
 (levels may be increased)

Platelet count and
Red blood cell (RBC) count and
White blood cell (WBC) count
 (may be increased or decreased, and abnormalities may be present)

### Medical considerations/Contraindications
The medical considerations/contraindications included have been selected on the basis of their potential clinical significance (reasons given in parentheses where appropriate)—not necessarily inclusive (» = major clinical significance).

*Risk-benefit should be considered when the following medical problems exist:*

Hepatic function impairment
(dosage reduction may be required in patients with severe hepatic disease because of the prolonged plasma half-life of lansoprazole)

Sensitivity to lansoprazole

## Side/Adverse Effects

The following side/adverse effects have been selected on the basis of their potential clinical significance (possible signs and symptoms in parentheses where appropriate)—not necessarily inclusive:

**Those indicating need for medical attention**
Incidence more frequent
  *Diarrhea; skin rash or itching*
Incidence less frequent
  *Abdominal or stomach pain; increased or decreased appetite; nausea*
Incidence rare
  *Anxiety; constipation; flu syndrome* (flu-like symptoms); *increased cough; mental depression; myalgia* (muscle pain); *thrombocytopenia* (unusual bleeding or bruising); *ulcerative colitis* (diarrhea, abdominal pain, rectal bleeding); *upper respiratory tract inflammation or infection* (cold symptoms)

**Those indicating need for medical attention only if they continue or are bothersome**
Incidence more frequent
  *Dizziness; headache*

## Overdose

For information on the management of overdose or unintentional ingestion, **contact a Poison Control Center** (see *Poison Control Center Listing*).

**Clinical effects of overdose**
Experience with lansoprazole overdose is limited. In one case in which a patient consumed 600 mg of lansoprazole, no adverse reaction was noted.

**Treatment of overdose**
There is no specific antidote for lansoprazole. Treatment is essentially symptomatic and supportive. Hemodialysis does not remove an appreciable fraction of the total quantity of lansoprazole or its metabolites.

Patients in whom intentional overdose is confirmed or suspected should be referred for psychiatric consultation.

## Patient Consultation

As an aid to patient consultation, refer to *Advice for the Patient, Lansoprazole (Systemic)*.

In providing consultation, consider emphasizing the following selected information (» = major clinical significance):

**Before using this medication**
» Conditions affecting use, especially:
  Sensitivity to lansoprazole
  Breast-feeding—Distributed into milk in rat studies; may cause potentially serious adverse effects in nursing infants
  Use in children—Safety and efficacy not established in children up to 18 years of age
  Other medications, especially sucralfate

**Proper use of this medication**
» Importance of taking before a meal, preferably in the morning
» Swallowing capsule whole without crushing, breaking, or chewing; however, if patient cannot swallow whole, capsule may be opened and intact granules sprinkled on one tablespoon of applesauce and swallowed immediately; granules should not be chewed or crushed
» Compliance with therapy
» Proper dosing
  Missed dose: Taking as soon as possible; not taking if almost time for next dose; not doubling doses
» Proper storage

**Precautions while using this medication**
» Regular visits to physician to check progress

**Side/adverse effects**
Signs of potential side effects, especially diarrhea, skin rash or itching, abdominal or stomach pain, increased or decreased appetite, nausea, anxiety, constipation, flu syndrome; increased cough, mental depression, myalgia, thrombocytopenia, ulcerative colitis, upper respiratory tract inflammation or infection

## General Dosing Information

Since lansoprazole is acid-labile, it is administered as a capsule containing enteric-coated granulesto prevent gastric decomposition and to increase bioavailability. Capsules should be swallowed whole, and not chewed or crushed. However, if the patient has difficulty swallowing capsules, the capsule may be opened and the intact granules may be sprinkled on one tablespoon of applesauce and swallowed immediately; granules should not be chewed or crushed. For patients who have a nasogastric tube in place, lansoprazole capsules may be opened and the intact granules mixed in 40 milliliters (mL) of apple juice and administered through the tube into the stomach. After administration, the tube should be flushed with additional apple juice to clear the tube.

Symptomatic response to therapy does not preclude the presence of gastric malignancy.

In patients with hypersecretory conditions such as Zollinger-Ellison syndrome, dosing should be adjusted according to individual needs and should continue for as long as clinically indicated. In general, treatment goals are to maintain basal acid output below 10 mEq per hour (<10 mmol/hr). Doses up to 90 mg two times a day have been administered, in some cases for as long as four years.

Lansoprazole may be taken with antacids.

**Diet/Nutrition**
Lansoprazole capsules should be taken before breakfast.

## Oral Dosage Forms

Note: Bracketed uses in the *Dosage Forms* section refer to categories of use and/or indications that are not included in U.S. product labeling.

### LANSOPRAZOLE DELAYED-RELEASE CAPSULES

**Usual adult dose**
Gastroesophageal reflux disease—
  Oral, 15 mg once a day for the relief of heartburn and regurgitation. For the treatment of erosive esophagitis, 30 mg once a day for eight weeks is recommended. An additional eight-week course may be helpful for patients who do not heal in the first eight weeks. For recurrence of erosive esophagitis, a third eight-week course of treatment may be considered. In patients requiring maintenance therapy, a dose of 15 mg once a day is recommended.
Ulcer, gastric—
  Oral, 15 to 30 mg once a day, preferably in the morning before breakfast, for up to eight weeks.
Ulcer, duodenal—
  Oral, 15 to 30 mg once a day, preferably in the morning before a meal, for up to four weeks. In patients requiring maintenance therapy, doses of 15 mg once a day have been used.
Ulcer, duodenal, associated with *H. pylori* infection—
  Oral, triple therapy regimens of lansoprazole 30 mg, plus amoxicillin 1 gram, plus clarithromycin 500 mg, in which all three medications are taken twice a day for fourteen days. For dual therapy regimens, lansoprazole 30 mg plus amoxicillin 1 gram, with both medications taken three times a day for fourteen days.

  Note: For the eradication of *H. pylori*, amoxicillin and clarithromycin should not be administered to patients with renal impairment since the appropriate dosage in this patient population has not yet been established.

Hypersecretory conditions, gastric, including Zollinger-Ellison syndrome—
  Oral, initially 60 mg once a day, preferably in the morning before a meal, the dosage being increased as needed, and therapy continued for as long as clinically indicated. Some patients have received doses as high as 90 mg two times a day for as long as four years. Daily dosages greater than 120 mg should be administered in divided doses.

Note: Dosage reduction should be considered in patients with severe hepatic function impairment; the dose generally should not exceed 30 mg a day in these patients.

**Usual adult prescribing limits**
For duodenal and gastric ulcers—
  30 mg a day.
For hypersecretory conditions—
  180 mg a day.

**Usual pediatric dose**
Safety and efficacy in children up to 18 years of age have not been established.

**Usual geriatric dose**
See *Usual adult dose*.

USP DI

**Usual geriatric prescribing limits**
30 mg a day.

**Strength(s) usually available**
U.S.—
  15 mg (Rx) [*Prevacid*].
  30 mg (Rx) [*Prevacid*].
Canada—
  15 mg (Rx) [*Prevacid*].
  30 mg (Rx) [*Prevacid*].

**Packaging and storage**
Store below 40 °C (104 °F), preferably between 15 and 30 °C (59 and 86 °F), unless otherwise specified by manufacturer. Store in a tight container.

**Auxiliary labeling**
• Take before a meal.

Developed: 05/29/96
Interim revision: 08/14/98

---

# LATANOPROST Ophthalmic—INTRODUCTORY VERSION

VA CLASSIFICATION (Primary): OP116
Commonly used brand name(s): *Xalatan*.
Note: For a listing of dosage forms and brand names by country availability, see *Dosage Forms* section(s).

## Category
Antiglaucoma agent (ophthalmic); antihypertensive, ocular.

## Indications

**Accepted**
Glaucoma, open-angle (treatment) or
Hypertension, ocular (treatment)—Latanoprost is indicated in the treatment of open-angle glaucoma or ocular hypertension in patients who are intolerant of other intraocular pressure (IOP)–lowering medications or insufficiently responsive (i.e., failed to achieve target IOP after multiple measurements over time) to another IOP-lowering medication. Latanoprost may be used alone or in combination with other antiglaucoma agents.

**Acceptance not established**
There is limited experience with latanoprost in the treatment of angle-closure, inflammatory, or neovascular glaucoma.

## Pharmacology/Pharmacokinetics

**Physicochemical characteristics**
Chemical group—Latanoprost is a prostaglandin $F_{2\text{-alpha}}$ analog.
Molecular weight—432.58.
pH—Approximately 6.7.

**Mechanism of action/Effect**
Latanoprost is a prostaglandin $F_{2\text{-alpha}}$ analog. It is believed to reduce intraocular pressure by increasing the outflow of aqueous humor. Studies suggest that the main mechanism of action is increased uveoscleral outflow.

**Absorption**
Latanoprost is an isopropyl ester prodrug. It is absorbed into the cornea, where it is hydrolyzed by esterases to latanoprost acid, which is biologically active.

**Distribution**
$Vol_D$—$0.16 \pm 0.02$ L per kg (L/kg). Latanoprost acid has been measured in aqueous humor during the first 4 hours and in plasma only during the first hour, following ophthalmic administration.

**Biotransformation**
Latanoprost is an isopropyl ester prodrug. It is hydrolyzed by esterases in the cornea to latanoprost acid, which is biologically active. The portion of the latanoprost acid that reaches the systemic circulation is metabolized primarily by the liver to 1,2-dinor and 1,2,3,4-tetranor metabolites by fatty acid beta-oxidation.

**Half-life**
The elimination of latanoprost acid from plasma is rapid (half-life 17 minutes) after either ophthalmic or intravenous administration.

**Onset of action**
Approximately 3 to 4 hours after administration.

**Time to peak concentration**
Peak concentration in the aqueous humor is reached approximately 2 hours after ophthalmic administration.

**Time to peak effect**
8 to 12 hours after administration.

**Elimination**
Metabolites are eliminated mainly via the kidneys. Approximately 88 or 98% of the administered dose can be recovered in the urine after ophthalmic or intravenous dosing, respectively.

## Precautions to Consider

**Carcinogenicity**
Latanoprost was not carcinogenic in mice and rats that were administered oral doses of up to 170 mcg per kg of body weight (mcg/kg) a day (approximately 2800 times the recommended maximum human dose) for up to 20 and 24 months, respectively.

**Mutagenicity**
Latanoprost was not mutagenic in bacteria, mouse lymphoma, or mouse micronucleus tests. *In vitro* and *in vivo* studies of unscheduled DNA synthesis in rats were negative. However, *in vitro* tests using human lymphocytes showed chromosome aberrations.

**Pregnancy/Reproduction**
Fertility—In animal studies, latanoprost was not found to have any effect on male or female fertility.
Pregnancy—Adequate and well-controlled studies in humans have not been done. Risk-benefit should be carefully considered when latanoprost is used during pregnancy.
In rabbits, 4 of 16 dams had no viable fetuses after receiving a dose approximately 80 times the maximum recommended human dose. The highest nonembryocidal dose in rabbits was approximately 15 times the maximum recommended human dose.
FDA Pregnancy Category C.

**Breast-feeding**
It is not known whether latanoprost or its metabolites are distributed into breast milk. Caution should be exercised when latanoprost is administered to nursing women.

**Pediatrics**
Appropriate studies on the relationship of age to the effects of latanoprost have not been performed in the pediatric population. Safety and efficacy have not been established.

**Geriatrics**
No information is available on the relationship of age to the effects of latanoprost in geriatric patients.

**Drug interactions and/or related problems**
The following drug interactions and/or related problems have been selected on the basis of their potential clinical significance (possible mechanism in parentheses where appropriate)—not necessarily inclusive (» = major clinical significance):

Note: Combinations containing any of the following medications, depending on the amount present, may also interact with this medication.

» Thimerosal-containing ophthalmic medications
  (precipitation occurs when latanoprost is applied concurrently with thimerosal-containing ophthalmic medications; an interval of at least 5 minutes should elapse between applications of these medications)

**Medical considerations/Contraindications**
The medical considerations/contraindications included have been selected on the basis of their potential clinical significance (reasons given in parentheses where appropriate)—not necessarily inclusive (» = major clinical significance).

*Except under special circumstances, this medication should not be used when the following medical problems exist:*
» Hypersensitivity to latanoprost
» Hypersensitivity to benzalkonium chloride

*Risk-benefit should be considered when the following medical problems exist:*
» Aphakia or
» Macular edema, including cystoid macular edema, risk factors for or
» Pseudophakia
(macular edema, including cystoid macular edema, has been reported during treatment with latanoprost, mainly in patients with aphakia, in patients with pseudophakia who have a torn posterior lens capsule, or in patients with known risk factors for macular edema; latanoprost should be used with caution in these patients)

Hepatic function impairment or
Renal function impairment
(studies have not been done in patients with hepatic or renal function impairment; therefore, caution should be used when administering latanoprost in these patients)

Iritis or
Uveitis
(latanoprost should be used with caution in patients with active intraocular inflammation [iritis/uveitis])

**Patient monitoring**
The following may be especially important in patient monitoring (other tests may be warranted in some patients, depending on condition; » = major clinical significance):

Ophthalmic examinations
(patients should be examined regularly and, depending on the clinical situation, treatment may be stopped if increased brown pigmentation of iris occurs)

## Side/Adverse Effects

Note: Changes in pigmented tissues may occur with use of latanoprost. Latanoprost may gradually change eye color by increasing the number of melanosomes (pigment granules) in the melanocytes, thereby increasing the amount of brown pigment in the iris. The mechanism of this increased pigmentation is probably not associated with proliferation of the melanocytes, but rather with stimulation of melanin production within the melanocytes of the iris stroma. The long-term effects on the melanocytes, the consequences of potential injury to the melanocytes, and the possibility of deposition of pigment granules to other areas of the eye are not known. The change in iris color occurs slowly and may not be noticeable for several months to years. Patients with mixed-color irides, such as blue-brown, gray-brown, green-brown, or yellow-brown, appear to be predisposed to the iris pigmentation changes. In addition, latanoprost has been reported to cause increased pigmentation of the periorbital tissue (eyelid). Also, latanoprost may gradually change eyelashes. The changes to the lashes include increased length, thickness, pigmentation, and the number of lashes. Patients should be advised of all the effects listed above and informed that if only one eye is treated with the medication, only one eye will be affected (heterochromia between the eyes). The changes in pigmentation and eyelash growth may be permanent.

Macular edema, including cystoid macular edema, has been reported during treatment with latanoprost, mainly in patients with aphakia, in patients with pseudophakia who have a torn posterior lens capsule, or in patients with known risk factors for macular edema. It is recommended that latanoprost be used with caution in these patients.

The following side/adverse effects have been selected on the basis of their potential clinical significance (possible signs and symptoms in parentheses where appropriate)—not necessarily inclusive:

**Those indicating need for medical attention**
Incidence more frequent
*Blurred vision; increased length, thickness, pigmentation, and number of eyelashes* (longer, thicker, and darker eyelashes); *increased pigmentation of iris* (increase in brown color in colored part of eye); *increased pigmentation of periorbital tissue* (darkening of eyelid skin color); *punctate epithelial keratopathy* (blurred vision, eye irritation, or tearing)

Incidence less frequent
*Allergic skin reaction* (skin rash); *angina pectoris or other chest pain; eye pain; eyelid crusting, redness, swelling, discomfort, or pain; pain in muscles, joints, or back; upper respiratory tract infection, cold, or flu* (cold or flu symptoms)

Incidence rare
*Conjunctivitis* (redness of eye or inside of eyelid); *diplopia* (double vision); *discharge from the eye; intraocular inflammation, such as iritis or uveitis* (eye pain, tearing, sensitivity of eye to light, redness of eye, or blurred vision or other change in vision); *macular edema, including cystoid macular edema* (blurred vision or other change in vision); *toxic epidermal necrolysis* (fever; pain in muscles; skin rash; sore throat)

**Those indicating need for medical attention only if they continue or are bothersome**
Incidence more frequent
*Burning of eye; conjunctival hyperemia* (redness of eye or inside of eyelid); *foreign body sensation* (feeling of something in eye); *itching of eye; stinging of eye*

Incidence less frequent
*Dryness of eye; photophobia* (increased sensitivity of eyes to light); *tearing*

## Overdose

For more information on the management of overdose or unintentional ingestion, **contact a Poison Control Center** (see *Poison Control Center Listing*).

**Clinical effects of overdose**
Other than ocular irritation or conjunctival or episcleral hyperemia, the ocular effects of high doses of latanoprost are not known.

Following intravenous doses of 3 mcg per kg of body weight (mcg/kg) in healthy volunteers (which produced mean plasma concentrations that were 200 times the mean plasma concentrations produced by the usual clinical dose), no adverse reactions were observed. However, intravenous doses of 5.5 to 10 mcg/kg caused abdominal pain, dizziness, fatigue, hot flushes, nausea, and sweating.

**Treatment of overdose**
Treatment of overdose should be symptomatic.

## Patient Consultation

As an aid to patient consultation, refer to *Advice for the Patient, Latanoprost (Ophthalmic)—Introductory Version*.

In providing consultation, consider emphasizing the following selected information (» = major clinical significance):

**Before using this medication**
» Conditions affecting use, especially:
Hypersensitivity to latanoprost, benzalkonium chloride, or any other ingredient in the product

Mutagenicity—*In vitro* tests using human lymphocytes showed chromosome aberrations

Breast-feeding—Caution should be exercised when latanoprost is administered to nursing women, since it is not known whether latanoprost or its metabolites are distributed into breast milk

Other medications, especially thimerosal-containing ophthalmic medications

Other medical problems, especially aphakia; macular edema, including cystoid macular edema, risk factors for; and pseudophakia

**Proper use of this medication**
» Using medication only as directed; not using more of it or using it more often than directed; to do so may increase absorption and the chance of side effects

If physician ordered two different eye drops to be used together, waiting at least 5 minutes between applications of medications to prevent second medication from "washing out" the first one

» Importance of regular visits to physician to check eye pressure during therapy

Removing contact lenses prior to administration of latanoprost; reinserting lenses, if desired, at least 15 minutes after administration

» Proper administration technique; preventing contamination; not touching applicator tip to any surface; keeping container tightly closed

» Proper dosing
Missed dose: Applying as soon as possible; not applying if not remembered until next day; applying regularly scheduled dose

» Proper storage

**Precautions while using this medication**
» Possibility of iris of eye becoming more brown in color; change in color of iris is usually noticeable within several months to years while using medication; in addition, possibility of the darkening of eyelid skin color; also, possibility of increased length, thickness, pigmentation, and the number of lashes; iris, eyelid, and lash pigmentation and other lash changes may be permanent even if medication is stopped; the color and lash changes will occur only to the eye being treated; if only one eye is treated, there is a possibility of having differently colored eyes and differently appearing eyelashes

Possibility of medication causing eyes to become more sensitive to light than they are normally; wearing sunglasses and avoiding too much exposure to bright light may help lessen discomfort

### Side/adverse effects
Signs of potential side effects, especially blurred vision; increased length, thickness, pigmentation, and number of eyelashes; increased pigmentation of iris; increased pigmentation of periorbital tissue; punctate epithelial keratopathy; allergic skin reaction; angina pectoris or other chest pain; eye pain; eyelid crusting, redness, swelling, discomfort, or pain; pain in muscles, joints, or back; upper respiratory tract infection, cold, or flu; conjunctivitis; diplopia; discharge from the eye; intraocular inflammation, such as iritis or uveitis; macular edema, including cystoid macular edema; or toxic epidermal necrolysis

## General Dosing Information
Latanoprost may be used alone or in combination with other antiglaucoma agents. If more than one ophthalmic medication is used, the medications should be administered at least 5 minutes apart.

Latanoprost contains benzalkonium chloride, which may be absorbed by contact lenses. Contact lenses should be removed prior to administration of latanoprost. Lenses may be reinserted 15 minutes after administration.

Once-daily dosing of latanoprost should not be exceeded. More frequent administration may decrease the intraocular pressure–lowering effect of the medication.

## Ophthalmic Dosage Forms
### LATANOPROST OPHTHALMIC SOLUTION
**Usual adult and adolescent dose**
Antiglaucoma agent (ophthalmic)
Antihypertensive, ocular—
  Topical, to the conjunctiva, 1 drop in the affected eye(s) once a day in the evening.

**Usual adult prescribing limits**
No more than one dose per day.

**Usual pediatric dose**
Safety and efficacy have not been established.

**Strength(s) usually available**
U.S.—
  0.005% (50 mcg per mL) (Rx) [*Xalatan* (benzalkonium chloride 0.02%; sodium chloride; sodium dihydrogen phosphate monohydrate; disodium hydrogen phosphate anhydrous; water for injection)].

Note: One drop contains approximately 1.5 mcg of latanoprost.

**Packaging and storage**
Store the unopened bottle between 2 and 8 °C (36 and 46 °F), unless otherwise specified by manufacturer. Protect from light.

**Stability**
Once the container has been opened, the medication may be stored at room temperature (up to 25 °C [77 °F]) for up to 6 weeks before discarding.

**Incompatibilities**
A precipitation occurs when latanoprost is applied concurrently with thimerosal-containing ophthalmic medications; an interval of at least 5 minutes should elapse between applications of these medications.

**Auxiliary labeling**
• For the eye.
• Keep container tightly closed.

Developed: 6/12/97
Interim revision: 08/13/98

---

**LAXATIVES**—The *Laxatives (Local)* monograph is not included in this published version of the USP DI database. Copies of the monograph are available on request from Micromedex, Inc. - Reprint Requests, 6200 S. Syracuse Way, Suite 300, Englewood, CO 80111; telephone (303) 486-6400; telefax (303) 486-6464; Email: USPDI@MDX.COM.

---

# LEPIRUDIN  Systemic—INTRODUCTORY VERSION

VA CLASSIFICATION (Primary): BL113
Commonly used brand name(s): *Refludan*.
Another commonly used name is hirudin, recombinant.
Note: For a listing of dosage forms and brand names by country availability, see *Dosage Forms* section(s).

## Category
Anticoagulant.

## Indications
**Accepted**
Thromboembolism, heparin-induced (treatment)—Lepirudin is indicated for anticoagulation in patients with heparin-induced thrombocytopenia and associated thromboembolic disease in order to prevent further thromboembolic complications.

## Pharmacology/Pharmacokinetics
Note: Pharmacokinetic behavior follows a two-compartment model.

**Physicochemical characteristics**
Source—Synthetic. Recombinant form of hirudin (a naturally occurring family of highly homologous isopolypeptides produced by the leech *Hirudo medicinalis*) that is produced by a recombinant DNA process involving yeast cells. A polypeptide composed of 65 amino acids, which differs from naturally occurring hirudin by substitution of leucine for isoleucine at the N-terminal end of the molecule and by absence of a sulfate group on the tyrosine at position 63.
Molecular weight—6979.5 daltons.
pH—Approximately 7.
Solubility—Freely soluble in water for injection or 0.9% sodium chloride injection.

**Mechanism of action/Effect**
A highly specific inhibitor of the thrombogenic activity of thrombin; one molecule of lepirudin binds to one molecule of thrombin. Produces dose-dependent increases in activated partial thromboplastin time (aPTT). Its action is independent of antithrombin III and it is not inhibited by platelet factor 4.

The pharmacodynamic response is directly related to lepirudin concentrations. No saturable effect has been observed at intravenous doses up to 500 mcg (0.5 mg) per kg of body weight.

**Distribution**
Essentially confined to extracellular fluids.

**Biotransformation**
Although conclusive data are not available, biotransformation is thought to involve release of amino acids via catabolic hydrolysis of the parent drug.

**Half-life**
Distribution—
  10 minutes.
Elimination—
  Young healthy volunteers: About 1.3 hours.
  Renal function impairment, severe (creatinine clearance less than 15 mL per minute): Up to 2 days.
  Hemodialysis: Up to 2 days.
Note: Elimination follows a first-order kinetics process.

**Elimination**
Renal, about 48% (35% unchanged).
  In dialysis—
    May be removable by hemofiltration or hemodialysis.
Note: Systemic clearance of lepirudin is proportional to the glomerular filtration rate (GFR) or creatinine clearance. Systemic clearance is about 25% lower in women than in men and about 20% lower in the elderly than in younger patients.

## Precautions to Consider

**Cross-sensitivity and/or related problems**
Patients sensitive to other hirudins may also be sensitive to lepirudin.

**Carcinogenicity**
Long-term studies in animals have not been done.

**Mutagenicity**
Lepirudin was not found to be genotoxic in the Ames test, the Chinese hamster cell (V79/HGPRT) forward mutation test, the A549 human cell line unscheduled DNA synthesis (UDS) test, the Chinese hamster V79 cell chromosome aberration test, or the mouse micronucleus test.

## Pregnancy/Reproduction

Fertility—Studies in male and female rats given intravenous doses up to 30 mg per kg of body weight (mg/kg) per day (180 mg per square meter of body surface area [mg/m$^2$] per day or 1.2 times the recommended maximum human total daily dose based on body surface area of 1.45 m$^2$ for a 50-kg subject) found no effect on fertility or reproductive performance.

Pregnancy—Adequate and well-controlled studies in humans have not been done.

Lepirudin has been found to cross the placenta after intravenous administration to pregnant rats. It is not known whether lepirudin crosses the placenta in humans.

Studies in rats and rabbits at intravenous doses up to 30 mg/kg per day (180 and 360 mg/m$^2$ per day or 1.2 and 2.4 times, respectively, the maximum recommended human total daily dose based on body surface area) found no evidence of fetal toxicity. However, an increase in maternal mortality due to undetermined causes was found in pregnant rats given 30 mg/kg per day during organogenesis and perinatal-postnatal periods.

FDA Pregnancy Category B.

## Breast-feeding

It is not known whether lepirudin is distributed into human breast milk. However, risk-benefit should be considered.

## Pediatrics

Safety and efficacy in pediatric patients have not been established. However, two children (11 and 12 years of age) were treated with lepirudin at doses ranging from 0.15 to 0.22 mg/kg per hour for 8 days, and 0.1 to 0.7 mg/kg per hour for 58 days, respectively, without serious adverse events.

## Geriatrics

Appropriate studies performed to date have not demonstrated geriatrics-specific problems that would limit the usefulness of lepirudin in the elderly. However, elderly patients are more likely to have age-related renal function impairment, which may require adjustment of dosage in patients receiving lepirudin.

Systemic clearance in elderly patients is about 20% lower than in younger patients.

## Drug interactions and/or related problems

The following drug interactions and/or related problems have been selected on the basis of their potential clinical significance (possible mechanism in parentheses where appropriate)—not necessarily inclusive (» = major clinical significance):

Note: Combinations containing any of the following medications, depending on the amount present, may also interact with this medication.

» Anticoagulants, coumarin- or indandione-derivative or
» Platelet aggregation inhibitors
 (concurrent use may increase the risk of bleeding; gradual reduction in dose/rate of lepirudin is recommended prior to switching to an oral anticoagulant)

» Thrombolytics, such as:
  Alteplase, recombinant
  Anistreplase
  Reteplase
  Streptokinase
  Urokinase
  (concurrent use may considerably increase the effect of lepirudin on activated partial thromboplastin time [aPTT] prolongation and increase the risk of bleeding complications such as intracranial bleeding)

## Laboratory value alterations

The following have been selected on the basis of their potential clinical significance (possible effect in parentheses where appropriate)—not necessarily inclusive (» = major clinical significance):

With physiology/laboratory test values
 Activated partial thromboplastin time (aPTT)
  (lepirudin dose-related increases occur)
 Thrombin time (TT)
  (increased even at low doses of lepirudin)

## Medical considerations/Contraindications

The medical considerations/contraindications included have been selected on the basis of their potential clinical significance (reasons given in parentheses where appropriate)—not necessarily inclusive (» = major clinical significance):

*Risk-benefit should be considered when the following medical problems exist:*

» Conditions associated with a possible increased risk of bleeding, including
  Anomaly of vessels or organs
  Bacterial endocarditis
  Bleeding, recent major (e.g., intracranial, gastrointestinal, intraocular, or pulmonary bleeding)
  Cerebrovascular accident, stroke, intracerebral surgery, or other neuraxial procedures, recent
  Hemorrhagic diathesis
  Hypertension, severe uncontrolled
  Puncture of large vessels or organ biopsy, recent
  Renal function impairment, severe
  Surgery, recent major
   (careful assessment of risk-benefit is recommended before initiation of treatment with lepirudin, because of the risk of life-threatening intracranial bleeding)

» Hepatic function impairment, severe, including cirrhosis
   (may increase the anticoagulant effect of lepirudin as a result of reduced generation of vitamin K–dependent coagulation factors)

» Renal function impairment, known or suspected (creatinine clearance less than 60 mL per minute or serum creatinine greater than 1.5 mg per deciliter)
   (dosage reduction of both the bolus intravenous injection and the intravenous infusion rate is recommended to prevent possible overdosage that may occur even with the standard dosing regimen)

» Sensitivity to lepirudin or other hirudins

## Patient monitoring

The following may be especially important in patient monitoring (other tests may be warranted in some patients, depending on condition; » = major clinical significance):

» Activated partial thromboplastin time (aPTT)
   (recommended prior to initiation of therapy, 4 hours after the start of the lepirudin infusion, and at least once a day during treatment; it is recommended that frequency of monitoring be increased in patients with renal function impairment, severe hepatic injury, or an increased risk of bleeding; the goal is to maintain the aPTT ratio [the patient's aPTT at a given time over an aPTT reference value, usually the median of the laboratory normal range for aPTT] between 1.5 and 2.5; it is recommended that lepirudin treatment not be initiated in patients with an aPTT ratio over 2.5 to avoid initial overdosing)

Note: At plasma lepirudin concentrations of 1500 nanograms per mL, the following aPTT ratios have been observed: nearly 3 for healthy volunteers, 2.3 for patients with heparin-induced thrombocytopenia, and 2.1 for patients with deep venous thrombosis.

Thrombin time (TT) is not suitable for routine monitoring of lepirudin therapy because TT has been found to exceed 200 seconds even at low plasma concentrations of lepirudin.

## Side/Adverse Effects

Note: Formation of *antihirudin antibodies* has been observed in about 40% of heparin-induced thrombocytopenia patients treated with lepirudin, which may increase the anticoagulant effect of lepirudin as a result of delayed renal elimination of active lepirudin-antihirudin complexes. Strict monitoring of aPTT is recommended during prolonged therapy. However, neither neutralization of lepirudin's effects nor allergic reactions associated with positive antibody test results have been observed.

*Intracranial bleeding* has been reported, but only in patients with acute myocardial infarction who were treated with both lepirudin and thrombolytic therapy (rt-PA or streptokinase). It has not been reported in patients treated with lepirudin alone.

The following side/adverse effects have been selected on the basis of their potential clinical significance (possible signs and symptoms in parentheses where appropriate)—not necessarily inclusive:

### Those indicating need for medical attention

Incidence more frequent
 ***Bleeding complications; including bleeding from puncture sites and wounds; and hematoma*** (collection of blood under the skin)

Incidence less frequent
 ***Allergic reaction*** (skin rash or itching); ***bleeding complications; including anemia*** (unusual tiredness); ***hematuria*** (blood in urine); ***gastrointestinal and rectal bleeding*** (black, tarry stools; blood in stools; vomiting of blood or material that looks like coffee grounds); ***coughing up blood; nosebleed; and vaginal bleeding; fever; heart failure*** (swell-

ing of feet or lower legs); *pneumonia* (fever or chills; cough; shortness of breath)

## Overdose

For more information on the management of overdose or unintentional ingestion, **contact a Poison Control Center** (see *Poison Control Center Listing*).

### Clinical effects of overdose
The following effects have been selected on the basis of their potential clinical significance (possible signs and symptoms in parentheses where appropriate)—not necessarily inclusive:

Acute
  *Bleeding complications*

### Treatment of overdose
Discontinue lepirudin immediately.

Determine aPTT and other coagulation factor levels as appropriate.

Determine hemoglobin and prepare for blood transfusion if necessary.

Treat patient for shock as necessary and appropriate.

There is some evidence that hemofiltration or hemodialysis (using high-flux dialysis membranes with a cutoff point of 50,000 daltons, e.g., AN/69) may be effective.

## General Dosing Information

In general, the dosage or infusion rate is adjusted according to the activated partial thromboplastin time (aPTT) ratio, which is the patient's aPTT at a given time over an aPTT reference value (usually the median of the laboratory normal range for aPTT). The target range for the aPTT ratio during treatment is 1.5 to 2.5, above which the risk of bleeding increases without an incremental increase in clinical efficacy.

It is recommended that lepirudin treatment not be initiated in patients with an aPTT ratio of over 2.5, to avoid initial overdosing.

Unless there is a clinical need to react immediately, it is recommended that any aPTT ratio that is out of the target range be confirmed at least once before altering the dose of lepirudin.

If the aPTT ratio is confirmed to be above 2.5, it is recommended that the lepirudin infusion be discontinued for 2 hours and the rate decreased by 50% when it is reinstituted (without repeating the initial bolus injection), followed by another determination of aPTT ratio 4 hours later.

If the aPTT ratio is confirmed to be below 1.5, it is recommended that the infusion rate be increased in increments of 20%, with determination of the aPTT ratio 4 hours after each increase.

When switching to oral anticoagulation, it is recommended that the dose of lepirudin be gradually reduced to produce an aPTT ratio just above 1.5 before initiation of oral anticoagulant therapy. Lepirudin may be discontinued as soon as the international normalized ratio (INR) reaches 2.

Lepirudin is almost exclusively excreted in the kidneys; therefore, the patient's renal function should be considered prior to administration. The initial intravenous injection and the continuous infusion rate must be reduced in case of known or suspected renal function impairment. Dosage adjustments should be based on creatinine clearance values, whenever available, as obtained from a reliable method (24-hour urine sampling). If creatinine clearance is not available, dosage adjustments should be based on serum creatinine values.

### Dosage adjustment in renal function impairment
The initial intravenous injection should be reduced to 0.2 mg per kg of body weight.

Adjustment of infusion rate:

| Creatinine clearance (mL/min) | Serum creatinine (mg/dL) | % of standard initial infusion rate | Infusion rate (mg/kg/hour) |
|---|---|---|---|
| 45 - 60 | 1.6 - 2 | 50% | 0.075 |
| 30 - 44 | 2.1 - 3 | 30% | 0.045 |
| 15 - 29 | 3.1 - 6 | 15% | 0.0225 |
| < 15 | > 6 | avoid or stop infusion | |

In hemodialysis patients or in case of acute renal failure, the lepirudin infusion should be avoided or stopped. Additional intravenous bolus injections at a dose of 0.1 mg per kg of body weight may be considered every other day, only if the aPTT ratio falls below the lower therapeutic limit of 1.5.

### Concomitant use with thrombolytic therapy
There is limited information on the combined use of lepirudin and thrombolytic agents. The following dosage regimen of lepirudin was used in nine patients with heparin-induced thrombocytopenia who presented with thromboembolic complications at baseline and were started on both lepirudin and thrombolytic therapy:
- Initial intravenous injection: 0.2 mg per kg of body weight
- Continuous intravenous infusion: 0.1 mg per kg of body weight per hour.

Concomitant treatment with thrombolytic agents may increase the risk of bleeding complications, including potentially life-threatening intracranial bleeding, and considerably enhance the effect of lepirudin on aPTT prolongation.

## Parenteral Dosage Forms

### LEPIRUDIN FOR INJECTION

#### Usual adult dose
Thromboembolism, heparin-induced (treatment)—
  Initial: Intravenous (slowly, for example over fifteen to twenty seconds), 400 mcg (0.4 mg) per kg of body weight (up to 44 mg), followed by—
  Intravenous infusion, at a rate of 150 mcg (0.15 mg) per kg of body weight per hour (up to 16.5 mg per hour, initially) for two to ten days or longer.

Note: Basing the initial dosage on the patient's body weight is valid for patients weighing up to 110 kg. However, for patients weighing more than 110 kg, the initial dosage should not be increased above 44 mg or the maximum infusion rate above 16.5 mg per hour.

Dosage is adjusted according to activated partial thromboplastin time (aPTT) ratio determinations.

Dosage adjustment in renal function impairment is recommended. See *General Dosing Information*.

Although lepirudin has been used in a few patients in combination with thrombolytic therapy, the dosage in such combination has not been established. See *General Dosing Information*.

#### Usual adult prescribing limits
In general, it is recommended that the infusion rate not exceed 0.21 mg per kg of body weight per hour without checking for coagulation abnormalities that might prevent an appropriate aPTT response.

#### Usual pediatric dose
Safety and efficacy have not been established.

Note: Two children (11 and 12 years of age) were treated with lepirudin at doses ranging from 150 to 220 mcg (0.15 to 0.22 mg) per kg of body weight per hour for eight days and 100 to 700 mcg (0.1 to 0.7 mg) per kg of body weight per hour for fifty-eight days, respectively, without serious adverse events.

#### Size(s) usually available
U.S.—
  50 mg (Rx) [*Refludan* (mannitol 40 mg; sodium hydroxide)].

#### Packaging and storage
Store unopened vials between 2 and 25 °C (36 and 77 °F).

#### Preparation of dosage form
Lepirudin for injection is reconstituted by adding 1 mL of water for injection or 0.9% sodium chloride injection to the 50-mg vial and shaking gently, producing a clear, colorless solution within a few seconds to less than 3 minutes.

For administration by intravenous injection (bolus), the reconstituted solution is further diluted by transferring the solution to a sterile, single-use syringe (of at least 10 mL capacity) and adding sufficient water for injection, 0.9% sodium chloride injection, or 5% dextrose injection to produce a total volume of 10 mL of a solution containing 5 mg of lepirudin per mL.

For administration by continuous intravenous infusion, the contents of two vials of reconstituted solution (total of 100 mg of lepirudin) are transferred into an infusion bag containing 500 mL or 250 mL of 0.9% sodium chloride injection or 5% dextrose injection, producing a solution containing 0.2 or 0.4 mg of lepirudin per mL, respectively.

#### Stability
It is recommended that any unused portion of a vial be discarded and that the reconstituted solution be used immediately. For administration by intravenous infusion, the reconstituted solution is stable for up to 24 hours at room temperature.

#### Incompatibilities
Mixing with other drugs is not recommended.

Developed: 08/07/98

# LETROZOLE Systemic—INTRODUCTORY VERSION

VA CLASSIFICATION (Primary): AN500
Commonly used brand name(s): *Femara*.
Note: For a listing of dosage forms and brand names by country availability, see *Dosage Forms* section(s).

## Category
Antineoplastic.

## Indications

**Accepted**

Carcinoma, breast (treatment)—Letrozole is indicated for treatment of advanced breast cancer in postmenopausal women with disease progression following antiestrogen therapy.

## Pharmacology/Pharmacokinetics

**Physicochemical characteristics**
Molecular weight—285.31.
Solubility—Freely soluble in dichloromethane, slightly soluble in ethanol, and practically insoluble in water.

**Mechanism of action/Effect**
Letrozole is a nonsteroidal competitive inhibitor of aromatase and thus, in postmenopausal women, inhibits conversion of adrenal androgens (primarily androstenedione and testosterone) to estrogens (estrone and estradiol) in peripheral tissues and cancer tissue. As a result, letrozole interferes with estrogen-induced stimulation or maintenance of growth of hormonally responsive (estrogen and/or progesterone receptor positive or receptor unknown) breast cancers.

**Other actions/effects**
In human liver microsomes, letrozole strongly inhibits the cytochrome P450 (CYP) isoenzyme 2A6 (CYP 2A6) and moderately inhibits the CYP isoenzyme 2C19 (CYP 2C19).
Letrozole has not been shown to affect synthesis of adrenal corticosteroids, aldosterone, or thyroid hormones.

**Absorption**
Rapidly and completely absorbed. Absorption is not affected by food.

**Distribution**
The volume of distribution ($Vol_D$) is approximately 1.9 liters per kg of body weight.

**Biotransformation**
Hepatic, by the CYP isoenzymes 3A4 and 2A6 (CYP 3A4 and CYP 2A6), to an inactive carbinol metabolite and its ketone analog.

**Half-life**
Terminal—
Approximately 2 days.

**Time to steady-state concentration**
Plasma—2 to 6 weeks.
Note: Steady-state plasma concentrations are 1.5 to 2 times higher than would be predicted on the basis of single-dose measurements, indicating some nonlinearity in letrozole's pharmacokinetics with daily administration. However, steady-state concentrations are maintained for extended periods, without further accumulation of letrozole.

**Elimination**
Renal, approximately 90% of a dose (approximately 75% as the glucuronide conjugate of the inactive metabolite, 9% as two unidentified metabolites, and 6% unchanged).

## Precautions to Consider

**Carcinogenicity**
A study in mice given doses of 0.6 to 60 mg per kg of body weight (mg/kg) per day by oral gavage (approximately 1 and 100 times, respectively, the maximum recommended daily human dose [MRHD] on a mg per square meter of body surface area [mg/m²] basis) for up to 2 years found a dose-related increase in the incidence of benign ovarian stromal tumors. When the high-dose group was excluded because of low survival rates, a significant trend in the incidences of hepatocellular adenoma and carcinoma was shown in females. A study in rats given oral doses of 0.1 to 10 mg/kg per day (approximately 0.4 and 40 times the MRHD on a mg/m² basis, respectively) for up to 2 years found an increase in the incidence of benign ovarian stromal tumors with 10 mg/kg per day. Ovarian hyperplasia was also seen in female rats given 0.1 mg/kg or more per day.

**Mutagenicity**
Letrozole demonstrated no mutagenic effects in *in vitro* tests (Ames and *E. coli* bacterial tests), but was found to be a potential clastogen in *in vitro* assays (CHO K1 and CCL 61 Chinese hamster ovary cells). It was not clastogenic *in vivo* (micronucleus test in rats).

**Pregnancy/Reproduction**
Fertility—Fertility studies in animals have not been done. However, in male and female mice, rats, and dogs receiving repeated dosing with 0.6, 0.1, and 0.03 mg/kg, respectively (approximately 1, 0.4, and 0.4 times the MRHD on a mg/m² basis, respectively), letrozole caused sexual inactivity in females and atrophy of the reproductive tract in males and females.

Pregnancy—Studies in humans have not been done. Letrozole is indicated for use in postmenopausal women only. However, if a pregnant woman is exposed to the medication, she should be apprised of the possibility of fetal harm and/or loss of the pregnancy.
Studies in rats given doses of 0.003 mg/kg (approximately 1/100 of the MHRD on a mg/m² basis) or more during the period of organogenesis found embryotoxicity and fetotoxicity, including intrauterine mortality, increased resorption, increased postimplantation loss, decreased numbers of live fetuses, and fetal anomalies including absence and shortening of renal papilla, dilation of ureter, edema, and incomplete ossification of frontal skull and metatarsals. Also, letrozole was teratogenic in rats, causing fetal domed head and cervical/centrum vertebral fusion at a dose of 0.03 mg/kg (approximately 1/20 of the MRHD on a mg/m² basis). Studies in rabbits found fetotoxicity at doses of 0.02 mg/kg (approximately 1/10,000 of the MRHD on a mg/m² basis) and embryotoxicity at doses of 0.002 mg/kg or greater (about 1/100,000 of the MRHD on a mg/m² basis). Fetal anomalies included incomplete ossification of the skull, sternebrae, and fore- and hindlegs.

FDA Pregnancy Category D.

**Breast-feeding**
It is not known whether letrozole is distributed into breast milk.

**Pediatrics**
No information is available on the relationship of age to the effects of letrozole in pediatric patients. Safety and efficacy have not been established.

**Geriatrics**
Clinical trials with letrozole included geriatric patients; the mean age in two randomized trials was 64 years, and 30% of the patients were 70 years of age or older. There were no differences in response between patients 70 years of age or older and younger patients. Also, no age-related effects on the pharmacokinetics of letrozole were found in studies that included patients ranging in age from 35 years to more than 80 years.

**Laboratory value alterations**
The following have been selected on the basis of their potential clinical significance (possible effect in parentheses where appropriate)—not necessarily inclusive (» = major clinical significance):

With physiology/laboratory test values
Calcium, serum
(concentrations may be increased in some patients)

Cholesterol, serum
(concentrations may be increased in some patients)

Alanine aminotransferase (ALT [SGPT]) and
Aspartate aminotransferase (AST [SGOT]) and
Gamma glutamyl transferase
(increases in serum values have been seen, but are most often associated with hepatic metastases)

**Medical considerations/Contraindications**
The medical considerations/contraindications included have been selected on the basis of their potential clinical significance (reasons given in parentheses where appropriate)—not necessarily inclusive (» = major clinical significance).

*Risk-benefit should be considered when the following medical problems exist:*
Hepatic function impairment
(although modest increases in letrozole blood concentrations have been observed in individuals with hepatic function impairment due to cirrhosis, no dosage adjustment is recommended in mild to moderate hepatic function impairment; studies in patients with severe hepatic function impairment have not been done but, since letrozole is eliminated by hepatic metabolism, caution is recommended)

Renal function impairment
(no dosage adjustment is necessary when creatinine clearance is 10 mL per minute or more)
Sensitivity to letrozole

### Side/Adverse Effects

Note: Most side effects are mild to moderate.

The following side/adverse effects have been selected on the basis of their potential clinical significance (possible signs and symptoms in parentheses where appropriate)—not necessarily inclusive:

**Those indicating need for medical attention**
Incidence less frequent (< 10%)
*Chest pain; dyspnea* (shortness of breath); *edema, peripheral* (swelling of feet or lower legs); *hypertension*—usually asymptomatic; *mental depression*
Incidence rare
*Thromboembolism* (pain in chest, groin, or legs, especially the calves; severe, sudden headache; slurred speech; sudden, unexplained shortness of breath; sudden loss of coordination; sudden, severe weakness or numbness in arm or leg; vision changes)—specific symptoms dependent on site of thromboembolism; *vaginal bleeding*

**Those indicating need for medical attention only if they continue or are bothersome**
Incidence more frequent (> 10%)
*Nausea*
Incidence less frequent (< 10%)
*Anorexia* (loss of appetite); *anxiety; arthralgia* (joint pain); *asthenia* (weakness); *constipation; cough; diarrhea; dizziness; headache; hot flashes* (sudden sweating and feeling of warmth); *increased sweating; myalgia* (muscle pain); *skin rash or itching; sleepiness; stomach pain or upset; unusual tiredness; vomiting; weight gain*

**Those not indicating need for medical attention**
Incidence less frequent (< 5%)
*Alopecia* (loss of hair)

### Overdose

For more information on the management of overdose or unintentional ingestion, **contact a Poison Control Center** (see *Poison Control Center Listing*).

**Clinical effects of overdose**
There is no human experience with overdose.
In mice and rats, lethality associated with reduced motor activity, ataxia, and dyspnea occurred with single oral doses of 2000 mg per kg of body weight (mg/kg) or over (approximately 4000 to 8000 times the maximum recommended daily human dose [MRHD] on a mg per square meter of body surface area [mg/m$^2$] basis). In cats, death preceded by depressed blood pressure and arrhythmias was caused by single intravenous doses of 10 mg/kg or greater (approximately 50 times the MRHD on a mg/m$^2$ basis).

**Treatment of overdose**
No specific treatment is recommended, although emesis could be induced if the patient is alert. Supportive care with frequent monitoring of vital signs is recommended.

### Patient Consultation

As an aid to patient consultation, refer to *Advice for the Patient, Letrozole (Systemic)—Introductory version*.
In providing consultation, consider emphasizing the following selected information (» = major clinical significance):

**Before using this medication**
» Conditions affecting use, especially:
Sensitivity to letrozole
Pregnancy—Intended for postmenopausal women only; accidental exposure during pregnancy may result in fetotoxicity and/or loss of the pregnancy

**Proper use of this medication**
» Compliance with prescribed regimen
» Proper dosing
Missed dose
» Proper storage

**Precautions while using this medication**
Importance of close monitoring by physician

**Side/adverse effects**
Stopping treatment and getting emergency help immediately if symptoms of thromboembolism occur
Signs of other potential side effects, especially chest pain, dyspnea, edema, hypertension, mental depression, and vaginal bleeding
Possibility of hair loss

### General Dosing Information

Letrozole has no effect on cortisol or aldosterone secretion; therefore, glucocorticoid or mineralocorticoid replacement therapy is not required.

### Oral Dosage Forms

**LETROZOLE TABLETS**

**Usual adult dose**
Carcinoma, breast—
Oral, 2.5 mg once a day.

**Usual geriatric dose**
Carcinoma, breast—
See *Usual adult dose*.

**Strength(s) usually available**
U.S.—
2.5 mg (Rx) [*Femara* (lactose monohydrate)].

**Packaging and storage**
Store between 15 and 30 °C (59 and 86 °F), preferably at 27 °C (81 °F).

Developed: 09/30/97

---

# LEUCOVORIN   Systemic

VA CLASSIFICATION (Primary/Secondary): VT102/AD900; BL400; AN400

Commonly used brand name(s): *Wellcovorin*.

Other commonly used names are citrovorum factor and folinic acid.

Note: For a listing of dosage forms and brand names by country availability, see *Dosage Forms* section(s).

### Category

Antidote (to folic acid antagonists); antianemic; antineoplastic adjunct.

### Indications

**Accepted**
Methotrexate toxicity (prophylaxis and treatment)
Pyrimethamine toxicity (prophylaxis and treatment) or
Trimethoprim toxicity (prophylaxis and treatment)—Leucovorin is indicated as an antidote to the toxic effects of folic acid antagonists such as methotrexate, pyrimethamine, or trimethoprim. Leucovorin also is indicated as a rescue after high-dose methotrexate therapy in osteosarcoma and as a part of chemotherapeutic treatment programs in the management of several forms of cancer.
Anemia, megaloblastic (treatment)—Leucovorin is indicated to treat megaloblastic anemias associated with sprue, nutritional deficiency, pregnancy, and infancy when oral folic acid therapy is not feasible.
Leucovorin is not recommended for use in the treatment of pernicious anemia or other megaloblastic anemias secondary to lack of vitamin B$_{12}$, since it may produce a hematologic remission while neurologic manifestations continue to progress.
Carcinoma, colorectal (treatment adjunct)—Leucovorin is indicated for use in combination with fluorouracil to prolong survival in the palliative treatment of patients with advanced colorectal cancer.

### Pharmacology/Pharmacokinetics

**Physicochemical characteristics**
Molecular weight—511.51.

**Mechanism of action/Effect**
Antidote (to folic acid antagonists)—Leucovorin is a reduced form of folic acid, which is readily converted to other reduced folic acid derivatives (e.g., tetrahydrofolate). Because it does not require reduction by dihy-

drofolate reductase as does folic acid, leucovorin is not affected by blockage of this enzyme by folic acid antagonists (dihydrofolate reductase inhibitors). This allows purine and thymidine synthesis, and thus DNA, RNA, and protein synthesis, to occur. Leucovorin may limit methotrexate action on normal cells by competing with methotrexate for the same transport processes into the cell. Leucovorin given at the appropriate time rescues bone marrow and gastrointestinal cells from methotrexate but has no apparent effect on pre-existing methotrexate nephrotoxicity.

**Absorption**
Rapidly absorbed after oral administration; saturation of absorption is reached at doses greater than 25 mg. Bioavailability is approximately 97% for a 25-mg dose, 75% for a 50-mg dose, and 37% for a 100-mg dose.

**Distribution**
Crosses blood-brain barrier in moderate amounts; largely concentrated in liver.

**Biotransformation**
Hepatic and intestinal mucosal, mainly to 5-methyltetrahydrofolate (active). After oral administration, leucovorin is substantially (greater than 90%) and rapidly (within 30 minutes) metabolized. Metabolism is less extensive (about 66% after intravenous and 72% after intramuscular administration) and slower with parenteral administration.

**Half-life**
Terminal half-life for total reduced folates—6.2 hours.

**Onset of action**
Oral—20 to 30 minutes.
Intramuscular—10 to 20 minutes.
Intravenous—Less than 5 minutes.

**Time to peak serum reduced folate concentration**
Oral—1.72 ± 0.8 hours.
Intramuscular—0.71 ± 0.09 hour.

**Peak serum reduced folate concentration**
After 15 mg dose—
  Oral: 268 ± 18 nanograms per mL (approximately 1 micromolar [$1 \times 10^{-6}$ Molar]).
  Intramuscular: 241 ± 17 nanograms per mL (approximately 1 micromolar [$1 \times 10^{-6}$ Molar]).

**Duration of action**
All routes—3 to 6 hours.

**Elimination**
Renal—80 to 90%.
Fecal—5 to 8%.

## Precautions to Consider

**Pregnancy/Reproduction**
Pregnancy—Studies have not been done in either animals or humans.
FDA Pregnancy Category C.
Recommended for treatment of megaloblastic anemia caused by pregnancy.

**Breast-feeding**
It is not known whether leucovorin is distributed into breast milk. However, problems in humans have not been documented.

**Pediatrics**
Leucovorin may increase the frequency of seizures in susceptible pediatric patients by counteracting the anticonvulsant effects of barbiturates, hydantoin anticonvulsants, and primidone.

**Geriatrics**
No information is available on the relationship of age to the effects of leucovorin in geriatric patients. However, elderly patients are more likely to have age-related renal function impairment, which may require adjustment of dosage in patients receiving leucovorin as a rescue from the effects of high-dose methotrexate.

**Drug interactions and/or related problems**
The following drug interactions and/or related problems have been selected on the basis of their potential clinical significance (possible mechanism in parentheses where appropriate)—not necessarily inclusive (» = major clinical significance):

Note: Combinations containing any of the following medications, depending on the amount present, may also interact with this medication.

Anticonvulsants, barbiturate or
Anticonvulsants, hydantoin or
Primidone
  (large doses of leucovorin may counteract the anticonvulsant effects of these medications)

Fluorouracil
  (concurrent use of leucovorin may increase the therapeutic and toxic effects of fluorouracil; although the two medications may be used together for therapeutic advantage, caution is necessary)

Sulfamethoxazole and trimethoprim
  (concurrent use of leucovorin may be associated with increased morbidity rates and treatment failure when used for the treatment of pneumonia due to *Pneumocystis carinii* in patients with human immunodeficiency virus (HIV) infection)

**Medical considerations/Contraindications**
The medical considerations/contraindications included have been selected on the basis of their potential clinical significance (reasons given in parentheses where appropriate)—not necessarily inclusive (» = major clinical significance).

*Except under special circumstances, this medication should not be used when the following medical problems exist:*

For treatment of anemia (as the sole agent)
» Pernicious anemia or
» Vitamin $B_{12}$ deficiency
  (may produce a partial hematologic response while neurologic manifestations continue to progress)

*This medication should be used with caution when the following medical problems exist:*

Sensitivity to leucovorin

**Patient monitoring**
The following may be especially important in patient monitoring (other tests may be warranted in some patients, depending on condition; » = major clinical significance):

*For patients receiving high-dose methotrexate*

» Creatinine clearance determinations
  (recommended prior to initiation of high-dose methotrexate with leucovorin rescue therapy or if serum creatinine concentrations increase by 50% or more)

» Creatinine concentrations, serum
  (recommended prior to and every 24 hours after each methotrexate dose, until plasma or serum methotrexate concentrations are less than $5 \times 10^{-8}$ Molar, to detect developing renal function impairment and predict methotrexate toxicity. An increase of greater than 50% over the pretreatment concentration at 24 hours is associated with severe renal toxicity)

» Methotrexate concentrations, plasma or serum
  (recommended by some clinicians every 12 to 24 hours after high-dose methotrexate administration to determine dose and duration of leucovorin treatment needed to maintain rescue. May aid in identifying patients with delayed methotrexate clearance; toxicity appears to be related at least as much to the length of time that methotrexate concentrations are elevated as to the peak concentrations achieved. In general, monitoring should continue until concentrations are less than $5 \times 10^{-8}$ Molar)

» pH determinations, urine
  (recommended prior to each dose of high-dose methotrexate therapy and about every 6 hours throughout leucovorin rescue, until plasma or serum methotrexate concentrations are less than $5 \times 10^{-8}$ Molar, to ensure that pH remains greater than 7 so as to minimize the risk of methotrexate nephropathy from precipitation of methotrexate or metabolites in urine)

## Side/Adverse Effects

The following side/adverse effects have been selected on the basis of their potential clinical significance (possible signs and symptoms in parentheses where appropriate)—not necessarily inclusive:

**Those indicating need for medical attention**
Incidence rare
  *Allergic reaction* (skin rash, hives, or itching; wheezing); *seizures*—reported with use in cancer chemotherapy

## Patient Consultation

As an aid to patient consultation, refer to *Advice for the Patient, Leucovorin (Systemic)*.

In providing consultation, consider emphasizing the following selected information (» = major clinical significance):

**Before using this medication**
» Conditions affecting use, especially:
  Sensitivity to leucovorin
  Use in children—May increase frequency of seizures in susceptible pediatric patients

Other medical problems, especially pernicious anemia or vitamin $B_{12}$ deficiency (for treatment of anemia as the sole agent)

**Proper use of this medication**
» Importance of taking as directed and not missing doses; taking at evenly spaced times
» Checking with physician before discontinuing medication or if vomiting occurs shortly after dose is taken
» Proper dosing
  Missed dose: Checking with physician right away; possible need for additional leucovorin; importance of not increasing dose unless directed by physician
» Proper storage

**Side/adverse effects**
Signs of potential side effects, especially allergic reaction and seizures

## General Dosing Information

A 15-mg dose produces a serum reduced folate concentration of approximately 1 micromolar ($1 \times 10^{-6}$ Molar).

**For use as an antidote to folic acid antagonists**
Patients receiving leucovorin as a "rescue" from the toxic effects of methotrexate should be under supervision of a physician experienced in high-dose methotrexate therapy.

Leucovorin should be administered orally or parenterally. Leucovorin should not be administered intrathecally for the treatment of accidental overdoses of intrathecally administered folic acid antagonists. *Leucovorin may be harmful or fatal if administered intrathecally.*

Parenteral administration of leucovorin is recommended if it appears that absorption may be impaired as a result of nausea and vomiting.

*High-dose methotrexate administration should not be initiated unless leucovorin is physically present and ready to be administered, since rescue is critical.*

A variety of dosage schedules of leucovorin in combination with high-dose methotrexate have been used. Since this regimen is still largely investigational, the prescriber should consult the medical literature in choosing a specific dosage. Alkalinization of urine (with bicarbonate and/or acetazolamide) and intravenous hydration (1000 mL per square meter of body surface area over six hours prior to beginning the methotrexate infusion and 3000 mL per square meter of body surface area per day during the methotrexate infusion and for two days after the infusion is completed) are also important to prevent renal toxicity caused by methotrexate and/or its metabolites.

Administration of leucovorin should be consecutive to rather than simultaneous with methotrexate administration so as not to interfere with methotrexate's antineoplastic effects. However, leucovorin has been administered simultaneously with pyrimethamine and trimethoprim in oral or intramuscular doses ranging from 400 mcg (0.4 mg) to 5 mg to prevent megaloblastic anemia due to high doses of these medications.

In general, it is recommended that the first dose of leucovorin be administered within the first 24 to 42 hours of starting a high-dose methotrexate infusion (within 1 hour of an overdose), in a dosage to produce blood concentrations equal to or greater than methotrexate blood concentrations (leucovorin in a dose of 15 mg produces peak plasma concentrations of approximately 1 micromolar [$1 \times 10^{-6}$ Molar]). Duration of leucovorin administration varies with the dosage of methotrexate and plasma concentrations achieved (including rate of elimination); in general, leucovorin administration is continued until methotrexate concentrations fall to less than $5 \times 10^{-8}$ Molar.

A larger dose and/or longer duration of leucovorin treatment may be required in patients with aciduria, ascites, dehydration, gastrointestinal obstruction, renal function impairment, or pleural or peritoneal effusions because excretion of methotrexate is slowed and the length of time for plasma methotrexate concentrations to decrease to nontoxic levels ($<5 \times 10^{-8}$ Molar) is increased. It is recommended that duration of leucovorin administration in these patients be based on determination of plasma methotrexate concentrations.

**For use as an adjunct to fluorouracil for colorectal carcinoma**
Patients receiving leucovorin in combination with fluorouracil should be under supervision of a physician experienced in cancer chemotherapy.

## Oral Dosage Forms

Note: The dosing and strengths of the dosage forms available are expressed in terms of leucovorin base (not the calcium salt).

### LEUCOVORIN CALCIUM TABLETS USP

**Usual adult and adolescent dose**
Antidote (to folic acid antagonists)—
  To methotrexate—
    Oral, 10 mg (base) per square meter of body surface area every six hours until methotrexate blood concentrations fall to less than $5 \times 10^{-8}$ M.
  To pyrimethamine or trimethoprim—
    Prevention—Oral, 400 mcg (0.4 mg) to 5 mg (base) with each dose of the folic acid antagonist.
    Treatment—Oral, 5 to 15 mg (base) per day.
Megaloblastic anemia, secondary to folate deficiency—
  Oral, up to 1 mg (base) per day.
Note: Doses higher than 25 mg should be given parenterally because oral absorption is saturable at doses above 25 mg.

**Usual pediatric dose**
See *Usual adult and adolescent dose.*

**Strength(s) usually available**
U.S.—
  5 mg (base) (Rx) [*Wellcovorin* (scored) [GENERIC (scored)].
  15 mg (base) (Rx) [GENERIC (scored)].
  25 mg (base) (Rx) [*Wellcovorin* (scored)].
Canada—
  5 mg (base) (Rx) [GENERIC (scored)].
  15 mg (base) (Rx) [GENERIC (scored)].

**Packaging and storage**
Store below 40 °C (104 °F), preferably between 15 and 30 °C (59 and 86 °F), in a well-closed container. Protect from light.

## Parenteral Dosage Forms

Note: The dosing and strengths of the dosage forms available are expressed in terms of leucovorin base (not the calcium salt).

### LEUCOVORIN CALCIUM INJECTION USP

**Usual adult and adolescent dose**
Antidote (to folic acid antagonists)—
  To methotrexate (inadvertent overdose)—
    Intramuscular or intravenous, 10 mg (base) per square meter of body surface area every six hours until methotrexate blood concentrations fall to less than $5 \times 10^{-8}$ Molar.
Note: If, at 24 hours following methotrexate administration, the serum creatinine is increased by 50% or greater over baseline or serum methotrexate is greater than $5 \times 10^{-6}$ Molar, the dose of leucovorin should be 100 mg (base) per square meter of body surface area every three hours intravenously until methotrexate concentrations are reduced to appropriate levels.
  To pyrimethamine or trimethoprim—
    Prevention—Intramuscular, 400 mcg (0.4 mg) to 5 mg (base) with each dose of the folic acid antagonist.
    Treatment—Intramuscular, 5 to 15 mg (base) per day.
Megaloblastic anemia, secondary to folate deficiency—
  Intramuscular, up to 1 mg (base) per day.
Note: Because of its calcium content, leucovorin calcium injection should be administered by intravenous injection slowly, at a rate that does not exceed 160 mg of leucovorin per minute.

**Usual pediatric dose**
See *Usual adult and adolescent dose.*

**Strength(s) usually available**
U.S.—
  Not commercially available.
Canada—
  10 mg (base) per mL (Rx) [GENERIC (without preservative)].

**Packaging and storage**
Store in the refrigerator between 2 and 8 °C (36 and 46 °F). Protect from light.

**Stability**
Intravenous solutions containing leucovorin calcium in lactated Ringer's injection, Ringer's injection, or 0.9% sodium chloride injection are stable for up to 24 hours at room temperature. When diluted in 5% dextrose in water injection or 10% dextrose injection, intravenous solutions containing leucovorin calcium are stable for 12 hours at room temperature. When diluted in 10% dextrose in 0.9% sodium chloride injection, solutions are stable for 6 hours at room temperature.

**Incompatibilities**
Leucovorin calcium injection is incompatible with fluorouracil; precipitation will occur if these agents are combined in the same infusion solution.

## LEUCOVORIN CALCIUM FOR INJECTION

### Usual adult and adolescent dose
Antidote (to folic acid antagonists)—
  To methotrexate (inadvertent overdose)—
    Intramuscular or intravenous, 10 mg (base) per square meter of body surface area every six hours until methotrexate blood concentrations fall to less than $5 \times 10^{-8}$ Molar.
  Note: If, at 24 hours following methotrexate administration, the serum creatinine is increased 50% over baseline or serum methotrexate is greater than $5 \times 10^{-6}$ Molar, the dose of leucovorin should be 100 mg (base) per square meter of body surface area every three hours intravenously until methotrexate concentrations are reduced to appropriate levels. *Only solutions prepared with sterile water for injection (i.e., without benzyl alcohol) should be used for doses greater than 10 mg per square meter of body surface area.*
  To pyrimethamine or trimethoprim—
    Prevention—Intramuscular, 400 mcg (0.4 mg) to 5 mg (base) with each dose of the folic acid antagonist.
    Treatment—Intramuscular, 5 to 15 mg (base) per day.
Megaloblastic anemia, secondary to folate deficiency—
  Intramuscular, up to 1 mg (base) per day.
Carcinoma, colorectal (treatment adjunct)—
  Intravenous, 200 mg per square meter of body surface area over a minimum of three minutes, followed by fluorouracil 370 mg per square meter of body surface area intravenously, or
  Intravenous, 20 mg per square meter of body surface area, followed by fluorouracil 425 mg per square meter of body surface area intravenously.
  Either regimen is given daily for five days, and the course may be repeated at four-week intervals for two courses and then at four- to five-week intervals, as determined by toxicity to the previous course.
  Note: Only solutions prepared with sterile water for injection (i.e., without benzyl alcohol) should be used, since the dose is greater than 10 mg per square meter of body surface area.
    Because of its calcium content, leucovorin calcium for injection should be administered by intravenous injection slowly, at a rate that does not exceed 160 mg of leucovorin per minute.

### Usual pediatric dose
Antidote (to folic acid antagonists) or
Megaloblastic anemia—See *Usual adult and adolescent dose*.
Carcinoma, colorectal (treatment adjunct)—Dosage has not been established.

### Size(s) usually available
U.S.—
  50 mg (base) (Rx) [GENERIC (without preservative)].
  100 mg (base) (Rx) [*Wellcovorin* (without preservative) [GENERIC (without preservative)].
  350 mg (base) (Rx) [GENERIC (without preservative)].
Canada—
  50 mg (base) (Rx) [GENERIC (without preservative)].
  100 mg (base) (Rx) [GENERIC (without preservative)].
  350 mg (base) (Rx) [GENERIC (without preservative)].

### Packaging and storage
Prior to reconstitution, store below 40 °C (104 °F), preferably between 20 and 25 °C (68 and 77 °F), unless otherwise specified by manufacturer. Protect from light.

### Preparation of dosage form
Leucovorin calcium for injection is prepared for parenteral use by adding 5 or 10 mL of bacteriostatic water for injection (preserved with benzyl alcohol) to the vial containing 50 or 100 mg (base), respectively, producing a solution containing 10 mg per mL. If doses greater than 10 mg per square meter of body surface area are to be used, sterile water for injection should be used for reconstitution and the resulting solution used immediately.
Caution: Use of diluents containing benzyl alcohol is not recommended for preparation of medications for use in neonates. A fatal toxic syndrome consisting of metabolic acidosis, CNS depression, respiratory problems, renal failure, hypotension, and possibly seizures and intracranial hemorrhages has been associated with this use.

### Stability
Reconstituted solutions prepared with bacteriostatic water for injection (preserved with benzyl alcohol) should be used within 7 days. Intravenous solutions containing leucovorin calcium in 10% dextrose injection, 10% dextrose in 0.9% sodium chloride injection, lactated Ringer's injection, or Ringer's injection have been found to maintain at least 90% of labeled potency when used within twenty-four hours.

### Incompatibilities
Leucovorin calcium for injection is incompatible with fluorouracil; precipitation will occur if these agents are combined in the same infusion solution.

Revised: 07/23/92
Interim revision: 11/17/93; 07/05/94; 04/11/95; 09/30/97

# LEUPROLIDE Systemic

INN: Leuprorelin
BAN: Leuprorelin
VA CLASSIFICATION (Primary/Secondary): HS900/AN500
Commonly used brand name(s): *Lupron; Lupron Depot; Lupron Depot-3 Month 11.25 mg; Lupron Depot-3 Month 22.5 mg; Lupron Depot-4 Month 30 mg; Lupron Depot-Ped; Lupron-3 Month SR Depot 22.5 mg.*
Note: For a listing of dosage forms and brand names by country availability, see *Dosage Forms* section(s).

## Category
Gonadotropin-releasing hormone analog; antiendometriotic agent; antineoplastic; gonadotropin inhibitor.

## Indications
Bracketed information in the *Indications* section refers to uses that are not included in U.S. product labeling.

### Accepted
Anemia due to uterine leiomyomas (treatment)[1]—Leuprolide, in conjunction with iron supplement therapy, is indicated for the preoperative hematologic improvement of patients with anemia caused by uterine leiomyomas (fibroids). Because some patients respond to iron supplementation alone, a 1-month trial period with iron should be considered prior to initiation of leuprolide therapy. Leuprolide may then be added if the response to iron supplementation is inadequate.
Carcinoma, prostatic (treatment)—Leuprolide is indicated for the palliative treatment of advanced prostatic cancer, especially as an alternative to orchiectomy or estrogen administration.
Endometriosis (treatment)—Leuprolide is indicated for management of endometriosis, including pain relief and reduction of endometriotic lesions.
Puberty, precocious, central (treatment)—Leuprolide is indicated for the treatment of central precocious puberty (CPP, idiopathic or neurogenic) in children with the onset of secondary sexual characteristics before the age of 8 years in females and 9 years in males. Prior to initiation of leuprolide therapy, clinical diagnosis should be confirmed by a prepubertal response to a gonadorelin stimulation test and by bone age that is advanced 1 year beyond the chronological age. Diagnosis of CPP should be confirmed before initiation of treatment with leuprolide by measuring serum sex steroids, height and weight, and basal gonadotropin levels, and by testing stimulation response to gonadorelin, assessing diagnostic imaging of the brain (including pituitary and hypothalamus), and performing pelvic ultrasound examinations.
Before beginning treatment for CPP with leuprolide, it is especially important to confirm that the patient is willing to comply with dosing requirements and the frequent monitoring required by the physician during the first 6 to 8 weeks of treatment to assure that suppression of gonadal-pituitary function is rapid.
[Carcinoma, breast (treatment)][1]—Leuprolide is indicated in the palliative treatment of advanced breast carcinoma in premenopausal and perimenopausal women.

[1]Not included in Canadian product labeling.

## Pharmacology/Pharmacokinetics
Note: Pharmacokinetic studies of leuprolide use in children have not been done.

### Physicochemical characteristics
Source—Synthetic gonadotropin-releasing hormone (GnRH) analog.
Molecular weight—Leuprolide acetate: 1269.48.

### Mechanism of action/Effect
Like naturally occurring luteinizing hormone–releasing hormone (LHRH), initial or intermittent administration of leuprolide stimulates release of luteinizing hormone (LH) and follicle-stimulating hormone (FSH) from the anterior pituitary.

Prostatic carcinoma—LH and FSH release from the anterior pituitary transiently increases testosterone and dihydrotestosterone concentrations in males. However, continuous administration of leuprolide in the treatment of prostatic carcinoma suppresses secretion of gonadotropin-releasing hormone, with a resultant fall in testosterone concentrations and a pharmacologic castration.

Anemia due to uterine leiomyomas; endometriosis; or breast carcinoma— Initial stimulation of gonadotropins from the anterior pituitary is followed by prolonged suppression. Gonadotropin release from the anterior pituitary transiently increases estrone and estradiol concentrations in premenopausal females. However, continuous administration of leuprolide produces a decrease in estradiol, estrone, and progesterone concentrations to postmenopausal levels. As a consequence of suppression of ovarian function, both normal and ectopic endometrial tissues become inactive and atrophic. As a result, amenorrhea occurs.

Central precocious puberty—After an initial stimulation of gonadotropins and increase in the rate of pubertal development, testosterone and estradiol concentrations in males and females, respectively, decrease to prepubertal levels with continuous administration of therapeutic doses of leuprolide in children. Stimulated and basal gonadotropin concentrations also are reduced to prepubertal levels. As a result, menses stop, reproductive organ development decreases, and bone age velocity approaches normal, improving the child's chance of attaining the predicted adult height. Upon discontinuation of leuprolide, gonadotropins return to pubertal levels and natural maturation resumes.

### Other actions/effects
Leuprolide also has some androgenic effects in females.

### Absorption
Bioavailability after intramuscular injection of the depot formulation is estimated to be about 90%.

### Distribution
The mean steady-state volume of distribution following a single intravenous dose in healthy male volunteers was 27 L.

### Protein binding
Moderate (46%).

### Biotransformation
Metabolized to smaller inactive peptides, Metabolite I (a pentapeptide), Metabolites II and III (tripeptides), and Metabolite IV (a dipeptide).

### Half-life
Approximately 3 hours following a 1-mg intravenous dose in healthy male volunteers.

### Onset of action
Transient increases in testosterone and estradiol concentrations occur within the first week of therapy; a decline to castrate and postmenopausal levels, respectively, occurs within 2 to 4 weeks.

### Time to peak concentration
3.75-mg depot—4 hours.
7.5-mg depot—4 hours.
22.5-mg depot—4 hours.

### Peak plasma concentration
3.75-mg depot—4.6 to 10.2 nanograms per mL (nanograms/mL).
7.5-mg depot—20 nanograms/mL.
22.5-mg depot—48.9 nanograms/mL.

### Time to peak effect
Amenorrhea—Usually occurs after 1 to 2 months of therapy.

### Duration of action
Pituitary-gonadal system—Normal function is usually restored within 4 to 12 weeks after therapy is withdrawn.
Amenorrhea—Cyclic bleeding usually returns within 60 to 90 days after therapy is withdrawn.

### Elimination
Less than 5% of a 3.75-mg dose was recovered in the urine as parent drug and Metabolite I.

## Precautions to Consider

### Cross-sensitivity and/or related problems
Patients sensitive to gonadorelin (GnRH) or to gonadotropin-releasing hormone analogs (GnRHa), such as buserelin, goserelin, histrelin, and nafarelin, may be sensitive to leuprolide also.

### Carcinogenicity
Adults treated with doses of leuprolide as high as 10 mg a day for up to 3 years and 20 mg a day for up to 2 years have not shown clinical abnormalities of the pituitary.

Studies in rats and mice for 2 years at daily subcutaneous doses of 0.6 to 4 mg per kg of body weight (mg/kg) and up to 60 mg/kg, respectively, found an increased incidence of benign pituitary hyperplasia and benign pituitary adenomas at 24 months in the rats. Also, there was a significant, but not dose-related, increase of pancreatic islet-cell adenomas in female rats and, at the lower dose, interstitial cell adenomas in the testes of male rats.

### Mutagenicity
Mutagenicity studies in bacterial and mammalian systems found no evidence of mutagenic effects.

### Pregnancy/Reproduction
Fertility—In adult males: Suppression of testosterone secretion results in impairment of fertility. However, studies in adults administered leuprolide and similar analogs have shown reversal of fertility suppression when the medications were discontinued after continuous administration for periods of up to 24 weeks.

In adult females: Leuprolide usually induces anovulation and amenorrhea. This effect is reversible and the average time to return of menses is about 60 to 90 days following withdrawal of therapy. A nonhormonal contraceptive method should be used during leuprolide therapy.

Male and female children: Long-term posttreatment follow-up studies of fertility in children treated for central precocious puberty (CPP) have not been done.

Animal studies of adult and prepubertal rats and monkeys given leuprolide or other GnRH analogs showed functional reproductive recovery. Immature male and female rats given leuprolide in one study were normal when compared with controls, even though the histologic investigation showed that tubular degeneration in the testes occurred after a recovery period. The offspring of both sexes appeared normal.

Pregnancy—Leuprolide is not recommended for use during pregnancy; spontaneous abortion may occur.

Studies in rabbits at doses of 0.00024, 0.0024, and 0.024 mg/kg (1/600 to 1/6 the human adult dose; 1/1200 to 1/12 the human pediatric dose) on day 6 of pregnancy found a dose-related increase in major fetal abnormalities; these effects did not occur at similar doses in rats. The two higher doses in rabbits and the highest dose in rats were associated with increased fetal mortality and decreased fetal weights.

FDA Pregnancy Category X.

### Breast-feeding
It is not known whether leuprolide passes into breast milk. However, because of potential adverse effects in the infant, breast-feeding is usually not recommended during treatment with leuprolide.

### Pediatrics
Studies performed to date have not demonstrated pediatrics-specific problems that would limit the usefulness of leuprolide in children.

### Geriatrics
Appropriate studies on the relationship of age to the effects of leuprolide have not been performed in the geriatric population. However, this medication is frequently used in elderly patients, especially for treatment of prostatic carcinoma, and geriatrics-specific problems that would limit the usefulness of this medication in the elderly are not expected.

### Laboratory value alterations
The following have been selected on the basis of their potential clinical significance (possible effect in parentheses where appropriate)—not necessarily inclusive (» = major clinical significance):

With diagnostic test results
» Gonadal function testing and
» Pituitary gonadotropic function testing
(therapeutic doses of leuprolide suppress the pituitary-gonadal feedback regulatory system; baseline function usually is restored within 3 months after discontinuation of treatment)

With physiology/laboratory test values
Acid phosphatase
(transient increases in values may occur early in treatment of prostatic carcinoma, but usually decrease to or near baseline by the fourth week)

Alanine aminotransferase (ALT [SGPT]) and
Alkaline phosphatase and
Aspartate aminotransferase (AST [SGOT]) and
Lactate dehydrogenase (LDH)
(values may be increased)
Estradiol
(serum concentrations usually are increased during the first weeks of therapy in adult females but then decrease to postmenopausal levels)
Low-density liproprotein (LDL) cholesterol and
Total cholesterol and
Triglycerides
(concentrations may be increased)
Platelet counts and
White blood cell counts
(may decrease; platelet count decrease may be transient, returning to normal during treatment)
Testosterone
(serum concentrations are usually increased during the first week of therapy for prostatic carcinoma but then decrease; castrate levels are reached within 2 to 4 weeks)

**Medical considerations/Contraindications**
The medical considerations/contraindications included have been selected on the basis of their potential clinical significance (reasons given in parentheses where appropriate)—not necessarily inclusive (» = major clinical significance).

*Risk-benefit should be considered when the following medical problems exist:*
Sensitivity to gonadorelin (synthetic gonadotropin-releasing hormone [GnRH]); gonadotropin-releasing hormone analogs (GnRHa), such as buserelin, goserelin, histrelin, leuprolide, and nafarelin; or benzyl alcohol
*For treatment of endometriosis or of anemia due to uterine leiomyomas*
Conditions causing decrease in bone density or
Osteoporosis, or history of, or family history of
(hypoestrogenism-induced loss of bone mineral density may occur in females treated with leuprolide and may be irreversible; major risk factors include chronic alcohol and/or tobacco abuse, family history of severe osteoporosis, and chronic use of medications, such as anticonvulsants or corticosteroids, that decrease bone mineral density; leuprolide should be used with caution in these patients)
» Uterine bleeding, undiagnosed abnormal
(use of leuprolide may delay diagnosis)
*For treatment of prostatic carcinoma*
» Urinary tract obstruction or history of
(existing urinary tract obstruction should be treated before beginning treatment with leuprolide; for patients with a history of urinary tract obstruction, there is an increased incidence of disease flare during initial leuprolide treatment because of the initial increase in serum testosterone concentrations; close monitoring is recommended during the first month of treatment; catheterization may be necessary on occurrence)
» Vertebral metastases
(worsening of symptoms during first few weeks of leuprolide therapy, with risk of neurologic problems, including paralysis)

**Patient monitoring**
The following may be especially important in patient monitoring (other tests may be warranted in some patients, depending on condition; » = major clinical significance):
Bone density assessment
(recommended as needed to monitor patient's response during long-term use of leuprolide, including treatment of endometriosis for longer than 6 months)
*For treatment of central precocious puberty*
Bone linear growth velocity and bone age velocity determinations and
Imaging studies
(recommended prior to treatment initiation and periodically during treatment, beginning 3 to 6 months after treatment initiation; diagnostic imaging studies should include radiography of the left hand and wrist [or nondominating hand and wrist] for bone age determination, pelvic ultrasonography, and magnetic resonance imaging of the brain)
Dehydroepiandrosterone concentrations, serum and/or
Estradiol concentrations, serum and/or
Follicle-stimulating hormone concentrations, serum and/or
Human chorionic gonadotropin concentrations, serum and/or
Hydroxyprogesterone concentrations, serum and/or
Luteinizing hormone concentrations, serum and/or
Prolactin concentrations, serum and/or
Testosterone concentrations, serum
(recommended prior to treatment initiation to establish prepubertal gonadotropin response. If gonadal-pituitary function suppression is not apparent within 6 to 8 weeks after therapy with leuprolide is initiated and lack of patient compliance is ruled out, leuprolide should be discontinued and the diagnosis of gonadotropin-independent sexual precocity should be reconsidered. Other possible causes of sexual precocity include adrenal hyperplasia, testoxicosis, and hypothalamic or testicular tumors)
Gonadotropin-releasing hormone stimulation test
(recommended prior to treatment initiation to establish prepubertal gonadotropin response)
Pregnancy test
(recommended if treatment is not started during menstruation and in patients with irregular menstrual cycles)
*For treatment of endometriosis*
Pregnancy test
(recommended for females of reproductive potential if treatment is not started during menstruation, if irregular menstrual cycles exist, or if a scheduled dose is delayed)
*For treatment of prostatic carcinoma*
Acid phosphatase concentrations, plasma prostatic or serum and/or
Prostate-specific antigen (PSA) concentrations, serum and/or
Testosterone concentrations, serum
(recommended at periodic intervals to monitor response)
Bone scans
(recommended as needed to monitor response in patients at risk for vertebral metastases)
Imaging studies
(intravenous pyelogram, computerized tomography [CT] scan, and/or ultrasonography may be used to diagnose or assess patients at risk for obstructive uropathy; these are especially useful during the first week of therapy)

## Side/Adverse Effects

Note: Many of the side/adverse effects of leuprolide are related to hypoestrogenism in females and hypotestosteronism in males. The reversibility of clinical hypogonadism produced by leuprolide has not been established for long-term use.

There is a risk of increased loss of vertebral trabecular bone density during treatment for endometriosis or for anemia due to uterine leiomyomas; this loss may be irreversible. However, the loss usually is small when the treatment period is limited to 3 months (for fibroids) or 6 months (for endometriosis), except in patients with existing risk factors (e.g., history of osteoporosis). Compared to pretreatment bone density values, bone density values measured by dual energy x-ray absorptiometry (DEXA) decreased by 3.9% for patients treated for endometriosis at 6 months; a 12-month measurement, 6 months after leuprolide discontinuation, showed the decrease as 2% in these patients. Decreased bone density also has been reported in men who have had orchiectomy or who have been treated with a gonadotropin–releasing hormone analog.

The following side/adverse effects have been selected on the basis of their potential clinical significance (possible signs and symptoms in parentheses where appropriate)—not necessarily inclusive:

**Those indicating need for medical attention**
Incidence less frequent—> 5%
*In adult females and males*
***Cardiac arrhythmias or palpitations*** (fast or irregular heartbeat)— up to 19% in males

Incidence rare—< 5%
*In adult females and males*
***Anaphylaxis*** (changes in facial skin color; fast or irregular breathing; puffiness or swelling of the eyelids or around the eyes; shortness of breath, troubled breathing, tightness in chest, and/or wheezing; skin rash, hives, and/or itching; sudden, severe decrease in blood pressure and collapse); ***bone, muscle, or joint pain, continuing; paresthesias*** (numbness or tingling of hands or feet); ***syncope*** (fainting)

*In adult females only*
***Androgenic effects*** (deepening of voice; increased hair growth); ***personality or behavioral changes*** (anxiety; mental depression; mood changes; nervousness)

*In adult males only*
***Angina or myocardial infarction*** (pains in chest); ***pulmonary em-***

bolism (sudden shortness of breath); ***thrombophlebitis*** (pains in groin or legs, especially calves of legs)

*In pediatric females and males*
   ***Body pain; injection site reactions*** (burning, itching, redness, or swelling at place of injection); ***skin rash***

*In pediatric females—expected within first few weeks*
   ***Uterine bleeding, continuing*** (vaginal bleeding); ***vaginal discharge, continuing*** (white vaginal discharge)

**Those indicating need for medical attention only if they continue or are bothersome**
Incidence more frequent—> 50%

*In adult females and males*
   ***Hot flashes*** (sudden sweating and feelings of warmth)

*In adult females only*
   ***Amenorrhea*** (stopping of menstrual periods); *or* ***spotting*** (light, irregular vaginal bleeding)

Incidence less frequent–5 to 13%

*In adult females and males*
   ***Blurred vision; decreased libido*** (decreased interest in sexual intercourse); ***dizziness; edema*** (swelling of feet or lower legs); ***headache; injection site reaction*** (burning, itching, redness, or swelling at place of injection); ***nausea or vomiting; swelling or increased tenderness of breasts; trouble in sleeping; weight gain***

*In adult females only*
   ***Endometriotic disease flare, transient*** (pelvic pain); ***vaginitis*** (burning, dryness, or itching of vagina)

Note: *An endometriotic disease flare*, with a transient increase in symptoms (pelvic pain, dysmenorrhea, dyspareunia, pelvic tenderness, induration), may occur shortly after initiation of therapy for endometriosis as a result of the temporary increase in serum estradiol.

*In adult males only*
   ***Constipation; decreased size of testicles; prostatic carcinoma disease flare, transient*** (bone pain); ***impotence*** (inability to have or keep an erection)

Note: *A prostatic carcinoma disease flare*, with a transient, sometimes severe, increase in bone or tumor pain, may occur shortly after initiation of therapy for prostatic carcinoma, usually associated with the increase in serum testosterone, but usually subsides with continued leuprolide treatment. Analgesics may be required during this time. Other signs and symptoms of prostatic carcinoma, including difficult urination and spinal compression, may also worsen transiently. In addition, worsening of neurologic signs and symptoms in patients with vertebral metastases may result in temporary weakness and paresthesias of the lower extremities; paralysis, with or without fatal complications, is possible.

## Patient Consultation

As an aid to patient consultation, refer to *Advice for the Patient, Leuprolide (Systemic)*.

In providing consultation, consider emphasizing the following selected information (» = major clinical significance):

### Before using this medication
» Conditions affecting use, especially:
   Sensitivity to gonadorelin (GnRH), leuprolide or other GnRH analogs (GnRHa), or to other ingredients in the product's formulation, such as benzyl alcohol
   Pregnancy/reproduction
      For females and males: May impair fertility by suppressing sperm production in males and causing anovulation in most females, usually reversible after discontinuation
      For females: Not recommended for use during pregnancy; may cause spontaneous abortion, causes birth defects in animals
   Breast-feeding—Not recommended for use in nursing mothers
   Other medical problems, especially undiagnosed abnormal vaginal bleeding (for endometriosis or uterine leiomyomas), urinary tract obstruction (for prostatic carcinoma), or vertebral metastases (for prostatic carcinoma)

### Proper use of this medication
» Carefully reading patient instruction sheet contained in package
   Using disposable syringes provided in kit
» Importance of not using more or less medication than the amount prescribed
» Importance of continuing medication despite side effects
» Proper dosing
   Missed dose:
      For daily dosing—Using as soon as remembered; not using if not remembered until next day; not doubling doses
      For monthly or every 3 to 4 months dosing—Receiving as soon as remembered; returning to normal dosing schedule
» Proper storage

### Precautions while using this medication
» Importance of close monitoring by the physician
*For treatment of endometriosis or of anemia due to uterine leiomyomas*
   Possibility of amenorrhea or irregular menstrual periods; checking with physician if regular menstruation does not occur within 60 to 90 days after discontinuation of medication
   Notifying physician if regular menstruation persists during treatment; however, missing one or more successive doses of leuprolide may result in breakthrough menstrual bleeding
   Advisability of using nonhormonal forms of contraception during therapy; not using oral contraceptives
» Stopping medication and checking with physician if pregnancy is suspected

### Side/adverse effects
Signs of potential side effects, especially cardiac arrhythmias or palpitations (adults); anaphylaxis (adults); bone, muscle, or joint pain (adults); paresthesias (adults); syncope (adults); androgenic effects in females (adults); personality or behaviorial changes in females (adults); angina or myocardial infarction in males (adults); pulmonary embolism in males (adults); thrombophlebitis in males (adults); body pain (children); injection site reactions (children); skin rash (children); uterine bleeding in females, continuing (children); and vaginal discharge, continuing (children)

## General Dosing Information

It is recommended that the intramuscular depot injection be administered by the physician. Parents or guardians may be instructed in how to give the subcutaneous injections at home to their child. Injection sites should be rotated periodically.

Leuprolide has approximately 15 to 50 times the activity of naturally occurring luteinizing hormone–releasing hormone (LHRH), and 80 to 100 times that of gonadotropin–releasing hormone (gonadorelin).

### For treatment of anemia due to uterine leiomyomas
Therapy should continue uninterrupted for 3 months. Re-treatment is not recommended. However, if re-treatment is contemplated, bone density should be assessed prior to beginning treatment to verify that values are in the normal range.

### For treatment of central precocious puberty
Dose must be individualized for each patient and titrated upward until patient's pituitary-gonadal axis is suppressed, according to clinical and/or laboratory parameters. Usually the dose that adequately suppresses the pituitary-gonadal axis is appropriate for the entire therapy; however, there are insufficient data to guide dosage adjustments as a child's weight changes, a special concern for children who started therapy at a very early age at a low dose. Careful monitoring for suppression of the pituitary-gonadal axis is required, especially 1 or 2 months after treatment initiation or following changes in dose.

If the patient responds and tolerates leuprolide therapy, treatment should continue until resumption of puberty is desired. Discontinuation of leuprolide therapy should be considered before the age of 11 years in females and 12 years in males. Normal function of pituitary-gonadal axis is restored within 4 to 12 weeks after treatment discontinuation.

### For treatment of endometriosis
It is recommended that therapy begin with the first day of the menstrual cycle after pregnancy has been ruled out.

Development of amenorrhea is usually evidence of a clinical response, although spotting or bleeding from the atrophic endometrium can still occur.

Therapy should continue uninterrupted for 6 months. Re-treatment is not recommended. However, if re-treatment is contemplated, bone density should be assessed prior to beginning treatment to verify that values are in the normal range.

### For treatment of prostatic carcinoma
Patients receiving leuprolide should be under supervision of a physician experienced in cancer chemotherapy.

Isolated short-term worsening of neurologic symptoms may contribute to paralysis with or without fatal complications in patients with vertebral metastases. For patients at risk, therapy may be initiated with daily leuprolide injection for the first 2 weeks to observe patient reaction, since worsening of symptoms occasionally requires discontinuation of therapy and possible surgical intervention.

**1844   Leuprolide (Systemic)**

**For treatment of adverse effects**
Recommended treatment:
- Bone pain—Mild oral analgesics with rest or, if severe, parenteral narcotics. Bone pain usually subsides after 2 weeks.
- Urinary obstruction, worsening of, in treatment of prostatic carcinoma—Catheterization. Urinary obstruction usually disappears after the first week of leuprolide therapy.

## Parenteral Dosage Forms

### LEUPROLIDE ACETATE INJECTION

**Usual adult dose**
Carcinoma, prostatic—
  Subcutaneous, 1 mg per day.

**Usual pediatric dose**
Puberty, precocious, central—
  Subcutaneous, initially 50 mcg per kg of body weight per day as a single injection, increased as needed by increments of 10 mcg per kg of body weight per day to a maintenance dose. Younger children require larger doses on a mcg per kg of body weight basis; dose should be increased as weight increases throughout treatment.

**Strength(s) usually available**
U.S.—
  5 mg per mL (Rx) [*Lupron* (sodium chloride 6.3 mg; benzyl alcohol 9 mg; water for injection)].
Note: Packaging is labeled as *Lupron 14 Day Patient Administration Kit* (2.8 mL multiple dose vial and 1/2 cc 28-gauge 1/2-inch syringes) or *Lupron 28 Day Patient Administration Kit* (double the supplies of *Lupron 14 Day Patient Administration Kit*). Insulin syringes may be used also if volume is appropriately adjusted.
Canada—
  5 mg per mL (Rx) [*Lupron* (benzyl alcohol)].
  Note: Packaging includes multiple dose vial of 2.8 mL.

**Packaging and storage**
In U.S.: Store below 25 °C (77 °F), unless otherwise specified by manufacturer. In Canada: Store between 2 and 8 °C (36 and 46 °F) before dispensing and between 15 and 30 °C (59 and 86 °F) after dispensing, unless otherwise specified by manufacturer. Protect from freezing. Protect from light.

**Stability**
Do not use if cloudy or discolored.

**Auxiliary labeling**
- Do not freeze.

### LEUPROLIDE ACETATE FOR INJECTION

Note: Due to different release characteristics, a fractional dose of the 3-month or 4-month depot formulations is not equivalent to the same dose of the 1-month depot formulation and should not be given in its place.

**Usual adult dose**
Anemia due to uterine leiomyomas[1]—
  Intramuscular, 3.75 mg once a month for a maximum duration of three months or one 11.25-mg injection.
Carcinoma, prostatic—
  Intramuscular, 7.5 mg once a month, 22.5 mg once every three months (eighty-four days), or 30 mg every four months.
Endometriosis—
  Intramuscular, 3.75 mg once a month or 11.25 mg every three months for a maximum duration of six months.

**Usual pediatric dose**
Puberty, precocious, central—
  Initial:
    Intramuscular, 0.3 mg per kg of body weight every four weeks, using a minimum total dose of 7.5 mg every four weeks.
    For children weighing ≤ 25 kg—Intramuscular, 7.5 mg every four weeks.
    For children weighing 25 to 37.5 kg—Intramuscular, 11.25 mg every four weeks.
    For children weighing > 37.5 kg—Intramuscular, 15 mg every four weeks.
  Maintenance:
    The dose may be increased as needed by increments of 3.75 mg every four weeks, up to a maximum total dose of 15 mg every four weeks.

**Size(s) usually available**
U.S.—
  1-month release formulation
    3.75 mg vial [*Lupron Depot*].
    7.5 mg vial (Rx) [*Lupron Depot; Lupron Depot-Ped*].
    11.25 mg vial (Rx) [*Lupron Depot-Ped*].
    15 mg vial (Rx) [*Lupron Depot-Ped*].
Note: Packaged as single-use vial kits for *Lupron Depot 7.5 mg* and single-use vial kits and prefilled dual-chamber syringe kits for *Lupron Depot 3.5 mg* and for all pediatric formulations. Kits include alcohol swabs and syringes. All packaging includes the diluent. Inactive ingredients may differ among products and their diluents.
  3-month release formulation
    11.25 mg vial [*Lupron Depot-3 Month 11.25 mg*].
    22.5 mg vial (Rx) [*Lupron Depot-3 Month 22.5 mg*].
  4-month release formulation
    30 mg vial (Rx) [*Lupron Depot-4 Month 30 mg*].
Canada—
  1-month release formulation
    3.75 mg vial [*Lupron Depot*].
    7.5 mg vial (Rx) [*Lupron Depot*].
    11.25 mg vial (Rx) [*Lupron Depot*].
    15 mg vial (Rx) [*Lupron Depot*].
  3-month release formulation
    22.5 mg vial (Rx) [*Lupron-3 Month SR Depot 22.5 mg*].
Note: Packaging of single-use vial kits includes alcohol swabs and syringes. All packaging includes the diluent. Inactive ingredients may differ among products and their diluents.

**Packaging and storage**
Store between 15 and 30 °C (59 and 86 °F), unless otherwise specified by manufacturer. Protect from freezing.

**Preparation of dosage form**
Vial and ampule—Leuprolide acetate for injection is reconstituted with an appropriate volume of diluent provided by the manufacturer; the suspension should be shaken thoroughly to disperse particles evenly.
Prefilled dual-chamber syringe—For reconstitution, the manufacturer's instructions should be followed to release the diluent into the chamber of lyophilized microspheres. The suspension is then shaken gently to disperse the particles evenly.

**Stability**
Since leuprolide for injection and the diluent contain no preservatives, the reconstituted suspension should be used immediately after preparation and any unused portion should be discarded.

**Auxiliary labeling**
- Do not freeze.
- Shake well (after reconstitution).

---

[1]Not included in Canadian product labeling.

Revised: 07/07/98

# LEVAMISOLE   Systemic

VA CLASSIFICATION (Primary/Secondary): IM700/AN400
Commonly used brand name(s): *Ergamisol*.
Note: For a listing of dosage forms and brand names by country availability, see *Dosage Forms* section(s).

## Category
Biological response modifier; antineoplastic adjunct.

## Indications

### Accepted
Carcinoma, colorectal (treatment adjunct)—Levamisole is indicated, in combination with fluorouracil, for treatment of Dukes C adenocarcinoma of the colon (i.e., with regional lymph node involvement) after complete resection of primary tumor, with no gross or microscopic evidence of residual disease and no evidence of distant metastases or remaining local metastases that could not be removed en bloc with the

primary resection. It is not useful for therapy of advanced and metastatic disease.

## Pharmacology/Pharmacokinetics

**Physicochemical characteristics**
Molecular weight—240.75.

**Mechanism of action/Effect**
Not precisely known. Levamisole appears to act as an immunorestorative agent in the presence of immunosuppression resulting from recent surgery and chemotherapy, but does not stimulate the immune response to above normal levels. May be related to T-cell activation and proliferation, augmentation of monocyte and macrophage activity (including phagocytosis and chemotaxis), and an increase in neutrophil mobility, adherence, and chemotaxis. Does not have cytotoxic effects.

**Other actions/effects**
Anthelmintic. Also has cholinergic, mood-elevating, and, at high doses, convulsant effects. Inhibits alkaline phosphatase in animals.

**Absorption**
Rapidly absorbed from gastrointestinal tract.

**Biotransformation**
Hepatic, extensive.

**Half-life**
Levamisole—3 to 4 hours.
Metabolites—16 hours.

**Time to peak plasma concentration**
1.5 to 2 hours.

**Elimination**
Renal, 70% over 3 days (less than 5% unchanged); fecal, 5% (less than 0.2% unchanged).

## Precautions to Consider

**Carcinogenicity**
Adequate studies in animals have not been done. Studies at doses of 5, 20, and 80 mg per kg of body weight (mg/kg) per day for up to 18 months in mice and up to 24 months in rats found no evidence of carcinogenicity; however, these studies were not conducted at the maximum tolerated dose, and there is a possibility that the animals may not have been exposed to a reasonable drug challenge. Chronic administration of high doses (25 mg/kg) in New Zealand Black mice increased the rate and intensity of spontaneous lymphomas. No carcinogenic effect was found in 12- to 18-month studies in dogs.

**Mutagenicity**
Levamisole was not found to be mutagenic in dominant lethal studies in male and female mice, in an Ames test, and in a study to detect chromosomal aberrations in cultured peripheral human lymphocytes.

**Pregnancy/Reproduction**
Fertility—Administration through 3 generations of rats and rabbits did not affect fertility. No adverse effects on male or female fertility were noted in rats given oral doses of 2.5, 10, 40, and 160 mg/kg. In a rat gavage study at doses of 20, 60, and 180 mg/kg, the copulation period was increased, the duration of pregnancy was slightly increased, and fertility, pup viability and weight, lactation index, and number of fetuses were decreased at a dose of 60 mg/kg. No adverse reproductive effects occurred when the offspring were allowed to mate and litter.

Pregnancy—Adequate and well-controlled studies in humans have not been done.

Studies in rats and rabbits at oral doses up to 180 mg/kg found no evidence of fetal malformations. Embryotoxicity occurred at doses of 160 mg/kg in rats and was significant in rabbits at doses of 180 mg/kg.

FDA Pregnancy Category C.

**Breast-feeding**
It is not known whether levamisole is distributed into human breast milk; however, it is distributed into cows' milk.

**Pediatrics**
No information is available on the relationship of age to the effects of levamisole in pediatric patients. Safety and efficacy have not been established.

**Geriatrics**
Appropriate studies on the relationship of age to the effects of levamisole have not been performed in the geriatric population. However, clinical trials were conducted in older patients and geriatrics-specific problems that would limit the usefulness of this medication in the elderly are not expected.

**Dental**
The leukopenic effects of levamisole may result in an increased incidence of microbial infection, delayed healing, and gingival bleeding. If leukopenia occurs, dental work should be deferred until blood counts have returned to normal and patients should be instructed in proper oral hygiene, including caution in use of regular toothbrushes, dental floss, and toothpicks.

Levamisole may also cause mild stomatitis associated with discomfort (severe stomatitis may occur during combination therapy with fluorouracil).

**Drug interactions and/or related problems**
The following drug interactions and/or related problems have been selected on the basis of their potential clinical significance (possible mechanism in parentheses where appropriate)—not necessarily inclusive (» = major clinical significance):

Note: Combinations containing any of the following medications, depending on the amount present, may also interact with this medication.

Anticoagulants, coumarin
(there have been reports of prolongation of the prothrombin time beyond the therapeutic range with concurrent use; monitoring of prothrombin time and adjustment of anticoagulant dose, if necessary, are recommended)

Bone marrow depressants (see *Appendix II*) or
Radiation therapy
(leukopenic and/or thrombocytopenic effects of bone marrow depressants or radiation may be increased with concurrent or recent therapy if levamisole causes the same effects; dosage adjustment of the bone marrow depressant, if necessary, should be based on blood counts)

**Medical considerations/Contraindications**
The medical considerations/contraindications included have been selected on the basis of their potential clinical significance (reasons given in parentheses where appropriate)—not necessarily inclusive (» = major clinical significance).

*Risk-benefit should be considered when the following medical problems exist:*
» Bone marrow depression
(may be increased)
» Infection
(may be worsened because of bone marrow depression)
Seizure disorder
(incidence of seizures associated with levamisole therapy may be increased)
» Sensitivity to levamisole

**Patient monitoring**
The following may be especially important in patient monitoring (other tests may be warranted in some patients, depending on condition; » = major clinical significance):

Alanine aminotransferase (ALT [SGPT]) values, serum and
Alkaline phosphatase values, serum, and
Aspartate aminotransferase (AST [SGOT]) values, serum and
Bilirubin values, serum
(recommended prior to initiation of therapy and at 3, 6, 9, and 12 months after initiation of therapy)

» Complete blood counts, including differential and platelets
(recommended prior to initiation of therapy and before each dose of fluorouracil; although leukopenia is not an indication for withdrawal of levamisole, it is an indication for delaying administration of fluorouracil)

Electrolyte concentrations, serum
(recommended prior to initiation of therapy and 3, 6, 9, and 12 months after initiation of therapy)

Monitoring for tumor recurrence or second primary, which may include:
Carcinoembryonic antigen (CEA)
Chest x-ray
Computed tomographic (CT) scan of abdomen and pelvis
» Colonoscopy or double contrast barium enema x-ray
» History and physical examination
Proctosigmoidoscopy
(prior to initiation of therapy and at periodic intervals during therapy)

## Side/Adverse Effects

Note: Frequency of side effects listed is for levamisole alone. Side effects are usually mild. Incidence of most side effects, especially hematological and gastrointestinal effects, is more frequent with combination treatment with fluorouracil, although not more frequent than would be expected with fluorouracil alone.

The following side/adverse effects have been selected on the basis of their potential clinical significance (possible signs and symptoms in parentheses where appropriate)—not necessarily inclusive:

### Those indicating need for medical attention
Incidence less frequent
  **Blood dyscrasias, including agranulocytosis or leukopenia** (fever or chills; cough or hoarseness; lower back or side pain; painful or difficult urination); *or thrombocytopenia* (unusual bleeding or bruising; black, tarry stools; blood in urine or stools; pinpoint red spots on skin)—usually asymptomatic; *flu-like syndrome* (fever; chills; unusual feeling of discomfort or weakness); *mild stomatitis* (sores in mouth and on lips)—more frequent with combination treatment with fluorouracil

  Note: *Agranulocytosis* is an idiosyncratic-allergic effect. Sudden onset; commonly preceded by and associated with flu-like syndrome, but may be asymptomatic. Reversible, usually within 7 to 10 days, after levamisole therapy is withdrawn. Sometimes fatal.

  *Leukopenia* is not associated with bone marrow function impairment. Usually does not develop into agranulocytosis and leukocyte counts usually recover even with continued levamisole therapy (does not apply to combination therapy with fluorouracil).

  The *flu-like syndrome* is commonly associated with agranulocytosis and may be an early sign of agranulocytosis, but may also occur in the absence of agranulocytosis; also an allergic-type reaction; usually occurs within hours of a dose; may be mild and transient or severe and progressive.

Incidence rare
  **Central nervous system toxicity, specifically ataxia** (trouble in walking); *blurred vision; confusion; paranoia; paresthesias* (numbness, tingling, or pain in face, hands, or feet); *seizures; tardive dyskinesia* (lip smacking or puckering; puffing of cheeks; rapid or worm-like movements of tongue; uncontrolled movements of arms and legs); *or tremors; cerebrospinal fluid (CSF) pleiocytosis* (blurred vision; fever); *hepatotoxicity*—not symptomatic

### Those indicating need for medical attention only if they continue or are bothersome
Incidence more frequent
  *Diarrhea; metallic taste; nausea*

Incidence less frequent
  *Arthralgia or myalgia* (pain in joints or muscles); *central nervous system (CNS) effects, specifically anxiety or nervousness; dizziness; headache; insomnia; mental depression; nightmares; or unusual tiredness or sleepiness; dermatitis* (skin rash or itching); *vomiting*

  Note: A life-threatening *exfoliative dermatitis* has been reported.

### Those not indicating need for medical attention
Incidence less frequent
  *Alopecia* (loss of hair)

## Overdose
For more information on the management of overdose or unintentional ingestion, **contact a Poison Control Center** (see *Poison Control Center Listing*).

### Treatment of overdose
Recommended treatment of overdose includes gastric lavage with symptomatic and supportive treatment.

## Patient Consultation
As an aid to patient consultation, refer to *Advice for the Patient, Levamisole (Systemic)*.

In providing consultation, consider emphasizing the following selected information (» = major clinical significance):

### Before using this medication
» Conditions affecting use, especially:
    Sensitivity to levamisole
    Other medical problems, especially infection

### Proper use of this medication
» Importance of not taking more or less medication than the amount prescribed
  Checking with physician if vomiting occurs shortly after dose is taken
» Proper dosing
  Missed dose: Not taking at all; not doubling doses; checking with physician
» Proper storage

### Precautions while using this medication
» Importance of close monitoring by the physician

### Side/adverse effects
  Signs of potential side effects, especially leukopenia, agranulocytosis, flu-like syndrome, stomatitis, and thrombocytopenia
  Physician or nurse can help in dealing with side effects

## General Dosing Information
Patients receiving levamisole should be under supervision of a physician experienced in cancer therapy.

If agranulocytosis occurs in patients receiving levamisole alone, it is recommended that levamisole be discontinued. However, if leukopenia (leukocyte count of 2500–3500) occurs, single-agent levamisole therapy may be continued with careful monitoring.

Patients who develop leukopenia should be observed carefully for signs of infection. Antibiotic support may be required. In neutropenic patients who develop fever, broad-spectrum antibiotic coverage should be initiated empirically, pending bacterial cultures and appropriate diagnostic tests.

Special precautions are recommended in patients who develop thrombocytopenia as a result of administration of levamisole. These may include extreme care in performing invasive procedures; regular inspection of intravenous sites, skin (including perirectal area), and mucous membrane surfaces for signs of bleeding or bruising; limiting frequency of venipuncture and avoiding intramuscular injections; testing urine, emesis, stool, and secretions for occult blood; care in use of regular toothbrushes, dental floss, toothpicks, safety razors, and fingernail and toenail cutters; avoiding constipation; and using caution to prevent falls and other injuries. Such patients should avoid alcohol and aspirin intake because of the risk of gastrointestinal bleeding. Platelet transfusions may be required.

### For use in combination with fluorouracil for colorectal carcinoma
Fluorouracil therapy should be discontinued promptly if the patient develops stomatitis or diarrhea. If stomatitis or diarrhea develops during weekly therapy, the next dose of fluorouracil should be withheld until it has resolved. If these effects are moderate to severe, a 20% reduction in dosage is recommended when fluorouracil therapy is resumed.

If leukopenia occurs, the following adjustments in fluorouracil therapy are recommended:
• If the leukocyte count is 2500–3500, the fluorouracil dose should be withheld until the count exceeds 3500.
• If the leukocyte count is less than 2500, the fluorouracil dose should be withheld until the count exceeds 3500, then resumed with a dosage reduction of 20%. If the leukocyte count remains below 2500 for over 10 days despite withholding of fluorouracil, administration of both levamisole and fluorouracil should be discontinued.

If thrombocytopenia occurs, it is recommended that both levamisole and fluorouracil be withheld until platelet counts exceed 100,000.

## Oral Dosage Forms

### LEVAMISOLE HYDROCHLORIDE TABLETS
Note: The dosing and strengths are expressed in terms of levamisole base.

#### Usual adult dose
Colorectal carcinoma—
  Oral, beginning seven to thirty days after surgery, 50 mg (base) every eight hours for three days, repeated every two weeks for one year. It is given in combination with fluorouracil 450 mg per square meter of body surface by rapid intravenous push once a day for five days concomitant with a three-day course of levamisole, followed by 450 mg per square meter of body surface once a week beginning twenty-eight days after initiation of the five-day course and continued for a total treatment time of one year. Fluorouracil therapy should be initiated between twenty-one and thirty-five days after surgery. If levamisole treatment is initiated from seven to twenty days after surgery, fluorouracil should be initiated with the second course of levamisole (i.e., at twenty-one to thirty-four days). If levamisole is initiated from twenty-one to thirty days after surgery, fluorouracil should be initiated with the first course of levamisole.

Note: Although fluorouracil dosages are based on the patient's actual weight, use of estimated lean body mass (dry weight) is recommended in obese patients or those with weight gain due to edema, ascites, or other abnormal fluid retention.

#### Usual pediatric dose
Safety and efficacy have not been established.

**Strength(s) usually available**
U.S.—
  50 mg (base) (Rx) [*Ergamisol* (lactose)].
Canada—
  50 mg (base) (Rx) [*Ergamisol* (lactose)].

**Packaging and storage**
Store below 40 °C (104 °F), preferably between 15 and 30 °C (59 and 86 °F), unless otherwise specified by manufacturer.

Revised: 08/12/92
Interim revision: 07/08/94; 09/30/97

**LEVOBUNOLOL**—See *Beta-adrenergic Blocking Agents (Ophthalmic)*.

**LEVOCABASTINE**—The *Levocabastine (Ophthalmic)* monograph is not included in this published version of the USP DI database. Copies of the monograph are available on request from Micromedex, Inc. - Reprint Requests, 6200 S. Syracuse Way, Suite 300, Englewood, CO 80111; telephone (303) 486-6400; telefax (303) 486-6464; Email: USPDI@MDX.COM.

# LEVOCARNITINE Systemic

VA CLASSIFICATION (Primary): TN900
Commonly used brand name(s): *Carnitor*.
Another commonly used name is L-Carnitine.

Note: For a listing of dosage forms and brand names by country availability, see *Dosage Forms* section(s).

## Category
Carnitine deficiency therapy agent.

## Indications
Note: Bracketed information in the *Indications* section refers to uses that are not included in U.S. product labeling.

**Accepted**
Carnitine deficiency (treatment)—Levocarnitine is indicated for treatment of primary systemic carnitine deficiency, a genetic impairment of normal biosynthesis or utilization of levocarnitine from dietary sources. It is also used for the treatment of secondary carnitine deficiency that accompanies several organic acidurias.

Deficiency of levocarnitine may lead to elevated triglyceride and free fatty acid concentrations, reduced ketogenesis, and lipid infiltration of liver and muscle. Severe, chronic deficiency may lead to hypoglycemia, progressive myasthenia, hypotonia, lethargy, hepatomegaly, hepatic encephalopathy, hepatic coma, cardiomegaly, congestive heart failure, cardiac arrest, neurologic disturbances, and impaired infant growth and development.

[Carnitine deficiency, secondary to valproic acid toxicity (prophylaxis and treatment)][1]—Levocarnitine oral solution is used for the prevention and treatment of carnitine deficiency secondary to valproic acid toxicity.

**Unaccepted**
Levocarnitine has not been proven effective for treatment of abnormal plasma lipoprotein patterns or cardiac conditions unrelated to systemic carnitine deficiency. It has also not been proven effective for improvement of athletic performance.

[1]Not included in Canadian product labeling.

## Pharmacology/Pharmacokinetics

**Physicochemical characteristics**
Molecular weight—161.20.

**Mechanism of action/Effect**
Levocarnitine is necessary for normal mammalian fat utilization and energy metabolism. It facilitates entry of long-chain fatty acids into cellular mitochondria, where they are used during oxidation and energy production. It also exports acyl groups from subcellular organelles and from cells to urine before they accumulate to toxic concentrations.

Only the L isomer of carnitine (sometimes called vitamin $B_T$) affects lipid metabolism. The "vitamin $B_T$" form actually contains D,L-carnitine, which competitively inhibits levocarnitine and can cause deficiency.

**Elimination**
Renal/fecal. Plasma carnitine concentrations may be increased in patients with renal failure.
In dialysis—Removable by hemodialysis; deficiency may occur.

## Precautions to Consider

**Carcinogenicity**
Studies have not been done in either animals or humans.

**Mutagenicity**
Studies in *Salmonella typhimurium*, *Saccharomyces cerevisiae*, and *Schizosaccharomyces pombe* found no evidence of mutagenicity.

**Pregnancy/Reproduction**
Pregnancy—Adequate and well-controlled studies have not been done in humans.
Studies in rats and rabbits at parenteral doses equivalent on a mg per kg of body weight (mg/kg) basis to the usual adult dose have not shown that levocarnitine causes adverse effects on the fetus.
FDA Pregnancy Category B.

**Breast-feeding**
It is not known whether levocarnitine is distributed into breast milk. Problems in humans have not been documented. Carnitine occurs naturally in human milk.

**Pediatrics**
Appropriate studies on the relationship of age to the effects of levocarnitine have not been performed in the pediatric population. However, pediatrics-specific problems that would limit the usefulness of this medicine in children are not expected.

**Geriatrics**
Appropriate studies on the relationship of age to the effects of levocarnitine have not been performed in the geriatric population. However, geriatrics-specific problems that would limit the usefulness of this medication in the elderly are not expected.

**Drug interactions and/or related problems**
The following drug interactions and/or related problems have been selected on the basis of their potential clinical significance (possible mechanism in parentheses where appropriate)—not necessarily inclusive (» = major clinical significance):

Valproic acid
    (requirements for carnitine may be increased in patients receiving valproic acid)

**Patient monitoring**
The following may be especially important in patient monitoring (other tests may be warranted in some patients, depending on condition; » = major clinical significance):

Carnitine concentrations and
Free fatty acid concentrations and
Triglyceride concentrations
    (plasma determinations recommended at periodic intervals to assess efficacy of levocarnitine)

## Side/Adverse Effects
Note: Side/adverse effects are dose-related and may be reduced by decreasing the dose of levocarnitine.

The following side/adverse effects have been selected on the basis of their potential clinical significance (possible signs and symptoms in parenthesis where appropriate)—not necessarily inclusive:

**Those indicating need for medical attention only if they continue or are bothersome**
Incidence more frequent
    *Body odor; diarrhea or stomach cramps; nausea or vomiting*

## Patient Consultation
As an aid to patient consultation, refer to *Advice for the Patient, Levocarnitine (Systemic)*.
In providing consultation, consider emphasizing the following selected information (» = major clinical significance):

### Description of use
Description should include caution against confusion with the D,L-carnitine form

### Proper use of this medication
Taking during or immediately following meals and consuming slowly to reduce gastrointestinal upset

Taking at evenly spaced times throughout day (every 3 or 4 hours)
» Proper dosing
Missed dose: Not taking at all and not doubling doses
» Proper storage

### Precautions while using this medication
Not changing brands or dosage forms of levocarnitine without checking with physician

## General Dosing Information
Even spacing of doses throughout the day (every 3 or 4 hours) will help increase tolerance of levocarnitine.

### Diet/Nutrition
Levocarnitine oral solution may be given alone. However, to reduce gastrointestinal side effects caused by overly rapid ingestion, it is recommended that the solution be dissolved in drinks or other liquid foods and that no more than 10 mL (1 gram) be taken at each dose.

Levocarnitine tablets should be taken with meals to minimize gastrointestinal upset.

### Bioequivalence information
There are no data showing the therapeutic equivalence of those levocarnitine products approved for drug use and those products sold as food supplements.

## Oral Dosage Forms

### LEVOCARNITINE ORAL SOLUTION USP

**Usual adult and adolescent dose**
Carnitine deficiency—
Oral/enteral, initially 1 gram once a day with food, the dosage being increased slowly as needed and tolerated. For a 50-kg patient, the usual dose is 1 gram one to three times a day with meals.

**Usual pediatric dose**
Carnitine deficiency—
Oral/enteral, initially 50 mg per kg of body weight a day with food, the dosage being increased slowly as needed and tolerated. The usual dose is 50 to 100 mg per kg of body weight a day with meals (maximum 3 grams a day).

**Strength(s) usually available**
U.S.—
100 mg per mL (Rx) [*Carnitor*].
Canada—
100 mg per mL (Rx) [*Carnitor*].

**Packaging and storage**
Store below 40 °C (104 °F), preferably between 15 and 30 °C (59 and 86 °F), unless otherwise specified by manufacturer. Store in a tight container. Protect from freezing.

**Stability**
Should be used immediately after opening. Any unused portion should be discarded.

**Auxiliary labeling**
• Take with meals.

**Note**
Not for parenteral use.

### LEVOCARNITINE TABLETS USP
Note: Certain levocarnitine tablets are labeled and sold as food supplements only. These products have not been approved as drugs by the Food and Drug Administration for use in the treatment of carnitine deficiency. When used on prescription, one levocarnitine product should not be substituted for another unless otherwise directed by the patient's physician. There are no data showing the therapeutic equivalence of those products approved for drug use and those products sold as food supplements.

**Usual adult and adolescent dose**
Carnitine deficiency—
Oral, 1 gram two or three times a day with meals.

**Usual pediatric dose**
Carnitine deficiency—
Oral, initially 50 mg per kg of body weight a day with food, the dosage being increased slowly as needed and tolerated. The usual dose is 50 to 100 mg per kg of body weight a day with meals (maximum 3 grams a day).

**Strength(s) usually available**
U.S.—
330 mg (Rx) [*Carnitor*].
Canada—
330 mg (Rx) [*Carnitor*].

**Packaging and storage**
Store below 40 °C (104 °F), preferably between 15 and 30 °C (59 and 86 °F), in a well-closed container, unless otherwise specified by manufacturer.

**Auxiliary labeling**
• Take with meals.

## Parenteral Dosage Forms

### LEVOCARNITINE INJECTION

**Usual adult dose**
Carnitine deficiency—
Intravenous, 50 mg per kg (mg/kg) of body weight a day.
For severe metabolic crisis—
Intravenous, loading dose of 50 mg/kg of body weight, followed by a total of 50 mg/kg every 3 or 4 hours for one day, then 50 mg/kg a day.

**Pediatric dose**—
See *Usual adult dose*.

**Strength(s) usually available**
U.S.—
200 mg per mL (Rx) [*Carnitor*].
Canada—
200 mg per mL (Rx) [*Carnitor*].

**Packaging and storage**
Store at 25 °C (77 °F). Keep ampuls in original container and protect from light.

Revised: 03/04/92
Interim revision: 08/10/92; 05/28/93; 08/29/94; 08/07/95

---

# LEVODOPA   Systemic

VA CLASSIFICATION (Primary): CN500

Commonly used brand name(s): *Dopar*; *Larodopa*.

Note: For a listing of dosage forms and brand names by country availability, see *Dosage Forms* section(s).

## Category
Antidyskinetic.

## Indications

### Accepted
Parkinsonism (treatment)—Levodopa is indicated to alleviate symptoms and allow more normal body movements with improved muscular control in the treatment of idiopathic Parkinson's disease (paralysis agitans), postencephalitic parkinsonism, or symptomatic parkinsonism that may follow injury to the nervous system by carbon monoxide intoxication or manganese intoxication. It is also indicated in parkinsonism associated with cerebral arteriosclerosis.

## Pharmacology/Pharmacokinetics

### Physicochemical characteristics
Molecular weight—197.19.

### Mechanism of action/Effect
The precise mechanism of action has not been established. It is believed that the small percentage of each dose crossing the blood-brain barrier is decarboxylated to dopamine. The dopamine then stimulates dopaminergic receptors in the basal ganglia to improve the balance between cholinergic and dopaminergic activity, resulting in the improved modulation of voluntary nerve impulses transmitted to the motor cortex.

### Other actions/effects
Levodopa's metabolite, dopamine, stimulates beta-adrenergic cardiac receptors, interacts with chemoreceptors in the medullary emetic center, and promotes release of pituitary growth hormone.

### Absorption
Rapidly absorbed from the small intestine by an active amino acid transport system, with 30 to 50% reaching general circulation. High gastric acidity, delayed stomach emptying time, and the presence of certain other amino acids, such as those that occur after digestion of a protein meal, may delay absorption of levodopa.

### Distribution
Widely distributed to most body tissues, but not to the central nervous system (CNS), which receives less than 1% of the dose because of extensive metabolism in the periphery.

### Biotransformation
95% converted to dopamine by L-aromatic amino acid decarboxylase enzyme in the lumen of the stomach and intestines and on first pass through liver.

### Half-life
1 to 3 hours.

### Onset of action
Significant improvement may occur in 2 to 3 weeks. Some patients may require up to 6 months of continuous levodopa therapy to obtain optimal therapeutic benefit.

### Time to peak concentration
1 to 3 hours (may be longer when taken with food).

### Duration of action
Up to 5 hours per dose.

### Elimination
Renal; 80% of dose eliminated within 24 hours as dopamine metabolites, mainly dihydroxyphenylacetic acid (DOPAC) and homovanillic acid (HVA). Some of the eliminated metabolites may color the urine red.

## Precautions to Consider

### Pregnancy/Reproduction
Pregnancy—Studies in humans have not been done.
Reproduction studies in rodents have shown that levodopa, when given in doses in excess of 200 mg per kg of body weight (mg/kg) per day, depresses fetal and postnatal growth and viability. Also, studies in rabbits have shown that levodopa alone or in combination with carbidopa causes visceral and skeletal malformations.

### Breast-feeding
Levodopa is distributed into breast milk. Although problems in humans have not been documented, breast-feeding is not recommended because of the potential for side effects in the infant.
Also, levodopa may inhibit lactation.

### Pediatrics
Appropriate studies on the relationship of age to the effects of levodopa have not been performed in children up to 12 years of age. Safety and efficacy have not been established.

### Geriatrics
Smaller doses may be required in geriatric patients since they may have a reduced tolerance to the effects of levodopa. Also, peripheral dopa decarboxylase, the enzyme responsible for decarboxylation, decreases with age, thus making large doses unnecessary.
Geriatric patients, especially those with osteoporosis, responsive to antiparkinsonian therapy should resume normal activity gradually and with caution because increased mobility may increase risk of fractures.
Psychic side effects, such as anxiety, confusion, or nervousness, occur more frequently in geriatric patients receiving other antiparkinsonian medications, especially anticholinergics.
Geriatric patients, especially those with pre-existing coronary disease, are more susceptible to levodopa's cardiac effects, such as arrhythmias. These cardiac effects are minimized or eliminated when levodopa is combined with carbidopa.

### Dental
Involuntary movements of jaws may result in poor retention of full dentures; dosage reduction may be required.

### Drug interactions and/or related problems
The following drug interactions and/or related problems have been selected on the basis of their potential clinical significance (possible mechanism in parentheses where appropriate)—not necessarily inclusive (» = major clinical significance):

Note: Combinations containing any of the following medications, depending on the amount present, may also interact with this medication.

Amantadine or
Benztropine or
Procyclidine or
Trihexyphenidyl
(concurrent use may result in increased efficacy of levodopa; however, concurrent use is not recommended if there is a history of psychosis)

» Anesthetics, hydrocarbon inhalation
(concurrent administration may result in cardiac arrhythmias because of increased endogenous dopamine concentration; levodopa should be discontinued 6 to 8 hours before administration of anesthetics, especially halothane)

» Anticonvulsants, hydantoin, or
Benzodiazepines or
Droperidol or
» Haloperidol or
Loxapine or
Metyrosine or
Papaverine or
» Phenothiazines or
Rauwolfia alkaloids or
Thioxanthenes
(concurrent use may decrease the therapeutic effects of levodopa; hydantoin anticonvulsants increase the metabolism of levodopa when used concurrently, thus decreasing its effect; since droperidol, haloperidol, loxapine, papaverine, phenothiazines, and the thioxanthenes block the dopamine receptors in the brain, they may induce extrapyramidal symptoms, thus aggravating parkinsonism and antagonizing the effects of levodopa; the rauwolfia alkaloids cause dopamine depletion in the brain, thus opposing the effects of levodopa)

Bromocriptine
(may produce additive effects, allowing reduction in levodopa dosage)

» Cocaine
(concurrent use with levodopa may increase the risk of cardiac arrhythmias; if use of cocaine is necessary in patients receiving levodopa, it is recommended that cocaine be administered with caution, in reduced dosage, and in conjunction with electrocardiographic monitoring)

Foods, especially high-protein
(concurrent or previous ingestion of food may decrease the absorption of levodopa from the gastrointestinal tract, consequently delaying its effect; in addition, proteins in food may be degraded into the amino acids that compete with levodopa for transport to the brain, thus decreasing and/or making erratic the response to levodopa; however, rather than cutting down on daily protein intake to avoid this effect on levodopa, it is recommended that the intake of proteins be distributed equally throughout the day)

Hypotension-producing medications, other (See *Appendix II*)
(concurrent use with levodopa may result in an increased hypotensive effect)

Methyldopa
(concurrent use with levodopa may alter the antiparkinsonian effects of levodopa and may also produce additive toxic CNS effects such as psychosis)

Metoclopramide
(gastric emptying of levodopa may be accelerated with concurrent use of metoclopramide, thus possibly increasing levodopa's rate and extent of absorption from the small intestine; the clinical significance of this interaction has not been determined)

Molindone
(concurrent use may inhibit antiparkinsonian effects of levodopa by blocking dopamine receptor in the brain; also, levodopa may counteract the antipsychotic effects of molindone)

» Monoamine oxidase (MAO) inhibitors, including furazolidone and procarbazine
(concurrent use with levodopa is not recommended as the combination may result in a hypertensive crisis; it is recommended that MAO inhibitors be discontinued for 2 to 4 weeks prior to initiation of levodopa therapy)

» Pyridoxine
(concurrent use with levodopa is not recommended since levodopa's antiparkinsonian effects are reversed by as little as 10 mg of orally administered pyridoxine)

» Selegiline
(although sometimes used in conjunction with levodopa or with carbidopa and levodopa combination, selegiline may enhance lev-

odopa-induced dyskinesias, nausea, orthostatic hypotension, confusion, and hallucinations; levodopa dosage should be reduced within 2 to 3 days after the initiation of selegiline therapy)

Sympathomimetics
(concurrent use with levodopa may increase the possibility of cardiac arrhythmias; dosage reduction of the sympathomimetic is recommended; the administration of carbidopa with levodopa reduces the tendency of sympathomimetics to cause dopamine-induced cardiac arrhythmias)

## Laboratory value alterations
The following have been selected on the basis of their potential clinical significance (possible effect in parentheses where appropriate)—not necessarily inclusive (» = major clinical significance):

With diagnostic test results
Coombs' (antiglobulin) test
(occasionally becomes positive after long-term levodopa therapy)
Glucose, urine
(tests using copper reduction methods may cause false-positive results; tests using glucose oxidase methods may cause false-negative results)
Gonadorelin test
(levodopa may elevate serum gonadotropin concentrations)
Ketones, urine
(tests using dipstick methods may cause false-positive results)
Norepinephrine, urine
(test shows false-positive results)
Pancreas imaging
(in animal studies, levodopa decreased pancreatic uptake of selenomethionine Se 75, probably because of levodopa-induced stimulation of growth hormone release by the pituitary; human data are not available)
Protein, urine
(use of the Lowery test may cause false-positive results)
Thyroid function determinations
(chronic use of levodopa may inhibit the TSH response to protirelin)
Uric acid, serum and urine
(tests may show high concentrations with colorimetric measurements, but not with uricase)

With physiology/laboratory test values
Alanine aminotransferase (ALT [SGPT]) and
Alkaline phosphatase and
Aspartate aminotransferase (AST [SGOT]) and
Bilirubin and
Lactate dehydrogenase (LDH) and
Protein-bound iodine (PBI)
(serum concentrations may be increased)
Blood urea nitrogen (BUN)
(concentrations may be increased)

## Medical considerations/Contraindications
The medical considerations/contraindications included have been selected on the basis of their potential clinical significance (reasons given in parentheses where appropriate)—not necessarily inclusive (» = major clinical significance).

*Risk-benefit should be considered when the following medical problems exist:*

» Bronchial asthma, emphysema, and other severe pulmonary diseases
(respiratory effects of levodopa may aggravate condition)
» Cardiovascular disease, severe
(increased risk of cardiac arrhythmias)
Convulsive disorders, history of
(use of levodopa may precipitate seizures)
Diabetes mellitus
(use of levodopa may adversely affect control of glucose in blood)
Endocrine diseases
(use of levodopa may adversely affect hypothalamus or pituitary function)
» Glaucoma, angle-closure, or predisposition to
(mydriatic effect resulting in increased intraocular pressure may precipitate an acute attack of angle-closure glaucoma)
Glaucoma, open-angle, chronic
(mydriatic effect may cause a slight increase in intraocular pressure; glaucoma therapy may need to be adjusted)
Hepatic function impairment
» Melanoma, history of or suspected
(use of levodopa may activate a malignant melanoma)
» Myocardial infarction, history of, with residual arrhythmias
(use of levodopa may precipitate or aggravate condition)
» Peptic ulcer, history of
(increased risk of upper gastrointestinal hemorrhage)
» Psychotic states
(increased risk of developing depression and suicidal tendencies)
» Renal function impairment
(use of levodopa may lead to urinary retention)
Sensitivity to levodopa
» Urinary retention
(use of levodopa may precipitate or aggravate condition)

## Patient monitoring
The following may be especially important in patient monitoring (other tests may be warranted in some patients, depending on condition; » = major clinical significance):

Blood cell counts and
Hemoglobin determinations and
Hepatic function determinations and
Ophthalmologic examinations for glaucoma and monitoring of intraocular pressure in patients with open-angle glaucoma and
Renal function determinations
(recommended at periodic intervals for patients on long-term levodopa therapy; also, blood cell counts and hepatic and renal function determinations are recommended after withdrawal of levodopa therapy as part of the evaluation of a patient with suspected neuroleptic malignant–like syndrome)
Cardiovascular monitoring for detection of arrhythmias or orthostatic hypotensive tendencies
(recommended during the period of initial dosage adjustment)
Creatine phosphokinase concentrations
(serum determinations recommended after discontinuation of levodopa therapy, especially if fever is present; an elevated serum creatine phosphokinase level may be an early indication of the presence of neuroleptic malignant–like syndrome)

# Side/Adverse Effects

Note: Patients receiving this medication for one to several years may experience sudden, unexpected akinesia, tremor, and rigidity, such as the "on-off" phenomenon. Emotional stress may precipitate akinesia paradoxica or "start hesitation" in these patients.

A syndrome resembling neuroleptic malignant syndrome, which includes intermittent dystonia alternating with substantial agitation, hyperthermia, and mental changes, has been reported after the abrupt discontinuation of levodopa therapy.

Convulsions have been reported but a causal relationship to the use of levodopa has not been established.

The following side/adverse effects have been selected on the basis of their potential clinical significance (possible signs and symptoms in parentheses where appropriate)—not necessarily inclusive:

### Those indicating need for medical attention
Incidence more frequent
**Difficult urination; irregular heartbeat; mental depression; mood or mental changes, such as aggressive behavior; nausea or vomiting, severe or continuing; orthostatic hypotension** (dizziness or lightheadedness when getting up from a lying or sitting position); **unusual and uncontrolled movements of the body, including the face, tongue, arms, hands, head, and upper body**—may indicate excessive concentration of dopamine in the striatum

Note: *Orthostatic hypotension* occurs in about 30% of patients at the initiation of levodopa therapy.

*Nausea and vomiting* occur in nearly 80% of patients in early levodopa therapy with tolerance being gradually achieved during continued use.

*Difficult urination, dizziness or lightheadedness, irregular heartbeat,* and *nausea and vomiting* may become less frequent when levodopa is combined with carbidopa because of the reduced dose requirements and unavailability of peripheral dopamine.

*Choreiform and other involuntary movements* occur in 50 to 80% of patients and are usually dose-related.

Incidence less frequent
**Spasm or closing of eyelids**—possible early sign of overdose

Incidence rare
*Duodenal ulcer* (stomach pain); ***hemolytic anemia*** (unusual tiredness or weakness); ***hypertension*** (high blood pressure)

**Those indicating need for medical attention only if they continue or are bothersome**
Incidence more frequent
*Anxiety, confusion, or nervousness*—especially in elderly patients receiving other antiparkinsonian medication; *constipation; nightmares*

Note: *Constipation* and *nightmares* may become less frequent when levodopa is combined with carbidopa because of the reduced dose requirements and unavailability of peripheral dopamine.

Incidence less frequent
*Anorexia* (loss of appetite); *diarrhea; dryness of mouth; flushing of skin; headache; insomnia* (trouble in sleeping); *muscle twitching; unusual tiredness or weakness*

**Those not indicating need for medical attention**
Incidence less frequent
*Darkening in color of urine or sweat*

## Overdose

For more information on the management of overdose or unintentional ingestion, **contact a Poison Control Center** (see *Poison Control Center Listing*).

**Clinical effects of overdose**
The following effects have been selected on the basis of their potential clinical significance (possible signs and symptoms in parentheses where appropriate)—not necessarily inclusive:

*Spasm or closing of eyelids*—possible early sign of overdose

**Treatment of overdose**
Since there is no specific antidote for acute overdose with levodopa, treatment is symptomatic and supportive, with possible utilization of the following:
To decrease absorption—Immediate gastric lavage.
The value of dialysis in the treatment of overdose is not known.
Specific treatment—Antiarrhythmic medication, if necessary.
Pyridoxine in oral doses of 10 to 25 mg has been reported to reverse toxic and therapeutic effects of levodopa; however, in the treatment of acute overdosage, its usefulness has not been established.
Supportive care—Patients in whom intentional overdose is confirmed or suspected should be referred for psychiatric consultation.

## Patient Consultation

As an aid to patient consultation, refer to *Advice for the Patient, Levodopa (Systemic)*.

In providing consultation, consider emphasizing the following selected information (» = major clinical significance):

**Before using this medication**
» Conditions affecting use, especially:
Sensitivity to levodopa
Pregnancy—No studies in humans; depressed growth and malformations in animal studies
Breast-feeding—Distributed into breast milk; may inhibit lactation
Use in the elderly—Reduced tolerance to effects of levodopa; caution in resuming normal activity, especially in patients with osteoporosis
Dental—Possible difficulty in retention of full dentures
Other medications, especially haloperidol, hydantoin anticonvulsants, hydrocarbon inhalation anesthetics, phenothiazines, cocaine, MAO inhibitors, pyridoxine, and selegiline
Other medical problems, especially severe cardiovascular disease, severe pulmonary diseases, glaucoma, melanoma (history of or suspected), peptic ulcer (history of), psychosis, renal function impairment, or urinary retention

**Proper use of this medication**
» Taking food shortly after taking medication to relieve gastric irritation; taking food before or concurrently may retard levodopa's effect
» Compliance with therapy; taking medication only as directed; not stopping medication unless ordered by physician
» Maximum effectiveness of medication may not occur for several weeks or months after therapy is initiated
» Proper dosing
Missed dose: Taking as soon as possible; skipping dose if next scheduled dose is within 2 hours; not doubling doses
» Proper storage

**Precautions while using this medication**
Caution if any kind of surgery (including dental surgery) or emergency treatment is required
Diabetics: May interfere with urine tests for sugar and ketones
» Caution if drowsiness occurs
» Caution when getting up suddenly from lying or sitting position; dizziness and fainting may occur
» Avoiding foods or vitamin products containing pyridoxine (vitamin B$_6$); diminished levodopa effect when used with pyridoxine
» Caution in resuming normal physical activities when condition has improved, especially for geriatric patients
Possibility of "on-off" phenomenon

**Side/adverse effects**
Signs of potential side effects, especially difficult urination, duodenal ulcer, hemolytic anemia, hypertension, irregular heartbeat, mental depression, mood or mental changes, severe nausea or vomiting, orthostatic hypotension, spasm or closing of eyelids, uncontrolled movements of body
Occasional darkening of urine or sweat may be alarming to patient although medically insignificant

## General Dosing Information

Titrated dosage is necessary to achieve the individual therapeutic blood concentration requirements and to minimize side effects. This is especially important for geriatric patients and patients receiving other medications.

Postencephalitic and geriatric patients often require and tolerate lower dosage levels than other parkinsonism patients.

The concurrent administration of carbidopa may permit the dose of levodopa to be reduced by up to 75% and yet achieve equal therapeutic results. Carbidopa also reduces the adverse effect of pyridoxine on levodopa.

Amantadine or anticholinergic medications are often used concurrently with levodopa in the more advanced cases of parkinsonism or when response to levodopa decreases. Gradual dosage reduction of these medications is recommended during initiation of therapy with levodopa and after optimum dosage is reached to maintain proper control of the patient's condition.

When levodopa is to be discontinued, dosage should be reduced gradually to prevent the occurrence of a syndrome that resembles the neuroleptic malignant syndrome. Careful patient monitoring after withdrawal of levodopa will allow early diagnosis and treatment of neuroleptic malignant-like syndrome.

**Diet/Nutrition**
Food should be eaten shortly after levodopa is taken to relieve gastric irritation; taking food before or concurrently may retard levodopa's effects.

High protein diets should be avoided, because amino acid degradation products compete with levodopa for transport to the brain, resulting in a decreased or erratic response to levodopa. It is recommended that intake of normal amounts of protein be distributed equally throughout the day.

In addition, pyridoxine (vitamin B$_6$) reverses the effects of levodopa. Vitamin products containing pyridoxine should be avoided; intake of foods containing large amounts of pyridoxine (such as avocado, bacon, beans, beef liver, dry skim milk, oatmeal, peas, pork, sweet potato, tuna, and certain health foods) may need to be limited.

**For treatment of adverse effects**
Immediate relief of nausea and vomiting may sometimes be obtained by reducing the daily dose, giving smaller individual doses at more frequent intervals, giving smaller doses concurrently with carbidopa, or having patient take food shortly after each dose; however, high-protein foods should be avoided since they may decrease levodopa's effect as well (see *Absorption; Drug interactions and/or related problems*). Since the nausea results primarily from the CNS effects of levodopa, non-phenothiazine antiemetics are sometimes successfully used. Phenothiazine antiemetics may be more effective but should not be used because of their tendency to negate levodopa's therapeutic effect.

The appearance of choreiform and other involuntary movements may require a reduction in dosage since tolerance usually does not develop.

Serious psychiatric disturbances, such as severe mental depression, with or without suicidal tendencies, may require reduction in dosage or complete withdrawal of levodopa.

Orthostatic hypotension may be controlled by the use of elastic hosiery and an increase in sodium intake. However, use of the carbidopa and levodopa combination reduces the incidence of this side effect.

The temporary withdrawal of levodopa has been used to prevent some of the complications of long-term therapy. Also, it has been used to enhance the efficacy of levodopa when therapy is reinstated since drug withdrawal presumably allows resensitization of the striatal dopamine receptors. However, full withdrawal of levodopa involves certain risks, such as worsening of parkinsonian symptoms, immobility, depression, pulmonary embolism, and thrombophlebitis. The patient, in most cases, will require nursing care and daily physical therapy during the temporary withdrawal.

After discontinuation of levodopa therapy, dantrolene and/or bromocriptine may be used in patients with evidence of neuroleptic malignant–like syndrome, to help reduce fever and thus avoid a potentially lethal complication.

## Oral Dosage Forms

### LEVODOPA CAPSULES USP

**Usual adult and adolescent dose**
Antidyskinetic—
　Oral, 250 mg two to four times a day initially, the dosage per day being increased by an additional 100 to 750 mg at three- to seven-day intervals as tolerated until the desired response is obtained.

Note: Postencephalitic patients may be more sensitive to the effects of the usual adult dose.

**Usual adult prescribing limits**
Up to 8 grams daily.

**Usual pediatric dose**
Children up to 12 years of age: Safety and efficacy have not been established.
Children 12 years of age and over: See *Usual adult and adolescent dose*.

**Usual geriatric dose**
See *Usual adult and adolescent dose*.

Note: Geriatric patients may be more sensitive to the effects of the usual adult dose.

**Strength(s) usually available**
U.S.—
　100 mg (Rx) [*Dopar; Larodopa*].
　250 mg (Rx) [*Dopar; Larodopa*].
　500 mg (Rx) [*Dopar; Larodopa*].
Canada—
　Not commercially available.

**Packaging and storage**
Store between 15 and 30 °C (59 and 86 °F), unless otherwise specified by manufacturer. Store in a tight, light-resistant container.

**Auxiliary labeling**
• May darken urine or sweat.

### LEVODOPA TABLETS USP

**Usual adult and adolescent dose**
See *Levodopa Capsules USP*.

**Usual adult prescribing limits**
See *Levodopa Capsules USP*.

**Usual pediatric dose**
See *Levodopa Capsules USP*.

**Usual geriatric dose**
See *Levodopa Capsules USP*.

**Strength(s) usually available**
U.S.—
　100 mg (Rx) [*Larodopa*].
　250 mg (Rx) [*Larodopa*].
　500 mg (Rx) [*Larodopa*].
Canada—
　250 mg (Rx) [*Larodopa* (scored)].

**Packaging and storage**
Store between 15 and 30 °C (59 and 86 °F), unless otherwise specified by manufacturer. Store in a tight, light-resistant container.

**Auxiliary labeling**
• May darken urine or sweat.

Revised: 08/18/92
Interim revision: 08/17/94

# LEVOFLOXACIN　Systemic—INTRODUCTORY VERSION

VA CLASSIFICATION (Primary): AM402

Note: For a listing of dosage forms and brand names by country availability, see *Dosage Forms* section(s).

## Category
Antibacterial (systemic).

## Indications

**Accepted**

Bronchitis, bacterial exacerbations (treatment)—Levofloxacin is indicated in the treatment of bacterial exacerbations of bronchitis caused by *Haemophilus influenzae*, *Haemophilus parainfluenzae*, *Moraxella catarrhalis*, *Staphylococcus aureus*, or *Streptococcus pneumoniae*.

Pneumonia, community-acquired (treatment)—Levofloxacin is indicated in the treatment of community-acquired pneumonia caused by *Chlamydia pneumoniae*, *H. influenzae*, *H. parainfluenzae*, *Klebsiella pneumoniae*, *Legionella pneumophila*, *M. catarrhalis*, *Mycoplasma pneumoniae*, *S. aureus*, or *S. pneumoniae*.

Pyelonephritis (treatment)—Levofloxacin is indicated in the treatment of pyelonephritis caused by *Escherichia coli*.

Sinusitis (treatment)—Levofloxacin is indicated in the treatment of sinusitis caused by *H. influenzae*, *M. catarrhalis*, or *S. pneumoniae*.

Skin and soft tissue infections (treatment)—Levofloxacin is indicated in the treatment of skin and soft tissue infections caused by *S. aureus* or *Streptococcus pyogenes*.

Urinary tract infections, bacterial, complicated (treatment)—Levofloxacin is indicated in the treatment of complicated bacterial urinary tract infections caused by *Enterobacter cloacae*, *Enterococcus faecalis*, *E. coli*, *K. pneumoniae*, *Proteus mirabilis*, or *Pseudomonas aeruginosa*.

## Pharmacology/Pharmacokinetics

**Physicochemical characteristics**
Chemical group—Fluoroquinolone; levofloxacin is the L-isomer of the racemic medication, ofloxacin.
Molecular weight—370.38.

**Mechanism of action/Effect**
Levofloxacin acts by inhibiting DNA gyrase (bacterial topoisomerase II), an enzyme required for DNA replication, transcription, repair, and recombination.

**Absorption**
Rapidly and almost completely absorbed after oral administration. Bioavailability is approximately 99%. Levofloxacin may be taken with or without food.

**Distribution**
Widely distributed. Levofloxacin penetrates well into blister fluid and lung tissues.
$Vol_D$—89 to 112 L after single and multiple 500-mg doses.

**Protein binding**
Moderate (24 to 38%).

**Biotransformation**
Levofloxacin is stereochemically stable and does not invert metabolically to its enantiomer, D-ofloxacin. It undergoes limited metabolism.

**Half-life**
Elimination—6 to 8 hours.

**Time to peak concentration**
Oral—Approximately 1 to 2 hours. Oral administration with food prolongs the time to peak concentration by approximately 1 hour; however, levofloxacin may be taken without regard to food consumption.

**Peak serum concentration**
Oral—Approximately 5.7 mcg per mL after multiple doses of 500 mg. Oral administration with food prolongs the peak concentration by approximately 14%.
Intravenous—Approximately 6.4 mcg per mL. The serum concentration profile of the intravenous infusion is similar and comparable to the

extent of exposure (area under the plasma concentration–time curve [AUC]) seen with the tablets when equal doses are administered. Therefore, oral and intravenous routes of administration are considered to be interchangeable.

### Elimination
Renal—Approximately 87% of an orally administered dose is excreted unchanged in the urine within 48 hours; renal clearance in excess of the glomerular filtration rate suggests that tubular secretion also occurs.
Fecal—Approximately 4% of an orally administered dose is excreted fecally within 72 hours.
In dialysis—
Levofloxacin is not efficiently removed by hemodialysis or peritoneal dialysis.

## Precautions to Consider

### Cross-sensitivity and/or related problems
Patients allergic to one fluoroquinolone or other chemically related quinolone derivatives (e.g., cinoxacin, nalidixic acid) may be allergic to other fluoroquinolones also.

### Carcinogenicity/Tumorigenicity
In a long-term study in rats, levofloxacin did not show carcinogenic or tumorigenic potential after daily dietary administration for 2 years. The highest dose was two times the recommended human dose or 10 times the recommended human dose based on body surface area or body weight, respectively.

### Mutagenicity
Levofloxacin was not mutagenic in the Ames test (*Salmonella typhimurium* and *Escherichia coli*), CHO/HGPRT forward mutation assay, mouse micronucleus test, mouse dominant lethal assay, rat unscheduled DNA synthesis assay, and the mouse sister chromatid exchange assay. It was positive in the *in vitro* chromosomal aberration (CHL cell line) and sister chromatid exchange (CHL/IU cell line) assays.

### Pregnancy/Reproduction
Fertility—Levofloxacin had no effect on the fertility or reproductive performance of male and female rats at oral doses of up to 360 mg per kg of body weight (mg/kg), or 2124 mg per square meter of body surface area (mg/m$^2$), per day, corresponding to 18 and 3 times the maximum recommended human dose (MRHD) based on body weight and body surface area, respectively, or at intravenous doses of up to 100 mg/kg, or 590 mg/m$^2$, per day, corresponding to 5 and 1 times the MRHD based on body weight and body surface area, respectively.

Pregnancy—Adequate and well-controlled studies in humans have not been done. Since levofloxacin has been shown to cause arthropathy in immature animals, use is recommended in pregnancy only if the potential benefit to the mother outweighs the potential risk to the fetus.

Levofloxacin was not teratogenic in rats at oral doses of up to 810 mg/kg, or 4779 mg/m$^2$, per day, corresponding to 82 and 14 times the MRHD based on body weight and body surface area, respectively, or at intravenous doses of up to 160 mg/kg, or 944 mg/m$^2$, per day, corresponding to 16 and 2.7 times the MRHD based on body weight and body surface area, respectively. Doses equivalent to 81 and 26 times the MRHD of levofloxacin, based on body weight and body surface area, respectively, caused decreased fetal body weight and increased fetal mortality in rats when administered orally at doses of 810 mg/kg, or 8910 mg/m$^2$, per day. No teratogenicity was observed when rabbits were given oral doses of up to 50 mg/kg, or 550 mg/m$^2$, per day, corresponding to 5 and 1.6 times the MRHD based on body weight and body surface area, respectively, or at intravenous doses of up to 25 mg/kg, or 275 mg/m$^2$, per day, corresponding to 2.5 and 0.8 times the MRHD based on body weight and body surface area, respectively.

FDA Pregnancy Category C.

### Breast-feeding
It is not known whether levofloxacin is distributed into breast milk; however, based on data for ofloxacin, it is expected that levofloxacin is distributed into human milk. Because of the potential for serious adverse effects in nursing infants, a decision should be made to either stop breast-feeding or discontinue taking levofloxacin.

### Pediatrics
Safety and efficacy have not been established in patients up to 18 years of age. Fluoroquinolones have been shown to cause arthropathy and osteochondrosis in immature animals of several species.

### Geriatrics
The pharmacokinetics of levofloxacin are not altered in elderly patients with normal renal function. Following a 500-mg oral dose of levofloxacin, the mean elimination half-life was approximately 7.6 hours in healthy elderly subjects, as compared with 6 hours in younger adults.

The difference was attributed to variation in renal function and was not believed to be clinically significant.

### Drug interactions and/or related problems
The following drug interactions and/or related problems have been selected on the basis of their potential clinical significance (possible mechanism in parentheses where appropriate)—not necessarily inclusive (» = major clinical significance):

Note: Unlike other fluoroquinolones, levofloxacin does not alter the pharmacokinetics of cyclosporine, digoxin, theophylline, or warfarin.
Combinations containing any of the following medications, depending on the amount present, may also interact with this medication.

» Antacids, aluminum-, calcium-, and/or magnesium-containing or
» Ferrous sulfate or
» Sucralfate or
» Zinc
(antacids, ferrous sulfate, sucralfate, and zinc may reduce absorption of levofloxacin by chelation, resulting in lower serum and urine concentrations; therefore, concurrent use is not recommended; it is recommended that levofloxacin be taken at least 2 hours before or 2 hours after taking any of these agents)

» Antidiabetic agents
(concurrent administration has resulted in hyperglycemia or hypoglycemia, usually in diabetic patients who are taking oral hypoglycemic agents or insulin; careful monitoring of blood glucose is recommended)

» Anti-inflammatory drugs, nonsteroidal
(concurrent use may increase the risk of central nervous system [CNS] stimulation and seizures)

Cimetidine or
Probenecid
(concurrent use of levofloxacin with cimetidine or probenecid increases the area under the plasma concentration–time curve [AUC] by 27 to 38% and 30%, respectively, and decreases the clearance by 21 to 35%; although these differences are statistically significant, the changes are not considered high enough to warrant a change in dose)

### Laboratory value alterations
The following have been selected on the basis of their potential clinical significance (possible effect in parentheses where appropriate)—not necessarily inclusive (» = major clinical significance):

With physiology/laboratory test values
» Glucose, blood
(concentrations may be increased or decreased)
Lymphocytes
(counts may be decreased)

### Medical considerations/Contraindications
The medical considerations/contraindications included have been selected on the basis of their potential clinical significance (reasons given in parentheses where appropriate)—not necessarily inclusive (» = major clinical significance).

*Except under special circumstances, this medication should not be used when the following medical problem exists:*

» Previous allergic reaction to fluoroquinolones or other chemically related quinolone derivatives

*Risk-benefit should be considered when the following medical problems exist:*

CNS disorders, including cerebral arteriosclerosis or epilepsy
(levofloxacin may cause CNS stimulation or toxicity, increasing the risk of seizures in patients with these conditions)

» Diabetes mellitus
(levofloxacin has been reported to cause hyperglycemia and hypoglycemia, usually in diabetic patients who are taking oral hypoglycemic agents or insulin; diabetic patients should be carefully monitored)

» Renal function impairment
(levofloxacin is renally excreted; it is recommended that patients with a creatinine clearance of less than 50 mL per minute receive a reduced dosage of levofloxacin)

## Side/Adverse Effects

Note: There have been reports of ruptures of the Achilles tendon and of tendons in the shoulder and hand that required surgical repair or resulted in prolonged disability in patients taking levofloxacin or other fluoroquinolones. Patients should discontinue levofloxacin if they experience pain, inflammation, or rupture of a tendon. They should rest and refrain from exercise until the diagnosis of tendinitis or tendon rupture has been excluded. Tendon rupture can occur at any time during or after levofloxacin therapy.

The following side/adverse effects have been selected on the basis of their potential clinical significance (possible signs and symptoms in parentheses where appropriate)—not necessarily inclusive:

### Those indicating need for medical attention
Incidence rare
*Central nervous system (CNS) stimulation* (agitation; confusion; hallucinations; psychosis, acute; tremors); *hypersensitivity reactions* (skin rash, itching, or redness); *phototoxicity* (blisters; itching; rash; redness; sensation of skin burning; swelling); *pseudomembranous colitis* (abdominal or stomach cramps and pain, severe; abdominal tenderness; diarrhea, watery and severe, which may also be bloody; fever); *tendinitis or tendon rupture* (pain, inflammation, or swelling in calves, shoulders, or hands)

### Those indicating need for medical attention only if they continue or are bothersome
Incidence less frequent
*CNS effects* (dizziness; drowsiness; headache; lightheadedness; nervousness; trouble in sleeping); *gastrointestinal effects* (abdominal or stomach pain or discomfort; constipation; diarrhea; nausea; vomiting); *taste perversion* (change in sense of taste); *vaginal candidiasis* (vaginal itching and discharge)

### Those indicating possible pseudomembranous colitis and the need for medical attention if they occur after medication is discontinued
Abdominal or stomach cramps and pain, severe; abdominal tenderness; diarrhea, watery and severe, which may also be bloody; fever

## Overdose
In the event of an acute levofloxacin overdose, the stomach should be emptied, the patient observed, and hydration maintained. Levofloxacin is not efficiently removed by hemodialysis or peritoneal dialysis.

Levofloxacin exhibits a low potential for acute toxicity. Mice, rats, dogs, and monkeys exhibited the following signs after receiving a single high dose of levofloxacin: ataxia, decreased locomotor activity, dyspnea, prostration, ptosis, seizures, and tremors. Doses greater than 1500 mg per kg of body weight (mg/kg) orally and 250 mg/kg intravenously produced significant morbidity in rodents.

For more information on the management of overdose or unintentional ingestion, **contact a Poison Control Center** (see *Poison Control Center Listing*).

### Treatment of overdose
Supportive care—Patients in whom intentional overdose is confirmed or suspected should be referred for psychiatric consultation.

## Patient Consultation
As an aid to patient consultation, refer to *Advice for the Patient, Levofloxacin (Systemic)—Introductory Version*.

In providing consultation, consider emphasizing the following selected information (» = major clinical significance):

### Before using this medication
» Conditions affecting use, especially:
  Allergy to fluoroquinolones or other quinolone derivatives
  Pregnancy—Levofloxacin is recommended for use during pregnancy only if the potential benefit to the mother outweighs the potential risk to the fetus, because levofloxacin has been shown to cause arthropathy in immature animals
  Breast-feeding—It is not known whether levofloxacin is distributed into breast milk; however, caution should be exercised in making the decision whether to breast-feed, since levofloxacin has been shown to cause arthropathy in immature animals
  Use in children—Safety and efficacy have not been established in children up to 18 years of age; levofloxacin has been shown to cause arthropathy in immature animals
  Other medications, especially antidiabetic agents; aluminum-, calcium-, and/or magnesium-containing antacids; ferrous sulfate; nonsteroidal anti-inflammatory drugs; sucralfate; or zinc
  Other medical problems, especially diabetes mellitus or renal function impairment

### Proper use of this medication
» Levofloxacin may be taken with or without food
  Importance of maintaining adequate fluid intake
» Proper dosing
  Missed dose: Taking as soon as possible; not taking if almost time for next dose; not doubling doses
» Proper storage

### Precautions while using this medication
Checking with physician if no improvement within a few days
» Avoiding concurrent use of antacids, ferrous sulfate, sucralfate, or zinc and levofloxacin; taking these products at least 2 hours before or 2 hours after administration of levofloxacin
» Possible phototoxicity reactions
» Discontinuing levofloxacin at the first sign of skin rash or other allergic reaction
» Caution when driving or doing anything else requiring alertness because of possible dizziness, drowsiness, or lightheadedness
» Discontinuing levofloxacin and notifying physician if pain, inflammation, or rupture of a tendon is experienced; resting and refraining from exercise until the diagnosis of tendinitis or tendon rupture has been excluded
» Discontinuing levofloxacin and contacting physician if patient is a diabetic being treated with insulin or an oral hypoglycemic agent and a hypoglycemic episode occurs

### Side/adverse effects
Signs of potential side effects, especially central nervous system stimulation, hypersensitivity reactions, phototoxicity, pseudomembranous colitis, and tendinitis or tendon rupture

## General Dosing Information

### For parenteral dosage forms only
Because rapid intravenous injection may result in hypotension, levofloxacin should be administered only by slow intravenous infusion over a period of 60 minutes.

Levofloxacin concentrate for injection must be diluted prior to parenteral administration.

### Diet/Nutrition
Levofloxacin may be taken with or without food.

### Bioequivalenence information
The profile of serum levofloxacin concentration observed after intravenous administration is comparable to the extent of exposure (area under the plasma concentration–time curve) observed for oral administration of tablets when equal doses are administered (mg/mg). Therefore, the oral and intravenous routes of administration are considered to be interchangeable.

### For treatment of adverse effects
For antibiotic-associated pseudomembranous colitis (AAPMC)
• Some patients may develop antibiotic-associated pseudomembranous colitis (AAPMC), caused by *Clostridium difficile* toxin, during or after administration of levofloxacin. Mild cases may respond to discontinuation of the drug alone. Moderate to severe cases may require fluid, electrolyte, and protein replacement.
• In cases not responding to the above measures or in more severe cases, oral doses of an antibacterial medication effective against *C. difficile* should be administered.
• In addition, AAPMC may result in severe watery diarrhea, which may occur during therapy or up to several weeks after therapy is discontinued. If diarrhea occurs, administration of antiperistaltic antidiarrheals (e.g., diphenoxylate and atropine combination, loperamide, opiates) is not recommended since they may delay the removal of toxins from the colon, thereby prolonging and/or worsening the condition.

## Oral Dosage Forms

### LEVOFLOXACIN TABLETS

#### Usual adult dose
Bronchitis, bacterial exacerbations, treatment—
  Oral, 500 mg every twenty-four hours for seven days.
Pneumonia, community-acquired, treatment—
  Oral, 500 mg every twenty-four hours for seven to fourteen days.
Pyelonephritis, treatment—
  Oral, 250 mg every twenty-four hours for ten days.
Sinusitis, treatment—
  Oral, 500 mg every twenty-four hours for ten to fourteen days.
Skin and soft tissue infections, treatment—
  Oral, 500 mg every twenty-four hours for seven to ten days.
Urinary tract infections, bacterial, complicated, treatment—
  Oral, 250 mg every twenty-four hours for ten days.

#### Usual pediatric dose
Safety and efficacy have not been established.

#### Strength(s) usually available
U.S.—
  250 mg (Rx) [*Levaquin*].
  500 mg (Rx) [*Levaquin*].

**Packaging and storage**
Store below 40 °C (104 °F), preferably between 15 and 30 °C (59 and 86 °F), unless otherwise specified by manufacturer.

**Auxiliary labeling**
- Continue medicine for the full time of treatment.
- Avoid too much sun exposure or use of sunlamp.
- Take with full glass of water.
- May cause dizziness, drowsiness, or lightheadedness.

## Parenteral Dosage Forms

### LEVOFLOXACIN CONCENTRATE FOR INJECTION

**Usual adult dose**
Bronchitis, bacterial exacerbations, treatment—
   Intravenous infusion, 500 mg, administered over a 60-minute period, every twenty-four hours for seven days.
Pneumonia, community-acquired, treatment—
   Intravenous infusion, 500 mg, administered over a 60-minute period, every twenty-four hours for seven to fourteen days.
Pyelonephritis, treatment—
   Intravenous infusion, 250 mg, administered over a 60-minute period, every twenty-four hours for ten days.
Sinusitis, treatment—
   Intravenous infusion, 500 mg, administered over a 60-minute period, every twenty-four hours for ten to fourteen days.
Skin and soft tissue infections, treatment—
   Intravenous infusion, 500 mg, administered over a 60-minute period, every twenty-four hours for seven to ten days.
Urinary tract infections, bacterial, complicated, treatment—
   Intravenous infusion, 250 mg, administered over a 60-minute period, every twenty-four hours for ten days.

**Usual pediatric dose**
Safety and efficacy have not been established.

**Strength(s) usually available**
U.S.—
   500 mg per 20 mL (Rx) [*Levaquin*].

**Packaging and storage**
Store below 40 °C (104 °F), preferably between 15 and 30 °C (59 and 86 °F), unless otherwise specified by the manufacturer. Protect from light.

**Preparation of dosage form**
To prepare a 250-mg dose for intravenous infusion, withdraw 10 mL of levofloxacin concentrate for injection from the vial and dilute with 40 mL of a compatible intravenous solution, for a total volume of 50 mL. To prepare a 500-mg dose, withdraw 20 mL of levofloxacin concentrate for injection from the vial and dilute with 80 mL of a compatible intravenous solution, for a total volume of 100 mL.

**Stability**
When diluted to a concentration of 5 mg per mL, levofloxacin concentrate for injection is stable for 72 hours when stored at or below 25 °C (77 °F) and for 14 days when refrigerated (5 °C [41 °F]) in plastic intravenous containers. Diluted solutions that are frozen in glass bottles or plastic containers are stable for 6 months when stored at -20 °C (-4 °F). Frozen solutions should be thawed at room temperature or in a refrigerator. They should not be thawed in a microwave or by water bath immersion. Do not refreeze after initial thawing.

**Incompatibilities**
Because there are only limited data on the compatibility of other substances with levofloxacin concentrate for injection, additives or other medications should not be added to levofloxacin concentrate for injection in the single-use vials or infused simultaneously through the same intravenous line.

**Note**
This product should be inspected visually for any particulate matter before administration. Samples with visible particles should be discarded.
Levofloxacin concentrate for injection contains no preservative or bacteriostatic agent. Because of this, the vials are for single use only; any unused portion remaining in the vial should be discarded.

### LEVOFLOXACIN INJECTION

**Usual adult dose**
See *Levofloxacin Concentrate for Injection*.

**Usual pediatric dose**
See *Levofloxacin Concentrate for Injection*.

**Strength(s) usually available**
U.S.—
   250 mg per 50 mL (Rx) [*Levaquin*].
   500 mg per 100 mL (Rx) [*Levaquin*].

**Packaging and storage**
Store at or below 25 °C (77 °F); however, brief exposure up to 40 °C (104 °F) does not adversely affect the product. Protect from excessive heat, freezing, and light.

**Incompatibilities**
Because there are only limited data on the compatibility of other substances with levofloxacin injection, additives or other medications should not be added to levofloxacin injection in the single-use vials or infused simultaneously through the same intravenous line.

**Note**
This product should be inspected visually for any particulate matter before administration. Samples with visible particles should be discarded.
Levofloxacin injection vials are for single use only; any unused portion should be discarded.

Developed: 07/31/97

---

# LEVOMETHADYL Systemic†

INN: Levomethadyl acetate—Levacetylmethadol.
VA CLASSIFICATION (Primary): CN101
Note: Controlled substance classification—
   U.S.—II.
Commonly used brand name(s): *Orlaam*.
Other commonly used names are LAAM, LAM, levacetylmethadol, levo-alpha-acetylmethadol, levomethadyl acetate, and MK790.
Note: For a listing of dosage forms and brand names by country availability, see *Dosage Forms* section(s).

†Not commercially available in Canada.

## Category
Opioid (narcotic) abuse therapy adjunct.
Note: Levomethadyl is an opioid (narcotic) analgesic, but is not used for relief of pain.

## Indications

**General considerations**
In the U.S., levomethadyl is permitted to be dispensed only through opioid addiction treatment programs approved by the Food and Drug Administration (FDA), Drug Enforcement Administration (DEA), and designated state authorities. Use of levomethadyl in such programs is subject to treatment requirements stipulated in Federal regulations.

**Accepted**
Opioid (narcotic) drug use, illicit (treatment adjunct)—Levomethadyl is indicated as an adjunct to other measures, which may include psychological and social counseling and medical and rehabilitative services, in the treatment of opioid dependence. It may be used in detoxification programs (to assist withdrawal from illicit opioids) and in maintenance programs (to discourage illicit use of other opioids). Appropriate evaluation, planning, counseling, and follow-up are essential components of successful treatment. There is no evidence that administration of an opioid alone is effective treatment for opioid addiction.

Note: In the U.S., Federal regulations permit specific opioids (levomethadyl and methadone) to be used in approved detoxification and interim or comprehensive maintenance treatment programs. Levomethadyl is administered only 3 times a week and may be particularly useful for patients who do not require daily visits to the clinic, whereas methadone must be administered every day and may be more useful for patients who benefit from the support of daily clinic visits. Also, because some patients experience effects perceived as aversive during treatment with one opioid or the other, the selection of a particular opioid may depend on patient acceptance.

   Short-term (up to 30 days) or long-term (up to 180 days) detoxification programs use an opioid to alleviate adverse physiological or psychological consequences of withdrawal from illicit opioids, with dosage gradually being decreased until a drug-free state is achieved. After 180 days, patients who have not achieved a drug-free state are considered to be receiving maintenance treatment. Patients may also be enrolled directly into a maintenance program without first attempting detoxification. In maintenance treatment programs, relatively stable doses of opioid are given on a continuing basis as a substitute for illicit opioids.

Detoxification and comprehensive maintenance programs must include a full range of medical and rehabilitative services in addition to opioid administration. However, patients who are awaiting admission to a comprehensive maintenance program may receive up to 120 days of interim maintenance treatment, which consists only of opioid administration and needed medical services.

## Pharmacology/Pharmacokinetics

### Physicochemical characteristics
Chemical group—Opioid analgesic; chemically related to both oxymorphone and naloxone.
Molecular weight—Levomethadyl acetate hydrochloride: 389.97.
Octanol:water partition coefficient—405:1.

### Mechanism of action/Effect
Levomethadyl is a mu-receptor opioid agonist. It substitutes for opioids of the morphine type, thereby suppressing withdrawal symptoms in individuals who are addicted to such agents. With chronic use, levomethadyl produces cross-tolerance to the effects of other mu-receptor agonists, including the subjective "high" they produce, and decreases the addict's desire for such drugs.

### Other actions/effects
Levomethadyl produces effects characteristic of mu-receptor opioid analgesics, including analgesia, respiratory depression, sedation, pupillary constriction, and physical dependence.

### Absorption
Rapid.

### Distribution
Extensive. The volume of distribution is about 20 L per kg of body weight (L/kg).

### Protein binding
High (approximately 80%); primarily to an alpha globulin. Studies in heroin addicts have demonstrated that levomethadyl, levomethadyl's active metabolites, and methadone bind to, compete for, and displace each other from the same protein-binding sites.

### Biotransformation
Levomethadyl undergoes extensive first-pass metabolism to the active demethylated metabolite nor-levomethadyl (nor-LAAM), which is further demethylated to a second active metabolite, dinor-levomethadyl (dinor-LAAM). Smaller quantities of levomethadyl are also deacetylated to methadol, nor-methadol, and dinor-methadol. The rate of biotransformation is subject to interindividual variability. Although biotransformation to nor-LAAM generally occurs more slowly in males than in females, the differences are not as great as the interindividual differences.

### Half-life
Distribution—
  Levomethadyl: Approximately 6 hours.
Elimination—
  Levomethadyl: Approximately 2.6 days.
  nor-LAAM: Approximately 2 days.
  dinor-LAAM: Approximately 4 days.

### Onset of action
Although some opioid analgesic effects are apparent 2 to 4 hours after an oral dose, suppression of opioid withdrawal symptoms occurs after a delay of at least several days, during which levomethadyl's active metabolites are forming and accumulating.

### Time to peak concentration
Levomethadyl—Usually 1.5 to 2 hours, but up to 4 hours in some studies.
nor-LAAM—Usually 4 to 7 hours, but up to 10 hours in some individuals.
dinor-LAAM—Usually 5 to 7 hours, but 24 to 48 hours in some individuals.

### Peak serum concentration
One study in 12 patients reported substantial interindividual variability in the peak concentrations of levomethadyl and its active metabolites after single and multiple doses. Plasma concentrations of levomethadyl, nor-LAAM, and dinor-LAAM were higher after multiple doses than after single doses, but the concentrations of the metabolites, especially dinor-LAAM, were increased to a greater extent than those of levomethadyl.

Studies of peak and trough steady-state concentrations showed that there is great interindividual variability in levomethadyl concentrations over a 72-hour dosing interval. Also, although the concentration of levomethadyl itself decreased considerably during the 72-hour interval, the concentrations of the active metabolites, especially dinor-LAAM, decreased to a much lesser extent.

### Time to steady state
Three-times-per-week dosing schedule—1 to 2 weeks (approximately 9, 8, and 12.5 days for levomethadyl, nor-LAAM, and dinor-LAAM, respectively).

### Time to peak effect
Suppression of opioid withdrawal symptoms—Approximately 7 to 10 days after initiation of treatment.

### Duration of action
Suppression of opioid withdrawal symptoms—
  Single 30- to 60-mg dose: 24 to 48 hours.
  Single 80-mg or higher dose: 48 to 72 hours.

### Elimination
Approximately 27% of a dose is eliminated in the urine as levomethadyl and various metabolites (nor-LAAM, dinor-LAAM, methadol, nor-methadol, and dinor-methadol). The disposition of the remainder of the dose has not been determined in humans, but extensive biliary elimination has been demonstrated in animal studies.

## Precautions to Consider

### Carcinogenicity
Levomethadyl was not carcinogenic in 2-year studies in rats given 13 mg per kg of body weight (mg/kg) (77 mg per square meter of body surface area [mg/m$^2$]) or in mice given 30 mg/kg (90 mg/m$^2$).

### Mutagenicity
Levomethadyl was not mutagenic in the Ames test, the unscheduled DNA synthesis and repair test, *in vitro* mouse lymphoma cell studies, or *in vivo* rat chromosomal aberration tests. However, levomethadyl exhibited mutagenic activity in the ad-3 forward mutation assay in *N. crassa* in concentrations of 150 mcg per mL (mcg/mL) *in vitro* and in the heritable translocation assay in mice receiving 21 mg/kg (63 mg/m$^2$). The significance of these findings to clinical use in humans is not known.

### Pregnancy/Reproduction
Pregnancy—Methadone is the agent of choice for pregnant women in comprehensive maintenance treatment programs. There are no clinical data on the safety of levomethadyl during pregnancy. Levomethadyl administration should not be started or continued during pregnancy except by the written order of a physician who determines levomethadyl to be the best choice of therapy for an individual patient. In the U.S., Federal regulations require that women of childbearing potential receive a pregnancy test prior to initiation of, and monthly during, levomethadyl maintenance treatment.

Animal reproduction studies have not been completed. However, in one study administration of 0.2 or 2 mg/kg per day to rats prior to and throughout gestation caused opioid dependence in both the dams and pups. The larger dose also produced high incidences of premature delivery, stillbirths, and decreased pup weights. However, there were no differences in the rates of implantation, resorption, or morphological abnormalities between treated and control groups.

FDA Pregnancy Category C.

Labor and delivery—The effects of levomethadyl on labor and delivery are not known.

Postpartum—Use of levomethadyl during pregnancy may result in respiratory depression and/or physical dependence with delayed emergence of withdrawal symptoms in the neonate.

### Breast-feeding
It is not known whether levomethadyl is distributed into breast milk in quantities sufficient to affect the nursing infant.

### Pediatrics
In the U.S., Federal regulations prohibit use of levomethadyl in addicts younger than 18 years of age.

### Geriatrics
No information is available on the relationship of age to the effects of levomethadyl in geriatric patients.

### Dental
Opioid analgesics may decrease or inhibit salivary flow, thus contributing to the development of caries, periodontal disease, oral candidiasis, and discomfort.

## Drug interactions and/or related problems
The following drug interactions and/or related problems have been selected on the basis of their potential clinical significance (possible mechanism in parentheses where appropriate)—not necessarily inclusive (» = major clinical significance):

Note: Combinations containing any of the following medications, depending on the amount present, may also interact with this medication.

» Alcohol or
» CNS depression–producing medications, other (See *Appendix II*)
(concurrent use may increase the CNS depressant, respiratory depressant, and hypotensive effects of these medications and/or levomethadyl; a reduction in dosage of levomethadyl and/or other prescribed CNS depressants may be required if concurrent use is necessary; also, opioid addicts should be warned of the risk of additive effects and potential for serious toxicity if they abuse alcohol or other CNS depressants while receiving levomethadyl)

» Enzyme inducers, hepatic, cytochrome P450 (see *Appendix II*)
(induction of the hepatic cytochrome P450 enzyme system may increase the rate of levomethadyl metabolism to its active metabolites and enhance its peak effectiveness, but may also shorten its duration of action)

» Enzyme inhibitors, hepatic (see *Appendix II*)
(inhibition of hepatic enzymes may slow the onset, lower the peak activity, and/or increase the duration of action of levomethadyl; adjustment of levomethadyl dosage and/or the interval between doses may be required)

» Opioid analgesics, mixed agonist/antagonist, such as:
   Butorphanol
   Nalbuphine
   Pentazocine

» Opioid analgesics, partial mu-receptor agonist, such as:
   Buprenorphine
   Dezocine or

» Opioid antagonists, such as:
   Naloxone
   Naltrexone
(these medications may precipitate withdrawal symptoms if administered to a patient receiving levomethadyl therapy; the severity of withdrawal symptoms will depend on the potency and dose of the antagonist or partial agonist and on the degree to which physical dependence is present)

(opioid analgesics such as levomethadyl will be ineffective if treatment is initiated in a patient receiving naltrexone, which blocks the therapeutic effects of opioids)

» Opioid analgesics, mu-receptor agonist, other, such as:
   Alfentanil
   Anileridine
   Codeine
   Fentanyl
   Heroin
   Hydrocodone
   Hydromorphone
   Levorphanol
   Meperidine
   Methadone
   Morphine
   Opium
   Oxycodone
   Oxymorphone
   Propoxyphene
   Sufentanil
(chronic use of levomethadyl produces cross-tolerance to the therapeutic effects, but not necessarily to the toxic effects, of other mu-receptor opioid agonists, leading to a considerably higher-than-normal dosage requirement for other mu-receptor agonists and a substantial risk of additive toxicity; deaths have occurred early in levomethadyl treatment in opioid addicts who continued to use illicit opioids during the 1- to 2-week delay in levomethadyl's onset of action. Administration of a mu-receptor opioid analgesic to levomethadyl-treated patients, if necessary for therapeutic purposes, requires extreme caution and careful monitoring. Opioid agonists that are *N*-demethylated to long-acting, excitatory metabolites [e.g., meperidine, propoxyphene] should not be used because the high dosage requirement also leads to an unacceptably high risk of metabolite-induced toxicity)

## Laboratory value alterations
The following have been selected on the basis of their potential clinical significance (possible effect in parentheses where appropriate)—not necessarily inclusive (» = major clinical significance):

Note: The following laboratory value alterations have not been documented with levomethadyl. However, they are commonly produced by other mu-receptor opioid agonists and should be considered potential effects of levomethadyl also.

Because of the long half-life of levomethadyl and its active metabolites, effects on laboratory values may persist for several days after treatment has been discontinued.

With diagnostic test results
   Gastric emptying studies
      (opioid analgesics may delay gastric emptying, thereby invalidating test results)
   Hepatobiliary imaging using technetium Tc 99m disofenin
      (delivery of technetium Tc 99m disofenin to the small bowel may be prevented because of opioid analgesic–induced constriction of the sphincter of Oddi and increased biliary tract pressure; these actions result in delayed visualization and thus resemble obstruction of the common bile duct)

With physiology/laboratory test values
   Amylase, plasma and
   Lipase, plasma
      (values may be increased because opioid analgesics can cause contractions of the sphincter of Oddi and increased biliary tract pressure)
   Cerebrospinal fluid (CSF) pressure
      (may be increased; effect is secondary to respiratory depression–induced carbon dioxide retention)

## Medical considerations/Contraindications
The medical considerations/contraindications included have been selected on the basis of their potential clinical significance (reasons given in parentheses where appropriate)—not necessarily inclusive (» = major clinical significance).

*Risk-benefit should be considered when the following medical problems exist:*
   Abdominal conditions, acute
      (diagnosis or clinical course may be obscured)
   » Asthma, acute attack or
   » Respiratory depression, acute or
   » Respiratory impairment or disease, chronic
      (risk of apnea because opioids decrease respiratory drive and increase airway resistance)
   Cardiac dysrhythmias
      (levomethadyl may cause QT interval prolongation; careful monitoring is recommended during therapy)
   Dependence on or abuse of nonopioid medications, history of, including alcoholism or
   Emotional instability or
   Suicidal ideation or attempts
      (addicts often attempt suicide using combinations of opioids and other drugs of abuse. Patients who continue to use illicit opioids or other CNS-active medications despite adequate levomethadyl therapy require individualized evaluation and treatment planning; hospitalization may be necessary)
   Diagnostic, surgical, or other procedure requiring general anesthesia or sedation
      (levomethadyl-induced alterations in patient response to medications that may be used in conjunction with general anesthesia or sedation [e.g., tolerance to the therapeutic effects of mu-receptor opioid agonists; increased risk of severe CNS and/or respiratory depression with anesthetics, sedatives, and opioid analgesics] and the risk of precipitating withdrawal via use of opioid antagonists, mixed agonists/antagonists, or partial mu-receptor agonists must be taken into consideration when selecting medications and dosages to be administered)
   Diarrhea associated with pseudomembranous colitis caused by antibiotics or
   Diarrhea caused by poisoning
      (opioids may slow the elimination of toxic material, and it is generally recommended that they not be administered until after toxins have been cleared from the gastrointestinal tract; however, levomethadyl administration should not be interrupted if these conditions occur during treatment)
   Gallbladder disease or gallstones
      (opioids may cause biliary colic)

Gastrointestinal tract surgery, recent
   (opioids may alter gastrointestinal motility)
Head injury or
Increased intracranial pressure, pre-existing or
Intracranial lesions
   (increased risk of respiratory depression and further elevation of cerebrospinal fluid pressure; also, opioids may cause sedation and pupillary changes that may obscure the clinical course of head injury)
Hepatic function impairment or
Renal function impairment
   (although studies have not been done in patients with clinically significant hepatic or renal function impairment, the possibility must be considered that formation of levomethadyl's active metabolites and/or elimination of levomethadyl and its active metabolites may be substantially altered; because of its less complex metabolic profile, methadone may be preferable for such patients)
Hypothyroidism
   (risk of respiratory depression and prolonged CNS depression is greatly increased)
» Inflammatory bowel disease, severe
   (risk of toxic megacolon may be increased)
Prostatic hypertrophy or obstruction or
Urethral stricture or
Urinary tract surgery, recent
   (increased risk of urinary retention, which may be induced by these conditions as well as by opioids)
Sensitivity to levomethadyl, history of

**Patient monitoring**
The following may be especially important in patient monitoring (other tests may be warranted in some patients, depending on condition; » = major clinical significance):
» Drug screen
   (in the U.S., Federal regulations mandate screening for drugs of abuse [amphetamines, barbiturates, cocaine, other opioids, and any other agents known to be abused in the program's locality] at the time a prospective patient first appears at the treatment center. Further testing is not required for patients undergoing detoxification from opioid drugs. Patients receiving interim maintenance treatment must be tested at least twice during a 120-day interim program, and patients receiving comprehensive maintenance treatment must be tested at least 8 times at random intervals during the first year of treatment and at least quarterly thereafter)
» Pregnancy test
   (in the U.S., Federal regulations require that women of childbearing potential receive a pregnancy test prior to initiation of, and monthly during, levomethadyl maintenance therapy because levomethadyl administration should not be started or continued during pregnancy except by the written order of a physician who determines levomethadyl to be the best choice of therapy for an individual patient)

## Side/Adverse Effects

Note: Many symptoms typical of opioid withdrawal (listed below) occur during levomethadyl treatment. Early in treatment, while levomethadyl's active metabolites are forming and accumulating, such symptoms probably indicate withdrawal from illicit opioid analgesics. However, they may continue to occur many weeks after treatment has begun, especially on the days between doses. Adjustment of levomethadyl dosage, supplemental low doses of methadone, and/or a suppressant such as clonidine or guanabenz may be needed.

In addition to the side/adverse effects listed below, the following have been reported in patients receiving levomethadyl (although a causal relationship has not been established): Amenorrhea; electrocardiographic irregularities, including prolongation of the QT interval and nonspecific ST-T wave changes; hepatitis; liver function test abnormalities; and pyuria.

The following side/adverse effects have been selected on the basis of their potential clinical significance (possible signs and symptoms in parentheses where appropriate)—not necessarily inclusive:

**Those indicating need for medical attention**
Incidence less frequent (1 to 3%)
   *Edema* (swelling of face, fingers, feet, and/or lower legs; weight gain); *mental depression; skin rash*

**Those indicating need for medical attention only if they continue or are bothersome**
Incidence more frequent (3% or higher)
   *Abdominal pain; constipation; general feeling of discomfort or illness; joint pain; nervousness; sexual problems in males; sweating; trouble in sleeping; weakness*
Incidence less frequent (1 to 3%)
   *Back pain; blurred vision; chills; CNS symptoms* (anxiety; decreased sensitivity to stimulation; drowsiness; false sense of well-being; headache; unusual dreams); *coughing; decreased desire for sex; diarrhea; dry mouth; flu-like syndrome; hot flashes; nausea and vomiting; runny nose; yawning*

Note: In some clinical trials, a significant number of patients experienced symptoms of stimulation, such as anxiety and nervousness, on the day of administration. Some patients continued to experience these symptoms on the days between doses, whereas others experienced symptoms such as lack of energy, dysphoria, and depression.
   Patients should be advised to report severe *drowsiness* or stimulation (e.g., feeling "wired") at the next visit to the clinic, because dosage adjustment may be needed.

Incidence less than 1%
   *Hypotension, postural* (dizziness, lightheadedness, or feeling faint when rising from a lying or sitting position); *muscle pain; watery eyes*

**Those indicating possible withdrawal and/or the need for dosage adjustment or other treatment if they occur during therapy or after medication is discontinued**
   *Body aches; diarrhea; fast heartbeat; gooseflesh; increased sweating; loss of appetite; nausea or vomiting; nervousness, restlessness, or irritability; runny nose; shivering or trembling; sneezing; stomach cramps; trouble in sleeping; unexplained fever; unusually large pupils of eyes; weakness; yawning*

## Overdose

For specific information on the agents used in the management of levomethadyl overdose, see:
- *Naloxone (Systemic)* monograph; and/or
- *Charcoal, Activated (Oral-Local)* monograph.

For more information on the management of overdose, **contact a Poison Control Center** (see *Poison Control Center Listing*).

Levomethadyl toxicity is more likely to develop when therapy is started in patients who have not developed tolerance to the effects of opioids. In nontolerant patients, initial doses of 20 to 40 mg may cause somnolence, and larger initial doses may cause serious toxicity. Opioid-tolerant individuals may also experience symptoms, but at higher initial doses.

Although overdose with levomethadyl alone has been reported rarely, as a result of too-frequent (daily) administration, most overdoses have involved ingestion of other opioids in addition to levomethadyl. Deaths have occurred when patients continued to use illicit opioids after initiation of levomethadyl treatment.

**Clinical effects of overdose**
The following effects have been selected on the basis of their potential clinical significance (possible signs and symptoms in parentheses where appropriate)—not necessarily inclusive:
   *Cold, clammy skin; confusion; low blood pressure; pinpoint pupils of eyes; respiratory depression* (blue lips, fingernails, or skin; slow or troubled breathing); *severe dizziness, drowsiness, muscle weakness, nervousness, or restlessness; slow heartbeat; unconsciousness*

Note: In severe overdosage, extreme CNS and respiratory depression may result in apnea, shock, pulmonary edema, cardiac arrest, and death.

**Treatment of overdose**
Primary importance should be given to maintaining adequate ventilation. Assessing the patient's respiratory status and, if necessary, administering oxygen or otherwise assisting respiration are essential. Provision of an artificial airway may be necessary.

To decrease absorption—Emptying the stomach by inducing emesis and/or administering activated charcoal. The initial dose of charcoal should be followed by a cathartic, such as magnesium citrate, if the charcoal is not pre-mixed with sorbitol. Gastric lavage may also be performed. During these procedures, care should be taken to protect the airway of any patient who is not fully alert. However, treatment of respiratory depression or other life-threatening complications must take precedence.

To enhance elimination—Forced diuresis, peritoneal dialysis, hemoperfusion, and hemodialysis are not likely to be effective for removal of levomethadyl because of its lipophilicity and large volume of distribution.

Specific treatment—Administering naloxone, keeping in mind that rapid reversal of opioid effects may precipitate severe withdrawal symptoms, which may rarely lead to cardiac instability, in this patient population. Administration of several doses of naloxone, starting with considerably lower-than-usual quantities that may be increased gradually, if necessary, until the desired effect has been achieved is preferable to administration of large, single doses. Prolonged naloxone treatment, via repeated injections or continuous intravenous infusion, is likely to be necessary because of levomethadyl's long duration of action. Oral administration of the long-acting opioid antagonist naltrexone may precipitate prolonged withdrawal symptoms and is not recommended. See the package insert or *Naloxone (Systemic)* for specific dosing guidelines for use of this product.

Monitoring—

Respiration, oxygenation, patient alertness, and vital signs should be monitored. Because of levomethadyl's long duration of action, prolonged observation will be needed.

A screen for other medications, especially other drugs of abuse, should be performed and additional treatment instituted as required.

Supportive care—

Supportive measures include establishing intravenous lines, hydration, and administering vasopressors if necessary.

## Patient Consultation

As an aid to patient consultation, refer to *Advice for the Patient, Levomethadyl (Systemic)*.

In providing consultation, consider emphasizing the following selected information (» = major clinical significance):

### Before using this medication
» Conditions affecting use, especially:
   Sensitivity to levomethadyl
   Pregnancy—Not starting levomethadyl during pregnancy; methadone is preferred medication for treating pregnant opioid addicts
   Use in children—Use in patients up to 18 years of age not permitted by U.S. Federal regulations
   Other medications, especially alcohol or other CNS depressants, hepatic enzyme inducers or inhibitors, other opioid analgesics, and opioid antagonists
   Other medical problems, especially diarrhea caused by antibiotics or by poisoning, asthma or other respiratory problems, and severe inflammatory bowel disease

### Proper use of this medication
» Medication must be taken at clinic, usually 3 times per week
» Proper dosing

### Precautions while using this medication
» Importance of compliance with other measures necessary for rehabilitation, e.g., counseling, attending support group meetings, making lifestyle changes
» Avoiding use of alcoholic beverages and illicit opioids or other CNS depressants during therapy, even if experiencing withdrawal symptoms and cravings, because of the risk of potentially fatal additive toxicity or overdose
» Caution if severe drowsiness occurs, especially when treatment initiated or dosage adjusted
» Getting up slowly from a lying or sitting position; lying down for a while may relieve symptoms associated with postural hypotension, such as dizziness, lightheadedness, or feeling faint
» Need to inform physicians and dentists of levomethadyl use, particularly if any kind of surgery (including dental surgery) or emergency treatment is required
   Possible need for regimen to prevent severe constipation
   Possible dryness of mouth; using sugarless gum or candy, ice, or saliva substitute for relief; checking with dentist if dry mouth continues for more than 2 weeks
» Female patients only: Not becoming pregnant during treatment; discussing planned pregnancy with counselor ahead of time; informing counselor if pregnancy suspected
» If transferring to methadone: Not taking first dose of methadone for at least 48 hours after last dose of levomethadyl
» Suspected overdose: Getting emergency help at once; need to inform emergency practitioners that the patient is physically dependent on a long-acting opioid, naloxone is likely to precipitate withdrawal, and prolonged observation and monitoring are needed

### Side/adverse effects
Getting emergency help immediately if respiratory depression or other symptoms of overdose occur

Signs and symptoms of other potential side effects, especially edema, mental depression, and skin rash
Informing counselor at clinic if severe drowsiness, severe stimulation, or withdrawal symptoms occurred after previous dose

## General Dosing Information

In the U.S., levomethadyl is available only through treatment programs that have been approved by the Food and Drug Administration, Drug Enforcement Agency, and designated state authorities.

Levomethadyl is given only by the oral route. The commercially available oral solution must be diluted before being administered to the patient. Treatment centers that dispense both levomethadyl and methadone (which must also be dispensed as a dilute liquid) should use liquids of different colors for preparing each medication, so that they can be distinguished from each other readily.

Levomethadyl is to be ingested by the patient at the treatment center. Take-home doses are not permitted.

Levomethadyl treatment should be initiated using a dose that suppresses withdrawal symptoms and decreases craving for illicit opioids without inducing excessive opioid effects. Interpatient variability in levomethadyl kinetics and each patient's level of tolerance to opioids must be taken into account when selecting initial dosage. However, because of levomethadyl's slow onset of action and the risk of toxicity if dosage is increased too rapidly, elimination of withdrawal symptoms and craving may not be possible during the first 1 or 2 weeks of therapy. Patients may need extra counseling and support and/or administration of a withdrawal suppressant, preferably a nonopioid such as clonidine or guanabenz, during this time. Alternatively, treatment may be initiated with methadone (especially if the patient's degree of tolerance to opioids is not known), since effective dosage can be achieved more rapidly, and the patient transferred to levomethadyl after a few weeks. The changeover from methadone to levomethadyl may be accomplished in a single dose.

Levomethadyl is usually administered 3 times a week (on Monday, Wednesday, and Friday or on Tuesday, Thursday, and Saturday), but some patients experience withdrawal symptoms during the 72-hour Friday-to-Monday or Saturday-to-Tuesday interval. Administration of a higher dose on Friday or Saturday prevents or minimizes this problem in most patients. However, in a clinical trial patients receiving such a regimen reported feeling overmedicated on the day that the higher dose was given and undermedicated after the next (lower) dose. For some patients, use of a withdrawal suppressant such as clonidine or guanabenz; provision of a low take-home dose of methadone (if the patient meets the criteria specified in U.S. Federal regulations for take-home methadone); arranging the patient's schedule so that the 72-hour interval occurs during the week, so that a small dose of methadone can be administered to the patient at the clinic if necessary; or administration of levomethadyl on an every-other-day basis may be necessary. **Levomethadyl should not be administered daily** because rapid accumulation of the medication and its active metabolites may lead to an overdose.

Patients receiving levomethadyl may be transferred directly to methadone, although some patients may experience mild withdrawal symptoms during the first 1 or 2 weeks. The initial dose of methadone, which should be taken at least 48 hours after the last dose of levomethadyl, should be 80% of the patient's lower levomethadyl dose. For example, a patient receiving three-times-a week treatment with 80, 80, and 100 mg of levomethadyl would be given 64 mg of methadone per day, initially. The daily dose of methadone may be increased or decreased by 5 or 10 mg if symptoms of withdrawal or opioid excess occur. This regimen may also be used, provided that the regulations and requirements for take-home methadone are met, when a levomethadyl-treated patient who is unable to attend the clinic regularly for a period of time (for example, because of illness or travel) requires a temporary transfer to take-home methadone. The risk of the methadone's being diverted to illicit use must be considered. The number of take-home methadone doses should be 2 fewer than the number of days of expected absence, but must not exceed the maximum number of take-home doses specified in U.S. Federal regulations. When the patient returns to the clinic levomethadyl may be resumed, following the same dosage regimen as before the temporary change in treatment. However, if the last methadone dose was taken more than 48 hours previously, levomethadyl should be reintroduced at a dose based on clinical and/or toxicological evaluation of the patient.

Patients who miss a single dose of levomethadyl and who arrive at the clinic the next day should receive their usual dose on an every-other-day basis for the remainder of the week, then resume their normal dosing schedule the following week. For example, a missed Monday dose would be administered on Tuesday, after which the remaining doses for the week would be given on Thursday and Saturday and the normal Monday, Wednesday, and Friday schedule resumed the following Monday. Although most patients who miss a single dose and return to the clinic on their next regularly scheduled day should be able to tolerate the usual dose of levomethadyl, some individuals may require a reduced dose. After 2 doses have been missed, treatment should be restarted using only one-half to three-fourths of the previous maintenance dose for the first dose and increasing each subsequent dose by 5 or 10 mg until the previous maintenance dose is reached. After a lapse of 3 doses (1 week) or more, therapy should be reinstituted with induction doses.

Discontinuation of levomethadyl maintenance therapy may be considered after the patient has achieved behavioral objectives outlined in the patient's comprehensive treatment plan, i.e., stopped using illicit drugs, reached social and occupational goals, and changed his or her lifestyle to decrease the risk of relapse. Treatment should not be stopped prematurely, and appropriate nonpharmacological support should be provided to reduce further the risk of relapse. Stable long-term treatment is preferable to cycles of discontinuation of therapy followed by recidivism. Treatment has been successfully discontinued by abrupt withdrawal or by reducing dosage gradually (by 5 to 10% per week). One study comparing both methods of detoxification found that withdrawal symptoms were not more severe, and a significantly higher number of patients were successfully withdrawn from maintenance treatment without returning to illicit opioid use, when levomethadyl was stopped abruptly.

**Safety considerations for handling this medication**

Because of the risk of diversion of this potent opioid, security measures stipulated in the U.S. Federal Code of Regulations should be taken to safeguard supplies of the medication.

There are no known hazards associated with dermal or aerosol exposure to levomethadyl. However, if the medication is spilled onto an individual, contaminated clothing should be removed and the exposed skin rinsed with cool water.

## Oral Dosage Forms

### LEVOMETHADYL ACETATE HYDROCHLORIDE ORAL SOLUTION

**Usual adult dose**

Opioid (narcotic) abuse therapy adjunct—
Induction—
  Patients not receiving prior methadone maintenance treatment—Oral, 20 to 40 mg for the first dose. Subsequent doses, given at forty-eight- or seventy-two-hour intervals, may be increased by 5 to 10 mg until the desired effects (absence of withdrawal symptoms and decreased craving for illicit opioids) have been achieved or decreased by the same amount if undue sedation or other symptoms of opioid excess occur.
  Patients transferred from methadone maintenance treatment—Oral, a quantity of levomethadyl equivalent to 1.2 to 1.3 times the patient's daily methadone dose, up to a maximum of 120 mg, for the first dose. Subsequent doses, administered at forty-eight- or seventy-two-hour intervals, should be adjusted according to the response of the individual patient, using caution not to increase the dose too rapidly because of the risk of toxicity. Dosage is generally increased by 5 to 10 mg every second or third dose.
Maintenance—
  Dosage must be individualized according to the patient's tolerance and response. Most patients can be stabilized on 60 to 80 mg, administered three times a week at forty-eight- or seventy-two-hour intervals. However, maintenance doses as low as 10 mg and as high as 140 mg, administered three times a week, have been used in clinical trials. If necessary to prevent withdrawal over a seventy-two-hour interdose interval, the dose prior to this interval may be increased, in 6- to 10-mg increments, to up to forty percent higher than the doses given prior to a forty-eight-hour interval. At least two weeks are required to achieve a new clinical plateau after each adjustment of levomethadyl dosage.

Note: U.S. Federal regulations require that single doses of 140 mg or more be justified in the patient's record.

**Usual adult prescribing limits**

Initial induction dose—40 mg (if the patient's level of opioid tolerance is unknown) or 120 mg (if the patient's level of tolerance, based on methadone dosage requirements, is known).

Maintenance—Dosage should not exceed 140 mg three times a week or every other day, or two 130-mg doses and one 180-mg dose per week.

**Usual pediatric dose**

U.S. Federal regulations prohibit use of levomethadyl in patients younger than 18 years of age.

**Usual geriatric dose**

See *Usual adult dose*.

**Strength(s) usually available**

U.S.—
  10 mg per mL (Rx) [*Orlaam* (methylparaben 1.8 mg; and propylparaben 0.2 mg per mL)].
Canada—
  Not commercially available.

**Packaging and storage**

Store between 15 and 30 °C (59 and 86 °F), protected from freezing, unless otherwise specified by manufacturer.

**Preparation of dosage form**

U.S. Federal regulations stipulate that the oral solution must be diluted before being administered to the patient. The liquid used for dilution should be colored differently than a liquid used to prepare methadone solutions in the same clinic.

## Selected Bibliography

Tennant FS, Rawson RA, Pumphrey E, et al. Clinical experiences with 959 opioid-dependent patients treated with levo-alpha-acetylmethadol (LAAM). J Subst Abuse Treat 1986; 3: 195-202.

Ling W, Blakis M, Holmes ED, et al. Restabilization with methadone after methadyl acetate maintenance. Arch Gen Psychiatry 1980; 37: 194-6.

Judson BA, Goldstein A, Inturrisi CE. Methadyl acetate (LAAM) in the treatment of heroin addicts. II. Double-blind comparison of graduated and abrupt detoxification. Arch Gen Psychiatry 1983; 40: 834-40.

Developed: 08/11/95

**LEVONORGESTROL**—See *Progestins (Systemic)*

**LEVORPHANOL**—See *Opioid (Narcotic) Analgesics (Systemic)*

**LEVOTHYROXINE**—See *Thyroid Hormones (Systemic)*

**LIDOCAINE**—See *Anesthetics (Mucosal-Local); Anesthetics (Parenteral-Local); Anesthetics (Topical); Lidocaine (Systemic)*

# LIDOCAINE Systemic

VA CLASSIFICATION (Primary): CV300

Commonly used brand name(s): *Xylocaine; Xylocard.*

Note: For a listing of dosage forms and brand names by country availability, see *Dosage Forms* section(s).

## Category

Antiarrhythmic.

## Indications

**Accepted**

Arrhythmias, ventricular (treatment)—Lidocaine (systemic) is indicated and is the drug of choice in the acute management of ventricular arrhythmias, such as those resulting from acute myocardial infarction, digitalis toxicity, cardiac surgery, or cardiac catheterization.

# Pharmacology/Pharmacokinetics

**Physicochemical characteristics**
pKa—7.86.

**Mechanism of action/Effect**
Antiarrhythmic—Lidocaine decreases the depolarization, automaticity, and excitability in the ventricles during the diastolic phase by a direct action on the tissues, especially the Purkinje network, without involvement of the autonomic system. Neither contractility, systolic arterial blood pressure, atrioventricular (AV) conduction velocity, nor absolute refractory period is altered by usual therapeutic doses. In the Vaughan Williams classification of antiarrhythmics, lidocaine is a class IB agent.

**Distribution**
Rapid. Volume of distribution (Vol$_D$)—About 1 liter per kg of body weight (L/kg); reduced in heart failure patients.

**Protein binding**
Moderate to high (60 to 80%; dependent on drug concentration).

**Biotransformation**
90% hepatic; active metabolites, monoethylglycinexylidide and glycinexylidide, may contribute to therapeutic and toxic effects, especially after infusions lasting 24 hours or more.

**Half-life**
1 to 2 hours (average about 100 minutes); dose-dependent (tends to be biphasic with the distribution phase of 7 to 9 minutes causing the short duration of action following an intravenous loading dose); increased to 3 hours or longer during prolonged intravenous infusions (longer than 24 hours).

**Onset of action**
Intravenous—Immediate (45 to 90 seconds).

**Time to steady-state plasma concentration**
Continuous intravenous infusion—3 to 4 hours (8 to 10 hours in patients with acute myocardial infarction).

**Therapeutic plasma concentration**
1.5 to 5 mcg/mL (concentrations exceeding 5 mcg/mL are considered to be in the toxic range).

**Duration of action**
Intravenous—10 to 20 minutes.

**Elimination**
Renal, 10% unchanged.
In dialysis—Very little removable by dialysis.

# Precautions to Consider

**Cross-sensitivity and/or related problems**
Patients sensitive to other amide-type anesthetics or flecainide or tocainide may be sensitive to lidocaine also. Cross-sensitivity with procainamide or quinidine has not been reported.

**Carcinogenicity/Mutagenicity**
Long-term animal studies evaluating the carcinogenic or mutagenic potential of lidocaine have not been done.

**Pregnancy/Reproduction**
Pregnancy—Lidocaine crosses the placenta. Adequate and well-controlled studies in humans have not been done.
Studies in rats given doses up to 6.6 times the maximum human dose have not shown that lidocaine causes adverse effects in the fetus. However, lidocaine has been shown to constrict uterine arteries in sheep and in experimentally isolated uterine artery segments. Furthermore, studies in sheep have shown that lidocaine causes significant increases in fetal blood pressure and increases or decreases in fetal heart rate related to the rate of lidocaine infusion.
FDA Pregnancy Category B.

**Breast-feeding**
It is not known whether lidocaine is distributed into human breast milk. However, problems in humans have not been documented.

**Pediatrics**
Appropriate studies on the relationship of age to the effects of lidocaine have not been performed in the pediatric population. However, no pediatrics-specific problems have been documented to date.

**Geriatrics**
Elderly patients are more prone to the adverse effects of lidocaine. In patients over 65 years of age, dose and rate of infusion should be reduced by one half and adjusted slowly as needed and tolerated. In addition, elderly patients are more likely to have age-related renal function impairment, which may require dosage adjustment.

**Drug interactions and/or related problems**
The following drug interactions and/or related problems have been selected on the basis of their potential clinical significance (possible mechanism in parentheses where appropriate)—not necessarily inclusive (» = major clinical significance):

Note: Combinations containing any of the following medications, depending on the amount present, may also interact with this medication.

Antiarrhythmics, other
(although some antiarrhythmic agents may be used in combination for therapeutic advantage, combined use may sometimes potentiate risk of adverse cardiac effects)

» Anticonvulsants, hydantoin
(concurrent use with lidocaine may have additive cardiac depressant effects; hydantoin anticonvulsants may also promote increased hepatic metabolism of lidocaine, reducing its intravenous concentration)

Beta-adrenergic blocking agents, systemic and ophthalmic (if systemic absorption occurs)
(concurrent use may slow hepatic metabolism and increase the risk of toxicity of lidocaine because of reduced hepatic blood flow)

Cimetidine
(concurrent administration with lidocaine may result in reduced hepatic clearance of lidocaine, possibly resulting in delayed elimination and increased blood concentrations; monitoring of blood concentrations and clinical parameters as a guide to dosage is recommended)

Neuromuscular blocking agents
(effects may be potentiated when used concurrently with large doses [such as those over 5 mg per kg] of intravenous lidocaine)

**Laboratory value alterations**
The following have been selected on the basis of their potential clinical significance (possible effect in parentheses where appropriate)—not necessarily inclusive (» = major clinical significance):

With diagnostic test results
Bentiromide
(concurrent administration of lidocaine during a bentiromide test period will invalidate test results since lidocaine is also metabolized to arylamines and will thus increase the percent of PABA recovered; discontinuation of lidocaine at least 3 days prior to the administration of bentiromide is recommended)

**Medical considerations/Contraindications**
The medical considerations/contraindications included have been selected on the basis of their potential clinical significance (reasons given in parentheses where appropriate)—not necessarily inclusive (» = major clinical significance).

*Except under special circumstances, this medication should not be used when the following medical problems exist:*

» Adams-Stokes syndrome or
» Heart block, severe, including atrioventricular, intraventricular, or sinoatrial blocks
(heart block may be worsened)

*Risk-benefit should be considered when the following medical problems exist:*

» Congestive heart failure or
Hepatic function impairment or
» Reduced hepatic blood flow or
Renal function impairment
(accumulation may occur; dose and rate of infusion should be reduced by one half)

» Heart block, incomplete or
» Hypovolemia and shock or
» Sinus bradycardia or
» Wolff-Parkinson-White syndrome
(may be aggravated)

Sensitivity to lidocaine

**Patient monitoring**
The following may be especially important in patient monitoring (other tests may be warranted in some patients, depending on condition; » = major clinical significance):

Blood pressure determinations and
» Electrocardiograph (ECG) determinations
(recommended throughout therapy to help adjust dosage and detect toxicity; intravenous infusion of lidocaine should be promptly discontinued if ECG determinations show a prolonged PR interval and QRS complex or if arrhythmias occur or become worse)

Electrolyte concentrations, serum
  (periodic to allow imbalance corrections during prolonged infusions)

Lidocaine concentrations, serum
  (useful to avoid toxicity during prolonged or high-dose infusions or in patients receiving drugs that alter lidocaine clearance)

## Side/Adverse Effects

Note: Adverse effects are dose- and age-related; incidence is increased in patients over 65 years of age.

Adverse cardiovascular effects at therapeutic doses are rare, except in patients with existing compromised ventricular function. Cardiac conduction disturbances are extremely rare. High plasma lidocaine concentrations may lead to hypotension, arrhythmias, heart block, and respiratory and cardiac arrest.

The following side/adverse effects have been selected on the basis of their potential clinical significance (possible signs and symptoms in parentheses where appropriate)—not necessarily inclusive:

**Those indicating need for medical attention**
Incidence rare
  *Allergic reaction* (difficulty in breathing; itching; skin rash; swelling of skin)

**Those indicating need for medical attention only if they continue or are bothersome**
Incidence less frequent or rare
  *Pain at site of injection*—with prolonged intravenous use
Incidence dose-related
  *With serum lidocaine concentrations of 1.5 to 6 mcg/mL*
    *Anxiety or nervousness; dizziness; drowsiness; feelings of coldness, heat, or numbness*

## Overdose

For more information on the management of overdose or unintentional ingestion, **contact a Poison Control Center** (see *Poison Control Center Listing*).

**Clinical effects of overdose**
The following effects have been selected on the basis of their potential clinical significance (possible signs and symptoms in parentheses where appropriate)—not necessarily inclusive:

With serum lidocaine concentrations of 6 to 8 mcg/mL
  *Blurred or double vision; nausea or vomiting; ringing in ears; tremors or twitching*

With serum lidocaine concentrations of > 8 mcg/mL
  *Difficulty in breathing; dizziness, severe, or fainting; seizures; slow heartbeat*

**Treatment of overdose (for severe reactions)**
Stopping administration of lidocaine; monitoring patient closely.
Maintenance of airway and administration of oxygen.
  Specific treatment—
    For circulatory depression—Administration of a vasopressor (such as ephedrine or metaraminol) and intravenous fluids if necessary.
    For seizures—If no satisfactory response to respiratory support is obtained, diazepam in 2.5-mg increments, or an ultra-short-acting barbiturate (such as thiopental or thiamylal) in 50- to 100-mg increments, is often beneficial. Caution must be maintained because of possible additive circulatory depression. If patient is under anesthesia, a short-acting muscle relaxant (such as succinylcholine) administered intravenously is sometimes helpful. When such relaxants are used, ability to provide artificial respiration is mandatory.

## General Dosing Information

See also *Patient monitoring*.

Dosage should be adjusted to meet the individual requirements of each patient, on the basis of clinical response.

The use of lidocaine necessitates concurrent ECG monitoring and the availability of oxygen, resuscitation equipment, and emergency medications for the management of possible adverse reactions involving the cardiovascular system and/or central nervous system (CNS) as well as possible allergic reactions.

**For intravenous administration**
Lidocaine for intravenous administration must *not* contain preservatives or other medications such as epinephrine.

The preferred diluent for lidocaine infusion is 5% dextrose injection.

Lidocaine must *not* be added to blood transfusions.

To achieve optimal control of lidocaine dosage and rate of administration, it is recommended that lidocaine be administered intravenously by means of an infusion pump, a microdrip regulator, or a similar device that allows precise adjustment of the flow rate.

A loading dose of lidocaine is commonly administered for the initial intravenous dose to partially compensate for its rapid perfusion and distribution, which tend to delay attainment of a therapeutic serum concentration. If the initial loading dose does not provide the desired effect within 5 minutes, a second loading dose reduced to one half to one third of the first dose may be given.

Dosage reduction may be required with prolonged intravenous infusions (longer than 24 hours) because of the risk of accumulation.

## Parenteral Dosage Forms

### LIDOCAINE HYDROCHLORIDE INJECTION (FOR CONTINUOUS INTRAVENOUS INFUSION) USP

**Usual adult dose**
Antiarrhythmic—
  Continuous intravenous infusion (usually following a loading dose), 20 to 50 mcg (0.02 to 0.05 mg) per kg of body weight at a rate of 1 to 4 mg per minute.

Note: Geriatric patients may be more sensitive to the effects of the usual adult dose.

**Usual adult prescribing limits**
300 mg (about 4.5 mg per kg of body weight) in any one-hour period.

**Usual pediatric dose**
Antiarrhythmic—
  Continuous intravenous infusion (usually following a loading dose), 30 mcg (range, 20 to 50 mcg) (0.03 mg; range, 0.02 to 0.05 mg) per kg of body weight per minute.

**Strength(s) usually available**
U.S.—
  4% w/v (40 mg per mL [1 gram per 25 mL or 2 grams per 50 mL]) (Rx) [*Xylocaine* (preservative-free) [GENERIC (may contain methylparaben)].
  10% w/v (100 mg per mL [1 gram per 10 mL]) (Rx) [GENERIC (may contain methylparaben)].
  20% w/v (200 mg per mL [1 gram per 5 mL or 2 grams per 10 mL]) (Rx) [*Xylocaine* (preservative-free) [GENERIC (may contain methylparaben)].
Canada—
  2% (20 mg per mL [1 gram per 50 mL]) (Rx) [*Xylocard*].
  20% (200 mg per mL [1 gram per 5 mL]) (Rx) [*Xylocard*].

**Packaging and storage**
Store below 40 °C (104 °F), preferably between 15 and 30 °C (59 and 86 °F). Protect from freezing.

**Preparation of dosage form**
To prepare solution for intravenous infusion, add 1 gram of lidocaine hydrochloride (25 mL of 4% or 5 mL of 20% Lidocaine Hydrochloride Injection USP) to 1 liter of 5% dextrose injection; the resultant concentration will be 1 mg per mL. Check manufacturer's package insert for additional dilution information.

**Stability**
After dilution in the appropriate intravenous solution for infusion, lidocaine hydrochloride is stable for at least 24 hours.

**Auxiliary labeling**
Following dilution, a label stating the concentration of the lidocaine hydrochloride contents with time and date of dilution should be placed on the infusion solution container.

### LIDOCAINE HYDROCHLORIDE INJECTION (FOR DIRECT INTRAVENOUS INJECTION) USP

**Usual adult dose**
Antiarrhythmic—
  Direct intravenous injection, 1 mg per kg of body weight (usually 50 to 100 mg) as a loading dose at a rate of about 25 to 50 mg per minute, the dose being repeated after five minutes if necessary; usually followed by continuous intravenous infusion of lidocaine to maintain antiarrhythmic effects.

Note: Geriatric patients may be more sensitive to the effects of the usual adult dose.

**Usual adult prescribing limits**
300 mg (about 4.5 mg per kg of body weight) in any one-hour period.

**Usual pediatric dose**
Antiarrhythmic—
  Direct intravenous injection, 1 mg per kg of body weight as a loading dose at a rate of about 25 to 50 mg per minute, the dose being repeated after five minutes if necessary but not exceeding a total dose of 3 mg per kg; usually followed by continuous intravenous infusion of lidocaine to maintain antiarrhythmic effects.

**Strength(s) usually available**
U.S.—
  1% w/v (10 mg per mL [50 mg per 5 mL or 100 mg per 10 mL]) (Rx) [*Xylocaine* (preservative-free) [GENERIC (may contain methylparaben)].
  2% w/v (20 mg per mL [100 mg per 5 mL]) (Rx) [*Xylocaine* (preservative-free) [GENERIC (may contain methylparaben)].
Canada—
  2% w/v (20 mg per mL [100 mg per 5 mL]) (Rx) [*Xylocard* [GENERIC].

**Packaging and storage**
Store below 40 °C (104 °F), preferably between 15 and 30 °C (59 and 86 °F). Protect from freezing.

**Stability**
When dilution is required, it should be done immediately prior to direct intravenous administration.

### STERILE LIDOCAINE HYDROCHLORIDE USP

**Usual adult dose**
Antiarrhythmic—
  Continuous intravenous infusion (usually following a loading dose), 20 to 50 mcg (0.02 to 0.05 mg) per kg of body weight at a rate of 1 to 4 mg per minute.
Note: Geriatric patients may be more sensitive to the effects of the usual adult dose.

**Usual adult prescribing limits**
300 mg (about 4.5 mg per kg of body weight) in any one-hour period.

**Usual pediatric dose**
Antiarrhythmic—
  Continuous intravenous infusion (usually following a loading dose), 30 mcg (0.03 mg) (range, 20 to 50 mcg) per kg of body weight per minute.

**Size(s) usually available**
U.S.—
  1 gram (Rx) [GENERIC].
  2 grams (Rx) [GENERIC].
Canada—
  Not commercially available.

**Packaging and storage**
Store below 40 °C (104 °F), preferably between 15 and 30 °C (59 and 86 °F).

**Preparation of dosage form**
Sterile Lidocaine Hydrochloride USP is prepared for continuous intravenous infusion by adding 1 or 2 grams to 1000 mL of 5% dextrose injection, producing a solution containing 1 or 2 mg of lidocaine hydrochloride per mL, respectively. Check manufacturer's package insert for additional dilution information.

**Stability**
After dilution in the appropriate intravenous solution for infusion, lidocaine hydrochloride is stable for at least 24 hours.

**Auxiliary labeling**
Following dilution, a label stating the concentration of the lidocaine hydrochloride contents with time and date of dilution should be placed on the infusion solution container.

### LIDOCAINE HYDROCHLORIDE AND DEXTROSE INJECTION (FOR CONTINUOUS INTRAVENOUS INFUSION) USP

**Usual adult dose**
Antiarrhythmic—
  Continuous intravenous infusion (usually following a loading dose), 20 to 50 mcg (0.02 to 0.05 mg) of lidocaine hydrochloride per kg of body weight at a rate of 1 to 4 mg per minute.
Note: Geriatric patients may be more sensitive to the effects of the usual adult dose.

**Usual adult prescribing limits**
300 mg (about 4.5 mg per kg of body weight) in any one-hour period.

**Usual pediatric dose**
Antiarrhythmic—
  Continuous intravenous infusion (usually following a loading dose), 30 mcg (range, 20 to 50 mcg) (0.03 mg; range, 0.02 to 0.05 mg) of lidocaine hydrochloride per kg of body weight per minute at a rate of 1 to 4 mg per minute.

**Strength(s) usually available**
U.S.—
  Lidocaine Hydrochloride
  0.1% w/v (1 mg per mL [250 mg per 250 mL, 500 mg per 500 mL, or 1 gram per 1000 mL]) (Rx) [[GENERIC]].
  0.2% w/v (2 mg per mL [500 mg per 250 mL, 1 gram per 500 mL or 2 grams per 1000 mL]) (Rx) [[GENERIC]].
  0.4% w/v (4 mg per mL [1 gram per 250 mL, 2 grams per 500 mL, or 4 grams per 1000 mL]) (Rx) [[GENERIC]].
  0.8% w/v (8 mg per mL [2 grams per 250 mL, 4 grams per 500 mL, 8 grams per 1000 mL]) (Rx) [[GENERIC]].
Canada—
  Lidocaine Hydrochloride
  0.1% w/v (1 mg per mL [250 mg per 250 mL, 500 mg per 500 mL, or 1 gram per 1000 mL]) (Rx) [[GENERIC]].
  0.2% w/v (2 mg per mL [500 mg per 250 mL, 1 gram per 500 mL or 2 grams per 1000 mL]) (Rx) [[GENERIC]].
  0.4% w/v (4 mg per mL [1 gram per 250 mL, 2 grams per 500 mL, or 4 grams per 1000 mL]) (Rx) [[GENERIC]].
  0.8% w/v (8 mg per mL [2 grams per 250 mL or 4 grams per 500 mL]) (Rx) [[GENERIC]].

**Packaging and storage**
Store below 40 °C (104 °F), preferably between 15 and 30 °C (59 and 86 °F). Protect from freezing.

## Selected Bibliography
Anderson JL. Current understanding of lidocaine as an antiarrhythmic agent: a review. Clin Ther 1984; 1986(2): 125-44.

Revised: 10/21/92
Interim revision: 10/27/93; 08/19/97

---

**LIDOCAINE AND PRILOCAINE**—The *Lidocaine and Prilocaine (Topical)* monograph is not included in this published version of the USP DI database. Copies of the monograph are available on request from Micromedex, Inc. - Reprint Requests, 6200 S. Syracuse Way, Suite 300, Englewood, CO 80111; telephone (303) 486-6400; telefax (303) 486-6464; Email: USPDI@MDX.COM.

---

# LINCOMYCIN  Systemic

VA CLASSIFICATION (Primary): AM350
Commonly used brand name(s): *Lincocin*; *Lincorex*.
Note: For a listing of dosage forms and brand names by country availability, see *Dosage Forms* section(s).

## Category
Antibacterial (systemic).

## Indications
**Accepted**
Lincomycin has been used in the treatment of serious infections caused by susceptible strains of streptococci, pneumococci, and staphylococci. However, lincomycin generally has been replaced by safer and more effective agents.

Not all species or strains of a particular organism may be susceptible to lincomycin.

## Pharmacology/Pharmacokinetics

### Physicochemical characteristics
Molecular weight—461.01.

### Mechanism of action/Effect
Antibacterial (systemic)—Lincomycin inhibits protein synthesis in susceptible bacteria by binding to the 50 S subunits of bacterial ribosomes and preventing peptide bond formation. It is usually considered bacteriostatic, but may be bactericidal in high concentrations or when used against highly susceptible organisms.

### Absorption
Rapidly absorbed from the gastrointestinal tract following oral administration. Approximately 20 to 30% absorbed orally in fasting state; absorption decreased when taken with food.

### Distribution
Widely and rapidly distributed to most fluids and tissues, except cerebrospinal fluid (CSF); high concentrations in bone, bile, and urine; lincomycin may reach significant concentrations in the eye following parenteral administration.

Readily crosses the placenta. Up to 25% of maternal serum concentrations. Also distributed into breast milk.

### Protein binding
Protein binding decreases with increased plasma concentrations. Range, 28 to 86% (average, 70 to 75%). Albumin is not thought to be the primary binding component.

### Biotransformation
Presumed to be hepatic; metabolites have not been fully characterized.

### Half-life
Normal renal function—5.4 hours (range, 4 to 6 hours).
End-stage renal disease—10 to 20 hours.
Impaired hepatic function—Half-life almost doubled.

### Time to peak serum concentration
Oral: 2 to 4 hours.
Intramuscular: 0.5 hour.
Intravenous: End of infusion.

### Elimination
Renal, biliary. Mean urinary recovery of unchanged drug over a 24-hour period ranges from 10–47% after an intramuscular dose, 13–72% after an intravenous dose, and 3–13% after a fasting oral dose. Approximately 30–40% of an oral dose is excreted unchanged in the feces within 72 hours.

In dialysis—Not removed from the blood by hemodialysis or peritoneal dialysis.

## Precautions to Consider

### Cross-sensitivity and/or related problems
Patients hypersensitive to clindamycin may be hypersensitive to lincomycin also. A case of apparent cross-sensitivity has also been reported with doxorubicin.

### Pregnancy/Reproduction
Lincomycin crosses the placenta and may be concentrated in the fetal liver. However, problems in humans have not been documented.

### Breast-feeding
Lincomycin is distributed into breast milk; reported concentrations range from 0.5 to 2.4 mcg per mL. However, problems in humans have not been documented.

### Pediatrics
Lincomycin hydrochloride injection contains benzyl alcohol, which has been associated with a fatal gasping syndrome in premature infants.

### Geriatrics
No information is available on the relationship of age to the effects of lincomycin in geriatric patients.

### Drug interactions and/or related problems
The following drug interactions and/or related problems have been selected on the basis of their potential clinical significance (possible mechanism in parentheses where appropriate)—not necessarily inclusive (» = major clinical significance):

Note: Combinations containing any of the following medications, depending on the amount present, may also interact with this medication.

» Anesthetics, hydrocarbon inhalation, such as:
  Chloroform
  Cyclopropane
  Enflurane
  Halothane
  Isoflurane
  Methoxyflurane
  Trichloroethylene or
» Neuromuscular blocking agents
  (concurrent use of these medications with lincomycin, if necessary, should be carefully monitored since neuromuscular blockade may be enhanced, resulting in skeletal muscle weakness and respiratory depression or paralysis [apnea]; caution is also recommended when these medications are used concurrently with lincomycin during surgery or in the postoperative period; treatment with anticholinesterase agents or calcium salts may help reverse the blockade)

» Antidiarrheals, adsorbent
  (concurrent use of kaolin- or attapulgite-containing antidiarrheals with oral lincomycin may significantly decrease absorption of oral lincomycin; concurrent use should be avoided or patients should be advised to take adsorbent antidiarrheals not less than 2 hours before or 3 to 4 hours after oral lincomycin)

» Antidiarrheals, antiperistaltic
  (antiperistaltic agents, such as opiates, difenoxin, diphenoxylate, or loperamide, may prolong or worsen pseudomembranous colitis by delaying toxin elimination)

Antimyasthenics
  (concurrent use of medications with neuromuscular blocking action may antagonize the effect of antimyasthenics on skeletal muscle; temporary dosage adjustments of antimyasthenics may be necessary to control symptoms of myasthenia gravis during and following concurrent use)

» Chloramphenicol or
» Erythromycins
  (may displace lincomycin from or prevent its binding to 50 S subunits of bacterial ribosomes, thus antagonizing the effects of lincomycin; concurrent use is not recommended)

Opioid (narcotic) analgesics
  (respiratory depressant effects of drugs with neuromuscular blocking activity may be additive to central respiratory depressant effects of opioid analgesics, possibly leading to increased or prolonged respiratory depression or paralysis [apnea]; caution and careful monitoring of the patient are recommended)

### Laboratory value alterations
The following have been selected on the basis of their potential clinical significance (possible effect in parentheses where appropriate)—not necessarily inclusive (» = major clinical significance):

With physiology/laboratory test values
  Alanine aminotransferase (ALT [SGPT]), serum and
  Alkaline phosphatase, serum and
  Aspartate aminotransferase (ALT [SGOT]), serum
    (values may be increased)

### Medical considerations/Contraindications
The medical considerations/contraindications included have been selected on the basis of their potential clinical significance (reasons given in parentheses where appropriate)—not necessarily inclusive (» = major clinical significance).

*Risk-benefit should be considered when the following medical problems exist:*

» Gastrointestinal disease, history of, especially ulcerative colitis, regional enteritis, or antibiotic-associated colitis
  (lincomycin may cause pseudomembranous colitis)

» Hepatic function impairment, severe
  (the half-life of lincomycin is prolonged in patients with severe hepatic function impairment; this may require an adjustment in dosage)

Hypersensitivity to lincomycins or doxorubicin

» Renal function impairment, severe
  (patients with impaired renal function do not generally require a reduction in dose unless the impairment is severe; patients receiving lincomycin with severely impaired renal function should receive 25 to 30% of the usual dose of patients with normal renal function)

### Patient monitoring
The following may be especially important in patient monitoring (other tests may be warranted in some patients, depending on condition; » = major clinical significance):

*For antibiotic-associated pseudomembranous colitis (AAPMC)*
  Proctosigmoidoscopy and/or
  Colonoscopy
    (proctosigmoidoscopy and/or colonoscopy may be required in selected, severely ill patients with persistant symptoms of AAPMC to

document the presence of pseudomembranes; it is no longer recommended as a routine monitoring parameter)

Stool examinations
(cytotoxin assays of stool samples for the presence of *Clostridium difficile* and its cytotoxin, neutralizable by *C. sordellii* antitoxin, may be required prior to treatment in patients with AAPMC to document the presence of *C. difficile* and/or its cytotoxin; however, *C. difficile* and its cytotoxin may persist following treatment with oral vancomycin despite clinical improvement; follow-up cytotoxin assays are generally not recommended with complete clinical improvement)

## Side/Adverse Effects

The following side/adverse effects have been selected on the basis of their potential clinical significance (possible signs and symptoms in parentheses where appropriate)—not necessarily inclusive:

**Those indicating need for medical attention**
Incidence more frequent
*Pseudomembranous colitis* (abdominal or stomach cramps and pain, severe; abdominal tenderness; diarrhea, watery and severe, which may also be bloody; fever)
Incidence less frequent
*Hypersensitivity* (skin rash, redness, and itching); *neutropenia* (sore throat and fever); *thrombocytopenic purpura* (unusual bleeding or bruising)

**Those indicating need for medical attention only if they continue or are bothersome**
Incidence more frequent
*Gastrointestinal disturbances* (abdominal pain; diarrhea; nausea and vomiting)
Incidence less frequent
*Fungal overgrowth* (itching of rectal or genital areas)

**Those indicating possible pseudomembranous colitis and the need for medical attention if they occur after medication is discontinued**
*Abdominal or stomach cramps and pain, severe; abdominal tenderness; diarrhea, watery and severe, which may also be bloody; fever*

## Patient Consultation

As an aid to patient consultation, refer to *Advice for the Patient, Lincomycin (Systemic)*.
In providing consultation, consider emphasizing the following selected information (» = major clinical significance):

**Before using this medication**
» Conditions affecting use, especially:
Hypersensitivity to lincomycin, clindamycin, or doxorubicin
Pregnancy—Lincomycin crosses the placenta
Breast-feeding—Lincomycin is distributed into breast milk
Use in children—Lincomycin is not recommended in infants up to 1 month of age; lincomycin injection contains benzyl alcohol, which has been associated with a fatal gasping syndrome in premature infants
Other medications, especially hydrocarbon inhalation anesthetics, neuromuscular blocking agents, antiperistaltic and adsorbent antidiarrheals, chloramphenicol, or erythromycins
Other medical problems, especially a history of gastrointestinal disease, particularly ulcerative colitis, severe renal function impairment, or severe hepatic function impairment

**Proper use of this medication**
» Taking on an empty stomach with an 8 ounce glass of water
» Compliance with full course of therapy, especially in streptococcal infections
» Importance of not missing doses and taking at evenly spaced times
» Proper dosing
Missed dose: Taking as soon as possible; not taking if almost time for next dose; not doubling doses
» Proper storage

**Precautions while using this medication**
Regular visits to physician to check progress
Checking with physician if no improvement within a few days
» For severe diarrhea, checking with physician before taking any antidiarrheals; for mild diarrhea, taking kaolin- or attapulgite-containing antidiarrheals at least 2 hours before or 3 to 4 hours after taking oral lincomycin; other antidiarrheals may worsen or prolong the diarrhea; checking with physician or pharmacist if mild diarrhea continues or worsens
Caution if surgery with general anesthesia is required

**Side/adverse effects**
Signs of potential side effects, especially hypersensitivity, neutropenia, thrombocytopenic purpura, and pseudomembranous colitis

## General Dosing Information

Therapy should be continued for at least 10 days in group A beta-hemolytic streptococcal infections to help prevent the occurrence of acute rheumatic fever.

**For oral dosage forms only**
Lincomycin should preferably be taken with a full glass (240 mL) of water on an empty stomach (either 1 hour before or 2 hours after meals) to obtain optimum serum concentrations.

**For intravenous administration**
Lincomycin should be infused over a period of at least one hour. Rare instances of cardiopulmonary arrest and hypotension have been reported after administration at greater-than-recommended concentration and rate.

**For treatment of adverse effects**
For antibiotic-associated pseudomembranous colitis (AAPMC)
• Some patients may develop AAPMC, caused by *Clostridium difficile* toxin, during or following administration of lincomycins. Mild cases may respond to discontinuation of the drug alone. Moderate to severe cases may require fluid, electrolyte, and protein replacement.
• In cases not responding to the above measures or in more severe cases, oral doses of metronidazole, bacitracin, cholestyramine, or vancomycin may be used. Oral vancomycin is effective in doses of 125 to 500 mg every 6 hours for 5 to 10 days. The dose of metronidazole is 250 to 500 mg every 8 hours; cholestyramine, 4 grams four times a day; and bacitracin, 25,000 units, orally, four times a day. Recurrences may be treated with a second course of these medications.
• Cholestyramine and colestipol resins have been shown to bind *C. difficile* toxin *in vitro*. If cholestyramine or colestipol resin is administered in conjunction with oral vancomycin, the medications should be administered several hours apart since the resins have been shown to bind oral vancomycin also.
• In addition, antibiotic-associated pseudomembranous colitis may result in severe watery diarrhea, which may occur during therapy or up to several weeks after therapy is discontinued. If diarrhea occurs, administration of antiperistaltic antidiarrheals (e.g., opiates, diphenoxylate and atropine combination, loperamide) is not recommended since they may delay the removal of toxins from the colon, thereby prolonging and/or worsening the condition.

## Oral Dosage Forms

Note: The dosing and strengths of the dosage forms available are expressed in terms of lincomycin base (not the hydrochloride salt).

### LINCOMYCIN HYDROCHLORIDE CAPSULES USP

**Usual adult and adolescent dose**
Antibacterial—
Oral, 500 mg (base) every six to eight hours.

**Usual pediatric dose**
Antibacterial—
Infants up to 1 month of age: Use is not recommended.
Infants 1 month of age and over: Oral, 7.5 to 15 mg (base) per kg of body weight every six hours; or 10 to 20 mg per kg of body weight every eight hours.

**Strength(s) usually available**
U.S.—
250 mg (base) (Rx) [*Lincocin*].
500 mg (base) (Rx) [*Lincocin*].
Canada—
500 mg (Rx) [*Lincocin*].

**Packaging and storage**
Store below 40 °C (104 °F), preferably between 15 and 30 °C (59 and 86 °F), unless otherwise specified by manufacturer. Store in a tight container.

**Auxiliary labeling**
• Take on empty stomach.
• Continue medicine for full time of treatment.

## Parenteral Dosage Forms

Note: The dosing and strengths of the dosage forms available are expressed in terms of lincomycin base (not the hydrochloride salt).

### LINCOMYCIN HYDROCHLORIDE INJECTION USP

**Usual adult and adolescent dose**
Antibacterial—
   Intramuscular, 600 mg (base) every twelve to twenty-four hours.
   Intravenous, 600 mg to 1 gram (base), administered over at least one hour, every eight to twelve hours.
   Subconjunctival, 75 mg (base).

**Usual adult prescribing limits**
Intravenous, up to 8 grams (base) daily.

**Usual pediatric dose**
Antibacterial—
   Infants up to 1 month of age:
      Use is not recommended.
   Infants 1 month of age and over:
      Intramuscular, 10 mg (base) per kg of body weight every twelve to twenty-four hours.
      Intravenous, administered over at least one hour: 3.3 to 6.7 mg (base) per kg of body weight every eight hours; or 5 to 10 mg per kg of body weight every twelve hours.

**Strength(s) usually available**
U.S.—
   600 mg (base) in 2 mL (Rx) [*Lincocin* (benzyl alcohol 9.45 mg per mL)].
   3000 mg (base) in 10 mL (Rx) [*Lincorex*].
Canada—
   600 mg (base) in 2 mL (Rx) [*Lincocin* (benzyl alcohol 9.45 mg per mL)].

**Packaging and storage**
Store below 40 °C (104 °F), preferably between 15 and 30 °C (59 and 86 °F), unless otherwise specified by manufacturer. Protect from freezing.

**Preparation of dosage form**
To prepare initial dilution for intravenous use, each dose must be diluted as follows:

| Dose (grams) | Diluent (mL) | Duration of Administration (hr) |
| --- | --- | --- |
| ≤1 | 125 | 1 |
| 2 | 200 | 2 |
| 3 | 300 | 3 |
| 4 | 400 | 4 |

**Stability**
Lincomycin is physically compatible for 4 hours at room temperature with intravenous solutions containing penicillin G sodium or colistimethate.
Lincomycin is physically compatible for 24 hours at room temperature with 5 and 10% dextrose injection, 5 or 10% dextrose and 0.9% sodium chloride injection, Ringer's injection, M/6 sodium lactate injection, 6% dextran and 0.9% sodium chloride injection, or 10% invert sugar and electrolytes injection, and with intravenous solutions containing vitamin B complex, vitamin B complex and ascorbic acid, cephalothin, cephoranide, tetracycline hydrochloride, ampicillin, methicillin, chloramphenicol, or polymyxin B sulfate.

**Incompatibilities**
Lincomycin is physically incompatible with novobiocin and kanamycin.

Revised: 10/06/92
Interim revision: 03/24/94

---

# LINDANE  Topical

VA CLASSIFICATION (Primary/Secondary): AP300/AP900
[Former name—Gamma Benzene Hexachloride]

Commonly used brand name(s): *Bio-Well; G-well; GBH; Hexit; Kildane; Kwell; Kwellada; Kwildane; PMS Lindane; Scabene; Thionex.*

Another commonly used name is gamma benzene hexachloride

Note: For a listing of dosage forms and brand names by country availability, see *Dosage Forms* section(s).

## Category

Pediculicide—Lindane Shampoo; Lindane Cream; Lindane Lotion.
Scabicide—Lindane Cream; Lindane Lotion.

## Indications

Note: Bracketed information in the *Indications* section refers to uses that are not included in U.S. product labeling.

**Accepted**
Pediculosis capitis (treatment) or
Pediculosis pubis (treatment)—Lindane shampoo, [cream], and [lotion] are indicated for the treatment of pediculosis (lice) infestations caused by *Pediculus humanus* var. *capitis* (head louse) and *Phthirus pubis* (pubic or crab louse) and their ova.
Scabies (treatment)—Lindane cream and lotion are indicated for the treatment of scabies infestation caused by *Sarcoptes scabiei*.

**Unaccepted**
In the U.S., lindane cream and lotion are no longer indicated for the treatment of pediculosis capitis (head lice) or pediculosis pubis (pubic or crab lice).

## Pharmacology/Pharmacokinetics

**Physicochemical characteristics**
Molecular weight—290.83.

**Mechanism of action/Effect**
Lindane is a central nervous system (CNS) stimulant when absorbed systemically. Following absorption through the chitinous exoskeleton of arthropods, lindane is presumed to stimulate the nervous system, resulting in convulsions and death.

**Absorption**
Lindane is absorbed significantly through the skin.
Lotion—In one study, a mean peak blood concentration of 28 nanograms per mL occurred in infants and children 6 hours after total body application of lindane lotion for scabies.
Shampoo—In one study, a mean peak blood concentration of 3 nanograms per mL occurred in persons 6 hours after topical use of lindane shampoo.

**Half-life**
In one study, the half-life of lindane was 18 hours in infants and children treated for scabies using total body application of lindane lotion.

## Precautions to Consider

**Carcinogenicity**
Studies in animals have not shown lindane to have carcinogenic properties.

**Tumorigenicity**
In one study, despite the high incidence of tumors in the control group, lindane was thought to be associated with a significant increase in the incidence of hepatoma.

**Mutagenicity**
Studies have not shown lindane to have mutagenic properties.

**Pregnancy/Reproduction**
Pregnancy—Adequate and well-controlled studies in humans have not been done. Because lindane is absorbed through the skin and has the potential for causing CNS toxicity, some clinicians do not recommend the use of lindane during pregnancy. If lindane is used, however, the recommended dosage should not be exceeded in pregnant women, and these women should not be treated more than twice during pregnancy.
Studies in animals have not shown that lindane causes adverse effects on the fetus.
FDA Pregnancy Category B.

**Breast-feeding**
Problems in humans have not been documented; however, lindane is systemically absorbed and is distributed into breast milk. Although the concentrations found in human blood following topical application of lindane make it unlikely that breast milk will contain amounts of lindane sufficient to cause toxicity, an alternate method of feeding the infant should be used for 2 days.

### Pediatrics
Caution is recommended in infants and children, since studies have shown that the potential for toxic effects of topically applied lindane is greater in the young than in adults.

Lindane is not recommended for use in premature neonates, because their skin is likely to be more permeable than that of full-term neonates and their liver enzymes may not be sufficiently developed to metabolize the medication.

### Geriatrics
Although appropriate studies on the relationship of age to the effects of lindane have not been performed in the geriatric population, no geriatrics-specific problems have been documented to date. However, some experts believe that absorption of lindane may be increased in the elderly because of possible increased permeability of their skin. In addition, elderly patients with a history of seizure activity may be especially sensitive to the CNS toxicity effects of lindane.

### Drug interactions and/or related problems
The following drug interactions and/or related problems have been selected on the basis of their potential clinical significance (possible mechanism in parentheses where appropriate)—not necessarily inclusive (» = major clinical significance):

Skin, scalp, or hair preparations, other, such as creams, lotions, ointments, or oils
 (simultaneous application may increase the percutaneous absorption of lindane)

### Medical considerations/Contraindications
The medical considerations/contraindications included have been selected on the basis of their potential clinical significance (reasons given in parentheses where appropriate)—not necessarily inclusive (» = major clinical significance).

*Risk-benefit should be considered when the following medical problems exist:*

Convulsive disorders
 (sufficient systemic absorption of lindane may induce seizures)

Sensitivity to lindane

Skin rash or raw or broken skin
 (possible increased absorption of lindane)

## Side/Adverse Effects
Note: Lindane is absorbed through the skin and has the potential for CNS toxicity, especially in infants, children, and possibly the elderly.

The following side/adverse effects have been selected on the basis of their potential clinical significance (possible signs and symptoms in parentheses where appropriate)—not necessarily inclusive:

**Those indicating need for medical attention**
Incidence rare
 *Skin irritation not present before therapy*—if lindane is applied incorrectly or repeatedly, the incidence of skin irritation is increased; *skin rash*

Symptoms of CNS toxicity
 *Convulsions; dizziness, clumsiness, or unsteadiness; fast heartbeat; muscle cramps; nervousness, restlessness, or irritability; vomiting*

**Those indicating need for medical attention if they occur and continue or are bothersome after medication is discontinued**
Itching of skin—acquired sensitivity to mites and their products; may continue for one to several weeks

## Patient Consultation
As an aid to patient consultation, refer to *Advice for the Patient, Lindane (Topical)*.
In providing consultation, consider emphasizing the following selected information (» = major clinical significance):

### Before using this medication
» Conditions affecting use, especially:
 Sensitivity to lindane
 Pregnancy—Lindane is absorbed through the skin and has the potential for causing toxic effects in the CNS of the fetus; not increasing the amount, frequency, or length of therapy that physician ordered; not being treated more than twice during a pregnancy
 Breast-feeding—Lindane is distributed into breast milk; another method of feeding infant should be used for 2 days after use of lindane
 Use in children—Caution is recommended, since infants and children are especially sensitive to the effects of lindane; in addition, use is not recommended in premature infants
 Use in the elderly—Absorption may be increased in the elderly because of increased permeability of their skin; elderly patients with a history of seizure activity may be especially sensitive to the CNS toxicity effects of lindane

### Proper use of this medication
» Poison; importance of keeping away from mouth
» Importance of not using more lindane than the amount prescribed
» Avoiding contact with the eyes
» Not using on open wounds, such as cuts or sores on skin or scalp, to minimize systemic absorption
 When applying lindane to another person: Wearing plastic disposable or rubber gloves to prevent systemic absorption, especially if you are pregnant or are breast-feeding

Proper administration:
 Reading patient directions carefully before using
 If necessary, treating sexual partner or partners, especially, and all members of household, since infestation may spread to persons in close contact; checking with doctor if these persons have not been checked or if there are any questions

*For cream or lotion dosage form*
 For scabies
  Washing, rinsing, and drying skin well before using lindane if skin has any cream, lotion, ointment, or oil on it
  Drying skin well if warm bath or shower is taken before using lindane
  Applying enough lindane to dry skin to cover entire skin surface from neck down; rubbing in well
  Leaving lindane on skin for 8 hours
  Removing lindane by washing thoroughly

*For shampoo dosage form*
 For lice
  Shampooing, rinsing, and drying hair and scalp well before using lindane if hair or scalp has any cream, lotion, ointment, or oil-based product on it
» If applying shampoo in the shower or in the bathtub, making sure shampoo does not run down on other parts of body; also, not applying shampoo in a bathtub where shampoo may run into bath water in which patient is sitting; this minimizes systemic absorption; when rinsing out the shampoo, thoroughly rinsing entire body to remove any shampoo that may have gotten on it
  Applying enough to dry hair (1 ounce or less for short hair, 1½ ounces for medium length hair and 2 ounces or less for long hair) to thoroughly wet the hair and skin or scalp of affected and surrounding hairy areas
  Rubbing thoroughly into hair and skin or scalp; allowing to remain in place for 4 minutes
  Using just enough water to work up a good lather
  Rinsing thoroughly; drying with clean towel
  When hair is dry, combing with fine-toothed comb to remove any remaining nits or nit shells
» Not using as a regular shampoo
» Proper dosing
» Proper storage

### Precautions while using this medication
To help prevent reinfestation or spreading of the infestation to other persons:
 For scabies—Washing in very hot water or dry-cleaning all recently worn underwear and pajamas and used sheets, pillowcases, and towels
 For lice—Washing in very hot water or dry-cleaning all recently worn clothing and used bed linens and towels

### Side/adverse effects
Risk of systemic absorption greater in infants and children than in adults; use not recommended in premature neonates, because risk of systemic absorption greater than in older infants
Signs of potential side effects, especially skin irritation or rash not present before therapy or CNS toxicity

## General Dosing Information
Since lindane has no continuing effect after treatment, it is not effective as a prophylaxis against possible future infestation.

### For scabies (using the cream or lotion)
Sexual partners and persons living in the same household should receive prophylactic treatment for scabies, since the signs of scabies can appear as late as 1 to 2 months after exposure and scabies can be transmitted during this period of time.

Although a total body application is considered to be from the neck down including the soles of the feet, scabies may also affect the heads of infants (scabies rarely affects the heads of children or adults). Consideration should be given to treating the head also if the patient is an infant.

If the skin has any cream, lotion, ointment, or oil on it, the skin should be washed, rinsed, and dried well before application of the medication.

If a warm bath or shower is taken before the cream or lotion is used, the skin should be well dried prior to application. The cream or lotion should be applied to dry skin in an amount sufficient to cover the entire body surface from the neck down including the soles of the feet (usually 1 to 2 ounces for an adult). The medication should be left on for 8 hours, then removed by thorough washing.

To help prevent reinfestation or spreading of the infestation, all recently worn underwear and pajamas and used sheets, pillowcases, and towels should be washed in very hot water or dry-cleaned.

**For pediculosis (using the shampoo)**
Sexual partners and other persons in close contact or living in the same household should be checked for infestation and treated if necessary, since the infestation may spread to persons in close contact.

If the hair or scalp has any cream, lotion, ointment, or oil-based product on it, shampoo, rinse, and dry hair and scalp well before the application of lindane.

A sufficient amount of shampoo should be used on dry hair (1 ounce or less for short hair, 1½ ounces for medium length hair, and 2 ounces or less for long hair) to thoroughly wet the hair and skin or scalp of the affected and surrounding hairy areas. The shampoo should be rubbed thoroughly into the hair and skin or scalp and allowed to remain in place for 4 minutes. Then, just enough water should be used to work up a good lather. The hair and skin or scalp should be rinsed thoroughly and dried with a clean towel. When the hair is dry, patient should use a fine-toothed comb to remove any remaining nits or nit shells.

Lindane shampoo should not be used as a regular shampoo.

For treatment of eyelashes, petroleum jelly can be applied 3 times a day for 1 week.

To help prevent reinfestation or spreading of the infestation, all recently worn clothing and used bed linens and towels should be washed in very hot water or dry-cleaned.

**For treatment of toxicity**
Recommended treatment includes
- If accidental ingestion occurs, it may be life threatening and prompt gastric lavage is recommended.
- Since oils favor absorption, saline cathartics should be administered rather than oily cathartics for intestinal evacuation.
- If CNS manifestations occur, they may be treated by the administration of pentobarbital, phenobarbital, or diazepam.

## Topical Dosage Forms

Note: Bracketed uses in the *Dosage Forms* section refer to categories of use and/or indications that are not included in U.S. product labeling

### LINDANE CREAM USP

**Usual adult and adolescent dose**
[Pediculicide] or
Scabicide—
　Topical, to the skin, as a 1% cream for one application.

**Usual pediatric dose**
[Pediculicide] or
Scabicide—
　Premature neonates: Use is not recommended.
　Infants and children: See *Usual adult and adolescent dose*.

**Strength(s) usually available**
U.S.—
　1% (Rx) [*Kwell*].
Canada—
　1% (Rx) [*Kwellada*].

**Packaging and storage**
Store below 40 °C (104 °F), preferably between 15 and 30 °C (59 and 86 °F), unless otherwise specified by manufacturer. Store in a tight container. Protect from freezing.

**Auxiliary labeling**
- Poison.
- For external use only.

**Note**
When dispensing, include patient instructions.

### LINDANE LOTION USP

**Usual adult and adolescent dose**
[Pediculicide] or
Scabicide—
　Topical, to the skin, as a 1% lotion for one application.

**Usual pediatric dose**
[Pediculicide] or
Scabicide—
　Premature neonates: Use is not recommended.
　Infants and children: See *Usual adult and adolescent dose*.

**Strength(s) usually available**
U.S.—
　1% (Rx) [*Bio-Well; G-well; Kildane; Kwell; Kwildane; Scabene; Thionex* GENERIC].
Canada—
　1% (Rx) [*GBH; Kwellada; PMS Lindane;* GENERIC].

**Packaging and storage**
Store below 40 °C (104 °F), preferably between 15 and 30 °C (59 and 86 °F), unless otherwise specified by manufacturer. Store in a tight container. Protect from freezing.

**Auxiliary labeling**
- Poison.
- For external use only.
- Shake well.

**Note**
When dispensing, include patient instructions.

### LINDANE SHAMPOO USP

**Usual adult and adolescent dose**
Pediculicide—
　Topical, to the scalp or skin, as a 1% shampoo for one application, repeated after seven days if necessary.

**Usual pediatric dose**
Pediculicide—
　Premature neonates: Use is not recommended.
　Infants and children: See *Usual adult and adolescent dose*.

**Strength(s) usually available**
U.S.—
　1% (Rx) [*Bio-Well; GBH; G-well; Kildane; Kwell; Kwildane; Scabene;* GENERIC].
Canada—
　1% (Rx) [*GBH; Hexit; Kwellada; PMS Lindane* GENERIC].

**Packaging and storage**
Store below 40 °C (104 °F), preferably between 15 and 30 °C (59 and 86 °F), unless otherwise specified by manufacturer. Store in a tight container. Protect from freezing.

**Auxiliary labeling**
- Poison.
- For external use only.
- Shake well.

**Note**
When dispensing, include patient instructions.

Revised: 08/15/94

---

# LIOTHYRONINE—See *Thyroid Hormones (Systemic)*

---

# LIOTRIX—See *Thyroid Hormones (Systemic)*

---

# LISINOPRIL—See *Angiotensin-converting Enzyme (ACE) Inhibitors (Systemic)*

# LITHIUM Systemic

VA CLASSIFICATION (Primary/Secondary): CN750/CN900; BL400

Commonly used brand name(s): *Carbolith; Cibalith-S; Duralith; Eskalith; Eskalith CR; Lithane; Lithizine; Lithobid; Lithonate; Lithotabs.*

Note: For a listing of dosage forms and brand names by country availability, see *Dosage Forms* section(s).

## Category

Antimanic; antidepressant therapy adjunct; granulopoietic; vascular headache prophylactic.

## Indications

Note: Bracketed information in the *Indications* section refers to uses that are not included in U.S. product labeling.

### Accepted

Bipolar disorder (treatment)—Lithium is indicated as the primary agent in the treatment of acute manic and hypomanic episodes in bipolar disorder, and for maintenance therapy to help diminish the intensity and frequency of subsequent manic episodes in patients with a history of mania.

Lithium is used in some patients as the agent of choice in the prevention of bipolar depression. Clinicians have observed a diminished intensity and frequency of severe depressive episodes.

[Depression, mental (treatment)][1]—Lithium is used alone for maintenance therapy in unipolar depression, and for acute and maintenance therapy in schizoaffective disorder. It is also used to augment the antidepressant effect of tricyclic or monoamine oxidase (MAO) inhibitor antidepressants in the treatment of major unipolar depression in patients not responsive to antidepressants alone.

[Headache, vascular (prophylaxis)][1]—Lithium is used to reduce the frequency of the occurrence of episodic and chronic cluster headaches.

[Neutropenia (treatment)][1]—Lithium is used to reduce the incidence of infection in patients with chemotherapy-induced neutropenia and in patients with chronic or acquired neutropenia.

[1] Not included in Canadian product labeling.

## Pharmacology/Pharmacokinetics

### Physicochemical characteristics

Molecular weight—Lithium carbonate: 73.89.
Lithium citrate: 282.00.

Other characteristics—A monovalent cation easily assayed in biological fluids; salts share some chemical characteristics with salts of sodium and potassium

### Mechanism of action/Effect

Antimanic—Has not been established. The mood-stabilizing effect has been postulated to relate to a reduction of catecholamine neurotransmitter concentration, possibly mediated by lithium ion ($Li^+$) effect on $Na^+K^+$ adenosine triphosphatase ($Na^+K^+ATPase$) to produce improved transneuronal membrane transport of sodium ion. An alternate postulate is that lithium may decrease cyclic adenosine monophosphate (cyclic AMP) concentrations, which would result in decreased sensitivity of hormonal-sensitive adenylcyclase receptors. Another hypothesis is the "second messenger" theory of lithium's interference with lipid inositol metabolism. This theory postulates that a group of improperly regulated neurons may be the underlying cause of manic symptoms. A phospholipase C-type enzyme hydrolyzes the plasma membrane–located lipid, phosphatidylinositol biphosphate, to diacyglycerol and inositol triphosphate, postsynaptic second messengers that contribute to chronic cell stimulation by altering electrical activity in the neuron. Inositol formed during this process is recycled by the inositol phospholipid–synthesizing enzymes in the CNS. There is evidence that cells in the CNS do not have access to plasma sources of inositol but, instead, depend on the synthesis of inositol for the transduction of neuronal signals. Lithium, in therapeutic concentrations, blocks the activity of the enzyme, inositol-1-phosphatase, resulting in a depletion of neuronal inositol and ultimately a decrease in the levels of phosphatidylinositol biphosphate. The lipid will no longer be able to stimulate the formation of adequate quantities of the second messengers or alter electrical activity. Subsequent cells in the CNS become relatively insensitive to the agonist stimulation, and clinical improvement results.

Granulopoietic—The exact mechanism of action has not been established; however, studies have shown that lithium stimulates granulopoiesis, enhances marrow proliferation, elevates neutrophil production, and increases the granulocyte pool.

Vascular headache prophylactic—Specific mechanism has not been established. It has been postulated that the action of lithium in cluster headaches may be directly related to changes in platelet serotonin and histamine concentrations.

Antidepressant—Has not been established. However, the mechanism may involve enhancement of serotonergic activity and downregulation of beta-receptors.

### Absorption

Rapid; complete within 6 to 8 hours. Absorption rate of slow-release capsules is slower and the total amount of lithium absorbed is lower than with other dosage forms.

### Protein binding

Not bound to plasma proteins.

### Biotransformation

None.

### Half-life (average)

Elimination—
  Adults: 24 hours.
  Adolescents: 18 hours.
  Elderly patients: Up to 36 hours.
  Note: When therapy is initiated, the serum concentration decreases rapidly during the initial 5 or 6 hours, followed by a more gradual decline over the next 24 hours.

### Time to peak serum concentration

Syrup—0.5 hours.
Capsules or tablets—1 to 3 hours.
Extended-release tablets—4 hours.
Slow-release capsules—3 hours.
Steady-state serum concentrations—4 days.

### Therapeutic serum concentration

Bipolar disorder—
  Acute: 0.8 to 1.2 mEq per liter, occasionally up to 1.5 mEq per liter.
  Maintenance: 0.5 to 1.0 mEq per liter. Occasionally may require same concentration range as acute illness.

### Onset of therapeutic action

Clinical improvement—1 to 3 weeks.

### Elimination

Renal—
  95% unchanged; rapid initially, slower with extended therapy; 80% may be actively reabsorbed in the proximal tubule; rate of excretion decreases with age.
Fecal—
  <1%.
Sweat—
  4 to 5%.

## Precautions to Consider

### Pregnancy/Reproduction

Pregnancy—First trimester: Use of lithium is not recommended during pregnancy, especially in the first trimester, because of possible teratogenicity. Lithium crosses the placenta and is present in almost equal concentrations in the fetal and maternal serum. Data from lithium birth registers suggest an increased incidence of neonatal goiter and congenital cardiovascular malformations, especially Ebstein's anomaly.

FDA Pregnancy Category D.

Delivery—Lithium toxicity may be manifested as hypotonia, lethargy, and cyanosis in newborn infants of mothers taking lithium at term. Risk-benefit must be considered.

### Breast-feeding

Lithium is excreted in breast milk at a concentration about one-half that in maternal serum. Signs and symptoms of lithium toxicity such as hypotonia, hypothermia, cyanosis, and electrocardiogram (ECG) changes have been reported in some infants. With rare exceptions, infants should not be breast-fed while the mother is receiving lithium therapy.

### Pediatrics

Appropriate studies on the relationship of age to the effects of lithium have not been performed in the pediatric population. However, lithium may decrease bone formation or density in children by altering parathyroid hormone concentrations. Also, lithium is deposited in bone, replacing calcium in hydroxyapatite, an effect more pronounced in immature bone.

### Geriatrics

Geriatric patients and patients with organic mental disease usually require lower lithium dosage, lower serum concentration, and more frequent monitoring than younger adults because renal clearance rate and distribution volume are reduced. Lithium is more toxic to the central nervous system (CNS) in the elderly, even when serum lithium concentrations are within the therapeutic range for younger adults. Also, the elderly possibly may be more prone to develop lithium-induced goiter and clinical hypothyroidism. Excessive thirst and larger volume of urine as early side effects of lithium therapy may be more frequent in the elderly.

### Drug interactions and/or related problems

The following drug interactions and/or related problems have been selected on the basis of their potential clinical significance (possible mechanism in parentheses where appropriate)—not necessarily inclusive (» = major clinical significance):

Note: Combinations containing any of the following medications, depending on the amount present, may also interact with this medication.

Amphetamines
(concurrent use with lithium may antagonize the CNS stimulating effects of amphetamines)

Angiotensin-converting enzyme (ACE) inhibitors
(reversible increases in serum lithium concentrations and toxicity have been reported during concurrent use with ACE inhibitors; frequent monitoring of serum lithium concentrations is recommended during concurrent use)

Antidepressants, tricyclic
(since tricyclics may cause a swing into mania and a rapid recycling between mania and depression, lithium plasma concentrations at or greater than 0.8 mEq per liter may be needed to prevent the tricyclic switch process)

» Anti-inflammatory drugs, nonsteroidal (NSAIDs)
(concurrent use may increase the toxic effects of lithium by decreasing its renal excretion, thereby increasing the steady-state plasma lithium concentration by 39 to 50%; patient should be observed for symptoms of lithium toxicity, and increased monitoring of lithium plasma concentrations is recommended during concurrent use)

Atracurium or
Pancuronium or
Succinylcholine
(neuromuscular blocking effects may be potentiated or prolonged when these medications are used concurrently with chronic lithium therapy)

Calcium channel blocking agents
(concurrent use with lithium may increase the risk of neurotoxicity in the form of ataxia, tremors, nausea, vomiting, diarrhea, and/or tinnitus; caution is recommended)

» Calcium iodide or
» Iodinated glycerol or
» Potassium iodide
(concurrent use with lithium may potentiate the hypothyroid and goitrogenic effects of either these medications or lithium)

Carbamazepine or
Desmopressin or
Lypressin or
Posterior pituitary or
Vasopressin
(lithium may decrease the antidiuretic effect of these medications when used concurrently)

(lithium may prevent or decrease carbamazepine-induced leukopenia with a possible increase in therapeutic effect when carbamazepine is used to treat psychotic disorders or bipolar conditions)

» Chlorpromazine and possibly other phenothiazines
(concurrent use with lithium may reduce gastrointestinal absorption of the phenothiazine, thereby decreasing its serum concentrations by as much as 40%; phenothiazines, especially chlorpromazine, increase intracellular lithium concentration; concurrent use may increase rate of renal excretion of lithium; extrapyramidal symptoms, delirium, and cerebellar function impairment may be increased, especially in elderly patients; also, nausea and vomiting, early indications of lithium toxicity, may be masked by the antiemetic effect of some phenothiazines; admixture of lithium citrate syrup with any liquid forms of phenothiazines may form a precipitate of the free phenothiazine)

» Diuretics
(concurrent use with lithium may provoke severe lithium toxicity by delaying renal excretion of lithium and consequently increasing serum and red blood cell lithium concentrations; close monitoring of lithium plasma concentrations is essential since sodium and lithium reabsorption in the proximal tubule is increased, due to the body sodium deficit; a reduction in lithium dosage may be necessary)

Fludrocortisone
(in one published case report, lithium antagonized the mineralocorticoid effects of fludrocortisone; increased fludrocortisone dose and dietary sodium supplementation were required during concurrent use)

Fluoxetine
(lithium concentrations may be altered, leading to toxicity; close monitoring of lithium concentrations is recommended)

» Haloperidol
(lithium is frequently used concurrently with haloperidol during the first 1 or 2 weeks of treatment for acute manic episodes, but lithium alone may be adequate thereafter. However, concurrent use with lithium has been reported, in a few cases, to be associated with irreversible neurological toxicity and brain damage, especially in patients with organic mental syndrome or other CNS impairment, although this interaction is controversial; extrapyramidal symptoms may be increased by enhancement of dopamine blockade by haloperidol; patients should be monitored closely during concurrent use; dosage adjustments may be necessary)

(admixture of the liquid forms of lithium and haloperidol may precipitate free haloperidol)

Methyldopa
(concurrent use may increase the risk of lithium toxicity even though serum lithium concentrations remain within the recommended therapeutic range)

Metronidazole
(concurrent use may promote renal retention of lithium, leading to lithium toxicity; reducing the dose or discontinuing the use of lithium may be necessary during metronidazole therapy; if not feasible to discontinue, frequent monitoring of serum creatinine, electrolyte and lithium concentrations, and urine osmolality to detect possible nephrogenic diabetes insipidus are recommended)

» Molindone
(concurrent use with lithium may produce neurotoxic symptoms such as confusion, delirium, seizures, somnambulism, or abnormal electroencephalogram [EEG] changes)

Norepinephrine
(concurrent use with lithium may decrease the pressor response to norepinephrine; a higher dose of norepinephrine may be required to achieve the desired effect)

Sodium-containing medications or foods, especially sodium bicarbonate or sodium chloride
(high sodium intake enhances lithium excretion, possibly resulting in decreased efficacy)

Urea
(may increase the renal excretion of lithium, thereby decreasing its effects)

Xanthines such as:
Aminophylline
Caffeine
Dyphylline
Oxtriphylline
Theophylline
(concurrent use of these medications with lithium increases urinary excretion of lithium, thereby possibly reducing its therapeutic effect)

### Laboratory value alterations

The following have been selected on the basis of their potential clinical significance (possible effect in parentheses where appropriate)—not necessarily inclusive (» = major clinical significance):

With physiology/laboratory test values
Glucose, blood
(may be increased during treatment with lithium; concentrations return to normal when lithium administration is discontinued)

Parathyroid hormone, immunoreactive and
Calcium
(serum concentrations may rise above normal after long-term therapy)

### Medical considerations/Contraindications

The medical considerations/contraindications included have been selected on the basis of their potential clinical significance (reasons given in parentheses where appropriate)—not necessarily inclusive (» = major clinical significance).

*Except under special circumstances, this medication should not be used when the following medical problem exists:*

» Leukemia, history of
(leukemia may be reactivated by lithium)

*Risk-benefit should be considered when the following medical problems exist:*

» Cardiovascular disease
(may be exacerbated; possible interference with lithium excretion)

» CNS disorders, such as epilepsy and parkinsonism
(may be exacerbated; lithium-induced neurotoxicity may be masked)

» Dehydration, severe
(risk of toxicity is increased; the loss of large volumes of body fluid as in prolonged vomiting, diarrhea, or profuse perspiration due to fever, exercise, saunas, or hot baths may result in increased serum lithium concentration; such loss of body fluid may necessitate dosage adjustment of lithium and/or the supplemental intake of sodium and fluids until hydration status and electrolytes are stable)

Diabetes mellitus
(serum insulin concentration may be increased)

Goiter or
Hypothyroidism
(latent hypothyroidism may be induced in predisposed or elderly patients)

Hyperparathyroidism
(calcium metabolism may be altered after long-term use)

» Infections, severe
(fever with prolonged sweating, diarrhea, or vomiting may necessitate a decrease in lithium dosage to prevent lithium toxicity)

Organic mental disease or
Schizophrenia
(patients may be hypersensitive to lithium and exhibit increased confusion, seizures, or electroencephalogram [EEG] changes at normal serum lithium concentrations)

Psoriasis
(may be aggravated by lithium; dosage adjustments of lithium and/or other medications may be necessary)

» Renal insufficiency or
» Urinary retention
(lithium excretion may be delayed, leading to toxicity)

Sensitivity to lithium

Caution should be used also in severely debilitated patients or in patients on a sodium-restricted diet because these conditions may increase the risk of toxicity by delaying renal excretion of lithium.

**Patient monitoring**

The following may be especially important in patient monitoring (other tests may be warranted in some patients, depending on condition; » = major clinical significance):

Calcium concentrations, serum and
Phosphate concentrations, serum
(determinations recommended in children under 12 years of age prior to initiation of therapy and periodically during treatment since lithium increases parathyroid hormone concentrations and risk of hypercalcemia and hypophosphatemia)

» Electrocardiogram (ECG)
(recommended at least once prior to therapy in all patients, and especially in patients over 40 years of age and those with a history suggestive of cardiovascular disease; should be repeated if symptoms such as palpitations, irregular pulse, weight gain with edema, or diminished consciousness occur; also, lithium may cause the benign effect of flattening of T-waves and prominent U-waves)

Electrolyte concentrations, serum
(determinations recommended prior to therapy to detect pre-existing hyponatremia, which will decrease lithium excretion)

Height and
Weight evaluation
(baseline weight measurement prior to therapy and every 3 months are recommended; weight gain, possibly due to a high intake of calorie-containing liquids as a result of lithium-induced polydipsia or to fluid retention to balance the increase in cations, may lead to a patient's noncompliance with lithium therapy; in children, height and weight charts should be maintained, and lithium therapy reevaluated or discontinued if there is any decrease in growth rate)

» Lithium concentrations, serum
(determinations recommended once or twice weekly during treatment of acute manic episode until serum concentrations and patient's clinical condition have stabilized; recommended at least every 2 to 3 months during remission when patient is stabilized; blood samples should be drawn in the morning immediately prior to the next dose, 10 to 14 hours following the previous dose, when there is maximal stability in serum concentration. Some side effects may occur at serum lithium concentrations below 1.5 mEq per liter, and mild to moderate toxic reactions are likely to occur at concentrations from 1.5 to 2.5 mEq per liter. Serum lithium concentrations should not be permitted to exceed 1.5 mEq per liter during the acute treatment phase; concentrations above 2.0 mEq per liter in chronic consumption of lithium can produce complex and serious clinical problems. Severe toxicity can occur at 2.5 mEq per liter. Close monitoring is recommended if lithium is used during the last trimester of pregnancy, used concurrently with any other medication, and used in the elderly when renal clearance rate and distribution volume are reduced)

Pregnancy test, beta-HCG
(recommended prior to initiation of therapy in all women of childbearing potential)

» Renal function determinations
(close assessment recommended prior to initiation of lithium therapy and periodically thereafter, even in asymptomatic patients with stable serum lithium concentrations; blood urea nitrogen [BUN]; serum creatinine; and urinalysis should be performed prior to initiating therapy to determine hydration status, renal flow, and presence of pre-existing renal concentrating defect)

Thyroid function determinations
(serum thyroxine and thyroxine-stimulating hormone [TSH] should be evaluated at baseline before lithium therapy is initiated and at 6-month intervals during therapy; patient should be monitored for symptoms of hypothyroidism; maintenance of adequate thyroid function is important in children to maintain a satisfactory growth rate)

» White blood cell count, total and differential
(recommended prior to therapy and repeated if signs of unusual tiredness or weakness develop because of possible rare leukemia that may develop during lithium therapy; however, the association of lithium with leukemia is controversial; benign leukocytosis may be reversible on discontinuation of therapy)

## Side/Adverse Effects

The following side/adverse effects have been selected on the basis of their potential clinical significance (possible signs and symptoms in parentheses where appropriate)—not necessarily inclusive:

**Those indicating need for medical attention**
Incidence less frequent
*Cardiovascular problems* (fainting; fast or slow heartbeat; irregular pulse; troubled breathing [dyspnea] on exertion); *leukocytosis* (unusual tiredness or weakness); *weight gain*

Note: *Sinus node function impairment, sinoatrial block,* or v*entricular irritability* may occur at therapeutic serum lithium concentrations; possibly reversible when lithium is discontinued.

*Leukocytosis* is usually reversible upon discontinuation of lithium, but a rare leukemia may develop during lithium therapy.

Incidence rare
*Blue color and pain in fingers and toes; coldness of arms and legs; pseudotumor cerebri* (dizziness; eye pain; headache; nausea or vomiting; noises in ears; vision problems)

Note: If undetected, *pseudotumor cerebri* may result in enlargement of blind spot, constriction of visual fields, and eventual blindness, due to optic atrophy.

Symptoms of hypothyroidism
*Dry, rough skin; hair loss; hoarseness; mania* (unusual excitement); *mental depression; sensitivity to cold; swelling of feet or lower legs; swelling of neck*

**Those indicating need for medical attention only if they continue or are bothersome**
Incidence more frequent
*Diarrhea; increased thirst; nausea, mild; stress incontinence or urinary urgency* (increased frequency of urination; loss of bladder control); *trembling of hands, slight*

Note: *Stress incontinence* or *urinary urgency* is dose-related; more common in women; usually begins 2 to 7 years after start of treatment with lithium.

Incidence less frequent
*Acne or skin rash; bloated feeling or pressure in the stomach; muscle twitching, slight*

## Overdose

For specific information on the agents used in the management of lithium overdose, see:
- *Acetazolamide* in *Carbonic Anhydrase Inhibitors (Systemic)* monograph; and/or
- *Mannitol (Systemic)* monograph.

For more information on the management of overdose or unintentional ingestion, **contact a Poison Control Center** (see *Poison Control Center Listing*).

### Clinical effects of overdose

The following effects have been selected on the basis of their potential clinical significance (possible signs and symptoms in parentheses where appropriate)—not necessarily inclusive:

Early symptoms of toxicity
   *Diarrhea; drowsiness; loss of appetite; muscle weakness; nausea or vomiting; slurred speech; trembling*

Late symptoms of toxicity
   *Blurred vision; clumsiness or unsteadiness; confusion; convulsions; dizziness; increase in amount of urine; trembling, severe*

### Treatment of overdose

No specific antidote is available. Early toxic symptoms can usually be treated by reducing or stopping administration of lithium and resuming treatment at a lower dosage after 24 to 48 hours.

Treatment of more severe toxicity or acute overdose may include the following:
   To decrease absorption—
      Inducing vomiting or using small volume (100 mL) gastric lavage (in acute overdose).
   To enhance elimination—
      Utilizing intermittent hemodialysis if plasma lithium does not drop more than 10% every 3 hours or half-life is greater than 36 hours. Since plasma lithium determinations immediately after dialysis do not take into account the rebound increase that occurs as lithium redistributes from tissue to blood, determinations must be obtained 6 hours later.
      Possibly increasing lithium excretion with single dose of intravenous acetazolamide or using mannitol as an osmotic diuretic.
   Monitoring—
      Measuring plasma lithium concentrations every 3 hours until lithium is less than 1.0 mEq per liter.
      Monitoring patient closely.
   Supportive care—
      Maintaining electrolyte balance and body fluids.
      Regulating kidney function.
      Maintaining adequate respiration.
      Preventing infection.
      Patients in whom intentional overdose is known or suspected should be referred for psychiatric consultation.

## Patient Consultation

As an aid to patient consultation, refer to *Advice for the Patient, Lithium (Systemic)*.

In providing consultation, consider emphasizing the following selected information (» = major clinical significance):

### Before using this medication

» Conditions affecting use, especially:
   Sensitivity to lithium
   Pregnancy—Lithium crosses placenta; contraindicated in first trimester because of possible neonatal goiter and cardiovascular malformations; at delivery, hypotonia, lethargy, and cyanosis in newborns of mothers taking lithium at term
   Breast-feeding—Excreted in breast milk; may cause hypotonia, hypothermia, cyanosis, and ECG changes in some babies
   Use in children—May decrease bone formation or density
   Use in the elderly—Elderly more prone to develop CNS toxicity, hypothyroidism and goiter; lower doses and more frequent monitoring required
   Other medications, especially iodine-containing preparations, nonsteroidal anti-inflammatory drugs, chlorpromazine (and possibly other phenothiazines), diuretics, haloperidol, or molindone
   Other medical problems, especially history of leukemia, cardiovascular disease, epilepsy, parkinsonism, severe dehydration, renal insufficiency, urinary retention, or severe infections with prolonged sweating, vomiting, or diarrhea

### Proper use of this medication

Taking after a meal or snack to prevent laxative action and to decrease the severity of stomach upset, tremors, or weakness by slowing absorption rate

» Importance of adequate fluid (2.5 to 3 liters each day) and sodium intake
» Importance of not taking more medication than the amount prescribed
» Compliance with therapy; improvement in condition may require 1 to 3 weeks; importance of maintaining adequate blood levels even though symptoms improved
» Proper dosing
   Missed dose: Taking as soon as possible, unless within 4 hours (6 hours for extended-release tablets or slow-release capsules) of next scheduled dose; not doubling doses
» Proper storage

*For extended-release or slow-release dosage form*
   Swallowing tablet or capsule whole
   Not breaking, crushing, or chewing

*For syrup dosage form*
   Diluting dose with fruit juice or other flavored beverage before taking

### Precautions while using this medication

» Regular visits to physician to check progress during therapy; importance of serum lithium monitoring
   Caution in drinking large amounts of coffee, tea, or colas because of diuretic effect
» Possible drowsiness or dizziness; caution if driving or doing jobs requiring alertness
» Caution during exercise, saunas, and hot weather
» Caution during illnesses that cause high fevers with profuse sweating, vomiting, or diarrhea
» Caution on self-imposed dieting
» Importance of patient and family knowing early symptoms of overdose or toxicity

*For slow-release dosage form*
» Not using interchangeably with any other dosage form

### Side/adverse effects

» Early symptoms of lithium overdose or toxicity:
   Diarrhea
   Drowsiness
   Loss of appetite
   Muscle weakness
   Nausea or vomiting
   Slurred speech
   Trembling
   Side effects are more likely to occur in the elderly
   Signs of potential side effects, especially cardiovascular problems, leukocytosis, weight gain, blue color and pain in fingers and toes, coldness of arms and legs, pseudotumor cerebri, symptoms of hypothyroidism

## General Dosing Information

Warning—Lithium toxicity can occur with doses at or near therapeutic serum concentrations. Facilities for prompt and accurate serum lithium determinations must be available during therapy. Accurate patient evaluation requires both clinical and laboratory analysis.

During the acute manic phase, the patient may have a greater ability to tolerate lithium. This tolerance decreases as the manic symptoms subside and often necessitates a corresponding dosage adjustment.

During the acute manic phase, lithium administration of 300 (8 mEq) to 600 mg three times a day should usually produce effective serum concentrations ranging from 0.8 to 1.2 mEq per liter, with weekly adjustments based on plasma lithium concentrations. An increase of 8 mEq a day will increase plasma concentrations by $0.3 \pm 0.1$ mEq per liter. The maintenance dose of 300 mg three or four times a day usually produces effective serum concentrations ranging from 0.5 to 1.0 mEq per liter.

If a satisfactory therapeutic response to lithium at the highest tolerated serum concentrations within the therapeutic range is not achieved within 3 weeks, lithium therapy should be discontinued.

Slow-release lithium carbonate capsules and tablets are not bioequivalent to other lithium dosage forms and should not be used interchangeably with them.

### Diet/Nutrition

Since lithium decreases sodium reabsorption by the renal tubules, a normal diet with an average consumption of salt and adequate fluid intake, 2.5 to 3 liters of fluid per day, is essential to prevent sodium depletion leading to lithium toxicity.

This medication may be taken with food, juice, or milk, if necessary, to lessen laxative action, stomach irritation, tremors, or weakness, by slowing absorption of lithium. The syrup must be diluted in juice or other flavored beverage before administration.

### For treatment of adverse effects

Early side effects—If slight hand tremor, mild nausea or diarrhea, unusual drowsiness, or acne do not subside with continued treatment, a reduction in lithium dosage may be necessary. If hand tremor is especially bothersome, shifting a majority of the dose to bedtime, decreasing caffeine intake, or adding a beta-blocker such as propranolol may be helpful.

Suppression of thyroid activity—May necessitate thyroid hormone replacement therapy.

Urinary incontinence—Lowering dose of lithium whenever possible, adding an anticholinergic agent or an antidepressant with anticholinergic properties, or switching to another medication for treatment of bipolar disorder.

Polyuria—Lowering dose of lithium alone, whenever possible. If the lower plasma lithium concentration is inadequate to maintain a response, adding a thiazide diuretic and reducing the lithium dose by 50%, then readjusting it to reproduce the original plasma lithium concentration, may be effective. Alternatively, extended-release or slow-release lithium products can improve the patient's renal concentrating ability.

Weight gain—May be safely and effectively treated by limiting calorie intake with emphasis on adequate fluid and sodium intake.

## Oral Dosage Forms

### LITHIUM CARBONATE CAPSULES USP

**Usual adult and adolescent dose**
Antimanic—
  Acute mania: Oral, initially 300 to 600 mg (8 to 16 mEq) three times a day, the dosage being adjusted as needed and tolerated at weekly intervals.
  Maintenance: Oral, 300 mg three or four times a day, the dosage being adjusted as needed and tolerated.

Note: Geriatric or debilitated patients usually require a lower dosage.

**Usual adult prescribing limits**
Up to 2.4 grams a day.

**Usual pediatric dose**
Antimanic—
  Children up to 12 years of age: Oral, initially 15 to 20 mg (0.4 to 0.5 mEq) per kg of body weight a day in two or three divided doses, the dosage being adjusted at weekly intervals, based on plasma lithium concentrations.
  Children 12 to 18 years of age: See *Usual adult and adolescent dose*.

**Strength(s) usually available**
U.S.—
  150 mg (Rx) [GENERIC].
  300 mg (Rx) [*Eskalith*; *Lithonate*; GENERIC].
  600 mg (Rx) [GENERIC].
Canada—
  150 mg (Rx) [*Carbolith*].
  300 mg (Rx) [*Carbolith*; *Lithane*].

**Packaging and storage**
Store below 40 °C (104 °F), preferably between 15 and 30 °C (59 and 86 °F), unless otherwise specified by manufacturer. Store in a well-closed container.

**Auxiliary labeling**
• May cause drowsiness.
• Take after a meal or snack.

### LITHIUM CARBONATE SLOW-RELEASE CAPSULES

**Usual adult and adolescent dose**
Antimanic—
  Acute mania: Oral, initially 600 to 900 mg a day on the first day, the dosage being increased, thereafter, to 1200 to 1800 mg a day in three divided doses, as needed and tolerated.
  Maintenance: Oral, 900 to 1200 mg a day in three divided doses, the dosage being adjusted as needed and tolerated.

**Usual adult prescribing limits**
Up to 2.4 grams a day.

**Usual pediatric dose**
Antimanic—
  Children up to 12 years of age: Dosage has not been established.
  Children 12 to 18 years of age: See *Usual adult and adolescent dose*.

**Usual geriatric dose**
Antimanic—
  Oral, 600 to 1200 mg a day in three divided doses.

**Strength(s) usually available**
U.S.—
  Not commercially available.
Canada—
  150 mg (Rx) [*Lithizine*].
  300 mg (Rx) [*Lithizine*].

Note: Not bioequivalent to other lithium dosage forms and should not be used interchangeably with them.

**Packaging and storage**
Store below 40 °C (104 °F), preferably between 15 and 30 °C (59 and 86 °F), unless otherwise specified by manufacturer. Store in a well-closed container.

**Auxiliary labeling**
• Swallow whole.
• May cause drowsiness.

### LITHIUM CARBONATE TABLETS USP

**Usual adult and adolescent dose**
See *Lithium Carbonate Capsules USP*.

**Usual adult prescribing limits**
See *Lithium Carbonate Capsules USP*.

**Usual pediatric dose**
See *Lithium Carbonate Capsules USP*.

**Strength(s) usually available**
U.S.—
  300 mg (Rx) [*Eskalith* (scored); *Lithane* (tartrazine); *Lithotabs*; GENERIC].
Canada—
  300 mg (Rx) [*Lithane*].

**Packaging and storage**
Store below 40 °C (104 °F), preferably between 15 and 30 °C (59 and 86 °F), unless otherwise specified by manufacturer. Store in a well-closed container.

**Auxiliary labeling**
• May cause drowsiness.
• Take after a meal or snack.

### LITHIUM CARBONATE EXTENDED-RELEASE TABLETS

**Usual adult and adolescent dose**
Antimanic—
  Acute mania: Oral, 450 to 900 mg two times a day or 300 to 600 mg three times a day, the dosage being adjusted as needed and tolerated.
  Maintenance: Oral, 450 mg two times a day or 300 mg three times a day, the dosage being adjusted as needed and tolerated.

Note: Geriatric or debilitated patients usually require a lower dosage.

**Usual adult prescribing limits**
Up to 2.4 grams a day.

**Usual pediatric dose**
Antimanic—
  Children up to 12 years of age: Dosage has not been established.
  Children 12 to 18 years of age: See *Usual adult and adolescent dose*.

**Strength(s) usually available**
U.S.—
  300 mg (Rx) [*Lithobid*].
  450 mg (Rx) [*Eskalith CR* (scored)].
Canada—
  300 mg (Rx) [*Duralith* (scored)].

**Packaging and storage**
Store below 40 °C (104 °F), preferably between 15 and 30 °C (59 and 86 °F), in a well-closed container, unless otherwise specified by manufacturer.

**Auxiliary labeling**
• Swallow whole.
• May cause drowsiness.
• Take after a meal or snack.

### LITHIUM CITRATE SYRUP USP

**Usual adult and adolescent dose**
Antimanic—
  Acute mania: Oral, the equivalent of 300 to 600 mg (8 to 16 mEq) of lithium carbonate three times a day, the dosage being adjusted as needed and tolerated.
  Maintenance: Oral, the equivalent of 300 mg of lithium carbonate three or four times a day, the dosage being adjusted as needed and tolerated.

Note: Geriatric or debilitated patients usually require a lower dosage.

## Lithium (Systemic)

**Usual adult prescribing limits**
Up to the equivalent of 2.4 grams of lithium carbonate a day.

**Usual pediatric dose**
Antimanic—
  Children up to 12 years of age: Oral, initially the equivalent of 15 to 20 mg (0.4 to 0.5 mEq) of lithium carbonate per kg of body weight a day in two or three divided doses, the dosage being adjusted at weekly intervals, based on plasma lithium concentrations.
  Children 12 to 18 years of age: See *Usual adult and adolescent dose*.

**Strength(s) usually available**
U.S.—
  8 mEq of lithium ion (equivalent to approximately 300 mg of lithium carbonate) per 5 mL (Rx) [*Cibalith-S;* GENERIC].
Canada—
  Not commercially available.

**Packaging and storage**
Store between 15 and 30 °C (59 and 86 °F), unless otherwise specified by manufacturer. Store in a tight container. Protect from freezing.

**Incompatibilities**
Lithium citrate syrup should not be mixed with or administered at the same time as other medication, solid or liquid, that contains a basic form, such as chlorpromazine concentrate, haloperidol, thioridazine, or trifluoperazine, and tricyclic antidepressants.

**Auxiliary labeling**
- May cause drowsiness.
- Take after a meal or snack.
- Dilute with juice or other beverage before taking.

Revised: 03/09/93

---

**LODOXAMIDE**—The *Lodoxamide (Ophthalmic)* monograph is not included in this published version of the USP DI database. Copies of the monograph are available on request from Micromedex, Inc. - Reprint Requests, 6200 S. Syracuse Way, Suite 300, Englewood, CO 80111; telephone (303) 486-6400; telefax (303) 486-6464; Email: USPDI@MDX.COM.

---

**LOMEFLOXACIN**—See *Fluoroquinolones (Systemic)*

---

# LOMUSTINE  Systemic

VA CLASSIFICATION (Primary): AN100
Commonly used brand name(s): *CeeNU*.
Another commonly used name is CCNU.
Note: For a listing of dosage forms and brand names by country availability, see *Dosage Forms* section(s).

## Category
Antineoplastic.

## Indications
Note: Bracketed information in the *Indications* section refers to uses that are not included in U.S. product labeling.

**Accepted**
Tumors, brain, primary (treatment)
[Carcinoma, colorectal (treatment)][1]
[Carcinoma, lung, non-small cell (treatment)] or
[Carcinoma, breast (treatment)]—Lomustine is indicated for treatment of both primary and metastatic brain tumors, in patients who have already received appropriate surgical or radiotherapeutic procedures. It is also indicated for treatment of colorectal carcinoma, non–small-cell lung carcinoma, and advanced breast carcinoma after conventional therapy has failed.
Lymphomas, Hodgkin's (treatment)—Lomustine is indicated for treatment of Hodgkin's disease, as secondary therapy in combination with other drugs in patients who relapse while being treated with primary therapy or in patients who fail to respond to primary therapy.
[Multiple myeloma (treatment)][1]—Lomustine is also indicated for treatment of multiple myeloma.
[Melanoma, malignant (treatment)]—Lomustine is indicated for treatment of malignant melanoma, alone or in combination with other drugs.

[1]Not included in Canadian product labeling.

## Pharmacology/Pharmacokinetics

**Physicochemical characteristics**
Molecular weight—233.70.

**Mechanism of action/Effect**
Lomustine is an alkylating agent of the nitrosourea type. Lomustine (and/or its metabolites) interferes with the function of DNA and RNA. It is cell cycle–phase nonspecific. Lomustine also acts to inhibit DNA synthesis by inhibiting key enzymatic processes.

**Absorption**
Well and rapidly absorbed from the gastrointestinal tract.

**Distribution**
Crosses the blood-brain barrier.

**Protein binding**
Moderate (50%; metabolites).

**Biotransformation**
Hepatic; rapid and complete (active metabolites).

**Half-life**
Biologic—Approximately 94 minutes.
Chemical—Approximately 15 minutes.
Metabolites—Prolonged; 16 to 48 hours.

**Elimination**
Renal (totally as metabolites); some enterohepatic circulation is believed to occur.
Fecal (less than 5%).
Respiratory (10%).

## Precautions to Consider

**Carcinogenicity/Mutagenicity**
Secondary malignancies are potential delayed effects of many antineoplastic agents, although it is not clear whether the effect is related to their mutagenic or immunosuppressive action. The effect of dose and duration of therapy is also unknown, although risk seems to increase with long-term use. Although information is limited, available data seem to indicate that the carcinogenic risk is greatest with the alkylating agents.
Long-term use of nitrosoureas in humans has been reported to be possibly associated with development of secondary malignancies (acute leukemia) and bone marrow dysplasias.
Lomustine is carcinogenic in rats and mice at the approximate clinical dose and, like other alkylating agents, is probably carcinogenic in humans.

**Pregnancy/Reproduction**
Fertility— Gonadal suppression, resulting in amenorrhea or azoospermia, may occur in patients taking antineoplastic therapy, especially with the alkylating agents. In general, these effects appear to be related to dose and length of therapy and may be irreversible. Prediction of the degree of testicular or ovarian function impairment is complicated by the common use of combinations of several antineoplastics, which makes it difficult to assess the effects of individual agents.
Lomustine suppresses gonadal function in male rats (at higher than the human dose) and in humans.

Pregnancy—Adequate and well-controlled studies in humans have not been done.
First trimester: It is usually recommended that use of antineoplastics, especially combination chemotherapy, be avoided whenever possible, especially during the first trimester. Although information is limited because of the relatively few instances of antineoplastic administration during pregnancy, the mutagenic, teratogenic, and carcinogenic potential of these medications must be considered.
Other hazards to the fetus include adverse reactions seen in adults.
In general, use of a contraceptive is recommended during cytotoxic drug therapy.
Lomustine is embryotoxic in rats and rabbits and teratogenic in rats at doses approximately equivalent to the human dose.

FDA Pregnancy Category D.

### Breast-feeding
Lomustine is distributed into breast milk. Breast-feeding is not recommended during chemotherapy because of the risks to the infant (adverse effects, mutagenicity, carcinogenicity).

### Pediatrics
Appropriate studies on the relationship of age to the effects of lomustine have not been performed in the pediatric population. However, pediatrics-specific problems that would limit the usefulness of this medication in children are not expected.

### Geriatrics
No information is available on the relationship of age to the effects of lomustine in geriatric patients. However, elderly patients are more likely to have age-related renal function impairment, which may require caution in patients receiving lomustine.

### Dental
The bone marrow depressant effects of lomustine may result in an increased incidence of microbial infection, delayed healing, and gingival bleeding. Dental work, whenever possible, should be completed prior to initiation of therapy or deferred until blood counts have returned to normal. Patients should be instructed in proper oral hygiene during treatment, including caution in use of regular toothbrushes, dental floss, and toothpicks.

Lomustine may also cause stomatitis that is associated with considerable discomfort.

### Drug interactions and/or related problems
The following drug interactions and/or related problems have been selected on the basis of their potential clinical significance (possible mechanism in parentheses where appropriate)—not necessarily inclusive (» = major clinical significance):

Blood dyscrasia–causing medications (see *Appendix II*)
(leukopenic and/or thrombocytopenic effects of lomustine may be increased with concurrent or recent therapy if these medications cause the same effects; dosage adjustment of lomustine, if necessary, should be based on blood counts)

» Bone marrow depressants, other (see *Appendix II*) or
Radiation therapy
(additive bone marrow depression may occur; dosage reduction may be required when two or more bone marrow depressants, including radiation, are used concurrently or consecutively)

Vaccines, killed virus
(because normal defense mechanisms may be suppressed by lomustine therapy, the patient's antibody response to the vaccine may be decreased. The interval between discontinuation of medications that cause immunosuppression and restoration of the patient's ability to respond to the vaccine depends on the intensity and type of immunosuppression-causing medication used, the underlying disease, and other factors; estimates vary from 3 months to 1 year)

» Vaccines, live virus
(because normal defense mechanisms may be suppressed by lomustine therapy, concurrent use with a live virus vaccine may potentiate the replication of the vaccine virus, may increase the side/adverse effects of the vaccine virus, and/or may decrease the patient's antibody response to the vaccine; immunization of these patients should be undertaken only with extreme caution after careful review of the patient's hematologic status and only with the knowledge and consent of the physician managing the lomustine therapy. The interval between discontinuation of medications that cause immunosuppression and restoration of the patient's ability to respond to the vaccine depends on the intensity and type of immunosuppression-causing medication used, the underlying disease, and other factors; estimates vary from 3 months to 1 year. Immunization with oral poliovirus vaccine should also be postponed in persons in close contact with the patient, especially family members)

### Laboratory value alterations
The following have been selected on the basis of their potential clinical significance (possible effect in parentheses where appropriate)—not necessarily inclusive (» = major clinical significance):

With physiology/laboratory test values
Hepatic function tests
(may be elevated transiently and reversibly)

### Medical considerations/Contraindications
The medical considerations/contraindications included have been selected on the basis of their potential clinical significance (reasons given in parentheses where appropriate)—not necessarily inclusive (» = major clinical significance).

*Risk-benefit should be considered when the following medical problems exist:*
» Bone marrow depression
» Chickenpox, existing or recent (including recent exposure) or
» Herpes zoster
(risk of severe generalized disease)
» Infection
» Pulmonary function impairment, especially with a baseline below 70% of the forced vital capacity (FVC) or carbon monoxide diffusion capacity ($DL_{CO}$)
(increased risk of pulmonary toxicity)
» Renal function impairment
» Sensitivity to lomustine
» Caution should be used also in patients who have had previous cytotoxic drug therapy and radiation therapy.

### Patient monitoring
The following may be especially important in patient monitoring (other tests may be warranted in some patients, depending on condition; » = major clinical significance):

Alanine aminotransferase (ALT [SGPT]) values, serum and
Aspartate aminotransferase (AST [SGOT]) values, serum and
Bilirubin values, serum and
Lactate dehydrogenase (LDH) values, serum
(recommended prior to initiation of therapy and at periodic intervals during therapy; frequency varies according to clinical state, agent, dose, and other agents being used concurrently)

» Blood urea nitrogen (BUN) concentrations and
» Creatinine concentrations, serum
(recommended prior to initiation of therapy and at periodic intervals during therapy; frequency varies according to clinical state, agent, dose, and other agents being used concurrently)

» Hematocrit or hemoglobin and
» Leukocyte count, total and, if appropriate, differential and
» Platelet count
(determinations recommended prior to initiation of therapy and at periodic intervals during and after therapy; frequency varies according to clinical state, agent, dose, and other agents being used concurrently)

Pulmonary function tests
(recommended prior to initiation of therapy and at periodic intervals during therapy)

## Side/Adverse Effects
Note: Many "side effects" of antineoplastic therapy are unavoidable and represent the medication's pharmacologic action. Some of these (for example, leukopenia and thrombocytopenia) are actually used as parameters to aid in individual dosage titration.

The following side/adverse effects have been selected on the basis of their potential clinical significance (possible signs and symptoms in parentheses where appropriate)—not necessarily inclusive:

### Those indicating need for medical attention
Incidence more frequent
***Immunosuppression or leukopenia or infection*** (fever or chills; cough or hoarseness; lower back or side pain; painful or difficult urination)—usually asymptomatic; ***thrombocytopenia*** (unusual bleeding or bruising; black, tarry stools; blood in urine or stools; pinpoint red spots on skin)—usually asymptomatic

Note: Maximum *thrombocytopenia* occurs about 4 weeks after a dose and persists for 1 to 2 weeks. Maximum *leukopenia* occurs about 4 to 6 weeks after a dose and persists for 1 to 2 weeks. Recovery usually occurs within 6 to 7 weeks after administration. Severity of bone marrow depression varies and determines subsequent dosage of lomustine.

Incidence less frequent
***Anemia*** (unusual tiredness or weakness); ***neurotoxicity*** (awkwardness; confusion; slurred speech; unusual tiredness)—not definitely attributed to medication; ***renal toxicity and failure*** (decrease in urination; swelling of feet or lower legs)—especially with long-term therapy; ***stomatitis*** (sores in mouth and on lips)

Incidence rare
***Hepatotoxicity***—usually asymptomatic; ***pulmonary infiltrates and/or fibrosis*** (cough; shortness of breath)

Note: Pulmonary toxicity has occurred after cumulative doses ranging from 600 to 1240 mg or therapy of 6 months or more.

# Lomustine (Systemic)

Those indicating need for medical attention only if they continue or are bothersome
Incidence more frequent
*Loss of appetite; nausea and vomiting*
Note: *Loss of appetite* may persist for 2 to 3 days after a dose.
*Nausea and vomiting* occur 3 to 6 hours after a dose and usually persist less than 24 hours.
Incidence less frequent
*Darkening of skin; diarrhea; skin rash and itching*

Those not indicating need for medical attention
Incidence less frequent
*Loss of hair*

Those indicating the need for medical attention if they occur after medication is discontinued
*Bone marrow depression* (black, tarry stools; blood in urine or stools; cough or hoarseness; fever or chills; lower back or side pain; painful or difficult urination; pinpoint red spots on skin; unusual bleeding or bruising)
Note: Cumulative myelosuppression may occur with repeated doses.

## Patient Consultation

As an aid to patient consultation, refer to *Advice for the Patient, Lomustine (Systemic)*.

In providing consultation, consider emphasizing the following selected information (» = major clinical significance):

### Before using this medication
» Conditions affecting use, especially:
Sensitivity to lomustine
Pregnancy—Use not recommended because of mutagenic, teratogenic, and carcinogenic potential; advisability of using contraception; telling physician immediately if pregnancy is suspected
Breast-feeding—Not recommended because of risk of serious side effects
Other medications, especially other bone marrow depressants or previous cytotoxic drug or radiation therapy
Other medical problems, especially chickenpox, herpes zoster, infection, pulmonary function impairment, or renal function impairment

### Proper use of this medication
» Importance of not taking more or less medication than the amount prescribed
Explanation of different kinds of capsules included in one container
Caution in taking combination therapy; taking each medication at the right time
Frequency of nausea and vomiting, which usually lasts less than 24 hours; taking on an empty stomach to reduce nausea
Checking with physician if vomiting occurs shortly after dose is taken
» Proper dosing

### Precautions while using this medication
» Importance of close monitoring by the physician
» Avoiding immunizations unless approved by physician; other persons in patient's household should avoid immunizations with oral poliovirus vaccine; avoiding other persons who have taken oral poliovirus vaccine or wearing a protective mask that covers nose and mouth

*Caution if bone marrow depression occurs*
» Avoiding exposure to persons with infections, especially during periods of low blood counts; checking with physician immediately if fever or chills, cough or hoarseness, lower back or side pain, or painful or difficult urination occurs
» Checking with physician immediately if unusual bleeding or bruising; black, tarry stools; blood in urine or stools; or pinpoint red spots on skin occur
Caution in use of regular toothbrush, dental floss, or toothpick; physician, dentist, or nurse may suggest alternatives; checking with physician before having dental work done
Not touching eyes or inside of nose unless hands washed immediately before
Using caution to avoid accidental cuts with use of sharp objects such as safety razor or fingernail or toenail cutters
Avoiding contact sports or other situations where bruising or injury could occur

### Side/adverse effects
May cause adverse effects such as blood problems, loss of hair, and cancer; importance of discussing possible effects with physician
Signs of potential side effects, especially immunosuppression, leukopenia, infection, thrombocytopenia, anemia, neurotoxicity, renal toxicity, stomatitis, hepatotoxicity, and pulmonary infiltrates and/or fibrosis
Physician or nurse can help in dealing with side effects

## General Dosing Information

Patients receiving lomustine should be under supervision of a physician experienced in cancer chemotherapy.

A variety of dosage schedules and regimens of lomustine, alone or in combination with other antitumor agents, are used. The prescriber may consult the medical literature as well as the manufacturer's literature in choosing a specific dosage.

Treatment with lomustine is continued as long as the medication is effective. If no response occurs after 1 or 2 courses, a response is unlikely.

Some cross-resistance has been reported between lomustine and carmustine.

Frequency and duration of nausea and vomiting may be reduced in some patients by administration of antiemetics prior to dosing and by administration of lomustine to fasting patients.

Dosage subsequent to the initial dose should be adjusted to meet the individual requirements of each patient based on the hematological response of the patient to the previous dose. An additional course of lomustine should be given only after circulating blood elements have returned to acceptable levels (leukocytes above 4000 per cubic millimeter and platelets above 100,000 per cubic millimeter).

Because of the delayed and cumulative bone marrow suppression caused by lomustine, the medication should be given no more frequently than every 6 weeks.

Special precautions are recommended in patients who develop thrombocytopenia as a result of administration of lomustine. These may include extreme care in performing invasive procedures; regular inspection of intravenous sites, skin (including perirectal area), and mucous membrane surfaces for signs of bleeding or bruising; limiting frequency of venipuncture and avoiding intramuscular injections; testing urine, emesis, stool, and secretions for occult blood; care in use of regular toothbrushes, dental floss, toothpicks, safety razors, and fingernail and toenail cutters; avoiding constipation; and using caution to prevent falls and other injuries. Such patients should avoid alcohol and any aspirin intake because of the risk of gastrointestinal bleeding. Platelet transfusions may be required.

Patients who develop leukopenia should be observed carefully for signs of infection. Antibiotic support may be required. In neutropenic patients who develop fever, broad-spectrum antibiotic coverage should be initiated empirically, pending bacterial cultures and appropriate diagnostic tests.

### Combination chemotherapy

Lomustine may be used in combination with other agents in various regimens. As a result, incidence and/or severity of side effects may be altered and different dosages (usually reduced) may be used. For example, lomustine is part of the following chemotherapeutic combinations (some commonly used acronyms are in parentheses):
—lomustine, doxorubicin, and vinblastine (CAVE).
—cyclophosphamide, methotrexate, and lomustine (CMC).

For specific dosages and schedules, consult the literature. For information regarding each agent, consult the individual monographs.

## Oral Dosage Forms

Note: Bracketed uses in the *Dosage Forms* section refer to categories of use and/or indications that are not included in U.S. product labeling.

### LOMUSTINE CAPSULES

**Usual adult and adolescent dose**
Tumors, brain, primary or
[Carcinoma, colorectal][1] or
[Carcinoma, lung, non–small cell] or
[Carcinoma, breast] or
Lymphomas, Hodgkin's or
[Multiple myeloma][1] or
[Melanoma, malignant]—
Initial: As a single agent—Oral, 100 to 130 mg per square meter of body surface area as a single dose, repeated every six weeks. A lower dose is used when lomustine is combined with other agents.

Note: In patients with suppressed bone marrow function, dosage is reduced to 100 mg per square meter of body surface area as a single dose, repeated every six weeks.

A suggested dosage adjustment schedule for subsequent doses is:

| Nadir after Prior Dose (cells per cubic millimeter) || % of Prior Dose To Be Given |
|---|---|---|
| Leukocytes | Platelets | |
| >4000 | >100,000 | 100 |
| 3000–3999 | 75,000–99,999 | 100 |
| 2000–2999 | 25,000–74,999 | 70 |
| <2000 | <25,000 | 50 |

**Usual pediatric dose**
See *Usual adult and adolescent dose*.

**Strength(s) usually available**
U.S.—
   10 mg (Rx) [*CeeNU* (mannitol)].
   40 mg (Rx) [*CeeNU* (mannitol)].
   100 mg (Rx) [*CeeNU* (mannitol)].
Note: Available only in a dose pack that contains a total of 300 mg (2 capsules of each strength) and provides enough medication for titration of a single dose. The total prescribed dose, to within 10 mg, can be obtained using the appropriate combination of capsules.
Canada—
   10 mg (Rx) [*CeeNU* (mannitol)].
   40 mg (Rx) [*CeeNU* (mannitol)].
   100 mg (Rx) [*CeeNU* (mannitol)].
Note: Available also in a dose pack that contains a total of 300 mg (2 capsules of each strength) and will provide enough medication for titration of a single dose. The total prescribed dose, to within 10 mg, can be obtained using the appropriate combination of capsules.

**Packaging and storage**
Store below 40 °C (104 °F), preferably between 15 and 30 °C (59 and 86 °F), in a well-closed container, unless otherwise specified by manufacturer.

**Auxiliary labeling**
• There may be two or more different types of capsules in this container. This is not an error. It is important that you take all of the capsules so that you receive the right dose of the medicine.
• Take on an empty stomach.

**Note**
A patient information label should be attached, explaining the difference in appearance of the capsules and advising the patient that all of the capsules together constitute one dose.
No more than one dose should be dispensed at a time and refills supplied only after direct verbal or written order by the physician.

[1]Not included in Canadian product labeling.

Revised: 08/09/92
Interim revision: 06/21/94; 09/30/97

# LOPERAMIDE    Oral-Local

VA CLASSIFICATION (Primary): GA208
Commonly used brand name(s): *Apo-Loperamide*; *Diarr-Eze*; *Imodium*; *Imodium A-D*; *Imodium A-D Caplets*; *Kaopectate II*; *Loperacap*; *Maalox Anti-Diarrheal*; *Nu-Loperamide*; *PMS-Loperamide*; *Pepto Diarrhea Control*; *Rho-Loperamide*.
Note: For a listing of dosage forms and brand names by country availability, see *Dosage Forms* section(s).

## Category
Antidiarrheal.

## Indications
Note: Bracketed information in the *Indications* section refers to uses that not included in U.S. product labeling.

Note: The efficacy of any antidiarrheal medication for treatment of most cases of nonspecific diarrhea is questionable. Preferred treatment consists of fluid and electrolyte replacement, nutritional therapy, and, if possible, elimination of the underlying cause of the diarrhea.

**Accepted**
Diarrhea (treatment)—Loperamide is indicated in adults for the control and symptomatic relief of acute nonspecific diarrhea and of chronic diarrhea associated with inflammatory bowel disease. Loperamide is also indicated to reduce the volume of discharge from ileostomies, colostomies, and other intestinal resections.
[Loperamide may be used in children to treat diarrhea caused by rapid transit when the anatomy of the bowel has been altered by disease or by surgical procedures.][1]
Traveler's diarrhea (treatment)—Loperamide is indicated for symptomatic relief of secretory diarrhea produced by bacteria, viruses, and parasites.

**Unaccepted**
Loperamide is not recommended for use in children up to 6 years of age unless directed by a physician. Loperamide is also not recommended for routine use or as the first line of therapy for treatment of diarrhea resulting from infection or food allergy in otherwise healthy, older children.
Loperamide should not be used if diarrhea is accompanied by fever or if there is blood or mucus in the stool.

[1]Not included in Canadian product labeling.

## Pharmacology/Pharmacokinetics
**Physicochemical characteristics**
Molecular weight—513.51.
pKa—8.6.

**Mechanism of action/Effect**
Loperamide acts on receptors along the small intestine to decrease circular and longitudinal muscle activity. Loperamide exerts its antidiarrheal action by slowing intestinal transit and increasing contact time, and perhaps also by directly inhibiting fluid and electrolyte secretion and/or stimulating salt and water absorption.

**Other actions/effects**
High doses may inhibit gastric acid secretion.

**Absorption**
Not well absorbed from gastrointestinal tract.

**Protein binding**
Very high (97%).

**Biotransformation**
Hepatic.

**Half-life**
9.1 to 14.4 (average 10.8) hours.

**Time to peak concentration**
Capsules—5 hours.
Oral solution—2.5 hours.

**Duration of action**
Up to 24 hours.

**Elimination**
Fecal/renal.

## Precautions to Consider
**Carcinogenicity**
Carcinogenic potential was not documented in a study using rats administered doses up to 133 times the maximum human dose.

**Pregnancy/Reproduction**
Fertility—Reproduction studies in rats and rabbits have shown that loperamide administered in doses up to 30 times the human therapeutic dose does not interfere with fertility.
Pregnancy—Adequate and well-controlled studies have not been done in humans.
Reproduction studies in rats and rabbits have shown that loperamide administered in doses up to 30 times the human therapeutic dose did not cause harm to the offspring, or produce teratogenic effects. Higher doses, however, impaired maternal and neonate survival.
FDA Pregnancy Category B.

**Breast-feeding**
It is not known whether loperamide is distributed into breast milk. However, in a pre- and post-natal study, loperamide administered to female nursing rats at a dose of 40 mg per kg of body weight caused a decrease in pup survival.

# Loperamide (Oral-Local)

### Pediatrics
Loperamide is not recommended for use in children up to 6 years of age unless directed by a physician, or for routine use or as initial therapy in children older than 6 years of age.

Oral rehydration therapy is the preferred treatment for children with diarrhea because loperamide may mask dehydration and depletion of electrolytes. Dehydration may further increase the variability in the response to loperamide.

Children, especially those under 3 years of age, are more susceptible to the opiate-like effects (CNS effects) of loperamide.

### Geriatrics
In geriatric patients with diarrhea, caution is recommended because loperamide may mask dehydration and depletion of electrolytes. Dehydration may further increase the variability in the response to loperamide.

### Drug interactions and/or related problems
The following drug interactions and/or related problems have been selected on the basis of their potential clinical significance (possible mechanism in parentheses where appropriate)—not necessarily inclusive (» = major clinical significance):

» Opioid (narcotic) analgesics
(concurrent use of loperamide with an opioid analgesic may increase the risk of severe constipation)

### Medical considerations/Contraindications
The medical considerations/contraindications included have been selected on the basis of their potential clinical significance (reasons given in parentheses where appropriate)—not necessarily inclusive (» = major clinical significance).

*Except under special circumstances, this medication should not be used when the following medical problems exist:*

» Colitis, severe
(patient may develop toxic megacolon)

» Diarrhea associated with *Clostridium difficile* resulting from treatment with broad-spectrum antibiotics
(loperamide may prolong transit time, causing a delay in the removal of toxins from the colon, thereby prolonging and/or worsening the diarrhea)

» Dysentery, acute, characterized by bloody stools and elevated temperature
(sole treatment with loperamide may be inadequate; antibiotic therapy may be required)

» Previous allergic reaction to loperamide

*Risk-benefit should be considered when the following medical problems exist:*

» Dehydration
(rehydration therapy is essential if signs or symptoms of dehydration, such as dryness of mouth, excessive thirst, wrinkled skin, decreased urination, and dizziness or lightheadedness, are present; fluid loss may have serious consequences, such as circulatory collapse and renal failure, especially in young children)

Diarrhea caused by infectious organisms
(bacterial diarrhea may, on rare occasions, worsen due to the increased contact time between the mucosa and the penetrating microorganism; however, there is no evidence of this occurring in actual practice)

Hepatic function impairment
(loperamide undergoes extensive first pass metabolism in the liver; therefore, patients with hepatic function impairment may have an increased risk of developing CNS toxicity)

## Side/Adverse Effects
Note: Adverse effects may be difficult to distinguish from the diarrheal syndrome itself and are usually self-limited.

The following side/adverse effects have been selected on the basis of their potential clinical significance (possible signs and symptoms in parentheses where appropriate)—not necessarily inclusive:

### Those indicating need for medical attention
Incidence rare
*Allergic reaction* (skin rash); *toxic megacolon* (bloating; constipation; loss of appetite; severe stomach pain with nausea and vomiting)

### Those indicating need for medical attention only if they continue or are bothersome
Incidence rare
*Dizziness or drowsiness; dryness of mouth*

## Overdose
For specific information on the agents used in the management of loperamide, see:
- *Charcoal, Activated (Oral-Local)* monograph; and/or
- *Naloxone (Systemic)* monograph.

For more information on the management of overdose or unintentional ingestion, **contact a Poison Control Center** (see *Poison Control Center Listing*).

### Clinical effects of overdose
Although human data are inconclusive, animal pharmacological and toxicological data indicate that overdosage may result in CNS depression, constipation, and gastrointestinal irritation.

### Treatment of overdose
Note: Treatment of loperamide overdose is similar to treatment for narcotic overdosage and involves the following:

To decrease absorption—Administration of activated charcoal promptly after ingestion. If vomiting has occurred spontaneously after ingestion of loperamide overdose, a slurry of 100 grams of activated charcoal should be administered as soon as fluids can be retained. Gastric lavage if vomiting has not occurred.

Specific treatment—Use of narcotic antagonists (e.g., naloxone), if necessary.

Monitoring—Prolonged and careful monitoring.

Supportive care—Support of respiration. Patients in whom intentional overdose is confirmed or suspected should be referred for psychiatric consultation.

## Patient Consultation
As an aid to patient consultation, refer to *Advice for the Patient, Loperamide (Oral)*.

In providing consultation, consider emphasizing the following selected information (» = major clinical significance):

### Before using this medication
» Conditions affecting use, especially:
Allergy to loperamide
Use in children—Not recommended for use in children unless directed by a physician; may mask symptoms of dehydration; variability in response to loperamide; increased susceptibility to CNS effects
Use in the elderly—May mask symptoms of dehydration; variability in response to loperamide
Other medical problems, especially acute dysentery, dehydration, diarrhea caused by antibiotics, or severe colitis

### Proper use of this medication
» Not using if diarrhea is accompanied by fever or blood or mucus in the stool; contacting physician
» Importance of not taking more medication than the amount prescribed
Proper administration technique for oral solution
» Importance of maintaining adequate hydration and proper diet
» Proper dosing
Missed dose: Not taking missed dose; not doubling doses
» Proper storage

### Precautions while using this medication
Regular visits to physician to check progress during prolonged therapy
» Consulting physician if diarrhea is not controlled within 48 hours and/or fever develops

### Side/adverse effects
Signs of potential side effects, especially allergic reaction or toxic megacolon

## General Dosing Information
Reduction of intestinal motility in patients with traveler's diarrhea may result in prolonged fever by slowing expulsion of infectious organisms that penetrate intestinal mucosa (for example, *Shigella, Salmonella,* and certain strains of *Escherichia coli*).

Inhibition of peristalsis may produce fluid retention in the bowel, which may aggravate and mask dehydration and depletion of electrolytes, especially in young children, and may also increase variability in the response to the medication. If dehydration or electrolyte imbalance occurs, loperamide therapy should be withheld until appropriate corrective therapy has begun.

In patients with acute ulcerative colitis, treatment with loperamide should be discontinued promptly in the event of abdominal distention or other symptoms that may indicate impending toxic megacolon.

Neither tolerance to the antidiarrheal effects nor physical dependence on loperamide has been reported in humans, although a morphine-like dependence has occurred in monkeys receiving high doses.

In acute diarrhea, treatment with loperamide should be discontinued after 48 hours if improvement does not occur. In chronic diarrhea, if no improvement has occurred after at least 10 days of treatment with the maximum dose, loperamide is unlikely to be effective, although further administration may be the only alternative when diet and specific treatment are inadequate.

## Oral Dosage Forms

### LOPERAMIDE HYDROCHLORIDE CAPSULES USP

**Usual adult and adolescent dose**
Acute diarrhea; or
Traveler's diarrhea—
  Oral, 4 mg after first loose bowel movement, followed by 2 mg after each subsequent loose bowel movement.
Chronic diarrhea—
  Initial: Oral, 4 mg, followed by 2 mg after each subsequent loose bowel movement until diarrhea is controlled.
  Maintenance: Oral, 4 to 8 mg a day in divided daily doses as needed.

**Usual adult prescribing limits**
16 mg per day.
Note: Maximum daily dosage for self-medication with loperamide using the over-the-counter product is 8 mg.

**Usual pediatric dose**
Note: Although loperamide is not recommended for routine use in children, the following pediatric doses have been used to treat diarrhea caused by specific motility disorders.
Acute diarrhea; or
Traveler's diarrhea—
  Children up to 6 years of age:
    Use is not recommended unless directed by a physician.
  Children 6 to 12 years of age:
    Initial:
      Oral, 80 to 240 mcg (0.08 to 0.24 mg) per kg of body weight a day in two or three divided doses; or, for
      Children 6 to 8 years of age: Oral, 2 mg two times a day.
      Children 8 to 12 years of age: Oral, 2 mg three times a day.
    Maintenance:
      Oral, 1 mg per 10 kg of body weight administered only after a loose stool.
  Children older than 12 years of age:
    See *Usual adult and adolescent dose*.
Chronic diarrhea—
  Dosage has not been established.
Note: In general, oral rehydration therapy and dietary treatment of diarrhea in children are preferred whenever possible.

**Strength(s) usually available**
U.S.—
  2 mg (Rx) [*Imodium* (lactose); GENERIC].
Canada—
  2 mg (OTC) [*Imodium* (lactose); *Loperacap*].

**Packaging and storage**
Store below 40 °C (104 °F), preferably between 15 and 30 °C (59 and 86 °F), in a well-closed, light-resistant container, unless otherwise specified by manufacturer.

### LOPERAMIDE HYDROCHLORIDE ORAL SOLUTION

**Usual adult and adolescent dose**
See *Loperamide Hydrochloride Capsules USP*.

**Usual adult prescribing limits**
8 mg per day for no more than two days.

**Usual pediatric dose**
Note: Although loperamide is not recommended for routine use in children, the following pediatric doses have been used to treat diarrhea caused by specific motility disorders.
Acute diarrhea; or
Traveler's diarrhea—
  Children up to 2 years of age:
    Use is not recommended unless directed by a physician.
  Children 2 to 11 years of age:
    Initial:
      Oral, 80 to 240 mcg (0.08 to 0.24 mg) per kg of body weight a day in two or three divided doses; or, for
      Children 2 to 5 years of age: Oral, only under the direction of a physician, 1 mg after first loose bowel movement, followed by 1 mg after each subsequent loose bowel movement, not to exceed a total daily dose of 3 mg.
      Children 6 to 8 years of age: Oral, 2 mg after first loose bowel movement, followed by 1 mg after each subsequent loose bowel movement, not to exceed a total daily dose of 4 mg.
      Children 9 to 11 years of age: Oral, 2 mg after first loose bowel movement, followed by 1 mg after each subsequent loose bowel movement, not to exceed a total daily dose of 6 mg.
    Maintenance:
      Oral, 1 mg per 10 kg of body weight administered only after a loose stool.
  Children 12 years of age and older:
    See *Usual adult and adolescent dose*.
Note: In general, oral rehydration therapy and dietary treatment of diarrhea in children are preferred whenever possible.

**Strength(s) usually available**
U.S.—
  1 mg per 5 mL (OTC) [*Imodium A-D* (alcohol 5.25%); *Maalox Anti-Diarrheal*; *Pepto Diarrhea Control* (alcohol 5.25%); GENERIC].
Canada—
  1 mg per 5 mL (OTC) [*Diarr-Eze*; *Imodium* (alcohol 4.07%); *PMS-Loperamide*].

**Packaging and storage**
Store below 40 °C (104 °F), preferably between 15 and 30 °C (59 and 86 °F), unless otherwise specified by manufacturer. Protect from freezing.

### LOPERAMIDE HYDROCHLORIDE TABLETS USP

**Usual adult and adolescent dose**
See *Loperamide Hydrochloride Capsules USP*.

**Usual adult prescribing limits**
8 mg per day for no more than two days.

**Usual pediatric dose**
Note: Although loperamide is not recommended for routine use in children, the following pediatric doses have been used to treat diarrhea caused by specific motility disorders.
Acute diarrhea; or
Traveler's diarrhea—
  Children up to 6 years of age:
    Use is not recommended unless directed by a physician.
  Children 6 to 11 years of age:
    Initial:
      Oral, 80 to 240 mcg (0.08 to 0.24 mg) per kg of body weight a day in two or three divided doses; or, for
      Children 6 to 8 years of age: Oral, 2 mg after first loose bowel movement, followed by 1 mg after each subsequent loose bowel movement, not to exceed a total daily dose of 4 mg.
      Children 9 to 11 years of age: Oral, 2 mg after first loose bowel movement, followed by 1 mg after each subsequent loose bowel movement, not to exceed a total daily dose of 6 mg.
    Maintenance:
      Oral, 1 mg per 10 kg of body weight administered only after a loose stool.
  Children 12 years of age and older:
    See *Usual adult and adolescent dose*.
Note: In general, oral rehydration therapy and dietary treatment of diarrhea in children are preferred whenever possible.

**Strength(s) usually available**
U.S.—
  2 mg (OTC) [*Imodium A-D Caplets* (lactose); *Kaopectate II* (lactose); *Maalox Anti-Diarrheal*; *Pepto Diarrhea Control* (lactose); GENERIC].
Canada—
  2 mg (OTC) [*Apo-Loperamide*; *Diarr-Eze*; *Imodium*; *Nu-Loperamide*; *PMS-Loperamide* (scored); *Rho-Loperamide*; GENERIC].

**Packaging and storage**
Store below 40 °C (104 °F), preferably between 15 and 30 °C (59 and 86 °F), in a well-closed, light-resistant container.

## Selected Bibliography

Brownlee HJ. Family practitioner's guide to patient self-treatment of acute diarrhea. Am J Med 1990; 88(6A Suppl): 27S-29S.
Ericsson CD, DuPont HL. Travelers' diarrhea: approaches to prevention and treatment. Clin Infect Dis 1993; 16: 616-26.
Ericsson CD, Johnson PC. Safety and efficacy of loperamide. Am J Med 1990; 88(6A Suppl): 10S-14S.

Revised: 01/25/95
Interim revision: 08/14/98

# LORACARBEF Systemic†

VA CLASSIFICATION (Primary): AM119
Commonly used brand name(s): *Lorabid*.
Note: For a listing of dosage forms and brand names by country availability, see *Dosage Forms* section(s).

†Not commercially available in Canada.

## Category
Antibacterial (systemic).

## Indications

**General considerations**
Loracarbef is the first of a new class of beta-lactam antibiotics called carbacephems. Carbacephems are related structurally to cephalosporins. Loracarbef is chemically identical to cefaclor except that the sulfur atom in the dihydrothiazine ring has been replaced by a methylene group. Carbacephems have greater chemical stability than cephalosporins.

Loracarbef has *in vitro* activity against most pathogens responsible for upper respiratory tract infections. It is active *in vitro* against *Streptococcus pneumoniae*, as well as beta-lactamase positive and negative *Haemophilus influenzae* and *Moraxella catarrhalis*. Loracarbef may not be active against bacteria such as penicillin-resistant *S. pneumoniae* and nonbeta-lactamase–producing ampicillin-resistant *H. influenzae*. Loracarbef has good activity *in vitro* against *S. pyogenes* (group A streptococci), and groups B, C, and G streptococci. *Enterococcus* species (group D streptococci) are resistant. Most strains of *Staphylococcus aureus* are susceptible to loracarbef; however, beta-lactamase–producing strains may be less susceptible and methicillin-resistant staphylococci are resistant.

Some gram-negative bacteria have *in vitro* susceptibility to loracarbef, including *Escherichia coli*, *Salmonella* species, *Klebsiella pneumoniae*, *Proteus mirabilis*, and *Citrobacter diversus*. However, strains of *E. coli* and *K. pneumoniae* with high production of beta-lactamase may be resistant. *Citrobacter freundii*, *Proteus vulgaris*, *Klebsiella oxytoca*, *Serratia marcescens*, *Morganella morganii*, *Enterobacter* species, *Providencia* species, and *Pseudomonas* species are all resistant to loracarbef.

**Accepted**
Bronchitis, bacterial exacerbation of (treatment)—Loracarbef is indicated in the treatment of bacterial exacerbations of bronchitis caused by susceptible organisms.

Otitis media (treatment)—Loracarbef is indicated in the treatment of otitis media caused by susceptible organisms.

Pharyngitis, streptococcal (treatment)—Loracarbef is indicated in the treatment of streptococcal pharyngitis caused by susceptible organisms.

Pneumonia (treatment)—Loracarbef is indicated in the treatment of pneumonia caused by susceptible organisms.

Sinusitis (treatment)—Loracarbef is indicated in the treatment of sinusitis caused by susceptible organisms.

Skin and soft tissue infections (treatment)—Loracarbef is indicated in the treatment of skin and soft tissue infections caused by susceptible organisms.

Urinary tract infections, bacterial (treatment)—Loracarbef is indicated in the treatment of bacterial urinary tract infections caused by susceptible organisms.

## Pharmacology/Pharmacokinetics

**Physicochemical characteristics**
Chemical group—Carbacephems are chemically similar to cephalosporins.
Molecular weight—367.8.

**Mechanism of action/Effect**
Bactericidal; binds to essential target proteins of the bacterial cell wall, leading to inhibition of cell wall synthesis and cellular lysis.

**Absorption**
Well absorbed (90%) from the gastrointestinal tract. When administered with food, the peak plasma concentration ($C_{max}$) decreases by 50 to 60%, and the time to peak plasma concentration ($T_{max}$) increases by 30 to 60 minutes; however, the total absorption remains unchanged.

**Distribution**
Concentrations in middle ear fluid, skin-blister fluid, and tonsillar tissue are approximately 40 to 50% of the simultaneous plasma concentration. Concentration in urine is still in the therapeutic range for most organisms 6 to 12 hours after administration. Cerebrospinal fluid (CSF) levels are not available.

**Protein binding**
Approximately 25%.

**Biotransformation**
There is no evidence of metabolism in humans.

**Half-life**
Single dose—
  Normal renal function:
    Approximately 1 hour.
  Creatinine clearance:
    10 to 50 mL/min (0.17 to 0.83 mL/sec)—Approximately 5.6 hours.
    <10 mL/min (0.17 mL/sec)—Approximately 32 hours.

**Time to peak concentration**
Capsules—Approximately 1.2 hours.
Suspension—0.5 to 0.8 hour.

**Peak serum concentration**
Single dose—
  Capsule:
    200 mg—Approximately 8 mcg/mL.
    400 mg—Approximately 14 mcg/mL.
  Suspension:
    400 mg—Approximately 17 mcg/mL.
    7.5 mg/kg—Approximately 13 mcg/mL.
    15 mg/kg—Approximately 19 mcg/mL.

**Elimination**
Renal; virtually all of loracarbef (87 to 97%) is excreted unchanged in the urine.
In dialysis—Hemodialysis reduces the half-life of loracarbef to approximately 4 hours.

## Precautions to Consider

**Cross-sensitivity and/or related problems**
Patients allergic to cephalosporins or penicillins may be allergic to loracarbef. Loracarbef should be administered with caution to penicillin-allergic patients since the cross-reactivity among beta-lactam antibiotics is approximately 10%.

**Carcinogenicity**
Lifetime carcinogenic studies in animals have not been performed.

**Mutagenicity**
No mutagenic potential was found in bacterial mutation tests or in *in vitro* and *in vivo* mammalian systems.

**Pregnancy/Reproduction**
Fertility—Fertility and reproductive performance were not affected in rats given doses of loracarbef up to 33 times the maximum human exposure in mg per kg of body weight (mg/kg).

Pregnancy—Adequate and well-controlled studies in humans have not been done.
Studies in mice, rats, and rabbits given doses up to 33 times the maximum human exposure of loracarbef in mg/kg have revealed no evidence of harm to the fetus.
FDA Pregnancy Category B.

**Breast-feeding**
It is not known whether loracarbef is distributed into breast milk.

**Pediatrics**
Appropriate studies on the relationship of age to the effects of loracarbef have not been performed in children up to 6 months of age. The pharmacokinetics and clinical response to loracarbef in children 6 months to 17 years of age are very similar to those in adults.

**Geriatrics**
Appropriate studies performed to date have not demonstrated geriatrics-specific problems that would limit the usefulness of loracarbef in the elderly. However, elderly patients are more likely to have age-related renal function impairment, which may require a dosage adjustment in patients receiving loracarbef.

**Drug interactions and/or related problems**
The following drug interactions and/or related problems have been selected on the basis of their potential clinical significance (possible mechanism in parentheses where appropriate)—not necessarily inclusive (» = major clinical significance):

Note: Combinations containing any of the following medications, depending on the amount present, may also interact with this medication.
» Probenecid
(probenecid decreases the renal tubular secretion of loracarbef, increasing the area-under-the-curve [AUC] by approximately 80% and the half-life from 1 hour to 1.5 hours)

### Laboratory value alterations
The following have been selected on the basis of their potential clinical significance (possible effect in parentheses where appropriate)—not necessarily inclusive (» = major clinical significance):

With physiology/laboratory test values
  Alanine aminotransferase (ALT [SGPT]), serum or
  Alkaline phosphatase, serum or
  Aspartate aminotransferase (AST [SGOT]), serum
    (values may be increased transiently)
  Blood urea nitrogen (BUN) or
  Creatinine, serum
    (concentrations may be increased transiently)
  Leukocyte count and
  Platelet count
    (may be decreased; transient leukopenia, thrombocytopenia, eosinophilia have been seen on rare occasion)

### Medical considerations/Contraindications
The medical considerations/contraindications included have been selected on the basis of their potential clinical significance (reasons given in parentheses where appropriate)—not necessarily inclusive (» = major clinical significance).

*Except under special circumstances, this medication should not be used when the following medical problem exists:*
» Previous allergic reaction (anaphylaxis) to penicillins or cephalosporins

*Risk-benefit should be considered when the following medical problem exists:*
» Renal function impairment
  (loracarbef is excreted renally; patients with renal function impairment may require a reduced dosage)

## Side/Adverse Effects
The following side/adverse effects have been selected on the basis of their potential clinical significance (possible signs and symptoms in parentheses where appropriate)—not necessarily inclusive:

### Those indicating need for medical attention
Incidence less frequent
  *Hypersensitivity* (itching; skin rash)

### Those indicating need for medical attention only if they continue or are bothersome
Incidence more frequent
  *Gastrointestinal disturbances* (abdominal pain; anorexia; diarrhea; nausea and vomiting)
Incidence rare
  *Central nervous system disturbances* (dizziness; headache; drowsiness; insomnia; nervousness); *vaginitis* (vaginal itching and discharge)

## Patient Consultation
As an aid to patient consultation, refer to *Advice for the Patient, Loracarbef (Systemic).*
In providing consultation, consider emphasizing the following selected information (» = major clinical significance):

### Before using this medication
» Conditions affecting use, especially:
  Allergy to penicillins or cephalosporins
  Other medications, especially probenecid
  Other medical problems, especially renal function impairment

### Proper use of this medication
  Taking at least 1 hour before or 2 hours after meals
» Compliance with full course of therapy, especially in streptococcal infections
» Importance of not missing doses and taking at evenly spaced times
» Proper dosing
  Missed dose: Taking as soon as possible; not taking if almost time for next dose; not doubling doses
» Proper storage

### Precautions while using this medication
  Checking with physician if no improvement within a few days
» May cause diarrhea—
  For severe diarrhea, checking with physician before taking any antidiarrheals
  For mild diarrhea, kaolin- or attapulgite-containing, but not other, antidiarrheals may be tried
  Checking with physician or pharmacist if mild diarrhea continues or worsens

### Side/adverse effects
  Signs of potential side effects, especially hypersensitivity reactions

## General Dosing Information
Therapy should be continued for at least 10 days in group A beta-hemolytic streptococcal infections to prevent acute rheumatic fever or glomerulonephritis.

Because loracarbef has a high degree of chemical stability, refrigeration of the reconstituted oral suspension is not required.

Adults and children with renal function impairment require a reduction in dose as follows:

| Creatinine Clearance (mL/min)/(mL/sec) | Dose |
| --- | --- |
| ≥50/0.83 | See *Usual adult and adolescent dose* |
| 10–49/0.17–0.82 | One-half the *Usual adult and adolescent dose* or administer the *Usual adult and adolescent dose* at twice the regular dosing interval |
| <10/0.17 | *Usual adult and adolescent dose* given every 3 to 5 days |
| Hemodialysis patients | Administer after hemodialysis |

### Diet/Nutrition
Loracarbef should be taken on an empty stomach (1 hour before or 2 hours after meals).

## Oral Dosage Forms
### LORACARBEF CAPSULES
#### Usual adult and adolescent dose
Bronchitis, bacterial exacerbations—
  Oral, 200 to 400 mg every twelve hours for seven days.
Pharyngitis, streptococcal—
  Oral, 200 mg every twelve hours for ten days.
Pneumonia, caused by *S. pneumoniae* or *H. influenzae*—
  Oral, 400 mg every twelve hours for fourteen days.
Sinusitis—
  Oral, 400 mg every twelve hours for ten days.
Skin and soft tissue infections—
  Oral, 200 mg every twelve hours for seven days.
Urinary tract infections—
  Uncomplicated cystitis—Oral, 200 mg every twenty-four hours for seven days.
  Uncomplicated pyelonephritis—Oral, 400 mg every twelve hours for fourteen days.

#### Usual pediatric dose
Otitis media—
  Oral, 15 mg per kg of body weight every twelve hours for ten days.
Pharyngitis, streptococcal: Oral, 7.5 mg per kg of body weight every twelve hours for ten days.
Skin and soft tissue infections—
  Oral, 7.5 mg per kg of body weight every twelve hours for seven days.

#### Strength(s) usually available
U.S.—
  200 mg (Rx) [*Lorabid*].
  400 mg (Rx) [*Lorabid*].
Canada—
  Not commercially available.

#### Packaging and storage
Store below 40 °C (104 °F), preferably between 15 and 30 °C (59 and 86 °F), unless otherwise specified by manufacturer. Store in a tight container.

#### Auxiliary labeling
• Continue medicine for full time of treatment.
• Take on an empty stomach.

### LORACARBEF FOR ORAL SUSPENSION
#### Usual adult and adolescent dose
See *Loracarbef Capsules*.

#### Usual pediatric dose
See *Loracarbef Capsules*.

# 1882  Loracarbef (Systemic)

**Strength(s) usually available**
U.S.—
  100 mg per 5 mL (when reconstituted according to the manufacturer's instructions) (Rx) [*Lorabid*].
  200 mg per 5 mL (when reconstituted according to the manufacturer's instructions) (Rx) [*Lorabid*].
Canada—
  Not commercially available.

**Packaging and storage**
Store below 40 °C (104 °F), preferably between 15 and 30 °C (59 and 86 °F), unless otherwise specified by manufacturer. Store in a tight container. Discard reconstituted suspension after 14 days.

**Auxiliary labeling**
- Continue medicine for full time of treatment.
- Shake well.
- Take on an empty stomach.

Revised: 08/18/93
Interim revision: 06/09/94; 06/20/95

---

## LORATADINE—See *Antihistamines (Systemic)*

---

## LORAZEPAM—See *Benzodiazepines (Systemic)*

---

# LOSARTAN  Systemic†

VA CLASSIFICATION (Primary/Secondary): CV805/CV409
Commonly used brand name(s): *Cozaar*.
Other commonly used names are DuP 753 and MK594.
Note: For a listing of dosage forms and brand names by country availability, see *Dosage Forms* section(s).

†Not commercially available in Canada.

## Category
Antihypertensive; angiotensin II receptor antagonist.

## Indications

**Accepted**
Hypertension—Losartan is indicated for the treatment of hypertension. It may be used alone or in combination with other antihypertensive agents.

## Pharmacology/Pharmacokinetics

**Physicochemical characteristics**
Molecular weight—Losartan potassium: 461.01.

**Mechanism of action/Effect**
Losartan is a nonpeptide angiotensin II receptor antagonist with high affinity and selectivity for the $AT_1$ receptor. Losartan blocks the vasoconstrictor and aldosterone-secreting effects of angiotensin II by inhibiting the binding of angiotensin II to the $AT_1$ receptor. $AT_1$ receptor blockade results in an increase in plasma renin activity (PRA) followed by increases in plasma angiotensin II concentration. The potential clinical consequences of these increases are not clear. Angiotensin II agonist effects have not been demonstrated.

**Other actions/effects**
*In vitro* platelet aggregometry shows that losartan appears to be a weak antagonist to human platelet thromboxane $A_2$/prostaglandin $H_2$ (TP) receptors. The clinical relevance of this effect is presently unclear. Losartan also appears to have a uricosuric effect. However, the clinical significance of this effect has not been delineated.

**Absorption**
Well-absorbed following oral administration. Bioavailability is approximately 33%.

**Protein binding**
Losartan—Very high (98.7%).
Carboxylic acid metabolite—Very high (99.8%).

**Biotransformation**
Losartan undergoes substantial first-pass metabolism by the cytochrome P450 system. Biotransformation results in a major active carboxylic acid metabolite that is 10 to 40 times more potent than the parent compound and is responsible for most of the pharmacologic activity. In addition, there are 5 minor metabolites that are much less active than the parent compound.

**Half-life**
Elimination—
  Losartan: Approximately 2 hours.
  Carboxylic acid metabolite: Approximately 6 to 9 hours.

**Time to peak concentration**
Losartan—Approximately 1 hour.
Carboxylic acid metabolite—Approximately 2 to 4 hours.

**Time to peak effect**
Approximately 6 hours.

**Duration of action**
Single dose—24 hours or more.

**Elimination**
Renal—Approximately 35% (4% of dose as parent and 6% of dose as active metabolite).
Fecal (biliary)—Approximately 60%.
In dialysis—Losartan and its carboxylic acid metabolite are not removable by hemodialysis.

## Precautions to Consider

**Carcinogenicity**
Losartan was not carcinogenic in rats and mice given maximally tolerated doses of 270 mg per kg of body weight (mg/kg) per day and 200 mg/kg per day, respectively, for 105 and 92 weeks, respectively. However, female rats had a slightly higher incidence of pancreatic acinar adenoma. The maximally tolerated doses of losartan provided systemic exposures of up to 160 times (rats) and 30 times (mice) the exposure of a 50 kg human given 100 mg per day.

**Mutagenicity**
Losartan was not mutagenic in a number of *in vitro* and *in vivo* assays.

**Pregnancy/Reproduction**
Fertility—Studies in male rats given oral doses of up to 150 mg/kg per day did not reveal adverse effects on fertility or reproductive performance. However, toxic doses of 300 and 200 mg/kg per day given to females resulted in significant decreases in the number of corpora lutea, implants, and live fetuses. The relationship of these findings to losartan is uncertain.

Pregnancy—Medications affecting the renin-angiotensin system, such as losartan, can cause fetal and neonatal morbidity and mortality when administered to pregnant women. Losartan should be discontinued as soon as possible when pregnancy is detected.

Fetal exposure to medications affecting the renin-angiotensin system during the second and third trimesters of pregnancy have been associated with hypotension, neonatal skull hypoplasia, anuria, renal failure, and even death in the newborn. Maternal oligohydramnios has also been reported, probably reflecting decreasing fetal renal function. Oligohydramnios in this setting has been associated with fetal limb contractures, craniofacial deformation, and hypoplastic lung development. Prematurity, intrauterine growth retardation, and patent ductus arteriosus also have been reported. However, it is not clear that these occurrences were related to drug exposure.

It is recommended that infants exposed *in utero* to losartan be closely observed for hypotension, oliguria, and hyperkalemia. Oliguria should be treated with support of blood pressure and renal perfusion. If oligohydramnios is observed, losartan should be discontinued unless it is considered lifesaving for the mother. Oligohydramnios, however, may not appear until after the fetus has sustained irreversible damage.

Losartan exposure during late gestation at doses approximately 3 times the maximum recommended human dose on a mg per square meter of body surface area basis produced adverse effects in rat fetuses and neonates, including decreased body weight, delayed physical and behavioral development, mortality, and renal toxicity.

FDA Pregnancy Category C (first trimester) and D (second and third trimesters).

**Breast-feeding**
It is not known whether losartan is distributed into breast milk. However, significant concentrations of losartan and its active metabolite are present in the milk of rats.

**Pediatrics**
No information is available on the relationship of age to the effects of losartan in pediatric patients. Safety and efficacy have not been established.

**Geriatrics**
Use of losartan in a limited number of patients 65 years of age and over has not demonstrated geriatrics-specific problems that would limit the usefulness of losartan in the elderly.

**Drug interactions and/or related problems**
The following drug interactions and/or related problems have been selected on the basis of their potential clinical significance (possible mechanism in parentheses where appropriate)—not necessarily inclusive (» = major clinical significance):

Note: Combinations containing any of the following medications, depending on the amount present, may also interact with this medication.

Anti-inflammatory drugs, nonsteroidal (NSAIDs), especially indomethacin
  (NSAIDs may antagonize the antihypertensive effect of losartan by inhibiting renal prostaglandin synthesis and/or causing sodium and fluid retention; the patient should be carefully monitored to confirm that the desired effect is being obtained)

Blood from blood bank (may contain up to 30 mEq [mmol] of potassium per L of plasma or up to 65 mEq [mmol] per L of whole blood when stored for more than 10 days) or
Cyclosporine or
Diuretics, potassium-sparing or
Low-salt milk (may contain up to 60 mEq [mmol] of potassium per liter) or
Potassium-containing medications or
Potassium supplements or substances containing high concentrations of potassium or
Salt substitutes (most contain substantial amounts of potassium)
  (concurrent administration with losartan may result in hyperkalemia since reduction of aldosterone production induced by losartan may lead to elevation of serum potassium; determination of serum potassium concentrations is recommended if concurrent use of these agents is necessary)

» Diuretics
  (symptomatic hypotension may occur after initiation of losartan therapy in patients taking a diuretic; caution and a lower starting dose are recommended)

Hypotension-producing medications, other (See *Appendix II*)
  (concurrent use with losartan may produce additive hypotensive effects)

Sympathomimetics
  (concurrent use of these agents may reduce the antihypertensive effects of losartan; the patient should be carefully monitored to confirm that the desired effect is being obtained)

**Laboratory value alterations**
The following have been selected on the basis of their potential clinical significance (possible effect in parentheses where appropriate)—not necessarily inclusive (» = major clinical significance):

With physiology/laboratory test values
  Alanine aminotransferase (ALT) and
  Aspartate aminotransferase (AST)
    (transient increases have been reported rarely; these increases were infrequently greater than 2 or 3 times the upper limit of normal)
  Bilirubin, serum
    (concentrations may be increased)
  Hemoglobin and
  Hematocrit
    (small increases occur frequently, but are rarely of clinical significance)
  Potassium, serum
    (concentrations may be slightly increased as a result of reduced aldosterone concentrations)
  Uric acid, serum
    (concentrations may be decreased, reflecting losartan's uricosuric effect)
  Uric acid, urine
    (concentrations may be increased; losartan appears to significantly increase uric acid excretion; this effect appears to be related to the parent compound, losartan, and not the carboxylic acid metabolite)

**Medical considerations/Contraindications**
The medical considerations/contraindications included have been selected on the basis of their potential clinical significance (reasons given in parentheses where appropriate)—not necessarily inclusive (» = major clinical significance).

*Risk-benefit should be considered when the following medical problems exist:*

» Hepatic function impairment
  (increased plasma concentrations may occur; total plasma clearance of losartan may be 50% lower and oral bioavailability about 2 times higher than in individuals with normal hepatic function; lower dosages are recommended)

» Renal artery stenosis, bilateral or in a solitary kidney
  (increased risk of renal function impairment)

Renal function impairment, moderate to severe
  (losartan area under the curve [AUC] may be increased by approximately 50%; however, dosage adjustments are not necessary unless patient is volume-depleted)
  (in patients whose renal function is dependent on the renin-angiotensin-aldosterone system, especially those with congestive heart failure, there may be a risk of losartan-induced renal failure)

Sensitivity to losartan

» Caution is recommended in patients who are sodium- or volume-depleted. Symptomatic hypotension may occur following initiation of losartan therapy. Sodium- or volume-depletion should be corrected or a lower starting dose is recommended in these patients.

**Patient monitoring**
The following may be especially important in patient monitoring (other tests may be warranted in some patients, depending on condition; » = major clinical significance):

» Blood pressure measurements
  (recommended at periodic intervals; selected patients may be taught to monitor their blood pressure at home and report the results at regular physician visits)

Renal function determinations
  (recommended at periodic intervals, especially in patients who are sodium- and volume-depleted as a result of diuretic therapy or who have severe congestive heart failure)

## Side/Adverse Effects

Note: A case of angioedema has been reported in a patient being treated with losartan.

The following side/adverse effects have been selected on the basis of their potential clinical significance (possible signs and symptoms in parentheses where appropriate)—not necessarily inclusive:

**Those indicating need for medical attention**
Incidence less frequent
  *Dizziness; upper respiratory infection* (cough, fever, or sore throat)

**Those indicating need for medical attention only if they continue or are bothersome**
Incidence more frequent
  *Headache*
Incidence less frequent
  *Back pain; diarrhea; fatigue; nasal congestion*
Incidence rare
  *Cough, dry; insomnia* (trouble in sleeping); *leg pain; muscle cramps or pain; sinus problems*

## Overdose

For more information on the management of overdose or unintentional ingestion, **contact a Poison Control Center** (see *Poison Control Center Listing*).

**Clinical effects of overdose**
The following effects have been selected on the basis of their potential clinical significance (possible signs and symptoms in parentheses where appropriate)—not necessarily inclusive:
  *Bradycardia due to vagal stimulation; hypotension; tachycardia*

**Treatment of overdose**
Symptomatic and supportive.

# Losartan (Systemic)

## Patient Consultation
As an aid to patient consultation, refer to *Advice for the Patient, Losartan (Systemic).*

In providing consultation, consider emphasizing the following selected information (» = major clinical significance):

**Before using this medication**
- » Conditions affecting use, especially:
  - Sensitivity to losartan
  - Pregnancy—Can cause fetal and neonatal morbidity and mortality; not recommended for use during pregnancy
  - Other medications, especially diuretics
  - Other medical problems, especially hepatic and renal function impairment, renal artery stenosis, or sodium or volume depletion

**Proper use of this medication**
- Compliance with therapy; taking medication at the same time(s) each day to maintain the therapeutic effect
- Possible need for control of weight and diet, especially sodium intake; risks associated with sodium depletion; not taking salt substitutes or using low-salt milk unless approved by physician
- » Patient may not experience symptoms of hypertension; importance of taking medication even if feeling well
- » Does not cure, but helps control hypertension; possible need for lifelong therapy; checking with physician before discontinuing medication; serious consequences of untreated hypertension
- May be taken with or without food
- » Proper dosing
- Missed dose: Taking as soon as possible; not taking if almost time for next dose; not doubling doses
- » Proper storage

**Precautions while using this medication**
- » Notifying physician immediately if pregnancy is suspected
- Making regular visits to physician to check progress
- » Not taking other medications, especially nonprescription sympathomimetics, unless discussed with physician
- Caution when driving or doing other things requiring alertness, because of possible dizziness, especially after initial dose of losartan in patients taking diuretics
- To prevent dehydration and hypotension, checking with physician if severe nausea, vomiting, or diarrhea occurs and continues
- Caution when exercising or during hot weather because of the risk of dehydration and hypotension due to reduced fluid volume
- » Caution in using alcohol because of the risk of dehydration and hypotension due to reduced fluid volume

**Side/adverse effects**
- Signs of potential side effects, especially dizziness or upper respiratory infection

## General Dosing Information
Dosage must be adjusted to meet the individual requirements of each patient, on the basis of clinical response.

Although there does not appear to be a rebound effect after abrupt withdrawal of losartan, gradual dosage reduction is recommended to minimize any risk of a rebound effect.

Recent evidence suggests that withdrawal of antihypertensive therapy prior to surgery may be undesirable. However, the anesthesiologist must be aware of such therapy.

**Diet/Nutrition**
Losartan may be taken with or without food.

## Oral Dosage Forms

### LOSARTAN POTASSIUM TABLETS

**Usual adult dose**
Antihypertensive—
  Initial—
    Oral, 50 mg once a day.
Note: In patients with possible volume depletion and patients with a history of hepatic function impairment an initial dose of 25 mg once a day is recommended.
  Maintenance—
    Oral, 25 to 100 mg a day. Dose may be given once a day or divided into two doses.
Note: If adequate blood pressure control is not achieved by losartan alone, a low dose of a diuretic may be added for an additive effect.

**Usual pediatric dose**
Safety and efficacy have not been established.

**Strength(s) usually available**
U.S.—
  25 (Rx) [*Cozaar* (potassium 2.12 mg [0.054 mEq])].
  50 (Rx) [*Cozaar* (potassium 4.24 mg [0.108 mEq])].
Canada—
  Not commercially available.

**Packaging and storage**
Store below 40 °C (104 °F), preferably between 15 and 30 °C (59 and 86 °F), in a tightly closed container. Protect from light.

**Auxiliary labeling**
- Do not take other medicines without your doctor's advice.

## Selected Bibliography
Goldberg AI, Dunlay MC, Sweet CS. Safety and tolerability of losartan potassium, an angiotensin II receptor antagonist, compared with hydrochlorothiazide, atenolol, felodipine ER, and angiotensin-converting enzyme inhibitors for the treatment of systemic hypertension. Am J Cardiol 1995; 75: 793-5.

Developed: 08/15/95
Interim revision: 09/21/95; 08/19/98

---

# LOSARTAN AND HYDROCHLOROTHIAZIDE Systemic—INTRODUCTORY VERSION

VA CLASSIFICATION (Primary): CV401

Commonly used brand name(s): *Hyzaar*.

Note: For a listing of dosage forms and brand names by country availability, see *Dosage Forms* section(s).

## Category
Antihypertensive.

## Indications

**Accepted**
Hypertension (treatment)—Losartan and hydrochlorothiazide combination is indicated for the treatment of hypertension.

  Fixed-dosage combinations are generally not recommended for initial therapy and are useful for subsequent therapy only when the proportion of the component agents corresponds to the dose of the individual agents, as determined by titration.

## Pharmacology/Pharmacokinetics

**Physicochemical characteristics**
Molecular weight—Losartan potassium: 461.01.
Hydrochlorothiazide: 297.72.

**Mechanism of action/Effect**
Losartan—Losartan is a nonpeptide angiotensin II receptor antagonist with high affinity and selectivity for the $AT_1$ receptor. Losartan blocks the vasoconstrictor and aldosterone-secreting effects of angiotensin II by inhibiting the binding of angiotensin II to the $AT_1$ receptor. $AT_1$ receptor blockade results in an increase in plasma renin activity (PRA) followed by increases in plasma angiotensin II concentration. The potential clinical consequences of these increases are not clear. Angiotensin II agonist effects have not been demonstrated.

Hydrochlorothiazide—Hydrochlorothiazide is a thiazide diuretic. Thiazide diuretics increase urinary excretion of sodium and water by inhibiting sodium reabsorption in the early distal tubule. The diuretic action of hydrochlorothiazide decreases plasma volume, resulting in increases in plasma renin activity, increases in aldosterone secretion, increases in urinary potassium loss, and decreases in serum potassium. Since the renin-aldosterone link is mediated by angiotensin II, coadministration of losartan tends to reverse the potassium loss associated with hydrochlorothiazide.

**Absorption**
Losartan—Well-absorbed following oral administration. Bioavailability is approximately 33%.

**Protein binding**
Losartan—Very high (98.7%).
Carboxylic acid metabolite—Very high (99.8%).

**Biotransformation**
Losartan—Losartan undergoes substantial first-pass metabolism by the cytochrome P450 system. Biotransformation results in a major active carboxylic acid metabolite that is responsible for most of the angiotensin II receptor antagonism. In addition, several inactive metabolites are formed.
Hydrochlorothiazide—Hydrochlorothiazide is not metabolized.

**Half-life**
Elimination—
  Losartan: Approximately 2 hours.
  Carboxylic acid metabolite: Approximately 6 to 9 hours.
  Hydrochlorothiazide: 5.6 to 14.8 hours.

**Time to peak concentration**
Losartan—Approximately 1 hour.
Carboxylic acid metabolite—Approximately 3 to 4 hours.
Hydrochlorothiazide—Approximately 4 hours.

**Elimination**
Losartan—
  Renal: Approximately 35% (4% of dose as parent and 6% of dose as active metabolite).
  Fecal (biliary): Approximately 60%.
  In dialysis: Losartan and its carboxylic acid metabolite are not removable by hemodialysis.
Hydrochlorothiazide—
  Renal.

## Precautions to Consider

### Cross-sensitivity and/or related problems
Patients sensitive to sulfonamide-type medications may be sensitive to this medication also.

### Carcinogenicity
No carcinogenicity studies have been conducted with losartan and hydrochlorothiazide combination.
*Losartan*—Losartan was not carcinogenic in rats and mice given maximally tolerated doses of 270 mg per kg of body weight (mg/kg) per day and 200 mg/kg per day, respectively, for 105 and 92 weeks, respectively. However, female rats had a slightly higher incidence of pancreatic acinar adenoma. The maximally tolerated doses of losartan provided systemic exposures of up to 160 times (rats) and 30 times (mice) the exposure of a 50 kg human given 100 mg per day.
*Hydrochlorothiazide*—No evidence of carcinogenicity was found in two-year feeding studies at doses of up to approximately 600 mg/kg per day in female mice and 100 mg/kg per day in male and female rats. However, evidence was equivocal for hepatocarcinogenicity in male mice.

### Mutagenicity
Losartan and hydrochlorothiazide combination was not mutagenic when tested at a weight ratio of 4:1 in the Ames microbial mutagenesis assay and the V-79 Chinese hamster lung cell mutagenesis assay. In addition, there was no evidence of direct genotoxicity in the *in vitro* alkaline elution assay in rat hepatocytes and *in vitro* chromosomal aberration assay in Chinese hamster ovary cells at noncytotoxic concentrations.
*Losartan*—Losartan was not mutagenic in a number of *in vitro* and *in vivo* assays.
*Hydrochlorothiazide*—Positive test results were obtained in the *in vitro* CHO Sister Chromatid Exchange (clastogenicity) and in the Mouse Lymphoma Cell (mutagenicity) assays at hydrochlorothiazide concentrations from 43 to 1300 mcg per mL, and in the *Aspergillus nidulans* non-disjunction assay at an unspecified concentration. Other mutagenicity tests were negative.

### Pregnancy/Reproduction
Fertility—Losartan and hydrochlorothiazide combination did not affect fertility or mating behavior of male rats at dosages up to 135 mg/kg per day of losartan and 33.75 mg/kg per day of hydrochlorothiazide. These doses reflect systemic exposures (AUCs) of approximately 60, 60, and 30 times, respectively, for losartan, its active metabolite, and hydrochlorothiazide, greater than those achieved in humans with losartan and hydrochlorothiazide combination (100 mg/25 mg). However, administration of losartan and hydrochlorothiazide combination to female rats at doses as low as 10 mg/kg per day of losartan and 2.5 mg/kg per day of hydrochlorothiazide resulted in slight but statistically significant decreases in fecundity and fertility indices. These doses were approximately 6, 2, and 2 times, respectively, for losartan, its active metabolite, and hydrochlorothiazide, greater than those achieved in humans with 100 mg of losartan and 25 mg of hydrochlorothiazide.
*Losartan*: Studies in male rats given oral doses of up to 150 mg/kg per day did not reveal adverse effects on fertility or reproductive performance. However, toxic doses of 300 and 200 mg/kg per day given to females resulted in significant decreases in the number of corpora lutea, implants, and live fetuses. The relationship of these findings to losartan is uncertain.
*Hydrochlorothiazide*: Hydrochlorothiazide did not produce adverse effects on the fertility of mice and rats of either sex at doses up to 100 mg/kg and 4 mg/kg, respectively.
Pregnancy—Medications affecting the renin-angiotensin system, such as losartan, can cause fetal and neonatal morbidity and mortality when administered to pregnant women. Losartan and hydrochlorothiazide combination should be discontinued as soon as possible when pregnancy is detected.
Fetal exposure to medications affecting the renin-angiotensin system during the second and third trimesters of pregnancy have been associated with hypotension, neonatal skull hypoplasia, anuria, renal failure, and even death in the newborn. Maternal oligohydramnios has also been reported, probably reflecting decreasing fetal renal function. Oligohydramnios in this setting has been associated with fetal limb contractures, craniofacial deformation, and hypoplastic lung development. Prematurity, intrauterine growth retardation, and patent ductus arteriosus also have been reported. However, it is not clear that these occurrences were related to drug exposure.
It is recommended that infants exposed *in utero* to losartan and hydrochlorothiazide combination be closely observed for hypotension, oliguria, and hyperkalemia. Oliguria should be treated with support of blood pressure and renal perfusion. If oligohydramnios is observed, losartan and hydrochlorothiazide combination should be discontinued unless it is considered lifesaving for the mother. Oligohydramnios, however, may not appear until after the fetus has sustained irreversible damage.
Losartan and hydrochlorothiazide combination was not teratogenic in rats or rabbits given a maximum dose of 10 mg/kg per day of losartan and 2.5 mg/kg per day of hydrochlorothiazide. In female rats treated prior to and throughout gestation with 10 mg/kg per day of losartan and 2.5 mg/kg per day of hydrochlorothiazide, a slight increase in supernumerary ribs was observed.
Losartan and hydrochlorothiazide combination exposure during late gestation at doses of 50 mg/kg per day of losartan and 12.5 mg/kg per day of hydrochlorothiazide produced adverse fetal and neonatal effects in rats, including decreased body weight, renal toxicity, and mortality.
*Hydrochlorothiazide*: Thiazide diuretics cross the placenta and appear in cord blood. There is a risk of fetal or neonatal jaundice, thrombocytopenia, and possibly other adverse effects.
FDA Pregnancy Category C (first trimester) and D (second and third trimesters).

### Breast-feeding
It is not known whether losartan is distributed into breast milk. However, significant concentrations of losartan and its active metabolite are present in the milk of rats. Thiazide diuretics are distributed into breast milk.

### Pediatrics
No information is available on the relationship of age to the effects of losartan and hydrochlorothiazide combination in pediatric patients. Safety and efficacy have not been established.

### Geriatrics
Studies of losartan and hydrochlorothiazide combination have included a limited number of patients 65 years of age and over. No geriatrics-specific problems that would limit the usefulness of losartan and hydrochlorothiazide combination in the elderly have been identified.

### Drug interactions and/or related problems
The following drug interactions and/or related problems have been selected on the basis of their potential clinical significance (possible mechanism in parentheses where appropriate)—not necessarily inclusive (» = major clinical significance):

Note: Combinations containing any of the following medications, depending on the amount present, may also interact with this medication.

  Alcohol or
  Analgesics, narcotic or
  Barbiturates
    (concurrent administration with losartan and hydrochlorothiazide combination may potentiate orthostatic hypotension)

Antidiabetic agents, sulfonylurea or
Insulin
(hydrochlorothiazide may increase blood glucose concentrations; dosage adjustment of the antidiabetic medication may be necessary)

Anti-inflammatory drugs, nonsteroidal (NSAIDs)
(may antagonize the diuretic, natriuretic, and antihypertensive effects of hydrochlorothiazide; patients should be carefully monitored to confirm that the desired effect is being obtained)

Cholestyramine or
Colestipol
(cholestyramine or colstipol may inhibit gastrointestinal absorption of hydrochlorothiazide by up to 85% and 43%, respectively)

Corticosteroids
(concurrent use with hydrochlorothiazide may intensify electrolyte depletion, particularly hypokalemia)

Hypotension-producing medications, other (See *Appendix II*)
(concurrent use with losartan and hydrochlorothiazide combination may produce additive hypotensive effects)

» Lithium
(concurrent use with losartan and hydrochlorothiazide combination is not recommended; hydrochlorothiazide may reduce the renal clearance of lithium and increase the risk of lithium toxicity)

Neuromuscular blocking agents, nondepolarizing
(hydrochlorothiazide may enhance the blockade of nondepolarizing neuromuscular blocking agents)

Sympathomimetics, such as norepinephrine
(losartan and hydrochlorothiazide combination may decrease the response to sympathomimetic agents; patients should be carefully monitored to confirm that the desired effect is being obtained)

## Laboratory value alterations
The following have been selected on the basis of their potential clinical significance (possible effect in parentheses where appropriate)—not necessarily inclusive (» = major clinical significance):

With physiology/laboratory test values
Bilirubin
(concentrations may be increased)

Calcium, serum
(concentrations may be increased; losartan and hydrochlorothiazide combination should be discontinued before parathyroid function tests are performed)

Cholesterol and
Triglycerides
(serum concentrations may be increased)

Hemoglobin and
Hematocrit
(small increases occur frequently, but are rarely of clinical significance)

Liver function tests
(occasional elevations have been reported)

Magnesium, serum
Sodium, serum
(concentrations may be decreased)

Potassium, serum
(concentrations may be decreased; in clinical trials the incidence of hypokalemia [< 3.5 mEq per L] was 6.7% for patients receiving losartan and hydrochlorothiazide combination versus 3.5% for patients receiving placebo)

## Medical considerations/Contraindications
The medical considerations/contraindications included have been selected on the basis of their potential clinical significance (reasons given in parentheses where appropriate)—not necessarily inclusive (» = major clinical significance).

*Except under special circumstances, this medication should not be used when the following medical problems exist:*

» Anuria or
» Renal function impairment, severe
(may precipitate azotemia; may produce cumulative effects; use is not recommended)

» Hepatic function impairment
(increased plasma concentrations may occur; total plasma clearance of losartan may be 50% lower and oral bioavailability about 2 times higher than in individuals with normal hepatic function; losartan and hydrochlorothiazide combination is not recommended in these patients since dosage titration with losartan is needed; the lower recommended starting doses of losartan cannot be given with this combination)

(risk of dehydration and electrolyte imbalance, which may precipitate hepatic coma)

*Risk-benefit should be considered when the following medical problems exist:*

Allergy or
Asthma, bronchial
(hypersensitivity reactions to hydrochlorothiazide may be more likely in these patients)

Electrolyte imbalance
(condition may be exacerbated; correction of electrolyte imbalance prior to administration of losartan and hydrochlorothiazide combination is recommended)

» Renal artery stenosis, bilateral or in a solitary kidney
(increased risk of renal function impairment)

Renal function impairment, moderate
(losartan's area under the curve [AUC] may be increased by approximately 50%)
(in patients whose renal function is dependent on the renin-angiotensin-aldosterone system, especially those with severe congestive heart failure, there may be a risk of losartan-induced renal failure)

Sensitivity to losartan, thiazide diuretics, or sulfonamide-derived medications

Sympathectomy
(antihypertensive effects may be enhanced)

Systemic lupus erythematosus
(hydrochlorothiazide may exacerbate or activate systemic lupus erythematosus)

» Caution is recommended in patients who are sodium- or volume-depleted. Symptomatic hypotension may occur following initiation of losartan and hydrochlorothiazide combination therapy. Sodium- or volume-depletion should be corrected prior to administration of losartan and hydrochlorothiazide combination.

## Patient monitoring
The following may be especially important in patient monitoring (other tests may be warranted in some patients, depending on condition; » = major clinical significance):

Blood pressure measurements
(recommended at periodic intervals; selected patients may be taught to perform blood pressure measurements at home and report the results at regular physician visits)

Electrolyte concentrations, serum
(determinations recommended periodically to detect possible electrolyte imbalance)

Renal function determinations
(recommended at periodic intervals)

# Side/Adverse Effects
Note: A case of angioedema has been reported in a patient being treated with losartan.

The following side/adverse effects have been selected on the basis of their potential clinical significance (possible signs and symptoms in parentheses where appropriate)—not necessarily inclusive:

## Those indicating need for medical attention
Incidence less frequent
*Dizziness; electrolyte imbalance, especially hypokalemia* (dryness of mouth; increased thirst; irregular heartbeat; muscle cramps or pain; nausea or vomiting; unusual tiredness or weakness; weak pulse); *upper respiratory tract infection* (cough, fever, or sore throat)

Incidence rare
*Agranulocytosis* (cough or hoarseness; fever or chills; lower back or side pain; painful or difficult urination); *cholecystitis or pancreatitis* (severe stomach pain with nausea and vomiting); *edema* (swelling of feet or lower legs); *palpitations* (pounding heartbeat); *skin rash; thrombocytopenia* (black, tarry stools; blood in urine or stools; pinpoint red spots on skin; unusual bleeding or bruising)

## Those indicating need for medical attention only if they continue or are bothersome
Incidence less frequent
*Abdominal pain* (stomach pain); *back pain; headache; photosensitivity* (increased sensitivity of skin to sunlight)

Incidence rare
*Cough; sinusitis* (sinus problems)

## Overdose

For more infomation on the management of overdose or unintentional ingestion, **contact a Poison Control Center** (see *Poison Control Center Listing*).

**Clinical effects of overdose**
The following effects have been selected on the basis of their potential clinical significance (possible signs and symptoms in parentheses where appropriate)—not necessarily inclusive:
*Bradycardia due to vagal stimulation; dehydration; electrolyte depletion; hypotension; tachycardia*

**Treatment of overdose**
Symptomatic and supportive.

## Patient Consultation

As an aid to patient consultation, refer to *Advice for the Patient, Losartan and Hydrochlorothiazide (Systemic)—Introductory Version*.

In providing consultation, consider emphasizing the following selected information (» = major clinical significance):

**Before using this medication**
» Conditions affecting use, especially:
   Sensitivity to losartan, thiazide diuretics, or sulfonamide-type medications
   Pregnancy—Not recommended for use during pregnancy; can cause fetal and neonatal morbidity and mortality
   Breast-feeding—Hydrochlorothiazide is distributed into breast milk
   Other medications, especially lithium
   Other medical problems, especially anuria, hepatic function impairment, renal artery stenosis, or renal function impairment

**Proper use of this medication**
Compliance with therapy; taking medication at the same time each day to maintain the therapeutic effect
Possible need for control of weight and diet, especially sodium intake; risks associated with sodium depletion; not taking salt substitutes or using low-salt milk unless approved by physician
» Patient may not experience symptoms of hypertension; importance of taking medication even if feeling well
» Does not cure, but helps control, hypertension; possible need for lifelong therapy; checking with physician before discontinuing medication; serious consequences of untreated hypertension
May be taken with or without food
» Proper dosing
Missed dose: Taking as soon as possible; not taking if almost time for next dose; not doubling doses
» Proper storage

**Precautions while using this medication**
» Notifying physician immediately if pregnancy is suspected
Making regular visits to physician to check progress
» Not taking other medications, especially nonprescription sympathomimetics, unless discussed with physician
Caution when driving or doing other things requiring alertness, because of possible dizziness, especially after first dose of losartan and hydrochlorothiazide combination
To prevent dehydration and hypotension, checking with physician if severe nausea, vomiting, or diarrhea occurs and continues
Caution when exercising or during hot weather because of the risk of dehydration and hypotension due to reduced fluid volume
» Caution in using alcohol because of the risk of dehydration and hypotension due to reduced fluid volume
Diabetics: May increase blood sugar levels

**Side/adverse effects**
Signs of potential side effects, especially dizziness, electrolyte imbalance, upper respiratory tract infection, agranulocytosis, cholecystitis, pancreatitis, edema, palpitations, skin rash, or thrombocytopenia

## General Dosing Information

Although there does not appear to be a rebound effect after abrupt withdrawal of losartan and hydrochlorothiazide combination, gradual dosage reduction is recommended to minimize any risk of a rebound effect.

Losartan and hydrochlorothiazide combination is recommended for therapy only after dosage titration with the individual components.

## Oral Dosage Forms

### LOSARTAN POTASSIUM AND HYDROCHLOROTHIAZIDE TABLETS

**Usual adult dose**
Antihypertensive—
   Oral, 1 or 2 tablets once a day as determined by individual titration with the component agents.

**Usual adult prescribing limits**
2 tablets a day.

**Usual pediatric dose**
Safety and efficacy have not been established.

**Strength(s) usually available**
U.S.—
   50 mg of losartan potassium and 12.5 mg of hydrochlorothiazide (Rx) [*Hyzaar*].

**Packaging and storage**
Store at room temperature, preferably between 15 and 30 °C (59 and 86 °F), in a tightly closed container. Protect from light.

**Auxiliary labeling**
• Do not take other medicines without your doctor's advice.

Developed: 09/28/95
Interim revision: 08/11/98

---

# LOTEPREDNOL    Ophthalmic—INTRODUCTORY VERSION

VA CLASSIFICATION (Primary): OP301
Commonly used brand name(s): *Alrex; Lotemax*.
Note: For a listing of dosage forms and brand names by country availability, see *Dosage Forms* section(s).

## Category

Corticosteroid (ophthalmic); anti-inflammatory (steroidal), ophthalmic.

## Indications

**Accepted**
Conjunctivitis, seasonal allergic (treatment)—Ophthalmic loteprednol 0.2% is indicated for temporary relief of the signs and symptoms of seasonal allergic conjunctivitis.
Inflammation, postoperative (treatment)—Ophthalmic loteprednol 0.5% is indicated for the treatment of postoperative inflammation following ocular surgery.
Ocular conditions, inflammatory (treatment)—Ophthalmic loteprednol 0.5% is indicated for treatment of steroid-responsive inflammatory ocular conditions of the palpebral and bulbar conjunctiva, cornea, and anterior segment of the globe, including allergic conjunctivitis, acne rosacea, superficial punctate keratitis, herpes zoster keratitis, iritis, cyclitis, and selected infective conjunctivitides when the benefits in terms of diminished edema and inflammation outweigh the risk of corticosteroid use.

## Pharmacology/Pharmacokinetics

**Physicochemical characteristics**
Source—Synthetic. Structurally similar to other corticosteroids, except for the absence of the number 20 position ketone group.
Molecular weight—466.96.
pH—Ophthalmic suspension: 5.3 to 5.6.
Tonicity—250 to 310 milliosmoles per kg of body weight (mOsmol/kg).

**Mechanism of action/Effect**
Corticosteroids suppress the inflammatory response to a variety of inciting agents and probably delay or slow healing. They inhibit edema, fibrin deposition, capillary dilation, leukocyte migration, capillary proliferation, fibroblast proliferation, deposition of collagen, and scar formation, all of which are associated with inflammation. While the exact mechanism of action of ocular corticosteroids is not known, they are thought to act by induction of phospholipase $A_2$ inhibitory proteins, collectively called lipocortins, which are postulated to control the biosynthesis of potent mediators of inflammation, such as prostaglandins and leukotrienes by inhibiting the release of their common precursor, arachidonic acid.

**Other actions/effects**
Corticosteroids may increase intraocular pressure.

## Absorption

A bioavailability study with administration of one drop of 0.5% loteprednol in each eye eight times a day for 2 days or four times a day for 42 days found that plasma concentrations of loteprednol etabonate and its primary inactive metabolite were below the limit of quantitation at all sampling times, which suggests limited (less than 1 nanogram per mL) systemic absorption.

## Biotransformation

Extensive, to inactive carboxylic acid metabolites.

# Precautions to Consider

### Cross-sensitivity and/or related problems
Patients sensitive to other corticosteroids may be sensitive to loteprednol.

### Carcinogenicity
Long-term animal studies have not been done.

### Mutagenicity
Loteprednol was not found to be mutagenic *in vitro* in the Ames test, the mouse lymphoma tk assay, or in a chromosome aberration test in human lymphocytes, or *in vivo* in the single dose mouse micronucleus assay.

### Pregnancy/Reproduction
Fertility—Studies in male and female rats administered loteprednol etabonate (route of administration not specified) prior to and during mating in doses of up to 50 and 25 mg per kg of body weight (mg/kg) per day, respectively (1500 and 750 times, respectively, the maximum daily dose of the 0.2% ophthalmic suspension or 600 and 300 times, respectively, the maximum daily dose of the 0.5% ophthalmic suspension), found no impairment of fertility.

Pregnancy—Studies in rabbits administered loteprednol etabonate in oral doses of 3 mg/kg per day (85 and 35 times the maximum daily clinical dose of the 0.2% and 0.5% ophthalmic suspension, respectively) during the period of organogenesis found loteprednol to be embryotoxic (delayed ossification) and teratogenic (increased incidence of meningocele, abnormal left common carotid artery, and limb flexures). The no-observed-effect level (NOEL) for these effects was 0.5 mg/kg per day (15 and 6 times the maximum daily clinical dose of the 0.2% and 0.5% ophthalmic suspension, respectively). Oral administration of loteprednol etabonate to rats during the period of organogenesis also produced teratogenicity (absent innominate artery at doses of ≥ 5 mg/kg per day and cleft palate and umbilical hernia at doses of ≥ 50 mg/kg per day) and embryotoxicity (increased post-implantation losses at 100 mg/kg per day and decreased fetal body weight and skeletal ossification at doses of ≥ 50 mg/kg per day). Treatment of rats with loteprednol etabonate (route of administration not specified) at doses of 0.5 mg/kg per day (15 and 6 times the maximum clinical dose of the 0.2% and 0.5% ophthalmic suspension, respectively) during organogenesis did not result in any reproductive toxicity. Maternal toxicity (significantly reduced body weight gain during treatment) occurred in rats at doses of ≥ 5 mg/kg per day (route of administration not specified) during the period of organogenesis. Oral administration of 50 mg/kg per day (a maternally toxic dose) to rats from the start of the fetal period through the end of lactation produced decreased growth and survival and retarded development in the offspring during lactation; the NOEL for these effects was 5 mg/kg per day. No effect on the duration of parturition or gestation was observed in rats with oral doses of up to 50 mg/kg per day during the fetal period.

FDA Pregnancy Category C.

### Breast-feeding
It is not known whether ophthalmic corticosteroids could result in sufficient systemic absorption to produce detectable quantities in human breast milk. Caution should be exercised when ophthalmic corticosteroids are administered to women who breast-feed.

### Pediatrics
Safety and efficacy have not been established.

### Geriatrics
No information is available on the relationship of age to the effects of loteprednol in geriatric patients.

### Medical considerations/Contraindications
The medical considerations/contraindications included have been selected on the basis of their potential clinical significance (reasons given in parentheses where appropriate)—not necessarily inclusive (» = major clinical significance).

*Except under special circumstances, this medication should not be used when the following medical problems exist:*

- » Fungal diseases, ocular, or
- » Herpes simplex keratitis, epithelial (dendritic keratitis) or
- » Infections of the eye, other, including acute, purulent infections or
- » Mycobacterial infection, ocular or
- » Viral diseases, such as vaccinia, varicella, and other viral diseases of the cornea and conjunctiva
  (corticosteroids decrease resistance to bacterial, fungal, and viral infections; application may mask or exacerbate existing infections and encourage the development of new or secondary infections)

*Risk-benefit should be considered when the following medical problems exist:*

Cataract surgery
(use of corticosteroids after cataract surgery may delay healing and increase the incidence of bleb formation)

» Diseases causing thinning of the cornea or sclera
(use may result in perforation)

Glaucoma
(prolonged use of corticosteroids may result in glaucoma, with damage to the optic nerve and defects in visual acuity and visual fields; corticosteroids should be used with caution in the presence of glaucoma)

Sensitivity to loteprednol or other corticosteroids

### Patient monitoring
The following may be especially important in patient monitoring (other tests may be warranted in some patients, depending on condition; » = major clinical significance):

Intraocular pressure determinations
(recommended if loteprednol is administered for 10 days or longer)

Ophthalmologic examinations, including slit-lamp biomicroscopy and, if appropriate, fluorescein staining
(recommended before continuing therapy beyond 14 days)

# Side/Adverse Effects

Note: Prolonged use of corticosteroids may result in glaucoma, damage to the optic nerve, defects in visual acuity and visual fields, and posterior subcapsular cataract formation.

Prolonged use of corticosteroids may also result in secondary ocular infections, including herpes simplex, due to suppression of host response, and perforation of the globe where there is thinning of the cornea or sclera.

Fungal infections of the cornea are prone to develop during long-term corticosteroid treatment. Fungal invasion should be considered in any persistent corneal ulceration where a corticosteroid is, or was, in use. Fungal cultures are recommended when appropriate.

Some side/adverse effects reported with ophthalmic loteprednol may resemble the disease being treated.

The following side/adverse effects have been selected on the basis of their potential clinical significance (possible signs and symptoms in parentheses where appropriate)—not necessarily inclusive:

### Those indicating need for medical attention
Incidence more frequent—5 to 15%
*Blurred vision or other change in vision; chemosis* (swelling of the membrane covering the white part of the eye); *injection* (redness or swelling of the eye)

Incidence less frequent—< 5%
*Conjunctivitis or keratoconjunctivitis* (redness of eye, eyelid, or inner lining of eyelid); *corneal abnormalities; eyelid erythema* (redness of eyelid); *eye discomfort, irritation, or pain; increased intraocular pressure; ocular discharge* (discharge from the eye); *papillae* (tiny bumps on the inner lining of eyelid); *uveitis* (eye pain, tearing, sensitivity of eye to light, redness of eye, or blurred vision or other change in vision)

### Those indicating need for medical attention only if they continue or are bothersome
Incidence more frequent—5 to 15%
*Burning when medicine is applied; dry eye; epiphora* (watery eye); *foreign body sensation* (feeling of something in the eye); *headache; itching; pharyngitis* (sore throat); *photophobia* (increased sensitivity of eyes to light); *rhinitis* (runny nose)

# Patient Consultation

As an aid to patient consultation, refer to *Advice for the Patient, Loteprednol (Ophthalmic)—Introductory Version.*

In providing consultation, consider emphasizing the following selected information (» = major clinical significance):

### Before using this medication
» Conditions affecting use, especially:
Sensitivity to loteprednol or other corticosteroids
Pregnancy—Teratogenic and embryotoxic in animals

Other medical problems, especially diseases causing thinning of the cornea or sclera; fungal diseases, ocular; herpes simplex keratitis, epithelial (dendritic keratitis); infections of the eye, other, including acute, purulent infections or mycobacterial infection, ocular; or viral diseases, such as vaccinia, varicella, and other viral diseases of the cornea and conjunctiva

**Proper use of this medication**
Shaking suspension well before instilling
» If using the 0.5% strength, not wearing soft contact lenses while using medication
» If using the 0.2% strength, not wearing soft contact lenses if eyes are red; if eyes are not red, removing soft contact lenses before administration and waiting 10 minutes afterward before reinserting lenses
» Proper administration technique; preventing contamination; not touching applicator tip to any surface
» Proper dosing
Missed dose: Using as soon as remembered; not using if almost time for next dose; not doubling doses
» Proper storage

**Precautions while using this medication**
Need for ophthalmologic examinations during long-term therapy
» Checking with physician if symptoms do not improve or if condition becomes worse

**Side/adverse effects**
Signs of potential side effects, especially blurred vision or other change in vision; chemosis; injection; conjunctivitis or keratoconjunctivitis; corneal abnormalities; eyelid erythema; eye discomfort, irritation, or pain; increased intraocular pressure; ocular discharge; papillae; or uveitis

## General Dosing Information

If signs and symptoms fail to improve after 2 days of therapy, the patient should be re-evaluated.

For the 0.2% ophthalmic solution—Patients should not wear contact lenses if their eyes are red. Patients whose eyes are not red should remove soft contact lenses while administering loteprednol and wait at least 10 minutes afterward before reinserting the lenses.

For the 0.5% ophthalmic solution—Patients should not wear soft contact lenses while being treated with loteprednol.

## Ophthalmic Dosage Forms

### LOTEPREDNOL OPHTHALMIC SUSPENSION
**Usual adult dose**
Seasonal allergic conjunctivitis—
Topical, to the conjunctiva, 1 drop of the 0.2% ophthalmic suspension in the affected eye(s) four times a day.
Ocular disorders, inflammatory—
Topical, to the conjunctiva, 1 or 2 drops of the 0.5% ophthalmic suspension in the affected eye(s) four times a day.
Note: During the first week of treatment, the dose may be increased, if necessary, up to 1 drop every hour. Therapy should not be discontinued prematurely.
Postoperative inflammation—
Topical, to the conjunctiva, 1 or 2 drops of the 0.5% ophthalmic suspension in the affected eye(s) four times a day beginning twenty-four hours after surgery and continuing throughout the first two weeks of the postoperative period.

**Usual pediatric dose**
Seasonal allergic conjunctivitis or
Ocular disorders, inflammatory or
Postoperative inflammation—
Safety and efficacy have not been established.

**Strength(s) usually available**
U.S.—
0.2% (Rx) [*Alrex* (benzalkonium chloride 0.01%; edetate disodium; glycerin; povidone; tyloxapol; hydrochloric acid and/or sodium hydroxide)].
0.5% (Rx) [*Lotemax* (benzalkonium chloride 0.01%; edetate disodium; glycerin; povidone; tyloxapol; hydrochloric acid and/or sodium hydroxide)].

**Packaging and storage**
Store container upright between 15 and 25 °C (59 and 77 °F). Keep from freezing.

**Auxiliary labeling**
• For the eye.
• Shake well.

Developed: 08/14/98

---

**LOVASTATIN**—See *HMG-CoA Reductase Inhibitors (Systemic)*

---

# LOXAPINE  Systemic

VA CLASSIFICATION (Primary/Secondary): CN709/CN900
Commonly used brand name(s): *Loxapac; Loxitane; Loxitane C; Loxitane IM.*
Note: For a listing of dosage forms and brand names by country availability, see *Dosage Forms* section(s).

## Category

Antipsychotic; antianxiety agent–antidepressant.

## Indications

Note: Bracketed information in the *Indications* section refers to uses that are not included in U.S. product labeling.

**Accepted**
Psychotic disorders (treatment)—Loxapine is indicated for the management of symptoms and characteristics of psychotic conditions.
[Anxiety associated with mental depression (treatment)][1]—Loxapine has been used to treat anxiety neurosis with depression.

[1]Not included in Canadian product labeling.

## Pharmacology/Pharmacokinetics

Note: The pharmacological effects of loxapine are similar to those of phenothiazines.

**Physicochemical characteristics**
Chemical group—A tricyclic dibenzoxazepine derivative.
Molecular weight—
Loxapine: 327.81.
Loxapine succinate: 445.90.
pKa—6.6.

**Mechanism of action/Effect**
Although the exact mechanism of action has not been completely established, loxapine is thought to improve psychotic conditions by blocking dopamine at postsynaptic receptor sites in the brain.

**Other actions/effects**
Antiemetic—Inhibits the medullary chemoreceptor trigger zone.
Sedative—May cause indirect reduction of stimuli to the brain reticular activating system.

**Biotransformation**
Hepatic. Major active metabolites are 8-hydroxyloxapine, 7-hydroxyloxapine, and 8-hydroxyamoxapine.

**Half-life**
Oral—3 to 4 hours.
Intramuscular—12 hours.

**Onset of action**
30 minutes.

**Time to peak effect**
1½ to 3 hours.

**Duration of action**
Up to 12 hours.

**Elimination**
Biliary, as unconjugated metabolites. Renal, as conjugated metabolites.

# Loxapine (Systemic)

## Precautions to Consider

### Cross-sensitivity and/or related problems
Patients sensitive to amoxapine (a dibenzoxazepine derivative) may be sensitive to loxapine also.

### Carcinogenicity/Tumorigenicity
Most neuroleptic medications have been found to cause increased serum prolactin concentrations. Although the clinical significance of this increase is not known for most patients, *in vitro* studies have shown approximately ⅓ of human breast cancers to be prolactin dependent. Additionally, an increase in mammary neoplasms has been found in rodents after chronic administration of neuroleptics. However, a definite association between the chronic administration of these medications and mammary tumorigenesis is considered inconclusive because of limited evidence available.

### Pregnancy/Reproduction
Pregnancy—Problems in humans have not been documented.
Fetotoxic effects, such as increased fetal resorptions and decreased fetal weight, were seen in rats and mice given doses within the range of the human therapeutic dose.
FDA Pregnancy Category C.

### Breast-feeding
It is not known whether loxapine is excreted in breast milk. However, loxapine and its metabolites have been found in the milk of lactating dogs.

### Pediatrics
Appropriate studies on the relationship of age to the effects of loxapine have not been performed in the pediatric population. Safety and efficacy have not been established.

### Geriatrics
Geriatric patients tend to develop higher plasma concentrations of loxapine because of changes in distribution due to decreases in lean body mass, total body water, and albumin, and often an increase in total body fat composition. These patients usually require lower initial dosage and a more gradual titration of dose.

Elderly patients also appear to be more prone to orthostatic hypotension and exhibit an increased sensitivity to the anticholinergic and sedative effects of loxapine. In addition, they are more prone to develop extrapyramidal side effects, such as tardive dyskinesia and parkinsonism. The signs of tardive dyskinesia are persistent, difficult to control, and, in some patients, appear to be irreversible. There is no known effective treatment. The symptoms may be masked during long treatment but may appear if loxapine is discontinued. Careful observation during treatment for early signs of tardive dyskinesia and reduction of dosage or discontinuation of medication may prevent a more severe manifestation of the syndrome.

### Dental
The peripheral anticholinergic effects of loxapine may decrease or inhibit salivary flow, especially in middle-aged or elderly patients, thus contributing to the development of caries, periodontal disease, oral candidiasis, and discomfort.

Extrapyramidal reactions induced by loxapine will result in increased motor activity of the head, face, and neck. Occlusal adjustments, bite registrations, and treatment for bruxism may be made less reliable.

The leukopenic and thrombocytopenic effects of loxapine may result in an increased incidence of microbial infection, delayed healing, and gingival bleeding. Although the occurrence is rare with loxapine, if leukopenia or thrombocytopenia occurs, dental work should be deferred until blood counts have returned to normal. Patients should be instructed in proper oral hygiene, including caution in use of regular toothbrushes, dental floss, and toothpicks.

### Drug interactions and/or related problems
The following drug interactions and/or related problems have been selected on the basis of their potential clinical significance (possible mechanism in parentheses where appropriate)—not necessarily inclusive (» = major clinical significance):

Note: Combinations containing any of the following medications, depending on the amount present, may also interact with this medication.

Although not all of the following interactions have been documented specifically for loxapine, a potential exists for their occurrence because of loxapine's close pharmacological similarity to phenothiazine medications.

» Alcohol or
» Central nervous system (CNS) depression–producing medications, other, especially anesthetics, barbiturates, and opioid (narcotic) analgesics (See *Appendix II*)
(concurrent use may potentiate and prolong the CNS depressant effects of either these medications or loxapine; dosage adjustments to approximately ½ to ¼ of the usual dose may be necessary)

Amphetamines
(concurrent use may decrease the effects of amphetamines since loxapine produces alpha-adrenergic blockade)

Antacids or
Antidiarrheals, adsorbent
(concurrent use may inhibit the absorption of orally administered loxapine)

Anticholinergics or other medications with anticholinergic activity (See *Appendix II*) or
Antidyskinetic agents
(concurrent use with loxapine may intensify anticholinergic effects of both medications; patients should be advised to report gastrointestinal problems since paralytic ileus may occur; antidyskinetic agents should not be used for prophylaxis of pseudoparkinsonism during therapy with loxapine)

Anticonvulsants
(loxapine may lower the seizure threshold; dosage adjustment of anticonvulsant medications may be necessary; potentiation of anticonvulsant effects does not occur)

Antidepressants, tricyclic or
Monoamine oxidase (MAO) inhibitors, including furazolidone, procarbazine, and more than 10 mg of selegiline a day
(concurrent use may prolong and intensify the sedative and anticholinergic effects of either these medications or loxapine; serum concentrations of the antidepressant may be increased when it is administered concomitantly with loxapine; dosage reduction of antidepressant may be necessary)

Bromocriptine
(concurrent use with loxapine may antagonize effects of bromocriptine on serum prolactin activity; dosage adjustment of bromocriptine may be necessary)

Carbamazepine
(in addition to enhancement of CNS depressant effects and lowering of seizure threshold, the concurrent use of carbamazepine with loxapine, and possibly other neuroleptics, may decrease plasma concentrations of the neuroleptic; patient should be observed for clinical signs of ineffectiveness of loxapine and dosage adjusted accordingly)

Dopamine
(when dopamine is used concurrently with loxapine, alpha-adrenergic blocking action of loxapine may antagonize peripheral vasoconstriction produced by high doses of dopamine)

Ephedrine
(when used concurrently with loxapine, alpha-adrenergic blocking action of loxapine may decrease the pressor response to ephedrine)

Epinephrine
(alpha-adrenergic effects of epinephrine may be blocked when epinephrine is used concurrently with loxapine, possibly resulting in severe hypotension and tachycardia)

» Extrapyramidal reaction–causing medications, other (See *Appendix II*)
(concurrent use with loxapine may increase the severity and frequency of extrapyramidal effects)

» Guanadrel or
» Guanethidine
(concurrent use with loxapine may decrease the hypotensive effects of these agents because of their displacement from and inhibition of uptake by adrenergic neurons)

Levodopa
(concurrent use may inhibit the antiparkinsonian effects of levodopa by blocking dopamine receptors in the brain)

Metaraminol
(concurrent use usually decreases, but does not reverse or completely block, the pressor effect of metaraminol)

Methoxamine
(prior administration of alpha-adrenergic blocking agents such as loxapine may block the pressor effect and decrease the duration of action of methoxamine)

Ototoxic medications, especially ototoxic antibiotics
(concurrent use with loxapine may mask the symptoms of ototoxicity such as tinnitus, dizziness, or vertigo)

Phenylephrine or
Norepinephrine
(prior administration of loxapine may decrease the pressor response to phenylephrine or norepinephrine because of the alpha-adrenergic

blocking action of loxapine, but severe hypotension associated with overdosage of loxapine would be expected to respond to either agent)

**Medical considerations/Contraindications**
The medical considerations/contraindications included have been selected on the basis of their potential clinical significance (reasons given in parentheses where appropriate)—not necessarily inclusive (» = major clinical significance).

*Except under special circumstances, this medication should not be used when the following medical problems exist:*
» CNS depression, drug-induced, severe or
» Comatose states
　(may be exacerbated)

*Risk-benefit should be considered when the following medical problems exist:*
» Alcoholism, active
　(CNS depression may be potentiated)
　Cardiovascular disease
　(increased risk of arrhythmias and hypotension)
　Glaucoma, or predisposition to or
　Parkinson's disease or
　Urinary retention
　(may be exacerbated)
» Hepatic function impairment
　(metabolism may be altered)
　Prostatic hypertrophy, symptomatic
　(risk of urinary retention)
　Seizure disorders
　(seizure threshold may be lowered)
　Sensitivity to amoxapine or loxapine

**Patient monitoring**
The following may be especially important in patient monitoring (other tests may be warranted in some patients, depending on condition; » = major clinical significance):

　Blood cell counts
　(may be required at periodic intervals during high-dose or prolonged therapy)
　Careful observation for early symptoms of tardive dyskinesia
　(recommended at periodic intervals, especially in the elderly and patients on high or extended maintenance dosage; loxapine should be discontinued if early symptoms of tardive dyskinesia appear, since there is no known effective treatment)
　Hepatic function determinations and
　Urine tests for bilirubin and bile
　(may be required if jaundice or grippe-like symptoms occur)
　Ophthalmologic examination
　(may be advisable at periodic intervals during high-dose or prolonged therapy since deposition of particulate matter in the lens and cornea has occurred with some other antipsychotic medications)

## Side/Adverse Effects

The following side/adverse effects have been selected on the basis of their potential clinical significance (possible signs and symptoms in parentheses where appropriate)—not necessarily inclusive:

**Those indicating need for medical attention**
Incidence more frequent
　*Akathisia* (restlessness or need to keep moving); *extrapyramidal effects, parkinsonian* (difficulty in speaking or swallowing; loss of balance control; mask-like face; shuffling walk; slowed movements; stiffness of arms and legs; trembling and shaking of fingers and hands); *tardive dyskinesia, persistent* (lip smacking or puckering; puffing of cheeks; rapid or worm-like movements of tongue; uncontrolled movements of the arms and legs; uncontrolled chewing movements)

　Note: *Parkinsonian extrapyramidal effects* are more common during first few days of treatment or following dosage increases.
　　*Tardive dyskinesia* is initially dose related, but may increase with long-term treatment and total cumulative dose; may persist after discontinuation of loxapine.

Incidence less frequent
　*Allergic reaction* (skin rash); *anticholinergic effect* (difficult urination); *constipation, severe*—may lead to paralytic ileus; *extrapyramidal effects, dystonic* (difficulty in swallowing; inability to move eyes; muscle spasms, especially of the neck and back; twisting movements of body)—may be severe

Incidence rare
　*Agranulocytosis* (sore throat and fever; unusual bleeding or bruising); *jaundice, obstructive* (yellow eyes or skin); *neuroleptic malignant syndrome [NMS]* (convulsions; difficult or unusually fast breathing; fast heartbeat or irregular pulse; high fever; high or low [irregular] blood pressure; increased sweating; loss of bladder control; severe muscle stiffness or rigidity; unusual tiredness or weakness; unusually pale skin); *tardive dystonia* (increased blinking or spasms of eyelid; unusual facial expressions or body positions; uncontrolled twisting movements of neck, trunk, arms, or legs)

　Note: *NMS* may occur at any time during neuroleptic therapy, but is more commonly seen soon after start of therapy, or after patient has switched from one neuroleptic to another, during combined therapy with another psychotropic medication, or after a dosage increase. Along with the overt signs of skeletal muscle rigidity, hyperthermia, autonomic dysfunction, and altered consciousness, differential diagnosis may reveal leukocytosis (9500 to 26,000 cells per cubic millimeter), elevated liver function tests, and elevated creatine phosphokinase (CPK).

**Those indicating need for medical attention only if they continue or are bothersome**
Incidence more frequent
　*Blurred vision; confusion; drowsiness; dryness of mouth; hypotension, orthostatic* (dizziness, lightheadedness, or fainting)
Incidence less frequent
　*Constipation, mild; decreased sexual ability; enlargement of breasts, in males and females; headache; increased sensitivity of skin to sun; missing menstrual periods; nausea or vomiting; trouble in sleeping; unusual secretion of milk; weight gain*

**Those indicating the need for medical attention if they occur after the medication is discontinued**
　*Dizziness; dyskinesia, withdrawal emergent* (uncontrolled, repetitive movements of mouth, tongue, and jaw); *nausea and vomiting; stomach upset or pain; trembling of fingers and hands*

## Overdose

For specific information on the agents used in the management of loxapine overdose, see:
• *Norepinephrine* and *Phenylephrine* in *Sympathomimetic Agents—Cardiovascular Use (Parenteral-Systemic)* monograph.

For more information on the management of overdose or unintentional ingestion, **contact a Poison Control Center** (see *Poison Control Center Listing*).

**Clinical effects of overdose**
The following effects have been selected on the basis of their potential clinical significance (possible signs and symptoms in parentheses where appropriate)—not necessarily inclusive:

　*Dizziness; drowsiness, severe, or comatose state; muscle trembling, jerking, stiffness, or uncontrolled movements, severe; troubled breathing, severe; unusual tiredness or weakness, severe*

**Treatment of overdose**
No specific antidote for loxapine is available. Treatment is symptomatic and supportive.
Specific treatment—
　In event of severe hypotension, epinephrine should not be used, since it may further lower blood pressure in presence of partial adrenergic blockade. Norepinephrine or phenylephrine may be effective.
Supportive care—
　Oxygen, intravenous fluids, anticonvulsant therapy, and anticholinergic agents may be indicated.
　Patients in whom intentional overdose is known or suspected should be referred for psychiatric consultation.
Note: Because of the antiemetic effect of loxapine, centrally acting emetics, such as syrup of ipecac, may have little effect.

## Patient Consultation

As an aid to patient consultation, refer to *Advice for the Patient, Loxapine (Systemic)*.
In providing consultation, consider emphasizing the following selected information (» = major clinical significance):

**Before using this medication**
» Conditions affecting use, especially:
　Sensitivity to loxapine or amoxapine
　Pregnancy—Studies in rats showed an increased number of fetal resorptions and decreased fetal weight

Use in the elderly—Elderly patients are more likely to develop extrapyramidal, anticholinergic, hypotensive, and sedative effects; reduced dosage recommended

Dental—Loxapine-induced blood dyscrasias may result in infections, delayed healing, and bleeding; dry mouth may cause caries and candidiasis; increased motor activity of face, head, and neck may interfere with some dental procedures

Other medications, especially alcohol, other CNS depression–producing medications, other extrapyramidal reaction–producing medications, guanadrel, or guanethidine

Other medical problems, especially severe CNS depression, active alcoholism, or hepatic function impairment

**Proper use of this medication**

Taking with food, milk, or water to reduce stomach irritation

Measuring oral solution only with dropper provided by manufacturer

Mixing oral solution with orange or grapefruit juice just before each dose

» Compliance with therapy; not taking more or less medicine, nor taking more often, than directed

» Proper dosing

Missed dose: Taking as soon as possible; not taking if within 1 hour of next dose; returning to regular dosing schedule; not doubling doses

» Proper storage

**Precautions while using this medication**

Regular visits to physician to check progress of therapy

» Checking with physician before discontinuing medication; gradual dosage reduction may be needed

» Avoiding use of alcoholic beverages or other CNS depressants during therapy

Avoiding use of antacids or antidiarrheal medication within 2 hours of taking loxapine

» Possible drowsiness; caution when driving, using machines, or doing other things requiring alertness while taking loxapine

Possible dizziness or lightheadedness; caution when getting up suddenly from a lying or sitting position

Possible skin photosensitivity; avoiding unprotected exposure to sun; using protective clothing; using a sun block product that includes protection against both UVA-caused photosensitivity reactions and UVB-caused sunburn reactions; avoiding use of sunlamp, tanning bed, or tanning booth

Possible dryness of the mouth: using sugarless gum or candy, ice, or saliva substitute for relief; checking with physician or dentist if dry mouth continues for more than 2 weeks

» Caution if any kind of surgery, dental treatment, or emergency treatment is required

**Side/adverse effects**

Side effects are more likely to occur in the elderly

Signs of potential side effects, especially tardive dyskinesia, akathisia, dystonias, parkinsonian effects, anticholinergic effects, allergic skin reactions, agranulocytosis, obstructive jaundice, neuroleptic malignant syndrome (NMS), constipation (severe)

» Stopping medication and notifying physician immediately if symptoms of NMS appear, especially muscle rigidity, fever, difficult or fast breathing, seizures, fast heartbeat, increased sweating, loss of bladder control, unusually pale skin, unusual tiredness or weakness

» Notifying physician immediately if early symptoms of tardive dyskinesia appear, such as fine worm-like movements of the tongue or other uncontrolled movements of the mouth, tongue, jaw, or arms and legs; dosage adjustment or discontinuation may be needed to prevent irreversibility

Possibility of withdrawal symptoms

## General Dosing Information

Dosage must be individualized by titration from the lower dose range over the first 7 to 10 days of therapy until effective control of psychotic symptoms is obtained. After such control is established, the dosage is gradually decreased to the lowest level that will maintain an adequate clinical response.

Loxapine has an antiemetic effect that may mask signs of overdose of other medication or may obscure diagnosis of conditions whose main symptoms include nausea. However, since the antiemetic effect of loxapine is central, nausea is not affected when it results from vestibular stimulation or local gastrointestinal irritation.

Upon cessation of extended maintenance therapy, a gradual reduction in loxapine dosage is recommended since abrupt withdrawal may cause some patients to experience transient dyskinetic signs, nausea, vomiting, gastritis, trembling, and dizziness.

**For oral dosage forms only**

The oral solution should be measured only with the dropper provided by the manufacturer and diluted with orange or grapefruit juice just before each dose.

**For parenteral dosage form only**

Because hypotension is a possible side effect of loxapine, intramuscular administration is used for bedfast patients or for appropriate acute ambulatory patients who can be closely monitored. Patients should remain lying down for at least ½ hour after the injection to avoid possible acute orthostatic hypotensive effects.

**Diet/Nutrition**

This medication may be taken with food or a full glass (240 mL) of water or milk if necessary to lessen stomach irritation.

**For treatment of adverse effects**

Neuroleptic malignant syndrome—

Treatment is essentially symptomatic and supportive and includes the following
  • *Discontinuing loxapine immediately.*
  • Hyperthermia—Administering antipyretics (aspirin or acetaminophen); using cooling blanket.
  • Dehydration—Restoring fluids and electrolytes.
  • Cardiovascular instability—Monitoring blood pressure and cardiac rhythm closely.
  • Hypoxia—Administering oxygen; consider airway insertion and assisted ventilation.
  • Muscle rigidity—Dantrolene sodium may be administered (100 to 300 mg a day in divided doses; 1.25 to 1.5 mg per kg of body weight intravenously). Bromocriptine (5 to 7.5 mg every eight hours) has been used to reverse hyperpyrexia and muscle rigidity.

Parkinsonism—

Many authorities advise that the only appropriate treatment of extrapyramidal symptoms is reduction of the antipsychotic dosage, if possible. Oral antidyskinetic agents such as trihexyphenidyl, 2 mg three times a day, or benztropine, may be effective in treating more severe parkinsonism and acute motor restlessness but should be used sparingly, only when side effects appear, and then usually for no longer than 3 months. Milder effects may be treated by adjusting dosage. In the elderly patient, the use of amantadine, 100 to 200 mg at bedtime, minimizes severe anticholinergic effects that may occur with other antidyskinetics.

Akathisia—

May respond to antiparkinsonian drugs or propranolol (30 to 80 mg a day); nadolol (40 mg a day); pindolol (5 to 60 mg a day), lorazepam (1 or 2 mg two or three times a day), or diazepam (2 mg two or three times a day), but often requires dosage reduction of loxapine.

Dystonia—

Acute dystonic postures or oculogyric crisis may be relieved by parenteral administration of benztropine (2 mg intramuscularly); diphenhydramine (50 mg intramuscularly); or diazepam (5 to 7.5 mg intravenously), to be followed by oral antidyskinetic medication for one or two days to prevent recurrent dystonic episodes. Dosage adjustments of loxapine may control these effects, and discontinuation of loxapine may reverse severe symptoms.

Tardive dyskinesia or tardive dystonia—

No known effective treatment. Dosage of loxapine should be lowered or medication discontinued, if clinically feasible, at earliest signs of tardive dyskinesia or tardive dystonia, to prevent irreversible effects.

## Oral Dosage Forms

Note: The dosing and strengths of the dosage forms available are expressed in terms of loxapine base.

### LOXAPINE HYDROCHLORIDE ORAL SOLUTION

**Usual adult dose**

Antipsychotic—

Initial: Oral, 10 mg (base) two times a day, the dosage being increased gradually during the first seven to ten days as needed for symptomatic control and as tolerated.

Maintenance: Oral, 15 to 25 mg (base) two to four times a day.

Note: This dosage form is intended primarily for institutional use.

Dose to be measured only with calibrated dropper provided by manufacturer.

Severely disturbed patients—Initial: Oral, 10 to 25 mg (base) two times a day.

**Usual adult prescribing limits**

Up to 250 mg (base) a day.

**Usual pediatric dose**
Children up to 16 years of age—Safety and efficacy have not been established.

**Usual geriatric dose**
Initial, oral, 3 to 5 mg (base) two times a day.

**Strength(s) usually available**
U.S.—
- 25 mg (base) per mL (Rx) [*Loxitane C* (propylene glycol)].

Canada—
- 25 mg (base) per mL (Rx) [*Loxapac*].

**Packaging and storage**
Store below 40 °C (104 °F), preferably between 15 and 30 °C (59 and 86 °F), in a well-closed container, unless otherwise specified by manufacturer. Protect from freezing.

**Auxiliary labeling**
- Take by mouth.
- May cause drowsiness.
- Avoid alcoholic beverages.
- Must be diluted before use.

**Note**
When dispensing, include the manufacturer-provided graduated dropper for dose measuring.
Explain administration technique and the necessary dilution in orange or grapefruit juice.

### LOXAPINE SUCCINATE CAPSULES
**Usual adult dose**
See *Loxapine Hydrochloride Oral Solution*.

**Usual pediatric dose**
See *Loxapine Hydrochloride Oral Solution*.

**Strength(s) usually available**
U.S.—
- 5 mg (base) (Rx) [*Loxitane;* GENERIC].
- 10 mg (base) (Rx) [*Loxitane;* GENERIC].
- 25 mg (base) (Rx) [*Loxitane;* GENERIC].
- 50 mg (base) (Rx) [*Loxitane;* GENERIC].

Canada—
Not commercially available.

**Packaging and storage**
Store below 40 °C (104 °F), preferably between 15 and 30 °C (59 and 86 °F), in a well-closed container, unless otherwise specified by manufacturer.

**Auxiliary labeling**
- May cause drowsiness.
- Avoid alcoholic beverages.

### LOXAPINE SUCCINATE TABLETS
**Usual adult dose**
See *Loxapine Hydrochloride Oral Solution*.

**Usual pediatric dose**
See *Loxapine Hydrochloride Oral Solution*.

**Strength(s) usually available**
U.S.—
Not commercially available.

Canada—
- 5 mg (base) (Rx) [*Loxapac*].
- 10 mg (base) (Rx) [*Loxapac*].
- 25 mg (base) (Rx) [*Loxapac*].
- 50 mg (base) (Rx) [*Loxapac*].

**Packaging and storage**
Store below 40 °C (104 °F), preferably between 15 and 30 °C (59 and 86 °F), in a well-closed container, unless otherwise specified by manufacturer.

**Auxiliary labeling**
- May cause drowsiness.
- Avoid alcoholic beverages.

## Parenteral Dosage Forms

Note: The dosing and strengths of the dosage forms available are expressed in terms of loxapine base.

### LOXAPINE HYDROCHLORIDE INJECTION
**Usual adult dose**
Intramuscular, 12.5 to 50 mg (base) every four to six hours as needed and tolerated.

Note: For intramuscular administration only. Not for intravenous use.

**Usual adult prescribing limits**
Up to 250 mg (base) a day.

**Usual pediatric dose**
Children up to 16 years of age—Safety and efficacy have not been established.

**Strength(s) usually available**
U.S.—
- 50 mg (base) per mL (Rx) [*Loxitane IM* (polysorbate 80 [5% w/v]; propylene glycol [70% v/v])].

Canada—
- 50 mg (base) per mL (Rx) [*Loxapac*].

**Packaging and storage**
Store below 40 °C (104 °F), preferably between 15 and 30 °C (59 and 86 °F), unless otherwise specified by manufacturer. Protect from light. Protect from freezing.

**Stability**
A darkening of the solution to a light amber will not alter potency or effectiveness. Do not use if markedly discolored or if a precipitate is present.

**Note**
Advise patient to remain lying down for ½ hour following administration to avoid severe orthostatic hypotension.

Revised: 01/29/93

---

# LYPRESSIN   Systemic

VA CLASSIFICATION (Primary/Secondary): HS702/CV900

Commonly used brand name(s): *Diapid*.

Note: For a listing of dosage forms and brand names by country availability, see *Dosage Forms* section(s).

## Category
Antidiuretic (central diabetes insipidus).

## Indications
**Accepted**
Diabetes insipidus, central (treatment)—Lypressin is indicated for the prevention or control of polydipsia, polyuria, and dehydration associated with central diabetes insipidus caused by insufficient antidiuretic hormone.
Lypressin may be useful in patients who are unresponsive to other forms of therapy or who have shown various adverse reactions to other preparations of antidiuretic hormone of animal origin.
Lypressin is ineffective in the treatment of polyuria associated with nephrogenic or psychogenic diabetes insipidus, renal disease, hypokalemia, hypercalcemia, or the administration of demeclocycline or lithium.

## Pharmacology/Pharmacokinetics

**Physicochemical characteristics**
Source—Lypressin is a synthetic vasopressin analog.
Molecular weight—1056.22.

**Mechanism of action/Effect**
Increases water reabsorption in the kidney by increasing the cellular permeability of the collecting ducts, resulting in an increase in urine osmolality with a concurrent decrease in urine output.

**Other actions/effects**
Little pressor activity.

**Absorption**
Rapid from nasal mucosa.

**Biotransformation**
Renal and hepatic.

**Half-life**
Approximately 15 minutes.

**Onset of action**
Within 1 hour.

**Time to peak effect**
30 to 120 minutes.

**Duration of action**
3 to 4 hours.

**Elimination**
Renal, a small amount unchanged.

## Precautions to Consider

**Cross-sensitivity and/or related problems**
Patients sensitive to vasopressin may also be sensitive to lypressin.

**Carcinogenicity**
Studies have not been done.

**Pregnancy/Reproduction**
Pregnancy—Studies have not been done in either animals or humans.
FDA Pregnancy Category C.

**Breast-feeding**
It is not known whether lypressin is distributed into breast milk. However, problems in humans have not been documented.

**Pediatrics**
Appropriate studies on the relationship of age to the effects of lypressin have not been performed in the pediatric population. However, pediatrics-specific problems that would limit the usefulness of this medication in children are not expected.

**Geriatrics**
No information is available on the relationship of age to the effects of lypressin in geriatric patients.

**Drug interactions and/or related problems**
The following drug interactions and/or related problems have been selected on the basis of their potential clinical significance (possible mechanism in parentheses where appropriate)—not necessarily inclusive (» = major clinical significance):

Note: Combinations containing any of the following medications, depending on the amount present, may also interact with this medication.

Carbamazepine or
Chlorpropamide or
Clofibrate
(may potentiate the antidiuretic effect of lypressin when used concurrently)

Demeclocycline or
Lithium or
Norepinephrine
(may decrease the antidiuretic effect of lypressin when used concurrently)

**Medical considerations/Contraindications**
The medical considerations/contraindications included have been selected on the basis of their potential clinical significance (reasons given in parentheses where appropriate)—not necessarily inclusive (» = major clinical significance).

*Risk-benefit should be considered when the following medical problems exist:*

Allergic rhinitis or
Nasal congestion or
Upper respiratory infection
(may interfere with absorption of lypressin through the nasal mucosa)
Hypertensive cardiovascular disease
(although pressor effects of lypressin are minimal)
Sensitivity to lypressin

## Side/Adverse Effects

The following side/adverse effects have been selected on the basis of their potential clinical significance (possible signs and symptoms in parentheses where appropriate)—not necessarily inclusive:

**Those indicating need for medical attention**
Incidence rare
*Inadvertent inhalation* (continuing cough; feeling of tightness in chest; shortness of breath; troubled breathing); *water intoxication and overdose* (coma; confusion; continuing headache; drowsiness; problems with urination; seizures; weight gain)

**Those indicating need for medical attention only if they continue or are bothersome**
Incidence less frequent or rare
*Abdominal or stomach cramps; excessive administration with drippage into pharynx* (heartburn); *headache; increased bowel movements; irritation or pain in the eye; itching, irritation, or sores inside nose; runny or stuffy nose*

## Overdose

For specific information on the agents used in the management of lypressin overdose, see *Furosemide* in *Diuretics, Loop (Systemic)* monograph.

For more information on the management of overdose or unintentional ingestion, **contact a Poison Control Center** (see *Poison Control Center Listing*).

**Treatment of overdose**
To enhance elimination—Diuresis with furosemide and hypertonic saline if there is a risk of congestive heart failure.

Supportive care—Withdrawal of lypressin and restriction of fluid intake. Correction of electrolyte imbalance. Patients in whom intentional overdose is known or suspected should be referred for psychiatric consultation.

## Patient Consultation

As an aid to patient consultation, refer to *Advice for the Patient, Lypressin (Systemic)*.

In providing consultation, consider emphasizing the following selected information (» = major clinical significance):

**Before using this medication**
» Conditions affecting use, especially:
Allergies to lypressin or vasopressin

**Proper use of this medication**
» Importance of not using more medication than the amount prescribed
Proper administration technique
» Proper dosing
Missed dose: Using as soon as possible; not using at all if almost time for next dose; not doubling doses
» Proper storage

**Side/adverse effects**
Signs of potential side effects, especially inadvertent inhalation or water intoxication

## General Dosing Information

Lypressin is administered intranasally; it should not be inhaled.

Patients with nasal congestion, allergic rhinitis, and upper respiratory infections may experience decreased efficacy because of a decrease in absorption through the nasal mucosa. Larger doses of lypressin or adjunctive therapy may be required in such patients.

Since more than 2 or 3 sprays per nostril usually results in wastage, it is recommended that the time interval between sprays be reduced rather than increasing the number of sprays if a patient requires more than 3 sprays.

## Nasal Dosage Forms

### LYPRESSIN NASAL SOLUTION USP

**Usual adult and adolescent dose**
Antidiuretic—
Intranasal, 1 or 2 sprays in each nostril four times a day.

Note: Whenever the frequency of urination increases or increased thirst develops, the patient may administer 1 or 2 sprays to control these symptoms.

If the regular daily dosage of lypressin does not control nocturia, an additional dose may be given at bedtime.

The dosage has ranged from 1 spray per day at bedtime to 10 sprays in each nostril every three to four hours.

**Usual pediatric dose**
Children up to 6 weeks of age—Safety and efficacy have not been established in children less than 6 weeks of age.
Children 6 weeks of age and over— See *Usual adult and adolescent dose*.

**Strength(s) usually available**
U.S.—
0.185 mg (equivalent to 50 USP Posterior Pituitary Units) per mL; or approximately 0.007 mg (equivalent to 2 Posterior Pituitary Units) per spray (Rx) [*Diapid* (methylparaben; propylparaben)].

**Packaging and storage**
Store below 40 °C (104 °F), preferably between 15 and 30 °C (59 and 86 °F), unless otherwise specified by manufacturer. Protect from freezing.

**Auxiliary labeling**
• For the nose.

**Note**
Instruct patient to assume a vertical position with head upright and to hold bottle upright when administering the spray.

Revised: 07/01/93

**MAFENIDE**—The *Mafenide (Topical)* monograph is not included in this published version of the USP DI database. Copies of the monograph are available on request from Micromedex, Inc. - Reprint Requests, 6200 S. Syracuse Way, Suite 300, Englewood, CO 80111; telephone (303) 486-6400; telefax (303) 486-6464; Email: USPDI@MDX.COM.

**MAGALDRATE**—See *Antacids (Oral-Local)*

**MAGNESIUM CHLORIDE**—See *Magnesium Supplements (Systemic)*

**MAGNESIUM CITRATE**—See *Laxatives (Local)*; *Magnesium Supplements (Systemic)*

**MAGNESIUM GLUCEPTATE**—See *Magnesium Supplements (Systemic)*

**MAGNESIUM GLUCONATE**—See *Magnesium Supplements (Systemic)*

**MAGNESIUM HYDROXIDE**—See *Antacids (Oral-Local)*; *Laxatives (Local)*; *Magnesium Supplements (Systemic)*

**MAGNESIUM LACTATE**—See *Magnesium Supplements (Systemic)*

**MAGNESIUM OXIDE**—See *Antacids (Oral-Local)*; *Laxatives (Local)*; *Magnesium Supplements (Systemic)*

**MAGNESIUM PIDOLATE**—See *Magnesium Supplements (Systemic)*

**MAGNESIUM SALICYLATE**—See *Salicylates (Systemic)*

**MAGNESIUM SULFATE**—See *Laxatives (Local)*; *Magnesium Sulfate (Systemic)*; *Magnesium Supplements (Systemic)*

# MAGNESIUM SULFATE Systemic

VA CLASSIFICATION (Primary/Secondary): TN406/CN400; GU900; CV300

Note: For a listing of dosage forms and brand names by country availability, see *Dosage Forms* section(s).

## Category
Anticonvulsant; electrolyte replenisher; tocolytic; antiarrhythmic.

## Indications
Note: Bracketed information in the *Indications* section refers to uses that are not included in U.S. product labeling.

**Accepted**

Seizures, in toxemia of pregnancy (prophylaxis and treatment)—Intravenous magnesium sulfate is indicated for the prevention and immediate control of life-threatening seizures in the treatment of severe toxemias (pre-eclampsia and eclampsia) of pregnancy.

Hypomagnesemia (prophylaxis and treatment)—Magnesium sulfate is indicated for replacement therapy in magnesium deficiency, especially in acute hypomagnesemia accompanied by signs of tetany similar to those of hypocalcemia.

In patients receiving total parenteral nutrition, magnesium sulfate is added to the nutrient admixture to prevent or treat magnesium deficiency.

[Premature labor (treatment)][1]—Magnesium sulfate may be used as a tocolytic agent in the management of premature labor.

[Tachycardia, ventricular, polymorphous (treatment)][1]—Magnesium sulfate is used in the treatment of torsades de pointes. It is not effective in congenital QT interval prolongation syndromes.

**Acceptance not established**

Early studies seemed to show that intravenous magnesium sulfate administered in the setting of *acute myocardial infarction* reduced the mortality rate. Pooled data from 8 randomized controlled trials showed that intravenous magnesium administered within 24 to 48 hours after onset of symptoms decreased ventricular tachycardia and fibrillation by 49% and the incidence of cardiac arrest by 58% in patients who had not been treated with thrombolytic agents. Intravenous magnesium also reduced the early mortality rate in patients with suspected myocardial infarction in the second Leicester Intravenous Magnesium Intervention Trial (LIMIT-2). Magnesium's efficacy appeared to be independent of that of thrombolytic or antiplatelet therapy. In this study, little effect was seen on arrhythmic events, but the incidence of left ventricular failure was reduced in the treatment group.

However, recent data from the large randomized controlled trial, the Fourth International Study of Infarct Survival (ISIS-4), seems to challenge these earlier studies. ISIS-4 showed that intravenous magnesium was ineffective in significantly reducing mortality, independent of thrombolytic or antiplatelet therapy, in patients with suspected acute myocardial infarction. There was no significant evidence that magnesium had any effect on 5-week mortality and follow-up at one year did not indicate any beneficial effect. In direct contrast to the results of some earlier studies, administration of intravenous magnesium was associated with small but significant increases in heart failure, cardiogenic shock, and in deaths attributed to cardiogenic shock.

Differences in study design, particularly between ISIS-4 and LIMIT-2, may explain the conflicting results. Intravenous magnesium was administered later in the course of myocardial infarction in ISIS-4, as compared to LIMIT-2. The ISIS-4 study was not designed to detect a highly time-dependent effect of magnesium on reperfusion injury. Therefore, there is conflicting evidence that the **routine** use of intravenous magnesium sulfate in the setting of acute myocardial infarction is beneficial.

[1]Not included in Canadian product labeling.

## Pharmacology/Pharmacokinetics

**Physicochemical characteristics**

Molecular weight—246.47.

Other characteristics—Magnesium sulfate, as the hydrated salt, contains approximately 10% of the labeled weight as magnesium and 49% as anhydrous magnesium sulfate. Doses are calculated based on the hydrate weight unless otherwise stated. One gram of magnesium sulfate heptahydrate ($MgSO_4$ $7H_2O$) is equivalent to 8.12 mEq of magnesium.

**Mechanism of action/Effect**

Anticonvulsant—Exact mechanism is not clearly understood. Magnesium may decrease the amount of acetylcholine released at the myoneuronal junction, resulting in depression of neuromuscular transmission. Magnesium also may have a direct depressant effect on smooth muscle and may cause central nervous system (CNS) depression.

Antiarrhythmic—The exact mechanism of magnesium's antiarrhythmic effect is not clear. Magnesium may decrease myocardial cell excitability by contributing to the re-establishment of ionic equilibrium and stabilizing cell membranes. Magnesium also appears to modulate the sodium

current, the slow inward calcium current, and at least one potassium current.
Myocardial infarction—Possible mechanisms include antiarrhythmic action or direct cardioprotection. Magnesium's cardioprotective action may involve coronary vasodilation, reduction in peripheral vascular resistance, platelet aggregation inhibition, and an effect on the calcium current.
Tocolytic—The exact mechanism is not known. It is speculated that magnesium may decrease myometrial contractility by altering calcium uptake, binding, and distribution in smooth muscle cells. Magnesium has been shown to increase uterine blood flow secondary to vasodilation of uterine vessels.

**Onset of action**
Intramuscular—About 1 hour.
Intravenous—Nearly immediate.

**Therapeutic serum concentrations**
Anticonvulsant—4 to 7 mEq per L (2 to 3.5 mmol per L).

**Duration of action**
Intramuscular—3 to 4 hours.
Intravenous—About 30 minutes.

**Elimination**
Renal, at a rate proportional to the plasma concentration and glomerular filtration rate.

# Precautions to Consider

### Pregnancy/Reproduction
Pregnancy—Parenteral magnesium sulfate has been administered to pregnant women in the treatment of pre-eclampsia and eclampsia (toxemia) of pregnancy and as a tocolytic agent. It readily crosses the placenta and rapidly attains fetal serum concentrations that approximate those in the mother. Magnesium's effects in the neonate may be similar to those in the mother and may include hypotonia, drowsiness, and respiratory depression. Bony abnormalities and congenital rickets have been reported in neonates born to mothers treated with parenteral magnesium sulfate for prolonged periods of time (4 to 13 weeks' duration).

FDA Pregnancy Category A.

### Breast-feeding
Magnesium sulfate is distributed into breast milk. Milk concentrations are approximately twice those in maternal serum.

### Pediatrics
Appropriate studies on the relationship of age to the effects of magnesium sulfate have not been performed in the pediatric population. However, no pediatrics-specific problems have been documented to date.

### Geriatrics
Appropriate studies on the relationship of age to the effects of magnesium sulfate have not been performed in the geriatric population. However, elderly patients are more likely to have age-related renal function impairment, which may require dosage reduction in patients receiving magnesium sulfate.

### Drug interactions and/or related problems
The following drug interactions and/or related problems have been selected on the basis of their potential clinical significance (possible mechanism in parentheses where appropriate)—not necessarily inclusive (» = major clinical significance):

Note: Combinations containing any of the following medications, depending on the amount present, may also interact with this medication.

Calcium (intravenous salts)
(concurrent use may neutralize effects of parenteral magnesium sulfate; calcium gluconate and calcium gluceptate are used to antagonize the toxic effects of hypermagnesemia; also, calcium sulfate may precipitate when a calcium salt is admixed with magnesium sulfate in the same intravenous solution; however, calcium salts and magnesium sulfate may be administered concurrently through separate intravenous lines if required in post-parathyroidectomy "hungry bones" syndrome or tetany associated with hypocalcemia and hypomagnesemia)

CNS depression–producing medications, other (see *Appendix II*)
(CNS depressant effects may be potentiated when these medications are used concurrently with parenteral magnesium sulfate)

Digitalis glycosides
(parenteral magnesium sulfate must be administered with extreme caution in digitalized patients, especially if intravenous calcium salts are also employed; cardiac conduction changes and heart block may occur)

Neuromuscular blocking agents or
Nifedipine
(concurrent use with parenteral magnesium sulfate may result in severe and unpredictable potentiation of neuromuscular blockade)
(concurrent use of parenteral magnesium sulfate with nifedipine may produce an exaggerated hypotensive response)

### Laboratory value alterations
The following have been selected on the basis of their potential clinical significance (possible effect in parentheses where appropriate)—not necessarily inclusive (» = major clinical significance):

With diagnostic test results
Reticuloendothelial cell imaging
(parenteral magnesium sulfate may impair reticuloendothelial cell imaging with technetium Tc 99m sulfur colloid by causing clumping of colloidal particles with subsequent entrapment in the vasculature of the lungs rather than in the liver, spleen, and bone marrow)

### Medical considerations/Contraindications
The medical considerations/contraindications included have been selected on the basis of their potential clinical significance (reasons given in parentheses where appropriate)—not necessarily inclusive (» = major clinical significance).

*Except under special circumstances, this medication should not be used when the following medical problems exist:*

» Heart block
(magnesium may exacerbate this condition)
» Renal failure (creatinine clearance <20 mL per minute)
(clearance of magnesium decreased; risk of magnesium toxicity)

*Risk-benefit should be considered when the following medical problems exist:*

Myasthenia gravis
(magnesium sulfate may precipitate an acute myasthenic crisis by decreasing the sensitivity of the motor endplate to acetylcholine)
» Renal function impairment, severe
(risk of developing hypermagnesemia and magnesium toxicity; patients with severely impaired renal function should receive no more than 20 grams of magnesium sulfate [162 mEq of magnesium] within a 48-hour period; caution is recommended against administering intravenous magnesium too rapidly in patients with oliguria or severe renal failure; close monitoring of serum magnesium concentration is recommended)

Respiratory disease
(increased risk of respiratory depression)
Sensitivity to magnesium sulfate

### Patient monitoring
The following may be especially important in patient monitoring (other tests may be warranted in some patients, depending on condition; » = major clinical significance):

Blood pressure monitoring
(recommended at periodic intervals)

Cardiac function monitoring (ECG) and
Magnesium concentrations, serum
(recommended at periodic intervals during therapy as indicated by the clinical situation; normal average serum magnesium concentrations are 1.6 to 2.6 mEq per L [0.8 to 1.2 mmol per L])

Deep tendon reflexes, especially patellar reflex or knee jerk determinations
(used as an indication of CNS depression prior to administration of repeated doses; suppression of reflex may be related to impending respiratory arrest. The patellar reflex should be tested before each dose and, if the reflex is absent, no additional doses should be given until a positive response is obtained. The disappearance of the reflex is a useful sign for detecting excessive magnesium serum concentrations)

Renal function determinations, especially urine output
(recommended at periodic intervals; urine output should be at least 100 mL per 4 hours)

Respiration rate determination
(rate should be at least 16 per minute prior to each parenteral dose of magnesium sulfate, since respiratory depression is the most critical side effect of this medication, rapidly proceeding to fatal respiratory paralysis)

# Side/Adverse Effects

The following side/adverse effects have been selected on the basis of their potential clinical significance (possible signs and symptoms in parentheses where appropriate)—not necessarily inclusive:

Note: Although the side/adverse effects are stratified according to serum magnesium concentrations and early signs and symptoms of hypermagnesemia, these effects may occur early or late in the course of hypermagnesemia and may not always correlate with serum magnesium concentrations.

### Those indicating need for prompt medical attention
*Signs of hypermagnesemia*—in order of increasing serum magnesium concentrations:

| Effect | Serum magnesium concentration (mEq per L) |
|---|---|
| *Deep tendon reflexes present, but possibly hypoactive* | 4 to 7 |
| *Prolonged PQ interval; widened QRS interval on ECG* | 5 to 10 |
| *Loss of deep tendon reflexes* | 8 to 10 |
| *Respiratory paralysis* | 10 to 13 |
| *Altered cardiac conduction* | 15 |
| *Cardiac arrest* | 25 |

Early signs and symptoms of hypermagnesemia
*Bradycardia; diplopia; flushing; headache; hypotension; nausea; shortness of breath; slurred speech; vomiting; weakness*

## Overdose
For more information on the management of overdose or unintentional ingestion, **contact a Poison Control Center** (see *Poison Control Center Listing*).

### Treatment of overdose
Blood pressure and respiratory support; artificial respiration is often required.

Slow injection of intravenous calcium gluconate, 5 to 10 mEq of calcium or 10 to 20 mL of a 10% solution (diluted if desirable with 0.9% sodium chloride injection) to reverse heart block or respiratory depression.

Subcutaneous administration of physostigmine (0.5 to 1 mg) may be helpful; however, routine use is not recommended because of its toxicity.

Dialysis may be required to remove magnesium sulfate if renal function is reduced.

## General Dosing Information
Magnesium sulfate injection 50% must be diluted to a concentration of 20% or less prior to intravenous infusion.

The rate of intravenous injection should generally not exceed 150 mg per minute, except in severe eclampsia with seizures.

## Parenteral Dosage Forms
Note: Bracketed uses in the *Dosage Forms* section refer to categories of use and/or indications that are not included in U.S. product labeling.

### MAGNESIUM SULFATE INJECTION USP
#### Usual adult and adolescent dose
Seizures, in toxemia of pregnancy—
Intravenous, 4 to 5 grams (32 to 40 mEq [16 to 20 mmol] of magnesium) in 250 mL of 5% dextrose injection USP or 0.9% sodium chloride infused over thirty minutes. Simultaneously, intramuscular doses of up to 10 grams (5 grams or 10 mL of undiluted 50% solution in each buttock) are given. Alternatively, the initial intravenous dose of 4 grams may be given by diluting the 50% solution to a 10 or 20% concentration; the diluted fluid (40 mL of a 10% solution or 20 mL of a 20% solution) may then be injected intravenously over a period of three to four minutes. Subsequently, 4 to 5 grams are injected intramuscularly into alternate buttocks every four hours as needed. Alternatively, after the initial intravenous dose, some clinicians administer 1 or 2 grams per hour as an intravenous infusion.

Hypomagnesemia—
Severe deficiency:
Intramuscular, 250 mg (2 mEq [1 mmol] of magnesium) per kg of body weight administered within a four-hour period.
Intravenous infusion, 5 grams (40 mEq [20 mmol] of magnesium) in 1 L of 5% dextrose injection or 0.9% sodium chloride injection, administered slowly over a three-hour period.
Mild deficiency:
Intramuscular, 1 gram (8 mEq [4 mmol] of magnesium) as a 50% solution, administered every six hours for four doses (a total of 32.5 mEq of magnesium) per twenty-four hours.

Total parenteral nutrition (TPN)—
Intravenous infusion, 1 to 3 grams (8 to 24 mEq [4 to 12 mmol] of magnesium) a day.

Note: Up to 6 grams a day may be necessary in selected patients, such as in patients with short bowel syndrome.

[Ventricular tachycardia, polymorphous][1]—
Intravenous, 2 grams (16 mEq [8 mmol] of magnesium) given over one to two minutes; the dose may be repeated if the arrhythmia is not controlled after five to fifteen minutes. Additionally, an intravenous infusion of 3 to 20 mg per minute may be needed.

[Premature labor][1]—
Initial: Intravenous, 4 to 6 grams (32 to 48 mEq [16 to 24 mmol] of magnesium) infused over twenty to thirty minutes.
Maintenance: Intravenous infusion, 1 to 3 grams (8 to 24 mEq [4 to 12 mmol] of magnesium) per hour until contractions abate.

Note: Extreme care must be used in the parenteral administration of magnesium sulfate in order to avoid toxic serum concentrations.
Geriatric patients often require lower dosages because of reduced renal function.
An intravenous preparation of a calcium salt (e.g., 10% calcium gluconate or gluceptate) should be readily available when magnesium sulfate is administered.

#### Usual adult prescribing limits
Up to 40 grams (320 mEq [160 mmol] of magnesium) a day.

#### Usual pediatric dose
Total parenteral nutrition (TPN)—
Intravenous infusion, 0.25 to 1.25 grams (2 to 10 mEq [1 to 5 mmol] of magnesium) a day.

#### Strength(s) usually available
U.S.—
10% w/v (1 gram [8 mEq of magnesium] per 10 mL) (Rx) [GENERIC].
12.5% w/v (1.25 grams [10 mEq of magnesium] per 10 mL) (Rx) [GENERIC].
50% w/v (5 grams [40 mEq of magnesium] per 10 mL) (Rx) [GENERIC].
Canada—
20% w/v (2 grams [16 mEq of magnesium] per 10 mL) (Rx) [GENERIC].
50% w/v (5 grams [40 mEq of magnesium] per 10 mL) (Rx) [GENERIC].

#### Packaging and storage
Store below 40 °C (104 °F), preferably between 15 and 30 °C (59 and 86 °F), unless otherwise specified by manufacturer. Protect from freezing.

#### Incompatibilities
Formation of a precipitate may result when magnesium sulfate is mixed with solutions containing:
Alcohol (in high concentrations)
Alkali carbonates and bicarbonates
Alkali hydroxides
Arsenates
Barium
Calcium
Clindamycin phosphate
Heavy metals
Hydrocortisone sodium succinate
Phosphates
Polymyxin B sulfate
Procaine hydrochloride
Salicylates
Strontium
Tartrates

The potential for incompatibility will often be influenced by changes in the concentration of reactants and the pH of the solutions.

Separation of intravenous fat emulsions may occur with concentrations of magnesium greater than 20 mEq per mL in total parenteral nutrition admixtures.

It has been reported that magnesium may reduce the antibiotic activity of streptomycin, tetracycline, and tobramycin when given together.

[1]Not included in Canadian product labeling.

## Selected Bibliography
Chau AC, Gabert HA, Miller JM. A prospective comparison of terbutaline and magnesium for tocolysis. Obstet Gynecol 1992; 80: 847-51.
Sibai BM. Magnesium sulfate is the ideal anticonvulsant in preeclampsia-eclampsia. Am J Obstet Gynecol 1990; 162: 1141-5.

Revised: 08/03/94
Interim revision: 08/15/95

# MAGNESIUM SUPPLEMENTS  Systemic

This monograph includes information on the following: 1) Magnesium Chloride†; 2) Magnesium Citrate§; 3) Magnesium Gluceptate*; 4) Magnesium Gluconate; 5) Magnesium Hydroxide‡§; 6) Magnesium Lactate†; 7) Magnesium Oxide‡§; 8) Magnesium Pidolate*; 9) Magnesium Sulfate#.

INN:
Magnesium gluceptate—Magnesium glucoheptonate
Magnesium pidolate—Magnesium pyroglutamate

VA CLASSIFICATION (Primary): TN406

Commonly used brand name(s): *Almora*[4]; *Chloromag*[1]; *Citro-Mag*[2]; *Citroma*[2]; *Concentrated Phillips' Milk of Magnesia*[5]; *MGP*[4]; *Mag 2*[8]; *Mag-200*[8]; *Mag-L-100*[1]; *Mag-Ox 400*[7]; *Mag-Tab SR*[6]; *Maglucate*[4]; *Magnesium-Rougier*[3]; *Magonate*[4]; *Magtrate*[4]; *Maox*[7]; *Phillips' Chewable Tablets*[5]; *Phillips' Magnesia Tablets*[5]; *Phillips' Milk of Magnesia*[5]; *Slow-Mag*[1]; *Uro-Mag*[7].

Note: For a listing of dosage forms and brand names by country availability, see *Dosage Forms* section(s).

*Not commercially available in U.S.
†Not commercially available in Canada.
‡See *Antacids (Oral-Local)* for antacid use of magnesium hydroxide and magnesium oxide.
§See *Laxatives (Local)* for laxative use of magnesium citrate, magnesium hydroxide, magnesium oxide, and magnesium sulfate.
#See *Magnesium Sulfate (Systemic)* for use in seizures and uterine tetany.

## Category

Antihypomagnesemic—Magnesium Chloride; Magnesium Citrate; Magnesium Gluceptate; Magnesium Gluconate; Magnesium Hydroxide; Magnesium Lactate; Magnesium Oxide; Magnesium Pidolate; Magnesium Sulfate.

Electrolyte replenisher—Magnesium Chloride Injection; Magnesium Sulfate.

Nutritional supplement (mineral)—Magnesium Chloride; Magnesium Citrate; Magnesium Gluceptate; Magnesium Gluconate; Magnesium Hydroxide; Magnesium Lactate; Magnesium Oxide; Magnesium Pidolate; Magnesium Sulfate.

## Indications

Note: Bracketed information in the *Indications* section refers to uses that are not included in U.S. product labeling.

### Accepted

Electrolyte depletion (treatment)—Parenteral magnesium chloride and magnesium sulfate are used in conditions that require an increase in magnesium ions for electrolyte adjustment.

Hypomagnesemia (prophylaxis and treatment)—Magnesium supplements are indicated for correction of hypomagnesemia in patients with low or restricted oral intake or conditions in which requirements for magnesium are increased, such as chronic alcoholism, diabetic ketoacidosis, gastrointestinal disease (chronic diarrhea, Crohn's, ulcerative colitis), hyperaldosteronism, hypercalcemia, hypomagnesemic hypocalcemia, hypomagnesemic hypokalemia, hyperparathyroidism, hyperthyroidism, pancreatic insufficiency, renal tubular acidosis, stress, or possibly patients who are receiving thiazide or loop diuretics, cisplatin, amphotericin B therapy, cyclosporine, gentamicin, or digitalis glycosides, or are on total parenteral nutrition (TPN) therapy. For prophylaxis of magnesium deficiency, dietary improvement, rather than supplementation, is advisable. For treatment of magnesium deficiency, supplementation is preferred.

Deficiency of magnesium may lead to irritability, mental derangement, muscle weakness, tetany, and cardiac arrhythmias.

Recommended intakes for all vitamins and most minerals are increased during pregnancy. Many physicians recommend that pregnant women receive multivitamin and mineral supplements, especially those pregnant women who do not consume an adequate diet and those in high-risk categories (i.e., women carrying more than one fetus, heavy cigarette smokers, and alcohol and drug abusers). Taking excessive amounts of a multivitamin and mineral supplement may be harmful to the mother and/or fetus and should be avoided.

Recommended intakes for all vitamins and most minerals are increased during breast-feeding.

Antacid—See *Antacids (Oral-Local)*.
Laxative—See *Laxatives (Local)*.

Seizures (treatment)—See *Magnesium Sulfate (Systemic)*.
[Tachycardia, ventricular, atypical (treatment)]—See *Magnesium Sulfate (Systemic)*.
Tetany, uterine (treatment)—See *Magnesium Sulfate (Systemic)*.

## Pharmacology/Pharmacokinetics

### Physicochemical characteristics
Molecular weight—
 Elemental magnesium: 24.3.
 Magnesium chloride: 203.3.
 Magnesium citrate: 451.1.
 Magnesium gluceptate: 474.7.
 Magnesium gluconate: 450.6.
 Magnesium hydroxide: 58.3.
 Magnesium lactate: 202.4.
 Magnesium oxide: 40.3.
 Magnesium pidolate: 280.5.
 Magnesium sulfate: 246.47.

### Mechanism of action/Effect
Magnesium is necessary for the proper functioning of over 300 enzymes, including several in glycolysis and the Krebs cycle, adenyl cyclase, which forms cyclic-AMP, and various phosphatase reactions in protein and nucleic acid synthesis. Magnesium is also necessary for neuromuscular transmission and activity, bone mineralization, and parathyroid hormone function.

### Other effects
Calcium homeostasis is dependent on magnesium, with hypomagnesemia often being accompanied by hypocalcemia. Magnesium is necessary for secretion of parathyroid hormone (PTH) and also for the action of PTH at the site of its target organs. High doses of magnesium have been found to inhibit calcium absorption due to suppression of PTH secretion. Hypokalemia is frequently found with hypomagnesemia, possibly due to magnesium deficiency enhancing renal excretion of potassium or magnesium deficiency effecting the sodium-potassium pump.

### Absorption
Approximately 35 to 40% of dietary magnesium is absorbed through the jejunum and ileum. Some magnesium is reabsorbed from bile and pancreatic and intestinal juices. High fat diets or fat malabsorption syndromes have been found to interfere with magnesium absorption.

### Protein binding
Approximately 30% of magnesium is bound intracellularly to protein and energy-rich phosphates.

### Storage
Primarily bone, skeletal muscle, kidney, liver, and heart; small amounts found in extracellular fluid and erythrocytes.

### Time to peak concentration
Oral—4 hours.

### Duration of action
Oral—4 to 6 hours.

### Elimination
Parenteral magnesium is eliminated renally. Oral magnesium is eliminated renally and fecally.

## Precautions to Consider

### Pregnancy/Reproduction
Pregnancy—
 *Parenteral magnesium sulfate*—
  When magnesium sulfate is parenterally administered in the treatment of eclampsias (toxemias) of pregnancy, it readily crosses the placenta and rapidly attains fetal serum concentrations that approximate those of the mother. The effects of magnesium on the neonate are similar to those on the mother and may include hypotonia, hyporeflexia, hypotension, and respiratory depression when the mother has received magnesium sulfate prior to delivery. It is therefore usually not administered to the mother during the 2 hours preceding delivery unless it is the only therapy available to prevent eclamptic seizures. Magnesium sulfate can be administered continuously by intravenous drip at a rate of 1 to 2 grams every hour, provided the patient is closely monitored for magnesium plasma concentrations, blood pressure, respiratory rate, and deep tendon reflexes.
 FDA Pregnancy Category D.

*Other magnesium salts and oral magnesium sulfate—*
   Problems in humans have not been documented with intake of normal daily recommended amounts.
   FDA pregnancy categories have not been assigned.

**Breast-feeding**
Problems in humans have not been documented with intake of normal daily recommended amounts.

**Pediatrics**
Problems in pediatrics have not been documented with intake of normal daily recommended amounts.

Magnesium chloride injection that contains benzyl alcohol as a preservative should not be used in newborn and immature infants. The use of benzyl alcohol in neonates has been associated with a fatal toxic syndrome consisting of metabolic acidosis and CNS, respiratory, circulatory, and renal function impairment.

**Geriatrics**
Problems in geriatrics have not been documented with intake of normal daily recommended amounts.

The elderly may be at risk of developing a magnesium deficiency due to poor food selection, decreased absorption, diseases that cause magnesium depletion, or medications that may increase urinary loss of magnesium.

**Drug interactions and/or related problems**
The following drug interactions and/or related problems have been selected on the basis of their potential clinical significance (possible mechanism in parentheses where appropriate)—not necessarily inclusive (» = major clinical significance):

Note: Combinations containing any of the following medications, depending on the amount present, may also interact with magnesium supplements.

Alcohol or
Glucose
   (high alcohol or glucose intake has been found to increase urinary excretion of magnesium)

Amphotericin B or
Cisplatin or
Cyclosporine or
Gentamicin
   (magnesium requirements may be increased in patients receiving these nephrotoxic medications due to renal magnesium wasting)

Calcium (intravenous salts)
   (concurrent use may neutralize effects of parenteral magnesium sulfate; however, calcium gluconate and calcium gluceptate are used to antagonize the toxic effects of hypermagnesemia, also, calcium sulfate may precipitate when a calcium salt is admixed with magnesium sulfate in the same intravenous solution; calcium salts and magnesium sulfate may be administered through separate intravenous lines if required in post-parathyroidectomy "hungry bones" syndrome or tetany associated with hypocalcemia and hypomagnesemia)

Calcium-containing medications, oral
   (concurrent use with magnesium supplements may increase serum calcium or magnesium concentrations in susceptible patients, primarily patients with renal insufficiency)

» Cellulose sodium phosphate
Edetate disodium
   (concurrent use with magnesium supplements may result in binding of magnesium; patients should be advised not to take magnesium supplements within 1 hour of cellulose sodium phosphate or edetate disodium)

CNS depression–producing medications, other (See *Appendix II*)
   (CNS depressant effects may be potentiated when these medications are used concurrently with parenteral magnesium)

Digitalis glycosides
   (hypomagnesemia has been reported in patients receiving digitalis glycosides and may lead to digitalis toxicity; therefore, serum magnesium concentrations should be monitored in patients receiving digitalis glycosides, as magnesium supplements may be necessary)
   (concurrent use with magnesium supplements may inhibit absorption, possibly decreasing plasma concentrations of digitalis glycosides; magnesium salts in digitalized patients must be administered with extreme caution, especially if intravenous calcium salts are also employed; cardiac conduction changes and heart block may occur)

Diuretics, loop or
Diuretics, thiazide
   (long-term use of loop or thiazide diuretics may impair the magnesium-conserving ability of the kidneys and lead to hypomagnesemia; serum magnesium levels should be monitored in patients receiving thiazide or loop diuretics)

Diuretics, potassium-sparing
   (long-term use of potassium-sparing diuretics has been found to increase renal tubular reabsorption of magnesium; use with magnesium supplements may cause hypermagnesemia, especially in patients with renal insufficiency)

Etidronate, oral
   (concurrent use with oral magnesium supplements may prevent absorption of oral etidronate; patients should be advised to avoid using magnesium supplements within 2 hours of etidronate)

» Magnesium-containing preparations, other, such as:
Antacids
Laxatives
   (concurrent use with magnesium supplements may cause magnesium toxicity, especially in patients with renal insufficiency)

Misoprostol
   (concurrent use with magnesium supplements may aggravate misoprostol-induced diarrhea)

Neuromuscular blocking agents
   (concurrent use with parenteral magnesium may result in severe and unpredictable potentiation of neuromuscular blockade)

» Sodium polystyrene sulfonate
   (sodium polystyrene sulfonate may bind with oral magnesium supplements; concurrent use is not recommended, although the risk may be less with rectal administration of sodium polystyrene sulfonate)

» Tetracyclines, oral
   (concurrent use with magnesium supplements may decrease absorption of tetracyclines because of possible formation of nonabsorbable complexes; patients should be advised not to take magnesium supplements within 1 to 3 hours of taking an oral tetracycline)

**Medical considerations/Contraindications**
The medical considerations/contraindications included have been selected on the basis of their potential clinical significance (reasons given in parentheses where appropriate)—not necessarily inclusive (» = major clinical significance).

*Risk-benefit should be considered when the following medical problems exist:*

Heart block or
Myocardial damage
   (conditions may be exacerbated; magnesium should be infused at a slower rate with careful monitoring of serum magnesium concentrations)

Renal function impairment, severe
   (may cause high levels of magnesium; reduction of magnesium supplement dosage may be necessary)

Sensitivity to parenteral magnesium
   (sensitivity has been reported with use of parenteral magnesium in higher doses; sensitivity to oral magnesium supplements in recommended doses has not been reported)

**Patient monitoring**
The following may be especially important in patient monitoring (other tests may be warranted in some patients, depending on condition; » = major clinical significance):

Magnesium concentrations, serum and urinary
   (recommended daily for severe deficiency and monthly for chronic deficiency to determine status; magnesium equilibrates slowly with the intracellular compartment; thus serum magnesium concentrations may not be reliable indicators of normal tissue levels)

## Side/Adverse Effects

The following side/adverse effects have been selected on the basis of their potential clinical significance (possible signs and symptoms in parentheses where appropriate)—not necessarily inclusive:

**Those indicating need for medical attention**
Incidence rare (with parenteral magnesium only)
   ***Flushing; hypotension*** (dizziness or fainting); ***irritation and pain at injection site***—for intramuscular administration only; ***muscle paralysis; respiratory depression*** (troubled breathing)

**Those indicating need for medical attention only if they continue or are bothersome**
Incidence less frequent (with oral magnesium)
   ***Diarrhea***

## Overdose

For specific information on the agents used in the management of magnesium overdose, see
- Calcium Gluconate in *Calcium Supplements* monograph.

For more information on the management of overdose or unintentional ingestion, **contact a Poison Control Center** (see *Poison Control Center Listing*).

**Clinical effects of overdose**
The following effects have been selected on the basis of their potential clinical significance (possible signs and symptoms in parentheses where appropriate)—not necessarily inclusive:

Symptoms of overdose (rare in patients with normal renal function)
*Asystole; bradycardia* (slow heartbeat); *CNS depression* (severe drowsiness); *coma; hypotension* (dizziness or fainting); *muscle paralysis; renal failure* (blurred or double vision; increased or decreased urination); *respiratory failure* (troubled breathing)

**Treatment of overdose**
Discontinue magnesium-containing preparations.
Supportive care—
 Maintain respiration.
Specific treatment—
 If serum magnesium levels exceed 5 mEq per liter and adult patient is symptomatic, giving 10 mL of 10% calcium gluconate over several minutes. The dose may be repeated one time.

## Patient Consultation

As an aid to patient consultation, refer to *Advice for the Patient, Magnesium Supplements (Systemic)*.
In providing consultation, consider emphasizing the following selected information (» = major clinical significance):

**Description of use**
 Description should include function in the body; signs of deficiency

**Importance of diet**
 Importance of proper nutrition; supplement may be needed because of inadequate dietary intake
 Food sources of magnesium; effects of processing
 Recommended daily intake for magnesium

**Before using this medication**
» Conditions affecting use, especially:
 Sensitivity to magnesium
 Use in the elderly—More likely to develop magnesium deficiency
 Other medications, especially cellulose sodium phosphate, oral tetracyclines, other magnesium-containing preparations, or sodium polystyrene sulfonate
 Other medical problems, especially heart block, renal function impairment, hypotension, or respiratory depression

**Proper use of this medication**
» Proper dosing
 Taking with meals to prevent diarrhea
*Proper administration technique*
 Not crushing or chewing extended-release dosage forms, unless otherwise directed
 Proper mixing for powder form
 Missed dose: No cause for concern because of length of time necessary for depletion; remembering to take as directed
» Proper storage

**Side/adverse effects**
 Signs of potential side effects, especially dizziness or fainting, flushing, irritation and pain at injection site for intramuscular injection only, muscle paralysis, or troubled breathing (with injection)

## General Dosing Information

Magnesium supplements should be taken with meals because taking them on an empty stomach may cause diarrhea.

The action of magnesium supplements depends upon their content of magnesium ion. There are 12.2 mg of elemental magnesium per 1 mEq elemental magnesium. The various magnesium salts contain the following amounts of elemental magnesium:

| Magnesium salt | Magnesium (mg/gram) | Magnesium (mEq/gram) | Magnesium (mM/gram) | % Magnesium |
|---|---|---|---|---|
| Magnesium chloride (hydrous) | 120 | 9.8 | 4.9 | 12 |
| Magnesium citrate (anhydrous) | 162 | 4.4 | 2.2 | 16.2 |
| Magnesium gluceptate (anhydrous) | 51.3 | 4.2 | 2.1 | 5.1 |
| Magnesium gluconate (hydrous) | 54 | 4.4 | 2.2 | 5.4 |
| Magnesium hydroxide (anhydrous) | 417 | 34.3 | 17.2 | 41.7 |
| Magnesium lactate (anhydrous) | 120 | 9.8 | 4.9 | 12 |
| Magnesium oxide (anhydrous) | 603 | 49.6 | 24.8 | 60.3 |
| Magnesium pidolate (anhydrous) | 87 | 7.2 | 3.6 | 8.7 |
| Magnesium sulfate (hydrous) | 99 | 8.1 | 4.1 | 9.9 |

**For parenteral dosage forms only**
In most cases, parenteral administration is indicated only when oral administration is not acceptable (for example, in nausea, vomiting, preoperative and postoperative conditions) or possible (for example, in malabsorption syndromes or following gastric resection).

**Diet/Nutrition**
Recommended dietary intakes for magnesium are defined differently worldwide.
For U.S.—
 The Recommended Dietary Allowances (RDAs) for vitamins and minerals are determined by the Food and Nutrition Board of the National Research Council and are intended to provide adequate nutrition in most healthy persons under usual environmental stresses. In addition, a different designation may be used by the FDA for food and dietary supplement labeling purposes, as with Daily Value (DV). DVs replace the previous labeling terminology United States Recommended Daily Allowances (USRDAs).
For Canada—
 Recommended Nutrient Intakes (RNIs) for vitamins, minerals, and protein are determined by Health and Welfare Canada and provide recommended amounts of a specific nutrient while minimizing the risk of chronic diseases.
Daily recommended intakes for elemental magnesium are generally defined as follows:

| Persons | U.S. (mg) | Canada (mg) |
|---|---|---|
| Infants and children | | |
| Birth to 3 years of age | 40–80 | 20–50 |
| 4 to 6 years of age | 120 | 65 |
| 7 to 10 years of age | 170 | 100–135 |
| Adolescent and adult males | 270–400 | 130–250 |
| Adolescent and adult females | 280–300 | 135–210 |
| Pregnant females | 320 | 195–245 |
| Breast-feeding females | 340–355 | 245–265 |

The best dietary sources of magnesium include green leafy vegetables, nuts, legumes, and cereal grains in which the germ or outer layers have not been removed. Hard water has a higher concentration of magnesium than soft water. The magnesium content of food is reduced by refining and cooking.

---

### MAGNESIUM CHLORIDE

## Summary of Differences

Category: Injection may also be used as an electrolyte replenisher.
Precautions: Drug interactions and/or related problems—Possible additive effects when parenteral calcium chloride given with CNS depression–producing medications and neuromuscular blocking agents.

## Oral Dosage Forms

### MAGNESIUM CHLORIDE TABLETS

**Usual adult and adolescent dose**
Hypomagnesemia (prophylaxis)—
  Oral, amount based on normal daily recommended intakes of elemental magnesium:

| Persons | U.S. (mg) | Canada (mg) |
|---|---|---|
| Adolescent and adult males | 270–400 | 130–250 |
| Adolescent and adult females | 280–300 | 135–210 |
| Pregnant females | 320 | 195–245 |
| Breast-feeding females | 340–355 | 245–265 |

Hypomagnesemia (treatment)—
  Treatment dose is individualized by prescriber based on severity of deficiency.

**Usual pediatric dose**
Hypomagnesemia (prophylaxis)—
  Oral, amount based on normal daily recommended intakes of elemental magnesium:

| Persons | U.S. (mg) | Canada (mg) |
|---|---|---|
| Infants and children | | |
| Birth to 3 years of age | 40–80 | 20–50 |
| 4 to 6 years of age | 120 | 65 |
| 7 to 10 years of age | 170 | 100–135 |

Hypomagnesemia (treatment)—
  Treatment dose is individualized by prescriber based on severity of deficiency.

**Strength(s) usually available**
U.S.—
  64 mg elemental magnesium (OTC) [*Slow-Mag*].
Canada—
  Not commercially available.

Note: The strength of this magnesium preparation may exceed the dosage range recommended by USP DI Advisory Panels based on the amount necessary to meet normal nutritional needs.

**Packaging and storage**
Store below 40 °C (104 °F), preferably between 15 and 30 °C (59 and 86 °F), unless otherwise specified by manufacturer.

### MAGNESIUM CHLORIDE ENTERIC-COATED TABLETS

**Usual adult and adolescent dose**
See *Magnesium Chloride Tablets*.

**Usual pediatric dose**
Dosage form not appropriate for use in children.

**Strength(s) usually available**
U.S.—
  100 mg elemental magnesium (833 mg magnesium chloride) (OTC) [*Mag-L-100*].
Canada—
  Not commercially available.

Note: The strength of this magnesium preparation may exceed the dosage range recommended by USP DI Advisory Panels based on the amount necessary to meet normal nutritional needs.

**Packaging and storage**
Store below 40 °C (104 °F), preferably between 15 and 30 °C (59 and 86 °F), unless otherwise specified by manufacturer.

### MAGNESIUM CHLORIDE EXTENDED-RELEASE TABLETS

**Usual adult and adolescent dose**
See *Magnesium Chloride Tablets*.

**Usual pediatric dose**
Dosage form not appropriate for use in children.

**Strength(s) usually available**
U.S.—
  64 mg elemental magnesium (535 mg magnesium chloride) (OTC) [*Slow-Mag*].
Canada—
  Not commercially available.

Note: The strength of this magnesium preparation may exceed the dosage range recommended by USP DI Advisory Panels based on the amount necessary to meet normal nutritional needs.

**Packaging and storage**
Store below 40 °C (104 °F), preferably between 15 and 30 °C (59 and 86 °F), unless otherwise specified by manufacturer.

## Parenteral Dosage Forms

### MAGNESIUM CHLORIDE INJECTION

**Usual adult and adolescent dose**
Electrolyte replenisher—
  For intravenous infusion, 4 grams of magnesium chloride (39.2 mEq of elemental magnesium) diluted in 250 mL of dextrose 5% and infused at a rate not to exceed 3 mL per minute.
Hypomagnesemia (prophylaxis)—
  Intravenous infusion, as part of total parenteral nutrition solution, the specific amount determined by individual patient need.

**Usual adult prescribing limits**
40 grams a day.

**Usual pediatric dose**
Hypomagnesemia (prophylaxis)—
  Intravenous infusion, as part of total parenteral nutrition solution, the specific amount determined by individual patient need.

Note: Magnesium chloride injection that contains benzyl alcohol as a preservative should not be used in newborn and immature infants. The use of benzyl alcohol in neonates has been associated with a fatal toxic syndrome consisting of metabolic acidosis and CNS, respiratory, circulatory, and renal function impairment.

**Strength(s) usually available**
U.S.—
  200 mg magnesium chloride per mL (Rx) [*Chloromag;* GENERIC].
Canada—
  Not commercially available.

**Packaging and storage**
Store below 40 °C (104 °F), preferably between 15 and 30 °C (59 and 86 °F), unless otherwise specified by manufacturer.

---
### *MAGNESIUM CITRATE*
---

## Oral Dosage Forms

### MAGNESIUM CITRATE ORAL SOLUTION USP

**Usual adult dose**
Hypomagnesemia (prophylaxis)—
  Oral, amount based on normal daily recommended intakes of elemental magnesium:

| Persons | U.S. (mg) | Canada (mg) |
|---|---|---|
| Adolescent and adult males | 270–400 | 130–250 |
| Adolescent and adult females | 280–300 | 135–210 |
| Pregnant females | 320 | 195–245 |
| Breast-feeding females | 340–355 | 245–265 |

Hypomagnesemia (treatment)—
  Treatment dose is individualized by prescriber based on severity of deficiency.

**Usual pediatric dose**
Hypomagnesemia (prophylaxis)—
  Oral, amount based on normal daily recommended intakes of elemental magnesium:

| Persons | U.S. (mg) | Canada (mg) |
|---|---|---|
| Infants and children | | |
| Birth to 3 years of age | 40–80 | 20–50 |
| 4 to 6 years of age | 120 | 65 |
| 7 to 10 years of age | 170 | 100–135 |

Hypomagnesemia (treatment)—
  Treatment dose is individualized by prescriber based on severity of deficiency.

**Strength(s) usually available**
U.S.—
  47 mg elemental magnesium (290 mg magnesium citrate) per 5 mL (OTC) [*Citroma;* GENERIC].
Canada—
  40.5 mg elemental magnesium (250 mg magnesium citrate) per 5 mL (OTC) [*Citro-Mag*].

**Note:** Some strengths of these magnesium preparations may exceed the dosage range recommended by USP DI Advisory Panels based on the amount necessary to meet normal nutritional needs.

**Packaging and storage**
Store below 40 °C (104 °F), preferably between 15 and 30 °C (59 and 86 °F), unless otherwise specified by manufacturer.

## MAGNESIUM GLUCEPTATE

# Oral Dosage Forms
### MAGNESIUM GLUCEPTATE ORAL SOLUTION

**Usual adult and adolescent dose**
Hypomagnesemia (prophylaxis)—
  Oral, amount based on normal daily recommended intakes of elemental magnesium:

| Persons | U.S. (mg) | Canada (mg) |
|---|---|---|
| Adolescent and adult males | 270–400 | 130–250 |
| Adolescent and adult females | 280–300 | 135–210 |
| Pregnant females | 320 | 195–245 |
| Breast-feeding females | 340–355 | 245–265 |

Hypomagnesemia (treatment)—
  Treatment dose is individualized by prescriber based on severity of deficiency.

**Usual pediatric dose**
Hypomagnesemia (prophylaxis)—
  Oral, amount based on normal daily recommended intakes of elemental magnesium:

| Persons | U.S. (mg) | Canada (mg) |
|---|---|---|
| Infants and children | | |
| Birth to 3 years of age | 40–80 | 20–50 |
| 4 to 6 years of age | 120 | 65 |
| 7 to 10 years of age | 170 | 100–135 |

Hypomagnesemia (treatment)—
  Treatment dose is individualized by prescriber based on severity of deficiency.

**Strength(s) usually available**
U.S.—
  Not commercially available.
Canada—
  25 mg elemental magnesium (500 mg magnesium gluceptate) per 5 mL (OTC) [*Magnesium-Rougier*].

**Note:** The strength of this magnesium preparation may exceed the dosage range recommended by USP DI Advisory Panels based on the amount necessary to meet normal nutritional needs.

**Packaging and storage**
Store below 40 °C (104 °F), preferably between 15 and 30 °C (59 and 86 °F), unless otherwise specified by manufacturer.

## MAGNESIUM GLUCONATE

# Oral Dosage Forms
### MAGNESIUM GLUCONATE ORAL SOLUTION

**Usual adult and adolescent dose**
Deficiency (prophylaxis)—
  Oral, amount based on normal daily recommended intakes of elemental magnesium:

| Persons | U.S. (mg) | Canada (mg) |
|---|---|---|
| Adolescent and adult males | 270–400 | 130–250 |
| Adolescent and adult females | 280–300 | 135–210 |
| Pregnant females | 320 | 195–245 |
| Breast-feeding females | 340–355 | 245–265 |

Deficiency (treatment)—
  Treatment dose is individualized by prescriber based on severity of deficiency.

**Usual pediatric dose**
Deficiency (prophylaxis)—
  Oral, amount based on normal daily recommended intakes of elemental magnesium:

| Persons | U.S. (mg) | Canada (mg) |
|---|---|---|
| Infants and children | | |
| Birth to 3 years of age | 40–80 | 20–50 |
| 4 to 6 years of age | 120 | 65 |
| 7 to 10 years of age | 170 | 100–135 |

Deficiency (treatment)—
  Treatment dose is individualized by prescriber based on severity of deficiency.

**Strength(s) usually available**
U.S.—
  54 mg elemental magnesium (1 gram magnesium gluconate) per 5 mL (OTC) [*Magonate*].
Canada—
  Not commercially available.

**Note:** The strength of this magnesium preparation may exceed the dosage range recommended by USP DI Advisory Panels based on the amount necessary to meet normal nutritional needs.

### MAGNESIUM GLUCONATE TABLETS USP

**Usual adult and adolescent dose**
See *Magnesium Gluconate Oral Solution*.

**Usual pediatric dose**
See *Magnesium Gluconate Oral Solution*.

**Strength(s) usually available**
U.S.—
  27 mg elemental magnesium (500 mg magnesium gluconate) [*Almora* (OTC); *Magonate* (OTC); *Magtrate* (OTC); *MGP* (Rx); GENERIC].
  29 mg elemental magnesium (550 mg magnesium gluconate) (Rx) [GENERIC].
Canada—
  29.3 mg elemental magnesium (500 mg magnesium gluconate) (OTC) [*Maglucate*].

**Note:** Some strengths of these magnesium preparations may exceed the dosage range recommended by USP DI Advisory Panels based on the amount necessary to meet normal nutritional needs.

**Packaging and storage**
Store below 40 °C (104 °F), preferably between 15 and 30 °C (59 and 86 °F), unless otherwise specified by manufacturer.

## MAGNESIUM HYDROXIDE

# Oral Dosage Forms
### MAGNESIA TABLETS USP

**Usual adult and adolescent dose**
Hypomagnesemia (prophylaxis)—
  Oral, amount based on normal daily recommended intakes of elemental magnesium:

| Persons | U.S. (mg) | Canada (mg) |
|---|---|---|
| Adolescent and adult males | 270–400 | 130–250 |
| Adolescent and adult females | 280–300 | 135–210 |
| Pregnant females | 320 | 195–245 |
| Breast-feeding females | 340–355 | 245–265 |

Hypomagnesemia (treatment)—
  Treatment dose is individualized by prescriber based on severity of deficiency.

**Usual pediatric dose**
Hypomagnesemia (prophylaxis)—
  Oral, amount based on intake of normal daily recommended intakes of elemental magnesium:

| Persons | U.S. (mg) | Canada (mg) |
|---|---|---|
| Infants and children | | |
| Birth to 3 years of age | 40–80 | 20–50 |
| 4 to 6 years of age | 120 | 65 |
| 7 to 10 years of age | 170 | 100–135 |

Hypomagnesemia (treatment)—
    Treatment dose is individualized by prescriber based on severity of deficiency.

**Strength(s) usually available**
U.S.—
    135 mg elemental magnesium (325 mg magnesium hydroxide) (OTC) [GENERIC].
Canada—
    Not commercially available.

Note: Some strengths of these magnesium preparations may exceed the dosage range recommended by USP DI Advisory Panels based on the amount necessary to meet normal nutritional needs.

**Packaging and storage**
Store below 40 °C (104 °F), preferably between 15 and 30 °C (59 and 86 °F), unless otherwise specified by manufacturer.

### MAGNESIA TABLETS (CHEWABLE) USP

**Usual adult and adolescent dose**
See *Magnesium Tablets USP*.

**Usual pediatric dose**
See *Magnesia Tablets USP*.

**Strength(s) usually available**
U.S.—
    130 mg elemental magnesium (311 mg magnesium hydroxide) (OTC) [*Phillips' Chewable Tablets*].
Canada—
    129 mg elemental magnesium (310 mg magnesium hydroxide) (OTC) [*Phillips' Magnesia Tablets*].

Note: Some strengths of these magnesium preparations may exceed the dosage range recommended by USP DI Advisory Panels based on the amount necessary to meet normal nutritional needs.

**Packaging and storage**
Store below 40 °C (104 °F), preferably between 15 and 30 °C (59 and 86 °F), unless otherwise specified by manufacturer.

### MILK OF MAGNESIA USP

**Usual adult and adolescent dose**
See *Magnesia Tablets USP*.

**Usual pediatric dose**
See *Magnesia Tablets USP*.

**Strength(s) usually available**
U.S.—
    164 mg elemental magnesium (400 mg magnesium hydroxide) per 5 mL (OTC) [*Phillips' Milk of Magnesia*; GENERIC].
    328 mg elemental magnesium (800 mg magnesium hydroxide) per 5 mL (OTC) [*Concentrated Phillips' Milk of Magnesia*].
Canada—
    170 mg elemental magnesium (408 mg magnesium hydroxide) per 5 mL (OTC) [*Phillips' Milk of Magnesia*].

Note: Some strengths of these magnesium preparations may exceed the dosage range recommended by USP DI Advisory Panels based on the amount necessary to meet normal nutritional needs.

**Packaging and storage**
Store below 40 °C (104 °F), preferably between 15 and 30 °C (59 and 86 °F), unless otherwise specified by manufacturer.

---

## MAGNESIUM LACTATE

## Oral Dosage Forms

### MAGNESIUM LACTATE EXTENDED-RELEASE TABLETS

**Usual adult and adolescent dose**
Hypomagnesemia (prophylaxis)—
    Oral, amount based on normal daily recommended intakes of elemental magnesium:

| Persons | U.S. (mg) | Canada (mg) |
|---|---|---|
| Adolescent and adult males | 270–400 | 130–250 |
| Adolescent and adult females | 280–300 | 135–210 |
| Pregnant females | 320 | 195–245 |
| Breast-feeding females | 340–355 | 245–265 |

Hypomagnesemia (treatment)—
    Treatment dose is individualized by prescriber based on severity of deficiency.

**Usual pediatric dose**
Dosage form not appropriate for use in children.

**Strength(s) usually available**
U.S.—
    84 mg elemental magnesium (840 mg magnesium lactate) (OTC) [*Mag-Tab SR*].
Canada—
    Not commercially available.

Note: The strength of this magnesium preparation may exceed the dosage range recommended by USP DI Advisory Panels based on the amount necessary to meet normal nutritional needs.

**Packaging and storage**
Store below 40 °C (104 °F), preferably between 15 and 30 °C (59 and 86 °F), unless otherwise specified by manufacturer.

---

## MAGNESIUM OXIDE

## Oral Dosage Forms

### MAGNESIUM OXIDE CAPSULES USP

**Usual adult and adolescent dose**
Hypomagnesemia (prophylaxis)—
    Oral, amount based on normal daily recommended intakes of elemental magnesium:

| Persons | U.S. (mg) | Canada (mg) |
|---|---|---|
| Adolescent and adult males | 270–400 | 130–250 |
| Adolescent and adult females | 280–300 | 135–210 |
| Pregnant females | 320 | 195–245 |
| Breast-feeding females | 340–355 | 245–265 |

Hypomagnesemia (treatment)—
    Treatment dose is individualized by prescriber based on severity of deficiency.

**Usual pediatric dose**
Hypomagnesemia (prophylaxis)—
    Oral, amount based on normal daily recommended intakes of elemental magnesium:

| Persons | U.S. (mg) | Canada (mg) |
|---|---|---|
| Infants and children | | |
| Birth to 3 years of age | 40–80 | 20–50 |
| 4 to 6 years of age | 120 | 65 |
| 7 to 10 years of age | 170 | 100–135 |

Hypomagnesemia (treatment)—
    Treatment dose is individualized by prescriber based on severity of deficiency.

**Strength(s) usually available**
U.S.—
    84.5 mg elemental magnesium (140 mg magnesium oxide) (OTC) [*Uro-Mag*; GENERIC].
Canada—
    Not commercially available.

Note: The strengths of these magnesium preparations may exceed the dosage range recommended by USP DI Advisory Panels based on the amount necessary to meet normal nutritional needs.

**Packaging and storage**
Store below 40 °C (104 °F), preferably between 15 and 30 °C (59 and 86 °F), unless otherwise specified by manufacturer.

### MAGNESIUM OXIDE TABLETS USP

**Usual adult and adolescent dose**
See *Magnesium Oxide Capsules USP*.

**Usual pediatric dose**
See *Magnesium Oxide Capsules USP*.

**Strength(s) usually available**
U.S.—
    200 mg elemental magnesium (332 mg magnesium oxide) [*Mag-200*].
    241.3 mg elemental magnesium (400 mg magnesium oxide) (OTC) [*Mag-Ox 400* (scored); GENERIC].
    250 mg elemental magnesium (420 mg magnesium oxide) (OTC) [*Maox* (tartrazine); GENERIC].
    302 mg elemental magnesium (500 mg magnesium oxide) (OTC) [GENERIC].

Canada—
  50 mg elemental magnesium (OTC) [GENERIC].

Note: Some strengths of these magnesium preparations may exceed the dosage range recommended by USP DI Advisory Panels based on the amount necessary to meet normal nutritional needs.

**Packaging and storage**
Store below 40 °C (104 °F), preferably between 15 and 30 °C (59 and 86 °F), unless otherwise specified by manufacturer.

---

### *MAGNESIUM PIDOLATE*

## Oral Dosage Forms

### MAGNESIUM PIDOLATE FOR ORAL SOLUTION

**Usual adult and adolescent dose**
Hypomagnesemia (prophylaxis)—
  Oral, amount based on normal daily recommended intakes of elemental magnesium:

| Persons | U.S. (mg) | Canada (mg) |
|---|---|---|
| Adolescent and adult males | 270–400 | 130–250 |
| Adolescent and adult females | 280–300 | 135–210 |
| Pregnant females | 320 | 195–245 |
| Breast-feeding females | 340–355 | 245–265 |

Hypomagnesemia (treatment)—
  Treatment dose is individualized by prescriber based on severity of deficiency.

**Usual pediatric dose**
Hypomagnesemia (prophylaxis)—
  Oral, amount based on normal daily recommended intakes of elemental magnesium:

| Persons | U.S. (mg) | Canada (mg) |
|---|---|---|
| Infants and children | | |
| Birth to 3 years of age | 40–80 | 20–50 |
| 4 to 6 years of age | 120 | 65 |
| 7 to 10 years of age | 170 | 100–135 |

Hypomagnesemia (treatment)—
  Treatment dose is individualized by prescriber based on severity of deficiency.

**Strength(s) usually available**
U.S.—
  Not commercially available.
Canada—
  122 mg elemental magnesium (1500 mg magnesium pidolate) per 4 grams (OTC) [*Mag 2*].

Note: The strength of this magnesium preparation may exceed the dosage range recommended by USP DI Advisory Panels based on the amount necessary to meet normal nutritional needs.

**Packaging and storage**
Store below 40 °C (104 °F), preferably between 15 and 30 °C (59 and 86 °F), unless otherwise specified by manufacturer.

**Preparation of dosage form**
Pour contents of one pouch into a glass, add some water and stir quickly.

**Auxiliary labeling**
• Take before meals.

---

### *MAGNESIUM SULFATE*

## Summary of Differences

Category: Injection may also be used as an electrolyte replenisher.
Precautions: Drug interactions and/or related problems—Parenteral magnesium sulfate may form a precipitate when mixed with calcium salts. Possible additive effects when given with CNS depression–producing medications and neuromuscular blocking agents.

## Oral Dosage Forms

### MAGNESIUM SULFATE CRYSTALS

**Usual adult and adolescent dose**
Hypomagnesemia (prophylaxis)—
  Oral, amount based on normal daily recommended intakes of elemental magnesium:

| Persons | U.S. (mg) | Canada (mg) |
|---|---|---|
| Adolescent and adult males | 270–400 | 130–250 |
| Adolescent and adult females | 280–300 | 135–210 |
| Pregnant females | 320 | 195–245 |
| Breast-feeding females | 340–355 | 245–265 |

Hypomagnesemia (treatment)—
  Treatment dose is individualized by prescriber based on severity of deficiency.

**Usual pediatric dose**
Hypomagnesemia (prophylaxis)—
  Oral, amount based on normal daily recommended intakes of elemental magnesium:

| Persons | U.S. (mg) | Canada (mg) |
|---|---|---|
| Infants and children | | |
| Birth to 3 years of age | 40–80 | 20–50 |
| 4 to 6 years of age | 120 | 65 |
| 7 to 10 years of age | 170 | 100–135 |

Hypomagnesemia (treatment)—
  Treatment dose is individualized by prescriber based on severity of deficiency.

**Strength(s) usually available**
U.S.—
  40 mEq per 5 mg (OTC) [GENERIC].
Canada—
  Not commercially available.

Note: The strength of this magnesium preparation may exceed the dosage range recommended by USP DI Advisory Panels based on the amount necessary to meet normal nutritional needs.

**Packaging and storage**
Store below 40 °C (104 °F), preferably between 15 and 30 °C (59 and 86 °F), unless otherwise specified by manufacturer.

## Parenteral Dosage Forms

### MAGNESIUM SULFATE INJECTION USP

**Usual adult and adolescent dose**
Antihypomagnesemic or
Electrolyte replenisher—
  Intramuscular, 1 to 2 grams of a 50% solution (8.1 to 16.2 mEq elemental magnesium) four times a day until serum magnesium is within normal limits.
  Intravenous infusion, 5 grams (40.5 mEq elemental magnesium) in 1000 mL of dextrose 5% or sodium chloride 0.9% infused over 3 hours.
Hypomagnesemia (prophylaxis)—
  Intravenous infusion, as part of total parenteral nutrition solution, the specific amount determined by individual patient need.

**Usual pediatric dose**
Antihypomagnesemic or
Electrolyte replenisher—
  Intramuscular, 20 to 40 mg (0.16 to 0.32 mEq elemental magnesium) per kg of body weight in a 20% solution, repeated as necessary.
  Hypomagnesemia (prophylaxis)—Intravenous infusion, as part of total parenteral nutrition solutions, the specific amount determined by individual patient need.

**Strength(s) usually available**
U.S.—
  10% w/v (100 mg, 0.8 mEq, 0.8 mOsm per mL) (Rx) [GENERIC].
  12.5% w/v (125 mg, 1 mEq, 1 mOsm per mL) (Rx) [GENERIC].
  25% w/v (250 mg, 2 mEq per mL) (Rx) [GENERIC].
  50% w/v (500 mg, 4 mEq, 4 mOsm per mL) (Rx) [GENERIC].
Canada—
  50% w/v (500 mg per mL) (Rx) [GENERIC].

**Packaging and storage**
Store below 40 °C (104 °F), preferably between 15 and 30 °C (59 and 86 °F), unless otherwise specified by manufacturer.

**Incompatibilities**

Magnesium sulfate in solution may form a precipitate when mixed with solutions containing:

| | |
|---|---|
| Alcohol (in high concentrations) | Heavy metals |
| Alkali carbonates and bicarbonates | Hydrocortisone sodium succinate |
| Alkali hydroxides | Phosphates |
| Arsenates | Polymyxin B sulfate |
| Barium | Procaine hydrochloride |
| Calcium | Salicylates |
| Clindamycin phosphate | Sodium bicarbonate |
| Dobutamine | Strontium |
| Fat emulsions | Tartrates |

The potential incompatibility will often be influenced by changes in the concentration of reactants and the pH of the solution.

It has been reported that magnesium may reduce the antibiotic activity of streptomycin, tetracycline, and tobramycin when any of those medicines and magnesium are given together.

**Selected Bibliography**

Wester P. Magnesium. Am J Clin Nutr 1987; 45: 1305-12.
Gums J. Clinical significance of magnesium: a review. DICP 1987; 21: 240-6.

Revised: 12/03/92
Interim revision: 03/28/93; 08/23/94; 07/11/95

---

**MALATHION**—The *Malathion (Topical)* monograph is not included in this published version of the USP DI database. Copies of the monograph are available on request from Micromedex, Inc. - Reprint Requests, 6200 S. Syracuse Way, Suite 300, Englewood, CO 80111; telephone (303) 486-6400; telefax (303) 486-6464; Email: USPDI@MDX.COM.

---

**MALT SOUP EXTRACT**—See *Laxatives (Local)*

---

**MANGANESE CHLORIDE**—See *Manganese Supplements (Systemic)*

---

**MANGANESE SULFATE**—See *Manganese Supplements (Systemic)*

---

# MANGANESE SUPPLEMENTS   Systemic†

This monograph includes information on the following: 1) Manganese Chloride†; 2) Manganese Sulfate†.

VA CLASSIFICATION (Primary): TN499

Note:  For a listing of dosage forms and brand names by country availability, see *Dosage Forms* section(s).

†Not commercially available in Canada.

## Category

Nutritional supplement (mineral).

## Indications

**Accepted**

Manganese deficiency (prophylaxis and treatment)—Manganese supplements are indicated in the prevention and treatment of manganese deficiency, which may result from inadequate nutrition or intestinal malabsorption but does not occur in healthy individuals receiving an adequate balanced diet. For prophylaxis of manganese deficiency, dietary improvement, rather than supplementation, is advisable. For treatment of manganese deficiency, supplementation is preferred.

Although deficiency in humans has not been documented, deficiency of manganese in animals may lead to poor reproductive performance, growth retardation, congenital malformations in the offspring, abnormal formation of bone and cartilage, dermatitis, and impaired glucose tolerance.

Some unusual diets (e.g., reducing diets that drastically restrict food selection) may not supply minimum daily requirements of manganese. Supplementation may be necessary in patients receiving total parenteral nutrition (TPN) or undergoing rapid weight loss or in those with malnutrition, because of inadequate dietary intake.

## Pharmacology/Pharmacokinetics

**Physicochemical characteristics**
Molecular weight—
    Manganese chloride: 203.3.
    Manganese sulfate: 169.01.
    Elemental manganese: 54.9.

**Mechanism of action/Effect**
Manganese is an activator for enzymes such as polysaccharide polymerase, liver arginase, cholinesterase, and pyruvate carboxylase. It may also be a cofactor in lipid, protein, and carbohydrate metabolism.

**Absorption**
Variable, ranging from 3 to 50%. Manganese does undergo enterohepatic circulation.

**Protein binding**
Bound to a specific transport protein, transmanganin, a beta-1-globulin.

**Storage**
Manganese is concentrated in mitochondria-rich tissues such as brain, kidney, pancreas, and liver.

**Elimination**
Primarily through bile, but may be eliminated in pancreatic juice or returned to the lumen of duodenum, jejunum, or ileum in the event of biliary obstruction. Urinary excretion is negligible.

## Precautions to Consider

**Pregnancy/Reproduction**

Pregnancy—Studies have not been done in humans and problems in humans have not been documented with intake of normal daily recommended amounts.

Studies have not been done in animals.

FDA Pregnancy Category C (parenteral manganese).

**Breast-feeding**

Problems in humans have not been documented with intake of normal daily recommended amounts.

**Pediatrics**

Problems in pediatrics have not been documented with intake of normal daily recommended amounts.

Manganese sulfate injection that contains benzyl alcohol as a preservative should not be used in newborn and immature infants. The use of benzyl alcohol in neonates has been associated with a fatal toxic syndrome consisting of metabolic acidosis and CNS, respiratory, circulatory, and renal function impairment.

**Geriatrics**

Problems in geriatrics have not been documented with intake of normal daily recommended amounts.

**Medical considerations/Contraindications**

The medical considerations/contraindications included have been selected on the basis of their potential clinical significance (reasons given in parentheses where appropriate)—not necessarily inclusive (» = major clinical significance).

*Risk-benefit should be considered when the following medical problems exist:*

Biliary tract dysfunction or
Hepatic dysfunction
    (increased manganese blood concentrations may result because manganese is excreted in the bile)

**Patient monitoring**

The following may be especially important in patient monitoring (other tests may be warranted in some patients, depending on condition; » = major clinical significance):

Manganese concentrations, plasma
    (determinations may be recommended at monthly intervals; how-

ever, some clinicians do not recommend monitoring manganese concentrations because deficiency is rare)

## Side/Adverse Effects

There have been no reports of toxicity or side effects from oral manganese supplements.

## Patient Consultation

As an aid to patient consultation, refer to *Advice for the Patient, Manganese Supplements (Systemic)*.

In providing consultation, consider emphasizing the following selected information (» = major clinical significance):

**Description of use**
  Description should include function in the body, signs of deficiency
**Importance of diet**
  Importance of proper nutrition; supplement may be needed because of inadequate dietary intake
  Food sources of manganese
  Recommended daily intake for manganese
**Proper use of this dietary supplement**
  » Proper dosing
  Missed dose: No cause for concern because of length of time necessary for depletion; remembering to take as directed
  » Proper storage

## General Dosing Information

Because of the infrequency of manganese deficiency occurring alone, combinations of several vitamins and/or minerals are commonly administered. Many commercial vitamin-mineral complexes are available.

**For parenteral dosage forms only**
In most cases, parenteral administration is indicated only when oral administration is not acceptable (for example, in nausea, vomiting, preoperative and postoperative conditions) or possible (for example, in malabsorption syndromes or following gastric resection).

**Diet/Nutrition**
Recommended dietary intakes for manganese are defined differently worldwide.
For U.S.—
  The Recommended Dietary Allowances (RDAs) for vitamins and minerals are determined by the Food and Nutrition Board of the National Research Council and are intended to provide adequate nutrition in most healthy persons under usual environmental stresses. In addition, a different designation may be used by the FDA for food and dietary supplement labeling purposes, as with Daily Value (DV). DVs replace the previous labeling terminology United States Recommended Daily Allowances (USRDAs).
For Canada—
  Recommended Nutrient Intakes (RNIs) for vitamins, minerals, and protein are determined by Health and Welfare Canada and provide recommended amounts of a specific nutrient while minimizing the risk of chronic diseases.
There is no RDA or RNI established for manganese. The following daily intakes are considered adequate for all individuals:
  Infants and children:
    Birth to 3 years of age: 0.3 to 1.5 mg.
    4 to 6 years of age: 1.5 to 2 mg.
    7 to 10 years of age: 2 to 3 mg.
  Adolescents and adults:
    2 to 5 mg.

The best dietary sources of manganese include whole grains, cereal products, lettuce, dry beans, and peas.

---

### MANGANESE CHLORIDE

## Parenteral Dosage Forms

**MANGANESE CHLORIDE INJECTION USP**

**Usual adult and adolescent dose**
Deficiency (prophylaxis and treatment)—
  Intravenous, 200 mcg (0.2 mg) of elemental manganese a day, added to total parenteral nutrition (TPN).

**Usual pediatric dose**
Deficiency (prophylaxis and treatment)—
  Intravenous, 2 to 10 mcg (0.002 to 0.01 mg) of elemental manganese a day, added to total parenteral nutrition (TPN).

**Strength(s) usually available**
U.S.—
  360 mcg (0.36 mg) (0.1 mg elemental manganese) per mL (Rx) [GENERIC].
Canada—
  Not commercially available.

**Packaging and storage**
Store below 40 °C (104 °F), preferably between 15 and 30 °C (59 and 86 °F), unless otherwise specified by manufacturer.

---

### MANGANESE SULFATE

## Parenteral Dosage Forms

**MANGANESE SULFATE INJECTION USP**

**Usual adult and adolescent dose**
See *Manganese Chloride Injection USP*.

**Usual pediatric dose**
See *Manganese Chloride Injection USP*.

Note: Injection that contains benzyl alcohol as a preservative should not be used in newborn and immature infants. The use of benzyl alcohol in neonates has been associated with a fatal toxic syndrome consisting of metabolic acidosis and CNS, respiratory, circulatory, and renal function impairment.

**Strength(s) usually available**
U.S.—
  308 mcg (0.308 mg) (0.1 mg elemental manganese) per mL (Rx) [GENERIC].
Canada—
  Not commercially available.

**Packaging and storage**
Store below 40 °C (104 °F), preferably between 15 and 30 °C (59 and 86 °F), unless otherwise specified by manufacturer.

**Preparation of dosage form**
Manganese sulfate is compatible with amino acids, dextrose, electrolytes, and vitamins usually used for total parenteral nutrition (TPN).

Revised: 02/01/92
Interim revision: 08/07/92; 08/15/94; 04/25/95

---

# MANNITOL Systemic

VA CLASSIFICATION (Primary/Secondary): CV709/OP140

Commonly used brand name(s): *Osmitrol*.

Note: For a listing of dosage forms and brand names by country availability, see *Dosage Forms* section(s).

## Category

Diuretic; antiglaucoma agent (systemic); antihemolytic.

## Indications

Note: Bracketed information in the *Indications* section refers to uses that are not included in U.S. product labeling.

**Accepted**
Acute renal failure, oliguric phase (prophylaxis and treatment)—Mannitol, administered intravenously, is indicated to promote diuresis in the prevention and/or treatment of the oliguric phase of acute renal failure before irreversible renal failure becomes established.

Edema, cerebral (treatment) or
Intracranial pressure, elevated (treatment)—Mannitol, administered intravenously, is indicated to reduce intracranial pressure and treat cerebral edema by reducing brain mass.

Intraocular pressure, elevated (treatment)—Mannitol, administered intravenously, is indicated to reduce elevated intraocular pressure after other methods have failed or in preparation for intraocular surgery.

Toxicity, nonspecific (treatment)—Mannitol, administered intravenously, is indicated to promote urinary excretion of and prevent renal damage due to toxic substances (for example, salicylates, barbiturates, bromides, lithium).

Hemolysis (prophylaxis)—Mannitol, when used as an irrigating solution, is indicated to prevent hemolysis and hemoglobin buildup during transurethral prostatic resection or other transurethral surgical procedures. [It has also been used to prevent hemolysis during cardiopulmonary bypass procedures.][1]

**Unaccepted**

Mannitol has been used to measure glomerular filtration rate (GFR) in acute oliguria but has generally been replaced by more accurate tests.

[1]Not included in Canadian product labeling.

## Pharmacology/Pharmacokinetics

**Physicochemical characteristics**
Molecular weight—182.17.

**Mechanism of action/Effect**
Mannitol is an osmotic diuretic that is metabolically inert in humans and occurs naturally, as a sugar, in fruits and vegetables.

Osmotic agent (systemic)—
  Mannitol elevates blood plasma osmolality, resulting in enhanced flow of water from tissues, including the brain and cerebrospinal fluid, into interstitial fluid and plasma. As a result, cerebral edema, elevated intracranial pressure, and cerebrospinal fluid volume and pressure may be reduced.

Diuretic—
  Induces diuresis because mannitol is not reabsorbed in the renal tubule, thereby increasing the osmolality of the glomerular filtrate, facilitating excretion of water, and inhibiting the renal tubular reabsorption of sodium, chloride, and other solutes. It may, therefore, promote the urinary excretion of toxic materials and protect against nephrotoxicity by preventing the concentration of toxic substances in the tubular fluid.

Antiglaucoma agent—
  Elevates blood plasma osmolarity, resulting in enhanced flow of water from the eye into plasma and a consequent reduction in intraocular pressure.

Antihemolytic—
  When used as an irrigating solution in transurethral prostatic resection, dilute solutions of mannitol may minimize the hemolytic effect of water used alone. The entrance of hemolyzed blood into the circulation and the resultant hemoglobinemia may also be reduced.

Diagnostic aid (renal function)—
  Mannitol is freely filtered by the glomeruli with less than 10% tubular reabsorption. Therefore, its urinary excretion rate may serve as a measurement of glomerular filtration rate (GFR).

**Absorption**
Intravascular absorption during irrigation for transurethral prostatic resection is variable and depends primarily on the extent of the surgery.

**Distribution**
Mannitol remains in the extracellular compartment. If very high concentrations of mannitol are present in the plasma or the patient has acidosis, then mannitol may cross the blood-brain barrier and cause a rebound increase in intracranial pressure.

**Biotransformation**
Mannitol is metabolized only slightly, if at all, to glycogen in the liver.

**Half-life**
Approximately 100 minutes (may be increased to 36 hours in acute renal failure).

**Onset of action**
Diuresis—1 to 3 hours.
Reduction in cerebrospinal and intraocular fluid pressure—Within 15 minutes after start of infusion.

**Time to peak effect**
Reduction in intraocular pressure—30 to 60 minutes after injection.

**Duration of action**
Reduction in cerebrospinal fluid pressure—persists for 3 to 8 hours after infusion is discontinued.
Reduction in intraocular pressure—persists for 4 to 8 hours.

**Elimination**
Renal; 80% of a 100-gram intravenous dose appears in the urine within 3 hours.

## Precautions to Consider

**Carcinogenicity**
An early study with 1%, 5%, and 10% mannitol given for 94 weeks to Wistar rats found a low incidence of benign thymomas in females. However, a subsequent lifetime study at similar doses in Sprague-Dawley, Fischer, and Wistar rats found no evidence of carcinogenicity.

**Mutagenicity**
*In vivo* and *in vitro* mutagenicity studies were negative.

**Pregnancy/Reproduction**
Pregnancy—Adequate and well-controlled studies have not been done in humans.
Studies in mice, rats, and rabbits at oral doses up to 1600 mg per kg of body weight (mg/kg) did not find adverse effects on the fetus.
FDA Pregnancy Category B.

**Breast-feeding**
It is not known whether mannitol is distributed into breast milk. However, problems in humans have not been documented.

**Pediatrics**
Appropriate studies on the relationship of age to the effects of mannitol have not been performed in the pediatric population. Although mannitol has been used in this population and no pediatrics-specific problems have been documented to date, safety and efficacy have not been established in children younger than 12 years of age.

**Geriatrics**
No information is available on the relationship of age to the effects of mannitol in geriatric patients. However, elderly patients are more likely to have age-related renal function impairment, which may require caution in patients receiving mannitol.

**Drug interactions and/or related problems**
The following drug interactions and/or related problems have been selected on the basis of their potential clinical significance (possible mechanism in parentheses where appropriate)—not necessarily inclusive (» = major clinical significance):

Note: Combinations containing any of the following medications, depending on the amount present, may also interact with this medication.

» Digitalis glycosides
  (concurrent use with mannitol may enhance the possibility of digitalis toxicity associated with hypokalemia)

Diuretics, other, including carbonic anhydrase inhibitors
  (diuretic and intraocular pressure–reducing effects may be potentiated when these medications are used concurrently with mannitol; dosage adjustments may be necessary)

**Laboratory value alterations**
The following have been selected on the basis of their potential clinical significance (possible effect in parentheses where appropriate)—not necessarily inclusive (» = major clinical significance):

With physiology/laboratory test values
  Phosphate or
  Potassium or
  Sodium
    (serum concentrations may be decreased by excessive and prolonged use)

**Medical considerations/Contraindications**
The medical considerations/contraindications included have been selected on the basis of their potential clinical significance (reasons given in parentheses where appropriate)—not necessarily inclusive (» = major clinical significance).

*Except under special circumstances, this medication should not be used when the following medical problems exist:*

» Anuria, with well-established acute tubular necrosis due to severe renal disease
  (if patients do not respond to test dose; accumulation may lead to overexpansion of extracellular fluid and circulatory overload)

» Dehydration, severe
  (may be exacerbated by fluid loss caused by mannitol; may result in serious electrolyte imbalances)

» Heart failure or pulmonary congestion, progressive, after beginning mannitol therapy

» Intracranial bleeding, active, except during craniotomy
  (mannitol may increase bleeding by increasing cerebral blood flow)

» Pulmonary congestion or pulmonary edema, severe

» Renal damage or dysfunction, progressive, after beginning mannitol therapy, including worsening oliguria and azotemia

*Risk-benefit should be considered when the following medical problems exist:*

» Cardiopulmonary function impairment, significant
(sudden expansion of extracellular fluid may lead to congestive heart failure)

Hyperkalemia or
Hyponatremia or
Hypovolemia
(mannitol-induced sudden changes in fluid balance may further aggravate depleted or excessive electrolyte concentrations or fluid volume; serum sodium concentrations may be further diluted in hyponatremic patients by the shift of sodium-free intracellular fluid into the extracellular compartment; rapid or prolonged administration of mannitol, causing a loss of water in excess of electrolytes, may result in hypernatremia; mannitol-induced sustained diuresis may obscure or aggravate hypovolemia)

» Renal function impairment, significant
(accumulation of mannitol may lead to overexpansion of extracellular fluid and circulatory overload)

Sensitivity to mannitol

**Patient monitoring**

The following may be especially important in patient monitoring (other tests may be warranted in some patients, depending on condition; » = major clinical significance):

Blood pressure measurements and
» Electrolyte measurements, serum, including potassium and sodium, and
» Renal function determinations and
» Urine output determinations
(recommended during administration of mannitol, especially with large or repeated doses)

## Side/Adverse Effects

Note: The most serious side/adverse effect of mannitol is fluid and electrolyte imbalance. Rapid administration of large doses may lead to accumulation of mannitol, overexpansion of extracellular fluid, dilutional hyponatremia and occasional hyperkalemia, and circulatory overload, especially in patients with acute or chronic renal failure. Inadequate hydration or hypovolemia may be obscured by the diuresis produced by mannitol, which may lead to tissue dehydration, promotion of oliguria, and intensification of pre-existing hemoconcentration. Extravasation of mannitol may result in edema and skin necrosis.

When mannitol is used as an irrigating solution during transurethral prostatectomy, a systemic effect, from the entry of large volumes of mannitol into the systemic circulation, can occur, which can result in a significant alteration of cardiopulmonary and renal dynamics.

The following side/adverse effects have been selected on the basis of their potential clinical significance (possible signs and symptoms in parentheses where appropriate)—not necessarily inclusive:

**Those indicating need for medical attention**
Incidence rare
*Chest pain or fast heartbeat; chills or fever; difficult urination; electrolyte imbalance* (confusion; irregular heartbeat; muscle cramps or pain; numbness, tingling, pain, or weakness in hands or feet; seizures; trembling; unusual tiredness or weakness; weakness and heaviness of legs); *pulmonary congestion* (coughing; troubled breathing; wheezing); *renal failure* (sudden decrease in amount of urine; swelling of face, feet, or lower legs; skin rash; unusual weight gain; shortness of breath; troubled breathing; wheezing; tightness in chest; increase in blood pressure; unusual thirst; *swelling of feet or lower legs; thrombophlebitis* (redness, swelling, or pain at injection site)

**Those indicating need for medical attention only if they continue or are bothersome**
Incidence more frequent
*Dryness of mouth or increased thirst; headache; increased urination; nausea or vomiting*
Incidence less frequent
*Blurred vision; dizziness; skin rash or hives*

Note: In some cases, *headache, nausea* or *vomiting, blurred vision,* and *dizziness* may be symptoms of subdural or subarachnoid hemorrhage as a result of dehydration of the brain.

## General Dosing Information

One gram of mannitol is equivalent to approximately 5.5 milliosmole (mOsm).

The number of mOsm of mannitol per liter of sterile water for injection is as follows:

| Mannitol (%) | mOsm/liter (approx) |
|---|---|
| 5 | 275 |
| 10 | 550 |
| 15 | 825 |
| 20 | 1100 |
| 25 | 1375 |

Mannitol must be administered by intravenous infusion.

The administration set should include a filter when mannitol solutions with concentrations of 15% or above are infused, since these solutions have a greater tendency to crystallize when exposed to low temperatures.

The total dosage, concentration, and rate of administration should be determined by the nature and severity of the condition being treated, fluid requirement, and urinary output. The rate is usually adjusted to maintain an adequate urine flow (at least 30 to 50 mL per hour). Mannitol infusion should be discontinued promptly if urine output is low.

A test dose of mannitol is recommended prior to therapy in patients with marked oliguria or possible inadequate renal function. The test dose is given as an intravenous infusion, 200 mg per kg of body weight (mg/kg) as a 15 to 25% solution, administered over a period of three to five minutes. In children the dose is 200 mg/kg or 6 grams per square meter of body surface area as a 15 to 25% solution, administered over a period of three to five minutes. If urine flow does not increase to at least 30 to 50 mL per hour for two to three hours after this or a second test dose, mannitol should be withheld until the patient is re-evaluated.

If renal failure, heart failure, or pulmonary congestion progresses after starting mannitol therapy, mannitol should be discontinued.

Alkalinization of the urine with sodium bicarbonate may be necessary to aid in treatment of salicylate or barbiturate poisonings.

## Parenteral Dosage Forms

### MANNITOL INJECTION USP

**Usual adult dose:**

Note: As a general guide to therapy, the usual adult dose ranges from 50 to 200 grams in a twenty-four hour period, but in most cases an adequate response will be achieved at a usual dosage of approximately 100 grams in twenty-four hours.

Acute renal failure (oliguria), prophylaxis—
During surgery, immediately postoperatively, or following trauma: Intravenous infusion, 50 to 100 grams as a 5 to 25% solution, the concentration and amount depending upon the fluid requirements of the patient. Following suspected or actual hemolytic transfusion reactions to provoke diuresis: Intravenous infusion, 20 grams, over a period of five minutes. If diuresis does not occur, the 20-gram dose may be repeated. If urine flow is adequate (30 to 50 mL per hour), intravenous fluids containing not more than 50 to 75 milliequivalents (mEq) of sodium per liter should be given in sufficient volume to match the desired urine flow (100 mL per hour) until the patient can take fluids orally.

Acute renal failure (oliguria), treatment—
Intravenous infusion, 50 to 100 grams as a 15 to 25% solution.

Cerebral edema or
Elevated intracranial pressure or
Elevated intraocular pressure—
Intravenous infusion, 0.25 to 2 grams per kg of body weight as a 15 to 25% solution, administered over a period of thirty to sixty minutes. The patient's fluid and electrolyte balance, body weight, and total input and output should be closely monitored before and after infusion of mannitol. Evidence of reduced cerebral-spinal fluid pressure may be observed within fifteen minutes after starting the infusion. Maximal reduction of intraocular pressure occurs thirty to sixty minutes after the injection. When used preoperatively, the dose should be given sixty to ninety minutes before surgery to achieve maximum reduction of pressure before operation.

Note: In small or debilitated patients, a dose of 500 mg per kg of body weight may be sufficient.

Toxicity, nonspecific (to promote urinary excretion of toxic substances)—
Intravenous infusion, as a 5 to 25% solution (the concentration dependent upon the patient's fluid requirement and urinary output), as long as indicated if the level of urinary output remains high. Intravenous water and electrolytes must be given to replace the loss of these substances in the urine, sweat, and expired air. If benefits are not observed after administering 200 grams, mannitol should be discontinued.

Antihemolytic (urologic irrigation)—
   Mannitol may be used as a 2.5% irrigating solution for the bladder during transurethral prostatic resection or other transurethral surgical procedures.

**Usual adult prescribing limits**
6 grams per kg of body weight per twenty-four hours.

**Usual pediatric dose**
Diuretic—
   Intravenous infusion, 0.25 to 2 grams per kg of body weight or 60 grams per square meter of body surface area as a 15 to 20% solution, administered over a period of two to six hours.
Cerebral edema or
Elevated intracranial pressure or
Elevated intraocular pressure—
   Intravenous infusion, 1 to 2 grams per kg of body weight or 30 to 60 grams per square meter of body surface area as a 15 to 20% solution, administered over a period of thirty to sixty minutes.
Note: In small or debilitated patients, a dose of 500 mg per kg of body weight may be sufficient.
Toxicity, nonspecific—
   Intravenous infusion, up to 2 grams per kg of body weight or 60 grams per square meter of body surface area as a 5 to 10% solution.

**Strength(s) usually available**
U.S.—
   5% (Rx) [*Osmitrol;* GENERIC].
   10% (Rx) [*Osmitrol;* GENERIC].
   15% (Rx) [*Osmitrol;* GENERIC].
   20% (Rx) [*Osmitrol;* GENERIC].
   25% (Rx) [*Osmitrol;* GENERIC].
Canada—
   5% (Rx) [*Osmitrol*].
   10% (Rx) [*Osmitrol*].
   15% (Rx) [*Osmitrol*].
   20% (Rx) [*Osmitrol*].
   25% (Rx) [GENERIC].

**Packaging and storage**
Store below 40 °C (104 °F), preferably between 15 and 30 °C (59 and 86 °F), unless otherwise specified by manufacturer. Protect from freezing.

**Preparation of dosage form**
To prepare a 2.5% irrigating solution, add the contents of two 50-mL ampuls of 25% Mannitol Injection USP to 900 mL of sterile water for injection.

**Stability**
Solutions of mannitol may crystallize, especially if chilled. To dissolve crystals, see manufacturer's package insert for directions. If all crystals cannot be completely dissolved, the solution should not be used.
The contents of opened containers should be used promptly. Unused contents should be discarded.

**Incompatibilities**
Electrolyte-free mannitol solutions should not be given conjointly with blood. If blood must be administered simultaneously with mannitol, at least 20 mEq (mmol) of sodium chloride should be added to each liter of mannitol solution to prevent pseudoagglutination.

## Selected Bibliography
Nissenson AR, Weston RE, Kleeman CR. Mannitol. West J Med 1979 Oct; 131: 277-84.
Warren SE, Blantz RC. Mannitol. Arch Intern Med 1981 Mar; 141: 493-7.

Revised: 07/15/98

---

# MAPROTILINE  Systemic

VA CLASSIFICATION (Primary/Secondary): CN609/CN103
Commonly used brand name(s): *Ludiomil*.
Note: For a listing of dosage forms and brand names by country availability, see *Dosage Forms* section(s).

## Category
Antidepressant; antineuralgic.

## Indications
Note: Bracketed information in the *Indications* section refers to uses that are not included in U.S. product labeling.

**Accepted**
Bipolar disorder, depressed type (treatment)
Depressive disorder, major (treatment) or
Dysthymia (treatment)—Maprotiline is indicated for the treatment of depressive illness in patients with major depressive disorder, dysthymic disorder, or bipolar disorder, depressed type.
Anxiety associated with mental depression (treatment)—Maprotiline is also indicated for the management of anxiety associated with mental depression.
[Pain, neurogenic (treatment)][1]—Maprotiline is used to treat some types of chronic pain.

[1] Not included in Canadian product labeling.

## Pharmacology/Pharmacokinetics

**Physicochemical characteristics**
Molecular weight—313.87.

**Mechanism of action/Effect**
A tetracyclic antidepressant, maprotiline is thought to increase the synaptic concentration of norepinephrine in the central nervous system (CNS) by blocking its re-uptake by the presynaptic neuronal membrane. No effect on serotonin re-uptake has been observed. Recent research has suggested that after long-term treatment with antidepressants, changes in postsynaptic beta-adrenergic receptor sensitivity and enhancement of response to alpha-adrenergic and serotonergic stimulation may contribute to the mechanism of antidepressant action. Antidepressants may produce a downregulation (desensitization) of presynaptic $alpha_2$ receptors, equilibrating the noradrenergic system, and thus correcting the dysregulated output of depressed patients.

**Absorption**
Completely absorbed following oral administration.

**Protein binding**
High (88%).

**Biotransformation**
Hepatic.

**Half-life**
Elimination—27 to 58 hours (average 43 hours).
Active metabolite—60 to 90 hours.

**Onset of action**
For desired therapeutic effect, up to 2 or 3 weeks, but sometimes within 7 days.

**Time to peak concentration**
12 hours.

**Elimination**
Biliary—About 30%, in feces.
Renal—About 65%, mostly as glucuronide metabolites.

## Precautions to Consider
Note: The similarity of pharmacological effects of maprotiline and tricyclic antidepressants suggests that the same considerations and precautions be observed in the use of both medications. Therefore, until additional specific clinical information on maprotiline is available, certain precautionary guidelines for tricyclic antidepressants are included for consideration.

**Carcinogenicity**
No evidence of carcinogenicity was found in studies of animals given large daily doses of maprotiline for up to 1 year.

**Mutagenicity**
No evidence of mutagenicity was found in offspring of female mice mated with male mice treated with up to 60 times the maximum daily human dose.

**Pregnancy/Reproduction**
Pregnancy—Adequate and well-controlled studies in humans have not been done.
Studies in animals have not shown that maprotiline causes adverse effects on the fetus.
FDA Pregnancy Category B.

## Breast-feeding
Maprotiline is distributed into breast milk in the same concentration as in blood.

## Pediatrics
Appropriate studies on the relationship of age to the effects of maprotiline have not been performed in children up to 18 years of age. Safety and efficacy have not been established.

## Geriatrics
Elderly patients are more likely to exhibit increased dose sensitivity to the anticholinergic, sedative, and hypotensive effects of maprotiline; therefore, a lower initial dose should usually be used and the dosage maintained at the lowest effective level. Careful monitoring is necessary to maintain optimum therapeutic serum concentrations in the elderly. Orthostatic hypotension, although rare, may occur in elderly patients and caution must be observed to prevent falls.

## Dental
The peripheral anticholinergic effects of maprotiline may decrease or inhibit salivary flow, especially in middle-aged or elderly patients, thus contributing to the development of caries, periodontal disease, oral candidiasis, and discomfort.

Although rarely reported, the blood dyscrasia–causing effects of maprotiline may result in an increased incidence of microbial infection, delayed healing, and gingival bleeding. If agranulocytosis, eosinophilia, purpura, or thrombocytopenia occurs, dental work should be deferred until blood counts have returned to normal. Patient instruction in proper oral hygiene should include caution in use of regular toothbrushes, dental floss, and toothpicks.

## Drug interactions and/or related problems
The following drug interactions and/or related problems have been selected on the basis of their potential clinical significance (possible mechanism in parentheses where appropriate)—not necessarily inclusive (» = major clinical significance):

Note: Combinations containing any of the following medications, depending on the amount present, may also interact with this medication.

Although not all of the following interactions have been documented to pertain specifically to maprotiline, a potential exists for their occurrence because of the close similarity of maprotiline's pharmacological effects to those of tricyclic antidepressants.

» Alcohol or
» CNS depression–producing medications, other (see *Appendix II*)
(concurrent use with maprotiline may result in serious potentiation of CNS depressant effects)

Anticholinergics or other medications with anticholinergic activity (see *Appendix II*) or
Antihistamines
(concurrent use may potentiate the anticholinergic effects of either these medications or maprotiline; dosage adjustments may be necessary)

Anticonvulsants
(maprotiline may enhance CNS depression, lower the seizure threshold, and decrease the effects of the anticonvulsant medication)

Antidepressants, tricyclic or
Bupropion or
Clozapine or
Haloperidol or
Loxapine or
Molindone or
Phenothiazines or
Pimozide or
Thioxanthenes or
Trazodone
(concurrent use may prolong and intensify the anticholinergic and sedative effects of either these medications or maprotiline; in addition, these medications may increase the risk of seizures by lowering the seizure threshold, and should be added or withdrawn with caution)

Cimetidine
(concurrent use may increase plasma concentrations of maprotiline; dosage adjustment of maprotiline may be necessary when cimetidine therapy is initiated or discontinued)

Clonidine or
Guanadrel or
Guanethidine
(antihypertensive effects may be decreased when these medications are used concurrently with maprotiline)

(concurrent use of clonidine with maprotiline may result in serious potentiation of CNS depressant effects)

Contraceptives, oral, estrogen-containing or
Estrogens
(concurrent use of large doses of estrogens with tricyclic antidepressants may potentiate antidepressant side effects and reduce the therapeutic effects of the tricyclic antidepressants; although not documented, similar effects may occur with maprotiline, a tetracyclic antidepressant)

Fluoxetine
(plasma concentrations of tricyclic antidepressants may be increased twofold or more when fluoxetine is used concurrently; although not documented, similar increases may occur with maprotiline, a tetracyclic antidepressant; some clinicians recommend dosage reductions of maprotiline of 50% or greater if used concomitantly with fluoxetine)

» Monoamine oxidase (MAO) inhibitors, including furazolidone, procarbazine, and selegiline
(concurrent use with maprotiline is generally not recommended, especially on an outpatient basis, as hyperpyretic episodes, severe convulsions, hypertensive crises, and death have resulted in a small number of patients from concurrent use with tricyclic antidepressants; a minimum of 14 days should elapse between discontinuing MAO inhibitors and initiating maprotiline therapy)

Naphazoline, ophthalmic or
Oxymetazoline, nasal or
Phenylephrine, nasal or ophthalmic or
Xylometazoline, nasal
(if significant systemic absorption occurs, concurrent use with maprotiline may potentiate pressor effects of these medications)

» Sympathomimetics
(concurrent use with maprotiline may potentiate cardiovascular effects, possibly resulting in arrhythmias, tachycardia, or severe hypertension or hyperpyrexia; phentolamine can control the adverse reaction)

(significant systemic absorption of ophthalmic epinephrine may also potentiate cardiovascular effects; also, local anesthetics with vasoconstrictors should be avoided or a minimal amount of the vasoconstrictor should be used with the local anesthetic)

(concurrent use with maprotiline may decrease the pressor effects of ephedrine and mephentermine)

Thyroid hormones
(concurrent use with maprotiline may enhance the possibility of cardiac arrhythmias; dosage adjustments may be necessary)

## Medical considerations/Contraindications
The medical considerations/contraindications included have been selected on the basis of their potential clinical significance (reasons given in parentheses where appropriate)—not necessarily inclusive (» = major clinical significance).

*Except under special circumstances, this medication should not be used when the following medical problems exist:*

» Myocardial infarction, during the acute recovery period
» Seizure disorders, including epilepsy, or history of seizures
(risk of seizures is increased)

*Risk-benefit should be considered when the following medical problems exist:*

» Alcoholism, active
(increased risk of seizures and CNS depression)
» Asthma or
» Blood disorders or
» Glaucoma, angle-closure or
» Increased intraocular pressure or
» Urinary retention, or history of
(may be exacerbated)
» Bipolar disorder
(swing to hypomanic or manic phase may be accelerated and rapid cycling between mania and depression may be induced by maprotiline)
» Cardiovascular disorders
(increased risk of conduction defects, arrhythmias, myocardial infarction, strokes, and tachycardia)

Gastrointestinal disorders
(risk of paralytic ileus)
» Hepatic function impairment
(metabolism may be altered)
» Hyperthyroidism
(increased risk of cardiovascular toxicity)

» Myocardial infarction, history of
(increased risk of recurrence)
Prostatic hypertrophy
(risk of urinary retention)
» Schizophrenia
(psychosis may be aggravated)
Sensitivity to maprotiline or tricyclic antidepressants

**Patient monitoring**
The following may be especially important in patient monitoring (other tests may be warranted in some patients, depending on condition; » = major clinical significance):
Blood cell counts
(may be required at periodic intervals during long-term therapy; in patients with sore throat and fever, leukocyte and differential counts may be necessary; maprotiline should be discontinued if there is evidence of pathologic neutrophil depression)
Blood pressure determinations and
Cardiac function monitoring and
Hepatic function determinations
(may be required at periodic intervals during therapy to detect development of adverse effects that may not be evident to the patient)
Careful observation for possibility of drug-induced acceleration to hypomania or mania
(recommended periodically although most patients respond favorably to maprotiline when it is used to treat the depressed phase of bipolar disorder)
Careful observation for possibility of suicide attempt
(suicidal tendencies may persist in some severely depressed patients during the early phases of therapy until significant remission of depression occurs)

## Side/Adverse Effects

Note: Although not all of the following side effects have been attributed specifically to maprotiline, a potential exists for their occurrence as with the tricyclic antidepressants.

The following side/adverse effects have been selected on the basis of their potential clinical significance (possible signs and symptoms in parentheses where appropriate)—not necessarily inclusive:

**Those indicating need for medical attention**
Incidence more frequent
*Skin rash, redness, swelling, or itching*
Incidence less frequent
*Constipation, severe*—may lead to paralytic ileus; *nausea or vomiting; seizures; shakiness or trembling; unusual excitement; weight loss*
Note: *Seizures* may occur in patients with or without a history of seizures, usually with doses above 200 mg a day. The lowest effective maintenance dose is recommended to reduce further risk. Drugs that alter seizure threshold should be added to or withdrawn from maprotiline regimen with caution.
Incidence rare
*Agranulocytosis* (sore throat and fever)—rarely reported for maprotiline, but has occurred with tricyclic antidepressants; *anticholinergic effect* (difficulty in urinating); *breast enlargement*—in males and females; *confusion*—especially in elderly; *hallucinations; hypotension* (fainting); *inappropriate secretion of milk*—in females; *irregular heartbeat; jaundice, cholestatic* (yellow eyes or skin); *swelling of testicles*

**Those indicating need for medical attention only if they continue or are bothersome**
Incidence more frequent
*Blurred vision; dizziness or lightheadedness*—especially in the elderly; *drowsiness; dryness of mouth; headache; impotence* (decreased sexual ability); *increased or decreased sexual drive; tiredness or weakness*
Incidence less frequent
*Constipation, mild; diarrhea; heartburn; increased appetite and weight gain*—related to carbohydrate craving; *increased sensitivity of skin to sunlight; increased sweating; insomnia* (trouble in sleeping); *weight loss*

## Overdose
For specific information on the agents used in the management of maprotiline overdose, see:
• *Barbiturates (Systemic)* monograph;
• *Benzodiazepines (Systemic)* monograph;
• *Charcoal, Activated (Oral-Local)* monograph;
• *Corticosteroids—Glucocorticoid Effects (Systemic)* monograph;
• *Digitalis Glycosides (Systemic)* monograph;
• *Phenytoin* in *Anticonvulsants, Hydantoin (Systemic)* monograph;
• *Propranolol* in *Beta-adrenergic Blocking Agents (Systemic)* monograph; and/or
• *Sodium Bicarbonate (Systemic)* monograph.

For more information on the management of overdose or unintentional ingestion, **contact a Poison Control Center** (see *Poison Control Center Listing*).

**Clinical effects of overdose**
The following effects have been selected on the basis of their potential clinical significance (possible signs and symptoms in parentheses where appropriate)—not necessarily inclusive:

*Coma; convulsions; dizziness, severe; drowsiness, severe; fast or irregular heartbeat; fever; muscle stiffness or weakness, severe; restlessness or agitation; trouble in breathing; vomiting*

Note: Risk of *seizures, respiratory complications,* and *cardiotoxicity* is greater with maprotiline than with tricyclic antidepressants, and duration of comatose state and QRS complex is longer.

**Treatment of overdose**
There is no specific antidote for maprotiline overdose. The following steps of supportive and symptomatic treatment may be considered:
To decrease absorption—
Emptying stomach with emetic and/or lavage.
Administering activated charcoal slurry followed by a stimulant cathartic.
Specific treatment—
For circulatory collapse—Administering intravenous fluids, oxygen, and corticosteroids.
For congestive heart failure—Digitalizing rapidly.
For cardiac arrhythmias—Alkalinizing blood with sodium bicarbonate. Arrhythmias refractory to sodium bicarbonate may be treated with phenytoin. Propranolol may be used with caution.
For seizures and hyperirritability—Administering carefully titrated parenteral benzodiazepines or barbiturates. However, barbiturates should not be used if monoamine oxidase inhibitors have been used in recent therapy. Also, barbiturates may cause respiratory depression, especially in children. Equipment should be available to provide artificial ventilation and resuscitation. Administration of physostigmine salicylate is not recommended because of an increase in the risk of seizures.
Supportive care—
Controlling hyperpyrexia by any available means, including ice packs if necessary.
Patients in whom intentional overdose is known or suspected should be referred for psychiatric consultation.
Note: Dialysis of maprotiline has not been successful because of its high protein binding.

## Patient Consultation

As an aid to patient consultation, refer to *Advice for the Patient, Maprotiline (Systemic)*.
In providing consultation, consider emphasizing the following selected information (» = major clinical significance):

**Before using this medication**
» Conditions affecting use, especially:
Sensitivity to maprotiline or tricyclic antidepressants
Use in the elderly—Elderly patients may be more prone to develop anticholinergic, sedative, and hypotensive effects
Dental—Dry mouth may cause caries, oral candidiasis, periodontal disease, and discomfort; rare blood dyscrasias may result in increased incidence of microbial infection, delayed healing, and gingival bleeding
Other medications, especially alcohol or other CNS depression–producing medications, MAO inhibitors, or sympathomimetics
Other medical problems, especially active alcoholism, asthma, bipolar disorder, blood disorders, cardiovascular disorders, glaucoma, hepatic function impairment, hyperthyroidism, increased intraocular pressure, schizophrenia, seizure disorders, or urinary retention

**Proper use of this medication**
» Compliance with therapy
» May require up to 2 to 3 weeks of therapy to obtain optimal antidepressant effects
» Proper dosing
Missed dose: If dosing schedule is:

More than one dose a day—Taking as soon as possible; if almost time for next dose, skipping missed dose; going back to regular dosing schedule; not doubling doses

One dose a day at bedtime—Not taking missed dose following morning; checking with doctor

» Proper storage

**Precautions while using this medication**
Regular visits to physician to check progress during therapy
» Avoiding the use of alcohol or other CNS depressants during maprotiline therapy
» Possible drowsiness; caution when driving, using machines, or doing other things requiring alertness
» Possible dizziness or lightheadedness; caution when getting up suddenly from a lying or sitting position
» Possible dryness of mouth; using sugarless gum or candy, ice, or saliva substitute for relief; checking with physician or dentist if dry mouth continues for more than 2 weeks
» Caution if any kind of surgery, dental treatment, or emergency treatment is required
» Checking with physician before discontinuing medication; gradual dosage reduction may be needed

**Side/adverse effects**
Anticholinergic, sedative, and hypotensive effects more likely to occur in the elderly
Precautions followed for 3 to 7 days after discontinuing medication
Signs of potential side effects, especially skin rash, redness, swelling, or itching; severe constipation; convulsions; nausea or vomiting; shakiness or trembling; unusual excitement; weight loss; agranulocytosis; anticholinergic effect; breast enlargement; confusion; hallucinations; hypotension; inappropriate secretion of milk; irregular heartbeat; jaundice; or swelling of testicles

## General Dosing Information

Dosage of maprotiline must be individualized for each patient by titration.

Correlations between plasma concentration, clinical response, side effects, and toxicity have not been established.

Some clinicians recommend that for maintenance therapy, the optimal daily dose may be reduced somewhat, sometimes given as a single dose at bedtime, and often continued for 6 months to 1 year. (A divided dose may be preferred for geriatric, adolescent, or cardiovascular patients.) In patients with recurrent depression, however, continuation of the full treatment dose during maintenance therapy may be optimal.

The single daily dose at bedtime is useful when side effects such as excessive drowsiness or dizziness might be bothersome or dangerous during working hours.

A gradual reduction in dosage is recommended when this medication is to be discontinued.

Potentially suicidal patients should not have access to large quantities of this medication since depressed patients, particularly those who may use alcohol excessively, may continue to exhibit suicidal tendencies until significant improvement occurs. Some clinicians recommend that the patient be supplied with the least amount of medication necessary for satisfactory patient management.

## Oral Dosage Forms

### MAPROTILINE HYDROCHLORIDE TABLETS USP

**Usual adult and adolescent dose**
Antidepressant—
Oral, initially 25 to 75 mg a day, in divided doses, for at least two weeks, the dosage being adjusted gradually by 25 mg a day as needed and tolerated.

Note: The effective maintenance dose is usually about 150 mg a day, often given once a day at bedtime.

**Usual adult prescribing limits**
Outpatients: Up to 150 mg a day.
Hospitalized patients: Up to 225 mg a day.

**Usual pediatric dose**
Children up to 18 years of age: Safety and efficacy have not been established.

**Usual geriatric dose**
Initial: Oral, 25 mg a day.
Maintenance: Oral, 50 to 75 mg a day.

**Strength(s) usually available**
U.S.—
  25 mg (Rx) [*Ludiomil* (lactose); GENERIC].
  50 mg (Rx) [*Ludiomil* (lactose); GENERIC].
  75 mg (Rx) [*Ludiomil* (lactose); GENERIC].
Canada—
  10 mg (Rx) [*Ludiomil* (lactose)].
  25 mg (Rx) [*Ludiomil* (lactose; tartrazine)].
  50 mg (Rx) [*Ludiomil* (lactose)].
  75 mg (Rx) [*Ludiomil* (scored; lactose)].

**Packaging and storage**
Store below 40 °C (104 °F), preferably between 15 and 30 °C (59 and 86 °F), unless otherwise specified by manufacturer. Store in a well-closed container.

**Auxiliary labeling**
• May cause drowsiness.
• Avoid alcoholic beverages.

Revised: 08/29/94
Interim revision: 08/07/98

---

# MASOPROCOL Topical†

VA CLASSIFICATION (Primary): DE600
Commonly used brand name(s): *Actinex*.
Note: For a listing of dosage forms and brand names by country availability, see *Dosage Forms* section(s).

†Not commercially available in Canada.

## Category
Antineoplastic (topical).

## Indications

**Accepted**
Actinic keratoses, multiple (treatment)—Topical masoprocol is indicated for treatment of actinic (solar) keratoses.

## Pharmacology/Pharmacokinetics

**Physicochemical characteristics**
Molecular weight—302.37.

**Mechanism of action/Effect**
Unknown. Masoprocol is a potent 5-lipoxygenase inhibitor and has antiproliferative activity against keratinocytes in tissue culture, but the relationship between this activity and its effectiveness in actinic keratoses is unknown.

**Absorption**
Less than 2%.

## Precautions to Consider

**Cross-sensitivity and/or related problems**
Patients sensitive to sulfites may be sensitive to topical masoprocol because of the sulfite preservatives present.

**Carcinogenicity**
Studies in animals have not been done.

**Mutagenicity**
Masoprocol was mutagenic in the Ames assay (negative in three strains of *Salmonella* and positive in one). In an *in vivo* mouse estrogenic activity assay, a subcutaneous dose of 2 mg of masoprocol per kg of body weight (mg/kg) per day for 4 days produced no more estrogenic activity than did vehicle controls.

**Pregnancy/Reproduction**
Fertility—Studies in animals have not been done.

Pregnancy—Adequate and well-controlled studies in humans have not been done.

Studies in rabbits and rats at doses up to 6 and 16 times the human dose (on a mg per square meter of body surface basis), respectively, found no evidence of teratogenicity.

FDA Pregnancy Category B.

**Breast-feeding**
It is not known whether masoprocol is distributed into breast milk. However, because some systemic absorption occurs, caution is recommended while topical masoprocol is being administered.

**Pediatrics**
Appropriate studies on the relationship of age to the effects of topical masoprocol have not been performed in the pediatric population.

**Geriatrics**
Appropriate studies on the relationship of age to the effects of topical masoprocol have not been performed in the geriatric population.

**Medical considerations/Contraindications**
The medical considerations/contraindications included have been selected on the basis of their potential clinical significance (reasons given in parentheses where appropriate)—not necessarily inclusive (» = major clinical significance).

*Risk-benefit should be considered when the following medical problem exists:*
» Sensitivity to masoprocol

**Patient monitoring**
The following may be especially important in patient monitoring (other tests may be warranted in some patients, depending on condition; » = major clinical significance):
  Biopsy
    (may be recommended to confirm diagnosis if solar keratoses do not respond or if they recur after treatment)

## Side/Adverse Effects

Note: Local skin reactions usually resolve within two weeks after withdrawal of masoprocol.

The following side/adverse effects have been selected on the basis of their potential clinical significance (possible signs and symptoms in parentheses where appropriate)—not necessarily inclusive:

**Those indicating need for medical attention**
Incidence more frequent
  *Contact dermatitis* (redness and swelling of normal skin; redness, soreness, swelling, itching, dryness, and flaking of skin where medication is applied)
  Note: Allergic *contact dermatitis*, confirmed by patch testing, has been reported in up to 10% of patients, usually within 3 weeks after initiation of treatment. In patients rechallenged with masoprocol cream, both frequency and severity of reactions increased.
Incidence less frequent
  *Blistering or oozing at site of application*
Signs and symptoms of allergic reaction to sulfites
  *Bluish coloration of skin; dizziness, severe, or feeling faint; wheezing or trouble in breathing*

**Those indicating need for medical attention only if they continue or are bothersome**
Incidence more frequent
  *Burning feeling at site of application*
Incidence less frequent
  *Leathery feeling to skin; skin roughness; wrinkles*

## Patient Consultation

As an aid to patient consultation, refer to *Advice for the Patient, Masoprocol (Topical)*.

In providing consultation, consider emphasizing the following selected information (» = major clinical significance):

**Before using this medication**
» Conditions affecting use, especially:
    Sensitivity to masoprocol or sulfite preservatives
    Pregnancy—Caution recommended; some systemic absorption occurs
    Breast-feeding—Caution recommended; some systemic absorption occurs

**Proper use of this medication**
» Compliance with therapy; applying enough medication to cover affected areas
  Washing area to be treated with mild soap and water and drying thoroughly; using fingertips to apply
» Washing hands immediately after application to prevent accidental transfer of medication from fingertips to eyes or mouth
  Possible unsightly reaction during and for about 2 weeks after therapy is completed; checking with physician before discontinuing medication
» Proper dosing
  Missed dose: Applying as soon as remembered; not applying if not remembered within a few hours; checking with physician if more than one dose is missed
» Proper storage

**Precautions while using this medication**
» Importance of close monitoring by physician
» Caution in applying medication; avoiding eyes, nose, and mouth
» Possibility of allergic reaction to sulfites contained in the preparation; checking with physician immediately if signs of allergic reaction occur

**Side/adverse effects**
Signs of potential side effects, especially contact dermatitis

## General Dosing Information

Patients using topical masoprocol should be under supervision of a physician experienced in use of the medication.

Masoprocol has not been shown to produce necrosis, scarring, or ulceration during the initial course of therapy. Therapeutic efficacy does not rely on production of a local inflammatory skin reaction.

Use of occlusive dressings is not recommended.

It is recommended that treatment with masoprocol be discontinued if contact dermatitis occurs or if an excessive inflammatory response occurs on normal skin.

## Topical Dosage Forms

### MASOPROCOL CREAM

**Usual adult dose**
Actinic (solar) keratoses—
  Topical, to the skin, as a 10% cream twice a day in a sufficient amount to cover the lesions.

**Usual pediatric dose**
Safety and efficacy have not been established.

**Strength(s) usually available**
U.S.—
  10% (Rx) [*Actinex* (methylparaben; propylparaben; sodium metabisulfite)].
Canada—
  Not commercially available.

**Packaging and storage**
Store between 15 and 30 °C (59 and 86 °F), unless otherwise specified by manufacturer.

**Auxiliary labeling**
• For the skin.
• Continue medicine for full course of treatment.

## Selected Bibliography

Olsen EA, Abernethy ML, Kulp-Shorten C, et al. A double-blind, vehicle-controlled study evaluating masoprocol cream in the treatment of actinic keratoses on the head and neck. J Am Acad Dermatol 1991 May; 24(5 Pt 1): 738-43.

Developed: 07/31/95

---

**MAZINDOL** — See *Appetite Suppressants (Systemic)*

# MEASLES, MUMPS, AND RUBELLA VIRUS VACCINE LIVE Systemic

VA CLASSIFICATION (Primary): IM100

Note: This monograph is specific for the sterile lyophilized preparation of a more attenuated line of measles virus, derived from Enders' attenuated Edmonston strain and grown in cell cultures of chick embryo, the Jeryl Lynn (B level) strain of mumps virus grown in cell cultures of chick embryo, and the Wistar RA 27/3 strain of live attenuated rubella virus grown in human diploid cell (WI-38) culture.

Commonly used brand name(s): *M-M-R II*.

Note: For a listing of dosage forms and brand names by country availability, see *Dosage Forms* section(s).

## Category

Immunizing agent (active).

## Indications

### General considerations

Although serologic tests may be conducted to determine the susceptibility of persons of unknown immunity, studies have indicated there are no serious adverse effects from vaccinating persons already immune to rubella.

Previously nonimmunized children of susceptible pregnant women should receive live attenuated rubella vaccine, because an immunized child is less likely to acquire natural rubella and introduce the virus into the household.

Monovalent measles vaccine should be used to immunize infants 6 to 12 months of age during measles epidemics.

Persons should be considered immune to measles, mumps, and/or rubella only if they have documentation of immunization with measles, mumps, and/or rubella vaccines on or after their first birthdays, if they have laboratory evidence of measles, mumps, and/or rubella immunity, or if they have a physician's diagnosis of previous measles and/or mumps infection. Since the clinical diagnosis of rubella infection is unreliable, it should not be considered in assessing immune status to rubella.

Administration of measles, mumps, and rubella virus vaccine live yields results similar to those from administration of individual measles, mumps, and rubella vaccines at different sites. Therefore, there is no medical basis for administering these vaccines separately for routine vaccination instead of the preferred measles, mumps, and rubella virus combined vaccine. Measles, mumps, and rubella virus vaccine should be used for vaccinating individuals who are likely to be susceptible to more than one of these viruses, unless otherwise contraindicated.

Vaccines containing measles antigen should be administered to persons 12 to 15 months of age or older under routine conditions. Most individuals born before 1957 generally can be considered immune to measles and mumps because of probable previous infection, even though, in the case of mumps, they may not have had clinically recognizable disease.

### Accepted

Measles, mumps, and rubella (prophylaxis)—Measles, mumps, and rubella virus vaccine is indicated for simultaneous immunization against measles (rubeola; morbilli; coughing, hard, red, or 10-day measles), mumps, and rubella (German measles) in persons 12 to 15 months of age or older.

The main objectives of measles, mumps, and rubella immunization are:
- To prevent severe complications, such as pneumonia, ear infections, sinusitis, encephalitis, subacute sclerosing panencephalitis, gastroenteritis, and death, which may arise from a measles infection. The risk of serious complications and death from natural measles infection is greater for adults and infants than for children and adolescents.
- To prevent intrauterine infection of the fetuses of women exposed to rubella, which can result in miscarriage, abortion, stillbirth, or in congenital rubella syndrome in the neonate.
- To prevent complications, such as orchitis, which may occur in up to 20% of postpubescent and adult men infected with mumps virus, and meningoencephalitis, which may occur in up to 15% of persons infected with mumps virus. In addition, mumps infection during the first trimester of pregnancy may increase the rate of spontaneous abortion.

Unless otherwise contraindicated, all susceptible persons 12 months of age or older should be immunized against measles, mumps, and rubella, including:
- Women of childbearing potential, if they are not pregnant and if they are counseled not to become pregnant for 3 months following vaccination. Since there is an increased risk of acquiring rubella while traveling outside the U.S., women of childbearing age should be immunized before leaving the country.
- Postpartum women who do not plan to breast-feed, preferably before discharge from the hospital. Although problems in humans have not been documented, postpartum women who plan to breast-feed should consult their physicians to consider risk-benefit before receiving immunization with measles, mumps, and rubella virus vaccine.
- Persons traveling outside the U.S. These persons should receive measles, mumps, and rubella virus vaccine prior to international travel.

## Pharmacology/Pharmacokinetics

### Physicochemical characteristics

Source—Measles, mumps, and rubella virus vaccine live contains a sterile lyophilized preparation of a more attenuated line of measles virus, derived from Enders' attenuated Edmonston strain and grown in cell cultures of chick embryo, the Jeryl Lynn (B level) strain of mumps virus grown in cell cultures of chick embryo, and the Wistar RA 27/3 strain of live attenuated rubella virus grown in human diploid cell (WI-38) culture. The vaccine viruses are the same as those used in the manufacture of measles virus vaccine live, mumps virus vaccine live, and rubella virus vaccine live. The three viruses are mixed before being lyophilized.

### Mechanism of action/Effect

Following subcutaneous injection, measles, mumps, and rubella virus vaccine live produces a modified, noncommunicable measles, mumps, and rubella infection and provides active immunity to measles, mumps, and rubella.

### Protective effect

Clinical studies of 279 triple seronegative children, 11 months to 7 years of age, demonstrated that measles, mumps, and rubella virus vaccine live is highly immunogenic and generally well tolerated. In these studies, a single injection of measles, mumps, and rubella virus vaccine live induced measles hemagglutinin-inhibition (HI) antibodies in 95%, mumps neutralizing antibodies in 96%, and rubella HI antibodies in 99% of susceptible individuals. The presence of these antibodies has been correlated with clinical protection and their absence considered indicative of susceptibility.

Studies have shown that measles, mumps, and rubella virus vaccine live is as effective in producing immunity as each of the separate vaccines, and that the immunity induced by immunization with measles, mumps, and rubella virus vaccine is long-lasting and may even be lifelong.

The RA 27/3 rubella strain in measles, mumps, and rubella virus vaccine live elicits higher immediate postvaccination HI, complement-fixing, and neutralizing antibody levels than does other strains of rubella vaccine and has been shown to induce a broader profile of circulating antibodies, including anti-theta and anti-iota precipitating antibodies. The RA 27/3 rubella strain immunologically simulates natural infection more closely than other rubella vaccine viruses. The increased levels and broader profile of antibodies produced by RA 27/3 strain rubella virus vaccine appear to correlate with greater resistance to subclinical reinfection with the wild virus, and provide greater confidence for lasting immunity.

### Duration of protective effect

The immunity conferred by measles, mumps, and rubella virus vaccine appears to be long-lasting. Vaccine-induced antibody levels following administration of measles, mumps, and rubella virus vaccine live have been shown to persist for up to 11 years without substantial decline. Protective antibodies have been observed 21 years after measles vaccination and 18 years after rubella vaccination. Administration of a second dose of vaccine some years after the first dose may ensure that protective antibody titers are maintained. Continued surveillance will be necessary to determine further duration of antibody persistence. Continuous serosurveillance is important to monitor the immunity status in the population and especially to ensure that the immunity is sufficient during childbearing years.

## Precautions to Consider

### Cross-sensitivity and/or related problems

Patients allergic to systemic or topical neomycin may be allergic to the measles, mumps, and rubella virus vaccine live because each 0.5-mL dose contains approximately 25 mcg of neomycin, which is used in the production of the vaccine to prevent bacterial overgrowth in the viral culture. A history of hypersensitivity reactions (such as delayed-type allergic reaction or contact dermatitis), other than anaphylaxis, to neomycin or to eggs generally does not preclude immunization.

There is no evidence to indicate that persons with allergies to chicken or chicken feathers are at increased risk of reaction to the vaccine.

### Pregnancy/Reproduction

Pregnancy—Although adequate studies have not been done in humans, use in pregnant women is not recommended. Considerable complications, including increased rates of spontaneous abortion, premature births, low-birth-weight neonates, and possibly, congenital defects, have been observed with natural measles infection during pregnancy, and the possibility exists that the measles vaccine may cause similar effects.

Although mumps vaccine virus has not been isolated from electively aborted fetuses of women who were vaccinated during pregnancy, the vaccine virus may infect the placenta. In addition, natural mumps infection can infect the placenta and fetus, but there is no evidence that natural mumps infection during pregnancy causes congenital malformations. Therefore, there is no reason to suspect or evidence to indicate that mumps vaccine would cause congenital malformations.

Rubella vaccine virus crosses the placenta and has been recovered from the products of conception of some aborted fetuses of women who received the vaccine just prior to or during pregnancy; however, from 1971 through 1988, the Centers for Disease Control (CDC) monitored 210 pregnant women who had received the RA 27/3 strain of rubella virus vaccine 3 months before or after conception and carried their pregnancies to term. Although some neonates had serological evidence of rubella virus infection, none had malformations associated with congenital rubella syndrome. Therefore, vaccination of a pregnant woman should not in itself indicate the need for abortion, although the final decision rests with the woman and her physician. The risk of congenital rubella syndrome associated with maternal infection with the wild virus during the first trimester of pregnancy is at least 20%. Since the risk of teratogenicity is not known, and appears to be minimal, there is still a theoretical risk of fetal abnormality caused by the vaccine virus.

In addition, it is recommended that pregnancy be avoided for 3 months following vaccination.

Studies have not been done in animals.

FDA Pregnancy Category C.

### Breast-feeding

It is not known whether measles or mumps vaccine is distributed into breast milk. Although rubella vaccine may be distributed into breast milk and infants may subsequently show serological evidence of rubella infection or mild clinical illness typical of acquired rubella, studies have not shown that these effects cause serious clinical problems.

### Pediatrics

Infants younger than 15 months of age may fail to respond to the measles component of the vaccine due to the presence of residual circulating measles antibody of maternal origin. This effect usually starts to wane after the child reaches 6 months of age. However, children born to younger mothers might respond well to measles vaccine administered at 12 months of age. In one study, children randomly received measles vaccine at either 12 or 15 months of age. The measles antibody response to measles, mumps, and rubella virus vaccine was 93 to 95% when the vaccine was administered at 12 months of age, and 98% when it was administered at 15 months of age. Among children of mothers born after 1961, who probably had received a measles vaccine and were less likely to have had measles infection than women born in previous years, the seroconversion rate was 96% among children vaccinated at 12 months of age and 98% among those vaccinated at 15 months of age. Based on these findings, the Committee on Infectious Diseases of the American Academy of Pediatrics (AAP) and the Advisory Committee on Immunization Practices (ACIP) recommend administration of the first dose of measles, mumps, and rubella virus vaccine live at 12 to 15 months of age. Both AAP and ACIP recommend that all children receive a second dose of measles-containing vaccine. The second dose of measles, mumps, and rubella virus vaccine live is routinely recommended at 4 to 6 years of age or at 11 to 12 years of age, but may be administered at any visit, provided at least 1 month has elapsed since receipt of the first dose. Children who were vaccinated when younger than 12 months of age should be revaccinated at 15 months of age. Children who received monovalent measles vaccine rather than measles, mumps, and rubella virus vaccine on or after their first birthdays also should receive a primary dose of mumps and rubella vaccines, and doses of measles, mumps, and rubella virus vaccine or other measles-containing vaccines should be separated by at least 1 month.

If exposure to measles infection has occurred within 72 hours or is imminent, children between 6 and 15 months of age can be vaccinated, provided that those vaccinated before their first birthdays are revaccinated at 15 months of age. There is some evidence to suggest, however, that infants immunized at less than 12 months of age may not develop sustained antibody levels when later reimmunized. The advantage of early protection must be weighed against the chance for failure to respond adequately on reimmunization.

It is also very important to vaccinate HIV-infected children against measles. Children with end-stage renal disease receiving maintenance hemodialysis have a degree of immunosuppression that reduces their response to vaccination. One small trial showed that 80% of these vaccinated children developed antibodies to measles and rubella, while only 50% developed mumps antibodies. Moreover, only 30% developed antibodies to all three viruses. Therefore, it may be necessary to monitor postvaccination antibody levels in children with end-stage renal disease, and to revaccinate those children who have failed to demonstrate seroconversion.

AAP recommends the routine use of measles vaccine (including measles, mumps, and rubella virus vaccine live) in patients with nonanaphylactic allergy to eggs and in patients with allergies to chicken and chicken-feathers. One recent study showed that measles, mumps, and rubella virus vaccine live can be administered safely in a single dose to children with allergy to eggs, even those with severe hypersensitivity.

### Drug interactions and/or related problems

The following drug interactions and/or related problems have been selected on the basis of their potential clinical significance (possible mechanism in parentheses where appropriate)—not necessarily inclusive (» = major clinical significance):

Note: Combinations containing any of the following medications, depending on the amount present, may also interact with this medication.

Blood products or
Immune globulins
  (concurrent administration with measles, mumps, and rubella virus vaccine live may interfere with the patient's immune response to the vaccine because of the possibility of antibodies to measles, mumps, and rubella viruses in these products; measles, mumps, and rubella virus vaccine live should be administered at least 14 days before, or more than 5 to 6 months after, administration of blood products or immune globulins)

» Immunosuppressive agents or
» Radiation therapy
  (because normal host defense mechanisms are suppressed, concurrent use with measles, mumps, and rubella virus vaccine live may potentiate the replication of the vaccine virus, increase the side/adverse effects of the vaccine virus, and/or decrease the patient's antibody response to measles, mumps, and rubella virus vaccine live. The reaction may be severe enough to cause death. The interval between discontinuing medications that cause immunosuppression and regaining the ability to respond to measles, mumps, and rubella virus vaccine live depends on the intensity and type of immunosuppressive medication being used, the underlying disease, and other factors; estimates vary from 3 months to 1 year. Patients with leukemia that is in remission should not receive measles, mumps, and rubella virus vaccine live until at least 3 months after their last dose of chemotherapy. This precaution does not apply to corticosteroids used as replacement therapy, for short-term [less than 2 weeks] systemic therapy, or for other routes of administration that do not cause immunosuppression)

Live virus vaccines, other
  (although data are lacking on impairment of antibody responses to rubella, measles, mumps, or oral polio vaccine when these vaccines are administered on different days within 1 month of each other, the chance exists that the immune responses may be impaired when live virus vaccines are administered in this manner; therefore, when feasible, live virus vaccines should be given at least 1 month apart or simultaneously)

### Laboratory value alterations

The following have been selected on the basis of their potential clinical significance (possible effect in parentheses where appropriate)—not necessarily inclusive (» = major clinical significance):

With diagnostic test results
» Tuberculin skin test
  (short-term suppression lasting several weeks may occur and may result in false-negative tests; if required, tuberculin skin tests should be done before, simultaneously with, or at least 8 weeks after administration of measles, mumps, and rubella virus vaccine)

Skin tests, other
  (decreased responsiveness to skin test antigens may occur because of vaccine-induced transient suppression of delayed-type hypersensitivity; the period of time for which responsiveness is decreased depends upon the particular skin test used)

With physiology/laboratory test values
Platelets, blood
(counts may be decreased)

### Medical considerations/Contraindications
The medical considerations/contraindications included have been selected on the basis of their potential clinical significance (reasons given in parentheses where appropriate)—not necessarily inclusive (» = major clinical significance).

*Except under special circumstances, this medication should not be used when the following medical problems exist:*

» Febrile illness, severe
(manifestations of illness may be confused with possible side/adverse effects of vaccine; however, minor illnesses, such as upper respiratory infection, do not preclude administration of vaccine)

» Immune deficiency conditions, congenital or hereditary, family history of, or

» Immune deficiency conditions, primary or acquired
(because of reduced or suppressed defense mechanisms, the use of live virus vaccines, including measles, mumps, and rubella virus vaccine live, may potentiate the replication of the vaccine virus, and/or may decrease the patient's antibody response to measles, mumps, and rubella)

(persons with leukemia that is in remission may receive live virus vaccines if at least 3 months have passed since the last chemotherapy treatment)

(persons infected with human immunodeficiency virus [HIV] may receive measles, mumps, and rubella virus vaccine live if they are not severely lymphopenic)

(when there is a family history of congenital or hereditary immune deficiency conditions, the patient should not be vaccinated until immune competence is demonstrated)

*Risk-benefit should be considered when the following medical problems exist:*

Allergy to eggs
(patients allergic to eggs also may be allergic to measles, mumps, and rubella virus vaccine live, since measles and mumps virus vaccines are produced in chick embryo cell cultures. A history of hypersensitivity reactions other than anaphylaxis generally does not preclude immunization. In addition, no allergy to measles, mumps, and rubella virus vaccine live has been found in patients allergic to chicken feathers or chicken)

Allergy to gelatin
(patients allergic to gelatin also may be allergic to measles, mumps, and rubella virus vaccine live, since gelatin is used as a stabilizer in the production of the vaccine)

Sensitivity to measles, mumps, and rubella virus vaccine

Thrombocytopenia or history of vaccine-associated thrombocytopenia
(persons who experienced thrombocytopenia with the first dose of vaccine may develop thrombocytopenia with additional doses. These persons should have serological testing performed in order to determine the need for additional doses of vaccine. The risk-benefit ratio should be evaluated before considering vaccination in such cases)

### Patient monitoring
The following may be especially important in patient monitoring (other tests may be warranted in some patients, depending on condition; » = major clinical significance):

Seroconversion test
(may be performed 6 to 8 weeks following vaccination in patients for whom immunity is considered crucial [e.g., persons traveling outside the U.S. or women in high-risk areas who intend to become pregnant], since vaccination with measles, mumps, and rubella virus vaccine live may not result in seroconversion in all susceptible patients)

## Side/Adverse Effects

Note: The side/adverse effects associated with the use of measles, mumps, and rubella virus vaccine live are the same as those expected to follow administration of the monovalent vaccines given separately. However, it is very important to differentiate between vaccine-induced side/adverse effects and natural infection.

Revaccination of prior vaccinees appears to be associated with relatively low side/adverse effect rates.

The incidence of side/adverse effects increases with age and is generally higher in females.

A history of hypersensitivity reactions other than anaphylaxis, such as delayed-type allergic reaction (contact dermatitis), generally does not preclude immunization. There is a very small chance of an adverse reaction in any child, and a study showed that measles, mumps, and rubella virus vaccine live can be administered safely in a single dose to children allergic to eggs, even those with severe hypersensitivity.

Encephalitis and encephalopathy have been temporally related to measles vaccine administration and occur in one per million doses administered; however, no causal relationship has been established. The incidence of these diseases after a natural measles infection is one per thousand persons. These reactions also have been temporally related to mumps vaccine administration, but no causal relationship has been established. The incidence of these disorders in patients vaccinated with mumps vaccine is no more frequent than the incidence found in the general population.

Although there is a temporal relationship, no definite causal relationship has been established between the isolated reports of Guillain-Barré syndrome (GBS) or ocular palsies following the administration of measles vaccine. Isolated incidents of GBS also have been reported after immunization with rubella vaccine.

It is not known whether some of the cases of subacute sclerosing panencephalitis (SSPE) attributed to the measles vaccine were actually due to unrecognized natural measles infection during the first year of life. However, the use of measles vaccine has reduced the incidence of SSPE from 5 to 10 cases per million cases of natural measles infection to 1 case per million doses of measles vaccine.

Persons who are immune to measles, mumps, and/or rubella virus because of past vaccination or infection usually do not experience side/adverse effects from the vaccine.

Excretion of small amounts of the live attenuated rubella virus from the nose or throat has occurred in the majority of susceptible individuals 7 to 28 days after vaccination. There is, however, no confirmed evidence to indicate that the vaccine virus is transmitted to susceptible persons who are in contact with the vaccinated individuals.

The following side/adverse effects have been selected on the basis of their potential clinical significance (possible signs and symptoms in parentheses where appropriate)—not necessarily inclusive:

### Those indicating need for medical attention
Incidence more frequent
*Fever higher than 39.4 ºC (103 ºF)*

Incidence less frequent
*Optic neuritis* (pain or tenderness of eyes)—may occur from 1 to 4 weeks after immunization, lasting less than 1 week

Incidence rare
*Anaphylactic reaction* (difficulty in breathing or swallowing; hives; itching, especially of soles or palms; reddening of skin, especially around ears; swelling of eyes, face, or inside of nose; unusual tiredness or weakness, sudden and severe); *encephalitis or meningoencephalitis* (confusion; headache, severe or continuing; irritability; stiff neck; or vomiting); *ocular palsies* (double vision); *orchitis in postpubescent and adult men* (pain, tenderness, or swelling in testicles and scrotum); *peripheral neuropathy, polyneuritis, or polyneuropathy* (pain, numbness, or tingling of hands, arms, legs, or feet)—may occur from 1 to 4 weeks after immunization, lasting less than 1 week; *seizures* (convulsions); *thrombocytopenic purpura* (bruising or purple spots on skin)

### Those indicating need for medical attention only if they continue or are bothersome
Incidence more frequent
*Fever between 37.7 and 39.4 ºC (100 and 103 ºF); lymphadenopathy or parotitis* (swelling of glands in neck)—may occur from 1 to 4 weeks after immunization, lasting less than 1 week; *reaction to acid pH of vaccine* (burning or stinging at injection site); *skin rash*

Incidence less frequent
*Allergic reaction, delayed-type, cell-mediated* (itching, swelling, redness, tenderness, or hard lump at injection site); *arthralgia or arthritis* (aches or pain in joints)—may occur from 1 to 10 weeks after immunization, lasting less than 1 week; *malaise* (vague feeling of bodily discomfort)—may occur from 1 to 4 weeks after immunization, lasting less than 1 week; *mild headache, sore throat, or runny nose*—may occur from 1 to 4 weeks after immunization, lasting less than 1 week; *nausea*

Note: One study showed that the RA 27/3 strain of rubella vaccine administered to susceptible adult women is not associated with clinically important acute or chronic joint disease. Therefore, rubella vaccination should continue to be used to protect susceptible adult women from rubella in order to advance the goal of eliminating the congenital rubella syndrome. The incidence of *arthralgia or arthritis* is increased greatly in women of child-bearing age. Generally the older the woman, the greater the incidence, severity, and duration of arthralgia or arthritis. However, even in older women, the symptoms generally are well tolerated and rarely interfere with normal activities. No persistent joint disorders have been reported.

## Patient Consultation

As an aid to patient consultation, refer to *Advice for the Patient, Measles, Mumps, and Rubella Virus Vaccine Live (Systemic)*.
In providing consultation, consider emphasizing the following selected information (» = major clinical significance):

### Before receiving this vaccine
Conditions affecting use, especially:
  Sensitivity to measles, mumps, and rubella virus vaccine live, or allergy to eggs, gelatin or neomycin
  Pregnancy—Use of measles, mumps, and rubella virus vaccine during pregnancy or pregnancy within 3 months of immunization is not recommended
  Breast-feeding—Consulting physician if breast-feeding is considered
  Use in children—Use is not recommended for infants younger than 12 months of age
  Other medications, especially immunosuppressive agents or radiation therapy
  Other medical problems, especially severe febrile illness, family history of congenital or hereditary immune deficiency conditions, or primary or acquired immune deficiency conditions

### Proper use of this medication
» Proper dosing

### Precautions after receiving this vaccine
» Not becoming pregnant for 3 months without first checking with physician, because of possible problems during pregnancy
  Checking with physician before receiving:
  Tuberculin skin test within 8 weeks of this vaccine, since the results of the test may be affected by the vaccine
  Any other live-virus vaccines within 1 month of this vaccine
  Blood transfusions or other blood products within 2 weeks of this vaccine
  Gamma globulin or other globulins within 2 weeks of this vaccine

### Side/adverse effects
Signs of potential side effects, especially fever higher than 39.4 °C (103 °F), optic neuritis, anaphylactic reaction, encephalitis or meningoencephalitis, ocular palsies, orchitis in postpubescent and adult males, peripheral neuropathy, polyneuritis, or polyneuropathy, seizures, and thrombocytopenic purpura

## General Dosing Information

The dosage of measles, mumps, and rubella virus vaccine live is the same for both children and adults.

Measles, mumps, and rubella virus vaccine live is administered subcutaneously. It should not be injected intravenously.

When sterilizing syringes and skin before vaccination, care should be taken to avoid preservatives, antiseptics, detergents, and disinfectants, because the vaccine virus is easily inactivated by these substances.

To prevent inactivation of the vaccine, it is recommended that only the diluent provided by the manufacturer be used.

A 25-gauge, 5/8th-inch needle is recommended for administration of the vaccine.

Although measles, mumps, and rubella vaccines are available as a combination vaccine (measles, mumps, and rubella virus vaccine live) and, as such, are administered as a single injection, the commercially available individual vaccines should not be mixed in the same syringe or administered at the same body site.

Although the fourth dose of diphtheria-tetanus-pertussis (DTP) vaccine and the third dose of oral poliovirus vaccine (OPV) traditionally have been administered to children 18 months of age and measles, mumps, and rubella virus vaccine live traditionally has been administered to children 12 to 15 months of age, it is now recommended that DTP, OPV, and measles, mumps, and rubella virus vaccine live be administered concurrently to children 12 to 15 months of age. Measles, mumps, and rubella virus vaccine live should not be postponed in order to administer all of these vaccines concurrently at 18 months of age.

Measles, mumps, and rubella virus vaccine live, a live virus vaccine, may be administered concurrently with the following, using separate body sites, separate syringes, and the precautions that apply to each immunizing agent:
- Polysaccharide vaccines, such as haemophilus b polysaccharide vaccine, haemophilus b conjugate vaccine, meningococcal polysaccharide vaccine, or pneumococcal polyvalent vaccine
- Influenza vaccine, whole or split virus
- Diphtheria toxoid, tetanus toxoid, and/or pertussis vaccine
- Live virus vaccines, other, such as varicella and OPV, only if the vaccines are administered on the same day; otherwise they should be administered at least 1 month apart
- Inactivated poliovirus vaccine (IPV) or enhanced potency inactivated poliovirus vaccine (enhanced-potency IPV)
- Hepatitis B recombinant or plasma-derived vaccine
- Inactivated vaccines, other, except cholera, typhoid, and plague. It is recommended that cholera, typhoid, and plague vaccines be administered on separate occasions because of these vaccines' propensity to cause side/adverse effects.

### For treatment of adverse effects
Recommended treatment consists of the following:
- For mild hypersensitivity reaction—Administering antihistamines, and, if necessary, corticosteroids.
- For severe hypersensitivity or anaphylactic reaction—Administering epinephrine. Antihistamines or corticosteroids also may be administered as required.

## Parenteral Dosage Forms

### MEASLES, MUMPS, AND RUBELLA VIRUS VACCINE LIVE (FOR INJECTION) USP

#### Usual adult and adolescent dose
Immunizing agent (active)—
  Subcutaneous, 0.5 mL, preferably into the outer aspect of the upper arm.

#### Usual pediatric dose
Immunizing agent (active)—
  Infants up to 12 months of age: Use is not recommended.
  Infants and children 12 months of age and older: See *Usual adult and adolescent dose*.

Note: The Committee on Infectious Diseases of the American Academy of Pediatrics (AAP) and the Advisory Committee on Immunization Practices (ACIP) recommend that all children receive a second dose of measles-containing vaccine. The second dose of measles, mumps, and rubella virus vaccine live is routinely recommended at 4 to 6 years of age or at 11 to 12 years of age, but may be administered at any visit, provided at least 1 month has elapsed since receipt of the first dose.

#### Strength(s) usually available
U.S.—
  Not less than the equivalent of 1000 TCID$_{50}$ of the U.S. Reference Measles Virus, not less than the equivalent of 20,000 TCID$_{50}$ of the U.S. Reference Mumps Virus, and not less than the equivalent of 1000 TCID$_{50}$ of the U.S. Reference Rubella Virus in each 0.5-mL dose (Rx) [*M-M-R II* (neomycin approximately 25 mcg)].
Canada—
  Not less than the equivalent of 1000 TCID$_{50}$ of the U.S. Reference Measles Virus, not less than the equivalent of 20,000 TCID$_{50}$ of the U.S. Reference Mumps Virus, and not less than the equivalent of 1000 TCID$_{50}$ of the U.S. Reference Rubella Virus in each 0.5-mL dose (Rx) [*M-M-R II* (neomycin approximately 25 mcg)].

#### Packaging and storage
Store the lyophilized form of the vaccine, the diluent, and the reconstituted form of the vaccine between 2 and 8 °C (36 and 46 °F), unless otherwise specified by manufacturer.
Alternatively, the diluent for the single-dose vials may be stored between 15 and 30 °C (59 and 86 °F).
Protect both the lyophilized form and the reconstituted form of the vaccine from light.

#### Preparation of dosage form
To reconstitute, use only the diluent provided by the manufacturer, since it is free of preservatives and other substances that might inactivate the vaccine.
Single-dose vial—The entire volume of diluent (approximately 0.5 mL) should be withdrawn into the syringe. All the diluent in the syringe should be injected into the vial of lyophilized vaccine and agitated to mix thoroughly. The entire contents of the vial should be withdrawn into the syringe and the total volume of restored vaccine injected subcutaneously.

10-dose vial (in U.S., available only to government agencies/institutions)—
The entire contents (7 mL) of the diluent vial should be withdrawn into the syringe to be used for reconstitution. All of the diluent in the syringe should be injected into the 10-dose vial of lyophilized vaccine and agitated to mix thoroughly. The 10-dose container can be used with either syringes or a jet injector. Since the vaccine and diluent do not contain preservatives, special care should be taken to prevent contamination of the multiple-dose vial of vaccine. In addition, the vial should be stored properly until the reconstituted vaccine is used. Unused vaccine should be discarded after 8 hours.

### Stability
Both the lyophilized and the reconstituted vaccine should be stored between 2 and 8 °C (36 and 46 °F) and protected from light. Improper storage and protection may inactivate the vaccine.

The reconstituted vaccine should be used as soon as possible. Unused reconstituted vaccine should be discarded after 8 hours.

The reconstituted vaccine is clear yellow. It should not be used if it is discolored.

### Incompatibilities
Preservatives or other substances may inactivate the vaccine; therefore, only the diluent supplied by the manufacturer should be used for reconstitution.

A sterile syringe free of preservatives, antiseptics, disinfectants, and detergents should be used for each injection and/or reconstitution of the vaccine. These substances may inactivate the live virus vaccine.

### Auxiliary labeling
- Protect from light.
- Store in refrigerator.
- Discard reconstituted vaccine if not used within 8 hours.

Note: The date and the time of reconstitution should be indicated on the vial if the reconstituted vaccine is not used at once.

Developed: 01/27/97

# MEASLES AND RUBELLA VIRUS VACCINE LIVE   Systemic†

VA CLASSIFICATION (Primary): IM100

Note: This monograph is specific for the sterile lyophilized preparation of a more attenuated line of measles virus, derived from Enders' attenuated Edmonston strain and grown in cell cultures of chick embryos, and the Wistar RA 27/3 strain of live attenuated rubella virus grown in human diploid cell (WI-38) culture.

Commonly used brand name(s): *M-R-VAX II*.

Note: For a listing of dosage forms and brand names by country availability, see *Dosage Forms* section(s).

†Not commercially available in Canada.

## Category
Immunizing agent (active).

## Indications

### General considerations
Persons generally can be considered immune to measles and/or rubella only if they have documentation of adequate immunization with measles and/or rubella vaccines on or after their first birthdays, if they have laboratory evidence of measles and/or rubella immunity, or if they have a physician's diagnosis of previous measles infection. Since the clinical diagnosis of rubella infection is unreliable, it should not be considered in assessing immune status to rubella.

Most individuals born before 1957 can generally be considered immune to measles and mumps because of probable previous infection, even though, in the case of mumps, they may not have had clinically recognizable disease. However, birth before 1957 provides only presumptive evidence of immunity; measles can occur in some persons born before 1957.

Although serologic tests may be conducted to determine the susceptibility of persons of unknown immunity, studies have indicated there is no evidence of increased risk of adverse reactions due to vaccination with live measles and/or rubella vaccine virus in persons already immune to measles and/or rubella.

Previously nonimmunized children of susceptible pregnant women should receive live attenuated rubella vaccine because an immunized child is less likely to acquire natural rubella and introduce the virus into the household.

Monovalent measles vaccine should be used to immunize infants 6 to 12 months of age during measles epidemics, although combined measles, mumps, and rubella or measles and rubella vaccines can be used if monovalent measles vaccine is not available.

Measles, mumps, and rubella virus vaccine live should be used for vaccinating individuals who are likely to be susceptible to more than one of these viruses, unless otherwise contraindicated.

Vaccines containing measles antigen should be administered routinely to persons 12 to 15 months of age or older under routine conditions.

### Accepted
Measles and rubella (prophylaxis)—Measles and rubella virus vaccine live is indicated for simultaneous immunization against measles (rubeola; morbilli; coughing, hard, red, or 10-day measles) and rubella (German measles) in persons 12 to 15 months of age or older who already have evidence of immunity to mumps.

The main objectives of measles immunization are to prevent transmission of measles virus and to prevent severe complications, such as pneumonia, ear infections, sinusitis, encephalitis, subacute sclerosing panencephalitis, gastroenteritis, and death, which may arise from a measles infection. The risk of serious complications and death from a natural measles infection is greater for adults and infants than for children and adolescents.

The main objective of rubella immunization is to prevent intrauterine infection of the fetuses of women exposed to rubella, which can result in miscarriage, abortion, stillbirth, or in congenital rubella syndrome in the neonate.

Unless otherwise contraindicated, all susceptible persons 12 months of age or older should be immunized against measles and rubella, including:
- Women of childbearing potential, if they are not pregnant and if they are counseled not to become pregnant for 3 months following vaccination. Since there is an increased risk of acquiring rubella while traveling outside the U.S., women of childbearing age should be immunized before leaving the country.
- Postpartum women, preferably before discharge from the hospital. Breast-feeding is not a contraindication to vaccination. Although rubella vaccine virus can be distributed into breast milk, breast-fed newborns generally remain asymptomatic.
- Persons traveling outside the U.S. These persons should receive measles and rubella virus vaccine live prior to international travel.

## Pharmacology/Pharmacokinetics

### Physicochemical characteristics
Source—Measles and rubella virus vaccine live contains a sterile lyophilized preparation of a more attenuated line of measles virus, derived from Enders' attenuated Edmonston strain and grown in cell cultures of chick embryos, and the Wistar RA 27/3 strain of live attenuated rubella virus grown in human diploid cell (WI-38) culture. The vaccine viruses are the same as those used in the manufacture of measles virus vaccine live, and rubella virus vaccine live. The two viruses are mixed before they are lyophilized.

### Mechanism of action/Effect
Following subcutaneous injection, measles and rubella virus vaccine live produces a modified, noncommunicable measles and rubella infection and provides active immunity to measles and rubella.

### Protective effect
Clinical studies of 237 double seronegative children, 10 months to 10 years of age, demonstrated that measles and rubella virus vaccine live is highly immunogenic and generally well tolerated. In these studies, a single injection of measles and rubella virus vaccine live induced measles hemagglutinin-inhibition (HI) antibodies in 95%, and rubella HI antibodies in 99%, of susceptible individuals. The presence of these antibodies has been correlated with clinical protection and their absence considered indicative of susceptibility.

The RA 27/3 rubella strain in measles and rubella virus vaccine live elicits higher immediate postvaccination HI, complement-fixing, and neutralizing antibody levels than other strains of rubella vaccine and has been shown to induce a broader profile of circulating antibodies, including anti-theta and anti-iota precipitating antibodies. The RA 27/3 rubella strain immunologically simulates natural infection more closely than other rubella vaccine viruses. The increased levels and broader profile of antibodies produced by the RA 27/3 strain of rubella virus vaccine appear to correlate with greater resistance to subclinical reinfection with the wild virus, and provide greater confidence for lasting immunity.

**Duration of protective effect**
Vaccine-induced antibody levels following administration of measles and rubella virus vaccine live have been shown to persist for up to 11 years without substantial decline. Protective antibodies have been observed 21 years after measles vaccination and 18 years after rubella vaccination. Continued surveillance will be necessary to determine further duration of antibody persistence. Continuous serosurveillance is important to monitor the immunity status in the population and especially to ensure that the immunity is sufficient during childbearing years.

## Precautions to Consider

### Cross-sensitivity and/or related problems
Patients allergic to systemic or topical neomycin may be allergic to the measles and rubella virus vaccine live because each 0.5-mL dose contains approximately 25 mcg of neomycin, which is used in the production of the vaccine to prevent bacterial overgrowth in the viral culture. A history of hypersensitivity reactions (such as delayed-type allergic reaction or contact dermatitis) to neomycin generally does not preclude immunization. Anaphylaxis due to topically or systemically administered neomycin precludes immunization.

Patients allergic to gelatin also may be allergic to measles and rubella virus vaccine live, since gelatin is used as a stabilizer in the production of the vaccine.

Patients allergic to eggs also may be allergic to the measles and rubella virus vaccine live, since measles virus vaccine is produced in chick embryo cell cultures. However, the vaccine may be administered to egg-allergic children without prior skin testing or the use of protocols requiring gradually increasing doses of vaccine. There is no evidence to indicate that persons with allergies to chicken or chicken feathers are at increased risk of reaction to the vaccine.

### Pregnancy/Reproduction
Pregnancy—Although adequate studies have not been done in humans, use in pregnant women is not recommended. Considerable complications, including increased rates of spontaneous abortion, premature births, low-birth-weight neonates, and possibly, congenital defects, have been observed with natural measles infection during pregnancy. The possibility exists that the measles virus vaccine may cause similar effects.

Rubella vaccine virus crosses the placenta and has been recovered from the products of conception of some aborted fetuses of women who received the vaccine just prior to or during pregnancy. However, from 1971 through 1988, the Centers for Disease Control and Prevention (CDC) monitored 210 pregnant women who had received the RA 27/3 strain of rubella virus vaccine 3 months before or after conception and who carried their pregnancies to term. Although some neonates had serologic evidence of rubella virus infection, none had malformations associated with congenital rubella syndrome. Therefore, vaccination of a pregnant woman should not in itself indicate the need for abortion, although the final decision rests with the woman and her physician. The risk of congenital rubella syndrome associated with maternal infection with the wild virus during the first trimester of pregnancy is at least 20%. The risk of teratogenicity is not fully known; although it appears to be minimal, there is still a theoretical risk of fetal abnormality caused by the vaccine virus.

In addition, it is recommended that pregnancy be avoided for 3 months following vaccination.

Studies have not been done in animals.

FDA Pregnancy Category C.

### Breast-feeding
It is not known whether measles vaccine is distributed into breast milk. Although rubella vaccine may be distributed into breast milk and infants may subsequently show serologic evidence of rubella infection or mild clinical illness typical of acquired rubella, studies have not shown that these effects cause serious clinical problems.

### Pediatrics
Infants up to 15 months of age may fail to respond to the measles component of the vaccine due to the presence of residual circulating measles antibody of maternal origin. This effect usually starts to wane after the child reaches 6 months of age. However, children born to younger mothers might respond well to measles vaccine administered at 12 months of age. In one study, children randomly received measles vaccine at either 12 or 15 months of age. The measles antibody response to measles, mumps, and rubella virus vaccine was 93 to 95% when the vaccine was administered at 12 months of age, and 98% when it was administered at 15 months of age. Among children of mothers born after 1961, who probably had received a measles vaccine and were less likely to have had measles infection than women born in previous years, the seroconversion rate was 96% among children vaccinated at 12 months of age, and 98% among those vaccinated at 15 months of age. Based on these findings, the Committee on Infectious Diseases of the American Academy of Pediatrics (AAP) and the Advisory Committee on Immunization Practices (ACIP) recommend administration of the first dose of measles-containing vaccine at 12 to 15 months of age. Both AAP and ACIP recommend that all children receive a second dose of measles-containing vaccine. The second dose of measles-containing vaccine (preferably administered as measles, mumps, and rubella virus vaccine live) is routinely recommended at 4 to 6 years of age or at 11 to 12 years of age, but may be administered at any visit, provided at least 1 month has elapsed since receipt of the first dose. Children who were vaccinated when younger than 12 months of age should be revaccinated at 12 to 15 months of age, provided at least 1 month has elapsed since the previous dose of the vaccine was administered. Children who received the monovalent measles vaccine rather than the combination measles, mumps, and rubella vaccine live on or after their first birthdays also should receive a primary dose of mumps and rubella vaccines. Doses of measles, mumps, and rubella vaccine live or other measles-containing vaccines should be separated by at least 1 month.

If exposure to measles infection has occurred within 72 hours or is imminent, children between 6 and 15 months of age can be vaccinated, provided that those vaccinated before their first birthdays are revaccinated at 15 months of age. There is some evidence to suggest that infants immunized at younger than 12 months of age may not develop sustained antibody levels when later reimmunized. The advantage of early protection must be weighed against the chance for failure to respond adequately on reimmunization.

It is also very important to vaccinate children infected with human immunodeficiency virus (HIV) against measles.

Children with end-stage renal disease receiving hemodialysis have a degree of immunosuppression that reduces their response to vaccination. Therefore, it may be necessary to monitor postvaccination antibody levels in children with end-stage renal disease, and to revaccinate those children who have failed to demonstrate seroconversion.

### Drug interactions and/or related problems
The following drug interactions and/or related problems have been selected on the basis of their potential clinical significance (possible mechanism in parentheses where appropriate)—not necessarily inclusive (» = major clinical significance):

Note:  Combinations containing any of the following medications, depending on the amount present, may also interact with this medication.

Blood products or
Immune globulins
(concurrent administration with measles and rubella virus vaccine live may interfere with the patient's immune response to the vaccine because of the possibility of antibodies to measles and rubella viruses in these products; measles and rubella virus vaccine live should be administered at least 14 days before, or 3 to 11 months after administration of blood products or immune globulins, depending on the product and dose received)

» Immunosuppressive agents or
» Radiation therapy
(because normal host defense mechanisms are suppressed, concurrent use with measles and rubella vaccine live may potentiate the replication of the vaccine virus, increase the side/adverse effects of the vaccine virus, and/or decrease the patient's antibody response to measles and rubella virus vaccine live. The interaction may be severe enough to cause death. The interval between discontinuing medications that cause immunosuppression and regaining the ability to respond to measles and rubella virus vaccine live depends on the intensity and type of immunosuppressive medication used, the underlying disease, and other factors; estimates vary from 3 months to 1 year. Patients with leukemia that is in remission should not receive measles and rubella virus vaccine live until at least 3 months after the last dose of chemotherapy. The precaution does not apply to corticosteroids used as replacement therapy, for short-term [less than 2 weeks] systemic therapy, or by other routes of administration that do not cause immunosuppression)

Live virus vaccines, other
(data are lacking on impairment of antibody responses to rubella, measles, mumps, or oral poliovirus vaccine (OPV) when these vaccines are administered on different days within 1 month of each other; however, OPV and measles, mumps, and rubella virus vaccine [or its component vaccines] can be administered at any time before, with, or after each other, if indicated)

**Laboratory value alterations**
The following have been selected on the basis of their potential clinical significance (possible effect in parentheses where appropriate)—not necessarily inclusive (» = major clinical significance):

With diagnostic test results
» Tuberculin skin test
(short-term suppression of tuberculin skin test results lasting several weeks may occur and may result in false-negative tests; if required, tuberculin skin tests should be done before, simultaneously with, or at least 4 to 6 weeks after administration of measles and rubella virus vaccine live)

Skin tests, other
(decreased responsiveness to skin test antigens may occur because of vaccine-induced transient suppression of delayed-type hypersensitivity; the period of time for which responsiveness is decreased depends upon the particular skin test used)

With physiology/laboratory test values
Platelets, blood
(counts may be decreased)

**Medical considerations/Contraindications**
The medical considerations/contraindications included have been selected on the basis of their potential clinical significance (reasons given in parentheses where appropriate)—not necessarily inclusive (» = major clinical significance).

*Except under special circumstances, this medication should not be used when the following medical problems exist:*
» Febrile illness, severe
(manifestations of illness may be confused with possible side/adverse effects of vaccine; however, minor illnesses, such as upper respiratory infection, do not preclude administration of vaccine)
» Immune deficiency conditions, congenital or hereditary, family history of or
» Immune deficiency conditions, primary or acquired
(because of reduced or suppressed defense mechanisms, the use of live virus vaccines, including measles and rubella virus vaccine live, may potentiate the replication of the vaccine virus, and/or may decrease the patient's antibody response to measles and rubella)
(persons with leukemia in remission may receive live virus vaccines if at least 3 months have passed since the last chemotherapy treatment)
(persons infected with HIV may receive measles and rubella virus vaccine live if they are not severely lymphopenic)
(when there is a family history of congenital or hereditary immune deficiency conditions, the patient should not be vaccinated until immunocompetence is demonstrated)

*Risk-benefit should be considered when the following medical problems exist:*
Allergy to eggs or
Allergy to neomycin
(a history of hypersensitivity reactions generally does not preclude immunization. Anaphylaxis due to topically or systemically administered neomycin precludes immunization. The vaccine may be administered to egg-allergic children without prior skin testing or the use of protocols requiring gradually increasing doses of vaccine. In addition, no allergy to measles and rubella virus vaccine has been found in patients allergic to chicken feathers or chicken)

Allergy to gelatin
(patients allergic to gelatin also may be allergic to measles and rubella virus vaccine live, since gelatin is used as a stabilizer in the production of the vaccine)

Sensitivity to measles and rubella virus vaccine live
Thrombocytopenia or history of vaccine-associated thrombocytopenia
(persons who experienced thrombocytopenia with the first dose of vaccine may develop thrombocytopenia with additional doses. These persons should have serologic testing performed in order to determine the need for additional doses of vaccine. The risk-benefit ratio should be evaluated before considering vaccination in such cases)

**Patient monitoring**
The following may be especially important in patient monitoring (other tests may be warranted in some patients, depending on condition; » = major clinical significance):

Seroconversion test
(may be performed 6 to 8 weeks following vaccination in patients for whom immunity is considered crucial [e.g., persons traveling outside the U.S. or women in high-risk areas who intend to become pregnant], since vaccination with measles and rubella virus vaccine may not result in seroconversion in all susceptible patients)

## Side/Adverse Effects

Note: The side/adverse effects associated with the use of measles and rubella virus vaccine live are those expected to follow administration of the monovalent vaccines given separately. However, it is very important to differentiate between vaccine-induced side/adverse effects and natural infection.

Revaccination of prior vaccinees appears to be associated with relatively low side/adverse effect rates.

The incidence of side/adverse effects increases with age and is generally higher in females.

A history of hypersensitivity reactions other than anaphylaxis, such as delayed-type allergic reaction (contact dermatitis), generally does not preclude immunization. There is a very small chance of an adverse reaction in any child, and a study showed that measles- and rubella-containing combined vaccines such as measles, mumps, and rubella virus vaccine live can be administered safely in a single dose to children allergic to eggs, even those with severe hypersensitivity.

Encephalitis and encephalopathy have been temporally related to measles vaccine administration and occur in one per million doses administered; however, no causal relationship has been established. The incidence of these diseases after a natural measles infection is one per thousand persons.

Although there is a temporal relationship, no definite causal relationship has been established between the isolated reports of the occurrence of Guillain-Barré syndrome (GBS) or ocular palsies following the administration of measles vaccine. Isolated incidents of GBS also have been reported after immunization with rubella-containing vaccines.

It is not known whether some of the cases of subacute sclerosing panencephalitis (SSPE) attributed to the measles virus vaccine were actually due to unrecognized natural measles infection during the first year of life. However, the use of measles virus vaccine has reduced the incidence of SSPE from between 5 and 10 cases per million cases of natural measles infection to 1 case per million doses of measles virus vaccine.

Persons who are immune to measles and/or rubella virus because of past vaccination or infection usually do not experience side/adverse effects from the vaccine.

Excretion of small amounts of the live attenuated rubella virus from the nose or throat has occurred in the majority of susceptible individuals 7 to 28 days after vaccination. There is, however, no confirmed evidence to indicate that the vaccine virus is transmitted to susceptible persons who are in contact with the vaccinated individuals.

The following side/adverse effects have been selected on the basis of their potential clinical significance (possible signs and symptoms in parentheses where appropriate)—not necessarily inclusive:

### Those indicating need for medical attention
Incidence more frequent
*Fever over 39.4 °C (103 °F)*

Incidence less frequent
*Optic neuritis* (pain or tenderness of eyes)—may occur from 1 to 4 weeks after immunization, lasting less than 1 week

Incidence rare
*Anaphylactic reaction* (difficulty in breathing or swallowing; hives; itching, especially of feet and hands; reddening of skin, especially around ears; swelling of eyes, face, or inside of nose; unusual tiredness or weakness, sudden and severe); *encephalitis or meningoencephalitis* (confusion; headache, severe or continuing; irritability; stiff neck; vomiting); *ocular palsies* (double vision); *peripheral neuropathy, polyneuritis, or polyneuropathy* (pain, numbness, or tingling of hands, arms, legs, or feet)—may occur from 1 to 4 weeks after immunization, lasting less than 1 week; *thrombocytopenic purpura* (bruising or purple spots on skin)

### Those indicating need for medical attention only if they continue or are bothersome
Incidence more frequent
*Fever between 37.7 and 39.4 °C (100 and 103 °F); lymphadenopathy or parotitis* (swelling of glands in neck)—may occur from 1 to 4 weeks after immunization, lasting less than 1 week; *reaction to acid pH of vaccine* (burning or stinging at injection site); *skin rash*

Incidence less frequent
*Allergic reaction, delayed-type, cell-mediated* (itching, swelling, redness, tenderness, or hard lump at place of injection); *arthralgia or ar-*

*thritis* (aches or pain in joint)—may occur from 1 to 10 weeks after immunization, lasting less than 1 week; *malaise* (vague feeling of bodily discomfort)—may occur from 1 to 4 weeks after immunization, lasting less than 1 week; *mild headache, sore throat, or runny nose*—may occur from 1 to 4 weeks after immunization, lasting less than 1 week; *nausea*

Note: One study showed that the RA 27/3 strain of rubella vaccine administered to susceptible adult women is not associated with clinically important acute or chronic joint disease. Therefore, rubella vaccination should continue to be used to protect susceptible adult women from rubella in order to advance the goal of eliminating the congenital rubella syndrome. The incidence of *arthralgia or arthritis* is greatly increased in women of childbearing age. Generally the older the female, the greater the incidence, severity, and duration of arthralgia or arthritis. However, even in older women, the symptoms are generally well tolerated and rarely interfere with normal activities. No persistent joint disorders have been reported.

## Patient Consultation

As an aid to patient consultation, refer to *Advice for the Patient, Measles and Rubella Virus Vaccine Live (Systemic)*.

In providing consultation, consider emphasizing the following selected information (» = major clinical significance):

### Before receiving this vaccine
» Conditions affecting use, especially:
- Sensitivity to measles and rubella virus vaccine live, or allergy to eggs, gelatin, or neomycin
- Pregnancy—Use of measles and rubella virus vaccine live during pregnancy or pregnancy within 3 months of immunization is not recommended
- Use in children—Use is not recommended for infants up to 12 months of age, unless risk of measles infection is high
- Other medications, especially immunosuppressive agents or radiation therapy
- Other medical problems, especially severe febrile illness, family history of congenital or hereditary immune deficiency conditions, or primary or acquired immune deficiency conditions

### Proper use of this medication
Waiting at least 14 days after receiving vaccine before receiving blood products or immune globulins
Waiting at least 3 to 11 months after administration of blood products or immune globulins before receiving vaccine, depending on the product and dose received
» Proper dosing

### Precautions after receiving this vaccine
» Not becoming pregnant for 3 months without first checking with physician, because of theoretical possibility of birth defects
Checking with physician before receiving tuberculin skin test within 4 to 6 weeks of this vaccine, since the results of the test may be affected by the vaccine

### Side/adverse effects
Signs of potential side effects, especially fever over 39.4 °C (103 °F); optic neuritis; anaphylactic reaction; encephalitis or meningoencephalitis; ocular palsies; peripheral neuropathy, polyneuritis, or polyneuropathy; and thrombocytopenic purpura

## General Dosing Information

The dosage of measles and rubella virus vaccine live is the same for both children and adults.

Measles and rubella virus vaccine live is administered subcutaneously. It should not be injected intravenously.

When sterilizing syringes and skin before vaccination, care should be taken to avoid preservatives, antiseptics, detergents, and disinfectants because the vaccine virus is easily inactivated by these substances.

To prevent inactivation of the vaccine, it is recommended that only the diluent provided by the manufacturer be used.

A 25-gauge, 5/8th-inch needle is recommended for administration of the vaccine.

Although measles and rubella vaccines are available as a combination vaccine (measles and rubella virus vaccine live) and, as such, are administered as a single injection, the commercially available individual vaccines should not be mixed in the same syringe or administered at the same body site.

Although the fourth dose of diphtheria, tetanus, and pertussis (DTP) vaccine and the third dose of oral poliovirus vaccine (OPV) traditionally have been administered to children 18 months of age and a measles-containing vaccine (preferably as measles, mumps, and rubella virus vaccine live) traditionally has been administered to children 15 months of age, it is now recommended that DTP, OPV, and measles, mumps, and rubella virus vaccine live be administered concurrently to children 12 to 15 months of age. Measles, mumps, and rubella virus vaccine live should not be postponed in order to administer all of these vaccines concurrently at 18 months of age.

Measles and rubella virus vaccine, a live virus vaccine, may be administered concurrently with the following, using separate body sites, separate syringes, and the precautions that apply to each immunizing agent:
- Polysaccharide vaccines, such as Haemophilus b conjugate vaccine, Haemophilus b polysaccharide vaccine, meningococcal polysaccharide vaccine, or pneumococcal polyvalent vaccine.
- Influenza vaccine, whole or split virus.
- Diphtheria toxoid, tetanus toxoid, and/or pertussis vaccine.
- Live virus vaccines, other, such as OPV and varicella. OPV and measles, mumps, and rubella virus vaccine (or its component vaccines) can be administered at any time before, with, or after each other, if indicated.
- Inactivated poliovirus vaccine (IPV) or enhanced-potency inactivated poliovirus vaccine (enhanced-potency IPV).
- Hepatitis B recombinant or plasma-derived vaccine.
- Inactivated vaccines, other, except cholera, plague, and typhoid. It is recommended that cholera, plague, and typhoid vaccines be administered on separate occasions because of these vaccines' propensity to cause side/adverse effects.

### For treatment of adverse effects
Recommended treatment consists of the following:
- For mild hypersensitivity reaction—Administering antihistamines, and, if necessary, corticosteroids.
- For severe hypersensitivity or anaphylactic reaction—Administering epinephrine. Antihistamines or corticosteroids also may be administered as required.

## Parenteral Dosage Forms

### MEASLES AND RUBELLA VIRUS VACCINE LIVE (FOR INJECTION) USP

#### Usual adult and adolescent dose
Immunizing agent (active)—
Subcutaneous, 0.5 mL, preferably into the outer aspect of the upper arm.

#### Usual pediatric dose
Immunizing agent (active)—
Infants up to 12 months of age: Use is not recommended.
Infants and children 12 to 15 months of age and older: See *Usual adult and adolescent dose*.

Note: The Committee on Infectious Diseases of the American Academy of Pediatrics (AAP) and the Advisory Committee on Immunization Practices (ACIP) recommend that all children receive a second dose of measles-containing vaccine. The second dose of measles-containing vaccine (preferably as measles, mumps, and rubella virus vaccine live) is routinely recommended at 4 to 6 years of age, but may be administered at any visit, provided at least one month has elapsed since receipt of the first dose. The preadolescent health visit at 11 to 12 years of age can serve as a catch up opportunity to verify vaccination status and administer the vaccine to those children who have not yet received two doses of a measles-containing vaccine.

#### Strength(s) usually available
U.S.—
Not less than the equivalent of 1000 median tissue culture infective dose [TCID$_{50}$] of the U.S. Reference Measles Virus and not less than the equivalent of 1000 TCID$_{50}$ of the U.S. Reference Rubella Virus in each 0.5-mL dose (Rx) [*M-R-VAX II* (neomycin approximately 25 mcg)].
Canada—
Not commercially available.

#### Packaging and storage
Store the lyophilized form of the vaccine, the diluent, and the reconstituted form of the vaccine between 2 and 8 °C (36 and 46 °F), unless otherwise specified by manufacturer.
Alternatively, the diluent for the single-dose vials may be stored between 15 and 30 °C (59 and 86 °F).
Protect both the lyophilized form and the reconstituted form of the vaccine from light.

#### Preparation of dosage form
To reconstitute, use only the diluent provided by the manufacturer, since it is free of preservatives and other substances that might inactivate the vaccine.

Single-dose vial—The entire volume of diluent (approximately 0.5 mL) should be withdrawn into the syringe. All the diluent in the syringe should be injected into the vial of lyophilized vaccine and agitated to mix thoroughly. The entire contents of the vial should be withdrawn into the syringe and the total volume of restored vaccine injected subcutaneously.

10-dose vial (in U.S., available only to government agencies/institutions)— The entire contents (7 mL) of the diluent vial should be withdrawn into the syringe to be used for reconstitution. All of the diluent in the syringe should be injected into the 10-dose vial of lyophilized vaccine and agitated to mix thoroughly. The 10-dose container can be used with either syringes or a jet injector. Since the vaccine and diluent do not contain preservatives, special care should be taken to prevent contamination of the multiple-dose vial of vaccine. In addition, the vial should be stored properly until the reconstituted vaccine is used. Unused vaccine should be discarded after 8 hours.

50-dose vial (in U.S., available only to government agencies/institutions)— The entire contents (30 mL) of the diluent vial should be withdrawn into the syringe to be used for reconstitution. All of the diluent in the syringe should be injected into the 50-dose vial of lyophilized vaccine and agitated to mix thoroughly. The 50-dose container is designed to be used only with a jet injector. Since the vaccine and diluent do not contain preservatives, special care should be taken to prevent contamination of the multiple-dose vial of vaccine. In addition, the vial should be stored properly until the reconstituted vaccine is used. Unused vaccine should be discarded after 8 hours.

**Stability**
Both the lyophilized and the reconstituted vaccine should be stored between 2 and 8 °C (36 and 46 °F) and protected from light. Improper storage and protection may inactivate the vaccine.
The reconstituted vaccine should be used as soon as possible. Unused reconstituted vaccine should be discarded after 8 hours.
The reconstituted vaccine is clear yellow. It should not be used if it is discolored.

**Incompatibilities**
Preservatives or other substances may inactivate the vaccine; therefore, only the diluent supplied by the manufacturer should be used for reconstitution.
A sterile syringe free of preservatives, antiseptics, disinfectants, and detergents should be used for each injection and/or reconstitution of the vaccine. These substances may inactivate the live virus vaccine.

**Auxiliary labeling**
- Protect from light.
- Store in refrigerator.
- Discard reconstituted vaccine if not used within 8 hours.

**Note**
The date and the time of reconstitution should be indicated on the vial if the reconstituted vaccine is not used at once.

Developed: 04/29/97

# MEASLES VIRUS VACCINE LIVE   Systemic

VA CLASSIFICATION (Primary): IM100
Note: This monograph is specific for the measles virus vaccine live derived from Enders' attenuated Edmonston strain and grown in cell cultures of chick embryos.
Commonly used brand name(s): *Attenuvax*.
Note: For a listing of dosage forms and brand names by country availability, see *Dosage Forms* section(s).

## Category
Immunizing agent (active).

## Indications

**General considerations**
Persons can generally be considered immune to measles only if they have documentation of adequate immunization with measles vaccine on or after their first birthdays, if they have laboratory evidence of measles immunity, or if they have a physician's diagnosis of measles infection.

Most individuals born before 1957 can generally be considered immune to measles because of probable previous infection. However, birth before 1957 provides only presumptive evidence of immunity, and measles can still occur in some persons born before 1957.

Although serologic tests may be conducted to determine the susceptibility of persons of unknown immunity, studies have indicated, no evidence of increased risk of adverse reactions to vaccination with measles virus vaccine live in persons already immune to measles.

Monovalent measles vaccine should be used to immunize infants 6 to 12 months of age during measles epidemics, although the combined measles-mumps-rubella or measles-rubella vaccines can be used if the monovalent measles vaccine is not available.

Measles, mumps, and rubella virus vaccine should be used for vaccinating individuals who are likely to be susceptible to more than one of these viruses, unless otherwise contraindicated.

Vaccines containing the measles antigen should be administered to persons 12 to 15 months of age or older under routine conditions.

**Accepted**
Measles (prophylaxis)—Measles virus vaccine live is indicated for immunization against measles (rubeola; morbilli; coughing, hard, red, or ten-day measles). The main objective of measles immunization is to prevent transmission of measles virus and to prevent severe complications, such as pneumonia, ear infections, sinusitis, encephalitis, subacute sclerosing panencephalitis, and death, which may develop from a measles infection. The risk of serious complications and death from a natural measles infection is greater for adults and infants than for children and adolescents.

Unless otherwise contraindicated, all susceptible persons should be immunized against measles, including:
- Children 12 to 15 months of age. All children 12 to 15 months of age should receive measles virus vaccine live, preferably as measles, mumps, and rubella virus vaccine live, as part of the routine childhood immunization schedule. The slightly lower response to the first dose of measles virus vaccine live when administered at 12 months of age compared with administration at 15 months of age has limited clinical importance because a second dose of the measles, mumps, and rubella virus vaccine live is recommended routinely for all children, enhancing the likelihood of seroconversion among children who do not respond to the first dose. Both the American Academy of Pediatrics (AAP) and the Advisory Committee on Immunization Practices (ACIP) recommend administration of measles virus vaccine live, preferably as the measles, mumps, and rubella virus vaccine live, at 12 to 15 months of age and a second dose prior to elementary school entery. Infants up to 12 months of age may retain maternal measles-neutralizing antibodies that may interfere with the immune response to measles virus vaccine live. Therefore, children vaccinated when younger than 12 months of age should be revaccinated with two additional doses of measles-containing vaccine.
- Adolescents who didn't receive a second dose of measles-containing vaccine. Because the recommendation for a second dose of measles, mumps, and rubella virus vaccine was made in 1989, many children born before 1985 (and some children born after 1985, depending on local policy) may not have received the second vaccine dose. Therefore, a second dose of measles-containing vaccine (preferably as measles, mumps, and rubella virus vaccine) is recommended for all adolescents who have not received two doses of the measles, mumps, and rubella virus vaccine at ≥ 12 months of age.
- International travelers. Persons without evidence of measles immunity who travel abroad should be vaccinated against measles because measles is endemic and even epidemic in many countries throughout the world. From 1985 to 1991, 993 reported cases of measles in the U.S. were attributable to exposure in foreign countries, and additional cases occurred in contacts of these imported cases. Therefore, vaccination against measles is especially important for international travelers. These persons should receive either a single antigen vaccine or a combined antigen vaccine as appropriate prior to international travel. However, the measles, mumps, and rubella virus vaccine live is preferred for persons likely to be susceptible to more than one of these viruses; and if a single-antigen measles vaccine is not readily available, travelers should receive the measles, mumps, and rubella virus vaccine live regardless of their immune status to mumps and rubella. Infants 6 to 12 months of age should receive a dose of monovalent measles vaccine before departure. If a single-antigen measles vaccine is not readily available, these infants should receive the measles, mumps, and rubella virus vaccine live. They should be revaccinated at 12 to 15 months of age with the measles, mumps, and rubella virus vaccine live, at least 1 month after the initial measles vaccination, so that children 16 months

of age or older should have received two doses of measles-containing vaccine to assure immunity.

## Pharmacology/Pharmacokinetics

### Mechanism of action/Effect
Vaccination with measles virus vaccine live induces measles hemagglutination inhibiting (HI) antibodies, which provide active immunity against measles infection.

### Protective effect
A single injection of the vaccine has been shown to induce measles HI antibodies in 97% or more of susceptible persons. In one recent study in which children randomly received the measles, mumps, and rubella virus vaccine live at either 12 or 15 months of age, the measles antibody response to the vaccine was 93% among children vaccinated at 12 months of age and 98% among those vaccinated at 15 months of age. Among children of mothers born after 1961, who probably had received measles vaccine and were less likely to have had measles infection than women born in previous years, the seroconversion rate was 96% among children vaccinated at 12 months of age and 98% among those vaccinated at 15 months of age.

### Duration of protective effect
Vaccine-induced antibody levels have been shown to persist for at least 13 years without substantial decline. However, continued surveillance will be necessary to determine further duration of antibody persistence.

## Precautions to Consider

Note: In the past, persons who had a history of anaphylactic reactions following egg ingestion were considered to be at increased risk for serious reactions after receipt of measles-containing vaccines, which are produced in chick embryo fibroblasts. Protocols for skin testing were developed for persons receiving the vaccine who had had anaphylactic reactions after egg ingestion. However, the predictive value of such skin testing and the need for special protocols when vaccinating egg-allergic persons with measles-containing vaccines is uncertain. The results of recent studies suggest that anaphylactic reactions to measles-containing vaccines are not associated with hypersensitivity to egg antigens, but with some other component of the vaccines. The risk for serious allergic reaction to these vaccines in egg-allergic patients is extremely low, and skin testing is not necessarily predictive of vaccine hypersensitivity.

### Cross-sensitivity and/or related problems
Patients allergic to systemic or topical neomycin may be allergic to the measles virus vaccine live because each 0.5-mL dose contains approximately 25 mcg of neomycin, which is used in the production of the vaccine to prevent bacterial overgrowth in the viral culture. A history of hypersensitivity reactions, such as delayed-type allergic reaction (contact dermatitis), to neomycin generally does not preclude immunization. However, anaphylaxis from topically or systemically administered neomycin precludes immunization.

Patients allergic to gelatin also may be allergic to measles virus vaccine live, since gelatin is used as a stabilizer in the production of measles, mumps, and rubella virus vaccine and its component vaccines. The literature contains a single case report of a person with an anaphylactic sensitivity to gelatin who had an anaphylactic reaction after receipt of the measles, mumps, and rubella virus vaccine licensed in the U.S. Similar cases have occurred in Japan. Therefore, such persons should be vaccinated with measles, mumps, and rubella virus vaccine and its component vaccines with extreme caution.

### Pregnancy/Reproduction
Pregnancy—Live measles vaccine, when given as a component of measles and rubella virus vaccine live or measles, mumps, and rubella virus vaccine live should not be given to women known to be pregnant or who are considering becoming pregnant within the next 3 months. Women who are given monovalent measles vaccine should not become pregnant for at least 30 days after vaccination. This precaution is based on the theoretical risk of fetal infection, although no evidence substantiates this theoretical risk. In considering the importance of protecting adolescents and young adults against measles, asking women if they are pregnant, excluding those who are, and explaining the theoretical risks to others before vaccination should be sufficient precautions.

Studies have not been done in animals.

FDA Pregnancy Category C.

### Breast-feeding
It is not known whether this vaccine is distributed into breast milk. However, problems in humans have not been documented.

### Pediatrics
Infants up to 15 months of age may fail to respond to measles virus vaccine live due to the presence of residual circulating measles antibody of maternal origin. This effect usually starts to wane after the child reaches 6 months of age. However, children born to younger mothers might respond well to measles vaccine administered at 12 months of age. In one study, children randomly received measles vaccine at either 12 or 15 months of age. The antibody response to measles virus vaccine live was 93 to 95% when the vaccine was administered at 12 months of age, and 98% when it was administered at 15 months of age. Among children of mothers born after 1961, who probably had received a measles vaccine and who therefore were less likely to have had measles infection than women born in previous years, the seroconversion rate was 96% among those children vaccinated at 12 months of age and 98% among those vaccinated at 15 months of age. Based on these findings, the Committee on Infectious Diseases of the American Academy of Pediatrics (AAP) and the Advisory Committee on Immunization Practices (ACIP) of the Centers for Disease Control and Prevention recommend administration of the first dose of measles-containing vaccine at 12 to 15 months of age. Both AAP and ACIP recommend that all children receive a second dose of measles-containing vaccine. The second dose of measles-containing vaccine (preferably as measles, mumps, and rubella virus vaccine live) is routinely recommended at 4 to 6 years of age, but may be administered at any visit, provided at least 1 month has elapsed since receipt of the first dose. The preadolescent health visit at 11 to 12 years of age can serve as a catch up opportunity to verify vaccination status and administer the vaccine to those children who have not yet received two doses of a measles-containing vaccine. Children who received the monovalent measles vaccine rather than the measles, mumps, and rubella virus vaccine live on or after their first birthdays also should receive a primary dose of mumps and rubella vaccines, and doses of measles, mumps, and rubella virus vaccine live or other measles-containing vaccines should be separated by at least 1 month.

If exposure to measles infection has occurred within 72 hours or is imminent, children between 6 and 15 months of age can be vaccinated, provided that those vaccinated before their first birthdays are revaccinated at 15 months of age. There is some evidence to suggest, however, that infants immunized at less than 12 months of age may not develop sustained antibody levels when reimmunized later. The advantage of early protection must be weighed against the chance for failure to respond adequately on reimmunization.

Children with end-stage renal disease receiving maintenance hemodialysis have a degree of immunosuppression that reduces their response to vaccination. Therefore, it may be necessary to monitor postvaccination antibody levels in children with end-stage renal disease, and to revaccinate those children who have failed to demonstrate seroconversion.

It is also very important to vaccinate human immunodeficiency virus (HIV)-infected children against measles.

### Adolescents
The sustained decline of measles in the U.S. has been associated with a shift in occurrence from children to infants and young adults. From 1990 to 1994, 47% of reported cases occurred in persons aged 10 years or older, compared with only 10% from 1960 to 1964. During the 1980s, outbreaks of measles occurred among school-age children in schools with measles vaccination levels of ≥ 98%. Primary vaccine failure was considered the principal contributing factor in these outbreaks. As a result, beginning in 1989, a two-dose measles-vaccination schedule for students in primary schools, secondary schools, and colleges and universities was recommended. This two-dose vaccination schedule provides protection to ≥ 98% of persons vaccinated.

### Drug interactions and/or related problems
The following drug interactions and/or related problems have been selected on the basis of their potential clinical significance (possible mechanism in parentheses where appropriate)—not necessarily inclusive (» = major clinical significance):

Note: Combinations containing any of the following medications, depending on the amount present, may also interact with this medication.

Blood products or
Immune globulins
(concurrent administration with measles virus vaccine live may interfere with the patient's immune response to the virus because of the possibility of antibodies to measles virus in these products. Measles virus vaccine live should be administered at least 14 days before, or 3 to 11 months after, administration of blood products or immune globulins, depending on the product and dose received)

» Immunosuppressive agents or
» Radiation therapy
(because normal defense mechanisms are suppressed, concurrent use with measles virus vaccine live may potentiate the replication of the vaccine virus, may increase the side/adverse effects of the vaccine, and/or may decrease the patient's antibody response to measles vaccine. The interaction may be severe enough to cause

death. The interval between discontinuing medications that cause immunosuppression and regaining the ability to respond to measles virus vaccine live depends on the intensity and type of immunosuppressive medication used, the underlying disease, and other factors; estimates vary from 3 months to 1 year. Patients with leukemia in remission should not receive measles virus vaccine live until at least 3 months after their last chemotherapy. The precaution does not apply to corticosteroids used as replacement therapy, for short-term [less than 2 weeks] systemic therapy, or by other routes of administration that do not cause immunosuppression)

Live virus vaccines, other
(data are lacking on impairment of antibody responses to rubella, measles, mumps, or oral poliovirus vaccine (OPV) when these vaccines are administered on different days within 1 month of each other; however, OPV and measles, mumps, and rubella virus vaccine live [or its individual component vaccines] can be administered at any time before, with, or after each other, if indicated)

**Laboratory value alterations**
The following have been selected on the basis of their potential clinical significance (possible effect in parentheses where appropriate)—not necessarily inclusive (» = major clinical significance):

With diagnostic test results
» Tuberculin skin test
(short-term suppression lasting several weeks may occur, starting 4 to 7 days after vaccination, and may result in false-negative tests; if required, tuberculin skin tests should be done before, simultaneously with, or at least 4 to 6 weeks after administration of measles vaccine)

Skin tests, other
(decreased responsiveness to skin test antigens may occur because of vaccine-induced transient suppression of delayed-type hypersensitivity; the period of time for which responsiveness is decreased depends upon the particular skin test used)

**Medical considerations/Contraindications**
The medical considerations/contraindications included have been selected on the basis of their potential clinical significance (reasons given in parentheses where appropriate)—not necessarily inclusive (» = major clinical significance).

*Except under special circumstances, this medication should not be used when the following medical problems exist:*

» Febrile illness
(the decision to administer or delay vaccination because of a current or recent febrile illness depends largely on the cause of the illness and the severity of symptoms; minor illnesses, such as upper respiratory infection, do not preclude administration of vaccine; for persons whose compliance with medical care cannot be assured, every opportunity should be taken to provide appropriate vaccinations)

(children with moderate or severe febrile illnesses can be vaccinated as soon as they have recovered from the acute phase of the illness; this wait avoids superimposing adverse effects of vaccination on the underlying illness or mistakenly attributing a manifestation of the underlying illness to the vaccine; performing routine physical examinations or measuring temperatures are not prerequisites for vaccinating infants and children who appear to be in good health; Asking the parent or guardian if the child is ill, postponing vaccination for children with moderate or severe febrile illnesses, and vaccinating those without contraindications are appropriate procedures in childhood immunization programs)

» Immune deficiency conditions, congenital or hereditary, family history of, or
» Immune deficiency conditions, primary or acquired
(replication of vaccine viruses can be enhanced in persons with immune-deficiency diseases and in persons with immunosuppression, as occurs with leukemia, lymphoma, generalized malignancy, or therapy with alkylating agents, antimetabolites, radiation, or large doses of corticosteroids; evidence based on case reports has linked measles vaccine and measles infection to subsequent death in some severely immunocompromised children; of the more than 200 million doses of measles vaccine administered in the U.S., fewer than five such deaths have been reported; patients who have such conditions or are undergoing such therapies [excluding most HIV-infected patients] should not be given measles virus vaccine live)

(patients with leukemia in remission who have not received chemotherapy for at least 3 months may receive live virus vaccines; the exact amount of systemically absorbed corticosteroids and the duration of administration needed to suppress the immune system of an otherwise healthy child are not well defined; most experts agree that corticosteroid therapy usually does not contraindicate administration of live virus vaccine when such therapy is short-term [i.e., less than 2 weeks], low to moderate dose, long-term alternate-day treatment with short-acting preparations, maintenance physiologic doses [replacement therapy], or administered topically [skin or eyes], by aerosol, or by intraarticular, bursal, or tendon injection; although of recent theoretical concern, no evidence of increased severe reactions to live vaccines has been reported among persons receiving corticosteroid therapy by aerosol, and such therapy is not in itself a reason to delay vaccination)

(the immunosuppressive effects of corticosteroid treatment vary, but many clinicians consider a dose equivalent to either 2 mg per kg (mg/kg) of body weight or a total of 20 mg per day of prednisone as sufficiently immunosuppressive to raise concern about the safety of vaccination with live virus vaccines; corticosteroids used in greater than physiologic doses also can reduce the immune response to vaccines; physicians should wait at least 3 months after discontinuation of therapy before administering a live-virus vaccine to patients who have received high systemically absorbed doses of corticosteroids for ≥ 2 weeks)

(measles-containing vaccine is recommended for HIV-infected persons without evidence of measles immunity who are not severely immunocompromised; because of a reported case of pneumonitis in a measles vaccinee who had an advanced case of acquired immunodeficiency syndrome (AIDS), and because of other evidence indicating a diminished antibody response to measles vaccination among severely immunocompromised persons, it is important to withhold measles-containing vaccines from HIV-infected persons with evidence of severe immunosuppression)

*Risk-benefit should be considered when the following medical problems exist:*

Hypersensitivity to neomycin
(patients allergic to systemic or topical neomycin may be allergic to the measles virus vaccine live because each 0.5-mL dose contains approximately 25 mcg of neomycin, which is used in the production of the vaccine to prevent bacterial overgrowth in the viral culture. A history of hypersensitivity reactions, such as delayed-type allergic reaction (contact dermatitis), to neomycin generally does not preclude immunization. However, a history of anaphylaxis due to topically or systemically administered neomycin precludes immunization)

Allergy to gelatin
(patients allergic to gelatin also may be allergic to measles virus vaccine live, since gelatin is used as a stabilizer in the production of the vaccine)

Thrombocytopenia or vaccine-associated thrombocytopenia
(persons who experienced thrombocytopenia with the first dose of vaccine may develop thrombocytopenia with additional doses. These persons should have serological testing performed in order to determine the need for additional doses of vaccine. The risk-benefit ratio should be evaluated before vaccination is considered in such cases)

Conditions requiring avoidance of fever, such as cerebral injury or history of febrile seizures
(because of possible vaccine-induced fever)

Sensitivity to measles virus vaccine live

**Patient monitoring**
The following may be especially important in patient monitoring (other tests may be warranted in some patients, depending on condition; » = major clinical significance):

Seroconversion test
(may be performed at 4 or more weeks following vaccination in patients in whom immunity is considered crucial [e.g., persons traveling outside the U.S. or women in high-risk areas who intend to become pregnant], since vaccination with measles virus vaccine live may not result in seroconversion in all susceptible patients)

# Side/Adverse Effects

Note: More than 240 million doses of measles vaccine were distributed in the U.S. from 1963 through 1993. The vaccine has an excellent record of safety. From 5 to 15% of vaccinees develop a temperature of 103 °F (39.4 °C) or higher beginning 5 to 12 days after vaccination and usually lasting several days. Most persons with fever are otherwise asymptomatic.

Transient rashes have been reported in approximately 5% of vaccinees. Central nervous system (CNS) conditions, including encephalitis and encephalopathy, have been reported with a frequency of less than one per million doses administered. The incidence of encephalitis or encephalopathy after measles vaccination of healthy children is lower than the observed incidence of encephalitis of unknown etiology. This finding suggests that the reported severe neurologic disorders that have been temporally associated with measles vaccination were not caused by the vaccine. These adverse events should be anticipated only in susceptible vaccinees and do not appear to be age-related. After revaccination, most reactions should be expected to occur only among the small proportion of persons who failed to respond on the first dose.

Measles vaccine significantly reduces the likelihood of developing subacute sclerosing panencephalitis (SSPE), as evidenced by the near elimination of SSPE cases after widespread measles vaccination began. SSPE has been reported rarely in children who do not have a history of natural measles infection but who have received measles vaccine. The available evidence suggests that at least some of these children may have had an unidentified measles infection before vaccination and that the SSPE probably resulted from the natural measles infection. The administration of live measles vaccine does not increase the risk for SSPE, regardless of whether the vaccinee has had measles infection or has previously received live measles vaccine.

The following side/adverse effects have been selected on the basis of their potential clinical significance (possible signs and symptoms in parentheses where appropriate)—not necessarily inclusive:

**Those indicating need for medical attention**
Incidence more frequent—5 to 15%
  *Fever over 39.4 °C (103 °F)*
Incidence rare
  *Anaphylactic reaction* (difficulty in breathing or swallowing; hives; itching, especially of soles or palms; reddening of skin, especially around ears; swelling of eyes, face, or inside of nose; unusual tiredness or weakness, sudden and severe); *encephalitis or meningoencephalitis* (confusion, severe or continuing headache, irritability, stiff neck, or vomiting); *ocular palsies* (double vision); *thrombocytopenic purpura* (bruising or purple spots on skin); *Lymphadenopathy* (swelling of glands in neck); *swelling, blistering, or pain at injection site, severe and extensive*

**Those indicating need for medical attention only if they continue or are bothersome**
Incidence more frequent
  *Burning or stinging at injection site*—due to acid pH of vaccine; *fever of 37.7 °C (100 °F) or less*
Incidence less frequent
  *Allergic reaction, delayed-type, cell-mediated* (itching, swelling, redness, tenderness, or hard lump at injection site); *fever between 37.7 and 39.4 °C (100 and 103 °F); skin rash*

## Patient Consultation

As an aid to patient consultation, refer to *Advice for the Patient, Measles Virus Vaccine Live (Systemic)*.
In providing consultation, consider emphasizing the following selected information (» = major clinical significance):

**Before receiving this vaccine**
» Conditions affecting use, especially:
  Sensitivity to measles vaccine or allergy to gelatin or neomycin
  Pregnancy—Use of measles vaccine during pregnancy or pregnancy within 3 months of immunization is not recommended
  Use in children—Use is not recommended for infants up to 12 months of age, unless risk of measles infection is high
  Other medications, especially immunosuppressive agents or radiation therapy
  Other medical problems, especially febrile illness, primary or acquired immune deficiency conditions, or family history of congenital or hereditary immune deficiency conditions

**Proper use of this vaccine**
  Waiting at least 14 days after receiving vaccine before receiving blood products or immune globulin
  Waiting at least 3 to 11 months after administration of blood products or immune globulins before receiving vaccine, depending on the product and dose received
» Proper dosing

**Precautions after receiving this vaccine**
» Not becoming pregnant for 3 months without first checking with physician, because of theoretical risk of birth defects
  Checking with physician before receiving tuberculin skin test within 4 to 6 weeks of this vaccine, since the results of the test may be affected by the measles vaccine

**Side/adverse effects**
  Fever and skin rash may occur from 5 to 12 days after vaccination and usually last several days
  Signs of potential side effects, especially fever over 39.4 °C (103 °F), anaphylactic reaction, encephalitis, meningoencephalitis, ocular palsies, or thrombocytopenic purpura

## General Dosing Information

The American Academy of Pediatrics (AAP) and the Advisory Committee on Immunization Practices (ACIP) recommend that all children 12 to 15 months of age receive two doses of measles-containing vaccine, preferably as measles, mumps, and rubella virus vaccine live. Children who received monovalent measles vaccine rather than the measles, mumps, and rubella virus vaccine live on or after their first birthdays also should receive a primary dose of mumps and rubella vaccines; and doses of measles, mumps, and rubella virus vaccine live or other measles-containing vaccines should be separated by at least 1 month.

The dosage of measles vaccine is the same for both children and adults.

When sterilizing syringes and skin before vaccination, care should be taken to avoid preservatives, antiseptics, detergents, and disinfectants, since the vaccine virus is easily inactivated by these substances.

To prevent inactivation of the vaccine, it is recommended that only the diluent provided by the manufacturer be used for vaccine reconstitution.

A 25-gauge, 5/8th-inch needle is recommended for administration of the vaccine.

Measles vaccine is administered subcutaneously. It should not be injected intravenously.

Previous recommendations, based on data from persons who received low doses of immune globulin (IG) preparations, stated that measles, mumps, and rubella virus vaccine live and its individual component vaccines could be administered as early as 6 weeks to 3 months after administration of IG. However, recent evidence suggests that high doses of IG can inhibit the immune response to measles vaccine for more than 3 months. The duration of interference of IG preparations with the immune response to the measles virus vaccine live is dose-related. Therefore, measles virus vaccine live should be administered at least 14 days before, or 3 to 11 months after administration of IG.

Measles virus vaccine live generally should not be administered simultaneously with IG preparations. However, if administration of an IG preparation becomes necessary because of imminent exposure to disease, measles, mumps, and rubella virus vaccine live or its component vaccines can be administered simultaneously with the IG preparation, although vaccine-induced immunity might be compromised. The vaccine should be administered at a site remote from that chosen for the IG inoculation. Unless serologic testing indicates that specific antibodies have been produced, vaccination should be repeated after the recommended interval.

If administration of an IG preparation becomes necessary after measles, mumps, and rubella virus vaccine live or its individual component vaccines have been administered, interference may occur. Usually, vaccine virus replication and stimulation of immunity will occur 1 to 2 weeks after vaccination. Therefore, if the interval between administration of any of these vaccines and subsequent administration of an IG preparation is less than 14 days, vaccination should be repeated after the recommended interval, unless serologic testing indicates that antibodies have been produced.

Although measles, mumps, and rubella vaccines are commercially available as a combination vaccine (measles, mumps, and rubella virus vaccine live) and, as such, are administered as a single injection, the commercially available individual vaccines should not be mixed in the same syringe or administered at the same body site.

ACIP continues to recommend measles, mumps, and rubella virus vaccine live for HIV-infected persons without evidence of measles immunity. Severely immunocompromised and other symptomatic HIV-infected patients who are exposed to measles should receive IG, regardless of prior vaccination status. In addition, health-care providers should weigh the risks and benefits of measles vaccination or IG prophylaxis for severely immunocompromised HIV-infected patients who are at risk for measles exposure because of outbreaks or international travel.

Because the immunologic response to both live and killed antigen vaccines may decrease as HIV disease progresses, vaccination early in the course of HIV infection may be more likely to induce an immune response. Therefore, HIV-infected infants without severe immunosuppression should routinely receive measles, mumps, and rubella virus vaccine live as soon as possible upon reaching their first birthday. Evaluation and testing of asymptomatic persons to detect HIV infection are not necessary before deciding to administer measles, mumps, and rubella virus vaccine live or other measles-containing vaccine.

## Measles Virus Vaccine Live (Systemic)

Because of a reported case of pneumonitis in a measles vaccinee who had an advanced case of acquired immunodeficiency syndrome (AIDS), and because of other evidence indicating a diminished antibody response to measles vaccination among severely immunocompromised persons, ACIP is re-evaluating the recommendations for vaccination of severely immunocompromised HIV-infected persons.

In the interim, it may be prudent to withhold measles-containing vaccines from HIV-infected persons with evidence of severe immunosuppression, defined by one of the following criteria:
- CD4+ T-lymphocyte count < 750 for children < 12 months of age, < 500 for children 1 to 5 years of age, or < 200 for persons ≥ 6 years of age; or
- CD4+ T-lymphocytes constituting < 15 % of total lymphocytes for children < 13 years of age, or < 14 % for persons ≥ 13 years of age.

If immediate protection against measles is required for persons with contraindications to measles vaccination, passive immunization with IG, 0.25 mL per kg (mL/kg) [0.11 mL per pound] of body weight (maximum dose 15 mL), should be given as soon as possible after known exposure. Exposed symptomatic HIV-infected and other immunocompromised persons should receive IG regardless of their previous vaccination status; however, IG in usual doses may not be effective in such patients. For immunocompromised persons, the recommended dose is 0.5 mL/kg of body weight if IG is administered intramuscularly (maximum dose 15 mL). This corresponds to a dose of protein approximately 82.5 mg per kg (mg/kg) (maximum dose 2475 mg). Intramuscular IG may not be needed if a patient with HIV infection is receiving 100 to 400 mg/kg intravenous IG (IGIV) at regular intervals and the last dose was given within 3 weeks of exposure to measles. Because the amounts of protein administered are similar, high-dose IGIV may be as effective as IG given intramuscularly. However, no data are available concerning the effectiveness of IGIV in preventing measles.

In general, simultaneous administration of the most widely used live and inactivated vaccines does not impair antibody responses or increase rates of adverse effects. Vaccines recommended for administration at 12 to 15 months of age can be administered at either one or two visits. There are equivalent antibody responses and no clinically significant increases in the frequency of adverse events when diphtheria toxoid, tetanus toxoid, and pertussis vaccine (DTP), measles, mumps, and rubella virus vaccine live, oral poliovirus vaccine (OPV) or inactivated poliovirus vaccine (IPV) and *H. influenzae* type b conjugate vaccine (HbCV) are administered either simultaneously at different sites or at separate times. If a child might not be brought back for future vaccinations, all vaccines (including DTP [or DTaP], measles, mumps, and rubella virus vaccine live, OPV [or IPV], varicella, HbCV, and hepatitis B vaccines may be administered simultaneously, as appropriate to the child's age and previous vaccination status.

### For treatment of adverse effects
Recommended treatment includes
- For mild hypersensitivity reaction—Administering antihistamines and, if necessary, corticosteroids.
- For severe hypersensitivity or anaphylactic reaction—Administering epinephrine. Antihistamines or corticosteroids may also be administered as required.

## Parenteral Dosage Forms

### MEASLES VIRUS VACCINE LIVE (FOR INJECTION) USP

### Usual adult and adolescent dose
Immunizing agent (active)—
 Subcutaneous, 0.5 mL, preferably into the outer aspect of the upper arm:
  First dose—At initial visit.
  Second dose—At least one month after the first dose.

### Usual pediatric dose
Immunizing agent (active)—
 Infants up to 12 months of age—Use is not recommended.
 Infants and children 12 months of age and older—See *Usual adult and adolescent dose*.

Note: The Committee on Infectious Diseases of the American Academy of Pediatrics (AAP) and the Advisory Committee on Immunization Practices (ACIP) recommend that all children receive a second dose of measles-containing vaccine. The second dose of measles-containing vaccine (preferably as measles, mumps, and rubella virus vaccine live) is routinely recommended at 4 to 6 years of age, but may be administered at any visit, provided at least one month has elapsed since receipt of the first dose. The preadolescent health visit at 11 to 12 years of age can serve as a catch up opportunity to verify vaccination status and administer the vaccine to those children who have not yet received two doses of a measles containing vaccine.

### Strength(s) usually available
U.S.—
 Not less than the equivalent of 1000 median tissue culture infective dose [TCID$_{50}$] of the U.S. Reference Measles Virus in each 0.5 mL dose (Rx) [*Attenuvax* (neomycin approximately 25 mcg)].
Canada—
 Not less than the equivalent of 1000 median tissue culture infective dose [TCID$_{50}$] of a reference measles virus in each 0.5 mL dose (Rx) [GENERIC (may contain neomycin)].

### Packaging and storage
Store the lyophilized form of the vaccine, the diluent, and the reconstituted form of the vaccine between 2 and 8 °C (36 and 46 °F), unless otherwise specified by the manufacturer.
Alternatively, the diluent for the single-dose vials may be stored between 15 and 30 °C (59 and 86 °F).
Protect both the lyophilized form and the reconstituted form of the vaccine from light.

### Preparation of dosage form
To reconstitute, only the diluent provided by the manufacturer should be used, since it is free of preservatives and other substances that might inactivate the vaccine.
The entire volume of diluent (approximately 0.5 mL) should be withdrawn into the syringe. All the diluent in the syringe is injected into the vial of lyophilized vaccine and agitated to mix thoroughly. The entire contents should be withdrawn into the syringe and the total volume of restored vaccine injected subcutaneously.

### Stability
Both the lyophilized and the reconstituted vaccine should be protected from light, which may inactivate the virus.
Use the reconstituted vaccine as soon as possible. Discard unused reconstituted vaccine after 8 hours.
The reconstituted vaccine is clear yellow. It should not be used if it is discolored.

### Incompatibilities
Preservatives or other substances may inactivate the vaccine; therefore, only the diluent supplied by the manufacturer should be used for reconstitution.
Also, a sterile syringe free of preservatives, antiseptics, and detergents should be used for each injection and/or reconstitution of the vaccine because these substances may inactivate the live virus vaccine.

### Auxiliary labeling
- Protect from light.
- Store in refrigerator.
- Discard reconstituted vaccine if not used within 8 hours.

### Note
The date and time of reconstitution should be indicated on the vial if the reconstituted vaccine is not used at once.

Revised: 07/23/97

---

# MEBENDAZOLE   Systemic

VA CLASSIFICATION (Primary): AP200
Commonly used brand name(s): *Vermox*.
Note: For a listing of dosage forms and brand names by country availability, see *Dosage Forms* section(s).

## Category
Anthelmintic (systemic).

## Indications
Note: Bracketed information in the *Indications* section refers to uses that are not included in U.S. product labeling.

## Accepted

Ascariasis (treatment)—Mebendazole is indicated as a primary agent for ascariasis caused by *Ascaris lumbricoides* (common roundworm).

Enterobiasis (treatment)—Mebendazole is indicated as a primary agent for enterobiasis caused by *Enterobius vermicularis* (pinworm).

Hookworm infection (treatment)—Mebendazole is indicated as a primary agent for hookworm disease caused by *Ancylostoma duodenale* (common hookworm; Old World hookworm) and *Necator americanus* (American hookworm; New World hookworm).

Intestinal roundworm, multiple (treatment)—Mebendazole is indicated in the treatment of multiple intestinal roundworm infections.

Trichuriasis (treatment)—Mebendazole is indicated as a primary agent for trichuriasis caused by *Trichuris trichiura* (whipworm).

[Capillariasis (treatment)][1]—Mebendazole is used in the treatment of capillariasis caused by *Capillaria philippinensis*.

[Gnathostomiasis (treatment)][1]—Mebendazole is used in the treatment of gnathostomiasis caused by *Gnathostoma spinigerum*.

[Hydatid disease, alveolar (treatment)][1]—Mebendazole is used in the treatment of alveolar hydatid disease caused by *Echinococcus multilocularis* (*E. alveolaris*).

[Hydatid disease, unilocular (treatment)][1]—Mebendazole is used in the treatment of unilocular hydatid disease caused by *E. granulosus*. Mebendazole is used as a secondary agent in patients in whom surgery is contraindicated or has failed, in after-spill during surgery, or in recurrences. Very high doses may be effective.

[Trichinosis (treatment)][1]—Mebendazole is used as a secondary agent in the treatment of trichinosis (trichinellosis) caused by *Trichinella spiralis* (pork worm). Systemic corticosteroids are used concurrently, especially in patients with severe symptoms, to minimize inflammatory reactions to *Trichinella* larvae.

Not all species or strains of a particular helminth may be susceptible to mebendazole. In addition, efficacy varies with respect to pre-existing diarrhea, gastrointestinal transit time, and degree of infection.

[1]Not included in Canadian product labeling.

## Pharmacology/Pharmacokinetics

### Physicochemical characteristics
Molecular weight—295.30.

### Mechanism of action/Effect
Vermicidal; may also be ovicidal for ova of most helminths; mebendazole causes degeneration of parasite's cytoplasmic microtubules and thereby selectively and irreversibly blocks glucose uptake in susceptible adult intestine-dwelling helminths and their tissue-dwelling larvae; inhibition of glucose uptake apparently results in depletion of the parasite's glycogen stores; this, in turn, results in reduced formation of adenosine triphosphate (ATP) required for survival and reproduction of the helminth; corresponding energy levels are gradually reduced until death of the parasite ensues; mebendazole does not appear to affect serum glucose concentrations in humans, however.

### Absorption
Poorly absorbed (approximately 5 to 10%) from gastrointestinal tract; absorption may be increased when taken with food, especially fatty food.

### Distribution
Distributed to serum, cyst fluid, liver, omental fat, and pelvic, pulmonary, and hepatic cysts; highest concentrations found in liver; relatively high concentrations also found in muscle-encysted *Trichinella spiralis* larvae; also crosses the placenta.

### Protein binding
High to very high (90–95%).

### Biotransformation
Primarily hepatic; metabolized to inactive amino, hydroxy, and hydroxyamino metabolites; primary metabolite is 2-amino-5-benzoylbenzimidazole.

### Half-life
Normal hepatic function—2.5 to 5.5 hours (range: 2.5 to 9 hours).
Impaired hepatic function (cholestasis)—Approximately 35 hours.

### Time to peak serum concentration
2 to 5 hours (range—0.5 to 7 hours).

### Peak serum concentration
Following a dose of 100 mg twice a day for 3 days—
  Mebendazole: Not more than 0.03 mcg per mL.
  2-Amino metabolite: Not more than 0.09 mcg per mL.
Serum concentrations up to 0.5 mcg per mL have been reported in chronic, high-dose therapy.

### Elimination
Fecal—Approximately 95% excreted unchanged or as the primary metabolite (2-amino derivative) in feces.
Renal—Approximately 2 to 5% excreted unchanged or as the primary metabolite in urine.

## Precautions to Consider

### Carcinogenicity
Carcinogenicity studies in mice and rats given doses as high as 40 mg per kg of body weight (mg/kg) daily for over two years have not shown mebendazole to be carcinogenic.

### Mutagenicity
Dominant lethal mutation studies in mice given single doses as high as 640 mg/kg have not shown that mebendazole is mutagenic. The spermatocyte test, the $F_1$ translocation test, and the Ames test produced negative results.

### Pregnancy/Reproduction
Fertility—Studies in mice given doses of up to 40 mg/kg for 60 days prior to gestation in males and 14 days in females have not shown that mebendazole causes adverse effects on the fetus or offspring. However, mebendazole has been shown to cause slight maternal toxicity at this dose.

Pregnancy—Mebendazole crosses the placenta. A post-marketing survey in pregnant women who inadvertently took mebendazole during the first trimester has not shown an incidence of spontaneous abortion or malformation greater than that of the general population. In a total of 170 deliveries at term, mebendazole has not been shown to be teratogenic in humans.

Studies in rats given single oral doses as low as 10 mg/kg have shown that mebendazole is teratogenic and embryotoxic.

FDA Pregnancy Category C.

### Breast-feeding
It is not known whether mebendazole is distributed into breast milk. However, problems in humans have not been documented.

### Pediatrics
Appropriate studies on the relationship of age to the effects of mebendazole have not been performed in children up to 2 years of age. However, no pediatrics-specific problems have been documented to date in children over the age of 2.

### Geriatrics
No information is available on the relationship of age to the effects of mebendazole in geriatric patients.

### Drug interactions and/or related problems
The following drug interactions and/or related problems have been selected on the basis of their potential clinical significance (possible mechanism in parentheses where appropriate)—not necessarily inclusive (» = major clinical significance):

Note: Combinations containing any of the following medications, depending on the amount present, may also interact with this medication.

Carbamazepine
  (in patients receiving high doses of mebendazole for treatment of tissue-dwelling organisms such as *Echinococcus multilocularis* or *E. granulosus* [hydatid disease], carbamazepine has been shown to lower mebendazole plasma concentrations by induction of hepatic microsomal enzymes and to impair the therapeutic response; if carbamazepine is being used for seizures, replacement with valproic acid is recommended; treatment of intestinal helminths such as whipworms or hookworms does not appear to be affected by the rate of hepatic metabolism of mebendazole)

### Laboratory value alterations
The following have been selected on the basis of their potential clinical significance (possible effect in parentheses where appropriate)—not necessarily inclusive (» = major clinical significance):

With physiology/laboratory test values
» Alanine aminotransferase (ALT [SGPT]), serum, and
» Alkaline phosphatase, serum, and
» Aspartate aminotransferase (AST [SGOT]), serum, and
  Blood urea nitrogen (BUN)
    (values may be transiently increased)

  Hemoglobin, serum
    (concentration may be decreased)

### Medical considerations/Contraindications
The medical considerations/contraindications included have been selected on the basis of their potential clinical significance (reasons given in

parentheses where appropriate)—not necessarily inclusive (» = major clinical significance).

*Risk-benefit should be considered when the following medical problems exist:*

Crohn's ileitis or
Ulcerative colitis
(may increase absorption and toxicity of mebendazole, especially in high-dose therapy)
» Hepatic function impairment
(mebendazole is metabolized primarily in liver; prolonged half-life and drug accumulation may occur, with an increased incidence of side effects; dosage may need to be decreased)
Hypersensitivity to mebendazole

**Patient monitoring**

The following may be especially important in patient monitoring (other tests may be warranted in some patients, depending on condition; » = major clinical significance):

*For pinworms*
» Perianal examinations
(cellophane tape swabs of the perianal area to detect the presence of eggs may be required prior to and starting 1 week following treatment with mebendazole, especially in patients with persisting symptoms; swabs should be taken every morning prior to defecation and bathing for at least 3 days to determine efficacy or proof of cure; perianal examinations may also be required to detect the presence of adult worms in the perianal area; no patient should be considered cured unless perianal swabs have been negative for 7 consecutive days)

*For roundworms, whipworms, and capillariasis*
» Stool examinations
(may be required prior to and approximately 1 to 3 weeks following treatment with mebendazole to determine efficacy or proof of cure; because of colonic mixing, eggs may persist in the stool for up to 1 week following cure)

*For patients on high-dose therapy*
» Complete blood counts (CBCs)
(may be required prior to and periodically during the first month of treatment with mebendazole since high-dose mebendazole may cause granulocytopenia, neutropenia, and/or leukopenia; CBC's performed two or three times a week from day 10 through day 25, and weekly thereafter, are recommended)

## Side/Adverse Effects

The following side/adverse effects have been selected on the basis of their potential clinical significance (possible signs and symptoms in parentheses where appropriate)—not necessarily inclusive:

**Those indicating need for medical attention**
Incidence rare
***Hypersensitivity*** (fever; skin rash or itching); ***neutropenia*** (sore throat and fever; unusual tiredness and weakness)—with high doses, reversible

**Those indicating need for medical attention only if they continue or are bothersome**
Incidence less frequent
***Gastrointestinal disturbances*** (abdominal pain or upset; diarrhea; nausea or vomiting)
Incidence rare
***Alopecia*** (hair loss)—with high doses; ***dizziness; headache***

## Overdose

For more information on the management of overdose or unintentional ingestion, **contact a Poison Control Center** (see *Poison Control Center Listing*).

In accidental overdose, gastrointestinal symptoms may occur and may last up to a few hours.

**Treatment of overdose**
Supportive care—
Supportive therapy necessary to maintain the vital functions of the patient may be administered.

## Patient Consultation

As an aid to patient consultation, refer to *Advice for the Patient, Mebendazole (Systemic)*.

In providing consultation, consider emphasizing the following selected information (» = major clinical significance):

**Before using this medication**
» Conditions affecting use, especially:
Hypersensitivity to mebendazole
Pregnancy—Mebendazole crosses the placenta
Other medical problems, especially hepatic function impairment

**Proper use of this medication**
Reading patient instructions before taking medication
No special preparations or other measures (e.g., dietary restrictions or fasting, concurrent medications, purging, or cleansing enemas) required before, during, or immediately after therapy
Chewing tablets, swallowing whole, or crushing tablets and mixing with food
» Compliance with full course of therapy; second course may be required in some infections
» Proper dosing
Missed dose: Taking as soon as possible; not taking if almost time for next dose; not doubling doses
» Proper storage
*For pinworms*
Treating all household members concurrently; treating again in 2 to 3 weeks
*For patients on high-dose therapy*
» Taking with meals, especially fatty ones, to increase absorption; checking with physician if on low-fat diet

**Precautions while using this medication**
Regular visits to physician to check progress, especially in high-dose therapy
Checking with physician if no improvement within a few days
*For hookworms or whipworms*
Importance of taking iron supplements daily during treatment and for up to 6 months following treatment if patient is anemic at the time of therapy
*For pinworms*
Washing (not shaking) all bedding and nightclothes after treatment to prevent reinfection
Other measures may be recommended by some physicians

**Side/adverse effects**
Signs of potential side effects, especially hypersensitivity and neutropenia

## General Dosing Information

No special preparations (e.g., dietary restrictions or fasting, concurrent medications, purging, or cleansing enemas) are required before, during, or immediately after treatment with mebendazole.

Mebendazole tablets may be chewed, swallowed whole, or crushed and mixed with food.

Patients who are heavily infected with helminths may require more prolonged treatment.

**For high-dose therapy**
In the treatment of tissue-dwelling helminth infections, the administration of much higher doses of mebendazole may be necessary because of poor absorption.

Mebendazole should preferably be taken with meals, especially fatty ones. This increases the bioavailability, absorption, and serum concentrations of mebendazole.

**For hookworms and whipworms**
In the treatment of hookworms and whipworms, especially in patients who are heavily infected or who have inadequate dietary intake of iron, concurrent iron therapy may be required if anemia is present. Iron therapy may need to be continued for up to 6 months to replenish iron stores.

**For pinworms**
Because of the high probability of transfer of pinworms, it is usually recommended that all members of the household be treated concurrently. Retreatment is recommended 2 to 3 weeks following initial treatment.

## Oral Dosage Forms

Note: Bracketed uses in the *Dosage Forms* section refer to categories of use and/or indications that are not included in U.S. product labeling.

### MEBENDAZOLE TABLETS (CHEWABLE) USP

**Usual adult and adolescent dose**
Ascariasis; or
Trichuriasis; or
Hookworm—
Oral, 100 mg two times a day, morning and evening, for three days. May be repeated in two to three weeks if required.

Enterobiasis—
  Oral, 100 mg as a single dose. Repeat in two to three weeks.
Intestinal roundworm, multiple—
  Oral, 100 mg two times a day, morning and evening, for three days.
[Capillariasis][1]—
  Oral, 200 mg two times a day for twenty days.
[Gnathostomiasis][1]—
  Oral, 200 mg every three hours for six days.
[Hydatid disease][1]—
  Oral, 13.3 to 16.7 mg per kg of body weight three times a day for up to three to six months.
[Trichinosis][1]—
  Oral, 200 to 400 mg three times a day for three days, then 400 to 500 mg three times a day for ten days.

### Usual adult prescribing limits
[Hydatid disease][1]—Doses up to 200 mg per kg of body weight daily have been used.

### Usual pediatric dose
Children up to 2 years of age—Dosage has not been established.
Children 2 years of age and over—Ascariasis, [capillariasis][1], enterobiasis, intestinal roundworm infections, trichuriasis, and uncinariasis: See *Usual adult and adolescent dose*.
Note: In the treatment of infections caused by tissue-dwelling organisms in which high doses are required, dosage should be based on the patient's body weight.

### Strength(s) usually available
U.S.—
  100 mg (Rx) [*Vermox;* GENERIC].
Canada—
  100 mg (Rx) [*Vermox* (scored)].

### Packaging and storage
Store below 40 °C (104 °F), preferably between 15 and 30 °C (59 and 86 °F), unless otherwise specified by manufacturer. Store in a well-closed container.

### Auxiliary labeling
• May be chewed, crushed, or swallowed whole.
• Take with meals (high-dose therapy).
• Continue medication for full time of treatment.

[1]Not included in Canadian product labeling.

Revised: 08/01/95

**MECAMYLAMINE**—The *Mecamylamine (Systemic)* monograph is not included in this published version of the USP DI database. Copies of the monograph are available on request from Micromedex, Inc. - Reprint Requests, 6200 S. Syracuse Way, Suite 300, Englewood, CO 80111; telephone (303) 486-6400; telefax (303) 486-6464; Email: USPDI@MDX.COM.

# MECHLORETHAMINE  Systemic

INN:  Chlormethine
VA CLASSIFICATION (Primary): AN100
Commonly used brand name(s): *Mustargen.*
Other commonly used names are chlormethine and nitrogen mustard.
Note: For a listing of dosage forms and brand names by country availability, see *Dosage Forms* section(s).

## Category
Antineoplastic.

## Indications
### Accepted
Lymphomas, Hodgkin's (treatment) or
Lymphomas, non-Hodgkin's (treatment)—Mechlorethamine is indicated for the palliative treatment of Hodgkin's disease (stages III and IV) and for treatment of some non-Hodgkin's lymphomas, including lymphosarcoma.
Malignant effusions, pericardial (treatment)
Malignant effusions, peritoneal (treatment) or
Malignant effusions, pleural (treatment)—Mechlorethamine is indicated by intracavitary administration for palliative treatment of metastatic carcinoma resulting in effusion.
Mycosis fungoides (treatment)—Mechlorethamine is indicated for treatment of mycosis fungoides.
Mechlorethamine has been used for bronchogenic carcinoma, chronic lymphocytic leukemia, chronic myelocytic leukemia, and polycythemia vera; however it *has been replaced* by safer and more effective agents.

## Pharmacology/Pharmacokinetics
### Physicochemical characteristics
Molecular weight—192.52.
pKa—6.1.

### Mechanism of action/Effect
Mechlorethamine is a bifunctional alkylating agent and is cell cycle–phase nonspecific. Activity occurs as a result of formation of an unstable ethylenimmonium ion, which alkylates or binds with many intracellular molecular structures, including nucleic acids. Its cytotoxic action is primarily due to cross-linking of strands of DNA and RNA, as well as inhibition of protein synthesis. With intracavitary use, mechlorethamine causes sclerosis and an inflammatory reaction on serous membranes, leading to adherence of serosal surfaces.

### Other actions/effects
Has weak immunosuppressive activity.

### Absorption
Mechlorethamine is incompletely absorbed following intracavitary administration, probably because of rapid deactivation by body fluids.

### Biotransformation
Rapidly deactivated in body fluids and tissues.

### Onset of action
Effects occur within a few seconds or minutes.

### Elimination
Apparently renal (less than 0.01% unchanged).

## Precautions to Consider
### Carcinogenicity/Mutagenicity
Secondary malignancies are potential delayed effects of many antineoplastic agents, although it is not clear whether the effect is related to their mutagenic or immunosuppressive action. The effect of dose and duration of therapy is also unknown, although risk seems to increase with long-term use. Although information is limited, available data seem to indicate that the carcinogenic risk is greatest with the alkylating agents.
Mechlorethamine has been associated with an increased risk of development of secondary carcinomas in animals and humans.

### Pregnancy/Reproduction
Fertility—Gonadal suppression, resulting in amenorrhea or azoospermia, may occur in patients taking antineoplastic therapy, especially with the alkylating agents. In general, these effects appear to be related to dose and length of therapy and may be irreversible. Prediction of the degree of testicular or ovarian function impairment is complicated by the common use of combinations of several antineoplastics, which makes it difficult to assess the effects of individual agents.
Mechlorethamine causes testicular atrophy and interferes with spermatogenesis.
Pregnancy—Although several successful pregnancies have been reported, there is evidence that mechlorethamine is teratogenic, especially when administered early in pregnancy.
First trimester: It is usually recommended that use of antineoplastics, especially combination chemotherapy, be avoided whenever possible, especially during the first trimester. Although information is limited because of the relatively few instances of antineoplastic administration during pregnancy, the mutagenic, teratogenic, and carcinogenic potential of these medications must be considered.
Other hazards to the fetus include adverse reactions seen in adults.
In general, use of a contraceptive is recommended during cytotoxic drug therapy.
FDA Pregnancy Category D.

## Breast-feeding
Although very little information is available regarding distribution of antineoplastic agents into breast milk, breast-feeding is not recommended while mechlorethamine is being administered because of the risks to the infant (adverse effects, mutagenicity, carcinogenicity). It is not known whether mechlorethamine is distributed into breast milk.

## Pediatrics
Appropriate studies on the relationship of age to the effects of mechlorethamine have not been performed in the pediatric population. However, pediatrics-specific problems that would limit the usefulness of this medication in children are not expected.

## Geriatrics
No information is available on the relationship of age to the effects of mechlorethamine in geriatric patients.

## Dental
The bone marrow depressant effects of mechlorethamine may result in an increased incidence of microbial infection, delayed healing, and gingival bleeding. Dental work, whenever possible, should be completed prior to initiation of therapy or deferred until blood counts have returned to normal. Patients should be instructed in proper oral hygiene during treatment, including caution in use of regular toothbrushes, dental floss, and toothpicks.

Mechlorethamine may also rarely cause stomatitis associated with considerable discomfort.

## Drug interactions and/or related problems
The following drug interactions and/or related problems have been selected on the basis of their potential clinical significance (possible mechanism in parentheses where appropriate)—not necessarily inclusive (» = major clinical significance):

Note: Combinations containing any of the following medications, depending on the amount present, may also interact with this medication.

Allopurinol or
Colchicine or
» Probenecid or
» Sulfinpyrazone
(mechlorethamine may raise the concentration of blood uric acid; dosage adjustment of antigout agents may be necessary to control hyperuricemia and gout; allopurinol may be preferred to prevent or reverse mechlorethamine-induced hyperuricemia because of risk of uric acid nephropathy with uricosuric antigout agents)

Blood dyscrasia–causing medications (see *Appendix II*)
(leukopenic and/or thrombocytopenic effects of mechlorethamine may be increased with concurrent or recent therapy if these medications cause the same effects; dosage adjustment of mechlorethamine, if necessary, should be based on blood counts)

» Bone marrow depressants, other (see *Appendix II*) or
Radiation therapy
(additive bone marrow depression may occur; dosage reduction may be required when two or more bone marrow depressants, including radiation, are used concurrently or consecutively)

Vaccines, killed virus
(because normal defense mechanisms may be suppressed by mechlorethamine therapy, the patient's antibody response to the vaccine may be decreased. The interval between discontinuation of medications that cause immunosuppression and restoration of the patient's ability to respond to the vaccine depends on the intensity and type of immunosuppression-causing medication used, the underlying disease, and other factors; estimates vary from 3 months to 1 year)

» Vaccines, live virus
(because normal defense mechanisms may be suppressed by mechlorethamine therapy, concurrent use with a live virus vaccine may potentiate the replication of the vaccine virus, may increase the side/adverse effects of the vaccine virus, and/or may decrease the patient's antibody response to the vaccine; immunization of these patients should be undertaken only with extreme caution after careful review of the patient's hematologic status and only with the knowledge and consent of the physician managing the mechlorethamine therapy. The interval between discontinuation of medications that cause immunosuppression and restoration of the patient's ability to respond to the vaccine depends on the intensity and type of immunosuppression-causing medication used, the underlying disease, and other factors; estimates vary from 3 months to 1 year. Immunization with oral poliovirus vaccine should also be postponed in persons in close contact with the patient, especially family members)

## Laboratory value alterations
The following have been selected on the basis of their potential clinical significance (possible effect in parentheses where appropriate)—not necessarily inclusive (» = major clinical significance):

With physiology/laboratory test values
Isocitric acid dehydrogenase (ICD)
(values may be increased, indicating hepatotoxicity)

Cholinesterase
(plasma values may be decreased)

Uric acid
(concentrations in blood and urine may be increased)

## Medical considerations/Contraindications
The medical considerations/contraindications included have been selected on the basis of their potential clinical significance (reasons given in parentheses where appropriate)—not necessarily inclusive (» = major clinical significance).

*Risk-benefit should be considered when the following medical problems exist:*

» Bone marrow depression
» Chickenpox, existing or recent (including recent exposure) or
» Herpes zoster
(risk of severe generalized disease)

Gout, history of or
Urate renal stones, history of
(risk of hyperuricemia)

» Infection
Sensitivity to mechlorethamine
» Tumor cell infiltration of bone marrow
» Caution should be used also in patients who have had previous cytotoxic drug therapy or radiation therapy.

## Patient monitoring
The following are especially important in patient monitoring (other tests may be warranted in some patients, depending on condition; » = major clinical significance):

Alanine aminotransferase (ALT [SGPT]) values, serum and
Aspartate aminotransferase (AST [SGOT]) values, serum and
Lactate dehydrogenase (LDH) values, serum
(determinations recommended prior to initiation of therapy and at periodic intervals during therapy; frequency varies according to clinical state, agent, dose, and other agents being used concurrently)

» Audiometric testing
(may be recommended at periodic intervals in patients receiving high doses)

» Hematocrit or hemoglobin and
» Leukocyte count, total and, if appropriate, differential and
» Platelet count
(determinations recommended prior to initiation of therapy and at periodic intervals during therapy; frequency varies according to clinical state, agent, dose, and other agents being used concurrently)

Bilirubin concentrations, serum and
Uric acid concentrations, serum
(determinations recommended prior to initiation of therapy and at periodic intervals during therapy; frequency varies according to clinical state, agent, dose, and other agents being used concurrently)

X-ray examination
(recommended after intracavitary administration to detect reaccumulation of fluid)

# Side/Adverse Effects
Note: Many "side effects" of antineoplastic therapy are unavoidable and represent the medication's pharmacologic action. Some of these (for example, leukopenia and thrombocytopenia) are actually used as parameters to aid in individual dosage titration.

Systemic effects are unpredictable following intracavitary administration.

Pain after intracavitary administration and nausea, vomiting, and diarrhea after intraperitoneal injection occur frequently and may persist for 2 or 3 days.

The following side/adverse effects have been selected on the basis of their potential clinical significance (possible cause in parentheses where appropriate)—not necessarily inclusive:

## Those indicating need for medical attention
Incidence more frequent
*Gonadal suppression* (missing menstrual periods); *idiosyncratic reaction or precipitation of herpes zoster* (painful rash); *leukopenia, im-*

munosuppression, or infection (fever or chills, cough or hoarseness, lower back or side pain, painful or difficult urination)—usually asymptomatic; *thrombocytopenia* (unusual bleeding or bruising; black, tarry stools; blood in urine or stools; pinpoint red spots on skin)—usually asymptomatic

Note: *Lymphocytopenia* usually occurs within 24 hours after the first dose. Significant granulocytopenia usually occurs within 6 to 8 days and lasts 10 days to 3 weeks.

Incidence more frequent with high doses or regional perfusion
*Ototoxicity* (dizziness; ringing in the ears; loss of hearing)

Incidence less frequent
*Hyperuricemia or uric acid nephropathy* (joint pain; lower back or side pain; swelling of feet or lower legs); *thrombosis, thrombophlebitis, or extravasation* (pain or redness at the site of injection)

Note: *Hyperuricemia or uric acid nephropathy* occurs most commonly during initial treatment of patients with leukemia or lymphoma, as a result of rapid cell breakdown that leads to elevated serum uric acid concentrations.

*Pain or redness at the site of injection* may persist for 4 to 6 weeks.

Incidence rare
*Allergic reaction* (shortness of breath, itching, wheezing); *hepatotoxicity* (yellow eyes or skin); *peptic ulcer* (black, tarry stools); *peripheral neuropathy* (numbness, tingling, or burning of fingers, toes, or face)

Note: An *allergic reaction* may also occur in patients previously treated with topical mechlorethamine.

**Those indicating need for medical attention only if they continue or are bothersome**
Incidence more frequent
*Nausea and vomiting*

Note: *Nausea and vomiting* occur in 90% of patients, usually within 1 to 3 hours of a dose; vomiting usually subsides within 8 hours, while nausea may persist for 24 hours.

Incidence less frequent
*Diarrhea; loss of appetite; metallic taste; neurotoxicity* (confusion; drowsiness; headache)—especially with high doses; *weakness*

**Those not indicating need for medical attention**
Incidence less frequent
*Loss of hair*

**Those indicating the need for medical attention if they occur after medication is discontinued**
*Bone marrow depression* (black, tarry stools; blood in urine or stools; cough or hoarseness; fever or chills; lower back or side pain; painful or difficult urination; pinpoint red spots on skin; unusual bleeding or bruising)

## Patient Consultation

As an aid to patient consultation, refer to *Advice for the Patient, Mechlorethamine (Systemic)*.

In providing consultation, consider emphasizing the following selected information (» = major clinical significance):

**Before using this medication**
» Conditions affecting use, especially:
Sensitivity to mechlorethamine
Pregnancy—Use not recommended because of mutagenic, teratogenic, and carcinogenic potential; advisability of using contraception; telling physician immediately if pregnancy is suspected
Breast-feeding—Not recommended because of risk of serious side effects
Other medications, especially other bone marrow depressants, probenecid, sulfinpyrazone, or other cytotoxic drug or radiation therapy
Other medical problems, especially chickenpox, herpes zoster, or infection

**Proper use of this medication**
Caution in taking combination therapy; taking each medication at the right time
Importance of ample fluid intake and subsequent increase in urine output to aid in excretion of uric acid
Frequency of nausea, vomiting, and loss of appetite; importance of continuing medication despite stomach upset
» Proper dosing

**Precautions while using this medication**
» Importance of close monitoring by the physician
» Avoiding immunizations unless approved by physician; other persons in patient's household should avoid immunizations with oral poliovirus vaccine; avoiding persons who have taken oral poliovirus vaccine or wearing a protective mask that covers nose and mouth

*Caution if bone marrow depression occurs*
» Avoiding exposure to persons with infections, especially during periods of low blood counts; checking with physician immediately if fever or chills, cough or hoarseness, lower back or side pain, or painful or difficult urination occurs
» Checking with physician immediately if unusual bleeding or bruising; black, tarry stools; blood in urine or stools; or pinpoint red spots on skin occur
Caution in use of regular toothbrush, dental floss, or toothpick; physician, dentist, or nurse may suggest alternatives; checking with physician before having dental work done
Not touching eyes or inside of nose unless hands are washed immediately before
Using caution to avoid accidental cuts with use of sharp objects such as safety razor or fingernail or toenail cutters
Avoiding contact sports or other situations where bruising or injury could occur
» Possibility of local tissue injury and scarring if infiltration of intravenous solution occurs; telling doctor or nurse right away about redness, pain, or swelling at injection site

**Side/adverse effects**
Importance of discussing possible effects, including cancer, with physician
Signs of potential side effects, especially gonadal suppression, idiosyncratic reaction, precipitation of herpes zoster, leukopenia, immunosuppression, infection, thrombocytopenia, ototoxicity, hyperuricemia, uric acid nephropathy, thrombosis, thrombophlebitis, extravasation, allergic reaction, hepatotoxicity, peptic ulcer, and peripheral neuropathy
Physician or nurse can help in dealing with side effects
Possibility of hair loss; normal hair growth should return after treatment has ended

## General Dosing Information

**For intravenous and intracavitary use**
Patients receiving mechlorethamine should be under supervision of a physician experienced in cancer chemotherapy or immunosuppressive therapy.

A variety of dosage schedules, regimens, and routes of administration of mechlorethamine, alone or in combination with other antitumor agents, are used. The prescriber may consult the medical literature as well as the manufacturer's literature in choosing a specific dosage.

Dosage must be adjusted to meet the individual requirements of each patient, based on clinical response and appearance or severity of toxicity.

Although dosages are based on the patient's actual weight, use of estimated lean body mass (dry weight) is recommended in obese patients or those with weight gain due to edema, ascites, or other abnormal fluid retention.

Because mechlorethamine may contribute to the development of amyloidosis, it is recommended that the medication be used only if foci of acute and chronic suppurative inflammation are absent.

Severity of nausea and vomiting may be reduced in some patients by administration of antiemetics, in addition to sedatives such as barbiturates or chlorpromazine, prior to dosing.

Administration of mechlorethamine at night is recommended if sedation for side effects is required.

Development of uric acid nephropathy in patients with leukemia or lymphoma may be prevented by adequate oral hydration and, in some cases, administration of allopurinol. Alkalinization of urine may be necessary if serum uric acid concentrations are elevated.

It is recommended that mechlorethamine therapy be withdrawn if leukocyte (particularly granulocyte) or platelet levels fall markedly. Therapy may be resumed at a lower dosage when leukocyte and platelet counts return to satisfactory levels.

Special precautions are recommended in patients who develop thrombocytopenia as a result of administration of mechlorethamine. These may include extreme care in performing invasive procedures; regular inspection of intravenous sites, skin (including perirectal area), and mucous membrane surfaces for signs of bleeding or bruising; limiting frequency of venipuncture and avoiding intramuscular injections; testing urine, emesis, stool, and secretions for occult blood; care in use of regular toothbrushes, dental floss, toothpicks, safety razors, and fingernail and toenail cutters; avoiding constipation; and using caution to prevent falls and other injuries. Such patients should avoid alcohol and aspirin intake because of the risk of gastrointestinal bleeding. Platelet transfusions may be required.

Patients who develop leukopenia should be observed carefully for signs of infection. Antibiotic support may be required. In neutropenic patients who develop fever, broad-spectrum antibiotic coverage should be initiated empirically, pending bacterial cultures and appropriate diagnostic tests.

**For intravenous use only**
Mechlorethamine may be administered by intravenous push, although injection into the tubing of a running intravenous infusion is preferred to reduce the risk of local toxicity. Administration by intravenous infusion is not recommended because of deactivation of the medication by the solution. The injection should be completed within a few minutes.

Avoid high concentration and prolonged contact with the medication, especially in cases of elevated pressure in the antebrachial vein.

If extravasation occurs, the reaction may be minimized by prompt infiltration of the area with sterile isotonic sodium thiosulfate (0.125 Molar) or 1% lidocaine and application of an ice compress for 6 to 12 hours.

**For intracavitary use only**
Administration of mechlorethamine by the intracavitary route is not recommended in patients receiving other systemic bone marrow depressants concurrently.

Prior removal of excess fluid (paracentesis) improves contact of the medication with the peritoneal and pleural linings.

Prior administration of analgesics usually is required to offset pain of treatment.

For intrapleural or intrapericardial injection, a thoracentesis needle is used. For intraperitoneal injection, mechlorethamine is given through a rubber catheter inserted into the trocar used for paracentesis or through an 18-gauge needle inserted at another site. Slow injection with frequent aspiration is recommended to prevent or detect extravasation and to ensure adequate dissemination of the medication.

Changing the position of the patient (prone, supine, right side, left side, knee-chest) every 5 to 10 minutes for an hour ensures uniform distribution of the medication in the serous cavity.

Remaining fluid is removed by paracentesis 24 to 36 hours later.

Intrapleural administration may produce increased pleural fluid as a result of pleural irritation by mechlorethamine.

**Safety considerations for handling this medication**
There is limited but increasing evidence and concern that personnel involved in preparation and administration of parenteral antineoplastics may be at some risk because of the potential mutagenicity, teratogenicity, and/or carcinogenicity of these agents, although the actual risk is unknown. USP advisory panels recommend cautious handling both in preparation and disposal of antineoplastic agents. Precautions that have been suggested include:
- Use of a biological containment cabinet during reconstitution and dilution of parenteral medications and wearing of disposable surgical gloves and masks.
- Use of proper technique to prevent contamination of the medication, work area, and operator during transfer between containers (including proper training of personnel in this technique).
- Cautious and proper disposal of needles, syringes, vials, ampuls, and unused medication.

A number of medical centers have developed detailed guidelines for handling of antineoplastic agents.

**Combination chemotherapy**
Mechlorethamine may be used in combination with other agents in various regimens. As a result, incidence and/or severity of side effects may be altered and different dosages (usually reduced) may be used. For example, mechlorethamine is part of the following chemotherapeutic combination (a commonly used acronym is in parentheses):
—mechlorethamine, vincristine, procarbazine, and prednisone (MOPP).

For specific dosages and schedules, consult the literature. For information regarding each agent, consult the individual monographs.

## Parenteral Dosage Forms

### MECHLORETHAMINE HYDROCHLORIDE FOR INJECTION USP

**Usual adult and adolescent dose**
Lymphomas, Hodgkin's or
Lymphomas, non-Hodgkin's or
Mycosis fungoides—
    Intravenous, total dose of 400 mcg (0.4 mg) per kg of body weight as a single dose or divided into two or four successive daily doses.

Malignant effusions, pericardial or
Malignant effusions, peritoneal or
Malignant effusions, pleural—
    Intracavitary, 400 mcg (0.4 mg) per kg of body weight, or 200 mcg (0.2 mg) per kg of body weight by the intrapericardial route.

Note: Total dosage in patients who have received prior cytotoxic drug therapy or radiation therapy should not exceed 200 to 300 mcg (0.2 to 0.3 mg) per kg of body weight.

**Usual adult prescribing limits**
Total intravenous dose exceeding 400 mcg (0.4 mg) per kg of body weight may result in severe bone marrow depression, bleeding, sepsis, and death, although 800 mcg (0.8 mg) of mechlorethamine per kg of body weight, as a single agent, is tolerated in some patients.

**Usual pediatric dose**
See *Usual adult and adolescent dose*.

**Size(s) usually available**
U.S.—
    10 mg (Rx) [*Mustargen*].
Canada—
    10 mg (Rx) [*Mustargen*].

**Packaging and storage**
Store below 40 °C (104 °F), preferably between 15 and 30 °C (59 and 86 °F), unless otherwise specified by manufacturer. Protect from light and humidity.

**Preparation of dosage form**
Mechlorethamine Hydrochloride for Injection USP is reconstituted for intravenous use by adding 10 mL of sterile water for injection or 0.9% sodium chloride injection to the vial and, with the needle still in the rubber stopper, shaking to dissolve, producing a clear, colorless solution containing 1 mg of mechlorethamine hydrochloride per mL.

Mechlorethamine Hydrochloride for Injection USP is reconstituted for intracavitary use by adding 10 mL of sterile water for injection or 0.9% sodium chloride injection to the vial (50 to 100 mL of 0.9% sodium chloride injection has also been used) and shaking to dissolve.

**Stability**
Solution should be freshly reconstituted immediately (less than 15 minutes) prior to each dose. Any unused portion should be discarded.

**Note**
Do not use if solution is discolored or if droplets of water appear in the vial.

Avoid inhalation of powder or vapors, If accidental contact with skin or mucous membranes occurs, immediately and thoroughly irrigate the affected part with a large volume of water for at least 15 minutes, followed by 2% sodium thiosulfate solution; if eye contact occurs, irrigation is performed with 0.9% sodium chloride solution or a balanced salt ophthalmic irrigating solution.

Any equipment used for administration of mechlorethamine (rubber gloves, tubing, glassware, etc.) should be neutralized immediately after use by soaking in an aqueous solution containing equal volumes of 5% sodium thiosulfate and 5% sodium bicarbonate for 45 minutes, washing away excess reagents and reaction products with water. Unused solution is neutralized by adding an equal volume of the sodium thiosulfate–bicarbonate solution and allowing the mixture to stand for 45 minutes. Vials that have contained mechlorethamine should be treated in the same way before disposal.

Revised: august 1990
Interim revision: 07/29/93; 12/15/93; 06/21/94; 09/30/97

**MECHLORETHAMINE**—The *Mechlorethamine (Topical)* monograph is not included in this published version of the USP DI database. Copies of the monograph are available on request from Micromedex, Inc. - Reprint Requests, 6200 S. Syracuse Way, Suite 300, Englewood, CO 80111; telephone (303) 486-6400; telefax (303) 486-6464; Email: USPDI@MDX.COM.

# MECLIZINE Systemic

INN: Meclozine
BAN: Meclozine
VA CLASSIFICATION (Primary/Secondary): GA605/CN550
Commonly used brand name(s): *Antivert; Antivert/25; Antivert/50; Bonamine; Bonine; D-Vert 15; D-Vert 30; Dramamine II; Meni-D*.

Note: For a listing of dosage forms and brand names by country availability, see *Dosage Forms* section(s).

## Category
Antiemetic; antivertigo agent.

## Indications
Note: Bracketed information in the *Indications* section refers to uses that are not included in U.S. product labeling.

**Accepted**

Motion sickness (prophylaxis and treatment)—Meclizine is indicated for the prophylaxis and treatment of nausea, vomiting, and dizziness associated with motion sickness or radiotherapy.

Vertigo (prophylaxis and treatment)—The U.S. Food and Drug Administration (FDA) has classified meclizine as possibly effective in the management of vertigo associated with diseases affecting the vestibular system, such as labyrinthitis and Meniere's disease. This classification requires the submission of adequate and well-controlled studies to provide substantial evidence of effectiveness.

[Nausea and vomiting, radiotherapy-induced (prophylaxis and treatment)]—Meclizine is indicated for the prophylaxis and treatment of nausea, vomiting, and dizziness associated with radiotherapy.

## Pharmacology/Pharmacokinetics

**Physicochemical characteristics**
Molecular weight—481.90.

**Mechanism of action/Effect**

Antiemetic; antivertigo agent—The mechanism by which meclizine exerts its antiemetic, antimotion sickness, and antivertigo effects is not precisely known but may be related to its central anticholinergic actions. It diminishes vestibular stimulation and depresses labyrinthine function. An action on the medullary chemoreceptive trigger zone may also be involved in the antiemetic effect.

**Other actions/effects**
Meclizine also has antihistaminic, anticholinergic, central nervous system (CNS) depressant, and local anesthetic effects.

**Half-life**
6 hours.

**Onset of action**
1 hour.

**Duration of action**
8 to 24 hours.

## Precautions to Consider

**Pregnancy/Reproduction**

Pregnancy—Epidemiological studies in pregnant women have not shown that meclizine causes an increase in the risk of fetal abnormalities. Studies in rats have shown that meclizine causes cleft palate when given in doses corresponding to 25 to 50 times the recommended human dose.

FDA Pregnancy Category B.

**Breast-feeding**

Meclizine may be distributed into breast milk. However, problems in humans have not been documented.

Because of its anticholinergic actions, meclizine may inhibit lactation.

**Pediatrics**

No information is available on the relationship of age to the effects of meclizine in pediatric patients. However, it is known that pediatric patients exhibit increased sensitivity to anticholinergics, which are related pharmacologically to meclizine.

**Geriatrics**

No information is available on the relationship of age to the effects of meclizine in geriatric patients. However, it is known that geriatric patients exhibit increased sensitivity to anticholinergics, which are related pharmacologically to meclizine. Therefore, constipation, dryness of mouth, and urinary retention (especially in males) are more likely to occur in the elderly.

**Drug interactions and/or related problems**

The following drug interactions and/or related problems have been selected on the basis of their potential clinical significance (possible mechanism in parentheses where appropriate)—not necessarily inclusive (» = major clinical significance):

Note: Combinations containing any of the following medications, depending on the amount present, may also interact with this medication.

» Alcohol or
» CNS depression–producing medications, other (See *Appendix II*)
 (concurrent use may potentiate the CNS depressant effects of either these medications or meclizine)

Anticholinergics or other medications with anticholinergic activity (See *Appendix II*)
 (concurrent use with meclizine may potentiate anticholinergic effects)

Apomorphine
 (prior administration of meclizine may decrease the emetic response to apomorphine)

**Laboratory value alterations**

The following have been selected on the basis of their potential clinical significance (possible effect in parentheses where appropriate)—not necessarily inclusive (» = major clinical significance):

With diagnostic test results
 Skin tests using allergen extracts
 (may inhibit the cutaneous histamine response, thus producing false-negative results; it is recommended that meclizine be discontinued at least 72 hours before testing begins)

**Medical considerations/Contraindications**

The medical considerations/contraindications included have been selected on the basis of their potential clinical significance (reasons given in parentheses where appropriate)—not necessarily inclusive (» = major clinical significance).

*Risk-benefit should be considered when the following medical problems exist:*

Bladder neck obstruction or
Prostatic hyperplasia, symptomatic
 (anticholinergic effects of meclizine may precipitate urinary retention)

Gastroduodenal obstruction
 (decrease in motility and tone may occur, aggravating obstruction and gastric retention)

Glaucoma, angle-closure, predisposition to
 (increased intraocular pressure may precipitate an acute attack of angle-closure glaucoma)

Pulmonary disease, chronic obstructive
 (reduction in bronchial secretion may cause inspissation and formation of bronchial plugs)

Sensitivity to meclizine

## Side/Adverse Effects

The following side/adverse effects have been selected on the basis of their potential clinical significance (possible signs and symptoms in parentheses where appropriate)—not necessarily inclusive:

**Those indicating need for medical attention only if they continue or are bothersome**

Incidence more frequent
 *Drowsiness*

Incidence less frequent or rare
 *Blurred vision; dryness of mouth, nose, and throat*

## Patient Consultation

As an aid to patient consultation, refer to *Advice for the Patient, Meclizine/Buclizine/Cyclizine (Systemic)*.

In providing consultation, consider emphasizing the following selected information (» = major clinical significance):

**Before using this medication**
» Conditions affecting use, especially:
 Sensitivity to meclizine

Pregnancy—No increase in fetal abnormalities in human studies; animal studies have shown meclizine to cause cleft palate at doses above recommended human dose

Breast-feeding—May be distributed into breast milk; may inhibit lactation due to anticholinergic effects

Use in children—Possible increased susceptibility to anticholinergic side effects

Use in the elderly—Possible increased susceptibility to anticholinergic side effects

Other medications, especially other CNS depressants

**Proper use of this medication**
Not taking more medication than the amount recommended
» Proper dosing
Missed dose (if on a regular dosing regimen): Taking as soon as possible; not taking if almost time for next dose; not doubling doses
» Proper storage

**Precautions while using this medication**
Possible interference with skin tests using allergens; need to inform physician of use of this medication
» Avoiding use of alcohol or other CNS depressants
» Caution if drowsiness occurs
Possible dryness of mouth; using sugarless candy or gum, ice, or saliva substitute for relief; checking with physician or dentist if dry mouth continues for more than 2 weeks

## General Dosing Information

For prophylaxis of motion sickness, this medication should be taken at least 1 hour before exposure to conditions that may precipitate motion sickness.

## Oral Dosage Forms

Note: Bracketed uses in the *Dosage Forms* section refer to categories of use and/or indications that are not included in U.S. product labeling.

### MECLIZINE HYDROCHLORIDE CAPSULES

**Usual adult and adolescent dose**
Motion sickness (prophylaxis and treatment)—Oral, 25 to 50 mg one hour before travel. Dose may be repeated every twenty-four hours as needed.
Vertigo (prophylaxis and treatment)—Oral, 25 to 100 mg a day as needed, in divided doses.
[Nausea and vomiting, radiotherapy-induced (prophylaxis and treatment)]—Oral, 50 mg two to twelve hours prior to radiotherapy.

**Usual pediatric dose**
Antiemetic or
Antivertigo agent—
Children up to 12 years of age: Use is not recommended unless directed by a physician.
Children 12 years of age or older: See *Usual adult and adolescent dose*.

**Usual geriatric dose**
See *Usual adult and adolescent dose*.

Note: Geriatric patients may be more sensitive to the effects of the usual adult dose.

**Strength(s) usually available**
U.S.—
  15 mg (OTC) [*D-Vert 15*].
  25 mg (Rx) [*Meni-D*].
  30 mg (OTC) [*D-Vert 30*].
Canada—
  Not commercially available.

**Packaging and storage**
Store below 40 °C (104 °F), preferably between 15 and 30 °C (59 and 86 °F), in a well-closed container, unless otherwise specified by manufacturer.

**Auxiliary labeling**
• May cause drowsiness.
• Avoid alcoholic beverages.

### MECLIZINE HYDROCHLORIDE TABLETS USP

**Usual adult and adolescent dose**
See *Meclizine Hydrochloride Capsules*.

**Usual pediatric dose**
See *Meclizine Hydrochloride Capsules*.

**Usual geriatric dose**
See *Meclizine Hydrochloride Capsules*.

**Strength(s) usually available**
U.S.—
  12.5 mg (Rx) [*Antivert*; GENERIC].
  25 mg [*Antivert/25 (Rx)*; *Dramamine II (OTC)*; GENERIC].
  50 mg (Rx) [*Antivert/50* (scored); GENERIC].
Canada—
  Not commercially available.

**Packaging and storage**
Store below 40 °C (104 °F), preferably between 15 and 30 °C (59 and 86 °F), unless otherwise specified by manufacturer. Store in a well-closed container.

**Auxiliary labeling**
• May cause drowsiness.
• Avoid alcoholic beverages.

### MECLIZINE HYDROCHLORIDE TABLETS (CHEWABLE) USP

**Usual adult and adolescent dose**
See *Meclizine Hydrochloride Capsules*.

**Usual pediatric dose**
See *Meclizine Hydrochloride Capsules*.

**Usual geriatric dose**
See *Meclizine Hydrochloride Capsules*.

**Strength(s) usually available**
U.S.—
  25 mg [*Bonine (OTC)*; GENERIC].
Canada—
  25 mg (Rx) [*Bonamine* (scored)].

**Packaging and storage**
Store between 15 and 30 °C (59 and 86 °F), unless otherwise specified by manufacturer. Store in a well-closed container.

**Auxiliary labeling**
• May cause drowsiness.
• Avoid alcoholic beverages.
• May be chewed or swallowed whole.

Revised: 01/03/96

---

**MECLOCYCLINE**—See *Tetracyclines (Topical)*

---

**MECLOFENAMATE**—See *Anti-inflammatory Drugs, Nonsteroidal (Systemic)*

---

**MEDROGESTONE**—See *Progestins (Systemic)*

---

**MEDROXYPROGESTERONE**—See *Progestins (Systemic)*

---

**MEDRYSONE**—See *Corticosteroids (Ophthalmic)*

---

**MEFENAMIC ACID**—See *Anti-inflammatory Drugs, Nonsteroidal (Systemic)*

# MEFLOQUINE Systemic†

VA CLASSIFICATION (Primary): AP101
Commonly used brand name(s): *Lariam*.
Note: For a listing of dosage forms and brand names by country availability, see *Dosage Forms* section(s).

†Not commercially available in Canada.

## Category
Antimalarial.

## Indications

### Accepted
Malaria (prophylaxis)—Mefloquine is indicated for the prophylaxis of malaria caused by chloroquine-resistant and multiple drug–resistant (including sulfadoxine and pyrimethamine–resistant) strains of *Plasmodium falciparum*. It is also effective as a prophylactic agent against malaria caused by *P. vivax, P. ovale,* and *P. malariae*.

Malaria (treatment)—Mefloquine is indicated for the treatment of chloroquine-resistant strains of *P. falciparum* malaria, usually as an alternative agent to quinine. It is also used for malaria caused by multiple drug–resistant (including sulfadoxine and pyrimethamine–resistant) strains of *P. falciparum*.

Since mefloquine does not eliminate the exoerythrocytic (intrahepatic) stages of *P. vivax* or *P. ovale* infection, subsequent treatment with primaquine is recommended to effect a radical cure and to avoid a relapse.

Not all species or strains of a particular organism may be susceptible to mefloquine.

### Unaccepted
Because of the potentially serious side effects caused by sulfadoxine and pyrimethamine combination, its use is not recommended concurrently with mefloquine for the prophylaxis of chloroquine-resistant *P. falciparum* malaria.

## Pharmacology/Pharmacokinetics

### Physicochemical characteristics
Chemical group—A 4-quinolinemethanol chemical structural analog of quinine.
Molecular weight—414.78.

### Mechanism of action/Effect
Exact mechanism of action unknown. However, mefloquine has been shown to act as a blood schizonticide. Inhibits replication of asexual erythrocytic parasites; has no effect on the gametocytes of *P. falciparum*. May bind weakly to DNA, resulting in inhibition of nucleic acid synthesis and protein synthesis. May also act as a weak base, raising the intravesicular pH of acid vesicles of the parasite and thus inhibiting parasitic growth. In addition, may have non–weak base effects on vesicular pH by means of a specific interaction between mefloquine and parasitic acid vesicles, resulting in swelling of secondary lysosomes (food vacuoles) of the parasite. Mefloquine does not eliminate the exoerythrocytic (intrahepatic) stages of *P. vivax* or *P. ovale* infection.

### Absorption
Well absorbed from the gastrointestinal tract; bioavailability greater than 85%. Rate of absorption is usually relatively rapid, but may be prolonged in some patients. Absorption may be incomplete in seriously ill patients, such as patients with cerebral malaria.

### Distribution
Distributed to blood, urine, cerebrospinal fluid (CSF), and tissues; concentrated in erythrocytes; also distributed to breast milk in low concentrations (approximately 3 to 4% of the ingested dose).
Apparent Vol$_D$=9 to 29 L/kg (median 20 L/kg).

### Protein binding
Very high (98 to 99%).

### Biotransformation
Hepatic (partial); metabolized primarily to the carboxylic acid metabolite.

### Half-life
Absorption—1 to 4 hours.
Elimination—13 to 33 days (median 20 days); may be shorter in seriously ill patients, such as patients with acute malaria.

### Time to peak concentration
7 to 24 hours (median 17 hours).

### Peak plasma concentration
Approximately 290 to 340 nanograms per mL following a single 250-mg dose.
Approximately 540 to 1240 nanograms per mL following a single 1-gram dose.
Mean steady state concentrations may vary from 560 to 1250 nanograms per mL in healthy adults following a 250-mg dose once a week for up to 21 weeks. Steady state concentrations may be significantly lower in pregnant women.

### Elimination
Biliary/fecal; eliminated very slowly, primarily through bile into the feces. Subtherapeutic concentrations may persist in the blood for up to several months or more.
Renal; approximately 5% of the oral dose is excreted unchanged in the urine.

## Precautions to Consider

### Cross-sensitivity and/or related problems
Patients hypersensitive to quinidine, quinine, or related medications may be hypersensitive to this medication also.

### Carcinogenicity
Two-year feeding studies in rats and mice, fed doses of up to 30 mg per kg of body weight (mg/kg) daily, have not shown that mefloquine is carcinogenic.

### Mutagenicity
Mefloquine has not been shown to be mutagenic in the Ames test, host-mediated assays in mice, fluctuation tests, and mouse micronucleus assays, with or without prior metabolic activation. In addition, mefloquine has not been shown to be mutagenic in modified Ames tests utilizing *Salmonella typhimurium* strains, with or without microsomal activation.

### Pregnancy/Reproduction
Fertility—Studies in adult human males, at doses of 250 mg once a week for 22 weeks, have not shown that mefloquine causes any adverse effects on spermatozoa.

However, studies in rats given doses of 5, 20, and 50 mg/kg daily have shown that mefloquine causes adverse effects on fertility in males at doses of 50 mg/kg daily and in females at doses of 20 and 50 mg/kg daily. In addition, degenerative lesions in the epididymides of male rats have been reported at doses of 20 and 50 mg/kg daily for 13 weeks.

Pregnancy—Adequate and well-controlled studies in humans have not been done. However, malaria in pregnant women may be more severe than in nonpregnant women and may result in maternal death. The risk of adverse pregnancy outcomes, including premature births, stillbirths, and abortion, may be increased. Although mefloquine is not recommended for use during pregnancy and its safety has not been proven, it has been used in women at high risk from falciparum malaria during the second and third trimester of pregnancy with no complications, and no adverse effects in development of their children to date.

If possible, pregnant women should avoid traveling to areas where chloroquine-resistant falciparum malaria is endemic. If travel to the malarious area and mefloquine chemoprophylaxis are considered necessary, women of child-bearing potential should be warned to take reliable contraceptive precautions while taking mefloquine and for 2 months after the last dose.

Studies in rats given doses of 5, 20, and 50 mg/kg daily have shown that mefloquine causes reduced litter size and reduced growth of offspring at the two higher dosage levels. Mefloquine also has been shown to cause an increased incidence of externally visible soft tissue and skeletal abnormalities in rats given doses of 100 mg/kg daily from day 6 to 15 of gestation. Studies utilizing similar doses in mice have shown that mefloquine causes reduced fetal growth and cleft palate. Other studies in rats and mice given doses of 100 mg/kg daily have shown that mefloquine is teratogenic. Studies in rabbits have shown that mefloquine is teratogenic at doses of 80 mg/kg daily and is both embryotoxic and teratogenic at doses of 160 mg/kg daily.

FDA Pregnancy Category C.

### Breast-feeding
Mefloquine is distributed into breast milk in low concentrations (approximately 3 to 4%) following administration of a 250-mg dose. Although the effects of mefloquine distribution into breast milk in nursing infants have not been studied, and the amount the infant is exposed to is small, caution should be exercised.

### Pediatrics
Although the safety and efficacy of mefloquine have not been well studied, it has been effective in preventing and treating malaria caused by *P. falciparum* in children. As in adults, nausea, vomiting, and dizziness have been the reported side effects of mefloquine use in children living in endemic malarious areas. Use is not recommended in infants and children up to 2 years of age or less than 15 kg of body weight.

### Geriatrics
No information is available on the relationship of age to the effects of mefloquine in geriatric patients.

### Drug interactions and/or related problems
The following drug interactions and/or related problems have been selected on the basis of their potential clinical significance (possible mechanism in parentheses where appropriate)—not necessarily inclusive (» = major clinical significance):

Note: Combinations containing any of the following medications, depending on the amount present, may also interact with this medication.

- » Beta-adrenergic blocking agents or
- » Calcium channel blocking agents or
- » Quinidine or
- » Quinine
  (concurrent use of these agents with mefloquine may result in sinus bradycardia, prolonged QT intervals, or cardiac arrest; the risk of seizures may also be increased with quinine; concurrent use should be avoided; if concurrent use is necessary, close monitoring of patient response is recommended; in addition, patients should be advised to take mefloquine at least 12 hours after the last dose of quinidine or quinine)
- » Chloroquine
  (concurrent use of chloroquine with mefloquine may increase the risk of seizures)
- » Divalproex or
- » Valproic acid
  (concurrent use of divalproex or valproic acid with mefloquine may result in low valproic acid serum concentrations and loss of seizure control; monitoring of valproic acid serum concentrations is recommended and dosage adjustments may be necessary during and after therapy with mefloquine)
- Typhoid vaccine, oral
  (concurrent use of the oral typhoid vaccine with mefloquine may decrease the effectiveness of the oral typhoid vaccine; doses of the two medications should be separated by 7 to 10 days)

### Laboratory value alterations
The following have been selected on the basis of their potential clinical significance (possible effect in parentheses where appropriate)—not necessarily inclusive (» = major clinical significance):

With physiology/laboratory test values
  Alanine aminotransferase (ALT [SGPT]), serum, and
  Aspartate aminotransferase (AST [SGOT]), serum
    (values may be transiently increased in patients taking mefloquine)

### Medical considerations/Contraindications
The medical considerations/contraindications included have been selected on the basis of their potential clinical significance (reasons given in parentheses where appropriate)—not necessarily inclusive (» = major clinical significance).

*Risk-benefit should be considered when the following medical problems exist:*
  Epilepsy or
  Seizure disorder, history of
    (mefloquine may rarely cause seizures)
- » Heart block, first or second degree
- » Psychiatric disorders, history of
    (mefloquine may cause psychosis, hallucinations, confusion, anxiety, or mental depression)
  Sensitivity to mefloquine, quinidine, quinine, or related medications
- » Caution is also required in any patient whose occupation requires fine coordination and spatial discrimination, such as airline pilots or neurosurgeons

## Side/Adverse Effects
Note: Some side/adverse effects of mefloquine may be difficult to distinguish from the symptoms of acute malaria infection. However, side effects are thought to be dose-related and may occur more frequently in therapeutic regimens (greater than 15 mg per kg of body weight [mg/kg]) than in prophylactic regimens. In therapeutic regimens, vomiting of doses has resulted in low plasma mefloquine concentrations and treatment failure. The incidence of vomiting may be reduced by dividing the dose into parts to be given at 8 to 24 hour intervals.

The following side/adverse effects have been selected on the basis of their potential clinical significance (possible signs and symptoms in parentheses where appropriate)—not necessarily inclusive:

### Those indicating need for medical attention
Incidence rare
  *Bradycardia* (slow heartbeat); *neuropsychiatric toxicity* (anxiety confusion, seizures, hallucinations, mental depression, psychosis, or restlessness)

### Those indicating need for medical attention only if they continue or are bothersome
Incidence more frequent
  *CNS toxicity* (difficulty concentrating; dizziness; headache; insomnia; lightheadedness; vertigo); *gastrointestinal disturbances* (abdominal or stomach pain, diarrhea, loss of appetite, or nausea or vomiting); *visual disturbances*

## Overdose
For more information on the management of overdose or unintentional ingestion, **contact a Poison Control Center** (see *Poison Control Center Listing*).

### Treatment of overdose
Since there is no known specific antidote, treatment of mefloquine overdose should include the following:
  To decrease absorption—
    Standard gastric decontamination procedures.
  Specific treatment—
    Symptomatic treatment may be given.
  Supportive care—
    Supportive measures such as maintaining an open airway, respiration, and circulation may be necessary. Patients in whom intentional overdose is known or suspected should be referred for psychiatric consultation.

## Patient Consultation
As an aid to patient consultation, refer to *Advice for the Patient, Mefloquine (Systemic)*.

In providing consultation, consider emphasizing the following selected information (» = major clinical significance):

### Before using this medication
- » Conditions affecting use, especially:
  Allergies to mefloquine, quinidine, quinine, or related medications
  Pregnancy—Not recommended for use during pregnancy; however, the risk of maternal and fetal morbidity and mortality from malaria must be considered for women who are at high risk from falciparum malaria
  Breast-feeding—Distributed into breast milk in low concentrations
  Use in children—Not recommended for use in infants and children up to 2 years of age or less than 15 kg of body weight
  Other medications, especially beta-adrenergic blocking agents, calcium channel blocking agents, chloroquine, divalproex, quinidine, quinine, or valproic acid
  Other medical problems, especially a history of psychiatric disorders or heart block

### Proper use of this medication
- » Not giving to infants and children up to 2 years of age or less than 15 kg of body weight
  Taking with full glass (240 mL) of water and with food
- » Proper storage

*For suppression of malaria symptoms*
  Starting medication 1 week before entering malarious area to ascertain response and allow time to substitute another medication if reactions occur
- » Continuing medication while staying in area and for 4 weeks after leaving area
- » Checking with physician immediately if fever or "flu-like" symptoms develop while traveling in, or within several months after departure from, endemic area
- » Importance of not missing doses and taking medication on a regular schedule
- » Proper dosing
  Missed dose: Taking as soon as possible; not taking if almost time for next dose; not doubling doses

*For treatment of malaria*
- » Compliance with therapy

### Precautions while using this medication
» Caution if visual disturbances, dizziness, lightheadedness, or hallucinations occur
Mosquito-control measures to help prevent malaria:
Sleeping under mosquito netting
Wearing long-sleeved shirts or blouses and long trousers to protect arms and legs when mosquitoes are out
Applying mosquito repellant to uncovered areas of skin when mosquitoes are out
Using a pyrethrum-containing flying insect spray to kill mosquitoes
» Taking mefloquine at least 12 hours after the last dose of quinidine or quinine
*For treatment of malaria*
Checking with physician if no improvement within a few days

### Side/adverse effects
Signs of potential side effects, especially bradycardia and neuropsychiatric toxicity

## General Dosing Information

Malaria prophylaxis should be started 1 week before the patient enters a malarious area, while in the malarious area, and for 4 weeks after the patient leaves the area. Starting the medication in advance will help to determine the patient's tolerance to the medication and allow time to substitute other antimalarials if the patient develops allergies to the medication or other adverse effects.

Mefloquine is also available in combination with sulfadoxine and pyrimethamine as a tablet, but because of toxicity, its use is not recommended. These medications were combined to try to prevent the development of mefloquine resistance to *P. falciparum*; however, in some countries, such as Thailand, *P. falciparum* is already resistant to sulfadoxine and pyrimethamine. *In vitro* mefloquine resistance has also been reported in Thailand, and may be related to the routine use of quinine.

In the treatment of serious, overwhelming, or life-threatening *P. falciparum* malaria, patients should be given intravenous antimalarial agents during the acute phase. Following this, oral mefloquine may be given to complete the course of therapy. Allow at least 12 hours between the last dose of quinine or quinidine and the start of mefloquine.

In the treatment of acute *P. vivax* or *P. ovale* malaria, it is recommended that mefloquine therapy be followed by treatment with primaquine to effect a radical cure and avoid a relapse since mefloquine does not eliminate the exoerythrocytic (intrahepatic) stages of *P. vivax* or *P. ovale* infection.

The *salt/base equivalence* of mefloquine products differs between the U.S. product and that of other countries. In the U.S., a 250 mg Lariam tablet contains 250 mg of mefloquine salt, which is equivalent to 228 mg of mefloquine base. In Canada and other countries, a 250 mg Lariam tablet contains 250 mg of mefloquine base, which is equivalent to 274 mg of mefloquine salt. This should be considered when dosing a patient with mefloquine.

Patients with impaired renal function do not generally require a reduction in dose since the urinary clearance of mefloquine is very low.

### Diet/Nutrition
Mefloquine should preferably be taken with a full glass (240 mL) of water and with food.

## Oral Dosage Forms

### MEFLOQUINE HYDROCHLORIDE TABLETS

Note: The dosing below is based on the product available in the U.S., in which a 250 mg tablet is equivalent to 228 mg of mefloquine base. The product available in Canada and other countries is 250 mg of mefloquine base, equivalent to 274 mg of mefloquine hydrochloride.

### Usual adult and adolescent dose
Antimalarial—
Prophylaxis: Oral, 250 mg (228 mg base) once a week, starting one week before travel, then weekly during travel in malarious areas and for four weeks after leaving endemic areas.
Therapeutic: Chloroquine-resistant *P. falciparum* malaria: Oral, 1250 mg (1140 mg base) as a single dose, or 16.5 mg (15 mg base) per kg of body weight as a single dose.

### Usual pediatric dose
Antimalarial—
Prophylaxis:
Infants and children up to 15 kg of body weight—Use is not recommended.
Children 15 to 19 kg of body weight—Oral, 62.5 mg (57 mg base) (¼ tablet) once a week, starting one week before travel, then weekly during travel in malarious areas and for four weeks after leaving endemic areas.
Children 20 to 30 kg of body weight—Oral, 125 mg (114 mg base) (½ tablet) once a week, starting one week before travel, then weekly during travel in malarious areas and for four weeks after leaving endemic areas.
Children 31 to 45 kg of body weight—Oral, 187.5 mg (171 mg base) (¾ tablet) once a week, starting one week before travel, then weekly during travel in malarious areas and for four weeks after leaving endemic areas.
Children over 45 kg of body weight—See *Usual adult and adolescent dose*.
Therapeutic:
Oral, 16.5 mg (15 mg base) per kg of body weight as a single dose.

### Usual pediatric prescribing limits
Prophylaxis—Up to 250 mg (228 mg base) once a week.

### Usual geriatric dose
See *Usual adult and adolescent dose*.

### Strength(s) usually available
U.S.—
250 mg (228 mg base) (Rx) [*Lariam* (scored; lactose)].
Canada—
Not commercially available; however, those who wish to prescribe mefloquine should contact the medical department of Hoffmann-LaRoche to obtain the name of the nearest principal investigator to arrange to become a co-investigator and for a supply of the drug.

### Packaging and storage
Store between 15 and 30 °C (59 and 86 °F), unless otherwise specified by manufacturer.

### Auxiliary labeling
• Take with food and full glass of water.
• May cause dizziness or vision problems.
• Continue medication for full time of treatment.

## Selected Bibliography

Anonymous. Change of dosing regimen for malaria prophylaxis with mefloquine. JAMA 91; 265(7): 849.
Keystone JS. Prevention of malaria. Drugs 1990; 39(3): 337-54.
Krogstad DJ, Herwaldt BL, Schlesinger PH. Antimalarial agents: specific treatment regimens. Antimicrob Agents Chemother 1988; 32: 957-61.
Lobel HO, et al. Effectiveness and tolerance of long-term malaria prophylaxis with mefloquine. JAMA 1991; 265(3): 361-4.
Panisko DM, Keystone JS. Treatment of malaria-1990. Drugs 1990; 39(2): 160-89.

Revised: 10/06/92
Interim revision: 08/26/94

---

**MEGESTROL**—See *Progestins (Systemic)*

---

**MEGLUMINE ANTIMONIATE**—The *Meglumine Antimoniate (Systemic)* monograph is not included in this published version of the USP DI database. Copies of the monograph are available on request from Micromedex, Inc. - Reprint Requests, 6200 S. Syracuse Way, Suite 300, Englewood, CO 80111; telephone (303) 486-6400; telefax (303) 486-6464; Email: USPDI@MDX.COM.

---

**MELARSOPROL**—The *Melarsoprol (Systemic)* monograph is not included in this published version of the USP DI database. Copies of the monograph are available on request from Micromedex, Inc. - Reprint Requests, 6200 S. Syracuse Way, Suite 300, Englewood, CO 80111; telephone (303) 486-6400; telefax (303) 486-6464; Email: USPDI@MDX.COM.

# MELPHALAN  Systemic

VA CLASSIFICATION (Primary): AN100
Commonly used brand name(s): *Alkeran*.
Other commonly used names are L-PAM and phenylalanine mustard.
Note: For a listing of dosage forms and brand names by country availability, see *Dosage Forms* section(s).

## Category
Antineoplastic.

## Indications
Note: Bracketed information in the *Indications* section refers to uses that are not included in U.S. product labeling.

### Accepted
Carcinoma, ovarian, epithelial (treatment) or
[Carcinoma, breast (treatment)][1]—Melphalan is indicated for the palliative treatment of nonresectable epithelial carcinoma of the ovary. It is also indicated for treatment of breast carcinoma.

[Melanoma, malignant (treatment)]—Melphalan is indicated for regional limb perfusion as an adjuvant to surgery to treat metastatic melanoma of the extremity.

Multiple myeloma (treatment) or
[Waldenström's macroglobulinemia (treatment)][1]—Melphalan is indicated for the palliative treatment of multiple myeloma and Waldenström's macroglobulinemia.

[Lymphomas, Hodgkin's (treatment)][1]—Melphalan is indicated as a component of conventional-dose salvage combination therapy for relapsed, resistant Hodgkin's lymphomas.

[1]Not included in Canadian product labeling.

## Pharmacology/Pharmacokinetics

### Physicochemical characteristics
Molecular weight—305.21.

### Mechanism of action/Effect
Melphalan is an alkylating agent of the nitrogen mustard type. Melphalan is a bifunctional alkylating agent and is cell cycle–phase nonspecific. Activity occurs as a result of formation of an unstable ethylenimmonium ion, which alkylates or binds with many intracellular molecular structures including nucleic acids. Its cytotoxic action is primarily due to cross-linking of strands of DNA and RNA, as well as inhibition of protein synthesis.

### Absorption
Variably and incompletely absorbed from the gastrointestinal tract. Absorption is decreased in the presence of food.

### Distribution
Apparent volume of distribution ($Vol_D$)—steady-state: 0.5 liter per kg of body weight (L/kg).

### Protein binding
Moderate to high (60 to 90%), primarily to albumin and alpha$_1$-acid glycoprotein; 30% is irreversibly bound to plasma proteins.

### Biotransformation
Deactivated in plasma by hydrolysis.

### Half-life
Distribution—Approximately 10 minutes.
Terminal—Approximately 90 minutes; the average terminal half-life of melphalan in the perfusion circuit during regional hyperthermic perfusion is 26 to 53 minutes.

### Elimination
Primarily nonrenal.
In dialysis—Not removable by hemodialysis or hemoperfusion.

## Precautions to Consider

### Cross-sensitivity and/or related problems
Patients sensitive to chlorambucil may also be sensitive (in form of skin rash) to melphalan.

### Carcinogenicity/Mutagenicity
Secondary malignancies are potential delayed effects of many antineoplastic agents, although it is not clear whether the effect is related to their mutagenic or immunosuppressive action. The risk may increase with increasing dose and duration of therapy. In one study, the 10-year risk of developing secondary acute leukemia or myeloproliferative syndrome was less than 2% for cumulative doses under 600 mg, but 19.5% for cumulative doses of 730 to 9652 mg. Although information is limited, available data seem to indicate that the highest carcinogenic risk is with the alkylating agents.

Melphalan has been associated with an increased risk of development of secondary malignancies, including acute nonlymphocytic leukemia and myeloproliferative syndrome, in humans. The risk of development of secondary leukemia may be increased by increased cumulative dose of melphalan.

Melphalan produces chromosomal aberrations in human cells both *in vitro* and *in vivo*.

### Pregnancy/Reproduction
Fertility—Gonadal suppression, resulting in amenorrhea or azoospermia, may occur in patients taking melphalan. These effects may be related to the dose and length of therapy and may be irreversible. Prediction of the degree of testicular or ovarian function impairment is complicated by the common use of combinations of several antineoplastics, which makes it difficult to assess the effects of individual agents.

Pregnancy—Adequate and well-controlled studies in humans have not been done. However, melphalan is believed to be potentially harmful to the fetus.

In a study in rats, oral administration of melphalan at a dose of 6 to 18 mg per square meter of body surface area per day (mg/m$^2$/day) resulted in abnormalities in the development of the brain, eyes, mandible, and tail.

FDA Pregnancy Category D.

In general, use of a contraceptive is recommended during cytotoxic drug therapy.

### Breast-feeding
It is not known whether melphalan is distributed into breast milk. Breast-feeding is not recommended while melphalan is being administered because of the risks to the infant (adverse effects, mutagenicity, carcinogenicity).

### Pediatrics
Appropriate studies on the relationship of age to the effects of melphalan have not been performed in the pediatric population. Safety and efficacy in pediatric patients have not been established.

### Geriatrics
No information is available on the relationship of age to the effects of melphalan in geriatric patients. However, geriatric patients are more likely to have age-related renal function impairment, which may require adjustment of dosage.

### Dental
The bone marrow depressant effects of melphalan may result in an increased incidence of microbial infection, delayed healing, and gingival bleeding. Dental work, whenever possible, should be completed prior to initiation of therapy or deferred until blood counts have returned to normal. Patients should be instructed in proper oral hygiene during treatment, including caution in use of regular toothbrushes, dental floss, and toothpicks.

Melphalan may cause stomatitis, especially when high doses are used.

### Drug interactions and/or related problems
The following drug interactions and/or related problems have been selected on the basis of their potential clinical significance (possible mechanism in parentheses where appropriate)—not necessarily inclusive (» = major clinical significance):

Note: Combinations containing any of the following medications, depending on the amount present, may also interact with this medication.

Blood dyscrasia–causing medications (see *Appendix II*)
(leukopenic and/or thrombocytopenic effects of melphalan may be increased with concurrent or recent therapy if these medications cause the same effects; dosage adjustment of melphalan, if necessary, should be based on blood counts)

» Bone marrow depressants, other (see *Appendix II*) or
Radiation therapy
(additive bone marrow depression may occur; dosage reduction may be required when two or more bone marrow depressants, including radiation, are used concurrently or consecutively)

Carmustine
(intravenous melphalan may be synergistic with carmustine in causing lung toxicity)

Cimetidine
(reduced serum concentration of melphalan may result, perhaps due to decreased absorption)

Cyclosporine
(increased risk of nephrotoxicity)
Interferons, alpha
(increased elimination of melphalan may occur, perhaps due to fever induced by alpha interferons)
Nalidixic acid
(increased incidence of hemorrhagic necrotic enterocolitis in pediatric patients)
Vaccines, killed virus
(because normal defense mechanisms may be suppressed by melphalan therapy, the patient's antibody response to the vaccine may be decreased. The interval between discontinuation of medications that cause immunosuppression and restoration of the patient's ability to respond to the vaccine depends on the intensity and type of immunosuppression-causing medication used, the underlying disease, and other factors; estimates vary from 3 months to 1 year)
» Vaccines, live virus
(because normal defense mechanisms may be suppressed by melphalan therapy, concurrent use with a live virus vaccine may potentiate the replication of the vaccine virus, may increase the side/adverse effects of the vaccine virus, and/or may decrease the patient's antibody response to the vaccine; immunization of these patients should be undertaken only with extreme caution after careful review of the patient's hematologic status and only with the knowledge and consent of the physician managing the melphalan therapy. The interval between discontinuation of medications that cause immunosuppression and restoration of the patient's ability to respond to the vaccine depends on the intensity and type of immunosuppression-causing medication used, the underlying disease, and other factors; estimates vary from 3 months to 1 year. Patients with leukemia in remission should not receive live virus vaccine until at least 3 months after their last chemotherapy. Oral poliovirus vaccine should not be administered to persons in close contact with the patient, especially family members)

**Laboratory value alterations**
The following have been selected on the basis of their potential clinical significance (possible effect in parentheses where appropriate)—not necessarily inclusive (» = major clinical significance):
With physiology/laboratory test values
Uric acid concentrations in blood and urine
(may be increased)
Urinary 5-hydroxyindoleacetic acid (5-HIAA) concentrations
(may be increased, possibly as a result of tumor cell destruction with accompanying release of metabolites)

**Medical considerations/Contraindications**
The medical considerations/contraindications included have been selected on the basis of their potential clinical significance (reasons given in parentheses where appropriate)—not necessarily inclusive (» = major clinical significance).

*Except under special circumstances, this medication should not be used when the following medical problem exists:*
» Hypersensitivity to melphalan

*Risk-benefit should be considered when the following medical problems exist:*
» Bone marrow depression
» Chickenpox, existing or recent (including recent exposure) or
» Herpes zoster
(risk of severe generalized disease)
Gout, history of or
Urate renal stones, history of
(risk of hyperuricemia)
» Infection
» Renal function impairment
(effect on toxicity difficult to predict; possible increased risk of bone marrow depression)
» Caution should be used also in patients who have had previous cytotoxic drug therapy or radiation therapy within 3 to 4 weeks.

**Patient monitoring**
The following are especially important in patient monitoring (other tests may be warranted in some patients, depending on condition; » = major clinical significance):
» Blood counts, complete (CBC), including
Hematocrit
Hemoglobin
Platelet count
(recommended prior to initiation of therapy and at periodic intervals during therapy; frequency varies according to the patient's condition, the dose of melphalan administered, and other drugs being administered concurrently)
Blood urea nitrogen (BUN) concentrations and
Serum creatinine concentrations
(recommended prior to initiation of therapy and at periodic intervals during therapy)
Serum uric acid concentrations
(recommended prior to initiation of therapy and at periodic intervals during therapy)

## Side/Adverse Effects

The following side/adverse effects have been selected on the basis of their potential clinical significance (possible cause in parentheses where appropriate)—not necessarily inclusive:

**Those indicating need for medical attention**
Incidence more frequent—dose-related
*Neutropenia, with or without infection* (fever or chills; cough or hoarseness; lower back or side pain; painful or difficult urination)—usually asymptomatic; uncommon after limb perfusion; *thrombocytopenia* (unusual bleeding or bruising; black, tarry stools; blood in urine or stools; pinpoint red spots on skin)—usually asymptomatic

Note: *Myelosuppression* usually occurs within 2 to 3 weeks of initiation of therapy, although *neutropenia* may occur within 5 days in a few patients. The nadir of leukocyte and platelet counts usually occurs within 3 to 5 weeks, and leukocyte and platelet counts usually return to normal within 4 to 8 weeks.

Incidence less frequent or rare
*Allergic reaction* (sudden skin rash or itching); *hyperuricemia or uric acid nephropathy* (joint pain; lower back or side pain; swelling of feet or lower legs); *mucositis* (diarrhea; difficulty in swallowing)—dose-related; *pulmonary fibrosis* (shortness of breath); *skin or soft tissue injury* (redness and/or soreness in arm or leg)—with isolated limb perfusion; *stomatitis* (sores in mouth and on lips); *vasculitis, severe, recurrent* (redness and/or soreness at the infusion site)

Note: *Hyperuricemia or uric acid nephropathy* occurs most commonly during initial treatment of patients with leukemia or lymphoma, as a result of rapid cell breakdown which leads to elevated serum uric acid concentrations.

**Those indicating need for medical attention only if they continue or are bothersome**
Incidence less frequent
*Nausea and vomiting*—dose-related

**Those indicating the need for medical attention if they occur after medication is discontinued**
*Bone marrow depression* (black, tarry stools; blood in urine or stools; cough or hoarseness; fever or chills; lower back or side pain; painful or difficult urination; pinpoint red spots on skin; unusual bleeding or bruising)

Note: Cumulative *myelosuppression* may occur with repeated dosing.

## Overdose

For specific information on the agents used in the management of melphalan overdose, see:
• *Colony Stimulating Factors (Systemic)* monograph.

For more information on the management of overdose or unintentional ingestion, **contact a Poison Control Center** (see *Poison Control Center Listing*).

**Clinical effects of overdose**
The following effects have been selected on the basis of their potential clinical significance (possible signs and symptoms in parentheses where appropriate)—not necessarily inclusive:

Acute and chronic
*Anemia* (unusual bleeding or bruising; unusual tiredness or weakness); *colitis* (abdominal cramping and pain); *mucositis, severe* (difficulty in swallowing; diarrhea); *nausea and vomiting; neutropenia, possibly with infection* (chills; cough or hoarseness; lower back or side pain; painful or difficult urination); *stomatitis* (painful sores in the mouth); *thrombocytopenia* (unusual bleeding or bruising; black, tarry stools; blood in urine or stools; pinpoint red spots on skin)

**Supportive care**
There is no specific antidote to melphalan; care of patients with melphalan overdose should be supportive. One pediatric patient who was inadvertently administered a dose of 254 mg per square meter of body surface area (mg/m$^2$) of melphalan survived with standard supportive care. Melphalan can not be removed from the plasma by hemodialysis or hemoperfusion.

The patient's blood count parameters should be monitored closely for 3 to 6 weeks following the overdose, and supportive therapy should be given as needed. Severe bone marrow depression may require transfusion of needed blood components. Patients who develop leukopenia should be observed carefully for signs of infection. Antibiotic support may be required. Treatment with colony stimulating factors may shorten the duration of pancytopenia. Nutritional support with parenteral nutrition may be used in cases of overdose if mucositis prevents the oral intake of nutrition.

## Patient Consultation

As an aid to patient consultation, refer to *Advice for the Patient, Melphalan (Systemic).*

Consider advising the patient on the following (» = major clinical significance):

**Before using this medication**
» Conditions affecting use, especially:
    Hypersensitivity to melphalan
    Carcinogenicity—Increased risk of secondary malignancies
    Pregnancy—Advisability of using contraception; telling physician immediately if pregnancy is suspected
    Breast-feeding—Not recommended because of the potential risk to the infant
    Other medications, especially other bone marrow depressants and live virus vaccines, or previous cytotoxic drug therapy or radiation therapy within 3 to 4 weeks
    Other medical problems, especially bone marrow depression, chickenpox or recent exposure, herpes zoster, infection, or renal function impairment

**Proper use of this medication**
» Importance of not taking more or less medication than the amount prescribed
    Importance of ample fluid intake and subsequent increase in urine output to aid in excretion of uric acid
» Frequency of nausea and vomiting; importance of continuing medication despite stomach upset
    Checking with physician if vomiting occurs shortly after dose is taken
» Proper dosing
    Missed dose: Not taking at all; not doubling doses
» Proper storage

**Precautions while using this medication**
» Importance of close monitoring by the physician
» Avoiding immunizations unless approved by physician; other persons in patient's household should avoid immunizations with oral poliovirus vaccine; avoiding other persons who have taken oral poliovirus vaccine or wearing a protective mask that covers nose and mouth

*Caution if bone marrow depression occurs*
» Avoiding exposure to persons with infections, especially during periods of low blood counts; checking with physician immediately if fever, chills, cough, hoarseness, lower back or side pain, or painful or difficult urination occurs
» Checking with physician immediately if unusual bleeding or bruising; black, tarry stools; blood in urine or stools; or pinpoint red spots on skin occur
    Caution in use of regular toothbrush, dental floss, or toothpick; checking with physician before having dental work done
    Not touching eyes or inside of nose unless hands washed immediately before
    Using caution to avoid accidental cuts with use of sharp objects such as safety razor or fingernail or toenail cutters
    Avoiding contact sports or other situations where bruising or injury could occur

**Side/adverse effects**
    May cause adverse effects such as blood problems and cancer; importance of discussing possible effects with physician
    Signs of potential side effects, especially neutropenia, with or without infection; thrombocytopenia; allergic reaction; hyperuricemia or uric acid nephropathy; mucositis; pulmonary fibrosis; skin or soft tissue injury; stomatitis; severe, recurrent vasculitis

## General Dosing Information

Patients receiving melphalan should be under the supervision of a physician experienced in cancer chemotherapy.

Although systemic complications are less common with isolated limb perfusion of melphalan as compared with orally or intravenously administered melphalan, severe local reactions, rarely requiring amputation, are possible. Isolated limb perfusion should be used only by physicians well-trained in the technique.

A variety of dosage schedules and regimens of melphalan, alone or in combination with other antitumor agents, are used. The prescriber may consult the medical literature as well as the manufacturer's literature in choosing a specific dosage.

Dosage must be adjusted to meet the individual requirements of each patient, based on clinical response and degree of bone marrow depression. This is especially important because of unreliable absorption of orally administered melphalan.

Although melphalan is eliminated primarily by nonrenal mechanisms, increased bone marrow toxicity has been observed in patients with renal function impairment who receive melphalan. The manufacturer recommends consideration of dosage reduction in patients with renal function impairment receiving melphalan intravenously, and careful observation of patients with renal function impairment receiving melphalan orally.

Development of uric acid nephropathy in patients with leukemia or lymphoma may be prevented by adequate oral hydration and, in some cases, administration of allopurinol. Alkalinization of urine may be necessary if serum uric acid concentrations are elevated.

It is recommended that melphalan therapy be discontinued if marked leukopenia (particularly granulocytopenia) or thrombocytopenia occurs. Therapy may be resumed at a lower dosage when the clinical and laboratory examinations are satisfactory.

Special precautions are recommended in patients who develop thrombocytopenia as a result of administration of melphalan. These may include extreme care in performing invasive procedures; regular inspection of intravenous sites, skin (including perirectal area), and mucous membrane surfaces for signs of bleeding or bruising; limiting frequency of venipuncture and avoiding intramuscular injections; testing urine, emesis, stool, and secretions for occult blood; care in use of regular toothbrushes, dental floss, toothpicks, safety razors, and fingernail and toenail cutters; avoiding constipation; and using caution to prevent falls and other injuries. Such patients should avoid alcohol and any aspirin intake because of the risk of gastrointestinal bleeding. Platelet transfusions may be required.

Patients who develop leukopenia should be observed carefully for signs of infection. Antibiotic support may be required.

**Safety considerations for handling this medication**

There is evidence that personnel involved in preparation and administration of parenteral antineoplastics may be at some risk because of the potential mutagenicity, teratogenicity, and/or carcinogenicity of these agents, although the actual risk is unknown. USP advisory panels recommend cautious handling both in preparation and disposal of antineoplastic agents. Precautions that have been suggested include:
• Use of a biological containment cabinet during reconstitution and dilution of parenteral medications and wearing of disposable surgical gloves and masks.
• Use of proper technique to prevent contamination of the medication, work area, and operator during transfer between containers (including proper training of personnel in this technique).
• Cautious and proper disposal of needles, syringes, vials, ampuls, and unused medication.

Detailed guidelines for the handling of cytotoxic and hazardous antineoplastic agents have been developed by various groups, including the American Society of Health-System Pharmacists (ASHP) and the Office of Occupational Medicine, Occupational Safety and Health Administration (OSHA).

Direct contact of skin or mucosa with melphalan requires immediate washing with soap and water or thoroughly flushing with water, respectively.

**Combination chemotherapy**

Melphalan may be used in combination with other agents in various regimens. As a result, incidence and/or severity of side effects may be altered and different dosages may be used. For specific dosages and schedules, consult the literature. For information regarding each agent, consult the individual monographs.

## Oral Dosage Forms

### MELPHALAN TABLETS USP

**Usual adult dose**
Multiple myeloma—
    Oral, 150 mcg (0.15 mg) per kg of body weight a day for seven days, followed by a rest period of at least three weeks, during which time the leukocyte count will fall. When white cell and platelet counts are rising, a maintenance dose of 50 mcg (0.05 mg) per kg of body weight a day may be instituted, or

Oral, 100 to 150 mcg (0.1 to 0.15 mg) per kg of body weight a day for two to three weeks, or 250 mcg (0.25 mg) per kg of body weight a day for four days, followed by a rest period of two to four weeks. When leukocyte counts rise above 3000 to 4000 per cubic millimeter and platelet counts above 100,000 per cubic millimeter, a maintenance dose of 2 to 4 mg a day may be instituted, or

Oral, 7 mg per square meter of body surface area or 250 mcg (0.25 mg) per kg of body weight a day for five days every five to six weeks, adjusted to produce mild leukopenia and thrombocytopenia.

Ovarian carcinoma, epithelial—
   Oral, 200 mcg (0.2 mg) per kg of body weight a day for five days, repeated every four to five weeks if blood counts return to normal.

### Usual pediatric dose
Children up to 12 years of age—Safety and efficacy have not been established.

### Usual geriatric dose
See *Usual adult dose*.

### Strength(s) usually available
U.S.—
   2 mg (Rx) [*Alkeran* (scored; lactose; sucrose)].
Canada—
   2 mg (Rx) [*Alkeran* (scored)].

### Packaging and storage
Store below 40 °C (104 °F), preferably between 15 and 30 °C (59 and 86 °F), unless otherwise specified by manufacturer. Store in a well-closed, light-resistant container.

### Note
Dispense in a glass container.

## Parenteral Dosage Forms

Note: Bracketed uses in the *Dosage Forms* section refer to categories of use and/or indications that are not included in U.S. product labeling.

### MELPHALAN HYDROCHLORIDE FOR INJECTION

#### Usual adult dose
Multiple myeloma—
   Intravenous infusion, 16 mg per square meter of body surface area (mg/m$^2$) administered over 15 to 20 minutes at two-week intervals for four doses; then at four-week intervals after recovery from toxicity. Dosage adjustments may be made, based on blood cell counts at the nadir.

[Malignant melanoma]—
   Upper extremity—
     Arterial infusion, by hyperthermic isolated limb perfusion technique, 1 mg per kg of body weight, not to exceed 80 mg, in three equally divided doses at five-minute intervals, or
   Lower extremity—
     Arterial infusion, by hyperthermic isolated limb perfusion technique, 1.5 mg per kg of body weight, not to exceed 120 mg, in three equally divided doses at five-minute intervals.

Note: The following perfusion guidelines are recommended by the manufacturer:

- Temperature of the perfusate should not exceed 42.5 °C (108.5 °F)
- Temperature of the limb should not exceed 42 °C (107.6 °F)
- Flow-rate—250 to 600 mL per minute (mL/min)
- Perfusate—650 to 750 mL of heparinized whole blood or an equal mixture of lactated Ringer's solution and washed packed red blood cells
- Perfusion duration—Not to exceed one hour

#### Usual pediatric dose
Safety and efficacy have not been established.

#### Usual geriatric dose
See *Usual adult dose*.

#### Strength(s) usually available
U.S.—
   50 mg (Rx) [*Alkeran* (lyophilized powder; povidone 20 mg)].
Canada—
   50 mg (Rx) [*Alkeran* (lyophilized powder; povidone 20 mg)].

#### Packaging and storage
Store between 15 and 30 °C (59 and 86 °F). Protect from light.

#### Preparation of dosage form
For intravenous infusion—
   Reconstitute the vial of melphalan with 10 mL of the diluent supplied by the manufacturer, for a concentration of 5 mg per mL (mg/mL). Immediately dilute the dose to be administered in 0.9% sodium chloride injection to a final concentration no greater than 2 mg/mL.

For isolated limb perfusion—
   Reconstitute the vial of melphalan with 10 mL of the diluent supplied by the manufacturer, for a concentration of 5 mg per mL (mg/mL).

#### Stability
Melphalan reconstituted as directed to a concentration of 5 mg/mL is stable for up to two hours at 30 °C (86 °F). The reconstituted solution should not be refrigerated because refrigeration will cause a precipitate to form.
Melphalan infusions prepared to a final concentration of 0.1 to 0.45 mg/mL in 0.9% sodium chloride injection are stable for up to 50 minutes when stored at 30 °C (86 °F), and up to four hours at 20 °C (68 °F).
Unused portions of melphalan should be discarded.

#### Incompatibilities
Melphalan 0.1 mg per mL (mg/mL) in 0.9% sodium chloride injection is incompatible for Y-site administration with amphotericin B, chlorpromazine hydrochloride, daunorubicin hydrochloride, idarubicin hydrochloride, lorazepam, methylprednisolone sodium succinate, and prochlorperazine edisylate.

#### Auxiliary labeling
- Do not refrigerate.
- Protect from light.

Revised: 10/01/97

---

# MENADIOL — See *Vitamin K (Systemic)*

---

# MENINGOCOCCAL POLYSACCHARIDE VACCINE    Systemic

VA CLASSIFICATION (Primary): IM100

Note: This monograph refers to the vaccine containing the polysaccharides from *Neisseria meningitidis* serogroups A, C, Y, and W-135.

Commonly used brand name(s): *Menomune*.

Note: For a listing of dosage forms and brand names by country availability, see *Dosage Forms* section(s).

## Category
Immunizing agent (active).

## Indications

### Accepted
Meningitis, meningococcal (prophylaxis)—Meningococcal polysaccharide vaccine consists of purified bacterial capsular polysaccharides and contains no viable components. It is indicated for immunization against meningococcal disease caused by *Neisseria meningitidis*, Group A, Group C, Group Y, or Group W-135. *N. meningitidis* is the second most common cause of bacterial meningitis in the U.S., affecting approximately 3000 to 4000 persons each year. The serogroups protected against by this vaccine are responsible for approximately 50% of these cases. The fatality rate from disease caused by all serogroups of *N. meningitidis* is approximately 10% for persons with meningococcal meningitis and 30% for persons with meningococcemia, despite appropriate treatment with antimicrobial agents. The incidence of endemic meningococcal disease peaks in late winter to early spring in the U.S.

Meningococcal polysaccharide vaccine is indicated primarily for persons 2 years of age and older at risk in epidemic or highly endemic areas, including:

- Military recruits. Before the advent of routine administration of meningococcal vaccine to military personnel in 1971, military recruits were at high risk, especially from the serogroup C disease.
- Persons with anatomic or functional asplenia. Asplenic persons seem to be at increased risk of developing meningococcal disease and experience particularly severe infections. Persons who have had their spleens removed because of trauma or non-lymphoid tumors have acceptable antibody responses to the vaccine, although clinical efficacy has not been documented.

In addition, immunization should be considered for:
- Household or institutional contacts of persons with meningococcal disease as an adjunct to antibiotic chemoprophylaxis.
- Medical and laboratory personnel at risk of exposure to meningococcal disease.
- Travelers to countries having epidemic meningococcal disease, particularly travelers who will have prolonged contact with the local populace. One area of the world recognized as having recurrent epidemics of meningococcal disease is the part of sub-Saharan Africa that extends from Mauritania in the west to Ethiopia in the east.
- Immunosuppressed persons. It is uncertain whether persons with diseases associated with immunosuppression (other than asplenia listed above) are at higher risk of acquiring meningococcal disease, as they are of acquiring disease caused by other encapsulated bacteria.

Revaccination may be indicated for persons in the above high risk categories, particularly children at high-risk who were first immunized when under 4 years of age; such children should be considered for revaccination after 2 or 3 years if they remain at high risk. The purpose of this revaccination is to reinstate the primary immune response of the vaccine if it has declined; the revaccination will not evoke a booster response.

**Unaccepted**
Because this vaccine protects against only *Neisseria meningitidis* serogroups A, C, Y, and W-135, protection against other serogroups, such as serogroup B, is not an indication for immunization with this vaccine.

## Pharmacology/Pharmacokinetics

### Mechanism of action/Effect
Meningococcal bacteria are surrounded by polysaccharide capsules, which make the bacteria resistant to attack by white blood cells. However, human blood serum contains antibodies, which render the bacteria vulnerable to attack. The vaccine, which is composed of the purified capsular polysaccharides from bacterial cells, stimulates production of these antibodies and provides active immunity to the 4 serogroups of *N. meningitidis* bacteria represented in the vaccine.

The vaccine will not stimulate protection against infections caused by organisms other than those in Groups A, C, Y, and W-135.

### Protective effect
The antibody response to each of the 4 polysaccharides in the vaccine is independent of the antibody responses to the other polysaccharides.

In a study of children 2 to 12 years of age, seroconversion rates as measured by bactericidal antibody were 72% for Group A, 58% for Group C, 90% for Group Y, and 82% for Group W-135. In the same study, seroconversion rates as measured by solid phase radioimmunoassay were 99% for Group A, 99% for Group C, 97% for Group Y, and 89% for Group W-135.

### Time to protective effect
Adequate antibody titers are achieved within 10 to 14 days after vaccination.

### Duration of protective effect
Antibodies against Group A and C polysaccharides decline markedly over the first 3 years following a single dose of vaccine. This antibody decline is more rapid in infants and young children than in adults. One study, conducted with Group A vaccine in children who were under 4 years of age at the time of vaccination, showed a decline in efficacy from greater than 90% to less than 10% within 3 years; in older children, efficacy was 67% 3 years after vaccination. Vaccine-induced clinical protection probably persists in school children and adults for at least 3 years.

## Precautions to Consider

### Cross-sensitivity and/or related problems
Patients allergic to thimerosal or lactose may be allergic to the meningococcal polysaccharide vaccine available in the U.S. and Canada because it may contain a small amount of thimerosal and lactose.

### Pregnancy/Reproduction
Pregnancy—Adequate and well-controlled studies have not been done in humans. Even though there is no convincing evidence of risk to the fetus from immunization of pregnant women using bacterial vaccines, it is recommended that the vaccine not be used in pregnant women, unless there is a substantial risk of infection. Evaluation of meningococcal polysaccharide vaccine used in pregnant women during an epidemic in Brazil demonstrated no adverse effects. In addition, antibody studies in these women showed good antibody levels in maternal and cord blood following vaccination during any given trimester. Furthermore, antibody titers in the neonates declined over the first few months and did not affect their subsequent response to immunization.

Studies have not been done in animals.

FDA Pregnancy Category C.

### Breast-feeding
Problems in humans have not been documented.

### Pediatrics
Meningococcal polysaccharide vaccine is not recommended for use in children up to 2 years of age, because children in this age group are unlikely to have an adequate antibody response to the vaccine.

Revaccination may be indicated for children at high risk who were first immunized when under 4 years of age; such children should be considered for revaccination after 2 or 3 years if they remain at high risk. The purpose of this revaccination is to reinstate the primary immune response of the vaccine if it has declined; the revaccination will not evoke a booster response.

### Geriatrics
Appropriate studies on the relationship of age to the effects of this vaccine have not been performed in the geriatric population. However, no geriatrics-specific problems have been documented to date.

### Drug interactions and/or related problems
The following drug interactions and/or related problems have been selected on the basis of their potential clinical significance (possible mechanism in parentheses where appropriate)—not necessarily inclusive (» = major clinical significance):

Note: Combinations containing any of the following medications, depending on the amount present, may also interact with this medication.

Immunosuppressive agents or
Radiation therapy
(because normal defense mechanisms are suppressed, the patient's antibody response to the meningococcal polysaccharide vaccine may be decreased. The precaution does not apply to corticosteroids used as replacement therapy, for short-term [less than 2 weeks] systemic therapy, or by other routes of administration that do not cause immunosuppression)

### Medical considerations/Contraindications
The medical considerations/contraindications included have been selected on the basis of their potential clinical significance (reasons given in parentheses where appropriate)—not necessarily inclusive (» = major clinical significance).

***Risk-benefit should be considered when the following medical problems exist:***

Febrile illness, severe
(to avoid confusing manifestations of illness with possible side/adverse effects of vaccine; minor illnesses, such as upper respiratory infection, do not preclude administration of vaccine)

Sensitivity to meningococcal polysaccharide vaccine

## Side/Adverse Effects

The following side/adverse effects have been selected on the basis of their potential clinical significance (possible signs and symptoms in parentheses where appropriate)—not necessarily inclusive:

### Those indicating need for medical attention
Incidence rare
  ***Anaphylactic reaction*** (difficulty in breathing or swallowing; hives; itching, especially of soles or palms; reddening of skin, especially around ears; swelling of eyes, face, or inside of nose; unusual tiredness or weakness, sudden and severe)

### Those indicating need for medical attention only if they continue or are bothersome
Incidence more frequent
  ***Erythema at injection site*** (redness)—lasting 1 or 2 days; ***tenderness, soreness, or pain at injection site***
Incidence less frequent
  ***Chills; fatigue*** (tiredness or weakness); ***fever over 37.8 °C (100 °F)*** (over 38.3° C [101° F])—rare; ***headache; induration at injection site*** (hard lump); ***malaise*** (general feeling of discomfort or illness)

## Patient Consultation

As an aid to patient consultation, refer to *Advice for the Patient, Meningococcal Polysaccharide Vaccine (Systemic)*.

In providing consultation, consider emphasizing the following selected information (» = major clinical significance):

## Before receiving this vaccine
» Conditions affecting use, especially:
> Sensitivity to meningococcal vaccine, thimerosal, or lactose; the vaccine contains thimerosal and lactose
>> Use in children—Not recommended for use in children up to 2 years of age

## Proper use of this vaccine
» Proper dosing

## Side/adverse effects
> Signs of potential side effects, especially anaphylactic reaction

## General Dosing Information
The dosage of meningococcal polysaccharide vaccine is the same for all persons—children and adults.

Meningococcal polysaccharide vaccine is administered by subcutaneous injection. The vaccine should not be administered intramuscularly, intradermally, or intravenously.

Meningococcal polysaccharide vaccine may be administered concurrently with the following, using separate body sites, separate syringes, and the precautions that apply to each immunizing agent:
- Polysaccharide vaccines, other, such as haemophilus b conjugate, haemophilus b polysaccharide, and pneumococcal polyvalent vaccines.
- Influenza vaccine, whole or split virus.
- Diphtheria toxoid, tetanus toxoid, and/or pertussis vaccine.
- Live virus vaccines, such as measles, mumps, or rubella vaccines.
- Poliovirus vaccines (oral [OPV], inactivated [IPV], or enhanced-potency inactivated [enhanced-potency IPV]).
- Hepatitis B recombinant or plasma-derived vaccine.
- Immune globulin and disease-specific immune globulins.
- Inactivated vaccines, except cholera, typhoid, and plague. It is recommended that cholera, typhoid, and plague vaccines be administered on separate occasions because of these vaccines' propensity to cause side/adverse effects.

Revaccination may be indicated for persons at high risk of infection, particularly children at high risk who were first immunized when under 4 years of age; such children should be considered for revaccination after 2 or 3 years if they remain at high risk.

In the U.S. and Canada, the vaccine is available in a 10-dose vial for use with either a needle and syringe or a jet injector and in a 50-dose vial for use only with a jet injector. However, although the manufacturer gives instructions and cautions for using a jet injector to administer the immunizing agent, it is recommended that jet injectors not be used to administer any medication until there is clarification of the risk of transmission of hepatitis B virus, human immunodeficiency virus (HIV), or other infectious agents by jet injectors.

## For treatment of adverse effects
Recommended treatment includes
- For mild hypersensitivity reaction—Administering antihistamines, and, if necessary, corticosteroids.
- For severe hypersensitivity or anaphylactic reaction—Administering epinephrine. Antihistamines or corticosteroids may also be administered as required.

## Parenteral Dosage Forms

### MENINGOCOCCAL POLYSACCHARIDE VACCINE FOR INJECTION

**Usual adult and adolescent dose**
Immunizing agent (active)—
> Subcutaneous, 0.5 mL.

**Usual pediatric dose**
Immunizing agent (active)—
> Children up to 2 years of age: Use is not recommended.
> Children 2 years of age and older: See *Usual adult and adolescent dose*.

**Strength(s) usually available**
U.S.—
> 50 mcg of polysaccharide from each of the 4 serogroups of meningococci represented in the vaccine in each 0.5 mL dose (Rx) [*Menomune* (thimerosal 1:10,000; lactose 2.5 to 5 mg)].

Canada—
> 50 mcg of polysaccharide from each of the 4 serogroups of meningococci represented in the vaccine in each 0.5 mL dose (Rx) [*Menomune* (thimerosal 1:10,000; lactose 2.5 to 5 mg)].

**Packaging and storage**
Store both the freeze-dried and the reconstituted vaccine between 2 and 8 °C (35 and 46 °F), unless otherwise specified by manufacturer. Protect from freezing.

**Preparation of dosage form**
- Reconstitute the vaccine using only the diluent supplied by the manufacturer.
- Draw up the appropriate amount of diluent into a suitably sized syringe and inject the diluent into the vial containing the vaccine.
- Shake the vial until the vaccine is dissolved.

**Stability**
Solution should not be used if there is extraneous particulate matter and/or discoloration prior to administration.

The date of reconstitution should be recorded on the label of the vaccine vial.

Single-dose vials of vaccine should be used within 24 hours of reconstitution.

Multidose vials of vaccine that have been reconstituted for administration by syringe should be discarded after 5 days.

Multidose vials of vaccine that have been reconstituted for administration by jet injector should be administered promptly. Partially used vials of vaccine should be discarded immediately.

## Selected Bibliography
Centers for Disease Control and Prevention. ACIP: Meningococcal vaccines: recommendation of the ACIP. MMWR 1985 May 10: 255-9.

Menomune-A/C/Y/W-135 package insert (Connaught—US), Rev 1/83, Rec 6/90.

Cadoz M, et al. Tetravalent (A, C, Y, W 135) meningococcal vaccine in children: immunogenicity and safety. Vaccine 1985 Sep; 3: 340-2.

Revised: 07/12/94

---

# MENOTROPINS  Systemic

BAN: Menotrophin
VA CLASSIFICATION (Primary): HS106
Note: Controlled substance in some states in the U.S.—Schedule IV
Commonly used brand name(s): *Humegon; Pergonal.*
Other commonly used names are human menopausal gonadotropins (hMG), human gonadotropins, and menotrophin.
Note: For a listing of dosage forms and brand names by country availability, see *Dosage Forms* section(s).

## Category
Gonadotropin; infertility therapy adjunct.

## Indications

### Accepted
Infertility, female (treatment)—Menotropins are indicated, in conjunction with chorionic gonadotropin, for stimulation of ovulation and pregnancy in patients with ovulatory dysfunction not due to primary ovarian failure. In general, menotropins are the treatment of choice for induction of ovulation in patients with hypothalamic hypogonadism or those who do not respond to clomiphene.

Reproductive technologies, assisted[1]—Menotropins are indicated, in conjunction with chorionic gonadotropin (hCG), to stimulate the development of multiple oocytes in ovulatory patients who are attempting to conceive by means of assisted reproductive technologies, such as gamete intrafallopian transfer (GIFT) or *in vitro* fertilization (IVF).

Infertility, male (treatment)—Menotropins are also indicated in combination with chorionic gonadotropin for stimulation of spermatogenesis in men with primary or secondary hypogonadotropic hypogonadism.

[1]Not included in Canadian product labeling.

## Pharmacology/Pharmacokinetics

**Physicochemical characteristics**
Source—Extracted from urine of postmenopausal women.

### Mechanism of action/Effect
Menotropins contain follicle-stimulating hormone (FSH) and luteinizing hormone (LH).
> For induction of ovulation and assisted reproductive technologies (ART)—
>> Menotropins prepare the ovarian follicle for ovulation. The combination of FSH and LH stimulates follicular growth and maturation. Chorionic gonadotropin, whose actions are nearly identical to those of LH, is administered following menotropins treatment to mimic the naturally occurring surge of LH that triggers ovulation.
> For treatment of male infertility—
>> Following administration of chorionic gonadotropin to increase testosterone concentrations in men with hypogonadotropic hypogonadism, administration of menotropins induces spermatogenesis.

### Elimination
Renal, 8% unchanged.

## Precautions to Consider

### Carcinogenicity
Long-term studies have not been done in animals to evaluate the carcinogenic potential of menotropins.

### Pregnancy/Reproduction
Fertility—Use of menotropins to induce ovulation is associated with a high incidence of multiple gestations and multiple births. As a result, this may increase the risk of neonatal prematurity, as well as other complications associated with multiple gestations.

Pregnancy—Although problems in humans have not been documented, use of menotropins during pregnancy is unnecessary.

Ovarian hyperstimulation syndrome (OHS), which may be induced by menotropins therapy, is more common, more severe, and protracted in patients who conceive.

FDA Pregnancy Category X.

### Breast-feeding
It is not known whether menotropins are distributed into breast milk. However, menotropins are not indicated during the course of breast-feeding.

### Medical considerations/Contraindications
The medical considerations/contraindications included have been selected on the basis of their potential clinical significance (reasons given in parentheses where appropriate)—not necessarily inclusive (» = major clinical significance).

*Except under special circumstances, this medication should not be used when the following medical problems exist:*

*For females only*
» Abnormal vaginal bleeding, undiagnosed
  (may indicate the presence of endometrial hyperplasia or carcinoma, which may be exacerbated by menotropins-induced increases in estrogen serum concentrations; other possible endocrinopathies should also be ruled out)
» Ovarian cyst or enlargement not associated with polycystic ovarian syndrome
  (risk of further enlargement)

### Patient monitoring
The following may be especially important in patient monitoring (other tests may be warranted in some patients, depending on condition; » = major clinical significance):

*For females only*
» Estradiol
  (measurement of serum concentrations is recommended as needed, continuing through the day of chorionic gonadotropin administration; recommended to determine optimal dose and to lessen the risk of ovarian hyperstimulation)
» Ultrasound examination
  (recommended during menotropins therapy and prior to administration of chorionic gonadotropin to provide information on the number and size of mature follicles, to follow follicular development, and to lessen the risk of ovarian hyperstimulation syndrome and multiple gestation)

Daily basal body temperature
  (can be used in ovulation induction to determine if ovulation has occurred; if basal body temperature following a cycle of treatment is biphasic and is not followed by menses, a pregnancy test is recommended)

Progesterone
  (measurement of serum or urine concentrations can be used prior to menotropins therapy to confirm anovulation; serum concentrations can be used after therapy to detect luteinized ovarian follicles)

*For males only*
Sperm count and determinations of sperm motility
  (to evaluate success of treatment)
Testosterone
  (measurement of baseline serum concentrations recommended prior to therapy, to rule out other causes of infertility and following therapy to evaluate success of treatment; should increase)

## Side/Adverse Effects
Note: Arterial thromboembolism has been reported in patients who have received menotropins and chorionic gonadotropin, both in association with and separate from ovarian hyperstimulation syndrome. Complications resulting from thromboembolism have included venous thrombophlebitis, pulmonary embolism, pulmonary infarction, stroke, arterial occlusion necessitating limb amputation, and (rarely) death.

Serious respiratory complications have occurred with menotropins therapy. These conditions included atelectasis and acute respiratory distress syndrome. Rarely, death has resulted.

The following side/adverse effects have been selected on the basis of their potential clinical significance (possible signs and symptoms in parentheses where appropriate)—not necessarily inclusive:

### Those indicating need for medical attention
Incidence more frequent—about 20%
  *For females only*
  **Uncomplicated, mild to moderate, ovarian enlargement or ovarian cysts** (mild bloating, abdominal or pelvic pain)—usually mild to moderate and abate within 7 to 10 days; ***pain, swelling, or irritation at injection site; rash at injection site or on body***

Incidence less frequent or rare
  *For females only*
  **Severe ovarian hyperstimulation syndrome** (severe abdominal or stomach pain; feeling of indigestion; moderate to severe bloating; decreased amount of urine; continuing or severe nausea, vomiting, or diarrhea; severe pelvic pain; rapid weight gain; swelling of lower legs; shortness of breath)

Note: In clinical trials, *ovarian hyperstimulation syndrome (OHS)* occurred in 0.4% of patients treated with 150 Units or less each of FSH and LH and in 1.3% of patients treated with higher doses of menotropins. OHS may often occur 7 to 10 days after ovulation or completion of therapy. OHS differs from uncomplicated ovarian enlargement and can progress rapidly to cause serious medical problems. With OHS, a marked increase in vascular permeability results in rapid accumulation of fluid in the peritoneal, pleural, and pericardial cavities (third spacing of fluids). Medical complications ultimately arising from this increased vascular permeability may include hypovolemia, hemoconcentration, electrolyte imbalance, ascites, hemoperitoneum, pleural effusions, hydrothorax, acute pulmonary distress, and thromboembolic events. OHS is more common, more severe, and protracted in patients who conceive.

  *For males only*
  **Erythrocytosis** (shortness of breath; irregular heartbeat; dizziness; loss of appetite; headache; fainting; more frequent nosebleeds)—has been reported in one patient

### Those indicating need for medical attention only if they continue or are bothersome
Incidence less frequent
  *For males only*
  **Gynecomastia** (enlargement of breasts)

## Patient Consultation
As an aid to patient consultation, refer to *Advice for the Patient, Menotropins (Systemic)*.
In providing consultation, consider emphasizing the following selected information (» = major clinical significance):

### Before using this medication
» Conditions affecting use, especially:
  Sensitivity to menotropins or gonadotropins
  Other medical problems, especially abnormal vaginal bleeding or ovarian cyst or enlargement

### Proper use of this medication
» Proper dosing

**Precautions while using this medication**
» Importance of close monitoring by physician
*For females only*
» Importance of recording of basal body temperature and timing of intercourse, when recommended by physician

**Side/adverse effects**
Signs of potential side effects, especially ovarian cysts, enlargement, or hyperstimulation syndrome or skin reactions (for ovulation induction) and erythrocytosis (for males)

## General Dosing Information
Patients receiving menotropins should be under supervision of a physician experienced in the treatment of gynecologic or endocrine disorders.

**For females only**
Dosage varies considerably and must be adjusted to meet the individual requirements of each patient, on the basis of clinical response.

Conception should be attempted within 48 hours of ovulation. It is recommended that the couple have intercourse or insemination performed daily beginning the day after chorionic gonadotropin is administered until ovulation is thought to have occurred.

If ovulation does not occur after any cycle of therapy, the therapeutic regimen employed should be re-evaluated. If ovulation does not occur after 3 cycles of menotropins therapy, the appropriateness of continuing use of menotropins for ovulation induction should be reconsidered.

**For treatment of adverse effects**
Ovarian enlargement or ovarian cyst formation
• Discontinuing therapy until ovarian size has returned to baseline. Human chorionic gonadotropin should also be withheld for that cycle.
• Prohibiting intercourse until ovarian size has returned to baseline to prevent cyst rupture.
• Reducing dosage in next course of therapy.

Ovarian hyperstimulation syndrome (OHS)
Acute phase
• Discontinuing therapy.
• Prohibiting intercourse until ovarian size has returned to baseline to prevent cyst rupture.
• Most cases of OHS will spontaneously resolve when menses begins. In selected cases, hospitalization of the patient with bed rest may be necessary.
• Utilizing therapy to prevent hemoconcentration and minimize risk of thromboembolism and renal injury.
• Correcting (cautiously) electrolyte imbalance while maintaining acceptable intravascular volume; in the acute phase, intravascular volume deficit cannot be completely corrected without increasing third space fluid volume.
• Monitoring fluid intake and output, body weight, hematocrit, serum and urine electrolytes, urine specific gravity, blood urea nitrogen (BUN), creatinine, and abdominal girth daily or as often as required.
• Monitoring serum potassium concentrations for development of hyperkalemia.
• Limiting performance of pelvic examinations since they may result in rupture of ovarian cysts and hemoperitoneum.
• Administering intravenous fluids, electrolytes, and human serum albumin as needed to maintain adequate urine output and to avoid hemoconcentration.
• Administering analgesics as needed.
• Avoiding diuretic use since it reduces intravascular volume further.
• Removing ascitic, pleural, or pericardial fluid *only* if it is imperative for relief of symptoms such as respiratory distress or cardiac tamponade; to do so may increase risk of injury to the ovary.
• In patients who require surgery to control bleeding from ovarian cyst rupture, employing surgical measures that also maximally conserve ovarian tissue.

Intermediate phase
• Once patient is stabilized, minimizing third spacing of fluids by cautiously replacing potassium, sodium, and fluids as required, based on monitoring of serum electrolyte concentrations.
• Avoiding diuretic use.

Resolution phase
• The third space fluid shifts to intravascular compartment, resulting in decreased hematocrit value and increased urinary output.
• Peripheral and/or pulmonary edema may result if third space fluid volume mobilized exceeds renal output.
• Administering diuretics when required, to manage pulmonary edema.

## Parenteral Dosage Forms
### MENOTROPINS FOR INJECTION USP

**Usual adult dose**
Induction of ovulation—
Intramuscular, 75 Units of FSH and 75 Units of LH activity once a day for usually seven or more days, followed by 5000 to 10,000 Units of chorionic gonadotropin one day after the last dose of menotropins. If necessary, the dose of menotropins may be increased by 75 to 150 Units FSH and 75 to 150 Units LH every four or five days. Up to 450 Units FSH and 450 Units LH a day may be required.

Assisted reproductive technologies[1]—
Intramuscular, 150 Units of FSH and 150 Units of LH activity once a day for usually seven or more days, followed by 5000 to 10,000 Units of chorionic gonadotropin one day after the last dose of menotropins. If necessary, the dose of menotropins may be increased by 75 to 150 Units FSH and 75 to 150 Units LH every four or five days.

Note: Dosage regimen may vary according to physician preference or patient response.
If the ovaries are abnormally enlarged or the serum estradiol concentration is excessively elevated on the last day of menotropins therapy, human chorionic gonadotropin should not be given for that cycle.

Male infertility (hypogonadotropic hypogonadism)—
Intramuscular, 75 Units of FSH and 75 Units of LH activity three times a week (plus chorionic gonadotropin 2000 Units twice a week) for at least four months following pretreatment with chorionic gonadotropin (5000 Units three times a week for up to four to six months). If an increase in spermatogenesis has not occurred after four months, the dose may be increased to 150 Units FSH and 150 Units LH three times a week (with no change in dose of chorionic gonadotropin).

**Size(s) usually available**
U.S.—
75 Units of FSH and 75 Units of LH activity (Rx) [*Humegon; Pergonal*].
150 Units of FSH and 150 Units of LH activity (Rx) [*Humegon; Pergonal*].
Canada—
75 Units of FSH and 75 Units of LH activity (Rx) [*Humegon; Pergonal*].

**Packaging and storage**
Store below 40 °C (104 °F), preferably between 15 and 30 °C (59 and 86 °F), unless otherwise specified by manufacturer.

**Preparation of dosage form**
Using standard aseptic technique, reconstitute by adding 1 to 2 mL of 0.9% Sodium Chloride Injection USP to each ampul of Menotropins for Injection USP.

**Stability**
Use immediately after reconstitution; discard any unused portion.

---
[1]Not included in Canadian product labeling.

---
Revised: 07/07/92
Interim revision: 06/30/94; 08/04/97

---

# MEPENZOLATE — See *Anticholinergics/Antispasmodics (Systemic)*

---

# MEPERIDINE — See *Opioid (Narcotic) Analgesics (Systemic)*

---

# MEPHENTERMINE — See *Sympathomimetic Agents—Cardiovascular Use (Parenteral-Systemic)*

---

# MEPHENYTOIN — See *Anticonvulsants, Hydantoin (Systemic)*

1946    Mephobarbital

**MEPHOBARBITAL**—See *Barbiturates (Systemic)*

**MEPIVACAINE**—See *Anesthetics (Parenteral-Local)*

**MEPROBAMATE**—The *Meprobamate (Systemic)* monograph is not included in this published version of the USP DI database. Copies of the monograph are available on request from Micromedex, Inc. - Reprint Requests, 6200 S. Syracuse Way, Suite 300, Englewood, CO 80111; telephone (303) 486-6400; telefax (303) 486-6464; Email: USPDI@MDX.COM.

**MEPROBAMATE AND ASPIRIN**—The *Meprobamate and Aspirin (Systemic)* monograph is not included in this published version of the USP DI database. Copies of the monograph are available on request from Micromedex, Inc. - Reprint Requests, 6200 S. Syracuse Way, Suite 300, Englewood, CO 80111; telephone (303) 486-6400; telefax (303) 486-6464; Email: USPDI@MDX.COM.

# MERCAPTOPURINE    Systemic

VA CLASSIFICATION (Primary/Secondary): AN300/IM600; MS105; GA900

Commonly used brand name(s): *Purinethol*.

Another commonly used name is 6-MP.

Note: For a listing of dosage forms and brand names by country availability, see *Dosage Forms* section(s).

## Category
Antineoplastic; immunosuppressant.

## Indications
Note: Bracketed information in the *Indications* section refers to uses that are not included in U.S. product labeling.

**Accepted**

Leukemia, acute lymphocytic (treatment) or

Leukemia, acute nonlymphocytic (treatment)—Mercaptopurine is indicated for remission induction and maintenance therapy of acute lymphocytic and acute nonlymphocytic leukemia.

[Leukemia, chronic myelocytic (treatment)]—Mercaptopurine is indicated for treatment of chronic myelocytic leukemia.

[Lymphomas, non-Hodgkin's (treatment)][1]—Mercaptopurine is indicated for treatment of some pediatric non-Hodgkin's lymphomas.

[Bowel disease, inflammatory (treatment)][1]—Mercaptopurine is also used in the treatment of regional enteritis (Crohn's disease) and ulcerative colitis.

[Arthritis, psoriatic (treatment)][1]—Mercaptopurine is used in the treatment of selected cases of severe psoriatic arthritis.

Extreme caution is recommended in use of mercaptopurine for non-neoplastic conditions because of potential carcinogenicity with long-term use of this agent.

[1]Not included in Canadian product labeling.

## Pharmacology/Pharmacokinetics

**Physicochemical characteristics**
Molecular weight—170.19.
pKa—7.6.

**Mechanism of action/Effect**
Mercaptopurine is an antimetabolite of the purine analog type. Mercaptopurine is cell cycle–specific for the S phase of cell division. Activity occurs as the result of activation in the tissues and may include inhibition of DNA synthesis with a lesser effect on RNA synthesis.

**Absorption**
Variably and incompletely (up to 50%) absorbed from the gastrointestinal tract.

**Distribution**
Crosses the blood-brain barrier, but in insufficient amounts to treat meningeal leukemia.

**Protein binding**
Low (20%).

**Biotransformation**
Hepatic (activation and catabolism); degradation primarily by xanthine oxidase.

**Half-life**
Triphasic—45 minutes, 2.5 hours, and 10 hours.

**Elimination**
Renal (7 to 39% unchanged).
In dialysis—Removable by dialysis.

## Precautions to Consider

**Carcinogenicity/Mutagenicity**
Secondary malignancies are potential delayed effects of many antineoplastic agents, although it is not clear whether the effect is related to their mutagenic or immunosuppressive action. The effect of dose and duration of therapy is also unknown, although risk seems to increase with long-term use. Although information is limited, available data seem to indicate that the carcinogenic risk is greatest with the alkylating agents.

Antimetabolites have been shown to be carcinogenic in animals and may be associated with an increased risk of development of secondary carcinomas in humans, although the risk appears to be less than with alkylating agents.

Mercaptopurine causes chromosome abnormalities in animals and humans and dominant-lethal mutations in male mice.

**Pregnancy/Reproduction**

Fertility—Gonadal suppression, resulting in amenorrhea or azoospermia, may occur in patients taking antineoplastic therapy, especially with the alkylating agents. In general, these effects appear to be related to dose and length of therapy and may be irreversible. Prediction of the degree of testicular or ovarian function impairment is complicated by the common use of combinations of several antineoplastics, which makes it difficult to assess the effects of individual agents.

Pregnancy—Mercaptopurine is not recommended during pregnancy.

First trimester: It is usually recommended that use of antineoplastics, especially combination chemotherapy, be avoided whenever possible, especially during the first trimester. Although information is limited because of the relatively few instances of antineoplastic administration during pregnancy, the mutagenic, teratogenic, and carcinogenic potential of these medications must be considered.

Other hazards to the fetus include adverse reactions seen in adults.

In general, use of a contraceptive is recommended during cytotoxic drug therapy.

Mercaptopurine is embryopathic in rats and has been associated with an increased risk of abortion or premature births in humans; the risk of teratogenicity in surviving offspring has not been studied.

FDA Pregnancy Category D.

**Breast-feeding**
Although very little information is available regarding distribution of antineoplastic agents into breast milk, breast-feeding is not recommended while mercaptopurine is being administered because of the risks to the infant (adverse effects, mutagenicity, carcinogenicity). It is not known whether mercaptopurine is distributed into breast milk.

**Pediatrics**
Appropriate studies on the relationship of age to the effects of mercaptopurine have not been performed in the pediatric population. However, pediatrics-specific problems that would limit the usefulness of this medication in children are not expected.

**Geriatrics**
No information is available on the relationship of age to the effects of mercaptopurine in geriatric patients. However, elderly patients are more likely to have age-related renal function impairment, which may require dosage reduction in patients receiving mercaptopurine.

**Dental**
The bone marrow depressant effects of mercaptopurine may result in an increased incidence of microbial infection, delayed healing, and gingival bleeding. Dental work, whenever possible, should be completed

prior to initiation of therapy or deferred until blood counts have returned to normal. Patients should be instructed in proper oral hygiene during treatment, including caution in use of regular toothbrushes, dental floss, and toothpicks.

Mercaptopurine may also cause stomatitis that is associated with considerable discomfort.

**Drug interactions and/or related problems**

The following drug interactions and/or related problems have been selected on the basis of their potential clinical significance (possible mechanism in parentheses where appropriate)—not necessarily inclusive (» = major clinical significance):

Note: Combinations containing any of the following medications, depending on the amount present, may also interact with this medication.

» Allopurinol or
  Colchicine or
» Probenecid or
» Sulfinpyrazone
   (concurrent use with allopurinol may result in greatly increased mercaptopurine activity and toxicity because of inhibition of metabolism; careful monitoring is recommended. It is recommended that mercaptopurine dosage be reduced to one-third to one-fourth of the usual dosage in patients receiving 300 to 600 mg of allopurinol a day concurrently to reduce or prevent hyperuricemia or to slow the metabolism of mercaptopurine. In addition, mercaptopurine may raise the concentration of blood uric acid; dosage adjustment of antigout agents may be necessary to control hyperuricemia and gout; concurrent use of uricosuric antigout agents should be avoided because of the risk of uric acid nephropathy)

Anticoagulants, coumarin- or indandione-derivative
   (mercaptopurine may increase anticoagulant activity and/or increase the risk of hemorrhage as a result of decreased hepatic synthesis of procoagulant factors and interference with platelet formation or may reduce anticoagulant activity by means of increased prothrombin synthesis or activation)

Blood dyscrasia–causing medications (see *Appendix II*)
   (leukopenic and/or thrombocytopenic effects of mercaptopurine may be increased with concurrent or recent therapy if these medications cause the same effects; dosage adjustment of mercaptopurine, if necessary, should be based on blood counts)

» Bone marrow depressants, other (see *Appendix II*) or
  Radiation therapy
   (additive bone marrow depression may occur; dosage reduction may be required when two or more bone marrow depressants, including radiation, are used concurrently or consecutively)

» Hepatotoxic medications, other (see *Appendix II*)
   (concurrent use may increase the risk of hepatotoxicity and should be avoided)

» Immunosuppressants, other, such as:
  Azathioprine
  Chlorambucil
  Corticosteroids, glucocorticoid
  Corticotropin (ACTH)
  Cyclophosphamide
  Cyclosporine
  Muromonab-CD3
   (concurrent use with mercaptopurine may increase the risk of infection and development of neoplasms)

Vaccines, killed virus
   (because normal defense mechanisms may be suppressed by mercaptopurine therapy, the patient's antibody response to the vaccine may be decreased. The interval between discontinuation of medications that cause immunosuppression and restoration of the patient's ability to respond to the vaccine depends on the intensity and type of immunosuppression-causing medication used, the underlying disease, and other factors; estimates vary from 3 months to 1 year)

» Vaccines, live virus
   (because normal defense mechanisms may be suppressed by mercaptopurine therapy, concurrent use with a live virus vaccine may potentiate the replication of the vaccine virus, may increase the side/adverse effects of the vaccine virus, and/or may decrease the patient's antibody response to the vaccine; immunization of these patients should be undertaken only with extreme caution after careful review of the patient's hematologic status and only with the knowledge and consent of the physician managing the mercaptopurine therapy. The interval between discontinuation of medications that cause immunosuppression and restoration of the patient's ability to respond to the vaccine depends on the intensity and type of immunosuppression-causing medication used, the underlying disease, and other factors; estimates vary from 3 months to 1 year. Patients with leukemia in remission should not receive live virus vaccine until at least 3 months after their last chemotherapy. Immunization with oral poliovirus vaccine should also be postponed in persons in close contact with the patient, especially family members)

**Laboratory value alterations**

The following have been selected on the basis of their potential clinical significance (possible effect in parentheses where appropriate)—not necessarily inclusive (» = major clinical significance):

With diagnostic test results
  Glucose and
  Uric acid
   (serum concentrations may be falsely increased when the sequential multiple analyzer [SMA] is used)

With physiology/laboratory test values
  Uric acid
   (concentrations in blood and urine may be increased)

**Medical considerations/Contraindications**

The medical considerations/contraindications included have been selected on the basis of their potential clinical significance (reasons given in parentheses where appropriate)—not necessarily inclusive (» = major clinical significance).

*Risk-benefit should be considered when the following medical problems exist:*

» Bone marrow depression
» Chickenpox, existing or recent (including recent exposure) or
» Herpes zoster
   (risk of severe generalized disease)
  Gout, history of or
  Urate renal stones, history of
   (risk of hyperuricemia)
» Hepatic function impairment
   (lower dosage recommended)
» Infection
» Renal function impairment
   (lower dosage recommended)
  Sensitivity to mercaptopurine
» Caution should be used also in patients who have had previous cytotoxic drug therapy and radiation therapy.

**Patient monitoring**

The following are especially important in patient monitoring (other tests may be warranted in some patients, depending on condition; » = major clinical significance):

» Alanine aminotransferase (ALT [SGPT]) values, serum and
» Aspartate aminotransferase (AST [SGOT]) values, serum and
» Bilirubin concentrations, serum and
» Lactate dehydrogenase (LDH) values, serum
   (recommended prior to initiation of therapy and at periodic intervals during therapy; frequency varies according to clinical state, agent, dose, and other agents being used concurrently)

Blood urea nitrogen (BUN) concentrations and
Creatinine concentrations, serum
   (recommended prior to initiation of therapy and at periodic intervals during therapy; frequency varies according to clinical state, agent, dose, and other agents being used concurrently)

» Hematocrit or hemoglobin and
» Leukocyte count, total and, if appropriate, differential and
» Platelet count
   (determinations recommended prior to initiation of therapy and at periodic intervals during therapy; frequency varies according to clinical state, agent, dose, and other agents being used concurrently)

Uric acid concentrations, serum
   (recommended prior to initiation of therapy and at periodic intervals during therapy; frequency varies according to clinical state, agent, dose, and other agents being used concurrently)

Note: In patients with acute leukemia and high total leukocyte counts, a rapid fall in leukocyte count may occur with mercaptopurine therapy. Daily blood counts are recommended in these patients.

## Side/Adverse Effects

Note: Many "side effects" of antineoplastic therapy are unavoidable and represent the medication's pharmacologic action. Some of these (for example, leukopenia and thrombocytopenia) are actually used as parameters to aid in individual dosage titration.

The following side/adverse effects have been selected on the basis of their potential clinical significance (possible signs and symptoms in parentheses where appropriate)—not necessarily inclusive:

**Those indicating need for medical attention**
Incidence more frequent
*Anemia* (unusual tiredness or weakness); *hepatotoxicity or biliary stasis* (yellow eyes or skin); *immunosuppression, leukopenia, or infection* (fever or chills; cough or hoarseness; lower back or side pain; painful or difficult urination)—usually asymptomatic; *thrombocytopenia* (unusual bleeding or bruising; black, tarry stools; blood in urine or stools; pinpoint red spots on skin)—usually asymptomatic

Note: *Anemia* occurs with high doses.

*Leukopenia* and *thrombocytopenia* (usually mild) may begin 5 to 6 days after initiation of therapy and persist about 7 days after withdrawal.

Incidence less frequent
*Hyperuricemia or uric acid nephropathy* (joint pain; lower back or side pain; swelling of feet or lower legs); *loss of appetite or nausea and vomiting*

Note: *Hyperuricemia and uric acid nephropathy* occur most commonly during initial treatment of patients with leukemia or lymphoma, as a result of rapid cell breakdown which leads to elevated serum uric acid concentrations.

Crystals of mercaptopurine have been found in urine of children receiving high dosage (1000 mg per square meter of body surface daily).

*Loss of appetite or nausea and vomiting* may be symptoms of overdosage.

Incidence rare
*Gastrointestinal ulceration* (black, tarry stools; stomach pain); *stomatitis* (sores in mouth and on lips)

Note: *Stomatitis* is common with large doses.

**Those indicating need for medical attention only if they continue or are bothersome**
Incidence less frequent
*Darkening of skin; diarrhea; headache; skin rash and itching; weakness*

**Those indicating need for medical attention if they occur after medication is discontinued**
*Bone marrow depression* (black, tarry stools; blood in urine or stools; cough or hoarseness; fever or chills; lower back or side pain; painful or difficult urination; pinpoint red spots on skin; unusual bleeding or bruising); *hepatotoxicity* (yellow eyes or skin)

## Patient Consultation

As an aid to patient consultation, refer to *Advice for the Patient, Mercaptopurine (Systemic)*.

In providing consultation, consider emphasizing the following selected information (» = major clinical significance):

**Before using this medication**
» Conditions affecting use, especially:
  Sensitivity to mercaptopurine
  Pregnancy—Use not recommended because of mutagenic, teratogenic, and carcinogenic potential; advisability of using contraception; telling physician immediately if pregnancy is suspected
  Breast-feeding—Not recommended because of risk of serious side effects
  Other medications, especially allopurinol, other bone marrow depressants, other hepatotoxic medications, other immunosuppressants, probenecid, sulfinpyrazone, or previous cytotoxic drug or radiation therapy
  Other medical problems, especially chickenpox, herpes zoster, hepatic function impairment, infection, or renal function impairment

**Proper use of this medication**
» Importance of not taking more or less medication than the amount prescribed
  Caution in taking combination therapy; taking each medication at the right time
  Importance of ample fluid intake and subsequent increase in urine output to aid in excretion of uric acid
  Checking with physician if vomiting occurs shortly after dose is taken
» Proper dosing
  Missed dose: Not taking at all; not doubling doses
» Proper storage

**Precautions while using this medication**
» Importance of close monitoring by the physician
» Possibility of increased toxicity if alcohol is ingested
» Avoiding immunizations unless approved by physician; other persons in patient's household should avoid immunizations with oral poliovirus vaccine; avoiding persons who have taken oral poliovirus vaccine or wearing a protective mask that covers nose and mouth

*Caution if bone marrow depression occurs*
» Avoiding exposure to persons with infections, especially during periods of low blood counts; checking with physician immediately if fever or chills, cough or hoarseness, lower back or side pain, or painful or difficult urination occurs
» Checking with physician immediately if unusual bleeding or bruising; black, tarry stools; blood in urine or stools; or pinpoint red spots on skin occur
  Caution in use of regular toothbrush, dental floss, or toothpick; physician, dentist, or nurse may suggest alternatives; checking with physician before having dental work done
  Not touching eyes or inside of nose unless hands washed immediately before
  Using caution to avoid accidental cuts with use of sharp objects such as safety razor or fingernail or toenail cutters
  Avoiding contact sports or other situations where bruising or injury could occur
  Caution if any laboratory tests required; possible interference with serum glucose and uric acid values measured by sequential multiple analyzer (SMA)

**Side/adverse effects**
Importance of discussing possible effects, including cancer, with physician
Signs of potential side effects, especially anemia, hepatotoxicity, biliary stasis, immunosuppression, leukopenia, infection, thrombocytopenia, hyperuricemia, uric acid nephropathy, loss of appetite, nausea and vomiting, gastrointestinal ulceration, and stomatitis
Physician or nurse can help in dealing with side effects

## General Dosing Information

Patients receiving mercaptopurine should be under supervision of a physician experienced in immunosuppressive and antimetabolite chemotherapy.

A variety of dosage schedules and regimens of mercaptopurine, alone or in combination with other antitumor agents, are used. The prescriber may consult the medical literature as well as the manufacturer's literature in choosing a specific dosage.

Dosage must be adjusted to meet the individual requirements of each patient, based on clinical response and appearance or severity of toxicity.

Development of uric acid nephropathy in patients with leukemia or lymphoma may be prevented by adequate oral hydration. Alkalinization of urine may be necessary if serum uric acid concentrations are elevated. Allopurinol should be administered with caution and only if uric acid concentrations are unacceptably high.

It is recommended that mercaptopurine dosage be reduced to one-third to one-fourth of the usual dosage in patients receiving 300 to 600 mg of allopurinol a day concurrently to reduce or prevent hyperuricemia or to slow the metabolism of mercaptopurine.

Because the actions of mercaptopurine may be delayed, it is recommended that mercaptopurine therapy be discontinued promptly at the first sign of marked leukopenia (particularly granulocytopenia) or thrombocytopenia, hemorrhage or bleeding tendencies, or jaundice. Therapy may be resumed at one-half the previous dosage when the leukocyte count remains constant for 2 or 3 days, or rises.

In acute leukemia, mercaptopurine may be administered despite the presence of thrombocytopenia and bleeding; stoppage of bleeding and increase in platelet count have occurred during treatment in some cases and platelet transfusions may be useful in others.

Special precautions are recommended in patients who develop thrombocytopenia as a result of administration of mercaptopurine. These may include extreme care in performing invasive procedures; regular inspection of intravenous sites, skin (including perirectal area), and mucous membrane surfaces for signs of bleeding or bruising; limiting frequency of venipuncture and avoiding intramuscular injections; testing urine, emesis, stool, and secretions for occult blood; care in use of regular toothbrushes, dental floss, toothpicks, safety razors, and fingernail and toenail cutters; avoiding constipation; and using caution to prevent falls and other injuries. Such patients should avoid alcohol and aspirin intake because of the risk of gastrointestinal bleeding. Platelet transfusions may be required.

Patients who develop leukopenia should be observed carefully for signs of infection. Antibiotic support may be required. In neutropenic patients who develop fever, broad-spectrum antibiotic coverage should be initiated empirically, pending bacterial cultures and appropriate diagnostic tests.

**Combination chemotherapy**
Mercaptopurine may be used in combination with other agents in various regimens. As a result, incidence and/or severity of side effects may be altered and different dosages (usually reduced) may be used.

## Oral Dosage Forms

Note: Bracketed uses in the *Dosage Forms* section refer to categories of use and/or indications that are not included in U.S. product labeling.

### MERCAPTOPURINE TABLETS USP

**Usual adult dose**
Leukemia, acute lymphocytic or
Leukemia, acute nonlymphocytic—
 Initial: Oral, 2.5 mg per kg of body weight or 80 to 100 mg per square meter of body surface area (to the nearest 25 mg) a day in single or divided doses. If there is no clinical improvement and no leukocyte depression after four weeks at this dosage, an increase in dosage to 5 mg per kg of body weight a day may be attempted.
 Maintenance: Oral, 1.5 to 2.5 mg per kg of body weight or 50 to 100 mg per square meter of body surface area a day.
[Inflammatory bowel disease][1]—
 Oral, 1.5 mg per kg of body weight per day, the dosage being adjusted as necessary. If there is no clinical improvement and no leukocyte depression after two to three months at this dosage, a gradual increase in dosage to 2.5 mg per kg of body weight per day may be attempted.

**Usual pediatric dose**
Leukemia, acute lymphocytic or
Leukemia, acute nonlymphocytic—
 Oral, 2.5 mg per kg of body weight or 75 mg per square meter of body surface area (to the nearest 25 mg) a day in single or divided doses.

**Strength(s) usually available**
U.S.—
 50 mg (Rx) [*Purinethol* (scored; lactose)].
Canada—
 50 mg (Rx) [*Purinethol* (scored)].

**Packaging and storage**
Store below 40 °C (104 °F), preferably between 15 and 30 °C (59 and 86 °F), unless otherwise specified by manufacturer. Store in a well-closed container.

[1]Not included in Canadian product labeling.

Revised: 8/90
Interim revision: 07/29/93; 12/10/93; 06/21/94; 09/29/97

---

# MEROPENEM  Systemic—INTRODUCTORY VERSION

VA CLASSIFICATION (Primary): AM119
Commonly used brand name(s): *Merrem I.V.*
Note: For a listing of dosage forms and brand names by country availability, see *Dosage Forms* section(s).

## Category
Antibacterial (systemic).

## Indications

**General considerations**
Meropenem is a carbapenem antibiotic. It has significant stability to hydrolysis by penicillinases and cephalosporinases produced by gram-positive and gram-negative organisms, with the exception of metallo–beta-lactamases.
Cross-resistance is sometimes seen with strains resistant to other carbapenems.
Meropenem has been shown to act synergistically with aminoglycosides *in vitro* against some isolates of *Pseudomonas aeruginosa*.

**Accepted**
Intra-abdominal infections (treatment)—Meropenem is indicated as a single agent in the treatment of intra-abdominal infections, including complicated appendicitis and peritonitis caused by susceptible organisms, in adults and children 3 months of age and older.
Meningitis, bacterial (treatment)—Meropenem is indicated as a single agent in the treatment of bacterial meningitis caused by susceptible organisms, in children 3 months of age and older. Meropenem has been found to be effective in eliminating concurrent bacteremia associated with bacterial meningitis.

**Unaccepted**
Meropenem should not be used to treat methicillin-resistant staphylococci.

## Pharmacology/Pharmacokinetics

**Physicochemical characteristics**
Chemical group—Carbapenem antibiotic.
Molecular weight—437.52.
pH—Between 7.3 and 8.3 after reconstitution.

**Mechanism of action/Effect**
Bactericidal; meropenem inhibits cell wall synthesis by penetrating the cell wall of most gram-positive and gram-negative bacteria to reach penicillin-binding–protein (PBP) targets. Its strongest affinity is toward PBPs 2, 3, and 4 of *Escherichia coli* and *Pseudomonas aeruginosa*, and PBPs 1, 2, and 4 of *Staphylococcus aureus*. Bactericidal concentrations are typically one to two times the bacteriostatic concentrations; the exception is *Listeria monocytogenes*, against which lethal activity has not been observed.

**Distribution**
Well distributed into most body fluids and tissues, including the cerebrospinal fluid (CSF); CSF concentrations match or exceed those concentrations required to inhibit most susceptible bacteria.

**Protein binding**
Low (approximately 2%).

**Biotransformation**
Meropenem is primarily excreted unchanged; however, there is one metabolite which is microbiologically inactive.

**Half-life**
Approximately 1 hour in adults and children 2 years of age and older with normal renal function.
Approximately 1.5 hours in children 3 months to 2 years of age.

**Time to peak concentration**
Approximately 1 hour after the start of the infusion.

**Peak serum concentration**
500 mg at the end of a 30-minute infusion—Approximately 23 mcg per mL (mcg/mL).
1 gram at the end of a 30-minute infusion—Approximately 49 mcg/mL.
500 mg at the end of a 5-minute injection—Approximately 45 mcg/mL.
1 gram at the end of a 5-minute injection—Approximately 112 mcg/mL.

**Elimination**
Renal—Approximately 70% of an administered dose is recovered in the urine as unchanged meropenem over 12 hours.
In dialysis—Meropenem and its metabolite are hemodialyzable; however, there is inadequate information on the use of meropenem in patients receiving hemodialysis and no information on the usefulness of hemodialysis to treat an overdose. There is also no information with regard to the effectiveness of peritoneal dialysis in the removal of meropenem.

## Precautions to Consider

**Cross-sensitivity and/or related problems**
Patients allergic to other beta-lactam antibacterials (e.g., penicillins, cephalosporins, imipenem) may be allergic to meropenem also.

**Carcinogenicity**
Carcinogenicity studies have not been performed.

**Mutagenicity**
No evidence of mutagenic potential was found when the bacterial reverse mutation test, the Chinese hamster ovary HGPRT assay, cultured human lymphocytes cytogenic assay, and the mouse micronuclear test were performed with meropenem.

**Pregnancy/Reproduction**
Fertility—No impairment of fertility was seen when meropenem was studied in rats at doses of up to 1000 mg per kg of body weight (mg/kg) per day, and in cynomolgus monkeys at doses of up to 360 mg/kg per day. These doses are comparable to 1.8 and 3.7 times, respectively, the

human exposure at the usual dose of 1 gram every 8 hours, based on area under the plasma concentration–time curve (AUC).

Pregnancy—Adequate and well-controlled studies in humans have not been done.

Studies have been performed in rats at doses of up to 1000 mg/kg per day, and cynomolgus monkeys at doses of up to 360 mg/kg per day. These doses are comparable to 1.8 and 3.7 times, respectively, the human exposure at the usual dose of 1 gram every 8 hours, based on AUC. These studies showed no harm to the fetus due to meropenem, although there were slight changes in fetal body weight at doses of 250 mg/kg per day (0.4 times the human exposure at the usual dose of 1 gram every 8 hours, based on AUC) and higher in rats.

FDA Pregnancy Category B.

**Breast-feeding**
It is not known whether meropenem is distributed into breast milk.

**Pediatrics**
Safety and efficacy have not been established in children less than 3 months of age. However, use of meropenem in children 3 months of age and older with bacterial meningitis is supported by evidence from adequate and well-controlled studies. Use of meropenem in children 3 months of age and older with intra-abdominal infections is supported by evidence from adequate and well-controlled studies in adults, with additional data from pediatric pharmacokinetics studies and controlled clinical trials in pediatric patients.

**Geriatrics**
No information is available on the relationship of age to the effects of meropenem in geriatric patients. However, elderly patients are more likely to have an age-related decrease in renal function, which may require a reduction of dosage in patients receiving meropenem.

**Drug interactions and/or related problems**
The following drug interactions and/or related problems have been selected on the basis of their potential clinical significance (possible mechanism in parentheses where appropriate)—not necessarily inclusive (» = major clinical significance):

Note: Combinations containing the following medication, depending on the amount present, may also interact with this medication.

» Probenecid
(probenecid competes with meropenem for active tubular secretion, inhibiting the renal excretion of meropenem; this results in a 38% increase in the elimination half-life and a 56% increase in the extent of systemic exposure to meropenem; concurrent administration is not recommended)

**Laboratory value alterations**
The following have been selected on the basis of their potential clinical significance (possible effect in parentheses where appropriate)—not necessarily inclusive (» = major clinical significance):

With diagnostic test results
Partial thromboplastin time and
Prothrombin time
(may be shortened or prolonged)
Positive direct or indirect antiglobulin (Coombs') tests

With physiology/laboratory test values
Alanine aminotransferase (ALT [SGPT]) and
Alkaline phosphatase and
Aspartate aminotransferase (AST [SGOT]) and
Bilirubin and
Lactate dehydrogenase (LDH)
(serum values may be increased)
Blood urea nitrogen (BUN) and
Creatinine, serum
(concentrations may be transiently increased)
Hematocrit and
Hemoglobin concentrations and
White blood count
(may be decreased)
Platelet count
(may be increased or decreased)

**Medical considerations/Contraindications**
The medical considerations/contraindications included have been selected on the basis of their potential clinical significance (reasons given in parentheses where appropriate)—not necessarily inclusive (» = major clinical significance).

*Except under special circumstances, this medication should not be used when the following medical problem exists:*
» Allergy to meropenem or other beta-lactam antibacterials (e.g., penicillins, cephalosporins, imipenem)

*Risk-benefit should be considered when the following medical problems exist:*
» Central nervous system (CNS) disorders (e.g., brain lesions or history of seizures) or
» Meningitis, bacterial
(seizures are more likely to occur in patients with CNS lesions, a history of seizure disorders, bacterial meningitis, and/or renal function impairment)
» Renal function impairment
(because meropenem is primarily excreted through the kidneys, it must be administered in a reduced dosage to patients with impaired renal function; dosage adjustment is also recommended in elderly patients; also, thrombocytopenia has been observed in patients with renal function impairment, but no clinical bleeding has been reported)

**Patient monitoring**
The following may be especially important in patient monitoring (other tests may be warranted in some patients, depending on condition; » = major clinical significance):

Alanine aminotransferase (ALT [SGPT]), serum and
Alkaline phosphatase, serum and
Aspartate aminotransferase (AST [SGOT]), serum and
Bilirubin, serum and
Lactate dehydrogenase (LDH), serum
(periodic monitoring is advisable during prolonged therapy)
Blood urea nitrogen (BUN) concentrations and
Creatinine, serum
(periodic monitoring is advisable during prolonged therapy)
Hematocrit and
Hemoglobin concentrations and
Platelet count
White blood count
(periodic monitoring is advisable during prolonged therapy)

## Side/Adverse Effects

Note: The incidence of seizures was reported to be 0.5% in patients treated for infections outside the CNS during clinical trials. All patients who experienced seizures had pre-existing contributing factors, including a prior history of seizures or CNS abnormality and concurrent administration of medications with seizure potential. Adherence to the recommended dose is strongly recommended, especially in patients with known factors that predispose them to seizure activity.

Thrombocytopenia has been seen in patients with renal dysfunction; however, no clinical bleeding has been reported.

The following side/adverse effects have been selected on the basis of their potential clinical significance (possible signs and symptoms in parentheses where appropriate)—not necessarily inclusive:

**Those indicating need for medical attention**
Incidence more frequent
*Inflammation at site of injection* (redness and swelling at site of injection)
Incidence less frequent
*Skin rash and itching; thrombophlebitis* (pain at site of injection)
Incidence rare
*Bleeding events* (black, bloody stools; black, bloody vomit; nosebleed); *pseudomembranous colitis* (abdominal or stomach cramps and pain, severe; diarrhea, watery and severe, which may also be bloody; fever); *seizures* (convulsions)

**Those indicating need for medical attention only if they continue or are bothersome**
Incidence more frequent
*Gastrointestinal disturbances* (constipation; diarrhea; nausea and vomiting)
Incidence less frequent
*Headache*

**Those indicating the need for medical attention if they occur after medication is discontinued**
*Pseudomembranous colitis* (abdominal or stomach cramps and pain, severe; diarrhea, watery and severe, which may also be bloody; fever)

## Overdose
No cases of overdose have been reported in humans to date. The largest dose of meropenem administered in clinical trials has been 2 grams every 8 hours and no increased safety risks have been seen.

Large doses (2200 to 4000 mg per kg of body weight) of meropenem were administered to rats and mice; toxicities included ataxia, dyspnea, convulsions, and mortalities.

For more information on the management of overdose or unintentional ingestion, **contact a Poison Control Center** (see *Poison Control Center Listing*).

**Treatment of overdose**
There is no specific information available for the treatment of meropenem overdose. In the event of an overdose, the medication should be discontinued and supportive care administered until meropenem can be eliminated through the kidneys. Meropenem and its metabolite are dialyzable; however, there is no information available on the use of hemodialysis in the event of an overdose.

Supportive care—Patients in whom intentional overdose is confirmed or suspected should be referred for psychiatric consultation.

## Patient Consultation
As an aid to patient consultation, refer to *Advice for the Patient, Meropenem (Systemic)—Introductory Version*.

In providing consultation, consider emphasizing the following selected information (» = major clinical significance)

**Before using this medication**
» Conditions affecting use, especially:
   Hypersensitivity to meropenem or other beta-lactam antibiotics
   Other medications, especially probenecid
   Other medical problems, especially bacterial meningitis, central nervous system disorders, or renal function impairment

**Proper use of this medication**
» Importance of receiving medication for full course of therapy and on regular schedule
» Proper dosing

**Precautions while using this medication**
» Continuing anticonvulsant therapy in patients with a history of seizures
» For severe diarrhea, checking with physician before taking any antidiarrheals; for mild diarrhea, taking kaolin- or attapulgite-containing, but not other, antidiarrheals; checking with physician or pharmacist if mild diarrhea continues or worsens

**Side/adverse effects**
Signs of potential side effects, especially inflammation at site of injection, skin rash and itching, thrombophlebitis, bleeding events, pseudomembranous colitis, and seizures

## General Dosing Information

**For treatment of adverse effects**
Anticonvulsants should be continued in the treatment of patients receiving meropenem who have known seizure disorders. In patients who develop symptoms of CNS toxicity (e.g., focal tremors, myoclonus, or seizures) during treatment with meropenem, anticonvulsant therapy (e.g., phenytoin or benzodiazepines) should be initiated, and the dosage of meropenem should be reduced or the drug should be discontinued.

For serious anaphylactic reactions, emergency treatment should include epinephrine, oxygen, intravenous corticosteroids, and airway management.

For antibiotic-associated pseudomembranous colitis (AAPMC)—
Some patients may develop AAPMC, caused by *Clostridium difficile* toxin, during or following administration of meropenem. Mild cases may respond to discontinuation of the drug alone. Moderate to severe cases may require fluid, electrolyte, and protein replacement. In cases not responding to the above measures or in more severe cases, treatment with an antibacterial medication effective against AAPMC may be necessary.

## Parenteral Dosage Forms

### MEROPENEM FOR INJECTION

**Usual adult and adolescent dose**
Antibacterial—
Intravenous, 1 gram, administered by intravenous infusion over fifteen to thirty minutes or by rapid intravenous injection over three to five minutes, every eight hours.

Note: Adults with impaired renal function may require a reduction in dose as given below:

| Creatinine Clearance (mL/min)/(mL/sec) | Dose |
|---|---|
| ≥ 51/0.85 | See *Usual adult and adolescent dose* |
| 26–50/0.43–0.83 | 1 gram every 12 hours |
| 10–25/0.17–0.42 | 500 mg every 12 hours |
| < 10/0.17 | 500 mg every 24 hours |

**Usual pediatric dose**
Intra-abdominal infections—
Children 3 months of age and older and weighing 50 kg of body weight and over: Intravenous, 1 gram, administered by intravenous infusion over fifteen to thirty minutes or by rapid intravenous injection over three to five minutes, every eight hours.
Children 3 months of age and older and weighing up to 50 kg of body weight: Intravenous, 20 mg per kg of body weight, administered by intravenous infusion over fifteen to thirty minutes or by rapid intravenous injection over three to five minutes, every eight hours.
Infants up to 3 months of age: Safety and efficacy have not been established.

Meningitis—
Children 3 months of age and older and weighing 50 kg of body weight and over: Intravenous, 2 grams, administered by intravenous infusion over fifteen to thirty minutes or by rapid intravenous injection over three to five minutes, every eight hours.
Children 3 months of age and older and weighing up to 50 kg of body weight: Intravenous, 40 mg per kg of body weight, administered by intravenous infusion over fifteen to thirty minutes or by rapid intravenous injection over three to five minutes, every eight hours.
Infants up to 3 months of age: Safety and efficacy have not been established.

**Usual pediatric prescribing limits**
2 grams every eight hours.

**Strength(s) usually available**
U.S.—
500 mg per 20 mL (Rx) [*Merrem I.V.* (sodium 45.1 mg)].
1 gram per 30 mL (Rx) [*Merrem I.V.* (sodium 90.2 mg)].
500 mg per 100 mL (Rx) [*Merrem I.V.* (sodium 45.1 mg)].
1 gram per 100 mL (Rx) [*Merrem I.V.* (sodium 90.2 mg)].

**Packaging and storage**
Store at controlled temperature between 20 and 25 °C (68 and 77 °F).

**Preparation of dosage form**
For rapid intravenous injection—Add 10 mL of sterile water for injection to the 500-mg-in-20-mL vial and 20 mL of sterile water for injection to the 1-gram-in-30-mL vial, for a final concentration of approximately 50 mg per mL. Shake to dissolve and let stand until clear.
For intravenous infusion—The infusion bottles (500 mg in 100 mL and 1 gram in 100 mL) may be reconstituted with 0.45% sodium chloride injection, 0.9% sodium chloride injection, or 5% dextrose injection. Alternatively, a 500-mg or 1-gram injection vial may be reconstituted, the resultant solution added to an intravenous container and further diluted with an appropriate infusion fluid.

**Stability**
For rapid intravenous injection—Reconstituted meropenem with sterile water for injection maintains its potency at controlled room temperature between 15 and 25 °C (59 and 77 °F) for up to 2 hours or for up to 12 hours under refrigeration at 4 °C (39 °F).
For intravenous infusion—Reconstituted meropenem with 0.9% sodium chloride injection maintains its potency at controlled room temperature between 15 and 25 °C (59 and 77 °F) for up to 2 hours or for up to 18 hours under refrigeration at 4 °C (39 °F). Reconstituted meropenem with 5% dextrose injection maintains its potency at controlled room temperature between 15 and 25 °C (59 and 77 °F) for up to 1 hour or for up to 8 hours under refrigeration at 4 °C (39 °F).

**Incompatibilities**
Compatibility of meropenem with other medications has not been established. Meropenem should not be mixed with or physically added to solutions containing other medications.

**Note**
Reconstituted meropenem should be visually inspected for particulate matter and discoloration prior to administration.

Developed: 02/27/97
Interim revision: 08/07/98

# MESALAMINE Oral-Local

INN: Mesalazine.
BAN: Mesalazine.
VA CLASSIFICATION (Primary): GA400
Commonly used brand name(s): *Asacol; Mesasal; Pentasa; Salofalk.*
Other commonly used names are 5-aminosalicylic acid and 5-ASA.
Note: For a listing of dosage forms and brand names by country availability, see *Dosage Forms* section(s).

## Category
Bowel disease (inflammatory) suppressant.

## Indications
Note: Bracketed information in the *Indications* section refers to uses that are not included in U.S. product labeling.

**Accepted**
Bowel disease, inflammatory (prophylaxis and treatment)—Mesalamine is indicated to treat and to maintain remission of mild to moderate ulcerative colitis or [Crohn's disease].

## Pharmacology/Pharmacokinetics

**Physicochemical characteristics**
Molecular weight—153.14.

**Mechanism of action/Effect**
Bowel disease (inflammatory) suppressant—
Uncertain. Mucosal production of arachidonic acid metabolites, both through the cyclooxygenase and lipoxygenase pathways, is increased in patients with inflammatory bowel disease. Mesalamine appears to diminish inflammation by inhibiting cyclooxygenase and lipoxygenase, thereby decreasing the production of prostaglandins, and leukotrienes and hydroxyeicosatetraenoic acids (HETEs), respectively.

It is also believed that mesalamine acts as a scavenger of oxygen-derived free radicals, which are produced in greater numbers in patients with inflammatory bowel disease.

**Absorption**
20 to 30% absorbed following oral administration. The site of mesalamine release and absorption within the gastrointestinal tract varies among the different formulations.
*Asacol*—Coated with an acrylic-based resin, Eudragit S, which dissolves at pH 7 or greater, releasing mesalamine into the distal ileum and the colon.
*Mesasal* and *Salofalk*—Coated with an acrylic-based resin, Eudragit L, which dissolves at pH 6 or greater, releasing mesalamine into the distal ileum and the colon.
*Pentasa*—Microgranules of mesalamine individually coated with ethylcellulose, which allows continuous release of mesalamine into the small (jejunum and ileum) and large (colon) bowel, independent of luminal pH.

**Biotransformation**
Absorbed mesalamine is rapidly acetylated to *N*-acetyl-5-aminosalicylic acid (Ac-5-ASA) in the intestinal mucosal wall and the liver.

**Half-life**
Elimination—
  Asacol:
    Mesalamine—3 hours.
    Ac-5-ASA—10 hours.
  Pentasa:
    Because of the continuous release and absorption of mesalamine throughout the gastrointestinal tract, the true elimination half-life cannot be determined following oral administration.
  Salofalk:
    Ac-5-ASA—5 to 10 hours.

**Time to peak concentration**
*Asacol*—4 to 12 hours.
*Mesasal*—6.5 to 7 hours.
*Pentasa*—3 hours.

**Peak serum concentration**
Mesasal—
  Mesalamine: 1.2 mcg per mL following a single 500-mg oral dose.
  Ac-5-ASA: 1.9 mcg per mL following a single 500-mg oral dose.
Pentasa—
  Mesalamine: 1 mcg per mL following a single 1-gram oral dose.
  Ac-5-ASA: 1.8 mcg per mL following a single 1-gram oral dose.

**Elimination**
Fecal—
  *Asacol:* Approximately 80% of an administered dose is recovered in the feces.
  *Pentasa:* Approximately 13% of an administered dose is recovered in the feces.
  *Salofalk:* Partially recovered unchanged in the feces.
Renal—
  Excreted in the urine as the Ac-5-ASA metabolite.

## Precautions to Consider

**Cross-sensitivity and/or related problems**
Patients sensitive to olsalazine, sulfasalazine, or salicylates may be sensitive to mesalamine also.

**Carcinogenicity**
Long-term studies in animals have not been performed to evaluate the carcinogenic potential of mesalamine.

**Mutagenicity**
No evidence of mutagenicity was observed in an *in vitro* Ames test or in an *in vivo* mouse micronucleus test.

**Pregnancy/Reproduction**
Fertility—Oligospermia and infertility in men, which have been reported in association with sulfasalazine, have not been seen with mesalamine.
Mesalamine was found to have no effect on the fertility and reproductive performance of male and female rats when given orally at a dose corresponding to 7 times the maximum human dose.

Pregnancy—Mesalamine crosses the placenta. Adequate and well-controlled studies have not been done in humans.
Studies in pregnant rats and rabbits given doses of 1000 and 800 mg per kg of body weight (mg/kg) per day, respectively, have not shown that mesalamine causes adverse effects in the fetus.
FDA Pregnancy Category B.

**Breast-feeding**
Mesalamine and its metabolite, *N*-acetyl-5-aminosalicylic acid, are distributed into breast milk. However, problems in humans have not been documented.

**Pediatrics**
Appropriate studies on the relationship of age to the effects of mesalamine have not been performed in the pediatric population. Safety and efficacy have not been established.

**Geriatrics**
No information is available on the relationship of age to the effects of mesalamine in geriatric patients. However, elderly patients are more likely to have age-related renal function impairment, which may require caution in patients receiving mesalamine.

**Drug interactions and/or related problems**
The following drug interactions and/or related problems have been selected on the basis of their potential clinical significance (possible mechanism in parentheses where appropriate)—not necessarily inclusive (» = major clinical significance):

Note: Combinations containing any of the following medications, depending on the amount present, may also interact with this medication.

Lactulose
  (acidification of the colonic lumen by lactulose may impair release of mesalamine from delayed- or extended-release formulations)
Omeprazole
  (omeprazole may increase gastrointestinal pH; concurrent use may result in an increase in the absorption of mesalamine)

**Laboratory value alterations**
The following have been selected on the basis of their potential clinical significance (possible effect in parentheses where appropriate)—not necessarily inclusive (» = major clinical significance):

With physiology/laboratory test values
  Alanine aminotransferase (ALT [SGPT]) and
  Alkaline phosphatase and
  Aspartate aminotransferase (AST [SGOT])
    (values may be increased, but return to normal with either continuation or discontinuation of therapy)

Bilirubin, serum
(concentration may be increased, but returns to normal with either continuation or discontinuation of therapy)

**Medical considerations/Contraindications**
The medical considerations/contraindications included have been selected on the basis of their potential clinical significance (reasons given in parentheses where appropriate)—not necessarily inclusive (» = major clinical significance).

*Risk-benefit should be considered when the following medical problems exist:*
Renal function impairment
(increased risk of interstitial nephritis and nephrotic syndrome)
Sensitivity to mesalamine, olsalazine, sulfasalazine, or salicylates
Stenosis, pyloric
(prolonged gastric retention may delay release of mesalamine)

**Patient monitoring**
The following may be especially important in patient monitoring (other tests may be warranted in some patients, depending on condition; » = major clinical significance):
Blood urea nitrogen (BUN) and
Creatinine, serum and
Urinalysis
(determinations recommended prior to, and periodically during, therapy)

## Side/Adverse Effects

The following side/adverse effects have been selected on the basis of their potential clinical significance (possible signs and symptoms in parentheses where appropriate)—not necessarily inclusive:

**Those indicating need for medical attention**
Incidence less frequent
*Acute intolerance syndrome* (abdominal or stomach cramps or pain, severe; bloody diarrhea; fever; headache, severe; skin rash and itching)
Note: Prompt withdrawal of mesalamine is recommended at the first signs of *acute intolerance syndrome*.

Incidence rare
*Hepatitis* (yellow eyes or skin); *pancreatitis* (back or stomach pain, severe; fast heartbeat; fever; nausea or vomiting; swelling of the stomach); *pericarditis* (anxiety; blue or pale skin; chest pain, possibly moving to the left arm, neck, or shoulder; chills; shortness of breath; unusual tiredness or weakness)

**Those indicating need for medical attention only if they continue or are bothersome**
Incidence more frequent
*Abdominal or stomach cramps or pain, mild; diarrhea, mild; dizziness; headache, mild; nausea or vomiting; rhinitis* (runny or stuffy nose or sneezing); *unusual tiredness or weakness*

Incidence less frequent or rare
*Acne; alopecia* (loss of hair); *anorexia* (loss of appetite); *back or joint pain; dyspepsia* (indigestion); *gas or flatulence*

## Overdose

For specific information on the agents used in the management of mesalamine overdose, see:
- *Charcoal, Activated (Oral-Local)* monograph;
- *Ipecac (Oral-Local)* monograph; and/or
- *Salicylates (Systemic)* monograph.

For more information on the management of overdose or unintentional ingestion, **contact a Poison Control Center** (see *Poison Control Center Listing*).

**Clinical effects of overdose**
The following effects have been selected on the basis of their potential clinical significance (possible signs and symptoms in parentheses where appropriate)—not necessarily inclusive:

Acute effects
*Confusion; diarrhea, severe or continuing; dizziness or lightheadedness; drowsiness, severe; fast or deep breathing; headache, severe or continuing; hearing loss or ringing or buzzing in ears, continuing; nausea or vomiting, continuing*

**Treatment of overdose**
There has been no clinical experience with mesalamine overdosage. However, because mesalamine is an aminosalicylate, the symptoms of overdose may mimic the symptoms of salicylate overdose; therefore, measures used to treat salicylate overdose may be applied to mesalamine overdose.

To decrease absorption—The stomach may be emptied by induction of emesis with ipecac syrup (with care being taken to guard against aspiration) or by gastric lavage. Activated charcoal may also be administered.

Supportive care—Fluid and electrolyte imbalance should be corrected by the administration of appropriate intravenous therapy. Vital functions should be monitored and supported. Patients in whom intentional overdose is confirmed or suspected should be referred for psychiatric consultation.

## Patient Consultation

As an aid to patient consultation, refer to *Advice for the Patient, Mesalamine (Oral)*.
In providing consultation, consider emphasizing the following selected information (» = major clinical significance):

**Before using this medication**
» Conditions affecting use, especially:
Sensitivity to mesalamine, olsalazine, sulfasalazine, or salicylates
Pregnancy—Crosses the placenta
Breast-feeding—Distributed into breast milk

**Proper use of this medication**
Swallowing capsules or tablets whole without breaking, crushing, or chewing
Taking medicine before meals and at bedtime with a full glass (8 ounces) of water
» Compliance with full course of therapy
» Not switching brands without consulting physician
» Proper dosing
Missed dose: Taking as soon as possible; not taking if almost time for next dose; not doubling doses
» Proper storage

**Precautions while using this medication**
Regular visits to physician to check progress
Patient may notice small beads or empty tablet in stool left over after medication is absorbed

**Side/adverse effects**
Signs of potential side effects, especially acute intolerance syndrome, hepatitis, pancreatitis, and pericarditis

## General Dosing Information

Mesalamine should be taken before meals and at bedtime with a full glass (8 ounces) of water.

## Oral Dosage Forms

Note: Bracketed uses in the *Dosage Forms* section refer to categories of use and/or indications that are not included in U.S. product labeling.

### MESALAMINE EXTENDED-RELEASE CAPSULES

**Usual adult dose**
Ulcerative colitis; or
[Crohn's disease]—
1 gram four times a day for up to eight weeks.

**Usual pediatric dose**
Safety and efficacy have not been established.

**Usual geriatric dose**
See *Usual adult dose*.

**Strength(s) usually available**
U.S.—
250 mg (Rx) [*Pentasa* (acetylated monoglyceride; castor oil; colloidal silicon dioxide; ethylcellulose; hydroxypropyl methylcellulose; starch; stearic acid; sugar; talc; white wax)].
Canada—
250 mg (Rx) [*Pentasa*].

**Packaging and storage**
Store at controlled room temperature between 15 and 30 °C (59 and 86 °F).

**Auxiliary labeling**
• Take with a full glass (8 ounces) of water.

### MESALAMINE DELAYED-RELEASE TABLETS

Note: There are differences in the rate and site of absorption among the various brands of mesalamine delayed-release tablets; therefore, these preparations are not bioequivalent, and one brand should not be substituted for another unless otherwise directed by the patient's physician.

### Usual adult dose
Ulcerative colitis; or
[Crohn's disease]—
  *Asacol:* 800 mg three times a day for six weeks.
  *Mesasal:* 1.5 to 3 grams daily in divided doses.
  *Salofalk:* 1 gram three or four times a day.
Maintenance of remission of ulcerative colitis—
  *Asacol:* 1.6 grams daily in divided doses.

### Usual pediatric dose
Safety and efficacy have not been established.

### Usual geriatric dose
See *Usual adult dose.*

### Strength(s) usually available
U.S.—
  400 mg (Rx) [*Asacol* (Eudragit S)].
Canada—
  250 mg (Rx) [*Salofalk* (Eudragit L)].
  400 mg (Rx) [*Asacol* (Eudragit S)].
  500 mg (Rx) [*Mesasal* (Eudragit L); *Salofalk* (Eudragit L)].

### Packaging and storage
Store at controlled room temperature between 15 and 30 °C (59 and 86 °F).

### Auxiliary labeling
• Take with a full glass (8 ounces) of water.

## MESALAMINE EXTENDED-RELEASE TABLETS

### Usual adult dose
See *Mesalamine Extended-release Capsules.*

### Usual pediatric dose
Safety and efficacy have not been established.

### Usual geriatric dose
See *Mesalamine Extended-release Capsules.*

### Strength(s) usually available
U.S.—
  Not commercially available.
Canada—
  250 mg (Rx) [*Pentasa*].
  500 mg (Rx) [*Pentasa*].

### Packaging and storage
Store at controlled room temperature between 15 and 30 °C (59 and 86 °F).

### Auxiliary labeling
• Take with a full glass (8 ounces) of water.

## Selected Bibliography
Thomson ABR. Review article: new developments in the use of 5-aminosalicylic acid in patients with inflammatory bowel disease. Aliment Pharmacol Ther 1991; 5: 449-70.

Developed: 03/17/95
Interim revision: 08/14/98

# MESALAMINE  Rectal-Local

INN:  Mesalazine
BAN:  Mesalazine
VA CLASSIFICATION (Primary): RS100
Commonly used brand name(s): *Rowasa; Salofalk.*
Other commonly used names are 5-aminosalicylic acid and 5-ASA.
Note:  For a listing of dosage forms and brand names by country availability, see *Dosage Forms* section(s).

## Category
Bowel disease (inflammatory) suppressant.

## Indications
Note:  Bracketed information in the *Indications* section refers to uses that are not included in U.S. product labeling.

### Accepted
Bowel disease, inflammatory (treatment)—Mesalamine is indicated for the treatment of mild to moderate distal ulcerative colitis, proctosigmoiditis, and proctitis.

[Bowel disease, inflammatory (prophylaxis)]—Mesalamine rectal suspension is indicated to help maintain remission of distal ulcerative colitis.

## Pharmacology/Pharmacokinetics

### Physicochemical characteristics
Molecular weight—153.14.
pKa—5.8.

### Mechanism of action/Effect
Bowel disease (inflammatory) suppressant—
  Uncertain. Mucosal production of arachidonic acid metabolites, both through the cyclooxygenase and lipoxygenase pathways, is increased in patients with inflammatory bowel disease. Mesalamine appears to diminish inflammation by inhibiting cyclooxygenase and lipoxygenase, thereby decreasing the production of prostaglandins, and leukotrienes and hydroxyeicosatetraenoic acids (HETEs), respectively.
  It is also believed that mesalamine acts as a scavenger of oxygen-derived free radicals, which are produced in greater numbers in patients with inflammatory bowel disease.

### Absorption
Ten to 35% absorbed from the colon; extent of absorption is determined by the length of time the drug is retained in the colon.

### Distribution
The distribution of absorbed mesalamine is not known.

### Biotransformation
Absorbed mesalamine is acetylated to *N*-acetyl-5-ASA(Ac-5-ASA); however, it is not known whether acetylation takes place at colonic or systemic sites. Ac-5-ASA is further acetylated (deactivated) in at least 2 sites, the colonic epithelium and the liver.

### Half-life
Elimination—
  Mesalamine: 0.5 to 1.5 hours.
  Ac-5-ASA: 5 to 10 hours.

### Elimination
Unabsorbed—Fecal.
Absorbed—Renal; 10 to 30% of administered dose is excreted in the urine within 24 hours as the Ac-5-ASA metabolite.

## Precautions to Consider

### Cross-sensitivity and/or related problems
Patients sensitive to olsalazine, sulfasalazine, or salicylates may be sensitive to mesalamine also.

### Carcinogenicity/Tumorigenicity
In a 2-year study in rats given mesalamine orally in doses up to 320 mg per kg of body weight (mg/kg) per day, no increase in the incidence of neoplastic lesions was found.

### Mutagenicity
No evidence of mutagenicity was observed in an Ames mutagen test using *Salmonella typhimurium*. In addition, there was neither evidence of reverse mutations in an assay using an *Escherichia coli* strain, nor evidence of adverse chromosomal effects in an *in vivo* mouse micronucleus assay in doses of 600 mg/kg or in an *in vivo* sister chromatid exchange test in doses up to 610 mg/kg.

### Pregnancy/Reproduction
Fertility—Oligospermia and infertility in men, which have been reported in association with sulfasalazine, have not been seen with mesalamine. Mesalamine was found to have no effect on the fertility of rats when given orally in doses up to 320 mg/kg per day.

Pregnancy—Adequate and well-controlled studies in humans have not been done.
Studies in rats and rabbits at oral doses 5 to 8 times the maximum recommended human dose, respectively, have not shown that mesalamine causes adverse effects in the embryo or the fetus.
FDA Pregnancy Category B.

### Breast-feeding
It is not known whether rectally administered mesalamine or its metabolites are distributed into breast milk. Orally administered mesalamine and its metabolite, *N*-acetyl-5-aminosalicylic acid, are distributed into breast milk.

### Pediatrics
Appropriate studies on the relationship of age to the effects of mesalamine have not been performed in the pediatric population. Safety and efficacy have not been established.

### Geriatrics
No information is available on the relationship of age to the effects of mesalamine in geriatric patients. However, elderly patients are more likely to have age-related renal function impairment, which may require caution in patients receiving mesalamine.

### Medical considerations/Contraindications
The medical considerations/contraindications included have been selected on the basis of their potential clinical significance (reasons given in parentheses where appropriate)—not necessarily inclusive (» = major clinical significance).

*Risk-benefit should be considered when the following medical problems exist:*
> Renal function impairment
>> (although absorption of mesalamine is limited, the possibility of increased risk of renal damage should be considered)
>
> Sensitivity to mesalamine, olsalazine, sulfasalazine, or salicylates

### Patient monitoring
The following may be especially important in patient monitoring (other tests may be warranted in some patients, depending on condition; » = major clinical significance):
> Blood urea nitrogen (BUN) and
> Creatinine, serum and
> Urinalysis
>> (determinations may be required in patients with renal function impairment and in patients concurrently using oral medications, such as sulfasalazine, that liberate mesalamine)

## Side/Adverse Effects

The following side/adverse effects have been selected on the basis of their potential clinical significance (possible signs and symptoms in parentheses where appropriate)—not necessarily inclusive:

**Those indicating need for medical attention**
Incidence rare
> *Acute intolerance syndrome* (abdominal or stomach cramps or pain, severe; bloody diarrhea; fever; headache, severe; skin rash); *anal irritation*; *hepatitis* (yellow eyes or skin); *pancreatitis* (back or stomach pain, severe; fast heartbeat; fever; nausea or vomiting; swelling of the stomach); *pericarditis* (anxiety; blue or pale skin; chest pain, possibly moving to the left arm, neck, or shoulder; chills; shortness of breath; unusual tiredness or weakness)

Note: Prompt withdrawal of mesalamine is recommended at the first signs of the *acute intolerance syndrome*, particularly in patients with a known allergy to sulfasalazine.

**Those indicating need for medical attention only if they continue or are bothersome**
Incidence more frequent
> *Abdominal or stomach cramps or pain, mild; gas or flatulence; headache, mild; nausea*

Incidence less frequent or rare
> *Alopecia* (loss of hair)

## Patient Consultation

As an aid to patient consultation, refer to *Advice for the Patient, Mesalamine (Rectal)*.
In providing consultation, consider emphasizing the following selected information (» = major clinical significance):

**Before using this medication**
» Conditions affecting use, especially:
> Sensitivity to mesalamine, olsalazine, sulfasalazine, or salicylates

**Proper use of this medication**
> Carefully reading and following patient directions for enema or suppository dosage forms
> Emptying bowel immediately prior to enema or suppository, for best results

» Compliance with full course of therapy
» Proper dosing
> Missed dose
>> Mesalamine enema—Using as soon as possible if remembered same night; using next dose at regularly scheduled time; not doubling doses
>> Mesalamine suppository—Using as soon as possible unless almost time for next dose; not doubling doses

» Proper storage

**Precautions while using this medication**
> Regular visits to physician to check progress
> Checking with physician if signs of rectal irritation occur
> Enema may stain clothing, fabrics, painted surfaces, marble, granite, vinyl, or other surfaces with which it comes into contact

**Side/adverse effects**
> Signs of potential side effects, especially acute intolerance syndrome, anal irritation, hepatitis, pancreatitis, and pericarditis

## General Dosing Information

The mesalamine enema should be used at bedtime with the objective of retaining the rectal suspension for at least 8 hours. The mesalamine suppository should be used two to three times a day with the objective of retaining it for at least 3 hours.

For best results, bowel should be emptied immediately prior to the rectal administration of mesalamine.

Response to therapy with mesalamine may occur within 3 to 21 days; however, the usual course of therapy is from 3 to 6 weeks depending on symptoms and sigmoidoscopic examinations.

After remission, some patients may be maintained on mesalamine enema on a less than nightly schedule; however, the possibility of relapse increases as the frequency of mesalamine enema administration is decreased.

Studies to date have not determined if mesalamine suppositories modify the relapse rate after remission; however, it is recommended that abrupt discontinuation be avoided.

## Rectal Dosage Forms

Note: Bracketed uses in the *Dosage Forms* section refer to categories of use and/or indications that are not included in U.S. product labeling.

### MESALAMINE RECTAL SUSPENSION

**Usual adult and adolescent dose**
Bowel disease, inflammatory (treatment)—
> Rectal, 4 grams as a retention enema each night for three to six weeks.

[Bowel disease, inflammatory (prophylaxis)]—
> Rectal, 2 grams as a retention enema each night. Alternatively, 4 grams every other, or every third night.

**Usual pediatric dose**
Safety and efficacy have not been established.

**Usual geriatric dose**
See *Usual adult and adolescent dose*.

**Strength(s) usually available**
U.S.—
> 4 grams per 60-mL unit (Rx) [*Rowasa* (potassium metabisulfite; carbomer 943P; edetate disodium; potassium acetate; water; xanthan gum; sodium benzoate)].

Canada—
> 2 grams per 60-mL unit (Rx) [*Salofalk* (potassium metabisulfite; sodium benzoate)].
> 4 grams per 60-mL unit (Rx) [*Salofalk* (potassium metabisulfite; sodium benzoate)].

**Packaging and storage**
Store between 15 and 30 °C (59 and 86 °F), unless otherwise specified by manufacturer.

**Stability**
Mesalamine rectal suspension may darken with time. Slight darkening will not affect potency; however, enemas with a dark brown color should be discarded.

**Auxiliary labeling**
• For rectal use.
• Shake well.

### MESALAMINE SUPPOSITORIES

**Usual adult and adolescent dose**
Bowel disease, inflammatory (treatment)—
> Rectal, 500 mg two or three times a day for three to six weeks. For best results, suppositories should be retained for at least 3 hours.

**Usual pediatric dose**
Safety and efficacy have not been established.

**Usual geriatric dose**
See *Usual adult and adolescent dose*.

**Strength(s) usually available**
U.S.—
> 500 mg (Rx) [*Rowasa* (hard fat)].

# Mesalamine (Rectal-Local)

Canada—
 250 mg (Rx) [*Salofalk* (hard fat)].
 500 mg (Rx) [*Salofalk* (hard fat)].

**Packaging and storage**
Store between 19 and 26 °C (66 and 79 °F).

**Auxiliary labeling**
- For rectal use.

## Selected Bibliography

Biddle WL, Greenberger NJ, Swan JT, et al. 5-Aminosalicylic acid enemas: effective agent in maintaining remission in left-sided ulcerative colitis. Gastroenterology 1988; 94: 1075-9.

Guarino J, Chatzinoff M, Berk T, et al. 5-Aminosalicylic acid enemas in refractory distal ulcerative colitis: long-term results. Am J Gastroenterol 1987; 82: 732-7.

Revised: 01/30/96

# MESNA  Systemic

VA CLASSIFICATION (Primary): AD900
Commonly used brand name(s): *MESNEX; Uromitexan*.

Note: For a listing of dosage forms and brand names by country availability, see *Dosage Forms* section(s).

## Category
Hemorrhagic cystitis prophylactic.

## Indications
Note: Bracketed information in the *Indications* section refers to uses that are not included in U.S. product labeling.

**Accepted**
Hemorrhagic cystitis, oxazaphosphorine-induced (prophylaxis)—Mesna is indicated to reduce the incidence of ifosfamide-induced or [cyclophosphamide-induced] hemorrhagic cystitis. Mesna is not effective in preventing hematuria due to other pathologic conditions such as thrombocytopenia, and does not affect other toxicities of oxazaphosphorines.

## Pharmacology/Pharmacokinetics

**Physicochemical characteristics**
Molecular weight—164.18.
Other characteristics—Mesna injection: pH is 6.5 to 8.5.

**Mechanism of action/Effect**
Mesna disulfide, which is physically inert, is reduced in the kidney (in the renal tubular epithelium) to mesna, which binds to and detoxifies urotoxic metabolites of oxazaphosphorines (for ifosfamide, 4-hydroxyifosfamide and acrolein).

**Distribution**
Apparent volume of distribution ($Vol_D$)—0.652 liter per kg.

**Biotransformation**
Rapid, by oxidation to one metabolite, mesna disulfide (dimesna).

**Half-life**
Mesna—0.36 hour.
Dimesna—1.17 hours.

**Elimination**
Renal, rapid, by glomerular filtration; 32% as mesna and 33% as dimesna.

## Precautions to Consider

**Carcinogenicity**
Studies have not been done.

**Mutagenicity**
Mesna was not found to be mutagenic in the Ames *Salmonella typhimurium* test, mouse micronucleus assay, and frequency of sister chromatid exchange and chromosomal aberrations in PHA-stimulated lymphocytes in *in vitro* assays.

**Pregnancy/Reproduction**
Pregnancy—Studies in humans have not been done.
Studies in rats and rabbits at oral doses up to 1000 mg per kg of body weight (mg/kg) have not shown that mesna causes adverse effects on the fetus.
FDA Pregnancy Category B.

**Breast-feeding**
It is not known whether mesna is distributed into breast milk. However, problems in humans have not been documented.

**Pediatrics**
Appropriate studies on the relationship of age to the effects of mesna have not been performed in the pediatric population. However, no pediatrics-specific problems have been documented to date.

**Geriatrics**
No information is available on the relationship of age to the effects of mesna in geriatric patients.

**Laboratory value alterations**
The following have been selected on the basis of their potential clinical significance (possible effect in parentheses where appropriate)—not necessarily inclusive (» = major clinical significance):

With physiology/laboratory test values
 Ketones, urinary
  (false-positive results may be produced; in this test, a red-violet color develops, which returns to violet with the addition of glacial acetic acid)

**Medical considerations/Contraindications**
The medical considerations/contraindications included have been selected on the basis of their potential clinical significance (reasons given in parentheses where appropriate)—not necessarily inclusive (» = major clinical significance).

*Risk-benefit should be considered when the following medical problems exist:*
» Sensitivity to mesna
» Sensitivity to other thiol compounds

**Patient monitoring**
The following may be especially important in patient monitoring (other tests may be warranted in some patients, depending on condition; » = major clinical significance):

Examination of urine for microscopic hematuria
 (recommended prior to administration of each dose of ifosfamide or cyclophosphamide and mesna)

## Side/Adverse Effects

Note: Since mesna is used in combination with ifosfamide and other chemotherapeutic agents with documented toxicities, it is difficult to distinguish the adverse reactions that may be due to mesna from those caused by the concomitantly administered cytostatic agents.

The following side/adverse effects have been selected on the basis of their potential clinical significance (possible signs and symptoms in parentheses where appropriate)—not necessarily inclusive:

**Those indicating need for medical attention**
Incidence rare
 *Allergic reaction* (skin rash or itching)

**Those indicating need for medical attention only if they continue or are bothersome**
Incidence less frequent
 *Diarrhea; nausea or vomiting; unpleasant taste*

## Patient Consultation

As an aid to patient consultation, refer to *Advice for the Patient, Mesna (Systemic)*.
In providing consultation, consider emphasizing the following selected information (» = major clinical significance):

**Before using this medication**
» Conditions affecting use, especially:
 Sensitivity to mesna or other thiol compounds

**Proper use of this medication**
» Proper dosing

**Side/adverse effects**
 Signs of potential side effects, especially allergic reaction

## General Dosing Information

Patients receiving mesna should be under supervision of a physician experienced in cancer chemotherapy.

Mesna injection has been developed as an agent to prevent ifosfamide-induced hemorrhagic cystitis. It will not prevent or alleviate any of the other adverse reactions or toxicities associated with ifosfamide therapy.

Mesna does not prevent hemorrhagic cystitis in all patients. Up to 6% of patients treated with mesna have developed hematuria. If hematuria develops when mesna is given with ifosfamide according to the recommended dosage schedule, depending on the severity of the hematuria, dosage reductions or discontinuation of ifosfamide therapy may be initiated.

## Parenteral Dosage Forms

### MESNA INJECTION

**Usual adult and adolescent dose**
Prophylaxis of ifosfamide-induced hemorrhagic cystitis—
Intravenous injection, rapid, in a dosage equal to 20% of the ifosfamide dosage (w/w) at the time of ifosfamide administration and four and eight hours after each dose of ifosfamide (i.e., the total daily dose of mesna is equal to 60% of the total daily dose of ifosfamide) each day that ifosfamide is administered. For example, patients receiving a daily ifosfamide dose of 1.2 grams per square meter of body surface area should receive 240 mg of mesna per square meter of body surface area at zero, four, and eight hours after administration of each dose of ifosfamide.

Note: If the dose of ifosfamide is adjusted, the dose of mesna should be adjusted accordingly.

**Usual pediatric dose**
Dosage has not been established.

**Strength(s) usually available**
U.S.—
  100 mg per mL (Rx) [*MESNEX*].
Canada—
  100 mg per mL (Rx) [*Uromitexan*].

**Packaging and storage**
Store below 40 °C (104 °F), preferably between 15 and 30 °C (59 and 86 °F), unless otherwise specified by the manufacturer.

**Preparation of dosage form**
Mesna injection is prepared for intravenous administration by adding it to a sufficient quantity of 5% dextrose injection, 5% dextrose and sodium chloride injection, 0.9% sodium chloride injection, or lactated Ringer's injection to produce a solution containing 20 mg of mesna per mL.

**Stability**
Diluted solutions of mesna are chemically and physically stable for 24 hours at 25 °C (77 °F). However, it is recommended that diluted solutions be refrigerated and used within 6 hours. Because exposure to oxygen causes mesna to be oxidized to dimesna, any unused portion of an ampul should be discarded.

**Incompatibilities**
Mesna injection is incompatible with cisplatin injection.

Revised: 09/26/97

---

**MESORIDAZINE**—See *Phenothiazines (Systemic)*

---

**METAPROTERENOL**—See *Bronchodilators, Adrenergic (Inhalation-Local)*; *Bronchodilators, Adrenergic (Systemic)*

---

**METARAMINOL**—See *Sympathomimetic Agents—Cardiovascular Use (Parenteral-Systemic)*

---

**METAXALONE**—See *Skeletal Muscle Relaxants (Systemic)*

---

# METFORMIN  Systemic

JAN: Metformin Hydrochloride
VA CLASSIFICATION (Primary): HS503
Commonly used brand name(s): *Glucophage*; *Novo-Metformin*.

Note: For a listing of dosage forms and brand names by country availability, see *Dosage Forms* section(s).

## Category
Antihyperglycemic agent.

## Indications

**Accepted**
Non–insulin-dependent diabetes mellitus (NIDDM) (treatment)—Metformin is indicated in NIDDM patients to control hyperglycemia that cannot be controlled by diet management, exercise, or weight reduction, or when insulin therapy is not required or feasible. It is used as monotherapy or as an adjunct to sulfonylureas when the sulfonylurea alone does not achieve adequate glycemic control. It can be tried if primary or secondary failure of sulfonylureas occurs. Caution and clinical judgment should be used when combining metformin with maximum doses of sulfonylureas for treating non-obese NIDDM patients who clearly are not responding to the sulfonylureas when insulin may be the preferred treatment.

## Pharmacology/Pharmacokinetics

**Physicochemical characteristics**
Chemical group—Biguanide.
Molecular weight—165.63.
pKa—2.8 and 11.5.

**Mechanism of action/Effect**
Metformin potentiates the effect of insulin by mechanisms not fully understood. Metformin does not stimulate pancreatic beta cells to increase secretion of insulin; insulin secretion must be present for metformin to work properly. It is postulated that metformin decreases hepatic glucose production and improves insulin sensitivity by increasing peripheral glucose uptake and utilization.

Specifically, it is thought that metformin may increase the number and/or affinity of insulin receptors on cell surface membranes, especially at peripheral receptor sites, and help to correct down regulation of the insulin receptor. This effect increases the sensitivity to insulin at receptor and postreceptor binding sites and increases glucose uptake peripherally. Insulin concentrations remain unchanged or are slightly reduced as glucose metabolism improves. At therapeutic doses, metformin does not cause hypoglycemia in diabetic or nondiabetic individuals. In addition, metformin's metabolic effects increase hepatic glycogen stores in diabetic patients (but not in nondiabetic patients), may decrease intestinal glucose absorption, and reduce fatty acid oxidation and acetyl coenzyme A formation. Glucose uptake or free fatty acid oxidation are effects considered to be caused by non–insulin-mediated mechanisms. Some studies have shown lipid-lowering effects in both diabetics and nondiabetics, while others have shown no clear evidence that metformin decreases lipid concentrations in all diabetics. These effects could manifest as weight reduction with nominal disturbance of the metabolic rate.

**Other actions/effects**
Metformin interferes with the absorption of vitamin $B_{12}$ by competitive inhibition of calcium-dependent binding of the intrinsic factor-vitamin $B_{12}$ complex to its receptor; anemia in predisposed individuals may be possible.

**Absorption**
Absorbed over 6 hours; bioavailability is 50 to 60% under fasting conditions. Food delays absorption (lowers peak concentration by 40%) and decreases the extent absorbed (lowers area under the concentration-time curve [AUC] by 25%).

**Distribution**
Apparent volume of distribution is 654±358 L. Main sites of concentration without accumulation are the intestinal mucosa and the salivary glands; also, the erythrocyte mass may be a compartment of distribution.

**Protein binding**
Negligible.

**Biotransformation**
Metformin is not metabolized.

**Half-life**
Plasma elimination—6.2 hours, mean, based on an initial elimination of 1.7 to 3 hours and terminal elimination of 9 to 17 hours.

**Time to peak concentration**
$2.25 \pm 0.44$ hours.

**Peak serum concentration**
At steady-state—Approximately 1 to 2 mcg/mL (6.04 to 12.08 mmol/L).

**Elimination**
Renal—Up to 90% of a dose, eliminated unchanged. The renal clearance is 450 to 513 mL/min.
Feces—Up to 30% of a dose.
In dialysis—Hemodialysis with clearance of 170 mL per minute prevents accumulation of metformin.

# Precautions to Consider

### Carcinogenicity
A study in rats and in mice for 104 weeks and 91 weeks, respectively, at 3 times the recommended human daily dose showed no evidence of carcinogenicity.

### Tumorigenicity
A study in male rats showed no evidence of tumorigenicity; however, female rats given 3 times the recommended human daily dose on a mg/kg weight basis, or 900 mg a day, had an increased incidence of benign stromal uterine polyps.

### Mutagenicity
Metformin was not found to be mutagenic in the Ames test, gene mutation test (mouse lymphoma cells), chromosome aberration test (human lymphocytes), or *in vivo* micronuclei formation test (mouse bone marrow).

### Pregnancy/Reproduction
Fertility—Problems in humans have not been documented.
No evidence of impairment of fertility was found in male or female rats given twice the recommended human daily dose of metformin.

Pregnancy—Adequate and well-controlled studies in humans have not been done. Control of blood glucose during pregnancy with diet alone or a combination of diet and insulin is recommended, while use of all oral antidiabetic agents is discouraged. Use of insulin rather than metformin for the treatment of NIDDM and gestational diabetes mellitus (GDM) permits maintenance of blood glucose at concentrations as close to normal as possible. High blood glucose concentrations have been associated with a higher incidence of major congenital abnormalities early in pregnancy (5 to 8 weeks gestation) and high perinatal morbidity and mortality later in pregnancy. A study reported infant malformation rates of 35, 12.9 and 4.8% when initial hemoglobin $A_{1c}$ (an indicator of blood glucose control for the preceding 3 months) was 10% or more, 8 to 9.9%, and below 8%, respectively. The malformation rate in infants born to nondiabetic mothers is approximately 2%.
Teratological studies in albino rats found no abnormalities.

FDA Pregnancy Category B.

### Breast-feeding
Problems in humans have not been documented. Metformin is distributed into breast milk.

### Pediatrics
No information is available on the relationship of age to the effects of metformin in pediatric patients. Safety and efficacy have not been established.

### Adolescents
No information is available on the relationship of age to the effects of metformin in adolescent patients. Safety and efficacy have not been established.

### Geriatrics
Appropriate studies performed to date have not demonstrated geriatrics-specific problems that would limit the usefulness of metformin in the elderly. However, because of possible gastrointestinal intolerance, it is recommended that treatment be initiated with low doses that are adjusted gradually, according to renal clearance. Maximum doses should not be used. Elderly patients are more likely to have age-related renal function impairment or peripheral vascular disease, which may require adjustment of dosage or dosage interval, or discontinuation of treatment when appropriate.

### Drug interactions and/or related problems
The following drug interactions and/or related problems have been selected on the basis of their potential clinical significance (possible mechanism in parentheses where appropriate)—not necessarily inclusive (» = major clinical significance):

Note: Combinations containing any of the following medications, depending on the amount present, may also interact with this medication.

Administration of any medication that may affect metabolic or glycemic control of diabetes mellitus requires careful monitoring of blood glucose concentrations by the patient or health care professional. This is particularly important when any medication is added to or removed from an established treatment regimen. Subsequent adjustments in diet or in dose of antidiabetic agent or both may be necessary; these adjustments may differ depending on the severity of the diabetes.

» Alcohol, acute or chronic ingestion of
(excessive intake may elevate blood lactate concentrations or increase the risk of developing hypoglycemia, especially when alcohol is ingested without meals)

» Cimetidine or
» Other cationic medications excreted by renal tubular transport, such as:
Amiloride
Calcium channel blocking agents, especially nifedipine
Digoxin
Morphine
Procainamide
Quinidine
Quinine
Ranitidine
Triamterene
Trimethoprim
Vancomycin
(cimetidine inhibits the renal tubular secretion of metformin, decreases renal clearance of metformin by 27% over 24 hours, and can significantly increase plasma concentrations of metformin by 60% for up to 6 hours when cimetidine and metformin are taken together; clinical significance is not known, but dosage reduction of metformin potentially may be needed)
(nifedipine increased absorption of metformin in a single-dose study, resulting in a 9% increase of area under the concentration-time curve [AUC] and a 20% increase in peak serum concentration with no change in half-life and urinary excretion; clinical significance is not known; it is not known whether similar effects are produced by other calcium channel blocking agents)
(other cationic medications excreted by renal tubular transport have the potential to increase metformin's plasma concentration or interfere with renal clearance; careful monitoring of blood glucose would be especially appropriate when these medications are given concurrently with metformin)

» Furosemide
(in one study, furosemide increased metformin's AUC by 15% in normal healthy volunteers; renal clearance was not affected; clinical significance is not known, but dosage reduction of metformin potentially may be needed)

Hyperglycemia-causing medications, such as:
Contraceptives, estrogen-containing, oral
Corticosteroids
Diuretics, thiazide
Estrogens
Isoniazid
Nicotinic acid
Phenothiazines, especially chlorpromazine
Phenytoin
Sympathomimetics
Thyroid hormones
(these medications may contribute to hyperglycemia; an increased dose of metformin or a change to another antidiabetic agent may be needed)

Hypoglycemia-causing medications, such as:
Clofibrate
Monoamine oxidase inhibitors
Probenecid
Propranolol
Rifabutin
Rifampin
Salicylates
Sulfonamides, long-acting

Sulfonylureas
(these medications may cause hypoglycemia and decrease the dosage of metformin needed; although studies with many of these agents in combination with metformin have not been done, it is expected that those medications that are highly protein-bound will cause fewer problems when used with metformin than when used with some of the sulfonylurea antidiabetic agents)

**Laboratory value alterations**
The following have been selected on the basis of their potential clinical significance (possible effect in parentheses where appropriate)—not necessarily inclusive (» = major clinical significance):

With diagnostic test results
Ketones, urine
(may produce false positive tests)

With physiology/laboratory test values
Cholesterol, total, serum or
Low-density lipoproteins (LDL), serum or
Triglycerides, serum
(the effects of metformin on these lipid subfractions in NIDDM patients are inconsistent and may depend on weight control; further studies are needed to fully characterize these effects. Generally, concentrations of cholesterol, low-density lipoproteins, or triglycerides may be lowered or unchanged in metformin users. This is thought to be independent of metformin's glucose lowering effect; it may involve suppression of free fatty acid oxidation and lipid oxidation or reduction in the triglyceride content of the LDL and VLDL fractions by metformin)

Lactate, fasting, serum
(may increase to the upper range of normal, 2 mEq/L [2 mmol/L], or show no change with therapeutic doses; although the source is unknown, any small increase is thought to be due to glucose metabolism in the splanchnic beds, not in skeletal muscle)

Lipoproteins, high-density (HDL), serum
(may be slightly increased or unchanged)

**Medical considerations/Contraindications**
The medical considerations/contraindications included have been selected on the basis of their potential clinical significance (reasons given in parentheses where appropriate)—not necessarily inclusive (» = major clinical significance).

*Except under special circumstances, this medication should not be used when the following medical problems exist:*

» Any condition needing close blood glucose control, such as:
  Burns, severe
  Dehydration
  Diabetic coma
  Diabetic ketoacidosis
  Hyperosmolar nonketotic coma
  Infection, severe
  Surgery, major
  Trauma, severe
  (risks of side effects related to uncontrolled blood glucose or lactic acidosis may be increased, and metformin should be discontinued; insulin controls blood glucose best in patients with these conditions; also, metformin should be discontinued 2 days prior to surgery)

» Conditions associated with hypoxemia, such as:
  Cardiorespiratory insufficiency
  Cardiovascular collapse
  Congestive heart failure
  Myocardial infarction, acute or

» Hepatic disease, severe, acute, or chronic or
» Lactic acidosis, active or history of or
» Renal function impairment or renal disease
  (lactic acidosis is associated with these conditions and the risk is further increased when metformin is given concurrently)
  (risk of lactic acidosis increases with the degree of renal dysfunction, impairment of renal clearance, and age of patient; patients who have demonstrated fasting serum lactate values above the upper limit of normal should not receive metformin)

» Diagnostic or medical examinations using contrast media such as:
  Angiography
  Pyelography
  (metformin should be discontinued 2 days prior to medical or diagnostic examinations requiring use of contrast media that can cause functional oliguria because of the increased risk of lactic acidosis; metformin therapy should not be reinstated until after renal function evaluation)

» Hypersensitivity to metformin

*Risk-benefit should be considered when the following medical problems exist:*

» Diarrhea or
» Gastroparesis or
» Intestinal obstruction or
» Vomiting or
» Other conditions causing delayed food absorption
  (conditions that decrease or delay stomach emptying may require a modification of metformin dose or a change to insulin)

» Hyperglycemia-causing conditions, such as:
  Female hormonal changes
  Fever, high
  Hypercortisolism, not optimally treated
  Psychological stress
  (these conditions, by increasing blood glucose, may increase the need for more frequent glucose monitoring and increase the need for a temporary or permanent dose increase of metformin or a change to insulin if blood glucose is uncontrolled)

» Hyperthyroidism, not optimally controlled
  (hyperthyroidism aggravates diabetes mellitus by increasing plasma glucose concentrations and glucose absorption and impairing glucose tolerance; thyroid hormone has dose-dependent biphasic effects on glycogenolysis and glycogeneogenesis, which can make glycemic control difficult until the patient is euthyroid; patients with hyperthyroidism may require an increased dose of metformin until euthyroidism is achieved)

» Hypoglycemia-causing conditions, such as:
  Adrenal insufficiency, not optimally controlled
  Debilitated physical condition
  Malnutrition
  Pituitary insufficiency, not optimally controlled
  (these conditions, which inherently predispose patients to the risk of developing hypoglycemia, increase the patient's risk of developing severe hypoglycemia during metformin treatment; reduction of metformin dose or more frequent blood glucose monitoring may be required)

» Hypothyroidism, not optimally controlled
  (this condition is associated with reduced glucose absorption and altered glucose and lipoprotein metabolism; lower-than-normal doses of metformin may be needed when hypothyroid conditions exist, although an increase in metformin dose may be required when initiating thyroid treatment; glucose control may be difficult until the patient is euthyroid)

**Patient monitoring**
The following may be especially important in patient monitoring (other tests may be warranted in some patients, depending on condition; » = major clinical significance):

Folic acid concentrations, serum and
Vitamin $B_{12}$ concentrations, serum
(recommended every 1 or 2 years during long-term metformin therapy because metformin may interfere with their absorption)

» Glucose concentration, blood or serum
(blood or serum glucose reflects the current degree of metabolic control and should be routinely self-monitored by the patient at home and by the physician [every 3 months or more often when patient is not stabilized] to confirm that blood glucose concentration is maintained within agreed upon targets by the selected diet and dosing regimen; this is particularly important during dosage adjustments. Self-monitoring of blood glucose by the patient may require testing several times a day or once to several times a week)

(caution in interpreting blood glucose concentrations is needed because normal whole blood glucose values are approximately 15% lower than serum glucose values; it is also laboratory- and method-specific. Normal fasting whole blood glucose for adults of all ages is 65 to 95 mg/dL [3.6 to 5.3 mmol/L]. Normal fasting serum glucose is 70 to 105 mg/dL [3.9 to 5.8 mmol/L] for adults younger than 60 years of age and 80 to 115 mg/dL [4.4 to 6.4 mmol/L] for adults 60 years of age and older. For pregnant diabetic women, a normal fasting serum glucose is less than 105 mg/dL [5.8 mmol/L] and a fasting whole blood glucose is less than 120 mg/dL [6.7 mmol/L].)

(capillary blood glucose measurement provides important information when done properly, but caution is warranted because of potential errors in technique and readings; it has been suggested that the values be relied upon only if the reported glucose concentration

for stable diabetics is between 75 mg/dL and 325 mg/dL [4.12 mmol/L and 17.88 mmol/L, respectively])
Glucose concentrations, urine and
Ketone concentrations, urine
(if blood glucose concentrations exceed 200 mg/dL [11.1 mmol/L], monitoring of urine for the presence of glucose and ketones may be necessary; normalization of glucose in the urine generally lags quantitatively behind serum glucose concentrations; test methods are generally capable of detecting glucose concentrations in the urine greater than 180 mg/dL [10 mmol/L])

» Glycosylated hemoglobin (hemoglobin $A_{1c}$) determinations
(monitoring should be done every 3 months or as often as necessary; assessment of this parameter does not eliminate the need for daily blood glucose monitoring. Hemoglobin $A_{1c}$ values reflect the blood glucose control over the preceding 3 months. Normal whole blood hemoglobin $A_{1c}$ is approximately 4 to 6% of total hemoglobin; specific values are laboratory-dependent. Hemoglobin $A_{1c}$ is falsely elevated in unstable diabetics when the intermediate precursor is elevated [i.e., in alcoholism] and falsely lowered in conditions of shortened red blood cell lifespan [i.e., in anemia and acute or chronic blood loss] or in patients with hemoglobinopathies [i.e., sickle cell])

Physical examinations
(regular examinations as often as necessary to reassess appropriateness of continuation of metformin therapy)

» Renal function assessment
(recommended annually, more often for at-risk patients)

## Side/Adverse Effects

The following side/adverse effects have been selected on the basis of their potential clinical significance (possible signs and symptoms in parentheses where appropriate)—not necessarily inclusive:

**Those indicating need for medical attention**
Incidence rare
*Anemia, megaloblastic* (tiredness; weakness); **hypoglycemia** (anxiousness; cold sweats; concentration difficulties; confusion; cool, pale skin; drowsiness; excessive hunger; headache; nausea; nervousness; rapid pulse; shakiness; unusual tiredness or weakness; vision changes); *lactic acidosis* (diarrhea; fast, shallow breathing; muscle pain or cramping; sleepiness; unusual tiredness or weakness)

Note: *Hypoglycemia* does not usually occur with use of metformin unless predisposing conditions or factors are present, such as unusual fasting, concurrent use of other antidiabetic agents, or toxic doses of metformin. Metformin, in combination with sulfonylureas, has been reported to lower basal glucose concentrations typically by at least 20% more than do sulfonylureas used alone.

*Lactic acidosis* is a potentially fatal complication. Twenty-eight cases have been reported in 600,000 users of metformin worldwide, and in each case a contraindication existed; otherwise, the risk is minimal with use of metformin. Patients usually presented not with symptoms of lactic acidosis but rather with acute symptoms of other problems that resulted in metformin accumulation because of renal function impairment or failure in conditions, such as myocardial infarction or renal or hepatic disease.

**Those indicating need for medical attention only if they continue or are bothersome**
Incidence more frequent
*Anorexia; dyspepsia* (stomachache); *flatulence* (gas in stomach or intestines); *headache; metallic taste; nausea; vomiting; weight loss*

Note: *Nausea, dyspepsia,* and *diarrhea* are less frequent when small doses are used initially and, along with *metallic taste* and *headache*, are transient. If *diarrhea* occurs after several months of metformin therapy, lactic acidosis should be considered.

## Overdose

For more information on the management of overdose or unintentional ingestion, **contact a Poison Control Center** (see *Poison Control Center Listing*).

**Clinical effects of overdose**
The following effects have been selected on the basis of their potential clinical significance (possible signs and symptoms in parentheses where appropriate)—not necessarily inclusive:
*Hypoglycemia; lactic acidosis*

## Patient Consultation

As an aid to patient consultation, refer to *Advice for the Patient, Metformin (Systemic)*.
In providing consultation, consider emphasizing the following selected information (» = major clinical significance):

**Before using this medication**
» Conditions affecting use, especially:
Hypersensitivity to metformin
Pregnancy—Use of any oral antidiabetic medicine is discouraged during pregnancy, while diet or diet/insulin is recommended to prevent maternal and fetal problems; importance of controlling and monitoring blood glucose during pregnancy; alerting physician to plans before becoming pregnant when possible
Breast-feeding—Metformin is distributed into breast milk
Use in the elderly—Age-related renal function impairment or peripheral vascular disease may require discontinuation of metformin treatment or special precautions in the elderly
Other medications, especially alcohol, amiloride, calcium channel blocking agents, cimetidine, digoxin, furosemide, morphine, procainamide, quinidine, quinine, ranitidine, triamterene, trimethoprim, vancomycin, or any other cationic medication excreted by renal transport
Other medical problems, especially hepatic disease (severe, acute, or chronic); hyper- or hypothyroidism (not optimally controlled); lactic acidosis (active or history of); renal function impairment or renal disease; conditions associated with hypoxemia; conditions causing delayed food absorption (e.g., diarrhea, gastroparesis, intestinal obstruction, or vomiting); conditions causing hyper- or hypoglycemia; or conditions needing close blood glucose control

**Proper use of this medication**
» Compliance with therapy, including not taking more or less medication than directed; alternative dosing or therapy changes for modifications in blood glucose testing, diet, exercise, fluid replacement, and sick day management
» Proper dosing
Missed dose: Taking as soon as possible; not taking if almost time for next dose; not doubling doses
» Proper storage

**Precautions while using this medication**
» Regular visits to physician to check progress
» Carefully following special instructions of health care team:
Discussing use of alcohol
Not taking other medications unless discussed with physician
Getting counseling for family to help assist diabetic; also, special counseling for pregnancy planning and contraception
Travel considerations
» Preparing for and understanding what to do in case of an emergency; having or wearing medical identification and keeping a glucagon kit and needles and quick-acting source of sugar close by
» Informing physician when medical examinations that require administration of contrast media or when surgery are scheduled; metformin should be discontinued 2 days before surgery or appropriate medical tests
» Recognizing symptoms of lactic acidosis, such as diarrhea, severe muscle pain or cramping, shallow and fast breathing, unusual tiredness and weakness, unusual sleepiness
» Knowing what to do if symptoms of lactic acidosis occur, such as checking blood glucose and getting immediate emergency medical help
» Checking with physician if vomiting occurs
» Recognizing what brings on symptoms of hypoglycemia, such as delaying or missing a meal, exercising more than usual, drinking significant amounts of alcohol, taking certain medicines, using too much antidiabetic medication (insulin or a sulfonylurea), illness, especially with vomiting or diarrhea
» Knowing what to do if symptoms of hypoglycemia occur, such as using glucagon, eating glucose tablets or gel, corn syrup, honey, or sugar cubes, or drinking fruit juice, nondiet soft drink, or dissolved sugar in water; also, eating small snack, such as crackers or half sandwich, when scheduled meal is longer than 1 hour away; not eating foods high in fat, such as chocolate, since fat slows gastric emptying
» Recognizing symptoms of hyperglycemia and ketoacidosis, such as blurred vision; drowsiness; dry mouth; flushed, dry skin; fruit-like breath odor; increased urination (frequency and volume); ketones in urine; loss of appetite; nausea or vomiting; stomachache; tiredness; somnolence (sleepiness); troubled breathing (rapid and deep); unconsciousness; unusual thirst

» Recognizing what brings on symptoms of hyperglycemia, such as fever or infection; not taking enough or missing a dose of antidiabetic medication; exercising less than usual; taking certain medicines; overeating or not following meal plan
» Knowing what to do if symptoms of hyperglycemia occur, such as checking blood glucose and contacting a member of the health care team

**Side/adverse effects**
Signs and symptoms of potential side effects, especially megaloblastic anemia, hypoglycemia, or lactic acidosis

## General Dosing Information

Individual determination of the minimum dose of metformin that lowers blood glucose adequately is recommended. Short-term treatment during periods of transient loss of glucose control may be sufficient for some patients. Some clinicians recommend that metformin be discontinued annually or semi-annually to assess its continued contribution to the control of blood glucose concentrations, especially if there are progressive signs of secondary failure. Metformin should be discontinued if it is not significantly contributing to disease management.

Metformin should be withdrawn or the dose reduced temporarily if vomiting occurs. Treatment may be resumed cautiously after the possibility of lactic acidosis has been excluded.

When transferring a patient from a sulfonylurea to metformin, no transition period is necessary, except when chlorpropamide has been used for treatment. Chlorpropamide's prolonged action requires more frequent monitoring for hypoglycemia during the first 2 weeks following the transition.

When adding a sulfonylurea to maximum doses of metformin or metformin to maximum doses of a sulfonylurea, even if primary or secondary failure of a sulfonylurea has occurred, the new medication should be added gradually and titrated to the lowest effective dose. Both agents should be discontinued and insulin should be initiated if the patient does not respond to maximum doses within 3 months (or less, depending on clinician's decision).

**Diet/Nutrition**
Metformin should be taken with food to reduce nausea or diarrhea.

**For treatment of adverse effects and/or overdose**
Recommended treatment consists of the following:
For treatment of lactic acidosis
- Hemodialysis with sodium bicarbonate has been used but is controversial because there is a lack of published information concerning outcome and lack of cases of metformin-induced lactic acidosis; peritoneal dialysis also has been used, but hemodialysis is thought to be the preferred method when dialysis is needed, such as in patients with shock syndrome. Dialysis is probably not necessary when renal function can be restored because of metformin's rapid renal elimination. Dialysis solutions commonly contain lactate as the buffering agent and these should not be used in cases of metformin-induced lactic acidosis.

For mild to moderate hypoglycemia
- Treating with immediate ingestion of a source of glucose, such as glucose gel, glucose tablets, fruit juice, corn syrup, non-diet soft drinks, honey, sugar cubes, or table sugar dissolved in water. A frequently used source of glucose is a glassful of orange juice containing 2 or 3 teaspoonfuls of table sugar.
- Documenting blood glucose and rechecking in 15 minutes.
- Counseling patient to seek medical assistance promptly.
- Possible adjustment of metformin dosage.
- Possible adjustment of meal pattern.

For severe hypoglycemia or acute overdose, including coma
Note: Dextrose administration is the basis for treatment of hypoglycemia; however, an exposure to sudden hyperglycemia caused by a rapid injection of hypertonic dextrose injection may further stimulate the sulfonylurea-primed pancreas when sulfonylureas are used with metformin to release more insulin, worsening the hypoglycemia.
- Counseling patient to obtain emergency medical assistance immediately.
- Immediately treating with 50 mL of 50% dextrose given intravenously to stabilize the patient. Then, administering a continuous infusion of 5 to 10% dextrose in water to maintain slight hyperglycemia (approximately 100 mg/dL [5.55 mmol/L] blood glucose concentration) for up to 12 days. Intravenous dextrose therapy should not be terminated suddenly. Oral dextrose cannot be relied upon to maintain euglycemia because 60% of an oral dextrose dose is stored as hepatic glycogen with only 15% left for brain utilization and 15% for insulin-dependent tissues.
- Glucagon, 1 to 2 mg administered intramuscularly, is useful for fast onset of action to mobilize hepatic glucose stores but may be ineffective or variable in its effect if glycogen stores are depleted. Therefore, glucagon should be administered after dextrose administration.
- Diazoxide (200 mg orally every 4 hours or 300 mg intravenously over a 30-minute period every 4 hours) can be used for nonresponders to dextrose therapy or for patients in a coma as an aid to dextrose infusion to reduce hypoglycemia; patient must be monitored for sodium concentration and hypotension.
- Emesis can be induced with ipecac syrup if the metformin overdose is recent (within the past 30 minutes) and if the patient is alert, has an intact gag reflex, and is not obtunded or convulsing. Otherwise, gastric lavage after endotracheal tube placement is required.
- Gastric decontamination by administration of repeated doses of oral activated charcoal with appropriate cathartic may be attempted, although the usefulness of this has not been established.
- Monitoring vital signs, arterial blood gases, blood glucose, and serum electrolytes (especially calcium, potassium, and sodium) as required. Initially, blood glucose concentrations should be monitored as frequently as every 1 to 3 hours. Blood urea nitrogen and serum creatinine concentrations should also be obtained.
- Cerebral edema—Managing with mannitol and dexamethasone.
- Hypokalemia—Managing with potassium supplements.
- Hospitalization for 6 to 91 hours (mean, 24 hours), because the hypoglycemia may be recurrent and prolonged.
- Other supportive measures should also be employed as needed.

## Oral Dosage Forms

### METFORMIN HYDROCHLORIDE TABLETS

**Usual adult dose**
Antihyperglycemic agent—
Initial: Oral, 500 mg two times a day, taken with morning and evening meals. The daily dose may be increased by 500 mg at weekly intervals as needed. An alternative dose is 850 mg a day, taken with the morning meal. The daily dose may be increased by 850 mg at fourteen-day intervals.
Maintenance: Oral, 500 or 850 mg two to three times a day, taken with meals.

**Usual adult prescribing limits**
2550 mg a day.

**Usual pediatric dose**
Safety and efficacy have not been established.

**Usual geriatric dose**
See *Usual adult dose*. For some sensitive individuals, lower initial doses may be needed. Maximum doses are not advised for use in the elderly.

**Strength(s) usually available**
U.S.—
500 mg (Rx) [*Glucophage* (scored)].
850 mg (Rx) [*Glucophage* (scored)].
Canada—
500 mg (Rx) [*Glucophage* (scored); *Novo-Metformin* (scored)].

**Packaging and storage**
Store below 40 °C (104 °F), preferably between 15 and 30 °C (59 and 86 °F), unless otherwise specified by manufacturer.

**Auxiliary labeling**
- Take with food.
- Do not drink alcohol.

## Selected Bibliography

Watkins PJ. Guidelines for good practice in the diagnosis and treatment of non-insulin–dependent diabetes mellitus. Report of a joint working party of the British Diabetic Association, the Research Unit of the Royal College of Physicians, and the Royal College of General Practitioners. J R Coll Physicians Lond 1993 Jul; 27(3): 259-66.

Aguilar C, Reza A, Garcia JE, et al. Biguanide related lactic acidosis: incidence and risk factors. Arch Med Res 1992 Spring; 23(1): 19-24.

Developed: 07/26/95

**METHADONE**—See *Opioid (Narcotic) Analgesics (Systemic)*

**METHAMPHETAMINE**—See *Amphetamines (Systemic)*

**METHANTHELINE**—See *Anticholinergics/Antispasmodics (Systemic)*

**METHARBITAL**—See *Barbiturates (Systemic)*

**METHAZOLAMIDE**—See *Carbonic Anhydrase Inhibitors (Systemic)*

**METHDILAZINE**—See *Antihistamines, Phenothiazine-derivative (Systemic)*

**METHENAMINE**—The *Methenamine (Systemic)* monograph is not included in this published version of the USP DI database. Copies of the monograph are available on request from Micromedex, Inc. - Reprint Requests, 6200 S. Syracuse Way, Suite 300, Englewood, CO 80111; telephone (303) 486-6400; telefax (303) 486-6464; Email: USPDI@MDX.COM.

**METHICILLIN**—See *Penicillins (Systemic)*

**METHIMAZOLE**—See *Antithyroid Agents (Systemic)*

**METHOCARBAMOL**—See *Skeletal Muscle Relaxants (Systemic)*

**METHOHEXITAL**—See *Anesthetics, Barbiturate (Systemic)*

# METHOTREXATE—FOR CANCER Systemic

VA CLASSIFICATION (Primary): AN300
Another commonly used name is amethopterin.
Note: For a listing of dosage forms and brand names by country availability, see *Dosage Forms* section(s).

## Category
Antineoplastic.

## Indications
Note: Bracketed information in the *Indications* section refers to uses that are not included in U.S. product labeling.

### Accepted
Carcinoma, breast (treatment)
Carcinoma, head and neck (treatment)
Carcinoma, lung, non–small cell (treatment)[1]
Carcinoma, lung, small cell (treatment)[1] or
Tumors, trophoblastic, gestational (treatment)—Methotrexate is indicated for treatment of breast carcinoma, head and neck cancers (epidermoid), non–small cell lung carcinoma (especially squamous cell types), small cell lung carcinoma, and gestational trophoblastic tumors (gestational choriocarcinoma, chorioadenoma destruens, hydatidiform mole).

[Carcinoma, cervical (treatment)][1]
[Carcinoma, ovarian, epithelial (treatment)][1]
[Carcinoma, bladder (treatment)]
[Carcinoma, colorectal (treatment)][1]
[Carcinoma, esophageal (treatment)][1]
[Carcinoma, gastric (treatment)]
[Carcinoma, pancreatic (treatment)][1] or
[Carcinoma, penile (treatment)][1]—Methotrexate is indicated for treatment of cervical carcinoma, ovarian carcinoma, bladder carcinoma, colorectal carcinoma, esophageal carcinoma, gastric carcinoma, pancreatic carcinoma, and penile carcinoma.

Leukemia, acute lymphocytic (treatment) or
Leukemia, meningeal (prophylaxis and treatment)—Methotrexate is indicated for treatment of acute lymphocytic leukemia and prophylaxis and treatment of meningeal leukemia.

[Leukemia, acute nonlymphocytic (treatment)][1]—Methotrexate is indicated for treatment of acute nonlymphocytic leukemia.

Lymphomas, non-Hodgkin's (treatment)—Methotrexate is indicated for treatment of non-Hodgkin's lymphomas, including advanced cases of lymphosarcoma (particularly in children) and Burkitt's lymphoma.

[Lymphomas, Hodgkin's (treatment)][1]—Methotrexate is indicated for treatment of Hodgkin's disease.

Mycosis fungoides (treatment)—Methotrexate is indicated for treatment of advanced cases of mycosis fungoides.

Osteosarcoma (treatment)—Methotrexate is indicated in high doses along with leucovorin rescue, in combination with other agents, for treatment of nonmetastatic osteosarcoma in patients who have undergone primary surgical treatment.

[Sarcomas, soft tissue (treatment)][1]—Methotrexate is indicated for treatment of soft tissue sarcomas.

[Carcinomatous meningitis (treatment)][1]—Methotrexate is indicated for treatment of carcinomatous menigitis (intrathecal and intraventricular administration)(Evidence rating: IIID).

Note: Although methotrexate has been used for treatment of multiple myeloma, the USP Division of Information Development Hematology-Oncology Advisory Panel believes there is insufficient evidence to support the effectiveness of methotrexate in the treatment of multiple myeloma.

[1]Not included in Canadian product labeling.

## Pharmacology/Pharmacokinetics

### Physicochemical characteristics
Molecular weight—454.44.

### Mechanism of action/Effect
Methotrexate is an antimetabolite of the folic acid analog type. Methotrexate is cell cycle–specific for the S phase of cell division. Activity is due to inhibition of DNA synthesis, repair, and cellular replication; inhibition occurs as a result of relatively irreversible binding of methotrexate with dihydrofolate reductase, which prevents reduction of dihydrofolate to the active tetrahydrofolate. Growth of rapidly proliferating cells (malignant cells, bone marrow, fetal cells, buccal and intestinal mucosa, cells of the urinary bladder, spermatogonia) is affected more severely than growth of most normal tissues and skin.

### Other actions/effects
Also has mild immunosuppressant activity.

### Absorption
Widely variable and dose-dependent. At doses of 30 mg per square meter of body surface area (mg/m$^2$), the mean bioavailability of methotrexate is approximately 60%. At doses greater than 80 mg/m$^2$, absorption is significantly decreased, possibly due to a saturation effect. Food may delay absorption and decrease the peak concentration.

### Distribution
Methotrexate crosses the blood-brain barrier (from blood to central nervous system [CNS]) in only limited amounts when administered orally or parenterally (dose-related); however, high concentrations can be found in cerebrospinal fluid following its intrathecal administration.
Following intravenous administration—Initial Vol$_D$ is approximately 0.18 L per kg (L/kg).
Steady state Vol$_D$ is approximately 0.4 to 0.8 L/kg.

**Protein binding**
Moderate (approximately 50%), primarily to albumin.

**Biotransformation**
Hepatic; intracellular, to active polyglutamated forms, small amounts of which are retained in tissues for extended periods of time.

**Half-life**
Terminal—
  Low doses: 3 to 10 hours.
  High doses: 8 to 15 hours.

Note: There is wide interindividual variation in clearance rates. Small amounts of methotrexate and its metabolites are protein-bound and may remain in tissues (kidneys, liver) for weeks to months; the presence of fluid loads, such as ascites or pleural effusion, and renal function impairment will also delay clearance.

**Time to peak serum concentration**
Oral—Approximately 40 minutes to 4 hours, following a dose of 15 mg/m$^2$.
Intramuscular—30 to 60 minutes.

**Elimination**
Single dose—
  Renal (unchanged), 80 to 90% in the first 24 hours; some accumulation of polyglutamates in tissues occurs with repeated doses.
  Biliary, 10% or less.

## Precautions to Consider

### Carcinogenicity/Mutagenicity
Secondary malignancies are potential delayed effects of many antineoplastic agents, although it is not clear whether the effect is related to their mutagenic or immunosuppressive action. The effect of dose and duration of therapy is also unknown, although risk seems to increase with long-term use.

Antimetabolites have been shown to be carcinogenic in animals, and may be associated with an increased risk of development of secondary carcinomas in humans, although the risk appears to be less than with alkylating agents.

Carcinogenicity studies with methotrexate in animals have been inconclusive. However, there is evidence that methotrexate causes chromosomal damage to animal somatic cells and human bone marrow cells.

### Pregnancy/Reproduction
Fertility—Gonadal suppression, resulting in amenorrhea or azoospermia, may occur in patients taking antineoplastic therapy, especially with the alkylating agents. In general, these effects appear to be related to dose and length of therapy and may be irreversible. Prediction of the degree of testicular or ovarian function impairment is complicated by the common use of combinations of several antineoplastics, which makes it difficult to assess the effects of individual agents. Methotrexate appears to have only a slight effect on gonadal function; however, reversible impairment of fertility, defective oogenesis and spermatogenesis, and menstrual function impairment have been reported.

Pregnancy—Methotrexate crosses the placenta and has been shown to cause adverse effects in the fetus. Methotrexate is a potent abortifacient.

First trimester: It is usually recommended that use of antineoplastics, especially combination chemotherapy, be avoided whenever possible, especially during the first trimester. Although information is limited because of the relatively few instances of antineoplastic administration during pregnancy, the mutagenic, teratogenic, and carcinogenic potential of these medications must be considered.

Other hazards to the fetus include adverse reactions seen in adults.

In general, use of a contraceptive is recommended during cytotoxic drug therapy.

FDA Pregnancy Category X.

### Breast-feeding
Methotrexate is distributed into breast milk; breast-feeding is not recommended while methotrexate is being administered because of the risks to the infant (adverse effects, mutagenicity, carcinogenicity).

### Pediatrics
Caution should be used in neonates and infants because of reduced renal and hepatic function.

### Geriatrics
Although appropriate studies with methotrexate have not been performed in the geriatric population, caution should be used in the elderly because of possible reduced renal and hepatic functions and reduced folate stores. Dosage adjustment, especially on the basis of renal function status, may be necessary.

### Dental
The bone marrow depressant effects of methotrexate may result in an increased incidence of microbial infection, delayed healing, and gingival bleeding. Dental work, whenever possible, should be completed prior to initiation of therapy or deferred until blood counts have returned to normal. Patients should be instructed in proper oral hygiene during treatment, including caution in use of regular toothbrushes, dental floss, and toothpicks.

Methotrexate also commonly causes ulcerative stomatitis associated with considerable discomfort.

### Drug interactions and/or related problems
The following drug interactions and/or related problems have been selected on the basis of their potential clinical significance (possible mechanism in parentheses where appropriate)—not necessarily inclusive (» = major clinical significance):

Note: Combinations containing any of the following medications, depending on the amount present, may also interact with this medication.

» Acyclovir, parenteral
  (concurrent administration of intrathecal methotrexate with acyclovir may result in neurological abnormalities; use with caution)

» Alcohol or
» Hepatotoxic medications, other (see *Appendix II*)
  (concurrent use may increase the risk of hepatotoxicity)

Allopurinol or
Colchicine or
» Probenecid or
» Sulfinpyrazone
  (methotrexate may raise the concentration of blood uric acid; dosage adjustment of antigout agents may be necessary to control hyperuricemia and gout; allopurinol may be preferred to prevent or reverse methotrexate-induced hyperuricemia because of risk of uric acid nephropathy with uricosuric antigout agents)

Anticoagulants, coumarin- or indandione-derivative
  (methotrexate may increase anticoagulant activity and/or increase the risk of hemorrhage as a result of decreased hepatic synthesis of procoagulant factors and interference with platelet formation)

» Anti-inflammatory drugs, nonsteroidal (NSAIDs)
  (concurrent use of phenylbutazone with methotrexate may increase the risk of agranulocytosis or bone marrow depression and is not recommended; also, phenylbutazone may displace methotrexate from its protein-binding sites and decrease its renal clearance, leading to increased methotrexate plasma concentration and risk of toxicity, especially during high-dose methotrexate infusion therapy. If concurrent use with phenylbutazone cannot be avoided, especially careful monitoring of the patient for plasma methotrexate concentrations or signs of methotrexate toxicity and/or adequacy of renal function is recommended; also, phenylbutazone therapy should be discontinued for 7 to 12 days prior to, and for at least 12 hours [depending on plasma methotrexate concentrations] following, administration of a high-dose methotrexate infusion)

  (administration of high-dose methotrexate infusions to patients receiving diflunisal or ketoprofen has resulted in severe and [with ketoprofen] sometimes fatal methotrexate toxicity; a few fatalities have also occurred in patients receiving intermediate-dose methotrexate infusions concurrently with indomethacin, possibly because of decreased methotrexate excretion leading to increased and prolonged methotrexate plasma concentration; however, severe methotrexate toxicity did not occur when ketoprofen was administered 12 hours following completion of the methotrexate infusion. It is recommended that NSAID therapy be discontinued for 24 to 48 hours [for diflunisal] or 12 to 24 hours [for ketoprofen] prior to, and for at least 12 hours [depending on plasma methotrexate concentrations] following, a high-dose methotrexate infusion and that indomethacin be discontinued for 24 to 48 hours prior to, and for at least 12 hours [depending on plasma methotrexate concentrations] following, administration of an intermediate- or high-dose methotrexate infusion)

  (although not well documented, the possibility exists that other NSAIDs may also decrease methotrexate excretion and increase its plasma concentration to potentially toxic levels; it is recommended that NSAID therapy be discontinued for 12 to 24 hours [for NSAIDs with a short elimination half-life] to up to 10 days [for piroxicam] prior to, and for at least 12 hours [depending on plasma methotrexate concentrations] following, administration of a high-dose methotrexate infusion)

  (severe, sometimes fatal, methotrexate toxicity has also been reported with low to moderate doses in patients receiving diclofenac, indomethacin, naproxen, or phenylbutazone; it is recommended that use of NSAIDs with low to moderate doses of methotrexate be undertaken with caution, with methotrexate dosage being adjusted

» Asparaginase
(concurrent use may block the effects of methotrexate by inhibiting cell replication; this inhibition of methotrexate's action appears to correlate with suppression of asparagine concentrations. Some studies indicate that administration of asparaginase 9 to 10 days before or within 24 hours after methotrexate does not produce this inhibition of antineoplastic effect and may reduce the gastrointestinal and hematological effects of methotrexate)

Blood dyscrasia–causing medications (see *Appendix II*)
(leukopenic and/or thrombocytopenic effects of methotrexate may be increased with concurrent or recent therapy if these medications cause the same effects; dosage adjustment of methotrexate, if necessary, should be based on blood counts)

» Bone marrow depressants, other (see *Appendix II*) or
Radiation therapy
(additive bone marrow depression may occur; dosage reduction may be required when two or more bone marrow depressants, including radiation, are used concurrently or consecutively)
(leukoencephalopathy has been reported following intravenous methotrexate administration to patients who have received craniospinal irradiation)

Cytarabine
(administration of cytarabine 48 hours before or 10 minutes after initiation of methotrexate therapy may result in a synergistic cytotoxic effect; however, evidence is inconclusive and dosage adjustment based on routine hematologic monitoring is recommended)

Folic acid
(may interfere with the antifolate effects of methotrexate)

Neomycin, oral
(may decrease absorption of oral methotrexate)

Penicillins
(concurrent use with methotrexate has resulted in decreased clearance of methotrexate and in methotrexate toxicity; this is thought to be due to competition for renal tubular secretion; patients should be closely monitored; leucovorin doses may need to be increased and administered for longer periods of time)

Phenytoin
(concurrent use may result in increased methotrexate toxicity; this is thought to be due to displacement of methotrexate from serum albumin by phenytoin)

» Probenecid
(concurrent use may inhibit renal excretion of methotrexate and result in toxic plasma concentrations; if used concurrently with probenecid, methotrexate dosage should be decreased, the patient observed for signs of toxicity, and/or plasma methotrexate concentrations monitored)

Pyrimethamine or
Triamterene or
Trimethoprim
(concurrent use may rarely increase the toxic effects of methotrexate because of similar folic acid antagonist actions)

» Salicylates and other weak organic acids
(concurrent use may inhibit renal tubular secretion of methotrexate and result in toxic plasma concentrations; salicylates may also increase plasma concentrations by displacing methotrexate from binding sites; if methotrexate is used concurrently with these medications, the patient should be observed for signs of toxicity and/or methotrexate plasma concentration monitored. In addition, it is recommended that salicylate therapy be discontinued for 24 to 48 hours prior to, and for at least 12 hours [depending on plasma methotrexate concentrations] following, administration of a high-dose methotrexate infusion)

Sulfonamides
(in addition to increased risk of hepatotoxicity that may occur when sulfonamides are used concurrently with other hepatotoxic medications, medications that cause displacement from plasma protein binding may theoretically produce toxic plasma concentrations of methotrexate when used concurrently, although clinical significance has not been established)

Theophylline
(methotrexate may decrease theophylline clearance. Monitoring of serum theophylline concentrations is recommended when it is used concurrently with methotrexate)

Vaccines, killed virus
(because normal defense mechanisms may be suppressed by methotrexate therapy, the patient's antibody response to the vaccine may be decreased. The interval between discontinuation of medications that cause immunosuppression and restoration of the patient's ability to respond to the vaccine depends on the intensity and type of immunosuppression-causing medication used, the underlying disease, and other factors; estimates vary from 3 months to 1 year)

» Vaccines, live virus
(because normal defense mechanisms may be suppressed by methotrexate therapy, concurrent use with a live virus vaccine may potentiate the replication of the vaccine virus, may increase the side/adverse effects of the vaccine virus, and/or may decrease the patient's antibody response to the vaccine; immunization of these patients should be undertaken only with extreme caution after careful review of the patient's hematologic status and only with the knowledge and consent of the physician managing the methotrexate therapy. The interval between discontinuation of medications that cause immunosuppression and restoration of the patient's ability to respond to the vaccine depends on the intensity and type of immunosuppression-causing medication used, the underlying disease, and other factors; estimates vary from 3 months to 1 year. Patients with leukemia in remission should not receive live virus vaccine until at least 3 months after their last chemotherapy. Immunization with oral poliovirus vaccine should also be postponed in persons in close contact with the patient, especially family members)

**Laboratory value alterations**
The following have been selected on the basis of their potential clinical significance (possible effect in parentheses where appropriate)—not necessarily inclusive (» = major clinical significance):

With diagnostic test results
Assay for folate
(methotrexate may inhibit the organism used in the assay and interfere with detection of folic acid deficiency)

With physiology/laboratory test values
Isocitric acid dehydrogenase (ICD)
(values may be increased, indicating hepatotoxicity)

Serum aspartate aminotransferase (AST [SGOT])
(values may be increased transiently during high-dose therapy)

Uric acid concentrations in blood and urine
(may be increased)

**Medical considerations/Contraindications**
The medical considerations/contraindications included have been selected on the basis of their potential clinical significance (reasons given in parentheses where appropriate)—not necessarily inclusive (» = major clinical significance).

*Except under special circumstances, this medication should not be used when the following medical problem exists:*
» Immunodeficiency

*Risk-benefit should be considered when the following medical problems exist:*

Aciduria (urine pH less than 7) or
» Ascites or
Dehydration or
Gastrointestinal obstruction or
» Pleural or peritoneal effusions or
» Renal function impairment
(risk of methotrexate toxicity is increased because elimination of methotrexate may be impaired and accumulation may occur; even small doses may lead to severe myelosuppression and mucositis; larger doses and/or increased duration of leucovorin treatment, if used, may be necessary, along with careful monitoring of methotrexate concentrations)

(a lower dosage of methotrexate and careful monitoring of plasma or serum methotrexate concentrations are recommended for patients with impaired renal function)

» Bone marrow depression
» Chickenpox, existing or recent (including recent exposure) or
» Herpes zoster
(risk of severe generalized disease)

Gout, history of or
Urate renal stones, history of
(risk of hyperuricemia)

» Hepatic function impairment
» Infection
» Mucositis, oral

Nausea and vomiting
(inadequate hydration secondary to severe nausea and vomiting may result in increased methotrexate toxicity)
» Peptic ulcer
Sensitivity to methotrexate
» Ulcerative colitis
» Caution should be used also in patients who have had previous cytotoxic drug therapy and radiation therapy, and in cases of general debility.

**Patient monitoring**
The following are especially important in patient monitoring (other tests may be warranted in some patients, depending on condition; » = major clinical significance):
» Blood urea nitrogen (BUN) concentrations and
Creatinine clearance and/or
» Serum creatinine concentrations
(recommended prior to initiation of therapy and at periodic intervals during therapy; frequency varies according to clinical state, agent, dose, and other agents being used concurrently)
Bone marrow aspiration studies and
Liver biopsy
(may be useful during high-dose or long-term therapy or if hematologic or hepatic function test results are abnormal; also recommended in patients who have received a cumulative dose of 1500 mg)
Examination of patient's mouth for ulceration
(recommended before administration of each dose)
» Hematocrit or hemoglobin and
» Platelet count and
» Total and, if appropriate, differential leukocyte count
(determinations recommended prior to initiation of therapy and at periodic intervals during therapy; frequency varies according to clinical state, agent, dose, and other agents being used concurrently)
» Serum alanine aminotransferase (ALT [SGPT]) and
» Serum aspartate aminotransferase (AST [SGOT]) and
» Serum lactate dehydrogenase (LDH)
(determinations recommended prior to initiation of therapy and at periodic intervals during therapy; frequency varies according to clinical state, agent, dose, and other agents being used concurrently)
» Serum bilirubin concentrations and
Serum uric acid concentrations
(recommended prior to initiation of therapy and at periodic intervals during therapy; frequency varies according to clinical state, agent, dose, and other agents being used concurrently)

*For patients receiving high-dose methotrexate*
» Creatinine clearance determinations
(recommended prior to initiation of high-dose methotrexate with leucovorin rescue therapy or if serum creatinine concentrations increase by 50% or more)
» Plasma or serum methotrexate concentrations
(recommended by some clinicians every 12 to 24 hours after high-dose methotrexate administration to determine dose and duration of leucovorin treatment needed to maintain rescue. May aid in identifying patients with delayed methotrexate clearance; toxicity appears to be related at least as much to the length of time that methotrexate concentrations are elevated as to the peak concentrations achieved. In general, monitoring should continue until concentrations are less than $5 \times 10^{-8}$ Molar [M])
» Serum creatinine concentrations
(recommended prior to and every 24 hours after each methotrexate dose, until plasma or serum methotrexate concentrations are less than $5 \times 10^{-8}$ M, to detect developing renal function impairment and predict methotrexate toxicity. An increase of greater than 50% over the pretreatment concentration at 24 hours is associated with severe renal toxicity)
» Urine pH determinations
(recommended prior to each dose of high-dose methotrexate therapy and about every 6 hours throughout leucovorin rescue, until plasma or serum methotrexate concentrations are less than $5 \times 10^{-8}$ M, to ensure that pH remains greater than 7, so as to minimize the risk of methotrexate nephropathy due to precipitation of methotrexate or its metabolites in the urine)

## Side/Adverse Effects

Note: Many "side effects" of antineoplastic therapy are unavoidable and represent the medication's pharmacologic action. Some of these (for example, leukopenia and thrombocytopenia) are actually used as parameters to aid in individual dosage titration.

Incidence and severity of side effects, particularly hepatotoxicity, appear to be related to dosage frequency and duration of methotrexate therapy. Toxicity tends to occur less frequently and be less severe with a total dose administered as intermittent weekly dosage than with prolonged daily dosage.

The following side/adverse effects have been selected on the basis of their potential clinical significance (possible signs and symptoms in parentheses where appropriate)—not necessarily inclusive:

**Those indicating need for medical attention**
Incidence more frequent
*Gastrointestinal ulceration and bleeding, enteritis, or intestinal perforation, which may be fatal* (black, tarry stools; bloody vomit; diarrhea; stomach pain); *leukopenia, bacterial infection, or septicemia* (fever or chills; cough or hoarseness; lower back or side pain; painful or difficult urination)—usually asymptomatic; *thrombocytopenia* (unusual bleeding or bruising; black, tarry stools; blood in urine or stools; pinpoint red spots on skin)—usually asymptomatic; *stomatitis, ulcerative* (sores in mouth and on lips)

Note: With development of *leukopenia* and *thrombocytopenia*, the nadir of the leukocyte and platelet counts occurs after 7 to 10 days, with recovery 7 days later.

Incidence more frequent (with high-dose therapy)
*Renal failure, azotemia, hyperuricemia, or severe nephropathy* (blood in urine; joint pain; swelling of feet or lower legs); *severe acute methotrexate toxicity, cutaneous vasculitis, or reactivation of sunburn or increased erythematous response to ultraviolet therapy* (reddening of skin)

Note: *Hyperuricemia* and *uric acid nephropathy* occur most commonly during initial treatment of patients with leukemia or lymphoma, as a result of rapid cell breakdown which leads to elevated serum uric acid concentrations. With high-dose methotrexate therapy, symptoms resembling uric acid nephropathy may also be due to renal tubular damage resulting from precipitation of methotrexate or metabolites in the urine.

Incidence less frequent, more frequent with prolonged, daily therapy
*Hepatotoxicity, including liver atrophy, necrosis, cirrhosis, fatty changes, periportal fibrosis* (dark urine; yellow eyes or skin); *pneumonitis, potentially fatal, or pulmonary fibrosis* (cough; shortness of breath)

Incidence less frequent, more frequent with intrathecal or prolonged high-dose administration
*Central nervous system (CNS) effects, increased cerebrospinal fluid pressure, leukoencephalopathy, demyelination, or chemical arachnoiditis* (back pain; blurred vision; confusion; convulsions; dizziness; drowsiness; fever; headache; unusual tiredness or weakness)

**Those indicating need for medical attention only if they continue or are bothersome**
Incidence more frequent
*Loss of appetite; nausea or vomiting*
Incidence less frequent
*Acne; boils; pale skin; skin rash or itching*

**Those not indicating need for medical attention**
Incidence less frequent
*Alopecia* (loss of hair)

**Those indicating need for medical attention if they occur after medication is discontinued**
*CNS toxicity (encephalopathy, especially after intrathecal administration, or CNS leukemia)* (back pain; blurred vision; confusion; convulsions; dizziness; drowsiness; fever; headache; unusual tiredness or weakness)

## Overdose

For specific information on the agents used in the management of methotrexate overdose, see: *Leucovorin (Systemic)*.

For more information on the management of overdose or unintentional ingestion, **contact a Poison Control Center** (see *Poison Control Center Listing*).

**Treatment of overdose**
Leucovorin should be administered as soon as possible following accidental methotrexate overdosage. The efficacy of leucovorin in reducing methotrexate toxicity decreases as the time between methotrexate administration and the initiation of leucovorin therapy increases.

Specific treatment—Preventing precipitation of methotrexate and metabolites in renal tubules by systemic hydration and urinary alkalization.

High dose leucovorin therapy, alkaline diuresis, rapid cerebrospinal fluid drainage, and ventriculolumbar perfusion may be necessary for treating intrathecal overdosage.

Monitoring—Monitoring of serum methotrexate concentration is necessary to determine the required dose and duration of treatment with leucovorin.

Supportive care—Intensive systemic supportive care is necessary following intrathecal overdose.

Patients in whom intentional overdose is confirmed or suspected should be referred for psychiatric consultation.

Note: Dialysis is of limited value in the treatment of overdose.

## Patient Consultation

As an aid to patient consultation, refer to *Advice for the Patient, Methotrexate—For Cancer (Systemic)*.

In providing consultation, consider emphasizing the following selected information (» = major clinical significance):

### Before using this medication
» Conditions affecting use, especially:
   Sensitivity to methotrexate
   Pregnancy—Use not recommended because of mutagenic, teratogenic, and carcinogenic potential; advisability of using contraception; telling physician immediately if pregnancy is suspected
   Breast-feeding—Not recommended because of risk of serious side effects
   Use in children—Newborns and other infants may be more sensitive to effects
   Use in the elderly—Side/adverse effects may be more frequent
   Other medications, especially acyclovir, alcohol or other hepatotoxic medications, asparaginase, live virus vaccines, nonsteroidal anti-inflammatory drugs (NSAIDs), other bone marrow depressants, previous cytotoxic drug therapy or radiation therapy, probenecid, sulfinpyrazone, or salicylates
   Other medical problems, especially chickenpox, herpes zoster, hepatic function impairment, renal function impairment, infection, oral mucositis, peptic ulcer, or ulcerative colitis

### Proper use of this medication
» Importance of not taking more or less medication than the amount prescribed
   Caution in taking combination therapy; taking each medication at the right time
   Importance of ample fluid intake and subsequent increase in urine output to prevent nephrotoxicity and aid in excretion of uric acid
» Frequency of nausea and vomiting; importance of continuing medication despite stomach upset
   Checking with physician if vomiting occurs shortly after dose is taken
» Proper dosing
   Missed dose: Not taking at all; not doubling doses
» Proper storage

### Precautions while using this medication
» Importance of close monitoring by physician
» Avoiding alcoholic beverages, which may increase hepatotoxicity
   Possible photosensitivity reactions; avoiding too much unprotected exposure to sun or overuse of sunlamp
» Avoiding salicylate-containing products and NSAIDs, which may increase toxicity
» Avoiding immunizations unless approved by physician; other persons in patient's household should avoid immunizations with oral poliovirus vaccine; avoiding other persons who have taken oral poliovirus vaccine or wearing a protective mask that covers nose and mouth

*Caution if bone marrow depression occurs*
» Avoiding exposure to persons with infections, especially during periods of low blood counts; checking with physician immediately if fever or chills, cough or hoarseness, lower back or side pain, or painful or difficult urination occurs
» Checking with physician immediately if unusual bleeding or bruising; black, tarry stools; blood in urine or stools; or pinpoint red spots on skin occur
   Caution in use of regular toothbrush, dental floss, or toothpick; physician, dentist, or nurse may suggest alternatives; checking with physician before having dental work done
   Not touching eyes or inside of nose unless hands are washed immediately before
   Using caution to avoid accidental cuts with use of sharp objects such as safety razor or fingernail or toenail cutters
   Avoiding contact sports or other situations where bruising or injury could occur

### Side/adverse effects
May cause adverse effects such as blood problems; stomach, kidney, or liver problems; or cancer; importance of discussing possible effects with physician

Signs of potential side effects, especially gastrointestinal ulceration and bleeding, enteritis, intestinal perforation, leukopenia, bacterial infection, septicemia, thrombocytopenia, ulcerative stomatitis, renal failure, azotemia, hyperuricemia, severe nephropathy, severe acute methotrexate toxicity, cutaneous vasculitis, reactivation of sunburn or reaction to ultraviolet light, hepatotoxicity, pneumonitis, pulmonary fibrosis, and CNS effects

Physician or nurse can help in dealing with side effects

Possibility of hair loss; normal hair growth should resume after treatment has ended

## General Dosing Information

Patients receiving methotrexate should be under supervision of a physician experienced in antineoplastic chemotherapy.

A variety of dosage schedules and regimens of methotrexate, alone or in combination with other antitumor agents, are used. The prescriber may consult the medical literature as well as the manufacturer's literature in choosing a specific dosage.

Dosage must be adjusted to meet the individual requirements of each patient, based on clinical response and appearance or severity of toxicity.

In general, use of intermittent courses of methotrexate is associated with less risk of serious toxicity than prolonged, daily dosage.

A significant amount of methotrexate passes into systemic circulation after intrathecal administration and may produce toxic levels in patients also receiving systemic methotrexate therapy; an adjustment in systemic dosage may be necessary.

Development of uric acid nephropathy in patients with leukemia or lymphoma may be prevented by adequate oral hydration and, in some cases, administration of allopurinol. Alkalinization of urine may be necessary if serum uric acid concentrations are elevated.

If severe bone marrow depression occurs, withdrawal of methotrexate may be necessary. However, in some patients with acute leukemia, methotrexate may be administered despite the presence of thrombocytopenia and bleeding; stoppage of bleeding and increase in platelet count have occurred during treatment in some cases and platelet transfusions may be useful in others.

Special precautions are recommended in patients who develop thrombocytopenia as a result of administration of methotrexate. These may include extreme care in performing invasive procedures; regular inspection of intravenous sites, skin (including perirectal area), and mucous membrane surfaces for signs of bleeding or bruising; limiting frequency of venipuncture and avoiding intramuscular injections; testing urine, emesis, stool, and secretions for occult blood; care in use of regular toothbrushes, dental floss, toothpicks, safety razors, and fingernail and toenail cutters; avoiding constipation; and using caution to prevent falls and other injuries. Such patients should avoid alcohol and any aspirin intake because of the risk of gastrointestinal bleeding. Platelet transfusions may be required.

Patients who develop leukopenia should be observed carefully for signs of infection. Antibiotic support may be required. In neutropenic patients who develop fever, broad-spectrum antibiotic coverage should be initiated empirically, pending bacterial cultures and appropriate diagnostic tests.

It is recommended that methotrexate therapy be interrupted if diarrhea or ulcerative stomatitis occurs, because of the risk of hemorrhagic enteritis and fatal intestinal perforation.

It is recommended that methotrexate therapy be interrupted if pulmonary symptoms (especially a dry, unproductive cough) occur, because of the risk of potentially irreversible pulmonary toxicity.

### For use in high-dose methotrexate therapy

Because of its ability to bypass the effects of methotrexate, leucovorin calcium (folinic acid, citrovorum factor) is administered as a "rescue" from the hematologic and gastrointestinal effects of high-dosage methotrexate.

*High-dose methotrexate administration should not be initiated unless leucovorin is physically present and ready to be administered, since rescue is critical.*

Methotrexate administration should not be initiated unless creatinine clearance is greater than 60 mL per minute and serum creatinine concentrations are normal. If renal function impairment develops during therapy, methotrexate should be withdrawn until creatinine clearance improves to acceptable levels.

Methotrexate administration also should not be initiated if:
—White blood cell count is less than 1500 per microliter
—Neutrophil count is less than 200 per microliter
—Platelet count is less than 75,000 per microliter

—Bilirubin is greater than 1.2 mg per dL
—Alanine aminotransferase (ALT [SGPT]) values are greater than 450 units

Methotrexate administration also should be delayed until healing of stomatitis is evident and until after complete drainage of persistent pleural effusions.

A variety of dosage schedules of leucovorin in combination with high-dose methotrexate have been used. The prescriber should consult the medical literature in choosing a specific dosage. Alkalinization of urine (with bicarbonate and/or acetazolamide) and intravenous hydration (1000 mL per square meter of body surface area over 6 hours prior to beginning the methotrexate infusion and 3000 mL per square meter of body surface area per day during the methotrexate infusion and for 2 days after the infusion is completed) are also important to prevent renal toxicity caused by methotrexate and/or its metabolites.

Administration of leucovorin should be consecutive to rather than simultaneous with methotrexate administration so as not to interfere with methotrexate's antineoplastic effects.

In general, it is recommended that the first dose of leucovorin be administered 24 hours after a high-dose methotrexate infusion is started (within 1 hour of an overdose), in a dosage to produce blood concentrations equal to or greater than methotrexate blood concentrations (leucovorin in a dose of 15 to 25 mg per square meter of body surface area produces peak plasma concentrations of approximately 1 micromolar or $1 \times 10^{-6}$ M). Duration of leucovorin administration varies with the dosage of methotrexate and plasma concentrations achieved (including rate of elimination); in general, leucovorin administration is continued until methotrexate concentrations fall to less than $5 \times 10^{-8}$ M.

A larger dose and/or longer duration of leucovorin treatment may be required in patients with aciduria, ascites, dehydration, gastrointestinal obstruction, renal function impairment, or pleural or peritoneal effusions because excretion of methotrexate is slowed and the length of time for plasma methotrexate concentrations to decrease to nontoxic levels ($< 5 \times 10^{-8}$ M) is increased. It is recommended that duration of leucovorin administration in these patients be based on determination of plasma methotrexate concentrations.

### For parenteral use
Methotrexate may be administered intramuscularly, intravenously (rapid or continuous infusion), intrathecally, intra-arterially, or intraventricularly.

Caution is recommended in making sure that the appropriate diluent for the intended route of administration is used when preparing methotrexate for administration.

### Safety considerations for handling this medication
There is limited but increasing evidence and concern that personnel involved in preparation and administration of parenteral antineoplastics may be at some risk because of the potential mutagenicity, teratogenicity, and/or carcinogenicity of these agents, although the actual risk is unknown. USP advisory panels recommend cautious handling both in preparation and disposal of antineoplastic agents. Precautions that have been suggested include:
- Use of a biological containment cabinet during reconstitution and dilution of parenteral medications and wearing of disposable surgical gloves and masks.
- Use of proper technique to prevent contamination of the medication, work area, and operator during transfer between containers (including proper training of personnel in this technique).
- Cautious and proper disposal of needles, syringes, vials, ampuls, and unused medication.

A number of medical centers have developed detailed guidelines for handling of antineoplastic agents.

### Combination chemotherapy
Methotrexate may be used in combination with other agents in various regimens. As a result, incidence and/or severity of side effects may be altered and different dosages (usually reduced) may be used. For example, methotrexate is part of the following chemotherapeutic combinations (some commonly used acronyms are in parentheses):
—cyclophosphamide, doxorubicin, methotrexate, and procarbazine (CAMP).
—cyclophosphamide, methotrexate, and fluorouracil (CMF).
—cyclophosphamide, methotrexate, fluorouracil, vincristine, and prednisone (CMFVP).

For specific dosages and schedules, consult the literature. For information regarding each agent, consult the individual monographs.

## Oral Dosage Forms

Note: Bracketed uses in the *Dosage Forms* section refer to categories of use and/or indications that are not included in U.S. product labeling.

## METHOTREXATE TABLETS USP
### Usual adult dose
Choriocarcinoma or
Chorioadenoma destruens or
Hydatidiform mole—
  Oral, 15 to 30 mg per day for five days, the course being repeated three to five times, with one to two weeks between courses. Usually, one or two courses are given after normalization of urinary human chorionic gonadotropin (HCG) concentrations.
Acute lymphocytic leukemia—
  Induction: Oral, 3.3 mg per square meter of body surface area per day in combination with prednisone or other agents.
  Maintenance: Oral, 30 mg per square meter of body surface area per week in two divided doses.
Burkitt's lymphoma—
  Stages I–II: Oral, 10 to 25 mg per day for four to eight days, the course being repeated several times, with seven to ten days between courses.
  Stage III: Oral, as for Stage I–II, in combination with other agents.
Lymphosarcoma (Stage III)—
  Oral, 625 mcg (0.625 mg) to 2.5 mg per kg of body weight per day.
Mycosis fungoides—
  Oral, 2.5 to 10 mg a day for weeks or months.
Carcinoma, breast or
Carcinoma, head and neck or
Carcinoma, lung, non–small cell[1] or
Carcinoma, lung, small cell[1] or
[Carcinoma, cervical][1] or
[Carcinoma, ovarian, epithelial][1] or
[Carcinoma, bladder] or
[Carcinoma, colorectal][1] or
[Carcinoma, esophageal][1] or
[Carcinoma, gastric] or
[Carcinoma, pancreatic][1] or
[Carcinoma, penile][1] or
[Leukemia, acute nonlymphocytic][1] or
[Lymphomas, Hodgkin's][1] or
[Sarcomas, soft tissue][1]—
  Consult medical literature or manufacturer's literature for specific dosage.

### Usual pediatric dose
Antineoplastic—
  Oral, 20 to 40 mg per square meter of body surface area, once a week.

### Strength(s) usually available
U.S.—
  2.5 mg (Rx) [GENERIC (lactose; magnesium stearate; pregelatinized starch)].
Canada—
  2.5 mg (Rx) [GENERIC].

### Packaging and storage
Store below 40 °C (104 °F), preferably between 15 and 30 °C (59 and 86 °F), unless otherwise specified by manufacturer. Store in a well-closed container. Protect from light.

### Auxiliary labeling
- Avoid alcoholic beverages.
- Do not take other medicines without advice from your doctor.
- Avoid overexposure to sun.

## Parenteral Dosage Forms

Note: Bracketed uses in the *Dosage Forms* section refer to categories of use and/or indications that are not included in U.S. product labeling.

The dosing and strengths of dosage forms available are expressed in terms of methotrexate base.

## METHOTREXATE SODIUM INJECTION USP
### Usual adult dose
Choriocarcinoma or
Chorioadenoma destruens or
Hydatidiform mole—
  Intramuscular, 15 to 30 mg (base) per day for five days, the course being repeated three to five times with one to two weeks between courses. Usually, one or two courses are given after normalization of urinary human chorionic gonadotropin (HCG) concentrations.
Acute lymphocytic leukemia—
  Induction—
    Intravenous or intramuscular, 3.3 mg (base) per square meter of body surface area per day in combination with prednisone or other agents.

Maintenance—
> Intramuscular, 30 mg (base) per square meter of body surface area per week in two divided doses; or
> Intravenous, 2.5 mg (base) per kg of body weight every fourteen days.

Osteosarcoma—
> Intravenous infusion (over four hours), 12 grams (base) per square meter of body surface area, followed by leucovorin rescue (usually 15 mg orally every six hours for ten doses starting at twenty-four hours after the methotrexate infusion is started), on weeks 4, 5, 6, 7, 11, 12, 15, 16, 29, 30, 44, and 45 after surgery on a combination chemotherapy schedule that also includes doxorubicin, cisplatin, bleomycin, cyclophosphamide, and dactinomycin. The dose may be increased, if necessary, to 15 grams (base) per square meter of body surface area to achieve a peak serum methotrexate concentration of $1 \times 10^{-3}$ M per liter.

Note: *High-dose methotrexate administration should not be initiated unless leucovorin is physically present and ready to be administered, since rescue is critical.*

> If the patient is vomiting or cannot take oral medication, leucovorin may be administered intravenously or intramuscularly at the same dose as the oral dose.

Mycosis fungoides—
> Intramuscular, 50 mg (base) once a week or 25 mg (base) two times a week.

Carcinoma, breast or
Carcinoma, head and neck or
Carcinoma, lung, non–small cell[1] or
Carcinoma, lung, small cell[1] or
[Carcinoma, cervical][1] or
[Carcinoma, ovarian, epithelial][1] or
[Carcinoma, bladder] or
[Carcinoma, colorectal][1] or
[Carcinoma, esophageal][1] or
[Carcinoma, gastric] or
[Carcinoma, pancreatic][1] or
[Carcinoma, penile][1] or
[Leukemia, acute nonlymphocytic][1] or
[Lymphomas, Hodgkin's][1] or
[Sarcomas, soft tissue][1]—
> Consult medical literature or manufacturer's literature for specific dosage.

**Usual pediatric dose**
Antineoplastic—
> Intramuscular, 20 to 40 mg (base) per square meter of body surface area, once a week.

**Strength(s) usually available**
U.S.—
> 25 mg (base) per mL (Rx) [GENERIC (with and without preservative)].

Canada—
> 2.5 mg (base) per mL (Rx) [GENERIC (with and without preservative)].
> 10 mg (base) per mL (Rx) [GENERIC (without preservative)].
> 25 mg (base) per mL (Rx) [GENERIC (with and without preservative)].

**Packaging and storage**
Store below 40 °C (104 °F), preferably between 15 and 30 °C (59 and 86 °F), unless otherwise specified by the manufacturer. Protect from light.

**Preparation of dosage form**
Methotrexate Sodium Injection USP may be further diluted with an appropriate preservative-free medium such as 0.9% sodium chloride injection or 5% dextrose injection.

**Stability**
If stored for 24 hours at a temperature of 21 to 25 °C (70 to 77 °F), a diluted solution of methotrexate sodium injection maintains 90% of its labeled potency. However, preservative-free solutions should be diluted immediately prior to use and any unused portion discarded.

## METHOTREXATE SODIUM FOR INJECTION USP

**Usual adult dose**
Meningeal leukemia—
> Induction: Intrathecal, 12 mg (base) every two to five days until the cell count of the cerebrospinal fluid (CSF) returns to normal.
> Prophylaxis: Intrathecal, 12 mg (base) at an interval determined by consultation of the medical literature.

Choriocarcinoma or
Chorioadenoma destruens or
Hydatidiform mole—
> Intramuscular, 15 to 30 mg (base) per day for five days, the course being repeated three to five times, with one to two weeks between courses. Usually, one or two courses are given after normalization of urinary human chorionic gonadotropin (HCG) concentrations.

Acute lymphocytic leukemia—
Induction—
> Intravenous or intramuscular, 3.3 mg (base) per square meter of body surface area per day in combination with prednisone or other agents.

Maintenance—
> Intramuscular, 30 mg (base) per square meter of body surface area per week in two divided doses; or
> Intravenous, 2.5 mg (base) per kg of body weight every fourteen days.

Osteosarcoma—
> Intravenous infusion (over four hours), 12 grams (base) per square meter of body surface area, followed by leucovorin rescue (usually 15 mg orally every six hours for ten doses starting at twenty-four hours after the methotrexate infusion is started), on weeks 4, 5, 6, 7, 11, 12, 15, 16, 29, 30, 44, and 45 after surgery on a combination chemotherapy schedule that also includes doxorubicin, cisplatin, bleomycin, cyclophosphamide, and dactinomycin. The dose may be increased, if necessary, to 15 grams (base) per square meter of body surface area to achieve a peak serum methotrexate concentration of $1 \times 10^{-3}$ M per liter.

Note: *High-dose methotrexate administration should not be initiated unless leucovorin is physically present and ready to be administered, since rescue is critical.*

> If the patient is vomiting or cannot take oral medication, leucovorin may be administered intravenously or intramuscularly in the same dose as the oral dose.

Mycosis fungoides—
> Intramuscular, 50 mg (base) once a week or 25 mg (base) two times a week.

[Carcinomatous meningitis][1]—
> Intrathecal or intraventricular; consult medical literature or manufacturer's literature for specific dosage.

Carcinoma, breast or
Carcinoma, head and neck or
Carcinoma, lung, non–small cell[1] or
Carcinoma, lung, small cell[1] or
[Carcinoma, cervical][1] or
[Carcinoma, ovarian, epithelial][1] or
[Carcinoma, bladder] or
[Carcinoma, colorectal][1] or
[Carcinoma, esophageal][1] or
[Carcinoma, gastric] or
[Carcinoma, pancreatic][1] or
[Carcinoma, penile][1] or
[Leukemia, acute nonlymphocytic][1] or
[Lymphomas, Hodgkin's][1] or
[Sarcomas, soft tissue][1]—
> Consult medical literature or manufacturer's literature for specific dosage.

**Usual pediatric dose**
Meningeal leukemia—
> For children up to 1 year of age: Intrathecal, 6 mg (base) every two to five days until the cell count of the CSF returns to normal.
> For children 1 year of age: Intrathecal, 8 mg (base) every two to five days until the cell count of the CSF returns to normal.
> For children 2 years of age: Intrathecal, 10 mg (base) every two to five days until the cell count of the CSF returns to normal.
> For children 3 years of age and over: Intrathecal, 12 mg (base) every two to five days until the cell count of the CSF returns to normal.

Antineoplastic, other—
> Intramuscular, 20 to 40 mg (base) per square meter of body surface area, once a week.

**Size(s) usually available**
U.S.—
> 20 mg (base) (Rx) [GENERIC (without preservative)].
> 1 gram (base) (Rx) [GENERIC (without preservative)].

Canada—
> 20 mg (base) (Rx) [GENERIC (without preservative)].

**Packaging and storage**
Store below 40 °C (104 °F), preferably between 15 and 30 °C (59 and 86 °F), unless otherwise specified by manufacturer. Protect from light.

**Preparation of dosage form**
For intrathecal use, methotrexate sodium for injection (containing no preservative) is recommended. It must be reconstituted immediately prior to use with an appropriate volume of a sterile, preservative-free medium such as 0.9% sodium chloride injection to yield a solution containing 1 mg (base) per mL.

For intravenous or intramuscular use, the 20-mg vial of methotrexate sodium for injection is diluted with an appropriate volume of a sterile, preservative-free medium, such as 5% dextrose injection or 0.9% sodium chloride injection, to yield a solution containing not more than 25 mg (base) per mL. The 1-gram vial should be diluted with 19.4 mL of 5% dextrose injection or 0.9% sodium chloride injection to yield a solution containing 50 mg (base) per mL. For high dose intravenous use, methotrexate sodium for injection should only be diluted in 5% dextrose injection.

**Stability**
Solutions without preservative should be freshly reconstituted immediately prior to each dose; any unused portion should be discarded.

[1]Not included in Canadian product labeling.

Revised: 07/02/98

# METHOTREXATE—FOR NONCANCEROUS CONDITIONS Systemic

VA CLASSIFICATION (Primary): DE801/MS105
Commonly used brand name(s): *Folex; Folex PFS; Mexate; Mexate-AQ; Rheumatrex.*
Another commonly used name is amethopterin.

Note: For a listing of dosage forms and brand names by country availability, see *Dosage Forms* section(s).

## Category
Antipsoriatic (systemic); antirheumatic (disease-modifying).

## Indications
Note: Bracketed information in the *Indications* section refers to uses that are not included in U.S. product labeling.

**Accepted**
Psoriasis (treatment)—Methotrexate is indicated only for treatment of severe, recalcitrant, disabling psoriasis not adequately responsive to other forms of therapy, as confirmed by biopsy and/or dermatologic consultation. Methotrexate is contraindicated in pregnant psoriatic patients and those with existing severe renal or hepatic disease or pre-existing blood dyscrasias.

Arthritis, rheumatoid (treatment)—Methotrexate tablets are indicated [and the parenteral dosage forms are used][1] in the treatment of selected cases of severe rheumatoid arthritis not adequately responsive to other forms of therapy, as confirmed by rheumatologic consultation. Methotrexate is contraindicated in pregnant rheumatoid arthritis patients and those with existing renal or hepatic disease or pre-existing blood dyscrasias.

[Arthritis, psoriatic (treatment)][1]—Methotrexate is being used in the treatment of selected cases of active severe psoriatic arthritis.

[Dermatomyositis, systemic (treatment)][1]—Methotrexate is used for treatment of systemic dermatomyositis (polymyositis).

Caution is recommended in use of methotrexate for non-neoplastic conditions because of potential toxicity with long-term use of this agent.

[1]Not included in Canadian product labeling.

## Pharmacology/Pharmacokinetics

**Physicochemical characteristics**
Molecular weight—454.44.

**Mechanism of action/Effect**
Methotrexate is an antimetabolite of the folic acid analog type. Methotrexate is cell cycle–specific for the S phase of cell division. Activity is due to inhibition of DNA, RNA, thymidylate, and protein synthesis as a result of relatively irreversible binding with dihydrofolate reductase, which prevents reduction of dihydrofolate to the active tetrahydrofolate. Growth of rapidly proliferating cells (epithelial cells in psoriasis, bone marrow, fetal cells, buccal and intestinal mucosa, cells of the urinary bladder, spermatogonia) is affected more than growth of most normal tissues and skin.

**Other actions/effects**
Also has mild immunosuppressant activity.

**Absorption**
Widely variable.

**Distribution**
Crosses the blood-brain barrier (from blood to central nervous system [CNS]) in only limited amounts (dose-related); however, passes significantly into systemic circulation after intrathecal administration.

**Protein binding**
Moderate (approximately 50%), primarily to albumin.

**Biotransformation**
Hepatic; intracellular (to polyglutamates, which are retained in the cells).

**Half-life**
Terminal—
　Low doses: 3 to 10 hours.
　High doses: 8 to 15 hours.

Note: There is wide interindividual variation in clearance rates. Small amounts of methotrexate and metabolites are bound and may remain in tissues (kidneys, liver) for weeks to months; the presence of fluids such as ascites or pleural effusion will also delay clearance.

**Time to peak serum concentration**
Oral—1 to 2 hours.
Intramuscular—30 to 60 minutes.

**Elimination**
Single dose—
　Renal (unchanged), 80 to 90% in the first 24 hours; some accumulation of polyglutamates in tissues occurs with repeated doses.
　Biliary, 10% or less.

## Precautions to Consider

**Carcinogenicity/Mutagenicity**
Secondary malignancies are potential delayed effects of many antineoplastic agents, although it is not clear whether the effect is related to their mutagenic or immunosuppressive action. The effect of dose and duration of therapy is also unknown, although risk seems to increase with long-term use. Although information is limited, available data seem to indicate that the carcinogenic risk is greatest with the alkylating agents.

Antimetabolites have been shown to be carcinogenic in animals, and may be associated with an increased risk of development of secondary carcinomas in humans, although the risk appears to be less than with alkylating agents.

Carcinogenicity studies with methotrexate in animals have been inconclusive. However, there is evidence that methotrexate causes chromosomal damage to animal somatic cells and human bone marrow cells.

**Pregnancy/Reproduction**
Fertility—Methotrexate appears to have only a slight effect on gonadal function; however, reversible impairment of fertility, defective oogenesis and spermatogenesis, and menstrual function impairment have been reported.

Pregnancy—Methotrexate crosses the placenta and has been shown to cause adverse effects on the fetus. Methotrexate is a potent abortifacient.

Use as an antipsoriatic or antiarthritic agent is contraindicated in pregnant women.

FDA Pregnancy Category X.

**Breast-feeding**
Methotrexate is excreted in breast milk; breast-feeding is not recommended while methotrexate is being administered because of the risks to the infant (adverse effects, mutagenicity, carcinogenicity).

**Pediatrics**
Caution should be used in neonates and infants because of reduced renal and hepatic function.

**Geriatrics**
Although appropriate studies with methotrexate have not been performed in the geriatric population, caution should be used in the elderly because of possible reduced renal and hepatic function and reduced folate stores. Dosage adjustment, especially on the basis of renal function, may be necessary.

**Dental**
The bone marrow depressant effects of methotrexate may result in an increased incidence of microbial infection, delayed healing, and gingival bleeding. Dental work, whenever possible, should be completed prior to initiation of therapy or deferred until blood counts have returned to normal. Patients should be instructed in proper oral hygiene during treatment, including caution in use of regular toothbrushes, dental floss, and toothpicks.

Methotrexate also commonly causes ulcerative stomatitis, gingivitis, and pharyngitis associated with considerable discomfort.

**Drug interactions and/or related problems**

The following drug interactions and/or related problems have been selected on the basis of their potential clinical significance (possible mechanism in parentheses where appropriate)—not necessarily inclusive (» = major clinical significance):

Note: Combinations containing any of the following medications, depending on the amount present, may also interact with this medication.

» Alcohol or
» Hepatotoxic medications, other (See *Appendix II* )
   (concurrent use may increase the risk of hepatotoxicity)

Anticoagulants, coumarin- or indandione-derivative
   (methotrexate may increase anticoagulant activity and/or increase the risk of hemorrhage as a result of decreased hepatic synthesis of procoagulant factors and interference with platelet formation)

» Anti-inflammatory analgesics, nonsteroidal (NSAIAs)
   (concurrent use of phenylbutazone with methotrexate may increase the risk of agranulocytosis or bone marrow depression and is not recommended; also, phenylbutazone may displace methotrexate from its protein-binding sites and decrease its renal clearance, leading to increased methotrexate plasma concentration and risk of toxicity. If concurrent use with phenylbutazone cannot be avoided, especially careful monitoring of the patient for plasma methotrexate concentrations or signs of methotrexate toxicity and/or adequacy of renal function is recommended)

   (although not well documented, the possibility exists that other NSAIAs may also decrease methotrexate excretion and increase its plasma concentration to potentially toxic levels)

   (severe, sometimes fatal, methotrexate toxicity has also been reported with low to moderate doses in patients receiving diclofenac, indomethacin, naproxen, or phenylbutazone; it is recommended that use of NSAIAs with low to moderate doses of methotrexate be undertaken with caution, with methotrexate dosage being adjusted by monitoring plasma methotrexate concentrations and/or adequacy of renal function)

Blood dyscrasia–causing medications (See *Appendix II*)
   (leukopenic and/or thrombocytopenic effects of methotrexate may be increased with concurrent or recent therapy if these medications cause the same effects; dosage adjustment of methotrexate, if necessary, should be based on blood counts)

» Bone marrow depressants, other (See *Appendix II*) or
   Radiation therapy
   (additive bone marrow depression may occur; dosage reduction may be required when two or more bone marrow depressants, including radiation, are used concurrently or consecutively)

Folic acid
   (may interfere with the antifolate effects of methotrexate)

Neomycin, oral
   (may decrease absorption of oral methotrexate)

» Probenecid
   (concurrent use may inhibit renal excretion of methotrexate and result in toxic plasma concentrations; if used concurrently with probenecid, methotrexate dosage should be decreased, the patient observed for signs of toxicity, and/or plasma methotrexate concentrations monitored)

Pyrimethamine or
Triamterene or
Trimethoprim
   (concurrent use may rarely increase the toxic effects of methotrexate because of similar folic acid antagonist actions)

» Salicylates and other weak organic acids
   (concurrent use may inhibit renal tubular secretion of methotrexate and result in toxic plasma concentrations; salicylates may also increase plasma concentrations by displacing methotrexate from binding sites; if methotrexate is used concurrently with these medications, the patient should be observed for signs of toxicity and/or methotrexate plasma concentration monitored)

Sulfonamides
   (in addition to increased risk of hepatotoxicity that may occur when sulfonamides are used concurrently with other hepatotoxic medications, medications that cause displacement from plasma protein binding may theoretically produce toxic plasma concentrations of methotrexate when used concurrently, although clinical significance has not been established)

Vaccines, killed virus
   (because normal defense mechanisms may be suppressed by methotrexate therapy, the patient's antibody response to the vaccine may be decreased. The interval between discontinuation of medications that cause immunosuppression and restoration of the patient's ability to respond to the vaccine depends on the intensity and type of immunosuppression-causing medication used, the underlying disease, and other factors; estimates vary from 3 months to 1 year)

» Vaccines, live virus
   (because normal defense mechanisms may be suppressed by methotrexate therapy, concurrent use with a live virus vaccine may potentiate the replication of the vaccine virus, may increase the side/adverse effects of the vaccine virus, and/or may decrease the patient's antibody response to the vaccine; immunization of these patients should be undertaken only with extreme caution after careful review of the patient's hematologic status and only with the knowledge and consent of the physician managing the methotrexate therapy. The interval between discontinuation of medications that cause immunosuppression and restoration of the patient's ability to respond to the vaccine depends on the intensity and type of immunosuppression-causing medication used, the underlying disease, and other factors; estimates vary from 3 months to 1 year. Immunization with oral poliovirus vaccine should also be postponed in persons in close contact with the patient, especially family members)

**Laboratory value alterations**

The following have been selected on the basis of their potential clinical significance (possible effect in parentheses where appropriate)—not necessarily inclusive (» = major clinical significance):

With diagnostic test results
   Assay for folate
      (methotrexate may inhibit the organism used in the assay and interfere with detection of folic acid deficiency)

With physiology/laboratory test values
   Isocitric acid dehydrogenase (ICD) concentrations
      (may be increased, indicating hepatotoxicity)

**Medical considerations/Contraindications**

The medical considerations/contraindications included have been selected on the basis of their potential clinical significance (reasons given in parentheses where appropriate)—not necessarily inclusive (» = major clinical significance).

*Except under special circumstances, this medication should not be used when the following medical problems exist:*

» Bone marrow depression
» Hepatic function impairment, severe
» Immunodeficiency
» Renal function impairment, severe

*Risk-benefit should be considered when the following medical problems exist:*

» Ascites or
   Gastrointestinal obstruction or
» Pleural or peritoneal effusions or
» Renal function impairment
   (risk of methotrexate toxicity is increased because elimination of methotrexate may be impaired and accumulation may occur; even small doses may lead to severe myelosuppression and mucositis)

   (a lower dosage of methotrexate and careful monitoring of plasma or serum methotrexate concentrations are recommended for patients with impaired renal function)

» Chickenpox, existing or recent (including recent exposure) or
» Herpes zoster
   (risk of severe generalized disease)
» Hepatic function impairment
» Infection
» Mucositis, oral
   Nausea and vomiting
      (inadequate hydration secondary to severe nausea and vomiting may result in increased methotrexate toxicity)
» Peptic ulcer
   Sensitivity to methotrexate
» Ulcerative colitis
» Caution should be used also in patients who have had previous cytotoxic drug therapy and radiation therapy, and in cases of general debility.

## Patient monitoring

The following are especially important in patient monitoring (other tests may be warranted in some patients, depending on condition; » = major clinical significance):

Blood urea nitrogen (BUN) concentrations and

Creatinine clearance and/or

Serum creatinine concentrations
(recommended prior to initiation of therapy and at periodic intervals during therapy; frequency varies according to clinical state, agent, dose, and other agents being used concurrently)

Examination of patient's mouth for ulceration
(recommended before administration of each dose)

» Hematocrit or hemoglobin and
» Platelet count and
» Total and, if appropriate, differential leukocyte count
(determinations recommended prior to initiation of therapy and at periodic intervals during therapy; frequency varies according to clinical state, agent, dose, and other agents being used concurrently)

Liver biopsy
(may be useful during long-term therapy or if hepatic function test results are abnormal; also recommended in patients who have received a cumulative dose of 1500 mg)

» Serum alanine aminotransferase (ALT [SGPT]) concentrations and
» Serum aspartate aminotransferase (AST [SGOT]) concentrations and
» Serum bilirubin concentrations and
» Serum lactate dehydrogenase (LDH) concentrations
(recommended prior to initiation of therapy and at periodic intervals during therapy; frequency varies according to clinical state, agent, dose, and other agents being used concurrently)

## Side/Adverse Effects

Note: Incidence and severity of side effects, particularly hepatotoxicity, appear to be related to dosage frequency and duration of methotrexate therapy. Toxicity tends to occur less frequently and be less severe with a total dose administered as intermittent weekly dosage than with prolonged daily dosage.

The following side/adverse effects have been selected on the basis of their potential clinical significance (possible signs and symptoms in parentheses where appropriate)—not necessarily inclusive:

### Those indicating need for medical attention
Incidence less frequent

*Gastrointestinal ulceration and bleeding, enteritis, or intestinal perforation, which may be fatal* (diarrhea; stomach pain); *leukopenia, bacterial infection, or septicemia* (usually asymptomatic; rarely, fever or chills; cough or hoarseness; lower back or side pain; painful or difficult urination); *thrombocytopenia* (usually asymptomatic; rarely, unusual bleeding or bruising; black, tarry stools; blood in urine or stools; pinpoint red spots on skin); *severe acute methotrexate toxicity, cutaneous vasculitis, or reactivation of sunburn or increased erythematous response to ultraviolet therapy* (reddening of skin); *ulcerative stomatitis, gingivitis, or pharyngitis* (sores in mouth and on lips)

Note: With *leukopenia* and *thrombocytopenia*, the nadir of the leukocyte and platelet counts occurs after 7 to 10 days, with recovery 7 days later.

Incidence rare—dose-related

*Central nervous system (CNS) effects, increased cerebrospinal fluid pressure, leukoencephalopathy, demyelination, or chemical arachnoiditis* (back pain; blurred vision; convulsions; dizziness; drowsiness; fever; headache; unusual tiredness or weakness); *hepatotoxicity, including liver atrophy; necrosis; cirrhosis; fatty changes; periportal fibrosis* (yellow eyes or skin); *pneumonitis, potentially fatal, or pulmonary fibrosis* (cough; shortness of breath)

### Those indicating need for medical attention only if they continue or are bothersome
Incidence less frequent or rare

*Acne; boils; loss of appetite; nausea; pale skin; skin rash or itching; vomiting*

### Those not indicating need for medical attention
Incidence less frequent or rare

*Loss of hair*

## Patient Consultation

As an aid to patient consultation, refer to *Advice for the Patient, Methotrexate—For Noncancerous Conditions (Systemic)*.

In providing consultation, consider emphasizing the following selected information (» = major clinical significance):

## Before using this medication

» Conditions affecting use, especially:

Sensitivity to methotrexate

Pregnancy—Use not recommended because of teratogenic, abortifacient, and carcinogenic potential; advisability of using contraception; telling physician immediately if pregnancy is suspected

Breast-feeding—Not recommended because of risk of serious side effects

Use in children—Newborns and other infants may be more sensitive to effects

Use in the elderly—Side/adverse effects may be more frequent

Other medications, especially alcohol or other hepatotoxic medications, nonsteroidal anti-inflammatory drugs (NSAIDs), other bone marrow depressants, probenecid, salicylates, or previous cytotoxic drug therapy or radiation therapy

Other medical problems, especially hepatic function impairment, renal function impairment, chickenpox, herpes zoster, infection, oral mucositis, peptic ulcer, or ulcerative colitis

## Proper use of this medication

» Importance of not taking more or less medication than the amount prescribed
» Frequency of nausea; importance of continuing medication despite stomach upset; checking with physician if vomiting occurs

Checking with physician if vomiting occurs shortly after dose is taken
» Proper dosing

Missed dose: Not taking at all; not doubling doses
» Proper storage

## Precautions while using this medication

» Importance of close monitoring by the physician
» Avoiding alcoholic beverages, which may increase hepatotoxicity

Possible photosensitivity reactions; avoiding too much unprotected exposure to sun or overuse of sunlamp
» Avoiding salicylate-containing products and NSAIDs, which may increase toxicity
» Avoiding immunizations unless approved by physician; other persons in patient's household should avoid immunizations with oral poliovirus vaccine; avoiding other persons who have taken oral poliovirus vaccine or wearing a protective mask that covers nose and mouth

*Caution if bone marrow depression occurs*
» Avoiding exposure to persons with bacterial infections, especially during periods of low blood counts; checking with physician immediately if fever or chills, cough or hoarseness, lower back or side pain, or painful or difficult urination occurs
» Checking with physician immediately if unusual bleeding or bruising; black, tarry stools; blood in urine or stools; or pinpoint red spots on skin occur

Caution in use of regular toothbrush, dental floss, or toothpick; physician, dentist, or nurse may suggest alternatives; checking with physician before having dental work done

Not touching eyes or inside of nose unless hands washed immediately before

Using caution to avoid accidental cuts with use of sharp objects such as safety razor or fingernail or toenail cutters

Avoiding contact sports or other situations where bruising or injury could occur

### Side/adverse effects

May cause adverse effects such as blood problems; stomach, kidney, or liver problems; loss of hair; or cancer; importance of discussing possible effects with physician

Signs of potential side effects, especially gastrointestinal ulceration and bleeding, enteritis, intestinal perforation, leukopenia, bacterial infection, septicemia, thrombocytopenia, severe acute methotrexate toxicity, cutaneous vasculitis, reactivation of sunburn or reaction to ultraviolet light, ulcerative stomatitis, gingivitis, pharyngitis, CNS effects, hepatotoxicity, pneumonitis, and pulmonary fibrosis

Physician or nurse can help in dealing with side effects

Possibility of hair loss; should return after treatment has ended

## General Dosing Information

Patients receiving methotrexate should be under supervision of a physician experienced in antimetabolite chemotherapy.

In general, use of intermittent courses of methotrexate is associated with less risk of serious toxicity than prolonged daily dosage.

It is recommended that methotrexate therapy be interrupted if diarrhea or ulcerative stomatitis occurs, because of the risk of hemorrhagic enteritis and fatal intestinal perforation.

# Methotrexate—For Noncancerous Conditions (Systemic)

It is recommended that methotrexate therapy be interrupted if pulmonary symptoms (especially a dry, unproductive cough) occur, because of the risk of potentially irreversible pulmonary toxicity.

If bone marrow depression occurs, withdrawal of methotrexate is recommended. The following precautions may also be useful:
- Special precautions are recommended in patients who develop thrombocytopenia as a result of administration of methotrexate. These may include extreme care in performing invasive procedures; regular inspection of intravenous sites, skin (including perirectal area), and mucous membrane surfaces for signs of bleeding or bruising; limiting frequency of venipuncture and avoiding intramuscular injections; testing urine, emesis, stool, and secretions for occult blood; care in use of regular toothbrushes, dental floss, toothpicks, safety razors, and fingernail and toenail cutters; avoiding constipation; and using caution to prevent falls and other injuries. Such patients should avoid alcohol and any aspirin intake because of the risk of gastrointestinal bleeding. Platelet transfusions may be required.
- Patients who develop leukopenia should be observed carefully for signs of infection. Antibiotic support may be required. In neutropenic patients who develop fever, broad-spectrum antibiotic coverage should be initiated empirically, pending bacterial cultures and appropriate diagnostic tests.

### For use as an antipsoriatic
After a favorable response is obtained, it is recommended that the dosage be decreased gradually to the lowest dosage and longest rest period that will maintain an adequate clinical response. To reduce the methotrexate requirement, it is recommended that an attempt be made to return to conventional therapy or to concomitant topical conventional therapy as soon as possible.

### For use as an antirheumatic
Methotrexate appears to be effective by the oral, intramuscular, or intravenous route; however, oral administration is associated with less toxicity.

### For parenteral use
Methotrexate may be administered intramuscularly or intravenously (rapid or continuous infusion).

### Safety considerations for handling this medication
There is limited but increasing evidence and concern that personnel involved in preparation and administration of parenteral cytotoxic agents may be at some risk because of the potential mutagenicity, teratogenicity, and/or carcinogenicity of these agents, although the actual risk is unknown. USP advisory panels recommend cautious handling both in preparation and disposal of antineoplastic agents. Precautions that have been suggested include:
- Use of a biological containment cabinet during reconstitution and dilution of parenteral medications and wearing of disposable surgical gloves and masks.
- Use of proper technique to prevent contamination of the medication, work area, and operator during transfer between containers (including proper training of personnel in this technique).
- Cautious and proper disposal of needles, syringes, vials, ampuls, and unused medication.

A number of medical centers have developed detailed guidelines for handling of antineoplastic agents.

## Oral Dosage Forms
Note: Bracketed uses in the *Dosage Forms* section refer to categories of use and/or indications that are not included in U.S. product labeling.

### METHOTREXATE TABLETS USP
**Usual adult dose**
Psoriasis or
Rheumatoid arthritis or
[Psoriatic arthritis][1]—
  Oral, initially 2.5 to 5 mg every twelve hours for three doses once a week, the dosage being increased as necessary in increments of 2.5 mg per week up to a maximum of 20 mg per week; or
  Oral, initially 10 mg once a week, the dosage being increased as necessary up to 25 mg once a week.

Note: Some clinicians recommend an initial test dose at the lowest dosage level because of interindividual variation in sensitivity to methotrexate.

**Usual pediatric dose**
Dosage has not been established.

**Strength(s) usually available**
U.S.—
  2.5 mg (Rx) [*Rheumatrex*; GENERIC].
Canada—
  2.5 mg (Rx) [*Rheumatrex*; GENERIC].

**Packaging and storage**
Store below 40 °C (104 °F), preferably between 15 and 30 °C (59 and 86 °F), unless otherwise specified by manufacturer. Store in a well-closed container.

**Auxiliary labeling**
- Avoid alcoholic beverages.
- Do not take other medicines without advice from your doctor.
- Avoid overexposure to sun.

## Parenteral Dosage Forms

### METHOTREXATE SODIUM INJECTION USP
**Usual adult dose**
Psoriasis or
[Rheumatoid arthritis][1]—Intramuscular or intravenous, initially 10 mg (base) once a week, the dosage being increased as necessary up to 25 mg (base) once a week.

Note: Some clinicians recommend an initial test dose of 10 mg because of interindividual variation in sensitivity to methotrexate.

**Usual pediatric dose**
Dosage has not been established.

**Strength(s) usually available**
U.S.—
  2.5 mg (base) per mL (Rx) [GENERIC (with preservative)].
  25 mg (base) per mL (Rx) [*Folex PFS* (without preservative); *Mexate-AQ* (with or without preservative) [GENERIC (with and without preservative)].
Canada—
  2.5 mg (base) per mL (Rx) [GENERIC (with and without preservative)].
  10 mg (base) per mL (Rx) [GENERIC (without preservative)].
  25 mg (base) per mL (Rx) [GENERIC (with and without preservative)].

**Packaging and storage**
Store below 40 °C (104 °F), preferably between 15 and 30 °C (59 and 86 °F), unless otherwise specified by manufacturer. Protect from light.

**Preparation of dosage form**
Methotrexate Sodium Injection USP may be further diluted with an appropriate preservative-free medium such as 0.9% sodium chloride injection or 5% dextrose injection.

**Stability**
If stored for 24 hours at a temperature of 21 to 25 °C (70 to 77 °F), a diluted solution of methotrexate sodium injection maintains 90% of its labeled potency. However, preservative-free solutions should be diluted immediately prior to use and any unused portion discarded.

### METHOTREXATE SODIUM FOR INJECTION USP
**Usual adult dose**
Psoriasis or
[Rheumatoid arthritis][1]—Intramuscular or intravenous, initially 10 mg (base) once a week, the dosage being increased as necessary up to 25 mg (base) once a week.

Note: Some clinicians recommend an initial test dose of 10 mg because of interindividual variation in sensitivity to methotrexate.

**Usual pediatric dose**
Dosage has not been established.

**Size(s) usually available**
U.S.—
  20 mg (base) (Rx) [*Mexate* [GENERIC (without preservative)].
  25 mg (base) (Rx) [*Folex* (without preservative)].
  50 mg (base) (Rx) [*Folex* (without preservative); *Mexate* [GENERIC (without preservative)].
  100 mg (base) (Rx) [*Folex* (without preservative); *Mexate* [GENERIC (without preservative)].
  250 mg (base) (Rx) [*Folex* (without preservative); *Mexate* [GENERIC (without preservative)].
  1 gram (base) [ (without preservative)].
Canada—
  20 mg (base) (Rx) [GENERIC (without preservative)].

**Packaging and storage**
Store below 40 °C (104 °F), preferably between 15 and 30 °C (59 and 86 °F), unless otherwise specified by manufacturer. Protect from light.

**Preparation of dosage form**
For intravenous or intramuscular use, methotrexate sodium for injection is diluted with 2 to 25 mL (depending on route of administration) of 0.9% sodium chloride injection (for *Folex*) or with 2 to 10 mL of sterile water

for injection, 0.9% sodium chloride injection, or bacteriostatic water for injection with parabens or benzyl alcohol (for *Mexate*).

**Stability**
Solutions without preservative should be freshly reconstituted immediately prior to each dose; any unused portion should be discarded. Solutions (for *Mexate*) prepared with Bacteriostatic Water for Injection USP with parabens or benzyl alcohol are stable for 4 weeks at 25 °C (77 °F) or for 3 months at 4 °C (39 °F) or −15 °C (5 °F).

[1] Not included in Canadian product labeling.

Revised: 08/90
Interim revision: 07/08/93; 07/05/94

**METHOTRIMEPRAZINE**—See *Phenothiazines (Systemic)*

**METHOXAMINE**—See *Sympathomimetic Agents—Cardiovascular Use (Parenteral-Systemic)*

# METHOXSALEN  Systemic

VA CLASSIFICATION (Primary/Secondary): DE801/DE890; AN900

Note: **Methoxsalen soft gelatin capsules should not be used interchangeably with the hard gelatin capsules, since the soft gelatin capsule dosage form exhibits significantly greater bioavailability and earlier photosensitization onset time than does the hard gelatin capsule dosage form.**

Commonly used brand name(s): *8-MOP; Oxsoralen; Oxsoralen-Ultra; Ultra MOP*.

Note: For a listing of dosage forms and brand names by country availability, see *Dosage Forms* section(s).

## Category

Repigmenting agent (systemic); antipsoriatic (systemic); antineoplastic; hair growth stimulant, alopecia areata (systemic).

Note: Methoxsalen is used in conjunction with ultraviolet light A (UVA). This mode of treatment is known as PUVA (psoralen plus ultraviolet light A).

**Methoxsalen soft gelatin capsules should not be used interchangeably with the hard gelatin capsules,** since the soft gelatin capsule dosage form exhibits significantly greater bioavailability and earlier photosensitization onset time than does the hard gelatin capsule dosage form.

## Indications

Note: Bracketed information in the *Indications* section refers to uses that are not included in U.S. product labeling.

**Accepted**
Mycosis fungoides (treatment)[1]—Photopheresis, using methoxsalen hard gelatin capsules [or soft gelatin capsules] with ultraviolet radiation of white blood cells, is indicated for use with the UVAR System in the palliative treatment of the skin manifestations of mycosis fungoides (also known as cutaneous T-cell lymphoma) in persons who have not been responsive to other forms of treatment. [PUVA is also used in the treatment of mycosis fungoides.][1]

Psoriasis (treatment)—PUVA, using methoxsalen hard gelatin capsules or soft gelatin capsules, is indicated in the treatment of severe, refractory, disabling psoriasis that has not responded to other therapy.

Vitiligo (treatment)—PUVA, using methoxsalen hard gelatin capsules [or soft gelatin capsules], is indicated for repigmentation in the treatment of vitiligo. PUVA is not effective in producing pigmentation in leukoderma of infectious origin or in albinism. Patients with albinism or patients who are intolerant to sunlight still may benefit from methoxsalen's ability to increase their tolerance to sunlight.

[Alopecia areata (treatment)][1]
[Dermatitis, atopic (treatment)]
[Dermatoses, inflammatory (treatment)][1]
[Eczema (treatment)][1]
[Lichen planus (treatment)][1] or
[Skin intolerance to sunlight]—PUVA is also used in the treatment of alopecia areata, atopic dermatitis, inflammatory dermatoses, eczema, and lichen planus. Methoxsalen, with natural light or with UVA light, also is used to increase skin tolerance to sunlight.

**Unaccepted**
The unsupervised use of methoxsalen to promote tanning is dangerous and should be discouraged.

[1] Not included in Canadian product labeling.

## Pharmacology/Pharmacokinetics

**Physicochemical characteristics**
Molecular weight—216.19.

**Mechanism of action/Effect**
Methoxsalen is a psoralen derivative with photosensitizing activity. Exact mechanism of erythemogenic, melanogenic, and cytotoxic response in the epidermis is unknown, but may involve increased tyrosinase activity in melanin-producing cells, as well as inhibition of DNA synthesis, cell division, and epidermal turnover. Successful pigmentation requires the presence of functioning melanocytes.

**Absorption**
Methoxsalen is variably (approximately 95%) absorbed from the gastrointestinal tract. It has been postulated that poor response in some patients may be due to poor absorption.

**Protein binding**
High.

**Biotransformation**
Activated by long-wavelength UVA in the range of 320 to 400 nanometers (nm). Further metabolism: hepatic.

**Half-life**
Hard gelatin capsule—1.1 hours.
Soft gelatin capsule—Approximately 2 hours.

**Onset of action**
Vitiligo—Up to 6 months or longer.
Psoriasis—30 treatments (10 weeks or longer).
For intolerance of skin to sunlight—1 hour.
Tanning—Within a few days.

**Time to peak photosensitivity**
Hard gelatin capsule—3.9 to 4.25 hours.
Soft gelatin capsule—1.5 to 2.1 hours.

**Mean minimal erythema dose (MED)**
Substantially fewer Joules per square cm are required with the soft gelatin capsule dosage form than with the hard gelatin capsule dosage form.

**Peak serum concentration**
Hard gelatin capsule—1.5 to 6 hours (mean of 3 hours), when administered with 8 ounces of milk.
Soft gelatin capsule—0.5 to 4 hours (mean of 1.8 hours), when administered with 8 ounces of milk.

**Duration of action**
Increased sensitivity of skin to sunlight—Approximately 8 hours.

**Elimination**
Renal—As metabolites (80 to 90% in 8 hours; 95% in 24 hours).
Fecal—4 to 10%.

## Precautions to Consider

**Carcinogenicity**
Psoralens have been found to augment UVA-induced carcinogenicity in laboratory animals. In addition, studies in humans treated with systemic methoxsalen plus UVA have shown an increase in the risk of squamous cell carcinoma. The possibility of increased risk may exist also for topical methoxsalen and systemic trioxsalen. This risk appears to be greatest in patients with predisposing risk factors, such as fair skin or a hypersensitivity to sunlight; a history of skin cancer, exposure to ionizing radiation, or excessive exposure to sunlight; or a history of treatment with tar and UVB (prolonged), arsenicals, or topical nitrogen mustard.

## Pregnancy/Reproduction
Pregnancy—Studies have not been done in humans.
Studies have not been done in animals.
FDA Pregnancy Category C.

## Breast-feeding
It is not known whether methoxsalen is distributed into breast milk. However, problems in humans have not been documented.

## Pediatrics
Children up to 12 years of age—Appropriate studies on the relationship of age to the effects of methoxsalen have not been performed; however, some side effects are more likely to occur in children up to 12 years of age, since these children may be more sensitive to the effects of methoxsalen.

Children 12 years of age and over—Appropriate studies on the relationship of age to the effects of methoxsalen have not been performed in this age group. However, no problems specific to this age group have been documented to date.

## Geriatrics
Although appropriate studies on the relationship of age to the effects of methoxsalen have not been performed in the geriatric population, no geriatrics-specific problems have been documented to date.

## Drug interactions and/or related problems
The following drug interactions and/or related problems have been selected on the basis of their potential clinical significance (possible mechanism in parentheses where appropriate)—not necessarily inclusive (» = major clinical significance):

Note: Combinations containing any of the following medications, depending on the amount present, may also interact with this medication.

Furocoumarin-containing foods, such as limes, figs, parsley, parsnips, mustard, carrots, and celery
(although there have been no reports of serious reactions, caution and avoidance of these foods are recommended because of the risk of additive phototoxicity)

Photosensitizing medications, other
(concurrent use of methoxsalen with these medications, systemic or topical, may cause additive photosensitizing effects; concurrent use with coal tar or coal tar derivatives or with trioxsalen is not recommended)

(concurrent use of systemic methoxsalen with phenothiazines may potentiate intraocular photochemical damage to the choroid, retina, and lens)

» Caution should be used also in evaluating for treatment and subsequently treating patients with a history of having taken arsenicals or having received x-rays, cytotoxic therapy, or coal tar and ultraviolet light B (UVB) therapy because of the increased risk of skin cancer

## Laboratory value alterations
The following have been selected on the basis of their potential clinical significance (possible effect in parentheses where appropriate)—not necessarily inclusive (» = major clinical significance):

With physiology/laboratory test values
Hepatic function tests
(abnormal hepatic function tests have been reported, but the relationship to the medication is not clear)

## Medical considerations/Contraindications
The medical considerations/contraindications included have been selected on the basis of their potential clinical significance (reasons given in parentheses where appropriate)—not necessarily inclusive (» = major clinical significance).

*Risk-benefit should be considered when the following medical problems exist:*

» Albinism or
» Hydroa or
» Leukoderma of infectious origin or
» Lupus erythematosus, acute or
Polymorphic light eruptions or
» Porphyria or
» Xeroderma pigmentosum
(these conditions are associated with photosensitization)
» Aphakia
(increased risk of retinal damage due to lack of lenses)
Cardiovascular disease, severe
(because of the potential heat stress or the prolonged standing associated with each UVA treatment, patients with this problem should be carefully monitored and, if possible, not treated in a vertical UVA chamber)
» Cataracts
Gastrointestinal diseases
Hepatic function impairment
(metabolism may be impaired)
Infection, chronic
Sensitivity to methoxsalen
» Skin cancer, history of
Sunlight allergy, or family history of
(PUVA may cause photoallergic contact dermatitis or precipitate sunlight allergy)
» Caution should be used also in evaluating for treatment and subsequently treating patients with a history of having taken arsenicals or having received x-rays, cytotoxic therapy, or coal tar and ultraviolet light B (UVB) therapy because of the increased risk of skin cancer

## Patient monitoring
The following may be especially important in patient monitoring (other tests may be warranted in some patients, depending on condition; » = major clinical significance):

Antinuclear antibodies test and
Complete blood count and
Hepatic function tests and
Renal function tests
(recommended prior to initiation of therapy)
Monitoring for melanoma and other skin carcinomas
(recommended in patients receiving methoxsalen for prolonged periods, since long-term safety has not been established)
Ophthalmic examination
(recommended prior to initiation of therapy and yearly thereafter during therapy)

# Side/Adverse Effects

Note: Cataracts have been reported with psoralen use; however, risk is very low in patients who wear UVA-absorbing, wraparound sunglasses when exposed to sunlight or ultraviolet light during the 24 hours after taking methoxsalen.

There is an increased risk of skin cancer with psoralen use. This risk appears to be greatest in patients with predisposing risk factors, such as fair skin or a hypersensitivity to sunlight; a history of skin cancer, exposure to ionizing radiation, or excessive exposure to sunlight; or a history of treatment with tar and UVB (prolonged), arsenicals, or topical nitrogen mustard.

Premature aging of the skin may occur as a result of prolonged PUVA therapy. This effect is permanent and is similar to the results of excessive exposure to sunlight.

Toxic hepatitis has been reported in patients treated with methoxsalen, but the relationship to the medication is not clear.

The following side/adverse effects have been selected on the basis of their potential clinical significance (possible signs and symptoms in parentheses where appropriate)—not necessarily inclusive:

## Those indicating need for medical attention
Symptoms of overdose or overexposure to ultraviolet light
*Blistering and peeling of skin; reddened, sore skin; swelling, especially in feet or lower legs*

## Those indicating need for medical attention only if they continue or are bothersome
Incidence more frequent
*Itching of skin; nausea*
Incidence less frequent
*Dizziness; headache; mental depression; nervousness; trouble in sleeping*

# Overdose

For more information on the management of overdose or unintentional ingestion, **contact a Poison Control Center** (see *Poison Control Center Listing*).

## Clinical effects of overdose
The following effects have been selected on the basis of their potential clinical significance (possible signs and symptoms in parentheses where appropriate)—not necessarily inclusive:

*Blistering and peeling of skin; reddened, sore skin; swelling, especially in feet or lower legs*

### Treatment of overdose
To decrease absorption—
  Inducing emesis, if it can be accomplished within the first 2 to 3 hours after ingestion, since maximum blood levels are reached by that time.
Specific treatment—
  For overdosage of methoxsalen: Keeping patient in a darkened room for at least 24 hours following methoxsalen ingestion to prevent the possibility of sun exposure and subsequent burn injury.
  For overexposure to sunlight or ultraviolet light: Keeping patient in a darkened room for at least 24 hours following ingestion of methoxsalen to prevent the possibility of further sun exposure and subsequent burn injury while assessment of the extent of damage is made.
Monitoring—
  Observing patient for erythema greater than Grade 2 (Grade 2 being marked erythema with no edema) occurring within 24 hours, which may signal the beginning of a potentially serious burn, since peak erythemal reaction to PUVA usually occurs approximately 48 hours following methoxsalen ingestion.
Supportive Care—
  Treating patient symptomatically for burns, depending on their extent and severity.

## Patient Consultation
As an aid to patient consultation, refer to *Advice for the Patient, Methoxsalen (Systemic)*.
In providing consultation, consider emphasizing the following selected information (» = major clinical significance):

### Before using this medication
» Conditions affecting use, especially:
  Sensitivity to methoxsalen
  Diet—Avoiding eating furocoumarin-containing foods (limes, figs, parsley, parsnips, mustard, carrots, celery)
  Other medical problems, especially acute lupus erythematosus; albinism; aphakia; cataracts; hydroa; leukoderma of infectious origin; porphyria; xeroderma pigmentosum; history of skin cancer; history of having taken arsenicals; history of having received x-rays, cytotoxic therapy, or coal tar and ultraviolet light B (UVB) therapy
  Not using for suntanning purposes

### Proper use of this medication
Usually comes with patient instructions; reading carefully before using medication
» May take 6 to 8 weeks to work; importance of not increasing the dosage of medication or exposure to ultraviolet light because of the risk of serious burns
The hard capsule dosage form may be taken with food or milk (the soft capsule dosage form may be taken with low-fat food or low-fat milk) to reduce gastrointestinal irritation
» Proper dosing
  Late or missed dose: Notifying physician for rescheduling of light treatment
» Proper storage

### Precautions while using this medication
Importance of regular visits to physician to have progress checked, including eye examinations
» Protecting skin from sunlight, even through window glass or on cloudy days, for at least 24 hours before and 8 hours following treatment; protecting lips with sun block lipstick that has a skin protection factor (SPF) of at least 15
  Possibility of continued skin sensitivity to sunlight because of medication; using extra precautions for at least 48 hours following each treatment; not sunbathing anytime during course of treatment
» Wearing special sunglasses during daylight hours (even in indirect light, such as through window glass or on cloudy days) for 24 hours following each dose of medication
» Possibility of dry skin or itching; checking with physician before treating
» Possible long-term effects (cataracts, premature skin aging, carcinogenesis)

### Side/adverse effects
Slight reddening of skin 24 to 48 hours after treatment is normal response to therapy
There is an increased risk of developing skin cancer. The body should be examined regularly and the physician shown skin sores that do not heal, new skin growths, and skin growths that have changed in appearance or feel
Premature aging of the skin may occur as a result of prolonged PUVA therapy. This effect is permanent and is similar to the results of excessive exposure to sunlight
Signs of potential side effects, especially blistering and peeling of skin; reddened, sore skin; swelling, especially in feet or lower legs
Note: Some side effects are more likely to occur in children.

## General Dosing Information
Patients receiving methoxsalen should be under the supervision of a physician experienced in PUVA therapy.

Although dosage of methoxsalen is generally based on body weight, usually no change in dose is necessary if the patient's weight changes. However, if the physician believes the weight change to be significant enough to warrant an alteration, adjustment of UVA exposure time should be made instead of adjustment of methoxsalen dosage.

Exposure to sunlight or ultraviolet light should be carefully controlled and adjusted on an individual basis according to skin type and tolerance. Exposure time to sunlight should be reduced at high altitudes or at midday.

Skin should be protected from sunlight, even through window glass or on a cloudy day, for at least 24 hours before and 8 hours following oral PUVA treatment by protective clothing, such as long-sleeved shirts, full-length slacks, wide-brimmed hat, and gloves and by using a sun block product that has a skin protection factor of at least 15 on body areas that cannot be covered by clothing. In addition, lips should be protected with a sun block lipstick that has a skin protection factor of at least 15. Also, since the skin continues to be sensitive to sunlight for some time after treatment, the patient should avoid overexposure to sunlight for 48 hours following administration of methoxsalen. In addition, the patient should not sunbathe anytime during the course of treatment.

If a scheduled treatment is missed, the dose of UVA at the next treatment should not be increased; if more than one treatment is missed, the subsequent dose of UVA should be reduced in proportion to the number of treatments missed to reduce the risk of painful erythema.

Repigmentation occurs most rapidly on fleshy areas (face, abdomen, buttocks) and more slowly on the extremities and bony areas (hands and feet).

Tolerance to the effects of methoxsalen may occur when pigmentation precedes erythema by a long period of time. Hyperpigmentation reduces subsequent responsiveness.

Use of psoralen derivatives to promote suntanning has resulted in serious reactions, including acute generalized dermatitis, blistering, and edema; residual edema of the legs and cutaneous damage have been reported.

### For skin intolerance to sunlight
Treatment should be limited to 14 days, since methoxsalen's effect to stimulate any new pigment production will have been accomplished by that time.

### For treatment of psoriasis
Some clinicians recommend an increased dose in the treatment of psoriasis if there is no response after 15 treatments at the recommended dose. A lower-than-recommended dose eventually may produce the same effect, but it usually occurs more slowly.

Lack of response in psoriasis may be associated with a general phototoxic reaction; this may be confirmed by temporary withdrawal for 2 weeks, with subsequent improvement in the condition. If improvement does not occur, treatment with methoxsalen is considered to be a failure.

Patients with pre-existing erythrodermic psoriasis require special care because the erythema may obscure a possible treatment-related phototoxic erythema. These patients should be treated similar to patients with sun-sensitive skin types.

### Diet/Nutrition
Methoxsalen hard gelatin capsules may be taken with food or milk (the soft gelatin capsules may be taken with low-fat food or low-fat milk) to reduce gastrointestinal irritation, or the dose may be split in two and the two halves taken one-half hour apart.

### Bioequivalenence information
Methoxsalen soft gelatin capsules should not be used interchangeably with the hard gelatin capsules, since the soft gelatin capsule dosage form exhibits significantly greater bioavailability and earlier photosensitization onset time than does the hard gelatin capsule dosage form.

### For treatment of adverse effects
Recommended treatment consists of the following:
• Burning or blistering of skin—Temporary withdrawal of therapy is recommended.
• Hepatic function impairment—Reduction in dosage or withdrawal of methoxsalen therapy.

## Oral Dosage Forms

Note: Bracketed uses in the *Dosage Forms* section refer to categories of use and/or indications that are not included in U.S. product labeling.

### METHOXSALEN CAPSULES (XXI) (HARD GELATIN) USP

**Usual adult and adolescent dose**
[Dermatitis, atopic] or
Psoriasis or
Mycosis fungoides[1]—
 Oral, 600 mcg (0.6 mg) per kg of body weight, two hours before measured periods of high-intensity UVA exposure, two or three times a week or as determined by the patient's schedule for UVA exposures (at least forty-eight hours apart). Dose may be increased by 10 mg after the fifteenth treatment, according to directions in the manufacturer's labeling. Exposure time should be based on skin type and response to therapy, according to the manufacturer's directions for the specific light source being used. Frequency of exposure may be gradually reduced for maintenance treatment; UVA exposure may be adjusted according to response.

Note: A commonly used dosage schedule according to weight is:

| Weight (kg) | Dose (mg) |
|---|---|
| < 30 | 10 |
| 30–50 | 20 |
| 51–65 | 30 |
| 66–80 | 40 |
| 81–90 | 50 |
| 91–115 | 60 |
| > 115 | 70 |

Vitiligo—
 Oral, 20 mg a day, two to four hours before measured periods of UVA exposure, two or three times a week (at least forty-eight hours apart).
 Sunlight—Initial exposure time should not exceed fifteen minutes for light skin colors, twenty minutes for medium skin colors, or twenty-five minutes for dark skin colors; may subsequently be increased five minutes each treatment, based on erythema and tenderness.
 Artificial light—Initial exposure time should not exceed one-half of that producing erythema after sunlight exposure, or should be based on the minimal phototoxic dose (MPD) and manufacturer's directions for the specific light source being used. The MPD can be determined by irradiating several areas of skin 2 cm in diameter; a range of light exposure times is used and the time that produces erythema at seventy-two hours after exposure is the MPD.

[Skin intolerance to sunlight]—
 Orally, 20 mg a day one hour before measured exposure to sunlight or to ultraviolet A light, for up to fourteen days.
 Sunlight—Initial exposure time should not exceed fifteen minutes for light skin colors, twenty minutes for medium skin colors, or twenty-five minutes for dark skin colors; subsequently may be increased by five minutes for each treatment, depending on degree of erythema and tenderness.

Note: A commonly used dosage schedule according to weight is:

| Weight (kg) | Dose (mg) |
|---|---|
| < 30 | 10 |
| 30–50 | 20 |
| 51–65 | 30 |
| 66–80 | 40 |
| 81–90 | 50 |

**Usual pediatric dose**
Children up to 12 years of age—Dosage has not been established.
Children 12 years of age and over—See *Usual adult and adolescent dose*.

**Strength(s) usually available**
U.S.—
 10 mg (Rx) [*8-MOP* (tartrazine)].
Canada—
 10 mg (Rx) [*Oxsoralen*].

**Packaging and storage**
Store below 40 °C (104 °F), preferably between 15 and 30 °C (59 and 86 °F) unless otherwise specified by manufacturer. Store in a tight, light-resistant container.

**Auxiliary labeling**
• Take with food or milk.

**Note**
Methoxsalen soft gelatin capsules should not be used interchangeably with the hard gelatin capsules.

### METHOXSALEN CAPSULES (XXII) (SOFT GELATIN) USP

**Usual adult and adolescent dose**
[Dermatitis, atopic] or
Psoriasis—
 Oral, 400 mcg (0.4 mg) per kg of body weight, one and one-half to two hours before measured periods of high-intensity UVA exposure, two or three times a week or as determined by the patient's schedule for UVA exposures (at least forty-eight hours apart). Exposure time should be based on skin type and response to therapy, according to the manufacturer's directions for the specific light source being used. Frequency of exposure may be gradually reduced for maintenance treatment; UVA exposure may be adjusted according to response.

Note: **The soft capsule dosage form exhibits significantly greater bioavailability and earlier photosensitization onset time than the hard capsule dosage form.** When this dosage form is used, the patient's minimum phototoxic dose (MPD) and phototoxic peak time after drug administration should be determined prior to initiation of photochemotherapy. The manufacturer's directions should be consulted for full information concerning dosage and administration.

[Skin intolerance to sunlight]—
 Orally, 20 mg a day one hour before measured exposure to sunlight or to ultraviolet A light, for up to fourteen days.
 Sunlight—Initial exposure time should not exceed fifteen minutes for light skin colors, twenty minutes for medium skin colors, or twenty-five minutes for dark skin colors; subsequently may be increased by five minutes for each treatment, depending on degree of erythema and tenderness.

Note: A commonly used dosage schedule according to weight is:

| Weight (kg) | Dose (mg) |
|---|---|
| < 30 | 10 |
| 30–50 | 20 |
| 51–65 | 30 |
| 66–80 | 40 |
| 81–90 | 50 |

[Vitiligo]—
 Oral, 20 mg a day, one hour before measured periods of ultraviolet light exposure or black fluorescent light, two or three times a week (at least forty-eight hours apart).
 Sunlight—Initial exposure time should not exceed fifteen minutes for light skin colors, twenty minutes for medium skin colors, or twenty-five minutes for dark skin colors; subsequently may be increased five minutes each treatment, based on degree of erythema and tenderness.
 Artificial light—Initial exposure time should not exceed one half of that producing erythema after sunlight exposure, or should be based on the minimal phototoxic dose (MPD) and manufacturer's directions for the specific light source being used. The MPD can be determined by irradiating several areas of skin 2 cm in diameter; a range of light exposure times is used and the time that produces erythema at seventy-two hours after exposure is the MPD.

**Usual pediatric dose**
Children up to 12 years of age—Dosage has not been established.
Children 12 years of age and over—See *Usual adult and adolescent dose*.

**Strength(s) usually available**
U.S.—
 10 mg (Rx) [*Oxsoralen-Ultra*].
Canada—
 10 mg (Rx) [*Ultra MOP*; *Oxsoralen-Ultra*].

**Packaging and storage**
Store below 40 °C (104 °F), preferably between 15 and 30 °C (59 and 86 °F), in a tight container, unless otherwise specified by manufacturer. Protect from light.

**Auxiliary labeling**
• Take with low-fat food or milk.

**Note**
Methoxsalen soft gelatin capsules should not be used interchangeably with the hard gelatin capsules.

[1] Not included in Canadian product labeling.

Revised: 06/24/94
Interim revision: 07/08/98

# METHOXSALEN Topical

VA CLASSIFICATION (Primary/Secondary): DE900/DE802
Commonly used brand name(s): *Oxsoralen Lotion; UltraMOP Lotion.*
Note: For a listing of dosage forms and brand names by country availability, see *Dosage Forms* section(s).

## Category
Repigmenting agent (topical); hair growth stimulant, alopecia areata (topical); antipsoriatic (topical).
Note: Methoxsalen is used in conjunction with ultraviolet light A (UVA). This mode of treatment is known as PUVA (psoralen plus ultraviolet light A).

## Indications
Note: Bracketed information in the *Indications* section refers to uses that are not included in U.S. product labeling.

**Accepted**
Vitiligo (treatment)—PUVA is indicated for repigmentation in the treatment of vitiligo. It is not effective in producing pigmentation in leukoderma of infectious origin or in albinism.
[Skin, increased tolerance to sunlight][1]—PUVA has been used to increase skin tolerance to sunlight.
[Psoriasis (treatment)]—PUVA has been used in the treatment of severe psoriasis that has not responded to other therapy.
[Mycosis fungoides (treatment)][1]—PUVA is used in the treatment of mycosis fungoides.
[Alopecia areata (treatment)][1]
[Dermatoses, inflammatory (treatment)][1]
[Eczema (treatment)][1] or
[Lichen planus (treatment)][1]—PUVA is used in the treatment of alopecia areata, inflammatory dermatoses, eczema, and lichen planus.

**Unaccepted**
The unsupervised use of methoxsalen to promote tanning is dangerous and should be discouraged.

[1] Not included in Canadian product labeling.

## Pharmacology/Pharmacokinetics

**Physicochemical characteristics**
Chemical group—Psoralen derivative.
Molecular weight—216.19.

**Mechanism of action/Effect**
Exact mechanism of erythemogenic, melanogenic, and cytotoxic response in the epidermis is unknown, but may involve increased tyrosinase activity in melanin-producing cells, as well as inhibition of DNA synthesis, cell division, and epidermal turnover. Successful pigmentation requires the presence of functioning melanocytes.

**Absorption**
Extent of systemic absorption is unknown.

**Biotransformation**
Activated by long-wavelength UVA in the range of 320 to 400 (maximal effect at 365) nanometers (nm).

**Onset of action**
Vitiligo—Up to 6 months.
For increased sensitivity of skin to sunlight—1 hour.
Tanning—Within a few days.

**Time to peak effect**
Increased sensitivity of skin to sunlight—2 hours (peak erythematous response may not occur for 2 days).

**Duration of action**
Increased sensitivity of skin to sunlight—Several days.

## Precautions to Consider

**Carcinogenicity**
Psoralens have been found to augment UVA-induced carcinogenicity in laboratory animals. In addition, studies in humans treated with systemic methoxsalen plus UVA have shown an increase in the risk of squamous cell carcinoma. The possibility of increased risk may exist also for topical methoxsalen and systemic trioxsalen. This risk appears to be greatest in patients with predisposing risk factors, such as fair skin or a hypersensitivity to sunlight; a history of skin cancer, exposure to ionizing radiation, or excessive exposure to sunlight; or a history of treatment with tar and UVB (prolonged), arsenicals, or topical nitrogen mustard.

**Pregnancy/Reproduction**
Pregnancy—Studies have not been done in humans.
Studies have not been done in animals.
FDA Pregnancy Category C.

**Breast-feeding**
It is not known whether topical methoxsalen is distributed into breast milk. However, problems in humans have not been documented.

**Pediatrics**
Appropriate studies on the relationship of age to the effects of topical methoxsalen have not been performed in children up to 12 years of age. Safety and efficacy have not been established.

**Geriatrics**
Appropriate studies on the relationship of age to the effects of topical methoxsalen have not been performed in the geriatric population. However, no geriatrics-specific problems have been documented to date.

**Drug interactions and/or related problems**
The following drug interactions and/or related problems have been selected on the basis of their potential clinical significance (possible mechanism in parentheses where appropriate)—not necessarily inclusive (» = major clinical significance):

Note: Combinations containing any of the following medications, depending on the amount present, may also interact with this medication.

Furocoumarin-containing foods, such as limes, figs, parsley, parsnips, mustard, carrots, and celery
(although there have been no reports of serious reactions, caution and avoidance of these foods are recommended because of the risk of additive phototoxicity)

Photosensitizing medications, other
(concurrent use of methoxsalen with other photosensitizing medications, systemic or topical, may cause additive photosensitizing effects; concurrent use with coal tar or coal tar derivatives or with trioxsalen is not recommended)

**Laboratory value alterations**
The following have been selected on the basis of their potential clinical significance (possible effect in parentheses where appropriate)—not necessarily inclusive (» = major clinical significance):

With physiology/laboratory test values
Liver function tests
(Abnormal liver function tests have been reported, but the relationship to the medication is not clear)

**Medical considerations/Contraindications**
The medical considerations/contraindications included have been selected on the basis of their potential clinical significance (reasons given in parentheses where appropriate)—not necessarily inclusive (» = major clinical significance).

*Risk-benefit should be considered when the following medical problems exist:*

» Albinism or
» Hydroa or
» Leukoderma of infectious origin or
» Lupus erythematosus, acute or
» Polymorphic light eruptions or
» Porphyria or
» Xeroderma pigmentosum
(these conditions are associated with photosensitization)

Cardiovascular disease, severe
(because of the potential heat stress or the prolonged standing associated with each UVA treatment, patients with severe cardiovascular disease should be carefully monitored and if possible not be treated in a vertical UVA chamber)

Infection, chronic

Sensitivity to methoxsalen

» Skin cancer, history of

Sunlight allergy, or family history of
(PUVA may cause photoallergic contact dermatitis or precipitate sunlight allergy)

» Caution should be used in evaluating for treatment and subsequently treating patients with a history of having taken arsenicals or having received x-rays, cytotoxic therapy, or coal tar and ultraviolet light B (UVB) therapy because of the increased risk of skin cancer.

**Patient monitoring**

The following may be especially important in patient monitoring (other tests may be warranted in some patients, depending on condition; » = major clinical significance):

Monitoring for melanoma and other skin carcinomas (recommended in patients receiving methoxsalen for prolonged periods, since long-term safety has not been established)

## Side/Adverse Effects

Note: There is an increased risk of skin cancer with systemic methoxsalen plus UVA. The possibility of increased risk may exist also with topical methoxsalen. This risk appears to be greatest in patients with predisposing risk factors, such as fair skin or a hypersensitivity to sunlight; a history of skin cancer, exposure to ionizing radiation, or excessive exposure to sunlight; or a history of treatment with tar and UVB (prolonged), arsenicals, or topical nitrogen mustard.

Premature aging of the skin may occur as a result of prolonged treatment with systemic methoxsalen plus UVA. The possibility of risk may exist also with topical methoxsalen. This effect is permanent and is similar to the results of excessive exposure to sunlight.

The following effects have been selected on the basis of their potential clinical significance (possible signs and symptoms in parentheses where appropriate)—not necessarily inclusive:

**Those indicating need for medical attention**

Symptoms of overdose or overexposure to ultraviolet light

*Blistering and peeling of skin; reddened, sore skin; swelling, especially in feet or lower legs*

## Overdose

For more information on the management of overdose or unintentional ingestion, **contact a Poison Control Center** (see *Poison Control Center Listing*).

**Clinical effects of overdose**

The following effects have been selected on the basis of their potential clinical significance (possible signs and symptoms in parentheses where appropriate)—not necessarily inclusive:

*Blistering and peeling of skin; reddened, sore skin; swelling, especially in feet or lower legs*

**Treatment of overdose**

To decrease absorption—
Inducing emesis.

Specific treatment—
For ingestion of topical methoxsalen solution: Keeping patient in a darkened room for at least 24 hours following methoxsalen ingestion to prevent the possibility of sun exposure and subsequent burn injury.

For overexposure to sunlight or ultraviolet light: Keeping patient in a darkened room for at least 24 hours following ingestion of methoxsalen to prevent the possibility of further sun exposure and subsequent burn injury while assessment of the extent of damage is made. With topical methoxsalen, erythema may not begin for several hours following overexposure and may not peak for 2 or 3 days or longer.

Supportive care—
Treating patient symptomatically for burns, depending on their extent and severity. Patients in whom intentional overdose is known or suspected should be referred for psychiatric consultation.

## Patient Consultation

As an aid to patient consultation, refer to *Advice for the Patient, Methoxsalen (Topical)*.

In providing consultation, consider emphasizing the following selected information (» = major clinical significance):

**Before using this medication**

» Conditions affecting use, especially:
Sensitivity to methoxsalen
Carcinogenicity—Possibility of increased risk of squamous cell carcinoma, especially in patients with predisposing risk factors such as fair skin and those with increased sensitivity to sunlight
Use in children—Not recommended for use in children up to 12 years of age

Diet—Avoiding eating furocoumarin-containing foods (limes, figs, parsley, parsnips, mustard, carrots, celery)

Other medical problems, especially acute lupus erythematosus; albinism; hydroa; leukoderma of infectious origin; polymorphic light eruptions; porphyria; xeroderma pigmentosum; history of skin cancer; history of having taken arsenicals; history of having received x-rays, cytotoxic therapy, or coal tar and ultraviolet light B (UVB) therapy

**Proper use of this medication**

Using medication only under the direct supervision of the physician
» Proper dosing

**Precautions while using this medication**

Importance of regular visits to physician for treatments and to have progress checked

» Protecting skin from sunlight, even through window glass or on a cloudy day, for at least 12 to 48 hours following treatment; washing treated areas after light treatment

Possibility of continued skin sensitivity to sunlight because of medication; using extra precautions for at least 72 hours following each treatment; not sunbathing anytime during course of treatment

» Possibility of dry skin or itching; checking with physician before treating

**Side/adverse effects**

There is an increased risk of developing skin cancer when treated with systemic methoxsalen. The possibility of increased risk may exist also with topical methoxsalen. The treated areas should be examined regularly and the physician shown skin sores that do not heal, new skin growths, and skin growths that have changed in appearance or feel.

Premature aging of the skin may occur as a result of prolonged treatment with systemic methoxsalen. The possibility of risk may exist also with topical methoxsalen. This effect is permanent and is similar to the results of excessive exposure to sunlight.

Signs of potential side effects, especially symptoms of overdose or overexposure to ultraviolet light

## General Dosing Information

Topical application should be performed only by or under the direct supervision of a physician familiar with the use of PUVA therapy.

Topical application causes a greater and less predictable photosensitizing response than does oral administration.

It is recommended that methoxsalen be applied only to small, well-defined lesions (less than 10 square cm) and that it be removed from the skin following exposure to sunlight or ultraviolet light.

Exposure to sunlight or ultraviolet light should be carefully controlled and adjusted on an individual basis according to skin type and tolerance. Exposure time to sunlight should be reduced at high altitudes or at midday.

Because topical application results in a higher concentration of methoxsalen in the epidermis than does oral administration, the dose of UVA is generally lower with topical application.

Following topical administration of methoxsalen, the treated skin should be protected from sunlight, even through window glass or on a cloudy day, for at least 12 to 48 hours by protective clothing or a sun block product that has a protection factor of at least 15. Furthermore, since the treated skin continues to be sensitive to sunlight for some time after treatment, the patient should avoid overexposure to sunlight for 72 hours following application of methoxsalen. In addition, the patient should not sunbathe anytime during the course of treatment.

Pigmentation may begin after a few weeks of treatment, but significant repigmentation may require 6 to 9 months. Periodic retreatment may be necessary to retain all of the new pigment. Repigmentation occurs most rapidly and is more predictable on fleshy areas (face, abdomen, buttocks) and occurs more slowly and is less effective on the extremities and bony areas (hands and feet).

Tolerance to the effects of methoxsalen may occur when pigmentation precedes erythema by a long period of time. Hyperpigmentation reduces subsequent responsiveness.

Use of psoralen derivatives to promote suntanning has resulted in serious reactions, including acute generalized dermatitis, blistering, and edema; residual edema of the legs and cutaneous damage have been reported.

Temporary withdrawal of therapy is recommended if burning or blistering of skin occurs.

Dilution to a strength of 1:1000 or 1:10,000 is sometimes necessary to avoid serious reactions.

## Topical Dosage Forms

### METHOXSALEN TOPICAL SOLUTION USP

**Usual adult and adolescent dose**
Repigmenting agent (topical)—
  The topical solution should be applied to a small, well-defined vitiliginous lesion, allowed to dry for one to two minutes, then reapplied. This is done two to two and one-half hours before measured periods of UVA exposure. Following exposure, the lesions should be washed with soap and water and protected with an opaque sunscreen.
  Sunlight—Initial exposure time should not exceed one minute and should be increased subsequently with caution.
  Artificial light—Initial exposure time should not exceed one-half of the time that produces erythema after sunlight exposure, or should be based on the minimal phototoxic dose (MPD) and manufacturer's directions for the specific light source being used. The MPD can be determined by irradiating several areas of skin 2 cm in diameter; a range of light-exposure times is used and the time that produces erythema at seventy-two hours after exposure is the MPD.
Note: The manufacturer recommends once-weekly treatment; however, some clinicians recommend treatment every three to five days.

**Usual pediatric dose**
Repigmenting agent (topical)—
  Children up to 12 years of age: Dosage has not been established.
  Children 12 years of age and over: See *Usual adult and adolescent dose*.

**Strength(s) usually available**
U.S.—
  1% (Rx) [*Oxsoralen Lotion* (alcohol 71%; acetone)].
Canada—
  1% (Rx) [*Oxsoralen Lotion*; *UltraMOP Lotion*].

**Packaging and storage**
Store below 40 °C (104 °F), preferably between 15 and 30 °C (59 and 86 °F), unless otherwise specified by manufacturer. Store in a tight, light-resistant container. Protect from freezing.

**Note**
Do not dispense to the patient for use at home.

Revised: 05/26/94

---

**METHOXYFLURANE**—See *Anesthetics, Inhalation (Systemic)*

---

**METHSCOPOLAMINE**—See *Anticholinergics/Antispasmodics (Systemic)*

---

**METHYCLOTHIAZIDE**—See *Diuretics, Thiazide (Systemic)*

---

**METHYLCELLULOSE**—See *Laxatives (Local)*

---

# METHYLDOPA  Systemic

VA CLASSIFICATION (Primary): CV409

Commonly used brand name(s): *Aldomet*; *Apo-Methyldopa*; *Dopamet*; *Novomedopa*; *Nu-Medopa*.

Note: For a listing of dosage forms and brand names by country availability, see *Dosage Forms* section(s).

## Category
Antihypertensive.

## Indications

**Accepted**
Hypertension (treatment)—Methyldopa is indicated in the treatment of moderate to severe hypertension, including that complicated by renal disease.
  Methyldopate may be used intravenously in the treatment of hypertensive crises. However, because of its slow onset of action, methyldopate is generally not recommended as sole initial therapy in hypertensive crises.

## Pharmacology/Pharmacokinetics

**Physicochemical characteristics**
Molecular weight—Methyldopa: 238.24.
Methyldopate hydrochloride: 275.73.

**Mechanism of action/Effect**
The exact mechanism of antihypertensive action has not been conclusively demonstrated. However, the major antihypertensive effect appears to result from conversion to alpha-methylnorepinephrine, a potent alpha-2 adrenergic agonist. Alpha-methylnorepinephrine acts centrally to stimulate alpha receptors. This results in a decrease in sympathetic outflow and decreased blood pressure.

**Absorption**
Absorption of methyldopa from the gastrointestinal tract is variable but averages approximately 50%.

**Protein binding**
Methyldopa—Low (less than 20%).
Sulfate conjugate—Moderate.

**Biotransformation**
Extensive.
Converted to alpha-methylnorepinephrine in central adrenergic neurons; methyldopate hydrochloride is hydrolyzed to methyldopa.
Hepatic; sulfate conjugation occurs to a greater extent after oral than after intravenous administration.

**Half-life**
Normal—Alpha: 1.7 hours.
Anuric—Alpha: 3.6 hours.

**Time to peak effect**
Single dose—4 to 6 hours.
Multiple doses—2 to 3 days.

**Duration of action**
Variable.
Oral—
  Single dose—12 to 24 hours.
  Multiple doses—24 to 48 hours.
Intravenous—
  10 to 16 hours.

**Elimination**
Renal; approximately 70% of absorbed drug is excreted in urine as methyldopa and its mono-0-sulfate metabolite. Unabsorbed oral methyldopa is excreted unchanged in the feces.
In dialysis—Methyldopa is removable by both hemodialysis and peritoneal dialysis.

## Precautions to Consider

**Cross-sensitivity and/or related problems**
Patients sensitive to sulfites may be sensitive to some methyldopa products because of the sulfite preservatives present.

**Tumorigenicity**
No evidence of a tumorigenic effect was seen in mice given doses up to 1800 mg per kg of body weight (mg/kg) per day (30 times the maximum recommended human dose) for 2 years or in rats given doses up to 240 mg/kg per day (4 times the maximum recommended human dose) for 2 years.

**Mutagenicity**
Methyldopa was not mutagenic in the Ames test with or without metabolic activation. There was no increase in chromosomal aberration or sister chromatid exchanges in Chinese hamster ovary cells.

## Pregnancy/Reproduction
Fertility—Methyldopa did not affect fertility in male and female rats given doses of 100 mg/kg per day (1.7 times the maximum daily human dose). However, at doses of 200 mg/kg and 400 mg/kg per day (3.3 and 6.7 times the maximum daily human dose) methyldopa decreased sperm count, sperm motility, the number of late spermatids, and the male fertility index.

Pregnancy—Methyldopa crosses the placenta. Adequate and well-controlled studies of methyldopa use in pregnant women during the first and second trimesters have not been done. Studies of methyldopa use in pregnant women during the third trimester have not been associated with adverse effects.

Studies in rabbits at doses of 200 mg/kg per day (3.3 times the maximum daily human dose), mice at doses of 1000 mg/kg per day (16.6 times the maximum daily human dose), and rats at doses of 100 mg/kg per day (1.7 times the maximum daily human dose) showed no adverse effects.

FDA Pregnancy Category B.

## Breast-feeding
Methyldopa is distributed into breast milk. However, problems in humans have not been documented.

## Pediatrics
Appropriate studies on the relationship of age to the effects of methyldopa have not been performed in the pediatric population. However, pediatrics-specific problems that would limit the usefulness of this medication in children are not expected.

## Geriatrics
Although appropriate studies on the relationship of age to the effects of methyldopa have not been performed in the geriatric population, the elderly may be more sensitive to the hypotensive and sedative effects. In addition, elderly patients are more likely to have age-related renal function impairment, which may require lower doses in patients receiving methyldopa.

## Dental
Use of methyldopa may decrease or inhibit salivary flow, thus contributing to the development of caries, periodontal disease, oral candidiasis, and discomfort.

## Drug interactions and/or related problems
The following drug interactions and/or related problems have been selected on the basis of their potential clinical significance (possible mechanism in parentheses where appropriate)—not necessarily inclusive (» = major clinical significance):

Note: Combinations containing any of the following medications, depending on the amount present, may also interact with this medication.

Alcohol or
Central nervous system (CNS) depression–producing medications (See *Appendix II*)
(concurrent use may enhance the CNS depressant effects of either these medications or methyldopa)

Anticoagulants, coumarin- or indandione-derivative
(concurrent use with methyldopa may increase the anticoagulant effect of these medications; adjustment of anticoagulant dosage based on prothrombin-time determinations is recommended)

Antidepressants, tricyclic
(may reduce antihypertensive effects of methyldopa; the patient should be carefully monitored to confirm that the desired effect is being obtained)

Anti-inflammatory drugs, nonsteroidal (NSAIDs), especially indomethacin
(antihypertensive effects of methyldopa may be reduced when it is used concurrently with these medications; indomethacin, and possibly other NSAIDs, may antagonize the antihypertensive effect by inhibiting renal prostaglandin synthesis and/or by causing sodium and fluid retention; the patient should be carefully monitored to confirm that the desired effect is being obtained)

Appetite suppressants, with the exception of fenfluramine
(concurrent use may decrease the hypotensive effects of methyldopa)

Bromocriptine
(methyldopa may increase serum prolactin concentrations and interfere with effects of bromocriptine; dosage adjustment of bromocriptine may be necessary)

Fenfluramine
(concurrent use may increase the hypotensive effects of methyldopa)

Haloperidol
(concurrent use of haloperidol with methyldopa may cause unwanted mental effects such as disorientation and slowed or difficult thought process)

Hypotension-producing medications, other (See *Appendix II*)
(hypotensive effects may be potentiated when these medications are used concurrently with methyldopa; although some antihypertensive and/or diuretic combinations are frequently used for therapeutic advantage, dosage adjustments may be necessary during concurrent use)

Levodopa
(concurrent use with methyldopa may alter the antiparkinsonian effects of levodopa and may also produce additive toxic CNS effects such as psychosis)

Lithium
(concurrent use with methyldopa may increase the risk of lithium toxicity, even though serum lithium concentrations remain within the recommended therapeutic range)

» Monoamine oxidase (MAO) inhibitors, including furazolidone, procarbazine, and selegiline
(methyldopa may cause hyperexcitability in patients receiving MAO inhibitors; headache, severe hypertension, and hallucinations have been reported)

Sympathomimetics, such as:
» Cocaine
  Dobutamine
  Dopamine
  Ephedrine
  Epinephrine
  Mephentermine
  Metaraminol
  Methoxamine
» Norepinephrine
» Phenylephrine or
  Phenylpropanolamine
(concurrent use with sympathomimetic pressor amines may decrease the hypotensive effect of methyldopa and potentiate the pressor effect of these medications; if concurrent use of cocaine, norepinephrine, or phenylephrine is indicated, caution is required, and only very small initial doses should be administered)

## Laboratory value alterations
The following have been selected on the basis of their potential clinical significance (possible effect in parentheses where appropriate)—not necessarily inclusive (» = major clinical significance):

With diagnostic test results
Aspartate aminotransferase (AST [SGOT]) measurement, serum, using colorimetric methods
(methyldopa may interfere with measurement of AST)

Creatinine measurement, serum, using the alkaline picrate method
(methyldopa may interfere with measurement of serum creatinine)

Urinary catecholamine measurement
(methyldopa may produce falsely elevated results since it causes fluorescence at the same wavelengths as catecholamines; methyldopa does not interfere with urinary vanillylmandelic acid [VMA] determinations)

Urinary uric acid measurement, using the phosphotungstate method
(methyldopa may interfere with measurement of urinary uric acid)

With physiology/laboratory test values
Alanine aminotransferase (ALT [SGPT]) and
Alkaline phosphatase and
Aspartate aminotransferase (AST [SGOT]) and
Bilirubin
(serum concentrations may be increased, indicating possible hepatotoxicity)

Blood urea nitrogen (BUN) and
Potassium and sodium, serum and
Prolactin, serum and
Uric acid, serum
(concentrations may be increased)

Positive direct antiglobulin (Coombs') tests
(may be produced in 10 to 20% of patients on prolonged methyldopa therapy and usually occur after 6 to 12 months of therapy; rarely, these are associated with hemolytic anemia; the positive Coombs' test may not revert to normal until weeks or months after methyldopa is discontinued; less frequently, a positive indirect Coombs' test may occur, which may interfere with crossmatching of blood; lowest incidence is with daily doses of 1 gram or less)

Prothrombin time
  (may be prolonged indicating possible hepatotoxicity)

**Medical considerations/Contraindications**
The medical considerations/Contraindications included have been selected on the basis of their potential clinical significance (reasons given in parentheses where appropriate)—not necessarily inclusive (» = major clinical significance).

*Except under special circumstances, this medication should not be used when the following medical problem exists:*
» Hepatic disease, active, such as acute hepatitis and active cirrhosis

*Risk-benefit should be considered when the following medical problems exist:*
Cerebrovascular disease, severe bilateral
  (rarely, involuntary choreoathetotic movements have been observed during methyldopa therapy)
Coronary insufficiency, including angina pectoris
  (may be aggravated)
» Hemolytic anemia, autoimmune, history of
» Hepatic disease, history of, in conjunction with past use of methyldopa
Hepatic function impairment
  (reduced biotransformation; lower doses may be required)
Mental depression, history of
Parkinson's disease
  (may be exacerbated)
» Pheochromocytoma
  (interference with tests for catecholamines; in addition, pressor responses have been reported)
Renal function impairment
  (increased sensitivity to effects of methyldopa, possibly due to accumulation of the sulfate conjugate; lower doses may be required)
Sensitivity to methyldopa

**Patient monitoring**
The following may be especially important in patient monitoring (other tests may be warranted in some patients, depending on condition; » = major clinical significance):
Antinuclear antibody (ANA) titer and
Complete blood counts and
Lupus erythematosus cell preparations
  (may be indicated if patient develops arthralgia, continued malaise, or other symptoms of systemic lupus erythematosus (SLE)–like syndrome)
Blood cell counts, including hematocrit, hemoglobin, or red cell count
  (recommended prior to initiation of therapy to establish a baseline for determination of development of hemolytic anemia; may also be required at periodic intervals during therapy)
» Blood pressure measurements
  (recommended at periodic intervals in patients being treated for hypertension; selected patients may be trained to perform blood pressure measurements at home and report the results at regular physician visits)
Direct Coombs' test
  (recommended before initiation of treatment and after 6 and 12 months of treatment)
Hepatic function determinations
  (recommended at baseline and at periodic intervals during therapy, especially during the first 6 to 12 weeks of therapy or whenever an unexplained fever occurs)

## Side/Adverse Effects

Note: Darkening of urine on exposure to air, caused by breakdown of methyldopa or its metabolites, may occur rarely.

The following side/adverse effects have been selected on the basis of their potential clinical significance (possible signs and symptoms in parentheses where appropriate)—not necessarily inclusive:

**Those indicating need for medical attention**
Incidence more frequent
  *Edema, peripheral* (swelling of feet or lower legs)
Incidence less frequent
  *Drug fever* (fever, shortly after onset of therapy); *mental status changes* (mental depression or anxiety, nightmares or unusually vivid dreams)
  Note: *Drug fever* usually occurs within the first 3 months of therapy and is sometimes accompanied by eosinophilia or hepatic function test changes. The hepatic reaction to methyldopa appears to be immunologic or hypersensitive in nature.
Incidence rare
  *Cholestasis or hepatitis and hepatocellular injury* (dark or amber urine; pale stools; yellow eyes or skin); *colitis* (severe or continuing diarrhea or stomach cramps); *hemolytic anemia, autoimmune* (continuing tiredness or weakness after having taken this medication for several weeks); *leukopenia, reversible, or granulocytopenia, reversible; myocarditis* (fever, chills, troubled breathing, and fast heartbeat); *pancreatitis* (severe stomach pain with nausea and vomiting); *systemic lupus erythematosus (SLE)–like syndrome* (general feeling of discomfort or illness or weakness; joint pain; skin rash or itching); *thrombocytopenia*
  Note: *Hemolytic anemia* occurs in less than 5% of patients showing a positive Coombs' test.
  Rarely, fatal *hepatic necrosis* has been reported.

**Those indicating need for medical attention only if they continue or are bothersome**
Incidence more frequent—more than 5%
  *Drowsiness; dryness of mouth; headache*
  Note: *Drowsiness* is especially likely to occur at initiation of therapy and after dosage increases.
Incidence less frequent or rare
  *Decreased sexual ability or interest in sex*—more common in men than in women; *diarrhea; hyperprolactinemia* (swelling of breasts or unusual milk production); *nausea or vomiting; orthostatic hypotension* (dizziness or lightheadedness when getting up from a lying or sitting position); *paresthesias* (numbness, tingling, pain, or weakness in hands or feet); *sinus bradycardia* (slow heartbeat); *stuffy nose*

## Overdose

For more information on the management of overdose or unintentional ingestion, **contact a Poison Control Center** (See *Poison Control Center Listing*).

**Clinical effects of overdose**
The following effects have been selected on the basis of their potential clinical significance (possible signs and symptoms in parentheses where appropriate)—not necessarily inclusive:
  *Bradycardia; constipation; diarrhea; dizziness; flatus; gastric distention; hypotension, acute; lightheadedness; nausea; sedation, excessive; vomiting; weakness*

**Treatment of overdose**
To decrease absorption—
  If clinically indicated and ingestion is recent, gastric lavage or emesis may reduce absorption.
Specific treatment—
  Management is mostly symptomatic and supportive. This includes particular attention to heart rate and cardiac output, blood volume, electrolyte balance, paralytic ileus, urinary function, and cerebral activity. Sympathomimetic agents may be indicated.

## Patient Consultation

As an aid to patient consultation, refer to *Advice for the Patient, Methyldopa (Systemic)*.
In providing consultation, consider emphasizing the following selected information (» = major clinical significance):

**Before using this medication**
» Conditions affecting use, especially:
  Sensitivity to methyldopa
  Breast-feeding—Distributed into breast milk
  Use in the elderly—Increased sensitivity to hypotensive and sedative effects
  Other medications, especially MAO inhibitors
  Other medical problems, especially active hepatic disease, history of hepatic disease associated with methyldopa, history of autoimmune hemolytic anemia, or pheochromocytoma

**Proper use of this medication**
Possible need for control of weight and diet, especially sodium intake
» Patient may not experience symptoms of hypertension; importance of taking medication even if feeling well
» Does not cure, but helps control hypertension; possible need for lifelong therapy; checking with physician before discontinuing medication; serious consequences of untreated hypertension
Compliance with therapy; taking medication at the same times each day to maintain the therapeutic effect

» Proper dosing
  Missed dose: Taking as soon as possible; not taking if almost time for next dose; not doubling doses
» Proper storage

**Precautions while using this medication**
Making regular visits to physician to check progress
» Not using other medications, especially nonprescription sympathomimetics, unless ordered by physician
» Reporting fever to physician
  Caution if any kind of surgery (including dental surgery) or emergency treatment is required
» Caution when driving or doing things requiring alertness, because of possible drowsiness
  Caution when getting up suddenly from a lying or sitting position
  Possible dryness of mouth; using sugarless candy or gum, ice, or saliva substitute for relief; checking with physician or dentist if dry mouth continues for more than 2 weeks
  Caution if any laboratory tests required; possible interference with test results

**Side/adverse effects**
Signs of potential side effects, especially edema, drug fever, mental status changes, cholestasis, hepatitis, hepatocellular injury, colitis, hemolytic anemia, leukopenia, granulocytopenia, myocarditis, pancreatitis, SLE-like syndrome, and thrombocytopenia

## General Dosing Information

If methyldopa is added to a thiazide diuretic regimen, the dosage of the thiazide need not be changed. If methyldopa is to be given with other antihypertensives, the initial dosage of methyldopa for an adult should be limited to 500 mg daily.

Any increase in dosage should be initiated with the evening dose of methyldopa to minimize the effects of sedation.

Tolerance to methyldopa may develop within 2 or 3 months after initiation of therapy as a result of fluid retention and expanded plasma volume. Adding a diuretic or increasing the dosage of methyldopa may restore control. Addition of thiazide diuretics to the regimen is recommended if therapy has not been started with a thiazide or if a daily dose of 2 grams of methyldopa does not maintain control.

If orthostatic hypotension occurs, dosage reduction is recommended.

Recent evidence suggests that withdrawal of antihypertensive therapy prior to surgery is not necessary, but that the anesthesiologist must be aware of such therapy.

It is recommended that methyldopa be discontinued if Coombs' positive hemolytic anemia occurs. Although the anemia usually remits promptly, corticosteroids may be administered if necessary. If this effect is shown to be due to methyldopa, therapy with the drug should not be reinstituted.

If a blood transfusion is needed in a patient receiving methyldopa, both a direct and indirect Coombs' test are recommended. If hemolytic anemia is not present, usually only the direct Coombs' test will be positive, which will not interfere with typing or positive crossmatching. However, a positive indirect Coombs' test may interfere with the major crossmatch, and a hematologist or transfusion expert will be needed.

It is recommended that methyldopa be withdrawn if fever, abnormal liver function tests, or jaundice occurs. If these effects are shown to be due to methyldopa, therapy with the drug should not be reinstituted.

**For parenteral dosage forms only**
Intramuscular or subcutaneous administration is not recommended because of unreliable absorption.

Following stabilization of blood pressure using intravenous methyldopate, the patient should be transferred to methyldopa tablets at the same dosage as was used parenterally.

## Oral Dosage Forms

### METHYLDOPA ORAL SUSPENSION USP

**Usual adult dose**
Antihypertensive—
  Initial: Oral, 250 mg two or three times a day for two days, the dosage then being adjusted, preferably at intervals of not less than two days, until the desired response is obtained.
  Maintenance: Oral, 500 mg to 2 grams a day, divided into two to four doses.
Note: Geriatric patients may be more sensitive to the effects of the usual adult dose and may require a lower dose to prevent syncope.

**Usual adult prescribing limits**
3 grams a day.

**Usual pediatric dose**
Antihypertensive—
  Oral, initially 10 mg per kg of body weight or 300 mg per square meter of body surface, divided into two to four doses, the dosage then being adjusted, preferably at intervals of not less than two days, until the desired response is obtained, but not exceeding 65 mg per kg of body weight or 3 grams daily, whichever is less.

**Strength(s) usually available**
U.S.—
  50 mg per mL (Rx) [*Aldomet* (alcohol 1%; benzoic acid; sodium bisulfite; sugar; polysorbate)].
Canada—
  Not commercially available.

**Packaging and storage**
Store below 26 °C (79 °F), unless otherwise specified by manufacturer. Store in a tight, light-resistant container. Protect from freezing.

**Auxiliary labeling**
• Shake well before using.
• May cause drowsiness.
• Do not take other medicines without your doctor's advice.

**Note**
Check refill frequency to determine compliance in hypertensive patients.

### METHYLDOPA TABLETS USP

**Usual adult dose**
Antihypertensive—
  Initial: Oral, 250 mg two or three times a day for two days, the dosage then being adjusted, preferably at intervals of not less than two days, until the desired response is obtained.
  Maintenance: Oral, 500 mg to 2 grams a day, divided into two to four doses.
Note: Geriatric patients may be more sensitive to the effects of the usual adult dose and may require a lower dose to prevent syncope.

**Usual adult prescribing limits**
3 grams a day.

**Usual pediatric dose**
Antihypertensive—
  Oral, initially 10 mg per kg of body weight or 300 mg per square meter of body surface, divided into two to four doses, the dosage then being adjusted, preferably at intervals of not less than two days, until the desired response is obtained, but not exceeding 65 mg per kg of body weight or 3 grams daily, whichever is less.

**Strength(s) usually available**
U.S.—
  125 mg (Rx) [*Aldomet* (without sodium metabisulfite preservative)] [GENERIC (with or without sodium metabisulfite preservative)].
  250 mg (Rx) [*Aldomet* (without sodium metabisulfite preservative)] [GENERIC (with or without sodium metabisulfite preservative)].
  500 mg (Rx) [*Aldomet* (without sodium metabisulfite preservative)] [GENERIC (with or without sodium metabisulfite preservative)].
Canada—
  125 mg (Rx) [*Aldomet; Apo-Methyldopa; Dopamet; Novomedopa; Nu-Medopa*].
  250 mg (Rx) [*Aldomet; Apo-Methyldopa; Dopamet; Novomedopa; Nu-Medopa*].
  500 mg (Rx) [*Aldomet; Apo-Methyldopa; Dopamet; Novomedopa; Nu-Medopa*].

**Packaging and storage**
Store below 40 °C (104 °F), preferably between 15 and 30 °C (59 and 86 °F), unless otherwise specified by manufacturer. Store in a well-closed container.

**Auxiliary labeling**
• May cause drowsiness.
• Do not take other medicines without your doctor's advice.

**Note**
Check refill frequency to determine compliance in hypertensive patients.

## Parenteral Dosage Forms

### METHYLDOPATE HYDROCHLORIDE INJECTION USP

**Usual adult dose**
Antihypertensive—
  Intravenous infusion, 250 to 500 mg in 100 mL of 5% dextrose injection, administered slowly over a thirty- to sixty-minute period, every six hours if necessary.
Note: Geriatric patients may be more sensitive to the effects of the usual adult dose and may require a lower dose to prevent syncope.

**Usual adult prescribing limits**
1 gram every 6 hours.

**Usual pediatric dose**
Antihypertensive—
  Intravenous infusion, 20 to 40 mg per kg of body weight in 5% dextrose injection, administered slowly over a thirty- to sixty-minute period, every six hours if necessary, but not exceeding 65 mg per kg of body weight or 3 grams daily, whichever is less.

**Strength(s) usually available**
U.S.—
  50 mg per mL (Rx) [*Aldomet* (sodium bisulfite; methylparaben; propylparaben)] [GENERIC (may contain sodium metabisulfite, methylparaben, propylparaben)].

Canada—
  50 mg per mL (Rx) [*Aldomet* (sodium bisulfite; methylparaben; propylparaben)].

**Packaging and storage**
Store below 40 °C (104 °F), preferably between 15 and 30 °C (59 and 86 °F), unless otherwise specified by manufacturer. Protect from freezing.

## Selected Bibliography
The fifth report of the Joint National Committee on Detection, Evaluation, and Treatment of High Blood Pressure (JNC V). Arch Intern Med 1993; 153(2): 154-83.

Revised: 07/22/96
Interim revision: 08/19/98

# METHYLDOPA AND THIAZIDE DIURETICS  Systemic

This monograph includes information on the following: 1) Methyldopa and Chlorothiazide; 2) Methyldopa and Hydrochlorothiazide.

VA CLASSIFICATION (Primary): CV401

NOTE:  The *Methyldopa and Thiazide Diuretics (Systemic)* monograph is maintained on the USP DI electronic data base. For a printed copy of the most recent revision of the complete monograph, contact Micromedex, Inc. - Reprint Requests, 6200 S. Syracuse Way, Suite 300, Englewood, CO 80111; telephone (303) 486-6400; telefax (303) 486-6464; Email: USPDI@MDX.COM.

For information on the specific components of this combination, see the USP DI monographs for) *Diuretics, Thiazide (Systemic)* and *Methyldopa (Systemic)*.

The information that follows is selectively abstracted from the complete monograph and is provided to facilitate drug use review and patient counseling.

Note:  For a listing of dosage forms and brand names by country availability, see *Dosage Forms* section(s).

## Category
Antihypertensive.

## Indications
**Accepted**
Hypertension (treatment)—This combination is indicated for treatment of hypertension.
  Fixed-dosage combinations are generally not recommended for initial therapy and are useful for subsequent therapy only when the proportion of the component agents corresponds to the dose of the individual agents, as determined by titration.

## Patient Consultation
As an aid to patient consultation, refer to *Advice for the Patient, Methyldopa and Thiazide Diuretics (Systemic)*.
In providing consultation, consider emphasizing the following selected information (» = major clinical significance):

**Before using this medication**
» Conditions affecting use, especially:
  Sensitivity to methyldopa, thiazide diuretics, other sulfonamide-type medications, bumetanide, furosemide, or carbonic anhydrase inhibitors
  Pregnancy—Thiazide diuretics not recommended for routine use; may cause jaundice, thrombocytopenia, hypokalemia in infant
  Breast-feeding—Excreted in breast milk; recommended that nursing mothers avoid thiazides during first month of breast-feeding because of reports of suppression of lactation
  Use in the elderly—Increased sensitivity to hypotensive, sedative, and electrolyte effects
  Other medications, especially MAO inhibitors, digitalis glycosides, or lithium
  Other medical problems, especially cerebrovascular disease, active hepatic disease, history of hemolytic anemia, history of hepatic disease associated with methyldopa, pheochromocytoma, or anuria or severe renal function impairment

**Proper use of this medication**
  Possible need for control of weight and diet, especially sodium intake
» Patient may not experience symptoms of hypertension; importance of taking medication even if feeling well
» Does not cure, but helps control hypertension; possible need for lifelong therapy; checking with physician before discontinuing medication; serious consequences of untreated hypertension
  Diuretic effects of the medication and timing of doses to minimize inconvenience of diuresis
  Compliance with therapy; taking medication at the same time(s) each day to maintain the therapeutic effect
» Proper dosing
  Missed dose: Taking as soon as possible; not taking if almost time for next dose; not doubling doses
» Proper storage

**Precautions while using this medication**
  Making regular visits to physician to check progress
» Not using other medications, especially nonprescription sympathomimetics, unless ordered by physician
» Possibility of hypokalemia; possible need for additional potassium in diet; not changing diet without first checking with physician
  To prevent dehydration, checking with physician if severe nausea, vomiting, or diarrhea occurs and continues
  Caution if any kind of surgery (including dental surgery) or emergency treatment is required
» Reporting fever to physician
» Caution when driving or doing things requiring alertness because of possible drowsiness
  Caution when getting up suddenly from a lying or sitting position
» Caution in using alcohol, while standing for long periods or exercising, and during hot weather because of enhanced orthostatic hypotensive effects
  For diabetic patients: May increase blood sugar levels
  Possible dryness of mouth; using sugarless candy or gum, ice, or saliva substitute for relief; checking with physician or dentist if dry mouth continues for more than 2 weeks
» Possible photosensitivity; avoiding unprotected exposure to sun; using protective clothing and sun block product; avoiding use of sunlamp, tanning bed, or tanning booth
  Caution if any laboratory tests required; possible interference with test results

**Side/adverse effects**
  Signs of potential side effects, especially drug fever, hypokalemia, mental changes, agranulocytosis, leukopenia, granulocytopenia, allergic reaction, cholestasis, hepatitis, cholecystitis, pancreatitis, colitis, hemolytic anemia, hyperuricemia, gout, myocarditis, SLE-like syndrome, and thrombocytopenia

## Oral Dosage Forms
### METHYLDOPA AND CHLOROTHIAZIDE TABLETS USP
**Usual adult dose**
Antihypertensive—
  Oral, 2 to 4 tablets a day in single or divided daily doses, as determined by individual titration with the component agents.

Note:  Geriatric patients may be more sensitive to the effects of the usual adult dose and may require a lower dose to prevent syncope.

**Usual pediatric dose**
Oral, as determined by individual titration with the component agents.

**Strength(s) usually available**

U.S.—
- 250 mg of methyldopa and 150 mg of chlorothiazide (Rx) [*Aldoclor-150*; GENERIC].
- 250 mg of methyldopa and 250 mg of chlorothiazide (Rx) [*Aldoclor-250*; GENERIC].

Canada—
- 250 mg of methyldopa and 150 mg of chlorothiazide (Rx) [*Supres-150*].
- 250 mg of methyldopa and 250 mg of chlorothiazide (Rx) [*Supres-250*].

**Auxiliary labeling**
- May cause drowsiness.
- Do not take other medicines without your doctor's advice.

## METHYLDOPA AND HYDROCHLOROTHIAZIDE TABLETS USP

**Usual adult dose**
Antihypertensive—
  Oral, 2 to 4 tablets a day in single or divided daily doses, as determined by individual titration with the component agents.

Note: Geriatric patients may be more sensitive to the effects of the usual adult dose and may require a lower dose to prevent syncope.

**Usual pediatric dose**
Oral, as determined by individual titration with the component agents.

**Strength(s) usually available**

U.S.—
- 250 mg of methyldopa and 15 mg of hydrochlorothiazide (Rx) [*Aldoril-15*; GENERIC].
- 250 mg of methyldopa and 25 mg of hydrochlorothiazide (Rx) [*Aldoril-25*; GENERIC].
- 500 mg of methyldopa and 30 mg of hydrochlorothiazide (Rx) [*Aldoril D30*; GENERIC].
- 500 mg of methyldopa and 50 mg of hydrochlorothiazide (Rx) [*Aldoril D50*; GENERIC].

Canada—
- 250 mg of methyldopa and 15 mg of hydrochlorothiazide (Rx) [*Aldoril-15; Novodoparil; PMS Dopazide*].
- 250 mg of methyldopa and 25 mg of hydrochlorothiazide (Rx) [*Aldoril-25; Novodoparil; PMS Dopazide*].

**Auxiliary labeling**
- May cause drowsiness.
- Do not take other medicines without your doctor's advice.

Revised: 04/13/93
Interim revision: 08/19/98

---

**METHYLENE BLUE**—The *Methylene Blue (Systemic)* monograph is not included in this published version of the USP DI database. Copies of the monograph are available on request from Micromedex, Inc. - Reprint Requests, 6200 S. Syracuse Way, Suite 300, Englewood, CO 80111; telephone (303) 486-6400; telefax (303) 486-6464; Email: USPDI@MDX.COM.

---

# METHYLERGONOVINE   Systemic†

INN: Methylergometrine
VA CLASSIFICATION (Primary): GU600
Commonly used brand name(s): *Methergine*.
Another commonly used name is methylergometrine.

Note: For a listing of dosage forms and brand names by country availability, see *Dosage Forms* section(s).

†Not commercially available in Canada.

## Category
Uterine stimulant.

## Indications

Note: Bracketed information in the *Indications* section refers to uses that are not included in U.S. product labeling.

**Accepted**

Hemorrhage, postpartum and postabortal (prophylaxis and treatment)—Methylergonovine is indicated in the prevention or treatment of postpartum or postabortal uterine bleeding due to uterine atony or subinvolution. Its use is not recommended prior to delivery of the placenta since placental entrapment may occur.

[Abortion, incomplete (treatment)]—In cases of incomplete abortion, methylergonovine may be used to hasten expulsion of uterine contents.

**Unaccepted**

Methylergonovine is not as effective in treatment of migraine as other ergot alkaloids and use is not recommended.

Methylergonovine is not indicated for induction or augmentation of labor, to induce abortion, or in cases of threatened spontaneous abortion because of its propensity to produce nonphysiologic, tetanic contractions and its long duration of action.

## Pharmacology/Pharmacokinetics

**Physicochemical characteristics**
Chemical group—Amine ergot alkaloid.
Molecular weight—455.51.

**Mechanism of action/Effect**
Uterine stimulant—
  Methylergonovine directly stimulates the uterine muscle to increase force and frequency of contractions. When usual doses of methylergonovine are used, these contractions precede periods of relaxation; when larger doses are used, basal uterine tone is elevated and these relaxation periods will be decreased. Contraction of the uterine wall around bleeding vessels at the placental site produces hemostasis. The sensitivity of the uterus to the oxytocic effect is much greater toward the end of pregnancy. The oxytocic actions of methylergonovine are greater than its vascular effects.

Vasoconstriction—
  Methylergonovine, like other ergot alkaloids, produces arterial vasoconstriction by stimulation of alpha-adrenergic and serotonin receptors and inhibition of endothelial-derived relaxation factor release. It is a less potent vasoconstrictor than ergotamine.

**Other actions/effects**
Methylergonovine has minor actions on the central nervous system (CNS). In the CNS, methylergonovine is a partial agonist and partial antagonist at some serotonin and dopamine receptors. Methylergonovine also possesses weak dopaminergic antagonist actions in certain blood vessels and partial agonist actions at serotonin receptors in umbilical and placental blood vessels. It does not possess significant alpha-adrenergic blocking activity.

**Absorption**
Absorption is rapid after oral (60%) and intramuscular (78%) administration.

**Distribution**
Rapidly, primarily to plasma and extracellular fluid following intravenous administration; distribution to tissues also occurs rapidly.
In a study in women who had received 125 mcg of methylergonovine orally 3 times a day for 5 days, concentrations in breast milk ranged from less than 0.5 (limit of detection) to 1.3 nanograms per mL at 1 hour after a 250 mcg oral dose and from 0 to 1.2 nanograms per mL at 8 hours.

**Biotransformation**
Likely hepatic, with extensive first-pass metabolism.

**Half-life**
Intravenous—
  2 to 3 minutes or less (alpha phase).
  20 to 30 minutes or longer (beta phase).

**Onset of action**
Contraction of uterus, postpartum—
  Oral: 5 to 10 minutes.
  Intramuscular: 2 to 5 minutes.
  Intravenous: Immediate.

**Time to peak concentration**
In a study in postpartum patients, peak plasma concentrations occurred at 3 hours after a 250 mcg oral dose. In a study in healthy fasting males, peak plasma concentrations occurred at 30 minutes.

**Peak serum concentration**
In a study in postpartum patients, peak plasma concentrations were 3 nanograms per mL after a 250 mcg oral dose. In a study in healthy fasting males, similar concentrations were achieved. Women given 125 mcg

by mouth 3 times a day for 5 days had plasma concentrations within the range of 0.6 to 4.4 nanograms per mL at 1 hour after a 250 mcg oral dose and from 0 to 0.6 nanograms per mL at 8 hours.

**Duration of action**
Contraction of uterus, postpartum—
 Oral: Approximately 3 hours.
 Intramuscular: Approximately 3 hours.
 Intravenous: 45 minutes (although rhythmic contractions may persist for up to 3 hours).

**Elimination**
Primarily renal excretion of metabolites; some fecal. Renal elimination of unchanged drug is responsible for less than 5% of total elimination. Methylergonovine does not appear to accumulate after multiple doses.

## Precautions to Consider

### Cross-sensitivity and/or related problems
Patients sensitive to other ergot derivatives may be sensitive to this medication also, although there is some degree of variation among ergot alkaloids in their ability to elicit oxytocic, CNS, or vasoconstrictive effects.

### Pregnancy/Reproduction
Pregnancy—Methylergonovine is contraindicated during pregnancy. Tetanic contractions may result in decreased uterine blood flow and fetal distress.

Labor and delivery—High doses of methylergonovine administered prior to delivery may cause uterine tetany and fetal distress. Methylergonovine should *not* be administered prior to delivery of the placenta. Administration prior to delivery of the placenta may cause captivation of the placenta or missed diagnosis of twin gestation, due to excessive uterine contraction.

### Breast-feeding
Problems in humans have not been documented. Ergot alkaloids are excreted in breast milk. However, very little passes into breast milk in humans. In a study in women who had received 125 mcg of methylergonovine orally 3 times a day for 5 days, concentrations in breast milk ranged from less than 0.5 (limit of detection) to 1.3 nanograms per mL at 1 hour after a 250 mcg oral dose and from 0 to 1.2 nanograms per mL at 8 hours.

Inhibition of lactation has not been reported for methylergonovine. However, studies have shown that methylergonovine may interfere with the secretion of prolactin (to a lesser degree than bromocriptine) in the immediate postpartum period. This could result in delayed or diminished lactation with prolonged use.

Ergot alkaloids have the potential to cause chronic ergot poisoning in the infant only if used in the mother in higher-than-recommended doses or if used for a longer period of time than is generally recommended.

### Pediatrics
In newborns, elimination of methylergonovine may be prolonged. Neonates inadvertently administered ergonovine in overdose amounts have developed respiratory depression, myoclonic movements, purpuric symptoms, mild jaundice, and severe peripheral vasoconstriction.

### Geriatrics
No information is available on the effects of methylergonovine in geriatric patients.

### Drug interactions and/or related problems
The following drug interactions and/or related problems have been selected on the basis of their potential clinical significance (possible mechanism in parentheses where appropriate)—not necessarily inclusive (» = major clinical significance):

Note: Combinations containing any of the following medications, depending on the amount present, may also interact with this medication.

 Anesthetics, general, especially halothane
  (peripheral vasoconstriction may be potentiated by the concurrent use of general anesthetics with methylergonovine)
  (concurrent use of halothane in concentrations greater than 1% may interfere with the oxytocic actions of methylergonovine, resulting in severe uterine hemorrhage)

 Bromocriptine or
 Ergot alkaloids, other
  (the incidence of rare cases of hypertension, strokes, seizures, and myocardial infarction associated with the postpartum use of bromocriptine or other ergot alkaloids may be increased with the use of ergot alkaloids)

 Nicotine or
 Smoking, tobacco
  (nicotine absorption from heavy smoking may result in enhanced vasoconstriction)

 Nitroglycerin or
 Antianginal agents, other
  (ergot alkaloids may induce coronary vasospasm, lowering the efficacy of nitroglycerin or other antianginal agents; increased doses of nitroglycerin or antianginal agents and/or use of intracoronary nitroglycerin may be necessary)

 Vasoconstrictors, other, including those present in local anesthetics or
 Vasopressors
  (concurrent use may result in enhanced vasoconstriction; dosage adjustments may be necessary)
  (the pressor effect of sympathomimetic pressor amines may be potentiated, resulting in potentially severe hypertension, headache, and rupture of cerebral blood vessels; gangrene developed in a patient receiving both dopamine and ergonovine infusions)

### Laboratory value alterations
The following have been selected on the basis of their potential clinical significance (possible effect in parentheses where appropriate)—not necessarily inclusive (» = major clinical significance):

With physiology/laboratory test values
 Blood pressure or
 Central venous pressure
  (may be elevated due to peripheral vasoconstriction primarily of postcapillary vessels; less likely with methylergonovine than ergonovine; has sometimes been associated with preeclampsia, history of hypertension, intravenous administration of methylergonovine, or concurrent use of local anesthetics containing vasoconstrictors; hypotension has also been reported)

 Heart rate
  (may be decreased due primarily to an increase in vagal tone, and possibly to decreased central sympathetic activity and direct depression of the myocardium)

 Prolactin
  (serum concentrations may be decreased)

### Medical considerations/Contraindications
The medical considerations/contraindications included have been selected on the basis of their potential clinical significance (reasons given in parentheses where appropriate)—not necessarily inclusive (» = major clinical significance).

*Except under special circumstances, this medication should not be used when the following medical problems exist:*

» Angina pectoris, unstable or
» Myocardial infarction, recent
  (vasospasm caused by methylergonovine may precipitate angina or myocardial infarction)

» Cardiovascular disease or
» Coronary artery disease
  (patients may be more susceptible to angina or myocardial infarction caused by methylergonovine-induced vasospasm)

» Cerebrovascular accident, history of or
» Transient ischemic attack, history of
  (patients may be susceptible to recurrence due to increases in blood pressure)

» Eclampsia or
» Preeclampsia
  (may be exacerbated; patients may be more likely to develop methylergonovine-induced hypertension; headaches, severe cardiac arrhythmias, seizures, and cerebrovascular accidents have occurred)

» Hypertension, severe, or history of
  (may be exacerbated)

» Occlusive peripheral vascular disease or
» Raynaud's phenomenon, severe
  (may be exacerbated; a patient with Raynaud's phenomenon developed impalpable arterial pulses with use of ergonovine)

*Risk-benefit should be considered when the following medical problems exist:*

 Allergy or sensitivity to methylergonovine or other ergot alkaloids
» Hepatic function impairment
  (impaired metabolism of methylergonovine may result in ergot overdose)

Hypocalcemia
(oxytocic response to methylergonovine may be reduced; cautious use of intravenous calcium gluconate may restore oxytocic response to methylergonovine)
» Mitral valve stenosis or
» Venoatrial shunts
(vasospasm caused by methylergonovine may precipitate angina or myocardial infarction)
» Renal function impairment
» Sepsis
(possible increased sensitivity to effects of methylergonovine)

**Patient monitoring**
The following may be especially important in patient monitoring (other tests may be warranted in some patients, depending on condition; » = major clinical significance):

Blood pressure determinations and
Pulse rate determinations and
Uterine response
(recommended at frequent intervals after parenteral therapy to monitor for adverse reactions; especially important with intravenous administration or before repeating doses)

## Side/Adverse Effects

Note: Because the duration of therapy with methylergonovine is generally short, many of the side effects seen with other ergot alkaloids do not occur.

The following side/adverse effects have been selected on the basis of their potential clinical significance (possible signs and symptoms in parentheses where appropriate)—not necessarily inclusive:

**Those indicating need for medical attention**
Incidence less frequent
*Bradycardia* (slow heartbeat); *coronary vasospasm* (chest pain)
Incidence rare
*Allergic reaction, including shock; cardiac arrest or ventricular arrhythmias, including fibrillation and tachycardia* (irregular heartbeat); *dyspnea* (unexplained shortness of breath); *hypertension, sudden and severe* (sudden, severe headache; blurred vision; seizures); *myocardial infarction* (crushing chest pain; unexplained shortness of breath)—has occurred with the use of ergot preparations in the postpartum period; *peripheral vasospasm* (itching of skin; pain in arms, legs, or lower back; pale or cold hands or feet; weakness in legs)—dose-related

**Those indicating need for medical attention only if they continue or are bothersome**
Incidence more frequent
*Nausea*—especially after intravenous use; *uterine cramping; vomiting*—especially after intravenous use
Note: *Uterine cramping* will occur to some degree in all patients and is indicative of efficacy. However, dosage reduction may be required in occasional patients with severe or intolerable uterine cramps.
Incidence less frequent
*Abdominal or stomach pain; diarrhea; dizziness; sweating; tinnitus* (ringing in the ears)

## Overdose

For specific information on the agents used in the management of methylergonovine overdose, see:
- *Charcoal, Activated (Oral-Local)* monograph;
- *Chlorpromazine* in *Phenothiazines (Systemic)* monograph;
- *Diazepam* in *Benzodiazepines (Systemic)* monograph;
- *Hydralazine (Systemic)* monograph;
- *Laxatives (Local)* monograph;
- *Nitroglycerin* in *Nitrates (Systemic)* monograph;
- *Nitroprusside (Systemic)* monograph;
- *Phentolamine (Systemic)* monograph;
- *Phenytoin* in *Anticonvulsants, Hydantoin (Systemic)* monograph; and/or
- *Tolazoline (Parenteral-Systemic)* monograph.

For more information on the management of overdose or unintentional ingestion, **contact a Poison Control Center** (see *Poison Control Center Listing*).

**Clinical effects of overdose**
The following effects have been selected on the basis of their potential clinical significance (possible signs and symptoms in parentheses where appropriate)—not necessarily inclusive:

Acute
*Angina* (chest pain); *bradycardia* (slow heartbeat); *confusion; drowsiness; fast, weak pulse; miosis* (small pupils); *peripheral vasoconstriction, severe* (coolness, paleness, or numbness of arms or legs; muscle pain; weak or absent arterial pulse in arms or legs; tingling, itching, and coolness of skin); *respiratory depression* (decreased breathing rate or trouble in breathing; bluish color of skin or inside of nose or mouth); *seizures; tachycardia* (fast heartbeat); *unconsciousness; unusual thirst; uterine tetany* (severe cramping of the uterus)
Chronic
*Formication* (false feeling of insects crawling on the skin); *gangrene* (dry, shriveled appearance of skin on hands, lower legs, or feet); *hemiplegia* (paralysis of one side of the body); *thrombophlebitis* (pain and redness in an arm or leg)
Note: Chronic overdose symptoms are unlikely with proper use since treatment is of short duration.

**Treatment of overdose**
Immediate discontinuation of methylergonovine. Since there is no specific antidote for the management of methylergonovine overdose, treatment is primarily supportive and symptomatic and may include the following:
To decrease absorption—
Gastrointestinal decontamination for oral overdose, preferably with multiple doses of activated charcoal and an appropriate cathartic. Gastric lavage may also be considered.
Specific treatment—
Use of nitroglycerin for treatment of myocardial ischemia. Intracoronary nitroglycerin may be necessary.
Use of diazepam or phenytoin for treatment of seizures.
Use of sodium nitroprusside, tolazoline, or phentolamine for treatment of peripheral ischemia.
Use of sodium nitroprusside, chlorpromazine 15 mg, or hydralazine for treatment of severe hypertension.
Monitoring—
Frequent monitoring of vital signs, arterial blood gases, and electrolytes. Electrocardiogram monitoring to assess cardiac function and perfusion. Monitoring of serum methylergonovine levels is not predictive of the outcome of overdose.
Supportive care—
May include maintaining an open airway and breathing, maintaining proper fluid and electrolyte balance, correcting hypertension, and controlling seizures. Patients in whom intentional overdose is known or suspected should be referred for psychiatric consultation.

## Patient Consultation

As an aid to patient consultation, refer to *Advice for the Patient, Ergonovine/Methylergonovine (Systemic)*.

In providing consultation, consider emphasizing the following selected information (» = major clinical significance):

**Before using this medication**
» Conditions affecting use, especially:
Allergies or sensitivity to methylergonovine or other ergot alkaloids
Pregnancy—Should not be used prior to delivery or delivery of the placenta
Breast-feeding—Ergot alkaloids are excreted in breast milk
Other medical problems, especially cardiac or vascular disease, hepatic function impairment, severe hypertension or history of hypertension, renal function impairment, and sepsis

**Proper use of this medication**
» Importance of not using more medication or using for longer than prescribed; risk of ergotism and gangrene with prolonged use
» Proper dosing
Missed dose: Not taking missed dose; not doubling doses
» Proper storage

**Precautions while using this medication**
Notifying physician if infection develops, since infection may cause increased sensitivity to medication

**Side/adverse effects**
Signs of potential side effects, especially allergic reaction, coronary vasospasm or other cardiovascular complications, dyspnea, severe hypertension, or peripheral vasospasm

## General Dosing Information

Antiemetic medications such as prochlorperazine may be administered prior to use of methylergonovine.

**For parenteral dosage forms only**
Because the risk of severe adverse effects is increased with intravenous use of methylergonovine, such use is recommended only for emergencies such as excessive uterine bleeding.

If intravenous use is warranted, administration must be done slowly, over a period of at least 1 minute; some clinicians recommend dilution of the solution with normal saline before administration.

In some patients who do not respond to methylergonovine because of hypocalcemia, cautious intravenous administration of calcium gluconate (provided the patient is not receiving digitalis) may restore the oxytocic action.

## Oral Dosage Forms

### METHYLERGONOVINE MALEATE TABLETS USP

**Usual adult and adolescent dose**
Uterine stimulant—
  Oral, 200 to 400 mcg (0.2 to 0.4 mg) two to four times a day (every six to twelve hours) until the danger of uterine atony and hemorrhage has passed.

Note:  Generally, a treatment course of 48 hours is sufficient. However, in some patients, treatment for up to 7 days may be necessary, especially when used for treatment of incomplete abortion. Oral administration usually follows an initial parenteral dose.

**Strength(s) usually available**
U.S.—
  200 mcg (0.2 mg) (Rx) [*Methergine*].
Canada—
  Not commercially available.

**Packaging and storage**
Store below 40 °C (104 °F), preferably between 15 and 30 °C (59 and 86 °F), unless otherwise specified by manufacturer. Store in a tight container. Protect from light.

## Parenteral Dosage Forms

### METHYLERGONOVINE MALEATE INJECTION USP

**Usual adult and adolescent dose**
Uterine stimulant—
  Intramuscular or intravenous, 200 mcg (0.2 mg), repeated in two to four hours if necessary, up to five doses.

**Strength(s) usually available**
U.S.—
  200 mcg (0.2 mg) per mL (Rx) [*Methergine*].
Canada—
  Not commercially available.

**Packaging and storage**
Store below 40 °C (104 °F), preferably between 15 and 30 °C (59 and 86 °F), unless otherwise specified by manufacturer. Protect from light. Protect from freezing.

**Stability**
Discolored solutions or solutions containing visible particles should not be used.

Revised: 06/07/93

# METHYLPHENIDATE   Systemic

VA CLASSIFICATION (Primary): CN802
Note:  Controlled substance classification—
  U.S.—Canada—
Note:  Controlled substance in the U.S. and Canada.
Commonly used brand name(s): *PMS-Methylphenidate; Ritalin; Ritalin SR; Ritalin-SR*.
Note:  For a listing of dosage forms and brand names by country availability, see *Dosage Forms* section(s).

## Category
Central nervous system stimulant.

## Indications
Note:  Bracketed information in the *Indications* section refers to uses that are not included in U.S. product labeling.

**Accepted**
Attention-deficit hyperactivity disorder (treatment)—Methylphenidate is used as the primary agent in a total treatment program that includes other remedial measures (psychological, educational, and social) to stabilize some children [and adults] with attention-deficit hyperactivity disorder (ADHD). This complex behavioral syndrome has been known in the past as hyperkinetic child syndrome, minimal brain damage, minimal cerebral dysfunction, or minor cerebral dysfunction.

Narcolepsy (treatment)—Methylphenidate is indicated in the management of the symptoms of narcolepsy.

[Depression, mental, secondary to medical illness (treatment)][1]—Methylphenidate may be useful in selected patients whose medical condition complicates treatment with conventional antidepressants.

**Unaccepted**
Methylphenidate is *not* recommended for the treatment of mental depression amenable to treatment with conventional antidepressants, for the prevention or treatment of normal fatigue states, or for children who exhibit symptoms secondary to environmental factors and/or psychiatric disorders, including psychosis.

[1]Not included in Canadian product labeling.

## Pharmacology/Pharmacokinetics

**Physicochemical characteristics**
Molecular weight—269.77.

**Mechanism of action/Effect**
Central nervous system (CNS) stimulant—Although the primary mechanism is largely unknown, the effects of methylphenidate appear to be mediated by blockage of the reuptake mechanism of dopaminergic neurons. In children with attention deficit disorder, methylphenidate decreases motor restlessness and enhances the ability to pay attention. In narcolepsy, methylphenidate appears to act at the cerebral cortex and subcortical structures, including the thalamus, to produce CNS stimulation, resulting in increased motor activity, increased mental alertness, diminished sense of fatigue, brighter spirits, and mild euphoria.

**Time to peak serum concentration**
Extended-release tablets—
  4.7 hours (range, 1.3 to 8.2 hours) in children.
Tablets—
  1.9 hours (range, 0.3 to 4.4 hours) in children.

**Elimination**
Renal—
  An average of 67% of the methylphenidate in an extended-release tablet is excreted by children (as compared to 86% by adults).

## Precautions to Consider

**Carcinogenicity/Tumorigenicity**
In a lifetime carcinogenicity study in a mouse strain that is sensitive to the development of hepatic tumors (B6C3F1 mice), methylphenidate caused an increase in hepatocellular adenomas (benign tumors) at a dose of approximately 60 mg per kg of body weight (mg/kg) a day, or approximately 2.5 times a human dose of 60 mg a day on a mg per square meter of body surface area (mg/m$^2$) basis. In the same study, male mice showed an increase in hepatoblastomas (rare malignant tumors). There was no increase in total malignant hepatic tumors. A similar study in F344 rats showed no increase in tumors. The significance of these findings to humans is unknown.

**Mutagenicity**
No mutagenic potential was found in the Ames reverse mutation assay or in the *in vitro* mouse lymphoma cell forward mutation assay. A weak clastogenic response was found in an *in vitro* assay in cultured Chinese Hamster Ovary cells. *In vivo* assays of genotoxic potential of methylphenidate have not been performed. The significance of these findings to humans is unknown.

**Pregnancy/Reproduction**
Pregnancy—Studies have not been done in humans.
Studies have not been done in animals.

**Breast-feeding**
It is not known whether methylphenidate is distributed into breast milk.

**Pediatrics**
Long-term effects of methylphenidate in children are not well established. Children are more prone than adults to develop anorexia, insomnia, stomach pain, tachycardia, and weight loss. Monitoring of growth (both

height and weight gain) has been recommended during long-term therapy since chronic administration of methylphenidate may be associated with growth inhibition, although data are inadequate to determine this conclusively. Some clinicians may recommend medication-free periods during methylphenidate treatment to evaluate the need for continued therapy.

### Geriatrics
No information is available on the relationship of age to the effects of methylphenidate in geriatric patients.

### Drug interactions and/or related problems
The following drug interactions and/or related problems have been selected on the basis of their potential clinical significance (possible mechanism in parentheses where appropriate)—not necessarily inclusive (» = major clinical significance):

Note: Combinations containing any of the following medications, depending on the amount present, may also interact with this medication.

Anticholinergics or other medications with anticholinergic activity (See *Appendix II*)
(concurrent use may intensify anticholinergic effects because of secondary anticholinergic effects of methylphenidate)

Anticonvulsants, especially phenytoin, phenobarbital, and primidone or
Anticoagulants, coumarin- or indandione-derivative or
Phenylbutazone
(serum concentrations may be increased when these medications are used concurrently with methylphenidate because of metabolism inhibition, possibly resulting in toxicity; dosage adjustments may be necessary)

Antidepressants, tricyclic, especially desipramine and imipramine
(serum concentrations may be increased when these medications are used concurrently with methylphenidate because of inhibition of metabolism; also, concurrent use may antagonize the effects of methylphenidate)

Antihypertensives or
Diuretics used as antihypertensives
(hypotensive effects may be reduced when these medications are used concurrently with methylphenidate; the patient should be carefully monitored to confirm that the desired effect is being obtained)

» CNS stimulation–producing medications, other (See *Appendix II*)
(concurrent use with methylphenidate may result in additive CNS stimulation to excessive levels, causing nervousness, irritability, insomnia, or possibly seizures or cardiac arrhythmias; close observation is recommended)

» Monoamine oxidase (MAO) inhibitors, including furazolidone, procarbazine, and selegiline
(concurrent use may potentiate the effects of methylphenidate, possibly resulting in a hypertensive crisis; methylphenidate should not be administered during or within 14 days following the administration of MAO inhibitors)

» Pimozide
(concurrent use with methylphenidate may mask the cause of tics since methylphenidate itself may provoke tics; before therapy with pimozide is initiated, methylphenidate should be withdrawn)

Vasopressors
(pressor effects may be potentiated when vasopressors are used concurrently with methylphenidate)

### Medical considerations/Contraindications
The medical considerations/contraindications included have been selected on the basis of their potential clinical significance (reasons given in parentheses where appropriate)—not necessarily inclusive (» = major clinical significance).

*Except under special circumstances, this medication should not be used when the following medical problems exist:*

» Anxiety, tension, or agitation, severe or
» Depression, mental, which is amenable to treatment with conventional antidepressants or
» Glaucoma or
» Motor tics other than Tourette's disorder
(may be exacerbated)

*Risk-benefit should be considered when the following medical problems exist:*

Emotional instability, including history of drug dependence or alcoholism
(increased potential for addiction or abuse)

Epilepsy or other seizure disorders
(seizure threshold may be lowered)

» Gilles de la Tourette's syndrome, family history or diagnosis of
(motor and vocal tics may be exacerbated; however, some patients, under close supervision, may benefit from cautious trials)
» Hypertension
(may be exacerbated)
Psychosis
(symptoms of behavior disturbance and thought disorder may be exacerbated in psychotic children)
Sensitivity to methylphenidate

### Patient monitoring
The following may be especially important in patient monitoring (other tests may be warranted in some patients, depending on condition; » = major clinical significance):

Assessment of amount and frequency of medication use
(recommended at periodic intervals to detect signs of dependence or abuse during long-term therapy)

Blood pressure determinations
(recommended at periodic intervals during therapy, especially for patients with hypertension)

Complete blood cell, differential, and platelet counts
(recommended at periodic intervals for patients on prolonged therapy)

Monitoring of growth, both height and weight gain, in children
(recommended during long-term therapy, since data are inadequate to determine whether chronic administration of methylphenidate may be associated with growth inhibition)

Reassessment of need for therapy for behavioral syndrome in children
(interruption of therapy at periodic intervals is recommended to determine if a recurrence of behavioral symptoms is sufficient to continue therapy; tapering of dose may be necessary to prevent withdrawal symptoms)

## Side/Adverse Effects

The following side/adverse effects have been selected on the basis of their potential clinical significance (possible signs and symptoms in parentheses where appropriate)—not necessarily inclusive:

**Those indicating need for medical attention**
Incidence more frequent
*Hypertension* (increased blood pressure); *tachycardia* (fast heartbeat)—especially with doses greater than 0.5 mg per kg of body weight (mg/kg)

Incidence less frequent
*Angina* (chest pain); *arthralgia* (joint pain); *dyskinesia* (uncontrolled movements of the body); *fever; skin rash or hives; thrombocytopenic purpura* (rarely, unusual bleeding or bruising; black tarry stools; blood in urine or stools; pinpoint red spots on skin)—usually asymptomatic

Note: *Arthralgia, fever, skin rash or hives, and thrombocytopenic purpura* may be indicative of a hypersensitivity reaction to methylphenidate.

Incidence rare
*Blurred vision or any change in vision; Tourette's syndrome* (uncontrolled vocal outbursts and tics [uncontrolled repeated body movements])

With prolonged use or at high doses
*Psychosis, toxic* (mood or mental changes); *weight loss*—possibly more frequent in children

**Those indicating need for medical attention only if they continue or are bothersome**
Incidence more frequent
*Anorexia* (loss of appetite)—possibly more frequent in children; *CNS stimulation* (nervousness; trouble in sleeping)—possibly more frequent in children

Incidence less frequent
*Dizziness; drowsiness; headache; nausea; stomach pain*—possibly more frequent in children

**Those indicating possible withdrawal and the need for medical attention if they occur after medication is discontinued**
*Mental depression, severe; unusual behavior; unusual tiredness or weakness*

## Overdose

For specific information on the agents used in the management of methylphenidate overdose, see:
• *Barbiturates (Systemic)* monograph.

For more information on the management of overdose or unintentional ingestion, **contact a Poison Control Center** (see *Poison Control Center Listing*).

### Clinical effects of overdose
The following effects have been selected on the basis of their potential clinical significance (possible signs and symptoms in parentheses where appropriate)—not necessarily inclusive:

*Agitation; cardiac arrhythmias* (fast or irregular heartbeat); *confusion; delirium* (extreme confusion); *dryness of mouth or mucous membranes; euphoria* (false sense of well-being); *fever; hallucinations* (seeing, hearing, or feeling things that are not there); *headache, severe; hyperreflexia* (overactive reflexes); *increased blood pressure; increased sweating; muscle twitching; mydriasis* (large pupils); *palpitations* (fast, pounding, or irregular heartbeat); *seizures*—may be followed by coma; *tachycardia* (fast heartbeat); *trembling or tremors; vomiting*

### Treatment of overdose
Since there is no specific antidote for overdose with methylphenidate, treatment is symptomatic and supportive with possible utilization of the following:

To decrease absorption—
  Emptying stomach by emesis or gastric lavage.
Specific treatment—
  For severe overdose, administering a short-acting barbiturate using carefully titrated dosage.
Supportive care—
  Maintaining quiet, protective surroundings.
  Maintaining adequate circulatory and respiratory function.
  Using external cooling procedures for hyperpyrexia.
  Patients in whom intentional overdose is known or suspected should be referred for psychiatric consultation.

Note: Usefulness of peritoneal dialysis or extracorporeal hemodialysis has not been established.

## Patient Consultation

As an aid to patient consultation, refer to *Advice for the Patient, Methylphenidate (Systemic)*.

In providing consultation, consider emphasizing the following selected information (» = major clinical significance):

### Before using this medication
» Conditions affecting use, especially:
    Sensitivity to methylphenidate
    Use in children—In attention-deficit hyperactivity disorder (ADHD), drug-free periods may be recommended during treatment; monitoring of height and weight recommended; children more likely to develop stomach pain, trouble in sleeping, and loss of appetite and weight
    Other medications, especially other CNS stimulation–producing medications, MAO inhibitors, or pimozide
    Other medical problems, especially severe anxiety, tension, or agitation; depression amenable to conventional treatment; glaucoma; hypertension; motor tics; or Tourette's syndrome

### Proper use of this medication
» Importance of not using more medication than the amount prescribed because of possible habit-forming potential
  Taking with or after a meal or snack
  Taking the last dose of the short-acting tablets for each day before 6 p.m. to minimize the possibility of insomnia
  Not increasing dose if medication seems less effective after a few weeks; checking with physician
  Proper administration for extended-release dosage form: Swallowing whole; not breaking, crushing, or chewing
» Proper dosing
  Missed dose: Taking as soon as possible; taking any remaining doses for that day at regularly spaced intervals; not doubling doses
» Proper storage

### Precautions while using this medication
  Regular visits to physician to check progress during therapy
» Checking with physician before discontinuing medication after long-term and high-dose therapy; gradual dosage reduction may be necessary to avoid possibility of withdrawal symptoms
» Suspected psychological or physical dependence; checking with physician

### Side/adverse effects
  Possibility of withdrawal effects
  Signs of potential side effects, especially hypertension, tachycardia, angina, arthralgia, dyskinesia, fever, skin rash or hives, thrombocytopenic purpura, blurred vision or any change in vision, Tourette's syndrome, toxic psychosis, or weight loss

## General Dosing Information

To reduce the possibility of insomnia, the last dose of methylphenidate tablets for each day should be administered before 6 p.m.

When symptoms of attention-deficit hyperactivity disorder are controlled in children, dosage reduction or interruption in therapy may be possible during the summer months and at other times when the child is under less stress; medication may be given on each of the 5 school days during the week, with medication-free weekends and school holidays. However, some children may require daily dosing and summer use.

Prolonged use of methylphenidate may result in psychological or physical dependence.

When the medication is to be discontinued following high-dose and long-term administration, the dosage should be reduced gradually in order to avoid the possibility of withdrawal symptoms.

### Diet/Nutrition
Methylphenidate should be taken with or after a meal or snack.

## Oral Dosage Forms

### METHYLPHENIDATE HYDROCHLORIDE TABLETS USP

#### Usual adult and adolescent dose
For narcolepsy or attention-deficit hyperactivity disorder—
  Oral, 5 to 20 mg two or three times a day, preferably with or after meals.

#### Usual adult prescribing limits
90 mg a day.

#### Usual pediatric dose
Attention-deficit hyperactivity disorder—
  Children up to 6 years of age: Dosage has not been established.
  Children 6 years of age and over: Oral, 5 mg two times a day, with or after breakfast and lunch, the dosage being increased as needed and tolerated by 5 to 10 mg at one-week intervals up to a maximum of 60 mg a day.

Note: If improvement in condition does not occur after appropriate dosage adjustment over a one-month period, it is recommended that the medication be discontinued.

#### Strength(s) usually available
U.S.—
  5 mg (Rx) [*Ritalin;* GENERIC].
  10 mg (Rx) [*Ritalin* (scored); GENERIC].
  20 mg (Rx) [*Ritalin* (scored); GENERIC].
Canada—
  10 mg (Rx) [*PMS-Methylphenidate* (scored); *Ritalin* (scored)].
  20 mg (Rx) [*PMS-Methylphenidate* (scored); *Ritalin* (scored)].

#### Packaging and storage
Store below 30 °C (86 °F), preferably between 15 and 30 °C (59 and 86 °F), protected from light, unless otherwise specified by manufacturer. Store in a tight container.

#### Note
Controlled substance in the U.S. and Canada.

### METHYLPHENIDATE HYDROCHLORIDE EXTENDED-RELEASE TABLETS USP

Note: Extended-release tablets have a duration of action of 8 hours, and may be used in place of the conventional tablets when the 8-hour dosage of the extended-release tablets corresponds to the titrated 8-hour dosage of the tablets.

#### Usual adult and adolescent dose
For narcolepsy or attention-deficit hyperactivity disorder—
  Oral, 20 mg one to three times a day at eight-hour intervals.

#### Usual pediatric dose
Attention-deficit hyperactivity disorder—
  Children up to 6 years of age: Dosage has not been established.
  Children 6 years of age and over: Oral, 20 mg one to three times a day at eight-hour intervals.

#### Strength(s) usually available
U.S.—
  20 mg (Rx) [*Ritalin-SR;* GENERIC].
Canada—
  20 mg (Rx) [*Ritalin SR*].

## Methylphenidate (Systemic)

**Packaging and storage**
Store below 30 °C (86 °F), preferably between 15 and 30 °C (59 and 86 °F), protected from light, unless otherwise specified by manufacturer. Store in a tight container.

**Auxiliary labeling**
- Swallow tablets whole.

**Note**
Controlled substance in the U.S. and Canada.

Revised: 08/15/95
Interim revision: 06/26/96

---

**METHYLPREDNISOLONE**— See *Corticosteroids—Glucocorticoid Effects (Systemic)*

---

**METHYLTESTOSTERONE**— See *Androgens (Systemic)*

---

**METHYPRYLON**— The *Methyprylon (Systemic)* monograph is not included in this published version of the USP DI database. Copies of the monograph are available on request from Micromedex, Inc. - Reprint Requests, 6200 S. Syracuse Way, Suite 300, Englewood, CO 80111; telephone (303) 486-6400; telefax (303) 486-6464; Email: USPDI@MDX.COM.

---

# METHYSERGIDE  Systemic

VA CLASSIFICATION (Primary): CN105
Commonly used brand name(s): *Sansert*.

Note: For a listing of dosage forms and brand names by country availability, see *Dosage Forms* section(s).

## Category
Vascular headache prophylactic.

## Indications

**Accepted**

Headache, vascular (prophylaxis)—Methysergide is indicated for prevention of vascular headaches such as migraine and cluster headaches in patients with frequent and/or disabling headaches not responsive to other treatment.

**Unaccepted**

Methysergide is not recommended for treatment of acute attacks or tension headaches.

## Pharmacology/Pharmacokinetics

**Physicochemical characteristics**
Molecular weight—469.54.

**Mechanism of action/Effect**
Antiserotonin; actions on central nervous system (CNS); direct stimulation of smooth muscle leading to vasoconstriction. Little alpha-adrenergic blocking activity. The exact mechanism of action in preventing migraine is unknown, although it may be related to the antiserotonin effect.

**Absorption**
Rapid after oral administration.

**Biotransformation**
Probably hepatic.

**Onset of action**
1 to 2 days.

**Duration of action**
1 to 2 days.

**Elimination**
Renal, 56%, as unchanged drug and metabolites.

## Precautions to Consider

**Cross-sensitivity and/or related problems**
Patients sensitive to other ergot derivatives may be sensitive to this medication also.

**Pregnancy/Reproduction**
Problems in humans have not been documented. However, methysergide is not recommended during pregnancy due to its oxytocic properties.
FDA Pregnancy Category X.

**Breast-feeding**
Problems in humans have not been documented; however, ergot alkaloids are distributed into breast milk. Ergot alkaloids inhibit lactation and may cause ergotism (vomiting, diarrhea, weak pulse, unstable blood pressure, seizures) in the infant.

**Pediatrics**
Because of the hazards of long-term use of this medication, use in pediatric patients is not recommended.

**Geriatrics**
Caution is recommended in the elderly, who are more likely to have occlusive peripheral vascular disease, and are therefore more likely to be adversely affected by peripheral vasoconstriction, than are younger adults. This increases the risk of hypothermia and other ischemic complications. Elderly patients are also more likely to have age-related renal function impairment, which requires caution in patients receiving methysergide.

**Drug interactions and/or related problems**
The following drug interactions and/or related problems have been selected on the basis of their potential clinical significance (possible mechanism in parentheses where appropriate)—not necessarily inclusive (» = major clinical significance):

Note: Combinations containing any of the following medications, depending on the amount present, may also interact with this medication.

Ergot alkaloids, other or
Sumatriptan or
Vasoconstrictors, systemic, other, such as:
  Cocaine
  Epinephrine, parenteral
  Metaraminol
  Methoxamine
  Norepinephrine
  Phenylephrine, parenteral or
Vasoconstrictor-containing local anesthetic solutions
  (concurrent use with methysergide may result in enhanced vasoconstriction; a reduced dosage of ergot alkaloids may be necessary when they are used to treat an acute attack)

Opioid (narcotic) analgesics
  (concurrent use with methysergide may reverse the activity of the opioid)

Smoking, tobacco
  (administration of methysergide to patients who smoke heavily may increase the risk of peripheral vascular ischemia because nicotine also constricts blood vessels)

**Laboratory value alterations**
The following have been selected on the basis of their potential clinical significance (possible effect in parentheses where appropriate)—not necessarily inclusive (» = major clinical significance):

With physiology/laboratory test values
  Blood urea nitrogen (BUN)
    (may be increased, indicating renal failure, if retroperitoneal fibrosis occurs)

**Medical considerations/Contraindications**
The medical considerations/contraindications included have been selected on the basis of their potential clinical significance (reasons given in parentheses where appropriate)—not necessarily inclusive (» = major clinical significance).

*Risk-benefit should be considered when the following medical problems exist:*

» Coronary artery disease, especially:
» Angina, unstable or vasospastic
    (vasospasm may aggravate existing angina, or cause angina or myocardial infarction)

» Hepatic function impairment
    (impaired metabolism may result in ergot poisoning)
» Hypertension, severe
    (may be aggravated)
Peptic ulcer
    (methysergide may elevate gastric hydrochloric acid concentrations)
» Peripheral vascular disease, occlusive or
» Pruritus, severe, especially when associated with hepatic disease or
» Sepsis or other severe infection
    (sensitivity to vascular effects may be increased)
» Pulmonary disease or
» Rheumatoid arthritis or other collagen diseases or
» Valvular heart disease
    (risk of retroperitoneal, pleuropulmonary, or cardiac fibrosis)
» Renal function impairment
Sensitivity to methysergide or other ergot alkaloids, history of

**Patient monitoring**
The following may be especially important in patient monitoring (other tests may be warranted in some patients, depending on condition; » = major clinical significance):

Retroperitoneal imaging
    (recommended prior to initiation of anticipated long-term therapy and at 6- to 12-month intervals during therapy to detect early signs of retroperitoneal fibrosis; may also be indicated if signs of urinary obstruction occur)

## Side/Adverse Effects

Note: Most side effects are dose-related and are usually relieved by a reduction in dosage or withdrawal of the medication.

The following side/adverse effects have been selected on the basis of their potential clinical significance (possible signs and symptoms in parentheses where appropriate)—not necessarily inclusive:

**Those indicating need for medical attention**
Incidence more frequent
    *Ischemia, peripheral vasospasm–induced* (abdominal pain; chest pain; itching of skin; numbness and tingling of fingers, toes, or face; pain in arms, legs, or lower back; pale or cold hands or feet; weakness in legs)—specific symptoms are dependent on the blood vessel(s) involved, and may also rarely be caused by vascular insufficiency

Incidence less frequent or rare—dose-related
    *Changes in vision; clumsiness or unsteadiness; CNS stimulation, mild* (excitement or difficulty in thinking; feeling of being outside the body; hallucinations; nightmares); *convulsions; edema, peripheral* (swelling of hands, ankles, feet, or lower legs); *fast or slow heartbeat; leukopenia* (rarely, fever or chills; cough or hoarseness; lower back or side pain; painful or difficult urination)—usually asymptomatic; *mental depression; redness or flushing of face; skin rash; telangiectasia* (raised red spots on skin); *weight gain, unusual*

    Note: Although methysergide is chemically related to the hallucinogen lysergic acid diethylamide (LSD), some of the listed CNS symptoms may be associated with vascular headaches rather than an effect of the medication.

Incidence rare—dependent on duration of therapy
    *Fibrosis* (chest pain; difficult or painful urination; fever; large increase or decrease in amount of urine; leg cramps; loss of appetite; lower back, side, or groin pain; shortness of breath or difficult breathing; swelling of hands, ankles, feet, or lower legs; tightness in chest; weight loss)—fibrosis may occur in cardiac, penile, pleuropulmonary, and/or retroperitoneal tissues; specific symptoms depend on the site involved and the occurrence of associated complications, such as ureteral obstruction and vascular insufficiency

**Those indicating need for medical attention only if they continue or are bothersome**
Incidence more frequent
    *CNS effects or hypotension, orthostatic* (dizziness or lightheadedness, especially when getting up from a lying or sitting position); *diarrhea; drowsiness; nausea, vomiting, or stomach pain*

Incidence less frequent or rare
    *Alopecia* (hair loss); *constipation; heartburn; trouble in sleeping*

**Those indicating possible withdrawal and the need for medical attention if they occur after medication is discontinued**
    *Headache*

## Overdose

For specific information on the agents used in the management of methysergide overdose, see:
• *Anesthetics, Barbiturate (Systemic)* monograph;
• *Diazepam* in *Benzodiazepines (Systemic)* monograph; and/or
• *Neuromuscular Blocking Agents (Systemic)*.

For more information on the management of overdose or unintentional ingestion, **contact a Poison Control Center** (see *Poison Control Center Listing*).

**Clinical effects of overdose**
The following effects have been selected on the basis of their potential clinical significance (possible signs and symptoms in parentheses where appropriate)—not necessarily inclusive:
Acute and chronic
    *Cold and pale hands or feet; dizziness, severe; excitement*

**Treatment of overdose**
Discontinuing methysergide administration.
To decrease absorption—Gastric lavage.
Specific treatment—
    For treatment of convulsions:
        If convulsions do not respond to respiratory support, administration of a benzodiazepine such as diazepam or an ultrashort-acting barbiturate such as thiopental or thiamylal is recommended. The fact that these agents, especially the barbiturates, may cause circulatory depression when administered intravenously must be kept in mind. Administration of a neuromuscular blocking agent has also been recommended to decrease the muscular manifestations of persistent convulsions; artificial respiration is mandatory if such an agent is used. See the package inserts or *Diazepam* in *Benzodiazepines (Systemic)*, *Anesthetics, Barbiturate (Systemic)*, or *Neuromuscular Blocking Agents (Systemic)* for specific dosing guidelines for use of these products.
    For treatment of peripheral vasospasm:
        Treat by applying warmth (but avoiding excessive heat) to ischemic extremities and, in some cases, by use of prazosin or sodium nitroprusside (the risk of hypotension being kept in mind). Also, careful nursing technique designed to prevent tissue damage should be instituted.
Monitoring—Prolonged and careful monitoring is recommended.
Supportive care—Support of respiration is recommended. Patients in whom intentional overdose is confirmed or suspected should be referred for psychiatric consultation.

## Patient Consultation

As an aid to patient consultation, refer to *Advice for the Patient, Methysergide (Systemic)*.
In providing consultation, consider emphasizing the following selected information (» = major clinical significance):

**Before using this medication**
» Conditions affecting use, especially:
    Sensitivity to ergot derivatives
    Pregnancy—Not recommended during pregnancy because of oxytocic properties
    Breast-feeding—Ergot alkaloids inhibit lactation; also, they are distributed into breast milk and may cause ergotism in the infant
    Use in children—Use is not recommended, because of the hazards associated with long-term use of methysergide
    Use in the elderly—Increased risk of hypothermia and other adverse effects associated with peripheral vasoconstriction
    Other medical problems, especially cardiovascular disease, hepatic function impairment, hypertension, peripheral vascular disease, severe pruritus (especially when associated with hepatic disease), severe infection, pulmonary disease, rheumatoid arthritis, valvular heart disease, and renal function impairment

**Proper use of this medication**
» Importance of not using more medication than the amount prescribed; risk of ergotism and gangrene with overdosage
» Taking with meals or milk to reduce gastrointestinal irritation
    Missed dose: Not taking at all; not doubling doses
» Proper dosing
» Proper storage

**Precautions while using this medication**
» Checking with physician before discontinuing medication; withdrawal headache may occur
» Not taking for longer than 6 months at a time

» Caution in driving or doing jobs requiring alertness because of possible dizziness, lightheadedness, or drowsiness
   Caution when getting up suddenly from a lying or sitting position
   Avoiding alcohol, which aggravates headache
   Avoiding smoking, since nicotine constricts blood vessels
   Avoiding exposure to excessive cold, which may aggravate peripheral vasoconstriction
   Notifying physician if infection develops, since infection may cause increased sensitivity to medication

**Side/adverse effects**
Signs of potential side effects, especially changes in vision, clumsiness or unsteadiness, CNS stimulation, convulsions, fast or slow heartbeat, fibrosis, ischemia, leukopenia, mental depression, peripheral edema, peripheral ischemia, redness or flushing of face, skin rash, telangiectasia, and unusual weight gain

## General Dosing Information

Methysergide is not as potent a vasoconstrictor as ergotamine.

Because of the risk of fibrosis, methysergide should be administered for no longer than 6 months, with a drug-free interval of 3 to 4 weeks between each course.

Incidence and severity of some of the side effects may be minimized if the dosage is increased slowly to its therapeutic concentration and methysergide is given with meals.

If a response has not occurred after 3 weeks of treatment, further treatment is unlikely to produce an effect.

Gradual withdrawal of methysergide over 2 to 3 weeks is recommended to prevent rebound headache.

It is recommended that methysergide be withdrawn immediately and diagnostic tests performed if signs of retroperitoneal, pleuropulmonary, or cardiac fibrosis occur. Partial to complete regression may occur after the medication is discontinued, although surgery may be necessary in some patients.

Methysergide should be withdrawn at the first sign of vascular insufficiency.

## Oral Dosage Forms

### METHYSERGIDE MALEATE TABLETS USP

**Usual adult dose**
Oral, 4 to 8 mg a day in divided doses.

**Strength(s) usually available**
U.S.—
   2 mg (Rx) [*Sansert* (lactose; tartrazine)].
Canada—
   2 mg (Rx) [*Sansert* (lactose; tartrazine)].

**Packaging and storage**
Store below 40 °C (104 °F), preferably between 15 and 30 °C (59 and 86 °F), unless otherwise specified by manufacturer. Store in a tight container.

**Auxiliary labeling**
• Take with meals or milk.

Revised: 07/07/97
Interim revision: 08/17/94

---

**METIPRANOLOL**—See *Beta-adrenergic Blocking Agents (Ophthalmic)*

---

# METOCLOPRAMIDE   Systemic

VA CLASSIFICATION (Primary/Secondary): AU300/GA605

Commonly used brand name(s): *Apo-Metoclop; Maxeran; Metoclopramide Intensol; Octamide; PMS-Metoclopramide; Reglan.*

Note:  For a listing of dosage forms and brand names by country availability, see *Dosage Forms* section(s).

## Category

Dopaminergic blocking agent; gastrointestinal emptying (delayed) adjunct; peristaltic stimulant; antiemetic.

## Indications

Note:  Bracketed information in the *Indications* section refers to uses that are not included in U.S. product labeling.

**Accepted**
Radiography, gastrointestinal, adjunct and
Intubation, intestinal—Metoclopramide injection is indicated to facilitate intestinal intubation in adults and children, and to stimulate gastric emptying and intestinal transit of barium in cases where delayed emptying interferes with radiological examinations of stomach or small intestine.
Gastroparesis (treatment)[1]—Metoclopramide is indicated for the relief of symptoms of acute and recurrent diabetic gastroparesis.
Nausea and vomiting, cancer chemotherapy–induced (prophylaxis)—Metoclopramide injection is indicated in high doses for the prevention of nausea and vomiting associated with emetogenic cancer chemotherapy.
   Some clinicians may prefer ondansetron to high-dose metoclopramide for prophylaxis of cancer chemotherapy–induced nausea and vomiting because ondansetron is less toxic, and in some studies, has been proven more effective than high-dose metoclopramide.
Nausea and vomiting, postoperative (prophylaxis)—Metoclopramide is indicated for the prophylaxis of postoperative nausea and vomiting in cases where nasogastric suction is undesirable.
Reflux, gastroesophageal (treatment)[1]—Oral metoclopramide is indicated in adults for the symptomatic short-term treatment of heartburn and reflux esophagitis due to delayed gastric emptying. [In infants, it is used in the treatment of chronic vomiting and recurrent bronchopulmonary manifestations associated with gastroesophageal reflux.]
[Nausea and vomiting, postoperative, drug-related (treatment)]—Metoclopramide is used in the treatment of drug-related postoperative nausea and vomiting.
[Gastric emptying, slow (treatment)] or
[Gastric stasis, in preterm infants (treatment)]—Metoclopramide is used for correcting the slow gastric emptying in postvagotomy stasis, in idiopathic stasis, and in various collagen diseases such as scleroderma. In addition, it is used for persistent functional feeding intolerance and gastric stasis in preterm infants.
[Pneumonitis, aspiration (prophylaxis)][1]—Metoclopramide is used prior to general anesthesia to promote gastric emptying and reduce the risk of aspiration, especially in emergency surgery, cesarean sections, or delivery.
[Headache, vascular (treatment adjunct)][1]—Metoclopramide is used to counteract the gastric stasis and nausea associated with migraine, and to promote the absorption of orally administered analgesics given in the treatment of migraine.
[Hiccups, persistent (treatment)][1]—Metoclopramide is used in the control of persistent hiccups.
[Metoclopramide has been used in the treatment of lactation deficiency; however, it has generally been replaced by more effective medications.]

[1]Not included in Canadian product labeling.

## Pharmacology/Pharmacokinetics

**Physicochemical characteristics**
pKa—0.6 and 9.3.

**Mechanism of action/Effect**
Dopaminergic blocking agents—Gastrointestinal emptying (delayed) adjunct; peristaltic stimulant: Exact mechanism of action is unknown; however, it is believed that metoclopramide inhibits gastric smooth muscle relaxation produced by dopamine, thus enhancing cholinergic responses of the gastrointestinal smooth muscle. Accelerates intestinal transit and gastric emptying by preventing relaxation of gastric body and increasing the phasic activity of antrum. At the same time, this action is accompanied by relaxation of the upper small intestine, resulting in an improved coordination between the body and antrum of the stomach and the upper small intestine. Decreases reflux into the esophagus by increasing the resting pressure of the lower esophageal sphincter and improves acid clearance from the esophagus by increasing amplitude of esophageal peristaltic contractions.
Antiemetic—Dopamine antagonist action raises the threshold of activity in the chemoreceptor trigger zone and decreases the input from afferent visceral nerves. High doses of metoclopramide have been found to an-

tagonize 5-hydroxytryptamine (5-HT) receptors in the peripheral nervous system in animals.

**Other actions/effects**
Metoclopramide stimulates prolactin secretion and causes a transient increase in circulating aldosterone levels, which may be associated with transient fluid retention.

**Absorption**
Rapid.

**Protein binding**
Approximately 30%.

**Biotransformation**
Hepatic.

**Half-life**
4 to 6 hours.

**Onset of action**
Intramuscular—10 to 15 minutes.
Intravenous—1 to 3 minutes.
Oral—30 to 60 minutes.

**Time to peak serum concentrations**
1 to 2 hours after a single oral dose.

**Duration of action**
1 to 2 hours.

**Elimination**
Renal; approximately 85% of an oral dose appears in the urine within 72 hours as unchanged drug and sulfate and glucuronide conjugates.

## Precautions to Consider

**Cross-sensitivity and/or related problems**
Patients sensitive to procaine and procainamide may be sensitive to this medication also.

**Mutagenicity/Tumorigenicity**
An Ames mutagenicity test performed on metoclopramide was negative. Dopaminergic blocking medications produce an elevation in prolactin concentrations, which persists during long-term administration. Tissue culture experiments indicate that approximately one third of human breast cancers are prolactin-dependent *in vitro*, a factor of potential importance if the prescription of these medications is contemplated in a patient with a previously detected breast cancer. Although disturbances such as galactorrhea, amenorrhea, gynecomastia, and impotence have been reported, the clinical significance of elevated serum prolactin concentrations is unknown for most patients. An increase in mammary neoplasms has been found in rodents after long-term administration of dopaminergic blocking medications. However, neither clinical studies nor epidemiologic studies conducted to date have shown an association between long-term administration of these medications and mammary tumorigenesis; the available evidence is considered too limited to be conclusive at this time.

**Pregnancy/Reproduction**
Fertility—Studies in rats, mice, and rabbits at doses from 12 to 250 times the human dose have shown that metoclopramide does not impair fertility.

Pregnancy—Extensive studies in humans have not been done.
Studies in animals have not shown that metoclopramide causes adverse effects in the fetus.

FDA Pregnancy Category B.

**Breast-feeding**
Problems in humans have not been documented; however, risk-benefit must be considered since metoclopramide is distributed into breast milk.

**Pediatrics**
Extrapyramidal effects, especially dystonic reactions, of metoclopramide are more likely to occur in children shortly after initiation of therapy, and usually with doses higher than 0.5 mg per kg of body weight (mg/kg) per day. Methemoglobinemia has been reported in premature and full-term neonates receiving metoclopramide intramuscularly at a dose of 1 to 2 mg/kg a day for 3 days or more.

**Geriatrics**
Extrapyramidal effects, especially parkinsonism and tardive dyskinesia, of metoclopramide are more likely to occur in elderly patients following usual or high doses over a long period of time.

**Drug interactions and/or related problems**
The following drug interactions and/or related problems have been selected on the basis of their potential clinical significance (possible mechanism in parentheses where appropriate)—not necessarily inclusive (» = major clinical significance):

Note: Only specific interactions between metoclopramide and other oral medications have been identified in this monograph. However, because of increased gastrointestinal motility and decreased gastric emptying time caused by metoclopramide, absorption of oral medications from the stomach may be decreased, while absorption from the small intestine may be enhanced.

Combinations containing any of the following medications, depending on the amount present, may also interact with this medication.

» Alcohol
(concurrent use may increase the central nervous system [CNS] depressant effects of either alcohol or metoclopramide; concurrent use also may accelerate gastric emptying of alcohol, thus possibly increasing its rate and extent of absorption from the small intestine)

Anticholinergics or other medications with anticholinergic activity (see *Appendix II*) or

Opioid-containing medications
(concurrent use may antagonize the effects of metoclopramide on gastrointestinal motility)

Apomorphine
(prior administration of metoclopramide may decrease the emetic response to apomorphine; also, concurrent use may potentiate the CNS depressant effects of either apomorphine or metoclopramide)

Bromocriptine
(metoclopramide may increase serum prolactin concentrations and interfere with effects of bromocriptine; dosage adjustment of bromocriptine may be necessary)

Cimetidine
(concurrent use may decrease the effect of cimetidine due to decreased absorption)

» CNS depression–producing medications, other (see *Appendix II*)
(concurrent use may increase the sedative effects of either these medications or metoclopramide)

Cyclosporine
(the decrease in gastric emptying time caused by metoclopramide may increase the bioavailability of cyclosporine; monitoring of cyclosporine concentrations may be necessary)

Digoxin
(concurrent use may decrease absorption of digoxin from stomach; dosage adjustment of digoxin may be necessary)

Extrapyramidal reaction–causing medications (see *Appendix II*)
(concurrent use with metoclopramide may increase the frequency and severity of extrapyramidal effects)

Hepatotoxic medications (see *Appendix II*)
(concurrent use with metoclopramide may increase the risk of hepatotoxicity)

Levodopa
(metoclopramide has been reported to decrease the effectiveness of levodopa with concurrent use)

Mexiletine
(concurrent use with metoclopramide may accelerate absorption of mexiletine)

Monoamine oxidase (MAO) inhibitors, including furazolidine and procarbazine
(metoclopramide releases catecholamines in patients with essential hypertension and should be used cautiously in patients receiving MAO inhibitors)

Pergolide
(dopamine antagonists such as metoclopramide may decrease the effectiveness of pergolide)

Succinylcholine
(metoclopramide has been reported to prolong succinylcholine block; dosage reduction of succinylcholine may be necessary with concurrent use)

**Laboratory value alterations**
The following have been selected on the basis of their potential clinical significance (possible effect in parentheses where appropriate)—not necessarily inclusive (» = major clinical significance):

With diagnostic test results
Gonadorelin test
(concurrent use with metoclopramide may blunt the response to gonadorelin by increasing serum prolactin concentrations)

Hepatic function test
(results may be altered)

With physiology/laboratory test values
Aldosterone and
Prolactin, serum
(concentrations may be increased)

### Medical considerations/Contraindications

The medical considerations/contraindications included have been selected on the basis of their potential clinical significance (reasons given in parentheses where appropriate)—not necessarily inclusive (» = major clinical significance).

*Except under special circumstances, this medication should not be used when the following medical problems exist:*

» Epilepsy
(severity and frequency of seizures or extrapyramidal effects may be increased)
» Gastrointestinal hemorrhage, mechanical obstruction, or perforation
(stimulation of gastrointestinal motility may aggravate condition)
» Pheochromocytoma
(may cause hypertensive crisis)

*Risk-benefit should be considered when the following medical problems exist:*

Asthma
(administration of metoclopramide may increase risk of bronchospasm)
Depression, mental
(condition may be exacerbated)
Hypertension
(administration of intravenous metoclopramide may worsen condition due to release of catecholamines)
Parkinson's disease
(symptoms may be exacerbated)
» Renal failure, severe, chronic
(risk of extrapyramidal effects may be increased; reduced dosage is recommended)
Sensitivity to metoclopramide, procaine, or procainamide

## Side/Adverse Effects

Note: Methemoglobinemia has been reported in premature and full-term neonates receiving metoclopramide at a dose of 1 to 4 mg per kg of body weight (mg/kg) a day for 1 to 3 days or more.

The following side/adverse effects have been selected on the basis of their potential clinical significance (possible signs and symptoms in parentheses where appropriate)—not necessarily inclusive:

### Those indicating need for medical attention
Incidence rare
*Agranulocytosis* (chills; fever; sore throat; general feeling of tiredness or weakness); *cardiovascular effects, specifically hypotension* (dizziness or fainting); *hypertension* (dizziness; severe or continuing headaches; increase in blood pressure); *tachycardia* (fast or irregular heartbeat); *extrapyramidal effects, dystonic* (muscle spasms of face, neck, and back; tic-like or twitching movements; twisting movements of body; inability to move eyes; weakness of arms and legs); *extrapyramidal effects, parkinsonian* (difficulty in speaking or swallowing; loss of balance control; mask-like face; shuffling walk; stiffness of arms or legs; trembling and shaking of hands and fingers); *tardive dyskinesia* (lip smacking or puckering; puffing of cheeks; rapid or worm-like movements of tongue; uncontrolled chewing movements; uncontrolled movements of arms and legs)—usually occurs after at least one year of continuous treatment and may persist after discontinuation of metoclopramide

Note: *Extrapyramidal effects* may occur at therapeutic doses in any age group. However, they occur more frequently in children and young adults, and at the higher doses used in prophylaxis of vomiting due to cancer chemotherapy. *Dystonic* reactions may start within minutes after start of intravenous therapy and disappear within 24 hours after discontinuation of metoclopramide. Onset of *parkinsonian* symptoms may vary from a few weeks to several months after initiation of therapy; symptoms are reversible upon discontinuation of metoclopramide.

With high doses
*Agitation* (unusual nervousness, restlessness, or irritability); *panic-like sensation; restless legs syndrome* (aching or discomfort in lower legs or sensation of crawling in legs)

Note: These effects may occur within minutes of receiving high doses of metoclopramide and may last for 2 to 24 hours.

### Those indicating need for medical attention only if they continue or are bothersome
Incidence more frequent
*Diarrhea*—with high doses; *drowsiness; restlessness; unusual tiredness or weakness*
Incidence less frequent or rare
*Breast tenderness and swelling; changes in menstruation; constipation; dizziness; headache; insomnia* (trouble in sleeping); *mental depression; prolactin stimulation* (increased flow of breast milk); *nausea; skin rash; unusual dryness of mouth; unusual irritability*

## Overdose

For specific information on the agents used in the management of metoclopramide overdose, see:
• *Diphenhydramine* in *Antihistamines (Systemic)* monograph; and/or
• *Methylene Blue (Systemic)* monograph.

For more information on the management of overdose or unintentional ingestion, **contact a Poison Control Center** (see *Poison Control Center Listing*).

### Clinical effects of overdose
Symptoms are self-limiting and usually disappear within 24 hours.
The following have been selected on the basis of their potential clinical significance (possible signs and symptoms in parentheses where appropriate)—not necessarily inclusive:

*Confusion; drowsiness, severe; extrapyramidal effects, severe; seizures*

### Treatment of overdose
To decrease absorption—
Dialysis is not likely to be an effective method of drug removal in overdose situations; hemodialysis and continuous ambulatory peritoneal dialysis do not remove significant amounts of metoclopramide.
Specific treatment—
Anticholinergic or antiparkinson drugs or antihistamines with anticholinergic properties (50 mg of diphenhydramine administered intramuscularly in adults and 1 mg per kg of body weight [mg/kg] intramuscularly or intravenously in infants and children) to help in controlling the extrapyramidal reactions.
Methylene blue (1 to 2 mg/kg of a 1% solution injected intravenously over a 5-minute period) is used to reverse methemoglobinemia resulting from metoclopramide administration in premature and full-term infants.
Supportive care—
Patients in whom intentional overdose is confirmed or suspected should be referred for psychiatric consultation.

## Patient Consultation

As an aid to patient consultation, refer to *Advice for the Patient, Metoclopramide (Systemic)*.
In providing consultation, consider emphasizing the following selected information (» = major clinical significance):

### Before using this medication
» Conditions affecting use, especially:
Sensitivity to metoclopramide, procaine, or procainamide
Breast-feeding—Distributed into breast milk
Use in children—Extrapyramidal effects more likely; increased risk of methemoglobinemia in premature and full-term infants
Use in the elderly—Extrapyramidal effects more likely
Other medications, especially alcohol and CNS depressants
Other medical problems, especially epilepsy; gastrointestinal bleeding, mechanical obstruction, or perforation; pheochromocytoma; or severe renal function impairment

### Proper use of this medication
» Taking 30 minutes before meals and at bedtime (for oral dosage forms)
» Not taking more medication than the amount prescribed
» Proper administration of metoclopramide oral solution (concentrate):
Mix with liquid or semi-solid food, such as water, juices, soda or soda-like beverages, applesauce, and puddings
» Proper dosing
Missed dose: Using as soon as possible; not using if almost time for next dose
» Proper storage

### Precautions while using this medication
» Avoiding use of alcohol or other CNS depressants
» Caution if drowsiness occurs

### Side/adverse effects
Signs of potential side effects, especially agranulocytosis, cardiovascular effects, extrapyramidal effects, and tardive dyskinesia

## General Dosing Information

In patients with severe renal function impairment (i.e., creatinine clearance < 40 mL per minute), the normally prescribed dose should be reduced by 50%, since adverse effects are more likely to be exacerbated.

### For parenteral dosage forms only

Intravenous injections of metoclopramide should be made *slowly* over a 1- to 2-minute period, since a transient but intense feeling of anxiety and restlessness followed by drowsiness may occur with rapid administration.

Intravenous infusion should be made *slowly* over a period of not less than 15 minutes. Metoclopramide injection may be diluted for intravenous infusion with 50 mL of 5% dextrose in water, sodium chloride injection, 5% dextrose in 0.45% sodium chloride, Ringer's injection, or lactated Ringer's injection.

### For treatment of adverse effects and/or overdose

Recommended treatment for metoclopramide's adverse effects and/or overdose includes:
- Anticholinergic or antiparkinson drugs or antihistamines with anticholinergic properties (50 mg of diphenhydramine administered intramuscularly in adults and 1 mg per kg of body weight [mg/kg] intramuscularly or intravenously in infants and children) to help in controlling the extrapyramidal reactions.
- Methylene blue (1 to 2 mg/kg of a 1% solution injected intravenously over a 5-minute period) is used to reverse methemoglobinemia resulting from metoclopramide administration in premature and full-term infants.

## Oral Dosage Forms

Note: Bracketed uses in the *Dosage Forms* section refer to categories of use and/or indications that are not included in U.S. product labeling. The dosing and strengths of the dosage forms available are expressed in terms of metoclopramide base.

### METOCLOPRAMIDE ORAL SOLUTION USP

**Usual adult and adolescent dose**
Treatment of diabetic gastroparesis[1]—
  Oral, 10 mg (base) thirty minutes before symptoms are likely to occur or before each meal and at bedtime, up to four times a day.
  Note: In the initial treatment of diabetic gastroparesis, the parenteral route of administration is recommended if severe symptoms are present. Therapy may begin at 10 mg (base) administered intramuscularly or intravenously three or four times a day, the dose adjusted as needed.
Treatment of gastroesophageal reflux[1]—
  Oral, 10 to 15 mg (base) thirty minutes before symptoms are likely to occur or before each meal and at bedtime, up to four times a day.
  Note: Intermittent symptoms may be treated by taking 20 mg of metoclopramide prior to the provoking situation.
[Treatment of hiccups][1]—
  Oral, 10 to 20 mg (base) four times a day for seven days. An initial dose of 10 mg intramuscularly may be given if necessary.
Note: In patients with renal function impairment whose creatinine clearance is less than 40 mL per minute, initial dosage should be reduced by approximately one half.

**Usual adult and adolescent prescribing limits**
500 mcg (0.5 mg) per kg of body weight per day.

**Usual pediatric dose**
Gastrointestinal emptying (delayed) adjunct or
Peristaltic stimulant—
  Oral, 0.1 to 0.2 mg per kg of body weight per dose, given thirty minutes before meals and at bedtime.

**Strength(s) usually available**
U.S.—
  5 mg (base) per 5 mL (Rx) [*Reglan*; GENERIC].
Canada—
  5 mg (base) per 5 mL (Rx) [*Maxeran; Reglan*].

**Packaging and storage**
Store between 20 and 25 °C (68 and 77 °F), in a tight container, unless otherwise specified by manufacturer. Protect from light. Protect from freezing.

**Auxiliary labeling**
- May cause drowsiness.
- Avoid alcoholic beverages.

### METOCLOPRAMIDE HYDROCHLORIDE ORAL SOLUTION (CONCENTRATE)

**Usual adult and adolescent dose**
See *Metoclopramide Oral Solution USP*.

**Usual adult and adolescent prescribing limits**
See *Metoclopramide Oral Solution USP*.

**Usual pediatric dose**
See *Metoclopramide Oral Solution USP*.

**Strength(s) usually available**
U.S.—
  10 mg (base) per 1 mL (Rx) [*Metoclopramide Intensol* (calibrated dropper enclosed; sodium benzoate; sorbitol)].
Canada—
  Not commercially available.

**Packaging and storage**
Store between 15 and 30 °C (59 and 86 °F), in a tight container, unless otherwise specified by manufacturer. Protect from light. Protect from freezing.

**Preparation of dosage form**
Each dose should be mixed with liquid or semi-solid food such as water, juices, soda or soda-like beverages, applesauce, or puddings.

**Auxiliary labeling**
- Dilute before use.
- May cause drowsiness.
- Avoid alcoholic beverages.

### METOCLOPRAMIDE TABLETS USP

**Usual adult and adolescent dose**
See *Metoclopramide Oral Solution USP*.

**Usual adult and adolescent prescribing limits**
See *Metoclopramide Oral Solution USP*.

**Usual pediatric dose**
See *Metoclopramide Oral Solution USP*.

**Usual geriatric dose**
See *Metoclopramide Oral Solution USP*.

**Strength(s) usually available**
U.S.—
  5 mg (Rx) [*Reglan* (scored); GENERIC].
  10 mg (Rx) [*Octamide; Reglan* (scored); GENERIC].
Canada—
  5 mg (Rx) [*Apo-Metoclop; Maxeran; PMS-Metoclopramide; Reglan*].
  10 mg (Rx) [*Apo-Metoclop; Maxeran* (scored); *PMS-Metoclopramide; Reglan*].

**Packaging and storage**
Store between 20 and 25 °C (68 and 77 °F), unless otherwise specified by manufacturer. Store in a tight, light-resistant container.

**Auxiliary labeling**
- May cause drowsiness.
- Avoid alcoholic beverages.

## Parenteral Dosage Forms

Note: Bracketed uses in the *Dosage Forms* section refer to categories of use and/or indications that are not included in U.S. product labeling.

### METOCLOPRAMIDE INJECTION USP

**Usual adult and adolescent dose**
Gastrointestinal emptying (delayed) adjunct or
Peristaltic stimulant—
  Intravenous, 10 mg as a single dose.
[Treatment of hiccups][1]—
  Intramuscular, 10 mg initially, followed by oral metoclopramide at a dose of 10 to 20 mg four times a day for seven days.
Antiemetic: For prevention of cancer chemotherapy–induced emesis—
  Intravenous infusion, 2 mg per kg of body weight, administered thirty minutes before cisplatin or other highly emetogenic chemotherapeutic agent; may be repeated as needed every two or three hours.
  Note: For prevention of emesis induced by chemotherapeutic agents with low emetic potential—Intravenous infusion, 1 mg per kg of body weight.
Continuous intravenous infusion, 3 mg per kg of body weight before chemotherapy, followed by 0.5 mg per kg of body weight per hour for eight hours.
Antiemetic: For prevention of postoperative emesis—
  Intramuscular, 10 to 20 mg near the end of surgery.

**Usual pediatric dose**
Antiemetic—For prevention of cancer chemotherapy–induced emesis or
Gastrointestinal emptying (delayed) adjunct or
Peristaltic stimulant—
  Intravenous, 1 mg per kg of body weight as a single dose. May be repeated one time after sixty minutes.

Note: To reduce the chance of increased adverse reactions, dosages should not exceed 2 mg per kg of body weight. Some clinicians recommend concurrent therapy with diphenhydramine at an intravenous dose of 1 mg per kg of body weight 15 minutes prior to metoclopramide infusion to limit side effects that may occur with doses of less than 2 mg per kg of body weight.

**Strength(s) usually available**
U.S.—
  5 mg per mL (Rx) [Reglan; GENERIC].
Canada—
  5 mg per mL (Rx) [Reglan].

**Packaging and storage**
Store between 15 and 30 °C (59 and 86 °F), unless otherwise specified by manufacturer. Protect from light (if injection does not contain an antioxidant).

**Preparation of dosage form**
Doses of Metoclopramide Injection USP in excess of 10 mg may be mixed with 50 mL of 0.9% sodium chloride injection, 5% dextrose injection, 5% dextrose in 0.45% sodium chloride injection, Ringer's injection, or lactated Ringer's injection.

**Stability**
Unused portion should be discarded.
Dilutions of metoclopramide injection may be stored for up to 48 hours after preparation if protected from light, or 24 hours if not protected from light.
Dilutions of metoclopramide and 0.9% sodium chloride may be stored frozen for up to 4 weeks after preparation.

**Incompatibilities**
Metoclopramide injection is incompatible with calcium gluconate, cephalothin sodium, chloramphenicol sodium, cisplatin, erythromycin lactobionate, furosemide, methotrexate, penicillin G potassium, and sodium bicarbonate.

[1]Not included in Canadian product labeling.

Revised: 08/12/98

---

**METOCURINE**—See Neuromuscular Blocking Agents (Systemic)

---

**METOLAZONE**—See Diuretics, Thiazide (Systemic)

---

**METOPROLOL**—See Beta-adrenergic Blocking Agents (Systemic)

---

**METRIZAMIDE**—The Metrizamide (Systemic) monograph is not included in this published version of the USP DI database. Copies of the monograph are available on request from Micromedex, Inc. - Reprint Requests, 6200 S. Syracuse Way, Suite 300, Englewood, CO 80111; telephone (303) 486-6400; telefax (303) 486-6464; Email: USPDI@MDX.COM.

---

# METRONIDAZOLE  Systemic

VA CLASSIFICATION (Primary/Secondary): AM900/AP109; AP200; GA900

Commonly used brand name(s): Apo-Metronidazole; Flagyl; Flagyl I.V.; Flagyl I.V. RTU; Metric 21; Metro I.V.; Novonidazol; Protostat; Trikacide.

Note: For a listing of dosage forms and brand names by country availability, see Dosage Forms section(s).

## Category
Antibacterial (systemic); antiprotozoal; bowel disease (inflammatory) suppressant; anthelmintic (systemic).

## Indications
Note: Bracketed information in the Indications section refers to uses that are not included in U.S. product labeling.

**Accepted**

Amebiasis, extraintestinal (treatment)—Metronidazole is indicated in the treatment of extraintestinal amebiasis, including amebic liver abscess, caused by Entamoeba histolytica. When used in the treatment of invasive amebiasis, metronidazole should be administered concurrently or sequentially with a luminal amebicide (e.g., iodoquinol, paromomycin, tetracycline, diloxanide furoate).

Amebiasis, intestinal (treatment)—Oral metronidazole is indicated in the treatment of acute intestinal amebiasis caused by Entamoeba histolytica. Metronidazole may not eradicate intestinal amebic infections, requiring treatment with a luminal amebicide.

Bone and joint infections (treatment)—Metronidazole is indicated in the treatment of bone and joint infections caused by Bacteroides species, including the B. fragilis group (B. fragilis, B. distasonis, B. ovatus, B. thetaiotaomicron, B. vulgatus).

Brain abscess (treatment)—Metronidazole is indicated in the treatment of brain abscess caused by Bacteroides species, including the B. fragilis group.

Central nervous system (CNS) infections (treatment)—Metronidazole is indicated in the treatment of CNS infections, including meningitis, caused by Bacteroides species, including the B. fragilis group.

Endocarditis, bacterial (treatment)—Metronidazole is indicated in the treatment of endocarditis caused by Bacteroides species, including the B. fragilis group.

Intra-abdominal infections (treatment)—Metronidazole is indicated in the treatment of intra-abdominal infections, including peritonitis, intra-abdominal abscess, and liver abscess, caused by Bacteroides species, including the B. fragilis group, Clostridium species, Eubacterium species, Peptococcus species, and Peptostreptococcus species.

Pelvic infections, female (treatment)—Metronidazole is indicated in the treatment of female pelvic infections, including endometritis, endomyometritis, tubo-ovarian abscess, and postsurgical vaginal cuff infections, caused by Bacteroides species, including the B. fragilis group, Clostridium species, Peptococcus species, and Peptostreptococcus species.

Perioperative infections, colorectal (prophylaxis)—Intravenous metronidazole is indicated for the prophylaxis of perioperative infections during colorectal surgery.

Pneumonia, Bacteroides species (treatment)—Metronidazole is indicated in the treatment of lower respiratory tract infections, including pneumonia, empyema, and lung abscess, caused by Bacteroides species, including the B. fragilis group.

Septicemia, bacterial (treatment)—Metronidazole is indicated in the treatment of bacterial septicemia caused by Bacteroides species, including the B. fragilis group, and Clostridium species.

Skin and soft tissue infections (treatment)—Metronidazole is indicated in the treatment of skin and soft tissue infections caused by Bacteroides species, including the B. fragilis group, Clostridium species, Fusobacterium species, Peptococcus species, and Peptostreptococcus species.

Trichomoniasis (treatment)—Oral metronidazole is indicated in the treatment of symptomatic and asymptomatic trichomoniasis, in males and females, caused by Trichomonas vaginalis.

[Balantidiasis (treatment)][1]—Metronidazole is used in the treatment of Balantidium coli infection.

[Bowel disease, inflammatory (treatment)][1]—Metronidazole is used in the treatment of inflammatory bowel disease.

[Colitis, antibiotic-associated (treatment)][1]—Metronidazole is used in the treatment of antibiotic-associated diarrhea and colitis caused by C. difficile.

[Dracunculiasis (treatment)][1]—Metronidazole is used in the treatment of dracunculiasis (guinea worm infection) caused by Dracunculus medinensis. It decreases the inflammation around the ulcer, increasing the ease of removing the worm.

[Gastritis, Helicobacter pylori–associated (treatment adjunct)][1] or
[Ulcer, duodenal, Helicobacter pylori–associated (treatment adjunct)][1]—Some studies indicate that metronidazole may be effective, in combination with bismuth subsalicylate or colloidal bismuth subcitrate, and other oral antibiotic therapy, such as ampicillin or amoxicillin, in the

treatment of *Helicobacter pylori*–associated gastritis and duodenal ulcer. However, metronidazole resistance may occur, especially in patients who have been previously exposed to metronidazole.

[Giardiasis (treatment)][1]—Oral metronidazole is used in the treatment of giardiasis caused by *Giardia lamblia*.

[Periodontal infections (treatment)][1]—Metronidazole is used in the treatment of periodontal infections caused by *Bacteroides* species.

[Vaginosis, bacterial (treatment)][1]—Oral metronidazole is used in the treatment of bacterial vaginosis caused by *Gardnerella vaginalis*.

Not all species or strains of a particular organism may be equally susceptible to metronidazole.

**Unaccepted**
Metronidazole is not effective against facultative anaerobes, obligate aerobes, *Propionibacterium acnes*, *Actinomyces* species, or *Candida albicans*.

[1]Not included in Canadian product labeling.

## Pharmacology/Pharmacokinetics

**Physicochemical characteristics**
Molecular weight—Metronidazole: 171.16.
Metronidazole hydrochloride: 207.62.

**Mechanism of action/Effect**
Antibacterial (systemic); antiprotozoal—Microbicidal; active against most obligate anaerobic bacteria and protozoa by undergoing intracellular chemical reduction via mechanisms unique to anaerobic metabolism. Reduced metronidazole, which is cytotoxic but short-lived, interacts with DNA to cause a loss of helical structure, strand breakage, and resultant inhibition of nucleic acid synthesis and cell death.

**Absorption**
Well absorbed orally; bioavailability at least 80%.

**Distribution**
Distributed to saliva, bile, seminal fluid, breast milk, bone, liver and liver abscesses, lungs, and vaginal secretions; crosses the placenta and blood-brain barrier, also.
 $Vol_D$—
  In adults: Approximately 0.55 L/kg.
  In neonates: 0.54–0.81 L/kg.

**Protein binding**
Low (<20%).

**Biotransformation**
Hepatic; metabolized primarily by side-chain oxidation and glucuronide conjugation to 2-hydroxymethyl (also active) and other metabolites.

**Half-life**
In adults—
 Normal liver function: 8 hours (range, 6 to 12 hours).
 Alcoholic liver disease: 18 hours (range, 10 to 29 hours).
In neonates—
 28 to 30 weeks gestational age: Approximately 75 hours.
 32 to 35 weeks gestational age: Approximately 35 hours.
 36 to 40 weeks gestational age: Approximately 25 hours.

**Time to peak serum concentration**
1 to 2 hours (oral).

**Peak serum concentration**
Peak serum concentrations following a 250-mg, 500-mg, and 2-gram oral dose are approximately 6, 12, and 40 mcg/mL, respectively.
At recommended intravenous doses, peak steady-state serum concentrations are approximately 25 mcg/mL; trough concentrations are approximately 18 mcg/mL.

**Elimination**
Renal—60 to 80%; of this amount, approximately 20% excreted unchanged in urine. Renal clearance approximately 10 mL/min/1.73 $M^2$.
Fecal—6 to 15%; inactive metabolites also present in feces.
In dialysis—
 Hemodialysis: Metronidazole and primary metabolites rapidly removed from the blood by hemodialysis (half-life shortened to approximately 2.6 hours).
 Peritoneal dialysis: Metronidazole is not significantly removed by peritoneal dialysis.

## Precautions to Consider

**Carcinogenicity/Tumorigenicity**
Metronidazole has been shown to be carcinogenic in a number of studies in mice. Pulmonary tumorigenesis has been reported in six studies in mice, including one study in which the animals were dosed on an intermittent schedule (every four weeks). Malignant hepatic tumors have also been reported in male mice given very high doses (approximately 500 mg/kg/day). Malignant lymphomas have been reported in one lifetime feeding study in mice.

Metronidazole has also been shown to be carcinogenic in rats. Several long-term, oral-dosing studies in rats have shown that metronidazole causes a statistically significant increase in the incidence of various neoplasms, especially mammary and hepatic tumors, in female rats.

Two lifetime tumorigenicity studies in hamsters have given negative results.

Metronidazole has not been shown to be carcinogenic or tumorigenic in humans.

**Mutagenicity**
Studies have shown that metronidazole is mutagenic in bacteria and fungi, although this has not been confirmed in mammals.

**Pregnancy/Reproduction**
Fertility; pregnancy—
Metronidazole crosses the placenta and enters the fetal circulation rapidly. Adequate and well-controlled studies in humans have not been done. Studies in rats, given doses of up to 5 times the human dose, have not shown that metronidazole causes impaired fertility or birth defects in the fetus. Metronidazole, administered intraperitoneally to pregnant mice at approximately the human dose, has been shown to cause fetotoxicity. When administered orally, no fetotoxicity was seen in pregnant mice. However, the use of metronidazole in the treatment of trichomoniasis is not recommended during the first trimester. If metronidazole is used during the second and third trimesters for trichomoniasis, it is recommended that its use be limited to those patients whose symptoms are not controlled by local palliative treatment. Also, the 1-day course of therapy should not be used since this results in higher maternal and fetal serum concentrations.

Studies in rats given doses of up to 5 times the usual human dose have not shown that metronidazole causes impaired fertility or birth defects in the fetus. Metronidazole, administered intraperitoneally to pregnant mice at approximately the human dose, has been shown to cause fetotoxicity. When metronidazole was administered orally, no fetotoxicity was seen in pregnant mice.

FDA Pregnancy Category B.

**Breast-feeding**
Metronidazole is distributed into breast milk; concentrations are similar to those found in the maternal plasma. Use is not recommended in nursing mothers since some studies in rats and mice have shown that metronidazole is carcinogenic and may cause adverse effects in the infant. However, use in the treatment of anaerobic bacterial infections or a short course of treatment with metronidazole for amebiasis, severe periodontal infections, or trichomoniasis may be necessary in nursing mothers. During treatment with metronidazole, the breast milk should be expressed and discarded. Breast-feeding may be resumed 24 to 48 hours after treatment is completed.

**Pediatrics**
When used for the treatment of anaerobic infections and amebiasis, metronidazole has not demonstrated any pediatrics-specific problems that would limit its usefulness in children.

**Geriatrics**
No information is available on the relationship of age to the effects of metronidazole in geriatric patients. However, elderly patients are more likely to have an age-related decrease in hepatic function, which may require an adjustment in dosage in patients receiving metronidazole.

**Dental**
Metronidazole may cause dry mouth, an unpleasant or sharp metallic taste, and alteration of taste sensation. Dry mouth may contribute to the development of caries, periodontal disease, oral candidiasis, and discomfort.

**Drug interactions and/or related problems**
The following drug interactions and/or related problems have been selected on the basis of their potential clinical significance (possible mechanism in parentheses where appropriate)—not necessarily inclusive (» = major clinical significance):

Note: Combinations containing any of the following medications, depending on the amount present, may also interact with this medication.

» Alcohol
  (it is recommended that metronidazole not be used concurrently with, or for at least 1 day following, ingestion of alcohol; accumulation of acetaldehyde by interference with the oxidation of alcohol may occur, resulting in disulfiram-like effects such as abdominal cramps, nausea, vomiting, headache, or flushing; in addition, modifications in the taste of alcoholic beverages have been reported during concurrent use)

» Anticoagulants, coumarin- or indandione-derivative
  (effects may be potentiated when these agents are used concurrently with metronidazole, because of inhibition of enzymatic metabolism of anticoagulants; periodic prothrombin time determinations may be required during therapy to determine if dosage adjustments of anticoagulants are necessary)
Cimetidine
  (hepatic metabolism of metronidazole may be decreased when metronidazole and cimetidine are used concurrently, possibly resulting in delayed elimination and increased serum metronidazole concentrations; monitoring of serum concentrations as a guide to dosage is recommended since dosage adjustments of metronidazole may be necessary during and after cimetidine therapy)
» Disulfiram
  (it is recommended that metronidazole not be used concurrently with, or for 2 weeks following, disulfiram in alcoholic patients; such use may result in confusion and psychotic reactions because of combined toxicity)
Neurotoxic medications, other (See *Appendix II*)
  (concurrent use of metronidazole with other neurotoxic medications may increase the potential for neurotoxicity)
Phenobarbital
  (phenobarbital may induce microsomal liver enzymes, increasing metronidazole's metabolism and resulting in a decrease in half-life and plasma concentration)
Phenytoin
  (metronidazole may impair the clearance of phenytoin, increasing phenytoin's plasma concentration)

**Laboratory value alterations**
The following have been selected on the basis of their potential clinical significance (possible effect in parentheses where appropriate)—not necessarily inclusive (» = major clinical significance):

With diagnostic test results
Alanine aminotransferase (ALT [SGPT]), serum and
Aspartate aminotransferase (AST [SGOT]), serum and
Lactate dehydrogenase (LDH)
  (metronidazole has a high absorbance at the wavelength at which nicotinamide-adenine dinucleotide [NADH] is determined; therefore, elevated liver enzyme concentrations may appear to be suppressed by metronidazole when measured by continuous-flow methods based on endpoint decrease in reduced NADH; unusually low liver enzyme concentrations, including zero values, have been reported)

**Medical considerations/Contraindications**
The medical considerations/contraindications included have been selected on the basis of their potential clinical significance (reasons given in parentheses where appropriate)—not necessarily inclusive (» = major clinical significance).

*Risk-benefit should be considered when the following medical problems exist:*
» Active organic disease of the CNS, including epilepsy
  (metronidazole may cause CNS toxicity, including seizures with high doses, and peripheral neuropathy)
» Blood dyscrasias, or history of
  (metronidazole may cause leukopenia)
Cardiac function impairment
  (parenteral dosage forms—because of sodium content)
» Hepatic function impairment, severe
  (metabolized in the liver; hepatic dysfunction may lead to decreased plasma clearance and accumulation of metronidazole and its metabolites; dosage may need to be reduced with severe hepatic function impairment)
Hypersensitivity to metronidazole

**Patient monitoring**
The following may be especially important in patient monitoring (other tests may be warranted in some patients, depending on condition; » = major clinical significance):

*For giardiasis*
» Stool examinations
  (3 stool examinations, taken several days apart, beginning 3 to 4 weeks following treatment are recommended if symptoms persist; however, in some successfully treated patients, the lactose intolerance brought on by the infection may persist for a period of some weeks or months, mimicking the symptoms of giardiasis; in cases of treatment failure, alternate drugs may be used)

## Side/Adverse Effects
The following side/adverse effects have been selected on the basis of their potential clinical significance (possible signs and symptoms in parentheses where appropriate)—not necessarily inclusive:

**Those indicating need for medical attention**
Incidence less frequent
  *Peripheral neuropathy* (numbness, tingling, pain, or weakness in hands or feet)—usually with high doses or prolonged use; *seizures*—usually with high doses
Incidence rare
  *CNS toxicity* (ataxia—clumsiness or unsteadiness; encephalopathy—mood or other mental changes); *hypersensitivity* (skin rash, hives, redness, or itching); *leukopenia* (sore throat and fever); *pancreatitis* (severe abdominal and back pain; anorexia; nausea and vomiting); *thrombophlebitis* (pain, tenderness, redness, or swelling at site of injection); *vaginal candidiasis* (any vaginal irritation, discharge, or dryness not present before therapy)

**Those indicating need for medical attention only if they continue or are bothersome**
Incidence more frequent
  *CNS effects* (dizziness or lightheadedness; headache); *gastrointestinal disturbance* (diarrhea; loss of appetite; nausea or vomiting; stomach pain or cramps)
Incidence less frequent or rare
  *Change in taste sensation; dryness of mouth; unpleasant or sharp metallic taste*

**Those not indicating need for medical attention**
Incidence less frequent or rare
  *Dark urine*

## Overdose
For more information on the management of overdose or unintentional ingestion, **contact a Poison Control Center** (see *Poison Control Center Listing*).

**Treatment of overdose**
Since there is no specific antidote, treatment for metronidazole overdose should be symptomatic and supportive.

## Patient Consultation
As an aid to patient consultation, refer to *Advice for the Patient, Metronidazole (Systemic)*.
In providing consultation, consider emphasizing the following selected information (» = major clinical significance):

**Before using this medication**
» Conditions affecting use, especially:
  Hypersensitivity to metronidazole
  Pregnancy—Metronidazole crosses the placenta; use is not recommended during the first trimester of pregnancy
  Breast-feeding—Metronidazole is distributed into breast milk; metronidazole is not recommended during breast-feeding
  Dental—Metronidazole may cause dry mouth, an unpleasant or sharp metallic taste, and alteration of taste sensation
  Other medications, especially alcohol, coumarin- or indandione-derivative anticoagulants, or disulfiram
  Other medical problems, especially active organic disease of the CNS, a history of blood dyscrasias, or severe hepatic function impairment

**Proper use of this medication**
Taking with meals or a snack to minimize gastrointestinal irritation
» Compliance with full course of therapy
» Importance of not missing doses and taking at evenly spaced times
» Proper dosing
  Missed dose: Taking as soon as possible; not taking if almost time for next dose; not doubling doses
» Proper storage

**Precautions while using this medication**
Follow-up visit to physician after treatment for giardiasis to ensure that infection has been eradicated.
Checking with physician if no improvement within a few days
» Avoiding use of alcoholic beverages or other alcohol-containing preparations while taking and for at least 1 day after discontinuing this medication
Possible dryness of mouth; using sugarless candy or gum, ice, or saliva substitute for relief; checking with dentist if dry mouth continues for more than 2 weeks

» Caution if dizziness or lightheadedness occurs
  Prevention of reinfection in trichomoniasis; possible need for concurrent treatment of male sexual partner and use of a condom

**Side/adverse effects**
  Signs of potential side effects, especially CNS toxicity, hypersensitivity, leukopenia, pancreatitis, seizures, peripheral neuropathy, vaginal candidiasis, and thrombophlebitis
  Dark urine may be alarming to patient although medically insignificant

## General Dosing Information

Patients with severely impaired hepatic function metabolize metronidazole slowly. Close monitoring for toxicity, as well as reduction in dose, may be required.

Anuric patients do not generally require a reduction in dose since metabolites of metronidazole may be rapidly removed by hemodialysis. Also, reduced renal function does not significantly affect single-dose pharmacokinetics of metronidazole.

**For oral dosage forms only**
Metronidazole may be taken with meals or a snack to lessen gastrointestinal irritation.

When metronidazole is used in the treatment of trichomoniasis, sexual partners should receive concurrent therapy since asymptomatic trichomoniasis in the male partner is a frequent source of reinfection in the female. The male partner should be advised to use a condom for the duration of treatment.

**For parenteral dosage forms only**
Parenteral metronidazole should be administered by slow intravenous infusion only, either continuously or intermittently over a 1-hour period.

If metronidazole is administered concurrently with a primary intravenous solution, the primary solution should be discontinued while metronidazole is being infused.

## Oral Dosage Forms

Note: Bracketed uses in the *Dosage Forms* section refer to categories of use and/or indications that are not included in U.S. product labeling.

### METRONIDAZOLE CAPSULES

**Usual adult and adolescent dose**
Antibacterial (systemic)—
  Anaerobic infections: Oral, 7.5 mg (base) per kg of body weight, up to a maximum of 1 gram, every six hours for seven days or longer.
  [Bowel disease, inflammatory][1]: Oral, 500 mg (base) four times a day.
  [Colitis, antibiotic-associated][1]: Oral, 500 mg (base) three or four times a day.
  [Gastritis, *Helicobacter pylori*–associated (treatment adjunct)][1] or
  [Ulcer, duodenal, *Helicobacter pylori*–associated (treatment adjunct)][1]—Oral, 500 mg (base) three times a day, in conjunction with bismuth subsalicylate or colloidal bismuth subcitrate and other oral antibiotic therapy, such as ampicillin or amoxicillin, for one to two weeks.
  [Vaginosis, bacterial][1]: Oral, 500 mg (base) two times a day for seven days.
Antiprotozoal—
  Amebiasis: Oral, 500 to 750 mg (base) three times a day for five to ten days.
  [Balantidiasis][1]: Oral, 750 mg (base) three times a day for five or six days.
  [Giardiasis][1]: Oral, 2 grams (base) once a day for three days; or 250 mg three times a day for five to seven days.
  Trichomoniasis: Oral, 2 grams (base) as a single dose; 1 gram two times a day for one day; or 250 mg three times a day for seven days.
Anthelmintic (systemic)—
  [Dracunculiasis][1]: Oral, 250 mg (base) three times a day for ten days.

**Usual adult prescribing limits**
Antibacterial (systemic)—
  Up to a maximum of 4 grams (base) daily.

**Usual pediatric dose**
Antibacterial (systemic)—
  Anaerobic infections[1]: Oral, 7.5 mg (base) per kg of body weight every six hours, or 10 mg per kg of body weight every eight hours.
Antiprotozoal—
  Amebiasis: Oral, 11.6 to 16.7 mg (base) per kg of body weight three times a day for ten days.
  [Balantidiasis][1]: Oral, 11.6 to 16.7 mg (base) per kg of body weight three times a day for five days.
  [Giardiasis][1]: Oral, 5 mg (base) per kg of body weight three times a day for five to seven days.
  Trichomoniasis: Oral, 5 mg (base) per kg of body weight three times a day for seven days.
Anthelmintic (systemic)—
  [Dracunculiasis][1]: Oral, 8.3 mg (base) per kg of body weight, up to a maximum of 250 mg, three times a day for ten days.

**Strength(s) usually available**
U.S.—
  Not commercially available.
Canada—
  500 mg (base) (Rx) [*Flagyl* (sodium 5.47 mg); *Trikacide*].

**Packaging and storage**
Store below 40 °C (104 °F), preferably between 15 and 30 °C (59 and 86 °F), in a well-closed container, unless otherwise specified by manufacturer. Store in a light-resistant container.

**Auxiliary labeling**
• Avoid alcoholic beverages.
• May cause dizziness.
• Continue medicine for full time of treatment.

### METRONIDAZOLE TABLETS USP

**Usual adult and adolescent dose**
See *Metronidazole Capsules*.

**Usual adult prescribing limits**
See *Metronidazole Capsules*.

**Usual pediatric dose**
See *Metronidazole Capsules*.

**Strength(s) usually available**
U.S.—
  250 mg (base) (Rx) [*Flagyl; Metric 21; Protostat* (scored; lactose); GENERIC].
  500 mg (base) (Rx) [*Flagyl; Protostat* (scored; lactose); GENERIC].
Canada—
  250 mg (base) (Rx) [*Apo-Metronidazole; Flagyl* (sodium 3.1 mg); *Novonidazol* (scored; sodium 2.2 mg); *Trikacide*].

**Packaging and storage**
Store below 40 °C (104 °F), preferably between 15 and 30 °C (59 and 86 °F), unless otherwise specified by manufacturer. Store in a well-closed, light-resistant container.

**Preparation of dosage form**
For patients who cannot take oral solids—According to the primary manufacturer, the tablets may be crushed and suspended in Cherry Syrup NF to prepare a pediatric dosage form. The recommended concentration per 5 mL is the dose calculated for a particular pediatric patient. The suspension is stable for 30 days if stored at ambient room temperature or refrigerated. Dispense with "shake well" instructions.

**Auxiliary labeling**
• Avoid alcoholic beverages.
• May cause dizziness.
• Continue medicine for full time of treatment.

## Parenteral Dosage Forms

Note: Bracketed uses in the *Dosage Forms* section refer to categories of use and/or indications that are not included in U.S. product labeling.

Note: The dosing and dosage forms available are expressed in terms of metronidazole base.

### METRONIDAZOLE INJECTION USP

**Usual adult and adolescent dose**
Antibacterial (systemic)—
  Anaerobic infections: Intravenous infusion, 15 mg (base) per kg of body weight initially, then 7.5 mg per kg of body weight, up to a maximum of 1 gram, every six hours for seven days or longer.
  Perioperative infections, colonic (prophylaxis): Intravenous infusion, 15 mg (base) per kg of body weight one hour prior to the start of surgery; and 7.5 mg per kg of body weight six and twelve hours after the initial dose.
[Antiprotozoal—Amebiasis][1]—
  Intravenous infusion, 500 to 750 mg (base) every eight hours for five to ten days.

**Usual adult prescribing limits**
Antibacterial (systemic)—
  Up to a maximum of 4 grams (base) daily.

**Usual pediatric dose**
Antibacterial (systemic)—Anaerobic infections:—
  Preterm infants—Intravenous infusion, 15 mg per kg of body weight (base) as an initial dose, then 7.5 mg per kg of body weight every twelve hours starting 48 hours after the initial dose.

Term infants—Intravenous infusion, 15 mg (base) per kg of body weight as an initial dose, then 7.5 mg per kg of body weight every twelve hours starting 24 hours after the initial dose.

Infants greater than 7 days of age and children—Intravenous infusion, 15 mg (base) per kg of body weight as an initial dose, then 7.5 mg per kg of body weight every six hours.

### Strength(s) usually available
U.S.—
500 mg in 100 mL (base) (Rx) [*Flagyl I.V. RTU* (sodium 14 mEq); *Metro I.V.* (sodium 13.5 mEq); GENERIC].

Canada—
500 mg in 100 mL (base) (Rx) [*Flagyl;* GENERIC].

### Packaging and storage
Store below 40 °C (104 °F), preferably between 15 and 30 °C (59 and 86 °F), unless otherwise specified by manufacturer. Protect from light during storage. Protect from freezing.

### Incompatibilities
Intravenous admixtures of metronidazole and other medications are not recommended.

### Additional information
Metronidazole Injection USP is an isotonic (297 to 310 mOsm per liter), ready-to-use solution, requiring no dilution or buffering prior to administration.

Metronidazole Injection USP in prefilled plastic minibags should not be used in series connections. This may result in air embolism because of residual air (approximately 15 mL), which may be drawn from the primary plastic bag before administration of the infusion from the secondary plastic bag is completed.

## METRONIDAZOLE HYDROCHLORIDE FOR INJECTION

### Usual adult and adolescent dose
See *Metronidazole Injection USP*.

### Usual adult prescribing limits
See *Metronidazole Injection USP*.

### Usual pediatric dose
See *Metronidazole Injection USP*.

### Size(s) usually available
U.S.—
500 mg (base) (Rx) [*Flagyl I.V.* (sodium 5 mEq)].

Canada—
Not commercially available.

### Packaging and storage
Prior to reconstitution, store below 30 °C (86 °F), in a light-resistant container, unless otherwise specified by manufacturer.

### Preparation of dosage form
Metronidazole hydrochloride for injection must not be given by direct intravenous injection since the initial dilution has an extremely low pH (0.5 to 2.0). It must be diluted further and neutralized prior to administration.

To prepare initial dilution for intravenous infusion, add 4.4 mL of sterile water for injection, bacteriostatic water for injection, 0.9% sodium chloride injection, or bacteriostatic sodium chloride injection to each 500-mg vial to provide a concentration of 100 mg per mL (pH 0.5 to 2.0). The resulting solution should be further diluted in 100 mL of 0.9% sodium chloride injection, 5% dextrose injection, or lactated Ringer's injection. The final dilution must be neutralized with approximately 5 mEq of sodium bicarbonate injection per 500 mg of metronidazole (final pH 6 to 7). Since carbon dioxide gas is produced during neutralization, it may be necessary to relieve the pressure in the final container. The final concentration should not exceed 8 mg per mL since neutralization decreases the solubility of metronidazole and precipitation may occur.

### Stability
After reconstitution, solutions retain their potency for 96 hours if stored below 30 °C (86 °F) in room light. Diluted and neutralized solutions retain their potency for 24 hours.

Do not refrigerate neutralized solutions since precipitation may occur.

### Incompatibilities
Do not use with aluminum needles or hubs.

Intravenous admixtures of metronidazole with other medications are not recommended.

---

[1]Not included in Canadian product labeling.

Revised: 10/20/92
Interim revision: 03/24/94

---

# METRONIDAZOLE Topical

VA CLASSIFICATION (Primary): DE752
Commonly used brand name(s): *MetroGel; MetroGel.*

Note: For a listing of dosage forms and brand names by country availability, see *Dosage Forms* section(s).

## Category
Antirosacea agent (topical).

## Indications
Note: Bracketed information in the *Indications* section refers to uses that are not included in U.S. product labeling.

### Accepted
Rosacea (treatment)—Topical metronidazole is indicated [as a primary agent] in the treatment of the inflammatory papules, pustules, and erythema of rosacea (acne rosacea; "adult acne") [in adults].

### Unaccepted
Topical metronidazole is not effective against the accompanying telangiectasias seen in rosacea patients.

## Pharmacology/Pharmacokinetics

### Physicochemical characteristics
Chemical group—Nitroimidazole.
Molecular weight—171.16.

### Mechanism of action/Effect
Unknown, but apparently not due to an antiparasitic effect on the mite *Demodex folliculorum*, found in hair follicles and sebaceous secretions, or to any effect on sebum production. Topical metronidazole may have an antioxidant effect. It has been shown to significantly reduce the concentrations of neutrophil-generated reactive oxygen species, hydroxyl radicals and hydrogen peroxide, which are potent oxidants capable of causing tissue injury at the site of inflammation. Topical metronidazole may also have an effect on neutrophil cellular functions, which is partly attributable to its direct anti-inflammatory effect.

### Absorption
Minimal; only trace amounts found in the serum following topical application of a 0.75% gel.

### Distribution
Absorbed metronidazole crosses the placenta and the blood-brain barrier.

### Peak serum concentration
Minimal; up to 66 nanograms per mL following application of 1 gram of gel (equivalent to 7.5 mg of metronidazole) to the face of rosacea patients. Serum concentrations were reported to be undetectable in some patients.

## Precautions to Consider

### Cross-sensitivity and/or related problems
Patients sensitive to parabens may be sensitive to metronidazole topical gel also since it contains methyl- and propylparabens.

### Carcinogenicity/Tumorigenicity
Carcinogenicity studies have not been done using topical formulations of metronidazole.

A number of studies using chronic, oral administration of metronidazole in mice and rats have shown that metronidazole is carcinogenic and tumorigenic. However, metronidazole has not been shown to be carcinogenic or tumorigenic in humans (See *Metronidazole [Systemic]*).

### Mutagenicity
Studies have shown that metronidazole is mutagenic in bacteria and fungi, although this has not been confirmed in mammals.

### Pregnancy/Reproduction
Fertility—Adequate and well-controlled studies using topical metronidazole in humans have not been done. However, studies using oral metronidazole in rats or mice have not shown that metronidazole causes impaired fertility.

Pregnancy—Absorbed metronidazole crosses the placenta and enters the fetal circulation rapidly. Adequate and well-controlled studies using topical metronidazole in humans have not been done.

Studies using oral metronidazole in rats and mice have not shown that metronidazole causes adverse effects on the fetus.

FDA Pregnancy Category B.

### Breast-feeding
Metronidazole, applied topically, is minimally absorbed. Only trace amounts appear in the serum following topical application. Therefore, topical metronidazole is unlikely to be distributed into breast milk in significant amounts since the topical dose is small. In addition, it is unlikely that the nursing infant would absorb significant amounts of metronidazole or that it would cause serious problems in the nursing infant.

### Pediatrics
Safety and efficacy have not been established. Since rosacea is considered primarily an adult-onset disease, topical metronidazole is not indicated in the treatment of pediatric patients.

### Geriatrics
No information is available on the relationship of age to the effects of topical metronidazole in geriatric patients.

### Medical considerations/Contraindications
The medical considerations/contraindications included have been selected on the basis of their potential clinical significance (reasons given in parentheses where appropriate)—not necessarily inclusive (» = major clinical significance).

*Risk-benefit should be considered when the following medical problem exists:*
Sensitivity to topical metronidazole

## Side/Adverse Effects
Note: Because metronidazole is minimally absorbed, with only trace amounts appearing in the serum following topical application, those side/adverse effects reported with systemic use of metronidazole have not been reported with topical use of the medication.

If local irritation occurs, metronidazole topical gel should be applied less frequently or discontinued.

The following side/adverse effects have been selected on the basis of their potential clinical significance (possible signs and symptoms in parentheses where appropriate)—not necessarily inclusive:

**Those indicating need for medical attention only if they continue or are bothersome**
Incidence less frequent
*Dry skin; redness or other signs of skin irritation not present before therapy; stinging or burning of the skin; watering of eyes*

## Patient Consultation
As an aid to patient consultation, refer to *Advice for the Patient, Metronidazole (Topical)*.
In providing consultation, consider emphasizing the following selected information (» = major clinical significance):

### Before using this medication
» Conditions affecting use, especially:
Sensitivity to topical metronidazole or to methyl- and propylparabens
Pregnancy—Absorbed metronidazole crosses the placenta and enters fetal circulation rapidly

### Proper use of this medication
» Not using medication in or near the eyes; tearing may occur
Washing eyes out immediately with large amounts of cool tap water if medication gets into eyes; checking with physician if eyes continue to burn or are painful
Before applying, thoroughly washing affected area(s) with a mild, nonirritating cleanser, rinsing well, and gently patting dry

*To use*
After washing affected area(s), applying medication with fingertips; washing medication off hands afterward
» Importance of applying medication to entire affected area
» Compliance with full course of therapy, which may take 9 weeks or longer
» Proper dosing
Missed dose: Applying as soon as possible; not applying if almost time for next dose
» Proper storage

### Precautions while using this medication
Checking with physician if no improvement within 3 weeks; may take up to 9 weeks before full therapeutic benefit is seen
Possibility of stinging or burning of the skin after application; checking with physician if irritation continues
Using only "oil-free" cosmetics to avoid worsening rosacea

## General Dosing Information
Topical metronidazole has also been used as a 1% cream formulation in the treatment of rosacea.

Before this medication is applied, the affected area(s) should be washed thoroughly with a mild, nonirritating cleanser, rinsed well, and gently patted dry.

After washing the affected area(s), a thin film of the gel should be applied and rubbed into the entire affected area.

Metronidazole topical gel should not be used in or near the eyes. Tearing has been reported when the gel is applied too close to the eyes.

If local irritation occurs, metronidazole topical gel should be applied less frequently or discontinued.

## Topical Dosage Forms
### METRONIDAZOLE TOPICAL GEL
**Usual adult dose**
Rosacea—
Topical, to the affected area(s) two times a day, morning and evening, for nine weeks.

**Usual pediatric dose**
Safety and efficacy have not been established. Since rosacea is considered primarily an adult-onset disease, topical metronidazole is not needed in the treatment of pediatric patients.

**Strength(s) usually available**
U.S.—
0.75% (Rx) [*MetroGel* (methylparaben; propylparaben; propylene glycol; edetate disodium)].
Canada—
0.75% (Rx) [*MetroGel* (methylparaben; propylparaben)].

**Packaging and storage**
Store between 15 and 30 °C (59 and 86 °F), in a well-closed container, unless otherwise specified by manufacturer. Protect from freezing.

**Auxiliary labeling**
• For external use only.
• Continue medication for full time of treatment.

**Additional information**
Metronidazole topical gel is an aqueous, nongreasy, invisible, and nonstaining preparation.

## Selected Bibliography
Bleicher PA, Charles HJ, Sober AJ. Topical metronidazole therapy for rosacea. Arch Dermatol 1987 May; 123: 609-14.
Aronson IK, Rumsfield JA, West DP, Alexander J, Fischer JH, Paloucek FP. Evaluation of topical metronidazole gel in acne rosacea. Drug Intell Clin Pharm 1987 Apr; 21: 348-51.
Nielsen PG. Metronidazole treatment in rosacea. Int J Dermatol 1988 Jan-Feb; 27: 1-5.

Revised: 06/24/94

# METRONIDAZOLE  Vaginal

VA CLASSIFICATION (Primary): GU301
Commonly used brand name(s): *Flagyl; MetroGel-Vaginal; Nidagel.*
Note: For a listing of dosage forms and brand names by country availability, see *Dosage Forms* section(s).

## Category
Anti-infective (vaginal).

## Indications

Note: Bracketed information in the *Indications* section refers to uses that are not included in U.S. product labeling.

### Accepted

Vaginosis, bacterial (treatment)—Vaginal metronidazole is indicated in the local treatment of bacterial vaginosis (previously known as *Haemophilus* vaginitis, *Gardnerella* vaginitis, nonspecific vaginitis, *Corynebacterium* vaginitis, or anaerobic vaginosis).

There are only limited clinical data regarding metronidazole gel's efficacy in treating bacterial vaginosis during pregnancy.

[Trichomoniasis (treatment)]—Metronidazole vaginal tablets and vaginal cream are indicated in the local treatment of trichomoniasis.

Not all species or strains of a particular organism may be equally susceptible to metronidazole.

### Unaccepted

Vaginal metronidazole is not effective against aerobic or facultative anaerobic bacteria, or in the treatment of vulvovaginitis caused by *Chlamydia trachomatis*, *Neisseria gonorrhoeae*, *Candida albicans*, or *Herpes simplex* virus. Metronidazole vaginal gel has not been proven to be clinically effective in the treatment of *Trichomonas vaginalis*.

## Pharmacology/Pharmacokinetics

### Physicochemical characteristics

Chemical group—Imidazole.
Molecular weight—171.16.

### Mechanism of action/Effect

The exact mechanism of action has not been completely established. Metronidazole is thought to be microbicidal against most obligate anaerobic bacteria and protozoa. To be active, it must undergo intracellular chemical reduction via mechanisms unique to anaerobic metabolism. The short-lived reduced forms are cytotoxic and interact with DNA to cause a loss of helical structure and strand breakage resulting in inhibition of nucleic acid synthesis and cell death.

Note: Metronidazole permits natural vaginal flora recovery because it has little effect on *Lactobacillus sp*.

### Other actions/effects

Metronidazole may produce a local antioxidant and anti-inflammatory effect on inflamed tissue by affecting neutrophil function.

### Absorption

Vaginal cream or
Vaginal tablets—Approximately 20% of the administered dose of metronidazole (500 mg) is absorbed systemically, producing plasma concentrations approximately 12% of that resulting from a single 500-mg oral dose. The rate of absorption is less predictable with the vaginal tablets than with the cream.
Vaginal gel—Approximately 56% of the administered dose of metronidazole (37.5 mg) is absorbed systemically, producing plasma concentrations approximately 2% of that resulting from a single 500-mg oral dose.

### Distribution

Systemically absorbed metronidazole may be distributed into breast milk and to most tissues. It crosses the blood-brain barrier and placenta.

### Protein binding

Low (< 20%).

### Biotransformation

Systemically absorbed metronidazole is metabolized primarily by side-chain oxidation by the hepatic cytochrome P450 enzyme system to two active metabolites, 1-[2-hydroxyethyl]-2-hydroxymethyl-5-nitroimidazole and 1-acetic acid-2-methyl-5-nitroimidazole. The hydroxylated metabolite is approximately 30% as potent as the parent compound while the acetic acid metabolite is 5% as potent. Small amounts of other metabolites (including glucuronide and sulfide conjugates) are also formed.

### Half-life

Elimination (determined with systemic administration)—Normal hepatic function: 8 hours (range, 6 to 12 hours) for unchanged metronidazole.

### Time to peak serum concentration:

Vaginal cream—11 hours.
Vaginal gel—6 to 12 hours.
Vaginal tablet—20 hours.

### Peak serum concentration

Vaginal cream—1.86 mg per liter (mg/L) (10.87 micromole/L).
Vaginal gel—0.152 to 0.368 mg/L (0.89 to 2.15 micromole/L).
Vaginal tablet—1.89 mg/L (11.04 micromole/L).

### Elimination

Renal—60 to 80% of a systemic dose; of this amount, approximately 20% is excreted unchanged.
Fecal—6 to 15% of a systemic dose.

## Precautions to Consider

Note: Some of the following information relates to the oral formulation. Depending on the vaginal product's strength and formulation, the vaginal administration of metronidazole may yield 2 to 12% of the blood concentrations achieved after a single 500-mg oral dose. The possibility of systemic effects may need to be considered until further studies quantify the degree of clinical significance.

### Carcinogenicity

Carcinogenicity studies have not been done using vaginal formulations of metronidazole. Systemic metronidazole has not been shown to be carcinogenic in humans.

Systemic metronidazole has been shown to be carcinogenic in a number of studies in mice and rats, including a study in which it produced malignant lymphomas in mice.

### Tumorigenicity

Tumorigenicity studies have not been done using vaginal formulations of metronidazole. Systemic metronidazole has not been shown to be tumorigenic in humans.

Pulmonary tumorigenesis has been reported in six studies in mice, including a study in which the animals were dosed every 4 weeks. Malignant hepatic tumors have also been reported in male mice given very high doses (approximately 500 mg per kg of body weight [mg/kg] per day). Several long-term oral-dose studies in rats have shown that metronidazole causes a statistically significant increase in the incidence of various neoplasms, especially mammary and hepatic tumors in female rats. Two lifetime tumorigenicity studies in hamsters using oral formulations have given negative results.

### Mutagenicity

Studies have shown that metronidazole is mutagenic in bacteria and fungi, although this has not been confirmed in mammals.

### Pregnancy/Reproduction

Fertility—No evidence of impaired fertility was found in mice.

Pregnancy—Metronidazole crosses the placenta, entering the fetal circulation rapidly. Adequate and well-controlled studies in humans have not been done.

Tumorigenicity has been demonstrated in animal studies, which may suggest that metronidazole should be withheld during pregnancy until more clinical data regarding vaginal administration are available.

A small study reported that intrauterine deaths resulted when metronidazole was administered intraperitoneally to pregnant mice in doses comparable to the oral human dose. No fetotoxicity or teratogenicity occurred with orally administered metronidazole.

FDA Pregnancy Category B.

### Breast-feeding

Metronidazole is distributed into breast milk; concentrations are similar to those found in the maternal plasma. Use in nursing mothers is not recommended. The theoretical risk is based on tumorigenicity studies in animals; human data have not supported this. Also, metronidazole may change the taste of the breast milk. If a nursing mother is treated with metronidazole, the breast milk may be expressed and discarded and breast-feeding resumed 24 to 48 hours after treatment is completed.

### Pediatrics

No information is available on the relationship of age to the effects of vaginal metronidazole in pediatric patients.

### Geriatrics

No information is available on the relationship of age to the effects of vaginal metronidazole in geriatric patients. However, elderly patients are more likely to have an age-related decrease in hepatic function, which may affect metronidazole elimination.

### Drug interactions and/or related problems

The following drug interactions and/or related problems have been selected on the basis of their potential clinical significance (possible mechanism in parentheses where appropriate)—not necessarily inclusive (» = major clinical significance):

Note: Combinations containing any of the following medications, depending on the amount present, may also interact with this medication.

» Alcohol
(caution in concurrent use with vaginal metronidazole and for at least 1 day following completion of treatment is advisable because systemic metronidazole may interfere with the oxidation of alcohol; such use may result in disulfiram-like effects such as abdominal

cramps, nausea, vomiting, headache, or flushing of the face from acetaldehyde accumulation; changes in the taste of alcoholic beverages also have been reported during concurrent use)
» Anticoagulants, coumarin- or indandione-derivative
(anticoagulant effects may be potentiated when these agents are used concurrently with metronidazole because of inhibition of enzymatic metabolism of anticoagulants; periodic prothrombin time determinations may be required during and following concurrent therapy to determine if dosage adjustments of anticoagulants are necessary)
Cimetidine
(hepatic metabolism of metronidazole may be decreased when metronidazole and cimetidine are used concurrently, possibly resulting in delayed elimination and increased serum metronidazole concentrations)
» Disulfiram
(it is recommended that metronidazole not be used concurrently with, or for 2 weeks following, disulfiram in alcoholic patients; such use may result in confusion and psychotic reactions because of combined toxicity)
Lithium
(concurrent use of systemic metronidazole with lithium has resulted in decreased renal clearance of lithium and lithium toxicity; adjustments of lithium dosage may be required)
Neurotoxic medications, other (see *Appendix II*)
(concurrent use of systemic metronidazole with other neurotoxic medications may increase the potential for neurotoxicity)
Phenytoin
(systemic metronidazole may impair the metabolism of phenytoin by inhibiting microsomal enzymes and increasing phenytoin's plasma concentration; the extent to which intravaginal metronidazole affects phenytoin is not presently known)

**Laboratory value alterations**
The following have been selected on the basis of their potential clinical significance (possible effect in parentheses where appropriate)—not necessarily inclusive (» = major clinical significance):
With diagnostic test results
Alanine aminotransferase (ALT [SGPT]) and
Aspartate aminotransferase (AST [SGOT]) and
Hexokinase glucose and
Lactate dehydrogenase (LDH) and
Triglycerides
(metronidazole has a high absorbance at the wavelength at which nicotinamide-adenine dinucleotide [NADH] is determined; therefore, falsely low values may occur when these substances are measured by continuous-flow methods based on endpoint decrease in reduced NADH)
White blood cell count
(may be increased or decreased)

**Medical considerations/Contraindications**
The medical considerations/contraindications included have been selected on the basis of their potential clinical significance (reasons given in parentheses where appropriate)—not necessarily inclusive (» = major clinical significance).

*Risk-benefit should be considered when the following medical problems exist:*
» Epilepsy or
» Other neurologic disease
(systemic metronidazole has caused CNS toxicity, including seizures and peripheral neuropathy)
» Hepatic function impairment, severe
(metronidazole is metabolized in the liver; hepatic function impairment may lead to decreased plasma clearance and accumulation of metronidazole and its metabolites and increased risk of side effects; dosage may need to be reduced in patients with severe hepatic function impairment)
Hypersensitivity to metronidazole
Leukopenia, or history of
(oral metronidazole has caused leukopenia; the possibility should be considered that vaginal metronidazole may induce or exacerbate leukopenia, especially with prolonged or multiple courses of therapy)

**Patient monitoring**
The following may be especially important in patient monitoring (other tests may be warranted in some patients, depending on condition; » = major clinical significance):

Leukocyte count, total and differential
(determinations recommended when metronidazole is used for longer than 10 days or if a second course of therapy is needed)

## Side/Adverse Effects
Note: Convulsions, peripheral neuropathy, and ataxia have been reported rarely with systemic administration of metronidazole. The possibility should be considered that these effects may also occur with vaginal administration, especially with the higher-potency formulations available in Canada or with prolonged use. If neurological symptoms occur, the medication should be discontinued. Severe symptoms may require immediate medical attention.

The incidences of side effects listed below are those reported in studies with the 0.75% gel. Although specific information about the incidence of side effects with the vaginal tablet or vaginal cream is not available, it is possible that some adverse effects could occur more frequently with these higher-potency formulations than with the gel. Also, the possibility of systemic effects may need to be considered since vaginal administration of metronidazole may yield 2 to 12% of the blood concentrations achieved after a single oral 500-mg dose.

The following side/adverse effects have been selected on the basis of their potential clinical significance (possible signs and symptoms in parentheses where appropriate)—not necessarily inclusive:

**Those indicating need for medical attention**
Incidence more frequent
*Candida cervicitis or vaginitis* (itching in the vagina; pain during sexual intercourse; thick, white vaginal discharge without odor or with mild odor)—incidence 6 to 15%
Incidence less frequent
*Abdominal cramping or pain*—incidence 3.4%; *burning or irritation of penis of sexual partner; burning or increased frequency of urination; vulvitis* (itching, stinging or redness of genital area)

**Those indicating need for medical attention only if they continue or are bothersome**
Incidence less frequent
*Altered taste sensation including metallic taste; CNS effects* (dizziness or lightheadedness; headache; *dryness of mouth; furry tongue; gastrointestinal disturbances* (diarrhea, nausea or vomiting); *loss of appetite*

**Those not indicating need for medical attention**
Incidence less frequent
*Dark urine*

**Those indicating possible need for medical attention if they occur after medication is discontinued**
*Vaginal candidiasis* (itching of the vagina or outside genitals; pain during sexual intercourse; thick, white vaginal discharge without odor or with mild odor)

## Patient Consultation
As an aid to patient consultation, refer to *Advice for the Patient, Metronidazole (Vaginal).*
In providing consultation, consider emphasizing the following selected information (» = major clinical significance):

**Before using this medication**
» Conditions affecting use, especially:
Sensitivity to metronidazole
Pregnancy—Metronidazole crosses the placenta; discussing use of medicine with physician before using during pregnancy
Breast-feeding—Metronidazole is distributed into breast milk and is not recommended during breast-feeding
Other medications, especially alcohol, coumarin- or indandione-derivative anticoagulants, or disulfiram
Other medical problems, especially epilepsy or other neurologic disease or severe hepatic function impairment

**Proper use of this medication**
» Washing hands immediately before and after vaginal administration
Avoiding getting medication into the eyes; washing with large amounts of cool tap water immediately if medication does get into eyes; checking with physician if eyes continue to be painful
Reading patient directions carefully before use
*Proper administration technique*
Following directions regarding filling the applicator, insertion technique, and cleaning the applicator after each use
*For cream or gel dosage forms*
Puncturing metal tamper-resistant seal on tube with top of cap

*For vaginal tablet dosage form*
- Placing vaginal tablet into the applicator, immersing exposed tablet in tap water for a few seconds before vaginal insertion to facilitate disintegration
» Compliance with full course of therapy, even during menstruation
» Proper dosing
- Missed dose: Inserting as soon as possible; not inserting if almost time for next dose
» Proper storage

**Precautions while using this medication**
- Checking with physician if no improvement within a few days
- Follow-up visit to physician after treatment for bacterial vaginosis to ensure that infection has been eradicated
» Avoiding use of alcoholic beverages or other alcohol-containing preparations while using and for at least 1 day after discontinuing this medication
» Caution if dizziness or lightheadedness occurs
- Protecting clothing because of possible soiling with vaginal metronidazole; avoiding use of tampons
» Using hygienic measures to cure infection and prevent reinfection, e.g., wearing freshly washed cotton panties instead of synthetic panties
» Sexual abstinence is recommended during treatment to prevent cross-infection, reinfection, or dilution of the dose. If this recommendation is not followed, use of the vaginal cream and vaginal tablets should be avoided with latex contraceptive devices, such as cervical caps, condoms, or diaphragms, since these products contain oils that damage latex

*For trichomoniasis*
» Using condoms to prevent reinfection with trichomoniasis after treatment; possible need for concurrent treatment of male partner for trichomoniasis

**Side/adverse effects**
- Signs of potential side effects, especially candida cervicitis or vaginitis, abdominal cramping or pain, burning or irritation of penis of sexual partner, increased frequency of urination, vulvitis, altered taste sensation, CNS effects, dryness of mouth, furry tongue, gastrointestinal disturbances, loss of appetite
- Dark urine may be alarming to patient although medically insignificant
- Possibility of vaginal candidiasis occurring after medication has been discontinued

## General Dosing Information

If sensitization or irritation occurs, treatment with vaginal metronidazole should be discontinued.

The cream and the vaginal tablet (but not the gel) may contain oils that may damage latex contraceptive devices, such as cervical caps, condoms, or diaphragms, and reduce their efficacy.

Vaginal applicators should be used with caution after the sixth month of pregnancy.

If there is no response to therapy, the presence of pathogens unresponsive to metronidazole should be ruled out by potassium hydroxide (KOH) wet mounts before a second course of therapy is initiated.

In treating bacterial vaginosis, concurrent treatment of the male partner generally is unnecessary.

In treating trichomoniasis, both sexual partners should receive metronidazole therapy concurrently since asymptomatic trichomoniasis in the male partner is a frequent source of reinfection in the female.

## Vaginal Dosage Forms

Note: Bracketed uses in the *Dosage Forms* section refer to categories of use and/or indications that are not included in U.S. product labeling.

### METRONIDAZOLE VAGINAL CREAM

**Usual adult and adolescent dose**
Bacterial vaginosis or
[Trichomoniasis]—
Intravaginal, 500 mg (one applicatorful) one or two times a day for ten or twenty consecutive days.

**Usual pediatric dose**
Safety and efficacy have not been established.

**Strength(s) usually available**
U.S.—
Not commercially available.
Canada—
10% w/w (Rx) [*Flagyl* (methylparaben; propylparaben)].

**Packaging and storage**
Store below 40 °C (104 °F), preferably between 15 and 30 °C (59 and 86 °F), unless otherwise specified by manufacturer. Protect from freezing.

**Auxiliary labeling**
- May cause dizziness.
- Continue medicine for full time of treatment.
- For vaginal use only.
- Avoid alcoholic beverages.

**Note**
Include patient package insert (PPI) when dispensing.

### METRONIDAZOLE VAGINAL GEL

**Usual adult and adolescent dose**
Bacterial vaginosis—
Intravaginal, 37.5 mg (one applicatorful) one or two times a day for five days.

**Usual pediatric dose**
Safety and efficacy have not been established.

**Strength(s) usually available**
U.S.—
0.75% (Rx) [*MetroGel-Vaginal* (EDTA; methylparaben; propylparaben; propylene glycol)].
Canada—
0.75% (Rx) [*Nidagel* (EDTA; methylparaben; propylparaben; propylene glycol)].

**Packaging and storage**
Store below 40 °C (104 °F), preferably between 15 and 30 °C (59 and 86 °F), unless otherwise specified by manufacturer. Protect from freezing. Keep out of reach of children.

**Auxiliary labeling**
- May cause dizziness.
- Continue medicine for full time of treatment.
- For vaginal use only.
- Avoid alcoholic beverages.

**Note**
Include patient package insert (PPI) when dispensing.

### METRONIDAZOLE VAGINAL TABLETS

**Usual adult and adolescent dose**
Bacterial vaginosis or
[Trichomoniasis]—
Intravaginal, 500 mg placed high into the vagina every night for ten or twenty consecutive days.

**Usual pediatric dose**
Safety and efficacy have not been established.

**Strength(s) usually available**
U.S.—
Not commercially available.
Canada—
500 mg (Rx) [*Flagyl*].

**Packaging and storage**
Store below 40 °C (104 °F), preferably between 15 and 30 °C (59 and 86 °F), unless otherwise specified by manufacturer. Protect from light.

**Auxiliary labeling**
- May cause dizziness.
- Continue medicine for full time of treatment.
- For vaginal use only.
- Avoid alcoholic beverages.

**Note**
Include patient package insert (PPI) when dispensing.
Patient should be instructed on technique for placement including immersing the vaginal tablet (in applicator) in tap water for a few seconds before insertion to facilitate disintegration.

## Selected Bibliography

Alper MM, Barwin N, McLean WM, et al. Systemic absorption of metronidazole by the vaginal route. Obstet Gynecol 1985 Jun; 65(6): 781-4.

Hillier SL, Lipinski C, Briseldene A, et al. Efficacy of intravaginal 0.75% metronidazole gel for the treatment of bacterial vaginosis. Obstet Gynecol 1993 June; 81(6): 963-7.

Revised: 08/13/98

**METYRAPONE**—The *Metyrapone (Systemic)* monograph is not included in this published version of the USP DI database. Copies of the monograph are available on request from Micromedex, Inc. - Reprint Requests, 6200 S. Syracuse Way, Suite 300, Englewood, CO 80111; telephone (303) 486-6400; telefax (303) 486-6464; Email: USPDI@MDX.COM.

**METYROSINE**—The *Metyrosine (Systemic)* monograph is not included in this published version of the USP DI database. Copies of the monograph are available on request from Micromedex, Inc. - Reprint Requests, 6200 S. Syracuse Way, Suite 300, Englewood, CO 80111; telephone (303) 486-6400; telefax (303) 486-6464; Email: USPDI@MDX.COM.

# MEXILETINE Systemic

VA CLASSIFICATION (Primary/Secondary): CV300
Commonly used brand name(s): *Mexitil*.
Note: For a listing of dosage forms and brand names by country availability, see *Dosage Forms* section(s).

## Category
Antiarrhythmic.

## Indications
**Accepted**
Arrhythmias, ventricular (treatment)—Mexiletine is indicated for the treatment of documented, life-threatening ventricular arrhythmias, such as ventricular tachycardia.

**Unaccepted**
Mexiletine is not recommended for use in the treatment of lesser arrhythmias, such as asymptomatic premature ventricular contractions following an acute myocardial infarction. Although the Cardiac Arrhythmias Suppression Trial (CAST) showed that treatment of asymptomatic, non–life-threatening arrhythmias following an acute myocardial infarction with encainide or flecainide was deleterious, the extrapolation of these results to other patient populations or antiarrhythmic agents remains uncertain.

## Pharmacology/Pharmacokinetics
**Physicochemical characteristics**
Molecular weight—215.72.
pKa—8.4.

**Mechanism of action/Effect**
Blocks the fast sodium channel in cardiac tissues, especially the Purkinje network, without involvement of the autonomic system. Reduces the rate of rise and amplitude of the action potential and decreases automaticity (increases the threshold of excitability) in the Purkinje fibers. Shortens the action potential duration and, to a lesser extent, decreases the effective refractory period in the Purkinje fibers. Does not usually alter conduction velocity, although it may slow conduction in patients with pre-existing conduction abnormalities. Does not significantly affect resting membrane potential or sinus node automaticity, left ventricular function, systolic arterial blood pressure, atrioventricular (AV) conduction velocity, or QRS or QT intervals. In the Vaughan Williams classification of antiarrhythmics, mexiletine is considered to be a class IB agent.

**Other actions/effects**
Also has local anesthetic and anticonvulsant properties.

**Absorption**
Well absorbed (approximately 90%) from upper intestinal section of gastrointestinal tract; low first-pass metabolism. Rate of absorption, but not bioavailability, is reduced in conditions in which gastric emptying time is increased (e.g., acute myocardial infarction) or with concurrent use of narcotics, atropine, or alumina and magnesia; metoclopramide may accelerate absorption.

**Protein binding**
Moderate (60 to 75%).

**Biotransformation**
Hepatic, approximately 85%, to inactive metabolites.

**Half-life**
Normal—
  10 to 12 hours.
In moderate to severe hepatic disease—
  25 hours.
In severely reduced cardiac output—
  25 hours.
In renal disease—
  Creatinine clearance less than 10 mL per minute: 15.7 hours.
  Creatinine clearance 11 to 40 mL per minute: 13.4 hours.
In acute myocardial infarction—
  15 to 17 hours.

**Onset of action**
30 minutes to 2 hours.

**Time to peak concentration**
2 to 3 hours.

**Therapeutic plasma concentration**
0.5 to 2 mcg per mL; however, toxicity may occur even at therapeutic plasma concentrations.

**Elimination**
Biliary.
Renal, approximately 10%, unchanged; excretion is accelerated in markedly acid urine and retarded in markedly alkaline urine.
Mexiletine is excreted in breast milk in concentrations similar to maternal plasma concentrations.
In dialysis—May be removable by hemodialysis; supplementary dose may be required on day of dialysis. Not removable by peritoneal dialysis.

## Precautions to Consider
**Cross-sensitivity and/or related problems**
Patients sensitive to other amide-type anesthetics (e.g., lidocaine) may be sensitive to mexiletine also.

**Tumorigenicity**
Studies in rats and mice for 24 months and 18 months, respectively, found no evidence of tumorigenicity.

**Mutagenicity**
Results of mutagenicity studies using the Ames test were negative.

**Pregnancy/Reproduction**
Fertility—Studies in rats, mice, and rabbits at doses up to 4 times the maximum human oral dose found no impairment of fertility.
Pregnancy—Adequate and well-controlled studies have not been done in humans.
Studies in rats, mice, and rabbits at doses up to 4 times the maximum human oral dose found an increased incidence of fetal resorption but not teratogenicity.
FDA Pregnancy Category C.

**Breast-feeding**
Mexiletine is distributed into human breast milk in concentrations similar to maternal plasma concentrations. Because of the potential for serious adverse effects in nursing infants, breast-feeding is generally not recommended while mexiletine is being administered.

**Pediatrics**
Appropriate studies on the relationship of age to the effects of mexiletine have not been performed in the pediatric population. Safety and efficacy have not been established.

**Geriatrics**
No information is available on the relationship of age to the effects of mexiletine in geriatric patients.

**Drug interactions and/or related problems**
The following drug interactions and/or related problems have been selected on the basis of their potential clinical significance (possible mechanism in parentheses where appropriate)—not necessarily inclusive (» = major clinical significance).
Note: Combinations containing any of the following medications, depending on the amount present, may also interact with this medication.

Acidifiers, urinary, such as:
  Ammonium chloride
  Ascorbic acid

Potassium or sodium phosphates
(marked acidification of urine may accelerate renal excretion of mexiletine)

Alkalizers, urinary, such as:
Antacids, calcium- and/or magnesium-containing
Carbonic anhydrase inhibitors
Citrates
Sodium bicarbonate
(marked alkalinization of urine may retard renal excretion of mexiletine)

Antiarrhythmics, other
(concurrent use with mexiletine may produce additive cardiac effects; although some combinations are used for therapeutic advantage, when used concurrently dosage adjustments may be necessary)

Hepatic enzyme inducers (see *Appendix II*)
(may accelerate metabolism and result in decreased plasma concentrations of mexiletine; plasma concentrations of mexiletine should be monitored during concurrent use to ensure that efficacy is maintained)

Metoclopramide
(may accelerate absorption of mexiletine)

Smoking, tobacco
(may induce hepatic metabolism and reduce the half-life of mexiletine)

Theophylline
(concurrent use may decrease theophylline clearance, resulting in prolonged elimination half-life, increased serum theophylline concentrations, and increased risk of theophylline-related CNS toxicity; serum theophylline concentrations should be monitored and dosage adjustments may be required)

**Laboratory value alterations**
The following have been selected on the basis of their potential clinical significance (possible effect in parentheses where appropriate)—not necessarily inclusive (» = major clinical significance):

With physiology/laboratory test values
Antinuclear antibody (ANA) titers
(positive test results may occur infrequently)
Aspartate aminotransferase (AST [SGOT]), serum
(values may be increased to as much as 3 times or greater the upper limit of normal in 1 to 2% of patients; usually asymptomatic and transient)

**Medical considerations/Contraindications**
The medical considerations/contraindications included have been selected on the basis of their potential clinical significance (reasons given in parentheses where appropriate)—not necessarily inclusive (» = major clinical significance).

*Risk-benefit should be considered when the following medical problems exist:*

» Atrioventricular (AV) block, pre-existing 2nd or 3rd degree, without pacemaker
(risk of complete heart block)

» Cardiogenic shock
(risk of further reduction of blood pressure)

Congestive heart failure, severe or
Myocardial infarction, acute
(may reduce hepatic metabolism and result in prolongation of effect)
(congestive heart failure may be aggravated by mexiletine)

Hepatic function impairment
(possible prolongation of effect)

Hypotension
(may be exacerbated)

Intraventricular conduction abnormalities or
Sinus node function impairment
(use of mexiletine has been reported to result in depression of sinus rate, prolongation of sinus node recovery time, decreased conduction velocity, and increased effective refractory period of the intraventricular conduction system)

Seizure disorders
(mexiletine may precipitate seizures)

Sensitivity to mexiletine

**Patient monitoring**
The following may be especially important in patient monitoring (other tests may be warranted in some patients, depending on condition; » = major clinical significance):

Aspartate aminotransferase (AST [SGOT]) values, serum
(recommended prior to initiation of therapy and at periodic intervals during therapy; if persistent or worsening elevation occurs, withdrawal of mexiletine may be necessary)

» Electrocardiogram (ECG)
(recommended continuously via Holter monitoring during therapy to assess efficacy and aid in dosage adjustment; intermittent chest x-rays may also be useful)

Mexiletine concentrations, plasma
(may be useful in some cases to aid in dosage adjustment)

## Side/Adverse Effects

Note: In the National Heart, Lung and Blood Institute's Cardiac Arrhythmias Suppression Trial (CAST), treatment with encainide or flecainide was found to be associated with excessive mortality or increased nonfatal cardiac arrest rate, as compared with placebo, in patients with asymptomatic, non–life-threatening arrhythmias who had a recent myocardial infarction. The implications of these results for other patient populations or other antiarrhythmic agents are uncertain.

Incidence of side effects, especially some central nervous system (CNS) side effects, is related to plasma mexiletine concentrations and is greatest at concentrations exceeding 2 mcg per mL.

Exacerbation of ventricular arrhythmias, including torsade de pointes, may occur.

Hepatic necrosis has occurred rarely.

A fatal overdose caused gastrointestinal disturbances, respiratory failure, and asystole.

Pulmonary changes, including pulmonary fibrosis, have been reported in patients receiving other medications or having other conditions known to result in pulmonary toxicity; therefore, the relationship to mexiletine is unknown.

The following side/adverse effects have been selected on the basis of their potential clinical significance (possible signs and symptoms in parentheses where appropriate)—not necessarily inclusive:

**Those indicating need for medical attention**
Incidence less frequent
*Chest pain; premature ventricular contractions* (fast or irregular heartbeat); *shortness of breath*

Incidence rare
*Leukopenia or agranulocytosis* (fever or chills); *or thrombocytopenia* (unusual bleeding or bruising); *seizures*

Note: *Thrombocytopenia* occurs within a few days after initiation of therapy, and blood counts usually return to normal within 1 month after withdrawal of mexiletine.

**Those indicating need for medical attention only if they continue or are bothersome**
Incidence more frequent
*CNS effects* (dizziness or lightheadedness, nervousness; trembling or shaking of hands; unsteadiness or trouble in walking); *heartburn; nausea and vomiting*

Note: *Nausea* and *vomiting* usually occur within 2 hours after a dose and tend to lessen with continued treatment.

Incidence less frequent
*Blurred vision; confusion; constipation or diarrhea; headache; numbness or tingling of fingers and toes; ringing in the ears; skin rash; slurred speech; trouble in sleeping; unusual tiredness or weakness*

## Overdose

For more information on the management of overdose or unintentional ingestion, **contact a Poison Control Center** (see *Poison Control Center Listing*).

**Treatment of overdose**
Treatment is primarily supportive and symptomatic and may include acidification of urine to accelerate excretion of mexiletine. Administration of atropine may be indicated if hypotension or bradycardia occurs.

## Patient Consultation

As an aid to patient consultation, refer to *Advice for the Patient, Mexiletine (Systemic)*.

In providing consultation, consider emphasizing the following selected information (» = major clinical significance):

**Before using this medication**
» Conditions affecting use, especially:
Sensitivity to amide-type anesthetics

Pregnancy—Increased incidence of fetal resorptions in animals
Breast-feeding—Distributed into breast milk
Medical problems, especially atrioventricular (AV) block, pre-existing 2nd or 3rd degree, without pacemaker or cardiogenic shock

**Proper use of this medication**
» Compliance with therapy; taking as directed even if feeling well
Taking with food, milk, or an antacid to reduce stomach upset
» Importance of not missing doses and taking at evenly spaced intervals
» Proper dosing
Missed dose: Taking as soon as possible if remembered within 4 hours; not taking if remembered later; not doubling doses
» Proper storage

**Precautions while using the medication**
Regular visits to physician to check progress
Carrying medical identification card or bracelet
» Caution if any kind of surgery (including dental surgery) or emergency treatment is required
» Caution when driving or doing things requiring alertness, because of possible dizziness

**Side/adverse effects**
Signs of adverse effects, especially chest pain, premature ventricular contractions, shortness of breath, leukopenia, agranulocytosis, thrombocytopenia, and seizures

## General Dosing Information

When mexiletine is replacing other antiarrhythmic therapy, the first dose may be given 6 to 12 hours after the last dose of quinidine sulfate or disopyramide, 3 to 6 hours after the last dose of procainamide, or 8 to 12 hours after the last dose of tocainide. In patients being transferred from parenteral lidocaine to oral mexiletine, substantial reduction of dose or withdrawal of lidocaine is recommended 1 to 2 hours after initiation of mexiletine therapy; lower initial doses of mexiletine (e.g., 100 to 200 mg every eight hours) may also be appropriate. In patients at risk of life-threatening arrhythmias, transfer to mexiletine therapy should take place in the hospital.

Mexiletine should be taken with food, milk, or antacid to reduce gastrointestinal irritation.

Patients with impaired hepatic function or severe congestive heart failure may require lower or less frequent doses of mexiletine.

It is recommended that dosage adjustments be made no more frequently than every 2 to 3 days.

It is recommended that the patient be evaluated carefully and mexiletine therapy may need to be withdrawn if significant leukopenia or thrombocytopenia occurs.

## Oral Dosage Forms

### MEXILETINE HYDROCHLORIDE CAPSULES USP

**Usual adult dose**
Arrhythmias, ventricular (treatment)—
Oral, initially 200 mg every eight hours, the dosage being increased or decreased in increments or decrements of 50 to 100 mg per dose every two to three days as needed and tolerated.
Note: For rapid control of ventricular arrhythmias, a loading dose of 400 mg may be administered, followed by a 200-mg dose eight hours later.

Some patients may tolerate twice-a-day dosing. For patients adequately maintained on a dose of 300 mg or less every eight hours, the total daily dose may be given in divided doses every twelve hours.

Patients not adequately controlled by dosing every eight hours (i.e., those experiencing breakthrough ectopy two hours before the next dose) may respond to dosing four times a day.

**Usual adult prescribing limits**
Up to 1200 mg per day when given every eight hours (i.e., 400 mg per dose) or 900 mg per day when given every twelve hours (i.e., 450 mg per dose).

**Usual pediatric dose**
Safety and efficacy have not been established.

**Strength(s) usually available**
U.S.—
150 mg (Rx) [*Mexitil*].
200 mg (Rx) [*Mexitil*].
250 mg (Rx) [*Mexitil*].
Canada—
100 mg (Rx) [*Mexitil*].
200 mg (Rx) [*Mexitil*].

**Packaging and storage**
Store below 40 °C (104 °F), preferably between 15 and 30 °C (59 and 86 °F), unless otherwise specified by manufacturer. Store in a tight container.

**Auxiliary labeling**
• Take with food, milk, or antacid.

## Selected Bibliography

Schrader BJ, Bauman JL. Mexiletine: a new type I antiarrhythmic agent. Drug Intell Clin Pharm 1986 Apr; 20: 255-60.
Fenster PE, Comess KA. Pharmacology and clinical use of mexiletine. Pharmacother 1986 Jan/Feb; 6: 1-9.

Revised: 10/06/92
Interim revision: 07/14/94

---

**MEZLOCILLIN**—See *Penicillins (Systemic)*

---

**MICONAZOLE**—See *Antifungals, Azole (Systemic)*; *Antifungals, Azole (Vaginal)*; *Miconazole (Systemic)*; *Miconazole (Topical)*

---

**MICONAZOLE**—The *Miconazole (Topical)* monograph is not included in this published version of the USP DI database. Copies of the monograph are available on request from Micromedex, Inc. - Reprint Requests, 6200 S. Syracuse Way, Suite 300, Englewood, CO 80111; telephone (303) 486-6400; telefax (303) 486-6464; Email: USPDI@MDX.COM.

---

# MIDAZOLAM  Systemic

VA CLASSIFICATION (Primary/Secondary): CN302/CN206
Note: Controlled substance classification—
U.S.—Schedule IV
Commonly used brand name(s): *Versed*.
Note: For a listing of dosage forms and brand names by country availability, see *Dosage Forms* section(s).

## Category

Sedative-hypnotic; anesthetic, general, adjunct; anesthetic, local, adjunct.

## Indications

Note: Bracketed information in the *Indications* section refers to uses that are not included in U.S. product labeling.

**WARNING: Intravenous midazolam should be used only in hospital or ambulatory care settings, including physicians' and dentists' offices, that provide for continuous monitoring of respiratory and cardiac function; also, resuscitative drugs and age- and size-appropriate resuscitative equipment, and personnel trained in their use, should be immediately available.** Midazolam administered intravenously has been associated with respiratory depression and respiratory arrest, especially when used concomitantly with opioid analgesics for conscious sedation or when rapidly administered; in some cases, death or hypoxic encephalopathy has occurred.

**Accepted**
Sedation and amnesia—Midazolam, used intramuscularly, is indicated for preoperative sedation (induction of sleepiness or drowsiness and relief of apprehension) and to impair memory of perioperative events.

Sedation, conscious—Midazolam, used intravenously either alone or in conjunction with a narcotic, is indicated to produce sedation, anxiolysis, and amnesia prior to short diagnostic procedures or endoscopic procedures, such as bronchoscopy, gastroscopy, cystoscopy, coronary angiography, and cardiac catheterization.

Midazolam also is indicated intravenously for sedation, anxiolysis, and amnesia prior to certain dental and minor surgical[1] procedures. This medication may be preferable to diazepam for intravenous sedation because of its faster onset of action, more consistent anterograde amnesia, and virtual lack of venous complications.

Sedation—Midazolam, administered as a continuous intravenous infusion, is indicated for the sedation of patients in intensive care settings, including intubated patients receiving mechanical ventilation.

Anesthesia, general, adjunct—Midazolam, used intravenously, is indicated for induction of general anesthesia prior to administration of other anesthetic agents. It may be used in conjunction with narcotic premedication, thereby achieving induction of anesthesia within a relatively narrow dose range and in a short period of time. It may also be used for intravenous supplementation of nitrous oxide and oxygen (balanced anesthesia) for short surgical procedures; however, the recovery time may be prolonged compared to that of thiopental. The use of midazolam in longer surgical procedures has not been studied.

[Anesthesia, local, adjunct][1]—Midazolam, administered intravenously, is indicated as an adjunct to local or regional anesthesia for some diagnostic and therapeutic procedures. It may be used for sedation of healthy patients receiving subarachnoid or epidural anesthesia.

[1]Not included in Canadian product labeling.

## Pharmacology/Pharmacokinetics

### Physicochemical characteristics
Molecular weight—362.24.
pKa—Midazolam base: 6.

### Mechanism of action/Effect
Midazolam is a relatively short-acting benzodiazepine central nervous system (CNS) depressant. Its effects on the CNS are dependent on the dose administered, the route of administration, and whether it is used concomitantly with other medications.

Midazolam has anxiolytic, hypnotic, anticonvulsant, muscle relaxant, and anterograde amnestic effects, which are characteristic of benzodiazepines.

Although the exact mechanisms of the actions of benzodiazepines have not been completely established, it has been postulated that the actions of benzodiazepines are mediated through the inhibitory neurotransmitter gamma-aminobutyric acid (GABA), which is one of the major inhibitory neurotransmitters in the brain. Benzodiazepines are believed to increase the activity of GABA, thereby calming the patient, relaxing skeletal muscles, and, in high doses, producing sleep.

Benzodiazepines act as agonists at the benzodiazepine receptors, which have been shown to form a component of the benzodiazepine-GABA receptor-chloride ionophore complex. Most anxiolytics appear to act through at least one component of this complex to enhance the inhibitory action of GABA. Other actions of benzodiazepines, such as sedative, anticonvulsant, and muscle relaxant effects, may be mediated through a similar mechanism, although different receptor subtypes may be involved.

The hypnotic effect of midazolam appears to be related to GABA accumulation and occupation of the benzodiazepine receptor. Midazolam has a relatively high affinity (about twice that of diazepam) for the benzodiazepine receptor. It is believed that there are separate benzodiazepine and GABA receptors coupled to a common ionophore (chloride) channel, and that occupation of both receptors produces membrane hyperpolarization and neuronal inhibition. Midazolam interferes with reuptake of GABA, thereby causing accumulation of GABA. Also, it is postulated that the action of midazolam in induction of anesthesia involves excess GABA at neuronal synapses.

The site and mechanism of the amnestic action of midazolam are not known; however, the degree of amnesia usually, but not always, parallels the degree of drowsiness produced by midazolam.

### Other actions/effects
Midazolam causes a moderate decrease in cerebrospinal fluid pressure (lumbar puncture measurements), similar to that produced by thiopental, when it is used for induction of anesthesia in patients without intracranial lesions.

In intracranial surgical patients with normal intracranial pressure but decreased compliance (subarachnoid screw measurements), midazolam attenuates the increase in intracranial pressure due to intubation to a degree comparable to that of thiopental.

Studies have shown that intraocular pressure is lowered moderately when midazolam is used for induction of anesthesia in patients without eye disease; studies have not been done in patients with glaucoma.

Respiratory depression is produced; however, the respiratory depressant effect of midazolam is dose-related.

The cardiovascular effects of midazolam appear to be minimal. Cardiac hemodynamic studies have shown midazolam to cause a slight to moderate decrease in mean arterial pressure, cardiac output, stroke volume, and systemic vascular resistance when used for induction of anesthesia. In a study comparing the systemic vascular effects of midazolam and lorazepam in patients on cardiopulmonary bypass, midazolam was more effective than lorazepam in attenuating the increase in systemic vascular resistance accompanying cardiopulmonary bypass. Midazolam may cause slow heart rates (less than 65 per minute) to rise slightly, especially in patients taking propranolol for angina; it may cause faster heart rates (e.g., 85 per minute) to slow slightly.

### Absorption
Mean absolute bioavailability of midazolam following intramuscular administration is greater than 90%.

### Distribution
Widely distributed in body, including the cerebrospinal fluid and brain. The volume of distribution (Vol$_D$) usually averages between 1 and 3.1 (range, 0.95 to 6.6) liters per kg of body weight in the majority of patients.

Note: In patients with congestive heart failure—A twofold to threefold increase in Vol$_D$ has been shown in a small group of patients, following a single intravenous dose of 5 mg.

In obese patients—Significant increase in Vol$_D$ because of greatly enhanced distribution of midazolam into peripheral adipose tissue.

### Protein binding
Plasma—Very high, 97% in healthy individuals and 93.5% in patients with renal failure.

### Biotransformation
Rapidly metabolized by cytochrome P450 3A4 enzymes to 1-hydroxymethyl midazolam and 4-hydroxymidazolam. These metabolites may have some pharmacologic activity but less than that of the parent compound.

### Half-life
Distribution—
 15 minutes.
Elimination—
 Midazolam: Approximately 2.5 (range, 1 to 5; rarely up to 12.3) hours in healthy patients.

Note: In patients with congestive heart failure—A twofold to threefold increase in elimination half-life has been shown in a small group of patients; however, total body clearance appeared to remain unchanged.

In patients with chronic renal failure—Elimination half-life does not appear to be significantly altered.

In obese patients—Because of greatly enhanced distribution of midazolam into peripheral adipose tissue, the elimination half-life is prolonged but there is no change in total body clearance.

In pediatric patients—The weight-adjusted clearance of midazolam in pediatric patients older than 1 year of age is the same as or higher than in adult patients. Clearance is slower and the terminal elimination half-life is longer (6.5 to 12 hours) in critically ill neonates as compared with those rates in other pediatric patients or adult patients.

1-Hydroxymethyl midazolam and 4-hydroxymidazolam: Elimination half-life is similar to that of midazolam.

### Onset of action
Sedation:
 Intramuscular: Within 15 minutes.
 Intravenous: Within 1.5 to 5 minutes.
Anesthesia, induction:
 Intravenous: With narcotic premedication—Approximately 0.75 to 1.5 minutes.
 Without narcotic premedication—2 to 2.5 minutes.
Amnesia:
 Intramuscular: In one study—30 minutes after administration, no recall shown in 73% of patients; 60 minutes after administration, no recall shown in 40% of patients.
 Intravenous: For sedation in endoscopy studies—71% of patients had no recall of introduction of endoscope and 82% of patients had no recall of withdrawal of endoscope.

Note: Time of onset is affected by total dose administered and whether narcotic premedication is used concurrently.

Rapid onset of action after intravenous administration is due to the high lipophilicity of midazolam at physiologic pH.

**Peak serum concentration**
The peak serum concentration achieved with intramuscular administration of midazolam is about one-half that achieved with intravenous administration.

**Time to peak effect**
Intramuscular—15 to 60 minutes. The time to attain peak effect may be longer in geriatric patients.

**Duration of action**
The relatively short duration of action of midazolam is due in part to its very high metabolic clearance and rapid rate of elimination. The termination of action after single doses is caused by both distribution into peripheral tissues and metabolic transformation.

The duration of the amnestic action appears to be directly dose-related.

**Time to recovery**
Usually within 2 hours, but may take up to 6 hours.
Note: Patients who receive midazolam usually recover at a slower rate than patients who receive thiopental.

**Elimination**
Renal; following intravenous administration, less than 0.03% of dose is excreted in urine as unchanged drug; 1-hydroxymethyl midazolam and 4-hydroxymidazolam metabolites are excreted in the urine as glucuronide conjugates.
Note: Elimination following intramuscular administration is comparable to that following intravenous administration.

## Precautions to Consider

### Cross-sensitivity and/or related problems
Patients sensitive to other benzodiazepines may be sensitive to this medication also.

### Carcinogenicity/Tumorigenicity
In 2-year studies in mice, midazolam was administered with the diet in doses of 1, 9, and 80 mg per kg of body weight (mg/kg) per day. At doses of 80 mg/kg per day, midazolam greatly increased the incidence of hepatic tumors in female mice and caused a small but significant increase in benign thyroid follicular cell tumors in male mice. These tumors occurred after chronic administration of midazolam, whereas only a single or several doses are usually used in humans. When midazolam was administered at doses of 9 mg/kg per day (25 times a human dose of 0.35 mg/kg per day), there was no increase in the incidence of tumors.

### Mutagenicity
Midazolam was shown to have no mutagenic activity in *Salmonella typhimurium* (5 bacterial strains), Chinese hamster lung cells (V79), human lymphocytes, or in the micronucleus test in mice.

### Pregnancy/Reproduction
Fertility—A reproduction study in male and female rats did not show midazolam to cause any impairment of fertility when given at doses up to 10 times the human intravenous dose of 0.35 mg/kg.

Pregnancy—Midazolam crosses the placenta. Since chlordiazepoxide and diazepam have been reported to increase the risk of congenital malformations when used during the first trimester of pregnancy, midazolam may be associated with this increased risk also.

Segment II teratology studies in rabbits and rats did not show midazolam to cause teratogenic effects when the medication was administered in doses 5 to 10 times the human dose of 0.35 mg/kg. In addition, studies in rats did not show midazolam to cause any adverse effects during gestation and lactation when administered at doses approximately 10 times the human dose of 0.35 mg/kg.

FDA Pregnancy Category D.

Labor and delivery—In humans, measurable concentrations of midazolam have been found in maternal venous serum, umbilical venous and arterial serum, and amniotic fluid, indicating placental transfer of the medication. Following intramuscular administration of 0.05 mg/kg of midazolam, both the venous and umbilical arterial serum concentrations were lower than maternal concentrations.

Midazolam was compared with thiopental for rapid-sequence intubation in women delivering babies by cesarean section. The neonates whose mothers received midazolam were more likely than the neonates whose mothers received thiopental to require tracheal intubation. In a second similar study, neonates whose mothers received midazolam were more likely to experience hypothermia and reduced body tone as compared with neonates whose mothers received thiopental. Additionally, midazolam is usually not recommended for induction of anesthesia prior to cesarean section because of the secondary CNS depressant effects on the neonate. Administration of other benzodiazepines during the last weeks of pregnancy has caused neonatal CNS depression.

Also, use of benzodiazepines just prior to or during labor may cause neonatal flaccidity.

### Breast-feeding
Midazolam is distributed into breast milk. Midazolam received in the breast milk by neonates may be eliminated slowly because of their immature organ function. Neonates may be more susceptible to respiratory depression than older pediatric patients.

### Pediatrics
The weight-adjusted clearance of midazolam in pediatric patients older than 1 year of age is the same as or higher than in adult patients. Clearance is slower and the terminal elimination half-life is longer in critically ill neonates than in other pediatric patients or adult patients.

Neonates are more likely than other pediatric patients or adult patients to experience respiratory depression following administration of midazolam.

Midazolam injection contains benzyl alcohol. Administration of excessive amounts of benzyl alcohol to neonates has been associated with toxicity, including death. Although midazolam administered to neonates in the recommended doses does not contain amounts of benzyl alcohol associated with toxicity, the total load of benzyl alcohol from all sources must be considered. The 1-mg-per-mL and the 5-mg-per-mL vials of midazolam contain equal amounts of benzyl alcohol. The amount of benzyl alcohol the neonates receive may be decreased by diluting the 5-mg-per-mL vials to prepare neonatal dosages.

### Geriatrics
The clearance of midazolam is reduced in geriatric patients as compared with that in younger adults.

When midazolam is used intravenously to produce sedation, anxiolysis, and amnesia in patients 60 years of age and older, debilitated, and/or chronically ill, dosage increments should be smaller and the rate of injection slower than in younger adults because the risk of underventilation or apnea is greater and the time to peak effect may be longer in older patients. Also, if concomitant CNS depressant premedication is used, the dose of midazolam should be reduced by at least 50%.

When midazolam is used for induction of anesthesia, patients older than 55 years of age, whether premedicated or not, usually require lower doses.

Also, time to complete recovery after midazolam administration for the induction of anesthesia may be prolonged in the elderly.

In addition, elderly patients are more likely to have age-related chronic renal failure, which may require reduction of dosage in patients receiving midazolam.

### Drug interactions and/or related problems
The following drug interactions and/or related problems have been selected on the basis of their potential clinical significance (possible mechanism in parentheses where appropriate)—not necessarily inclusive (» = major clinical significance):

Note: Combinations containing any of the following medications, depending on the amount present, may also interact with this medication.

» Alcohol or
» CNS depression–producing medications, other, including those commonly used for preanesthetic medication or induction or supplementation of anesthesia (see *Appendix II*)
(concurrent use may increase the CNS depressant, respiratory depressant, and hypotensive effects of either these medications or midazolam; decrease dosage requirements of either these medications or midazolam; and prolong recovery from anesthesia; midazolam dosage may be reduced by at least 50% in elderly or debilitated patients receiving other CNS depression–producing medications)

(when midazolam is used as an intramuscular premedication prior to use of thiopental as an induction agent, a reduction in thiopental dosage of about 15% may be required)

(severe hypotension may occur in neonates receiving a continuous infusion of midazolam followed by a rapid injection of fentanyl)

Cimetidine or
Diltiazem or
Erythromycin or
Indinavir or
Itraconazole or
Ketoconazole or
Ritonavir or
Verapamil or
Cytochrome P450 3A inhibitors, other
(inhibition of the cytochrome P450 3A enzyme system may cause a decrease in the metabolism of midazolam, which may result in

delayed elimination and increased blood concentration; interaction with cytochrome P450 3A inhibitors is more likely when midazolam is administered orally than when it is administered parenterally)

Grapefruit or
Grapefruit juice
(decreased metabolism of midazolam, with resulting increased blood concentrations of midazolam, may occur; there may be an increased risk of toxicity)

Hypotension-producing medications, other (see *Appendix II*)
(hypotensive effects may be potentiated when these medications are used concurrently with midazolam; patients should be monitored for excessive fall in blood pressure during and following concurrent use)

Rifampin or
Cytochrome P450 3A inducers, other
(induction of the cytochrome P450 3A enzyme system may cause an increase in the metabolism of midazolam, which may result in its accelerated elimination and decreased blood concentration; the interaction is more likely when midazolam is administered orally than when it is administered parenterally)

**Medical considerations/Contraindications**
The medical considerations/contraindications included have been selected on the basis of their potential clinical significance (reasons given in parentheses where appropriate)—not necessarily inclusive (» = major clinical significance).

*Except under special circumstances, this medication should not be used when the following medical problem exists:*
» Allergy to midazolam, history of

*Risk-benefit should be considered when the following medical problems exist:*
Alcohol intoxication, acute, with depressed vital signs
(potential additive CNS depression)
Coma or
Shock
(hypnotic or hypotensive effects may be intensified or prolonged)
Congestive heart failure
(possible twofold to threefold increase in elimination half-life and a 40% increase in the volume of distribution)
Hepatic function impairment
(midazolam is metabolized by the liver; in one study, patients with cirrhosis of the liver had reduced clearance and a longer elimination half-life of midazolam than healthy control subjects)
» Myasthenia gravis or
Neuromuscular disorders, other, such as muscular dystrophies and myotonias
(condition may be exacerbated)
Obesity
(midazolam's elimination half-life may be prolonged and volume of distribution may be increased)
» Pulmonary disease, obstructive, chronic, severe or
» Pulmonary insufficiency, acute
(midazolam has respiratory depressant effects; sedation and respiratory depression may be prolonged; patients with chronic obstructive pulmonary disease are unusually sensitive to the respiratory depressant effects of midazolam)
Renal failure, chronic
(peak concentration of midazolam may be higher in these patients than in healthy patients; induction of anesthesia may occur more rapidly, and recovery may be prolonged)
Sensitivity to other benzodiazepines
Caution is recommended in geriatric or debilitated patients and in higher risk surgical patients, whether premedicated or not, because they may require lower doses for induction of anesthesia; caution should be used when intravenous midazolam is administered to patients with uncompensated acute illnesses, such as electrolyte disturbances
Also, caution should be used in ophthalmology patients during surgery because some patients may be confused or disoriented if they awaken during the procedure. This is especially important in patients with an open globe for cataract surgery or in patients for whom movement might be critical

**Patient monitoring**
The following may be especially important in patient monitoring (other tests may be warranted in some patients, depending on condition; » = major clinical significance):

» Blood oxygenation (pulse oximetry) and
» Blood pressure and
» Respiratory status and
» Vital signs, other
(it is recommended that patients be monitored continuously; when midazolam is used by non-anesthesiologists to produce deep sedation for surgical or diagnostic procedures, it is recommended that the patient be monitored continuously by someone not involved in conducting the surgical or diagnostic procedure; patients should be monitored for early signs of hypoventilation or apnea).

Note: Various organizations, including the American Society of Anesthesiologists and the American Academy of Pediatrics, have established guidelines for pre-, intra-, and post-procedural care, evaluation, and monitoring of patients receiving sedation for diagnostic and therapeutic procedures. The level of monitoring should be appropriate to the level of sedation and the procedure being performed. When midazolam is used for light sedation (i.e., the patient is able to tolerate unpleasant procedures without cardiorespiratory compromise and is able to respond purposefully to verbal commands) by non-anesthesiologists, the American Society of Anesthesiologists recommends that a designated individual, other than the person performing the procedure, be present to monitor the patient. That designated person would be permitted to assist with other minor, interruptible tasks. However, when midazolam is used to produce deep sedation, the patient should be monitored continuously by someone not involved in conducting the surgical or diagnostic procedure. For deeply sedated patients, the person monitoring the patient should not assist with other tasks, even if the tasks are minor and interruptible.

## Side/Adverse Effects

Note: The most frequent side/adverse effects of midazolam during anesthesia and surgery include decreased tidal volume and/or respiratory rate (in 23.3% of patients following intravenous administration and in 10.8% of patients following intramuscular administration) and apnea (in 15.4% of patients following intravenous administration). In addition, variations in blood pressure and pulse rate may occur.

**Serious cardiorespiratory side/adverse effects have occurred primarily in older, chronically ill patients, with concomitant administration of other cardiorespiratory depressants (such as opioid [narcotic] analgesics), and with rapid administration of midazolam; these side/adverse effects have included respiratory depression, apnea, respiratory arrest, and/or cardiac arrest, sometimes resulting in death. Patients undergoing procedures involving the upper airway (e.g., upper endoscopy or dental procedures) are more likely than patients undergoing other types of procedures to experience respiratory depression, apnea, and respiratory arrest.**

**Midazolam administered intravenously has been associated with respiratory depression and respiratory arrest, especially when used concomitantly with opioid analgesics for conscious sedation or when rapidly administered; in some cases, death or hypoxic encephalopathy has occurred.**

Impairment of psychomotor skills may occur following midazolam sedation or anesthesia and may persist for varying lengths of time, depending upon the combination of medications and total dosages administered. Possible adverse effects on the patient's ability to drive or perform other tasks requiring alertness and coordination should be kept in mind when midazolam is administered for an outpatient procedure. It is recommended that patients not operate hazardous machinery or a motor vehicle until the effects of midazolam, such as drowsiness and amnesia, have subsided or until the day after anesthesia and surgery, whichever is longer.

The following side/adverse effects have been selected on the basis of their potential clinical significance (possible signs and symptoms in parentheses where appropriate)—not necessarily inclusive:

**Those indicating need for medical attention**
Incidence more frequent
*Apnea; hypotension*—especially in patients premedicated with narcotic; *respiratory depression*

Incidence rare— < 1%, primarily following intravenous administration
*Emergence delirium; hyperventilation; irregular or fast heartbeat; muscle tremor; phlebitis; skin rash, hives, or itching; uncontrolled or jerky movements of body; unusual excitement, irritability, or restlessness; wheezing or difficulty in breathing*

Note: *Muscle tremor, uncontrolled or jerky movements of body, unusual excitement, irritability, or restlessness* possibly are due to inadequate or excessive dosing or improper administration of medication; also, the possibility of cerebral hypoxia or paradoxical reaction should be considered.

*Those indicating need for medical attention only if they continue or are bothersome*
Incidence more frequent
> *Hiccups; pain at intramuscular injection site; pain during intravenous injection; tenderness at intravenous injection site*

Incidence less frequent or rare
> *Blurred vision or other changes in vision; coughing; dizziness, lightheadedness, or feeling faint; drowsiness, prolonged; headache; lumps or hardness at injection site; muscle stiffness at intramuscular injection site; nausea; numbness, tingling, pain, or weakness in hands or feet; redness at injection site; vomiting*

## Overdose

For specific information on the agents used in the management of midazolam overdose, see:
- *Flumazenil (Systemic)* monograph; and/or
- *Sympathomimetic Agents—Cardiovascular Use (Parenteral-Systemic)* monograph.

For more information on the management of overdose or unintentional ingestion, **contact a Poison Control Center** (see *Poison Control Center Listing*).

**Clinical effects of overdose**
The following effects have been selected on the basis of their potential clinical significance (possible signs and symptoms in parentheses where appropriate)—not necessarily inclusive:

Acute
> *Cardiovascular depression; respiratory depression*

**Treatment of overdose**
To enhance elimination—
> It is not known if peritoneal dialysis, forced diuresis, or hemodialysis is useful in the treatment of midazolam overdose.

Specific treatment—
> Administering flumazenil. See the package insert or the *Flumazenil (Systemic)* monograph for specific dosing guidelines for the use of this product.
> For hypotension: Treatment may include intravenous fluid therapy, repositioning, vasopressors (if indicated), and other appropriate countermeasures.

Monitoring—
> Monitoring of respiration, pulse rate, and blood pressure.

Supportive care—
> General supportive measures.
> Maintenance of a patent airway and support of ventilation.

## Patient Consultation

As an aid to patient consultation, refer to *Advice for the Patient, Midazolam (Systemic)*.

Note: The capacity of midazolam to cause anterograde amnesia should be considered when providing consultation to patients. Patients counseled after receiving midazolam may not remember being counseled.

In providing consultation, consider emphasizing the following selected information (» = major clinical significance):

**Before receiving this medication**
» Conditions affecting use, especially:
  Sensitivity to midazolam or other benzodiazepines
  Carcinogenicity—In 2-year studies in mice, chronic administration of midazolam at doses of 80 mg per kg of body weight (mg/kg) per day greatly increased incidence of hepatic tumors in female mice and caused a small but significant increase in benign thyroid follicular cell tumors in male mice
  Pregnancy—Risk of congenital malformations may be increased when midazolam is used during first trimester
  Labor and delivery—Midazolam is usually not recommended for induction of anesthesia prior to cesarean section because of secondary CNS depressant effects on neonate; use of benzodiazepines just prior to or during labor may cause neonatal flaccidity
  Breast-feeding—Midazolam is distributed into breast milk; neonates may have difficulty eliminating the midazolam received in breast milk; neonates may experience respiratory depression after receiving midazolam in breast milk
  Use in children—Critically ill neonates have reduced clearance of midazolam, and they are more likely than older pediatric patients or adult patients to experience respiratory depression after receiving midazolam; midazolam contains benzyl alcohol, excessive amounts of benzyl alcohol can cause toxicity in neonates
  Pediatric patients may require a higher dose of midazolam on a weight-adjusted basis than required for adult patients
  Use in the elderly—When midazolam is used intravenously to produce sedation, anxiolysis, and amnesia in patients 60 years of age and older, dosage increments should be smaller and the rate of injection slower than in younger adults because risk of underventilation or apnea is greater and the time to peak effect may be longer in older patients; if concomitant CNS depressant premedication is used, dosage of midazolam should be reduced by at least 50%; time to complete recovery after midazolam administration for induction of anesthesia may be prolonged in the elderly
  Other medications, especially alcohol or other CNS depression–producing medications
  Other medical problems, especially myasthenia gravis, severe chronic obstructive pulmonary disease, or acute pulmonary insufficiency

**Precautions after receiving this medication**
» Possibility of psychomotor impairment following use of midazolam; using caution in driving or performing other tasks requiring alertness and coordination until the effects of midazolam have subsided or until the day after receiving midazolam, whichever is longer
» Avoiding use of alcohol or other CNS depressants within 24 hours after receiving midazolam, except as directed by doctor

## General Dosing Information

Midazolam has been shown to be three to four times as potent per mg as diazepam.

**The dosage of midazolam must be individualized for each patient.** Lower doses are usually required for elderly, debilitated, or high-risk surgical patients. The dosage of intravenously administered midazolam should be adjusted according to the type and amount of premedication used. Additionally, the dose requirement of midazolam of each patient may vary. The dose always should be individualized and titrated slowly. The doses given in *Usual adult and adolescent dose* and *Usual pediatric dose* should be regarded as general guidelines only.

**Intravenous midazolam should be used only in hospital or ambulatory care settings, including physicians' and dentists' offices,** that provide for continuous monitoring of respiratory and cardiac function.

**Prior to intravenous administration of midazolam in any dose, age- and size-appropriate resuscitative equipment, oxygen, and skilled personnel for the maintenance of a patent airway and support of ventilation must be immediately available. When midazolam is used intravenously to produce deep sedation for surgical or diagnostic procedures, it is recommended that the patient be monitored continuously by someone not involved in conducting the surgical or diagnostic procedure.**

**Midazolam should be administered intravenously as an induction agent only by a person trained in general anesthesia and should be used for conscious sedation only when a person skilled in maintaining a patent airway and supporting ventilation is present,** because of possible respiratory depression.

**When midazolam is administered intravenously for conscious sedation, it should be injected slowly in multiple small injections to attain the desired effect; it should not be administered by rapid or single bolus intravenous injection** because of the risk of respiratory depression and/or arrest, especially in elderly or debilitated patients. Three to five minutes should elapse between each small injection, so the full effect of the injection can be assessed before another injection is administered.

To facilitate slower intravenous injection of midazolam, the 1-mg-per-mL solution or dilution of the 1-mg-per-mL or 5-mg-per-mL solution is recommended.

During intravenous administration of midazolam, patients should be monitored continuously for early signs of underventilation or apnea, which can lead to hypoxia/cardiac arrest unless effective countermeasures are immediately taken. Also, monitoring of vital signs should be continued during the recovery period. In one case series, respiratory arrest occurred in patients 30 to 120 minutes after administration of midazolam. Patients should be monitored for several hours following use of midazolam.

Adult and pediatric patients undergoing procedures involving the upper airway (e.g., upper endoscopy or dental procedures) are more likely than patients undergoing other types of procedures to experience respiratory depression, apnea, and respiratory arrest when midazolam is used.

Caution should be taken to avoid intra-arterial injection because adverse effects of intra-arterial administration of intravenous midazolam in humans are not known. Extravasation should also be avoided.

Midazolam contains benzyl alcohol, and so may not be administered by the intrathecal or epidural routes.

Administration of excessive amounts of benzyl alcohol to neonates has been associated with toxicity, including death. Although midazolam administered to neonates in the recommended doses does not contain amounts of benzyl alcohol associated with toxicity, the total load of benzyl alcohol from all sources must be considered. The 1-mg-per-mL and the 5-mg-per-mL vials of midazolam contain equal amounts of benzyl alcohol. The amount of benzyl alcohol may be decreased for neonatal patients by diluting the 5-mg-per-mL vials to prepare neonatal dosages.

When midazolam is administered intramuscularly, it is recommended that the medication be injected deep into a large muscle mass.

When midazolam is used for peroral endoscopic procedures, a topical anesthetic agent and the availability of necessary countermeasures are recommended because an increase in cough reflex and laryngospasm may occur.

When midazolam is used for bronchoscopic procedures, a narcotic premedication is recommended.

When midazolam is administered intravenously, it usually produces partial or complete impairment of recall for up to several hours, depending on the dose.

Although midazolam is approved by the Food and Drug Administration (FDA) for administration by the intramuscular and intravenous routes only, the intranasal, oral, rectal, and sublingual routes are sometimes used in pediatric patients. The 5-mg-per-mL midazolam injection has been used intranasally and sublingually for preoperative sedation and amnesia and sedation, anxiolysis, and amnesia prior to diagnostic or short therapeutic procedures by placing midazolam into a small syringe (with the needle removed) and administering it intranasally or sublingually. In one study, pediatric patients receiving intranasal midazolam were more likely to cry and cried longer than pediatric patients receiving the drug sublingually.

Patients receiving midazolam for sedation in the intensive care unit also may require appropriate analgesia. Administration of an opioid analgesic in addition to midazolam will reduce the dose requirement for midazolam.

Abrupt discontinuation of long-term midazolam therapy may result in precipitation of symptoms of withdrawal. Midazolam should be tapered gradually if it has been administered for more than a few days.

**Diet/Nutrition**
Bioavailability of orally administered midazolam may be increased by ingestion of grapefruit or grapefruit juice, resulting in higher blood concentrations of midazolam.

## Oral Dosage Forms

Note: Bracketed uses in the *Dosage Forms* section refer to categories of use and/or indications that are not included in U.S. product labeling. The dosing and dosage forms available are expressed in terms of midazolam base.

### MIDAZOLAM HYDROCHLORIDE ORAL SOLUTION

**Usual pediatric dose**
[Sedation, preoperative, and amnesia][1] or
[Sedation, conscious (sedation, anxiolysis, and amnesia)][1]—
   Children 1 year of age and older: Oral, 0.2 to 0.5 mg (base) per kg of body weight thirty to forty-five minutes prior to induction of anesthesia or to the diagnostic or therapeutic procedure.

**Usual pediatric prescribing limits**
15 to 20 mg.

Note: When midazolam is administered concomitantly with narcotic analgesics or other CNS depressants, the dosage of midazolam should be reduced.

U.S.—
   Dosage form not commercially available. Compounding required for prescriptions.
Canada—
   Dosage form not commercially available. Compounding required for prescriptions.

**Packaging and storage**
Package in a tight, light-resistant container.
Store between 15 and 30 °C (59 and 86 °F). Protect from excessive heat.

**Preparation of dosage form**
An oral solution containing 2.5 mg/mL midazolam can be prepared by combining equal quantities of midazolam hydrochloride injection 5 mg/mL and a flavored, dye-free syrup.

**Stability**
The solution is stable for at least 56 days.

**Auxiliary labeling**
- Protect from light.
- Shake well

## Parenteral Dosage Forms

Note: Bracketed uses in the *Dosage Forms* section refer to categories of use and/or indications that are not included in U.S. product labeling. The dosing and dosage forms available are expressed in terms of midazolam base.

### MIDAZOLAM HYDROCHLORIDE INJECTION

**Usual adult dose**
Sedation, preoperative, and amnesia—
   Patients younger than 60 years of age—
      ASA I or II (good risk surgical patients):
         Intramuscular, 70 to 80 mcg (0.07 to 0.08 mg) (base) per kg of body weight, approximately thirty to sixty minutes before surgery.
      ASA III or IV (patients with severe systemic disease or debilitation):
         Intramuscular, 20 to 50 mcg (0.02 to 0.05 mg) (base) per kg of body weight, approximately thirty to sixty minutes before surgery.
   Patients 60 years of age and older—
      Intramuscular, 20 to 50 mcg (0.02 to 0.05 mg) (base) per kg of body weight, approximately thirty to sixty minutes before surgery

Note: Lower doses may be sufficient in elderly or debilitated patients.
   Midazolam may be administered concurrently with atropine or scopolamine hydrochloride and reduced doses of narcotics.

Sedation, conscious (sedation, anxiolysis, and amnesia)—
   Unpremedicated patients younger than 60 years of age—
      Intravenous, initially no more than 2.5 mg (base), administered slowly over a period of at least two minutes, immediately prior to the procedure; after an additional two or more minutes to allow for clinical effect, dosage may be further titrated in small increments of the initial dose (with intervals of two or more minutes being allowed after each increment) to the desired effect. A total dose of more than 5 mg is not usually necessary. Additional maintenance doses may be administered, if necessary, in increments of 25% of initial dose to maintain desired level of sedation.

Note: When midazolam is administered concomitantly with narcotic analgesics or other CNS depressants, the dosage of midazolam should be reduced by approximately 30%.

Unpremedicated patients 60 years of age and older, and debilitated or chronically ill patients—
   Intravenous, initially no more than 1.5 mg (base), administered slowly over a period of at least two minutes, immediately prior to procedure; after an additional two or more minutes to allow for clinical effect, dosage may be further titrated, if necessary, but the rate of administration should not exceed 1 mg over a two-minute period (intervals of two or more minutes should be allowed each time). A total dose of more than 3.5 mg is not usually necessary. Additional maintenance doses may be administered, if necessary, in increments of 25% of initial dose to maintain desired level of sedation.

Note: When midazolam is administered concomitantly with narcotic analgesics or other CNS depressants, the dosage of midazolam should be reduced by 50%.

   Also, dosage increments should be smaller and the rate of injection slower because the danger of underventilation or apnea is greater in elderly patients and patients with chronic disease states or decreased pulmonary reserve; also, it may take longer to achieve the peak effect in these patients.

Note: The desired endpoint for conscious sedation can usually be attained within 3 to 6 minutes, depending on the total dose administered and whether or not narcotic premedication is used concomitantly.

   The therapeutic dosage range between sedation and unconsciousness or disorientation appears to be narrower than for other benzodiazepines (e.g., diazepam, lorazepam).

Anesthesia, general, adjunct (prior to administration of other general anesthetics)—
   Unpremedicated patients—
      Younger than 55 years of age—Intravenous, initially 200 to 350 mcg (0.2 to 0.35 mg)(base) per kg of body weight, administered over a period of five to thirty seconds and allowing two minutes for effect.

Note: If necessary to complete induction, additional doses may be given in increments of about 25% of initial dose, or inhalation general anesthetics may be used.

Up to 600 mcg (0.6 mg) (base) per kg of body weight as a total dose may be used for induction, if necessary; however, larger doses may prolong recovery.

55 years of age and older—ASA I or II (good risk surgical patients): Intravenous, initially 150 to 300 mcg (0.15 to 0.3 mg) (base) per kg of body weight, administered over a period of twenty to thirty seconds.

ASA III or IV (patients with severe systemic disease or debilitation): Intravenous, initially 150 to 250 mcg (0.15 to 0.25 mg) (base) per kg of body weight, administered over a period of twenty to thirty seconds.

Premedicated (sedative or narcotic) patients—

Younger than 55 years of age—Intravenous, 150 to 350 mcg (0.15 to 0.35 mg) (base) per kg of body weight, administered over a period of twenty to thirty seconds and allowing two minutes for effect. A dose of 250 mcg (0.25 mg) per kg of body weight is usually sufficient.

55 years of age and older—ASA I or II: Intravenous, initially 200 mcg (0.2 mg) (base) per kg of body weight.

ASA III or IV: Intravenous, 150 mcg (0.15 mg) (base) per kg of body weight may be sufficient.

Note: When sedative or, especially, narcotic premedication has been administered, the recommended dose range of midazolam is 150 to 250 mcg (0.15 to 0.25 mg) (base) per kg of body weight.

Additional doses may be given in increments of about 25% of induction dose in response to signs of lightening anesthesia, repeated as necessary.

Narcotic premedications frequently used include: fentanyl (1.5 to 2 mcg [0.0015 to 0.002 mg] per kg of body weight intravenously five minutes before induction); morphine (up to 150 mcg [0.15 mg] per kg of body weight intramuscularly, the dosage being individualized); meperidine (up to 1 mg per kg of body weight intramuscularly, the dosage being individualized); and fentanyl citrate and droperidol combination (0.02 mL per kg of body weight intramuscularly).

Sedative premedications frequently used include: hydroxyzine pamoate (100 mg orally) and secobarbital sodium (200 mg orally).

Premedications should be administered at least thirty to sixty minutes prior to midazolam induction, with the exception of narcotic analgesics (e.g., fentanyl), which should be administered two to five minutes before induction.

Sedation in critical care settings—

Intravenous infusion, 20 to 100 mcg (0.02 to 0.1 mg) (base) per kg of body weight per hour, initially, then titrated to the desired level of sedation. If a loading dose is needed, 10 to 50 mcg (0.01 to 0.05 mg) per kg of body weight may be administered over several minutes prior to initiation of the continuous infusion.

[Anesthetic, local, adjunct (epidural or axillary block)][1]—

Intravenous, 30 to 60 mcg (0.03 to 0.06 mg) (base) per kg of body weight, the dosage being slowly titrated.

## Usual pediatric dose

Sedation, preoperative, and amnesia or
Sedation, conscious (sedation, anxiolysis, and amnesia)—

Infants younger than 6 months of age:

The dose is not clearly established because there is variability in when pediatric patients progress from neonatal to infant physiology in terms of their abilities to tolerate, metabolize, and eliminate midazolam. Pediatric patients younger than 6 months of age are especially vulnerable to airway obstruction and hypoventilation. Titration with small increments and careful monitoring are especially important when midazolam is used in pediatric patients younger than 6 months of age.

Infants and children 6 months to 5 years of age:

Intravenously by intermittent injection, 50 to 100 mcg (0.05 to 0.1 mg) (base) per kg of body weight; sometimes up to 600 mcg (0.6 mg) per kg of body weight may be necessary, but usually no more than a total of 6 mg is needed to reach the desired endpoint.

Intramuscular, 100 to 150 mcg (0.1 to 0.15 mg) (base) per kg of body weight. Doses of up to 500 mcg (0.5 mg) per kg of body weight have been used for deep sedation.

Children 6 to 12 years of age:

Intravenously by intermittent injection, 25 to 50 mcg (0.025 to 0.05 mg) (base) per kg of body weight; sometimes up to 400 mcg (0.4 mg) per kg of body weight may be necessary, but usually no more than a total of 10 mg is needed to reach the desired endpoint.

Intramuscular, 100 to 150 mcg (0.1 to 0.15 mg) (base) per kg of body weight. Doses of up to 500 mcg (0.5 mg) per kg of body weight have been used for deep sedation.

Adolescents 12 to 16 years of age:

See *Usual adult dose*. Some adolescents may require higher doses than adults, but usually no more than a total of 10 mg is needed to reach the desired endpoint.

Note: In obese pediatric patients, the dose should be calculated based on ideal body weight.

Anesthesia, general, adjunct (prior to administration of other general anesthetics)—

Infants younger than 6 months of age:

The dose is not clearly established because there is variability in when pediatric patients progress from neonatal to infant physiology in terms of their abilities to tolerate, metabolize, and eliminate midazolam. Pediatric patients younger than 6 months of age are especially vulnerable to airway obstruction and hypoventilation. Titration with small increments and careful monitoring are especially important when midazolam is used in pediatric patients younger than 6 months of age.

Infants and children 6 months to 5 years of age:

Intravenously by intermittent injection, 50 to 100 mcg (0.05 to 0.1 mg) (base) per kg of body weight; sometimes up to 600 mcg (0.6 mg) per kg of body weight may be necessary, but usually no more than a total of 6 mg is needed to reach the desired endpoint.

Children 6 to 12 years of age:

Intravenously by intermittent injection, 25 to 50 mcg (0.025 to 0.05 mg) (base) per kg of body weight; sometimes up to 400 mcg (0.4 mg) per kg of body weight may be necessary, but usually no more than a total of 10 mg is needed to reach the desired endpoint.

Adolescents 12 to 16 years of age:

See *Usual adult dose*. Some adolescents may require higher doses than adults, but usually no more than a total of 10 mg is needed to reach the desired endpoint.

Sedation in critical care settings—

Neonates younger than 32 weeks gestation:

Intravenous infusion in patients whose trachea is intubated, 30 mcg (0.03 mg) (base) per kg of body weight per hour.

Note: Intravenous loading doses should not be administered to neonatal patients.

Neonates older than 32 weeks gestation:

Intravenous infusion in patients whose trachea is intubated, 60 mcg (0.06 mg) (base) per kg of body weight per hour.

Note: Intravenous loading doses should not be administered to neonatal patients.

Infants and children:

Intravenous infusion in patients whose trachea is intubated, initially, 60 to 120 mcg (0.06 to 0.12 mg) (base) per kg of body weight per hour, then titrated to desired effect. An intravenous loading dose of 50 to 200 mcg (0.05 to 0.2 mg) per kg of body weight administered over at least two to three minutes can be used prior to initiation of the continuous infusion.

## Strength(s) usually available

U.S.—

1 mg (base) per mL (Rx) [*Versed* (benzyl alcohol 1%; disodium edetate 0.01%; sodium chloride 0.8%)].

5 mg (base) per mL (Rx) [*Versed* (benzyl alcohol 1%; disodium edetate 0.01%; sodium chloride 0.8%)].

Canada—

5 mg (base) per mL (Rx) [*Versed* (benzyl alcohol 10.45 mg; disodium edetate 0.1 mg; sodium chloride 8 mg)].

## Packaging and storage

Store between 15 and 30 °C (59 and 86 °F), unless otherwise specified by manufacturer. Protect from freezing.

## Preparation of dosage form

Midazolam injection is compatible with 5% dextrose in water, 0.9% sodium chloride, and lactated Ringer's solution.

Midazolam injection may be mixed in same syringe with frequently used premedicants, such as morphine sulfate, meperidine hydrochloride, atropine sulfate, or scopolamine hydrobromide.

## Stability

Midazolam injection should not be used if it contains a precipitate or is discolored.

When midazolam injection is mixed in the same syringe with frequently used premedicants, such as morphine sulfate, meperidine hydrochloride, atropine sulfate, or scopolamine hydrobromide, the solution is stable for 30 minutes.

When midazolam injection is diluted in 5% dextrose in water or 0.9% sodium chloride, the solution is stable for 24 hours; if mixed with lactated Ringer's solution (Hartmann's solution), the solution should be used within 4 hours.

**Note**
Controlled substance in the U.S.

[1]Not included in Canadian product labeling.

Revised: 07/23/98

# MIDODRINE   Systemic—INTRODUCTORY VERSION

VA CLASSIFICATION (Primary): CV900
Commonly used brand name(s): *ProAmatine*.
Note:  For a listing of dosage forms and brand names by country availability, see *Dosage Forms* section(s).

## Category
Antihypotensive, idiopathic orthostatic; vasopressor.

## Indications
**Accepted**
Hypotension (treatment)—Midodrine is indicated for the treatment of symptomatic orthostatic hypotension. Midodrine should be used in patients who are considerably impaired and for whom standard clinical care, including nonpharmacologic treatment (such as support stockings), fluid expansion, and lifestyle changes, has not been successful.

## Pharmacology/Pharmacokinetics
**Physicochemical characteristics**
Molecular weight—290.7.
pH—3.5 to 5.5 (5% aqueous solution).
pKa—7.8 (0.3% aqueous solution).
Solubility—
  Water: Soluble.
  Methanol: Sparingly soluble.

**Mechanism of action/Effect**
Midodrine is a prodrug for desglymidodrine, the active metabolite. Desglymidodrine, an alpha$_1$-agonist, increases blood pressure and vascular tone by stimulating the alpha-adrenergic receptors of the arteriolar and venous vasculature. It does not stimulate cardiac beta-adrenergic receptors. Desglymidodrine does not have effects on the central nervous system because it diffuses poorly across the blood-brain barrier. Desglymidodrine increases standing, sitting, and supine systolic and diastolic blood pressure in patients with orthostatic hypotension of various etiologies.

**Other actions/effects**
Desglymidodrine may have a bradycardiac effect, primarily due to vagal reflex.

**Absorption**
Rapidly absorbed. Absolute bioavailability of desglymidodrine is 93% and is not affected by food. The amount of desglymidodrine formed after oral or intravenous administration is about the same.

**Protein binding**
Not significant for midodrine or desglymidodrine.

**Biotransformation**
Studies have not been done. Deglycination of midodrine to desglymidodrine occurs in various tissues. Both midodrine and desglymidodrine are metabolized in part by the liver.

**Half-life**
Elimination—
  Midodrine—Approximately 25 minutes.
  Desglymidodrine—3 to 4 hours.

**Time to peak concentration**
Midodrine—30 minutes.
Desglymidodrine—1 to 2 hours.

**Duration of action**
Approximately 2 to 3 hours after a 10-mg dose.

**Elimination**
Desglymidodrine—Renal: Approximately 80% by active renal tubular secretion.
  In dialysis—
    Desglymidodrine is dialyzable.

## Precautions to Consider
**Carcinogenicity**
No evidence of carcinogenicity was found in long-term studies in rats and mice given daily doses of 3 to 4 times the maximum recommended human dose (MRHD) on a mg per square meter of body surface area (mg/m$^2$) basis.

**Mutagenicity**
No evidence of mutagenicity was found in investigational studies.

**Pregnancy/Reproduction**
Fertility—No impaired fertility was observed in the dominant lethal assay in male mice. No other fertility studies have been done.
Pregnancy—Adequate and well-controlled studies in humans have not been done.
Reproduction studies in rats and rabbits given doses 13 and 7 times the maximum recommended human dose, respectively, on a mg/m$^2$ basis showed an increased rate of embryo resorption and reduced fetal body weight. Fetal survival in rabbits was also decreased at doses of 7 times the maximum recommended human dose. No teratogenic effects were observed in studies in rats and rabbits.

FDA Pregnancy Category C.

**Breast-feeding**
It is not known whether midodrine is distributed into breast milk. However, problems in humans have not been documented.

**Pediatrics**
No information is available on the relationship of age to the effects of midodrine in pediatric patients. Safety and efficacy have not been established.

**Geriatrics**
Studies performed in patients 65 years of age and older have not demonstrated geriatrics-specific problems that would limit the usefulness of midodrine in the elderly. Serum concentrations of midodrine and desglymidodrine in patients 65 years of age and older are similar to those of patients younger than 65.

**Drug interactions and/or related problems**
The following drug interactions and/or related problems have been selected on the basis of their potential clinical significance (possible mechanism in parentheses where appropriate)—not necessarily inclusive (» = major clinical significance):

Note:  Combinations containing any of the following medications, depending on the amount present, may also interact with this medication.

  Alpha-adrenergic blocking agents, such as:
    Doxazosin
    Prazosin
    Terazosin
      (concurrent use may antagonize the antihypotensive effects of midodrine)

  Bradycardia-causing medications, such as:
    Beta-adrenergic blocking agents
» Digitalis glycosides
      (concurrent use may have additive bradycardiac effects; digitalis glycosides may exacerbate or precipitate atrioventricular [AV] block or arrhythmia)

  Medications eliminated by active renal tubular secretion, such as:
    Cimetidine
    Flecainide
    Metformin
    Procainamide
    Quinidine
    Ranitidine
    Triamterene
      (concurrent use may interfere with renal clearance of these medications or of desglymidodrine because of competition for active renal tubular secretion)

» Sodium-retaining corticosteroids, such as fludrocortisone
  (concurrent use may increase sodium retention and cause supine hypertension; decreasing salt intake prior to initiation of midodrine therapy or reducing the dose of the corticosteroid may minimize this effect)
» Vasoconstricting medications, such as:
  Dihydroergotamine
  Ephedrine
  Phenylephrine
  Phenylpropanolamine
  Pseudoephedrine
  (effects on blood pressure may be additive with concurrent use; blood pressure should be monitored carefully)

### Medical considerations/Contraindications

The medical considerations/contraindications included have been selected on the basis of their potential clinical significance (reasons given in parentheses where appropriate)—not necessarily inclusive (» = major clinical significance).

*Except under special circumstances, this medication should not be used when the following medical problems exist:*

» Cardiac disease, severe or
» Hypertension, supine, persistent and excessive or
» Pheochromocytoma or
» Thyrotoxicosis
  (increases in blood pressure due to midodrine therapy may aggravate these conditions)
» Renal function impairment, acute
  (decreased elimination may increase serum concentrations of desglymidodrine)
» Urinary retention
  (condition may be exacerbated because of the action of desglymidodrine on the alpha-adrenergic receptors of the bladder neck)

*Risk-benefit should be considered when the following medical problems exist:*

Hepatic function impairment
  (metabolism of midodrine and desglymidodrine may be decreased)
Renal function impairment
  (elimination of desglymidodrine may be decreased; renal function should be assessed prior to midodrine therapy)
Sensitivity to midodrine
Visual problems, diabetes-associated or
Visual problems, history of
  (increases in blood pressure from midodrine therapy may aggravate this condition, particularly with concurrent use of fludrocortisone, a corticosteroid known to cause an increase in intraocular pressure and glaucoma)

### Patient monitoring

The following may be especially important in patient monitoring (other tests may be warranted in some patients, depending on condition; » = major clinical significance):

Blood pressure measurements
  (supine and sitting blood pressure should be monitored during midodrine therapy)
Hepatic function determinations and
Renal function determinations
  (because desglymidodrine is metabolized by the liver and eliminated by the kidneys, it may be necessary to evaluate renal and hepatic function prior to initiation of and during midodrine therapy)

## Side/Adverse Effects

The following side/adverse effects have been selected on the basis of their potential clinical significance (possible signs and symptoms in parentheses where appropriate)—not necessarily inclusive:

### Those indicating need for medical attention

Incidence more frequent
  *Hypertension, supine* (blurred vision; cardiac awareness; headache; pounding in the ears)
  Note: *Supine hypertension* is the most serious adverse effect that may occur with midodrine therapy. In clinical trials, patients experienced both sitting and supine hypertension. Approximately 13.4% of patients administered 10 mg of midodrine experienced systolic blood pressures of about 200 mm Hg. This was most commonly seen in patients with relatively elevated systolic blood pressures prior to treatment.

Incidence rare
  *Bradycardia* (fainting; increased dizziness; slow pulse)

**Those indicating need for medical attention only if they continue or are bothersome**

Incidence more frequent
  *Burning, itching, or prickling of the scalp; chills; piloerection* (goosebumps); *urinary frequency, retention, or urgency*

Incidence less frequent
  *Anxiety or nervousness; confusion; dry mouth; flushing of face or vasodilation; headache or feeling of pressure in the head; skin rash*

Incidence rare
  *Backache; canker sores; dizziness; dry skin; gastrointestinal effects, including flatulence; gastrointestinal distress; heartburn; and nausea; insomnia* (trouble in sleeping); *leg cramps; pain or sensitivity of skin to touch; somnolence* (drowsiness); *visual field defects; weakness*

## Overdose

For specific information on the agents used in the management of midodrine overdose, see the *Phentolamine (Systemic)* monograph.

For more information on the management of overdose or unintentional ingestion, **contact a Poison Control Center** (see *Poison Control Center Listing*).

### Clinical effects of overdose

The following effects have been selected on the basis of their potential clinical significance (possible signs and symptoms in parentheses where appropriate)—not necessarily inclusive:

Acute and chronic
  *Hypertension* (blurred vision; cardiac awareness; headache; pounding in the ears); *piloerection* (goosebumps); *sensation of coldness; urinary retention*

### Treatment of overdose

To decrease absorption—Emesis may be induced.

Specific treatment—Administration of alpha-sympatholytic medications, such as phentolamine.

Supportive care—Patients in whom intentional overdose is confirmed or suspected should be referred for psychiatric consultation.

## Patient Consultation

As an aid to patient consultation, refer to *Advice for the Patient, Midodrine (Systemic)—Introductory Version*.

In providing consultation, consider emphasizing the following selected information (» = major clinical significance):

### Before using this medication
» Conditions affecting use, especially:
  Sensitivity to midodrine
  Other medications, especially digitalis glycosides, sodium-retaining corticosteroids, or vasoconstricting medications
  Other medical problems, especially acute renal function impairment, persistent and excessive supine hypertension, pheochromocytoma, severe cardiac disease, thyrotoxicosis, or urinary retention

### Proper use of this medication
» Not taking last daily dose after the evening meal or less than 3 to 4 hours before bedtime
» Not taking dose if patient will be supine for any length of time
» Proper dosing
  Missed dose: Taking as soon as possible; not taking if almost time for next dose; not doubling doses
» Proper storage

### Precautions while using this medication
Not taking other medications, especially nonprescription sympathomimetic agents, unless discussed with physician

### Side/adverse effects
Signs of potential side effects, especially supine hypertension and bradycardia

## General Dosing Information

After initial treatment, midodrine should be continued only in patients who have significant symptomatic improvement.

It is not recommended that midodrine be used in patients with initial supine systolic pressure above 180 mm Hg.

### For treatment of adverse effects

To control supine hypertension, it may be helpful for the patient to avoid becoming fully supine, such as by sleeping with the head of the bed elevated. If supine hypertension persists, midodrine should be discontinued.

## Dosage Forms

### MIDODRINE HYDROCHLORIDE TABLETS

**Usual adult dose**
Hypotension, idiopathic orthostatic (treatment)—
  Oral, 10 mg three times a day in approximately four-hour intervals during the daytime hours, taken shortly before or upon rising in the morning, at midday, and in the late afternoon (not later than six p.m.). Doses may be administered in three-hour intervals, if necessary, to control symptoms. However, midodrine should not be administered more frequently than in three-hour intervals and should not be administered after the evening meal or less than four hours before bedtime.
  Note: Single doses up to 20 mg are associated with severe and persistent systolic supine hypertension, occurring in 45% of patients.
    An initial dose of 2.5 mg is recommended for patients with abnormal renal function.

**Usual adult prescribing limits**
Doses greater than 30 mg have been tolerated, but their safety and efficacy have not been studied or established.

**Usual pediatric dose**
Safety and efficacy have not been established.

**Strength(s) usually available**
U.S.—
  2.5 mg (Rx) [*ProAmatine*].
  5 mg (Rx) [*ProAmatine*].

**Packaging and storage**
Store between 15 and 25 °C (59 and 77 °F), unless otherwise specified by manufacturer.

**Auxiliary labeling**
• Do not take other medicines without your doctor's advice.

Developed: 04/02/97

---

# MILRINONE   Systemic

VA CLASSIFICATION (Primary): CV052
Commonly used brand name(s): *Primacor*.
Note: For a listing of dosage forms and brand names by country availability, see *Dosage Forms* section(s).

## Category
Cardiotonic.

## Indications

**Accepted**
Congestive heart failure (treatment)—Milrinone is indicated for the short-term management of congestive heart failure. Milrinone has been used primarily in patients concurrently receiving digoxin and diuretics.

## Pharmacology/Pharmacokinetics

**Physicochemical characteristics**
Molecular weight—211.22.

**Mechanism of action/Effect**
Milrinone is a phosphodiesterase inhibitor that has direct positive inotropic and vasodilatory actions. Milrinone increases cardiac contractility which results in an increase in cardiac output. Milrinone also relaxes both arterial and venous smooth muscle, thereby reducing both preload and afterload. These effects are mediated by an increase in cytoplasmic cyclic adenosine monophosphate (cAMP) resulting from phosphodiesterase III inhibition in cardiac and smooth muscle.

**Other actions/effects**
Milrinone slightly increases atrioventricular (AV) conduction velocity. Milrinone may also have a favorable effect on ventricular diastolic function.

**Protein binding**
High (70%).

**Half-life**
Elimination—2.3 to 2.7 hours. Elimination half-life is significantly increased in patients with renal function impairment.

**Duration of action**
3 to 6 hours.

**Elimination**
Renal.

## Precautions to Consider

**Cross-sensitivity and/or related problems**
Patients sensitive to amrinone may also be sensitive to milrinone.

**Carcinogenicity**
Twenty-four-month oral administration of milrinone to mice at doses of up to 40 mg per kg of body weight (mg/kg) per day (50 times the human oral therapeutic dose in a 50 kg patient) or to rats at doses of up to 5 mg/kg per day (about 6 times the human oral therapeutic dose) did not reveal carcinogenic potential.

**Mutagenicity**
Positive results were observed in the presence of a metabolic activation system with the Chinese hamster ovary chromosome aberration assay. However, negative results were observed in the Ames test, mouse lymphoma assay, micronucleus test, and the *in vivo* rat bone marrow metaphase analysis.

**Pregnancy/Reproduction**
Fertility—No effect on male or female fertility was observed when milrinone was studied in rats at oral doses of up to 32 mg/kg per day.

Pregnancy—Adequate and well-controlled studies have not been done in humans.
Studies in pregnant rats and rabbits given milrinone during organogenesis revealed no evidence of teratogenicity at oral doses of up to 40 mg/kg per day and 12 mg/kg per day, respectively. Lack of teratogenic effect was also observed in rats and rabbits given milrinone intravenously at doses of up to 3 mg/kg per day and 12 mg/kg per day, respectively. However, an increased resorption rate was observed in rabbits at doses at or above 8 mg/kg per day.
FDA Pregnancy Category C.

**Breast-feeding**
It is not known whether milrinone is distributed into breast milk.

**Pediatrics**
No information is available on the relationship of age to the effects of milrinone in pediatric patients. Safety and efficacy have not been established.

**Geriatrics**
Although appropriate studies on the relationship of age to the effects of milrinone have not been performed in the geriatric population, patients given milrinone in clinical trials included patients up to 80 years of age (mean age 57 to 61). These trials have not demonstrated geriatrics-specific problems that would limit the usefulness of milrinone in the elderly. However, elderly patients are more likely to have age-related renal function impairment, which may require adjustment of dosage in patients receiving milrinone.

**Drug interactions and/or related problems**
The following drug interactions and/or related problems have been selected on the basis of their potential clinical significance (possible mechanism in parentheses where appropriate)—not necessarily inclusive (» = major clinical significance):

Note: Combinations containing any of the following medications, depending on the amount present, may also interact with this medication.

  Hypotension-producing medications (see *Appendix II*)
    (concurrent use with milrinone may produce additive hypotensive effects)

**Medical considerations/Contraindications**
The medical considerations/contraindications included have been selected on the basis of their potential clinical significance (reasons given in parentheses where appropriate)—not necessarily inclusive (» = major clinical significance).

*Except under special circumstances, this medication should not be used when the following medical problem exists:*
» Hypersensitivity to milrinone

*Risk-benefit should be considered when the following medical problems exist:*
» Aortic or pulmonic valve disease, severe, including Hypertrophic subaortic stenosis

(inotropic agents, such as milrinone, should not be used as a substitute for surgery in patients with aortic or pulmonic valve disease; in patients with hypertrophic subaortic stenosis, inotropic agents may aggravate left ventricular outflow tract obstruction)

» Myocardial infarction, acute
(clinical studies have not been done in patients with acute myocardial infarction; use of milrinone in these patients is not recommended)

Renal function impairment
(milrinone elimination is reduced in these patients; a dosage adjustment may be necessary)

**Patient monitoring**
The following may be especially important in patient monitoring (other tests may be warranted in some patients, depending on condition; » = major clinical significance):

» Blood pressure and
» Heart rate
(determinations recommended at periodic intervals; milrinone infusion should be slowed or stopped if an excessive fall in blood pressure occurs)

» Body weight/fluid status and
» Renal function determinations and
» Electrolyte, especially potassium, concentrations, serum
(careful monitoring is recommended; hypokalemia due to excessive diuresis may increase the risk of arrhythmias in patients taking digitalis glycosides)

» Cardiac index and
Central venous pressure and
» Pulmonary capillary wedge pressure (PCWP)
(in most patients, milrinone administration increases cardiac output and reduces PCWP, signs of improved hemodynamics)

Electrocardiogram (ECG), continuous
(recommended throughout infusion period to monitor for potential arrhythmias)

Platelet counts
(recommended prior to initiation of therapy and at periodic intervals during milrinone therapy)

## Side/Adverse Effects

Although milrinone has not been shown to be arrhythmogenic electrophysiologically, supraventricular and ventricular arrhythmias have occurred in patients treated with milrinone. In some patients, milrinone has been shown to increase ventricular ectopic beats, including nonsustained ventricular tachycardia. Milrinone slightly decreases atrioventricular (AV) nodal conduction time, which may cause an increase in the ventricular response rate in patients with atrial flutter or atrial fibrillation if the rate is not controlled with digitalis therapy. In clinical trials, ventricular arrhythmias were reported in 12.1% of patients (2 patients experienced more than one type of arrhythmia): ventricular ectopic activity—8.5%; nonsustained ventricular tachycardia—2.8%; sustained ventricular tachycardia—1%; and ventricular fibrillation—0.2%. Life-threatening arrhythmias, although infrequent, have occurred with milrinone therapy and have been associated with underlying conditions, such as pre-existing arrhythmias, hypokalemia or other metabolic abnormalities, abnormal digoxin levels, and catheter insertion. Supraventricular arrhythmias have been reported in 3.8% of patients receiving milrinone. The incidence of supraventricular and ventricular arrhythmias does not appear to be dose-related.

The following side/adverse effects have been selected on the basis of their potential clinical significance (possible signs and symptoms in parentheses where appropriate)—not necessarily inclusive:

**Those indicating need for medical attention**
Incidence less frequent
*Arrhythmias; hypotension*
Incidence rare
*Angina; thrombocytopenia*
Note: *Thrombocytopenia* has been reported in approximately 0.4% of patients; in some cases, decreases in platelet counts were judged to be only possibly related to milrinone therapy.

**Those indicating need for medical attention only if they continue or are bothersome**
Incidence less frequent
*Headache*

## Overdose

For more information on the management of overdose or unintentional ingestion, **contact a Poison Control Center** (see *Poison Control Center Listing*).

**Clinical effects of overdose**
The following effect has been selected on the basis of its potential clinical significance (possible signs and symptoms in parentheses where appropriate)—not necessarily inclusive:

*Hypotension*

**Treatment of overdose**
Treatment of overdose consists of general measures for circulatory support.

## General Dosing Information

Pretreatment with digitalis is recommended in patients with atrial flutter or atrial fibrillation since milrinone's slight enhancement of atrioventricular (AV) conduction may increase ventricular response rates.

Patients who have received vigorous diuretic therapy may need cautiously liberalized fluid and electrolyte intake to ensure an adequate cardiac filling pressure for response to milrinone.

Caution is recommended to avoid extravasation of milrinone infusion.

It is recommended that a calibrated electronic infusion device be used to administer milrinone.

## Parenteral Dosage Forms

Note: The available dosage form contains milrinone lactate, but dosages and strengths are expressed in terms of the base.

### MILRINONE INJECTION

**Usual adult dose**
Congestive heart failure—
Milrinone should be administered with a loading dose followed by a continuous infusion (maintenance dose) according to the following guidelines:
Loading dose: Intravenous, 50 mcg (0.05 mg) (base) per kg of body weight, administered slowly over ten minutes. The following table provides the loading dose volume (mL) of milrinone injection (1 mg/mL) for a given patient body weight (kg):

Loading dose volume (mL) using 1 mg/mL concentration for a given patient body weight (kg)

| Patient body weight (kg) | 30 | 40 | 50 | 60 | 70 | 80 | 90 | 100 | 110 | 120 |
|---|---|---|---|---|---|---|---|---|---|---|
| Loading dose (mL) | 1.5 | 2 | 2.5 | 3 | 3.5 | 4 | 4.5 | 5 | 5.5 | 6 |

Maintenance dose: Intravenous infusion, continuous

| | Infusion rate (mcg/kg/min) | Total daily (24 hour) dose (mg/kg) |
|---|---|---|
| Minimum | 0.375 | 0.59 |
| Standard | 0.5 | 0.77 |
| Maximum | 0.75 | 1.13 |

The infusion rate should be adjusted according to the patient's hemodynamic and clinical response. Milrinone drawn from vials should be diluted prior to maintenance dose administration.

The maintenance dose in mL per hour by patient body weight (kg) may be determined by referencing one of the following three tables:

Milrinone infusion rate (mL/hr) using 100 mcg/mL concentration

| Maintenance dose (mcg/kg/min) | \multicolumn{10}{c}{Patient body weight (kg)} |
|---|---|---|---|---|---|---|---|---|---|---|
| | 30 | 40 | 50 | 60 | 70 | 80 | 90 | 100 | 110 | 120 |
| 0.375 | 6.8 | 9 | 11.3 | 13.5 | 15.8 | 18 | 20.3 | 22.5 | 24.8 | 27 |
| 0.4 | 7.2 | 9.6 | 12 | 14.4 | 16.8 | 19.2 | 21.6 | 24 | 26.4 | 28.8 |
| 0.5 | 9 | 12 | 15 | 18 | 21 | 24 | 27 | 30 | 33 | 36 |
| 0.6 | 10.8 | 14.4 | 18 | 21.6 | 25.2 | 28.8 | 32.4 | 36 | 39.6 | 43.2 |
| 0.7 | 12.6 | 16.8 | 21 | 25.2 | 29.4 | 33.6 | 37.8 | 42 | 46.2 | 50.4 |
| 0.75 | 13.5 | 18 | 22.5 | 27 | 31.5 | 36 | 40.5 | 45 | 49.5 | 54 |

## Milrinone (Systemic)

Milrinone infusion rate (mL/hr) using 150 mcg/mL concentration

| Maintenance dose (mcg/kg/min) | Patient body weight (kg) |||||||||
|---|---|---|---|---|---|---|---|---|---|
| | 30 | 40 | 50 | 60 | 70 | 80 | 90 | 100 | 110 | 120 |
| 0.375 | 4.5 | 6 | 7.5 | 9 | 10.5 | 12 | 13.5 | 15 | 16.5 | 18 |
| 0.4 | 4.8 | 6.4 | 8 | 9.6 | 11.2 | 12.8 | 14.4 | 16 | 17.6 | 19.2 |
| 0.5 | 6 | 8 | 10 | 12 | 14 | 16 | 18 | 20 | 22 | 24 |
| 0.6 | 7.2 | 9.6 | 12 | 14.4 | 16.8 | 19.2 | 21.6 | 24 | 26.4 | 28.8 |
| 0.7 | 8.4 | 11.2 | 14 | 16.8 | 19.6 | 22.4 | 25.2 | 28 | 30.8 | 33.6 |
| 0.75 | 9 | 12 | 15 | 18 | 21 | 24 | 27 | 30 | 33 | 36 |

Milrinone infusion rate (mL/hr) using 200 mcg/mL concentration

| Maintenance dose (mcg/kg/min) | Patient body weight (kg) |||||||||
|---|---|---|---|---|---|---|---|---|---|
| | 30 | 40 | 50 | 60 | 70 | 80 | 90 | 100 | 110 | 120 |
| 0.375 | 3.4 | 4.5 | 5.6 | 6.8 | 7.9 | 9 | 10.1 | 11.3 | 12.4 | 13.5 |
| 0.4 | 3.6 | 4.8 | 6 | 7.2 | 8.4 | 9.6 | 10.8 | 12 | 13.2 | 14.4 |
| 0.5 | 4.5 | 6 | 7.5 | 9 | 10.5 | 12 | 13.5 | 15 | 16.5 | 18 |
| 0.6 | 5.4 | 7.2 | 9 | 10.8 | 12.6 | 14.4 | 16.2 | 18 | 19.8 | 21.6 |
| 0.7 | 6.3 | 8.4 | 10.5 | 12.6 | 14.7 | 16.8 | 18.9 | 21 | 23.1 | 25.2 |
| 0.75 | 6.8 | 9 | 11.3 | 13.5 | 15.8 | 18 | 20.3 | 22.5 | 24.8 | 27 |

Note: In patients with renal function impairment, infusion rates may need to be reduced to compensate for a prolonged elimination half-life. The following infusion rates are recommended:

| Creatinine clearance (mL/min/1.73m$^2$) | Infusion rate (mcg/kg/min) |
|---|---|
| 5 | 0.20 |
| 10 | 0.23 |
| 20 | 0.28 |
| 30 | 0.33 |
| 40 | 0.38 |
| 50 | 0.43 |

**Usual adult prescribing limits**
1.13 mg (base) per kg of body weight per day. Duration of therapy should depend upon patient responsiveness.

**Usual pediatric dose**
Safety and efficacy have not been established.

**Strength(s) usually available**
U.S.—
  1 mg (base [as the lactate]) per mL (Rx) [*Primacor* (available in 10- and 20-mL single-dose vials and 5-mL cartridges)].
  200 mcg (base [as the lactate]) per mL in 5% dextrose injection (Rx) [*Primacor* (available in 100- and 200-mL flexible containers)].

Canada—
  1 mg (base [as the lactate]) per mL (Rx) [*Primacor* (available in 10- and 20-mL single-dose vials)].

**Packaging and storage**
Vials and cartridges of milrinone should be stored at controlled room temperature, between 15 and 30 °C (59 and 86 °F). Flexible containers should be stored at room temperature, 25 °C (77 °F); however, brief exposure to temperatures up to 40 °C (104 °F) does not adversely affect the product. Protect either product from excessive heat and freezing.

**Preparation of dosage form**
When given as a loading dose, milrinone drawn from vials may be administered undiluted, although diluting to a rounded total volume of 10 or 20 mL may simplify the visualization of the injection rate. When given as a maintenance dose, milrinone drawn from vials should be diluted. Milrinone may be diluted with 0.45% or 0.9% Sodium Chloride Injection USP or 5% Dextrose Injection USP. The table below shows the volume of diluent that must be used to achieve concentrations recommended for infusion:

| Desired infusion concentration (mcg/mL) | Volume (mL) of milrinone 1 mg/mL | Volume (mL) of diluent | To make a total volume (mL) of |
|---|---|---|---|
| 100 | 10 | 90 | 100 |
| 100 | 20 | 180 | 200 |
| 150 | 10 | 56.7 | 66.7 |
| 150 | 20 | 113 | 133 |
| 200 | 10 | 40 | 50 |
| 200 | 20 | 80 | 100 |

Milrinone in 100 mL and 200 mL flexible containers (200 mcg/mL in 5% dextrose injection) need not be diluted prior to use.

**Stability**
Milrinone injection should not be used if particulate matter is present or the solution is discolored.

**Incompatibilities**
Milrinone should not be administered in intravenous lines containing furosemide, since an immediate precipitate is formed. Supplementary medication should not be added to milrinone flexible containers.

### Selected Bibliography
Hilleman DE, Forbes WP. Role of milrinone in the management of congestive heart failure. DICP, Ann Pharmacother 1989; 23: 357-62.
Young RA, Ward A. Milrinone. A preliminary review of its pharmacological properties and therapeutic use. Drugs 1988; 36: 158-92.

Revised: 06/01/98

---

**MINERAL OIL**—See *Laxatives (Local)*

---

**MINOCYCLINE**—See *Tetracyclines (Systemic)*

---

# MINOXIDIL  Systemic

VA CLASSIFICATION (Primary): CV409
Commonly used brand name(s): *Loniten*.
Note: For a listing of dosage forms and brand names by country availability, see *Dosage Forms* section(s).

## Category
Antihypertensive.

## Indications
**Accepted**
Hypertension (treatment)—Minoxidil is indicated for treatment of hypertension.

Because of its serious side effects, minoxidil is not considered to be a primary agent in the treatment of essential hypertension. It is recommended for use only in patients with symptomatic or organ-damaging hypertension not responsive to other treatment.

**Unaccepted**
Use of extemporaneous topical preparations from minoxidil oral tablets is not recommended for treatment of male pattern baldness because there is lack of data on the best formulation and the risks associated with possible systemic absorption. A topical product is commercially available for this indication.

## Pharmacology/Pharmacokinetics
**Physicochemical characteristics**
Molecular weight—209.25.
pKa—Approximately 4.6.

**Mechanism of action/Effect**
The exact cellular mechanism of antihypertensive action is unknown. The predominant effect of minoxidil is direct vasodilation of arterioles with

little effect on veins. It reduces peripheral resistance and causes a reflex increase in heart rate and cardiac output.

**Absorption**
At least 90% absorbed from the gastrointestinal tract.

**Biotransformation**
Hepatic, at least 90%; metabolites have much less pharmacologic activity than minoxidil.

**Half-life**
Drug and metabolites—4.2 hours; not altered in impaired renal function.

**Onset of action**
30 minutes.

**Time to peak concentration**
1 hour.

**Time to peak effect**
Single dose—2 to 3 hours.
Multiple doses—Maximum blood pressure response with continued use usually occurs within 3 to 7 days (patients receiving the largest doses respond in the shortest period of time and vice versa).

**Duration of action**
Usually 24 to 48 hours; up to 75 hours in some patients.

**Elimination**
Fecal—3% (may be increased to up to 20% in severe renal function impairment).
Renal—97%, mostly as metabolites.
In dialysis—Removable by hemodialysis; however, this does not rapidly reverse the pharmacologic effect.

## Precautions to Consider

### Carcinogenicity
Twenty-two-month studies in rats at doses 15 times the human dose revealed no evidence of tumorigenicity.

### Mutagenicity
In Ames test, no evidence of mutagenicity was found.

### Pregnancy/Reproduction
Fertility—A reduction in conception rate occurred in rats receiving minoxidil at doses 5 times the human dose.
Pregnancy—Minoxidil crosses the placenta. Studies in humans have not been done. However, hypertrichosis has been reported in newborns following maternal minoxidil administration.
Studies in rats and rabbits did not reveal teratogenic effects; however, there was an increased incidence of fetal resorptions in rabbits given minoxidil at 5 times the human dose.
FDA Pregnancy Category C.

### Breast-feeding
Minoxidil passes into breast milk. However, problems in humans have not been documented.

### Pediatrics
Appropriate studies on the relationship of age to the effects of minoxidil have not been performed in the pediatric population. However, pediatrics-specific problems that would limit the usefulness of this medication in children are not expected.

### Geriatrics
Although appropriate studies on the relationship of age to the effects of minoxidil have not been performed in the geriatric population, the elderly may be more sensitive to the hypotensive effects. In addition, the risk of minoxidil-induced hypothermia may be increased in elderly patients. Elderly patients are also more likely to have age-related renal function impairment, which may require reduction of dosage in patients receiving minoxidil.

### Drug interactions and/or related problems
The following drug interactions and/or related problems have been selected on the basis of their potential clinical significance (possible mechanism in parentheses where appropriate)—not necessarily inclusive (» = major clinical significance):

Note: Combinations containing any of the following medications, depending on the amount present, may also interact with this medication.

» Antihypertensives, potent parenteral, such as diazoxide or nitroprusside or
» Guanethidine or
» Nitrates
(concurrent use with minoxidil may result in a severe, additive hypotensive effect; patients should be continuously observed for excessive fall in blood pressure for several hours after concurrent administration of potent peripheral antihypertensives or nitrates; concurrent use with guanethidine is not recommended)

Anti-inflammatory drugs, nonsteroidal (NSAIDs), especially indomethacin
(may reduce antihypertensive effects of minoxidil; indomethacin, and possibly other NSAIDs, may antagonize the antihypertensive effect by inhibiting renal prostaglandin synthesis and/or by causing sodium and fluid retention; the patient should be carefully monitored to confirm that the desired effect is being obtained)

Hypotension-producing medications, other (see *Appendix II*)
(hypotensive effects may be potentiated when these medications are used concurrently with minoxidil)
(although some antihypertensive and/or diuretic combinations are used for therapeutic advantage, dosage adjustments may be necessary during concurrent use)

Sympathomimetics
(may reduce antihypertensive effects of minoxidil; the patient should be carefully monitored to confirm that the desired effect is being obtained)

### Laboratory value alterations
The following have been selected on the basis of their potential clinical significance (possible effect in parentheses where appropriate)—not necessarily inclusive (» = major clinical significance):

With physiology/laboratory test values
Alkaline phosphatase concentrations, serum and
Plasma renin activity (PRA) and
Sodium concentrations, serum
(may be increased)

Blood urea nitrogen (BUN) and
Creatinine
(serum concentrations may be increased initially, but decline to pretreatment levels with continued treatment)

Erythrocyte count and
Hematocrit and
Hemoglobin concentrations
(may be decreased as a result of hemodilution; usually recover to pretreatment levels with continued treatment)

### Medical considerations/Contraindications
The medical considerations/contraindications included have been selected on the basis of their potential clinical significance (reasons given in parentheses where appropriate)—not necessarily inclusive (» = major clinical significance).

*Risk-benefit should be considered when the following medical problems exist:*

Cerebrovascular disease or accident or
Myocardial infarction
(a reduction in arterial pressure caused by minoxidil may further limit blood flow to the ischemic area)

» Congestive heart failure not due to hypertension
(may be exacerbated secondary to fluid retention caused by minoxidil)

» Coronary insufficiency, including angina pectoris
(may be exacerbated)

» Pericardial effusion
(minoxidil may aggravate this condition)

» Pheochromocytoma
(use may stimulate release of catecholamines from the tumor)

» Renal function impairment
(reduced elimination; lower doses may be required)

Sensitivity to minoxidil

### Patient monitoring
The following may be especially important in patient monitoring (other tests may be warranted in some patients, depending on condition; » = major clinical significance):

» Blood pressure measurements
(recommended at periodic intervals in patients being treated for hypertension; selected patients may be trained to perform blood pressure measurements at home and report the results at regular physician visits)

» Weight measurements
(daily weight measurements by the patient are recommended to detect excessive sodium and water retention)

## Side/Adverse Effects

Note: Minoxidil has been shown to cause severe myocardial toxicity in dogs. However, this effect has not been observed in other animals or in humans at this time, although nonspecific electrocardiogram (ECG) changes are commonly seen, pericardial effusion (sometimes progressing to cardiac tamponade) occurs in about 3% of patients, and pericarditis has been reported.

The following side/adverse effects have been selected on the basis of their potential clinical significance (possible signs and symptoms in parentheses where appropriate)—not necessarily inclusive:

**Those indicating need for medical attention**
Incidence more frequent
*Reflex sympathetic activation* (fast or irregular heartbeat; flushing or redness of skin); *sodium and water retention* (bloating; swelling of feet or lower legs; rapid weight gain of more than 5 pounds [2 kg] in adults or 2 pounds [1 kg] in children)
Incidence less frequent
*Angina, new or exacerbated, or pericarditis* (chest pain)
Incidence rare
*Allergic reaction or Stevens-Johnson syndrome* (skin rash and itching)
With long-term use
*Paresthesia* (numbness or tingling of hands, feet, or face); *pericardial effusion or pulmonary hypertension* (shortness of breath)

**Those indicating need for medical attention only if they continue or are bothersome**
Incidence more frequent—occurs in most patients
*Hypertrichosis* (excessive hair growth, usually on face, arms, and back)
Note: *Hypertrichosis* usually develops within 3 to 6 weeks after initiation of minoxidil therapy, and return to pretreatment appearance occurs approximately 1 to 6 months after the medication is withdrawn. The increased hair growth may be extensive and may be especially disturbing to women and children; various depilatory methods may help.
Incidence less frequent or rare
*Breast tenderness in males and females; vasodilation* (headache)

## Overdose

For more information on the management of overdose or unintentional ingestion, **contact a Poison Control Center** (see *Poison Control Center Listing*).

**Treatment of overdose**
Administration of intravenous sodium chloride injection is recommended to maintain blood pressure and facilitate urine formation.
Sympathomimetics such as norepinephrine or epinephrine should be avoided because of the risk of excessive cardiac stimulation.
Hypotension may be treated with phenylephrine, vasopressin, or dopamine, but they are recommended only if lack of perfusion of a vital organ occurs.

## Patient Consultation

As an aid to patient consultation, refer to *Advice for the Patient, Minoxidil (Systemic)*.
In providing consultation, consider emphasizing the following selected information (» = major clinical significance):

**Before using this medication**
» Conditions affecting use, especially:
   Sensitivity to minoxidil
   Pregnancy—Decreased conception and increased resorption in animals; hypertrichosis reported in newborns
   Breast-feeding—Passes into breast milk
   Other medications, especially guanethidine or nitrates
   Other medical problems, especially congestive heart failure, coronary insufficiency, pericardial effusion, pheochromocytoma, or renal function impairment

**Proper use of this medication**
Possible need for control of weight and diet, especially sodium intake
» Patient may not experience symptoms of hypertension; importance of taking medication even if feeling well
» Does not cure, but helps control hypertension; possible need for lifelong therapy; serious consequences of untreated hypertension
Compliance with therapy; taking medication at the same time(s) each day to maintain the therapeutic effect
Caution in taking combination therapy; taking each drug at the right time
» Proper dosing
   Missed dose: Taking as soon as remembered if within a few hours; not taking if forgotten until next day; not doubling doses
» Proper storage

**Precautions while using this medication**
Making regular visits to physician to check progress
» Checking resting pulse as directed; checking with physician if an increase of 20 or more beats per minute above normal occurs
» Checking weight daily; weight gain of 2 to 3 lb (approximately 1 kg) in adults is normal and is usually lost with continued treatment; checking with physician if rapid weight gain of more than 5 lb (2 lb in children) or signs of fluid retention occur
» Not taking other medications, especially nonprescription sympathomimetics, unless discussed with physician

**Side/adverse effects**
Probability of hypertrichosis, which is reversible when medication is withdrawn
Signs of potential side effects, especially sodium and water retention, reflex sympathetic activation, angina, pericarditis, allergic reaction, Stevens-Johnson syndrome, paresthesia, and pulmonary hypertension

## General Dosing Information

Sodium and water retention occurs rapidly in almost all patients receiving minoxidil and is difficult to control. Concomitant use of a diuretic (usually a loop diuretic) is recommended to prevent serious fluid accumulation and possible development of tolerance due to expansion of plasma volume.

Reflex tachycardia also occurs very commonly and may be less pronounced if a beta-adrenergic blocking agent or other sympathetic nervous system suppressant is used concurrently. The usual dose of beta-adrenergic blocker recommended is the equivalent of 80 to 160 mg of propranolol a day in divided doses. If beta-adrenergic blocking agents cannot be used, methyldopa in a dose of 250 to 750 mg twice a day may be substituted. Some investigators have used clonidine in a dose of 100 to 200 mcg (0.1 to 0.2 mg) twice a day.

If pericardial effusion occurs and does not respond to therapeutic measures, it is recommended that minoxidil therapy be withdrawn.

Because a few cases of rebound hypertension have been reported following abrupt withdrawal of minoxidil, caution is recommended when discontinuing the medication.

## Oral Dosage Forms

### MINOXIDIL TABLETS USP

**Usual adult and adolescent dose**
Antihypertensive—
   Initial: Oral, 5 mg a day as a single dose or as two divided doses, the dosage being adjusted in 100% increments as required (i.e., up to 10, 20, 40 mg, etc.).
   Maintenance: Oral, 10 to 40 mg a day, as a single dose or in divided daily doses.
Note: It is recommended that an interval of at least three days be allowed between each dosage adjustment, in order for the full effect of each dose to be obtained. In some patients, dosage adjustment may be made every six hours with careful monitoring.
   Geriatric patients may be more sensitive to effects of the usual adult dose.

**Usual adult prescribing limits**
100 mg a day.

**Usual pediatric dose**
Antihypertensive—
   Children up to 12 years of age:
      Initial—Oral, 200 mcg (0.2 mg) per kg of body weight a day as a single dose or as two divided doses, the dosage being adjusted as required (i.e., in increments of 100, 150, 200 mcg per kg of body weight, etc.), up to 50 mg a day.
      Maintenance—Oral, 250 mcg (0.25 mg) to 1 mg per kg of body weight a day, as a single dose or in divided daily doses, up to 50 mg a day.
   Children over 12 years of age:
      See *Usual adult and adolescent dose*.
Note: It is recommended that an interval of at least three days be allowed between each dosage adjustment, in order for the full effect of each dose to be obtained. When more rapid control of blood pressure is required, dosage adjustment may be made every six hours with careful monitoring.

**Strength(s) usually available**
U.S.—
    2.5 mg (Rx) [*Loniten* (scored)] [GENERIC (scored)].
    10 mg (Rx) [*Loniten* (scored)] [GENERIC (scored)].
Canada—
    2.5 mg (Rx) [*Loniten* (scored)].
    10 mg (Rx) [*Loniten* (scored)].

**Packaging and storage**
Store below 40 °C (104 °F), preferably between 15 and 30 °C (59 and 86 °F) unless otherwise specified by manufacturer. Store in a tight container.

**Auxiliary labeling**
- Do not take other medicines without your doctor's advice.

**Note**
Check refill frequency to determine compliance in hypertensive patients.

**Selected Bibliography**
The fifth report of the Joint National Committee on Detection, Evaluation, and Treatment of High Blood Pressure (JNC V). Arch Intern Med 1993; 153(2): 154-83.

Revised: 05/26/93
Interim revision: 08/19/98

---

# MINOXIDIL    Topical

VA CLASSIFICATION (Primary): DE900
Commonly used brand name(s): *Apo-Gain; Gen-Minoxidil; Minoxigaine; Rogaine; Rogaine Extra Strength For Men; Rogaine For Men; Rogaine For Women*.

Note: For a listing of dosage forms and brand names by country availability, see *Dosage Forms* section(s).

## Category
Hair growth stimulant, alopecia androgenetica, topical.

## Indications

**Accepted**

Alopecia androgenetica (treatment)—Minoxidil topical solution is indicated for treatment of alopecia androgenetica (also called male pattern baldness in men) in both adult males and females for the 2% strength and in adult males only for the 5% strength. Alopecia androgenetica is expressed in males as baldness of the vertex of the scalp and/or as frontal hair recession. In females, it is expressed as diffuse hair loss or thinning in the frontoparietal areas. Topical minoxidil is less likely to be effective in men with predominantly frontal hair loss than in patients with the other forms of alopecia androgenetica.

**Acceptance not established**

There are *insufficient data* to show that 2% minoxidil is effective in the treatment of alopecia areata.

## Pharmacology/Pharmacokinetics

**Physicochemical characteristics**
Molecular weight—209.25.
pKa—4.6.

**Mechanism of action/Effect**
Topical minoxidil stimulates hair growth in some persons with alopecia androgenetica. The mechanism by which minoxidil stimulates hair growth is not established, but possible mechanisms include increased cutaneous blood flow as a result of vasodilation, stimulation of resting hair follicles (telogen phase) into active growth (anagen phase), and stimulation of hair follicle cells.

**Other actions/effects**
Most studies have not found changes in blood pressure. In one report of 30 patients using 3% topical minoxidil for 15 months, seven normotensive patients absorbed a sufficient amount of minoxidil to decrease their systolic blood pressure by 60 mm of mercury and their diastolic blood pressure by 24 mm of mercury. The patients were asymptomatic and tachycardia did not occur. Systemically absorbed oral minoxidil may cause peripheral arterial vasodilation, reduced peripheral resistance, a reflex increase in heart rate and cardiac output, and fluid retention.

**Absorption**
Low percutaneous absorption; 1.6 to 3.9% of the total applied topical dose is absorbed systemically; however, absorption may increase if medication is applied to inflamed skin. Applying a 5-microliter-per-squared-centimeter dose to the entire scalp is expected to yield a systemic dose of 1.2 mg for the 1% topical solution of minoxidil and 2.7 mg for the 5% solution of minoxidil. Applying a 1 or 2% topical concentration of minoxidil to up to 50% of the scalp is unlikely to cause systemic side effects, since the average absorbed dose is less than 1.2 mg of minoxidil.

**Onset of action**
At least 4 months with twice-daily applications for the 2% strength, and 2 months for the 5% strength (although in some patients effect still takes 4 months).

**Duration of action**
In one study with continuous treatment using topical minoxidil for alopecia androgenetica, hair regrowth tended to peak at one year, with a slow decline in regrowth over subsequent years. Even so, after 4½ to 5 years of treatment, there were still more nonvellus hairs than there were at the beginning of the treatment.

New hair growth achieved during therapy may be expected to be lost 3 to 4 months after withdrawal of minoxidil, and progressive hair loss will resume.

**Elimination**
Renal—Approximately 95% of systemically absorbed minoxidil is eliminated within 4 days.

## Precautions to Consider

**Carcinogenicity**
A 1-year study of minoxidil applied topically in rats and rabbits showed no evidence of carcinogenicity.

**Mutagenicity**
Minoxidil was not found to be mutagenic in the Salmonella (Ames) test, the DNA damage/alkaline elution assay, or the rat micronucleus test.

**Pregnancy/Reproduction**
Fertility—There was a dose-dependent decreased conception rate in male and female rats given 1 or 5 times the maximum recommended oral antihypertensive human dose.

Pregnancy—Adequate and well-controlled studies in humans have not been done.

With oral administration of minoxidil, no teratogenic effects occurred in rats or rabbits, but there was evidence of increased fetal resorption in rabbits (but not rats) at 5 times the maximum recommended antihypertensive human dose.

Labor and delivery—The effects of minoxidil on labor or delivery are unknown.

**Breast-feeding**
Orally administered minoxidil is distributed into breast milk. It is not known whether topical minoxidil is distributed into breast milk. However, because of the potential for adverse effects, topical minoxidil should not be administered to women who are breast-feeding.

**Pediatrics**
No information is available on the relationship of age to the effects of topical minoxidil in pediatric patients. Safety and efficacy have not been established for pediatric patients up to 18 years of age. Use in infants is not recommended.

**Geriatrics**
No information is available on the relationship of age to the effects of this medication in geriatric patients. Safety and efficacy have not been established in patients older than 65 years of age.

Older patients up to 65 years of age have not demonstrated geriatric-specific problems that would limit the usefulness of topical minoxidil; however, the best results are shown in younger patients with a short history of hair loss.

**Drug interactions and/or related problems**
The following drug interactions and/or related problems have been selected on the basis of their potential clinical significance (possible mechanism in parentheses where appropriate)—not necessarily inclusive (» = major clinical significance):

Note: Combinations containing any of the following medications, depending on the amount present, may also interact with this medication.

- » Corticosteroids, topical or
- » Petrolatum, topical or
- » Retinoids, topical
    (concurrent use on the same area may enhance cutaneous absorption of topical minoxidil because of increased stratum corneum permeability and is not recommended; in one patient, concurrent use of a topical retinoid on the same area as topical minoxidil caused a lesion consisting of granulation tissue similar to pyogenic granuloma)

    Guanethidine
    (concurrent use may increase the chance of orthostatic hypotension)

**Medical considerations/Contraindications**
The medical considerations/contraindications included have been selected on the basis of their potential clinical significance (reasons given in parentheses where appropriate)—not necessarily inclusive (» = major clinical significance).

*Risk-benefit should be considered when the following medical problems exist:*

Allergy to minoxidil or propylene glycol

Cardiovascular disease or
Hypertension
(patients with these conditions were excluded from the clinical trials of topical minoxidil because of the potential that adverse systemic effects could occur for the rare patient who might receive significant systemic absorption from its use; although their deaths were not attributable to topical minoxidil treatment, unexplained sudden death occurred in two patients with underlying undetected, untreated cardiovascular conditions who used topical minoxidil)

Skin irritation or abrasion, including scalp psoriasis or severe sunburn
(systemic absorption may be increased)

**Patient monitoring**
The following may be especially important in patient monitoring (other tests may be warranted in some patients, depending on condition; » = major clinical significance):

Blood pressure and
Heart rate and
Weight
(if a patient's history indicates a potential problem, determinations are recommended prior to initiation of therapy and at periodic intervals during therapy to check for possible systemic effects; if systemic effects occur, it is recommended that minoxidil be discontinued; minimal effects on blood pressure are expected in normotensive patients)

## Side/Adverse Effects

Note: Although their deaths were not attributed to topical minoxidil therapy, sudden death has been reported in two patients treated with topical minoxidil who had underlying cardiovascular conditions—one patient had undetected Wolff-Parkinson-White syndrome and the other patient had untreated hypertension and cardiosclerotic cardiovascular disease.

The following side/adverse effects have been selected on the basis of their potential clinical significance (possible signs and symptoms in parentheses where appropriate)—not necessarily inclusive:

**Those indicating need for medical attention**
Incidence less frequent
*Contact dermatitis* (itching or skin rash)
Incidence rare
*Allergic reaction* (reddened skin; skin rash; swelling of face); *alopecia, increased* (increased hair loss); *burning of scalp*; *folliculitis* (acne; inflammation or soreness at root of hair)—at site of application
Signs and symptoms of systemic absorption—Rare
*Chest pain; fast or irregular heartbeat; headache; hypotension*—usually not symptomatic; *lightheadedness*; *neuritis* (numbness or tingling of hands, feet, or face); *reflex hypertension; sexual dysfunction* (decrease of sexual ability or desire); *sodium and water retention* (swelling of face, hands, feet, or lower legs; rapid weight gain); *vasodilation* (flushing; headache); *visual disturbances, including decreased visual acuity* (blurred vision or other changes in vision)

Note: Signs and symptoms of toxicity resulting from systemic absorption are unlikely unless a patient applies minoxidil too frequently to a large surface area (such as that occurring in a woman who had alopecia totalis) or unless the product is ingested orally (as was the case of one man attempting suicide by consuming topical minoxidil).

## Overdose

For specific information on the agents used in the management of oral ingestion of topical minoxidil overdose, see:
- *Phenylephrine* or *Dopamine* in *Sympathomimetic Agents—Cardiovascular Use (Parenteral-Systemic)* monograph; and/or
- *Vasopressin (Systemic)* monograph.

For more information on the management of overdose or unintentional ingestion, **contact a Poison Control Center** (see *Poison Control Center Listing*).

**Clinical effects of overdose**
The following effects have been selected on the basis of their potential clinical significance (possible signs and symptoms in parentheses where appropriate)—not necessarily inclusive:

*Chest pain; fast or irregular heartbeat; hypotension*—usually not symptomatic; *neuritis* (numbness or tingling of hands, feet, or face); *reflex hypertension; sodium and water retention* (swelling of face, hands, feet, or lower legs; rapid weight gain); *vasodilation* (flushing; headache)

**Treatment of overdose**
If systemic toxicity occurs as a result of overdose by oral ingestion of topical minoxidil, treatment may include the following:

To enhance elimination—Hemodialysis. Minoxidil and its metabolites are hemodialyzable.

Specific treatment—Hypotension may be treated with phenylephrine, angiotensin II, vasopressin, or dopamine, but these medications are recommended only if lack of perfusion of a vital organ occurs. Sympathomimetic medications, such as norepinephrine or epinephrine, should be avoided because of the risk of excessive cardiac stimulation.

Supportive care—Administration of intravenous sodium chloride injection is recommended to maintain blood pressure and facilitate urine formation. Patients in whom intentional overdose is known or suspected should be referred for psychiatric consultation.

## Patient Consultation

As an aid to patient consultation, refer to *Advice for the Patient, Minoxidil (Topical)*.

In providing consultation, consider emphasizing the following selected information (» = major clinical significance):

**Before using this medication**
» Conditions affecting use, especially:
    Allergy to minoxidil or propylene glycol (an inactive component of the preparation)
    Pregnancy—Animal studies using oral minoxidil have shown problems during pregnancy, but not birth defects
    Breast-feeding—Not recommended, since medication may cause problems in nursing babies
    Other medications, especially topical corticosteroids, petrolatum, or retinoids

**Proper use of this medication**
Reading patient instructions carefully
» Not using more medication or more frequently than prescribed; not applying to other parts of body; risk of adverse systemic effects with excessive use
» Not using other skin products on treated skin; hair colorings, hair permanents, and hair relaxers may be used during the course of minoxidil therapy, but minoxidil should be washed from scalp before their use; avoid using minoxidil 24 hours before and after hair products are applied, and do not double doses to make up for these missed minoxidil doses

Proper administration technique
    Applying to affected area of dry scalp, beginning at the center of the balding area; not shampooing hair for 4 hours after minoxidil application
    Method of application depends on applicator used (spray, extended spray tip, dropper, and/or rub-on assembly)
    Washing hands immediately after application to remove any medication that may be on them
    Allowing full drying for 2 to 4 hours; minoxidil can stain clothing, hats, or bed linens if not allowed to fully dry; however, not using hairdryer to speed drying, since this could decrease efficacy of the medication by removing product from the hair or scalp
    Avoiding transfer of medication to other parts of body or onto bed linens by allowing complete drying of medication before retiring
    Checking with physician before applying to abraded, irritated, or sunburned scalp

» Avoiding contact with eyes, nose, or mouth; flushing area with large amounts of cool tap water if accidental contact occurs; avoiding inhalation of pump spray
» Proper dosing
  Missed dose: Using as soon as remembered if within a few hours; not using if almost time for next dose; not doubling amount used
» Proper storage

**Precautions while using this medication**
Regular visits to physician to check progress
Telling physician if itching, burning, or redness occurs after application; if reaction is severe, washing minoxidil off and checking with physician before using again
Hair loss may continue for 2 weeks after initiating minoxidil therapy, but if it continues, patient should discuss continuation of medication with physician. If hair growth does not increase in 4 months, patient should discuss continuation of medication with physician

**Side/adverse effects**
Signs of potential side effects, especially contact dermatitis, allergic reaction, burning of scalp, folliculitis, increased alopecia, and systemic absorption (chest pain, fast or irregular heartbeat, hypotension, lightheadedness, neuritis, reflex hypertension, sexual dysfunction, sodium and water retention, vasodilation, and visual disturbances, including decreased visual acuity)

## General Dosing Information

If systemic effects occur, topical minoxidil should be discontinued and the patient should be seen by a physician.

Females are advised not to use the 5% solution because it does not work any better in females than the 2% solution and has caused excessive or unusual facial hair growth in females. Minoxidil will not work in males or females who experience hair loss caused by endocrine or nutritional problems or caused by skin damage that can occur from scarring, burns, or severe hair grooming methods, such as hair loss from ponytails or cornrowing. Minoxidil will not work for sudden or patchy hair loss.

If dermatologic reactions occur, it is recommended that discontinuation of topical minoxidil therapy be considered. Patients should not apply minoxidil if skin is red, infected, irritated, or painful.

Hair loss may continue for 2 weeks after initiation of minoxidil therapy, but if it continues past 2 weeks, patient should notify physician. If hair growth has not improved in 4 months of therapy, patient should reconsider continuing the use of topical minoxidil.

Patient should be instructed about proper administration of topical minoxidil, including the avoidance of inhaling the spray mist. In the event of accidental contact with sensitive areas (eye, abraded skin, mucous membranes), the sensitive area that is burning or irritated should be washed with copious amounts of cool water. Application should be restricted to the thinning or balding area of the scalp, and hands should be washed afterwards to avoid inadvertent translocation of minoxidil to inappropriate areas of the body. Waiting 2 to 4 hours for the minoxidil to dry before retiring is also recommended to avoid translocation of medication and to avoid rubbing it off inadvertently onto bed linens. Minoxidil may stain bed linens, hats, or clothing if it has not fully dried.

Topical minoxidil should be applied to the dry skin of the scalp. A hairdryer should not be used after application, as it might interfere with the efficacy of minoxidil. At least 4 hours should be allowed after minoxidil application before shampooing.

Hair colorings, hair permanents, and hair relaxers may be used with topical minoxidil; however, to avoid skin irritation, patient should wash minoxidil from scalp first before having hair treatments, avoid using minoxidil 24 hours before and 24 hours after having chemical treatments, and avoid making up missed doses by using more minoxidil when treatment is reinitiated.

## Topical Dosage Forms

### MINOXIDIL TOPICAL SOLUTION

**Usual adult dose**
Hair growth stimulant—
  Adults up to 65 years of age: Topical, to the scalp, 1 mL two times a day.
  Adults 65 years of age and older: Use and dose have not been established.
Note: The same dose is used regardless of the size of the area being treated.

**Usual pediatric dose**
Hair growth stimulant—
  Infants: Use is not recommended.
  Children up to 18 years of age: Use and dose have not been established.

**Strength(s) usually available**
U.S.—
  2% (20 mg per mL) (OTC) [*Rogaine For Men* (alcohol 60% v/v; propylene glycol; water); *Rogaine For Women* (alcohol 60% v/v; propylene glycol; water) [GENERIC].
  5% (50 mg per mL) (OTC) [*Rogaine Extra Strength For Men* (alcohol 30% v/v; propylene glycol 50% v/v; water)].
Canada—
  2% (20 mg per mL) (Rx) [*Apo-Gain* (alcohol 63%; propylene glycol; water); *Gen-Minoxidil* (alcohol; propylene glycol; water); *Minoxigaine* (alcohol 63%; propylene glycol; water); *Rogaine* (alcohol 63%)].
Note: Packaging may include spray, extended spray, dropper, and/or rub-on tips for application.

**Packaging and storage**
Store between 15 and 30 °C (59 and 86 °F), unless otherwise specified by manufacturer. Store in a tight container. Protect from light. Protect from freezing.

**Auxiliary labeling**
• For external use only.

## Selected Bibliography

Rumsfield JA, West DP, Fiedler-Weiss VC, et al. Topical minoxidil therapy for hair regrowth. Clin Pharm 1987 May; 6(5): 386-92.
Clissold SP, Heel RC. Topical minoxidil. A preliminary review of its pharmacodynamic properties and therapeutic efficacy in alopecia areata and alopecia androgenetica [review]. Drugs 1987 Feb; 33(2): 107-22.

Revised: 07/20/98

---

# MIRTAZAPINE    Systemic—INTRODUCTORY VERSION

VA CLASSIFICATION (Primary): CN609
Commonly used brand name(s): *Remeron*.
Note: For a listing of dosage forms and brand names by country availability, see *Dosage Forms* section(s).

## Category

Antidepressant.

## Indications

**Accepted**
Depressive disorder, major (treatment)—Mirtazapine is indicated for the treatment of depression. The effectiveness of using mirtazapine for longer than 6 weeks has not been evaluated in controlled trials.

## Pharmacology/Pharmacokinetics

**Physicochemical characteristics**
Chemical group—Piperazinoazepine. Mirtazapine has a tetracyclic structure. It is structurally unrelated to selective serotonin reuptake inhibitors, tricyclic antidepressants, or monoamine oxidase inhibitors.
Molecular weight—265.36.
Solubility—Slightly soluble in water.

**Mechanism of action/Effect**
The exact mechanism of action is unknown. Evidence indicates that mirtazapine may enhance central noradrenergic and serotonergic activity, possibly through its antagonist activity at central presynaptic alpha$_2$-adrenergic inhibitory autoreceptors and heteroreceptors. Mirtazapine shows no significant affinity for serotonin 5-HT$_{1A}$ or 5-HT$_{1B}$ receptors.

**Other actions/effects**
Mirtazapine is a potent antagonist at serotonin 5-HT$_2$ and 5-HT$_3$ receptors, and a moderate antagonist at muscarinic receptors. Mirtazapine produces sedative effects due to potent histamine H$_1$ receptor antagonism,

and orthostatic hypotension due to moderate peripheral alpha$_1$-adrenergic receptor antagonism.

**Absorption**
Rapid and complete; however, due to first-pass metabolism, absolute bioavailability is about 50%. The rate and extent of mirtazapine absorption are minimally affected by food.

**Protein binding**
High (85%).

**Biotransformation**
Mirtazapine is extensively metabolized after oral administration by demethylation and hydroxylation followed by glucuronide conjugation. *In vitro* testing indicates that cytochrome P450 2D6 (CYP2D6) and cytochrome P450 1A2 (CYP1A2) are involved in formation of the 8-hydroxy metabolite of mirtazapine, and cytochrome P450 3A (CYP3A) is responsible for the formation of the *N*-desmethyl and *N*-oxide metabolites. Several metabolites possess pharmacological activity, but plasma levels are very low.

**Half-life**
Elimination—
About 20 to 40 hours across age and gender subgroups. In females of all ages, the elimination half-life is significantly longer than in males (mean 37 hours versus 26 hours).
The half-life of the (−)-enantiomer is about twice that of the (+)-enantiomer.

**Time to peak concentration**
About 2 hours.

**Steady-state plasma concentration**
Attained within 5 days. Dose and plasma levels are linearly related over a dose range of 15 to 80 mg. Because of the difference in elimination half-life, the plasma level of the (−)-enantiomer is about three times as high as the plasma level of the (+)-enantiomer.

**Elimination**
Renal—
75%.
Fecal—
15%.

## Precautions to Consider

**Carcinogenicity/Tumorigenicity**
Carcinogenicity studies in mice given doses of 2, 20, and 200 mg per kg of body weight per day (mg/kg/day), which is up to 20 times the maximum recommended human dose (MRHD) of 45 mg per day (mg/day) on a mg per square meter of body surface area (mg/m$^2$) basis, found an increase in hepatocellular adenomas and carcinomas in male mice in the high dose group. Carcinogenicity studies in rats given doses of 2, 20, and 60 mg/kg/day, which is up to 12 times the MRHD on a mg/m$^2$ basis, found an increase in hepatocellular adenomas in females at the middle and high doses, and an increase in hepatocellular tumors and thyroid follicular adenomas/cystadenomas and carcinomas in males at the high dose. These effects may have been mediated by nongenotoxic mechanisms, the relevance of which to humans is unknown.

**Mutagenicity**
Mirtazapine had no mutagenic or clastogenic effects, and did not induce general DNA damage based on the Ames test, the *in vitro* gene mutation assay in Chinese hamster V 79 cells, the *in vitro* sister chromatid exchange assay in cultured rabbit lymphocytes, the *in vivo* bone marrow micronucleus test in rats, and the unscheduled DNA synthesis assay in HeLa cells.

**Pregnancy/Reproduction**
Fertility—When given mirtazapine doses that were three or more times the MRHD of 45 mg/day on a mg/m$^2$ basis, rats showed disrupted estrous cycling. Also, in rats given mirtazapine doses that were 20 times the MRHD on a mg/m$^2$ basis, preimplantation fetal losses occurred. Mating and conception in rats were not affected by mirtazapine.
Pregnancy—Adequate and well-controlled studies in humans have not been done.
Studies in pregnant rats and rabbits given mirtazapine doses of up to 20 and 17 times the MRHD on a mg/m$^2$ basis, respectively, showed no teratogenic effects. However, in rats receiving 20 times the MRHD on a mg/m$^2$ basis, there were an increase in postimplantation fetal losses, a decrease in pup birth weights, and an increase in pup deaths during the first 3 days of lactation. The cause of these deaths is unknown.
FDA Pregnancy Category C.
Labor and delivery—The effect of mirtazapine on labor and delivery is unknown.

**Breast-feeding**
It is not known whether mirtazapine is distributed into breast milk.

**Pediatrics**
No information is available on the relationship of age to the effects of mirtazapine in pediatric patients. Safety and efficacy have not been established.

**Geriatrics**
No geriatrics-specific problems that would limit the usefulness of mirtazapine in the elderly were seen in studies that included elderly subjects. However, mirtazapine clearance was reduced by 40% in elderly males, and by 10% in elderly females as compared with younger males and younger females, respectively. Also, elderly patients are more likely to have age-related renal function impairment, which may decrease mirtazapine clearance.

**Pharmacogenetics**
Mirtazapine exhibits a longer half-life in females than in males across all age groups. The mean elimination half-life was found to be 37 hours in females, and 26 hours in males. Also, in elderly females, mirtazapine clearance was reduced by 10%, while in elderly males clearance was reduced by 40%. However, responsiveness to mirtazapine therapy showed no age or gender differences, and initial dosing recommendations are the same for all adult patients.

**Dental**
Prolonged use of mirtazapine may decrease or inhibit salivary flow, thus contributing to the development of caries, periodontal disease, oral candidiasis, and discomfort.

**Drug interactions and/or related problems**
The following drug interactions and/or related problems have been selected on the basis of their potential clinical significance (possible mechanism in parentheses where appropriate)—not necessarily inclusive (» = major clinical significance):

Note: Combinations containing any of the following medications, depending on the amount present, may also interact with this medication.

» Alcohol or
» CNS depression–producing medications, other (see *Appendix II*)
(CNS depressant effects of these medications and mirtazapine are additive; concurrent use is not recommended)

Antihypertensive medications
(hypotensive effect of these medications or mirtazapine may be enhanced)

Enzyme inducers, hepatic, cytochrome P450 (see *Appendix II*) or
Enzyme inhibitors, hepatic, various (see *Appendix II*)
(*in vitro* studies have shown mirtazapine to be a substrate for cytochrome P450 isoenzymes CYP2D6, CYP1A2, and CYP3A4; metabolism and pharmacokinetics of mirtazapine may be affected by induction or inhibition of these isoenzymes)

» Monoamine oxidase (MAO) inhibitors, including furazolidone, procarbazine, and selegiline
(serious, sometimes fatal reactions have occurred in patients taking MAO inhibitors in combination with, or soon after discontinuing, other antidepressant medications; symptoms have included autonomic instability with rapid fluctuation of vital signs, diaphoresis, dizziness, flushing, hyperthermia, mental status changes ranging from agitation to coma, myoclonus, nausea, rigidity, seizures, tremor, and vomiting; although there is no experience with the combination in humans, use of mirtazapine concurrently with an MAO inhibitor, or within 14 days of discontinuing therapy with an MAO inhibitor is **contraindicated**; also, MAO inhibitor therapy should not be initiated within 14 days of the discontinuation of mirtazapine)

**Laboratory value alterations**
The following have been selected on the basis of their potential clinical significance (possible effect in parentheses where appropriate)—not necessarily inclusive (» = major clinical significance):

With physiology/laboratory test values
Alanine aminotransferase (ALT [SGPT])
(during premarketing studies, increases in ALT [SGPT] to ≥ three times the upper limit of normal were seen in 2% of patients receiving mirtazapine as compared with 0.3% of patients receiving placebo; while these increases were clinically significant, and led to discontinuation of mirtazapine in some patients, most of these patients did not develop signs or symptoms of decreased hepatic function; in some patients, ALT [SGPT] levels returned to normal with continued use of mirtazapine)

Cholesterol, total
(during premarketing studies, increases in nonfasting cholesterol to ≥ 20% above the upper limits of normal were seen in 15% of

patients receiving mirtazapine as compared with 7% of patients receiving placebo)

Triglycerides, serum
(during premarketing studies, increases in nonfasting triglyceride to ≥ 500 mg per deciliter were seen in 6% of patients receiving mirtazapine as compared with 3% of patients receiving placebo)

**Medical considerations/Contraindications**
The medical considerations/contraindications included have been selected on the basis of their potential clinical significance (reasons given in parentheses where appropriate)—not necessarily inclusive (» = major clinical significance).

*Except under special circumstances, this medication should not be used when the following medical problem exists:*
» Hypersensitivity to mirtazapine

*Risk-benefit should be considered when the following medical problems exist:*

Cardiovascular or cerebrovascular disease that could be exacerbated by hypotension, such as history of myocardial infarction, angina, or ischemic stroke or

Conditions that would predispose patients to hypotension, such as dehydration or hypovolemia
(mirtazapine showed a significant orthostatic hypotensive effect in early trials with normal volunteers; however, during premarketing studies, this effect was seen less frequently in depressed patients)

Drug abuse or dependence, or history of
(patients with a history of drug abuse should be observed closely for signs of misuse or abuse of mirtazapine, as with any new central nervous system [CNS] drug)

» Hepatic function impairment
(significant alanine aminotransferase [ALT (SPGT)] elevations [≥ three times the upper limit of normal] occurred in some patients with normal liver function while they were receiving mirtazapine in premarketing studies; most of these patients did not develop signs or symptoms of decreased hepatic function, but the increases in ALT [SGPT] levels led to discontinuation of mirtazapine in some patients; in other patients, ALT [SGPT] levels returned to normal with continued use of mirtazapine; mirtazapine should be used with caution in patients with impaired hepatic function)
(clearance of a single 15-mg oral dose of mirtazapine was reduced by 30% in patients with hepatic function impairment as compared with clearance in patients with normal hepatic function)

Mania or hypomania, or history of
(mania or hypomania has occurred rarely in patients treated with mirtazapine)

Renal function impairment
(the clearance of a single 15-mg oral dose of mirtazapine was reduced by about 30% in patients with moderate renal function impairment [glomerular filtration rate (GFR) = 11 to 39 mL per minute per 1.73 square meters of body surface area (mL/min/1.73m$^2$)], and by about 50% in patients with severe renal function impairment [GFR < 10 mL/min/1.73m$^2$])

Seizures, history of
(one patient experienced a seizure during premarketing clinical trials of mirtazapine; there are no controlled studies of mirtazapine use in patients who have a history of seizures)

**Patient monitoring**
The following may be especially important in patient monitoring (other tests may be warranted in some patients, depending on condition; » = major clinical significance):

Careful supervision of depressed patients with suicidal tendencies
(recommended especially during early treatment phase before peak effectiveness of mirtazapine is achieved; prescribing the smallest number of tablets necessary for good patient management is recommended to decrease the risk of overdose)

## Side/Adverse Effects

The following side/adverse effects have been selected on the basis of their potential clinical significance (possible signs and symptoms in parentheses where appropriate)—not necessarily inclusive:

**Those indicating need for medical attention**
Incidence less frequent
*Dyspnea* (shortness of breath); *edema* (swelling); *flu-like symptoms; hyperkinesia* (increased movement); *hypokinesia* (decreased movement); *mood or mental changes, including abnormal thinking; agitation; anxiety; apathy; and confusion; skin rash*

Incidence rare
*Agranulocytosis or neutropenia* (chills; fever; sore throat; sores in mouth)—may be asymptomatic; *facial edema* (swelling of face); *impotence* (decreased sexual ability); *menstrual changes* (painful menstruation; absence of menstruation); *mood or mental changes, including delusions; depersonalization; emotional lability; hallucinations; hostility; and mania; seizures*

Note: Use of mirtazapine was associated with *agranulocytosis* in two, and severe *neutropenia* in one of 2796 patients treated in premarketing clinical studies. Recovery occurred in all three patients after mirtazapine was discontinued. Mirtazapine treatment should be discontinued in any patient who develops fever, sore throat, stomatitis, or other signs of infection and who has a low white blood cell (WBC) count. The patient should then be closely monitored.

**Those indicating need for medical attention only if they continue or are bothersome**
Incidence more frequent
*Constipation; dizziness; drowsiness; dryness of mouth; increased appetite; weight gain*

Note: *Weight gain* led to discontinuation of mirtazapine treatment in 8% of patients enrolled in U.S. premarketing studies.

Incidence less frequent
*Abdominal pain; abnormal dreams; asthenia* (weakness); *back pain; hyperesthesia* (increased sensitivity to touch); *hypotension* (low blood pressure); *increased thirst; myalgia* (pain in muscles); *nausea; orthostatic hypotension* (dizziness or fainting when getting up suddenly from a sitting or lying position); *tremor* (trembling or shaking); *urinary frequency* (increased need to urinate); *vertigo* (sense of constant movement of self or surroundings); *vomiting*

## Overdose

For specific information on the agents used in the management of mirtazapine overdose, see the *Charcoal, Activated (Oral-Local)* monograph.

For more information on the management of overdose or unintentional ingestion, **contact a Poison Control Center** (see *Poison Control Center Listing*).

**Clinical effects of overdose**
The following effects have been selected on the basis of their potential clinical significance (possible signs and symptoms in parentheses where appropriate)—not necessarily inclusive:

Acute
*Disorientation; drowsiness; impaired memory; tachycardia* (fast heartbeat)

Note: Experience with mirtazapine overdose is very limited.

**Treatment of overdose**
Note: The possibility of multiple drug involvement should be considered in managing overdose.

There is no specific antidote for mirtazapine. General measures used in the treatment of overdose with any antidepressant should be employed.

To decrease absorption—Induction of emesis and/or gastric lavage and the use of activated charcoal should be considered.

Monitoring—Monitoring of cardiac and vital signs is recommended.

Supportive care—Establish and maintain an airway if the patient is unconscious. Employ general symptomatic and supportive measures. Patients in whom intentional overdose is confirmed or suspected should be referred for psychiatric consultation.

## Patient Consultation

In providing consultation, consider emphasizing the following selected information (» = major clinical significance):

**Before using this medication**
» Conditions affecting use, especially:
Use in the elderly—Elderly patients, especially males, may have reduced clearance
Dental—Possible dryness of mouth; using sugarless candy or gum, ice, or saliva substitute for relief; checking with physician or dentist if dry mouth continues for more than 2 weeks
Contraindicated medications—Monoamine oxidase (MAO) inhibitors
Other medications, especially alcohol or CNS depression–producing medications
Other medical problems, especially hypersensitivity to mirtazapine or hepatic function impairment

### Proper use of this medication
Taking with or without food, as directed by physician
» Proper dosing
» Proper storage

### Precautions while using this medication
» Not using concurrently or within 14 days of discontinuing therapy with an MAO inhibitor; not beginning MAO inhibitor therapy within 14 days of discontinuing therapy with mirtazapine
» Avoiding use of alcohol or other CNS depression–producing medications
Regular visits to physician to check progress during therapy
» Checking with physician immediately if any symptoms of infection, especially fever, chills, sore throat, or mucus membrane ulcerations, occur
» Possible drowsiness, impairment of judgement, thinking, or motor skills; caution when driving, using machinery, or doing other jobs requiring alertness
Possible orthostatic hypotension; getting up slowly from a lying or sitting position

### Side/adverse effects
Signs of potential side effects, especially dyspnea, edema, flu-like symptoms, hyperkinesia, hypokinesia, mood or mental changes, skin rash, agranulocytosis or neutropenia, facial edema, impotence, menstrual changes, and seizures

## General Dosing Information
Any symptoms of infection, especially flu-like symptoms, such as fever, chills, or sore throat, or mucous membrane ulcerations, occurring during mirtazapine treatment should be reported to the physician immediately. The patient should be evaluated for possible agranulocytosis.

Long-term efficacy of mirtazapine has not been evaluated in controlled trials, and its usefulness as long-term therapy for an individual patient should be evaluated periodically.

### Diet/Nutrition
Food has a minimal effect on mirtazapine absorption.

## Oral Dosage Forms
### MIRTAZAPINE TABLETS
#### Usual adult dose
Antidepressant—
Oral, initially 15 mg once a day, preferably in the evening prior to sleep. The dose may be increased, as needed and tolerated, at intervals of not less than one to two weeks.

#### Usual adult prescribing limits
Up to 45 mg a day.

#### Usual pediatric dose
Safety and efficacy have not been established.

#### Usual geriatric dose
See *Usual adult dose*.

Note: Plasma mirtazapine levels may be higher in elderly patients and in patients with moderate to severe renal or hepatic function impairment than in younger adults without renal or hepatic function impairment because of decreased clearance.

#### Strength(s) usually available
U.S.—
15 mg (Rx) [*Remeron* (scored; corn starch; hydroxypropyl cellulose; magnesium stearate; colloidal silicon dioxide; lactose)].
30 mg (Rx) [*Remeron* (scored; corn starch; hydroxypropyl cellulose; magnesium stearate; colloidal silicon dioxide; lactose)].

#### Packaging and storage
Store between 20 and 25 °C (68 and 77 °F), unless otherwise specified by manufacturer.

#### Auxiliary labeling
• Avoid alcoholic beverages.
• May cause dizziness or drowsiness.

Developed: 02/26/97
Interim revision: 08/07/98

# MISOPROSTOL  Systemic

VA CLASSIFICATION (Primary): HS200
Commonly used brand name(s): *Cytotec*.
Note: For a listing of dosage forms and brand names by country availability, see *Dosage Forms* section(s).

## Category
Gastric mucosa protectant; antiulcer agent.

## Indications
Note: Bracketed information in the *Indications* section refers to uses that are not included in U.S. product labeling.

### Accepted
Ulcer, gastric, nonsteroidal anti-inflammatory drug–induced (prophylaxis)—Misoprostol is indicated for the prevention of gastric ulcer associated with the use of nonsteroidal anti-inflammatory drugs (NSAIDs), including aspirin, in patients at high risk of complications from gastric ulcer, such as the elderly, and in patients with concomitant disease or patients at high risk of developing gastric ulceration, such as those with a history of ulcer.

[Ulcer, duodenal (treatment)]—Misoprostol is indicated in the short-term treatment of duodenal ulcer.

## Pharmacology/Pharmacokinetics

### Physicochemical characteristics
Molecular weight—382.54.

### Mechanism of action/Effect
Cytoprotective—Misoprostol enhances natural gastromucosal defense mechanisms and healing in acid-related disorders, probably by increasing production of gastric mucus and mucosal secretion of bicarbonate.
Antisecretory—Misoprostol inhibits basal and nocturnal gastric acid secretion by direct action on the parietal cells; also inhibits gastric acid secretion stimulated by food, histamine, and pentagastrin. It decreases pepsin secretion under basal, but not histamine stimulation. Misoprostol has no significant effect on fasting or postprandial gastrin or intrinsic factor output.

### Absorption
Rapidly absorbed following oral administration.

### Protein binding
High (approximately 85%).

### Biotransformation
Rapidly de-esterified to misoprostol acid (primary biologically active metabolite). The de-esterified metabolite undergoes further metabolism by beta and omega oxidation, which can take place in various tissues in the body.

### Half-life
Terminal—20–40 minutes.

### Time to peak concentration
12 ± 3 minutes.

### Peak serum concentration
<1 mcg (0.001 mg) per liter.

### Duration of action
3–6 hours.

### Elimination
Renal (64 to 73% of the oral dose excreted within the first 24 hours).
Fecal (15% of the oral dose).

## Precautions to Consider

### Cross-sensitivity and/or related problems
Patients sensitive to other prostaglandins or prostaglandin analogs may be sensitive to misoprostol also.

### Carcinogenicity/Mutagenicity
Animal studies have not shown misoprostol to be carcinogenic or mutagenic.

### Pregnancy/Reproduction
Pregnancy—**Misoprostol is contraindicated during pregnancy**. Studies in humans have shown that misoprostol causes an increase in the frequency and intensity of uterine contractions. Misoprostol administration has also been associated with a higher incidence of uterine bleeding and expulsion of uterine contents. Miscarriages caused by misoprostol are likely to be incomplete, resulting in very serious medical compli-

cations, sometimes requiring hospitalization and surgery, and possibly causing infertility.

FDA Pregnancy Category X.

Patients of childbearing potential may use misoprostol if nonsteroidal anti-inflammatory drug (NSAID) therapy is required and patient is at high risk of complications from gastric ulcers associated with the use of NSAIDs, or is at high risk of developing gastric ulceration. Such patients must comply with effective contraceptive measures, must have had a negative serum pregnancy test within 2 weeks prior to initiation of therapy, and must start misoprostol therapy only on the second or third day of the next normal menstrual period.

### Breast-feeding
It is unlikely that misoprostol is distributed into breast milk since it is rapidly metabolized throughout the body. However, it is not known if the active metabolite, misoprostol acid, is distributed into breast milk. Therefore, administration of misoprostol to nursing women is not recommended because of the potential distribution of misoprostol acid, which could cause significant diarrhea in the nursing infant.

### Pediatrics
Appropriate studies on the relationship of age to the effects of misoprostol have not been performed in patients up to 18 years of age.

### Geriatrics
Studies performed in approximately 500 ulcer patients 65 years of age or older have not demonstrated geriatrics-specific problems that would limit the usefulness of misoprostol in the elderly.

### Drug interactions and/or related problems
The following drug interactions and/or related problems have been selected on the basis of their potential clinical significance (possible mechanism in parentheses where appropriate)—not necessarily inclusive (» = major clinical significance):

Note: Combinations containing any of the following medications, depending on the amount present, may also interact with this medication.

Magnesium-containing antacids
(concurrent use with misoprostol may aggravate misoprostol-induced diarrhea)

### Medical considerations/Contraindications
The medical considerations/contraindications included have been selected on the basis of their potential clinical significance (reasons given in parentheses where appropriate)—not necessarily inclusive (» = major clinical significance).

***Risk-benefit should be considered when the following medical problems exist:***

Cerebral vascular disease or
Coronary artery disease
(although the effect has not been reported with misoprostol, prostaglandins and prostaglandin analogs have been reported to cause hypotension, thus increasing the risk of severe complications in these conditions)

Epilepsy
(although the effect has not been reported with misoprostol, prostaglandins and prostaglandin analogs have been reported to cause epileptic seizures when given by routes other than oral; it is recommended that misoprostol be used in epileptics only when their condition is adequately controlled)

Sensitivity to prostaglandins or prostaglandin analogs

## Side/Adverse Effects
The following side/adverse effects have been selected on the basis of their potential clinical significance (possible signs and symptoms in parentheses where appropriate)—not necessarily inclusive:

### Those indicating need for medical attention only if they continue or are bothersome
Incidence more frequent
***Abdominal or stomach pain, mild; diarrhea***—13 to 40%

Note: *Diarrhea* is dose-related; usually developing early in the course of therapy. Self-limiting, often resolving after 8 days. However, some patients (<2%) have required discontinuation of misoprostol because of continuing severe diarrhea.

Incidence less frequent or rare
***Constipation***—1.1%; ***flatulence***—2.9%; ***headache***—2.4%; ***nausea and/or vomiting; uterine stimulation*** (cramps in lower abdomen or stomach area); ***vaginal bleeding***

## Patient Consultation
As an aid to patient consultation, refer to *Advice for the Patient, Misoprostol (Systemic)*.

In providing consultation, consider emphasizing the following selected information (» = major clinical significance):

### Before using this medication
» Conditions affecting use, especially:
Sensitivity to prostaglandins or prostaglandin analogs
Pregnancy—Contraindicated during pregnancy because of risk of miscarriage; patients of childbearing potential must take measures to assure they are not pregnant prior to therapy and to prevent pregnancy during therapy
Breast-feeding—Not recommended because of possibility of causing diarrhea in nursing infant

### Proper use of this medication
Taking with or after meals and at bedtime
» Proper dosing
Missed dose: Taking as soon as possible; not taking if almost time for next dose; not doubling doses
» Proper storage
*For use in the treatment of duodenal ulcer*
Taking antacids for relief of ulcer pain; not taking magnesium-containing antacids
Compliance with full course of therapy and keeping appointments for check-ups
» Not taking for more than 4 weeks unless otherwise directed by physician

### Precautions while using this medication
Stopping medication and checking with physician immediately if pregnancy is suspected
Consulting physician if diarrhea develops and continues for more than a week

### Side/adverse effects
Signs of potential side effects, especially continuing and severe diarrhea

## General Dosing Information
Misoprostol therapy should be started at the onset of treatment with nonsteroidal anti-inflammatory drugs (NSAIDs).

Misoprostol should be taken with or after meals and at bedtime, for maximum effectiveness.

### For treatment of duodenal ulcer
If required, antacids may be administered before or after misoprostol for the relief of pain. However, magnesium-containing antacids are not recommended since they may aggravate the misoprostol-induced diarrhea.

Therapy with misoprostol should continue for a total of 4 weeks unless healing has been documented by endoscopic examination. If necessary, treatment may continue for an additional 4 weeks if ulcers have not fully healed after the initial 4 weeks.

## Oral Dosage Forms
Note: Bracketed uses in the *Dosage forms* section refer to categories of use and/or indications that are not included in U.S. product labeling.

### MISOPROSTOL TABLETS
#### Usual adult dose
Prevention of nonsteroidal anti-inflammatory drug–induced gastric ulcer or
[Treatment of duodenal ulcer]—
Oral, 200 mcg (0.2 mg) four times a day with or after meals and at bedtime; or 400 mcg (0.4 mg) two times a day with the last dose taken at bedtime.

Note: Dose may be reduced to 100 mcg (0.1 mg) in those patients sensitive to higher doses.

#### Usual pediatric and adolescent dose
Dosage has not been established.

#### Usual geriatric dose
See *Usual adult dose*.

#### Strength(s) usually available
U.S.—
0.1 mg (Rx) [*Cytotec* (scored)].
0.2 mg (Rx) [*Cytotec* (scored)].
Canada—
0.1 mg (Rx) [*Cytotec* (scored)].
0.2 mg (Rx) [*Cytotec* (scored)].

# MITOMYCIN Systemic

VA CLASSIFICATION (Primary/Secondary): AN200/DE600

Commonly used brand name(s): *Mutamycin*.

Another commonly used name is mitomycin-C.

Note: For a listing of dosage forms and brand names by country availability, see *Dosage Forms* section(s).

## Category
Antineoplastic.

## Indications

Note: Bracketed information in the *Indications* section refers to uses that are not included in U.S. product labeling.

**Accepted**

Carcinoma, gastric (treatment)
[Carcinoma, esophageal (treatment)][1]
Carcinoma, pancreatic (treatment)
[Carcinoma, anal (treatment)][1]
[Carcinoma, colorectal (treatment)][1]
[Carcinoma, breast (treatment)][1]
[Carcinoma, head and neck (treatment)][1]
[Carcinoma, biliary (treatment)][1]
[Carcinoma, lung, non–small cell (treatment)][1]
[Carcinoma, cervical (treatment)][1]—Mitomycin is indicated, in combination with other agents, for palliative treatment of adenocarcinoma of the stomach or pancreas unresponsive to surgery and/or radiotherapy. Mitomycin is also used for treatment of anal or esophageal carcinomas, adenocarcinoma of the colon or breast; some head and neck tumors; and advanced biliary, non–small-cell lung, and cervical squamous cell carcinomas.

[Carcinoma, bladder (treatment)]—Mitomycin is used for topical treatment of superficial transitional cell carcinoma of the urinary bladder.

[Leukemia, chronic myelocytic (treatment)][1]—Mitomycin is used for treatment of chronic myelocytic leukemia.

[1]Not included in Canadian product labeling.

## Pharmacology/Pharmacokinetics

**Physicochemical characteristics**
Molecular weight—334.34.

**Mechanism of action/Effect**
Mitomycin is classified as an antibiotic but is not useful as an antimicrobial agent because of its toxicity. Mitomycin is cell cycle–phase nonspecific, although it is most active in the G and S phases of cell division. After enzyme activation in the tissues, it functions as a bifunctional or trifunctional alkylating agent. Mitomycin causes cross-linking of DNA and inhibits DNA synthesis and, to a lesser extent, also inhibits RNA and protein synthesis.

**Distribution**
Does not cross the blood-brain barrier.

**Biotransformation**
Hepatic (primarily); some in other tissues.

**Half-life**
Initial, following 30-mg bolus injection—17 minutes.

**Elimination**
Renal (10% unchanged); the percentage of a dose excreted in urine increases with increasing doses due to saturation of metabolic pathways at relatively low doses.

## Precautions to Consider

**Carcinogenicity/Mutagenicity**
Secondary malignancies are potential delayed effects of many antineoplastic agents, although it is not clear whether the effect is related to their mutagenic or immunosuppressive action. The effect of dose and duration of therapy is also unknown, although risk seems to increase with long-term use. Although information is limited, available data seem to indicate that the carcinogenic risk is greatest with the alkylating agents.

Mitomycin is carcinogenic in rats and mice.

**Pregnancy/Reproduction**

Fertility—Gonadal suppression, resulting in amenorrhea or azoospermia, may occur in patients taking antineoplastic therapy, especially with the alkylating agents. In general, these effects appear to be related to dose and length of therapy and may be irreversible. Prediction of the degree of testicular or ovarian function impairment is complicated by the common use of combinations of several antineoplastics, which makes it difficult to assess the effects of individual agents. The effects of mitomycin on fertility are not known.

Pregnancy—First trimester: It is usually recommended that use of antineoplastics, especially combination chemotherapy, be avoided whenever possible, especially during the first trimester. Although information is limited because of the relatively few instances of antineoplastic administration during pregnancy, the mutagenic, teratogenic, and carcinogenic potential of these medications must be considered.

Other hazards to the fetus include adverse reactions seen in adults.

In general, use of a contraceptive is recommended during cytotoxic drug therapy.

Mitomycin is reported to cause teratogenicity in animals.

**Breast-feeding**
Although very little information is available regarding distribution of antineoplastic agents into breast milk, breast-feeding is not recommended while mitomycin is being administered because of the risks to the infant (adverse effects, mutagenicity, carcinogenicity).

**Pediatrics**
Appropriate studies on the relationship of age to the effects of mitomycin have not been performed in the pediatric population. However, pediatrics-specific problems that would limit the usefulness of this medication in children are not expected.

**Geriatrics**
No information is available on the relationship of age to the effects of mitomycin in geriatric patients. However, elderly patients are more likely to have age-related renal function impairment, which may require caution in patients receiving mitomycin.

**Dental**
The bone marrow depressant effects of mitomycin may result in an increased incidence of microbial infection, delayed healing, and gingival bleeding. Dental work, whenever possible, should be completed prior to initiation of therapy or deferred until blood counts have returned to normal. Patients should be instructed in proper oral hygiene during treatment, including caution in use of regular toothbrushes, dental floss, and toothpicks.

Mitomycin may also cause stomatitis associated with considerable discomfort.

**Drug interactions and/or related problems**
The following drug interactions and/or related problems have been selected on the basis of their potential clinical significance (possible mechanism in parentheses where appropriate)—not necessarily inclusive (» = major clinical significance):

---

# Misoprostol (Systemic) [continued]

**Packaging and storage**
Store below 30 °C (86 °F), in a well-closed container, unless otherwise specified by manufacturer.

**Stability**
Misoprostol tablets have an expiration date of 18 months following the date of manufacture.

**Auxiliary labeling**
- Continue medicine for full time of treatment.
- Do not give medication to any other persons.

## Selected Bibliography

Knodell RG, et.al. Stress-related mucosal damage: critical evaluation of potential new therapeutic agents. Pharmacotherapy 1987; 7(6 Pt 2): 104S-9S.

Garris RE, Kirkwood CF. Misoprostol: a prostaglandin $E_1$ analogue. Clin Pharm 1989; 8: 627–41.

Jones J, Baily R. Misoprostol: a prostaglandin $E_1$ analog with antisecretory and cytoprotective properties. DICP 1989; 23: 276-281.

Revised: 04/14/92
Interim revision: 08/10/94

Note: Combinations containing any of the following medications, depending on the amount present, may also interact with this medication.

Blood dyscrasia–causing medications (see *Appendix II*)
(leukopenic and/or thrombocytopenic effects of mitomycin may be increased with concurrent or recent therapy if these medications cause the same effects; dosage adjustment of mitomycin, if necessary, should be based on blood counts)

» Bone marrow depressants, other (see *Appendix II*) or
Radiation therapy
(additive bone marrow depression may occur; dosage reduction may be required when two or more bone marrow depressants, including radiation, are used concurrently or consecutively)

Doxorubicin
(concurrent use may result in increased cardiotoxicity; it is recommended that the total dose of doxorubicin not exceed 450 mg per square meter of body surface)

Vaccines, killed virus
(because normal defense mechanisms may be suppressed by mitomycin therapy, the patient's antibody response to the vaccine may be decreased. The interval between discontinuation of medications that cause immunosuppression and restoration of the patient's ability to respond to the vaccine depends on the intensity and type of immunosuppression-causing medication used, the underlying disease, and other factors; estimates vary from 3 months to 1 year)

» Vaccines, live virus
(because normal defense mechanisms may be suppressed by mitomycin therapy, concurrent use with a live virus vaccine may potentiate the replication of the vaccine virus, may increase the side/adverse effects of the vaccine virus, and/or may decrease the patient's antibody response to the vaccine; immunization of these patients should be undertaken only with extreme caution after careful review of the patient's hematologic status and only with the knowledge and consent of the physician managing the mitomycin therapy. The interval between discontinuation of medications that cause immunosuppression and restoration of the patient's ability to respond to the vaccine depends on the intensity and type of immunosuppression-causing medication used, the underlying disease, and other factors; estimates vary from 3 months to 1 year. Patients with leukemia in remission should not receive live virus vaccine until at least 3 months after their last chemotherapy. Immunization with oral poliovirus vaccine should also be postponed in persons in close contact with the patient, especially family members)

**Laboratory value alterations**
The following have been selected on the basis of their potential clinical significance (possible effect in parentheses where appropriate)—not necessarily inclusive (» = major clinical significance):

With physiology/laboratory test values
Blood urea nitrogen (BUN) and
Creatinine, serum
(concentrations may be increased, indicating renal toxicity)

**Medical considerations/Contraindications**
The medical considerations/contraindications included have been selected on the basis of their potential clinical significance (reasons given in parentheses where appropriate)—not necessarily inclusive (» = major clinical significance).

*Risk-benefit should be considered when the following medical problems exist:*

» Bone marrow depression
» Chickenpox, existing or recent (including recent exposure) or
» Herpes zoster
(risk of severe generalized disease)
» Coagulation disorders
» Infection
» Renal function impairment
(use is not recommended in patients with a serum creatinine greater than 1.7 mg per 100 mL)
Sensitivity to mitomycin
» Caution should be used also in patients who have received previous cytotoxic drug therapy or radiation therapy.

**Patient monitoring**
» Blood urea nitrogen (BUN) concentrations and
» Creatinine concentrations, serum
(recommended prior to initiation of therapy and at periodic intervals during therapy; frequency varies according to clinical state, agent, dose, and other agents being used concurrently)

» Hematocrit or hemoglobin and
» Leukocyte count, total and, if appropriate, differential and
» Observation for fragmented red blood cells on peripheral blood smears and
» Platelet count
(determinations recommended prior to initiation of therapy and at periodic intervals during therapy; frequency varies according to clinical state, agent, dose, and other agents being used concurrently)

Note: It is recommended that renal and hematologic function be followed during and for at least 8 weeks after mitomycin therapy, especially in patients receiving doses of 60 mg or more, to detect possible hemolytic-uremic syndrome or bone marrow depression.

## Side/Adverse Effects

Note: Many "side effects" of antineoplastic therapy are unavoidable and represent the medication's pharmacologic action. Some of these (for example, leukopenia and thrombocytopenia) are actually used as parameters to aid in individual dosage titration.

The following side/adverse effects have been selected on the basis of their potential clinical significance (possible signs and symptoms in parentheses where appropriate)—not necessarily inclusive:

**Those indicating need for medical attention**
Incidence more frequent
*Leukopenia* (fever or chills; cough or hoarseness; lower back or side pain; painful or difficult urination)—usually asymptomatic; *thrombocytopenia* (unusual bleeding or bruising; black, tarry stools; blood in urine or stools; pinpoint red spots on skin)—usually asymptomatic

Note: *Leukopenia and thrombocytopenia* occur up to 8 weeks after initiation of therapy (average, 4 weeks), and counts return to normal within 10 weeks after therapy is stopped, although in about 25% of episodes counts do not recover. Severity of bone marrow depression varies and determines subsequent dosage of mitomycin.

Incidence less frequent
*Pneumopathy* (cough; shortness of breath); *renal toxicity* (blood in urine; decreased urination; shortness of breath; swelling of feet or lower legs); *stomatitis* (sores in mouth and on lips)

Note: *Pneumopathy* usually occurs after several doses; it can be severe and may be life-threatening.

*Renal toxicity* has included a hemolytic-uremic syndrome (consisting of microangiopathic hemolytic anemia [hematocrit 25% or less], irreversible renal failure, thrombocytopenia [platelet count less than 100,000], and less frequently, pulmonary hypertension, neurologic abnormalities, and hypertension), which is fatal in greater than 50% of cases. Renal failure without hemolysis has also been reported. The syndrome may occur at any time during therapy with mitomycin, alone or in combination with other chemotherapy. Use of blood product transfusions may exacerbate the symptoms in some patients. Incidence appears to be greatest in patients receiving doses of mitomycin of 60 mg or greater.

Incidence rare
*Bloody vomit; thrombophlebitis or cellulitis* (redness or pain, especially at site of injection)—caused by extravasation

Note: Extravasation may also occur without accompanying burning or stinging. Delayed erythema and ulceration have occurred weeks to months after mitomycin administration, at or distant from the injection site.

**Those indicating need for medical attention only if they continue or are bothersome**
Incidence more frequent
*Loss of appetite; nausea and vomiting*

Note: *Nausea and vomiting* usually occur within 1 to 2 hours; vomiting usually stops in 3 to 4 hours, while nausea may persist for 2 or 3 days.

Incidence less frequent
*Numbness or tingling in fingers and toes; purple-colored bands on nails*—occur with repeated doses; *skin rash; unusual tiredness or weakness*—may last several days to 3 weeks

**Those not indicating need for medical attention**
Incidence less frequent
*Loss of hair*

**Those indicating the need for medical attention if they occur after medication is discontinued**
*Bone marrow depression* (black, tarry stools; blood in urine or stools; cough or hoarseness; fever or chills; lower back or side pain; painful or difficult urination; pinpoint red spots on skin; unusual bleeding or

bruising); ***possible hemolytic-uremic syndrome*** (blood in urine, decreased urination, shortness of breath, swelling of feet or lower legs); ***delayed skin reaction*** (red or painful skin)

Note: Cumulative *myelosuppression* may occur with repeated doses.

## Patient Consultation
As an aid to patient consultation, refer to *Advice for the Patient, Mitomycin (Systemic)*.

As an aid to patient consultation, consider emphasizing the following selected information (» = major clinical significance):

### Before using this medication
» Conditions affecting use, especially:
  Sensitivity to mitomycin
  Pregnancy—Use not recommended because of mutagenic, teratogenic, and carcinogenic potential; advisability of using contraception; telling physician immediately if pregnancy is suspected
  Breast-feeding—Not recommended because of risk of serious side effects
  Other medications, especially other bone marrow depressants or previous cytotoxic drug or radiation therapy
  Other medical problems, especially chickenpox, coagulation disorders, herpes zoster, other infections, or renal function impairment

### Proper use of this medication
  Caution in taking combination therapy; taking each medication at the right time
  Frequency of nausea and vomiting; importance of continuing medication despite stomach upset
» Proper dosing

### Precautions while using this medication
» Importance of close monitoring by physician
» Avoiding immunizations unless approved by physician; other persons in patient's household should avoid immunizations with oral poliovirus vaccine; avoiding persons who have taken oral poliovirus vaccine or wearing a protective mask that covers nose and mouth

*Caution if bone marrow depression occurs*
» Avoiding exposure to persons with infections, especially during periods of low blood counts; checking with physician immediately if fever or chills, cough or hoarseness, lower back or side pain, or painful or difficult urination occurs
» Checking with physician immediately if unusual bleeding or bruising; black, tarry stools; blood in urine or stools; or pinpoint red spots on skin occur
  Caution in use of regular toothbrush, dental floss, or toothpick; physician, dentist, or nurse may suggest alternatives; checking with physician before having dental work done
  Not touching eyes or inside of nose unless hands washed immediately before
  Using caution to avoid accidental cuts with use of sharp objects such as safety razor or fingernail or toenail cutters
  Avoiding contact sports or other situations where bruising or injury could occur
» Possibility of local tissue injury and scarring if infiltration of intravenous solution occurs or as delayed reaction; telling doctor or nurse right away about redness, pain, or swelling at injection or any other site

### Side/adverse effects
  Importance of discussing possible effects, including cancer, with physician
  Signs of potential side effects, especially leukopenia, thrombocytopenia, pneumopathy, renal toxicity, stomatitis, bloody vomit, thrombophlebitis, or cellulitis caused by extravasation
  Physician or nurse can help in dealing with side effects
  Possibility of hair loss; should return after treatment has ended

## General Dosing Information
Patients receiving mitomycin should be under supervision of a physician experienced in cancer chemotherapy.

A variety of dosage schedules and regimens of mitomycin in combination with other antitumor agents are used. The prescriber may consult the medical literature as well as the manufacturer's literature in choosing a specific dosage.

Mitomycin is usually administered intravenously via a functioning intravenous catheter.

Care must be taken to avoid extravasation during intravenous administration because of the risk of severe ulceration and necrosis. Extravasation may occur with or without an accompanying stinging or burning sensation and even if there is adequate blood return when the injection needle is aspirated. Delayed erythema and ulceration occurring either at or distant from the injection site have been reported weeks to months following mitomycin administration, even when no evidence of extravasation was observed during administration. Skin grafting has been required in some of the cases.

Mitomycin must not be administered intramuscularly or subcutaneously because it will cause local tissue necrosis.

Mitomycin has also been administered intra-arterially (for example, into hepatic artery) for treatment of some tumors.

Dosage of mitomycin subsequent to the initial course should be adjusted to meet the individual requirements of each patient, on the basis of hematological response of the patient to the previous dose. An additional course of mitomycin should be given only after circulating blood elements have returned to acceptable levels (leukocytes above 3000 per cubic millimeter and platelets above 75,000 per cubic millimeter).

Patients who have not responded after two courses of mitomycin are unlikely to show a response.

Special precautions are recommended in patients who develop thrombocytopenia as a result of administration of mitomycin. These may include extreme care in performing invasive procedures; regular inspection of intravenous sites, skin (including perirectal area), and mucous membrane surfaces for signs of bleeding or bruising; limiting frequency of venipuncture and avoiding intramuscular injections; testing urine, emesis, stool, and secretions for occult blood; care in use of regular toothbrushes, dental floss, toothpicks, safety razors, and fingernail and toenail cutters; avoiding constipation; and using caution to prevent falls and other injuries. Such patients should avoid alcohol and any aspirin intake because of the risk of gastrointestinal bleeding. Platelet transfusions may be required.

Patients who develop leukopenia should be observed carefully for signs of infection. Antibiotic support may be required. In neutropenic patients who develop fever, broad-spectrum antibiotic coverage should be initiated empirically, pending bacterial cultures and appropriate diagnostic tests.

Topical bladder instillations with 20 to 40 mg of mitomycin in a strength of 1 mg per mL in distilled water, which is retained for as long as possible (usually 2 to 3 hours), are used once weekly for 8 procedures per course in the treatment of small bladder papillomas.

### Safety considerations for handling this medication
There is limited but increasing evidence and concern that personnel involved in preparation and administration of parenteral antineoplastics may be at some risk because of the potential mutagenicity, teratogenicity, and/or carcinogenicity of these agents, although the actual risk is unknown. USP advisory panels recommend cautious handling both in preparation and disposal of antineoplastic agents. Precautions that have been suggested include:

• Use of a biological containment cabinet during reconstitution and dilution of parenteral medications and wearing of disposable surgical gloves and masks.

• Use of proper technique to prevent contamination of the medication, work area, and operator during transfer between containers (including proper training of personnel in this technique).

• Cautious and proper disposal of needles, syringes, vials, ampuls, and unused medication.

A number of medical centers have developed detailed guidelines for handling of antineoplastic agents.

### Combination chemotherapy
Mitomycin may be used in combination with other agents in various regimens. As a result, incidence and/or severity of side effects may be altered and different dosages (usually reduced) may be used.

## Parenteral Dosage Forms
Note: Bracketed uses in the *Dosage Forms* section refer to categories of use and/or indications that are not included in U.S. product labeling.

### MITOMYCIN FOR INJECTION USP
**Usual adult and adolescent dose**
Carcinoma, gastric or
Carcinoma, pancreatic or
[Carcinoma, colorectal]—
  Intravenous, 20 mg per square meter of body surface area as a single dose repeated every six to eight weeks.

A suggested dosage adjustment schedule for subsequent doses is:

| Nadir after Prior Dose (cells per cubic millimeter) | | Percentage of Prior Dose to Be Given |
|---|---|---|
| Leukocytes | Platelets | |
| >4000 | >100,000 | 100 |
| 3000–3999 | 75,000–99,999 | 100 |
| 2000–2999 | 25,000–74,999 | 70 |
| <2000 | <25,000 | 50 |

**Usual adult prescribing limits**
Doses greater than 20 mg per square meter of body surface area appear to be no more effective than lower doses and increase the risk of toxicity.

**Usual pediatric dose**
See *Usual adult and adolescent dose*.

**Size(s) usually available**
U.S.—
  5 mg (Rx) [*Mutamycin* (mannitol 10 mg)].
  20 mg (Rx) [*Mutamycin* (mannitol 20 mg)].
  40 mg (Rx) [*Mutamycin* (mannitol 80 mg)].
Canada—
  5 mg (Rx) [*Mutamycin* (mannitol 10 mg)].
  20 mg (Rx) [*Mutamycin* (mannitol 20 mg)].
  40 mg (Rx) [*Mutamycin* (mannitol 80 mg)].

**Packaging and storage**
Store below 40 °C (104 °F), preferably between 15 and 30 °C (59 and 86 °F), unless otherwise specified by manufacturer. Protect from light.

**Preparation of dosage form**
Mitomycin for Injection USP is reconstituted for intravenous use by adding 10 mL (5-mg vial), 40 mL (10-mg vial), or 80 mL (40-mg vial) of sterile water for injection to the vial and shaking to dissolve, allowing to stand at room temperature if necessary until solution occurs; a blue-gray solution is produced.
Reconstituted solutions may be further diluted with 5% dextrose injection, 0.9% sodium chloride injection, or sodium lactate injection for administration by intravenous infusion.

**Stability**
Reconstituted solutions of mitomycin are stable for 14 days refrigerated or 7 days at room temperature, when protected from light. When further diluted for administration by intravenous infusion, reconstituted solutions are stable for 3 hours in 5% dextrose injection, 12 hours in 0.9% sodium chloride injection, or 24 hours in sodium lactate injection at room temperature.

Revised: 06/90
Interim revision: 07/30/93; 12/13/93; 07/05/94; 09/29/97

# MITOTANE  Systemic

VA CLASSIFICATION (Primary/Secondary): AN900/HS900
Commonly used brand name(s): *Lysodren*.
Another commonly used name is o,p′-DDD.
Note: For a listing of dosage forms and brand names by country availability, see *Dosage Forms* section(s).

## Category
Antineoplastic; antiadrenal.

## Indications
Note: Bracketed information in the *Indications* section refers to uses that are not included in U.S. product labeling.

**Accepted**
Carcinoma, adrenocortical (treatment)—Mitotane is indicated in the treatment of inoperable functional and nonfunctional adrenocortical carcinoma.

[Cushing's syndrome (treatment)][1]—Mitotane is used in the treatment of Cushing's syndrome.

[1]Not included in Canadian product labeling.

## Pharmacology/Pharmacokinetics

**Physicochemical characteristics**
Molecular weight—320.05.

**Mechanism of action/Effect**
Mitotane apparently suppresses the activity of the adrenal cortex. Mechanism of cytotoxic action is unknown, but may be related to adrenal suppression.

**Absorption**
Approximately 35 to 40% absorbed from the gastrointestinal tract.

**Distribution**
To all body tissues; stored in fat; small amount (as metabolite) crosses blood-brain barrier.

**Biotransformation**
Hepatic and renal, to water-soluble metabolite.

**Half-life**
18 to 159 days.

**Onset of action**
Reduced concentrations of 17-hydroxycorticosteroid usually occur within 2 or 3 days after initiation of therapy; tumor response may occur within 6 weeks.

**Time to peak plasma concentration**
3 to 5 hours.

**Elimination**
Renal, 10 to 25% (as metabolite); bile, 1 to 17% (as metabolite). Measurable plasma concentrations persist for 6 to 9 weeks after withdrawal of mitotane.

## Precautions to Consider

**Carcinogenicity/Mutagenicity**
Studies have not been done.

**Pregnancy/Reproduction**
Pregnancy—Studies have not been done in either animals or humans. Problems in humans have not been documented. However, caution is recommended, especially during the first trimester.
FDA Pregnancy Category C.

**Breast-feeding**
It is not known whether mitotane is distributed into breast milk. However, problems in humans have not been documented.

**Pediatrics**
Appropriate studies with mitotane have not been performed in the pediatric population. However, pediatrics-specific problems that would limit the usefulness of this medication in children are not expected.

**Geriatrics**
No geriatrics-specific information is available on the use of mitotane in geriatric patients.

**Drug interactions and/or related problems**
The following drug interactions and/or related problems have been selected on the basis of their potential clinical significance (possible mechanism in parentheses where appropriate)—not necessarily inclusive (» = major clinical significance):

Note: Combinations containing any of the following medications, depending on the amount present, may also interact with this medication.

» Central nervous system (CNS) depression–producing medications (see *Appendix II*)
  (concurrent use may produce additive CNS depressant effects)

Corticosteroids, glucocorticoid and mineralocorticoid
  (higher dosage may be required to treat adrenal insufficiency since mitotane alters metabolism of these steroids)

Corticotropin (ACTH)
  (mitotane may inhibit the adrenal response to ACTH; this may interfere with the therapeutic response to ACTH)

**Laboratory value alterations**
The following have been selected on the basis of their potential clinical significance (possible effect in parentheses where appropriate)—not necessarily inclusive (» = major clinical significance):

With physiology/laboratory test values
  Plasma cortisol concentrations and
  Urinary 17-hydroxycorticosteroid concentrations
    (may be decreased as a result of adrenocortical inhibition)
  Protein-bound iodine (PBI) concentrations
    (may be decreased as a result of mitotane binding to thyroid-binding globulin)
  Serum uric acid concentrations
    (may be decreased)

## Medical considerations/Contraindications
The medical considerations/contraindications included have been selected on the basis of their potential clinical significance (reasons given in parentheses where appropriate)—not necessarily inclusive (» = major clinical significance).

*Risk-benefit should be considered when the following medical problems exist:*
- » Hepatic function impairment other than metastatic lesion of the adrenal cortex
  (reduced metabolism and possible accumulation; reduction in dosage may be required)
- » Infection
  Sensitivity to mitotane

## Patient monitoring
The following may be especially important in patient monitoring (other tests may be warranted in some patients, depending on condition; » = major clinical significance):

Neurological assessments
  (recommended at periodic intervals in patients receiving mitotane for longer than 2 years)
- » 8 a.m. plasma cortisol concentrations or
- » 24-hour urinary 17-hydroxycorticosteroid concentrations
  (recommended at periodic intervals to aid in assessing clinical response and to determine if steroid supplement therapy is necessary)

## Side/Adverse Effects
The following side/adverse effects have been selected on the basis of their potential clinical significance (possible signs and symptoms in parentheses where appropriate)—not necessarily inclusive:

**Those indicating need for medical attention**
Incidence more frequent—40 to 80%
  *Adrenocortical insufficiency* (darkening of skin; diarrhea; dizziness; drowsiness; loss of appetite; mental depression; nausea and vomiting; skin rash; unusual tiredness)
Incidence less frequent
  *Double vision; hemorrhagic cystitis* (blood in urine); *lens opacity or toxic retinopathy* (blurred vision)
Incidence rare
  *Allergic reaction* (shortness of breath; wheezing)

**Those indicating need for medical attention only if they continue or are bothersome**
Incidence less frequent
  *Aching muscles; fever; flushing or redness of skin; muscle twitching; orthostatic hypotension* (dizziness or lightheadedness when getting up from a lying or sitting position)

## Patient Consultation
As an aid to patient consultation, refer to *Advice for the Patient, Mitotane (Systemic)*.
In providing consultation, consider emphasizing the following selected information (» = major clinical significance):

**Before using this medication**
- » Conditions affecting use, especially:
    Sensitivity to mitotane
    Pregnancy—Caution is recommended, especially during the first trimester
    Other medications, especially CNS depressants
    Other medical problems, especially hepatic function impairment other than metastatic lesion of the adrenal cortex or infection

**Proper use of this medication**
- » Importance of not taking more or less medication than the amount prescribed
- » Checking with physician before discontinuing medication because of risk of adrenal suppression
- » Proper dosing
    Missed dose: Taking as soon as possible; not taking if almost time for next dose; not doubling doses; checking with physician
- » Proper storage

**Precautions while using this medication**
- » Importance of close monitoring by the physician
    Carrying medical identification card
- » Caution in taking alcohol or other CNS depressants
- » Caution if dizziness or drowsiness occurs, especially if driving, using machines, or doing other things that require alertness
- » Checking with physician immediately if injury, infection, or other illness occurs, because of the risk of adrenal insufficiency; physician may prescribe steroid supplement

**Side/adverse effects**
Signs of potential side effects, especially adrenocortical insufficiency, double vision, hemorrhagic cystitis, lens opacity, toxic retinopathy, and allergic reaction

## General Dosing Information
Patients receiving mitotane should be under supervision of a physician experienced in cancer chemotherapy.

Initial treatment often occurs in the hospital until dosage is stabilized.

Dosage must be adjusted to the maximum dose tolerated to meet the individual requirements of each patient, based on appearance of adverse reactions and improvement in clinical response.

Glucocorticoid therapy is usually required in patients being treated with mitotane; mineralocorticoid therapy may also be required, especially with prolonged therapy. Because metabolism of exogenous corticosteroids may be altered in patients receiving mitotane, higher than normal replacement doses may be required. Steroid therapy may have to be continued after mitotane is withdrawn, until adrenocortical function returns to normal.

Continuous treatment with the maximum tolerated dosage of mitotane appears to be more effective than intermittent courses.

Duration of treatment depends on clinical response. Only 10% of patients showing no response after 3 months of treatment at the maximum tolerated dosage will show a response to continued therapy.

It is recommended that mitotane be temporarily withdrawn immediately following shock or severe trauma and that steroids be administered, because adrenal suppression may prevent the normal response to stress.

## Oral Dosage Forms
Note: Bracketed uses in the *Dosage Forms* section refer to categories of use and/or indications that are not included in U.S. product labeling.

### MITOTANE TABLETS USP
**Usual adult dose**
Carcinoma, adrenocortical—
  Initial: Oral, 2 to 6 grams per day in three or four divided doses; the dosage may be increased until adverse reactions occur.
  Note: The maximum tolerated dosage may vary from 2 to 16 grams per day, with an average dosage of 9 to 10 grams per day.
[Cushing's syndrome][1]—
  Initial: Oral, 3 to 6 grams per day in three or four divided doses.
  Maintenance: Oral, 500 mcg (0.5 mg) two times a week to 2 grams per day.

**Usual pediatric dose**
Carcinoma, adrenocortical—
  Oral, 100 to 500 mcg (0.1 to 0.5 mg) per kg of body weight; or initially, 1 to 2 grams per day in divided doses, the dosage being gradually increased to 5 to 7 grams per day.

**Strength(s) usually available**
U.S.—
  500 mg (Rx) [*Lysodren* (scored)].
Canada—
  500 mg (Rx) [*Lysodren* (scored)].

**Packaging and storage**
Store below 40 °C (104 °F), preferably between 15 and 30 °C (59 and 86 °F), unless otherwise specified by the manufacturer. Store in a tight, light-resistant container.

**Auxiliary labeling**
- May cause drowsiness.

---
[1]Not included in Canadian product labeling.

---
Revised: 08/90
Interim revision: 06/30/94; 09/30/97; 07/08/98

# MITOXANTRONE Systemic

VA CLASSIFICATION (Primary): AN900

Commonly used brand name(s): *Novantrone*.

Note: For a listing of dosage forms and brand names by country availability, see *Dosage Forms* section(s).

## Category

Antineoplastic.

## Indications

Note: Bracketed information in the *Indications* section refers to uses that are not included in U.S. product labeling.

**Accepted**

Cancer, prostate, advanced hormone-refractory (treatment)[1]—Mitoxantrone, in combination with corticosteroids, is indicated as initial palliative treatment of patients with pain related to advanced hormone-refractory prostate cancer.

Leukemia, acute nonlymphocytic (treatment)—Mitoxantrone is indicated, in combination with other agents, for the treatment of acute nonlymphocytic (including myelocytic, promyelocytic, monocytic, and erythroid) leukemia in adults.

[Leukemia, acute lymphocytic (treatment)]—Mitoxantrone is used for the treatment of recurrent acute lymphocytic leukemia in adults.

[Carcinoma, breast (treatment)]—Mitoxantrone is indicated, alone or in combination with other agents, for treatment of breast carcinoma, including locally advanced and metastatic disease.

[Lymphomas, non-Hodgkin's (treatment)]—Mitoxantrone is used for treatment of non-Hodgkin's lymphomas.

[1]Not included in Canadian product labeling.

## Pharmacology/Pharmacokinetics

**Physicochemical characteristics**

Molecular weight—517.41.

**Mechanism of action/Effect**

Mitoxantrone appears to be most active in the late S phase of cell division, but is not cycle phase–specific. Although the exact mechanism of action is unknown, evidence seems to indicate involvement of two effects—binding to DNA by intercalation between base pairs, and a non-intercalative electrostatic interaction—resulting in inhibition of DNA and RNA synthesis.

**Other actions/effects**

Also has antiviral, antibacterial, antiprotozoal, and immunosuppressant effects.

**Distribution**

Rapid and extensive; largest concentrations are in the thyroid, liver, heart, and red blood cells.

**Protein binding**

High (78%).

**Biotransformation**

Hepatic.

**Half-life**

Mean, 5.8 days (range, 2.3–13.0 days).

**Elimination**

Biliary/fecal, up to 25% in 5 days.

Renal, 6-11% (65% unchanged).

Extensive tissue uptake and binding accounts for most of a dose, which is then thought to be gradually released.

In dialysis—Because of extensive tissue binding, unlikely to be significantly removed by hemodialysis or peritoneal dialysis.

## Precautions to Consider

**Carcinogenicity**

Secondary malignancies are potential delayed effects of many antineoplastic agents, although it is not clear whether the effect is related to their mutagenic or immunosuppressive action. The effect of dose and duration of therapy is also unknown, although the risk seems to increase with long-term use. Although information is limited, available data seem to indicate that the carcinogenic risk is greatest with the alkylating agents.

**Mutagenicity**

Mitoxantrone may cause chromosomal aberrations in animals and is mutagenic in bacterial systems. It has been reported to cause DNA damage and sister chromatid exchanges *in vitro*.

**Pregnancy/Reproduction**

Fertility—Gonadal suppression, resulting in amenorrhea or azoospermia, may occur in patients taking antineoplastic therapy, especially with the alkylating agents. In general, these effects appear to be related to dose and length of therapy and may be irreversible. Prediction of the degree of testicular or ovarian function impairment is complicated by the common use of combinations of several antineoplastics, which makes it difficult to assess the effects of individual agents.

Pregnancy—Adequate and well-controlled studies in humans have not been done.

First trimester: It is usually recommended that use of antineoplastics, especially combination chemotherapy, be avoided whenever possible, especially during the first trimester. Although information is limited because of the relatively few instances of antineoplastic administration during pregnancy, the mutagenic, teratogenic, and carcinogenic potential of these medications must be considered.

Other hazards to the fetus include adverse reactions seen in adults.

In general, use of a contraceptive is recommended during cytotoxic drug therapy.

Studies in rats found an increased incidence of low fetal birth weight and retarded development of the fetal kidney, and studies in rabbits found an increased incidence of premature delivery. Mitoxantrone was not found to be teratogenic in rabbits.

FDA Pregnancy Category D.

**Breast-feeding**

Although very little information is available regarding distribution of antineoplastic agents into breast milk, breast-feeding is not recommended while mitoxantrone is being administered because of the risks to the infant (adverse effects, mutagenicity, carcinogenicity). It is not known whether mitoxantrone is distributed into breast milk.

**Pediatrics**

Appropriate studies on the relationship of age to the effects of mitoxantrone have not been performed in the pediatric population.

**Geriatrics**

Appropriate studies on the relationship of age to the effects of mitoxantrone have not been performed in the geriatric population. However, no geriatrics-specific problems have been documented to date.

**Dental**

The bone marrow depressant effects of mitoxantrone may result in an increased incidence of microbial infection, delayed healing, and gingival bleeding. Dental work, whenever possible, should be completed prior to initiation of therapy or deferred until blood counts have returned to normal. Patients should be instructed in proper oral hygiene during treatment, including caution in use of regular toothbrushes, dental floss, and toothpicks.

Mitoxantrone also causes stomatitis or mucositis, which may be associated with considerable discomfort.

**Drug interactions and/or related problems**

The following drug interactions and/or related problems have been selected on the basis of their potential clinical significance (possible mechanism in parentheses where appropriate)—not necessarily inclusive (» = major clinical significance):

Note: Combinations containing any of the following medications, depending on the amount present, may also interact with this medication.

  Allopurinol or
  Colchicine or
» Probenecid or
» Sulfinpyrazone
   (mitoxantrone may raise the concentration of blood uric acid; dosage adjustment of antigout medications may be necessary to control hyperuricemia and gout; allopurinol may be preferred to prevent or reverse mitoxantrone-induced hyperuricemia because of risk of uric acid nephropathy with uricosuric antigout agents)

  Blood dyscrasia–causing medications (See *Appendix II*)
   (leukopenic and/or thrombocytopenic effects of mitoxantrone may be increased with concurrent or recent therapy if these medications cause the same effects; dosage adjustment of mitoxantrone, if necessary, should be based on blood counts)

» Bone marrow depressants, other (See *Appendix II*) or
  Radiation therapy
    (additive bone marrow depression may occur; dosage reduction may be required when two or more bone marrow depressants, including radiation, are used concurrently or consecutively)
  Daunorubicin or
  Doxorubicin or
  Radiation therapy to mediastinal area
    (use of mitoxantrone in a patient who has previously received any of these increases the risk of cardiotoxicity)
  Vaccines, killed virus
    (because normal defense mechanisms may be suppressed by mitoxantrone therapy, the patient's antibody response to the vaccine may be decreased. The interval between discontinuation of medications that cause immunosuppression and restoration of the patient's ability to respond to the vaccine depends on the intensity and type of immunosuppression-causing medication used, the underlying disease, and other factors; estimates vary from 3 months to 1 year)
  Vaccines, live virus
    (because normal defense mechanisms may be suppressed by mitoxantrone therapy, concurrent use with a live virus vaccine may potentiate the replication of the vaccine virus, may increase the side/adverse effects of the vaccine virus, and/or may decrease the patient's antibody response to the vaccine; immunization of these patients should be undertaken only with extreme caution after careful review of the patient's hematologic status and only with the knowledge and consent of the physician managing the mitoxantrone therapy. The interval between discontinuation of medications that cause immunosuppression and restoration of the patient's ability to respond to the vaccine depends on the intensity and type of immunosuppression-causing medication used, the underlying disease, and other factors; estimates vary from 3 months to 1 year. Patients with leukemia in remission should not receive live virus vaccine until at least 3 months after their last chemotherapy. Immunization with oral poliovirus vaccine should also be postponed in persons in close contact with the patient, especially family members)

**Laboratory value alterations**
The following have been selected on the basis of their potential clinical significance (possible effect in parentheses where appropriate)—not necessarily inclusive (» = major clinical significance):

With physiology/laboratory test values
  Alanine aminotransferase (ALT [SGPT]) values, serum and
  Aspartate aminotransferase (AST [SGOT]) values, serum and
  Bilirubin concentrations, serum
    (may be increased, indicating hepatotoxicity)
  Uric acid
    (concentrations in blood and urine may be increased)

**Medical considerations/Contraindications**
The medical considerations/contraindications included have been selected on the basis of their potential clinical significance (reasons given in parentheses where appropriate)—not necessarily inclusive (» = major clinical significance).

*Risk-benefit should be considered when the following medical problems exist:*
» Bone marrow depression
» Chickenpox, existing or recent (including recent exposure) or
» Herpes zoster
    (risk of severe generalized disease)
  Gout, history of or
  Urate renal stones, history of
    (risk of hyperuricemia)
» Heart disease
    (increased risk of cardiotoxicity)
  Hepatic function impairment, severe
    (mitoxantrone clearance may be reduced; dosage adjustment may be necessary)
» Infection
  Sensitivity to mitoxantrone
» Caution should be used also in patients with inadequate bone marrow reserves due to previous cytotoxic drug or radiation therapy.

**Patient monitoring**
The following may be especially important in patient monitoring (other tests may be warranted in some patients, depending on condition; » = major clinical significance):

  Alanine aminotransferase (ALT [SGPT]) values, serum and
  Aspartate aminotransferase (AST [SGOT]) values, serum and
  Bilirubin concentrations, serum and
  Lactate dehydrogenase (LDH) values, serum
    (determinations recommended prior to initiation of therapy and at periodic intervals during therapy; frequency varies according to clinical state, agent, dose, and other agents being used concurrently)
» Chest x-ray and
» Echocardiography and
  Electrocardiogram (ECG) studies and
» Radionuclide angiography determination of ejection fraction
    (recommended prior to initiation of therapy and at periodic intervals during therapy)
» Hematocrit or hemoglobin and
» Leukocyte count, total and, if appropriate, differential and
» Platelet count
    (determinations recommended prior to initiation of therapy and at periodic intervals during therapy; frequency varies according to clinical state, agent, dose, and other agents being used concurrently)
  Uric acid concentrations, serum
    (recommended prior to initiation of therapy and at periodic intervals during therapy)

## Side/Adverse Effects

Note: Many "side effects" of antineoplastic therapy are unavoidable and represent the medication's pharmacologic action. Some of these (for example, leukopenia and thrombocytopenia) are actually used as parameters to aid in individual dosage titration.

Cardiotoxicity has been reported, including decreased left ventricular ejection fraction, congestive heart failure, ECG changes, arrhythmias such as tachycardia, and, rarely, myocardial infarction. The risk of cardiotoxicity seems to be increased at cumulative mitoxantrone doses exceeding 140 mg per square meter of body surface (100 mg per square meter of body surface in patients with risk factors such as previous treatment with anthracyclines or mediastinal radiation or existing heart disease).

The following side/adverse effects have been selected on the basis of their potential clinical significance (possible signs and symptoms in parentheses where appropriate)—not necessarily inclusive:

**Those indicating need for medical attention**
Incidence more frequent
  *Cough or shortness of breath; gastrointestinal bleeding* (black, tarry stools); *leukopenia or infection* (fever or chills; cough or hoarseness; lower back or side pain; painful or difficult urination)—usually asymptomatic; *stomach pain; stomatitis or mucositis* (sores in mouth and on lips)

  Note: *Cough or shortness of breath* may be associated with congestive heart failure.

  In *leukopenia*, the nadir of the leukocyte count usually occurs within 10 days and usually recovers within 21 days.

  *Stomatitis or mucositis* usually occurs within 1 week after the start of treatment.

Incidence less frequent
  *Arrhythmias* (fast or irregular heartbeat); *congestive heart failure* (swelling of feet and lower legs); *conjunctivitis* (sore, red eyes); *jaundice* (yellow eyes or skin); *renal failure* (decrease in urination); *seizures; thrombocytopenia* (unusual bleeding or bruising; black, tarry stools; blood in urine or stools; pinpoint red spots on skin)—usually asymptomatic

Incidence rare
  *Allergic reaction, possible* (skin rash); *extravasation* (blue skin at site of injection, pain or redness at site of injection); *local irritation or phlebitis* (pain or redness at site of injection)

  Note: Tissue necrosis has been reported in only a few cases after *extravasation*.

**Those indicating need for medical attention only if they continue or are bothersome**
Incidence more frequent
  *Diarrhea; headache; nausea and vomiting*

  Note: *Nausea and vomiting* are usually mild to moderate.

**Those not indicating need for medical attention**
Incidence more frequent
  *Blue-green urine; loss of hair*
Incidence less frequent
  *Blue color in whites of eyes*

## Patient Consultation

As an aid to patient consultation, refer to *Advice for the Patient, Mitoxantrone (Systemic)*.

In providing consultation, consider emphasizing the following selected information (» = major clinical significance):

### Before using this medication
» Conditions affecting use, especially:
   Sensitivity to mitoxantrone
   Pregnancy—Use not recommended because of mutagenic, teratogenic, and carcinogenic potential; advisability of using contraception; telling physician immediately if pregnancy is suspected
   Breast-feeding—Not recommended because of risk of serious side effects
   Other medications, especially other bone marrow depressants, probenecid, or sulfinpyrazone
   Other medical problems, especially chickenpox, herpes zoster, heart disease, or other infection

### Proper use of this medication
Caution in taking combination therapy; taking each medication at the right time
Importance of ample fluid intake and subsequent increase in urine output to aid in excretion of uric acid
Frequency of nausea and vomiting; importance of continuing medication despite stomach upset
» Proper dosing

### Precautions while using this medication
» Importance of close monitoring by the physician
» Avoiding immunizations unless approved by physician; other persons in patient's household should avoid immunizations with oral poliovirus vaccine; avoiding persons who have taken oral poliovirus vaccine or wearing a protective mask that covers nose and mouth

*Caution if bone marrow depression occurs*
» Avoiding exposure to persons with infections, especially during periods of low blood counts; checking with physician immediately if fever or chills, cough or hoarseness, lower back or side pain, or painful or difficult urination occurs
» Checking with physician immediately if unusual bleeding or bruising; black, tarry stools; blood in urine or stools; or pinpoint red spots on skin occur
Caution in use of regular toothbrush, dental floss, or toothpick; physician, dentist, or nurse may suggest alternatives; checking with physician before having dental work done
Not touching eyes or inside of nose unless hands washed immediately before
Using caution to avoid accidental cuts with use of sharp objects such as safety razor or fingernail or toenail cutters
Avoiding contact sports or other situations where bruising or injury could occur

### Side/adverse effects
Importance of discussing possible effects with physician
Signs of potential side effects, especially cough, shortness of breath, gastrointestinal bleeding, leukopenia, infection, stomach pain, stomatitis, mucositis, arrhythmias, congestive heart failure, conjunctivitis, jaundice, renal failure, seizures, thrombocytopenia, allergic reaction, extravasation, local irritation, and phlebitis
Physician or nurse can help in dealing with side effects
Urine may have blue-green color and whites of eyes may have a blue color during treatment
Possibility of hair loss; normal hair growth should return after treatment has ended

## General Dosing Information

Patients receiving mitoxantrone should be under supervision of a physician experienced in cancer chemotherapy.

A variety of dosage schedules of mitoxantrone, alone or in combination with other antitumor agents, are used. The prescriber may consult the medical literature as well as the manufacturer's literature in choosing a specific dosage.

Dosage must be adjusted to meet the individual requirements of each patient, on the basis of clinical response and appearance or severity of toxicity.

Mitoxantrone hydrochloride injection should not be administered intrathecally; paralysis has occurred after administration by this route. Safety of administration by any route other than the intravenous route has not been established.

*Mitoxantrone hydrochloride concentrate for injection must be diluted prior to intravenous administration.*

An additional course of mitoxantrone should be given only after toxic hematological effects from the first course have subsided.

Although mitoxantrone is nonvesicant and does not usually cause a severe local reaction, if extravasation occurs during intravenous administration, the injection and infusion should be stopped immediately and resumed, completing the dose, in another vein.

Development of uric acid nephropathy in patients with leukemia or lymphoma may be prevented by adequate oral hydration and, in some cases, administration of allopurinol. Alkalinization of urine may be necessary if serum uric acid concentrations are elevated.

Special precautions are recommended in patients who develop thrombocytopenia as a result of administration of mitoxantrone. These may include extreme care in performing invasive procedures; regular inspection of intravenous sites, skin (including perirectal area), and mucous membrane surfaces for signs of bleeding or bruising; limiting frequency of venipuncture and avoiding intramuscular injections; testing urine, emesis, stool, and secretions for occult blood; care in use of regular toothbrushes, dental floss, toothpicks, safety razors, and fingernail and toenail cutters; avoiding constipation; and using caution to prevent falls and other injuries. Such patients should avoid alcohol and any aspirin intake because of the risk of gastrointestinal bleeding. Platelet transfusions may be required.

Patients who develop leukopenia should be observed carefully for signs of infection. Antibiotic support may be required. In neutropenic patients who develop fever, broad-spectrum antibiotic coverage should be initiated empirically, pending bacterial cultures and appropriate diagnostic tests.

### Safety considerations for handling this medication

There is limited but increasing evidence and concern that personnel involved in preparation and administration of parenteral antineoplastics may be at some risk because of the potential mutagenicity, teratogenicity, and/or carcinogenicity of these agents, although the actual risk is unknown. USP advisory panels recommend cautious handling both in preparation and disposal of antineoplastic agents. Precautions that have been suggested include:

- Use of a biological containment cabinet during reconstitution and dilution of parenteral medications and wearing of disposable surgical gloves and masks.
- Use of proper technique to prevent contamination of the medication, work area, and operator during transfer between containers (including proper training of personnel in this technique).
- Cautious and proper disposal of needles, syringes, vials, ampuls, and unused medication.

A number of medical centers have developed detailed guidelines for handling of antineoplastic agents.

## Parenteral Dosage Forms

Note: Bracketed uses in the *Dosage Forms* section refer to categories of use and/or indications that are not included in U.S. product labeling.

### MITOXANTRONE FOR INJECTION CONCENTRATE USP

Note: Although Mitoxantrone for Injection Concentrate USP is available as the hydrochloride salt, dosing and strengths are expressed in terms of the base.

**Usual adult dose**
Cancer, prostate, advanced hormone-refractory[1]—
   Intravenous infusion, over a short period of time, 12 to 14 mg (base) per square meter of body surface area every twenty-one days
Leukemia, acute nonlymphocytic—
   Initial—
      Intravenous infusion (introduced slowly into the tubing of a freely running intravenous infusion of 0.9% sodium chloride injection or 5% dextrose injection over a period of not less than 3 minutes), 12 mg (base) per square meter of body surface area daily on days 1 to 3, in combination with 100 mg of cytarabine (cytosine arabinoside) per square meter of body surface area daily given as a continuous twenty-four hour intravenous infusion on days 1 to 7.
   Note: If response to the initial course is inadequate, a second induction course at the same dosage may be given.
      If severe or life-threatening nonhematologic toxicity occurs during the first induction course, it is recommended that the second course not be administered until the toxicity has resolved.
   Maintenance—
      Intravenous infusion (introduced slowly into the tubing of a freely running intravenous infusion of 0.9% sodium chloride injection

or 5% dextrose injection over a period of not less than 3 minutes), 12 mg (base) per square meter of body surface area daily on days 1 and 2, in combination with 100 mg of cytarabine (cytosine arabinoside) per square meter of body surface area daily given as a continuous twenty-four hour intravenous infusion on days 1 to 5.

- Note: The maintenance or consolidation course should not be initiated until leukocyte and platelet counts have returned to pretreatment levels. The maintenance course is usually given approximately six weeks after the first induction course. A second consolidation course may be given four weeks after the first.

[Carcinoma, breast] or
[Lymphomas, non-Hodgkin's]—
Intravenous infusion (introduced slowly into the tubing of a freely running intravenous infusion of 0.9% sodium chloride injection or 5% dextrose injection over a period of not less than three minutes), 14 mg (base) per square meter of body surface area every twenty-one days.

Note: A lower initial dose (12 mg [base] per square meter of body surface area is recommended in patients with inadequate bone marrow reserves. Each subsequent dose should not be given until leukocyte and platelet counts have recovered after the previous dose; dosage reduction may be necessary if severe bone marrow depression occurs.

### Usual pediatric dose
Dosage has not been established.

### Strength(s) usually available
U.S.—
  2 mg (base) per mL (10-, 12.5-, and 15-mL vials) (Rx) [*Novantrone*].
Canada—
  2 mg (base) per mL (10- and 12.5-mL vials) (Rx) [*Novantrone*].

### Packaging and storage
Store between 15 and 25 °C (59 and 77 °F). Protect from freezing.

### Preparation of dosage form
Mitoxantrone for Injection Concentrate USP must be diluted for administration by intravenous infusion. The dose of mitoxantrone for injection concentrate should be diluted to at least 50 mL in 0.9% sodium chloride injection or 5% dextrose injection.

### Stability
Mitoxantrone for Injection Concentrate USP contains no preservative. Unused portions of solution prepared for intravenous infusion should be discarded. After penetration of the stopper, remaining portions of undiluted mitoxantrone for injection concentrate may be stored for no longer than 7 days at room temperature (15 to 25 °C [59 to 77 °F]) or 14 days in the refrigerator.

### Incompatibilities
Mitoxantrone should not be mixed with heparin, since a precipitate may form.

### Note
Any mitoxantrone solution that comes in contact with the skin or mucosa should be washed off thoroughly with warm water.

---

[1]Not included in Canadian product labeling.

## Selected Bibliography
Faulds D, Balfour JA, Chrisp P, et al. Mitoxantrone. A review of its pharmacodynamic and pharmacokinetic properties, and therapeutic potential in the chemotherapy of cancer. Drugs 1991; 41: 400-49.
Koeller J, Eble M. Mitoxantrone: a novel anthracycline derivative. Clin Pharm 1988; 7: 574-81.
Shenkenberg TD, Von Hoff DD. Mitoxantrone: a new anticancer drug with significant clinical activity. Ann Intern Med 1986; 105: 67-81.

Revised: 03/16/95
Interim revision: 09/30/97

# MIVACURIUM  Systemic†

VA CLASSIFICATION (Primary): MS300
Commonly used brand name(s): *Mivacron*.
Note: For a listing of dosage forms and brand names by country availability, see *Dosage Forms* section(s).

†Not commercially available in Canada.

## Category
Neuromuscular blocking agent.
Note: Mivacurium is a nondepolarizing neuromuscular blocking agent with a short duration of action.

## Indications
### Accepted
Muscle (skeletal) relaxation, for surgery—Mivacurium is indicated as an adjunct to anesthesia to facilitate endotracheal intubation and to induce skeletal muscle relaxation in the surgical field.

### Unaccepted
Mivacurium has not been adequately studied for facilitating prolonged mechanical ventilation in intensive care patients.

## Pharmacology/Pharmacokinetics
### Physicochemical characteristics
Source—Synthetic.
Chemical group—bis-Benzylisoquinolinium diester compound.
Molecular weight—1100.18.

Note: Mivacurium is a mixture of 3 stereoisomers, the trans-trans, cis-trans, and cis-cis diesters. The mixture contains about 57% of the trans-trans diester and about 36% of the cis-trans diester. These stereoisomers have neuromuscular blocking activities that are approximately equal to each other and to the mixture as a whole. In animals, the cis-cis diester is approximately one-tenth as potent as the other stereoisomers. Interconversion of the isomers does not occur *in vivo*.

### Mechanism of action/Effect
Mivacurium is a nondepolarizing (competitive) neuromuscular blocking agent. Nondepolarizing neuromuscular blocking agents inhibit neuromuscular transmission by competing with acetylcholine for the cholinergic receptors of the motor end plate, thereby reducing the response of the end plate to acetylcholine. This type of neuromuscular block is usually antagonized by anticholinesterase agents. Because mivacurium is hydrolyzed by plasma cholinesterase, the possibility that anticholinesterase agents might prolong, rather than reverse, the effects of mivacurium has been considered. However, both neostigmine and edrophonium have been shown to reverse the effects of mivacurium.
Neuromuscular blocking agents have no clinically significant effect on consciousness or the pain threshold.

### Other actions/effects
Mivacurium may cause histamine release, especially when relatively large doses are administered rapidly, leading to a decrease in blood pressure and an increase in heart rate.

### Distribution
Volume of distribution—0.15 (range, 0.06 to 0.24), 0.27 (range, 0.08 to 0.56), and 0.31 (range, 0.18 to 0.46) L per kg of body weight, for the trans-trans, cis-trans, and cis-cis diesters, respectively.

### Biotransformation
Extensive and rapid; via enzymatic hydrolysis catalyzed by plasma cholinesterase. Biotransformation may be significantly slowed in patients with abnormal or decreased plasma cholinesterase activity, especially individuals with a homozygous atypical cholinesterase gene abnormality.

### Half-life
Elimination—5 to 10 minutes, estimated using the premise that doubling the dose of a medication prolongs the duration of action by the length of its elimination half-life. Half-life values of 2.3 (range, 1.4 to 3.6) and 2.1 (range, 0.8 to 4.8) minutes have been reported for the trans-trans and cis-trans stereoisomers, respectively. A value of 55 (range, 32 to 102) minutes has been reported for the cis-cis diester, but this isomer is not likely to contribute significantly to the effects of the mixture. The half-life is not significantly prolonged in geriatric patients.

### Onset of action
Time to achieve intubating conditions:
  150 mcg per kg of body weight (mcg/kg): About 2.5 minutes.
  200 or 250 mcg/kg: About 2 minutes.

### Time to peak effect
Note: The time to maximal suppression of the twitch response to peripheral nerve stimulation is dependent on dosage and the age of the patient. Also, administration of a volatile inhalation agent (specified

below when applicable) may produce a dose-dependent decrease in the time to peak effect.
Children 2 to 12 years of age—
110 to 120 mcg/kg: 2.8 (range, 1.2 to 4.6) minutes.
200 mcg/kg: 1.9 (range, 1.3 to 3.3) minutes.
250 mcg/kg: 1.6 (range, 1.0 to 2.2) minutes.
Nongeriatric adults with normal hepatic and renal function—
70 to 100 mcg/kg: 4.9 (range, 2.0 to 7.6) minutes.
150 mcg/kg: 3.3 (range, 1.5 to 8.8) minutes.
200 mcg/kg: 2.5 (range, 1.2 to 6.0) minutes.
250 mcg/kg: 2.3 (range, 1.0 to 4.8) minutes.
Nongeriatric adults with end-stage renal failure undergoing renal transplantation—
150 mcg/kg (isoflurane/nitrous oxide/oxygen anesthesia): 2.6 (range, 1.0 to 4.5) minutes.
Nongeriatric adults with end-stage hepatic disease undergoing hepatic transplantation—
150 mcg/kg (isoflurane/oxygen anesthesia): 2.1 (range, 1 to 4) minutes.
Geriatric adults 68 to 77 years of age—
100 mcg/kg (isoflurane/nitrous oxide/oxygen anesthesia): 4.8 (range, 3 to 7) minutes; about 1.5 minutes longer than for nongeriatric adults receiving this dose under the same anesthetic regimen.

**Duration of action**

Note: Mivacurium's duration of action is dependent on the patient's age and plasma cholinesterase activity. In addition, the duration of action is more prolonged during anesthesia with a volatile inhalation anesthetic (specified below when applicable) than during other types of anesthesia. Although studies in a limited number of individuals have shown prolonged effects in patients with impaired hepatic or renal function, the contribution of these medical problems to the prolongation of effect, independent of decreased plasma cholinesterase activity and/or the anesthesia given, has not been ascertained.

The duration of mivacurium's clinical effect (time to 25% spontaneous recovery) is influenced by the dose to a significantly lesser extent than that of other nondepolarizing neuromuscular blocking agents. In children, increasing the dose from 110 to 200 mcg/kg, or from 120 to 250 mcg/kg, extends the duration of clinical effect by only 2 to 4 minutes. In adults, the duration of clinical effect of a 200 mcg/kg dose is about 25% longer, and that of a 300 mcg/kg dose is about 50% longer, than that of a 100 mcg/kg dose. In clinical studies, cumulative effects on the duration or depth of neuromuscular blockade did not occur when single supplemental doses were injected after 25% recovery from the previous dose or after cessation of a continuous infusion that was administered at a rate titrated to maintain 95% inhibition of the twitch response to peripheral stimulation.

Duration of clinical effect (time for spontaneous recovery of a single-twitch response to peripheral nerve stimulation to 25% of the control value [$T_{25}$])
Children 2 to 12 years of age:
110 to 120 mcg/kg—7 (range, 4 to 10) minutes.
200 mcg/kg—10 (range, 6 to 15) minutes.
250 mcg/kg—9 (range, 5 to 12) minutes.
Nongeriatric adults with normal hepatic and renal function:
70 to 100 mcg/kg—13 (range, 8 to 24) minutes.
150 mcg/kg—16 (range, 9 to 38) minutes.
200 mcg/kg—20 (range, 10 to 36) minutes.
250 mcg/kg—23 (range, 14 to 38) minutes.
Nongeriatric adults with end-stage renal disease undergoing renal transplantation:
150 mcg/kg (isoflurane/nitrous oxide/oxygen anesthesia)—30 (range, 19 to 58) minutes.
Nongeriatric adults with end-stage hepatic disease undergoing hepatic transplantation:
150 mcg/kg (isoflurane/oxygen anesthesia)—57 (range, 29 to 80) minutes.
Geriatric adults 68 to 77 years of age:
100 mcg/kg (isoflurane/nitrous oxide/oxygen anesthesia)—20 (range, 14 to 28) minutes; about 3 minutes longer than for nongeriatric adults receiving this dose under the same anesthetic regimen.

Recovery index (time for the twitch response to peripheral stimulation to increase spontaneously from 25 to 75% of the control value [$T_{25-75}$])
Children 2 to 10 years of age:
200 mcg/kg—About 5 minutes.
Nongeriatric adults with normal hepatic and renal function:
150 mcg/kg—About 6 minutes.
200 or 250 mcg/kg—About 7 to 8 minutes.

Time to spontaneous 95% recovery of the twitch response to peripheral stimulation ($T_{95}$)
Children 2 to 12 years of age:
110 mcg/kg—About 8 minutes.
200 mcg/kg—19 (range, 14 to 26) minutes.
Nongeriatric adults with normal hepatic and renal function:
70 to 100 mcg/kg—21 (range, 10 to 36) minutes.
150 mcg/kg—26 (range, 16 to 41) minutes.
200 mcg/kg—31 (range, 15 to 51) minutes.
250 mcg/kg—34 (range, 22 to 64) minutes.
Geriatric adults 65 to 80 years of age:
100 mcg/kg (isoflurane/nitrous oxide/oxygen anesthesia)—Approximately 37 minutes; about 5 minutes longer than for nongeriatric adults receiving this dose under the same anesthetic regimen.

Time to spontaneous recovery of the $T_4$:$T_1$ ratio (train-of-four stimulation) to 0.75
Children 2 to 12 years of age:
200 mcg/kg—16 (range, 12 to 23) minutes.
Nongeriatric adults with normal hepatic and renal function:
70 to 100 mcg/kg—21 (range, 10 to 36) minutes.
150 mcg/kg—26 (range, 15 to 45) minutes.
200 mcg/kg—34 (range, 19 to 56) minutes.
250 mcg/kg—43 (range, 26 to 75) minutes.

**Elimination**
Renal and biliary, as inactive metabolites, following biotransformation (enzymatic hydrolysis catalyzed by plasma cholinesterase). Plasma clearances of the 3 stereoisomers are 53 (range, 32 to 105), 99 (range, 52 to 230), and 4.2 (range, 2.4 to 5.4) mL per kg of body weight per minute for the trans-trans, cis-trans, and cis-cis diesters, respectively.

## Precautions to Consider

**Carcinogenicity**
Studies in animals have not been done.

**Mutagenicity**
Mivacurium displayed no mutagenicity in the Ames *Salmonella* assay, the mouse lymphoma assay, the human lymphocyte assay, or the *in vivo* rat bone marrow cytogenetic assay.

**Pregnancy/Reproduction**
Pregnancy—Adequate and well-controlled studies have not been done in pregnant women. However, the possibility of a prolonged response should be considered, because plasma cholinesterase activity may be reduced during pregnancy.
In animal studies, no maternal or fetal toxicity or teratogenicity occurred with subcutaneous administration of maximal subparalyzing doses to nonventilated pregnant rats or mice.
FDA Pregnancy Category C.
Labor and delivery—Use of mivacurium during labor, vaginal delivery, or cesarean section has not been studied. Whether administration during labor and delivery has any effects in the fetus has not been determined.
In animal studies, administration of 80 or 200 mcg per kg of body weight (mcg/kg) of mivacurium to female beagles undergoing cesarean section produced negligible concentrations of mivacurium in neonatal umbilical vessel blood. No deleterious effects on the puppies were observed.

**Breast-feeding**
It is not known whether mivacurium is distributed into human breast milk.

**Pediatrics**
Infants and children younger than 2 years of age—Appropriate studies on the relationship of age to the effects of mivacurium have not been performed in patients up to 2 years of age.
Children 2 to 12 years of age—Appropriate studies performed to date have not shown that mivacurium causes different, or more severe, adverse effects than have been reported in adults, or that the risk of adverse effects is increased in children. However, the $ED_{95}$ of mivacurium (dose required to produce 95% suppression of the adductor pollicis muscle twitch response to ulnar nerve stimulation) and the average infusion rate required to maintain a given degree of neuromuscular blockade are higher in children than in adults. The inverse relationship between mivacurium dosage requirement and the patient's age is significant among children of different ages (as well as between children and adults) when dosage is calculated on an mcg/kg basis, but not when it is calculated on an mcg per square meter of body surface area basis. Also, the onset of action of mivacurium is more rapid, and its duration of action is shorter, in children than in adults. Recovery after administration of a reversal agent also occurs more rapidly in children than in adults.

**Geriatrics**
Mivacurium has been studied in geriatric patients, some of whom had significant cardiovascular disease. No geriatrics-specific problems have

been documented to date. Although the duration of effect may be about 15 to 20% longer in elderly patients than in younger adults, studies have not shown significant variability in the pharmacokinetics of mivacurium (e.g., elimination half-life or clearance rate) that would account for the observed differences.

**Drug interactions and/or related problems**

The following drug interactions and/or related problems have been selected on the basis of their potential clinical significance (possible mechanism in parentheses where appropriate)—not necessarily inclusive (» = major clinical significance):

Note: Combinations containing any of the following medications, depending on the amount present, may also interact with this medication.

Some of the following interactions have not been documented with mivacurium. However, because they have been reported to occur with other nondepolarizing neuromuscular blocking agents, the possibility of a significant interaction with mivacurium must be considered.

Interactions reported below that may lead to enhanced neuromuscular blockade may result in prolonged paralysis, prolonged respiratory insufficiency, and/or difficulty in reversal. These interactions are of minimal clinical significance while the patient is being mechanically ventilated. With the exception of medications that can reduce the concentration or activity of plasma cholinesterase, these interactions may be less significant with a short-acting neuromuscular blocking agent such as mivacurium than with longer-acting agents. However, caution and careful monitoring of the patient are recommended during and following concurrent or sequential use of mivacurium with a medication that may significantly potentiate its effects, especially if there is a possibility of incomplete reversal of neuromuscular blockade postoperatively.

» Aminoglycosides, possibly including oral neomycin (if significant quantities are absorbed by patients with renal function impairment) or
Anesthetics, parenteral-local (large doses leading to significant plasma concentrations) or
Bacitracin or
» Capreomycin or
» Citrate-anticoagulated blood (massive transfusions) or
» Clindamycin or
Colistin or
Colistimethate sodium or
Lidocaine (systemic use, with intravenous doses > 5 mg/kg) or
» Lincomycin or
» Polymyxins or
Procaine (systemic use) or
Tetracyclines or
Trimethaphan (large doses)
(neuromuscular blocking activity of these medications may be additive to that of neuromuscular blocking agents; reversal agents have sometimes been ineffective in reversing neuromuscular blockade potentiated by aminoglycosides, clindamycin, lincomycin, or polymyxins)

Analgesics, opioid (narcotic), especially those commonly used as adjuncts to anesthesia
(central respiratory depressant effects of opioid analgesics may be additive to the respiratory insufficiency induced by neuromuscular blocking agents)
(concurrent use of a neuromuscular blocking agent prevents or reverses muscle rigidity induced by sufficiently high doses of most opioid analgesics, especially alfentanil, fentanyl, or sufentanil)

Anesthetics, hydrocarbon inhalation, such as:
Chloroform
Cyclopropane
Desflurane
Enflurane
Ether
Halothane
Isoflurane
Methoxyflurane
Trichloroethylene
(neuromuscular blocking activity of inhalation hydrocarbon anesthetics, especially desflurane, enflurane, or isoflurane, may be additive to that of nondepolarizing neuromuscular blocking agents, with the degree of potentiation being increased as the concentration of the anesthetic is increased; a reduction of mivacurium dosage may be necessary when it is given after steady-state anesthesia with one of these anesthetics has been established; with enflurane or isoflurane anesthesia, it is recommended that mivacurium dosage be decreased by about 25% for initial single doses and about 35 to 40% for administration by continuous infusion; although specific recommendations for altering mivacurium dosage during desflurane anesthesia are not currently available, desflurane has been shown to decrease the $ED_{95}$ of other nondepolarizing neuromuscular blocking agents [specifically, atracurium and pancuronium] by approximately 50%)
(halothane potentiates the effects of mivacurium to a lesser extent than enflurane or isoflurane; prior halothane administration may not decrease initial mivacurium dosage requirements, but halothane may decrease maintenance dose [infusion rate] requirements by about 20%, decrease mivacurium's onset of action, and prolong mivacurium's duration of action)

Antihypertensives or other hypotension-inducing medications or
Bradycardia-inducing medications
(although histamine release induced by rapid injection of large doses of mivacurium may increase heart rate, this effect is generally of brief duration, so that mivacurium should not significantly counteract bradycardia induced by other medications or vagal stimulation; however, mivacurium-induced histamine release may cause a temporary decrease in blood pressure, and it is possible that the risk of severe hypotension may be increased in patients receiving other hypotension-inducing medications; therefore, the incidence and/or severity of these effects may be higher with mivacurium than with a neuromuscular blocking agent that has significant vagolytic activity, especially in patients with compromised cardiac function and in patients receiving 2 or more medications that may decrease heart rate and/or blood pressure [e.g., benzodiazepines, beta-adrenergic blocking agents, calcium channel blocking agents, opioid analgesics] prior to and/or during surgery)

Antimyasthenics or
Edrophonium
(these agents antagonize the effects of nondepolarizing neuromuscular blocking agents; parenteral neostigmine, pyridostigmine, or edrophonium are indicated to reverse neuromuscular blockade following surgery, if necessary)
(neuromuscular blocking agents may antagonize the effects of antimyasthenics on skeletal muscle; temporary dosage adjustment may be required to control symptoms of myasthenia gravis following surgery)

Any medication that may reduce plasma cholinesterase concentrations or activity, such as:
Cytotoxic antineoplastic agents
» Demecarium
» Echothiophate
» Insecticides, neurotoxic, recent exposure to, possibly including large quantities of topical malathion
» Isoflurophate
Metoclopramide
Phenelzine
Procaine (systemic)
(reduction of plasma concentrations or activity of cholinesterase, the enzyme that catalyzes hydrolysis of mivacurium, to 50% or less of normal, may enhance and prolong mivacurium's effects; reduction of plasma cholinesterase activity may persist for weeks or months after therapy with demecarium, echothiophate, or isoflurophate has been discontinued)

Calcium channel blocking agents
(although an interaction with mivacurium has not been documented, verapamil and nifedipine have been shown to potentiate the effects of several other neuromuscular blocking agents; also, difficulty in reversing verapamil-potentiated neuromuscular blockade with a single dose of neostigmine has been reported)

Calcium salts
(calcium salts may reverse the effects of nondepolarizing neuromuscular blocking agents)

Carbamazepine and/or
Phenytoin
(although an interaction with mivacurium has not been documented, resistance to the effects of other nondepolarizing neuromuscular agents has occurred in patients receiving chronic carbamazepine and/or phenytoin therapy, leading to a lengthening of the time needed to achieve adequate skeletal muscle relaxation and to significantly accelerated recovery from an initial or supplemental dose)

Dantrolene or
Furosemide or
Lithium or
Magnesium salts, parenteral, or

» Procainamide or
» Quinidine
  (these medications may enhance and/or prolong the effects of neuromuscular blocking agents)

Neuromuscular blocking agents, other
  (prior administration of succinylcholine [for endotracheal intubation] has caused potentiation of some of the other nondepolarizing neuromuscular blocking agents; although the effect of succinylcholine administration on subsequent administration of mivacurium has not been studied, it is recommended that mivacurium not be administered until after spontaneous recovery from succinylcholine has begun)
  (use of subparalyzing doses of mivacurium prior to succinylcholine, to attenuate some of succinylcholine's adverse effects, has not been studied)
  (administration of mivacurium in conjunction with other nondepolarizing neuromuscular blocking agents has not been studied)

**Medical considerations/Contraindications**
The medical considerations/contraindications included have been selected on the basis of their potential clinical significance (reasons given in parentheses where appropriate)—not necessarily inclusive (» = major clinical significance).

Note: Medical problems that may lead to enhanced neuromuscular blockade may result in prolonged paralysis, prolonged respiratory impairment, and/or difficulty in reversal. With the exception of medical conditions associated with a reduction of the concentration or activity of plasma cholinesterase, such medical problems may be less troublesome with a short-acting neuromuscular blocking agent such as mivacurium than with longer-acting agents. However, some patients may require unexpectedly prolonged monitoring and ventilatory assistance postoperatively.

*Except under special circumstances, this medication should not be used when the following medical problem exists:*

» Genetic abnormality, homozygous for atypical cholinesterase gene
  (patients with homozygous atypical cholinesterase gene abnormality are extremely sensitive to the effects of mivacurium; in 3 such patients, a dose of only 30 mcg/kg produced complete neuromuscular block lasting from 26 to 128 minutes, although administration of conventional doses of neostigmine after spontaneous recovery began effectively antagonized the remaining block; in a fourth patient, a dose of 180 mcg/kg produced complete neuromuscular block for about 4 hours, and the patient was not extubated until 8 hours after administration [reversal was not attempted]; it is recommended that an alternative nondepolarizing neuromuscular blocking agent be used instead)

*Risk-benefit should be considered when the following medical problems exist:*

Allergy, including asthma, or other conditions predisposing to complications associated with histamine release or
Cardiovascular disease or other conditions in which histamine release–induced hypotension or tachycardia would be particularly hazardous
  (it is recommended that initial dosage of mivacurium not exceed 150 mcg/kg, administered over 60 seconds, to decrease the risk of histamine release–related adverse effects)

Burns
  (although resistance to the effects of nondepolarizing neuromuscular blocking agents has been reported in burn patients, the reduction in plasma cholinesterase activity that may occur in burn patients may prolong the effect of mivacurium; because the effect of mivacurium in these patients may be unpredictable, it is recommended that the response to a test dose of 15 to 20 mcg/kg, as determined via peripheral nerve stimulation, be used as a guide to appropriate dosage)

Carcinoma, bronchogenic, or other malignancy
  (the duration of action of nondepolarizing neuromuscular agents may be prolonged in patients with bronchogenic carcinoma; also, the reduction in plasma cholinesterase activity that may occur in patients with malignancy may prolong the effect of mivacurium)

Dehydration or
Electrolyte or acid-base imbalance, especially:
  Hypokalemia
  (action of neuromuscular blocking agents may be altered; neuromuscular blockade is usually counteracted by alkalosis and enhanced by acidosis, but mixed imbalances may be present, leading to unpredictable responses; also, the reduction in plasma cholinesterase activity that may occur in dehydrated patients may prolong the effect of mivacurium)
  (serum potassium determinations may be advisable prior to administration of a nondepolarizing neuromuscular blocking agent, because hypokalemia tends to enhance the blockade produced by these medications; adjustment of dosage of the neuromuscular blocking agent, or correction of potassium concentration prior to administration, may be needed)

» Familial periodic paralysis, hypokalemic or hyperkalemic, or
» Muscular dystrophy or
» Myasthenia gravis or
» Myasthenic syndrome (Eaton-Lambert syndrome) or
» Other neuromuscular disease leading to muscle weakness
  (risk of severe and prolonged muscle paralysis or weakness is increased; neuromuscular blocking agents are best avoided in patients with familial periodic paralysis or myasthenia gravis [and may not be needed in patients with myasthenia gravis if a volatile anesthetic with potent relaxant properties, such as enflurane or isoflurane, is administered in sufficient quantities]; if a neuromuscular blocking agent is needed for these patients, mivacurium may be preferable to longer-acting agents, but caution is recommended; patient response to a test dose of 15 to 20 mcg/kg, as determined via peripheral nerve stimulation, should be used as a guide to appropriate dosage)

» Genetic abnormality, heterozygous for atypical cholinesterase gene, or
Other conditions in which plasma cholinesterase activity may be substantially reduced, such as:
  Anemia, severe
  Exposure to neurotoxic insecticides or other cholinesterase inhibitors
  Hepatic disease, severe or chronic, including hepatic cirrhosis
  Malnutrition
  Pregnancy
  (effects of mivacurium may be enhanced and/or prolonged, especially when plasma cholinesterase activity is reduced to 50% or less of normal; in most patients, the time to 25% recovery of the twitch response to peripheral stimulation [$T_{25}$] is prolonged [by 8 to 11 minutes following doses of 100 to 200 mcg/kg in patients with heterozygous gene abnormality, compared with genotypically normal patients], but not the time from 25% to 75% recovery [$T_{25-75}$]; although mivacurium has been used safely in patients with reduced plasma cholinesterase activity, it is recommended that the response to a test dose of 15 to 20 mcg/kg, as determined via peripheral nerve stimulation, be used as a guide to appropriate dosage)

Hypothermia
  (intensity and duration of action of nondepolarizing neuromuscular blocking agents may be increased)

Obesity
  (the risk of a > 30% decrease in mean arterial blood pressure is increased in obese patients receiving doses calculated on the basis of actual body weight; it is recommended that dosage for these patients be calculated on the basis of ideal body weight)

Pulmonary function impairment or
Respiratory depression
  (risk of additive respiratory depression or impairment)

Sensitivity to mivacurium

## Side/Adverse Effects

Note: Mivacurium failed to trigger malignant hyperthermia in a study in malignant hyperthermia–susceptible swine. Whether mivacurium may precipitate malignant hyperthermia in susceptible humans has not been assessed.

Bradycardia may occur during mivacurium-assisted anesthesia, but is not likely to be a direct effect of the medication. Because mivacurium (unlike gallium and pancuronium) does not have vagolytic activity, it does not counteract bradycardia induced by other medications (e.g., anesthetics, opioid analgesics) or vagal stimulation.

The following side/adverse effects have been selected on the basis of their potential clinical significance (possible signs and symptoms in parentheses where appropriate)—not necessarily inclusive:

**Those indicating need for medical attention**
Incidence less frequent
  *Hypotension*

Incidence rare (1% or less)
  *Bronchospasm; cardiac arrhythmia; erythema; hypoxemia; injection site reaction; phlebitis; skin rash; tachycardia; urticaria; wheezing*

Note: Hypotension, tachycardia, bronchospasm, and/or wheezing may result from mivacurium-induced histamine release, which may occur when large initial doses of the medication are administered rapidly. In most patients, these effects last only a few minutes and do not require treatment. In clinical trials, *hypotension* requiring treatment occurred in 1 to 2% of patients receiving > 200 mcg per kg of body weight (mcg/kg) of mivacurium over 5 to 15 seconds, and 2 to 4% of cardiac surgery patients receiving > 200 mcg/kg over 60 seconds, but did not occur with doses of 150 mcg/kg or less.

*Hypotension* may also occur during mivacurium-assisted surgery because mivacurium does not counteract the hypotensive effects of other medications or vagal stimulation.

**Those indicating need for medical attention only if they continue or are bothersome**
Incidence less frequent or rare
   *Dizziness; muscle spasm*

**Those not indicating need for medical attention**
Incidence more frequent
   *Flushing*—incidence 15 to 20%
   Note: *Flushing* occurs mostly when initial doses of 150 mcg/kg or higher are administered over 5 to 15 seconds. It usually appears within 1 to 2 minutes after administration and persists for 3 to 5 minutes.

## Overdose

For specific information on the agents used in the management of mivacurium overdose, see:
- *Atropine* in *Anticholinergics/Antispasmodics (Systemic)* monograph;
- *Edrophonium (Systemic)* monograph;
- *Glycopyrrolate* in *Anticholinergics/Antispasmodics (Systemic)* monograph; and/or
- *Neostigmine* in *Antimyasthenics (Systemic)* monograph.

For more information on the management of overdose or unintentional ingestion, **contact a Poison Control Center** (see *Poison Control Center Listing*).

**For treatment of overdose**
Specific treatment—
   Because of mivacurium's short duration of action, administration of a reversal agent may not be necessary, or may not speed recovery to a clinically significant extent. However, an anticholinesterase agent, e.g., neostigmine or edrophonium, may be administered if needed. Use of an antagonist is an adjunct to, and not a substitute for, measures to ensure adequate ventilation. Ventilatory assistance must be continued until the patient can maintain an adequate ventilatory exchange unassisted. A suitable antimuscarinic agent (e.g., atropine, glycopyrrolate) should be administered prior to or concurrently with the antagonist to counteract its muscarinic side effects. It is recommended that reversal agents be administered only after some spontaneous recovery, as demonstrated using a peripheral nerve stimulator, has taken place. In adults, doses of 30 to 64 mcg/kg of neostigmine or 500 mcg/kg of edrophonium, administered at 10% recovery from neuromuscular block, generally produce 95% recovery of the single twitch response, and 75% recovery of the $T_4:T_1$ ratio (train-of-four stimulation), in about 10 minutes. In children younger than 12 years of age, 300 mcg/kg of edrophonium, administered at 11% or more recovery, produces 95% recovery of the single twitch response in less than 4 minutes. However, recovery may be delayed if the reversal agent is administered in the presence of medications or medical conditions that tend to prolong the effects of mivacurium.

Monitoring—
   Determining the degree of the neuromuscular blockade with a peripheral nerve stimulator.

Supportive care—
   For hypotension or other adverse hemodynamic effects—Cardiovascular support, e.g., fluid administration, proper positioning of the patient, and/or administration of a vasopressor may be needed.
   For apnea or prolonged paralysis—Maintaining an adequate airway and assisting or controlling ventilation. If prolonged paralysis occurs, checking the patient's plasma cholinesterase activity (via determination of dibucaine number and activity). If the patient's cholinesterase activity is found to be significantly reduced, continued respiratory support, rather than administration of a reversal agent, is recommended.

## General Dosing Information

Neuromuscular blocking agents have no clinically significant effect on consciousness or the pain threshold; therefore, when used as an adjunct to surgery, they should always be used with adequate anesthesia or sedation.

Because neuromuscular blocking agents suppress respiration, they should be used only by individuals experienced in tracheal intubation, artificial respiration, and the administration of oxygen under positive pressure; facilities for these procedures should be immediately available.

Mivacurium is intended for intravenous administration only.

The stated doses are intended as a guideline. Actual dosage must be individualized. It is recommended that a peripheral nerve stimulator be used to monitor response, need for additional doses, and reversal.

The $ED_{95}$ (dose required to produce maximum [95%] suppression of the adductor pollicis muscle twitch response to ulnar nerve stimulation) is about 70 (range, 60 to 90) mcg per kg of body weight (mcg/kg) in adults and about 100 to 110 mcg/kg in children 2 to 12 years of age (opioid/nitrous oxide/oxygen anesthesia).

A reduction in initial and maintenance doses of a nondepolarizing neuromuscular blocking agent may be required when it is administered after steady-state anesthesia has been established with a volatile (hydrocarbon) inhalation anesthetic. Halothane may cause less potentiation of mivacurium than desflurane, enflurane, or isoflurane.

A reduction of initial dosage may be advisable for patients in whom histamine release may be hazardous; patients with decreased plasma cholinesterase activity, hepatic or renal disease, burns, severe electrolyte abnormalities, or neuromuscular disease; and other patients in whom there is a risk of potentiation of neuromuscular blockade or difficulty with reversal. Supplemental doses should be titrated according to patient response. A slower rate of administration (i.e., administration of initial doses over 30 to 60 seconds) and/or pretreatment with antihistamines (both $H_1$- and $H_2$-receptor blockers) may also decrease the risk to patients who may be harmed by histamine release.

For obese patients (> 30% above ideal body weight for height), dosage of mivacurium should be calculated on the basis of ideal body weight.

## Parenteral Dosage Forms

### MIVACURIUM INJECTION

Note: Mivacurium injection contains mivacurium chloride, but the dosing and strengths are expressed in terms of mivacurium base.

**Usual adult dose**
Neuromuscular blocking agent—
   Initial (for endotracheal intubation and surgical relaxation)—
      Intravenous, 150 to 200 mcg (0.15 to 0.2 mg) per kg of body weight, administered over five to fifteen seconds, to provide intubating conditions in about two to two and one-half minutes and about fifteen to twenty minutes of clinically effective neuromuscular block (opioid/nitrous oxide/oxygen anesthesia).
      Note: Satisfactory intubating conditions are attained more slowly when initial doses lower than 150 mcg per kg of body weight are administered.
         For patients with cardiovascular disease or other patients who may be especially sensitive to histamine release, it is recommended that initial doses of 150 mcg per kg of body weight, or lower, be administered over at least sixty seconds. In most other patients, higher initial doses may be administered when a more rapid onset of action is needed, although the risk of inducing hypotension in some patients must be kept in mind. However, administration of higher initial doses may not reduce the onset of action sufficiently to permit emergency intubation. Initial doses higher than 250 mcg (0.25 mg) per kg of body weight are not recommended.
         Initial dosage may be decreased by 25% or more when mivacurium is administered after anesthesia with enflurane or isoflurane has been established. The need for a reduction in initial dosage should also be anticipated after anesthesia with desflurane has been established, but studies to determine the extent to which dosage should be reduced have not been done. A reduction in the initial mivacurium dose may not be needed after anesthesia with halothane has been established.
   Maintenance:
      Intravenous, to be administered after the twitch response to a previous dose has returned to about 10 to 25% of the control value, or after reappearance of the second twitch response to train-of-four stimulation—About 100 mcg (0.1 mg) per kg of body weight, to provide about fifteen additional minutes of clinically effective block (opioid/nitrous oxide/oxygen anesthesia). Smaller or larger doses may be given as needed to provide shorter or longer durations of action.
      Note: Maintenance dosage requirements may be reduced by 25% or more when enflurane or isoflurane is being administered,

and by a smaller amount when halothane is being administered. The need for a reduction in maintenance dosage should also be anticipated when desflurane is being administered, but studies to determine the extent to which dosage should be reduced have not been done.

Maintenance doses of mivacurium injection may also be given by intravenous infusion. See *Mivacurium in dextrose injection* for recommended doses. The manufacturer's prescribing information contains a table showing infusion delivery rate requirements (in mL per hour) for administration of various doses (in mcg per kg of body weight per minute) to patients of different weights.

**Usual pediatric dose**
Neuromuscular blocking agent—
    Children up to 2 years of age:
        Dosage has not been established.
    Children 2 to 12 years of age:
        Initial—Intravenous, 200 to 250 mcg (0.2 to 0.25 mg) per kg of body weight, administered over five to fifteen seconds, to provide maximum blockade in about two minutes and about ten minutes of clinically effective block (opioid/nitrous oxide/oxygen anesthesia).
        Maintenance—Intravenous, as required by clinical circumstances and the desired duration of clinically effective block. Additional doses may be required more frequently than in adults.

Note: No information is available about the effect of desflurane, enflurane, or isoflurane anesthesia on dosage requirements and/or the duration of clinical effect of mivacurium in pediatric patients. However, in two studies, the duration of clinical effect with nitrous oxide/halothane/oxygen anesthesia was not significantly different from that produced by the same dose under nitrous oxide/opioid/oxygen anesthesia.

Maintenance doses of mivacurium injection may also be given by intravenous infusion. See *Mivacurium in dextrose injection* for recommended doses. The manufacturer's prescribing information contains a table showing infusion delivery rate requirements (in mL per hour) for administration of various doses (in mcg per kg of body weight per minute) to patients of different weights.

**Strength(s) usually available**
U.S.—
    2 mg per mL (Rx) [*Mivacron*].
Canada—
    Not commercially available.

**Packaging and storage**
Store between 15 and 25 °C (59 and 77 °F), protected from exposure to direct ultraviolet light and from freezing, unless otherwise specified by manufacturer.

**Stability**
Mivacurium injection is physically and chemically stable for up to 24 hours when diluted to 500 mcg (0.5 mg) per mL with 5% dextrose injection, 5% dextrose and 0.9% sodium chloride injection, 0.9% sodium chloride injection, lactated Ringer's injection, or 5% dextrose in lactated Ringer's injection and stored in polyvinyl chloride bags at 5 to 25 °C (4 to 77 °F). After preparation, the diluted solution should be used within 24 hours. Also, the solution should be used for one patient only, and unused portions discarded.

**Incompatibilities**
Mivacurium injection should not be admixed with other medications (except for preparation of an infusion solution using a diluent listed under *Stability*, above). Mivacurium injection is acidic (pH 3.5 to 5.0) and may not be compatible with alkaline solutions (pH > 8.5), such as barbiturate solutions.

## MIVACURIUM IN DEXTROSE INJECTION

Note: Mivacurium in dextrose injection contains mivacurium chloride, but the dosing and strengths are expressed in terms of mivacurium base.

**Usual adult dose**
Neuromuscular blocking agent—
    Maintenance: Intravenous infusion, started after some evidence of recovery from an initial dose—Initially 9 to 10 mcg (0.009 to 0.01 mg) per kg of body weight per minute (opioid/nitrous oxide/oxygen anesthesia), then adjusted according to clinical conditions and response to peripheral nerve stimulation. Infusion rate requirements are generally significantly higher during the first fifteen minutes of infusion, after which an average dose of 6 to 7 mcg (0.006 to 0.007) per kg of body weight per minute is usually sufficient. Although infusion rate requirements are subject to wide interindividual variability (ranging from 1 to 15 mcg [0.001 to 0.015 mg] per kg of body weight per minute), dosage requirements for an individual patient, after the first fifteen-minute adjustment period, remain fairly stable.

Note: A lower initial infusion rate, e.g., 4 mcg (0.004 mg) per kg of body weight per minute, is recommended when an intravenous infusion is started simultaneously with administration of an initial dose.

Infusion rate requirements are reduced after anesthesia with a volatile hydrocarbon anesthetic has been established. Enflurane or isoflurane, depending on the concentration being administered, may reduce the infusion rate requirement by 35 to 40% or more. Halothane may reduce the infusion rate requirement by about 20%.

The manufacturer's prescribing information contains a table showing infusion delivery rate requirements (in mL per hour) for administration of various doses (in mcg per kg of body weight per minute) to patients of different weights.

**Usual pediatric dose**
Neuromuscular blocking agent—
    Maintenance: Infants and children up to 2 years of age—Dosage has not been established.
    Children 2 to 12 years of age—Intravenous infusion, about 14 mcg (0.014 mg) per kg of body weight per minute (average for opioid/nitrous oxide/oxygen anesthesia) or as required. In general, higher infusion rates are required for pediatric patients than for adults.

Note: The manufacturer's prescribing information contains a table showing infusion delivery rate requirements (in mL per hour) for administration of various doses (in mcg per kg of body weight per minute) to patients of different weights.

**Strength(s) usually available**
U.S.—
    500 mcg (0.5 mg) of mivacurium and 5% of dextrose per mL (Rx) [*Mivacron*].
Canada—
    Not commercially available.

**Packaging and storage**
Store between 15 and 25 °C (59 and 77 °F), protected from exposure to direct ultraviolet light and from freezing, unless otherwise specified by manufacturer.

**Stability**
Mivacurium in dextrose injection is intended for single-patient use only. Unused portions of the solution should be discarded.

For Y-site administration, mivacurium in dextrose injection is compatible with 5% dextrose injection, 0.9% sodium chloride injection, 5% dextrose and 0.9% sodium chloride injection, lactated Ringer's injection, 5% dextrose in lactated Ringer's injection, and, when the following are diluted for intravenous injection as directed, with alfentanil hydrochloride injection, fentanyl citrate injection, midazolam hydrochloride injection, and droperidol injection.

**Incompatibilities**
Mivacurium in dextrose injection is acidic (pH 3.5 to 5.0) and may not be compatible with alkaline solutions (pH > 8.5), such as barbiturate solutions.

Mivacurium in dextrose injection should not be admixed with other medications or used in series connections with other medications.

## Selected Bibliography

Savarese JJ, Ali HH, Basta SJ, et al. The clinical neuromuscular pharmacology of mivacurium chloride (BW B1090U). Anesthesiology 1988; 68: 723-32.

Sarner JB, Brandom BW, Woelfel SK, et al. Clinical pharmacology of mivacurium chloride (BW B1090U) in children during nitrous oxide–halothane and nitrous oxide–narcotic anesthesia. Anesth Analg 1989; 68: 116-21.

Choi WW, Mehta MP, Murray DJ, et al. Neuromuscular and cardiovascular effects of mivacurium chloride in surgical patients receiving nitrous oxide–narcotic or nitrous oxide–isoflurane anaesthesia. Can J Anaesth 1989; 36: 641-50.

Revised: 01/18/93

# MOEXIPRIL Systemic†

VA CLASSIFICATION (Primary/Secondary): CV800/CV409; CV900
Commonly used brand name(s): *Univasc*.
Note: For a listing of dosage forms and brand names by country availability, see *Dosage Forms* section(s).

†Not commercially available in Canada.

## Category
Antihypertensive.

## Indications
**Accepted**
Hypertension (treatment)—Moexipril is indicated, alone or in combination with a thiazide diuretic, in the treatment of hypertension.

## Pharmacology/Pharmacokinetics
**Physicochemical characteristics**
Molecular weight—Moexipril hydrochloride: 535.04.
Moexiprilat: 470.53.

**Mechanism of action/Effect**
Moexipril is a nonsulfhydryl-containing angiotensin-converting enzyme (ACE) inhibitor. It is a prodrug for moexiprilat, the active metabolite. Moexiprilat lowers blood pressure by competitively inhibiting ACE activity. ACE catalyzes the conversion of angiotensin I to angiotensin II. Angiotensin II, a vasoconstrictor, stimulates aldosterone secretion by the adrenal cortex and directly suppresses renin release. Inhibition of ACE decreases angiotensin II formation, resulting in reduced peripheral arterial resistance, increased plasma renin activity, and decreased aldosterone secretion. The decrease in aldosterone secretion results in diuresis and natriuresis and a slight increase in serum potassium concentrations.

**Other actions/effects**
ACE is also known as kininase II, an enzyme that degrades bradykinin. After ACE inhibition, local kinin concentrations may increase and the formation of prostaglandins may be enhanced. Both bradykinin and prostaglandins have local vasodilatory effects that may contribute to moexipril's antihypertensive effects.

**Absorption**
Incompletely absorbed. Bioavailability of moexipril is approximately 13% and is significantly affected by food, which reduces the peak plasma concentration ($C_{max}$) and area under the plasma concentration–time curve (AUC). An open, randomized, crossover trial found that bioavailability of moexipril was reduced by 40% when administered with food. Food appears to decrease the rate of absorption more than the extent of absorption. The decrease in bioavailability may not be clinically significant, especially during long-term dosing.

**Distribution**
$Vol_D$ of moexiprilat— 183 L.

**Protein binding**
Moexiprilat—Moderate (50%).

**Biotransformation**
Moexipril—Rapidly converted to moexiprilat, the active metabolite. Conversion to the active metabolite is thought to require carboxyesterases and is likely to occur in organs or tissues, other than the gastrointestinal tract, in which carboxyesterases occur. The liver is thought to be one site of conversion, but not the primary site.

**Half-life**
Elimination:
  Moexipril—
    Approximately 1 hour.
  Moexiprilat—
    2 to 9 hours.
    Effective elimination half-life: Approximately 12 hours.

**Onset of action**
Approximately 1 hour.

**Time to peak concentration**
Moexipril—1.5 hours.
Moexiprilat—3 to 4 hours.

**Elimination**
Fecal—53% (52% as moexiprilat and 1% as moexipril).
Renal—13% (1% as moexipril, 7% as moexiprilat, and 5% as other metabolites).
In dialysis—It is not known whether moexipril is dialyzable.

## Precautions to Consider

**Cross-sensitivity and/or related problems**
Patients hypersensitive to other angiotensin-converting enzyme (ACE) inhibitors may also be hypersensitive to moexipril.

**Carcinogenicity**
No evidence of carcinogenicity was found in long-term studies in mice and rats at doses up to 14 or 27.3 times the maximum recommended human dose (MRHD) on a mg per square meter of body surface area ($mg/m^2$) basis.

**Mutagenicity**
No evidence of mutagenicity was found in the Ames test and microbial reverse mutation assay, with and without activation, or in an *in vivo* nucleus anomaly test. However, at a 20-hour harvest time, increased chromosomal aberration frequency in Chinese hamster ovary cells was detected under metabolic activation conditions.

**Pregnancy/Reproduction**
Fertility—No evidence of impaired fertility, reproductive toxicity, or teratogenicity was detected in reproduction studies performed in rabbits and rats at doses up to 0.7 and 90.9 times the MRHD, respectively, on a $mg/m^2$ basis.

Pregnancy—ACE inhibitors, including moexipril, can cause fetal and neonatal morbidity and mortality when administered to pregnant women during the second and third trimesters. Moexipril should be discontinued as soon as possible when pregnancy is detected unless no alternative therapy can be used. In the latter instance, serial ultrasound examinations should be performed to assess the intra-amniotic environment. If oligohydramnios is observed, moexipril should be discontinued unless it is considered lifesaving for the mother. Perinatal diagnostics, such as contraction-stress testing (CST), a non-stress test (NST), or biophysical profiling (BPP) may also be appropriate during the applicable week of pregnancy. Oligohydramnios may not appear until after the fetus has sustained irreversible damage.

Fetal exposure to ACE inhibitors limited to the first trimester is not associated with fetal or neonatal morbidity. Fetal exposure to ACE inhibitors during the second and third trimesters can cause hypotension, renal failure, anuria, skull hypoplasia, and death in the fetus or neonate. Maternal oligohydramnios, which may result from decreased fetal renal function, has been reported, and has been associated with fetal limb contractures, craniofacial deformation, and hypoplastic lung development. Prematurity, intrauterine growth retardation, and patent ductus arteriosus have also been reported, although the relationship of these occurrences to drug exposure is not clear.

Infants exposed *in utero* to moexipril should be closely observed for hypotension, oliguria, and hyperkalemia. Oliguria should be treated with support of blood pressure and renal perfusion.

Embryotoxic, fetotoxic, or teratogenic effects were not observed in rats or rabbits given up to 90.9 and 0.7 times the MRHD, respectively, on a $mg/m^2$ basis.

FDA Pregnancy Category C (first trimester).
FDA Pregnancy Category D (second and third trimesters).

**Breast-feeding**
It is not known whether moexipril is distributed into breast milk. However, problems in humans have not been documented.

**Pediatrics**
No information is available on the relationship of age to the effects of moexipril in pediatric patients. Safety and efficacy have not been established.

**Geriatrics**
Use of moexipril in a limited number of patients 65 years of age and over (33% of patients in clinical studies) has not demonstrated geriatrics-specific problems that would limit the usefulness of moexipril in the elderly. However, moexipril plasma concentrations are slightly higher and renal clearance is reduced in these patients as compared with younger individuals.

**Pharmacogenetics**
Black hypertensive patients may be less responsive to the antihypertensive effects of moexipril, possibly because these patients may have low-renin hypertension. Black patients also may have a greater risk of developing ACE inhibitor–induced angioedema, or may have more severe angioedema, than white patients.

**Surgical**

It is recommended that ACE inhibitors be withheld before surgery because of reports of abnormal responses to the induction of anesthesia and poor tolerance of hypovolemia with concurrent administration of ACE inhibitors.

**Drug interactions and/or related problems**

The following drug interactions and/or related problems have been selected on the basis of their potential clinical significance (possible mechanism in parentheses where appropriate)—not necessarily inclusive (» = major clinical significance):

Note: Combinations containing any of the following medications, depending on the amount present, may also interact with this medication.

Alcohol
(use with ACE inhibitors may produce postural hypotensive effects shortly after drinking alcohol, especially when initiating ACE inhibitor therapy)

Allopurinol
(concurrent use with another ACE inhibitor, captopril, has been reported to cause hypersensitivity reactions in two cases; however, the basis for this interaction cannot be determined)

Antacids that contain both aluminum and magnesium
(concurrent use with another ACE inhibitor, captopril, has resulted in reduced bioavailability)

Anti-inflammatory drugs, nonsteroidal (NSAIDs)
(concurrent and, especially, long-term use of NSAIDs can decrease the effectiveness of ACE inhibitors, presumably by counteracting the effect of ACE inhibitor–stimulated prostaglandin biosynthesis; concurrent use in patients with low renal perfusion can lead to further renal deterioration)

Digoxin
(pharmacokinetic interactions have not been reported with concurrent use of moexipril; however, increases in serum digoxin concentrations have been reported with concurrent use of another ACE inhibitor, captopril)

» Diuretics or
Hypotension-producing medications, other (see *Appendix II*)
(concurrent use may produce additive hypotensive effects, especially when initiating moexipril therapy; if diuretics are used concurrently, withdrawal of diuretic therapy for several days, reducing the initial dose of moexipril, or cautiously increasing salt intake before initiation of moexipril therapy may minimize hypotensive effects)

» Diuretics, potassium-sparing or
» Potassium-containing medications or
» Potassium supplements or substances containing high concentrations of potassium or
» Salt substitutes that contain substantial amounts of potassium
(concurrent use may lead to further increases in serum potassium; caution and monitoring of serum potassium concentrations are recommended)

Lithium
(increases in serum lithium concentrations and symptoms of lithium toxicity have been reported during concurrent use with ACE inhibitors; caution and frequent monitoring of serum lithium concentrations are recommended)

Sympathomimetics
(concurrent use of these agents may counteract the antihypertensive effects of moexipril; the patient should be carefully monitored to confirm that the desired therapeutic effect is obtained)

**Laboratory value alterations**

The following have been selected on the basis of their potential clinical significance (possible effect in parentheses where appropriate)—not necessarily inclusive (» = major clinical significance):

With physiology/laboratory test values
Alkaline phosphatase, serum and
Bilirubin, serum and
Transaminases, serum
(significant increases may be a sign of ACE inhibitor–associated hepatotoxicity)

Antinuclear antibody (ANA) titer
(a positive ANA titer has been associated rarely with use of other ACE inhibitors, although it has not been associated with moexipril)

Blood urea nitrogen (BUN) and
Creatinine, serum
(concentrations may be transiently increased, especially in patients who are currently taking diuretics and in patients with renal function impairment)

Potassium, serum
(concentrations may be increased secondary to reduced circulating aldosterone concentrations, especially in patients with renal function impairment and/or diabetes mellitus)

Protein, urine
(protein in urine has been reported with use of other ACE inhibitors; however, ACE inhibitors may have a beneficial antiproteinuric effect in patients with renal diseases associated with proteinuria, such as diabetic nephropathy)

Uric acid, serum
(concentration increases have been reported)

**Medical considerations/Contraindications**

The medical considerations/contraindications included have been selected on the basis of their potential clinical significance (reasons given in parentheses where appropriate)—not necessarily inclusive (» = major clinical significance):

*Except under special circumstances, this medication should not be used when the following medical problems exist:*

» Angioedema, history of, related to previous ACE inhibitor therapy
(increased risk for development of moexipril-related angioedema)
» Hypersensitivity to moexipril

*Risk-benefit should be considered when the following medical problems exist:*

» Angioedema, hereditary or
» Angioedema, idiopathic, history of
(increased risk for development of angioedema)

Aortic stenosis or
Cerebrovascular disease or
Ischemic heart disease
(reduction in blood pressure from ACE inhibitor therapy could result in cerebrovascular accident or myocardial infarction)

Collagen-vascular disease, such as systemic lupus erythematosus (SLE) or scleroderma
(increased risk for development of neutropenia or agranulocytosis with ACE inhibitor therapy)

Congestive heart failure
(ACE inhibitor therapy may interfere with the compensatory mechanisms of the renin-angiotensin-aldosterone system in heart failure patients. The glomerular filtration rate [GFR] may be further reduced in patients with poor renal perfusion, leading to oliguria and/or progressive azotemia and, possibly, acute renal failure and/or death)

» Dehydration (sodium or volume depletion due to excessive perspiration, vomiting, diarrhea, prolonged diuretic therapy, dialysis, or dietary salt restriction)
(increased risk of symptomatic hypotension; sodium-depleted patients, usually as a result of diuretic therapy, are at increased risk of developing ACE inhibitor–induced acute renal dysfunction and/or failure. Renal insufficiency caused by ACE inhibition is, in nearly all cases, reversible after discontinuing the ACE inhibitor)

Diabetes mellitus
(increased risk of hyperkalemia; increased insulin sensitivity and/or increased glucose tolerance has been reported in diabetic patients receiving ACE inhibitors)

» Dialysis with high-flux membranes or
Low-density lipoprotein apheresis with dextran sulfate absorption
(anaphylactoid reactions have been reported in patients undergoing these procedures who are concurrently taking an ACE inhibitor)

Hepatic function impairment
(peak plasma concentration [$C_{max}$] and area under the plasma concentration–time curve [AUC] may be increased for moexipril; $C_{max}$ may be decreased and AUC may be increased for moexiprilat)

» Hymenoptera venom desensitizing treatment
(life-threatening anaphylactoid reactions have been reported in two patients undergoing desensitizing treatment with hymenoptera venom while receiving ACE inhibitors)

» Hyperkalemia
(further increases in serum potassium concentrations may occur secondary to decreased aldosterone secretion)

» Renal artery stenosis, bilateral or in a single kidney or
» Renal function impairment
(plasma concentrations of moexipril and moexiprilat may be increased due to decreased elimination; increased risk of agranulocytosis and neutropenia, hyperkalemia, and ACE inhibitor–induced

acute renal insufficiency and/or failure; increases in blood urea nitrogen [BUN] and serum creatinine may occur, especially in those patients pretreated with a diuretic; renal function should be monitored during the first few weeks of moexipril therapy; dosage adjustment and/or discontinuation of the diuretic may be necessary)

### Patient monitoring
The following may be especially important in patient monitoring (other tests may be warranted in some patients, depending on condition; » = major clinical significance):

» Blood pressure measurements
(antihypertensive effect of moexipril may diminish towards the end of the dosing interval; blood pressure measurements should be taken just before dosing to adjust the dose of moexipril according to the patient's response)

Leukocyte count
(determinations recommended periodically in patients at risk for neutropenia, particularly those with renal function impairment and/or a collagen-vascular disease)

Potassium, serum
(determinations recommended periodically, especially in patients concurrently receiving potassium supplements or potassium-sparing diuretics)

Renal function
(determinations recommended during the first few weeks of therapy in patients with renal function impairment)

## Side/Adverse Effects
The following side/adverse effects have been selected on the basis of their potential clinical significance (possible signs and symptoms in parentheses where appropriate)—not necessarily inclusive:

Note: *Asymptomatic acute renal insufficiency* has occurred in patients taking ACE inhibitors. In clinical trials, increases in serum creatinine concentrations to at least 140% of baseline occurred in 1% of patients treated with moexipril and in 2% of patients treated with moexipril and hydrochlorothiazide. These hypertensive patients had no apparent pre-existing renal disease. Acute renal insufficiency is usually reversible after discontinuing the ACE inhibitor.

### Those indicating need for medical attention
Incidence less frequent
*Hypotension* (lightheadedness or fainting)—especially during the first few days of therapy or in sodium- or volume-depleted patients as a result of prolonged diuretic therapy, dialysis, diarrhea, dietary salt restriction, or vomiting; *skin rash*

Incidence rare
*Anemia, hemolytic* (bleeding gums, nosebleeds, or pale skin); *angioedema of the face, extremities, lips, tongue, glottis, and/or larynx* (hoarseness; sudden trouble in swallowing or breathing; swelling of face, mouth, hands, or feet); *chest pain; hepatotoxicity* (yellow eyes or skin); *hyperkalemia* (confusion; irregular heartbeat; nervousness; numbness or tingling of hands, feet, or lips; shortness of breath or trouble breathing; weakness or heaviness of legs); *neutropenia or agranulocytosis* (chills; fever; sore throat); *pancreatitis* (bloating or pain of the stomach; fever; nausea; vomiting); *peripheral edema* (swelling of ankles, feet, or legs)

Note: *Angioedema* involving the tongue, glottis, or larynx may cause airway obstruction, which could be fatal. Angioedema may develop at any time during angiotensin-converting enzyme (ACE) inhibitor therapy. In placebo-controlled trials, symptoms suggestive of angioedema or facial edema were reported in less than 0.5% of patients treated with moexipril. None of the cases was life-threatening. Black patients may have an increased risk of developing ACE inhibitor–induced angioedema or may have more severe angioedema. In cases of angioedema, moexipril therapy should be discontinued and the patient carefully observed until the swelling resolves.

*Hepatotoxicity* has been reported rarely in patients receiving ACE inhibitors. The syndrome begins with cholestatic jaundice and progresses to fulminant hepatic necrosis and sometimes death. The mechanism of this effect is not fully understood. Patients who develop jaundice or significant elevations of hepatic enzymes should discontinue therapy with moexipril and receive appropriate medical follow-up.

ACE inhibitor–associated *neutropenia or agranulocytosis* and bone marrow depression have been reported. These conditions have occurred rarely in patients with uncomplicated hypertension, but more frequently in hypertensive patients with renal function impairment, especially if a collagen-vascular disease, such as systemic lupus erythematosus or scleroderma, exists.

### Those indicating need for medical attention only if they continue or are bothersome
Incidence more frequent
*Cough, dry, persistent; dizziness; flushing*

Note: In clinical trials, persistent, nonproductive *cough* was reported in 6.1% of moexipril-treated patients versus 2.2% of patients given placebo. The mechanism of this effect is probably the inhibition of endogenous bradykinin degradation. Cough usually resolves following discontinuation of moexipril therapy.

Incidence less frequent
*Diarrhea; dry mouth; fatigue* (unusual tiredness); *headache; loss of taste; myalgia* (muscle pain); *nausea; palpitations* (heartbeat sensations); *photosensitivity* (increased sensitivity to the sun); *pruritus* (itching); *unusual sweating*

## Overdose
For more information on the management of overdose or unintentional ingestion, **contact a Poison Control Center** (see *Poison Control Center Listing*).

### Clinical effects of overdose
The following effects have been selected on the basis of their potential clinical significance (possible signs and symptoms in parentheses where appropriate)—not necessarily inclusive:

Acute and chronic
*Hypotension* (dizziness, lightheadedness or fainting)

### Treatment of overdose
Symptomatic and supportive; may include volume expansion for correction of hypotension and monitoring of renal function and serum potassium.

## Patient Consultation
As an aid to patient consultation, refer to *Advice for the Patient, Moexipril (Systemic)*.

In providing consultation, consider emphasizing the following selected information (» = major clinical significance):

### Before using this medication
» Conditions affecting use, especially:
Hypersensitivity to moexipril or other angiotensin-converting enzyme (ACE) inhibitors
Pregnancy—ACE inhibitor–associated fetal and neonatal morbidity and mortality have been reported in humans; moexipril should be discontinued as soon as possible when pregnancy is detected
Other medications, especially diuretics (particularly potassium-sparing), potassium-containing medications or substances, potassium supplements, or salt substitutes
Other medical problems, especially angioedema, history of, idiopathic, or hereditary; dehydration (sodium or volume depletion); dialysis with high-flux membranes; hymenoptera venom desensitizing treatment; hyperkalemia; renal artery stenosis; or renal function impairment
Surgical—Withholding moexipril before surgery because of possible interaction with anesthesia induction and risk of hypovolemia

### Proper use of this medication
Taking medication at the same time each day to maintain the therapeutic effect of moexipril
Taking medication 1 hour before a meal
» Compliance with therapy; treatment period may be indefinite and necessary to prevent more serious consequences of hypertension; not stopping therapy without consulting physician
» Proper dosing
Missed dose: Taking as soon as possible; not taking if almost time for next dose; not doubling doses
» Proper storage

### Precautions while using this medication
Regular visits to physician to check progress
Notifying physician immediately if pregnancy is suspected
» Not taking other medications, especially nonprescription sympathomimetics, potassium-containing salt substitutes, or potassium supplements, unless discussed with physician
Caution when driving or doing other things requiring alertness, because of possible dizziness, especially after the initial dose of moexipril and in patients concurrently taking diuretics
Reporting any signs of infection (chills, fever, or sore throat) to physician because of risk of neutropenia
Reporting any signs of facial or extremity swelling and difficulty in swallowing or breathing because of risk of angioedema

To prevent dehydration and hypotension, checking with physician if severe nausea, vomiting, or diarrhea occurs and continues

Caution when exercising or during hot weather because of the risk of dehydration and hypotension due to reduced fluid volume

Avoiding alcoholic beverages because of increased risk of additive hypotensive effect

Caution if any kind of surgery (including dental surgery) or emergency treatment is required

### Side/adverse effects
Signs of potential side effects, especially hypotension, skin rash, hemolytic anemia, angioedema, chest pain, hepatotoxicity, hyperkalemia, neutropenia or agranulocytosis, pancreatitis, and peripheral edema

## General Dosing Information
As an aid to treatment of hypertension, refer to *Appendix III* for a summary of therapeutic guidelines.

Dosage must be adjusted to meet the individual requirements of each patient, on the basis of clinical response.

Black hypertensive patients may be less responsive to the antihypertensive effects of moexipril, possibly because these patients may have low-renin hypertension.

The antihypertensive effect of moexipril may diminish towards the end of the dosing period. If blood pressure is not controlled, it may be necessary to divide the dose into a twice-daily regimen or increase the dose, as appropriate.

### For treatment of adverse effects
For angioedema with swelling confined to the face and lips, treatment other than withdrawal of the medication is usually not necessary, although antihistamines may relieve the symptoms.

Treatment of angioedema involving the tongue, glottis, or larynx may include the following:
- Withdrawal of the angiotensin-converting enzyme (ACE) inhibitor and close observation of the patient to ensure full resolution of the symptoms.
- Subcutaneous epinephrine.
- Intravenous antihistamines, such as chlorpheniramine or diphenhydramine.
- Intravenous corticosteroids.

Note: The exact mechanism of angioedema is not known, but it may involve ACE inhibitor–induced inhibition of bradykinin degradation and not immunoglobulin E (IgE). Therefore, administration of epinephrine, antihistamines, and corticosteroids may not be effective in severe cases of angioedema and it may be necessary to ensure an open airway.

## Oral Dosage Forms
### MOEXIPRIL HYDROCHLORIDE TABLETS
#### Usual adult dose
Antihypertensive—
Oral, initially 7.5 mg once a day, taken one hour before a meal.

The recommended dose range is 7.5 to 30 mg a day, taken one hour before a meal. Dose may be taken once a day or divided into two doses.

Note: It is recommended that diuretic therapy be withdrawn two to three days before moexipril therapy is initiated to reduce the likelihood of hypotension. If hypertension is not controlled by moexipril alone, the diuretic may be reinstated. If diuretic therapy cannot be discontinued, an initial moexipril dose of 3.75 mg, given under medical supervision, is recommended until the blood pressure has stabilized.

An initial dose of 3.75 mg once a day is recommended for patients with a creatinine clearance ≤ forty mL/min. Dosage may be cautiously titrated upward to a maximum daily dose of 15 mg.

#### Usual adult prescribing limits
Antihypertensive—
30 mg per day; 15 mg per day for patients with a creatinine clearance ≤ forty mL/min. Doses above 60 mg per day have not been studied.

#### Usual pediatric dose
Safety and efficacy have not been established.

#### Strength(s) usually available
U.S.—
7.5 mg (Rx) [*Univasc* (scored; lactose)].
15 mg (Rx) [*Univasc* (scored)].
Canada—
Not commercially available.

#### Packaging and storage
Store at controlled room temperature, between 20 and 25 °C (68 and 77 °F) in a tightly closed container, unless otherwise specified by manufacturer. Protect from excessive moisture.

#### Auxiliary labeling
- Do not take other medicines without your doctor's advice.

Developed: 08/19/97

---

# MOEXIPRIL AND HYDROCHLOROTHIAZIDE   Systemic—INTRODUCTORY VERSION

VA CLASSIFICATION (Primary): CV401
Commonly used brand name(s): *Uniretic*.
Note: For a listing of dosage forms and brand names by country availability, see *Dosage Forms* section(s).

## Category
Antihypertensive.

## Indications
### Accepted
Hypertension (treatment)—Moexipril and hydrochlorothiazide combination is indicated for the treatment of hypertension. However, it is not indicated as initial therapy of hypertension and only should be used in patients who have failed to achieve the desired antihypertensive effect with one or the other as single therapy.

## Pharmacology/Pharmacokinetics
### Physicochemical characteristics
Molecular weight—Moexipril hydrochloride: 535.04.
Hydrochlorothiazide: 297.75.

### Mechanism of action/Effect
Moexipril is a nonsulfhydryl-containing angiotensin-converting enzyme (ACE) inhibitor. It is a prodrug of moexiprilat, the active metabolite. Moexiprilat lowers blood pressure by competitively inhibiting ACE activity. ACE catalyzes the conversion of angiotensin I to angiotensin II. Angiotensin II, a vasoconstrictor, stimulates aldosterone secretion by the adrenal cortex and directly suppresses renin release. Inhibition of ACE decreases angiotensin II formation, resulting in reduced peripheral arterial resistance, increased plasma renin activity, and decreased aldosterone secretion. The decrease in aldosterone secretion results in diuresis and natriuresis and a slight increase in serum potassium.

Hydrochlorothiazide is a thiazide diuretic. The exact mechanism by which hydrochlorothiazide reduces blood pressure is not known. It increases excretion of sodium and chloride by acting directly on the distal renal tubular mechanisms of electrolyte reabsorption. This results in a reduction in plasma volume, causing an increase in plasma renin activity, aldosterone secretion, and urinary potassium loss, and a decrease in serum potassium.

When moexipril is given in combination with hydrochlorothiazide, the antihypertensive effects are additive. The effects of ACE inhibition on the renin-angiotensin-aldosterone system by moexipril may reduce the potassium loss that occurs with hydrochlorothiazide.

### Other actions/effects
ACE is also known as kininase II, an enzyme that degrades bradykinin. After ACE inhibition, local kinin concentrations may increase and the formation of prostaglandins may be enhanced. Both bradykinin and prostaglandins have local vasodilatory effects that may contribute to the antihypertensive effects of moexipril.

### Absorption
Moexipril is incompletely absorbed. Bioavailability of moexipril is approximately 13% and is significantly affected by food, which reduces the peak plasma concentration ($C_{max}$) and area under the plasma concentration–time curve (AUC) by approximately 70% and 40%, respectively, after a low-fat breakfast or by approximately 80% and 50%, respectively, after a high-fat breakfast.

Hydrochlorothiazide is 60 to 80% absorbed, but in patients with congestive heart failure, absorption may be reduced by 50%.

**Distribution**
Moexiprilat—Volume of distribution ($Vol_D$): 2.8 L/kg.
Hydrochlorothiazide—Apparent $Vol_D$: 1.5 to 4.2 L/kg.

**Protein binding**
Moexiprilat—Moderate (50%).
Hydrochlorothiazide—Low (21 to 24%).

**Biotransformation**
Moexipril—Rapidly converted to moexiprilat, the active metabolite. Moexipril and moexiprilat are converted to diketopiperazine derivatives and unidentified metabolites.
Hydrochlorothiazide is not metabolized.

**Half-life**
Elimination—
  Moexipril:
    Approximately 1 hour.
  Moexiprilat:
    Terminal: 2 to 9 hours.
    Effective: Approximately 12 hours, may be increased in patients with impaired renal function by a factor of 3 or 4.
  Hydrochlorothiazide:
    5.6 to 14.8 hours, may be increased to 21 hours in patients with impaired renal function.

**Time to peak concentration**
Moexipril—0.8 hour.
Moexiprilat—1.6 hours.

**Elimination**
Moexipril—
  Fecal: 53% (52% as moexiprilat and 1% as moexipril).
  Renal: 13% (1% as moexipril, 7% as moexiprilat, and 5% as other metabolites).
  In dialysis: It is not known whether moexipril is dialyzable.
Hydrochlorothiazide—
  Renal: Approximately 60%.

## Precautions to Consider

**Cross-sensitivity and/or related problems**
Patients hypersensitive to other angiotensin-converting enzyme (ACE) inhibitors may also be hypersensitive to moexipril. Patients hypersensitive to sulfonamide-derived medications may also be hypersensitive to hydrochlorothiazide.

**Carcinogenicity**
No evidence of carcinogenicity of moexipril was found in long-term studies in mice and rats given doses of up to 14 or 27.3 times the maximum recommended human dose (MRHD) on a mg per square meter of body surface area (mg/m²) basis.
No evidence of carcinogenicity was found in female mice given daily dietary doses of up to 600 mg per kg of body weight (mg/kg) of hydrochlorothiazide for 2 years, or in rats given daily dietary doses of up to 100 mg/kg of hydrochlorothiazide for 2 years. However, evidence of hepatocarcinogenicity occurred in male mice given the same dose as that given to the female mice.

**Mutagenicity**
No evidence of mutagenicity of moexipril was found in the Ames test and microbial reverse mutation assay, with and without activation, or in an *in vivo* nucleus anomaly test. However, under metabolic activation conditions at a 20-hour harvest time, increased chromosomal aberration frequency in Chinese hamster ovary cells was detected.
No evidence of genotoxicity of hydrochlorothiazide was found in *in vitro* assays using strains TA 98, TA 100, TA 1535, TA 1537, or TA 1538 of *Salmonella typhimurium* (the Ames test); in the CHO test for chromosomal aberrations; or in *in vivo* assays using mouse germinal cell chromosomes, Chinese hamster bone marrow chromosomes, and the *Drosophila* sex-linked recessive lethal trait gene. Hydrochlorothiazide was found to be clastogenic in the *in vitro* CHO sister chromatid exchange test and mutagenic in the mouse lymphoma cell assays, using concentrations of hydrochlorothiazide of 43 to 1300 micrograms per mL (mcg/mL). Positive test results were also obtained in the *Aspergillus nidulans* nondisjunction assay, using hydrochlorothiazide at an unspecified concentration.

**Pregnancy/Reproduction**
Fertility—No evidence of impaired fertility, reproductive toxicity, or teratogenicity was detected in studies performed in rabbits and rats given oral doses of moexipril of up to 0.7 and 90.9 times the MRHD, respectively, on a mg/m² basis.
No evidence of impaired fertility was found in studies in mice and rats given daily dietary doses prior to mating and throughout gestation of up to 100 and 4 mg/kg of hydrochlorothiazide, respectively.
Pregnancy—ACE inhibitors, including moexipril, can cause fetal and neonatal morbidity and mortality when administered to pregnant women during the second and third trimesters. Moexipril should be discontinued as soon as possible when pregnancy is detected unless no alternative therapy can be used. In the latter instance, serial ultrasound examinations should be performed to assess the intra-amniotic environment. If oligohydramnios is observed, moexipril should be discontinued unless it is considered lifesaving for the mother. Perinatal diagnostics, such as contraction-stress testing (CST), a non-stress test (NST), or biophysical profiling (BPP) also may be appropriate during the applicable week of pregnancy. Oligohydramnios may not appear until after the fetus has sustained irreversible damage.
Fetal exposure to ACE inhibitors that is limited to the first trimester is not associated with fetal or neonatal morbidity. Fetal exposure to ACE inhibitors during the second and third trimesters can cause hypotension, reversible or irreversible renal failure, anuria, skull hypoplasia, and death in the fetus or neonate. Maternal oligohydramnios, which may result from decreased fetal renal function, has been reported, and has been associated with fetal limb contractures, craniofacial deformation, and hypoplastic lung development. Prematurity, intrauterine growth retardation, and patent ductus arteriosus also have been reported, although the relationship of these occurrences to drug exposure is not clear.
Infants exposed *in utero* to moexipril should be closely observed for hypotension, oliguria, and hyperkalemia. Oliguria should be treated with support of blood pressure and renal perfusion. Peritoneal dialysis or exchange transfusion may be necessary to reverse hypotension and/or substitute for disordered renal function, although there is no experience with the latter procedure.
Hydrochlorothiazide crosses the placenta. Intrauterine exposure to thiazide diuretics is associated with fetal or neonatal jaundice and/or thrombocytopenia. Other adverse reactions may also occur.
Moexipril and hydrochlorothiazide combination was not teratogenic in rats given up to the lethal dose of 800 mg/kg per day, or in rabbits given up to the maternotoxic dose of 160 mg/kg per day.
FDA Pregnancy Category C (first trimester).
FDA Pregnancy Category D (second and third trimesters).

**Breast-feeding**
It is not known whether moexipril or moexiprilat is distributed into breast milk. Thiazide diuretics are distributed into breast milk. Moexipril and hydrochlorothiazide combination is not recommended in nursing mothers because of the potential for adverse effects in the nursing infant.

**Pediatrics**
No information is available on the relationship of age to the effects of moexipril and hydrochlorothiazide combination in pediatric patients. Safety and efficacy have not been established.

**Geriatrics**
Use of moexipril and hydrochlorothiazide combination in a limited number of patients 65 years of age and over (24% of patients in clinical studies) has not demonstrated geriatrics-specific problems that would limit the usefulness of this combination in the elderly. However, moexipril plasma concentrations are slightly higher, moexipril renal clearance is reduced, and the area under the plasma concentration–time curve (AUC) and peak plasma concentrations ($C_{max}$) of moexiprilat are about 30% greater in elderly patients than in younger individuals.

**Pharmacogenetics**
Black hypertensive patients are less responsive to the antihypertensive effects of moexipril, although the combination of moexipril and hydrochlorothiazide does not appear to be less effective in black patients. Black patients also may have a greater risk of developing ACE inhibitor–induced angioedema.

**Surgical**
Patients receiving moexipril and hydrochlorothiazide combination and undergoing major surgery or receiving anesthesia with agents that produce hypotension may experience excessive hypotension. If hypotension in these patients is thought to be the result of ACE inhibition, it can be corrected by volume expansion.

**Drug interactions and/or related problems**
The following drug interactions and/or related problems have been selected on the basis of their potential clinical significance (possible mechanism in parentheses where appropriate)—not necessarily inclusive (» = major clinical significance):

Note: Combinations containing any of the following medications, depending on the amount present, may also interact with this medication.

Alcohol or
Barbiturates or
Narcotics
    (concurrent use with hydrochlorothiazide may produce postural hypotensive effects)

Antidiabetic agents, oral or
Insulin
    (thiazide diuretics may reduce glucose tolerance; a dosage adjustment may be necessary)

Antihypertensive agents, such as
Ganglionic blocking agent, trimethaphan or
Adrenergic blocking agents, peripheral, which include
» Alpha-adrenergic blocking agents and
» Beta-adrenergic blocking agents
    (antihypertensive effects may be potentiated with concurrent thiazide diuretic use)

Anti-inflammatory drugs, nonsteroidal (NSAIDs)
    (concurrent use may reduce the diuretic, natriuretic, and antihypertensive effects of thiazide diuretics; the patient should be monitored to assure that the desired therapeutic effect is obtained)

Cholestyramine or
Colestipol
    (a single dose of either cholestyramine or colestipol binds hydrochlorothiazide and decreases its absorption by up to 85% and 43%, respectively)

Corticosteroids or
Corticotropin (ACTH)
    (concurrent use with thiazide diuretics may increase depletion of electrolytes, especially potassium)

» Digitalis glycosides
    (hypokalemia associated with thiazide diuretic therapy may potentiate digitalis toxicity)

» Diuretics, potassium-sparing, such as:
    Amiloride or
    Spironolactone or
    Triamterene or
» Potassium supplements or
» Salt substitutes that contain potassium
    (although hydrochlorothiazide, when given concurrently with ACE inhibitors, tends to counteract the slight hyperkalemic effects of ACE inhibitors, concurrent use of moexipril and hydrochlorothiazide combination with these agents still may lead to increases in serum potassium; caution and monitoring of serum potassium concentrations are recommended)

Guanabenz or
Propantheline
    (concurrent use may increase hydrochlorothiazide absorption)

» Lithium
    (increases in serum lithium concentrations and symptoms of lithium toxicity have been reported during concurrent use with ACE inhibitors; thiazide diuretics reduce renal clearance of lithium, increasing the risk of toxicity; caution should be used and serum lithium concentrations should be monitored frequently)

Neuromuscular blocking agents, nondepolarizing, especially tubocurarine
    (thiazide diuretics may enhance the blockade action of nondepolarizing neuromuscular blocking agents)

Sympathomimetic agents, such as norepinephrine
    (concurrent use with thiazide diuretics may blunt the arterial responsiveness to sympathomimetic agents)

## Laboratory value alterations
The following have been selected on the basis of their potential clinical significance (possible effect in parentheses where appropriate)—not necessarily inclusive (» = major clinical significance):

With physiology/laboratory test values
Bilirubin, serum and
Transaminases, serum
    (significant increases may be a sign of ACE inhibitor–associated hepatotoxicity)

Blood urea nitrogen (BUN) and
Creatinine, serum
    (minor and transient concentration increases may occur with moexipril therapy, especially when given concurrently with a thiazide diuretic; increases are more likely to occur in patients with renal function impairment; concentration increases are reversible upon discontinuation of therapy; in hypertensive patients treated with moexipril and hydrochlorothiazide combination, increases occurred in less than 1% of patients)

Cholesterol, serum and
Triglycerides, serum
    (thiazide diuretics may increase concentrations)

Electrolytes, serum, such as:
    Calcium
    Chloride
    Magnesium
    Sodium
    (thiazide diuretics deplete serum sodium, chloride, and magnesium and reduce depletion of serum calcium; occasionally, patients on prolonged thiazide therapy may have pathological changes in the parathyroid gland, with hypercalcemia and hypophosphatemia; depletion of chloride is usually small, but may require treatment in cases of liver or renal function impairment; serum electrolyte concentrations should be monitored initially and periodically to detect imbalances)

Glucose, serum
    (hyperglycemia has occurred with moexipril and hydrochlorothiazide combination therapy; thiazide diuretics may reduce glucose tolerance and may precipitate overt diabetes in susceptible individuals)

Potassium, serum
    (although the effects of moexipril and hydrochlorothiazide on serum potassium may counterbalance each other, serum potassium concentrations should be monitored initially and periodically to detect imbalances; in patients treated with moexipril alone, increases in serum potassium occurred in 1.3% of hypertensive patients; patients treated with thiazide diuretics may experience decreases in serum potassium)

Uric acid, serum
    (concentration increases have been associated with thiazide diuretic use and may precipitate gout in susceptible individuals)

## Medical considerations/Contraindications
The medical considerations/contraindications included have been selected on the basis of their potential clinical significance (reasons given in parentheses where appropriate)—not necessarily inclusive (» = major clinical significance).

*Except under special circumstances, this medication should not be used when the following medical problems exist:*
» Angioedema, history of, related to previous ACE inhibitor therapy
    (increased risk for development of moexipril-related angioedema)
» Anuria
    (hydrochlorothiazide may aggravate this condition)
» Hypersensitivity to moexipril or other ACE inhibitors, hydrochlorothiazide, or other sulfonamide-derived medications like hydrochlorothiazide

*Risk-benefit should be considered when the following medical problems exist:*
Allergy, history of or
Asthma, bronchial
    (hypersensitivity reactions are more likely to occur in these patients)

Aortic stenosis or
Cerebrovascular disease or
Ischemic heart disease
    (excessive reduction in blood pressure could result in a cerebrovascular accident or a myocardial infarction)

Collagen-vascular disease, such as:
Systemic lupus erythematosus (SLE) or
Scleroderma
    (increased risk of development of neutropenia or agranulocytosis with ACE inhibitor therapy, especially if accompanied by renal function impairment; thiazide diuretics have been reported to cause activation or exacerbation of SLE)

» Congestive heart failure, with or without associated renal function impairment
    (ACE inhibitor therapy may cause excessive hypotension or, in patients with severe congestive heart failure, may interfere with the compensatory mechanisms of the renin-angiotensin-aldosterone system, possibly leading to oliguria and/or progressive azotemia and, possibly, acute renal failure and/or death; the patient should be under close medical supervision during initiation of therapy, the first 2 weeks of therapy, and dosage increases)

Dehydration (sodium or volume depletion due to excessive perspiration, vomiting, diarrhea, prolonged diuretic therapy, dialysis, or dietary salt restriction)
(increased risk of symptomatic hypotension; volume- and/or sodium-depletion should be corrected before initiating treatment with an ACE inhibitor)

Diabetes mellitus
(increased risk of hyperkalemia with ACE inhibitor therapy)

Dialysis with high-flux membranes or
Low-density lipoprotein apheresis with dextran sulfate absorption
(anaphylactoid reactions have been reported in patients undergoing these procedures who are concurrently taking an ACE inhibitor)

Diuresis, brisk or
Potassium intake, inadequate
(increased risk of hypokalemia with hydrochlorothiazide therapy)

Hepatic function impairment or
Liver disease, progressive
(minor alterations of fluid and electrolyte balance may precipitate hepatic coma in these patients; increased risk of hypokalemia with thiazide diuretic use; moexipril peak plasma concentration [$C_{max}$] and area under the plasma concentration–time curve [AUC] may be increased by approximately 50% and 120%, respectively; moexiprilat $C_{max}$ may be decreased and AUC may be increased by approximately 50% and 300%, respectively; caution should be used)

Hymenoptera venom desensitizing treatment
(life-threatening anaphylactoid reactions have been reported in two patients undergoing desensitizing treatment with hymenoptera venom while receiving ACE inhibitors)

» Renal artery stenosis, bilateral or unilateral or
» Renal function impairment
(there is no clinical experience in treating hypertension with moexipril and hydrochlorothiazide combination in these patients; plasma concentrations of moexipril and moexiprilat may be increased due to decreased elimination; ACE inhibitors may potentiate hyperkalemia; ACE inhibitors may increase the risk of agranulocytosis and neutropenia; increases in blood urea nitrogen [BUN] and serum creatinine have occurred with ACE inhibitor therapy, especially when given with a thiazide diuretic; thiazide diuretics may precipitate azotemia; a dosage adjustment of the ACE inhibitor and/or discontinuation of the diuretic may be necessary; renal function should be monitored during the first few weeks of moexipril and hydrochlorothiazide combination therapy)

Sympathectomy
(antihypertensive effect of thiazide diuretics may be enhanced)

**Patient monitoring**
The following may be especially important in patient monitoring (other tests may be warranted in some patients, depending on condition; » = major clinical significance):

» Blood pressure measurements
(periodic monitoring is necessary for titration of dose according to the patient's response; the adequacy of the dose of moexipril should be determined based on trough blood pressure measurements)

» Electrolytes, serum, including
Potassium, serum
(determinations recommended initially and periodically at appropriate intervals)

Leukocyte count
(determinations recommended periodically with ACE inhibitor therapy in patients at risk for neutropenia, particularly those with renal function impairment and/or a collagen-vascular disease, such as SLE or scleroderma)

Renal function
(determinations recommended during the first few weeks of ACE inhibitor therapy in patients with renal function impairment)

## Side/Adverse Effects

The following side/adverse effects have been selected on the basis of their potential clinical significance (possible signs and symptoms in parentheses where appropriate)—not necessarily inclusive:

**Those indicating need for medical attention**
Incidence less frequent
*Abdominal pain; chest pain; edema, peripheral* (swelling of ankles, feet, or legs); *hypochloremia, hypokalemia, or hyponatremia* (decreased urine output; drowsiness; dryness of mouth; fast heart rate; muscle pains or cramps; muscular fatigue; nausea or vomiting; thirst; weakness); *hypotension* (lightheadedness or fainting)—especially during the first few days of therapy or in sodium- or volume-depleted patients as a result of prolonged diuretic therapy, dialysis, diarrhea, dietary salt restriction, or vomiting; *skin rash*

Note: *Hypokalemia* has been reported with use of thiazide diuretics. Patients with liver function impairment, patients who do not receive adequate oral intake of potassium, and patients who experience a brisk diuresis are at risk of developing hypokalemia. Concurrent use of corticosteroids or corticotropin (ACTH) is also a risk factor for development of hypokalemia.

Incidence rare
*Anaphylactoid reactions* (abnormal, high-pitched, breathing sounds; anxiety; blueness of the skin, including the lips or nail beds; confusion; generalized itching; heartbeat sensations; hives; wheezing or difficulty breathing); *anemia* (pale skin; tiredness); *angioedema of the face, extremities, lips, tongue, glottis, and/or larynx* (hoarseness; sudden trouble in swallowing or breathing; swelling of face, mouth, hands, or feet); *hepatotoxicity* (yellow eyes or skin); *hyperkalemia* (confusion; irregular heartbeat; nervousness; numbness or tingling in hands, feet, or lips; shortness of breath or difficulty breathing; weakness or heaviness of legs); *impotence; neutropenia or agranulocytosis* (chills; fever; sore throat)

Note: *Angioedema* involving the tongue, glottis, or larynx may cause airway obstruction, which may be fatal. Angioedema usually occurs within the first month of therapy. In cases of angioedema, moexipril and hydrochlorothiazide combination therapy should be discontinued and the patient carefully observed until the swelling resolves. In clinical trials, symptoms resembling angioedema or facial edema were reported in less than 0.5% of patients treated with moexipril alone, and none of the cases were life-threatening. Black patients may have an increased risk of developing angiotensin-converting enzyme (ACE) inhibitor–induced angioedema. Laryngeal edema developed in one patient treated with hydrochlorothiazide alone.

*Hepatotoxicity* has been reported rarely in patients receiving ACE inhibitors. The syndrome begins with cholestatic jaundice and progresses to fulminant hepatic necrosis and sometimes death. The mechanism of this effect is not fully understood. Patients who develop jaundice or significant elevations of hepatic enzymes should discontinue ACE inhibitor therapy and receive appropriate medical follow-up.

ACE inhibitor–associated *neutropenia or agranulocytosis* and bone marrow depression have been reported. These conditions have occurred rarely in patients with uncomplicated hypertension, but more frequently in hypertensive patients with renal function impairment, especially if a collagen-vascular disease, such as systemic lupus erythematosus or scleroderma, exists.

In clinical trials with moexipril alone, persistent *hyperkalemia* occurred in approximately 1.3% of hypertensive patients. Patients with renal function impairment and patients with diabetes mellitus may be at risk for hyperkalemia. Patients using potassium-sparing diuretics, potassium supplements, and/or potassium-containing salt substitutes are also at risk for hyperkalemia.

**Those indicating need for medical attention only if they continue or are bothersome**
Incidence more frequent
*Cough, dry, persistent*—incidence 15%; *dizziness*—incidence 7%; *fatigue*—incidence 5%

Note: *Cough* usually resolves following discontinuation of the ACE inhibitor. The mechanism of this effect may be due to the inhibition of the degradation of endogenous bradykinin, resulting from kininase II inhibition by ACE inhibitor therapy.

Incidence less frequent
*Back pain; constipation; diarrhea; dyspepsia* (belching; heartburn; stomach discomfort); *headache; insomnia* (trouble in sleeping); *unusual sweating*

## Overdose

For more information on the management of overdose or unintentional ingestion, **contact a Poison Control Center** (see *Poison Control Center Listing*).

**Clinical effects of overdose**
The following effects have been selected on the basis of their potential clinical significance (possible signs and symptoms in parentheses where appropriate)—not necessarily inclusive:

Acute and chronic
*Hypotension* (lightheadedness or fainting); *dehydration; electrolyte depletion, such as hypochloremia; hypokalemia; and hyponatremia*

## Treatment of overdose
No specific information is available on the treatment of overdose with moexipril and hydrochlorothiazide combination. The medication should be discontinued and treatment of the patient should be symptomatic and supportive, which may include the following:

To decrease absorption—Emesis and/or gastric lavage.

For ACE inhibitor–associated hypovolemia—Infusion of normal saline solution.

Monitoring—Observing the patient and monitoring renal function and serum electrolytes, including serum potassium.

Supportive care—Correcting electrolyte imbalance and hypotension by established procedures. Patients in whom intentional overdose is confirmed or suspected should be referred for psychiatric consultation.

## Patient Consultation
As an aid to patient consultation, refer to *Advice for the Patient, Moexipril and Hydrochlorothiazide (Systemic)—Introductory Version.*

In providing consultation, consider emphasizing the following selected information (» = major clinical significance):

### Before using this medication
» Conditions affecting use, especially:
Hypersensitivity to moexipril or other angiotensin-converting enzyme (ACE) inhibitors, hydrochlorothiazide, or other sulfonamide-derived medications

Pregnancy—ACE inhibitors cause fetal and neonatal morbidity and mortality; thiazide diuretic use is associated with fetal or neonatal jaundice and/or thrombocytopenia and possibly other adverse reactions

Breast-feeding—Thiazide diuretics are distributed into breast milk; not recommended in nursing mothers

Pharmacogenetics—Black patients may be less responsive to moexipril and have a greater risk of developing ACE inhibitor–induced angioedema

Surgical—Patients undergoing major surgery or receiving anesthesia with agents that produce hypotension may experience excessive hypotension

Other medications, especially digitalis glycosides; lithium; potassium-sparing diuretics, such as amiloride, spironolactone, or triamterene; potassium supplements; or salt substitutes that contain potassium

Other medical problems, especially anuria, bilateral or unilateral renal artery stenosis, congestive heart failure with or without associated renal function impairment, history of angioedema related to previous ACE inhibitor therapy, or renal function impairment

### Proper use of this medication
Taking medication at the same time each day to maintain the therapeutic effect

Taking medication 1 hour before a meal

» Compliance with therapy; an indefinite treatment period may be necessary to prevent more serious consequences of hypertension; not stopping therapy without consulting physician

» Proper dosing
Missed dose: Taking as soon as possible; not taking if almost time for next dose; not doubling doses

» Proper storage

### Precautions while using this medication
Regular visits to physician to check progress

Notifying physician immediately if pregnancy is suspected because of possibility of fetal or neonatal injury and/or death

» Not taking other medications, especially potassium-containing salt substitutes or potassium supplements, unless discussed with physician

Caution when driving or doing other things requiring alertness because of possible lightheadedness or fainting due to symptomatic hypotension, especially during the first few days of therapy; notifying physician if fainting occurs

Reporting any signs of infection (chills, fever, or sore throat) to physician because of risk of neutropenia

Reporting any signs of facial or extremity swelling and difficulty in swallowing or breathing because of risk of angioedema

Checking with physician if severe nausea, vomiting, or diarrhea occurs and continues because of risk of dehydration and hypotension

Caution when exercising or during exposure to hot weather because of the risk of dehydration and hypotension due to reduced fluid volume

Avoiding alcoholic beverages because of increased risk of additive hypotensive effects

Caution if any kind of surgery (including dental surgery) or emergency treatment is required because concurrent use of agents that produce hypotension may cause excessive hypotension

### Side/adverse effects
Signs of potential side effects, especially abdominal pain; chest pain; peripheral edema; hypochloremia, hypokalemia, or hyponatremia; hypotension; skin rash; anaphylactoid reactions; anemia; angioedema of the face, extremities, lips, tongue, glottis, and/or larynx; hepatotoxicity; hyperkalemia; impotence; neutropenia or agranulocytosis

## General Dosing Information
Combination moexipril and hydrochlorothiazide therapy should only be used in patients who have failed to achieve the desired antihypertensive effect with one or the other medication as single therapy. For dosage ranges for the individual agents when given as single therapy, see
- *Moexipril (Systemic)* monograph; and/or
- *Hydrochlorothiazide* in *Diuretics, Thiazide (Systemic)* monograph.

In clinical trials, patients who received 3.75/6.25 mg or 7.5/12.5 mg of moexipril and hydrochlorothiazide combination experienced almost no change in serum potassium. Patients who received 15/25 mg of the combination experienced a mild decrease in serum potassium, similar to that experienced by patients who received 25 mg of hydrochlorothiazide alone.

Patients whose blood pressure is adequately controlled with 25 mg of hydrochlorothiazide daily, but who experience significant potassium loss with this regimen, may achieve blood-pressure control without electrolyte disturbance if they are switched to 3.75/6.25 mg of moexipril and hydrochlorothiazide combination (equivalent to one half of the 7.5/12.5 mg tablet).

The antihypertensive effect of moexipril is usually seen within 2 weeks of treatment; maximum effects are seen after 4 weeks. The efficacy of the dose of moexipril should be determined based on trough blood-pressure measurements. If control of diastolic blood pressure is not sufficient at the end of the dosing interval, the dose of moexipril may be increased or given as a divided, twice-daily, regimen.

Moexipril and hydrochlorothiazide combination therapy is not recommended in patients with a creatinine clearance of $\leq 40$ mL per minute (mL/min) (serum creatinine approximately $> 3$ mg per dL or 265 micromole per L).

### For treatment of adverse effects
Recommended treatment consists of the following:
- Treatment of symptomatic hypotension involves placing the patient in a supine position and, if needed, administering normal saline intravenously.
- For treatment of ACE inhibitor–associated angioedema—Medication should be discontinued immediately and the patient monitored until the swelling resolves. If swelling is confined to the face and lips, treatment, other than withdrawal of the medication, is usually not necessary, although antihistamines may relieve the symptoms.
- For treatment of ACE inhibitor–associated angioedema with swelling involving the tongue, glottis, or larynx, possibly causing airway obstruction—Withdrawal of the medication and appropriate treatment, such as subcutaneous epinephrine or measures to ensure an open airway, should be initiated immediately. The patient should be monitored until full resolution of the symptoms.

## Oral Dosage Forms

### MOEXIPRIL HYDROCHLORIDE AND HYDROCHLOROTHIAZIDE TABLETS

#### Usual adult dose
Antihypertensive—
Oral, 1 to 2 tablets daily, one hour before a meal, as determined by individual titration with the component agents and according to clinical response. The hydrochlorothiazide dose should not be increased until two or three weeks after initiation of treatment.

One-half tablet may be used in patients who experience excessive reduction in blood pressure with the 7.5/12.5 mg tablet.

#### Usual adult prescribing limits
30 mg moexipril and 50 mg hydrochlorothiazide.

#### Usual pediatric dose
Antihypertensive—
Safety and efficacy have not been established.

#### Strength(s) usually available
U.S.—
7.5 mg of moexipril hydrochloride and 12.5 mg of hydrochlorothiazide (Rx) [*Uniretic* (scored)].
15 mg of moexipril hydrochloride and 25 mg of hydrochlorothiazide (Rx) [*Uniretic* (scored)].

**Packaging and storage**
Store at controlled room temperature, between 20 and 25 °C (68 and 77 °F) in a tightly closed container. Protect from excessive moisture.

**Auxiliary labeling**
- Do not take other medicines without your doctor's advice.

Developed: 11/10/97

# MOLINDONE  Systemic†

VA CLASSIFICATION (Primary): CN709
Commonly used brand name(s): *Moban; Moban Concentrate*.
Note: For a listing of dosage forms and brand names by country availability, see *Dosage Forms* section(s).

†Not commercially available in Canada.

## Category
Antipsychotic.

## Indications

**Accepted**

Psychotic disorders (treatment)—Molindone is indicated for the management of the manifestations of psychotic conditions, especially in patients with chronic schizophrenia, brief reactive psychosis, or schizophreniform disorders.

**Unaccepted**

Molindone is *not* recommended for management of behavioral complications in mentally retarded patients.

## Pharmacology/Pharmacokinetics

**Physicochemical characteristics**
Molecular weight—312.84.
pKa—6.94.

**Mechanism of action/Effect**
The exact mechanism has not been established; however, based on electroencephalogram (EEG) studies, molindone is thought to act by occupying dopamine ($D_2$) receptor sites in the reticular activating and limbic systems in the brain, thus decreasing dopamine activity.

**Other actions/effects**
Causes changes in resting and sleeping EEG readings.
May decrease the duration of sleep.
May have an antiemetic effect.

**Absorption**
Rapidly absorbed from the gastrointestinal tract after oral administration.

**Biotransformation**
Probably hepatic; 36 recognized metabolites, some of which may be active.

**Time to peak serum concentration**
1.5 hours.

**Duration of action**
24 to 36 hours.

**Elimination**
More than 90% of a single dose is excreted as metabolites in urine and feces within 24 hours. Less than 2 to 3% is excreted unchanged. Small amount excreted via lungs as carbon dioxide.

## Precautions to Consider

**Cross-sensitivity and/or related problems**
Patients sensitive to other antipsychotic agents, such as phenothiazines, thioxanthenes, haloperidol, and loxapine, may be sensitive to this medication also.

**Carcinogenicity/Tumorigenicity**
Most antipsychotic medications have been found to cause increased serum prolactin concentrations. Although the clinical significance of this increase is not known for most patients, *in vitro* studies have shown approximately ⅓ of human breast cancers to be prolactin-dependent. In addition, an increase in mammary neoplasms has been found in rodents after chronic administration of antipsychotics. However, a definite association between the chronic administration of these medications and mammary tumorigenesis has not been established, because of limited evidence currently available.

**Pregnancy/Reproduction**
Pregnancy—Adequate and well-controlled studies in humans have not been done.
Studies in animals have not shown that molindone causes birth defects. Studies in mice have shown that molindone at oral doses of 20 and 40 mg per kg of body weight (mg/kg) per day for 10 days caused a slight increase in resorptions.

**Breast-feeding**
It is not known if molindone is excreted in breast milk. However, problems in humans have not been documented.

**Pediatrics**
Appropriate studies on the relationship of age to the effects of molindone have not been performed in children up to 12 years of age. Safety and efficacy have not been established.

**Geriatrics**
Geriatric patients tend to develop higher plasma concentrations of molindone because of changes in distribution due to decreases in lean body mass, total body water, and albumin, and often an increase in total body fat composition. Therefore, these patients usually require lower initial dosage and a more gradual titration of dose.
Elderly patients appear to be more prone to orthostatic hypotension and exhibit an increased sensitivity to the anticholinergic and sedative effects of molindone. In addition, they are more prone to develop extrapyramidal side effects, such as tardive dyskinesia and parkinsonism. The symptoms of tardive dyskinesia are persistent, difficult to control, and, in some patients, appear to be irreversible. There is no known effective treatment. Careful observation during treatment for early signs of tardive dyskinesia and reduction of dosage or discontinuation of medication may prevent a more severe manifestation of the syndrome.
It has been suggested that elderly patients should receive half the usual adult dose. A periodic attempt should be made to discontinue medication as soon as the patient improves.

**Dental**
The peripheral anticholinergic effects of molindone may decrease or inhibit salivary flow, especially in middle-aged or elderly patients, thus contributing to the development of caries, periodontal disease, candidiasis, or discomfort.
Extrapyramidal reactions induced by molindone will result in increased motor activity of the head, face, and neck. Occlusal adjustments, bite registrations, and treatment for bruxism may be made less reliable.

**Drug interactions and/or related problems**
The following drug interactions and/or related problems have been selected on the basis of their potential clinical significance (possible mechanism in parentheses where appropriate)—not necessarily inclusive (» = major clinical significance):

Note: Combinations containing any of the following medications, depending on the amount present, may also interact with this medication.

Although not all of the following interactions have been documented specifically for molindone, a potential exists for their occurrence because of the close similarity of molindone's pharmacological effects to those of phenothiazines and other antipsychotic medications.

» Alcohol or
» Central nervous system (CNS) depression–producing medications, other, especially anesthetics, barbiturates, benzodiazepines, and opioid (narcotic) analgesics (See *Appendix II*)
  (concurrent use may potentiate and prolong the CNS depressant effects of either these medications or molindone)

Amphetamines
  (concurrent use with molindone may antagonize the stimulant effects of amphetamines and counteract the antipsychotic effects of molindone)

Antacids or
Antidiarrheals, adsorbent
(concurrent use may inhibit the absorption of molindone; these medications should not be taken within 1 to 2 hours of molindone)
Anticholinergics or other medications with anticholinergic activity (See *Appendix II*) or
Antidyskinetic agents or
Antihistamines
(concurrent use with molindone may potentiate anticholinergic effects, such as urinary retention, blurred vision, dry mouth, and constipation)
Antidepressants, tricyclic or
Maprotiline or
Monoamine oxidase (MAO) inhibitors, including furazolidone and procarbazine or
Trazodone
(concurrent use may prolong and intensify the sedative or anticholinergic effects of these medications or molindone)
Antidiabetic agents, oral or
Insulin
(high doses of molindone, when added to an existing antidiabetic regimen, may increase plasma glucose concentrations, leading to loss of control of diabetes)
Beta-adrenergic blocking agents, especially metoprolol or propranolol
(concurrent use may increase the effects of beta-blockers by decreasing first-pass metabolism; reduction in dosage of beta-blocking agent may be required)
Bromocriptine
(molindone may increase serum prolactin concentrations and interfere with therapeutic effects of bromocriptine; dosage increase of bromocriptine may be necessary)
» Extrapyramidal reaction–causing medications, other (See *Appendix II*)
(concurrent use with molindone may increase the severity and frequency of extrapyramidal effects)
Levodopa
(concurrent use may inhibit antiparkinsonian effects of levodopa by blocking dopamine receptors in the brain and may counteract the antipsychotic effects of molindone)
» Lithium
(concurrent use with molindone may produce neurotoxic symptoms, such as confusion, delirium, seizures, somnambulism, or abnormal EEG changes; extrapyramidal symptoms may be increased; also, antiemetic effect of molindone may mask nausea and vomiting, which are early signs of lithium toxicity)
Phenytoin or
Tetracycline
(calcium ions from the excipient in molindone may interfere with the absorption of these medications)

**Laboratory value alterations**
The following have been selected on the basis of their potential clinical significance (possible effect in parentheses where appropriate)—not necessarily inclusive (» = major clinical significance):
With physiology/laboratory test values
Blood urea nitrogen (BUN) and
Glucose, serum and
Red blood cell counts
(alterations may occur but are not considered clinically significant)
Electrocardiogram (ECG) readings
(rare, transient, nonspecific T-wave changes have been reported)
Prolactin
(serum concentrations may be persistently elevated during chronic administration)
White blood cell counts
(may be increased or decreased, but molindone therapy may be continued if clinical symptoms of leukopenia or leukocytosis are absent; however, it has been suggested that if the white blood cell count is below 4000 without clinical symptoms, molindone should be discontinued until white blood cell counts increase; then therapy should be re-evaluated)

**Medical considerations/Contraindications**
The medical considerations/contraindications included have been selected on the basis of their potential clinical significance (reasons given in parentheses where appropriate)—not necessarily inclusive (» = major clinical significance).

*Except under special circumstances, this medication should not be used when the following medical problems exist:*
» CNS depression, severe, drug-induced
» Comatose states

*Risk-benefit should be considered when the following medical problems exist:*
Brain tumor or
Intestinal obstruction
(antiemetic effect of molindone may mask early signs of brain tumor or intestinal obstruction and interfere with diagnosis)
Glaucoma or
Hepatic function impairment or
Prostatic hypertrophy or
Urinary retention
(may be aggravated)
Parkinson's disease
(potentiation of extrapyramidal effects)
Sensitivity to molindone or other antipsychotic medications

**Patient monitoring**
The following may be especially important in patient monitoring (other tests may be warranted in some patients, depending on condition; » = major clinical significance):
Careful observation for early symptoms of tardive dyskinesia
(recommended at periodic intervals, especially in the elderly and those patients on high or extended maintenance dosage, although symptoms may appear when doses are small and treatment periods brief; since there is no known effective treatment if syndrome should develop, molindone should be discontinued, if clinically feasible, at the appearance of early symptoms, such as unusual tongue and mouth movements)
Careful observation for early symptoms of tardive dystonia
(recommended at periodic intervals; since there is no known effective treatment if syndrome should develop, molindone should be discontinued, if clinically feasible, at the earliest signs)
Liver function tests
(may be required periodically during therapy)
Ophthalmologic examinations
(may be required at periodic intervals during high-dose or prolonged therapy since deposition of particulate matter in the lens and cornea has occurred with some phenothiazines, although not reported with molindone)

## Side/Adverse Effects

The following side/adverse effects have been selected on the basis of their potential clinical significance (possible signs and symptoms in parentheses where appropriate)—not necessarily inclusive:

**Those indicating need for medical attention**
Incidence more frequent
*Akathisia* (severe restlessness or need to keep moving)—may be more frequent in elderly patients; *extrapyramidal effects, dystonic* (muscle spasms of face, neck, and back; tic-like or twitching movements; twisting movements of body; inability to move eyes; weakness of arms and legs); *extrapyramidal effects, parkinsonian* (difficulty in talking; loss of balance control; mask-like face; shuffling walk; stiffness of arms and legs; trembling and shaking of hands); *tardive dyskinesia, persistent* (lip smacking or puckering; puffing of cheeks; rapid or worm-like movements of tongue; uncontrolled movements of arms and legs; uncontrolled chewing movements)

Note: *Akathisia* or *dystonic extrapyramidal effects* may occur within 24 to 48 hours of first dose; more frequent in young and male patients.

*Parkinsonian extrapyramidal effects* may appear in the first few days of treatment; frequency usually increases with increase of dosage; may be more frequent in elderly patients.

*Tardive dyskinesia* occurs more frequently in elderly females; initially dose-related, but may appear when doses are small and treatment periods are brief; may increase with long-term treatment and total cumulative dose; may be masked when dosage is increased or treatment reinitiated, or may persist after molindone is discontinued.

Incidence less frequent
*Mental depression*
Incidence rare
*Allergic reaction* (skin rash); *heat stroke* (hot, dry skin; inability to sweat; muscle weakness; confusion); *hepatitis or jaundice, cholestatic* (yellow eyes or skin); *neuroleptic malignant syndrome (NMS)* (con-

vulsions; fast heartbeat; fever; high or low [irregular] blood pressure; increased sweating; loss of bladder control; severe muscle stiffness; troubled breathing; unusually pale skin; unusual tiredness); *tardive dystonia* (increased blinking or spasms of eyelid; unusual facial expressions or body positions; uncontrolled twisting movements of neck, trunk, arms, or legs)

Note: *Heat stroke* may occur in environmental conditions of high heat and high humidity; caused by molindone-induced suppression of central and peripheral temperature regulation in the hypothalamus. The effectiveness of sweating as a cooling mechanism may be reduced by humid conditions and by the anticholinergic effects of molindone or its combination with other anticholinergic medications such as nonprescription cold medications or antihistamines. Adequate interior temperature control (air conditioning) must be maintained for institutionalized patients during hot weather because of the increased risk of heat stroke and NMS. Patients should be advised to avoid exertion, stay in cool areas, and avoid dehydration and other anticholinergic medications.

*NMS* may occur at any time during neuroleptic therapy, but is more commonly seen soon after start of therapy, or after patient has switched from one neuroleptic to another, during combined therapy with another psychotropic medication, or after a dosage increase. Along with the overt signs of skeletal muscle rigidity, hyperthermia, autonomic dysfunction, and altered consciousness, differential diagnosis may reveal leukocytosis (9500 to 26,000 cells per cubic millimeter), elevated liver function tests, and elevated creatine phosphokinase (CPK).

**Those indicating need for medical attention only if they continue or are bothersome**
Incidence more frequent
*Blurred vision; constipation; decreased sweating; difficult urination; drowsiness; dryness of mouth; headache; hypotension, orthostatic* (dizziness or lightheadedness, especially when getting up suddenly from a lying or sitting position); *nausea; stuffy nose*
Incidence less frequent
*Changes in menstrual periods; decreased sexual ability; false sense of well-being; swelling of breasts; unusual secretion of milk*

**Those indicating the need for medical attention if they occur after medication is discontinued**
*Tardive dyskinesia, withdrawal emergent* (lip smacking or puckering; puffing of cheeks; rapid or worm-like movements of tongue; uncontrolled chewing movements; uncontrolled movements of arms and legs)

## Patient Consultation
As an aid to patient consultation, refer to *Advice for the Patient, Molindone (Systemic)*.
In providing consultation, consider emphasizing the following selected information (» = major clinical significance):

**Before using this medication**
» Conditions affecting use, especially:
  Sensitivity to molindone or other antipsychotic medications
  Pregnancy—Studies in mice have shown a slight increase in resorptions
  Use in the elderly—Elderly patients are more likely to develop extrapyramidal, anticholinergic, hypotensive, and sedative effects; reduced dosage recommended
  Dental—Dry mouth may cause caries, candidiasis, periodontal disease, and discomfort; increased motor activity of face, head, and neck may interfere with some dental procedures
  Other medications, especially alcohol, other CNS depression–producing medications, other extrapyramidal reaction–producing medications, or lithium
  Other medical problems, especially severe drug-induced CNS depression

**Proper use of this medication**
Taking with food or a full glass (8 ounces) of water or milk to reduce gastric irritation
Taking liquid form of medicine undiluted or mixed with water, milk, fruit juice, or carbonated beverage
» Compliance with therapy: importance of not taking more or less medication than the amount prescribed
» May require several weeks of therapy to obtain optimal effects
  Proper dosing
  Missed dose: Taking as soon as possible; not taking if within 2 hours of next scheduled dose; resuming regular schedule; not doubling doses
» Proper storage

**Precautions while using this medication**
Regular visits to physician to check progress of therapy
» Checking with physician before discontinuing medication; gradual dosage reduction may be needed
» Avoiding use of antacids or antidiarrheal medication within 2 hours of taking molindone
» Avoiding use of alcoholic beverages or other CNS depressants during therapy
  Avoiding the use of over-the-counter medications for colds or allergies, to prevent increased anticholinergic effects and risk of heat stroke
» Possible drowsiness; caution when driving, using machinery, or doing other things that require alertness
» Possible dizziness or lightheadedness; caution when getting up suddenly from a lying or sitting position
» Possible heat stroke: caution during exercise, hot weather, or hot baths or saunas
  Possible dryness of mouth; using sugarless gum or candy, ice, or saliva substitute for relief; checking with physician or dentist if dry mouth continues for more than 2 weeks

**Side/adverse effects**
» Stopping medication and notifying physician immediately if symptoms of neuroleptic malignant syndrome (NMS) appear
» Notifying physician as soon as possible if early signs of tardive dyskinesia appear
  Possibility of withdrawal emergent dyskinesia
  Signs of potential side effects, especially akathisia, dystonias, parkinsonism, tardive dyskinesia, mental depression, allergic reaction, heat stroke, cholestatic jaundice or hepatitis, neuroleptic malignant syndrome (NMS), or tardive dystonia

## General Dosing Information

**Diet/Nutrition**
Molindone should be taken with food or a full glass (8 ounces) of water or milk to reduce gastric irritation.

**For treatment of adverse effects**
Neuroleptic malignant syndrome—
  Treatment is essentially symptomatic and supportive and includes the following:
  • *Discontinuing molindone immediately.*
  • Hyperthermia—Administering antipyretics (aspirin or acetaminophen); using cooling blanket.
  • Dehydration—Restoring fluids and electrolytes.
  • Cardiovascular instability—Monitoring blood pressure and cardiac rhythm closely.
  • Hypoxia—Administering oxygen; consider airway insertion and assisted ventilation.
  • Muscle rigidity—Dantrolene sodium may be administered (100 to 300 mg per day in divided doses; 1.25 to 1.5 mg per kg, intravenously). Bromocriptine (5 to 7.5 mg every eight hours) has also been used.
Parkinsonism, severe—
  Many authorities advise that the only appropriate treatment of extrapyramidal symptoms is reduction of the antipsychotic dosage, if possible. Oral antidyskinetics such as trihexyphenidyl, 2 mg three times per day, benztropine, or diphenhydramine may be effective in treating more severe parkinsonism and acute motor restlessness but should be used sparingly, only when side effects appear, and then usually for no longer than 3 months. In the elderly patient, the use of amantadine, 100 to 200 mg at bedtime, minimizes severe anticholinergic effects that may occur with other antidyskinetics.
Akathisia—
  May respond to antiparkinsonian medications, or propranolol (30 to 120 mg per day), nadolol (40 mg per day), pindolol (5 to 60 mg per day), lorazepam (1 or 2 mg two or three times a day), or diazepam (2 mg two or three times a day), but often requires dosage reduction of molindone.
Dystonia—
  Acute dystonic postures or oculogyric crisis may be relieved by parenteral administration of benztropine, 2 mg intramuscularly; diphenhydramine, 50 mg intramuscularly; or diazepam, 5 to 7.5 mg intravenously, to be followed by oral antidyskinetic medication for one or two days to prevent recurrent dystonic episodes. Dosage adjustments of molindone may control these effects, and discontinuation of molindone may reverse severe symptoms in weeks to months.
Tardive dyskinesia or tardive dystonia—
  No known effective treatment. Dosage of molindone should be lowered or medication discontinued, if clinically feasible, at earliest signs of

tardive dyskinesia or tardive dystonia, to prevent irreversible effects.

## Oral Dosage Forms

### MOLINDONE HYDROCHLORIDE ORAL SOLUTION

**Usual adult dose**
Antipsychotic—
  Initial:
    Oral, 50 to 75 mg a day, in three or four divided doses, the dose being increased to 100 mg a day in three to four days as needed and tolerated.
  Maintenance:
    Mild psychosis—Oral, 5 to 15 mg three or four times a day.
    Moderate psychosis—Oral, 10 to 25 mg three or four times a day.
    Severe psychosis—Oral, 225 mg a day in divided doses.
Note: Elderly or debilitated patients usually require a lower initial dose, the dose being adjusted gradually as needed and tolerated.

**Usual adult prescribing limits**
225 mg a day.

**Usual pediatric dose**
Children up to 12 years of age—Safety and efficacy have not been established.

**Strength(s) usually available**
U.S.—
  20 mg per mL (Rx) [*Moban Concentrate* (alcohol; artificial cherry flavor; artificial cover flavor; edetate sodium; glycerin; liquid sugar; methylparaben; propylparaben; sodium metabisulfite; sorbitol solution; hydrochloric acid)].
Canada—
  Not commercially available.

**Packaging and storage**
Store below 40 °C (104 °F), preferably between 15 and 30 °C (59 and 86 °F), in a tight container, unless otherwise specified by manufacturer. Protect from freezing.

**Auxiliary labeling**
- May cause drowsiness.
- Avoid alcoholic beverages.

**Additional information**
Studies have shown that oral doses of the tablet and solution are equivalent in bioavailability.

### MOLINDONE HYDROCHLORIDE TABLETS

**Usual adult dose**
See *Molindone Hydrochloride Oral Solution*.

**Usual adult prescribing limits**
See *Molindone Hydrochloride Oral Solution*.

**Usual pediatric dose**
See *Molindone Hydrochloride Oral Solution*.

**Strength(s) usually available**
U.S.—
  5 mg (Rx) [*Moban* (calcium sulfate; lactose; magnesium stearate; microcrystalline cellulose; povidone; alginic acid; colloidal silicon dioxide; FD&C Yellow No. 6)].
  10 mg (Rx) [*Moban* (calcium sulfate; lactose; magnesium stearate; microcrystalline cellulose; povidone; alginic acid; colloidal silicon dioxide; FD&C Blue No. 2; FD&C Red No. 40)].
  25 mg (Rx) [*Moban* (calcium sulfate; lactose; magnesium stearate; microcrystalline cellulose; povidone; alginic acid; colloidal silicon dioxide; FD&C Blue No. 2; FD&C Yellow No. 6; D&C Yellow No. 10)].
  50 mg (Rx) [*Moban* (calcium sulfate; lactose; magnesium stearate; microcrystalline cellulose; povidone; FD&C Blue No. 2; starch)].
  100 mg (Rx) [*Moban* (calcium sulfate; lactose; magnesium stearate; microcrystalline cellulose; povidone; FD&C Blue No. 2; FD&C Yellow No. 6; sodium starch glycolate)].
Canada—
  Not commercially available.

**Packaging and storage**
Store below 40 °C (104 °F), preferably between 15 and 30 °C (59 and 86 °F), in a tight container, unless otherwise specified by manufacturer. Protect from light.

**Auxiliary labeling**
- May cause drowsiness.
- Avoid alcoholic beverages.

**Additional information**
Studies have shown that oral doses of the tablet and solution are equivalent in bioavailability.

Revised: 03/19/93

---

# MOLYBDENUM SUPPLEMENTS   Systemic†

VA CLASSIFICATION (Primary): TN499

Commonly used brand name(s): *Molypen*.

Note: For a listing of dosage forms and brand names by country availability, see *Dosage Forms* section(s).

†Not commercially available in Canada.

## Category
Nutritional supplement (mineral).

## Indications

**Accepted**
Molybdenum deficiency (prophylaxis and treatment)—Molybdenum is indicated in the prevention and treatment of molybdenum deficiency, which is rare but may result from inadequate nutrition or intestinal malabsorption. Molybdenum deficiency does not occur in healthy individuals receiving an adequate balanced diet. For prophylaxis of molybdenum deficiency, dietary improvement, rather than supplementation, is advisable. For treatment of molybdenum deficiency supplementation is preferred.

Deficiency of molybdenum is rare, but when it occurs it may lead to an intolerance of sulfur-containing amino acids.

Some unusual diets (e.g., reducing diets that drastically restrict food selection) may not supply minimum daily requirements of molybdenum. Supplementation may be necessary in patients receiving total parenteral nutrition (TPN) or undergoing rapid weight loss or in those with malnutrition, because of inadequate dietary intake.

## Pharmacology/Pharmacokinetics

**Physicochemical characteristics**
Molecular weight—Ammonium molybdate: 1235.86.
Elemental molybdenum: 95.94.

**Mechanism of action/Effect**
Molybdenum is a component of the enzymes xanthine oxidase, sulfite oxidase, and aldehyde oxidase. These enzymes are responsible for conversion of xanthine and hypoxanthine to uric acid, conversion of sulfite to sulfate, and detoxification of several harmful organic molecules, respectively.

**Absorption**
Dietary molybdenum is well absorbed in the gastrointestinal tract.

**Storage**
Molybdenum is stored in the liver, kidneys, spleen, lung, brain, and muscles.

**Elimination**
Primarily in urine, with small amounts excreted in bile.

## Precautions to Consider

**Pregnancy/Reproduction**
Pregnancy—Studies have not been done in humans and problems have not been documented with intake of normal daily recommended amounts.
Studies have not been done in animals.
FDA Pregnancy Category C (parenteral molybdenum).

**Breast-feeding**
Problems in humans have not been documented with intake of normal daily recommended amounts.

**Pediatrics**
Problems in pediatrics have not been documented with intake of normal daily recommended amounts.

**Geriatrics**
Problems in geriatrics have not been documented with intake of normal daily recommended amounts.

**Drug interactions and/or related problems**
The following drug interactions and/or related problems have been selected on the basis of their potential clinical significance (possible mechanism in parentheses where appropriate)—not necessarily inclusive (» = major clinical significance):

Note: Combinations containing any of the following medications, depending on the amount present, may also interact with this medication.

Copper supplements
(excessive amounts of molybdenum may mobilize copper from tissue and increase urinary excretion of copper; copper supplements may be recommended with molybdenum therapy)

**Medical considerations/Contraindications**
The medical considerations/contraindications included have been selected on the basis of their potential clinical significance (reasons given in parentheses where appropriate)—not necessarily inclusive (» = major clinical significance).

*Risk-benefit should be considered when the following medical problems exist:*

Biliary obstruction or
Renal dysfunction
(may cause an accumulation of molybdenum, since molybdenum is normally eliminated in bile and urine; a reduction in molybdenum dosage may be necessary)

Copper deficiency
(condition may be exacerbated due to the mobilization of tissue copper and increased urinary excretion of copper by thiomolybdate)

**Patient monitoring**
The following may be especially important in patient monitoring (other tests may be warranted in some patients, depending on condition; » = major clinical significance):

Copper
(serum copper concentrations may be decreased by thiomolybdate; monitoring of copper every six months may be required with long-term use of molybdenum)

Molybdenum, blood or urinary
(monitoring every six months by atomic absorption spectrophotometric method may be recommended by some clinicians to determine molybdenum status if deficiency or toxicity of molybdenum is suspected)

Purine and sulfur metabolic profiles
(monitoring every six months may be recommended by some clinicians if deficiency or toxicity of molybdenum is suspected)

## Side/Adverse Effects

No side effects have been reported with molybdenum with recommended dosages.

## Overdose

For information on the management of overdose or unintentional ingestion, **contact a Poison Control Center** (see *Poison Control Center Listing*).

**Clinical effects of overdose**
The following effects have been selected on the basis of their potential clinical significance (possible signs and symptoms in parentheses where appropriate)—not necessarily inclusive:

*Hyperuricemia* (joint pain; side, lower back, or stomach pain; swelling of feet or lower legs)—rarely has been reported from consumption of foods grown in molybdeniferous soil

## Patient Consultation

As an aid to patient consultation, refer to *Advice for the Patient, Molybdenum Supplements (Systemic)*.

In providing consultation, consider emphasizing the following selected information (» = major clinical significance):

**Description of use**
Description should include function in the body, signs of deficiency

**Importance of diet**
Importance of proper nutrition; supplement may be needed because of inadequate dietary intake

Food sources of molybdenum
Recommended daily intake for molybdenum

**Proper use of this dietary supplement**
» Proper dosing
Missed dose: No cause for concern because of length of time necessary for depletion; remembering to take as directed
» Proper storage

**Precautions while taking this dietary supplement**
Importance of taking copper supplement

## General Dosing Information

Because of the infrequency of molybdenum deficiency alone, combinations of several vitamins and/or minerals are commonly administered. In the oral form, molybdenum is available only as a vitamin/mineral combination.

**For parenteral dosage forms only**
In most cases, parenteral administration is indicated only when oral administration is not acceptable (for example, in nausea, vomiting, preoperative and postoperative conditions) or possible (for example, in malabsorption syndromes or following gastric resection).

**Diet/Nutrition**
Recommended dietary intakes for molybdenum are defined differently worldwide.
For U.S.—
The Recommended Dietary Allowances (RDAs) for vitamins and minerals are determined by the Food and Nutrition Board of the National Research Council and are intended to provide adequate nutrition in most healthy persons under usual environmental stresses. In addition, a different designation may be used by the FDA for food and dietary supplement labeling purposes, as with Daily Value (DV). DVs replace the previous labeling terminology United States Recommended Daily Allowances (USRDAs).
For Canada—
Recommended Nutrient Intakes (RNIs) for vitamins, minerals, and protein are determined by Health and Welfare in Canada and provide recommended amounts of a specific nutrient while minimizing the risk of chronic diseases.

There is no RDA or RNI established for molybdenum. The following daily intakes are considered adequate for all individuals—
Infants and children:
Birth to 3 years of age: 15 to 50 mcg.
4 to 6 years of age: 30 to 75 mcg.
7 to 10 years of age: 50 to 150 mcg.
Adolescents and adults:
75 to 250 mcg.

The amount of molybdenum in foods varies, depending on the environment in which the food is grown. Legumes, grain products, leafy vegetables, and low-fat milk are good sources of molybdenum.

## Parenteral Dosage Forms

### AMMONIUM MOLYBDATE INJECTION USP

**Usual adult and adolescent dose**
Deficiency (treatment)—
Intravenous, 163 mcg (0.163 mg) elemental molybdenum a day, added to total parenteral nutrition (TPN).
Deficiency (prophylaxis)—
Intravenous, 20 to 120 mcg (0.02 to 0.12 mg) elemental molybdenum a day, added to total parenteral nutrition (TPN).

**Strength(s) usually available**
U.S.—
46 mcg (0.046 mg) (25 mcg elemental molybdenum) per mL (Rx) [*Molypen*; GENERIC].
Canada—
Not commercially available.

**Packaging and storage**
Store below 40 °C (104 °F), preferably between 15 and 30 °C (59 and 86 °F), unless otherwise specified by manufacturer.

**Preparation of dosage form**
Ammonium molybdate is physically compatible with amino acid solutions, dextrose solutions, electrolytes, and other trace elements.

Revised: 03/02/92
Interim revision: 07/31/92; 08/10/94; 04/25/95

MOMETASONE—See *Corticosteroids (Topical)*

# MOMETASONE Nasal—INTRODUCTORY VERSION

VA CLASSIFICATION (Primary): NT201
Commonly used brand name(s): *Nasonex*.
Note: For a listing of dosage forms and brand names by country availability, see *Dosage Forms* section(s).

## Category
Anti-inflammatory (steroidal), nasal; corticosteroid (nasal).

## Indications
### Accepted
Rhinitis, perennial allergic (treatment)
Rhinitis, seasonal allergic (prophylaxis) or
Rhinitis, seasonal allergic (treatment)—Mometasone nasal is indicated for the treatment of perennial allergic and seasonal allergic rhinitis. It is also indicated for the prophylaxis of seasonal allergic rhinitis.

## Pharmacology/Pharmacokinetics
### Physicochemical characteristics
Chemical group—Corticosteroids.
Molecular weight—Mometasone furoate: 521.44.
Mometasone furoate monohydrate: 539.45.
pH—Nasal suspension: 4.3 to 4.9.
Solubility—Practically insoluble in water; slightly soluble in methanol, ethanol, and isopropanol; soluble in acetone and chloroform; freely soluble in tetrahydrofuran.
Partition coefficient—Between octanol and water: Greater than 5000.

### Mechanism of action/Effect
The precise mechanism by which corticosteroids affect allergic rhinitis symptoms is not known. Corticosteroids have been shown to have a wide range of effects on multiple cell types (e.g., eosinophils, lymphocytes, macrophages, mast cells, and neutrophils) and mediators (e.g., histamine, eicosanoids, cytokines, and leukotrienes) involved in inflammation.

A number of studies have been done to assess the efficacy and safety of mometasone furoate nasal spray in the treatment of perennial or seasonal allergic rhinitis. Doses ranged from 50 to 800 mcg of mometasone furoate nasal spray per day. However, most of the studies used 200 mcg of mometasone furoate nasal spray per day. These studies evaluated total nasal symptom scores that included stuffiness, rhinorrhea, itching, and sneezing. Patients treated with 200 mcg a day of mometasone furoate nasal spray had a significant decrease in total nasal symptom scores compared with patients given the placebo. No additional benefit was observed for doses greater than 200 mcg of mometasone furoate nasal spray a day.

Two clinical studies assessing 200 mcg of mometasone furoate nasal spray per day for the prophylaxis of seasonal allergic rhinitis were done in 284 patients 12 years of age and older. These patients received up to 4 weeks of prophylaxis with mometasone furoate nasal spray prior to the anticipated onset of the pollen season. Compared to patients receiving the placebo, patients receiving 2 to 4 weeks of prophylaxis demonstrated a statistically significant smaller mean increase in total nasal symptom scores at the onset of the pollen season.

### Other actions/effects
In two clinical studies using nasal antigen challenge, intranasal mometasone furoate (dosage unknown) decreased certain markers of the early- and late-phase allergic response. These markers included decreases in histamine and eosinophil cationic protein levels compared to the levels observed with administration of the placebo, and reductions in eosinophils, neutrophils, and epithelial cell adhesion proteins compared to baseline values. The clinical significance of these findings is not clear.

Following 12 months of treatment with intranasal mometasone furoate (dosage unknown) in 46 patients with allergic rhinitis, there was a marked reduction in intraepithelial eosinophilia and inflammatory cell infiltration (e.g., eosinophils, lymphocytes, monocytes, neutrophils, and plasma cells).

In preclinical trials, mometasone furoate demonstrated no mineralocorticoid, androgenic, antiandrogenic, or estrogenic activity.

Three clinical pharmacology studies were conducted in humans to assess the effect of various doses of mometasone furoate on adrenal function. In the first study, daily doses of 200 or 400 mcg of intranasal mometasone furoate were administered for 36 days to 64 patients with allergic rhinitis. Adrenal function was assessed before and after the 36 days by measuring plasma cortisol concentrations following a 6-hour Cortrosyn (ACTH) infusion and by measuring 24-hour urinary free cortisol concentrations. Compared to placebo, intranasal mometasone furoate demonstrated no statistically significant decrease in concentrations with either measurement. In the second study, daily doses of 400 or 1600 mcg of intranasal mometasone furoate were administered for 29 days to 48 male volunteers. Adrenal function was assessed before and after the 29 days by measuring the 24-hour plasma cortisol area under the curve ($AUC_{0-24}$) during and after an 8-hour Cortrosyn infusion and by measuring 24-hour urinary free cortisol concentrations. Compared to the placebo, intranasal mometasone furoate demonstrated no statistically significant differences in adrenal function. In the third study, single daily increasing doses of 1000, 2000, and 4000 mcg of intranasal mometasone furoate or 200, 400, and 800 mcg of oral mometasone furoate were administered to 24 male volunteers. Dose administrations were separated by at least 72 hours. A placebo was administered at the end of both series of drug doses. Determinations of serial plasma cortisol concentrations at 8 a.m. and for the 24-hour period following each treatment were used to calculate the plasma cortisol $AUC_{0-24}$. In addition, 24-hour urinary free cortisol concentrations were collected prior to initial treatment and during the period immediately following each dose. Compared to the placebo, oral or intranasal mometasone furoate demonstrated no statistically significant differences in plasma cortisol AUC, 8 a.m. cortisol levels, or 24-hour urinary free cortisol levels.

### Absorption
Using an assay with a lower quantitation limit (LOQ) of 50 picograms per mL, mometasone furoate monohydrate administered as a nasal spray was virtually undetectable in plasma.

### Distribution
In adult male rats administered a single dose of intranasal mometasone furoate, the highest drug concentrations were seen in the esophagus, trachea, nasal passage, and mouth.

### Biotransformation
Studies have shown that any portion of a dose of intranasal mometasone furoate that is swallowed and absorbed undergoes extensive metabolism to multiple metabolites.

### Half-life
Following intravenous administration, the effective plasma elimination half-life of mometasone furoate is 5.8 hours.

### Onset of action
Seasonal allergic rhinitis—Usually occurs within 2 days after the first dose.

### Time to peak effect
Seasonal allergic rhinitis—Maximum benefit usually occurs within 1 or 2 weeks.

### Elimination
Following intranasal administration, any absorbed drug is excreted as metabolites mostly via the bile and, to a limited extent, into the urine.

## Precautions to Consider
### Tumorigenicity
There was no statistically significant increase in the incidence of tumors in Sprague Dawley rats given an inhalation dose of 67 mcg per kg of body weight (mcg/kg) of mometasone furoate (approximately three times the maximum recommended daily [MRD] intranasal dose in humans on a mcg-per-square-meter of body surface area [$mcg/m^2$] basis).

Also, there was no statistically significant increase in the incidence of tumors in Swiss CD-1 mice given an inhalation dose of 160 mcg/kg of mometasone furoate (approximately four times the MRD intranasal dose in humans on a $mcg/m^2$ basis).

### Mutagenicity
At cytotoxic doses, mometasone furoate produced an increase in chromosome aberrations *in vitro* in Chinese hamster ovary cell cultures in the nonactivation phase, but not in the presence of rat liver S9 fraction. Mometasone furoate was not mutagenic in the mouse lymphoma assay and the *Salmonella/Escherichia coli*/mammalian microsome mutation assay, a Chinese hamster lung cell (CHL) chromosomal aberrations assay, an *in vivo* mouse bone marrow erythrocyte micronucleus assay, a rat bone marrow clastogenicity assay, and the mouse male germ cell

clastogenicity assay. Mometasone furoate did not induce unscheduled DNA synthesis *in vivo* in rat hepatocytes.

**Pregnancy/Reproduction**

In rats, mometasone furoate caused prolonged gestation, prolonged and difficult labor, reduced offspring survival, and reduced maternal body weight gain when given in subcutaneous doses of 15 mcg/kg (approximately three fourths of the MRD intranasal dose in humans on a mcg/m² basis).

In mice, mometasone furoate caused reduced offspring survival when given in subcutaneous doses of 180 mcg/kg (approximately four times the MRD intranasal dose in humans on a mcg/m² basis).

In mice, rabbits, and rats, there were reductions in maternal body weight gain and effects on fetal growth (lower fetal body weights and/or delayed ossification) when mometasone furoate was given at doses of 60 and 180 mcg/kg subcutaneously to mice, 150 mcg/kg topically to rabbits, and 600 mcg/kg topically to rats.

In rabbits, pregnancy failure was observed in most rabbits given mometasone furoate orally at a dose of 2800 mcg/kg (approximately 270 times the MRD intranasal dose in humans on a mcg/m² basis).

Fertility—In rats, impairment of fertility did not occur when mometasone furoate was given in subcutaneous doses of up to 15 mcg/kg.

Pregnancy—Adequate and well-controlled studies in humans have not been done. Corticosteroids, including intranasal mometasone furoate, should be used during pregnancy only if the potential benefits justify the potential risk to the fetus.

In mice, mometasone furoate caused cleft palate when given in subcutaneous doses of 60 and 180 mcg/kg. The nonteratogenic subcutaneous dose level in mice was 20 mcg/kg.

In rabbits, mometasone furoate was teratogenic and caused flexed front paws when given in a topical dermal dose of 150 mcg/kg.

In rats, mometasone furoate produced umbilical hernia, cleft palate, and delayed ossification when given in a topical dermal dose of 600 mcg/kg (approximately 30 times the MRD intranasal dose in humans on a mcg/m² basis). At a topical dermal dose of 1200 mcg/kg (approximately 60 times the MRD intranasal dose in humans on a mcg/m² basis), microphthalmia, umbilical hernias, and delayed ossification were observed in rat pups.

In rabbits given mometasone furoate orally at a dose of 700 mcg/kg, increased incidences of resorptions and malformations, including cleft palate and/or head malformations (hydrocephaly or domed head) were observed.

FDA Pregnancy Category C.

Postpartum—Infants born to women receiving corticosteroids should be carefully monitored, since hypoadrenalism may occur.

**Breast-feeding**

It is not known whether mometasone furoate is distributed into breast milk. However, since other corticosteroids are distributed into breast milk, caution should be used when intranasal mometasone furoate is administered to breast-feeding women.

**Pediatrics**

Safety and efficacy have not been established in children up to 12 years of age.

**Geriatrics**

The effects of age on the pharmacokinetics of mometasone furoate have not been adequately investigated.

Appropriate studies on the relationship of age to the effects of intranasal mometasone furoate have not been performed in the geriatric population. However, clinical trials included a limited number of older patients (203 patients; age range 64 to 85) and the adverse reactions reported were similar to those of younger adults; therefore, geriatrics-specific problems that would limit the usefulness of the medication in the elderly are not expected.

**Medical considerations/Contraindications**

The medical considerations/contraindications included have been selected on the basis of their potential clinical significance (reasons given in parentheses where appropriate)—not necessarily inclusive (» = major clinical significance).

*Risk-benefit should be considered when the following medical problems exist:*

Cataracts or
Glaucoma
(intranasal corticosteroids have been associated with the development of cataracts and/or glaucoma and also rarely may increase intraocular pressure; however, one controlled 12-week study (141 patients) and one uncontrolled 12-month study (139 patients) of patients using 200 mcg a day of intranasal mometasone did not find any cataract formation or significant change from baseline in mean intraocular pressure measurements as compared to placebo)

Hepatic function impairment or
Renal function impairment
(effects of hepatic or renal function impairment on the pharmacokinetics of mometasone furoate have not been adequately investigated)

» Infections, fungal, bacterial, or systemic viral
(corticosteroids may mask the infection; in addition, some infections, such as chickenpox or measles, may have a more serious course in patients on immunosuppressant doses of corticosteroids)

Intolerance to mometasone furoate or other corticosteroids

Nasal septal ulcers, recent or
Nasal surgery, recent or
Nasal trauma, recent
(corticosteroids inhibit wound healing; patients should not use a nasal corticosteroid until healing has occurred)

» Ocular herpes simplex
(corticosteroids may mask the infection)

Sensitivity to any ingredient in the product, such as benzalkonium chloride or phenylethyl alcohol

» Tuberculosis, latent or active, of respiratory tract
(corticosteroids may mask or activate the infection)

**Patient monitoring**

The following may be especially important in patient monitoring (other tests may be warranted in some patients, depending on condition; » = major clinical significance):

Adrenal function assessment
(assessment of hypothalamic-pituitary-adrenal (HPA) axis function may be advisable at periodic intervals in patients receiving long-term nasal corticosteroid therapy)

Otolaryngologic examination
(should be performed in patients on long-term therapy to monitor nasal mucosa and nasal passages for infection, nasal septal perforation, nasal membrane ulceration, or other histologic changes; as determined by the condition of the mucosa, it may be advisable periodically to discontinue the medication for a week or more)

## Side/Adverse Effects

Note: Following 12 months of treatment with 50 mcg of intranasal mometasone furoate in 46 patients with allergic rhinitis, there was no evidence of atrophy of the nasal mucosa.

Extremely rare instances of wheezing have been reported with use of intranasal mometasone furoate. In addition, nasal septum perforation and increased intraocular pressure rarely have been reported with other corticosteroids.

The following side/adverse effects have been selected on the basis of their potential clinical significance (possible signs and symptoms in parentheses where appropriate)—not necessarily inclusive:

**Those indicating need for medical attention**
Incidence less frequent
*Asthma* (shortness of breath, troubled breathing, tightness in chest, or wheezing); *bronchitis* (cough); *chest pain; conjunctivitis* (redness of the eye, eyelid, or inner lining of eyelid); *dysmenorrhea* (increased abdominal pain and cramping at menstrual periods); *earache; epistaxis* (bloody mucus or unexplained nosebleeds); *sinusitis* (stuffy or runny nose or headache); *upper respiratory tract infection* (cold or flu-like symptoms)

Incidence rare
*Nasal or oral candidiasis* (white patches inside nose or mouth); *nasal ulcers* (sores inside nose)

**Those indicating need for medical attention only if they continue or are bothersome**
Incidence less frequent
*Arthralgia or myalgia* (joint or muscle ache or pain); *cough; diarrhea; dyspepsia* (stomach discomfort following meals; upset stomach); *headache; nausea; pharyngitis* (sore throat); *rhinitis* (runny or stuffy nose); *sneezing*

## Overdose

For more information on the management of overdose or unintentional ingestion, **contact a Poison Control Center** (see *Poison Control Center Listing*).

**Treatment of overdose**

One bottle of mometasone nasal spray contains approximately 8.5 mg of mometasone furoate.

For acute overdose—Because of low systemic bioavailability of intranasal mometasone, an absence of acute drug-related systemic findings in clinical studies, and the small quantity of corticosteroid contained in each spray bottle, acute overdose with mometasone nasal spray is unlikely to require any therapy other than observation.

For chronic overdose—Chronic overdosage with mometasone nasal spray may result in signs or symptoms of hypercorticism. If symptoms of chronic overdose occur, nasal corticosteroids should be discontinued slowly.

Supportive care—Patients in whom intentional overdose is confirmed or suspected should be referred for psychiatric consultation.

## Patient Consultation

As an aid to patient consultation, refer to *Advice for the Patient, Mometasone (Nasal)—Introductory Version.*
In providing consultation, consider emphasizing the following selected information (» = major clinical significance):

### Before using this medication
» Conditions affecting use, especially:
  Intolerance to mometasone furoate or other corticosteroids; sensitivity to any ingredient in the product, such as benzalkonium chloride or phenylethyl alcohol
  Pregnancy—Risk-benefit must be considered; studies in animals have demonstrated embryotoxicity, fetotoxicity, and teratogenicity; infants born to mothers who received substantial doses of corticosteroids during pregnancy should be observed for hypoadrenalism
  Breast-feeding—Although it is not known whether mometasone furoate is distributed into breast milk, some other corticosteroids are; caution should be used when intranasal mometasone furoate is administered to breast-feeding women
  Other medical problems, especially fungal, bacterial, or systemic viral infections; latent or active tuberculosis of respiratory tract; or ocular herpes simplex

### Proper use of this medication
» Reading patient instructions carefully before using medication
  Proper administration technique; blowing nose to clear nasal passages before administration; aiming spray away from nasal septum by aiming spray toward the inner corner of eye
» Compliance with therapy; may require up to 2 weeks for full benefit
» Importance of not using more medication than the amount prescribed and not using it more than once a day
» Checking with physician before using medication for other nasal problems
» Proper dosing
  Missed dose: Using as soon as possible; if not remembered until next day, skipping missed dose and going back to regular dosing schedule; not doubling doses
» Proper storage

### Precautions while using this medication
» Avoiding exposure to chickenpox or measles if taking immunosuppressant doses of corticosteroids; checking with physician if exposure is suspected
  Checking with physician if symptoms do not improve or if condition gets worse

### Side/adverse effects
Signs of potential side effects, especially asthma, bronchitis, chest pain, conjunctivitis, dysmenorrhea, earache, epistaxis, sinusitis, upper respiratory tract infection, nasal or oral candidiasis, and nasal ulcers

## General Dosing Information

Patients with known seasonal allergic rhinitis should initiate prophylaxis with intranasal mometasone 2 to 4 weeks prior to the anticipated start of the pollen season.

Patients may be intolerant of or adverse to the odor of the product.

With the treatment of seasonal allergic rhinitis, improvement in nasal symptoms usually occurs within 2 days after the first dose of intranasal mometasone. Maximum benefit usually occurs within 1 or 2 weeks.

It is recommended that intranasal mometasone be used at a frequency of once daily only. In addition, no additional benefit has been observed for doses greater than 200 mcg of intranasal mometasone a day.

Prior to initial use of mometasone nasal spray, the pump should be primed ten times or until a fine spray appears. The pump may be stored unused for up to 1 week without repriming. If unused for more than 1 week, the pump should be reprimed two times or until a fine spray appears.

Caution is recommended if a systemic corticosteroid is replaced with a nasal corticosteroid, such as mometasone, since adrenal insufficiency may occur. In addition, some patients may experience symptoms of withdrawal, such as joint or muscular pain, lassitude, or depression. It is recommended that patients previously treated for prolonged periods with systemic corticosteroids and transferred to nasal corticosteroids be carefully monitored for acute adrenal insufficiency in response to stress.

The dosage of other corticosteroids being administered concurrently by other routes of administration, including oral inhalation, should be taken into account when determining the usual adult prescribing limits of nasal corticosteroids.

## Nasal Dosage Forms

### MOMETASONE FUROATE NASAL SUSPENSION

**Usual adult and adolescent dose**
Rhinitis, perennial allergic (treatment) or
Rhinitis, seasonal allergic (prophylaxis) or
Rhinitis, seasonal allergic (treatment)—
  Nasal, 200 mcg (0.2 mg) a day, administered as 2 metered sprays in each nostril once a day. Each metered spray delivers 50 mcg (0.05 mg).

**Usual adult and adolescent prescribing limits**
200 mcg (0.2 mg) a day.

**Usual pediatric dose**
Rhinitis, perennial allergic (treatment) or
Rhinitis, seasonal allergic (prophylaxis) or
Rhinitis, seasonal allergic (treatment)—
  For children up to 12 years of age: Safety and efficacy have not been established.
  For children 12 years of age and older: See *Usual adult and adolescent dose*.

**Strength(s) usually available**
U.S.—
  50 mcg per metered spray (as mometasone furoate) (Rx) [*Nasonex* (glycerin; microcrystalline cellulose; carboxymethylcellulose sodium; sodium citrate 0.25%; phenylethyl alcohol; citric acid; benzalkonium chloride; polysorbate 80)].

Note:  The container holds 120 metered sprays.

**Packaging and storage**
Store between 2 and 25 °C (36 and 77 °F). Protect from light.

**Auxiliary labeling**
• Shake well before each use.
• For the nose.
• Do not spray into the eyes.
• Keep out of direct light.

**Note**
Include patient instructions when dispensing.

Developed: 03/26/98
Interim revision: 08/12/98

---

**MONOCTANOIN**—The *Monoctanoin (Local)* monograph is not included in this published version of the USP DI database. Copies of the monograph are available on request from Micromedex, Inc. - Reprint Requests, 6200 S. Syracuse Way, Suite 300, Englewood, CO 80111; telephone (303) 486-6400; telefax (303) 486-6464; Email: USPDI@MDX.COM.

---

# MONTELUKAST   Systemic—INTRODUCTORY VERSION

VA CLASSIFICATION (Primary): RE108
Commonly used brand name(s): *Singulair*.
Note:  For a listing of dosage forms and brand names by country availability, see *Dosage Forms* section(s).

## Category

Antiasthmatic (leukotriene receptor antagonist).

# Montelukast (Systemic)—Introductory Version

## Indications

### Accepted
**Asthma, bronchial, chronic (prophylaxis and treatment)**—Montelukast is indicated for prophylaxis and chronic treatment of asthma.

### Unaccepted
Montelukast is not indicated for treatment of bronchospasm in acute asthma attacks, including status asthmaticus.

## Pharmacology/Pharmacokinetics

### Physicochemical characteristics
Molecular weight—608.18.
Solubility—Freely soluble in ethanol, methanol, and water and practically insoluble in acetonitrile.

### Mechanism of action/Effect
Montelukast inhibits bronchoconstriction due to antigen challenge. Montelukast is a selective leukotriene receptor antagonist of the cysteinyl leukotriene $CysLT_1$ receptor. The cysteinyl leukotrienes ($LTC_4$, $LTD_4$, $LTE_4$) are products of arachidonic acid metabolism that are released from various cells, including mast cells and eosinophils. They bind to cysteinyl leukotriene receptors (CysLT) found in the human airway. Binding of cysteinyl leukotrienes to leukotriene receptors has been correlated with the pathophysiology of asthma, including airway edema, smooth muscle contraction, and altered cellular activity associated with the inflammatory process, factors that contribute to the signs and symptoms of asthma. Montelukast binding to the $CysLT_1$ receptor is high-affinity and selective, preferring the $CysLT_1$ receptor to other pharmacologically important airway receptors, such as the prostanoid, cholinergic, or beta-adrenergic receptor. Montelukast inhibits physiologic actions of $LTD_4$ at the $CysLT_1$ receptors, without any agonist activity.

### Absorption
Rapid.
For the 10-mg tablets—Mean oral bioavailability is 64%. Bioavailability is not affected by a standard meal in the morning.
For the 5-mg chewable tablet—Mean oral bioavailability is 73% in the fasted state versus 63% when administered with a standard meal in the morning.

### Distribution
Steady-state volume of distribution averages 8 to 11 liters.

### Protein binding
Plasma proteins—Very high (more than 99%).

### Biotransformation
Hepatic, extensive. Involves cytochrome P450 3A4 and 2C9.

### Half-life
Range, 2.7 to 5.5 hours in healthy young adults.

### Onset of action
In clinical trials, the treatment effect was achieved after the first dose.

### Time to peak concentration
10-mg tablet—3 to 4 hours.
5-mg chewable tablet—2 to 2.5 hours.

### Peak plasma concentration
The peak plasma concentration is not affected by administration with a standard meal in the morning.

### Duration of action
Single dose—24 hours.
Note: There was no rebound worsening of asthma following withdrawal of montelukast after 12 weeks of therapy.

### Elimination
Biliary/fecal, 86%.
Renal, less than 0.2%.
Plasma clearance averages 45 mL per minute in healthy adults.
In dialysis—
It is not known whether montelukast is removable by peritoneal dialysis or hemodialysis.
Note: The pharmacokinetics of montelukast are nearly linear at doses of up to 50 mg.

## Precautions to Consider

### Carcinogenicity
A 2-year study in Sprague Dawley rats at oral (gavage) doses of up to 200 mg per kg of body weight per day (mg/kg/day) (approximately 160 and 190 times the maximum recommended daily oral dose in adults and children, respectively, on a mg per square meter of body surface area basis) and a 92-week study in mice at oral doses of up to 100 mg/kg/day (approximately 40 and 50 times the maximum recommended daily oral dose in adults and children, respectively, on a mg per square meter of body surface area basis) found no evidence of carcinogenicity or tumorigenicity.

### Mutagenicity
Montelukast was not found to be mutagenic or clastogenic in the microbial mutagenesis assay, the V-79 mammalian cell mutagenesis assay, the alkaline elution assay in rat hepatocytes, the chromosomal aberration assay in Chinese hamster ovary cells, and the *in vivo* mouse bone marrow chromosomal aberration assay.

### Pregnancy/Reproduction
Fertility—A reduction in fertility was seen in female rats on oral doses of montelukast of 200 mg/kg (approximately 160 times the maximum recommended daily oral dose in adults, on a mg per square meter of body surface area basis). However, no effects on fertility were seen in female rats on oral doses of montelukast of 100 mg/kg (approximately 80 times the maximum recommended daily oral dose in adults, on a mg per square meter of body surface area basis). No reduction in fertility was seen in male rats at oral doses of up to 800 mg/kg (approximately 650 times the maximum recommended daily oral dose in adults, on a mg per square meter of body surface area basis).

Pregnancy—Adequate and well-controlled studies in humans have not been done.
Studies in rats at oral doses of up to 400 mg/kg/day (approximately 320 times the maximum recommended daily oral dose in adults on a mg per square meter of body surface area basis) and in rabbits at oral doses of up to 300 mg/kg/day (approximately 490 times the maximum recommended daily oral dose in adults on a mg per square meter of body surface area basis) found no evidence of teratogenicity. Montelukast crosses the placenta in rats and rabbits.

Risk-benefit should be considered before use of montelukast during pregnancy.

FDA Pregnancy Category B.

### Breast-feeding
It is not known whether montelukast is distributed into breast milk in humans. However, it is distributed into breast milk in rats. Risk-benefit should be considered before breast-feeding during treatment with montelukast.

### Pediatrics
Safety and efficacy in children younger than 6 years of age have not been established. Studies in children 6 to 14 years of age have found a similar efficacy and side effects profile to that in adults. Adverse reactions, such as diarrhea, laryngitis, pharyngitis, nausea, otitis, sinusitis, and viral infection were slightly more frequent in the pediatric group. The pharmacokinetics of the 5-mg chewable tablet in children 6 to 14 years of age are similar to the pharmacokinetics of the 10-mg tablet in adults; use of the 5-mg chewable tablet is recommended for children 6 to 14 years of age. The chewable tablet contains aspartame, which has phenylalanine as a component. Individuals with phenylketonuria should be informed that there is 0.842 mg of phenylalanine per 5-mg tablet.

### Adolescents
The pharmacokinetics of the 10-mg tablet are similar in adolescents 15 years of age and older and young adults; the pharmacokinetics of the 5-mg chewable tablet in children 6 to 14 years of age are similar to those of the 10-mg tablet in adults. The 5-mg chewable tablet is recommended for children 6 to 14 years of age and the 10-mg tablet is recommended for adolescents 15 years of age and older.

### Geriatrics
The pharmacokinetics and oral bioavailability of montelukast are similar in elderly and younger adults. The plasma half-life is slightly longer in the elderly, but no dosage adjustment is necessary.
No information is available comparing the use of montelukast in elderly patients with its use in younger adults. However, a small percentage of the patients in clinical trials were 65 years of age and over, and no differences in efficacy or adverse effects were observed.

### Drug interactions and/or related problems
The following drug interactions and/or related problems have been selected on the basis of their potential clinical significance (possible mechanism in parentheses where appropriate)—not necessarily inclusive (» = major clinical significance):

Note: Although studies have not been done, because of the potential for interactions, monitoring is recommended during concurrent use with potent cytochrome P450 enzyme inducers, such as rifampin.

Studies have not found that montelukast causes significant changes in the pharmacokinetics of theophylline, warfarin, immunoreactive digoxin, terfenadine, fexofenadine, oral contraceptives containing norethindrone 1 mg and ethinyl estradiol 35 mcg, prednisone, or prednisolone.

Combinations containing any of the following medications, depending on the amount present, may also interact with this medication.

Phenobarbital
(concurrent use results in significant decreases [approximately 40%] in the area under the curve [AUC] for montelukast, as a result of induction of hepatic metabolism; however, no dosage adjustment is necessary)

**Laboratory value alterations**
The following have been selected on the basis of their potential clinical significance (possible effect in parentheses where appropriate)—not necessarily inclusive (» = major clinical significance):

With physiology/laboratory test values
Alanine aminotransferase (ALT [SGPT]) and
Aspartate aminotransferase (AST [SGOT])
(serum values may infrequently be increased)

Eosinophils
(mean peripheral eosinophils may be increased by approximately 13 to 15% from baseline)

**Medical considerations/Contraindications**
The medical considerations/contraindications included have been selected on the basis of their potential clinical significance (reasons given in parentheses where appropriate)—not necessarily inclusive (» = major clinical significance).

*Risk-benefit should be considered when the following medical problems exist:*

Hepatic function impairment
(metabolism of montelukast may be decreased in patients with mild to moderate hepatic function impairment and clinical evidence of cirrhosis; half-life may be slightly prolonged [to a mean of 7.4 hours]; however, dosage adjustment is not necessary; montelukast has not been evaluated in patients with severe hepatic function impairment)

Sensitivity to montelukast

## Side/Adverse Effects

The following side/adverse effects have been selected on the basis of their potential clinical significance (possible signs and symptoms in parentheses where appropriate)—not necessarily inclusive:

**Those indicating need for medical attention**
Incidence less frequent
*Elevated hepatic enzymes* (asymptomatic)
Note: *Elevated hepatic enzymes* included alanine aminotransferase (ALT [SGPT]) and aspartate aminotransferase (AST [SGOT]).

Incidence rare
*Pyuria* (pus in the urine)

**Those indicating need for medical attention only if they continue or are bothersome**
Incidence more frequent
*Headache*
Incidence less frequent
*Abdominal or stomach pain; asthenia or fatigue* (weakness or unusual tiredness); *cough; dental pain; dizziness; dyspepsia* (heartburn); *fever; gastroenteritis, infectious* (abdominal or stomach pain); *nasal congestion* (stuffy nose); *skin rash*

## Overdose

**Clinical effects of overdose**
No information is available on the clinical effects of overdose.

**Treatment of overdose**
Treatment may include removal of unabsorbed material from the gastrointestinal tract, clinical monitoring, and supportive therapy if required.

It is not known if montelukast can be removed by peritoneal dialysis or hemodialysis.

Patients in whom intentional overdose is confirmed or suspected should be referred for psychiatric consultation.

## Patient Consultation

As an aid to patient consultation, refer to *Advice for the Patient, Montelukast (Systemic)—Introductory Version*.

In providing consultation, consider emphasizing the following selected information (» = major clinical significance):

**Before using this medication**
» Conditions affecting use, especially:
Sensitivity to montelukast

**Proper use of this medication**
» Importance of not using this medicine to treat acute asthma symptoms
» Proper dosing
Missed dose: Taking as soon as remembered; not taking if almost time for next dose; not doubling doses
» Proper storage

**Precautions while using this medication**
» Compliance with therapy; using every day, even during symptom-free periods
» Importance of not discontinuing montelukast without discussing with physician
» Checking with physician if condition becomes worse
» Importance of not discontinuing any concurrent antiasthmatic medication without physician's advice

**Side/adverse effects**
Signs of potential side effects, especially pus in the urine

## General Dosing Information

Patients should be instructed to have appropriate rescue treatment available while being treated with montelukast. Therapy with montelukast may be continued during acute exacerbations of asthma.

Montelukast should not be abruptly substituted for inhaled or oral corticosteroids. If appropriate, the dose of corticosteroids should be tapered gradually under medical supervision. Rarely, the reduction of systemic corticosteroids in patients on another leukotriene antagonist has been followed by the occurrence of eosinophilia, vasculitic rash, worsening pulmonary symptoms, cardiac complications, and/or neuropathy sometimes presenting as Churg-Strauss syndrome, a systemic eosinophilic vasculitis. A causal relationship between this phenomenon and leukotriene receptor antagonism has not been established and the problem was not observed during clinical trials with montelukast. However, caution and appropriate clinical monitoring is recommended when systemic corticosteroid dose reduction is considered in patients receiving montelukast.

Montelukast should not be used as monotherapy for the treatment or management of exercise-induced bronchospasm. The patient should be instructed to continue with the usual regimen of an inhaled beta-agonist for prophylaxis of exercise-induced bronchospasm and have a short-acting inhaled beta-agonist available for rescue treatment.

## Oral Dosage Forms

### MONTELUKAST SODIUM TABLETS

Note: The chewable tablets are recommended for use in children 6 to 15 years of age and the tablets are recommended for use in children 15 years of age and over and in adults.

**Usual adult and adolescent dose**
Asthma, bronchial, chronic—
Oral, 10 mg once a day in the evening.

**Usual pediatric dose**
Asthma, bronchial, chronic—
Children younger than 6 years of age: Safety and efficacy have not been established.
Children 6 to 15 years of age: See *Montelukast Sodium Chewable Tablets*.
Children 15 years of age and over: See *Usual adult and adolescent dose*.

**Usual geriatric dose**
Asthma, bronchial, chronic—
See *Usual adult and adolescent dose*.

**Strength(s) usually available**
U.S.—
10 mg (Rx) [*Singulair* (lactose monohydrate)].

Note: This product contains 10.4 mg of montelukast sodium which is equivalent to 10 mg of the free acid.

**Packaging and storage**
Store between 15 and 30 °C (59 and 86 °F). Protect from light. Protect from moisture.

### MONTELUKAST SODIUM CHEWABLE TABLETS

Note: The chewable tablets are recommended for use in children 6 to 15 years of age and the tablets are recommended for use in children 15 years of age and over and in adults.

**Usual adult and adolescent dose**
Asthma, bronchial, chronic—
See *Montelukast Sodium Tablets*.

**Usual pediatric dose**
Asthma, bronchial, chronic—
Children younger than 6 years of age: Safety and efficacy have not been established.
Children 6 to 15 years of age: Oral, 5 mg once a day in the evening.
Children 15 years of age and over: See *Montelukast Sodium Tablets*.

**Usual geriatric dose**
Asthma, bronchial, chronic—
See *Montelukast Sodium Tablets*.

**Strength(s) usually available**
U.S.—
5 mg (Rx) [*Singulair* (aspartame [contains 0.842 mg of phenylalanine]; cherry flavor)].
Note: This product contains 5.2 mg of montelukast sodium which is equivalent to 5 mg of the free acid.

**Packaging and storage**
Store between 15 and 30 °C (59 and 86 °F). Protect from light. Protect from moisture.

Developed: 08/12/98

---

# MORICIZINE   Systemic†

INN: Moracizine
VA CLASSIFICATION (Primary): CV300
Commonly used brand name(s): *Ethmozine*.
Note: For a listing of dosage forms and brand names by country availability, see *Dosage Forms* section(s).

†Not commercially available in Canada.

## Category
Antiarrhythmic.

## Indications

**Accepted**
Arrhythmias, ventricular (treatment)—Moricizine is indicated for suppression of documented life-threatening ventricular arrhythmias, including sustained ventricular tachycardia.

**Unaccepted**
Use of moricizine is not accepted for treatment of less severe arrhythmias such as nonsustained ventricular tachycardias or frequent premature ventricular contractions, even if patients are symptomatic. In these cases, there is a possibility that proarrhythmic potential may outweigh any beneficial effect. In the National Heart, Lung and Blood Institute's Cardiac Arrhythmia Suppression Trial (CAST), encainide or flecainide treatment was associated with excessive mortality or increased nonfatal cardiac arrest rate as compared with placebo in patients with asymptomatic, non–life-threatening arrhythmias who had a recent myocardial infarction; and, therefore, the encainide and flecainide arms of CAST were prematurely terminated. The CAST protocol was modified and continued as CAST-II with the moricizine arm compared to placebo. However, CAST-II was subsequently terminated prematurely because of excessive cardiac mortality during the first 2 weeks of moricizine exposure as compared to placebo. Furthermore, it appeared unlikely that moricizine would improve long-term survival.

## Pharmacology/Pharmacokinetics

**Physicochemical characteristics**
Source—Phenothiazine derivative.
Molecular weight—Moricizine hydrochloride: 427.52.
pKa—6.4.

**Mechanism of action/Effect**
Inhibits the rapid inward sodium current across myocardial cell membranes. Has potent local anesthetic activity and membrane stabilizing effect. Decreases excitability, conduction velocity, and automaticity as a result of slowed atrioventricular (AV) nodal and His-Purkinje conduction. Decreases the action potential duration (APD) in Purkinje fibers; also decreases the effective refractory period (ERP) but to a lesser extent than the APD, so the ERP/APD ratio is increased. Decreases the maxiumum rate of Phase 0 depolarization ($V_{max}$), but does not affect action potential amplitude or maximum diastolic potential. Does not affect atrial, AV nodal, or left ventricular refractory periods and has minimal effect on ventricular repolarization (evidenced by the overall decrease in JT interval). Has no effect on sinoatrial (SA) nodal or intra-atrialconduction and only minimal effect on sinus cycle length and sinus node recovery time. In the Vaughan Williams classification of antiarrhythmics, moricizine is considered to be a class I agent. It has properties of class IA, IB, and IC agents but does not clearly belong to any of the three subclasses. It has less effect on the slope of phase 0 and a greater effect on action potential duration and effective refractory period than class IC agents.

**Other actions/effects**
Causes a small but consistent increase in resting blood pressure and heart rate. May inhibit platelet aggregation. May have anticholinergic effects.

**Absorption**
Well absorbed; absorption is complete within 2 to 3 hours. Significant first-pass metabolism results in an absolute bioavailability of approximately 38%. Administration within 30 minutes after a meal slows the rate, but does not affect the extent, of absorption, although peak plasma concentrations are reduced.

**Protein binding**
Very high (approximately 95%).

**Biotransformation**
Hepatic, extensive, to at least 26 metabolites, none accounting for as much as 1% of the administered dose. Two metabolites may be pharmacologically active but are present in extremely small quantities.
Moricizine induces its own metabolism (it induces hepatic cytochrome P-450 activity). Average plasma concentrations decline with continued dosing, but the clinical effect does not appear to be altered.

**Half-life**
1.5 to 3.5 (usually 2) hours. Duration of action is longer than would be predicted on the basis of this figure.

**Onset of action**
Prolongation of PR interval—Occurs promptly but normalization occurs within 2 hours.
Effect on ventricular premature depolarization (VPD) rates—Within 2 hours.

**Time to peak concentration**
0.5 to 2 hours; plasma concentration is directly dose-related.

**Time to peak effect**
Shortening of JT interval—6 hours.
Effect on VPD rates—10 to 14 hours.

**Duration of action**
Shortening of JT interval—At least 10 hours.
Effect on VPD rates—In full for more than 10 hours and continues to be significant at 24 hours.

**Elimination**
Biliary/fecal, 56%; renal, 39%. Less than 1% of a dose is excreted unchanged. Some enterohepatic recycling occurs.
In dialysis—Not significantly removable by hemodialysis.

## Precautions to Consider

**Carcinogenicity**
A 24-month study in mice at oral doses up to 320 mg per kg of body weight (mg/kg) per day produced a borderline statistically significant incidence of ovarian tubular adenomas and granulosa cell tumors. A 24-month study in rats at oral doses of 25, 50, and 100 mg/kg per day produced a Zymbal's gland carcinoma in one mid-dose and two high-dose males. A dose-related increase in hepatocellular cholangioma (also described as bile ductile cystadenoma or cystic hyperplasia), along with fatty metamorphosis, possibly due to disruption of hepatic choline utilization for phospholipid biosynthesis, also occurred in rats of both sexes (the rat is uniquely sensitive to alteration in choline metabolism).

**Mutagenicity**
Moricizine was not found to be mutagenic in *in vitro* bacterial (Ames test) and mammalian (Chinese hamster ovary/hypoxanthine-guanine phosphoribosyl transferase and sister chromatid exchange) cell systems or in *in vivo* mammalian systems (rat bone cytogenicity and mouse micronucleus).

**Pregnancy/Reproduction**

Fertility—Studies in male and female rats at doses of up to 6.7 times the maximum recommended human dose found no evidence of impaired fertility.

Pregnancy—Adequate and well-controlled studies in humans have not been done.

Teratogenicity studies in rats and rabbits at doses of up to 6.7 and 4.7 times the maximum recommended human dose, respectively, have not shown that moricizine causes adverse effects in the fetus.

A study in rats at doses of 3.4 and 6.7 times the maximum recommended human dose given prior to mating, during mating, and throughout gestation found a dose-related decrease in both pup and maternal weight gain, possibly related to a larger litter size; a study in which doses of 6.7 times the maximum recommended human dose were begun on Day 15 of gestation found retardation of maternal weight gain but no effect on pup growth.

FDA Pregnancy Category B.

**Breast-feeding**

Moricizine has been reported to be present in human breast milk and is distributed into the milk of laboratory animals.

**Pediatrics**

Appropriate studies on the relationship of age to the effects of moricizine have not been performed in the pediatric population. However, moricizine was used in 12 children with atrial ectopic tachycardia and did not demonstrate pediatrics-specific problems that would limit the usefulness of moricizine in children.

**Geriatrics**

One study found a decreased incidence of neurological side/adverse effects in patients over 65 years of age; there were no other age-related differences in incidence of side/adverse effects. In addition, elderly patients are more likely to have age-related renal function impairment, which, when significant, may require dosage reduction in patients receiving moricizine.

**Drug interactions and/or related problems**

The following drug interactions and/or related problems have been selected on the basis of their potential clinical significance (possible mechanism in parentheses where appropriate)—not necessarily inclusive (» = major clinical significance):

Antiarrhythmics, other
  (although some antiarrhythmic agents may be used in combination for therapeutic advantage, combined use may potentiate risk of adverse cardiac effects)

Cimetidine
  (concurrent use of cimetidine has been reported to decrease clearance of moricizine by about 49% and increase plasma concentrations 1.4 fold; although clinical effects of moricizine do not appear to be changed, caution is recommended if concurrent use with cimetidine is necessary)

Theophylline
  (concurrent use with moricizine significantly increases clearance and decreases half-life of theophylline, with a resultant decrease in plasma theophylline concentrations, possibly as a result of hepatic microsomal enzyme induction; monitoring of plasma theophylline concentrations is recommended when moricizine therapy is initiated or discontinued)

**Laboratory value alterations**

The following have been selected on the basis of their potential clinical significance (possible effect in parentheses where appropriate)—not necessarily inclusive (» = major clinical significance):

With physiology/laboratory test values

Electrocardiogram (ECG) changes such as:
  JT interval
    (slight shortening occurs)
  QRS widening and
  PR prolongation
    (occur in most patients; dose-related)
    (PR interval prolongation occurs promptly after single doses, but the interval returns to normal within 2 hours)
  QT prolongation
    (may occur secondary to QRS widening, but usually is not significant)
    Note: ECG changes produced by moricizine do not necessarily indicate efficacy, toxicity, or overdose.

**Medical considerations/Contraindications**

The medical considerations/contraindications included have been selected on the basis of their potential clinical significance (reasons given in parentheses where appropriate)—not necessarily inclusive (» = major clinical significance).

*Except under special circumstances, this medication should not be used when the following medical problems exist:*

» Atrioventricular (AV) block, pre-existing second or third degree without pacemaker, or
» Right bundle branch block associated with a left hemiblock (bifascicular block) without pacemaker
  (risk of complete heart block)

*Risk-benefit should be considered when the following medical problems exist:*

» Cardiogenic shock
  Cardiomegaly
    (incidence of moricizine-induced arrhythmias is increased; the possibility of proarrhythmic effects should be kept in mind during moricizine therapy)
  Congestive heart failure, severe
    (worsening has been reported; incidence of moricizine-induced arrhythmias is increased; absorption, half-life, and clearance of moricizine are not affected)
  Coronary artery disease
    (incidence of moricizine-induced arrhythmias is increased; the possibility of proarrhythmic effects should be kept in mind during moricizine therapy)
  Hepatic function impairment
    (reduced clearance and increased half-life of moricizine; lower doses of moricizine and close monitoring are recommended)
  Hypokalemia or hyperkalemia or
  Hypomagnesemia
    (effects of moricizine may be altered; any electrolyte imbalance should be corrected prior to beginning therapy with moricizine)
  Myocardial infarction, history of
    (incidence of moricizine-induced arrhythmias is increased; the possibility of proarrhythmic effects should be kept in mind during moricizine therapy)
  Renal function impairment
    (reduced elimination; if significant, dosage reduction and close monitoring are recommended)
» Sensitivity to moricizine
» Sick sinus syndrome
    (sinus node recovery time prolonged; sinus bradycardia, sinus pause, or sinus arrest may occur)
  Caution is also recommended in patients with existing pacemakers because the risk of moricizine-induced arrhythmias may be increased; the effect of moricizine on endocardial pacing thresholds has not been studied.

**Patient monitoring**

The following may be especially important in patient monitoring (other tests may be warranted in some patients, depending on condition; » = major clinical significance):

» ECG, 24-hour Holter monitoring and
» Exercise testing and/or
  Programmed electrical stimulation
    (may be recommended prior to initiation of therapy and at periodic intervals during therapy to help assess efficacy and detect possible proarrhythmic effects)

## Side/Adverse Effects

Note: In the National Heart, Lung and Blood Institute's Cardiac Arrhythmia Suppression Trial (CAST), encainide or flecainide treatment was found to be associated with excessive mortality or increased nonfatal cardiac arrest rate as compared with placebo in patients with asymptomatic, non–life-threatening arrhythmias who had a recent myocardial infarction. CAST-II comparing moricizine to placebo was discontinued because of excessive cardiac mortality during the first 2 weeks of moricizine exposure as compared to placebo. Furthermore, it appeared unlikely that moricizine would improve long-term survival.

Adverse cardiac effects reported with moricizine administration include new or exacerbated ventricular arrhythmias in about 3.7% of patients and, in 1% or less of patients, new or exacerbated congestive heart failure, second or third degree atrioventricular (AV) block, sinus bradycardia, sinus pause, or sinus arrest.

Side/adverse effects are usually mild and transient. However, deaths have been reported from overdosage of moricizine.

The following side/adverse effects have been selected on the basis of their potential clinical significance (possible signs and symptoms in parentheses where appropriate)—not necessarily inclusive:

**Those indicating need for medical attention**
Incidence less frequent
*Chest pain; congestive heart failure* (shortness of breath; swelling of feet or lower legs); *ventricular tachyarrhythmias* (fast or irregular heartbeat)
Note: *Ventricular tachyarrhythmias* are potentially fatal; incidence is increased in patients with coronary artery disease, sustained ventricular tachycardia, cardiomegaly, congestive heart failure, or history of myocardial infarction. Proarrhythmic effects usually occur during the first week of therapy and are not dose-related.

Incidence rare
*Drug fever* (sudden high fever); *hepatotoxicity* (not symptomatic)

**Those indicating need for medical attention only if they continue or are bothersome**
Incidence more frequent
*Dizziness*—dose-related
Incidence less frequent
*Blurred vision; diarrhea; dryness of mouth; headache; hypesthesias or paresthesias* (numbness or tingling in arms or legs or around mouth); *nausea or vomiting; nervousness; pain in arms or legs; stomach pain; trouble in sleeping; unusual tiredness or weakness*

## Overdose

For more information on the management of overdose or unintentional ingestion, **contact a Poison Control Center** (see *Poison Control Center Listing*).

**Clinical effects of overdose**
The following effects have been selected on the basis of their potential clinical significance (possible signs and symptoms in parentheses where appropriate)—not necessarily inclusive:

*Conduction disturbances; hypotension; exacerbation of congestive heart failure; myocardial infarction; sinus arrest; arrhythmias* (including junctional bradycardia, ventricular tachycardia, ventricular fibrillation, and asystole); *emesis; lethargy; coma; syncope; respiratory failure*

**Treatment of overdose**
Treatment is primarily supportive and symptomatic and includes immediate evacuation of the stomach, with special care to avoid aspiration; cardiac, respiratory, and CNS monitoring.

## Patient Consultation

As an aid to patient consultation, refer to *Advice for the Patient, Moricizine (Systemic)*.

In providing consultation, consider emphasizing the following selected information (» = major clinical significance):

**Before using this medication**
» Conditions affecting use, especially:
   Sensitivity to moricizine
   Other medical problems, especially second or third degree atrioventricular (AV) block, right bundle branch block associated with a left hemiblock, cardiogenic shock, or sick sinus syndrome

**Proper use of this medication**
» Compliance with therapy; taking as directed even if feeling well
» Importance of not missing doses and taking at evenly spaced intervals
» Proper dosing
   Missed dose: Taking as soon as possible if remembered within 4 hours; not taking if remembered later; not doubling doses
» Proper storage

**Precautions while using this medication**
Regular visits to physician to check progress
Carrying medical identification card or bracelet
» Caution if any kind of surgery (including dental surgery) or emergency treatment is required

Caution when driving or doing things requiring alertness because of possible dizziness

**Side/adverse effects**
Signs of potential side effects, especially chest pain, congestive heart failure, ventricular tachyarrhythmias, and drug fever

## General Dosing Information

It is recommended that treatment be initiated in the hospital because of the risk of proarrhythmic effects associated with moricizine administration.

In general, it is recommended that previous antiarrhythmic therapy be withdrawn 1 to 2 plasma half-lives before initiation of moricizine therapy. However, individual circumstances must be taken into consideration.

If second- or third-degree AV block occurs, moricizine therapy should be withdrawn unless a ventricular pacemaker is in place.

## Oral Dosage Forms

### MORICIZINE HYDROCHLORIDE TABLETS

**Usual adult dose**
Antiarrhythmic—
   Oral, 600 to 900 mg per day in three divided doses given every eight hours, the dosage being increased, if necessary, in increments of 150 mg per day at three-day intervals up to a total dose of 900 mg per day.
Note: In patients with hepatic function impairment or significant renal function impairment, an initial dose of 600 mg per day or less is recommended with close monitoring, including ECG intervals, before dosage adjustment.
   Some patients whose arrhythmias are well-controlled may be changed to every-twelve-hour dosing if necessary to aid in compliance. Incidence of dizziness and nausea may be increased with higher doses.

**Usual pediatric dose**
Safety and efficacy have not been established.
Note: One study involving 12 pediatric patients used a daily dose of 200 mg per square meter of body surface divided into three equal doses, increased as necessary up to a maximum of 600 mg per square meter of body surface per day.

**Strength(s) usually available**
U.S.—
   200 mg (Rx) [*Ethmozine* (lactose)].
   250 mg (Rx) [*Ethmozine* (lactose)].
   300 mg (Rx) [*Ethmozine* (lactose)].
Canada—
   Not commercially available.

**Packaging and storage**
Store between 15 and 30 °C (59 and 86 °F), unless otherwise specified by manufacturer. Store in a tight container. Protect from light.

## Selected Bibliography

Carnes CA, Coyle JD. Moricizine: a novel antiarrhythmic agent. DICP 1990 Jul/Aug; 24: 745-53.
Fitton A, Buckley MM. Moricizine: A review of its pharmacological properties, and therapeutic efficacy in cardiac arrhythmias. Drugs 1990; 40(1): 138-67.
Morganroth J, Bigger JT, editors. A symposium: pharmacologic management of ventricular arrhythmias—current status in the role of moricizine HCl. Am J Cardiol 1990; 65(8): 1D-71D.

Revised: 09/27/92
Interim revision: 06/30/94

---

**MORPHINE**—See *Opioid (Narcotic) Analgesics (Systemic)*

---

# MUMPS VIRUS VACCINE LIVE   Systemic

VA CLASSIFICATION (Primary): IM100
Note: This monograph is specific for the sterile lyophilized preparation of the Jeryl Lynn (B level) strain of mumps virus grown in cell cultures of chick embryo.
Commonly used brand name(s): *Mumpsvax*.

Note: For a listing of dosage forms and brand names by country availability, see *Dosage Forms* section(s).

## Category
Immunizing agent (active).

## Indications

### General considerations
Persons generally can be considered immune to mumps only if they have documentation of adequate immunization with mumps vaccine on or after their first birthdays, if they have laboratory evidence of mumps immunity, or if they have a physician's diagnosis of mumps infection.

Most individuals born before 1957 can generally be considered immune to mumps because of probable previous infection. However, birth before 1957 provides only presumptive evidence of immunity; mumps can occur in some persons born before 1957.

Although serologic tests may be conducted to determine the susceptibility of persons with unknown immunity, studies have not indicated an increased risk of adverse reactions from live mumps vaccinations in persons already immune to mumps.

The combined measles, mumps, and rubella virus vaccine live should be used for vaccinating individuals who are likely to be susceptible to more than one of these viruses, unless otherwise contraindicated.

Children vaccinated with mumps virus vaccine live at less than 12 months of age should be revaccinated. Based on available evidence, there is no reason to routinely revaccinate persons who were vaccinated originally when 12 months of age or older. However, persons should be revaccinated if there is evidence to suggest that the initial immunization was ineffective.

### Accepted
Mumps (prophylaxis)—Mumps virus vaccine live is indicated for immunization against mumps. The main objective of mumps immunization is to prevent complications, such as orchitis, which may occur in up to 20% of postpubescent and adult males infected with mumps virus, and meningoencephalitis, which may occur in up to 15% of persons infected with mumps virus. In addition, mumps infection during the first trimester of pregnancy may increase the rate of spontaneous abortion.

Unless otherwise contraindicated, all susceptible persons 12 months of age or older should be immunized against mumps, including:
- Children 12 months of age and older. All children 12 months of age and older should receive mumps virus vaccine live, preferably as the combined measles, mumps, and rubella virus vaccine live, as part of the routine childhood immunization schedule. Infants less than 12 months of age may retain maternal mumps-neutralizing antibodies that may interfere with the immune response to mumps virus vaccine live. Therefore, children vaccinated when less than 12 months of age should be revaccinated.
- International travelers. Persons without evidence of mumps immunity who travel abroad should be vaccinated against mumps because mumps is endemic throughout most of the world. These persons should receive either a single-antigen vaccine or a combined-antigen vaccine as appropriate prior to international travel. However, the combined measles, mumps, and rubella virus vaccine live is preferred for persons likely to be susceptible to more than one of these viruses; if a single-antigen mumps vaccine is not readily available, travelers should receive measles, mumps, and rubella virus vaccine live regardless of their immune status to measles and rubella.

## Pharmacology/Pharmacokinetics

### Mechanism of action/Effect
Following subcutaneous injection, mumps vaccine produces a modified, noncommunicable mumps infection and provides active immunity to mumps.

### Protective effect
A single injection of the vaccine has been shown to induce mumps-neutralizing antibodies in approximately 97% of susceptible children and approximately 93% of susceptible adults. The pattern of antibody response closely resembles that observed following natural mumps.

### Duration of protective effect
Although the antibody level following mumps virus vaccination is significantly lower than that attained following natural infection, it provides long lasting protection against the disease. Vaccine-induced antibody levels have been shown to persist for at least 15 years with a rate of decline comparable to that seen in natural infection. If the pattern of comparable immunity continues, permanent immunity following vaccination may be expected. Continued surveillance will be required to demonstrate this.

## Precautions to Consider

Note: In the past, persons with a history of anaphylactic reaction following egg ingestion were considered to be at increased risk for serious reactions after receipt of mumps-containing vaccines, which are produced in chick embryo fibroblasts. Protocols requiring caution were developed for skin testing and vaccinating these persons. However, the predictive value of such skin testing and the need for special protocols when vaccinating egg-allergic persons with mumps-containing vaccines is uncertain. The results of recent studies suggest that anaphylactic reactions to mumps-containing vaccines are not associated with hypersensitivity to egg antigens but with some other component of the vaccines. The risk for serious allergic reaction to these vaccines in egg-allergic patients is extremely low, and skin testing is not necessarily predictive of vaccine hypersensitivity.

### Pregnancy/Reproduction
Pregnancy—Although mumps virus vaccine live has been shown to infect the placenta and fetus, there is no evidence that it causes congenital malformations in humans. However, because of the theoretical risk of fetal damage, it is important to avoid giving live virus vaccines to pregnant women. Live mumps vaccine, when combined with rubella virus vaccine live, should not be administered to women known to be pregnant or who are considering becoming pregnant within the next 3 months. Women vaccinated with monovalent mumps virus vaccine live should avoid becoming pregnant for 30 days after the vaccination. Routine precautions for vaccinating postpubertal women include asking if they are or may be pregnant, excluding those who say they are, and explaining the theoretical risk to those who plan to receive the vaccine.

Studies have not been done in animals.

FDA Pregnancy Category C.

### Breast-feeding
It is not known whether mumps virus vaccine live is distributed into breast milk. However, problems in humans have not been documented.

### Pediatrics
Mumps vaccination is a part of routine childhood immunization. Therefore, children 12 months of age and older should receive the combined measles, mumps, and rubella virus vaccine instead of a single-antigen vaccine. Children who received monovalent mumps virus vaccine live rather than combined measles, mumps, and rubella virus vaccine live on or after their first birthdays also should receive a primary dose of measles and rubella virus vaccines. The American Academy of Pediatrics (AAP) and the Advisory Committee on Immunization Practices (ACIP) recommend that all children receive a second dose of measles-containing vaccine (preferably as the combined measles, mumps, and rubella virus vaccine live). Doses of the combined measles, mumps, and rubella virus vaccine live or other measles-containing vaccines should be separated by at least 1 month.

Children with end-stage renal disease receiving maintenance hemodialysis have a degree of immunosuppression that reduces their response to vaccination. One small trial showed that only 50% of these vaccinated children developed mumps antibodies. Therefore, it may be necessary to monitor postvaccination antibody levels in children with end-stage renal disease, and to revaccinate those children who have failed to demonstrate seroconversion.

### Drug interactions and/or related problems
The following drug interactions and/or related problems have been selected on the basis of their potential clinical significance (possible mechanism in parentheses where appropriate)—not necessarily inclusive (» = major clinical significance):

Note: Combinations containing any of the following medications, depending on the amount present, may also interact with this medication.

Blood products or
Immune globulins
(concurrent administration with mumps virus vaccine live may interfere with the patient's immune response to the virus because of the possibility of antibodies to mumps virus in these products. Mumps virus vaccine live should be administered at least 14 days before, or more than 3 months after, administration of blood products or immune globulins)

» Corticosteroids or
» Immunosuppressive agents or
» Radiation therapy
(because normal defense mechanisms are suppressed, concurrent use with mumps virus vaccine live may potentiate the replication of the vaccine virus, may increase the side/adverse effects of the vaccine virus, and/or may decrease the patient's antibody response to mumps virus vaccine live. The interval between discontinuation

of medications that cause immunosuppression and restoration of the patient's ability to respond to mumps virus vaccine live depends on the intensity and type of immunosuppression-causing medication used, the underlying disease, and other factors; estimates vary from 3 months to 1 year. Patients with leukemia in remission should not receive mumps virus vaccine live until at least 3 months after their last chemotherapy. This precaution does not apply to corticosteroids used as replacement therapy, for short-term [less than 2 weeks] systemic therapy, or by other routes of administration that do not cause immunosuppression)

- Live virus vaccines, other
  (data are lacking on impairment of antibody responses to rubella, measles, mumps, or oral poliovirus vaccine [OPV] when these vaccines are administered on different days within 1 month of each other; however, OPV and measles, mumps, and rubella virus vaccine live [or its individual component vaccines] can be administered at any time before, with, or after each other, if indicated)

**Laboratory value alterations**
The following have been selected on the basis of their potential clinical significance (possible effect in parentheses where appropriate)—not necessarily inclusive (» = major clinical significance):

With diagnostic test results
  Tuberculin skin test
    (short-term suppression of tuberculin skin test results lasting several weeks may occur, which may yield false-negative results; if required, tuberculin skin tests should be administered before, simultaneously with, or at least 4 to 6 weeks after administration of mumps virus vaccine live)

**Medical considerations/Contraindications**
The medical considerations/contraindications included have been selected on the basis of their potential clinical significance (reasons given in parentheses where appropriate)—not necessarily inclusive (» = major clinical significance).

*Except under special circumstances, this medication should not be used when the following medical problems exist:*

» Febrile illness, severe
  (the decision to administer or delay vaccination because of current or recent febrile illness depends largely on the cause of the illness and the severity of symptoms; minor illnesses, such as upper respiratory infection, do not preclude administration of the vaccine; for persons whose compliance with medical care cannot be assured, every opportunity should be taken to provide appropriate vaccination)

  (children with moderate or severe febrile illnesses can be vaccinated as soon as they have recovered from the acute phase of the illness; this wait avoids superimposing adverse effects of vaccination on the underlying illness or mistakenly attributing a manifestation of the underlying illness to the vaccine; routine physical examinations or measurements of temperatures are not prerequisites for vaccinating infants and children who appear to be in good health; asking the parent or guardian if the child is ill, postponing vaccination for children with moderate or severe febrile illnesses, and vaccinating those without contraindications are appropriate procedures in childhood immunization programs)

» Immune deficiency conditions, congenital or hereditary, family history of, or
» Immune deficiency conditions, primary or acquired
  (replications of live vaccine viruses can be enhanced in persons with immunodeficiency diseases and in persons with immunosuppression, as occurs with leukemia, lymphoma, generalized malignancy, or therapy with alkylating agents, antimetabolites, radiation, or large doses of corticosteroids)

  (patients with leukemia in remission who have not received chemotherapy for at least 3 months may receive live-virus vaccines; the exact amount of systemically absorbed corticosteroids and the duration of administration needed to suppress the immune system of an otherwise healthy child are not well defined; most experts agree that short term [i.e., less than 2 weeks], low- to moderate-dose corticosteroid therapy, or long-term alternate-day treatment with short-acting preparations, maintenance physiologic doses [replacement therapy], or administration of corticosteroids topically [skin or eyes], by aerosol, or by intra-articular, bursal, or tendon injection usually does not contraindicate administration of live virus vaccine; although a theoretical concern has been raised, no evidence of increased severe reactions to live vaccines has been reported among persons receiving corticosteroid therapy by aerosol, and such therapy is not in itself a reason to delay vaccination)

  (the immunosuppressive effects of corticosteroid treatment vary with its dosage, but many clinicians consider a dose equivalent to either 2 mg per kg of body weight (mg/kg) or a total of 20 mg per day of prednisone sufficiently immunosuppressive to raise concern about the safety of vaccination with live virus vaccines; corticosteroids used in greater-than-physiologic doses also can reduce the immune response to vaccines; physicians should wait at least 3 months after discontinuation of therapy to administer a live-virus vaccine in patients who have received systemically absorbed high doses of corticosteroids for ≥ 2 weeks)

*Risk-benefit should be considered when the following medical problems exist:*

Allergy to neomycin
  (patients allergic to systemic or topical neomycin may be allergic to the mumps virus vaccine live because each 0.5-mL vaccine dose contains approximately 25 mcg of neomycin, which is used in the production of the vaccine to prevent bacterial overgrowth in the viral culture. A history of hypersensitivity reactions, such as delayed-type allergic reaction (contact dermatitis) to neomycin, generally does not preclude immunization. However, a history of anaphylaxis due to topically or systemically administered neomycin precludes immunization with this vaccine)

Allergy to gelatin
  (patients allergic to gelatin also may be allergic to mumps virus vaccine live, since gelatin is used as a stabilizer in the production of the vaccine. The literature records a single case report of a person with an anaphylactic sensitivity to gelatin having an anaphylactic reaction after receipt of the combined measles, mumps, and rubella virus vaccine licensed in the U.S.; similar cases have been reported in Japan. Therefore, such persons should be vaccinated with the combined measles, mumps and rubella virus vaccine and its component vaccines with extreme caution)

Thrombocytopenia or vaccine-associated thrombocytopenia
  (persons who experienced thrombocytopenia with the first dose of vaccine may develop thrombocytopenia with additional doses. These persons should be tested serologically to determine the need for additional doses of vaccine. The risk-benefit ratio should be evaluated before vaccination is considered in such cases)

Sensitivity to mumps virus vaccine live

## Side/Adverse Effects

Note: In field trials before licensure, illness did not occur more frequently in vaccinees than in unvaccinated controls. Illnesses reported following mumps virus vaccination have been mainly episodes of parotitis and low-grade fever. Allergic reactions including rash, pruritus, and purpura have been temporally associated with mumps vaccination, but are uncommon and usually mild and of brief duration. The reported occurrence of encephalitis within 30 days of receipt of a mumps-containing vaccine (0.4 instances per million doses) was not greater than the observed background incidence rate of central nervous system (CNS) dysfunction in the general population. No association has been established between mumps virus vaccination and pancreatic damage or subsequent development of diabetes mellitus.

The following side/adverse effects have been selected on the basis of their potential clinical significance (possible signs and symptoms in parentheses where appropriate)—not necessarily inclusive:

**Those indicating need for medical attention**
Incidence rare
  *Anaphylactic reaction* (difficulty in breathing or swallowing; hives; itching, especially of feet or hands; reddening of skin, especially around ears; swelling of eyes, face, or inside of nose; unusual tiredness or weakness, sudden and severe); *encephalitis or meningoencephalitis* (confusion; severe or continuing headache; irritability; stiff neck; or vomiting); *fever over 39.4 °C (103 °F); orchitis in postpubescent and adult males* (pain, tenderness, or swelling in testicles and scrotum); *thrombocytopenic purpura* (bruising or purple spots on skin)

**Those indicating need for medical attention only if they continue or are bothersome**
Incidence more frequent
  *Burning or stinging at injection site*—due to acid pH of vaccine
Incidence less frequent or rare
  *Delayed-type, cell-mediated, allergic reaction* (itching, swelling, redness, tenderness or hard lump at place of injection); *fever of 37.7 °C (100 °F) or less; parotitis* (swollen glands on side of face or neck); *skin rash*

## Patient Consultation

As an aid to patient consultation, refer to *Advice for the Patient, Mumps Virus Vaccine Live (Systemic)*.

In providing consultation, consider emphasizing the following selected information (» = major clinical significance):

### Before receiving this vaccine
» Conditions affecting use, especially:
- Sensitivity to mumps virus vaccine live or allergy to gelatin or neomycin
- Pregnancy—Use of mumps virus vaccine live during pregnancy or pregnancy within 30 days of immunization is not recommended
- Use in children—Use is not recommended for infants up to 12 months of age
- Other medications, especially immunosuppressive agents or radiation therapy
- Other medical problems, especially severe febrile illness; primary or acquired immune deficiency conditions; or family history of congenital or hereditary immune deficiency conditions

### Proper use of this vaccine
- Waiting at least 14 days after receiving vaccine before receiving blood products or immune globulins
- Waiting at least 3 months after administration of blood products or immune globulins before receiving vaccine
» Proper dosing

### Precautions after receiving this vaccine
» Not becoming pregnant for 3 months after receiving rubella and mumps virus vaccine live or 30 days after receiving monovalent mumps virus vaccine live without first checking with physician, because of possible problems during pregnancy
- Checking with physician before receiving tuberculin skin test within 4 to 6 weeks of this vaccine, since the results of the test may be affected by mumps vaccine

### Side/adverse effects
Signs of potential side effects, especially anaphylactic reaction, encephalitis or meningoencephalitis, fever over 39.4 °C, orchitis in postpubescent and adult males, or thrombocytopenic purpura

## General Dosing Information

The American Academy of Pediatrics (AAP) and the Advisory Committee on Immunization Practices (ACIP) recommend that all children 12 to 15 months of age receive two doses of measles, mumps, and rubella virus vaccine live. Children who received monovalent mumps virus vaccine live rather than the combined measles, mumps, and rubella virus vaccine live on or after their first birthdays also should receive a primary dose of measles and rubella virus vaccines. Doses of the combined measles, mumps, and rubella virus vaccine live or other measles-containing vaccines should be separated by at least 1 month.

The dosage of mumps vaccine is the same for both children and adults.

When sterilizing syringes before vaccination, care should be taken to avoid preservatives, antiseptics, detergents, and disinfectants, since the vaccine virus is easily inactivated by these substances.

To prevent inactivation of the vaccine, it is recommended that only the diluent provided by the manufacturer be used.

A 25-gauge, 5/8th-inch needle is recommended for administration of the vaccine.

Mumps vaccine is administered subcutaneously. While not routinely recommended, intramuscular administration is considered effective and safe also. The vaccine should not be injected intravenously.

Although measles, mumps, and rubella vaccines are commercially available as a combination vaccine (measles, mumps, and rubella virus vaccine live) and, as such, are administered as a single injection, the commercially available individual vaccines should not be mixed in the same syringe or administered at the same body site.

ACIP continues to recommend measles, mumps, and rubella virus vaccine live for human immunodeficiency virus (HIV)-infected persons without evidence of immunity to these viruses. Because the immunologic response to both live and killed antigen vaccines may decrease as HIV disease progresses, vaccination early in the course of HIV infection may be more likely to induce an immune response. Therefore, HIV-infected infants without severe immunosuppression should receive measles, mumps, and rubella virus vaccine live as soon as possible upon reaching their first birthday. Evaluation and testing of asymptomatic persons to identify HIV infection are not necessary before deciding to administer measles, mumps, and rubella virus vaccine live.

In general, simultaneous administration of the most widely used live and inactivated vaccines does not impair antibody responses or increase rates of adverse effects. Vaccines recommended for administration at 12 to 15 months of age can be administered at either one or two visits. There are equivalent antibody responses and no clinically significant increases in frequency of adverse events when diphtheria toxoid, tetanus toxoid, and pertussis vaccine (DTP); measles, mumps, and rubella virus vaccine live; oral poliovirus vaccine (OPV) or inactivated poliovirus vaccine (IPV); and *Haemophilus influenzae* type b conjugate vaccine (HbCV) are administered either simultaneously at different sites or at separate times. If a child might not be brought back for future vaccinations, all vaccines (including DTP [or DTaP]; measles, mumps, and rubella virus vaccine live; OPV [or IPV]; varicella; HbCV; and hepatitis B vaccines may be administered simultaneously, as appropriate to the child's age and previous vaccination status.

### For treatment of adverse effects
Recommended treatment includes:
- For mild hypersensitivity reaction—Administering antihistamines, and, if necessary, corticosteroids.
- For severe hypersensitivity or anaphylactic reaction—Administering epinephrine. Antihistamines or corticosteroids also may be administered as required.

## Parenteral Dosage Forms

### MUMPS VIRUS VACCINE LIVE (FOR INJECTION) USP

**Usual adult and adolescent dose**
Immunizing agent (active)—
Subcutaneous, 0.5 mL, preferably into the outer aspect of the upper arm.

**Usual pediatric dose**
Immunizing agent (active)—
Infants up to 12 months of age: Use is not recommended.
Infants and children 12 months of age and older: See *Usual adult and adolescent dose*.

**Strength(s) usually available**
U.S.—
Not less than the equivalent of 20,000 median tissue culture infective doses [TCID$_{50}$] of the U.S. Reference Mumps Virus in each 0.5-mL dose (Rx) [*Mumpsvax* (neomycin 25 mcg)].
Canada—
Not less than the equivalent of 5000 median tissue culture infective doses [TCID$_{50}$] of the U.S. Reference Mumps Virus in each 0.5-mL dose (Rx) [*Mumpsvax* (neomycin 17.5 mcg)].

**Packaging and storage**
Store the lyophilized form of the vaccine, the diluent, and the reconstituted form of the vaccine between 2 and 8 °C (36 and 46 °F), unless otherwise specified by the manufacturer.
Alternatively, the diluent for the single-dose vials only may be stored between 15 and 30 °C (59 and 86 °F).
Protect both the lyophilized form and the reconstituted form of the vaccine from light.

**Preparation of dosage form**
To reconstitute, use only the diluent provided by the manufacturer, since it is free of preservatives or other substances that might inactivate the vaccine.
Single-dose vial—Withdraw the entire volume of diluent (approximately 0.5 mL) into the syringe. Inject all the diluent in the syringe into the vial of lyophilized vaccine and agitate to mix thoroughly. Withdraw the entire contents into the syringe and inject the total volume of restored vaccine subcutaneously.
10-dose vial (in U.S., available only to government agencies/institutions)—Withdraw the entire contents (7 mL) of the diluent vial into the syringe to be used for reconstitution. Inject all of the diluent in the syringe into the 10-dose vial of lyophilized vaccine and agitate to mix thoroughly. The 10-dose container can be used with either syringes or a jet injector. Since the vaccine and diluent do not contain preservatives, special care should be taken to prevent contamination of the multiple-dose vial of vaccine. In addition, the vial should be stored properly until the reconstituted vaccine is used. Discard unused vaccine after 8 hours.
50-dose vial (in U.S., available only to government agencies/institutions)—Withdraw the entire contents (30 mL) of the diluent vial into the syringe to be used for reconstitution. Inject all of the diluent in the syringe into the 50-dose vial of lyophilized vaccine and agitate to mix thoroughly. The 50-dose container is designed to be used only with a jet injector. Since the vaccine and diluent do not contain preservatives, special care should be taken to prevent contamination of the multiple-dose vial of vaccine. In addition, the vial should be stored properly until the reconstituted vaccine is used. Discard unused vaccine after 8 hours.

# MUPIROCIN  Nasal—INTRODUCTORY VERSION

VA CLASSIFICATION (Primary): NT900
Commonly used brand name(s): *Bactroban Nasal*.
Note: For a listing of dosage forms and brand names by country availability, see *Dosage Forms* section(s).

## Category
Antibacterial (nasal).

## Indications

### Accepted
*Staphylococcus aureus*, methicillin-resistant (treatment)—Intranasal mupirocin calcium is indicated for the eradication of nasal colonization with methicillin-resistant *S. aureus* in adult patients and health care workers as part of a comprehensive infection control program to reduce the risk of infection among patients at high risk of methicillin-resistant *S. aureus* infection during institutional outbreaks of infections with this pathogen.

In clinical trials, more than 90% of persons treated with intranasal mupirocin had eradication of nasal colonization 2 to 4 days after completion of therapy, as compared with 5 to 30% of persons administered the vehicle only. In one study, recolonization in approximately 30% of patients was reported within 4 weeks after completion of therapy as compared with 85 to 100% cases of recolonization with administration of the vehicle only.

### Acceptance not established
There are insufficient data to establish that intranasal mupirocin calcium is safe and effective as part of an intervention program to prevent autoinfection of high-risk patients from their own nasal colonization with *S. aureus*.
There are insufficient data to recommend use of intranasal mupirocin calcium for general prophylaxis of any infection in any patient population.

### Unaccepted
The safety and efficacy of using intranasal mupirocin calcium for more than 5 days have not been established. There are no human clinical or animal data to support the use of this product for more than 5 days or in ways not described in this monograph.

## Pharmacology/Pharmacokinetics

### Physicochemical characteristics
Source—Produced by fermentation of *Pseudomonas fluorescens*.
Molecular weight—Mupirocin calcium: 1075.36.
Mupirocin free acid: 500.6.

### Mechanism of action/Effect
Mupirocin inhibits bacterial protein synthesis by reversibly and specifically binding to bacterial isoleucyl transfer-RNA synthetase. Because of this process, mupirocin does not demonstrate *in vitro* cross-resistance with other classes of antimicrobial agents.
The type of mupirocin resistance that may occur appears to result from the production of a modified isoleucyl transfer-RNA synthetase. High-level plasmid-mediated resistance (minimum inhibitory concentration [MIC] > 1024 mcg per mL) has been reported in some strains of *Staphylococcus aureus* and coagulase-negative staphylococci.
Mupirocin is bactericidal at concentrations achieved by topical intranasal administration. However, the minimum bactericidal concentration (MBC) against relevant intranasal pathogens is generally eightfold to thirtyfold higher than the MIC. In addition, mupirocin is highly protein-bound, and the effect of nasal secretions on the MIC of intranasal mupirocin has not been determined.

Mupirocin has been shown to be active against most strains of methicillin-resistant *S. aureus*, both *in vitro* and in clinical studies of the eradication of nasal colonization.

### Absorption
Repeated intranasal applications of 0.2 gram of mupirocin calcium ointment three times a day for 3 days to five adult males resulted in no evidence of systemic absorption of mupirocin. For up to 72 hours after the nasal applications, concentrations of mupirocin in urine and of monic acid in urine and serum were below the limits of determination of the assay. The lower detectable limits of the assay were 50 nanograms per mL of mupirocin in urine, 75 nanograms per mL of monic acid in urine, and 10 nanograms per mL of monic acid in serum. Extrapolation of the detectable limit of the urine assay for monic acid yields a mean of 3.3% (range, 1.2 to 5.1%) of the applied dose that could possibly be absorbed systemically from the nasal mucosa of adults.

### Protein binding
Very high (> 97%).

### Biotransformation
Mupirocin is rapidly metabolized following intravenous or oral administration. The principal metabolite is monic acid, which has no antibacterial activity.

### Half-life
A study of seven men who were administered intravenous mupirocin reported an elimination half-life of 20 to 40 minutes for mupirocin and 30 to 80 minutes for monic acid.

### Elimination
Predominately renal as monic acid after intravenous administration of mupirocin.

## Precautions to Consider

### Carcinogenicity
Long-term animal studies have not been done.

### Mutagenicity
The following *in vitro* or *in vivo* tests, using either mupirocin calcium or mupirocin sodium, did not show any mutagenic potential: rat primary hepatocyte unscheduled DNA synthesis, sediment analysis for DNA strand breaks, *Salmonella* reversion test (Ames), *Escherichia coli* mutation assay, metaphase analysis of human lymphocytes, mouse lymphoma assay, and bone marrow micronuclei assay in mice.

### Pregnancy/Reproduction
Fertility—No evidence of impaired fertility was found in reproductive studies in rats administered mupirocin sodium subcutaneously at doses that were comparable (on a mg-per-square-meter [mg/m²] basis) to up to 40 times the human intranasal dose of approximately 20 mg of mupirocin per day.
Pregnancy—Adequate and well-controlled studies in humans have not been done.
No evidence of harm to the fetus was found in reproductive studies in rats and rabbits administered mupirocin (salt not disclosed) subcutaneously at doses that were comparable (on a mg-per-square-meter [mg/m²] basis) to up to 65 and 130 times, respectively, the human intranasal dose of approximately 20 mg of mupirocin per day.
FDA Pregnancy Category B.

### Breast-feeding
It is not known whether mupirocin is distributed into breast milk. However, problems in humans have not been documented.

### Pediatrics
Safety and efficacy have not been established. Appropriate studies on the relationship of age to the effects of mupirocin have not been performed in children up to 12 years of age. However, a report of a pharmacokinetic study in neonates and premature infants indicated that significant systemic absorption occurred following administration of intranasal mupirocin.

### Geriatrics
Appropriate studies on the relationship of age to the effects of mupirocin have not been performed in the geriatric population. However, no geriatrics-specific problems have been documented to date.

### Drug interactions and/or related problems
The following drug interactions and/or related problems have been selected on the basis of their potential clinical significance (possible mechanism in parentheses where appropriate)—not necessarily inclusive (» = major clinical significance):

Note: Combinations containing any of the following medications, depending on the amount present, may also interact with this medication.

» Intranasal products, other
(concurrent use of mupirocin with other intranasal products has not been studied and is not recommended until studies are done)

### Medical considerations/Contraindications
The medical considerations/contraindications included have been selected on the basis of their potential clinical significance (reasons given in parentheses where appropriate)—not necessarily inclusive (» = major clinical significance).

*Except under special circumstances, this medication should not be used when the following medical problem exists:*

» Sensitivity to mupirocin

## Side/Adverse Effects
The following side/adverse effects have been selected on the basis of their potential clinical significance (possible signs and symptoms in parentheses where appropriate)—not necessarily inclusive:

### Those indicating need for medical attention
Incidence less frequent
*Cough; respiratory disorder, including upper respiratory tract congestion* (chest congestion)

Incidence rare
*Ear pain*

### Those indicating need for medical attention only if they continue or are bothersome
Incidence more frequent
*Headache*

Incidence less frequent or rare
*Burning or stinging in the nose; pharyngitis* (sore throat); *pruritus* (itching); *rhinitis* (stuffy or runny nose); *taste perversion* (change in taste)

## Overdose
There was no evidence of systemic absorption following repeated intranasal applications of mupirocin calcium in adults. (See *Absorption*.) In addition, intravenous infusions of 252 mg of mupirocin and single oral doses of 500 mg of mupirocin have been well tolerated in adults.

## Patient Consultation
As an aid to patient consultation, refer to *Advice for the Patient, Mupirocin (Nasal)—Introductory Version*.

In providing consultation, consider emphasizing the following selected information (» = major clinical significance):

### Before using this medication
» Conditions affecting use, especially:
Sensitivity to mupirocin
Use in children—Safety and efficacy have not been established in children up to 12 years of age; in addition, a report of a pharmacokinetic study in neonates and premature infants indicated that significant systemic absorption occurred following administration of intranasal mupirocin
Other medications, especially other intranasal products

### Proper use of this medication
» Proper administration: First washing hands; applying approximately one half of the ointment from single-use tube directly from tube into nostril; applying the remainder of ointment directly into other nostril; closing nostrils by pressing sides of nose together and then releasing them repeatedly for approximately 1 minute to help spread medication throughout inside of nostrils; another method is pressing sides of nose together and gently massaging nose; being careful not to touch eyes; discarding tube after using; washing hands afterwards to remove any medication that may be on them

» Proper dosing
Missed dose: Using as soon as possible; not using if almost time for next dose; not doubling doses

» Proper storage

### Precautions while using this medication
» Keeping medication away from eyes; medication may cause severe burning and tearing of eyes that may last days or weeks; contacting physician if this occurs

» Not using any other medication in your nose without checking with physician

» Discontinuing medication and checking with physician if severe nasal irritation occurs

### Side/adverse effects
Signs of potential side effects, especially cough; respiratory disorder, including upper respiratory tract congestion; and ear pain

## General Dosing Information
The single-use tube should not be reused, but should be discarded immediately after use.

If sensitization or a severe local irritation develops, treatment with mupirocin should be discontinued.

Patients should be cautioned to keep mupirocin away from the eyes. Under test conditions, application of mupirocin nasal ointment to the eye caused severe symptoms, such as burning and tearing, that resolved over days to weeks.

## Nasal Dosage Forms

### MUPIROCIN CALCIUM NASAL OINTMENT

**Usual adult and adolescent dose**
Antibacterial, nasal—
Intranasal, approximately one half of the ointment from a single-use tube applied into each nostril two times a day (morning and evening) for five days.

**Usual adult and adolescent prescribing limits**
Five days of twice-daily treatment.

**Usual pediatric dose**
Antibacterial, nasal—
Children up to 12 years of age: Safety has not been established.
Children 12 years of age and older: See *Usual adult and adolescent dose*.

**Usual geriatric dose**
Antibacterial, nasal—
See *Usual adult and adolescent dose*.

**Strength(s) usually available**
U.S.—
2% (Rx) [*Bactroban Nasal* (2.15% w/w mupirocin calcium equivalent to 2% mupirocin free acid; paraffin; glycerin esters mixture [Softisan 649])].

**Packaging and storage**
Store at or below 25 °C (77 °F). Protect from freezing.

**Auxiliary labeling**
• For the nose.
• Keep away from eyes.

Developed: 11/4/97

---

**MUPIROCIN**—The *Mupirocin (Topical)* monograph is not included in this published version of the USP DI database. Copies of the monograph are available on request from Micromedex, Inc. - Reprint Requests, 6200 S. Syracuse Way, Suite 300, Englewood, CO 80111; telephone (303) 486-6400; telefax (303) 486-6464; Email: USPDI@MDX.COM.

# MUROMONAB-CD3 Systemic

VA CLASSIFICATION (Primary): IM600
Commonly used brand name(s): *Orthoclone OKT3*.
Note: For a listing of dosage forms and brand names by country availability, see *Dosage Forms* section(s).

## Category
Monoclonal antibody; immunosuppressant.

## Indications
### Accepted
Transplant rejection, organ (treatment)—Muromonab-CD3 is indicated, usually in combination with azathioprine, cyclosporine, and/or corticosteroids, for treatment of acute rejection of renal transplants (allografts). It is also indicated for treatment of steroid-resistant acute rejection of hepatic and cardiac transplants.

## Pharmacology/Pharmacokinetics
### Mechanism of action/Effect
Muromonab-CD3, a murine monoclonal antibody, reacts with a T3 (CD3) molecule that is linked to an antigen receptor on the surface membrane of human T-lymphocytes and thereby blocks both the generation and function of the T-cells in response to antigenic challenge. Initially, binding of muromonab-CD3 to T-lymphocytes leads to early activation of T-cells and subsequent cytokine release; however, ultimately, T-cell functions are blocked. Muromonab-CD3 does not cause myelosuppression.

### Onset of action
Number of circulating CD3 positive T-cells is reduced within minutes after administration.

### Time to steady-state serum trough concentration
3 days.

### Steady-state trough serum concentration
With dose of 5 mg per day—0.9 mcg per mL.

### Duration of action
Number of circulating CD3 positive T-cells returns to pretreatment levels, and T-cell function returns to normal, within 1 week after muromonab-CD3 is withdrawn.

## Precautions to Consider
### Cross-sensitivity and/or related problems
Patients sensitive to any product of murine (mouse) origin may also be sensitive to muromonab-CD3. Muromonab-CD3 may induce human anti-mouse antibody production and hypersensitivity in patients.

### Carcinogenicity
Studies have not been done in either animals or humans; however, suppression of cell-mediated immunity in organ transplant patients is associated with an increased risk of benign and malignant lymphoproliferative disorders, lymphomas, and skin cancers. Lymphomas have developed in humans treated with muromonab-CD3, although a definite causal relationship has not been established. Other infrequently reported neoplasms have included multiple myeloma, leukemia, breast carcinoma, adenocarcinoma, cholangiocarcinoma, and recurrences of pre-existing hepatoma and renal cell carcinoma.

### Pregnancy/Reproduction
Pregnancy—Studies have not been done in humans. However, muromonab-CD3 is an immunoglobulin G (IgG) antibody that may cross the human placenta; the effect of cytokine release and immunosuppression on the fetus is unknown.
Studies have not been done in animals.
FDA Pregnancy Category C.

### Breast-feeding
Problems in humans have not been documented. However, breast-feeding is generally not recommended while muromonab-CD3 is being administered because of the potential risks to the infant (adverse effects, carcinogenicity). It is not known whether muromonab-CD3 is distributed into breast milk.

### Pediatrics
Appropriate studies on the relationship of age to the effects of muromonab-CD3 have not been performed in the pediatric population. Muromonab-CD3 has been used in children, with appropriate dosage adjustments. Small children may be at increased risk of dehydration as a result of gastrointestinal fluid loss from diarrhea and/or vomiting with the cytokine release syndrome. The risk of long-term adverse sequelae to high fever, seizures, central nervous system (CNS) infections, aseptic meningitis, etc., is unknown.

### Geriatrics
No information is available on the relationship of age to the effects of muromonab-CD3 in geriatric patients.

### Dental
The immunosuppressant effects of muromonab-CD3 may result in an increased incidence of microbial infection and delayed healing. Dental work, whenever possible, should be completed prior to initiation of therapy and undertaken only with great caution during therapy. Patients should be instructed in proper oral hygiene during treatment, including caution in use of regular toothbrushes, dental floss, and toothpicks.

### Drug interactions and/or related problems
The following drug interactions and/or related problems have been selected on the basis of their potential clinical significance (possible mechanism in parentheses where appropriate)—not necessarily inclusive (» = major clinical significance):

» Immunosuppressant agents, other, such as:
  Azathioprine
  Chlorambucil
  Corticosteroids, glucocorticoid
  Cyclophosphamide
  Cyclosporine
  Cytarabine
  Mercaptopurine
    (although muromonab-CD3 is often administered in conjunction with azathioprine, cyclosporine, and/or corticosteroids, concurrent use may increase the risk of infection and development of lymphoproliferative disorders; reduced dosage of corticosteroids and azathioprine is recommended when muromonab-CD3 therapy is begun; continued use of cyclosporine is recommended only with extreme caution and in reduced dosage)
    (concurrent use of other immunosuppressant agents with muromonab-CD3 has been shown to alter the time course of anti-mouse antibody development as well as the specificity [idiotypic, isotypic, allotypic] of the antibodies formed)

  Vaccines, killed virus
    (because normal defense mechanisms may be suppressed by muromonab-CD3 therapy, the patient's antibody response to the vaccine may be decreased. The interval between discontinuation of medications that cause immunosuppression and restoration of the patient's ability to respond to the vaccine depends on the intensity and type of immunosuppression-causing medication used, the underlying disease, and other factors; estimates vary from 3 months to 1 year)

» Vaccines, live virus
    (because normal defense mechanisms may be suppressed by muromonab-CD3 therapy, concurrent use with a live virus vaccine may potentiate the replication of the vaccine virus, may increase the side/adverse effects of the vaccine virus, and/or may decrease the patient's antibody response to the vaccine; immunization of these patients should be undertaken only with extreme caution after careful review of the patient's immunologic status and only with the knowledge and consent of the physician managing the muromonab-CD3 therapy. The interval between discontinuation of medications that cause immunosuppression and restoration of the patient's ability to respond to the vaccine depends on the intensity and type of immunosuppression-causing medication used, the underlying disease, and other factors; estimates vary from 3 months to 1 year. Immunization with oral poliovirus vaccine should also be postponed in persons in close contact with the patient, especially family members)

### Laboratory value alterations
The following have been selected on the basis of their potential clinical significance (possible effect in parentheses where appropriate)—not necessarily inclusive (» = major clinical significance):

With physiology/laboratory test values
  Hepatic transaminase
    (serum values may be increased transiently after the first few doses of muromonab-CD3)

### Medical considerations/Contraindications
The medical considerations/contraindications included have been selected on the basis of their potential clinical significance (reasons given in

parentheses where appropriate)—not necessarily inclusive (» = major clinical significance).

*Except under special circumstances, this medication should not be used when the following medical problems exist:*
- » Anti-mouse antibody titre of 1:1000 or more
  (increased risk of hypersensitivity to muromonab-CD3)
- » Fever greater than 37.8 °C (100 °F)
  (should be lowered by antipyretics, after infection has been ruled out, before administration of muromonab-CD3)
- » Fluid overload, as seen on chest x-ray or as a weight gain of greater than 3% within 1 week before administration is planned or
- » Heart failure, uncompensated
  (risk of severe and potentially fatal pulmonary edema)

*Risk-benefit should be considered when the following medical problems exist:*
- » Angina, unstable or
- » Cerebrovascular disease or
- » Chronic obstructive pulmonary disease or
- » Heart failure of any etiology or
- » Intravascular volume overload or depletion of any etiology (e.g., excessive dialysis, recent intensive diuresis, blood loss, etc.) or
- » Ischemic heart disease, symptomatic or
- » Myocardial infarction, recent or
- » Neuropathy, advanced symptomatic or
- » Pulmonary edema of any etiology or
- » Seizures, history of or
- » Septic shock or
- » Vascular disease, advanced symptomatic
  (increased risk of serious complications from cytokine release syndrome; condition should be corrected or stabilized prior to initiation of muromonab-CD3 therapy)
- » Chickenpox, existing or recent (including recent exposure) or
- » Herpes zoster
  (risk of severe generalized disease)
- » Infection
  Sensitivity to muromonab-CD3
  Thrombosis, history of
  (arterial or venous thromboses of allografts and other vascular beds [e.g., heart, lungs, brain, bowel] have been reported in patients treated with muromonab-CD3)

**Patient monitoring**
The following may be especially important in patient monitoring (other tests may be warranted in some patients, depending on condition; » = major clinical significance):
- » Assay for circulating T-cells expressing the CD3 antigen or
- » Muromonab-CD3 concentrations, plasma, as determined by enzyme-linked immunosorbent assay (ELISA)
  (recommended at periodic intervals during therapy to assess efficacy)
    Note: Recommended targets are fewer than 25 CD3-positive T-cells per cubic millimeter or muromonab-CD3 concentrations of 800 nanograms per mL (ng/mL) or more.
  Blood counts, complete, including differential and leukocytes and Platelet counts
  (recommended at periodic intervals during therapy)
- » Body temperature determinations
  (recommended prior to administration and at frequent intervals for several hours after administration, especially with the first two doses)
  Hepatic function determinations, including serum transaminase and alkaline phosphatase values and bilirubin concentrations and
  Renal function determinations, including blood urea nitrogen and serum creatinine concentrations
  (recommended at periodic intervals during therapy)

# Side/Adverse Effects

Note: Neutralizing antibodies, primarily of the IgG class, have been detected in most patients during or following the second week of muromonab-CD3 therapy and may potentially reduce subsequent effectiveness by blocking the ability of muromonab-CD3 to bind to the CD3 antigen on T-lymphocytes. Development of neutralizing antibodies has been linked to reappearance of CD3 positive T-cells prior to withdrawal of muromonab-CD3.

The following side/adverse effects have been selected on the basis of their potential clinical significance (possible signs and symptoms in parentheses where appropriate)—not necessarily inclusive:

**Those indicating need for medical attention**
Incidence more frequent
  *Cytokine release syndrome, mild* (diarrhea; dizziness or faintness; fever [often spiking and up to 42 °C or 107 °F] and chills; headache; malaise; muscle or joint pain; nausea and vomiting)
  Note: Symptoms of the *cytokine release syndrome* occur in most patients, usually 30 minutes to 48 hours after the first dose, and last several hours; both frequency and severity seem to decrease with each subsequent dose; fever and chills occurring later may be due to infection; cytokine release syndrome may also occur with dosage increases or resumption of dosing after a period of withdrawal.

Incidence less frequent
  *Anaphylaxis* (rapid or irregular heartbeat; shortness of breath or wheezing; swelling of face or throat); *or hypersensitivity* (itching or tingling; skin rash); *cytokine release syndrome, severe* (chest pain; rapid or irregular heartbeat; shortness of breath or wheezing; trembling and shaking of hands; weakness); *neuropsychiatric reactions, including seizures; encephalopathy* (confusion; hallucinations; unusual tiredness; coma); *cerebral edema; aseptic meningitis syndrome* (fever; headache; stiff neck; unusual sensitivity of eyes to light; rarely, seizures); *and headache*
  Note: *Anaphylactic reactions*, which are serious and occasionally fatal, usually occur within 10 minutes after a dose, and may be difficult to differentiate from the cytokine release syndrome. Such reactions may include cardiovascular collapse, cardiorespiratory arrest, loss of consciousness, hypotension/shock, tachycardia, tingling, angioedema (including laryngeal, pharyngeal, or facial edema), airway obstruction, bronchospasm, dyspnea, urticaria, and pruritus.

  Symptoms of the *cytokine release syndrome* occur in most patients, usually 30 minutes to 48 hours after the first dose, and last several hours; both frequency and severity seem to decrease with each subsequent dose; fever and chills occurring later may be due to infection; cytokine release syndrome may also occur with dosage increases or resumption of dosing after a period of withdrawal.

  Cardiorespiratory findings with the *cytokine release syndrome* may include tachypnea; respiratory distress, failure, or arrest; cardiovascular collapse; cardiac arrest; myocardial infarction; tachycardia; hypertension; hemodynamic instability; hypotension including profound shock; heart failure; cardiogenic and noncardiogenic pulmonary edema; adult respiratory distress syndrome; hypoxemia; apnea; and arrhythmias. Of these, severe, potentially fatal pulmonary edema is the most serious.

  An acute and transient decline in the glomerular filtration rate and diminished urine output, manifested as an increase in the serum creatinine concentration, may occur as a result of *cytokine release*, and may lead to reversible renal function impairment.

  *Neuropsychiatric reactions* may be caused partly by T-cell activation resulting in systemic release of cytokines.

  *Neurologic* signs and symptoms are usually reversible, even with continued treatment, but are sometimes irreversible.

  Symptoms of *aseptic meningitis syndrome* usually occur within the first 3 days of therapy. Examination of cerebrospinal fluid may show leukocytosis, elevated protein, or reduced glucose concentrations.

  Other *neurologic events* that have been reported occasionally include impaired vision, irreversible blindness, para- or quadriparesis/plegia, cerebrovascular accident [hemiparesis/plegia], aphasia, transient ischemic attack, subarachnoid hemorrhage, palsy of the VI cranial nerve, and hearing loss.

**Those indicating possible need for medical attention if they occur after medication is discontinued**
  *Infection* (fever and chills)

# Patient Consultation
As an aid to patient consultation, refer to *Advice for the Patient, Muromonab-CD3 (Systemic)*.

In providing consultation, consider emphasizing the following selected information (» = major clinical significance):

**Before using this medication**
- » Conditions affecting use, especially:
  Sensitivity to muromonab-CD3
  Pregnancy—May cross placenta; risk of adverse effects unknown
  Breast-feeding—Not recommended because of risk of serious side effects

Use in children—Possible increased risk of dehydration as a result of diarrhea and/or vomiting associated with cytokine release syndrome

Other medications, especially other immunosuppressants

Other medical problems, especially unstable angina, cerebrovascular disease, chickenpox, chronic obstructive pulmonary disease, fever, heart failure, herpes zoster, infection, symptomatic ischemic heart disease, recent myocardial infarction, advanced symptomatic neuropathy, pulmonary edema, history of seizures, septic shock, or advanced symptomatic vascular disease

**Proper use of this medication**
» Proper dosing

**Precautions while using this medication**
» Importance of close monitoring by physician
» Avoiding immunizations unless approved by physician; other persons in patient's household should avoid immunizations with oral poliovirus vaccine; avoiding persons who have taken oral poliovirus vaccine or wearing a protective mask that covers nose and mouth

Avoiding exposure to persons with bacterial infections; telling physician if signs of bacterial infection occur

» Possible cytokine release syndrome, which should be reduced after second and subsequent doses; telling doctor or nurse immediately if symptoms of angioedema, cardiac effects, or pulmonary edema occur

**Side/adverse effects**
Signs of potential side effects, especially cytokine release syndrome, anaphylaxis or hypersensitivity, and neuropsychiatric reactions

## General Dosing Information

Patients receiving muromonab-CD3 should be under supervision of a physician experienced in immunosuppressive therapy.

It is recommended that equipment and medications necessary for cardiopulmonary resuscitation be immediately available during administration of each dose of muromonab-CD3.

Muromonab-CD3 should be administered by intravenous push over a period of less than 1 minute.

Acetaminophen and antihistamines may be used to reduce or treat early reactions. Patient temperature should be maintained below 37.8 °C (100 °F) at administration of each dose.

Dosage reduction of other immunosuppressive therapy is recommended when muromonab-CD3 therapy is begun. Dosage should be returned to maintenance levels approximately 3 days before muromonab-CD3 therapy is completed.

Initiation of anti-infective prophylaxis may be warranted in patients at high risk for infection or viral-induced lymphoproliferative disorders. If an infection develops, it must be treated promptly; withdrawal of muromonab-CD3 may be necessary.

**For treatment of adverse effects**
Intensive treatment with oxygen, intravenous fluids, corticosteroids, pressor amines, antihistamines, intubation, etc., may be required for serious manifestations of the cytokine release syndrome.

Subcutaneous aqueous epinephrine (0.3 to 0.5 mL of the 1:1000 dilution), along with other resuscitative measures, may be required for severe anaphylaxis.

## Parenteral Dosage Forms

### MUROMONAB-CD3 INJECTION

**Usual adult and adolescent dose**
Immunosuppressant—
Intravenous (rapid), 5 mg per day for ten to fourteen days.
Note: Intravenous administration of methylprednisolone sodium succinate (8 mg per kg of body weight) one to four hours prior to the first dose of muromonab-CD3 is recommended to reduce the incidence and severity of the cytokine release syndrome.

**Usual pediatric dose**
Immunosuppressant—
Children less than 12 years of age: Intravenous (rapid), 100 mcg (0.1 mg) per kg of body weight per day for ten to fourteen days.

**Strength(s) usually available**
U.S.—
1 mg per mL (Rx) [*Orthoclone OKT3* (polysorbate 80)].
Canada—
1 mg per mL (Rx) [*Orthoclone OKT3*].

**Packaging and storage**
Store between 2 and 8 °C (36 and 46 °F), unless otherwise specified by manufacturer. Protect from freezing.

**Preparation of dosage form**
Sterile muromonab-CD3 is prepared for intravenous administration by drawing the solution into a syringe through a low protein–binding 0.2 or 0.22 micrometer filter, then discarding the filter and attaching an appropriate needle.

**Stability**
Because the product contains no bacteriostatic agent, muromonab-CD3 injection should be used immediately after the ampule is opened and any unused portion should be discarded. In addition, muromonab-CD3 injection, like other protein solutions, may develop a few fine translucent particles, which have not been shown to affect potency.

**Incompatibilities**
Muromonab-CD3 should not be administered by intravenous infusion or in conjunction with other drug solutions.

**Auxiliary labeling**
• Do not shake.

Revised: 08/08/95

---

# MYCOPHENOLATE   Systemic—INTRODUCTORY VERSION

VA CLASSIFICATION (Primary): IM600
Commonly used brand name(s): *CellCept*.
Note: For a listing of dosage forms and brand names by country availability, see *Dosage Forms* section(s).

## Category
Immunosuppressant.

## Indications

**Accepted**
Transplant rejection, organ (prophylaxis)—Mycophenolate is indicated, in combination with cyclosporine and corticosteroids, for prevention of rejection of allogeneic cardiac and renal transplants.

## Pharmacology/Pharmacokinetics

**Physicochemical characteristics**
Molecular weight—Mycophenolate mofetil: 433.5.
pKa—Morpholino group: 5.6.
 Phenolic group: 8.5.

**Mechanism of action/Effect**
Mycophenolate mofetil inhibits immunologically-mediated inflammatory responses in animal models and inhibits tumor development and prolongs survival in murine tumor transplant models. As a potent, selective, noncompetitive, and reversible inhibitor of inosine monophosphate dehydrogenase (IMPDH), mycophenolic acid (MPA), the active metabolite, inhibits the *de novo* synthesis pathway of guanosine nucleotide synthesis without being incorporated into DNA. Because T and B lymphocytes are critically dependent for their proliferation on *de novo* synthesis of purines, while other cell types can utilize salvage pathways, MPA has potent cytostatic effects on lymphocytes. MPA inhibits proliferative responses of T and B lymphocytes to both mitogenic and allospecific stimulation. The addition of guanosine or deoxyguanosine reverses the cytostatic effects of MPA on lymphocytes. MPA also suppresses antibody formation by B lymphocytes. MPA prevents the glycosylation of lymphocyte and monocyte glycoproteins that are involved in intercellular adhesion to endothelial cells and may inhibit recruitment of leukocytes into sites of inflammation and graft rejection. Mycophenolate mofetil does not inhibit early events in the activation of human peripheral blood mononuclear cells, such as the production of interleukin-1 and interleukin-2, but does block the coupling of these events to DNA synthesis and proliferation.

**Absorption**

Rapid and extensive after oral administration. Mean absolute bioavailability in 12 healthy volunteers was 94%.

Observations that a secondary peak in plasma MPA concentrations occurs 6 to 12 hours after a dose and that concurrent administration of cholestyramine results in an approximately 40% decrease in MPA concentrations suggest that enterohepatic recirculation is involved.

Food had no effect on the extent of absorption of mycophenolate when administered at doses of 1.5 grams two times a day; however, the maximum plasma concentrations of MPA were decreased by 40% in the presence of food.

**Distribution**

Mean apparent volume of distribution—In healthy volunteers: Approximately 3.6 and 4 liters per kg of body weight (L/kg), following intravenous and oral administration, respectively. Studies comparing mean blood to plasma ratios of radioactivity concentrations indicate that MPA and mycophenolic acid glucuronide (MPAG), the phenolic glucuronide metabolite, do not extensively distribute into the cellular fractions of blood.

**Protein binding**

To plasma albumin—High (97% for MPA at clinically relevant concentrations, and 82% for MPAG at concentration ranges normally seen in stable renal transplant patients). At higher MPAG concentrations, (e.g., in patients with renal impairment or delayed graft function), binding of MPA may be decreased as a result of competition between MPA and MPAG for binding sites.

**Biotransformation**

Mycophenolate mofetil is hydrolyzed presystemically and completely to mycophenolic acid (MPA), the active metabolite, which is then metabolized primarily by glucuronyl transferase to the inactive phenolic glucuronide (MPAG); other metabolites include those of the 2-hydroxy-ethyl-morpholino moiety. Evidence suggests that enterohepatic recirculation contributes to MPA plasma concentrations.

Plasma clearance is approximately 193 mL per minute after oral administration and 177 mL per minute after intravenous administration.

**Half-life**

For MPA—Mean apparent: Approximately 17.9 hours after oral administration and 16.6 hours after intravenous administration.

**Time to peak plasma concentration**

Adults—
  Cardiac transplant:
    Early (day before hospital discharge post–cardiac transplant)—Approximately 1.8 hours.
    Late (more than 6 months post–cardiac transplant)—1.1 hours.
  Renal transplant:
    Early (less than 40 days post–renal transplant)—Approximately 1.31 hours.
    Late (more than 3 months post–renal transplant)—0.9 hour.
  Children (based on limited data 21 days post–renal transplant):
    3 months to 6 years of age: Approximately 1.25 hours.
    6 to 12 years of age: 0.5 hour.
    12 to 18 years of age: 0.5 to approximately 1.1 hours (dose-related).

**Peak plasma concentration**

Adults—
  Cardiac transplant:
    Early (day before hospital discharge post–cardiac transplant)—Approximately 11.5 mcg per mL (mcg/mL).
    Late (more than 6 months post–cardiac transplant)—20 mcg/mL.
  Renal transplant:
    Early (less than 40 days post–renal transplant)—Approximately 8.16 and 13.5 mcg/mL in studies of multiple doses of 1 and 1.5 grams two times a day, respectively.
    Late (more than 3 months post–renal transplant)—Approximately 24.1 mcg/mL in studies of multiple doses of 1.5 grams two times a day.

Note: In single-dose studies in patients with chronic or severe renal insufficiency, increased plasma concentrations of mycophenolate mofetil metabolites (75% increase in MPA and 3- to 6-fold increase in MPAG) have been observed.

Children (based on limited data 21 days post–renal transplant)—
  3 months to 6 years of age:
    At doses of 15 mg per kg of body weight (mg/kg) two times a day—Approximately 3.7 mcg/mL.
  6 to 12 years of age:
    At doses of 15 mg/kg two times a day—Approximately 13.5 mcg/mL.
  12 to 18 years of age:
    At doses of 15 mg/kg two times a day—Approximately 13.2 mcg/mL.
    At doses of 23 mg/kg two times a day—Approximately 10.6 mcg/mL.

**Elimination**

Renal—93% (less than 1% as MPA; 87% as MPAG). Renal clearance occurs by renal tubular secretion and glomerular filtration.

Fecal—6%.

In dialysis—MPA and MPAG usually are not removed by hemodialysis, although small amounts of MPAG are removed at high plasma MPAG concentrations (greater than 100 mcg per mL).

## Precautions to Consider

### Carcinogenicity/Tumorigenicity

No evidence of tumorigenicity was found in carcinogenicity studies in mice and rats given daily oral doses of up to 180 mg per kg of body weight (mg/kg) and 15 mg/kg, respectively, for 104 weeks. In mice, the highest dose tested was 0.5 times the recommended clinical dose (2 grams per day) when corrected for differences in body surface area (BSA); in rats the highest dose was 0.08 times the recommended clinical dose when corrected for BSA. Although lower than doses given to patients, these doses were considered adequate to evaluate potential risk to humans.

Suppression of cell-mediated immunity in organ transplant patients is associated with an increased risk of benign and malignant lymphoproliferative disorders, lymphomas, and skin cancers. Lymphomas have developed in humans treated with mycophenolate, although a definite causal relationship has not been established. Other neoplasms have been reported infrequently.

### Mutagenicity

No evidence of genotoxicity, with or without metabolic activation, was found in the bacterial mutation assay, the yeast mitotic gene conversion assay, the mouse micronucleus aberration assay, or the Chinese hamster ovary cell (CHO) chromosomal aberration assay.

### Pregnancy/Reproduction

Fertility—Studies in male rats at oral doses of up to 20 mg per kg of body weight (mg/kg) a day (0.1 times the recommended clinical dose when corrected for BSA) found no effect on fertility. A study in female rats at oral doses of 4.5 mg/kg a day (0.02 times the recommended clinical dose when corrected for BSA) found no effect on fertility or reproductive parameters in the dams or in the offspring.

Pregnancy—Adequate and well-controlled studies in humans have not been done. However, because of the teratogenic effects of mycophenolate in animals, it is recommended that two reliable forms of contraception be used simultaneously before, during, and for 6 weeks after discontinuing mycophenolate therapy, including for women with a history of infertility (unless the result of hysterectomy). Mycophenolate should not be initiated in women of childbearing potential without a negative serum or urine pregnancy test with a sensitivity of at least 50 million International Units (mIU) per mL obtained within one week prior to beginning therapy.

A study in female rats at oral doses of 4.5 mg/kg a day (0.02 times the recommended clinical dose when corrected for BSA) found that mycophenolate caused malformations (primarily of the head and eyes) in the first generation offspring in the absence of maternal toxicity. Studies in rats and rabbits at oral doses of 6 mg/kg a day and 90 mg/kg a day (equivalent to 0.03 and 0.92 times the recommended clinical dose when corrected for BSA), respectively, found fetal resorptions and malformations in the absence of maternal toxicity.

FDA Pregnancy Category C.

### Breast-feeding

It is not known whether mycophenolate is distributed into breast milk in humans.

However, studies in rats treated with mycophenolate have shown mycophenolic acid (MPA) to be distributed into milk.

### Pediatrics

No information is available on the relationship of age to the effects of this medication in pediatric patients. Safety and efficacy have not been established.

### Geriatrics

No information is available on the relationship of age to the effects of mycophenolate in geriatric patients.

### Dental

The immunosuppressive effects of mycophenolate may result in an increased incidence of certain microbial infections and delayed healing. Dental work, whenever possible, should be completed prior to initiation of therapy and undertaken with caution during therapy. Patients should be instructed in proper oral hygiene.

### Drug interactions and/or related problems
The following drug interactions and/or related problems have been selected on the basis of their potential clinical significance (possible mechanism in parentheses where appropriate)—not necessarily inclusive (» = major clinical significance):

Note: Combinations containing any of the following medications, depending on the amount present, may also interact with this medication.

Acyclovir or
Ganciclovir
  (in the presence of renal impairment, acyclovir or ganciclovir may compete with MPAG for tubular secretion, thus further increasing plasma concentrations of each)

Antacids, magnesium- or aluminum hydroxide–containing
  (concurrent administration may result in decreased absorption of mycophenolate; it is recommended that simultaneous administration be avoided)

Cholestyramine
  (plasma concentrations of MPA may be decreased as a result of interruption of enterohepatic recirculation of MPAG possibly caused by intestinal binding with cholestyramine)

Medications that alter gastrointestinal flora
  (may disrupt enterohepatic circulation; interference with MPAG hydrolysis may result in less MPA available for absorption)

» Immunosuppressants, other, such as:
  Antithymocyte globulin
  Azathioprine
  Chlorambucil
  Corticosteroids, glucocorticoid
  Cyclophosphamide
  Cyclosporine
  Mercaptopurine
  Muromonab-CD3
  Tacrolimus
    (increased risk of development of lymphomas and other malignancies of the skin or increased susceptibility to infection due to increased intensity and duration of immunosuppression)

Probenecid or
Medications that undergo renal tubular secretion
  (probenecid may inhibit renal tubular secretion and result in increased plasma concentrations of the metabolites of mycophenolate; other medications known to undergo renal tubular secretion may also compete with MPAG to raise plasma concentrations of either drug undergoing tubular secretion)

### Laboratory value alterations
The following have been selected on the basis of their potential clinical significance (possible effect in parentheses where appropriate)—not necessarily inclusive (» = major clinical significance):

With physiology/laboratory test values
  Alanine aminotransferase (ALT [SGPT]) and
  Alkaline phosphatase and
  Aspartate aminotransferase (AST [SGOT])
    (values may be increased)
  Calcium and
  Phosphate and
  Potassium, serum
    (concentrations may be increased or decreased)
  Chloride, serum
    (concentration may be decreased)
  Cholesterol, serum
    (values may be increased)
  Creatinine, serum
    (concentration may be increased)
  Glucose, blood
    (concentration may be increased or decreased)
  Leukocytes (neutrophils [WBC])
    (blood counts may be increased or decreased)

### Medical considerations/Contraindications
The medical considerations/contraindications included have been selected on the basis of their potential clinical significance (reasons given in parentheses where appropriate)—not necessarily inclusive (» = major clinical significance):

*Risk-benefit should be considered when the following medical problems exist:*

  Delayed renal graft function posttransplant
    (increased MPAG concentrations reported, as well as increased incidence of some adverse events [anemia, thrombocytopenia, hyperkalemia], as compared with patients without delayed graft function; observation, but not dosage reduction, is recommended)

» Digestive system disease, active
    (risk of gastrointestinal ulceration, hemorrhage, or perforation, possibly associated with mycophenolate administration)

» Renal function impairment, severe
    (reduced elimination)

» Sensitivity to mycophenolate
    (allergic reactions to mycophenolate may occur)

### Patient monitoring
The following may be especially important in patient monitoring (other tests may be warranted in some patients, depending on condition; » = major clinical significance):

» Complete blood count (CBC)
    (recommended weekly during the first month of therapy, twice a month for the second and third months of treatment, and then once a month through the remainder of the first year)

## Side/Adverse Effects
The following side/adverse effects have been selected on the basis of their potential clinical significance (possible signs and symptoms in parentheses where appropriate)—not necessarily inclusive:

### Those indicating need for medical attention
Incidence more frequent
  *Anemia*—asymptomatic; *chest pain; cough, increased*—more common in patients receiving mycophenolate for cardiac transplantation than in patients receiving mycophenolate for renal transplantation; *dyspnea* (shortness of breath)—more common in patients receiving mycophenolate for cardiac transplantation than in patients receiving mycophenolate for renal transplantation; *hematuria* (blood in urine); *hypertension*—asymptomatic; *leukopenia (neutropenia) or infection* (fever or chills, cough or hoarseness, lower back or side pain, painful or difficult urination); *peripheral edema* (swelling of feet or lower legs)

Note: Neutropenia occurs most frequently 31 to 180 days posttransplant. Incidence of fatal infections or sepsis (usually cytomegalovirus [CMV] viremia) in three controlled studies was similar (less than 2%) between patients receiving mycophenolate and those receiving control therapy in combination with other immunosuppressants.

Incidence less frequent
  *Arrhythmia* (irregular heartbeat); *arthralgia* (joint pain); *colitis* (abdominal pain)—sometimes caused by cytomegalovirus; *gastrointestinal hemorrhage* (bloody vomit); *gingival hyperplasia* (enlarged gums); *gingivitis* (red, inflamed, bleeding gums); *myalgia* (muscle pain); *neutropenia, severe; oral moniliasis* (white patches on mouth, tongue, or throat); *pancreatitis* (abdominal pain); *stomatitis* (sores inside mouth); *thrombocytopenia* (unusual bleeding or bruising; black, tarry stools; blood in urine or stools; pinpoint red spots on skin)—usually asymptomatic; *tremor* (trembling or shaking of hands or feet)

Note: Severe neutropenia is defined as an absolute neutrophil count (ANC) of less than 500 cells per microliter.

### Those indicating need for medical attention only if they continue or are bothersome
Incidence more frequent
  *Abdominal or stomach pain; constipation or diarrhea; dyspepsia* (heartburn); *headache; nausea; vomiting; weakness*

Incidence less frequent
  *Acne; dizziness; insomnia* (trouble in sleeping); *skin rash*

## Overdose
For more information on the management of overdose or unintentional ingestion, **contact a Poison Control Center** (see *Poison Control Center Listing*).

### Treatment of overdose
Although overdose has not been reported with mycophenolate, mycophenolic acid (MPA) could be removed by bile acid sequestrants such as cholestyramine, which would increase excretion of mycophenolate.

## Patient Consultation
As an aid to patient consultation, refer to *Advice for the Patient, Mycophenolate (Systemic)—Introductory version*.

In providing consultation, consider emphasizing the following selected information (» = major clinical significance):

**Before using this medication**
» Conditions affecting use, especially:
  Sensitivity to mycophenolate
  Pregnancy—Causes birth defects in animals; two forms of effective birth control recommended before, during, and for 6 weeks after discontinuing mycophenolate
  Breast-feeding—Distributed into milk of lactating rats
  Dental—Dental work should be completed prior to initiation of therapy whenever possible
  Other medications, especially other immunosuppressants
  Other medical problems, especially active digestive system disease or renal function impairment

**Proper use of this medication**
  Taking on empty stomach
» Proper dosing
  Importance of not using more or less medication than the amount prescribed
  Getting into the habit of taking at the same time each day
  Checking with physician before discontinuing or changing medication
  Swallowing capsule or tablet whole
  Missed dose: Taking as soon as possible; not taking if almost time for next dose; not doubling doses
» Proper storage

**Precautions while using this medication**
» Importance of close monitoring by physician
  Maintaining good dental hygiene and seeing dentist regularly for teeth cleaning
  Avoiding contact with people with colds or other infections

**Side/adverse effects**
  Signs of potential side effects, especially anemia, chest pain, increased cough, dyspnea, hematuria, hypertension, leukopenia or infection, peripheral edema, arrhythmia, arthralgia, colitis, gastrointestinal hemorrhage, gingival hyperplasia, gingivitis, myalgia, severe neutropenia, oral moniliasis, pancreatitis, stomatitis, thrombocytopenia, and tremor

## General Dosing Information

Patients receiving mycophenolate should be under the supervision of a physician experienced in immunosuppressive therapy.

If neutropenia (absolute neutrophil count [ANC] less than 1300 cells per microliter) develops, dosage reduction or interruption of mycophenolate, along with appropriate diagnostic tests, is recommended.

**Diet/Nutrition**
Administration on an empty stomach is recommended.

## Oral Dosage Forms

### MYCOPHENOLATE MOFETIL CAPSULES
**Usual adult dose**
Transplant rejection, prophylaxis—
Cardiac—
  Oral, 1.5 grams two times a day as soon as possible following cardiac transplant surgery, in combination with cyclosporine and corticosteroids.

Renal—
  Oral, 1 gram two times a day as soon as possible following renal transplant surgery, in combination with cyclosporine and corticosteroids.
Note: In patients with severe chronic renal function impairment beyond the immediate posttransplant period, doses greater than 1 gram twice a day should be avoided and patients observed carefully.

**Usual pediatric dose**
Safety and efficacy have not been established.

**Strength(s) usually available**
U.S.—
  250 mg (Rx) [*CellCept*].

**Packaging and storage**
Store between 15 and 30 °C (59 and 86 °F). Protect from light.

**Auxiliary labeling**
• Take on empty stomach.
• Swallow capsule whole. Do not open or crush.

**Note**
Because of potential teratogenicity, mycophenolate capsules should not be opened or crushed. Great care should be taken to prevent inhalation of mycophenolate powder and exposure of the skin to it. Any powder that comes in contact with the skin or mucosae should be washed off thoroughly with soap and water (eyes should be rinsed with plain water).

### MYCOPHENOLATE MOFETIL TABLETS
**Usual adult dose**
See *Mycophenolate Mofetil Capsules*.

**Usual pediatric dose**
See *Mycophenolate Mofetil Capsules*.

**Strength(s) usually available**
U.S.—
  500 mg (Rx) [*CellCept* (film-coated)].

**Packaging and storage**
Store between 15 and 30 °C (59 and 86 °F). Protect from light.

**Auxiliary labeling**
• Take on empty stomach.
• Swallow tablet whole. Do not crush.

**Note**
Because of potential teratogenicity, mycophenolate tablets should not be crushed.

Developed: 09/28/95
Revised: 03/18/98

# NABILONE Systemic*

VA CLASSIFICATION (Primary): GA605

Note: Controlled substance classification—
Canada—N.

Commonly used brand name(s): *Cesamet*.

Note: For a listing of dosage forms and brand names by country availability, see *Dosage Forms* section(s).

*Not commercially available in U.S.

## Category
Antiemetic.

## Indications

**Accepted**

*Nausea and vomiting, cancer chemotherapy–induced* (prophylaxis)—Nabilone is indicated in selected patients for the prevention of nausea and vomiting associated with emetogenic cancer chemotherapy when other antiemetic medications are not effective.

## Pharmacology/Pharmacokinetics

**Physicochemical characteristics**
Chemical group—Synthetic 9-ketocannabinoid; resembles the cannabinols but is not a tetrahydrocannabinol.
Molecular weight—372.55.

**Mechanism of action/Effect**
The exact mechanism of nabilone's antiemetic action is not known. However, animal studies with other cannabinoids suggest it may be due to inhibition of the vomiting control mechanism in the medulla oblongata.

**Other actions/effects**
Central nervous system (CNS) depression and stimulation; may increase supine and standing heart rates (dose-dependent); may inhibit prolactin release.

**Absorption**
Rapidly absorbed from the gastrointestinal tract after oral administration.

**Biotransformation**
Hepatic.

**Half-life**
Elimination—
  Terminal phase:
    Nabilone—2 hours.
    Other metabolites—35 hours.

**Time to peak concentration**
2 hours.

**Elimination**
Primarily fecal (biliary); approximately 65% of an oral dose appears in the feces and 20% in the urine.

## Precautions to Consider

**Cross-sensitivity and/or related problems**
Patients sensitive to other marijuana products may be sensitive to this preparation also.

**Carcinogenicity**
Studies to evaluate the carcinogenic potential of nabilone have not been performed.

**Pregnancy/Reproduction**
Pregnancy—Adequate and well-controlled studies in humans have not been done.
Studies in rats and rabbits at doses 150 and 40 times, respectively, the usual human adult dose have shown that nabilone decreases litter size, and increases the incidence of fetal resorptions and stillborn pups.

**Breast-feeding**
It is not known whether nabilone is distributed into breast milk. However, use of nabilone in nursing mothers is not recommended since dronabinol, another synthetic cannabinoid closely related to nabilone, is concentrated and distributed into breast milk.

**Pediatrics**
Appropriate studies on the relationship of age to the effects of nabilone have not been performed in children up to 18 years of age. Safety and efficacy have not been established.

**Geriatrics**
Although appropriate studies on the relationship of age to the effects of nabilone have not been performed in the geriatric population, the elderly may be more sensitive to the cardiac effects and orthostatic hypotension produced by nabilone.

Also, because of this medication's psychoactive effects and potential for dependence, therapy could be more troublesome in the elderly and should be used with caution, after less toxic alternatives have been considered and found ineffective. Recommended doses should not be exceeded, and the elderly patient should be carefully monitored during therapy.

**Drug interactions and/or related problems**
The following drug interactions and/or related problems have been selected on the basis of their potential clinical significance (possible mechanism in parentheses where appropriate)—not necessarily inclusive (» = major clinical significance):

Note: Combinations containing any of the following medications, depending on the amount present, may also interact with this medication.

» Alcohol or
» CNS depression–producing medications, other (See *Appendix II*)
  (concurrent use may potentiate the CNS depressant effects of either these medications or nabilone)

Apomorphine
  (prior administration of nabilone may decrease the emetic response to apomorphine; also, concurrent use may potentiate the CNS depressant effects of either apomorphine or nabilone)

**Medical considerations/Contraindications**
The medical considerations/contraindications included have been selected on the basis of their potential clinical significance (reasons given in parentheses where appropriate)—not necessarily inclusive (» = major clinical significance):

*Risk-benefit should be considered when the following medical problems exist:*

Cardiac disorders
  (nabilone may elevate supine and standing heart rates)

Drug abuse or dependence, history of, including active or treated alcoholism
  (increased risk of nabilone abuse and dependence)

Hepatic function impairment, severe
  (increased risk of toxic effects because of decreased metabolism of nabilone)

Hypertension
  (hypertensive effects of nabilone may cause an increase in blood pressure)

Hypotension
  (hypotensive effects of nabilone may further decrease blood pressure)

» Manic or depressive states or
» Schizophrenia
  (symptoms may be exacerbated)

Sensitivity to nabilone or other marijuana products

**Patient monitoring**
The following may be especially important in patient monitoring (other tests may be warranted in some patients, depending on condition; » = major clinical significance):

Blood pressure determinations and
Cardiac function monitoring
  (recommended for early detection of tachycardia and changes in blood pressure, especially in patients with hypertension or cardiac disease)

## Side/Adverse Effects

Note: Overdose may occur either with therapeutic doses or at higher, nontherapeutic, doses.

The following side/adverse effects have been selected on the basis of their potential clinical significance (possible signs and symptoms in parentheses where appropriate)—not necessarily inclusive:

**Those indicating need for medical attention**
*Psychiatric effects* (changes in mood; confusion, possibly including delusions and feelings of depersonalization or unreality; hallucinations; mental depression; nervousness or anxiety); **difficulty in breathing; hypotension** (severe dizziness or fainting); **fast, slow, irregular, or**

pounding heartbeat; increase in blood pressure; unusual tiredness or weakness, severe

Note: *Psychiatric effects* usually resolve by themselves within 72 hours after discontinuation of nabilone.

**Those indicating need for medical attention only if they continue or are bothersome**
Incidence more frequent
*Clumsiness or unsteadiness; difficulty concentrating; dizziness; drowsiness; dryness of mouth; false sense of well-being; headache*
Incidence less frequent or rare
*Blurred vision or any changes in vision; dizziness or lightheadedness, especially when getting up from a lying or sitting position* (orthostatic hypotension)—more frequent with high doses; *loss of appetite; muscle pain or weakness*

## Overdose

Note: Overdose may occur either with therapeutic doses or at higher, nontherapeutic, doses.

For more information on the management of overdose or unintentional ingestion, **contact a Poison Control Center** (see *Poison Control Center Listing*).

**Clinical effects of overdose**
The following effects have been selected on the basis of their potential clinical significance (possible signs and symptoms in parentheses where appropriate)–not necessarily inclusive:

*Psychiatric effects* (changes in mood; confusion, possibly including delusions and feelings of depersonalization or unreality; hallucinations; mental depression; nervousness or anxiety); *difficulty in breathing; hypotension* (severe dizziness or fainting); *fast, slow, irregular, or pounding heartbeat; increase in blood pressure; unusual tiredness or weakness, severe*

Note: *Psychiatric effects* usually resolve by themselves within 72 hours after discontinuation of nabilone.

**Treatment of overdose**
Specific treatment—Observation of patient in a quiet environment. Verbal support and comforting if psychotic episodes occur; in severe cases, antipsychotic drugs may be used with careful attention being paid to possible CNS-depressant additive effects. Treatment of hypertension or hypotension, if necessary.

Monitoring—Continuous blood pressure monitoring; cardiac monitoring.

Supportive care—Supportive therapy. Patients in whom intentional overdose is confirmed or suspected should be referred for psychiatric consultation.

## Patient Consultation

As an aid to patient consultation, refer to *Advice for the Patient, Nabilone (Systemic)*.

In providing consultation, consider emphasizing the following selected information (» = major clinical significance):

**Before using this medication**
» Conditions affecting use, especially:
   Sensitivity to nabilone or other marijuana products
   Pregnancy—No studies in humans; increased risk of fetal resorptions and stillbirths in animal studies with doses many times the usual human dose
   Breast-feeding—Use not recommended; although not known if distributed into breast milk, possibility exists
   Use in the elderly—Increased sensitivity to cardiac effects and orthostatic hypotension; caution recommended because of psychoactive effects and potential for dependence
   Other medications, especially CNS depressants
   Other medical problems, especially manic depression and schizophrenia

**Proper use of this medication**
» Importance of not taking more medication than the amount prescribed because of danger of overdose
» Proper dosing
   Missed dose: Taking as soon as possible; not taking if almost time for next dose; not doubling doses
» Proper storage

**Precautions while using this medication**
» Avoiding use of alcohol or other CNS depressants during therapy
» Suspected overdose: Getting emergency help at once
» Caution if dizziness, drowsiness, lightheadedness, or false sense of well-being occurs
   Caution when getting up suddenly from a lying or sitting position

Possible dryness of mouth; using sugarless candy or gum, ice, or saliva substitute for relief

**Side/adverse effects**
Signs of potential side effects, especially psychiatric effects, difficulty in breathing, hypotension, tachycardia, hypertension, and unusual tiredness or weakness

## General Dosing Information

Amount of nabilone dispensed should be limited to the amount necessary for a single cycle of chemotherapy.

Patients on nabilone therapy should be closely observed, if possible within an inpatient setting. Since response and tolerance to the effects of nabilone vary with each patient, the period of patient supervision required should be determined by the physician on an individual basis.

Adequate and well-controlled studies have not been done to determine whether psychological and physical dependence will develop with chronic administration of nabilone. However, like other similar cannabinoids, nabilone has a high potential for abuse and for production of psychological dependence.

**For treatment of adverse effects**
Recommended treatment includes
• Observation of patient in a quiet environment.
• Verbal support and comforting if psychotic episodes occur; in severe cases, antipsychotic drugs may be used with careful attention being paid to possible CNS depressant additive effects.
• Supportive therapy.
• Continuous blood pressure monitoring.
• Cardiac monitoring.
• Treatment of hypertension or hypotension, if necessary.

## Oral Dosage Forms

**NABILONE CAPSULES**

**Usual adult and adolescent dose**
Antiemetic—
   Oral, 1 or 2 mg two times a day. A dose of 1 or 2 mg may be given the night before chemotherapy is initiated. On the day of chemotherapy, the initial dose of nabilone should be given one to three hours before the chemotherapeutic agent. The dose of nabilone may be administered two or three times a day during the course of chemotherapy and, if needed, for forty-eight hours after the last dose of the chemotherapeutic cycle.

Note: The lower starting dose should be used to minimize side effects. Dosage may be increased as necessary if side effects are not significant.

**Usual adult prescribing limits**
Up to 6 mg daily, in divided doses three times a day.

**Usual pediatric dose**
Safety and efficacy have not been established.

**Usual geriatric dose**
See *Usual adult and adolescent dose*.

Note: Geriatric patients may be more sensitive to the effects of the usual adult dose.

**Strength(s) usually available**
U.S.—
   Not commercially available.
Canada—
   1 mg (Rx) [*Cesamet*].

**Packaging and storage**
Store between 15 and 30 °C (59 and 86 °F), unless otherwise specified by manufacturer.

**Auxiliary labeling**
• May cause drowsiness.
• Avoid alcoholic beverages.

**Note**
Controlled substance in Canada.

Revised: 06/17/93

---

**NABUMETONE**—See *Anti-inflammatory Drugs, Nonsteroidal (Systemic)*

---

**NADOLOL**—See *Beta-adrenergic Blocking Agents (Systemic)*

# NAFARELIN  Systemic

VA CLASSIFICATION (Primary): HS900

Commonly used brand name(s): *Synarel*.

Note: For a listing of dosage forms and brand names by country availability, see *Dosage Forms* section(s).

## Category

Gonadotropin-releasing hormone analog; gonadotropin inhibitor; antiendometriotic agent.

## Indications

### Accepted

Endometriosis (treatment)—Nafarelin is indicated for the management of endometriosis, including treatment of pelvic pain associated with all stages of endometriosis and reduction in the size and number of endometriotic implants. Nafarelin may also have a modest effect on infertility in patients who have moderate endometriosis. Preoperative use of nafarelin in infertile patients with severe endometriosis may also facilitate the surgical procedure.

Nafarelin has been shown to be as effective as danazol in decreasing the size and extent of endometriotic implants as well as in reducing clinical symptoms of endometriosis.

Generally, the use of nafarelin or other gonadotropin-releasing hormone (GnRH) analogs for the treatment of endometriosis is limited to short-term, single courses of therapy of 6 months, and to those patients who cannot tolerate the androgenic side effects of danazol or who are not candidates for surgery, because its use is associated with significant, but largely reversible, decreases in bone mass. The long-term clinical significance and safety of these changes on bone mass are unknown.

Puberty, central precocious (treatment)—Nafarelin is indicated for the treatment of central precocious puberty (CPP) in children of both genders. Children suspected of having CPP usually develop secondary sexual characteristics at an earlier stage than cohorts (up to 8 years of age in girls; up to 9 years of age in boys). They also show a significantly advanced bone age that can result in poor adult height attainment. Diagnosis of CPP should be confirmed before initiation of treatment with nafarelin by measuring serum sex steroids and basal gonadotropins levels, testing stimulation response to gonadotropin-releasing hormone (GnRH), assessing diagnostic imaging of the brain (including pituitary and hypothalamus), and performing pelvic ultrasound examination in girls.

Before beginning treatment for CPP with nafarelin, it is especially important that the patient is willing to comply with dosing and frequent monitoring by the physician during the first 6 to 8 weeks of treatment to assure that suppression of gonadal-pituitary function is rapid.

## Pharmacology/Pharmacokinetics

### Physicochemical characteristics

Chemical group—Nafarelin acetate is a decapeptide, which is an agonistic analog of the hypothalamic hormone, gonadotropin-releasing hormone (GnRH). Substitution of a naphthylalanine group for glycine at the sixth amino acid position results in higher affinity for the GnRH receptor in the pituitary gland (approximately 200 times greater than GnRH), resistance to degradation by endopeptidases, and increased lipophilicity.

Molecular weight—1322.51 (anhydrous free decapeptide).

### Mechanism of action/Effect

Like GnRH, initial or intermittent administration of nafarelin acetate stimulates release of the gonadotropins luteinizing hormone (LH) and follicle-stimulating hormone (FSH) from the pituitary gland, which in turn transiently increases production of estradiol in females and testosterone in both sexes. However, with continuous daily administration, nafarelin continuously occupies the GnRH receptor. A reversible down-regulation of the GnRH receptors in the pituitary gland and desensitization of the pituitary gonadotropes occur. This causes a significant and sustained decline in the production of LH and FSH. A decline in gonadotropin production and release causes a dramatic reversible decrease in synthesis of estradiol, progesterone, and testosterone by the ovaries or testes.

Antiendometriotic agent—Like normal endometrium, endometriotic implants contain estrogen receptors. Estrogen stimulates the growth of endometrium. Use of nafarelin induces anovulation and amenorrhea and decreases serum concentrations of estradiol to the postmenopausal range, which induces atrophy of endometriotic implants. Nafarelin does not abolish the underlying pathophysiology of endometriosis, however. After nafarelin therapy is discontinued, pituitary and ovarian function normalize and estradiol serum concentrations increase to pretreatment levels. Recurrences of endometriosis are frequent after cessation of any hormonal therapy and after surgery that leaves the ovaries and/or uterus intact.

Gonadotropin inhibitor—When used regularly in boys and girls for treatment of central precocious puberty, nafarelin suppresses LH response to gonadotropin-releasing hormone to prepubertal LH levels of less than 15 milli-international units (mIU) within 1 month of treatment. As a result, serum concentrations of the sex steroids estrogen and testosterone decrease. Consequently, secondary sexual development of breasts in 82% of girls and genital development in 100% of boys regresses or ceases; however, pubic hair development, a function of adrenal androgens, regresses in only 54% of boys and girls. Also, linear growth velocity slows to 5 to 6 centimeters (cm) per year or less. Although bone age velocity approaches the normal rate after 1 year of nafarelin treatment, the gap that exists before treatment between bone age and chronological age continues to narrow for 2 to 3 years during nafarelin treatment, improving the chance of attaining the predicted adult height.

### Absorption

Rapidly absorbed across nasal mucosa.

Bioavailability—2.8% (average, relative; range, 1.2 to 5.6%) after a 400-mcg dose.

### Protein binding

78 to 84% (*in vitro* estimation), primarily to albumin.

### Biotransformation

Enzymatic hydrolysis.

### Half-life

Elimination—3 hours (range, 2 to 4 hours).

### Onset of action

Within approximately 4 weeks, complete suppression of gonadal steroids occurs.

For treatment of endometriosis—Amenorrhea occurred in 65% of adult patients using 400 mcg of nafarelin a day within 60 days, 80% within 90 days, and 100% within 120 days. After the end of their treatment, 60% of patients were free of symptoms for endometriosis, 32% had mild symptoms, 7% had moderate symptoms, and 1% had severe symptoms. Of the 60% of patients who had complete relief of symptoms, 50% of patients remained symptom-free after 6 months, 33% had mild symptoms, 17% had moderate symptoms, and no patient had severe symptoms.

### Time to peak concentration

10 to 45 minutes.

### Peak serum concentration

200-mcg dose—0.6 nanograms per mL (average).
400-mcg dose—1.8 to 2.2 nanograms per mL.
600-mcg dose—6.6 nanograms per mL.

### Time to peak effect

Maximal suppression of estradiol serum concentrations—20 days, with use of 400 to 800 mcg per day.

### Duration of action

Relief from symptoms of endometriosis may persist for up to 3 to 6 months after discontinuance of nafarelin therapy.

### Elimination

In one study in three males given a single subcutaneous dose of radiolabeled nafarelin, 44 to 55% of the radiolabel appeared in urine and 19 to 44% appeared in stool over 7 days following administration. Most of the radioactivity was recovered within the first 48 hours. Approximately 3% appears in the urine unchanged.

## Precautions to Consider

### Carcinogenicity/Tumorigenicity

In studies conducted in rats and mice, use of nafarelin at proportionately high doses (100 to 500 mcg per kg of body weight [mcg/kg], corresponding to 110 to 560 times the maximum recommended human intranasal dose) and for prolonged periods induced hyperplasia and/or neoplasia of endocrine organs. Increases in pancreatic islet cell adenomas, benign adrenal medullary tumors, Harderian gland tumors, benign testicular and ovarian tumors, pituitary adenomas, and carcinomas were noted in some animal treatment groups. No metastases of these tumors were observed. Generally, tumorigenicity in rodents is particularly sensitive to hormonal stimulation.

No evidence of tumorigenicity has been reported in monkeys or humans.

**Mutagenicity**
No evidence of mutagenic potential was found in mutagenicity studies conducted in bacterial, yeast, and mammalian systems.

**Pregnancy/Reproduction**
Fertility—Nafarelin induces anovulation and amenorrhea in most adult females. This effect is reversible and the average time until the return of menses after discontinuance of therapy is about 45 days. A nonhormonal contraceptive method should be used during nafarelin therapy if conception is likely or possible. If an inadequate dose is used or successive doses are missed, breakthrough bleeding or ovulation may occur.

In one study of adult females using nafarelin for treatment of endometriosis, serum progesterone concentrations indicated that ovulation occurred in less than 18% of menstrual cycles over 3 to 6 months of dosing with 100 or 200 mcg per day. At a dose of 500 mcg twice a day, ovulation was completely suppressed.

Long-term posttreatment follow-up studies of fertility in children treated for central precocious puberty (CPP) have not been done. At 1 year posttreatment, serum sex steroid and gonadotropin levels in girls and boys returned to normal; menses returned in girls and semen analyses were normal in two boys who were examined.

Pregnancy—Nafarelin should not be given during the course of pregnancy. It is not known what effects nafarelin may have on the embryo if administered during pregnancy. The pre-existence of a pregnancy should be ruled out prior to its use. A nonhormonal contraceptive method should be used during nafarelin therapy.

Major fetal abnormalities were observed in one study in rats, but not in mice or rabbits, after administration of nafarelin throughout gestation. A similar, repeat study in rats failed to show an increase in fetal abnormalities. A dose-related increase in fetal mortality and a decrease in fetal weight occurred in rabbits and rats. The effects on rat fetal mortality were expected results of the changes in gonadal steroid levels induced by nafarelin.

FDA Pregnancy Category X.

**Breast-feeding**
It is not known whether nafarelin is distributed into breast milk. However, it is recommended that nafarelin not be used by nursing mothers.

**Pediatrics**
No information is available on the relationship of age to the effects of nafarelin for treatment of endometriosis in patients younger than 18 years of age. Safety and efficacy have not been established.

It is not known if ovarian cysts, a potential side effect that can occur in adult females taking nafarelin for treatment of endometriosis, could also occur in children treated for CPP.

Reversal of the suppressive effects of nafarelin for treatment of CPP in 69 pediatric patients studied 1 year posttreatment has been demonstrated by return of secondary sexual development, menses, and pubertal concentrations of serum gonadotropins and sex steroids. Semen analyses were normal in a few boys after treatment discontinuation; fertility studies in girls have not been done, and nafarelin's potential effect on fertility is not known.

**Drug interactions and/or related problems**
The following drug interactions and/or related problems have been selected on the basis of their potential clinical significance (possible mechanism in parentheses where appropriate)—not necessarily inclusive (» = major clinical significance):

Note: Combinations containing any of the following medications, depending on the amount present, may also interact with this medication.

Decongestants, nasal, topical
(it is not known whether use of topical nasal decongestants will interfere with the absorption of nafarelin; it is recommended that patients allow at least 2 hours to pass after the use of nafarelin before using a topical nasal decongestant)

**Laboratory value alterations**
The following have been selected on the basis of their potential clinical significance (possible effect in parentheses where appropriate)—not necessarily inclusive (» = major clinical significance):

With diagnostic test results
» Pituitary gonadotropic function testing and
» Gonadal function testing
(therapeutic doses of nafarelin suppress the pituitary-gonadal system; baseline function is usually restored within 4 to 8 weeks of discontinuance of nafarelin)

With physiology/laboratory test values
Alkaline phosphatase, serum and
Calcium-to-creatinine ratio, urine and
Hydroxyproline-to-creatinine ratio, urine and
Phosphate, serum and
Phosphorous, plasma
(values are increased to postmenopausal levels for adults during use of nafarelin, indicating increased bone remodeling; generally reversible within 3 to 6 months of discontinuation of nafarelin therapy)

Androstenedione and
» Estradiol and
Follicle-stimulating hormone and
Luteinizing hormone and
» Progesterone and
Sex-hormone binding globulin and
» Testosterone, total and free
(serum concentrations are transiently increased at the onset of therapy; with continued use, serum concentrations will be suppressed. Estradiol serum concentrations will decline to postmenopausal levels in adults. Effects are reversible within 4 to 8 weeks upon discontinuation of nafarelin)

» Bone mineral content
(hypoestrogenism-induced loss of bone mineral content occurs in most adult patients during use of nafarelin, which is especially evident in those skeletal regions that are composed mostly of trabecular bone, such as the spinal vertebrae. Bone mineral content decreases reported range from 0 to 2% for the forearm [mostly cortical bone] and from 6 to 11% for the spinal vertebrae, after 6 months of therapy. In the 6 months following discontinuation of therapy, this effect has been reported to be largely reversible, with a net overall loss of approximately one to one and one-half percent. The long-term clinical significance of these changes on bone mass are unknown, and their importance in the selection of therapy is controversial)
(decreased bone density is not seen in children treated with nafarelin for central precocious puberty)

Calcium
(serum concentrations are decreased in adults during nafarelin therapy)

Eosinophil count
(asymptomatic eosinophilia has occurred in approximately 10 to 15% of adult patients during nafarelin therapy in clinical trials)

Triglycerides, serum
(increased above the upper limit of 150 mg per dL in 12% of adult patients in one study)

White blood cell count
(asymptomatic leukopenia has occurred in approximately 10 to 15% of adult patients during nafarelin therapy in clinical trials)

**Medical considerations/Contraindications**
The medical considerations/contraindications included have been selected on the basis of their potential clinical significance (reasons given in parentheses where appropriate)—not necessarily inclusive (» = major clinical significance).

*Except under special circumstances, this medication should not be used when the following medical problem exists:*
» Uterine bleeding, abnormal, undiagnosed
(may delay diagnosis by masking underlying condition)

*Risk-benefit should be considered when the following medical problems exist:*
Allergy to nafarelin acetate

Hypersensitivity to gonadotropin-releasing hormone or agonists or other ingredients in product formulation

Significant risk factors for low bone mineral content
(nafarelin may additionally increase the risk for development of osteopenia or osteoporosis in adult females; repeat courses of gonadotropin-releasing hormone analog therapy for treatment of endometriosis are not advisable. Additional bone loss can occur in adult females using nafarelin for longer than 6 months or when adult females have other known osteoporotic risk factors, such as alcohol and/or tobacco abuse, family history of severe osteoporosis, or long-term use of medications that decrease bone mineral density, including anticonvulsants or corticosteroids)

**Patient monitoring**
The following may be especially important in patient monitoring (other tests may be warranted in some patients, depending on condition; » = major clinical significance):

*For treatment of CPP*
Bone linear growth velocity and bone age velocity determinations and Imaging studies
(recommended prior to treatment initiation and periodically during

treatment, beginning 3 to 6 months after treatment initiation; diagnostic imaging studies should include radiography of the left hand and wrist [or nondominating hand and wrist] for bone age determination, pelvic ultrasonography in females, and magnetic resonance imaging of the brain)

Dehydroepiandrosterone concentrations, serum and/or
Estradiol concentrations, serum and/or
Follicle-stimulating hormone concentrations, serum and/or
Human chorionic gonadotropin concentrations, serum and/or
Hydroxyprogesterone concentrations, serum and/or
Luteinizing hormone concentrations, serum and/or
Prolactin concentrations, serum and/or
Testosterone concentrations, serum
(recommended prior to treatment initiation to establish prepubertal gonadotropin response. If gonadal-pituitary function suppression is not apparent within 6 to 8 weeks after therapy with nafarelin is initiated and lack of patient compliance is ruled out, nafarelin should be discontinued and the diagnosis of gonadotropin-independent sexual precocity should be reconsidered. Other possible causes of sexual precocity include adrenal hyperplasia, testoxicosis, and hypothalamic or testicular tumors)

Gonadotropin-releasing hormone stimulation test
(recommended prior to treatment initiation to establish prepubertal gonadotropin response)

Pregnancy test
(recommended if treatment is not started during menstruation and in patients with irregular menstrual cycles)

*For treatment of endometriosis*
Bone density determination
(recommended if a second course of nafarelin therapy is considered)

Pregnancy test
(recommended if treatment is not started during menstruation and in patients with irregular menstrual cycles)

## Side/Adverse Effects

Note: Some signs of puberty, including uterine bleeding and breast enlargement in girls, are expected and will occur in the first month with use of nafarelin for treatment of central precocious puberty (CPP) until the hypothalamic-pituitary axis becomes suppressed. Suppression usually occurs within 4 weeks.

Relevance of reported pituitary enlargement and asymmetry and pituitary adenoma during nafarelin treatment is not known. In children, regular examinations of the pituitary gland by magnetic resonance imaging (MRI) or computerized axial tomography (CAT) scanning during and after nafarelin treatment showed changes in pituitary shape and size. A pituitary adenoma was discovered in one male child.

The following side/adverse effects have been selected on the basis of their potential clinical significance (possible signs and symptoms in parentheses where appropriate)—not necessarily inclusive:

**Those indicating need for medical attention**
Incidence more frequent
*For female patients treated for endometriosis*
**Loss of bone mineral density**

Note: Hypoestrogenism-induced *loss of bone mineral density* may occur in adult females who are using nafarelin for treatment of endometriosis. This loss may not be completely reversible. The risk may be greatest with adult females who use nafarelin for longer than 6 months and for those adult females with additional osteoporotic risk factors, such as alcohol and/or tobacco abuse, family history of severe osteoporosis, and long-term use of medications that decrease bone mineral density, such as anticonvulsants or corticosteroids.

*For female patients treated for endometriosis or CPP*
**Breast enlargement**—incidence of 8% for patients with CPP; **changes in uterine bleeding patterns, including breakthrough bleeding** (vaginal bleeding between regular menstrual periods); **menorrhagia** (longer or heavier menstrual periods); **spotting** (light vaginal bleeding between regular menstrual periods)—may be transient in the treatment of CPP

Note: In the first 2 months after beginning nafarelin therapy, most adult females experience *changes in uterine bleeding patterns*. However, the continuing occurrence of irregular uterine bleeding may indicate noncompliance with the prescribed therapeutic regimen, the need for an increase in dose, or a pathologic process. *Menorrhagia* has been reported with low doses (≤ 200 mcg per day).

*For male or female patients treated for CPP*
**Body odor**—incidence of 4%; **growth of pubic hair**—incidence of 5%

Note: *Growth of pubic hair* may continue throughout treatment with nafarelin since it is caused by adrenal androgens.

Incidence less frequent or rare
*For female patients treated for endometriosis and for male or female patients treated for CPP*
**Anaphylaxis or hypersensitivity reaction, immediate** (shortness of breath; chest pain; hives)—incidences of 0.2% in the treatment of endometriosis and 2.4% in the treatment of CPP

*For female patients treated for endometriosis*
**Arthralgia** (joint pain); **asthenia** (unusual tiredness or weakness); **chloasma** (patchy brown or dark brown discoloration of skin); **eye pain; galactorrhea** (unexpected or excess milk flow from breasts); **ovarian cysts; ovarian enlargement; or ovarian hyperstimulation, mild** (pelvic bloating or tenderness); **palpitations** (fast or irregular heartbeat); **paresthesia** (numbness or tingling of hands or feet)

Note: *Ovarian cysts, enlargement, or hyperstimulation* have been reported in adult patients using low doses (≤ 200 mcg per day) or in the first 2 months of therapy. Ovarian cysts have occurred primarily in adult patients with polycystic ovary disease. Most ovarian cysts resolve spontaneously, within 4 to 6 weeks of initiating therapy, but some cases may require discontinuation of nafarelin and/or surgery.

**Those indicating need for medical attention only if they continue or are bothersome**
Incidence more frequent
*For female patients treated for endometriosis and for male or female patients treated for CPP*
**Acne; emotional lability** (mood swings); **seborrhea** (dandruff; oily skin)

*For female patients treated for endometriosis or CPP*
**Hot flashes**—common in adults, occurring transiently in the treatment of CPP

*For female patients treated for endometriosis*
**Amenorrhea** (stopping of menstrual periods); **edema** (rapid weight gain; swelling of feet or lower legs); **hirsutism** (increased hair growth, often abnormally distributed); **hypoestrogenism** (dyspareunia; reduced breast size; vaginal dryness; oily skin)—occurs in almost all patients; **increased or decreased libido** (increase or decrease in sexual desire); **myalgia** (muscle pain)

Incidence less frequent or rare
*For female patients treated for endometriosis and for male or female patients treated for CPP*
**Rhinitis** (irritated or runny nose)—incidence of 5 to 10%

*For female patients treated for CPP*
**Vaginal discharge** (white or brownish vaginal discharge)

*For female patients treated for endometriosis*
**Headache, mild and transient; maculopapular rash** (skin rash); **mastalgia** (breast pain); **mental depression, mild and transient**

## Patient Consultation

As an aid to patient consultation, refer to *Advice for the Patient, Nafarelin (Systemic)*.

In providing consultation, consider emphasizing the following selected information (» = major clinical significance):

**Before using this medication**
» Conditions affecting use, especially:
Allergy to nafarelin acetate or hypersensitivity to gonadotropin-releasing hormone or agonists or other ingredients in product formulation
Pregnancy—Pregnancy should be ruled out prior to use of nafarelin; nonhormonal contraceptive should be used during therapy if conception is likely or possible; stopping medication and alerting physician if pregnancy is suspected
Breast-feeding—Not recommended for use during breast-feeding
Use in children—It is not known if the potential side effect of ovarian cysts that can occur in adult women treated for endometriosis is relevant to children treated for central precocious puberty (CPP); long-term effect on fertility in boys and girls who used nafarelin for treatment of CPP is not known; reversal of nafarelin's suppressive effects and resumption of puberty in pediatric patients has been demonstrated
Other medications, especially topical nasal decongestants; waiting 30 minutes after use of nafarelin to apply nasal decongestant

Other medical conditions, especially significant risk factors for low bone mineral content (for adult females) and uterine bleeding (abnormal and undiagnosed)

**Proper use of this medication**
Carefully reading patient instruction sheet contained in the package
Proper administration technique
Avoiding sneezing during administration or immediately afterwards to receive the best absorption
Importance of not using more or less medication than amount prescribed
Importance of parents helping children adhere to a regular dosing schedule
» Proper dosing
Missed dose: Using as soon as remembered; not using if not remembered until next day; not doubling doses
» Proper storage

**Precautions while using this medication**
Importance of regular follow-up visits to monitor progress
*For children treated for central precocious puberty*
Importance of close monitoring by the physician, during and after nafarelin treatment for central precocious puberty
Telling physician if pubertal symptoms are not suppressed within 6 to 8 weeks, expecting that symptoms may continue or increase for the first few weeks after nafarelin therapy is initiated until medication begins to work
*For adult females treated for endometriosis*
Possibility of amenorrhea or irregular menstrual periods; checking with physician if regular menstruation does not occur within 60 to 90 days after discontinuation of medication
Advisability of using nonhormonal forms of contraception during therapy
Using a water-based vaginal lubricant if painful sexual intercourse or vaginal dryness is a problem
» Stopping medication and checking with physician if pregnancy is suspected

**Side/adverse effects**
Signs of potential side effects, especially:
*For female patients treated for endometriosis and for male or female patients treated for CPP*—Loss of bone mineral density or anaphylaxis or immediate hypersensitivity reaction
*For female patients treated for endometriosis or CPP*—Breast enlargement or changes in uterine bleeding pattern
*For male or female patients treated for CPP*—Body odor or growth of pubic hair
*For female patients treated for endometriosis*—Arthralgia; asthenia; chloasma; eye pain; galactorrhea; ovarian cysts, ovarian enlargement, or ovarian hyperstimulation (mild); palpitations; or paresthesia
Some signs of puberty, including uterine bleeding and breast enlargement in girls, are expected and will occur in the first month of treatment with nafarelin until the hypothalamic-pituitary axis becomes suppressed. Suppression usually occurs within 4 weeks

## General Dosing Information

After administration of a dose, the head should be slightly tilted backwards for 30 seconds to allow the medication to reach the back of the nose. Sneezing during or immediately after administering nafarelin may decrease drug absorption and should be avoided when possible.

**Diet/Nutrition**
Supplementation with calcium has not been shown to help to prevent the loss of bone mineral content associated with the use of GnRH analogs.

**For treatment of central precocious puberty**
If the patient responds and tolerates nafarelin therapy, treatment should continue until resumption of puberty is desired.
After priming, a nafarelin metered dose inhaler provides 56 sprays or a 7-day supply at a dose of 1600 mcg a day.

**For treatment of endometriosis**
Information on re-treatment with nafarelin after 6 months of use or use beyond 6 months is not available. If re-treatment with nafarelin is contemplated, bone density should be assessed with respect to the normal range before the second course is initiated.
After priming, a nafarelin metered dose inhaler provides 60 sprays or a 30-day supply at a dose of 400 mcg a day.

## Nasal Dosage Forms

Note: The dosing and strengths of the dosage forms available are expressed in terms of nafarelin base (not the acetate).

### NAFARELIN ACETATE NASAL SOLUTION

**Usual adult dose**
Endometriosis—
Intranasal, 200 mcg (base) into one nostril in the morning and 200 mcg into the other nostril in the evening (total daily dose of 400 mcg) for up to six months. Treatment should begin on Days 2 to 4 of the menstrual cycle.
In an occasional patient, a total daily dose of 400 mcg does not produce amenorrhea. If regular menstrual cycles persist after two months of therapy, the total daily dose may be increased to 800 mcg, administered by applying 200 mcg into each nostril in the morning and 200 mcg into each nostril in the evening.

**Usual pediatric dose**
Endometriosis—
Safety and efficacy have not been established for children up to 18 years of age.
Puberty, central precocious—
Intranasal, 2 sprays into each nostril (200 mcg [base] each spray) two times a day, morning and evening, giving a total daily dose of 1600 mcg (8 sprays). The dose can be increased to a total daily dose of 1800 mcg (9 sprays), achieved by giving 3 sprays (600 mcg) into alternating nostrils three times a day.

**Strength(s) usually available**
U.S.—
2 mg (base) per mL (200 mcg per metered spray) (Rx) [*Synarel* (benzalkonium chloride; glacial acetic acid; sodium hydroxide or hydrochloric acid; sorbitol; water [purified])].
Canada—
2 mg (base) per mL (200 mcg per metered spray) (Rx) [*Synarel* (benzalkonium chloride; glacial acetic acid; sodium hydroxide or hydrochloric acid; sorbitol; water [purified])].

**Packaging and storage**
Store bottle upright between 15 and 30 °C (59 and 86 °F), unless otherwise specified by manufacturer. Protect from light. Protect from freezing.

**Auxiliary labeling**
• For nasal use only.

**Note**
Dispense manufacturer's patient information.

### Selected Bibliography

Barbieri RL. Endometriosis 1990: current treatment approaches [review]. Drugs 1990; 39(4): 502-10.
Henzl MR, Corson SL, Moghissi K, et al. Administration of nasal nafarelin as compared with oral danazol for endometriosis: a multicenter double-blind comparative clinical trial. N Engl J Med 1988; 318(8): 485-9.
Letassy NA, Thompson DF, Britton ML, et al. Nafarelin acetate: a gonadotropin-releasing hormone agonist for the treatment of endometriosis [review]. DICP 1990; 24: 1204-9.

Revised: 05/27/98

---

**NAFCILLIN**—See *Penicillins (Systemic)*

---

**NAFTIFINE**—The *Naftifine (Topical)* monograph is not included in this published version of the USP DI database. Copies of the monograph are available on request from Micromedex, Inc. - Reprint Requests, 6200 S. Syracuse Way, Suite 300, Englewood, CO 80111; telephone (303) 486-6400; telefax (303) 486-6464; Email: USPDI@MDX.COM.

---

**NALBUPHINE**—See *Opioid (Narcotic) Analgesics (Systemic)*

---

**NALIDIXIC ACID**—The *Nalidixic Acid (Systemic)* monograph is not included in this published version of the USP DI database. Copies of the monograph are available on request from Micromedex, Inc. - Reprint Requests, 6200 S. Syracuse Way, Suite 300, Englewood, CO 80111; telephone (303) 486-6400; telefax (303) 486-6464; Email: USPDI@MDX.COM.

# NALMEFENE Systemic

VA CLASSIFICATION (Primary): AD800

Commonly used brand name(s): *Revex*.

Note: For a listing of dosage forms and brand names by country availability, see *Dosage Forms* section(s).

## Category
Opioid (narcotic) antagonist.

## Indications

**Accepted**

Opioid (narcotic) overdose (treatment)—Nalmefene is indicated in the management of known or suspected opioid overdose.

Opioid depression, postoperative (treatment)—Nalmefene is indicated for the complete or partial reversal of the effects induced by natural or synthetic opioids, including respiratory depression.

## Pharmacology/Pharmacokinetics

**Physicochemical characteristics**
Molecular weight—339.44.

**Mechanism of action/Effect**
Nalmefene antagonizes the effects of opioids by competing for the opioid receptors in the central nervous system (CNS). This results in reversal of the effects of the opioid, including reversal of respiratory depression, sedation, and hypotension. Reversal of the analgesic effects of opioids may also occur. Reversal of buprenorphine-induced respiratory depression may be incomplete because buprenorphine has high affinity for opioid receptors, and is displaced from these receptors slowly.

**Other actions/effects**
Nalmefene can precipitate withdrawal in patients who are physically dependent on opioid drugs.

**Absorption**
Variable in rate, but complete.

**Distribution**
At steady state, the volume of distribution is 8.6 L per kg of body weight (L/kg). Nalmefene is distributed centrally.

**Protein binding**
Moderate (45%).

**Biotransformation**
Hepatic, primarily by glucuronide conjugation, but also by dealkylation.

**Half-life**
Distribution—
  41 (range, 7 to 75) minutes.
Elimination—
  10.8 (range, 5.6 to 16) hours.

**Onset of action**
Intramuscular and subcutaneous—5 to 15 minutes.
Intravenous—2 to 5 minutes.

**Time to peak concentration**
Intramuscular—2.3 hours.
Subcutaneous—1.5 hours.

Note: A secondary plasma peak may occur hours after intravenous injection with nalmefene, perhaps due to enterohepatic recycling.

**Time to peak effect**
Dose- and route-dependent.

**Duration of action**
Dose- and route-dependent. The duration of action of nalmefene is longer than that of most opioid analgesics and anesthetics. However, partially reversing doses of nalmefene (1 mcg per kg of body weight) have a duration of only 30 to 60 minutes, the time required for nalmefene to redistribute. Fully reversing doses (1 mg per 70 kg of body weight) have a duration of action of many hours. The intramuscular and subcutaneous routes of administration provide an extended duration of action as compared to intravenous administration.

**Elimination**
Renal (83%) and fecal (17%).
  In dialysis—
    Removed by dialysis; plasma clearance is reduced 25% during dialysis as compared to clearance in patients with normal renal function.

## Precautions to Consider

**Carcinogenicity/Tumorigenicity**
Studies have not been done to determine the carcinogenic and tumorigenic potential of nalmefene.

**Mutagenicity**
No mutagenic or clastogenic effect was observed in the Ames test, the mouse micronucleus test, or in the mouse lymphoma assay. Weak clastogenic activity was observed in the human lymphocyte metaphase assay in the absence of exogenous metabolic activation.

**Pregnancy/Reproduction**
Fertility—Adequate and well-controlled studies in humans have not been done.

In a study in rats, ingestion of 1200 mg per square meter of body surface per day (mg/m$^2$/day) did not affect fertility. Rabbits given up to 2400 mg/m$^2$/day orally or 96 mg/m$^2$/day intravenously did not show impaired fertility.

Pregnancy—Adequate and well-controlled studies in humans have not been done.

No adverse effects were seen in the fetuses of rats and rabbits in studies in which nalmefene was administered orally or intravenously in doses up to 114 times the human dose.

FDA Pregnancy Category B.

**Breast-feeding**
It is not known if nalmefene is distributed into breast milk. Problems in humans have not been documented.

Nalmefene and its metabolites were distributed into the milk of lactating rats. The concentration of nalmefene in rat milk was about three times the concentration in the plasma 1 hour after a bolus injection, and about one-half the concentration in the plasma 24 hours after the injection.

**Pediatrics**
No information is available on the relationship of age to the effects of nalmefene in pediatric patients. Safety and efficacy have not been established.

**Geriatrics**
In a premarketing study comparing the pharmacokinetics of nalmefene in geriatric patients and younger adult patients, no differences were observed in half-life, plasma clearance, or steady-state volume of distribution. However, initial nalmefene serum concentrations were increased in geriatric patients as compared with younger adult patients. Dosing adjustments for age are not recommended in geriatric patients.

**Drug interactions and/or related problems**
The following drug interactions and/or related problems have been selected on the basis of their potential clinical significance (possible mechanism in parentheses where appropriate)—not necessarily inclusive (» = major clinical significance):

Note: Combinations containing any of the following medications, depending on the amount present, may also interact with this medication.

Opioid agonist analgesics, including alfentanil, fentanyl, and sufentanil (nalmefene reverses the analgesic and side effects of opioid agonist analgesics and may precipitate withdrawal symptoms in physically dependent patients being treated for opioid dependence with methadone)

**Laboratory value alterations**
The following have been selected on the basis of their potential clinical significance (possible effect in parentheses where appropriate)—not necessarily inclusive (» = major clinical significance):

With physiology/laboratory test values
  Aspartate aminotransferase (AST [SGOT])
    (increases in serum values have been reported)
  Creatine kinase (CK)
    (serum values may be transiently increased; the increases in CK may be related to surgery and not to the administration of nalmefene)

**Medical considerations/Contraindications**
The medical considerations/contraindications included have been selected on the basis of their potential clinical significance (reasons given in parentheses where appropriate)—not necessarily inclusive (» = major clinical significance).

*Except under special circumstances, this medication should not be used when the following medical problem exists:*

» Hypersensitivity to nalmefene, history of

*Risk-benefit should be considered when the following medical problems exist:*

Cardiac disease
(cardiovascular instability, hypotension, hypertension, pulmonary edema, ventricular fibrillation, and ventricular tachycardia have been reported rarely in connection with opioid reversal in both emergency and postoperative settings, perhaps as a result of abrupt reversal of opioid effects)

Opioid dependence or addiction, current
(nalmefene may precipitate withdrawal)

Renal function impairment
(dizziness and hypertension may occur following rapid administration of nalmefene in patients with renal function impairment; slow administration of nalmefene is recommended)
(duration of action of nalmefene may be prolonged)

**Patient monitoring**
The following may be especially important in patient monitoring (other tests may be warranted in some patients, depending on condition; » = major clinical significance):

Patient alertness
(although nalmefene has a longer duration of action than other opioid antagonists, resedation is possible, especially when nalmefene is used to reverse the effects of long-acting opioid agonists such as methadone or levomethadyl)

» Vital signs
(monitoring of blood pressure, heart rate, and respiratory rate is recommended; patients treated with nalmefene should be monitored until there is no reasonable risk of recurrent respiratory depression; the length of this period of observation depends on the duration of action of the opioid administered)

## Side/Adverse Effects

Note: Nalmefene caused no serious adverse effects when administered in large intravenous doses to healthy volunteers who had not received an opioid agonist. Many of the side/adverse effects (e.g., agitation, hypertension, nausea, postoperative pain, tachycardia, vomiting) may be caused by the abrupt reversal of the effects of the opioid.

Withdrawal symptoms may be precipitated in patients without previous opioid dependence or addiction when nalmefene is used following surgery for which high doses of opioids were administered.

The following side/adverse effects have been selected on the basis of their potential clinical significance (possible signs and symptoms in parentheses where appropriate)—not necessarily inclusive:

**Those indicating need for medical attention**
Incidence more frequent
*Hypertension; tachycardia* (fast heartbeat)
Incidence less frequent
*Fever; hypotension; vasodilatation*
Incidence rare
*Agitation; arrhythmia* (irregular heartbeat); *bradycardia* (slow heartbeat); *confusion; hallucinations* (seeing, hearing, or feeling things that are not there); *myoclonus* (rhythmic movement of muscles); *pharyngitis* (sore throat); *pruritus* (itching); *urinary retention* (difficult urination)

**Those indicating need for medical attention only if they continue or are bothersome**
Incidence more frequent
*Dizziness; nausea; pain, postoperative; vomiting*
Incidence less frequent
*Chills; headache*

## Overdose

Healthy volunteers injected with 24 mg of nalmefene did not experience overdose effects. Treatment of patients dependent on opioids with nalmefene can cause adverse effects, but the adverse effects are caused by reversal of opioid effects. This is most likely to occur if fully blocking doses are administered. Treatment of withdrawal reactions should be symptomatic and supportive. Use of opioids to overcome full blockade is not recommended because this has resulted in adverse respiratory and cardiovascular effects.

For more information on the management of overdose, **contact a Poison Control Center** (see *Poison Control Center Listing*).

## General Dosing Information

Treatment with nalmefene for ventilatory failure should not precede usual emergency measures such as securing a patent airway, administering oxygen, assisting ventilation, and establishing circulatory access.

Nalmefene is available in two concentrations, in ampuls with color-coded labels: the 100-mcg-per-mL (mcg/mL) concentration has a blue label, and the 1-mg-per-mL (mg/mL) concentration has a green label. The 100-mcg/mL concentration is suitable for routine postoperative use, and the 1-mg/mL concentration is suitable for the management of overdose.

Lack of clinical response in sedation and/or respiratory depression after administration of nalmefene in sufficient dosage usually indicates that the conditions are not caused by an opioid. It is recommended that nalmefene be administered to reverse sedation and hypoventilation only when it is likely that opioid administration is responsible. However, in preclinical animal testing, nalmefene did not completely reverse the analgesic effects of buprenorphine, even when very high doses of nalmefene were administered. Nalmefene may not be effective in reversing buprenorphine-induced sedation and respiratory depression.

Nalmefene may cause withdrawal symptoms in patients tolerant to or dependent on opioids. If nalmefene is used when there is concern about opioid dependency, a test dose of 0.1 mg per 70 kg of body weight should be administered. If there is no evidence of withdrawal after 2 minutes, the full dose may be administered. Following each injection of nalmefene, patients should be observed closely for withdrawal symptoms. Subsequent doses should be administered after 2 to 5 minutes to allow the full effect of each incremental dose to be reached.

When nalmefene is used to reverse the effects of opioid agonists used as anesthesia adjuncts, the dosage of nalmefene must be carefully titrated in order to achieve the desired effect without interfering with control of postoperative pain or causing other adverse effects.

The duration of action of nalmefene exceeds the duration of action of most opioids. However, if recurrence of sedation and/or respiratory depression occurs, nalmefene should be administered and titrated to clinical effect.

The long duration of action of nalmefene could cause patients to be without opiate analgesia for an extended period of time if fully reversing doses of nalmefene are administered after surgical procedures. Additionally, patients may experience increased sensitivity to pain after receiving nalmefene, possibly due to blocking of endogenous neuropeptides.

In premarketing clinical trials, intravenous nalmefene was effective in reversing respiratory depression in patients given intrathecal morphine. Administration of nalmefene at the recommended doses did not prevent analgesia with subsequently administered opioids.

## Parenteral Dosage Forms

Note: The dosing and strengths of the dosage form available are expressed in terms of nalmefene base (not the hydrochloride salt).

### NALMEFENE HYDROCHLORIDE INJECTION

**Usual adult dose**
Management of opioid overdose—
Intravenous, 0.5 mg (base) per 70 kg of body weight initially. If needed, a second dose of 1 mg per 70 kg of body weight can be administered two to five minutes later. Nalmefene may be administered by intramuscular or subcutaneous injection if intravenous access is lost or cannot be obtained. Intramuscular or subcutaneous injections should be effective within five to fifteen minutes.

Reversal of postoperative opioid depression—
Intravenous, 0.25 mcg (base) per kg of body weight at two- to five-minute intervals, stopping when the desired degree of reversal is achieved.

Note: Nalmefene should be carefully titrated. The recommended doses of nalmefene balance the need for rapid onset of action and reasonable duration of action against achieving a controlled reversal. Using higher doses or shorter intervals between incremental doses increases the likelihood of reversing analgesia and causing the patient to experience symptoms related to acute withdrawal, such as nausea, vomiting, increased blood pressure, and agitation. Once adequate reversal has been established, additional administration is not recommended.

For patients with increased risk of cardiovascular complications, it is recommended that the dose of nalmefene be diluted in an equal amount of normal saline or sterile water, and administered in increments of 0.1 mcg per kg of body weight.

**Usual adult prescribing limits**
Management of opioid overdose—
1.5 mg per 70 kg of body weight.

## Nalmefene (Systemic)

Reversal of postoperative opioid depression—
  1 mcg per kg of body weight.

**Usual pediatric dose**
Safety and efficacy have not been established.

**Usual geriatric dose**
See *Usual adult dose*.

**Strength(s) usually available**
U.S.—
  100 mcg (base) per mL (Rx) [*Revex*].
  1 mg (base) per mL (Rx) [*Revex*].
Canada—
  100 mcg (base) per mL (Rx) [*Revex*].
  1 mg (base) per mL (Rx) [*Revex*].

**Packaging and storage**
Store between 15 and 30 °C (59 and 86 °F).

### Selected Bibliography
Kaplan J, Marx J. Effectiveness and safety of intravenous nalmefene for emergency department patients with suspected narcotic overdose: a pilot study. Ann Emerg Med 1993; 22: 187-90.
Glass P, Jhaveri R, Smith L, et al. Comparison of potency and duration of action of nalmefene and naloxone. Anesth Analg 1994; 78: 536-41.

Developed: 01/14/97
Interim revision: 08/12/97

# NALOXONE   Systemic

VA CLASSIFICATION (Primary): AD800
Commonly used brand name(s): *Narcan*.
Note: For a listing of dosage forms and brand names by country availability, see *Dosage Forms* section(s).

## Category
Opioid (narcotic) antagonist.

## Indications
Note: Bracketed information in the *Indications* section refers to uses that are not included in U.S. product labeling.

**Accepted**
Toxicity, opioid (narcotic) (diagnosis and treatment) or
Respiratory depression, opioid (narcotic)-induced (treatment)—Naloxone is considered the drug of choice to reverse respiratory depression caused by opioid drugs, including those with mixed agonist/antagonist activity such as buprenorphine (although the effects of buprenorphine are especially resistant to reversal by naloxone), butorphanol, nalbuphine, and pentazocine, and other effects due to known or suspected opioid overdose, including sedation, coma, excitation, or convulsions. Naloxone will not increase respiratory depression caused by nonopioid medications or disease processes and may therefore be used when the cause is unknown. A satisfactory response to naloxone confirms the diagnosis of opioid toxicity.
  When naloxone is given to reverse postoperative opioid depression, the dose must be carefully titrated to avoid interfering with control of postoperative pain or causing other adverse effects.
  Naloxone is also indicated in neonates to reverse respiratory depression caused by opioids given to the mothers during labor and delivery.

Shock, septic (treatment adjunct)[1]—Naloxone is indicated as an adjunctive agent to treat hypotension in the management of septic shock.

[Opioid dependence (diagnosis)][1]—Naloxone is used to diagnose opioid dependence or suspected illicit opioid use because it precipitates withdrawal symptoms in patients who are physically dependent on opioids (except for buprenorphine). Use of laboratory methods to detect an opioid drug in the urine of the suspected addict may be preferable. However, a naloxone challenge test is recommended to detect possible opioid use or dependence prior to initiation of naltrexone therapy in opioid addicts who have completed a detoxification regimen.

[1]Not included in Canadian product labeling.

## Pharmacology/Pharmacokinetics

**Physicochemical characteristics**
Molecular weight—Naloxone hydrochloride: 363.84.

**Mechanism of action/Effect**
The precise mechanism by which naloxone reverses most of the effects of opioid analgesics has not been fully determined. It has been proposed that there are multiple subtypes of opioid receptors within the central nervous system (CNS), each mediating different therapeutic and/or side effects of opioid drugs. At least two of these types of receptors (mu and kappa) mediate analgesia as well as side effects. A third type of receptor (sigma) may not mediate analgesia; actions at this receptor may produce the subjective and psychotomimetic effects characteristic of opioids with mixed agonist/antagonist activity (i.e., butorphanol, nalbuphine, and pentazocine). Naloxone apparently displaces previously administered opioid analgesics from all of these types of receptors and competitively inhibits their actions. Antagonism of opioid actions may precipitate withdrawal symptoms in patients who are physically dependent on opioid drugs (except for buprenorphine). Naloxone has no opioid agonist activity of its own.

**Biotransformation**
Hepatic.

**Half-life**
64 (range, 30 to 81) minutes.

**Onset of action**
Intravenous: 1 or 2 minutes.
Intramuscular: 2 to 5 minutes.

**Time to peak effect**
5 to 15 minutes.

**Duration of action**
Dose- and route-dependent. In one study, effects persisted for 45 minutes following a 400-mcg (0.4-mg) intravenous dose. Intramuscular administration results in a prolonged duration of action.

**Elimination**
Renal; about 70% of a dose is excreted within 72 hours.

## Precautions to Consider

**Pregnancy/Reproduction**
Fertility—Reproduction studies in mice and rats receiving up to 1000 times the human dose have not shown that naloxone impairs fertility.
Pregnancy—Naloxone crosses the placenta. Adequate and well-controlled studies in humans have not been done.
  Studies in rats and mice receiving up to 1000 times the human dose have not shown teratogenic or other harmful effects in the fetus.
  Risk-benefit must be considered before naloxone is administered to a pregnant woman who is known or suspected to be opioid-dependent because maternal dependence leads to fetal dependence. Naloxone crosses the placenta and may precipitate withdrawal in the fetus as well as in the mother.
FDA Pregnancy Category B.
Labor and delivery—It is generally not advisable to give naloxone to a pregnant woman just prior to delivery. Endogenous endorphins may help the fetus withstand the stress of delivery. Blocking these endogenous endorphins usually is not desirable.

**Breast-feeding**
It is not known if naloxone is distributed into breast milk. Problems in humans have not been documented.

**Pediatrics**
Studies have not demonstrated pediatrics-specific problems that would limit the usefulness of naloxone in children.
Naloxone should be administered cautiously to neonates of mothers who are physically dependent on opioids.

**Geriatrics**
Appropriate studies with naloxone have not been performed in the geriatric population. However, geriatrics-specific problems that would limit the usefulness of this medication in the elderly are not expected.

**Drug interactions and/or related problems**
The following drug interactions and/or related problems have been selected on the basis of their potential clinical significance (possible mechanism in parentheses where appropriate)—not necessarily inclusive (» = major clinical significance):

Note: Combinations containing any of the following medications, depending on the amount present, may also interact with this medication.

Butorphanol or
Nalbuphine or
Pentazocine
(naloxone reverses the analgesic and side effects of these opioid agonist/antagonist analgesics and may precipitate withdrawal symptoms in physically dependent patients)

Opioid agonist analgesics, including alfentanil, fentanyl, remifentanil, and sufentanil
(naloxone reverses the analgesic and side effects of opioid agonist analgesics and may precipitate withdrawal symptoms in physically dependent patients, including patients being treated for opioid dependence with methadone)

(when naloxone is used to reverse the effects of opioid agonists used as anesthesia adjuncts, the dose of naloxone must be carefully titrated to achieve the desired effect without interfering with control of postoperative pain or causing other adverse effects)

### Medical considerations/Contraindications
The medical considerations/contraindications included have been selected on the basis of their potential clinical significance (reasons given in parentheses where appropriate)—not necessarily inclusive (» = major clinical significance).

*Risk-benefit should be considered when the following medical problems exist:*
Allergic reaction to naloxone, history of

Cardiovascular disease or
Pulmonary disease
(sudden exacerbation of underlying cardiovascular or pulmonary disease may occur)

Opioid dependence or addiction, current
(naloxone may precipitate withdrawal)

## Side/Adverse Effects

The following side/adverse effects have been selected on the basis of their potential clinical significance (possible signs and symptoms in parentheses where appropriate)—not necessarily inclusive:

**Those indicating need for medical attention**
*Convulsions; fast or irregular heartbeat; increased or decreased blood pressure; pulmonary edema; ventricular arrhythmia; violent behavior*

**Those indicating need for medical attention only if they continue or are bothersome**
*Increased sweating; nausea or vomiting; nervousness, restlessness, excitement, or irritability; trembling*

**Those indicating possible precipitation of withdrawal in a patient physically dependent on opioids**
In all patients except neonates
*Body aches; diarrhea; fever, runny nose, or sneezing; gooseflesh; increased sweating; increased yawning; nausea or vomiting; nervousness, restlessness, or irritability; shivering or trembling; stomach cramps; tachycardia; weakness*

Note: A degree of physical dependence may occur during prolonged administration of an opioid analgesic as an adjunct to anesthesia. It has been proposed that adverse effects occurring after administration of naloxone for reversal of opioid effects following lengthy surgical procedures may be manifestations of an induced withdrawal syndrome in acutely dependent individuals. Alternatively, adverse effects occurring after administration of naloxone may be due to the abrupt reversal of analgesia in patients with significant acute postoperative pain.

In neonates
*Convulsions; diarrhea; excessive crying; fever; hyperactive reflexes; sneezing; tremors; unusual irritability; vomiting; yawning*

## General Dosing Information

When naloxone is used to antagonize the effects of buprenorphine, butorphanol, nalbuphine, or pentazocine, larger doses may be needed than are required to antagonize the effects of most opioids having only agonist activity. Propoxyphene overdose may also require larger doses of naloxone.

Use of naloxone should be supplemented by other resuscitative procedures, such as administration of oxygen and/or vasopressors, artificial respiration, mechanical ventilation, and/or cardiac massage.

When naloxone is used to treat opioid toxicity, continued monitoring of the patient is necessary after naloxone is administered. If the duration of action of the opioid exceeds that of naloxone, re-emergence of opioid toxicity following initial reversal is likely.

Lack of significant improvement of CNS depression and/or respiratory depression following administration of an adequate dose (10 mg) of naloxone usually indicates that the condition is either due to a nonopioid CNS depressant not affected by the antagonist or to disease processes. However, the effects of buprenorphine (a partial mu-receptor opioid agonist with high affinity for the mu receptor) are especially resistant to reversal by naloxone; doses of naloxone as high as 16 mg have been ineffective.

When naloxone is administered to a patient known or suspected to be physically dependent on an opioid analgesic, the dose should be carefully titrated. Withdrawal symptoms may occur within a few minutes and may last up to 2 hours. The duration and severity of the withdrawal syndrome depend upon the dose of the antagonist, the specific opioid involved, and the degree to which dependence has developed. However, naloxone does not precipitate withdrawal symptoms in buprenorphine-dependent individuals.

The naloxone challenge test (recommended prior to initiation of naltrexone therapy in detoxified opioid addicts) should *not* be administered if withdrawal symptoms are present or the patient's urine contains opioids. Naloxone may be administered intravenously or subcutaneously. If the intravenous route is used, one fourth of the total dose should be administered and the patient observed for 30 seconds for withdrawal symptoms; if none occurs, the remainder of the dose should be administered and the patient observed for 20 minutes. If the subcutaneous route is used, the full dose should be administered and the patient observed for 45 minutes for withdrawal symptoms. If withdrawal symptoms occur, the naloxone challenge should be repeated at 24-hour intervals until absence of opioid dependence is confirmed.

## Parenteral Dosage Forms

Note: Bracketed uses in the *Dosage Forms* section refer to categories of use and/or indications that are not included in U.S. product labeling.

### NALOXONE HYDROCHLORIDE INJECTION USP

**Usual adult and adolescent dose**
Toxicity, opioid (narcotic)—
[Endotracheal][1], intravenous (preferred in emergencies), intramuscular, or subcutaneous, 400 mcg (0.4 mg) to 2 mg as a single dose. The intravenous dose may be repeated at two- to three-minute intervals as needed.

Note: If the patient is suspected of being physically dependent on an opioid medication and is not in immediate danger, the dose may be reduced to 100 to 200 mcg (0.1 to 0.2 mg). This dose may be repeated at two- to three-minute intervals as needed.

Additional single doses of naloxone may be administered intravenously as needed. However, longer-lasting effects may be obtained if supplemental doses are administered via the intramuscular route. Also, initial treatment may be followed by continuous intravenous infusion of naloxone, with adjustment of the infusion rate according to the response of the patient.

Respiratory depression, opioid (narcotic)-induced—
Intravenous, 100 to 200 mcg (0.1 to 0.2 mg) every two to three minutes until adequate ventilation and alertness without significant pain are obtained. If necessary, the dose may be repeated at one- or two-hour intervals.

Note: The dose should be titrated to avoid interference with control of postoperative pain; initial doses as low as 0.5 mcg (0.0005 mg) per kg of body weight have been recommended.

Shock, septic[1]—
Intravenous, 30 mcg (0.03 mg) to 200 mcg (0.2 mg) per kg of body weight initially, followed by an intravenous infusion of 0.03 to 0.3 mg per kg of body weight per hour for one to twenty-four hours.

Note: The optimal dose of naloxone in the treatment of hypotension due to septic shock has not been established. Some patients unresponsive to fluids and pressor agents experience an immediate, transient increase in blood pressure after receiving naloxone. The effectiveness of naloxone appears to be greater if it is administered early in the course of septic shock. The use of naloxone as an adjunctive treatment for hypotension in septic shock has not been shown to reduce mortality.

[Opioid dependence diagnosis][1]—
Intravenous, 200 mcg (0.2 mg) initially, followed by 600 mcg (0.6 mg) thirty seconds later if withdrawal symptoms are not apparent; or
Subcutaneous, 800 mcg (0.8 mg).
If necessary to confirm that the patient is not opioid-dependent, a rechallenge with 1.6 mg of naloxone intravenously may be performed.

## Naloxone (Systemic)

**Usual pediatric dose**

Toxicity, opioid (narcotic)—
[Endotracheal][1], intravenous (preferred in emergencies), intramuscular, or subcutaneous, 10 mcg (0.01 mg) per kg of body weight. If this dose does not result in improvement in the condition of the patient, an additional 100 mcg (0.1 mg) per kg of body weight may be given.

Note: Doses higher than those listed above have been used to treat opioid toxicity. The American Academy of Pediatrics (AAP) recommends an initial dose of 0.1 mg per kg of body weight for infants and children up to 5 years of age and weighing less than twenty kg. For children 5 years of age and older or weighing more than twenty kg, an initial dose of 2 mg is recommended by AAP.

Respiratory depression, opioid (narcotic)-induced—
Intravenous, 5 to 10 mcg (0.005 to 0.01 mg) every two to three minutes until adequate ventilation and alertness without significant pain are obtained. If necessary, the dose may be repeated at one- or two-hour intervals.

Respiratory depression, opioid (narcotic)-induced, neonatal—
Intravenous via the umbilical vein (preferred), intramuscular, or subcutaneous, 10 mcg (0.01 mg) per kg of body weight. The intravenous dose may be repeated at two- to three-minute intervals until the desired response is obtained.

**Strength(s) usually available**

U.S.—
With preservatives (methylparaben and propylparaben)
400 mcg (0.4 mg) per mL (Rx) [*Narcan;* GENERIC].
1 mg per mL (Rx) [*Narcan;* GENERIC].
Without preservatives
20 mcg (0.02 mg) per mL (Rx) [*Narcan;* GENERIC].
400 mcg (0.4 mg) per mL (Rx) [*Narcan;* GENERIC].
1 mg per mL (Rx) [*Narcan;* GENERIC].

Canada—
With preservatives (methylparaben and propylparaben)
20 mcg (0.02 mg) per mL (Rx) [*Narcan*].
400 mcg (0.4 mg) per mL (Rx) [*Narcan*].
1 mg per mL (Rx) [*Narcan*].

**Packaging and storage**

Store below 40 °C (104 °F), preferably between 15 and 30 °C (59 and 86 °F), unless otherwise specified by the manufacturer. Protect from light. Protect from freezing.

**Preparation of dosage form**

When given by intravenous injection, naloxone may be diluted with sterile water for injection if a larger volume is needed.

For continuous intravenous infusion—Add 2 mg (5 mL of solution containing 400 mcg [0.4 mg] per mL or 2 mL of solution containing 1 mg per mL) of naloxone hydrochloride to 500 mL of 0.9% sodium chloride injection or 5% dextrose injection to prepare a solution containing 4 mcg (0.004 mg) per mL.

**Stability**

After dilution for intravenous infusion, the solution should be used within 24 hours. Any unused solution should be discarded after 24 hours.

Naloxone should not be mixed with any preparation containing bisulfite, metabisulfite, or long-chain or high molecular weight anions, or with any solution having an alkaline pH.

---

[1]Not included in Canadian product labeling.

Revised: 08/12/97

# NALTREXONE Systemic

VA CLASSIFICATION (Primary/Secondary): AD800/AD100

Commonly used brand name(s): *ReVia*.

Note: For a listing of dosage forms and brand names by country availability, see *Dosage Forms* section(s).

## Category

Opioid (narcotic) antagonist; opioid (narcotic) abuse therapy adjunct; alcohol abuse therapy adjunct.

## Indications

**Accepted**

Opioid (narcotic) drug use, illicit (treatment adjunct)—Naltrexone is indicated as an adjunct to other measures, including psychological and social counseling, in the treatment of detoxified, formerly opioid-dependent individuals. Naltrexone assists in maintaining an opioid-free state in these individuals; however, an unequivocally beneficial effect on recidivism rates has not been demonstrated.

Alcoholism (treatment)—Naltrexone is indicated as an adjunct to other measures, including psychological and social counseling, in the treatment of alcohol dependence.

**Unaccepted**

Naltrexone is *not* effective in treating dependency on cocaine or other non-opioid drugs.

## Pharmacology/Pharmacokinetics

**Physicochemical characteristics**

Molecular weight—Naltrexone: 341.41.

**Mechanism of action/Effect**

Naltrexone binds to opioid receptors in the central nervous system (CNS) and competitively inhibits the actions of opioid drugs (both pure agonists and agonist/antagonists) and endogenous opioids. Naltrexone markedly attenuates or completely blocks opioid-induced euphoria and physical dependence; with continued use it may therefore reduce the patient's craving for opioid drugs. Naltrexone may be more effective in blocking the subjective effects (such as euphoria) than the objective effects (such as respiratory depression or miosis) of opioids.

The mechanism of action whereby naltrexone reduces alcohol craving and consumption is not completely understood. Naltrexone may attenuate alcohol-induced euphoria, thereby reducing the patient's craving for alcohol.

**Other actions/effects**

Naltrexone precipitates withdrawal symptoms in individuals who are physically dependent on opioid drugs. It also blocks the therapeutic (e.g., analgesic, antidiarrheal, and antitussive) actions of opioids. Although naltrexone has few if any actions other than opioid blockade, it produces some pupillary constriction via an unknown mechanism.

**Absorption**

Rapid and almost complete.

**Protein binding**

Low (21%).

**Biotransformation**

Hepatic; approximately 98% of a dose is metabolized. Naltrexone is subject to extensive first-pass hepatic metabolism. The major metabolite, 6-beta-naltrexol, has opioid antagonist activity and may contribute to the therapeutic effect.

**Half-life**

Elimination—
Naltrexone: Approximately 4 hours; independent of dose.
6-Beta-naltrexol: Approximately 13 hours; independent of dose.

**Time to peak concentration**

For both naltrexone and 6-beta-naltrexol—1 hour; independent of dose.

**Peak serum concentration**

Following a single 50-mg dose—
Naltrexone: 8.6 nanograms per mL.
6-Beta-naltrexol: 99.3 nanograms per mL.

Note: Naltrexone and 6-beta-naltrexol do not accumulate with long-term administration of 100 mg of naltrexone a day.

**Duration of action**

Dose-dependent; as determined by blockade of the effects of 25 mg of intravenously administered heroin—
50-mg dose: 24 hours.
100-mg dose: 48 hours.
150-mg dose: 72 hours.

**Elimination**

Primarily renal; 60% of a dose is excreted in the urine within 48 hours. Less than 2% of a dose is excreted in the urine as unchanged naltrexone; about 43% of a dose is excreted as unchanged or conjugated 6-beta-naltrexol.

## Precautions to Consider

**Carcinogenicity/Tumorigenicity**

Studies in rats have shown that naltrexone caused small increases in the numbers of mesotheliomas in males and tumors of vascular origin in both sexes. However, only the incidence of vascular tumors in females (4%) exceeded the maximum (2%) reported in historical control groups.

**Mutagenicity**
Naltrexone produced weakly positive findings in the *Drosophila* recessive lethal assay and in nonspecific DNA repair tests with *E. coli*. However, no positive findings were reported in 20 other tests using bacterial, mammalian, and tissue culture systems. The significance of these findings is not known.

**Pregnancy/Reproduction**
Fertility—Studies in rats given doses of 100 mg per kg (approximately 100 times the human therapeutic dose) have shown that naltrexone causes a significant increase in pseudopregnancy and a decrease in the pregnancy rate of mated females. The relevance of these findings to humans is not known.

Pregnancy—Adequate and well-controlled studies in humans have not been done.

Naltrexone has been shown to have embryocidal and fetotoxic effects in rats (doses of 30 times the human dose equivalent prior to and throughout gestation) and rabbits (doses of 60 times the human dose equivalent during the period of organogenesis).

FDA Pregnancy Category C.

**Breast-feeding**
It is not known whether naltrexone is distributed into breast milk. However, problems in humans have not been documented.

**Pediatrics**
Appropriate studies on the relationship of age to the effects of naltrexone have not been performed in the pediatric population. However, no pediatrics-specific problems have been documented.

**Geriatrics**
Appropriate studies on the relationship of age to the effects of naltrexone have not been performed in the geriatric population. However, no geriatrics-specific problems have been documented.

**Drug interactions and/or related problems**
The following drug interactions and/or related problems have been selected on the basis of their potential clinical significance (possible mechanism in parentheses where appropriate)—not necessarily inclusive (» = major clinical significance):

Note: Combinations containing any of the following medications also interact with this medication.

Hepatotoxic medications(see *Appendix II*)
(additive hepatotoxicity may occur)

» Opioid (narcotic) medications
(administration of naltrexone to a patient physically dependent on opioid drugs will precipitate withdrawal symptoms; symptoms may appear within 5 minutes of naltrexone administration, persist for up to 48 hours, and be difficult to reverse; opioid-dependent patients should be detoxified before treatment with naltrexone; a naloxone challenge test usually is administered before naltrexone therapy is started to verify abstinence [see *General Dosing Information*])

(naltrexone blocks the therapeutic effects of opioids [i.e., analgesic, antidiarrheal, and antitussive]; naltrexone therapy should not be initiated in patients receiving these agents for therapeutic purposes; also, patients receiving naltrexone should be advised to use alternative medications when necessary)

(administration of increased doses of opioids to override naltrexone-induced blockade of opioid receptors may result in increased and more prolonged respiratory depression and/or circulatory collapse)

(naltrexone should be discontinued several days prior to elective surgery if administration of an opioid medication prior to, during, or following surgery is unavoidable)

(the efficacy of naltrexone in antagonizing opioid effects not mediated via opioid receptors [i.e., those which may be caused by histamine release, such as facial swelling, itching, generalized erythema, hives, and, to some extent, hypotension] has not been fully determined; naltrexone may not antagonize these effects completely)

Thioridazine
(lethargy and somnolence have been reported rarely when patients taking thioridazine have begun naltrexone therapy)

**Laboratory value alterations**
The following have been selected on the basis of their potential clinical significance (possible effect in parentheses where appropriate)—not necessarily inclusive (» = major clinical significance):

With physiology/laboratory test values
Serum transaminase (ALT [SGPT]; AST [SGOT]) activity
(excessive doses of naltrexone may cause hepatocellular damage in a dose-dependent manner; elevation of serum transaminase activity may occur; although mild abnormalities occur frequently in patients with alcohol or drug addiction, and are not necessarily related to naltrexone-induced hepatotoxicity, significant abnormalities indicative of the medication's hepatotoxic potential have occurred in subjects receiving about five times the recommended daily dose; in one placebo-controlled study, 5 of 26 subjects developed elevations of serum transaminases 3 to 19 times the baseline value; the abnormalities were reversible upon discontinuation of naltrexone, and symptomatic hepatotoxicity with clinical use has not been reported)

**Medical considerations/Contraindications**
The medical considerations/contraindications included have been selected on the basis of their potential clinical significance (reasons given in parentheses where appropriate)—not necessarily inclusive (» = major clinical significance).

*Except under special circumstances, this medication should not be used when the following medical problems exist:*

» Allergic reaction to naltrexone, history of
» Dependence on opioid drugs, current, as demonstrated by presence of withdrawal symptoms, detection of opioid drugs in urine, or failure to pass naloxone challenge test
(naltrexone will precipitate or exacerbate withdrawal symptoms)
» Hepatic failure or
» Hepatitis, acute
(increased risk of hepatotoxicity)

*Risk-benefit should be considered when the following medical problems exist:*

» Hepatic disease, current or recent history of, excluding mild liver function abnormalities known to be associated with opioid or alcohol dependence
(increased risk of hepatotoxicity; naltrexone may cause hepatocellular damage in a dose-dependent manner)

**Patient monitoring**
The following may be especially important in patient monitoring (other tests may be warranted in some patients, depending on condition; » = major clinical significance):

» Hepatic function tests
(recommended prior to initiation of therapy to detect hepatic injury and/or to determine baseline values, then periodically thereafter; naltrexone should be discontinued if significant abnormalities occur)

## Side/Adverse Effects

The following side/adverse effects have been selected on the basis of their potential clinical significance (possible signs and symptoms in parentheses where appropriate)—not necessarily inclusive:

**Those indicating need for medical attention**
Incidence less frequent
*Skin rash*

Incidence rare
*Blurred vision or aching, burning, or swollen eyes; chest pain; confusion; discomfort while urinating and/or frequent urination; edema* (swelling of face, fingers, feet, or lower legs; weight gain); *fever; gastrointestinal ulceration* (abdominal or stomach pain, severe); *hallucinations; increased blood pressure; itching; mental depression or other mood or mental changes; ringing or buzzing in ears; shortness of breath*

**Those indicating need for medical attention only if they continue or are bothersome**
Incidence more frequent
*Abdominal cramping or pain, mild to moderate; anxiety, nervousness, restlessness, and/or trouble in sleeping; headache; joint or muscle pain; nausea or vomiting; unusual tiredness*

Incidence less frequent or rare
*Chills; constipation; cough; diarrhea; dizziness; fast or pounding heartbeat; hoarseness; increased thirst; irritability; loss of appetite; runny or stuffy nose; sexual problems in males; sinus problems; sneezing; sore throat*

Note: In some individuals, *loss of appetite* has led to substantial weight loss requiring discontinuation of therapy.

Some of the above-listed side/adverse effects are identical to symptoms of *opioid withdrawal* (see list below). Several of them, such as *abdominal pain, anxiety, joint or muscle pain, nausea or vomiting,* and *unusual tiredness,* may lessen or disappear during continued use. It has been suggested that such effects may be mild withdrawal symptoms in some patients.

**Those indicating possible withdrawal in patients physically dependent on opioid drugs**

Note: These side effects may occur within 5 minutes after administration of naltrexone and may persist for up to 48 hours.

*Abdominal or stomach cramps; anxiety, nervousness, restlessness, or irritability; diarrhea; fast heartbeat; fever, continuing runny nose, or sneezing; gooseflesh; increased sweating; increased yawning; joint or muscle pain; loss of appetite; nausea or vomiting; shivering or trembling; trouble in sleeping; weakness*

## Overdose

For more information on the management of overdose or unintentional ingestion, **contact a Poison Control Center** (see *Poison Control Center Listing*).

**Treatment of overdose**

Clinical experience with overdose is lacking. It is recommended that the patient be closely monitored and the observed symptoms treated as required.

## Patient Consultation

As an aid to patient consultation, refer to *Advice for the Patient, Naltrexone (Systemic)*.

In providing consultation, consider emphasizing the following selected information (» = major clinical significance):

### Before using this medication
» Conditions affecting use, especially:
   Allergic reaction to naltrexone, history of
   Other medications, especially opioids
   Other medical problems, especially hepatic failure; hepatitis, acute; or other hepatic disease

### Proper use of this medication
» Importance of taking each dose as scheduled
» Proper dosing
   Missed dose: If dosing schedule is—
      One tablet every day—
         Taking as soon as possible; not taking if not remembered until the next day; not doubling the next day's dose
      One tablet every weekday and two tablets on Saturday—
         If weekday dose missed—Following missed dose directions as for one tablet every day
         If Saturday dose missed—Taking two tablets as soon as possible if remembered the same day, or taking one tablet if not remembered until Sunday, then returning to regular dosing schedule on Monday
      Two tablets every other day—
         Taking two tablets as soon as remembered, skipping a day, then continuing every other day; or
         Taking two tablets as soon as possible if remembered the same day, or taking one tablet if not remembered until the next day, then returning to the regular dosing schedule
      Two tablets on Monday and Wednesday and three tablets on Friday—
         If Monday or Wednesday dose missed—Taking two tablets as soon as possible if remembered the same day, or taking one tablet if not remembered until the next day, then returning to the regular dosing schedule
         If Friday dose missed—Taking three tablets as soon as possible if remembered the same day; taking two tablets if not remembered until Saturday or one tablet if not remembered until Sunday; returning to the regular dosing schedule on Monday
      Three tablets every three days—
         Taking three tablets as soon as remembered, skipping two days, then continuing every three days; or
         Taking three tablets as soon as possible if remembered the same day; taking two tablets if not remembered until the next day, or one tablet if not remembered until the following day, then returning to the regular dosing schedule
» Proper storage

### Precautions while using this medication
» Regular visits to physician or clinic; blood tests may be needed to detect possible hepatotoxicity
» Importance of compliance with all components of a comprehensive treatment program, including attending counseling sessions and/or support group meetings; naltrexone is intended only as an aid to other forms of therapy that discourage return to alcohol or opioid use
» Not attempting to overcome effects of naltrexone by taking opioids; such attempts may lead to coma or death; therapy with naltrexone may lead to increased sensitivity to the effects of narcotics
» Not using opioid medications to relieve pain, diarrhea, or cough because naltrexone also prevents therapeutic effects of opioids
» Not taking naltrexone to perform activities (for example, driving) while under the influence of alcohol
» Never sharing medication with others, especially those dependent on opioids
» Notifying all physicians, dentists, and pharmacists of use of naltrexone
» Carrying identification card indicating use of medication

### Side/adverse effects
Signs of potential side effects, especially skin rash; blurred vision or aching, burning, or swollen eyes; chest pain; confusion; discomfort while urinating and/or frequent urination; edema; fever; gastrointestinal ulceration; hallucinations; itching; mental depression or other mood or mental changes; ringing or buzzing in ears; shortness of breath

## General Dosing Information

When naltrexone is used as adjunct therapy to treat opioid (narcotic) abuse, naltrexone therapy should not be initiated until the patient has been completely detoxified, is free of withdrawal symptoms, and has remained opioid-free for 7 to 10 days (following use of a relatively short-acting opioid such as heroin) or longer (following use of a longer-acting opioid such as methadone). Abstinence should be verified by examination of the urine for opioids and/or a naloxone challenge test.

Clonidine or methadone may be used to prevent or attenuate withdrawal symptoms during detoxification; however, if methadone is used, initiation of naltrexone therapy must be delayed until there is no risk of precipitating withdrawal symptoms.

The naloxone challenge test should not be administered if withdrawal symptoms are present or the patient's urine contains opioids. Naloxone may be administered intravenously or subcutaneously. If the intravenous route is used, an initial dose of 200 mcg (0.2 mg) should be administered and the patient observed for 30 seconds for withdrawal symptoms; if none occurs, an additional 600 mcg (0.6 mg) of naloxone should be administered and the patient observed for 20 minutes. If the subcutaneous route is used, 800 mcg (0.8 mg) of naloxone should be administered and the patient observed for 20 minutes for withdrawal symptoms. If withdrawal symptoms occur, the naloxone challenge should be repeated at 24-hour intervals until absence of opioid dependence is confirmed.

It is recommended that naltrexone therapy be initiated with a low dose (e.g., 25 mg), which may be increased to 50 mg a day if no signs or symptoms of withdrawal occur. Alternatives to daily administration include several maintenance dosing regimens permitting administration of higher doses every second or third day on an occasional or regular basis (e.g., over weekends). It has been suggested that less frequent dosing, scheduled to suit the individual patient, may improve compliance. The alternative dosing schedules have not been studied in the treatment of alcoholism.

In emergency situations requiring an opioid analgesic, naltrexone's effects can be overcome by administering sufficiently high doses of the analgesic. It is recommended that a rapidly acting analgesic with minimal potential for respiratory depression be administered in doses carefully titrated to the needs of the patient. Since high doses of analgesic are required, the risk of adverse effects, including severe, prolonged respiratory depression and circulatory collapse, is greatly increased. Therefore, such treatment must be carried out in a hospital setting, where the patient can be carefully monitored by trained personnel. Some patients on naltrexone therapy may be sensitive to low doses of opioids. In these patients, adverse effects may occur even with low doses of opioids.

Naltrexone does not cause physical or psychological dependence.

Tolerance to the opioid-blocking action of naltrexone has not been reported.

Long-term success with naltrexone-based regimens for the treatment of alcoholism or opioid drug dependence has not been established. Compliance may be improved if the medication is administered as a component of an integrated program including psychosocial therapy.

### For treatment of adverse effects

Precipitation of withdrawal symptoms in physically dependent patients: Symptoms may be very difficult to reverse. It is recommended that the patient be monitored closely and treated for observed symptoms as required.

## Oral Dosage Forms

### NALTREXONE HYDROCHLORIDE TABLETS

**Usual adult dose**
Opioid (narcotic) drug use, illicit (treatment adjunct)—
   Initial—
      Oral, 25 mg for the first dose; an additional 25 mg may be given one hour later if no withdrawal symptoms occur.
   Maintenance—
      Oral, 50 mg every twenty-four hours. Alternatively, the weekly dose of 350 mg may be administered using an intermittent dosing schedule, such as:
      Oral, 50 mg every twenty-four hours on weekdays and 100 mg on Saturday; or
      Oral, 100 mg every forty-eight hours; or
      Oral, 100 mg every Monday and Wednesday and 150 mg on Friday; or
      Oral, 150 mg every seventy-two hours.
Alcoholism (treatment)—
   Oral, 50 mg every twenty-four hours for up to twelve weeks.

**Usual pediatric dose**
Dosage in patients up to 18 years of age has not been established.

**Strength(s) usually available**
U.S.—
   50 mg (Rx) [*ReVia* (scored; lactose; microcrystalline cellulose; crospovidone; colloidal silicon dioxide; magnesium stearate; hydroxypropyl methylcellulose; titanium dioxide; polyethylene glycol; polysorbate 80; yellow iron oxide; red iron oxide); GENERIC].
Canada—
   50 mg (Rx) [*ReVia* (scored; lactose monohydrate; microcrystalline cellulose; crospovidone; colloidal silicon dioxide; magnesium stearate; microcrystalline methylcellulose; Pale Yellow Opadry® YS-1-6378-G)].

**Packaging and storage**
Store below 40 °C (104 °F), preferably between 15 and 30 °C (59 and 86 °F), in a tight, light-resistant container, unless otherwise specified by manufacturer.

Revised: 08/13/97
Interim revision: 07/07/98

---

**NANDROLONE**—See *Anabolic Steroids (Systemic)*

---

**NAPHAZOLINE**—The *Naphazoline (Ophthalmic)* monograph is not included in this published version of the USP DI database. Copies of the monograph are available on request from Micromedex, Inc.-Reprint Requests, 6200 S. Syracuse Way, Suite 300, Englewood, CO 80111; telephone (303) 486-6400; telefax (303) 486-6464; Email: USPDI@MDX.COM.

---

**NAPROXEN**—See *Anti-inflammatory Drugs, Nonsteroidal (Systemic)*

---

# NARATRIPTAN   Systemic—INTRODUCTORY VERSION

VA CLASSIFICATION (Primary): CN105
Note: For a listing of dosage forms and brand names by country availability, see *Dosage Forms* section(s).

## Category
Antimigraine agent.

## Indications

**General considerations**
Naratriptan should only be prescribed for patients who have an established clear diagnosis of migraine.

**Accepted**
Headache, migraine (treatment)—Naratriptan is indicated to relieve (abort) acute migraine headaches (with or without aura).

**Unaccepted**
Naratriptan is not recommended for treatment of basilar artery migraine or hemiplegic migraine.

Naratriptan is not recommended for treatment of cluster headaches. Efficacy and safety of naratriptan in these conditions have not been established.

## Pharmacology/Pharmacokinetics

**Physicochemical characteristics**
Molecular weight—371.93.

**Mechanism of action/Effect**
Naratriptan's mechanism of action has not been established. It is thought that agonist activity at the 5-hydroxytryptamine $(5\text{-HT})_{1D}$ and $5\text{-HT}_{1B}$ receptor subtypes provides relief of headaches. Naratriptan is a highly selective agonist at these receptor subtypes; it has no significant activity at $5\text{-HT}_2$, $5\text{-HT}_3$, or $5\text{-HT}_4$ receptor subtypes or at adrenergic, dopaminergic, histamine, muscarinic, or benzodiazepine receptors. It has been proposed that constriction of cerebral blood vessels resulting from $5\text{-HT}_{1D/1B}$ receptor stimulation reduces the pulsation that may be responsible for the pain of migraine headaches. It has also been proposed that naratriptan may relieve migraine headaches by decreasing the release of pro-inflammatory neuropeptides.

**Absorption**
Oral—Rapid; bioavailability is 70%. The rate and extent of the absorption of naratriptan are not affected by administration with food. The rate of absorption is slower during a migraine attack.

**Protein binding**
Low (28 to 31%), at plasma concentrations of 50 to 1000 nanograms per mL (nanograms/mL).

**Biotransformation**
Hepatic. *In vitro* studies indicate that naratriptan is metabolized by cytochrome P450 isoenzymes into inactive metabolites.

**Half-life**
Approximately 6 hours.

**Time to peak concentration**
Within 2 to 3 hours (3 to 4 hours during a migraine attack).

**Elimination**
Renal—80% (50% of the dose as unchanged; 30% as metabolites).

## Precautions to Consider

**Carcinogenicity/Tumorigenicity**
Lifetime carcinogenicity studies were done in mice and rats receiving naratriptan by oral gavage. In mice receiving doses of 200 mg per kg of body weight (mg/kg) per day (reflects an area under the plasma concentration–time curve [AUC] exposure of 110 times the exposure in humans receiving the maximum recommended human dose [MRHD]), no evidence of tumorigenicity was found. Two studies were done in rats, one receiving a standard diet and the other a nitrate-supplemented diet. Rats receiving the standard and nitrate-supplemented diet with doses of naratriptan 5, 20, and 90 mg/kg per day reflected plasma concentration AUC exposures of 7, 40, and 236 times the MRHD and 7, 29, 180 times the MRHD at week 13, respectively. There was an increase in the incidence of thyroid follicular hyperplasia and thyroid follicular adenomas in high-dosed male rats in both studies. However, there was only an increase in thyroid follicular hyperplasia in the high-dosed female rats. Also, in the standard and nitrate supplement studies, the exposure to achieve the no-effect dose for thyroid tumors was 40 and 29 times the MRHD, respectively. In the standard study, there was an increase in the incidence of the benign c-cell adenomas in the thyroid of the high-dosed male rats. The incidence of benign lymphocytic thymoma was increased in all of the females in the nitrate-supplemented diet study.

**Mutagenicity**
Naratriptan demonstrated no mutagenic effects in the Ames test or in the *in vitro* thymidine locus mouse lymphoma gene mutation assays. There was no evidence of clastogenic activity in the *in vitro* human lymphocyte assay or in the *in vivo* mouse micronucleus cytogenetics assay. A mutagenic product (WHO nitrosation assay) is formed *in vitro* from

nitrosated naratriptan, and has been found in stomachs of rats receiving a nitrate-supplemented diet. It was not determined in the two rat studies whether the nitrosated product is systemically absorbed. However, no changes were found in the stomachs of the rats.

**Pregnancy/Reproduction**

Fertility—A reproductive toxicity study in male and female rats receiving doses of naratriptan up to 10, 60, 170, or 340 mg/kg per day (AUC exposure approximately 11, 70, 230, and 470 times the MRHD) found a treatment-related decrease in the number of females exhibiting normal estrous cycles at doses of 170 mg/kg per day or greater. In female rats receiving doses up to 60 mg/kg per day or greater, an increase in preimplantation loss was observed. In the high-dose group males, testicular and/or epididymal atrophy along with spermatazoa depletion resulted in reduced mating success. Also, the preimplantation loss in females may have been due to the testicular and/or epididymal atrophy. However, the exposures achieved at approximately 11, 70, and 230 times the MRHD of naratriptan resulted in no preimplantation loss, anestrus, and testicular effects, respectively.

A study in rats receiving 10, 60, or 340 mg/kg per day for 6 months found changes in the female reproductive tract including atrophic or cystic ovaries at the highest dose. However, in rats receiving 60 mg/kg per day (85 times the MRHD) of naratriptan, no effect was observed.

Pregnancy—Adequate and well-controlled trials have not been done in pregnant women.

In a reproductive toxicity study, rats and rabbits receiving oral doses of naratriptan equivalent to maternal plasma exposure of 11, 70, and 230 times the MRHD had evidence of developmental toxicity, such as embryo lethality, fetal abnormalities, pup mortality, and offspring growth retardation.

In pregnant rats doses of naratriptan of up to 10, 60, or 340 mg/kg per day (maternal plasma exposures [AUC] approximately 11, 70, and 470 times the MRHD, respectively) given during the organogenesis period resulted in an increase in dose-related embryonic death. The increased incidence of embryo lethality was statistically significant at the highest dose only. However, the incidence of fetal structural variations, such as incomplete or irregular ossification of skull bones, sternebrae, and ribs were increased at all the doses. The highest dose was found to be maternally toxic, which resulted in a lower than normal maternal weight gain during gestation.

In pregnant Dutch rabbits receiving doses of naratriptan of up to 1, 5, or 30 mg/kg per day (approximately 4, 20, and 120 times the MRHD on a mg per square meter of body surface area [mg/m$^2$] basis, respectively), during the organogenesis period, an increase in incidences of fused sternebrae at the highest dose was observed. In addition, at all the doses there was evidence of an increase in embryonic death, and fetal variations, such as major blood vessel variations, incomplete skeletal ossification, and supernumary ribs. The highest dose in this study was also found to be maternally toxic, which resulted in a lower maternal weight gain during gestation. A study in pregnant New Zealand white rabbits, during the organogenesis period, receiving naratriptan doses of 1, 5, or 30 mg/kg (maternal exposure approximately 2.5, 19, and 140 times the MRHD) per day found decreased fetal weights and increased incidences of fetal skeletal variations at all doses. In contrast with the Dutch rabbits, the maternal weight gain in the New Zealand white rabbits was lower at doses of naratriptan of 5 mg/kg or greater.

In female rats receiving 10, 60, 340 mg/kg doses of naratriptan during late gestation and lactation, behavioral impairment, such as tremors, was observed. At doses of 60 mg/kg per day or greater of naratriptan, a decrease in offspring viability and growth was observed. However, maternal toxicity occurred only at the highest doses. The maternal exposure achieved at approximately 11 times the MRHD of naratriptan did not cause any developmental effects.

FDA Pregnancy Category C.

**Breast-feeding**

It is not known whether naratriptan is distributed into human breast milk. Naratriptan is distributed in the milk of lactating rats.

**Pediatrics**

No information is available on the relationship of age to the effects of naratriptan in pediatric patients. Safety and efficacy have not been established.

**Adolescents**

In clinical trials, 300 children 12 to 17 years of age have been treated with naratriptan (0.25- to 1.5-mg doses); adverse effects were similar to those occurring in patients older than 17 years of age. However, the safety and efficacy of naratriptan in children up to 18 years of age have not been established.

**Geriatrics**

Use of naratriptan in elderly patients is not recommended.

**Drug interactions and/or related problems**

The following drug interactions and/or related problems have been selected on the basis of their potential clinical significance (possible mechanism in parentheses where appropriate)—not necessarily inclusive (» = major clinical significance):

Note: Combinations containing any of the following medications, depending on the amount present, may also interact with this medication.

Dihydroergotamine or
Ergotamine or
Methysergide or
Other 5-hydroxytryptamine (5HT$_1$) agonists such as:
  Sumatriptan or
  Zolmitriptan
  (a delay of 24 hours between administration of dihydroergotamine, ergotamine, methysergide, or other 5HT$_1$ and naratriptan is recommended because of the possibility of additive and/or prolonged vasoconstriction)

Serotonergics (see *Appendix II*), such as:
  Fluoxetine
  Fluvoxamine
  Paroxetine
  Sertraline
  (concurrent use may result in weakness, hyperreflexia, and incoordination; monitoring is recommended)

**Medical considerations/Contraindications**

The medical considerations/contraindications included have been selected on the basis of their potential clinical significance (reasons given in parentheses where appropriate)—not necessarily inclusive (» = major clinical significance).

*Except under special circumstances, this medication should not be used when the following medical problems exist:*

» Coronary artery disease, especially:
  Angina pectoris
  Myocardial infarction, history of
  Myocardial ischemia, silent, documented
  Prinzmetal's angina or

» Other conditions in which coronary vasoconstriction would be detrimental
  (naratriptan may cause coronary vasospasms)

» Hypertension, uncontrolled
  (may be exacerbated)

» Peripheral vascular disease, including:
  Ischemic bowel disease
    (may be exacerbated)

*Risk-benefit should be considered when the following medical problems exist:*

» Cerebrovascular accident, history of
  (5HT$_1$ agonists may precipitate a cerebrovascular syndrome; caution should be used when administering to patients at risk for cerebrovascular events)

» Coronary artery disease, predisposition to
  (naratriptan may cause serious coronary adverse effects; patients in whom coronary artery disease is a possibility on the basis of age or the presence of other risk factors, such as diabetes, hypercholesterolemia, obesity, a strong family history of coronary artery disease, or tobacco smoking should be evaluated for the presence of cardiovascular disease before naratriptan is prescribed; even after a satisfactory evaluation, the advisability of administering the patient's first dose under medical supervision should be considered)

» Hepatic function impairment, severe or
» Renal function impairment, severe
  (studies have shown a decrease in naratriptan clearance in patients with moderate hepatic and renal impairment; caution is recommended; a dosage adjustment is recommended in patients with severe hepatic and renal impairment)

» Hypersensitivity to naratriptan
» Hypertension, controlled
  (may precipitate an increase in systolic and diastolic pressure)

**Patient monitoring**

The following may be especially important in patient monitoring (other tests may be warranted in some patients, depending on condition; » = major clinical significance):

Electrocardiogram (ECG)
  (monitoring is recommended for long-term intermittent users of naratriptan)

## Side/Adverse Effects

The following side/adverse effects have been selected on the basis of their potential clinical significance (possible signs and symptoms in parentheses where appropriate)—not necessarily inclusive:

**Those indicating need for medical attention**
Incidence more frequent
  *Chest pain, severe; heaviness, tightness, or pressure in chest, throat, and/or neck; paresthesias* (sensation of burning, warmth or heat, numbness, tightness, or tingling)
Incidence less frequent or rare
  *Arrythmias* (irregular heartbeat); *bradycardia* (slow heartbeat); *convulsions; decreased blood pressure; increased blood pressure*

**Those indicating need for medical attention only if they continue or are bothersome**
Incidence more frequent
  *Dizziness; drowsiness; malaise* (increased tiredness); *nausea and/or vomiting*
Incidence less frequent
  *Anxiety; arthralgia* (joint pain); *blurred vision; chills and/or fever; constipation; diarrhea; gastroenteritis* (diarrhea; nausea; stomach pain); *increased thirst; muscle or joint stiffness, tightness, or rigidity; muscle pain or spasms; palpitations* (pounding heartbeat); *polyuria* (sudden, large increase in frequency and quantity of urine); *pruritus* (itching of the skin); *sleep disorders* (difficulty sleeping); *skin rash; stomach discomfort and/or pain; syncope* (fainting); *tremors* (trembling or shaking of hands or feet)
Incidence rare
  *Acne; anemia* (unusual tiredness or weakness); *bone or skeletal pain; confusion; eye problems, including dry eyes; eye pain and/or discomfort; fluid imbalance; mood or mental changes, including agitation; hallucinations; and panic disorders; restlessness; taste perversion* (change in taste sensation)

## Overdose

For more information on the management of overdose or unintentional ingestion, **contact a Poison Control Center** (see *Poison Control Center Listing*).

**Clinical effects of overdose**
The following effects have been selected on the basis of their potential clinical significance (possible signs and symptoms in parentheses where appropriate)—not necessarily inclusive:

Acute and/or chronic
  *Increased blood pressure; lightheadedness; loss of coordination; tension in neck; tiredness*

**Treatment of overdose**
Monitoring—
  Electrocardiogram (ECG) monitoring should be performed in patients who present with symptoms of chest pain or other symptoms consistent with angina.
  Patients should be monitored for at least 24 hours after an overdose of naratriptan.
Supportive care—
  Maintaining an open airway and breathing, maintaining proper fluid and electrolyte balance and/or correcting hypertension. Patients in whom intentional overdose is confirmed or suspected should be referred for psychiatric consultation.

## Patient Consultation

As an aid to patient consultation, refer to *Advice for the Patient, Naratriptan (Systemic)—Introductory Version*.
In providing consultation, consider emphasizing the following selected information (» = major clinical significance):

**Before using this medication**
» Conditions affecting use, especially:
    Hypersensitivity to naratriptan
    Use in the elderly—Use is not recommended
    Other medical problems, especially cerebrovascular accident (history of), coronary artery disease, predisposition to coronary artery disease, or other conditions that may be adversely affected by coronary artery constriction, hepatic function impairment (severe), peripheral vascular disease, renal function impairment (severe), hypertension

**Proper use of this medication**
» Not administering if atypical headache symptoms are present; checking with physician instead
    Administering after onset of headache pain
    Additional benefit may be obtained if the patient lies down in a quiet, dark room after administering medication
» Not taking additional doses if first dose does not provide substantial relief; taking alternate medication as previously advised by physician, then checking with physician as soon as possible
» Taking additional doses, if needed, for return of migraine headache after initial relief was obtained, provided that prescribed limits (quantity used and frequency of administration) are not exceeded
» Compliance with prophylactic therapy, if prescribed
» Proper dosing
» Proper storage

**Precautions while using this medication**
  Avoiding alcohol, which aggravates headache
» Caution when driving or doing anything else requiring alertness because of possible drowsiness, dizziness, lightheadedness, impairment of physical or mental abilities

**Side/adverse effects**
  Signs of potential side effects, especially chest pain, severe; heaviness, tightness, or pressure in chest and/or neck; paresthesias; upper respiratory tract infection; arrythmias; hypertension; bradycardia; and convulsions

## Oral Dosage Forms

### NARATRIPTAN HYDROCHLORIDE TABLETS

**Usual adult dose:**
Note:  The dosing and strengths of the dosage form available are expressed in terms of naratriptan base (not the hydrochloride salt).
Antimigraine agent—
  Oral, 1 or 2.5 mg (base) as a single dose. If necessary, additional doses may be taken at intervals of at least four hours.
  A starting dose of less than 2.5 mg is recommended for patients with mild to moderate hepatic or renal impairment.

**Usual adult prescribing limits**
5 mg in twenty-four hours.
2.5 mg in patients with mild or moderate hepatic or renal impairment.

**Usual pediatric dose**
Safety and efficacy have not been established in children up to 18 years of age.

**Usual geriatric dose**
Use is not recommended.

**Strength(s) usually available**
U.S.—
  1 mg (base) (Rx) [*Amerge* (croscarmellose sodium; hydroxypropyl methylcellulose; lactose; magnesium stearate; microcrystalline cellulose; triacetin; titanium dioxide; iron oxide yellow; indigo carmine aluminum lake (FD&C Blue No. 2))].
  2.5 mg (base) (Rx) [*Amerge* (croscarmellose sodium; hydroxypropyl methylcellulose; lactose; magnesium stearate; microcrystalline cellulose; triacetin; titanium dioxide; iron oxide yellow; indigo carmine aluminum lake (FD&C Blue No. 2))].

**Packaging and storage**
Store below 25 °C (77 °F).

**Auxiliary labeling**
• Take with a full glass of water.

Developed: 07/07/98

---

**NATAMYCIN**—The *Natamycin (Ophthalmic)* monograph is not included in this published version of the USP DI database. Copies of the monograph are available on request from Micromedex, Inc. - Reprint Requests, 6200 S. Syracuse Way, Suite 300, Englewood, CO 80111; telephone (303) 486-6400; telefax (303) 486-6464; Email: USPDI@MDX.COM.

# NEDOCROMIL Inhalation-Local

VA CLASSIFICATION (Primary/Secondary): RE101/RE109

Commonly used brand name(s): *Tilade*.

Note: For a listing of dosage forms and brand names by country availability, see *Dosage Forms* section(s).

## Category

Anti-inflammatory, nonsteroid (inhalation); asthma prophylactic; antiallergic (inhalation).

## Indications

Note: Bracketed information in the *Indications* section refers to indications that are not included in U.S. product labeling.

**Accepted**

Asthma, bronchial (prophylaxis)—Nedocromil is indicated for prevention of airway inflammation and bronchoconstriction in patients with bronchial asthma who require daily therapy. It may be used alone as primary therapy or with other asthma medications, such as bronchodilators and/or corticosteroids. In mild or moderate asthma, nedocromil may be used instead of corticosteroids, inhaled or systemic.

[Bronchospasm (prophylaxis)]—Nedocromil is indicated for prevention of bronchospasm in patients with reversible obstructive airways disease. It may be used regularly or occasionally just prior to an anticipated exposure to such provocation as inhaled allergens, exercise, cold air, or atmospheric pollutants.

**Unaccepted**

Nedocromil is not a bronchodilator and, therefore, is not indicated for the reversal or relief of acute bronchospasm, especially in status asthmaticus.

## Pharmacology/Pharmacokinetics

**Physicochemical characteristics**

Chemical group—Pyranoquinoline.
Molecular weight—415.31.
pKa—2.

**Mechanism of action/Effect**

Nedocromil inhibits activation and release of inflammatory mediators from a variety of cell types in the lumen and mucosa of the bronchial tree. These mediators, which include the leukotrienes, histamine, and prostaglandins, are preformed or derived from arachidonic acid metabolism through the lipoxygenase and cyclo-oxygenase pathways. A range of human cells associated with asthma, such as eosinophils, neutrophils, macrophages, monocytes, mast cells, and platelets, may be involved. Nedocromil exhibits specific anti-inflammatory properties when administered directly to the bronchial mucosa. It has demonstrated a significant inhibitory effect on allergen-induced early and late asthmatic reactions and on bronchial hyperresponsiveness. Nedocromil may also affect sensory nerves in the lung. The mechanism of action of nedocromil may be due partly to inhibition of axon reflexes and release of sensory neuropeptides, such as substance P, neurokinin A, and calcitonin-gene–related peptides. The result is inhibition of bradykinin-induced bronchoconstriction. Nedocromil does not posess any bronchodilator, antihistamine, or corticosteroid activity. At recommended doses, inhaled nedocromil has no known systemic activity.

**Absorption**

The extent of absorption is about 7 to 9% of a single inhaled dose of 3.5 to 4 mg and 17% of multiple inhaled doses, with absorption largely from the respiratory tract.

Gastrointestinal tract—Although most of an inhaled dose of nedocromil is subsequently swallowed, only 2 to 3% of it is absorbed from the gastrointestinal tract.

Respiratory tract—5 to 6% of an inhaled dose of nedocromil is absorbed slowly from the respiratory tract.

**Distribution**

Distributed into plasma. With repeated dosing, nedocromil seems to exert a residual effect that allows for twice-a-day dosing for some patients.

**Protein binding**

Approximately 89% is reversibly bound to plasma proteins when plasma concentrations range between 0.5 and 50 mcg/mL.

**Biotransformation**

Nedocromil is not metabolized.

**Half-life**

Approximately 1.5 to 3.3 hours.

**Onset of action**

Nedocromil has been shown to prevent bronchospasm when administered up to 30 minutes before exposure to a chemical irritant, an allergen, or exercise.

When nedocromil is used as maintenance therapy, clinical improvement in symptoms and lung function usually occurs within 2 to 4 weeks of the beginning of treatment. In some patients, improvement of symptoms can occur within a few days.

**Time to peak concentration**

Following single-dose or multiple-dose inhalation—In asthmatic patients: 5 to 90 minutes.

**Peak serum concentration**

Following single-dose or multiple-dose inhalation—In asthmatic patients: 2.8 nanograms per mL.

**Duration of action**

When a single dose is administered prior to an allergen challenge, nedocromil inhibits the late reactions of bronchoconstriction occurring 6 to 12 hours after provocation.

**Elimination**

Rapidly excreted as unchanged drug, in the bile and urine.

## Precautions to Consider

**Cross-sensitivity and/or related problems**

Patients sensitive to fluorocarbons may be sensitive to the fluorocarbons, dichlorotetrafluoroethane and dichlorodifluoromethane, contained in this preparation.

**Carcinogenicity/Mutagenicity**

Various animal studies and *in vitro* studies using human cells showed no evidence of mutagenic or carcinogenic potential.

**Pregnancy/Reproduction**

Fertility—The results of fertility studies of nedocromil in rats and mice showed no effect on male or female fertility.

Pregnancy—Adequate and well controlled studies in humans have not been done.

In reproduction studies in rats and mice, small amounts of nedocromil crossed the placenta but did not cause teratogenic or embryotoxic effects.

FDA Pregnancy Category B.

**Breast-feeding**

It is not known whether nedocromil is distributed into human breast milk. However, problems in humans have not been documented. In animal studies, small amounts of nedocromil were distributed into milk but did not cause adverse effects.

**Pediatrics**

Appropriate studies have been performed in children 6 years of age and older, although data regarding use of nedocromil in treatment of childhood asthma remain limited to date. These studies have not demonstrated pediatrics-specific problems that would limit the usefulness of nedocromil in children. The types and frequency of side effects associated with nedocromil use in children were similar to those observed in adults.

Nedocromil appeared to offset the increase of symptoms of asthma when used in pediatric patients who experience seasonal exacerbations of asthma.

**Geriatrics**

No information is available on the relationship of age to the effects of nedocromil in geriatric patients.

**Drug interactions and/or related problems**

The following drug interactions and/or related problems have been selected on the basis of their potential clinical significance (possible mechanism in parentheses where appropriate)—not necessarily inclusive (» = major clinical significance):

Note: Nedocromil has not shown an increase in frequency of adverse reactions or lab abnormalities with concomitant use of other anti-asthma medications, such as inhaled or oral bronchodilators, or inhaled corticosteriods; however, no formal drug interaction studies have been conducted.

**Medical considerations/Contraindications**

The medical considerations/contraindications included have been selected on the basis of their potential clinical significance (reasons given in parentheses where appropriate)—not necessarily inclusive (» = major clinical significance).

Risk-benefit should be considered when the following medical problem exists:
   Sensitivity to nedocromil

## Side/Adverse Effects
The following side/adverse effects have been selected on the basis of their potential clinical significance (possible signs and symptoms in parentheses where appropriate)—not necessarily inclusive:

**Those indicating need for medical attention**
Incidence less frequent
   *Abdominal pain; bronchospasm, increased* (increased wheezing, tightness in chest, or difficulty in breathing)—may be due to sensitivity to nedocromil or fluorocarbon propellants
Incidence rare
   *Arthritis* (pain, stiffness, or swelling of joints); *neutropenia or leukopenia* (signs of infection, such as fever, sore throat, body aches, or chills)

**Those indicating need for medical attention only if they continue or are bothersome**
Incidence less frequent—(about 4 to 7%)
   *Cough; headache; nausea or vomiting; rhinitis* (runny or stuffy nose); *throat irritation*
Incidence rare
   *Sensation of warmth; tremor*

**Those not indicating need for medical attention**
Incidence more frequent—(about 12% or more)
   *Unpleasant taste after inhalation*

## Overdose
**Clinical effects of overdose**
Overdosage of necrodomil is unlikely to result in any clinical manifestations which would require more than the observation of the patient and discontinuation of the medication where appropriate.

## Patient Consultation
As an aid to patient consultation, refer to *Advice for the Patient, Nedocromil (Inhalation)*.
In providing consultation, consider emphasizing the following selected information (» = major clinical significance):

**Before using this medication**
» Conditions affecting use, especially:
   Sensitivity to nedocromil

**Proper use of this medication**
» Helps prevent, but does not relieve, acute attacks of asthma or bronchospasm
   Reading patient instructions carefully before using
   Using metered dose inhaler; checking periodically with doctor, nurse, or pharmacist for proper use of inhaler to prevent incorrect dosage
   Priming inhaler with three actuations before using for the first time or if inhaler has not been used for more than seven days
   Proper administration technique
» Proper dosing
   Importance of not increasing or decreasing dose without physician's supervision
   Proper administration technique if spacer device used
   Proper cleaning procedure for inhaler
   Missed dose: If used regularly, using as soon as possible; using any remaining doses for that day at regularly spaced intervals
» Proper storage
   Importance of storing canister at room temperature before use for best results
   Keeping out of the reach of children
*For patients on scheduled dosing regimen*
» Compliance with therapy; 2 to 4 weeks usually required for maximum therapeutic benefit after the beginning of nedocromil therapy

**Precautions while using this medication**
» Checking with physician if symptoms do not improve within 2 to 4 weeks; checking with physician immediately if condition becomes worse
» Importance of not discontinuing any concurrent antiasthmatic medication without physician's advice
   Gargling or rinsing mouth after inhalation to relieve throat irritation and unpleasant taste

**Side/adverse effects**
   Signs of potential side effects, especially abdominal pain, increased bronchospasm, arthritis, or neutropenia or leukopenia

## General Dosing Information
In maintenance therapy, nedocromil must be used regularly, even during symptom-free periods, to achieve benefit.

It is essential that patients be properly instructed in the use of the inhaler, and that the correct method be reinforced periodically.

A decrease in severity of clinical symptoms or in the need for concomitant therapy is a sign of improvement that usually will be evident in the first 2 to 4 weeks of therapy if patient responds to nedocromil therapy.

After a patient becomes stabilized on nedocromil, the frequency of administration may be slowly decreased to a frequency that maintains freedom from exacerbations of asthma. The frequency of administration is usually no less than twice a day.

When nedocromil is added to an existing regimen of bronchodilators and/or inhaled or systemic corticosteroids, a reduction in dosage of the corticosteroid or bronchodilator may be achieved in some patients. However, the reduction should be gradual and under close medical supervision to avoid an exacerbation of asthma, since nedocromil has a very limited capacity to effectively substitute for inhaled or systemic corticosteroids.

Nedocromil therapy should be continued during acute exacerbations, unless the patient becomes intolerant to the use of inhaled dosage forms.

When nedocromil is added to as-needed usage of beta$_2$-adrenergic bronchodilators, symptom control and pulmonary function improve after approximately 2 weeks of therapy.

Studies were conducted comparing both two-times-a-day and four-times-a-day nedocromil dosing regimens. The medication was found to be more effective when used four times a day; however, if good control of symptoms has been maintained on the four-times-daily regimen, a less frequent dosing schedule may be considered.

Nedocromil inhaler requires priming with three actuations before the initial use and when the inhaler has not been used for more than 7 days.

**For treatment of adverse effects**
Recommended treatment consists of the following:
• Discontinue nedocromil and substitute alternative therapy if bronchospasm occurs after administration of nedocromil.

## Inhalation Dosage Forms
Note: Bracketed uses in the *Dosage Forms* section refer to categories of use and/or indications that are not included in U.S. product labeling.

### NEDOCROMIL INHALATION AEROSOL
**Usual adult and adolescent dose**
Asthma, bronchial (prophylaxis)—
   Oral inhalation, 3.5 or 4 mg (2 inhalations) four times a day at regular intervals. Dosage frequency may be reduced to three times a day and then two times a day when patient's asthma is under good control.
[Bronchospasm (prophylaxis)]—
   Oral inhalation, 4 mg (2 inhalations) as a single dose up to thirty minutes before exercise or exposure to any precipitating factor.

**Usual adult prescribing limits**
14 mg or 16 mg of nedocromil per twenty-four-hour period (2 inhalations four times daily at evenly spaced intervals).

Note: If the patient's asthma is well-controlled, as demonstrated by the absence of serious exacerbations and only occasional use of inhaled or oral beta$_2$-adrenergic bronchodilators, a less frequent dosing schedule may be effective.

**Usual pediatric dose**
Children up to 6 years of age: Safety and efficacy have not been established.
Children 6 years of age and older: See *Usual adult and adolescent dose*.

**Usual geriatric dose**
See *Usual adult and adolescent dose*.

**Strength(s) usually available**
U.S.—
   1.75 mg per metered spray (Rx) [*Tilade*].
Note: Each 16.2 gm canister contains 210 gm of nedocromil and provides 104 actuations. Use of the inhaler should not exceed 104 actuations as the dose may be inaccurate for subsequent doses.
Canada—
   2 mg per metered spray (Rx) [*Tilade*].
Note: Each 17 mL canister contains 112 actuations.
   In Canada, metered dose inhalers are labeled according to the amount of nedocromil delivered at the valve; in the U.S., metered dose inhalers are labeled according to the amount of nedocromil delivered at the mouthpiece or actuator. Therefore, 2 mg of nedo-

cromil delivered at the valve is equivalent to 1.75 mg delivered at the mouthpiece.

**Packaging and storage**
Store between 2 and 30 °C (36 and 86 °F), unless otherwise specified by manufacturer. Protect from freezing.
Canister contents are under pressure, therefore the canister should not be punctured, incinerated, or placed near sources of heat. The product should not be exposed to temperatures above 49 °C (120 ° F).

**Auxiliary labeling**
- For oral inhalation only.
- Shake well before using.
- Store away from heat and direct sunlight.
- Do not use with other mouthpieces.

**Note**
Include patient instructions when dispensing.
Demonstrate inhalation technique to patient when dispensing.

**Additional information**
This product contains dichlorotetrafluoroethane and dichlorodifluoromethane, substances that harm public health and the environment by destroying ozone in the upper atmosphere.

## Selected Bibliography
Parish RC, Miller LJ. Nedocromil sodium. Ann Pharmacother 1993; 27: 599-606.
Brogden RN, Sorkin EM. Nedocromil sodium. An updated review of its pharmacological properties and therapeutic efficacy in asthma. Drugs 1993; 45(5): 693-715.

Revised: 08/14/98

# NEFAZODONE    Systemic—INTRODUCTORY VERSION

VA CLASSIFICATION (Primary): CN609
Commonly used brand name(s): *Serzone*.
Note:  For a listing of dosage forms and brand names by country availability, see *Dosage Forms* section(s).

## Category
Antidepressant.

## Indications
**Accepted**
Depressive disorder, major (treatment)—Nefazodone is indicated for the treatment of depression.

## Pharmacology/Pharmacokinetics
**Physicochemical characteristics**
Structurally related to trazodone; structurally unrelated to selective serotonin reuptake inhibitors, tricyclic, tetracyclic, or monoamine oxidase inhibitors.
Chemical group—Phenylpiperazine.
Molecular weight—Nefazodone hydrochloride: 506.5.

**Mechanism of action/Effect**
The mechanism of action of nefazodone is unknown. However, nefazodone inhibits neuronal uptake of serotonin and norepinephrine. Nefazodone occupies central 5-$HT_2$ receptors at nanomolar concentrations, where it acts as an antagonist. It has also been shown to antagonize $alpha_1$-adrenergic receptors, a property which may be associated with postural hypotension.
In *in vitro* studies, nefazodone has not demonstrated significant affinity for $alpha_2$-adrenergic, beta-adrenergic, 5-$HT_{1A}$, cholinergic, dopaminergic, or benzodiazepine receptors.

**Absorption**
Rapid and complete. However, due to extensive metabolism, absolute bioavailability is low (about 20%) and variable. Food delays absorption and decreases the bioavailability by approximately 20%.

**Distribution**
Nefazodone is widely distributed in body tissues, including the central nervous system (CNS). The volume of distribution of nefazodone in humans ranges from 0.22 to 0.87 liters per kilogram (L/kg).

**Protein binding**
Very high (99%).

**Biotransformation**
Nefazodone is extensively metabolized after oral administration by *N*-dealkylation and aliphatic and aromatic hydroxylation. Three metabolites have been identified in the plasma: hydroxynefazodone (HO-NEF), meta-chlorophenylpiperazine (mCPP), and a triazole-dione metabolite. HO-NEF has a pharmacological profile qualitatively and quantitatively similar to that of nefazodone. Meta-chlorophenylpiperazine (mCPP) has some similarities to nefazodone, but also has agonist activity at some serotonergic receptor subtypes. The pharmacological profile of the triazole-dione metabolite has not been well characterized. Several other metabolites have been identified but not tested for pharmacological activity.

**Half-life**
2 to 4 hours.

**Onset of action**
Full antidepressant effect may take several weeks to achieve.

**Time to peak concentration**
About 1 hour.

**Plasma concentrations**
Both nefazodone and HO-NEF exhibit nonlinear kinetics for both dose and time, with area under the plasma concentration–time curve (AUC) and peak plasma concentrations ($C_{max}$) increasing more than proportionally with dose increases.

**Steady-state plasma concentrations**
Attained within 4 to 5 days after initiation of twice-daily dosing or upon dosage increase or decrease. In studies involving 29 patients with renal function impairment (creatinine clearances ranging from 7 to 60 mL/min/1.73 m$^2$), no effect on steady-state plasma concentrations was observed. In a study of patients with liver cirrhosis, the AUC values for nefazodone and HO-NEF at steady-state were approximately 25% greater than those observed in normal volunteers. In studies comparing single 300 mg doses of nefazodone in younger and older patients, AUC and $C_{max}$ were increased up to two-fold in older patients. However, with multiple doses, increases were only 10 to 20% greater in the older patients. Similarly, women exhibited a higher AUC and $C_{max}$ after single doses of nefazodone, but no differences after multiple dosing.

**Elimination**
Following oral administration of radiolabeled nefazodone, approximately 55% of administered radioactivity was excreted in the urine and about 20 to 30% in feces.

## Precautions to Consider
**Cross-sensitivity and/or related problems**
Patients sensitive to other phenylpiperazine antidepressants (e.g., trazodone) may be sensitive to nefazodone also.

**Carcinogenicity/Tumorigenicity**
There is no evidence of carcinogenicity with nefazodone. No increased incidence of tumors was demonstrated after two years of administration of nefazodone to rats and mice at daily doses of up to 200 and 800 mg per kg of body weight (mg/kg), respectively. (These doses correlate to approximately 3 and 6 times, respectively, the maximum human daily dose on a mg per square meter of body surface area [mg/m$^2$] basis.)

**Mutagenicity**
Nefazodone has been shown to have no genotoxic effects based on the following assays: bacterial mutation assays, a DNA repair assay in cultured rat hepatocytes, a mammalian mutation assay in Chinese hamster ovary cells, an *in vivo* cytogenetics assay in rat bone marrow cells, and a rat dominant lethal study.

**Pregnancy/Reproduction**
Fertility—A fertility study in rats showed a slight decrease in fertility when nefazodone was administered at a dose of 200 mg/kg per day (approximately 3 times the maximum human daily dose on a mg/m$^2$ basis); however, this effect was not demonstrated at a dose of 100 mg/kg per day (approximately 1.5 times the maximum human daily dose on a mg/m$^2$ basis).

Pregnancy—There are no adequate and well-controlled studies in pregnant women.
No malformations attributable to nefazodone were observed in the offspring of rabbits and rats receiving daily doses up to 200 and 300 mg/kg, respectively (approximately 6 and 5 times, respectively, the maximum

human daily dose on a mg/m² basis). Increased early pup mortality was seen in rats at a dose approximately five times the maximum human dose, and decreased pup weights were seen at this and lower doses, when dosing began during pregnancy and continued until weaning; the cause of these deaths is unknown. The no-effect dose for rat pup mortality was 1.3 times the human dose on a mg/m² basis.

FDA Pregnancy Category C.

Labor and delivery—The effect of nefazodone on labor and delivery in humans is unknown.

**Breast-feeding**
It is not known if nefazodone or its metabolites are distributed into human breast milk.

**Pediatrics**
No information is available on the relationship of age to the effects of nefazodone in pediatric patients. Safety and efficacy in children up to 18 years of age have not been established.

**Geriatrics**
Appropriate studies on the relationship of age to the effects of nefazodone have not been performed in geriatric patients. However, elderly patients who were included in premarketing clinical trials demonstrated increases in the AUC and $C_{max}$ as compared to younger patients. Therefore, decreases in initial dosing in geriatric patients are recommended.

**Pharmacogenetics**
About 3 to 10% of the population have reduced activity of the drug-metabolizing enzyme cytochrome P450 2D6 (CYP2D6) and are referred to as poor metabolizers of drugs such as debrisoquin, dextromethorphan, and the tricyclic antidepressants. The pharmacokinetics of nefazodone and its major metabolite HO-NEF are not altered in this population, but plasma concentrations of the mCPP metabolite are increased. However, dosage adjustment of nefazodone in poor metabolizers is not necessary.

**Dental**
Because nefazodone has the potential to decrease or inhibit salivary flow, it may contribute to the development of caries, periodontal disease, oral candidiasis, and discomfort.

**Surgical**
Since little is known about the potential for interaction between nefazodone and general anesthetics, nefazodone should be discontinued for as long as clinically feasible prior to elective surgery.

**Drug interactions and/or related problems**
The following drug interactions and/or related problems have been selected on the basis of their potential clinical significance (possible mechanism in parentheses where appropriate)—not necessarily inclusive (» = major clinical significance):

Note: Nefazodone has been shown *in vitro* to be an an inhibitor of cytochrome P450 3A4 (CYP3A4), and caution is indicated in the combined use of nefazodone with any drugs known to be metabolized by CYP3A4.

Nefazodone and its metabolites have been shown *in vitro* to be extremely weak inhibitors of CYP2D6; therefore, it is unlikely that nefazodone will decrease the metabolic clearance of drugs metabolized by this isoenzyme.

Nefazodone and its metabolites have been shown *in vitro* not to inhibit CYP1A2; metabolic interactions between nefazodone and drugs metabolized by this isoenzyme are unlikely.

Because of nefazodone's high degree of binding to plasma proteins, concurrent administration with another highly protein-bound medication may displace that agent and cause increased free concentrations of that agent, potentially resulting in adverse effects. Conversely, displacement of nefazodone by other highly protein-bound medications may result in adverse effects.

Combinations containing any of the following medications, depending on the amount present, may also interact with this medication.

Alcohol or
CNS-active medications
(although nefazodone did not potentiate the cognitive and psychomotor effects of alcohol in normal subjects, the concomitant use of nefazodone with alcohol in depressed patients is not advised)
(the use of nefazodone in combination with other CNS-active agents has not been systematically evaluated; caution is advised)

» Alprazolam or
» Triazolam
(triazolobenzodiazepines metabolized by CYP3A4 have demonstrated significantly increased plasma concentrations when administered concomitantly with nefazodone; initial alprazolam dosage should be reduced by 50%; initial triazolam dosage should be reduced by 75%, and many patients [e.g., the elderly] should not receive triazolam and nefazodone concurrently; coadministration of nefazodone potentiated the effects of triazolam on psychomotor performance tests)

Antihypertensives
(potential hypotensive effects of these medications can enhance hypotensive effects of nefazodone)

» Astemizole or
» Cisapride or
» Terfenadine
(as an inhibitor of CYP3A4, nefazodone can block the metabolism of these medications, resulting in increased plasma concentrations, which are associated with QT prolongation; rare cases of cardiovascular adverse effects, including death, principally due to *torsades de pointes*, have been reported with other inhibitors of CYP3A4; concomitant use with nefazodone is **contraindicated**)

Digoxin
(coadministration of nefazodone and digoxin to male volunteers who were phenotyped as extensive metabolizers of CYP2D6 substrates resulted in elevated plasma concentrations of digoxin; because of digoxin's narrow therapeutic index, caution should be exercised and monitoring of digoxin plasma concentrations is recommended)

Haloperidol
(concomitant administration of a single oral 5-mg dose of haloperidol with nefazodone [200 mg twice a day] at steady-state resulted in a 35% decrease in apparent clearance of haloperidol with no significant increase in peak concentrations or time to peak concentration; pharmacodynamic effects of haloperidol were generally not altered significantly; the clinical significance of decreased clearance is unknown, but dosage adjustments of haloperidol may be necessary during coadministration)

» Monoamine oxidase (MAO) inhibitors
(serious and sometimes fatal reactions have occurred in patients receiving an MAO inhibitor in combination with antidepressants with pharmacological properties similar to those of nefazodone; reactions have included hyperthermia, rigidity, myoclonus, autonomic instability with possible rapid fluctuations of vital signs, and mental status changes including extreme agitation progressing to delirium and coma; some cases presented with features resembling neuroleptic malignant syndrome, such as severe hyperthermia and seizures, sometimes fatal)
(the effects of nefazodone combined with MAO inhibitors have not been evaluated in humans or animals; however, because nefazodone is an inhibitor of both serotonin and norepinephrine reuptake, concomitant use is not recommended; in addition, at least 14 days should elapse between discontinuation of an MAO inhibitor and initiation of therapy with nefazodone; at least 7 days should elapse between discontinuation of nefazodone and initiation of therapy with an MAO inhibitor)

Propranolol
(coadministration of propranolol and nefazodone to healthy male volunteers [3 poor and 15 extensive CYP2D6 metabolizers] resulted in significant decreases in AUC and $C_{max}$ of propranolol and in $C_{max}$ of the metabolite 4-hydroxypropranolol; the kinetics of nefazodone, HO-NEF, and the triazole-dione metabolite were unaffected; however, the peak and nadir plasma concentrations and AUC of mCPP were increased; no change in the initial dose of either drug is necessary, and dosage adjustments should be made on the basis of clinical response)

**Laboratory value alterations**
The following have been selected on the basis of their potential clinical significance (possible effect in parentheses where appropriate)—not necessarily inclusive (» = major clinical significance):

With diagnostic test results
Electrocardiogram (ECG)
(during premarketing studies, a statistically significant difference in the incidence of sinus bradycardia was observed in 1.5% of patients receiving nefazodone as compared with 0.4% of patients receiving placebo who met the defined criteria of a potentially important decrease in heart rate: ≤ 50 bpm and a decrease of ≥ 15 bpm; there was no obvious clinical significance of the observed changes in these patients)

With physiology/laboratory test values
Hematocrit
(during premarketing studies, a potentially important decrease in hematocrit [≤ 37% in males or ≤ 32% in females] was reported in

2.8% of patients receiving nefazodone as compared to 1.5% of patients receiving placebo; decreases in hematocrit, presumably dilutional, have been reported with other medications that block alpha$_1$-adrenergic receptors; there was no apparent clinical significance of the observed changes in these patients)

**Medical considerations/Contraindications**
The medical considerations/contraindications included have been selected on the basis of their potential clinical significance (reasons given in parentheses where appropriate)—not necessarily inclusive (» = major clinical significance).

*Risk-benefit should be considered when the following medical problems exist:*
» Cardiovascular disease, including angina, ischemic stroke, or history of myocardial infarction or
» Cerebrovascular disease
  (may be exacerbated by potential hypotensive effects of nefazodone)
» Dehydration or
» Hypovolemia
  (nefazodone-induced hypotension may be exacerbated)
  Drug abuse or dependence, or history of
  (patients with a history of drug abuse should be observed closely for signs of misuse or abuse, as with any new central nervous system [CNS] drug)
» Mania or hypomania, history of
  (condition may be activated)
» Seizures, history of
  (although not documented to occur with nefazodone, as with other antidepressants, the condition potentially may be exacerbated)
» Sensitivity to nefazodone or other phenylpiperazine antidepressants

**Patient monitoring**
The following may be especially important in patient monitoring (other tests may be warranted in some patients, depending on condition; » = major clinical significance):
  Careful supervision of depressed patients with suicidal tendencies
  (recommended especially during early treatment phase before peak effectiveness of nefazodone is achieved; prescribing the smallest number of tablets necessary for good patient management is recommended to decrease the risk of overdose)

## Side/Adverse Effects

Note: Although priapism has not been reported in premarketing studies with nefazodone, it has been reported with a structurally related antidepressant, trazodone. If priapism occurs, the medication should be immediately discontinued and the physician consulted. If the condition persists for longer than 24 hours, a urologist should be consulted to determine appropriate management.

The following side/adverse effects have been selected on the basis of their potential clinical significance (possible signs and symptoms in parentheses where appropriate)—not necessarily inclusive:

**Those indicating need for medical attention**
Incidence more frequent
  *Abnormal gait or ataxia* (clumsiness or unsteadiness); *abnormal vision, including blurred vision; scotoma; visual trails; or visual field defects* (changes in vision); *hypotension or postural hypotension* (lightheadedness or fainting); *skin rash or itching; tinnitus* (ringing in the ears)
Note: *Abnormal vision* and *tinnitus* appear to be dose-related.
Incidence less frequent
  *Bronchitis* (shortness of breath, tightness in chest, or wheezing); *dyspnea* (troubled breathing); *eye pain; gastroenteritis* (diarrhea; nausea; stomach pain)
Incidence rare
  *Allergic reactions, including photosensitivity* (increased sensitivity to sun); *facial edema* (swelling of face); *and urticaria* (hives); *anemia* (unusual tiredness or weakness); *arthritis, bursitis, tenosynovitis, or muscle stiffness* (joint or muscle pain or stiffness); *asthma; cardiovascular effects, including angina pectoris* (chest pain); *hypertension; syncope* (fainting); *or tachycardia* (fast heartbeat); *CNS effects, including abnormal thinking; apathy; decreased concentration; depersonalization; derealization; hostility or paranoid reaction* (mood or mental changes); *dysarthria* (problems in speaking); *euphoria* (unusual feeling of well-being); *hallucinations* (seeing, hearing, or feeling things that are not there); *mania or hypomania* (talking, feeling, and acting with excitement and activity you cannot control); *neuralgia* (nerve pain); *or twitching; ear pain or hyperacusis* (increased sense of hearing); *ecchymosis* (unusual bleeding or bruising); *eye problems, including dryness of eyes; abnormality of accommodation* (blurred vision); *diplopia* (double vision); *conjunctivitis or keratoconjunctivitis* (red or irritated eyes); *mydriasis* (large pupils); *photophobia* (sensitivity of eyes to light); *gout* (joint pain; lower back or side, or stomach pain); *leukopenia* (fever, chills, or sore throat); *lymphadenopathy* (swollen glands); *menstrual problems, including amenorrhea; menorrhagia; metrorrhagia; or vaginal hemorrhage* (menstrual changes); *mouth ulcers or stomatitis* (irritation or soreness of mouth); *pelvic pain; rectal hemorrhage* (bleeding from the rectum); *sexual dysfunction, including increased or decreased libido; impotence; or abnormal ejaculation* (change in sexual desire or performance); *urinary effects, including cystitis; urinary urgency; polyuria; hematuria; nocturia; urinary incontinence* (problems with urination); *or kidney calculus* (kidney stones)

**Those indicating need for medical attention only if they continue or are bothersome**
Incidence more frequent
  *Abnormal dreams; agitation; confusion; constipation; diarrhea; dizziness; drowsiness; dryness of mouth; dyspepsia* (heartburn); *fever or chills; flushing or a feeling of warmth; headache; increased appetite; increased cough; insomnia* (trouble in sleeping); *memory impairment; nausea; paresthesias* (tingling, burning, or prickly sensations); *peripheral edema* (swelling of arms or legs); *pharyngitis* (sore throat); *tremor; vomiting*
Note: *Confusion, constipation, dizziness, drowsiness,* and *nausea* are dose-related.
Incidence less frequent
  *Arthralgia* (joint pain); *breast pain; increased thirst*

## Overdose

For more information on the management of overdose or unintentional ingestion, **contact a Poison Control Center** (see *Poison Control Center Listing*).

**Clinical effects of overdose**
The following effects have been selected on the basis of their potential clinical significance (possible signs and symptoms in parentheses where appropriate)—not necessarily inclusive:
Acute effects
  *Hypotension; nausea; somnolence; vomiting*
Note: Overdosage of nefazodone may cause an increase in incidence or severity of any of the reported adverse reactions.

**Treatment of overdose**
Note: The possibility of multiple drug involvement should be considered in managing overdose.
  There is no specific antidote for nefazodone. Treatment is essentially symptomatic and supportive.
  To decrease absorption—Gastric lavage should be initiated in any patient suspected of having taken an overdose of nefazodone.
  Supportive care—Patients in whom intentional overdose is known or suspected should be referred for psychiatric consultation.

## Patient Consultation

In providing consultation, consider emphasizing the following selected information (» = major clinical significance):

**Before using this medication**
» Conditions affecting use, especially:
  Sensitivity to nefazodone or trazodone
  Pregnancy—In studies in rats, increased early pup mortality was seen at a dose approximately five times the maximum human dose, and decreased pup weights were seen at this and lower doses, when dosing began during pregnancy and continued until weaning; the cause of these deaths is unknown
  Contraindicated medications
    Astemizole, cisapride, and terfenadine
  Other medications, especially alprazolam, monoamine oxidase (MAO) inhibitors, and triazolam
  Other medical problems, especially cardiovascular or cerebrovascular disease, dehydration or hypovolemia, history of mania or hypomania, or history of seizures

**Proper use of this medication**
» Compliance with therapy; not taking more or less medicine than prescribed
» Several weeks of treatment may be required before antidepressant effects are achieved

» Proper dosing
  Missed dose: Taking as soon as possible; continuing on regular schedule with next dose; not doubling doses
» Proper storage

**Precautions while using this medication**
Regular visits to physician to check progress of therapy
» Not taking astemizole, cisapride, or terfenadine because of possible life-threatening cardiac arrhythmias
» Not taking an MAO inhibitor with or less than 7 days after taking nefazodone; not taking nefazodone less than 14 days after taking an MAO inhibitor
» Avoiding use of alcoholic beverages; not taking other CNS-active agents unless prescribed by physician
» Possible blurred vision, drowsiness, impairment of judgment, thinking, or motor skills; caution when driving or doing jobs requiring alertness
» Possible dizziness or lightheadedness; caution when getting up suddenly from a lying or sitting position
» Possible dryness of mouth; using sugarless gum or candy, ice, or saliva substitute for relief; checking with physician or dentist if dry mouth continues for more than 2 weeks

**Side/adverse effects**
Signs of potential side effects, especially abnormal gait or ataxia; abnormal vision; hypotension or postural hypotension; skin rash or itching; tinnitus; bronchitis; dyspnea; eye pain; gastroenteritis; allergic reactions; anemia; arthritis, bursitis, tenosynovitis, or muscle stiffness; asthma; cardiovascular effects; CNS effects; ear pain or hyperacusis; ecchymosis; eye problems; gout; leukopenia; lymphadenopathy; menstrual problems; mouth ulcers or stomatitis; pelvic pain; rectal hemorrhage; sexual dysfunction; and urinary effects

## General Dosing Information

There is no body of evidence from controlled trials to indicate how long a depressed patient should be treated with nefazodone. It is generally agreed, however, that pharmacological treatment for acute episodes of depression should continue for up to six months or longer. It is unknown whether the dose of antidepressant needed to induce remission is identical to the dose needed to maintain euthymia.

Potentially suicidal patients should not have access to large quantities of this medication since depressed patients, particularly those who may use alcohol excessively, may continue to exhibit suicidal tendencies until significant improvement occurs. Some clinicians recommend that the patient be supplied with the smallest quantity of medication necessary for satisfactory patient management.

Activation of hypomania or mania has been reported in depressed patients treated with nefazodone.

## Oral Dosage Forms

### NEFAZODONE HYDROCHLORIDE TABLETS

**Usual adult dose**
Antidepressant—
Oral, initially 200 mg a day, administered in two divided doses. The dosage may be increased, as needed and tolerated, in increments of 100 to 200 mg a day at intervals of no less than one week. The effective dosage range in clinical trials was generally 300 to 600 mg a day.

Note: For dosage for debilitated patients, see *Usual geriatric dose*.

**Usual pediatric dose**
Safety and efficacy in children up to 18 years of age have not been established.

**Usual geriatric dose**
Antidepressant—
Oral, initially 100 mg a day administered in two divided doses. Since these patients may have reduced nefazodone clearance and/or increased sensitivity to the CNS side effects, the subsequent titration rate of nefazodone dosage may need to be modified. Final dosage determination should be based on the patient's clinical response; since steady-state plasma levels do not change with age, the target dose may be similar in healthy younger and older patients.

**Strength(s) usually available**
U.S.—
  50 mg (Rx) [*Serzone* (microcrystalline cellulose; povidone; sodium starch glycolate; colloidal silicon dioxide; magnesium stearate; iron oxides)].
  100 mg (Rx) [*Serzone* (scored; microcrystalline cellulose; povidone; sodium starch glycolate; colloidal silicon dioxide; magnesium stearate; iron oxides)].
  150 mg (Rx) [*Serzone* (scored; microcrystalline cellulose; povidone; sodium starch glycolate; colloidal silicon dioxide; magnesium stearate; iron oxides)].
  200 mg (Rx) [*Serzone* (microcrystalline cellulose; povidone; sodium starch glycolate; colloidal silicon dioxide; magnesium stearate; iron oxides)].
  250 mg (Rx) [*Serzone* (microcrystalline cellulose; povidone; sodium starch glycolate; colloidal silicon dioxide; magnesium stearate; iron oxides)].

**Packaging and storage**
Store below 40 °C (104 °F) unless otherwise specified by manufacturer. Dispense in a tight container.

**Auxiliary labeling**
• Avoid alcoholic beverages.
• May cause dizziness or drowsiness.

Developed: 09/27/95
Interim revision: 08/07/98; 08/14/98

---

# NELFINAVIR Systemic—INTRODUCTORY VERSION

VA CLASSIFICATION (Primary): AM803
Commonly used brand name(s): *Viracept*.
Note: For a listing of dosage forms and brand names by country availability, see *Dosage Forms* section(s).

## Category
Antiviral (systemic).

## Indications

**General considerations**
Nelfinavir is a human immunodeficiency virus (HIV) protease inhibitor. Cross-resistance between nelfinavir and reverse transcriptase inhibitors is unlikely because different enzyme targets are involved. Clinical HIV isolates exhibiting zidovudine or pyridinone resistance retain *in vitro* susceptibility to nelfinavir. The potential for cross-resistance between nelfinavir and other protease inhibitors has not been fully explored. A clinical HIV isolate exhibiting reduced susceptibility to saquinavir (sevenfold) did not show reduced susceptibility to nelfinavir. However, several isolates exhibiting ritonavir resistance (eight- to one hundred thirteenfold) were also less sensitive to nelfinavir (five- to fortyfold). Therapy with nelfinavir (ranging from 2 to 52 weeks) is associated with reduced sensitivity to nelfinavir, ranging from a five- to a ninety-threefold loss of sensitivity in *in vitro* phenotypic assays. The most frequent site of mutation associated with reduced nelfinavir sensitivity is codon 30. After 12 to 16 weeks of therapy, the incidence of mutation at this site was 56% in patients receiving nelfinavir monotherapy and 6% in patients receiving triple therapy with nelfinavir, lamivudine, and zidovudine. The clinical relevance of phenotypic and genotypic changes in the virus associated with nelfinavir therapy has not been established.

**Accepted**
Human immunodeficiency virus (HIV) infection (treatment)—Nelfinavir is indicated in the treatment of HIV infection when antiretroviral therapy is warranted.

## Pharmacology/Pharmacokinetics

Note: No substantial differences were observed between the pharmacokinetic properties of nelfinavir in healthy volunteers and in patients infected with human immunodeficiency virus (HIV).

**Physicochemical characteristics**
Molecular weight—Nelfinavir: 567.79.
Nelfinavir mesylate: 663.9.

### Mechanism of action/Effect
Nelfinavir inhibits HIV type 1 protease. HIV protease cleaves the viral precursor proteins gag and pol, which are required to produce mature, infectious virus particles. Inhibition of HIV protease results in the production of immature, noninfectious virus particles.

### Absorption
Maximum plasma concentration and area under the plasma concentration–time curve (AUC) values were two to three times higher under fed conditions than under fasting conditions.

### Distribution
Apparent $Vol_D$—2 to 7 liters per kilogram.

### Protein binding
Very high (> 98%).

### Biotransformation
Following a single oral 750-mg dose, 82 to 86% of the total plasma nelfinavir remains unchanged; one major and several minor metabolites are found in plasma; the major oxidative metabolite has *in vitro* antiviral activity comparable to that of the parent drug. Nelfinavir is metabolized *in vitro* by multiple cytochrome P450 isoforms, including CYP3A.

### Half-life
Terminal half-life in plasma—3.5 to 5 hours.

### Time to peak concentration
Following single and multiple oral doses of 500 to 750 mg with food—2 to 4 hours.

### Peak plasma concentration
Following multiple dosing with 750 mg three times a day for 28 days (steady state)—Average, 3 to 4 mcg per mL.

### Elimination
Fecal—87% of an oral 750-mg dose is recovered in feces; 22% of this portion consists of unchanged nelfinavir, while 78% of this portion consists of numerous oxidative metabolites.

Renal—1 to 2% of an oral 750-mg dose is recovered in urine; unchanged nelfinavir is the major component.

## Precautions to Consider

### Carcinogenicity
Studies have not been done.

### Mutagenicity
Nelfinavir is not mutagenic *in vitro* in the Ames test, the mouse lymphoma assay, or in human lymphocytes, or *in vivo* in the rat micronucleus assay.

### Pregnancy/Reproduction
Fertility—Nelfinavir did not affect mating or fertility in male or female rats; reproductive performance of offspring born to female rats that had been exposed to nelfinavir from midpregnancy through lactation also was not affected.

Pregnancy—Adequate and well-controlled studies have not been done in humans.

In pregnant rats, nelfinavir was not maternally toxic when administered in doses that resulted in systemic exposure (based on the steady-state area under the plasma concentration–time curve [AUC]) comparable to that observed in humans receiving the recommended therapeutic dose. Exposure of female rats to nelfinavir from midpregnancy through lactation had no effect on the survival, growth, or development of the offspring to weaning. In pregnant rabbits, fetal development was not affected by administration of nelfinavir at doses up to the level at which a slight decrease in maternal body weight was observed; however, even at the highest dose evaluated, systemic exposure in rabbits was significantly lower than comparable human exposure.

FDA Pregnancy Category B.

### Breast-feeding
It is not known whether nelfinavir is distributed into breast milk. However, the U.S. Public Health Service Centers for Disease Control and Prevention advises HIV-infected women not to breast-feed, to avoid postnatal transmission of HIV to an uninfected child.

Nelfinavir is distributed into milk in rats.

### Pediatrics
Nelfinavir has been studied in one open-label, uncontrolled trial in pediatric patients ranging from 2 to 13 years of age; the adverse event profile observed during the pediatric clinical trial with nelfinavir was similar to that observed in adult patients.

The safety, effectiveness, and pharmacokinetics of nelfinavir have not been studied in patients up to 2 years of age.

### Geriatrics
No information is available on the relationship of age to the effects of nelfinavir in geriatric patients.

### Drug interactions and/or related problems
The following drug interactions and/or related problems have been selected on the basis of their potential clinical significance (possible mechanism in parentheses where appropriate)—not necessarily inclusive (» = major clinical significance):

Note: Based on known metabolic profiles of these agents, clinically significant medication interactions are not expected between nelfinavir and azithromycin, clarithromycin, dapsone, erythromycin, fluconazole, itraconazole, or sulfamethoxazole/trimethoprim.

It is recommended that nelfinavir be taken with food, and that didanosine be taken on an empty stomach. Therefore, nelfinavir should be taken more than 2 hours before or 1 hour after didanosine is taken.

Combinations containing any of the following medications, depending on the amount present, may also interact with this medication.

» Amiodarone or
» Astemizole or
» Cisapride or
» Ergot derivatives or
» Midazolam or
» Quinidine or
» Terfenadine or
» Triazolam
(competition for the cytochrome P450 enzyme CYP3A by nelfinavir may inhibit the metabolism of these medications and create the potential for serious and/or life-threatening cardiac arrhythmias or prolonged sedation; concurrent use is not recommended)

Carbamazepine or
Phenobarbital or
Phenytoin
(concurrent use may cause a decrease in the plasma concentration of nelfinavir)

Indinavir
(concurrent use causes an 83% increase in the AUC of nelfinavir; the AUC for indinavir increases by 51%; the safety of this combination has not been established)

Ketoconazole
(concurrent use causes a 35% increase in the AUC of nelfinavir; no dose adjustment is needed)

Lamivudine
(concurrent use causes a 10% increase in the AUC of lamivudine)

Oral contraceptives, such as:
» Ethinyl estradiol or
» Norethindrone
(concurrent administration with nelfinavir causes a decrease in the plasma concentrations of these medications; alternate or additional contraceptive measures should be used)

» Rifabutin
(concurrent use causes a 32% decrease in the AUC of nelfinavir; the AUC for rifabutin increases by 207%; it is recommended that the dose of rifabutin be reduced to one half the usual dose when administered concurrently with nelfinavir)

» Rifampin
(concurrent use causes an 82% decrease in the AUC of nelfinavir; concurrent use is not recommended)

Ritonavir
(concurrent use causes a 152% increase in the AUC of nelfinavir; the safety of this combination has not been established)

Saquinavir
(concurrent use causes an 18% increase in the AUC of nelfinavir; the AUC for saquinavir increases by 392%; no dose adjustments are needed)

Zidovudine
(concurrent use causes a 35% decrease in the AUC of zidovudine; no dose adjustments are needed)

### Medical considerations/Contraindications
The medical considerations/contraindications included have been selected on the basis of their potential clinical significance (reasons given in parentheses where appropriate)—not necessarily inclusive (» = major clinical significance).

*Except under special circumstances, this medication should not be used when the following medical problems exist:*
» Hypersensitivity to nelfinavir
» Hepatic impairment
(nelfinavir is metabolized primarily by the liver; caution should be exercised when administering nelfinavir to patients with hepatic impairment)

*Risk-benefit should be considered when the following medical problem exists:*
Phenylketonuria
(the oral powder form of nelfinavir contains 11.2 grams of phenylalanine per gram of powder)

**Patient monitoring**
The following may be especially important in patient monitoring (other tests may be warranted in some patients, depending on condition; » = major clinical significance):
Blood glucose determinations
(development of hyperglycemia or diabetes may be associated with the use of protease inhibitors; close monitoring of patient glucose concentrations is recommended; new cases of diabetes or hyperglycemia that might be associated with use of protease inhibitors should be reported to the FDA or the pharmaceutical manufacturer)

## Side/Adverse Effects

Note: There have been reports of increased bleeding, including spontaneous skin hematomas and hemarthrosis, in HIV-infected patients with hemophilia type A or B who are receiving protease inhibitor therapy. A causal relationship has not been established.

The following side/adverse effects have been selected on the basis of their potential clinical significance (possible signs and symptoms in parentheses where appropriate)—not necessarily inclusive:

**Those indicating need for medical attention**
*Diabetes, or hyperglycemia* (dry or itchy skin; fatigue; hunger, increased; thirst, increased; unexplained weight loss; urination, increased); *ketoacidosis* (confusion; dehydration; fruity mouth odor; nausea; vomiting; weight loss)

**Those indicating need for medical attention only if they continue or are bothersome**
Incidence more frequent
*Diarrhea*
Incidence less frequent
*Flatulence* (intestinal gas); *nausea; skin rash*

## Overdose

For specific information on the agents used in the management of Nelfinavir overdose, see:
• *Charcoal, Activated (Oral-Local)* monograph.

For more information on the management of overdose or unintentional ingestion, **contact a Poison Control Center** (see *Poison Control Center Listing*).

**Treatment of overdose**
There is no specific antidote for overdose with nelfinavir.
To decrease absorption—Activated charcoal may be used to aid removal of unabsorbed nelfinavir.
To enhance elimination—Emesis or gastric lavage may be used.
Supportive care—Patients in whom intentional overdose is confirmed or suspected should be referred for psychiatric consultation.

## Patient Consultation

As an aid to patient consultation, refer to *Advice for the Patient, Nelfinavir (Systemic)—Introductory Version.*
In providing consultation, consider emphasizing the following selected information (» = major clinical significance):

**Before using this medication**
» Conditions affecting use, especially:
Hypersensitivity to nelfinavir
Breast-feeding—Not recommended for HIV-infected mothers
Use in children—Safety and efficacy have not been established in children up to 2 years of age
Other medications, especially amiodarone, astemizole, cisapride, ergot derivatives, ethinyl estradiol, midazolam, norethindrone, quinidine, rifabutin, rifampin, terfenadine, and triazolam
Other medical problems, especially hepatic impairment

**Proper use of this medication**
» Importance of taking nelfinavir with food
» Importance of not taking more medication than prescribed
» Compliance with full course of therapy
» Importance of not missing doses and of taking at evenly spaced times
Not sharing medication with others
» Proper dosing
Missed dose: Taking as soon as possible; not taking if almost time for next dose; not doubling doses
» Proper storage

**Precautions while using this medication**
» Not taking any other medications (prescription or nonprescription) without first consulting your physician
Taking nelfinavir more than 2 hours before or 1 hour after taking didanosine
» Using alternate or additional contraceptive measures if oral contraceptives are taken during nelfinavir therapy
» Regular visits to physician for blood tests and monitoring of blood glucose concentrations

**Side/adverse effects**
Signs of potential side effects, especially diabetes or hyperglycemia and ketoacidosis

## General Dosing Information

**Diet/Nutrition**
For optimal absorption, nelfinavir should be taken with food.
The oral powder form of nelfinavir contains 11.2 grams of phenylalanine per gram of powder.

**For treatment of adverse effects**
Recommended treatment consists of the following:
• Diarrhea may be controlled with nonprescription medications that slow gastrointestinal motility, such as loperamide.

## Oral Dosage Forms

Note: The dosing and strength of dosing forms available are expressed in terms of nelfinavir base (not the mesylate salt).

### NELFINAVIR MESYLATE ORAL POWDER

Note: Nelfinavir Mesylate Oral Powder contains 11.2 grams of phenylalanine per gram of powder.

**Usual adult and adolescent dose**
The oral powder usually is used only in children. See *Nelfinavir Mesylate Tablets.*

**Usual pediatric dose**
Human immunodeficiency virus (HIV) infection—
Children 2 to 13 years of age: Oral, 20 to 30 mg per kg of body weight three times a day with food.

| Body weight | | Pediatric dose to be administered three times a day | | |
|---|---|---|---|---|
| Kilograms | Pounds | Number of level 1-gram scoopfuls | Number of level teaspoonfuls | Number of tablets |
| 7 to < 8.5 | 15.5 to < 18.5 | 4 | 1 | — |
| 8.5 to < 10.5 | 18.5 to < 23 | 5 | 1 1/4 | — |
| 10.5 to < 12 | 23 to < 26.5 | 6 | 1 1/2 | — |
| 12 to < 14 | 26.5 to < 31 | 7 | 1 3/4 | — |
| 14 to < 16 | 31 to < 35 | 8 | 2 | — |
| 16 to < 18 | 35 to < 39.5 | 9 | 2 1/4 | — |
| 18 to < 23 | 39.5 to < 50.5 | 10 | 2 1/2 | 2 |
| ≥ 23 | ≥ 50.5 | 15 | 3 3/4 | 3 |

Children up to 2 years of age: Dosage has not been established.

**Usual pediatric prescribing limits**
750 mg three times a day.

**Strength(s) usually available**
U.S.—
50 mg (base) per gram (Rx) [*Viracept* (phenylalanine, 11.2 mg per gram)].

**Packaging and storage**
Store at 15 to 30 °C (59 to 86 °F), unless otherwise specified by manufacturer.

**Preparation of dosage form**
The oral powder form of nelfinavir may be mixed with a small amount of water, milk, formula, soy formula, soy milk, or dietary supplements. Acidic foods or juices (e.g., apple juice, applesauce, orange juice) are not recommended because the combination may result in a bitter taste. The oral powder should not be reconstituted with water in its original

container. Once mixed, the entire contents must be consumed to obtain the full dose.

**Stability**
Once reconstituted, nelfinavir should be taken within 6 hours.

**Auxiliary labeling**
• Take with food.

## NELFINAVIR MESYLATE TABLETS

**Usual adult and adolescent dose**
Human immunodeficiency virus (HIV) infection—
   Oral, 750 mg three times a day with food in combination with nucleoside analogs.

**Usual pediatric dose**
See *Nelfinavir Mesylate Oral Powder*.

**Usual geriatric dose**
See *Usual adult and adolescent dose*.

**Strength(s) usually available**
U.S.—
   250 mg (base) (Rx) [*Viracept*].

**Packaging and storage**
Store at 15 to 30 ºC (59 to 86 ºF), unless otherwise specified by manufacturer.

**Auxiliary labeling**
• Take with food.

Developed: 11/10/97

---

**NEOMYCIN**—See *Aminoglycosides (Systemic)*; *Neomycin (Ophthalmic)*; *Neomycin (Oral-Local)*; *Neomycin (Topical)*

---

**NEOMYCIN**—The *Neomycin (Ophthalmic)* monograph is not included in this published version of the USP DI database. Copies of the monograph are available on request from Micromedex, Inc. - Reprint Requests, 6200 S. Syracuse Way, Suite 300, Englewood, CO 80111; telephone (303) 486-6400; telefax (303) 486-6464; Email: USPDI@MDX.COM.

---

**NEOMYCIN**—The *(Neomycin Oral-Local)* monograph is not included in this published version of the USP DI database. Copies of the monograph are available on request from Micromedex, Inc. - Reprint Requests, 6200 S. Syracuse Way, Suite 300, Englewood, CO 80111; telephone (303) 486-6400; telefax (303) 486-6464; Email: USPDI@MDX.COM.

---

**NEOMYCIN**—The *Neomycin (Topical)* monograph is not included in this published version of the USP DI database. Copies of the monograph are available on request from Micromedex, Inc. - Reprint Requests, 6200 S. Syracuse Way, Suite 300, Englewood, CO 80111; telephone (303) 486-6400; telefax (303) 486-6464; Email: USPDI@MDX.COM.

---

**NEOMYCIN AND POLYMYXIN B**—The *Neomycin and Polymyxin B (Topical)* monograph is not included in this published version of the USP DI database. Copies of the monograph are available on request from Micromedex, Inc. - Reprint Requests, 6200 S. Syracuse Way, Suite 300, Englewood, CO 80111; telephone (303) 486-6400; telefax (303) 486-6464; Email: USPDI@MDX.COM.

---

**NEOMYCIN, POLYMYXIN B, AND BACITRACIN**—The *Neomycin, Polymyxin B, and Bacitracin (Ophthalmic)* monograph is not included in this published version of the USP DI database. Copies of the monograph are available on request from Micromedex, Inc. - Reprint Requests, 6200 S. Syracuse Way, Suite 300, Englewood, CO 80111; telephone (303) 486-6400; telefax (303) 486-6464; Email: USPDI@MDX.COM.

---

**NEOMYCIN, POLYMYXIN B, AND BACITRACIN**—The *Neomycin, Polymyxin B, and Bacitracin (Topical)* monograph is not included in this published version of the USP DI database. Copies of the monograph are available on request from Micromedex, Inc. - Reprint Requests, 6200 S. Syracuse Way, Suite 300, Englewood, CO 80111; telephone (303) 486-6400; telefax (303) 486-6464; Email: USPDI@MDX.COM.

---

**NEOMYCIN, POLYMYXIN B, AND GRAMICIDIN**—The *Neomycin, Polymyxin B, and Gramicidin (Ophthalmic)* monograph is not included in this published version of the USP DI database. Copies of the monograph are available on request from Micromedex, Inc. - Reprint Requests, 6200 S. Syracuse Way, Suite 300, Englewood, CO 80111; telephone (303) 486-6400; telefax (303) 486-6464; Email: USPDI@MDX.COM.

---

**NEOMYCIN, POLYMYXIN B, AND HYDROCORTISONE**—The *Neomycin, Polymyxin B, and Hydrocortisone (Ophthalmic)* monograph is not included in this published version of the USP DI database. Copies of the monograph are available on request from Micromedex, Inc. - Reprint Requests, 6200 S. Syracuse Way, Suite 300, Englewood, CO 80111; telephone (303) 486-6400; telefax (303) 486-6464; Email: USPDI@MDX.COM.

---

**NEOMYCIN, POLYMYXIN B, AND HYDROCORTISONE**—The *Neomycin, Polymyxin B, and Hydrocortisone (Otic)* monograph is not included in this published version of the USP DI database. Copies of the monograph are available on request from Micromedex, Inc. - Reprint Requests, 6200 S. Syracuse Way, Suite 300, Englewood, CO 80111; telephone (303) 486-6400; telefax (303) 486-6464; Email: USPDI@MDX.COM.

---

**NEOSTIGMINE**—See *Antimyasthenics (Systemic)*

---

**NETILMICIN**—See *Aminoglycosides (Systemic)*

---

# NEUROMUSCULAR BLOCKING AGENTS   Systemic

This monograph includes information on the following: 1) Atracurium Besylate; 2) Gallamine; 3) Metocurine; 4) Pancuronium; 5) Succinylcholine; 6) Tubocurarine; 7) Vecuronium

Note: See also the individual *Doxacurium (Systemic)*, *Mivacurium (Systemic)*, and *Pipecuronium (Systemic)* monographs.

INN:
   Atracurium Besylate—Atracurium besilate
   Succinylcholine—Suxamethonium

VA CLASSIFICATION (Primary/Secondary):
   Atracurium—MS300
   Gallamine—MS300
   Metocurine—MS300
   Pancuronium—MS300
   Succinylcholine—MS300
   Tubocurarine—MS300/DX900
   Vecuronium—MS300

Commonly used brand name(s): *Anectine*[5]; *Anectine Flo-Pack*[5]; *Flaxedil*[2]; *Metubine Iodide*[3]; *Norcuron*[7]; *Pavulon*[4]; *Quelicin*[5]; *Sucostrin*[5]; *Sucostrin High Potency*[5]; *Tracrium*[1]; *Tubarine*[6].

Other commonly used names are: Atracurium besilate [Atracurium Besylate], Curare [Tubocurarine], Suxamethonium [Succinylcholine].

Note: For a listing of dosage forms and brand names by country availability, see *Dosage Forms* section(s).

## Category
Neuromuscular blocking agent

Note: Depolarizing neuromuscular blocking agent—Succinylcholine.

Nondepolarizing neuromuscular blocking agent—Atracurium, Gallamine, Metocurine, Pancuronium, Tubocurarine, Vecuronium.

## Indications
Note: Bracketed information in the *Indications* section refers to uses that are not included in U.S. product labeling.

### Accepted
Muscle (skeletal) relaxation, for surgery—The neuromuscular blocking agents are indicated as adjuncts to anesthesia to induce skeletal muscle relaxation and to facilitate the management of patients undergoing mechanical ventilation.

Generally, a relatively short-acting nondepolarizing neuromuscular blocking agent or a single dose of the depolarizing neuromuscular blocking agent succinylcholine is used to facilitate endotracheal intubation. Continuous infusion of succinylcholine may be used for short surgical procedures requiring muscle relaxation. Nondepolarizing neuromuscular blocking agents, or, less commonly, succinylcholine administered by continuous infusion, are used for surgical procedures requiring an intermediate or prolonged duration of muscle relaxant action and to facilitate controlled ventilation.

Convulsions (treatment)—[Atracurium][1], [gallamine], metocurine, [pancuronium][1], [succinylcholine], tubocurarine, and [vecuronium][1] are indicated to reduce the intensity of muscle contractions of pharmacologically or electrically induced convulsions. Succinylcholine is generally preferred because of its short duration of action.

[Neuromuscular blocking agents are also used to decrease the muscular manifestations of persistent convulsions associated with toxic reactions to other medications.][1]

Myasthenia gravis (diagnosis)—Tubocurarine is indicated as a diagnostic aid for myasthenia gravis when the results of tests with neostigmine or edrophonium are inconclusive.

[1]Not included in Canadian product labeling.

## Pharmacology/Pharmacokinetics
See *Table 1*, page 2107 and *Table 2*, page 2107.

### Physicochemical characteristics
Molecular weight—
Atracurium besylate: 1243.49.
Gallamine triethiodide: 891.54.
Metocurine iodide: 906.64.
Pancuronium bromide: 732.68.
Succinylcholine chloride: 397.34 (dihydrate); 361.31 (anhydrous).
Tubocurarine chloride: 771.73 (pentahydrate); 681.65 (anhydrous).
Vecuronium bromide: 637.74.

### Mechanism of action/Effect
Neuromuscular blocking agents produce skeletal muscle paralysis by blocking neural transmission at the myoneural junction. The paralysis is selective initially and usually appears in the following muscles consecutively: levator muscles of eyelids, muscles of mastication, limb muscles, abdominal muscles, muscles of the glottis, and finally, the intercostal muscles and the diaphragm. Neuromuscular blocking agents have no known effect on consciousness or the pain threshold.

*Depolarizing neuromuscular blocking agents* compete with acetylcholine for the cholinergic receptors of the motor end plate and, like acetylcholine, combine with these receptors to produce depolarization; however, because of their high affinity for the cholinergic receptors and their resistance to acetylcholinesterase, they produce a more prolonged depolarization than does acetylcholine. This results initially in transient muscle contractions, usually visible as fasciculations, followed by inhibition of neuromuscular transmission. This type of neuromuscular block is not antagonized, and may even be enhanced, by anticholinesterase agents.

With prolonged or repeated use of depolarizing neuromuscular blocking agents, neuromuscular blockade resembling a nondepolarization block may be produced, resulting in prolonged respiratory depression or apnea.

*Nondepolarizing neuromuscular blocking agents* inhibit neuromuscular transmission by competing with acetylcholine for the cholinergic receptors of the motor end plate, thereby reducing the response of the end plate to acetylcholine. This type of neuromuscular block is usually antagonized by anticholinesterase agents.

### Other actions/effects
Tubocurarine and, to a lesser extent, atracurium, metocurine, and succinylcholine may cause histamine release. Gallamine, pancuronium, and vecuronium are least likely to cause histamine release.

Gallamine and pancuronium also have vagolytic activity.

## Precautions to Consider

### Cross-sensitivity and/or related problems
Patients sensitive to bromides may be sensitive to the bromide salts of pancuronium or vecuronium also.

Patients sensitive to iodine or iodides may be sensitive to the iodide salts of gallamine or metocurine also.

### Mutagenicity
For atracurium—Mutagenic activity was observed in the mouse lymphoma assay under conditions in which more than 80% of the treated cells were killed, i.e., a relatively strong effect with concentrations of 80 and 100 mcg per mL in the absence of metabolic activation and a much weaker effect with concentrations of 1.2 mg per mL or higher in the presence of metabolic activation. However, mutagenic activity has not been demonstrated in the Ames test or in a rat bone marrow cytogenicity assay.

### Pregnancy/Reproduction
Pregnancy—For atracurium: Adequate and well-controlled studies have not been done in humans. However, studies in rabbits (doses of 0.15 mg per kg of body weight (mg/kg) once a day or 0.1 mg/kg twice a day on Day 6 through Day 18 of gestation) have shown that atracurium causes visceral and skeletal anomalies. Also, postimplantation losses were greater in the group given 0.15 mg/kg once daily than in controls.

FDA Pregnancy Category C.

For gallamine: Problems in humans have not been documented. However, it has been determined that gallamine crosses the placenta.

For metocurine: Adequate and well-controlled studies have not been done in humans. However, it has been determined that metocurine crosses the placenta. Six minutes after intravenous injection in the mother, the fetal plasma concentration is approximately one-tenth of that in the mother.

FDA Pregnancy Category C.

For pancuronium: Studies have not been done in either animals or humans. However, problems in humans have not been documented.

FDA Pregnancy Category C.

For succinylcholine: Studies have not been done in humans. However, succinylcholine has been shown to cause intrauterine growth retardation and limb deformities resembling clubfoot when administered to the rat fetus between the 16th and 19th days of gestation or when injected in chick embryos from the 5th to 15th days of incubation.

For tubocurarine: Although adequate and well-controlled studies have not been done in humans, it has been determined that tubocurarine crosses the placenta. In animal studies, intramuscular injection of tubocurarine into the intercapsular region of the rat fetus on the 16th and 19th days of gestation caused growth retardation (incidence 21–23%) and limb deformity (incidence 7–8%), respectively. Tubocurarine has also caused growth retardation and limb deformities when injected into chick embryos from the 5th to the 15th day of incubation.

FDA Pregnancy Category C.

Tubocurarine may cause congenital fetal contractures if large and repeated doses are administered during the early months of pregnancy, possibly by immobilizing the fetus at the time of joint formation.

For vecuronium: Vecuronium crosses the placenta. Studies have not been done in either animals or humans.

FDA Pregnancy Category C.

Labor and delivery—Atracurium has been shown to cross the placenta in small quantities following administration to pregnant women for delivery by cesarean section. Although no adverse effects in the neonates were reported with atracurium, tubocurarine has been reported to cause diminished skeletal muscle activity leading to respiratory difficulty in the newborn when large and repeated doses are given near delivery. The possibility of neonatal respiratory depression or reduced skeletal muscle activity should be considered when any of these agents is used near delivery.

### Breast-feeding
Problems in humans have not been documented.

### Pediatrics
Specific products that contain benzyl alcohol, or that are diluted with bacteriostatic water for injection (which contains benzyl alcohol), should

not be administered to premature neonates because the preservative has been associated with a fatal "gasping syndrome" in these patients.

*For atracurium, gallamine, metocurine, pancuronium, and tubocurarine*—
Neonates up to 1 month of age may be more sensitive to the effects of nondepolarizing neuromuscular blocking agents. However, studies with atracurium have not been done in this age group.
No other pediatrics-specific problems have been documented in studies done to date.

*For succinylcholine*—
Pediatric patients may be especially susceptible to succinylcholine-induced myoglobinemia, myoglobinuria, and cardiac effects such as transient bradycardia, hypotension, cardiac arrhythmias, and/or sinus arrest.

*For vecuronium*—
Pediatric patients 7 weeks to 1 year of age are more sensitive to the effects of vecuronium (on a mg-per-kg basis) than are adults. Recovery time may be 1½ times that of adults.

### Geriatrics
Although appropriate studies with neuromuscular blocking agents have not been performed in the geriatric population, geriatrics-specific problems that would limit the usefulness of these medications in the elderly are not expected. However, elderly patients are more likely to have age-related renal function impairment, which may decrease the rate of clearance of gallamine, metocurine, pancuronium, succinylcholine, or tubocurarine from the body and thereby prolong their effects.

### Drug interactions and/or related problems
The following drug interactions and/or related problems have been selected on the basis of their potential clinical significance (possible mechanism in parentheses where appropriate)—not necessarily inclusive (» = major clinical significance):
See *Table 3*, page 2108.

### Laboratory value alterations
The following have been selected on the basis of their potential clinical significance (possible effect in parentheses where appropriate)—not necessarily inclusive (» = major clinical significance):

With physiology/laboratory test values

*For succinylcholine*
Serum potassium concentrations
(may be increased; increase may cause cardiac arrest or arrhythmias in patients with severe trauma, burns, or neurologic disorders; this effect may persist for several weeks or months after the initial trauma)

### Medical considerations/Contraindications
The medical considerations/contraindications included have been selected on the basis of their potential clinical significance (reasons given in parentheses where appropriate)—not necessarily inclusive (» = major clinical significance).
See *Table 4*, page 2111.

## Side/Adverse Effects
See *Table 5*, page 2112.

Note: Overdose of the neuromuscular blocking agents may result in prolonged respiratory depression or apnea and cardiovascular collapse.

## Overdose
For specific information on the agents used in the management of a neuromuscular blocking agent overdose, see:
- *Atropine* in *Anticholinergics/Antispasmodics (Systemic)* monograph;
- *Edrophonium (Systemic)* monograph;
- *Neostigmine* in *Antimyasthenics (Systemic)* monograph; and/or
- *Pyridostigmine* in *Antimyasthenics (Systemic)* monograph.

For more information on the management of overdose or unintentional ingestion, **contact a Poison Control Center** (see *Poison Control Center Listing*).

### Clinical effects of overdose
The following effects have been selected on the basis of their potential clinical significance (possible signs and symptoms in parentheses where appropriate)—not necessarily inclusive:

Acute
**Apnea; hypotension, severe; paralysis, prolonged; shock**

### Treatment of overdose
Specific treatment—
Administering anticholinesterase agents, such as edrophonium, neostigmine, or pyridostigmine, to antagonize the action of the nondepolarizing neuromuscular blocking agents. It is recommended that atropine or another suitable anticholinergic agent be administered prior to or concurrently with the antagonist to counteract its cholinergic side effects.

The depolarization block produced by succinylcholine is not antagonized by anticholinesterase agents such as edrophonium, neostigmine, and pyridostigmine. However, if succinylcholine has been administered over a prolonged period of time and the characteristic depolarization block has gradually changed to a nondepolarization block, as determined with a peripheral nerve stimulator, small doses of the anticholinesterase agent may be tried as an antagonist. If an anticholinesterase agent is used as an antagonist, it is recommended that atropine be administered prior to or concurrently with the antagonist to counteract its cholinergic side effects. Patients should be closely observed for at least 1 hour after reversal of nondepolarization block for possible return of muscle relaxation.

The antagonists are merely adjuncts to, and are not to be substituted for, the institution of measures to ensure adequate ventilation. Ventilatory assistance must be continued until the patient can maintain an adequate ventilatory exchange unassisted.

Monitoring—
Determining the nature and degree of the neuromuscular blockade, using a peripheral nerve stimulator.

Supportive care—
For apnea or prolonged paralysis—maintaining an adequate airway and administering manual or mechanical ventilation. Artificial respiration should be continued until complete recovery of normal respiration is assured.

For severe hypotension or shock—administering fluids and vasopressors as needed to treat.

## General Dosing Information
Neuromuscular blocking agents have no known effect on consciousness or the pain threshold; therefore, when used as an adjunct to surgery, the neuromuscular blocking agent should always be used with adequate anesthesia.

Since neuromuscular blocking agents may cause respiratory depression, they should be used only by those individuals experienced in the techniques of tracheal intubation, artificial respiration, and the administration of oxygen under positive pressure; facilities for these procedures should be immediately available.

The stated doses are intended as a guideline. Actual dosage must be individualized. To minimize the risk of overdosage, it is recommended that a peripheral nerve stimulator be used to monitor response to the neuromuscular blocking agents.

When nondepolarizing neuromuscular blocking agents are administered concurrently with potent general anesthetics such as enflurane, ether, isoflurane, methoxyflurane, or cyclopropane, the dosage of vecuronium should be decreased by 15%, and that of the other neuromuscular blocking agents should be reduced by 33 to 50%, or as determined with a peripheral nerve stimulator. Halothane causes less potentiation of neuromuscular blockade than either enflurane or isoflurane; therefore, a smaller reduction in the dosage of the neuromuscular blocking agent may be considered.

---

### *ATRACURIUM*

## Summary of Differences
Pharmacology/pharmacokinetics:
Mechanism of action/effect—
A nondepolarizing neuromuscular blocking agent.
Action is usually antagonized by anticholinesterase agents.
Other actions/effects—
May cause histamine release.
Protein-binding—
High.
Biotransformation—
In plasma, by ester hydrolysis and by Hofmann elimination; independent of hepatic or renal function or plasma pseudocholinesterase activity.
Half-life—
Distribution: 2–3.4 minutes.
Elimination: 20 minutes.
Onset of action—
Initial effect within 2 minutes; intubation conditions in 2–2.5 minutes.
Time to peak effect—
1.7–10 (average 3–5) minutes.

Duration of peak effect—
  20–35 minutes (balanced anesthesia); not changed by repeated dosing, provided that recovery from the prior dose begins before subsequent doses are given.
Time to recovery—
  From time of injection (balanced anesthesia):
    25% of twitch response achieved in 35–45 minutes and 95% of twitch response achieved in 60–70 minutes.
  From beginning of recovery—
    Balanced anesthesia—95% of twitch response achieved in 30 minutes.
    Inhalation anesthesia—95% of twitch response achieved in 40 minutes.
Elimination—
  Renal and biliary; less than 10% of the quantity excreted via the biliary route as unchanged atracurium.
Precautions:
  Pregnancy—
    Teratogenic and embryotoxic effects have been demonstrated in rabbits.
    Has been shown to cross the human placenta.
  Drug interactions and/or related problems—
    May increase incidence and severity of bradycardia and hypotension when used together with opioid analgesics; also, histamine release may be additive to that induced by many opioids.
    Use with digitalis glycosides not reported to cause cardiac arrhythmias or other undesirable cardiac effects.
    Effects may be enhanced or prolonged in patients receiving chronic lithium therapy.
    Effects not prolonged by cholinesterase inhibitors or hexafluorenium.
    Serious side effects with concurrent use of methotrimeprazine have not been reported.
    Additive effects with physostigmine have not been reported.
  Medical considerations/contraindications—
    Lower risk of problems than with gallamine or pancuronium if used in patients with cardiac conditions in which tachycardia would be undesirable.
    Efficacy not reduced by hepatic function impairment.
    Caution required in patients with pre-existing hypotension.
    Effects not prolonged in patients with renal function impairment or shock.
Side/adverse effects:
  Moderate risk of side effects associated with histamine release.
  More likely than other neuromuscular blocking agents to cause flushing of skin.
  Hives and laryngospasm have been reported.

## Additional Dosing Information

See also *General Dosing Information*.

Atracurium must be administered intravenously because intramuscular injection may cause tissue irritation and because there are no clinical data to support intramuscular administration.

A reduction in dosage and rate of administration is recommended for patients in whom histamine release may be hazardous. Also, patients with neuromuscular disease, severe electrolyte disorders, or carcinomatosis should receive lower doses because of potential enhancement of neuromuscular blockade or difficulties with reversal.

Bradycardia occurring during atracurium administration may be treated by intravenous administration of atropine.

## Parenteral Dosage Forms

### ATRACURIUM BESYLATE INJECTION

**Usual adult and adolescent dose**
Initial—
  Intravenous, 400 to 500 mcg (0.4 to 0.5 mg) per kg of body weight; or
    For patients in whom histamine release might be hazardous:
      Intravenous, 300 to 400 mcg (0.3 to 0.4 mg) per kg of body weight, administered slowly or in divided doses over a period of one minute.
    For administration after steady-state enflurane or isoflurane anesthesia has been established:
      Intravenous, 250 to 350 mcg (0.25 to 0.35 mg) per kg of body weight, or approximately one-third less than the usual initial dose. Halothane causes less potentiation of neuromuscular blockade; therefore, a smaller reduction in atracurium dosage may be considered.
    After succinylcholine-assisted endotracheal intubation under balanced anesthesia:
      Intravenous, 300 to 400 mcg (0.3 to 0.4 mg) per kg of body weight. If a potent inhalation anesthetic is being administered, even lower doses may be required. The effects of succinylcholine, as determined using a peripheral nerve stimulator, should be permitted to subside prior to administration of atracurium.
Supplemental—
  Intravenous, 80 to 100 mcg (0.08 to 0.1 mg) per kg of body weight twenty to forty-five minutes following the initial dose, then every fifteen to twenty-five minutes or as required by clinical conditions; or
  Intravenous infusion (initiated after recovery from the effects of an initial intravenous dose of 300 to 500 mcg [0.3 to 0.5 mg])
Balanced anesthesia—
  9 to 10 mcg (0.009 to 0.01 mg) per kg of body weight per minute until the desired degree of neuromuscular blockade is re-established, after which the rate of infusion may be adjusted according to clinical requirements and patient response. Most patients require 5 to 9 mcg (0.005 to 0.009 mg) per kg of body weight per minute, although some may require as little as 2 mcg (0.002 mg) per kg of body weight per minute and others may require as much as 15 mcg (0.015 mg) per kg of body weight per minute.
After steady-state enflurane or isoflurane anesthesia has been established—
  The required rate of infusion may be reduced by approximately 33%. A smaller reduction in the rate of infusion may be considered for patients anesthetized with halothane.
For cardiopulmonary bypass procedures in which hypothermia is induced—
  The required rate of infusion may be reduced by approximately 50%.

**Usual pediatric dose**
Neonates up to 1 month of age—
  Dosage has not been established.
Children 1 month to 2 years of age (under halothane anesthesia)—
  Intravenous, 300 to 400 mcg (0.3 to 0.4 mg) per kg of body weight, initially.
Children 2 years of age and over—
  See *Usual adult and adolescent dose*.
Note: Maintenance doses may be required somewhat more frequently than in adults.

**Strength(s) usually available**
U.S.—
  10 mg per mL (Rx) [*Tracrium* (benzyl alcohol [multiple-dose vials only]); GENERIC].
Canada—
  10 mg per mL (Rx) [*Tracrium;* GENERIC].

**Packaging and storage**
Store between 2 and 8 °C (36 and 46 °F), unless otherwise specified by manufacturer. Protect from freezing.

**Preparation of dosage form**
For intravenous infusion—Atracurium besylate injection may be diluted with 0.9% sodium chloride injection, 5% dextrose injection, or 5% dextrose in 0.9% sodium chloride injection. Lactated Ringer's injection should *not* be used (see *Incompatibilities,* below). A solution prepared by adding 2 mL of atracurium besylate injection (10 mg per mL) to 98 mL of diluent contains 200 mcg (0.2 mg) of atracurium besylate per mL; a solution prepared by adding 5 mL of atracurium besylate injection (10 mg per mL) to 95 mL of diluent contains 500 mcg (0.5 mg) per mL.

**Stability**
Intravenous infusion solutions prepared with 5% dextrose injection, 0.9% sodium chloride injection, or 5% dextrose in 0.9% sodium chloride injection may be stored in a refrigerator or at room temperature for up to 24 hours without significant loss of potency. Unused portions of such solutions should be discarded after 24 hours.
Atracurium besylate injection should be used within 14 days if stored at room temperature (25 °C [77 °F]), even if later refrigerated.

**Incompatibilities**
Alkaline solutions such as barbiturate injections should not be mixed in the same syringe, or administered simultaneously through the same intravenous needle, with atracurium. Alkaline solutions may change the pH of the acidic atracurium solution, resulting in inactivation of atracurium or precipitation of a free acid.
Spontaneous degradation of atracurium has been shown to occur more rapidly when the medication is diluted with lactated Ringer's injection than when the medication is diluted with 0.9% sodium chloride injection. Therefore, it is recommended that lactated Ringer's injection not be used to prepare intravenous infusion solutions containing atracurium.

## GALLAMINE

### Summary of Differences
Pharmacology/pharmacokinetics:
   Mechanism of action/effect—
      A nondepolarizing neuromuscular blocking agent.
      Action is usually antagonized by anticholinesterase agents.
   Other actions/effects—
      Has vagolytic activity.
      Less likely than most other neuromuscular blocking agents to cause histamine release.
   Biotransformation—
      Essentially none.
   Half-life—
      Distribution: 16 minutes.
      Elimination: 150 minutes.
   Onset of action—
      Initial effect within 1–2 minutes.
   Time to peak effect—
      3–5 minutes.
   Duration of peak effect—
      15–30 minutes; increased by repeated dosing.
   Elimination—
      Renal, almost completely as unchanged gallamine.
Precautions:
   Cross-sensitivity and/or related problems—
      Cross-sensitivity may occur in patients sensitive to iodine or iodides.
   Drug interactions and/or related problems—
      Vagolytic activity may decrease risk of opioid analgesic–induced bradycardia and/or hypotension, but may increase risk of tachycardia and/or hypertension in some patients.
      Use with digitalis glycosides not reported to cause cardiac arrhythmias or other undesirable cardiac effects.
      Effects may be enhanced or prolonged by beta-adrenergic blocking agents.
   Medical considerations/contraindications—
      More likely than most other neuromuscular blocking agents to cause problems in patients with cardiac conditions in which tachycardia would be undesirable.
      Less likely than other neuromuscular blocking agents to cause problems in patients for whom histamine release would be hazardous.
      Caution required in patients with pre-existing hypertension.
      Prolongation of effects in patients with renal function impairment or shock more likely and/or more severe than with other neuromuscular blocking agents.
Side/adverse effects:
   Side effects caused by histamine release have not been reported.
   More likely than other neuromuscular blocking agents to cause hypertension and/or tachycardia.

### Additional Dosing Information
See also *General Dosing Information*.

In usual doses, gallamine has a slightly shorter duration of action than tubocurarine; however, in very large doses, its duration of action may be longer.

### Parenteral Dosage Forms
#### GALLAMINE TRIETHIODIDE INJECTION USP
**Usual adult and adolescent dose**
Intravenous, initially 1 mg per kg of body weight, not to exceed 100 mg per dose; then 500 mcg (0.5 mg) to 1 mg per kg of body weight after an interval of thirty to forty minutes, if necessary, for prolonged procedures.

Note: A dose of 1 mg per kg of body weight produces a 50% reduction in respiratory minute volume; a dose of 1.5 mg per kg of body weight produces a 75% reduction in respiratory minute volume.

**Usual pediatric dose**
See *Usual adult and adolescent dose*.

Note: Caution in use is recommended, especially for patients weighing less than 5 kg.

**Strength(s) usually available**
U.S.—
   20 mg per mL (Rx) [*Flaxedil* (edetate disodium; sodium bisulfite)].
Canada—
   20 mg per mL (Rx) [*Flaxedil* (potassium metabisulfite; sodium sulfite)].

**Packaging and storage**
Store below 40 °C (104 °F), preferably between 15 and 30 °C (59 and 86 °F), unless otherwise specified by manufacturer. Protect from light. Protect from freezing.

## METOCURINE

### Summary of Differences
Pharmacology/pharmacokinetics:
   Mechanism of action/effect—
      A nondepolarizing neuromuscular blocking agent.
      Action is usually antagonized by anticholinesterase agents.
   Other actions/effects—
      May cause histamine release.
   Protein-binding—
      Moderate; primarily to beta and gamma globulins.
   Half-life—
      Distribution: 1.9 minutes.
      Elimination: 216 minutes.
   Onset of action—
      Initial effect within 1–4 minutes.
   Time to peak effect—
      1.5–10 (average 3–5) minutes.
   Duration of peak effect—
      35–60 minutes (maximum effect); average duration of relaxation 60 (range 25–90) minutes; increased by repeated dosing.
   Time to recovery:
      From time of injection—
         50% of twitch response achieved in >360 minutes.
   Elimination—
      Renal (50% within 48 hours as unchanged metocurine) and biliary (2% as unchanged metocurine).
Precautions:
   Cross-sensitivity and/or related problems—
      Cross-sensitivity may occur in patients sensitive to iodine or iodides.
   Drug interactions and/or related problems—
      May increase incidence and severity of bradycardia and hypotension when used together with opioid analgesics; also, histamine release may be additive to that induced by many opioids.
      Use with digitalis glycosides not reported to cause cardiac arrhythmias or other undesirable cardiac effects.
      Effects not prolonged by cholinesterase inhibitors or hexafluorenium.
      Serious side effects with concurrent use of methotrimeprazine have not been reported.
      Additive effects with physostigmine have not been reported.
   Medical considerations/contraindications—
      Caution required in patients with cardiovascular function impairment.
      Efficacy may be reduced by hepatic function impairment.
      Caution required in patients with pre-existing hypotension.
      Effects may be prolonged by renal function impairment or shock, but to a lesser extent than for gallamine.
Side/adverse effects:
   Moderate risk of side effects associated with histamine release.

### Additional Dosing Information
See also *General Dosing Information*.

Metocurine is approximately twice as potent as tubocurarine; 1 mg of metocurine may be expected to produce a therapeutic response comparable to that obtained with 1.8 mg of tubocurarine.

Rapid intravenous injection and/or large doses of metocurine may cause an increased release of histamine, resulting in hypotension and in decreased respiratory capacity due to bronchospasm combined with drug-induced paralysis of the respiratory muscles. Hypotension may also occur because of ganglionic blockade or as a complication of positive pressure respiration.

Intramuscular administration of metocurine iodide injection is not recommended.

### Parenteral Dosage Forms
#### METOCURINE IODIDE INJECTION USP
**Usual adult and adolescent dose**
Intravenous, 150 to 400 mcg (0.15 to 0.4 mg) per kg of body weight, administered over thirty to sixty seconds, initially. Supplemental doses of 500 mcg (0.5 mg) to 1 mg may be administered every thirty to ninety minutes as required.

Enfluorane or isoflurane anesthesia—A 33% to 50% reduction in dosage may be required. A reduction in dosage may also be required during halothane anesthesia.

In electroshock therapy—Intravenous, 2 to 3 mg (range, 1.75 to 5.5 mg).

**Usual pediatric dose**
Dosage has not been established.

**Strength(s) usually available**
U.S.—
 2 mg per mL (Rx) [*Metubine Iodide* (phenol); GENERIC].
Canada—
 2 mg per mL (Rx) [*Metubine Iodide* (phenol)].

**Packaging and storage**
Store below 40 °C (104 °F), preferably between 15 and 30 °C (59 and 86 °F), unless otherwise specified by manufacturer. Protect from freezing.

**Stability**
Metocurine iodide is unstable in alkaline solutions. When metocurine iodide injection is mixed with a barbiturate solution such as methohexital sodium or thiopental sodium, a precipitate may form because of the high pH of the barbiturate solution. Solutions containing barbiturates, meperidine, or morphine sulfate should not be administered from the same syringe as metocurine.

---

## *PANCURONIUM*

## Summary of Differences
Pharmacology/pharmacokinetics:
 Mechanism of action/effect—
  A nondepolarizing neuromuscular blocking agent.
  Action is usually antagonized by anticholinesterase agents.
 Other actions/effects—
  Has vagolytic activity.
  Less likely than most other neuromuscular blocking agents to cause histamine release.
 Protein-binding—
  Very low.
 Biotransformation—
  Hepatic, in small quantities.
 Half-life—
  Distribution: 10–13 minutes.
  Elimination: 114–116 minutes.
 Onset of action—
  Initial effect within 1 minute; intubation conditions in 2–3 minutes.
 Time to peak effect—
  3–4.5 minutes, depending on dose.
 Duration of peak effect—
  35–45 minutes; increased by repeated dosing.
 Time to recovery—
  From time of injection: 90% of twitch response achieved in <60 minutes.
 Elimination—
  Renal (about 80% as unchanged pancuronium); about 10% biliary (up to 10% as unchanged pancuronium).
Precautions:
 Cross-sensitivity and/or related problems—
  Cross-sensitivity may occur in patients sensitive to bromides.
 Drug interactions and/or related problems—
  Vagolytic activity may decrease risk of opioid analgesic–induced bradycardia and/or hypotension, but may increase risk of tachycardia and/or hypertension in some patients.
  Use with digitalis glycosides may cause cardiac arrhythmias or other undesirable cardiac effects.
  Effects may be enhanced or prolonged by beta-adrenergic blocking agents.
  Effects may be enhanced or prolonged in patients receiving chronic lithium therapy.
  Effects not prolonged by cholinesterase inhibitors or hexafluorenium.
  Serious side effects with concurrent use of methotrimeprazine have not been reported.
  Additive effects with physostigmine have not been reported.
  Effects may be decreased by hydrocortisone or prednisone.
 Medical considerations/contraindications—
  More likely than most other neuromuscular blocking agents to cause problems in patients with cardiac conditions in which tachycardia would be undesirable.
  Caution required in patients for whom histamine release would be hazardous.
  Effects may be prolonged by hepatic function impairment.
  Effects may be prolonged by renal function impairment, but to a lesser extent than for gallamine.
Side/adverse effects:
 Relatively low risk of side effects associated with histamine release.
 May cause itching of skin more frequently than other neuromuscular blocking agents.
 Excessive salivation has been reported.

## Additional Dosing Information
See also *General Dosing Information*.
Pancuronium is approximately 5 times as potent as tubocurarine.

## Parenteral Dosage Forms
### PANCURONIUM BROMIDE INJECTION

**Usual adult and adolescent dose**
Initial—
 Intravenous, 40 to 100 mcg (0.04 to 0.1 mg) per kg of body weight. Incremental doses starting at 10 mcg (0.01 mg) per kg of body weight may then be administered, generally every twenty to sixty minutes, the dosage being adjusted as needed.
For administration after steady-state enflurane or isoflurane anesthesia has been established and/or after succinylcholine-assisted endotracheal intubation—
 Intravenous, 40 mcg (0.04 mg) per kg of body weight, initially, then adjusted according to patient response.
For endotracheal intubation—
 Intravenous, 60 to 100 mcg (0.06 to 0.1 mg) per kg of body weight.

**Usual pediatric dose**
Neonates up to 1 month of age—
 Dosage must be individualized by the physician. Dosage may be based on the patient's response to a test dose of 20 mcg (0.02 mg) per kg of body weight.
Children 1 month of age and over—
 See *Usual adult and adolescent dose*.

**Strength(s) usually available**
U.S.—
 1 mg per mL (Rx) [*Pavulon* (benzyl alcohol); GENERIC].
 2 mg per mL (Rx) [*Pavulon* (benzyl alcohol); GENERIC].
Canada—
 1 mg per mL (Rx) [*Pavulon*].
 2 mg per mL (Rx) [*Pavulon*].

**Packaging and storage**
Store between 2 and 8 °C (36 and 46 °F), unless otherwise specified by manufacturer. Protect from freezing.

---

## *SUCCINYLCHOLINE*

## Summary of Differences
Pharmacology/pharmacokinetics:
 Mechanism of action/effect—
  A depolarizing neuromuscular blocking agent.
  Action not antagonized by anticholinesterase agents.
 Other actions/effects—
  May cause histamine release.
 Biotransformation—
  In plasma; rapidly hydrolyzed by pseudocholinesterase.
 Onset of action —
  Intravenous: Initial effect within 0.5–1 minute.
  Intramuscular: Initial effect within 3 minutes.
 Time to peak effect—
  Intravenous: 1–2 minutes.
 Duration of peak effect—
  Intravenous: 4–10 minutes.
  Intramuscular: 10–30 minutes.
 Elimination—
  Renal; about 10% as unchanged succinylcholine.
Precautions:
 Pediatrics—
  Pediatric patients may be especially susceptible to succinylcholine-induced myoglobinemia, myoglobinuria, and cardiac effects.
 Drug interactions and/or related problems—
  May increase incidence and severity of bradycardia and hypotension when used together with opioid analgesics; also, histamine release may be additive to that induced by many opioids.
  Potentiation of effect by hydrocarbon inhalation anesthetics less than for nondepolarizing neuromuscular blocking agents.

Effects not enhanced or prolonged by beta-adrenergic blocking agents.
Effects not reversed by calcium salts.
Effects prolonged by cholinesterase inhibitors or hexafluorenium.
Use with digitalis glycosides may cause cardiac arrhythmias or other undesirable cardiac effects.
Effects may be enhanced or prolonged in patients receiving chronic lithium therapy.
Serious side effects with concurrent use of methotrimeprazine have been reported.
Additive effects with physostigmine have been reported.
Effects may be enhanced by potassium-depleting medications.
Laboratory value alterations—
  Serum potassium concentration may be increased.
Medical considerations/contraindications—
  Caution required in patients with cardiovascular function impairment.
  Effects may be prolonged in patients with renal function impairment, but to a lesser extent than for gallamine.
  Caution also required in:
    Conditions that may be adversely affected by increased potassium concentrations (severe burns, digitalis toxicity or recent digitalization, degenerative or dystrophic neuromuscular disease, paraplegia, pre-existing hyperkalemia, spinal cord injury, severe trauma).
    Conditions that may lead to low plasma pseudocholinesterase activity (severe anemia, dehydration, exposure to neurotoxic insecticides or other cholinesterase inhibitors, severe hepatic disease or cirrhosis, malnutrition, pregnancy, recessive hereditary trait).
    Conditions that may be adversely affected by increase in intraocular pressure (open eye injury, glaucoma, ocular surgery).
    Fractures or muscle spasm.
    Malignant hyperthermia, history of in patient or close relative.
Side/adverse effects:
  Moderate risk of side effects associated with histamine release.
  More likely than other neuromuscular blocking agents to cause bradycardia or cardiac arrhythmias.
  Increased intraocular pressure, malignant hyperthermia, rhabdomyolysis leading to myoglobinemia and myoglobinuria, postoperative muscle pains and stiffness, and excessive salivation have been reported.

## Additional Dosing Information

See also *General Dosing Information*.

Succinylcholine is usually administered intravenously but may be administered intramuscularly if necessary.

When administered intramuscularly, the injection should be deep and high into the deltoid muscle.

An initial test dose of 10 mg may be administered to determine the sensitivity of the patient and recovery time.

Patients with low levels of pseudocholinesterase activity may require reduced doses, because they may be unusually sensitive to the effects of succinylcholine.

If low pseudocholinesterase activity is suspected, a test dose of 5 to 10 mg may be administered.

Premedication with atropine or scopolamine is recommended to prevent excessive salivation.

To reduce the severity of muscle fasciculations, a small dose of a nondepolarizing agent may be administered prior to administration of succinylcholine.

Following administration, succinylcholine may cause transient bradycardia accompanied by hypotension, cardiac arrhythmias, and possibly a short period of sinus arrest due to vagal stimulation, especially with repeated administration and in children. These effects may be inhibited by prior administration of atropine or thiopental sodium.

Succinylcholine may cause myoglobinemia and myoglobinuria, especially in children. Administration of small doses of tubocurarine prior to succinylcholine has been shown to decrease the incidence of myoglobinuria.

Repeated doses of succinylcholine may result in tachyphylaxis.

## Parenteral Dosage Forms

### SUCCINYLCHOLINE CHLORIDE INJECTION USP

**Usual adult and adolescent dose**
For short surgical procedures—
  Intravenous, usually 600 mcg (0.6 mg) (range 300 mcg [0.3 mg] to 1.1 mg) per kg of body weight, initially. Repeated doses may be administered, if necessary, calculated on the basis of response to the first dose.
  Intramuscular, 3 to 4 mg per kg of body weight, not to exceed a total dose of 150 mg.
For prolonged surgical procedures—
  Intravenous, initially 600 mcg (0.6 mg) to 1.1 mg per kg of body weight; subsequent doses to be individualized for maintaining degree of relaxation required.
  Note: Administration of repeated fractional doses is generally not recommended because of possible tachyphylaxis and prolonged apnea; continuous infusion is preferred for prolonged surgical procedures.
  Intravenous infusion, as a 0.1 to 0.2% solution in 5% dextrose injection, sodium chloride injection, or other appropriate diluent, administered at a rate of 500 mcg (0.5 mg) to 10 mg per minute, depending on patient response and degree of relaxation required, for up to one hour.
  Note: When succinylcholine is administered by infusion, careful monitoring of neuromuscular function with a peripheral nerve stimulator is recommended to avoid overdose and to detect development of a nondepolarizing block.
Electroshock therapy—
  Intravenous, 10 to 30 mg administered approximately one minute before the shock, although dosage must be individualized according to the size and physical condition of the patient.
  Intramuscular, up to 2.5 mg per kg of body weight, not to exceed a total dose of 150 mg.

**Usual pediatric dose**
Endotracheal intubation—
  Intramuscular, up to 2.5 mg per kg of body weight, not to exceed a total dose of 150 mg.
  Intravenous, 1 to 2 mg per kg of body weight. Repeated doses may be administered, if necessary, calculated on the basis of response to the first dose.
  Note: Administration of succinylcholine by continuous intravenous infusion is considered to be unsafe in neonates and children because of the risk of malignant hyperpyrexia.

**Strength(s) usually available**
U.S.—
  20 mg per mL (Rx) [*Anectine* (methylparaben); *Quelicin* (methylparaben; propylparaben); *Sucostrin* (methylparaben; propylparaben); GENERIC].
  50 mg per mL (Rx) [*Quelicin*].
  100 mg per mL (Rx) [*Sucostrin High Potency* (methylparaben; propylparaben)].
Canada—
  20 mg per mL (Rx) [*Anectine* (methylparaben [multiple-dose vials only]); *Quelicin* (methylparaben; propylparaben); GENERIC].
  100 mg per mL (Rx) [*Quelicin*].

**Packaging and storage**
Store between 2 and 8 °C (36 and 46 °F). Protect from freezing.

**Stability**
Do not use if the solution is not absolutely clear.
Only freshly prepared solutions of succinylcholine should be used.
The stability of diluted solutions may vary, depending on the specific product. See the manufacturer's prescribing information for product-specific information.
Succinylcholine is rapidly hydrolyzed, quickly loses potency, and may cause formation of a precipitate when mixed with alkaline solutions of other medications. Therefore, succinylcholine should not be mixed in the same syringe or administered simultaneously through the same needle with solutions of short-acting barbiturates such as thiopental sodium or other medications that have an alkaline pH. It should be injected separately.

### SUCCINYLCHOLINE CHLORIDE STERILE USP

**Usual adult and adolescent dose**
Intravenous infusion, as a 0.1 to 0.2% solution in 5% dextrose injection, sodium chloride injection, or other appropriate diluent, administered at a rate of 500 mcg (0.5 mg) to 10 mg per minute, depending on patient response and degree of relaxation required, for up to one hour.

Note: When succinylcholine is administered by infusion, careful monitoring of neuromuscular function with a peripheral nerve stimulator is recommended to avoid overdose and to detect development of a nondepolarizing block.

**Usual pediatric dose**
Use of succinylcholine by continuous intravenous infusion is not recommended, because of the risk of malignant hyperpyrexia.

**Size(s) usually available**
U.S.—
   500 mg (Rx) [*Anectine Flo-Pack*].
   1 gram (Rx) [*Anectine Flo-Pack*].
Canada—
   500 mg (Rx) [*Anectine Flo-Pack*].
   1 gram (Rx) [*Anectine Flo-Pack*].

**Packaging and storage**
Prior to reconstitution, store below 40 °C (104 °F), preferably between 15 and 30 °C (59 and 86 °F), unless otherwise specified by manufacturer.

**Preparation of dosage form**
For intravenous infusion, sterile succinylcholine chloride may be dissolved in 0.9% sodium chloride injection, 5% dextrose injection, or other appropriate infusion solution.

**Stability**
Only freshly prepared solutions of succinylcholine should be used.
The reconstituted solution should be used within 24 hours.
Succinylcholine is rapidly hydrolyzed, quickly loses potency, and may cause formation of a precipitate when mixed with alkaline solutions of other medications. Therefore, succinylcholine should not be mixed in the same syringe or administered simultaneously through the same needle with solutions of short-acting barbiturates such as thiopental sodium or other medications that have an alkaline pH. It should be injected separately.

---

## *TUBOCURARINE*

## Summary of Differences
Indications:
   Also indicated as a diagnostic aid for myasthenia gravis.
Pharmacology/pharmacokinetics:
   Mechanism of action/effect—
      A nondepolarizing neuromuscular blocking agent.
      Action is usually antagonized by anticholinesterase agents.
   Other actions/effects—
      Most likely of the neuromuscular blocking agents to cause histamine release.
   Protein-binding—
      Moderate.
   Biotransformation—
      Hepatic.
   Half-life—
      Distribution: 4.8–6.4 minutes.
      Elimination: 84–120 minutes.
   Onset of action—
      Intravenous: Initial effect within 1 minute.
      Intramuscular: Initial effect within 15–25 minutes.
   Time to peak effect—
      Intravenous: 2–5 minutes.
   Duration of peak effect—
      20–40 minutes; increased with repeated dosing.
   Time to recovery—
      From time of injection: 50% of twitch response achieved in 50 minutes and 95% of twitch response achieved in 74–90 minutes.
   Elimination—
      Renal (about 40% as unchanged tubocurarine) and biliary (about 12% as unchanged tubocurarine).
Precautions:
   Pregnancy—
      May cause congenital fetal contractures if large and repeated doses are administered during the early months of pregnancy.
      Also, diminished skeletal muscle activity of the newborn may occur if large and repeated doses are administered near delivery.
   Drug interactions and/or related problems—
      May increase incidence and severity of bradycardia and hypotension when used together with opioid analgesics; also, histamine release may be additive to that induced by many opioids.
      Use with digitalis glycosides not reported to cause cardiac arrhythmias or other undesirable cardiac effects.
      Effects not prolonged by cholinesterase inhibitors or hexafluorenium.
      Effects may be prolonged or enhanced by calcium salts.
      Serious side effects with concurrent use of methotrimeprazine have not been reported.
      Additive effects with physostigmine have not been reported.
   Medical considerations/contraindications—
      Caution required in patients with cardiovascular function impairment.
      Effects may be reduced by hepatic function impairment.
      Caution required in patients with pre-existing hypotension.
      Effects may be prolonged in patients with renal function impairment or shock, but to a lesser extent than for gallamine.
Side/adverse effects:
   Relatively high risk of side effects associated with histamine release.
   Decrease in blood pressure occurs more frequently than with other neuromuscular blocking agents.

## Additional Dosing Information
See also *General Dosing Information*.

Tubocurarine is usually administered intravenously as a sustained injection over a period of 1 to 1.5 minutes. It may also be administered intramuscularly, if necessary, but is slowly and irregularly absorbed.

Rapid intravenous injection and/or large doses of tubocurarine may cause an increased release of histamine, resulting in hypotension and in decreased respiratory capacity due to bronchospasm combined with drug-induced paralysis of the respiratory muscles. Hypotension may also occur because of ganglionic blockade or as a complication of positive pressure respiration.

## Parenteral Dosage Forms
### TUBOCURARINE CHLORIDE INJECTION USP
**Usual adult and adolescent dose**
Neuromuscular blocking agent—
   Adjunct to surgical anesthesia:
      Intramuscular or intravenous, 6 to 9 mg initially, then 3 to 4.5 mg in three to five minutes if necessary. For prolonged procedures, supplemental doses of 3 mg may be administered.
      Note: Dosage may generally be calculated on the basis of 165 mcg (0.165 mg) per kg of body weight.
   Aid to controlled respiration:
      Intravenous, initially 16.5 mcg (0.0165 mg) per kg of body weight, the subsequent doses being adjusted as needed.
   Electroshock therapy:
      Intravenous, 165 mcg (0.165 mg) per kg of body weight, administered over a period of thirty to ninety seconds.
      Note: Initially, a dose of 3 mg less than the calculated total dose should be used.
Diagnostic aid (myasthenia gravis)—
   Intravenous, 4 to 33 mcg (0.004 to 0.033 mg) per kg of body weight.
   Note: It is recommended that the test be terminated within two to three minutes by intravenous injection of 1.5 mg of neostigmine, since the marked exaggeration of myasthenia gravis symptoms may result in prolonged respiratory paralysis.

**Usual pediatric dose**
Neuromuscular blocking agent—Adjunct to surgical anesthesia:
   Neonates up to 4 weeks of age—Intravenous, 250 to 500 mcg (0.25 to 0.5 mg) per kg of body weight initially; then subsequent doses in increments of one-fifth or one-sixth of the initial doses, if necessary.
   Infants and children—Intravenous, 500 mcg (0.5 mg) per kg of body weight.

**Strength(s) usually available**
U.S.—
   3 mg (20 Units) per mL (Rx) [GENERIC].
Canada—
   3 mg (20 Units) per mL (Rx) [*Tubarine;* GENERIC].

**Packaging and storage**
Store below 40 °C (104 °F), preferably between 15 and 30 °C (59 and 86 °F), unless otherwise specified by manufacturer. Protect from freezing.

**Stability**
When tubocurarine is mixed with a barbiturate solution such as methohexital sodium or thiopental sodium, a precipitate may form because of the high pH of the barbiturate solution. Each medication should be given in a separate syringe.

## VECURONIUM

### Summary of Differences
Pharmacology/pharmacokinetics:
  Mechanism of action/effect—
    A nondepolarizing neuromuscular blocking agent.
    Action is usually antagonized by anticholinesterase agents.
  Other actions/effects—
    Less likely than most other neuromuscular blocking agents to cause histamine release.
  Protein-binding—
    Moderate to high.
  Biotransformation—
    Hepatic; only 5–10% of a dose is metabolized. One metabolite has some neuromuscular blocking activity.
  Half-life—
    Distribution: 2–3.4 minutes.
    Elimination: 20 minutes.
  Onset of action—
    Initial effect within 1 minute; intubation conditions in 2.5–3 minutes.
  Time to peak effect—
    3–5 minutes.
  Duration of peak effect—
    25–30 minutes (balanced anesthesia); not changed by repeated dosing, provided that recovery from the prior dose begins before subsequent doses are given.
  Time to recovery—
    From time of injection (balanced anesthesia): 25% of twitch response achieved in 25–40 minutes and 95% of twitch response achieved in 45–65 minutes.
  Elimination—
    Biliary (25–50% of a dose) and renal (3–35% of a dose).
Precautions:
  Cross-sensitivity and/or related problems—
    Cross-sensitivity may occur in patients sensitive to bromides.
  Pregnancy/reproduction—
    Has been shown to cross the human placenta.
  Pediatrics—
    Patients 7 weeks to 1 year of age are more sensitive to the effects of vecuronium than are adults; recovery time may be 1½ times that of adults.
  Drug interactions and/or related problems—
    May increase incidence and severity of bradycardia and hypotension when used together with opioid analgesics.
    Use with digitalis glycosides not reported to cause cardiac arrhythmias or other undesirable cardiac effects.
    Effects not prolonged by cholinesterase inhibitors or hexafluorenium.
    Serious side effects with concurrent use of methotrimeprazine have not been reported.
    Additive effects with physostigmine have not been reported.
  Medical considerations/contraindications—
    Caution required in patients with cardiovascular function impairment.
    Effects may be prolonged by hepatic function impairment.
Side/adverse effects:
  Relatively low risk of side effects caused by histamine release.

### Additional Dosing Information
See also *General Dosing Information*.

Vecuronium is to be administered by intravenous injection only.

### Parenteral Dosage Forms
#### VECURONIUM BROMIDE FOR INJECTION
**Usual adult and adolescent dose**
Initial—
  For intubation:
    Intravenous, 80 to 100 mcg (0.08 to 0.1 mg) per kg of body weight.
  For administration after the patient has been anesthetized with enflurane or isoflurane (i.e., more than 5 minutes after anesthesia has been instituted or after steady state has been achieved):
    Intravenous, 60 to 85 mcg (0.06 to 0.085 mg) per kg of body weight, or approximately 15% less than the usual initial dose.
  For administration after succinylcholine-assisted endotracheal intubation:
    Intravenous, 40 to 60 mcg (0.04 to 0.06 mg) per kg of body weight under inhalation anesthesia, or 50 to 60 mcg (0.05 to 0.06 mg) per kg of body weight under balanced anesthesia. The effects of succinylcholine, as determined with a peripheral nerve stimulator, should be permitted to subside prior to administration of vecuronium.
  Note: If larger initial doses are required by the individual patient, initial doses ranging from 150 to 280 mcg (0.15 to 0.28 mg) per kg of body weight have been administered during surgery with halothane anesthesia without adverse effects on the cardiovascular system occurring, provided that adequate ventilation was maintained.
Supplemental—
  Intravenous, 10 to 15 mcg (0.01 to 0.015 mg) per kg of body weight, administered twenty-five to forty minutes following the initial dose, then every twelve to fifteen minutes or as required by clinical conditions; or
  Intravenous infusion (initiated after recovery from the effects of an initial intravenous dose of 80 to 100 mcg per kg of body weight has begun): 1 mcg (0.001 mg) per kg of body weight per minute, initially, then adjusted according to clinical requirements and patient response. Average infusion rates may range from 0.8 to 1.2 mcg (0.0008 to 0.0012 mg) per kg of body weight per minute.
  After steady-state enflurane or isoflurane anesthesia has been established—
    The required rate of infusion may be reduced by 25 to 60%. This reduction may not be required for patients anesthetized with halothane.

**Usual pediatric dose**
Neonates—
  Dosage has not been established.
Patients 7 weeks to 1 year of age—
  Dosage must be individualized.
Patients 1 to 10 years of age—
  Dosage must be individualized. These patients may require a slightly higher initial dose and slightly more frequent supplemental doses than adults.
Patients 10 years of age and older—
  Initial:
    See *Usual adult and adolescent dose*.
  Supplemental:
    Intravenous—See *Usual adult and adolescent dose*.
    Intravenous infusion—Dosage has not been established.

**Size(s) usually available**
U.S.—
  10 mg (Rx) [*Norcuron;* GENERIC].
Canada—
  10 mg (Rx) [*Norcuron;* GENERIC].
  20 mg (Rx) [GENERIC].

**Packaging and storage**
Prior to reconstitution, store between 15 and 30 °C (59 and 86 °F), protected from light, unless otherwise specified by manufacturer.

**Preparation of dosage form**
Reconstitute using bacteriostatic water for injection (provided by the manufacturer in some packages of vecuronium bromide for injection) or another compatible intravenous solution, such as 5% dextrose injection, 0.9% sodium chloride injection, 5% dextrose in sodium chloride injection, or lactated Ringer's injection. For direct intravenous injection, the medication is generally reconstituted using 5 or 10 mL of diluent. For intravenous infusion, the medication is diluted to a convenient concentration, such as 10 or 20 mg per 100 mL of infusion solution.

**Stability**
After reconstitution with bacteriostatic water for injection, the solution may be stored at room temperature or in a refrigerator; it should be used within 5 days. After reconstitution with other compatible intravenous solutions, the solution should be stored in a refrigerator and used within 24 hours. Reconstituted solutions are intended to be used only once; unused portions should be discarded.

**Incompatibilities**
Alkaline solutions such as barbiturate injections should not be mixed in the same syringe, or administered simultaneously through the same intravenous needle, with vecuronium.

Revised: September 1990
Interim revision: 07/30/97

## Table 1. Pharmacology/Pharmacokinetics

| Drug | Protein Binding | Biotransformation | Half-life Distribution/ Elimination (min) | Elimination Primary (% excreted unchanged)/Secondary (% excreted unchanged) |
|---|---|---|---|---|
| **Depolarizing** | | | | |
| Succinylcholine | — | In plasma, by pseudocholinesterase* | — | Renal (about 10) |
| **Nondepolarizing** | | | | |
| Atracurium | High | In plasma† | 2–3.4/20 | Renal and biliary (<10) |
| Gallamine | — | Essentially none | 16/150 | Renal (almost 100) |
| Metocurine | Moderate‡ | — | 1.9/216 | Renal (about 50 within 48 hr)/ biliary (2) |
| Pancuronium | Very low | Hepatic (in small quantities) | 10–13/114–116 | Renal (about 80)/10% biliary (up to 10) |
| Tubocurarine | Moderate§ | Hepatic | 4.8–6.4/84–120 | Renal (about 40)/biliary (12) |
| Vecuronium | Moderate to high# | Hepatic** | 4/65–75†† | 25–50% Biliary within 42 hr/3– 35% renal within 24 hr‡‡ |

*Hydrolyzed rapidly to succinylmonocholine (a weak nondepolarizing neuromuscular blocking agent that is one-twentieth as potent as succinylcholine), then more slowly to succinic acid and choline.
†Metabolized by ester hydrolysis catalyzed by nonspecific esterases and by Hofmann elimination, a nonenzymatic chemical process that occurs at plasma pH; is independent of hepatic or renal function or plasma pseudocholinesterase activity.
‡Bound primarily to beta and gamma globulins.
§With plasma concentrations of 5 to 50 mcg/mL.
#With doses of 40 to 100 mcg per kg of body weight.
**Only 5 to 10% of a dose is metabolized. However, one metabolite, 3-deacetyl vecuronium, has been shown in animal studies to have neuromuscular blocking activity that is 50% as potent as that of vecuronium.
††May be decreased to 35 to 40 minutes in late pregnancy and prolonged in patients with cirrhosis or cholestasis.
‡‡Up to 25% of a dose may be excreted in bile, and up to 10% of a dose may be excreted in urine, as 3-deacetyl vecuronium.

## Table 2. Pharmacology/Pharmacokinetics*

| Drug | Initial Dose (mg/kg) | Onset of Initial Action (Time to Intubation Conditions) (min) | Time to Peak Effect (min) | Duration of Peak Effect (min)/Effect of Repeated Dosing | Time to Recovery in min (% of twitch response attained) |
|---|---|---|---|---|---|
| **Depolarizing** | | | | | |
| Succinylcholine | | | | | |
| Intramuscular | 3–4 | Up to 3 | — | 10–30† | — |
| Intravenous | 0.3–1.0 | 0.5–1 | 1–2 | 4–10† | — |
| **Nondepolarizing** | | | | | |
| Atracurium | | | | | From time of injection— |
| Intravenous | 0.4–0.5 | Within 2 (2–2.5) | 3–5 (range 1.7–10) | 20–35 under balanced anesthesia/no change‡ | balanced anesthesia‡: 35–45 (25); 60–70 (95) From beginning of recovery§— balanced anesthesia: 30 (95) inhalation anesthesia: 40 (95) |
| Gallamine | | | | | |
| Intravenous | 1.0 | 1–2 | 3–5 | 15–30/increased# | — |
| Metocurine | | | | | From time of injection#: |
| Intravenous | 0.2–0.4 | 1–4 | 1.5–10; usually 3–5 | 35–60(maximum effect); average duration of relaxation 60 (range 25–90)/increased | >360 (50); may be decreased with lower doses |

*Onset of initial action and of effective skeletal muscle relaxation (peak effect) are dose-dependent and decrease with increasing doses. Duration of effective skeletal muscle relaxation and time to recovery are also dose-dependent and increase with increasing doses. Other factors, especially administration of hydrocarbon inhalation anesthetics or other potentiating medications, also influence the duration of effective skeletal muscle relaxation and time to recovery.
†Duration of action and time to recovery with succinylcholine may be increased when plasma pseudocholinesterase activity is decreased.
‡The duration of peak effect and time to recovery with atracurium or vecuronium are not affected by repeated administration of recommended maintenance doses, provided that recovery from the effects of the previous dose begins prior to administration of a subsequent dose.
§Once recovery begins, the rate of recovery is independent of atracurium dosage; however, it is affected by the type of anesthesia administered.
#Following a single dose, the action of the medication is terminated by redistribution into inactive sites. However, following multiple doses, the inactive sites of uptake become saturated, and factors of degradation and/or elimination then directly influence the duration of action and time to recovery.

## Table 2. Pharmacology/Pharmacokinetics* (continued)

| Drug | Initial Dose (mg/kg) | Onset of Initial Action (Time to Intubation Conditions) (min) | Time to Peak Effect (min) | Duration of Peak Effect (min)/Effect of Repeated Dosing | Time to Recovery in min (% of twitch response attained) |
|---|---|---|---|---|---|
| Pancuronium Intravenous | 0.04<br>0.06<br>0.08 | Within 0.75<br>(2–3)<br>0.5 | 4.5<br>—<br>Within 3 | —/increased#<br>35–45/increased#<br>—/increased# | From time of injection#:<br><60 (90)<br>—<br>— |
| Tubocurarine Intramuscular<br>Intravenous | 0.1–0.3<br>0.1–0.3 | 15–25<br>Within 1 | —<br>2–5 | —<br>20–40/increased# | —<br>From time of injection:<br>50 (50); 74–90 (95) |
| Vecuronium Intravenous | 0.08–0.1 | 1 (2.5–3) | 3–5 | 25–30 under balanced anesthesia/ no change‡ | From time of injection—balanced anesthesia‡:<br>25–40 (25); 45–65 (95) |

*Onset of initial action and of effective skeletal muscle relaxation (peak effect) are dose-dependent and decrease with increasing doses. Duration of effective skeletal muscle relaxation and time to recovery are also dose-dependent and increase with increasing doses. Other factors, especially administration of hydrocarbon inhalation anesthetics or other potentiating medications, also influence the duration of effective skeletal muscle relaxation and time to recovery.
†Duration of action and time to recovery with succinylcholine may be increased when plasma pseudocholinesterase activity is decreased.
‡The duration of peak effect and time to recovery with atracurium or vecuronium are not affected by repeated administration of recommended maintenance doses, provided that recovery from the effects of the previous dose begins prior to administration of a subsequent dose.
§Once recovery begins, the rate of recovery is independent of atracurium dosage; however, it is affected by the type of anesthesia administered.
#Following a single dose, the action of the medication is terminated by redistribution into inactive sites. However, following multiple doses, the inactive sites of uptake become saturated, and factors of degradation and/or elimination then directly influence the duration of action and time to recovery.

## Table 3. Drug Interactions and/or Related Problems

| The following drug interactions and/or related problems have been selected on the basis of their potential clinical significance (possible mechanism in parentheses where appropriate)—not necessarily inclusive (» = major clinical significance):<br><br>Note: Combinations containing any of the following medications, depending on the amount present, may also interact with this medication. | Depolarizing<br>Legend:<br>I=Succinylcholine | Nondepolarizing<br>II=Atracurium  V=Pancuronium<br>III=Gallamine  VI=Tubocurarine<br>IV=Metocurine  VII=Vecuronium | | | | | |
|---|---|---|---|---|---|---|---|
| | I | II | III | IV | V | VI | VII |
| » Aminoglycosides, possibly including oral neomycin (if significant quantities are absorbed in patients with renal function impairment), or<br>» Anesthetics, parenteral-local (large doses leading to significant plasma concentrations) or<br>» Capreomycin or<br>» Citrate-anticoagulated blood (massive transfusions) or<br>» Clindamycin or<br>   Lidocaine (intravenous doses > 5 mg per kg) or<br>» Lincomycin or<br>» Polymyxins or<br>   Procaine (intravenous) or<br>   Trimethaphan (large doses)<br>   (neuromuscular blocking activity of these medications may be additive to that of neuromuscular blocking agents)* | ✔ | ✔ | ✔ | ✔ | ✔ | ✔ | ✔ |

## Table 3. Drug Interactions and/or Related Problems (continued)

| The following drug interactions and/or related problems have been selected on the basis of their potential clinical significance (possible mechanism in parentheses where appropriate)—not necessarily inclusive (» = major clinical significance):<br><br>Note: Combinations containing any of the following medications, depending on the amount present, may also interact with this medication. | Depolarizing<br>Legend:<br>I=Succinyl-<br>choline | Nondepolarizing ||||||
|---|---|---|---|---|---|---|---|
| | | II=Atracurium<br>III=Gallamine<br>IV=Metocurine ||| V=Pancuronium<br>VI=Tubocurarine<br>VII=Vecuronium |||
| | I | II | III | IV | V | VI | VII |
| Analgesics, opioid (narcotic), especially those commonly used as adjuncts to anesthesia | | | | | | | |
| (central respiratory depressant effects of opioid analgesics may be additive to the respiratory depressant effects of neuromuscular blocking agents)* | ✓ | ✓ | ✓ | ✓ | ✓ | ✓ | ✓ |
| (high doses of sufentanil may reduce the initial dosage requirements for a nondepolarizing neuromuscular blocking agent; it is recommended that a peripheral nerve stimulator be used to determine dosage) | | ✓ | ✓ | ✓ | ✓ | ✓ | ✓ |
| (concurrent use of a neuromuscular blocking agent prevents or reverses muscle rigidity induced by sufficiently high doses of most opioid analgesics, especially alfentanil, fentanyl, or sufentanil) | ✓ | ✓ | ✓ | ✓ | ✓ | ✓ | ✓ |
| (gallamine and pancuronium, because of their vagolytic activity, may decrease the risk of opioid analgesic–induced bradycardia or hypotension [especially in patients receiving chronic therapy with beta-adrenergic blocking agents and/or vasodilators for treatment of coronary artery disease], but may also increase the risk of tachycardia or hypertension in some patients) | | | ✓ | | ✓ | | |
| (a nonvagolytic neuromuscular blocking agent will not decrease the risk of opioid analgesic-induced bradycardia or hypotension; in some patients [especially patients with compromised cardiac function and/or those receiving a beta-adrenergic blocking agent preoperatively], the incidence and/or severity of these effects may be increased) | ✓ | ✓ | | ✓ | | ✓ | ✓ |
| (histamine release induced by tubocurarine or, to a lesser extent, atracurium, metocurine, or succinylcholine, may be additive to that induced by many opioid analgesics [except alfentanil, fentanyl, and sufentanil, which do not cause histamine release], leading to increased risk of hypotension; administration of histamine [both H$_1$ and H$_2$] receptor–blocking agents may prevent or reduce this effect) | ✓ | ✓ | | ✓ | | ✓ | |
| Anesthetics, hydrocarbon inhalation, such as:<br>Chloroform<br>Cyclopropane<br>Enflurane<br>Ether<br>Halothane<br>Isoflurane<br>Methoxyflurane<br>Trichloroethylene | | | | | | | |
| (concurrent use with succinylcholine may increase the potential for malignant hyperthermia; also, repeated concurrent use may enhance the initial transient bradycardia produced by succinylcholine) | ✓ | | | | | | |
| (neuromuscular blocking activity of inhalation anesthetics, especially enflurane or isoflurane, may be additive to that of the nondepolarizing neuromuscular blocking agents; dosage of vecuronium should be reduced by 15%, and dosage of other neuromuscular blocking agents should be reduced by ⅓ to ½ of the usual dose or as determined with a peripheral nerve stimulator)* | | ✓ | ✓ | ✓ | ✓ | ✓ | ✓ |
| (halogenated hydrocarbon anesthetics may also potentiate succinylcholine-induced neuromuscular blockade, but to a lesser extent than they potentiate the effects of nondepolarizing neuromuscular blocking agents)* | ✓ | | | | | | |
| Antimyasthenics or Edrophonium | | | | | | | |
| (these agents may antagonize the effects of nondepolarizing neuromuscular blocking agents; parenteral neostigmine or pyridostigmine are indicated to reverse neuromuscular blockade following surgery; although the usefulness of edrophonium for this purpose has been considered to be limited because of its brief duration of action, recent studies indicate that edrophonium is equivalent to neostigmine in reversing the effects of tubocurarine) | | ✓ | ✓ | ✓ | ✓ | ✓ | ✓ |
| (these agents may prolong phase I block when used concurrently with succinylcholine*; however, if succinylcholine has been used for a prolonged period of time and the depolarization block has changed to a nondepolarization block, edrophonium, neostigmine, or pyridostigmine may reverse the nondepolarization block) | ✓ | | | | | | |
| (neuromuscular blocking agents may antagonize the effects of antimyasthenics on skeletal muscle; temporary dosage adjustment may be required to control symptoms of myasthenia gravis following surgery) | ✓ | ✓ | ✓ | ✓ | ✓ | ✓ | ✓ |

*Increased or prolonged respiratory depression or paralysis (apnea) may occur but is of minor clinical significance while the patient is being mechanically ventilated. However, caution and careful monitoring of the patient are recommended during and following concurrent or sequential use, especially if there is a possibility of incomplete reversal of neuromuscular blockade postoperatively.

## Table 3. Drug Interactions and/or Related Problems (continued)

| The following drug interactions and/or related problems have been selected on the basis of their potential clinical significance (possible mechanism in parentheses where appropriate)—not necessarily inclusive (» = major clinical significance):<br><br>Note: Combinations containing any of the following medications, depending on the amount present, may also interact with this medication. | Depolarizing<br>Legend:<br>I=Succinyl-choline<br>**I** | Nondepolarizing<br>II=Atracurium<br>III=Gallamine<br>IV=Metocurine<br>**II** | <br><br><br><br>**III** | <br><br><br><br>**IV** | V=Pancuronium<br>VI=Tubocurarine<br>VII=Vecuronium<br>**V** | <br><br><br>**VI** | <br><br><br>**VII** |
|---|---|---|---|---|---|---|---|
| Beta-adrenergic blocking agents<br>(concurrent use may enhance or prolong the blockade of the nondepolarizing neuromuscular blocking agents)* | | | ✓ | ✓ | ✓ | ✓ | |
| Calcium salts<br>(calcium salts usually reverse the effects of nondepolarizing neuromuscular blocking agents) | | ✓ | ✓ | ✓ | ✓ | ✓ | ✓ |
| (concurrent use has been reported to enhance or prolong the neuromuscular blocking action of tubocurarine)* | | | | | | ✓ | |
| » Cholinesterase inhibitors, especially echothiophate, demecarium, and isoflurophate, or<br>Cyclophosphamide or<br>» Insecticides, neurotoxic, exposure to, possibly including large quantities of topical malathion, or<br>Phenelzine or<br>Thiotepa<br>(may decrease plasma concentrations or activity of pseudocholinesterase, the enzyme that metabolizes succinylcholine, thereby enhancing the neuromuscular blockade of succinylcholine; effects of echothiophate, demecarium, or isoflurophate may persist for weeks or months after the cholinesterase inhibitor has been discontinued)* | ✓ | | | | | | |
| » Digitalis glycosides<br>(cardiac effects may be increased when digitalis glycosides are used concurrently with succinylcholine and, to a lesser extent, with pancuronium, possibly resulting in cardiac arrhythmias) | ✓ | | | | ✓ | | |
| Doxapram<br>(the residual effects of neuromuscular blocking agents may be masked temporarily by doxapram when it is used post-anesthesia) | ✓ | ✓ | ✓ | ✓ | ✓ | ✓ | |
| Hexafluorenium<br>(concurrent use may prolong the action of succinylcholine and may minimize or prevent the muscle fasciculations and pain that may occur when succinylcholine is used alone; however, concurrent use may increase the potential for development of a dual block)* | ✓ | | | | | | |
| Lithium (chronic therapy)<br>(concurrent use may enhance or prolong the neuromuscular blockade of atracurium, succinylcholine, or pancuronium)* | ✓ | ✓ | | | ✓ | | |
| Magnesium salts, parenteral, or<br>» Procainamide or<br>» Quinidine<br>(concurrent use may enhance the blockade of the neuromuscular blocking agents)* | ✓ | ✓ | ✓ | ✓ | ✓ | ✓ | ✓ |
| Methotrimeprazine<br>(concurrent use with succinylcholine may cause tachycardia, a fall in blood pressure, CNS stimulation and delirium, and an aggravation of extrapyramidal effects) | ✓ | | | | | | |
| Neuromuscular blocking agents, depolarizing<br>(prior administration may enhance the blockade of nondepolarizing neuromuscular blocking agents; if a depolarizing agent is used before a nondepolarizing agent, administration of the nondepolarizing agent should be delayed until the effects of the depolarizing agent have decreased) | | ✓ | ✓ | ✓ | ✓ | ✓ | ✓ |
| Neuromuscular blocking agents, nondepolarizing<br>(concurrent use may enhance the blockade of depolarizing neuromuscular blocking agents if they have been administered over a prolonged period of time and the depolarized block has gradually changed to a nondepolarized block) | ✓ | | | | | | |
| (concurrent use of pancuronium and another nondepolarizing neuromuscular blocking agent may substantially reduce the required dose of both medications) | | ✓ | | ✓ | ✓ | ✓ | ✓ |
| » Physostigmine<br>(concurrent use with succinylcholine is not recommended since high doses of physostigmine may cause muscle fasciculation and ultimately, a depolarization block, which may be additive to that produced by succinylcholine) | ✓ | | | | | | |

## Table 3. Drug Interactions and/or Related Problems (continued)

| The following drug interactions and/or related problems have been selected on the basis of their potential clinical significance (possible mechanism in parentheses where appropriate)—not necessarily inclusive (» = major clinical significance):<br><br>Note: Combinations containing any of the following medications, depending on the amount present, may also interact with this medication. | Depolarizing<br><br>Legend:<br>I=Succinyl-choline | Nondepolarizing ||||||
|---|---|---|---|---|---|---|---|
| | | II=Atracurium<br>III=Gallamine<br>IV=Metocurine ||| V=Pancuronium<br>VI=Tubocurarine<br>VII=Vecuronium |||
| | **I** | **II** | **III** | **IV** | **V** | **VI** | **VII** |
| Potassium-depleting medications, such as:<br>  Amphotericin B<br>  Bumetanide<br>  Carbonic anhydrase inhibitors<br>  Corticosteroids, glucocorticoid, especially with significant mineralocorticoid activity<br>  Corticosteroids, mineralocorticoid<br>  Corticotropin, chronic therapeutic use<br>  Ethacrynic acid<br>  Furosemide<br>  Indapamide<br>  Thiazide diuretics<br>    (hypokalemia induced by these medications may enhance the blockade of nondepolarizing neuromuscular blocking agents; serum potassium determinations and correction of serum potassium concentration may be necessary prior to administration of nondepolarizing neuromuscular blocking agents)* | | ✓ | ✓ | ✓ | ✓ | ✓ | ✓ |
|     (hydrocortisone and prednisone have also been reported to decrease the efficacy of pancuronium by an unknown mechanism; increased dosage of pancuronium or use of an alternate neuromuscular blocking agent may be necessary) | | | | | ✓ | | |

*Increased or prolonged respiratory depression or paralysis (apnea) may occur but is of minor clinical significance while the patient is being mechanically ventilated. However, caution and careful monitoring of the patient are recommended during and following concurrent or sequential use, especially if there is a possibility of incomplete reversal of neuromuscular blockade postoperatively.

## Table 4. Medical Considerations/Contraindications

Note: A blank space usually signifies lack of information; it is not necessarily an indication that a given medical problem is of no concern. However, the pharmacologic similarity of the nondepolarizing neuromuscular blocking agents may suggest that if caution is required in particular medical problems for one agent, then it may be required for the others as well.

| | Depolarizing<br><br>Legend:<br>I=Succinyl-choline | Nondepolarizing ||||||
|---|---|---|---|---|---|---|---|
| The medical considerations/contraindications included have been selected on the basis of their potential clinical significance (reasons given in parentheses where appropriate)—not necessarily inclusive (» = major clinical significance).<br>***Risk-benefit should be considered when the following medical problems exist*** | | II=Atracurium<br>III=Gallamine<br>IV=Metocurine ||| V=Pancuronium<br>VI=Tubocurarine<br>VII=Vecuronium |||
| | **I** | **II** | **III** | **IV** | **V** | **VI** | **VII** |
| Allergic reaction to the neuromuscular blocker considered for use, history of | ✓ | ✓ | ✓ | ✓ | ✓ | ✓ | ✓ |
| Burns, severe, or<br>Digitalis toxicity or in patients recently digitalized or<br>Neuromuscular disease, degenerative or dystrophic, or<br>Paraplegia or<br>Spinal cord injury or<br>Trauma, severe<br>  (serious cardiac arrhythmias or cardiac arrest may occur as a result of increased serum potassium concentrations) | ✓ | | | | | | |
| Carcinoma, bronchogenic<br>  (action of neuromuscular blocking agent may be enhanced) | ✓ | ✓ | ✓ | ✓ | ✓ | ✓ | ✓ |
| Cardiac conditions in which tachycardia would be undesirable<br>  (gallamine and pancuronium may cause tachycardia) | | | ✓ | | ✓ | | |
| Cardiovascular function impairment | ✓ | | | | ✓ | ✓ | ✓ |
| Conditions in which histamine release would be hazardous<br>  (these neuromuscular blocking agents may cause histamine release) | ✓ | ✓ | | | ✓ | ✓ | ✓ |
| Conditions in which low levels of plasma pseudocholinesterase activity may exist, such as:<br>  Anemia, severe<br>  Dehydration<br>  Exposure to neurotoxic insecticides or other cholinesterase inhibitors<br>  Hepatic disease, severe, or cirrhosis<br>  Malnutrition<br>  Pregnancy<br>  Recessive hereditary trait<br>    (prolonged respiratory depression or apnea may occur) | ✓ | | | | | | |
| Dehydration or<br>Electrolyte or acid-base imbalance<br>  (action of neuromuscular blocking agent may be altered) | ✓ | ✓ | ✓ | ✓ | ✓ | ✓ | ✓ |

## Table 4. Medical Considerations/Contraindications (continued)

Note: A blank space usually signifies lack of information; it is not necessarily an indication that a given medical problem is of no concern. However, the pharmacologic similarity of the nondepolarizing neuromuscular blocking agents may suggest that if caution is required in particular medical problems for one agent, then it may be required for the others as well.

| The medical considerations/contraindications included have been selected on the basis of their potential clinical significance (reasons given in parentheses where appropriate)—not necessarily inclusive (» = major clinical significance).<br>*Risk-benefit should be considered when the following medical problems exist* | Depolarizing<br>Legend:<br>**I**=Succinyl-<br>choline | \multicolumn{6}{c}{Nondepolarizing} |
|---|---|---|---|---|---|---|---|
| | | **II**=Atracurium<br>**III**=Gallamine<br>**IV**=Metocurine | | | **V**=Pancuronium<br>**VI**=Tubocurarine<br>**VII**=Vecuronium | | |
| | **I** | **II** | **III** | **IV** | **V** | **VI** | **VII** |
| Eye injury, open, or<br>Glaucoma or<br>Ocular surgery<br>(succinylcholine may increase intraocular pressure) | ✔ | | | | | | |
| Fractures or muscle spasm<br>(initial muscle fasciculations may cause additional trauma) | ✔ | | | | | | |
| Hepatic function impairment<br>(patients may have decreased levels of pseudocholinesterase activity, possibly resulting in prolonged respiratory depression or apnea)<br>(effect of metocurine, panuronium, or tubocurarine may be reduced)<br>(effect of vecuronium may be prolonged) | ✔ | | | ✔ | ✔ | ✔ | ✔ |
| Hyperkalemia, preexisting<br>(may be exacerbated by succinylcholine-induced increases in serum potassium concentration) | ✔ | | | | | | |
| Hypertension<br>(gallamine may increase blood pressure) | | | ✔ | | | | |
| Hyperthermia<br>(intensity and duration of action of depolarizing agents may be decreased and that of nondepolarizing agents may be increased) | ✔ | | ✔ | ✔ | ✔ | ✔ | |
| Hypotension<br>(rapid IV administration and/or large doses of atracurium, metocurine, and tubocurarine may cause hypotension) | | ✔ | | ✔ | | ✔ | |
| Hypothermia<br>(intensity and/or duration of action of succinylcholine and atracurium may be increased and that of gallamine, metocurine, pancuronium, and tubocurarine may be decreased) | ✔ | ✔ | ✔ | ✔ | ✔ | ✔ | |
| » Malignant hyperthermia, history of in patient or close relative, or suspected predisposition to<br>(may be induced by succinylcholine) | ✔ | | | | | | |
| Myasthenia gravis, except when tubocurarine is used as a diagnostic agent | ✔ | ✔ | ✔ | ✔ | ✔ | ✔ | ✔ |
| Pulmonary function impairment or<br>Respiratory depression<br>(risk of additive respiratory depression) | ✔ | ✔ | ✔ | ✔ | ✔ | ✔ | ✔ |
| Renal function impairment<br>(eliminated by kidneys; prolonged neuromuscular blockade may occur) | ✔ | | | ✔ | ✔ | ✔ | |
| » Renal function impairment<br>(eliminated by kidneys primarily as unchanged drug; prolonged neuromuscular blockade may occur) | | | | ✔ | | | |
| » Shock<br>(action of gallamine may be prolonged) | | | ✔ | | | | |
| Shock<br>(action of metocurine and tubocurarine may be prolonged) | | | | ✔ | | ✔ | |

## Table 5. Side/Adverse Effects*

| The following side/adverse effects have been selected on the basis of their potential clinical significance (possible signs and symptoms in parentheses where appropriate)—not necessarily inclusive: | Depolarizing<br>Legend:<br>**I**=Succinyl-<br>choline | \multicolumn{6}{c}{Nondepolarizing} |
|---|---|---|---|---|---|---|---|
| | | **II**=Atracurium<br>**III**=Gallamine<br>**IV**=Metocurine | | | **V**=Pancuronium<br>**VI**=Tubocurarine<br>**VII**=Vecuronium | | |
| | **I** | **II** | **III** | **IV** | **V** | **VI** | **VII** |
| **Medical attention needed**<br>*Anaphylactic, anaphylactoid, or other hypersensitivity reaction* | R | R | R | R | R | R | R |
| *Bradycardia* | L† | R‡ | U | U | U | R | R‡ |
| *Bronchospasm* | R§ | R§ | U | R§ | R§ | R§ | R§ |
| *Cardiac arrhythmias* | L† | U | U | U | U | R | U |

## Table 5. Side/Adverse Effects* (continued)

| The following side/adverse effects have been selected on the basis of their potential clinical significance (possible signs and symptoms in parentheses where appropriate)—not necessarily inclusive: | Depolarizing Legend: I=Succinylcholine | Nondepolarizing II=Atracurium III=Gallamine IV=Metocurine | | | V=Pancuronium VI=Tubocurarine VII=Vecuronium | | |
|---|---|---|---|---|---|---|---|
| | **I** | **II** | **III** | **IV** | **V** | **VI** | **VII** |
| *Circulatory depression or collapse*—may occur in overdose | R§ | R§ | U | R§ | R§ | R§ | R§ |
| *Decreased blood pressure*—may reach hypotensive levels; with usual doses of metocurine or tubocurarine, or larger-than-recommended doses of atracurium, may be caused by ganglionic blockade; may also occur as a complication of high-dose positive pressure respiration | R†§ | L§ | U | L§ | R§ | M§ | R§ |
| *Edema* | R§ | R§ | U | R§ | R§ | R§ | R§ |
| *Erythema* | R§ | R§ | U | R§ | R§ | R§ | R§ |
| *Flushing of skin* | R§ | M§ | U | R§ | R§ | R§ | R§ |
| *Hives* | U | R | U | U | U | U | U |
| *Increased blood pressure*—may reach hypertensive levels; with gallamine or pancuronium, may be caused by vagolytic activity | R† | L | M | U | L | U | U |
| *Increased intraocular pressure*—possibly caused by contraction of extraocular muscle; occurs immediately after injection and during the fasciculation phase | M | U | U | U | U | U | U |
| *Laryngospasm* | U | R | U | U | U | U | U |
| *Malignant hyperthermic crisis* | R | U | U | U | U | U | U |
| *Myoglobinemia and myoglobinuria caused by rhabdomyolysis*—especially in children; may lead to myoglobinuric acute renal failure | R | U | U | U | U | U | U |
| *Tachycardia*—with gallamine, occurs after doses of 500 mcg (0.5 mg) per kg of body weight and reaches a maximum within 3 minutes, then declines gradually to the control level; with gallamine and pancuronium, may be due to vagolytic activity | L†§ | L§ | M | R§ | L§ | R§ | R§ |
| **Medical attention needed only if continuing or bothersome** *Itching of skin* | R§ | R§ | U | R§ | L§ | R§ | R§ |
| *Muscle pain and stiffness, postoperative*—possibly caused by muscle fasciculations that occur immediately following injection; incidence may vary from 10% in patients maintained on bed rest for 1 day to 70% in ambulatory patients; symptoms usually appear 12 to 24 hours following administration and last for several hours to a few days | M | — | — | — | — | — | — |
| *Salivation, excessive* | L | U | U | U | L | U | U |
| *Skin rash* | R§ | R§ | U | R§ | L§ | R§ | R§ |

*Differences in frequency of occurrence may reflect either lack of clinical-use data or actual pharmacologic distinctions among agents (although their pharmacologic similarity suggests that side effects occurring with one may occur with the others). M=more frequent; L=less frequent; R=rare; U=unknown.

†Succinylcholine may cause transient bradycardia accompanied by hypotension, cardiac arrhythmias, and possibly a short period of sinus arrest due to increased vagal stimulation, especially with repeated administration and in children. Following these effects, tachycardia and hypertension may occur due to asphyxial pressor response and mild sympathetic ganglion stimulation.

‡Atracurium and vecuronium have little or no direct effect on heart rate; bradycardia may occur because these medications do not counteract the bradycardia caused by other medications (e.g., anesthetics, opioid analgesics) or vagal stimulation.

§May be caused by histamine release, especially following rapid intravenous injection and/or large doses, or an overdose. The risk of clinically significant histamine release is highest with tubocurarine; moderate with atracurium, metocurine, or succinylcholine; relatively low with pancuronium or vecuronium; and least with gallamine.

# NEVIRAPINE Systemic—INTRODUCTORY VERSION

VA CLASSIFICATION (Primary): AM800
Commonly used brand name(s): *Viramune*.
Note: For a listing of dosage forms and brand names by country availability, see *Dosage Forms* section(s).

## Category
Antiviral (systemic).

## Indications

### General considerations
Nevirapine monotherapy results in the rapid emergence of resistant human immunodeficiency virus (HIV). Therefore, nevirapine should always be administered in combination with at least one other antiretroviral agent.

### Accepted
Human immunodeficiency virus (HIV) infection (treatment) or Immunodeficiency syndrome, acquired (AIDS) (treatment)—Nevirapine is indicated, in combination with other antiretroviral agents, for the treatment of HIV infection or AIDS in patients who have experienced clinical and/or immunologic deterioration.

## Pharmacology/Pharmacokinetics

### Physicochemical characteristics
Chemical group—Dipyridodiazepinone.
Molecular weight—266.3.

### Mechanism of action/Effect
Nevirapine is a nonnucleoside reverse transcriptase inhibitor that binds directly to reverse transcriptase and blocks RNA-dependent and DNA-dependent polymerase activities of human immunodeficiency virus–1 (HIV-1). This causes disruption of the enzyme's catalytic site. Nevirapine does not compete with template or nucleoside triphosphates. HIV-2 reverse transcriptase and eukaryotic DNA polymerases are not inhibited by nevirapine.

### Absorption
Readily absorbed. Bioavailability was 93% for single-dose administration of a 50-mg tablet. When nevirapine was administered with a high-fat

breakfast or an antacid, the extent of absorption was comparable to that seen under fasting conditions. Nevirapine may be administered with or without food.

**Distribution**
Vol$_D$—1.2 L per kg. Highly lipophilic and widely distributed.
Nevirapine crosses the placenta and is distributed into breast milk. Concentrations in the cerebrospinal fluid (n=6) were 45% of those seen in plasma, which is a ratio that is approximately equal to the fraction not bound to plasma protein.

**Protein binding**
Moderate (60%).

**Biotransformation**
Extensive oxidative metabolism by the cytochrome P450 enzyme system (primarily isozymes from the CYP3A family) to several hydroxylated metabolites.

**Half-life**
Approximately 45 hours after a single dose, and 25 to 30 hours following multiple dosing with 200 to 400 mg per day.

**Time to peak concentration**
4 hours after a single 200-mg dose.

**Peak serum concentration**
2 micrograms per mL after a single 200-mg dose.

**Elimination**
Renal; approximately 91% of a radiolabeled dose was recovered in the urine, with > 80% of that made up of glucuronide conjugates of hydroxylated metabolites. Less than 5% of the recovered radiolabeled dose was made up of the parent drug.
Fecal; approximately 10% of a radiolabeled dose was recovered in the feces.

## Precautions to Consider

**Carcinogenicity**
Long-term carcinogenicity studies in animals are currently in progress.

**Mutagenicity**
Nevirapine showed no evidence of mutagenic or clastogenic activity in a battery of in vitro and in vivo genetic toxicology assays. These included microbial assays for gene mutation (Ames: *Salmonella* strains and *Escherichia coli*), mammalian cell gene mutation assays (CHO/HGPRT), cytogenetic assays using a Chinese hamster ovary cell line, and a mouse bone marrow micronucleus assay following oral administration.

**Pregnancy/Reproduction**
Fertility—Evidence of impaired fertility was seen in female rats at doses providing systemic exposure (based on the area under the plasma concentration–time curve [AUC]) approximately equivalent to that attained with the recommended clinical dose of nevirapine.
Pregnancy—Nevirapine crosses the placenta; however, adequate and well-controlled studies have not been done in humans.
Teratogenicity was not seen in reproductive studies performed in pregnant rats and rabbits. A significant decrease in fetal body weight was seen in rats given doses providing systemic exposure approximately 50% higher than that seen at the recommended human clinical dose, based on AUC values. The maternal and developmental no-observable-effect level dosages in rats and rabbits produced systemic exposures approximately equivalent to or approximately 50% higher than, respectively, those seen at the recommended daily human dose, based on AUC values.

FDA Pregnancy Category C.

**Breast-feeding**
Nevirapine is distributed into breast milk. It is recommended that HIV-infected mothers not breast-feed to avoid the risk of transmitting HIV to their infants.

**Pediatrics**
Safety and effectiveness have not been established. However, nevirapine was studied in a small number of children (ages 0.1 to 15 years) and 7 of the 37 patients developed rash. In another study, 1 of 288 patients developed Stevens-Johnson syndrome. Single-dose pharmacokinetic studies done in nine HIV-infected children (ages 9 months to 14 years) who were administered an oral suspension form of nevirapine showed a twofold greater clearance than studies in adults.

**Geriatrics**
No information is available on the relationship of age to the effects of nevirapine in geriatric patients. Nevirapine has not been extensively evaluated in patients older than 55 years of age.

**Drug interactions and/or related problems**
The following drug interactions and/or related problems have been selected on the basis of their potential clinical significance (possible mechanism in parentheses where appropriate)—not necessarily inclusive (» = major clinical significance):

Note: Combinations containing any of the following medications, depending on the amount present, may also interact with this medication.

Nevirapine is an inducer of cytochrome P450 enzymes, particularly CYP3A. Autoinduction occurs with nevirapine and it has been found to increase the apparent oral clearance by 1.5 to 2 times as treatment continues from a single dose to multiple dosing at 2 to 4 weeks. Autoinduction also results in a decrease in the terminal half-life of nevirapine from approximately 45 hours after a single dose to approximately 25 to 30 hours after multiple dosing with 200 to 400 mg per day. Medications that are metabolized by CYP3A should be monitored carefully when they are administered concurrently with nevirapine.

Cimetidine
(concurrent use of nevirapine with cimetidine, a known inhibitor of CYP3A, resulted in elevated steady-state nevirapine trough concentrations when studied in a small number of patients)

» Contraceptives, estrogen-containing, oral
(nevirapine may decrease the plasma concentration of oral contraceptives due to induction of CYP3A by nevirapine; however, clinical studies have not been conducted; concurrent use is not recommended)

Didanosine or
Zalcitabine or
Zidovudine
(clinically significant pharmacokinetic changes were not seen when nevirapine was administered concurrently with didanosine, zalcitabine, or zidovudine; no dosage adjustments are recommended)

» Ketoconazole
(concurrent use with nevirapine results in significantly reduced plasma concentrations of ketoconazole; concurrent use is not recommended)

Macrolide antibiotics
(concurrent use of nevirapine with macrolide antibiotics, known inhibitors of CYP3A, showed elevated steady-state nevirapine trough concentrations when studied in a small number of patients)

» Protease inhibitors, such as:
Indinavir
Ritonavir
Saquinavir
(nevirapine decreases the plasma concentration of indinavir and saquinavir due to induction of cytochrome P450 enzymes; the clinical significance of these interactions is not known; dosage adjustment of these medications may be necessary)

» Rifabutin or
» Rifampin
(the plasma concentration of nevirapine may be decreased by rifabutin or rifampin due to induction of CYP3A; these medications should be used in combination only if clearly indicated and with careful monitoring)

**Laboratory value alterations**
The following have been selected on the basis of their potential clinical significance (possible effect in parentheses where appropriate)—not necessarily inclusive (» = major clinical significance):

With physiology/laboratory test values
» Alanine aminotransferase (ALT [SGPT]), serum and
» Aspartate aminotransferase (AST [SGOT]), serum and
Gamma-glutamyltransferase (GGT)
(values may be increased; hepatitis has been reported occasionally)

**Medical considerations/Contraindications**
The medical considerations/contraindications included have been selected on the basis of their potential clinical significance (reasons given in parentheses where appropriate)—not necessarily inclusive (» = major clinical significance).

*Except under special circumstances, this medication should not be used when the following medical problem exists:*

» Hypersensitivity to nevirapine

*Risk-benefit should be considered when the following medical problems exist:*

» Hepatic function impairment
(abnormal liver function tests and hepatitis have been reported, some in the first few weeks of therapy; administration should be interrupted in patients who develop moderate to severe liver function test abnormalities until they return to baseline values; nevira-

pine therapy should be discontinued permanently if liver function test abnormalities recur on readmission)

Renal function impairment
(nevirapine metabolites are extensively eliminated by the kidney; although no studies have been done, nevirapine should be used with caution in patients with renal function impairment)

**Patient monitoring**

The following may be especially important in patient monitoring (other tests may be warranted in some patients, depending on condition; » = major clinical significance):

» Alanine aminotransferase (ALT [SGPT]), serum and
» Aspartate aminotransferase (AST [SGOT]), serum and Gamma-glutamyltransferase (GGT)
(abnormal liver function tests and hepatitis have been reported, some in the first few weeks of therapy; administration should be interrupted in patients who develop moderate to severe liver function test abnormalities until they return to baseline values; nevirapine therapy should be discontinued permanently if liver function test abnormalities recur on readmission)

## Side/Adverse Effects

Note: Severe and life-threatening skin reactions, including Stevens-Johnson syndrome and toxic epidermal necrolysis, have occurred in patients taking nevirapine. It usually occurs within the first 6 weeks of therapy. Nevirapine must be discontinued immediately in patients who develop a severe rash or a rash accompanied by constitutional symptoms. Nevirapine therapy is initiated with a 14-day lead-in period of 200 mg per day before increasing the dose to 400 mg per day in divided doses. This has been found to decrease the incidence of rash. If rash is seen during the lead-in period, the dose should not be increased to 400 mg per day until the rash resolves.

Severe or life-threatening hepatotoxicity, including fatal fulminant hepatitis, has been reported with nevirapine therapy. Some of these cases began in the first few weeks of therapy, and some were accompanied by rash. Nevirapine treatment should be interrupted in patients who develop moderate or severe liver function test abnormalities until they return to normal values. Nevirapine should be discontinued if liver function abnormalities recur upon the resumption of therapy.

The following side/adverse effects have been selected on the basis of their potential clinical significance (possible signs and symptoms in parentheses where appropriate)—not necessarily inclusive:

**Those indicating need for medical attention**
Incidence more frequent
*Skin rash*
Note: Skin rash occurred in 17% of patients receiving nevirapine in combination regimens. Severe or life-threatening rash occurred in 7.6% of patients treated with nevirapine compared to 1.2% of those in the control groups. Rash is usually a mild to moderate, maculopapular erythematous eruption, with or without itching, located primarily on the trunk, face, and extremities. Most severe rashes occur within the first 28 days of therapy.

Incidence less frequent
*Fever; hepatitis* (yellow skin or eyes); *ulcerative stomatitis* (sores or ulcers in the mouth)

**Those indicating need for medical attention only if they continue or are bothersome**
Incidence more frequent
*Gastrointestinal effects* (abdominal or stomach pain; diarrhea; nausea); *headache*

## Overdose

Cases of nevirapine overdosage ranging from 800 to 1800 mg per day for up to 15 days have been reported. These patients experienced edema, erythema nodosum, fatigue, fever, headache, insomnia, nausea and vomiting, pulmonary infiltrates, rash, vertigo, and weight decrease. There is no known antidote for nevirapine overdose.

For more information on the management of overdose or unintentional ingestion, **contact a Poison Control Center** (see *Poison Control Center Listing*).

## Patient Consultation

As an aid to patient consultation, refer to *Advice for the Patient, Nevirapine (Systemic)—Introductory Version.*

In providing consultation, consider emphasizing the following selected information (» = major clinical significance)

**Before using this medication**
» Conditions affecting use, especially:
Hypersensitivity to nevirapine
Pregnancy—Decreased fetal body weight was seen in rats administered high doses
Breast-feeding—Nevirapine is distributed into breast milk
Other medications, especially estrogen-containing oral contraceptives, ketoconazole, protease inhibitors, rifabutin, or rifampin
Other medical problems, especially hepatic function impairment

**Proper use of this medication**
Nevirapine may be taken with or without food
» Importance of not taking more medication than prescribed; importance of not discontinuing nevirapine without checking with physician
» Compliance with full course of therapy
» Importance of not missing doses and taking doses at evenly spaced times
Not sharing medication with others
» Proper dosing
Missed dose: Taking as soon as possible; not taking if almost time for next dose; not doubling doses
» Proper storage

**Precautions while using this medication**
» Because nevirapine interacts with so many medications, not taking any other medications (prescription or nonprescription) without first consulting your physician
» Regular visits to physician for blood tests
» Using an additional method of contraception if taking estrogen-containing oral contraceptives concurrently

**Side/adverse effects**
Signs of potential side effects, especially, skin rash, fever, hepatitis, and ulcerative stomatitis

## General Dosing Information

Nevirapine therapy is initiated with a 14-day period of 200 mg per day before increasing the dose to 400 mg per day. This has been found to decrease the incidence of rash, which can be severe and life-threatening. Rash usually occurs within the first 28 days of therapy. The dose of nevirapine should not be increased to 400 mg per day until the rash has resolved. Nevirapine must be discontinued immediately in patients who develop a severe rash or a rash accompanied by constitutional symptoms.

Nevirapine therapy should be interrupted in patients who develop moderate or severe liver function test abnormalities. Therapy may be restarted with a 14-day period of 200 mg per day before increasing the dose to 400 mg per day when liver function tests return to baseline. Nevirapine should be discontinued permanently if moderate or severe liver function test abnormalities recur.

Patients who interrupt nevirapine therapy for more than 7 days should restart dosing with 200 mg once a day for the first 14 days, then increase the dose to 200 mg twice a day.

No data are available on the recommended dosage of nevirapine for patients with hepatic function impairment, renal function impairment, or patients undergoing dialysis.

## Oral Dosage Forms

### NEVIRAPINE TABLETS

**Usual adult dose**
Antiviral—
Oral, 200 mg once a day for the first fourteen days, then 200 mg two times a day, in combination with nucleoside analogs.

**Usual pediatric dose**
Safety and effectiveness have not been established.

**Strength(s) usually available**
U.S.—
200 mg (Rx) [*Viramune*].

**Packaging and storage**
Store between 15 and 30 °C (59 and 86 °F). Store in a tight container.

**Auxiliary labeling**
• Take for full time of treatment.

Developed: 01/27/97
Interim revision: 08/24/98

# NIACIN Systemic

This monograph includes information on the following: 1) Niacin; 2) Niacinamide.

INN:
- Niacin—Nicotinic acid
- Niacinamide—Nicotinamide

VA CLASSIFICATION (Primary/Secondary): VT103/CV609

Commonly used brand name(s): *Endur-Acin*[1]; *Nia-Bid*[1]; *Niac*[1]; *Niacels*[1]; *Niacor*[1]; *Nico-400*[1]; *Nicobid Tempules*[1]; *Nicolar*[1]; *Nicotinex Elixir*[1]; *Novo-Niacin*[1]; *Slo-Niacin*[1].

Other commonly used names are: Nicotinamide [Niacinamide], Nicotinic acid [Niacin], Vitamin $B_3$ [Niacin; Niacinamide].

Note: For a listing of dosage forms and brand names by country availability, see *Dosage Forms* section(s).

## Category

Note: Niacin and niacinamide (vitamin $B_3$) are water-soluble vitamins.

Nutritional supplement (vitamin)—Niacin; Niacinamide.
Antihyperlipidemic—Niacin.

## Indications

### Accepted

Niacin deficiency (prophylaxis and treatment)—Niacin and niacinamide are indicated for prevention and treatment of vitamin $B_3$ deficiency states. Vitamin $B_3$ deficiency may occur as a result of inadequate nutrition or intestinal malabsorption but does not occur in healthy individuals receiving an adequate balanced diet. Simple nutritional deficiency of individual B vitamins is rare since dietary inadequacy usually results in multiple deficiencies. For prophylaxis of niacin deficiency, dietary improvement, rather than supplementation, is advisable. For treatment of niacin deficiency, supplementation is preferred.

Deficiency of niacin may lead to pellagra.

Recommendended intakes may be increased and/or supplementation may be necessary in the following persons or conditions (based on documented niacin deficiency):
- Diabetes mellitus
- Fever, chronic
- Gastrectomy
- Hartnup disease
- Hepatic-biliary tract disease—cirrhosis
- Hyperthyroidism
- Infection, chronic
- Intestinal diseases—celiac disease, persistent diarrhea, tropical sprue, regional enteritis
- Malabsorption syndromes associated with pancreatic insufficiency
- Malignancy
- Oropharyngeal lesions
- Stress, continuing

Some unusual diets (e.g., reducing diets that drastically restrict food selection) may not supply minimum daily requirements of niacin. Supplementation is necessary in patients receiving total parenteral nutrition (TPN) or undergoing rapid weight loss or in those with malnutrition, because of inadequate dietary intake.

Recommended intakes for all vitamins and most minerals are increased during pregnancy. Many physicians recommend that pregnant women receive multivitamin and mineral supplements, especially those pregnant women who do not consume an adequate diet and those in high-risk categories (i.e., women carrying more than one fetus, heavy cigarette smokers, and alcohol and drug abusers). However, taking excessive amounts of a multivitamin and mineral supplement may be harmful to the mother and/or fetus and should be avoided.

Recommended intakes for all vitamins and most minerals are increased during breast-feeding.

Hyperlipidemia (treatment)—Niacin (but not niacinamide) is also indicated in the treatment of hyperlipidemia. Niacin is recommended for use only in patients with primary hyperlipidemia (type IIa, IIb, III, IV, or V hyperlipoproteinemia) and a significant risk of coronary artery disease who have not responded to other measures alone. It is one of the drugs of first choice for initiating therapy to reduce low density lipoprotein (LDL)–cholesterol concentrations and triglycerides, and to increase high density lipoprotein (HDL)–cholesterol concentrations.

Studies have suggested that control of elevated cholesterol and triglycerides may not lessen the danger of cardiovascular disease and mortality, although incidence of nonfatal myocardial infarctions may be decreased.

For additional information on initial therapeutic guidelines related to the treatment of hyperlipidemia, see *Appendix III*.

### Unaccepted

Niacin is not useful for treatment of schizophrenia and other mental disorders not related to niacin deficiency. Niacin also has not been proven effective for treatment of acne, alcohol dependence, drug-induced hallucinations, hyperkinesis, leprosy, livedoid vasculitis, peripheral vascular disease, motion sickness, or for prevention of heart attacks.

## Pharmacology/Pharmacokinetics

### Physicochemical characteristics

Molecular weight—
- Niacin: 123.11.
- Niacinamide: 122.13.

pKa—
- Niacin: 4.85.
- Niacinamide: 0.5 and 3.35.

### Mechanism of action/Effect

Nutritional supplement—Niacin, after conversion to niacinamide, is a component of two coenzymes, nicotinamide adenine dinucleotide (NAD) and nicotinamide adenine dinucleotide phosphate (NADP), which are necessary for tissue respiration; glycogenolysis; and lipid, amino acid, protein, and purine metabolism.

Antihyperlipidemic—Niacin lowers serum cholesterol and triglyceride concentrations by inhibiting the synthesis of very low density lipoproteins (VLDL), which are precursors to the formation of low-density lipoproteins, the principal carrier of blood cholesterol.

### Other actions/effects

Niacin (but not niacinamide) causes direct peripheral vasodilation.

### Absorption

The B vitamins, including niacin and niacinamide, are readily absorbed from the gastrointestinal tract, except in malabsorption syndromes.

### Biotransformation

Hepatic. Dietary tryptophan is converted by intestinal bacteria to niacin and niacinamide (about 60 mg of tryptophan is equivalent to 1 mg of niacin). Niacin is also converted to niacinamide as needed.

### Half-life

Elimination—Approximately 45 minutes.

### Onset of action

Reduced cholesterol concentrations—Oral: Several days.
Reduced triglyceride concentrations—Oral: Several hours.

### Time to peak serum concentration

Oral—45 minutes.

### Elimination

Renal (almost entirely as metabolites). Excess beyond daily needs is excreted, largely unchanged, in urine.

## Precautions to Consider

### Pregnancy/Reproduction

Problems in humans have not been documented with intake of normal daily recommended amounts. Studies have not been done in humans.
Studies have not been done in animals.

### Breast-feeding

Problems in humans have not been documented with intake of normal daily recommended amounts.

### Pediatrics

Problems in pediatrics have not been documented with intake of normal daily recommended amounts. Appropriate studies of niacin as an antihyperlipidemic have not been performed in the pediatric population. However, use of niacin as an antihyperlipidemic in children under 2 years of age is not recommended since cholesterol is required for normal development.

### Geriatrics

Problems in geriatrics have not been documented with intake of normal daily recommended amounts.

### Drug interactions and/or related problems

The following drug interactions and/or related problems have been selected on the basis of their potential clinical significance (possible mechanism in parentheses where appropriate)—not necessarily inclusive (» = major clinical significance):

Chenodiol or
Ursodiol
(effect may be decreased when chenodiol or ursodiol is used concurrently with antihyperlipidemics, which tend to increase cholesterol saturation of bile)

HMG-CoA reductase inhibitors
(concurrent use with niacin may be associated with an increased risk of rhabdomyolysis and acute renal failure; combined therapy with lovastatin, pravastatin, or simvastatin should include careful monitoring for symptoms of myopathy or rhabdomyolysis)

**Laboratory value alterations**
The following have been selected on the basis of their potential clinical significance (possible effect in parentheses where appropriate)—not necessarily inclusive (» = major clinical significance):

Note: Usually occur only with large doses.

With diagnostic test results
Urinary catecholamine concentration, measurements by fluorimetric methods
(niacin may produce fluorescent substances and falsely elevated results)

Urine glucose determinations using cupric sulfate (Benedict's reagent)
(niacin may produce false-positive reactions)

With physiology/laboratory test values
Uric acid concentrations in blood
(may be increased by large doses of niacin)

**Medical considerations/Contraindications**
The medical considerations/contraindications included have been selected on the basis of their potential clinical significance (reasons given in parentheses where appropriate)—not necessarily inclusive (» = major clinical significance).

*Risk-benefit should be considered when the following medical problems exist:*
» Arterial bleeding or hemorrhage or
Glaucoma
(these conditions may be exacerbated)
» Diabetes mellitus
(large doses of niacin may cause impaired glucose tolerance)
Gout
(large doses may cause hyperuricemia)
» Hepatic disease
(large doses may cause hepatic damage)
Hypotension
(may worsen due to vasodilating effects of niacin)
» Peptic ulcer
(large doses may activate peptic ulcer)
Sensitivity to niacin or niacinamide

**Patient monitoring**
The following may be especially important in patient monitoring (other tests may be warranted in some patients, depending on condition; » = major clinical significance):

Cholesterol concentrations, serum
(determinations recommended at periodic intervals during antihyperlipidemic therapy)

Glucose concentrations, blood and
Hepatic function determinations and
Uric acid concentrations
(determinations recommended at periodic intervals in patients receiving high doses of niacin or niacinamide for prolonged periods)

## Side/Adverse Effects

Note: Flushing and pruritus may be reduced with the extended-release dosage form of niacin.

The following side/adverse effects have been selected on the basis of their potential clinical significance (possible signs and symptoms in parentheses where appropriate)—not necessarily inclusive:

**Those indicating need for medical attention**
Incidence rare
*Allergic reaction, anaphylactic* (skin rash or itching; wheezing)—after intravenous administration

With long-term use of extended-release niacin
*Hepatotoxicity or cholestasis* (darkening of urine; light gray-colored stools; loss of appetite; severe stomach pain; yellow eyes or skin)

**Those indicating need for medical attention only if they continue or are bothersome**
Incidence less frequent—with niacin only
*Feeling of warmth; flushing or redness of skin, especially on face and neck; headache*

With high oral doses
*Cardiac arrhythmias* (unusually fast, slow, or irregular heartbeat); *diarrhea; dizziness or faintness; dryness of skin or eyes; hyperglycemia* (frequent urination or unusual thirst)—may occasionally be fatal; *hyperuricemia* (joint pain; side, lower back, or stomach pain; swelling of feet or lower legs); *myalgia* (fever; muscle aching or cramping; unusual tiredness or weakness); *nausea or vomiting; peptic ulcer, aggravation of* (stomach pain); *pruritus* (itching of skin)—may be severe

Note: Rarely, along with markedly elevated creatine kinase (CK) concentrations, fever, muscle aching or cramping, or unusual tiredness or weakness may be symptoms of myositis or rhabdomyolysis; incidence may be increased in patients treated concurrently with lovastatin, pravastatin, or simvastatin.

## Patient Consultation

As an aid to patient consultation, refer to *Advice for the Patient, Niacin (Vitamin B$_3$) (Systemic)* or *Niacin—For High Cholesterol (Systemic)*.

In providing consultation, consider emphasizing the following selected information (» = major clinical significance):

**Description of use**
Description should include function in the body, signs of deficiency, and unproven uses

**Importance of diet**
*For use as a vitamin supplement*
Importance of proper nutrition; supplement may be needed because of inadequate dietary intake
Food sources of niacin; effects of processing
Not using vitamins as substitute for balanced diet
Recommended daily intake for niacin

**Before using this medication**
*For use as a vitamin supplement*
See *Indications* for conditions and medications affecting requirements.

*For use as an antihyperlipidemic (niacin only)*
Diet as preferred therapy
» Conditions affecting use, especially:
Sensitivity to niacin or niacinamide
Use in children—Not recommended as antihyperlipidemic in children under 2 years of age since cholesterol is required for normal development
Other medical problems, especially arterial bleeding or hemorrhage, diabetes mellitus, hepatic disease, or peptic ulcer

**Proper use of this medication**
Possibility of stomach upset; taking with meals or milk; checking with physician if stomach upset continues
Proper administration of extended-release dosage forms: Swallowing whole without crushing, breaking, or chewing; contents of capsule may be mixed with jam or jelly and swallowed without chewing
» Proper storage

*For use as a vitamin supplement*
» Proper dosing
Missed dose: No cause for concern because of length of time necessary for depletion; remembering to take as directed

*For use as an antihyperlipidemic (niacin only)*
» Importance of not taking more or less medication than prescribed
Niacin does not cure the condition but instead helps control it
» Importance of following prescribed diet
Missed dose: Taking as soon as possible; not taking if almost time for next dose; not doubling doses

**Precautions while using this medication**
Caution if dizziness or faintness occurs
*For use as an antihyperlipidemic (niacin only)*
» Importance of close monitoring by physician to check progress
» Checking with physician before discontinuing medication; blood lipid concentrations may increase significantly

**Side/adverse effects**
Signs of potential side effects, especially anaphylactic reaction with injection only; hepatotoxicity or cholestasis with high doses of extended-release niacin

## General Dosing Information

Dosages of niacin and niacinamide as vitamin supplements are equal; some clinicians prefer niacinamide because of its lack of vasodilating effect.

Because of the infrequency of single B vitamin deficiencies, combinations are commonly administered. Many commercial combinations of B vitamins are available.

When used for treatment of pellagra, niacin or niacinamide is usually given in combination with 5 mg each of thiamine, riboflavin, and pyridoxine.

**For parenteral dosage forms only**

In most cases, parenteral administration is indicated only when oral administration is not acceptable (for example, in nausea, vomiting, and preoperative and postoperative conditions) or possible (for example, in malabsorption syndromes or following gastric resection).

When administered intravenously, niacin or niacinamide should be given at a rate not exceeding 2 mg per minute.

**Diet/Nutrition**

Niacin or niacinamide may be taken with meals or milk if nausea, vomiting, or diarrhea occurs. A physician should be consulted if stomach upset continues.

Recommended dietary intakes for niacin are defined differently worldwide.

For U.S.—
The Recommended Dietary Allowances (RDAs) for vitamins and minerals are determined by the Food and Nutrition Board of the National Research Council and are intended to provide adequate nutrition in most healthy persons under usual environmental stresses. In addition, a different designation may be used by the FDA for food and dietary supplement labeling purposes, as with Daily Value (DV). DVs replace the previous labeling terminology United States Recommended Daily Allowances (USRDAs).

For Canada—
Recommended Nutrient Intakes (RNIs) for vitamins, minerals, and protein are determined by Health and Welfare Canada and provide recommended amounts of a specific nutrient while minimizing the risk of chronic diseases.

Daily recommended intakes for niacin are generally defined as follows:

| Persons | U.S. (mg) | Canada (mg) |
|---|---|---|
| Infants and children | | |
| Birth to 3 years of age | 5–9 | 4–9 |
| 4 to 6 years of age | 12 | 13 |
| 7 to 10 years of age | 13 | 14–18 |
| Adolescent and adult males | 15–20 | 14–23 |
| Adolescent and adult females | 13–15 | 14–16 |
| Pregnant females | 17 | 14–16 |
| Breast-feeding females | 20 | 14–16 |

These are usually provided by adequate diets.

Best dietary sources of niacin include meats, eggs, and milk and dairy products; dietary tryptophan (from protein) is converted to niacin. There is little loss of niacin from foods with ordinary cooking.

**For treatment of adverse effects**

Tolerance to the vasodilating and gastrointestinal effects of niacin usually occurs within 2 weeks.

The severe flushing, pruritus, and gastrointestinal effects may be minimized by starting therapy with a low dose and increasing the dosage gradually, and by taking niacin with meals or milk.

Persistent flushing may sometimes be controlled with 300 mg of aspirin taken 30 minutes before each niacin dose.

---

## NIACIN

## Oral Dosage Forms

### NIACIN EXTENDED-RELEASE CAPSULES

Note: Dose-related hepatotoxicity may be more prevalent with high doses of the extended-release dosage form of niacin.

Flushing and pruritus may be reduced with the extended-release dosage form of niacin.

**Usual adult and adolescent dose**

Antihyperlipidemic—
Initial: Oral, 1 gram three times a day, the dosage being increased in increments of 500 mg a day every two to four weeks as needed.

Note: Some clinicians may begin with 500 mg per day and gradually increase the dosage to 4 grams a day.

Maintenance: Oral, 1 to 2 grams three times a day.

Deficiency (prophylaxis)—
Oral, amount based on normal daily recommended intakes:

| Persons | U.S. (mg) | Canada (mg) |
|---|---|---|
| Adolescent and adult males | 15–20 | 14–23 |
| Adolescent and adult females | 13–15 | 14–16 |
| Pregnant females | 17 | 14–16 |
| Breast-feeding females | 20 | 14–16 |

Deficiency (treatment)—
Treatment dose is individualized by prescriber based on severity of deficiency.

**Usual adult prescribing limits**
Oral, 6 grams a day.

**Usual pediatric dose**
Dosage form is not recommended for use in children.

**Strength(s) usually available**

U.S.—
125 mg (OTC) [*Nicobid Tempules*; GENERIC].
250 mg [*Nicobid Tempules (OTC)*; GENERIC].
300 mg (OTC) [*Niac*].
400 mg [*Nia-Bid (OTC); Niacels (OTC); Nico-400 (OTC)*; GENERIC].
500 mg [*Nicobid Tempules (OTC)*; GENERIC].

Canada—
Not commercially available.

Note: For use as a dietary supplement, some strengths of these niacin preparations may exceed the dosage range recommended by USP DI Advisory Panels based on the amount necessary to meet normal nutritional needs.

**Packaging and storage**
Store below 40 °C (104 °F), preferably between 15 and 30 °C (59 and 86 °F), in a well-closed container, unless otherwise specified by manufacturer.

**Auxiliary labeling**
- Swallow capsules whole.
- Take with meals or milk.

**Note**
Contents of capsule may be mixed with jelly or jam and swallowed without chewing.

### NIACIN ORAL SOLUTION

**Usual adult and adolescent dose**

Antihyperlipidemic—
Initial: Oral, 1 gram three times a day, the dosage being increased in increments of 500 mg a day every two to four weeks as needed.
Maintenance: Oral, 1 to 2 grams three times a day.

Deficiency (prophylaxis or treatment)—
See *Niacin Extended-release Capsules*.

**Usual adult prescribing limits**
Oral, 6 grams a day.

**Usual pediatric dose**
Deficiency (prophylaxis)—
Oral, amount based on normal daily recommended intakes:

| Persons | U.S. (mg) | Canada (mg) |
|---|---|---|
| Infants and children | | |
| Birth to 3 years of age | 5–9 | 4–9 |
| 4 to 6 years of age | 12 | 13 |
| 7 to 10 years of age | 13 | 14–18 |

Deficiency (treatment)—
Treatment dose is individualized by prescriber based on severity of deficiency.

**Strength(s) usually available**

U.S.—
50 mg per 5 mL (OTC) [*Nicotinex Elixir* (alcohol 14%)].

Canada—
Not commercially available.

Note: For use as a dietary supplement, the strength of this niacin preparation may exceed the dosage range recommended by USP DI Advisory Panels based on the amount necessary to meet normal nutritional needs.

**Packaging and storage**
Store below 40 °C (104 °F), preferably between 15 and 30 °C (59 and 86 °F), in a tight container, unless otherwise specified by manufacturer. Protect from freezing.

**Auxiliary labeling**
- Take with meals or milk.

### NIACIN TABLETS USP

**Usual adult and adolescent dose**
Antihyperlipidemic—
  Initial: Oral, 1 gram three times a day, the dosage being increased in increments of 500 mg a day every two to four weeks as needed.
  Note: Some clinicians may begin with 100 mg per day and gradually increase the dosage to 4 grams per day.
  Maintenance: Oral, 1 to 2 grams three times a day.
Deficiency (prophylaxis or treatment)—
  See *Niacin Extended-release Capsules*.

**Usual adult prescribing limits**
Oral, 6 grams a day.

**Usual pediatric dose**
Deficiency (prophylaxis or treatment)—
  See *Niacin Oral Solution*.

**Strength(s) usually available**
U.S.—
  25 mg (OTC) [GENERIC].
  50 mg (OTC) [GENERIC].
  100 mg (OTC) [GENERIC].
  125 mg (OTC) [GENERIC].
  250 mg (OTC) [GENERIC].
  400 mg (OTC) [GENERIC].
  500 mg [*Niacor (Rx)* (scored); *Nicolar (Rx)* (scored; tartrazine); GENERIC].
Canada—
  50 mg (OTC) [*Novo-Niacin*; GENERIC].
  100 mg (OTC) [GENERIC].
  500 mg (OTC) [GENERIC].
Note: For use as a dietary supplement, some strengths of these niacin preparations may exceed the dosage range recommended by USP DI Advisory Panels based on the amount necessary to meet normal nutritional needs.

**Packaging and storage**
Store below 40 °C (104 °F), preferably between 15 and 30 °C (59 and 86 °F), unless otherwise specified by manufacturer. Store in a well-closed container.

**Auxiliary labeling**
- Take with meals or milk.

### NIACIN EXTENDED-RELEASE TABLETS

Note: Dose-related hepatotoxicity may be more prevalent with high doses of the extended-release dosage form.
  Flushing and pruritus may be reduced with the extended-release dosage form of niacin.

**Usual adult and adolescent dose**
Antihyperlipidemic—
  Initial: Oral, 1 gram three times a day, the dosage being increased in increments of 500 mg a day every two to four weeks as needed and tolerated.
  Note: Some clinicians may begin with 500 mg per day and gradually increase the dosage to 3 grams a day.
  Maintenance: Oral, 1 to 2 grams three times a day.
  Note: Some clinicians may use a maintenance dose of 500 mg to 1 gram two to three times a day.
Deficiency (prophylaxis and treatment)—
  See *Niacin Extended-release Capsules*.

**Usual adult prescribing limits**
Oral, 6 grams a day.

**Usual pediatric dose**
Dosage form is not recommended for use in children.

**Strength(s) usually available**
U.S.—
  125 mg (Rx) [GENERIC].
  250 mg [*Endur-Acin (OTC)*; *Slo-Niacin (OTC)* (scored); GENERIC].
  400 mg (OTC) [GENERIC].
  500 mg [*Endur-Acin (OTC)*; *Slo-Niacin (OTC)* (scored); GENERIC].
  750 mg [*Slo-Niacin (OTC)* (scored); GENERIC].
  1000 mg (OTC) [GENERIC].
Canada—
  500 mg (OTC) [GENERIC].
Note: For use as a dietary supplement, some strengths of these niacin preparations may exceed the dosage range recommended by USP DI Advisory Panels based on the amount necessary to meet normal nutritional needs.

**Packaging and storage**
Store below 40 °C (104 °F), preferably between 15 and 30 °C (59 and 86 °F), in a well-closed container, unless otherwise specified by manufacturer.

**Auxiliary labeling**
- Swallow tablets whole.
- Take with meals or milk.

**Note**
If tablets are scored, they may be broken, but not crushed or chewed, before swallowing.

## Parenteral Dosage Forms

### NIACIN INJECTION USP

**Usual adult and adolescent dose**
Deficiency (prophylaxis)—
  Intravenous infusion, as part of total parenteral nutrition solutions, the specific amount determined by individual patient need.
Deficiency (treatment)—
  Intramuscular, 50 to 100 mg five or more times a day.
  Intravenous (slow), 25 to 100 mg two or more times a day.

**Usual pediatric dose**
Deficiency (prophylaxis)—
  Intravenous infusion, as part of total parenteral nutrition solutions, the specific amount determined by individual patient need.
Deficiency (treatment)—
  Intravenous (slow), up to 300 mg a day.

**Strength(s) usually available**
U.S.—
  100 mg per mL (Rx) [GENERIC].
Canada—
  Not commercially available.

**Packaging and storage**
Store below 40 °C (104 °F), preferably between 15 and 30 °C (59 and 86 °F), unless otherwise specified by manufacturer. Protect from freezing.

**Preparation of dosage form**
For administration by the intravenous route, niacin injection should be diluted to a strength of 2 mg per mL or added to 500 mL of sodium chloride injection and administered at a rate not exceeding 2 mg per minute.

---

### NIACINAMIDE

## Oral Dosage Forms

### NIACINAMIDE TABLETS USP

**Usual adult and adolescent dose**
Deficiency (prophylaxis)—
  Oral, amount based on normal daily recommended intakes:

| Persons | U.S. (mg) | Canada (mg) |
|---|---|---|
| Adolescent and adult males | 15–20 | 14–23 |
| Adolescent and adult females | 13–15 | 14–16 |
| Pregnant females | 17 | 14–16 |
| Breast-feeding females | 20 | 14–16 |

Deficiency (treatment)—
  Treatment dose is individualized by prescriber based on severity of deficiency.

**Usual pediatric dose**
Deficiency (prophylaxis)—
  Oral, amount based on normal daily recommended intakes:

| Persons | U.S. (mg) | Canada (mg) |
|---|---|---|
| Infants and children | | |
| Birth to 3 years of age | 5–9 | 4–9 |
| 4 to 6 years of age | 12 | 13 |
| 7 to 10 years of age | 13 | 14–18 |

Deficiency (treatment)—
  Treatment dose is individualized by prescriber based on severity of deficiency.

# Niacin (Systemic)

**Strength(s) usually available**
U.S.—
  50 mg (OTC) [GENERIC].
  100 mg (OTC) [GENERIC].
  125 mg (OTC) [GENERIC].
  250 mg (OTC) [GENERIC].
  500 mg (Rx/OTC) [GENERIC].
Canada—
  100 mg (OTC) [GENERIC].
  500 mg (OTC) [GENERIC].

Note: For use as a dietary supplement, some strengths of these niacinamide preparations may exceed the dosage range recommended by USP DI Advisory Panels based on the amount necessary to meet normal nutritional needs.

**Packaging and storage**
Store below 40 °C (104 °F), preferably between 15 and 30 °C (59 and 86 °F), unless otherwise specified by manufacturer. Store in a tight container.

## Parenteral Dosage Forms

### NIACINAMIDE INJECTION USP

**Usual adult and adolescent dose**
Deficiency (prophylaxis)—
  Intravenous infusion, as part of total parenteral nutrition solutions, the specific amount determined by individual patient need.
Deficiency (treatment)—
  Intramuscular, 50 to 100 mg five or more times a day.
  Intravenous (slow), 25 to 100 mg two or more times a day.

**Usual pediatric dose**
Deficiency (prophylaxis)—
  Intravenous infusion, as part of total parenteral nutrition solutions, the specific amount determined by individual patient need.
Deficiency (treatment)—
  Intravenous (slow), up to 300 mg a day.

**Strength(s) usually available**
U.S.—
  100 mg per mL (Rx) [GENERIC].
Canada—
  Not commercially available.

**Packaging and storage**
Store below 40 °C (104 °F), preferably between 15 and 30 °C (59 and 86 °F), unless otherwise specified by manufacturer. Protect from freezing.

Revised: 11/09/91
Interim revision: 08/10/94; 05/26/95; 07/11/95

---

**NIACINAMIDE**—See *Niacin (Systemic)*

---

**NICARDIPINE**—See *Calcium Channel Blocking Agents (Systemic)*

---

**NICLOSAMIDE**—The *Niclosamide (Oral-Local)* monograph is not included in this published version of the USP DI database. Copies of the monograph are available on request from Micromedex, Inc. - Reprint Requests, 6200 S. Syracuse Way, Suite 300, Englewood, CO 80111; telephone (303) 486-6400; telefax (303) 486-6464; Email: USPDI@MDX.COM.

---

# NICOTINE   Inhalation-Systemic—INTRODUCTORY VERSION

VA CLASSIFICATION (Primary): AD600
Commonly used brand name(s): *Nicotrol Inhaler*.
Note: For a listing of dosage forms and brand names by country availability, see *Dosage Forms* section(s).

## Category
Smoking cessation adjunct.

## Indications

**Accepted**
Nicotine dependence (treatment adjunct)—The nicotine inhaler is indicated as a temporary aid for cigarette smokers who want to give up smoking. It serves as an alternative source of nicotine and provides relief of nicotine withdrawal symptoms in nicotine-dependent individuals who are acutely withdrawing from cigarette smoking. It is recommended that the nicotine inhaler be used in conjunction with a comprehensive behavioral smoking cessation program.

## Pharmacology/Pharmacokinetics

**Physicochemical characteristics**
Source—Tobacco plant.
Molecular weight—162.23.
pKa—At 15 °C (59 °F): $pKa_1$—7.84; $pKa_2$—3.04.
Solubility—Freely soluble in water.
Octanol-water partition coefficient—15:1 at pH 7.

**Mechanism of action/Effect**
Nicotine acts as an agonist at the nicotinic-cholinergic receptors in the autonomic ganglia, adrenal medulla, neuromuscular junctions, and brain. Nicotine's positive reinforcing properties are believed to be the result of the release of neurotransmitters including acetylcholine, beta-endorphin, dopamine, norepinephrine, serotonin, and others that mediate pleasure, arousal, mood, appetite, and other desirable psychological states.

**Other actions/effects**
Cardiovascular effects include peripheral vasoconstriction, tachycardia, and elevated blood pressure.

**Absorption**
Nicotine is absorbed rapidly through the mucous membranes and respiratory tract, and slowly through the buccal mucosa.
The high, rapid rise and decline in nicotine plasma concentrations that occur with cigarette smoking do not occur with the use of the nicotine inhaler.

**Distribution**
Most of the nicotine released from the inhaler is deposited in the mouth. Less than 5% of a dose reaches the lower respiratory tract.
Nicotine is distributed into breast milk; the milk-to-plasma ratio average is 2.9:1.
The volume of distribution following intravenous administration is approximately 2 to 3 L per kg.

**Protein binding**
Very low (< 5%).

**Biotransformation**
Primarily hepatic; also metabolized in the kidneys and lungs. More than 20 metabolites have been identified; all are less active than the parent compound. The primary urinary metabolites are cotinine, which comprises 15% of a dose; and trans-3-hydroxycotinine, which comprises 45% of a dose.

**Half-life**
Elimination—
  Nicotine: 1 to 2 hours.
  Cotinine: 15 to 20 hours.

**Time to peak concentration**
Within 15 minutes of the end of an inhalation.

**Peak plasma concentration (at steady-state)**
Following an intensive inhalation regimen (80 deep inhalations over 20 minutes) every hour for 10 hours—
  At 20 °C (68 °F): 22.5 nanograms per mL (nanograms/mL), range 11.1 to 40.4 nanograms/mL.
  At 30 °C (86 °F): 29.7 nanograms/mL, range 17.6 to 47.2 nanograms/mL.
  At 40 °C (104 °F): 34 nanograms/mL, range 24.1 to 48.6 nanograms/mL.
Following as-needed use—
  6 to 8 nanograms/mL (approximately one third the concentration achieved with cigarette smoking).

### Elimination
Renal, approximately 10% excreted unchanged; up to 30% may be excreted in acidified urine (pH < 5) and with a high urine flow rate. The average plasma clearance is approximately 1.2 L per minute in a healthy adult smoker.

## Precautions to Consider

### Carcinogenicity
Nicotine does not appear to be carcinogenic in laboratory animals. Inconclusive evidence suggests that its metabolite, cotinine, may be carcinogenic in rats.

### Tumorigenicity
When given in conjunction with tumor initiators, nicotine and its metabolites increased the incidence of tumors in hamsters and rats.

### Mutagenicity
Neither nicotine nor its metabolite, cotinine, was shown to be mutagenic in the Ames *Salmonella* test. Nicotine induced reparable DNA damage in an *Escherichia coli* test system and was shown to be genotoxic in Chinese hamster ovary cells.

### Pregnancy/Reproduction
Fertility—In rats and rabbits, nicotine caused a reduction in DNA synthesis, resulting in delayed or inhibited implantation. Rats treated with nicotine during the time of gestation have produced decreased litter sizes.

Pregnancy—The nicotine inhaler is not recommended for use during pregnancy and should be used only if the likelihood of smoking cessation justifies the potential risk in pregnant patients who continue to smoke. Pregnant smokers should be encouraged to attempt smoking cessation using educational and behavioral interventions before using pharmacological measures. Cigarette smoking may cause low birth weight, increased risk of spontaneous abortion, and increased perinatal mortality. Spontaneous abortion during nicotine replacement therapy has been reported and possibly may be due to the nicotine.

Studies in pregnant rhesus monkeys have shown that nicotine administered intravenously reduced maternal uterine blood flow and produced acidosis, hypercarbia, and hypotension in the fetus. Nicotine administered intravenously to pregnant ewes reduced breathing movements in the fetal lamb. Teratogenicity has been demonstrated in the offspring of mice given toxic doses (25 mg per kg of body weight) of nicotine.

FDA Pregnancy Category D.

Labor—The nicotine inhaler is not recommended for use during labor because its effect on the mother and fetus is not known.

Delivery—The nicotine inhaler is not recommended for use during delivery.

### Breast-feeding
Nicotine is distributed into breast milk. The ability of infants to clear nicotine via hepatic first-pass metabolism is probably lowest at birth. Nicotine concentrations in breast milk may be expected to be lower with the nicotine inhaler than with cigarette smoking. The risk of exposing the infant to nicotine from the inhaler should be weighed against the risk associated with exposing the infant to nicotine from continued smoking by the mother.

### Pediatrics
Small amounts of nicotine can cause poisoning in children. Even used nicotine inhaler cartridges contain enough nicotine to cause serious harm in children. The cartridges also are small enough to cause choking if they are swallowed.

Safety and efficacy in children younger than 18 years of age have not been established. However, there are no specific medical problems that would limit the usefulness of the nicotine inhaler in adolescent smokers. The nicotine inhaler may be used in older adolescents only if the potential benefit justifies the potential risk.

### Geriatrics
One hundred thirty-two patients 60 years of age or older have participated in clinical trials, and geriatrics-specific problems that would limit the usefulness of this medication in the elderly are not expected. However, elderly patients are more likely to have cardiac function impairment, which may require caution in patients receiving the nicotine inhaler.

### Drug interactions and/or related problems
The following drug interactions and/or related problems have been selected on the basis of their potential clinical significance (possible mechanism in parentheses where appropriate)—not necessarily inclusive (» = major clinical significance):

Note: Combinations containing any of the following medications, depending on the amount present, may also interact with this medication.

» Antidepressants, tricyclic or
» Theophylline
(smoking cessation, with or without nicotine replacement, may alter the pharmacokinetics of these agents; dosage adjustment may be necessary)

### Medical considerations/Contraindications
The medical considerations/contraindications included have been selected on the basis of their potential clinical significance (reasons given in parentheses where appropriate)—not necessarily inclusive (» = major clinical significance).

*Except under special circumstances, this medication should not be used when the following medical problems exist:*

» Allergy or hypersensitivity to nicotine or to menthol
» Angina pectoris, severe or worsening or
» Cardiac arrhythmias, life-threatening or
» Myocardial infarction, recent
(use is not recommended)

*Risk-benefit should be considered when the following medical problems exist:*

Angina pectoris or
Cardiac arrhythmias or
Myocardial infarction, history of or
Vasospastic disease, such as:
  Buerger's disease
  Prinzmetal's angina
  Raynaud's phenomena
  (patients should be evaluated carefully before beginning therapy with the nicotine inhaler)
» Asthma or
» Chronic obstructive pulmonary disease (COPD)
(use of the nicotine inhaler has not been studied in patients with these conditions; however, nicotine is an airway irritant and may cause bronchospasm; other forms of nicotine replacement may be preferable in patients with severe bronchospastic airway disease, but if the nicotine inhaler is used, caution is recommended)

Diabetes mellitus, type 1 or
Hyperthyroidism or
Pheochromocytoma
(nicotine causes release of catecholamines from the adrenal medulla; caution is recommended)

Hepatic function impairment
(nicotine is extensively metabolized in the liver, and its total system clearance is dependent upon hepatic blood flow; therefore, reduced clearance should be anticipated)

» Hypertension, accelerated
(risk of progression to malignant hypertension is increased; caution is recommended)

Peptic ulcer disease, active
(nicotine delays healing; caution is recommended)

## Side/Adverse Effects

The following side/adverse effects have been selected on the basis of their potential clinical significance (possible signs and symptoms in parentheses where appropriate)—not necessarily inclusive:

### Those indicating need for medical attention
Incidence less frequent
*Allergic reaction* (fever with or without chills; headache; nausea with or without vomiting; runny nose; shortness of breath, tightness in chest, trouble in breathing, or wheezing; skin rash, itching, or hives; tearing of eyes); *fast or irregular heartbeat*

Note: If *fast or irregular heartbeat* occurs, use of the nicotine inhaler should be discontinued.

### Those indicating need for medical attention only if they continue or are bothersome
Incidence more frequent
*Coughing*—incidence 32%; *dyspepsia* (indigestion)—incidence 18%; *headache*—incidence 26%; *mouth and throat irritation*—incidence 40%; *rhinitis* (stuffy nose)—incidence 23%

Note: The frequency of *coughing* and *mouth and throat irritation* decreases with continued use.

Incidence less frequent
*Back pain; change in taste; diarrhea; fever; flatulence* (passing of gas); *flu-like symptoms; hiccups; nausea; nicotine withdrawal* (anxiety; dizziness; feelings of drug dependence; mental depression; pain in muscles; trouble in sleeping; unusual tiredness or weakness); *pain, general; pain in jaw and neck; paresthesias* (sensation of burning, numb-

ness, tightness, tingling, warmth or heat); *sinusitis* (stuffy nose); *tooth disorders*

## Overdose

For specific information on the agents used in the management of nicotine overdose, see:
- *Atropine* in *Anticholinergics/Antispasmodics (Systemic)* monograph;
- *Barbiturates (Systemic)* monograph;
- *Charcoal, Activated (Oral-Local)* monograph;
- *Lorazepam* in *Benzodiazepines (Systemic)* monograph; and/or
- *Sympathomimetic Agents—Cardiovascular Use (Parenteral-Systemic)* monograph.

For more information on the management of overdose or unintentional ingestion, **contact a Poison Control Center** (see *Poison Control Center Listing*).

The minimum lethal oral dose of nicotine for adults is reported to be 40 to 60 mg.

**Clinical effects of overdose**
The following effects have been selected on the basis of their potential clinical significance (possible signs and symptoms in parentheses where appropriate)—not necessarily inclusive:

*Abdominal pain; bradycardia; cold sweat; confusion; death*—due to respiratory paralysis or cardiac failure; *diarrhea; disturbed hearing and vision; dizziness; extreme exhaustion*—with large overdoses; *headache; hypotension*—with large overdoses; *nausea; pale skin; respiratory failure*—with large overdoses; *salivation; seizures*—at lethal doses; *tremors; vomiting; weakness*

**Treatment of overdose**
To decrease absorption—Following ingestion of a nicotine inhaler cartridge, activated charcoal should be administered (via nasogastric tube if the patient is unconscious). A saline cathartic or sorbitol may be added to the first dose of activated charcoal. Repeated doses of charcoal should be administered as long as the cartridge remains in the gastrointestinal tract because it will continue to release nicotine. The cartridge may be visualized using a radiograph.

Supportive care—Administration of lorazepam or barbiturates for seizures, and atropine for excess bronchial secretions, diarrhea, bradycardia, or hypotension; respiratory support for respiratory failure; vigorous fluid support for hypotension and cardiovascular collapse. Vasopressors may be administered if hypotension does not respond to atropine and fluids. Patients in whom intentional overdose is confirmed or suspected should be referred for psychiatric consultation.

## Patient Consultation

As an aid to patient consultation, refer to *Advice for the Patient, Nicotine (Inhalation-Systemic)—Introductory Version.*

In providing consultation, consider emphasizing the following selected information (» = major clinical significance):

**Before using this medication**
» Conditions affecting use, especially:
  Allergy or hypersensitivity to nicotine or to menthol
  Pregnancy—Use is not recommended; spontaneous abortions have been reported; use only if likelihood of smoking cessation justifies the potential risk in pregnant patients who continue to smoke
  Breast-feeding—Distributed into breast milk
  Use in children—A small amount of nicotine from a nicotine inhaler cartridge can cause poisoining in children; cartridge also can cause choking if swallowed
  Other medications, especially theophylline or tricyclic antidepressants
  Other medical problems, especially accelerated hypertension, asthma, chronic obstructive pulmonary disease (COPD), life-threatening cardiac arrhythmias, recent myocardial infarction, or severe or worsening angina pectoris

**Proper use of this medication**
» Reading patient directions carefully before using
  Using the nicotine inhaler at or above room temperature (60 °F [16 °C]) because cold temperatures decrease the amount of nicotine inhaled
» Participating in a comprehensive behavioral smoking cessation program
  Gradually reducing use of the nicotine inhaler by keeping a tally of, and steadily reducing, daily usage or setting a planned date for stopping use
» Proper dosing
» Proper storage

**Precautions while using this medication**
» Not smoking during treatment with the nicotine inhaler
» Not using the nicotine inhaler for longer than 6 months
» Not using the nicotine inhaler during pregnancy
» Prevention of unintentional ingestion of nicotine by children or pets to prevent poisoning or choking

**Side/adverse effects**
  Signs of potential side effects, especially allergic reaction and fast or irregular heartbeat

## General Dosing Information

It must be emphasized that smoking should be stopped upon initiation of therapy. Continued smoking while using the nicotine inhaler may cause adverse effects as a result of peak nicotine concentrations higher than concentrations found after smoking alone.

If a patient is unable to stop smoking by the fourth week of therapy, treatment should be discontinued because the patient is unlikely to quit on that attempt.

The safety and efficacy of the use of the nicotine inhaler for longer than 6 months has not been evaluated and is not recommended.

To minimize the risk of becoming dependent on the nicotine inhaler, gradual withdrawal from therapy should begin after 3 months of use. Suggested strategies include keeping a tally of, and steadily reducing, daily usage or setting a planned date for stopping use of the nicotine inhaler.

## Inhalation Dosage Forms

### NICOTINE FOR INHALATION

**Usual adult and adolescent dose**
Smoking cessation adjunct—
  Oral inhalation, initially 6 to 16 cartridges (24 to 64 mg) per day for up to twelve weeks followed by a gradual reduction in dosage over a period of up to twelve weeks.

Note: An inhalation regimen consisting of frequent, continuous puffing for 20 minutes is recommended.

**Usual adult and adolescent prescribing limits**
16 cartridges per day.

**Usual pediatric dose**
Safety and efficacy have not been established.

**Strength(s) usually available**
U.S.—
  10 mg (4 mg delivered) per cartridge in a kit containing 42 cartridges (Rx) [*Nicotrol Inhaler*].

**Packaging and storage**
Store below 30 °C (86 °F). Protect from light.

**Auxiliary labeling**
- For oral inhalation only.
- Include patient information when dispensing.

Developed: 07/06/98

# NICOTINE Nasal—INTRODUCTORY VERSION

VA CLASSIFICATION (Primary): AD600

Commonly used brand name(s): *Nicotrol NS*.

Note: For a listing of dosage forms and brand names by country availability, see *Dosage Forms* section(s).

## Category

Smoking cessation adjunct.

## Indications

**Accepted**
Nicotine dependence (treatment adjunct)—Nicotine nasal spray is indicated as a temporary aid for cigarette smokers who want to give up smoking. It serves as an alternate source of nicotine and provides relief from nicotine withdrawal symptoms in nicotine-dependent individuals acutely withdrawing from cigarette smoking. It is recommended that

nicotine nasal spray be used in conjunction with a comprehensive behavioral smoking cessation program.

## Pharmacology/Pharmacokinetics

### Physicochemical characteristics
Source—Tobacco plant.
Molecular weight—162.23.
pH—7.
pKa—At 15 °C (59 °F): $pKa_1$—7.84; $pKa_2$—3.04.
Solubility—Freely soluble in water.

### Mechanism of action/Effect
Nicotine acts as an agonist at the nicotine receptors in the autonomic ganglia, adrenal medulla, neuromuscular junctions, and brain. Nicotine's positive reinforcing properties are believed to be the result of the release of neurotransmitters including acetylcholine, beta-endorphin, dopamine, norepinephrine, serotonin, and others that mediate pleasure, arousal, mood, appetite, and other desirable psychological states.

### Other actions/effects
Cardiovascular effects include peripheral vasoconstriction, tachycardia, and elevated blood pressure.

### Absorption
Nicotine is absorbed rapidly through the mucous membranes and respiratory tract.
Following administration of two sprays, one in each nostril, approximately 53% enters the systemic circulation.

### Distribution
Nicotine is distributed into breast milk; the milk-to-plasma ratio average is 2.9:1.
The volume of distribution following intravenous administration is approximately 2 to 3 L per kg.

### Protein binding
Very low (< 5%).

### Biotransformation
Primarily hepatic; also metabolized in the kidneys and lungs. More than 20 metabolites have been identified; all are less active than the parent compound. The primary urinary metabolites are cotinine, which comprises 15% of a dose; and trans-3-hydroxycotinine, which comprises 45% of a dose.

### Half-life
Elimination—
  Nicotine: 1 to 3 hours.
  Cotinine: 15 to 20 hours.
Absorption—
  Nicotine: Approximately 3 minutes.

### Time to peak concentration
4 to 15 minutes.

### Peak arterial plasma concentration
5 to 15 nanograms per mL. However, individual plasma nicotine concentrations following administration of nicotine nasal spray may vary widely.

### Elimination
Renal, approximately 10% excreted unchanged; up to 30% may be excreted in acidified urine (pH < 5) or with a high urine flow rate. The average plasma clearance is approximately 1.2 L per minute in a healthy adult smoker.

## Precautions to Consider

### Carcinogenicity
Nicotine does not appear to be carcinogenic in laboratory animals. Inconclusive evidence suggests that cotinine may be carcinogenic in rats.

### Tumorigenicity
When given in conjunction with tumor initiators, nicotine and its metabolites increased the incidence of tumors in hamsters and rats.

### Mutagenicity
Neither nicotine nor its metabolite, cotinine, was shown to be mutagenic in the Ames *Salmonella* test. Nicotine induced reparable DNA damage in an *Escherichia coli* test system and was shown to be genotoxic in Chinese hamster ovary cells.

### Pregnancy/Reproduction
Fertility—In rats and rabbits, nicotine caused a reduction in DNA synthesis, resulting in delayed or inhibited implantation. Rats treated with nicotine during the time of gestation have produced decreased litter sizes.
Pregnancy—Nicotine replacement therapy is not recommended for use during pregnancy and should be used only if the likelihood of smoking cessation justifies the potential risk in pregnant patients who continue to smoke. Pregnant smokers should be encouraged to attempt smoking cessation using educational and behavioral interventions before using pharmacological measures.
Cigarette smoking may cause low birth weight, increased risk of spontaneous abortion, and increased perinatal mortality. Spontaneous abortion during nicotine replacement therapy has been reported, and possibly may be due to the nicotine.
Studies in pregnant rhesus monkeys have shown that nicotine administered intravenously produces acidosis, hypercarbia, and hypotension in the fetus. Nicotine administered intravenously to pregnant ewes reduced breathing movements in the fetal lamb. Teratogenicity has been demonstrated in offspring of mice given toxic doses of nicotine.

FDA Pregnancy Category D.

Labor—Nicotine nasal spray is not recommended for use during labor because its effect on the mother and fetus is not known.
Delivery—Nicotine nasal spray is not recommended for use during delivery.

### Breast-feeding
Nicotine is distributed into breast milk. The ability of infants to clear nicotine via hepatic first-pass metabolism is probably lowest at birth. Nicotine concentrations in breast milk may be expected to be lower with nicotine nasal spray than with cigarette smoking. The risk of exposing the infant to nicotine from the nasal spray should be weighed against the risk associated with exposing the infant to nicotine from continued smoking by the mother.

### Pediatrics
The amount of nicotine that is tolerated by adult smokers can cause poisoning in children. Use in children is not recommended.

### Geriatrics
Appropriate studies on the relationship of age to the effects of nicotine nasal spray have not been performed in the geriatric population. However, 41 patients 60 years of age and older participated in clinical trials, and geriatrics-specific problems that would limit the usefulness of this medication in the elderly are not expected.

### Drug interactions and/or related problems
The following drug interactions and/or related problems have been selected on the basis of their potential clinical significance (possible mechanism in parentheses where appropriate)—not necessarily inclusive (» = major clinical significance):

Note: Combinations containing any of the following medications, depending on the amount present, may also interact with this medication.

  Acetaminophen or
» Beta-adrenergic blocking agents, such as propranolol or
  Caffeine or
  Imipramine or
  Oxazepam or
  Pentazocine or
» Theophylline
    (smoking cessation may increase the therapeutic effects of these agents by decreasing metabolism; a decrease in dosage may be necessary)

» Insulin
    (smoking cessation may increase the therapeutic effects of insulin by increasing absorption; a decrease in dosage may be necessary)

  Nasal decongestants, topical, such as xylometazoline
    (concurrent use by patients with rhinitis may prolong the time to peak nicotine concentration by approximately 40%)

### Medical considerations/Contraindications
The medical considerations/contraindications included have been selected on the basis of their potential clinical significance (reasons given in parentheses where appropriate)—not necessarily inclusive (» = major clinical significance).

*Except under special circumstances, this medication should not be used when the following medical problems exist:*

» Allergy or hypersensitivity to nicotine or any component of the nasal spray
» Angina pectoris, severe or worsening or
» Cardiac arrhythmias, life-threatening or
» Myocardial infarction, recent
    (use is not recommended)

» Chronic nasal disorders, such as:
    Allergy
    Polyps, nasal
    Rhinitis

Sinusitis
(safety and efficacy have not been established; use is not recommended)

*Risk-benefit should be considered when the following medical problems exist:*
Angina pectoris or
Cardiac arrhythmias or
Myocardial infarction, history of or
Vasospastic disease, such as:
  Buerger's disease
  Prinzmetal's angina
  Raynaud's phenomena
    (patients should be evaluated carefully before beginning therapy with nicotine nasal spray)
Common cold or
Rhinitis, acute
(extent of absorption may be reduced by approximately 10%; peak plasma concentration may be reduced by approximately 20%, and time to peak concentration may be prolonged by approximately 30% in patients with rhinitis)
Diabetes, type 1 or
Hyperthyroidism or
Pheochromocytoma
(nicotine causes release of catecholamines from the adrenal medulla; caution is recommended)
Hepatic function impairment
(nicotine is extensively metabolized in the liver, and its total system clearance is dependent upon blood flow; therefore, reduced clearance should be anticipated)
» Hypertension, accelerated
(risk of progression to malignant hypertension is increased by cigarette smoking; caution is recommended)
Peptic ulcer disease, active
(nicotine delays healing; caution is recommended)

## Side/Adverse Effects

The following side/adverse effects have been selected on the basis of their potential clinical significance (possible signs and symptoms in parentheses where appropriate)—not necessarily inclusive:

**Those indicating need for medical attention**
Incidence more frequent
*Feelings of physical dependence*—incidence 32%; *pain in joints; shortness of breath; swelling of gums, mouth, or tongue; tightness in chest; tingling in arms, legs, hands, or feet*
Incidence less frequent
*Confusion; fast or irregular heartbeat; nasal blister or ulcer; numbness of nose or mouth; pain in muscles; paresthesias of nose, mouth, or head* (burning, tingling, or prickly sensations); *pharyngitis* (difficulty in swallowing; dryness or pain in throat)
Note: If *fast or irregular heartbeat* occurs, use of nicotine nasal spray should be discontinued.
Incidence rare
*Amnesia; bronchitis; bronchospasm; difficulty in speaking; edema* (swelling of feet or lower legs); *migraine headache; purpura* (blood-containing blisters on skin); *skin rash*

**Those indicating need for medical attention only if they continue or are bothersome**
Incidence more frequent
*Back pain; constipation; cough; headache; indigestion; nasal irritation, moderate or severe*—incidence 94%; *nausea; runny nose; sneezing; throat irritation; watery eyes*
Note: The severity of *nasal irritation* usually declines with continued use.
Incidence less frequent
*Abdominal pain; acne; burning or irritation in eyes; change in sense of smell, transient; change in sense of taste, transient; dysmenorrhea or menstrual disorders; earache; flatulence; flushing of face; gum problems; hoarseness; itching; nasal congestion; nosebleed, transient; sinus irritation*
Incidence rare
*Changes in vision; diarrhea; dryness of mouth; hiccups; increased sputum production*

## Overdose

For specific information on the agents used in the management of nicotine overdose, see:
- *Atropine* in *Anticholinergics/Antispasmodics (Systemic)* monograph;
- *Barbiturates (Systemic)* monograph;
- *Lorazepam* in *Benzodiazepines (Systemic)* monograph; and/or
- *Sympathomimetic Agents—Cardiovascular Use (Parenteral-Systemic)* monograph.

For more information on the management of overdose or unintentional ingestion, **contact a Poison Control Center** (see *Poison Control Center Listing*).

The minimum lethal oral dose of nicotine for adults is reported to be 40 to 60 mg.

**Clinical effects of overdose**
The following effects have been selected on the basis of their potential clinical significance (possible signs and symptoms in parentheses where appropriate)—not necessarily inclusive:
*Abdominal pain; bradycardia; cold sweat; confusion; death*—due to respiratory paralysis or cardiac failure; *diarrhea; disturbed hearing and vision; dizziness; excessive salivation; extreme exhaustion; fast or irregular heartbeat; headache; hypotension; nausea; pale skin; seizures*—at lethal doses; *tremors; vomiting; weakness*

**Treatment of overdose**
To decrease absorption—
Following eye contact: Flushing the eyes with a gentle stream of water for 20 minutes.
Supportive care—
Administration of lorazepam or barbiturates for seizures, and atropine for excess bronchial secretions, diarrhea, bradycardia, or hypotension; respiratory support for respiratory failure; vigorous fluid support for hypotension and cardiovascular collapse. Vasopressors may be administered if hypotension does not respond to atropine and fluids. Patients in whom intentional overdose is confirmed or suspected should be referred for psychiatric consultation.

## Patient Consultation

As an aid to patient consultation, refer to *Advice for the Patient, Nicotine (Nasal)—Introductory Version*.
In providing consultation, consider emphasizing the following selected information (» = major clinical significance):

**Before using this medication**
» Conditions affecting use, especially:
  Allergy or hypersensitivity to nicotine or any component of the nasal spray
  Pregnancy—Not recommended during pregnancy; spontaneous abortions have been reported; use only if likelihood of smoking cessation justifies the potential risk in pregnant patients who continue to smoke
  Breast-feeding—Distributed into breast milk
  Use in children—Use is not recommended
  Other medications, especially beta-adrenergic blocking agents, insulin, or theophylline
  Other medical problems, especially angina pectoris, severe or worsening; cardiac arrhythmias, life-threatening; chronic nasal disorders; hypertension, accelerated; or myocardial infarction, recent

**Proper use of this medication**
» Reading patient instructions carefully before using
» Participating in a comprehensive behavioral smoking cessation program
Tapering off use of nicotine nasal spray by using only one half of a dose at a time, skipping doses by not medicating every hour, keeping tally of and steadily reducing daily usage, or setting date for stopping use of nicotine nasal spray
» Proper dosing
» Proper storage

**Precautions while using this medication**
» Not recommended for use by nonsmokers because of potential for addiction
» Continuing use of nicotine nasal spray for at least 1 week to adapt to the irritant effects of the spray; contacting physician if irritant effects do not lessen after 1 week
» Avoiding contact of nicotine nasal spray with skin, mouth, eyes, and ears
» Not using nicotine nasal spray for longer than 3 months
» Not using nicotine nasal spray during pregnancy
» Prevention of unintentional ingestion of nicotine nasal spray by children or pets to prevent poisoning

### Side/adverse effects
Signs of potential side effects, especially feelings of physical dependence; pain in joints; shortness of breath; swelling of gums, mouth, or tongue; tightness in chest; tingling in arms, legs, hands, or feet; confusion; fast or irregular heartbeat; nasal blister or ulcer; numbness of nose or mouth; pain in muscles; paresthesias of nose, mouth, or head; pharyngitis; amnesia; bronchitis; bronchospasm; difficulty in speaking; edema; migraine headache; purpura; and skin rash

## General Dosing Information
The necessity for immediate cessation of smoking upon initiation of therapy must be emphasized. Continued smoking while using nicotine nasal spray may cause adverse effects as a result of peak nicotine concentrations higher than concentrations found after smoking alone.

If a patient is unable to stop smoking by the fourth week of therapy, treatment should be discontinued because the patient is unlikely to quit on that attempt.

Because of the risk of addiction, nicotine nasal spray should not be used by nonsmokers.

No optimal strategy for tapering off use of nicotine nasal spray was found during clinical trials. However, suggested strategies include using only one half of a dose at a time, skipping doses by not medicating every hour, keeping a tally of and steadily reducing daily usage, or setting a planned date for stopping use of nicotine nasal spray.

### Safety considerations for handling this medication
If even a small amount of nicotine nasal spray comes into contact with the skin, mouth, eyes, or ears, the affected area should be immediately rinsed with water only.

## Nasal Dosage Forms

### Nicotine Nasal Solution

#### Usual adult dose
Smoking cessation adjunct—
Intranasal, initially 1 or 2 mg per hour. Dosage then should be individualized based upon degree of nicotine dependence and occurrence of symptoms of nicotine excess.

Note: One mg of nicotine is delivered by two sprays, one in each nostril.

#### Usual adult prescribing limits
The minimum recommended dose is 8 mg per day. The maximum recommended dose is 5 mg per hour or 40 mg per day. The maximum recommended duration of therapy is three months.

#### Usual pediatric dose
Use is not recommended.

#### Strength(s) usually available
U.S.—
0.5 mg per 50 microliter metered spray (Rx) [*Nicotrol NS* (disodium phosphate; sodium dihydrogen phosphate; citric acid; methylparaben; propylparaben; edetate disodium; sodium chloride; polysorbate 80; aroma; water)].

#### Packaging and storage
Store below 30 ºC (86 ºF), unless otherwise specified by manufacturer.

#### Auxiliary labeling
• For the nose.
• Include patient information when dispensing.

Revised: 08/05/98

---

# NICOTINE Systemic

VA CLASSIFICATION (Primary): AD900

Commonly used brand name(s): *Habitrol; Nicoderm; Nicorette; Nicorette Plus; Nicotrol; ProStep*.

Note: For a listing of dosage forms and brand names by country availability, see *Dosage Forms* section(s).

## Category
Smoking cessation adjunct.

## Indications

### Accepted
Nicotine dependence (treatment adjunct)—Nicotine chewing gum and nicotine transdermal systems are indicated as temporary aids to the cigarette smoker who wants to give up smoking while participating in a behavior modification program. They provide an alternate source of nicotine for nicotine-dependent individuals acutely withdrawing from cigarette smoking.

Behavior modification encompasses supervised programs of education, counseling, and psychological support. The efficacy of these nicotine products without concomitant participation in such a program has not been established.

Generally, smokers who have a strong physical nicotine dependence are more likely to benefit from the use of these nicotine products. Smoking withdrawal effects such as irritability, drowsiness, fatigue, headache, and nicotine craving are lessened with their use.

Nicotine chewing gum has not been shown to be beneficial for longer than 3 months. The use of nicotine transdermal systems for longer than 12 to 20 weeks, depending on the product, has not been evaluated and is not recommended.

### Unaccepted
Nicotine chewing gum and transdermal systems are not recommended for use by nonsmokers because increase in heart rate and blood pressure and central nervous system (CNS)–mediated symptoms such as hiccups, nausea, and vomiting are associated with even small doses of nicotine from these products. Also, nicotine in these products may cause dependence in nonsmokers.

## Pharmacology/Pharmacokinetics

### Physicochemical characteristics
Molecular weight—Nicotine: 162.2.

### Mechanism of action/Effect
Nicotine acts as an agonist at the nicotinic receptors in the peripheral and central nervous systems, producing both stimulant and depressant phases of action on all autonomic ganglia.

When the gum is chewed, nicotine is displaced from polacrilex by alkaline saliva.

### Other actions/effects
Has actions on the chemoreceptors of the aortic and carotid bodies, resulting in reflex vasoconstriction, tachycardia, elevated blood pressure, and stimulation of respiration.

Stimulates sympathetic ganglia and adrenal medulla, causing release of catecholamines, resulting in direct sympathomimetic effects on the heart and peripheral vasculature.

Has actions that tend to reduce blood pressure and heart rate. In low concentrations, stimulates certain chemoreceptors in the pulmonary and coronary circulation, leading to reflex bradycardia and hypotension.

Causes release of antidiuretic hormone (ADH) by stimulation of hypothalamus.

Stimulation of emetic chemoreceptor trigger zone of medulla oblongata and vagal reflex activation may result in vomiting.

Parasympathetic stimulation increases tone and motor activity of the gastrointestinal tract, leading to nausea, vomiting, and occasionally diarrhea.

Effects of nicotine on exocrine glands cause an initial stimulation followed by inhibition of salivary and bronchial secretions.

Action on CNS may result in respiratory failure due to both central paralysis and peripheral blockade of muscles of respiration.

### Absorption
Chewing gum:
Buccal mucosa: Absorption enhanced by buffering of gum to pH 8.5; rate of absorption is slower than from lungs during smoking.
Stomach: Not absorbed in significant amounts when gum is swallowed because of poor release of nicotine from gum in acidic pH of stomach.
Transdermal systems:
Skin: Well absorbed.

### Distribution
Nicotine passes into breast milk.

### Biotransformation
Primarily hepatic; smaller amounts are metabolized in the kidneys and lungs; metabolites include cotinine and nicotine-1′-N-oxide.

**Half-life**
Nicotine—1 to 2 hours.
Cotinine—15 to 20 hours.

**Time to peak concentration**
Chewing gum:
  15 to 30 minutes after start of chewing.
Transdermal systems (at steady state):
  *Habitrol*: 5 to 6 hours after application.
  *Nicoderm*: 4 hours after application.
  *ProStep*: 9 hours after application.

**Peak serum concentration**
Average steady-state—
  Chewing gum:
    7.9 to 10.8 nanograms per mL.
  Transdermal systems:
    *Habitrol*—17 nanograms per mL following application of the 21 mg/day patch.
    *Nicoderm*—23 nanograms per mL following application of the 21 mg/day patch; 17 nanograms per mL following application of the 14 mg/day patch; 8 nanograms per mL following application of the 7 mg/day patch.
    *ProStep*—16 nanograms per mL following application of the 22 mg/day patch.

**Elimination**
Renal, 10 to 20% unchanged; up to 30% may be excreted in acidified urine (pH <5) and with high urine flow rate.

## Precautions to Consider

**Carcinogenicity**
Nicotine does not appear to be carcinogenic in laboratory animals. Inconclusive evidence suggests that cotinine, an oxidized metabolite, may be carcinogenic in rats.

**Tumorigenicity**
When given in combination with tumor initiators, nicotine and its metabolites increased the incidence of tumors in hamsters and rats.

**Mutagenicity**
Neither nicotine nor its metabolite, cotinine, was shown to be mutagenic in the Ames *Salmonella* test. Nicotine induced repairable DNA damage in an *E. coli* test system. Nicotine was shown to be genotoxic in Chinese hamster ovary cells.

**Pregnancy/Reproduction**
Fertility—Impaired fertility has been demonstrated in mice. In addition, implantation was delayed or inhibited in rats and rabbits by reduction in DNA synthesis that appears to be caused by nicotine. Rats treated with nicotine during the time of gestation have produced decreased litter sizes.

Pregnancy—Nicotine replacement therapy is not recommended during pregnancy and should be used only if the likelihood of smoking cessation justifies the potential risk in pregnant patients who continue to smoke. Pregnant smokers should be encouraged to attempt smoking cessation using education and behavioral interventions before using pharmacological measures.

Cigarette smoking may cause low birth weight, increased risk of spontaneous abortion, and increased perinatal mortality. Spontaneous abortion during nicotine replacement therapy has been reported, and possibly may be due to the nicotine.

Studies in pregnant rhesus monkeys have shown that nicotine administered intravenously produces acidosis, hypoxia, and hypercarbia in the fetus. Teratogenicity has been demonstrated in offspring of mice given toxic doses of nicotine.

Nicotine chewing gum—FDA Pregnancy Category X.
Nicotine transdermal systems—FDA Pregnancy Category D.

**Breast-feeding**
Nicotine is distributed into breast milk. Problems in humans have not been documented; however, because of the potential for serious adverse effects, risk-benefit must be considered.

**Pediatrics**
Small amounts of nicotine can cause serious harm in children. Even used nicotine transdermal systems contain enough nicotine to cause potential problems in children.

**Geriatrics**
Appropriate studies on the relationship of age to the effects of nicotine have not been performed in the geriatric population. However, evidence to date from a limited number of geriatric patients has not indicated geriatrics-specific problems.

**Dental**
When used over an extended period of time, nicotine gum may cause severe occlusal stress because its viscosity is heavier than ordinary chewing gum. This can cause loosening of inlays or fillings, can stick to dentures, and can cause damage to oral mucosa and natural teeth. The use of hard sugarless candy between doses of gum is recommended to help alleviate mucosal discomfort and to provide oral stimulation required by some patients. Also, some temporomandibular joint dysfunction and pain have been associated with excessive chewing.

**Drug interactions and/or related problems**
The following drug interactions and/or related problems have been selected on the basis of their potential clinical significance (possible mechanism in parentheses where appropriate)—not necessarily inclusive (» = major clinical significance):

Note: Combinations containing any of the following medications, depending on the amount present, may also interact with this medication.

» Bronchodilators, xanthine-derivative, except dyphylline or
» Propoxyphene or
» Propranolol, and possibly other beta-adrenergic blocking agents
    (smoking cessation may increase therapeutic effects of these agents by decreasing metabolism, thereby increasing serum concentrations; dosage adjustments may be necessary)

» Insulin
    (smoking cessation and concurrent therapy with nicotine chewing gum, transdermal systems, or other smoking deterrents, such as lobeline sulfate and silver acetate, may increase the therapeutic effects of insulin by increasing absorption, thereby increasing serum concentrations; dosage reduction of insulin may be necessary when an insulin-dependent diabetic patient suddenly stops smoking)

**Medical considerations/Contraindications**
The medical considerations/contraindications included have been selected on the basis of their potential clinical significance (reasons given in parentheses where appropriate)—not necessarily inclusive (» = major clinical significance).

*Except under special circumstances, this medication should not be used when the following medical problems exist:*
» Angina pectoris, severe or
» Cardiac arrhythmias, life-threatening or
» Post-myocardial infarction
    (may be exacerbated by action on heart of catecholamines released from adrenal medulla; tolerance to this effect does not develop)

*Risk-benefit should be considered when the following medical problems exist:*
Angina pectoris or
Cardiac arrhythmias or
Diabetes mellitus, insulin-dependent or
Hypertension or
Hyperthyroidism or
Myocardial infarction, history of or
Pheochromocytoma or
Vasospastic diseases, such as Buerger's disease and Prinzmetal's (or variant) angina
    (increases in blood pressure, heart rate, and plasma glucose concentrations may result from effects of nicotine-induced catecholamine release)

Peptic ulcer disease, history of
    (may be exacerbated)

Sensitivity to nicotine

*For the chewing gum only (in addition to the above)*
Dental problems or
Temporomandibular joint (TMJ) disorder
    (injury to teeth or aggravation of TMJ may result from mechanical effects of chewing gum)

Esophagitis, history of or
Inflammation of mouth or throat
    (may be exacerbated)

*For the transdermal systems only (in addition to the above)*
Skin diseases
    (may be exacerbated)

**Patient monitoring**
The following may be especially important in patient monitoring (other tests may be warranted in some patients, depending on condition; » = major clinical significance):

» Evaluation of progress of smoking cessation
    (recommended periodically during therapy to assess therapeutic efficacy of nicotine replacement products and to re-evaluate their use)

## Side/Adverse Effects

Note: Side effects are dose-dependent; extremely high doses can produce toxic symptoms, even in nicotine-tolerant individuals.

The following side/adverse effects have been selected on the basis of their potential clinical significance (possible signs and symptoms in parentheses where appropriate)—not necessarily inclusive:

**Those indicating need for medical attention**
Incidence more frequent
  *For chewing gum only*
    **Injury to mouth, teeth, or dental work**
    Note: Nicotine gum is stickier and of heavier viscosity than ordinary gum, making it harder to chew.
Incidence rare
  *For all nicotine replacement products*
    **Atrial fibrillation, reversible** (irregular heartbeat); **hypersensitivity reactions, local or generalized, including edema** (swelling); **erythema** (redness); **pruritus** (itching); **rash; or urticaria** (hives)

**Those indicating need for medical attention only if they continue or are bothersome**
Incidence more frequent
  *For all nicotine replacement products*
    **Fast heartbeat; headache, mild; increased appetite**
  *For chewing gum only*
    **Belching**—may be minimized by modifying chewing technique; **increased watering of mouth, mild; jaw muscle ache; sore mouth or throat**
  *For transdermal systems only*
    **Erythema, pruritus, and/or burning at site of application** (redness, itching, and/or burning)—usually subsides within an hour
Incidence less frequent or rare
  *For all nicotine replacement products*
    **Constipation; coughing, increased; diarrhea; dizziness or light-headedness, mild; drowsiness; dryness of mouth; dysmenorrhea** (menstrual pain); **insomnia** (trouble in sleeping); **or abnormal dreams; loss of appetite; muscle or joint pain; stomach upset or indigestion, mild; sweating, increased; unusual irritability or nervousness**
  *For chewing gum only*
    **Hiccups; hoarseness**

## Overdose

For specific information on the agents used in the management of nicotine overdose, see:
- *Atropine* in *Anticholinergics/Antispasmodics (Systemic)* monograph;
- *Barbiturates (Systemic)* monograph;
- *Charcoal, Activated (Oral-Local)* monograph;
- *Diazepam* in *Benzodiazepines (Systemic)* monograph; and/or
- *Ipecac (Oral-Local)* monograph.

For more information on the management of overdose or unintentional ingestion, **contact a Poison Control Center** (see *Poison Control Center Listing*).

**Clinical effects of overdose**
The following effects have been selected on the basis of their potential clinical significance (possible signs and symptoms in parentheses where appropriate)—not necessarily inclusive:

Early effects of overdose (in possible order of occurrence)
  **Nausea and/or vomiting; increased watering of mouth, severe; abdominal pain, severe; diarrhea, severe; cold sweat; headache, severe; dizziness, severe; drooling; disturbed hearing and vision; confusion; weakness, severe**

Late effects of overdose (in possible order of occurrence)
  **Fainting; hypotension; difficulty in breathing, severe; fast, weak, or irregular pulse; convulsions**
  Note: *Overdose* may occur if many pieces of gum are chewed simultaneously or in rapid succession, or may occur after a single piece of gum in some patients; absorption may be reduced by the early nausea and vomiting known to occur with excessive nicotine intake; if gum is swallowed without chewing, little nicotine will be released or absorbed in significant amounts because of acid pH of stomach.

**Treatment of overdose**
For chewing gum only—
  To decrease absorption—In a conscious patient, if emesis has not occurred, induction of vomiting with ipecac syrup. In an unconscious patient with a clear airway, gastric lavage followed by a suspension of activated charcoal left in the stomach.
  To enhance elimination—A saline cathartic will hasten the gastrointestinal passage of the gum.
For transdermal systems only—
  To decrease absorption—Remove patch and flush skin surface with water and dry. Do not use soap, because it may increase nicotine absorption. If patch has been ingested, administer activated charcoal. Repeated doses of charcoal should be administered as long as the patch remains in the gastrointestinal tract because it will continue to release nicotine.
  To enhance elimination—A saline cathartic or sorbitol may be added to the first dose of activated charcoal to speed passage of the patch.
For all nicotine replacement products—
  Supportive care—Respiratory support for respiratory failure. Intensive treatment of hypotension and cardiovascular collapse. Anticonvulsants such as diazepam or barbiturates for seizures. Administration of atropine for excessive bronchial secretions or diarrhea. Patients in whom intentional overdose is confirmed or suspected should be referred for psychiatric consultation.

## Patient Consultation

As an aid to patient consultation, refer to *Advice for the Patient, Nicotine (Systemic)*.

In providing consultation, consider emphasizing the following selected information (» = major clinical significance):

**Before using this medication**
» Conditions affecting use, especially:
    Pregnancy—Not recommended during pregnancy; spontaneous abortions have been reported; use only if the likelihood of smoking cessation justifies the potential risk in pregnant patients who continue to smoke
    Breast-feeding—Distributed into breast milk
    Use in children—Small amounts of nicotine can cause serious harm in children
    Dental—Chewing gum may cause severe occlusive stress resulting in damage to teeth, dentures, or dental work
    Other medications, especially insulin, propoxyphene, propranolol, or xanthine-derivative bronchodilators (except dyphylline)
    Other medical problems, especially severe angina pectoris, life-threatening cardiac arrhythmias, postmyocardial infarction state

**Proper use of this medication**
*Proper administration of the chewing gum*
» Reading patient instructions carefully before using
» Participating in a supervised stop-smoking program
» Using gum only when there is an urge to smoke
» Chewing gum slowly and intermittently for 30 minutes
» Not chewing too fast, not chewing more than one piece of gum at a time, and not chewing one piece too soon after another, to avoid adverse effects or overdose
*Compliance with chewing gum therapy*
» Reducing number of pieces chewed each day over a 2- to 3-month period
» Importance of carrying gum at all times during therapy
» Using hard sugarless candy between doses of gum to help alleviate mucosal discomfort
*Proper administration of the transdermal systems*
» Reading patient instructions carefully before using
» Participating in a supervised stop-smoking program
» Keeping patch in sealed pouch until ready to apply to skin
» Not trimming or cutting patch
» Applying to clean, dry skin area on upper arm or torso free of oil, hair, scars, cuts, burns, or irritation
» Pressing the patch firmly in place with palm for about 10 seconds; making sure there is good contact, especially around edges
» Keeping patch in place even during showering, bathing, or swimming; replacing systems that have fallen off
» Washing hands with plain water after handling patches; soap will enhance transdermal absorption of nicotine
» Alternating application sites
» Folding used patches in half with adhesive sides together, and replacing in protective pouch or aluminum foil; disposing of patch carefully, out of reach of children or pets
» Getting into the habit of changing patch at the same time each day to help increase compliance
» Proper dosing
» Proper storage

## Precautions while using this medication
» Regular visits to physician to check progress in smoking cessation
» Not smoking during treatment with nicotine replacement products
» Not using nicotine replacement products during pregnancy
» Prevention of accidental ingestion of nicotine replacement products by children or pets to prevent poisoning

*For the chewing gum only*
» Not chewing more than 24 pieces of gum a day
» Not using gum for longer than 6 months to avoid physical dependence
» Discontinuing use and consulting physician or dentist if excessive sticking to dental work occurs; gum may damage dental work or dentures

*For the transdermal systems only*
» Calling physician and not applying new patch if evidence of allergic reaction; knowing that allergic reaction to nicotine patch could cause reaction to use of cigarettes or other products containing nicotine
» Not using patches for longer than 20 weeks

### Side/adverse effects
Signs of potential side effects, especially injury to mouth, teeth, or dental work (with gum only); irregular heartbeat; or hypersensitivity reaction (with transdermal systems only)

## General Dosing Information
The necessity of immediate cessation of smoking upon initiation of therapy must be emphasized.

Overdose of nicotine can be fatal, especially in small children. Immediate treatment is necessary.

### For chewing gum only
When there is an urge to smoke, one piece of gum is chewed very slowly and intermittently for about 30 minutes until most (90%) of the nicotine is released.

The amount of nicotine released depends on the rate of chewing and the amount of time the saliva is in contact with the resin.

The use of nicotine polacrilex for longer than 3 months may be an indication that this medication is being used as a substitute source of nicotine to maintain nicotine dependence. If gum consumption has not been spontaneously reduced within 6 months, a gradual withdrawal should be initiated.

### For transdermal systems only
If a patient is unable to stop smoking by the 4th week of therapy, treatment should be discontinued, as the patient is unlikely to quit on that attempt.

The use of nicotine patches for longer than 12 to 20 weeks (depending on the product) in patients who have stopped smoking has not been evaluated and is not recommended because chronic use of nicotine can be harmful and addictive.

Most manufacturers supply supportive instructional materials and provide telephone information accessible by patients.

## Oral Dosage Forms

### NICOTINE POLACRILEX GUM USP

**Usual adult and adolescent dose**
Smoking cessation adjunct—
    Oral, 2 or 4 mg as a chewing gum, the dose being repeated as determined by individual's urge to smoke and rate of chewing.

Note: Most patients require approximately 20 mg a day during first month of treatment.

Some clinicians maintain that patients initially need at least 12 pieces daily and recommend regular dosing, such as 1 piece per hour while awake, in addition to doses taken in response to an individual's urge to smoke.

**Usual adult prescribing limits**
96 mg a day.

**Usual pediatric dose**
Safety and efficacy have not been established.

**Strength(s) usually available**
U.S.—
    2 mg (OTC) [*Nicorette* (flavors; glycerin; gum base; sodium bicarbonate; sodium carbonate; sorbitol)].
    4 mg (OTC) [*Nicorette* (flavors; glycerin; gum base; sodium carbonate; sorbitol; D&C Yellow No. 10)].
Canada—
    2 mg (OTC) [*Nicorette* (gum; menthol; magnesium oxide; peppermint oil; sodium bicarbonate; sodium carbonate; xylitol)].
    4 mg (Rx) [*Nicorette Plus* (gum; magnesium oxide; menthol; peppermint oil; sodium carbonate; xylitol; D&C Yellow No. 10)].

**Packaging and storage**
Store below 40 °C (104 °F), preferably between 15 and 30 °C (59 and 86 °F), unless otherwise specified by manufacturer. Protect from light.

**Auxiliary labeling**
• Chew slowly.
• Do not chew more than 24 pieces in one day.

## Topical Dosage Forms

### NICOTINE TRANSDERMAL SYSTEM

**Usual adult dose**
Smoking cessation adjunct; depending on the product—
    Patients weighing more than 100 pounds, smoking more than 10 cigarettes a day, and without cardiovascular disease:
        16-hour system: Topical, to intact skin—
            *Nicotrol*: Initially one 15-mg system applied for sixteen hours per day for four to twelve weeks. Patients who have successfully abstained from smoking should have their dose reduced to one 10-mg system applied for sixteen hours per day for the next two to four weeks, and then to one 5-mg system applied for sixteen hours per day for the following two to four weeks.
        24-hour system: Topical, to intact skin—
            *Habitrol*: Initially one 21-mg system per day for four to eight weeks. Patients who have successfully abstained from smoking should have their dose reduced to one 14-mg system per day for the next two to four weeks. The dosage should be further reduced to one 7-mg system per day for the following two to four weeks.
            *Nicoderm*: Initially one 21-mg system per day for six weeks. Patients who have successfully abstained from smoking should have their dose reduced to one 14-mg system per day for two weeks. The dosage should be further reduced to one 7-mg system per day for two weeks.
            *ProStep*: Initially one 22-mg system per day for four to eight weeks. Patients who have successfully abstained from smoking should have their dose reduced to one 11-mg system per day for two to four weeks.
    Patients weighing less than 100 pounds, smoking less than 10 cigarettes a day, or with cardiovascular disease:
        24-hour system: Topical, to intact skin—
            *Habitrol*: Initially one 14-mg system per day for four to eight weeks. Patients who have successfully abstained from smoking should have their dose reduced to one 7-mg system per day for the next two to four weeks.
            *Nicoderm*: Initially one 14-mg system per day for six weeks. Patients who have successfully abstained from smoking should have their dose reduced to one 7-mg system per day for two to four weeks.
            *ProStep*: Initially one 11-mg system per day for four to eight weeks.

**Usual pediatric dose**
Safety and efficacy have not been established.

**Usual geriatric dose**
See *Usual adult dose*.

**Strength(s) usually available**
U.S.—
    16-hour Systems
        5 mg (Rx) [*Nicotrol*].
        10 mg (Rx) [*Nicotrol*].
        15 mg (Rx) [*Nicotrol*].
    24-hour Systems
        7 mg (Rx) [*Habitrol; Nicoderm*].
        11 mg (Rx) [*ProStep*].
        14 mg (Rx) [*Habitrol; Nicoderm*].
        21 mg (Rx) [*Habitrol; Nicoderm*].
        22 mg (Rx) [*ProStep*].
Canada—
    16-hour Systems
        5 mg (Rx) [*Nicotrol*].
        10 mg (Rx) [*Nicotrol*].
        15 mg (Rx) [*Nicotrol*].
    24-hour Systems
        7 mg (Rx) [*Habitrol; Nicoderm*].
        11 mg (Rx) [*ProStep*].
        14 mg (Rx) [*Habitrol; Nicoderm*].
        21 mg (Rx) [*Habitrol; Nicoderm*].
        22 mg (Rx) [*ProStep*].

Note: Nicotine transdermal systems are designed to release a constant, controlled dose of nicotine over the period during which they are applied to the skin. Systems are labeled by the dose actually absorbed by the patient, not by the total nicotine content.

**Packaging and storage**
Store below 30 °C (86 °F), in the intact pouch. Because nicotine is volatile, the system may lose strength if removed from pouch prematurely.

**Auxiliary labeling**
- For external use only.
- Follow the manufacturer's directions carefully.

Revised: 09/08/92
Interim revision: 05/19/94; 07/11/96

---

**NICOTINYL ALCOHOL**—The *Nicotinyl Alcohol (Systemic)* monograph is not included in this published version of the USP DI database. Copies of the monograph are available on request from Micromedex, Inc. - Reprint Requests, 6200 S. Syracuse Way, Suite 300, Englewood, CO 80111; telephone (303) 486-6400; telefax (303) 486-6464; Email: USPDI@MDX.COM.

---

**NIFEDIPINE**—See *Calcium Channel Blocking Agents (Systemic)*

---

**NIFURTIMOX**—The *Nifurtimox (Systemic)* monograph is not included in this published version of the USP DI database. Copies of the monograph are available on request from Micromedex, Inc. - Reprint Requests, 6200 S. Syracuse Way, Suite 300, Englewood, CO 80111; telephone (303) 486-6400; telefax (303) 486-6464; Email: USPDI@MDX.COM.

---

**NILUTAMIDE**—See *Antiandrogens, Nonsteroidal (Systemic)*

---

**NIMODIPINE**—See *Calcium Channel Blocking Agents (Systemic)*

---

# NITRATES  Systemic

This monograph includes information on the following: 1) Erythrityl Tetranitrate; 2) Isosorbide Dinitrate; 3) Isosorbide Mononitrate†; 4) Nitroglycerin; 5) Pentaerythritol Tetranitrate.

INN:
  Erythrityl Tetranitrate—Eritrityl Tetranitrate
  Pentaerythritol Tetranitrate—Pentaerithrityl Tetranitrate

VA CLASSIFICATION (Primary/Secondary):
  Erythrityl tetranitrate—CV250/CV900
  Isosorbide dinitrate—CV250/CV900
  Isosorbide mononitrate—CV250
  Nitroglycerin—CV250/CV490; CV900
  Pentaerythritol tetranitrate—CV250/CV900

Commonly used brand name(s): *Apo-ISDN*[2]; *Cardilate*[1]; *Cedocard-SR*[2]; *Coronex*[2]; *Deponit*[4]; *Dilatrate-SR*[2]; *Duotrate*[5]; *IMDUR*[3]; *ISMO*[3]; *Iso-Bid*[2]; *Isonate*[2]; *Isorbid*[2]; *Isordil*[2]; *Isotrate*[2]; *Klavikordal*[4]; *Minitran*[4]; *Monoket*[3]; *Niong*[4]; *Nitro-Bid*[4]; *Nitro-Dur*[4]; *Nitrocap*[4]; *Nitrocap T.D*[4]; *Nitrodisc*[4]; *Nitrogard*[4]; *Nitrogard SR*[4]; *Nitroglyn*[4]; *Nitroject*[4]; *Nitrol*[4]; *Nitrolin*[4]; *Nitrolingual*[4]; *Nitronet*[4]; *Nitrong*[4]; *Nitrong SR*[4]; *Nitrospan*[4]; *Nitrostat*[4]; *Novosorbide*[2]; *Pentylan*[5]; *Peritrate*[5]; *Peritrate Forte*[5]; *Peritrate SA*[5]; *Sorbitrate*[2]; *Sorbitrate SA*[2]; *Transderm-Nitro*[4]; *Tridil*[4].

Other commonly used names are: Eritrityl tetranitrate [Erythrityl Tetranitrate] [Erythrityl Tetranitrate] Glyceryl trinitrate [Nitroglycerin] [Pentaerythritol Tetranitrate] [Pentaerythritol Tetranitrate]

Note: For a listing of dosage forms and brand names by country availability, see *Dosage Forms* section(s).

†Not commercially available in Canada.

## Category

Note: All of the nitrates have similar pharmacologic actions; however, clinical uses among specific agents may vary because of actual pharmacokinetic differences, availability of specific testing, and/or availability of clinical-use data.

Antianginal—Erythrityl Tetranitrate; Isosorbide Dinitrate; Isosorbide Mononitrate; Nitroglycerin; Pentaerythritol Tetranitrate.
Antihypertensive—Nitroglycerin Injection.
Vasodilator, congestive heart failure—Erythrityl Tetranitrate; Isosorbide Dinitrate; Nitroglycerin; Pentaerythritol Tetranitrate.

## Indications

See *Table 1*, page 2137.

**Accepted**

Angina pectoris, acute (treatment)—The sublingual, lingual, and extended-release buccal[1] dosage forms of nitroglycerin and the sublingual[1] and chewable dosage forms of isosorbide dinitrate are indicated for the relief of pain of an acute episode of angina pectoris due to coronary artery disease. Sublingual or lingual nitroglycerin is preferred; isosorbide dinitrate should be used in patients intolerant of or unresponsive to nitroglycerin. Sublingual isosorbide dinitrate[1] or sublingual or lingual nitroglycerin may be administered to relieve acute anginal attacks that may occur while the patient is on oral prophylactic therapy.

Angina pectoris, acute (prophylaxis)—The sublingual, lingual[1], and extended-release buccal dosage forms of nitroglycerin; the sublingual dosage form of erythrityl tetranitrate; and the sublingual or chewable dosage forms of isosorbide dinitrate are indicated for prophylaxis of acute angina attacks in situations (such as stress or exertion) likely to provoke such attacks.

Angina pectoris, chronic (treatment)—The oral/sublingual dosage form of erythrityl tetranitrate; the regular, chewable, sublingual, and extended-release oral dosage forms of isosorbide dinitrate; the regular and extended-release oral dosage forms of isosorbide mononitrate; and the extended-release oral and buccal dosage forms of nitroglycerin are indicated for the prophylaxis and long-term treatment of angina pectoris due to coronary artery disease, but not in the treatment of acute anginal attacks (except for chewable isosorbide dinitrate and buccal nitroglycerin). Rapid first-pass hepatic destruction of nitroglycerin may increase the dosage requirements of the oral extended-release capsules and tablets in the prophylaxis and treatment of angina.

FDA has classified the oral dosage forms of pentaerythritol tetranitrate as *possibly effective* in the prophylaxis of angina pectoris, but not in the treatment of acute attacks. This classification requires the submission of adequate and well-controlled studies in order to provide substantial evidence of effectiveness.

Nitroglycerin injection is indicated in the treatment of unstable angina pectoris in patients who have not responded to recommended doses of other organic nitrates and/or a beta-blocker.

Nitroglycerin ointment and nitroglycerin transdermal systems are indicated for the prophylaxis and long-term treatment of angina pectoris but are not indicated for the relief of an acute angina episode.

Hypertension (treatment) or
Hypotension, controlled—Nitroglycerin injection is indicated for blood pressure control during certain surgical procedures and for controlled hypotension during surgery to reduce bleeding into the surgical field.

Myocardial infarction (treatment adjunct) or
Congestive heart failure (treatment)—Nitroglycerin injection is indicated in the adjunctive therapy for congestive heart failure associated or not associated with acute myocardial infarction. (Treatment of congestive heart failure not associated with acute myocardial infarction is not included in Canadian product labeling.) [Sublingual][1], [lingual][1], and [topical][1] nitroglycerin; [regular oral and sublingual erythrityl tetranitrate][1]; [regular oral][1], [chewable], and [sublingual][1] isosorbide dinitrate; and [regular oral pentaerythritol tetranitrate][1] are also being used for treatment of congestive heart failure, whether or not it is associated with acute myocardial infarction. In general, the oral extended-release dosage forms are not recommended because the effects are difficult to terminate if excessive hypotension or tachycardia develops, although these dosage forms may be acceptable once the patient is stabilized.

[1]Not included in Canadian product labeling.

## Pharmacology/Pharmacokinetics

### Physicochemical characteristics
Molecular weight—
- Erythrityl tetranitrate: 302.11.
- Isosorbide dinitrate: 236.14.
- Isosorbide mononitrate: 191.14.
- Nitroglycerin: 227.09.
- Pentaerythritol tetranitrate: 316.14.

### Mechanism of action/Effect
Antianginal or cardiac load–reducing agent—Not specifically known but thought to cause a reduction of myocardial oxygen demand. This is attributed to a reduction in left ventricular preload and afterload because of venous (predominantly) and arterial dilation with a more efficient redistribution of blood flow within the myocardium.

Antihypertensive—Peripheral vasodilation.

### Absorption
Erythrityl tetranitrate—Readily absorbed after oral or sublingual administration.

Isosorbide dinitrate—Bioavailability is 59% after sublingual administration and 22% after oral administration.

Isosorbide mononitrate—Nearly 100%.

### Protein binding
Nitroglycerin—Moderate (60%).
Isosorbide mononitrate—Very low (< 4%).

### Biotransformation
Hepatic (very rapid and nearly complete) and in blood (enzymatically). Oral dosage forms undergo extensive first-pass metabolism.

### Half-life
Isosorbide dinitrate—
- Sublingual: 60 minutes.
- Oral: 4 hours.

Isosorbide mononitrate—
- 5 hours.

Nitroglycerin—
- 1 to 4 minutes.

### Onset of action
Note: Although information is limited, pharmacokinetics of sublingual tablets administered buccally are probably similar to those after sublingual administration.

Erythrityl tetranitrate—
- Oral tablets: 15 to 30 minutes.
- Sublingual tablets: 5 minutes.

Isosorbide dinitrate—
- Oral capsules and tablets: 15 to 40 minutes.
- Chewable tablets: 2 to 5 minutes.
- Extended-release capsules and tablets: 30 minutes.
- Sublingual tablets: 2 to 5 minutes.

Isosorbide mononitrate—
- Oral tablets: 1 hour.

Nitroglycerin—
- Buccal tablets: 3 minutes.
- Lingual aerosol: 2 to 4 minutes.
- Intravenous infusion: Immediate.
- Sublingual tablets: 1 to 3 minutes.
- Ointment: Within 30 minutes.
- Transdermal systems: Within 30 minutes.

Pentaerythritol tetranitrate—
- Oral tablets: 30 minutes.
- Extended-release capsules and tablets: Slow.

### Duration of action
Note: Although information is limited, pharmacokinetics of sublingual tablets administered buccally are probably similar to those after sublingual administration.

Erythrityl tetranitrate—
- Oral tablets: Up to 6 hours.
- Sublingual tablets: 2 to 3 hours.

Isosorbide dinitrate—
- Oral capsules and tablets: 4 to 6 hours.
- Chewable tablets: 1 to 2 hours.
- Extended-release capsules and tablets: 12 hours.
- Sublingual tablets: 1 to 2 hours.

Nitroglycerin—
- Buccal extended-release tablets: Approximately 5 hours.
- Extended-release capsules and tablets: 8 to 12 hours.
- Intravenous infusion: Several minutes (dose-dependent).
- Sublingual tablets: 30 to 60 minutes.
- Ointment: 4 to 8 hours.
- Transdermal systems: 8 to 24 hours.

Pentaerythritol tetranitrate—
- Oral tablets: 4 to 5 hours.
- Extended-release capsules and tablets: 12 hours.

### Elimination
Renal (after nearly total metabolism).

## Precautions to Consider

### Cross-sensitivity and/or related problems
Patients sensitive to one nitrate may be sensitive to other nitrates also, although the reaction is rare.

Patients sensitive to nitrites may be sensitive to nitrates also, although the reaction is rare.

### Carcinogenicity
Studies with erythrityl tetranitrate, isosorbide dinitrate, or nitroglycerin have not been done. Studies in mice given oral isosorbide mononitrate at doses of up to 900 mg per kg of body weight (mg/kg) per day (102 times the human exposure comparing body surface area) did not reveal evidence of carcinogenicity.

### Pregnancy/Reproduction
Fertility—*Isosorbide dinitrate:* Studies in rats given isosorbide dinitrate at doses of 25 or 100 mg/kg per day found no impairment of fertility.

*Isosorbide mononitrate:* No adverse effect on fertility was observed in male and female rats given isosorbide mononitrate at doses of up to 500 mg/kg per day (125 times the human exposure comparing body surface area).

Pregnancy—Adequate and well-controlled studies in humans have not been done.

Studies in rabbits given isosorbide dinitrate in oral doses of 35 and 150 times the maximum daily recommended human dose have shown a dose-related increase in embryotoxicity. Administration of isosorbide mononitrate to rats at doses of 500 mg/kg per day (125 times the human exposure comparing body surface area) was associated with increased rates of prolonged gestation, prolonged parturition, stillbirths and neonatal death, and decreases in birth weight, live litter size, and pup survival. No evidence of developmental abnormalities, fetal abnormalities, or other effects on reproductive performance was observed in rats and rabbits given isosorbide mononitrate at doses of 250 mg/kg per day.

FDA Pregnancy Category C.

### Breast-feeding
It is not known whether nitrates are distributed into breast milk. However, problems in humans have not been documented.

### Pediatrics
Appropriate studies on the relationship of age to the effects of nitrates have not been performed in the pediatric population.

### Geriatrics
Appropriate studies on the relationship of age to the effects of nitrates have not been performed in the geriatric population. However, elderly patients may be more sensitive to the hypotensive effects of nitrates. In addition, elderly patients are more likely to have age-related renal function impairment, which may require caution in patients receiving nitrates.

### Drug interactions and/or related problems
The following drug interactions and/or related problems have been selected on the basis of their potential clinical significance (possible mechanism in parentheses where appropriate)—not necessarily inclusive (» = major clinical significance):

Note: Combinations containing any of the following medications, depending on the amount present, may also interact with this medication.

Acetylcholine or
Histamine or
Norepinephrine (levarterenol)
(effects of these medications may be decreased when they are used concurrently with nitrates)

» Alcohol, moderate or excessive amounts or
» Antihypertensives or
Hypotension-producing medications, other (see *Appendix II*) or
Opioid (narcotic) analgesics or
» Vasodilators, other
(concurrent use may intensify the orthostatic hypotensive effects of nitrates; dosage adjustments may be necessary)

Heparin
(the anticoagulant effect of heparin may be decreased in patients receiving nitroglycerin via intravenous infusion; adjustment of heparin dosage may be required to maintain the desired degree of an-

ticoagulation during and following administration of a nitroglycerin infusion)
Sympathomimetics
(concurrent use may reduce the antianginal effects of nitrates)
(nitrates may counteract the pressor effect of sympathomimetics, possibly resulting in hypotension)

**Laboratory value alterations**
The following have been selected on the basis of their potential clinical significance (possible effect in parentheses where appropriate)—not necessarily inclusive (» = major clinical significance):

With diagnostic test results
Serum cholesterol determinations by the Zlatkis-Zak color reaction method
(may be falsely decreased)

With physiology/laboratory test values
Methemoglobin concentrations in blood
(may be increased by excessive doses of nitrates)
Urine catecholamine concentrations (epinephrine and norepinephrine) and
Urine vanillylmandelic acid (VMA) concentrations
(may be markedly increased by nitroglycerin)

**Medical considerations/Contraindications**
The medical considerations/contraindications included have been selected on the basis of their potential clinical significance (reasons given in parentheses where appropriate)—not necessarily inclusive (» = major clinical significance).

*Except under special circumstances, this medication should not be used when the following medical problems exist:*
For nitroglycerin injection only
» Cerebral hemorrhage or
» Head trauma, recent
(nitroglycerin may increase cerebrospinal fluid pressure)
» Pericardial tamponade
» Pericarditis, constrictive

*Risk-benefit should be considered when the following medical problems exist:*
For all nitrates
» Anemia, severe
» Cerebral hemorrhage or
» Head trauma, recent
(nitrates may increase cerebrospinal fluid pressure)
» Glaucoma
(nitrates may increase intraocular pressure)
Hepatic function impairment, severe
(increased risk of methemoglobinemia)
» Hyperthyroidism
Hypertrophic cardiomyopathy
(angina may be aggravated)
Hypotension, with low systolic pressure
(may be aggravated, accompanied by paradoxical bradycardia and increased angina pectoris)
» Myocardial infarction, recent
(risk of hypotension and tachycardia, which may aggravate ischemia)
Renal function impairment, severe
Sensitivity to the nitrate prescribed
*For oral dosage forms only (in addition to the above)*
Gastrointestinal hypermotility or
Malabsorption syndrome
(use of extended-release dosage forms should be avoided because they may not dissolve and may be excreted intact)
*For nitroglycerin injection only (in addition to the above)*
» Hypovolemia
(risk of producing severe hypotension and shock; should be corrected prior to use of nitroglycerin)
» Normal or low pulmonary capillary wedge pressure
(patients may be unusually sensitive to hypotensive effects)

**Patient monitoring**
The following may be especially important in patient monitoring (other tests may be warranted in some patients, depending on condition; » = major clinical significance):

Blood pressure determinations and
Heart rate determinations
(recommended at periodic intervals in patients using nitrates regularly to aid in dosage adjustment)

## Side/Adverse Effects

The following side/adverse effects have been selected on the basis of their potential clinical significance (possible signs and symptoms in parentheses where appropriate)—not necessarily inclusive:

**Those indicating need for medical attention**
Incidence rare
*Blurred vision; dryness of mouth; headache, severe or prolonged; skin rash*

**Those indicating need for medical attention only if they continue or are bothersome**
Incidence more frequent—dose-related
*Flushing of face and neck; headache; nausea or vomiting; orthostatic hypotension* (dizziness or lightheadedness, especially when getting up from a lying or sitting position); *restlessness; tachycardia* (fast heartbeat)
Incidence less frequent
*Sore, reddened skin*—topical nitroglycerin dosage forms

## Overdose

For more information on the management of overdose or unintentional ingestion, **contact a Poison Control Center** (see *Poison Control Center Listing*).

**Clinical effects of overdose**
The following effects have been selected on the basis of their potential clinical significance (possible signs and symptoms in parentheses where appropriate)—not necessarily inclusive:
Signs and symptoms of overdose (in order of occurrence)
*Bluish-colored lips, fingernails, or palms of hands; dizziness, extreme, or fainting; feeling of extreme pressure in head; shortness of breath; unusual tiredness or weakness; weak and fast heartbeat; fever; convulsions*

Note: Cyanosis may occur at blood methemoglobin concentrations of 1.5 grams per 100 mL. More pronounced signs of methemoglobinemia (pressure in head, tiredness or weakness, shortness of breath) occur at concentrations of 20 to 50 grams per 100 mL.

**Treatment of overdose**
Any remaining nitroglycerin should be removed (e.g., ointment, transdermal system). Buccal or sublingual tablets should be removed and the gum wiped clean at the site of insertion.

If excessive hypotension occurs, elevate the legs to aid venous return.

The rapid metabolism of nitroglycerin usually makes additional measures unnecessary. However, if additional correction of severe hypotension is required, administration of an intravenous alpha-adrenergic agonist such as methoxamine or phenylephrine may be considered; epinephrine should be avoided since it aggravates the shock-like reaction.

Methemoglobin concentrations in blood should be monitored and methemoglobinemia treated with high-flow oxygen and intravenous methylene blue.

## Patient Consultation
See *Table 2*, page 2138.

## General Dosing Information

Dosage must be adjusted to the needs and tolerance of the individual patient. Dosage requirements may be increased by a worsening of the patient's condition or a loss of medication potency.

Tolerance to the pharmacologic and therapeutic effects of nitrate medications may occur. Nitrate tolerance manifests as a decrease in patient response to the nitrate or as a need for progressively higher doses to maintain therapeutic effect. The development of nitrate tolerance may occur with any nitrate dosage form that maintains continuous medication blood levels. Tolerance can be managed by adjustments in dosing strategy. Intermittent nitrate therapy appears to be effective. An optimal nitrate-free period of at least 8 to 12 hours appears to be effective in preventing attenuation of nitrate effect. Careful monitoring is recommended to make sure that the desired therapeutic effect is being maintained.

Nitrate therapy should be discontinued if blurred vision or dry mouth continues or is severe.

When this medication is to be discontinued following high-dose or long-term administration, dosage should be reduced gradually to prevent possible withdrawal rebound angina.

**For oral dosage forms only**
There have been reports of patients finding intact or partially dissolved extended-release isosorbide dinitrate or pentaerythritol tetranitrate tablets in the stool. Some patients may benefit by a change from the extended-release tablet to the extended-release capsule or the regular oral tablet and an increase in dosage to an effective level for each individual patient.

**For buccal extended-release nitroglycerin tablets or sublingual tablets administered buccally only**
The tablet should be placed between upper lip and gum (above the incisors) or between cheek and upper gum, and allowed to dissolve in place. Tablet placement sites may be alternated as patient desires.

The dissolution time of the buccal extended-release tablet may vary from 3 to 5 hours in most patients. The dissolution rate is increased when the tablet is touched with the tongue or the patient drinks hot liquids. The buccal extended-release tablet utilizes an inert polymer vehicle which enables a metered nitroglycerin release not affected by pH, food, or drink (placement is suggested behind the upper lip if food and drink are to be taken during dosing).

Use at bedtime is not recommended because of the risk of aspiration.

Sublingual erythrityl tetranitrate, isosorbide dinitrate, and nitroglycerin tablets may also be administered buccally. Although information is limited, onset and duration of action are probably similar to sublingual dosing.

**Diet/Nutrition**
The regular oral dosage forms of this medication should preferably be taken with a glass of water on an empty stomach (either 1 hour before or 2 hours after meals) for faster absorption.

---
### ERYTHRITYL TETRANITRATE
---

## Summary of Differences
Indications: Although available in sublingual dosage form, is not useful for treatment of acute angina attacks.

## Oral Dosage Forms
### ERYTHRITYL TETRANITRATE TABLETS USP
**Usual adult dose**
Antianginal—
  Oral, sublingual, or buccal, 5 to 10 mg three or four times a day, the dosage being adjusted as needed and tolerated.
Note: The regular tablet of erythrityl tetranitrate currently marketed may be utilized for oral, sublingual, or buccal dosage.

**Usual adult prescribing limits**
Up to 100 mg daily.

**Usual pediatric dose**
Dosage has not been established.

**Strength(s) usually available**
U.S.—
  10 mg (Rx) [*Cardilate*].
Canada—
  10 mg (Rx) [*Cardilate*].

**Packaging and storage**
Store below 40 °C (104 °F), preferably between 15 and 30 °C (59 and 86 °F), unless otherwise specified by manufacturer. Store in a tight container.

**Stability**
Loss of potency is accelerated by exposure to heat and moisture.

**Auxiliary labeling**
• Caution with alcoholic beverages.
• Keep container tightly closed.
• Store in a cool, dry place.

---
### ISOSORBIDE DINITRATE
---

## Oral Dosage Forms
### ISOSORBIDE DINITRATE CAPSULES
**Usual adult dose**
Antianginal—
  Oral, 5 to 20 mg every six hours, the dosage being adjusted as needed and tolerated. The dosage range is 5 to 40 mg four times a day, with the usual dosage range being 20 to 40 mg four times a day.

**Usual pediatric dose**
Dosage has not been established.

**Strength(s) usually available**
U.S.—
  40 mg (Rx) [GENERIC].
Canada—
  Not commercially available.

**Packaging and storage**
Store below 40 °C (104 °F), preferably between 15 and 30 °C (59 and 86 °F), in a well-closed container, unless otherwise specified by manufacturer.

**Stability**
Loss of potency is accelerated by exposure to heat and moisture.

**Auxiliary labeling**
• Caution with alcoholic beverages.
• Store in a cool, dry place.

### ISOSORBIDE DINITRATE EXTENDED-RELEASE CAPSULES USP
**Usual adult dose**
Antianginal—
  Oral, 40 to 80 mg every eight to twelve hours.

**Usual pediatric dose**
Dosage has not been established.

**Strength(s) usually available**
U.S.—
  40 mg (Rx) [*Dilatrate-SR; Iso-Bid; Isorbid; Isordil; Isotrate;* GENERIC].
Canada—
  Not commercially available.

**Packaging and storage**
Store below 40 °C (104 °F), preferably between 15 and 30 °C (59 and 86 °F), unless otherwise specified by manufacturer. Store in a well-closed container.

**Stability**
Loss of potency is accelerated by exposure to heat and moisture.

**Auxiliary labeling**
• Caution with alcoholic beverages.
• Swallow capsules whole.
• Store in a cool, dry place.

### ISOSORBIDE DINITRATE TABLETS USP
**Usual adult dose**
Antianginal—
  Oral, 5 to 20 mg every six hours, the dosage being adjusted as needed and tolerated. The dosage range is 5 to 40 mg four times a day, with the usual dosage range being 20 to 40 mg four times a day.

**Usual pediatric dose**
Dosage has not been established.

**Strength(s) usually available**
U.S.—
  2.5 mg (Rx) [GENERIC].
  5 mg (Rx) [*Isonate; Isorbid; Isordil; Sorbitrate;* GENERIC].
  10 mg (Rx) [*Isonate; Isorbid; Isordil; Sorbitrate;* GENERIC].
  20 mg (Rx) [*Isonate; Isorbid; Isordil; Sorbitrate;* GENERIC].
  30 mg (Rx) [*Isonate; Isorbid; Isordil; Sorbitrate;* GENERIC].
  40 mg (Rx) [*Isordil; Sorbitrate*].
Canada—
  10 mg (Rx) [*Apo-ISDN; Coronex; Isordil; Novosorbide*].
  30 mg (Rx) [*Apo-ISDN; Coronex; Isordil; Novosorbide*].

**Packaging and storage**
Store below 40 °C (104 °F), preferably between 15 and 30 °C (59 and 86 °F), unless otherwise specified by manufacturer. Store in a well-closed container.

**Stability**
Loss of potency is accelerated by exposure to heat and moisture.

**Auxiliary labeling**
- Caution with alcoholic beverages.
- Store in a cool, dry place.

### ISOSORBIDE DINITRATE CHEWABLE TABLETS USP

**Usual adult dose**
Antianginal—
  Oral, 5 mg chewed well every two to three hours, the dosage being adjusted as needed and tolerated.
Note: Chewed tablet is to be held in mouth for one or two minutes to allow time for absorption through buccal tissues.

**Usual pediatric dose**
Dosage has not been established.

**Strength(s) usually available**
U.S.—
  5 mg (Rx) [*Sorbitrate*].
  10 mg (Rx) [*Sorbitrate*].
Canada—
  Not commercially available.

**Packaging and storage**
Store below 40 °C (104 °F), preferably between 15 and 30 °C (59 and 86 °F), unless otherwise specified by manufacturer. Store in a well-closed container.

**Stability**
Loss of potency is accelerated by exposure to heat and moisture.

**Auxiliary labeling**
- Caution with alcoholic beverages.
- Chew well before swallowing.
- Store in a cool, dry place.

**Note**
Chewable tablets up to 10 mg each are exempt from child-resistant container regulations.

### ISOSORBIDE DINITRATE EXTENDED-RELEASE TABLETS USP

**Usual adult dose**
Antianginal—
  Oral, 20 to 80 mg every eight to twelve hours.

**Usual pediatric dose**
Dosage has not been established.

**Strength(s) usually available**
U.S.—
  40 mg (Rx) [*Isonate; Isorbid; Isordil; Sorbitrate SA;* GENERIC].
Canada—
  20 mg (Rx) [*Cedocard-SR*].

**Packaging and storage**
Store below 40 °C (104 °F), preferably between 15 and 30 °C (59 and 86 °F), unless otherwise specified by manufacturer. Store in a well-closed container.

**Stability**
Loss of potency is accelerated by exposure to heat and moisture.

**Auxiliary labeling**
- Caution with alcoholic beverages.
- Swallow tablets whole.
- Store in a cool, dry place.

## Sublingual Dosage Forms

### ISOSORBIDE DINITRATE SUBLINGUAL TABLETS USP

**Usual adult dose**
Antianginal—
  Sublingual or buccal, 2.5 to 5 mg every two to three hours as needed.

**Usual pediatric dose**
Dosage has not been established.

**Strength(s) usually available**
U.S.—
  2.5 mg (Rx) [*Isonate; Isorbid; Isordil; Sorbitrate;* GENERIC].
  5 mg (Rx) [*Isonate; Isorbid; Isordil; Sorbitrate;* GENERIC].
  10 mg (Rx) [*Isonate; Isorbid; Isordil; Sorbitrate;* GENERIC].
Canada—
  5 mg (Rx) [*Apo-ISDN; Coronex; Isordil*].

**Packaging and storage**
Store below 40 °C (104 °F), preferably between 15 and 30 °C (59 and 86 °F), unless otherwise specified by manufacturer. Store in a well-closed container.

**Stability**
Loss of potency is accelerated by exposure to heat and moisture.

**Auxiliary labeling**
- Caution with alcoholic beverages.
- Dissolve tablets under tongue.
- Store in a cool, dry place.

**Note**
Do not dispense sublingual tablets in child-resistant containers. Sublingual tablets up to 10 mg each are exempt from child-resistant container regulations.

---

## ISOSORBIDE MONONITRATE

## Summary of Differences
Pharmacology/pharmacokinetics:
  Protein binding—Very low.
  Half-life—5 hours.

## Oral Dosage Form

### ISOSORBIDE MONONITRATE TABLETS

**Usual adult dose**
Antianginal—
  Oral, 20 mg two times a day, with the two doses given seven hours apart.
Note: An initial dose of 5 mg may be appropriate for patients of particularly small stature; the dosage being increased to at least 10 mg by the second or third day of therapy.

**Usual pediatric dose**
Safety and efficacy have not been established.

**Strength(s) usually available**
U.S.—
  10 mg (Rx) [*Monoket* (scored)].
  20 mg (Rx) [*ISMO; Monoket* (scored)].
Canada—
  Not commercially available.

**Packaging and storage**
Store below 40 °C (104 °F), preferably between 15 and 30 °C (59 and 86 °F) in a tight container, unless otherwise specified by manufacturer.

**Stability**
Loss of potency is accelerated by exposure to heat and moisture.

**Auxiliary labeling**
- Caution with alcoholic beverages.
- Store in a cool, dry place.

### ISOSORBIDE MONONITRATE EXTENDED-RELEASE TABLETS

**Usual adult dose**
Antianginal—
  Oral, 30 or 60 mg once a day, the dosage being increased after several days to 120 mg once a day, as needed and tolerated. Rarely, 240 mg once a day may be needed.

**Usual pediatric dose**
Safety and efficacy have not been established.

**Strength(s) usually available**
U.S.—
  60 mg (Rx) [*IMDUR* (scored; ethanol, trace)].
Canada—
  Not commercially available.

**Packaging and storage**
Store between 2 and 30 °C (36 and 86 °F) in a tight container.

**Stability**
Loss of potency is accelerated by exposure to heat and moisture.

**Auxiliary labeling**
- Caution with alcoholic beverages.
- Store in a cool, dry place.
- Do not crush or chew.

## NITROGLYCERIN

### Summary of Differences
Category:
    Antihypertensive; cardiac load–reducing agent.
Indications:
    Hypertension (parenteral dosage form); hypotension, controlled (parenteral dosage form); acute myocardial infarction; congestive heart failure.
Pharmacology/pharmacokinetics:
    Half-life—1 to 4 minutes.
Precautions:
    Medical considerations/contraindications—Contraindicated in increased intracranial pressure, constrictive pericarditis (parenteral dosage form); caution needed in hypovolemia or severe hepatic or renal function impairment (parenteral dosage form).

### Additional Dosing Information
See also *General Dosing Information*.

#### For sublingual tablets only
Judging the ability of a sublingual tablet to relieve angina by the presence of a tingling or burning sensation after a tablet has been dissolved under the tongue, is not completely reliable since some patients may be unable to detect these effects. Newer, stabilized sublingual nitroglycerin tablets are making such potency testing less useful, since the stabilized tablets may be less likely to produce these detectable effects.

Nitroglycerin tablets should maintain their potency through the expiration date on the bottle, provided the cap is tightly replaced after each use and proper storage instructions are adhered to.

A supplementary stainless steel container has been developed and approved for temporary storage of small quantities of nitroglycerin tablets. The pendant-type container on a chain, which can be worn around the patient's neck, is intended to provide a convenient source of nitroglycerin for emergency use.

#### For intravenous infusion form only
Special nitroglycerin infusion sets made of non-PVC plastic cause minimal absorption; therefore, nearly all the calculated dose will be delivered to the patient. When these sets are used, *dosage instructions should be followed with care*, as changing from a standard set (PVC) to a special set (non-PVC) may result in excessive nitroglycerin dosage unless allowances are made for the difference in the amount of nitroglycerin actually delivered to the patient.

#### For ointment dosage form only
The dose should be individualized starting with ½ to 1 inch of ointment as squeezed from the tube and then increasing the dose by ½ inch at each application until the desired clinical effect and the greatest asymptomatic decrease in resting blood pressure occur. The largest dose that does not cause symptomatic hypotension is used as the patient's individualized dose.

The ointment is applied with the dose-measuring application papers supplied with the medicine. The ointment is squeezed onto the measuring scale printed on the paper. The paper is then used to spread the ointment onto the skin in a thin, even layer, covering an area (at least 2 by 3 inches) of the same size at each dose without rubbing or massage.

The site of ointment application may be the non-hairy skin of the chest, stomach, front of the thighs, or any other accessible area of clean, dry skin. Application to the chest is commonly preferred since the patient also benefits psychologically from applying medication to the area where the pain is experienced.

#### For transdermal dosage forms only
Application should preferably be made at the same time each day (after removal of the previous system) to areas of clean, dry, hairless skin on the chest, inner side of the upper arm, or shoulders; application to extremities below the knee or elbow should be avoided. Skin areas with extensive scarring, calluses, or irritation should also be avoided. Application sites should be varied to avoid causing skin irritation.

All available transdermal systems provide therapeutic effects within 30 minutes and sustain the required plasma concentration of nitroglycerin for 8 to 24 hours.

The transdermal units *should not* be cut or trimmed in an attempt to adjust dosage.

A new dosage unit should be applied if the first becomes loosened or falls off.

Removal of the transdermal unit before defibrillation or cardioversion is recommended because of the potential for altered electrical conductivity and enhanced risk of arcing associated with use of defibrillators.

### Buccal Dosage Forms
#### NITROGLYCERIN EXTENDED-RELEASE BUCCAL TABLETS
**Usual adult dose**
Antianginal—
    Buccal, 1 mg dissolved in place on the oral mucosa every five hours during waking hours, the dosage being increased by frequency and/or strength as required.

**Usual pediatric dose**
Dosage has not been established.

**Strength(s) usually available**
U.S.—
    1 mg (Rx) [*Nitrogard*].
    2 mg (Rx) [*Nitrogard*].
    3 mg (Rx) [*Nitrogard*].
Canada—
    1 mg (Rx) [*Nitrogard SR*].
    2 mg (Rx) [*Nitrogard SR*].
    3 mg (Rx) [*Nitrogard SR*].
    5 mg (Rx) [*Nitrogard SR*].

**Packaging and storage**
Store between 15 and 30 °C (59 and 86 °F), unless otherwise specified by manufacturer. Store in a glass container with a tight screw cap.

**Stability**
Loss of potency is accelerated by exposure to heat and moisture.

**Auxiliary labeling**
- Caution with alcoholic beverages.
- Dissolve tablet between lip or cheek and upper gum.
- Do not chew or swallow.
- Keep in original container, tightly closed.
- Store in a cool, dry place.

### Lingual Dosage Forms
#### NITROGLYCERIN LINGUAL AEROSOL
**Usual adult dose**
Antianginal—
    On or under the tongue, 1 or 2 metered doses (400 or 800 mcg [0.4 or 0.8 mg]) repeated at five-minute intervals as needed for relief of angina attack.
Note: If relief is not obtained after a total of 3 metered doses in a fifteen-minute period, the physician should be contacted or the patient taken to a hospital.

**Usual adult prescribing limits**
Up to 1.2 mg per day.

**Usual pediatric dose**
Dosage has not been established.

**Strength(s) usually available**
U.S.—
    400 mcg (0.4 mg) per metered dose (Rx) [*Nitrolingual*].
Canada—
    400 mcg (0.4 mg) per metered dose (Rx) [*Nitrolingual*].

**Packaging and storage**
Store below 40 °C (104 °F), preferably between 15 and 30 °C (59 and 86 °F), unless otherwise specified by manufacturer. Protect from freezing.

**Auxiliary labeling**
- Do not shake.
- Caution with alcoholic beverages.
- Store in a cool place.

### Oral Dosage Forms
#### NITROGLYCERIN EXTENDED-RELEASE CAPSULES
**Usual adult dose**
Antianginal—
    Oral, 2.5, 6.5, or 9 mg every twelve hours, the dosage being increased to every eight hours if needed and tolerated.

**Usual pediatric dose**
Dosage has not been established.

**Strength(s) usually available**
U.S.—
    2.5 mg (Rx) [*Nitrocap T.D; Nitroglyn; Nitrolin; Nitrospan;* GENERIC].
    6.5 mg (Rx) [*Nitrocap; Nitroglyn; Nitrolin; Nitrospan;* GENERIC].
    9 mg (Rx) [*Nitroglyn; Nitrolin;* GENERIC].

Canada—
　Not commercially available.

**Packaging and storage**
Store between 15 and 30 °C (59 and 86 °F), unless otherwise specified by manufacturer. Store in a container with a tight screw cap.

**Stability**
Loss of potency is accelerated by exposure to heat and moisture.

**Auxiliary labeling**
- Caution with alcoholic beverages.
- Swallow capsules whole.
- Keep container tightly closed.
- Store in a cool, dry place.

## NITROGLYCERIN EXTENDED-RELEASE TABLETS

**Usual adult dose**
Antianginal—
　Oral, 1.3, 2.6, or 6.5 mg every twelve hours, the dosage being increased to every eight hours as needed and tolerated.

**Usual pediatric dose**
Dosage has not been established.

**Strength(s) usually available**
U.S.—
　2.6 mg (Rx) [*Klavikordal; Niong; Nitronet; Nitrong*].
　6.5 mg (Rx) [*Klavikordal; Niong; Nitronet; Nitrong*].
　9 mg (Rx) [*Nitrong*].
Canada—
　2.6 mg (Rx) [*Nitrong SR*].

**Packaging and storage**
Store between 15 and 30 °C (59 and 86 °F), unless otherwise specified by manufacturer. Store in a glass container with a tight screw cap.

**Stability**
Loss of potency is accelerated by exposure to heat and moisture.

**Auxiliary labeling**
- Caution with alcoholic beverages.
- Swallow tablets whole.
- Keep container tightly closed.
- Store in a cool, dry place.

# Parenteral Dosage Forms

## NITROGLYCERIN INJECTION USP

**Usual adult dose**
Antianginal or
Antihypertensive or
Cardiac load–reducing agent—
　Intravenous infusion, initially administered at a rate of 5 mcg (0.005 mg) per minute, the dosage being increased by increments of 5 mcg per minute at three- to five-minute intervals until an effect is obtained or until the rate is 20 mcg (0.02 mg) per minute. If no effect is obtained at 20 mcg per minute, the dosage may be increased further by increments of 10 mcg (0.01 mg) per minute at the same time intervals, and later increased by increments of 20 mcg (0.02 mg) per minute if necessary to obtain an effect. The dosage increments should be reduced and the time interval between dosage increases lengthened when a partial effect is observed, to attain the desired response cautiously.

Note:　Close attention must be given to manufacturers' instructions for dilution, dosage, and administration because concentrations and/or volume per vial of nitroglycerin may differ among the several products available from different manufacturers.

　Stated dosage is based on use of special, non-polyvinylchloride (non-PVC) intravenous infusion sets. Dosage requirements may vary when standard infusion sets of polyvinyl chloride (PVC) are used. Continuous concurrent monitoring of blood pressure and heart rate in *all patients* must be performed to establish the correct effective dose.

　To achieve optimal control of dosage and effects, it is recommended that nitroglycerin be administered intravenously by means of an infusion pump, a micro-drip regulator, or a similar device to allow precise adjustment of the flow rate.

　Standard intravenous infusion sets made of PVC plastic may unpredictably absorb 40 to 80% of the nitroglycerin from a diluted solution for infusion.

　Some intravenous filters may also absorb nitroglycerin, but the effect is variable; since nitroglycerin dosage is titrated according to response, no precaution is necessary.

　Extra caution should be observed when non-PVC infusion sets are used to administer intravenous nitroglycerin. Some infusion pumps—

- When turned off may not completely stop the flow of infusion solution with these non-PVC sets.
- May not accurately deliver the infusion solution at low rates of flow.
- Require extension sets and other connecting equipment made of PVC, thus partially negating the advantage of the non-PVC infusion set.

Close monitoring of patient hemodynamic response is required. All infusion pumps should be tested with the infusion set being used to ensure accurate delivery of nitroglycerin at low flow rates and complete interruption of flow when the set is turned off.

**Usual adult prescribing limits**
No fixed maximum dose established. Dosage is titrated to individual patient response beginning with small doses (to which hypersensitive patients may respond).

**Usual pediatric dose**
Dosage has not been established.

**Strength(s) usually available**
U.S.—
　500 mcg (0.5 mg) per mL (Rx) [*Tridil*].
　800 mcg (0.8 mg) per mL (Rx) [*Nitrol; Nitrostat*].
　1 mg per mL (Rx) [*Nitroject*].
　5 mg per mL (Rx) [*Nitro-Bid; Nitroject; Nitrol; Nitrostat; Tridil;* GENERIC].
　10 mg per mL (Rx) [*Nitro-Bid; Nitrostat*].
Canada—
　800 mcg (0.8 mg) per mL (Rx) [*Nitrostat*].
　1 mg per mL (Rx) [*Nitroject*].
　5 mg per mL (Rx) [*Nitro-Bid; Nitroject; Nitrostat; Tridil;* GENERIC].

**Packaging and storage**
Store between 15 and 30 °C (59 and 86 °F), unless otherwise specified by manufacturer. Protect from light. Protect from freezing.

**Preparation of dosage form**
- *Not for direct intravenous injection.*
- Must be diluted prior to infusion. Dilution may be in 5% dextrose injection or 0.9% sodium chloride injection, followed by thorough mixing. Dilution and storage of nitroglycerin injection should be made only in glass parenteral solution bottles, to avoid absorption of nitroglycerin into plastic containers.
- *Must not be admixed with other medications.*

**Stability**
It is recommended that diluted solutions of nitroglycerin not be kept or used longer than 24 hours, unless otherwise specified by the manufacturer. Solution is *not* explosive either before or after dilution.

**Note**
Manufacturer's package information must be checked for dilution, administration, and dosage because of product differences.

Some products contain substantial amounts of propylene glycol or ethanol.

# Sublingual Dosage Forms

## NITROGLYCERIN TABLETS (SUBLINGUAL) USP

**Usual adult dose**
Antianginal—
　Sublingual or buccal, 150 to 600 mcg (0.15 to 0.6 mg) repeated at five-minute intervals as needed for relief of angina attack.

Note:　If relief is not obtained after a total of 3 tablets used over a fifteen-minute period, the physician should be contacted or the patient taken to a hospital.

**Usual adult prescribing limits**
Up to 10 mg per day.

**Usual pediatric dose**
Dosage has not been established.

**Strength(s) usually available**
U.S.—
　150 mcg (0.15 mg) (Rx) [*Nitrostat;* GENERIC].
　300 mcg (0.3 mg) (Rx) [*Nitrostat;* GENERIC].
　400 mcg (0.4 mg) (Rx) [*Nitrostat;* GENERIC].
　600 mcg (0.6 mg) (Rx) [*Nitrostat;* GENERIC].
Canada—
　300 mcg (0.3 mg) (Rx) [*Nitrostat;* GENERIC].
　600 mcg (0.6 mg) (Rx) [*Nitrostat;* GENERIC].

**Packaging and storage**
Store between 15 and 30 °C (59 and 86 °F), unless otherwise specified by manufacturer. Store in original container with tight metal screw cap.

### Stability
Loss of potency through volatilization of nitroglycerin from tablets is accelerated by exposure to air, heat, and moisture. After the bottle is opened, stabilized tablets will maintain potency through the expiration date provided the bottle cap is replaced tightly after each use.

### Auxiliary labeling
- Caution with alcoholic beverages.
- Dissolve tablets under tongue.
- Keep in original container, tightly closed.
- Store in a cool, dry place.

### Note
Do not dispense sublingual nitroglycerin tablets in child-resistant containers.

Suggest to the patient that the cotton be removed from the container *before* the tablets are required for angina attack.

USP requires that sublingual forms of nitroglycerin be dispensed in the original unopened manufacturer's container.

Sublingual nitroglycerin tablets should not be placed in containers with other medications.

## Topical Dosage Forms

### NITROGLYCERIN OINTMENT USP

#### Usual adult dose
Antianginal—
Topical, to the skin, 15 to 30 mg of nitroglycerin (contained in 2.5 to 5 cm [1 to 2 inches] of ointment as squeezed from the tube) every eight hours during the day and at bedtime. If angina occurs between doses, frequency of application may be increased to every six hours.

Note: Ointment is applied in a thin, even layer covering an area of the same size (measuring at least 2 by 3 inches) at each use, but is not to be rubbed or massaged into the skin.

#### Usual adult prescribing limits
Up to 75 mg of nitroglycerin (contained in 12.5 cm [5 inches] of ointment as squeezed from the tube) per application. Rarely, application as frequently as every four hours may be necessary.

#### Usual pediatric dose
Dosage has not been established.

#### Strength(s) usually available
U.S.—
  2% (Rx) [*Nitro-Bid; Nitrol; Nitrong; Nitrostat;* GENERIC].
Canada—
  2% (Rx) [*Nitro-Bid; Nitrol; Nitrong*].

#### Packaging and storage
Store between 15 and 30 °C (59 and 86 °F), unless otherwise specified by manufacturer. Store in a tight container.

#### Auxiliary labeling
- Caution with alcoholic beverages.
- For external use only.
- Store in a cool place.
- Keep tightly closed.

#### Note
Dispense ointment in original manufacturer's tube together with patient instructions and dose-measuring papers.

### NITROGLYCERIN TRANSDERMAL SYSTEM

#### Usual adult dose
Antianginal—
Topical, to the intact skin, 1 transdermal dosage system, delivering the smallest available dose of nitroglycerin in its dosage series, every twenty-four hours. Dosage adjustments may be made by changing to the next larger dosage system in the series or to a combination of systems.

Note: To prevent tolerance, it is recommended that the patch be left on only 12 to 14 hours a day, with a patch-off period of 10 to 12 hours before the next daily patch is applied.

#### Usual pediatric dose
Dosage has not been established.

#### Strength(s) usually available
U.S.—
  Dose of nitroglycerin delivered per hour:
    0.1 mg (Rx) [*Minitran; Nitro-Dur; Transderm-Nitro*].
    0.2 mg (Rx) [*Deponit; Minitran; Nitrodisc; Nitro-Dur; Transderm-Nitro;* GENERIC].
    0.3 mg (Rx) [*Nitrodisc; Nitro-Dur*].
    0.4 mg (Rx) [*Deponit; Minitran; Nitrodisc; Nitro-Dur; Transderm-Nitro;* GENERIC].
    0.6 mg (Rx) [*Minitran; Nitro-Dur; Transderm-Nitro;* GENERIC].
    0.8 mg (Rx) [*Nitro-Dur; Transderm-Nitro;* GENERIC].
Canada—
  Dose of nitroglycerin delivered per hour:
    0.2 mg (Rx) [*Minitran; Nitro-Dur; Transderm-Nitro*].
    0.3 mg (Rx) [*Nitro-Dur*].
    0.4 mg (Rx) [*Minitran; Nitro-Dur; Transderm-Nitro*].
    0.6 mg (Rx) [*Minitran; Nitro-Dur; Transderm-Nitro*].
    0.8 mg (Rx) [*Minitran; Nitro-Dur; Transderm-Nitro*].

#### Packaging and storage
Store between 15 and 30 °C (59 and 86 °F), unless otherwise specified by manufacturer.

#### Auxiliary labeling
- Caution with alcoholic beverages.
- For external use only.
- Store in a cool place.

#### Note
Include patient instructions when dispensing.

---

## *PENTAERYTHRITOL TETRANITRATE*

## Oral Dosage Forms

### PENTAERYTHRITOL TETRANITRATE EXTENDED-RELEASE CAPSULES

#### Usual adult dose
Antianginal—
Oral, 30 to 80 mg two times a day.

#### Usual adult prescribing limits
Up to 160 mg daily.

#### Usual pediatric dose
Dosage has not been established.

#### Strength(s) usually available
U.S.—
  30 mg (Rx) [*Duotrate*].
  45 mg (Rx) [*Duotrate*].
  80 mg (Rx) [GENERIC].
Canada—
  Not commercially available.

#### Packaging and storage
Store below 40 °C (104 °F), preferably between 15 and 30 °C (59 and 86 °F), unless otherwise specified by manufacturer. Store in a tight container.

#### Stability
Loss of potency is accelerated by exposure to heat and moisture.

#### Auxiliary labeling
- Caution with alcoholic beverages.
- Swallow capsules whole.
- Keep container tightly closed.
- Store in a cool, dry place.

### PENTAERYTHRITOL TETRANITRATE TABLETS USP

#### Usual adult dose
Antianginal—
Oral, 10 to 20 mg four times a day, the dosage being adjusted as needed and tolerated.

#### Usual adult prescribing limits
Up to 160 mg daily.

#### Usual pediatric dose
Dosage has not been established.

#### Strength(s) usually available
U.S.—
  10 mg (Rx) [*Pentylan;* GENERIC].
  20 mg (Rx) [*Pentylan; Peritrate;* GENERIC].
  80 mg (Rx) [GENERIC].
Canada—
  10 mg (Rx) [*Peritrate*].
  20 mg (Rx) [*Peritrate*].
  80 mg (Rx) [*Peritrate Forte*].

#### Packaging and storage
Store below 40 °C (104 °F), preferably between 15 and 30 °C (59 and 86 °F), unless otherwise specified by manufacturer. Store in a tight container.

## Stability
Loss of potency is accelerated by exposure to heat and moisture.

### Auxiliary labeling
- Caution with alcoholic beverages.
- Keep container tightly closed.
- Store in a cool, dry place.

## PENTAERYTHRITOL TETRANITRATE EXTENDED-RELEASE TABLETS

### Usual adult dose
Antianginal—
  Oral, up to 80 mg two times a day.

### Usual adult prescribing limits
Oral, up to 160 mg daily.

### Usual pediatric dose
Dosage has not been established.

### Strength(s) usually available
U.S.—
  80 mg (Rx) [*Peritrate SA;* GENERIC].

Canada—
  80 mg (Rx) [*Peritrate SA*].

### Packaging and storage
Store below 40 °C (104 °F), preferably between 15 and 30 °C (59 and 86 °F), unless otherwise specified by manufacturer. Store in a tight container.

### Stability
Loss of potency is accelerated by exposure to heat and moisture.

### Auxiliary labeling
- Caution with alcoholic beverages.
- Swallow tablets whole.
- Keep container tightly closed.
- Store in a cool, dry place.

Revised: 10/06/93
Interim revision: 02/22/94; 06/06/95; 08/19/97

---

## Table 1. Indications

Note: Bracketed information in the *Indications* section refers to uses that are not included in U.S. product labeling.

Legend:
**I** = Angina pectoris, acute (treatment)
**II** = Angina pectoris, acute (prophylaxis)
**III** = Angina pectoris, chronic (treatment)
**IV** = Hypertension (treatment); or Hypotension, controlled
**V** = Myocardial infarction (treatment adjunct)
**VI** = Congestive heart failure (treatment)

| | I | II | III | IV | V | VI |
|---|---|---|---|---|---|---|
| **Erythrityl tetranitrate** <br> Oral/Sublingual | | ✔ | ✔ | | [✔][1] | [✔][1] |
| **Isosorbide dinitrate** <br> Oral <br>    Capsules and tablets, regular | | | ✔ | | [✔][1] | [✔][1] |
|    Extended-release capsules or tablets | | | ✔ | | | |
|    Chewable tablets | ✔ | ✔ | ✔ | | [✔] | [✔] |
|    Sublingual | ✔[1] | ✔ | ✔ | | [✔][1] | [✔][1] |
| **Isosorbide mononitrate** <br> Oral <br>    Tablets, regular | | | ✔ | | | |
| **Nitroglycerin** <br> Buccal, extended-release | ✔[1] | ✔ | ✔ | | | |
|    Lingual, aerosol | ✔ | ✔[1] | | | [✔][1] | [✔][1] |
|    Oral, extended-release | | | ✔ | | | |
|    Parenteral | | | ✔ | ✔ | ✔ | ✔ |
|    Sublingual | ✔ | ✔ | | | [✔][1] | [✔][1] |
| **Topical** <br>    Ointment | | | ✔ | | [✔][1] | [✔][1] |
|    Transdermal systems | | | ✔ | | [✔] | [✔] |
| **Pentaerythritol tetranitrate** <br> Oral <br>    Tablets, regular | | | ✔ | | [✔][1] | [✔][1] |
|    Extended-release capsules and tablets | | | ✔ | | | |

[1] Not included in Canadian product labeling

## Table 2. Patient Consultation

As an aid to patient consultation, refer to *Advice for the Patient, Nitrates—Lingual Aerosol (Systemic), Nitrates—Oral (Systemic), Nitrates—Sublingual, Chewable, or Buccal (Systemic), or Nitrates—Topical (Systemic)*.
Consider advising the patient on the following:

Legend:
- **I** = Extended-release nitroglycerin
- **II** = Aerosol nitroglycerin
- **III** = Regular
- **IV** = Chewable
- **V** = Extended-release
- **VI** = Erythrityl tetranitrate
- **VII** = Isosorbide dinitrate
- **VIII** = Nitroglycerin
- **IX** = Nitroglycerin ointment
- **X** = Transdermal nitroglycerin

| | Buccal | Lingual | Oral | | | Sublingual | | | Topical | |
|---|---|---|---|---|---|---|---|---|---|---|
| | I | II | III | IV | V | VI | VII | VIII | IX | X |
| **Before using this medication** — See *Precautions to Consider*. | ✔ | ✔ | ✔ | ✔ | ✔ | ✔ | ✔ | ✔ | ✔ | ✔ |
| **Proper use of this medication** | | | | | | | | | | |
| » Compliance with therapy | ✔ | ✔ | ✔ | ✔ | ✔ | ✔ | ✔ | ✔ | ✔ | ✔ |
| » Reading patient instructions carefully | | ✔ | | | | | | | ✔ | ✔ |
| Proper administration: | | | | | | | | | | |
| » Regular or extended-release capsule or tablet—Taking with full glass of water on empty stomach | | | ✔ | | ✔ | | | | | |
| » Buccal— | | | | | | | | | | |
|     Under upper lip (above incisors) against gum or between cheek and upper gum; placing between upper lip (above incisors) and gum if food or drink to be taken within 3 to 5 hours; patients with dentures may place anywhere between cheek and gum | ✔ | | | | | ✔ | ✔ | ✔ | | |
|     Touching with tongue or drinking hot liquids may increase rate of dissolution | ✔ | | | | | ✔ | ✔ | ✔ | | |
|     Bedtime use not recommended because of risk of aspiration | ✔ | | | | | ✔ | ✔ | ✔ | | |
|     Replacing tablet if inadvertently swallowed | ✔ | | | | | ✔ | ✔ | ✔ | | |
|     Not using chewing tobacco while tablet in place | ✔ | | | | | | | | | |
| » Chewable tablet—Chewing well and holding in mouth for approximately 2 minutes | | | | ✔ | | | | | | |
| » Lingual aerosol— | | | | | | | | | | |
|     Removing plastic cover; not shaking container | | ✔ | | | | | | | | |
|     Holding container vertically and spraying onto or under tongue; not inhaling spray | | ✔ | | | | | | | | |
|     Closing mouth after each spray; not swallowing immediately | | ✔ | | | | | | | | |
| » Sublingual tablet—Under the tongue; avoiding eating, drinking, smoking, or using chewing tobacco while tablet is dissolving | | | | | | ✔ | ✔ | ✔ | | |
| » Ointment—Cleansing skin before applying; measuring; using applicator; spreading evenly over same size of skin area in each application; not rubbing into skin; applying to skin free of hair, in different areas; proper application of occlusive dressing, if ordered | | | | | | | | | ✔ | |
|     Transdermal—Not trimming or cutting patch; applying to clean, dry skin free of hair, scars, cuts, or irritation (after removal of previous system); replacing systems that have loosened or fallen off; alternating application sites | | | | | | | | | | ✔ |
| » Not chewing, crushing, or swallowing | ✔ | | | | | ✔ | ✔ | ✔ | | |
| » Not breaking, crushing, or chewing before swallowing | | | | | ✔ | | | | | |
| *For use in treating acute angina attacks* | | | | | | | | | | |
| » Sitting down and using medication at first sign of angina attack; caution if dizziness or faintness occurs | ✔ | ✔ | | ✔ | | ✔ | ✔ | | | |
|     Remaining calm until medicine has opportunity to work | ✔ | ✔ | | ✔ | | ✔ | ✔ | | | |
| » Relief usually occurs within 5 minutes— | ✔ | ✔ | | ✔ | | ✔ | ✔ | | | |
|     Dose may be repeated if pain not relieved in 5 to 10 minutes; calling physician or going to emergency room if angina pain not relieved by 3 doses in 15 minutes | | ✔ | | ✔ | | ✔ | ✔ | | | |
|     Not repeating dose; using sublingual nitroglycerin and calling physician or going to emergency room if angina pain not relieved in 15 minutes | ✔ | | | | | | | | | |

## Table 2. Patient Consultation (continued)

Consider advising the patient on the following:

Legend:
- **I** = Extended-release nitroglycerin (Buccal)
- **II** = Aerosol nitroglycerin (Lingual)
- **III** = Regular, **IV** = Chewable, **V** = Extended-release (Oral)
- **VI** = Erythrityl tetranitrate, **VII** = Isosorbide dinitrate, **VIII** = Nitroglycerin (Sublingual)
- **IX** = Nitroglycerin ointment, **X** = Transdermal nitroglycerin (Topical)

| | I | II | III | IV | V | VI | VII | VIII | IX | X |
|---|---|---|---|---|---|---|---|---|---|---|
| *For use in preventing angina* » This dosage form does not relieve angina attacks but rather prevents them (exceptions are chewable and sublingual isosorbide dinitrate) | | | | ✔ | ✔ | ✔ | ✔ | | ✔ | ✔ |
| Using 5 to 10 minutes prior to anticipated stress to prevent attack | ✔ | ✔ | | | ✔ | | ✔ | ✔ | | |
| Missed dose: Taking/using as soon as possible unless next scheduled dose is within: | | | | | | | | | | |
| —2 hours (exception is oral extended-release) | ✔ | | ✔ | ✔ | | ✔ | ✔ | ✔ | ✔ | |
| —6 hours (for oral extended-release) | | | | | ✔ | | | | | |
| Returning to regular dosing schedule; not doubling doses | ✔ | | ✔ | ✔ | ✔ | ✔ | ✔ | ✔ | ✔ | |
| » Proper storage | ✔ | ✔ | | | | | | | | |
| Protecting from freezing | | ✔ | | | | | | | | |
| Not puncturing, breaking, or burning aerosol container | | ✔ | | | | | | | | |
| Storing in cool place, tightly closed | | | | | | | | | ✔ | |
| Lack of reliability of flushing or headache as test of potency | | | | | | | | ✔ | | |
| » Keeping sublingual nitroglycerin in original glass, screw-cap bottle (unless using special nitroglycerin container) with cotton plug removed; avoiding handling tablets; capping quickly and tightly after each use; not storing in same container as other medications; not carrying close to body or in auto glove compartment; not storing in refrigerator or bathroom medicine cabinet | | | | | | | | ✔ | | |
| **Precautions while using this medication** | | | | | | | | | | |
| » Checking with physician before discontinuing medication; gradual dosage reduction may be needed | ✔ | ✔ | ✔ | ✔ | ✔ | ✔ | ✔ | ✔ | ✔ | ✔ |
| » Caution when getting up suddenly from a lying or sitting position | ✔ | ✔ | ✔ | ✔ | ✔ | ✔ | ✔ | ✔ | ✔ | ✔ |
| » Caution in using alcohol, while standing for long periods or exercising, and during hot weather because of enhanced orthostatic hypotensive effects | ✔ | ✔ | ✔ | ✔ | ✔ | ✔ | ✔ | ✔ | ✔ | ✔ |
| » Headache as a common effect; should decrease with continuing therapy; checking with physician if continuing or severe | ✔ | ✔ | ✔ | ✔ | ✔ | ✔ | ✔ | ✔ | ✔ | ✔ |
| Notifying physician if undigested extended-release tablets are found in stools (for isosorbide dinitrate and pentaerythritol tetranitrate only) | | | | | ✔ | | | | | |
| **Side/adverse effects** Signs of potential side effects, especially blurred vision, dryness of mouth, severe or prolonged headache, and skin rash | ✔ | ✔ | ✔ | ✔ | ✔ | ✔ | ✔ | ✔ | ✔ | ✔ |

---

**NITRAZEPAM** — See *Benzodiazepines (Systemic)*

---

# NITROFURANTOIN Systemic

VA CLASSIFICATION (Primary): AM600

Commonly used brand name(s): *Apo-Nitrofurantoin; Furadantin; Furalan; Furatoin; Macrobid; Macrodantin; Nitrofuracot.*

Note: For a listing of dosage forms and brand names by country availability, see *Dosage Forms* section(s).

## Category
Antibacterial (systemic).

## Indications
Note: Bracketed information in the *Indications* section refers to uses that are not included in U.S. product labeling.

**Accepted**

Urinary tract infections, bacterial (treatment)—Nitrofurantoin is indicated in the treatment of urinary tract infections caused by susceptible strains of *Escherichia coli*, enterococci, *Staphylococcus aureus*, *S. saprophyticus*, *Klebsiella* species, *Enterobacter* species, and *Proteus* species.

[Urinary tract infections, bacterial (prophylaxis)][1]—Nitrofurantoin is used in the prophylaxis of urinary tract infections.

Not all species or strains of a particular organism may be susceptible to nitrofurantoin.

[1] Not included in Canadian product labeling.

# Nitrofurantoin (Systemic)

## Pharmacology/Pharmacokinetics

**Physicochemical characteristics**
Molecular weight—238.16.

**Mechanism of action/Effect**
Nitrofurantoin, a synthetic, broad-spectrum, weakly acidic antibacterial, is generally bactericidal at therapeutic concentrations. Therapeutic concentrations are achieved only in the urine. The mechanism of antimicrobial action is unique among antibacterials. Nitrofurantoin is reduced by bacterial flavoproteins to reactive intermediates, which inactivate or alter bacterial ribosomal proteins and other macromolecules.

**Absorption**
Microcrystalline—Rapidly and completely absorbed in the small intestine.
Macrocrystalline—More slowly absorbed and usually causes less gastrointestinal irritation.
The presence of food can increase the bioavailability of both forms of nitrofurantoin; this also increased the duration of therapeutic urinary concentrations.

**Distribution**
High concentrations are achieved in urine and the kidneys; serum concentrations are very low; crosses the placenta and blood-brain barrier.

**Protein binding**
Moderate (60%).

**Biotransformation**
Approximately two-thirds of the drug is rapidly metabolized and inactivated in most body tissues, including the liver.

**Half-life**
0.3 to 1 hour.

**Elimination**
Renal—Primarily excreted by glomerular filtration with some tubular secretion and reabsorption; 30 to 40% rapidly excreted unchanged; the macrocrystalline form is excreted more slowly; active drug accumulates in patients with impaired renal function and may reach toxic concentrations.
Biliary—May also be excreted in the bile.
In dialysis—Nitrofurantoin is dialyzable.

## Precautions to Consider

**Cross-sensitivity and/or related problems**
Patients hypersensitive to one nitrofuran may be hypersensitive to other nitrofurans also.

**Carcinogenicity**
Nitrofurantoin, given as 0.3% of the diet to female Holtzman rats for up to 44.5 weeks or given as 0.1% to 0.187% of the diet to female Sprague-Dawley rats for 75 weeks, has not been shown to be carcinogenic. No evidence of carcinogenicity was found in 2 chronic rodent bioassays in male and female Sprague-Dawley rats and 2 chronic bioassays in Swiss mice and in $BDF_1$ mice. Increased incidences of tubular adenomas, benign mixed tumors, and granulosa cell tumors of the ovary were seen in female $B6C3F_1$ mice. There was an increased incidence of uncommon kidney tubular cell neoplasms, osteosarcomas, and neoplasms of the subcutaneous tissue in male F344/N rats. Lung papillary adenomas of unknown significance were observed in the F1 generation of pregnant mice given 75 mg per kg of body weight (mg/kg) of nitrofurantoin by subcutaneous injection.

**Mutagenicity**
Nitrofurantoin has induced point mutations in certain strains of *Salmonella typhimurium* and forward mutations in L5178Y mouse lymphoma cells. It has also induced increased numbers of sister chromatid exchanges and chromosomal aberrations in Chinese hamster ovary cells but not in human cells in culture. Results of the sex-linked recessive lethal assay in *Drosophila* were negative after oral or parenteral administration of nitrofurantoin. The medication did not induce heritable mutation in the rodent models examined.

**Pregnancy/Reproduction**
Fertility—Nitrofurantoin, given in high doses in rats, has been shown to cause temporary spermatogenic arrest, which was reversible upon discontinuation of the medication. Nitrofurantoin, in doses of 10 mg/kg per day or greater, may produce slight to moderate spermatogenic arrest, with decreased sperm counts, in human males.
Pregnancy—Nitrofurantoin crosses the placenta. Use is contraindicated in pregnancy at term and during labor and delivery, or when the onset of labor is imminent, because of the possibility of hemolytic anemia due to immature enzyme systems in the fetus.
Reproduction studies have been performed in rabbits and rats given doses up to 6 times the human dose; these studies have revealed no evidence of impaired fertility or harm to the fetus due to nitrofurantoin. In a single study conducted in mice given 68 times the human dose (based on mg/kg administered to the dam), growth retardation and a low incidence of minor and common malformations were observed. However, fetal malformations were not observed at 25 times the human dose.
FDA Pregnancy Category B.

**Breast-feeding**
Nitrofurantoin is excreted in breast milk in trace amounts. Hemolytic anemia may occur, especially in glucose-6-phosphate dehydrogenase (G6PD)–deficient infants.

**Pediatrics**
Use of nitrofurantoin is contraindicated in infants up to 1 month of age because of the possibility of hemolytic anemia due to immature enzyme systems.

**Geriatrics**
No information is available on the relationship of age to the effects of nitrofurantoin in geriatric patients. However, elderly patients are more likely to have an age-related decrease in renal function, which may require a decrease in dosage or change in medication. Side effects, such as acute pneumonitis and peripheral polyneuropathy, may also occur more frequently in elderly patients.

**Drug interactions and/or related problems**
The following drug interactions and/or related problems have been selected on the basis of their potential clinical significance (possible mechanism in parentheses where appropriate)—not necessarily inclusive (» = major clinical significance):

Note: Combinations containing any of the following medications, depending on the amount present, may also interact with this medication.

» Hemolytics, other (See *Appendix II*)
(concurrent use with nitrofurantoin may increase the potential for toxic side effects)

Hepatotoxic medications, other (See *Appendix II*)
(concurrent use of nitrofurantoin with other hepatotoxic medications may increase the potential for hepatotoxicity)

Magnesium trisilicate
(magnesium trisilicate reduces both the rate and extent of absorption of nitrofurantoin, probably by adsorption of nitrofurantoin to its surface)

Nalidixic acid
(nitrofurantoin interferes with the therapeutic effects of nalidixic acid)

» Neurotoxic medications, other (See *Appendix II*)
(concurrent use of nitrofurantoin with other neurotoxic medications may increase the potential for neurotoxicity)

» Probenecid or
» Sulfinpyrazone
(these medications may inhibit renal tubular secretion of nitrofurantoin, resulting in increased serum concentrations and/or toxicity, prolonged elimination half-life, and reduced urinary concentrations and effectiveness; dosage adjustment of probenecid may be necessary)

**Laboratory value alterations**
The following have been selected on the basis of their potential clinical significance (possible effect in parentheses where appropriate)—not necessarily inclusive (» = major clinical significance):

With diagnostic test results
Glucose, urine
(nitrofurantoin may produce metabolites in the urine that may give false-positive results with copper sulfate reduction tests, such as *Benedict's* solution)

**Medical considerations/Contraindications**
The medical considerations/contraindications included have been selected on the basis of their potential clinical significance (reasons given in parentheses where appropriate)—not necessarily inclusive (» = major clinical significance).

*Risk-benefit should be considered when the following medical problems exist:*

» Glucose-6-phosphate dehydrogenase (G6PD) deficiency
(hemolysis may occur in patients with G6PD deficiency who take nitrofurantoin)

Hypersensitivity to nitrofurans

» Neuropathy, peripheral
(nitrofurantoin may cause peripheral neuropathy)

» Pulmonary disease
  (nitrofurantoin may cause acute, subacute, and chronic pulmonary reactions, including pneumonitis)
» Renal function impairment
  (because nitrofurantoin is excreted through the kidneys, it is recommended that nitrofurantoin not be given to patients with a creatinine clearance of less than 40 to 60 mL per minute [0.67 to 1.00 mL per second]; nitrofurantoin loses its effectiveness in patients with renal function impairment, and toxic effects are increased)

**Patient monitoring**
The following may be especially important in patient monitoring (other tests may be warranted in some patients, depending on condition; » = major clinical significance):

Hepatic function determinations
  (may be required periodically during long-term therapy to detect changes in hepatic function; if hepatitis occurs, nitrofurantoin should be discontinued immediately and appropriate measures taken)
» Pulmonary function determinations
  (may be required periodically during long-term therapy if pulmonary reactions [e.g., diffuse interstitial pneumonitis, pulmonary fibrosis] occur; if pulmonary reactions occur, nitrofurantoin should be discontinued and appropriate measures taken)

## Side/Adverse Effects

Note: Acute pneumonitis is more common in the elderly; symptoms usually occur within the first week of therapy. The pneumonitis is often reversible with discontinuation of the drug; corticosteroids may be beneficial in severe cases. Chronic pulmonary reactions, including diffuse interstitial pneumonitis and fibrosis, are insidious in onset and are more likely to occur in patients who have been on nitrofurantoin therapy for at least 6 months. Pulmonary function may be permanently impaired even after the drug has been stopped, especially if pulmonary reactions are not recognized early.

Peripheral polyneuropathy is an ascending sensorimotor neuropathy, which may be progressive if the drug is not discontinued immediately. Polyneuropathy occurs more frequently in patients with renal dysfunction and in the elderly; however, it also occurs in patients with normal renal function who have received nitrofurantoin for prolonged periods of time. Demyelination and degeneration of both sensory and motor nerves occur. Nitrofurantoin should be stopped at the first signs of neuritis.

The following side/adverse effects have been selected on the basis of their potential clinical significance (possible signs and symptoms in parentheses where appropriate)—not necessarily inclusive:

**Those indicating need for medical attention**
Incidence more frequent
  *Pneumonitis* (chest pain; chills; cough; fever; troubled breathing)
Incidence less frequent
  *Hematologic reactions, specifically granulocytopenia* (sore throat and fever); *leukopenia* (sore throat and fever); *or megaloblastic anemia* (unusual tiredness or weakness); *neurotoxicity* (dizziness; drowsiness; headache; unusual tiredness or weakness); *polyneuropathy* (numbness, tingling, or burning of face or mouth; unusual muscle weakness)
Incidence rare
  *Hemolytic anemia* (pale skin; unusual tiredness or weakness); *hepatitis* (yellow eyes or skin); *hypersensitivity* (skin rash; itching; arthralgia; fever; chills)

**Those indicating need for medical attention only if they continue or are bothersome**
Incidence more frequent
  *Gastrointestinal disturbances* (abdominal or stomach pain or upset; diarrhea; loss of appetite; nausea or vomiting)

**Those not indicating need for medical attention**
  *Rust-yellow to brown discoloration of urine*

## Overdose

For more information on the management of overdose or unintentional ingestion, **contact a Poison Control Center** (see *Poison Control Center Listing*).

**Treatment of overdose**
Recommended treatment consists of the following:
To decrease absorption—Induction of emesis if vomiting has not already occurred.
Specific treatment—Maintaining a high fluid intake to promote urinary excretion of nitrofurantoin.

Supportive care—Patients in whom intentional overdose is known or suspected should be referred for psychiatric consultation.

## Patient Consultation

As an aid to patient consultation, refer to *Advice for the Patient, Nitrofurantoin (Systemic)*.
In providing consultation, consider emphasizing the following selected information (» = major clinical significance):

**Before using this medication**
» Conditions affecting use, especially:
  Hypersensitivity to nitrofurans
  Pregnancy—Nitrofurantoin is contraindicated at term and during labor and delivery because of the possibility of hemolytic anemia in the fetus
  Breast-feeding—Not recommended since hemolytic anemia may occur in G6PD-deficient infants
  Use in children—Nitrofurantoin is contraindicated in infants up to 1 month of age because of the possibility of hemolytic anemia
  Use in the elderly—Side effects, such as acute pneumonitis and peripheral polyneuropathy, may occur more frequently in elderly patients
  Other medications, especially other hemolytics, other neurotoxic medications, probenecid, or sulfinpyrazone
  Other medical problems, especially G6PD deficiency, peripheral neuropathy, pulmonary disease, or renal function impairment

**Proper use of this medication**
» Not giving to infants up to 1 month of age
  Taking with food or milk
*Proper administration technique for oral liquid:*
  Shaking well before each dose
  Using a specially marked measuring spoon or other device
  May be mixed with water, milk, fruit juices, or infants' formulas
  Proper administration technique for extended-release tablets: Swallowing tablet whole; not breaking, crushing, or chewing before swallowing
» Compliance with full course of therapy
» Proper dosage
  Missed dose: Taking as soon as possible; not taking if almost time for next dose; not doubling doses
» Proper storage

**Precautions while using this medication**
  Regular visits to physician to check progress if on long-term therapy
  Checking with physician if no improvement within a few days
» Diabetics: False-positive reactions with copper sulfate urine glucose tests may occur

**Side/adverse effects**
  Rust-yellow to brown discoloration of urine may be alarming to patient although medically insignificant
  Signs of potential side effects, especially hemolytic anemia, jaundice, neurotoxicity, pneumonitis, and polyneuropathy

## General Dosing Information

Nitrofurantoin should preferably be taken with food or milk. This minimizes gastrointestinal irritation, delays and increases absorption of both the macrocrystalline and microcrystalline forms, increases the peak concentration of the macrocrystalline form, and prolongs the duration of therapeutic concentrations in the urine.

Patients on long-term suppressive therapy require a reduction in dose.

Patients with impaired renal function (creatinine clearance less than 40 to 60 mL per minute [0.67 to 1.00 mL per second]) should not receive nitrofurantoin since increased toxicity due to possible accumulation of toxic metabolites may occur. Also, nitrofurantoin is ineffective in patients whose creatinine clearance is less than 40 mL per minute.

## Oral Dosage Forms

Note: Bracketed uses in the *Dosage Forms* section refer to categories of use and/or indications that are not included in U.S. product labeling.

### NITROFURANTOIN CAPSULES USP

**Usual adult and adolescent dose**
Antibacterial—
  Oral, 50 to 100 mg every six hours.
Note: [Urinary tract infections, bacterial (prophylaxis)][1]—Oral, 50 to 100 mg once a day at bedtime.
  Most uncomplicated infections caused by susceptible bacteria are adequately treated with 50 mg three times a day.

**Usual adult prescribing limits**
Up to 600 mg daily; or up to 10 mg per kg of body weight daily.

**Usual pediatric dose**
Antibacterial—
    Infants up to 1 month of age: Use is contraindicated because of the possibility of hemolytic anemia due to immature enzyme systems.
    Infants and children 1 month of age and over: Oral, 0.75 to 1.75 mg per kg of body weight every six hours.
Note:  [Urinary tract infections, bacterial (prophylaxis)][1]—Oral, 1 mg per kg of body weight once a day at bedtime.
    Therapeutic doses up to 10 mg per kg of body weight daily in four evenly divided doses have been used.

**Strength(s) usually available**
U.S.—
    25 mg (Rx) [*Macrodantin* (macrocrystalline)].
    50 mg (Rx) [*Macrodantin* (macrocrystalline) [GENERIC (macrocrystalline and microcrystalline)].
    100 mg (Rx) [*Macrodantin* (macrocrystalline) [GENERIC (macrocrystalline and microcrystalline)].
Canada—
    25 mg (Rx) [*Macrodantin* (macrocrystalline)].
    50 mg (Rx) [*Macrodantin* (macrocrystalline)].
    100 mg (Rx) [*Macrodantin* (macrocrystalline)].

**Packaging and storage**
Store below 40 °C (104 °F), preferably between 15 and 30 °C (59 and 86 °F), unless otherwise specified by manufacturer. Store in a tight, light-resistant container.

**Auxiliary labeling**
• Continue medicine for full time of treatment.
• Take with food or milk.
• May discolor urine.

## NITROFURANTOIN EXTENDED-RELEASE CAPSULES

**Usual adult and adolescent dose**
Antibacterial—
    Oral, 100 mg every twelve hours for seven days.

**Usual pediatric dose**
Antibacterial—
    Safety and efficacy have not been established in children up to 12 years of age.

**Strength(s) usually available**
U.S.—
    100 mg (Rx) [*Macrobid* (macrocrystalline 25 mg, monohydrate 75 mg)].
Canada—
    Not commercially available.

**Packaging and storage**
Store below 40 °C (104 °F), preferably between 15 and 30 °C (59 and 86 °F), unless otherwise specified by manufacturer. Store in a tight, light-resistant container.

**Auxiliary labeling**
• Continue medicine for full time of treatment.
• Take with food or milk.
• May discolor urine.

## NITROFURANTOIN ORAL SUSPENSION USP

**Usual adult and adolescent dose**
See *Nitrofurantoin Capsules USP*.

**Usual adult prescribing limits**
See *Nitrofurantoin Capsules USP*.

**Usual pediatric dose**
See *Nitrofurantoin Capsules USP*.

**Strength(s) usually available**
U.S.—
    25 mg per 5 mL (Rx) [*Furadantin* (methylparaben; propylparaben; saccharin; sorbitol)].
Canada—
    Not commercially available.

**Packaging and storage**
Store below 40 °C (104 °F), preferably between 15 and 30 °C (59 and 86 °F), unless otherwise specified by manufacturer. Store in a tight, light-resistant container. Protect from freezing.

**Incompatibilities**
Nitrofurantoin and its solutions are discolored by alkalis and by exposure to strong light and decompose upon contact with metals other than stainless steel or aluminum.

**Auxiliary labeling**
• Shake well.
• Continue medicine for full time of treatment.
• Take with food or milk.
• May discolor urine.

**Note**
Dispense in amber bottles.
When dispensing, include a calibrated liquid-measuring device.

**Additional information**
The oral suspension dosage form is readily miscible with water, milk, fruit juices, or infants' formulas.

## NITROFURANTOIN TABLETS USP

**Usual adult and adolescent dose**
See *Nitrofurantoin Capsules USP*.

**Usual adult prescribing limits**
See *Nitrofurantoin Capsules USP*.

**Usual pediatric dose**
See *Nitrofurantoin Capsules USP*.

**Strength(s) usually available**
U.S.—
    50 mg (Rx) [*Furalan*; *Furatoin*; *Nitrofuracot* [GENERIC].
    100 mg (Rx) [*Furalan* [GENERIC].
Canada—
    50 mg (Rx) [*Apo-Nitrofurantoin*].
    100 mg (Rx) [*Apo-Nitrofurantoin*].

**Packaging and storage**
Store below 40 °C (104 °F), preferably between 15 and 30 °C (59 and 86 °F), unless otherwise specified by manufacturer. Store in a tight, light-resistant container.

**Incompatibilities**
Nitrofurantoin and its solutions are discolored by alkalis and by exposure to strong light and decompose upon contact with metals other than stainless steel or aluminum.

**Auxiliary labeling**
• Continue medicine for full time of treatment.
• Take with food or milk.
• May discolor urine.

**Note**
Dispense in amber bottles.

---
[1]Not included in Canadian product labeling.

Revised: 01/19/93

---

**NITROFURAZONE**—The *Nitrofurazone (Topical)* monograph is not included in this published version of the USP DI database. Copies of the monograph are available on request from Micromedex, Inc. - Reprint Requests, 6200 S. Syracuse Way, Suite 300, Englewood, CO 80111; telephone (303) 486-6400; telefax (303) 486-6464; Email: USPDI@MDX.COM.

---

**NITROGLYCERIN**—See *Nitrates (Systemic)*

---

# NITROPRUSSIDE   Systemic

VA CLASSIFICATION (Primary/Secondary): CV402/CV500; CV900; AD900

Commonly used brand name(s): *Nipride*; *Nitropress*.

Note:  For a listing of dosage forms and brand names by country availability, see *Dosage Forms* section(s).

## Category
Antihypertensive; vasodilator, congestive heart failure; myocardial infarction therapy adjunct; antidote (to ergot alkaloid poisoning).

## Indications
Note:  Bracketed information in the *Indications* section refers to uses that are not included in U.S. product labeling.

### Accepted

Congestive heart failure (treatment)[1]—Nitroprusside is indicated for the management of acute congestive heart failure.

Hypertension (treatment)—Nitroprusside is indicated for the immediate reduction of blood pressure of patients in hypertensive crisis.

Hypotension, controlled (induction and maintenance)—Nitroprusside is indicated for producing controlled hypotension during surgery to reduce bleeding into the surgical field.

[Hypertension, paroxysmal, in surgery for pheochromocytoma (treatment)][1]—Nitroprusside is used to control paroxysmal hypertension prior to and during surgery for pheochromocytoma.

[Myocardial infarction (treatment adjunct)][1]—Use of nitroprusside to reduce afterload is also recommended in patients with acute myocardial infarction who are hypertensive with persistent chest pain or left ventricular failure.

[Valvular regurgitation (treatment adjunct)][1]—Nitroprusside is also used as an adjunct to standard treatment of aortic or mitral regurgitation prior to surgical intervention.

[Toxicity, ergot alkaloid (treatment)][1]—Nitroprusside is also used for treatment of peripheral vasospasm caused by ergot alkaloid overdose.

### Unaccepted

Nitroprusside should *not* be used in the treatment of compensatory hypertension (such as in arteriovenous shunt or coarctation of the aorta).

[1] Not included in Canadian product labeling.

## Pharmacology/Pharmacokinetics

### Physicochemical characteristics
Molecular weight—297.95.

### Mechanism of action/Effect

Antihypertensive—Hypertension or controlled hypotension: Causes vasodilation by a direct effect on arterial and venous smooth muscle, with no effect on uterine or duodenal smooth muscle or on myocardial contractility; regional distribution of blood flow is only marginally affected. Reduces peripheral resistance and has a variable effect on cardiac output. Is more active on veins than arteries (but less markedly so than nitroglycerin). Increases renin activity.

Vasodilator, congestive heart failure—Beneficial effects in congestive heart failure are due to decreased systemic resistance, preload and afterload reduction, and improved cardiac output.

Myocardial infarction therapy adjunct—The effect of nitroprusside on ischemic myocardial areas is not totally known. It dilates coronary arteries. The medication reportedly reduces myocardial oxygen consumption and relieves persistent chest pain but has also been found to aggravate ischemia by redistributing blood flow away from ischemic myocardium.

Valvular regurgitation therapy adjunct—In the treatment of valvular regurgitation, nitroprusside reduces aortic and left ventricular impedance.

Antidote (to ergot alkaloid poisoning)—Causes vasodilation.

### Other actions/effects
Slightly increases heart rate. Decreases platelet aggregation.

### Biotransformation

By intraerythrocytic reaction with hemoglobin to produce cyanmethemoglobin and cyanide ion. Exogenous cyanide is sequestered by erythrocyte methemoglobin as cyanmethemoglobin until intraerythrocytic methemoglobin is saturated. Some cyanide ion is eliminated from the body as expired hydrogen cyanide, but most is enzymatically converted to thiocyanate, which is eliminated in the urine; this reaction requires a hepatic mitochondrial enzyme, rhodanase (thiosulfate-cyanide sulfur transferase), and a sulfur donor, especially thiosulfate, cystine, and cysteine. Cyanide not removed by any of these methods binds to mitochondrial cytochromes and prevents oxidative metabolism; cells either are forced to provide for their energy needs via anaerobic pathways, generating lactic acid, or die hypoxic deaths.

Cyanide is normally found in serum and is derived from dietary substrates and tobacco smoke. Normal cyanide ion concentrations in packed erythrocytes are less than 1 micromole per liter (25 mg per liter); these concentrations are doubled in heavy smokers.

At healthy steady state, less than 1% of hemoglobin is in the form of methemoglobin. Nitroprusside metabolism leads to methemoglobin formation either through dissociation of cyanmethemoglobin formed in the original reaction of nitroprusside with hemoglobin or by direct oxidation of hemoglobin by the released nitroso group. A patient with normal red-cell mass and normal methemoglobin concentrations can buffer about 175 mcg of cyanide ion per kg of body weight (mcg/kg), corresponding to a little less than 500 mcg/kg of infused sodium nitroprusside.

Thiosulfate is a normal constituent of serum, produced by cysteine. Normal physiological concentrations of 0.1 millimole per liter (11 mg per liter) are approximately double in children and in adults who are not eating. When thiosulfate is being supplied only by normal physiologic mechanisms, conversion of cyanide ion to thiocyanate generally occurs at about 1 mcg/kg per minute. This rate of cyanide clearance corresponds to steady-state processing of a sodium nitroprusside infusion of slightly more than 2 mcg/kg per minute. Cyanide begins to accumulate when sodium nitroprusside infusions exceed this rate.

### Half-life
Nitroprusside—Circulatory: About 2 minutes.
Thiosulfate—After intravenous infusion: About 20 minutes.
Thiocyanate—About 3 days; may be doubled or tripled in renal failure.

### Onset of action
Hypotensive—Within 1 to 2 minutes after start of an adequate infusion.

### Time to peak effect
Hypotensive—Almost immediate.

### Duration of action
Hypotensive—1 to 10 minutes after infusion is stopped.

### Elimination
Thiocyanate and infused thiosulfate—Renal.

## Precautions to Consider

### Carcinogenicity/Mutagenicity
Studies have not been done in either animals or humans.

### Pregnancy/Reproduction

Pregnancy—Adequate and well-controlled studies in humans have not been done. Birth of a stillborn infant without any obvious anomalies was reported after one woman was given nitroprusside to control gestational hypertension; however, cyanide concentrations in the infant's liver were well below usual toxic levels and the mother demonstrated no cyanide toxicity.

Teratogenicity studies in laboratory animals have not been done. In three studies in pregnant ewes, nitroprusside was shown to cross the placenta; fetal cyanide levels were dose-related to maternal levels; fatal cyanide levels could be produced in fetuses by using high rates of nitroprusside administration to the pregnant ewes.

FDA Pregnancy Category C.

### Breast-feeding
It is not known whether nitroprusside is excreted in breast milk. Problems in humans have not been documented.

### Pediatrics
Appropriate studies on the relationship of age to the effects of nitroprusside have not been performed in the pediatric population. However, pediatrics-specific problems that would limit the usefulness of this medication in children are not expected.

### Geriatrics
Although appropriate studies on the relationship of age to the effects of nitroprusside have not been performed in the geriatric population, the elderly may be more sensitive to the hypotensive effects. In addition, elderly patients are more likely to have age-related renal function impairment, which may require caution in patients receiving nitroprusside.

### Drug interactions and/or related problems
The following drug interactions and/or related problems have been selected on the basis of their potential clinical significance (possible mechanism in parentheses where appropriate)—not necessarily inclusive (» = major clinical significance):

Note: Combinations containing any of the following medications, depending on the amount present, may also interact with this medication.

Dobutamine
(concurrent use with nitroprusside may result in a higher cardiac output and a lower pulmonary wedge pressure)

Hypotension-producing medications, other (see *Appendix II*)
(concurrent use may result in increased hypotensive effects which may be severe; dosage adjustment based on careful blood pressure monitoring is recommended)

Sympathomimetics
(hypotensive effects of nitroprusside may be reduced when it is used concurrently with sympathomimetics)

### Laboratory value alterations
The following have been selected on the basis of their potential clinical significance (possible effect in parentheses where appropriate)—not necessarily inclusive (» = major clinical significance):

With physiology/laboratory test values
Bicarbonate concentrations, blood and
$PCO_2$ and
pH
(may be decreased, indicating metabolic acidosis, during cyanide toxicity; however, may not be present until an hour or more after toxic cyanide concentrations are reached)

Cyanide, serum
(concentrations increased with excessive rate of nitroprusside infusion; except at low nitroprusside infusion rates [less than 2 mcg per kg of body weight (mcg/kg) per minute] or with brief use, concentrations produced are significant, potentially reaching toxic or lethal levels; venous blood appears bright red because of hyperoxemia)

Lactate, arterial blood
(concentrations may be increased in overdose, indicating metabolic acidosis, during cyanide toxicity; however, may not be present until an hour or more after toxic cyanide concentrations are reached)

Methemoglobin, blood
(concentrations may rarely be increased if amount of nitroprusside administered exceeds rate at which back-conversion of methemoglobin to hemoglobin can occur; blood appears chocolate brown, without color change on exposure to air)

Oxygen, venous blood
(concentrations increased in cyanide toxicity; venous blood appears bright red)

Thiocyanate, serum
(concentrations increased as a result of cyanide enzymatic reaction with thiosulfate; with prolonged infusions, the steady-state concentration is increased with increased infusion rate)

## Medical considerations/Contraindications

The medical considerations/contraindications included have been selected on the basis of their potential clinical significance (reasons given in parentheses where appropriate)—not necessarily inclusive (» = major clinical significance).

*Risk-benefit should be considered when the following medical problems exist:*

Anemia—for use in producing controlled hypotension during anesthesia only; patient's capacity to compensate may be diminished; should be corrected prior to use of nitroprusside

» Cerebrovascular or coronary artery insufficiency
(reduced tolerance of hypotension)

» Encephalopathy or other conditions where intracranial pressure is elevated
(intracranial pressure may be further increased; nitroprusside should be used only with extreme caution)

» Hepatic function impairment
(hepatic enzyme is involved in metabolism of nitroprusside)

Hypothyroidism
(thiocyanate, one of the metabolic products of nitroprusside, inhibits both uptake and binding of iodine)

Hypovolemia—for use in producing controlled hypotension during anesthesia only; patient's capacity to compensate may be diminished; should be corrected prior to use of nitroprusside

» Leber's hereditary optic atrophy or
» Tobacco amblyopia
(deficiency or absence of enzyme [rhodanase] needed for metabolism of nitroprusside)

Pulmonary function impairment
(aggravation of hypoxemia)

» Renal function impairment
(reduced excretion of thiocyanate)

Sensitivity to nitroprusside

» Vitamin $B_{12}$ deficiency
(related to metabolism)

## Patient monitoring

The following may be especially important in patient monitoring (other tests may be warranted in some patients, depending on condition; » = major clinical significance):

Acid-base balance and

Oxygen concentrations, venous
(may indicate metabolic acidosis resulting from cyanide toxicity; however, because measurable effects may be delayed an hour or more after toxic cyanide concentrations are reached, these values should not be used to decide when to treat for cyanide toxicity)

» Blood pressure determinations
(should be made continuously, either with a continually reinflated sphygmomanometer or, preferably, an intra-arterial pressure sensor)
(pulmonary artery diastolic or wedge pressure determinations may be required in patients with acute myocardial infarction)

Cyanide concentrations, serum
(may be determined; however, not particularly useful because the cyanide assay is technically difficult and cyanide concentrations in body fluids other than packed red cells are difficult to interpret)

Methemoglobin concentrations, blood
(recommended in patients who have received more than 10 mg of nitroprusside per kg of body weight and who exhibit signs of impaired oxygen delivery despite adequate cardiac output and adequate arterial $pO_2$)

Thiocyanate concentrations, serum
(recommended at daily intervals in patients receiving prolonged nitroprusside infusions at a rate greater than 3 mcg per kg of body weight [mcg/kg] per minute [1 mcg/kg per minute in anuric patients]; should not exceed 1 millimole per liter)

*For congestive heart failure*
Invasive hemodynamic monitoring and
Urine output
(recommended to guide titration of infusion rate)

## Side/Adverse Effects

Note: A severe rebound hypertension has been reported after discontinuation of an infusion used to produce controlled hypotension during surgery.

The following side/adverse effects have been selected on the basis of their potential clinical significance (possible signs and symptoms in parentheses where appropriate)—not necessarily inclusive:

### Those indicating need for medical attention

Signs and/or symptoms of excessively rapid fall in blood pressure (appear to be related to rate of administration rather than total dose)
*Abdominal pain* (stomach pain); *dizziness; excessive sweating; headache; muscle twitching; nervousness or anxiety; restlessness; retching; tachycardia, reflex*

Note: Excessive *hypotension*, sometimes to levels low enough to compromise perfusion of vital organs, may be produced by small transient excesses in the infusion rate. Excessively rapid decreases in blood pressure can lead to irreversible ischemic injuries or death if patients are not properly monitored.

Signs and/or symptoms of thiocyanate toxicity
*Ataxia; blurred vision; delirium; dizziness; headache; loss of consciousness; nausea and vomiting; shortness of breath; tinnitus* (ringing in ears)

Note: Mild neurotoxicity (*tinnitus, miosis, hyperreflexia*) occurs at serum thiocyanate concentrations of 1 millimole per liter (60 mg per liter). Thiocyanate toxicity becomes life-threatening at serum concentrations of 200 mg per liter.

Signs and/or symptoms of cyanide toxicity
*Absence of reflexes; coma; distant heart sounds; hypotension; imperceptible pulse; metabolic acidosis; pink color; very shallow breathing; widely dilated pupils*

Note: Nitroprusside infusion rates greater than 2 mcg per kg of body weight (mcg/kg) per minute generate cyanide ion faster than the body can normally eliminate it (administration of thiosulfate greatly increases the body's capacity for cyanide elimination). The capacity of methemoglobin to buffer cyanide is exhausted from about 500 mcg/kg of nitroprusside (the amount administered in less than an hour at a rate of 10 mcg/kg per minute). Above this level, toxic effects of cyanide may be rapid, serious, and lethal.

Elevated cyanide concentrations, metabolic acidosis, and marked clinical deterioration have occasionally been reported in patients given infusions at recommended rates for only a few hours (in one case, for only 35 minutes).

Incidence less frequent or rare
*Flushing; hypothyroidism; ileus; increased intracranial pressure; methemoglobinemia*—concentrations greater than 10%; *pain or redness at site of injection; skin rash*

Note: *Hypothyroidism*—Thiocyanate interferes with iodine uptake by the thyroid.

*Methemoglobinemia* is usually rare, because the back-conversion process returning methemoglobin to hemoglobin is normally rapid. Even in patients congenitally incapable of back-converting methemoglobin, a cumulative dose of 10 mg of nitroprusside per kg of body weight (mg/kg) (e.g., given at a rate of 10 mcg/kg per minute for 16 hours) would be required to produce 10% methemoglobinemia.

## General Dosing Information

Nitroprusside should be administered *only* by intravenous infusion by means of an infusion pump, preferably a volumetric pump.

It is recommended that patients receiving nitroprusside be in a setting with available equipment and personnel to allow blood pressure to be monitored continuously.

Care should be taken to avoid extravasation because of possible irritation.

Larger than ordinary doses may be required for hypotensive anesthesia in young, vigorous males.

It is recommended that administration of nitroprusside be discontinued immediately if administration of 10 mcg (0.01 mg) (sodium nitroprusside dihydrate) per kg of body weight per minute for 10 minutes does not produce adequate reduction of blood pressure.

Concurrent administration of sodium thiosulfate (at 5 to 10 times the rate of sodium nitroprusside administration) may reduce the risk of cyanide toxicity by increasing the rate of cyanide conversion. However, it has not been extensively studied, and in one study appeared to potentiate nitroprusside's hypotensive effect. Caution is necessary to avoid prolonged or high doses of sodium nitroprusside with sodium thiosulfate, which could lead to thiocyanate toxicity and hypovolemia.

Apparent tolerance has occurred occasionally. Although a correlation between tachyphylaxis and concomitant cyanide toxicity has been proposed, no correlation has been demonstrated.

### For use in treatment of hypertension
It is recommended that oral antihypertensive therapy be instituted while the patient is receiving nitroprusside and that nitroprusside be withdrawn as soon as the patient has stabilized. Patients receiving concomitant antihypertensive medication require lower doses of nitroprusside.

### For use in treatment of congestive heart failure
Addition of a potent inotropic medication such as dopamine or dobutamine may be useful when doses of nitroprusside that are effective in restoring pump function in left ventricular congestive heart failure cause excessive hypotension.

### For treatment of adverse effects/overdose
For methemoglobinemia
- Intravenous administration of methylene blue in a dose of 1 to 2 mg per kg of body weight (mg/kg) given over several minutes. Extreme caution is necessary in patients likely to have substantial amounts of cyanide bound to methemoglobin as cyanmethemoglobin.

For excessive hypotension
- Slowing or discontinuation of infusion; symptoms disappear quickly (within 1 to 10 minutes). Placement of the patient in the Trendelenberg position to maximize venous return may be helpful.

For thiocyanate toxicity
- Hemodialysis; clearance rates during dialysis can approach the blood flow rate of the dialyzer.

For cyanide toxicity
- Discontinuation of nitroprusside administration. Because metabolic acidosis may not be evident until more than an hour after the appearance of dangerous cyanide concentrations, laboratory test results should not be awaited; treatment should be initiated with reasonable suspicion of cyanide toxicity.
- Intravenous administration of sodium nitrite (as a 3% solution), in a dose of 4 to 6 mg/kg over 2 to 4 minutes. Sodium nitrite provides a buffer for cyanide by converting as much hemoglobin into methemoglobin as the patient can safely tolerate; this dose can be expected to convert about 10% of the patient's hemoglobin, and this level of methemoglobinemia is not associated with any known hazards. Sodium nitrite infusion may cause transient vasodilation and hypotension, which should be managed as necessary. Amyl nitrite inhalations may be used in environments where intravenous administration of sodium nitrite may be delayed.
- Immediately following sodium nitrite infusion, intravenous infusion of sodium thiosulfate in a sufficient amount to convert the cyanide into thiocyanate. The recommended dose of sodium thiosulfate is 150 to 200 mg/kg; a typical adult dose is 50 mL of a 25% solution (sodium thiosulfate is also available as a 50% solution). Thiocyanate concentrations will be raised in acutely cyanide-toxic patients, but not to a dangerous level.
- Hemodialysis is not effective in removing cyanide.
- If necessary, the nitrite/thiosulfate regimen may be repeated, at half the original doses, after 2 hours.

## Parenteral Dosage Forms

### STERILE SODIUM NITROPRUSSIDE

**Usual adult and adolescent dose**
Antihypertensive—
   Intravenous infusion, initially, 0.3 mcg (0.0003 mg) (sodium nitroprusside dihydrate) per kg of body weight per minute, adjusted every few minutes according to response; usual dose is 3 mcg (0.003 mg) per kg of body weight per minute.

Note: Geriatric patients may be more sensitive to the usual adult dose of nitroprusside.

**Usual adult prescribing limits**
10 mcg (0.01 mg) per kg of body weight per minute for a maximum period of 10 minutes, or a total dose of 3.5 mg per kg of body weight (500 mcg [0.5 mg] per kg of body weight during short-term infusions such as in controlled hypotension during surgery). To keep the steady-state thiocyanate concentration below 1 millimole per liter, the rate of a prolonged infusion should be no more than 3 mcg per kg of body weight per minute (1 mcg per kg of body weight per minute in anuric patients).

**Usual pediatric dose**
Antihypertensive—
   See *Usual adult and adolescent dose.*

**Size(s) usually available**
U.S.—
   50 mg (sodium nitroprusside dihydrate) (Rx) [*Nitropress;* GENERIC].
Canada—
   50 mg (sodium nitroprusside dihydrate) (Rx) [*Nipride*].

**Packaging and storage**
Store below 40 °C (104 °F), preferably between 15 and 30 °C (59 and 86 °F), unless otherwise specified by manufacturer. Protect from light.

**Preparation of dosage form**
Nitroprusside is prepared for intravenous infusion by dissolving the contents of a 50-mg vial in 2.3 mL of 5% dextrose injection only and shaking gently to dissolve. The reconstituted solution must be diluted further in 250 to 1000 mL of 5% dextrose injection to achieve the desired concentration and the container is wrapped in a supplied opaque sleeve, aluminum foil, or other opaque material to protect it from light (it is not necessary to wrap the infusion drip chamber or the tubing).

**Stability**
Solutions of nitroprusside should be freshly prepared and any unused portion discarded. A freshly prepared solution has a slight brownish tint and should be discarded if the color is dark brown, orange, or blue.

It is recommended that solutions of nitroprusside not be kept or used longer than 24 hours, unless otherwise specified by the manufacturer.

No other medications should be added to infusion fluid containing nitroprusside.

Sodium nitroprusside solution is rapidly degraded by trace contaminants, often with resulting color changes. A change in color to blue, green, or bright red indicates reaction of nitroprusside ion with another substance, and the solution must be replaced and discarded.

Sodium nitroprusside solution is sensitive to certain wavelengths of light and therefore must be protected from light. After preparation of the medication, the container should be promptly wrapped in the supplied opaque sleeve, aluminum foil, or other opaque material (it is not necessary to wrap the infusion drip chamber or the tubing).

## Selected Bibliography

Kreye VAW. Sodium nitroprusside. In: Scriabine A, ed. Pharmacology of antihypertensive drugs. New York: Raven Press, 1980: 373-96.

Gaskins JD, Holt RJ, Kessler C. Comparative review of intravenous nitroglycerin and nitroprusside sodium. Hosp Form 1982 Jul; 928-34.

---

Revised: 08/07/92
Interim revision: 08/20/98

**NITROUS OXIDE**—See *Anesthetics, Inhalation (Systemic)*

**NIZATIDINE**—See *Histamine H$_2$-receptor Antagonists (Systemic)*

**NOREPINEPHRINE**—See *Sympathomimetic Agents—Cardiovascular Use (Parenteral-Systemic)*

**NORETHINDRONE**—See *Progestins (Systemic)*

**NORFLOXACIN**—See *Fluoroquinolones (Systemic); Norfloxacin (Ophthalmic)*

**NORFLOXACIN**—The *Norfloxacin (Ophthalmic)* monograph is not included in this published version of the USP DI database. Copies of the monograph are available on request from Micromedex, Inc. - Reprint Requests, 6200 S. Syracuse Way, Suite 300, Englewood, CO 80111; telephone (303) 486-6400; telefax (303) 486-6464; Email: USPDI@MDX.COM.

**NORGESTREL**—See *Progestins (Systemic)*

**NORTRIPTYLINE**—See *Antidepressants, Tricyclic (Systemic)*

**NYLIDRIN**—The *Nylidrin (Systemic)* monograph is not included in this published version of the USP DI database. Copies of the monograph are available on request from Micromedex, Inc. - Reprint Requests, 6200 S. Syracuse Way, Suite 300, Englewood, CO 80111; telephone (303) 486-6400; telefax (303) 486-6464; Email: USPDI@MDX.COM.

# NYSTATIN  Oral-Local

VA CLASSIFICATION (Primary): AM700

Commonly used brand name(s): *Mycostatin; Nadostine; Nilstat; Nystex; PMS Nystatin.*

Note: For a listing of dosage forms and brand names by country availability, see *Dosage Forms* section(s).

## Category
Antifungal (oral-local).

## Indications
Note: Bracketed information in the *Indications* section refers to uses that are not included in U.S. product labeling.

**Accepted**

Candidiasis, oropharyngeal (treatment)—Nystatin lozenges (pastilles), nystatin oral suspension, and nystatin for oral suspension are indicated in the local treatment of fungal infections of the oral cavity caused by *Candida albicans* and other *Candida* species.

[Candidiasis, oropharyngeal (prophylaxis)]—Nystatin oral suspension, lozenges (pastilles), and nystatin for oral suspension are used in the prophylaxis of oropharyngeal candidiasis.

Not all species or strains of a particular organism may be susceptible to nystatin.

**Unaccepted**

Nystatin is not indicated in the treatment of systemic fungal infections since it is not absorbed from the gastrointestinal tract.

USP medical experts do not recommend nystatin oral tablets for any indication.

## Pharmacology/Pharmacokinetics

**Mechanism of action/Effect**

Binds to sterols in the fungal cell membrane, resulting in the cell membrane's inability to function as a selective barrier, thus allowing loss of essential cellular constituents.

**Absorption**

Not absorbed from the gastrointestinal tract.

**Saliva concentrations**

Saliva concentrations of nystatin are maintained above those required *in vitro* to inhibit the growth of clinically significant *Candida* species for approximately 2 hours after the start of oral dissolution of 2 nystatin lozenges (400,000 units).

**Elimination**

Fecal. Orally administered nystatin is excreted almost entirely as unchanged drug.

## Precautions to Consider

**Carcinogenicity/Mutagenicity**

Studies have not been done to evaluate the carcinogenic or mutagenic potential of nystatin.

**Pregnancy/Reproduction**

Fertility—Studies have not been done to evaluate the effect of nystatin on fertility in either males or females.

Pregnancy—Studies in humans have not shown that nystatin causes adverse effects on the fetus.

**Breast-feeding**

It is not known whether oral nystatin is excreted in breast milk. However, problems in humans have not been documented.

**Pediatrics**

Use of nystatin lozenges is not recommended in infants and children up to 5 years of age since this age group may not be capable of using the lozenges or tablets safely. However, no pediatrics-specific problems have been documented to date with nystatin oral suspension.

**Geriatrics**

No information is available on the relationship of age to the effects of oral nystatin in geriatric patients.

**Dental**

Patients with full or partial dentures who have symptomatic oral candidiasis may need to soak their dentures nightly in reconstituted nystatin for oral suspension to eliminate *Candida* species from the dentures. In rare cases when this does not eliminate the fungus, it may be necessary to have new dentures made.

**Medical considerations/Contraindications**

The medical considerations/contraindications included have been selected on the basis of their potential clinical significance (reasons given in parentheses where appropriate)—not necessarily inclusive (» = major clinical significance).

*Risk-benefit should be considered when the following medical problem exists:*

Intolerance to nystatin

## Side/Adverse Effects

The following side/adverse effects have been selected on the basis of their potential clinical significance (possible signs and symptoms in parentheses where appropriate)—not necessarily inclusive:

**Those indicating need for medical attention only if they continue or are bothersome**

Incidence less frequent

*Gastrointestinal disturbances* (diarrhea; nausea or vomiting; stomach pain)

## Patient Consultation

As an aid to patient consultation, refer to *Advice for the Patient, Nystatin (Oral)*.

In providing consultation, consider emphasizing the following selected information (» = major clinical significance):

### Before using this medication
» Conditions affecting use, especially:
   Intolerance to nystatin
   Use in children—Nystatin lozenges or tablets are not recommended in infants and children up to 5 years of age since this age group may not be capable of using the lozenges or tablets safely

### Proper use of this medication
Proper administration technique for dry powder, lozenges, and oral suspension
» Compliance with full course of therapy
» Proper dosing
   Missed dose: Taking as soon as possible; not taking if almost time for next dose; not doubling doses
» Proper storage

### Side/adverse effects
Signs of potential side effects, especially gastrointestinal disturbance

## General Dosing Information

The oral suspension should be administered by placing ½ of the dose in each side of the mouth. The patient should hold the suspension in the mouth or swish it throughout the mouth for as long as possible, then gargle and swallow.

Lozenges (pastilles) should be allowed to dissolve slowly and completely in the mouth. They should not be chewed or swallowed whole.

To prevent relapse, therapy should be continued for 48 hours after symptoms have disappeared and the cultures have returned to normal.

## Oral Dosage Forms

### NYSTATIN LOZENGES (PASTILLES)

**Usual adult and adolescent dose**
Candidiasis—
   Oral, as a lozenge dissolved slowly and completely in the mouth, 200,000 to 400,000 Units four or five times a day for up to fourteen days.

**Usual pediatric dose**
Candidiasis—
   Infants and children up to 5 years of age: Use is not recommended since this age group may not be capable of using the lozenges safely.
   Children 5 years of age and over: See *Usual adult and adolescent dose*.

**Strength(s) usually available**
U.S.—
   200,000 Units (Rx) [*Mycostatin*].
Canada—
   Not commercially available.

**Packaging and storage**
Store between 2 and 8 °C (36 and 46 °F), in a well-closed container, unless otherwise specified by manufacturer.

**Auxiliary labeling**
- Refrigerate.
- Dissolve slowly in mouth.
- Continue medicine for full time of treatment.

### NYSTATIN ORAL SUSPENSION USP

**Usual adult and adolescent dose**
Candidiasis—
   Oral, 400,000 to 600,000 Units four times a day.

**Usual pediatric dose**
Candidiasis—
   Premature and low-birth-weight infants: Oral, 100,000 Units four times a day.
   Older infants: Oral, 200,000 Units four times a day.
   Children: See *Usual adult and adolescent dose*.

**Strength(s) usually available**
U.S.—
   100,000 Units per mL (Rx) [*Mycostatin; Nilstat; Nystex;* GENERIC].
Canada—
   100,000 Units per mL (Rx) [*Mycostatin; Nadostine; Nilstat; PMS Nystatin*].

**Packaging and storage**
Store below 40 °C (104 °F), preferably between 15 and 30 °C (59 and 86 °F), unless otherwise specified by manufacturer. Store in a tight, light-resistant container. Protect from freezing.

**Auxiliary labeling**
- Shake well.
- Continue medicine for full time of treatment.

**Note**
When dispensing, include a calibrated liquid-measuring device.

### NYSTATIN FOR ORAL SUSPENSION USP

**Usual adult and adolescent dose**
See *Nystatin Oral Suspension USP*.

**Usual pediatric dose**
See *Nystatin Oral Suspension USP*.

**Size(s) usually available**
U.S.—
   50,000,000 Units (Rx) [GENERIC].
   150,000,000 Units (Rx) [GENERIC].
   500,000,000 Units (Rx) [GENERIC].
   1,000,000,000 Units (Rx) [*Nilstat;* GENERIC].
   2,000,000,000 Units (Rx) [*Nilstat;* GENERIC].
   5,000,000,000 Units (Rx) [GENERIC].
   10,000,000,000 Units (Rx) [GENERIC].
Canada—
   1,000,000,000 Units (Rx) [*Nilstat*].
   2,000,000,000 Units (Rx) [*Nilstat*].

Note: One-eighth (⅛) teaspoonful of nystatin for oral suspension is approximately equal to 500,000 units.

**Packaging and storage**
Prior to reconstitution, store below 40 °C (104 °F), preferably between 15 and 30 °C (59 and 86 °F), unless otherwise specified by manufacturer. Store in a tight container.

**Preparation of dosage form**
Add ⅛ teaspoonful (approximately 500,000 Units) of dry powder to approximately 120 mL of water. Stir well.

**Stability**
After mixing, suspension should be used immediately since nystatin for oral suspension contains no preservatives.

**Auxiliary labeling**
- Dissolve in water immediately before taking.
- Continue medicine for full time of treatment.

**Note**
Explain administration technique.

### NYSTATIN TABLETS USP

**Usual adult and adolescent dose**
Candidiasis—
   Oral, 500,000 to 1,000,000 Units three times a day.

**Usual pediatric dose**
Candidiasis—
   Infants and children up to 5 years of age: Use is not recommended since this age group may not be capable of using the tablet safely.
   Children 5 years of age and over: Oral, 500,000 Units four times a day.

**Strength(s) usually available**
U.S.—
   500,000 Units (Rx) [*Mycostatin* (film-coated); *Nilstat* (film-coated); GENERIC].
Canada—
   500,000 Units (Rx) [*Mycostatin* (film-coated); *Nadostine* (film-coated); *Nilstat* (film-coated)].

**Packaging and storage**
Store below 40 °C (104 °F), preferably between 15 and 30 °C (59 and 86 °F), unless otherwise specified by manufacturer. Store in a tight, light-resistant container.

**Auxiliary labeling**
- Continue medicine for full time of treatment.

---

Revised: 01/19/93
Interim revision: 04/14/95

# NYSTATIN Topical

VA CLASSIFICATION (Primary): DE102

Commonly used brand name(s): *Mycostatin; Nadostine; Nilstat; Nyaderm; Nyaderm; Nystex.*

Note: For a listing of dosage forms and brand names by country availability, see *Dosage Forms* section(s).

## Category
Antifungal (topical).

## Indications
Note: Bracketed information in the *Indications* section refers to uses that are not included in U.S. product labeling.

**Accepted**
Candidiasis, cutaneous (treatment) or
Candidiasis, mucocutaneous, chronic (treatment)—Topical nystatin is indicated in the treatment of cutaneous and chronic mucocutaneous candidiasis caused by *Candida (Monilia) albicans* and other *Candida* species.

[Tinea barbae (treatment)] or
[Tinea capitis (treatment)]—Topical nystatin is used in the treatment of tinea barbae and tinea capitis.

Not all species or strains of a particular organism may be susceptible to nystatin.

## Pharmacology/Pharmacokinetics

**Mechanism of action/Effect**
Topical nystatin binds to sterols in the fungal cell membrane, resulting in the cell membrane's inability to function as a selective barrier, allowing loss of essential cellular constituents.

**Absorption**
Not absorbed following topical application to intact skin or mucous membranes.

## Precautions to Consider

**Pregnancy/Reproduction**
Pregnancy—Problems in humans have not been documented.

**Breast-feeding**
It is not known whether topically applied nystatin is distributed into breast milk. However, problems in humans have not been documented.

**Pediatrics**
Appropriate studies on the relationship of age to the effects of topical nystatin have not been performed in the pediatric population. However, no pediatrics-specific problems have been documented to date. When this medication is used in the treatment of candidiasis, occlusive dressings (e.g., tight-fitting diaper, plastic pants) should be avoided since they provide conditions that favor growth of yeast and release of its irritating endotoxin.

**Geriatrics**
No information is available on the relationship of age to the effects of topical nystatin in geriatric patients.

**Medical considerations/Contraindications**
The medical considerations/contraindications included have been selected on the basis of their potential clinical significance (reasons given in parentheses where appropriate)—not necessarily inclusive (» = major clinical significance).

*Risk-benefit should be considered when the following medical problem exists:*
Hypersensitivity to nystatin

## Side/Adverse Effects
The following side/adverse effects have been selected on the basis of their potential clinical significance (possible signs and symptoms in parentheses where appropriate)—not necessarily inclusive:

**Those indicating need for medical attention**
*Skin irritation not present before therapy*

## Patient Consultation
As an aid to patient consultation, refer to *Advice for the Patient, Nystatin (Topical).*

In providing consultation, consider emphasizing the following selected information (» = major clinical significance):

**Before using this medication**
» Conditions affecting use, especially:
Hypersensitivity to nystatin

**Proper use of this medication**
Not for ophthalmic use
Applying sufficient medication to cover affected area
Proper administration technique for topical powder
» Not applying occlusive dressing over this medication unless directed to do so by physician; avoiding tight-fitting diapers and plastic pants on diaper area of children
» Compliance with full course of therapy
» Proper dosing
Missed dose: Applying as soon as possible
» Proper storage

**Side/adverse effects**
Signs of potential side effects, especially skin irritation not present before therapy

## General Dosing Information
The cream is usually preferred to the ointment for candidiasis involving intertriginous areas. However, very moist lesions involving intertriginous areas are usually best treated with the topical powder.

For fungal infection of the feet, the powder should be dusted freely on the feet as well as in the shoes and socks.

Symptomatic relief usually occurs within 24 to 72 hours following initiation of therapy.

Therapy for a period of 2 weeks is usually sufficient, but more prolonged treatment may be necessary.

When this medication is used in the treatment of candidiasis, occlusive dressings should be avoided since they provide conditions that favor growth of yeast and release of its irritating endotoxin. An oleaginous ointment, a thin film of polyethylene, a bandage, a tight-fitting diaper, plastic pants, or tape may constitute an occlusive dressing.

## Topical Dosage Forms

### NYSTATIN CREAM USP

**Usual adult and adolescent dose**
Candidiasis—
Topical, to the skin, two or three times a day.

**Usual pediatric dose**
See *Usual adult and adolescent dose*.

**Strength(s) usually available**
U.S.—
100,000 Units per gram (Rx) [*Mycostatin; Nilstat; Nystex;* GENERIC].
Canada—
100,000 Units per gram (OTC) [*Mycostatin; Nadostine; Nilstat; Nyaderm*].

**Packaging and storage**
Store below 40 °C (104 °F), in a collapsible tube, or in other tight container. Protect from freezing.

**Auxiliary labeling**
• For external use only.
• Continue medication for full time of treatment.

### NYSTATIN OINTMENT USP

**Usual adult and adolescent dose**
See *Nystatin Cream USP*.

**Usual pediatric dose**
See *Nystatin Cream USP*.

**Strength(s) usually available**
U.S.—
100,000 Units per gram (Rx) [*Mycostatin; Nilstat; Nystex;* GENERIC].
Canada—
100,000 Units per gram (OTC) [*Mycostatin; Nadostine; Nilstat; Nyaderm*].

**Packaging and storage**
Store in a well-closed container, preferably between 15 and 30 °C (59 and 86 °F), unless otherwise specified by manufacturer. Protect from freezing.

**Auxiliary labeling**
- For external use only.
- Continue medication for full time of treatment.

### NYSTATIN TOPICAL POWDER USP

**Usual adult and adolescent dose**
See *Nystatin Cream USP*.

**Usual pediatric dose**
See *Nystatin Cream USP*.

**Strength(s) usually available**
U.S.—
    100,000 Units per gram (Rx) [*Mycostatin*].

Canada—
    100,000 Units per gram (OTC) [*Mycostatin*].

**Packaging and storage**
Store in a well-closed container below 40 °C (104 °F), preferably between 15 and 30 °C (59 and 86 °F), unless otherwise specified by manufacturer.

**Auxiliary labeling**
- For external use only.
- Keep container tightly closed.
- Continue medication for full time of treatment.

Revised: 07/25/94

---

# NYSTATIN   Vaginal

VA CLASSIFICATION (Primary): GU302
Commonly used brand name(s): *Mycostatin; Nadostine; Nilstat; Nyaderm*.

Note: For a listing of dosage forms and brand names by country availability, see *Dosage Forms* section(s).

## Category
Antifungal (vaginal).

## Indications
Note: Bracketed information in the *Indications* section refers to uses that are not included in U.S. product labeling.

**Accepted**
Candidiasis, vulvovaginal (treatment)—Vaginal nystatin is indicated in the local treatment of vulvovaginal candidiasis caused by *Candida albicans* and other *Candida* species.

[Candidiasis, oropharyngeal (treatment)]—Nystatin vaginal tablets are used as lozenges to treat oropharyngeal candidiasis since their slow dissolution rate provides prolonged oral contact.

Not all species or strains of a particular organism may be susceptible to nystatin.

**Unaccepted**
Nystatin is not effective against *Trichomonas vaginalis* or *Gardnerella vaginalis (Haemophilus vaginalis)*.

## Pharmacology/Pharmacokinetics

**Physicochemical characteristics**
Source—Derived from *Streptomyces noursei*.
Chemical group—Polyene antifungal.

**Mechanism of action/Effect**
Binds to sterols in the fungal cell membrane, resulting in the cell membrane's inability to function as a selective barrier, which allows loss of essential cellular constituents.

## Precautions to Consider

**Carcinogenicity/Mutagenicity**
Long-term studies in animals have not been done to evaluate the carcinogenic or mutagenic potential of nystatin.

**Pregnancy/Reproduction**
Fertility—Long-term studies in animals have not been done to evaluate the effect of nystatin on fertility in females.

Pregnancy—Studies in animals have not been done. However, studies in humans have not shown that nystatin causes adverse effects on the fetus.

FDA Pregnancy Category A.

**Breast-feeding**
It is not known whether vaginal nystatin is distributed into breast milk. However, problems in humans have not been documented.

**Pediatrics**
No information is available on the relationship of age to the effects of vaginal nystatin in pediatric patients.

**Geriatrics**
No information is available on the relationship of age to the effects of vaginal nystatin in geriatric patients.

**Medical considerations/Contraindications**
The medical considerations/contraindications included have been selected on the basis of their potential clinical significance (reasons given in parentheses where appropriate)—not necessarily inclusive (» = major clinical significance).

*Risk-benefit should be considered when the following medical problem exists:*
Sensitivity to nystatin

## Side/Adverse Effects
The following side/adverse effects have been selected on the basis of their potential clinical significance (possible signs and symptoms in parentheses where appropriate)—not necessarily inclusive:

**Those indicating need for medical attention**
Incidence rare
    *Vaginal irritation not present before therapy* (vaginal burning or itching)

## Patient Consultation
As an aid to patient consultation, refer to *Advice for the Patient, Nystatin (Vaginal)*.

In providing consultation, consider emphasizing the following selected information (» = major clinical significance):

**Before using this medication**
» Conditions affecting use, especially:
    Sensitivity to nystatin

**Proper use of this medication**
Reading patient instructions before using medication
Using applicator cautiously during pregnancy
Using medication during menstual periods if they start during treatment period
» Compliance with full course of therapy
» Proper dosing
    Missed dose: Inserting as soon as possible; not inserting if almost time for next dose
» Proper storage

**Precautions while using this medication**
» Using hygienic measures to control sources of infection or reinfection
Checking with physician about douching or intercourse during therapy
Protection of clothing because of possible vaginal drainage

**Side/adverse effects**
Signs of potential side effects, especially vaginal irritation not present before therapy

## General Dosing Information
Therapy for a period of 2 weeks is usually sufficient, but more prolonged treatment may be necessary. Treatment of resistent infections may be supplemented with oral products.

To prevent thrush in the newborn, it is suggested that nystatin vaginal tablets be administered to pregnant patients with vulvovaginal candidiasis in a dosage of 100,000 to 200,000 Units daily for 3 to 6 weeks prior to delivery.

## Vaginal Dosage Forms

### NYSTATIN VAGINAL CREAM

**Usual adult and adolescent dose**
Antifungal—
    Intravaginal, 1 (100,000-Unit) applicatorful one or two times a day for two weeks; or 1 (500,000-Unit) applicatorful once daily.

**2150   Nystatin (Vaginal)**

Note: For severe infections, the dose of 500,000-Units of vaginal cream may be increased to every 12 hours.

**Usual pediatric dose**
Dosage has not been established.

**Strength(s) usually available**
U.S.—
  Not commercially available.
Canada—
  25,000 Units per gram (100,000 Units per applicatorful) (Rx) [*Mycostatin; Nadostine; Nyaderm*].
  100,000 Units per gram (500,000 Units per applicatorful) (Rx) [*Nilstat*].

**Packaging and storage**
Store below 40 °C (104 °F), preferably between 15 and 30 °C (59 and 86 °F), unless otherwise specified by manufacturer. Store in a tight, light-resistant container.

**Auxiliary labeling**
• Continue medicine for full time of treatment.
• For vaginal use only.

**Note**
Include patient instructions when dispensing.
Explain administration technique.

## NYSTATIN VAGINAL TABLETS USP

**Usual adult and adolescent dose**
Antifungal—
  Intravaginal, 100,000 Units one or two times a day for two weeks.

**Usual pediatric dose**
Dosage has not been established.

**Strength(s) usually available**
U.S.—
  100,000 Units (Rx) [GENERIC].
Canada—
  100,000 Units (Rx) [*Mycostatin; Nadostine; Nilstat*].

**Packaging and storage**
Store below 40 °C (104 °F), preferably between 15 and 30 °C (59 and 86 °F), unless otherwise specified by manufacturer. Store in a tight, light-resistant container.

Note: Some manufacturers recommend storage in a refrigerator.

**Auxiliary labeling**
• Continue medicine for full time of treatment.
• For vaginal use only.
• Refrigerate.

**Note**
Include patient instructions when dispensing.
Explain administration technique (for use as oral lozenge).

Revised: 08/11/98

# NYSTATIN AND TRIAMCINOLONE   Topical

**VA CLASSIFICATION (Primary):** DE250

**NOTE:** The *Nystatin and Triamcinolone (Topical)* monograph is maintained on the USP DI electronic data base. For a printed copy of the most recent revision of the complete monograph, contact Micromedex, Inc. - Reprint Requests, 6200 S. Syracuse Way, Suite 300, Englewood, CO 80111; telephone (303) 486-6400; telefax (303) 486-6464; Email: USPDI@MDX.COM.

For information on the specific components of this combination, see the *USP DI* monographs for *Corticosteroids (Topical)* and *Nystatin (Topical)*.

The information that follows is selectively abstracted from the complete monograph and is provided to facilitate drug use review and patient counseling.

Note: For a listing of dosage forms and brand names by country availability, see *Dosage Forms* section(s).

## Category
Antifungal-corticosteroid (topical).

## Indications
Note: Bracketed information in the *Indications* section refers to uses that are not included in U.S. product labeling.

**Accepted**
Candidiasis, cutaneous (treatment)—Nystatin and triamcinolone combination is indicated as a secondary agent in the topical treatment of cutaneous candidiasis, [accompanied by inflammation], caused by *Candida albicans (Monilia albicans)* and other *Candida* species.

The use of nystatin and triamcinolone combination has been shown to provide greater benefit than nystatin alone during the first few days of treatment [or for as long as inflammation persists. After this time, USP medical experts recommend the use of plain nystatin or other topical antifungal agents. Also, nystatin and triamcinolone combination is recommended only for short-term (less than 2 weeks) treatment of inflammatory candidiasis confined to limited areas of the skin].

Not all species or strains of a particular organism may be susceptible to nystatin.

**Unaccepted**
Nystatin and triamcinolone combination is not recommended in the treatment of mucocutaneous candidiasis. In addition, nystatin is not effective against bacteria, protozoa, trichomonads, or viruses.

## Patient Consultation
As an aid to patient consultation, refer to *Advice for the Patient, Nystatin and Triamcinolone (Topical)*.

In providing consultation, consider emphasizing the following selected information (» = major clinical significance):

**Before using this medication**
» Conditions affecting use, especially:
  Sensitivity to nystatin or corticosteroids
  Pregnancy—Topical corticosteroids may be systemically absorbed; potent corticosteroids have been shown to be teratogenic in animals following topical application
  Breast-feeding—Systemic corticosteroids are distributed into breast-milk and may cause growth suppression in the infant; topical corticosteroids may be systemically absorbed
  Use in children—Children may absorb a proportionately larger amount of topical corticosteroid than adults, making them more susceptible to HPA axis suppression and Cushing's syndrome
  Other medical problems, especially Herpes simplex; tubercular infections of the skin; vaccinia, eczema vaccinatum, varicella, or other viral infections of the skin

**Proper use of this medication**
» Not for ophthalmic use
» Checking with physician before using medication on other skin problems
  Applying a thin layer of medication to affected area and rubbing in gently and thoroughly
» Not applying occlusive dressing over this medication unless directed to do so by physician; wearing loose-fitting clothing when using on inguinal area; avoiding tight-fitting diapers and plastic pants on diaper area of children
» Compliance with full course of therapy; not using more often or longer than directed by physician; excessive use on thin skin areas may result in skin atrophy and stretch marks
» Proper dosing
  Missed dose: Applying as soon as possible; not applying if almost time for next dose
» Proper storage

**Precautions while using this medication**
» Using hygienic measures to cure infection or prevent reinfection; keeping affected area as cool and dry as possible
  Checking with physician if no improvement within 2 or 3 weeks
» May be more likely to cause systemic toxicity in children; chronic use may interfere with growth and development also; having children closely monitored by their physician
» Diabetics: May rarely cause hyperglycemia and glucosuria; checking with physician before changing diet or dosage of antidiabetic medication

### Side/adverse effects
Side effects more likely to occur in children
Signs of potential side effects, especially hypersensitivity; acne or oily skin; increased hair growth especially on the face; increased loss of hair, especially on the scalp; reddish purple lines on arms, face, legs, trunk, or groins; skin atrophy

## Topical Dosage Forms

### NYSTATIN AND TRIAMCINOLONE ACETONIDE CREAM USP

**Usual adult and adolescent dose**
Antifungal—
Topical, to the skin, two times a day, morning and evening.

**Usual pediatric dose**
See *Usual adult and adolescent dose*.

**Strength(s) usually available**
U.S.—
100,000 Units of nystatin and 1 mg of triamcinolone acetonide per gram [*Dermacomb; Myco II; Mycobiotic II; Mycogen II; Mycolog II; Myco-Triacet II; Mykacet II; Mytrex; Tristatin II;* GENERIC].
Canada—
Not commercially available.

**Auxiliary labeling**
• For external use only.
• Continue medication for full time of treatment.
• Do not use in or around the eyes.

### NYSTATIN AND TRIAMCINOLONE ACETONIDE OINTMENT USP

**Usual adult and adolescent dose**
Antifungal—
Topical, to the skin, two or three times a day.

**Usual pediatric dose**
See *Usual adult and adolescent dose*.

**Strength(s) usually available**
U.S.—
100,000 Units of nystatin and 1 mg of triamcinolone acetonide per gram [*Myco II; Mycobiotic II; Mycogen II; Mycolog II; Myco-Triacet II; Mykacet; Mytrex; Tristatin II;* GENERIC].
Canada—
Not commercially available.

**Auxiliary labeling**
• For external use only.
• Continue medication for full time of treatment.
• Do not use in or around the eyes.

Revised: 08/15/94

# OCTREOTIDE Systemic

VA CLASSIFICATION (Primary/Secondary): GA250/CV900; HS900
Commonly used brand name(s): *Sandostatin*.

Note: For a listing of dosage forms and brand names by country availability, see *Dosage Forms* section(s).

## Category

Antidiarrheal (gastrointestinal tumor; acquired immune deficiency syndrome [AIDS]); antihypotensive (carcinoid crisis); growth hormone suppressant (acromegaly); antihypoglycemic (pancreatic tumor).

## Indications

Note: Bracketed information in the *Indications* section refers to uses that are not included in U.S. product labeling.

**Accepted**

Tumors, gastrointestinal (treatment adjunct)—Octreotide is indicated for palliative management of gastrointestinal endocrine tumors, such as:
Carcinoid tumors—To suppress or inhibit the associated severe diarrhea and facial flushing episodes.
Vasoactive intestinal peptide tumors (VIPomas)—For the treatment of the profuse watery diarrhea associated with vasoactive intestinal peptide (VIP)–secreting tumors.

[Hypotension (treatment)][1]—Octreotide is used to reverse life-threatening hypotension due to carcinoid crisis during induction of anesthesia.

Acromegaly (treatment)[1]—Octreotide is used to decrease secretion of growth hormone from pituitary tumors and decrease blood concentrations of insulin-like growth factor-I (IGF-I or somatomedin-C) in patients with acromegaly who have not optimally responded to or cannot be treated with surgical resection or pituitary irradiation, or have been unable to tolerate bromocriptine. Octreotide may be used as adjunctive therapy with irradiation treatment to help relieve symptoms of acromegaly and possibly suppress the rate of tumor growth.

[Tumors, pancreatic (treatment adjunct)][1]—Octreotide is used as palliative treatment of the symptoms resulting from hyperinsulinemia from severe refractory metastatic insulinoma.

[Diarrhea, AIDS-associated (treatment)][1]—Octreotide is used in AIDS patients with severe secretory diarrhea who have failed to respond to antimicrobial or antimotility agents.

[1] Not included in Canadian product labeling.

## Pharmacology/Pharmacokinetics

**Physicochemical characteristics**
Molecular weight—1019.26.

**Mechanism of action/Effect**
Action similar to naturally occurring somatostatin, but with a prolonged duration of action. Like the naturally occurring hormone, octreotide suppresses secretion of serotonin and the gastroenteropancreatic peptides. Stimulates fluid and electrolyte absorption from the gastrointestinal tract, and prolongs intestinal transit time. It blocks the carcinoid flush, decreases circulating levels of serotonin metabolite 5-hydroxyindoleacetic acid (5-HIAA), and controls other symptoms associated with the carcinoid syndrome.

**Other actions/effects**
Suppresses growth hormone, insulin, and glucagon. Decreases splanchnic blood flow. Inhibits gallbladder contractions. Slows gastrointestinal transit time.

**Absorption**
Absorbed rapidly and completely from injection site.

**Protein binding**
High (65%, to lipoproteins and to a lesser extent to albumin).

**Half-life**
Elimination—1.5 hours.

**Time to peak concentration**
≤0.5 hours.

**Peak serum concentration**
5.5 nanograms/mL (with 100-mcg dose).

**Duration of action**
Up to 12 hours (depending on type of tumor).

**Elimination**
Renal (32% of dose).

## Precautions to Consider

**Carcinogenicity/Mutagenicity**
No long-term studies to assess carcinogenic potential of octreotide have been completed in animals or humans. Studies in animals have demonstrated no mutagenic potential.

**Pregnancy/Reproduction**
Pregnancy—Appropriate studies in humans have not been performed. Studies in rats and rabbits at doses up to 30 times the maximum human dose have not shown that octreotide causes adverse effects on the fetus.
FDA Pregnancy Category B.

**Breast-feeding**
It is not known whether octreotide is distributed into breast milk. However, problems in humans have not been documented.

**Pediatrics**
Appropriate studies with octreotide have not been performed in the pediatric population. However, doses of 1 to 10 mcg per kg of body weight, given to children as young as 1 month old, were well tolerated. One case in which an infant (a case of nesidioblastosis) suffered a seizure while undergoing octreotide therapy was thought to be unrelated to octreotide administration.

**Geriatrics**
Studies performed to date in patients as old as 83 years of age have not demonstrated geriatrics-specific problems that would limit the usefulness of this medication in the elderly.

**Drug interactions and/or related problems**
The following drug interactions and/or related problems have been selected on the basis of their potential clinical significance (possible mechanism in parentheses where appropriate)—not necessarily inclusive (» = major clinical significance):

Note: Combinations containing any of the following medications, depending on the amount present, may also interact with this medication.

» Antidiabetic agents, sulfonlyurea or
» Glucagon or
» Growth hormone or
» Insulin
(use of these medications during octreotide therapy may result in hypo- or hyperglycemia; patient monitoring and dosage adjustment of these medications may be necessary)

Cyclosporine
(a single case of transplant rejection [renal/whole pancreas] in a patient who was receiving octreotide and who was immunosuppressed with cyclosporine has been reported; the use of octreotide to reduce exocrine secretion and close a fistula in this patient resulted in a decrease in the blood levels of cyclosporine, thus possibly contributing to the rejection episode)

**Laboratory value alterations**
The following have been selected on the basis of their potential clinical significance (possible effect in parentheses where appropriate)—not necessarily inclusive (» = major clinical significance):

With physiology/laboratory test values
Thyroid hormones
(serum concentration of thyroxine [$T_4$] may be decreased; hypothyroidism occurred in 1 clinical trial patient after 19 months of receiving 1.5 mg of octreotide daily)

**Medical considerations/Contraindications**
The medical considerations/contraindications included have been selected on the basis of their potential clinical significance (reasons given in parentheses where appropriate)—not necessarily inclusive (» = major clinical significance):

*Risk-benefit should be considered when the following medical problems exist:*

Diabetes mellitus
(therapy used to control glycemic states may need to be adjusted)
» Gallbladder disease or gallstones, or history of
(increased risk of cholelithiasis possibly due to alteration of fat absorption and decrease in gallbladder motility caused by octreotide)
Renal function impairment, severe
(half-life of octreotide may be increased; dosage adjustment may be necessary)
Sensitivity to octreotide

## Patient monitoring

The following may be especially important in patient monitoring (other tests may be warranted in some patients, depending on condition; » = major clinical significance):

Carotene, serum concentrations and
Fat content, fecal
(octreotide therapy may alter absorption of dietary fats; periodic 72-hour fecal fat and serum carotene determinations are recommended to assess possible aggravation of fat malabsorption)

Glucose
(measurement of blood concentrations is recommended at beginning of octreotide therapy and at each change of dosage if clinical signs of increase or decrease occur)

Plasma vasoactive intestinal peptide (VIP)
(determinations recommended periodically during therapy of patients with VIPomas to assess patient response)

Thyroid function determinations
(baseline and periodic thyroid function tests using total and free serum thyroxine [$T_4$] are recommended during chronic therapy)

» Ultrasonograms
(therapy with octreotide, like the natural hormone somatostatin, may be associated with cholelithiasis presumably due to an alteration of fat absorption and possibly to a decrease in the motility of the gallbladder; baseline and periodic ultrasonograms may be required to assess the presence of gallstones)

» Urinary 5-hydroxyindoleacetic acid (5-HIAA) and
Plasma substance P
(determinations recommended periodically during therapy of patients with carcinoid tumors to assess patient response)

## Side/Adverse Effects

Note: Isolated reports of hepatic dysfunctions associated with octreotide administration include acute hepatitis without cholestasis, slow development of hyperbilirubinemia, and gallstone formation.
The risk of cholelithiasis increases with long-term therapy, as is usually required in the treatment of acromegaly.

The following side/adverse effects have been selected on the basis of their potential clinical significance (possible signs and symptoms in parentheses where appropriate)—not necessarily inclusive:

### Those indicating need for medical attention
Incidence less frequent or rare
**Hyperglycemia** (drowsiness; dry mouth; flushed, dry skin; fruit-like breath odor; increased urination; loss of appetite; rapid weight loss; stomachache, nausea, or vomiting; trouble in breathing; unusual thirst; unusual tiredness); **hypoglycemia** (anxious feeling; chills; cool, pale skin; difficulty in concentrating; headache; hunger; nausea; nervousness; shakiness; sweating; unconsciousness; unusual tiredness; weakness)

Note: Octreotide therapy is occasionally associated with mild transient *hypo-* or *hyperglycemia* due to alteration in the balance between the counter regulatory hormones, insulin, glucagon, and growth hormone.

### Those indicating need for medical attention only if they continue or are bothersome
Incidence more frequent (3 to 10%)
*Gastrointestinal symptoms* (abdominal or stomach pain or discomfort; diarrhea; nausea and vomiting); *pain, stinging, tingling, or burning sensation at injection site, with redness and swelling*

Note: *Gastrointestinal symptoms* are usually self-limiting and usually are resolved after 2 to 3 weeks of therapy.

Incidence less frequent or rare (1 to 3%)
*Dizziness or lightheadedness; edema* (swelling of feet or lower legs); *fatigue; headache; redness or flushing of face; unusual weakness*

## Overdose

For more information on the management of overdose or unintentional ingestion, **contact a Poison Control Center** (see *Poison Control Center Listing*).

### Clinical effects of overdose
Although octreotide overdosage in humans has not been reported, based on the pharmacological properties of octreotide, acute overdosage may be expected to produce hyper- or hypoglycemia depending on the endocrine status of the patient and the type of tumor involved. Temporary withdrawal of octreotide and symptomatic treatment should alleviate this condition.

### Treatment of overdose
Supportive care—Recommended treatment consists of temporary withdrawal of octreotide and symptomatic treatment of hyper- or hypoglycemia.

## Patient Consultation

As an aid to patient consultation, refer to *Advice for the Patient, Octreotide (Systemic)*.
In providing consultation, consider emphasizing the following selected information (» = major clinical significance):

### Before using this medication
» Conditions affecting use, especially:
Sensitivity to octreotide
Other medications, especially oral antidiabetics, glucagon, growth hormone, insulin
Other medical problems, especially diabetes, severe renal function impairment, or gallbladder disease or gallstones

### Proper use of this medication
» Using medication only as directed by physician; taking in evenly spaced doses as ordered
» Reading directions in starter kit before using
» Proper dosing
Missed dose: Using as soon as possible unless almost time for next dose, then going back to regular dosing schedule; not doubling doses
» Proper storage

### Precautions while using this medication
» Importance of close monitoring by physician
» Carefully selecting and rotating injection sites

### Side/adverse effects
Signs of potential side effects, especially hyperglycemia or hypoglycemia

## General Dosing Information

Preferred sites for subcutaneous injection of octreotide are the hip, thigh, or abdomen.

Multiple injections at the same injection site within short periods of time are not recommended. This is to avoid irritating the area.

To avoid the occurrence of gastrointestinal side effects, injections of octreotide should be scheduled between meals and at bedtime.

Local reactions at injection site may be reduced by allowing the solution to reach room temperature before injection and by administering slowly.

## Parenteral Dosage Forms

Note: Bracketed uses in the *Dosage Forms* section refer to categories of use and/or indications that are not included in U.S. product labeling.

### OCTREOTIDE ACETATE INJECTION

**Usual adult and adolescent dose**
Antidiarrheal (gastrointestinal tumor)—
Subcutaneous, 50 mcg (0.05 mg) initially, administered one or two times a day, the dose being increased gradually according to patient tolerance and response. The following dosages are recommended for specific tumors:
Carcinoid tumors—Subcutaneous, 100 to 600 mcg (0.1 to 0.6 mg) per day, administered in two to four divided doses, for the first two weeks of therapy.
Vasoactive intestinal peptide tumors (VIPomas)—Subcutaneous, 200 to 300 mcg (0.2 to 0.3 mg) per day, administered in two to four divided doses, for the first two weeks of therapy.
[Antidiarrheal (AIDS)][1]—
Subcutaneous, 100 to 1800 mcg (0.1 to 1.8 mg) per day.
Growth hormone suppressant (acromegaly)[1]—
Subcutaneous or intravenous, initially 50 mcg (0.05 mg) injected two or three times a day. Dosage is titrated every two weeks as needed, according to IGF-I blood concentrations, to reach a dose of 100 mcg (0.1 mg) three times a day; or, for rapid titration, dosage increase may be based on multiple serum growth hormone concentrations taken at one- to four-hour intervals over eight to twelve hours. Doses up to 500 mcg (0.5 mg) three times a day have been used rarely.

Note: Octreotide injection may be administered subcutaneously (the preferred route) or intravenously. To help prevent pain at the injection site, octreotide should be given in the smallest volume needed to achieve the proper dose. In emergencies, intravenous injections may be used cautiously.

## Octreotide (Systemic)

[Antihypoglycemic (pancreatic tumor)][1]—
Subcutaneous, 50 to 150 mcg (0.05 to 0.15 mg) initially, administered two times a day thirty minutes before meals, the dose being increased gradually according to patient tolerance and response.

**Usual adult prescribing limits**
Up to 750 mcg (0.75 mg) daily.

**Usual pediatric dose**
Subcutaneous, 1 to 10 mcg (0.001 to 0.01 mg) per kg of body weight per day.

**Usual geriatric dose**
See *Usual adult and adolescent dose*.

**Strength(s) usually available**
U.S.—
  0.05 mg per mL (Rx) [*Sandostatin*].
  0.1 mg per mL (Rx) [*Sandostatin*].
  0.2 mg per mL (Rx) [*Sandostatin*].
  0.5 mg per mL (Rx) [*Sandostatin*].
  1 mg per mL (Rx) [*Sandostatin*].
Note: 0.05 mg per mL, 0.1 mg per mL, and 0.5 mg per mL are packaged as single-use ampules; the remaining strengths are packaged as multiple-dose vials.
Canada—
  0.05 mg per mL (Rx) [*Sandostatin*].
  0.1 mg per mL (Rx) [*Sandostatin*].
  0.5 mg per mL (Rx) [*Sandostatin*].

**Packaging and storage**
Store at 2 to 8 °C (36 to 46 °F), unless otherwise specified by manufacturer. Protect from freezing. Protect from light.

Note: Solution should be allowed to warm to room temperature before administration. Do not warm artificially before injection. Single-use ampules should be opened just prior to use and any unused portion discarded.

**Preparation of dosage form**
Octreotide is stable when diluted for intravenous use when diluted in 50 to 200 mL of either sterile 0.9% sodium chloride injection or 5% dextrose in sterile water for injection. The diluted solution can be infused intravenously and administered over a 15- to 30-minute period or administered via a direct intravenous injection over a 3-minute period. In emergencies, rapid intravenous injections may be used cautiously.

**Stability**
If protected from light, octreotide injection is stable at room temperature, preferably between 15 and 30 °C (59 and 86 °F), for 14 days. Octreotide should not be used if discolored or if particulate matter forms in solution.

**Incompatibilities**
Octreotide is not compatible with total parenteral nutrition (TPN) solutions; decreased efficacy may result if glycosyl octreotide conjugates form.

**Auxiliary labeling**
• Refrigerate.

**Note**
Subcutaneous injection sites should be rotated.

[1]Not included in Canadian product labeling.

### Selected Bibliography
Lamberts SW. A guide to the clinical use of the somatostatin analogue SMS 201-995 (Sandostatin). Acta Endrocrinol Suppl 1987; 286: 54-66.
O'Donnell LJ, Farthing MJ. Therapeutic potential of a long-acting somatostatin analogue in gastrointestinal diseases. Gut 1989; 30(9): 1165-72.

Revised: 12/15/92
Interim revision: 06/30/94; 08/08/95

---

**OFLOXACIN**—See *Fluoroquinolones (Systemic)*; *Ofloxacin (Ophthalmic)*.

---

**OFLOXACIN**—The *Ofloxacin (Ophthalmic)* monograph is not included in this published version of the USP DI database. Copies of the monograph are available on request from Micromedex, Inc. - Reprint Requests, 6200 S. Syracuse Way, Suite 300, Englewood, CO 80111; telephone (303) 486-6400; telefax (303) 486-6464; Email: USPDI@MDX.COM.

---

# OFLOXACIN  Otic—INTRODUCTORY VERSION

VA CLASSIFICATION (Primary): OT101
Commonly used brand name(s): *Floxin Otic*.
Note: For a listing of dosage forms and brand names by country availability, see *Dosage Forms* section(s).

## Category
Antibacterial (otic).

## Indications
**Accepted**
Otitis externa (treatment)
Otitis media, acute (treatment) or
Otitis media, chronic suppurative (treatment)—Otic ofloxacin is indicated for the treatment of otitis externa (in adults and children 1 year of age and older) caused by *Staphylococcus aureus* and *Pseudomonas aeruginosa*. In addition, otic ofloxacin is indicated for treatment of acute otitis media (in children 1 to 12 years of age with tympanostomy tubes) due to *Staphylococcus aureus*, *Streptococcus pneumoniae*, *Haemophilus influenzae*, *Moraxella catarrhalis*, and *Pseudomonas aeruginosa*. Otic ofloxacin is also indicated for treatment of chronic suppurative otitis media (in adults and children 12 years of age and older with perforated tympanic membranes) due to *Staphylococcus aureus*, *Proteus mirabilis*, and *Pseudomonas aeruginosa*.

## Pharmacology/Pharmacokinetics

**Physicochemical characteristics**
Chemical group—Fluoroquinolone.
Molecular weight—361.38.
pH—6.5.

**Mechanism of action/Effect**
Bactericidal; ofloxacin acts intracellularly by inhibiting DNA gyrase. DNA gyrase is an essential bacterial enzyme that is a critical catalyst in the replication, transcription, deactivation, and repair of bacterial DNA.

**Absorption**
In two single-dose studies in adults with tympanostomy tubes, with and without otorrhea, mean serum ofloxacin concentrations were low after otic administration of a 0.3% ofloxacin solution (4.1 nanograms per mL [n=3] and 5.4 nanograms per mL [n=5], respectively). In a study in adults with perforated tympanic membranes, the maximum serum ofloxacin concentration after otic administration of a 0.3% solution was 10 nanograms per mL. Concentrations of ofloxacin in the middle ear mucosa of adult patients with perforated tympanic membranes (detectable in 11 of 16 subjects) varied widely, ranging from 1.2 to 602 micrograms per gram after otic administration of a 0.3% solution. Concentrations of ofloxacin in otorrhea were found to be high (389 to 2850 micrograms per gram) 30 minutes after otic administration of a 0.3% solution to 13 subjects with chronic suppurative otitis media and perforated tympanic membranes; however, this measurement does not necessarily reflect the exposure of the middle ear to ofloxacin.

## Precautions to Consider

**Cross-sensitivity and/or related problems**
Patients sensitive to systemic ofloxacin or to other quinolones or their derivatives may be sensitive to otic ofloxacin also.

**Carcinogenicity**
Long-term studies have not been done.

**Mutagenicity**
Ofloxacin was not found to be mutagenic in the Ames test, the sister chromatid exchange assay (Chinese hamster and human cell lines), the unscheduled DNA synthesis (UDS) assay using human fibroblasts, the dominant lethal assay, or the mouse micronucleus assay. However, of-

loxacin was positive in the rat hepatocyte UDS assay and in the mouse lymphoma assay.

**Pregnancy/Reproduction**
Fertility—Studies in male and female rats administered oral doses of ofloxacin of up to 360 mg per kg of body weight (mg/kg) per day (over 1000 times the maximum recommended clinical dose in humans, based on body surface area, assuming total absorption from the ear of a patient treated with ofloxacin otic solution twice a day) found no effect on reproductive performance.

Pregnancy—Adequate and well-controlled studies in humans have not been done.

Studies in rats and rabbits administered oral doses of ofloxacin of 810 mg/kg per day and 160 mg/kg per day, respectively, found an embryocidal effect. These doses produced decreased fetal body weights and increased fetal mortality in rats and rabbits, respectively. Minor fetal skeletal variations were reported in rats administered oral doses of ofloxacin of 810 mg/kg per day. No teratogenic effects have been shown in pregnant rats and rabbits administered oral doses of ofloxacin as high as 810 mg/kg per day and 160 mg/kg per day, respectively. No adverse effects on the developing embryo or fetus have been found at doses relevant to the amount of ofloxacin that would be delivered topically to the ear at the recommended clinical doses. In addition, studies in rats administered oral doses of ofloxacin of up to 360 mg/kg per day during late gestation found no adverse effects on late fetal development, labor, delivery, lactation, neonatal viability, or growth of the newborn.

It is recommended that risk-benefit be considered before use of ofloxacin otic solution in pregnant women.

FDA Pregnancy Category C.

**Breast-feeding**
It is not known whether ofloxacin is distributed into human breast milk following topical otic administration. Administration of a single 200-mg oral dose in nursing women has been shown to produce an ofloxacin concentration in breast milk similar to that in plasma. Because of the potential for serious adverse reactions from ofloxacin in nursing infants, risk-benefit should be considered before making a decision about either continuing nursing or using the medication.

**Pediatrics**
A study of audiometric parameters in 30 pediatric patients treated with otic ofloxacin found no changes in hearing function. Safety and efficacy in children 1 year of age and older have been demonstrated. However, safety and efficacy in children younger than 1 year of age have not been established.

Although systemically administered quinolones, including ofloxacin, have been shown to cause arthropathy in immature animals, a study in which 0.3% ofloxacin otic solution was administered in the middle ear of young growing guinea pigs for 1 month found no systemic effects, quinolone-induced lesions, erosions of the cartilage in weight-bearing joints, or other signs of arthropathy.

**Geriatrics**
No information is available on the relationship of age to the effects of otic ofloxacin in geriatric patients.

**Medical considerations/Contraindications**
The medical considerations/contraindications included have been selected on the basis of their potential clinical significance (reasons given in parentheses where appropriate)—not necessarily inclusive (» = major clinical significance).

*Except under special circumstances, this medication should not be used when the following medical problem exists:*
» Sensitivity to ofloxacin or other quinolones or their derivatives (serious and occasionally fatal hypersensitivity [anaphylactic] reactions have been reported following systemic use of quinolones, including ofloxacin)

## Side/Adverse Effects

Note: Systemic administration of quinolones, including ofloxacin, at doses much higher than those given or absorbed by the otic route, has resulted in lesions or erosions of the cartilage in weight-bearing joints and other signs of arthropathy in immature animals of various species. However, a study in which 0.3% ofloxacin otic solution was administered in the middle ear of young growing guinea pigs for 1 month found no systemic effects, quinolone-induced lesions, erosions of the cartilage in weight-bearing joints, or other signs of arthropathy.

Serious and occasionally fatal hypersensitivity (anaphylactic) reactions have been reported with systemic administration of ofloxacin and other quinolones, some following the first dose. In some cases, the reactions were accompanied by cardiovascular collapse, loss of consciousness, angioedema (including laryngeal, pharyngeal, or facial edema), airway obstruction, dyspnea, urticaria, and itching. If an allergic reaction to otic ofloxacin is suspected, it is recommended that the medication be stopped.

The following side/adverse effects have been selected on the basis of their potential clinical significance (possible signs and symptoms in parentheses where appropriate)—not necessarily inclusive:

**Those indicating need for medical attention**
Incidence less frequent
*Application site reaction* (burning, itching, redness, skin rash, swelling, or other sign of irritation not present before use of this medicine); *dizziness or vertigo*
Incidence rare
*Fever; headache; otorrhagia* (bleeding from the ear); *pharyngitis* (sore throat); *rhinitis or sinusitis* (runny or stuffy nose); *tachycardia* (fast heartbeat); *tinnitus* (ringing in the ear)

**Those indicating need for medical attention only if they continue or are bothersome**
Incidence less frequent
*Change in taste; earache; numbness or tingling*

## Patient Consultation

As an aid to patient consultation, refer to *Advice for the Patient, Ofloxacin (Otic)—Introductory Version.*

In providing consultation, consider emphasizing the following selected information (» = major clinical significance):

**Before using this medication**
» Conditions affecting use, especially:
  Sensitivity to ofloxacin or other quinolones or their derivatives
  Pregnancy—Studies with otic ofloxacin have not been done; because of the embryocidal and fetotoxic effects of large systemic doses in animals, risk-benefit should be considered before using during pregnancy; however, ofloxacin has not been shown to cause problems when given in doses comparable to doses administered by the otic route
  Breast-feeding—It is not known whether otic ofloxacin is distributed into breast milk; however, oral ofloxacin is distributed into breast milk
  Use in children—Safety and efficacy have not been established in children up to 1 year of age

**Proper use of this medication**
» Reading patient medication guide before using eardrops; checking with physician if patient has questions
» Proper administration technique; not touching applicator tip to any surface, including the ear, in order to avoid contamination
» Compliance with full course of therapy
» Proper dosing
  Missed dose: Using as soon as possible; not using if almost time for next dose
» Proper storage

**Precautions while using this medication**
Checking with physician if no improvement within a few days
» Discontinuing medication and checking with physician immediately at the first sign of a rash or allergic reaction

**Side/adverse effects**
Signs of potential side effects, especially application site reaction, dizziness or vertigo, fever, headache, otorrhagia, pharyngitis, rhinitis or sinusitis, tachycardia, and tinnitus

## General Dosing Information

It is recommended that the bottle be held in the hand for 1 or 2 minutes before use to warm the solution; this will help prevent the dizziness that may occur following instillation of a cold solution into the ear. The patient should lie with the affected ear up for instillation of the drops and hold this position for 5 minutes after instillation. This procedure may then be repeated for the opposite ear, if necessary.

As with other antiinfectives, prolonged use may lead to overgrowth of nonsusceptible organisms, including fungi. It is recommended that cultures be obtained if the infection has not improved after 1 week, to aid in selection of further treatment.

If otorrhea persists after a full course of therapy, or occurs two or more times during a period of 6 months, it is recommended that further evaluation be undertaken to exclude underlying conditions, such as cholesteatoma, foreign body, or tumor.

Because of the serious anaphylactic reaction that has been reported with systemic ofloxacin, it is recommended that otic ofloxacin be discontinued at the first sign of an allergic reaction. Emergency medical treat-

## Ofloxacin (Otic)—Introductory Version

ment, including oxygen and airway management, including intubation, may be needed for serious acute hypersensitivity reactions.

Ofloxacin otic solution is not for ophthalmic use or for injection.

## Otic Dosage Forms

### OFLOXACIN OTIC SOLUTION

**Usual adult and adolescent dose**
Otitis externa—
  Topical, to the ear canal, 10 drops in the affected ear two times a day for ten days.
Otitis media, chronic suppurative (in patients with perforated tympanic membranes)—
  Topical, to the ear canal, 10 drops in the affected ear two times a day for fourteen days. It is recommended that the tragus be pumped four times during instillation, by pushing inward, to facilitate penetration of the solution into the middle ear.

**Usual pediatric dose**
Otitis externa—
  Children 12 years of age and older: See *Usual adult and adolescent dose*.
  Children 1 to 12 years of age: Topical, to the ear canal, 5 drops in the affected ear two times a day for ten days.
  Children younger than 1 year of age: Safety and efficacy have not been established.
Otitis media, acute (in pediatric patients with tympanostomy tubes)—
  Children 1 to 12 years of age: Topical, to the ear canal, 5 drops in the affected ear two times a day for ten days. It is recommended that the tragus be pumped four times during instillation, by pushing inward, to facilitate penetration of the solution into the middle ear.
  Children younger than 1 year of age: Safety and efficacy have not been established.

**Strength(s) usually available**
U.S.—
  0.3% (Rx) [*Floxin Otic* (benzalkonium chloride 0.0025%; sodium chloride 0.9%; hydrochloric acid; sodium hydroxide)].

**Packaging and storage**
Store between 15 and 25 °C (59 and 77 °F).

**Auxiliary labeling**
• For the ear.
• Continue medicine for full time of treatment.

Developed: 08/14/98
Interim revision: 08/27/98

# OLANZAPINE  Systemic—INTRODUCTORY VERSION

VA CLASSIFICATION (Primary): CN709
Commonly used brand name(s): *Zyprexa*.
Note: For a listing of dosage forms and brand names by country availability, see *Dosage Forms* section(s).

## Category
Antipsychotic.

## Indications

**Accepted**
Psychotic disorders (treatment)—Olanzapine is used to treat the manifestations of psychotic disorders. The effectiveness of olanzapine therapy for more than 6 weeks has not been evaluated in controlled trials.

## Pharmacology/Pharmacokinetics

**Physicochemical characteristics**
Chemical group—Thienobenzodiazepine.
Molecular weight—312.44.
Solubility—Practically insoluble in water.

**Mechanism of action/Effect**
The exact mechanism by which olanzapine exerts its antipsychotic effect is unknown. However, this effect may be mediated through a combination of dopamine and serotonin 5-HT$_2$ antagonism. Olanzapine is a selective monoaminergic antagonist with a strong affinity for serotonin 5-HT$_{2A}$ and 5-HT$_{2C}$ receptors, and dopamine D$_1$, D$_2$, D$_3$, and D$_4$ receptors.
Olanzapine binds weakly to gamma-aminobutyric acid type A (GABA$_A$), benzodiazepine (BZD), and beta-adrenergic receptors.
Olanzapine's high affinity binding to, and antagonism of, muscarinic M$_1$, M$_2$, M$_3$, M$_4$, and M$_5$ receptors may explain its anticholinergic effects. Olanzapine also binds with high affinity to histamine H$_1$ and alpha$_1$-adrenergic receptors. Antagonism of histamine H$_1$ and alpha$_1$-adrenergic receptors may be responsible for the occurrence of somnolence and orthostatic hypotension, respectively, seen with olanzapine use.

**Other actions/effects**
A modest elevation in prolactin levels persists during chronic olanzapine administration, probably due to antagonism of dopamine D$_2$ receptors. The clinical significance of elevated prolactin levels is unknown for most patients, although such effects as galactorrhea, amenorrhea, gynecomastia, and impotence have been reported in patients receiving prolactin-elevating medications. Also, studies have found approximately one third of human breast cancers to be prolactin-dependent *in vitro*.

**Absorption**
Well absorbed; however, 40% of the absorbed drug is metabolized before reaching systemic circulation. The rate and extent of olanzapine absorption are unaffected by food. Oral bioavailability of olanzapine was not affected by single doses of cimetidine (800 mg) or aluminum- and magnesium-containing antacids.

**Distribution**
Extensively distributed throughout the body, with a volume of distribution of approximately 1000 L.

**Protein binding**
High (93%); primarily to albumin and alpha$_1$-acid glycoprotein.

**Biotransformation**
Olanzapine is metabolized primarily through oxidation mediated by cytochrome P450 (CYP) enzymes and by direct glucuronidation. *In vitro* studies suggest that oxidation is mediated by cytochrome P450 isozymes IA$_2$ (CYP1A2) and IID$_6$ (CYP2D6), and by the flavin-containing monooxygenase system. However, studies in subjects who are deficient in CYP2D6 indicate that CYP2D6-mediated metabolism is a minor pathway of olanzapine metabolism.
The two major metabolites, 10-*N*-glucuronide and 4'-*N*-desmethyl olanzapine, are not pharmacologically active at the plasma levels achieved during normal therapeutic olanzapine dosing.
A study in six patients with clinically significant cirrhosis revealed little effect of hepatic function impairment on the pharmacokinetics of olanzapine.

**Half-life**
Elimination—
  Mean, 30 hours; range, 21 to 54 hours. Mean apparent plasma clearance is 25 L per hour (L/hr); range, 12 to 47 L/hr.

**Time to peak concentration**
Peak plasma concentration of olanzapine occurs approximately 6 hours following oral administration. Kinetics are linear over the therapeutic dosage range.

**Time to steady-state plasma concentration**
Steady-state plasma concentration of olanzapine, which is approximately twice the concentration seen after a single dose, is achieved in about 1 week with once-a-day dosing.

**Elimination**
Renal—
  Approximately 57% of an administered dose is renally excreted, 7% as unchanged drug. Pharmacokinetics of olanzapine were similar in patients with severe renal function impairment and in patients with normal renal function. Pharmacokinetics of the metabolites of olanzapine were not studied in patients with renal function impairment.
Fecal—
  Approximately 30% of an administered dose.
In dialysis—
  Olanzapine is not removed by dialysis.

## Precautions to Consider

**Carcinogenicity/Tumorigenicity**
In carcinogenicity studies, significant increases in the incidence of mammary gland adenomas and adenocarcinomas occurred in female mice receiving 0.5 times the maximum recommended human daily dose (MRHD) of 20 mg per day of olanzapine on a mg per square meter of body surface area (mg/m$^2$) basis and in female rats receiving two times

the MRHD of olanzapine on a mg/m² basis. A toxicity study in rats showed prolactin levels to be elevated up to fourfold at the same doses of olanzapine that were used in the carcinogenicity studies. The increased incidence of mammary gland neoplasms found in rodents after chronic administration of antipsychotic drugs is considered to be prolactin mediated. Drugs that antagonize dopamine $D_2$ receptors, including olanzapine, are associated with increased prolactin levels in humans. Because studies have found approximately one third of human breast cancers to be prolactin-dependent *in vitro*, this prolactin level elevation may be of importance when considering use of these medications in patients with previously detected breast cancers. However, there has been no association shown between chronic administration of medications that elevate prolactin levels and tumorigenesis in either epidemiological or clinical studies to date. Current evidence is too limited to be conclusive.

Two carcinogenicity studies were conducted in which mice received olanzapine for 78 weeks at doses ranging from 0.06 to 5 times the MRHD on a mg/m² basis (0.8 to 5 times the MRHD in one study, and 0.06 to 2 times the MRHD in the other study). In one of these studies, a significant increase in the incidence of liver hemangiomas and hemangiosarcomas was seen in female mice dosed at two times the MRHD. In the other study, this increased incidence of liver hemangiomas and hemangiosarcomas was not seen, but early mortality was increased in male mice receiving five times the MRHD.

**Mutagenicity**
Olanzapine demonstrated no mutagenic potential in the following tests: Ames reverse mutation test, *in vivo* micronucleus test in mice, the chromosomal aberration test in Chinese hamster ovary cells, unscheduled DNA synthesis test in rat hepatocytes, induction of forward mutation test in mouse lymphoma cells, or *in vivo* sister chromatid exchange test in bone marrow of Chinese hamsters.

**Pregnancy/Reproduction**
Fertility—The mating performance, but not the fertility, of male rats was impaired during administration of olanzapine at doses that were 11 times the maximum recommended human daily dose (MRHD) of 20 mg per day on a mg per square meter of body surface area (mg/m²) basis. The impairment of mating performance was reversed with discontinuation of olanzapine administration. Studies in female rats indicate that olanzapine may produce a delay in ovulation. When olanzapine was administered at doses that were 1.5 times the MRHD on a mg/m² basis, female rats showed a decrease in fertility. At doses that were 2.5 times the MRHD on a mg/m² basis, female rats showed an increased precoital period, and a reduced mating index.

Pregnancy—Adequate and well-controlled studies in humans have not been done.

Of seven pregnancies that occurred during clinical trials with olanzapine, two resulted in normal births, one resulted in neonatal death due to a cardiovascular defect, three ended in therapeutic abortions, and one ended in spontaneous abortion.

Olanzapine crosses the placenta in rats. No evidence of teratogenicity was seen in rats administered olanzapine at doses up to nine times the MRHD on a mg/m² basis, or in rabbits administered olanzapine at doses up to 30 times the MRHD on a mg/m² basis. At the maximum doses in these studies, early fetal resorptions and increased numbers of nonviable fetuses were observed in rats, and increased fetal resorptions and decreased fetal weight were observed in rabbits. The maximum dose used in the rabbit study was considered to be maternally toxic. Also, in rats, gestation was prolonged at a dose that was five times the MRHD on a mg/m² basis.

FDA Pregnancy Category C.

Labor and delivery—The effect of olanzapine on labor and delivery in humans is unknown. Olanzapine did not affect parturition in rats.

**Breast-feeding**
It is not known whether olanzapine is distributed into human breast milk. However, olanzapine is distributed into the milk of rats, and use in nursing mothers is not recommended.

**Pediatrics**
No information is available on the relationship of age to the effects of olanzapine in pediatric patients. Safety and efficacy have not been established in patients up to 18 years of age.

**Geriatrics**
No geriatrics-specific problems that would limit the usefulness of olanzapine in the elderly were seen in studies that included elderly subjects. However, the mean elimination half-life was found to be about 1.5 times greater in elderly subjects than in younger subjects in one study.

**Pharmacogenetics**
Olanzapine clearance is approximately 30% lower in females than in males. However, no differences in adverse effects or efficacy were seen in clinical studies, and dosage adjustments based on gender are not recommended.

Comparisons of pharmacokinetic data from studies conducted in Japan with data from studies conducted in the U.S. indicate a twofold higher exposure to olanzapine in Japanese subjects when doses are equivalent. However, no clinically significant differences in safety or efficacy were seen when comparisons were made among Caucasian, African-descent, and pooled Asian and Hispanic patient groups. Dosage adjustments based on race are not recommended.

**Drug interactions and/or related problems**
The following drug interactions and/or related problems have been selected on the basis of their potential clinical significance (possible mechanism in parentheses where appropriate)—not necessarily inclusive (» = major clinical significance):

Note: *In vitro* studies indicate that olanzapine has little potential to inhibit CYP1A2, CYP2C9, CYP2C19, CYP2D6, or CYP3A. Therefore, olanzapine is not expected to interfere with the metabolism of medications that are metabolized by these enzymes.

Combinations containing any of the following medications, depending on the amount present, may also interact with this medication.

Agents that induce CYP1A2 or glucuronyl transferase enzymes, such as carbamazepine, omeprazole, or rifampin
(olanzapine clearance may be increased; carbamazepine therapy at a dose of 200 mg two times a day increased olanzapine clearance by about 50%)

Agents that inhibit CYP1A2, such as fluvoxamine
(olanzapine clearance may be decreased, although, because multiple enzymes are involved in olanzapine metabolism, the effect of inhibiting one isozyme may not be significant)

» Alcohol or
» Central nervous system (CNS) depression–producing medications, other (See *Appendix II*)
(additive CNS depressant effects may occur; orthostatic hypotension may be potentiated)

» Anticholinergics, other (See *Appendix II*)
(anticholinergic effects of either these medications or olanzapine may be increased; disruption of the body's ability to reduce core temperature may be a special consideration)

Antihypertensive agents
(hypotensive effects of these medications or olanzapine may be enhanced)

Dopamine agonists or
Levodopa
(effects of these medications may be antagonized by olanzapine)

» Hepatotoxic medications (See *Appendix II*)
(asymptomatic but clinically significant alanine aminotransferase [ALT (SGPT)] value increases occurred in about 2% of patients in premarketing studies of olanzapine; about 1% of patients discontinued olanzapine treatment due to increased transaminase levels; caution is recommended when olanzapine is used concurrently with hepatotoxic medications)

Smoking, cigarette
(olanzapine clearance is increased by about 40%)

**Laboratory value alterations**
The following have been selected on the basis of their potential clinical significance (possible effect in parentheses where appropriate)—not necessarily inclusive (» = major clinical significance):

With physiology/laboratory test values
Alanine aminotransferase (ALT [SGPT]) values and
Aspartate transaminase (AST [SGOT]) values and
Gamma-glutamyl transpeptidase (GGT) values
(in premarketing studies, about 2% of patients with baseline ALT [SGPT] values ≤ 90 international units per L [IU/L] had ALT value increases to > 200 IU/L during treatment with olanzapine; none of these patients experienced symptoms of liver function impairment, and in most the ALT value returned to normal with continued olanzapine treatment; asymptomatic increases in AST and GGT were seen also; about 1% of patients in clinical trials discontinued olanzapine treatment due to increased transaminase values)

Prolactin concentration, serum
(sustained elevations occur during olanzapine therapy)

**Medical considerations/Contraindications**
The medical considerations/contraindications included have been selected on the basis of their potential clinical significance (reasons given in parentheses where appropriate)—not necessarily inclusive (» = major clinical significance).

*Except under special circumstances, this medication should not be used when the following medical problem exists:*

» Hypersensitivity to olanzapine

*Risk-benefit should be considered when the following medical problems exist:*

» Alzheimer's dementia
(dysphagia associated with olanzapine use may increase risk of aspiration pneumonia; possible increased risk of seizures because of lowered seizure threshold with Alzheimer's dementia)

» Breast cancer, or history of
(prolactin-dependent breast cancers may be exacerbated)

» Cardiovascular disease, including:
Conduction abnormalities or
Heart failure or
Myocardial infarction or ischemia, or history of, or

» Cerebrovascular disease or

» Conditions that would predispose to hypotension, including:
Dehydration or
Hypovolemia
(orthostatic hypotension may be exacerbated, or may exacerbate preexisting cardiovascular or cerebrovascular conditions)
(dehydration may predispose to increased core body temperature, and antipsychotic medications may disrupt the body's ability to lower core body temperature, thus increasing the risk of heatstroke)

Drug abuse or dependence, history of
(patients should be observed closely for signs of misuse or abuse of olanzapine, as with any new CNS medication)

» Glaucoma, narrow angle or
» Paralytic ileus, history of or
» Prostatic hypertrophy, clinically significant
(may be exacerbated due to cholinergic antagonism by olanzapine)

» Hepatic function impairment
(in premarketing studies, about 1% of patients discontinued olanzapine treatment due to increased transaminase levels; transaminase levels should be assessed periodically in patients with significant hepatic disease)

Seizures, or history of
(seizures occurred rarely in premarketing studies of olanzapine; it is recommended that olanzapine be used with caution in patients with a history of seizures or a decreased seizure threshold)

**Patient monitoring**

The following may be especially important in patient monitoring (other tests may be warranted in some patients, depending on condition; » = major clinical significance):

Alanine aminotransferase (ALT [SGPT]) values and
Aspartate transaminase (AST [SGOT]) values
(recommended periodically in patients with significant hepatic disease)

Careful supervision of patients with suicidal tendencies
(recommended in high-risk patients, since the possibility of a suicide attempt is inherent in schizophrenia)

## Side/Adverse Effects

Note: Disturbances of body temperature regulation have been associated with use of other antipsychotic agents. Caution is advised in administering olanzapine to patients who will be experiencing conditions that may contribute to an elevation in core body temperature, such as strenuous exercise, exposure to extreme heat, or dehydration.

The neuroleptic malignant syndrome (NMS) has been associated with the use of other antipsychotic agents. NMS is a potentially fatal symptom complex that may include hyperpyrexia, muscle rigidity, altered mental status, and autonomic instability seen as irregular pulse or blood pressure, tachycardia, diaphoresis, and cardiac dysrythmia. Elevated creatine kinase, myoglobinuria (rhabdomyolysis), and acute renal failure also may occur. Differential diagnosis should exclude serious medical illnesses, such as pneumonia or systemic infection presenting in conjunction with extrapyramidal effects, as well as central anticholinergic toxicity, heatstroke, drug fever, and primary CNS pathology.

The following side/adverse effects have been selected on the basis of their potential clinical significance (possible signs and symptoms in parentheses where appropriate)—not necessarily inclusive:

**Those indicating need for medical attention**

Incidence more frequent
*Agitation; akathesia* (restlessness or need to keep moving); *extrapyramidal effects, parkinsonian* (difficulty in speaking or swallowing; stiffness of arms or legs; trembling or shaking of hands and fingers); *personality disorder* (nonaggressive objectionable behavior)

Note: *Akathesia* and *extrapyramidal effects* are dose-related.

Incidence less frequent
*Chest pain; extrapyramidal effects, dystonic* (inability to move eyes; muscle spasms of face, neck, and back; twitching movements); *fever; flu-like symptoms; mood or mental changes, including amnesia, anxiety; euphoria; hostility; and nervousness; peripheral edema* (swelling of feet or ankles); *tardive dyskinesia* (lip smacking or puckering; puffing of cheeks; rapid or worm-like movements of tongue; uncontrolled chewing movements; uncontrolled movements of arms and legs)

Note: *Tardive dyskinesia* occurs more frequently in elderly patients, especially elderly women. The risk of developing the syndrome, and of experiencing irreversible effects, appears to increase with treatment duration and total cumulative dose, although it may develop at any time during antipsychotic therapy. There is no known treatment for tardive dyskinesia, although partial or complete remission may occur when the antipsychotic medication is withdrawn. Alternatively, the antipsychotic medication may suppress the signs of the syndrome, masking the underlying process. For these reasons, olanzapine should be used only in those patients with chronic illness that is responsive to antipsychotic medication, and for whom potentially less harmful treatments are unavailable or inappropriate. Also, the smallest effective dose of olanzapine should be used and the need for continuing treatment should be assessed periodically.

Incidence rare
*Dyspnea* (trouble in breathing); *facial edema* (swelling of face); *menstrual changes; skin rash; water intoxication* (confusion; mental or physical sluggishness)

**Those indicating need for medical attention only if they continue or are bothersome**

Incidence more frequent
*Amblyopia* (problems with vision); *asthenia* (weakness); *constipation; dizziness; drowsiness; dry mouth; headache; increased weight; postural hypotension* (dizziness or fainting when getting up suddenly from a lying or sitting position); *rhinitis* (runny nose); *tremor* (trembling or shaking)

Note: *Asthenia, drowsiness, dry mouth*, and *tremor* are dose-related. *Postural hypotension* is most likely to occur during the initial dose-titration period.

During premarketing long-term continuation treatment with olanzapine (median exposure 238 days), 56% of patients had *weight gain* > 7% of their baseline weight. The average weight gain was 5.4 kg.

Incidence less frequent
*Abdominal pain; articulation impairment* (speaking unclearly); *hypertonia* (tightness of muscles); *hypotension* (low blood pressure); *increased appetite; increased cough; increased salivation* (watering of mouth); *insomnia* (trouble in sleeping); *joint pain; nausea; pharyngitis* (sore throat); *stuttering; tachycardia* (fast heartbeat); *thirst; urinary incontinence* (trouble in controlling urine); *vomiting; weight loss*

Note: *Nausea* is dose related.

Incidence rare
*Decreased libido* (decrease in sexual desire); *diplopia* (double vision); *palpitation* (awareness of heartbeat); *photosensitivity* (increased sensitivity of skin to sunlight)

## Overdose

For specific information on the agents used in the management of olanzapine overdose, see:
- Charcoal, Activated (Oral-Local) monograph; and
- Sympathomimetic Agents—Cardiovascular Use (Parenteral-Systemic) monograph.

For more information on the management of overdose or unintentional ingestion, **contact a Poison Control Center** (see *Poison Control Center Listing*).

**Clinical effects of overdose**

The following effects have been selected on the basis of their potential clinical significance (possible signs and symptoms in parentheses where appropriate)—not necessarily inclusive:

Acute

Note: During premarketing trials, 67 cases of acute overdosage with olanzapine were identified. The highest reported ingestion was 300 mg. The only symptoms reported in this patient were drowsiness and slurred speech. Among overdose patients who were evaluated in hospitals, none showed changes in laboratory analyses or electrocardiograms (ECG), and vital signs were usually within normal limits.

### Treatment of overdose
Multiple drug involvement should be considered. There is no specific antidote to olanzapine.

To decrease absorption—Gastric lavage, after intubation if patient is unconscious, and administration of activated charcoal with a laxative should be considered. Activated charcoal has been shown to reduce absorption of olanzapine, and may be of use since olanzapine does not reach peak plasma levels for approximately 6 hours following ingestion. The risk of aspiration with induction of emesis may be increased by possible obtundation, seizures, or dystonic reaction of the head and neck.

Specific treatment—Hypotension and circulatory collapse may be treated with intravenous fluids and/or sympathomimetic agents. Because of olanzapine-induced alpha blockade, sympathomimetics with beta agonist activity, such as epinephrine and dopamine, may worsen hypotension and should not be used.

Monitoring—Continuous ECG monitoring should be employed to detect possible arrhythmias. Close medical supervision should continue until patient recovers.

Supportive care—Airway should be established and maintained to ensure adequate oxygenation and ventilation. Patients in whom intentional overdose is confirmed or suspected should be referred for psychiatric consultation.

Note: Olanzapine is not removed by dialysis.

## Patient Consultation
In providing consultation, consider emphasizing the following selected information (» = major clinical significance)

### Before using this medication
» Conditions affecting use, especially:

Carcinogenicity/Tumorigenicity—Increase in mammary gland neoplasias seen in animal studies; sustained prolactin level elevations with olanzapine use; one third of human breast cancers are prolactin-dependent *in vitro*; no association between chronic administration of prolactin level–increasing antipsychotic medications and tumorigenesis seen in epidemiological or clinical studies in humans; evidence inconclusive

Pregnancy—Seven pregnancies occurring during clinical trials ended in two normal births, one neonatal death due to cardiovascular defect, one spontaneous abortion, three therapeutic abortions

Breast-feeding—Distributed into the milk of rats; use in nursing mothers not recommended

Dental—Possible dryness of mouth

Other medications, especially alcohol, anticholinergics, CNS depression–producing medications, or hepatotoxic medications

Other medical problems, especially hypersensitivity to olanzapine, Alzheimer's dementia, breast cancer, cardiovascular disease, cerebrovascular disease, conditions that would predispose to hypotension, glaucoma, hepatic function impairment, paralytic ileus, or prostatic hypertrophy

### Proper use of this medication
Compliance with therapy; not taking more or less medicine than prescribed

Taking with or without food, on a full or empty stomach, as directed by physician

» Proper dosing
» Proper storage

### Precautions while using this medication
Possible drowsiness, impaired judgement, thinking, motor skills, or vision; caution when driving, operating machinery, or doing jobs requiring alertness, coordination, or clear vision

Possible orthostatic hypotension; rising slowly from a sitting or lying position

Possible impairment of ability to regulate core body temperature; avoiding overheating and dehydration

Avoiding use of alcoholic beverages; not taking other CNS depressants unless prescribed by physician

### Side/adverse effects
Signs of potential side effects, especially agitation, akathesia, extrapyramidal effects, personality disorder, chest pain, fever, flu-like symptoms, mood or mental changes, peripheral edema, tardive dyskinesia, dyspnea, facial edema, menstrual changes, skin rash, and water intoxication

## General Dosing Information
Since the possibility of suicide is inherent in schizophrenia, patients should not have access to large quantities of olanzapine. To reduce the risk of overdose, the patient should be supplied with the smallest quantity of medication necessary for satisfactory patient management.

### Diet/Nutrition
Olanzapine may be taken without regard to food.

### For treatment of adverse effects
Neuroleptic malignant syndrome (NMS)—Recommended treatment consists of the following:
- *Discontinuing olanzapine and other drugs not essential to current therapy.*
- Providing intensive symptomatic treatment and medical monitoring.
- Treating any concomitant serious medical problems for which specific treatments are available.
- After recovery, giving careful consideration to the reintroduction of antipsychotic drug therapy in patients with severe psychosis requiring treatment, because of possible recurrence of NMS; closely monitoring patients in whom antipsychotic drug therapy is reintroduced after recovery from NMS.

Tardive dyskinesia—There is no known effective treatment. If signs and symptoms of tardive dyskinesia appear, discontinuation of olanzapine treatment should be considered if clinically feasible. To minimize the occurrence of tardive dyskinesia, chronic antipsychotic treatment should be in the smallest effective dose for the shortest duration necessary to produce a satisfactory clinical response.

## Oral Dosage Forms
### OLANZAPINE TABLETS
#### Usual adult dose
Antipsychotic—

Oral, initially 5 to 10 mg once a day, with a target dose of 10 mg once a day within several days. Dosage may then be adjusted as needed and tolerated at increments or decrements of 5 mg a day, at intervals of not less than one week.

Note: The risk of orthostatic hypotension and syncope may be minimized by initiating therapy with 5 mg a day. If hypotension occurs, a more gradual titration to the target dose may be considered.

While individual factors that decrease olanzapine clearance do not necessitate dosage reduction, patients exhibiting a combination of these factors, such as an elderly female nonsmoker, should begin therapy with an initial dosage of 5 mg a day. Dosage should be increased cautiously in these patients if clinically necessary.

Debilitated patients, patients predisposed to hypotensive reactions, and patients who may be more pharmacodynamically sensitive to olanzapine should begin therapy with an initial dosage of 5 mg a day. Dosage should be increased cautiously in these patients if clinically necessary.

In clinical trials, dosages above 10 mg a day were not shown to be more efficacious than 10 mg a day.

#### Usual adult prescribing limits
20 mg a day.

#### Usual pediatric dose
Antipsychotic—
Safety and efficacy in children up to 18 years of age have not been established.

#### Usual geriatric dose
Antipsychotic—
See *Usual adult dose*.

#### Usual geriatric prescribing limits
See *Usual adult prescribing limits*.

#### Strength(s) usually available
U.S.—

5 mg (Rx) [*Zyprexa* (carnauba wax; color mixture white; crospovidone; FD&C Blue No. 2 Aluminum Lake; hydroxypropyl cellulose; hydroxypropyl methylcellulose; lactose; magnesium stearate; microcrystalline cellulose)].

7.5 mg (Rx) [*Zyprexa* (carnauba wax; color mixture white; crospovidone; FD&C Blue No. 2 Aluminum Lake; hydroxypropyl cellulose;

hydroxypropyl methylcellulose; lactose; magnesium stearate; microcrystalline cellulose)].
- 10 mg (Rx) [*Zyprexa* (carnauba wax; color mixture white; crospovidone; FD&C Blue No. 2 Aluminum Lake; hydroxypropyl cellulose; hydroxypropyl methylcellulose; lactose; magnesium stearate; microcrystalline cellulose)].

## Packaging and storage
Store between 20 and 25 °C (68 and 77 °F), unless otherwise specified by manufacturer. Protect from light and moisture.

### Auxiliary labeling
- Avoid alcoholic beverages.
- May cause dizziness or drowsiness.

Developed: 02/26/97
Interim revision: 08/25/97

# OLOPATADINE   Ophthalmic—INTRODUCTORY VERSION

VA CLASSIFICATION (Primary): OP801
Commonly used brand name(s): *Patanol*.

Note: For a listing of dosage forms and brand names by country availability, see *Dosage Forms* section(s).

## Category
Antihistaminic ($H_1$-receptor), ophthalmic; mast cell stabilizer, ophthalmic; antiallergic, ophthalmic.

## Indications
### Accepted
Conjunctivitis, allergic (treatment)—Ophthalmic olopatadine is indicated for temporary prevention of itching of the eye due to allergic conjunctivitis.

## Pharmacology/Pharmacokinetics
### Physicochemical characteristics
Molecular weight—Olopatadine hydrochloride: 373.88.

### Mechanism of action/Effect
Olopatadine is a relatively selective histamine $H_1$-receptor antagonist that inhibits the type 1 immediate hypersensitivity reaction *in vivo* and *in vitro*. Olopatadine also inhibits the release of histamine from mast cells. Olopatadine does not affect alpha-adrenergic, dopamine, muscarinic types 1 and 2, or serotonin receptors.

### Absorption
Ophthalmic use of olopatadine usually does not produce measurable plasma concentrations. Two studies in normal volunteers (total 24 subjects) administered olopatadine 0.15% ophthalmic solution in each eye once every 12 hours for 2 weeks found that plasma concentrations were generally below the quantitative limit of the assay (less than 0.5 nanograms per mL). Samples in which olopatadine was quantifiable were typically those taken within 2 hours of dosing and contained plasma concentrations ranging from 0.5 to 1.3 nanograms per mL.

### Biotransformation
The mono-desmethyl and the *N*-oxide metabolites have been detected at low concentrations in the urine.

### Half-life
Elimination—
  Plasma: Approximately 3 hours.

### Elimination
Renal (60 to 70% as unchanged drug). Also, low concentrations of 2 metabolites (mono-desmethyl and *N*-oxide) have been detected in the urine.

## Precautions to Consider
### Carcinogenicity
Studies in mice and rats given oral doses of olopatadine of up to 500 and 200 mg per kg of body weight (mg/kg) per day, respectively, which (based on a 40 microliter drop size) were 78,125 and 31,250 times, respectively, the maximum recommended ocular human dose (MROHD), found no evidence of carcinogenicity.

### Mutagenicity
Olopatadine was not found to be mutagenic in an *in vitro* bacterial reverse mutation (Ames) test, an *in vitro* mammalian chromosome aberration assay, or an *in vivo* mouse micronucleus test.

### Pregnancy/Reproduction
Fertility—Studies in male and female rats given oral doses of olopatadine that were 62,500 times the MROHD level found a slight decrease in the fertility index and a reduced implantation rate. No effects on fertility were observed at doses of 7800 times the MROHD.

Pregnancy—Adequate and well-controlled studies in humans have not been done.
Olopatadine was not found to be teratogenic in rats or rabbits. However, studies in rats given doses of 600 mg/kg per day (93,750 times the MROHD) and in rabbits given doses of 400 mg/kg per day (62,500 times the MROHD) during organogenesis resulted in a decrease in live fetuses.
It is recommended that risk-benefit be considered before using olopatadine during pregnancy.
FDA Pregnancy Category C.

### Breast-feeding
It is not known whether ophthalmic olopatadine is absorbed in sufficient quantities to be distributed into human breast milk. However, it has been found in the milk of nursing rats following oral administration.

### Pediatrics
Safety and efficacy in children up to 3 years of age have not been established.

### Geriatrics
No information is available on the relationship of age to the effects of ophthalmic olopatadine in geriatric patients.

### Medical considerations/Contraindications
The medical considerations/contraindications included have been selected on the basis of their potential clinical significance (reasons given in parentheses where appropriate)—not necessarily inclusive (» = major clinical significance).

*Except under special circumstances, this medication should not be used when the following medical problem exists:*
» Sensitivity to olopatadine

*Risk-benefit should be considered when the following medical problem exists:*
Sensitivity to benzalkonium chloride

## Side/Adverse Effects
The following side/adverse effects have been selected on the basis of their potential clinical significance (possible signs and symptoms in parentheses where appropriate)—not necessarily inclusive:

**Those indicating need for medical attention only if they continue or are bothersome**
Incidence more frequent
  *Headache*—7%

Incidence less frequent—Less than 5%
  *Asthenia* (unusual tiredness or weakness); ***burning, dryness, itching, or stinging of the eye; change in taste; cold-like symptoms, such as sore throat and runny nose; feeling of something in the eye;*** *hyperemia* (redness of eye or inside of eyelid); *keratitis* (eye redness, irritation, or pain); *lid edema* (swelling of eyelid); *pharyngitis* (sore throat); *rhinitis* (stuffy or runny nose); *sinusitis* (headache or runny nose)

## Patient Consultation
As an aid to patient consultation, refer to *Advice for the Patient, Olopatadine (Ophthalmic)—Introductory Version*.
In providing consultation, consider emphasizing the following selected information (» = major clinical significance):

### Before using this medication
» Conditions affecting use, especially:
    Sensitivity to olopatadine
    Pregnancy—Risk-benefit should be considered

### Proper use of this medication
   Removing contact lenses prior to administration; waiting at least 15 minutes after administration before reinserting lenses
» Proper administration; using a second drop if necessary; not touching applicator tip to any surface; keeping container tightly closed

» Proper dosing
　Missed dose: Using as soon as possible; not using if almost time for next dose; using next dose at regularly scheduled time; not doubling doses
» Proper storage

**Precautions while using this medication**
» Checking with physician if symptoms do not improve or if condition worsens

**Side/adverse effects**
Signs of potential side effects

## General Dosing Information

Olopatadine contains benzalkonium chloride, which may be absorbed by contact lenses. Contact lenses should be removed prior to administration of olopatadine. Lenses may be reinserted 15 minutes after administration.

Although some manufacturers recommend a dose of 2 drops of an ophthalmic solution at appropriate intervals, the conjunctival sac usually will hold 1 drop or less.

## Ophthalmic Dosage Forms

Note: The dosing and strength of the dosage form available are expressed in terms of olopatadine base.

### OLOPATADINE HYDROCHLORIDE OPHTHALMIC SOLUTION

**Usual adult and adolescent dose**
Allergic conjunctivitis—
　Topical, to the conjunctiva, 1 drop in each affected eye two times a day, separated by an interval of at least six to eight hours.

**Usual pediatric dose**
Allergic conjunctivitis—
　Children up to 3 years of age: Safety and efficacy have not been established.
　Children 3 years of age and older: See *Usual adult and adolescent dose*.

**Strength(s) usually available**
U.S.—
　0.1% (1 mg olopatadine [base] per mL) (Rx) [*Patanol* (benzalkonium chloride 0.01%; dibasic sodium phosphate; sodium chloride; hydrochloric acid/sodium hydroxide; purified water)].

**Packaging and storage**
Store between 4 and 30 °C (39 and 86 °F).

**Auxiliary labeling**
• For the eye.

Developed: 11/13/97
Interim revision: 08/13/98

---

# OLSALAZINE  Oral-Local

VA CLASSIFICATION (Primary): GA400
Commonly used brand name(s): *Dipentum*.
Other commonly used names are azodisal sodium and sodium azodisalicylate.
Note: For a listing of dosage forms and brand names by country availability, see *Dosage Forms* section(s).

## Category

Bowel disease (inflammatory) suppressant.

## Indications

Note: Bracketed information in the *Indications* section refers to uses that are not included in U.S. product labeling.

**Accepted**
Bowel disease, inflammatory (prophylaxis)—Olsalazine is indicated to maintain remission of ulcerative colitis in patients who are intolerant of sulfasalazine.

[Bowel disease, inflammatory (treatment)]—Olsalazine is indicated to treat acute ulcerative colitis of mild to moderate severity.

## Pharmacology/Pharmacokinetics

**Physicochemical characteristics**
Molecular weight—346.21.

**Mechanism of action/Effect**
Bowel disease (inflammatory) suppressant—
　Uncertain. Unabsorbed olsalazine is cleaved in the colon by colonic bacteria to form 2 molecules of mesalamine (5-aminosalicylic acid; 5-ASA), the therapeutically active moiety in the management of ulcerative colitis. Mucosal production of arachidonic acid metabolites, both through the cyclooxygenase and lipoxygenase pathways, is increased in patients with inflammatory bowel disease. Mesalamine appears to diminish inflammation by inhibiting cyclooxygenase and lipoxygenase, thereby decreasing the production of prostaglandins, and leukotrienes and hydroxyeicosatetraenoic acids (HETEs), respectively.
　It is also believed that mesalamine acts as a scavenger of oxygen-derived free radicals, which are produced in greater numbers in patients with inflammatory bowel disease.

**Absorption**
Limited systemic bioavailability; approximately 2.4% of a single 1-gram dose of olsalazine is absorbed.

**Distribution**
Approximately 99% of an oral dose (unabsorbed) of olsalazine reaches the colon.

**Protein binding**
Olsalazine—Very high (99%).
Olsalazine-O-sulfate (olsalazine-S)—Very high (99%).
Mesalamine (5-ASA)—High (74%).
*N*-acetyl-5-ASA (Ac-5-ASA)—High (81%).

**Biotransformation**
Absorbed—Approximately 0.1% of an oral dose of olsalazine is metabolized in the liver to olsalazine-S.
Unabsorbed—Each molecule of olsalazine that reaches the colon is rapidly converted into 2 molecules of mesalamine by colonic bacteria, and the low prevailing redox potential found in this environment. The liberated mesalamine is then absorbed slowly, resulting in very high local concentrations in the colon. The absorbed mesalamine is acetylated to Ac-5-ASA; however, it is not known whether acetylation takes place at colonic or systemic sites. Ac-5-ASA is further acetylated (deactivated) in at least 2 sites, the colonic epithelium and the liver.

**Half-life**
Elimination—
　Olsalazine: 0.9 hours.
　Olsalazine-S: 7 days.

**Time to peak concentration**
Olsalazine—Approximately 1 hour.
Mesalamine—4 to 8 hours.

**Peak serum concentration**
Following a single 1-gram dose of olsalazine, peak serum concentrations were—
　Olsalazine: 1.6 to 6.2 micromoles per L.
　Mesalamine: 0 to 4.3 micromoles per L.
　Ac-5-ASA: 1.7 to 8.7 micromoles per L.

**Elimination**
Renal—
　As olsalazine: <1% of administered dose.
　As Ac-5-ASA (major metabolite): Approximately 20% of the total mesalamine.
Fecal—
　Approximately 80% of the total mesalamine (partially acetylated).

## Precautions to Consider

**Cross-sensitivity and/or related problems**
Because olsalazine is a sodium salt of a salicylate derivative, patients sensitive to salicylates may be sensitive to olsalazine also. In addition, patients sensitive to mesalamine or sulfasalazine may be sensitive to this medication.

**Carcinogenicity**
In a 2-year study in male and female rats, olsalazine given orally in doses corresponding to 10 to 40 times the human dose caused an increase in

# Olsalazine (Oral-Local)

the incidence of urinary bladder transitional cell carcinomas in males receiving the highest dose.

**Mutagenicity**
No evidence of mutagenicity was observed in *in vitro* Ames tests, mouse lymphoma cell mutation assays, human lymphocyte chromosomal aberration tests, or an *in vivo* rat bone marrow cell chromosomal aberration test.

**Pregnancy/Reproduction**
Fertility—Oligospermia and infertility in men, which have been reported in association with sulfasalazine, have not been seen with olsalazine.
Olsalazine was found to have no effect on the fertility of male and female rats when given orally at a dose corresponding to 5 to 20 times the human dose.
Pregnancy—Adequate and well-controlled studies in humans have not been done.
Fetotoxic effects, such as decreased fetal weight, retarded ossification, and immaturity of the fetal visceral organs, were seen in rats given doses corresponding to 5 to 20 times the human dose.
FDA Pregnancy Category C.

**Breast-feeding**
It is not known whether olsalazine or its metabolites are distributed into breast milk. However, olsalazine administered to nursing rats at a dose corresponding to 5 to 20 times the human dose caused growth retardation in the pups.

**Pediatrics**
Appropriate studies on the relationship of age to the effects of olsalazine have not been performed in the pediatric population. Safety and efficacy have not been established.

**Geriatrics**
Appropriate studies on the relationship of age to the effects of olsalazine have not been performed in the geriatric population. However, geriatrics-specific problems that would limit the usefulness of this medication in the elderly are not expected.

**Drug interactions and/or related problems**
The following drug interactions and/or related problems have been selected on the basis of their potential clinical significance (possible mechanism in parentheses where appropriate)—not necessarily inclusive (» = major clinical significance):
Note: Combinations containing any of the following medications, depending on the amount present, may also interact with this medication.

Anticoagulants, coumarin- or indandione-derivative
(olsalazine may prolong the prothrombin time, which is used for dosage adjustments of anticoagulants)

**Medical considerations/Contraindications**
The medical considerations/contraindications included have been selected on the basis of their potential clinical significance (reasons given in parentheses where appropriate)—not necessarily inclusive (» = major clinical significance).

*Risk-benefit should be considered when the following medical problems exist:*

Renal function impairment
(increased risk of renal tubular damage)
Sensitivity to olsalazine, mesalamine, sulfasalazine, or salicylates

**Patient monitoring**
The following may be especially important in patient monitoring (other tests may be warranted in some patients, depending on condition; » = major clinical significance):

Blood urea nitrogen (BUN) and
Creatinine, serum and
Urinalysis
(determinations may be required in patients with renal function impairment)
Proctoscopy and
Sigmoidoscopy
(may be required periodically during treatment to determine patient response and dosage adjustments)

## Side/Adverse Effects

The following side/adverse effects have been selected on the basis of their potential clinical significance (possible signs and symptoms in parentheses where appropriate)—not necessarily inclusive:

**Those indicating need for medical attention**
Incidence rare
*Exacerbation of ulcerative colitis* (bloody diarrhea; fever; skin rash); *hepatitis* (yellow eyes or skin); *pancreatitis* (back or stomach pain, severe; fast heartbeat; fever; nausea or vomiting; swelling of the stomach)

**Those indicating need for medical attention only if they continue or are bothersome**
Incidence more frequent
*Gastrointestinal disturbances* (abdominal or stomach pain or upset; diarrhea; loss of appetite; nausea or vomiting)
Note: In controlled studies, diarrhea has been reported in approximately 11% of patients receiving olsalazine, resulting in treatment withdrawal in approximately 6% of patients. Diarrhea appeared to be dose-related and coincident with the start of olsalazine therapy; it was distinguishable from disease-related diarrhea by its watery appearance and absence of blood.

Incidence less frequent
*Aching joints and muscles; acne; anxiety or depression; dizziness or drowsiness; headache; insomnia* (trouble in sleeping)

## Patient Consultation

As an aid to patient consultation, refer to *Advice for the Patient, Olsalazine (Oral)*.
In providing consultation, consider emphasizing the following selected information (» = major clinical significance):

**Before using this medication**
» Conditions affecting use, especially:
Sensitivity to olsalazine, mesalamine, sulfasalazine, or salicylates

**Proper use of this medication**
Taking with food to lessen gastrointestinal irritation
» Compliance with full course of therapy
» Proper dosing
Missed dose: Taking as soon as possible; not taking if almost time for next dose; not doubling doses
» Proper storage

**Precautions while using this medication**
» Regular visits to physician to check progress in patients on long-term therapy

**Side/adverse effects**
Signs of potential side effects, especially exacerbation of ulcerative colitis, hepatitis, and pancreatitis

## General Dosing Information

Olsalazine should be taken with food to decrease gastrointestinal irritation.
The total daily dose should be taken in evenly divided doses.

## Oral Dosage Forms

Note: Bracketed uses in the *Dosage Forms* section refer to categories of use and/or indications that are not included in U.S. product labeling.

### OLSALAZINE SODIUM CAPSULES

**Usual adult and adolescent dose**
Bowel disease, inflammatory (prophylaxis)—
Oral, 500 mg two times a day.
[Bowel disease, inflammatory (treatment)]—
Oral, 500 mg four times a day.

**Usual pediatric dose**
Safety and efficacy have not been established.

**Usual geriatric dose**
See *Usual adult and adolescent dose*.

**Strength(s) usually available**
U.S.—
250 mg (Rx) [*Dipentum* (magnesium stearate)].
Canada—
250 mg (Rx) [*Dipentum*].

**Packaging and storage**
Store below 40 °C (104 °F), preferably between 15 and 30 °C (59 and 86 °F), unless otherwise specified by manufacturer. Store in a well-closed container.

**Auxiliary labeling**
• Continue medicine for full time of treatment.
• Take with food.

## Selected Bibliography

Ruderman WB. Newer pharmacologic agents for the therapy of inflammatory bowel disease. Med Clin North Am 1990; 74: 133-53.

Segars LW, Gales BJ. Mesalamine and olsalazine: 5-aminosalicylic acid agents for the treatment of inflammatory bowel disease. Clin Pharm 1992; 11: 514-28.

Wadworth AN, Fitton A. Olsalazine. A review of its pharmacodynamic and pharmacokinetic properties, and therapeutic potential in inflammatory bowel disease. Drugs 1991; 41: 647-64.

Revised: 03/15/95

# OMEPRAZOLE  Systemic

VA CLASSIFICATION (Primary): GA304

Commonly used brand name(s): *Losec; Prilosec.*

Note: For a listing of dosage forms and brand names by country availability, see *Dosage Forms* section(s).

## Category

Gastric acid pump inhibitor; antiulcer agent.

## Indications

Note: Bracketed information in the *Indications* section refers to uses that are not included in U.S. product labeling.

### Accepted

Gastroesophageal reflux disease [GERD] (prophylaxis and treatment)—Omeprazole is indicated for the treatment of heartburn and other symptoms associated with gastroesophageal reflux disease. Omeprazole is indicated for the short-term treatment of erosive esophagitis (associated with GERD) that has been diagnosed by endoscopy. Omeprazole also is indicated to maintain healing of erosive esophagitis.

Hypersecretory conditions, gastric (treatment)
Zollinger-Ellison syndrome (treatment)
Mastocytosis, systemic (treatment) or
Adenoma, multiple endocrine (treatment)—Omeprazole is indicated for the long-term treatment of pathologic gastric hypersecretion associated with Zollinger-Ellison syndrome (alone or as part of multiple endocrine neoplasia Type-1), systemic mastocytosis, and multiple endocrine adenoma.

Ulcer, peptic (treatment)—Omeprazole is indicated for the short-term treatment of active duodenal ulcer and active benign gastric ulcer.

Ulcer, peptic, *Helicobacter pylori*–associated (treatment adjunct)—Omeprazole is indicated in combination with clarithromycin [and amoxicillin or metronidazole] for the treatment of duodenal and gastric ulcer associated with *H. pylori* infection. Eradication of *H. pylori* has been shown to reduce the risk of ulcer recurrence.

[Ulcer, peptic, nonsteroidal anti-inflammatory drug–induced (treatment)]—Omeprazole is indicated for the treatment of duodenal or gastric ulcers associated with the use of nonsteroidal anti-inflammatory drugs (NSAIDs).

## Pharmacology/Pharmacokinetics

### Physicochemical characteristics

Molecular weight—345.42.
pKa—4 and 8.8.

### Mechanism of action/Effect

Omeprazole is activated at an acidic pH to a sulphenamide derivative that binds irreversibly to $H^+$, $K^+$-ATPase, an enzyme system found at the secretory surface of parietal cells. It thereby inhibits the final transport of hydrogen ions (via exchange with potassium ions) into the gastric lumen. Since the $H^+$, $K^+$-ATPase enzyme system is regarded as the acid (proton) pump of the gastric mucosa, omeprazole is known as a gastric acid pump inhibitor. Omeprazole inhibits both basal and stimulated acid secretion irrespective of the stimulus.

### Other actions/effects

Inhibits hepatic cytochrome P-450 mixed function oxidase system.

### Absorption

Rapid.

### Distribution

Distributed in tissue, particularly gastric parietal cells.

### Protein binding

Very high, approximately 95% bound to albumin and alpha$_1$-acid glycoprotein.

### Biotransformation

Hepatic, extensive.

### Half-life

Plasma—
 Normal hepatic function—30 minutes to 1 hour.
 Chronic hepatic disease—3 hours.

### Onset of action

Within one hour.

### Time to peak concentration

Within 30 minutes to 3.5 hours.

### Time to peak effect

Within 2 hours.

### Duration of action

Up to 72 hours or more (96 hours required for full restoration of acid production).

### Elimination

Renal—72 to 80%.
Fecal—18 to 23%.
In dialysis—Not readily dialyzable, because of extensive protein binding.

## Precautions to Consider

### Carcinogenicity/Tumorigenicity/Mutagenicity

In two 2-year studies in rats, omeprazole, given in doses corresponding to 4 to 352 times the human dose, caused end-life gastric carcinoid tumors and enterochromaffin-like (ECL) cell hyperplasia in a dose-related manner in both male and female animals. These ECL cell changes have been shown to be caused by high levels of gastrin (or hypergastrinemia). Pronounced acid inhibition at extremely high doses of gastric acid pump inhibitors or $H_2$-receptor antagonists results in the same feedback elevation of gastrin and subsequent ECL cell changes of the stomach.

### Pregnancy/Reproduction

Fertility—In a rat fertility and general reproductive performance test, omeprazole, in a dose 35 to 345 times the human dose, was not toxic or deleterious to the reproductive performance of parental animals.

Pregnancy—Adequate and well-controlled studies in humans have not been done.

Studies in pregnant rats did not show omeprazole to have any teratogenic potential at doses 345 times the human dose. Omeprazole produced dose-related increases in embryo-lethality, fetal resorptions, and pregnancy disruptions in rabbits receiving 17 to 172 times the human dose. In rats, dose-related embryo/fetal toxicity and postnatal developmental toxicity were observed in offspring resulting from parents treated with 35 to 345 times the human dose.

FDA Pregnancy Category C.

### Breast-feeding

It is not known whether omeprazole is distributed into human milk. However, because omeprazole has been shown to cause tumorigenic and carcinogenic effects in animals, a decision should be made on whether nursing should be discontinued or the medication withdrawn, taking into account the importance of the omeprazole to the mother.

### Pediatrics

Appropriate studies on the relationship of age to the effects of omeprazole have not been performed in the pediatric population.

### Geriatrics

No information is available on the relationship of age to the effects of omeprazole in geriatric patients. However, a somewhat decreased rate of elimination and an increased bioavailability are more likely to occur in geriatric patients taking omeprazole.

### Pharmacogenetics

Pharmacokinetic studies in Asian subjects receiving single 20-mg doses of omeprazole showed an approximately fourfold increase in the area under the plasma concentration-time curve (AUC) as compared to Caucasian subjects. Dosage adjustments should be considered for Asian patients, especially for prophylaxis of recurrence of erosive esophagitis.

### Drug interactions and/or related problems

The following drug interactions and/or related problems have been selected on the basis of their potential clinical significance (possible mechanism

in parentheses where appropriate)—not necessarily inclusive (» = major clinical significance):

Note: Only specific interactions between omeprazole and other medications have been identified in this monograph. However, omeprazole, by increasing gastric pH, has the potential to affect the bioavailability of any medication for which absorption is pH-dependent. Also, omeprazole may prevent the degradation of acid-labile drugs.

In addition, because of omeprazole's ability to inhibit hepatic microsomal drug metabolism, elimination of other medications that require hepatic metabolism via the cytochrome P-450 system or that are highly extracted by the liver may be decreased during concurrent use with omeprazole.

Combinations containing any of the following medications, depending on the amount present, may also interact with this medication.

Ampicillin esters
Iron salts or
Ketoconazole
(omeprazole may increase gastrointestinal pH; concurrent use with omeprazole may result in a reduction in absorption of ampicillin esters, iron salts, or ketoconazole)

» Anticoagulants, coumarin- or indandione-derivative or
» Diazepam or
» Phenytoin
(inhibition of the cytochrome P-450 enzyme system by omeprazole, especially in high doses, may cause a decrease in the hepatic metabolism of these medications, which may result in delayed elimination and increased blood concentrations, when these medications are used concurrently with omeprazole)
(monitoring of blood concentrations, or prothrombin time for anticoagulants, is recommended as a guide to dosage since dosage adjustment of these medications may be necessary during and after omeprazole therapy to prevent bleeding due to anticoagulant potentiation)

Bone marrow depressants (see *Appendix II*)
(concurrent use of omeprazole with these medications may increase the leukopenic and/or thrombocytopenic effects of both these medications; if concurrent use is required, close observation for toxic effects should be considered)

**Laboratory value alterations**
The following have been selected on the basis of their potential clinical significance (possible effect in parentheses where appropriate)—not necessarily inclusive (» = major clinical significance):

With physiology/laboratory test values
Alanine aminotransferase (ALT [SGPT]) and
Alkaline phosphatase and
Aspartate aminotransferase (AST [SGOT])
(serum values may be increased)

Gastrin, serum
(concentrations will increase during the first 1 to 2 weeks of omeprazole therapy and return to normal after the medication is discontinued; this increase is probably due to the inhibition of acid secretion, which eliminates the negative feedback effect of acid on gastrin secretion; in addition to stimulating gastric acid secretion, gastrin promotes the growth and proliferation of endocrine or enterochromaffin-like [ECL] cells in the gastric mucosa)

**Medical considerations/Contraindications**
The medical considerations/contraindications included have been selected on the basis of their potential clinical significance (reasons given in parentheses where appropriate)—not necessarily inclusive (» = major clinical significance).

*Risk-benefit should be considered when the following medical problems exist:*

» Hepatic disease, chronic, current or history of
(dosage reduction may be required due to increased half-life in chronic hepatic disease)
Sensitivity to omeprazole

## Side/Adverse Effects

Note: Gastric fundic gland polyps have occurred rarely in patients receiving omeprazole; these appear to be benign and reversible upon discontinuance of omeprazole.

Gastroduodenal carcinoids have been reported in patients with Zollinger-Ellison syndrome who have received long-term omeprazole therapy. These carcinoids are believed to be a manifestation of the underlying syndrome, which is known to be associated with such tumors.

Atrophic gastritis has been noted occasionally in gastric corpus biopsies from patient receiving long-term omeprazole therapy.

The following side/adverse effects have been selected on the basis of their potential clinical significance (possible signs and symptoms in parentheses where appropriate)—not necessarily inclusive:

**Those indicating need for medical attention**
Incidence rare
*Hematologic abnormalities, specifically anemia* (unusual tiredness or weakness); *eosinopenia; leukocytosis* (sore throat and fever); *neutropenia* (continuing ulcers or sores in mouth); *pancytopenia or thrombocytopenia* (unusual bleeding or bruising); *hematuria* (bloody urine); *proteinuria* (cloudy urine); *urinary tract infection* (bloody or cloudy urine; difficult, burning, or painful urination; frequent urge to urinate)

**Those indicating need for medical attention only if they continue or are bothersome**
Incidence more frequent
*Abdominal pain or colic*
Incidence less frequent
*Asthenia* (muscle pain; unusual tiredness); *central nervous system (CNS) disturbances, specifically dizziness, headache, somnolence* (unusual drowsiness); *or unusual tiredness; chest pain; gastrointestinal disturbances, specifically acid regurgitation* (heartburn); *constipation; diarrhea or loose stools; flatulence* (gas); *or nausea and vomiting; skin rash or itching*

## Overdose

For more information on the management of overdose or unintentional ingestion, **contact a Poison Control Center** (see *Poison Control Center Listing*).

**Clinical effects of overdose**
The following effects have been selected on the basis of their potential clinical significance (possible signs and symptoms in parentheses where appropriate)—not necessarily inclusive:

*Blurred vision; confusion; diaphoresis* (increased sweating); *drowsiness; dryness of mouth; flushing; headache; nausea; tachycardia* (fast or irregular heartbeat)

**Treatment of overdose**
Since there is no specific antidote for overdose with omeprazole, treatment should be symptomatic and supportive. Due to extensive protein binding, omeprazole is not readily dialyzable. Patients in whom intentional overdose is confirmed or suspected should be referred for psychiatric consultation.

## Patient Consultation

As an aid to patient consultation, refer to *Advice for the Patient, Omeprazole (Systemic)*.
In providing consultation, consider emphasizing the following selected information (» = major clinical significance):

**Before using this medication**
» Conditions affecting use, especially:
Sensitivity to omeprazole
Breast-feeding—May be distributed into breast milk; may cause potentially serious adverse effects in nursing infants
Other medications, especially anticoagulants, diazepam, or phenytoin
Other medical problems, especially chronic hepatic disease or history of

**Proper use of this medication**
Taking the capsule form of this medication immediately before a meal, preferably the morning meal
May take antacids for relief of pain, unless otherwise instructed by physician
Swallowing capsule whole; not crushing, breaking, chewing, or opening the capsule
» Compliance with full course of therapy
» Proper dosing
Missed dose: Taking as soon as possible; not taking if almost time for next dose; not doubling doses
» Proper storage

**Precautions while using this medication**
Checking with physician if condition does not improve or worsens

**Side/adverse effects**
Signs of potential side effects, especially hematologic abnormalities, hematuria, proteinuria, and urinary tract infection

## General Dosing Information

For therapy of gastrointestinal reflux disease, omeprazole usually is used for short-term (4- to 8-week) courses; however, additional 4- to 8-week courses of treatment may be considered if there is recurrence of severe or symptomatic gastroesophageal reflux poorly responsive to customary medical treatment. Controlled studies of omeprazole used as maintenance therapy to prevent erosive eophagitis recurrence have not been conducted beyond 12 months, although a limited number of patients have received continuous maintenance treatment for up to 6 years. Dosage adjustments should be considered for Asian patients, especially for prophylaxis of erosive esophagitis recurrence, since pharmacokinetic studies in Asian subjects receiving single 20-mg doses of omeprazole showed an approximately fourfold increase in the area under the plasma concentration-time curve (AUC) as compared to Caucasian subjects.

Although the symptoms of duodenal ulcers may subside within 1 or 2 weeks after initiation of therapy, unless healing has been documented by endoscopic examination or x-rays, therapy should be continued for at least 4 to 6 weeks.

Omeprazole may be taken with antacids, especially for the first few doses, to aid in the relief of pain.

Initial titration of doses and subsequent dosage adjustment of omeprazole is recommended in the long-term treatment of pathological hypersecretory conditions (e.g., Zollinger-Ellison syndrome, systemic mastocytosis, multiple endocrine adenomas). Doses of up to 120 mg three times a day have been administered. Patients may require at least one increase in dose per year. If the daily dose is greater than 80 mg, it should be administered in divided doses. Zollinger-Ellison syndrome has been treated continuously with omeprazole for more than 5 years.

### Diet/Nutrition
Omeprazole capsules should be taken immediately before meals. Omeprazole tablets may be taken with food or on an empty stomach.

## Oral Dosage Forms

Note: Dosing recommendations vary between dosage forms; please check the appropriate section for dosage form–specific dosing recommendations.

### OMEPRAZOLE DELAYED-RELEASE CAPSULES

**Usual adult dose**
Gastroesophageal reflux disease (treatment)—
   Oral, 20 mg once a day for four to eight weeks.
   Note: A dosage of 40 mg once a day has been used for esophagitis associated with gastroesophageal reflux disease refractory to other treatment regimens.
Erosive esophagitis (prophylaxis)—
   Oral, 20 mg once a day.
Gastric hypersecretory conditions (e.g., Zollinger-Ellison syndrome, systemic mastocytosis, multiple endocrine adenomas)—
   Oral, 60 mg once a day, the dosage being adjusted as needed, and therapy continued for as long as clinically indicated. Doses of up to 120 mg three times a day have been used. If the total daily dose is greater than 80 mg, it should be administered in divided doses.
Duodenal ulcer—
   Oral, 20 mg once a day.
   Note: The dosage can be increased to 40 mg once a day for duodenal ulcer refractory to other treatment regimens.
Gastric ulcer (treatment)—
   Oral, 40 mg once a day for four to eight weeks.
Peptic ulcer associated with *Helicobacter pylori* infection—
   Oral, omeprazole 40 mg once a day taken in combination with clarithromycin 500 mg three times a day for the first fourteen days. For days 15 through 28, further treatment with omeprazole 20 mg once a day follows.

**Usual pediatric dose**
Dosage has not been established.

**Strength(s) usually available**
U.S.—
   10 mg (Rx) [*Prilosec*].
   20 mg (Rx) [*Prilosec*].
   40 mg (Rx) [*Prilosec*].
Canada—
   Not commercially available.

**Packaging and storage**
Store between 15 and 30 °C (59 and 86 °F), in a tight container, unless otherwise specified by manufacturer. Protect from light.

**Auxiliary labeling**
• Take before meals.
• Swallow capsules whole.

### OMEPRAZOLE MAGNESIUM DELAYED-RELEASE TABLETS

Note: The dosing and dosage forms of omeprazole magnesium are expressed in terms of omeprazole base.

**Usual adult dose**
Gastroesophageal reflux disease (treatment)—
   Oral, 20 mg once a day for the relief of heartburn and regurgitation. Some patients respond adequately to a dose of 10 mg once a day. In patients requiring maintenance therapy, doses of 10 mg once a day have been used. For the treatment of reflux esophagitis, 20 mg once a day is recommended. The dosage may be increased to 40 mg once a day for esophagitis refractory to other treatment regimens. In patients requiring maintenance therapy, doses of 10 mg once a day have been used. If reflux esophagitis recurs, the dose may be increased to 20 or 40 mg once a day.
Gastric hypersecretory conditions (e.g., Zollinger-Ellison syndrome, systemic mastocytosis, multiple endocrine adenomas)—
   Oral, 60 mg once a day, the dosage being adjusted as needed, and therapy continued for as long as clinically indicated. Doses of up to 120 mg three times a day have been used. If the total daily dose is greater than 80 mg, it should be administered in divided doses.
Duodenal ulcer—
   Oral, 20 mg once a day. The dosage may be increased to 40 mg once a day for duodenal ulcer refractory to other treatment regimens. In patients requiring maintenance therapy, doses of 10 mg once a day, increased to 20 or 40 mg once a day as needed, have been used.
Gastric ulcer (treatment)—
   Oral, 20 mg once a day for four to eight weeks. The dosage may be increased to 40 mg once a day for gastric ulcer refractory to other treatment regimens. In patients requiring maintenance therapy, doses of 20 mg once a day, increased to 40 mg once a day as needed, have been used.
Peptic ulcer associated with *H. pylori* infection—
   Oral, triple therapy regimens of omeprazole 20 mg, plus clarithromycin 500 mg, plus either amoxicillin 1000 mg or metronidazole 500 mg, in which all three medications are taken twice a day for seven days. These regimens are followed by further treatment with omeprazole, 20 mg a day for up to three weeks for active duodenal ulcer, and 20 to 40 mg a day for up to twelve weeks for active gastric ulcer.
Peptic ulcer, nonsteroidal anti-inflammatory drug–induced (treatment)—
   Oral, 20 mg once a day for four to eight weeks. In patients requiring maintenance therapy, doses of 20 mg once a day for up to six months have been used.

**Usual pediatric dose**
Dosage has not been established.
U.S.—
   Not commercially available.
Canada—
   10 mg (base) (Rx) [*Losec*].
   20 mg (base) (Rx) [*Losec*].

**Packaging and storage**
Store between 15 and 30 °C (59 and 86 °F), in a tight container, unless otherwise specified by manufacturer.

**Auxiliary labeling**
• Swallow tablets whole.

Revised: 08/05/96
Interim revision: 08/27/97; 08/13/98

# ONDANSETRON  Systemic

VA CLASSIFICATION (Primary): GA605
Commonly used brand name(s): *Zofran*.
Note: For a listing of dosage forms and brand names by country availability, see *Dosage Forms* section(s).

## Category
Antiemetic.

# Indications

## Accepted
**Nausea and vomiting, cancer chemotherapy–induced (prophylaxis)**—Ondansetron is indicated for the prevention of nausea and vomiting associated with initial and repeat courses of moderately or highly emetogenic cancer chemotherapy, including high-dose cisplatin.

Studies done to date comparing ondansetron to high-dose metoclopramide have shown ondansetron to be more effective in preventing nausea and vomiting induced by emetogenic chemotherapy agents during the acute phase lasting 24 hours after the start of chemotherapy.

The combination of ondansetron plus dexamethasone has been shown to provide better emetic control over cisplatin-induced emesis than ondansetron alone.

**Nausea and vomiting, postoperative (prophylaxis and treatment)**—Ondansetron is indicated for the prevention and treatment of postoperative nausea and vomiting. Patients at greatest risk of developing postoperative nausea and vomiting include patients who have previously experienced postoperative nausea, patients predisposed to motion sickness, and patients with high levels of preoperative anxiety. The incidence of postoperative nausea and vomiting is also higher in women and children than in men and adults, respectively. Routine prophylaxis is not recommended for patients in whom there is little expectation that postoperative nausea and vomiting will occur, except in cases in which the stress of vomiting may damage the operation site.

**Nausea and vomiting, radiotherapy-induced (prophylaxis)**—Ondansetron tablets are indicated for the prevention of nausea and vomiting associated with radiotherapy in patients receiving total body irradiation, or single high-dose fraction or daily fractions to the abdomen.

## Unaccepted
Ondansetron is not effective in preventing motion-induced nausea and vomiting.

# Pharmacology/Pharmacokinetics

## Physicochemical characteristics
Molecular weight—365.86.
pH—Injection: 3.3 to 4.

## Mechanism of action/Effect
**Antiemetic**—Ondansetron is a competitive, highly selective antagonist of 5-hydroxytryptamine (serotonin) subtype 3 ($5-HT_3$) receptors. $5-HT_3$ receptors are present peripherally on vagal nerve terminals and centrally in the area postrema of the brain. It is not certain whether ondansetron's action is mediated peripherally, centrally, or both. Cytotoxic drugs and radiation appear to damage gastrointestinal mucosa, causing the release of serotonin from the enterochromaffin cells of the gastrointestinal tract. Stimulation of $5-HT_3$ receptors causes transmission of sensory signals to the vomiting center via vagal afferent fibers to induce vomiting. By binding to $5-HT_3$ receptors, ondansetron blocks vomiting mediated by serotonin release.

Ondansetron has no dopamine-receptor antagonist activity.

## Other actions/effects
Multiple oral doses or multiday intravenous doses of ondansetron administered to healthy volunteers slowed colonic transit time. However, following single intravenous doses of 0.15 mg of ondansetron per kg of body weight (mg/kg), no effects were observed on esophageal motility, gastric motility, lower esophageal sphincter pressure, small intestine transit time, or plasma prolactin concentrations.

## Absorption
Ondansetron is well absorbed after oral administration and undergoes limited first-pass metabolism. The extent and rate of ondansetron's absorption following a single oral dose is greater in women than in men. However, it is not known if this difference is clinically significant.

## Distribution
The volume of distribution ($Vol_D$) in healthy young males following administration of 8 mg of ondansetron as an intravenous infusion over 5 minutes was about 160 L. Patients 4 to 12 years of age reportedly have a $Vol_D$ somewhat larger than do adults.

Thirty-six percent of circulating ondansetron is distributed into erythrocytes.

## Protein binding
High (70 to 76%).

## Biotransformation
Hepatic; extensive. Primarily hydroxylation, followed by glucuronide or sulfate conjugation.

## Half-life
The mean elimination half-life in adult cancer patients is 4 hours. Elderly patients tend to have an increased elimination half-life, while most pediatric patients less than 15 years of age have shorter mean terminal half-lives (range, 2.5 to 3 hours) than patients older than 15 years of age. Adults with mild to moderate hepatic impairment had a mean half-life of 9.2 hours, while those with severe hepatic impairment had a mean half-life prolonged to 20.6 hours.

A study performed in normal volunteers to evaluate the pharmacokinetics of a single 4-mg dose of ondansetron administered as a 5-minute intravenous infusion and as a single intramuscular injection showed that the mean elimination half-life was not affected by route of administration.

## Peak plasma concentration
Following administration of a single intravenous dose of 0.15 mg/kg to healthy volunteers, peak plasma concentrations of 102 to 106 nanograms per mL were observed in those from 19 to 74 years of age, and 170 nanograms per mL in those ≥ 75 years of age. Mean peak plasma concentrations in volunteers who received a single 4-mg dose of ondansetron via a 5-minute intravenous infusion or as a single intramuscular injection were 42.9 nanograms/mL at 10 minutes following the infusion, and 31.9 nanograms/mL at 41 minutes after intramuscular injection.

Following administration of a single oral dose of 8 mg of ondansetron to healthy volunteers:

| Age group (years) | Gender | Peak plasma concentration (nanograms per mL) |
|---|---|---|
| 19–40 | M | 26.2 |
|  | F | 42.7 |
| 61–74 | M | 24.1 |
|  | F | 52.4 |
| ≥75 | M | 37 |
|  | F | 46.1 |

The higher plasma concentrations in females may be attributed to slower clearance, smaller apparent $Vol_D$ (adjusted for weight), and higher absolute bioavailability in females than in males.

## Elimination
Predominantly hepatic; less than 5% of an intravenous dose of ondansetron is recovered unchanged in the urine.

Following administration of a single intravenous dose of 0.15 mg/kg to healthy volunteers, plasma clearance values were 0.381 liters per hour per kg of body weight (L/hr/kg) in subjects 9 to 40 years of age, 0.319 L/hr/kg in subjects 61 to 74 years of age, and 0.262 L/hr/kg in subjects ≥ 75 years of age.

Elderly patients tended to have lower clearance values than did younger adults, while most pediatric patients 4 to 12 years of age had greater clearance values than adults.

# Precautions to Consider

## Cross-sensitivity and/or related problems
Patients sensitive to granisetron or dolasetron may also be sensitive to ondansetron.

## Carcinogenicity
Carcinogenic effects were not seen in 2-year studies in rats and mice given ondansetron orally in doses up to 10 and 30 mg per kg of body weight (mg/kg) per day, respectively.

## Mutagenicity
Standard tests showed no mutagenic activity of ondansetron.

## Pregnancy/Reproduction
**Fertility**—Ondansetron had no effect on the fertility or reproductive performance of male and female rats when given in oral doses up to 15 mg/kg per day.

**Pregnancy**—Adequate and well-controlled studies in humans have not been done.

Studies in pregnant rats and rabbits given intravenous doses of up to 4 mg/kg per day, and oral doses of up to 15 and 30 mg/kg per day, respectively, have not shown that ondansetron causes adverse effects in the fetus.

FDA Pregnancy Category B.

## Breast-feeding
It is not known whether ondansetron is distributed into human breast milk. However, ondansetron is distributed into the milk of rats.

## Pediatrics
Studies performed to date that included cancer patients 4 to 18 years of age and postoperative patients 2 to 12 years of age have not demonstrated pediatrics-specific problems that would limit the usefulness of ondansetron in children.

### Geriatrics
Studies performed to date that included cancer patients over 65 years of age have not demonstrated geriatrics-specific problems that would limit the usefulness of ondansetron in the elderly.

### Drug interactions and/or related problems
The following drug interactions and/or related problems have been selected on the basis of their potential clinical significance (possible mechanism in parentheses where appropriate)—not necessarily inclusive (» = major clinical significance):

Enzyme inducers, hepatic, cytochrome P450 (see *Appendix II*) or
Enzyme inhibitors, hepatic, various (see *Appendix II*)
   (because ondansetron is metabolized by hepatic cytochrome P450 enzymes, inducers or inhibitors of these enzymes potentially may alter its clearance and half-life; ondansetron does not appear to induce or inhibit the cytochrome P450 enzyme system of the liver)

### Laboratory value alterations
The following have been selected on the basis of their potential clinical significance (possible effect in parentheses where appropriate)—not necessarily inclusive (» = major clinical significance):

With physiology/laboratory test values
   Alanine aminotransferase (ALT [SGPT]) and
   Aspartate aminotransferase (AST [SGOT])
      (values may be increased; increases reportedly are transient and unrelated to dose or duration of therapy)
   Bilirubin, serum
      (concentrations may be increased; increases reportedly are transient and unrelated to dose or duration of therapy)

### Medical considerations/Contraindications
The medical considerations/contraindications included have been selected on the basis of their potential clinical significance (reasons given in parentheses where appropriate)—not necessarily inclusive (» = major clinical significance).

*Risk-benefit should be considered when the following medical problems exist:*

Hepatic function impairment
   (use of ondansetron may result in increases in hepatic enzymes)
Surgery, abdominal
   (use of ondansetron may mask a progressive ileus and/or gastric distension)
Sensitivity to ondansetron, granisetron, or dolasetron

## Side/Adverse Effects
Note: Since ondansetron is used in conjunction with cancer chemotherapeutic agents, it is difficult to attribute some side effects, such as diarrhea and fever, to ondansetron alone.

Signs and symptoms consistent with extrapyramidal effects have been reported in a very small number of patients receiving ondansetron; however, a causal relationship has not been established.

The following side/adverse effects have been selected on the basis of their potential clinical significance (possible signs and symptoms in parentheses where appropriate)—not necessarily inclusive:

**Those indicating need for medical attention**
Incidence rare
   *Anaphylaxis* (hypotension; skin rash, hives, and/or itching; troubled breathing); *bronchospasm* (shortness of breath, tightness in chest, troubled breathing, or wheezing); *chest pain; injection site reactions* (pain, redness, and burning at site of injection)

**Those indicating need for medical attention only if they continue or are bothersome**
Incidence more frequent
   *Constipation; diarrhea; fever; headache*
Incidence less frequent or rare
   *Abdominal pain or stomach cramps; cold sensation* (feeling cold); *dizziness or lightheadedness; drowsiness; dryness of mouth; paresthesias* (burning, tingling, or prickling sensations); *pruritus* (itching); *skin rash; unusual tiredness or weakness*

## Overdose
For information on the management of overdose or unintentional ingestion, **contact a Poison Control Center** (see *Poison Control Center Listing*).

### Clinical effects of overdose
Individual doses as large as 145 mg and total daily dosages as large as 252 mg have been administered intravenously without significant adverse events.

Hypotension and faintness occurred in a patient that ingested 48 mg of oral ondansetron. Sudden blindness (amaurosis) of 2 to 3 minutes' duration plus severe constipation occurred in another patient that was administered a single dose of 72 mg of ondansetron intravenously. A vasovagal episode with transient second degree heart block was observed in another patient following the infusion of 32 mg of ondansetron over a 4-minute period. In all cases, the events resolved completely.

### Treatment of overdose
There is no specific antidote for ondansetron overdose.

Supportive care—Patients should be managed with appropriate supportive therapy. Patients in whom intentional overdose is confirmed or suspected should be referred for psychiatric evaluation.

## Patient Consultation
As an aid to patient consultation, refer to *Advice for the Patient, Ondansetron (Systemic)*.

In providing consultation, consider emphasizing the following selected information (» = major clinical significance):

**Before using this medication**
» Conditions affecting use, especially:
   Sensitivity to ondansetron, granisetron, or dolasetron

**Proper use of this medication**
Taking additional dose if vomiting occurs within 30 minutes after a dose; checking with doctor if vomiting persists
» Proper dosing
   Missed dose: Taking missed dose as soon as possible if nausea or vomiting occurs
» Proper storage

**Side/adverse effects**
Signs of potential side effects, especially anaphylaxis, bronchospasm, chest pain, or injection site reactions

## Oral Dosage Forms
Note: The oral dosage form of ondansetron is indicated for prevention of nausea and vomiting induced by *moderately* emetogenic cancer chemotherapy. For prophylaxis against nausea and vomiting induced by *highly* emetogenic chemotherapeutic agents, the injection dosage form is recommended.

### ONDANSETRON HYDROCHLORIDE ORAL SOLUTION

**Usual adult and adolescent dose**
Nausea and vomiting, cancer chemotherapy–induced (prophylaxis)—
   Initial: Oral, 8 mg thirty minutes prior to chemotherapy.
   Post-chemotherapy: Oral, 8 mg eight hours after the initial dose, followed by 8 mg every twelve hours for one to two days.
Nausea and vomiting, postoperative (prophylaxis)—
   Oral, 16 mg one hour prior to induction of anesthesia.
Nausea and vomiting, radiotherapy-induced (prophylaxis)—
   Initial: Oral, 8 mg one to two hours prior to radiotherapy.
   Post-radiotherapy: Oral, 8 mg every eight hours.

Note: In patients with hepatic function impairment, the maximum recommended dose of ondansetron is 8 mg a day.

**Usual pediatric dose**
Nausea and vomiting, cancer chemotherapy–induced (prophylaxis)—
   Children up to 4 years of age:
      Dosage has not been established.
   Children 4 to 12 years of age:
      Initial—Oral, 4 mg thirty minutes prior to chemotherapy.
      Post-chemotherapy—Oral, 4 mg four and eight hours after the initial dose, followed by 4 mg every eight hours for one to two days.
   Children 12 years of age and older:
      See *Usual adult and adolescent dose*.
Nausea and vomiting, postoperative (prophylaxis) or
Nausea and vomiting, radiotherapy-induced (prophylaxis)—
   Dosage has not been established.

**Usual geriatric dose**
See *Usual adult and adolescent dose*.

U.S.—
   4 mg per 5 mL (Rx) [*Zofran* (strawberry flavored; sorbitol; citric acid anhydrous; sodium benzoate; sodium citrate)].

Canada—
   4 mg per 5 mL (Rx) [*Zofran* (strawberry flavored; sorbitol; citric acid anhydrous; sodium benzoate; sodium citrate dihydrate)].

**Packaging and storage**
Store between 15 and 30 °C (59 and 86 °F), unless otherwise specified by manufacturer. Protect from light. Store bottles upright in cartons.

## ONDANSETRON HYDROCHLORIDE TABLETS

**Usual adult and adolescent dose**
See *Ondansetron Hydrochloride Oral Solution.*

**Usual pediatric dose**
See *Ondansetron Hydrochloride Oral Solution.*

**Usual geriatric dose**
See *Ondansetron Hydrochloride Oral Solution.*

**Strength(s) usually available**
U.S.—
- 4 mg (Rx) [*Zofran* (lactose; microcrystalline cellulose; pregelatinized starch; hydroxypropyl methylcellulose; magnesium stearate; titanium dioxide; sodium benzoate)].
- 8 mg (Rx) [*Zofran* (lactose; microcrystalline cellulose; pregelatinized starch; hydroxypropyl methylcellulose; magnesium stearate; titanium dioxide; iron oxide)].

Canada—
- 4 mg (Rx) [*Zofran* (lactose; microcrystalline cellulose; pregelatinized starch; magnesium stearate; methyl hydroxypropyl cellulose; Opadry yellow; Opaspray yellow [containing titanium dioxide and iron oxide yellow])].
- 8 mg (Rx) [*Zofran* (lactose; microcrystalline cellulose; pregelatinized starch; magnesium stearate; methyl hydroxypropyl cellulose; Opadry yellow; Opaspray yellow [containing titanium dioxide and iron oxide yellow])].

**Packaging and storage**
Store between 2 and 30 °C (36 and 86 °F), unless otherwise specified by manufacturer. Protect from light.

## Parenteral Dosage Forms

### ONDANSETRON HYDROCHLORIDE INJECTION

**Usual adult dose**
Nausea and vomiting, cancer chemotherapy–induced (prophylaxis)—
Intravenous, 32 mg administered over fifteen minutes prior to chemotherapy. Alternatively, three doses of 150 mcg (0.15 mg) per kg of body weight, each administered over fifteen minutes, with the initial dose beginning thirty minutes prior to chemotherapy, and subsequent doses administered four and eight hours after the first dose. Or, 8 mg administered over fifteen minutes beginning thirty minutes prior to chemotherapy, followed immediately by a continuous infusion of 1 mg per hour for up to twenty-four hours.

Nausea and vomiting, postoperative (prophylaxis)—
Intravenous, 4 mg administered over not less than thirty seconds and preferably over two to five minutes, beginning immediately prior to induction of anesthesia. Alternatively, 4 mg may be administered undiluted as a single intramuscular injection.

Nausea and vomiting, postoperative (treatment)—
Intravenous, 4 mg administered over not less than thirty seconds and preferably over two to five minutes, given postoperatively if nausea or vomiting occur. Alternatively, 4 mg may be administered undiluted as a single intramuscular injection.

Note: In patients with severe hepatic function impairment, the maximum recommended dose of ondansetron is 8 mg a day, infused over 15 minutes beginning 30 minutes before the start of emetogenic chemotherapy.

**Usual pediatric dose**
Nausea and vomiting, cancer chemotherapy–induced (prophylaxis)—
Children up to 4 years of age: Dosage has not been established.
Children 4 to 18 years of age: Intravenous, three doses of 150 mcg (0.15 mg) per kg of body weight, each administered over fifteen minutes, with the initial dose beginning thirty minutes prior to chemotherapy, and subsequent doses administered four and eight hours after the first dose. Alternatively, 3 to 5 mg per square meter of body surface area administered over fifteen minutes beginning immediately prior to chemotherapy, followed after therapy by oral ondansetron 4 mg every eight hours for up to five days.

Nausea and vomiting, postoperative—
Children up to 2 years of age: Dosage has not been established.
Children 2 to 12 years of age: Intravenous, a single dose of 150 mcg (0.15 mg) per kg of body weight for those weighing 40 kg or less, or a single 4-mg dose for those weighing more than 40 kg, administered over not less than thirty seconds and preferably over two to five minutes.

**Usual geriatric dose**
See *Usual adult dose.*

**Strength(s) usually available**
U.S.—
- 2 mg per mL (Rx) [*Zofran* (sodium chloride; citric acid monohydrate 0.5 mg; sodium citrate dihydrate 0.25 mg; [may contain methylparaben 1.2 mg, propylparaben 0.15 mg])].
- 32 mg per 50 mL (premixed) (Rx) [*Zofran* (dextrose 2500 mg; citric acid 26 mg; sodium citrate 11.5 mg)].

Canada—
- 2 mg per mL (Rx) [*Zofran*].

**Packaging and storage**
Store between 2 and 30 °C (36 and 86 °F), unless otherwise specified by manufacturer. Protect from light. Do not freeze.

**Preparation of dosage form**
For intravenous administration—The manufacturer recommends that the dose of ondansetron be diluted in 50 mL of 5% dextrose injection or 0.9% sodium chloride injection; however, ondansetron also has been shown to be stable in dextrose and sodium chloride injections, 3% sodium chloride injection, 10% mannitol injection, and Ringer's injection.

**Stability**
Intravenous infusions of ondansetron retain their potency for 48 hours at room temperature under normal lighting after dilution with 5% dextrose injection, dextrose and sodium chloride injections, 0.9% sodium chloride injection, and 3% sodium chloride injection.

**Incompatibilities**
The following medications may be incompatible with ondansetron and should be avoided in admixtures: acyclovir, allopurinol, aminophylline, amphotericin B, ampicillin, ampicillin and sulbactam, amsacrine, cefepime, cefoperazone, furosemide, ganciclovir, lorazepam, methylprednisolone, mezlocillin, piperacillin, and sargramostim. In addition, alkaline solutions and fluorouracil in concentrations greater than 0.8 mg per mL have been shown to be physically incompatible with ondansetron.

**Caution**
Occasionally, ondansetron precipitates at the stopper/vial interface in vials stored upright. If a precipitate is observed, resolubilize by shaking the vial vigorously. Potency and stability are not affected.

## Selected Bibliography

Markham A, Sorkin EM, Ondansetron. An update of its therapeutic use in chemotherapy-induced and postoperative nausea and vomiting. Drugs 1993; 45: 931-52.

Revised: 06/24/98

# OPIOID (NARCOTIC) ANALGESICS  Systemic

This monograph includes information on the following: 1) Butorphanol†; 2) Codeine; 3) Hydrocodone‡; 4) Hydromorphone; 5) Levorphanol; 6) Meperidine; 7) Methadone; 8) Morphine; 9) Nalbuphine; 10) Opium; 11) Oxycodone; 12) Oxymorphone; 13) Pentazocine; 14) Propoxyphene

Note: See also individual *Buprenorphine (Systemic)* and *Dezocine (Systemic)* monographs.
See also *Fentanyl Derivatives (Systemic)* for information on alfentanil, fentanyl, and sufentanil.

INN:
Meperidine—Pethidine
Propoxyphene—Dextropropoxyphene

VA CLASSIFICATION (Primary/Secondary):
Butorphanol—CN101/CN206
Codeine
    Oral—CN101/RE301; GA400
    Parenteral—CN101/GA400
Hydrocodone—CN101/RE301
Hydromorphone
    Oral—CN101/RE301
    Parenteral—CN101/CN206; RE301
    Rectal—CN101
Levorphanol
    Oral—CN101
    Parenteral—CN101/CN206

Meperidine
    Oral—CN101
    Parenteral—CN101/CN206
Methadone—CN101/AD900; RE301
Morphine
    Oral—CN101/RE301; GA400
    Parenteral—CN101/CN206; RE301; GA400
    Rectal—CN101/RE301
Nalbuphine—CN101/CN206
Opium
    Oral—GA400/CN101
    Parenteral—CN101
Oxycodone—CN101
Oxymorphone
    Parenteral—CN101/CN206
    Rectal—CN101
Pentazocine
    Oral—CN101
    Parenteral—CN101/CN206
Propoxyphene—CN101

Note: Controlled substance classification—

| Drug | U.S. | Canada |
|---|---|---|
| Butorphanol | II | †† |
| Codeine | II | N |
| Hydrocodone | ‡‡ | N |
| Hydromorphone | II | N |
| Levorphanol | II | N |
| Meperidine | II | N |
| Methadone | II | N§§ |
| Morphine | II | N |
| Nalbuphine | ** | C |
| Opium | II | N |
| Oxycodone | II | N |
| Oxymorphone | II | N |
| Pentazocine | IV | N |
| Propoxyphene | IV | N |

**Not a controlled substance in the U.S.
††Not commercially available in Canada.
‡‡Commercially available in the U.S. only in combination with other active ingredients.
§§Available in Canada only through practitioners authorized to treat opioid addicts.

Commonly used brand name(s): 642[14]; Astramorph PF[8]; Cotanal-65[14]; Darvon[14]; Darvon-N[14]; Demerol[6]; Dilaudid[4]; Dilaudid-5[4]; Dilaudid-HP[4]; Dolophine[7]; Duramorph[8]; Epimorph[8]; Hycodan[3]; Hydrostat IR[4]; Levo-Dromoran[5]; M S Contin[8]; M-Eslon[8]; M.O.S.[8]; M.O.S.-S.R[8]; MS IR[8]; MS/L[8]; MS/L Concentrate[8]; MS/S[8]; MSIR[8]; Methadose[7]; Morphine Extra-Forte[8]; Morphine Forte[8]; Morphine H.P[8]; Morphitec[8]; Nubain[9]; Numorphan[12]; OMS Concentrate[8]; Oramorph SR[8]; PMS-Hydromorphone[4]; PMS-Hydromorphone Syrup[4]; PP-Cap[14]; Pantopon[10]; Paveral[2]; RMS Uniserts[8]; Rescudose[8]; Robidone[3]; Roxanol[8]; Roxanol[8]; Roxanol 100[8]; Roxanol UD[8]; Roxicodone[11]; Roxicodone Intensol[11]; Stadol[1]; Statex[8]; Statex Drops[8]; Supeudol[11]; Talwin[13]; Talwin-Nx[13].

Other commonly used names are: Dextropropoxyphene [Propoxyphene] Dihydromorphinone [Hydromorphone] Laudanum [Opium Tincture] Levorphan [Levorphanol] Pethidine [Meperidine] Papaveretum [Opium (Parenteral)]

Note: For a listing of dosage forms and brand names by country availability, see *Dosage Forms* section(s).

‡Commercially available in the U.S. only in combination with other active ingredients. See *Cough/Cold Combinations (Systemic)*, *Opioid (Narcotic) Analgesics and Acetaminophen (Systemic)*, and *Opioid (Narcotic) Analgesics and Aspirin (Systemic)*.

†Not commercially available in Canada.

## Category

Note: All of the opioid analgesics have similar pharmacologic actions; however, clinical uses among specific agents may vary because of actual pharmacokinetic differences, differences in potential for causing adverse effects, lack of specific testing, and/or lack of clinical-use data.

Analgesic—Butorphanol; Codeine; Hydrocodone; Hydromorphone; Levorphanol; Meperidine; Methadone; Morphine; Nalbuphine; Opium; Oxycodone; Oxymorphone; Pentazocine; Propoxyphene

Note: Butorphanol, nalbuphine, and pentazocine are opioid agonist/antagonist analgesics; the other agents in this group are opioid agonist analgesics.

Anesthesia adjunct (opioid analgesic)—Parenteral dosage forms only: Butorphanol; Hydromorphone; Levorphanol; Meperidine; Morphine; Nalbuphine; Oxymorphone; Pentazocine

Note: For other opioids used primarily as anesthesia adjuncts, see *Fentanyl Derivatives (Systemic)*.

Antidiarrheal—Codeine; Morphine; Opium Tincture

Note: For other opioids used only as antidiarrheals, see individual monograph listings for *Difenoxin and Atropine*, *Diphenoxylate and Atropine*, *Loperamide*, and *Paregoric*.

Antitussive—Codeine (oral dosage forms only); Hydrocodone; Hydromorphone; Methadone; Morphine

Note: For use of hydromorphone as an antitussive, see *Cough-Cold Combinations (Systemic)—Hydromorphone and Guaifenesin*.

Suppressant (narcotic abstinence syndrome)—Methadone; Opium Tincture.

Pulmonary edema therapy adjunct—Morphine.

## Indications

Note: Bracketed information in the *Indications* section refers to uses that are not included in U.S. product labeling.

**Accepted**

Pain (treatment)—Morphine, methadone, and parenteral opium are indicated for relief of severe pain; codeine and propoxyphene are indicated for relief of mild to moderate pain; and the other opioid analgesics are indicated for relief of moderate to severe pain.

Epidural or intrathecal administration of small doses of opioid analgesics may provide prolonged pain relief. Although administration via these routes may decrease the risk of some side/adverse effects, respiratory depression may occur. Solutions containing a preservative must *not* be used. Only morphine sulfate is currently commercially available in a dosage form that is FDA–approved for administration via these routes.

For relief of pain due to acute myocardial infarction, morphine is usually considered the drug of choice. Butorphanol and pentazocine are less desirable than other opioid analgesics for this purpose because they have cardiovascular effects that tend to increase cardiac work. Although nalbuphine has not been reported to adversely affect cardiovascular function in patients with acute myocardial infarction (and may be less likely than morphine to cause hypotension), its effects in patients with severely compromised cardiac function caused by acute myocardial infarction have not been fully determined. Therefore, these agents should be used with caution in such patients.

Parenterally administered opioid analgesics (except for methadone) are indicated to provide obstetrical analgesia.

Controlled clinical studies have shown that intrathecal, but not epidural, administration of opioid analgesics provides adequate relief of labor pain. Only a preservative-free solution should be used. Morphine sulfate is the only opioid analgesic currently commercially available in a dosage form that is FDA–approved for administration via these routes.

Anesthesia, general or local, adjunct—Parenteral dosage forms of butorphanol, [hydromorphone], levorphanol, meperidine, morphine, nalbuphine, oxymorphone, and pentazocine are indicated to supplement general, regional, or local anesthesia. During surgery, they are often used in conjunction with other agents, such as a combination of an ultrashort-acting barbiturate, a neuromuscular blocking agent, and an inhalation anesthetic (usually nitrous oxide), for the maintenance of "balanced" anesthesia.

Parenteral dosage forms of most opioid analgesics are indicated to provide analgesic, antianxiety, and sedative effects as presurgical medication. However, other medications, such as benzodiazepines, are more commonly used if the patient is not in pain.

Diarrhea (treatment)—[Codeine][1], [morphine], and opium tincture are indicated for treatment of diarrhea. In diarrhea caused by poisoning, these agents should not be used until the toxic material has been eliminated from the gastrointestinal tract.

Cough (treatment)—Although only codeine (oral dosage forms), hydrocodone, and hydromorphone are indicated as antitussives, all opioid analgesics depress the cough reflex. Meperidine, oxymorphone, and propoxyphene have relatively less antitussive activity than other opioid analgesics, especially in low or moderate doses.

[Methadone and morphine are sometimes used as antitussives when severe pain is present and coughing cannot be relieved by other means.]

Opioid (narcotic) abstinence syndrome (prophylaxis and treatment); or

Opioid (narcotic) drug use, illicit (treatment)—Methadone is indicated as a suppressant to permit detoxification. Oral methadone is also indicated as maintenance therapy to discourage addicts from returning to illicit use of other opioid drugs.

Edema, pulmonary, acute (treatment adjunct)—Morphine is indicated as adjunctive therapy in the treatment of acute pulmonary edema secondary to left ventricular failure.

Oxymorphone is also FDA–approved as an adjunct in the treatment of acute pulmonary edema. However, oxymorphone is rarely if ever used for this indication; morphine is the preferred medication.

[Opioid (narcotic) dependence, neonatal (treatment)]—Opium tincture is used in diluted form in the treatment of neonatal opioid dependence.

### Unaccepted
Methadone is not recommended for obstetrical analgesia because its long duration of action increases the risk of neonatal respiratory depression.

[1]Not included in Canadian product labeling.

## Pharmacology/Pharmacokinetics
See *Table 1*, page 2190 and *Table 2* page 2191.

### Physicochemical characteristics
Molecular weight—
 Butorphanol tartrate: 477.55.
 Codeine phosphate: 406.37 (hemihydrate); 397.36 (anhydrous).
 Codeine sulfate: 750.86 (trihydrate); 696.81 (anhydrous).
 Hydrocodone bitartrate: 494.50 (hydrate); 449.46 (anhydrous).
 Hydromorphone hydrochloride: 321.80.
 Levorphanol tartrate: 443.49 (dihydrate); 407.46 (anhydrous).
 Meperidine hydrochloride: 283.80.
 Methadone hydrochloride: 345.91.
 Morphine sulfate: 758.83 (pentahydrate); 668.76 (anhydrous).
 Nalbuphine hydrochloride: 393.91.
 Oxycodone hydrochloride: 351.83.
 Oxymorphone hydrochloride: 337.80.
 Pentazocine hydrochloride: 321.89.
 Pentazocine lactate: 375.51.
 Propoxyphene hydrochloride: 375.94.
 Propoxyphene napsylate: 565.72 (monohydrate); 547.71 (anhydrous).

### Mechanism of action/Effect
Opioid analgesics bind with stereospecific receptors at many sites within the central nervous system (CNS) to alter processes affecting both the perception of pain and the emotional response to pain. Although the precise sites and mechanisms of action have not been fully determined, alterations in release of various neurotransmitters from afferent nerves sensitive to painful stimuli may be partially responsible for the analgesic effects. When these medications are used as adjuncts to anesthesia, analgesic actions may provide dose-related protection against hemodynamic responses to surgical stress.

It has been proposed that there are multiple subtypes of opioid receptors, each mediating various therapeutic and/or side effects of opioid drugs. The actions of an opioid analgesic may therefore depend upon its binding affinity for each type of receptor and on whether it acts as a full agonist or a partial agonist or is inactive at each type of receptor.

At least two types of opioid receptors (mu and kappa) mediate analgesia. A third type of receptor (sigma) may not mediate analgesia; actions at this receptor may produce the subjective and psychotomimetic effects characteristic of pentazocine and, to a lesser extent, butorphanol and nalbuphine. Morphine and other opioid agonists exert their agonist activity primarily at the mu receptor, whereas buprenorphine, nalbuphine, and pentazocine exert agonist activity at the kappa and sigma receptors. Mu receptors are widely distributed throughout the CNS, especially in the limbic system (frontal cortex, temporal cortex, amygdala, and hippocampus), thalamus, striatum, hypothalamus, and midbrain as well as laminae I, II, IV, and V of the dorsal horn in the spinal cord. Kappa receptors are localized primarily in the spinal cord and in the cerebral cortex.

Nalbuphine and pentazocine may displace opioids having only agonist activity from their receptor binding sites and competitively inhibit their actions. The medications may therefore precipitate withdrawal symptoms in patients who are physically dependent on such agonists. Butorphanol appears to have no significant antagonist activity at the mu receptor; in some studies, it failed to produce withdrawal symptoms in patients physically dependent on morphine. However, butorphanol does not substitute for mu-receptor agonists sufficiently to prevent or attenuate withdrawal symptoms caused by abrupt discontinuation of these agonists in physically dependent patients. Also, opioid agonist/antagonist drugs share several pharmacologic actions that differ from those of opioids having only agonist activity; i.e., different respiratory depressant, subjective, psychotomimetic, and hemodynamic effects; lower dependence liability; and reduced severity of withdrawal symptoms produced when they are discontinued after prolonged use.

Antidiarrheal—
 Act locally and possibly centrally to alter intestinal motility.

Antitussive—
 Suppress the cough reflex by a direct central action, probably in the medulla or pons.

Suppressant (narcotic abstinence syndrome)—
 Substitute for other opioid drugs when administered orally and prevent or attenuate withdrawal symptoms during detoxification. Withdrawal symptoms that may occur when the substituted opioid is discontinued are usually greatly reduced in severity. With continued administration, methadone may produce cross-tolerance to the euphoric effects of other opioid drugs, thereby reducing the patient's desire for such drugs.

### Biotransformation
Hepatic; also in intestinal mucosa.

## Precautions to Consider

### Pregnancy/Reproduction
Pregnancy—Risk-benefit must be considered because opioid analgesics cross the placenta. Regular use during pregnancy may cause physical dependence in the fetus, leading to withdrawal symptoms (convulsions, irritability, excessive crying, tremors, hyperactive reflexes, fever, vomiting, diarrhea, sneezing, and yawning) in the neonate. Use of methadone by pregnant women participating in methadone maintenance programs has also been associated with fetal distress in utero and low birth weight.

For butorphanol, nalbuphine, pentazocine, and propoxyphene: Although studies in humans have not been done, studies in animals have not shown that these agents cause adverse effects on fetal development (Pentazocine and naloxone tablets—FDA Pregnancy Category C).

For codeine, hydrocodone, hydromorphone, morphine, and opium: Although teratogenic effects in humans have not been documented, controlled studies have not been done. Studies in animals have shown codeine (single dose of 100 mg per kg) to cause delayed ossification in mice and (in doses of 120 mg per kg) increased resorptions in rats, and hydrocodone, hydromorphone, and morphine to be teratogenic in very high doses (FDA Pregnancy Category C).

For levorphanol, meperidine, methadone, oxycodone, and oxymorphone: Although teratogenic effects in humans have not been documented, controlled studies have not been done.

Labor and delivery—Opioid analgesics, including epidurally or intrathecally administered opioids, readily enter the fetal circulation when used during labor and may cause respiratory depression in the neonate, especially the premature neonate. These agents should be used with caution, if at all, during the delivery of a premature infant. Methadone is not recommended for obstetrical analgesia because its long duration of action increases the risk of neonatal respiratory depression. Also, morphine, hydromorphone, codeine, and possibly other opioids may prolong labor. Intrathecal administration of up to 1 mg of morphine sulfate has little effect on the first stage of labor but may prolong the second stage of labor.

### Breast-feeding
Problems in humans with most opioid analgesics have not been documented. Butorphanol, codeine, meperidine, methadone, morphine, and propoxyphene are distributed into breast milk. Information concerning the excretion of other opioid analgesics in breast milk is lacking. With usual analgesic doses, concentrations of those drugs known to be distributed into breast milk are generally low. However, risk-benefit must be considered when methadone is administered to a nursing mother in a methadone maintenance program because use of maintenance doses may cause physical dependence in the infant.

### Pediatrics
Children up to 2 years of age may be more susceptible to the effects, especially the respiratory depressant effects, of these medications.

Paradoxical excitation is especially likely to occur in pediatric patients receiving opioid analgesics.

### Geriatrics
Geriatric patients may be more susceptible to the effects, especially the respiratory depressant effects, of these medications. Also, geriatric patients are more likely to have prostatic hypertrophy or obstruction and age-related renal function impairment, and are therefore more likely to be adversely affected by opioid-induced urinary retention. In addition, geriatric patients may metabolize or eliminate these medications more slowly than younger adults. Lower doses or longer dosing intervals than those usually recommended for adults may be required, and are usually therapeutically effective, for these patients.

### Dental
Opioid analgesics may decrease or inhibit salivary flow, thus contributing to the development of caries, periodontal disease, oral candidiasis, and discomfort.

### Drug interactions and/or related problems
See *Table 3,* page 2193.

### Laboratory value alterations
The following have been selected on the basis of their potential clinical significance (possible effect in parentheses where appropriate)—not necessarily inclusive (» = major clinical significance):

With diagnostic test results
   Gastric emptying studies
      (opioid analgesics delay gastric emptying, thereby invalidating test results)
   Hepatobiliary imaging using technetium Tc 99m disofenin
      (delivery of technetium Tc 99m disofenin to the small bowel may be prevented because opioid analgesics [except for butorphanol] may cause constriction of the sphincter of Oddi and increased biliary tract pressure; these actions result in delayed visualization and thus resemble obstruction of the common bile duct)

With physiology/laboratory test values
   Cerebrospinal fluid (CSF) pressure
      (may be increased; effect is secondary to respiratory depression–induced carbon dioxide retention)
   Plasma amylase activity and
   Plasma lipase activity
      (may be increased because opioid analgesics [except butorphanol] can cause contractions of the sphincter of Oddi and increased biliary tract pressure; the diagnostic utility of determinations of these enzymes may be compromised for up to 24 hours after the medication has been given)
   Serum alanine aminotransferase (ALT [SGPT]) and
   Serum alkaline phosphatase and
   Serum aspartate aminotransferase (AST [SGOT]) and
   Serum bilirubin and
   Serum lactate dehydrogenase (LDH)
      (activity may be increased in patients receiving propoxyphene)

### Medical considerations/Contraindications
The medical considerations/contraindications included have been selected on the basis of their potential clinical significance (reasons given in parentheses where appropriate)—not necessarily inclusive (» = major clinical significance).

*Except under special circumstances, this medication should not be used when the following medical problems exist:*

*For all opioid analgesic usage*
» Diarrhea associated with pseudomembranous colitis caused by cephalosporins, lincomycins (possibly including topical clindamycin), or penicillins or
» Diarrhea caused by poisoning, until toxic material has been eliminated from gastrointestinal tract
      (opioid analgesics may slow elimination of toxic material, thereby worsening and/or prolonging the diarrhea)
» Respiratory depression, acute
      (may be exacerbated)

*For epidural or intrathecal administration*
» Any condition that precludes epidural or intrathecal administration, such as:
» Coagulation defects caused by anticoagulant therapy or hematologic disorders
      (trauma to a blood vessel during administration may result in uncontrollable CNS or soft tissue hemorrhage)
» Infection at or near site of administration
      (risk of spreading the infection into the CNS)

*Risk-benefit should be considered when the following medical problems exist:*

*For all opioid analgesics*
   Abdominal conditions, acute
      (diagnosis or clinical course may be obscured)
   Allergic reaction to the opioid analgesic considered for use, history of
» Asthma, acute attack or
» Respiratory impairment or disease, chronic
      (opioids may decrease respiratory drive and increase airway resistance in patients with these conditions)
   Cardiac arrhythmias or
   Convulsions, history of
      (may be induced or exacerbated by opioids; meperidine and propoxyphene may be especially likely to induce or exacerbate convulsions; with meperidine, the proconvulsant activity of its metabolite normeperidine may be responsible)
   Drug abuse or dependence, current or history of, including alcoholism, or
   Emotional instability or
   Suicidal ideation or attempts
      (patient predisposition to drug abuse)
   Gallbladder disease or gallstones
      (opioids [except butorphanol] may cause biliary contraction)
   Gastrointestinal tract surgery, recent
      (opioids may alter gastrointestinal motility)
   Head injury or
   Increased intracranial pressure, pre-existing or
   Intracranial lesions
      (risk of respiratory depression and further elevation of cerebrospinal fluid pressure is increased; also, opioids may cause sedation and pupillary changes that may obscure clinical course of head injury)
   Hepatic function impairment
      (opioids metabolized in liver)
   Hypothyroidism
      (risk of respiratory depression and prolonged CNS depression is greatly increased)
» Inflammatory bowel disease, severe
      (risk of toxic megacolon may be increased, especially with repeated dosing)
   Prostatic hypertrophy or obstruction or
   Urethral stricture or
   Urinary tract surgery, recent
      (opioids may cause urinary retention)
   Renal function impairment
      (increased risk of convulsions [with meperidine] or other adverse effects because opioids and/or their metabolites excreted primarily via kidneys; also, opioids may cause urinary retention)
   Caution is also advised in administration to very young, elderly, or very ill or debilitated patients, who may be more sensitive to the effects, especially the respiratory depressant effects, of these medications.

*For butorphanol, nalbuphine, or pentazocine only (in addition to those medical problems listed above)*
   Dependence on opioid agonist analgesics, current
      (nalbuphine and pentazocine may precipitate, and butorphanol does not prevent occurrence of, withdrawal symptoms)
   Hypertension
      (butorphanol may increase blood pressure in these patients when used as presurgical medication)
» Myocardial infarction, acute
      (pentazocine and butorphanol may increase cardiac work; effects of nalbuphine in patients with severely compromised cardiac function have not been fully evaluated)

*For epidural or intrathecal administration (in addition to those medical problems listed above as applying to all opioid analgesics)*
   Dependence on opioid analgesics, current
      (low doses of opioids administered via epidural or intrathecal injection will not prevent withdrawal symptoms from occurring in a physically dependent patient)

### Patient monitoring
The following may be especially important in patient monitoring (other tests may be warranted in some patients, depending on condition; » = major clinical significance):

» Respiratory function
      (monitoring recommended for at least 24 hours following epidural or intrathecal injection because delayed respiratory depression may occur up to 24 hours after administration via these routes)

## Side/Adverse Effects
See *Table 4,* page 2197.

Note: Physical dependence, with or without psychological dependence, may occur with chronic administration of opioid analgesics; an abstinence syndrome may occur when these drugs are discontinued. Specific withdrawal symptoms that may occur, and their severity, depend upon the specific drug used, the abruptness of withdrawal, and the degree to which dependence has developed. Butorphanol, nalbuphine, and pentazocine have lower dependence liability and potential for abuse than opioid agonists; codeine and propoxyphene have lower dependence liability and potential for abuse than other agonists because of their comparatively lower potency with usual doses.

Epidural or intrathecal administration does not eliminate the risk of severe side effects common to systemic opioid analgesics. Respiratory depression may occur shortly after administration because of direct venous redistribution to the respiratory centers in the CNS. Also, delayed respiratory depression may occur up to 24 hours after administration, possibly as the result of rostral spread of the medication. Intrathecal administration and/or injection into thoracic sites are more likely to cause respiratory depression than epidural administration and/or injection into lumbar sites.

Following epidural or intrathecal administration of morphine, urinary retention occurs very frequently (incidence about 90% in males and somewhat lower in females) and may persist for 10 to 20 hours following injection. Catheterization may be required. Also, dose-related generalized pruritus occurs frequently. Excessive sedation is uncommon, and loss of motor, sensory, or sympathetic function does not occur.

**Those indicating possible withdrawal and the need for medical attention if they occur after medication is discontinued**
*Body aches; diarrhea; fast heartbeat; fever, runny nose, or sneezing; gooseflesh; increased sweating; increased yawning; loss of appetite; nausea or vomiting; nervousness, restlessness, or irritability; shivering or trembling; stomach cramps; trouble in sleeping; unusually large pupils; weakness*

Note: *The signs and symptoms of withdrawal* listed above are characteristic of the abstinence syndrome produced by abrupt discontinuation of mu-receptor agonists such as morphine. The milder abstinence syndrome produced by abrupt discontinuation of opioids having mixed agonist/antagonist activity may also include some of these signs and symptoms.

It has been proposed that adverse effects (such as tachycardia, hypertension, hyperpnea, hyperalgesia, nausea, and vomiting) occurring (rarely) after naloxone is administered for postoperative reversal of opioid effects following a lengthy surgical procedure may be manifestations of an induced abstinence syndrome in acutely dependent individuals. However, other symptoms more commonly associated with an opioid withdrawal syndrome have not been reported.

## Overdose
For specific information on the agents used in the management of opioid (narcotic) analgesics overdose, see:
- *Naloxone (Systemic)* monograph.

For more information on the management of overdose or unintentional ingestion, **contact a Poison Control Center** (see *Poison Control Center Listing*).

**Clinical effects of overdose**
The following effects have been selected on the basis of their potential clinical significance (possible signs and symptoms in parentheses where appropriate)—not necessarily inclusive:

Acute and chronic
*Cold, clammy skin; confusion; convulsions; dizziness, severe; drowsiness, severe; low blood pressure; nervousness or restlessness, severe; pinpoint pupils of eyes; slow heartbeat; slow or troubled breathing; unconsciousness; weakness, severe*

Note: *Convulsions* are more likely to occur with meperidine or propoxyphene than with other opioids.

**Treatment of overdose**
To decrease absorption—Emptying the stomach via induction of emesis or gastric lavage (if the opioid was taken orally). However, treatment of respiratory depression or other potentially life-threatening adverse effects must take precedence.

Specific treatment—Administering the opioid antagonist naloxone. However, larger doses of naloxone may be required for treatment of overdose with butorphanol, nalbuphine, pentazocine, or propoxyphene. Naloxone injections may be repeated at two- to three-minute intervals as needed. The fact that naloxone may also antagonize the analgesic actions of opioid analgesics and may precipitate withdrawal symptoms in physically dependent patients must be kept in mind. For reversal of postoperative opioid depression, dosage of naloxone must be carefully titrated to avoid interference with control of postoperative pain or causing other adverse effects; hypertension and tachycardia, sometimes resulting in left ventricular failure and pulmonary edema, have occurred following naloxone administration in these circumstances (especially in cardiac patients). See the package insert or *Naloxone (Systemic)* for specific dosing guidelines for use of this product.

Monitoring—Continuing to monitor the patient (mandatory because the duration of action of the opioid analgesic may exceed that of the antagonist) and administering additional naloxone as needed. Alternatively, initial treatment may be followed by continuous intravenous infusion of naloxone, with the rate of infusion being adjusted according to patient response.

Supportive care—Establishing adequate respiratory exchange through provision of a patent airway and institution of assisted or controlled respiration. Administering intravenous fluids and/or vasopressors and using other supportive measures as needed. Patients in whom intentional overdose is known or suspected should be referred for psychiatric consultation.

## Patient Consultation
As an aid to patient consultation, refer to *Advice for the Patient, Narcotic Analgesics—For Pain Relief (Systemic), Narcotic Analgesics—For Surgery and Obstetrics (Systemic),* and *Opium Preparations (Systemic).*

In providing consultation, consider emphasizing the following selected information (» = major clinical significance):

**Before using this medication**
» Conditions affecting use, especially:
  Sensitivity to the opioid considered for use, history of
  Pregnancy—Opioids cross the placenta; regular use by pregnant women may cause physical dependence in the fetus and withdrawal symptoms in the neonate
  Breast-feeding—Butorphanol, codeine, meperidine, methadone, morphine, and propoxyphene are known to be distributed into breast milk; high-dose methadone may cause dependence in nursing infants
  Use in children—Children up to 2 years of age are more susceptible to the effects of opioids, especially respiratory depression; also, children may be more likely to experience paradoxical CNS excitation during therapy
  Use in the elderly—Geriatric patients are more susceptible to the effects of opioids, especially respiratory depression
  Dental—May cause dryness of mouth, which can lead to caries, periodontal disease, oral candidiasis, and discomfort
  Other medications, especially alcohol or other CNS depressants, monoamine oxidase inhibitors, naltrexone, rifampin, and zidovudine
  Other medical problems, especially diarrhea caused by antibiotics or poisoning, asthma or other respiratory problems, and severe inflammatory bowel disease

**Proper use of this medication**
*Proper administration of*
» Injections (if dispensed to the patient for home use)
» Meperidine syrup—Mixing with ½ glass (4 ounces) of water to lessen numbing effect in mouth and throat
» Methadone oral concentrate—Diluting with water to at least 1 ounce before taking, unless premixed at a methadone treatment center
» Methadone dispersible tablets—Must be dissolved in water or fruit juice before taking
  Morphine oral liquid—May be mixed with fruit juice to improve taste
» Morphine extended-release tablets—Swallowing tablets whole; not breaking, crushing, or chewing
  Suppository dosage forms—proper administration technique
*Proper administration of opium tincture*
  Medication may be diluted in water, which will cause it to turn milky
  Taking with food or meals if gastrointestinal irritation occurs
» Importance of not taking more medication than the amount prescribed because of danger of overdose and habit-forming potential
» Not increasing dose if medication is less effective after a few weeks; checking with physician
  Missed dose (if on scheduled dosing): Taking as soon as possible; not taking if almost time for next dose; not doubling doses
» Proper storage

**Precautions while using this medication**
  Regular visits to physician to check progress during long-term therapy
» Avoiding use of alcoholic beverages or other CNS depressants during therapy, unless prescribed or otherwise approved by physician
» Caution if dizziness, drowsiness, lightheadedness, or false sense of well-being occurs
» Caution when getting up suddenly from a lying or sitting position
  Lying down if nausea or vomiting, or dizziness or lightheadedness occurs
  Need to inform physician or dentist of use of medication if any kind of surgery (including dental surgery) or emergency treatment is required
  Possible dryness of mouth; using sugarless gum or candy, ice, or saliva substitute for relief; checking with dentist if dry mouth continues for more than 2 weeks

» Checking with physician before discontinuing medication after prolonged use of high doses; gradual dosage reduction may be necessary to avoid withdrawal symptoms
» Suspected overdose: Getting emergency help at once
*For opium tincture when used as antidiarrheal only*
» Consulting physician if diarrhea continues and/or fever develops

**Side/adverse effects**
Signs of potential side effects, especially respiratory depression or impairment; allergic reactions; confusion, convulsions, hallucinations, mental depression, or other signs of CNS toxicity; hepatotoxicity; hypertension; and paradoxical CNS excitation, especially in children

## General Dosing Information

These medications may suppress respiration, especially in very young, elderly, very ill, or debilitated patients and those with respiratory problems. Lower doses may be required for these patients. However, elderly patients may also be more sensitive to the analgesic effects of these medications so that lower doses or an increased dosing interval may be sufficient to provide effective analgesia.

Dosage and dosing intervals should be individualized on the basis of the potency and duration of action of the specific drug used, the severity of pain, the condition of the patient, other medications given concurrently, and patient response.

Concurrent administration of a nonopioid analgesic (such as aspirin or other salicylates, other nonsteroidal anti-inflammatory analgesics, or acetaminophen) with opioid analgesics provides additive analgesia and may permit lower doses of the opioid analgesic to be utilized.

Some clinicians recommend that patients in severe chronic pain receive opioid analgesics on a fixed dosage schedule so that they remain free of pain rather than on an as needed basis after pain recurs. The medication should be given orally if possible.

Tolerance to many of the effects of these medications may develop with repeated administration. The first sign of tolerance is usually a decrease in the duration of adequate analgesia. Tolerance to the respiratory depressant effects of opioid analgesics develops concurrently with tolerance to their analgesic effects. Careful adjustment of dosage as required to provide adequate analgesia is not likely to increase the risk of respiratory depression. Patients who become tolerant to one of these agents may be partially cross-tolerant to the others. However, when an alternate opioid analgesic is substituted for one to which tolerance has developed, it is recommended that one-half of the equianalgesic dose of the new medication be used initially. Dosage of the new medication may then be adjusted as necessary.

Psychological and physical dependence may occur with chronic administration of opioid analgesics, including epidurally or intrathecally administered opioid analgesics; an abstinence syndrome may occur when these drugs are discontinued. Physical dependence in patients receiving prolonged therapy for severe chronic pain rarely leads to true addiction, i.e., a desire to continue taking the drug (for its euphoric effect) after it is no longer required for treatment. Fear of causing addiction should not result in failure to provide adequate pain relief, although caution is advised if patient predisposition toward drug abuse is known or strongly suspected. Gradual withdrawal may minimize the development of withdrawal symptoms following prolonged use.

**For parenteral dosage forms only**
Rapid intravenous injection of most opioid analgesics has caused anaphylactoid reactions, severe respiratory depression, hypotension, peripheral circulatory collapse, and cardiac arrest. It is recommended that when an opioid analgesic must be given intravenously, dosage should be reduced and a dilute solution should be injected slowly over a period of several minutes. An opioid antagonist and equipment for artificial ventilation should be available.

When an opioid analgesic is administered parenterally, the patient usually should be lying down and should remain recumbent for a period of time to minimize side effects such as hypotension, dizziness, lightheadedness, nausea, and vomiting. If these side effects occur in an ambulatory patient, they may be relieved if the patient lies down.

In patients with shock, impaired perfusion may prevent complete absorption following intramuscular or subcutaneous injection. Repeated administration may result in overdose due to an excessive amount suddenly being absorbed when circulation is restored.

Opioid analgesics may not provide sufficient analgesia to prevent or overcome hemodynamic responses to surgical stress when used as the sole intravenous supplement to nitrous oxide for the maintenance of balanced anesthesia. Concurrent use of other medications, such as a benzodiazepine, an ultrashort-acting barbiturate, or a potent hydrocarbon inhalation anesthetic, may be required.

Epidural or intrathecal administration of opioid analgesics should be performed only by physicians experienced in these techniques. Solutions containing a preservative must *not* be injected via these routes. *Resuscitative equipment and medications should be immediately available for management of respiratory depression or other complications that may arise from inadvertent intrathecal or intravascular administration.* Also, facilities for adequate monitoring of the patient's respiratory status must be available.

For epidural or intrathecal administration, injection into the lumbar area may be preferred because of the increased risk of respiratory depression with injection into the thoracic area. Also, the epidural route is preferred, whenever possible, because of the increased risk of respiratory depression with intrathecal administration.

Prior to epidural administration, proper placement of the needle or catheter in the epidural space must be verified. Aspiration to check for blood in the cerebrospinal fluid may be performed; however, the fact that intravascular administration is possible even when aspiration for blood is negative must be kept in mind. Alternatively, administration of 5 mL (3 mL for obstetrical patients) of preservative-free 1.5% lidocaine hydrochloride with epinephrine 1:200,000 injection may be used to verify placement in the epidural space. Tachycardia occurring after injection of the test medication indicates that the medication has entered the circulation; sudden onset of segmental anesthesia indicates that the medication has been administered intrathecally.

Following epidural or intrathecal injection of an opioid analgesic, administration of low doses of naloxone via continuous intravenous infusion for 24 hours may decrease the incidence of potential side effects without interfering with the analgesic effectiveness of the medication.

## *BUTORPHANOL*

## Summary of Differences

Indications:
Caution required when used as analgesic to relieve pain due to acute myocardial infarction because of cardiovascular effects that tend to increase cardiac work.
Pharmacology/pharmacokinetics:
Mechanism of action/effect—
An opioid agonist/antagonist analgesic.
Agonist: Has agonist activity at the kappa and sigma receptors.
Antagonist: Probably has no direct antagonist activity at the mu receptor; antagonist effects may result from failure to substitute for mu-receptor agonists sufficiently to prevent or attenuate withdrawal symptoms in physically dependent patients.
Equivalence—
2 mg via intramuscular injection therapeutically equivalent to 10 mg of intramuscular morphine.
Protein binding—
High.
Half-life—
2.5–4 hours.
Onset of action—
Intramuscular: 10–30 minutes.
Intravenous: 2–3 minutes.
Time to peak concentration—
0.5–1 hour.
Peak plasma concentration—
2.2 nanograms/mL.
Time to peak effect—
Intramuscular: 30–60 minutes.
Intravenous: 30 minutes.
Duration of action (nontolerant patients only; decreases as tolerance develops during chronic therapy)—
Intramuscular: 3–4 hours.
Intravenous: 2–4 hours.
Elimination—
72% Renal, <5% as unchanged buprenorphine; 15% biliary.
Precautions:
Laboratory value alterations—
Does not intefere with hepatobiliary imaging.
Does not increase plasma amylase or lipase activity.
Medical considerations/contraindications—
Caution not required in gallbladder disease or gallstones.
Also, should be used with caution in patients physically dependent on opioid agonists, in hypertensive patients (when used preoperatively), and in patients with acute myocardial infarction.
Side/adverse effects:
Less likely to cause constipation than most other opioids.
Biliary spasm has not been reported.

# Opioid (Narcotic) Analgesics (Systemic)

Rarely, may cause subjective and psychotomimetic effects characteristic of sigma receptor agonists.
Has lower dependence liability than opioid agonists.
Withdrawal symptoms less severe than those produced by opioid agonist analgesics.

## Parenteral Dosage Forms
### BUTORPHANOL TARTRATE INJECTION USP
**Usual adult dose**
Analgesic—
  Intramuscular, 1 to 4 mg (usually 2 mg) every three to four hours as needed.
  Intravenous, 500 mcg (0.5 mg) to 2 mg (usually 1 mg) every three to four hours as needed.
Anesthesia adjunct—
  Preoperative:
    Intravenous, usually 2 mg sixty to ninety minutes prior to surgery, although dosage must be individualized.
  Balanced anesthesia:
    Intravenous, initially 1 to 4 mg, followed by supplemental doses of 500 mcg (0.5 mg) to 1 mg as needed.
    Note: Dosage must be individualized. Supplemental doses of up to 60 mcg (0.06 mg) per kg of body weight may be necessary in some patients.
    The total quantity of butorphanol required during surgery usually ranges between 60 and 180 mcg (0.06 and 0.18 mg) per kg of body weight.

**Usual pediatric dose**
Dosage in patients up to 18 years of age has not been established.

**Strength(s) usually available**
U.S.—
  With preservative (benzethonium chloride 0.1 mg/mL):
    2 mg per mL (Rx) [Stadol].
  Without preservative:
    1 mg per mL (Rx) [Stadol].
    2 mg per mL (Rx) [Stadol].
Canada—
  Not commercially available.

**Packaging and storage**
Store between 15 and 30 °C (59 and 86 °F), unless otherwise specified by manufacturer. Protect from light. Protect from freezing.

**Auxiliary labeling**
- May cause drowsiness.
- Avoid alcoholic beverages.

**Note**
Controlled substance in the U.S.

---

## CODEINE

## Summary of Differences
Indications:
  Oral dosage forms also indicated as antitussive.
  Also, used as antidiarrheal.
Pharmacology/pharmacokinetics:
  Mechanism of action/effect—
    An opioid agonist analgesic; exerts agonist activity primarily at the mu receptor, but with usual doses is relatively weak.
  Equivalence—
    120 mg via intramuscular injection or 200 mg via oral administration therapeutically equivalent to 10 mg of intramuscular morphine.
  Protein binding—
    Very low.
  Half-life—
    2.5–4 hours.
  Biotransformation—
    Hepatic; about 10% demethylated to morphine.
  Onset of action:
    Analgesic—
      Intramuscular—10–30 minutes.
      Subcutaneous—10–30 minutes.
      Oral—30–45 minutes.
  Time to peak effect:
    Analgesic—
      Intramuscular—30–60 minutes.
      Oral—1–2 hours.
  Duration of action—
    Analgesic (in nontolerant patients only; decreases as tolerance develops during chronic therapy): Intramuscular, subcutaneous, or oral—4 hours.
    Antitussive: Oral—4–6 hours.
  Elimination—
    Renal, 5–15% as unchanged codeine and 10% as unchanged or conjugated morphine.
Side/adverse effects:
  More likely than most other opioids to cause constipation, especially during chronic therapy.
  Has lower dependence liability than most other opioid agonists.
  Withdrawal symptoms less severe than those produced by stronger opioid agonist analgesics.

## Additional Dosing Information
See also *General Dosing Information*.

**For parenteral dosage forms only**
Local tissue irritation, pain, and induration may occur with repeated subcutaneous injection.

## Oral Dosage Forms
Note: Bracketed uses in the *Dosage Forms* section refer to categories of use and/or indications that are not included in U.S. product labeling.

### CODEINE PHOSPHATE ORAL SOLUTION
**Usual adult dose**
Analgesic—
  Oral, 15 to 60 mg (usually 30 mg) every three to six hours as needed.
[Antidiarrheal][1]—
  Oral, 30 mg up to four times a day.
Antitussive—
  Oral, 10 to 20 mg every four to six hours.

**Usual adult prescribing limits**
Antitussive—
  Up to 120 mg in twenty-four hours.

**Usual pediatric dose**
Analgesic—
  Premature infants: Use is not recommended.
  Newborn infants: Dosage has not been established.
  Infants and children: Oral, 500 mcg (0.5 mg) per kg of body weight or 15 mg per square meter of body surface every four to six hours as needed.
[Antidiarrheal][1]—
  Oral, 500 mcg (0.5 mg) per kg of body weight up to four times a day.
Antitussive—
  Children up to 2 years of age:
    Use is not recommended.
  Children 2 to 5 years of age:
    Oral, 1 mg per kg of body weight per day, administered in four equal divided doses, or for
    Children 2 years of age (average body weight 12 kg)—Oral, 3 mg every four to six hours, not to exceed 12 mg per day.
    Children 3 years of age (average body weight 14 kg)—Oral, 3.5 mg every four to six hours, not to exceed 14 mg per day.
    Children 4 years of age (average body weight 16 kg)—Oral, 4 mg every four to six hours, not to exceed 16 mg per day.
    Children 5 years of age (average body weight 18 kg)—Oral, 4.5 mg every four to six hours, not to exceed 18 mg per day.
  Children 6 to 12 years of age:
    Oral, 5 to 10 mg every four to six hours, not to exceed 60 mg per day.
Note: Use of a calibrated measure is recommended to prevent possible overdosage in children up to 6 years of age.

**Strength(s) usually available**
U.S.—
  15 mg per 5 mL (Rx) [GENERIC].
Canada—
  10 mg per mL (Rx) [Paveral].

**Packaging and storage**
Store below 40 °C (104 °F), preferably between 15 and 30 °C (59 and 86 °F), in a tight, light-resistant container, unless otherwise specified by manufacturer. Protect from freezing.

**Auxiliary labeling**
- May cause drowsiness.
- Avoid alcoholic beverages.
- May be habit-forming.

**Note**
Controlled substance in both the U.S. and Canada.

### CODEINE PHOSPHATE TABLETS USP

**Usual adult dose**
Analgesic—
  Oral, 15 to 60 mg (usually 30 mg) every three to six hours as needed.
[Antidiarrheal][1]—
  Oral, 30 mg up to four times a day.
Antitussive—
  Oral, 10 to 20 mg every four to six hours.

**Usual adult prescribing limits**
Antitussive—
  Up to 120 mg in twenty-four hours.

**Usual pediatric dose**
Analgesic—
  Premature infants: Use is not recommended.
  Newborn infants: Dosage has not been established.
  Infants and children: Oral, 500 mcg (0.5 mg) per kg of body weight or 15 mg per square meter of body surface every four to six hours as needed.
[Antidiarrheal][1]—
  Oral, 500 mcg (0.5 mg) per kg of body weight up to four times a day.
Antitussive—
  Children up to 2 years of age:
    Use is not recommended.
  Children 2 to 5 years of age:
    Oral, 1 mg per kg of body weight per day, administered in four equal divided doses, or for
    Children 2 years of age (average body weight 12 kg)—Oral, 3 mg every four to six hours, not to exceed 12 mg per day.
    Children 3 years of age (average body weight 14 kg)—Oral, 3.5 mg every four to six hours, not to exceed 14 mg per day.
    Children 4 years of age (average body weight 16 kg)—Oral, 4 mg every four to six hours, not to exceed 16 mg per day.
    Children 5 years of age (average body weight 18 kg)—Oral, 4.5 mg every four to six hours, not to exceed 18 mg per day.
  Children 6 to 12 years of age:
    Oral, 5 to 10 mg every four to six hours, not to exceed 60 mg per day.

**Strength(s) usually available**
U.S.—
  30 mg (Rx) [GENERIC].
  60 mg (Rx) [GENERIC].
Canada—
  15 mg (Rx) [GENERIC].
  30 mg (Rx) [GENERIC].
Note: Strengths of commercially available tablets do not correspond to recommended antitussive doses.

**Packaging and storage**
Store below 40 °C (104 °F), preferably between 15 and 30 °C (59 and 86 °F). Store in a well-closed, light-resistant container.

**Auxiliary labeling**
• May cause drowsiness.
• Avoid alcoholic beverages.
• May be habit-forming.

**Note**
Controlled substance in both the U.S. and Canada.

### CODEINE SULFATE TABLETS USP

**Usual adult dose**
Analgesic—
  Oral, 15 to 60 mg (usually 30 mg) every three to six hours as needed.
[Antidiarrheal]—
  Oral, 30 mg up to four times a day.
Antitussive—
  Oral, 10 to 20 mg every four to six hours.

**Usual pediatric dose**
Analgesic—
  Premature infants: Use is not recommended.
  Newborn infants: Dosage has not been established.
  Infants and children: Oral, 500 mcg (0.5 mg) per kg of body weight or 15 mg per square meter of body surface every four to six hours as needed.
[Antidiarrheal]—
  Oral, 500 mcg (0.5 mg) per kg of body weight up to four times a day.
Antitussive—
  Children up to 2 years of age:
    Use is not recommended.
  Children 2 to 5 years of age:
    Oral, 1 mg per kg of body weight per day, administered in four equal divided doses, or for
    Children 2 years of age (average body weight 12 kg)—Oral, 3 mg every four to six hours, not to exceed 12 mg per day.
    Children 3 years of age (average body weight 14 kg)—Oral, 3.5 mg every four to six hours, not to exceed 14 mg per day.
    Children 4 years of age (average body weight 16 kg)—Oral, 4 mg every four to six hours, not to exceed 16 mg per day.
    Children 5 years of age (average body weight 18 kg)—Oral, 4.5 mg every four to six hours, not to exceed 18 mg per day.
  Children 6 to 12 years of age:
    Oral, 5 to 10 mg every four to six hours, not to exceed 60 mg per day.

**Strength(s) usually available**
U.S.—
  15 mg (Rx) [GENERIC].
  30 mg (Rx) [GENERIC].
  60 mg (Rx) [GENERIC].
Canada—
  Not commercially available.
Note: Strengths of commercially available tablets do not correspond to recommended antitussive doses.

**Packaging and storage**
Store below 40 °C (104 °F), preferably between 15 and 30 °C (59 and 86 °F). Store in a well-closed container.

**Auxiliary labeling**
• May cause drowsiness.
• Avoid alcoholic beverages.
• May be habit-forming.

## Parenteral Dosage Forms

### CODEINE PHOSPHATE INJECTION USP

**Usual adult dose**
Analgesic—
  Intramuscular, intravenous, or subcutaneous, 15 to 60 mg (usually 30 mg) every four to six hours as needed.

**Usual pediatric dose**
Analgesic—
  Premature infants: Use is not recommended.
  Newborn infants: Dosage has not been established.
  Infants and children: Intramuscular or subcutaneous, 500 mcg (0.5 mg) per kg of body weight or 15 mg per square meter of body surface every four to six hours as needed.

**Strength(s) usually available**
U.S.—
  With preservative:
    30 mg per mL (Rx) [GENERIC].
    60 mg per mL (Rx) [GENERIC].
Canada—
  30 mg per mL (Rx) [GENERIC].
  60 mg per mL (Rx) [GENERIC].

**Packaging and storage**
Store below 40 °C (104 °F), preferably between 15 and 30 °C (59 and 86 °F), unless otherwise specified by manufacturer. Protect from light. Protect from freezing.

**Auxiliary labeling**
• May cause drowsiness.
• Avoid alcoholic beverages.
• May be habit-forming.

**Note**
Controlled substance in both the U.S. and Canada.

### CODEINE PHOSPHATE SOLUBLE TABLETS

**Usual adult dose**
Analgesic—
  Intramuscular or subcutaneous, 15 to 60 mg (usually 30 mg) every four to six hours as needed.

**Usual pediatric dose**
Analgesic—
  Premature infants: Use is not recommended.
  Newborn infants: Dosage has not been established.

## 2176  Opioid (Narcotic) Analgesics (Systemic)

Infants and children: Intramuscular or subcutaneous, 500 mcg (0.5 mg) per kg of body weight or 15 mg per square meter of body surface every four to six hours as needed.

**Strength(s) usually available**
U.S.—
  30 mg (Rx) [GENERIC].
  60 mg (Rx) [GENERIC].
Canada—
  Not commercially available.

**Packaging and storage**
Store between 15 and 30 °C (59 and 86 °F), in a tight, light-resistant container, unless otherwise specified by manufacturer.

**Preparation of dosage form**
For parenteral administration—Dissolve the required number of tablets in a suitable volume of sterile water for injection, then filter through a 0.22–micron membrane filter.

**Auxiliary labeling**
- May cause drowsiness.
- Avoid alcoholic beverages.
- May be habit-forming.

**Note**
Controlled substance in the U.S.

### CODEINE SULFATE SOLUBLE TABLETS

**Usual adult dose**
Analgesic—
  Intramuscular or subcutaneous, 15 to 60 mg (usually 30 mg) every four to six hours as needed.

**Usual pediatric dose**
Analgesic—
  Premature infants: Use is not recommended.
  Newborn infants: Dosage has not been established.
  Infants and children: Intramuscular or subcutaneous, 500 mcg (0.5 mg) per kg of body weight or 15 mg per square meter of body surface every four to six hours as needed.

**Strength(s) usually available**
U.S.—
  30 mg (Rx) [GENERIC].
  60 mg (Rx) [GENERIC].
Canada—
  Not commercially available.

**Packaging and storage**
Store between 15 and 30 °C (59 and 86 °F), in a tight, light-resistant container, unless otherwise specified by manufacturer.

**Preparation of dosage form**
For parenteral administration—Dissolve the required number of tablets in a suitable volume of sterile water for injection, then filter through a 0.22–micron membrane filter.

**Auxiliary labeling**
- May cause drowsiness.
- Avoid alcoholic beverages.
- May be habit-forming.

**Note**
Controlled substance in the U.S.

---
[1]Not included in Canadian product labeling.

---

### HYDROCODONE

## Summary of Differences

Indications:
  Also, indicated as an antitussive.
Pharmacology/pharmacokinetics:
  Mechanism of action/effect—
    An opioid agonist analgesic; exerts agonist activity primarily at the mu receptor.
  Half-life—
    3.8 hours.
  Onset of action—
    Analgesic: Oral 10–30 minutes.
  Time to peak effect—
    Analgesic: Oral 30–60 minutes.
  Duration of action—
    Analgesic (nontolerant patients only; decreases as tolerance develops during chronic therapy): Oral—4–6 hours.
    Antitussive: Oral—4–6 hours.
  Elimination—
    Renal.
Side/adverse effects:
  More likely than most other opioids to cause side effects associated with histamine release.

## Oral Dosage Forms

### HYDROCODONE BITARTRATE SYRUP

**Usual adult dose**
Antitussive—
  Oral, 5 mg every four to six hours as needed.

**Usual pediatric dose**
Dosage has not been established.

**Strength(s) usually available**
U.S.—
  Not commercially available.
Canada—
  5 mg per 5 mL (Rx) [*Hycodan* (sucrose); *Robidone* (alcohol 3.2%; sugar)].

Note: In Canada, *Hycodan* contains only hydrocodone bitartrate; in the U.S., *Hycodan* contains homatropine in addition to hydrocodone bitartrate.

**Packaging and storage**
Store below 40 °C (104 °F), preferably between 15 and 30 °C (59 and 86 °F), in a well-closed container, unless otherwise specified by manufacturer. Protect from freezing.

**Auxiliary labeling**
- May cause drowsiness.
- Avoid alcoholic beverages.
- May be habit-forming.

**Note**
Controlled substance in Canada.

### HYDROCODONE BITARTRATE TABLETS USP

**Usual adult dose**
Analgesic—
  Oral, 5 to 10 mg every four to six hours as needed.
Antitussive—
  Oral, 5 mg every four to six hours as needed.

**Usual pediatric dose**
Analgesic—
  Oral, 150 mcg (0.15 mg) per kg of body weight every six hours as needed.

**Strength(s) usually available**
U.S.—
  Not commercially available.
Canada—
  5 mg (Rx) [*Hycodan* (scored; lactose)].

Note: In Canada, *Hycodan* contains only hydrocodone bitartrate; in the U.S., *Hycodan* contains homatropine in addition to hydrocodone bitartrate.

**Packaging and storage**
Store below 40 °C (104 °F), preferably between 15 and 30 °C (59 and 86 °F). Store in a tight, light-resistant container.

**Auxiliary labeling**
- May cause drowsiness.
- Avoid alcoholic beverages.
- May be habit-forming.

**Note**
Controlled substance in Canada.

---

### HYDROMORPHONE

## Summary of Differences

Indications:
  Also, indicated as an antitussive; see also *Cough/Cold Combinations (Systemic)—Hydromorphone and Guaifenesin*.
Pharmacology/pharmacokinetics:
  Mechanism of action/effect—
    An opioid agonist analgesic; exerts agonist activity primarily at the mu receptor.

Equivalence—
  1.5 mg via intramuscular injection, 7.5 mg via oral administration, or 3 mg via rectal administration therapeutically equivalent to 10 mg of intramuscular morphine.
Half-life—
  2.6–4 hours.
Onset of action—
  Intramuscular: 15 minutes.
  Intravenous: 10–15 minutes.
  Oral: 30 minutes.
  Subcutaneous: 15 minutes.
Time to peak effect—
  Intramuscular: 30–60 minutes.
  Intravenous: 15–30 minutes.
  Oral: 90–120 minutes.
  Subcutaneous: 30–90 minutes.
Duration of action (nontolerant patients only; decreases as tolerance develops during chronic therapy)—
  Intramuscular: 4–5 hours.
  Intravenous: 2–3 hours.
  Oral: 4 hours.
  Subcutaneous: 4 hours.
Elimination—
  Renal.

## Oral Dosage Forms

### HYDROMORPHONE HYDROCHLORIDE ORAL SOLUTION

**Usual adult dose**
Oral, 2.5 to 10 mg every three to six hours, depending on the severity of pain and patient tolerance.

**Usual pediatric dose**
Dosage must be individualized by physician, depending on the severity of pain and the patient's age, size, and opioid tolerance.

**Strength(s) usually available**
U.S.—
  5 mg per 5 mL [*Dilaudid-5*].
Canada—
  5 mg per 5 mL [*Dilaudid* (sucrose); *PMS-Hydromorphone Syrup*].

### HYDROMORPHONE HYDROCHLORIDE TABLETS USP

**Usual adult dose**
Analgesic—
  Oral, 2 mg every three to six hours as needed.
Note:  Dosage may be increased to 4 mg or more every four to six hours, depending on the severity of pain and patient tolerance.

**Usual pediatric dose**
Dosage must be individualized by physician, depending on the severity of pain and the patient's age, size, and opioid tolerance.

**Strength(s) usually available**
U.S.—
  1 mg (Rx) [*Hydrostat IR*].
  2 mg (Rx) [*Dilaudid* (lactose); *Hydrostat IR*; GENERIC].
  3 mg (Rx) [*Hydrostat IR*].
  4 mg (Rx) [*Dilaudid* (lactose); *Hydrostat IR*; GENERIC].
  8 mg (Rx) [*Dilaudid*].
Canada—
  1 mg (Rx) [*Dilaudid; PMS-Hydromorphone*].
  2 mg (Rx) [*Dilaudid; PMS-Hydromorphone;* GENERIC].
  4 mg (Rx) [*Dilaudid; PMS-Hydromorphone;* GENERIC].
  8 mg (Rx) [*Dilaudid; PMS-Hydromorphone*].

**Packaging and storage**
Store below 40 °C (104 °F), preferably between 15 and 30 °C (59 and 86 °F), unless otherwise specified by manufacturer. Store in a tight, light-resistant container.

**Auxiliary labeling**
• May cause drowsiness.
• Avoid alcoholic beverages.
• May be habit-forming.

**Note**
Controlled substance in both the U.S. and Canada.

## Parenteral Dosage Forms

### HYDROMORPHONE HYDROCHLORIDE INJECTION USP

**Usual adult dose**
Analgesic—
  Intramuscular or subcutaneous, 1 to 2 mg every three to six hours as needed; may be increased to 3 or 4 mg every four to six hours if pain is severe.
Note:  For opioid-tolerant patients requiring high-dose therapy, the 10-mg-per-mL concentration may be substituted for lower strengths of hydromorphone hydrochloride injection or for other opioid analgesics. Dosage must be individualized, depending on the severity of pain, opioid requirements at the time therapy with the high-potency injection is initiated, and patient response. Although patients who have become tolerant to another opioid may be at least partially cross-tolerant to hydromorphone also, it is recommended that one-half of the equianalgesic dose of hydromorphone be used initially, then adjusted as necessary.
  Intravenous, 500 mcg (0.5 mg) to 1 mg every three hours as needed; administered slowly.

**Usual pediatric dose**
Dosage must be individualized by physician on the basis of patient's age and size.

**Strength(s) usually available**
U.S.—
  With preservatives:
    1 mg per mL (Rx) [GENERIC].
    2 mg per mL (Rx) [*Dilaudid* (methylparaben and propylparaben); GENERIC].
    3 mg per mL (Rx) [GENERIC].
    4 mg per mL (Rx) [GENERIC].
  Without preservative:
    1 mg per mL (Rx) [*Dilaudid*].
    2 mg per mL (Rx) [*Dilaudid*].
    4 mg per mL (Rx) [*Dilaudid*].
    10 mg per mL (Rx) [*Dilaudid-HP*].
Canada—
  Without preservative:
    2 mg per mL (Rx) [*Dilaudid*].
    10 mg per mL (Rx) [*Dilaudid-HP*].

**Packaging and storage**
Store below 40 °C (104 °F), preferably between 15 and 30 °C (59 and 86 °F), unless otherwise specified by manufacturer. Protect from light. Protect from freezing.

**Auxiliary labeling**
• May cause drowsiness.
• Avoid alcoholic beverages.
• May be habit-forming.

**Note**
Controlled substance in both the U.S. and Canada.

## Rectal Dosage Forms

### HYDROMORPHONE HYDROCHLORIDE SUPPOSITORIES

**Usual adult dose**
Analgesic—
  Rectal, 3 mg every four to eight hours as needed.

**Usual pediatric dose**
Dosage has not been established.

**Strength(s) usually available**
U.S.—
  3 mg (Rx) [*Dilaudid*].
Canada—
  3 mg (Rx) [*Dilaudid; PMS-Hydromorphone*].

**Packaging and storage**
Store between 2 and 8 °C (36 and 46 °F), in a well-closed container, unless otherwise specified by manufacturer. Protect from freezing.

**Auxiliary labeling**
• May cause drowsiness.
• Avoid alcoholic beverages.
• May be habit-forming.
• Store in refrigerator.

**Note**
Controlled substance in both the U.S. and Canada.

## LEVORPHANOL

### Summary of Differences
Pharmacology/pharmacokinetics:
  Mechanism of action/effect—
    An opioid agonist analgesic; exerts agonist activity primarily at the mu receptor.
  Equivalence—
    2 mg via intramuscular injection or 4 mg via oral administration therapeutically equivalent to 10 mg of intramuscular morphine.
  Protein binding—
    Moderate.
  Onset of action—
    Oral: 10–60 minutes.
  Time to peak effect—
    Intramuscular: 60 minutes.
    Intravenous: Within 20 minutes.
    Oral: 90–120 minutes.
    Subcutaneous: 60–90 minutes.
  Duration of action (nontolerant patients only; duration decreases as tolerance develops during chronic therapy)—
    Intramuscular, intravenous, oral, or subcutaneous: 4–5 hours.
  Elimination—
    Renal.

## Oral Dosage Forms

### LEVORPHANOL TARTRATE TABLETS USP

**Usual adult dose**
Analgesic—
  Oral, 2 mg; may be increased to 3 or 4 mg if pain is severe.

**Usual pediatric dose**
Dosage must be individualized by physician on the basis of patient's age and size.

**Strength(s) usually available**
U.S.—
  2 mg (Rx) [*Levo-Dromoran* (scored; lactose); GENERIC].
Canada—
  2 mg (Rx) [*Levo-Dromoran* (scored; lactose)].

**Packaging and storage**
Store between 15 and 30 °C (59 and 86 °F), in a light-resistant container, unless otherwise specified by manufacturer. Store in a well-closed container.

**Auxiliary labeling**
• May cause drowsiness.
• Avoid alcoholic beverages.
• May be habit-forming.

**Note**
Controlled substance in both the U.S. and Canada.

## Parenteral Dosage Forms

### LEVORPHANOL TARTRATE INJECTION USP

**Usual adult dose**
Analgesic—
  Subcutaneous, 2 mg; may be increased to 3 mg if pain is severe.
Note: The medication may also be given intravenously.
  For preoperative analgesia—Subcutaneous, 1 to 2 mg ninety minutes prior to surgery.

**Usual pediatric dose**
Dosage must be individualized by physician on the basis of patient's age and size.

**Strength(s) usually available**
U.S.—
  With preservatives:
    2 mg per mL (Rx) [*Levo-Dromoran* (methylparaben and propylparaben [1-mL ampuls]; or 0.45% phenol [10-mL vials])].
Canada—
  With preservatives:
    2 mg per mL (Rx) [*Levo-Dromoran* (0.45% phenol)].

**Packaging and storage**
Store below 40 °C (104 °F), preferably between 15 and 30 °C (59 and 86 °F), unless otherwise specified by manufacturer. Protect from freezing.

**Auxiliary labeling**
• May cause drowsiness.
• Avoid alcoholic beverages.
• May be habit-forming.

**Note**
Controlled substance in both the U.S. and Canada.

## MEPERIDINE

### Summary of Differences
Pharmacology/pharmacokinetics:
  Mechanism of action/effect—
    An opioid agonist analgesic; exerts agonist activity primarily at the mu receptor.
  Equivalence—
    75 mg via intramuscular injection or 300 mg via oral administration therapeutically equivalent to 10 mg of intramuscular morphine.
  Protein binding—
    High.
  Half-life—
    2.4–4 hours.
  Biotransformation—
    Metabolized to normeperidine, which is active and toxic.
  Onset of action—
    Intramuscular: 10–15 minutes.
    Intravenous: 1 minute.
    Oral: 15 minutes.
    Subcutaneous: 10–15 minutes.
  Time to peak effect—
    Intramuscular: 30–50 minutes.
    Intravenous: 5–7 minutes.
    Oral: 60–90 minutes.
    Subcutaneous: 30–50 minutes.
  Duration of action (nontolerant patients only; decreases as tolerance develops during chronic therapy)—
    Intramuscular, intravenous, oral, or subcutaneous: 2–4 hours.
  Elimination—
    Renal, 5% as unchanged meperidine.
Precautions:
  Drug interactions and/or related problems—
    May increase effects of coumarin- or indandione-derivative anticoagulants.
    Contraindicated in patients who have received a monoamine oxidase (MAO) inhibitor within past 14–21 days; concurrent use has produced serious, sometimes fatal, reactions.
    Concurrent use with amphetamines, which have some MAO inhibiting activity, not recommended because of risk of serious reactions similar to those reported with other MAO inhibitors.
Side/adverse effects:
  More likely than most other opioids to cause side effects associated with histamine release, convulsions, or constipation.

### Additional Dosing Information
See also *General Dosing Information*.

**For oral dosage forms only**
The syrup may be diluted with ½ glass (120 mL) of water to prevent a slight topical anesthetic effect on the mucous membranes.

**For parenteral dosage forms only**
Intramuscular administration is preferred when repeated doses are required. Repeated subcutaneous administration causes local tissue irritation and induration.
Inadvertent injection around a nerve trunk may cause sensory-motor paralysis, which is usually, but not always, transitory.

## Oral Dosage Forms

### MEPERIDINE HYDROCHLORIDE SYRUP USP

**Usual adult dose**
Analgesic—
  Oral, 50 to 150 mg (usually 100 mg) every three to four hours as needed.

**Usual pediatric dose**
Analgesic—
  Oral, 1.1 to 1.76 mg per kg of body weight, not to exceed 100 mg, every three to four hours as needed. Use of a calibrated measure is recommended to prevent possible overdosage in children up to 6 years of age.

**Strength(s) usually available**
U.S.—
  50 mg per 5 mL (Rx) [*Demerol* (glucose; saccharin sodium); GENERIC].

Canada—
    Not commercially available.

**Packaging and storage**
Store below 40 °C (104 °F), preferably between 15 and 30 °C (59 and 86 °F). Store in a tight, light-resistant container. Protect from freezing.

**Auxiliary labeling**
• May cause drowsiness.
• Avoid alcoholic beverages.
• May be habit-forming.

**Note**
Controlled substance in the U.S.

### MEPERIDINE HYDROCHLORIDE TABLETS USP

**Usual adult dose**
Analgesic—
    Oral, 50 to 150 mg (usually 100 mg) every three to four hours as needed.

**Usual pediatric dose**
Analgesic—
    Oral, 1.1 to 1.76 mg per kg of body weight, not to exceed 100 mg, every three to four hours as needed.

**Strength(s) usually available**
U.S.—
    50 mg (Rx) [*Demerol;* GENERIC].
    100 mg (Rx) [*Demerol;* GENERIC].
Canada—
    50 mg (Rx) [*Demerol* (scored)].

**Packaging and storage**
Store below 40 °C (104 °F), preferably between 15 and 30 °C (59 and 86 °F). Store in a well-closed, light-resistant container.

**Auxiliary labeling**
• May cause drowsiness.
• Avoid alcoholic beverages.
• May be habit-forming.

**Note**
Controlled substance in both the U.S. and Canada.

## Parenteral Dosage Forms

### MEPERIDINE HYDROCHLORIDE INJECTION USP

**Usual adult dose**
Analgesic—
    Intramuscular (preferred) or subcutaneous, 50 to 150 mg (usually 100 mg) every three to four hours as needed.
    Intravenous infusion, 15 to 35 mg per hour as required, administered using an infusion pump.
    Note: Dosage must be adjusted according to the severity of pain and patient response.
    Obstetrical analgesia: Intramuscular (preferred) or subcutaneous, 50 to 100 mg administered when pains become regular. May be repeated at one- to three-hour intervals as needed.
Anesthesia adjunct—
    Preoperative: Intramuscular (preferred) or subcutaneous, 50 to 100 mg thirty to ninety minutes prior to anesthesia.
    Intravenous, by repeated slow injection of fractional doses of a solution diluted to 10 mg per mL.
    Intravenous infusion, as a solution diluted to 1 mg per mL.
    Note: Dosage must be titrated to the needs of the patient, depending on the premedication given, the type of anesthesia, and the nature and duration of the surgical procedure.

**Usual pediatric dose**
Analgesic—
    Intramuscular (preferred) or subcutaneous, 1.1 to 1.76 mg per kg of body weight, not to exceed 100 mg, every three to four hours as needed.
Preoperative—
    Intramuscular (preferred) or subcutaneous, 1 to 2.2 mg per kg of body weight, not to exceed 100 mg, thirty to ninety minutes prior to anesthesia.

**Strength(s) usually available**
U.S.—
    With preservative:
        25 mg per mL (Rx) [GENERIC].
        50 mg per mL (Rx) [*Demerol* (metacresol); GENERIC].
        75 mg per mL (Rx) [GENERIC].
        100 mg per mL (Rx) [*Demerol* (metacresol); GENERIC].
    Without preservative:
        10 mg per mL (Rx) [GENERIC].
        25 mg per mL (Rx) [*Demerol;* GENERIC].
        50 mg per mL (Rx) [*Demerol;* GENERIC].
        75 mg per mL (Rx) [*Demerol;* GENERIC].
        100 mg per mL (Rx) [*Demerol;* GENERIC].
    Note: In addition to being available in single- or multiple-dose units containing the concentrations listed above, *Demerol* is available in single-dose ampuls that contain 0.5, 1.5, or 2 mL of the 50 mg per mL concentration (providing 25, 75, or 100 mg of meperidine hydrochloride, respectively).
Canada—
    With preservative:
        50 mg per mL (Rx) [*Demerol* (metacresol)].
        100 mg per mL (Rx) [*Demerol* (metacresol)].
    Without preservative:
        10 mg per mL (Rx) [GENERIC].
        25 mg per mL (Rx) [GENERIC].
        50 mg per mL (Rx) [*Demerol;* GENERIC].
        75 mg per mL (Rx) [*Demerol;* GENERIC].
        100 mg per mL (Rx) [*Demerol;* GENERIC].

**Packaging and storage**
Store below 40 °C (104 °F), preferably between 15 and 30 °C (59 and 86 °F), unless otherwise specified by manufacturer. Protect from light. Protect from freezing.

**Incompatibilities**
Solutions of meperidine are chemically incompatible with aminophylline, barbiturates, heparin, iodides, methicillin, phenytoin, sodium bicarbonate, sulfadiazine, and sulfisoxazole.

**Auxiliary labeling**
• May cause drowsiness.
• Avoid alcoholic beverages.
• May be habit-forming.

**Note**
Controlled substance in both the U.S. and Canada.

---

## METHADONE

## Summary of Differences

Note: In the U.S., methadone may be dispensed for treatment of opioid addiction only through treatment programs that have been approved by the Food and Drug Administration (FDA), Drug Enforcement Administration (DEA), and designated state authorities. Use of methadone in such programs is subject to treatment requirements stipulated in the Code of Federal Regulations.

In Canada, methadone is a controlled substance (Classification N). It is available only through physicians who have received special authorization to prescribe the medication for treatment of opioid addiction.

Indications:
    Also, indicated as narcotic abstinence syndrome suppressant.
    Also, used as antitussive.
    Not recommended for obstetrical analgesia.
Pharmacology/pharmacokinetics:
    Mechanism of action/effect—
        An opioid agonist analgesic; exerts agonist activity primarily at the mu receptor.
    Equivalence—
        10 mg via intramuscular injection or 20 mg via oral administration therapeutically equivalent to 10 mg of intramuscular morphine.
    Protein binding—
        High.
    Half-life—
        15–25 hours; increases with repeated administration.
    Onset of action—
        Intramuscular: 10–20 minutes.
        Oral: 30–60 minutes.
    Time to peak effect—
        Intramuscular: 1–2 hours.
        Intravenous: 15–30 minutes.
        Oral: 1.5–2 hours.

Duration of action (in nontolerant patients, may increase considerably with chronic use because of accumulation of methadone or active metabolites; may then decrease as tolerance develops during chronic therapy)—
  Intramuscular: 4–5 hours.
  Intravenous: 3–4 hours.
  Oral: 4–6 hours.
Elimination—
  Primarily renal (rate increased in acidic urine); also some biliary elimination.

Precautions:
Drug interactions and/or related problems—
  Urinary acidifiers may increase methadone elimination, thereby reducing the plasma concentration; withdrawal symptoms may occur in some physically dependent patients.
  Phenytoin or rifampin may increase methadone metabolism and precipitate withdrawal symptoms in physically dependent patients.

Side/adverse effects:
May be more likely than most other opioids to cause constipation.

## Additional Dosing Information

See also *General Dosing Information.*

U.S. Federal regulations permit methadone to be used in detoxification and maintenance treatment programs for opioid addiction. Short-term (up to 30 days) or long-term (up to 180 days) detoxification programs use methadone to alleviate adverse physiological or psychological consequences of withdrawal from illicit opioids, with dosage gradually being decreased until a drug-free state is achieved. After 180 days, patients who have not achieved a drug-free state are considered to be receiving maintenance treatment. Patients 18 years of age or older may also be enrolled directly into a maintenance program without first attempting detoxification. In maintenance treatment programs, relatively stable doses of opioid are given on a continuing basis as a substitute for illicit opioids.

Detoxification and comprehensive maintenance programs must include a full range of medical and rehabilitative services in addition to opioid administration. However, patients who are awaiting admission to a comprehensive maintenance program may receive up to 120 days of interim maintenance treatment, which consists only of opioid administration and needed medical services.

Oral administration is preferred for detoxification and mandatory for maintenance.

**For parenteral dosage forms only**
Intramuscular administration is recommended when repeated doses are required. Repeated subcutaneous administration causes local tissue irritation and induration.

## Oral Dosage Forms

### METHADONE HYDROCHLORIDE ORAL CONCENTRATE USP

**Usual adult dose**
Analgesic—
  Oral, 5 to 20 mg every four to eight hours. Dosage may be increased or the interval between doses decreased if pain is very severe or if the patient becomes tolerant to the medication.
Suppressant (narcotic abstinence syndrome)—
  Detoxification: Oral, 15 to 40 mg once a day or as needed to control observed withdrawal symptoms; dosage to be reduced at one- or two-day intervals according to patient response.
  Maintenance: Dosage must be individualized.

**Usual adult prescribing limits**
Up to 120 mg per day.

**Usual pediatric dose**
Analgesic—
  Dosage must be individualized by physician on the basis of patient's age and size. Use of a calibrated measure is recommended to prevent possible overdosage in children up to 6 years of age.
Suppressant (narcotic abstinence syndrome)—
  Dosage must be individualized by physician according to the needs of the specific patient. Dosage must not exceed 120 mg per day.
  Note: Patients younger than 18 years of age may be admitted to methadone maintenance programs only after 2 documented attempts at short-term (up to 30 days) detoxification or drug-free treatment have failed. A one-week waiting period is required between a detoxification attempt and admission to a methadone maintenance program. A parent, legal guardian, or other responsible adult designated by the State authority must complete and sign a consent to treatment form for all such minors.

**Strength(s) usually available**
U.S.—
  10 mg per mL (Rx) [*Methadose;* GENERIC].

**Packaging and storage**
Store between 15 and 30 °C (59 and 86 °F). Store in a tight container. Protect from light. Protect from freezing.

**Preparation of dosage form**
Each dose must be diluted with water or another liquid before administration. For use in the treatment of chronic pain, each dose should be diluted to at least 30 mL. U.S. Federal regulations stipulate that the oral concentrate be diluted with water or other suitable liquid before being administered to a patient undergoing treatment for opioid addiction. It is recommended that each dose be diluted to 90 mL or more as a deterrent to misuse by injection. Treatment centers that dispense both methadone and levomethadyl (which must also be dispensed as a diluted liquid) should use liquids of different colors for preparing each medication, so that they can be readily distinguished from each other.

**Auxiliary labeling**
• May cause drowsiness.
• Avoid alcoholic beverages.
• May be habit-forming.

**Note**
Controlled substance in the U.S.

When preparing the label, indicate that the medication must be diluted with water or another liquid to 30 mL or more prior to administration.

If the concentrate is being taken home, make sure the patient understands the dilution requirements.

### METHADONE HYDROCHLORIDE ORAL SOLUTION USP

**Usual adult dose**
Analgesic—
  Oral, 5 to 20 mg every four to eight hours. Dosage may be increased or the interval between doses decreased if pain is very severe or if the patient becomes tolerant to the medication.

**Usual pediatric dose**
Analgesic—
  Dosage must be individualized by physician on the basis of patient's age and size. Use of a calibrated measure is recommended to prevent possible overdosage in children up to 6 years of age.

**Strength(s) usually available**
U.S.—
  5 mg per 5 mL (Rx) [GENERIC].
  10 mg per 5 mL (Rx) [GENERIC].
Canada—
  Not commercially available.

**Packaging and storage**
Store between 15 and 30 °C (59 and 86 °F). Store in a tight container. Protect from light. Protect from freezing.

**Auxiliary labeling**
• May cause drowsiness.
• Avoid alcoholic beverages.
• May be habit-forming.

**Note**
Controlled substance in the U.S.

### METHADONE HYDROCHLORIDE TABLETS USP

**Usual adult dose**
Analgesic—
  Oral, 2.5 to 10 mg every three to four hours as needed initially. For chronic use, dose and dosing interval to be adjusted according to patient response.

**Usual pediatric dose**
Analgesic—
  Dosage must be individualized by physician on the basis of patient's age and size.

**Strength(s) usually available**
U.S.—
  5 mg (Rx) [*Dolophine* (lactose; sucrose); *Methadose;* GENERIC].
  10 mg (Rx) [*Dolophine* (lactose; sucrose); *Methadose;* GENERIC].
Canada—
  Not commercially available.

**Packaging and storage**
Store below 40 °C (104 °F), preferably between 15 and 30 °C (59 and 86 °F). Store in a well-closed container.

**Auxiliary labeling**
- May cause drowsiness.
- Avoid alcoholic beverages.
- May be habit-forming.

**Note**
Controlled substance in the U.S.

### METHADONE HYDROCHLORIDE TABLETS (DISPERSIBLE) USP

**Usual adult dose**
Suppressant (narcotic abstinence syndrome)—
  Detoxification: Oral, 15 to 40 mg once a day or as needed to control observed withdrawal symptoms; dosage to be reduced at one- or two-day intervals according to patient response.
  Maintenance: Dosage must be individualized.

**Usual adult prescribing limits**
Up to 120 mg per day.

**Usual pediatric dose**
Suppressant (narcotic abstinence syndrome)—
  Dosage must be individualized by physician according to the needs of the specific patient. Dosage must not exceed 120 mg per day.
Note: Patients younger than 18 years of age may be admitted to methadone maintenance programs only after 2 documented attempts at short-term (up to 30 days) detoxification or drug-free treatment have failed. A 1-week waiting period is required between a detoxification attempt and admission to a methadone maintenance program. A parent, legal guardian, or other responsible adult designated by the State authority must complete and sign a consent to treatment form for all such minors.

**Strength(s) usually available**
U.S.—
  40 mg (Rx) [*Methadose;* GENERIC].

**Packaging and storage**
Store between 15 and 30 °C (59 and 86 °F). Store in a well-closed container.

**Preparation of dosage form**
U.S. Federal regulations stipulate that the tablets must be dispersed in water or other suitable liquid before being administered to the patient. Treatment centers that dispense both methadone and levomethadyl (which must also be dispensed as a diluted liquid) should use liquids of different colors for preparing each medication, so that they can be readily distinguished from each other. The dispersible tablets have been formulated with insoluble excipients as a deterrent to misuse of the medication by injection.

**Auxiliary labeling**
- May cause drowsiness.
- Avoid alcoholic beverages.
- May be habit-forming.

**Note**
Controlled substance in the U.S.

## Parenteral Dosage Forms

### METHADONE HYDROCHLORIDE INJECTION USP

**Usual adult dose**
Analgesic—
  Intramuscular or subcutaneous, 2.5 to 10 mg every three to four hours as needed.
Suppressant (narcotic abstinence syndrome)—
  For detoxification only: Intramuscular or subcutaneous, 15 to 40 mg once a day or as needed to control observed withdrawal symptoms; dosage to be reduced at one- or two-day intervals according to patient response.
  Note: Parenteral administration in a detoxification regimen is recommended only for patients unable to take medication orally.

**Usual pediatric dose**
Analgesic—
  Dosage must be individualized by physician on the basis of patient's age and size.

**Strength(s) usually available**
U.S.—
  With preservative:
    10 mg per mL (Rx) [*Dolophine* (chlorobutanol)].
  Without preservative:
    10 mg per mL (Rx) [*Dolophine*].

**Packaging and storage**
Store below 40 °C (104 °F), preferably between 15 and 30 °C (59 and 86 °F), in a light-resistant container. Protect from freezing.

**Auxiliary labeling**
- May cause drowsiness.
- Avoid alcoholic beverages.
- May be habit-forming.

**Note**
Controlled substance in the U.S.

---

## MORPHINE

## Summary of Differences
Indications:
  Drug of choice to relieve pain due to acute myocardial infarction.
  Also, indicated as adjunctive therapy in the treatment of acute pulmonary edema secondary to left ventricular failure.
  Also, used as antitussive.
Pharmacology/pharmacokinetics:
  Mechanism of action/effect—
    An opioid agonist analgesic; exerts agonist activity primarily at the mu receptor.
  Equivalence—
    60 mg via oral administration therapeutically equivalent to 10 mg intramuscularly; however, with chronic use on a fixed schedule may decrease to 20–30 mg.
  Protein binding—
    Low.
  Half-life—
    2–3 hours.
  Onset of action—
    Epidural: 15–60 minutes.
    Intramuscular: 10–30 minutes.
    Intrathecal: 15–60 minutes.
    Rectal: 20–60 minutes.
    Subcutaneous: 10–30 minutes.
  Time to peak effect—
    Intramuscular: 30–60 minutes.
    Intravenous: 20 minutes.
    Oral (immediate-release dosage forms): 1–2 hours.
    Subcutaneous: 50–90 minutes.
  Duration of action (nontolerant patients only; may decrease as tolerance develops during chronic therapy)—
    Epidural: Up to 24 hours.
    Intramuscular: 4–5 hours.
    Intrathecal: Up to 24 hours.
    Intravenous: 4–5 hours.
    Oral: 4–5 hours with immediate-release dosage forms; 8 or 12 hours (depending on specific product) with extended-release dosage forms.
    Subcutaneous: 4–5 hours.
  Elimination—
    85% Renal, 9–12% as unchanged morphine; 7–10% biliary.
Precautions:
  Drug interactions and/or related problems—
    Also may decrease clearance of zidovudine; toxicity of either or both medications may be potentiated.
Side/adverse effects:
  More likely than most other opioids to cause constipation and to produce symptoms associated with histamine release.

## Additional Dosing Information
See also *General Dosing Information.*

**For oral dosage forms only**
The oral dosage forms are recommended for administration via a fixed dosage schedule to patients with severe, chronic pain. However, low doses of an immediate-release oral dosage form may be used on an as-needed basis to relieve "breakthrough" pain that occurs during chronic treatment with an extended-release dosage form.
Periodic attempts should be made to reduce the dosage after an initial response has been achieved and maintained for at least 3 days.
The oral liquid may be diluted in a glass of fruit juice just prior to ingestion, if desired, to improve the taste.
The extended-release tablets are to be swallowed whole. They should not be broken, crushed, or chewed.

### For parenteral dosage forms only
Intramuscular administration is recommended when repeated doses are required. Repeated subcutaneous administration causes local tissue irritation, pain, and induration.

The 25- or 50-mg per mL concentration of morphine sulfate injection available in Canada may be administered undiluted to opioid-tolerant patients requiring high-dose therapy. The 25-mg-per-mL concentration of morphine sulfate injection available in the U.S. is intended only for the preparation of intravenous infusion solutions and is not to be administered via other parenteral routes.

### Bioequivalenence information
Bioavailability or bioequivalence problems among different brands of Morphine Sulfate Tablets (immediate-release) and different brands of Morphine Sulfate Oral Solution have not been documented.

Morphine Sulfate Extended-release Capsules (available in Canada) should not be interchanged with other extended-release dosage forms containing morphine hydrochloride or morphine sulfate. Bioavailability or bioequivalence studies comparing the products have not been done.

## Oral Dosage Forms

### MORPHINE HYDROCHLORIDE SYRUP

#### Usual adult dose
Analgesic—
   Chronic pain: Dosage and dosing interval must be individualized by the physician according to the severity of pain and patient response. Initial oral doses of 10 to 30 mg every four hours are recommended by most manufacturers of oral morphine products. However, some patients receiving the medication via the recommended fixed dosing schedule may respond to lower doses, while others have required 75 mg or more.

#### Usual pediatric dose
Analgesic—
   Dosage must be individualized by the physician according to the severity of pain as well as on the basis of the patient's age and size. Use of calibrated measure is recommended to prevent possible overdosage in children up to 6 years of age.

#### Strength(s) usually available
U.S.—
   Not commercially available.
Canada—
   1 mg per mL (Rx) [*Morphitec* (alcohol 5%; tartrazine); *M.O.S*].
   5 mg per mL (Rx) [*Morphitec* (alcohol 5%; tartrazine); *M.O.S*].
   10 mg per mL (Rx) [*Morphitec* (alcohol 5%; tartrazine); *M.O.S*].
   20 mg per mL (Rx) [*Morphitec* (alcohol 5%; tartrazine); *M.O.S*].
   50 mg per mL (Rx) [*M.O.S*].

#### Packaging and storage
Store below 40 °C (104 °F), preferably between 15 and 30 °C (59 and 86 °F), in a well-closed container, unless otherwise specified by manufacturer. Protect from freezing.

#### Auxiliary labeling
- May cause drowsiness.
- Avoid alcoholic beverages.
- May be habit-forming.

#### Note
Controlled substance in Canada.

### MORPHINE HYDROCHLORIDE TABLETS

#### Usual adult dose
Analgesic—
   Chronic pain: Dosage and dosing interval must be individualized by the physician according to the severity of pain and patient response. Initial oral doses of 10 to 30 mg every four hours are recommended by most manufacturers of oral morphine products. However, some patients receiving the medication via the recommended fixed dosing schedule may respond to lower doses, while others have required 75 mg or more.

#### Usual pediatric dose
Analgesic—
   Dosage must be individualized by the physician according to the severity of pain as well as on the basis of the patient's age and size.

#### Strength(s) usually available
U.S.—
   Not commercially available.
Canada—
   10 mg (Rx) [*M.O.S*].
   20 mg (Rx) [*M.O.S*].
   40 mg (Rx) [*M.O.S*].
   60 mg (Rx) [*M.O.S*].

#### Packaging and storage
Store below 40 °C (104 °F), preferably between 15 and 30 °C (59 and 86 °F), in a well-closed container, unless otherwise specified by manufacturer. Protect from freezing.

#### Auxiliary labeling
- May cause drowsiness.
- Avoid alcoholic beverages.
- May be habit-forming.

#### Note
Controlled substance in Canada.

### MORPHINE HYDROCHLORIDE EXTENDED-RELEASE TABLETS

#### Usual adult dose
Analgesic—
   Chronic pain: Dosage must be individualized by the physician according to the severity of pain and patient response.

#### Usual pediatric dose
Dosage has not been established.

#### Strength(s) usually available
U.S.—
   Not commercially available.
Canada—
   30 mg (Rx) [*M.O.S.-S.R*].
   60 mg (Rx) [*M.O.S.-S.R*].

#### Packaging and storage
Store below 40 °C (104 °F), preferably between 15 and 30 °C (59 and 86 °F), in a well-closed container, unless otherwise specified by manufacturer.

#### Auxiliary labeling
- Swallow tablets whole.
- May cause drowsiness.
- Avoid alcoholic beverages.
- May be habit-forming.

#### Note
Controlled substance in Canada.

### MORPHINE SULFATE CAPSULES

#### Usual adult dose
Analgesic—
   Chronic pain: Dosage and dosing interval must be individualized by the physician according to the severity of pain and patient response. Initial oral doses of 10 to 30 mg every four hours are recommended by most manufacturers of oral morphine products. However, some patients receiving the medication via the recommended fixed dosing schedule may respond to lower doses, while others have required 75 mg or more.

#### Usual pediatric dose
Analgesic—
   Dosage must be individualized by the physician according to the severity of pain as well as on the basis of the patient's age and size.

#### Strength(s) usually available
U.S.—
   15 mg (Rx) [*MSIR*].
   30 mg (Rx) [*MSIR*].
Canada—
   Not commercially available.

### MORPHINE SULFATE EXTENDED-RELEASE CAPSULES

Note: The extended-release capsule dosage form has not been evaluated for bioequivalence with other extended-release dosage forms containing morphine hydrochloride or morphine sulfate and should not be interchanged with them.

#### Usual adult dose
Analgesic—
   Chronic pain: Oral, 30 mg every twelve hours, initially, with dosage then being adjusted according to the requirements of the individual patient.

Note: Patients being transferred from other opioid analgesics or other morphine dosage forms to the morphine sulfate extended-release capsules should receive a total daily dose of oral morphine sulfate equivalent to the established total daily dose of previously administered medication, administered in divided doses at twelve-hour intervals. The manufacturers' prescribing information contains recommendations for calculating equivalent dosage.

**Usual pediatric dose**
Dosage has not been established.

**Strength(s) usually available**
U.S.—
  Not commercially available.
Canada—
  10 mg (Rx) [*M-Eslon*].
  30 mg (Rx) [*M-Eslon*].
  60 mg (Rx) [*M-Eslon*].
  100 mg (Rx) [*M-Eslon*].

**Packaging and storage**
Store between 15 and 30 °C (59 and 86 °F).

**Auxiliary labeling**
• May cause drowsiness.
• Avoid alcoholic beverages.
• May be habit-forming.

**Note**
Controlled substance in Canada.

## MORPHINE SULFATE ORAL SOLUTION

Note: Bioavailability or bioequivalence problems among different brands of Morphine Sulfate Oral Solution have not been documented.

**Usual adult dose**
Analgesic—
  Chronic pain: Dosage and dosing interval must be individualized by the physician according to the severity of pain and patient response. Initial oral doses of 10 to 30 mg every four hours are recommended by most manufacturers of oral morphine products. However, some patients receiving the medication via the recommended fixed dosing schedule may respond to lower doses, while others have required 75 mg or more.

**Usual pediatric dose**
Analgesic—
  Dosage must be individualized by the physician according to the severity of pain as well as on the basis of the patient's age and size. Use of calibrated measure is recommended to prevent possible overdosage in children up to 6 years of age.

**Strength(s) usually available**
U.S.—
  10 mg per 2.5 mL (unit dose) (Rx) [*Rescudose*; *Roxanol UD*].
  10 mg per 5 mL (Rx) [*MSIR* (sucrose); *MS/L*; GENERIC].
  20 mg per 5 mL (Rx) [*MSIR*; *Roxanol UD*; GENERIC].
  20 mg per mL (Rx) [*MSIR*; *MS/L Concentrate*; *OMS Concentrate*; *Roxanol*].
  30 mg per 1.5 mL (Rx) [*Roxanol UD*].
  100 mg per 5 mL (Rx) [*Roxanol 100*].
Canada—
  2 mg per mL (Rx) [GENERIC].
  4 mg per mL (Rx) [GENERIC].
  20 mg per mL (Rx) [*Statex Drops*].
  50 mg per mL (Rx) [*Statex Drops*].

**Packaging and storage**
Store between 15 and 30 °C (59 and 86 °F), in a tight, light-resistant container, unless otherwise specified by manufacturer. Protect from freezing.

**Auxiliary labeling**
• May cause drowsiness.
• Avoid alcoholic beverages.
• May be habit-forming.

**Note**
Controlled substance in both the U.S. and Canada.

## MORPHINE SULFATE SYRUP

**Usual adult dose**
Analgesic—
  Chronic pain: Dosage and dosing interval must be individualized by the physician according to the severity of pain and patient response. Initial oral doses of 10 to 30 mg every four hours are recommended by most manufacturers of oral morphine products. However, some patients receiving the medication via the recommended fixed dosing schedule may respond to lower doses, while others have required 75 mg or more.

**Usual pediatric dose**
Analgesic—
  Dosage must be individualized by the physician according to the severity of pain as well as on the basis of the patient's age and size.

**Strength(s) usually available**
U.S.—
  Not commercially available.
Canada—
  1 mg per mL (Rx) [*Statex*].
  5 mg per mL (Rx) [*Statex*].
  10 mg per mL (Rx) [*Statex*].

**Packaging and storage**
Store below 40 °C (104 °F), preferably between 15 and 30 °C (59 and 86 °F), in a well-closed container, unless otherwise specified by manufacturer. Protect from freezing.

**Auxiliary labeling**
• May cause drowsiness.
• Avoid alcoholic beverages.
• May be habit-forming.

**Note**
Controlled substance in Canada.

## MORPHINE SULFATE TABLETS

Note: Bioavailability or bioequivalence problems among different brands of Morphine Sulfate Tablets have not been documented.

**Usual adult dose**
Analgesic—
  Chronic pain: Dosage and dosing interval must be individualized by the physician according to the severity of pain and patient response. Initial oral doses of 10 to 30 mg every four hours are recommended by most manufacturers of oral morphine products. However, some patients receiving the medication via the recommended fixed dosing schedule may respond to lower doses, while others have required 75 mg or more.

**Usual pediatric dose**
Analgesic—
  Chronic pain: Dosage must be individualized by the physician according to the severity of pain as well as on the basis of the patient's age and size.

**Strength(s) usually available**
U.S.—
  15 mg (Rx) [*MSIR* (scored); GENERIC].
  30 mg (Rx) [*MSIR* (scored); GENERIC].
Canada—
  5 mg (Rx) [*MS IR* (scored); *Statex* (scored)].
  10 mg (Rx) [*MS IR* (scored); *Statex* (scored)].
  15 mg (Rx) [GENERIC].
  20 mg (Rx) [*MS IR* (scored)].
  25 mg (Rx) [*Statex* (scored)].
  30 mg (Rx) [*MS IR* (scored); GENERIC].
  50 mg (Rx) [*Statex* (scored)].

**Packaging and storage**
Store below 40 °C (104 °F), preferably between 15 and 30 °C (59 and 86 °F), in a well-closed container, unless otherwise specified by manufacturer.

**Auxiliary labeling**
• May cause drowsiness.
• Avoid alcoholic beverages.
• May be habit-forming.

**Note**
Controlled substance in both the U.S. and Canada.

## MORPHINE SULFATE EXTENDED-RELEASE TABLETS

**Usual adult dose**
Analgesic—
  Chronic pain: Oral, 30 mg every twelve hours, initially, with dosage and dosing interval then being adjusted according to the requirements of the individual patient.

Note: Patients being transferred from other opioid analgesics or other morphine sulfate dosage forms to the morphine sulfate extended-release tablets should receive a total daily dose of oral morphine sulfate equivalent to the established total daily dose of previously administered medication, administered in divided doses at twelve-hour intervals. The manufacturers' prescribing information contains recommendations for calculating equivalent dosage.

### Usual pediatric dose
Dosage has not been established.

### Strength(s) usually available
U.S.—
- 15 mg (Rx) [*M S Contin*; GENERIC].
- 30 mg (Rx) [*M S Contin*; *Oramorph SR*; GENERIC].
- 60 mg (Rx) [*M S Contin*; *Oramorph SR*; GENERIC].
- 100 mg (Rx) [*M S Contin*; *Oramorph SR*; GENERIC].
- 200 mg (Rx) [*M S Contin*].

Canada—
- 15 mg (Rx) [*M S Contin*].
- 30 mg (Rx) [*M S Contin*; *Oramorph SR*].
- 60 mg (Rx) [*M S Contin*; *Oramorph SR*].
- 100 mg (Rx) [*M S Contin*; *Oramorph SR*].
- 200 mg (Rx) [*M S Contin* (scored)].

### Packaging and storage
Store below 40 °C (104 °F), preferably between 15 and 30 °C (59 and 86 °F), in a well-closed container, unless otherwise specified by manufacturer.

### Auxiliary labeling
- Swallow tablets whole.
- May cause drowsiness.
- Avoid alcoholic beverages.
- May be habit-forming.

### Note
Controlled substance in both the U.S. and Canada.

## Parenteral Dosage Forms

### MORPHINE SULFATE INJECTION USP

#### Usual adult dose
Analgesic—
Intramuscular or subcutaneous, 5 to 20 mg (usually 10 mg, initially) every four hours as needed. For severe, chronic pain the medication may also be administered by subcutaneous infusion, using a portable pump, at a rate titrated to the requirements and response of the individual patient.

Note: The recommendation of an initial 10-mg dose is based on a 70-kg person.

In Canada, the 25- or 50-mg-per-mL concentration may be substituted for lower strengths of morphine sulfate injection or for other opioid analgesics in opioid-tolerant patients requiring high-dose therapy. Dosage must be individualized, depending on the severity of pain, opioid requirements at the time therapy with the high-potency injection is initiated, and patient response. Although patients who have become tolerant to another opioid may be at least partially cross-tolerant to morphine also, it is recommended that one-half of the equianalgesic dose of morphine be used initially, then adjusted as necessary.

Intravenous, 4 to 10 mg diluted in 4 to 5 mL of sterile water for injection, administered slowly. For severe, chronic pain the medication may also be administered via intravenous infusion at a rate titrated to the requirements and response of the individual patient.

Epidural (in the lumbar region), 5 mg.

Note: If adequate pain relief is not achieved within one hour, incremental doses of 1 to 2 mg may be administered at intervals sufficient to assess effectiveness, up to a maximum of 10 mg per twenty-four hours.

Intrathecal, 200 mcg (0.2 mg) to 1 mg as a single dose.

Note: Clinical experience with repeated intrathecal injections is limited. Therefore, repeated administration via this route is not recommended. Alternate routes of administration should be considered for treating recurrent or chronic pain.

#### Usual pediatric dose
Analgesic—
Subcutaneous, 100 to 200 mcg (0.1 to 0.2 mg) per kg of body weight every four hours as needed, not to exceed 15 mg per dose.

Intravenous, 50 to 100 mcg (0.05 to 0.1 mg) per kg of body weight, administered very slowly.

Preoperative—
Intramuscular, 50 to 100 mcg (0.05 to 0.1 mg) per kg of body weight, not to exceed 10 mg per dose.

#### Strength(s) usually available
U.S.—
With preservative:
- 1 mg per mL (Rx) [GENERIC].
- 2 mg per mL (Rx) [GENERIC].
- 4 mg per mL (Rx) [GENERIC].
- 5 mg per mL (Rx) [GENERIC].
- 8 mg per mL (Rx) [GENERIC].
- 10 mg per mL (Rx) [GENERIC].
- 15 mg per mL (Rx) [GENERIC].
- 25 mg per mL (Rx) [GENERIC].
- 50 mg per mL (Rx) [GENERIC].

Without preservative:
- 500 mcg (0.5 mg) per mL (Rx) [*Astramorph PF*; *Duramorph*; GENERIC].
- 1 mg per mL (Rx) [*Astramorph PF*; *Duramorph*; GENERIC].
- 50 mg per mL (Rx) [GENERIC].

Canada—
With preservative:
- 1 mg per mL (Rx) [GENERIC].
- 2 mg per mL (Rx) [GENERIC].
- 5 mg per mL (Rx) [GENERIC].
- 10 mg per mL (Rx) [GENERIC].
- 15 mg per mL (Rx) [GENERIC].
- 25 mg per mL (Rx) [*Morphine Forte*].
- 50 mg per mL (Rx) [*Morphine Extra-Forte*].

Without preservative:
- 500 mcg (0.5 mg) per mL (Rx) [*Epimorph*; GENERIC].
- 1 mg per mL (Rx) [*Epimorph*; GENERIC].
- 2 mg per mL (Rx) [GENERIC].
- 25 mg per mL (Rx) [*Morphine H.P*; GENERIC].
- 50 mg per mL (Rx) [*Morphine H.P*; GENERIC].

#### Packaging and storage
Store below 40 °C (104 °F), preferably between 15 and 30 °C (59 and 86 °F), unless otherwise specified by manufacturer. Protect from light. Protect from freezing.

#### Stability
Do not autoclave the preservative-free injection.
Unused portion of preservative-free injection must be discarded.

#### Incompatibilities
Morphine Sulfate Injection USP is incompatible with soluble barbiturates.

#### Auxiliary labeling
- May cause drowsiness.
- Avoid alcoholic beverages.
- May be habit-forming.

#### Note
Controlled substance in both the U.S. and Canada.

### MORPHINE SULFATE SOLUBLE TABLETS

#### Usual adult dose
Analgesic—
Intramuscular or subcutaneous, 5 to 20 mg (usually 10 mg, initially) every four hours as needed.

Note: The recommendation of an initial 10-mg dose is based on a 70-kg person.

#### Usual pediatric dose
Analgesic—
Subcutaneous, 100 to 200 mcg (0.1 to 0.2 mg) per kg of body weight every four hours as needed, not to exceed 15 mg per dose.

#### Strength(s) usually available
U.S.—
- 10 mg (Rx) [GENERIC].
- 15 mg (Rx) [GENERIC].
- 30 mg (Rx) [GENERIC].

Canada—
Not commercially available.

#### Packaging and storage
Store between 15 and 30 °C (59 and 86 °F), in a tight, light-resistant container, unless otherwise specified by manufacturer.

#### Preparation of dosage form
For parenteral administration—Dissolve the required number of tablets in a suitable volume of sterile water for injection, then filter through a 0.22–micron membrane filter.

#### Auxiliary labeling
- May cause drowsiness.
- Avoid alcoholic beverages.
- May be habit-forming.

#### Note
Controlled substance in the U.S.

## Rectal Dosage Forms
### MORPHINE HYDROCHLORIDE SUPPOSITORIES
**Usual adult dose**
Analgesic—
   Rectal, 20 to 30 mg every four to six hours.

**Usual pediatric dose**
Analgesic—
   Dosage must be individualized by the physician according to the severity of pain as well as on the basis of the patient's age and size.

**Strength(s) usually available**
U.S.—
   Not commercially available.
Canada—
   10 mg (Rx) [*M.O.S*].
   20 mg (Rx) [*M.O.S*].
   30 mg (Rx) [*M.O.S*].

**Packaging and storage**
Store below 40 °C (104 °F), preferably between 15 and 30 °C (59 and 86 °F), in a well-closed container, unless otherwise specified by manufacturer. Protect from freezing.

**Auxiliary labeling**
- May cause drowsiness.
- Avoid alcoholic beverages.
- May be habit-forming.

**Note**
Controlled substance in Canada.

### MORPHINE SULFATE SUPPOSITORIES
**Usual adult dose**
Analgesic—
   Rectal, 10 to 30 mg every four hours or as required.
   Note: Dosage must be individualized according to the severity of pain and the response of the patient.

**Usual pediatric dose**
Analgesic—
   Dosage must be individualized by physician on the basis of the patient's age and size.

**Strength(s) usually available**
U.S.—
   5 mg (Rx) [*MS/S; RMS Uniserts; Roxanol;* GENERIC].
   10 mg (Rx) [*MS/S; RMS Uniserts; Roxanol;* GENERIC].
   20 mg (Rx) [*MS/S; RMS Uniserts; Roxanol;* GENERIC].
   30 mg (Rx) [*MS/S; RMS Uniserts; Roxanol;* GENERIC].
Canada—
   5 mg (Rx) [*Statex*].
   10 mg (Rx) [*MS IR; Statex*].
   20 mg (Rx) [*MS IR; Statex*].
   30 mg (Rx) [*MS IR; Statex*].

**Packaging and storage**
Store between 15 and 30 °C (59 and 86 °F), in a well-closed container, unless otherwise specified by manufacturer. Protect from freezing.

**Auxiliary labeling**
- May cause drowsiness.
- Avoid alcoholic beverages.
- May be habit-forming.

**Note**
Controlled substance in both the U.S. and Canada.

---

# *NALBUPHINE*

## Summary of Differences
Indications:
   Caution required when used as analgesic to relieve pain in patients with severely compromised cardiac function; cardiovascular effects in these patients have not been fully evaluated.
Pharmacology/pharmacokinetics:
   Mechanism of action/effect—
     An opioid agonist/antagonist analgesic.
     Agonist: Has agonist activity at the kappa and sigma receptors.
     Antagonist: Has antagonist activity at the mu receptor; may precipitate withdrawal symptoms in patients who are physically dependent on mu-receptor agonists.
   Equivalence—
     10 mg via intramuscular injection therapeutically equivalent to 10 mg of intramuscular morphine.
   Half-life—
     5 hours.
   Onset of action—
     Intramuscular: Within 15 minutes.
     Intravenous: 2–3 minutes.
     Subcutaneous: Within 15 minutes.
   Time to peak concentration—
     Intramuscular: 0.5 hour.
   Peak plasma concentration—
     48 nanograms per mL.
   Time to peak effect—
     Intramuscular: 60 minutes.
     Intravenous: 30 minutes.
   Duration of action (nontolerant patients only; decreases as tolerance develops during chronic therapy)—
     Intramuscular: 3–6 hours.
     Intravenous: 3–4 hours.
     Subcutaneous: 3–6 hours.
   Elimination—
     Renal.
Precautions:
   Drug interactions and/or related problems—
     May antagonize effects of mu-receptor agonists.
   Medical considerations/contraindications—
     Also should be used with caution in patients who are physically dependent on opioid agonists.
Side/adverse effects:
   Rarely, may cause subjective and psychotomimetic effects characteristic of sigma receptor agonists.
   Respiratory depression subject to a "ceiling effect," after which the depth of respiratory depression does not increase with dose.
   More likely than most other opioid analgesics to produce symptoms associated with histamine release.
   Has lower dependence liability than opioid agonists.
   Withdrawal symptoms less severe than those produced by opioid agonist analgesics.

## Parenteral Dosage Forms
### NALBUPHINE HYDROCHLORIDE INJECTION
**Usual adult dose**
Analgesic—
   Intramuscular, intravenous, or subcutaneous, 10 mg every three to six hours as needed.
   Note: The usual adult dose is based on a 70-kg person.
Anesthesia adjunct (balanced anesthesia)—
   Initial: Intravenous, 300 mcg (0.3 mg) to 3 mg per kg of body weight, administered over a ten- to fifteen-minute period.
   Supplemental: Intravenous, 250 to 500 mcg (0.25 to 0.5 mg) per kg of body weight, as required.

**Usual adult prescribing limits**
For nontolerant patients—
   Up to 20 mg as a single dose and up to 160 mg as a total daily dose.

**Usual pediatric dose**
Dosage has not been established.

**Strength(s) usually available**
U.S.—
   With preservatives:
     10 mg per mL (Rx) [*Nubain* (methylparaben; propylparaben; sodium metabisulfite); GENERIC].
     20 mg per mL (Rx) [*Nubain* (methylparaben; propylparaben; sodium metabisulfite); GENERIC].
   Without preservatives:
     10 mg per mL (Rx) [*Nubain*].
     20 mg per mL (Rx) [*Nubain*].
Canada—
   With preservatives:
     10 mg per mL (Rx) [*Nubain* (methylparaben; propylparaben; sodium metabisulfite)].
     20 mg per mL (Rx) [*Nubain* (methylparaben; propylparaben; sodium metabisulfite)].

**Packaging and storage**
Store between 15 and 30 °C (59 and 86 °F), unless otherwise specified by manufacturer. Protect from light. Protect from freezing.

**Auxiliary labeling**
- May cause drowsiness.
- Avoid alcoholic beverages.

**Note**
Controlled substance in Canada.

## OPIUM

## Summary of Differences
Indications:
  Oral dosage form—
    Indicated as antidiarrheal.
    Also, used as narcotic abstinence syndrome suppressant in neonates.
Pharmacology/pharmacokinetics:
  Mechanism of action/effect—
    An opioid agonist analgesic; has agonist activity primarily at the mu receptor.
  Equivalence—
    13.3 mg parenterally is therapeutically equivalent to 10 mg of intramuscular morphine.
  Elimination—
    Renal and biliary.

## Additional Dosing Information
See also *General Dosing Information*.
The effects of opium preparations are due primarily to the morphine component.

**For oral dosage form only**
Alteration of intestinal motility in patients with traveler's diarrhea may result in prolonged fever by slowing expulsion of infectious organisms that penetrate intestinal mucosa (for example, *Shigella*, *Salmonella*, and certain strains of *Escherichia coli*).

Opium may produce fluid retention in the bowel, which may mask dehydration and electrolyte depletion caused by severe diarrhea, especially in young children. Patients with severe or prolonged diarrhea should be monitored for signs of dehydration or electrolyte imbalance, and corrective therapy administered as required.

To reduce the risk of toxic megacolon in patients with acute inflammatory bowel disease, treatment with opium tincture should be discontinued promptly if abdominal distention or other gastrointestinal symptoms occur.

Tolerance to the antidiarrheal effects of opium tincture may develop with prolonged use.

Following prolonged administration of high doses, opium tincture should be withdrawn gradually in order to reduce the possibility of withdrawal symptoms.

Many clinicians have recommended use of diluted opium tincture instead of paregoric in the treatment of neonatal narcotic dependence, because of the risks associated with two of the components of the paregoric formulation. Opium tincture is diluted to produce the same concentration of morphine as paregoric and may be administered every 3 hours, with gradual withdrawal over 2 to 4 weeks when symptoms are controlled.

**For parenteral dosage form only**
This formulation contains all of the alkaloids of opium as the hydrochlorides.

## Oral Dosage Forms
### OPIUM TINCTURE (Laudanum) USP
**Usual adult dose**
Antidiarrheal—
  Oral, 0.3 to 1.0 mL (usually 0.6 mL) (the equivalent of morphine—3 to 10 mg) four times a day.

**Usual adult prescribing limits**
A single dose of 1 mL, or a total of 6 mL within twenty-four hours.

**Usual pediatric dose**
Dosage has not been established.

**Strength(s) usually available**
U.S.—
  10% of opium (the equivalent of 900 mg to 1.1 grams of anhydrous morphine per 100 mL) (Rx) [GENERIC (alcohol 17–21%)].
Canada—
  10% of opium (the equivalent of 900 mg to 1.1 grams of anhydrous morphine per 100 mL) (Rx) [GENERIC (alcohol 17–21%)].

**Packaging and storage**
Store below 40 °C (104 °F), preferably between 15 and 30 °C (59 and 86 °F), unless otherwise specified by manufacturer. Store in a tight, light-resistant container. Avoid exposure to direct sunlight and excessive heat. Protect from freezing.

**Auxiliary labeling**
- May cause drowsiness.
- Avoid alcoholic beverages.
- Do not take other medicines without your doctor's advice.
- Keep out of reach of children.
- May be habit-forming.

**Note**
Caution—Be careful not to confuse opium tincture with camphorated tincture of opium (paregoric).
Controlled substance in both the U.S. and Canada.
Refrigeration is not recommended because decreased solubility and precipitation of some of the ingredients may occur. If this occurs, the preparation must be discarded.

## Parenteral Dosage Forms
### OPIUM ALKALOIDS HYDROCHLORIDES INJECTION (Papaveretum)
**Usual adult dose**
Analgesic—
  Intramuscular or subcutaneous, 5 to 20 mg every four to five hours as needed.

**Usual pediatric dose**
Dosage has not been established.

**Strength(s) usually available**
U.S.—
  Not commercially available.
Canada—
  With preservatives:
    20 mg, as hydrochlorides of opium alkaloids, per mL (Rx) [*Pantopon* (methylparaben; propylparaben)].
Note: Contains 10 mg of anhydrous morphine per mL.

**Packaging and storage**
Store between 15 and 30 °C (59 and 86 °F), unless otherwise specified by manufacturer. Protect from freezing.

**Auxiliary labeling**
- May cause drowsiness.
- Avoid alcoholic beverages.
- May be habit-forming.

**Note**
Controlled substance in Canada.

## OXYCODONE

## Summary of Differences
Pharmacology/pharmacokinetics:
  Mechanism of action/effect—
    An opioid agonist analgesic; has agonist activity primarily at the mu receptor.
  Equivalence—
    30 mg via oral administration therapeutically equivalent to 10 mg of intramuscular morphine.
  Half-life—
    2–3 hours.
  Time to peak effect—
    Oral: 1 hour.
  Duration of action (nontolerant patients only; duration decreases as tolerance develops during chronic therapy)—
    Oral: 3–4 hours.
  Elimination—
    Renal.

## Oral Dosage Forms
### OXYCODONE HYDROCHLORIDE ORAL SOLUTION USP
**Usual adult dose**
Analgesic—
  Oral, 5 mg every three to six hours as needed; may be increased if severe pain is present.

Usual pediatric dose
Dosage must be individualized by physician on the basis of patient's age and size. Use of calibrated measure is recommended to prevent possible overdosage in children up to 6 years of age.

Strength(s) usually available
U.S.—
  5 mg per 5 mL (Rx) [*Roxicodone* (alcohol 7–9%)].
  20 mg per mL (Rx) [*Roxicodone Intensol*].
Canada—
  Not commercially available.

Packaging and storage
Store between 15 and 30 °C (59 and 86 °F), unless otherwise specified by manufacturer. Store in a tight, light-resistant container. Protect from freezing.

Auxiliary labeling
• May cause drowsiness.
• Avoid alcoholic beverages.
• May be habit-forming.

Note
Controlled substance in the U.S.

### OXYCODONE HYDROCHLORIDE TABLETS USP

Usual adult dose
Analgesic—
  Oral, 5 mg every three to six hours or 10 mg three or four times a day as needed; may be increased if severe pain is present.

Usual pediatric dose
Dosage must be individualized by physician on the basis of patient's age and size.

Strength(s) usually available
U.S.—
  5 mg (Rx) [*Roxicodone* (scored)].
Canada—
  5 mg (Rx) [*Supeudol*].
  10 mg (Rx) [*Supeudol*].

Packaging and storage
Store below 40 °C (104 °F), preferably between 15 and 30 °C (59 and 86 °F). Store in a tight, light-resistant container.

Auxiliary labeling
• May cause drowsiness.
• Avoid alcoholic beverages.
• May be habit-forming.

Note
Controlled substance in both the U.S. and Canada.

## Rectal Dosage Forms

### OXYCODONE HYDROCHLORIDE SUPPOSITORIES

Usual adult dose
Analgesic—
  Rectal, 10 to 40 mg three or four times a day.

Usual pediatric dose
Dosage must be individualized by physician on the basis of patient's age and size.

Strength(s) usually available
U.S.—
  Not commercially available.
Canada—
  10 mg (Rx) [*Supeudol*].
  20 mg (Rx) [*Supeudol*].

Packaging and storage
Store between 2 and 8 °C (36 and 46 °F), in a well-closed container, unless otherwise specified by manufacturer. Protect from freezing.

Auxiliary labeling
• May cause drowsiness.
• Avoid alcoholic beverages.
• May be habit-forming.
• Store in refrigerator. Protect from freezing.

Note
Controlled substance in Canada.

# OXYMORPHONE

## Summary of Differences
Indications:
  Also, FDA-approved, but rarely if ever used, as adjunctive therapy in the treatment of acute pulmonary edema secondary to left ventricular failure.
Pharmacology/pharmacokinetics:
  Mechanism of action/effect—
    An opioid agonist analgesic; has agonist activity primarily at the mu receptor.
  Equivalence—
    1 mg via intramuscular injection or 10 mg rectally therapeutically equivalent to 10 mg of intramuscular morphine.
  Onset of action—
    Intramuscular: 10–15 minutes.
    Intravenous: 5–10 minutes.
    Subcutaneous: 10–20 minutes.
    Rectal: 15–30 minutes.
  Time to peak effect—
    Intramuscular: 30–90 minutes.
    Intravenous: 15–30 minutes.
    Rectal: 2 hours.
  Duration of action (nontolerant patients only; duration decreases as tolerance develops during chronic therapy)—
    Intramuscular: 3–6 hours.
    Intravenous: 3–4 hours.
    Subcutaneous: 3–6 hours.
    Rectal: 3–6 hours.
  Elimination—
    Renal.

## Parenteral Dosage Forms

### OXYMORPHONE HYDROCHLORIDE INJECTION USP

Usual adult dose
Analgesic—
  Intramuscular or subcutaneous, 1 to 1.5 mg every three to six hours as needed.
  Intravenous, 500 mcg (0.5 mg).
Note: Doses may be cautiously increased, if necessary, if pain is severe.
  For obstetrical analgesia—Intramuscular, 500 mcg (0.5 mg) to 1 mg.

Usual pediatric dose
Dosage has not been established.

Strength(s) usually available
U.S.—
  With preservatives:
    1 mg per mL (Rx) [*Numorphan* (methylparaben; propylparaben)].
    1.5 mg per mL (Rx) [*Numorphan* (methylparaben; propylparaben)].
Canada—
  With preservatives:
    1.5 mg per mL (Rx) [*Numorphan* (methylparaben; propylparaben)].

Packaging and storage
Store below 40 °C (104 °F), preferably between 15 and 30 °C (59 and 86 °F), unless otherwise specified by manufacturer. Protect from light. Protect from freezing.

Auxiliary labeling
• May cause drowsiness.
• Avoid alcoholic beverages.
• May be habit-forming.

Note
Controlled substance in both the U.S. and Canada.

## Rectal Dosage Forms

### OXYMORPHONE HYDROCHLORIDE SUPPOSITORIES USP

Usual adult dose
Analgesic—
  Rectal, 5 mg every four to six hours as needed.

Usual pediatric dose
Dosage has not been established.

Strength(s) usually available
U.S.—
  5 mg (Rx) [*Numorphan*].

Canada—
 5 mg (Rx) [*Numorphan*].

**Packaging and storage**
Store between 2 and 8 °C (36 and 46 °F), in a well-closed container. Protect from freezing.

**Auxiliary labeling**
- May cause drowsiness.
- Avoid alcoholic beverages.
- May be habit-forming.
- Store in refrigerator. Protect from freezing.

**Note**
Controlled substance in both the U.S. and Canada.

## PENTAZOCINE

## Summary of Differences
Indications:
 Less desirable than morphine or other opioid agonist analgesics for relief of pain due to acute myocardial infarction because of cardiovascular effects that tend to increase cardiac work.
Pharmacology/pharmacokinetics:
 Mechanism of action/effect—
  An opioid agonist/antagonist analgesic.
  Agonist: Has agonist activity at the kappa and sigma receptors.
  Antagonist: Has antagonist activity at the mu receptor; may precipitate withdrawal symptoms in patients who are physically dependent on mu-receptor agonists.
 Equivalence—
  60 mg via intramuscular injection or 180 mg via oral administration therapeutically equivalent to 10 mg of intramuscular morphine.
 Protein binding—
  Moderate.
 Half-life—
  2–3 hours.
 Onset of action—
  Intramuscular: 15–20 minutes.
  Intravenous: 2–3 minutes.
  Oral: 15–30 minutes.
  Subcutaneous: 15–20 minutes.
 Time to peak effect—
  Intramuscular: 30–60 minutes.
  Intravenous: 15–30 minutes.
  Oral: 60–90 minutes.
  Subcutaneous: 30–60 minutes.
 Duration of action (nontolerant patients only; decreases as tolerance develops during chronic therapy)—
  Intramuscular: 2–3 hours.
  Intravenous: 2–3 hours.
  Oral: 3 hours.
  Subcutaneous: 2–3 hours.
 Elimination—
  Renal, 5–23% as unchanged pentazocine, and biliary.
Precautions:
 Drug interactions and/or related problems—
  May antagonize the effects of mu-receptor agonists.
 Medical considerations/contraindications—
  Also must be used with caution in patients physically dependent on opioid agonists and in patients with acute myocardial infarction.
Side/adverse effects:
 Although occurs rarely, more likely than butorphanol or nalbuphine to cause subjective and psychotomimetic effects characteristic of sigma receptor agonists.
 Respiratory depression subject to a "ceiling effect," after which the depth of respiratory depression does not increase with dose.
 Has lower dependence liability than opioid agonists.
 Withdrawal symptoms less severe than those produced by opioid agonist analgesics.

## Additional Dosing Information
See also *General Dosing Information*.

The naloxone present in the pentazocine and naloxone dosage formulation has no pharmacologic activity when administered orally. If the product is misused by injection, the naloxone antagonizes the effects of pentazocine. Also, injection of the medication will precipitate withdrawal symptoms if the patient is physically dependent on an opioid agonist.

For long-term administration, the oral form of the medication is preferred. If the parenteral form is used instead, dosage should be reduced gradually when the medication is to be discontinued to reduce the risk of withdrawal symptoms.

The extent to which pentazocine may produce withdrawal symptoms in patients who are physically dependent on opioid analgesics depends upon the dose of pentazocine, the specific opioid drug involved, and the degree to which physical dependence has developed.

**For parenteral dosage forms only**
Intravenous or intramuscular administration is recommended, especially when repeated doses are required. Subcutaneous administration may lead to severe tissue damage at the injection site. When the intramuscular route is used, rotation of injection sites is essential to prevent tissue damage.

## Oral Dosage Forms
### PENTAZOCINE HYDROCHLORIDE TABLETS USP
**Usual adult dose**
Analgesic—
 Oral, 50 mg of pentazocine (base) every three to four hours as needed. The dose may be increased to 100 mg (base) if necessary, but total daily dosage should not exceed 600 mg (base).

**Usual adult prescribing limits**
Analgesic—
 Up to 600 mg of pentazocine (base) per day

**Usual pediatric dose**
Dosage has not been established.

**Strength(s) usually available**
U.S.—
 Not commercially available.
Canada—
 50 mg (base) (Rx) [*Talwin* (scored; sulfites)].

**Packaging and storage**
Store below 40 °C (104 °F), preferably between 15 and 30 °C (59 and 86 °F), unless otherwise specified by manufacturer. Store in a tight, light-resistant container.

**Auxiliary labeling**
- May cause drowsiness.
- Avoid alcoholic beverages.
- May be habit-forming.

**Note**
Controlled substance in Canada.

### PENTAZOCINE AND NALOXONE HYDROCHLORIDES TABLETS USP
**Usual adult dose**
Analgesic—
 Oral, 50 mg of pentazocine (base) every three to four hours as needed. The dose may be increased to 100 mg (base) if necessary, but total daily dosage should not exceed 600 mg (base).

**Usual adult prescribing limits**
Analgesic—
 Up to 600 mg of pentazocine (base) per day.

**Usual pediatric dose**
Dosage has not been established.

**Strength(s) usually available**
U.S.—
 50 mg (base), with 500 mcg (0.5 mg) of naloxone hydrochloride (Rx) [*Talwin-Nx* (scored)].
Canada—
 Not commercially available.

**Packaging and storage**
Store below 40 °C (104 °F), preferably between 15 and 30 °C (59 and 86 °F), unless otherwise specified by manufacturer. Store in a tight, light-resistant container.

**Auxiliary labeling**
- May cause drowsiness.
- Avoid alcoholic beverages.
- May be habit-forming.

**Note**
Controlled substance in the U.S.

## Parenteral Dosage Forms
### PENTAZOCINE LACTATE INJECTION USP
**Usual adult dose**
Analgesic—
   Intramuscular, intravenous, or subcutaneous, 30 mg (base) every three to four hours as needed.
Obstetrical analgesia—
   Intramuscular, 30 mg (base) as a single dose; or
   Intravenous, 20 mg (base) administered when contractions become regular and repeated two or three times at two- to three-hour intervals as needed.

**Usual adult prescribing limits**
Up to 360 mg (base) daily.
As a single dose, up to 30 mg (base) intravenously or 60 mg (base) intramuscularly.

**Usual pediatric dose**
Dosage has not been established.

**Strength(s) usually available**
U.S.—
   With preservative:
      30 mg (base) per mL (Rx) [*Talwin* (acetone sodium bisulfite; methylparaben)].
   Without preservative:
      30 mg (base) per mL (Rx) [*Talwin* (may contain acetone sodium bisulfite)].
Canada—
   Without preservative:
      30 mg (base) per mL (Rx) [*Talwin*].

**Packaging and storage**
Store below 40 °C (104 °F), preferably between 15 and 30 °C (59 and 86 °F), unless otherwise specified by manufacturer. Protect from freezing.

**Incompatibilities**
Precipitation will occur if a soluble barbiturate is mixed in the same syringe as pentazocine.

**Auxiliary labeling**
• May cause drowsiness.
• Avoid alcoholic beverages.
• May be habit-forming.

**Note**
Controlled substance in both the U.S. and Canada.

---

## PROPOXYPHENE

## Summary of Differences
Pharmacology/pharmacokinetics:
   Mechanism of action/effect—
      An opioid agonist analgesic; has agonist activity at the mu receptor.
   Equivalence—
      Dose therapeutically equivalent to 10 mg of intramuscular morphine too toxic to administer.
   Protein binding—
      High.
   Biotransformation—
      Metabolite norpropoxyphene is toxic.
   Half-life—
      Propoxyphene: 6–12 hours.
      Norpropoxyphene: 30–36 hours.
   Onset of action—
      Oral: 15–60 minutes.
   Time to peak concentration—
      Oral: 2–2.5 hours.
   Peak plasma concentration—
      0.05–0.1 mcg per mL.
   Time to peak effect—
      Oral: 2 hours.
   Duration of action (nontolerant patients only; decreases as tolerance develops during chronic therapy)—
      Oral: 4–6 hours.
   Elimination—
      Renal, <10% as unchanged propoxyphene; biliary.
Precautions:
   Drug interactions and/or related problems—
      Risk of convulsions if overdose of propoxyphene administered to amphetamine-treated patients.
      May increase effects of coumarin- or indandione-derivative anticoagulants.
      Concurrent use with carbamazepine not recommended because may decrease carbamazepine metabolism, leading to increased risk of toxicity.
      Effects may be decreased in patients who smoke because tobacco smoking increases propoxyphene metabolism.
   Laboratory value alterations—
      May elevate levels of enzymes in liver function tests.
Side/adverse effects:
   May be more likely than most opioid analgesics to cause convulsions.
   Hepatotoxicity has been reported.
   Has lower dependence liability than other opioid agonists.
   Withdrawal symptoms less severe than those produced by stronger opioid agonist analgesics.

## Additional Dosing Information
See also *General Dosing Information*.
100 mg of propoxyphene napsylate are equivalent to 65 mg of propoxyphene hydrochloride.

## Oral Dosage Forms
### PROPOXYPHENE HYDROCHLORIDE CAPSULES USP
**Usual adult dose**
Analgesic—
   Oral, 65 mg every four hours as needed.

**Usual adult prescribing limits**
Up to 390 mg daily.

**Usual pediatric dose**
Dosage has not been established.

**Strength(s) usually available**
U.S.—
   65 mg (Rx) [*Cotanal-65*; *Darvon*; *PP-Cap*; GENERIC].
Canada—
   Not commercially available.

**Packaging and storage**
Store below 40 °C (104 °F), preferably between 15 and 30 °C (59 and 86 °F). Store in a tight container.

**Auxiliary labeling**
• May cause drowsiness.
• Avoid alcoholic beverages.
• May be habit-forming.

**Note**
Controlled substance in both the U.S. and Canada.

### PROPOXYPHENE HYDROCHLORIDE TABLETS
**Usual adult dose**
Analgesic—
   Oral, 65 mg every four hours as needed.

**Usual adult prescribing limits**
Analgesic—
   Oral, up to 390 mg daily.

**Usual pediatric dose**
Dosage has not been established.

**Strength(s) usually available**
U.S.—
   Not commercially available.
Canada—
   65 mg (Rx) [*642* (scored)].

**Packaging and storage**
Store below 40 °C (104 °F), preferably between 15 and 30 °C (59 and 86 °F), in a well-closed container, unless otherwise specified by manufacturer.

**Auxiliary labeling**
• May cause drowsiness.
• Avoid alcoholic beverages.
• May be habit-forming.

**Note**
Controlled substance in Canada.

### PROPOXYPHENE NAPSYLATE CAPSULES
**Usual adult dose**
Analgesic—
   Oral, 100 mg every four hours as needed.

**Usual adult prescribing limits**
Analgesic—
   Up to 600 mg daily.

**Usual pediatric dose**
Dosage has not been established.

**Strength(s) usually available**
U.S.—
  Not commercially available.
Canada—
  100 mg (Rx) [*Darvon-N*].

**Packaging and storage**
Store below 40 °C (104 °F), preferably between 15 and 30 °C (59 and 86 °F), unless otherwise specified by manufacturer. Store in a tight container.

**Auxiliary labeling**
• May cause drowsiness.
• Avoid alcoholic beverages.
• May be habit-forming.

**Note**
Controlled substance in Canada.

## PROPOXYPHENE NAPSYLATE ORAL SUSPENSION USP

**Usual adult dose**
Analgesic—
  Oral, 100 mg every four hours as needed.

**Usual adult prescribing limits**
Analgesic—
  Up to 600 mg daily.

**Usual pediatric dose**
Dosage has not been established.

**Strength(s) usually available**
U.S.—
  50 mg per 5 mL (Rx) [*Darvon-N* (butylparaben; methylparaben; propylparaben; saccharin; sucrose)].
Canada—
  Not commercially available.

**Packaging and storage**
Store below 40 °C (104 °F), preferably between 15 and 30 °C (59 and 86 °F), unless otherwise specified by manufacturer. Store in a tight container. Protect from light. Protect from freezing.

**Auxiliary labeling**
• Shake well.
• May cause drowsiness.
• Avoid alcoholic beverages.
• May be habit-forming.

**Note**
Controlled substance in the U.S.

## PROPOXYPHENE NAPSYLATE TABLETS USP

**Usual adult dose**
Analgesic—
  Oral, 100 mg every four hours as needed.

**Usual adult prescribing limits**
Analgesic—
  Up to 600 mg daily.

**Usual pediatric dose**
Dosage has not been established.

**Strength(s) usually available**
U.S.—
  100 mg (Rx) [*Darvon-N*; GENERIC].
Canada—
  Not commercially available.

**Packaging and storage**
Store below 40 °C (104 °F), preferably between 15 and 30 °C (59 and 86 °F), unless otherwise specified by manufacturer. Store in a tight container.

**Auxiliary labeling**
• May cause drowsiness.
• Avoid alcoholic beverages.
• May be habit-forming.

**Note**
Controlled substance in the U.S.

Revised: July 1990
Interim revision: 03/30/98

### Table 1. Pharmacology/Pharmacokinetics

| Drug | Protein Binding | Half-life (hr)* | Elimination Primary (% excreted unchanged)† | Secondary |
|---|---|---|---|---|
| Butorphanol | High | 2.5–4 | 72% Renal (<5) | 15% biliary |
| Codeine‡ | Very low | 2.5–4 | Renal (5–15); 10% as unchanged or conjugated morphine | |
| Hydrocodone | | 3.8 | Renal | |
| Hydromorphone | | 2.6–4 | Renal | |
| Levorphanol | Moderate | | Renal | |
| Meperidine§ | High | 2.4–4 | Renal (5) | |
| Methadone# | High | 15–25; increases with repeated administration | Renal; rate increased in acidic urine | Biliary |
| Morphine | Low | 2–3 | 85% Renal (9–12) | 7–10% Biliary |
| Nalbuphine | | 5 | Renal | |
| Opium | | | Renal | Biliary |
| Oxycodone | | 2–3 | Renal | |
| Oxymorphone | | | Renal | |
| Pentazocine | Moderate | 2–3 | Renal (5–23) | Biliary |
| Propoxyphene** | High | 6–12 (propoxyphene) 30–36 (norpropoxyphene) | Renal (<10) | Biliary |

*Half-life may be increased in geriatric patients because of decreased clearance rate. Also, significant increases have been reported in patients with hepatic cirrhosis for meperidine (6 to 7 hr), morphine, and pentazocine.
  †All opioid analgesics are excreted primarily as metabolites.
  ‡About 10% of a dose is demethylated to morphine, which may contribute to the therapeutic actions.
  §Metabolite normeperidine is active and toxic (having CNS excitatory [proconvulsant] activity) and accumulates in patients with renal function impairment.
  #Some metabolites are active; drug and/or metabolites may accumulate with repeated administration.
  **Metabolite norpropoxyphene may be toxic; it is not known whether this metabolite has analgesic activity.

## Table 2. Pharmacology/Pharmacokinetics

| Drug and Route* | Equivalence† | Time to Peak Concentration (hr) | Peak Plasma Concentration | Onset of Analgesic Action (min) | Peak Analgesic Effect (min) | Duration of Action Analgesic (hr)‡/Antitussive (hr) |
|---|---|---|---|---|---|---|
| **Butorphanol** | | | | | | |
| IM | 2 | 0.5–1 | 2.2 ng§/mL | 10–30 | 30–60 | 3–4 |
| IV | | | | 2–3 | 30 | 2–4 |
| **Codeine** | | | | | | |
| Oral | 200 | | | 30–45 | 60–120 | 4/4–6 |
| IM | 120 | | | 10–30 | 30–60 | 4 |
| SC | | | | 10–30 | | 4 |
| **Hydrocodone** | | | | | | |
| Oral | | | | 10–30 | 30–60 | 4–6/4–6 |
| **Hydromorphone** | | | | | | |
| Oral | 7.5 | | | 30 | 90–120 | 4 |
| IM | 1.5 | | | 15 | 30–60 | 4–5 |
| IV | | | | 10–15 | 15–30 | 2–3 |
| SC | | | | 15 | 30–90 | 4 |
| Rectal | 3 | | | | | |
| **Levorphanol** | | | | | | |
| Oral | 4 | | | 10–60 | 90–120 | 4–5 |
| IM | 2 | | | | 60 | 4–5 |
| IV | | | | | Within 20 | 4–5 |
| SC | | | | | 60–90 | 4–5 |
| **Meperidine** | | | | | | |
| Oral | 300 | | | 15 | 60–90 | 2–4 |
| IM | 75 | | | 10–15 | 30–50 | 2–4 |
| IV | | | | 1 | 5–7 | 2–4 |
| SC | | | | 10–15 | 30–50 | 2–4 |
| **Methadone** | | | | | | |
| Oral | 20 | | | 30–60 | 90–120 | 4–6# |
| IM | 10 | | | 10–20 | 60–120 | 4–5# |
| IV | | | | | 15–30 | 3–4# |
| **Morphine** | | | | | | |
| Oral | 60** | | | | | |
|   Extended-release tablets | | | | | | 8–12 |
|   Other oral dosage forms | | | | Slower than IM | 60–120 | 4–5 |
| IM | 10 | | | 10–30 | 30–60 | 4–5 |
| IV | | | | | 20 | 4–5 |
| SC | | | | 10–30 | 50–90 | 4–5 |
| Epidural | | | | 15–60 | | Up to 24 |
| Intrathecal | | | | 15–60 | | Up to 24 |
| Rectal | | | | 20–60 | | |
| **Nalbuphine** | | | | | | |
| IM | 10 | 0.5 | 48 ng§/mL | Within 15 | 60 | 3–6 |
| IV | | | | 2–3 | 30 | 3–4 |
| SC | | | | Within 15 | | 3–6 |
| **Opium** | | | | | | |
| Parenteral | 13.3 | | | | | |
| **Oxycodone** | | | | | | |
| Oral | 30 | | | | 60 | 3–4 |
| **Oxymorphone** | | | | | | |
| IM | 1 | | | 10–15 | 30–90 | 3–6 |
| IV | | | | 5–10 | 15–30 | 3–4 |
| SC | | | | 10–20 | | 3–6 |
| Rectal | 10 | | | 15–30 | 120 | 3–6 |

*IM=Intramuscular; IV=Intravenous; SC=Subcutaneous.

†Dose in mg therapeutically equivalent to a 10-mg intramuscular dose of morphine.

‡In nontolerant patients only. The first sign of tolerance is usually a decrease in the duration of adequate analgesia. Also, may be increased in geriatric patients because of decreased clearance rate.

§Nanograms.

#Increases with repeated dosing because of accumulation of drug and/or active metabolites.

**For single doses or occasional use only; with chronic dosing on a fixed schedule, may decrease to 20 or 30 mg.

††Dose equivalent to 10 mg of morphine would be too toxic to administer. Values reported under *time to peak concentration* and *peak plasma concentration* were determined following a 65-mg dose of propoxyphene hydrochloride or a 100-mg dose of propoxyphene napsylate.

## Table 2. Pharmacology/Pharmacokinetics (continued)

| Drug and Route* | Equivalence† | Time to Peak Concentration (hr) | Peak Plasma Concentration | Onset of Analgesic Action (min) | Peak Analgesic Effect (min) | Duration of Action Analgesic (hr)‡/Antitussive (hr) |
|---|---|---|---|---|---|---|
| Pentazocine | | | | | | |
|   Oral | 180 | | | 15–30 | 60–90 | 3 |
|   IM | 60 | | | 15–20 | 30–60 | 2–3 |
|   IV | | | | 2–3 | 15–30 | 2–3 |
|   SC | | | | 15–20 | 30–60 | 2–3 |
| Propoxyphene | | | | | | |
|   Oral | †† | 2–2.5 | 0.05–0.1 mcg/mL | 15–60 | 120 | 4–6 |

\*IM=Intramuscular; IV=Intravenous; SC=Subcutaneous.
†Dose in mg therapeutically equivalent to a 10-mg intramuscular dose of morphine.
‡In nontolerant patients only. The first sign of tolerance is usually a decrease in the duration of adequate analgesia. Also, may be increased in geriatric patients because of decreased clearance rate.
§Nanograms.
#Increases with repeated dosing because of accumulation of drug and/or active metabolites.
\*\*For single doses or occasional use only; with chronic dosing on a fixed schedule, may decrease to 20 or 30 mg.
††Dose equivalent to 10 mg of morphine would be too toxic to administer. Values reported under *time to peak concentration* and *peak plasma concentration* were determined following a 65-mg dose of propoxyphene hydrochloride or a 100-mg dose of propoxyphene napsylate.

*USP DI* — Opioid (Narcotic) Analgesics (Systemic) — 2193

## Table 3. Drug Interactions and/or Related Problems

The following drug interactions and/or related problems have been selected on the basis of their potential clinical significance (possible mechanism in parentheses where appropriate)—not necessarily inclusive (» = major clinical significance):

Note: Combinations containing any of the following medications, depending on the amount present, may also interact with this medication.

Legend:
I = Codeine
II = Hydrocodone
III = Hydromorphone
IV = Levorphanol

Agonist
V = Meperidine
VI = Methadone
VII = Morphine
VIII = Opium
IX = Oxycodone
X = Oxymorphone
XI = Propoxyphene

Agonist/Antagonist
XII = Butorphanol
XIII = Nalbuphine
XIV = Pentazocine

| Medication / Problem | I | II | III | IV | V | VI | VII | VIII | IX | X | XI | XII | XIII | XIV |
|---|---|---|---|---|---|---|---|---|---|---|---|---|---|---|
| Acidifiers, urinary, such as: Ammonium chloride, Ascorbic acid, Potassium or sodium phosphate (acidification of the urine by these medications increases methadone excretion, resulting in decreased methadone plasma concentrations; high doses of urinary acidifiers, such as several grams daily of ammonium chloride, may cause withdrawal symptoms in patients who are dependent on methadone) | | | | | | ✓ | | | | | | | | |
| » Alcohol or » CNS depression–producing medications, other (See *Appendix II*) (concurrent use with opioid analgesics may result in increased CNS depressant, respiratory depressant, and hypotensive effects; caution is recommended and dosage of one or both agents should be reduced. In addition, some phenothiazines increase, while others decrease, the effects of opioid analgesics used as adjuncts to anesthesia) | ✓ | ✓ | ✓ | ✓ | ✓ | ✓ | ✓ | ✓ | ✓ | ✓ | ✓ | ✓ | ✓ | ✓ |
| (concurrent use with other CNS depressants having habituation potential may increase the risk of habituation) | ✓ | ✓ | ✓ | ✓ | ✓ | ✓ | ✓ | ✓ | ✓ | ✓ | ✓ | | | |
| Amphetamines (amphetamines may potentiate the analgesic effects of meperidine; however, concurrent use of the 2 medications is not recommended because the monoamine oxidase inhibiting effect of amphetamines may increase the risk of hypotension, severe respiratory depression, coma, convulsions, hyperpyrexia, vascular collapse, and death) | | | | | ✓ | | | | | | | | | |
| (an overdose of propoxyphene may potentiate the CNS stimulating effects of amphetamines; fatal convulsions can result) | | | | | | | | | | | ✓ | | | |
| Anticholinergics or other medications with anticholinergic activity (See *Appendix II*) (concurrent use with opioid analgesics may result in increased risk of severe constipation, which may lead to paralytic ileus, and/or urinary retention) | ✓ | ✓ | ✓ | ✓ | ✓ | ✓ | ✓ | ✓ | ✓ | ✓ | ✓ | | | |
| Anticoagulants, coumarin- or indandione-derivative (meperidine and propoxyphene have been reported to increase the effects of these anticoagulants; although clinical significance has not been established, the possibility should be considered that adjustment of anticoagulant dosage based on prothrombin time determinations may be necessary during and following concurrent use) | | | | | ✓ | | | | | | ✓ | | | |
| Antidiarrheals, antiperistaltic, such as: Difenoxin and atropine, Diphenoxylate and atropine, Kaolin, pectin, belladonna alkaloids, and opium, Loperamide, Opium tincture, Paregoric (concurrent use with an opioid analgesic may increase the risk of severe constipation as well as central nervous system [CNS] depression) | ✓ | ✓ | ✓ | ✓ | ✓ | ✓ | ✓ | ✓ | ✓ | ✓ | ✓ | ✓ | ✓ | ✓ |

## Table 3. Drug Interactions and/or Related Problems (continued)

The following drug interactions and/or related problems have been selected on the basis of their potential clinical significance (possible mechanism in parentheses where appropriate)—not necessarily inclusive (» = major clinical significance):

Note: Combinations containing any of the following medications, depending on the amount present, may also interact with this medication.

Legend:
I = Codeine
II = Hydrocodone
III = Hydromorphone
IV = Levorphanol

V = Meperidine
VI = Methadone
VII = Morphine

VIII = Opium
IX = Oxycodone
X = Oxymorphone
XI = Propoxyphene

XII = Butorphanol
XIII = Nalbuphine
XIV = Pentazocine

| | I | II | III | IV | V | VI | VII | VIII | IX | X | XI | XII | XIII | XIV |
|---|---|---|---|---|---|---|---|---|---|---|---|---|---|---|
| Antihypertensives, especially ganglionic blockers such as guanadrel, guanethidine, and mecamylamine, or Diuretics or Hypotension-producing medications, other (See *Appendix II*) (hypotensive effects of these medications may be potentiated when used concurrently with opioid analgesics, leading to increased risk of orthostatic hypotension; patients should be monitored during concurrent use) | ↙ | ↙ | ↙ | ↙ | ↙ | ↙ | ↙ | ↙ | ↙ | ↙ | ↙ | ↙ | ↙ | ↙ |
| » Buprenorphine (buprenorphine is a partial mu-receptor agonist with high affinity for, and a slow rate of dissociation from, the mu receptor; if administered prior to another opioid agonist, it may reduce the therapeutic effects of the other opioid; in one study in opioid addicts receiving chronic administration of 8 mg of buprenorphine per day, the effects of large doses [up to 120 mg] of morphine were blocked during buprenorphine therapy and for at least 30 hours following the last dose of buprenorphine) | ↙ | | | | ↙ | ↙ | ↙ | ↙ | ↙ | ↙ | ↙ | | | |
| (buprenorphine may also have some antagonist activity at the kappa receptor; the possibility should be considered that it may also reduce the therapeutic effects of subsequently administered butorphanol, nalbuphine, or pentazocine) | | | | | | | | | | | | ↙ | ↙ | ↙ |
| (buprenorphine antagonizes the respiratory depressant effects of large doses of previously administered mu-receptor agonists; however, additive respiratory depression may occur if buprenorphine is administered in conjunction with low doses of other mu-receptor agonists or with kappa-receptor agonists) | ↙ | ↙ | ↙ | ↙ | ↙ | ↙ | ↙ | ↙ | ↙ | ↙ | ↙ | ↙ | ↙ | ↙ |
| (buprenorphine may precipitate withdrawal symptoms in physically dependent patients who are chronically receiving potent mu-receptor agonists; however, because of its partial agonist activity, buprenorphine may partially suppress spontaneous withdrawal symptoms caused by abrupt discontinuation of these agonists) | ↙ | ↙ | ↙ | ↙ | ↙ | ↙ | ↙ | ↙ | ↙ | ↙ | ↙ | | | |
| » Carbamazepine (concurrent use with propoxyphene may result in decreased carbamazepine metabolism and lead to increased carbamazepine blood concentration and toxicity; concurrent use is not recommended) | | | | | | | | | | | ↙ | | | |
| Hydroxyzine (concurrent use with opioid analgesics may result in increased analgesia as well as increased CNS depressant and hypotensive effects) | ↙ | ↙ | ↙ | ↙ | ↙ | ↙ | ↙ | ↙ | ↙ | ↙ | ↙ | ↙ | ↙ | ↙ |
| Metoclopramide (opioid analgesics may antagonize the effects of metoclopramide on gastrointestinal motility) | ↙ | ↙ | ↙ | ↙ | ↙ | ↙ | ↙ | ↙ | ↙ | ↙ | ↙ | ↙ | ↙ | ↙ |

## Table 3. Drug Interactions and/or Related Problems (continued)

The following drug interactions and/or related problems have been selected on the basis of their potential clinical significance (possible mechanism in parentheses where appropriate)—not necessarily inclusive (» = major clinical significance):

Note: Combinations containing any of the following medications, depending on the amount present, may also interact with this medication.

Legend:
I = Codeine
II = Hydrocodone
III = Hydromorphone
IV = Levorphanol
V = Meperidine
VI = Methadone
VII = Morphine
VIII = Opium
IX = Oxycodone
X = Oxymorphone
XI = Propoxyphene
XII = Butorphanol
XIII = Nalbuphine
XIV = Pentazocine

Agonist: I–XI
Agonist/Antagonist: XII–XIV

| | I | II | III | IV | V | VI | VII | VIII | IX | X | XI | XII | XIII | XIV |
|---|---|---|---|---|---|---|---|---|---|---|---|---|---|---|
| » Monoamine oxidase (MAO) inhibitors, including furazolidone, pargyline, and procarbazine (concurrent use with meperidine has resulted in unpredictable, severe, and sometimes fatal reactions, including immediate excitation, sweating, rigidity, and severe hypertension, or, in some patients, hypotension, severe respiratory depression, coma, seizures; hyperpyrexia, and cardiovascular collapse; meperidine is contraindicated in patients who have received an MAO inhibitor within 14 to 21 days) (other opioid analgesics may be used cautiously and in reduced dosage in patients receiving MAO inhibitors; however, it is recommended that a small test dose [¼ of the usual dose] or several small incremental test doses over a period of several hours first be administered to permit observation of any interaction) | | | | | ✓ | | | | | | | | | |
| Naloxone (antagonizes the analgesic, CNS, and respiratory depressant effects of opioid analgesics; however, larger doses may be required to reverse the effects of butorphanol, nalbuphine, pentazocine, or propoxyphene than are needed to reverse the effects of other opioids; also, because naloxone may precipitate withdrawal symptoms in physically dependent patients, dosage of naloxone should be carefully titrated when used to treat opioid overdosage in dependent patients) | ✓ | ✓ | ✓ | ✓ | ✓ | ✓ | ✓ | ✓ | ✓ | ✓ | ✓ | ✓ | ✓ | ✓ |
| » Naltrexone (administration of naltrexone to a patient physically dependent on opioid drugs will precipitate withdrawal symptoms; symptoms may appear within 5 minutes of naltrexone administration, persist for up to 48 hours, and be difficult to reverse) (naltrexone blocks the therapeutic effects of opioids [i.e., analgesic, antidiarrheal, and antitussive]; naltrexone therapy should not be initiated in patients receiving these agents for therapeutic purposes; also, patients receiving naltrexone should be advised to use alternative medications when necessary) (administration of increased doses of opioids to override naltrexone blockade of opioid receptors may result in increased and prolonged respiratory depression and/or circulatory collapse) (naltrexone should be discontinued several days prior to elective surgery if administration of an opioid prior to, during, or following surgery is unavoidable) (the efficacy of naltrexone in antagonizing opioid effects not mediated via opioid receptors [i.e., those that may be caused by histamine release, such as facial swelling, itching, generalized erythema, hives, and, to some extent, hypotension] has not been fully determined; naltrexone may not antagonize these effects completely) | ✓ | ✓ | ✓ | ✓ | ✓ | ✓ | ✓ | ✓ | ✓ | ✓ | ✓ | ✓ | ✓ | ✓ |

## Table 3. Drug Interactions and/or Related Problems (continued)

The following drug interactions and/or related problems have been selected on the basis of their potential clinical significance (possible mechanism in parentheses where appropriate)—not necessarily inclusive (» = major clinical significance):

Note: Combinations containing any of the following medications, depending on the amount present, may also interact with this medication.

Legend:
I=Codeine
II=Hydrocodone
III=Hydromorphone
IV=Levorphanol

V=Meperidine
VI=Methadone
VII=Morphine

VIII=Opium
IX=Oxycodone
X=Oxymorphone
XI=Propoxyphene

XII=Butorphanol
XIII=Nalbuphine
XIV=Pentazocine

| | I | II | III | IV | V | VI | VII | VIII | IX | X | XI | XII | XIII | XIV |
|---|---|---|---|---|---|---|---|---|---|---|---|---|---|---|
| Neuromuscular blocking agents and possibly other medications having some neuromuscular blocking activity (respiratory depressant effects of neuromuscular blockade may be additive to central respiratory depressant effects of opioid analgesics; increased or prolonged respiratory depression [apnea] or paralysis may occur but is of minor clinical significance if the patient is being mechanically ventilated; however, caution and careful monitoring of the patient are recommended during and following concurrent or sequential use, especially if there is a possibility of incomplete reversal of neuromuscular blockade postoperatively) | » | » | » | » | » | » | » | » | » | » | » | | | » |
| Nicotine chewing gum or Other smoking deterrents or Smoking, tobacco, or cessation of (tobacco smoking may increase the metabolism of propoxyphene leading to decreased therapeutic effects; also, smoking cessation by a patient receiving propoxyphene chronically may increase its effects) | | | | | | | | | | | » | | | |
| Opioid agonist analgesics, including alfentanil, fentanyl, and sufentanil (additive CNS depressant, respiratory depressant, and hypotensive effects may occur if two or more opioid agonist analgesics are used concurrently) | » | » | » | » | » | » | » | » | » | » | » | | | |
| (pentazocine and nalbuphine may partially antagonize the analgesic and CNS depressant effects of opioid agonists) | | | | | | | | | | | | » | » | » |
| (in patients who are not physically dependent on opioid agonists, concurrent use of butorphanol, nalbuphine, or pentazocine may result in additive side effects) | | | | | | | | | | | | » | » | » |
| (in patients who are physically dependent on opioid agonists, nalbuphine and pentazocine may precipitate, and butorphanol will not prevent or attenuate, withdrawal symptoms) | | | | | | | | | | | | » | » | » |
| » Phenytoin, chronic use of, or Rifampin (these medications may increase methadone metabolism, probably via induction of hepatic microsomal enzyme activity, and may precipitate withdrawal symptoms in patients being treated for opioid dependence; methadone dosage adjustments may be necessary when phenytoin or rifampin therapy is initiated or discontinued) | | | | | | » | | | | | | | | |
| » Zidovudine (morphine may competitively inhibit the hepatic glucuronidation and decrease the clearance of zidovudine; concurrent use should be avoided because the toxicity of either or both of these medications may be potentiated) | | | | | | | » | | | | | | | |

## Table 4. Side/Adverse Effects*

| The following side/adverse effects have been selected on the basis of their potential clinical significance (possible signs and symptoms in parentheses where appropriate)—not necessarily inclusive: | Legend:<br>I=Butorphanol<br>II=Codeine<br>III=Hydrocodone<br>IV=Hydromorphone | | | | V=Levorphanol<br>VI=Meperidine<br>VII=Methadone | | | VIII=Morphine<br>IX=Nalbuphine<br>X=Opium | | | XI=Oxycodone<br>XII=Oxymorphone<br>XIII=Pentazocine<br>XIV=Propoxyphene | | | |
|---|---|---|---|---|---|---|---|---|---|---|---|---|---|---|
| | I | II | III | IV | V | VI | VII | VIII | IX | X | XI | XII | XIII | XIV |
| **Medical attention needed** | | | | | | | | | | | | | | |
| ***Allergic reaction*** (skin rash, hives, and/or itching†; swelling of face) | R (<1%) | L | R | R | R | R | R | L | L | R | R | R | L | L |
| ***Atelectasis; bronchospastic allergic reaction; laryngeal edema, allergic; laryngospasm, allergic;* or *respiratory depression*‡** (shortness of breath, slow or irregular breathing, troubled breathing) | R (<1%) | L | L | L | L | L | L | L | R (<1%) | R | R | L | L | U |
| ***CNS stimulation, paradoxical*** (unusual excitement or restlessness)—especially in children | R | L | R | R | R | R | R | R | R | R | R | R | R | R |
| ***Confusion*** §—may include delusions and feelings of depersonalization or unreality | R (<1%) | L | L | L | L | L | L | L | R (<1%) | L | R | L | R | R |
| ***Convulsions*** | U | R | R | U | U | L | U | U | U | U | U | U | R | L |
| ***Fast, slow, or pounding heartbeat*** | R (<1%) | L | L | L | L | L | L | L | R (<1%) | | R | U | L | U |
| ***Hallucinations*** § | R (<1%) | R | R | R | R | R | R | R | R (<1%) | R | R | R | R | U |
| ***Hepatotoxicity*** (dark urine, pale stools, yellow eyes or skin) | U | U | U | U | U | U | U | U | U | U | U | U | U | R |
| ***Histamine release*** (decreased blood pressure, fast heartbeat, increased sweating, redness or flushing of face, wheezing or troubled breathing) | L | L | M | L | R | M | M | M | M | M | L | L | L | L |
| ***Increased blood pressure*** | R (<1%) | U | R | U | U | U | U | U | R | (U) | U | U | L | R |
| ***Mental depression*** | R (<1%) | R | R | R | R | R | R | R | R (<1%) | R | R | R | R | R |
| ***Muscle rigidity, especially in muscles of respiration***—with large doses | U | R | R | U | U | U | U | R | U | U | U | U | U | R |
| ***Paralytic ileus* or *toxic megacolon*** (severe constipation, bloating, nausea, stomach cramps or pain, vomiting)—in patients with inflammatory bowel disease | R | R | R | R | R | R | R | R | R | R | R | R | R | R |
| ***Ringing or buzzing in the ears*** | R | U | R | U | U | U | U | U | U | U | U | U | R | L |
| ***Trembling or uncontrolled muscle movements*** | U | R | R | L | U | L | U | L | U | L | U | U | R | L |
| **Medical attention needed only if continuing or bothersome** | | | | | | | | | | | | | | |
| ***Antidiuretic effect*** (decreased urination) | L | L | L | L | L | L | L | L | R (<1%) | L | L | L | L | L |
| ***Biliary spasm*** (stomach cramps or pain) | U | R | R | L | L | L | L (<1%) | L | R (<1%) | R | R | U | L | R |
| ***Blurred or double vision or other changes in vision*** | R (<1%) | L | L | L | L | L | L | L | R (<1%) | L | U | L | L | L |

*Differences in frequency of occurrence may reflect either lack of clinical-use data or actual pharmacologic distinctions among agents (although their pharmacologic similarity suggests that side effects occurring with one may occur with the others). M = more frequent; L = less frequent; R = rare; U = unknown.

†*Generalized or facial pruritus* may represent an opioid-induced dysesthesia rather than an allergic reaction, especially following epidural or intrathecal administration, and requires medical attention only if bothersome to the patient.

‡*Respiratory depression* induced by butorphanol, nalbuphine, and pentazocine differs from that due to other opioid analgesics in that the depth of respiratory depression is not increased with higher doses (ceiling effect); however, with butorphanol the duration of respiratory depression is increased with higher doses.

§Although these effects may occur with large doses of any opioid analgesic, with butorphanol, nalbuphine, and pentazocine they may be part of a group of subjective and psychotomimetic effects characteristic of opioids having sigma-receptor activity. These effects include *confusion, delusions, feelings of depersonalization or unreality, hallucinations* (usually visual), *dysphoria, nightmares,* and *nervousness or anxiety*. These effects generally occur with large doses of these drugs; although they occur rarely with any of them, they may be most likely to occur with pentazocine.

## Table 4. Side/Adverse Effects* (continued)

| The following side/adverse effects have been selected on the basis of their potential clinical significance (possible signs and symptoms in parentheses where appropriate)—not necessarily inclusive: | Legend:<br>I=Butorphanol<br>II=Codeine<br>III=Hydrocodone<br>IV=Hydromorphone | | | | V=Levorphanol<br>VI=Meperidine<br>VII=Methadone | | | VIII=Morphine<br>IX=Nalbuphine<br>X=Opium | | | XI=Oxycodone<br>XII=Oxymorphone<br>XIII=Pentazocine<br>XIV=Propoxyphene | | | |
|---|---|---|---|---|---|---|---|---|---|---|---|---|---|---|
| | I | II | III | IV | V | VI | VII | VIII | IX | X | XI | XII | XIII | XIV |
| *Constipation* | R | M | L | L | L | M | M | M | U | R | L | L | L | L |
| *Dizziness, feeling faint, or lightheadedness*—especially in ambulatory patients. | L | L | M | M | M | M | M | M | L | M | M | M | L | M |
| *Drowsiness* | M (40%) | M | M | M | M | M | M | M | M (36%) | M | M | M | M | M |
| *Dry mouth* | R (<1%) | L | L | L | L | L | L | L | L (4%) | L | L | L | L | L |
| *False sense of well-being* | R (<1%) | L | L | L | U | L | L | L | R (<1%) | L | U | L | M | L |
| *Gastrointestinal irritation* (stomach cramps or pain) | R | R | R | L | L | L | L | L | R | L | R | U | R | R |
| *General feeling of discomfort or illness§* | L | L | L | L | L | L | L | L | R (<1%) | L | L | L | L | L |
| *Headache* | L (3%) | L | L | L | L | L | L | L | L (3%) | L | L | L | L | L |
| *Hypotension* (dizziness, feeling faint, lightheadedness, unusual tiredness or weakness)—although hypotension may occur in recumbent patients, orthostatic hypotension commonly occurs in ambulatory patients | L | L | M | M | M | M | M | M | L | M | M | M | L | M |
| *Loss of appetite* | L | L | L | M | L | L | L | L | L | R | U | R | R | R |
| *Nausea or vomiting*—occurs more frequently in ambulatory patients; are more frequent with initial doses, and are less likely to occur with subsequent doses | L (6%) | L | L | L | M | M | M | M | L (6%) | R | M | M | M | M |
| *Nervousness or restlessness§* | R (<1%) | L | L | L | L | L | L | L | R (<1%) | L | L | L | L | L |
| *Nightmares or unusual dreams§* | R (<1%) | R | R | U | U | L | U | U | R (<1%) | U | U | U | L | L |
| *Redness, swelling, pain, or burning at site of injection* | R | L | — | L | L | R | L | L | L | L | — | L | L | — |
| *Unusual tiredness or weakness* | L | L | M | M | M | M | M | M | L | M | M | M | L | M |
| *Ureteral spasm* (difficult or painful urination, frequent urge to urinate) | L | L | L | L | L | L | L | L | R (<1%) | L | L | L | L | L |
| *Trouble in sleeping* | R | R | R | R | R | L | R | R | R | R | R | R | R | R |

*Differences in frequency of occurrence may reflect either lack of clinical-use data or actual pharmacologic distinctions among agents (although their pharmacologic similarity suggests that side effects occurring with one may occur with the others). M = more frequent; L = less frequent; R = rare; U = unknown.

†*Generalized or facial pruritus* may represent an opioid-induced dysesthesia rather than an allergic reaction, especially following epidural or intrathecal administration, and requires medical attention only if bothersome to the patient.

‡*Respiratory depression* induced by butorphanol, nalbuphine, and pentazocine differs from that due to other opioid analgesics in that the depth of respiratory depression is not increased with higher doses (ceiling effect); however, with butorphanol the duration of respiratory depression is increased with higher doses.

§Although these effects may occur with large doses of any opioid analgesic, with butorphanol, nalbuphine, and pentazocine they may be part of a group of subjective and psychotomimetic effects characteristic of opioids having sigma-receptor activity. These effects include *confusion, delusions, feelings of depersonalization or unreality, hallucinations* (usually visual), *dysphoria, nightmares, and nervousness or anxiety*. These effects generally occur with large doses of these drugs; although they occur rarely with any of them, they may be most likely to occur with pentazocine.

# OPIOID (NARCOTIC) ANALGESICS AND ACETAMINOPHEN    Systemic

This monograph includes information on the following: 1) Acetaminophen and Codeine; 2) Dihydrocodeine and Acetaminophen; 3) Hydrocodone and Acetaminophen; 4) Oxycodone and Acetaminophen; 5) Pentazocine and Acetaminophen; 6) Propoxyphene and Acetaminophen

Pharmacy Equivalent Name (PEN):
   Acetaminophen and Codeine—Co-codAPAP
   Hydrocodone and Acetaminophen—Co-hycodAPAP
   Oxycodone and Acetaminophen—Co-oxycodAPAP
   Propoxyphene napsylate and Acetaminophen—Co-proxAPAP

INN:
   Acetaminophen—Paracetamol
   Propoxyphene—Dextropropoxyphene

VA CLASSIFICATION (Primary): CN101

**NOTE:** The *Opioid (Narcotic) Analgesics and Acetaminophen (Systemic)* monograph is maintained on the USP DI electronic data base. For a printed copy of the most recent revision of the complete monograph, contact Micromedex, Inc. - Reprint Requests, 6200 S. Syracuse Way, Suite 300, Englewood, CO 80111; telephone (303) 486-6400; telefax (303) 486-6464; Email: USPDI@MDX.COM.

For information on the specific components of this combination, see the *USP DI* monographs for *Acetaminophen (Systemic)* and *Opioid (Narcotic) Analgesics (Systemic)*.

The information that follows is selectively abstracted from the complete monograph and is provided to facilitate drug use review and patient counseling.

Note: For a listing of dosage forms and brand names by country availability, see *Dosage Forms* section(s).

## Category
Analgesic

Note: Opioid agonist analgesics—Codeine, Dihydrocodeine, Hydrocodone, Oxycodone, and Propoxyphene.

Opioid agonist/antagonist analgesic—Pentazocine.

## Indications
### Accepted
Pain (treatment)—Indicated for the symptomatic relief of:

Mild to moderate pain—Pentazocine and acetaminophen; propoxyphene and acetaminophen.

Mild to severe pain (depending on the dose of codeine)—Acetaminophen and codeine.

Moderate to moderately severe pain—Dihydrocodeine and acetaminophen; hydrocodone and acetaminophen; oxycodone and acetaminophen.

## Patient Consultation
As an aid to patient consultation, refer to *Advice for the Patient, Narcotic Analgesics and Acetaminophen (Systemic)*.

In providing consultation, consider emphasizing the following selected information (» = major clinical significance):

### Before using this medication
» Conditions affecting use, especially:

Sensitivity to acetaminophen or to opioid analgesic considered for use, history of

Pregnancy—Acetaminophen and opioid analgesics cross the placenta; regular use of opioids by pregnant women may cause physical dependence in the fetus and withdrawal symptoms in the neonate

Breast-feeding—Acetaminophen, codeine, and propoxyphene are distributed into breast milk

Use in children—Children up to 2 years of age are more susceptible to the effects of opioids, especially respiratory depression; also, children may be more likely to experience paradoxical CNS excitation during therapy

Use in the elderly—Geriatric patients are more susceptible to the effects of opioids, especially respiratory depression

Other medications, especially alcohol or other CNS depressants, monoamine oxidase inhibitors, tricyclic antidepressants, zidovudine, and naltrexone

Other medical problems, especially alcoholism (active or in remission), diarrhea caused by antibiotics or poisoning, asthma or other respiratory problems, hepatic disease, viral hepatitis, and severe inflammatory bowel disease

### Proper use of this medication
» Importance of not taking more medication than the amount prescribed because of danger of overdose and habit-forming potential of opioid analgesics; also, acetaminophen may cause liver damage with long-term or high-dose use

» Not increasing dose if medication is less effective after a few weeks; checking with physician

» Missed dose (if on scheduled dosing): Taking as soon as possible; not taking if almost time for next dose; not doubling doses

» Proper storage

### Precautions while using this medication
Regular visits to physician to check progress during long-term or high-dose therapy

» Caution if other medications containing opioid analgesics or acetaminophen are used

» Avoiding use of alcohol or other central nervous system (CNS) depressants during therapy unless prescribed or otherwise approved by physician

Possibility that drinking large amounts of alcohol may increase risk of liver damage with acetaminophen

Not regularly taking aspirin or other salicylates or other nonsteroidal anti-inflammatory drugs concurrently, unless directed by physician or dentist

» Caution if dizziness, drowsiness, lightheadedness, or false sense of well-being occurs

Caution when getting up suddenly from a lying or sitting position

Lying down if nausea or vomiting, or dizziness or lightheadedness occurs

Caution if any kind of surgery (including dental surgery) or emergency treatment is required

Possible dryness of mouth; using sugarless gum or candy, ice, or saliva substitute for relief; checking with dentist if dry mouth continues for more than 2 weeks

» Checking with physician before discontinuing medication after prolonged use of high doses; gradual dosage reduction may be necessary to avoid withdrawal symptoms

» Suspected overdose: Getting emergency help at once

### Side/adverse effects
Signs of potential side effects, especially respiratory depression or impairment; allergic reactions; confusion, convulsions, hallucinations, mental depression, or other signs of CNS toxicity; agranulocytosis; hepatotoxicity; hypertension; paradoxical CNS excitation, especially in children; renal function impairment; and thrombocytopenia

---
### ACETAMINOPHEN AND CODEINE
---

## Oral Dosage Forms

### ACETAMINOPHEN AND CODEINE PHOSPHATE CAPSULES USP

**Usual adult dose**
Analgesic—
Oral, 1 or 2 capsules containing 325 mg of acetaminophen and 30 mg of codeine phosphate every four hours as needed; or
Oral, 1 capsule containing 325 mg of acetaminophen and 60 mg of codeine phosphate every four hours as needed.

**Usual pediatric dose**
Dosage must be individualized by the physician.

**Strength(s) usually available**
U.S.—
325 mg of acetaminophen and 30 mg of codeine phosphate (Rx) [*Phenaphen with Codeine No.3* (D&C Yellow 10; edible ink; FD&C Blue 1; FD&C Yellow 6; gelatin; magnesium stearate; sodium starch glycolate; stearic acid)].

325 mg of acetaminophen and 60 mg of codeine phosphate (Rx) [*Phenaphen with Codeine No.4* (lactose; cornstarch; D&C Yellow 10; edible ink; FD&C Green 3 or Blue 1; FD&C Yellow 6; gelatin; magnesium stearate; sodium starch glycolate; stearic acid)].

Canada—
Not commercially available.

Note: In Canada, *Phenaphen with Codeine* contains phenobarbital, aspirin, and codeine. See *Barbiturates and Analgesics (Systemic)*.

**Auxiliary labeling**
• May cause drowsiness.
• Avoid alcoholic beverages.
• May be habit-forming.

### ACETAMINOPHEN AND CODEINE PHOSPHATE ORAL SOLUTION USP

**Usual adult dose**
Analgesic—
Oral, 15 mL every four hours, as needed.

**Usual pediatric dose**
Analgesic—
Children up to 3 years of age: Dosage has not been established.
Children 3 to 7 years of age: Oral, 5 mL three or four times a day, as needed.
Children 7 to 12 years of age: Oral, 10 mL three or four times a day, as needed.

**Strength(s) usually available**
U.S.—
120 mg of acetaminophen and 12 mg of codeine phosphate, per 5 mL (Rx) [*Tylenol with Codeine Elixir* (alcohol 7%); GENERIC].

## Opioid (Narcotic) Analgesics and Acetaminophen (Systemic)

Canada—
- 160 mg of acetaminophen and 8 mg of codeine phosphate, per 5 mL (Rx) [*PMS-Acetaminophen with Codeine* (alcohol 7%); *Tylenol with Codeine Elixir* (alcohol 7%)].

**Auxiliary labeling**
- May cause drowsiness.
- Avoid alcoholic beverages.
- May be habit-forming.

### ACETAMINOPHEN AND CODEINE PHOSPHATE ORAL SUSPENSION USP

**Usual adult dose**
See *Acetaminophen and Codeine Phosphate Oral Solution USP*.

**Usual pediatric dose**
See *Acetaminophen and Codeine Phosphate Oral Solution USP*.

**Strength(s) usually available**
U.S.—
- 120 mg of acetaminophen and 12 mg of codeine phosphate, per 5 mL (Rx) [*Capital with Codeine*].

Canada—
- Not commercially available.

**Auxiliary labeling**
- May cause drowsiness.
- Avoid alcoholic beverages.
- Shake well.
- May be habit-forming.

### ACETAMINOPHEN AND CODEINE PHOSPHATE TABLETS USP

**Usual adult dose**
Analgesic—
- Oral, 1 or 2 tablets containing 300 mg of acetaminophen and 15 or 30 mg of codeine phosphate every four hours as needed; or
- Oral, 1 tablet containing 300 mg of acetaminophen and 60 mg of codeine phosphate every four hours as needed; or
- Oral, 1 tablet containing 650 mg of acetaminophen and 30 mg of codeine phosphate every four hours as needed.

**Usual pediatric dose**
Dosage must be individualized by the physician.

**Strength(s) usually available**
U.S.—
- 300 mg of acetaminophen and 15 mg of codeine phosphate (Rx) [*Tylenol with Codeine No.2* (sodium metabisulfite); GENERIC].
- 300 mg of acetaminophen and 30 mg of codeine phosphate (Rx) [*Pyregesic-C*; *Tylenol with Codeine No.3* (sodium metabisulfite); GENERIC].
- 300 mg of acetaminophen and 60 mg of codeine phosphate (Rx) [*Tylenol with Codeine No.4* (sodium metabisulfite); GENERIC].
- 650 mg of acetaminophen and 30 mg of codeine phosphate (Rx) [*EZ III*; *Margesic #3*].

Canada—
- 300 mg of acetaminophen and 30 mg of codeine phosphate (Rx) [*Acet Codeine 30* (scored); *Empracet-30* (scored); *Emtec-30*; *Triatec-30*].
- 300 mg of acetaminophen and 60 mg of codeine phosphate (Rx) [*Acet Codeine 60* (scored); *Empracet-60*; *Lenoltec with Codeine No.4*; *Tylenol with Codeine No.4*].

**Auxiliary labeling**
- May cause drowsiness.
- Avoid alcoholic beverages.
- May be habit-forming.

### ACETAMINOPHEN, CODEINE PHOSPHATE, AND CAFFEINE TABLETS

**Usual adult dose**
Analgesic—
- Oral, 1 or 2 tablets every four hours as needed.

**Usual pediatric dose**
Dosage must be individualized by the physician.

**Strength(s) usually available**
U.S.—
- Not commercially available.

Canada—
- 300 mg of acetaminophen, 8 mg of codeine phosphate, and 15 mg of caffeine (OTC) [*Lenoltec with Codeine No.1*; *Novo-Gesic C8*; *Tylenol with Codeine No.1* [GENERIC (may be scored)].
- 300 mg of acetaminophen, 8 mg of codeine phosphate, and 30 mg of caffeine citrate (OTC) [*Exdol-8* (scored)].
- 300 mg of acetaminophen, 15 mg of codeine phosphate, and 15 mg of caffeine (Rx) [*Acet-2* (scored); *Lenoltec with Codeine No.2*; *Novo-Gesic C15* (scored); *Tylenol with Codeine No.2*].
- 300 mg of acetaminophen, 30 mg of codeine phosphate, and 15 mg of caffeine (Rx) [*Acet-3* (scored); *Lenoltec with Codeine No.3*; *Novo-Gesic C30* (scored); *Tylenol with Codeine No.3*].
- 325 mg of acetaminophen, 8 mg of codeine phosphate, and 15 mg of caffeine (OTC) [*Cetaphen with Codeine*].
- 325 mg of acetaminophen, 8 mg of codeine phosphate, and 30 mg of caffeine citrate (OTC) [*Atasol-8* (scored); *Cotabs*; *Triatec-8*].
- 325 mg of acetaminophen, 15 mg of codeine phosphate, and 30 mg of caffeine citrate (Rx) [*Atasol-15* (scored)].
- 325 mg of acetaminophen, 30 mg of codeine phosphate, and 30 mg of caffeine citrate (Rx) [*Atasol-30* (scored)].
- 500 mg of acetaminophen, 8 mg of codeine phosphate, and 15 mg of caffeine (OTC) [*Cetaphen Extra Strength with Codeine*; *Tylenol with Codeine No.1 Forte* [GENERIC].
- 500 mg of acetaminophen, 8 mg of codeine phosphate, and 30 mg of caffeine citrate (OTC) [*Triatec-8 Strong*].

**Auxiliary labeling**
- May cause drowsiness.
- Avoid alcoholic beverages.
- May be habit-forming.

---

### DIHYDROCODEINE AND ACETAMINOPHEN

## Oral Dosage Forms

### DIHYDROCODEINE BITARTRATE, ACETAMINOPHEN, AND CAFFEINE CAPSULES

**Usual adult dose**
Analgesic—
- Oral, 2 capsules every four hours.

**Usual pediatric dose**
Dosage has not been established.

**Strength(s) usually available**
U.S.—
- 16 mg of dihydrocodeine bitartrate, 356.4 mg of acetaminophen, and 30 mg of caffeine (Rx) [*DHCplus* (croscarmellose sodium; FD&C Blue 1; FD&C Green 3; gelatin; silica gel; silicon dioxide; sodium lauryl sulfate; cornstarch; titanium dioxide; zinc stearate)].

Canada—
- Not commercially available.

**Auxiliary labeling**
- May cause drowsiness.
- Avoid alcoholic beverages.
- May be habit-forming.

---

### HYDROCODONE AND ACETAMINOPHEN

## Oral Dosage Forms

### HYDROCODONE BITARTRATE AND ACETAMINOPHEN CAPSULES

**Usual adult dose**
Analgesic—
- Oral, one capsule every four to six hours, as needed. Dosage may be increased to two capsules every six hours if necessary.

**Usual adult prescribing limits**
Analgesic—
- Up to eight capsules per 24 hours.

**Usual pediatric dose**
Dosage has not been established.

**Strength(s) usually available**
U.S.—
- 5 mg of hydrocodone bitartrate and 500 mg of acetaminophen (Rx) [*Allay*; *Anolor DH 5*; *Bancap-HC*; *Dolacet*; *Dolagesic*; *Hycomed*; *Hyco-Pap*; *Hydrocet*; *Hydrogesic*; *Lorcet-HD*; *Margesic-H*; *Panlor*; *Polygesic*; *Stagesic*; *T-Gesic*; *Ugesic*; *Vendone*; *Zydone* (FD&C Yellow 6); GENERIC].

Canada—
- Not commercially available.

**Auxiliary labeling**
- May cause drowsiness.
- Avoid alcoholic beverages.
- May be habit-forming.

## HYDROCODONE BITARTRATE AND ACETAMINOPHEN ORAL SOLUTION

### Usual adult dose
Analgesic—
Oral, 5 to 15 mL every four to six hours as needed.

### Usual pediatric dose
Dosage has not been established.

### Strength(s) usually available
U.S.—
2.5 mg of hydrocodone bitartrate and 167 mg of acetaminophen per 5 mL (Rx) [*Lortab* (alcohol 7%; citric acid; ethyl maltol; glycerin; methylparaben; propylene glycol; propylparaben; saccharin sodium; sorbitol solution; sucrose; D&C Yellow #10; FD&C Yellow #6)].

Canada—
Not commercially available.

### Auxiliary labeling
- May cause drowsiness.
- Avoid alcoholic beverages.
- May be habit-forming.

## HYDROCODONE BITARTRATE AND ACETAMINOPHEN TABLETS USP

### Usual adult dose
Analgesic—
Oral, 1 or 2 tablets containing 2.5 mg of hydrocodone bitartrate and 500 mg of acetaminophen every four to six hours; or

Oral, 1 tablet containing 5 mg of hydrocodone bitartrate and 500 mg of acetaminophen every four to six hours as needed, with dosage being increased to 2 tablets every six hours if necessary; or

Oral, 1 tablet containing 7.5 mg of hydrocodone bitartrate and 650 mg of acetaminophen every four to six hours as needed, with dosage being increased to 2 tablets every six hours if necessary; or

Oral, 1 tablet containing 7.5 mg of hydrocodone bitartrate and 750 mg of acetaminophen every four to six hours as needed; or

Oral, 1 tablet containing 10 mg of hydrocodone bitartrate and 650 mg of acetaminophen every four to six hours as needed.

### Usual adult prescribing limits
Up to 40 mg of hydrocodone bitartrate and 4 grams of acetaminophen in twenty-four hours.

### Usual pediatric dose
Dosage has not been established.

### Strength(s) usually available
U.S.—
2.5 mg of hydrocodone bitartrate and 500 mg of acetaminophen (Rx) [*Lortab 2.5/500* (scored); GENERIC].

5 mg of hydrocodone bitartrate and 500 mg of acetaminophen (Rx) [*Anexsia 5/500* (scored); *Co-Gesic* (scored); *Duocet* (scored); *HY-PHEN* (scored); *Lortab 5/500* (scored); *Oncet*; *Panacet 5/500* (scored); *Vanacet*; *Vicodin* (scored); GENERIC].

7.5 mg of hydrocodone bitartrate and 500 mg of acetaminophen (Rx) [*Lortab 7.5/500* (scored); GENERIC].

7.5 mg of hydrocodone bitartrate and 650 mg of acetaminophen (Rx) [*Anexsia 7.5/650* (scored); *Lorcet Plus* (scored); GENERIC].

7.5 mg of hydrocodone bitartrate and 750 mg of acetaminophen (Rx) [*Vicodin ES* (scored); GENERIC].

10 mg of hydrocodone bitartrate and 650 mg of acetaminophen (Rx) [*Lorcet 10/650* (scored; colloidal silicon dioxide; croscarmellose sodium; crospovidone; microcrystalline cellulose; povidone; pregelatinized starch; stearic acid; FD&C Blue #1 Lake)].

Canada—
Not commercially available.

### Auxiliary labeling
- May cause drowsiness.
- Avoid alcoholic beverages.
- May be habit-forming.

---

## OXYCODONE AND ACETAMINOPHEN

## Oral Dosage Forms

### OXYCODONE AND ACETAMINOPHEN CAPSULES USP

#### Usual adult dose
Analgesic—
Oral, 1 capsule every four to six hours as needed.

#### Usual pediatric dose
Dosage has not been established.

#### Strength(s) usually available
U.S.—
5 mg of oxycodone hydrochloride and 500 mg of acetaminophen (Rx) [*Roxilox*; *Tylox* (sodium metabisulfite); GENERIC].

Canada—
Not commercially available.

#### Auxiliary labeling
- May cause drowsiness.
- Avoid alcoholic beverages.
- May be habit-forming.

### OXYCODONE AND ACETAMINOPHEN ORAL SOLUTION

#### Usual adult dose
Analgesic—
Oral, 5 mL every four to six hours as needed.

#### Usual pediatric dose
Dosage has not been established.

#### Strength(s) usually available
U.S.—
5 mg of oxycodone hydrochloride and 325 mg of acetaminophen per 5 mL (Rx) [*Roxicet* (alcohol 0.4%; edetic acid; saccharin)].

Canada—
Not commercially available.

#### Auxiliary labeling
- May cause drowsiness.
- Avoid alcoholic beverages.
- May be habit-forming.

### OXYCODONE AND ACETAMINOPHEN TABLETS USP

#### Usual adult dose
Oral, 1 tablet every four to six hours as needed.

#### Usual pediatric dose
Dosage has not been established.

#### Strength(s) usually available
U.S.—
5 mg of oxycodone hydrochloride and 325 mg of acetaminophen (Rx) [*Endocet*; *Percocet* (scored); *Roxicet* (scored); GENERIC].

5 mg of oxycodone hydrochloride and 500 mg of acetaminophen (Rx) [*Roxicet 5/500* (scored); GENERIC].

Canada—
2.5 mg of oxycodone hydrochloride and 325 mg of acetaminophen (Rx) [*Percocet-Demi* (double-scored)].

5 mg of oxycodone hydrochloride and 325 mg of acetaminophen (Rx) [*Endocet* (scored); *Oxycocet* (scored); *Percocet* (scored); *Roxicet* (scored)].

#### Auxiliary labeling
- May cause drowsiness.
- Avoid alcoholic beverages.
- May be habit-forming.

---

## PENTAZOCINE AND ACETAMINOPHEN

## Oral Dosage Forms

### PENTAZOCINE HYDROCHLORIDE AND ACETAMINOPHEN TABLETS

#### Usual adult dose
Analgesic—
Oral, 1 tablet every four hours.

#### Usual adult prescribing limits
Up to 6 tablets daily.

#### Usual pediatric dose
Dosage has not been established.

#### Strength(s) usually available
U.S.—
650 mg of acetaminophen and 25 mg of pentazocine base (Rx) [*Talacen* (scored; colloidal silicon dioxide; FD&C Blue #1; gelatin; microcrystalline cellulose; potassium sorbate; pregelatinized starch; sodium lauryl sulfate; sodium metabisulfite; sodium starch glycolate; stearic acid)].

Canada—
Not commercially available.

**Auxiliary labeling**
- May cause drowsiness.
- Avoid alcoholic beverages.
- May be habit-forming.

---

### PROPOXYPHENE AND ACETAMINOPHEN

## Oral Dosage Forms

### PROPOXYPHENE HYDROCHLORIDE AND ACETAMINOPHEN TABLETS USP

**Usual adult dose**
Analgesic—
Oral, 1 tablet every four hours, as needed.

**Usual pediatric dose**
Dosage has not been established.

**Strength(s) usually available**
U.S.—
65 mg of propoxyphene hydrochloride and 650 mg of acetaminophen (Rx) [*E-Lor; Wygesic* (scored); GENERIC].
Canada—
Not commercially available.

**Auxiliary labeling**
- May cause drowsiness.
- Avoid alcoholic beverages.
- May be habit-forming.

### PROPOXYPHENE NAPSYLATE AND ACETAMINOPHEN TABLETS USP

**Usual adult dose**
Analgesic—
Oral, 2 tablets containing 50 mg of propoxyphene napsylate and 325 mg of acetaminophen every four hours, as needed; or
Oral, 1 tablet containing 100 mg of propoxyphene napsylate and 650 mg of acetaminophen every four hours, as needed.

**Usual pediatric dose**
Dosage has not been established.

**Strength(s) usually available**
U.S.—
50 mg of propoxyphene napsylate and 325 mg of acetaminophen (Rx) [*Darvocet-N 50;* GENERIC].
100 mg of propoxyphene napsylate and 650 mg of acetaminophen (Rx) [*Darvocet-N 100* ( cellulose; cornstarch; FD&C Yellow #6; magnesium stearate; stearic acid; titanium dioxide); *Propacet 100;* GENERIC].
Canada—
Not commercially available.

**Auxiliary labeling**
- May cause drowsiness.
- Avoid alcoholic beverages.
- May be habit-forming.

Revised: July 1990
Interim revision: 07/11/95

---

# OPIOID (NARCOTIC) ANALGESICS AND ASPIRIN   Systemic

This monograph includes information on the following: 1) Aspirin and Codeine‡; 2) Aspirin and Codeine, Buffered‡; 3) Aspirin and Dihydrocodeine; 4) Hydrocodone and Aspirin; 5) Oxycodone and Aspirin‡; 6) Pentazocine and Aspirin; 7) Propoxyphene and Aspirin‡.

Pharmacy Equivalent Name (PEN):
Aspirin and Codeine—Co-codaprin.
INN: Propoxyphene—Dextropropoxyphene
VA CLASSIFICATION (Primary): CN101
**NOTE:** The *Opioid (Narcotic) Analgesics and Aspirin (Systemic)* monograph is maintained on the USP DI electronic data base. For a printed copy of the most recent revision of the complete monograph, contact Micromedex, Inc. - Reprint Requests, 6200 S. Syracuse Way, Suite 300, Englewood, CO 80111; telephone (303) 486-6400; telefax (303) 486-6464; Email: USPDI@MDX.COM.

For information on the specific components of this combination, see the *USP DI* monographs for *Opioid (Narcotic) Analgesics (Systemic)* and *Salicylates (Systemic)*.

The information that follows is selectively abstracted from the complete monograph and is provided to facilitate drug use review and patient counseling.†**Aspirin** is a brand name in Canada; acetylsalicylic acid is the generic name. ASA, a commonly used designation for aspirin (or acetylsalicylic acid) in both the U.S. and Canada, is the term used in Canadian product labeling.

Note: For a listing of dosage forms and brand names by country availability, see *Dosage Forms* section(s).

‡*Aspirin* is a brand name in Canada; acetylsalicylic acid is the generic name. ASA, a commonly used designation for aspirin (or acetylsalicylic acid) in both the U.S. and Canada, is the term used in Canadian product labeling.

## Category

Analgesic.
Note: Opioid agonist analgesics—Codeine, dihydrocodeine, hydrocodone, oxycodone, and propoxyphene.
Opioid agonist/antagonist analgesic—Pentazocine.

## Indications

**Accepted**
Pain (treatment)—Indicated for symptomatic relief of
Mild to severe pain (depending on the dose of codeine)—Aspirin and codeine; buffered aspirin and codeine.
Mild to moderate pain—Propoxyphene and aspirin.
Moderate pain—Pentazocine and aspirin.
Moderate to moderately severe pain—Aspirin and dihydrocodeine; oxycodone and aspirin.
Moderate to severe pain—Hydrocodone and aspirin.

## Patient Consultation

As an aid to patient consultation, refer to *Advice for the Patient, Narcotic Analgesics and Aspirin (Systemic)*.
In providing consultation, consider emphasizing the following selected information (» = major clinical significance):

**Before using this medication**
» Conditions affecting use, especially:
Sensitivity to the opioid considered for use, to aspirin, or to nonsteroidal anti-inflammatory drugs (NSAIDs), history of
Pregnancy—Aspirin and opioid analgesics cross the placenta; high-dose chronic use or abuse of aspirin in the third trimester may be hazardous to the mother as well as the fetus and/or neonate, causing heart problems in fetus or neonate and/or bleeding in mother, fetus, or neonate; high-dose chronic use or abuse may also prolong and complicate labor and delivery; also, regular use of opioids by pregnant women may cause physical dependence in the fetus and withdrawal symptoms in the neonate; not taking aspirin during the third trimester unless prescribed by physician
Breast-feeding—Aspirin, codeine, and propoxyphene are distributed into breast milk
Use in children and in teenagers—Checking with physician before giving to children or teenagers with symptoms of acute febrile illness, especially influenza or varicella, because of the risk of Reye's syndrome; also, increased susceptibility to aspirin toxicity in children, especially with fever and dehydration; also, children up to 2 years of age are more susceptible to the effects of opioids, especially respiratory depression; in addition, children may be more likely to experience opioid-induced paradoxical CNS excitation during therapy
Use in the elderly—Increased risk of aspirin toxicity and of opioid-induced adverse effects, especially respiratory depression
Other medications, especially alcohol or other CNS depressants, anticoagulants, antidiabetic agents (oral), those cephalosporins that may cause hypoprothrombinemia, methotrexate, monoamine oxidase inhibitors, naltrexone, nonsteroidal anti-inflammatory drugs (NSAIDs), platelet aggregation inhibitors, plicamycin, probenecid, sulfinpyrazone, urinary alkalizers, valproic acid, vancomycin, and zidovudine

Other medical problems, especially coagulation or platelet function disorders, diarrhea caused by antibiotics or poisoning, asthma or other respiratory problems, and gastrointestinal problems such as ulceration or erosive gastritis (especially a bleeding ulcer) or other severe inflammatory bowel disease

**Proper use of this medication**
» Taking with food or a full glass (240 mL) of water to minimize stomach irritation
» Not taking medication if it has a strong vinegar-like odor
» Importance of not taking more medication than the amount prescribed because of danger of overdose of aspirin or opioid analgesics and habit-forming potential of opioid analgesics
» Not increasing dose if medication seems less effective after a few weeks; checking with physician instead
» Proper dosing
  Missed dose (if on scheduled dosing): Taking as soon as possible; not taking if almost time for next dose; not doubling doses
» Proper storage

**Precautions while using this medication**
Regular visits to physician to check progress during long-term therapy
» Caution if other medications containing aspirin or other salicylates or opioid analgesics are used
» Avoiding use of alcohol or other central nervous system (CNS) depressants during therapy unless prescribed or otherwise approved by physician; also, alcohol consumption may increase risk of aspirin-induced stomach problems
  Not taking acetaminophen or ibuprofen or other NSAIDs concurrently for more than a few days unless directed by physician or dentist
» Caution if dizziness, drowsiness, lightheadedness, or false sense of well-being occurs
  Caution when getting up suddenly from a lying or sitting position
  Lying down if nausea or vomiting, or dizziness or lightheadedness occurs
  Need to inform physician or dentist of use of medication if any kind of surgery (including dental surgery) or emergency treatment is required
  Caution if any kind of surgery is required; aspirin should be discontinued 5 days prior to surgery unless otherwise directed by physician or dentist
  Checking with pharmacist before using the buffered formulation (available in Canada) with any other oral medication; antacids in the formulation may interfere with absorption of many oral medications
  Diabetics: Aspirin may cause false urine sugar test results with prolonged use of 8 or more 325-mg (5-grain), or 4 or more 650-mg (10-grain), doses per day
  Possible dryness of mouth; using sugarless gum or candy, ice, or saliva substitute for relief; checking with dentist if dry mouth continues for more than 2 weeks
» Checking with physician before discontinuing medication after prolonged use of high doses; gradual dosage reduction may be necessary to avoid withdrawal symptoms
» Suspected overdose: Getting emergency help at once

**Side/adverse effects**
Signs of potential side effects, especially respiratory depression or impairment; allergic reactions; confusion, convulsions, hallucinations, mental depression, or other signs of CNS toxicity; gastrointestinal toxicity; hepatotoxicity; hypertension, and paradoxical CNS excitation, especially in children

---

### ASPIRIN AND CODEINE

## Oral Dosage Forms

### ASPIRIN AND CODEINE PHOSPHATE TABLETS USP

**Usual adult dose**
Oral, 1 or 2 tablets every four hours as needed.

**Usual pediatric dose**
Dosage has not been established.

**Strength(s) usually available**
U.S.—
  325 mg of aspirin and 15 mg of codeine phosphate (Rx) [GENERIC].
  325 mg of aspirin and 30 mg of codeine phosphate (Rx) [*Empirin with Codeine No.3;* GENERIC].
  325 mg of aspirin and 60 mg of codeine phosphate (Rx) [*Empirin with Codeine No.4;* GENERIC].
Canada—
  Not commercially available.

**Auxiliary labeling**
• May cause drowsiness.
• Avoid alcoholic beverages.
• Take with food or with a full glass of water.
• May be habit-forming.

### ASPIRIN, CODEINE PHOSPHATE, AND CAFFEINE TABLETS USP

**Usual adult dose**
Analgesic—
  Oral, 1 or 2 tablets every four hours as needed.

**Usual pediatric dose**
Dosage has not been established.

**Strength(s) usually available**
U.S.—
  Not commercially available.
Canada—
  325 mg of ASA, 8 mg of codeine phosphate, and 15 mg of caffeine (OTC) [*C2 with Codeine;* GENERIC].
  325 mg of ASA, 8 mg of codeine phosphate, and 32 mg of caffeine (OTC) [*Anacin with Codeine*].
  375 mg of ASA, 8 mg of codeine phosphate, and 30 mg of caffeine (OTC) [GENERIC].
  375 mg of ASA, 8 mg of codeine phosphate, and 30 mg of caffeine citrate (OTC) [*222* (double-scored)].
  375 mg of ASA, 15 mg of codeine phosphate, and 30 mg of caffeine citrate (Rx) [*282* (scored)].
  375 mg of ASA, 30 mg of codeine phosphate, and 30 mg of caffeine citrate (Rx) [*292* (scored)].
  400 mg of ASA, 8 mg of codeine phosphate, and 15 mg of caffeine (OTC) [*Novo-AC and C*].
  500 mg of ASA, 8 mg of codeine phosphate, and 15 mg of caffeine (OTC) [GENERIC].
Note: 30 mg of caffeine citrate are equivalent to 15 mg of caffeine base.

**Auxiliary labeling**
• May cause drowsiness.
• Avoid alcoholic beverages.
• Take with food or with a full glass of water.
• May be habit-forming.

---

### ASPIRIN AND CODEINE, BUFFERED

## Oral Dosage Forms

### ASPIRIN, CODEINE PHOSPHATE, CAFFEINE, ALUMINA, AND MAGNESIA TABLETS

**Usual adult dose**
Analgesic—
  Oral, 1 or 2 tablets every four hours as needed.

**Usual pediatric dose**
Dosage has not been established.

**Strength(s) usually available**
U.S.—
  Not commercially available.
Canada—
  325 mg of ASA, 8 mg of codeine phosphate, and 15 mg of caffeine, with 35 mg of aluminum hydroxide and 70 mg of magnesium hydroxide (OTC) [*C2 Buffered with Codeine*].

**Auxiliary labeling**
• May cause drowsiness.
• Avoid alcoholic beverages.
• Take with food or with a full glass of water.
• May be habit-forming.

---

### ASPIRIN AND DIHYDROCODEINE

## Oral Dosage Forms

### ASPIRIN, CAFFEINE, AND DIHYDROCODEINE BITARTRATE CAPSULES USP

**Usual adult dose**
Analgesic—
  Oral, 2 capsules every four hours as needed.

**Usual pediatric dose**
Dosage has not been established.

**Strength(s) usually available**
U.S.—
   356.4 mg of aspirin, 30 mg of caffeine, and 16 mg of dihydrocodeine bitartrate (Rx) [*Synalgos-DC*].
Canada—
   Not commercially available.

**Auxiliary labeling**
- May cause drowsiness.
- Avoid alcoholic beverages.
- Take with food or with a full glass of water.
- May be habit-forming.

---

## HYDROCODONE AND ASPIRIN

# Oral Dosage Forms
## HYDROCODONE BITARTRATE AND ASPIRIN TABLETS

**Usual adult dose**
Analgesic—
   Oral, 1 or 2 tablets every four to six hours as needed.

**Usual pediatric dose**
Dosage has not been established.

**Strength(s) usually available**
U.S.—
   5 mg of hydrocodone bitartrate and 500 mg of aspirin (Rx) [*Azdone* (scored); *Damason-P*; *Lortab ASA*; *Panasal 5/500*].
Canada—
   Not commercially available.

**Auxiliary labeling**
- May cause drowsiness.
- Avoid alcoholic beverages.
- Take with food or with a full glass of water.
- May be habit-forming.

---

## OXYCODONE AND ASPIRIN

# Oral Dosage Forms
## OXYCODONE AND ASPIRIN TABLETS USP

**Usual adult dose**
Analgesic—
   Oral, 1 or 2 half-strength tablets or 1 full-strength tablet, every four to six hours as needed. Dosage may be increased if necessary for severe pain.

**Usual pediatric dose**
Analgesic—
   Children up to 6 years of age—Use is not recommended.
   Children 6 to 12 years of age—Oral, ¼ half-strength tablet every six hours as needed.
   Children 12 years of age and over—Oral, ½ half-strength tablet every six hours as needed.

**Strength(s) usually available**
U.S.—
   Half-strength: 2.25 mg of oxycodone hydrochloride and 190 mcg (0.19 mg) of oxycodone terephthalate, with 325 mg of aspirin (Rx) [*Percodan-Demi* (scored)].
   Full-strength: 4.5 mg of oxycodone hydrochloride and 380 mcg (0.38 mg) of oxycodone terephthalate, with 325 mg of aspirin (Rx) [*Endodan*; *Percodan* (scored); *Roxiprin*; GENERIC].
Canada—
   Half-strength: 2.5 mg of oxycodone hydrochloride and 325 mg of ASA (Rx) [*Percodan-Demi* (scored)].
   Full-strength: 5 mg of oxycodone hydrochloride and 325 mg of ASA (Rx) [*Endodan* (scored); *Oxycodan* (scored); *Percodan* (scored)].

**Auxiliary labeling**
- May cause drowsiness.
- Avoid alcoholic beverages.
- Take with food or with a full glass of water.
- May be habit-forming.

---

## PENTAZOCINE AND ASPIRIN

# Oral Dosage Forms
## PENTAZOCINE HYDROCHLORIDE AND ASPIRIN TABLETS USP

**Usual adult dose**
Analgesic—
   Oral, 2 tablets three or four times a day as needed.

**Usual pediatric dose**
Dosage has not been established.

**Strength(s) usually available**
U.S.—
   12.5 mg of pentazocine (base) and 325 mg of aspirin (Rx) [*Talwin Compound*].
Canada—
   Not commercially available.

**Auxiliary labeling**
- May cause drowsiness.
- Avoid alcoholic beverages.
- Take with food or with a full glass of water.
- May be habit-forming.

---

## PROPOXYPHENE AND ASPIRIN

# Oral Dosage Forms
## PROPOXYPHENE HYDROCHLORIDE, ASPIRIN, AND CAFFEINE CAPSULES USP

**Usual adult dose**
Oral, 1 capsule every four hours, as needed.

**Usual adult prescribing limits**
Up to 390 mg of propoxyphene hydrochloride a day.

**Usual pediatric dose**
Dosage has not been established.

**Strength(s) usually available**
U.S.—
   65 mg of propoxyphene hydrochloride, 389 mg of aspirin, and 32.4 mg of caffeine (Rx) [*Darvon Compound-65*; *PC-Cap*; *Propoxyphene Compound-65*; GENERIC].
Canada—
   Not commercially available.

**Auxiliary labeling**
- May cause drowsiness.
- Avoid alcoholic beverages.
- Take with food or with a full glass of water.
- May be habit-forming.

## PROPOXYPHENE HYDROCHLORIDE, ASPIRIN, AND CAFFEINE TABLETS

**Usual adult dose**
Analgesic—
   Oral, 1 tablet every four hours, as needed.

**Usual adult prescribing limits**
Up to 390 mg of propoxyphene hydrochloride a day.

**Usual pediatric dose**
Dosage has not been established.

**Strength(s) usually available**
U.S.—
   Not commercially available.
Canada—
   65 mg of propoxyphene hydrochloride, 375 mg of ASA, and 30 mg of caffeine (Rx) [*692* (scored)].

**Auxiliary labeling**
- May cause drowsiness.
- Avoid alcoholic beverages.
- Take with food or with a full glass of water.
- May be habit-forming.

## PROPOXYPHENE NAPSYLATE AND ASPIRIN CAPSULES

**Usual adult dose**
Analgesic—
   Oral, 1 capsule every four hours, as needed.

### Usual adult prescribing limits
Up to 600 mg of propoxyphene napsylate a day.

### Usual pediatric dose
Dosage has not been established.

### Strength(s) usually available
U.S.—
   Not commercially available.
Canada—
   100 mg of propoxyphene napsylate and 325 mg of ASA (Rx) [*Darvon-N with A.S.A.*].

### Auxiliary labeling
- May cause drowsiness.
- Avoid alcoholic beverages.
- Take with food or with a full glass of water.
- May be habit-forming.

## PROPOXYPHENE NAPSYLATE, ASPIRIN, AND CAFFEINE CAPSULES

### Usual adult dose
Analgesic—
   Oral, 1 capsule every four hours, as needed.

### Usual adult prescribing limits
Up to 600 mg of propoxyphene napsylate a day.

### Usual pediatric dose
Dosage has not been established.

### Strength(s) usually available
U.S.—
   Not commercially available.
Canada—
   100 mg of propoxyphene napsylate, 375 mg of ASA, and 30 mg of caffeine (Rx) [*Darvon-N Compound*].

### Auxiliary labeling
- May cause drowsiness.
- Avoid alcoholic beverages.
- Take with food or with a full glass of water.
- May be habit-forming.

Revised: July 1990
Interim revision: 07/05/95

---

**OPIUM**—See *Opioid (Narcotic) Analgesics (Systemic)*

---

# OPRELVEKIN Systemic—INTRODUCTORY VERSION

VA CLASSIFICATION (Primary): BL400
Commonly used brand name(s): *Neumega*.
Other commonly used names are interleukin-11, recombinant; and rIL-11.
Note: For a listing of dosage forms and brand names by country availability, see *Dosage Forms* section(s).

## Category
Hematopoietic stimulant.

## Indications

### Accepted
Thrombocytopenia (prophylaxis)—Oprelvekin is indicated to prevent severe thrombocytopenia and reduce the need for platelet transfusions following myelosuppressive chemotherapy in patients with nonmyeloid malignancies who are at high risk of severe thrombocytopenia.
Note: Oprelvekin is not indicated following myeloablative chemotherapy.
   Use of oprelvekin has not been evaluated in patients receiving chemotherapy regimens of greater than 5 days duration or regimens including medications associated with delayed myelosuppression (e.g., nitrosoureas, mitomycin).

## Pharmacology/Pharmacokinetics

### Physicochemical characteristics
Source—Synthetic. Produced by a recombinant DNA process involving *Escherichia coli*. Oprelvekin differs from naturally occurring interleukin-11 (IL-11) in that it lacks the amino-terminal proline residue, so that the polypeptide is composed of 177 amino acids instead of 178 in the native chain. This variation has not been found to result in measurable differences in bioactivity either *in vitro* or *in vivo*.
Chemical group—Related to naturally occurring interleukins.
Molecular weight—Approximately 19,000 daltons.
pH—Reconstituted injection: 7.

### Mechanism of action/Effect
Naturally occurring IL-11 is produced by bone marrow stromal cells and is part of the cytokine family that shares the gp130 signal transducer. Primary osteoblasts and mature osteoclasts express messenger RNAs (mRNAs) for both IL-11 receptor (IL-11R alpha) and gp130. Both bone-forming and bone-resorbing cells are potential targets of IL-11.
Oprelvekin's primary hematopoietic action is to stimulate megakaryocytopoiesis and thrombopoiesis. Preclinical studies have shown that mature megakaryocytes developed during *in vivo* treatment with oprelvekin are ultrastructurally normal and that platelets developed during treatment are morphologically and functionally normal with a normal life span.
No change in platelet reactivity as measured by platelet activation in response to adenosine diphosphate (ADP) has been reported. Platelet aggregation in response to ADP, epinephrine, collagen, ristocetin, and arachidonic acid has not been reported in association with oprelvekin treatment.

### Other actions/effects
Nonhematopoietic actions in animals include regulation of intestinal epithelium growth (enhanced healing of gastrointestinal lesions), inhibition of adipogenesis, induction of acute phase protein synthesis, inhibition of pro-inflammatory cytokine production by macrophages, and stimulation of osteoclastogenesis and neurogenesis.
Mean 24-hour sodium excretion decreases during oprelvekin treatment.
Oprelvekin produces a mean increase in plasma volume of more than 20% (with all subjects having at least a 10% increase); red blood cell volume decreases similarly (as a result of repeated phlebotomy). As a result, whole blood volume increases approximately 10% and hemoglobin decreases approximately 10%.

### Biotransformation
Appears to be extensive (based on animal studies).

### Half-life
Elimination—
   $6.9 \pm 1.7$ hours.

### Onset of action
Increased platelet count—5 to 9 days after initiation of therapy in non-myelosuppressed patients.

### Time to peak concentration
$3.2 \pm 2.4$ hours after a single 50 mcg per kg of body weight (mcg/kg) dose.

### Peak serum concentration
$17.4 \pm 5.4$ nanograms per mL after a single 50 mcg/kg dose.
Note: No accumulation has been found to occur after multiple doses.

### Duration of action
Platelet count—Continues to increase for up to 7 days after therapy is discontinued, then returns to baseline within 14 days in non-myelosuppressed patients.

### Elimination
Renal (largely metabolized).
Note: Pharmacokinetic studies suggest that clearance decreases with age; clearance in infants and children (8 months to 11 years of age) is approximately 1.2- to 1.6-fold higher than in adults and adolescents (12 years of age and older).

## Precautions to Consider

### Carcinogenicity
Studies have not been done. However, oprelvekin was not found to stimulate *in vitro* growth of tumor colony–forming cells harvested from patients with a variety of human malignancies.

### Mutagenicity
*In vitro* studies found no evidence of genotoxicity.

### Pregnancy/Reproduction
Fertility—Studies in rats at doses of 2 to 20 times the human dose found prolonged estrus cycles, but no effect on fertility was found at doses of up to 1000 mcg per kg of body weight (mcg/kg) per day.

Pregnancy—Adequate and well-controlled studies in humans have not been done.

Studies in rats and rabbits given doses of 0.2 to 20 times the human dose found embryocidal effects. Studies in rats given doses of 2 to 20 times the human dose (100 mcg/kg per day or more) and in rabbits given doses of 0.02 to 2 times the human dose (1 mcg/kg per day or more) found parental toxicity. In rats, findings included transient hypoactivity and dyspnea after administration, prolonged estrus cycle, increased early embryonic deaths, and decreased numbers of live fetuses. In addition, in rats given 20 times the human dose, studies found low fetal body weights and a reduced number of ossified sacral and caudal vertebrae (i.e., retarded fetal development); however, no long-term behavioral or developmental abnormalities were detected. In rabbits, findings included decreased (fecal and urine) eliminations (the only toxicity noted at a dosage of 1 mcg/kg per day), decreased food consumption, body weight loss, abortion, increased embryonic and fetal death, and decreased numbers of live fetuses; no teratogenic effects were observed.

Risk-benefit should be considered before use of oprelvekin during pregnancy.

FDA Pregnancy Category C.

### Breast-feeding
It is not known whether oprelvekin is distributed into breast milk. Risk-benefit should be considered before breast-feeding during oprelvekin treatment.

### Pediatrics
Studies of efficacy have not been done in pediatric patients. However, based on a pharmacokinetic study, a dose of 75 to 100 mcg/kg will produce plasma concentrations consistent with those obtained in adults at a dose of 50 mcg/kg.

Incidence of adverse effects in children appears to be similar to or lower than that in adults, although the incidences of tachycardia and conjunctival injection were higher in the pediatric study than in studies in adults.

Long-term studies of the effects of oprelvekin on growth and development have not been done. Studies in growing rodents given doses of 100, 300, or 1000 mcg/kg per day for a minimum of 28 days found thickening of femoral and tibial growth plates, which did not completely resolve after a 28-day nontreatment period. A nonhuman primate toxicology study at doses of 10 to 1000 mcg/kg for 2 to 13 weeks found partially reversible joint capsule and tendon fibrosis and periosteal hyperostosis. One patient in the pediatric studies was found to have an asymptomatic, laminated periosteal reaction in the diaphyses of the femur, tibia, and fibula.

### Geriatrics
Appropriate studies performed to date have not demonstrated geriatrics-specific problems that would limit the usefulness of oprelvekin in the elderly.

### Laboratory value alterations
The following have been selected on the basis of their potential clinical significance (possible effect in parentheses where appropriate)—not necessarily inclusive (» = major clinical significance):

With physiology/laboratory test values
  Acute-phase proteins, such as
    Alpha$_1$-acid glycoprotein
    C-reactive protein
    Fibrinogen
    Serum amyloid A protein
      (plasma concentrations may be increased; the increase in plasma fibrinogen may be two-fold; concentrations return to normal after treatment with oprelvekin is discontinued)
  Albumin and
  Gamma globulins and
  Transferrin
      (serum concentrations may be decreased as a result of the increase in plasma volume)
  Calcium
      (serum concentrations may be decreased in parallel to the decrease in albumin concentrations)
  Hematocrit and
  Hemoglobin and
  Red blood cell count
      (serum concentrations may be moderately decreased [approximately 10 to 15%], without a decrease in red blood cell mass, predominantly as a result of the increase in plasma volume [dilutional anemia] that is primarily related to renal sodium and water retention; the decrease in hemoglobin concentrations typically begins within 3 to 5 days after initiation of oprelvekin therapy and reverses over approximately 1 week following discontinuation of oprelvekin)
  Von Willebrand factor
      (concentrations may be increased with a normal multimer pattern)

### Medical considerations/Contraindications
The medical considerations/contraindications included have been selected on the basis of their potential clinical significance (reasons given in parentheses where appropriate)—not necessarily inclusive (» = major clinical significance).

*Risk-benefit should be considered when the following medical problems exist:*

» Arrhythmias, atrial, history of
   (transient atrial arrhythmias have occurred during oprelvekin treatment; risk-benefit should be considered before use of oprelvekin in patients with a history of atrial arrhythmia)

» Congestive heart failure
   (oprelvekin may cause fluid retention; caution is recommended in patients with existing, or a predisposition to, congestive heart failure, as well as in those with a history of congestive heart failure who are well-compensated and receiving appropriate medical therapy)

» Fluid collections, pre-existing, including
   Ascites or
   Pleural effusions
      (may be increased as a result of fluid retention caused by oprelvekin; monitoring is recommended and drainage considered if clinically indicated)

Medical conditions associated with fluid retention or
Medical conditions exacerbated by fluid retention
   (oprelvekin may cause fluid retention)

Papilledema, existing or
Tumors involving the central nervous system
   (risk of worsening or development of papilledema during oprelvekin treatment)

Sensitivity to oprelvekin

### Patient monitoring
The following may be especially important in patient monitoring (other tests may be warranted in some patients, depending on condition; » = major clinical significance):

» Complete blood count and
» Platelet count
   (a complete blood count should be obtained prior to chemotherapy and at regular intervals during oprelvekin treatment; platelet counts should be monitored during the time of the expected nadir and until adequate recovery of platelets has occurred [post-nadir counts ≥ 50,000 cells per microliter])

» Electrolyte concentrations, serum and
» Fluid balance monitoring
   (recommended during treatment, with appropriate medical management for fluid retention; if a diuretic is used, it is recommended that fluid and electrolyte balance be carefully monitored; sudden deaths associated with severe hypokalemia have occurred in patients receiving chronic diuretic therapy and ifosfamide during oprelvekin treatment)

## Side/Adverse Effects
Note: Most side/adverse effects are mild to moderate and reversible when oprelvekin is discontinued.

Two cases of sudden death have been reported; both cases involved patients with severe hypokalemia (< 3 mEq per liter) who had received high doses of ifosfamide and daily doses of a diuretic.

The following side/adverse effects have been selected on the basis of their potential clinical significance (possible signs and symptoms in parentheses where appropriate)—not necessarily inclusive:

### Those indicating need for medical attention
Incidence more frequent
  ***Arrhythmias, atrial*** (irregular heartbeat)—may be asymptomatic; transient; ***fluid retention*** (shortness of breath; swelling of feet or lower legs)—mild to moderate; ***moniliasis, oral*** (sore mouth or tongue; white patches in mouth and/or on tongue); ***tachycardia*** (fast heartbeat)

  Note: Transient *atrial arrhythmias*, including atrial fibrillation or atrial flutter, have occurred in approximately 10% of patients treated with oprelvekin. In some patients, this effect may be related to increased plasma volume associated with fluid retention; oprelvekin is not directly arrhythmogenic. Arrhythmias are usually brief in duration, with conversion to sinus rhythm usually occurring either spontaneously or with rate-control medication therapy, and without clinical sequelae. Recurrence is unusual, even with continued oprelvekin treatment. Retrospective studies indicate a possible correlation between advancing age and other conditions associated with an increased risk of atrial arrhythmias (e.g., use of cardiac medications and a history of doxorubicin exposure) and the risk of development of atrial arrhythmias during oprelvekin therapy.

Weight gain is not commonly associated with *fluid retention*. In some patients, pre-existing pleural effusions increase during oprelvekin treatment. Capillary leak syndrome has not been observed.

*Fluid retention* is reversible within several days following withdrawal of oprelvekin.

Incidence less frequent
**Blurred vision; conjunctival hemorrhage** (bloody eye); **dehydration**—may be asymptomatic; **exfoliative dermatitis** (severe redness and peeling of skin)

Note: *Blurred vision* is usually transient and mild. However, papilledema has been reported in approximately 1.5% of patients following repeated treatment cycles. Papilledema not associated with inflammation or any other histologic abnormality has also been reported in nonhuman primates given doses of 1000 mcg per kg of body weight (mcg/kg) subcutaneously once a day for 4 to 13 weeks; it was reversible on discontinuation of oprelvekin.

**Those indicating need for medical attention only if they continue or are bothersome**
Incidence more frequent
**Asthenia, severe** (weakness); **conjunctival injection** (red eyes)
Incidence less frequent
**Paresthesia** (numbness or tingling of hands or feet); **skin discoloration; skin rash at injection site**

Note: Transient *skin rashes at the injection site* have occurred, as well as development of antibodies to oprelvekin (in about 1% of patients). However, presence of these antibodies or occurrence of the injection site reaction has not been associated with anaphylactoid reactions or loss of clinical response. No anaphylactoid or other severe allergic reactions have been reported with oprelvekin therapy.

## Overdose
For more information on the management of overdose or unintentional ingestion, **contact a Poison Control Center** (see *Poison Control Center Listing*).

**Clinical effects of overdose**
While doses higher than 100 mcg per kg of body weight (mcg/kg) have not been administered to humans and clinical experience is limited, doses above 50 mcg/kg may be associated with an increased incidence of cardiovascular effects in adults.

**Treatment of overdose**
Discontinue oprelvekin therapy and observe patient for signs of toxicity. Decisions about possible reinstitution of oprelvekin should be based on individual patient factors (e.g., evidence of toxicity, continued need for therapy).

## Patient Consultation
As an aid to patient consultation, refer to *Advice for the Patient, Oprelvekin (Systemic)*.

In providing consultation, consider emphasizing the following selected information (» = major clinical significance):

**Before using this medication**
» Conditions affecting use, especially:
　　Sensitivity to oprelvekin
　　Pregnancy—Embryocidal and toxic to parents in animal studies; risk-benefit should be considered
　　Use in children—Possible joint capsule and tendon fibrosis and periosteal hyperostosis with continuous dosing
　　Other medical problems, especially history of atrial arrhythmias, congestive heart failure, and pre-existing fluid retention states such as ascites or pleural effusions

**Proper use of this medication**
» Reading and following patient directions carefully with regard to: Preparation of the injection
　　Use of disposable syringes; safe handling and disposal of syringe and needle
　　Proper administration technique
　　Stability of the injection
　　Giving each dose at about the same time each day
» Proper dosing
　　Missed dose: Skip the missed dose and continue with the next scheduled dose
» Proper storage

**Precautions while using this medication**
» Importance of close monitoring by physician

**Side/adverse effects**
Signs of potential side effects, especially atrial arrhythmias, fluid retention, oral moniliasis, tachycardia, blurred vision, conjunctival hemorrhage, dehydration, and exfoliative dermatitis

## General Dosing Information
It is recommended that appropriate precautions be taken in the event that an allergic reaction occurs.

Oprelvekin therapy should be initiated 6 to 24 hours after the completion of chemotherapy and discontinued at least 2 days before starting the next planned cycle of chemotherapy. Safety and efficacy of administration of oprelvekin prior to or concurrently with cytotoxic chemotherapy have not been established.

## Parenteral Dosage Forms
### OPRELVEKIN FOR INJECTION
**Usual adult dose**
Thrombocytopenia (prophylaxis)—
　Subcutaneous, 50 mcg per kg of body weight once a day.

Note: It is recommended that oprelvekin be administered as a single subcutaneous injection into either the abdomen, thigh, or hip (or upper arm if the patient is not self-injecting).

It is recommended that dosing be initiated six to twenty-four hours after the completion of chemotherapy, and continued until the post-nadir platelet count is 50,000 cells per microliter or more. In clinical studies, doses were administered in courses of ten to twenty-one days.

It is recommended that a single treatment course not exceed twenty-one days.

It is recommended that treatment with oprelvekin be discontinued at least two days before the next planned cycle of chemotherapy.

**Usual pediatric dose**
Thrombocytopenia (prophylaxis)—
　Efficacy has not been established. However, a pharmacokinetic study has shown that a dose of 75 to 100 mcg per kg of body weight will produce a plasma concentration consistent with a dose of 50 mcg per kg of body weight in adults.

**Strength(s) usually available**
U.S.—
　5 mg (Rx) [*Neumega* (lyophilized powder)].

Note: The specific activity is approximately $8 \times 10^6$ Units per mg.

**Packaging and storage**
Store between 2 and 8 °C (36 and 46 °F). Protect from freezing.

**Preparation of dosage form**
Oprelvekin for injection is prepared for subcutaneous administration by adding 1 mL of sterile water for injection (without preservative), provided by the manufacturer, to the vial using aseptic technique, producing a solution containing 5 mg of oprelvekin per mL. The vial should be gently swirled until the powder is dissolved. The vial should not be shaken.

**Stability**
Any unused portion of a vial should be discarded. The single-use vial should not be re-entered.

The reconstituted solution can be stored for up to 3 hours either at 2 to 8 °C (36 to 46 °F) or at room temperature up to 25 °C (77 °F) before use. Reconstituted solution should not be stored in a syringe.

**Auxiliary labeling**
- Do not shake.
- Do not freeze.

Developed: 04/23/98

**ORAL REHYDRATION SALTS**—See *Carbohydrates and Electrolytes (Systemic)*

**ORPHENADRINE**—See *Skeletal Muscle Relaxants (Systemic)*

# ORPHENADRINE AND ASPIRIN Systemic

VA CLASSIFICATION (Primary): MS200

NOTE: The *Orphenadrine and Aspirin (Systemic)* monograph is maintained on the USP DI electronic data base. For a printed copy of the most recent revision of the complete monograph, contact Micromedex, Inc. - Reprint Requests, 6200 S. Syracuse Way, Suite 300, Englewood, CO 80111; telephone (303) 486-6400; telefax (303) 486-6464; Email: USPDI@MDX.COM.

For information on the specific components of this combination, see the *USP DI* monographs for *Salicylates (Systemic)* and *Skeletal Muscle Relaxants (Systemic)*.

The information that follows is selectively abstracted from the complete monograph and is provided to facilitate drug use review and patient counseling.

Note: For a listing of dosage forms and brand names by country availability, see *Dosage Forms* section(s).

## Category
Analgesic–skeletal muscle relaxant.

## Indications

**Accepted**
Spasm, skeletal muscle, accompanied by pain (treatment)—Indicated as an adjunct to other measures, such as rest and physical therapy, for relief of pain and muscle spasm associated with acute painful musculoskeletal conditions.

## Patient Consultation
As an aid to patient consultation, refer to *Advice for the Patient, Orphenadrine and Aspirin (Systemic)*.

In providing consultation, consider emphasizing the following selected information (» = major clinical significance):

**Before using this medication**
» Conditions affecting use, especially:
  Allergic reaction to orphenadrine, aspirin, or nonsteroidal anti-inflammatory drugs (NSAIDs), history of
  Pregnancy—High-dose chronic use or abuse of aspirin in third trimester may be hazardous to the mother as well as the fetus and/or neonate, causing heart problems in fetus or neonate and/or bleeding in mother, fetus, or neonate; high-dose chronic use or abuse may also prolong and complicate labor and delivery; not taking aspirin in third trimester unless prescribed by physician
  Use in children and teenagers—Checking with physician before giving to children or teenagers with symptoms of acute febrile illness, especially influenza or varicella, because of the risk of Reye's syndrome; also, increased susceptibility to aspirin toxicity in children, especially with fever and dehydration
  Use in the elderly—Increased risk of aspirin toxicity
  Other medications, especially anticoagulants, antidiabetic agents (oral), CNS depression–producing medications, those cephalosporins that may cause hypoprothrombinemia, moxalactam, plicamycin, valproic acid, methotrexate, NSAIDs, platelet aggregation inhibitors, probenecid, sulfinpyrazone, urinary alkalizers, vancomycin, and zidovudine
  Other medical problems, especially achalasia, bladder neck obstruction, coagulation or platelet function disorders, gastrointestinal problems such as ulceration or erosive gastritis (especially a bleeding ulcer or a stenosing peptic ulcer), glaucoma (or predisposition to), myasthenia gravis, prostatic hypertrophy, and pyloric or duodenal obstruction

**Proper use of this medication**
» Taking with food or full glass (240 mL) of water to minimize stomach irritation
» Not taking medication if it has a strong vinegar-like odor
» Importance of not taking more medication than the amount prescribed
» Proper dosing
  Missed dose: Taking if remembered within an hour; not taking if not remembered until later; not doubling doses
» Proper storage

**Precautions while using this medication**
  Regular visits to physician to check progress during prolonged therapy
» Caution if other medications containing aspirin or other salicylates or orphenadrine are used
  Not taking acetaminophen or ibuprofen or other nonsteroidal anti-inflammatory analgesics concurrently for more than a few days unless directed by physician
  Diabetics: May cause false urine sugar test results
  Caution if any kind of surgery is required; aspirin should be discontinued 5 days prior to surgery
» Avoiding use of alcohol or other central nervous system (CNS) depressants unless prescribed or otherwise approved by physician
  Alcohol consumption may increase probability of stomach problems
» Caution if blurred vision, drowsiness, dizziness, lightheadedness, or faintness occurs
  Possible dryness of mouth; using sugarless gum or candy, ice, or saliva substitute for relief; checking with dentist if dry mouth continues for more than 2 weeks
» Suspected overdose: Getting emergency help at once

**Side/adverse effects**
  Signs and symptoms of possible side effects, especially allergic reactions (including anaphylaxis and angioedema), blood dyscrasias, fainting, fast or pounding heartbeat, gastrointestinal toxicity, and hallucinations

## Oral Dosage Forms

### ORPHENADRINE CITRATE, ASPIRIN, AND CAFFEINE TABLETS

**Usual adult and adolescent dose**
Oral, 1 or 2 tablets containing 25 mg of orphenadrine citrate three or four times a day; or
Oral, ½ or 1 tablet containing 50 mg of orphenadrine citrate three or four times a day.

**Usual pediatric dose**
Dosage has not been established.

**Strength(s) usually available**
U.S.—
  25 mg of orphenadrine citrate, 385 mg of aspirin, and 30 mg of caffeine (Rx) [*Norgesic; Norphadrine; N3 Gesic; Orphenagesic*].
  50 mg of orphenadrine citrate, 770 mg of aspirin, and 60 mg of caffeine (Rx) [*Norgesic Forte; Norphadrine Forte; N3 Gesic Forte; Orphenagesic Forte*].
Canada—
  25 mg of orphenadrine citrate, 385 mg of ASA, and 30 mg of caffeine (OTC) [*Norgesic*].
  50 mg of orphenadrine citrate, 770 mg of ASA, and 60 mg of caffeine (OTC) [*Norgesic Forte*].
  Note: *Aspirin* is a brand name in Canada; acetylsalicylic acid is the generic name. ASA, a commonly used designation for aspirin (or acetylsalicylic acid) in both the U.S. and Canada, is the term used in Canadian product labeling.

**Auxiliary labeling**
• May cause drowsiness.
• Avoid alcoholic beverages.
• Take with food or with a full glass of water.

Revised: July 1990
Interim revision: 08/11/94

---

**OVULATION PREDICTION TEST KITS FOR HOME USE**—The *Ovulation Prediction Test Kits for Home Use* monograph is not included in this published version of the USP DI database. Copies of the monograph are available on request from Micromedex, Inc. - Reprint Requests, 6200 S. Syracuse Way, Suite 300, Englewood, CO 80111; telephone (303) 486-6400; telefax (303) 486-6464; Email: USPDI@MDX.COM.

**OXACILLIN**—See *Penicillins (Systemic)*

**OXAMNIQUINE**—The *Oxamniquine (Systemic)* monograph is not included in this published version of the USP DI database. Copies of the monograph are available on request from Micromedex, Inc. - Reprint Requests, 6200 S. Syracuse Way, Suite 300, Englewood, CO 80111; telephone (303) 486-6400; telefax (303) 486-6464; Email: USPDI@MDX.COM.

**OXANDROLONE**—See *Anabolic Steroids (Systemic)*

**OXAPROZIN**—See *Anti-inflammatory Drugs, Nonsteroidal (Systemic)*

**OXAZEPAM**—See *Benzodiazepines (Systemic)*

**OXICONAZOLE**—The *Oxiconazole (Topical)* monograph is not included in this published version of the USP DI database. Copies of the monograph are available on request from Micromedex, Inc. - Reprint Requests, 6200 S. Syracuse Way, Suite 300, Englewood, CO 80111; telephone (303) 486-6400; telefax (303) 486-6464; Email: USPDI@MDX.COM.

**OXPRENOLOL**—See *Beta-adrenergic Blocking Agents (Systemic)*

**OXTRIPHYLLINE**—See *Bronchodilators, Theophylline (Systemic)*

**OXTRIPHYLLINE AND GUAIFENESIN**—The *Oxtriphylline and Guaifenesin (Systemic)* monograph is not included in this published version of the USP DI database. Copies of the monograph are available on request from Micromedex, Inc. - Reprint Requests, 6200 S. Syracuse Way, Suite 300, Englewood, CO 80111; telephone (303) 486-6400; telefax (303) 486-6464; Email: USPDI@MDX.COM.

# OXYBUTYNIN Systemic

VA CLASSIFICATION (Primary): GU201

Commonly used brand name(s): *Ditropan*.

Note: For a listing of dosage forms and brand names by country availability, see *Dosage Forms* section(s).

## Category

Antispasmodic (urinary tract).

## Indications

**Accepted**

Urologic disorders, symptoms of (treatment) and

Irritative voiding, symptoms of (treatment)—Oxybutynin is indicated for the relief of symptoms associated with voiding, such as frequent urination, urgency, urge incontinence, nocturia, and incontinence in patients with uninhibited neurogenic bladder contractions and in those patients with reflex neurogenic bladder.

**Unaccepted**

Oxybutynin has been used as an antispasmodic in the symptomatic treatment of gastrointestinal disorders; however, its effectiveness has not been established.

## Pharmacology/Pharmacokinetics

**Physicochemical characteristics**

Molecular weight—393.95.

pKa—6.96.

**Mechanism of action/Effect**

Exerts direct antispasmodic effect on smooth muscle and inhibits the action of acetylcholine at postganglionic cholinergic sites, thus increasing bladder capacity and delaying the initial desire to void by reducing the number of motor impulses reaching the detrusor muscle. It does not block acetylcholine effects at skeletal myoneural junctions or at autonomic ganglia; neither does it have effect on the smooth muscle of blood vessels.

**Other actions/effects**

Oxybutynin has also shown (in animal studies) moderate antihistaminic, some local anesthetic, mild analgesic, and very low mydriatic and antisialagogue activity.

**Absorption**

Rapidly absorbed from gastrointestinal tract.

**Biotransformation**

Hepatic.

**Onset of action**

30 minutes to 1 hour.

**Time to peak effect**

3 to 6 hours.

**Duration of action**

6 to 10 hours (antispasmodic effect).

**Elimination**

Primarily renal.

## Precautions to Consider

**Pregnancy/Reproduction**

Fertility—Reproduction studies in the hamster, rabbit, rat, and mouse have not shown oxybutynin to impair fertility.

Pregnancy—Adequate and well-controlled studies in humans have not been done.

Reproduction studies in the hamster, rabbit, rat, and mouse have not shown oxybutynin to harm the fetus.

FDA Pregnancy Category B.

**Breast-feeding**

Problems in humans have not been documented. However, oxybutynin may inhibit lactation.

**Pediatrics**

Appropriate studies on the relationship of age to the effects of oxybutynin have not been performed in children up to 5 years of age.

**Geriatrics**

Geriatric patients may be more sensitive than younger adults to the anticholinergic effects of oxybutynin.

Oxybutynin may also exacerbate underlying disease states in these patients.

**Dental**

Prolonged use of oxybutynin may decrease or inhibit salivary flow, thus contributing to the development of caries, periodontal disease, oral candidiasis, and discomfort.

**Drug interactions and/or related problems**

The following drug interactions and/or related problems have been selected on the basis of their potential clinical significance (possible mechanism in parentheses where appropriate)—not necessarily inclusive (» = major clinical significance):

Note: Combinations containing any of the following medications, depending on the amount present, may also interact with this medication.

» Anticholinergics or other medications with anticholinergic activity (See *Appendix II*)
(concurrent use may intensify the anticholinergic effects of oxybutynin)

Central nervous system (CNS) depression–producing medications, other (See *Appendix II*)
(concurrent use may increase the sedative effects of either these medications or oxybutynin)

**Medical considerations/Contraindications**
The medical considerations/contraindications included have been selected on the basis of their potential clinical significance (reasons given in parentheses where appropriate)—not necessarily inclusive (» = major clinical significance).

*Risk-benefit should be considered when the following medical problems exist:*
» Cardiac disease, especially mitral stenosis, cardiac arrhythmias, congestive heart failure, coronary heart disease or
» Hemorrhage, acute, with unstable cardiovascular status
(increase in heart rate may be undesirable)
» Gastrointestinal tract obstructive disease as in achalasia and pyloroduodenal stenosis
(decrease in motility and tone may occur, resulting in obstruction and gastric retention)
» Glaucoma, angle-closure, or predisposition to
(possible mydriatic effect of oxybutynin resulting in increased intraocular pressure may precipitate an acute attack of angle-closure glaucoma)
Hepatic function impairment
(decreased metabolism of oxybutynin)
» Hernia, hiatal, associated with reflux esophagitis or
Hypertension
(may be aggravated)
Hyperthyroidism
(characterized by tachycardia, which may be increased)
» Intestinal atony in the elderly or debilitated patient or
» Paralytic ileus
(use of oxybutynin may lead to obstruction)
» Myasthenia gravis
(oxybutynin may aggravate condition because of inhibition of acetylcholine action)
Neuropathy, autonomic
(urinary retention and cycloplegia may be aggravated)
» Prostatic hypertrophy, nonobstructive
(reduction in tone of urinary bladder may lead to complete urinary retention)
Renal function impairment
(decreased excretion may increase the risk of side effects)
Sensitivity to oxybutynin
» Tachycardia
(may be increased)
Toxemia of pregnancy
(hypertension may be aggravated)
» Ulcerative colitis, severe
(large doses may suppress intestinal motility and may cause paralytic ileus; also, use may precipitate or aggravate the serious complication of toxic megacolon)
» Urinary retention or
» Uropathy, obstructive, such as bladder neck obstruction due to prostatic hypertrophy
(urinary retention may be precipitated or aggravated)
Xerostomia
(prolonged use may further reduce limited salivary flow)
Caution in use is also recommended in patients over 40 years of age because of danger of precipitating undiagnosed glaucoma.
In patients with diarrhea the possibility of intestinal obstruction should be excluded before oxybutynin is administered.

**Patient monitoring**
The following may be especially important in patient monitoring (other tests may be warranted in some patients, depending on condition; » = major clinical significance):
Cystometry
(recommended at periodic intervals to evaluate response to therapy)

## Side/Adverse Effects

Note: When oxybutynin is given to patients where the environmental temperature is high, there is risk of a rapid increase in body temperature because of suppression of sweat gland activity.

The following side/adverse effects have been selected on the basis of their potential clinical significance (possible signs and symptoms in parentheses where appropriate)—not necessarily inclusive:

**Those indicating need for medical attention**
Incidence rare
*Allergic reaction* (skin rash or hives); *increased intraocular pressure* (eye pain)

**Those indicating need for medical attention only if they continue or are bothersome**
Incidence more frequent
*Constipation; decreased sweating; drowsiness; dryness of mouth, nose, and throat*
Incidence less frequent or rare
*Decreased flow of breast milk; decreased saliva secretion* (difficulty in swallowing); *decreased sexual ability; difficult urination; difficulty in accommodation* (blurred vision); *headache; mydriatic effect* (increased sensitivity of eyes to light); *nausea or vomiting; trouble in sleeping; unusual tiredness or weakness*

## Overdose
For specific information on the agents used in the management of oxybutynin overdose, see:
• *Physostigmine (Systemic)* monograph

For more information on the management of overdose or unintentional ingestion, **contact a Poison Control Center** (see *Poison Control Center Listing*).

**Clinical effects of overdose**
The following effects have been selected on the basis of their potential clinical significance (possible signs and symptoms in parentheses where appropriate)—not necessarily inclusive:

*Clumsiness or unsteadiness; confusion; dizziness; severe drowsiness; fast heartbeat; fever; flushing or redness of face; hallucinations; respiratory depression* (shortness of breath or troubled breathing); *unusual excitement, nervousness, restlessness, or irritability*

**Treatment of overdose**
To decrease absorption—
Immediate gastric lavage.
Specific treatment—
*Slow* intravenous administration of 0.5 to 2 mg of physostigmine, repeated as needed up to a total of 5 mg.
Supportive care—
In the event of respiratory depression, starting and maintaining artificial respiration. Treating fever symptomatically with ice packs or alcohol sponging.

## Patient Consultation
As an aid to patient consultation, refer to *Advice for the Patient, Oxybutynin (Systemic)—Introductory Version*.
In providing consultation, consider emphasizing the following selected information » = major clinical significance):

**Before using this medication**
» Conditions affecting use, especially:
Sensitivity to oxybutynin
Use in the elderly—Increased sensitivity to anticholinergic effects
Dental—Possible development of dental problems because of decreased salivary flow
Other medications, especially other anticholinergics
Other medical problems, especially cardiac diseases, glaucoma, hemorrhage, hiatal hernia, intestinal atony, myasthenia gravis, paralytic ileus, prostatic hypertrophy, obstruction in gastrointestinal or urinary tract, tachycardia, ulcerative colitis, urinary retention

**Proper use of this medication**
Taking medication on an empty stomach with water, or with food or milk to reduce gastric irritation
» Importance of not taking more medication than the amount prescribed
» Proper dosing
Missed dose: Taking as soon as possible; if almost time for next dose, not taking at all; not doubling doses
» Proper storage

**Precautions while using this medication**
» Avoiding use of alcohol or other CNS depressants
Possible increased sensitivity of eyes to light
» Caution if drowsiness or blurred vision occurs
» Caution during exercise and hot weather; overheating may result in heat stroke

USP DI

Possible dryness of mouth, nose, and throat; using sugarless gum or candy, ice, or saliva substitute for relief of dry mouth; checking with physician or dentist if dry mouth continues for more than 2 weeks

**Side/adverse effects**
Signs of potential side effects, especially allergic reaction or increased intraocular pressure

## General Dosing Information

Oxybutynin may be taken on an empty stomach with water; however, if gastric irritation occurs it may be taken with food or milk.

Cystometry and other appropriate diagnostic procedures should precede treatment with oxybutynin.

If urinary tract infection is present, appropriate antibacterial therapy should be administered.

## Oral Dosage Forms

### OXYBUTYNIN CHLORIDE SYRUP USP

**Usual adult and adolescent dose**
Antispasmodic (urinary tract)—
  Oral, 5 mg two or three times a day, the dosage being adjusted as needed and tolerated.

**Usual adult prescribing limits**
Antispasmodic (urinary tract)—
  Oral, 5 mg four times a day or 20 mg daily.

**Usual pediatric dose**
Antispasmodic (urinary tract)—
  Children up to 5 years of age: Dosage has not been established.
  Children 5 years of age and over: Oral, 5 mg two or three times a day, not to exceed 15 mg per day.

**Usual geriatric dose**
See *Usual adult and adolescent dose*.

Note: Geriatric patients may be more sensitive to the effects of the usual adult dose.

**Strength(s) usually available**
U.S.—
  5 mg per 5 mL (Rx) [*Ditropan* (methylparaben; sucrose); GENERIC].
Canada—
  5 mg per 5 mL (Rx) [*Ditropan* (methylparaben; sucrose)].

**Packaging and storage**
Store below 40 °C (104 °F), preferably between 15 and 30 °C (59 and 86 °F), unless otherwise specified by manufacturer. Store in a tight, light-resistant container. Protect from freezing.

**Auxiliary labeling**
• May cause drowsiness or blurred vision.

### OXYBUTYNIN CHLORIDE TABLETS USP

**Usual adult and adolescent dose**
See *Oxybutynin Chloride Syrup USP*.

**Usual adult prescribing limits**
See *Oxybutynin Chloride Syrup USP*.

**Usual pediatric dose**
See *Oxybutynin Chloride Syrup USP*.

**Usual geriatric dose**
See *Oxybutynin Chloride Syrup USP*.

Note: Geriatric patients may be more sensitive to the effects of the usual adult dose.

**Strength(s) usually available**
U.S.—
  5 mg (Rx) [*Ditropan* (scored); GENERIC].
Canada—
  5 mg (Rx) [*Ditropan* (scored)].

**Packaging and storage**
Store below 40 °C (104 °F), preferably between 15 and 30 °C (59 and 86 °F), unless otherwise specified by manufacturer. Store in a tight, light-resistant container.

**Auxiliary labeling**
• May cause drowsiness or blurred vision.

Revised: 06/16/93
Interim revision: 04/30/98

---

**OXYCODONE** — See *Opioid (Narcotic) Analgesics (Systemic)*

---

**OXYMETAZOLINE** — The *Oxymetazoline (Nasal)* monograph is not included in this published version of the USP DI database. Copies of the monograph are available on request from Micromedex, Inc. - Reprint Requests, 6200 S. Syracuse Way, Suite 300, Englewood, CO 80111; telephone (303) 486-6400; telefax (303) 486-6464; Email: USPDI@MDX.COM.

---

**OXYMETAZOLINE** — The *Oxymetazoline (Ophthalmic)* monograph is not included in this published version of the USP DI database. Copies of the monograph are available on request from Micromedex, Inc. - Reprint Requests, 6200 S. Syracuse Way, Suite 300, Englewood, CO 80111; telephone (303) 486-6400; telefax (303) 486-6464; Email: USPDI@MDX.COM.

---

**OXYMETHOLONE** — See *Anabolic Steroids (Systemic)*

---

**OXYMORPHONE** — See *Opioid (Narcotic) Analgesics (Systemic)*

---

**OXYTETRACYCLINE** — See *Tetracyclines (Systemic)*

---

# OXYTOCIN   Systemic

VA CLASSIFICATION (Primary/Secondary): GU600/DX900; HS900
Commonly used brand name(s): *Pitocin; Syntocinon*.
Note: For a listing of dosage forms and brand names by country availability, see *Dosage Forms* section(s).

## Category

Oxytocic—Oxytocin.
Antihemorrhagic (postpartum and postabortal uterine bleeding)—Oxytocin Injection.
Lactation stimulant—Oxytocin Nasal Solution.
Diagnostic aid (utero-placental insufficiency; placental reserve)—Oxytocin Injection.

## Indications

Note: Bracketed information in the *Indications* section refers to uses that are not included in U.S. product labeling.

**Accepted**
Labor, medical induction of or
Labor, augmentation of or
Abortion, incomplete (treatment)—Parenterally administered oxytocin is indicated for induction and augmentation of labor. Parenteral oxytocin is also indicated for management of incomplete abortion. Oxytocin is sometimes used in combination with prostaglandins.
Abortion, therapeutic—Parenterally administered oxytocin is indicated for performance of therapeutic abortion. Oxytocin is sometimes used in combination with hypertonic sodium chloride, urea, or prostaglandins.
Hemorrhage, postabortion and postpartum (treatment)—Oxytocin is indicated in the management of postabortion and postpartum bleeding or hemorrhage.

Lactation deficiency (treatment)—Intranasally administered oxytocin is indicated for stimulation of impaired milk ejection (lack of let-down). Nasal oxytocin is recommended for short-term use, generally during the first week postpartum.

[Fetal distress (diagnosis)][1] or

[Utero-placental insufficiency (diagnosis)][1]—Oxytocin is administered parenterally to assess fetal-placental respiratory capabilities in high-risk pregnancies. This is also referred to as the oxytocin challenge test.

[1]Not included in Canadian product labeling.

## Pharmacology/Pharmacokinetics

### Physicochemical characteristics
Source—Synthetically produced pituitary hormone.
Molecular weight—1007.19.

### Mechanism of action/Effect
Uterine—
The uterine myometrium contains receptors specific to oxytocin. Oxytocin stimulates contraction of uterine smooth muscle by increasing intracellular calcium concentrations, thus mimicking contractions of normal, spontaneous labor and transiently impeding uterine blood flow. Amplitude and duration of uterine contractions are increased, leading to dilation and effacement of the cervix. The number of oxytocin receptors and, therefore, uterine response to oxytocin increases gradually throughout pregnancy, reaching its peak at term.

For diagnosis of fetal distress and utero-placental insufficiency: By comparing baseline and oxytocin-induced fetal heart rate patterns and uterine contraction patterns, the oxytocin challenge test may aid in determining if there is adequate placental reserve for continuation of a high-risk pregnancy. The occurrence of a fetal heart rate pattern exhibiting late decelerations with administration of oxytocin may indicate utero-placental insufficiency.

Lactation—
Stimulates smooth muscle to facilitate ejection of milk from breasts. Oxytocin does not increase milk production.

### Absorption
Rapidly absorbed through nasal mucous membranes; may be erratic.

### Protein binding
Low (30%).

### Biotransformation
Enzymatic hydrolysis, primarily by tissue oxytocinase. Oxytocinase is also found in placental tissue and plasma.

### Half-life
1 to 6 minutes (decreased in late pregnancy and lactation).

### Onset of action
Nasal—Within a few minutes.
Intramuscular—3 to 5 minutes.
Intravenous—Immediate.

### Duration of action
Nasal—20 minutes.
Intramuscular—2 to 3 hours.
Intravenous—Uterine activity generally subsides within one hour.

### Elimination
Only small amounts are excreted unchanged.

## Precautions to Consider

### Carcinogenicity/Mutagenicity
No animal or human studies have been conducted to evaluate the carcinogenic or mutagenic potential of oxytocin.

### Pregnancy/Reproduction
Pregnancy—
*For augmentation or stimulation of labor—*
Oxytocin is not indicated for use in the first trimester of pregnancy, other than for the treatment of incomplete abortion or therapeutic abortion.
Animal reproductive studies have not been conducted.

*For stimulation of lactation—*
Not recommended for use during pregnancy because its use may result in contractions and abortion.
FDA Pregnancy Category X.

Labor and delivery—Based on extensive clinical use and known pharmacologic properties of oxytocin, it is not expected to cause an increased risk of fetal abnormalities when used as indicated. Because of maternal and fetal risks, oxytocin must be administered with caution. It has been reported to cause fetal bradycardia, neonatal retinal hemorrhage, and neonatal jaundice, in addition to maternal effects.

Fetal deaths due to various causes have reportedly been associated with the parenteral use of oxytocics for induction or augmentation of labor.

Excessive dosage or administration of oxytocin to hypersensitive patients may cause uterine hypertonicity with spasm and tetanic contraction or uterine rupture. Abruptio placentae, impaired uterine blood flow, amniotic fluid embolism, and fetal trauma including cardiac arrhythmias, intracranial hemorrhage, and asphyxia may occur as a result.

Oxytocin may inhibit, rather than promote, expulsion of the placenta and increase the risk of hemorrhage and infection.

### Breast-feeding
For stimulation of milk ejection—Problems in humans have not been documented. Only minimal amounts pass into breast milk.

### Drug interactions and/or related problems
The following drug interactions and/or related problems have been selected on the basis of their potential clinical significance (possible mechanism in parentheses where appropriate)—not necessarily inclusive (» = major clinical significance):

Note: Combinations containing any of the following medications, depending on the amount present, may also interact with this medication.

Anesthetics, hydrocarbon inhalation, such as
  Cyclopropane
  Enflurane
  Halothane
  Isoflurane
  (cyclopropane anesthesia may lessen tachycardia but worsen hypotension caused by oxytocin; maternal sinus bradycardia and abnormal atrioventricular rhythms have been reported with concurrent use, although the correlation is controversial)
  (enflurane [concentrations > 1.5%], halothane [concentrations > 1%], and possibly isoflurane produce a dose-dependent decrease in the uterine response to oxytocics and may abolish the response if sufficient concentrations [> 3% of enflurane] are administered; uterine hemorrhage may result)

Caudal block anesthesia with a vasoconstrictor or
Vasopressors
  (concurrent use with oxytocin may potentiate the pressor effect of the sympathomimetic pressor amines with possible severe hypertension and rupture of cerebral blood vessels)
  (severe hypertension has been reported when oxytocin was given 3 to 4 hours after caudal block anesthesia with a vasoconstrictor)

» Sodium chloride, intra-amniotic for abortion or
» Urea, intra-amniotic for abortion or
» Oxytocics, other
  (concurrent use with oxytocin may result in uterine hypertonus, possibly causing uterine rupture or cervical laceration, especially in the absence of adequate cervical dilation; although combinations are sometimes used for therapeutic advantage, patient should be monitored closely during concurrent use; when used as an adjunct to abortifacients, it is recommended that oxytocin not be administered until the oxytocic effect of the abortifacient has subsided, to reduce the risk of uterine rupture and cervical laceration; water intoxication may also occur in patients given oxytocin following the use of intra-amniotic hypertonic saline for abortion)

### Laboratory value alterations
The following have been selected on the basis of their potential clinical significance (possible effect in parentheses where appropriate)—not necessarily inclusive (» = major clinical significance):

With physiology/laboratory test values
  Bilirubin, neonatal serum concentrations
    (neonatal jaundice has been reported, although it is not clear whether jaundice is due to oxytocin or labor process itself)
  Chloride and
  Sodium
    (antidiuretic effect of oxytocin may cause reduced maternal serum concentrations and water intoxication)

### Medical considerations/Contraindications
The medical considerations/contraindications included have been selected on the basis of their potential clinical significance (reasons given in parentheses where appropriate)—not necessarily inclusive (» = major clinical significance).

*Except under special circumstances, this medication should not be used when the following medical problems exist:*

*For all indications*
» Allergy to oxytocin, history of

*For augmentation or induction of labor*
» Absolute contraindications to vaginal delivery
» Hypertonic uterine patterns

**Risk-benefit should be considered when the following medical problems exist:**
For all indications, except for stimulation of lactation
Cardiac disease, especially involving fixed cardiac output or
Hypertension or
Renal function impairment
(increased susceptibility to fluid overload, arrhythmia, or hypotension and reflex tachycardia; reduction in dosage is recommended)
Exaggerated response to oxytocin or other oxytocics, history of
(excessive dosage or administration of oxytocin to hypersensitive patients may cause uterine hypertonicity with spasm and tetanic contraction, which can lead to uterine rupture, cervical lacerations, abruptio placentae, impaired uterine blood flow, amniotic fluid embolism, and fetal trauma including cardiac arrhythmias, intracranial hemorrhage, and asphyxia)

*For augmentation or induction of labor only, in addition to those problems listed above*
» Relative contraindications to vaginal delivery
» Uterine inertia
(*prolonged use* of oxytocin is not recommended; in cases of uterine inertia, it is recommended that oxytocin be administered for no longer than 6 to 8 hours)

**Patient monitoring**
The following may be especially important in patient monitoring (other tests may be warranted in some patients, depending on condition; » = major clinical significance):

Acid-base equilibrium determinations, fetal and
Contractions—frequency, duration, and force of and
Fetal heart rate monitoring, continuous and
Heart rate and blood pressure determinations, maternal and
Uterine tone, resting
(recommended at frequent intervals during labor and delivery)
Fluid intake and output determinations
(recommended to reduce the risk of water intoxication, especially during prolonged administration of oxytocin)

## Side/Adverse Effects

The following side/adverse effects have been selected on the basis of their potential clinical significance (possible signs and symptoms in parentheses where appropriate)—not necessarily inclusive:

**Those indicating need for medical attention**
Incidence rare
With nasal use
*Psychotic reaction*—one case reported; *seizures*—one case reported; *unexpected uterine bleeding or contractions*

With parenteral use
***Afibrinogenemia or pelvic hematoma or postpartum hemorrhage*** (increased or continuing vaginal bleeding); ***allergy or*** (skin rash or itching; hives); ***generalized anaphylaxis*** (difficulty in breathing; skin rash or itching; hives); ***cardiac arrhythmias or premature ventricular contractions*** (fast or irregular heartbeat); ***hypotension*** (weakness; dizziness); ***followed by hypertension and*** (continuing or severe headache); ***reflexive tachycardia*** (fast heartbeat); ***uterine rupture*** (increased or continuing vaginal bleeding; severe pelvic or abdominal pain); ***water intoxication*** (seizures; coma; confusion; continuing headache; rapid weight gain)

Note: Fatal *allergic reactions* have occurred with the use of oxytocin.
*Hypotension* may be caused by administration of large doses or rapid intravenous infusion.
Maternal death due to *uterine rupture* has been reported to be associated with the parenteral administration of oxytocics for the induction or augmentation of labor.
Because of its slight antidiuretic effect, prolonged intravenous administration of oxytocin (usually in doses of 40 to 50 milliunits or more per minute) with large volumes of fluid may produce severe *water intoxication*. Maternal deaths due to hypertensive episodes and subarachnoid hemorrhage have been reported.

**Those indicating need for medical attention only if they continue or are bothersome**
Incidence rare
With parenteral use
*Nausea; vomiting*
With nasal use
*Lacrimation* (tearing of the eyes); *nasal irritation; rhinorrhea* (runny nose)

## Patient Consultation

As an aid to patient consultation, refer to *Advice for the Patient, Oxytocin (Systemic)*.
In providing consultation, consider emphasizing the following selected information (» = major clinical significance):

**Before using this medication**
Conditions affecting use, especially:
Allergy to oxytocin

**Proper use of this medication**
For intranasal use only
Proper administration
» Proper dosing

**Precautions while using this medication**
Possible therapeutic failure of nasal spray when used as lactation stimulant

**Side/adverse effects**
Signs of potential side effects, especially:
For parenteral use—Water intoxication, afibrinogenemia, pelvic hematoma, postpartum hemorrhage, anaphylaxis, allergy, cardiac arrhythmias, premature ventricular contractions, hypotension, and uterine rupture
For nasal use—Unexpected uterine bleeding or contractions, psychotic reaction, and seizures

## General Dosing Information

Patients receiving oxytocin should be hospitalized and under the supervision of a physician experienced in its use.
Therapeutic failure frequently occurs with the administration of nasal spray for stimulation of lactation.

**For parenteral dosage forms only**
Oxytocin must be diluted and administered by intravenous infusion for induction or stimulation of labor. Intramuscular administration of oxytocin is not recommended for induction or stimulation of labor, since intramuscular administration is difficult to regulate and may lead to uterine hyperactivity and fetal distress.
It is recommended that oxytocin infusion be administered intravenously by means of an infusion pump, a microdrip regulator, or a similar device to allow precise adjustment of the flow rate.
Dosage must be adjusted to meet the individual requirements of each patient, on the basis of maternal and fetal response.
Oxytocin should not be used simultaneously by more than one route.

**For treatment of adverse effects**
Oxytocin infusion should be discontinued or the rate of infusion decreased at the first sign of uterine hyperactivity or fetal distress. Supportive care, including administration of oxygen to the mother, is also recommended.

## Nasal Dosage Forms

### OXYTOCIN NASAL SOLUTION USP

**Usual adult dose**
Lactation stimulant—
Intranasal, 1 spray into one or both nostrils two to three minutes before nursing or pumping of breasts.

**Strength(s) usually available**
U.S.—
40 Units per mL (Rx) [*Syntocinon*].
Canada—
40 Units per mL (Rx) [*Syntocinon*].

**Packaging and storage**
Store below 40 °C (104 °F), preferably between 15 and 30 °C (59 and 86 °F), unless otherwise specified by manufacturer.

## Parenteral Dosage Forms

Note: Bracketed uses in the *Dosage Forms* section refer to categories of use and/or indications that are not included in U.S. product labeling.

# OXYTOCIN INJECTION USP

**Usual adult dose**
Augmentation or
Induction of labor—
  Intravenous infusion, initially no more than 0.5 to 2 milliunits per minute, increased every fifteen to sixty minutes in increments of 1 to 2 milliunits per minute until adequate uterine activity is established, up to 20 milliunits per minute (usually 2 to 5 milliunits per minute). Occasionally, doses higher than 20 milliunits per minute may be required.
  The infusion rate may be reduced by similar increments, once labor is established.
Abortion, incomplete (treatment) or
Abortion, therapeutic—
  Intravenous infusion, 10 Units at a rate of 20 to 40 milliunits per minute.
Hemorrhage, postpartum (treatment)—
  Intravenous infusion, 10 Units at a rate of 20 to 40 milliunits per minute following delivery of the infant(s) and preferably the placenta(s).
  Intramuscular, 10 Units after delivery of the placenta(s).
Hemorrhage, postabortion (treatment)—
  Intravenous infusion, 10 Units at a rate of 20 to 100 milliunits per minute.
[Utero-placental insufficiency (diagnosis)][1]—
  Intravenous infusion, initially 0.5 milliunits per minute, doubled every twenty minutes as necessary to the effective dose (usually 5 to 6 milliunits per minute). When three moderate uterine contractions (duration of forty to sixty seconds) occur in one ten-minute interval, the infusion is discontinued and baseline and oxytocin-induced fetal heart rate and uterine contraction patterns are compared.

**Strength(s) usually available**
U.S.—
  10 Units per mL (Rx) [*Pitocin*; *Syntocinon*; GENERIC].
Canada—
  5 Units per mL (Rx) [*Syntocinon*].
  10 Units per mL (Rx) [*Syntocinon*].

**Packaging and storage**
Store below 40 °C (104 °F), preferably between 15 and 30 °C (59 and 86 °F), unless otherwise specified by manufacturer. Protect from freezing.

**Preparation of dosage form**
For augmentation or induction of labor—Using standard aseptic technique, add 10 units of Oxytocin Injection USP to 1000 mL of normal saline (0.9% sodium chloride injection), lactated Ringer's solution, or other nonhydrating diluent. Final solution concentration is 10 milliunits per mL.

For control of postabortion or postpartum uterine bleeding—Using standard aseptic technique, add 10 to 40 units of Oxytocin Injection USP to 1000 mL of a nonhydrating diluent. Final solution concentration is 10 to 40 milliunits per mL.

---
[1] Not included in Canadian product labeling.

Revised: 07/14/93
Interim revision: 06/30/94

# PACLITAXEL Systemic

VA CLASSIFICATION (Primary): AN900
Commonly used brand name(s): *Taxol*.
Note: For a listing of dosage forms and brand names by country availability, see *Dosage Forms* section(s).

## Category
Antineoplastic.

## Indications
Note: Bracketed information in the *Indications* section refers to uses that are not included in U.S. product labeling.

### Accepted
Carcinoma, ovarian, epithelial (treatment)—Paclitaxel is indicated for treatment of metastatic ovarian carcinoma after failure of first-line or subsequent chemotherapy.

Carcinoma, breast (treatment)—Paclitaxel is indicated for treatment of metastatic breast carcinoma after failure of combination chemotherapy or at relapse within 6 months of adjuvant chemotherapy.

Kaposi's sarcoma, acquired immunodeficiency syndrome (AIDS)–associated (treatment)[1]—Paclitaxel is indicated for second-line treatment of AIDS-associated Kaposi's sarcoma.

[Carcinoma, bladder (treatment)][1] or
[Carcinoma, head and neck (treatment)][1]—Paclitaxel is indicated for treatment of transitional-cell bladder carcinoma (Evidence rating: IIID) and head and neck carcinoma (Evidence rating: IIID).

[Carcinoma, cervical (treatment)][1]
[Carcinoma, esophageal (treatment)][1] or
[Carcinoma, endometrial (treatment)][1]—Paclitaxel is considered reasonable medical therapy at some point in the management of cervical carcinoma (Evidence rating: IIID), esophageal carcinoma (Evidence rating: IIID), and endometrial carcinoma (Evidence rating: IIID).

[Carcinoma, lung, non–small cell (treatment)][1]—Paclitaxel is indicated for treatment of non–small cell lung carcinoma, based upon reports of objective tumor responses, almost all of which were partial.

[Carcinoma, lung, small cell (treatment)][1]—Paclitaxel is indicated for treatment of small cell lung carcinoma.

[1]Not included in Canadian product labeling.

## Pharmacology/Pharmacokinetics
Note: Pharmacokinetic studies were conducted in adult cancer patients who received paclitaxel in single doses of 15 to 135 mg per square meter of body surface area (mg/m$^2$) given by 1-hour infusions (15 patients), 30 to 275 mg/m$^2$ given by 6-hour infusions (36 patients), and 200 to 275 mg/m$^2$ given by 24-hour infusions (54 patients). Pharmacokinetic studies were also conducted in ovarian cancer patients who received single doses of 135 mg/m$^2$ given by 3-hour infusions (seven patients), 135 mg/m$^2$ given by 24-hour infusions (two patients), 175 mg/m$^2$ given by 3-hour infusions (five patients), and 175 mg/m$^2$ given by 24-hour infusions (four patients).

### Physicochemical characteristics
Source—Semi-synthetic. Obtained from *Taxus baccata*.
Chemical group—Paclitaxel is a diterpenoid taxane.
Molecular weight—853.93.

### Mechanism of action/Effect
Paclitaxel belongs to the class of medications known as antimicrotubule agents. It promotes the assembly of microtubules from tubulin dimers and stabilizes microtubules by preventing depolymerization. This stability results in the inhibition of the normal dynamic reorganization of the microtubule network that is essential for vital interphase and mitotic cellular functions. In addition, paclitaxel induces abnormal arrays or "bundles" of microtubules throughout the cell cycle and multiple asters of microtubules during mitosis.

### Other actions/effects
Paclitaxel enhances the cytotoxic effects of ionizing radiation *in vitro*.

### Distribution
The mean steady state volume of distribution (Vol$_D$) ranged from 227 to 688 liters per square meter of body surface area following single doses of 135 and 175 mg/m$^2$ given over 24 hours. Similar Vol$_D$ were obtained following single doses of 15 to 135 mg/m$^2$ given over 1 hour and single doses of 30 to 275 mg/m$^2$ given over 6 hours. This indicates extensive extravascular distribution and/or tissue binding.

The mean area under the plasma concentration–time curve (AUC) (24-hour infusion) was 6300 and 7993 nanograms per hour per mL for doses of 135 and 175 mg/m$^2$, respectively. The mean maximum plasma concentration following a 24-hour infusion of paclitaxel was 195 and 365 nanograms per mL for doses of 135 and 175 mg/m$^2$, respectively.

The mean AUC (3-hour infusion) was 7952 and 15,007 nanograms per hour per mL for doses of 135 and 175 mg/m$^2$, respectively. The mean maximum plasma concentration following a 3-hour infusion of paclitaxel was 2170 and 3650 nanograms per mL for doses of 135 and 175 mg/m$^2$, respectively.

### Protein binding
Very high (89 to 98%).

### Biotransformation
Hepatic. Metabolized via the cytochrome P450 isoenzyme CYP2C8 to one major metabolite (6-alpha-hydroxypaclitaxel), and via the cytochrome P450 isoenzyme CYP3A4 to two minor metabolites (3-para-hydroxypaclitaxel and 6-alpha,3'-para-dihydroxypaclitaxel).

### Half-life
Terminal—Mean (standard deviation): Range 5.3 (4.6) to 17.4 (4.7) hours, following 1-hour and 6-hour infusions at doses of 15 to 275 mg per square meter of body surface area.

### Elimination
Not completely understood. Mean (standard deviation) values for urinary recovery of unchanged drug following 1-, 6-, and 24-hour infusions at doses of 15 to 275 mg per square meter of body surface area ranged from 1.3% (0.5%) to 12.6% (16.2%) of the dose, indicating extensive nonrenal clearance. High concentrations of paclitaxel and its metabolites have been reported in the bile.

The decline in plasma concentrations is biphasic; the initial rapid decline represents distribution to the peripheral compartment and significant elimination. The later phase is due, in part, to a relatively slow efflux from the peripheral compartment.

Mean values for total body clearance were 21.7 and 23.8 liters per hour per square meter of body surface area, following single doses of 135 and 175 mg/m$^2$ given by 24-hour infusions, respectively. Clearance values following single doses of 135 and 175 mg/m$^2$ given by 3-hour infusions were 17.7 and 12.2 liters per hour per square meter of body surface area, respectively.

## Precautions to Consider

### Cross-sensitivity and/or related problems
Patients sensitive to polyoxyethylated castor oil may be sensitive to paclitaxel also, since the injection contains a polyoxyethylated castor oil vehicle.

### Carcinogenicity
Studies with paclitaxel have not been done.

Secondary malignancies are potential delayed effects of many antineoplastic agents, although it is not clear whether the effect is related to their mutagenic or immunosuppressive action. The effect of dose and duration of therapy is also unknown, although risk seems to increase with long-term use.

### Mutagenicity
Paclitaxel is mutagenic in *in vitro* (chromosome aberrations in human lymphocytes) and in *in vivo* (micronucleus test in mice) mammalian test systems. However, it was not mutagenic in the Ames test or the CHO/HGPRT gene mutation assay.

### Pregnancy/Reproduction
Fertility—Studies in rats at doses of 1 mg per kg of body weight (mg/kg) (6 mg per square meter of body surface area) found that paclitaxel reduced fertility.

Pregnancy—Adequate and well-controlled studies in humans have not been done.

First trimester: It is usually recommended that use of antineoplastics, especially combination chemotherapy, be avoided whenever possible, especially during the first trimester. Although information is limited because of the relatively few instances of antineoplastic administration during pregnancy, the mutagenic, teratogenic, and carcinogenic potential of these medications must be considered.

Other hazards to the fetus include adverse reactions seen in adults.

In general, use of contraception is recommended during cytotoxic drug therapy.

Paclitaxel was found to cause maternal and embryo-fetal toxicity in rabbits at intravenous doses of 3 mg/kg (33 mg per square meter of body surface area) given during organogenesis. In rats and rabbits, paclitaxel was found to cause abortions, decreased corpora lutea, a decrease in implantations and live fetuses, and increased resorptions and embryo-fetal deaths. No gross external, soft tissue, or skeletal alterations occurred.

FDA Pregnancy Category D.

### Breast-feeding
Although very little information is available regarding distribution of antineoplastic agents into breast milk, breast-feeding is not recommended during chemotherapy because of the potential risks to the infant (adverse effects, mutagenicity, carcinogenicity). It is not known whether paclitaxel is distributed into breast milk.

### Pediatrics
No information is available on the relationship of age to the effects of paclitaxel in pediatric patients, although phase I studies in children have been reported. Safety and efficacy have not been established.

### Geriatrics
One retrospective study on the relationship of age to the effects of paclitaxel found no difference in dose intensity achieved in elderly patients.

### Dental
The bone marrow depressant effects of paclitaxel may result in an increased incidence of microbial infection, delayed healing, and gingival bleeding. Dental work, whenever possible, should be completed prior to initiation of therapy or deferred until blood counts have returned to normal. Patients should be instructed in proper oral hygiene during treatment, including caution in use of regular toothbrushes, dental floss, and toothpicks.

Paclitaxel also may cause mucositis, which is usually mild but which at high doses may be associated with considerable discomfort.

### Drug interactions and/or related problems
The following drug interactions and/or related problems have been selected on the basis of their potential clinical significance (possible mechanism in parentheses where appropriate)—not necessarily inclusive (» = major clinical significance):

Note: Combinations containing any of the following medications, depending on the amount present, may also interact with this medication.

Blood dyscrasia–causing medications (see *Appendix II*)
(leukopenic and/or thrombocytopenic effects of paclitaxel may be increased with concurrent or recent therapy if these medications cause the same effects; dosage adjustment of paclitaxel, if necessary, should be based on blood counts)

» Bone marrow depressants, other (see *Appendix II*) or
Radiation therapy
(additive bone marrow depression may occur; dosage reduction may be required when two or more bone marrow depressants, including radiation, are used concurrently or consecutively)

(severity of paclitaxel-induced neutropenia may be related to the extent of prior myelotoxic therapy)

(in one Phase I study, administration of cisplatin before paclitaxel, rather than after, was found to reduce paclitaxel clearance by approximately 25%)

Vaccines, killed virus
(because normal defense mechanisms may be suppressed by paclitaxel therapy, the patient's antibody response to the vaccine may be decreased. The interval between discontinuation of medications that cause immunosuppression and restoration of the patient's ability to respond to the vaccine depends on the intensity and type of immunosuppression-causing medication used, the underlying disease, and other factors; estimates vary from 3 months to 1 year)

» Vaccines, live virus
(because normal defense mechanisms may be suppressed by paclitaxel therapy, concurrent use with a live virus vaccine may potentiate the replication of the vaccine virus, may increase the side/adverse effects of the vaccine virus, and/or may decrease the patient's antibody response to the vaccine; immunization of these patients should be undertaken only with extreme caution after careful review of the patient's hematologic status and only with the knowledge and consent of the physician managing the paclitaxel therapy. The interval between discontinuation of medications that cause immunosuppression and restoration of the patient's ability to respond to the vaccine depends on the intensity and type of immunosuppression-causing medication used, the underlying disease, and other factors; estimates vary from 3 months to 1 year. In addition, immunization with oral poliovirus vaccine should be postponed in persons in close contact with the patient, especially family members)

### Laboratory value alterations
The following have been selected on the basis of their potential clinical significance (possible effect in parentheses where appropriate)—not necessarily inclusive (» = major clinical significance):

With physiology/laboratory test values
Alkaline phosphatase values, serum and
Aspartate aminotransferase (AST [SGOT]) values, serum and
Bilirubin concentrations, serum
(may be increased transiently; elevations of alkaline phosphatase and bilirubin may be dose-related)
Triglycerides
(elevations in serum concentrations have been reported)

### Medical considerations/Contraindications
The medical considerations/contraindications included have been selected on the basis of their potential clinical significance (reasons given in parentheses where appropriate)—not necessarily inclusive (» = major clinical significance):

*Risk-benefit should be considered when the following medical problems exist:*

» Bone marrow depression
(will be increased; it is recommended that paclitaxel not be administered to patients with solid tumors when baseline neutrophil counts are lower than 1500 cells per cubic millimeter, and that subsequent doses not be administered until neutrophil counts have returned to greater than 1500 cells per cubic millimeter and platelet counts to greater than 100,000 cells per cubic millimeter or to baseline values; it is also recommended that paclitaxel not be administered to patients with AIDS-associated Kaposi's sarcoma when baseline neutrophil counts are lower than 1000 cells per cubic millimeter)

Cardiac function impairment, including:
Angina
» Cardiac conduction abnormalities
Congestive heart failure, history of
Myocardial infarction within the past 6 months
(the patient's ability to tolerate the cardiovascular side effects of paclitaxel may be reduced)

» Chickenpox, existing or recent (including recent exposure) or
» Herpes zoster
(risk of severe generalized disease)

» Infection
» Sensitivity to paclitaxel
» Caution should be used also in patients who have had previous cytotoxic drug therapy or radiation therapy.

### Patient monitoring
The following may be especially important in patient monitoring (other tests may be warranted in some patients, depending on condition; » = major clinical significance):

Hematocrit or hemoglobin and
» Leukocyte count, total and, if appropriate, differential and
» Platelet count
(determinations recommended prior to initiation of therapy and at periodic intervals during therapy; frequency varies according to clinical state, agent, dose, and other agents being used concurrently)

» Vital signs
(recommended frequently, especially during the first hour of paclitaxel infusions)

## Side/Adverse Effects

Note: Neutropenia is the major dose-limiting effect.

The following side/adverse effects have been selected on the basis of their potential clinical significance (possible signs and symptoms in parentheses where appropriate)—not necessarily inclusive:

### Those indicating need for medical attention
Incidence more frequent
*Anemia* (unusual tiredness or weakness)—usually asymptomatic; *hypersensitivity reaction* (flushing of face; skin rash or itching; shortness of breath; rarely [with proper premedication], severe shortness of breath; severe skin reaction); *leukopenia or neutropenia, with or without infection* (fever or chills; cough or hoarseness; lower back or side pain; painful or difficult urination); *thrombocytopenia* (unusual bleeding or bruising; black, tarry stools; blood in urine or stools; pinpoint red spots on skin)—usually asymptomatic

Note: Incidence and severity of *anemia* seem to increase with increasing exposure to paclitaxel.

With proper premedication, *hypersensitivity reactions* are usually mild (flushing of face, skin rash, shortness of breath). However, severe reactions (hypotension requiring treatment, dyspnea requiring bronchodilators, angioedema or generalized urticaria, chest pain) can occur, even with premedication, and necessitate immediate discontinuation of paclitaxel and aggressive symptomatic therapy. Severe symptoms usually occur within the first 10 minutes of paclitaxel infusion, after the first or second dose of paclitaxel. A fatal reaction occurred in a patient who was not premedicated. In general, it is recommended that paclitaxel not be readministered to patients who have experienced a severe hypersensitivity reaction. However, in patients with objective tumor responses and without other options to paclitaxel therapy, re-treatment may be attempted with extreme caution and aggressive premedication by experienced practitioners.

Severe *neutropenia* (neutrophil count below 500 cells per cubic millimeter) is common but only infrequently persists for more than 7 days. The nadir of the neutrophil counts usually occurs at approximately day 11 of paclitaxel therapy; in general, neutropenia is rapidly reversible, with recovery by day 15 to 21. Cumulative neutropenia does not occur. The most common infections associated with neutropenia are urinary tract infections, upper respiratory infections, and sepsis. Fatalities have occurred from neutropenia-related sepsis.

In *thrombocytopenia*, the nadir of the platelet counts usually occurs at approximately day 8 or 9 of paclitaxel therapy. Platelet counts generally do not fall below 100,000 cells per cubic millimeter. Hemorrhagic episodes may also be disease-related.

Incidence less frequent
    ***Cardiovascular effects, including bradycardia; hypotension; or abnormal electrocardiogram (ECG)***—usually asymptomatic; ***elevated serum hepatic enzymes***—asymptomatic

    Note: *Cardiovascular effects* have also included more severe atrioventricular (AV) blocks, occasionally resulting in third-degree block requiring cardiac pacing. Atypical chest pains and a fatal myocardial infarction have also occurred, as well as asymptomatic bundle branch block and transient ventricular tachycardia, although the exact relationship to paclitaxel is unknown.

Incidence rare
    ***Extravasation, with phlebitis or cellulitis*** (pain or redness at site of injection); ***mucositis*** (sores in mouth and on lips)

    Note: Oropharyngeal *mucositis* is dose-related; it is infrequent or mild at usual recommended doses and usually resolves 5 to 7 days following treatment. However, esophageal and intestinal epithelial necrosis and ulceration have been reported.

**Those indicating need for medical attention only if they continue or are bothersome**
Incidence more frequent
    ***Arthralgias or myalgias*** (pain in joints or muscles, especially in arms or legs); ***diarrhea; nausea and vomiting; peripheral neuropathy, including mild paresthesia*** (numbness, burning, or tingling in hands or feet)

    Note: *Arthralgias or myalgias* usually begin 2 to 3 days after treatment and resolve within 5 days. Pain is usually relieved by analgesics, but occasionally may be severe enough to require narcotics.
    *Nausea and vomiting* are usually mild or moderate.
    Incidence and severity of *peripheral neuropathy* are dose-related; at usual doses, a sensory neuropathy in a glove-and-stocking distribution occurs. Only rarely is withdrawal of paclitaxel necessary. Symptoms usually appear after multiple doses and improve or resolve within several months after paclitaxel is discontinued. High doses (over 250 mg per square meter of body surface area) may cause dose-limiting motor and autonomic dysfunction, especially in patients with pre-existing neuropathies, beginning as early as 24 to 72 hours after treatment.

**Those not indicating need for medical attention**
Incidence more frequent
    ***Alopecia*** (loss of hair)

    Note: Complete loss of hair (including scalp hair, eyebrows, eyelashes, and pubic hair) occurs in almost all patients between days 14 and 21, but is reversible after therapy has ended.

## Patient Consultation

As an aid to patient consultation, refer to *Advice for the Patient, Paclitaxel (Systemic)*.
In providing consultation, consider emphasizing the following selected information (» = major clinical significance):

**Before using this medication**
» Conditions affecting use, especially:
    Sensitivity to paclitaxel
    Pregnancy—Use not recommended because of mutagenic, teratogenic, and carcinogenic potential; advisability of using contraception; telling physician immediately if pregnancy is suspected
    Breast-feeding—Not recommended because of risk of serious side effects
    Other medications, especially other bone marrow depressants, or other cytotoxic drugs or radiation therapy
    Other medical problems, especially cardiac conduction abnormalities, chickenpox, herpes zoster, or infection

**Proper use of this medication**
    Frequency of nausea and vomiting; importance of continuing medication despite stomach upset
» Proper dosing

**Precautions while using this medication**
» Importance of close monitoring by the physician
» Avoiding immunizations unless approved by physician; other persons in patient's household should avoid immunizations with oral poliovirus vaccine; avoiding other persons who have taken oral poliovirus vaccine or wearing a protective mask that covers nose and mouth

*Caution if bone marrow depression occurs*
» Avoiding exposure to persons with infections, especially during periods of low blood counts; checking with physician immediately if fever or chills, cough or hoarseness, lower back or side pain, or painful or difficult urination occurs
» Checking with physician immediately if unusual bleeding or bruising; black, tarry stools; blood in urine or stools; or pinpoint red spots on skin occur
    Caution in use of regular toothbrush, dental floss, or toothpick; physician, dentist, or nurse may suggest alternatives; checking with physician before having dental work done
    Not touching eyes or inside of nose unless hands are washed immediately before
    Using caution to avoid accidental cuts with use of sharp objects such as safety razor or fingernail or toenail cutters
    Avoiding contact sports or other situations where bruising or injury could occur

**Side/adverse effects**
    May cause adverse effects such as blood problems; importance of discussing possible effects with physician
    Signs of potential side effects, especially hypersensitivity reaction, leukopenia or neutropenia, thrombocytopenia, extravasation, and mucositis
    Asymptomatic side effects, including anemia, leukopenia or neutropenia, thrombocytopenia, cardiovascular effects, and elevated hepatic enzymes
    Physician or nurse can help in dealing with side effects
    Possibility of hair loss; normal hair growth should return after treatment has ended

## General Dosing Information

Patients receiving paclitaxel should be under supervision of a physician experienced in cancer chemotherapy.

A variety of dosage schedules and regimens of paclitaxel, alone or in combination with other antitumor agents, are used. The prescriber may consult the medical literature as well as the manufacturer's literature in choosing a specific dosage.

It is recommended that patients receiving paclitaxel be under continuous observation for at least the first 30 minutes of the infusion and at frequent intervals after that. Equipment and medications (including epinephrine and oxygen) necessary for treatment of a possible anaphylactic reaction should be immediately available during each administration of paclitaxel.

*Paclitaxel concentrate for injection must be diluted before administration by intravenous infusion.*

The needle should be carefully positioned in the vein to avoid extravasation and resulting phlebitis and cellulitis.

In order to prevent severe hypersensitivity reactions, it is recommended that all patients be premedicated with corticosteroids (such as dexamethasone), diphenhydramine, and histamine $H_2$-receptor antagonists (such as cimetidine or ranitidine) (see *Parenteral Dosage Forms* for specific dosing).

Mild hypersensitivity symptoms (flushing, skin reactions, dyspnea, hypotension, tachycardia) do not require interruption of paclitaxel therapy. However, severe reactions (hypotension requiring treatment, dyspnea requiring bronchodilators, angioedema, or generalized urticaria) require immediate withdrawal of paclitaxel and aggressive symptomatic therapy. It is generally recommended that paclitaxel administration not be repeated in patients who have experienced severe hypersensitivity reactions to the medication. However, in patients with objective tumor responses and without other options to paclitaxel therapy, re-treatment may be attempted with extreme caution and aggressive premedication by experienced practitioners.

If severe peripheral neuropathy occurs, it is recommended that subsequent dosage of paclitaxel be reduced by 20%.

If significant cardiac conduction abnormalities occur during administration of paclitaxel, appropriate therapy is recommended, along with continuous cardiac monitoring during subsequent paclitaxel administration.

If severe neutropenia (neutrophil counts of less than 500 cells per cubic millimeter for 7 days or more) occurs during a course of paclitaxel, it is recommended that the paclitaxel dose for subsequent courses be reduced by 20%.

Patients who develop leukopenia should be observed carefully for signs of infection. Antibiotic support may be required. In neutropenic patients who develop fever, broad-spectrum antibiotic coverage should be initiated empirically, pending bacterial cultures and appropriate diagnostic tests. Patients with advanced acquired immunodeficiency syndrome (AIDS) may require concomitant administration of a hematopoietic growth factor such as granulocyte colony stimulating factor (G-CSF).

Special precautions are recommended in patients who develop thrombocytopenia as a result of administration of paclitaxel. These may include extreme care in performing invasive procedures; regular inspection of intravenous sites, skin (including perirectal area), and mucous membrane surfaces for signs of bleeding or bruising; limiting frequency of venipuncture and avoiding intramuscular injections; testing urine, emesis, stool, and secretions for occult blood; care in use of regular toothbrushes, dental floss, toothpicks, safety razors, and fingernail and toenail cutters; avoiding constipation; and using caution to prevent falls and other injuries. Such patients should avoid alcohol and aspirin intake because of the risk of gastrointestinal bleeding. Platelet transfusions may be required.

**Safety considerations for handling this medication**
There is limited but increasing evidence and concern that personnel involved in preparation and administration of parenteral antineoplastics may be at some risk because of the potential mutagenicity, teratogenicity, and/or carcinogenicity of these agents, although the actual risk is unknown. USP advisory panels recommend cautious handling both in preparation and disposal of antineoplastic agents. Precautions that have been suggested include:
• Use of a biological containment cabinet during reconstitution and dilution of parenteral medications and wearing of disposable surgical gloves and masks.
• Use of proper technique to prevent contamination of the medication, work area, and operator during transfer between containers (including proper training of personnel in this technique).
• Cautious and proper disposal of needles, syringes, vials, ampuls, and unused medication.

A number of medical centers have developed detailed guidelines for handling of antineoplastic agents.

## Parenteral Dosage Forms

Note: Bracketed uses in the *Dosage Forms* section refer to categories of use and/or indications that are not included in U.S. product labeling.

### PACLITAXEL CONCENTRATE FOR INJECTION
**Usual adult dose**
Ovarian carcinoma—
   Intravenous (as a three- or twenty-four-hour infusion), 135 or 175 mg per square meter of body surface area, repeated every twenty-one days. (Canadian product labeling recommends a dose of 175 mg per square meter of body surface area as a three- or twenty-four-hour intravenous infusion, repeated every twenty-one days.)
Breast carcinoma—
   Intravenous (as a three- or twenty-four-hour infusion), 175 mg per square meter of body surface area, repeated every twenty-one days.
AIDS-associated Kaposi's sarcoma[1]—
   Intravenous (as a three- or twenty-four-hour infusion), 135 mg per square meter of body surface area, repeated every twenty-one days or
   Intravenous (as a three- or twenty-four-hour infusion), 100 mg per square meter of body surface area, repeated every fourteen days.
[Carcinoma, bladder][1] or
[Carcinoma, head and neck][1] or
[Carcinoma, cervical][1] or
[Carcinoma, esophageal][1] or
[Carcinoma, endometrial][1] or
[Carcinoma, lung, non–small cell][1] or
[Carcinoma, lung, small cell]—
   Consult medical literature and manufacturer's literature for specific dosage.

Note: To prevent severe hypersensitivity reactions, all patients should be premedicated with corticosteroids (e.g., dexamethasone 20 mg orally or intravenously [patients with solid tumors] or dexamethasone 10 mg orally [patients with AIDS-associated Kaposi's sarcoma] approximately twelve and six hours prior to paclitaxel administration); diphenhydramine (e.g., 50 mg intravenously, thirty to sixty minutes prior to paclitaxel) or its equivalent; and cimetidine (e.g., 300 mg intravenously, thirty to sixty minutes prior to paclitaxel), ranitidine (e.g., 50 mg intravenously, thirty to sixty minutes prior to paclitaxel), or famotidine (e.g., 20 mg intravenously, thirty to sixty minutes prior to paclitaxel).

Contact of paclitaxel with plasticized polyvinyl chloride (PVC) equipment or devices must be avoided because of the risk of patient exposure to the plasticizer DEHP (di-[2-ethylhexyl]phthalate), which may be leached from PVC infusion bags or sets. Paclitaxel solutions should be diluted and stored in glass or polypropylene bottles or in plastic bags (polypropylene, polyolefin) and administered through polyethylene-lined administration sets.

Paclitaxel intravenous infusion should be administered through an in-line filter with a microporous membrane not greater than 0.22 microns. Use of filter devices that incorporate short inlet and outlet PVC-coated tubing has not resulted in significant leaching of DEHP. Frequent changing of filters (e.g., every twelve hours) may be necessary because of clogging during the infusion.

**Usual pediatric dose**
Safety and efficacy in pediatric patients have not been established.

**Strength(s) usually available**
U.S.—
   6 mg per mL (5-, 16.7-, and 50-mL multidose vials) (Rx) [*Taxol* (polyoxyethylated castor oil 527 mg per mL; dehydrated alcohol USP 49.7% v/v)].
Canada—
   6 mg per mL (single-dose vials) (Rx) [*Taxol* (polyoxyethylated castor oil 527 mg per mL; dehydrated alcohol USP 49.7% v/v)].

**Packaging and storage**
Store between 2 and 25 °C (36 and 77 °F), unless otherwise specified by the manufacturer. Not adversely affected by freezing.

**Preparation of dosage form**
*Paclitaxel concentrate for injection must be diluted before administration.* Paclitaxel concentrate for injection is prepared for administration by intravenous infusion by diluting it to a concentration of 0.3 to 1.2 mg per mL in 5% dextrose injection, 0.9% sodium chloride injection, or 5% dextrose in Ringer's injection.

Note: Diluted solutions of paclitaxel may show haziness, which is attributed to the formulation vehicle.

**Stability**
Diluted solutions of paclitaxel are physically and chemically stable for up to 27 hours at ambient room temperature (approximately 25 °C [77 °F]) and room lighting conditions.

**Auxiliary labeling**
• Must be diluted prior to administration.

**Note**
If paclitaxel solution contacts the skin, the skin should be washed immediately and thoroughly with soap and water. If paclitaxel contacts mucous membranes, thorough flushing with water is recommended.

---
[1]Not included in Canadian product labeling.

Revised: 07/02/98
Interim revision: 07/14/98

# PALIVIZUMAB Systemic—INTRODUCTORY VERSION

VA CLASSIFICATION (Primary): IM500
Commonly used brand name(s): *Synagis*.
Note: For a listing of dosage forms and brand names by country availability, see *Dosage Forms* section(s).

## Category
Immunizing agent (passive).

## Indications

**Accepted**

Respiratory syncytial virus infection (prophylaxis)—Palivizumab is indicated for the prevention of serious lower respiratory tract infection caused by respiratory syncytial virus (RSV) in infants and children with bronchopulmonary dysplasia (BPD) and infants with a history of premature birth (gestation ≤ 35 weeks).

Note: The safety and efficacy of palivizumab have not been demonstrated for treatment of established RSV disease.

## Pharmacology/Pharmacokinetics

**Physicochemical characteristics**

Source—Palivizumab is a humanized monoclonal antibody (IgG1k) produced by recombinant DNA technology, directed to an epitope in the A antigenic site of the F protein of respiratory syncytial virus (RSV). It is a composite of 95% human and 5% murine antibody sequences. Palivizumab is supplied as a sterile lyophilized product.

Molecular weight—Approximately 148,000 Daltons.

**Mechanism of action/Effect**

Palivizumab exhibits neutralizing and fusion-inhibitory activity against RSV. These activities inhibit RSV replication in laboratory experiments. Although resistant RSV strains may be isolated in laboratory studies, a panel of 57 clinical RSV isolates were all neutralized by palivizumab.

Palivizumab serum concentrations of ≥ 40 mcg/mL have been shown to reduce pulmonary RSV replication in the cotton rat model of RSV infection by 100-fold.

The *in vivo* neutralizing activity of palivizumab was assessed in a randomized, placebo-controlled study of 35 pediatric patients tracheally intubated because of RSV disease. In these patients, palivizumab significantly reduced the quantity of RSV in the lower respiratory tract compared with that in control patients.

**Protective effect**

The safety and efficacy of palivizumab were assessed in a randomized, double blind, placebo controlled trial (IMpact-RSV Trial) of RSV disease prophylaxis among high-risk pediatric patients. This trial, conducted at 139 centers in the U.S., Canada, and the United Kingdom (U.K.), studied patients ≤ 24 months of age with bronchopulmonary dysplasia (BPD) and patients with premature birth (gestation ≤ 35 weeks) who were ≤ 6 months of age at study entry. Patients with uncorrected congenital heart disease were excluded from enrollment. In this trial, 500 patients were randomized to receive five monthly placebo injections and 1002 patients were randomized to receive five monthly injections of 15 mg per kg (mg/kg) of palivizumab. Subjects were randomized into the study for 28 days, and were followed for safety and efficacy for 150 days. Ninety-nine percent of all subjects completed the study and 93% received all five injections. The primary end point was the incidence of RSV hospitalization.

RSV hospitalization occurred among 53 of 500 (10.6%) patients in the placebo group and 48 of 1002 (4.8%) patients in the palivizumab group, a difference of 55%. The lower rate of RSV hospitalization was observed both in patients enrolled with a diagnosis of BPD and in patients enrolled with a diagnosis of prematurity without BPD. The lower rate of RSV hospitalization was observed throughout the course of the RSV season.

Among secondary end points, the incidence of intensive care unit (ICU) admission during hospitalization for RSV infection was lower among subjects receiving palivizumab (1.3%) than among those receiving placebo (3%), but there was no difference in the mean duration of ICU care. Overall, the data do not suggest that RSV illness was less severe among patients who received palivizumab and who required hospitalization due to RSV infection. Palivizumab did not alter the incidence and mean duration of hospitalization from non-RSV respiratory illness or the incidence of otitis media.

**Half-life**

Adults—18 days.
Children younger than 24 months of age—20 days.

## Precautions to Consider

**Carcinogenicity**

Carcinogenicity studies have not been performed with palivizumab.

**Tumorigenicity**

Tumorigenicity studies have not been performed with palivizumab.

**Pregnancy/Reproduction**

Fertility—Reproductive toxicity studies have not been performed with palivizumab.

Pregnancy—Studies have not been done in humans. However, palivizumab is not indicated for adult usage.

Studies have not been done in animals.

FDA Pregnancy Category C.

**Breast-feeding**

Problems in humans have not been documented.

**Pediatrics**

Safety and efficacy have been established in infants with bronchopulmonary dysplasia (BPD) and infants with a history of premature birth (gestation ≤ 35 weeks).

**Geriatrics**

No information is available on the relationship of age to the effects of palivizumab in geriatric patients. However, palivizumab is not indicated for adult usage.

**Medical considerations/Contraindications**

The medical considerations/contraindications included have been selected on the basis of their potential clinical significance (reasons given in parentheses where appropriate)—not necessarily inclusive (» = major clinical significance).

*Except under special circumstances, this medication should not be used when the following medical problem exists:*

» Hypersensitivity to palivizumab
(palivizumab should not be used in pediatric patients with a history of severe prior reaction to palivizumab or other components of the product)

## Side/Adverse Effects

Note: In the combined pediatric prophylaxis studies of pediatric patients with BPD or prematurity involving 420 subjects receiving placebo and 1168 subjects receiving palivizumab, the proportions of subjects in the placebo and palivizumab groups who experienced any adverse effect or any serious adverse effect were similar.

Most of the safety information was derived from the IMpact-RSV Trial. In this study, palivizumab was discontinued in five patients: two because of vomiting and diarrhea, one because of erythema and moderate induration at the site of the fourth injection, and two because of pre-existing medical conditions that required management (one with congenital anemia and one with pulmonary venous stenosis requiring cardiac surgery). Deaths in study patients occurred in 5 of 500 placebo recipients and 4 of 1002 palivizumab recipients. Sudden infant death syndrome (SIDS) was responsible for two of these deaths in the placebo group and one death in the palivizumab group.

The following side/adverse effects have been selected on the basis of their potential clinical significance (possible signs and symptoms in parentheses where appropriate)—not necessarily inclusive:

**Those indicating need for medical attention**
Incidence more frequent
*Otitis media* (ringing or buzzing in the ears); *rhinitis* (runny nose); *skin rash; upper respiratory tract infection* (difficulty in breathing)

## Overdose

No data from clinical studies are available on overdosage. No toxicity was observed in rabbits administered a single intramuscular or subcutaneous injection of palivizumab at a dose of 50 mg/kg. No data are available from human subjects who have received more than five monthly palivizumab doses during a single RSV season.

## Patient Consultation

As an aid to patient consultation, refer to *Advice for the Patient, Palivizumab (Systemic)—Introductory Version*.

In providing consultation, consider emphasizing the following selected information (» = major clinical significance):

**Before using this medication**
» Conditions affecting use, especially:
Other medical problems, especially hypersensitivity to palivizumab

**Proper use of this medication**
» Proper dosing

**Side/adverse effects**
Signs of potential side effects, especially otitis media, rhinitis, skin rash, and upper respiratory tract infection

## General Dosing Information

Although anaphylactoid reactions following the administration of palivizumab have not been observed, these reactions can occur following the administration of proteins. Therefore appropriate precautions should be taken prior to palivizumab injection to prevent allergic or other unwanted reactions. These precautions should include the ready availability of epinephrine 1:1000 and other appropriate agents used to control immediate allergic reactions.

The recommended dose of palivizumab is 15 mg/kg of body weight. Palivizumab should be administered intramuscularly, preferably in the anterolateral aspect of the thigh. Injection volumes over 1 mL should be given as a divided dose.

Patients, including those who develop a respiratory syncytial virus (RSV) infection, should receive monthly doses throughout the RSV season. The first dose should be administered prior to commencement of the RSV season. In the northern hemisphere, the RSV season typically commences in November and lasts through April, but it may begin earlier or persist later in certain communities.

**For treatment of adverse effects**
Recommended treatment consists of the following:
- For severe hypersensitivity or anaphylactic reaction—Administering epinephrine and providing supportive care as required.

## Parenteral Dosage Forms

### PALIVIZUMAB INJECTION

**Usual adult and adolescent dose**
Use is not recommended.

**Usual pediatric dose**
Respiratory syncytial virus infection (prophylaxis)—
Intramuscular, 15 mg per kg of body weight.

**Strength(s) usually available**
U.S.—
100 mg palivizumab per vial (Rx) [*Synagis* (47 mM histidine; 3 mM glycine; 5.6% mannitol)].

**Packaging and storage**
Store between 2 and 8 °C (36 and 46 °F), in its original container, unless otherwise specified by manufacturer.

**Preparation of dosage form**
To reconstitute, remove the tab portion of the vial cap and clean the rubber stopper with 70% ethanol or equivalent.
Slowly add 1 mL of sterile water for injection to a 100 mg vial. The vial should be gently swirled for 30 seconds to avoid foaming. **Do not shake vial.**
Reconstituted palivizumab should stand at room temperature for a minimum of 20 minutes until the solution clarifies.
Reconstituted palivizumab does not contain preservative and should be administered within 6 hours of reconstitution.

**Auxiliary labeling**
- Do not freeze.

Developed: 08/11/98

---

# PAMIDRONATE Systemic

VA CLASSIFICATION (Primary/Secondary): HS302/HS303
Commonly used brand name(s): *Aredia*.
Another commonly used name is APD.
Note: For a listing of dosage forms and brand names by country availability, see *Dosage Forms* section(s).

## Category

Bone resorption inhibitor; antihypercalcemic.

## Indications

**Accepted**

Hypercalcemia, associated with neoplasms (treatment)—Pamidronate disodium is indicated for the treatment of hypercalcemia of malignancy, with or without bone metastases, that is inadequately managed by oral hydration alone. It is used with saline hydration and may be used with loop diuretics.

Paget's disease of bone (treatment)—Pamidronate is indicated in the treatment of symptomatic Paget's disease (osteitis deformans), characterized by abnormal and accelerated bone metabolism in one or more bones. Signs and symptoms may include bone pain, deformity, and/or fractures; increased concentrations of serum alkaline phosphatase and/or urinary hydroxyproline; neurologic disorders associated with skull lesions and spinal deformities; and elevated cardiac output and other vascular disorders associated with increased vascularity of bones.

Metastases, osteolytic (treatment adjunct)[1]—Pamidronate is used in the treatment of osteolytic bone metastases sometimes found with breast cancer and myeloma.

**Unaccepted**

The safety and efficacy of pamidronate disodium in the treatment of hypercalcemia associated with hyperparathyroidism or other nontumor-related conditions have not been established.

---
[1]Not included in Canadian product labeling.

## Pharmacology/Pharmacokinetics

**Physicochemical characteristics**
Molecular weight—369.11.

**Mechanism of action/Effect**

Pamidronate inhibits bone resorption and is believed to accomplish this by several mechanisms. It adsorbs onto the surface of hydroxyapatite crystals in mineralized bone matrix, thus reducing the solubility of the mineralized matrix and rendering it more resistant to osteoclastic resorption. By impairing attachment of osteoclast precursors to mineralized matrix, pamidronate blocks their transformation into mature, functioning osteoclasts.

Hypercalcemia of malignancy—Bone resorption is increased in the presence of neoplastic tissue. Pamidronate inhibits abnormal bone resorption and reduces the flow of calcium from the resorbing bone into the blood, effectively decreasing total and ionized serum calcium. When kidney function is adequate for the fluid load, hydration with saline increases urine output and the use of loop diuretics increases the rate of calcium excretion.

Paget's disease—Pamidronate reduces the rate of bone turnover, by an initial blocking of bone resorption, resulting in decreases in serum alkaline phosphatase (reflecting decreased bone formation) and decreases in urinary hydroxyproline excretion (reflecting decreased bone resorption, i.e., breakdown of collagen).

Osteolytic metastases—Osteolytic metastases result from accelerated bone resorption induced by the tumor via an activation of osteoclasts. By inhibiting bone resorption, pamidronate may reduce morbidity of bone metastases from breast cancer and myeloma.

**Distribution**
In cancer patients, 45 to 53% of an intravenous dose of 60 mg infused over 24 hours is adsorbed to bone preferentially in areas of high turnover.

**Half-life**
Alpha—1.6 hours.
Beta—27.2 hours.

**Elimination**
51% of drug excreted unchanged in urine within 24 hours after an intravenous dose of 60 mg infused over 4 to 24 hours.

## Precautions to Consider

### Cross-sensitivity and/or related problems
Patients sensitive to any bisphosphonate may also be sensitive to pamidronate.

### Carcinogenicity
A 104-week carcinogenicity study with daily oral pamidronate administration in rats found a positive dose-response relationship for benign adrenal pheochromocytoma in males. The condition was observed in females, but was not statistically significant. Another 80-week study in mice found that daily oral pamidronate administration was not carcinogenic.

### Mutagenicity
Pamidronate was nonmutagenic in the Ames test, nucleus-anomaly test, sister-chromatid-exchange study, and point-mutation test.

### Pregnancy/Reproduction
Fertility—In rats, decreased fertility occurred in first-generation offspring of parents who had received 150 mg of oral pamidronate per kg of body weight (mg/kg). This occurred only when animals were mated with members of the same dose group.

Pregnancy—Adequate and well-controlled studies have not been done in pregnant women.

Adequate and well-controlled studies with intravenous pamidronate have not been done in animals. However, oral doses of 60 and 150 mg/kg of body weight a day increased the length of gestation and parturition in rats and increased pup mortality. Oral doses of 25 to 150 mg/kg a day during gestation failed to demonstrate any teratogenic, fetotoxic, or embryotoxic effects in rats or rabbits.

FDA Pregnancy Category C.

### Breast-feeding
It is not known if pamidronate is distributed into breast milk.

### Pediatrics
No information is available on the relationship of age to the effects of pamidronate in pediatric patients. Safety and efficacy have not been established.

### Geriatrics
Appropriate studies have not been performed in the geriatric population. However, elderly patients may be more prone to overhydration when treated with parenteral pamidronate in conjunction with hydration therapy. Careful monitoring of fluid and electrolyte status or infusing pamidronate in a smaller volume of fluid is recommended.

### Drug interactions and/or related problems
The following drug interactions and/or related problems have been selected on the basis of their potential clinical significance (possible mechanism in parentheses where appropriate)—not necessarily inclusive (» = major clinical significance):

Note: Combinations containing any of the following, depending on the amount present, may also interact with this medication.

» Calcium-containing preparations or
» Vitamin D, including calcifediol and calcitriol
 (concurrent use may antagonize the effects of pamidronate in the treatment of hypercalcemia)

### Medical considerations/Contraindications
The medical considerations/contraindications included have been selected on the basis of their potential clinical significance (reasons given in parentheses where appropriate)—not necessarily inclusive (» = major clinical significance).

*Risk-benefit should be considered when the following medical problems exist:*

» Cardiac failure
 (overhydration should be avoided when pamidronate is used in patients with cardiac failure; infusing pamidronate in a smaller volume of fluid is recommended)
» Renal function impairment when serum creatinine is 5 mg per dL or greater
 (pamidronate is excreted via the kidneys; use of pamidronate in patients with renal function impairment may require a lower dose and slower rate of infusion)

### Patient monitoring
The following may be especially important in patient monitoring (other tests may be warranted in some patients, depending on condition; » = major clinical significance):

Alkaline phosphatase concentrations serum
 (determinations recommended periodically during therapy for Paget's disease as a marker for disease activity)

Calcium, serum and
Magnesium, serum and
Phosphate, serum and
Potassium, serum
 (determinations recommended periodically during therapy; some clinicians recommend monitoring serum magnesium and potassium concentrations only with concurrent diuretic use; serum ionized calcium concentrations are preferable to determine free and bound calcium, but may not be available from a reliable lab)

Complete blood count with differential and
Hematocrit and
Hemoglobin
 (determinations recommended periodically during therapy, especially for patients who develop fever during pamidronate use; patients with pre-existing anemia, leukopenia, or thrombocytopenia should be carefully monitored for the first 2 weeks of therapy)

Creatinine, serum and
Renal function
 (determinations recommended periodically during therapy; if serum creatinine exceeds 5 mg per dL, risk-benefit of continued treatment or reduction of dosage should be considered)

## Side/Adverse Effects

Note: Fluid overload, hypokalemia, hypomagnesemia, and hypophosphatemia may occur due to concurrent fluid and diuretic use.

The following side/adverse effects have been selected on the basis of their potential clinical significance (possible signs and symptoms in parentheses where appropriate)—not necessarily inclusive:

### Those indicating need for medical attention
Incidence more frequent
 *Hypocalcemia* (abdominal cramps; confusion; muscle spasms); *leukopenia or lymphopenia* (fever, chills, or sore throat)

Note: Hypocalcemia occurs less frequently when doses of 60 mg, rather than 90 mg, are used.

### Those indicating need for medical attention only if they continue or are bothersome
Incidence more frequent—at higher doses
 *Fever, transient; nausea; pain and swelling at injection site*

Incidence less frequent
 *Muscle stiffness*

## Overdose

For specific information on the agents used in the management of pamidronate overdose, see:
• *Calcium Supplements (Systemic)* monograph.

For more information on the management of overdose or unintentional ingestion, **contact a Poison Control Center** (see *Poison Control Center Listing*).

### Specific treatment
Hypocalcemia resulting from overdose should be treated with intravenous calcium.

## Patient Consultation

As an aid to patient consultation, refer to *Advice for the Patient, Pamidronate (Systemic)*.

In providing consultation, consider emphasizing the following selected information (» = major clinical significance):

### Before using this medication
» Conditions affecting use, especially:
 Sensitivity to etidronate or pamidronate
 Use in the elderly—Elderly patients may be more prone to overhydration when treated with pamidronate in conjunction with hydration therapy
 Other medications, especially calcium- and vitamin D–containing preparations
 Other medical problems, especially cardiac failure and renal function impairment

### Proper use of this medication
» Proper dosing

### Precautions while using this medication
Importance of close monitoring by physician
*For patients with hypercalcemia*
 Possible need for calcium and vitamin D restriction, including calcifediol and calcitriol

**2222  Pamidronate (Systemic)**

### Side/adverse effects
Signs of potential adverse effects, especially hypocalcemia, leukopenia, and lymphopenia

## General Dosing Information
The U.S. product manufacturer recommends that the daily dose of pamidronate be reconstituted and diluted in 1000 mL of 0.45% or 0.9% sodium chloride or 5% dextrose injection. The Canadian products should be reconstituted and diluted in 0.9% sodium chloride or 5% dextrose injection to a maximum concentration of 30 mg of pamidronate per 250 mL of solution. The diluted dose should be administered over a period of 24 hours. However, some clinicians recommend that the daily dose be diluted in as little as 500 mL of fluid and administered over 4 to 24 hours.

Fluid overload, hypokalemia, hypomagnesemia, and hypophosphatemia may occur due to concurrent fluid and diuretic use.

## Parenteral Dosage Forms

### PAMIDRONATE DISODIUM FOR INJECTION

**Usual adult dose**
Hypercalcemia—
  Intravenous infusion, 60 mg administered over a period of four to twenty-four hours.
  Note: Patients with renal failure or mild hypercalcemia may receive 30 mg of pamidronate over a period of four to twenty-four hours.
  Patients with more severe hypercalcemia (corrected serum calcium greater than 13.5 mg per dL) may receive 90 mg of pamidronate over a period of twenty-four hours. Retreatment with pamidronate may be considered if hypercalcemia recurs; however, seven days should elapse before retreatment.
Paget's disease of bone (treatment)—
  Intravenous infusion, a total dose of 90 to 180 mg per treatment period, administered at a rate of 15 mg per hour. Dosage may be administered between the range of 30 mg per day on three consecutive days up to 30 mg once a week for six weeks. Alternatively, three doses of 60 mg may be administered every second week. The regimen may need to be repeated in some patients.
  Note: Some clinicians have found that a single dose of 60 to 90 mg is effective in some cases.

Osteolytic metastases (treatment adjunct)—
In breast cancer—
  Intravenous infusion, 90 mg over a period of two hours once every three or four weeks.
In myeloma—
  Intravenous infusion, 90 mg over a period of two to four hours once a month.

**Usual pediatric dose**
Safety and efficacy have not been established.

**Strength(s) usually available**
U.S.—
  30 mg per vial (Rx) [*Aredia*].
  60 mg per vial (Rx) [*Aredia*].
  90 mg per vial (Rx) [*Aredia*].
Canada—
  30 mg per vial (Rx) [*Aredia*].
  60 mg per vial (Rx) [*Aredia*].
  90 mg per vial (Rx) [*Aredia*].

**Packaging and storage**
Store below 40 °C (104 °F), preferably between 15 and 30 °C (59 and 86 °F), unless otherwise specified by manufacturer. Protect from freezing.

**Preparation of dosage form**
Each vial should be reconstituted with 10 mL of sterile water for injection. The daily dose should then be diluted in 1000 mL of 0.45% or 0.9% sodium chloride or 5% dextrose injection.

**Stability**
The diluted infusion solution is stable for twenty-four hours at room temperature.

**Incompatibilities**
Pamidronate should not be mixed with calcium-containing infusion solutions, such as Ringer's solution.

## Selected Bibliography
Fitton A, McTavish D. Pamidronate: a review of its pharmacological properties and therapeutic efficacy in resorptive bone diseases. Drugs 1991; 41[2]: 289-318.

Revised: 08/05/97

---

# PANCRELIPASE   Systemic

VA CLASSIFICATION (Primary): HS451/GA500

Commonly used brand name(s): *Cotazym; Cotazym E.C.S. 20; Cotazym E.C.S. 8; Cotazym-65 B; Cotazym-S; Enzymase-16; Ilozyme; Ku-Zyme HP; Pancoate; Pancrease; Pancrease MT 10; Pancrease MT 16; Pancrease MT 20; Pancrease MT 4; Panokase; Protilase; Ultrase MT 12; Ultrase MT 20; Viokase; Zymase.*

Another commonly used name is lipancreatin.

Note: For a listing of dosage forms and brand names by country availability, see *Dosage Forms* section(s).

## Category
Enzyme (pancreatic) replenisher; digestant; diagnostic aid (pancreatic function).

## Indications
Note: Bracketed information in the *Indications* section refers to uses that are not included in U.S. product labeling.

**Accepted**
Pancreatic insufficiency (treatment)—Pancrelipase is indicated as a pancreatic enzyme supplement and replacement therapy in conditions where pancreatic enzymes are either absent or deficient, resulting in inadequate fat and carbohydrate digestion. Such conditions are usually due to chronic pancreatitis, pancreatectomy, cystic fibrosis, gastrointestinal bypass surgery (Billroth II and total), and ductal obstruction from neoplasm (of the pancreas or common bile duct).

Steatorrhea (treatment)—Indicated for treating steatorrhea associated with the postgastrectomy syndrome and bowel resection, and for decreasing malabsorption in these patients.

[Pancreatic insufficiency (diagnosis)][1]—Pancrelipase is used as a presumptive test for pancreatic function, especially in pancreatic insufficiency due to chronic pancreatitis.

**Unaccepted**
Pancrelipase is not effective in the treatment of gastrointestinal disorders unrelated to pancreatic enzyme insufficiency.

[1]Not included in Canadian product labeling.

## Pharmacology/Pharmacokinetics

**Mechanism of action/Effect**
Proteolytic, amylolytic, and lipolytic enzymes in pancrelipase enhance the digestion of proteins, starches, and fats in the gastrointestinal tract, primarily in the duodenum and upper jejunum. The activity of pancrelipase is greater in neutral or faintly alkaline media. Pancrelipase has about 12 times the lipolytic activity, 4 times the proteolytic activity, and 4 times the amylolytic activity of pancreatin.

The efficacy of pancrelipase activity is dependent on how much of the enzyme reaches the small intestine. This can be influenced by the enzyme dose, the prevention of release of pancrelipase in the stomach, the microsphere size of the delayed-release product, and the pH at which the microsphere dissolves and releases the enzyme, with activity being greater at a neutral or alkaline pH.

## Precautions to Consider

**Cross-sensitivity and/or related problems**
Patients sensitive to pancreatin or pork protein may be sensitive to this medication also.

**Pregnancy/Reproduction**
Pregnancy—Studies have not been done in humans.
Studies have not been done in animals.

FDA Pregnancy Category C.

**Breast-feeding**
It is not known whether pancrelipase is distributed into breast milk. However, problems in humans have not been documented.

### Pediatrics
Appropriate studies on the relationship of age to the effects of pancrelipase have not been performed in children up to 6 months of age.

### Geriatrics
Appropriate studies on the relationship of age to the effects of pancrelipase have not been performed in the geriatric population. However, geriatrics-specific problems that would limit the usefulness of this medication in the elderly are not expected.

### Drug interactions and/or related problems
The following drug interactions and/or related problems have been selected on the basis of their potential clinical significance (possible mechanism in parentheses where appropriate)—not necessarily inclusive (» = major clinical significance):

Note: Combinations containing any of the following medications, depending on the amount present, may also interact with this medication.

Antacids, calcium carbonate– and/or magnesium hydroxide–containing
(concurrent administration of antacids may be required to prevent inactivation of pancrelipase [except the enteric-coated dosage forms] by gastric pepsin and acid pH; however, calcium carbonate– and/or magnesium hydroxide–containing antacids are not recommended since they may decrease the effectiveness of pancrelipase)

Iron, supplements or preparations
(iron absorption may be decreased when used concurrently with pancrelipase)

### Laboratory value alterations
The following have been selected on the basis of their potential clinical significance (possible effect in parentheses where appropriate)—not necessarily inclusive (» = major clinical significance):

With physiology/laboratory test values
Uric acid
(blood and urine concentrations may be increased; ribonuclease present in pancreatic extracts catalyzes the formation of purine precursors of uric acid, thus increasing the risk of hyperuricosuria, especially with large doses of the purine-rich older formulations of pancrelipase)

### Medical considerations/Contraindications
The medical considerations/contraindications included have been selected on the basis of their potential clinical significance (reasons given in parentheses where appropriate)—not necessarily inclusive (» = major clinical significance).

*Except under special circumstances, this medication should not be used if the following medical problems exist:*

» Pancreatitis, acute
» Sensitivity to pork protein, pancrelipase, or pancreatin

## Side/Adverse Effects
The following side/adverse effects have been selected on the basis of their potential clinical significance (possible signs and symptoms in parentheses where appropriate)—not necessarily inclusive:

### Those indicating need for medical attention
Incidence rare
*Allergic reaction* (skin rash or hives); *irritation of the mouth*—induced by enzymatic digestion of mucous membranes when tablet dosage form is retained in mouth; *sensitization* (shortness of breath; stuffy nose; troubled breathing; wheezing; tightness in chest)—induced by repeated inadvertent inhalation of powder dosage form or the powder from opened capsules

With high doses
*Gastrointestinal effects, specifically diarrhea; intestinal obstruction; nausea; stomach cramps or pain; hyperuricemia or hyperuricosuria* (blood in urine; joint pain; swelling of feet or lower legs)—more frequent with extremely high doses of the purine-rich older formulations of pancrelipase

Note: There have been reports of gastrointestinal stricture requiring surgery in cystic fibrosis patients receiving high potency pancrelipase for 12 months or longer. The pathogenesis is unknown at this time. The U. S. Food and Drug Administration has issued a voluntary recall of pancrelipase products that contain greater than 20,000 Units of lipase.

## Patient Consultation
As an aid to patient consultation, refer to *Advice for the Patient, Pancrelipase (Systemic)*.

In providing consultation, consider emphasizing the following selected information (» = major clinical significance):

### Before using this medication
» Conditions affecting use, especially:
Sensitivity to pork protein, pancrelipase, or pancreatin
Other medical problems, especially acute pancreatitis

### Proper use of this medication
Taking dose before or with meals for maximum effectiveness
» Importance of following diet ordered by physician
» Not chewing tablets; swallowing them quickly with liquid to lessen potential for mouth irritation
Not chewing or crushing capsules containing enteric-coated spheres
» Proper dosing
Missed dose: Taking as soon as possible; not taking if almost time for next dose; not doubling doses
» Proper storage

### Precautions while using this medication
Possible concurrent use with antacids that contain calcium carbonate and/or magnesium hydroxide
Not changing brands or dosage forms of pancrelipase without checking with physician
Possible sensitization resulting from repeated inhalation of powder, either from opened capsules or from powder dosage form

### Side/adverse effects
Signs of potential side effects, especially allergic reaction, hyperuricemia or hyperuricosuria (with extremely high doses); gastrointestinal effects; irritation of mucous membranes; and respiratory problems (with inhalation of powder)

## General Dosing Information
The destruction of pancrelipase's enzymes by gastric pepsin or their inactivation by acid pH may be prevented by the use of enteric-coated dosage forms, particularly the enteric-coated spheres. Or, if dosage forms of pancrelipase which are not enteric-coated are used, the gastric and duodenal pH may be raised instead by the concurrent administration of sodium bicarbonate, aluminum hydroxide, histamine H$_2$-receptor antagonists, misoprostol, or omeprazole (also, antacid, H$_2$-receptor antagonist, misoprostol, or omeprazole administration may be necessary in patients with deficient pancreatic bicarbonate secretion for the control of steatorrhea). An H$_2$-receptor antagonist administered with meals may be preferred instead of antacids, especially in patients with high rates of acid secretion.

Dosage should be individualized and determined by the degree of maldigestion and malabsorption, the fat content of the diet, and the enzyme activity of each preparation rather than by the weight of the extract. Ideally, a starting dose of 8,000 to 10,000 Units of lipase should be given with each meal.

To avoid irritation of the mouth, lips, and tongue, the tablets should not be chewed. Instead, the tablets should be swallowed quickly, preferably with some liquid, since proteolytic enzymes (trypsin and chymotrypsin) present in pancrelipase, when retained in the mouth may begin to digest the mucous membranes and cause ulcerations.

Retention of the tablet dosage form in the esophagus may occur in some patients with esophageal abnormalities or in patients taking the tablet in a recumbent position. To decrease the likelihood of mucous membrane digestion, 1 or 2 mouthfuls of solid food should be swallowed after each dose.

### Diet/Nutrition
Pancrelipase should preferably be taken before or with meals for maximum effectiveness.

In pancreatic insufficiency, a high-calorie diet which is high in protein and low in fat is recommended. In severe cases, higher doses of pancrelipase and dietary adjustment may be necessary. Some clinicians recommend that cystic fibrosis patients consume a liberal fat diet along with an increase in pancrelipase dosage to ensure adequate energy intake.

Capsule dosage forms may be opened and sprinkled on food for administration to young children. However, capsules containing the enteric-coated spheres should be taken with liquids or small amounts of soft foods (e.g., applesauce, gelatin) that do not require chewing.

### Bioequivalence information
The microsphere size of the delayed-release product, among other factors, determines how much of the enzyme reaches the small intestine. It has been found that some delayed-release pancrelipase products provide higher levels of enzyme activity than labeled. Since substitution of one manufacturer's delayed-release product for another may sometimes be accompanied by therapeutic failure, caution should be exercised in substituting.

# Oral Dosage Forms

## PANCRELIPASE CAPSULES USP

### Usual adult and adolescent dose
Enzyme (pancreatic) replenisher and
Digestant—
  Oral, 1 to 3 capsules before or with meals and snacks, the dosage being adjusted as needed and tolerated.

### Usual pediatric dose
Enzyme (pancreatic) replenisher and
Digestant—
  Oral, contents of 1 to 3 capsules with meals, the dosage being adjusted as needed and tolerated.

### Usual geriatric dose
See *Usual adult and adolescent dose*.

### Strength(s) usually available
U.S.—
  8000 USP Units of lipase, 30,000 USP Units of protease, and 30,000 USP Units of amylase, per capsule (Rx) [*Cotazym* (calcium carbonate 25 mg); *Ku-Zyme HP*].

Canada—
  8000 USP Units of lipase, 30,000 USP Units of protease, and 30,000 USP Units of amylase, per capsule (Rx) [*Cotazym; Cotazym-65 B* (bile salts 65 mg; cellulase 2 mg)].

### Packaging and storage
Store below 25 °C (77 °F), in a tight container, unless otherwise specified by manufacturer. Store with a desiccant.

### Auxiliary labeling
• Take before or with meals.
• If capsules are opened, do not inhale powder.

## PANCRELIPASE DELAYED-RELEASE CAPSULES

Note: Substitution of one manufacturer's delayed-release product for another has resulted in therapeutic failure.

### Usual adult and adolescent dose
Enzyme (pancreatic) replenisher and
Digestant—
  Oral, 1 or 2 capsules before or with meals and snacks, the dosage being adjusted as needed and tolerated.

### Usual pediatric dose
Enzyme (pancreatic) replenisher and
Digestant—
  Oral, contents of 1 or 2 capsules with meals, the dosage being adjusted as needed and tolerated.

Note: Contents of capsules containing the enteric-coated spheres should be taken with liquids or a small amount of soft foods that do not require chewing.

### Usual geriatric dose
See *Usual adult and adolescent dose*.

### Strength(s) usually available
U.S.—
  4000 USP Units of lipase, 12,000 USP Units of protease, and 12,000 USP Units of amylase, per capsule (Rx) [*Pancrease MT 4*].
  4000 USP Units of lipase, 25,000 USP Units of protease, and 20,000 USP Units of amylase, per capsule (Rx) [*Pancoate; Pancrease; Protilase;* GENERIC].
  5000 USP Units of lipase, 20,000 USP Units of protease, and 20,000 USP Units of amylase, per capsule (Rx) [*Cotazym-S*].
  10,000 USP Units of lipase, 30,000 USP Units of protease, and 30,000 USP Units of amylase, per capsule (Rx) [*Pancrease MT 10*].
  12,000 USP Units of lipase, 24,000 USP Units of protease, and 24,000 USP Units of amylase, per capsule (Rx) [*Zymase*].
  12,000 USP Units of lipase; 39,000 USP Units of protease, and 39,000 USP Units of amylase, per capsule (Rx) [*Ultrase MT 12*].
  16,000 USP Units of lipase, 48,000 USP Units of protease, and 48,000 USP Units of amylase, per capsule (Rx) [*Enzymase-16; Pancrease MT 16;* GENERIC].
  20,000 USP Units of lipase, 44,000 USP Units of protease, and 56,000 USP Units of amylase, per capsule (Rx) [*Pancrease MT 20*].
  20,000 USP Units of lipase, 65,000 USP Units of protease, and 65,000 USP Units of amylase, per capsule (Rx) [*Ultrase MT 20*].

Canada—
  4000 USP Units of lipase, 12,000 USP Units of protease, and 12,000 USP Units of amylase, per capsule (Rx) [*Pancrease MT 4*].
  4000 USP Units of lipase, 25,000 USP Units of protease, and 20,000 USP Units of amylase, per capsule (Rx) [*Pancrease*].
  8000 USP Units of lipase, 30,000 USP Units of protease, and 30,000 USP Units of amylase, per capsule (Rx) [*Cotazym E.C.S. 8*].
  10,000 USP Units of lipase, 30,000 USP Units of protease, and 30,000 USP Units of amylase, per capsule (Rx) [*Pancrease MT 10*].
  16,000 USP Units of lipase, 48,000 USP Units of protease, and 48,000 USP Units of amylase, per capsule (Rx) [*Pancrease MT 16*].
  20,000 USP Units of lipase, 55,000 USP Units of protease, and 55,000 USP Units of amylase, per capsule (Rx) [*Cotazym E.C.S. 20*].

### Packaging and storage
Store below 25 °C (77 °F), in a tight container, unless otherwise specified by manufacturer. Store with a desiccant.

### Auxiliary labeling
• Take before or with meals.
• Do not chew or crush (for capsules containing the enteric-coated spheres only).

## PANCRELIPASE POWDER

### Usual adult and adolescent dose
Enzyme (pancreatic) replenisher and
Digestant—
  Oral, 0.7 gram with meals and snacks, the dosage being adjusted as needed and tolerated.

### Usual pediatric dose
Enzyme (pancreatic) replenisher and
Digestant—
  Oral, 0.7 gram with meals, the dosage being adjusted as needed and tolerated.

### Usual geriatric dose
See *Usual adult and adolescent dose*.

### Strength(s) usually available
U.S.—
  16,800 USP Units of lipase, 70,000 USP Units of protease, and 70,000 USP Units of amylase, per 0.7 gram (Rx) [*Viokase*].

Canada—
  Not commercially available.

### Packaging and storage
Store below 25 °C (77 °F), unless otherwise specified by manufacturer.

### Auxiliary labeling
• Take with meals.
• Do not inhale.

## PANCRELIPASE TABLETS USP

### Usual adult and adolescent dose
Enzyme (pancreatic) replenisher and
Digestant—
  Oral, 1 to 3 tablets before or with meals and snacks, the dosage being adjusted as needed and tolerated.

### Usual pediatric dose
Enzyme (pancreatic) replenisher and
Digestant—
  Oral, 1 or 2 tablets with meals.

### Usual geriatric dose
See *Usual adult and adolescent dose*.

### Strength(s) usually available
U.S.—
  8000 USP Units of lipase, 30,000 USP Units of protease, and 30,000 USP Units of amylase, per tablet (Rx) [*Panokase; Viokase*].
  11,000 USP Units of lipase, 30,000 USP Units of protease, and 30,000 USP Units of amylase, per tablet (Rx) [*Ilozyme*].

Canada—
  Not commercially available.

### Packaging and storage
Store below 25 °C (77 °F), in a tight container, unless otherwise specified by manufacturer. Store with a desiccant.

### Auxiliary labeling
• Take before or with meals.
• Do not chew.

Revised: 02/13/92
Interim revision: 08/01/94; 08/01/95

---

**PANCURONIUM**—See *Neuromuscular Blocking Agents (Systemic)*

**PANTOTHENIC ACID**—The *Pantothenic Acid (Systemic)* monograph is not included in this published version of the USP DI database. Copies of the monograph are available on request from Micromedex, Inc. - Reprint Requests, 6200 S. Syracuse Way, Suite 300, Englewood, CO 80111; telephone (303) 486-6400; telefax (303) 486-6464; Email: USPDI@MDX.COM.

**PAPAVERINE**—The *Papaverine (Intracavernosal)* monograph is not included in this published version of the USP DI database. Copies of the monograph are available on request from Micromedex, Inc. - Reprint Requests, 6200 S. Syracuse Way, Suite 300, Englewood, CO 80111; telephone (303) 486-6400; telefax (303) 486-6464; Email: USPDI@MDX.COM.

**PAPAVERINE**—The *Papaverine (Systemic)* monograph is not included in this published version of the USP DI database. Copies of the monograph are available on request from Micromedex, Inc. - Reprint Requests, 6200 S. Syracuse Way, Suite 300, Englewood, CO 80111; telephone (303) 486-6400; telefax (303) 486-6464; Email: USPDI@MDX.COM.

**PARALDEHYDE**—The *Paraldehyde (Systemic)* monograph is not included in this published version of the USP DI database. Copies of the monograph are available on request from Micromedex, Inc. - Reprint Requests, 6200 S. Syracuse Way, Suite 300, Englewood, CO 80111; telephone (303) 486-6400; telefax (303) 486-6464; Email: USPDI@MDX.COM.

**PARAMETHASONE**—See *Corticosteroids—Glucocorticoid Effects (Systemic)*

**PAREGORIC**—The *Paregoric (Systemic)* monograph is not included in this published version of the USP DI database. Copies of the monograph are available on request from Micromedex, Inc. - Reprint Requests, 6200 S. Syracuse Way, Suite 300, Englewood, CO 80111; telephone (303) 486-6400; telefax (303) 486-6464; Email: USPDI@MDX.COM.

# PAROXETINE Systemic

VA CLASSIFICATION (Primary/Secondary): CN603/CN900
Commonly used brand name(s): *Paxil*.
Note: For a listing of dosage forms and brand names by country availability, see *Dosage Forms* section(s).

## Category
Antidepressant; antiobsessional agent; antipanic agent.

## Indications

### Accepted
Depressive disorder, major (treatment)—Paroxetine is indicated for the treatment of major depressive disorder. Treatment of acute depressive episodes typically requires 6 to 12 months of antidepressant therapy. Patients with recurrent or chronic depression may require long-term treatment. Paroxetine has shown effective maintenance of antidepressant response for up to 52 weeks of treatment in a placebo-controlled trial.

Obsessive-compulsive disorder (treatment)—Paroxetine is indicated for the treatment of obsessions and compulsions in patients with obsessive-compulsive disorder. Paroxetine has shown effective relapse prevention for up to 6 months of treatment in a placebo-controlled trial.

Panic disorder (treatment)—Paroxetine is indicated for the treatment of panic disorder, with or without agoraphobia.

## Pharmacology/Pharmacokinetics
Note: A wide range of intersubject variability has been observed in the pharmacokinetic parameters of paroxetine.

### Physicochemical characteristics
Chemical group—Phenylpiperidine. Chemically unrelated to other selective serotonin reuptake inhibitors (SSRIs), or to tricyclic, tetracyclic, or any other currently available antidepressants.
Molecular weight—
  Paroxetine hydrochloride: 374.8.
  Paroxetine base: 329.37.
Solubility—5.4 mg of paroxetine hydrochloride per mL water.

### Mechanism of action/Effect
Paroxetine potently and selectively inhibits neuronal serotonin reuptake through antagonism of the serotonin transporter. Its antidepressant, antiobsessional, and antipanic activities are presumed to be linked to potentiation of serotonergic activity in the central nervous system (CNS). Paroxetine inhibits the active membrane transport mechanism for reuptake of serotonin, which increases concentration of the neurotransmitter at the synaptic cleft and prolongs its activity at synaptic receptor sites. Inhibition of serotonin reuptake also enhances serotonergic neurotransmission by reducing turnover of the neurotransmitter via a negative feedback mechanism. Paroxetine inhibits serotonin reuptake *in vitro* more selectively and more potently than do fluoxetine, sertraline, fluvoxamine, zimeldine, or clomipramine. Paroxetine very weakly inhibits reuptake of norepinephrine and dopamine.

Receptor binding studies have demonstrated that paroxetine does not interact directly with central neurotransmitter receptor sites, including alpha$_1$-, alpha$_2$-, or beta-adrenoreceptors, and dopamine D$_2$, serotonin (5-hydroxytryptamine) 5HT$_1$ or 5HT$_2$, or histamine H$_1$ receptors. Paroxetine has very weak affinity for the muscarinic-cholinergic receptor, and does not inhibit monoamine oxidase.

### Other actions/effects
Paroxetine potently inhibits the P450 2D6 (CYP2D6) isoenzyme of the hepatic cytochrome P450 system. *In vitro* studies indicate that paroxetine is a very weak inhibitor of CYP3A4. This inhibition of isoenzyme CYP3A4 is not likely to be of clinical significance, and an *in vivo* study revealed no effect of paroxetine on the pharmacokinetics of terfenadine, a CYP3A4 substrate.

Paroxetine inhibits serotonin (5-HT) uptake by platelets as well as neurons. At therapeutic doses, paroxetine does not significantly impair psychomotor function and exerts no significant effects on heart rate, blood pressure, or electrocardiogram (ECG) parameters. Also, paroxetine does not appear to induce epileptiform activity or to lower the seizure threshold.

### Absorption
Paroxetine is well absorbed from both the suspension and tablet forms, with bioavailability for both dosage forms ranging from 50 to 100%. Bioavailability increases after multiple dosing due to partial saturation of first-pass metabolism. Absorption is not influenced by the presence of food, milk, or antacids.

### Distribution
Paroxetine is extensively distributed into tissues, with only 1% remaining in the systemic circulation. The volume of distribution (Vol$_D$) is large due to the lipophilic nature of paroxetine; values ranging from 3 to 28 L per kg of body weight (L/kg) have been reported. Paroxetine is distributed into breast milk in concentrations similar to plasma concentrations.

### Protein binding
Very high (95%). *In vitro*, protein binding of phenytoin and warfarin are not altered by paroxetine.

### Biotransformation
Paroxetine undergoes extensive first-pass metabolism in the liver. At least 85% of a paroxetine dose is oxidized to a catechol intermediate that undergoes subsequent methylation and conjugation to clinically inactive glucuronide and sulfate metabolites.

Metabolism is accomplished in part by cytochrome P450 2D6 (CYP2D6); saturation of this enzyme at clinical doses appears to account for the nonlinear kinetics observed with increasing dose and duration of paroxetine treatment. The elderly may be more susceptible to the saturation of hepatic metabolic capacity, leading to conversion to nonlinear kinetics, which results in increased plasma concentrations of paroxetine at lower-than-usual doses.

**Half-life**
Elimination—
About 24 hours (range, 3 to 65 hours) in healthy adults. Due to partially saturable kinetics, the elimination half-life may be increased in the elderly. However, there is wide intersubject variability. Half-life is prolonged in patients with severe hepatic or renal function impairment.

**Onset of action**
Antidepressant effects—Within 1 to 4 weeks, with improvement in sleep parameters usually occurring in 1 to 2 weeks.
Antiobsessional and antipanic effects—May require several weeks to occur.

**Time to peak concentration**
Range, 2 to 8 hours.

**Time to steady-state serum concentration**
Usually achieved in 7 to 14 days in most patients, although it may take considerably longer in some patients.

**Concentration**
Peak plasma—Following dosing at 30 mg a day for 30 days in healthy volunteers, peak paroxetine plasma concentrations ($C_{max}$) ranged from 8.6 to 105 mcg/L (0.02 to 0.28 micromoles per L). Peak plasma concentrations are subject to wide interpatient variability because of first-pass metabolism, and increase in a nonlinear fashion with increasing dose because of saturation of CYP2D6.
Steady-state serum—In nonelderly depressed patients receiving long-term dosing of 20 to 50 mg of paroxetine a day, mean steady-state serum concentrations ranged from 48.7 to 117 mcg/L (0.13 to 0.31 micromoles per L). In 15 normal male subjects, steady-state area under the plasma concentration–time curve (AUC) was about eight times greater than was predicted from single-dose kinetics. Nonlinearity is thought to be the result of increased systemic availability due to reduced first-pass metabolism, rather than a decrease in systemic clearance. There appears to be no correlation between paroxetine plasma concentrations and clinical efficacy or incidence of adverse effects.
Mean plasma concentrations in patients with creatinine clearances below 30 mL per minute (mL/min) were fourfold greater than those in healthy volunteers. Mean plasma concentrations in patients with creatinine clearances of 30 to 60 mL/min and in patients with hepatic function impairment were twofold greater.

**Elimination**
Renal—
In the 10-day period following administration of 30 mg of a paroxetine solution, approximately 64% of the dose was excreted in the urine, of which 2% or less was the parent compound.
Fecal—
In the 10-day period following administration of 30 mg of a paroxetine solution, about 36% of the dose was excreted in the feces, of which unchanged paroxetine comprised less than 1%.

## Precautions to Consider

**Carcinogenicity**
In 2-year carcinogenicity studies, a significantly greater number of male rats in the group receiving 3.9 times the maximum recommended human dose (MRHD) of 50 mg for depression (3.2 times the MRHD of 60 mg for obsessive-compulsive disorder and panic disorder) on a mg per square meter of body surface area (mg/m²) basis exhibited reticulum cell sarcomas than did rats receiving lower doses. Also, there was a significantly increased linear trend across dose groups for occurrence of lymphoreticular tumors in male rats. Female rats were unaffected. In mice receiving up to 2.4 times the MRHD for depression (2 times the MRHD for obsessive-compulsive disorder and panic disorder) on a mg/m² basis, there was a dose-related increase in the number of tumors in mice, but no drug-related increase in the number of mice with tumors. The relevance of these findings to humans is not known.

**Mutagenicity**
Paroxetine demonstrated no genotoxic effects in a battery of five *in vitro* and two *in vivo* assays, including the bacterial mutation assay, mouse lymphoma mutation assay, unscheduled DNA synthesis assay, tests for cytogenetic aberrations *in vivo* in mouse bone marrow and *in vitro* in human lymphocytes, and a dominant lethal test in rats.

**Pregnancy/Reproduction**
Fertility—Rats administered paroxetine at doses 2.9 times the MRHD for depression (2.4 times the MRHD for obsessive-compulsive disorder and panic disorder) on a mg/m² basis had reduced pregnancy rates.
Irreversible reproductive tract lesions occurred in male rats in toxicity studies of 2 to 52 weeks duration. These lesions comprised atrophic changes in the seminiferous tubules of the testes with arrested spermatogenesis at doses 4.9 times the MRHD for depression (4.1 times the MRHD for obsessive-compulsive disorder and panic disorder) on a mg/m² basis, and vacuolation of the epididymal tubular epithelium at doses 9.8 times the MRHD for depression (8.2 times the MRHD for obsessive-compulsive disorder and panic disorder) on a mg/m² basis.

Pregnancy—A prospective study compared birth outcomes of 267 pregnancies that were exposed to the selective serotonin reuptake inhibitors (SSRIs) sertraline (50 mg/day, range 25 to 250 mg/day), paroxetine (30 mg/day, range 10 to 60 mg/day), or fluvoxamine (50 mg/day, range 25 to 200 mg/day) with those of 267 pregnancies that were exposed to medications or medical treatments known to be nonteratogenic. Paroxetine was taken at some time during 97 of the SSRI-exposed pregnancies. Based on interviews with the mothers 6 to 9 months after the births, no differences in the infants' gestational ages or mean birth weights, or in the rates of major malformations, spontaneous or elective abortions, or stillbirths were found between the two groups. Also, no differences were found between infants exposed to SSRIs during the first trimester only and infants exposed to SSRIs throughout gestation. The behavioral effects of *in utero* paroxetine exposure were not examined.

No teratogenic effects or selective toxicity to the fetus were demonstrated in studies in rats and rabbits receiving 9.7 and 2.2 times, respectively, the MRHD for depression on a mg/m² basis. However, increased pup death during the first week postpartum occurred in rats given doses 0.19 times the MRHD for depression on a mg/m² basis during the last trimester and continuing throughout lactation.

FDA Pregnancy Category C.

Labor and delivery—The effect of paroxetine on labor and delivery is not known.

**Breast-feeding**
Paroxetine is distributed into breast milk in concentrations similar to those found in plasma.

**Pediatrics**
No information is available on the relationship of age to the effects of paroxetine in pediatric patients. Safety and efficacy have not been established.

**Geriatrics**
No geriatrics-specific problems have been documented to date in studies that included geriatric patients. However, paroxetine clearance is reduced in the elderly. Also, elderly patients are more likely to have age-related renal function impairment. Reduced paroxetine dosage is recommended for elderly patients.

**Pharmacogenetics**
Approximately 2 to 10% of the adult population are slow metabolizers of CYP2D6 substrates. These patients have a reduced ability to metabolize paroxetine and may be more likely to experience adverse effects. Paroxetine dosage reductions may be necessary in these patients.

**Drug interactions and/or related problems**
The following drug interactions and/or related problems have been selected on the basis of their potential clinical significance (possible mechanism in parentheses where appropriate)—not necessarily inclusive (» = major clinical significance):

Note: Paroxetine is a potent inhibitor of cytochrome P450 2D6 (CYP2D6), but a very weak inhibitor of CYP3A4. Caution should be exercised when paroxetine is coadministered with medications that are metabolized by CYP2D6, such as tricyclic antidepressants, phenothiazines (e.g., thioridazine), or type IC antiarrhythmics (e.g., encainide, flecainide, or propafenone), or medications that inhibit CYP2D6, such as quinidine. Dosage reductions of paroxetine and/or the other medication may be necessary. Interactions with medications metabolized by the CYP3A4 isoenzyme are unlikely.

At steady state with paroxetine, the CYP2D6 isoenzyme is saturated, and paroxetine metabolism is governed by other hepatic P450 enzymes, which appear to be nonsaturable. Interactions with hepatic enzyme inducers, hepatic enzyme inhibitors, and other medications that are metabolized by the hepatic P450 enzyme system, other than those listed below, have not been studied and the possibility of a significant interaction should be considered.

*In vitro* studies have shown little chance of paroxetine being displaced by other highly protein-bound agents; also, paroxetine is unlikely to displace other highly protein-bound medications. *In vivo*, however, the potential exists for displacement of one highly protein-bound medication by another; increased free concentrations of the displaced agent could result, increasing the likelihood of adverse effects.

Combinations containing any of the following medications, depending on the amount present, may also interact with this medication.

Alcohol
(although paroxetine has not been shown to alter alcohol metabolism and does not appear to potentiate cognitive and psychomotor effects of alcohol in normal subjects, concomitant use is not recommended)

» Antidepressants, tricyclic (TCAs)
(paroxetine may inhibit TCA metabolism, leading to increased TCA plasma concentrations, and possibly causing adverse effects; maximum plasma concentration, area under the plasma concentration–time curve, and elimination half-life of a single 100-mg dose of desipramine were increased twofold, fivefold, and threefold, respectively, in subjects at steady-state receiving 20 mg per day of paroxetine; plasma concentration of the TCA may need to be monitored, and dosage reduction of either the TCA or paroxetine may be required)

» Astemizole
(because paroxetine inhibits cytochrome P450 enzymes and may increase plasma concentrations of astemizole, thereby increasing the risk of cardiac arrhythmias, concurrent use is not recommended)

Cimetidine
(in one study, steady-state plasma concentrations of paroxetine were increased by approximately 50% during concurrent administration of cimetidine; although the clinical significance of this interaction has not been definitively established, initial dosage reductions are not thought to be necessary, but subsequent dose titration should be based on clinical effects)

Digoxin
(mean digoxin area under the plasma concentration–time curve [AUC] decreased 15% in the presence of paroxetine; since there is little clinical experience with this combination, concurrent administration should be undertaken with caution)

» Moclobemide
(because of the potentially fatal effects of concomitant use of paroxetine and nonselective, irreversible monoamine oxidase [MAO] inhibitors, and the increased risk of development of the serotonin syndrome with concomitant use of paroxetine and the selective, reversible MAO-A inhibitor moclobemide, concurrent use is not recommended; allowing 3 to 7 days to elapse between discontinuing moclobemide and initiating paroxetine therapy, and allowing 2 weeks to elapse between discontinuing paroxetine and initiating moclobemide therapy is advised)

» Monoamine oxidase (MAO) inhibitors, including furazolidone, procarbazine, and selegiline
(concurrent use of MAO inhibitors with paroxetine may result in potentially fatal reactions, which may include confusion, agitation, restlessness, and gastrointestinal symptoms, or possibly hyperpyretic episodes, severe convulsions, hypertensive crises, or the serotonin syndrome; concurrent use is **contraindicated**, and at least 14 days should elapse between discontinuation of one medication and initiation of the other)

Phenobarbital or
Primidone
(primidone is partially metabolized to phenobarbital, which induces many cytochrome P450 enzymes; administration of either of these agents concomitantly with paroxetine may reduce the systemic availability of paroxetine; no initial dosage adjustments are recommended, but subsequent titration should be based on clinical effects)

Phenytoin
(concomitant administration with paroxetine may decrease the systemic availability of either agent; no initial dosage adjustments are recommended, but subsequent titration should be based on clinical effects)

Procyclidine
(concurrent use may increase the systemic availability of procyclidine; if anticholinergic effects occur, the dosage of procyclidine should be reduced)

» Serotonergics or other medications or substances with serotonergic activity (see *Appendix II*)
(increased risk of developing the serotonin syndrome, a rare but potentially fatal hyperserotonergic state; symptoms typically occur shortly [hours to days] after the addition of a serotonergic agent, such as paroxetine, to a regimen that includes serotonin-enhancing drugs or an increase in dosage of a serotonergic agent; symptoms include agitation, diaphoresis, diarrhea, fever, hyperreflexia, incoordination, mental status changes [confusion, hypomania], myoclonus, shivering, or tremor; if recognized early, the syndrome usually resolves quickly upon withdrawal of the offending agents)

(concurrent use of tryptophan and paroxetine is not recommended)

Theophylline
(elevated theophylline concentrations have been reported during concurrent use; monitoring of theophylline serum concentrations during concurrent use is recommended)

» Warfarin
(although paroxetine does not alter *in vitro* protein binding of warfarin, a pharmacodynamic interaction may exist that causes an increased bleeding diathesis despite unaltered prothrombin time; since there is little clinical experience, caution is advised when these agents are used concomitantly)

**Laboratory value alterations**
The following have been selected on the basis of their potential clinical significance (possible effect in parentheses where appropriate)—not necessarily inclusive (» = major clinical significance):

With physiology/laboratory test values
Hematocrit or
Hemoglobin or
White blood cell counts
(may be decreased)

**Medical considerations/Contraindications**
The medical considerations/contraindications included have been selected on the basis of their potential clinical significance (reasons given in parentheses where appropriate)—not necessarily inclusive (» = major clinical significance).

*Risk-benefit should be considered when the following medical problems exist:*
» Hepatic function impairment, severe
(paroxetine plasma concentrations and elimination half-life are increased; initial dosage should be reduced, starting at 10 mg once a day, and intervals between dosage increases should be lengthened)

Mania, history of
(activation of hypomania or mania has been reported in depressed patients treated with paroxetine)

Neurological impairment, including developmental delay
(risk of seizures may be increased)

» Renal function impairment, severe
(in patients with creatinine clearance < 30 mL per minute [mL/min] and in patients with creatinine clearance between 30 and 60 mL/min, mean plasma paroxetine concentrations were four and two times, respectively, the plasma concentrations seen in healthy volunteers; initial dosage should be reduced, starting at 10 mg once a day, and intervals between dosage increases should be lengthened)

Seizures, history of
(as with other antidepressants, paroxetine should be introduced with caution; if seizures develop, paroxetine should be discontinued)

**Patient monitoring**
The following may be especially important in patient monitoring (other tests may be warranted in some patients, depending on condition; » = major clinical significance):

Careful supervision of patients with suicidal tendencies
(recommended especially during early treatment phase before peak effectiveness of paroxetine is achieved; prescribing the smallest number of tablets necessary for good patient management is recommended to decrease risk of overdose)

# Side/Adverse Effects

Note: Side effects are usually mild and transient, with evidence of dose-dependency for some of the most common adverse effects. In addition, there is evidence of adaptation with continuing therapy (over 4 to 6 weeks) to some effects, such as nausea and dizziness.

The following side/adverse effects have been selected on the basis of their potential clinical significance (possible signs and symptoms in parentheses where appropriate)—not necessarily inclusive:

**Those indicating need for medical attention**
Incidence less frequent
*Agitation; myalgia, myasthenia, or myopathy* (muscle pain or weakness); *palpitation* (fast or irregular heartbeat); *skin rash*

Incidence rare
*Abnormal bleeding* (red or purple patches on skin); *extrapyramidal symptoms; including akinesia or hypokinesia* (absence of or decrease in body movements); *dyskinesia* (unusual or incomplete body movements); *dystonia* (unusual or sudden body or facial movements; inability to move eyes); *and dysarthria* (difficulty in speaking); *hyponatremia* (confusion; drowsiness; dryness of mouth; increased thirst; lack of energy; seizures); *mania or hypomania* (talking, feeling, and acting

with excitement and activity you cannot control); *serotonin syndrome* (diarrhea; fever; increased sweating; mood or behavior changes; overactive reflexes; racing heartbeat; restlessness; shivering or shaking)

- Note: Reports of *abnormal bleeding* have included a report of impaired platelet aggregation, which could be caused by paroxetine-induced platelet serotonin depletion. However, a causal relationship between paroxetine and abnormal bleeding has not been established.

  *Hyponatremia* has been reported mostly in elderly patients, some of whom were taking diuretics or were otherwise volume-depleted.

  Activation of *mania/hypomania* occurred in about 1% of unipolar and in about 2% of a subset of bipolar patients during premarketing testing.

  The *serotonin syndrome* is most likely to occur shortly (within hours to days) after a paroxetine dosage increase or the addition of another serotonergic agent to the patient's regimen. The syndrome may include cardiac arrhythmias, coma, disseminated intravascular coagulation, hypertension or hypotension, renal failure, respiratory failure, seizures, or severe hyperthermia.

**Those indicating need for medical attention only if they continue or are bothersome**
Incidence more frequent
- *Asthenia* (unusual tiredness or weakness); *constipation; diarrhea; dizziness; drowsiness; dryness of mouth; headache; increased sweating; insomnia* (trouble in sleeping); *nausea; sexual dysfunction, especially ejaculatory disturbances or anorgasmia* (decreased sexual ability); *tremor* (trembling or shaking); *urinary frequency or retention* (problems in urinating); *vomiting*
- Note: *Dryness of mouth* is probably due to a direct effect on the serotonin system rather than cholinergic blockade.

Incidence less frequent
- *Anxiety or nervousness; blurred vision; decreased libido* (decreased sexual desire); *decreased or increased appetite; paresthesia* (tingling, burning, or prickling sensations); *taste perversion* (change in sense of taste); *weight loss or gain*
- Note: Paroxetine may cause less *weight loss* than fluoxetine or sertraline; also, it may cause less *weight gain* than imipramine, especially in females. Long-term paroxetine treatment may cause *increased appetite* and *weight gain*.

**Those indicating the need for medical attention if they occur after medication is discontinued**
- *Agitation, confusion, or restlessness; diarrhea; dizziness, vertigo, or lightheadedness; headache; increased sweating; insomnia* (trouble in sleeping); *migraine-like visual disturbances* (vision changes); *myalgia* (muscle pain); *nausea or vomiting; rhinorrhea* (runny nose); *tremor* (trembling or shaking); *unusual tiredness or weakness*
- Note: Discontinuation symptoms, if they occur, usually start 1 to 4 days after stopping paroxetine; however, some patients may experience effects immediately. Instances of withdrawal symptoms occurring in patients after paroxetine dosage was tapered over 7 to 10 days have been reported. Although most effects are generally mild and transient, some patients may experience more severe symptoms.

## Overdose

For specific information on the agents used in the management of paroxetine overdose, see *Charcoal, Activated (Oral-Local)* monograph.

For more information on the management of overdose or unintentional ingestion, **contact a Poison Control Center** (see *Poison Control Center Listing*).

**Clinical effects of overdose**
The following effects have been selected on the basis of their potential clinical significance (possible signs and symptoms in parentheses where appropriate)—not necessarily inclusive:

*Dilated pupils* (large pupils); *dizziness; drowsiness; dryness of mouth; flushing of face; irritability; nausea; sinus tachycardia* (racing heartbeat); *tremor* (trembling or shaking); *vomiting*

**Treatment of overdose**
There is no specific antidote for paroxetine. Treatment is essentially symptomatic and supportive.

To decrease absorption—Decontaminating gastrointestinal tract by induction of emesis, gastric lavage, or both, followed by administration of 20 to 30 grams of activated charcoal every 4 to 6 hours during the first 24 to 48 hours following ingestion.

Monitoring—Taking an electrocardiogram (ECG) and monitoring cardiac function if there is any sign of abnormality. Monitoring vital signs.

Supportive care—Establishing and monitoring airway. Patients in whom intentional overdose is confirmed or suspected should be referred for psychiatric consultation.

- Note: Due to the large volume of distribution of paroxetine, forced diuresis, hemodialysis, hemoperfusion, or exchange transfusions are not likely to be of benefit.

  If a tricyclic antidepressant has been coingested, the tricyclic toxicity may be prolonged due to inhibition of metabolism by paroxetine.

## Patient Consultation

As an aid to patient consultation, refer to *Advice for the Patient, Paroxetine (Systemic)*.

In providing consultation, consider emphasizing the following selected information (» = major clinical significance):

**Before using this medication**
» Conditions affecting use, especially:
　Sensitivity to paroxetine
　Pregnancy—No difference in birth outcome was found between 267 SSRI-exposed pregnancies (97 to paroxetine) and 267 pregnancies exposed to known nonteratogenic medications or procedures; behavioral effects were not studied
　Breast-feeding—Distributed into breast milk
　Contraindicated medications—Monoamine oxidase (MAO) inhibitors
　Other medications, especially astemizole, moclobemide, serotonergics or other medications or substances with serotonergic activity, tricyclic antidepressants, and warfarin
　Other medical problems, especially severe hepatic or renal function impairment

**Proper use of this medication**
» Compliance with therapy; not taking more or less medicine than prescribed
　Taking with or without food, on a full or empty stomach, as directed by physician
» Four or more weeks of therapy may be required before antidepressant effects are achieved; antiobsessional and antipanic effects may require several weeks to achieve
　For patients taking oral suspension dosage form—Shaking well before measuring dose; measuring dose with a calibrated measuring device
» Proper dosing
　Missed dose: Taking as soon as possible; continuing on regular schedule with next dose; not doubling doses
» Proper storage

**Precautions while using this medication**
　Regular visits to physician to check progress of therapy
　Checking with physician before discontinuing medication; gradual dosage reduction may be recommended
» Not taking paroxetine within 2 weeks of taking a monoamine oxidase (MAO) inhibitor; not starting an MAO inhibitor within 2 weeks of discontinuing paroxetine
　Avoiding use of alcoholic beverages
» Possible blurred vision, drowsiness, impairment of judgment, thinking, or motor skills; caution when driving or doing jobs requiring alertness until effects of medication are known

**Side/adverse effects**
　Possibility of discontinuation symptoms
　Signs of potential side effects, especially agitation; myalgia, myasthenia, or myopathy; palpitation; skin rash; abnormal bleeding; extrapyramidal symptoms; hyponatremia; mania or hypomania; serotonin syndrome

## General Dosing Information

Paroxetine may be administered once daily, usually in the morning, to diminish sleep disturbances and other adverse effects.

Potentially suicidal patients, particularly those who may use alcohol excessively, should not have access to large quantities of this medication. Some clinicians recommend that the patient have immediate access to the smallest total amount of medication necessary for satisfactory patient management.

Abrupt discontinuation of paroxetine may result in discontinuation symptoms. It is not known whether tapering the dose will prevent or reduce discontinuation symptoms.

**Diet/Nutrition**
Paroxetine may be taken with or without food. Some clinicians advise their patients to take this medication with food to lessen gastrointestinal side effects.

## For treatment of adverse effects
Serotonin syndrome—Serotonergic medications should be discontinued. Treatment is essentially symptomatic and supportive. The nonspecific serotonergic receptor antagonists cyproheptadine and methysergide have been reported to be of some use in shortening the duration of the syndrome.

# Oral Dosage Forms

## PAROXETINE HYDROCHLORIDE ORAL SUSPENSION

Note: The dosing and strength of the available dosage forms are expressed in terms of paroxetine base (not the hydrochloride salt).

### Usual adult dose
Antidepressant or
Antiobsessional agent—
  Oral, initially 20 mg (base) once a day, usually in the morning. The dosage may be increased, as needed and tolerated, by 10 mg a day at intervals of at least seven days.
Antipanic agent—
  Oral, initially 10 mg (base) once a day, usually in the morning. The dosage may be increased, as needed and tolerated, by 10 mg a day at intervals of at least seven days.

Note: For most patients, 20 mg a day is the optimal dosage for treatment of depression. For treatment of obsessive-compulsive disorder and panic disorder, 40 mg a day is the recommended dosage.

For all indications, debilitated patients and patients with severe renal or hepatic function impairment should receive an initial dosage of 10 mg (base) a day, with upward titration as needed, up to a maximum of 40 mg a day. Longer intervals should be allowed between dosage increases in patients with renal or hepatic function impairment.

### Usual adult prescribing limits
Antidepressant—
  50 mg (base) per day.
Antiobsessional agent or
Antipanic agent—
  60 mg (base) per day.

### Usual pediatric dose
Safety and efficacy have not been established.

### Usual geriatric dose
Antidepressant or
Antiobsessional agent or
Antipanic agent—
  Oral, initially 10 mg (base) once a day, usually in the morning. The dosage may be increased as needed and tolerated.

### Usual geriatric prescribing limits
Antidepressant or
Antiobsessional agent or
Antipanic agent—
  40 mg (base) a day.

### Strength(s) usually available
U.S.—
  10 mg (base) per 5 mL (Rx) [*Paxil* (citric acid anhydrate; FD&C Yellow No. 6; flavorings; glycerin; methylparaben; microcrystalline cellulose; polacrilin potassium; propylparaben; propylene glycol; Simethicone Emulsion USP; sodium citrate dihydrate; sodium saccharin; sorbitol)].
Canada—
  Not commercially available.

### Packaging and storage
Store at or below 25 °C (77 °F), unless otherwise specified by manufacturer.

### Auxiliary labeling
• Avoid alcoholic beverages.
• May cause drowsiness.
• Shake well before using.

### Additional information
Paroxetine hydrochloride oral suspension is orange flavored.

## PAROXETINE HYDROCHLORIDE TABLETS

Note: The dosing and strength of the available dosage forms are expressed in terms of paroxetine base (not the hydrochloride salt).

### Usual adult dose
See *Paroxetine Hydrochloride Oral Suspension*

### Usual adult prescribing limits
See *Paroxetine Hydrochloride Oral Suspension*

### Usual pediatric dose
See *Paroxetine Hydrochloride Oral Suspension*

### Usual geriatric dose
See *Paroxetine Hydrochloride Oral Suspension*

### Usual geriatric prescribing limits
See *Paroxetine Hydrochloride Oral Suspension*

### Strength(s) usually available
U.S.—
  10 mg (base) (Rx) [*Paxil* (dibasic calcium phosphate dihydrate; hydroxypropyl methylcellulose; magnesium stearate; polyethylene glycols; polysorbate 80; sodium starch glycolate; titanium dioxide; D&C Red No. 30; and/or D&C Yellow No. 10; and/or FD&C Blue No. 2; and/or FD&C Yellow No. 6)].
  20 mg (base) (Rx) [*Paxil* (scored; dibasic calcium phosphate dihydrate; hydroxypropyl methylcellulose; magnesium stearate; polyethylene glycols; polysorbate 80; sodium starch glycolate; titanium dioxide; D&C Red No. 30; and/or D&C Yellow No. 10; and/or FD&C Blue No. 2; and/or FD&C Yellow No. 6)].
  30 mg (base) (Rx) [*Paxil* (dibasic calcium phosphate dihydrate; hydroxypropyl methylcellulose; magnesium stearate; polyethylene glycols; polysorbate 80; sodium starch glycolate; titanium dioxide; D&C Red No. 30; and/or D&C Yellow No. 10; and/or FD&C Blue No. 2; and/or FD&C Yellow No. 6)].
  40 mg (base) (Rx) [*Paxil* (dibasic calcium phosphate dihydrate; hydroxypropyl methylcellulose; magnesium stearate; polyethylene glycols; polysorbate 80; sodium starch glycolate; titanium dioxide; D&C Red No. 30; and/or D&C Yellow No. 10; and/or FD&C Blue No. 2; and/or FD&C Yellow No. 6)].
Canada—
  10 mg (base) (Rx) [*Paxil* (scored; dibasic calcium phosphate dihydrate USP; sodium starch glycolate NF; hydroxypropyl methylcellulose USP; magnesium stearate NF; opadry yellow; opadry clear)].
  20 mg (base) (Rx) [*Paxil* (scored; dibasic calcium phosphate dihydrate USP; sodium starch glycolate NF; hydroxypropyl methylcellulose USP; magnesium stearate NF; opadry pink; opadry clear)].
  30 mg (base) (Rx) [*Paxil* (dibasic calcium phosphate dihydrate USP; sodium starch glycolate NF; hydroxypropyl methylcellulose USP; magnesium stearate NF; opadry blue; opadry clear)].

### Packaging and storage
Store between 15 and 30 °C (59 and 86 °F), unless otherwise specified by manufacturer.

### Auxiliary labeling
• Avoid alcoholic beverages.
• May cause drowsiness.

## Selected Bibliography
Caley CF, Weber SS. Paroxetine: a selective serotonin reuptake inhibiting antidepressant. Ann Pharmacother 1993 Oct; 27: 1212-22.
Nemeroff CB. The clinical pharmacology and use of paroxetine, a new selective serotonin reuptake inhibitor. Pharmacotherapy 1994; 14(2): 127-38.

Revised: 08/08/97
Interim revision: 03/25/98; 08/13/98

**PEGADEMASE**—The *Pegademase (Systemic)* monograph is not included in this published version of the USP DI database. Copies of the monograph are available on request from Micromedex, Inc. - Reprint Requests, 6200 S. Syracuse Way, Suite 300, Englewood, CO 80111; telephone (303) 486-6400; telefax (303) 486-6464; Email: USPDI@MDX.COM.

# PEGASPARGASE Systemic†

VA CLASSIFICATION (Primary): AN900

Commonly used brand name(s): *Oncaspar*.

Another commonly used name is PEG-L-asparaginase.

Note: For a listing of dosage forms and brand names by country availability, see *Dosage Forms* section(s).

†Not commercially available in Canada.

## Category
Antineoplastic.

## Indications

### Accepted
Leukemia, acute lymphoblastic (treatment)—Pegaspargase is indicated for patients with acute lymphoblastic leukemia who require L-asparaginase in their treatment regimen, but have developed hypersensitivity to the native forms of L-asparaginase.

## Pharmacology/Pharmacokinetics

### Physicochemical characteristics
Source—Pegaspargase is a modified version of the enzyme L-asparaginase. L-asparaginase is modified by covalently conjugating units of monomethoxypolyethylene glycol (PEG), which has a molecular weight of 5000, to the enzyme, forming the active ingredient PEG-L-asparaginase. The L-asparaginase used in the manufacture of pegaspargase is derived from *Escherichia coli*. Monomethoxypolyethylene glycol covalently linked with L-asparaginase decreases antigenicity and extends the plasma half-life, allowing lower doses and less frequent administration.

### Mechanism of action/Effect
The growth of malignant and normal cells depends on the availability of specific nutrients and cofactors required for protein synthesis. Some nutrients can be synthesized within the cell, whereas others, such as essential amino acids, require exogenous sources. L-asparagine is a nonessential amino acid synthesized by the transamination of L-aspartic acid by a reaction catalyzed by the enzyme L-asparagine synthetase. The ability to synthesize asparagine is notably lacking in malignancies of lymphoid origin; therefore, leukemic cells are dependent on an exogenous source of asparagine for survival. Asparaginase catalyzes the conversion of L-asparagine to aspartic acid and ammonia. The enzyme does not enter cells; instead, it degrades circulating asparagine to aspartic acid, which cannot be converted to asparagine by the leukemic cells. Rapid depletion of asparagine, which results from treatment with the enzyme L-asparaginase, kills the leukemic cells. Normal cells, however, are less affected by the rapid depletion due to their ability to synthesize asparagine. This therapeutic approach is based on a specific metabolic defect in some leukemic cells that do not produce asparagine synthetase.

In animal studies, pegaspargase is more effective than L-asparaginase when administered at the same dose. One unit of pegaspargase was as effective as 5 units of *E. coli* L-asparaginase in one tumor type and nearly twice as active as L-asparaginase in another tumor type. In studies of animals with non-Hodgkin's lymphoma, pegaspargase in doses of 10 to 30 International Units per kg (IU/kg) was as effective as L-asparaginase 400 IU/kg, and caused fewer side effects.

### Half-life
L-asparaginase levels are detectable for at least 15 days after intravenous treatment with pegaspargase. After a single intramuscular injection of pegaspargase (2500 International Units per square meter of body surface area [IU/m$^2$]) in children, the half-life was 5.73 days as compared with 1.24 days after *E. coli* L-asparaginase (25,000 IU/m$^2$) and 0.65 days after *Erwinia* L-asparaginase (25,000 IU/m$^2$).

Among adults treated with pegaspargase 2500 IU/m$^2$ every 2 weeks, the half-life was 3.24 days in patients previously hypersensitive to L-asparaginase and 5.69 days in nonhypersensitive patients.

### Peak serum concentration
Found in the lymph at about 20% of the concentration in plasma.

### Elimination
The metabolic fate and method of elimination of pegaspargase are unknown. Little is excreted in the urine. In one study, the results of serum and urine enzyme-linked immunoadsorbent assay (ELISA) suggest that pegaspargase activity and protein are cleared by mechanisms other than urinary excretion. Possible mechanisms that are consistent with the results of this study include proteolysis of the enzyme and/or removal by an organ other than the kidneys. Although previous reports suggest this may not be the case, pegaspargase may be metabolized by the liver, excreted in the bile, or filtered from the plasma by the reticuloendothelial system.

## Precautions to Consider

### Cross-sensitivity and/or related problems
Patients who are allergic to native forms of L-asparaginase may also be allergic to pegaspargase. During clinical trials, approximately 18% of patients experienced hypersensitivity reactions to pegaspargase. Sixty-five percent of the patients who had reactions previously experienced hypersensitivity reaction to *Escherichia coli* asparaginase. The other 35% had no prior hypersensitivity reaction to native asparaginase. Since these trials included patients who had previous hypersensitivity reactions to the native asparaginase, the possibility exists that cross-sensitivity played a role in the reported reactions. Documentation of cross-sensitivity between *E. coli* and *Erwina* asparaginase in leukemic children exists in which 33% of patients experiencing a reaction to *E. coli* asparaginase also become hypersensitive to *Erwina* asparaginase. Therefore, this phenomenon should also be considered as a possible factor when reviewing the incidence of reported hypersensitivity reactions to pegaspargase.

### Carcinogenicity
Long-term studies in animals have not been done.

### Mutagenicity
Pegaspargase did not exhibit a mutagenic effect when tested against *Salmonella typhimurium* strains in the Ames mutagenicity assay.

### Pregnancy/Reproduction
Fertility—Studies on the effects of pegaspargase on fertility have not been done.

Pregnancy—Studies have not been done in humans. However, pegaspargase should be avoided during pregnancy unless it is clearly needed. Studies have not been done in animals.

FDA Pregnancy Category C.

### Breast-feeding
It is not known whether pegaspargase is distributed into breast milk. However, because of the potential for serious adverse reactions due to pegaspargase in nursing infants, a decision should be made to either discontinue nursing or discontinue the medication, taking into account the importance of the medication to the welfare of the mother.

### Pediatrics
Infants up to 1 year of age—Safety and efficacy have not been established. The safety and efficacy of pegaspargase have been established in pediatric patients 1 year of age and older with known previous hypersensitivity to L-asparaginase. Pediatric patients treated with pegaspargase had a somewhat lower incidence of known L-asparaginase toxicities, except for hypersensitivity reactions, than the adult patients treated with pegaspargase.

### Adolescents
The safety and efficacy of pegaspargase have been established in adolescent and young adult patients 21 years of age and younger with known previous hypersensitivity to L-asparaginase.

### Geriatrics
No information is available on the relationship of age to the effects of pegaspargase in geriatric patients.

### Dental
The leukopenic and thrombocytopenic effects of pegaspargase may result in an increased incidence of certain microbial infections of the mouth, delayed healing, and gingival bleeding. If leukopenia or thrombocytopenia occurs, dental work should be deferred until blood counts have returned to normal. Patients should be instructed in proper oral hygiene, including caution in use of regular toothbrushes, dental floss, and toothpicks.

### Drug interactions and/or related problems
The following drug interactions and/or related problems have been selected on the basis of their potential clinical significance (possible mechanism in parentheses where appropriate)—not necessarily inclusive (» = major clinical significance):

Note: Combinations containing any of the following medications, depending on the amount present, may also interact with this medication.

- » Anti-inflammatory drugs, nonsteroidal (NSAIDs) or
- » Aspirin or
- » Dipyridamole or
- » Heparin or
- » Warfarin
    (patients treated with pegaspargase are at increased risk of bleeding complications, especially when administered concomitantly with agents with anticoagulant properties; imbalances in coagulation factors have been noted with the use of pegaspargase, predisposing the patient to bleeding and/or thrombosis; caution should be used when administering any concurrent anticoagulant therapy; it has also been suggested that blood coagulation factor XIII participates in the cross-linking between fibrins and between fibrin and asparaginase)

    Blood-dyscrasia causing medications (see *Appendix II*)
    (leukopenic and/or thrombocytopenic effects of pegaspargase may be increased with concurrent or recent therapy if these medications cause the same effects; dosage adjustment of pegaspargase, if necessary, should be based on blood counts)
- » Bone marrow depressants, other (see *Appendix II*)
    Radiation therapy
    (additive bone marrow depression, including severe dermatitis and/or mucositis, may occur; dosage reduction may be required when two or more bone marrow depressants, including radiation, are used concurrently or consecutively)

    Hepatotoxic medications, other (see *Appendix II*)
    (concurrent use may increase the risk of toxicity)

    Methotrexate
    (pegaspargase antagonizes the effects of methotrexate [antifolate] when given before methotrexate administration; however, if pegaspargase is given 24 hours after methotrexate, the action of the antifolate is abbreviated at that point and patients can tolerate large doses of methotrexate)

    Vaccines, killed virus
    (because normal defense mechanisms may be suppressed by pegaspargase therapy, the patient's antibody response to the vaccine may be decreased. The interval between discontinuation of medications that cause immunosuppression and restoration of the patient's ability to respond to the vaccine depends on the intensity and type of immunosuppression-causing medication used, the underlying disease, and other factors; estimates vary from 3 months to 1 year)
- » Vaccines, live virus
    (because normal defense mechanisms may be suppressed by pegaspargase therapy, concurrent use with a live virus vaccine may potentiate the replication of the vaccine virus, may increase the side/adverse effects of the vaccine virus, and/or may decrease the patient's antibody response to the vaccine; immunization of these patients should be undertaken only with extreme caution after careful review of the patient's hematologic status and only with the knowledge and consent of the physician managing the pegaspargase therapy. The interval between discontinuation of medications that cause immunosuppression and restoration of the patient's ability to respond to the vaccine depends on the intensity and type of immunosuppression-causing medication used, the underlying disease, and other factors; estimates vary from 3 months to 1 year. Patients with leukemia in remission should not receive live virus vaccine until at least 3 months after their last chemotherapy. In addition, immunization with oral poliovirus vaccine should be postponed in persons in close contact with the patient, especially family members)

**Laboratory value alterations**
The following have been selected on the basis of their potential clinical significance (possible effect in parentheses where appropriate)—not necessarily inclusive (» = major clinical significance):

With physiology/laboratory test values
- » Alanine aminotransferase (ALT [SGPT]) and
- » Alkaline phosphatase and
- » Amylase, serum and
- » Aspartate aminotransferase (AST [SGOT]) and
- » Bilirubin, serum concentrations and
- » Blood urea nitrogen (BUN) and
- » Glucose, serum and
- » Uric acid, serum concentrations
    (values may be increased)
- » Prothrombin time
    (may be prolonged)

**Medical considerations/Contraindications**
The medical considerations/contraindications included have been selected on the basis of their potential clinical significance (reasons given in parentheses where appropriate)—not necessarily inclusive (» = major clinical significance).

*Except under special circumstances, this medication should not be used when the following medical problems exist:*
- » Allergy to pegaspargase
- » Bleeding disorders, associated with previous asparaginase therapy
    (pegaspargase should not be used in patients who have experienced significant hemorrhagic events associated with prior asparaginase therapy [all preparations])
- » Pancreatitis, or history of
    (pegaspargase should not be used in patients with active pancreatitis or a history of pancreatitis)

*Risk-benefit should be considered when the following medical problems exist:*
- » Anticoagulant therapy, or
- » Bleeding disorders, history of
    (may cause platelet dysfunction and hemorrhage)
- » Chickenpox, existing or recent (including recent exposure) or
- » Herpes zoster
    (risk of severe generalized disease)
- » Diabetes mellitus
    (increased risk of hyperglycemia)
- » Hepatic function impairment
    (impaired metabolism of pegaspargase may result in fatty changes in the liver and liver failure)
- » Tumor cell infiltration of the bone marrow
- » Caution should be used also in patients with inadequate bone marrow reserves due to previous cytotoxic drug or radiation therapy

**Patient monitoring**
The following may be especially important in patient monitoring (other tests may be warranted in some patients, depending on condition; » = major clinical significance):
- » Amylase, concentrations, serum
    (recommended at periodic intervals throughout therapy to detect early evidence of pancreatitis)

    Blood counts, complete, including differential and leukocytes and platelet counts and
    Glucose, blood, concentrations and
    Hepatic function determinations, including serum transaminase and alkaline phosphatase values and bilirubin concentrations
    (recommended at periodic intervals throughout therapy)

## Side/Adverse Effects

Note: In studies, adult patients treated with pegaspargase had a higher incidence of adverse reactions than children. The exception was hypersensitivity reactions, which occurred more frequently in children.

Anaphylactic-type reactions have been described in three cancer patients receiving intravenous pegaspargase administered over 1 hour every 2 weeks. In two of these patients, anaphylaxis occurred after the second (500 International Units per square meter of body surface area [IU/m$^2$]) and third (2000 IU/m$^2$) doses, respectively. A sudden disappearance of plasma asparaginase preceded both reactions. Anti-asparaginase antibodies were seen in one of the patients, and this patient previously had developed a mild allergic reaction to the native enzyme. The second patient, who did not possess anti-asparaginase antibodies, had not previously received native asparaginase. The third patient, who developed bronchospasm following the first dose, had not received native asparaginase previously and had normal enzyme levels with no antibodies present. These results suggest that a sudden disappearance of plasma enzyme levels may predispose patients to hypersensitivity reactions during subsequent pegaspargase administration.

Some investigators described significant reduction in plasma asparaginase activity despite continued administration of *Escherichia coli* asparaginase. The investigators attributed this reduction in enzyme activity to specific immune globulin G (IgG) antibodies (anti-L-asparaginase antibodies) that destroy the enzyme and/or enhance its clearance. This has been referred to as "silent hypersensitivity," as it can occur prior to, or in the absence of, an observable clinical hypersensitivity reaction.

Hepatotoxicity occurs in most patients to some degree. It is manifested by decreases in serum albumin and serum lipoprotein levels, and increases in liver transaminase levels. Biopsy specimens and autopsies have shown fatty changes in the liver. Liver toxicity can be dose-limiting, but function generally returns to normal after the medication is discontinued.

Neurotoxicity may occur in some patients. L-asparaginase breaks down L-asparagine into aspartic acid and ammonia, and L-glutamine into L-glutamic acid. Central nervous system changes may result from a high level of ammonia in the blood or from a lack of L-asparagine or L-glutamine in the brain. These changes are characterized by confusion and, rarely, stupor, coma, or death. Neurotoxicity is less common in children.

The following side/adverse effects have been selected on the basis of their potential clinical significance (possible signs and symptoms in parentheses where appropriate)—not necessarily inclusive:

**Those indicating need for medical attention**
Incidence more frequent
*Allergic reaction* (skin rash); *hyperglycemia* (blurry vision; dry mouth and skin; fatigue; increased need to urinate; increased hunger or thirst; unexplained weight loss)—requiring insulin therapy; *liver damage; pancreatitis* (abdominal or stomach pain; constipation; nausea; vomiting)

Incidence less frequent
*Anaphylactic reaction* (difficulty in breathing or swallowing; hives; itching, especially of hands or feet; reddening of the skin, especially around ears; swelling of eyes, face, or inside of nose; unusual tiredness or weakness, sudden and severe)

Incidence rare
*Leukopenia, septicemia, thrombocytopenia, or bone marrow depression* (black, tarry stools; blood in urine; cough or hoarseness; fever or chills; lower back or side pain; painful or difficult urination; pinpoint red spots on skin; unusual bleeding or bruising)

**Those indicating need for medical attention only if they continue or are bothersome**
Incidence more frequent
*Fever; malaise* (general feeling of discomfort or illness); *nausea and vomiting*

Incidence less frequent
*Anorexia* (lack of appetite); *arthralgia or myalgia* (pain in joints or muscles); *convulsions* (seizures); *hypoglycemia* (anxiety; behavior change similar to drunkenness; blurred vision; cold sweats; confusion; cool pale skin; difficulty in concentrating; drowsiness; excessive hunger; fast heartbeat; headache; nausea; nervousness; nightmares; restless sleep; shakiness; slurred speech; unusual tiredness or weakness); *hypoproteinemia; hypotension reaction* (severe tiredness or weakness); *pain at place of injection; tachycardia* (fast heartbeat)

## Patient Consultation

As an aid to patient consultation, refer to *Advice for the Patient, Pegaspargase (Systemic)*.

In providing consultation, consider emphasizing the following selected information (» = major clinical significance):

**Before using this medication**
» Conditions affecting use, especially:
  Sensitivity to pegaspargase
  Pregnancy—Use is not recommended; women of childbearing age should be advised to avoid pregnancy during treatment
  Breast-feeding—Use is not recommended because of the potential for serious adverse effects in nursing infants
  Use in children—Safety and efficacy have not been established in infants up to 1 year of age.
  Dental—Patients who develop blood dyscrasias may be at increased risk of microbial infections of the mouth, delayed healing, and gingival bleeding
  Other medications, especially nonsteroidal anti-inflammatory drugs (NSAIDs), aspirin, dipyridamole, heparin, other bone marrow depressants, or warfarin
  Other medical problems, especially allergy to pegaspargase; anticoagulant therapy; bleeding disorders associated with previous asparaginase therapy; chickenpox; diabetes mellitus; hepatic function impairment; herpes zoster; history of bleeding disorders; pancreatitis or history of; or tumor cell infiltration of the bone marrow

**Proper use of this medication**
Caution in taking combination therapy; taking each medication at the right time
Importance of ample fluid intake and subsequent increase in urine output to aid in excretion of uric acid
Frequency of nausea and vomiting; importance of continuing medication despite stomach upset
» Proper dosing

**Precautions while using this medication**
» Importance of close monitoring by the physician
» Avoiding immunizations unless approved by physician; other persons in patient's household should avoid immunizations with oral poliovirus vaccine; avoiding persons who have taken oral poliovirus vaccine or wearing a protective mask that covers nose and mouth

*Caution if bone marrow depression occurs*
» Avoiding exposure to persons with infections, especially during periods of low blood counts; checking with physician immediately if fever or chills, cough or hoarseness, lower back or side pain, or painful or difficult urination occurs
» Checking with physician immediately if unusual bleeding or bruising; black, tarry stools; blood in urine or stools; or pinpoint red spots on skin occur
Caution in use of regular toothbrush, dental floss, or toothpick; physician, dentist, or nurse may suggest alternatives; checking with physician before having dental work done
Not touching eyes or inside of nose unless hands washed immediately before
Using caution to avoid accidental cuts with use of sharp objects such as safety razor or fingernail or toenail cutters
Avoiding contact sports or other situations where bruising or injury could occur
» Possibility of local tissue injury and scarring if infiltration of intravenous solution occurs; telling doctor or nurse right away about redness, pain, or swelling at injection site

**Side/adverse effects**
Signs of potential side effects, especially allergic reaction, hyperglycemia, liver damage, pancreatitis, anaphylactic reaction, leukopenia, septicemia, thrombocytopenia, and bone marrow depression

## General Dosing Information

Hypersensitivity reactions to pegaspargase, including life-threatening anaphylaxis, may occur during therapy. Therefore, appropriate precautions should be taken prior to pegaspargase administration to prevent allergic or other unwanted reactions, especially in patients with known hypersensitivity to the other forms of L-asparaginase. Precautions should include a review of the patient's history regarding possible sensitivity and the ready availability of epinephrine 1:1000, oxygen, intravenous corticosteroids, and other appropriate agents used for control of immediate allergic reactions. All patients should be observed for 1 hour after pegaspargase administration. Delayed hypersensitivity (more than 1 hour after administration) is possible, however, reactions are more likely to occur within 1 hour of administration.

The National Cancer Institute has developed Common Toxicity Criteria that can be used by health care providers to classify the severity of hypersensitivity reactions. These criteria are:
• Grade 1 or mild hypersensitivity reactions (transient rash).
• Grade 2 or moderate hypersensitivity reactions (mild bronchospasm).
• Grade 3 or severe hypersensitivity reactions (moderate bronchospasm and/or serum sickness).
• Grade 4 or life-threatening hypersensitivity reactions (hypotension and/or anaphylaxis).

Grade 2–4 reactions are considered dose-limiting and require discontinuation of asparaginase therapy.

Pegaspargase should be given under the supervision of an individual who is qualified by training and experience to administer cancer chemotherapeutic agents.

When administered intravenously, a solution of pegaspargase in water for injection or 0.9% sodium chloride injection should be given over a period of 1 to 2 hours in 100 mL of 0.9% sodium chloride injection or 5% dextrose injection, through an infusion that is already running. When pegaspargase is given intramuscularly, no more than 2 mL of a solution in sodium chloride injection should be injected at a single site. If the volume to be administered is greater than 2 mL, multiple injection sites should be used.

As a component of selected multiple agent regimens, the recommended dose of pegaspargase is 2500 International Units per square meter of body surface area (IU/m$^2$) every 14 days by either the intramuscular or intravenous route of administration. However, the preferred route of administration is the intramuscular route because of the lower incidence of hepatotoxicity, coagulopathy, and gastrointestinal and renal disorders as compared with the intravenous route of administration.

Pegaspargase, like native L-asparaginase, is used generally in combination with other chemotherapeutic agents, such as vincristine, methotrexate, cytarabine, daunorubicin, and doxorubicin. Multidrug chemotherapy now can cure about 70% of children and about 40% of adults with acute lymphoblastic leukemia. The usual drugs of choice for initial treatment ("induction") are vincristine, prednisone, and asparaginase with or without daunorubicin or doxorubicin, which produce a remission in more than 95% of children and about 75% of adults.

The use of pegaspargase as the sole induction agent should be undertaken only in an unusual situation in which a combined regimen, using other chemotherapeutic agents such as vincristine, methotrexate, cytarabine, daunorubicin, or doxorubicin, is inappropriate because of toxicity or other specific patient-related factors, or in patients refractory to other therapy. When pegaspargase is to be used as the sole induction agent, the recommended dosage regimen is also 2500 IU/m² every 14 days.

Recurrence of childhood acute lymphoblastic leukemia occurs in about 30 to 50% of patients and indicates irresistible progression of the disease. While systemic (i.e., hematologic) relapse is due to drug resistance of leukemic cells, pharmacologic barriers may be responsible for local relapses such as meningeal involvement, leukemic ophthalmopathy or testicular infiltration. L-asparaginase seems to be an important component of drug combinations for reinduction therapy for systemic relapse. Following reinduction therapy, modification of continuation therapy is necessary.

Local relapses require local treatment, i.e., radiotherapy and intrathecal administration of chemotherapy. Local relapse is almost always followed by hematologic relapse; therefore, intensification of systemic therapy is also recommended. Prevention of these relapses is much more important and probably more successful than treatment.

**Safety considerations for handling this medication**
There is limited but increasing evidence and concern that personnel involved in preparation and administration of parenteral antineoplastic agents may be at some risk because of the potential mutagenicity, teratogenicity, and/or carcinogenicity of these agents, although the actual risk is unknown. USP advisory panels recommend cautious handling both in preparation and disposal of antineoplastic agents. Precautions that have been suggested include:
• Use of a biological containment cabinet during reconstitution and dilution of parenteral medications and wearing of disposable surgical gloves and masks.
• Use of proper technique to prevent contamination of the medication, work area, and operator during transfer between containers (including proper training of personnel in this technique).
• Cautious and proper disposal of needles, syringes, vials, ampuls, and unused medication.

A number of medical centers have developed detailed guidelines for handling of antineoplastic agents.

Pegaspargase may be a contact irritant, and therefore the solution must be handled and administered with care. Gloves are recommended. Inhalation of vapors and contact with skin or mucous membranes, especially those of the eyes, must be avoided.

**For treatment of adverse effects**
Recommended treatment consists of the following:
• For mild hypersensitivity reaction—Administering antihistamines, and, if necessary, corticosteroids.
• For severe hypersensitivity or anaphylactic reaction—Administering epinephrine. Antihistamines or corticosteroids may also be administered as required.

## Parenteral Dosage Forms

### PEGASPARGASE INJECTION

**Usual adult and adolescent dose**
Leukemia, acute lymphoblastic (treatment)—
Adults and adolescents up to 21 years of age: Intramuscular or intravenous, 2500 International Units per square meter of body surface area administered every fourteen days.
Adults 21 years of age and older: Safety and efficacy have not been established.

**Usual pediatric dose**
Leukemia, acute lymphoblastic (treatment)—
Infants up to 1 year of age: Safety and efficacy have not been established.
Children with body surface area ≥ 0.6 square meter: Intramuscular or intravenous, 2500 International Units per square meter of body surface area administered every fourteen days.
Children with body surface area < 0.6 square meter: Intramuscular or intravenous, 82.5 International Units per kg of body weight administered every fourteen days.

Note: The safety and efficacy of pegaspargase have been established only in patients with known previous hypersensitivity to L-asparaginase who ranged in age from 1 to 21. Pegaspargase can be administered by intramuscular injection or intravenous infusion in these patients. However, the preferred route of administration is intramuscular injection because of decreased incidence of hypersensitivity reactions.

**Strength(s) usually available**
U.S.—
750 International Units (IU) per 5-mL vial (Rx) [*Oncaspar*].
Canada—
Not commercially available.

**Packaging and storage**
Store between 2 and 8 °C (36 and 46 °F), unless otherwise specified by the manufacturer. Protect from freezing.

**Stability**
Storage above or below the recommended temperature may reduce potency. Freezing destroys potency, and product should be discarded if freezing occurs.
• Use only one dose per vial; do not re-enter the vial. Discard unused portions. Do not save unused drug for later administration.
• Do not use if cloudy or if precipitate is present.
• Do not use if stored at room temperature for more than 48 hours.

**Auxiliary labeling**
• Avoid excessive agitation. Do not shake.
• Do not freeze; discard if freezing occurs.

Developed: 08/29/97
Interim revision: 07/01/98

---

# PEMOLINE Systemic

VA CLASSIFICATION (Primary): CN809
Note: Controlled substance classification—U.S.—Schedule IV.
Commonly used brand name(s): *Cylert; Cylert Chewable*.
Note: For a listing of dosage forms and brand names by country availability, see *Dosage Forms* section(s).

## Category
Central nervous system stimulant.

## Indications

**Accepted**
Attention-deficit hyperactivity disorder (treatment)—Pemoline is indicated in attention-deficit hyperactivity disorder (ADHD) as an integral part of a total treatment program that includes other remedial measures (psychological, educational, and social) for a stabilizing effect in some children with ADHD. However, pemoline is **not** considered a first-line agent due to its association with life-threatening hepatic failure.

ADHD has been known in the past as hyperkinetic child syndrome, minimal brain damage, minimal cerebral dysfunction, or minor cerebral dysfunction. The syndrome is characterized by moderate to severe distractibility, short attention span, hyperactivity, emotional lability, and impulsivity. The timing, severity, and age-inappropriateness of symptoms should be considered in determining the need for pharmacologic treatment.

## Pharmacology/Pharmacokinetics

**Physicochemical characteristics**
Chemical group—Oxazolidine. Pemoline is structurally different from amphetamines and methylphenidate.
Molecular weight—176.18.
Solubility—Pemoline is relatively insoluble (less than 1 mg per mL [mg/mL]) in water. Solubility of pemoline in 95% ethyl alcohol is 2.2 mg/mL.

**Mechanism of action/Effect**
Pemoline's mechanism and site of action have not been conclusively determined; however, animal studies suggest that pemoline may act through dopaminergic mechanisms. In children with attention-deficit hyperactivity disorder, pemoline decreases hyperactivity and prolongs attention span. However, the mechanism by which pemoline produces mental and behavioral effects in children has not been established.

**Protein binding**
Moderate (50%).

**Biotransformation**
Hepatic; metabolites include pemoline conjugate, pemoline dione, mandelic acid, and unidentified polar compounds.

**Half-life**
Serum—Approximately 12 hours.

**Time to peak serum concentration**
2 to 4 hours; steady state reached in 2 to 3 days.

**Time to peak effect**
3 to 4 weeks.

**Elimination**
Renal; about 50% is excreted unchanged.

## Precautions to Consider

### Carcinogenicity
There was no significant difference in the incidence of neoplasms in rats given doses as high as 150 mg per kg per day for 18 months from that in untreated rats.

### Mutagenicity
Data are not available concerning long-term effects on mutagenicity in humans or animals.

### Pregnancy/Reproduction
Fertility—Fertility was not impaired in male or female rats given doses of 18.75 and 37.5 mg per kg of body weight (mg/kg) a day.

Pregnancy—Adequate and well-controlled studies have not been done in humans.

No teratogenic effects were seen in animal studies. However, animal studies have shown an increased incidence of stillbirths when pemoline was administered at a dose of 37.5 mg/kg a day. Postnatal survival rate of offspring was reduced at doses of 18.75 and 37.5 mg/kg a day.

FDA Pregnancy Category B.

### Breast-feeding
It is not known whether pemoline is distributed into breast milk. However, problems in humans have not been documented.

### Pediatrics
Safety and efficacy of pemoline use in children less than 6 years of age have not been established.

Monitoring of growth should be conducted in children during long-term treatment with pemoline since suppression of growth has been reported with the use of central nervous system (CNS) stimulants in children.

Some medical authorities recommend drug-free periods during treatment to reassess the need for medication and to prevent growth suppression.

Pemoline may exacerbate symptoms of behavior disturbance and thought disorder in psychotic children.

### Drug interactions and/or related problems
The following drug interactions and/or related problems have been selected on the basis of their potential clinical significance (possible mechanism in parentheses where appropriate)—not necessarily inclusive (» = major clinical significance):

Note: Combinations containing any of the following medications, depending on the amount present, may also interact with this medication.

» Anticonvulsants
(pemoline may decrease the seizure threshold; therefore, dosage adjustments of the anticonvulsant may be necessary during concurrent use)

» CNS stimulation–producing medications, other (see *Appendix II*)
(concurrent use of other CNS stimulation–producing medications with pemoline may result in excessive CNS stimulation, causing nervousness, irritability, insomnia, or possibly convulsions or cardiac arrhythmias; close observation is recommended)

» Monoamine oxidase (MAO) inhibitors, including furazolidone, procarbazine, and selegiline
(concurrent use of MAO inhibitors with other CNS stimulation–producing medications has resulted in severe hypertensive and hyperpyretic crises, cardiac arrhythmias, convulsions, coma, headache, respiratory depression, vascular collapse, vomiting, and death; concurrent use of pemoline with an MAO inhibitor or use of pemoline within 14 days of discontinuing an MAO inhibitor is not recommended)

### Laboratory value alterations
The following have been selected on the basis of their potential clinical significance (possible effect in parentheses where appropriate)—not necessarily inclusive (» = major clinical significance):

With physiology/laboratory test values
Alanine aminotransferase (ALT [SGPT]) and
Aspartate aminotransferase (AST [SGOT]) and
Lactate dehydrogenase (LDH)
(values may be increased; increases often occur after several months of therapy; effects appear to be reversible upon withdrawal of pemoline in most patients; relationship to acute hepatic failure is unknown)

### Medical considerations/Contraindications
The medical considerations/contraindications included have been selected on the basis of their potential clinical significance (reasons given in parentheses where appropriate)—not necessarily inclusive (» = major clinical significance).

*Except under special circumstances, this medication should not be used if the following medical problem exists:*

» Hepatic function impairment
(acute hepatic failure, which resulted in death or liver transplantation in 11 of 13 reported cases, usually within 4 weeks of onset of symptoms, has been associated with pemoline use)

*Risk-benefit should be considered when the following medical problems exist:*

Drug abuse or dependence, history of
(increased potential for abuse of pemoline)

» Gilles de la Tourette's syndrome or other tics
(attacks may be precipitated)

» Psychosis
(symptoms of behavior disturbance and thought disorder may be exacerbated in psychotic children)

Renal function impairment
(excretion may be altered)

Sensitivity to pemoline

### Patient monitoring
The following may be especially important in patient monitoring (other tests may be warranted in some patients, depending on condition; » = major clinical significance):

Assessment of potential tolerance, dependence, or drug-seeking behavior
(recommended at periodic intervals during long-term therapy)

» Hepatic function determinations
(recommended prior to and at periodic intervals during therapy; pemoline therapy should be initiated only if baseline liver function tests are normal; if clinically significant abnormalities occur at any time during therapy, pemoline should be discontinued. It is not known whether reversible elevations in liver function tests are related to acute hepatic failure. Also, the onset of acute hepatic failure may not be predicted by liver function testing)

Monitoring for motor or vocal tics
(recommended prior to and at periodic intervals during therapy; in addition, family history of tic disorder should be assessed prior to initiation of pemoline therapy)

Monitoring of growth (both height and weight gain) in children
(recommended at periodic intervals during long-term therapy since suppression of growth has been reported with use of CNS stimulants in children)

Reassessment of need for therapy for attention-deficit hyperactivity disorder in children
(interruption of therapy at periodic intervals is recommended to determine if behavioral symptoms recur, requiring continuation of therapy)

## Side/Adverse Effects

Note: Acute hepatic failure, occurring at a rate of at least 4 to 17 times the rate expected in the general population, has been associated with pemoline use. Death or liver transplantation occurred in 11 of 13 reported cases, usually within 4 weeks of the onset of symptoms. In all cases, liver abnormalities were first seen 6 months or more after initiation of pemoline therapy. Jaundice may be the first sign of hepatic failure, although jaundice may be preceded by anorexia, dark urine, gastrointestinal symptoms, or malaise. Asymptomatic, reversible elevations in liver enzyme values also have occurred with pemoline use. The relationship between these enzyme value elevations and acute hepatic failure is unknown. If any sign of clinically significant hepatic dysfunction is seen, pemoline should be discontinued.

The following side/adverse effects have been selected on the basis of their potential clinical significance (possible signs and symptoms in parentheses where appropriate)—not necessarily inclusive:

**Those indicating need for medical attention**
Incidence rare
*Aplastic anemia* (shortness of breath, troubled breathing, wheezing, or tightness in chest; sores, ulcers, or white spots on lips or in mouth; swollen or painful glands; unusual bleeding or bruising); *dyskinesia* (uncontrolled movements of tongue, lips, face, arms, or legs); *hallucinations* (seeing, hearing, or feeling things that are not there); *hepatic dysfunction* (dark urine; loss of appetite; nausea and vomiting; unusual tiredness; yellow eyes or skin)—may be asymptomatic; *motor or vocal tics, or Tourette's syndrome* (movements or vocal sounds that you cannot control); *nystagmus* (uncontrolled side-to-side or circular movement of eyes); *seizures; skin rash*

**Those indicating need for medical attention only if they continue or are bothersome**
Incidence more frequent
*Anorexia* (loss of appetite); *insomnia* (trouble in sleeping); *weight loss*
Note: *Anorexia*, *insomnia*, and *weight loss* usually are reported early in therapy, and often resolve with continued pemoline therapy. For resolution of insomnia, a reduction of pemoline dosage may be required.

Incidence less frequent
*Dizziness; drowsiness; headache; increased irritability; mental depression; nausea; stomachache*

**Those indicating possible withdrawal and the need for medical attention if they occur after medication is discontinued**
*Abdominal pain; headache; mental depression; nausea; seizures; unusual behavior; unusual tiredness or weakness; vomiting*

## Overdose
For specific information on the agents used in the management of pemoline overdose, see:
- *Benzodiazepines (Systemic)* monograph;
- *Charcoal, Activated (Oral-Local)* monograph; and/or
- *Phentolamine (Systemic)* monograph.

For more information on the management of overdose or unintentional ingestion, **contact a Poison Control Center** (see *Poison Control Center Listing*).

**Clinical effects of overdose**
Note: The clinical effects of pemoline overdose are caused primarily by overstimulation of the central and sympathetic nervous systems.

The following effects have been selected on the basis of their potential clinical significance (possible signs and symptoms in parentheses where appropriate)—not necessarily inclusive:
Acute
*Agitation; confusion; euphoria* (false sense of well-being); *fast heartbeat; hallucinations* (seeing, hearing, or feeling things that are not there); *headache, severe; high fever; hypertension* (high blood pressure); *mydriasis* (large pupils); *muscle trembling or twitching; restlessness; seizures*—may be followed by coma; *sweating; vomiting*

**Treatment of overdose**
Treatment is symptomatic and supportive, and is essentially the same as that for an overdosage of any CNS stimulant.

To decrease absorption—Inducing emesis, using gastric lavage, and/or administering activated charcoal and a cathartic.

Specific treatment—Using a benzodiazepine to control excessive CNS stimulation and sympathomimetic effects if needed. Using intravenous phentolamine to control hypertension.

Monitoring—Monitoring cardiovascular and respiratory functioning.

Supportive care—Protecting patient from self-injury and from external stimuli. Patients in whom intentional overdose is confirmed or suspected should be referred for psychiatric consultation.

## Patient Consultation
As an aid to patient consultation, refer to Advice for the Patient, Pemoline (Systemic).

In providing consultation, consider emphasizing the following selected information (» = major clinical significance):

**Before using this medication**
» Conditions affecting use, especially:
   Sensitivity to pemoline
   Pregnancy—Animal studies have shown an increase in stillbirths and reduced postnatal survival rate

Use in children—Inhibition of growth has been reported with CNS stimulants, but data are inconclusive; drug-free periods are recommended; symptoms of behavior disturbance and thought disorder may be exacerbated in psychotic children

Other medications, especially anticonvulsants; monoamine oxidase inhibitors; or other CNS stimulation–producing medications

Other medical problems, especially hepatic function impairment, psychosis, or Tourette's syndrome

**Proper use of this medication**
Proper administration of chewable tablet: Tablet must be chewed
» May require 3 to 4 weeks of therapy to obtain optimal effects
» Importance of not taking more medication than the amount prescribed because of possible habit-forming potential
» Proper dosing
   Missed dose: Taking as soon as possible; if not remembered until the next day, skipping missed dose and continuing on schedule; not doubling doses
» Proper storage

**Precautions while using this medication**
Regular visits to physician to check progress during therapy
» Notifying physician immediately if darkening of urine or jaundice occurs
» Caution if dizziness occurs
» Suspected physical or psychological dependence; checking with physician

Checking with physician before discontinuing medication after long-term and high-dose therapy; gradual dosage reduction may be necessary to avoid possibility of withdrawal symptoms

**Side/adverse effects**
» Importance of discussing possible effects, including hepatic failure, with physician
   Signs of potential side effects, especially aplastic anemia, dyskinesia, hallucinations, hepatic dysfunction, motor or vocal tics or Tourette's syndrome, nystagmus, seizures, or skin rash

## General Dosing Information
Significant beneficial effects of pemoline may not be evident until the third or fourth week of therapy since clinical improvement is gradual.

Prolonged use of pemoline may result in psychological or physical dependence.

When symptoms of attention-deficit hyperactivity disorder are controlled in children, dosage reduction or interruption in therapy may be possible during the summer months and at other times when the child is under less stress; medication may be given on each of the 5 school days during the week, with medication-free weekends and school holidays.

When the medication is to be discontinued following high-dose and long-term administration, the dosage should be reduced gradually since abrupt withdrawal may result in extreme fatigue, mental depression, seizures, or unusual behavior.

**Diet/Nutrition**
Pemoline may be taken with or after meals to reduce anorexia.

## Oral Dosage Forms

### PEMOLINE TABLETS

**Usual pediatric dose**
Attention-deficit hyperactivity disorder—
Children up to 6 years of age: Safety and efficacy have not been established.
Children 6 years of age and older: Oral, initially 37.5 mg as a single dose each morning, the dosage being increased by 18.75 mg a day at one-week intervals until the desired response is obtained.

Note: The effective daily dosage for most patients ranges from 56.25 to 75 mg.

In small clinical studies of adults with attention-deficit hyperactivity disorder, some response to a daily dosage of 65 mg of pemoline was seen.

**Usual pediatric prescribing limits**
Attention-deficit hyperactivity disorder—
112.5 mg a day.

**Strength(s) usually available**
U.S.—
18.75 mg (Rx) [*Cylert* (scored; corn starch; gelatin; lactose; magnesium hydroxide; polyethylene glycol; talc)].
37.5 mg (Rx) [*Cylert* (scored; corn starch; FD&C Yellow No. 6; gelatin; lactose; magnesium hydroxide; polyethylene glycol; talc)].

75 mg (Rx) [*Cylert* (scored; corn starch; gelatin; iron oxide; lactose; magnesium hydroxide; polyethylene glycol; talc)].

Canada—
- 37.5 mg (Rx) [*Cylert* (scored; gelatin; lactose monohydrate; magnesium hydroxide; purified water; polyethylene glycol 8000; purified water; starch; talc; FD&C Yellow No. 6 aluminum lake)].
- 75 mg (Rx) [*Cylert* (scored; gelatin; iron oxide brown; lactose monohydrate; magnesium hydroxide; polyethylene glycol 8000; purified water; starch; talc)].

**Packaging and storage**
Store below 30 °C (86 °F), in a well-closed container, unless otherwise specified by manufacturer.

**Note**
Controlled substance in the U.S.

### PEMOLINE CHEWABLE TABLETS

**Usual pediatric dose**
See *Pemoline Tablets*.

**Usual pediatric prescribing limits**
See *Pemoline Tablets*.

**Strength(s) usually available**
U.S.—
- 37.5 mg (Rx) [*Cylert Chewable* (corn starch; FD&C Yellow No. 6; magnesium hydroxide; magnesium stearate; mannitol; polyethylene glycol; povidone; talc; artificial flavor)].

Canada—
Not commercially available.

**Packaging and storage**
Store below 30 °C (86 °F), in a well-closed container, unless otherwise specified by manufacturer.

**Auxiliary labeling**
- Must be chewed.

**Note**
Controlled substance in the U.S.

Revised: 01/07/98

**PENBUTOLOL**—See *Beta-adrenergic Blocking Agents (Systemic)*

# PENCICLOVIR   Topical—INTRODUCTORY VERSION

VA CLASSIFICATION (Primary): DE103

Commonly used brand name(s): *Denavir*.

Note: For a listing of dosage forms and brand names by country availability, see *Dosage Forms* section(s).

## Category
Antiviral (topical).

## Indications

**General considerations**
Penciclovir is an antiviral agent used to treat infections caused by herpes viruses. Penciclovir has *in vitro* inhibitory activity against herpes simplex virus types 1 and 2 (HSV-1 and HSV-2).

**Accepted**
Herpes labialis (treatment)—Topical penciclovir is indicated in the treatment of recurrent herpes labialis (cold sores) in adults.

## Pharmacology/Pharmacokinetics

**Physicochemical characteristics**
Chemical group—9-[4-hydroxy-3-(hydroxymethyl) butyl]guanine.
Molecular weight—253.26.
Solubility—At 20 °C 0.2 mg/mL in methanol; 1.3 mg/mL in propylene glycol; and 1.7 mg/mL in water; in aqueous buffer (pH 2) the solubility is 10 mg/mL.
Partition coefficient—In *n*-octanol/water at pH 7.5 penciclovir has a partition coefficient of 0.024 (logP = −1.62).

**Mechanism of action/Effect**
Penciclovir is phosphorylated by the enzyme thymidine kinase to a monophosphate form. The monophosphate is converted to penciclovir triphosphate by cellular phosphokinases. Studies show that penciclovir triphosphate inhibits herpes simplex virus polymerase competitively with deoxyguanosine triphosphate. This effect selectively inhibits herpes viral DNA synthesis and replication.

**Absorption**
Measurable concentrations of penciclovir have not been detected in plasma or urine following daily topical application in healthy male volunteers. Male volunteers were given doses approximately 67 times the estimated recommended clinical dose.
Systemic absorption of penciclovir following topical administration has not been studied in patients younger than 18 years of age.

## Precautions to Consider

**Carcinogenicity**
A 2-year study in mice and rats given famciclovir (the oral prodrug of penciclovir) in doses of 600 mg per kg of body weight (mg/kg) per day showed an increased incidence of mammary adenocarcinoma in female rats. This dose is approximately 395 times the maximum theoretical human exposure to penciclovir following application of the topical product, based on 24-hour area under the plasma concentration–time curve (AUC) comparisons.

A 2-year study in mice and rats given famciclovir in doses of up to 240 mg/kg per day found no increase of tumor incidence among male rats or in male and female mice at doses of up to 600 mg/kg per day. These doses are approximately 190 times and 100 times, respectively, the maximum theoretical human AUC for penciclovir.

**Mutagenicity**
*In vitro* studies found that penciclovir did not cause an increase in gene mutation in the Ames test or in unscheduled DNA repair in mammalian HeLaS3 cells. An increase in clastogenic response was seen with penciclovir in the mouse lymphoma cell assay and in human lymphocytes.
*In vivo* studies showed an increase in micronuclei in mouse bone marrow following intravenous administration of penciclovir at doses greater than or equal to 500 mg/kg, which is approximately 810 times the maximum recommended human dose.

**Pregnancy/Reproduction**
Fertility—Adequate and well controlled studies on the effects of topical penciclovir have not been done in humans. Intravenous administration of penciclovir at doses of 160 mg/kg per day and 100 mg/kg per day resulted in testicular toxicity in rats and dogs.

Pregnancy—Adequate and well-controlled studies have not been done in humans.

Studies done in rats and rabbits given intravenous doses of 80 mg/kg per day and 60 mg/kg per day, respectively, have shown no adverse effect on the course and outcome of pregnancy or on fetal development. The body surface area doses were 260 and 355 times, respectively, the maximum recommended human dose following topical application of penciclovir cream.

FDA Pregnancy Category B.

**Breast-feeding**
It is not known whether penciclovir is distributed into breast milk after topical application.
However, penciclovir was distributed into the milk of lactating rats at concentrations higher than those seen in plasma following oral administration of famciclovir (the oral prodrug of penciclovir).

**Pediatrics**
No information is available on the relationship of age to the effects of penciclovir in pediatric patients. Safety and efficacy have not been established.

**Geriatrics**
In patients 65 years of age and older, the adverse events profile was comparable to that observed in younger patients.

**Medical considerations/Contraindications**
The medical considerations/contraindications included have been selected on the basis of their potential clinical significance (reasons given in parentheses where appropriate)—not necessarily inclusive (» = major clinical significance).

*Except under special circumstances, this medication should not be used when the following problem exists:*
» Immune deficiency conditions in patients who are immunocompromised
   (the effect of penciclovir has not been established)

*Risk-benefit should be considered when the following medical problem exists:*
Sensitivity to penciclovir or other components of the formulation

## Side/Adverse Effects

The following side/adverse effects have been selected on the basis of their potential clinical significance (possible signs and symptoms in parentheses where appropriate)—not necessarily inclusive:

**Those indicating need for medical attention**
Incidence rare
   *Application site reaction*

**Those indicating need for medical attention only if they continue or are bothersome**
Incidence more frequent
   *Headache*—incidence 5.3%
Incidence less frequent
   *Hypoesthesia* (abnormally decreased sensitivity, particularly to touch); *skin rash, erythematous* (redness of the skin); *taste perversion* (change in sense of taste)

## Overdose

For more information on the management of overdose or unintentional ingestion, **contact a Poison Control Center** (see *Poison Control Center Listing*).
There is no information on overdose. Penciclovir is poorly absorbed following oral administration. Adverse reactions related to penciclovir ingestion are unlikely.

## Patient Consultation

As an aid to patient consultation, refer to *Advice for the Patient, Penciclovir (Topical)—Introductory Version*.
In providing consultation, consider emphasizing the following selected information (» = major clinical significance):

**Before using this medication**
» Conditions affecting use, especially:
   Sensitivity to penciclovir or other components of the formulation
   Other medical problems, especially immune deficiency conditions

**Proper use of this medication**
» Using only on herpes labialis on the lips and face

» Beginning as early as possible at the first signs of symptoms (during the prodrome stage or when lesion appears)
» Avoiding application in or near the eyes
» Avoiding application to mucous membranes or within oral cavity
» Proper dosing
   Missed dose: Applying as soon as possible; not applying if almost time for next dose
» Proper storage

**Side/adverse effects**
Signs of potential side effects, especially application site reaction

## General Dosing Information

Penciclovir cream is for external use only. Contact with eyes and mucous membranes should be avoided.
The effect of penciclovir has not been established in immunocompromised patients.

## Topical Dosage Forms

### PENCICLOVIR CREAM

**Usual adult dose**
Antiviral—
   Topical, to cold sores every two hours during waking hours for four days.

**Usual pediatric dose**
Safety and efficacy have not been established.

**Usual geriatric dose**
See *Usual adult dose*.

**Strength(s) usually available**
U.S.—
   1% (10 mg per gram) (Rx) [*Denavir* (cetomacrogol 1000 BP; cetostearyl alcohol; mineral oil; propylene glycol; purified water; white petrolatum)].

**Packaging and storage**
Store at or below 30 °C (86 °F). Protect from freezing.

**Auxiliary labeling**
• For external use only.
• Do not use in eyes.
• Continue medicine for full time of treatment.

Developed: 11/12/97
Revised: 08/12/98

# PENICILLAMINE  Systemic

VA CLASSIFICATION (Primary/Secondary): MS109/GU900; AD300
Commonly used brand name(s): *Cuprimine; Depen*.
Note:  For a listing of dosage forms and brand names by country availability, see *Dosage Forms* section(s).

## Category

Chelating agent; antirheumatic (disease-modifying); antiurolithic (cystine calculi); antidote (to heavy metals).

## Indications

Note:  Bracketed information in the *Indications* section refers to uses that are not included in U.S. product labeling.

**Accepted**
Wilson's disease (treatment)—Penicillamine is indicated in the treatment of symptomatic patients (those with tissue damage due to deposition of excessive copper in various tissues) and as prophylaxis against the development of tissue damage in asymptomatic patients.
Arthritis, rheumatoid (treatment);
[Felty's syndrome (treatment)][1] or
[Vasculitis, rheumatoid (treatment)][1]—Penicillamine is indicated in the treatment of patients with severe, active rheumatoid arthritis [including Felty's syndrome or rheumatoid vasculitis] who have not responded to other therapy.
Cystinuria (treatment) or
Renal calculi, cystine, recurrence (prophylaxis)—Penicillamine is indicated in the treatment of patients with excessive urinary cystine concentration and/or recurrent cystine stone formation who have not responded to or will not comply with other prophylactic measures.
[Toxicity, heavy metal (treatment)]—Penicillamine is less effective than other chelating agents (edetate calcium disodium or dimercaprol) for the treatment of severe lead poisoning. It is used as adjunctive treatment following initial therapy with another chelating agent. It may also be used as sole therapy in the treatment of asymptomatic patients with moderately elevated blood concentrations of lead. Penicillamine is also used in the treatment of poisoning due to other heavy metals, including mercury.

**Unaccepted**
Penicillamine is not effective in treating ankylosing spondylitis or psoriatic arthritis.

[1]Not included in Canadian product labeling.

## Pharmacology/Pharmacokinetics

**Physicochemical characteristics**
Molecular weight—149.21.

**Mechanism of action/Effect**
Chelating agent—
   Penicillamine chelates mercury, lead, copper, iron, and probably other heavy metals to form stable, soluble complexes that are readily excreted in the urine.
Antirheumatic—
   The mechanism of action of penicillamine in rheumatoid arthritis is not known, but may involve improvement of lymphocyte function. It markedly reduces IgM rheumatoid factor and immune complexes

in serum and synovial fluid, but does not significantly lower absolute concentrations of serum immunoglobulins. *In vitro*, penicillamine depresses T-cell but not B-cell activity. However, the relationship of these effects to the activity of penicillamine in rheumatoid arthritis is not known.

Antiurolithic (cystine calculi)—
Penicillamine combines chemically with cystine (cysteine–cysteine disulfide) to form penicillamine–cysteine disulfide, which is more soluble than cystine and is readily excreted. As a result, urinary cystine concentrations are lowered and the formation of cystine calculi is prevented. With prolonged treatment, existing cystine calculi may be gradually dissolved.

Antidote (to heavy metals)—
See *Chelating agent* above.

### Biotransformation
Hepatic.

### Onset of action
Wilson's disease—1 to 3 months.
Rheumatoid arthritis—2 to 3 months.

### Elimination
Renal and fecal.

## Precautions to Consider

### Cross-sensitivity and/or related problems
Patients sensitive to penicillin may be sensitive to this medication also.

### Carcinogenicity
Long-term animal carcinogenicity studies with penicillamine have not been done. However, in one study in autoimmune disease–prone NZB Hybrid mice receiving 400 mg per kg of body weight (mg/kg) intraperitoneally 5 days a week for 6 months, 5 of 10 of the animals tested developed lymphocytic leukemia.

### Pregnancy/Reproduction
Pregnancy—Controlled studies have not been done in pregnant women. However, birth defects have occurred in infants born to women who received penicillamine for rheumatoid arthritis or cystinuria during pregnancy.
In rheumatoid arthritis: It is recommended that penicillamine not be used in pregnant women with rheumatoid arthritis.
In cystinuria: It is recommended that penicillamine be avoided if possible in pregnant patients with cystinuria.
In Wilson's disease: Although birth defects have not been reported in infants of women receiving penicillamine for Wilson's disease, it is recommended that the daily dose be limited to 1 gram. Also, if cesarean section is planned, it is recommended that the daily dose be limited to 250 mg during the last 6 weeks of pregnancy and following surgery until wound healing is complete.
Studies in animals have shown that penicillamine causes skeletal defects, cleft palates, and an increased number of resorptions when administered to rats in doses 6 times the maximum recommended human dose.

### Breast-feeding
It is not known whether penicillamine is distributed into breast milk.

### Pediatrics
Appropriate studies with penicillamine have not been performed in the pediatric population. Efficacy for treatment of juvenile arthritis has not been established. However, pediatrics-specific problems that would limit the usefulness of this medication for other indications in children are not expected.

### Geriatrics
Patients 65 years of age or older may be more likely to develop hematologic toxicity with penicillamine. Also, elderly patients are more likely to have age-related renal function impairment, which increases the risk of adverse renal effects in patients receiving penicillamine for the treatment of rheumatoid arthritis.

### Dental
The leukopenic and thrombocytopenic effects of penicillamine may result in an increased incidence of microbial infection, delayed healing, and gingival bleeding. If leukopenia or thrombocytopenia occurs, dental work should be delayed until blood counts have returned to normal, and patients should be instructed in proper oral hygiene, including caution in use of regular toothbrushes, dental floss, and toothpicks.
Penicillamine may cause oral ulcerations, which in some cases have the appearance of aphthous stomatitis, and, rarely, cheilosis, glossitis, or gingivostomatitis.

### Drug interactions and/or related problems
The following drug interactions and/or related problems have been selected on the basis of their potential clinical significance (possible mechanism in parentheses where appropriate)—not necessarily inclusive (» = major clinical significance):

Note: Combinations containing any of the following medications, depending on the amount present, may also interact with this medication.

4-Aminoquinolines or
Bone marrow depressants (See *Appendix II*) or
» Gold compounds or
Immunosuppressants, except glucocorticoids or
» Phenylbutazone
(concurrent use with penicillamine may increase the potential for serious hematologic and/or renal adverse reactions; concurrent use with gold compounds or phenylbutazone is not recommended)
(concurrent use with 4-aminoquinolines may also increase the risk of severe dermatologic reactions)

Iron supplements
(concurrent use may decrease the effects of penicillamine; if necessary, iron may be administered in short courses, but a period of 2 hours should elapse between administration of penicillamine and iron)

Pyridoxine
(penicillamine may cause anemia or peripheral neuritis by acting as a pyridoxine antagonist or increasing renal excretion of pyridoxine; requirements for pyridoxine may be increased during penicillamine therapy)

### Laboratory value alterations
The following have been selected on the basis of their potential clinical significance (possible effect in parentheses where appropriate)—not necessarily inclusive (» = major clinical significance):

With physiology/laboratory test values
Renal imaging using technetium Tc 99m gluceptate
(penicillamine may cause transchelation of technetium Tc 99m gluceptate to a compound excreted through the hepatobiliary system, resulting in gallbladder visualization; gallbladder visualization may mimic abnormal kidney localization on posterior views of renal images)

### Medical considerations/Contraindications
The medical considerations/contraindications included have been selected on the basis of their potential clinical significance (reasons given in parentheses where appropriate)—not necessarily inclusive (» = major clinical significance).

*Risk-benefit should be considered when the following medical problems exist:*

» Agranulocytosis or aplastic anemia, penicillamine-related, history of (risk of recurrence)
Sensitivity to penicillamine, history of
*In rheumatoid arthritis patients*
Renal function impairment, current or history of (increased risk of adverse renal effects)

### Patient monitoring
The following may be especially important in patient monitoring (other tests may be warranted in some patients, depending on condition; » = major clinical significance):

Blood cell counts, white and differential and
Hemoglobin determinations and
Platelet counts, direct and
Urinalyses, especially for protein and cells
(recommended at least every 2 weeks during the first 6 months of therapy, then monthly thereafter during therapy; however, more frequent testing of blood cell count and urinalyses may be advisable during the first 6 weeks of therapy and for several weeks following an increase in maintenance dosage)

Hepatic function determinations
(recommended every 6 months during the first 18 months of therapy because of possible intrahepatic cholestasis and toxic hepatitis)

*In cystinuria*
X-ray for renal calculi
(recommended annually during therapy since cystine stones may form rapidly, sometimes within 6 months)

*In rheumatoid arthritis*
Urinary protein determinations, 24-hour
(recommended at 1- to 2-week intervals for those patients who develop moderate degrees of proteinuria)

*In Wilson's disease*
  Urinary copper analyses, 24-hour
    (recommended prior to and soon after initiation of therapy to determine optimal dosage; during continued therapy, recommended approximately every 3 months; urine specimens must be collected in copper-free glassware)

## Side/Adverse Effects

The following side/adverse effects have been selected on the basis of their potential clinical significance (possible signs and symptoms in parentheses where appropriate)—not necessarily inclusive:

### Those indicating need for medical attention
Incidence more frequent
  ***Allergic reaction*** (fever; joint pain; skin rash, hives, and/or itching; swelling of lymph glands); ***stomatitis*** (ulcers, sores, or white spots in mouth)

Incidence less frequent
  ***Agranulocytosis*** (sore throat and fever with or without chills; sores, ulcers, or white spots on lips or in mouth); ***aplastic anemia*** (shortness of breath, troubled breathing, tightness in chest, and/or wheezing; sores, ulcers, or white spots on lips or in mouth; swollen and/or painful glands; unusual bleeding or bruising; unusual tiredness or weakness); ***glomerulopathy, possible impending*** (bloody or cloudy urine; swelling of face, feet, or lower legs; weight gain)—glomerulopathy may progress to nephrotic syndrome; ***hemolytic anemia*** (troubled breathing, exertional; unusual tiredness or weakness); ***leukopenia*** (usually asymptomatic; fever or chills; cough or hoarseness; lower back or side pain; painful or difficult urination)—rarely; ***thrombocytopenia*** (usually asymptomatic; rarely, unusual bleeding or bruising; black, tarry stools; blood in urine or stools; pinpoint red spots on skin)

Incidence rare
  ***Bronchiolitis, obstructive*** (coughing, wheezing, or shortness of breath); ***dermatitis, exfoliative*** (fever with or without chills; red, thickened, or scaly skin; swollen and/or painful glands; unusual bruising); ***Goodpasture's syndrome*** (difficulty in breathing, spitting blood, unusual tiredness or weakness); ***jaundice, cholestatic*** (dark urine, itching, pale stools, yellow eyes or skin); ***myasthenia gravis syndrome*** (difficulty in breathing, chewing, talking, or swallowing; double vision; muscle weakness); ***necrolysis, toxic epidermal*** (redness, tenderness, itching, burning, or peeling of skin; sore throat; fever with or without chills; red or irritated eyes); ***neuritis, optic*** (eye pain, blurred vision, or any change in vision)—may be caused by pyridoxine deficiency; ***pancreatitis or peptic ulcer reactivation;*** (abdominal or stomach pain, severe); ***ringing or buzzing in ears; systemic lupus erythematosus (SLE)–like syndrome*** (skin rash, hives, and/or itching; blisters on skin; chest pain; general feeling of discomfort or illness; joint pain)

### Those indicating need for medical attention only if continuing or bothersome
Incidence more frequent
  ***Diarrhea; lessening or loss of taste sense; loss of appetite; nausea or vomiting; stomach pain, mild***

## Patient Consultation

As an aid to patient consultation, refer to *Advice for the Patient, Penicillamine (Systemic)*.

In providing consultation, consider emphasizing the following selected information (» = major clinical significance):

### Before using this medication
» Conditions affecting use, especially:
    Sensitivity to penicillamine or penicillin, history of
    Pregnancy—Has been reported to cause birth defects in humans
    Use in the elderly—Increased risk of hematologic toxicity
    Other medications, especially gold compounds and phenylbutazone
    Other medical problems, especially a history of penicillamine-induced agranulocytosis or aplastic anemia

### Proper use of this medication
*For patients with cystinuria*
  Importance of high fluid intake, especially at night
  Possible need for low-methionine diet
*For patients with rheumatoid arthritis*
  Taking medication on an empty stomach
  Improvement in condition may require 2 to 3 months of therapy
*For patients with Wilson's disease*
  Taking medication on an empty stomach
  Possible need for low-copper diet
  Improvement in condition may require 1 to 3 months of therapy
*For patients with lead poisoning*
  Taking medication on an empty stomach

*For all patients*
» Compliance with therapy; checking with physician before discontinuing medication since interruption of therapy may cause sensitivity reactions when therapy is reinstituted
» Proper dosing
  Missed dose: If dosing schedule is—
    Once a day: Taking as soon as possible; not taking if not remembered until next day; not doubling doses
    Two times a day: Taking as soon as possible; not taking if almost time for next dose; not doubling doses
    More than two times a day: Taking if remembered within an hour; not taking if not remembered until later; not doubling doses
» Proper storage

### Precautions while using this medication
Regular visits to physician to check progress during therapy
Caution if any kind of surgery (including dental surgery) is required because of the effects of penicillamine on collagen and elastin
Avoiding concurrent use of iron-containing medications

### Side/adverse effects
Signs of potential side effects, especially allergic reactions, stomatitis, blood dyscrasias, glomerulopathy, obstructive bronchiolitis, exfoliative dermatitis, Goodpasture's syndrome, jaundice, myasthenia gravis syndrome, toxic epidermal necrolysis, optic neuritis, pancreatitis, peptic ulcer reactivation, ringing or buzzing in ears, and SLE-like syndrome

## General Dosing Information

Penicillamine therapy should be continued on a daily basis because interruptions for even a few days may cause sensitivity reactions following reinstitution of therapy.

If surgery is necessary during penicillamine therapy, the dosage should be reduced to 250 mg daily because of the effects on collagen and elastin. Reinstitution of full therapy should be delayed until wound healing is complete.

In the treatment of cystinuria or Wilson's disease, a daily dose of 250 mg may be administered with the dosage being increased gradually to the optimum dosage if the patient cannot tolerate the usual initial dose of penicillamine. This may also help to reduce the incidence of adverse reactions.

Patients with rheumatoid arthritis (whose nutrition is impaired), cystinuria, or Wilson's disease should be given 25 mg of pyridoxine daily during therapy because penicillamine increases the intake requirement for this vitamin.

Impairment of taste may occur with penicillamine therapy. Except for patients with Wilson's disease, normal taste acuity may be restored while therapy with penicillamine is continued by administering 5 to 10 mg of copper daily (5 to 10 drops of a 4% cupric sulfate solution may be administered in fruit juice 2 times a day).

If therapy is interrupted for any reason, it should be reinstituted with a small dosage, which is gradually increased until full dosage is achieved.

### In cystinuria
The daily dosage of penicillamine may range from 1 to 4 grams.

The dosage of penicillamine should be based on measurements of urinary cystine excretion. Urinary cystine excretion should be maintained at less than 100 mg daily in patients with a history of renal calculi and/or pain, or at 100 to 200 mg daily in patients without a history of renal calculi.

If administration in 4 equally divided doses is not possible, the larger dose should be given at bedtime; or, if the occurrence of side effects requires dosage reduction, the bedtime dose should be one of the doses retained.

To help prevent the formation of cystine stones, a high fluid intake is recommended. The patient should drink 500 mL of water at bedtime and another 500 mL once during the night when the urine is more concentrated and more acidic than during the day. Usually the greater the fluid intake, the lower the required dose of penicillamine.

A diet low in methionine may be necessary to minimize cystine production. This diet is not recommended in growing children or during pregnancy because of its low protein content.

### In lead poisoning
Penicillamine should be administered on an empty stomach, 2 hours before meals or at least 3 hours after meals.

### In rheumatoid arthritis
Penicillamine should be given on an empty stomach (at least 1 hour before meals or 2 hours after meals) and at least 1 hour apart from any other medication, food, or milk in order to achieve maximum absorption and to reduce the possibility of inactivation by metal binding.

Dosage up to 500 mg per day may be given as a single dose. Dosage above 500 mg per day should be administered in divided doses.

During initial therapy, if the dosage has been increased up to 1 to 1.5 grams of penicillamine per day and after 3 to 4 months there is still no improvement in the patient's condition, the medication should be discontinued.

The maintenance dosage of penicillamine may need adjustment during the course of treatment. Changes in maintenance dosage levels may not be noticed clinically or in the erythrocytic sedimentation rate for 2 or 3 months after each dosage adjustment.

For those patients who require an increase in the maintenance dosage to achieve maximal disease suppression after the first 6 to 9 months of therapy, the daily dosage may be increased by 125 or 250 mg per day at 3-month intervals up to 1.5 grams per day.

**In Wilson's disease**

Dosage of penicillamine should be determined by measurements of urinary copper excretion to achieve and maintain a negative copper balance.

Penicillamine should be administered on an empty stomach (30 minutes to 1 hour before meals and at least 2 hours after the evening meal).

The dosage may be increased as indicated by urinary copper analyses, but dosage greater than 2 grams daily is usually not necessary.

In conjunction with penicillamine therapy, a low-copper diet of less than 2 mg daily should be maintained. Such a diet should exclude, most importantly, chocolate, nuts, shellfish, mushrooms, liver, molasses, broccoli, and cereals enriched with copper. Distilled or demineralized water should be used if the patient's drinking water contains more than 100 mcg (0.1 mg) of copper per liter.

Sulfurated potash (10 to 40 mg) may be administered with meals to minimize absorption of copper (capsules of sulfurated potash may be prepared by using light magnesium oxide as a diluent).

## Oral Dosage Forms

Note: Bracketed uses in the *Dosage Forms* section refer to categories of use and/or indications that are not included in U.S. product labeling.

### PENICILLAMINE CAPSULES USP

**Usual adult and adolescent dose**

Chelating agent—
 Oral, 250 mg four times a day.
Antirheumatic—
 Oral, initially 125 or 250 mg once a day as a single dose, the dosage being increased, if necessary and tolerated, by adding 125 or 250 mg per day at two- to three-month intervals up to a maximum of 1.5 grams per day.
 Note: Some clinicians recommend a maximum dose of 1 gram per day in rheumatoid arthritis.
Antiurolithic—
 Oral, 500 mg four times a day.
[Antidote (to heavy metals)]—
 Oral, 500 mg to 1.5 grams per day for one to two months.

**Usual pediatric dose**

Chelating agent—
 Infants over 6 months of age and young children: Oral, 250 mg as a single dose administered in fruit juice.
 Older children: See *Usual adult and adolescent dose*.
Antirheumatic—
 Efficacy and dosage have not been established.
Antiurolithic—
 Oral, 7.5 mg per kg of body weight four times a day.
[Antidote (to heavy metals)]—
 Oral, 30 to 40 mg per kg of body weight or 600 to 750 mg per square meter of body surface per day for one to six months.

**Usual geriatric dose**

Oral, initially 125 mg per day. Dosage may be increased, if necessary and tolerated, by adding 125 mg per day at two- to three-month intervals, up to a maximum of 750 mg per day.

**Strength(s) usually available**

U.S.—
 125 mg (Rx) [*Cuprimine* (lactose)].
 250 mg (Rx) [*Cuprimine* (lactose)].
Canada—
 125 mg (Rx) [*Cuprimine* (lactose)].
 250 mg (Rx) [*Cuprimine* (lactose)].

**Packaging and storage**

Store below 40 °C (104 °F), preferably between 15 and 30 °C (59 and 86 °F), unless otherwise specified by manufacturer. Store in a tight container.

**Auxiliary labeling**

• Take on an empty stomach.

### PENICILLAMINE TABLETS USP

**Usual adult and adolescent dose**

Chelating agent—
 Oral, 250 mg four times a day.
Antirheumatic—
 Oral, initially 125 or 250 mg once a day as a single dose, the dosage being increased, if necessary and tolerated, by adding 125 or 250 mg per day at two- to three-month intervals up to a maximum of 1.5 grams per day.
 Note: Some clinicians recommend a maximum dose of 1 gram per day in rheumatoid arthritis.
Antiurolithic—
 Oral, 500 mg four times a day.
[Antidote (to heavy metals)]—
 Oral, 500 mg to 1.5 grams per day for one to two months.

**Usual pediatric dose**

Chelating agent—
 Infants over 6 months of age and young children: Oral, 250 mg as a single dose administered in fruit juice.
 Older children: See *Usual adult and adolescent dose*.
Antirheumatic—
 Dosage has not been established.
Antiurolithic—
 Oral, 7.5 mg per kg of body weight four times a day.
[Antidote (to heavy metals)]—
 Oral, 30 to 40 mg per kg of body weight or 600 to 750 mg per square meter of body surface per day for one to six months.

**Usual geriatric dose**

Oral, initially 125 mg per day. Dosage may be increased, if necessary and tolerated, by adding 125 mg per day at two- to three-month intervals, up to a maximum of 750 mg per day.

**Strength(s) usually available**

U.S.—
 250 mg (Rx) [*Depen* (scored; lactose)].
Canada—
 250 mg (Rx) [*Depen* (scored; lactose)].

**Packaging and storage**

Store below 40 °C (104 °F), preferably between 15 and 30 °C (59 and 86 °F), unless otherwise specified by manufacturer. Store in a tight container.

**Auxiliary labeling**

• Take on an empty stomach.

Revised: July 1990
Interim revision: 09/01/94

---

**PENICILLIN G**—See *Penicillins (Systemic)*

---

# PENICILLINS  Systemic

This monograph includes information on the following: 1) Amoxicillin; 2) Ampicillin; 3) Bacampicillin; 4) Carbenicillin; 5) Cloxacillin; 6) Dicloxacillin†; 7) Flucloxacillin*; 8) Methicillin†; 9) Mezlocillin†; 10) Nafcillin; 11) Oxacillin†; 12) Penicillin G; 13) Penicillin V; 14) Piperacillin; 15) Pivampicillin*; 16) Pivmecillinam*; 17) Ticarcillin.

INN:
 Amoxicillin—Amoxicilline
 Carbenicillin indanyl sodium—Carindacillin
 Methicillin†—Meticillin
 Penicillin G benzathine—Benzathine benzylpenicillin
 Penicillin V—Phenoxymethylpenicillin

BAN:
 Amoxicillin—Amoxycillin
 Carbenicillin indanyl sodium—Carindacillin
 Penicillin G benzathine—Benzathine penicillin

Penicillin G procaine—Procaine penicillin
Penicillin V—Phenoxymethylpenicillin

VA CLASSIFICATION (Primary):
Amoxicillin—AM112
Ampicillin—AM112
Bacampicillin—AM112
Carbenicillin—AM114
Cloxacillin—AM113
Dicloxacillin—AM113
Flucloxacillin—AM113
Methicillin—AM113
Mezlocillin—AM114
Nafcillin—AM113
Oxacillin—AM113
Penicillin G—AM111
Penicillin V—AM111
Piperacillin—AM114
Pivampicillin—AM112
Pivmecillinam—AM112
Ticarcillin—AM114

Commonly used brand name(s): *Amoxil*[1]; *Ampicin*[2]; *Apo-Amoxi*[1]; *Apo-Ampi*[2]; *Apo-Cloxi*[5]; *Apo-Pen VK*[13]; *Ayercillin*[12]; *Bactocill*[11]; *Beepen-VK*[13]; *Betapen-VK*[13]; *Bicillin L-A*[12]; *Cloxapen*[5]; *Crysticillin 300 A.S*[12]; *Dycill*[6]; *Dynapen*[6]; *Fluclox*[7]; *Geocillin*[4]; *Geopen*[4]; *Geopen Oral*[4]; *Ledercillin VK*[13]; *Megacillin*[12]; *Mezlin*[9]; *Nadopen-V*[13]; *Nadopen-V 200*[13]; *Nadopen-V 400*[13]; *Nafcil*[10]; *Nallpen*[10]; *Novamoxin*[1]; *Novo-Ampicillin*[2]; *Novo-Cloxin*[5]; *Novo-Pen-VK*[13]; *Nu-Amoxi*[1]; *Nu-Ampi*[2]; *Nu-Cloxi*[5]; *Nu-Pen-VK*[13]; *Omnipen*[2]; *Omnipen-N*[2]; *Orbenin*[5]; *PVF*[13]; *PVF K*[13]; *Pathocil*[6]; *Pen Vee*[13]; *Pen Vee K*[13]; *Pen-Vee*[13]; *Penbritin*[2]; *Penglobe*[3]; *Pentids*[12]; *Permapen*[12]; *Pfizerpen*[12]; *Pfizerpen-AS*[12]; *Pipracil*[14]; *Polycillin*[2]; *Polycillin-N*[2]; *Polymox*[1]; *Pondocillin*[15]; *Principen*[2]; *Prostaphlin*[11]; *Pyopen*[4]; *Selexid*[16]; *Spectrobid*[3]; *Staphcillin*[8]; *Tegopen*[5]; *Ticar*[17]; *Totacillin*[2]; *Totacillin-N*[2]; *Trimox*[1]; *Unipen*[10]; *V-Cillin K*[13]; *Veetids*[13]; *Wycillin*[12]; *Wymox*[1].

Note: For a listing of dosage forms and brand names by country availability, see *Dosage Forms* section(s).

*Not commercially available in U.S.
†Not commercially available in Canada.

## Category
Antibacterial (systemic).

## Indications
Note: Bracketed information in the *Indications* section refers to uses that are not included in U.S. product labeling.

### General considerations
Penicillins can be classified into four broad categories, each covering a different spectrum of activity. The natural penicillins (penicillin G and penicillin V) have activity against many gram-positive organisms, gram-negative cocci, and some other gram-negative organisms. The aminopenicillins (ampicillin, amoxicillin, bacampicillin, and pivampicillin) have activity against penicillin-sensitive gram-positive bacteria, as well as *Escherichia coli*, *Proteus mirabilis*, *Salmonella* sp., *Shigella* sp., and *Haemophilus influenzae*. The antistaphylococcal penicillins (cloxacillin, dicloxacillin, flucloxacillin, methicillin, nafcillin, and oxacillin) are also active against beta-lactamase–producing staphylococci. The antipseudomonal penicillins (carbenicillin, mezlocillin, piperacillin, and ticarcillin) have less activity against gram-positive organisms than the natural penicillins or aminopenicillins; however, unlike the other penicillins, these penicillins are active against some gram-negative bacilli, including *Pseudomonas aeruginosa*.

Resistance to penicillins is thought to be due to 3 main mechanisms. The first is alteration of the antibiotic target sites' penicillin-binding proteins (PBPs); the second is inactivation of the penicillin by bacterially produced enzymes (beta-lactamases); and the third is decreased permeability of the cell wall to penicillins. Of these 3 mechanisms, production of beta-lactamase is the most common and the most important.

The spectrums of activity of penicillin G and penicillin V include *Staphylococcus* and *Streptococcus* species. However, most strains of *S. aureus* and *S. epidermidis* produce beta-lactamases, which destroy these penicillins. A small proportion of community-acquired strains (5 to 15%) of *S. aureus* remains susceptible to penicillin G. Penicillin G also has activity against the gram-negative cocci, *Neisseria meningitidis* and *N. gonorrhoeae*. However, resistance to penicillin G by beta-lactamase–producing *N. gonorrhoeae* has become a widespread problem in many parts of the world. Penicillin G is more active than penicillin V against *Haemophilus* and *Neisseria* species. Some other organisms for which penicillin G has good activity include *Actinomyces israelii*, *Bacillus anthracis*, oropharyngeal *Bacteroides* species, *Borrelia burgdorferi*, *Clostridium* sp., *Corynebacterium diphtheriae*, *Erysipelothrix rhusiopathiae*, *Listeria monocytogenes*, *Spirillium minor*, *Streptobacillus moniliformis*, and *Treponema pallidum*.

The aminopenicillins have activity against *H. influenzae*, *E. coli*, *P. mirabilis*, and *Salmonella* and some *Shigella* species, while also retaining activity against penicillin-sensitive gram-positive bacteria. However, many Enterobacteriaceae, *H. influenzae*, *Salmonella* and *Shigella* species are resistant to these penicillins because of beta-lactamase production by these organisms. Bacampicillin and pivampicillin are esters of ampicillin that are hydrolyzed during absorption to liberate ampicillin; this results in increased bioavailability and serum concentrations of ampicillin. Amoxicillin has the same *in vitro* activity as ampicillin, although amoxicillin has slightly better activity against *Enterococcus faecalis*, *E. coli*, and *Salmonella* sp.

The antistaphylococcal penicillins were developed to treat beta-lactamase–producing staphylococci. These penicillins are active against both penicillin-sensitive and penicillin-resistant staphylococci, as well as *S. pyogenes* and *S. pneumoniae*. However, they are less potent than penicillin G against penicillin-sensitive bacteria, and they have very little activity against *E. faecalis* and gram-negative organisms. Nafcillin has more intrinsic activity than methicillin against staphylococci and streptococci. The mechanism of methicillin-resistant *S. aureus* is not due to beta-lactamase production by the organism, but results from an alteration of penicillin binding proteins. Methicillin-resistant staphylococci are also resistant to the other penicillins in this category.

The antipseudomonal penicillins are active against a wide variety of gram-negative bacteria, including *Pseudomonas aeruginosa*, *Enterobacter*, *Morganella*, and *Providencia* species. These penicillins are less active than ampicillin against streptococci and enterococci; however, their activity against non-beta-lactamase–producing *Haemophilus*, *N. meningitidis*, and *N. gonorrhoeae* is similar to that of ampicillin. These agents are also destroyed by beta-lactamases produced by gram-positive and some gram-negative organisms. Ticarcillin is 2 to 4 times more active than carbenicillin against *P. aeruginosa*. Mezlocillin has a spectrum of activity similar to that of carbenicillin and ticarcillin; however, mezlocillin has better activity against non-beta-lactamase–producing strains of *Klebsiella*, *H. influenzae*, and *B. fragilis*. Piperacillin has excellent activity against streptococci, *Neisseria*, and *Haemophilus* species, and is the most active penicillin against *P. aeruginosa*.

Another penicillin, which does not neatly fit into any of these four categories, is pivmecillinam. Pivmecillinam is hydrolyzed during absorption to liberate the active agent, mecillinam. Mecillinam has poor activity against gram-positive organisms, *Haemophilus*, and *Neisseria* species; however, it has very good activity against many gram-negative bacteria, including *E. coli*, many *Klebsiella*, *Enterobacter*, and *Citrobacter* species. It has variable activity against *Proteus* sp. and does not inhibit *P. aeruginosa* or anaerobes, such as *B. fragilis* or *Clostridium* species.

### Accepted
Actinomycosis (treatment)— Penicillin G (parenteral) and [penicillin V][1] are indicated in the treatment of actinomycosis caused by *Actinomyces* sp.

Anthrax (treatment)—Penicillin G (parenteral), [penicillin V][1], and penicillin G procaine are indicated in the treatment of anthrax caused by *Bacillus anthracis*.

Arthritis, gonococcal (treatment)—Penicillin G (parenteral) is indicated in the treatment of infective arthritis caused by susceptible strains of *Neisseria gonorrhoeae*.

Bejel (treatment)—Penicillin G benzathine and penicillin G procaine are indicated in the treatment of bejel caused by *Treponema pallidum endemicum*.

Bone and joint infections (treatment)—Carbenicillin (parenteral), cloxacillin (parenteral), [methicillin][1], [nafcillin (parenteral)][1], [oxacillin (parenteral)][1], [penicillin G (parenteral)][1], and piperacillin are indicated in the treatment of bone and joint infections caused by susceptible organisms.

Bronchitis, bacterial exacerbations (treatment)—Amoxicillin, ampicillin, bacampicillin, cloxacillin (oral), dicloxacillin, penicillin V, and pivampicillin are indicated in the treatment of bronchitis caused by susceptible organisms.

Diphtheria (prophylaxis)—Penicillin G (parenteral), [penicillin G benzathine][1], penicillin G procaine, and penicillin V are indicated in the prophylaxis of diphtheria, caused by *Corynebacterium diphtheriae*, as an adjunct to antitoxin.

Endocarditis, bacterial (prophylaxis)—[Amoxicillin][1], [ampicillin][1], penicillin G (parenteral), and penicillin V are indicated in the prophylaxis of bacterial endocarditis caused by susceptible organisms.

Endocarditis, bacterial (treatment)—Ampicillin (parenteral), carbenicillin (parenteral), cloxacillin (parenteral), [methicillin]¹, [nafcillin (parenteral)]¹, [oxacillin (parenteral)], [penicillin G (parenteral)]¹ and penicillin G procaine are indicated in the treatment of bacterial endocarditis caused by susceptible organisms.

Erysipelas (treatment)—Penicillin G (parenteral), penicillin V, and penicillin G procaine are indicated in the treatment of erysipelas caused by susceptible strains of group A streptococci.

Erysipeloid (treatment)—Penicillin G (parenteral), [penicillin V]¹, [penicillin G benzathine]¹, and [penicillin G procaine]¹ are indicated in the treatment of erysipeloid, including endocarditis and septicemia, caused by *Erysipelothrix rhusiopathiae*.

Gingivitis, acute, necrotizing, ulcerative (treatment)—Penicillin G (oral and parenteral), penicillin V, and penicillin G procaine are indicated in the treatment of acute, necrotizing, ulcerative gingivitis, also called Vincent's angina or "trench mouth," a pharyngeal and tonsillar infection caused by anaerobes and spirochetes.

Gonorrhea, endocervical and urethral, uncomplicated (treatment)—Amoxicillin, in combination with probenecid, and [penicillin G (parenteral)]¹ are indicated in the treatment of gonorrhea caused by susceptible strains of *Neisseria gonorrhoeae*. However, because of resistance to penicillin, other agents, such as ceftriaxone, cefixime, or ciprofloxacin, are considered to be first-line agents.

Intra-abdominal infections (treatment)—Carbenicillin (parenteral), mezlocillin, [penicillin G (parenteral)]¹, piperacillin, and ticarcillin are indicated in the treatment of intra-abdominal infections caused by susceptible organisms.

Listeriosis (treatment)—[Ampicillin (parenteral)]¹ and penicillin G (parenteral) are indicated in the treatment of listeriosis caused by *Listeria monocytogenes*.

Meningitis, bacterial (treatment)—Ampicillin (parenteral), carbenicillin (parenteral), [nafcillin (parenteral)]¹, [oxacillin (parenteral)]¹, penicillin G (parenteral), [piperacillin]¹, and [ticarcillin]¹ are indicated in the treatment of bacterial meningitis caused by susceptible organisms.

Otitis media, acute (treatment)—Amoxicillin, ampicillin, bacampicillin, penicillin G procaine, penicillin G (oral), penicillin V, and pivampicillin are indicated in the treatment of acute otitis media caused by susceptible organisms.

*Pasteurella multocida* infections (treatment)—[Ampicillin (parenteral)]¹, penicillin G (parenteral), and [penicillin V]¹ are indicated in the treatment of infections caused by *Pasteurella multocida*.

Pelvic infections, female (treatment)—[Carbenicillin (parenteral)]¹, mezlocillin, piperacillin, and ticarcillin are indicated in the treatment of female pelvic infections caused by susceptible organisms.

Pericarditis, bacterial (treatment)—Penicillin G (parenteral), penicillin G procaine, and [nafcillin (parenteral)]¹ are indicated in the treatment of bacterial pericarditis caused by susceptible organisms.

Pharyngitis, bacterial (treatment)—Amoxicillin, ampicillin, bacampicillin, cloxacillin (oral), dicloxacillin, flucloxacillin, penicillin G benzathine, penicillin G (oral), penicillin V, and pivampicillin are indicated in the treatment of bacterial pharyngitis caused by susceptible organisms.

Pinta (treatment)—Penicillin G benzathine and penicillin G procaine are indicated in the treatment of pinta caused by *Treponema carateum*.

Pneumonia, bacterial (treatment)—Amoxicillin, ampicillin, bacampicillin, carbenicillin (parenteral), cloxacillin, dicloxacillin, mezlocillin, penicillin G (parenteral), penicillin G procaine, piperacillin, and ticarcillin are indicated in the treatment of bacterial pneumonia caused by susceptible organisms.

Prostatitis (treatment)—Carbenicillin (oral) is indicated in the treatment of prostatitis caused by susceptible organisms.

Rat-bite fever (treatment)—Penicillin G (parenteral), penicillin G procaine, and [penicillin V]¹ are indicated in the treatment of rat-bite fever caused by *Streptobacillus moniliformis* or *Spirillum minor*.

Rheumatic fever (prophylaxis)—Penicillin V, and penicillin G benzathine are indicated in the prophylaxis of rheumatic fever caused by group A streptococci.

Scarlet fever (treatment)—Penicillin V, penicillin G procaine, and [penicillin G (parenteral)]¹ are indicated in the treatment of scarlet fever caused by group A streptococci.

Septicemia, bacterial (treatment)—Ampicillin (parenteral), carbenicillin (parenteral), cloxacillin (parenteral), methicillin, mezlocillin, nafcillin (parenteral), oxacillin (parenteral), penicillin G (parenteral), penicillin G procaine, piperacillin, and ticarcillin are indicated in the treatment of bacterial septicemia caused by susceptible organisms.

Sinusitis (treatment)—Amoxicillin, ampicillin, bacampicillin, cloxacillin, flucloxacillin, methicillin, nafcillin, oxacillin, and penicillin V are indicated in the treatment of sinusitis caused by susceptible organisms.

Skin and soft tissue infections (treatment)—Carbenicillin (parenteral), cloxacillin, dicloxacillin, flucloxacillin, methicillin, mezlocillin, nafcillin, oxacillin, penicillin G procaine, [penicillin G (parenteral)]¹, penicillin V, piperacillin, pivampicillin, and ticarcillin are indicated in the treatment of skin and soft tissue infections caused by susceptible organisms.

Syphilis (treatment)—Penicillin G benzathine is indicated in the treatment of primary, secondary, and early and late latent syphilis. Penicillin G (parenteral) and penicillin G procaine, in combination with probenecid, are indicated in the treatment of tertiary syphilis. Penicillin G (parenteral) is indicated in the treatment of neurosyphilis. Penicillin G benzathine fails to achieve adequate concentrations in the cerebrospinal fluid.

Tetanus (treatment)—Penicillin G (parenteral) is indicated in the treatment of the infecting organism in tetanus, *Clostridium tetani*.

Urinary tract infections, bacterial (treatment)—Amoxicillin, ampicillin, bacampicillin, carbenicillin (oral and parenteral), mezlocillin, piperacillin, pivampicillin, pivmecillinam, and ticarcillin are indicated in the treatment of bacterial urinary tract infections caused by susceptible organisms.

Yaws (treatment)—Penicillin G benzathine, penicillin G procaine, and [penicillin G (parenteral)]¹ are indicated in the treatment of yaws caused by *Treponema pallidum pertenue*.

[Chlamydial infections in pregnant women (treatment)]¹—Amoxicillin and ampicillin are used in the treatment of chlamydial infections in pregnant women who cannot tolerate erythromycin.

[Gas gangrene infections (treatment)]¹—Penicillin G (parenteral) is used in the treatment of gas gangrene caused by *Clostridium* sp.

[Gastritis, *Helicobacter pylori*-associated (treatment adjunct)]¹ or

[Ulcer, peptic, *Helicobacter pylori*-associated (treatment adjunct)]¹—Amoxicillin is used, in combination with metronidazole and bismuth subsalicylate, in the treatment of gastritis and peptic ulcer disease caused by *H. pylori*.

[Leptospirosis (treatment)]¹—Ampicillin (parenteral) and penicillin G (parenteral) are used in the treatment of leptospirosis caused by *Leptospira* sp.

[Lyme disease (treatment)]¹—Amoxicillin and penicillin V are used in the treatment of early Lyme disease, caused by *Borrelia burgdorferi*. Amoxicillin, in combination with probenecid, and penicillin G (parenteral) are used to treat more advanced stages of Lyme disease, including mild neurological manifestations, cardiac manifestations, and arthritis.

[Typhoid fever (treatment)]¹—Amoxicillin and ampicillin are used in the treatment of typhoid fever caused by *Salmonella typhi*.

**Unaccepted**

For carbenicillin (oral)
 Since effective serum concentrations are not achieved with oral carbenicillin, it is indicated only for urinary tract infections and prostatitis.

For nafcillin (oral)
 The oral absorption of nafcillin is erratic and the resulting serum concentrations are low; therefore, use of oral nafcillin is not recommended.

For penicillin G benzathine (parenteral)
 Parenteral penicillin G benzathine is not indicated for the treatment of meningitis or neurosyphilis because it fails to achieve adequate concentrations in the cerebrospinal fluid (CSF).

For penicillin G (oral)
 Because of the low serum concentrations achieved with oral penicillin G, it is not indicated for the treatment of severe infections.

---

¹Not included in Canadian product labeling.

## Pharmacology/Pharmacokinetics

See *Table 1*, page 2261 and *Table 2*, page 2262.

**Physicochemical characteristics**

Chemical group—
 Amoxicillin: Aminopenicillin.
 Ampicillin: Aminopenicillin.
 Bacampicillin: Aminopenicillin.
 Carbenicillin: Carboxypenicillin.
 Cloxacillin: Isoxazolyl penicillin.
 Dicloxacillin: Isoxazolyl penicillin.
 Flucloxacillin: Isoxazolyl penicillin.
 Mezlocillin: Acylureidopenicillin.
 Oxacillin: Isoxazolyl penicillin.

Piperacillin: Acylureidopenicillin.
Pivampicillin: Aminopenicillin.
Ticarcillin: Carboxypenicillin.

Molecular weight—
Amoxicillin: 419.45.
Ampicillin: 349.40.
Ampicillin sodium: 371.39.
Bacampicillin hydrochloride: 501.98.
Carbenicillin disodium: 422.36.
Carbenicillin indanyl sodium: 516.54.
Cloxacillin sodium: 475.88.
Dicloxacillin sodium: 510.32.
Flucloxacillin: 453.87.
Methicillin sodium: 420.41.
Mezlocillin sodium: 561.56.
Nafcillin sodium: 454.47.
Oxacillin sodium: 441.43.
Penicillin G benzathine: 981.19.
Penicillin G potassium: 372.48.
Penicillin G procaine: 588.72.
Penicillin G sodium: 356.37.
Penicillin V potassium: 388.48.
Piperacillin sodium: 539.54.
Pivampicillin hydrochloride: 500.01.
Pivmecillinam: 439.57.
Ticarcillin disodium: 428.38.

**Mechanism of action/Effect**
Bactericidal; inhibit bacterial cell wall synthesis. Action is dependent on the ability of penicillins to reach and bind penicillin-binding proteins (PBPs) located on the inner membrane of the bacterial cell wall. PBPs (which include transpeptidases, carboxypeptidases, and endopeptidases) are enzymes that are involved in the terminal stages of assembling the bacterial cell wall and in reshaping the cell wall during growth and division. Penicillins bind to, and inactivate, PBPs, resulting in the weakening of the bacterial cell wall and lysis.

**Distribution**
Penicillins are widely distributed to most tissues and body fluids, including peritoneal fluid, blister fluid, urine (high concentrations), pleural fluid, middle ear fluid, intestinal mucosa, bone, gallbladder, lung, female reproductive tissues, and bile. Distribution into the cerebrospinal fluid (CSF) is low in subjects with noninflamed meninges, as is penetration into purulent bronchial secretions.
Penicillins also cross the placenta and are distributed into breast milk.

**Biotransformation**
Hepatic metabolism accounts for less than 30% of the biotransformation of most penicillins, with the exception of nafcillin and oxacillin.
Bacampicillin—A prodrug of ampicillin; bacampicillin is hydrolyzed by esterases in the intestinal wall during absorption to produce ampicillin. Bacampicillin provides earlier and higher peak concentrations of ampicillin than administration of ampicillin does.
Carbenicillin indanyl sodium—After absorption, carbenicillin indanyl sodium is rapidly converted to carbenicillin by hydrolysis of the ester linkage.
Penicillin G benzathine (intramuscular)—Slowly released from the intramuscular injection site and hydrolyzed to penicillin G, resulting in serum concentrations that are much lower but much more prolonged than other parenteral penicillins.
Penicillin G procaine—Dissolves slowly at the site of injection, giving a plateau-type blood level at 4 hours, which falls slowly over the next 15 to 20 hours.
Pivampicillin—A prodrug of ampicillin, which is converted during absorption to ampicillin, formaldehyde, and pivalic acid, by non-specific esterases in most body tissues. Pivampicillin provides earlier and higher peak concentrations of ampicillin than administration of ampicillin does.
Pivmecillinam—A prodrug of mecillinam, which is converted during absorption to mecillinam, formaldehyde, and pivalic acid, by non-specific esterases in most body tissues.

**Elimination**
Primarily renal (glomerular filtration and tubular secretion).
Hepatic metabolism accounts for less than 30% of the elimination of most penicillins, with the exception of nafcillin and oxacillin.
Biliary—Some penicillins may be excreted in the bile in high concentrations, such as ampicillin, mezlocillin, nafcillin, penicillin G, piperacillin, and pivmecillinam. Approximately 10% of cloxacillin, dicloxacillin, flucloxacillin, and oxacillin is recovered in the bile.

## Precautions to Consider

### Cross-sensitivity and/or related problems
Patients allergic to one penicillin may be allergic to other penicillins also. Patients allergic to cephalosporins or cephamycins may be allergic to penicillins also. Patients allergic to procaine or other ester-type local anesthetics may also be allergic to sterile penicillin G procaine suspension, which is an equimolar compound of procaine and penicillin G.

### Carcinogenicity
*Amoxicillin, ampicillin, bacampicillin, cloxacillin, dicloxacillin, methicillin, nafcillin, oxacillin, penicillin G, penicillin V*—Long-term studies have not been performed in animals.
*Carbenicillin*—Long-term studies have not been performed in animals. Rats given 25 to 100 mg per kg of body weight (mg/kg) per day of carbenicillin for 18 months developed mild liver pathology (bile duct hyperplasia) at all dose levels, but there was no evidence of drug-related neoplasia.

### Mutagenicity
*Amoxicillin, ampicillin, bacampicillin, cloxacillin, dicloxacillin, methicillin, nafcillin, oxacillin, penicillin G, penicillin V*—Long-term studies have not been performed in animals.

### Pregnancy/Reproduction
Fertility—*Amoxicillin:* Studies in mice and rats at doses up to 10 times the human dose of amoxicillin revealed no evidence of impaired fertility.
*Bacampicillin:* Studies in mice and rats given doses of up to 750 mg/kg (more than 25 times the usual human dose) showed no evidence of impaired fertility. Also, bacampicillin had no effect on the reproductive organs of rats or dogs receiving daily oral doses of up to 800 and 650 mg, respectively, for 6 months.
*Carbenicillin:* Administration of carbenicillin at doses of up to 1000 mg/kg had no apparent effect on the fertility or reproductive performance of rats.
*Cloxacillin, dicloxacillin, methicillin, nafcillin, oxacillin, penicillin G, penicillin V:* Reproductive studies performed in the mouse, rat, and rabbit given these penicillins have revealed no evidence of impaired fertility.
*Mezlocillin:* Studies in mice and rats given doses up to twice the usual human dose have not shown that mezlocillin impairs fertility.
*Piperacillin:* Studies in mice and rats given doses up to 4 times the human dose of piperacillin have shown no evidence of impaired fertility.
*Ticarcillin:* Reproductive studies done in mice and rats given ticarcillin have revealed no evidence of impaired fertility.

Pregnancy—Penicillins cross the placenta. Adequate and well-controlled studies in humans have not been done to determine whether penicillins are teratogenic; however, penicillins are widely used in pregnant women and problems have not been documented.
*Amoxicillin:* Studies in mice and rats at doses up to 10 times the human dose of amoxicillin revealed no evidence of harm to the fetus.

FDA Pregnancy Category B.
*Ampicillin:* Studies in animals given doses several times the human dose have revealed no evidence of adverse effects in the fetus.

FDA Pregnancy Category B.
*Bacampicillin:* Studies in mice and rats given doses of up to 750 mg/kg (more than 25 times the usual human dose) have not shown that bacampicillin causes adverse effects in the fetus.

FDA Pregnancy Category B.
*Carbenicillin:* Reproductive studies using doses of 500 or 1000 mg/kg in rats, 200 mg/kg in mice, and 500 mg/kg in monkeys showed no harm to the fetus.

FDA Pregnancy Category B.
*Cloxacillin, dicloxacillin, methicillin, nafcillin, oxacillin, penicillin G, penicillin V:* Reproductive studies performed in the mouse, rat, and rabbit given these penicillins have revealed no evidence of impaired fertility or harm to the fetus.

FDA Pregnancy Category B.
*Flucloxacillin, pivampicillin, pivmecillinam:* Safety during pregnancy has not been established.
*Mezlocillin:* Studies in mice and rats given doses up to twice the usual human dose have not shown that mezlocillin causes adverse effects in the fetus.

FDA Pregnancy Category B.
*Piperacillin:* Studies in mice and rats given doses up to 4 times the usual human dose have not shown that piperacillin causes adverse effects in the fetus.

FDA Pregnancy Category B.
*Ticarcillin:* Reproductive studies done in mice and rats given ticarcillin have not shown that ticarcillin causes adverse effects in the fetus.

FDA Pregnancy Category B.

### Breast-feeding
Penicillins are distributed into breast milk, some in low concentrations. Although significant problems in humans have not been documented, the use of penicillins by nursing mothers may lead to sensitization, diarrhea, candidiasis, and skin rash in the infant.

### Pediatrics
Many penicillins have been used in pediatric patients and no pediatrics-specific problems have been documented to date. However, the incompletely developed renal function of neonates and young infants may delay the excretion of renally eliminated penicillins.

Because pivampicillin and pivmecillinam have been associated with a decrease in serum carnitine, it is recommended that these penicillins be avoided in children less than 3 months of age.

### Geriatrics
Penicillins have been used in geriatric patients and no geriatrics-specific problems have been documented to date. However, elderly patients are more likely to have age-related renal function impairment, which may require an adjustment in dosage in patients receiving penicillins.

### Dental
Prolonged use of penicillins may lead to the development of oral candidiasis.

### Drug interactions and/or related problems
The following drug interactions and/or related problems have been selected on the basis of their potential clinical significance (possible mechanism in parentheses where appropriate)—not necessarily inclusive (» = major clinical significance):

Note: Combinations containing any of the following medications, depending on the amount present, may also interact with this medication.

Allopurinol
(concurrent use with ampicillin or bacampicillin may significantly increase the possibility of skin rash, especially in hyperuricemic patients; however, it has not been established that allopurinol, rather than the presence of hyperuricemia, is responsible for this effect)

» Aminoglycosides
(mixing penicillins with aminoglycosides *in vitro* has resulted in substantial mutual inactivation; if these groups of antibacterials are to be administered concurrently, they should be administered at separate sites at least 1 hour apart)

» Angiotensin-converting enzyme (ACE) inhibitors or
» Diuretics, potassium-sparing or
» Potassium-containing medications, other or
» Potassium supplements
(concurrent administration of these medications with parenteral penicillin G potassium may promote serum potassium accumulation with possible resultant hyperkalemia, especially in patients with renal insufficiency; concurrent administration with ACE inhibitors may result in hyperkalemia since reduction of aldosterone production induced by ACE inhibitors may lead to elevation of serum potassium)

» Anticoagulants, coumarin- or indandione-derivative or
» Heparin or
» Thrombolytic agents
(concurrent use of these medications with high-dose parenteral carbenicillin, piperacillin, or ticarcillin may increase the risk of hemorrhage because these penicillins inhibit platelet aggregation; patients should be monitored carefully for signs of bleeding; concurrent use of these penicillins with thrombolytic agents may increase the risk of severe hemorrhage and is not recommended)

Anti-inflammatory drugs, nonsteroidal (NSAIDs), especially aspirin or Diflunisal, very high doses or
Other salicylates or
» Platelet aggregation inhibitors, other (See *Appendix II*) or
» Sulfinpyrazone
(concurrent use of these medications with high-dose parenteral carbenicillin, piperacillin, or ticarcillin may increase the risk of hemorrhage because of additive inhibition of platelet function; in addition, hypoprothrombinemia induced by large doses of salicylates and the gastrointestinal ulcerative or hemorrhagic potential of NSAIDs, salicylates, or sulfinpyrazone may also increase the risk of hemorrhage when these medications are used concurrently with these penicillins)

Chloramphenicol or
Erythromycins or
Sulfonamides or
Tetracyclines
(since bacteriostatic drugs may interfere with the bactericidal effect of penicillins in the treatment of meningitis or in other situations in which a rapid bactericidal effect is necessary, it is best to avoid concurrent therapy; however, chloramphenicol and ampicillin are sometimes administered concurrently to pediatric patients)

» Cholestyramine or
» Colestipol
(may impair absorption of oral penicillin G when used concurrently; patients should be advised to take oral penicillin G and these medications several hours apart)

» Contraceptives, estrogen-containing, oral
(there have been case reports of reduced oral contraceptive effectiveness in women taking ampicillin, amoxicillin, and penicillin V, resulting in unplanned pregnancy. This is thought to be due to a reduction in enterohepatic circulation of estrogens. Although the association is weak, patients should be advised of this information and given the option to use an alternate or additional method of contraception while taking any of these penicillins)

Disulfiram
(metabolism of the ester moiety of bacampicillin yields acetaldehyde and ethanol, which are later converted to acetaldehyde; furthermore, since disulfiram blocks the hepatic conversion of acetaldehyde to nontoxic compounds, concurrent use with bacampicillin may result in nausea, vomiting, confusion, and cardiovascular abnormalities)

Hepatotoxic medications, other (See *Appendix II*)
(concurrent use of other hepatotoxic medications with cloxacillin, dicloxacillin, flucloxacillin, mezlocillin, nafcillin, oxacillin, or piperacillin may increase the potential for hepatotoxicity)

» Methotrexate
(concurrent use with penicillins has resulted in decreased clearance of methotrexate and in methotrexate toxicity; this is thought to be due to competition for renal tubular secretion; patients should be closely monitored; leucovorin doses may need to be increased and administered for longer periods of time)

» Probenecid
(probenecid decreases renal tubular secretion of penicillins when used concurrently; this effect results in increased and prolonged serum concentrations, prolonged elimination half-life, and increased risk of toxicity. Penicillins and probenecid are often used concurrently to treat sexually transmitted diseases [STDs] or other infections in which high and/or prolonged antibiotic serum and tissue concentrations are required)

### Laboratory value alterations
The following have been selected on the basis of their potential clinical significance (possible effect in parentheses where appropriate)—not necessarily inclusive (» = major clinical significance):

With diagnostic test results
» Glucose, urine
(high urinary concentrations of a penicillin may produce false-positive or falsely elevated test results with copper sulfate tests [Benedict's, *Clinitest*, or Fehling's]; glucose enzymatic tests [*Clinistix* or *Testape*] are not affected)

Direct antiglobulin (Coombs') tests
(false-positive result may occur during therapy with any penicillin)

Protein, urine
(high urinary concentrations of mezlocillin or ticarcillin may produce false-positive protein reactions [pseudoproteinuria] with the sulfosalicylic acid and boiling test, the acetic acid test, the biuret reaction, and the nitric acid test; bromophenol blue reagent test strips [*Multi-stix*] are reportedly unaffected)

With physiology/laboratory test values
Alanine aminotransferase (ALT [SGPT]) and
Alkaline phosphatase and
Aspartate aminotransferase (AST [SGOT]) and
Lactate dehydrogenase (LDH), serum
(values may be increased)

Bilirubin, serum
(an increase has been associated with mezlocillin, piperacillin, and ticarcillin)

Blood urea nitrogen (BUN) and
Creatinine, serum
(an increase has been associated with flucloxacillin, mezlocillin, and piperacillin)

Estradiol or
Estriol, total conjugated or
Estriol-glucuronide or
Estrone, conjugated
(concentrations may be transiently decreased in pregnant women following administration of ampicillin and bacampicillin)

» Partial thromboplastin time (PTT) and
» Prothrombin time (PT)
(an increase has been associated with intravenous carbenicillin, piperacillin, and ticarcillin)
Potassium, serum
(hyperkalemia may occur following administration of large doses of parenteral penicillin G potassium because of high potassium content; hypokalemia may occur following administration of parenteral carbenicillin, mezlocillin, piperacillin, or ticarcillin, which may act as a nonreabsorbable anion in the distal renal tubules; this may cause an increase in pH and result in increased urinary potassium loss; the risk of hypokalemia increases with use of larger doses)
Sodium, serum
(hypernatremia may occur following administration of large doses of parenteral carbenicillin, mezlocillin, penicillin G sodium, or ticarcillin because of the high sodium content of these medications)
Uric acid, serum
(flucloxacillin may transiently decrease the serum uric acid concentration in some patients)
White blood cell count
(leukopenia or neutropenia is associated with the use of all penicillins; the effect is more likely to occur with prolonged therapy and severe hepatic function impairment)

### Medical considerations/Contraindications
The medical considerations/contraindications included have been selected on the basis of their potential clinical significance (reasons given in parentheses where appropriate)—not necessarily inclusive (» = major clinical significance).

***Except under special circumstances, this medication should not be used when the following medical problem exists:***
» Allergy to penicillins

***Risk-benefit should be considered when the following medical problems exist:***
  Allergy, general, history of sensitivity to multiple allergens
» Bleeding disorders, history of
(some penicillins, especially carbenicillin, piperacillin, and ticarcillin, may cause platelet dysfunction and hemorrhage)
  Carnitine deficiency
(pivampicillin and pivmecillinam may reduce serum carnitine concentrations by increasing the urinary excretion of carnitine; use of these penicillins is not recommended in patients with carnitine deficiency or in infants up to 3 months of age)
» Congestive heart failure (CHF) or
  Hypertension
(the sodium content of high doses of parenteral carbenicillin and ticarcillin should be considered in patients who require sodium restriction)
» Cystic fibrosis
(patients with cystic fibrosis may be at increased risk of fever and skin rash when given piperacillin)
» Gastrointestinal disease, history of, especially antibiotic-associated colitis
(penicillins may cause pseudomembranous colitis)
» Mononucleosis, infectious
(a morbilliform skin rash may occur in a high percentage [43 to 100%] of patients taking ampicillin, bacampicillin, or pivampicillin)
» Renal function impairment
(because most penicillins are excreted through the kidneys, a reduction in dosage, or increase in dosing interval, is recommended in patients with renal function impairment; also, the sodium content of high doses of parenteral carbenicillin and ticarcillin, and the potassium content of high doses of penicillin G potassium, should be considered in patients with severe renal function impairment)

### Patient monitoring
The following may be especially important in patient monitoring (other tests may be warranted in some patients, depending on condition; » = major clinical significance):

*For carbenicillin (parenteral), piperacillin, ticarcillin*
» Partial thromboplastin time (PTT) and
» Prothrombin time (PT)
(may be required prior to and during prolonged therapy in patients with renal function impairment who are receiving high doses since hemorrhagic manifestations may occur, although this effect is rare)
» Potassium, serum or
» Sodium, serum
(determinations may be required periodically in patients with low potassium reserves and in patients receiving cytotoxic medications or diuretics who are also receiving high doses since hypokalemia may occur; also, because of the high sodium content of these medications, hypernatremia may occur)

*For methicillin*
» Renal function determinations
(may be required during prolonged therapy since methicillin may cause interstitial nephritis in up to 33% of patients treated with methicillin for more than 10 days)

*For mezlocillin*
  Potassium, serum
(may be required periodically during prolonged therapy in patients receiving high doses since hypokalemia may occur)

*For penicillin G (parenteral)*
  Potassium, serum or
» Sodium, serum
(may be required periodically during therapy in patients receiving high doses of penicillin G potassium or penicillin G sodium since hyperkalemia or hypernatremia may occur; very high doses of penicillin G potassium may cause severe or fatal hyperkalemia; very high doses of penicillin G sodium may cause congestive heart failure)

*For all penicillins (if Clostridium difficile colitis occurs)*
» Stool cytotoxin assays
(enzyme immunoassay of stool samples for the presence of *C. difficile* toxins may be required prior to treatment of patients with antibiotic-associated colitis to document the presence of *C. difficile* toxins; however, *C. difficile* and its toxins may persist following treatment with oral vancomycin, metronidazole, or cholestyramine, despite clinical improvement; follow-up cultures and toxin assays are not recommended if clinical improvement is complete)

## Side/Adverse Effects
The following side/adverse effects have been selected on the basis of their potential clinical significance (possible signs and symptoms in parentheses where appropriate)—not necessarily inclusive:

### Those indicating need for medical attention
Incidence less frequent
  ***Allergic reactions, specifically anaphylaxis*** (fast or irregular breathing; puffiness or swelling around face; shortness of breath; sudden, severe decrease in blood pressure); ***exfoliative dermatitis*** (red, scaly skin); ***serum sickness–like reactions*** (skin rash; joint pain; fever); ***skin rash, hives, or itching***

Incidence rare
  ***Clostridium difficile colitis*** (severe abdominal or stomach cramps and pain; abdominal tenderness; watery and severe diarrhea, which may also be bloody; fever); ***hepatotoxicity*** (fever; nausea and vomiting; yellow eyes or skin); ***interstitial nephritis*** (fever; possibly decreased urine output; skin rash); ***leukopenia or neutropenia*** (sore throat and fever); ***mental disturbances*** (anxiety; confusion; agitation or combativeness; depression; seizures; hallucinations; expressed fear of impending death); ***pain at site of injection; platelet dysfunction or thrombocytopenia*** (unusual bleeding or bruising); ***seizures***

Note: *Hepatotoxicity* has been associated with several penicillins, especially cloxacillin, dicloxacillin, flucloxacillin, and oxacillin; however, flucloxacillin appears to have a very high association with cholestatic jaundice, especially in older patients and those receiving flucloxacillin for more than 14 days. Also, one small study found HIV-infected patients to be more susceptible to oxacillin-hepatotoxicity (81%) than HIV-negative patients (4.5%).

*Interstitial nephritis* is seen primarily with methicillin, and to a lesser degree with nafcillin and oxacillin, but may occur with any penicillin.

*Mental disturbances* are toxic reactions to the procaine content of penicillin G procaine; this reaction may be seen in patients who receive a large single dose of the medication, as in the treatment of gonorrhea.

*Platelet dysfunction* is primarily associated with carbenicillin, piperacillin, and ticarcillin; it may be more pronounced in patients with renal insufficiency due to the prolongation of the penicillin's half-life and uremic platelet dysfunction.

*Clostridium difficile colitis* may occur up to several weeks after discontinuation of these medications.

*Seizures* are more likely to occur in patients receiving high doses of a penicillin and/or patients with severe renal function impairment.

## Those indicating need for medical attention only if they continue or are bothersome
Incidence more frequent
*Gastrointestinal reactions* (mild diarrhea; nausea or vomiting); *headache; oral candidiasis* (sore mouth or tongue; white patches in mouth and/or on tongue); *vaginal candidiasis* (vaginal itching and discharge)

## Overdose
For more information on the management of overdose or unintentional ingestion, **contact a Poison Control Center** (see *Poison Control Center Listing*).

### Treatment of overdose
Specific treatment—Hemodialysis may aid in the removal of penicillins from the blood.

Supportive care—Since there is no specific antidote, treatment of penicillin overdose should be symptomatic and supportive. Patients in whom intentional overdose is known or suspected should be referred for psychiatric consultation.

## Patient Consultation
As an aid to patient consultation, refer to *Advice for the Patient, Penicillins (Systemic)*.

In providing consultation, consider emphasizing the following selected information (» = major clinical significance):

### Before using this medication
» Conditions affecting use, especially:
   Allergy to penicillins, cephalosporins, or cephamycins
   Pregnancy—Penicillins cross the placenta
   Breast-feeding—Penicillins are distributed into breast milk
   Use in children—Neonates and young infants may have reduced elimination of renally eliminated penicillins due to incompletely developed renal function
   Other medications, especially aminoglycosides; angiotensin-converting enzyme inhibitors; cholestyramine; colestipol; coumarin- or indandione-derivative anticoagulants; estrogen-containing oral contraceptives; heparin; methotrexate; nonsteroidal anti-inflammatory drugs (NSAIDs), especially aspirin; other platelet aggregation inhibitors; other potassium-containing medications; potassium-sparing diuretics; potassium supplements; probenecid; sulfinpyrazone; or thrombolytic agents
   Other medical problems, especially a history of bleeding disorders; congestive heart failure; cystic fibrosis; active or history of gastrointestinal disease, especially antibiotic-associated colitis; infectious mononucleosis; or renal function impairment

### Proper use of this medication
   Taking on an empty stomach (for ampicillin, bacampicillin oral suspension, carbenicillin; cloxacillin, dicloxacillin, flucloxacillin, nafcillin, oxacillin, penicillin G)
   Taking on a full or empty stomach (for amoxicillin, bacampicillin tablets, penicillin V, pivampicillin, pivmecillinam)
   Taking amoxicillin suspension straight or mixed with formulas, milk, fruit juice, water, ginger ale, or other cold drinks; taking immediately after mixing; drinking full dose
   Not drinking acidic fruit juices or other acidic beverages within 1 hour of taking oral penicillin G
   Proper administration technique for oral liquids and/or pediatric drops
   Not using after expiration date
» Compliance with full course of therapy, especially in streptococcal infections
» Importance of not missing doses and taking at evenly spaced times
» Proper dosing
   Missed dose: Taking as soon as possible; not taking if almost time for next dose; not doubling doses
» Proper storage

### Precautions while using this medication
   Checking with physician if no improvement within a few days
» For severe diarrhea, checking with physician before taking any antidiarrheals; for mild diarrhea, kaolin- or attapulgite-containing antidiarrheals may be used, but antiperistaltic antidiarrheals should be avoided; checking with physician or pharmacist if mild diarrhea continues or worsens
» Possibly using an alternate or additional method of contraception if taking estrogen-containing oral contraceptives concurrently, especially with ampicillin, amoxicillin, or penicillin V
» Diabetics: False-positive reactions with copper sulfate urine glucose tests may occur
   Possible interference with diagnostic tests

### Side/adverse effects
Signs of potential side effects, especially allergic reactions, *Clostridium difficile* colitis, hepatotoxicity, interstitial nephritis, leukopenia or neutropenia, mental disturbances, pain at site of injection, platelet dysfunction or thrombocytopenia, and seizures

## General Dosing Information
Therapy should be continued for at least 10 days in Group A beta-hemolytic streptococcal infections to help prevent the occurrence of acute rheumatic fever.

### For oral dosage forms only
Penicillins, except amoxicillin, bacampicillin hydrochloride tablets, penicillin V, pivampicillin, and pivmecillinam should preferably be taken with a full glass (240 mL) of water on an empty stomach (either 1 hour before or 2 hours after meals) to obtain optimum serum and/or urine concentrations. Amoxicillin, bacampicillin hydrochloride tablets, penicillin V, pivampicillin, and pivmecillinam may be taken on a full or empty stomach.

### For treatment of adverse effects
Serious anaphylactoid reactions require immediate emergency treatment, which consists of the following:
• Parenteral epinephrine.
• Oxygen.
• Intravenous corticosteroids.
• Airway management (including intubation).

For *Clostridium difficile* colitis—
• Some patients may develop *Clostridium difficile* colitis during or following administration of penicillins.
• *C. difficile* colitis may result in severe watery diarrhea, which may occur during therapy or up to several weeks after therapy is discontinued. If diarrhea occurs, administration of antiperistaltic antidiarrheals (e.g., opioids, diphenoxylate and atropine combination, loperamide, paregoric) is not recommended since they may delay the removal of toxins from the colon, thereby prolonging and/or worsening the condition.
• Mild cases may respond to discontinuation of the medication alone. Moderate to severe cases may require fluid, electrolyte, and protein replacement.
• In cases not responding to the above measures or in more severe cases, oral doses of vancomycin, metronidazole, or cholestyramine may be used. Oral vancomycin is effective in doses of 125 mg every 6 hours for 5 to 10 days. The dose of metronidazole is 250 to 500 mg every 8 hours and the dose of cholestyramine is 4 grams four times a day. Recurrences, which occur in approximately 25% of patients treated with vancomycin or metronidazole, may be treated with a second course of these medications.
• Cholestyramine resin has been shown to bind *C. difficile* toxin *in vitro*. If cholestyramine resin is administered in conjunction with oral vancomycin, the medications should be administered several hours apart since the resin has been shown to bind oral vancomycin also.

---

### AMOXICILLIN

## Summary of Differences
Category:
   Aminopenicillin.
Pharmacology/pharmacokinetics:
   High oral absorption (75 to 90%).
Precautions:
   Drug interactions and/or related problems—May also interact with oral contraceptives.
   Medical considerations/Contraindications—Caution also needed in infectious mononucleosis.

## Additional Dosing Information
Patients with impaired renal function do not generally require a reduction in dose unless the impairment is severe.

### For oral dosage forms only
Amoxicillin may be taken on a full or empty stomach.
Amoxicillin may be taken with formulas, milk, fruit juice, water, ginger ale, or other cold drinks.

## Oral Dosage Forms
Note: Bracketed uses in the *Dosage Forms* section refer to categories of use and/or indications that are not included in U.S. product labeling.

### AMOXICILLIN CAPSULES USP
**Usual adult and adolescent dose**
Antibacterial—
   Oral, 250 to 500 mg every eight hours.

Endocarditis, bacterial (prophylaxis): Oral, 3 grams one hour before the procedure, then 1.5 grams six hours after the initial dose.

[Chlamydia, treatment in pregnant women][1]: Oral, 500 mg every eight hours for seven to ten days.

[Gastritis, *Helicobacter pylori*][1] or

[Ulcer, peptic, *Helicobacter pylori*][1]: Oral, 500 mg four times a day; or 750 mg three times a day.

[Lyme disease][1]: Oral, 250 to 500 mg three or four times a day for three to four weeks. Duration of therapy is based on clinical response. Treatment failures have occurred and retreatment may be necessary.

### Usual adult prescribing limits
Up to 4.5 grams a day.

### Usual pediatric dose
Antibacterial—

Gonorrhea, endocervical and urethral, uncomplicated: Oral, 50 mg per kg of body weight and 25 mg of probenecid per kg of body weight simultaneously as a single dose in prepubertal children. However, probenecid is not recommended in children under 2 years of age.

[Lyme disease][1]: Oral, 6.7 to 13.3 mg per kg of body weight every eight hours for ten to thirty days. Duration of therapy is based on clinical response. Treatment failures have occurred and retreatment may be necessary.

For all other indications: Infants and children up to 20 kg of body weight—A product of suitable strength is not available for infants and children up to 20 kg of body weight. See *Amoxicillin for Oral Suspension USP*.

Children 20 kg of body weight and over—See *Usual adult and adolescent dose*.

### Strength(s) usually available
U.S.—
  250 mg (Rx) [*Amoxil; Trimox; Wymox;* GENERIC].
  500 mg (Rx) [*Amoxil; Trimox; Wymox;* GENERIC].
Canada—
  250 mg (Rx) [*Amoxil; Apo-Amoxi; Novamoxin; Nu-Amoxi*].
  500 mg (Rx) [*Amoxil; Apo-Amoxi; Novamoxin; Nu-Amoxi*].

### Packaging and storage
Store between 15 and 30 °C (59 and 86 °F). Store in a tight container.

### Auxiliary labeling
- Continue medication for full time of treatment.

## AMOXICILLIN FOR ORAL SUSPENSION USP

### Usual adult and adolescent dose
See *Amoxicillin Capsules USP*.

### Usual adult prescribing limits
See *Amoxicillin Capsules USP*.

### Usual pediatric dose
Antibacterial—

Infants up to 6 kg of body weight: Oral, 25 to 50 mg every eight hours.
Infants 6 to 8 kg of body weight: Oral, 50 to 100 mg every eight hours.
Infants and children 8 to 20 kg of body weight: Oral, 6.7 to 13.3 mg per kg of body weight every eight hours.
Children 20 kg of body weight and over: See *Usual adult and adolescent dose*.

### Strength(s) usually available
U.S.—
  50 mg per mL (when reconstituted according to manufacturer's instructions) (Rx) [*Amoxil; Trimox; Polymox*].
  125 mg per 5 mL (when reconstituted according to manufacturer's instructions) (Rx) [*Amoxil; Polymox; Trimox; Wymox;* GENERIC].
  250 mg per 5 mL (when reconstituted according to manufacturer's instructions) (Rx) [*Amoxil; Polymox; Trimox; Wymox;* GENERIC].
Canada—
  50 mg per mL (when reconstituted according to manufacturer's instructions) (Rx) [*Amoxil*].
  125 mg per 5 mL (when reconstituted according to manufacturer's instructions) (Rx) [*Amoxil; Apo-Amoxi; Novamoxin; Nu-Amoxi*].
  250 mg per 5 mL (when reconstituted according to manufacturer's instructions) (Rx) [*Amoxil; Apo-Amoxi; Novamoxin; Nu-Amoxi*].

### Packaging and storage
Prior to reconstitution, store between 15 and 30 °C (59 and 86 °F). Store in a tight container.

### Stability
After reconstitution, suspensions retain their potency for up to 14 days at room temperature or for up to 14 days if refrigerated, depending on the manufacturer.

Note: Some manufacturers prefer refrigerated storage.

### Auxiliary labeling
- Refrigerate.
- Shake well.
- Continue medication for full time of treatment.
- Beyond-use date.
- Take by mouth only (pediatric drops).

### Note
Explain administration technique for pediatric drops (50 mg per mL).
When dispensing, include a calibrated liquid-measuring device.

## AMOXICILLIN TABLETS (CHEWABLE) USP

### Usual adult and adolescent dose
See *Amoxicillin Capsules USP*.

### Usual adult prescribing limits
See *Amoxicillin Capsules USP*.

### Usual pediatric dose
See *Amoxicillin Capsules USP*.

### Strength(s) usually available
U.S.—
  125 mg (Rx) [*Amoxil*].
  250 mg (Rx) [*Amoxil;* GENERIC].
Canada—
  125 mg (Rx) [*Amoxil*].
  250 mg (Rx) [*Amoxil*].

### Packaging and storage
Store between 15 and 30 °C (59 and 86 °F). Store in a tight container.

### Auxiliary labeling
- Should be chewed or crushed.
- Continue medication for full time of treatment.

---

[1]Not included in Canadian product labeling.

---

# AMPICILLIN

## Summary of Differences
Category:
  Aminopenicillin.
Precautions:
  Drug interactions and/or related problems—Also interacts with allopurinol and oral contraceptives.
  Medical considerations/contraindications—Caution also needed in infectious mononucleosis.

## Additional Dosing Information
Patients with impaired renal function do not generally require a reduction in dose unless the impairment is severe.

## Oral Dosage Forms
Note: Bracketed uses in the *Dosage Forms* section refer to categories of use and/or indications that are not included in U.S. product labeling.

## AMPICILLIN CAPSULES USP

### Usual adult and adolescent dose
Antibacterial—
  Oral, 250 to 500 mg every six hours.
  [Typhoid fever][1]: Oral, 25 mg per kg of body weight every six hours.

### Usual adult prescribing limits
Up to 4 grams a day.

### Usual pediatric dose
Antibacterial—
  Infants and children up to 20 kg of body weight: A product of suitable strength is not available for infants and children up to 20 kg of body weight. See *Ampicillin for Oral Suspension USP*.
  Children 20 kg of body weight and over: See *Usual adult and adolescent dose*.

### Strength(s) usually available
U.S.—
  250 mg (Rx) [*Omnipen; Principen; Totacillin;* GENERIC].
  500 mg (Rx) [*Omnipen; Principen; Totacillin;* GENERIC].
Canada—
  250 mg (Rx) [*Apo-Ampi; Novo-Ampicillin; Nu-Ampi; Penbritin*].
  500 mg (Rx) [*Apo-Ampi; Novo-Ampicillin; Nu-Ampi; Penbritin*].

### Packaging and storage
Store below 40 °C (104 °F), preferably between 15 and 30 °C (59 and 86 °F), unless otherwise specified by manufacturer. Store in a tight container.

## Penicillins (Systemic)

**Auxiliary labeling**
- Continue medication for full time of treatment.
- Take on empty stomach.

### AMPICILLIN FOR ORAL SUSPENSION USP

**Usual adult and adolescent dose**
See *Ampicillin Capsules USP*.

**Usual adult prescribing limits**
See *Ampicillin Capsules USP*.

**Usual pediatric dose**
Antibacterial—
   Infants and children up to 20 kg of body weight: Oral, 12.5 to 25 mg per kg of body weight every six hours; or 16.7 to 33.3 mg per kg of body weight every eight hours
   Children 20 kg of body weight and over: See *Usual adult and adolescent dose*.

**Strength(s) usually available**
U.S.—
   100 mg per mL (Rx) [*Polycillin*].
   125 mg per 5 mL (Rx) [*Omnipen; Polycillin; Principen; Totacillin;* GENERIC].
   250 mg per 5 mL (Rx) [*Omnipen; Polycillin; Principen; Totacillin;* GENERIC].
   500 mg per 5 mL (Rx) [*Polycillin*].
Canada—
   125 mg per 5 mL (Rx) [*Apo-Ampi; Novo-Ampicillin; Nu-Ampi*].
   250 mg per 5 mL (Rx) [*Apo-Ampi; Novo-Ampicillin; Nu-Ampi; Penbritin*].

**Packaging and storage**
Prior to reconstitution, store below 40 °C (104 °F), preferably between 15 and 30 °C (59 and 86 °F), unless otherwise specified by manufacturer. Store in a tight container.

**Stability**
After reconstitution, suspensions retain their potency for 7 days at room temperature or for 14 days if refrigerated, depending on manufacturer.

**Auxiliary labeling**
- Refrigerate.
- Shake well.
- Continue medication for full time of treatment.
- Beyond-use date.
- Take by mouth only (pediatric drops).
- Take on empty stomach.

**Note**
Explain administration technique for pediatric drops (100 mg per mL).
When dispensing, include a calibrated liquid-measuring device.

## Parenteral Dosage Forms

Note:  Bracketed uses in the *Dosage Forms* section refer to categories of use and/or indications that are not included in U.S. product labeling.

Note:  The dosing and strengths of the dosage forms available are expressed in terms of ampicillin base (not the sodium salt).

### AMPICILLIN SODIUM STERILE USP

**Usual adult and adolescent dose**
Antibacterial—
   Intramuscular or intravenous, 250 to 500 mg (base) every six hours.
   Endocarditis, bacterial
   Meningitis, bacterial or
   Septicemia, bacterial: Intramuscular or intravenous, 1 to 2 grams (base) every three to four hours.
   Listeriosis: Intramuscular or intravenous, 50 mg per kg of body weight every six hours.
   [Leptospirosis][1]: Intramuscular or intravenous, 500 mg to 1 gram every six hours.
   [Typhoid fever][1]: Intramuscular or intravenous, 25 mg per kg of body weight every six hours.

**Usual adult prescribing limits**
Up to 14 grams a day.

**Usual pediatric dose**
Antibacterial—
   Meningitis, bacterial:
      Neonates up to 2 kg of body weight—Intramuscular or intravenous, 25 to 50 mg per kg of body weight every twelve hours during the first week of life, then 50 mg per kg of body weight every eight hours thereafter.
      Neonates 2 kg of body weight and over—Intramuscular or intravenous, 50 mg per kg of body weight every eight hours during the first week of life, then 50 mg per kg of body weight every six hours thereafter.
   For all other indications:
      Infants up to 20 kg of body weight—Intramuscular or intravenous, 12.5 mg (base) per kg of body weight every six hours.
      Infants and children 20 kg of body weight and over—See *Usual adult and adolescent dose*.

**Strength(s) usually available**
U.S.—
   125 mg (base) (Rx) [*Omnipen-N; Polycillin-N;* GENERIC].
   250 mg (base) (Rx) [*Omnipen-N; Polycillin-N; Totacillin-N;* GENERIC].
   500 mg (base) (Rx) [*Omnipen-N; Polycillin-N; Totacillin-N;* GENERIC].
   1 gram (base) (Rx) [*Omnipen-N; Polycillin-N; Totacillin-N;* GENERIC].
   2 grams (base) (Rx) [*Omnipen-N; Polycillin-N; Totacillin-N;* GENERIC].
   10 grams (base) (Rx) [*Omnipen-N; Polycillin-N;* GENERIC].
Canada—
   125 mg (base) (Rx) [*Ampicin; Penbritin*].
   250 mg (base) (Rx) [*Ampicin; Penbritin*].
   500 mg (base) (Rx) [*Ampicin; Penbritin*].
   1 gram (base) (Rx) [*Ampicin; Penbritin*].
   2 grams (base) (Rx) [*Ampicin; Penbritin*].

**Packaging and storage**
Prior to reconstitution, store below 40 °C (104 °F), preferably between 15 and 30 °C (59 and 86 °F), unless otherwise specified by manufacturer. Protect the reconstituted solution from freezing.

**Preparation of dosage form**
To prepare initial dilution for intramuscular use, depending on the manufacturer, add 0.9 to 1.2 mL of sterile water for injection or bacteriostatic water for injection to each 125-mg vial, 0.9 to 1.9 mL of diluent to each 250-mg vial, 1.2 to 1.8 mL of diluent to each 500-mg vial, 2.4 to 7.4 mL of diluent to each 1-gram vial, and 6.8 mL of diluent to each 2-gram vial.
To prepare initial dilution for direct intermittent intravenous use, add 5 mL of sterile water for injection or bacteriostatic water for injection to each 125-, 250-, or 500-mg vial or at least 7.4 to 10 mL of diluent to each 1- or 2-gram vial. The resulting solution should be administered slowly over a 3- to 5-minute period for each 125- to 500-mg dose or over a 10- to 15-minute period for each 1- to 2-gram dose. More rapid administration may result in convulsive seizures.
Intravenous infusions of sterile ampicillin sodium should be administered in a suitable diluent in a concentration not exceeding 30 mg per mL (see manufacturer's package insert).
For reconstitution of pharmacy bulk vials or piggyback infusion bottles, see manufacturer's labeling for instructions.

**Stability**
After reconstitution for intramuscular or direct intravenous use, solutions retain their potency for 1 hour.
After reconstitution for intravenous infusion, solutions in concentrations up to 30 mg per mL retain at least 90% of their potency for 2 to 8 hours at room temperature or for up to 72 hours if refrigerated in suitable diluents (see manufacturer's package insert).
Concentrated solutions (100 mg per mL) prepared from pharmacy bulk vials retain their potency for 2 hours at room temperature or for 4 hours if refrigerated.
Diluted solutions (20 mg per mL or less) in 5% dextrose injection retain their potency for 2 hours at room temperature or for 3 hours if refrigerated.

**Incompatibilities**
Extemporaneous admixtures of beta-lactam antibacterials (penicillins and cephalosporins) and aminoglycosides may result in substantial mutual inactivation. If these groups of antibacterials are administered concurrently, they should be administered in separate sites at least 1 hour apart. Do not mix them in the same intravenous bag, bottle, or tubing.
When aminoglycosides and penicillins are administered separately by different routes, a reduction in aminoglycoside serum concentration may occur. Usually this is clinically significant only in patients with severely impaired renal function when the excretion of both medications is delayed.

**Additional information**
The sodium content is approximately 3.4 mEq (3.4 mmol) per gram of ampicillin, depending on the manufacturer. This must be considered in patients on a restricted sodium intake when calculating total daily sodium intake.

---

[1]Not included in Canadian product labeling.

## BACAMPICILLIN

### Summary of Differences
Category:
  Aminopenicillin.
Pharmacology/pharmacokinetics:
  Hydrolyzed to ampicillin during absorption.
Precautions:
  Drug interactions and/or related problems—Also interacts with allopurinol and disulfiram.
  Medical considerations/contraindications—Caution also needed in infectious mononucleosis.

### Additional Dosing Information
Bacampicillin is stable in the presence of gastric acid. Also, food does not delay or reduce absorption of bacampicillin hydrochloride tablets. Therefore, the tablets may be taken on a full or empty stomach. However, bacampicillin hydrochloride oral suspension should preferably be taken with a full glass (240 mL) of water on an empty stomach (either 1 hour before or 2 hours after meals) to obtain optimum serum and/or urine concentrations.

Patients with impaired renal function do not generally require a reduction in dose unless the impairment is severe. The serum half-life increases when the creatinine clearance is below 30 mL per minute (0.50 mL per second).

### Oral Dosage Forms
Note: The dosing and strengths of the dosage forms available are expressed in terms of bacampicillin hydrochloride (not the base).

#### BACAMPICILLIN HYDROCHLORIDE FOR ORAL SUSPENSION USP

**Usual adult and adolescent dose**
Antibacterial—
  Oral, 400 to 800 mg every twelve hours.

**Usual adult prescribing limits**
Up to 3.2 grams a day.

**Usual pediatric dose**
Antibacterial—
  Oral, 12.5 to 25 mg per kg of body weight every twelve hours.

**Strength(s) usually available**
U.S.—
  125 mg per 5 mL (Rx) [*Spectrobid*].
  Note: 125 mg of bacampicillin hydrochloride are equivalent to 87.5 mg of ampicillin.
Canada—
  Not commercially available.

**Packaging and storage**
Prior to reconstitution, store below 40 °C (104 °F), preferably between 15 and 30 °C (59 and 86 °F), unless otherwise specified by manufacturer. Store in a tight container.

**Stability**
After reconstitution, suspensions retain their potency for 10 days if refrigerated.

**Auxiliary labeling**
- Refrigerate.
- Shake well.
- Continue medication for full time of treatment.
- Beyond-use date.
- Take on empty stomach.

**Note**
When dispensing, include a calibrated liquid-measuring device.

#### BACAMPICILLIN HYDROCHLORIDE TABLETS USP

**Usual adult and adolescent dose**
See *Bacampicillin Hydrochloride for Oral Suspension USP*.

**Usual adult prescribing limits**
See *Bacampicillin Hydrochloride for Oral Suspension USP*.

**Usual pediatric dose**
Infants and children up to 25 kg of body weight—Use of the tablets is not recommended. See *Bacampicillin Hydrochloride for Oral Suspension USP*.
Children 25 kg of body weight and over—See *Usual adult and adolescent dose*.

**Strength(s) usually available**
U.S.—
  400 mg (Rx) [*Spectrobid*].
Canada—
  400 mg (Rx) [*Penglobe* (scored)].
  800 mg (Rx) [*Penglobe* (scored)].
Note: 400 mg of bacampicillin hydrochloride are equivalent to 280 mg of ampicillin.

**Packaging and storage**
Store below 40 °C (104 °F), preferably between 15 and 30 °C (59 and 86 °F), unless otherwise specified by manufacturer. Store in a tight container.

**Auxiliary labeling**
- Continue medication for full time of treatment.

## CARBENICILLIN

### Summary of Differences
Category:
  Antipseudomonal penicillin.
Pharmacology/pharmacokinetics:
  Renal elimination of oral carbenicillin is approximately 36%, and 75 to 95% for intravenous carbenicillin.
Precautions:
  Drug interactions and/or related problems—Parenteral carbenicillin also interacts with anticoagulants and other medications that affect blood clotting.
  Laboratory value alterations—May increase bleeding time; may also cause hypernatremia.
  Medical considerations/contraindications—Caution in patients with a history of bleeding disorders, congestive heart failure, or hypertension.
  Patient monitoring—Bleeding time and serum potassium and sodium determinations may be required (parenteral only).

### Additional Dosing Information

**For oral dosage forms only**
Patients with severely impaired renal function (creatinine clearance less than 10 mL per minute) will not achieve therapeutic urine concentrations of carbenicillin.

**For parenteral dosage forms only**
Intramuscular injections should not exceed 2 grams in each site.
Intermittent infusions may be administered over a 30- to 40-minute period.
Patients with impaired renal function may require a reduction in dose and should be observed for hemorrhagic complications.

### Oral Dosage Forms
Note: The dosing and strengths of the dosage forms available are expressed in terms of carbenicillin indanyl sodium (not the base).

#### CARBENICILLIN INDANYL SODIUM TABLETS USP

**Usual adult and adolescent dose**
Antibacterial—
  Oral, 500 mg to 1 gram every six hours.

**Usual pediatric dose**
Dosage has not been established.

**Strength(s) usually available**
U.S.—
  500 mg (Rx) [*Geocillin*].
Canada—
  500 mg (Rx) [*Geopen Oral*].
Note: 500 mg of carbenicillin indanyl sodium are equivalent to 382 mg of carbenicillin and 118 mg of indanyl sodium.

**Packaging and storage**
Store below 40 °C (104 °F), preferably between 15 and 30 °C (59 and 86 °F), unless otherwise specified by manufacturer. Store in a tight container.

**Auxiliary labeling**
- Continue medication for full time of treatment.

### Parenteral Dosage Forms
Note: The dosing and strengths of the dosage forms available are expressed in terms of carbenicillin disodium (not the base).

## CARBENICILLIN DISODIUM STERILE USP

**Usual adult and adolescent dose**
Antibacterial—
    Intramuscular or intravenous, 50 to 83.3 mg per kg of body weight every four hours.
    Urinary tract infections: Intramuscular or intravenous, 1 to 2 grams every six hours; or up to 50 mg per kg of body weight every six hours.

**Usual adult prescribing limits**
Up to 40 grams a day.

**Usual pediatric dose**
Antibacterial—
    Neonates up to 2 kg of body weight: Intramuscular or intravenous, 75 mg per kg of body weight every twelve hours during the first week of life; followed by 75 mg per kg of body weight every eight hours thereafter.
    Neonates 2 kg of body weight and over: Intramuscular or intravenous, 75 mg per kg of body weight every eight hours during the first week of life; followed by 75 mg per kg of body weight every six hours thereafter.
    Older infants and children: Intramuscular or intravenous, 25 to 75 mg per kg of body weight every six hours; or 16.7 to 50 mg per kg of body weight every four hours.

**Size(s) usually available**
U.S.—
    1 gram (Rx) [*Geopen*].
    2 grams (Rx) [*Geopen*].
    5 grams (Rx) [*Geopen*].
    10 grams (Rx) [*Geopen*].
    30 grams (Rx) [*Geopen*].
Canada—
    1 gram (Rx) [*Pyopen*].
    5 grams (Rx) [*Pyopen*].

**Packaging and storage**
Prior to reconstitution, store below 40 °C (104 °F), preferably between 15 and 30 °C (59 and 86 °F), unless otherwise specified by manufacturer.

**Preparation of dosage form**
To prepare initial dilution for intramuscular use, depending on the manufacturer, add 2 to 3.6 mL of sterile water for injection or bacteriostatic water for injection (preserved with 0.9% benzyl alcohol) to each 1-gram vial, 4 to 7.2 mL of diluent to each 2-gram vial, and 7 to 17 mL of diluent to each 5-gram vial. Lidocaine hydrochloride injection 0.5% (without epinephrine) may also be used as a diluent for intramuscular use.

To prepare initial dilution for direct intravenous use, reconstitute as directed above for intramuscular use. Each gram of carbenicillin should be further diluted with the addition of not less than 5 mL of diluent. The resulting solution should be administered as slowly as possible to avoid vein irritation.

For reconstitution of pharmacy bulk vials or piggyback infusion bottles, see manufacturer's labeling for instructions.

Caution—Use of diluents containing benzyl alcohol is not recommended for preparation of medications for use in neonates. A fatal toxic syndrome consisting of metabolic acidosis, CNS depression, respiratory problems, renal failure, hypotension, and possibly seizures and intracranial hemorrhages has been associated with this use.

**Stability**
After reconstitution for intramuscular or direct intravenous use, solutions retain their potency for 24 hours at room temperature or for 72 hours if refrigerated.

Intravenous infusions in suitable diluents (see manufacturer's package insert), concentrated solutions (200 mg per mL), or diluted solutions (10 to 100 mg per mL) prepared from pharmacy bulk vials retain their potency for 24 hours at room temperature or for 72 hours if refrigerated.

**Incompatibilities**
Extemporaneous admixtures of beta-lactam antibacterials (penicillins and cephalosporins) and aminoglycosides may result in substantial mutual inactivation. If these groups of antibacterials are administered concurrently, they should be administered in separate sites at least 1 hour apart. Do not mix them in the same intravenous bag, bottle, or tubing.

When aminoglycosides and penicillins are administered separately by different routes, a reduction in aminoglycoside serum concentration may occur. Usually this is clinically significant only in patients with severely impaired renal function when the excretion of both medications is delayed.

**Additional information**
The sodium content is approximately 4.7 to 5.3 mEq (4.7 to 5.3 mmol), but may be as high as 6.5 mEq (6.5 mmol), per gram of carbenicillin. This must be considered in patients on a restricted sodium intake when calculating total daily sodium intake.

## CLOXACILLIN

### Summary of Differences
Category: Penicillinase-resistant penicillin.
Pharmacology/pharmacokinetics: Very high plasma protein binding (95%).
Precautions: Drug interactions and/or related problems—May interact with other hepatotoxic medications.
Side/adverse effects: May be an increased risk of hepatotoxicity.

### Additional Dosing Information
Patients with impaired renal function do not generally require a reduction in dose unless the impairment is severe.

Cloxacillin should be taken on an empty stomach, preferably 1 hour before meals.

### Oral Dosage Forms
Note: The dosing and strengths of the dosage forms available are expressed in terms of cloxacillin base (not the sodium salt).

## CLOXACILLIN SODIUM CAPSULES USP

**Usual adult and adolescent dose**
Antibacterial—
    Oral, 250 to 500 mg (base) every six hours.

**Usual adult prescribing limits**
Up to 6 grams (base) a day.

**Usual pediatric dose**
Antibacterial—
    Infants and children up to 20 kg of body weight: Oral, 6.25 to 12.5 mg (base) per kg of body weight every six hours.
    Children 20 kg of body weight and over: See *Usual adult and adolescent dose*.

**Strength(s) usually available**
U.S.—
    250 mg (base) (Rx) [*Cloxapen*; GENERIC].
    500 mg (base) (Rx) [*Cloxapen*; GENERIC].
Canada—
    250 mg (base) (Rx) [*Apo-Cloxi*; *Novo-Cloxin*; *Nu-Cloxi*; *Orbenin*].
    500 mg (base) (Rx) [*Apo-Cloxi*; *Novo-Cloxin*; *Nu-Cloxi*; *Orbenin*].

**Packaging and storage**
Store below 40 °C (104 °F), preferably between 15 and 30 °C (59 and 86 °F), unless otherwise specified by manufacturer. Store in a tight container.

**Auxiliary labeling**
• Continue medication for full time of treatment.
• Take on empty stomach.

## CLOXACILLIN SODIUM FOR ORAL SOLUTION USP

**Usual adult and adolescent dose**
See *Cloxacillin Sodium Capsules USP*.

**Usual adult prescribing limits**
See *Cloxacillin Sodium Capsules USP*.

**Usual pediatric dose**
See *Cloxacillin Sodium Capsules USP*.

**Strength(s) usually available**
U.S.—
    125 mg per 5 mL (base) (Rx) [*Tegopen*; GENERIC].
Canada—
    125 mg per 5 mL (base) (Rx) [*Apo-Cloxi*; *Novo-Cloxin*; *Nu-Cloxi*; *Orbenin*].

**Packaging and storage**
Prior to reconstitution, store below 40 °C (104 °F), preferably between 15 and 30 °C (59 and 86 °F), unless otherwise specified by manufacturer. Store in a tight container.

**Stability**
After reconstitution, solutions retain their potency for 14 days if refrigerated.

**Auxiliary labeling**
• Refrigerate.
• Continue medication for full time of treatment.
• Beyond-use date.
• Take on empty stomach.

### Note
When dispensing, include a calibrated liquid-measuring device.

### Parenteral Dosage Forms
Note: The dosing and dosage forms available are expressed in terms of cloxacillin base (not the sodium salt).

#### CLOXACILLIN SODIUM INJECTION

**Usual adult and adolescent dose**
Antibacterial—
   Intravenous, 250 to 500 mg (base) every six hours.

**Usual adult prescribing limits**
Up to 6 grams (base) a day.

**Usual pediatric dose**
Antibacterial—
   Infants and children up to 20 kg of body weight: Intravenous, 6.25 to 12.5 mg (base) per kg of body weight every six hours.
   Children 20 kg of body weight and over: See *Usual adult and adolescent dose*.
Note: Cystic fibrosis patients: Intravenous, 25 mg (base) per kg of body weight every six hours.

**Strength(s) usually available**
U.S.—
   Not commercially available.
Canada—
   250 mg (base) (Rx) [*Orbenin; Tegopen*].
   500 mg (base) (Rx) [*Orbenin; Tegopen*].
   2 grams (base) (Rx) [*Orbenin; Tegopen*].

**Packaging and storage**
Prior to reconstitution, store between 15 and 30 °C (59 and 86 °F), unless otherwise specified by manufacturer.

**Preparation of dosage form**
To prepare for intramuscular injection, add 1.9 mL or 1.7 mL of sterile water for injection to each 250 mg or 500 mg vial, respectively, and shake to dissolve.
To prepare for intravenous injection, add 4.9 mL, 4.8 mL, or 6.8 mL of sterile water for injection to each 250 mg, 500 mg, or 2 gram vial, respectively, and shake to dissolve.
For direct intravenous use, the resulting solution should be administered slowly over a 2- to 4-minute period.
For intermittent intravenous use, the resulting solution should be further diluted with a suitable diluent (see manufacturer's package insert). It may be administered over a 30- to 40-minute period.

**Stability**
After reconstitution with suitable diluents (see manufacturer's package insert), solutions retain their potency for 24 hours at controlled room temperature (25 °C [77 °F]), or 72 hours if refrigerated.

**Incompatibilities**
Extemporaneous admixtures of beta-lactam antibacterials (penicillins and cephalosporins) and aminoglycosides may result in substantial mutual inactivation. If these groups of antibacterials are administered concurrently, they should be administered in separate sites at least 1 hour apart. Do not mix them in the same intravenous bag, bottle, or tubing.
When aminoglycosides and penicillins are administered separately by different routes, a reduction in aminoglycoside serum concentration may occur. Usually this is clinically significant only in patients with severely impaired renal function when the excretion of both medications is delayed.

---
## DICLOXACILLIN
---

### Summary of Differences
Category: Penicillinase-resistant penicillin.
Pharmacology/pharmacokinetics: Very high plasma protein binding (95 to 98%).
Precautions: Drug interactions and/or related problems—May react with other hepatotoxic medications.
Side/adverse effects: May be an increased risk of hepatotoxicity.

### Additional Dosing Information
Patients with impaired renal function do not generally require a reduction in dose unless the impairment is severe.
Dicloxacillin should be taken on an empty stomach, preferably 1 hour before meals.

### Oral Dosage Forms
Note: The dosing and strengths of the dosage forms available are expressed in terms of dicloxacillin base (not the sodium salt).

#### DICLOXACILLIN SODIUM CAPSULES USP

**Usual adult and adolescent dose**
Antibacterial—
   Oral, 125 to 250 mg (base) every six hours.

**Usual adult prescribing limits**
Up to 6 grams (base) a day.

**Usual pediatric dose**
Antibacterial—
   Infants and children up to 40 kg of body weight: Oral, 3.125 to 6.25 mg (base) per kg of body weight every six hours.
   Children 40 kg of body weight and over: See *Usual adult and adolescent dose*.
Note: Cystic fibrosis patients: Oral, 12.5 to 25 mg (base) per kg of body weight every six hours.

**Strength(s) usually available**
U.S.—
   125 mg (base) (Rx) [*Dynapen*].
   250 mg (base) (Rx) [*Dycill; Dynapen; Pathocil;* GENERIC].
   500 mg (base) (Rx) [*Dycill; Dynapen; Pathocil;* GENERIC].
Canada—
   Not commercially available.

**Packaging and storage**
Store below 40 °C (104 °F), preferably between 15 and 30 °C (59 and 86 °F), unless otherwise specified by manufacturer. Store in a tight container.

**Auxiliary labeling**
• Continue medication for full time of treatment.
• Take on empty stomach.

#### DICLOXACILLIN SODIUM FOR ORAL SUSPENSION USP

**Usual adult and adolescent dose**
See *Dicloxacillin Sodium Capsules USP*.

**Usual adult prescribing limits**
See *Dicloxacillin Sodium Capsules USP*.

**Usual pediatric dose**
See *Dicloxacillin Sodium Capsules USP*.

**Strength(s) usually available**
U.S.—
   62.5 mg per 5 mL (base) (Rx) [*Dynapen; Pathocil*].
Canada—
   Not commercially available.

**Packaging and storage**
Prior to reconstitution, store below 40 °C (104 °F), preferably between 15 and 30 °C (59 and 86 °F), unless otherwise specified by manufacturer. Store in a tight container.

**Stability**
After reconstitution, suspensions retain their potency for 7 days at room temperature or for 14 days if refrigerated.

**Auxiliary labeling**
• Refrigerate.
• Shake well.
• Continue medication for full time of treatment.
• Beyond-use date.
• Take on empty stomach.

### Note
When dispensing, include a calibrated liquid-measuring device.

---
## FLUCLOXACILLIN
---

### Summary of Differences
Category:
   Penicillinase-resistant penicillin.
Pharmacology/pharmacokinetics:
   Very high plasma protein binding (94%).
Precautions:
   Drug interactions and/or related problems—May react with other hepatotoxic medications.
   Laboratory value alterations—May transiently decrease the serum uric acid concentration in some patients.

Side/adverse effects:
    May be an increased risk of cholestatic jaundice.

## Additional Dosing Information
Patients with impaired renal function do not generally require a reduction in dose unless the impairment is severe.

Flucloxacillin should be taken on an empty stomach, preferably, 1 hour before meals.

## Oral Dosage Forms
Note: The dosing and strengths of the dosage forms available are expressed in terms of flucloxacillin sodium (not the base).

### FLUCLOXACILLIN SODIUM CAPSULES
**Usual adult and adolescent dose**
Antibacterial—
    Oral, 250 to 500 mg every six hours.

**Usual pediatric dose**
Antibacterial—
    Children less than 12 years of age and up to 40 kg of body weight: Oral, 125 to 250 mg every six hours; or 6.25 to 12.5 mg per kg of body weight every six hours
    Infants up to 6 months of age: Oral, 6.25 mg per kg of body weight every six hours.

**Strength(s) usually available**
U.S.—
    Not commercially available.
Canada—
    250 mg (Rx) [*Fluclox*].
    500 mg (Rx) [*Fluclox*].

**Packaging and storage**
Store between 15 and 30 °C (59 and 86 °F). Store in a tight container.

**Auxiliary labeling**
• Continue medication for full time of treatment.
• Take on empty stomach.

### FLUCLOXACILLIN FOR ORAL SUSPENSION USP
**Usual adult and adolescent dose**
See *Flucloxacillin Sodium Capsules*.

**Usual pediatric dose**
See *Flucloxacillin Sodium Capsules*.

**Strength(s) usually available**
U.S.—
    Not commercially available.
Canada—
    125 mg per 5 mL (Rx) [*Fluclox*].
    250 mg per 5 mL (Rx) [*Fluclox*].

**Packaging and storage**
Prior to reconstitution, store between 15 and 30 °C (59 and 86 °F). Store in a tight container.

**Stability**
After reconstitution, the suspension retains its potency for 7 days when refrigerated.

**Auxiliary labeling**
• Refrigerate.
• Shake well.
• Continue medication for full time of treatment.
• Beyond-use date.
• Take on empty stomach.

**Note**
When dispensing, include a calibrated liquid-measuring device.

---

## METHICILLIN

## Summary of Differences
Category: Penicillinase-resistant penicillin.
Precautions: Patient monitoring—Renal function determinations may be required because of interstitial nephritis.
Side/adverse effects—May be increased risk of interstitial nephritis.

## Additional Dosing Information
Methicillin sodium for injection should be administered by deep intragluteal injection or by intravenous injection only.

Patients with impaired renal function require a reduction in dose.

## Parenteral Dosage Forms
Note: The dosing and strengths of the dosage forms available are expressed in terms of methicillin sodium (not the base).

### METHICILLIN SODIUM FOR INJECTION USP
**Usual adult and adolescent dose**
Antibacterial—
    Intramuscular, 1 gram every four to six hours.
    Intravenous, 1 gram every six hours.

**Usual adult prescribing limits**
Up to 24 grams a day.

**Usual pediatric dose**
Antibacterial—
    Meningitis, bacterial:
        Neonates up to 2 kg of body weight—Intramuscular or intravenous, 25 to 50 mg per kg of body weight every twelve hours during the first week of life, then 50 mg per kg of body weight every eight hours thereafter.
        Neonates 2 kg of body weight and over—Intramuscular or intravenous, 50 mg per kg of body weight every eight hours during the first week of life, then 50 mg per kg of body weight every six hours thereafter.
    For all other indications:
        Infants and children up to 40 kg of body weight—Intramuscular or intravenous, 25 mg per kg of body weight every six hours.
        Children 40 kg of body weight and over—See *Usual adult and adolescent dose*.
Note: Cystic fibrosis patients—Intramuscular or intravenous, 50 mg per kg of body weight every six hours.

**Size(s) usually available**
U.S.—
    1 gram (Rx) [*Staphcillin*].
    4 grams (Rx) [*Staphcillin*].
    6 grams (Rx) [*Staphcillin*].
    10 grams (Rx) [*Staphcillin*].
Canada—
    Not commercially available.

**Packaging and storage**
Prior to reconstitution, store between 15 and 30 °C (59 and 86 °F).

**Preparation of dosage form**
To prepare initial dilution for intramuscular use, add 1.5 mL of sterile water for injection or 0.9% sodium chloride injection to each 1-gram vial, 5.7 mL of diluent to each 4-gram vial, and 8.6 mL of diluent to each 6-gram vial to provide a concentration of 500 mg per mL.

To prepare initial dilution for direct intravenous use, reconstitute as directed above for intramuscular use. Each mL (500 mg) of the resulting solution should be further diluted in 25 mL of 0.9% sodium chloride injection and administered at the rate of 10 mL per minute.

For reconstitution of pharmacy bulk vials or piggyback infusion bottles, see manufacturer's labeling for instructions.

**Stability**
After reconstitution for intramuscular use, solutions retain their potency for 24 hours at room temperature or for 4 days if refrigerated.

After reconstitution for intravenous use, solutions in concentrations of 2 to 20 mg per mL retain at least 90% of their potency for 8 hours at room temperature in suitable diluents (see manufacturer's package insert).

**Incompatibilities**
Extemporaneous admixtures of beta-lactam antibacterials (penicillins and cephalosporins) and aminoglycosides may result in substantial mutual inactivation. If these groups of antibacterials are administered concurrently, they should be administered in separate sites at least 1 hour apart. Do not mix them in the same intravenous bag, bottle, or tubing.

When aminoglycosides and penicillins are administered separately by different routes, a reduction in aminoglycoside serum concentration may occur. Usually this is clinically significant only in patients with severely impaired renal function when the excretion of both medications is delayed.

Extemporaneous admixtures of other drugs with methicillin sodium for injection are not recommended.

**Additional information**
The total sodium content is approximately 2.24 mEq (2.24 mmol) per gram of methicillin sodium. This must be considered in patients on a restricted sodium intake when calculating total daily sodium intake.

# MEZLOCILLIN

## Summary of Differences
Category:
   Antipseudomonal penicillin.
Precautions:
   Drug interactions and/or related problems—May also interact with other hepatotoxic medications.
   Laboratory value alterations—May produce false-positive protein reactions with various urine protein tests.
   Patient monitoring—Serum potassium determinations may be required.

## Additional Dosing Information
Intramuscular injections should not exceed 2 grams in each site.

Adults with impaired renal function may require a reduction in dose as follows:

| Creatinine Clearance (mL/min)/(mL/sec) | Dose |
|---|---|
| > 30/0.50 | See *Usual adult and adolescent dose* |
| 10–30/0.17–0.50 | 1.5 to 3 grams every 6 to 8 hours |
| < 10/0.17 | 1.5 to 2 grams every 8 hours |
| Hemodialysis patients | 3 to 4 grams after each dialysis, then every 12 hours |
| Peritoneal dialysis patients | 3 grams every 12 hours |

## Parenteral Dosage Forms
Note: The dosing and strengths of the dosage forms available are expressed in terms of mezlocillin sodium (not the base).

### MEZLOCILLIN SODIUM STERILE USP

**Usual adult and adolescent dose**
Antibacterial—
   Intramuscular or intravenous, 33.3 to 58.3 mg per kg of body weight every four hours; 50 to 87.5 mg per kg of body weight every six hours; or 3 to 4 grams every four to six hours.
   Urinary tract infections, complicated: Intravenous, 37.5 to 50 mg per kg of body weight every six hours; or 3 grams every six hours.
   Urinary tract infections, uncomplicated: Intramuscular or intravenous, 25 to 31.25 mg per kg of body weight every six hours; or 1.5 to 2 grams every six hours.

**Usual adult prescribing limits**
Up to 24 grams a day.

**Usual pediatric dose**
Antibacterial—
   Neonates up to 2 kg of body weight: Intramuscular or intravenous, 50 to 75 mg per kg of body weight every twelve hours during the first week of life, then 50 mg per kg of body weight every eight hours thereafter.
   Neonates 2 kg of body weight and over: Intramuscular or intravenous, 50 mg per kg of body weight every eight hours during the first week of life, then 50 mg per kg of body weight every six hours thereafter.
   Infants over 1 month of age and children up to 12 years of age: Intramuscular or intravenous, 50 mg per kg of body weight every four hours.

**Size(s) usually available**
U.S.—
   1 gram (Rx) [*Mezlin*].
   2 grams (Rx) [*Mezlin*].
   3 grams (Rx) [*Mezlin*].
   4 grams (Rx) [*Mezlin*].
   20 grams (Rx) [*Mezlin*].
Canada—
   Not commercially available.

**Packaging and storage**
Prior to reconstitution, store below 30 °C (86 °F). After reconstitution, if precipitation occurs during refrigeration, the solution may be warmed to 37 °C (98.6 °F) for 20 minutes in a water bath, and shaken well.

**Preparation of dosage form**
To prepare initial dilution for intramuscular use, add 3 to 4 mL of sterile water for injection or 0.5 or 1% lidocaine hydrochloride injection (without epinephrine) to each 1-gram vial and shake vigorously.

The resulting solution should be administered slowly over a 12- to 15-second period to minimize discomfort.

To prepare initial dilution for intravenous use, add at least 10 mL of sterile water for injection, 5% dextrose injection, or 0.9% sodium chloride injection to each 1-gram vial and shake vigorously. For direct intravenous use, the resulting solution should be administered slowly over a 3- to 5-minute period to minimize vein irritation. The concentration should not exceed 10% (100 mg per mL).

For intermittent intravenous use, the resulting solution should be further diluted in 50 to 100 mL of a suitable diluent (see manufacturer's package insert). It may be administered over a 30-minute period by direct infusion or by a Y-type hook-up.

For reconstitution of piggyback infusion bottles, see manufacturer's labeling for instructions. If the Y-type or piggyback method of administration is used, the primary infusion should be temporarily discontinued during infusion of mezlocillin.

**Stability**
After reconstitution with suitable diluents (see manufacturer's package insert), solutions at concentrations of 10 and 100 mg per mL retain at least 90% of their potency for 24 to 72 hours at controlled room temperature (15 to 30 °C [59 to 86 °F]) or for 1 to 7 days if refrigerated.

After reconstitution with sterile water for injection, 0.9% sodium chloride injection, or 5% dextrose injection, solutions at concentrations up to 100 mg per mL retain their potency for 4 weeks when frozen at −12 °C (10 °F).

After reconstitution with sterile water for injection, 0.9% sodium chloride injection, or 0.5 or 1% lidocaine hydrochloride injection (without epinephrine), solutions at concentrations up to 250 mg per mL retain their potency for 24 hours at room temperature.

Solutions range from clear and colorless to pale yellow in color. However, the powder and reconstituted solution may darken slightly during storage; this darkening does not affect their potency.

**Incompatibilities**
Extemporaneous admixtures of beta-lactam antibacterials (penicillins and cephalosporins) and aminoglycosides may result in substantial mutual inactivation. If these groups of antibacterials are administered concurrently, they should be administered in separate sites at least 1 hour apart. Do not mix them in the same intravenous bag, bottle, or tubing.

When aminoglycosides and penicillins are administered separately by different routes, a reduction in aminoglycoside serum concentration may occur. Usually this is clinically significant only in patients with severely impaired renal function when the excretion of both medications is delayed.

**Additional information**
The sodium content is approximately 1.9 mEq (43 mg) per gram of mezlocillin. This must be considered in patients on a restricted sodium intake when calculating total daily sodium intake.

---

# NAFCILLIN

## Summary of Differences
Category:
   Penicillinase-resistant penicillin.
Pharmacology/pharmacokinetics:
   Oral absorption—Erratic and poor.
   Protein binding—High (90%).
   Hepatic biotransformation—High (60–70%).
Precautions:
   Drug interactions and/or related problems—
     May also interact with other hepatotoxic medications.
Side/adverse effects:
   May be an increased risk of interstitial nephritis.

## Additional Dosing Information
Nafcillin sodium for injection should be administered by deep intragluteal injection or by intravenous injection only.

## Oral Dosage Forms
Note: The dosing and strengths of the dosage forms available are expressed in terms of nafcillin base (not the sodium salt).

### NAFCILLIN SODIUM CAPSULES USP

**Usual adult and adolescent dose**
Antibacterial—
   Oral, 250 mg to 1 gram (base) every four to six hours.

**Usual adult prescribing limits**
Up to 6 grams (base) daily.

### Usual pediatric dose
Antibacterial—
  Pharyngitis, bacterial:
    Oral, 250 mg (base) every eight hours.
  For all other indications:
    Neonates—Oral, 10 mg (base) per kg of body weight every six to eight hours.
    Older infants and children—Oral, 6.25 to 12.5 mg (base) per kg of body weight every six hours.

### Strength(s) usually available
U.S.—
  250 mg (base) (Rx) [*Unipen*].
Canada—
  Not commercially available.

### Packaging and storage
Store below 40 °C (104 °F), preferably between 15 and 30 °C (59 and 86 °F), unless otherwise specified by manufacturer. Store in a tight container.

### Auxiliary labeling
• Continue medication for full time of treatment.
• Take on empty stomach.

## NAFCILLIN SODIUM TABLETS USP

### Usual adult and adolescent dose
See *Nafcillin Sodium Capsules USP*.

### Usual adult prescribing limits
See *Nafcillin Sodium Capsules USP*.

### Usual pediatric dose
See *Nafcillin Sodium Capsules USP*.

### Strength(s) usually available
U.S.—
  500 mg (base) (Rx) [*Unipen*].
Canada—
  Not commercially available.

### Packaging and storage
Store below 40 °C (104 °F), preferably between 15 and 30 °C (59 and 86 °F), unless otherwise specified by manufacturer. Store in a tight, light-resistant container.

### Auxiliary labeling
• Continue medication for full time of treatment.
• Take on empty stomach.

## Parenteral Dosage Forms

Note: The dosing and strengths of the dosage forms available are expressed in terms of nafcillin base (not the sodium salt).

## NAFCILLIN SODIUM FOR INJECTION USP

### Usual adult and adolescent dose
Antibacterial—
  Bone and joint infections
  Endocarditis, bacterial
  Meningitis, bacterial or
  Pericarditis, bacterial:
    Intravenous, 1.5 to 2 grams every four to six hours.
  For all other indications:
    Intramuscular, 500 mg (base) every four to six hours.
    Intravenous, 500 mg to 1.5 grams (base) every four hours.

### Usual adult prescribing limits
Intramuscular—Up to 12 grams (base) a day.
Intravenous—Up to 20 grams (base) a day.

### Usual pediatric dose
Antibacterial—
  Meningitis, bacterial:
    Neonates up to 2 kg of body weight—
      Intramuscular or intravenous, 25 to 50 mg per kg of body weight every twelve hours during the first week of life, then 50 mg per kg of body weight every eight hours thereafter.
    Neonates 2 kg of body weight and over—
      Intramuscular or intravenous, 50 mg per kg of body weight every eight hours during the first week of life, then 50 mg per kg of body weight every six hours thereafter.
  For all other indications:
    Neonates—
      Intramuscular, 10 mg (base) per kg of body weight every twelve hours.
      Intravenous, 10 to 20 mg (base) per kg of body weight every four hours; or 20 to 40 mg per kg of body weight every eight hours.
    Older infants and children—
      Intramuscular, 25 mg (base) per kg of body weight every twelve hours.
      Intravenous, 10 to 20 mg (base) per kg of body weight every four hours; or 20 to 40 mg per kg of body weight every eight hours.

### Size(s) usually available
U.S.—
  500 mg (base) (Rx) [*Nafcil; Nallpen;* GENERIC].
  1 gram (base) (Rx) [*Nafcil; Nallpen; Unipen;* GENERIC].
  2 grams (base) (Rx) [*Nafcil; Nallpen; Unipen;* GENERIC].
  10 grams (base) (Rx) [*Nafcil; Nallpen; Unipen;* GENERIC].
Canada—
  500 mg (base) (Rx) [*Unipen*].

### Packaging and storage
Prior to reconstitution, store below 40 °C (104 °F), preferably between 15 and 30 °C (59 and 86 °F), unless otherwise specified by manufacturer.

### Preparation of dosage form
To prepare initial dilution for intramuscular use, depending on the manufacturer, add 1.7 to 1.8 mL of sterile water for injection or bacteriostatic water for injection to each 500-mg vial, 3.4 mL of diluent to each 1-gram vial, or 6.6 to 6.8 mL of diluent to each 2-gram vial to provide 250 mg (base) per mL.

To prepare initial dilution for direct intravenous use, reconstitute as directed above for intramuscular use. The resulting solution should be further diluted in 15 to 30 mL of sterile water for injection or 0.9% sodium chloride injection and administered over a 5- to 10-minute period.

For reconstitution of pharmacy bulk vials or piggyback infusion bottles, see manufacturer's labeling for instructions.

Intravenous infusions of nafcillin sodium for injection should be administered in suitable diluents (see manufacturer's package insert) in a concentration of 2 to 40 mg per mL. Infusions should be administered over at least a 30- to 60-minute period to avoid vein irritation.

### Stability
After reconstitution for intramuscular use, solutions retain their potency for 3 days at room temperature or for 7 days if refrigerated, depending on the manufacturer.

After reconstitution for intravenous use, solutions in concentrations of 2 to 40 mg per mL retain at least 90% of their potency for 24 hours at room temperature or for 96 hours if refrigerated (depending on the manufacturer) in suitable diluents (see manufacturer's package insert).

Concentrated solutions (100 mg per mL) prepared from pharmacy bulk vials retain their potency for 8 hours at room temperature or for 48 hours if refrigerated.

Concentrated solutions (250 mg per mL) retain their potency for 3 days at room temperature or for 7 days if refrigerated or frozen.

### Incompatibilities
Extemporaneous admixtures of beta-lactam antibacterials (penicillins and cephalosporins) and aminoglycosides may result in substantial mutual inactivation. If these groups of antibacterials are administered concurrently, they should be administered in separate sites at least 1 hour apart. Do not mix them in the same intravenous bag, bottle, or tubing.

When aminoglycosides and penicillins are administered separately by different routes, a reduction in aminoglycoside serum concentration may occur. Usually this is clinically significant only in patients with severely impaired renal function when the excretion of both medications is delayed.

### Additional information
The total sodium content is approximately 2.9 mEq (2.9 mmol) per gram of nafcillin. This must be considered in patients on a restricted sodium intake when calculating total daily sodium intake.

---

# OXACILLIN

## Summary of Differences
Category: Penicillinase-resistant penicillin.
Pharmacology/pharmacokinetics: High plasma protein binding (90%).
Precautions: Drug interactions and/or related problems—May also interact with other hepatotoxic medications.
Side/adverse effects: May be an increased risk of hepatotoxicity and interstitial nephritis.

## Additional Dosing Information
Patients with impaired renal function do not generally require a reduction in dose.

## Oral Dosage Forms
Note: The dosing and strengths of the dosage forms available are expressed in terms of oxacillin base (not the sodium salt).

### OXACILLIN SODIUM CAPSULES USP

**Usual adult and adolescent dose**
Antibacterial—
  Oral, 500 mg to 1 gram (base) every four to six hours.

**Usual adult prescribing limits**
Up to 6 grams (base) a day.

**Usual pediatric dose**
Antibacterial—
  Children up to 40 kg of body weight: Oral, 12.5 to 25 mg (base) per kg of body weight every six hours.
  Children 40 kg of body weight and over: See *Usual adult and adolescent dose*.

**Strength(s) usually available**
U.S.—
  250 mg (base) (Rx) [*Bactocill; Prostaphlin;* GENERIC].
  500 mg (base) (Rx) [*Bactocill; Prostaphlin;* GENERIC].
Canada—
  Not commercially available.

**Packaging and storage**
Store between 15 and 30 °C (59 and 86 °F). Store in a tight container.

**Auxiliary labeling**
• Continue medication for full time of treatment.
• Take on empty stomach.

### OXACILLIN SODIUM FOR ORAL SOLUTION USP

**Usual adult and adolescent dose**
See *Oxacillin Sodium Capsules USP*.

**Usual adult prescribing limits**
See *Oxacillin Sodium Capsules USP*.

**Usual pediatric dose**
See *Oxacillin Sodium Capsules USP*.

**Strength(s) usually available**
U.S.—
  250 mg per 5 mL (base) (Rx) [*Prostaphlin;* GENERIC].
Canada—
  Not commercially available.

**Packaging and storage**
Prior to reconstitution, store between 15 and 30 °C (59 and 86 °F). Store in a tight container.

**Stability**
After reconstitution, solutions retain their potency for 7 days at room temperature or for 14 days if refrigerated.

**Auxiliary labeling**
• Refrigerate.
• Continue medication for full time of treatment.
• Beyond-use date.
• Take on empty stomach.

**Note**
When dispensing, include a calibrated liquid-measuring device.

## Parenteral Dosage Forms

### OXACILLIN SODIUM FOR INJECTION USP

**Usual adult and adolescent dose**
Antibacterial—
  Intramuscular or intravenous, 250 mg to 1 gram (base) every four to six hours.
  Meningitis, bacterial: Intravenous, 1.5 to 2 grams every four hours.

**Usual pediatric dose**
Antibacterial—
  Meningitis, bacterial:
    Neonates up to 2 kg of body weight—Intramuscular or intravenous, 25 to 50 mg per kg of body weight every twelve hours during the first week of life, then 50 mg per kg of body weight every eight hours thereafter.
    Neonates 2 kg of body weight and over—Intramuscular or intravenous, 50 mg per kg of body weight every eight hours during the first week of life, then 50 mg per kg of body weight every six hours thereafter.
  For all other indications:
    Premature infants and neonates—Intramuscular or intravenous, 6.25 mg (base) every six hours.
    Children up to 40 kg of body weight—Intramuscular or intravenous, 12.5 to 25 mg (base) per kg of body weight every six hours; or 16.7 mg per kg of body weight every four hours.
    Children 40 kg of body weight and over—See *Usual adult and adolescent dose*.

**Size(s) usually available**
U.S.—
  250 mg (base) (Rx) [*Prostaphlin*].
  500 mg (base) (Rx) [*Bactocill; Prostaphlin;* GENERIC].
  1 gram (base) (Rx) [*Bactocill; Prostaphlin;* GENERIC].
  2 grams (base) (Rx) [*Bactocill; Prostaphlin;* GENERIC].
  4 grams (base) (Rx) [*Bactocill; Prostaphlin*].
  10 grams (base) (Rx) [*Bactocill; Prostaphlin;* GENERIC].
Canada—
  Not commercially available.

**Packaging and storage**
Prior to reconstitution, store between 15 and 30 °C (59 and 86 °F).

**Preparation of dosage form**
To prepare initial dilution for intramuscular use, depending on the manufacturer, add 1.4 mL of sterile water for injection to each 250-mg vial, 2.7 to 2.8 mL of diluent to each 500-mg vial, 5.7 mL of diluent to each 1-gram vial, 11.4 to 11.5 mL of diluent to each 2-gram vial, and 21.8 to 23 mL of diluent to each 4-gram vial to provide a concentration of 250 mg per 1.5 mL.
To prepare initial dilution for direct intravenous use, add 5 mL of sterile water for injection or 0.9% sodium chloride injection to each 250- or 500-mg vial, 10 mL of diluent to each 1-gram vial, 20 mL of diluent to each 2-gram vial, and 40 mL of diluent to each 4-gram vial. The resulting solution should be administered slowly over a 10-minute period.
Intravenous infusions of oxacillin sodium for injection should be administered in a suitable diluent in a concentration of up to 40 mg per mL (see manufacturer's package insert).
For reconstitution of pharmacy bulk vials, piggyback infusion bottles, and dual-compartment vials, see manufacturer's labeling for instructions.

**Stability**
After reconstitution for intramuscular use, solutions retain their potency for 4 days at room temperature or for 7 days if refrigerated.
Concentrated solutions (100 mg per mL) prepared from pharmacy bulk vials retain their potency for 48 hours at room temperature or for 7 days if refrigerated.
Diluted solutions (up to 40 mg per mL) retain their potency for 72 hours at room temperature, for 7 days if refrigerated, or for 30 days if frozen.
Solutions (10 to 50 mg per mL) prepared from piggyback infusion bottles retain their potency for 24 hours at room temperature.

**Incompatibilities**
Extemporaneous admixtures of beta-lactam antibacterials (penicillins and cephalosporins) and aminoglycosides may result in substantial mutual inactivation. If these groups of antibacterials are administered concurrently, they should be administered in separate sites at least 1 hour apart. Do not mix them in the same intravenous bag, bottle, or tubing.
When aminoglycosides and penicillins are administered separately by different routes, a reduction in aminoglycoside serum concentration may occur. Usually this is clinically significant only in patients with severely impaired renal function when the excretion of both medications is delayed.

**Additional information**
The total sodium content (derived from dibasic sodium phosphate buffer and oxacillin sodium) is approximately 2.8 to 3.1 mEq (64 to 71 mg) per gram of oxacillin. This must be considered in patients on a restricted sodium intake when calculating total daily sodium intake.

---

## PENICILLIN G

## Summary of Differences
Category:
  Natural penicillin.
Pharmacology/pharmacokinetics:
  Oral absorption low (15 to 30%).
  Time to peak serum concentration—
    Benzathine salt: 24 hours.
    Procaine salt: 4 hours.

**Precautions:**
Cross-sensitivity and/or related problems—
Cross-sensitivity with other ester-type local anesthetics may also occur with administration of penicillin G procaine.
Drug interactions and/or related problems—
Use of angiotensin-converting enzyme (ACE) inhibitors, potassium-sparing diuretics, other potassium-containing medications, or potassium supplements with parenteral penicillin G potassium may promote hyperkalemia; also oral penicillin G may interact with cholestyramine and colestipol.
Patient monitoring—
Serum potassium or sodium determinations may be required (parenteral only).
Side/adverse effects:
May be an increased risk of mental disturbances with administration of penicillin G procaine.

## Additional Dosing Information
Patients with impaired renal function do not generally require a reduction in dose unless the impairment is severe.
**For oral dosage forms only**
Oral administration of penicillin G commonly results in low serum concentrations. Therefore, severe infections should not be treated with oral penicillin during the acute stage.
Penicillin G is an acid-labile penicillin; therefore, concurrent administration with acidic fruit juices and other acidic beverages should be avoided.

## Oral Dosage Forms
Note: The dosing and strengths of the dosage forms available are expressed in terms of penicillin G benzathine (not the base).

### PENICILLIN G BENZATHINE SUSPENSION
**Usual adult and adolescent dose**
Antibacterial—
Oral, 200,000 to 500,000 Units (125 to 312 mg) every four to six hours.
Continuous prophylaxis of streptococcal infections in patients with a history of rheumatic heart disease: Oral, 200,000 to 250,000 Units (125 to 156 mg) every twelve hours.

**Usual adult prescribing limits**
Up to 2,000,000 Units a day.

**Usual pediatric dose**
Antibacterial—
Infants and children up to 12 years of age: Oral, 4167 to 15,000 Units per kg of body weight every four hours; 6250 to 22,500 Units per kg of body weight every six hours; or 8333 to 30,000 Units per kg of body weight every eight hours.
Children 12 years of age and over: See *Usual adult and adolescent dose*.

**Strength(s) usually available**
U.S.—
Not commercially available.
Canada—
250,000 Units (156 mg) per 5 mL (Rx) [*Megacillin*].
500,000 Units (312 mg) per 5 mL (Rx) [*Megacillin*].

**Packaging and storage**
Store between 15 and 30 °C (59 and 86 °F), unless otherwise specified by manufacturer.

**Stability**
The reconstituted suspension may be stored at room temperature until the labeled expiration date.

**Auxiliary labeling**
• Continue medication for full time of treatment.
• Take on empty stomach.
• Beyond-use date.

### PENICILLIN G POTASSIUM FOR ORAL SOLUTION USP
**Usual adult and adolescent dose**
See *Penicillin G Benzathine Suspension*.
**Usual adult prescribing limits**
See *Penicillin G Benzathine Suspension*.
**Usual pediatric dose**
See *Penicillin G Benzathine Suspension*.

**Strength(s) usually available**
U.S.—
400,000 Units (250 mg) per 5 mL (Rx) [GENERIC].
Canada—
Not commercially available.

**Packaging and storage**
Prior to reconstitution, store below 40 °C (104 °F), preferably between 15 and 30 °C (59 and 86 °F), unless otherwise specified by manufacturer. Store in a tight container.

**Stability**
After reconstitution, solutions retain their potency for 14 days if refrigerated.

**Auxiliary labeling**
• Refrigerate.
• Continue medication for full time of treatment.
• Beyond-use date.
• Take on empty stomach.

**Note**
When dispensing, include a calibrated liquid-measuring device.

### PENICILLIN G POTASSIUM TABLETS USP
**Usual adult and adolescent dose**
See *Penicillin G Benzathine for Oral Solution*.
**Usual adult prescribing limits**
See *Penicillin G Benzathine for Oral Solution*.
**Usual pediatric dose**
See *Penicillin G Benzathine for Oral Solution*.

**Strength(s) usually available**
U.S.—
200,000 Units (125 mg) (Rx) [GENERIC].
250,000 Units (156 mg) (Rx) [GENERIC].
400,000 Units (250 mg) (Rx) [*Pentids*; GENERIC].
800,000 Units (500 mg) (Rx) [GENERIC].
Canada—
500,000 Units (312 mg) (Rx) [*Megacillin* (scored)].

**Packaging and storage**
Store below 40 °C (104 °F), preferably between 15 and 30 °C (59 and 86 °F), unless otherwise specified by manufacturer. Store in a tight container.

**Auxiliary labeling**
• Continue medication for full time of treatment.
• Take on empty stomach.

## Parenteral Dosage Forms
Note: Bracketed uses in the *Dosage Forms* section refer to categories of use and/or indications that are not included in U.S. product labeling.
Note: The dosing and strengths of the dosage forms available are expressed in terms of penicillin G salt (not the base).

### STERILE PENICILLIN G BENZATHINE SUSPENSION USP
**Usual adult and adolescent dose**
Antibacterial—
Bejel
Pinta or
Yaws: Intramuscular, 1,200,000 Units as a single dose.
Continuous prophylaxis of streptococcal infections in patients with a history of rheumatic heart disease: Intramuscular, 1,200,000 Units every three to four weeks.
Pharyngitis, streptococcal: Intramuscular, 1,200,000 Units as a single dose.
Syphilis (primary, secondary, and early latent): Intramuscular, 2,400,000 Units as a single dose.
Syphilis (tertiary and late latent, excluding neurosyphilis): Intramuscular, 2,400,000 Units once a week for three weeks.

**Usual adult prescribing limits**
Up to 2,400,000 Units a day.

**Usual pediatric dose**
Antibacterial—
Pharyngitis, group A streptococcal:
Infants and children up to 27.3 kg of body weight—Intramuscular, 300,000 to 600,000 Units as a single dose.
Children 27.3 kg of body weight and over—Intramuscular, 900,000 Units as a single dose.
Rheumatic fever (prophylaxis):
Intramuscular, 1,200,000 Units every two or three weeks.
Syphilis (primary, secondary, and early latent):
Intramuscular, 50,000 Units per kg of body weight, up to 2,400,000 Units, as a single dose.
Syphilis (late latent or latent of unknown duration):
Intramuscular, 50,000 Units per kg of body weight once a week for three weeks.

**Strength(s) usually available**
U.S.—
  600,000 Units in 1 mL (Rx) [*Bicillin L-A; Permapen*].
  1,200,000 Units in 2 mL (Rx) [*Bicillin L-A*].
  2,400,000 Units in 4 mL (Rx) [*Bicillin L-A*].
  3,000,000 Units in 10 mL (Rx) [*Bicillin L-A*].
Canada—
  1,200,000 Units in 2 mL (Rx) [*Bicillin L-A*].

**Packaging and storage**
Store between 2 and 8 °C (36 and 46 °F).

**Additional information**
For deep intramuscular use only. Do not administer intravenously, intra-arterially, subcutaneously, by fat-layer injection, or into or near a nerve. Intravenous injection may cause embolic or toxic reactions. Intra-arterial injection may cause extensive necrosis of the extremity or organ, especially in children. Subcutaneous and fat-layer injection may cause pain and induration. Injection into or near a nerve may result in permanent neurological damage.

Injection of penicillin G benzathine should be made at a slow, steady rate to prevent blockage of the needle because of the high concentration of suspended material.

Intramuscular administration of penicillin G benzathine results in much lower and more prolonged serum concentrations than those attained with other parenteral penicillins.

## PENICILLIN G POTASSIUM FOR INJECTION USP

**Usual adult and adolescent dose**
Antibacterial—
  Intramuscular or intravenous, 1,000,000 to 5,000,000 Units every four to six hours.
  Actinomycosis: Intramuscular or intravenous, 10,000,000 to 20,000,000 Units a day for two to six weeks.
  Anthrax: Intramuscular or intravenous, 2,000,000 Units every six hours.
  Clostridial infections: Intramuscular or intravenous, 20,000,000 Units a day.
  Erysipelas: Intramuscular or intravenous, 600,000 to 2,000,000 Units every six hours.
  Erysipeloid endocarditis: Intramuscular or intravenous, 12,000,000 to 20,000,000 Units a day.
  Listeriosis: Intramuscular or intravenous, 300,000 Units per kg of body weight a day.
  Meningitis, bacterial: Intramuscular or intravenous, 50,000 Units per kg of body weight every four hours; or 24,000,000 Units daily divided every two to four hours.
  Neurosyphilis: Intravenous, 2,000,000 to 4,000,000 Units every four hours for ten to fourteen days.
  *Pasteurella multocida* septicemia and meningitis: Intramuscular or intravenous, 4,000,000 to 6,000,000 Units a day.
  Pericarditis, bacterial: Intramuscular or intravenous, 20,000,000 to 30,000,000 Units a day for four to six weeks.
  Rat-bite fever: Intramuscular or intravenous, 20,000,000 Units a day.
  [Leptospirosis][1]: Intramuscular or intravenous, 1,500,000 Units every six hours.
  [Lyme disease][1]: Intravenous, 20,000,000 to 24,000,000 Units a day for two to three weeks. Duration of therapy is based on clinical response. Treatment failures have occurred and retreatment may be necessary.

**Usual adult prescribing limits**
Up to 80,000,000 Units a day.

**Usual pediatric dose**
Antibacterial—
  Listeriosis in neonates:
    500,000 to 1,000,000 Units daily.
  Meningitis, bacterial:
    Neonates up to 2 kg of body weight—Intramuscular or intravenous, 25,000 to 50,000 Units per kg of body weight every twelve hours during the first week of life, then 50,000 Units per kg of body weight every eight hours thereafter.
    Neonates 2 kg of body weight and over—Intramuscular or intravenous, 50,000 Units per kg of body weight every eight hours during the first week of life, then 50,000 Units per kg of body weight every six hours thereafter.
  Syphilis, congenital:
    Intramuscular or intravenous, 50,000 Units per kg of body weight every twelve hours for the first week of life, then 50,000 Units per kg of body weight every eight hours for the next ten to fourteen days.
  [Lyme disease][1]:
    Intravenous, 250,000 to 400,000 Units per kg of body weight daily for two to three weeks. Duration of therapy is based on clinical response. Treatment failures have occurred and retreatment may be necessary.
  For all other indications:
    Premature and full-term neonates—Intramuscular or intravenous, 30,000 Units per kg of body weight every twelve hours.
    Older infants and children—Intramuscular or intravenous, 8333 to 16,667 Units per kg of body weight every four hours; or 12,500 to 25,000 Units per kg of body weight every six hours.

**Size(s) usually available**
U.S.—
  1,000,000 Units (Rx) [GENERIC].
  5,000,000 Units (Rx) [*Pfizerpen;* GENERIC].
  10,000,000 Units (Rx) [GENERIC].
  20,000,000 Units (Rx) [*Pfizerpen;* GENERIC].
Canada—
  1,000,000 Units (Rx) [GENERIC].
  5,000,000 Units (Rx) [GENERIC].
  10,000,000 Units (Rx) [GENERIC].

**Packaging and storage**
Prior to reconstitution, store below 40 °C (104 °F), preferably between 15 and 30 °C (59 and 86 °F), unless otherwise specified by manufacturer.

**Preparation of dosage form**
To prepare initial dilution for intramuscular or intravenous use, see manufacturer's labeling for instructions.
To prepare for further dilution for intravenous use, see manufacturer's labeling for instructions.

**Stability**
After reconstitution, solutions retain their potency for 24 hours at room temperature or for 7 days if refrigerated.

**Incompatibilities**
Penicillin G potassium is rapidly inactivated by oxidizing and reducing agents, such as alcohols and glycols.
Extemporaneous admixtures of beta-lactam antibacterials (penicillins and cephalosporins) and aminoglycosides may result in substantial mutual inactivation. If these groups of antibacterials are administered concurrently, they should be administered in separate sites at least 1 hour apart. Do not mix them in the same intravenous bag, bottle, or tubing.
When aminoglycosides and penicillins are administered separately by different routes, a reduction in aminoglycoside serum concentration may occur. Usually this is clinically significant only in patients with severely impaired renal function when the excretion of both medications is delayed.

**Additional information**
Daily doses of 10,000,000 Units or more should be administered by slow intravenous infusion or by intermittent piggyback infusion because of possible electrolyte imbalance.
The potassium content and sodium content (derived from sodium citrate buffer) of penicillin G potassium for injection are approximately 1.7 mEq (66.3 mg) and 0.3 mEq (6.9 mg) per 1,000,000 Units of penicillin G, respectively. The sodium content must be considered in patients on a restricted sodium intake when calculating total daily sodium intake.

## STERILE PENICILLIN G PROCAINE SUSPENSION USP

**Usual adult and adolescent dose**
Antibacterial—
  Intramuscular, 600,000 to 1,200,000 Units a day.
  Diphtheria: Intramuscular, 300,000 to 600,000 Units a day as adjunctive therapy to diphtheria antitoxin.
  Neurosyphilis: Intramuscular, 2,400,000 Units a day, and 500 mg of probenecid orally four times a day, for ten to fourteen days.
  Rat-bite fever: Intramuscular, 600,000 Units every twelve hours for ten to fourteen days.

**Usual pediatric dose**
Antibacterial—
  Syphilis, congenital: Intramuscular, 50,000 Units per kg of body weight a day for ten to fourteen days.

**Strength(s) usually available**
U.S.—
  600,000 Units in 1 mL (Rx) [*Wycillin*].
  1,200,000 Units in 2 mL (Rx) [*Wycillin*].
  2,400,000 Units in 4 mL (Rx) [*Wycillin*].
  3,000,000 Units in 10 mL (Rx) [*Crysticillin 300 A.S; Pfizerpen-AS*].
Canada—
  3,000,000 Units per 10 mL (Rx) [*Ayercillin* ( propylparaben 0.013%)].
  5,000,000 Units per 10 mL (base) (Rx) [*Wycillin*].

**Packaging and storage**
Store between 2 and 8 °C (36 and 46 °F).

### Additional information
For deep intramuscular use only. Do not administer intravenously, intra-arterially, or into or near a nerve. Intravenous injection may cause embolic or toxic reactions. Intra-arterial injection may cause extensive necrosis of the extremity or organ, especially in children.

Some patients may experience immediate toxic reactions to procaine, especially when administered in large single doses. These reactions, usually transient, may be characterized by anxiety, confusion, agitation or combativeness, depression, seizures, hallucinations, or expressed fear of impending death.

## PENICILLIN G SODIUM FOR INJECTION USP

### Usual adult and adolescent dose
See *Penicillin G Potassium for Injection USP*.

### Usual adult prescribing limits
See *Penicillin G Potassium for Injection USP*.

### Usual pediatric dose
See *Penicillin G Potassium for Injection USP*.

### Size(s) usually available
U.S.—
   5,000,000 Units (Rx) [GENERIC].
Canada—
   1,000,000 Units (Rx) [GENERIC].
   5,000,000 Units (Rx) [GENERIC].
   10,000,000 Units (Rx) [GENERIC].

### Packaging and storage
Prior to reconstitution, store below 40 °C (104 °F), preferably between 15 and 30 °C (59 and 86 °F), unless otherwise specified by manufacturer.

### Preparation of dosage form
To prepare initial dilution for intramuscular or intravenous use, see manufacturer's labeling for instructions.

### Stability
After reconstitution, solutions retain their potency for 24 hours at room temperature or for 7 days if refrigerated.

### Incompatibilities
Penicillin G sodium is rapidly inactivated by acids, alkalies, and oxidizing agents and in carbohydrate solutions at alkaline pH.

Extemporaneous admixtures of beta-lactam antibacterials (penicillins and cephalosporins) and aminoglycosides may result in substantial mutual inactivation. If these groups of antibacterials are administered concurrently, they should be administered in separate sites at least 1 hour apart. Do not mix them in the same intravenous bag, bottle, or tubing.

When aminoglycosides and penicillins are administered separately by different routes, a reduction in aminoglycoside serum concentration may occur. Usually this is clinically significant only in patients with severely impaired renal function when the excretion of both medications is delayed.

### Additional information
Daily doses of 10,000,000 Units or more should be administered by slow intravenous infusion to avoid causing possible electrolyte imbalance.

The sodium content is approximately 2 mEq (2 mmol) per million Units of penicillin G. This must be considered in patients on a restricted sodium intake when calculating total daily sodium intake.

[1]Not included in Canadian product labeling.

---

## PENICILLIN V

## Summary of Differences
Category: Penicillin G-related natural penicillin.
Precautions: Drug interactions and/or related problems—Also interacts with oral contraceptives.

## Additional Dosing Information
Penicillin V may be taken on a full or empty stomach.
Patients with impaired renal function do not generally require a reduction in dose unless the impairment is severe.

## Oral Dosage Forms
Note: Bracketed uses in the *Dosage Forms* section refer to categories of use and/or indications that are not included in U.S. product labeling.
Note: The dosing and strengths of the dosage forms available are expressed in terms of penicillin V salt (not the base).

## PENICILLIN V BENZATHINE SUSPENSION

### Usual adult and adolescent dose
Antibacterial—
   Oral, 200,000 to 500,000 Units every six to eight hours.
   Continuous prophylaxis of streptococcal infections in patients with a history of rheumatic heart disease: Oral, 200,000 Units every twelve hours.

### Usual pediatric dose
Antibacterial—
   Infants and children up 60 kg of body weight: Oral, 100,000 to 250,000 Units every six to eight hours.
   Children 60 kg of body weight and over: See *Usual adult and adolescent dose*.

### Strength(s) usually available
U.S.—
   Not commercially available.
Canada—
   250,000 Units (156 mg) per 5 mL (Rx) [*PVF*].
   300,000 Units (180 mg) per 5 mL (Rx) [*Pen-Vee*].
   500,000 Units (300 mg) per 5 mL (Rx) [*Pen-Vee; PVF*].

### Packaging and storage
Prior to reconstitution, store below 40 °C (104 °F), preferably between 15 and 30 °C (59 and 86 °F), unless otherwise specified by manufacturer. Store in a tight container.

### Stability
Store at room temperature.

### Auxiliary labeling
- Continue medication for full time of treatment.
- Beyond-use date.

### Note
When dispensing, include a calibrated liquid-measuring device.

## PENICILLIN V POTASSIUM FOR ORAL SOLUTION USP

### Usual adult and adolescent dose
Antibacterial—
   Oral, 125 to 500 mg (200,000 to 800,000 Units) every six to eight hours.
   Continuous prophylaxis of streptococcal infections in patients with a history of rheumatic heart disease: Oral, 125 to 250 mg (200,000 to 400,000 Units) every twelve hours.
   Erysipelas: Oral, 500 mg every six hours.
   Erysipeloid, uncomplicated: Oral, 250 mg every six hours for five to ten days.
   Gingivitis, acute, necrotizing, ulcerative: Oral, 500 mg every six hours.
   *Pasteurella* infections: Oral, 500 mg every six hours for ten to fourteen days.
   Rat-bite fever: Oral, 500 mg every six hours for fourteen days.
   [Lyme disease][1]: Oral, 250 to 500 mg three or four times a day for three to four weeks. Duration of therapy is based on clinical response. Treatment failures have occurred and retreatment may be necessary.

### Usual adult prescribing limits
Up to 7.2 grams (11,520,000 Units) a day.

### Usual pediatric dose
Antibacterial—
   [Lyme disease][1]:
     Oral, 5 to 12.5 mg per kg of body weight four times a day for three to four weeks. Duration of therapy is based on clinical response. Treatment failures have occurred and retreatment may be necessary.
   For all other indications:
     Infants and children up to 12 years of age—Oral, 2.5 to 8.3 mg (4167 to 13,280 Units) per kg of body weight every four hours; 3.75 to 12.5 mg (6250 to 20,000 Units) per kg of body weight every six hours; or 5 to 16.7 mg (8333 to 26,720 Units) per kg of body weight every eight hours.
     Children 12 years of age and over—See *Usual adult and adolescent dose*.

### Strength(s) usually available
U.S.—
   125 mg (200,000 Units) per 5 mL (Rx) [*Beepen-VK; Betapen-VK; Ledercillin VK; Pen Vee K; Veetids;* GENERIC].
   250 mg (400,000 Units) per 5 mL (Rx) [*Beepen-VK; Betapen-VK; Ledercillin VK; Pen Vee K; V-Cillin K; Veetids;* GENERIC].
Canada—
   125 mg (200,000 Units) per 5 mL (Rx) [*Apo-Pen VK; Nadopen-V 200; V-Cillin K*].
   250 mg (400,000 Units) per 5 mL (Rx) [*Nadopen-V 400; V-Cillin K*].
   300 mg (500,000 Units) per 5 mL (Rx) [*Apo-Pen VK; Novo-Pen-VK*].

### Packaging and storage
Prior to reconstitution, store below 40 °C (104 °F), preferably between 15 and 30 °C (59 and 86 °F), unless otherwise specified by manufacturer. Store in a tight container.

### Stability
After reconstitution, solutions retain their potency for 14 days if refrigerated.

### Auxiliary labeling
- Refrigerate.
- Continue medication for full time of treatment.
- Beyond-use date.
- Shake well.

### Note
When dispensing, include a calibrated liquid-measuring device.

## PENICILLIN V POTASSIUM TABLETS USP

### Usual adult and adolescent dose
See *Penicillin V Potassium for Oral Solution USP*.

### Usual adult prescribing limits
See *Penicillin V Potassium for Oral Solution USP*.

### Usual pediatric dose
See *Penicillin V Potassium for Oral Solution USP*.

### Strength(s) usually available
U.S.—
- 250 mg (400,000 Units) (Rx) [*Beepen-VK; Ledercillin VK; Pen Vee K; V-Cillin K; Veetids;* GENERIC].
- 500 mg (800,000 Units) (Rx) [*Beepen-VK; Ledercillin VK; Pen Vee K; V-Cillin K; Veetids;* GENERIC].

Canada—
- 250 mg (400,000 Units) (Rx) [*Ledercillin VK* (scored); *V-Cillin K*].
- 300 mg (500,000 Units) (Rx) [*Apo-Pen VK; Nadopen-V* (scored); *Novo-Pen-VK; Nu-Pen-VK; Pen Vee* (scored); *PVF K* (scored)].
- 500 mg (800,000 Units) (Rx) [*Ledercillin VK*].

### Packaging and storage
Store below 40 °C (104 °F), preferably between 15 and 30 °C (59 and 86 °F), unless otherwise specified by manufacturer. Store in a tight container.

### Auxiliary labeling
- Continue medication for full time of treatment.

[1]Not included in Canadian product labeling.

---

## PIPERACILLIN

## Summary of Differences
Category:
  Antipseudomonal penicillin.
Precautions:
  Drug interactions and/or related problems—Also interacts with anticoagulants and other medications that affect blood clotting, and other hepatotoxic medications.
  Laboratory value alterations—May increase bleeding time.
  Medical considerations/contraindications—Caution in patients with a history of bleeding disorders and cystic fibrosis.
  Patient monitoring—Serum potassium and sodium determinations may be required.

## Additional Dosing Information
Intramuscular injections should not exceed 2 grams in each site.

Adults with impaired renal function may require a reduction in dose as follows:

| Creatinine Clearance (mL/min)/(mL/sec) | Dose (base) |
|---|---|
| > 40/0.67 | See *Usual adult and adolescent dose* |
| 20–40/0.33–0.67 | 3 to 4 grams every 8 hours |
| < 20/0.33 | 3 to 4 grams every 12 hours |
| Hemodialysis patients | 1 gram after each dialysis, then 2 grams every 8 hours |

## Parenteral Dosage Forms
Note: The dosing and strengths of the dosage forms available are expressed in terms of piperacillin base (not the sodium salt).

### PIPERACILLIN SODIUM STERILE USP

#### Usual adult and adolescent dose
Antibacterial—
  Intramuscular or intravenous, 3 to 4 grams (base) every four to six hours.
  Meningitis, bacterial: Intravenous, 4 grams every four hours; or 75 mg per kg of body weight every six hours.
  Urinary tract infections, complicated: Intravenous, 3 to 4 grams (base) every six to eight hours.
  Urinary tract infections, uncomplicated: Intramuscular or intravenous, 1.5 to 2 grams (base) every six hours or 3 to 4 grams every twelve hours.

#### Usual adult prescribing limits
Up to 24 grams (base) a day.

#### Usual pediatric dose
Antibacterial—
  Meningitis, bacterial:
    Neonates up to 2 kg of body weight—Intramuscular or intravenous, 50 mg per kg of body weight every twelve hours during the first week of life, then 50 mg per kg of body weight every eight hours thereafter.
    Neonates 2 kg of body weight and over—Intramuscular or intravenous, 50 mg per kg of body weight every eight hours during the first week of life, then 50 mg per kg of body weight every six hours thereafter.
  For all other indications:
    Infants and children under 12 years of age—Dosage has not been established.
    Children 12 years of age and over—See *Usual adult and adolescent dose*.

Note: Cystic fibrosis patients—Intravenous, 350 to 450 mg per kg of body weight daily.

#### Size(s) usually available
U.S.—
- 2 grams (base) (Rx) [*Pipracil*].
- 3 grams (base) (Rx) [*Pipracil*].
- 4 grams (base) (Rx) [*Pipracil*].
- 40 grams (base) (Rx) [*Pipracil*].

Canada—
- 2 grams (base) (Rx) [*Pipracil*].
- 3 grams (base) (Rx) [*Pipracil*].
- 4 grams (base) (Rx) [*Pipracil*].

#### Packaging and storage
Prior to reconstitution, store below 40 °C (104 °F), preferably between 15 and 30 °C (59 and 86 °F), unless otherwise specified by manufacturer.

#### Preparation of dosage form
To prepare initial dilution for intramuscular use, add 4 mL of sterile water for injection or 0.5 or 1% lidocaine hydrochloride injection (without epinephrine) to each 2-gram vial, 6 mL of diluent to each 3-gram vial, and 7.8 mL of diluent to each 4-gram vial to provide a concentration of 1 gram (base) per 2.5 mL.

To prepare initial dilution for intravenous use, add at least 5 mL of a suitable diluent (see manufacturer's package insert) for each gram of piperacillin and shake well until dissolved. For direct intravenous use, the resulting solution should be administered slowly over a 3- to 5-minute period. For intermittent intravenous use, the resulting solution should be further diluted with a suitable diluent (see manufacturer's package insert) to at least 50 mL. It should be administered over approximately a 20- to 30-minute period.

For reconstitution of pharmacy bulk vials or piggyback infusion bottles, see manufacturer's labeling for instructions.

#### Stability
After reconstitution with suitable diluents (see manufacturer's package insert), solutions retain their potency for 24 hours at controlled room temperature, 7 days if refrigerated, or 1 month if frozen at −15 °C (5 °F).

#### Incompatibilities
Because of chemical instability, piperacillin should not be used for intravenous admixtures with solutions containing *only* sodium bicarbonate.

Extemporaneous admixtures of beta-lactam antibacterials (penicillins and cephalosporins) and aminoglycosides may result in substantial mutual inactivation. If these groups of antibacterials are administered concurrently, they should be administered in separate sites at least 1 hour apart. Do not mix them in the same intravenous bag, bottle, or tubing.

When aminoglycosides and penicillins are administered separately by different routes, a reduction in aminoglycoside serum concentration may occur. Usually this is clinically significant only in patients with severely impaired renal function when the excretion of both medications is delayed.

**Additional information**

The sodium content is approximately 1.98 mEq (45.5 mg) per gram of piperacillin. This must be considered in patients on a restricted sodium intake when calculating total daily sodium intake.

## PIVAMPICILLIN

### Summary of Differences

Category: Aminopenicillin.

Pharmacology/pharmacokinetics: Converted to ampicillin during absorption.

Pediatrics: Should be avoided in children up to 3 months of age since pivampicillin decreases serum carnitine concentrations.

Precautions: Medical considerations/contraindications—Caution in patients with carnitine deficiency.

### Additional Dosing Information

Patients with impaired renal function do not generally require a reduction in dose unless the impairment is severe.

Pivampicillin may be taken on a full or empty stomach.

### Oral Dosage Forms

Note: The dosing and strengths of the dosage forms available are expressed in terms of pivampicillin (not the ampicillin base).

#### PIVAMPICILLIN FOR ORAL SUSPENSION USP

**Usual adult and adolescent dose**
Antibacterial—
   Oral, 525 to 1050 mg two times a day.

**Usual pediatric dose**
Antibacterial—
   Infants 3 to 12 months of age: Oral, 20 to 30 mg per kg of body weight two times a day.
   Children 1 to 3 years of age: Oral, 175 mg two times a day.
   Children 4 to 6 years of age: Oral, 262.5 mg two times a day.
   Children 7 to 10 years of age: Oral, 350 mg two times a day
   Children 10 years of age and older: See *Usual adult and adolescent dose*.

**Strength(s) usually available**
U.S.—
   Not commercially available.
Canada—
   35 mg per mL (Rx) [*Pondocillin*].

Note: 35 mg of pivampicillin are equivalent to 26.4 mg of ampicillin.

**Packaging and storage**
Prior to reconstitution, store between 15 and 30 °C (59 and 86 °F). Store in a tight container.

**Auxiliary labeling**
• Shake well.
• Continue medication for full time of treatment.
• Beyond-use date.

**Note**
When dispensing, include a calibrated liquid-measuring device.

#### PIVAMPICILLIN TABLETS

**Usual adult and adolescent dose**
Antibacterial—
   Oral, 500 mg to 1 gram two times a day.

**Usual pediatric dose**
Antibacterial—
   Children 10 years of age and over: See *Usual adult and adolescent dose*.
   Children up to 10 years of age: A product of suitable strength is not available for infants and children up to 10 years of age. See *Pivampicillin for Oral Suspension USP*.

**Strength(s) usually available**
U.S.—
   Not commercially available.
Canada—
   500 mg (Rx) [*Pondocillin*].

Note: 500 mg of pivampicillin are equivalent to 377 mg of ampicillin.

**Packaging and storage**
Store between 15 and 30 °C (59 and 86 °F). Store in a tight container.

**Auxiliary labeling**
• Continue medication for full time of treatment.

## PIVMECILLINAM

### Summary of Differences

Category: Aminopenicillin.

Pharmacology/pharmacokinetics: Converted to mecillinam during absorption.

Pediatrics: Should be avoided in children up to 3 months of age since pivmecillinam decreases serum carnitine concentrations.

Precautions: Medical considerations/contraindications—Caution in patients with carnitine deficiency.

### Additional Dosing Information

Patients with impaired renal function do not generally require a reduction in dose unless the impairment is severe.

Pivmecillinam may be taken on a full or empty stomach.

### Oral Dosage Forms

Note: The dosing and strengths of the dosage forms available are expressed in terms of pivmecillinam hydrochloride (not the mecillin base).

#### PIVMECILLINAM HYDROCHLORIDE TABLETS

**Usual adult and adolescent dose**
Antibacterial—
   Oral, 200 mg two to four times a day for three days.

**Usual pediatric dose**
Antibacterial—
   Children up to 40 kg of body weight: Dosage has not been established.
   Children 40 kg of body weight and over: See *Usual adult and adolescent dose*.

**Strength(s) usually available**
U.S.—
   Not commercially available.
Canada—
   200 mg (Rx) [*Selexid*].

Note: 200 mg of pivmecillinam hydrochloride is equivalent to 137 mg of mecillinam.

**Packaging and storage**
Store between 15 and 30 °C (59 and 86 °F). Store in a tight container.

**Auxiliary labeling**
• Continue medication for full time of treatment.

## TICARCILLIN

### Summary of Differences

Category:
   Antipseudomonal penicillin.
Precautions:
   Drug interactions and/or related problems—Also interacts with anticoagulants and other medications that affect blood clotting.
   Laboratory value alterations—May increase bleeding time and may cause false-positive protein reaction for various urine protein tests.
   Medical considerations/contraindications—Caution in patients with a history of bleeding disorders, and congestive heart failure or hypertension.
   Patient monitoring—Bleeding time and serum potassium and sodium determinations may be required.

### Additional Dosing Information

Intramuscular injections should not exceed 2 grams in each site.

Patients with impaired renal function should be observed for hemorrhagic complications.

Note: After an initial intravenous loading dose of 3 grams (base), adults with impaired renal function may require a reduction in dose as follows:

| Creatinine Clearance (mL/min)/(mL/sec) | Dose (base) |
|---|---|
| > 60/1 | 3 grams every 4 hours |
| 30–60/0.5–1 | 2 grams every 4 hours |
| 10–30/0.17–0.5 | 2 grams every 8 hours |
| < 10/0.17 | 2 grams every 12 hours |
| < 10 with impaired hepatic function | 2 grams every 24 hours |
| Hemodialysis | 2 grams every 12 hours plus 3 grams after dialysis |
| Peritoneal dialysis | 3 grams every 12 hours |

## Parenteral Dosage Forms

Note: The dosing and strengths of the dosage forms available are expressed in terms of ticarcillin base (not the sodium salt).

### STERILE TICARCILLIN DISODIUM USP

**Usual adult and adolescent dose**
Antibacterial—
  Intravenous infusion, 3 grams (base) every four hours; or 4 grams every six hours.
  Meningitis, bacterial: Intravenous infusion, 75 mg per kg of body weight every six hours.
  Urinary tract infections, complicated: Intravenous infusion, 3 grams (base) every six hours.
  Urinary tract infections, uncomplicated: Intramuscular or intravenous, 1 gram (base) every six hours.

**Usual adult prescribing limits**
Up to 24 grams a day.

**Usual pediatric dose**
Antibacterial—
  Neonates up to 2 kg of body weight:
    Intramuscular or intravenous, 75 mg per kg of body weight every twelve hours during the first week of life; followed by 75 mg per kg of body weight every eight hours thereafter.
  Neonates 2 kg of body weight and over:
    Intramuscular or intravenous, 75 mg per kg of body weight every eight hours during the first week of life; followed by 75 mg per kg of body weight every six hours thereafter.
  Children up to 40 kg of body weight:
    Intravenous infusion, 33.3 to 50 mg (base) per kg of body weight every four hours; or 50 to 75 mg per kg of body weight every six hours.
    Urinary tract infections, bacterial (complicated)—Intravenous infusion, 25 to 33.3 mg (base) per kg of body weight every four hours; or 37.5 to 50 mg per kg of body weight every six hours.
    Urinary tract infections, bacterial (uncomplicated)—Intramuscular or intravenous, 12.5 to 25 mg (base) per kg of body weight every six hours; or 16.7 to 33.3 mg per kg of body weight every eight hours.
  Children 40 kg of body weight and over:
    See *Usual adult and adolescent dose*.

**Size(s) usually available**
U.S.—
  1 gram (base) (Rx) [*Ticar*].
  3 grams (base) (Rx) [*Ticar*].
  6 grams (base) (Rx) [*Ticar*].
  20 grams (base) (Rx) [*Ticar*].
  30 grams (base) (Rx) [*Ticar*].
Canada—
  1 gram (base) (Rx) [*Ticar*].
  3 grams (base) (Rx) [*Ticar*].
  6 grams (base) (Rx) [*Ticar*].
  20 grams (base) (Rx) [*Ticar*].

**Packaging and storage**
Prior to reconstitution, store below 40 °C (104 °F), preferably between 15 and 30 °C (59 and 86 °F), unless otherwise specified by manufacturer.

**Preparation of dosage form**
To prepare initial dilution for intramuscular use, add 2 mL of sterile water for injection, 1% lidocaine hydrochloride injection (without epinephrine), or sodium chloride injection to each 1-gram vial to provide a concentration of 1 gram per 2.6 mL.
To prepare initial dilution for direct intravenous use, add at least 4 mL of 5% dextrose, 0.9% sodium chloride, or lactated Ringer's injection to each 1-gram vial. Each gram of ticarcillin may be further diluted if desired. The resulting solution should be administered as slowly as possible to avoid vein irritation.
Intermittent infusions may be administered over a 30-minute to 2-hour period in adults. In neonates, intermittent infusions may be administered over a 10- to 20-minute period.
For reconstitution of pharmacy bulk vials or piggyback infusion bottles, see manufacturer's labeling for instructions.

**Stability**
After reconstitution for intramuscular use, solutions retain their potency for 12 hours at room temperature or for 24 hours if refrigerated.
After reconstitution for intravenous use, solutions in concentrations of 10 to 50 mg per mL retain at least 90% of their potency for 48 to 72 hours at room temperature or for 14 days if refrigerated in suitable diluents (see manufacturer's package insert).
If frozen after reconstitution with sterile water for injection, 0.9% sodium chloride injection, 5% dextrose injection, Ringer's injection, or lactated Ringer's injection, solutions in concentrations up to 100 mg per mL retain their potency up to 30 days at −18 °C (0 °F). Once thawed, solutions must be used within 24 hours.

**Incompatibilities**
Extemporaneous admixtures of beta-lactam antibacterials (penicillins and cephalosporins) and aminoglycosides may result in substantial mutual inactivation. If these groups of antibacterials are administered concurrently, they should be administered in separate sites at least 1 hour apart. Do not mix them in the same intravenous bag, bottle, or tubing.
When aminoglycosides and penicillins are administered separately by different routes, a reduction in aminoglycoside serum concentration may occur. Usually this is clinically significant only in patients with severely impaired renal function when the excretion of both medications is delayed.

**Additional information**
The sodium content is approximately 5.2 mEq (5.2 mmol), but may be as high as 6.5 mEq (6.5 mmol), per gram of ticarcillin. This must be considered in patients on a restricted sodium intake when calculating total daily sodium intake.

Revised: 08/25/94
Interim revision: 04/26/95

## Table 1. Pharmacology/Pharmacokinetics

| Drug | Oral Absorption (%) | Time to Peak Serum Concentration (hr) | Peak Serum Concentration Dose | mcg/mL | Half-life (hr) Creatinine Clearance > 50 mL/min (0.83 mL/sec) | Half-life (hr) Creatinine Clearance 10–30 mL/min (0.17–0.83 mL/sec) | Half-life (hr) Creatinine Clearance < 10 mL/min (0.17 mL/sec) |
|---|---|---|---|---|---|---|---|
| Amoxicillin | 75–90 | 1–2 (oral) | 250 mg (oral) | 3.5–5 | 1 | 4.5 | 12.6 |
| Ampicillin | 35–50 | 1.5–2 (oral) 1 (IM)* | 500 mg (oral) 500 mg (IM) 500 mg (IV)* | 3–6 7–14 12–29 | 1–1.5 | 3.4 | 19 |
| Bacampicillin | 35–50† | 0.5–1† (oral) | 400 mg (oral) | 7.9† | 1† | 4.5† | 12.6† |

*IV=intravenous; IM=intramuscular.
†As ampicillin.
‡As mecillinam.

## Table 1. Pharmacology/Pharmacokinetics (continued)

| Drug | Oral Absorption (%) | Time to Peak Serum Concentration (hr) | Peak Serum Concentration Dose | mcg/mL | Half-life (hr) Creatinine Clearance > 50 mL/min (0.83 mL/sec) | Creatinine Clearance 10–30 mL/min (0.17–0.83 mL/sec) | Creatinine Clearance < 10 mL/min (0.17 mL/sec) |
|---|---|---|---|---|---|---|---|
| Carbenicillin | 30 | 0.5–1 (oral and IM) | 500 mg (oral) 1 gram (IM) 2 grams (IV) | 6.5 20 241 | 1–1.5 | 9.6 | 18.2 |
| Cloxacillin | 50 | 1–2 (oral) | 500 mg (oral) 500 mg (IM) | 8 16 | 0.5–1 | | 2.5 |
| Dicloxacillin | 37–50 | 0.5–1 (oral) | 125 mg (oral) | 4.7 | 0.5–1 | | 1.8 |
| Flucloxacillin | 30–50 | 1 (oral) | 250 mg (oral) | 6–10 | 0.7–1.3 | | |
| Methicillin | | 0.5–1 (IM) | 1 gram (IM) 1 gram (IV) | 12 60 | 0.3–1 | | 4 |
| Mezlocillin | | 0.5–1 (IM) | 1 gram (IM) 4 grams (IV) | 35–45 254 | 0.8–1.1 | 2 | 2.6 |
| Nafcillin | Erratic; poor | 1–2 (oral) 0.5–1 (IM) | 1 gram (IM) | 7.6 | 0.5–1.5 | 1.9 | 2.1 |
| Oxacillin | 30–35 | 0.5–1 (oral and IM) | 500 mg (oral) 500 mg (IM) | 5–7 15 | 0.4–0.7 | | 0.8 |
| Penicillin G Oral IV Benzathine (IM) Procaine (IM) | 15–30 | 1–2 24 4 | 3,200,000 units (IV) 300,000 units (IM) | 2.2–17 0.03–0.05 | 0.5–0.7 | | 4.1 |
| Penicillin V | 60–73 | 0.5–1 (oral) | 250 mg (oral) | 2–3 | 0.5–1 | | 4.1 |
| Piperacillin | | 0.5 (IM) | 4 grams (IV) | 412 | 0.6–1.2 | 2 | 2.8 |
| Pivampicillin | 35–50† | 1†(oral) | 500 mg (oral) | 13† | 1† | | |
| Pivmecillinam | Poor‡ | 0.5–1.5‡ (oral) | 200 mg (oral) | 3.3‡ | 1‡ | | |
| Ticarcillin | | 0.5–1 (IM) | 3 grams (IV) | 190 | 1–1.2 | 5.2 | 8.9 |

*IV=intravenous; IM=intramuscular.
†As ampicillin.
‡As mecillinam.

## Table 2. Pharmacology/Pharmacokinetics

| Drug | Protein Binding (%) | Hepatic Biotransformation (%) | Renal Elimination (% unchanged) | Vol $_D$ (L/kg) | Removal by Hemodialysis |
|---|---|---|---|---|---|
| Amoxicillin | Low (20) | 10 | 60–75 | 0.36 | Yes |
| Ampicillin | Low (20) | 10 | 75–90 | 0.29 | Yes |
| Bacampicillin | Low (18–20)* | 10* | 70–75* | 0.29* | Yes |
| Carbenicillin | Moderate (50) | 0–2 | 36 (oral) 75–95 (intravenous) | 0.12 | Yes |
| Cloxacillin | Very high (95) | 20 | 30–60 | 0.11 | No |
| Dicloxacillin | Very high (95–98) | 10 | 50–70 | 0.08 | No |
| Flucloxacillin | Very high (94) | | 50–65 | | No |
| Methicillin | Low to moderate (40) | 10 | 60–80 | 0.36 | No |
| Mezlocillin | Low to moderate (16–42) | 20–30 | 55–60 | 0.23 | Yes |
| Nafcillin | High (90) | 60–70 | 11–30 | 1.1 | No |
| Oxacillin | High (90–94) | 45 | 55–60 | 0.4 | No |
| Penicillin G Oral Parenteral Benzathine IM Procaine | Moderate (60) | 20 | 20 60–90 | 0.5–0.7 | Yes |

## Table 2. Pharmacology/Pharmacokinetics (continued)

| Drug | Protein Binding (%) | Hepatic Biotransformation (%) | Renal Elimination (% unchanged) | Vol$_D$ (L/kg) | Removal by Hemodialysis |
|---|---|---|---|---|---|
| Penicillin V | High (80) | 55 | 20–40 | 0.5 | Yes |
| Piperacillin | Low (16) | 20–30 | 60–80 | 0.23 | Yes† |
| Pivampicillin | Low (20)* | 10* | 25–30* | | |
| Pivmecillinam | Low (5–10)‡ | | 60–80‡ | | Yes§ |
| Ticarcillin | Moderate (45–60) | 15 | 60–80 | 0.16 | Yes |

*As ampicillin.
†Hemodialysis removes 30–50% of piperacillin in 4 hours.
‡As mecillinam.
§Hemodialysis removes 50–70% of pivmecillinam in 4 hours.

# PENICILLINS AND BETA-LACTAMASE INHIBITORS  Systemic

This monograph includes information on the following: 1) Amoxicillin and Clavulanate; 2) Ampicillin and Sulbactam†; 3) Piperacillin and Tazobactam; 4) Ticarcillin and Clavulanate.

INN: Amoxicillin—Amoxicilline

BAN: Amoxicillin—Amoxycillin

VA CLASSIFICATION (Primary):
 Amoxicillin and Clavulanate—AM112
 Ampicillin and Sulbactam—AM112
 Piperacillin and Tazobactam—AM114
 Ticarcillin and Clavulanate—AM114

Commonly used brand name(s): Augmentin[1]; Clavulin-125F[1]; Clavulin-250[1]; Clavulin-250F[1]; Clavulin-500F[1]; Tazocin[3]; Timentin[4]; Unasyn[2]; Zosyn[3].

Note: For a listing of dosage forms and brand names by country availability, see Dosage Forms section(s).

†Not commercially available in Canada.

## Category
Antibacterial (systemic).

## Indications

Note: Bracketed information in the *Indications* section refers to uses that are not included in U.S. product labeling.

**General considerations**

Ampicillin and amoxicillin have activity against *Haemophilus influenzae*, *Escherichia coli*, and *Salmonella* and *Shigella* species, and also retain activity against penicillin-sensitive gram-positive bacteria. However, many Enterobacteriaceae and *H. influenzae* are resistant as a result of beta-lactamase production. Amoxicillin has the same spectrum of activity as ampicillin, although amoxicillin has slightly better activity against *Enterococcus faecalis*, *E. coli*, and *Salmonella* sp., and slightly less activity against *Shigella* sp.

Ticarcillin combines the gram-negative spectrum of ampicillin with activity against most species of *Enterobacter*, *Providencia*, and *Morganella* sp. It also has some activity against *Pseudomonas aeruginosa* and some indole-positive *Proteus* sp.

Piperacillin is more active than ticarcillin against *P. aeruginosa* and *Klebsiella* sp., but has activity similar to that of ticarcillin against most other gram-negative bacteria. Piperacillin also inhibits *P. cepacia*, *P. maltophilia*, and *P. fluorescens*.

Resistance to penicillins is thought to be due to 3 main mechanisms. The first is alteration of the antibiotic target sites' penicillin-binding proteins (PBPs); the second is inactivation of the penicillin by bacterially produced enzymes (beta-lactamases); and the third is decreased permeability of the cell wall to penicillins. Of these 3 mechanisms, production of beta-lactamase is the most common and the most important.

When combined with a penicillin, beta-lactamase inhibitors, which include clavulanic acid (clavulanate), sulbactam, and tazobactam, have effectively extended the penicillin's spectrum of activity. Like penicillins, the beta-lactamase inhibitors are beta-lactam compounds; however, they have minimal intrinsic antibacterial activity. Instead of being hydrolyzed by beta-lactamases, they irreversibly bind to these enzymes, thereby protecting the penicillin from hydrolysis ('suicide' inhibition). Beta-lactamase inhibitors only work when a beta-lactamase enzyme is present. They will not alter the susceptibility of organisms inherently resistant to the penicillin; nor will they alter resistance patterns due to other causes, e.g., alteration of the penicillin-binding proteins (PBPs) (the mechanism of resistance for methicillin-resistant staphylococci).

Clavulanate, sulbactam, and tazobactam are irreversible inhibitors of a wide variety of plasmid-mediated and some chromosomally mediated bacterial beta-lactamases. Clavulanate and tazobactam are highly active, and sulbactam is moderately active, against transferable plasmid-mediated beta-lactamases. The inhibitory effect on chromosomally mediated type I enzymes is variable. Any beta-lactam agent, including beta-lactamase inhibitors and penicillins, may induce beta-lactamase production. Therefore, organisms such as *Enterobacter*, *Serratia*, *Morganella*, and *Pseudomonas* species may produce more beta-lactamase enzyme when they are exposed to a penicillin or a beta-lactamase inhibitor. Clavulanate is a moderate inducer of the chromosomal enzymes in these organisms; sulbactam and tazobactam are weaker inducers. Also, if the complex with the beta-lactamase inhibitor is not stable, regeneration of the beta-lactamase may occur. If so, the enzyme must be repeatedly inactivated for inhibition to be maintained. It is also easier to protect a beta-lactam antibiotic against organisms that produce a small amount of enzyme than it is to protect against organisms producing a large amount.

All 3 beta-lactamase inhibitors inactivate staphylococcal penicillinase. Beta-lactamase inhibitors inactivate the chromosomally mediated beta-lactamases of *Proteus vulgaris* and *Bacteroides* sp., and the class IV beta-lactamases present in some *Klebsiella* sp. Resistance in *H. influenzae* and *Neisseria gonorrhoeae* that produce TEM beta-lactamases is rare since these organisms produce only a small quantity of enzyme and are very permeable to the inhibitor.

Clavulanate is a potent inhibitor of plasmid-mediated enzymes, most commonly found in Enterobacteriaceae. However, all beta-lactamases are not equally susceptible. The class I beta-lactamases of the Richmond-Sykes classification are often resistant, including beta-lactamases typically produced by *Enterobacter*, *Citrobacter*, and *Serratia* species, and *P. aeruginosa*. Clavulanic acid is available as a combined product with both amoxicillin and ticarcillin, resulting in products with broad-spectrum antibacterial activity against beta-lactamase–producing strains of *E. coli*, *H. influenzae*, *Moraxella (Branhamella) catarrhalis*, many *Klebsiella* sp., most *Bacteroides* sp., *S. aureus*, and *S. epidermidis*, except methicillin-resistant staphylococcal strains. Combining ticarcillin with clavulanic acid increases the activity of ticarcillin to include 60 to 80% of ticarcillin-resistant strains of Enterobacteriaceae and all beta-lactamase–producing strains of *Staphylococcus aureus*, *H. influenzae*, and *Bacteroides* sp. No increase in activity is provided against *P. aeruginosa*.

Sulbactam also inhibits many beta-lactamases, including those produced by *Bacteroides*, *Haemophilus*, and *Klebsiella* sp., and *N. gonorrhoeae*, but it appears to be less potent than clavulanic acid against several beta-lactamases, including staphylococcal beta-lactamases, TEM-type enzymes, especially strains of *E. coli* and other pathogens producing TEM-1 and TEM-2 beta-lactamases, and the beta-lactamases typically present in *B. fragilis*.

Tazobactam also has a broad spectrum of activity, and appears to be at least as effective as clavulanic acid against a wide variety of beta-lactamases. Tazobactam may have greater activity than clavulanate against some Enterobacteriaceae class I chromosomally mediated beta-lactamases, such as those of *Morganella morganii*, *E. coli*, *K. pneumoniae*, *Citro-*

*bacter diversus*, *P. mirabilis*, *Providencia stuartii*, and *Pseudomonas aeruginosa*. Both tazobactam and clavulanate have greater activity against these organisms than sulbactam has. The piperacillin and tazobactam combination also has good activity against staphylococci, streptococci, *H. influenzae*, *Moraxella catarrhalis*, *Enterococcus faecalis*, and *Listeria monocytogenes*. Greater resistance was seen with *E. faecium*, *Enterobacter* sp., *Citrobacter freundii*, *Serratia* sp., and *Xanthomonas maltophilia*.

### Accepted

Bone and joint infections (treatment)—Ticarcillin and clavulanate combination and [ampicillin and sulbactam combination][1] are indicated in the treatment of bone and joint infections caused by susceptible organisms.

Intra-abdominal infections (treatment)—Ampicillin and sulbactam combination, piperacillin and tazobactam combination, and ticarcillin and clavulanate combination are indicated in the treatment of intra-abdominal infections caused by susceptible organisms.

Otitis media, acute (treatment)—Amoxicillin and clavulanate combination is indicated in the treatment of acute otitis media caused by susceptible organisms.

Pelvic infections, female (treatment)—Ampicillin and sulbactam combination, piperacillin and tazobactam combination, and ticarcillin and clavulanate combination are indicated in the treatment of female pelvic infections caused by susceptible organisms.

Pneumonia, bacterial (treatment)—Amoxicillin and clavulanate combination, piperacillin and tazobactam combination, and ticarcillin and clavulanate combination are indicated in the treatment of bacterial pneumonia caused by susceptible organisms.

Septicemia, bacterial (treatment)—Ticarcillin and clavulanate combination and [piperacillin and tazobactam combination][1] are indicated in the treatment of bacterial septicemia caused by susceptible organisms.

Sinusitis (treatment)—Amoxicillin and clavulanate combination is indicated in the treatment of sinusitis caused by susceptible organisms.

Skin and soft tissue infections (treatment)—Amoxicillin and clavulanate combination, ampicillin and sulbactam combination, piperacillin and tazobactam combination, and ticarcillin and clavulanate combination are indicated in the treatment of skin and soft tissue infections caused by susceptible organisms.

Urinary tract infections, bacterial (treatment)—Amoxicillin and clavulanate combination and ticarcillin and clavulanate combination are indicated in the treatment of bacterial urinary tract infections caused by susceptible organisms.

[Bronchitis (treatment)][1]—Amoxicillin and clavulanate combination is used in the treatment of bronchitis caused by susceptible organisms.

[Chancroid (treatment)][1]—Amoxicillin and clavulanate combination is used in the treatment of chancroid caused by *Haemophilus ducreyi*.

[Gonorrhea, endocervical and urethral (treatment)][1]—Ampicillin and sulbactam combination is used in the treatment of uncomplicated endocervical and urethral gonorrhea caused by *Neisseria gonorrhoeae*.

[Perioperative infection prophylaxis for colorectal surgery, abdominal hysterectomy, and high-risk cesarean section]—Ticarcillin and clavulanate combination is used prophylactically to help prevent perioperative infections that may result from colorectal surgery, abdominal hysterectomy, and high-risk cesarean section; however, other agents (i.e., cefazolin for hysterectomy and high-risk cesarean section, and neomycin plus erythromycin base for colorectal surgery) are preferred for use as perioperative prophylaxis in these procedures.

### Unaccepted

Piperacillin and tazobactam combination should not be used for the treatment of complicated urinary tract infections because of inadequate efficacy at the usual dose (3.375 grams every six hours).

---

[1]Not included in Canadian product labeling.

## Pharmacology/Pharmacokinetics

### Physicochemical characteristics

Source—
  Clavulanate: Naturally occurring compound produced by *Streptomyces clavuligerus*.
  Sulbactam: Synthetic penicillanic acid sulfone.
  Tazobactam: Analog of sulbactam.
Chemical group—
  Amoxicillin: Aminopenicillin.
  Ampicillin: Aminopenicillin.
  Piperacillin: Acylureidopenicillin.
  Ticarcillin: Carboxypenicillin.
Molecular weight—
  Amoxicillin: 419.45.
  Ampicillin sodium: 371.39.
  Clavulanate potassium: 237.25.
  Piperacillin sodium: 539.54.
  Sulbactam sodium: 255.22.
  Tazobactam sodium: 322.27.
  Ticarcillin disodium: 428.39.

### Mechanism of action/Effect

Penicillins—Bactericidal; inhibit bacterial cell wall synthesis. Action is dependent on the ability of penicillins to reach and bind penicillin-binding proteins (PBPs) located on the inner membrane of the bacterial cell wall. PBPs (which include transpeptidases, carboxypeptidases, and endopeptidases) are enzymes that are involved in the terminal stages of assembling the bacterial cell wall and in reshaping the cell wall during growth and division. Penicillins bind to, and inactivate, PBPs, resulting in the weakening of the bacterial cell wall and lysis.

Beta-lactamase inhibitors—Act by irreversibly binding to the beta-lactamase enzyme, preventing hydrolysis of the beta-lactam ring of the penicillin. The inhibitor first forms a noncovalent complex, which is fully reversible, with a beta-lactam agent. Beta-lactamase inhibitors then act by recognizing the serine residue at the active site of the beta-lactamase enzyme. The structure of the inhibitor is opened and a covalent acyl-enzyme complex is formed with the serine residue. This prevents the beta-lactamase enzyme from hydrolyzing the penicillin and the liberation of the beta-lactamase enzyme.

### Absorption

Amoxicillin and clavulanate are both well absorbed after oral administration and are stable in the presence of gastric acid. Food does not affect absorption, and this combination product may be given without regard to meals. Oral bioavailability of amoxicillin and clavulanic acid is approximately 90% and 75%, respectively. Orally administered sulbactam is poorly absorbed.

### Distribution

The penicillins and beta-lactamase inhibitors are widely distributed to most tissues and body fluids, including peritoneal fluid, blister fluid, urine (high concentrations), pleural fluid, middle ear fluid, intestinal mucosa, bone, gallbladder, lung, female reproductive tissues, and bile. Distribution into the cerebrospinal fluid (CSF) is low in subjects with non-inflamed meninges, as is penetration into purulent bronchial secretions.

Penicillins also cross the placenta and are distributed into breast milk.

Volume of distribution (Vol$_D$)—
  Amoxicillin: 0.36 L/kg.
  Ampicillin: 0.29 L/kg.
  Piperacillin: 0.23 L/kg.
  Ticarcillin: 0.16 L/kg.

### Protein binding

Amoxicillin—Low (17 to 20%).
Ampicillin—Low (20 to 28%).
Clavulanic acid—Low (22 to 30%).
Piperacillin—Low (Approximately 16 to 30%).
Sulbactam—Moderate (38%).
Tazobactam—Low (Approximately 30%).
Ticarcillin—Moderate (45 to 60%).

### Biotransformation

Hepatic—
  Amoxicillin: Approximately 10% of a dose is metabolized.
  Ampicillin: Approximately 10% of a dose is metabolized to inactive penicilloic acid.
  Clavulanic acid: Less than 50% of a dose is metabolized.
  Piperacillin: Metabolized to the desethyl metabolite, which has minor activity.
  Sulbactam: Less than 25% of a dose is metabolized.
  Tazobactam: Metabolized to a single, inactive metabolite.
  Ticarcillin: Less than 15% of a dose is metabolized.

### Half-life

Normal renal function—
  Amoxicillin: Approximately 1.3 hours.
  Ampicillin: Approximately 1 hour.
  Clavulanic acid: Approximately 1 hour.
  Piperacillin: 0.7 to 1.2 hours.
  Sulbactam: Approximately 1 hour.
  Tazobactam: 0.7 to 1.2 hours.
  Ticarcillin: 1 to 1.2 hours.
Impaired renal function (severe)—
  Amoxicillin: Approximately 12 hours.
  Ampicillin: 9 to 19 hours.
  Clavulanic acid: Approximately 3 hours.
  Piperacillin: 1.4 to 2.8 hours.
  Sulbactam: Approximately 9 hours.

Tazobactam: 2.8 to 4.8 hours.
Ticarcillin: Approximately 9 hours.

**Time to peak serum concentration**
Amoxicillin and clavulanic acid combination—1 to 2 hours.
Ampicillin and sulbactam combination—End of infusion.
Piperacillin and tazobactam combination—End of infusion.
Ticarcillin and clavulanate combination—End of infusion.

**Peak serum concentration**
Amoxicillin and clavulanic acid combination—
  Chewable tablets and oral suspension: Approximately 6.9 mcg per mL (mcg/mL) amoxicillin and 1.6 mcg/mL clavulanic acid after an oral dose of 250 mg amoxicillin and 62.5 mg clavulanic acid.
  Tablets (film-coated): Approximately 4.4 to 4.7 mcg/mL amoxicillin and 2.3 to 2.5 mcg/mL clavulanic acid after an oral dose of 250 mg amoxicillin and 125 mg clavulanic acid.
Ampicillin and sulbactam combination—
  Intramuscular: Approximately 8 to 35 mcg/mL ampicillin and 6 to 25 mcg/mL sulbactam following an intramuscular dose of 1.5 grams (1 gram of ampicillin and 500 mg of sulbactam).
  Intravenous: Approximately 40 to 70 mcg/mL ampicillin and 20 to 40 mcg/mL sulbactam following an intravenous dose of 1.5 grams (1 gram of ampicillin and 500 mg of sulbactam).
Piperacillin and tazobactam combination—
  Approximately 242 mcg/mL piperacillin and 24 mcg/mL tazobactam following an intravenous dose of 3.375 grams (3 grams of piperacillin and 0.375 gram of sulbactam).
Ticarcillin and clavulanic acid combination—
  Approximately 330 mcg/mL ticarcillin and 8 mcg/mL clavulanic acid following an intravenous dose of 3.1 grams (3 grams of ticarcillin and 0.1 gram of clavulanic acid).

**Elimination**
Primarily renal (glomerular filtration and tubular secretion)—
  Amoxicillin and clavulanic acid combination:
    50 to 78%, and 25 to 40% of an administered dose of amoxicillin and clavulanic acid, respectively, are excreted unchanged in the urine within first 6 hours after administration.
  Ampicillin and sulbactam combination:
    75 to 85% of an administered dose of both ampicillin and sulbactam is excreted unchanged in the urine within first 8 hours after administration.
  Piperacillin and tazobactam combination:
    Approximately 68% and 80% of an administered dose of piperacillin and tazobactam, respectively, are excreted unchanged in the urine.
  Ticarcillin and clavulanic acid combination:
    60 to 70%, and 35 to 45% of an administered dose of ticarcillin and clavulanic acid, respectively, are excreted unchanged in the urine within first 6 hours after administration.
Biliary—
  Ampicillin and sulbactam:
    Less than 1%.
  Piperacillin and tazobactam combination:
    Less than 2%.
In dialysis—
  Hemodialysis:
    Hemodialysis removes amoxicillin, ampicillin, clavulanate, piperacillin, sulbactam, tazobactam, and ticarcillin from the blood.
    Piperacillin and tazobactam combination—30 to 40% of an administered dose is removed, plus an additional 5% of the tazobactam dose as the metabolite.
  Peritoneal dialysis:
    Piperacillin and tazobactam combination—6 to 21% of an administered dose is removed, plus an additional 16% of the tazobactam dose as the metabolite.

## Precautions to Consider

### Cross-sensitivity and/or related problems
Patients allergic to one penicillin may be allergic to other penicillins also.
Patients allergic to cephalosporins, cephamycins, or beta-lactamase inhibitors may be allergic to penicillin and beta-lactamase inhibitor combinations also.

### Carcinogenicity
Long-term carcinogenicity studies in animals have not been done on any of the penicillin and beta-lactamase inhibitor combinations.

### Mutagenicity
*Amoxicillin and clavulanic acid combination*—Long-term studies in animals have not been done to evaluate the mutagenic potential of this combination.

*Ampicillin and sulbactam combination*—Long-term studies in animals have not been done to evaluate the mutagenic potential of this combination.

*Piperacillin and tazobactam combination*—Microbial mutagenicity studies with piperacillin and tazobactam combination at concentrations of up to 14.84 and 1.86 mcg, respectively, per plate were negative. Negative results were also found in the unscheduled DNA synthesis (UDS) test at concentrations of up to 5689 and 711 mcg per mL (mcg/mL), respectively, in the mammalian point mutation (Chinese hamster ovary cell HPRT) assay at concentrations of up to 8000 and 1000 mcg/mL, respectively, and in the mammalian cell (BALB/c-3T3) transformation assay at concentrations of up to 8 and 1 mcg/mL, respectively. *In vivo*, piperacillin and tazobactam combination did not induce chromosomal aberrations in rats administered intravenous doses of 1500 and 187.5 mg per kg of body weight (mg/kg), respectively; this dose is similar to the maximum recommended human daily dose based on mg per square meter of body surface area (mg/m$^2$).

*Ticarcillin and clavulanic acid combination*—Studies performed *in vitro* and *in vivo* did not indicate a potential for mutagenicity.

### Pregnancy/Reproduction
Fertility—
*Amoxicillin and clavulanic acid combination:* Studies in rats and mice given doses up to 10 times the usual human dose have not shown that amoxicillin and clavulanate combination impairs fertility.

*Ampicillin and sulbactam combination:* Studies in mice, rats, and rabbits given doses up to 10 times the human dose have not shown that ampicillin and sulbactam combination causes adverse effects on fertility.

*Piperacillin and tazobactam combination:* Reproduction studies in rats revealed no evidence of impaired fertility when piperacillin and tazobactam combination was administered at doses similar to the maximum recommended human daily dose based on body surface area (mg/m$^2$). There was also no evidence of impaired fertility when tazobactam was administered at doses up to 3 times the maximum recommended human daily dose based on body surface area (mg/m$^2$).

*Ticarcillin and clavulanic acid combination:* Studies in rats given daily doses of up to 1050 mg/kg have not shown that ticarcillin and clavulanate combination impairs fertility.

Pregnancy—Penicillins cross the placenta. Clavulanic acid also crosses the placenta. Adequate and well-controlled studies in humans have not been done; however, problems in humans have not been documented.

*Amoxicillin and clavulanate combination:* Studies in rats and mice given doses up to 10 times the usual human dose have not shown that amoxicillin and clavulanate combination causes adverse effects in the fetus.
FDA Pregnancy Category B.

*Ampicillin and sulbactam combination:* Studies in mice, rats, and rabbits given doses up to 10 times the human dose have not shown that ampicillin and sulbactam combination causes adverse effects in the fetus.
FDA Pregnancy Category B.

*Piperacillin and tazobactam combination:* Teratology studies performed in mice and rats given piperacillin and tazobactam combination at doses 1 to 2 times, respectively, the human dose based on body surface area (mg/m$^2$) revealed no evidence of harm to the fetus. In addition, no evidence of harm to the fetus was found when tazobactam was administered to mice and rats at doses up to 6 and 14 times the human dose, respectively, based on body surface area (mg/m$^2$). Tazobactam crosses the placenta in mice; concentrations in the fetus are 10% or less those found in maternal plasma.
FDA Pregnancy Category B.

*Ticarcillin and clavulanate combination:* Studies in rats given daily doses of up to 1050 mg/kg have not shown that ticarcillin and clavulanate combination causes adverse effects in the fetus.
FDA Pregnancy Category B.

### Breast-feeding
Penicillins and sulbactam are distributed into breast milk in low concentrations; it is not known whether clavulanic acid and tazobactam are distributed into breast milk. Although significant problems in humans have not been documented, the use of penicillins by nursing mothers may lead to sensitization, diarrhea, candidiasis, and skin rash in the infant.

### Pediatrics
Many penicillins have been used in pediatric patients, and no pediatrics-specific problems have been documented to date. However, the incompletely developed renal function of neonates and young infants may delay the excretion of renally eliminated penicillins.

*Piperacillin and tazobactam combination:* Although safety and efficacy have not been established in pediatric patients, the results of one study found the clearance and elimination half-life to be increased in infants < 6 months of age. Piperacillin and tazobactam combination had no effect on bilirubin-albumin binding *in vitro*.

## Geriatrics
Penicillins have been used in geriatric patients and no geriatrics-specific problems have been documented to date. However, elderly patients are more likely to have an age-related decrease in renal function, which may require an adjustment in dosage in patients receiving penicillins.

## Dental
Prolonged use of penicillins may lead to the development of oral candidiasis.

## Drug interactions and/or related problems
The following drug interactions and/or related problems have been selected on the basis of their potential clinical significance (possible mechanism in parentheses where appropriate)—not necessarily inclusive (» = major clinical significance):

Note: Combinations containing any of the following medications, depending on the amount present, may also interact with this medication.

Allopurinol
(concurrent use with ampicillin may significantly increase the possibility of skin rash, especially in hyperuricemic patients; however, it has not been established that allopurinol, rather than the presence of hyperuricemia, is responsible for this effect)

» Aminoglycosides
(mixing penicillins with aminoglycosides *in vitro* has resulted in substantial mutual inactivation; concurrent administration of piperacillin and tazobactam combination with tobramycin decreased the urinary recovery of tobramycin by 38%; concurrent administration of tobramycin and ticarcillin resulted in a decrease in serum tobramycin concentration by 11%; if these groups of antibacterials are to be administered concurrently, they should be administered at separate sites at least 1 hour apart)

» Anticoagulants, coumarin- or indandione-derivative or
» Heparin or
» Thrombolytic agents
(concurrent use of these medications with high-dose piperacillin or ticarcillin may increase the risk of hemorrhage because these penicillins inhibit platelet aggregation; patients should be monitored carefully for signs of bleeding; concurrent use of piperacillin or ticarcillin with thrombolytic agents may increase the risk of severe hemorrhage and is not recommended)

» Anti-inflammatory drugs, nonsteroidal (NSAIDs), especially aspirin or
Diflunisal, very high doses or
Other salicylates or
» Platelet aggregation inhibitors, other, (See *Appendix II*) or
» Sulfinpyrazone
(concurrent use of these medications with high-dose piperacillin or ticarcillin may increase the risk of hemorrhage because of additive inhibition of platelet function; in addition, hypoprothrombinemia induced by large doses of salicylates and the gastrointestinal ulcerative or hemorrhagic potential of NSAIDs, salicylates, or sulfinpyrazone may also increase the risk of hemorrhage when these medicines are used concurrently with piperacillin or ticarcillin)

Chloramphenicol or
Erythromycins or
Sulfonamides or
Tetracyclines
(since bacteriostatic drugs may interfere with the bactericidal effect of penicillins in the treatment of meningitis or in other situations in which a rapid bactericidal effect is necessary, it is best to avoid concurrent therapy; however, chloramphenicol and ampicillin are sometimes administered concurrently in pediatric patients)

» Probenecid
(probenecid decreases renal tubular secretion of penicillins, sulbactam, and tazobactam [but not clavulanic acid, which is cleared primarily by glomerular filtration] when used concurrently; this effect results in increased and more prolonged serum concentrations, prolonged elimination half-life [half-life of piperacillin increased by 21%, that of tazobactam by 71%, and that of sulbactam by 40%], and increased risk of toxicity. Penicillins and probenecid are often used concurrently to treat sexually transmitted diseases [STDs] or other infections in which high and/or prolonged antibiotic serum and tissue concentrations are required)

## Laboratory value alterations
The following have been selected on the basis of their potential clinical significance (possible effect in parentheses where appropriate)—not necessarily inclusive (» = major clinical significance):

With diagnostic test results
» Glucose, urine
(high urinary concentrations of a penicillin may produce false-positive or falsely elevated test results with copper-reduction tests [Benedict's, *Clinitest*, or Fehling's]; glucose enzymatic tests [*Clinistix* or *Testape*] are not affected)

Direct antiglobulin (Coombs') tests
(false-positive result may occur during therapy with any penicillin)

Protein, urine
(high urinary concentrations of piperacillin or ticarcillin may produce false-positive protein reactions [pseudoproteinuria] with the sulfosalicylic acid and boiling test, the acetic acid test, the biuret reaction, and the nitric acid test; bromophenol blue reagent test strips [*Multi-stix*] are reportedly unaffected)

With physiology/laboratory test values
Alanine aminotransferase (ALT [SGPT]) and
Alkaline phosphatase and
Aspartate aminotransferase (AST [SGOT]) and
Bilirubin, serum
Lactate dehydrogenase (LDH), serum
(values may be increased)

Blood urea nitrogen (BUN) and
Creatinine, serum
(increased concentrations have been associated with ampicillin and sulbactam, piperacillin, and ticarcillin)

Estradiol or
Estriol, total conjugated or
Estriol-glucuronide or
Estrone, conjugated
(concentrations may be transiently decreased in pregnant women following administration of amoxicillin and ampicillin)

» Partial thromboplastin time (PTT) and
» Prothrombin time (PT)
(an increase has been associated with piperacillin and ticarcillin)

Potassium, serum
(hypokalemia may occur following administration of piperacillin or ticarcillin, either of which may act as a nonreabsorbable anion in the distal renal tubules; this may cause an increase in pH and result in increased urinary potassium loss; the risk of hypokalemia increases with use of larger doses)

Sodium, serum
(hypernatremia may occur following administration of large doses of ticarcillin because of the medication's high sodium content)

Uric acid, serum
(ticarcillin may transiently decrease the serum concentration in some patients)

White blood count
(leukopenia or neutropenia is associated with the use of all penicillins; the effect is more likely to occur with prolonged therapy and severe hepatic function impairment)

## Medical considerations/Contraindications
The medical considerations/contraindications included have been selected on the basis of their potential clinical significance (reasons given in parentheses where appropriate)—not necessarily inclusive (» = major clinical significance).

*Except under special circumstances, this medication should not be used when the following medical problem exists:*
» Allergy to penicillins or beta-lactamase inhibitors

*Risk-benefit should be considered when the following medical problems exist:*
Allergy, general, history of, such as asthma, eczema, hay fever, hives
» Bleeding disorders, history of
(some penicillins, especially piperacillin and ticarcillin, may cause platelet dysfunction and hemorrhage)
» Congestive heart failure (CHF) or
Hypertension
(the sodium content of high doses of ticarcillin should be considered in patients who require sodium restriction)
» Cystic fibrosis
(patients with cystic fibrosis may be at increased risk of fever and skin rash when given piperacillin)
» Gastrointestinal disease, active or a history of, especially antibiotic-associated colitis
(penicillins may cause pseudomembranous colitis)
» Mononucleosis, infectious
(a morbilliform skin rash may occur in a high percentage of patients taking ampicillin)

» Renal function impairment
(because most penicillins are excreted through the kidneys, a reduction in dosage, or an increase in dosing interval, is recommended in patients with renal function impairment; also, the sodium content of high doses of ticarcillin should be considered in patients with severe renal function impairment)

**Patient monitoring**
The following may be especially important in patient monitoring (other tests may be warranted in some patients, depending on condition; » = major clinical significance):

*For piperacillin and tazobactam combination and ticarcillin and clavulanate combination*
» Partial thromboplastin time (PTT) and
» Prothrombin time (PT)
(may be required prior to and during prolonged therapy in patients with renal function impairment who are receiving high doses, since hemorrhagic manifestations may occur, although the effect is rare)

*For piperacillin and ticarcillin*
Potassium, serum
(determinations may be required periodically during therapy in patients with low potassium reserves and in patients receiving cytotoxic medications or diuretics, since hypokalemia may occur)

*For all penicillin and beta-lactamase inhibitor combinations (if C. difficile colitis occurs)*
» Stool toxin assays
(enzyme immunoassay of stool samples for the presence of *Clostridium difficile* toxins may be required prior to treatment of patients with antibiotic-associated colitis to document the presence of *C. difficile* toxins; however, *C. difficile* and its toxins may persist following treatment with oral vancomycin, metronidazole, or cholestyramine, despite clinical improvement; follow-up cultures and toxin assays are not recommended if clinical improvement is complete)

## Side/Adverse Effects

The following side/adverse effects have been selected on the basis of their potential clinical significance (possible signs and symptoms in parentheses where appropriate)—not necessarily inclusive:

**Those indicating need for medical attention**
Incidence less frequent
*Allergic reactions, specifically anaphylaxis* (fast or irregular breathing; puffiness or swelling around face; shortness of breath; sudden, severe decrease in blood pressure); *serum sickness–like reactions* (skin rash; joint pain; fever); *skin rash, hives, or itching*
Incidence rare
*Leukopenia or neutropenia* (sore throat and fever); *pain at site of injection; platelet dysfunction* (unusual bleeding or bruising); *Clotridium difficile colitis* (severe abdominal or stomach cramps and pain; abdominal tenderness; watery and severe diarrhea, which may also be bloody; fever); *seizures*

Note: *Platelet dysfunction* is primarily associated with piperacillin and ticarcillin.
*Clotridium difficile* colitis may occur up to several weeks after discontinuation of these medications.
*Seizures* are more likely to occur in patients receiving high doses of a penicillin and/or patients with severe renal function impairment.

**Those indicating need for medical attention only if they continue or are bothersome**
Incidence more frequent
*Gastrointestinal reactions* (mild diarrhea; nausea or vomiting; stomach pain); *headache; oral candidiasis* (sore mouth or tongue; white patches in mouth and/or on tongue); *vaginal candidiasis* (vaginal itching and discharge)

## Overdose

For more information on the management of overdose or unintentional ingestion, **contact a Poison Control Center** (see *Poison Control Center Listing*).

**Treatment of overdose**
Since there is no specific antidote, treatment of penicillin overdose should be symptomatic and supportive.
Specific treatment—Hemodialysis may aid in the removal of penicillins from the blood.
Supportive care—Patients in whom intentional overdose is known or suspected should be referred for psychiatric consultation.

## Patient Consultation

As an aid to patient consultation, refer to *Advice for the Patient, Penicillins and Beta-lactamase Inhibitors (Systemic)*.
In providing consultation, consider emphasizing the following selected information (» = major clinical significance):

**Before using this medication**
» Conditions affecting use, especially:
Allergy to penicillins, cephalosporins, cephamycins, or beta-lactamase inhibitors
Pregnancy—Penicillins cross the placenta
Breast-feeding—Penicillins and sulbactam are distributed into breast milk
Use in children—Neonates and young infants may have reduced elimination of renally eliminated penicillins due to incompletely developed renal function
Other medications, especially aminoglycosides; coumarin- or indandione-derivative anticoagulants; heparin; nonsteroidal anti-inflammatory drugs (NSAIDs), especially aspirin; other platelet aggregation inhibitors; probenecid; sulfinpyrazone; or thrombolytic agents
Other medical problems, especially a history of bleeding disorders; congestive heart failure; cystic fibrosis; active or history of gastrointestinal disease, especially antibiotic-associated colitis; infectious mononucleosis; or renal function impairment

**Proper use of this medication**
Taking amoxicillin and clavulanate combination on a full or empty stomach; administration with food may decrease the incidence of gastrointestinal side effects (diarrhea, nausea and vomiting)
Proper administration technique for oral liquids
Not using after expiration date
» Importance of taking at evenly spaced times and not missing doses
» Proper dosing
Missed dose: Taking as soon as possible; not taking if almost time for next dose; not doubling doses
» Proper storage

**Precautions while using this medication**
Checking with physician if no improvement within a few days
» For severe diarrhea, checking with physician before taking any antidiarrheals; for mild diarrhea, kaolin- or attapulgite-containing, but not other, antidiarrheals may be tried; checking with physician or pharmacist if mild diarrhea continues or worsens
» Diabetics: False-positive reactions with copper sulfate urine glucose tests may occur, especially with amoxicillin and clavulanate, ampicillin and sulbactam, and piperacillin and tazobactam combinations
Possible interference with diagnostic tests

**Side/adverse effects**
Signs of potential side effects, especially allergic reactions, leukopenia or neutropenia, pain at site of injection, platelet dysfunction, pseudomembranous colitis, and seizures

## General Dosing Information

**For oral dosage forms only**
Amoxicillin and clavulanate combination may be taken on a full or empty stomach. Administration with food may decrease the incidence of gastrointestinal side effects (diarrhea, nausea and vomiting).

**For treatment of adverse effects**
Serious anaphylactoid reactions require immediate emergency treatment, which consists of the following:
• Parenteral epinephrine.
• Oxygen.
• Intravenous corticosteroids.
• Airway management (including intubation).

For *Clostridium difficile* colitis—
• Some patients may develop *C. difficile* colitis during or following administration of penicillins.
• *C. difficile* colitis may result in severe watery diarrhea, which may occur during therapy or up to several weeks after therapy is discontinued. If diarrhea occurs, administration of antiperistaltic antidiarrheals (e.g., opioids, diphenoxylate and atropine combination, loperamide, paregoric) is not recommended since they may delay the removal of toxins from the colon, thereby prolonging and/or worsening the condition.
• Mild cases may respond to discontinuation of the medication alone. Moderate to severe cases may require fluid, electrolyte, and protein replacement.
• In cases not responding to the above measures or in more severe cases, oral doses of vancomycin, metronidazole, or cholestyramine may be

used. Oral vancomycin is effective in doses of 125 mg every 6 hours for 5 to 10 days. The dose of metronidazole is 250 to 500 mg every 8 hours, and the dose of cholestyramine is 4 grams four times a day. Recurrences, which occur in approximately 25% of patients treated with vancomycin or metronidazole, may be treated with a second course of these medications.
• Cholestyramine resin has been shown to bind *C. difficile* toxin *in vitro*. If cholestyramine resin is administered in conjunction with oral vancomycin, the medications should be administered several hours apart since the resin has been shown to bind oral vancomycin also.

---

## AMOXICILLIN AND CLAVULANATE

## Summary of Differences
Precautions:
    Drug interactions and/or related problems—Clavulanic acid does not interact with probenecid.
    Laboratory value alterations—Amoxicillin may decrease total conjugated estriol, estriol-glucuronide, conjugated estrone, and estradiol concentrations in pregnant women.

## Additional Dosing Information
Absorption of amoxicillin and clavulanate combination is not affected by food. The medication may be taken on a full or empty stomach. Administration with food may decrease the incidence of gastrointestinal side effects (diarrhea, nausea and vomiting).

Amoxicillin and clavulanate 250-mg tablets and 250-mg chewable tablets do not contain the same amount of clavulanate. The 250-mg tablets contain 125 mg of clavulanate, and the 250-mg chewable tablets contain 62.5 mg of clavulanate. Therefore, these products should not be substituted for each other or used interchangeably. This is important to ensure that there is a sufficient concentration of clavulanate at the site of infection to inhibit the beta-lactamase that is present.

The 250-mg tablet should not be used in children who weigh less than 40 kg.

Since the 250-mg and the 500-mg strengths of amoxicillin and clavulanate combination tablets contain the same amount of clavulanate (125 mg), two 250-mg tablets are not equivalent to one 500-mg tablet.

Adults and adolescents with impaired renal function may receive the usual dose with the dosing interval increased as follows:

| Creatinine Clearance (mL/min)/(mL/sec) | Dosing interval (hours) |
|---|---|
| >30/0.50 | 8 |
| 10–30/0.17–0.50 | 12 |
| 2–10/0.03–0.17 | 24 |

## Oral Dosage Forms
Note: Bracketed uses in the *Dosage Forms* section refer to categories of use and/or indications that are not included in U.S. product labeling.

### AMOXICILLIN AND CLAVULANATE POTASSIUM FOR ORAL SUSPENSION USP

#### Usual adult and adolescent dose
Antibacterial—
    Pneumonia and other severe infections:
        Oral, 500 mg of amoxicillin and 125 mg of clavulanic acid every eight hours for seven to ten days.
    Other infections:
        Oral, 250 mg of amoxicillin and 62.5 mg of clavulanic acid every eight hours for seven to ten days.

#### Usual pediatric dose
Antibacterial—
    Infants and children up to 40 kg of body weight:
        Otitis media, acute
        Pneumonia
        Sinusitis
        Other severe infections—Oral, 13.3 mg of amoxicillin and 3.3 mg of clavulanic acid per kg of body weight every eight hours for seven to ten days.
        Other infections—Oral, 6.7 mg of amoxicillin and 1.7 mg of clavulanic acid per kg of body weight every eight hours for seven to ten days.
    Children 40 kg of body weight and over:
        See *Usual adult and adolescent dose*.

#### Strength(s) usually available
U.S.—
    125 mg of amoxicillin and 31.25 mg of clavulanic acid per 5 mL (when reconstituted according to manufacturer's instructions) (Rx) [*Augmentin*].
    250 mg of amoxicillin and 62.5 mg of clavulanic acid per 5 mL (when reconstituted according to manufacturer's instructions) (Rx) [*Augmentin*].
Canada—
    125 mg of amoxicillin and 31.25 mg of clavulanic acid per 5 mL (when reconstituted according to manufacturer's instructions) (Rx) [*Clavulin-125F*].
    250 mg of amoxicillin and 62.5 mg of clavulanic acid per 5 mL (when reconstituted according to manufacturer's instructions) (Rx) [*Clavulin-250F*].

#### Packaging and storage
Prior to reconstitution, store between 15 and 30 °C (59 and 86 °F). Store in a tight container.

#### Stability
After reconstitution, suspensions retain their potency for 10 days if refrigerated.

#### Auxiliary labeling
• Refrigerate.
• Shake well.
• Continue medication for full time of treatment.
• Beyond-use date.

#### Note
When dispensing, include a calibrated liquid-measuring device.

### AMOXICILLIN AND CLAVULANATE POTASSIUM TABLETS USP

#### Usual adult and adolescent dose
Antibacterial—
    Pneumonia and other severe infections:
        Oral, 500 mg of amoxicillin and 125 mg of clavulanic acid every eight hours for seven to ten days.
    Other infections:
        Oral, 250 mg of amoxicillin and 125 mg of clavulanic acid every eight hours for seven to ten days.
    [Chancroid][1]:
        Oral, 500 mg of amoxicillin and 125 mg of clavulanic acid, or 500 mg of amoxicillin and 250 mg of clavulanic acid every eight hours for three to seven days.

#### Usual pediatric dose
Antibacterial—
    Infants and children up to 40 kg of body weight:
        Otitis media, acute
        Pneumonia
        Sinusitis
        Other severe infections—Oral, 13.3 mg of amoxicillin and 3.3 mg of clavulanic acid per kg of body weight every eight hours for seven to ten days.
        Other infections—Oral, 6.7 mg of amoxicillin and 1.7 mg of clavulanic acid per kg of body weight every eight hours for seven to ten days.
    Children 40 kg of body weight and over:
        See *Usual adult and adolescent dose*.

#### Strength(s) usually available
U.S.—
    250 mg of amoxicillin and 125 mg of clavulanic acid (Rx) [*Augmentin*].
    500 mg of amoxicillin and 125 mg of clavulanic acid (Rx) [*Augmentin*].
Canada—
    250 mg of amoxicillin and 125 mg of clavulanic acid (Rx) [*Clavulin-250*].
    500 mg of amoxicillin and 125 mg of clavulanic acid (Rx) [*Clavulin-500F*].

Note: Two 250-mg tablets are not equivalent to one 500-mg tablet since both strengths contain equal amounts of clavulanate potassium.

#### Packaging and storage
Store below 40 °C (104 °F), preferably between 15 and 30 °C (59 and 86 °F), unless otherwise specified by manufacturer. Store in a tight container.

#### Auxiliary labeling
• Continue medication for full time of treatment.

## AMOXICILLIN AND CLAVULANATE POTASSIUM TABLETS (CHEWABLE) USP

**Usual adult and adolescent dose**
See *Amoxicillin and Clavulanate Potassium for Oral Suspension.*

**Usual pediatric dose**
See *Amoxicillin and Clavulanate Potassium for Oral Suspension.*

**Strength(s) usually available**
U.S.—
  125 mg of amoxicillin and 31.25 mg of clavulanic acid (Rx) [*Augmentin*].
  250 mg of amoxicillin and 62.5 mg of clavulanic acid (Rx) [*Augmentin*].
Canada—
  Not commercially available.

**Packaging and storage**
Store below 40 °C (104 °F), preferably between 15 and 30 °C (59 and 86 °F), unless otherwise specified by manufacturer. Store in a tight container.

**Auxiliary labeling**
- Should be chewed or crushed.
- Continue medication for full time of treatment.

[1]Not included in Canadian product labeling.

---

### AMPICILLIN AND SULBACTAM

## Summary of Differences

Precautions:
  Drug interactions and/or related problems—Concurrent use with allopurinol may increase the risk of skin rash.
  Laboratory value alterations—Ampicillin may decrease total conjugated estriol, estriol-glucuronide, conjugated estrone, and estradiol concentrations in pregnant women.
  Medical considerations/contraindications—Use in patients with infectious mononucleosis may increase the risk of skin rash.

## Additional Dosing Information

Ampicillin and sulbactam combination should be administered by deep intramuscular injection or by direct, slow intravenous injection over at least a 10- to 15-minute period. It may also be administered by intravenous infusion in 50 to 100 mL of a suitable diluent over a 15- to 30-minute period.

Adults with impaired renal function may require an increase in the dosing interval as follows:

| Creatinine Clearance (mL/min)/(mL/sec) | Dosing interval (hours) |
|---|---|
| ≥30/0.50 | 6 to 8 |
| 15–29/0.25–0.48 | 12 |
| 5–14/0.08–0.23 | 24 |
| <5/0.08 | 48 |

## Parenteral Dosage Forms

Note: Bracketed uses in the *Dosage Forms* section refer to categories of use and/or indications that are not included in U.S. product labeling.

### AMPICILLIN SODIUM AND SULBACTAM SODIUM STERILE USP

**Usual adult and adolescent dose**
Antibacterial—
  Intramuscular or intravenous, 1.5 to 3 grams (1 to 2 grams of ampicillin and 500 mg to 1 gram of sulbactam) every six hours.
  [Gonorrhea][1]—
  Intramuscular, 1.5 grams (1 gram of ampicillin and 500 mg of sulbactam) as a single dose with 1 gram of oral probenecid.

**Usual adult prescribing limits**
Up to 4 grams of sulbactam daily.

**Usual pediatric dose**
Antibacterial—
  Children up to 12 years of age: Dosage has not been established. However, doses of 200 to 400 mg per kg of body weight of ampicillin and 100 to 200 mg per kg of body weight of sulbactam per day, administered in divided doses, have been used.

**Size(s) usually available**
U.S.—
  1.5 grams (1 gram of ampicillin and 500 mg of sulbactam) (Rx) [*Unasyn* (sodium 5 mEq [5 mmol])].
  3 grams (2 grams of ampicillin and 1 gram of sulbactam) (Rx) [*Unasyn* (sodium 10 mEq [10 mmol])].
Canada—
  Not commercially available.

**Packaging and storage**
Prior to reconstitution, store below 30 °C (86 °F), unless otherwise specified by manufacturer.

**Preparation of dosage form**
To prepare initial dilution for intramuscular use, add 3.2 mL of sterile water for injection or of 0.5 or 2% lidocaine hydrochloride injection (without epinephrine) to each 1.5-gram vial and 6.4 mL of diluent to each 3-gram vial to provide an ampicillin concentration of 250 mg per mL and a sulbactam concentration of 125 mg per mL.

To prepare initial dilution for direct intermittent intravenous use, add 3.2 mL of sterile water for injection to each 1.5-gram vial and 6.4 mL of diluent to each 3-gram vial to provide an ampicillin concentration of 250 mg per mL and a sulbactam concentration of 125 mg per mL. The resulting solution should be immediately diluted with a suitable diluent (see manufacturer's package insert) to a final ampicillin concentration of 2 to 30 mg per mL and a final sulbactam concentration of 1 to 15 mg per mL.

Solutions should be allowed to stand following dissolution to allow any foaming to dissipate.

For reconstitution of piggyback infusion bottles, consult manufacturer's labeling.

**Stability**
After reconstitution for intramuscular use, solutions retain their potency for 1 hour.

After reconstitution for intravenous infusion, solutions containing 30 mg of ampicillin and 15 mg of sulbactam per mL retain their potency for 8 hours at 25 °C (77 °F) or for 48 hours at 4 °C (39 °F) in sterile water for injection or 0.9% sodium chloride injection. Solutions containing 20 mg of ampicillin and 10 mg of sulbactam per mL retain their potency for 72 hours at 4 °C (39 °F) in sterile water for injection or 0.9% sodium chloride injection. Solutions containing 20 mg of ampicillin and 10 mg of sulbactam per mL retain their potency for 2 hours at 25 °C (77 °F) or for 4 hours at 4 °C (39 °F) in 5% dextrose injection. Solutions containing 2 mg of ampicillin and 1 mg of sulbactam per mL retain their potency for 4 hours at 25 °C (77 °F) in 5% dextrose injection. For stability in other diluents, consult manufacturer's package insert.

Solutions (250 mg of ampicillin and 125 mg of sulbactam per mL) may vary in color from pale yellow to yellow. Dilute solutions (up to 30 mg of ampicillin and 15 mg of sulbactam per mL) may vary in color from colorless to pale yellow.

**Incompatibilities**
Extemporaneous admixtures of beta-lactam antibacterials (penicillins) and aminoglycosides may result in substantial mutual inactivation. If these groups of antibacterials are administered concurrently, they should be administered at separate sites at least 1 hour apart. Do not mix them in the same intravenous bag, bottle, or tubing.

When aminoglycosides and penicillins are administered separately by different routes, a reduction in aminoglycoside serum concentration may occur. Usually this is clinically significant only in patients with severely impaired renal function in whom the excretion of both medications is delayed.

**Additional information**
The sodium content (derived from ampicillin sodium and sulbactam sodium) is approximately 5 mEq (5 mmol) per 1.5 grams (1 gram of ampicillin and 500 mg of sulbactam). This must be considered in patients on a restricted sodium intake when calculating total daily sodium intake.

---

### PIPERACILLIN AND TAZOBACTAM

## Summary of Differences

Precautions:
  Drug interactions and/or related problems—Piperacillin also interacts with anticoagulants and other medications that affect blood clotting.
  Laboratory value alterations—May cause false-positive protein reaction in various urine protein tests; may decrease serum potassium concentrations; may increase prothrombin time and partial thromboplastin time.

Medical considerations/contraindications—Caution required in patients with history of bleeding problems; patients with cystic fibrosis may be at increased risk of fever and skin rash.

Side/adverse effects:
Increased risk of platelet dysfunction.

## Additional Dosing Information

Piperacillin and tazobactam combination should be administered by intravenous infusion over a 30-minute period.

The half-life of piperacillin and tazobactam is increased by 25% and 18%, respectively, in patients with hepatic cirrhosis. However, this difference does not warrant an adjustment in dose.

Patients with impaired renal function may require a reduction in dose and should be observed for hemorrhagic complications. Reductions in dose for adults and adolescents with impaired renal function are as follows:

| Creatinine Clearance (mL/min)/(mL/sec) | Dose/Dosing interval (piperacillin and tazobactam) |
| --- | --- |
| >40/0.67 | 3.375 grams every 6 hours |
| 20–40/0.33–0.67 | 2.25 grams every 6 hours |
| <20/0.33 | 2.25 grams every 8 hours |
| Hemodialysis patients | 2.25 grams every 8 hours and 0.75 grams after each dialysis |

## Parenteral Dosage Forms

### STERILE PIPERACILLIN SODIUM AND TAZOBACTAM SODIUM

**Usual adult and adolescent dose**
Antibacterial—
Intravenous infusion, 3.375 grams to 4.5 grams (3 to 4 grams of piperacillin and 0.375 to 0.5 grams of tazobactam) every six to eight hours for seven to ten days.

**Usual pediatric dose**
Antibacterial—
Infants and children up to 12 years of age: Dosage has not been established.
Children 12 years of age and older: See *Usual adult and adolescent dose*.

**Size(s) usually available**
U.S.—
2.25 grams (2 grams of piperacillin and 0.25 grams of tazobactam) (Rx) [*Zosyn* (sodium 4.7 mEq [4.7 mmol])].
3.375 grams (3 grams of piperacillin and 0.375 grams of tazobactam) (Rx) [*Zosyn* (sodium 7.1 mEq [7.1 mmol])].
4.5 grams (4 grams of piperacillin and 0.5 grams of tazobactam) (Rx) [*Zosyn* (sodium 9.4 mEq [9.4 mmol])].
Canada—
2.25 grams (2 grams of piperacillin and 0.25 grams of tazobactam) (Rx) [*Tazocin*].
3.375 grams (3 grams of piperacillin and 0.375 grams of tazobactam) (Rx) [*Tazocin*].
4.5 grams (4 grams of piperacillin and 0.5 grams of tazobactam) (Rx) [*Tazocin*].

**Packaging and storage**
Prior to reconstitution, store below 40 °C (104 °F), preferably between 15 and 30 °C (59 and 86 °F), unless otherwise specified by manufacturer.

**Preparation of dosage form**
To prepare initial dilution for intravenous use, add 5 mL of sterile water for injection, 5% dextrose injection, or sodium chloride injection to each vial and shake well until dissolved. This solution may be further diluted to the desired final volume with compatible intravenous diluents. Lactated Ringer's injection is *not* compatible as an initial diluent with piperacillin and tazobactam combination.

**Stability**
After reconstitution for intravenous use, solutions retain their potency for 24 hours at room temperature (21 to 24 °C [70 to 75 °F]) or for up to 7 days if refrigerated at 4 °C (39 °F). Lactated Ringer's injection is compatible with piperacillin and tazobactam combination for up to 2 hours when used as a diluent after initial reconstitution with 5% dextrose injection or sodium chloride injection.

**Incompatibilities**
Lactated Ringer's injection is *not* compatible as an initial diluent with piperacillin and tazobactam combination.
Extemporaneous admixtures of beta-lactam antibacterials (penicillins) and aminoglycosides may result in substantial mutual inactivation. If these groups of antibacterials are administered concurrently, they should be administered in separate sites at least 1 hour apart. Do not mix them in the same intravenous bag, bottle, or tubing.
When aminoglycosides and penicillins are administered separately by different routes, a reduction in aminoglycoside serum concentration may occur. Usually this is clinically significant only in patients with severely impaired renal function in whom the excretion of both medications is delayed.

**Additional information**
The sodium content is approximately 2.35 mEq (2.35 mmol) per gram of piperacillin. This must be considered in patients on a restricted sodium intake when calculating total daily sodium intake.

---

## TICARCILLIN AND CLAVULANATE

## Summary of Differences

Precautions:
Drug interactions and/or related problems—Ticarcillin interacts with anticoagulants and other medications that affect blood clotting; clavulanic acid does not interact with probenecid.
Laboratory value alterations—May cause false-positive protein reaction for various urine protein tests; may decrease serum potassium concentrations; may increase prothrombin time and partial thromboplastin time; may increase serum sodium concentrations; may decrease uric acid.
Medical considerations/contraindications—Caution required in patients with history of bleeding problems; caution also required in patients with congestive heart failure, hypertension, or renal function impairment because of sodium content.

Side/adverse effects:
Increased risk of platelet dysfunction.

## Additional Dosing Information

Sterile ticarcillin disodium and clavulanate potassium and ticarcillin disodium and clavulanate potassium injection should be administered by intravenous infusion over a 30-minute period.

Patients with impaired renal function may require a reduction in dose and should be observed for hemorrhagic complications. After an initial loading dose of 3 grams of ticarcillin and 100 mg of clavulanic acid, adults with impaired renal function may require a reduction in dose as follows:

| Creatinine Clearance (mL/min)/(mL/sec) | Dose/Dosing interval (based on ticarcillin content) |
| --- | --- |
| >60/1.0 | 3 grams every 4 hours |
| 30–60/0.50–1.0 | 2 grams every 4 hours |
| 10–30/0.17–0.50 | 2 grams every 8 hours |
| <10/0.17 | 2 grams every 12 hours |
| <10 with hepatic dysfunction | 2 grams every 24 hours |
| Peritoneal dialysis patients | 3 grams every 12 hours |
| Hemodialysis patients | 2 grams every 12 hours; and 3 grams after each dialysis |

## Parenteral Dosage Forms

Note: Bracketed uses in the *Dosage Forms* section refer to categories of use and/or indications that are not included in U.S. product labeling.

### TICARCILLIN DISODIUM AND CLAVULANATE POTASSIUM STERILE USP

**Usual adult and adolescent dose**
Antibacterial—
Treatment:
Adults and adolescents up to 60 kg of body weight—Intravenous infusion, 33.3 to 50 mg of ticarcillin and 1.1 to 1.7 mg of clavulanic acid per kg of body weight every four hours; or 50 to 75 mg of ticarcillin and 1.7 to 2.5 mg of clavulanic acid per kg of body weight every six hours.
Adults and adolescents 60 kg of body weight and over—Intravenous infusion, 3 grams of ticarcillin and 100 mg of clavulanic acid every four to six hours.
[Surgical prophylaxis]:
Intravenous infusion, 3 grams of ticarcillin and 100 mg of clavulanic acid one-half to one hour prior to the start of surgery, or (for cesarean section) as soon as the umbilical cord is clamped, then 3.1 grams at four-hour intervals for a total of three doses.

**Usual pediatric dose**
Antibacterial—
Infants less than 1 month of age:
Dosage has not been established.

Infants and children 1 month to 12 years of age:
  Intravenous infusion, 50 mg of ticarcillin and 1.7 mg of clavulanic acid per kg of body weight every four to six hours.
    Note: Children with cystic fibrosis—Intravenous infusion, 350 to 450 mg of ticarcillin and 11.7 to 17 mg of clavulanic acid per kg of body weight a day in divided doses.
Children 12 years of age and older:
  See *Usual adult and adolescent dose (Adults and adolescents up to 60 kg of body weight)*.

### Size(s) usually available
U.S.—
   3.1 grams (3 grams of ticarcillin and 100 mg of clavulanic acid) (Rx) [*Timentin* (sodium 4.75 mEq [4.75 mmol] per gram)].
   31 grams (30 grams of ticarcillin and 1 gram of clavulanic acid) (Rx) [*Timentin*].
Note: Although listed in the U.S. package insert, the 3.2-gram vial is not currently available, according to the manufacturer.
Canada—
   3.1 grams (3 grams of ticarcillin and 100 mg of clavulanic acid) (Rx) [*Timentin* (sodium 4.75 mEq [4.75 mmol] per gram)].

### Packaging and storage
Prior to reconstitution, store below 40 °C (104 °F), preferably between 15 and 30 °C (59 and 86 °F), unless otherwise specified by manufacturer.

### Preparation of dosage form
To prepare initial dilution for direct intravenous use, add 13 mL of sterile water for injection or sodium chloride injection to each 3.1-gram vial to provide a ticarcillin concentration of approximately 200 mg per mL and a clavulanic acid concentration of approximately 6.7 mg per mL. The resulting solution should be further diluted to desired volume in sodium chloride injection, 5% dextrose injection, or lactated Ringer's injection and administered over a 30-minute period.
For reconstitution of piggyback infusion bottles or pharmacy bulk vials, see manufacturer's labeling for instructions. If the Y-type method of administration is used, the primary infusion should be temporarily discontinued during infusion of ticarcillin and clavulanate combination.

### Stability
After reconstitution for intravenous use, solutions containing 200 mg of ticarcillin per mL retain their potency for 6 hours at room temperature (21 to 24 °C [70 to 75 °F]) or for up to 72 hours if refrigerated at 4 °C (39 °F).
Solutions containing 10 to 100 mg of ticarcillin per mL in sodium chloride injection or lactated Ringer's injection retain their potency for 24 hours at room temperature (21 to 24 °C [70 to 75 °F]) or for 7 days if refrigerated at 4 °C (39 °F). Solutions containing 10 to 100 mg of ticarcillin per mL in 5% dextrose injection retain their potency for 24 hours at room temperature or for 3 days if refrigerated.
After reconstitution, solutions containing 100 mg of ticarcillin or less per mL in sodium chloride injection or lactated Ringer's injection may be frozen and stored for up to 30 days. Solutions in 5% dextrose injection may be frozen for 7 days. Thawed solutions should be used within 8 hours.
Solutions may vary in color from colorless to pale yellow.

### Incompatibilities
Extemporaneous admixtures of beta-lactam antibacterials (penicillins) and aminoglycosides may result in substantial mutual inactivation. If these groups of antibacterials are administered concurrently, they should be administered in separate sites at least 1 hour apart. Do not mix them in the same intravenous bag, bottle, or tubing.
When aminoglycosides and penicillins are administered separately by different routes, a reduction in aminoglycoside serum concentration may occur. Usually this is clinically significant only in patients with severely impaired renal function in whom the excretion of both medications is delayed.
Sterile ticarcillin disodium and clavulanate potassium combination is incompatible with sodium bicarbonate.

### Additional information
The sodium content is approximately 4.75 mEq (4.75 mmol) per gram of ticarcillin. This must be considered in patients on a restricted sodium intake when calculating total daily sodium intake.
The potassium content is approximately 0.15 mEq (6 mg) per 100 mg of clavulanic acid.

## TICARCILLIN DISODIUM AND CLAVULANATE POTASSIUM INJECTION

### Usual adult and adolescent dose
See *Sterile Ticarcillin Disodium and Clavulanate Potassium USP*.

### Usual pediatric dose
See *Sterile Ticarcillin Disodium and Clavulanate Potassium USP*.

### Strength(s) usually available
U.S.—
   3.1 grams (3 grams of ticarcillin and 100 mg of clavulanic acid) in 50 mL (Rx) [*Timentin* (sodium 4.75 mEq [4.75 mmol] per gram)].
   3.1 grams (3 grams of ticarcillin and 100 mg of clavulanic acid) in 100 mL (Rx) [*Timentin* (sodium 4.75 mEq [4.75 mmol] per gram)].
Canada—
   Not commercially available.

### Packaging and storage
Do not store above -10 °C (14 °F), unless otherwise specified by manufacturer.

### Preparation of dosage form
Thaw container at room temperature before administration, making sure that all ice crystals have melted.
Minibags should not be used in series connections. Doing so may result in air embolism because of residual air being drawn from the primary container before administration of intravenous solution from the secondary container is complete.

### Stability
Thawed solutions should be used within 8 hours. Once thawed, solutions should not be refrozen.

### Incompatibilities
Extemporaneous admixtures of beta-lactam antibacterials (penicillins) and aminoglycosides may result in substantial mutual inactivation. If these groups of antibacterials are administered concurrently, they should be administered in separate sites at least 1 hour apart. Do not mix them in the same intravenous bag, bottle, or tubing.
When aminoglycosides and penicillins are administered separately by different routes, a reduction in aminoglycoside serum concentration may occur. Usually this is clinically significant only in patients with severely impaired renal function in whom the excretion of both medications is delayed.

### Additional information
The sodium content is approximately 4.75 mEq (4.75 mmol) per gram of ticarcillin. This must be considered in patients on a restricted sodium intake when calculating total daily sodium intake.
The potassium content is approximately 0.15 mEq (6 mg) per 100 mg of clavulanic acid.

Developed: 07/29/94
Revised: 04/19/95

**PENICILLIN V** — See *Penicillins (Systemic)*

**PENTAERYTHRITOL TETRANITRATE** — See *Nitrates (Systemic)*

**PENTAGASTRIN** — The *Pentagastrin (Systemic)* monograph is not included in this published version of the USP DI database. Copies of the monograph are available on request from Micromedex, Inc. - Reprint Requests, 6200 S. Syracuse Way, Suite 300, Englewood, CO 80111; telephone (303) 486-6400; telefax (303) 486-6464; Email: USPDI@MDX.COM.

# PENTAMIDINE Inhalation

VA CLASSIFICATION (Primary): AP109
Commonly used brand name(s): *NebuPent; Pentacarinat; Pneumopent.*
Note: For a listing of dosage forms and brand names by country availability, see *Dosage Forms* section(s).

## Category
Antiprotozoal.

## Indications
Note: Bracketed information in the *Indications* section refers to uses that are not included in U.S. product labeling.

**Accepted**
Pneumonia, *Pneumocystis carinii* (PCP) (prophylaxis)—Aerosolized pentamidine is indicated in both secondary prophylaxis (patients who have already had at least one episode of *Pneumocystis carinii* pneumonia), and primary prophylaxis (HIV-infected patients with a CD4 lymphocyte count less than or equal to 200 cells per cubic millimeter) of *Pneumocystis carinii* pneumonia.

[Pneumonia, *Pneumocystis carinii* (PCP) (treatment)][1]—Aerosolized pentamidine is used in the treatment of mild (A-a gradient < 30 mm Hg) *Pneumocystis carinii* pneumonia. However, preliminary studies have suggested that aerosolized pentamidine may be less effective than conventional systemic therapies; patients receiving this regimen should be followed closely for evidence of progressive disease.

[1]Not included in Canadian product labeling.

## Pharmacology/Pharmacokinetics

**Physicochemical characteristics**
Molecular weight—340.42.

**Mechanism of action/Effect**
Not clearly defined; pentamidine may interfere with incorporation of nucleotides into RNA and DNA and may inhibit oxidative phosphorylation, resulting in inhibition of DNA, RNA, phospholipid, and protein biosynthesis; may also interfere with folate transformation.

**Absorption**
Systemic absorption of inhaled pentamidine is minimal, with serum pentamidine concentrations less than 20 nanograms per mL after a nebulized dose of 4 mg per kg in most cases (versus 612 nanograms per mL after a single intravenous dose of 4 mg per kg). Peak systemic absorption occurs at, or near, completion of inhalation therapy.

**Distribution**
Aerosolized pentamidine produces concentrations approximately 10 to 100 times higher in the lungs than would a comparable dose of intravenous pentamidine.

**Elimination**
Unknown; in one study, cumulative percentage of total dose renally excreted was 0.4% over a 72-hour period.

## Precautions to Consider

**Carcinogenicity/Mutagenicity**
Pentamidine has not been shown to be mutagenic in Ames studies. Carcinogenicity studies have not been done.

**Pregnancy/Reproduction**
Fertility—Studies have not been done.
Pregnancy—Studies with aerosolized pentamidine have not been done in humans.
Studies with aerosolized pentamidine have not been done in animals. However, studies in rabbits have shown that systemic pentamidine was associated with an increased incidence of post-implantation losses and delayed fetal ossification.
FDA Pregnancy Category C.

**Breast-feeding**
It is not known whether pentamidine is distributed into breast milk.

**Pediatrics**
No information is available on the relationship of age to the effects of aerosolized pentamidine in pediatric patients. Safety and efficacy have not been established. However, if sulfamethoxazole and trimethoprim combination is not tolerated, aerosolized pentamidine is recommended for children 5 years of age and older.

**Geriatrics**
No information is available on the relationship of age to the effects of pentamidine in geriatric patients.

**Dental**
Pentamidine may cause a bitter or metallic taste, gingivitis, hypersalivation, or dry mouth.

**Drug interactions and/or related problems**
At this time, no clinically significant drug interactions and/or related problems have been documented in patients receiving prophylactic aerosolized pentamidine.

**Medical considerations/Contraindications**
The medical considerations/contraindications included have been selected on the basis of their potential clinical significance (reasons given in parentheses where appropriate)—not necessarily inclusive (» = major clinical significance).

*Except under special circumstances, this medication should not be used when the following medical problem exists:*
» Allergy to pentamidine
(aerosolized pentamidine is contraindicated in patients with a history of an anaphylactic reaction to inhaled or systemic pentamidine)

*Risk-benefit should be considered when the following medical problem exists:*
Asthma
(aerosolized pentamidine may induce acute bronchospasm, usually in patients with a history of asthma; this may be reduced by pretreatment with a bronchodilator)

**Patient monitoring**
The following may be especially important in patient monitoring (other tests may be warranted in some patients, depending on condition » = major clinical significance):
At this time, there are no particular laboratory tests or monitoring parameters recommended routinely for patients receiving prophylactic aerosolized pentamidine. However, baseline parameters, including pulmonary function tests, serum amylase and lipase, may be obtained for the first treatment, and then followed as needed.

## Side/Adverse Effects

Note: The prophylactic use of aerosolized pentamidine has a very low incidence of severe side effects. Many adverse reactions will be due to other medications, other concurrent infections, or the HIV disease itself, and may be difficult to differentiate.

Coughing and bronchospasm occur primarily in patients who are cigarette smokers and continue to smoke, or have an underlying pulmonary disease, such as asthma.

A number of cases of extrapulmonary pneumocystosis and pneumothorax have been reported in patients receiving aerosolized pentamidine. These are thought to be infectious complications due to subclinical, peripheral infection and poor systemic distribution of aerosolized pentamidine. Although the incidence is not known at this time, one study found that extrapulmonary pneumocystosis appears to occur more frequently in, but is not limited to, patients who have been diagnosed with AIDS for longer than 12 months. These patients usually have had prior episodes of *Pneumocystis carinii* pneumonia (PCP), often do not have concurrent pneumonia, are receiving concurrent zidovudine, and have had prolonged treatment with aerosolized pentamidine. It is suggested that use of zidovudine and prophylactic aerosolized pentamidine may allow for the emergence of extrapulmonary pneumocystosis.

The following side/adverse effects have been selected on the basis of their potential clinical significance (possible signs and symptoms in parentheses where appropriate)—not necessarily inclusive:

**Those indicating need for medical attention**
Incidence more frequent
*Chest pain or congestion; coughing; dyspnea* (difficulty in breathing); *pharyngitis* (burning pain, dryness, or sensation of lump in throat; difficulty in swallowing); *skin rash; wheezing*

Incidence rare
*Extrapulmonary pneumocystosis*—most frequent sites include the spleen, liver, lymph nodes, and eyes; *pancreatitis* (nausea; pain in upper abdomen, possibly radiating to the back; vomiting)—may occur more frequently with prolonged use; *pneumothorax* (sudden onset of severe breathing difficulty; severe pain in chest)

Incidence rare—with daily treatment doses only
> **Hypoglycemia, mild** (anxiety; chills; cold sweats; cool, pale skin; headache; increased hunger; nausea; nervousness; shakiness); **renal insufficiency** (decreased urination; loss of appetite; nausea; unusual tiredness)

**Those not indicating need for medical attention**
Incidence less frequent
> *Bitter or metallic taste*

## Patient Consultation

As an aid to patient consultation, refer to *Advice for the Patient, Pentamidine (Inhalation)*.

In providing consultation, consider emphasizing the following selected information (» = major clinical significance):

**Before using this medication**
» Conditions affecting use, especially:
  Allergy to pentamidine

**Proper use of this medication**
  Importance of receiving medication for full course of therapy and on regular schedule
» Proper dosing
  Missed dose: Receiving therapy as soon as possible

**Precautions while using this medication**
  If also using a bronchodilator inhaler, using about 5 to 10 minutes prior to aerosolized pentamidine
  Possible bitter or metallic taste; dissolving a hard candy in mouth after administration of medication
  Cigarette smokers who continue to smoke are more likely to experience coughing and bronchospasm during aerosolized pentamidine therapy

**Side/adverse effects**
  Signs of potential side effects, especially chest pain or congestion, coughing, dyspnea, pharyngitis, skin rash, wheezing, extrapulmonary pneumocystosis, pancreatitis, pneumothorax, hypoglycemia, and renal insufficiency
  A bitter or metallic taste may occur; however, it is medically insignificant

## General Dosing Information

Coughing and bronchospasm occur primarily in cigarette smokers who continue to smoke, or patients with an underlying pulmonary disease, such as asthma. A higher incidence of coughing and bronchospasm may be related to larger particle sizes; however, these symptoms appear to occur most frequently due to an increased particle load with larger doses. Pretreatment with a bronchodilator, e.g., albuterol, metaproterenol, or terbutaline, helps to alleviate this problem and may improve pentamidine distribution in the lung.

It is important that as much medication as possible reach the upper lobes of the lungs, since upper lobe *P. carinii* pneumonia relapses have occurred in patients while they were receiving aerosolized pentamidine. There appears to be a more uniform distribution of aerosolized pentamidine in the lungs when it is administered to patients in a supine or recumbent position.

Before aerosolized pentamidine treatment is started, a tuberculin skin test, chest x-ray, and sputum culture, if possible, should be performed to rule out tuberculosis due to *Mycobacterium tuberculosis*. A tuberculin skin test alone may not be useful because false negative readings often occur in AIDS patients. The risk of active disease or reactivation of latent tuberculosis infection is more prevalent in HIV-infected people. Also, the risk of transmission of tuberculosis to health care workers or others in the vicinity may exist.

Health care workers are advised to administer aerosolized pentamidine in a well-ventilated room if possible. Although one study found the environmental levels of pentamidine in a treatment room to be low, long-term occupational studies have not been done and the risk has not been established. Of primary concern is the previously mentioned risk of transmission of tuberculosis or other respiratory pathogens via aerosols, as well as anecdotal reports of a reversible decrease in pulmonary function testing parameters and chemical conjunctivitis due to ocular exposure to aerosolized pentamidine.

Two types of nebulizers have been shown to be effective in decreasing the incidence of *P. carinii* pneumonia. Respirgard II is a jet nebulizer and is used with NebuPent and Pentacarinat; Fisoneb is an ultrasonic nebulizer and is used with Pneumopent. Jet nebulizers use a high-flow gas to shear liquid strands from a thin layer of solution. The liquid strands hit a baffle, creating a wide variety of particle sizes. Larger particles generally fall by gravity and get reincorporated into the solution. Ultrasonic nebulizers generate an ultrahigh frequency sound, creating a geyser from which particles are expelled. When the flow through the nebulizer is interrupted, as with tidal breathing, the smaller particles coalesce into larger particles. Because of this, measurements of output and particle size will vary with different operating conditions.

Particle size produced by the nebulizer is an important factor in the location of aerosol deposition. The optimal size for deposition in the alveoli, where *Pneumocystis carinii* pneumonia (PCP) causes damage, is 1 to 2 microns; the optimal size for tracheobronchial deposition is 4 to 7 microns. Many factors can affect and limit aerosol deposition into the alveoli, including inspiratory flowrates, frequency of respiration, breath-holding, tidal volumes, and airway narrowing from bronchospasm, emphysema, mucus, and PCP.

Because of the differences in nebulizers and the efficacy with which they deliver aerosolized pentamidine, the nebulizers should not be utilized interchangeably with the different dosing regimens. The two regimens shown to be effective are described below.

## Inhalation Dosage Forms

Note: Bracketed uses in the *Dosage Forms* section refer to categories of use and/or indications that are not included in U.S. product labeling.

### PENTAMIDINE ISETHIONATE FOR INHALATION SOLUTION

**Usual adult and adolescent dose**
Pneumonia, *Pneumocystis carinii*—
  For *NebuPent* and *Pentacarinat* using the Respirgard II jet nebulizer:
    Prophylaxis—
      Oral inhalation, 300 mg every four weeks, administered via the Respirgard II nebulizer. The aerosol treatment should be continued over a period of approximately thirty to forty-five minutes, until the nebulizer chamber is empty.
    Note: A prophylactic dose of 150 mg every two weeks, administered via the Respirgard II nebulizer, has also been used if the patient cannot tolerate a single monthly dose. One study found that although patients who received 300 mg monthly had a lower rate of PCP than those receiving 150 mg every two weeks, the difference was not significant.
    [Treatment][1]—
      Oral inhalation, 600 mg a day, administered via the Respirgard II nebulizer for twenty-one days. Continue the aerosol treatment over a period of approximately twenty-five to thirty minutes.
    Note: The flow rate for the nebulizer should be 5 to 7 liters per minute from a 40- to 50-pounds-per-square-inch (PSI) air or oxygen source.
      Low pressure compressors (<20 PSI) should not be used.
  For *Pneumopent* using the Fisoneb ultrasonic nebulizer:
    Loading dose (prophylaxis)—
      Oral inhalation, 60 mg, administered via the Fisoneb ultrasonic nebulizer, every twenty-four to seventy-two hours for a total of 5 doses over a two week period. The aerosol treatment should be continued over a period of approximately fifteen minutes, until the nebulizer chamber is empty.
    Maintenance dose (prophylaxis)—
      Oral inhalation, 60 mg, administered via the Fisoneb ultrasonic nebulizer, every two weeks.
    Note: The flow rate of the nebulizer should be set at the mid-flow mark.

**Usual pediatric dose**
Pneumonia, *Pneumocystis carinii*—
  Prophylaxis: Dosage has not been established. However, 300 mg every four weeks has been used in children 5 years of age and older who cannot tolerate sulfamethoxazole and trimethoprim combination.

**Size(s) usually available**
U.S.—
  300 mg (Rx) [*NebuPent* (Respirgard II nebulizer)].
Canada—
  60 mg (Rx) [*Pneumopent* (Fisoneb nebulizer)].
  300 mg (Rx) [*Pentacarinat* (Respirgard II nebulizer)].

**Packaging and storage**
Prior to reconstitution, store between 15 and 30 °C (59 and 86 °F), unless otherwise specified by manufacturer.

### Preparation of dosage form
For *NebuPent* and *Pentacarinat*—
  To prepare pentamidine for oral inhalation *prophylaxis*, add 6 mL of sterile water for injection to each 300-mg vial of sterile pentamidine isethionate.
  To prepare pentamidine for oral inhalation *treatment*, add 6 mL of sterile water for injection to 600 mg of sterile pentamidine isethionate. For administration, place the entire reconstituted contents into the reservoir chamber of the Respirgard II nebulizer.

For *Pneumopent*—
  To prepare for oral inhalation, remove the rubber stopper and put it aside, upside down, on a clean surface for later use. Add 3 to 5 mL of sterile water for inhalation or sterile water for injection to the vial. Do not use tap water and do not use normal saline. Replace the rubber stopper. The powder should dissolve immediately; if it does not, gently shake the vial to mix it. It should form a clear, colorless solution; if the solution is cloudy, do not use it.
  For administration, place the entire reconstituted contents into the chamber of the Fisoneb ultrasonic nebulizer.

### Stability
For *NebuPent*:
  After reconstitution, solutions in concentrations of 93 mg per mL retain at least 90% of their potency for up to 4 months when frozen in plastic syringes at −20 °C. Do not defrost and refreeze.

For *Pentacarinat*:
  Store unopened vials at room temperature; protect from light.
  After reconstitution, solutions in concentrations of approximately 2 mg per mL are stable for up to 24 hours at room temperature.

For *Pneumopent*:
  Store unopened vials at room temperature.
  After reconstitution, solution may be stored for up to 24 hours at room temperature or up to 48 hours in a refrigerator. Do not freeze.

### Incompatibilities
Reconstitution of pentamidine with saline solutions may cause pentamidine to precipitate out of solution.

### Additional information
Pentamidine inhalation solution should not be mixed with any other medications.
Do not use the Respirgard II nebulizer to administer a bronchodilator.

[1]Not included in Canadian product labeling.

### Selected Bibliography
Monk JP, Benfield P. Inhaled pentamidine. An overview of its pharmacological properties and a review of its therapeutic use in Pneumocystis carinii pneumonia. Drugs 1990; 39(5): 741-56.

Revised: 03/03/92
Interim revision: 03/28/94

# PENTAMIDINE  Systemic

VA CLASSIFICATION (Primary): AP109

Commonly used brand name(s): *Pentacarinat; Pentam 300*.

Note: For a listing of dosage forms and brand names by country availability, see *Dosage Forms* section(s).

## Category
Antiprotozoal.

## Indications
Note: Bracketed information in the *Indications* section refers to uses that are not included in U.S. product labeling.

### Accepted
Pneumonia, *Pneumocystis carinii* (treatment)—Pentamidine is indicated in the treatment of *Pneumocystis carinii* pneumonia (PCP) in immunocompromised patients, including patients with acquired immunodeficiency syndrome (AIDS). Sulfamethoxazole and trimethoprim combination is considered to be the primary agent for PCP in patients who can tolerate it.

[Leishmaniasis, visceral (treatment)][1]—Pentamidine is used as a secondary agent in the treatment of visceral leishmaniasis (kala-azar) caused by *Leishmania donovani*. Stibogluconate sodium, a pentavalent antimony derivative, is considered to be the primary agent for visceral leishmaniasis.

[Leishmaniasis, cutaneous (treatment)][1]—Pentamidine is used as a secondary agent in the treatment of cutaneous leishmaniasis caused by *Leishmania tropica, L. major, L. mexicana, L. aethiopica, L. peruviana, L. guyanensis*, and *L. braziliensis*. Stibogluconate sodium, a pentavalent antimony derivative, is considered to be the primary agent for cutaneous leishmaniasis.

[Trypanosomiasis, African (treatment)][1]—Pentamidine is used as a secondary agent in the treatment of African trypanosomiasis (trypanosome fever; African sleeping sickness) caused by *Trypanosoma brucei gambiense* and *T. b. rhodesiense* in patients with early or hemolymphatic disease without central nervous system (CNS) involvement. Suramin is considered to be the primary agent for African trypanosomiasis in these patients.

In patients with late or chronic trypanosomiasis involving the CNS, melarsoprol, an arsenical complexed with dimercaprol, is considered the primary agent.

Not all species or strains of a particular organism may be susceptible to pentamidine.

### Unaccepted
Since pentamidine does not cross the blood-brain barrier, it is not useful in patients with late or chronic trypanosomiasis involving the CNS.

[1]Not included in Canadian product labeling.

## Pharmacology/Pharmacokinetics

### Physicochemical characteristics
Molecular weight—Pentamidine: 340.42.

### Mechanism of action/Effect
Not clearly defined; pentamidine may interfere with incorporation of nucleotides into RNA and DNA and inhibit oxidative phosphorylation and biosynthesis of DNA, RNA, protein, and phospholipid; may also interfere with folate transformation.

### Other actions/effects
May also have antifungal activity.

### Absorption
Poorly absorbed from the gastrointestinal tract; must be given parenterally.

### Distribution
Rapidly distributed after administration; distribution half-life of 5 to 15 minutes after intravenous administration, 0.9 hours after intramuscular administration. In humans, highest concentrations of pentamidine were found in the liver, kidneys, adrenal glands, and spleen; lung concentrations were lower than concentrations in these organs, and accumulated over a 4 to 5 day period. There were indications of very slow uptake into the CNS, with pentamidine being detected in brain tissue approximately 30 days after the start of daily therapy.

Apparent Vol $_D$ at steady state—3 to 32 liters per kg (L/kg).

### Protein binding
High (69%). Rapidly bound to tissues following administration.

### Storage
In humans, appears to be stored in the body to some extent, and slowly excreted; in mice, may be stored for months in the kidneys and liver.

### Biotransformation
In rats, metabolized to as many as 6 primary metabolic forms; human metabolism is unknown.

### Half-life
Intramuscular—9.1 to 13.2 hours.

Intravenous—Approximately 6.5 hours.

Terminal half-life—2 to 4 weeks.

Renal function impairment—Pentamidine half-life may be prolonged in patients with renal dysfunction; however, no correlation between renal function and plasma clearance of pentamidine has been found.

### Time to peak serum concentration
Intramuscular—0.5 to 1 hour.

Intravenous—End of infusion (1 to 2 hours).

### Peak serum concentration
Intramuscular—0.2 to 1.4 mcg per mL (mcg/mL) after 4 mg per kg of body weight (mg/kg).

Intravenous—0.5 to 3.4 mcg/mL after 4 mg/kg infused over 1 to 2 hours.

Multiple dosing results in progressive drug accumulation; this may occur even in patients with normal renal function who receive a reduced daily dose of intravenous pentamidine.

### Elimination
Renal—4 to 17% of intramuscular dose excreted in urine over 24 hours; approximately 2.5% of intravenous dose excreted in urine over 24 hours. Patients may continue to excrete decreasing amounts in urine for up to 8 weeks following discontinuation of therapy.

Fecal—In humans, no information available; in mice, excreted in feces in an amount approximately ¼ that in urine.

In dialysis—Neither peritoneal dialysis nor hemodialysis appears to significantly reduce plasma pentamidine concentrations.

## Precautions to Consider

### Carcinogenicity/Mutagenicity
No studies have been conducted to evaluate the potential of pentamidine as a carcinogen or mutagen.

### Pregnancy/Reproduction
Fertility—Studies have not been done.

Pregnancy—Adequate and well-controlled studies in humans have not been done.

Pentamidine has been found to cross the placenta in rats given high doses late in pregnancy. Studies in rabbits have also shown pentamidine to be mildly embryotoxic, with an increase in post-implantation losses and delayed fetal ossification at doses of 1, 3, and 8 mg per kg of body weight (mg/kg)

FDA Pregnancy Category C.

### Breast-feeding
It is not known whether pentamidine is distributed into breast milk. However, because of the potential risks to the newborn, breast-feeding is not recommended during pentamidine therapy.

### Pediatrics
Limited clinical and pharmacokinetic data are available in children; however, the mg/kg dose used in children is the same as that used in adults, and side effects seen in children are similar to those seen in adults. No pediatrics-specific problems have been documented to date.

### Geriatrics
No information is available on the relationship of age to the effects of pentamidine in geriatric patients.

### Dental
Systemic pentamidine may rarely cause an unpleasant metallic taste.

Pentamidine may cause leukopenia and thrombocytopenia, resulting in an increased incidence of certain microbial infections, delayed healing, and gingival bleeding. Dental work, whenever possible, should be completed prior to initiation of therapy or deferred until blood counts have returned to normal. Patients should be instructed in proper oral hygiene during treatment, including caution in use of regular toothbrushes, dental floss, and toothpicks.

### Drug interactions and/or related problems
The following drug interactions and/or related problems have been selected on the basis of their potential clinical significance (possible mechanism in parentheses where appropriate)—not necessarily inclusive (» = major clinical significance):

Note: Combinations containing any of the following medications, depending on the amount present, may also interact with this medication.

Blood dyscrasia–causing medications (See *Appendix II*) or
» Bone marrow depressants, other (See *Appendix II*) or
» Radiation therapy
(concurrent use with pentamidine may increase the abnormal hematologic effects of these medications and radiation therapy; dosage reduction may be required)

» Didanosine
(concurrent use with pentamidine may increase the potential for development of pancreatitis)

Erythromycin
(concurrent use of intravenous erythromycin with pentamidine may increase the potential for development of torsades de pointes)

» Foscarnet
(concurrent use with pentamidine may result in severe, but reversible, hypocalcemia, hypomagnesemia, and nephrotoxicity)

» Nephrotoxic medications, other (See *Appendix II*)
(concurrent use of other nephrotoxic medications with pentamidine may increase the potential for nephrotoxicity; renal function determinations, dosage reductions, and/or dosage interval adjustments may be required)

### Laboratory value alterations
The following have been selected on the basis of their potential clinical significance (possible effect in parentheses where appropriate)—not necessarily inclusive (» = major clinical significance):

With physiology/laboratory test values
Alanine aminotransferase (ALT [SGPT]) and
Alkaline phosphatase, serum, and
Aspartate aminotransferase (AST [SGOT]) and
Bilirubin, serum
(values may be increased)
» Blood urea nitrogen (BUN) and
» Creatinine, serum
(concentrations may be increased)
Calcium, serum and
Magnesium, serum
(concentrations may be decreased)
» Glucose, blood
(concentrations may be increased or decreased since both hypoglycemia and hyperglycemia have occurred)
Potassium, serum
(concentrations may be increased)

### Medical considerations/Contraindications
The medical considerations/contraindications included have been selected on the basis of their potential clinical significance (reasons given in parentheses where appropriate)—not necessarily inclusive (» = major clinical significance):

*Except under special circumstances, this medication should not be used when the following medical problem exists:*
» Previous allergic reaction to pentamidine
(pentamidine is contraindicated in patients with a history of an anaphylactic reaction to inhaled or systemic pentamidine)

*Risk-benefit should be considered when the following medical problems exist:*
Anemia or
» Bleeding disorders, history of, or
» Bone marrow depression
(pentamidine may cause hematologic abnormalities, resulting in anemia, leukopenia, and thrombocytopenia)
» Cardiac disease or arrhythmias
(pentamidine may cause fatal cardiac arrhythmias, tachycardia, torsades de pointes, or other cardiotoxicity)
» Dehydration or
» Renal function impairment
(pentamidine may cause azotemia or acute renal insufficiency; dehydration may contribute to renal toxicity)
» Diabetes mellitus or
» Hypoglycemia
(pentamidine may cause hypoglycemia or hyperglycemia and may aggravate diabetes mellitus)
Hepatic function impairment
(pentamidine may cause an increase in AST [SGOT], ALT [SGPT], bilirubin, and alkaline phosphatase)
» Hypotension
(pentamidine may cause sudden severe hypotension; this is seen most frequently after intramuscular injections and rapid intravenous infusions)
» Risk-benefit should also be considered in patients who have had previous cytotoxic drug therapy or radiation therapy.

### Patient monitoring
The following may be especially important in patient monitoring (other tests may be warranted in some patients, depending on condition; » = major clinical significance):

» Blood pressure determinations
(since sudden, severe hypotension may occur, even after a single intramuscular or intravenous dose of pentamidine, patients should be lying down and their blood pressure should be closely monitored during administration and several times thereafter until blood pressure is stable)

» Blood urea nitrogen (BUN) and
» Creatinine, serum
(concentrations may be required prior to and daily during therapy since pentamidine may be nephrotoxic; serum creatinine concentrations up to 6 mg per dL, as well as acute renal failure with even higher serum creatinine concentrations, have been reported; patients with severely impaired renal function may require a reduction in dose)

Calcium, serum and
Magnesium, serum
(concentrations may be required prior to and every 3 days during therapy since hypocalcemia and hypomagnesemia due to pentamidine-induced tubular injury may occur)
» Complete blood counts (CBCs) or
» Platelet counts
(may be required prior to and every 3 days during therapy since pentamidine may cause severe leukopenia, thrombocytopenia, and, occasionally, anemia)
» Electrocardiograms (ECGs)
(may be required at regular intervals during therapy since fatalities due to cardiac arrhythmias, tachycardia, torsades de pointes, or other cardiotoxicity have been reported; potassium and magnesium concentrations should also be monitored; patients who develop monomorphic and polymorphic ventricular tachycardia may benefit from rapid intravenous injection of magnesium sulfate)
» Glucose concentrations, blood
(pentamidine may cause hypoglycemia, which may be associated with pancreatic beta islet cell necrosis and inappropriately high plasma insulin concentrations; blood glucose concentrations below 20 mg per dL have been reported; hyperglycemia and permanent diabetes mellitus, with or without preceding hypoglycemia, have also occurred, sometimes up to several months after therapy is discontinued; therefore, blood glucose determinations may be required prior to therapy, daily during therapy, and up to several months following therapy)
Liver function tests
(hepatic function determinations, including bilirubin, alkaline phosphatase, AST [SGOT], and ALT [SGPT], may be required prior to and every 3 days during therapy since elevated hepatic function test results have been reported)

## Side/Adverse Effects

Note: Rapid intravenous infusion may result in a precipitous drop in blood pressure. The risk of hypotension is decreased if pentamidine is administered by slow intravenous infusion, over at least 60 minutes, and preferably over 2 hours.

Pentamidine can produce prolonged, severe hypoglycemia lasting from 1 day to several weeks. This hypoglycemia has been associated with a direct cytolytic effect on pancreatic beta islet cells, leading to insulin release. It usually occurs after 5 to 7 days of therapy; however, it may not occur until after pentamidine has been discontinued. One study found the risk of hypoglycemia to be increased with higher doses, longer duration of therapy, and retreatment within 3 months.

Hyperglycemia and diabetes mellitus may occur up to several months after pentamidine therapy has been discontinued.

The following side/adverse effects have been selected on the basis of their potential clinical significance (possible signs and symptoms in parentheses where appropriate)—not necessarily inclusive:

**Those indicating need for medical attention**
Incidence more frequent
*Diabetes mellitus or hyperglycemia* (drowsiness; flushed, dry skin; fruit-like breath odor; increased thirst; increased urination; loss of appetite); *elevated liver function tests; hypoglycemia* (anxiety; chills; cold sweats; cool, pale skin; headache; increased hunger; nausea; nervousness; shakiness); *hypotension* (blurred vision; confusion; dizziness; fainting; lightheadedness; unusual tiredness or weakness); *leukopenia or neutropenia* (sore throat and fever); *nephrotoxicity* (decreased frequency of urination; loss of appetite; weakness); *thrombocytopenia* (unusual bleeding or bruising)

Incidence less frequent
*Anemia* (unusual tiredness or weakness); *cardiac arrhythmias* (rapid or irregular pulse; ECG abnormalities; torsades de pointes)—primarily ventricular tachycardia; *hypersensitivity* (skin rash, redness, or itching; fever); *pancreatitis* (pain in upper abdomen; nausea and vomiting); *phlebitis* (pain at site of injection)—with intravenous injection; *sterile abscess* (pain, redness, and hardness at site of injection)—with intramuscular injection

**Those indicating need for medical attention only if they continue or are bothersome**
Incidence more frequent
*Gastrointestinal disturbances* (nausea and vomiting; loss of appetite; diarrhea)

**Those not indicating need for medical attention**
Incidence less frequent
*Unpleasant metallic taste*

Those indicating possible hyperglycemia or hypoglycemia and the need for medical attention if they occur after medication is discontinued
Signs of hyperglycemia
*Drowsiness; flushed, dry skin; fruit-like breath odor; increased thirst; increased urination; loss of appetite*
Signs of hypoglycemia
*Anxiety; chills and cold sweats; cool, pale skin; headache; increased hunger; nausea; nervousness; shakiness*

## Patient Consultation

As an aid to patient consultation, refer to *Advice for the Patient, Pentamidine (Systemic)*.

In providing consultation, consider emphasizing the following selected information (» = major clinical significance):

**Before using this medication**
» Conditions affecting use, especially:
Allergy to pentamidine
Pregnancy—Pentamidine crosses the placenta in animals; studies have found it to be mildly embryotoxic in rabbits
Use in children—There are limited data available on the use of pentamidine in children; however, the dose used in children is the same as that used in adults and the side effects seen appear to be similar to those seen in adults
Other medications, especially bone marrow depressants, didanosine, foscarnet, other nephrotoxic medications, or radiation therapy
Other medical problems, especially a history of bleeding disorders, bone marrow depression, cardiac disease, dehydration, diabetes mellitus, hypoglycemia, hypotension, or renal function impairment

**Proper use of this medication**
» Importance of receiving medication for full course of therapy and on regular schedule
» Proper dosing

**Precautions while using this medication**
» Severe hypotension may occur; patient should be lying down during administration; physician may need to monitor blood pressure during administration and several times thereafter until blood pressure stabilizes

*To reduce the risk of bleeding during periods of low blood counts:*
» Checking with physician immediately if unusual bleeding or bruising occurs
Using caution in use of regular toothbrushes, dental floss, and toothpicks; physician, dentist, or nurse may suggest alternative methods for cleaning teeth and gums; checking with physician before having dental work done
Avoiding use of safety razor; using electric shaver instead; using caution in use of fingernail or toenail cutters

*For visceral leishmaniasis or African trypanosomiasis*
*Measures for sandfly and tsetse fly control:*
Sleeping under fine-mesh netting
Wearing long-sleeved shirts or blouses and long trousers; wearing clothing of moderately heavy material to protect from tsetse fly bites
Applying insect repellant to uncovered areas of skin

**Side/adverse effects**
Unpleasant metallic taste may occur, although medically insignificant
Signs of potential side effects, especially diabetes mellitus, hyperglycemia, hypoglycemia, hypotension, leukopenia, neutropenia, nephrotoxicity, thrombocytopenia, anemia, cardiac arrhythmias, hypersensitivity, pancreatitis, phlebitis, and sterile abscess

## General Dosing Information

Slow intravenous infusion, over 1 to 2 hours, is the preferred route of administration. Intramuscular administration can cause a sterile abscess at the site of injection. If pentamidine must be given intramuscularly, it should be reserved for patients with adequate muscle mass, and the daily dose of pentamidine should be administered by deep injection only.

Pentamidine may cause sudden, severe hypotension, even after a single dose. Therefore, patients should be lying down and their blood pressure should be closely monitored during administration and several times thereafter until blood pressure is stable.

No adjustment of the pentamidine dose is needed in patients with renal impairment. Because less than 3% of a dose of pentamidine is excreted through the kidneys, no correlation has been seen between renal function and plasma drug clearance. Also, the renal excretion increased only marginally with repeated pentamidine dosing.

## Parenteral Dosage Forms

Note: Bracketed uses in the *Dosage Forms* section refer to categories of use and/or indications that are not included in U.S. product labeling.

### STERILE PENTAMIDINE ISETHIONATE

**Usual adult and adolescent dose**
Pneumonia, *Pneumocystis carinii*—
   Intravenous infusion, 4 mg per kg of body weight, administered over one to two hours, once a day for fourteen to twenty-one days, depending on clinical response.
   Note: In preliminary studies, a reduced intravenous dose of 3 mg per kg of body weight once a day was used successfully in the treatment of mild to moderate *P. carinii* pneumonia.
[Leishmaniasis, visceral][1]—
   Intravenous infusion, 2 to 4 mg per kg of body weight, administered over one to two hours, once a day for up to fifteen days. Administration may be repeated in one to two weeks if required.
[Leishmaniasis, cutaneous][1]—
   Intravenous infusion, 2 to 4 mg per kg of body weight, administered over one to two hours, once or twice a week until the lesions heal.
[Trypanosomiasis, African (without CNS involvement)][1]—
   Treatment: Intravenous infusion, 4 mg per kg of body weight, administered over one to two hours, once a day for ten days.
Note: The dose of pentamidine isethionate is based on the total weight of the salt, whereas the dose of pentamidine mesylate (methanesulfonate) is based on the weight of pentamidine base. Since both preparations are available in some countries, clinicians should calculate the dose for pentamidine preparations on the basis that 2.4 mg of pentamidine mesylate is equivalent to 4 mg of pentamidine isethionate.

**Usual adult prescribing limits**
Trypanosomiasis, African—
   3 to 5 mg per kg of body weight a day.

**Usual pediatric dose**
See *Usual adult and adolescent dose*.

**Size(s) usually available**
U.S.—
   300 mg (Rx) [*Pentam 300;* GENERIC].
Canada—
   200 mg (Rx) [*Pentacarinat*].
   300 mg (Rx) [*Pentacarinat;* GENERIC].

**Packaging and storage**
Prior to reconstitution, store between 2 and 8 °C (36 and 46 °F), unless otherwise specified by manufacturer. Protect dry powder and reconstituted solution from light.

**Preparation of dosage form**
To prepare initial dilution for intramuscular use, add 3 mL of sterile water for injection to each 300-mg vial.
To prepare initial dilution for intermittent intravenous use, add 2.1 mL of sterile water for injection to each 200-mg vial, or add 3 to 5 mL of sterile water for injection or 5% dextrose injection to each 300-mg vial. The solution may be further diluted in 50 to 250 mL of 5% dextrose injection and administered over a period of *at least 1 hour, and preferably up to 2 hours*.

**Stability**
After reconstitution in 5% dextrose injection, pentamidine solutions with concentrations of 1 and 2.5 mg per mL retain their potency for up to 24 hours at room temperature. Discard any unused portion. Reconstituted pentamidine should not be mixed with any solutions other than 5% dextrose.

---

[1]Not included in Canadian product labeling.

Revised: 05/27/94
Interim revision: 04/24/95

---

**PENTAZOCINE**—See *Opioid (Narcotic) Analgesics (Systemic)*

---

**PENTOBARBITAL**—See *Barbiturates (Systemic)*

---

# PENTOSAN Systemic

VA CLASSIFICATION (Primary): GU900
Commonly used brand name(s): *Elmiron*.
Note: For a listing of dosage forms and brand names by country availability, see *Dosage Forms* section(s).

## Category
Anti-inflammatory, local (interstitial cystitis).

## Indications

**Accepted**
Cystitis, interstitial (treatment)—Pentosan is indicated for the relief of bladder pain or discomfort associated with interstitial cystitis. It may improve symptoms such as urinary urgency and urinary frequency, including nocturia. Symptoms of interstitial cystitis exacerbate and remit, with days up to years between episodes.
   In clinical trials, approximately one fourth to one third of patients receiving pentosan reported an improvement in bladder pain and discomfort after 3 months of therapy.

## Pharmacology/Pharmacokinetics

**Physicochemical characteristics**
Molecular weight—4000 to 6000.

**Mechanism of action/Effect**
The exact mechanism of action is not known, but pentosan has been found to adhere to the bladder wall mucosal membrane, which may act as a buffer to prevent irritating solutes from reaching the cells.

**Other actions/effects**
Pentosan has anticoagulant (1/15 the activity of heparin) and fibrinolytic effects.

**Absorption**
Approximately 3% of different administered doses.

**Distribution**
Pentosan is distributed to the uroepithelium of the genitourinary tract, with lesser amounts found in the bone marrow, liver, lung, periosteum, skin, and spleen.

**Biotransformation**
Pentosan undergoes depolymerization in the kidney; 68% of the drug undergoes desulfation in the liver and the spleen 1 hour after intravenous administration; both depolymerization and desulfation can be saturated with continued dosing.

**Half-life**
Elimination—
   Intravenous: 24 hours after a 40-mg dose.
   Oral: 4.8 hours for the unchanged drug.

**Elimination**
Renal, 3.5% with a single dose; 11% with multiple doses, with 3% of that as the unchanged drug.

## Precautions to Consider

**Carcinogenicity**
Studies to determine the carcinogenic potential of pentosan have not been done in humans or animals.

**Mutagenicity**
Pentosan was not clastogenic or mutagenic when tested in the mouse micronucleus test or the Ames test.

**Pregnancy/Reproduction**
Fertility—Reproductive studies in mice and rats using intravenous daily doses of 15 mg per kg of body weight (mg/kg) and in rabbits using 7.5 mg/kg (0.42 and 0.14 times the daily oral human doses of pentosan based on body surface area, respectively) did not reveal evidence of impaired fertility.

Pregnancy—Studies have not been done in humans.
Reproductive studies in mice and rats using intravenous daily doses of 15 mg/kg and in rabbits using 7.5 mg/kg (0.42 and 0.14 times the daily oral human doses of pentosan based on body surface area, respectively)

did not reveal any harm to the fetus. Direct *in vitro* bathing of cultured mouse embryos with pentosan at a concentration of 1 mg per mL may cause reversible limb bud abnormalities.

FDA Pregnancy Category B.

**Breast-feeding**
It is not known whether pentosan is distributed into breast milk.

**Pediatrics**
No information is available on the relationship of age to the effects of pentosan in pediatric patients. Safety and efficacy have not been established.

**Geriatrics**
Studies performed in patients with interstitial cystitis have not demonstrated geriatrics-specific problems that would limit the usefulness of pentosan in the elderly.

**Drug interactions and/or related problems**
The following drug interactions and/or related problems have been selected on the basis of their potential clinical significance (possible mechanism in parentheses where appropriate)— not necessarily inclusive (» = major clinical significance):

Note: Combinations containing any of the following medications, depending on the amount present, may also interact with this medication.

» Medications/therapies that increase the risk of hemorrhage, such as:
  Alteplase, recombinant or
  Anticoagulants, coumarin-derivative or
  Aspirin, high dose or
  Heparin or
  Streptokinase
    (concurrent use with pentosan may increase the risk of hemorrhage; patients should be monitored for signs of hemorrhage; if hemorrhage occurs, pentosan should be discontinued)

**Laboratory value alterations**
The following have been selected on the basis of their potential clinical significance (possible effect in parentheses where appropriate)—not necessarily inclusive (» = major clinical significance):

With physiology/laboratory test values
  Alanine aminotransferase (ALT [SGPT]), serum and
  Alkaline phosphatase, serum and
  Aspartate aminotransferase (AST [SGOT]), serum and
  Gamma-glutamyl transpeptidase, serum and
  Lactate dehydrogenase, serum
    (increases in values of up to 2.5 times the normal values have occurred in 1.2% of patients taking pentosan; increases usually appeared 3 to 12 months after initiation of therapy, and were not associated with jaundice or other clinical signs or symptoms; these increases were transient, remained unchanged, or, rarely, progressed with continued use)
  Partial thromboplastin time (PTT) and
  Prothrombin time (PT)
    (increases have been reported in fewer than 1% of patients taking pentosan; however, PTT and PT were unaffected in one study using up to 1200 mg of pentosan a day for 8 days)

**Medical considerations/Contraindications**
The medical considerations/contraindications included have been selected on the basis of their potential clinical significance (reasons given in parentheses where appropriate)—not necessarily inclusive (» = major clinical significance).

*Risk-benefit should be considered when the following medical problems exist:*

» Any condition in which risk of hemorrhage is present, such as:
  Aneurysms or
  Diverticula or
  Gastrointestinal ulceration or
  Hemophilia or
  Polyps or
  Thrombocytopenia or thrombocytopenia, heparin-induced, history of
    (since pentosan has weak anticoagulant activity, an additive effect may occur; patients with these conditions should be evaluated carefully before beginning pentosan therapy)
  Hepatic insufficiency or
  Spleen disorders
    (since pentosan is desulfated by the liver and the spleen, bioavailability of the parent or active metabolites may be increased; pentosan should be used cautiously in patients with these conditions)
  Sensitivity to pentosan, structurally related compounds, or excipients

**Patient monitoring**
The following may be especially important in patient monitoring (other tests may be warranted in some patients, depending on condition; » = major clinical significance):
  Alanine aminotransferase (ALT [SGPT]), serum and
  Aspartate aminotransferase (AST [SGOT]), serum
    (determinations recommended every 6 months during treatment)

## Side/Adverse Effects

The following side/adverse effects have been selected on the basis of their potential clinical significance (possible signs and symptoms in parentheses where appropriate)—not necessarily inclusive:

**Those indicating need for medical attention**
Incidence rare—incidence ≤ 1%
  *Allergic reaction* (skin rash or hives); *amblyopia* (vision impairment); *anemia* (unusual tiredness and weakness); *dyspnea* (difficulty in breathing); *ecchymosis* (unusual bleeding or bruising); *leukopenia* (chills; fever; sore throat); *thrombocytopenia* (unusual bleeding or bruising)

**Those indicating need for medical attention only if they continue or are bothersome**
Incidence less frequent
  *Abdominal pain*—incidence 2%; *alopecia* (hair loss)—incidence 4%; *diarrhea*—incidence 4%; *dizziness*—incidence 1%; *dyspepsia* (stomach upset)—incidence 2%; *headache*—incidence 3%; *nausea*—incidence 4%; *skin rash*—incidence 3%

  Note: Alopecia may begin within the first 4 weeks of treatment; 97% of reported cases were limited to a single area on the scalp.

Incidence rare—incidence ≤ 1%
  *Anorexia* (loss of appetite); *conjunctivitis* (irritated or red eyes); *constipation; epistaxis* (nosebleed); *esophagitis* (difficulty in swallowing); *flatulence* (stomach gas); *gastritis* (stomach upset); *gum hemorrhage* (bleeding gums); *heartburn; mouth ulcer* (sores in mouth); *pharyngitis* (dryness of throat; pain upon swallowing); *photosensitivity* (increased sensitivity of skin to sunlight); *pruritus* (itching); *rhinitis* (runny nose); *tinnitus* (ringing in the ears); *urticaria* (skin rash); *vomiting*

## Overdose

For information on the management of overdose or unintentional ingestion, **contact a Poison Control Center** (see *Poison Control Center Listing*).

**Treatment of overdose**
To decrease absorption—Gastric lavage.

Supportive care—Patients in whom intentional overdose is confirmed or suspected should be referred for psychiatric consultation.

## Patient Consultation

As an aid to patient consultation, refer to *Advice for the Patient, Pentosan (Systemic)*.

In providing consultation, consider emphasizing the following selected information (» = major clinical significance):

**Before using this medication**
» Conditions affecting use, especially:
    Sensitivity to pentosan, structurally related compounds, or excipients
    Other medications, especially alteplase, recombinant; anticoagulants, coumarin-derivative; aspirin, high dose; heparin; or streptokinase
    Other medical problems, especially aneurysms, diverticula, gastrointestinal ulceration, hemophilia, polyps, or thrombocytopenia

**Proper use of this medication**
  Taking on empty stomach with a full glass (8 ounces) of water 1 hour before or 2 hours after meals
  May require up to 3 to 6 months of therapy to feel effects
» Proper dosing
  Missed dose: Taking as soon as possible; not taking if almost time for next dose; not doubling doses
» Proper storage

**Precautions while using this medication**
» Possibility of increased bleeding time
  Following any dietary instructions

**Side/adverse effects**
  Signs of potential side effects, especially allergic reaction, amblyopia, anemia, dyspnea, ecchymosis, leukopenia, thrombocytopenia, and alopecia

### General Dosing Information
The clinical value and risks of treatment for longer than 6 months are not known.

### Diet/Nutrition
Pentosan should be taken with a full glass (8 ounces) of water at least 1 hour before or 2 hours after meals.

Some patients with interstitial cystitis may benefit by avoiding acidic foods and beverages such as alcohol, caffeinated and citrus beverages, chocolate, spices, and tomatoes. However, this recommendation is not universal; patients should avoid foods or beverages that aggravate their condition.

## Oral Dosage Form

### PENTOSAN POLYSULFATE SODIUM Capsules

**Usual adult dose**
Cystitis, interstitial (treatment)—
   Oral, 100 mg three times a day. If there is no improvement and no side/adverse effects have been reported after three months, pentosan therapy may be continued for another three months.

**Usual pediatric dose**
Safety and efficacy have not been established.

**Strength(s) usually available**
U.S.—
   100 mg (Rx) [*Elmiron*].
Canada—
   100 mg (Rx) [*Elmiron*].

**Packaging and storage**
Store below 40 °C (104 °F), preferably between 15 and 30 °C (59 and 86 °F), unless otherwise specified by the manufacturer.

**Auxiliary labeling**
• Take on empty stomach.

Developed: 05/20/98

---

# PENTOSTATIN  Systemic

VA CLASSIFICATION (Primary): AN900
Commonly used brand name(s): *Nipent*.
Other commonly used names are 2'-deoxycoformycin and 2'DCF.
Note: For a listing of dosage forms and brand names by country availability, see *Dosage Forms* section(s).

## Category
Antineoplastic.

## Indications
Note: Bracketed information in the *Indications* section refers to uses that are not included in U.S. product labeling.

**Accepted**
Leukemia, hairy cell (treatment)—Pentostatin is indicated as a single agent for treatment of adult patients with hairy cell leukemia who have not responded to treatment with alpha interferons. [There is also some evidence that pentostatin is useful for treatment of hairy cell leukemia not refractory to interferon treatment.]

## Pharmacology/Pharmacokinetics

**Physicochemical characteristics**
Source—Isolated from fermentation cultures of *Streptomyces antibioticus*.
Chemical group—Pentostatin is a purine (deoxyinosine) analog.
Molecular weight—268.27.

**Mechanism of action/Effect**
Pentostatin is an antimetabolite. Its exact mechanism of action in hairy cell leukemia is unknown. Pentostatin is a potent transition state inhibitor of adenosine deaminase (ADA), the greatest activity of which is found in cells of the lymphoid system. T-cells have higher ADA activity than B-cells, and T-cell malignancies have higher activity than B-cell malignancies. The cytotoxicity that results from prevention of catabolism of adenosine or deoxyadenosine is thought to be due to elevated intracellular levels of dATP, which can block DNA synthesis through inhibition of ribonucleotide reductase. Inhibition of RNA synthesis may also contribute to the cytotoxic effect. Although pentostatin arrests cells in the $G_1$ or S phase of cell division, it is also reported to have cell cycle–phase nonspecific actions (including increased DNA strand breaks).

**Other actions/effects**
Pentostatin appears to have immunosuppressant activity; significant reductions in T- and B-cells occur during treatment and T4 reductions persist, sometimes for months or years, after treatment.

**Distribution**
Pentostatin crosses the blood-brain barrier; cerebrospinal fluid concentrations achieved are 10 to 12.5% of serum concentrations within 24 hours after a single dose.

**Protein binding**
Low (4%).

**Biotransformation**
Hepatic; however, only small amounts are metabolized.

**Half-life**
Distribution—
   11 minutes (following a single dose of 4 mg per square meter of body surface infused over 5 minutes). A range of 17 to 85 minutes has also been reported.
Terminal—
   Normal: 5.7 hours (following a single dose of 4 mg per square meter of body surface infused over 5 minutes). A range of 2.6 to 15 hours has been reported.
   Renal function impairment (creatinine clearance less than 50 mL per minute): 18 hours.

**Onset of action**
Time to achieve response—Median 4.7 months (range 2.9 to 24.1 months).

**Duration of action**
Pharmacologic—Inhibition of ADA: More than 1 week after a single dose.

**Elimination**
Renal, 90%, as unchanged drug and metabolites as measured by adenosine deaminase inhibitory activity. In two small studies, 32 to 73% was recovered unchanged.

## Precautions to Consider

**Carcinogenicity**
Secondary malignancies are potential delayed effects of many antineoplastic agents, although it is not clear whether the effect is related to their mutagenic or immunosuppressive action. The effect of dose and duration of therapy is also unknown, although risk seems to increase with long-term use. Although information is limited, available data seem to indicate that the carcinogenic risk is greatest with the alkylating agents. Antimetabolites have been shown to be carcinogenic in animals and may be associated with an increased risk of development of secondary carcinomas in humans, although the risk appears to be less than with alkylating agents.
Lymphoid neoplasms have been reported in humans.
Studies with pentostatin in animals have not been done.

**Mutagenicity**
Pentostatin was not found to be mutagenic in several strains of *Salmonella typhimurium*, including TA-98, TA-1535, TA-1537, and TA-1538. When tested with strain TA-100, a repeatable statistically significant response trend was observed with and without metabolic activation. The response was 2.1- to 2.2-fold higher than the background at 10 mg/plate, the maximum possible drug concentration. Formulated pentostatin was clastogenic in the *in vivo* mouse bone marrow micronucleus assay at 20, 120, and 240 mg per kg of body weight (mg/kg). Pentostatin was nonmutagenic to V79 Chinese hamster lung cells at the hypoxanthine-guanine-phosphororibosyltransferase (HGPRT) locus exposed for 3 hours to concentrations of 1 to 3 mg per mL, with or without metabolic activation. Pentostatin did not significantly increase chromosomal aberrations in V79 Chinese hamster lung cells exposed for 3 hours to 1 to 3 mg per mL in the presence or absence of metabolic activation.

**Pregnancy/Reproduction**
Fertility—Gonadal suppression, resulting in amenorrhea or azoospermia, may occur in patients taking antineoplastic therapy, especially with the alkylating agents. In general, these effects appear to be related to dose

and length of therapy and may be irreversible. Prediction of the degree of testicular or ovarian function impairment is complicated by the common use of combinations of several antineoplastics, which makes it difficult to assess the effects of individual agents. Fertility studies with pentostatin have not been done in animals; however, mild seminiferous tubular degeneration was observed in a 5-day intravenous toxicity study at doses of 1 and 4 mg/kg in dogs.

Pregnancy—Adequate and well-controlled studies in women have not been done.

First trimester: It is usually recommended that use of antineoplastics, especially combination chemotherapy, be avoided whenever possible, especially during the first trimester. Although information is limited because of the relatively few instances of antineoplastic administration during pregnancy, the mutagenic, teratogenic, and carcinogenic potential of these medications must be considered.

Other hazards to the fetus include adverse reactions seen in adults.

In general, use of contraception is recommended during cytotoxic drug therapy.

Studies in rats at intravenous doses of 0, 0.01, 0.1, or 0.75 mg/kg (0, 0.06, 0.6, or 4.5 mg per square meter of body surface, respectively) per day on days 6 through 15 of gestation found drug-related maternal toxicity at doses of 0.1 and 0.75 mg/kg per day (0.6 and 4.5 mg per square meter of body surface, respectively). Teratogenic effects (increased incidence of various skeletal malformations) were observed at doses of 0.75 mg/kg (4.5 mg per square meter of body surface per day). In a dose range–finding study in rats at intravenous doses of 0, 0.05, 0.1, 0.5, 0.75, or 1 mg/kg (0, 0.3, 0.6, 3, 4.5, or 6 mg per square meter of body surface, respectively, per day) on days 6 through 15 of gestation, fetal malformations were observed, including an omphalocele at 0.05 mg/kg (0.3 mg per square meter of body surface), gastroschisis at 0.75 mg/kg and 1 mg/kg (4.5 and 6 mg per square meter of body surface, respectively), and a flexure defect of the hindlimbs at 0.75 mg/kg (4.5 mg per square meter of body surface). Pentostatin was also teratogenic in mice in single intraperitoneal doses of 2 mg/kg (6 mg per square meter of body surface) on day 7 of gestation. Pentostatin was not teratogenic in rabbits at intravenous doses of 0, 0.005, 0.01, or 0.02 mg/kg per day (0, 0.015, 0.03, or 0.06 mg per square meter of body surface per day, respectively); however, maternal toxicity, abortions, early deliveries, and deaths occurred in all drug-treated groups.

FDA Pregnancy Category D.

**Breast-feeding**
Although very little information is available regarding distribution of antineoplastic agents into breast milk, breast-feeding is not recommended during chemotherapy because of the potential risks to the infant (adverse effects, mutagenicity, carcinogenicity). It is not known whether pentostatin is distributed into breast milk.

**Pediatrics**
No information is available on the relationship of age to the effects of pentostatin in pediatric patients. Safety and efficacy have not been established.

**Geriatrics**
Although appropriate studies on the relationship of age to the effects of pentostatin have not been performed in the geriatric population, clinical trials have included elderly patients and geriatrics-specific problems that would limit the usefulness of this medication in the elderly are not expected. However, elderly patients are more likely to have age-related renal function impairment, which may require caution in patients receiving pentostatin.

**Dental**
The bone marrow depressant effects of pentostatin may result in an increased incidence of microbial infection, delayed healing, and gingival bleeding. Dental work, whenever possible should be completed prior to initiation of therapy or deferred until blood counts have returned to normal. Patients should be instructed in proper oral hygiene during treatment, including caution in use of regular toothbrushes, dental floss, and toothpicks.

Pentostatin also sometimes causes stomatitis that is associated with considerable discomfort.

**Drug interactions and/or related problems**
The following drug interactions and/or related problems have been selected on the basis of their potential clinical significance (possible mechanism in parentheses where appropriate)—not necessarily inclusive (» = major clinical significance):

Note: Combinations containing any of the following medications, depending on the amount present, may also interact with this medication.

Allopurinol or
Colchicine or
» Probenecid or
» Sulfinpyrazone
   (pentostatin may raise the concentration of blood uric acid; dosage adjustment of antigout agents may be necessary to control hyperuricemia and gout; allopurinol may be preferred to prevent or reverse pentostatin-induced hyperuricemia because of risk of uric acid nephropathy with uricosuric antigout agents)
   (one case has been reported in which a patient receiving both allopurinol and pentostatin developed a fatal hypersensitivity vasculitis, although a definite connection with the combination has not been established)

Blood dyscrasia–causing medications (see *Appendix II*)
   (leukopenic and/or thrombocytopenic effects of pentostatin may be increased with concurrent or recent therapy if these medications cause the same effects; dosage adjustment of pentostatin, if necessary, should be based on blood counts)

» Bone marrow depressants, other (see *Appendix II*) or
Radiation therapy
   (additive bone marrow depression may occur; dosage reduction may be required when two or more bone marrow depressants, including radiation, are used concurrently or consecutively)

Fludarabine
   (concurrent use with pentostatin is not recommended because of a possible increased risk of fatal pulmonary toxicity)

Vaccines, killed virus
   (because normal defense mechanisms may be suppressed by pentostatin therapy, the patient's antibody response to the vaccine may be decreased. The interval between discontinuation of medications that cause immunosuppression and restoration of the patient's ability to respond to the vaccine depends on the intensity and type of immunosuppression-causing medication used, the underlying disease, and other factors; estimates vary from 3 months to 1 year)

» Vaccines, live virus
   (because normal defense mechanisms may be suppressed by pentostatin therapy, concurrent use with a live virus vaccine may potentiate the replication of the vaccine virus, may increase the side/adverse effects of the vaccine virus, and/or may decrease the patient's antibody response to the vaccine; immunization of these patients should be undertaken only with extreme caution after careful review of the patient's hematologic status and only with the knowledge and consent of the physician managing the pentostatin therapy. The interval between discontinuation of medications that cause immunosuppression and restoration of the patient's ability to respond to the vaccine depends on the intensity and type of immunosuppression-causing medication used, the underlying disease, and other factors; estimates vary from 3 months to 1 year. Patients with leukemia in remission should not receive live virus vaccine until at least 3 months after their last chemotherapy. In addition, immunization with oral poliovirus vaccine should be postponed in persons in close contact with the patient, especially family members)

Vidarabine
   (biochemical studies have shown an enhancement of vidarabine's effects by pentostatin, which could result in an increase in adverse effects of each)

**Laboratory value alterations**
The following have been selected on the basis of their potential clinical significance (possible effect in parentheses where appropriate)—not necessarily inclusive (» = major clinical significance):

With physiology/laboratory test values
   Alanine aminotransferase (ALT [SGPT]) and
   Alkaline phosphatase and
   Aspartate aminotransferase (AST [SGOT]) and
   Lactate dehydrogenase (LDH)
      (serum values are transiently increased in most patients)
   Creatinine
      (dose-related increases in serum concentrations may occur, indicating renal toxicity, but increases are usually minor and transient at recommended doses in patients with normal baseline renal function)
   Uric acid concentrations in blood and urine
      (may be increased)

**Medical considerations/Contraindications**
The medical considerations/contraindications included have been selected on the basis of their potential clinical significance (reasons given in parentheses where appropriate)—not necessarily inclusive (» = major clinical significance).

***Risk-benefit should be considered when the following medical problems exist:***
» Bone marrow depression
  Cardiovascular function impairment, including coronary artery disease, congestive heart failure, hypertension
    (cardiac effects of pentostatin may be more likely)
» Chickenpox, existing or recent (including recent exposure) or
» Herpes zoster
    (risk of severe generalized disease)
  Gout, history of or
  Urate renal stones, history of
    (risk of hyperuricemia)
» Infection
    (pentostatin should be withheld until active infection is controlled)
» Renal function impairment
    (reduced elimination; in patients with increased serum creatinine concentrations, pentostatin should be withheld and creatinine clearance determined)
» Sensitivity to pentostatin
» Caution should be used also in patients who have had previous cytotoxic drug therapy or radiation therapy.

**Patient monitoring**
The following may be especially important in patient monitoring (other tests may be warranted in some patients, depending on condition; » = major clinical significance):
» Creatinine clearance and/or
  Creatinine concentrations, serum
    (creatinine clearance and/or serum creatinine concentration determinations are recommended prior to initiation of therapy; serum creatinine concentration determinations are recommended before each dose and at other appropriate intervals during therapy)
» Hematocrit or hemoglobin and
» Leukocyte count, total and, if appropriate, differential and
» Platelet count
    (determinations recommended prior to initiation of therapy and at periodic intervals during therapy, especially during early courses; frequency varies according to clinical state, agent, dose, and other agents being used concurrently)
  Uric acid concentrations, serum
    (determinations recommended prior to initiation of therapy and at periodic intervals during therapy; frequency varies according to clinical state, agent, dose, and other agents being used concurrently)

## Side/Adverse Effects
Note: In patients with progressive hairy cell leukemia, neutropenia may worsen during the initial courses of pentostatin therapy.
  Most side/adverse effects decrease in severity with continued treatment.

The following side/adverse effects have been selected on the basis of their potential clinical significance (possible signs and symptoms in parentheses where appropriate)—not necessarily inclusive:

**Those indicating need for medical attention**
Incidence more frequent
  *Allergic reaction* (sudden skin rash or itching); *anemia*—usually asymptomatic; *central nervous system (CNS) toxicity* (unusual tiredness; anxiety or nervousness; confusion; mental depression; numbness or tingling of hands or feet; sleepiness; trouble in sleeping); *hepatic function impairment*—usually asymptomatic; *leukopenia or infection* (fever or chills; cough or hoarseness; lower back or side pain; painful or difficult urination); *pain; thrombocytopenia* (unusual bleeding or bruising; black, tarry stools; blood in urine or stools; pinpoint red spots on skin)—usually asymptomatic
  Note: *Unusual tiredness* has been reported to increase with repeated weekly dosing and has been reduced by limiting pentostatin to three weekly doses or giving it every other week.
    With high doses, *CNS toxicity* may lead to seizures, coma, and death.
    Although hepatic enzyme elevations are usually transient, severe *hepatotoxicity* requiring withdrawal of pentostatin has been reported.
    Severe *neutropenia* has occurred during early courses of treatment with pentostatin.
    *Infections* may be bacterial, viral, or fungal, may occur even in the absence of leukopenia, and may be life-threatening.

Incidence less frequent—less than 10%
  *Cardiac effects, including angina and myocardial infarction, congestive heart failure, and acute arrhythmias* (chest pain; swelling of feet or lower legs); *changes in vision; keratoconjunctivitis* (sore, red eyes); *pulmonary toxicity, including bronchitis, dyspnea, epistaxis, lung edema, pneumonia, pharyngitis, rhinitis, or sinusitis* (cough; nosebleed; shortness of breath); *renal toxicity*—asymptomatic; seen as increases in serum creatinine; *stomatitis* (sores in mouth or on lips); *stomach pain; thrombophlebitis* (cramps in lower legs)
  Note: *Cardiac effects* tend to occur in patients with preexisting cardiovascular conditions. Fatalities have occurred.
    *Keratoconjunctivitis* is transient but may recur with subsequent doses.

**Those indicating need for medical attention only if they continue or are bothersome**
Incidence more frequent
  *Diarrhea; headache; loss of appetite; muscle pain; nausea and vomiting; skin rash*
  Note: Maculopapular *skin rashes* are occasionally severe and may worsen with continued treatment, necessitating withdrawal of pentostatin. *Herpes simplex* and *herpes zoster* infections may also occur. Inflammation of multiple actinic (solar) keratoses has been reported.
Incidence less frequent—less than 10%
  *Back pain; constipation; dry skin; flatulence* (bloating or gas); *flu-like syndrome* (general feeling of discomfort or illness); *itching; joint pain; weakness; weight loss*

## Overdose
For more information on the management of overdose or unintentional ingestion, **contact a Poison Control Center** (see *Poison Control Center Listing*).

**Treatment of overdose**
Treatment consists of withdrawal of pentostatin and supportive therapy.

## Patient Consultation
As an aid to patient consultation, refer to *Advice for the Patient, Pentostatin (Systemic)*.
In providing consultation, consider emphasizing the following selected information (» = major clinical significance):

**Before using this medication**
» Conditions affecting use, especially:
    Sensitivity to pentostatin
    Pregnancy—Use not recommended because of mutagenic, teratogenic, and carcinogenic potential; advisability of using contraception; telling physician immediately if pregnancy is suspected
    Breast-feeding—Not recommended because of risk of serious side effects
    Other medications, especially probenecid, sulfinpyrazone, other bone marrow depressants, or other cytotoxic drug or radiation therapy
    Other medical problems, especially chickenpox, herpes zoster, renal function impairment, or infection

**Proper use of this medication**
  Frequency of nausea and vomiting; importance of continuing medication despite stomach upset
» Proper dosing

**Precautions while using this medication**
» Importance of close monitoring by the physician
» Avoiding immunizations unless approved by physician; other persons in patient's household should avoid immunizations with oral poliovirus vaccine; avoiding other persons who have taken oral poliovirus vaccine or wearing a protective mask that covers nose and mouth
*Caution if bone marrow depression occurs*
» Avoiding exposure to persons with infections, especially during periods of low blood counts; checking with physician immediately if fever or chills, cough or hoarseness, lower back or side pain, or painful or difficult urination occurs
» Checking with physician immediately if unusual bleeding or bruising; black, tarry stools; blood in urine or stools; or pinpoint red spots on skin occur
  Caution in use of regular toothbrush, dental floss, or toothpick; physician, dentist, or nurse may suggest alternatives; checking with physician before having dental work done
  Not touching eyes or inside of nose unless hands washed immediately before

Using caution to avoid accidental cuts with use of sharp objects such as safety razor or fingernail or toenail cutters

Avoiding contact sports or other situations where bruising or injury could occur

**Side/adverse effects**

May cause adverse effects such as blood problems; importance of discussing possible effects with physician

Signs of potential side effects, especially allergic reaction, CNS toxicity, leukopenia or infection, pain, thrombocytopenia, cardiac effects, changes in vision, keratoconjunctivitis, pulmonary toxicity, stomatitis, stomach pain, and thrombophlebitis

Asymptomatic side effects, including anemia, hepatic function impairment, thrombocytopenia, and renal function impairment

Physician or nurse can help in dealing with side effects

## General Dosing Information

Patients receiving pentostatin should be under supervision of a physician experienced in cancer chemotherapy.

It is recommended that antiemetics be prescribed for 48 to 74 hours after pentostatin administration.

If CNS toxicity occurs, it is recommended that pentostatin be withheld or discontinued.

If severe skin rash occurs, it is recommended that pentostatin be withheld.

If elevated serum creatinine occurs, it is recommended that pentostatin be withheld and creatinine clearance determined. No recommendations are available for dosage adjustment in renal function impairment (creatinine clearance less than 60 mL per minute).

Development of uric acid nephropathy in patients with leukemia or lymphoma may be prevented by adequate oral hydration and, in some cases, administration of allopurinol. Alkalinization of urine may be necessary if serum uric acid concentrations are elevated.

Special precautions are recommended in patients who develop thrombocytopenia as a result of administration of pentostatin. These may include extreme care in performing invasive procedures; regular inspection of intravenous sites, skin (including perirectal area), and mucous membrane surfaces for signs of bleeding or bruising; limiting frequency of venipuncture and avoiding intramuscular injections; testing urine, emesis, stool, and secretions for occult blood; care in use of regular toothbrushes, dental floss, toothpicks, safety razors, and fingernail and toenail cutters; avoiding constipation; and using caution to prevent falls and other injuries. Such patients should avoid alcohol and aspirin intake because of the risk of gastrointestinal bleeding. Platelet transfusions may be required.

It is recommended that pentostatin be temporarily withheld if the absolute neutrophil count (ANC) falls below 200 per cubic millimeter in patients who had an initial count of greater than 500 per cubic millimeter. Treatment with pentostatin may be resumed when the ANC returns to pretreatment levels.

Patients who develop leukopenia should be observed carefully for signs of infection. Antibiotic support may be required. In neutropenic patients who develop fever, broad-spectrum antibiotic coverage should be initiated empirically, pending bacterial cultures and appropriate diagnostic tests.

If active infection occurs during pentostatin treatment, it is recommended that pentostatin be withheld until the infection is controlled.

**Safety considerations for handling this medication**

There is limited but increasing evidence and concern that personnel involved in preparation and administration of parenteral antineoplastics may be at some risk because of the potential mutagenicity, teratogenicity, and/or carcinogenicity of these agents, although the actual risk is unknown. USP advisory panels recommend cautious handling both in preparation and disposal of antineoplastic agents. Precautions that have been suggested include:

- Use of a biological containment cabinet during reconstitution and dilution of parenteral medications and wearing of disposable surgical gloves and masks.

- Use of proper technique to prevent contamination of the medication, work area, and operator during transfer between containers (including proper training of personnel in this technique).

- Cautious and proper disposal of needles, syringes, vials, ampuls, and unused medication.

A number of medical centers have developed detailed guidelines for handling of antineoplastic agents.

## Parenteral Dosage Forms

### PENTOSTATIN FOR INJECTION

**Usual adult dose**

Hairy cell leukemia—
Intravenous (by rapid injection or diluted in a larger volume and given over twenty to thirty minutes), 4 mg per square meter of body surface area every other week.

Note: Hydration with 500 to 1000 mL of 5% dextrose in 0.45% sodium chloride injection or the equivalent before administration and 500 mL after administration is recommended.

Higher doses are not recommended because of the risk of renal, hepatic, pulmonary, and CNS toxicity.

It is recommended that pentostatin treatment be continued until two doses after a complete response is achieved. If the best response achieved is a partial response, it is recommended that pentostatin be discontinued after twelve months of treatment. If a complete or partial response is not achieved after six months of treatment, it is recommended that pentostatin be discontinued.

**Usual pediatric dose**

Safety and efficacy have not been established.

**Size(s) usually available**

U.S.—
10 mg (Rx) [*Nipent* (mannitol 50 mg; sodium hydroxide or hydrochloric acid)].

Canada—
10 mg (Rx) [*Nipent* (mannitol 50 mg; sodium hydroxide or hydrochloric acid)].

**Packaging and storage**

Store between 2 and 8 °C (36 and 46 °F), unless otherwise specified by manufacturer.

**Preparation of dosage form**

Pentostatin for injection is prepared for intravenous use by aseptically adding 5 mL of sterile water for injection to the 10-mg vial, producing a solution containing 2 mg of pentostatin per mL.

Pentostatin solutions may be given intravenously by rapid injection or further diluted in 25 to 50 mL of 5% dextrose injection or 0.9% sodium chloride injection (producing a solution containing 0.33 mg per mL or 0.18 mg per mL, respectively) for administration by intravenous infusion.

**Stability**

Reconstituted solutions contain no preservative and should be used within 8 hours of reconstitution.

**Note**

The manufacturer recommends that spills and wastes be treated with 5% sodium hypochlorite solution prior to disposal.

## Selected Bibliography

Kane BJ, Kuhn JG, Roush MK. Pentostatin: an adenosine deaminase inhibitor for the treatment of hairy cell leukemia. Ann Pharmacother 1992; 26: 939-47.

Revised: 05/06/93
Interim revision: 06/30/94; 09/30/97

---

# PENTOXIFYLLINE  Systemic

VA CLASSIFICATION (Primary): CV900

Commonly used brand name(s): *Trental*.

Another commonly used name is oxypentifylline.

Note: For a listing of dosage forms and brand names by country availability, see *Dosage Forms* section(s).

## Category

Blood viscosity–reducing agent.

## Indications

Note: Bracketed information in the *Indications* section refers to uses that are not included in U.S. product labeling.

### Accepted

**Vascular disease, peripheral (treatment)**—Pentoxifylline is indicated to provide symptomatic relief of intermittent claudication [and other signs and symptoms, including trophic ulcers] associated with chronic occlusive arterial disorders of the limbs. Although pentoxifylline may improve function as well as provide symptomatic relief, it is not intended as a replacement for more definitive therapy that may be needed, such as surgical bypass procedures or removal of arterial obstructions.

### Unaccepted

Pentoxifylline is used, in conjunction with other forms of treatment, to promote healing of stasis ulcers associated with venous insufficiency. However, further study is needed to determine the efficacy of the medication for this purpose.

## Pharmacology/Pharmacokinetics

### Physicochemical characteristics
Chemical group—A dimethylxanthine derivative.
Molecular weight—278.31.

### Mechanism of action/Effect
Pentoxifylline reduces blood viscosity and improves erythrocyte flexibility, microcirculatory flow, and tissue oxygen concentrations. Improvement in erythrocyte flexibility appears to be due to inhibition of phosphodiesterase and a resultant increase in cyclic AMP in red blood cells. Reduction of blood viscosity may be the result of decreased plasma fibrinogen concentrations and inhibition of red blood cell and platelet aggregation.

### Absorption
Almost completely absorbed; absorption is slowed but not reduced by food. Some first-pass metabolism occurs.

### Protein binding
Bound to erythrocyte membrane.

### Biotransformation
First by erythrocytes and then hepatic. Some metabolites are active.

### Half-life
Unchanged drug—0.4 to 0.8 hours.
Metabolites—1 to 1.6 hours.

### Onset of action
Multiple doses—2 to 4 weeks.

### Time to peak concentration
Within 2 to 4 hours.

### Elimination
Renal (as metabolites).
Fecal—Less than 4%.

## Precautions to Consider

### Cross-sensitivity and/or related problems
Patients sensitive to methylxanthines such as caffeine, theophylline, or theobromine may be sensitive to pentoxifylline also.

### Carcinogenicity
Studies in mice given pentoxifylline at doses up to 24 times the maximum recommended human dose for 18 months found no evidence of carcinogenicity.

### Tumorigenicity
Studies in rats given pentoxifylline at doses up to 24 times the maximum recommended human dose for 18 months, with a 6-month drug-free period, showed an increase in benign mammary fibroadenomas in females at the highest dose.

### Mutagenicity
Pentoxifylline was not found to be mutagenic in Ames tests in the presence and absence of metabolic activation.

### Pregnancy/Reproduction
Pregnancy—Adequate and well-controlled studies have not been done in humans.
Studies in rabbits and rats given up to about 10 and 25 times the maximum recommended human dose, respectively, have found an increased incidence of fetal resorptions in rats when pentoxifylline was given at the highest dose. No fetal malformations were observed.
FDA Pregnancy Category C.

### Breast-feeding
Pentoxifylline and its metabolites are distributed into breast milk. Although problems in humans have not been documented, breast-feeding during treatment is not recommended because pentoxifylline may be tumorigenic (as demonstrated by the occurrence of benign mammary fibroadenomas in animal studies).

### Pediatrics
No information is available on the relationship of age to the effects of pentoxifylline in pediatric patients. Safety and efficacy have not been established.

### Geriatrics
Bioavailability of pentoxifylline may be increased and excretion decreased in the elderly, with resulting increased potential for toxicity. In addition, elderly patients are more likely to have age-related renal function impairment, which may require caution in patients receiving pentoxifylline.

### Drug interactions and/or related problems
The following drug interactions and/or related problems have been selected on the basis of their potential clinical significance (possible mechanism in parentheses where appropriate)—not necessarily inclusive (» = major clinical significance):

Note: Combinations containing any of the following medications, depending on the amount present, may also interact with this medication.

Anticoagulants, coumarin- or indandione-derivative, or
Heparin or
Other medications that may interfere with blood clotting by interfering with platelet function and/or by causing hypoprothrombinemia, such as:
  Cefamandole
  Cefoperazone
  Cefotetan
  Plicamycin
  Valproic acid, or
Platelet aggregation inhibitors, other (See *Appendix II*), or
Thrombolytic agents
  (pentoxifylline inhibits platelet aggregation and has also caused prolongation of prothrombin time and bleeding; concurrent use with any of these medications may increase the risk of bleeding because of additive interferences with blood clotting; caution, increased monitoring of the patient for any indication of bleeding, and, when applicable, more frequent monitoring of the prothrombin time are recommended)

Antihypertensives
  (antihypertensive effects may be potentiated when these medications are used concurrently with pentoxifylline; dosage adjustments of both pentoxifylline and the antihypertensive may be necessary)

Cimetidine
  (cimetidine significantly increases the steady-state plasma concentration of pentoxifylline, which may increase the chance of side effects during concurrent use)

Smoking, tobacco
  (although pentoxifylline is not a peripheral vasodilator, smoking may interfere with the therapeutic effect because nicotine constricts blood vessels, which may worsen the condition for which pentoxifylline is being used; avoidance of smoking is recommended)

Sympathomimetic agents or
Xanthines, other
  (concurrent use with pentoxifylline may lead to excessive central nervous system [CNS] stimulation)

### Medical considerations/Contraindications
The medical considerations/contraindications included have been selected on the basis of their potential clinical significance (reasons given in parentheses where appropriate)—not necessarily inclusive (» = major clinical significance).

*Risk-benefit should be considered when the following medical problems exist:*

» Any condition in which there is a risk of bleeding, especially recent cerebral or retinal hemorrhage, or
Bleeding, active
  (pentoxifylline may cause or exacerbate bleeding; careful patient selection and monitoring of at risk patients via hematocrit and/or hemoglobin determinations are recommended)

Cerebrovascular disease or
Coronary artery disease
  (angina, arrhythmia, and/or hypotension have occurred in some patients with these medical problems during treatment with pentoxifylline)

» Hepatic function impairment or
» Renal function impairment
   (medication may accumulate; lower doses may be required; therapy may be inadvisable in patients with severe impairment; patients with mild to moderate impairment should be closely monitored)
   Sensitivity to pentoxifylline or other methylxanthines

## Side/Adverse Effects
The following side/adverse effects have been selected on the basis of their potential clinical significance (possible signs and symptoms in parentheses where appropriate)—not necessarily inclusive:

**Those indicating need for medical attention**
Incidence rare
   *Arrhythmias* (irregular heartbeat); *chest pain*

**Those indicating need for medical attention only if they continue or are bothersome**
Incidence less frequent—dose-related
   *Dizziness; headache; nausea or vomiting; stomach discomfort*

## Overdose
For more information on the management of overdose or unintentional ingestion, **contact a Poison Control Center** (see *Poison Control Center Listing*).

**Clinical effects of overdose**
The following effects have been selected on the basis of their potential clinical significance (possible signs and symptoms in parentheses where appropriate)—not necessarily inclusive:

Acute effects—in order of occurrence
   *Drowsiness; flushing; faintness; unusual excitement; convulsions*

**Treatment of overdose**
To decrease absorption—Immediate evacuation of the stomach.
Supportive care—Symptomatic and supportive treatment, including respiratory support, maintenance of blood pressure, and control of convulsions.

## Patient Consultation
As an aid to patient consultation, refer to *Advice for the Patient, Pentoxifylline (Systemic)*.
In providing consultation, consider emphasizing the following selected information (» = major clinical significance):

**Before using this medication**
» Conditions affecting use, especially:
   Sensitivity to pentoxifylline or other methylxanthines
   Breast-feeding—Passes into breast milk; breast-feeding may be inadvisable on the basis of tumorigenic effects in animal studies
   Use in the elderly—Increased risk of side effects because of decreased clearance
   Other medical problems, especially hepatic or renal function impairment or any condition in which there is a risk of bleeding

**Proper use of this medication**
Swallowing whole without crushing, breaking, or chewing
» Taking with meals and/or antacids to reduce gastrointestinal irritation
» Proper dosing
   Missed dose: Taking as soon as possible; not taking if almost time for next dose; not doubling doses
» Proper storage

**Precautions while using this medication**
Checking with physician before discontinuing medication; pentoxifylline may take several weeks to work
Avoiding smoking (nicotine constricts blood vessels)

**Side/adverse effects**
Signs of potential side effects, especially arrhythmias and chest pain

## General Dosing Information
Pentoxifylline should be administered with meals and/or with antacids to reduce gastrointestinal irritation.
It is recommended that dosage be reduced if gastrointestinal or central nervous system (CNS) side effects develop. If symptoms persist, pentoxifylline therapy should be withdrawn.

## Oral Dosage Forms

### PENTOXIFYLLINE EXTENDED-RELEASE TABLETS

**Usual adult dose**
Peripheral vascular disease—
   Oral, 400 mg three times a day with meals.
Note: Dosage should be reduced to 400 mg two times a day if gastrointestinal or CNS side effects occur.
   Geriatric patients may be more sensitive to the effects of the usual adult dose.

**Usual pediatric dose**
Safety and efficacy have not been established.

**Strength(s) usually available**
U.S.—
   400 mg (Rx) [*Trental*; GENERIC].
Canada—
   400 mg (Rx) [*Trental*; GENERIC].

**Packaging and storage**
Store below 40 °C (104 °F), preferably between 15 and 30 °C (59 and 86 °F), in a well-closed container, unless otherwise specified by manufacturer. Protect from light.

**Auxiliary labeling**
• Take with meals or food.
• Swallow tablets whole.

## Selected Bibliography
Ward A, Clissold SP. Pentoxifylline. A review of its pharmacodynamic and pharmacokinetic properties, and its therapeutic efficacy. Drugs 1987; 34: 50-97.

Revised: 07/13/93
Interim revision: 08/13/97

---

**PERFLUBRON**—The *Perflubron (Oral-Local)* monograph is not included in this published version of the USP DI database. Copies of the monograph are available on request from Micromedex, Inc. - Reprint Requests, 6200 S. Syracuse Way, Suite 300, Englewood, CO 80111; telephone (303) 486-6400; telefax (303) 486-6464; Email: USPDI@MDX.COM.

---

**PERFLUOROCHEMICAL EMULSION**—The *Perfluorochemical Emulsion (Systemic)* monograph is not included in this published version of the USP DI database. Copies of the monograph are available on request from Micromedex, Inc. - Reprint Requests, 6200 S. Syracuse Way, Suite 300, Englewood, CO 80111; telephone (303) 486-6400; telefax (303) 486-6464; Email: USPDI@MDX.COM.

---

# PERGOLIDE Systemic

VA CLASSIFICATION (Primary): CN500
Commonly used brand name(s): *Permax*.
Note: For a listing of dosage forms and brand names by country availability, see *Dosage Forms* section(s).

## Category
Antidyskinetic (dopamine agonist).

## Indications
**Accepted**
Parkinsonism (treatment adjunct)—Pergolide is indicated, as an adjunct to levodopa or levodopa/carbidopa therapy, for treatment of the signs and symptoms of idiopathic or postencephalitic Parkinson's disease to allow achievement of symptomatic relief with lower doses of levodopa or levodopa/carbidopa.

## Pharmacology/Pharmacokinetics

**Physicochemical characteristics**
Source—Pergolide is a semisynthetic ergot alkaloid derivative.
Molecular weight—410.59.

**Mechanism of action/Effect**
Stimulation of post-synaptic dopamine receptors (at both $D_1$ and $D_2$ receptor sites) in the nigrostriatal system. Unlike bromocriptine, but similar

to apomorphine and lysuride, postsynaptic dopamine agonist properties are independent of presynaptic dopamine synthesis or stores.

**Other actions/effects**
Inhibits secretion of prolactin; causes transient rise in serum concentration of growth hormone in normal patients while in patients with acromegaly it causes a decrease; causes decrease in serum concentrations of luteinizing hormone (LH).

**Absorption**
Significant amount may be absorbed (at present, data on systemic bioavailability is insufficient).

**Protein binding**
Very high (approximately 90%).

**Elimination**
Primarily renal.

## Precautions to Consider

**Cross-sensitivity and/or related problems**
Patients sensitive to other ergot derivatives may be sensitive to this medication also.

**Carcinogenicity**
Uterine neoplasms in rats and mice, and endometrial adenomas and carcinomas in rats, occurred with doses as high as 340 and 12 times (in mice and rats, respectively) the maximum human oral dose. It is believed that this was due to the high estrogen/progesterone ratio that may occur in rodents as a result of inhibition of prolactin secretion. Human data are not available.

**Pregnancy/Reproduction**
Pregnancy—Adequate and well-controlled studies in humans have not been done.
Reproduction studies in mice and rabbits with doses as high as 375 and 133 times, respectively, the maximum human dose administered in clinical trials (6 mg/day) have not shown that pergolide causes adverse effects on the fetus.
FDA Pregnancy Category B.

**Breast-feeding**
This medication should not be administered to mothers who intend to breast-feed, since pergolide may inhibit lactation.

**Pediatrics**
No published pediatrics-specific information is available. Safety and efficacy have not been established.

**Geriatrics**
Studies performed to date have not demonstrated geriatrics-specific problems that would limit the usefulness of pergolide in the elderly.

**Dental**
Pergolide may decrease or inhibit salivary flow, thus contributing to the development of caries, periodontal disease, oral candidiasis, and discomfort.

**Drug interactions and/or related problems**
The following drug interactions and/or related problems have been selected on the basis of their potential clinical significance (possible mechanism in parentheses where appropriate)—not necessarily inclusive (» = major clinical significance):

Note: Combinations containing any of the following medications, depending on the amount present, may also interact with this medication.

Droperidol or
Haloperidol or
Loxapine or
Methyldopa or
Metoclopramide or
Molindone or
Papaverine or
Phenothiazines or
Reserpine or
Thioxanthenes
  (dopamine antagonists may decrease the effectiveness of pergolide)
Hypotension-producing medications, other (See *Appendix II*)
  (concurrent use may result in additive hypotensive effects)

**Laboratory value alterations**
The following have been selected on the basis of their potential clinical significance (possible effect in parentheses where appropriate)—not necessarily inclusive (» = major clinical significance):

With physiology/laboratory test values
  Plasma growth hormone concentrations
    (may be transiently increased in individuals with normal concentrations; paradoxically reduced in patients with acromegaly)

**Medical considerations/Contraindications**
The medical considerations/contraindications included have been selected on the basis of their potential clinical significance (reasons given in parentheses where appropriate)—not necessarily inclusive (» = major clinical significance).

*Except under special circumstances, this medication should not be used when the following medical problem exists:*
» Sensitivity to pergolide or other ergot alkaloids

*Risk-benefit should be considered when the following medical problems exist:*
Cardiac dysrhythmias
  (increased risk of atrial premature contractions and sinus tachycardia)
Psychiatric disorders
  (pre-existing states of confusion and hallucinations may be exacerbated)

**Patient monitoring**
The following may be especially important in patient monitoring (other tests may be warranted in some patients, depending on condition; » = major clinical significance):

» Blood pressure measurements
  (pergolide commonly decreases or less frequently increases blood pressure)

## Side/Adverse Effects

The following side/adverse effects have been selected on the basis of their potential clinical significance (possible signs and symptoms in parentheses where appropriate)—not necessarily inclusive:

**Those indicating need for medical attention**
Incidence more frequent
  *CNS effects* (confusion; dyskinesias [uncontrolled movements of the body, such as the face, tongue, arms, hands, head, and upper body]; hallucinations); *urinary tract infections* (pain or burning while urinating)
Incidence less frequent
  *Hypertension*
Incidence rare
  *Cerebrovascular hemorrhage* (severe or continuing headache; seizures; vision changes, such as blurred vision or temporary blindness; sudden weakness); *myocardial infarction* (severe chest pain; fainting; fast heartbeat; increased sweating; continuing or severe nausea and vomiting; nervousness; unexplained shortness of breath; weakness)

**Those indicating need for medical attention only if they continue or are bothersome**
Incidence more frequent
  *Abdominal or stomach pain; constipation; dizziness or drowsiness; flu-like symptoms; hypotension* (dizziness or lightheadedness, especially when getting up from a lying or sitting position); *lower back pain; nausea; rhinitis* (runny nose); *weakness*

Note: Approximately 10% of patients experience *orthostatic hypotension* during initial treatment. Tolerance usually develops with gradual dosage titration.

Incidence less frequent
  *Chills; diarrhea; dryness of mouth; facial edema* (swelling of the face); *loss of appetite; vomiting*

## Overdose

For specific information on the agents used in the management of pergolide overdose, see:
• *Charcoal, Activated (Oral-Local)* monograph; and/or
• *Phenothiazines (Systemic)* monograph.

For more information on the management of overdose or unintentional ingestion, **contact a Poison Control Center** (see *Poison Control Center Listing*).

**Treatment of overdose**
Treatment is symptomatic and supportive, with possible utilization of the following:

To decrease absorption—Administration of activated charcoal instead of or in addition to gastric emptying.

## Pergolide (Systemic)

Specific treatment—Antiarrhythmic medication, if necessary. Phenothiazine or other neuroleptic agent, to treat CNS stimulation.

Monitoring—Monitoring of cardiac function.

Supportive care—Maintenance of arterial blood pressure. Patients in whom intentional overdose is confirmed or suspected should be referred for psychiatric consultation.

### Patient Consultation

As an aid to patient consultation, refer to *Advice for the Patient, Pergolide (Systemic)*.

In providing consultation, consider emphasizing the following selected information (» = major clinical significance):

**Before using this medication**
» Conditions affecting use, especially:
  Sensitivity to pergolide or other ergot alkaloids
  Breast-feeding—May prevent lactation in mothers who intend to breast-feed
  Dental—Reduced salivary flow may contribute to dental problems

**Proper use of this medication**
Taking with meals to reduce gastric effects
» Proper dosing
  Missed dose: Taking as soon as possible; not taking if almost time for next dose; not doubling doses
» Proper storage

**Precautions while using this medication**
Regular visits to physician to check progress
» Caution when driving or doing jobs requiring alertness, because of possible drowsiness or dizziness
  Dizziness may be more likely to occur after initial doses; taking first dose at bedtime or while lying down; getting up slowly from sitting or lying position
  Possible dryness of mouth; using sugarless gum or candy, ice, or saliva substitute for relief; checking with physician or dentist if dry mouth continues for more than 2 weeks
  Checking with physician before reducing dosage or discontinuing medication

**Side/adverse effects**
Signs of potential side effects, especially CNS effects, urinary tract infection, hypertension, cerebrovascular hemorrhage, and myocardial infarction

### General Dosing Information

Titrated dosage is necessary to achieve the individual therapeutic blood concentration requirements and to minimize the risk of side effects.

Nausea and dizziness associated with initiation of pergolide therapy usually resolve with continued therapy; however, incidence and severity of these side effects may be reduced with a decrease in pergolide dose. Dizziness and nausea may be better tolerated by administering the initial dose at bedtime or while lying down. Also, administration of pergolide with food may alleviate the nausea.

### Oral Dosage Forms

Note: The dosing and strengths of the dosage forms available are expressed in terms of pergolide base, not the mesylate salt.

**PERGOLIDE MESYLATE TABLETS**

**Usual adult and adolescent dose**
Parkinsonism—
  Oral, 50 mcg (0.05 mg) (base) a day for the first two days; the dosage being increased gradually by 100 or 150 mcg (0.1 or 0.15 mg) (base) every third day over the next twelve days of therapy. Afterwards, the dose may be increased by 250 mcg (0.25 mg) (base) every third day until optimum therapeutic effect is achieved.

Note: Usually administered in divided doses three times a day.
  During dosage titration of pergolide the concurrent dose of levodopa or levodopa/carbidopa may be decreased with caution according to clinical response.

**Usual adult prescribing limits**
Up to 5 mg daily.

**Usual pediatric dose**
Safety and efficacy have not been established.

**Usual geriatric dose**
See *Usual adult and adolescent dose*.

**Strength(s) usually available**
U.S.—
  50 mcg (0.05 mg) (base) (Rx) [*Permax* (scored; carboxymethylcellulose sodium; iron oxide; lactose; magnesium stearate; povidone)].
  250 mcg (0.25 mg) (base) (Rx) [*Permax* (scored; carboxymethylcellulose sodium; iron oxide; lactose; magnesium stearate; povidone; FD&C Blue No. 1)].
  1 mg (base) (Rx) [*Permax* (scored; carboxymethylcellulose sodium; iron oxide; lactose; magnesium stearate; povidone)].
Canada—
  50 mcg (0.05 mg) (base) (Rx) [*Permax* (scored; croscarmellose sodium; iron oxide yellow; lactose; magnesium stearate; povidine; FD &C Blue No. 2 Aluminum Lake)].
  250 mcg (0.25 mg) (base) (Rx) [*Permax* (scored; croscarmellose sodium; iron oxide yellow; lactose; l-methionine; magnesium stearate; povidine)].
  1 mg (base) (Rx) [*Permax* (scored; croscarmellose sodium; iron oxide red pure; lactose; magnesium stearate; povidine)].

**Packaging and storage**
Store between 15 and 30 °C (59 and 86 °F), unless otherwise specified by manufacturer.

**Auxiliary labeling**
• May cause drowsiness.

### Selected Bibliography

Lieberman AN, Goldstein M, Gopinathan G, et al. $D_1$ and $D_2$ agonists in Parkinson's disease. Can J Neurol Sci 1987 Aug; 14(3 Suppl): 466-73.

Lieberman AN, Gopinathan G, Neophytides A, et al. Management of levodopa failures: the use of dopamine agonists. Clin Neuropharmacol 1986; 9(Suppl 2): S9-21.

Factor SA, Sanchez-Ramos JR, Weiner WJ. Parkinson's disease: An open label trial of pergolide in patients failing bromocriptine therapy. J Neurol Neurosurg Psychiatry 1988 Apr; 51(4): 529-33.

Revised: 03/19/93

---

**PERICYAZINE**—See *Phenothiazines (Systemic)*

---

**PERMETHRIN**—The *Permethrin (Topical)* monograph is not included in this published version of the USP DI database. Copies of the monograph are available on request from Micromedex, Inc. - Reprint Requests, 6200 S. Syracuse Way, Suite 300, Englewood, CO 80111; telephone (303) 486-6400; telefax (303) 486-6464; Email: USPDI@MDX.COM.

---

**PERPHENAZINE**—See *Phenothiazines (Systemic)*

---

# PERPHENAZINE AND AMITRIPTYLINE Systemic

VA CLASSIFICATION (Primary): CN900

NOTE: The *Perphenazine and Amitriptyline (Systemic)* monograph is maintained on the USP DI electronic data base. For a printed copy of the most recent revision of the complete monograph, contact Micromedex, Inc. - Reprint Requests, 6200 S. Syracuse Way, Suite 300, Englewood, CO 80111; telephone (303) 486-6400; telefax (303) 486-6464; Email: USPDI@MDX.COM.

For information on the specific components of this combination, see the USP DI monographs for *Antidepressants, Tricyclic (Systemic)* and *Phenothiazines (Systemic)*.

The information that follows is selectively abstracted from the complete monograph and is provided to facilitate drug use review and patient counseling.

Note: For a listing of dosage forms and brand names by country availability, see *Dosage Forms* section(s).

### Category

Antipsychotic-antidepressant.

## Indications

### Accepted
Anxiety associated with mental depression (treatment)—Perphenazine and amitriptyline combination is indicated in the treatment of patients with moderate to severe anxiety and/or agitation and depression, anxiety and depression associated with chronic physical disease, anxiety and depression that cannot be differentiated, and symptoms of depression in schizophrenia.

## Patient Consultation

As an aid to patient consultation, refer to *Advice for the Patient, Perphenazine and Amitriptyline (Systemic)*.

In providing consultation, consider emphasizing the following selected information (» = major clinical significance):

### Before using this medication
» Conditions affecting use, especially:
- Sensitivity to phenothiazines, tricyclic antidepressants, or possibly maprotiline or trazodone
- Pregnancy—
  - Amitriptyline: Animal studies have shown teratogenic effects when amitriptyline was given in doses many times larger than the human dose; reports of cardiac problems, muscle spasms, respiratory distress, or urinary retention in neonates of mothers taking amitriptyline just prior to delivery
  - Perphenazine: Phenothiazines have been found to depress spermatogenesis in animals; not recommended for use during pregnancy, because of reports of prolonged jaundice, hypo- or hyperreflexia, and extrapyramidal effects in neonates
- Breast-feeding—Distributed into breast milk, possibly causing drowsiness, dystonias, and tardive dyskinesia in the baby; increased prolactin secretion in mother
- Use in children—Adolescents more sensitive to effects, requiring lower doses; children more prone to develop extrapyramidal reactions
- Use in the elderly—Elderly more likely to develop extrapyramidal, anticholinergic, hypotensive, and sedative effects; lower doses and more gradual increases required
- Dental—Decreased salivary flow contributes to caries, periodontal disease, candidiasis, and discomfort; blood dyscrasias may cause increased infections, delayed healing, and gingival bleeding; increased extrapyramidal motor activity of head, face, and neck may cause difficulty with occlusal and other procedures
- Other medications, especially alcohol and other CNS depressants, antithyroid agents, epinephrine, levodopa, lithium, cimetidine, other EPS-causing medications, MAO inhibitors, metrizamide, or sympathomimetics
- Other medical problems, especially alcoholism (active), bipolar disorder, blood disorders, cardiovascular disorders, gastrointestinal disorders, glaucoma, hepatic function impairment, renal function impairment, hyperthyroidism, prostatic hypertrophy, latent psychosis, Reye's syndrome, severe CNS depression, seizures, or urinary retention

### Proper use of this medication
Taking after meals or with food to reduce gastrointestinal irritation
» Compliance with therapy; not taking more or less medication than the amount prescribed
» Several weeks of therapy may be required to produce optimal therapeutic effects
» Proper dosing
- Missed dose: Taking as soon as possible; not taking at all if less than 2 hours to next dose; not doubling doses
» Proper storage

### Precautions while using this medication
Regular visits to physician to check progress of therapy
» Checking with physician before discontinuing medication; gradual dosage reduction may be needed
- Avoiding use of antacids or antidiarrheals within 2 hours of taking this medication
» Avoiding use of alcoholic beverages or other CNS depressants during therapy
» Caution if any kind of surgery, dental treatment, or emergency treatment is required
» Possible drowsiness or blurred vision; caution when driving, using machines or doing jobs requiring alertness or accurate vision
» Possible dizziness or lightheadedness; caution when getting up suddenly from a lying or sitting position
» Possible heat stroke: caution during exercise, hot weather, or hot baths or saunas
- Possible dryness of mouth; using sugarless gum or candy, ice, or saliva substitute for relief; checking with physician or dentist if dry mouth continues for more than 2 weeks
- Possible skin photosensitivity; avoiding unprotected exposure to sun; using protective clothing; using a sun block product that includes protection against both UVA-caused photosensitivity reactions and UVB-caused sunburn reactions; avoiding use of sunlamp, tanning bed, or tanning booth
- Observing precautions for 3 to 7 days after stopping medication

### Side/adverse effects
» Stopping medication and getting emergency treatment if symptoms of neuroleptic malignant syndrome (NMS) appear
» Notifying physician as soon as possible if early symptoms of tardive dyskinesia appear
- Possibility of withdrawal symptoms
- Signs of potential side effects, especially anticholinergic effects; hypotension; dystonias; fast, slow, or irregular heartbeat; tardive dyskinesia or Parkinsonian syndrome; akathisia; shakiness or tremors; NMS; heat stroke; testicular swelling; allergic reactions; alopecia; blood dyscrasias; cholestatic jaundice; photosensitivity; ophthalmologic effects; melanosis; priapism; seizures; SIADH; or tinnitus

## Oral Dosage Forms

### PERPHENAZINE AND AMITRIPTYLINE HYDROCHLORIDE TABLETS USP

**Usual adult dose**
Oral, 2 mg of perphenazine and 25 mg of amitriptyline hydrochloride to 4 mg of perphenazine and 25 mg of amitriptyline hydrochloride three or four times a day initially, the daily dosage being adjusted as needed and tolerated.

Note: Debilitated patients usually require a lower initial dose, which is then gradually increased as needed and tolerated.

**Usual adult prescribing limits**
Up to a total of 32 mg of perphenazine and 200 mg of amitriptyline hydrochloride daily.

**Usual pediatric dose**
Children up to 12 years of age—Safety and efficacy have not been established.

Children over 12 years of age—Adolescent patients usually require a lower initial dose, which is then gradually increased as needed and tolerated. Dosage must be individualized by physician.

**Usual geriatric dose**
Oral, 4 mg of perphenazine and 10 mg of amitriptyline hydrochloride three or four times a day initially, the dosage being adjusted as needed and tolerated.

**Strength(s) usually available**
U.S.—
- 2 mg of perphenazine and 10 mg of amitriptyline hydrochloride (Rx) [*Etrafon; Triavil;* GENERIC].
- 2 mg of perphenazine and 25 mg of amitriptyline hydrochloride (Rx) [*Etrafon; Triavil;* GENERIC].
- 4 mg of perphenazine and 10 mg of amitriptyline hydrochloride (Rx) [*Etrafon-A; Triavil;* GENERIC].
- 4 mg of perphenazine and 25 mg of amitriptyline hydrochloride (Rx) [*Etrafon-Forte; Triavil;* GENERIC].
- 4 mg of perphenazine and 50 mg of amitriptyline hydrochloride (Rx) [*Triavil;* GENERIC].

Canada—
- 2 mg of perphenazine and 10 mg of amitriptyline hydrochloride (Rx) [*Etrafon*].
- 2 mg of perphenazine and 25 mg of amitriptyline hydrochloride (Rx) [*Elavil Plus; Etrafon-D; PMS Levazine*].
- 3 mg of perphenazine and 15 mg of amitriptyline hydrochloride (Rx) [*Triavil*].
- 4 mg of perphenazine and 10 mg of amitriptyline hydrochloride (Rx) [*Etrafon-A*].
- 4 mg of perphenazine and 25 mg of amitriptyline hydrochloride (Rx) [*Etrafon-F; PMS Levazine*].

**Auxiliary labeling**
- May cause drowsiness.
- Avoid alcoholic beverages.

Revised: 01/27/92
Interim revision: 08/09/94

**PHENACEMIDE**—The *Phenacemide (Systemic)* monograph is not included in this published version of the USP DI database. Copies of the monograph are available on request from Micromedex, Inc. - Reprint Requests, 6200 S. Syracuse Way, Suite 300, Englewood, CO 80111; telephone (303) 486-6400; telefax (303) 486-6464; Email: USPDI@MDX.COM.

# PHENAZOPYRIDINE Systemic

VA CLASSIFICATION (Primary): GU100

Commonly used brand name(s): *Azo-Standard; Baridium; Eridium; Geridium; Phenazo; Phenazodine; Pyridiate; Pyridium; Urodine; Urogesic; Viridium.*

Note: For a listing of dosage forms and brand names by country availability, see *Dosage Forms* section(s).

## Category
Analgesic (urinary).

## Indications

**Accepted**

Urinary tract irritation (treatment)—Phenazopyridine is indicated for short-term use to relieve symptoms such as pain, burning, and urinary urgency and/or frequency caused by irritation of the lower urinary tract mucosa. The underlying cause of the irritation must be determined and treated (for example, antibacterial therapy for infection).

## Pharmacology/Pharmacokinetics

**Physicochemical characteristics**
Chemical group—Azo dye.
Molecular weight—249.70.

**Mechanism of action/Effect**
Exerts a topical analgesic or local anesthetic action on the urinary tract mucosa. The exact mechanism of action is unknown.

**Biotransformation**
Probably hepatic; also in other tissues. One of the metabolites is acetaminophen.

**Elimination**
Renal. Up to 90% of a dose is excreted within 24 hours, as unchanged drug and metabolites. About 18% of a dose is eliminated as acetaminophen. Up to 65% of a dose may be excreted unchanged.

## Precautions to Consider

**Carcinogenicity**
Long-term administration of phenazopyridine has caused neoplasia of the large intestine in rats and neoplasia of the liver in mice. No association between use of the medication in humans and development of neoplasia has been reported; however, studies in humans have not been done.

**Pregnancy/Reproduction**
Fertility—Studies in rats with doses up to 50 mg per kg of body weight (mg/kg) per day have not shown evidence of impaired fertility.

Pregnancy—Adequate and well-controlled studies have not been done in humans.
Studies in rats with doses up to 50 mg/kg per day have not shown evidence of harm to the fetus.

FDA Pregnancy Category B.

**Breast-feeding**
It is not known whether phenazopyridine or any of its metabolites are distributed into breast milk. However, problems in humans have not been documented.

**Pediatrics**
Appropriate studies with phenazopyridine have not been performed in the pediatric population. However, no pediatrics-specific problems have been documented to date.

**Geriatrics**
Although appropriate studies with phenazopyridine have not been performed in the geriatric population, no geriatrics-specific problems have been documented to date. However, elderly patients are more likely to have age-related renal function impairment, which may increase the risk of accumulation and toxicity in patients receiving phenazopyridine.

**Laboratory value alterations**
The following have been selected on the basis of their potential clinical significance (possible effect in parentheses where appropriate)—not necessarily inclusive (» = major clinical significance):

With physiology/laboratory test values
 Urinalyses based on color reaction or spectroscopy, for example:
  Bilirubin, urine, determined via foam test, talc-disk–Fouchetspot test, or Franklin's tablet-Fouchet test methods
  Glucose, urine, determined using glucose oxidase
  17-Hydroxycorticosteroids, urine, determined via Glenn-Nelson method
  Ketones, urine, determined using sodium nitroprusside or Gerhardt ferric chloride test
  17-Ketosteroids, urine, determined via Haltorff Koch modification of Zimmerman reaction
  Kidney function tested via phenolsulfonphthalein (PSP) excretion
  Protein, urine, determined using bromophenol blue test reagent strips or nitric acid ring test
  Urobilinogen, urine, determined using Ehrlich's reagent
   (phenazopyridine may interfere with test results by causing discoloration of the urine)

**Medical considerations/Contraindications**
The medical considerations/contraindications included have been selected on the basis of their potential clinical significance (reasons given in parentheses where appropriate)—not necessarily inclusive (» = major clinical significance).

*Risk-benefit should be considered when the following medical problems exist:*
 Allergic reaction to phenazopyridine, history of
 » Glucose-6-phosphate dehydrogenase (G6PD) deficiency
  (increased risk of severe hemolytic anemia)
 Hepatitis
  (increased risk of adverse effects)
 Renal function impairment
  (increased risk of accumulation and toxicity)

## Side/Adverse Effects

Note: In addition to the side effects reported below, an anaphylactoid-like reaction has been reported.

The following side/adverse effects have been selected on the basis of their potential clinical significance (possible signs and symptoms in parentheses where appropriate)—not necessarily inclusive:

**Those indicating need for medical attention**
Incidence rare
 *Anemia, hemolytic* (troubled breathing, exertional; unusual tiredness or weakness); *aseptic meningitis* (fever; confusion)—reported in 1 patient; causal relationship verified via rechallenge; *dermatitis, allergic* (skin rash); *hepatotoxicity* (yellow eyes or skin); *methemoglobinemia* (blue or blue-purple discoloration of skin; shortness of breath); *renal function impairment or failure* (increased blood pressure; shortness of breath; troubled breathing; tightness in chest, and/or wheezing; sudden decrease in amount of urine; swelling of face, fingers, feet, and/or lower legs; thirst, continuing; unusual tiredness or weakness; weight gain)

Note: *Hemolytic anemia* or *methemoglobinemia* may be more likely with an overdose or if the medication is administered to patients with renal function impairment, but have also been reported with therapeutic doses in patients with normal renal function. Also, *hemolytic anemia* is especially likely to occur in patients with glucose-6-phosphate dehydrogenase deficiency.

*Hepatotoxicity* has been reported in conjunction with impaired renal excretion of the medication; however, yellowish discoloration of eyes or skin may also occur independently of hepatotoxicity, indicating accumulation. Permanent staining of soft contact lenses has also been reported.

**Those indicating need for medical attention only if they continue or are bothersome**
Incidence less frequent or rare
*Dizziness; headache; indigestion; stomach cramps or pain*

## Patient Consultation

As an aid to patient consultation, refer to *Advice for the Patient, Phenazopyridine (Systemic)*.

In providing consultation, consider emphasizing the following selected information (» = major clinical significance):

**Before using this medication**
» Conditions affecting use, especially:
Allergic reaction to phenazopyridine, history of
Other medical problems, especially glucose-6-phosphate dehydrogenase (G6PD) deficiency

**Proper use of this medication**
Taking with or following food (a meal or a snack) to reduce gastric upset
» Not using any saved portion of medication in the future unless authorized by physician
» Proper dosing
Missed dose: Taking as soon as possible; not taking if almost time for next dose; not doubling doses
» Proper storage

**Precautions while using this medication**
» Informing physician if symptoms worsen
» Medication causes urine to turn reddish orange and may stain clothing
Not wearing soft contact lenses during therapy because of possible permanent staining
Diabetics: May cause false urine sugar and urine ketone test results
Possible interference with laboratory test results; notifying person in charge that medication is being used

**Side/adverse effects**
Signs of potential side effects, especially allergic dermatitis, aseptic meningitis, hemolytic anemia, hepatotoxicity, methemoglobinemia, and renal impairment or failure

## General Dosing Information

This medication should be taken with or following food to lessen gastric irritation.

When phenazopyridine is used concurrently with an antibacterial agent in the treatment of a urinary tract infection, the duration of phenazopyridine therapy should not exceed 2 days. Adequate evidence that more prolonged phenazopyridine therapy provides greater therapeutic benefit than is achieved with the antibacterial agent alone is not available.

**For treatment of adverse effects**
Recommended treatment consists of the following:
• For methemoglobinemia—Administering methylene blue (1 to 2 mg per kg of body weight (mg/kg), intravenously) or ascorbic acid (100 to 200 mg orally).

## Oral Dosage Forms

### PHENAZOPYRIDINE HYDROCHLORIDE TABLETS USP

**Usual adult and adolescent dose**
Analgesic (urinary)—
Oral, 200 mg three times a day, with or following food.

**Usual pediatric dose**
Analgesic (urinary)—
Oral, 4 mg per kg of body weight three times a day, with food.

**Strength(s) usually available**
U.S.—
100 mg (Rx) [*Azo-Standard; Baridium; Eridium; Geridium; Phenazodine; Pyridiate; Pyridium; Urodine; Urogesic;* GENERIC].
200 mg (Rx) [*Geridium; Phenazodine; Pyridiate; Pyridium; Urodine; Viridium;* GENERIC].
Canada—
100 mg (OTC) [*Phenazo; Pyridium*].
200 mg (OTC) [*Phenazo; Pyridium*].

**Packaging and storage**
Store below 40 °C (104 °F), preferably between 15 and 30 °C (59 and 86 °F), unless otherwise specified by manufacturer. Store in a tight container.

**Auxiliary labeling**
• May discolor urine.
• Take with food.

**Note**
Stains on clothing may be removed with a 0.25% solution of sodium dithionate or sodium hydrosulfite.

Revised: 06/08/92
Interim revision: 08/24/94

---

**PHENDIMETRAZINE**—See *Appetite Suppressants (Systemic)*

---

**PHENELZINE**—See *Antidepressants, Monoamine Oxidase (MAO) Inhibitor (Systemic)*

---

**PHENINDAMINE**—See *Antihistamines (Systemic)*

---

**PHENOBARBITAL**—See *Barbiturates (Systemic)*

---

**PHENOLPHTHALEIN**—See *Laxatives (Local)*

---

**PHENOLSULFONPHTHALEIN**—The *Phenolsulfonphthalein (Systemic)* monograph is not included in this published version of the USP DI database. Copies of the monograph are available on request from Micromedex, Inc. - Reprint Requests, 6200 S. Syracuse Way, Suite 300, Englewood, CO 80111; telephone (303) 486-6400; telefax (303) 486-6464; Email: USPDI@MDX.COM.

---

# PHENOTHIAZINES Systemic

This monograph includes information on the following: 1) Acetophenazine[†]; 2) Chlorpromazine; 3) Fluphenazine; 4) Mesoridazine; 5) Methotrimeprazine; 6) Pericyazine[*]; 7) Perphenazine; 8) Pipotiazine[*]; 9) Prochlorperazine; 10) Promazine; 11) Thiopropazate[*]; 12) Thioproperazine[*]; 13) Thioridazine; 14) Trifluoperazine; 15) Triflupromazine[†].

INN:
Methotrimeprazine—Levomepromazine
Pericyazine[*]—Periciazine

VA CLASSIFICATION (Primary/Secondary):
Acetophenazine—CN701
Chlorpromazine—CN701/GA700; AU350
Fluphenazine—CN701/CN103
Mesoridazine—CN701
Methotrimeprazine—CN701/CN103; CN309
Pericyazine—CN701
Perphenazine—CN701/GA700
Pipotiazine—CN701
Prochlorperazine—CN701/GA700
Promazine—CN701
Thiopropazate—CN701
Thioproperazine—CN701
Thioridazine—CN701/AU350
Trifluoperazine—CN701
Triflupromazine—CN701/GA700

Commonly used brand name(s): *Apo-Fluphenazine*[3]; *Apo-Perphenazine*[7]; *Apo-Thioridazine*[13]; *Apo-Trifluoperazine*[14]; *Chlorpromanyl-20*[2]; *Chlorpromanyl-40*[2]; *Chlorpromanyl-5*[2]; *Compa-Z*[9]; *Compazine*[9]; *Com-*

pazine Spansule[9]; Cotranzine[9]; Dartal[11]; Largactil[2]; Largactil Liquid[2]; Largactil Oral Drops[2]; Levoprome[5]; Majeptil[12]; Mellaril[13]; Mellaril Concentrate[13]; Mellaril-S[13]; Modecate[3]; Modecate Concentrate[3]; Moditen Enanthate[3]; Moditen HCl[3]; Moditen HCl-H.P.[3]; Neuleptil[6]; Novo-Chlorpromazine[2]; Novo-Flurazine[14]; Novo-Ridazine[13]; Nozinan[5]; Nozinan Liquid[5]; Nozinan Oral Drops[5]; Ormazine[2]; PMS Perphenazine[7]; PMS Prochlorperazine[9]; PMS Thioridazine[13]; PMS Trifluoperazine[14]; Permitil[3]; Permitil Concentrate[3]; Piportil L4[8]; Primazine[10]; Prolixin[3]; Prolixin Concentrate[3]; Prolixin Decanoate[3]; Prolixin Enanthate[3]; Prorazin[9]; Prozine-50[10]; Serentil[4]; Serentil Concentrate[4]; Solazine[14]; Sparine[10]; Stelazine[14]; Stelazine Concentrate[14]; Stemetil[9]; Stemetil Liquid[9]; Terfluzine[14]; Terfluzine Concentrate[14]; Thor-Prom[2]; Thorazine[2]; Thorazine Concentrate[2]; Thorazine Spansule[2]; Tindal[1]; Trilafon[7]; Trilafon Concentrate[7]; Ultrazine-10[9]; Vesprin[15].

Note: For a listing of dosage forms and brand names by country availability, see *Dosage Forms* section(s).

*Not commercially available in U.S.
†Not commercially available in Canada.

## Category

Antipsychotic—Acetophenazine; Chlorpromazine; Fluphenazine; Mesoridazine; Methotrimeprazine; Pericyazine; Perphenazine; Pipotiazine; Prochlorperazine; Promazine; Thiopropazate; Thioproperazine; Thioridazine; Trifluoperazine; Triflupromazine.
Antiemetic—Chlorpromazine; Perphenazine; Prochlorperazine; Triflupromazine.
Analgesic—Methotrimeprazine.
Sedative (preoperative)—Methotrimeprazine.
Antidyskinetic (Huntington's disease)—Chlorpromazine; Thioridazine.
Antineuralgia adjunct—Fluphenazine.

## Indications

Note: Bracketed information in the *Indications* section refers to uses that are not included in U.S. product labeling.

**Accepted**

Psychotic disorders (treatment)—Acetophenazine, chlorpromazine, fluphenazine, mesoridazine, [methotrimeprazine], pericyazine, perphenazine, pipotiazine, prochlorperazine, promazine, thiopropazate, thioproperazine, thioridazine, trifluoperazine, and triflupromazine are indicated in the management of psychotic conditions. They are clearly effective in schizophrenia, and for production of a quieting effect in hyperactive or excited psychotic patients.

Chlorpromazine, mesoridazine, and thioridazine are used for the treatment of children or adults with severe behavior problems associated with psychotic disorders or neurologic disease, who show combativeness and/or explosive, hyperexcitable behavior that is out of proportion to the immediate provocation. These agents are also used in the short-term treatment of hyperactive children who show excessive motor activity with accompanying conduct disorders such as impulsivity, mood lability, aggressiveness, short attention span, and poor frustration tolerance. Pericyazine is a more sedative phenothiazine with weak antipsychotic properties. It is indicated as an adjunctive medication in some psychotic patients for the control of residual prevailing hostility, impulsiveness, and aggressiveness.

Long-acting parenteral forms, fluphenazine decanoate and enanthate and pipotiazine palmitate, are indicated for the maintenance treatment of chronic, non-agitated schizophrenic patients stabilized with shorter-acting neuroleptics, who may benefit from a transfer to the longer-acting drug.

Thioridazine is indicated for the short-term treatment of adult patients with moderate to severe mental depression with varying degrees of anxiety and geriatric patients with multiple symptoms such as anxiety, agitation, depressed mood, tension, sleep disturbances, and fears. Chlorpromazine is used for anxiety, apprehension, and restlessness before surgery.

Nausea and vomiting (treatment)—Prochlorperazine, chlorpromazine, perphenazine, and triflupromazine are indicated in the control of severe nausea and vomiting in selected patients, with prochlorperazine being superior to other phenothiazines.

Pain (treatment)—Methotrimeprazine is indicated for the relief of moderate to severe pain in nonambulatory patients, and to produce obstetrical analgesia when respiratory depression should be avoided.

Sedation—Methotrimeprazine is indicated as a presurgical or obstetrical medication to produce sedation and somnolence.

[Anesthesia, general, adjunct]—Intravenous administration of methotrimeprazine is indicated as an adjunct to anesthesia, to increase the effects of anesthetics. The dose of a barbiturate or narcotic should be reduced by half when used with methotrimeprazine during surgery or labor.

Tetanus (treatment adjunct)—Chlorpromazine is indicated, usually in conjunction with a barbiturate, for the treatment of tetanus.

Porphyria, acute, intermittent (treatment)—Chlorpromazine is indicated in the treatment of acute intermittent porphyria.

Hiccups, intractable (treatment)—Chlorpromazine is indicated in the control of intractable hiccups.

[Pain, neurogenic (treatment adjunct)][1]—Fluphenazine has been used as an adjunct to tricyclic antidepressant therapy for some chronic pain states, as in patients trying to withdraw from narcotics, and in treatment of symptoms of diabetic neuropathy.

[Huntington's disease, choreiform movement of (treatment)][1]—Chlorpromazine and thioridazine are effective in reducing choreiform movement in Huntington's disease, and have been used as alternatives to haloperidol.

[1]Not included in Canadian product labeling.

## Pharmacology/Pharmacokinetics

**Physicochemical characteristics**
Chemical group—
  Aliphatic: Chlorpromazine; methotrimeprazine; promazine; triflupromazine.
  Piperazine: Acetophenazine; fluphenazine; perphenazine; prochlorperazine; thiopropazate; thioproperazine; trifluoperazine.
  Piperidine: Mesoridazine; pericyazine; pipotiazine; thioridazine.
Molecular weight—
  Acetophenazine maleate: 643.71.
  Chlorpromazine: 318.86.
  Chlorpromazine hydrochloride: 355.32.
  Fluphenazine decanoate: 591.8.
  Fluphenazine enanthate: 549.69.
  Fluphenazine hydrochloride: 510.44.
  Mesoridazine besylate: 544.74.
  Methotrimeprazine: 328.47.
  Pericyazine: 365.19.
  Perphenazine: 403.97.
  Pipotiazine palmitate: 714.08.
  Prochlorperazine: 373.94.
  Prochlorperazine edisylate: 564.13.
  Prochlorperazine maleate: 606.09.
  Prochlorperazine mesylate: 566.1.
  Promazine hydrochloride: 320.88.
  Thiopropazate hydrochloride: 518.94.
  Thioproperazine mesylate: 638.8.
  Thioridazine: 370.57.
  Thioridazine hydrochloride: 407.03.
  Trifluoperazine hydrochloride: 480.42.
  Triflupromazine: 352.42.
  Triflupromazine hydrochloride: 388.88.

**Mechanism of action/Effect**

Antipsychotic—Thought to improve psychotic conditions by blocking postsynaptic mesolimbic dopaminergic receptors in the brain. Phenothiazines also produce an alpha-adrenergic blocking effect and depress the release of hypothalamic and hypophyseal hormones. However, blockade of dopamine receptors increases prolactin release by the pituitary.

Antiemetic—Phenothiazines act centrally to inhibit or block the dopamine ($D_2$) receptors in the medullary chemoreceptor trigger zone (CTZ) and peripherally by blocking the vagus nerve in the gastrointestinal tract. The antiemetic effects of phenothiazines may be augmented by their anticholinergic, sedative, and antihistaminic effects.

Antianxiety—Thought to cause indirect reduction in arousal and increased filtering of internal stimuli to the brainstem reticular system.

Analgesic; sedative—Methotrimeprazine raises pain threshold and produces amnesia by suppression of sensory impulses. The alpha-adrenergic blocking effects of phenothiazines may produce sedation and tranquilization.

| Drug | Action* |||||
|---|---|---|---|---|---|
| | Legend:<br>I = Antiemetic<br>II = Anticholinergic<br>III = Extrapyramidal<br>IV = Hypotensive<br>V = Sedative |||||
| | I | II | III | IV | V |
| **Aliphatic** | | | | | |
| Chlorpromazine | S | M–S | W–M | S | S |
| Methotrimeprazine | W | M | W–M | S | S |
| Promazine | M | S | W | S | S |
| Triflupromazine | S | S | M–S | M | M–S |
| **Piperazine** | | | | | |
| Acetophenazine | W | W | M | W | M |
| Fluphenazine | W | W | S | W | W |
| Perphenazine | S | W–M | S | W | W–M |
| Prochlorperazine | S | W | S | W | W |
| Thiopropazate | W | W | S | W | W |
| Thioproperazine | W | W | S | W | W |
| Trifluoperazine | S | W | S | W | W |
| **Piperidine** | | | | | |
| Mesoridazine | W | M | W | M–S | S |
| Pericyazine | S | S | M | M | S |
| Pipotiazine | W | W | S | W | W |
| Thioridazine | W | M | W | M–S | M |

*S = strong; M = moderate; W = weak

**Protein binding**
Very high (90% or more).

**Biotransformation**
Hepatic.

**Onset of action**
Antipsychotic effect—
  Gradual (up to several weeks) and variable between patients.
Long-acting parenteral dosage forms—
  Fluphenazine decanoate injection—Antipsychotic effects usually begin between 24 and 72 hours after administration and become significant within 48 to 96 hours.
  Pipotiazine palmitate injection—Antipsychotic effects usually begin within the first 48 to 72 hours after administration and become significant within 1 week.

**Time to peak effect**
Antipsychotic effect—Approximately 4 to 7 days to achieve steady-state plasma concentrations; peak therapeutic effects may take from 6 weeks to 6 months.
Analgesic effect (methotrimeprazine)—Within 20 to 40 minutes after intramuscular injection, maintained for about 4 hours.

**Elimination**
Primarily renal; biliary.
In dialysis—Phenothiazines are not successfully dialyzed because of their high protein binding.

# Precautions to Consider

### Cross-sensitivity and/or related problems
Patients sensitive to one phenothiazine may be sensitive to other phenothiazines also.

### Tumorigenicity
Antipsychotic medications produce an elevation in prolactin concentrations, which persists during chronic administration. Tissue culture experiments indicate that approximately one-third of human breast cancers are prolactin-dependent *in vitro*, a factor of potential importance if the prescription of these medications is contemplated in a patient with a previously detected breast cancer. Although disturbances such as galactorrhea, amenorrhea, gynecomastia, and impotence have been reported, the clinical significance of elevated serum prolactin concentrations is unknown for most patients. An increase in mammary neoplasms has been found in rodents after chronic administration of antipsychotic medications. However, neither clinical studies nor epidemiologic studies conducted to date have shown an association between chronic administration of these medications and mammary tumorigenesis; the available evidence is considered too limited to be conclusive at this time.

### Pregnancy/Reproduction
Fertility—Phenothiazines have been found to depress spermatogenesis in animals at doses greatly exceeding the human dose.

Pregnancy—Although adequate and well-controlled studies in humans have not been done, there have been reports of prolonged jaundice, hypo- or hyperreflexia, and extrapyramidal effects in the neonates of mothers who received phenothiazines near term. Phenothiazines are not recommended for use during pregnancy.
For chlorpromazine: Chlorpromazine crosses the placenta. Reproductive studies in rodents have shown a potential for embryotoxicity, increased neonatal mortality and decreased performance. The possibility of permanent neurological damage in offspring of rodent mothers cannot be excluded.
For methotrimeprazine: Reproductive studies in animals and clinical experience have failed to show a teratogenic effect. However, a possible antifertility effect has been suggested since successive generations of animals administered methotrimeprazine have shown smaller litter sizes than those of controls.
For thioridazine: Reproductive studies in animals and clinical experience have failed to show a teratogenic effect.
For trifluoperazine: Reproductive studies in rats given 600 times the human dose showed an increased incidence of malformations and reduced weight and litter size linked to maternal toxicity.

### Breast-feeding
Phenothiazines are distributed into breast milk, possibly causing drowsiness and an increased risk of dystonias and tardive dyskinesia in the baby. Most phenothiazines increase prolactin secretion in the mother.

### Pediatrics
Children appear to be prone to develop neuromuscular or extrapyramidal reactions, especially dystonias, and should be closely monitored while receiving therapeutic doses of phenothiazines. Children with acute illnesses, such as chickenpox, CNS infections, measles, gastroenteritis, or dehydration, are especially at risk.

### Geriatrics
Geriatric patients tend to develop higher plasma concentrations of phenothiazines because of changes in distribution due to decreases in lean body mass, total body water, and albumin, and often an increase in total body fat composition. Therefore, these patients usually require lower initial dosage and a more gradual titration of dose.
Elderly patients appear to be more prone to orthostatic hypotension and exhibit an increased sensitivity to the anticholinergic and sedative effects of phenothiazines. In addition, they are more prone to develop extrapyramidal side effects, such as tardive dyskinesia and parkinsonism. The symptoms of tardive dyskinesia are persistent, difficult to control, and, in some patients, appear to be irreversible. There is no known effective treatment. Careful observation during treatment for early signs of tardive dyskinesia and reduction of dosage or discontinuation of medication may prevent a more severe manifestation of the syndrome.
It has been suggested that elderly patients receive half the usual adult dose. Patients with organic brain syndrome or acute confusional states, should initially receive one-third to one-half the usual adult dose, with the dose being increased no more frequently than every 2 or 3 days, preferably at intervals of 7 to 10 days, if possible. After clinical improvement occurs, periodic attempts should be made to discontinue medication.

### Dental
The peripheral anticholinergic effects of phenothiazines may decrease or inhibit salivary flow, especially in middle-aged or elderly patients, thus contributing to the development of caries, periodontal disease, oral candidiasis, and discomfort.
Extrapyramidal reactions induced by phenothiazines will result in increased motor activity of the head, face, and neck. Occlusal adjustments, bite registrations, and treatment for bruxism may be made less reliable.
The leukopenic and thrombocytopenic effects of phenothiazines may result in an increased incidence of microbial infection, delayed healing, and gingival bleeding. If leukopenia or thrombocytopenia occurs, dental work should be deferred until blood counts have returned to normal, and patients should be instructed in proper oral hygiene, including caution in use of regular toothbrushes, dental floss, and toothpicks.

### Drug interactions and/or related problems
The following drug interactions and/or related problems have been selected on the basis of their potential clinical significance (possible mechanism in parentheses where appropriate)—not necessarily inclusive (» = major clinical significance):
Note: Combinations containing any of the following medications, depending on the amount present, may also interact with this medication.
» Alcohol or
» CNS depression–producing medications other, (See *Appendix II*) (concurrent use with phenothiazines may result in increased CNS and respiratory depression and increased hypotensive effects; dosage reductions of either drug may be necessary during concurrent use or when sequence of use enhances CNS effects)

(alcohol may increase the risk of heat stroke when taken concurrently with phenothiazines)

(in addition, barbiturates increase the metabolism of chlorpromazine by induction of hepatic microsomal enzymes, thus decreasing plasma concentrations, and possibly the therapeutic effect, of chlorpromazine; conversely, thioridazine may reduce serum phenobarbital concentrations)

Amantadine or
Antidyskinetics or
Antihistamines or
Anticholinergics or other medications with anticholinergic action (See *Appendix II*)

(concurrent use with phenothiazines may intensify anticholinergic side effects, especially confusion, hallucinations, and nightmares, because of the phenothiazines' secondary anticholinergic effects; medications with anticholinergic effects may potentiate the hyperpyretic effect of phenothiazines, especially when environmental temperatures are high, by preventing sweating as a cooling mechanism; this effect could lead to heat stroke; also, patients should be advised to report occurrence of gastrointestinal problems since paralytic ileus may occur with concurrent therapy)

(trihexyphenidyl may decrease plasma phenothiazine concentrations by decreasing gastrointestinal motility and increasing metabolism of the phenothiazine; since the antipsychotic effectiveness may be reduced, dosage adjustment of the phenothiazine may be required)

(parenteral methotrimeprazine, used as preanesthetic medication, may be administered concurrently, but with caution, with lowered doses of atropine or scopolamine; tachycardia and a fall in blood pressure may occur, and CNS reactions, such as stimulation, delirium, and extrapyramidal reactions, may be aggravated)

Amphetamines
(stimulant effects may be decreased when amphetamines are used concurrently with phenothiazines since phenothiazines produce alpha-adrenergic blockade; also, the antipsychotic effectiveness of phenothiazines may be reduced)

Antacids, aluminum- or magnesium-containing or
Antidiarrheals, adsorbent
(concurrent use of these medications with phenothiazines may inhibit the absorption of orally administered phenothiazines, especially chlorpromazine; simultaneous use should be avoided)

Anticonvulsants, including barbiturates
(phenothiazines may lower the seizure threshold; dosage adjustment of anticonvulsant medications may be necessary)

(phenothiazines may inhibit phenytoin metabolism, leading to phenytoin toxicity)

» Antidepressants, tricyclic or
Maprotiline or
Monoamine oxidase (MAO) inhibitors, including furazolidone, procarbazine, and selegiline
(concurrent use may prolong and intensify the sedative and anticholinergic effects of either these medications or phenothiazines; phenothiazines may increase plasma concentrations of cyclic antidepressants by inhibiting metabolism; conversely, cyclic antidepressants may inhibit phenothiazine metabolism; also, the risk of neuroleptic malignant syndrome [NMS] may be increased)

» Antithyroid agents
(concurrent use with phenothiazines may increase the risk of agranulocytosis)

Apomorphine
(prior ingestion of phenothiazine antiemetics may decrease the emetic response to apomorphine; also, the CNS depressant effects of phenothiazine antiemetics are additive to those of apomorphine and may induce dangerous respiratory depression, circulatory system effects, or prolonged sleep)

Appetite suppressants
(concurrent use with phenothiazines may antagonize the anorectic effect of appetite suppressants, with the exception of fenfluramine and phenmetrazine)

Beta-adrenergic blocking agents
(concurrent use of beta-blockers, possibly including ophthalmics, with phenothiazines may result in an increased plasma concentration of each medication because of inhibition of metabolism; this may result in additive hypotensive effects, irreversible retinopathy, cardiac arrhythmias, and tardive dyskinesia)

Bromocriptine
(concurrent use may increase serum prolactin concentrations and interfere with effects of bromocriptine; dosage adjustments may be necessary)

Cimetidine
(concurrent use may decrease steady-state chlorpromazine concentrations by impairing its gastrointestinal absorption)

Diuretics, thiazide
(concurrent use may potentiate hyponatremia and water intoxication; alternate methods of hypertension control should be considered)

Dopamine
(concurrent use may antagonize the peripheral vasoconstriction produced by high doses of dopamine, because of the alpha-adrenergic blocking action of phenothiazines)

Ephedrine
(concurrent use with phenothiazines may decrease the pressor response to ephedrine)

» Epinephrine
(the use of epinephrine to treat phenothiazine-induced hypotension should be avoided because the alpha-adrenergic effects of epinephrine may be blocked, resulting in beta stimulation only and causing severe hypotension and tachycardia)

» Extrapyramidal reaction–causing medications, other (See *Appendix II*)
(concurrent use with phenothiazines may increase the severity and frequency of extrapyramidal effects)

Hepatotoxic medications, other (See *Appendix II*)
(concurrent use of phenothiazines with medications known to alter hepatic microsomal enzyme activity may result in an increased incidence of hepatotoxicity; patients, especially those on prolonged administration or with a history of liver disease, should be carefully monitored)

» Hypotension–producing medications, other (See *Appendix II*)
(concurrent use with phenothiazines may produce severe hypotension with postural syncope)

» Levodopa
(antiparkinsonian effects of levodopa may be inhibited when it is used concurrently with phenothiazines, because of blockade of dopamine receptors in brain; levodopa has not been shown to be effective in the treatment of phenothiazine-induced parkinsonism)

» Lithium
(concurrent use with chlorpromazine and possibly other phenothiazines may reduce gastrointestinal absorption of the phenothiazine, thereby decreasing its serum concentrations by as much as 40%; concurrent use may increase rate of renal excretion of lithium; extrapyramidal symptoms may be increased; also, nausea and vomiting, early indications of lithium toxicity, may be masked by the antiemetic effect of some phenothiazines)

Metaraminol
(concurrent use with phenothiazines usually decreases, but does not reverse or completely block, the pressor effect of metaraminol because of the alpha-adrenergic blocking action of phenothiazines)

Mephentermine
(concurrent use with phenothiazines, especially chlorpromazine, may antagonize the antipsychotic effect of the phenothiazine or the pressor effect of mephentermine by exerting opposing effects on monoaminergic functions in the central and peripheral nervous systems)

Methoxamine
(prior administration of phenothiazines may decrease the pressor effect and shorten the duration of action of methoxamine, because of the alpha-adrenergic blocking action of phenothiazines)

» Metrizamide
(concurrent use with phenothiazines may lower the seizure threshold; phenothiazines should be discontinued at least 48 hours before, and not resumed for at least 24 hours following, myelography)

Ototoxic medications, especially ototoxic antibiotics (See *Appendix II*)
(concurrent use with phenothiazines may mask some symptoms of ototoxicity such as tinnitus, dizziness, or vertigo)

Opioid (narcotic) analgesics
(in addition to increased CNS and respiratory depression, concurrent use with phenothiazines increases orthostatic hypotension and increases the risk of severe constipation, which may lead to paralytic ileus, and/or urinary retention)

Phenylephrine
(prior administration of phenothiazines may decrease the pressor effect and shorten the duration of action of phenylephrine)

Photosensitizing medications, other
(concurrent use with phenothiazines may cause additive photosensitizing effects)
(in addition, concurrent use of systemic methoxsalen, trioxsalen, or tetracyclines with phenothiazines may potentiate intraocular photochemical damage to the choroid, retina, or lens)

Probucol
(additive QT interval prolongation may increase the risk of ventricular tachycardia)

Succinylcholine
(concurrent use with methotrimeprazine may cause tachycardia and a fall in blood pressure, CNS stimulation and delirium, and an aggravation of extrapyramidal effects)

**Laboratory value alterations**
The following have been selected on the basis of their potential clinical significance (possible effect in parentheses where appropriate)—not necessarily inclusive (» = major clinical significance):

With diagnostic test results
Bilirubin tests, urine
(phenothiazine use may produce false-positive results)

Electrocardiogram (ECG) readings
(may cause Q- and T-wave changes, such as increased QT intervals, ST depression, and changes in AV conduction; these are usually reversible)

Gonadorelin test
(phenothiazines may blunt the response to gonadorelin by increasing serum prolactin concentrations)

Pregnancy tests, immunologic urine
(phenothiazines may produce false-positive or false-negative results, depending on the test used)

Metyrapone tests
(adrenocorticotropic hormone [ACTH] secretion may be reduced)

**Medical considerations/Contraindications**
The medical considerations/contraindications included have been selected on the basis of their potential clinical significance (reasons given in parentheses where appropriate)—not necessarily inclusive (» = major clinical significance).

*Except under special circumstances, this medicine should not be used when the following medical problems exist:*
» Cardiovascular disease, severe or
» CNS depression, severe or
» Comatose states
(may be exacerbated)

*Risk-benefit should be considered when the following medical problems exist:*
» Alcoholism, active
(CNS depression may be potentiated; risk of heat stroke may be increased; chronic alcohol abusers may be predisposed to hepatotoxic reactions during phenothiazine therapy)

Angina pectoris
(pain may be increased with use of trifluoperazine)

» Blood dyscrasias
(may be exacerbated; treatment may have to be discontinued)

Breast cancer
(potentially higher risk of disease progression and possible increased resistance to endocrine and cytotoxic treatment, due to phenothiazine-induced prolactin secretion)

Cardiovascular disease
(increased risk of hypotension; myocardial depression, cardiomegaly, congestive heart failure [CHF], and arrhythmias may be induced)

Glaucoma, or predisposition to
(may be potentiated)

» Hepatic function impairment
(metabolism may be decreased; higher serum phenothiazine concentrations may increase sensitivity to CNS effects)

Parkinson's disease
(potentiation of extrapyramidal effects)

Peptic ulcer or
Urinary retention
(may be exacerbated)

Prostatic hypertrophy, symptomatic
(increased risk of urinary retention)

Respiratory disorders, chronic, especially in children
(may be potentiated)

» Reye's syndrome
(increased risk of hepatotoxicity in children and adolescents whose signs and symptoms suggest Reye's syndrome)

Seizure disorders
(seizures may be precipitated)

Sensitivity to any phenothiazine
(may be potentiated upon re-exposure to any phenothiazine in patients with a history of phenothiazine-induced blood dyscrasias, jaundice, or skin reactions)

Vomiting
(antiemetic action of phenothiazines may mask vomiting caused by overdose of other medications)

Caution should also be used in geriatric, emaciated, and debilitated patients, who usually require a lower initial dose.

**Patient monitoring**
The following may be especially important in patient monitoring (other tests may be warranted in some patients, depending on condition; » = major clinical significance):

Abnormal-movement determinations
(recommended every 2 months during therapy for institutionalized patients, using the abnormal involuntary movement scale [AIMS], and again at 8 to 12 weeks after therapy has been discontinued)

Blood cell counts and differential in patients with sore throat and fever or infections
(may be required during high-dose or prolonged therapy when symptoms of infection develop; agranulocytosis is more likely to occur between the 4th and 10th weeks of therapy; if significant cellular depression occurs, medication should be discontinued and appropriate therapy initiated; rechallenge in recovered patients will usually cause a recurrence of agranulocytosis; use of alternate neuroleptics such as haloperidol or thioxanthenes is recommended)

Blood pressure measurements
(recommended periodically to detect hypotension)

Careful observation for early signs of tardive dyskinesia
(recommended at periodic intervals, especially in the elderly and other patients on high or extended maintenance dosage; since there is no known effective treatment if syndrome should develop, the phenothiazine should be discontinued at earliest signs, usually fine, worm-like movements of the tongue, to stop further development)

Hepatic function determinations and
Urine tests for bilirubin and bile
(may be required at periodic intervals during prolonged therapy, or if jaundice or grippe-like symptoms occur, to detect liver function impairment; these side effects are more likely to occur between the 2nd and 4th weeks of therapy; phenothiazine should be discontinued if bilirubinemia, bilirubinuria, or icterus occurs)

Ophthalmologic examinations
(recommended, if possible, prior to initiation of phenothiazine therapy as a baseline; initial screening should include measurement of visual acuity with and without refraction, a color vision test to detect possible central defects, and, if feasible, a slit-lamp microscopy study of the fundus and examination of the visual fields. Tests may be required at periodic intervals [usually every 6 to 12 months] during high-dose or prolonged therapy, since deposition of particulate matter in the lens and cornea has occurred with some phenothiazines; therapy should be discontinued if corneal, retinal, or lens changes are noticed; blurred vision, defective color vision, and night blindness are early symptoms of pigmentary retinopathy and may be reversible if detected and the phenothiazine discontinued in the early stages)

Phenothiazine concentrations, serum
(determinations recommended when toxicity or poor response occurs, or when noncompliance is suspected)

## Side/Adverse Effects

The following side/adverse effects have been selected on the basis of their potential clinical significance (possible signs and symptoms in parentheses where appropriate)—not necessarily inclusive:

**Those indicating need for medical attention**

Incidence more frequent
*Akathisia* (restlessness or need to keep moving); *blurred vision associated with anticholinergic effect; deposition of opaque material in lens, cornea, and retina* (blurred vision); *dystonic extrapyramidal effects* (muscle spasms of face, neck, and back; tic-like or twitching movements, twisting movements of body; inability to move eyes; weak-

ness of arms and legs); ***parkinsonian extrapyramidal effects*** (difficulty in speaking or swallowing; loss of balance control; mask-like face; shuffling walk; stiffness of arms or legs; trembling and shaking of hands and fingers); ***hypotension*** (fainting)—less common with the piperazine phenothiazines; ***pigmentary retinopathy*** (blurred vision; defective color vision; difficulty seeing at night)—more frequent with high doses of thioridazine; ***tardive dyskinesia*** (lip smacking or puckering; puffing of cheeks; rapid or worm-like movements of tongue; uncontrolled chewing movements; uncontrolled movements of arms and legs)—more frequent in elderly patients, women, and patients with brain damage

Note: *Parkinsonian* effects are more frequent in the elderly, whereas *dystonias* occur more often in younger patients. Symptoms may be seen in the first few days of treatment or after prolonged treatment, and can recur after even a single dose. The effects are more common with the piperazine phenothiazines.

Incidence less frequent
 ***Difficulty in urinating; increased sensitivity of skin to sun*** (rash; severe sunburn); ***skin rash***—associated with contact dermatitis (with liquid products), or other allergic reaction, or cholestatic jaundice

Incidence rare
 ***Agranulocytosis*** (sore throat; fever; unusual bleeding or bruising; unusual tiredness or weakness)—more frequent with aliphatic phenothiazines; ***cholestatic jaundice*** (abdominal or stomach pains; aching muscles and joints; fever and chills; severe skin itching; yellow eyes or skin; fatigue; nausea, vomiting, or diarrhea); ***heat stroke*** (hot dry skin; inability to sweat; muscle weakness; confusion); ***neuroleptic malignant syndrome (NMS)*** (convulsions; difficult or fast breathing; fast heartbeat or irregular pulse; fever; high or low [irregular] blood pressure; increased sweating; loss of bladder control; severe muscle stiffness; unusually pale skin; unusual tiredness or weakness); ***priapism*** (prolonged, painful, inappropriate penile erection); ***melanosis*** (tanning or blue-gray discoloration of skin)—more common with long-term, high-dose, low-potency chlorpromazine and thioridazine

Note: *Agranulocytosis* can develop within the first 3 months of treatment, with recovery within 1 to 2 weeks after medication is discontinued; may recur upon rechallenge in recovered patients.

Liver function tests may be abnormal without overt jaundice. *Jaundice* may appear about 2 weeks after severe pruritus and may progress to chronic active hepatitis. Discontinuing medication may be necessary.

*Heat stroke*, caused by phenothiazine-induced suppression of central and peripheral temperature regulation in the hypothalamus, may occur in environmental conditions of high heat and high humidity. The effectiveness of sweating as a cooling mechanism may be reduced by humid conditions and by the *anticholinergic effects* of phenothiazines or their combination with other anticholinergic medications such as nonprescription cold medications or antihistamines. Adequate interior temperature control (air-conditioning) must be maintained for institutionalized patients during hot weather because of the increased risk of *heat stroke* and *neuroleptic malignant syndrome (NMS)*. Patients should be advised to avoid exertion, stay in cool areas, and avoid dehydration and other anticholinergic medications. Phenothiazines may also cause hypothermia in cold weather, since the disruption of the thermoregulatory mechanisms results in a poikilothermic state.

*NMS* may occur at any time during neuroleptic therapy and is potentially fatal. It is more commonly seen soon after start of therapy or after patient has switched from one neuroleptic to another, during combined therapy with another psychotropic medication, or after a dosage increase. Along with the overt signs of skeletal muscle rigidity, hyperthermia, autonomic dysfunction, and altered consciousness, differential diagnosis may reveal leukocytosis (9500 to 26,000 cells per cubic millimeter), elevated liver enzyme tests, and elevated creatine phosphokinase (CPK).

**Those indicating need for medical attention only if they continue or are bothersome**
Incidence more frequent
 ***Anticholinergic effects*** (constipation; decreased sweating; dizziness [orthostatic hypotension]; drowsiness; dry mouth)—less frequent with piperazine phenothiazines; ***nasal congestion***

Incidence less frequent
 ***Changes in menstrual period; decreased sexual ability; secretion of milk, unusual; swelling or pain in breasts; weight gain, unusual***

**Those indicating need for medical attention if they occur after the medication is discontinued**
Incidence more frequent
 ***Tardive dyskinesia, persistent*** (lip smacking or puckering; puffing of cheeks; rapid or worm-like movements of tongue; uncontrolled chewing movements; uncontrolled movements of arms and legs)—more frequent in elderly patients, women, and patients with brain damage

Incidence less frequent
 ***Dizziness; nausea and vomiting; stomach pain; trembling of fingers and hands***

## Overdose

For specific information on the agents used in the management of phenothiazine overdose, see:
 *Benztropine* in *Antidyskinetics (Systemic)* monograph;
 *Charcoal, Activated (Oral-Local)* monograph;
 *Diazepam* in *Benzodiazepines (Systemic)* monograph;
 *Digitalis Glycosides (Systemic)* monograph;
 *Diphenhydramine* in *Antihistamines (Systemic)* monograph;
 *Norepinephrine* and/or *Phenylephrine* in *Sympathomimetic Agents—Cardiovascular Use (Parenteral-Systemic)* monograph; and/or
 *Phenytoin* in *Anticonvulsants, Hydantoin (Systemic)* monograph.

For more information on the management of overdose or unintentional ingestion, **contact a Poison Control Center** (see *Poison Control Center Listing*).

**Treatment of overdose**
Treatment is essentially symptomatic and supportive. The following may be considered:
 To decrease absorption—
  Attempting early gastric lavage; avoiding induction of vomiting because potential phenothiazine-induced dystonic reactions of the head and neck may result in aspiration of vomitus.
  Administering activated charcoal slurry.
  Administering saline cathartic.
 Specific treatment—
  Controlling cardiac arrhythmias with intravenous phenytoin, 9 to 11 mg per kg of body weight (mg/kg).
  Digitalizing for cardiac failure.
  Administering vasopressor such as norepinephrine or phenylephrine for hypotension (not using epinephrine, because it may cause paradoxical hypotension).
  Controlling convulsions with diazepam followed by phenytoin, 15 mg/kg, while monitoring ECG.
  Administering benztropine or diphenhydramine to manage acute, parkinson-like symptoms that may occur.
 Monitoring—
  Monitoring cardiovascular function for not less than 5 days.
 Supportive care—
  Maintaining respiratory function.
  Maintaining body temperature.
  Patients in whom intentional overdose is known or suspected should be referred for psychiatric consultation.

Note: Dialysis of phenothiazines has not been successful.

## Patient Consultation

As an aid to patient consultation, refer to *Advice for the Patient, Phenothiazines (Systemic)*.

In providing consultation, consider emphasizing the following selected information (» = major clinical significance):

**Before using this medication**
» Conditions affecting use, especially:
  Sensitivity to any phenothiazine
  Pregnancy—Not recommended for use during pregnancy because of reports of jaundice, hypo- or hyperreflexia, and extrapyramidal symptoms in neonates
  Breast-feeding—Distributed into breast milk; may cause drowsiness, dystonias, and tardive dyskinesia in the baby
  Use in children—Children, especially those with acute illnesses, are more prone to extrapyramidal symptoms
  Use in the elderly—Elderly patients are more likely to develop extrapyramidal, anticholinergic, hypotensive, and sedative effects; reduced dosage recommended
  Dental—Phenothiazine-induced blood dyscrasias may result in infections, delayed healing, and bleeding; dry mouth may cause caries and candidiasis; increased motor activity of face, head, and neck may interfere with some dental procedures
  Other medications, especially alcohol, other CNS depression-producing medications, tricyclic antidepressants, antithyroid agents, epinephrine, other hypotension-producing medications,

other extrapyramidal-producing medications, levodopa, lithium, or metrizamide

Other medical problems, especially cardiovascular disease, severe CNS depression, active alcoholism, blood dyscrasias, liver disease, or Reye's syndrome

**Proper use of this medication**
*Proper administration of this medication*
*For oral dosage forms*
Taking with food, milk, or water to reduce stomach irritation
» Diluting medication that comes in dropper bottle with recommended beverages prior to use
Swallowing the extended-release dosage form whole
*For rectal dosage forms*
Chilling suppository if too soft to insert
How to insert suppository
» Compliance with therapy; not taking more or less medication than prescribed
» Several weeks of therapy may be required to produce desired effects in treatment of nervous, mental, or emotional conditions
» Proper dosing
Missed dose: When dosing schedule is—
One dose a day: Taking as soon as possible unless almost time for next dose, then going back to regular dosing schedule; not doubling doses
More than one dose a day: Taking as soon as possible if within an hour or so of missed dose; skipping missed dose if not remembered until later; going back to regular dosing schedule; not doubling doses
» Proper storage

**Precautions while using this medication**
Regular visits to physician to check progress of therapy
» Checking with physician before discontinuing medication; gradual dosage reduction may be needed
Avoiding use of antacids or antidiarrheal medication within 2 hours of taking phenothiazine
» Avoiding use of alcoholic beverages or other CNS depressants during therapy
Avoiding the use of over-the-counter medications for colds or allergies, to prevent increased anticholinergic effects and risk of heat stroke
Caution if any laboratory tests required; possible interference with ECG readings, and with gonadorelin, immunologic urine pregnancy, metyrapone, and urine bilirubin test results
» Caution if any kind of surgery, dental treatment, or emergency treatment is required; telling physician or dentist in charge about phenothiazine because of possible drug interactions or blood dyscrasias
» Possible drowsiness or blurred vision; caution when driving, using machines, or doing other things requiring alertness or accurate vision
» Possible dizziness or lightheadedness (orthostatic hypotension); caution when getting up suddenly from a lying or sitting position
» Possible heat stroke: Caution during exercise, hot weather, or when taking hot baths
Possible hypothermia: Caution during prolonged exposure to cold
» Possible dryness of mouth; using sugarless gum or candy, ice, or saliva substitute for relief; checking with physician or dentist if dry mouth continues for more than 2 weeks
» Possible skin photosensitivity; avoiding unprotected exposure to sun; using protective clothing; using a sun block product that includes protection against both UVA-caused photosensitivity reactions and UVB-caused sunburn reactions; avoiding use of sunlamp, tanning bed, or tanning booth
» Possible eye photosensitivity; wearing sunglasses that block ultraviolet light
» Avoiding spilling liquid dosage form on skin or clothing; may cause skin irritation
» Observing precautions for up to 12 weeks with long-acting parenteral forms

**Side/adverse effects**
Side effects more likely to occur in the elderly
Signs of potential side effects, especially tardive dyskinesia, dystonias, parkinsonian effects, anticholinergic effects, blurred vision, possible pigmentary retinopathy, allergic skin reactions, photosensitivity, agranulocytosis, cholestatic jaundice, heat stroke, neuroleptic malignant syndrome, priapism, melanosis, dryness of mouth, orthostatic hypotension, or akathisia
» Stopping medication and notifying physician immediately if symptoms of neuroleptic malignant syndrome (NMS) appear, especially muscle rigidity, fever, difficult or fast breathing, seizures, fast heartbeat, increased sweating, loss of bladder control, unusually pale skin, unusual tiredness or weakness

» Notifying physician immediately if early symptoms of tardive dyskinesia appear, such as fine worm-like movements of the tongue or other uncontrolled movements of the mouth, tongue, jaw, or arms and legs; dosage adjustment or discontinuation may be needed to prevent irreversibility
Possibility of withdrawal symptoms

## General Dosing Information

Dosage must be individualized by titration from the lower dose range. After a favorable psychiatric response is noted (within several days to several months), that dosage should be continued for about 2 weeks, then gradually decreased to the lowest level that will maintain an adequate clinical response.

When extended therapy is discontinued, a gradual reduction in phenothiazine dosage over several weeks is recommended, since abrupt withdrawal may cause some patients on high or long-term dosage to experience transient dyskinetic signs, nausea, vomiting, gastritis, trembling, and dizziness.

The antiemetic effect of some phenothiazines may mask signs of drug toxicity or obscure diagnosis of conditions whose primary symptom is nausea. Phenothiazines have no antiemetic effect when nausea is a result of vestibular stimulation or local gastrointestinal irritation.

Antidyskinetic agents such as trihexyphenidyl or benztropine may be used concurrently to control phenothiazine-induced extrapyramidal symptoms. They should be used only when required (not prophylactically), and, generally, are only needed for a few weeks to two or three months.

Avoid skin contact with liquid forms of phenothiazine medication; contact dermatitis has resulted.

**For parenteral dosage forms only**
Because hypotension is a possible side effect of phenothiazines, parenteral administration should be used only in patients who are bedfast or for appropriate acute therapy in ambulatory patients who can be closely monitored. A possible exception may be those patients who are dose-stabilized on the extended-action injectable forms.

Intramuscular injections should be administered slowly and deeply into the upper outer quadrant of the buttock. Patient should remain lying down for at least ½ hour after injection to avoid possible hypotensive effects.

To prevent irritation or sterile abscesses at the site of intramuscular injection, rotation of the injection sites, dilution of the phenothiazine injection with sodium chloride injection, and/or addition of 2% procaine are recommended.

Effects of the extended-action injectable forms may last for up to 12 weeks in some patients. The side effects information and precautions apply during this period of time.

The dose of the extended-action injectable forms should *not* be increased to prolong the dosing interval. Each patient must be carefully supervised to determine the optimal dosing interval and lowest effective dose, depending on patient's response, age, physical condition, symptoms, severity of illness, and drug history.

Geriatric and pediatric patients, especially those acutely ill or dehydrated, should be monitored very carefully during parenteral therapy because of a higher incidence of hypotensive and extrapyramidal reactions in these age groups.

**Diet/Nutrition**
The oral dosage forms of this medication may be taken with food or a full glass (240 mL) of water or milk, if necessary, to lessen stomach irritation.

Requirements for riboflavin may be increased in patients receiving phenothiazines.

**For treatment of adverse effects**
Neuroleptic malignant syndrome (NMS)—
Treatment is essentially symptomatic and supportive and may include the following
• *Discontinuing phenothiazine immediately.*
• Hyperthermia—Administering antipyretics (aspirin or acetaminophen); using cooling blanket.
• Dehydration—Restoring fluids and electrolytes.
• Cardiovascular instability—Monitoring blood pressure and cardiac rhythm closely. Use of sodium nitroprusside may allow vasodilation with subsequent heat loss from the skin in patients with less dominant muscle rigidity.
• Hypoxia—Administering oxygen; considering airway insertion and assisted ventilation.
• Muscle rigidity—Administering dantrolene sodium (100 to 300 mg per day in divided doses or 1.25 to 1.5 mg/kg, intravenously) for muscle relaxation; or administering amantadine (100 mg twice daily) or bromocriptine (5 mg three times a day)

to restore central balance of dopamine and acetylcholine at the receptor site.
- If neuroleptics must be continued because of severe psychosis, rechallenge should consist of:
  —at least five days of neuroleptic abstinence before rechallenge.
  —a low-potency neuroleptic.
  —a neuroleptic of a different class from the one causing NMS.
  —a low dose.
  —using a neuroleptic only for controlling the psychosis.
  —avoiding parenteral and extended-action dosage forms.

Parkinsonism—
Treatment may include:
- Reducing the antipsychotic dosage, if possible, for treatment of milder effects.
- Administering oral antiparkinsonian agents (of the anticholinergic type) such as trihexyphenidyl, 2 mg three times per day, or benztropine for treatment of more severe parkinsonism and acute motor restlessness; using sparingly, only when side effects appear, and then usually for no longer than 3 months. Observing caution to prevent hyperpyrexia with concomitant use of phenothiazines and other medications with anticholinergic action.
- In the elderly patient, using amantadine, 100 to 200 mg at bedtime, to minimize severe anticholinergic effects that may occur with other antidyskinetics.
- Levodopa is *not* useful in the treatment of phenothiazine-induced parkinsonism because the dopamine receptors are blocked by the phenothiazine.

Restlessness (akathisia)—
May respond to antiparkinsonian drugs or propranolol, 30 to 80 mg per day; nadolol, 40 mg per day; or diazepam, 2 mg two or three times a day, but often requires dosage reduction of the phenothiazine or substitution of a less potent neuroleptic.

Dystonia—
Acute dystonic postures or oculogyric crisis may be relieved by parenteral administration of benztropine, 2 mg intramuscularly or intravenously; diphenhydramine, 50 mg intramuscularly; or diazepam, 5 to 7.5 mg intravenously, to be followed by oral antidyskinetic medication for one or two days to prevent recurrent dystonic episodes. Dosage adjustments of the phenothiazine may control these effects, and discontinuation of the phenothiazine may reverse severe symptoms.

Tardive dyskinesia—
No known effective treatment. Dosage of phenothiazine should be lowered or medication discontinued at earliest signs of tardive dyskinesia to prevent irreversible effects.

Pruritus associated with cholestasis—
- Topical treatment may include:
  —Topical adrenocorticoids combined with cool-water compresses, aluminum acetate solution, or calamine lotion.
  —For widespread itching, baths containing colloidal oatmeal or baking soda (2 cups per tubful).
  —For severe itching, topical anesthetics containing 20% benzocaine or 5% lidocaine; however, itching may be relieved for only 30 to 60 minutes.
- Oral treatment may include:
  —Initially, diphenhydramine, cyproheptadine, or hydroxyzine.
  —Bile acid sequestrants or cholestyramine, but only when topical and oral antipruritic agents fail to control symptoms.
  —Supplementation with fat-soluble vitamins (A, D, E, K) for patients with protracted jaundice.
  —Resuming therapy with a nonphenothiazine neuroleptic, such as loxapine, thioxanthenes, and molindone.

---

## ACETOPHENAZINE

## Summary of Differences
Pharmacology/pharmacokinetics:
  Chemical Group—
    Piperazine
  Actions—
    Antiemetic: Weak
    Anticholinergic: Weak
    Extrapyramidal: Moderate
    Hypotensive: Weak
    Sedative: Moderate

## Oral Dosage Forms

### ACETOPHENAZINE MALEATE TABLETS USP

**Usual adult and adolescent dose**
Psychotic disorders—
  Oral, 20 mg three times a day, the dosage being adjusted as needed and tolerated.

Note: Geriatric, emaciated, or debilitated patients usually require a lower initial dose, the dosage being gradually increased as needed and tolerated.

**Usual adult prescribing limits**
Up to 120 mg a day.

**Usual pediatric dose**
Psychotic disorders—
  Children up to 12 years of age: Dosage has not been established.
  Children 12 years of age and over: See *Usual adult and adolescent dose*.

**Strength(s) usually available**
U.S.—
  20 mg (Rx) [*Tindal*].
Canada—
  Not commercially available.

**Packaging and storage**
Store below 40 °C (104 °F), preferably between 15 and 30 °C (59 and 86 °F), unless otherwise specified by manufacturer. Store in a tight, light-resistant container.

**Auxiliary labeling**
- May cause drowsiness.
- Avoid alcoholic beverages.

---

## CHLORPROMAZINE

## Summary of Differences
Category:
  Includes antiemetic and antidyskinetic (Huntington's disease) uses.
Pharmacology/pharmacokinetics:
  Chemical group—
    Aliphatic
  Actions—
    Antiemetic: Strong
    Anticholinergic: Moderate to strong
    Extrapyramidal: Weak to moderate
    Hypotensive: Strong
    Sedative: Strong

## Additional Dosing Information
See also *General Dosing Information*.

For intractable hiccups, chlorpromazine is initially administered orally. If symptoms persist for 2 or 3 days, intramuscular administration is indicated, followed by slow intravenous infusion if hiccups continue.

*For parenteral use*
Chlorpromazine injection must not be administered subcutaneously, because it causes severe tissue necrosis.
For intramuscular injection, diluting chlorpromazine injection with sodium chloride injection and/or adding 2% procaine may prevent irritation at the injection site.
The intravenous route of administration is used only for severe hiccups, surgery, and tetanus.
Before intravenous injection, chlorpromazine hydrochloride injection should be diluted with sodium chloride injection.
Close monitoring of blood pressure for hypotension is necessary during parenteral administration.

## Oral Dosage Forms

Note: The dosing and strengths of the dosage forms available are expressed in terms of chlorpromazine base (not the hydrochloride salt).

### CHLORPROMAZINE HYDROCHLORIDE EXTENDED-RELEASE CAPSULES

**Usual adult and adolescent dose**
Psychotic disorders—
  Oral, 30 to 300 mg (base) one to three times a day, the dosage being adjusted as needed and tolerated.

Note: Geriatric, emaciated, or debilitated patients usually require a lower initial dose, the dosage being gradually increased as needed and tolerated.

The 300-mg extended-release capsules are used only in severe neuropsychiatric conditions.

### Usual adult prescribing limits
Up to 1 gram (base) a day.

Note: Although doses are sometimes gradually increased to 2 grams a day or more for short periods, 1 gram or less is usually sufficient for extended therapy.

### Usual pediatric dose
The extended-release dosage form is not recommended for use in children.

### Strength(s) usually available
U.S.—
- 30 mg (base) (Rx) [*Thorazine Spansule* (benzyl alcohol; calcium sulfate; cetylpyridinium chloride; FD&C Yellow No. 6; gelatin; glyceryl distearate; glyceryl monostearate; iron oxide; povidone; silicon dioxide; sodium lauryl sulfate; starch; sucrose; titanium dioxide; wax)].
- 75 mg (base) (Rx) [*Thorazine Spansule* (benzyl alcohol; calcium sulfate; cetylpyridinium chloride; FD&C Yellow No. 6; gelatin; glyceryl distearate; glyceryl monostearate; iron oxide; povidone; silicon dioxide; sodium lauryl sulfate; starch; sucrose; titanium dioxide; wax)].
- 150 mg (base) (Rx) [*Thorazine Spansule* (benzyl alcohol; calcium sulfate; cetylpyridinium chloride; FD&C Yellow No. 6; gelatin; glyceryl distearate; glyceryl monostearate; iron oxide; povidone; silicon dioxide; sodium lauryl sulfate; starch; sucrose; titanium dioxide; wax)].
- 200 mg (base) (Rx) [*Thorazine Spansule* (benzyl alcohol; calcium sulfate; cetylpyridinium chloride; FD&C Yellow No. 6; gelatin; glyceryl distearate; glyceryl monostearate; iron oxide; povidone; silicon dioxide; sodium lauryl sulfate; starch; sucrose; titanium dioxide; wax)].
- 300 mg (base) (Rx) [*Thorazine Spansule* (benzyl alcohol; calcium sulfate; cetylpyridinium chloride; FD&C Yellow No. 6; gelatin; glyceryl distearate; glyceryl monostearate; iron oxide; povidone; silicon dioxide; sodium lauryl sulfate; starch; sucrose; titanium dioxide; wax)].

Canada—
Not commercially available.

### Packaging and storage
Store below 40 °C (104 °F), preferably between 15 and 30 °C (59 and 86 °F), in a tight, light-resistant container, unless otherwise specified by manufacturer.

### Auxiliary labeling
- May cause drowsiness.
- Avoid alcoholic beverages.

## CHLORPROMAZINE HYDROCHLORIDE ORAL CONCENTRATE USP

### Usual adult and adolescent dose
Psychotic disorders—
Oral, 10 to 25 mg (base) two to four times a day, the dosage being increased by 20 to 50 mg a day every three or four days as needed and tolerated.
Nausea and vomiting—
Oral, 10 to 25 mg (base) every four hours, the dosage being increased as needed and tolerated.
Anxiety, presurgical—
Oral, 25 to 50 mg (base) two to three hours before surgery.
Hiccups or
Porphyria—
Oral, 25 to 50 mg (base) three or four times a day.

Note: Geriatric, emaciated, or debilitated patients usually require a lower initial dose, the dosage being gradually increased as needed and tolerated.

### Usual adult prescribing limits
Up to 1 gram (base) a day.

Note: Although doses are sometimes gradually increased to 2 grams a day or more for short periods, 1 gram or less is usually sufficient for extended therapy.

### Usual pediatric dose
Psychotic disorders or
Nausea and vomiting—
Children up to 6 months of age: Dosage has not been established.
Children 6 months of age and older: Oral, 550 mcg (0.55 mg) (base) per kg of body weight or 15 mg per square meter of body surface every four to six hours, the dosage being adjusted as needed and tolerated.
Anxiety, presurgical—
Oral, 550 mcg (0.55 mg) (base) per kg of body weight or 15 mg per square meter of body surface two or three hours before surgery.

### Strength(s) usually available
U.S.—
- 30 mg (base) per mL (Rx) [*Thorazine Concentrate;* GENERIC].
- 100 mg (base) per mL (Rx) [*Thorazine Concentrate; Thor-Prom;* GENERIC].

Canada—
- 40 mg (base) per mL (Rx) [*Chlorpromanyl-40; Largactil Oral Drops* (alcohol 17.5%)].

### Packaging and storage
Store below 40 °C (104 °F), preferably between 15 and 30 °C (59 and 86 °F), in a tight container, unless otherwise specified by manufacturer. Protect from light. Protect from freezing.

### Stability
A slight yellowing will not alter potency; however, do not use if markedly discolored or if a precipitate is present.

### Auxiliary labeling
- May cause drowsiness.
- Avoid alcoholic beverages.
- Do not spill on skin or clothing.
- Must be diluted before use.

### Note
Avoid skin contact with liquid forms of this medication; contact dermatitis has resulted.

Each dose must be diluted just before administration in a half glass (120 mL) of coffee, tea, milk, tomato or fruit juice, water, soup, or carbonated beverage.

Explain dilution and dosage measurement to patient if self-administered.

## CHLORPROMAZINE HYDROCHLORIDE SYRUP USP

### Usual adult and adolescent dose
Psychotic disorders—
Oral, 10 to 25 mg (base) two to four times a day, the dosage being increased by 20 to 50 mg a day every three or four days as needed and tolerated.
Nausea and vomiting—
Oral, 10 to 25 mg (base) every four hours, the dosage being increased as needed and tolerated.
Anxiety, presurgical—
Oral, 25 to 50 mg (base) two to three hours before surgery.
Hiccups or
Porphyria—
Oral, 25 to 50 mg (base) three or four times a day.

Note: Geriatric, emaciated, or debilitated patients usually require a lower initial dose, the dosage being gradually increased as needed and tolerated.

### Usual adult prescribing limits
Up to 1 gram (base) a day.

Note: Although doses are sometimes gradually increased to 2 grams a day or more for short periods, 1 gram or less is usually sufficient for extended therapy.

### Usual pediatric dose
Psychotic disorders or
Nausea and vomiting—
Children up to 6 months of age: Dosage has not been established.
Children 6 months of age and older: Oral, 550 mcg (0.55 mg) (base) per kg of body weight or 15 mg per square meter of body surface every four to six hours, the dosage being adjusted as needed and tolerated.
Anxiety, presurgical—
Oral, 550 mcg (0.55 mg) (base) per kg of body weight or 15 mg per square meter of body surface two or three hours before surgery.

### Strength(s) usually available
U.S.—
- 10 mg (base) per 5 mL (Rx) [*Thorazine;* GENERIC].

Canada—
- 25 mg (base) per 5 mL (Rx) [*Chlorpromanyl-5; Largactil Liquid* (alcohol 0.5%; sucrose)].
- 100 mg (base) per 5 mL (Rx) [*Chlorpromanyl-20; Largactil Liquid* (alcohol 0.5%; sucrose)].

### Packaging and storage
Store below 40 °C (104 °F), preferably between 15 and 30 °C (59 and 86 °F), unless otherwise specified by manufacturer. Store in a tight, light-resistant container. Protect from freezing.

### Stability
A slight yellowing will not alter potency; however, do not use if markedly discolored or if a precipitate is present.

### Auxiliary labeling
- May cause drowsiness.
- Avoid alcoholic beverages.
- Do not spill on skin or clothing.

### Note
Avoid skin contact with liquid forms of this medication; contact dermatitis has resulted.

## CHLORPROMAZINE HYDROCHLORIDE TABLETS USP

### Usual adult and adolescent dose
Psychotic disorders—
  Oral, 10 to 25 mg (base) two to four times a day, the dosage being increased by 20 to 50 mg a day every three to four days as needed and tolerated.
Nausea and vomiting—
  Oral, 10 to 25 mg (base) every four hours, the dosage being increased as needed and tolerated.
Anxiety, presurgical—
  Oral, 25 to 50 mg (base) two to three hours before surgery.
Hiccups or
Porphyria—
  Oral, 25 to 50 mg (base) three or four times a day.
Note: Geriatric, emaciated, or debilitated patients usually require a lower initial dose, the dosage being gradually increased as needed and tolerated.
  The 100- and 200-mg tablets are for use in severe neuropsychiatric conditions.

### Usual adult prescribing limits
Up to 1 gram (base) a day.
Note: Although doses are sometimes gradually increased to 2 grams a day or more for short periods, 1 gram or less is usually sufficient for extended therapy.

### Usual pediatric dose
Psychotic disorders or
Nausea and vomiting—
  Children up to 6 months of age: Dosage has not been established.
  Children 6 months of age and older: Oral, 550 mcg (0.55 mg) (base) per kg of body weight or 15 mg per square meter of body surface every four to six hours, the dosage being adjusted as needed and tolerated.
Anxiety, presurgical—
  Oral, 550 mcg (0.55 mg) (base) per kg of body weight or 15 mg per square meter of body surface two or three hours before surgery.
Note: Since tablets are not suitable for many pediatric patients' requirements, the oral solution or syrup dosage forms are usually preferred.

### Strength(s) usually available
U.S.—
  10 mg (base) (Rx) [*Thorazine; Thor-Prom;* GENERIC].
  25 mg (base) (Rx) [*Thorazine; Thor-Prom;* GENERIC].
  50 mg (base) (Rx) [*Thorazine; Thor-Prom;* GENERIC].
  100 mg (base) (Rx) [*Thorazine; Thor-Prom;* GENERIC].
  200 mg (base) (Rx) [*Thorazine; Thor-Prom;* GENERIC].
Canada—
  10 mg (base) (Rx) [*Largactil; Novo-Chlorpromazine*].
  25 mg (base) (Rx) [*Largactil; Novo-Chlorpromazine* [GENERIC].
  50 mg (base) (Rx) [*Largactil; Novo-Chlorpromazine* [GENERIC].
  100 mg (base) (Rx) [*Largactil; Novo-Chlorpromazine* [GENERIC].
  200 mg (base) (Rx) [*Largactil; Novo-Chlorpromazine*].

### Packaging and storage
Store below 40 °C (104 °F), preferably between 15 and 30 °C (59 and 86 °F), unless otherwise specified by manufacturer. Store in a well-closed, light-resistant container.

### Auxiliary labeling
- May cause drowsiness.
- Avoid alcoholic beverages.

## Parenteral Dosage Forms

Note: The dosing and strengths of the dosage forms available are expressed in terms of chlorpromazine base (not the hydrochloride salt).

## CHLORPROMAZINE HYDROCHLORIDE INJECTION USP

### Usual adult dose
Psychotic disorders (severe)—
  Intramuscular, 25 to 50 mg (base), the dose being repeated in one hour if needed, and every three to twelve hours thereafter as needed and tolerated. The dosage may be gradually increased over several days as needed and tolerated.
Nausea and vomiting—
  Intramuscular, 25 mg (base) in a single dose, the dosage being increased to 25 to 50 mg every three to four hours as needed and tolerated until vomiting stops.
Nausea and vomiting during surgery—
  Intramuscular: 12.5 mg (base) in a single dose, the dose being repeated in thirty minutes as needed and tolerated.
  Intravenous infusion: Up to 25 mg (base), diluted to a concentration of at least 1 mg per mL of 0.9% sodium chloride injection, administered at a rate of no more than 2 mg every 2 minutes.
Anxiety, presurgical—
  Intramuscular, 12.5 to 25 mg (base) one or two hours before surgery.
Hiccups—
  Intramuscular: 25 to 50 mg (base) three or four times a day.
  Intravenous infusion: 25 to 50 mg (base), diluted in 500 to 1000 mL sodium chloride injection, administered slowly at a rate of 1 mg per minute.
Porphyria—
  Intramuscular, 25 mg (base) every six or eight hours until patient can take oral therapy.
Tetanus—
  Intramuscular: 25 to 50 mg (base) three or four times a day, the dosage being increased gradually as needed and tolerated.
  Intravenous infusion: 25 to 50 mg (base), diluted to a concentration of at least 1 mg per mL with sodium chloride injection, administered at a rate of 1 mg per minute.
Note: Geriatric, emaciated, or debilitated patients usually require a lower initial dose, the dosage being gradually increased as needed and tolerated.

### Usual adult prescribing limits
Up to 1 gram (base) a day.
Note: Although antipsychotic doses are sometimes gradually increased to 2 grams a day or more for short periods, 1 gram or less is usually sufficient for extended therapy.

### Usual pediatric dose
Psychotic disorders or
Nausea and vomiting—
  Children up to 6 months of age: Dosage has not been established.
  Children 6 months of age and over: Intramuscular, 550 mcg (0.55 mg) (base) per kg of body weight or 15 mg per square meter of body surface every six to eight hours as needed.
Nausea and vomiting during surgery—
  Intramuscular: 275 mcg (0.275 mg) (base) per kg of body weight, the dosage being repeated in thirty minutes as needed and tolerated.
  Intravenous infusion: 275 mcg (0.275 mg) (base) per kg of body weight, diluted to a concentration of at least 1 mg per mL with 0.9% sodium chloride injection, administered at a rate of no more than 1 mg every 2 minutes.
Anxiety, presurgical—
  Intramuscular, 550 mcg (0.55 mg) (base) per kg of body weight one to two hours before surgery.
Tetanus—
  Intramuscular: 550 mcg (0.55 mg) (base) per kg of body weight every six to eight hours.
  Intravenous infusion: 550 mcg (0.55 mg) (base) per kg of body weight, diluted to a concentration of at least 1 mg per mL with 0.9% sodium chloride injection, administered at a rate of 1 mg per 2 minutes.
Note: Children 6 months to 5 years of age (up to 23 kg) should receive no more than 40 mg a day.
  Children 5 to 12 years of age (23 to 46 kg) should receive no more than 75 mg a day, except in unmanageable cases.

### Strength(s) usually available
U.S.—
  25 mg (base) per mL (Rx) [*Ormazine; Thorazine* (sulfite; vials, benzyl alcohol 2%); GENERIC].

Canada—
25 mg (base) per mL (Rx) [*Largactil* (sodium sulfite; potassium metabisulfite) [GENERIC].

**Packaging and storage**
Store below 40 °C (104 °F), preferably between 15 and 30 °C (59 and 86 °F), unless otherwise specified by manufacturer. Protect from light. Protect from freezing.

**Stability**
A slight yellowing will not alter potency; however, do not use if markedly discolored or if a precipitate is present.

**Incompatibilities**
A precipitate will form if chlorpromazine hydrochloride injection is mixed with thiopental, atropine, or solutions not having a pH of 4 to 5. Mixing chlorpromazine hydrochloride injection with other agents in the syringe is not recommended.

**Note**
Avoid skin contact with liquid forms of this medication; contact dermatitis has resulted.

## Rectal Dosage Forms
### CHLORPROMAZINE SUPPOSITORIES USP
**Usual adult and adolescent dose**
Nausea and vomiting—
Rectal, 50 to 100 mg every six to eight hours as needed.
Note: Geriatric, emaciated, or debilitated patients usually require a lower initial dose, the dosage being gradually increased as needed and tolerated.

**Usual adult prescribing limits**
Up to 400 mg a day.

**Usual pediatric dose**
Nausea and vomiting—
Children up to 6 months of age: Dosage has not been established.
Children 6 months of age and over: Rectal, 1 mg per kg of body weight every six to eight hours as needed.
Note: The 100-mg suppository dosage form is not recommended for pediatric use.

**Strength(s) usually available**
U.S.—
25 mg (Rx) [*Thorazine* (glycerin; glyceryl monopalmitate; glyceryl monostearate; hydrogenated coconut oil fatty acids; hydrogenated palm kernel oil fatty acids)].
100 mg (Rx) [*Thorazine* (glycerin; glyceryl monopalmitate; glyceryl monostearate; hydrogenated coconut oil fatty acids; hydrogenated palm kernel oil fatty acids)].
Canada—
100 mg (Rx) [*Largactil*].

**Packaging and storage**
Store between 15 and 30 °C (59 and 86 °F). Store in a well-closed, light-resistant container.

**Auxiliary labeling**
- May cause drowsiness.
- Avoid alcoholic beverages.
- For rectal use only.

**Note**
Explain administration technique.

---

## FLUPHENAZINE

## Summary of Differences
Category:
Includes use as antineuralgia adjunct in patients with chronic pain.
Pharmacology/pharmacokinetics:
Chemical group—
Piperazine
Actions—
Antiemetic: Weak
Anticholinergic: Weak
Extrapyramidal: Strong
Hypotensive: Weak
Sedative: Weak

## Additional Dosing Information
See also *General Dosing Information*.

**For long-acting parenteral dosage forms**
A dry syringe and needle (at least 21 gauge) should be used, since use of a wet needle may cause the solution to become cloudy.
After the initial dose of the decanoate or enanthate extended-action injection, dosages and dosing intervals are determined by the patient's response.

## Oral Dosage Forms
### FLUPHENAZINE HYDROCHLORIDE ELIXIR USP
**Usual adult and adolescent dose**
Psychotic disorders—
Initial: Oral, 2.5 to 10 mg a day in divided doses every six to eight hours, the dosage being increased gradually as needed and tolerated.
Maintenance: Oral, 1 to 5 mg a day as a single dose or in divided doses.
Note: Emaciated or debilitated patients usually require a lower initial dosage (1 to 2.5 mg daily), the dosage being gradually increased as needed and tolerated.

**Usual adult prescribing limits**
Up to 20 mg a day.

**Usual pediatric dose**
Psychotic disorders—
Oral, 250 to 750 mcg (0.25 to 0.75 mg) one to four times a day.

**Usual geriatric dose**
Psychotic disorders—
Oral, 1 to 2.5 mg a day, the dosage being gradually increased as needed and tolerated.

**Strength(s) usually available**
U.S.—
2.5 mg per 5 mL (0.5 mg per mL) (Rx) [*Prolixin* (alcohol 14%; FD&C Yellow No. 6; flavors; glycerin; polysorbate 40; purified water; sodium benzoate; sucrose)].
Canada—
2.5 mg per 5 mL (0.5 mg per mL) (Rx) [*Moditen HCl* (alcohol 14%)].

**Packaging and storage**
Store below 40 °C (104 °F), preferably between 15 and 30 °C (59 and 86 °F), unless otherwise specified by manufacturer. Store in a tight container. Protect from light. Protect from freezing.

**Auxiliary labeling**
- May cause drowsiness.
- Avoid alcoholic beverages.
- Do not spill on skin or clothing.
- Keep container tightly closed.

**Note**
Avoid skin contact with liquid forms of this medication; contact dermatitis has resulted.

### FLUPHENAZINE HYDROCHLORIDE ORAL SOLUTION USP
**Usual adult and adolescent dose**
Psychotic disorders—
Initial: Oral, 2.5 to 10 mg a day in divided doses every six to eight hours, the dosage being increased gradually as needed and tolerated.
Maintenance: Oral, 1 to 5 mg a day as a single dose or in divided doses.
Note: Emaciated or debilitated patients usually require a lower initial dosage (1 to 2.5 mg daily), the dosage being gradually increased as needed and tolerated.

**Usual adult prescribing limits**
Up to 20 mg a day.

**Usual pediatric dose**
Psychotic disorders—
Oral, 250 to 750 mcg (0.25 to 0.75 mg) one to four times a day.

**Usual geriatric dose**
Psychotic disorders—
Oral, 1 to 2.5 mg a day, the dosage being gradually increased as needed and tolerated.

**Strength(s) usually available**
U.S.—
5 mg per mL (Rx) [*Permitil Concentrate* (alcohol 1%); *Prolixin Concentrate* (alcohol 14%; sodium benzoate); GENERIC].
Canada—
Not commercially available.

**Packaging and storage**
Store below 40 °C (104 °F), preferably between 15 and 30 °C (59 and 86 °F), unless otherwise specified by manufacturer. Store in a tight container. Protect from light. Protect from freezing.

### Auxiliary labeling
- May cause drowsiness.
- Avoid alcoholic beverages.
- Do not spill on skin or clothing.
- Must be diluted before use.

### Note
Avoid skin contact with liquid forms of this medication; contact dermatitis has resulted.

Each dose must be diluted just before administration in a half (120 mL) to a full (240 mL) glass of milk, tomato or fruit juice, water, soup, or carbonated beverage.

Explain dilution and dosage measurement to patient if self-administered.

## FLUPHENAZINE HYDROCHLORIDE TABLETS USP

### Usual adult and adolescent dose
Psychotic disorders—
  Initial: Oral, 2.5 to 10 mg a day in divided doses every six to eight hours, the dosage being increased gradually as needed and tolerated.
  Maintenance: Oral, 1 to 5 mg a day as a single dose or in divided doses.
Note: Emaciated or debilitated patients usually require a lower initial dosage (1 to 2.5 mg daily), the dosage being gradually increased as needed and tolerated.

### Usual adult prescribing limits
Up to 20 mg a day.

### Usual pediatric dose
Psychotic disorders—
  Oral, 250 to 750 mcg (0.25 to 0.75 mg) one to four times a day.

### Usual geriatric dose
Psychotic disorders—
  Oral, 1 to 2.5 mg a day, the dosage being gradually increased as needed and tolerated.

### Strength(s) usually available
U.S.—
  1 mg (Rx) [*Prolixin;* GENERIC].
  2.5 mg (Rx) [*Permitil; Prolixin* (tartrazine); GENERIC].
  5 mg (Rx) [*Permitil; Prolixin* (tartrazine); GENERIC].
  10 mg (Rx) [*Permitil; Prolixin* (tartrazine); GENERIC].
Canada—
  1 mg (Rx) [*Apo-Fluphenazine; Moditen HCl; Permitil*].
  2 mg (Rx) [*Apo-Fluphenazine; Moditen HCl* (tartrazine)].
  5 mg (Rx) [*Apo-Fluphenazine; Moditen HCl; Permitil*].
  10 mg (Rx) [*Moditen HCl*].

### Packaging and storage
Store below 40 °C (104 °F), preferably between 15 and 30 °C (59 and 86 °F), unless otherwise specified by manufacturer. Store in a tight, light-resistant container.

### Auxiliary labeling
- May cause drowsiness.
- Avoid alcoholic beverages.

## Parenteral Dosage Forms

### FLUPHENAZINE DECANOATE INJECTION

#### Usual adult dose
Psychotic disorders—
  Initial: Intramuscular or subcutaneous, 12.5 to 25 mg, the dose being repeated or increased every one to three weeks as needed and tolerated.
  Maintenance: Intramuscular or subcutaneous, usually up to 50 mg every one to four weeks, as needed and tolerated.
Note: For doses greater than 50 mg, increases should be made cautiously in increments of 12.5 mg.

#### Usual adult prescribing limits
Up to 100 mg per dose.

#### Usual pediatric dose
Psychotic disorders—
  Children 5 to 12 years of age: Intramuscular or subcutaneous, 3.125 to 12.5 mg, the dosage being repeated every one to three weeks as needed and tolerated.
  Children 12 years of age and over: Intramuscular or subcutaneous, initially 6.25 to 18.75 mg a week, the dosage being increased to 12.5 to 25 mg and administered every one to three weeks as needed and tolerated.

#### Strength(s) usually available
U.S.—
  25 mg per mL (Rx) [*Prolixin Decanoate* (sesame oil; benzyl alcohol 1.2% w/v); GENERIC].
Canada—
  25 mg per mL (Rx) [*Modecate* (sesame oil; benzyl alcohol 1.2% w/v)].
  100 mg per mL (Rx) [*Modecate Concentrate* (sesame oil; benzyl alcohol 1.5% w/v)].

#### Packaging and storage
Store below 40 °C (104 °F), preferably between 15 and 30 °C (59 and 86 °F), unless otherwise specified by manufacturer. Protect from light. Protect from freezing.

#### Note
Avoid skin contact with liquid forms of this medication; contact dermatitis has resulted.

#### Additional information
The onset of action of the initial dose is generally between 24 and 72 hours after administration, and antipsychotic effects become significant within 48 to 96 hours.

The effects of a single injection of the extended-action injectable forms may last for up to 6 weeks in some patients. The side effects information and precautions apply during this period of time.

The time to steady-state from a dosage change requires 6 to 12 weeks or longer.

### FLUPHENAZINE ENANTHATE INJECTION USP

#### Usual adult and adolescent dose
Psychotic disorders—
  Intramuscular or subcutaneous, 25 mg, the dosage being repeated or increased every one to three weeks as needed and tolerated.
Note: For doses greater than 50 mg, increases should be made cautiously in increments of 12.5 mg.

#### Usual adult prescribing limits
Up to 100 mg per dose.

#### Usual pediatric dose
Psychotic disorders—
  Children up to 12 years of age: Dosage has not been established.
  Children 12 years of age and over: See *Usual adult and adolescent dose.*

#### Strength(s) usually available
U.S.—
  25 mg per mL (Rx) [*Prolixin Enanthate* (sesame oil; benzyl alcohol 1.5% w/v)].
Canada—
  25 mg per mL (Rx) [*Moditen Enanthate* (sesame oil; benzyl alcohol 1.5% w/v)].

#### Packaging and storage
Store below 40 °C (104 °F), preferably between 15 and 30 °C (59 and 86 °F), unless otherwise specified by manufacturer. Protect from light. Protect from freezing.

#### Note
Avoid skin contact with liquid forms of this medication; contact dermatitis has resulted.

#### Additional information
The effects of a single dose of the extended-action injectable forms may last for up to 6 weeks in some patients. The side effects information and precautions apply during this period of time.

### FLUPHENAZINE HYDROCHLORIDE INJECTION USP

#### Usual adult and adolescent dose
Psychotic disorders—
  Intramuscular, 1.25 to 2.5 mg every six to eight hours as needed and tolerated.
Note: Emaciated or debilitated patients usually require a lower initial dose (1 to 2.5 mg daily), the dosage being increased gradually as needed and tolerated.

#### Usual adult prescribing limits
Up to 10 mg a day.

#### Usual pediatric dose
Psychotic disorders—
  Children up to 12 years of age: Dosage has not been established.
  Children 12 years of age and over: See *Usual adult and adolescent dose.*

**Usual geriatric dose**
Psychotic disorders—
  Intramuscular, 1 to 2.5 mg a day, the dosage being increased gradually as needed and tolerated.

**Strength(s) usually available**
U.S.—
  2.5 mg per mL (Rx) [*Prolixin* (methylparaben 0.1%; propylparaben 0.01%); GENERIC].
Canada—
  10 mg per mL (Rx) [*Moditen HCl-H.P.* (benzyl alcohol 1.5%)].

**Packaging and storage**
Store below 40 °C (104 °F), preferably between 15 and 30 °C (59 and 86 °F), unless otherwise specified by manufacturer. Protect from light. Protect from freezing.

**Stability**
A slight yellowing to a light amber color will not alter potency; however, do not use if markedly discolored or if a precipitate is present.

**Note**
Avoid skin contact with liquid forms of this medication; contact dermatitis has resulted.

---
## MESORIDAZINE
---

## Summary of Differences
Pharmacology/pharmacokinetics:
  Chemical group—
    Piperidine
  Actions—
    Antiemetic: Weak
    Anticholinergic: Moderate
    Extrapyramidal: Weak
    Hypotensive: Strong
    Sedative: Strong

## Oral Dosage Forms
Note: The dosing and strengths of the dosage forms available are expressed in terms of mesoridazine base (not the besylate salt).

### MESORIDAZINE BESYLATE ORAL SOLUTION USP
**Usual adult and adolescent dose**
Psychotic disorders—
  Oral, 30 to 150 mg (base) a day in two or three divided doses, the dosage being adjusted as needed and tolerated.
Note: Geriatric, emaciated, or debilitated patients usually require a lower initial dose, the dosage being increased gradually as needed and tolerated.

**Usual pediatric dose**
Psychotic disorders—
  Children up to 12 years of age: Dosage has not been established.
  Children 12 years of age and over: See *Usual adult and adolescent dose*.

**Strength(s) usually available**
U.S.—
  25 mg (base) per mL (Rx) [*Serentil Concentrate* (alcohol 0.6% v/v)].
Canada—
  Not commercially available.

**Packaging and storage**
Store below 25 °C (77 °F). Store in a tight, light-resistant container. Protect from freezing.

**Auxiliary labeling**
• May cause drowsiness.
• Avoid alcoholic beverages.
• Do not spill on skin or clothing.
• Must be diluted before use.

**Note**
Avoid skin contact with liquid forms of this medication; contact dermatitis has resulted.

Each dose must be diluted just before administration in distilled water, acidified tap water, orange juice, or grapefruit juice. The recommended dilution is 25 mg in 2 teaspoonfuls of diluent. Higher doses require more diluent. Preparation and storage of bulk dilution is not recommended.

Explain dilution and dosage measurement to patient if self-administered.

### MESORIDAZINE BESYLATE TABLETS USP
**Usual adult and adolescent dose**
Psychotic disorders—
  Oral, 30 to 150 mg (base) a day in two or three divided doses, the dosage being adjusted as needed and tolerated.
Note: Geriatric, emaciated, or debilitated patients usually require a lower initial dose, the dosage being increased gradually as needed and tolerated.

**Usual pediatric dose**
Psychotic disorders—
  Children up to 12 years of age: Dosage has not been established.
  Children 12 years of age and older: See *Usual adult and adolescent dose*.

**Strength(s) usually available**
U.S.—
  10 mg (base) (Rx) [*Serentil* (acacia; carnauba wax; colloidal silicon dioxide; FD&C Red No. 40 aluminum lake; microcrystalline cellulose; povidone; sodium benzoate; stearic acid; sucrose; lactose; talc; titanium dioxide; starch)].
  25 mg (base) (Rx) [*Serentil* (acacia; carnauba wax; colloidal silicon dioxide; FD&C Red No. 40 aluminum lake; microcrystalline cellulose; povidone; sodium benzoate; stearic acid; sucrose; lactose; talc; titanium dioxide)].
  50 mg (base) (Rx) [*Serentil* (acacia; carnauba wax; colloidal silicon dioxide; FD&C Red No. 40 aluminum lake; microcrystalline cellulose; povidone; sodium benzoate; stearic acid; sucrose; lactose; talc; titanium dioxide; starch; gelatin)].
  100 mg (base) (Rx) [*Serentil* (acacia; carnauba wax; colloidal silicon dioxide; FD&C Red No. 40 aluminum lake; microcrystalline cellulose; povidone; sodium benzoate; stearic acid; sucrose; lactose; talc; titanium dioxide; starch; gelatin)].
Canada—
  10 mg (base) (Rx) [*Serentil* (cornstarch; lactose)].
  25 mg (base) (Rx) [*Serentil* (cornstarch; lactose)].
  50 mg (base) (Rx) [*Serentil* (cornstarch; lactose)].

**Packaging and storage**
Store below 30 °C (86 °F), unless otherwise specified by manufacturer. Store in a well-closed, light-resistant container.

**Auxiliary labeling**
• May cause drowsiness.
• Avoid alcoholic beverages.

## Parenteral Dosage Forms
Note: The dosing and strengths of the dosage forms available are expressed in terms of mesoridazine base (not the besylate salt).

### MESORIDAZINE BESYLATE INJECTION USP
**Usual adult and adolescent dose**
Psychotic disorders—
  Intramuscular, 25 mg (base), the dose being repeated in one-half to one hour as needed and tolerated.
Note: Geriatric, emaciated, or debilitated patients usually require a lower initial dose, the dosage being gradually increased as needed and tolerated.

**Usual pediatric dose**
Psychotic disorders—
  Children up to 12 years of age: Dosage has not been established.
  Children 12 years of age and older: See *Usual adult and adolescent dose*.

**Strength(s) usually available**
U.S.—
  25 mg (base) per mL (Rx) [*Serentil* (edetate sodium)].
Canada—
  Not commercially available.

**Packaging and storage**
Store below 30 °C (86 °F), unless otherwise specified by manufacturer. Protect from light. Protect from freezing.

**Stability**
A slight yellowing will not alter potency; however, do not use if markedly discolored or if a precipitate is present.

**Note**
Avoid skin contact with liquid forms of this medication; contact dermatitis has resulted.

## METHOTRIMEPRAZINE

### Summary of Differences
Category:
  In addition to being used as an antipsychotic, methotrimeprazine is used as an analgesic, antianxiety agent, and sedative.
Indications:
  Also indicated for relief of moderate to severe pain in nonambulatory patients, and for obstetrical pain and sedation when respiratory depression should be avoided; anxiety, apprehension, restlessness, and sedation before surgery; adjunctive therapy in general anesthesia to increase effects of anesthetics.
Pharmacology/pharmacokinetics:
  Chemical group—
    Aliphatic
  Actions—
    Antiemetic: Weak
    Anticholinergic: Moderate
    Extrapyramidal: Weak to moderate
    Hypotensive: Strong
    Sedative: Strong

## Oral Dosage Forms
Note:  The dosing and strengths of the dosage forms available are expressed in terms of methotrimeprazine base (not the hydrochloride or maleate salts).

### METHOTRIMEPRAZINE HYDROCHLORIDE ORAL SOLUTION

**Usual adult and adolescent dose**
Psychotic disorders or
Pain—
  Oral, initially, 6 to 25 mg (base) a day in three divided doses with meals (mild to moderate pain or psychosis), or 50 to 75 mg a day in two or three divided doses with meals (severe pain or psychosis), the dosage being gradually increased as needed and tolerated.
  Note:  If doses of 100 to 200 mg a day are required, the patient should be confined to bed for the first few days to prevent orthostatic hypotension.
Sedation, presurgical—
  Oral, initially, 6 to 25 mg (base) a day in three divided doses with meals, the dosage being increased gradually as needed and tolerated.

**Usual pediatric dose**
Psychotic disorders or
Pain or
Sedation, presurgical—
  Oral, initially, 250 mcg (0.25 mg) per kg (base) of body weight a day in two or three divided doses with meals, the dosage being increased gradually as needed and tolerated.
  Note:  Dosage must not exceed 40 mg a day in children under twelve years of age.

**Strength(s) usually available**
U.S.—
  Not commercially available.
Canada—
  40 mg (base) per mL (Rx) [*Nozinan Oral Drops* (alcohol 16.5%; sucrose)].

**Packaging and storage**
Store below 40 °C (104 °F), preferably between 15 and 30 °C (59 and 86 °F), protected from light, unless otherwise specified by manufacturer. Protect from freezing.

**Auxiliary labeling**
- May cause drowsiness.
- Avoid alcoholic beverages.
- Do not spill on skin or clothing.

**Note**
Avoid skin contact with liquid forms of this medication; contact dermatitis may result.

**Additional information**
Only enclosed calibrated dropper should be used for measuring dose.

### METHOTRIMEPRAZINE HYDROCHLORIDE SYRUP

**Usual adult and adolescent dose**
Psychotic disorders or
Pain—
  Oral, initially, 6 to 25 mg (base) a day in three divided doses with meals (mild to moderate pain or psychosis), or 50 to 75 mg a day in two or three divided doses with meals (severe pain or psychosis), the dosage being increased gradually as needed and tolerated.
  Note:  If doses of 100 to 200 mg a day are required, the patient should be confined to bed for the first few days to prevent orthostatic hypotension.
Sedation, presurgical—
  Oral, initially, 6 to 25 mg (base) a day in three divided doses with meals, the dosage being increased gradually as needed and tolerated.

**Usual pediatric dose**
Psychotic disorders or
Pain or
Sedation—
  Oral, initially, 250 mcg (0.25 mg) (base) per kg of body weight a day in two or three divided doses with meals, the dosage being increased gradually as needed and tolerated.
  Note:  Dosage must not exceed 40 mg a day in chidren under twelve years of age.

**Strength(s) usually available**
U.S.—
  Not commercially available.
Canada—
  25 mg (base) per 5 mL (Rx) [*Nozinan Liquid* (alcohol 2%; sucrose)].

**Packaging and storage**
Store below 40 °C (104 °F), preferably between 15 and 30 °C (59 and 86 °F), protected from light, unless otherwise specified by manufacturer. Protect from freezing.

**Auxiliary labeling**
- May cause drowsiness.
- Avoid alcoholic beverages.
- Do not spill on skin or clothing.

**Note**
Avoid skin contact with liquid forms of this medication; contact dermatitis may result.

### METHOTRIMEPRAZINE MALEATE TABLETS

**Usual adult and adolescent dose**
Psychotic disorders or
Pain—
  Oral, initially, 6 to 25 mg (base) a day in three divided doses with meals (mild to moderate pain or psychosis), or 50 to 75 mg a day in two or three divided doses with meals (severe pain or psychosis), the dosage being increased gradually as needed and tolerated.
  Note:  If doses of 100 to 200 mg a day are required, the patient should be confined to bed for the first few days to prevent orthostatic hypotension.
Sedation, presurgical—
  Oral, initially, 6 to 25 mg (base) a day in three divided doses with meals, the dosage being gradually increased as needed and tolerated.

**Usual pediatric dose**
Psychotic disorders or
Pain or
Sedation—
  Oral, initially, 250 mcg (0.25 mg) (base) per kg of body weight a day in two or three divided doses with meals, the dosage being increased gradually as needed and tolerated.
  Note:  Doses must not exceed 40 mg a day in children under twelve years of age.

**Strength(s) usually available**
U.S.—
  Not commercially available.
Canada—
  2 mg (base) (Rx) [*Nozinan*].
  5 mg (base) (Rx) [*Nozinan*].
  25 mg (base) (Rx) [*Nozinan*].
  50 mg (base) (Rx) [*Nozinan*].

**Packaging and storage**
Store below 40 °C (104 °F), preferably between 15 and 30 °C (59 and 86 °F), protected from light, unless otherwise specified by manufacturer.

**Auxiliary labeling**
- May cause drowsiness.
- Avoid alcoholic beverages.

## Parenteral Dosage Forms

Note: Bracketed uses in the *Dosage Forms* section refer to categories of use and/or indications that are not included in U.S. product labeling.

### METHOTRIMEPRAZINE INJECTION USP

**Usual adult and adolescent dose**
[Psychotic disorders, severe or]
Pain, acute or intractable—
    Intramuscular, initially, 10 to 20 mg at four- to six-hour intervals, the dosage being increased as needed for pain and sedation.
Pain, obstetrical—
    Intramuscular, initially 15 to 20 mg, the dose being adjusted and repeated as needed.
Pain, postoperative—
    Intramuscular, 2.5 to 7.5 mg immediately after surgery, the dosage being adjusted and repeated every three to four hours as needed.
    Note: After initial dose, the patient should be confined to bed or carefully supervised for at least 6 hours following administration, to prevent orthostatic hypotension, dizziness, or fainting.
    Residual effects of anesthetic agents may be additive to the effects of methotrimeprazine.
Sedation, preanesthetic—
    Intramuscular, 2 to 20 mg administered forty-five minutes to three hours before surgery.
[Anesthesia adjunct during surgery or labor]—
    Intravenous infusion, 10 to 25 mg in 500 mL of 5% dextrose injection administered at a rate of 20 to 40 drops a minute.

**Usual pediatric dose**
Pain—
    Intramuscular, 62.5 to 125 mcg (0.062 to 0.125 mg) per kg of body weight a day in single or divided doses.
[Anesthesia adjunct during surgery]—
    Intravenous infusion, 62.5 to 125 mcg (0.062 to 0.125 mg) per kg of body weight a day in 250 mL of 5% dextrose injection, administered at a rate of 20 to 40 drops a minute.

**Usual geriatric dose**
Pain—
    Intramuscular, initially, 5 to 10 mg every four to six hours, the dosage being increased gradually as needed and tolerated.

**Strength(s) usually available**
U.S.—
    20 mg per mL (Rx) [*Levoprome* (benzyl alcohol 0.9% w/v; disodium edetate; sodium metabisulfite)].
Canada—
    25 mg per mL (Rx) [*Nozinan* (sodium sulfite)].

**Packaging and storage**
Store below 40 °C (104 °F), preferably between 15 and 30 °C (59 and 86 °F), unless otherwise specified by manufacturer. Protect from light. Protect from freezing.

**Incompatibilities**
Methotrimeprazine should not be mixed in the same syringe with any drug except atropine sulfate or scopolamine hydrobromide.

**Note**
Avoid skin contact with liquid forms of this medication; contact dermatitis may result.

---

## PERICYAZINE

## Summary of Differences

Indications:
    Indicated in some psychotic patients for the control of residual prevailing hostility, impulsivity, and aggressiveness.
Pharmacology/pharmacokinetics:
    Chemical group—
        Piperidine
    Actions—
        Antiemetic: Strong
        Anticholinergic: Strong
        Extrapyramidal: Moderate
        Hypotensive: Moderate
        Sedative: Strong

## Oral Dosage Forms

### PERICYAZINE CAPSULES

**Usual adult dose**
Psychotic disorders—
    Initial: Oral, 5 to 20 mg in the morning and 10 to 40 mg in the evening as needed and tolerated.
    Maintenance: Oral, 2.5 to 15 mg in the morning and 5 to 30 mg in the evening.

**Usual pediatric dose**
Psychotic disorders—
    Children 5 years of age to adolescence: Oral, 2.5 to 10 mg in the morning and 5 to 30 mg in the evening as needed and tolerated.

**Usual geriatric dose**
Psychotic disorders—
    Oral, initially, 5 mg a day, the dosage being increased gradually as needed and tolerated, up to about 30 mg a day.

**Strength(s) usually available**
U.S.—
    Not commercially available.
Canada—
    5 mg (Rx) [*Neuleptil*].
    10 mg (Rx) [*Neuleptil*].
    20 mg (Rx) [*Neuleptil*].

**Packaging and storage**
Store below 40 °C (104 °F), preferably between 15 and 30 °C (59 and 86 °F), protected from light, unless otherwise specified by manufacturer.

**Auxiliary labeling**
- May cause drowsiness.
- Avoid alcoholic beverages.

### PERICYAZINE ORAL SOLUTION

**Usual adult dose**
Psychotic disorders—
    Initial: Oral, 5 to 20 mg in the morning and 10 to 40 mg in the evening as needed and tolerated.
    Maintenance: Oral, 2.5 to 15 mg in the morning and 5 to 30 mg in the evening.

**Usual pediatric dose**
Psychotic disorders—
    Children 5 years of age to adolescence: Oral, 2.5 to 10 mg in the morning and 5 to 30 mg in the evening as needed and tolerated.

**Usual geriatric dose**
Psychotic disorders—
    Oral, initially, 5 mg a day, the dosage being increased gradually as needed and tolerated up to about 30 mg a day.

**Strength(s) usually available**
U.S.—
    Not commercially available.
Canada—
    10 mg per mL (Rx) [*Neuleptil*].

**Packaging and storage**
Store below 40 °C (104 °F), preferably between 15 and 30 °C (59 and 86 °F), protected from light, unless otherwise specified by manufacturer.

**Auxiliary labeling**
- May cause drowsiness.
- Avoid alcoholic beverages.
- Do not spill on skin or clothing.

**Note**
Avoid skin contact with liquid forms of this medication; contact dermatitis may result.

**Additional information**
Only enclosed calibrated dropper should be used for measuring dose.

---

## PERPHENAZINE

## Summary of Differences

Category:
    Includes antiemetic use.
Pharmacology/pharmacokinetics:
    Chemical group—
        Piperazine
    Actions—
        Antiemetic: Strong
        Anticholinergic: Weak to moderate

# Phenothiazines (Systemic)

Extrapyramidal: Strong
Hypotensive: Weak
Sedative: Weak to moderate

## Oral Dosage Forms

Note: Bracketed uses in the *Dosage Forms* section refer to categories of use and/or indications that are not included in U.S. product labeling.

### PERPHENAZINE ORAL SOLUTION USP

**Usual adult and adolescent dose**
Psychotic disorders (hospitalized patients)—
  Oral, 8 to 16 mg two to four times a day, up to 64 mg a day, the dosage being adjusted as needed and tolerated.
Note: Geriatric, emaciated, or debilitated patients usually require a lower initial dose, the dosage being gradually increased as needed and tolerated.
  Adolescents usually require the lowest limit of the adult dose range.

**Usual pediatric dose**
Psychotic disorders—
  Children up to 12 years of age: Dosage has not been established.
  Children 12 years of age and over: See *Usual adult and adolescent dose*.

**Strength(s) usually available**
U.S.—
  16 mg per 5 mL (Rx) [*Trilafon Concentrate*].
Canada—
  16 mg per 5 mL (Rx) [*PMS Perphenazine; Trilafon Concentrate*].

**Packaging and storage**
Store below 40 °C (104 °F), preferably between 15 and 30 °C (59 and 86 °F), unless otherwise specified by manufacturer. Store in a well-closed, light-resistant container. Protect from freezing.

**Auxiliary labeling**
- May cause drowsiness.
- Avoid alcoholic beverages.
- Do not spill on skin or clothing.
- Must be diluted before use.

**Note**
The oral solution is intended primarily for institutional usage.
Avoid skin contact with liquid forms of this medication; contact dermatitis has resulted.
Each dose must be measured with accompanying dropper and diluted before administration in water, salt solution, milk, tomato or fruit juice (except apple juice), soup, or carbonated beverage. The oral solution should not be mixed with beverages containing caffeine or tannins (colas, coffee, or tea). The recommended dilution is 2 fluid ounces (60 mL) of diluent for each teaspoonful (5 mL) of perphenazine oral solution.
Explain dilution and dosage measurement to patient if self-administered.

### PERPHENAZINE SYRUP USP

**Usual adult and adolescent dose**
Psychotic disorders—
  Oral, 2 to 16 mg two to four times a day, the dosage being adjusted gradually as needed and tolerated.
Nausea and vomiting—
  Oral, 2 to 4 mg two to four times a day, the dosage being adjusted gradually as needed and tolerated.
Note: Geriatric, emaciated, or debilitated patients usually require a lower initial dose, the dosage being gradually increased as needed and tolerated.
  Adolescents usually require the lowest limit of the adult dose range.

**Usual pediatric dose**
Psychotic disorders or
Nausea and vomiting—
  Children up to 12 years of age: Dosage has not been established.
  Children 12 years of age and over: See *Usual adult and adolescent dose*.

**Strength(s) usually available**
U.S.—
  Not commercially available.
Canada—
  2 mg per 5 mL (Rx) [*Trilafon* (methylparaben; propylparaben; sorbitol; sucrose)].

**Packaging and storage**
Store below 40 °C (104 °F), preferably between 15 and 30 °C (59 and 86 °F), unless otherwise specified by manufacturer. Store in a well-closed, light-resistant container. Protect from freezing.

**Auxiliary labeling**
- May cause drowsiness.
- Avoid alcoholic beverages.
- Do not spill on skin or clothing.

**Note**
Avoid skin contact with liquid forms of this medication; contact dermatitis has resulted.

### PERPHENAZINE TABLETS USP

**Usual adult and adolescent dose**
Psychotic disorders—
  Oral, 4 to 16 mg two to four times a day, the dosage being adjusted gradually as needed and tolerated.
Nausea and vomiting—
  Oral, 8 to 16 mg a day in divided doses, the dosage being decreased as early as possible.
Note: Geriatric, emaciated, or debilitated patients usually require a lower initial dose, the dosage being increased gradually as needed and tolerated.
  Adolescents usually require the lowest limit of the adult dose range.

**Usual adult prescribing limits**
Psychotic disorders—
  Up to 64 mg a day.
Nausea and vomiting—
  Up to 24 mg a day.

**Usual pediatric dose**
Psychotic disorders or
Nausea and vomiting—
  Children up to 12 years of age: Dosage has not been established.
  Children 12 years of age and over: See *Usual adult and adolescent dose*.

**Strength(s) usually available**
U.S.—
  2 mg (Rx) [*Trilafon;* GENERIC].
  4 mg (Rx) [*Trilafon;* GENERIC].
  8 mg (Rx) [*Trilafon;* GENERIC].
  16 mg (Rx) [*Trilafon;* GENERIC].
Canada—
  2 mg (Rx) [*Apo-Perphenazine; PMS Perphenazine; Trilafon* [GENERIC].
  4 mg (Rx) [*Apo-Perphenazine; PMS Perphenazine; Trilafon* [GENERIC].
  8 mg (Rx) [*Apo-Perphenazine; PMS Perphenazine; Trilafon* [GENERIC].
  16 mg (Rx) [*Apo-Perphenazine; PMS Perphenazine; Trilafon* [GENERIC].

**Packaging and storage**
Store below 40 °C (104 °F), preferably between 15 and 30 °C (59 and 86 °F), unless otherwise specified by manufacturer. Store in a tight, light-resistant container.

**Auxiliary labeling**
- May cause drowsiness.
- Avoid alcoholic beverages.

## Parenteral Dosage Forms

### PERPHENAZINE INJECTION USP

**Usual adult and adolescent dose**
Psychotic disorders—
  Intramuscular, 5 to 10 mg every six hours, the dosage being adjusted as needed and tolerated.
Nausea and vomiting—
  Intramuscular, 5 mg, the dose being increased to 10 mg as needed and tolerated for rapid control of severe vomiting.
  Intravenous, up to 5 mg diluted to 0.5 mg per mL with 0.9% sodium chloride injection, in divided doses, not more than 1 mg administered not less than every one to two minutes; or administered as an infusion at a rate not to exceed 1 mg per minute.
Note: Geriatric, emaciated, or debilitated patients usually require a lower initial dose, the dosage being gradually increased as needed and tolerated.
  Adolescents usually require the lowest limit of the adult dose range.
  In psychotic conditions, most patients are controlled and amenable to oral therapy within a maximum of 24 to 48 hours.

**Usual adult prescribing limits**
Ambulatory patients: Up to 15 mg daily.
Institutionalized patients: Up to 30 mg daily.
Intravenous administration: Up to 5 mg.

**Usual pediatric dose**
Psychotic disorders—
  Children up to 12 years of age: Dosage has not been established.
  Children 12 years of age and over: See *Usual adult and adolescent dose*.

**Strength(s) usually available**
U.S.—
  5 mg per mL (Rx) [*Trilafon* (sodium bisulfite)].
Canada—
  5 mg per mL (Rx) [*Trilafon* (sodium bisulfite)].

**Packaging and storage**
Store below 40 °C (104 °F), preferably between 15 and 30 °C (59 and 86 °F), unless otherwise specified by manufacturer. Protect from light. Protect from freezing.

**Stability**
A slight yellowing will not alter potency; however, do not use if markedly discolored or if a precipitate is present.

**Note**
Avoid skin contact with liquid forms of this medication; contact dermatitis has resulted.

---

## PIPOTIAZINE

## Summary of Differences
Indications:
  For the maintenance treatment of chronic, non-agitated schizophrenic patients stabilized on shorter-acting neuroleptics.
Pharmacology/pharmacokinetics:
  Chemical group—
    Piperidine
  Actions—
    Antiemetic: Weak
    Anticholinergic: Weak
    Extrapyramidal: Strong
    Hypotensive: Weak
    Sedative: Weak

## Additional Dosing Information
See also *General Dosing Information*.
A dry syringe and needle (at least 21-gauge) should be used, since use of a wet needle or syringe may cause the solution to become cloudy.
After the initial dose of pipotiazine palmitate extended-action injection, dosages and dosing intervals are determined by the patient's response.

## Parenteral Dosage Forms

### PIPOTIAZINE PALMITATE INJECTION
**Usual adult and adolescent dose**
Psychotic disorders—
  Intramuscular, initially, 50 to 100 mg, the dosage being increased in increments of 25 mg every two to three weeks, as needed and tolerated, usually up to a maintenance dose of 75 to 150 mg every four weeks.
Note: Geriatric patients usually require lower initial doses and, after initial titration, dosage should be reduced to the lowest effective maintenance dosage as soon as possible.

**Usual pediatric dose**
Dosage has not been established.

**Strength(s) usually available**
U.S.—
  Not commercially available.
Canada—
  25 mg per mL (Rx) [*Piportil L*$_4$ (sesame oil)].
  50 mg per mL (Rx) [*Piportil L*$_4$ (sesame oil)].

**Packaging and storage**
Store below 40 °C (104 °F), preferably between 15 and 30 °C (59 and 86 °F), protected from light, unless otherwise specified by manufacturer. Protect from freezing.

**Note**
Avoid skin contact with liquid forms of this medication; contact dermatitis may result.

**Additional information**
The onset of action is usually within the first 2 or 3 days after injection, and antipsychotic effects become significant within 1 week.

The effects of a single injection may last from 3 to 6 weeks, but adequate symptom control may be maintained with one injection every 4 weeks.

---

## PROCHLORPERAZINE

## Summary of Differences
Category:
  Includes antiemetic use.
Pharmacology/pharmacokinetics:
  Chemical group—
    Piperazine
  Actions—
    Antiemetic: Strong
    Anticholinergic: Weak
    Extrapyramidal: Strong
    Hypotensive: Weak
    Sedative: Moderate

## Additional Dosing Information
See also *General Dosing Information*.
For parenteral dosage forms only
  • Must be injected deep into upper outer quadrant of the buttock.
  • Subcutaneous administration is not recommended because of irritation at injection site and a potential for sterile abscesses.

## Oral Dosage Forms
Note: The dosing and strengths of the dosage forms available are expressed in terms of prochlorperazine base (not the edisylate, maleate, or mesylate salts).

### PROCHLORPERAZINE EDISYLATE SYRUP USP
**Usual adult and adolescent dose**
Psychotic disorders—
  Oral, 5 to 10 mg (base) three or four times a day, the dosage being gradually increased every two to three days as needed and tolerated.
Anxiety—
  Oral, 5 mg (base) three or four times a day, up to 20 mg a day, for no longer than twelve weeks.
Nausea and vomiting—
  Oral, 5 to 10 mg (base) three or four times a day, up to 40 mg a day.
Note: Geriatric, emaciated, or debilitated patients usually require a lower initial dose, the dosage being gradually increased as needed and tolerated.

**Usual adult prescribing limits**
Up to 150 mg (base) a day.

**Usual pediatric dose**
Psychotic disorders—
  Children up to 2 years of age or 9 kg of body weight: Dosage has not been established.
  Children 2 to 12 years of age: Oral, 2.5 mg (base) two or three times a day.
  Children 12 years of age and over: See *Usual adult and adolescent dose*.
Nausea and vomiting—
  Children 9 to 13 kg of body weight: Oral, 2.5 mg (base) one or two times a day, not to exceed 7.5 mg per day.
  Children 14 to 17 kg of body weight: Oral, 2.5 mg (base) two or three times a day, not to exceed 10 mg per day.
  Children 18 to 39 kg of body weight: Oral, 2.5 mg (base) three times a day or 5 mg two times a day, not to exceed 15 mg per day.
Note: The total daily dose for any child should not exceed 10 mg the first day. On subsequent days the total daily dose should not exceed 20 mg for children 2 to 5 years of age or 25 mg for children 6 to 12 years of age.

**Strength(s) usually available**
U.S.—
  5 mg (base) per 5 mL (Rx) [*Compazine* (FD&C Yellow No. 6; flavors; polyoxyethylene polyoxypropylene glycol; sodium benzoate; sodium citrate; sucrose; water)].
Canada—
  Not commercially available.

**Packaging and storage**
Store below 40 °C (104 °F), preferably between 15 and 30 °C (59 and 86 °F), unless otherwise specified by manufacturer. Store in a tight, light-resistant container. Protect from freezing.

**Stability**
A slight yellowing will not affect potency; however, do not use if markedly discolored or if a precipitate is present.

**Auxiliary labeling**
- May cause drowsiness.
- Avoid alcoholic beverages.
- Do not spill on skin or clothing.

**Note**
Avoid skin contact with liquid forms of this medication; contact dermatitis has resulted.

## PROCHLORPERAZINE MALEATE EXTENDED-RELEASE CAPSULES

**Usual adult and adolescent dose**
Psychotic disorders—
  Oral, 5 to 10 mg (base) every three or four hours, the dosage being increased gradually every two or three days as needed and tolerated, up to 100 to 150 mg a day.
Anxiety—
  Oral, 15 mg (base) in the morning; or 10 mg every twelve hours, up to 20 mg a day for no longer than 12 weeks.
Nausea and vomiting—
  Oral, 15 to 30 mg (base) once a day in the morning; or 10 mg every twelve hours, up to 40 mg a day as needed and tolerated.
  Note: Daily dosages above 40 mg should be used only in resistant cases.
Note: Geriatric, emaciated, or debilitated patients usually require a lower initial dose, the dosage being gradually increased as needed and tolerated.

**Usual adult prescribing limits**
Psychotic disorders—
  Up to 150 mg (base) daily.

**Usual pediatric dose**
The extended-release dosage form is not recommended for use in children.

**Strength(s) usually available**
U.S.—
  10 mg (base) (Rx) [*Compazine Spansule* (benzyl alcohol; cetylpyridinium chloride; D&C Green No. 5; D&C Yellow No. 10; FD&C Blue No. 1; FD&C Red No. 40; FD&C Yellow No. 6; gelatin; glyceryl monostearate; sodium lauryl sulfate; starch; sucrose; wax)].
  15 mg (base) (Rx) [*Compazine Spansule* (benzyl alcohol; cetylpyridinium chloride; D&C Green No. 5; D&C Yellow No. 10; FD&C Blue No. 1; FD&C Red No. 40; FD&C Yellow No. 6; gelatin; glyceryl monostearate; sodium lauryl sulfate; starch; sucrose; wax)].
  30 mg (base) (Rx) [*Compazine Spansule* (benzyl alcohol; cetylpyridinium chloride; D&C Green No. 5; D&C Yellow No. 10; FD&C Blue No. 1; FD&C Red No. 40; FD&C Yellow No. 6; gelatin; glyceryl monostearate; sodium lauryl sulfate; starch; sucrose; wax)].
Canada—
  Not commercially available.

**Packaging and storage**
Store below 40 °C (104 °F), preferably between 15 and 30 °C (59 and 86 °F), in a well-closed container, unless otherwise specified by manufacturer. Protect from light.

**Auxiliary labeling**
- May cause drowsiness.
- Avoid alcoholic beverages.
- Swallow capsule whole.

## PROCHLORPERAZINE MALEATE TABLETS USP

**Usual adult and adolescent dose**
Psychotic disorders—
  Oral, 5 to 10 mg (base) three or four times a day, the dosage being gradually increased every two or three days as needed and tolerated.
Anxiety—
  Oral, 5 mg (base) three or four times a day, up to 20 mg a day, for no longer than twelve weeks.
Nausea and vomiting—
  Oral, 5 to 10 mg (base) three or four times a day, up to 40 mg a day.
  Note: Daily dosages above 40 mg should be used only in resistant cases.
Note: Geriatric, emaciated, or debilitated patients usually require a lower initial dose, the dosage being gradually increased as needed and tolerated.

**Usual adult prescribing limits**
Psychotic disorders—
  Up to 150 mg (base) a day.

**Usual pediatric dose**
Since tablets are not suitable for many pediatric patients' requirements, the oral syrup dosage form is usually preferred.

**Strength(s) usually available**
U.S.—
  5 mg (base) (Rx) [*Compazine*; GENERIC].
  10 mg (base) (Rx) [*Compazine*; GENERIC].
  25 mg (base) (Rx) [*Compazine*; GENERIC].
Canada—
  5 mg (base) (Rx) [*PMS Prochlorperazine; Prorazin; Stemetil*].
  10 mg (base) (Rx) [*PMS Prochlorperazine; Prorazin; Stemetil*].

**Packaging and storage**
Store below 40 °C (104 °F), preferably between 15 and 30 °C (59 and 86 °F), unless otherwise specified by manufacturer. Store in a well-closed container. Protect from light.

**Auxiliary labeling**
- May cause drowsiness.
- Avoid alcoholic beverages.

## PROCHLORPERAZINE MESYLATE SYRUP

**Usual adult and adolescent dose**
Psychotic disorders—
  Oral, 5 to 10 mg (base) three or four times a day, the dosage being gradually increased every two to three days as needed and tolerated.
Anxiety—
  Oral, 5 mg (base) three or four times a day, up to 20 mg a day, for no longer than twelve weeks.
Nausea and vomiting—
  Oral, 5 to 10 mg (base) three or four times a day, up to 40 mg a day.
Note: Geriatric, emaciated, or debilitated patients usually require a lower initial dose, the dosage being gradually increased as needed and tolerated.

**Usual pediatric dose**
Psychotic disorders—
  Children up to 2 years of age or 9 kg of body weight: Dosage has not been established.
  Children 2 to 12 years of age: Oral, 2.5 mg (base) two or three times a day.
  Children 12 years of age and older: See *Usual adult and adolescent dose*.
Nausea and vomiting—
  Children 9 to 13 kg of body weight: Oral, 2.5 mg (base) one or two times a day, not to exceed 7.5 mg a day.
  Children 14 to 17 kg of body weight: Oral, 2.5 mg (base) two or three times a day, not to exceed 10 mg a day.
  Children 18 to 39 kg of body weight: Oral, 2.5 mg (base) three times a day or 5 mg two times a day, not to exceed 15 mg a day.
Note: The total daily dose for any child should not exceed 10 mg the first day. On subsequent days the total daily dose should not exceed 20 mg for children 2 to 5 years of age or 25 mg for children 6 to 12 years of age.

**Strength(s) usually available**
U.S.—
  Not commercially available.
Canada—
  5 mg (base) per 5 mL (Rx) [*Stemetil Liquid* (sucrose)].

**Packaging and storage**
Store below 40 °C (104 °F), preferably between 15 and 30 °C (59 and 86 °F), in a tight container, protected from light, unless otherwise specified by manufacturer. Protect from freezing.

**Auxiliary labeling**
- May cause drowsiness.
- Avoid alcoholic beverages.
- Do not spill on skin or clothing.

**Note**
Avoid skin contact with liquid forms of this medication; contact dermatitis has resulted.

# Parenteral Dosage Forms

Note: The dosing and strengths of the dosage forms available are expressed in terms of prochlorperazine base (not the edisylate or mesylate salts).

## PROCHLORPERAZINE EDISYLATE INJECTION USP
### Usual adult and adolescent dose
Nausea and vomiting—
- Intramuscular, 5 to 10 mg (base), the dosage to be repeated every three to four hours as needed.
- Intravenous, 2.5 to 10 mg as a slow injection or infusion, at a rate not exceeding 5 mg per minute, up to 40 mg a day.
- Note: May be administered undiluted or diluted in isotonic solution.
  - Single dose should not exceed 10 mg.

Nausea and vomiting in surgery—
- Intramuscular, 5 to 10 mg (base) one to two hours before induction of anesthesia, or to control acute symptoms during or after surgery, the dose being repeated once in thirty minutes if needed.
- Intravenous, 5 to 10 mg (base), administered as a slow injection or infusion fifteen to thirty minutes before induction of anesthesia, or to control acute symptoms during or after surgery, at a rate not exceeding 5 mg per mL per minute, the dose being repeated once if needed.
- Note: May be administered undiluted or diluted in isotonic solution.
  - Single dose should not exceed 10 mg.

Psychotic disorders—
- Initial (for immediate control of severely disturbed patients): Intramuscular, 10 to 20 mg (base), the dose being repeated every two to four hours as needed, usually up to three or four doses.
- Maintenance: Intramuscular, 10 to 20 mg (base) every four to six hours.

Anxiety—
- Intramuscular, 5 to 10 mg (base), the dosage to be repeated every three to four hours as needed.
- Intravenous, 2.5 to 10 mg as a slow injection or infusion, at a rate not exceeding 5 mg per minute, up to 40 mg a day.
- Note: May be administered undiluted or diluted in isotonic solution.
  - Single dose should not exceed 10 mg.

Note: Geriatric, emaciated, or debilitated patients usually require a lower dose, the dosage being increased gradually as needed and tolerated.

### Usual adult prescribing limits
Nausea and vomiting or anxiety—
- Up to 40 mg (base) a day.

Psychotic disorders—
- Up to 200 mg (base) a day.

### Usual pediatric dose
Nausea and vomiting or
Psychotic disorders or anxiety—
- Children up to 2 years of age or 9 kg of body weight: Dosage has not been established.
- Children 2 to 12 years of age: Intramuscular, 132 mcg (0.132 mg) (base) per kg of body weight.
- Children 12 years of age and older: See *Usual adult and adolescent dose*.
- Note: Usual pediatric prescribing limits are 20 mg a day for children 2 to 5 years of age, and 25 mg a day for children 6 to 12 years old.
  - Control is usually obtained after one dose, after which patient may be switched to an oral dosage form at the same dosage level or higher.
  - Not recommended in pediatric surgery.

### Strength(s) usually available
U.S.—
- 5 mg (base) per mL (Rx) [*Compa-Z; Compazine* (ampuls: sulfite; vials: benzyl alcohol 0.75%); *Cotranzine; Ultrazine-10;* GENERIC].

Canada—
- Not commercially available.

### Packaging and storage
Store below 40 °C (104 °F), preferably between 15 and 30 °C (59 and 86 °F), unless otherwise specified by manufacturer. Protect from light. Protect from freezing.

### Stability
A slight yellowing will not alter potency; however, do not use if markedly discolored or if a precipitate is present.

### Incompatibilities
A white milky precipitate may form when prochlorperazine edisylate injection is mixed in the same syringe with morphine sulfate injection produced by certain manufacturers.

### Note
Avoid skin contact with liquid forms of this medication; contact dermatitis has resulted.

## PROCHLORPERAZINE MESYLATE INJECTION
### Usual adult and adolescent dose
Nausea and vomiting—
- Intramuscular, 5 to 10 mg (base), the dose being repeated every three to four hours if needed.

Nausea and vomiting in surgery—
- Intramuscular, 5 to 10 mg (base) one to two hours before induction of anesthesia, or to control acute symptoms during or after surgery, the dose being repeated once in thirty minutes if needed.
- Intravenous, 5 to 10 mg (base), administered fifteen to thirty minutes before induction of anesthesia, or to control acute symptoms during or after surgery, at a rate not to exceed 5 mg per mL per minute, the dose being repeated once if needed.
- Intravenous infusion, 20 mg (base) in no less than 1 liter of isotonic solution, administered fifteen to thirty minutes before induction of anesthesia.

Psychotic disorders—
- Initial (for immediate control of severely disturbed patients): Intramuscular, 10 to 20 mg (base), the dose being repeated every two to four hours as needed, usually up to three or four doses.
- Maintenance: Intramuscular, 10 to 20 mg (base) every four to six hours.

Anxiety—
- Intramuscular, 5 to 10 mg (base), the dose being repeated every three to four hours if needed.

Note: Geriatric, emaciated, or debilitated patients usually require a lower dose, the dosage being increased gradually as needed and tolerated.

### Usual adult prescribing limits
Nausea and vomiting—
- Up to 40 mg (base) a day.

Psychotic disorders—
- Up to 200 mg (base) a day.

### Usual pediatric dose
Nausea and vomiting or
Psychotic disorders or anxiety—
- Children up to 2 years of age or 9 kg of body weight: Dosage has not been established.
- Children 2 to 12 years of age: Intramuscular, 132 mcg (0.132 mg) (base) per kg of body weight, not exceeding 10 mg the first day, the dosage being increased, thereafter, as needed and tolerated.
- Children 12 years of age and over: See *Usual adult or adolescent dose*.
- Note: Usual pediatric prescribing limits are 20 mg a day for children 2 to 5 years of age, and 25 mg a day for children 6 to 12 years old.
  - Not recommended in pediatric surgery.

### Strength(s) usually available
U.S.—
- Not commercially available.

Canada—
- 5 mg (base) per mL (Rx) [*PMS Prochlorperazine; Stemetil* (sulfite) [GENERIC].

### Packaging and storage
Store below 40 °C (104 °F), preferably between 15 and 30 °C (59 and 86 °F), protected from light, unless otherwise specified by manufacturer. Protect from freezing.

### Stability
A slight yellowing will not alter potency; however, do not use if markedly discolored or if a precipitate is present.

### Note
Avoid skin contact with liquid forms of this medication; contact dermatitis has resulted.

# Rectal Dosage Forms
## PROCHLORPERAZINE SUPPOSITORIES USP
### Usual adult and adolescent dose
Nausea and vomiting—
- Rectal, 25 mg two times a day.

Psychotic disorders—
- Rectal, 10 mg three or four times a day, the dosage being increased gradually by 5 to 10 mg every two to three days as needed and tolerated.

Note: Geriatric, emaciated, or debilitated patients usually require a lower initial dose, the dosage being gradually increased as needed and tolerated.

**Usual pediatric dose**
Nausea and vomiting—
- Children up to 2 years of age or 9 kg of body weight: Dosage has not been established.
- Children 9 to 13 kg of body weight: Rectal, 2.5 mg one or two times a day, not to exceed 7.5 mg per day.
- Children 14 to 17 kg of body weight: Rectal, 2.5 mg two or three times a day, not to exceed 10 mg per day.
- Children 18 to 39 kg of body weight: Rectal, 2.5 mg three times a day or 5 mg two times a day, not to exceed 15 mg per day.

Note: The total daily dose for any child should not exceed 10 mg the first day. On subsequent days, the total daily dose should not exceed 20 mg for children 2 to 5 years of age or 25 mg for children 6 to 12 years of age.

The 25-mg suppository is not recommended for use in children.

**Strength(s) usually available**
U.S.—
- 2.5 mg (Rx) [*Compazine*].
- 5 mg (Rx) [*Compazine*].
- 25 mg (Rx) [*Compazine*; GENERIC].

Canada—
- 10 mg (Rx) [*PMS Prochlorperazine*; *Prorazin*; *Stemetil* [GENERIC]].

**Packaging and storage**
Store below 37 °C (98 °F). Store in a tight container. Protect from light.

**Auxiliary labeling**
- May cause drowsiness.
- Avoid alcoholic beverages.
- For rectal use only.

**Note**
Explain administration technique.

---

## *PROMAZINE*

## Summary of Differences
Pharmacology/pharmacokinetics:
  Chemical group—
    Aliphatic
  Actions—
    Antiemetic: Moderate
    Anticholinergic: Strong
    Extrapyramidal: Weak
    Hypotensive: Strong
    Sedative: Strong

## Oral Dosage Forms
### PROMAZINE HYDROCHLORIDE TABLETS USP

**Usual adult dose**
Psychotic disorders—
  Oral, 10 to 200 mg every four to six hours, the dosage being adjusted gradually as needed and tolerated.

Note: Geriatric, emaciated, or debilitated patients usually require a lower initial dose, the dosage being gradually increased as needed and tolerated.

**Usual adult prescribing limits**
Up to 1 gram a day.

**Usual pediatric dose**
Psychotic disorders—
  Children up to 12 years of age: Dosage has not been established.
  Children 12 years of age and over: Oral, 10 to 25 mg every four to six hours, the dosage being adjusted as needed and tolerated.

**Strength(s) usually available**
U.S.—
- 25 mg (Rx) [*Sparine* (tartrazine; sucrose)].
- 50 mg (Rx) [*Sparine* (sucrose)].
- 100 mg (Rx) [*Sparine* (sucrose)].

Canada—
  Not commercially available.

**Packaging and storage**
Store below 40 °C (104 °F), preferably between 15 and 30 °C (59 and 86 °F), unless otherwise specified by manufacturer. Store in a tight, light-resistant container.

**Auxiliary labeling**
- May cause drowsiness.
- Avoid alcoholic beverages.

## Parenteral Dosage Forms
### PROMAZINE HYDROCHLORIDE INJECTION USP

**Usual adult dose**
Psychotic disorders—
  Intramuscular:
    Initial—50 to 150 mg, the dosage being increased, if necessary, after thirty minutes.
    Maintenance—10 to 200 mg, the dose being repeated at four- to six-hour intervals as needed and tolerated.
  Intravenous:
    Administered slowly after being diluted to 25 mg or less per mL with 0.9% sodium chloride injection.

Note: Geriatric, emaciated, or debilitated patients usually require a lower initial dose, the dosage being gradually increased as needed and tolerated.
  Intravenous injection should be reserved for severely agitated hospitalized patients.
  In acutely inebriated patients, the initial dose should not exceed 50 mg.

**Usual adult prescribing limits**
Up to 1 gram a day.

Note: Although doses are sometimes gradually increased to 2 grams a day or more for short periods, extended therapy with 1 gram or less is usually sufficient.

**Usual pediatric dose**
Psychotic disorders—
  Children up to 12 years of age: Dosage has not been established.
  Children 12 years of age and over: Intramuscular, 10 to 25 mg every four to six hours, up to 1 gram a day.

**Strength(s) usually available**
U.S.—
- 50 mg per mL (Rx) [*Primazine*; *Prozine-50*; *Sparine*; GENERIC (syringe units; sulfite)].

Canada—
- 50 mg per mL (Rx) [GENERIC].

**Packaging and storage**
Store below 40 °C (104 °F), preferably between 15 and 30 °C (59 and 86 °F), unless otherwise specified by manufacturer. Protect from light. Protect from freezing.

**Stability**
A slight yellowing will not alter potency; however, do not use if markedly discolored or if a precipitate is present.

**Note**
Avoid skin contact with liquid forms of this medication; contact dermatitis has resulted.

---

## *THIOPROPAZATE*

## Summary of Differences
Pharmacology/pharmacokinetics:
  Chemical group—
    Piperazine
  Actions—
    Antiemetic: Weak
    Anticholinergic: Weak
    Extrapyramidal: Strong
    Hypotensive: Weak
    Sedative: Weak

## Oral Dosage Forms
### THIOPROPAZATE HYDROCHLORIDE TABLETS

**Usual adult and adolescent dose**
Psychotic disorders—
  Initial: Oral, 10 mg three times a day, the dosage being adjusted gradually by 10 mg every three or four days as needed and tolerated.
  Maintenance: Oral, 10 to 20 mg two to four times a day.

Note: Geriatric, emaciated, or debilitated patients usually require a lower initial dose, the dosage being increased gradually as needed and tolerated, and decreased to the lowest effective dose as soon as possible.

**Usual adult prescribing limits**
Up to 100 mg a day.

**Usual pediatric dose**
Dosage has not been established.

**Strength(s) usually available**
U.S.—
  Not commercially available.
Canada—
  5 mg (Rx) [*Dartal* (acacia; activated charcoal; cornstarch; lactose; light liquid parafin; magnesium stearate; sodium sulfate; talc; tapioca starch; sodium 3.5 mmol [80 mg])].

**Packaging and storage**
Store below 40 °C (104 °F), in a well-closed, light-resistant container, unless otherwise specified by manufacturer.

**Auxiliary labeling**
• May cause drowsiness.
• Avoid alcoholic beverages.

---
### THIOPROPERAZINE
---

## Summary of Differences
Pharmacology/pharmacokinetics:
  Chemical group—
    Piperazine
  Actions—
    Antiemetic: Weak
    Anticholinergic: Weak
    Extrapyramidal: Strong
    Hypotensive: Weak
    Sedative: Weak

## Oral Dosage Forms
Note: The dosing and strengths of the dosage forms available are expressed in terms of thioproperazine base (not the mesylate salt).

### THIOPROPERAZINE MESYLATE TABLETS

**Usual adult and adolescent dose**
Psychotic disorders—
  Oral, initially, 5 mg (base) a day, the dosage being adjusted gradually by 5 mg every two or three days as needed and tolerated.
Note: The usual effective dose is about 30 to 40 mg a day. In some patients, 90 mg or more a day may be necessary to control symptoms. Once symptoms are controlled, dosage should be reduced gradually to the lowest effective maintenance dose.

**Usual pediatric dose**
Dosage has not been established.

**Strength(s) usually available**
U.S.—
  Not commercially available.
Canada—
  10 mg (base) (Rx) [*Majeptil*].

**Packaging and storage**
Store below 40 °C (104 °F), in a well-closed, light-resistant container, unless otherwise specified by manufacturer.

**Auxiliary labeling**
• May cause drowsiness.
• Avoid alcoholic beverages.

---
### THIORIDAZINE
---

## Summary of Differences
Pharmacology/pharmacokinetics:
  Chemical group—
    Piperidine
  Actions—
    Antiemetic: Weak
    Anticholinergic: Moderate
    Extrapyramidal: Weak
    Hypotensive: Moderate to strong
    Sedative: Moderate
Side/adverse effects:
  In high doses, more likely to cause pigmentary retinopathy than other phenothiazines.

## Oral Dosage Forms

### THIORIDAZINE ORAL SUSPENSION USP

**Usual adult and adolescent dose**
Psychotic disorders—
  Initial: Oral, 25 to 100 mg (hydrochloride) three times a day, the dosage being adjusted gradually as needed and tolerated.
  Maintenance: Oral, 10 to 200 mg (hydrochloride) two to four times a day.
Note: Geriatric, emaciated, or debilitated patients usually require a lower initial dose, the dosage being gradually increased as needed and tolerated.

**Usual adult prescribing limits**
Up to 800 mg (hydrochloride) a day.

**Usual pediatric dose**
Psychotic disorders—
  Children up to 2 years of age: Dosage has not been established.
  Children 2 to 12 years of age: Oral, 250 mcg (0.25 mg) to 3 mg (hydrochloride) per kg of body weight or 7.5 mg per square meter of body surface four times a day; or 10 to 25 mg two or three times a day.
  Children 12 years of age and over: See *Usual adult and adolescent dose*.

**Strength(s) usually available**
U.S.—
  25 mg (hydrochloride) per 5 mL (Rx) [*Mellaril-S* (carbomer 934; flavor; polysorbate 80; purified water; sodium hydroxide; sucrose)].
  100 mg (hydrochloride) per 5 mL (Rx) [*Mellaril-S* (carbomer 934; flavor; polysorbate 80; purified water; sodium hydroxide; sucrose; D&C Yellow No. 10; FD&C Yellow No. 6)].
Canada—
  10 mg (hydrochloride) per 5 mL (Rx) [*Mellaril* (alcohol; parabens)].

**Packaging and storage**
Store below 30 °C (86 °F). Store in a tight, light-resistant container. Protect from freezing.

**Auxiliary labeling**
• Shake well before using.
• May cause drowsiness.
• Avoid alcoholic beverages.
• Do not spill on skin or clothing.

**Note**
Avoid skin contact with liquid forms of this medication; contact dermatitis has resulted.

### THIORIDAZINE HYDROCHLORIDE ORAL SOLUTION USP

**Usual adult and adolescent dose**
Psychotic disorders—
  Initial: Oral, 25 to 100 mg three times a day, the dosage being adjusted gradually as needed and tolerated.
  Maintenance: Oral, 10 to 200 mg two to four times a day.
Note: Geriatric, emaciated, or debilitated patients usually require a lower initial dose, the dosage being gradually increased as needed and tolerated.

**Usual adult prescribing limits**
Up to 800 mg a day.

**Usual pediatric dose**
Psychotic disorders—
  Children up to 2 years of age: Dosage has not been established.
  Children 2 to 12 years of age: Oral, 250 mcg (0.25 mg) to 3 mg per kg of body weight or 7.5 mg per square meter of body surface four times a day; or 10 to 25 mg two or three times a day.
  Children 12 years of age and over: See *Usual adult and adolescent dose*.

**Strength(s) usually available**
U.S.—
  30 mg per mL (Rx) [*Mellaril Concentrate* (alcohol 3%); GENERIC].
  100 mg per mL (Rx) [*Mellaril Concentrate* (alcohol 4.2%); GENERIC].
Canada—
  30 mg per mL (Rx) [*Mellaril* (alcohol 3%; parabens)].

**Packaging and storage**
Store between 15 and 30 °C (59 and 86 °F), unless otherwise specified by manufacturer. Store in a tight, light-resistant container. Protect from freezing.

**Auxiliary labeling**
- May cause drowsiness.
- Avoid alcoholic beverages.
- Do not spill on skin or clothing.
- Must be diluted before use.

**Note**

Avoid skin contact with liquid forms of this medication; contact dermatitis has resulted.

Each dose must be diluted just before administration in a half glass (120 mL) of distilled water, acidified tap water, orange juice, or grapefruit juice.

Explain dilution and dosage measurement to patient if self-administered.

### THIORIDAZINE HYDROCHLORIDE TABLETS USP

**Usual adult and adolescent dose**
Psychotic disorders—
   Initial: Oral, 25 to 100 mg three times a day, the dosage being adjusted gradually as needed and tolerated.
   Maintenance: Oral, 10 to 200 mg two to four times a day.
Note: Geriatric, emaciated, or debilitated patients usually require a lower initial dose, the dosage being gradually increased as needed and tolerated.

**Usual adult prescribing limits**
Up to 800 mg a day.

**Usual pediatric dose**
Psychotic disorders—
   Children up to 2 years of age: Dosage has not been established.
   Children 2 to 12 years of age: Oral, 250 mcg (0.25 mg) to 3 mg per kg of body weight or 7.5 mg per square meter of body surface four times a day; or 10 to 25 mg two or three times a day.
   Children 12 years of age and over: See *Usual adult and adolescent dose*.
Note: Since tablets are not suitable for many pediatric patients' requirements, the oral solution may be preferred.

**Strength(s) usually available**
U.S.—
   10 mg (Rx) [*Mellaril*; GENERIC].
   15 mg (Rx) [*Mellaril*; GENERIC].
   25 mg (Rx) [*Mellaril*; GENERIC].
   50 mg (Rx) [*Mellaril*; GENERIC].
   100 mg (Rx) [*Mellaril*; GENERIC].
   150 mg (Rx) [*Mellaril*; GENERIC].
   200 mg (Rx) [*Mellaril*; GENERIC].
Canada—
   10 mg (Rx) [*Apo-Thioridazine; Mellaril; Novo-Ridazine; PMS Thioridazine*].
   25 mg (Rx) [*Apo-Thioridazine; Mellaril; Novo-Ridazine; PMS Thioridazine*].
   50 mg (Rx) [*Apo-Thioridazine; Mellaril; Novo-Ridazine; PMS Thioridazine*].
   100 mg (Rx) [*Apo-Thioridazine; Mellaril; Novo-Ridazine; PMS Thioridazine*].
   200 mg (Rx) [*Mellaril; Novo-Ridazine*].

**Packaging and storage**
Store below 40 °C (104 °F), preferably between 15 and 30 °C (59 and 86 °F), unless otherwise specified by manufacturer. Store in a tight, light-resistant container.

**Auxiliary labeling**
- May cause drowsiness.
- Avoid alcoholic beverages.

---

## TRIFLUOPERAZINE

## Summary of Differences

Pharmacology/pharmacokinetics:
   Chemical group—
      Piperazine
   Actions—
      Antiemetic: Strong
      Anticholinergic: Weak
      Extrapyramidal: Strong
      Hypotensive: Weak
      Sedative: Weak

## Oral Dosage Forms

Note: The dosing and strengths of the dosage forms available are expressed in terms of trifluoperazine base (not the hydrochloride salt).

### TRIFLUOPERAZINE HYDROCHLORIDE ORAL SOLUTION

**Usual adult and adolescent dose**
Psychotic disorders—
   Oral, 2 to 5 mg (base) two times a day initially, the dosage being gradually increased as needed and tolerated.
Anxiety—
   1 to 2 mg (base) a day, up to a total of 6 mg a day, for no longer than twelve weeks.
Note: Geriatric, emaciated, or debilitated patients usually require a lower initial dose, the dosage being gradually increased as needed and tolerated.

**Usual adult prescribing limits**
Up to 40 mg (base) a day.

**Usual pediatric dose**
Psychotic disorders—
   Children up to 6 years of age: Dosage has not been established.
   Children 6 years of age and over: Oral, 1 mg (base) one or two times a day, the dosage being adjusted gradually as needed and tolerated.

**Strength(s) usually available**
U.S.—
   10 mg (base) per mL (Rx) [*Stelazine Concentrate* (sulfite); GENERIC].
Canada—
   10 mg (base) per mL (Rx) [*Stelazine Concentrate* (sulfite); *Terfluzine Concentrate*].

**Packaging and storage**
Store below 40 °C (104 °F), preferably between 15 and 30 °C (59 and 86 °F), in a tight, light-resistant container, unless otherwise specified by manufacturer. Protect from freezing.

**Stability**
A slight yellowing will not alter potency; however, do not use if markedly discolored or if a precipitate is present.

**Auxiliary labeling**
- May cause drowsiness.
- Avoid alcoholic beverages.
- Do not spill on skin or clothing.
- Must be diluted before use.

**Note**

The oral solution is intended primarily for institutional usage.

Avoid skin contact with liquid forms of this medication; contact dermatitis has resulted.

Each dose must be diluted just before administration in a half glass (120 mL) of milk, tomato or fruit juice, water, or soup.

Explain dilution and dosage measurement to patient if self-administered.

### TRIFLUOPERAZINE HYDROCHLORIDE SYRUP USP

**Usual adult and adolescent dose**
Psychotic disorders—
   Oral, 2 to 5 mg (base) two times a day initially, the dosage being gradually increased as needed and tolerated.
Anxiety—
   1 to 2 mg (base) a day, up to a total of 6 mg a day, for no longer than twelve weeks.
Note: Geriatric, emaciated, or debilitated patients usually require a lower initial dose, the dosage being gradually increased as needed and tolerated.

**Usual adult prescribing limits**
Up to 40 mg (base) a day.

**Usual pediatric dose**
Psychotic disorders—
   Children up to 6 years of age: Dosage has not been established.
   Children 6 years of age and over: Oral, 1 mg (base) one or two times a day, the dosage being adjusted gradually as needed and tolerated.

**Strength(s) usually available**
U.S.—
   Not commercially available.
Canada—
   1 mg (base) per mL (Rx) [*PMS Trifluoperazine*].
   10 mg (base) per mL (Rx) [*PMS Trifluoperazine; Terfluzine*].

**Packaging and storage**
Store below 40 °C (104 °F), preferably between 15 and 30 °C (59 and 86 °F), in a tight, light-resistant container, unless otherwise specified by manufacturer. Protect from freezing.

**Auxiliary labeling**
- May cause drowsiness.
- Avoid alcoholic beverages.

### TRIFLUOPERAZINE HYDROCHLORIDE TABLETS USP

**Usual adult and adolescent dose**
Psychotic disorders—
  Oral, 2 to 5 mg (base) two times a day initially, the dosage being gradually increased as needed and tolerated.
Anxiety—
  1 to 2 mg (base) a day, up to a total of 6 mg a day, for not longer than twelve weeks.
Note: Geriatric, emaciated, or debilitated patients usually require a lower initial dose, the dosage being gradually increased as needed and tolerated.

**Usual adult prescribing limits**
Up to 40 mg (base) a day.

**Usual pediatric dose**
Psychotic disorders—
  Children up to 6 years of age: Dosage has not been established.
  Children 6 years of age and over: Oral, 1 mg (base) one or two times a day, the dosage being adjusted gradually as needed and tolerated.

**Strength(s) usually available**
U.S.—
  1 mg (base) (Rx) [*Stelazine;* GENERIC].
  2 mg (base) (Rx) [*Stelazine;* GENERIC].
  5 mg (base) (Rx) [*Stelazine;* GENERIC].
  10 mg (base) (Rx) [*Stelazine;* GENERIC].
Canada—
  1 mg (base) (Rx) [*Apo-Trifluoperazine; Novo-Flurazine; PMS Trifluoperazine; Stelazine; Terfluzine*].
  2 mg (base) (Rx) [*Apo-Trifluoperazine; Novo-Flurazine; PMS Trifluoperazine; Solazine; Stelazine; Terfluzine*].
  5 mg (base) (Rx) [*Apo-Trifluoperazine; Novo-Flurazine; PMS Trifluoperazine; Solazine; Stelazine; Terfluzine*].
  10 mg (base) (Rx) [*Apo-Trifluoperazine; Novo-Flurazine; PMS Trifluoperazine; Solazine* (tartrazine); *Stelazine; Terfluzine*].
  20 mg (base) (Rx) [*Apo-Trifluoperazine; Novo-Flurazine; PMS Trifluoperazine*].

**Packaging and storage**
Store below 40 °C (104 °F), preferably between 15 and 30 °C (59 and 86 °F), unless otherwise specified by manufacturer. Store in a well-closed, light-resistant container.

**Auxiliary labeling**
- May cause drowsiness.
- Avoid alcoholic beverages.

## Parenteral Dosage Forms

Note: The dosing and strengths of the dosage forms available are expressed in terms of trifluoperazine base (not the hydrochloride salt).

### TRIFLUOPERAZINE HYDROCHLORIDE INJECTION USP

**Usual adult and adolescent dose**
Psychotic disorders—
  Intramuscular, 1 to 2 mg (base) every four to six hours as needed.
Note: Geriatric, emaciated, or debilitated patients usually require a lower initial dose, the dosage being increased gradually as needed and tolerated.

**Usual adult prescribing limits**
Up to 10 mg (base) a day.

**Usual pediatric dose**
Psychotic disorders—
  Children up to 6 years of age: Dosage has not been established.
  Children 6 years of age and over: Intramuscular, 1 mg (base) one or two times a day.

**Strength(s) usually available**
U.S.—
  2 mg (base) per mL (Rx) [*Stelazine* (benzyl alcohol 0.75%; sodium tartrate; sodium biphosphate; sodium saccharin); GENERIC].
Canada—
  1 mg (base) per mL (Rx) [*Stelazine* (sulfite; benzyl alcohol 0.75%)].

**Packaging and storage**
Store below 40 °C (104 °F), preferably between 15 and 30 °C (59 and 86 °F), unless otherwise specified by manufacturer. Protect from light. Protect from freezing.

**Stability**
A slight yellowing will not alter potency; however, do not use if markedly discolored or if a precipitate is present.

**Note**
Avoid skin contact with liquid forms of this medication; contact dermatitis has resulted.

---

## TRIFLUPROMAZINE

### Summary of Differences
Category:
  Includes antiemetic use.
Pharmacology/pharmacokinetics:
  Chemical group—
    Aliphatic
  Actions—
    Antiemetic: Strong
    Anticholinergic: Strong
    Extrapyramidal: Moderate to strong
    Hypotensive: Moderate
    Sedative: Moderate to strong

## Parenteral Dosage Forms

### TRIFLUPROMAZINE HYDROCHLORIDE INJECTION USP

**Usual adult and adolescent dose**
Psychotic disorders—
  Intramuscular, 60 mg as needed.
Nausea and vomiting—
  Intramuscular, 5 to 15 mg every four hours.
  Intravenous, 1 mg as needed.
Note: Geriatric, emaciated, or debilitated patients usually require a lower initial dose, the dosage being increased as needed and tolerated.

**Usual adult prescribing limits**
Psychotic disorders—
  Intramuscular, up to 150 mg a day.
Nausea and vomiting—
  Intramuscular, up to 60 mg a day.
  Intravenous, up to 3 mg a day.

**Usual pediatric dose**
Psychotic disorders or
Nausea and vomiting—
  Children up to 2½ years of age: Dosage has not been established.
  Children 2½ years of age and over: Intramuscular, 200 to 250 mcg (0.2 to 0.25 mg) per kg of body weight, not to exceed 10 mg per day.
Note: Intravenous administration is not recommended in children because of hypotension and rapid onset of severe extrapyramidal reactions.

**Strength(s) usually available**
U.S.—
  10 mg per mL (Rx) [*Vesprin* (benzyl alcohol 1.5%)].
  20 mg per mL (Rx) [*Vesprin* (benzyl alcohol 1.5%)].
Canada—
  Not commercially available.

**Packaging and storage**
Store between 15 and 30 °C (59 and 86 °F), unless otherwise specified by manufacturer. Protect from light. Protect from freezing.

**Stability**
A slight yellowing to a light amber color will not alter potency; however, do not use if markedly discolored or if a precipitate is present.

**Note**
Avoid skin contact with liquid forms of this medication; contact dermatitis has resulted.

Revised: 03/16/92
Interim revision: 08/23/94

# PHENOXYBENZAMINE Systemic

VA CLASSIFICATION (Primary/Secondary): CV150/CV409; GU900
Commonly used brand name(s): *Dibenzyline*.
Note: For a listing of dosage forms and brand names by country availability, see *Dosage Forms* section(s).

## Category
Antihypertensive (pheochromocytoma); benign prostatic hypertrophy therapy.

## Indications
Note: Bracketed information in the *Indications* section refers to uses that are not included in U.S. product labeling.

### Accepted
Pheochromocytoma (treatment)—Phenoxybenzamine is indicated to control episodes of hypertension and sweating in the treatment of pheochromocytoma as preoperative preparation for surgery, in management of patients when surgery is contraindicated, and in chronic management of patients with malignant pheochromocytoma.

[Benign prostatic hypertrophy (treatment)]—Phenoxybenzamine is used for the treatment of urinary symptoms associated with benign prostatic hypertrophy (BPH).

### Unaccepted
Phenoxybenzamine is not useful in the treatment of essential hypertension because of its side effects, particularly reflex tachycardia.

## Pharmacology/Pharmacokinetics

### Physicochemical characteristics
Molecular weight—340.29.
pKa—4.4.

### Mechanism of action/Effect
Nonselective alpha-adrenergic blockade; phenoxybenzamine combines irreversibly with postganglionic alpha-adrenergic receptor sites, preventing or reversing effects of endogenous or exogenous catecholamines; no effect on beta-adrenergic receptors.

### Absorption
Variable following oral administration. Approximately 20 to 30% absorbed in the active form.

### Biotransformation
Hepatic.

### Half-life
Approximately 24 hours.

### Onset of action
Alpha-adrenergic blockade—Several hours.

Note: Alpha-adrenergic blocking effects are cumulative over approximately 7 days with daily dosing.

### Duration of action
Alpha-adrenergic blockade—3 to 4 days after a single dose.

### Elimination
Renal/biliary.

## Precautions to Consider

### Carcinogenicity
Repeated intraperitoneal administration of phenoxybenzamine to rats and mice caused peritoneal sarcomas, and chronic oral dosing in rats caused malignant tumors of the gastrointestinal tract (primarily in the nonglandular stomach). Chronic oral studies in rats found probable drug-related development of ulcerative and/or erosive gastritis of the glandular stomach.

### Mutagenicity
Phenoxybenzamine has been found to be mutagenic *in vitro* in the Ames test and in the mouse lymphoma assay. However, it has not shown mutagenic activity in the micronucleus test in mice.

### Pregnancy/Reproduction
Pregnancy—Studies have not been done in humans.
Studies have not been done in animals.

FDA Pregnancy Category C.

### Breast-feeding
It is not known whether phenoxybenzamine is distributed into breast milk. However, problems in humans have not been documented.

### Pediatrics
Appropriate studies on the relationship of age to the effects of phenoxybenzamine have not been performed in the pediatric population. However, pediatrics-specific problems that would limit the usefulness of this medication in children are not expected.

### Geriatrics
Although appropriate studies on the relationship of age to the effects of phenoxybenzamine have not been performed in the geriatric population, no geriatrics-specific problems have been documented to date. However, the elderly may be more sensitive to the hypotensive effects and the risk of phenoxybenzamine-induced hypothermia may be increased in elderly patients. Furthermore, elderly patients are also more likely to have age-related renal function impairment, which may require caution in patients receiving phenoxybenzamine.

### Dental
Use of phenoxybenzamine may decrease or inhibit salivary flow, thus contributing to the development of caries, periodontal disease, oral candidiasis, and discomfort.

### Drug interactions and/or related problems
The following drug interactions and/or related problems have been selected on the basis of their potential clinical significance (possible mechanism in parentheses where appropriate)—not necessarily inclusive (» = major clinical significance):

Note: Combinations containing any of the following medications, depending on the amount present, may also interact with this medication.

Diazoxide
(concurrent use with phenoxybenzamine antagonizes the inhibition of insulin release by diazoxide)

Guanadrel or
Guanethidine
(concurrent use with phenoxybenzamine may cause an increased incidence of orthostatic hypotension or bradycardia)

Sympathomimetics, such as:
Dopamine
Ephedrine
» Epinephrine
» Metaraminol
» Methoxamine
» Phenylephrine
(concurrent use of dopamine with phenoxybenzamine antagonizes the peripheral vasoconstriction produced by high doses of dopamine)
(concurrent use of ephedrine with phenoxybenzamine may decrease the pressor response to ephedrine)
(concurrent use of epinephrine with phenoxybenzamine may block the alpha-adrenergic effects of epinephrine, possibly resulting in severe hypotension and tachycardia)
(alpha-adrenergic blocking agents such as phenoxybenzamine usually decrease, but do not reverse, pressor response to metaraminol)
(prior administration of phenoxybenzamine may block the pressor response to methoxamine, possibly resulting in severe hypotension)
(prior administration of phenoxybenzamine may decrease the pressor response to phenylephrine)

### Medical considerations/Contraindications
The medical considerations/contraindications included have been selected on the basis of their potential clinical significance (reasons given in parentheses where appropriate)—not necessarily inclusive (» = major clinical significance).

*Risk-benefit should be considered when the following medical problems exist:*

Cerebrovascular insufficiency
(reduced blood pressure may aggravate ischemia)
Congestive heart failure, compensated or
Coronary artery disease
(reflex tachycardia may precipitate frank congestive heart failure and angina)
Renal function impairment
Respiratory infection
(symptoms such as nasal congestion may be aggravated)
Sensitivity to phenoxybenzamine

### Patient monitoring
The following may be especially important in patient monitoring (other tests may be warranted in some patients, depending on condition; » = major clinical significance):
» Blood pressure measurements and
» Urinary catecholamine measurements
(recommended at periodic intervals during initial therapy to determine maximal dose)

### Side/Adverse Effects
The following side/adverse effects have been selected on the basis of their potential clinical significance (possible signs and symptoms in parentheses where appropriate)—not necessarily inclusive:

**Those indicating need for medical attention only if they continue or are bothersome**
Incidence more frequent—resulting from alpha-adrenergic blockade
*Miosis* (pinpoint pupils); *nasal congestion* (stuffy nose); *postural hypotension* (dizziness or lightheadedness, especially when getting up from a lying or sitting position); *tachycardia, reflex* (fast heartbeat)
Incidence less frequent
*Confusion; drowsiness; dryness of mouth; headache; inability to ejaculate; lack of energy; unusual tiredness or weakness*
Note: *Inability to ejaculate* is caused by alpha-adrenergic blockade.

### Overdose
For more information on the management of overdose or unintentional ingestion, **contact a Poison Control Center** (see *Poison Control Center Listing*).

**Treatment of overdose**
Treatment of circulatory failure, either by placing the patient in the recumbent position with legs elevated or additional measures if shock is present.
The usual pressor agents are not effective; epinephrine should not be used because of the risk of further hypotension.
Intravenous administration of levarterenol bitartrate may be useful.

### Patient Consultation
As an aid to patient consultation, refer to *Advice for the Patient, Phenoxybenzamine (Systemic)*.
In providing consultation, consider emphasizing the following selected information (»= major clinical significance):

**Before using this medication**
» Conditions affecting use, especially:
  Sensitivity to phenoxybenzamine
  Use in the elderly—Elderly patients may be more sensitive to the hypotensive effects; risk of phenoxybenzamine-induced hypothermia may be increased
  Dental—May decrease or inhibit salivary flow

**Proper use of this medication**
Compliance with therapy; taking medication at the same time(s) each day to maintain the therapeutic effect
» Proper dosing
  Missed dose: Taking as soon as possible; not taking if almost time for next dose; not doubling doses
» Proper storage

**Precautions while using this medication**
Making regular visits to physician to check progress during therapy
» Not taking other medications, especially nonprescription sympathomimetics, unless discussed with physician
» Caution when driving or doing things requiring alertness because of possible dizziness or drowsiness
» Caution when getting up suddenly from a lying or sitting position
» Caution in using alcohol, while standing for long periods or exercising, and during hot weather because of enhanced orthostatic hypotensive effects
» Caution if any kind of surgery (including dental surgery) or emergency treatment is required
Possible dryness of mouth; using sugarless candy or gum, ice, or saliva substitute for relief; checking with physician or dentist if dry mouth continues for more than 2 weeks

### General Dosing Information
Dosage must be adjusted to meet the individual requirements of each patient, on the basis of clinical response and urinary catecholamine determinations.

Incidence and severity of side effects may be reduced by initiating therapy at a low dose and increasing gradually to the minimum effective dose.
It is recommended that dosage increments be made no more frequently than every 4 days.
Concurrent administration of a beta-adrenergic blocker may be necessary if reflex tachycardia is severe.
If gastrointestinal irritation occurs, phenoxybenzamine may be administered with meals or milk; dosage reduction may be necessary.

### Oral Dosage Forms

**PHENOXYBENZAMINE HYDROCHLORIDE CAPSULES USP**

**Usual adult dose**
Antihypertensive (pheochromocytoma)—
  Initial: Oral, 10 mg twice a day, increased by increments of 10 mg every other day until an adequate response is achieved.
  Maintenance: Oral, 20 to 40 mg two or three times a day.
[Benign prostatic hypertrophy therapy]—
  10 to 20 mg per day.
Note: Geriatric patients may be more sensitive to the effects of the usual adult dose.

**Usual pediatric dose**
Antihypertensive (pheochromocytoma)—
  Initial: Oral, 200 mcg (0.2 mg) per kg of body weight or 6 mg per square meter of body surface, up to a maximum dose of 10 mg, once a day. Dosage is increased gradually at four-day intervals, until an adequate response is achieved.
  Maintenance: Oral, 400 mcg (0.4 mg) to 1.2 mg per kg of body weight or 12 to 36 mg per square meter of body surface a day in three or four divided doses.

**Strength(s) usually available**
U.S.—
  10 mg (Rx) [*Dibenzyline* (lactose)].

**Packaging and storage**
Store below 40 °C (104 °F), preferably between 15 and 30 °C (59 and 86 °F), unless otherwise specified by manufacturer. Store in a well-closed container.

Revised: 09/20/92
Interim revision: 07/20/94; 08/19/98

---

**PHENTERMINE**—See *Appetite Suppressants (Systemic)*

---

**PHENTOLAMINE**—The *Phentolamine (Intracavernosal)* monograph is not included in this published version of the USP DI database. Copies of the monograph are available on request from Micromedex, Inc. - Reprint Requests, 6200 S. Syracuse Way, Suite 300, Englewood, CO 80111; telephone (303) 486-6400; telefax (303) 486-6464; Email: USPDI@MDX.COM.

---

**PHENTOLAMINE**—The *Phentolamine (Systemic)* monograph is not included in this published version of the USP DI database. Copies of the monograph are available on request from Micromedex, Inc. - Reprint Requests, 6200 S. Syracuse Way, Suite 300, Englewood, CO 80111; telephone (303) 486-6400; telefax (303) 486-6464; Email: USPDI@MDX.COM.

---

**PHENYLBUTAZONE**—See *Anti-inflammatory Drugs, Nonsteroidal (Systemic)*

---

**PHENYLEPHRINE**—See *Phenylephrine (Nasal)*; *Sympathomimetic Agents—Cardiovascular Use (Parenteral-Systemic)*

**PHENYLEPHRINE**—The *Phenylephrine (Nasal)* monograph is not included in this published version of the USP DI database. Copies of the monograph are available on request from Micromedex, Inc. - Reprint Requests, 6200 S. Syracuse Way, Suite 300, Englewood, CO 80111; telephone (303) 486-6400; telefax (303) 486-6464; Email: USPDI@MDX.COM.

**PHENYLEPHRINE**—The *Phenylephrine (Ophthalmic)* monograph is not included in this published version of the USP DI database. Copies of the monograph are available on request from Micromedex, Inc. - Reprint Requests, 6200 S. Syracuse Way, Suite 300, Englewood, CO 80111; telephone (303) 486-6400; telefax (303) 486-6464; Email: USPDI@MDX.COM.

# PHENYLPROPANOLAMINE  Systemic†

VA CLASSIFICATION (Primary/Secondary): AU100/GA751; RE200

Commonly used brand name(s): *Acutrim 16 Hour; Acutrim II Maximum Strength; Acutrim Late Day; Control; Dexatrim Maximum Strength Caplets; Dexatrim Maximum Strength Capsules; Dexatrim Maximum Strength Tablets; Diet-Aid Maximum Strength; Efed II Yellow; Phenyldrine; Prolamine; Propagest.*

Another commonly used name is PPA.

Note: For a listing of dosage forms and brand names by country availability, see *Dosage Forms* section(s).

†Not commercially available in Canada.

## Category
Sympathomimetic (adrenergic) agent; appetite suppressant; decongestant, nasal (systemic).

## Indications
Note: Bracketed information in the *Indications* section refers to uses that are not included in U.S. product labeling.

**Accepted**

Obesity, exogenous (treatment)—Phenylpropanolamine (PPA) is indicated in the management of exogenous obesity for short-term use (6 to 12 weeks) in conjunction with a regimen of weight reduction based on caloric restriction, exercise, and behavior modification.

Nasal congestion (treatment)—Administered orally, phenylpropanolamine is indicated in the temporary, symptomatic relief of local swelling and congestion of nasal mucous membranes.

[Urinary incontinence (treatment)]—Phenylpropanolamine is used in the treatment of mild to moderate stress incontinence; it may be effective in up to 75% of patients with mild to moderate conditions. In females, phenylpropanolamine may be used in combination with estrogen therapy for a synergistic clinical effect.

## Pharmacology/Pharmacokinetics

**Physicochemical characteristics**
Molecular weight—187.67.
pKa—9.
Other characteristics—Similar in structure and action to ephedrine and amphetamine but with less central nervous system (CNS) stimulation

**Mechanism of action/Effect**

Appetite suppression—A mixed-acting sympathomimetic amine with predominantly alpha-adrenergic activity, phenylpropanolamine is believed to suppress the appetite control center in the hypothalamus. Other CNS actions and/or metabolic effects may also be involved. PPA acts as an agonist at central norepinephrine receptors and may also have dopamine agonist properties.

Decongestion, nasal—Phenylpropanolamine acts on alpha-adrenergic receptors in the mucosa of the respiratory tract to produce vasoconstriction, which temporarily reduces the swelling associated with inflammation of the mucous membranes lining the nasal passages.

Urinary incontinence—Phenylpropanolamine produces contraction of the bladder neck and of the smooth muscle of the urethra, possibly due to stimulation of alpha-adrenergic receptors.

**Other actions/effects**
Increases heart rate, force of contraction, and cardiac output and excitability, possibly by stimulating beta-adrenergic receptors in the heart.
Causes CNS stimulation by releasing norepinephrine from storage sites.
Produces mydriasis.

**Absorption**
Readily absorbed.

**Biotransformation**
Hepatic, to an active hydroxylated metabolite.

**Onset of action**
Nasal decongestion—15 to 30 minutes.

**Duration of action**
Capsules and tablets—3 hours.
Extended-release—12 to 16 hours.

**Elimination**
Renal; about 80 to 90% excreted unchanged within 24 hours.

## Precautions to Consider

**Cross-sensitivity and/or related problems**
Patients sensitive to other sympathomimetics (for example, amphetamines, ephedrine, epinephrine, isoproterenol, metaproterenol, norepinephrine, phenylephrine, pseudoephedrine, terbutaline) may be sensitive to this medication also.

**Pregnancy/Reproduction**
Pregnancy—Problems with teratogenicity in humans have not been documented.
Postpartum—Evidence shows that postpartum women may be at greater risk than the rest of the population of developing psychiatric disorders with the use of phenylpropanolamine at recommended doses and with overdose.

**Breast-feeding**
Problems in humans have not been documented.

**Pediatrics**
Appropriate studies have not been performed in children up to 12 years of age. However, recent evidence shows that children under 6 years of age may be at greater risk than the rest of the population of developing psychiatric disorders with the use of phenylpropanolamine at recommended doses and with overdose.
Phenylpropanolamine is not recommended as an appetite suppressant in children up to 12 years of age. In children between 12 and 18 years of age, the use of phenylpropanolamine as an appetite suppressant must be carefully supervised by a physician.

**Geriatrics**
No information is available on the relationship of age to the effects of phenylpropanolamine in geriatric patients.

**Drug interactions and/or related problems**
The following drug interactions and/or related problems have been selected on the basis of their potential clinical significance (possible mechanism in parentheses where appropriate)—not necessarily inclusive (» = major clinical significance):

Note: Combinations containing any of the following medications, depending on the amount present, may also interact with this medication.

» Anesthetics, hydrocarbon inhalation
 (chronic use of phenylpropanolamine prior to anesthesia with these agents may increase the risk of cardiac arrhythmias, since these medications may sensitize the myocardium to the effects of phenylpropanolamine; arrhythmias may respond to a beta-adrenergic blocking agent such as propranolol)

Antidepressants, tricyclic
 (tricyclic antidepressants may potentiate the response to sympathomimetic amines such as PPA by blocking the reuptake of biogenic amines by nerve terminals)

Antihypertensives or
Diuretics used as antihypertensives
 (hypotensive effects of these medications may be reduced during concurrent use with phenylpropanolamine; the patient should be carefully monitored to confirm that the desired effect is being obtained)

» Beta-adrenergic blocking agents
 (concurrent use with phenylpropanolamine may result in significant hypertension and excessive bradycardia with possible heart block; concurrent use requires careful monitoring)

» CNS stimulation–producing medications (see *Appendix II*) or

» Sympathomimetics, other
  (concurrent use with phenylpropanolamine may result in additive CNS stimulation to excessive levels, causing nervousness, irritability, insomnia, or possibly seizures or cardiac arrhythmias; close monitoring is recommended)
  (also, concurrent use of other sympathomimetics with phenylpropanolamine may increase pressor or cardiovascular effects of either medication)
» Digitalis glycosides
  (concurrent use may result in cardiac arrhythmias)
» Monoamine oxidase (MAO) inhibitors, including furazolidone, procarbazine, and selegiline
  (concurrent use may potentiate the pressor effect of phenylpropanolamine with resultant hypertensive crisis by releasing catecholamines, which accumulate during therapy with MAO inhibitors, from intraneuronal storage sites; phenylpropanolamine should not be administered during or within 14 days following administration of MAO inhibitors)
» Rauwolfia alkaloids
  (concurrent use may inhibit the indirect-acting sympathomimetic action of phenylpropanolamine by depleting catecholamine stores)

**Medical considerations/Contraindications**
The medical considerations/contraindications included have been selected on the basis of their potential clinical significance (reasons given in parentheses where appropriate)—not necessarily inclusive (» = major clinical significance).

*Except under special circumstances, this medication should not be used when the following medical problems exist:*
» Coronary artery disease, severe
  (phenylpropanolamine may increase heart rate and force of contraction, with resultant decreased cardiac efficiency)
» Hypertension, severe
  (pressor effect of phenylpropanolamine may result in hypertensive crisis)

*Risk-benefit should be considered when the following medical problems exist:*
» Cardiovascular disorders
  (phenylpropanolamine may cause cardiac excitation leading to arrhythmias)
  Diabetes mellitus
  (adrenergic properties of phenylpropanolamine may lead to increased blood glucose concentrations)
  Glaucoma, angle-closure
  (condition may be aggravated)
» Hypertension, mild
  (vasoconstrictive properties of phenylpropanolamine may exacerbate condition)
  Hyperthyroidism
  (symptoms may be exacerbated by cardiac stimulant properties of phenylpropanolamine)
  Prostatic hypertrophy
  (urinary retention may be precipitated)
  Psychosis or other psychiatric disorders, history of
  (phenylpropanolamine may precipitate psychiatric disorders)
  Sensitivity to phenylpropanolamine or other sympathomimetics

## Side/Adverse Effects

Note: The safety profile of phenylpropanolamine is controversial. Most controlled studies have demonstrated minimal side effects from PPA. Serious adverse reactions including hypertensive crises, stroke, arrhythmias, acute renal failure, rhabdomyolysis, psychotic disturbances, hallucinations, and seizures have been reported following consumption of PPA; however, case studies in many of these patients have revealed confounding factors such as pre-existing conditions and/or consumption of medications in addition to PPA.

Some investigators have suggested that serious cardiovascular side effects may be more likely to occur in patients prone to hypertension (such as obese patients, patients under stress, elderly patients, or female patients receiving oral contraceptives); in patients with eating disorders, such as anorexia nervosa or bulimia (these patients may tend to abuse weight control medications); and in females and children who, because of their smaller size, receive a greater dose per unit of body weight.

Similarly, serious CNS side effects may occur more frequently in patients with a history of pre-existing neurological or psychiatric conditions. In addition, one study noted that organic symptoms (such as dizziness, loss of motor coordination, confusion, and photophobia) that have occurred in many patients are comparable to CNS dysfunction due to increased blood pressure.

Increases in blood pressure and CNS toxicity may represent idiosyncratic reactions in some patients.

The following side/adverse effects have been selected on the basis of their potential clinical significance (possible signs and symptoms in parentheses where appropriate)—not necessarily inclusive:

**Those indicating need for medical attention**
Incidence rare
  *Headache, severe*—may be prodromal of severe side effects related to elevated blood pressure; *increased blood pressure; painful or difficult urination; tightness in chest*

**Those indicating need for medical attention only if they continue or are bothersome**
Incidence less frequent—more frequent with high doses
  *Dizziness; dryness of nose or mouth; false sense of well-being; headache, mild; insomnia* (trouble in sleeping); *nausea, mild; nervousness, mild; restlessness, mild*

## Overdose

For more information on the management of overdose or unintentional ingestion, **contact a Poison Control Center** (see *Poison Control Center Listing*).

**Clinical effects of overdose**
The following have been selected on the basis of their potential clinical significance (possible signs and symptoms in parentheses where appropriate)—not necessarily inclusive:

Early symptoms of overdose
  *Abdominal or stomach pain; fast, pounding, or irregular heartbeat; headache, severe; increased sweating not associated with exercise; nausea and vomiting, severe; nervousness or restlessness, severe*

Late symptoms of overdose
  *Confusion; convulsions; fast breathing; fast and irregular pulse; hallucinations; hostile behavior; muscle trembling*

**Treatment of overdose**
Since there is no specific antidote for overdosage with phenylpropanolamine, treatment is symptomatic and supportive with possible use of the following:
  Induction of emesis and/or use of gastric lavage is primary.
  Barbiturate sedatives are sometimes used to control excessive CNS stimulation.
  Cardiovascular and respiratory monitoring.
  Intravenous fluids to control hypotension.
  Intravenous phentolamine or nitrates to control hypertension.
  Acidification of urine and forced diuresis.
  Protecting patient from self-injury by use of restraints if necessary.

## Patient Consultation

As an aid to patient consultation, refer to *Advice for the Patient, Phenylpropanolamine (Systemic)*.
In providing consultation, consider emphasizing the following selected information (» = major clinical significance):

**Before using this medication**
» Conditions affecting use, especially:
  Sensitivity to phenylpropanolamine or other sympathomimetics
  Pregnancy—Psychiatric side effects more likely in postpartum women
  Use in children—Psychiatric side effects more likely in children up to 6 years of age; not recommended for use as appetite suppressant in children up to 12 years of age; in adolescents between 12 and 18 years of age, use for appetite suppression recommended only with doctor's supervision
  Other medications, especially beta-adrenergic blocking agents, CNS stimulation–producing medications, other sympathomimetics, digitalis glycosides, monoamine oxidase (MAO) inhibitors, or rauwolfia alkaloids
  Other medical problems, especially severe coronary artery disease, other cardiovascular disorders, or hypertension

**Proper use of this medication**
  Proper administration of extended-release dosage forms: swallowing whole; not breaking, crushing, or chewing; taking with a full glass of water; taking around 10 am if taking only one dose of medication a day
» Importance of not taking more medication than the amount recommended or for a longer period of time than directed

//
Taking the last dose of medication a few hours before bedtime to minimize the possibility of insomnia
» Proper dosing
» Proper storage
*For decongestant use only*
Missed dose: Taking as soon as possible; not taking within 2 hours (12 hours for extended-release dosage forms) of next scheduled dose; not doubling doses
*For appetite suppressant use only*
Not taking for longer than a few weeks without physician's permission

**Precautions while using this medication**
Not drinking large amounts of caffeine-containing coffee, tea, or colas
» Caution if dizziness occurs; not driving, using machines, or doing anything else that requires alertness while taking medication
*For decongestant use only*
» Checking with physician if cold symptoms do not improve within 7 days or if fever is present

**Side/adverse effects**
Signs of potential side effects, especially severe headache, increased blood pressure, painful or difficult urination, or tightness in chest

## General Dosing Information

To minimize the possibility of insomnia, the last dose of phenylpropanolamine for each day should be administered a few hours before bedtime.

With prolonged use or too frequent administration, tolerance to the therapeutic effects of phenylpropanolamine may develop. Phenylpropanolamine is effective as an appetite suppressant only for a few weeks.

## Oral Dosage Forms

Note: Bracketed uses in the *Dosage Forms* section refer to categories of use and/or indications not included in U.S. product labeling.

### PHENYLPROPANOLAMINE HYDROCHLORIDE CAPSULES

**Usual adult dose**
Appetite suppressant—
Oral, 25 mg three times a day, not to exceed 75 mg in twenty-four hours.
Decongestant—
Oral, 25 mg every four hours as needed, not to exceed 150 mg in twenty-four hours.
[Urinary incontinence]—
Oral, 50 to 150 mg a day, in divided doses.

**Usual pediatric dose**
Appetite suppressant—
Children up to 12 years of age: Use is not recommended.
Children 12 to 18 years of age: Dosage must be individualized by physician.
Decongestant—
Children up to 2 years of age: Dosage must be individualized by physician.
Children 2 to 6 years of age: Oral, 6.25 mg every four hours as needed, not to exceed 37.5 mg in twenty-four hours.
Children 6 to 12 years of age: Oral, 12.5 mg every four hours as needed, not to exceed 75 mg in twenty-four hours.
Children 12 to 18 years of age: See *Usual adult dose*.

**Strength(s) usually available**
U.S.—
25 mg (OTC) [*Efed II Yellow*].
37.5 mg (OTC) [*Prolamine*].
Canada—
Not commercially available.

**Packaging and storage**
Store below 40 °C (104 °F), preferably between 15 and 30 °C (59 and 86 °F), in a tight container, unless otherwise specified by manufacturer. Protect from light.

### PHENYLPROPANOLAMINE HYDROCHLORIDE EXTENDED-RELEASE CAPSULES USP

**Usual adult dose**
Appetite suppressant—
Oral, 75 mg once a day at mid-morning (10 a.m.) with a full glass of water.
Decongestant—
Oral, 75 mg every twelve hours.
[Urinary incontinence]—
Oral, 50 to 150 mg a day, in divided doses.

**Usual pediatric dose**
Appetite suppressant—
Children up to 12 years of age: Use is not recommended.
Children 12 to 18 years of age: Dosage must be individualized by physician.
Decongestant—
Dosage has not been established.

**Strength(s) usually available**
U.S.—
75 mg (OTC) [*Control; Dexatrim Maximum Strength Capsules; Diet-Aid Maximum Strength;* GENERIC].
Canada—
Not commercially available.

**Packaging and storage**
Store below 40 °C (104 °F), preferably between 15 and 30 °C (59 and 86 °F), unless otherwise specified by manufacturer. Store in a tight, light-resistant container.

**Auxiliary labeling**
• Swallow capsules whole.

### PHENYLPROPANOLAMINE HYDROCHLORIDE TABLETS

**Usual adult dose**
See *Phenylpropanolamine Hydrochloride Capsules*.

**Usual pediatric dose**
See *Phenylpropanolamine Hydrochloride Capsules*.

**Strength(s) usually available**
U.S.—
25 mg (OTC) [*Propagest;* GENERIC].
50 mg (OTC) [GENERIC].
Canada—
Not commercially available.

**Packaging and storage**
Store below 40 °C (104 °F), preferably between 15 and 30 °C (59 and 86 °F), in a tight container, unless otherwise specified by manufacturer. Protect from light.

### PHENYLPROPANOLAMINE HYDROCHLORIDE EXTENDED-RELEASE TABLETS

**Usual adult dose**
See *Phenylpropanolamine Hydrochloride Extended-release Capsules USP*.

**Usual pediatric dose**
See *Phenylpropanolamine Hydrochloride Extended-release Capsules USP*.

**Strength(s) usually available**
U.S.—
75 mg (OTC) [*Acutrim 16 Hour; Acutrim Late Day* (isopropyl alcohol); *Acutrim II Maximum Strength; Dexatrim Maximum Strength Caplets; Dexatrim Maximum Strength Tablets; Phenyldrine*].
Canada—
Not commercially available.

**Packaging and storage**
Store below 40 °C (104 °F), preferably between 15 and 30 °C (59 and 86 °F), in a tight container, unless otherwise specified by manufacturer. Protect from light.

**Auxiliary labeling**
• Swallow tablets whole.

Revised: 06/21/94

**PHENYTOIN**—See *Anticonvulsants, Hydantoin (Systemic)*

# PHOSPHATES Systemic

This monograph includes information on the following: 1) Potassium Phosphates; 2) Potassium and Sodium Phosphates; 3) Sodium Phosphates†.

**VA CLASSIFICATION** (Primary/Secondary): TN408/GU900

Commonly used brand name(s): *K-Phos M. F*[2]; *K-Phos Neutral*[2]; *K-Phos No. 2*[2]; *K-Phos Original*[1]; *Neutra-Phos*[2]; *Neutra-Phos-K*[1]; *Neutra-Phos*[2]; *Uro-KP-Neutral*[2].

Note: For a listing of dosage forms and brand names by country availability, see *Dosage Forms* section(s).

†Not commercially available in Canada.

## Category

Acidifier (urinary)—Monobasic Potassium Phosphate; Potassium and Sodium Phosphates.
Antiurolithic (calcium calculi)—Monobasic Potassium Phosphate; Potassium and Sodium Phosphates.
Electrolyte replenisher—Potassium Phosphates; Potassium and Sodium Phosphates; Sodium Phosphates.

## Indications

### Accepted

Hypophosphatemia (prophylaxis and treatment)—Phosphates, both oral and parenteral, provide supplemental ionic phosphorus for correction of hypophosphatemia in patients with low or restricted oral intake or conditions with increased requirements for phosphorus, such as premature infants fed human milk, or patients who have inadequately controlled diabetes mellitus, hyperparathyroidism, hyperthyroidism, chronic alcoholism, renal tubular defects leading to increased urinary phosphate loss, respiratory alkalosis, gastrectomy, vitamin D deficiency, total parenteral nutrition (TPN) therapy, or patients who use thiazide diuretics, intravenous dextrose solutions, or those who chronically use aluminum- or magnesium-containing antacids. For prophylaxis of phosphorus deficiency, dietary improvement, rather than supplementation, is advisable. For treatment of phosphorus deficiency, supplementation is preferred.

Requirements for all vitamins and most minerals are increased during pregnancy. Many physicians recommend that pregnant women receive multivitamin and mineral supplements, especially those pregnant women who do not consume an adequate diet and those in high-risk categories (i.e., women carrying more than one fetus, heavy cigarette smokers, and alcohol and drug abusers). Taking excessive amounts of a multivitamin and mineral supplement may be harmful to the mother and/or fetus and should be avoided.

Recommended intakes for all vitamins and most minerals are increased during breast-feeding.

Urinary tract infections (treatment adjunct)—Urinary acidification by potassium and sodium phosphates combination and monobasic potassium phosphate augments the efficacy of methenamine mandelate and methenamine hippurate, which are dependent upon an acid medium for antibacterial activity. Phosphates eliminate the odor, rash, and turbidity present with ammoniacal urine associated with urinary tract infections. However, use of phosphates for urea splitting urinary tract infections may predispose to struvite stones that form in alkaline urine.

Renal calculi, calcium (prophylaxis)—Potassium and sodium phosphates combination and monobasic potassium phosphate have been used to reduce urinary calcium concentration and help prevent precipitation of calcium deposits in the urinary tract.

### Unaccepted

Although sodium and/or potassium phosphates have been used in the treatment of hypercalcemia, USP medical advisory panels do not recommend this use since these medications have been replaced by safer and more effective agents.

## Pharmacology/Pharmacokinetics

### Physicochemical characteristics

Molecular weight—
Dibasic potassium phosphate: 174.18.
Dibasic sodium phosphate (heptahydrate): 268.07.
Monobasic potassium phosphate: 136.09.
Monobasic sodium phosphate (anhydrous): 119.98.

### Mechanism of action/Effect

Urinary acidification—At the renal distal tubule, the secretion of hydrogen by the tubular cell in exchange for sodium in the tubular urine converts dibasic phosphate salts to monobasic phosphate salts. Therefore, large amounts of acid can be excreted without lowering the pH of the urine to a degree that would block hydrogen transport by a high concentration gradient between the tubular cell and luminal fluid.

Antiurolithic—Phosphates inhibit spontaneous nucleation of calcium oxalate, thus reducing the possibility of calcium urolithiasis.

Electrolyte replenisher—Phosphorus modifies the steady state of calcium concentrations, has a buffering effect on acid-base equilibrium, and influences the renal excretion of hydrogen ion.

### Absorption

Ingested phosphates are absorbed from the gastrointestinal tract. However, the presence of large amounts of calcium or aluminum may lead to formation of insoluble phosphate and reduce the net absorption. Vitamin D stimulates phosphate absorption.

### Elimination

Renal (90%) and fecal (10%).

## Precautions to Consider

### Pregnancy/Reproduction

Pregnancy—Adequate and well-controlled studies have not been done in humans. However, problems in humans have not been documented with intakes of normal daily recommended amounts.
Studies have not been done in animals.
FDA Pregnancy Category C.

### Breast-feeding

It is not known if phosphates are distributed into breast milk. However, problems in nursing infants have not been documented with intake of normal daily recommended amounts.

### Pediatrics

Problems in pediatrics have not been documented with intake of normal daily recommended amounts. However, there have been several case reports of phosphate toxicity in pediatric patients from use of phosphate-containing enemas.

### Geriatrics

Problems in geriatrics have not been documented with intakes of normal daily recommended amounts.

### Drug interactions and/or related problems

The following drug interactions and/or related problems have been selected on the basis of their potential clinical significance (possible mechanism in parentheses where appropriate)—not necessarily inclusive (» = major clinical significance):

Note: Combinations containing any of the following, depending on the amount present, may also interact with this medication.

Anabolic steroids or
Androgens or
Estrogens
(concurrent use with sodium phosphates may increase the risk of edema, due to the sodium content)

» Angiotensin-converting enzyme (ACE) inhibitors or
» Anti-inflammatory drugs, nonsteroidal (NSAIDs) or
» Cyclosporine or
» Diuretics, potassium-sparing or
» Heparin, chronic use of or
» Low-salt milk or
» Potassium-containing medications, other or
» Salt substitutes
(concurrent use with potassium phosphate may result in hyperkalemia, especially in patients with renal impairment; patient should have serum potassium concentration determinations at periodic intervals)

» Antacids, aluminum- or magnesium-containing or
Oxalates, found in large quantities in rhubarb and spinach or
Phytates, in bran and whole-grain cereals
(concurrent use with phosphates may bind the phosphate and prevent its absorption)

» Calcium-containing medications, including dietary supplements and antacids
(concurrent use with phosphates may increase risk of deposition of calcium in soft tissues, if serum ionized calcium is high; also, phosphate absorption may be reduced because of formation of large amounts of insoluble phosphate)

» Corticosteroids, glucocorticoid, especially with significant mineralocorticoid activity or

- » Corticosteroids, mineralocorticoid or
- » Corticotropin (ACTH)
    (concurrent use with sodium phosphates may result in edema, due to the sodium content)
- » Digitalis glycosides
    (use of potassium phosphates injection in digitalized patients with severe or complete heart block is not recommended because of possible hyperkalemia)
- Iron supplements
    (concurrent use with foods or medicines containing phosphates will decrease iron absorption because of the formation of less soluble or insoluble complexes; iron supplements should not be taken within 1 hour before or 2 hours after ingestion of phosphates)
- » Phosphate-containing medication, other
    (concurrent use with other phosphate containing medications may increase the risk of hyperphosphatemia, especially in patients with renal disease)
- Salicylates
    (concurrent use with potassium and sodium phosphates combination or monobasic potassium phosphate may increase plasma concentrations of salicylates since salicylate excretion is decreased in acidified urine; addition of these phosphates to patients stabilized on a salicylate may lead to toxic salicylate concentrations)
- » Sodium-containing medications
    (concurrent use with sodium phosphates may increase the risk of edema, especially in patients with renal disease)
- Vitamin D, including calcifediol and calcitriol
    (concurrent use with phosphorus-containing medications in high doses may increase the potential for hyperphosphatemia because of vitamin D enhancement of phosphate absorption)
- Zinc supplements
    (concurrent use of phosphorus-containing medications with zinc supplements may reduce zinc absorption by formation of nonabsorbable complexes; phosphorus-containing medications should be taken 2 hours after zinc supplements)

**Laboratory value alterations**

The following have been selected on the basis of their potential clinical significance (possible effect in parentheses where appropriate)—not necessarily inclusive (» = major clinical significance):

*With diagnostic tests results*
Skeletal imaging
(saturation of bone binding sites by phosphorus ions in phosphates may cause decreased bone uptake of technetium Tc 99m–labeled diagnostic aids during bone imaging)

**Medical considerations/Contraindications**

The medical considerations/contraindications included have been selected on the basis of their potential clinical significance (reasons given in parentheses where appropriate)—not necessarily inclusive (» = major clinical significance).

*Except under special circumstances, this medication should not be used when the following medical problems exist:*

- » Hyperphosphatemia
    (phosphates may further increase serum phosphate concentrations, especially in patients with renal disease)
- » Renal function impairment, severe—less than 30% of normal
    (use may result in increased serum phosphate concentrations)
- Urinary tract infections caused by urea splitting organisms
    (use of phosphates may predispose to struvite stone formation)
- » Urolithiasis, magnesium ammonium phosphate, infected
    (condition may be exacerbated)

*Risk-benefit should be considered when the following medical problems exist:*

*For all phosphates*
- » Conditions in which high phosphate concentrations may be encountered, such as:
    Hypoparathyroidism
    Renal disease, chronic
    Rhabdomyolysis
    (administration of phosphates may further increase serum phosphate concentrations)
- » Conditions in which low calcium concentrations may be encountered, such as:
    Hypoparathyroidism
    Osteomalacia
    Pancreatitis, acute
    Renal disease, chronic
    Rhabdomyolysis
    Rickets
    (administration of phosphates may further decrease serum calcium concentrations)
- Sensitivity to potassium, sodium, or phosphates

*For potassium-containing phosphates only*
Cardiac disease, particularly in digitalized patients
    (condition may be exacerbated)
- » Conditions in which high potassium concentrations may be encountered, such as:
    Adrenal insufficiency, severe—Addison's disease
    Dehydration, acute
    Pancreatitis
    Physicial exercise, strenuous, in unconditioned persons
    Renal insufficiency, severe
    Rhabdomyolysis
    Tissue breakdown, extensive, such as severe burns
        (increased serum potassium concentrations leading to cardiac arrest may occur; exercise-induced hyperkalemia is transient and is a problem only in patients with renal insufficiency or those taking medications that increase serum potassium)
Myotonia congenita
    (condition may be exacerbated)

*For sodium-containing phosphates only*
Cardiac failure or
Cirrhosis of liver or severe hepatic disease or
Edema, peripheral and pulmonary or
» Hypernatremia or
Hypertension or
Renal function impairment or
Toxemia of pregnancy
    (sodium salts should be used cautiously in patients with these conditions to prevent exacerbation; also, patients on sodium restricted diets should not use sodium phosphates)

**Patient monitoring**

The following may be especially important in patient monitoring (other tests may be warranted in some patients, depending on condition; » = major clinical significance):

*For all phosphates*
Calcium concentrations, serum and
Phosphorus concentrations, serum and
Potassium concentrations, serum and
Renal function and
Sodium concentrations, serum
    (determinations may be required at frequent intervals during therapy, especially during intravenous therapy; high serum phosphate concentrations increase the incidence of extraskeletal calcification)

*For potassium phosphates injection only*
Electrocardiogram (ECG)
    (may be required at frequent intervals during intravenous therapy)

## Side/Adverse Effects

The following side/adverse effects have been selected on the basis of their potential clinical significance (possible signs and symptoms in parentheses where appropriate)—not necessarily inclusive:

**Those indicating need for medical attention**

Incidence less frequent or rare
*Fluid retention* (swelling of feet or lower legs; weight gain); *hyperkalemia* (confusion; tiredness or weakness; irregular or slow heartbeat; numbness or tingling around lips, hands, or feet; unexplained anxiety; weakness or heaviness of legs; shortness of breath or troubled breathing); *hypernatremia* (confusion; tiredness or weakness; convulsions; decrease in amount of urine or in frequency of urination; fast heartbeat; headache or dizziness; increased thirst); *hyperphosphatemia orhypocalcemic tetany* (convulsions, muscle cramps, numbness, tingling, pain, or weakness in hands or feet; shortness of breath, tremor or troubled breathing); *metastatic calcification*

**Those indicating need for medical attention only if they continue or are bothersome**

Incidence less frequent—for oral dosage forms only
*Laxative effect or diarrhea; nausea or vomiting; stomach pain*

## Patient Consultation

As an aid to patient consultation, refer to *Advice for the Patient, Phosphates (Systemic)*.

In providing consultation, consider emphasizing the following selected information (» = major clinical significance):

**Importance of diet**
　Importance of proper nutrition; supplement under physician's care may be needed because of inadequate dietary intake or increased requirements
　Food sources of phosphorus
　Recommended daily intake for phosphorus

**Before using this medication**
» Conditions affecting use, especially:
　Sensitivity to potassium, sodium, or phosphates
　Other medications, especially angiotensin-converting (ACE) inhibitors, antacids, calcium-containing medications, corticosteroids, corticotropin (ACTH), cyclosporine, digitalis glycosides, chronic use of heparin, low-salt milk, nonsteroidal anti-inflammatory drugs, potassium-containing medications, potassium-sparing diuretics, salt substitutes, or sodium-containing medicines
　Other medical problems, especially acute dehydration, acute pancreatitis, Addison's disease, edema, hypernatremia, hyperphosphatemia, hypoparathyroidism, infected urolithiasis, osteomalacia, rickets, severe dehydration, severe kidney disease

**Proper use of this medication**
　Taking dissolved in water
» Taking after meals or with food to minimize possible stomach upset or laxative action
» Importance of high fluid intake (8-ounce glass of water every hour) to prevent kidney stones
» Importance of not taking more medication than the amount recommended
» For patients taking sodium-containing phosphates: Importance of low-sodium diet
» Proper dosing
　Missed dose: Taking as soon as possible; not taking if within 1 or 2 hours of next dose; not doubling doses
» Proper storage

**Precautions while using this medication**
　Regular visits to physician to check progress during therapy
　Not taking iron supplements within 1 or 2 hours of phosphates
　Checking with physician before beginning exercise program if on potassium-containing phosphate
　Possible need for potassium or sodium restriction

**Side/adverse effects**
　Signs of potential side effects, especially hyperkalemia, hypernatremia, hyperphosphatemia, hypocalcemic tetany, or fluid retention

## General Dosing Information

The normal concentration of serum inorganic phosphate is 3 to 4.5 mg (0.1 to 0.15 mmol) per 100 mL in adults and 4 to 7 mg (0.13 to 0.2 mmol) per 100 mL in children.

**For oral dosage forms**
Before this medication is taken, it must be thoroughly dissolved in water.

**For parenteral dosage forms**
Before administration, the concentrated phosphates injection (3 mmol of phosphorus per mL) must be diluted and thoroughly mixed with a larger volume of fluid.

The dose and rate of administration must be individualized.

When used as an electrolyte replenisher, a dose of the equivalent of 10 to 15 mmol (310 mg or 465 mg) of phosphorus a day is usually sufficient to maintain normal serum phosphate, although larger amounts may be required in hypermetabolic states.

The solution should be infused slowly to avoid phosphate intoxication.

Intravenous infusion of phosphates in high concentrations may cause hypocalcemia.

**Diet/Nutrition**
This medication should be taken immediately after a meal or with food to minimize possible stomach upset or laxative action.

Recommended dietary intakes for phosphorus are defined differently worldwide.

For U.S.—
　The Recommended Dietary Allowances (RDAs) for vitamins and minerals are determined by the Food and Nutrition Board of the National Research Council and are intended to provide adequate nutrition in most healthy persons under usual environmental stresses. In addition, a different designation may be used by the FDA for food and dietary supplement labeling purposes, as with Daily Value (DV). DVs replace the previous labeling terminology United States Recommended Daily Allowances (USRDAs).

For Canada—
　Recommended Nutrient Intakes (RNIs) for vitamins, minerals, and protein are determined by Health and Welfare Canada and provide recommended amounts of a specific nutrient while minimizing the risk of chronic diseases.

Daily recommended intakes for phosphorus are generally defined as follows:

| Persons | U.S. (mg) | Canada (mg) |
| --- | --- | --- |
| Infants and children | | |
| 　Birth to 3 years of age | 300–800 | 150–350 |
| 　4 to 6 years of age | 800 | 400 |
| 　7 to 10 years of age | 800 | 500–800 |
| Adolescent and adult males | 800–1200 | 700–1000 |
| Adolescent and adult females | 800–1200 | 800–850 |
| Pregnant females | 1200 | 1050 |
| Breast-feeding females | 1200 | 1050 |

The best dietary sources of phosphorus include dairy products, meat, poultry, fish, and cereal products.

**For treatment of adverse effects**
Recommended treatment consists of the following:
- Withholding administration of phosphates.
- Correcting deficient serum electrolyte concentrations (such as that of calcium).

## POTASSIUM PHOSPHATES

## Oral Dosage Forms

### MONOBASIC POTASSIUM PHOSPHATE TABLETS FOR ORAL SOLUTION

**Usual adult and adolescent dose**
Acidifier (urinary) or
Antiurolithic or
Electrolyte replenisher—
　Oral, 1 gram (228 mg or 7.4 mmol of phosphorus) in 180 to 240 mL of water four times a day, with meals and at bedtime.

**Usual pediatric dose**
Electrolyte replenisher—
　Children up to 4 years of age: Oral, the equivalent of 200 mg (6.4 mmol) of phosphorus in 60 mL of water four times a day, after meals and at bedtime.
　Children 4 years of age and over: See *Usual adult and adolescent dose*.

**Strength(s) usually available**
U.S.—
　500 mg (114 mg [3.7 mmol] of phosphorus) (Rx) [K-Phos Original (scored)].
Canada—
　Not commercially available.

**Packaging and storage**
Store below 40 °C (104 °F), preferably between 15 and 30 °C (59 and 86 °F), in a well-closed container, unless otherwise specified by manufacturer.

**Preparation of dosage form**
Soak the tablets in 60 or 75 mL of water for 2 to 5 minutes. Stir well to dissolve completely before swallowing.

**Auxiliary labeling**
- Do not swallow tablet.
- Dissolve tablet in a full glass (8 ounces) of water.

**Additional information**
Each 500-mg tablet supplies 114 mg (3.7 mmol) of phosphorus and 3.7 mEq (144 mg) of potassium.

### POTASSIUM PHOSPHATES CAPSULES FOR ORAL SOLUTION

**Usual adult and adolescent dose**
Electrolyte replenisher—
　Oral, 1.45 grams (250 mg or 8 mmol of phosphorus) in 75 mL of water or juice four times a day, after meals and at bedtime.

**Usual pediatric dose**
Electrolyte replenisher—
　Children up to 4 years of age: Oral, the equivalent of 200 mg (6.4 mmol) of phosphorus in 60 mL of water or juice four times a day, after meals and at bedtime.
　Children 4 years of age and over: See *Usual adult and adolescent dose*.

**Strength(s) usually available**
U.S.—
  1.45 grams (250 mg [8 mmol] of phosphorus) (OTC) [*Neutra-Phos-K*].
Canada—
  Not commercially available.

**Packaging and storage**
Store below 40 °C (104 °F), preferably between 15 and 30 °C (59 and 86 °F), in a well-closed container, unless otherwise specified by manufacturer.

**Preparation of dosage form**
Empty contents of capsule into 60 or 75 mL of water or juice and stir well.

**Auxiliary labeling**
- Do not swallow filled capsule.
- Mix contents of each capsule with one-third glass of water or juice.

**Additional information**
Each 1.45-gram capsule supplies 250 mg (8 mmol) of phosphorus and 14.25 mEq (556 mg) of potassium, as monobasic and dibasic potassium phosphates per 75 mL of water or juice, or 200 mg (6.4 mmol) per 60 mL of water or juice, when reconstituted according to manufacturer's instructions.

### POTASSIUM PHOSPHATES FOR ORAL SOLUTION

**Usual adult and adolescent dose**
Electrolyte replenisher—
  Oral, the equivalent of 250 mg (8 mmol) of phosphorus four times a day, after meals and at bedtime.

**Usual pediatric dose**
Electrolyte replenisher—
  Children up to 4 years of age: Oral, the equivalent of 200 mg (6.4 mmol) of phosphorus four times a day, after meals and at bedtime.
  Children 4 years of age and over: See *Usual adult and adolescent dose*.

**Size(s) usually available**
U.S.—
  1.45 grams (250 mg [8 mmol] of phosphorus) (OTC) [*Neutra-Phos-K*].
  71 grams (250 mg [8 mmol] of phosphorus) (OTC) [*Neutra-Phos-K*].
Canada—
  Not commercially available.

**Packaging and storage**
Store below 40 °C (104 °F), preferably between 15 and 30 °C (59 and 86 °F), in a well-closed container, unless otherwise specified by manufacturer.

**Preparation of dosage form**
To prepare solution, add the contents of one bottle (71 grams) of powder concentrate, supplied by the manufacturer, to a sufficient amount of water to make 1 gallon (3.785 liters) of solution or the contents of one packet of powder concentrate to a sufficient amount of water to make 1/3 of a glass (approximately 2.5 ounces) of water. Shake the container for 2 or 3 minutes or until all the powder is dissolved. Solution should not be diluted.

**Stability**
Solution can be stored for 60 days.

**Additional information**
Each 75 mL of solution or the solution prepared from one packet, when constituted according to manufacturer's instructions, supplies 250 mg (8 mmol) of phosphorus and 14.25 mEq (556 mg) of potassium, as monobasic and dibasic potassium phosphates.

## Parenteral Dosage Forms

### POTASSIUM PHOSPHATES INJECTION USP

Note: **Potassium phosphates injection must be diluted prior to intravenous administration.**

**Usual adult and adolescent dose**
Electrolyte replenisher—
  Intravenous infusion, the equivalent of 10 mmol (310 mg) of phosphorus a day.

**Usual pediatric dose**
Electrolyte replenisher—
  Intravenous infusion, the equivalent of 1.5 to 2 mmol (46.5 to 62 mg) of phosphorus a day.

**Strength(s) usually available**
U.S.—
  224 mg of monobasic potassium phosphate and 236 mg of dibasic potassium phosphate (3 mmol [93 mg] of phosphorus) per mL (Rx) [GENERIC].

Canada—
  224 mg of monobasic potassium phosphate and 236 mg of dibasic potassium phosphate (3 mmol [93 mg] of phosphorus) per mL (Rx) [GENERIC].

**Packaging and storage**
Store between 15 and 30 °C (59 and 86 °F), unless otherwise specified by manufacturer.

**Incompatibilities**
Precipitate may form when phosphates are added to solution containing calcium or magnesium.

**Additional information**
Each mL of potassium phosphates injection supplies 283.5 mg of phosphate (approximately 3 mmol [93 mg] of phosphorus) and 4.4 mEq (170.2 mg) of potassium.

---
### POTASSIUM AND SODIUM PHOSPHATES
---

## Oral Dosage Forms

### MONOBASIC POTASSIUM AND SODIUM PHOSPHATES TABLETS FOR ORAL SOLUTION

**Usual adult and adolescent dose**
Acidifier (urinary) or
Antiurolithic or
Electrolyte replenisher—
  Oral, 250 mg (8 mmol) of phosphorus with a full glass (240 mL) of water four times a day, after meals and at bedtime.

Note: When the urine is difficult to acidify, a dose of the equivalent of 250 mg (8 mmol) of phosphorus may be administered every two hours, not to exceed 2 grams of phosphorus in a twenty-four-hour period.

**Usual pediatric dose**
Electrolyte replenisher—
  Children up to 4 years of age: Oral, 200 mg (6.4 mmol) of phosphorus in 60 mL of water four times a day, after meals and at bedtime.
  Children 4 years of age and over: See *Usual adult and adolescent dose*.

**Strength(s) usually available**
U.S.—
  155 mg of monobasic potassium phosphate and 350 mg of anhydrous monobasic sodium phosphate (125.6 mg [4 mmol] of phosphorus) (Rx) [*K-Phos M. F* (scored)].
  155 mg of monobasic potassium phosphate, 130 mg of hydrous monobasic sodium phosphate, and 852 mg of anhydrous dibasic sodium phosphate (250 mg [8 mmol] of phosphorus) (Rx) [*K-Phos Neutral*].
  305 mg of monobasic potassium phosphate and 700 mg of anhydrous monobasic sodium phosphate (250 mg [8 mmol] of phosphorus) (Rx) [*K-Phos No. 2*].
Canada—
  Not commercially available.

**Packaging and storage**
Store between 15 and 30 °C (59 and 86 °F), in a well-closed container, unless otherwise specified by manufacturer.

**Auxiliary labeling**
- Do not swallow tablet.
- Dissolve tablet in a full glass (8 ounces) of water.

**Additional information**
A dose of 155 mg of monobasic potassium phosphate and 350 mg of anhydrous monobasic sodium phosphate supplies 125.6 mg (4 mmol) of phosphorus, 1.14 mEq (44.5 mg) of potassium, and 2.9 mEq (67 mg) of sodium.
A dose of 305 mg of monobasic potassium phosphate and 700 mg of anhydrous monobasic sodium phosphate supplies 250 mg (8 mmol) of phosphorus, 2.3 mEq (88 mg) of potassium, and 5.8 mEq (134 mg) of sodium.
A dose of 155 mg of monobasic potassium phosphate, 130 mg of hydrous monobasic sodium phosphate, and 852 mg of anhydrous dibasic sodium phosphate supplies 250 mg (8 mmol) of phosphorus, 1.15 mEq (45 mg) of potassium, and 12.9 mEq (298 mg) of sodium.

### POTASSIUM AND SODIUM PHOSPHATES CAPSULES FOR ORAL SOLUTION

**Usual adult and adolescent dose**
Electrolyte replenisher—
  Oral, 1.25 grams (250 mg or 8 mmol of phosphorus) in 75 mL of water or juice four times a day, after meals and at bedtime.

**Usual pediatric dose**
Electrolyte replenisher—
Children up to 4 years of age: Oral, the equivalent of 200 mg (6.4 mmol) of phosphorus in 60 mL of water or juice four times a day, after meals and at bedtime.
Children 4 years of age and over: See *Usual adult and adolescent dose.*

**Strength(s) usually available**
U.S.—
1.25 grams (250 mg [8 mmol] of phosphorus) (OTC) [*Neutra-Phos*].
Canada—
Not commercially available.

**Packaging and storage**
Store below 40 °C (104 °F), preferably between 15 and 30 °C (59 and 86 °F), in a well-closed container, unless otherwise specified by manufacturer.

**Preparation of dosage form**
Empty contents of capsule into 75 mL of water or juice and stir well.

**Auxiliary labeling**
• Do not swallow filled capsule.
• Mix contents of each capsule with one-third glass of water or juice.

**Additional information**
Each 1.25-gram capsule supplies 250 mg (8 mmol) of phosphorus, 278 mg (7.125 mEq) of potassium, and 164 mg (7.125 mEq) of sodium.

## POTASSIUM AND SODIUM PHOSPHATES FOR ORAL SOLUTION

**Usual adult and adolescent dose**
Electrolyte replenisher—
Oral, 250 mg (8 mmol) of phosphorus four times a day, after meals and at bedtime.

**Usual pediatric dose**
Electrolyte replenisher—
Children up to 4 years of age: Oral, 200 mg (6.4 mmol) four times a day after meals and at bedtime.
Children 4 years of age and over: See *Usual adult and adolescent dose.*

**Size(s) usually available**
64 grams (250 mg or 8 mmol of phosphorus per 75 mL, when reconstituted according to manufacturer's instruction).
U.S.—
1.25 grams (250 mg [8mmol] of phosphorus) (OTC) [*NeutraPhos*].
64 grams (250 mg [8 mmol] of phosphorus) (OTC) [*Neutra-Phos*].
Canada—
Not commercially available.

**Packaging and storage**
Store between 15 and 30 °C (59 and 86 °F), in a well-closed container, unless otherwise specified by manufacturer.

**Preparation of dosage form**
To prepare solution, add the contents of one bottle (64 grams) of dibasic potassium and sodium phosphates and monobasic potassium sodium phosphates powder concentrate, supplied by the manufacturer, to a sufficient amount of water to make 1 gallon (3.785 liters) of solution or the contents of one packet, supplied by the manufacturer, to a sufficient amount of water to make 1/3 glass of water (approximately 2.5 ounces) of solution. Shake for 2 or 3 minutes or until all the powder is dissolved. Solution should not be diluted.

**Stability**
Solution can be stored for 60 days.

**Additional information**
Each 75 mL of solution or solution prepared from one packet supplies 250 mg (8 mmol) of phosphorus, 7.125 mEq (278 mg) of potassium, and 7.125 mEq (164 mg) of sodium.

## POTASSIUM AND SODIUM PHOSPHATES TABLETS FOR ORAL SOLUTION

**Usual adult and adolescent dose**
Electrolyte replenisher—
Oral, the equivalent of 250 mg (8 mmol) of phosphorus with a full glass (240 mL) of water four times a day.

**Usual pediatric dose**
Electrolyte replenisher—
Children up to 4 years of age: Oral, 200 mg (6.4 mmol) of phosphorus in 60 mL of water four times a day, after meals and at bedtime.
Children 4 years of age and over: See *Usual adult and adolescent dose.*

**Strength(s) usually available**
U.S.—
250 mg (8 mmol) of phosphorus (Rx) [*Uro-KP-Neutral*].
Canada—
250 mg (8 mmol) of phosphorus (Rx) [*Uro-KP-Neutral*].

**Packaging and storage**
Store below 40 °C (104 °F), preferably between 15 and 30 °C (59 and 86 °F), in a well-closed container, unless otherwise specified by manufacturer.

**Auxiliary labeling**
• Do not swallow tablet.
• Dissolve tablet in a full glass (8 ounces) of water.

**Additional information**
Each tablet supplies 250 mg (8 mmol) of phosphorus, 1.28 mEq (50 mg) of potassium, and 10.8 mEq (250 mg) of sodium, as anhydrous dibasic sodium phosphate, anhydrous dibasic potassium phosphate, and anhydrous monobasic sodium phosphate.

## SODIUM PHOSPHATES

## Parenteral Dosage Forms

Note: **Sodium phosphates injection must be diluted prior to intravenous administration.**

### SODIUM PHOSPHATES INJECTION USP

**Usual adult and adolescent dose**
Electrolyte replenisher—
Intravenous infusion, 10 to 15 mmol (310 to 465 mg) of phosphorus a day.

**Usual pediatric dose**
Electrolyte replenisher—
Intravenous infusion, 1.5 to 2 mmol of phosphorus per kg of body weight a day.

**Strength(s) usually available**
U.S.—
276 mg of hydrous monobasic sodium phosphate and 142 mg of anhydrous dibasic sodium phosphate (3 mmol [93 mg] of phosphorus) per mL (Rx) [GENERIC].
Canada—
Not commercially available.

**Packaging and storage**
Store below 40 °C (104 °F), preferably between 15 and 30 °C (59 and 86 °F), unless otherwise specified by manufacturer. Protect from freezing.

**Incompatibilities**
Precipitate may form when sodium phosphates injection is added to solution containing calcium or magnesium.

**Additional information**
Each mL of sodium phosphates injection supplies 285 mg of phosphate (approximately 3 mmol [93 mg] of phosphorus) and 4 mEq (92 mg) of sodium.

Revised: 04/16/92
Interim revision: 08/30/94; 07/18/95

**PHYSOSTIGMINE**—The *Physostigmine (Ophthalmic)* monograph is not included in this published version of the USP DI database. Copies of the monograph are available on request from Micromedex, Inc. - Reprint Requests, 6200 S. Syracuse Way, Suite 300, Englewood, CO 80111; telephone (303) 486-6400; telefax (303) 486-6464; Email: USPDI@MDX.COM.

# PHYSOSTIGMINE  Systemic

VA CLASSIFICATION (Primary): AU300
Commonly used brand name(s): *Antilirium*.
Another commonly used name is eserine.

Note: For a listing of dosage forms and brand names by country availability, see *Dosage Forms* section(s).

## Category

Cholinergic (cholinesterase inhibitor); antidote (to anticholinergics).

## Indications

Note: Bracketed information in the *Indications* section refers to uses that are not included in U.S. product labeling.

**Accepted**

Toxicity, anticholinergic agent (treatment)—Physostigmine is indicated to reverse toxic effects on the central nervous system (CNS) caused by drugs and plants capable of producing anticholinergic poisoning in clinical or toxic dosages. Physostigmine is not recommended for treatment of routine anticholinergic poisoning or those not responding to less toxic alternatives because of potential complications such as bradycardia, seizures, and asystole.

[Ataxias, hereditary (treatment)][1]—FDA has granted physostigmine an orphan drug designation for use in Friedreich's and other inherited ataxias.

**Unaccepted**

Physostigmine has been reported to antagonize the CNS depressant effects of benzodiazepines; however, physostigmine should not be used in benzodiazepine overdosage because of its nonspecific action and potential toxicity.

[1]Not included in Canadian product labeling.

## Pharmacology/Pharmacokinetics

**Mechanism of action/Effect**

Antidote (to anticholinergics)—
  Antagonizes action of anticholinergics, which block the postsynaptic receptor sites of acetylcholine, by reversibly inhibiting the destruction of acetylcholine by acetylcholinesterase, thereby increasing the concentration of acetylcholine at sites of cholinergic transmission.
  Since physostigmine is a lipid-soluble tertiary amine, which (unlike the quaternary amines neostigmine and pyridostigmine) can cross the blood-brain barrier, it acts against both central and peripheral anticholinergic effects.

**Distribution**

Easily penetrates the blood-brain barrier.

**Biotransformation**

Rapidly hydrolyzed by cholinesterases.

**Time to peak effect**

Intramuscular—20 to 30 minutes.
Intravenous—Within 5 minutes.

**Duration of action**

Intramuscular and intravenous—30 to 60 minutes.

**Elimination**

Very small amounts eliminated in urine; largely destroyed in body by hydrolysis.

## Precautions to Consider

**Pregnancy/Reproduction**

Pregnancy—Studies in humans have not been done. Physostigmine crosses the blood-brain barrier and would be expected to cross the placenta.

**Breast-feeding**

It is not known whether physostigmine is excreted in breast milk.

**Pediatrics**

No information is available on the relationship of age to the effects of physostigmine in pediatric patients. However, physostigmine should be used in children only in life-threatening situations.

Physostigmine injection that contains benzyl alcohol as a preservative should not be used in newborn and immature infants. The use of benzyl alcohol in neonates has been associated with a fatal toxic syndrome consisting of metabolic acidosis and CNS, respiratory, circulatory, and renal function impairment.

**Geriatrics**

No information is available on the relationship of age to the effects of physostigmine in geriatric patients.

**Drug interactions and/or related problems**

The following drug interactions and/or related problems have been selected on the basis of their potential clinical significance (possible mechanism in parentheses where appropriate)—not necessarily inclusive (» = major clinical significance):

Note: Combinations containing any of the following medications, depending on the amount present, may also interact with this medication.

» Choline esters (acetylcholine, bethanechol, carbachol, methacholine)
  (effects of acetylcholine and methacholine are markedly enhanced by prior administration of physostigmine, since these medications are hydrolyzed by acetylcholinesterase; physostigmine produces only additive effects when used concurrently with carbachol or bethanechol)

» Succinylcholine
  (concurrent use with physostigmine is not recommended since high doses of physostigmine may cause muscle fasciculation and ultimately, a depolarization block, which may be additive to that produced by the depolarizing neuromuscular blocking agents)

**Medical considerations/Contraindications**

The medical considerations/contraindications included have been selected on the basis of their potential clinical significance (reasons given in parentheses where appropriate)—not necessarily inclusive (» = major clinical significance).

*Risk-benefit should be considered when the following medical problems exist:*

» Asthma
  (increase in bronchial secretions and other respiratory effects of physostigmine may aggravate condition)

» Cardiovascular disease or
» Gangrene or
» Intestinal or urogenital tract obstruction, mechanical, or any vagotonic state
  (these conditions may be exacerbated by physostigmine)

  Parkinsonism
  (akinesia, rigidity, and tremor may be increased)

» Organophosphate poisoning
  (physostigmine may potentiate anticholinesterase activity)

  Sensitivity to physostigmine

**Patient monitoring**

The following may be especially important in patient monitoring (other tests may be warranted in some patients, depending on condition; » = major clinical significance):

Blood pressure and
Heart rate and rhythm
  (monitoring is recommended because physostigmine has been reported to cause bradycardia and hypotension)

## Side/Adverse Effects

The following side/adverse effects have been selected on the basis of their potential clinical significance (possible signs and symptoms in parentheses where appropriate)—not necessarily inclusive:

**Those indicating need for medical attention**

Incidence less frequent or rare
  *Irregular heartbeat; muscle twitching; shortness of breath, troubled breathing, wheezing, or tightness in chest; unusual tiredness or weakness*

With too rapid intravenous administration
  *Convulsions; difficulty in breathing; slow heartbeat*

**Those indicating need for medical attention only if they continue or are bothersome**

Incidence more frequent
  *Diarrhea; increased sweating; increased watering of mouth; nausea or vomiting; stomach cramps or pain*

Incidence less frequent
  *Frequent urge to urinate; increase in bronchial secretions; nervousness or restlessness; unusually small pupils; unusual watering of eyes*

## Overdose

For specific information on the agents used in the management of physostigmine overdose, see:
- **Atropine** in *Anticholinergics/Antispasmodics (Systemic)* monograph.

For more specific information on the management of overdose or unintentional ingestion, **contact a Poison Control Center** (see *Poison Control Center Listing*).

**Treatment of overdose**
Specific treatment—
Use of the antagonist atropine sulfate injection. See the package insert or *Atropine* in *Anticholinergic/Antispasmodics (Systemic)* for specific dosing guidelines for use of this product.

Use of intravenous administration of pralidoxime chloride to counteract ganglionic and skeletal muscle effects. See the package insert for specific dosing guidelines for use of this product.

Treatment of convulsions or shock as appropriate.

Monitoring— May include monitoring of cardiac function.

Supportive care—Maintenance of open airway (possible suction of bronchial secretions); use of assisted respiration.

## General Dosing Information

The dosage of physostigmine should be reduced if excessive sweating or nausea occurs.

Physostigmine should be discontinued if excessive symptoms of salivation, vomiting, urination, or diarrhea occur.

Rapid intravenous administration may cause bradycardia, hypersalivation resulting in breathing difficulties, and possibly convulsions.

## Parenteral Dosage Forms

### PHYSOSTIGMINE SALICYLATE INJECTION USP

**Usual adult and adolescent dose**
Antidote—
Intramuscular or intravenous, 500 mcg (0.5 mg) to 2 mg, administered at a rate of not more than 1 mg per minute; doses of 1 to 4 mg may be repeated, if necessary, at intervals of 20 to 30 minutes as life-threatening signs recur.

**Usual pediatric dose**
Antidote—
Intravenous, initially no more than 20 mcg (0.02 mg) per kilogram of body weight administered over a period of at least one minute; if toxic effects persist and there is no sign of cholinergic effects, dose may be repeated at five- to ten-minute intervals, if necessary, up to a maximum dose of 2 mg.

Note: Use should be reserved for life-threatening situations only.

Physostigmine injection that contains benzyl alcohol as a preservative should not be used in newborn and immature infants. The use of benzyl alcohol in neonates has been associated with a fatal toxic syndrome consisting of metabolic acidosis and CNS, respiratory, circulatory, and renal function impairment.

**Strength(s) usually available**
U.S.—
1 mg per mL (Rx) [*Antilirium* (benzyl alcohol 2%); GENERIC].
Canada—
1 mg per mL (Rx) [*Antilirium* (benzyl alcohol 2%)].

**Packaging and storage**
Store below 40 °C (104 °F), preferably between 15 and 30 °C (59 and 86 °F), unless otherwise specified by manufacturer. Protect from light. Protect from freezing.

Revised: 08/21/92

---

**PHYTONADIONE**—See *Vitamin K (Systemic)*

---

**PILOCARPINE**—The *Pilocarpine (Ophthalmic)* monograph is not included in this published version of the USP DI database. Copies of the monograph are available on request from Micromedex, Inc. - Reprint Requests, 6200 S. Syracuse Way, Suite 300, Englewood, CO 80111; telephone (303) 486-6400; telefax (303) 486-6464; Email: USPDI@MDX.COM.

---

# PILOCARPINE  Systemic†

VA CLASSIFICATION (Primary): AU300
Commonly used brand name(s): *Salagen*.
Note: For a listing of dosage forms and brand names by country availability, see *Dosage Forms* section(s).

†Not commercially available in Canada.

## Category
Cholinergic.

## Indications

**Accepted**
Xerostomia (treatment)—Pilocarpine is indicated for the treatment of xerostomia from salivary gland hypofunction caused by radiotherapy for cancer of the head and neck.

## Pharmacology/Pharmacokinetics

**Physicochemical characteristics**
Molecular weight—Pilocarpine hydrochloride: 244.72.
pKa—7.15.

**Mechanism of action/Effect**
Pilocarpine is a cholinergic parasympathomimetic agent that exerts a broad spectrum of pharmacologic effects with predominantly muscarinic action, including stimulation of exocrine function. This stimulation results in increased secretion by the exocrine glands, including the salivary glands.

**Other actions/effects**
Other exocrine glands, such as the sweat, lacrimal, gastric, pancreatic, and intestinal glands, may be stimulated.

Pulmonary effects may include stimulation of the mucous cells of the respiratory tract, increased airway resistance, and increased bronchial smooth muscle tone and secretions.

Cardiovascular effects may include changes in hemodynamics and cardiac rhythm. However, pilocarpine may have paradoxical effects. Instead of the expected muscarinic effect of vasodepression occurring, pilocarpine may produce short-lived hypotension followed by hypertension. In addition, both bradycardia and tachycardia have been reported.

Gastrointestinal effects include smooth muscle stimulation of the intestinal tract that may result in increased tone and motility, spasm, and tenesmus. The tone and motility of the urinary tract, gallbladder, and biliary duct smooth muscle may be enhanced.

**Biotransformation**
Not fully understood; inactivation of pilocarpine is thought to occur at the neuronal synapses and in the plasma.

**Half-life**
Elimination—0.76 hours after 2 days of 5 mg of pilocarpine administered orally 3 times daily; 1.35 hours after 2 days of 10 mg of pilocarpine administered orally 3 times daily.

**Onset of action**
20 minutes.

**Time to peak concentration**
1.25 or 0.85 hours, after 2 days of 5 or 10 mg, respectively, of pilocarpine administered orally 3 times daily.

**Peak serum concentration**
15 or 41 nanograms per mL (72 or 196.8 nanomoles per L), after 2 days of 5 or 10 mg, respectively, of pilocarpine administered orally 3 times daily.

Pharmacokinetic studies were done in young men and men and women over 65 years of age after administration of 5 or 10 mg oral pilocarpine 3 times daily for 2 days. The pharmacokinetics were comparable in men under and over 65 years. However, all 5 of the women over 65 years of age in the study had mean maximum concentrations ($C_{max}$) that were approximately twice as high as the men's values. The men's $C_{max}$ values were 15 and 41 nanograms per mL (72 and 196.8 nanomoles per L) after the 5 and 10 mg dosage, respectively. No pharmacokinetic values are available for younger women.

**Time to peak effect**
1 hour.

**Duration of action**
3 to 5 hours.

**Elimination**
Not fully understood; in the urine, as unchanged pilocarpine and its minimally active or inactive degradation products, such as pilocarpic acid.
In dialysis—It is not known if pilocarpine is dialyzable.

## Precautions to Consider

### Cross-sensitivity and/or related problems
Patients sensitive to ophthalmic pilocarpine may be sensitive to oral pilocarpine also.

### Carcinogenicity
Studies have not been done.

### Mutagenicity
Pilocarpine did not cause genetic toxicity in bacterial assays (*Salmonella* and *E. coli*) for reverse gene mutations, *in vitro* chromosome aberration assay (micronucleus test) in mice, and primary DNA damage assay (unscheduled DNA synthesis) in rat hepatocyte primary cultures.

### Pregnancy/Reproduction
Fertility—Studies have not been done in humans.
Male rats given 39 mg per kg of body weight (mg/kg) per day of pilocarpine (approximately 10 times the usual human dose) exhibited morphologic evidence of reduced spermatogenesis.

Pregnancy—Studies have not been done in humans.
Fetuses of pregnant rats given 90 mg/kg per day of pilocarpine (approximately 26 times the maximum recommended human dose) had reduced mean body weight and an increased incidence of skeletal variations. However, these effects may have been secondary to maternal toxicity.

FDA Pregnancy Category C.

### Breast-feeding
It is not known whether pilocarpine is distributed into breast milk. However, problems in humans have not been documented.

### Pediatrics
Appropriate studies on the relationship of age to the effects of oral pilocarpine have not been performed in the pediatric population. Safety and efficacy have not been established.

### Geriatrics
Appropriate studies performed to date have not demonstrated geriatric-specific problems that would limit the usefulness of oral pilocarpine in the elderly.
Clinical trials were conducted in both men and women under and over 65 years of age. The adverse events reported by these 4 groups were comparable. In addition, pharmacokinetic studies were done in young men and men and women over 65 years of age after administration of 5 or 10 mg oral pilocarpine 3 times daily for 2 days. The pharmacokinetics were comparable in men under and over 65 years. However, all 5 of the women over 65 years of age in the study had mean maximum concentrations ($C_{max}$) and trapezoidal values of the areas under the curve (AUC) that were approximately twice as high as the men's values. The men's $C_{max}$ values were 15 and 41 nanograms per mL (72 and 196.8 nanomoles per L) after the 5 and 10 mg dosage, respectively. The men's AUC trapezoidal values were 33 and 108 h (nanograms per mL) after the 5 and 10 mg dosage, respectively.

### Drug interactions and/or related problems
The following drug interactions and/or related problems have been selected on the basis of their potential clinical significance (possible mechanism in parentheses where appropriate)—not necessarily inclusive (» = major clinical significance):

Note: Combinations containing any of the following medications, depending on the amount present, may also interact with this medication.

» Anticholinergics or other medications with anticholinergic activity (See *Appendix II*)
(concurrent use may cause an antagonism of pilocarpine's therapeutic cholinergic effect)

(concurrent use may cause an antagonism of the anticholinergic drug's anticholinergic effects; this may be important not only when the drug is being used therapeutically for its anticholinergic effects, but also when the drug has other therapeutic effects and its anticholinergic side effects are being used as indicators of impending adverse effects)

» Antiglaucoma agents, cholinergic, long acting, ophthalmic or
» Antiglaucoma agents, cholinergic, short acting, ophthalmic or
» Bethanechol or

» Cholinergics, other, or other medications with cholinergic activity, such as antimyasthenics
(concurrent use with pilocarpine may result in additive cholinergic effects)

» Beta-adrenergic blocking agents, systemic and ophthalmic
(concurrent use with pilocarpine may increase the possibility of conduction disturbances)

### Medical considerations/Contraindications
The medical considerations/contraindications included have been selected on the basis of their potential clinical significance (reasons given in parentheses where appropriate)—not necessarily inclusive (» = major clinical significance).

*Except under special circumstances, this medication should not be used when the following medical problems exist:*

» Asthma, uncontrolled
(pilocarpine may stimulate the mucous cells of the respiratory tract and may increase airway resistance and bronchial smooth muscle tone)

» Glaucoma, angle closure or
» Iritis, acute
(pilocarpine may cause miosis)

» Sensitivity to pilocarpine

*Risk-benefit should be considered when the following medical problems exist:*

» Asthma, controlled or
» Bronchitis, chronic or
» Chronic obstructive pulmonary disease
(pilocarpine may stimulate the mucous cells of the respiratory tract and may increase airway resistance and bronchial smooth muscle tone)

» Biliary tract disease or
» Cholelithiasis, known or suspected
(pilocarpine may cause contractions of the gallbladder or biliary smooth muscle and cholecystitis, cholangitis, or biliary obstruction may occur)

» Cardiovascular disease
(patients with significant cardiovascular disease may be unable to compensate for the transient changes in hemodynamics or heart rhythm that are induced by pilocarpine; pulmonary edema has occurred as a complication of pilocarpine toxicity from high ophthalmic doses and may occur with oral pilocarpine also)

» Cognitive disturbances or
» Psychiatric disturbances
(pilocarpine may have central nervous system effects, which may exacerbate these conditions)

Nephrolithiasis
(pilocarpine may increase ureteral smooth muscle tone and may theoretically precipitate renal colic, especially in patients with nephrolithiasis)

» Retinal detachment, predisposition to or
» Retinal disease
(an association between use of ophthalmic pilocarpine and retinal detachment has been reported in patients with pre-existing retinal disease; it is not known whether this association may occur with oral pilocarpine)

### Patient monitoring
The following may be especially important in patient monitoring (other tests may be warranted in some patients, depending on condition; » = major clinical significance):

Fundus examination
(should be performed periodically in patients with pre-existing retinal disease, since an association between use of ophthalmic pilocarpine and retinal detachment has been reported in patients with pre-existing retinal disease; it is not known whether this association may occur with oral pilocarpine)

## Side/Adverse Effects

Note: Pilocarpine toxicity is characterized by an exaggeration of its parasympathomimetic effects.

The following side/adverse effects have occurred in less than 1% of patients treated with pilocarpine; however, the causal relationship is unknown: anorexia, anxiety, deafness, depression, dysuria, electrocardiogram abnormality, esophagitis, eye pain, glaucoma, hyperkinesia, hypoesthesia, hypothermia, leukopenia, lymphadenopathy, metrorrhagia, paresthesias, seborrhea, speech disorder, stridor, syncope, and urinary impairment. In addition, 1 patient experienced a myocardial infarction and 1 patient had an episode of syncope; both patients had underlying cardiovascular disease.

The following side/adverse effects have occurred rarely in patients treated with ophthalmic pilocarpine: agitation, atrioventricular block, ciliary congestion, confusion, delusion, depression, dermatitis, iris cysts, macular hole, malignant glaucoma, middle ear disturbance, shock, and visual hallucination.

The following side/adverse effects have been selected on the basis of their potential clinical significance (possible signs and symptoms in parentheses where appropriate)—not necessarily inclusive:

**Those indicating need for medical attention only if they continue or are bothersome**
Incidence more frequent
*Sweating*

Incidence less frequent or rare
*Amblyopia* (trouble seeing); *asthenia* (unusual weak feeling); *chills; diarrhea; dizziness; dyspepsia* (indigestion); *dysphagia* (trouble swallowing); *edema* (holding more body water; swelling of face, fingers, ankles, or feet); *epistaxis* (nosebleeds); *flushing* (redness of face or feeling of warmth); *headache; hypertension; nausea; rhinitis* (runny nose); *tachycardia* (fast heartbeat); *tremors* (trembling or shaking); *urinary frequency* (passing urine more often); *voice change; vomiting*

## Overdose

For specific information on the agents used in the management of systemic pilocarpine overdose, see:
- *Atropine* in *Anticholinergics/Antispasmodics (Systemic)* monograph; and/or
- *Epinephrine* in *Bronchodilators, Adrenergic (Systemic)* monograph.

For more information on the management of overdose or unintentional ingestion, **contact a Poison Control Center** (see *Poison Control Center Listing*).

Pilocarpine toxicity is characterized by an exaggeration of its parasympathomimetic effects. One hundred mg of pilocarpine is considered to be potentially fatal.

**Clinical effects of overdose**
The following effects have been selected on the basis of their potential clinical significance (possible signs and symptoms in parentheses where appropriate)—not necessarily inclusive:

Acute and chronic
*Arrhythmia* (irregular heartbeat, continuing or severe); *atrioventricular block* (chest pain or fainting); *bradycardia* (slow heartbeat, continuing or severe); *confusion; diarrhea, continuing or severe; gastrointestinal spasm* (stomach cramps or pain); *headache, continuing or severe; hypertension; hypotension* (tiredness or weakness, continuing or severe); *nausea, continuing or severe; respiratory distress* (shortness of breath or troubled breathing); *shock* (fainting or tiredness or weakness, continuing or severe); *tachycardia* (fast heartbeat, continuing or severe); *tremors* (trembling or shaking, continuing or severe); *visual disturbance, continuing or severe* (trouble seeing, continuing or severe); *vomiting, continuing or severe*

**Treatment of overdose**
0.5 to 1 mg of atropine should be administered subcutaneously or intravenously.

Supportive measures to maintain respiration and circulation should be used.

For severe cardiovascular depression or bronchoconstriction, 0.3 to 1 mg of epinephrine should be administered subcutaneously or intramuscularly.

## Patient Consultation

As an aid to patient consultation, refer to *Advice for the Patient, Pilocarpine (Systemic)*.

In providing consultation, consider emphasizing the following selected information (» = major clinical significance):

**Before using this medication**
» Conditions affecting use, especially:
   Sensitivity to ophthalmic or oral pilocarpine
   Use in children—Safety and efficacy have not been established
   Other medications, especially anticholinergics or other medications with anticholinergic activity; antiglaucoma agents, cholinergic, long acting, ophthalmic; antiglaucoma agents, cholinergic, short acting, ophthalmic; beta-adrenergic blocking agents, systemic and ophthalmic; bethanechol; or cholinergics, other, or other medications with cholinergic activity

Other medical problems, especially asthma, controlled; asthma, uncontrolled; biliary tract disease; bronchitis, chronic; cardiovascular disease; cholelithiasis, known or suspected; chronic obstructive pulmonary disease; cognitive disturbances; glaucoma, angle closure; iritis, acute; psychiatric disturbances; retinal detachment, predisposition to; or retinal disease

**Proper use of this medication**
» Taking medication only as directed; not taking it more often and not taking larger dose than directed; doing so may increase chance of side/adverse effects

Importance of seeing dentist regularly to prevent dental and other mouth problems, which are more likely to occur in patients with xerostomia
» Proper dosing
   Missed dose: Taking as soon as possible; skipping missed dose if it is almost time for next dose; not doubling doses
» Proper storage

**Precautions while using this medication**
» Caution if difficulty in reading or other vision problems occur; caution if dizziness or lightheadedness occurs; not driving, using machines, or doing anything else that could be dangerous if not alert or able to see well; checking with physician if reactions are especially bothersome
» Importance of drinking enough liquids to offset the sweating that medication may cause

**Side/adverse effects**
Signs of potential side effects, especially signs of overdose

## General Dosing Information

The lowest dosage that is effective should be used, since the incidence of side/adverse effects is dose dependent.

## Oral Dosage Forms

### PILOCARPINE HYDROCHLORIDE TABLETS

**Usual adult and adolescent dose**
Xerostomia (treatment)—
   Oral, 5 mg three times a day. Dosage may be increased up to 10 mg three times a day for patients who do not respond to lower doses; however, increasing the dose also increases the incidence of side/adverse effects. The lowest dose that is tolerated and effective should be used for maintenance.

**Usual pediatric dose**
Safety and efficacy have not been established.

**Strength(s) usually available**
U.S.—
   5 mg (Rx) [*Salagen*].
Canada—
   Not commercially available.

**Packaging and storage**
Store at controlled room temperature between 15 and 30 °C (59 and 86 °F).

## Selected Bibliography

LeVeque FG, Montgomery M, Potter D, et al. A multicenter, randomized, double-blind, placebo-controlled, dose-titration study of oral pilocarpine for treatment of radiation-induced xerostomia in head and neck cancer patients. J Clin Oncol 1993 Jun; 11(6): 1124-31.

Johnson JT, Ferretti GA, Nethery WJ, et al. Oral pilocarpine for post-irradiation xerostomia in patients with head and neck cancer. N Engl J Med 1993 Aug 5; 329(6): 390-5.

Wolff A, Atkinson JC, Macynski AA, et al. Oral complications of cancer therapies. Pretherapy interventions to modify salivary dysfunction. NCI Monogr 1990; (9): 87-90.

Developed: 01/17/95
Interim revision: 03/15/95

# PIMOZIDE Systemic

VA CLASSIFICATION (Primary/Secondary): CN900/CN709
Commonly used brand name(s): *Orap*.

Note: For a listing of dosage forms and brand names by country availability, see *Dosage Forms* section(s).

## Category
Antidyskinetic (Gilles de la Tourette's syndrome); antipsychotic.

## Indications
Note: Bracketed information in the *Indications* section refers to uses that are not included in U.S. product labeling.

### Accepted
Gilles de la Tourette's syndrome (treatment)[1]—Pimozide is indicated for the suppression of motor and vocal tics in patients with Tourette's disorder whose symptoms are severe and who cannot tolerate or have failed to respond satisfactorily to haloperidol.

[Psychotic disorders (treatment)]—Pimozide is used for maintenance therapy in the management of *chronic* schizophrenic patients *without* symptoms of excitement, agitation, or hyperactivity.

### Unaccepted
Pimozide must not be used for simple tics or tics that are not associated with Tourette's disorder, because of the high risk of cardiovascular and extrapyramidal effects.

Pimozide is ineffective and should not be used for the management of patients with mania or acute schizophrenia.

[1]Not included in Canadian product labeling.

## Pharmacology/Pharmacokinetics

### Physicochemical characteristics
Chemical group—A diphenylbutylpiperidine analog of butyrophenone and a derivative of the meperidine-like analgesics.
Molecular weight—461.56.
Solubility—Less than 0.01 mg per mL in water.

### Mechanism of action/Effect
Pimozide's exact mechanism of action has not been established; however, pimozide is thought to block dopamine $D_2$ receptors in the central nervous system (CNS). Secondary changes in central dopamine function and metabolism, including increased brain turnover of dopamine, may contribute to both the therapeutic and the adverse effects of pimozide. Pimozide also appears to block voltage-operated calcium channels and to interact with opiate receptors, probably as an antagonist.

Pimozide is thought to have more specific dopamine receptor blocking activity and less alpha-adrenergic receptor antagonism than other neuroleptic agents. This results in less potential for inducing sedation and hypotension.

### Other actions/effects
Electrocardiographic changes, including QT interval prolongation; flattening, notching, and inversion of the T wave; and the appearance of U waves have been observed with pimozide use.

Prolactin levels are elevated with antipsychotic drug therapy, probably due to antagonism of dopamine receptors. The clinical significance of elevated prolactin levels is unknown for most patients, although such effects as galactorrhea, amenorrhea, gynecomastia, and impotence have been reported in patients receiving prolactin-elevating medications. Also, studies have found approximately one third of human breast cancers to be prolactin-dependent *in vitro*.

Pimozide possesses anticholinergic activity and a substantial antiemetic effect.

### Absorption
Approximately 50% absorbed after oral administration.

### Biotransformation
Significant first-pass metabolism, primarily by *N*-dealkylation in the liver; *in vitro* data indicate that pimozide is metabolized, at least in part, by the cytochrome P450 3A (CYP3A) and CYP2D6 isoenzymes, producing two major metabolites of undetermined neuroleptic activity.

### Half-life
Elimination—
Mean, $29 \pm 10$ hours in a single-dose study of healthy volunteers.
Mean, $55 \pm 20$ hours in a repeat-dose study of short duration in schizophrenic patients.
Mean, $111 \pm 57$ hours in a single-dose study of seven adults with Tourette's syndrome.
Mean, $66 \pm 49$ hours in a single-dose study of four male children, 6 to 13 years of age, with Tourette's syndrome.

### Time to peak concentration
6 to 8 hours (range, 4 to 12 hours).

### Elimination
Renal—
40 to 50% within one week in a single-dose study in healthy volunteers, mostly as metabolites.
Fecal—
20% within one week in a single-dose study in healthy volunteers, at least half as unchanged drug.

## Precautions to Consider

### Cross-sensitivity and/or related problems
Patients sensitive to neuroleptic agents such as haloperidol, loxapine, molindone, phenothiazines, or thioxanthenes may also be sensitive to pimozide.

### Carcinogenicity
In a 24-month carcinogenicity study of rats receiving up to 50 times the maximum recommended human dose (MRHD), no increased incidence of tumors overall or at any site was observed in either sex. The meaning of these results is unclear because of the limited number of animals that survived the study.

### Tumorigenicity
Studies in mice have shown that pimozide causes a dose-related increase in benign pituitary and mammary gland tumors. The mechanism of tumor induction is unknown, but may be related to elevated prolactin synthesis and release. The pituitary gland tumors, which developed in female mice only, developed as hyperplasia at doses approximating the human dose, and as adenoma at doses about 15 times the MRHD on a mg per kg of body weight (mg/kg) basis.

Mammary gland tumors increased in female mice treated with pimozide, which elevates serum prolactin concentrations. Prolactin concentrations increase in humans, also, with chronic administration of antipsychotic agents. Tissue culture experiments indicate that approximately one third of human breast cancers are prolactin-dependent *in vitro*, a factor of potential importance if the prescription of these drugs is contemplated in a patient with previously detected breast cancer or if the patient is young and chronic use of the medication is anticipated.

### Mutagenicity
Pimozide did not have mutagenic activity in the Ames test with four bacterial test strains, in the mouse dominant lethal test, or in the micronucleus test in rats.

### Pregnancy/Reproduction
Fertility—Studies in rats have shown prolonged estrus cycles and fewer pregnancies. These effects are thought to be due to an inhibition of or delay in implantation, which has also been observed in rodents administered other antipsychotic agents.

Pregnancy—Adequate and well-controlled studies in humans have not been done.

Studies in rats given doses eight times the maximum recommended human dose showed retarded fetal development. In rabbits, maternal toxicity, mortality, decreased weight gain, and embryotoxicity, including increased incidence of resorptions, were dose-related.

FDA Pregnancy Category C.

### Breast-feeding
It is not known whether pimozide is distributed into breast milk. Problems in humans have not been documented, although there is potential for maternal mammary gland tumor formation and unknown cardiovascular effects in the infant.

### Pediatrics
Because its use and safety have not been evaluated in other childhood disorders, pimozide currently is not recommended for use in children with conditions other than Tourette's disorder.

A gradual initiation of pimozide therapy in patients up to 12 years of age is recommended since information on safety and efficacy in this age group is very limited.

Children may be especially sensitive to the effects of pimozide.

### Geriatrics
Geriatric patients tend to develop higher plasma concentrations because of changes in distribution due to decreases in lean body mass, total body water, and albumin, and often an increase in total body fat composition. These patients usually require a lower initial dosage and a more gradual dosage titration than do younger patients.

Elderly patients are more prone to the development of transient hypotension and exhibit an increased sensitivity to the anticholinergic and sedative effects of pimozide. Also, older patients tend to develop extrapyramidal side effects more frequently, especially parkinsonism and tardive dyskinesia.

**Dental**

The peripheral anticholinergic effects of pimozide may decrease or inhibit salivary flow, especially in middle-aged or elderly patients, thus contributing to the development of caries, periodontal disease, oral candidiasis, and discomfort.

Extrapyramidal reactions induced by pimozide will result in increased motor activity of the head, face, and neck. Occlusal adjustments, bite registrations, and treatment for bruxism may be made less reliable.

The blood dyscrasia–causing effects of pimozide may result in an increased incidence of microbial infection, delayed healing, and gingival bleeding. If leukopenia or thrombocytopenia occurs, dental work should be deferred until blood counts have returned to normal. Patients should be instructed in proper oral hygiene, including caution in use of regular toothbrushes, dental floss, and toothpicks.

**Drug interactions and/or related problems**

The following drug interactions and/or related problems have been selected on the basis of their potential clinical significance (possible mechanism in parentheses where appropriate)—not necessarily inclusive (» = major clinical significance):

Note: *In vitro* data indicate that pimozide is metabolized, at least in part, by the isoenzymes CYP3A and CYP2D6. Possible interactions with medications that inhibit these isoenzymes, other than those listed below, should be considered.

Combinations containing any of the following medications, depending on the amount present, may also interact with this medication.

» Alcohol or
» CNS depression–producing medications, other (see *Appendix II*)
   (concurrent use with pimozide may potentiate the CNS depressant effects of these medications)

» Amphetamines or
» Methylphenidate or
» Pemoline
   (these medications may provoke tics; before therapy with pimozide is initiated, these medications should be withdrawn to determine the underlying cause of observed tics; pimozide is not indicated for the treatment of tics caused by other medications)
   (pimozide may block the effects of amphetamines)

» Anticholinergics or other medications with anticholinergic activity (see *Appendix II*)
   (concurrent use with pimozide may intensify anticholinergic effects, especially those of dry mouth, constipation, and unusual excitability, because of secondary anticholinergic effects of pimozide; symptoms of tardive dyskinesia may be worsened)

Anticonvulsants
   (although there has been no primary documentation for a drug interaction with pimozide and anticonvulsants, the potential exists for a lowering of the convulsive threshold by pimozide; dosage adjustment of the anticonvulsant may be necessary when pimozide treatment is initiated or discontinued or when the dose is reduced)

Antidepressants, monoamine oxidase (MAO) inhibitor
   (concurrent use may prolong and intensify the sedative, hypotensive, and anticholinergic effects of MAO inhibitors and pimozide)

» Azithromycin or
» Clarithromycin or
» Dirithromycin or
» Erythromycin
   (pimozide prolongs the QT interval, and macrolide antibiotic use in patients with prolonged QT intervals has been associated with ventricular arrhythmias; sudden deaths have occurred when clarithromycin was added to pimozide therapy, probably due to inhibition of pimozide metabolism by clarithromycin; concurrent use is **contraindicated**)

» Extrapyramidal reaction–causing medications, other (see *Appendix II*)
   (concurrent use of these agents with pimozide may increase the anticholinergic, CNS depressant, and extrapyramidal effects of both medications)

» QT interval–prolonging medications, other, such as:
   Antidepressants, tricyclic or
   Disopyramide or
   Maprotiline or
   Phenothiazines or
   Probucol or
   Procainamide or
   Quinidine
   (concurrent use of these agents with pimozide may potentiate cardiac arrhythmias through an additive prolongation of the QT interval; concurrent use is **contraindicated**)

» Ritonavir
   (although there is no clinical experience with the combination, because ritonavir inhibits CYP3A and CYP2D6, it is expected to produce large increases in the plasma concentration of pimozide, which could result in cardiac arrhythmias; concurrent use is **contraindicated**)

**Laboratory value alterations**

The following have been selected on the basis of their potential clinical significance (possible effect in parentheses where appropriate)—not necessarily inclusive (» = major clinical significance):

With diagnostic test results
» Electrocardiogram [ECG]
   (pimozide use may result in prolongation of the QT interval; flattening, notching, and inversion of the T-wave; and the appearance of U-waves)

Pregnancy tests, immunologic urine
   (pimozide may produce false-positive results)

**Medical considerations/Contraindications**

The medical considerations/contraindications included have been selected on the basis of their potential clinical significance (reasons given in parentheses where appropriate)—not necessarily inclusive (» = major clinical significance).

*Except under special circumstances, this medication should not be used when the following medical problems exist:*

» Cardiac arrhythmias, history of or
» Long QT syndrome, congenital or acquired
   (may be aggravated by use of pimozide, predisposing patients to ventricular arrhythmias)

» CNS depression, severe or
» Comatose states
   (may be potentiated)

» Tics, motor or vocal, other than those caused by Tourette's disorder
   (efficacy has not been established and risk of cardiovascular and extrapyramidal effects may outweigh potential benefit)

*Risk-benefit should be considered when the following medical problems exist:*

» Breast cancer, history of
   (may be aggravated by increased serum prolactin concentrations)

Glaucoma, narrow angle or
Paralytic ileus, history of or
Prostatic hypertrophy, clinically significant
   (condition may be exacerbated by secondary anticholinergic effects of pimozide)

Hepatic function impairment or
Renal function impairment
   (metabolism and excretion of pimozide may be altered)

» Hypokalemia
   (potassium deficiency, such as from diarrhea or use of diuretics, should be corrected before initiation of pimozide therapy because of risk of ventricular arrhythmias)

Seizures, or history of
   (pimozide may lower seizure threshold; increased incidence of epileptic seizures has been reported)

Sensitivity to pimozide or other neuroleptics, such as haloperidol, loxapine, molindone, phenothiazines, or thioxanthenes

**Patient monitoring**

The following may be especially important in patient monitoring (other tests may be warranted in some patients, depending on condition; » = major clinical significance):

» Electrocardiogram [ECG]
   (recommended at initiation of therapy as baseline, and periodically thereafter, especially during dosage adjustment; any indication of prolongation of the QTc interval beyond an absolute limit of 0.47 seconds in children, 0.52 seconds in adults, or more than 25% of the patient's original baseline should be considered a basis for stopping increase of dosage or for reducing dosage)

Careful observation for early signs of tardive dyskinesia, especially in the elderly or patients on high or extended maintenance dosage
   (recommended at least every 3 months; since there is no known effective treatment if syndrome should develop, pimozide should

be discontinued, if clinically feasible, at earliest signs, usually fine, worm-like movements of the tongue, to stop further development)

Careful observation for early signs of tardive dystonia (recommended at periodic intervals; since there is no known effective treatment if syndrome should develop, pimozide should be discontinued, if clinically feasible, at the earliest signs)

## Side/Adverse Effects

Note: Sudden, unexplained deaths have occurred in patients receiving pimozide, mainly at dosages above 20 mg a day. These deaths may be related to the prolonged QT interval associated with pimozide use.

The following side/adverse effects have been selected on the basis of their potential clinical significance (possible signs and symptoms in parentheses where appropriate)—not necessarily inclusive:

### Those indicating need for medical attention
Incidence more frequent
  *Akathisia* (restlessness or need to keep moving); ***arrhythmias, ventricular*** (dizziness or fainting; fast or irregular heartbeat)—seen on ECG as prolonged QT interval as well as lowered and inverted T-wave and S-T segment changes; *extrapyramidal effects, parkinsonian* (difficulty in speaking; loss of balance control; lack of facial expression; shuffling walk; slowed movements; stiffness of arms and legs; trembling and shaking of fingers and hands); *mood or behavior changes; swelling or soreness of breasts*—less frequent in males; *unusual secretion of milk*—rare in males

  Note: In children, *akathisia* may appear to be a worsening of Tourette's syndrome symptoms and may improve with a decrease in dosage. *Mood or behavior changes* in children may occur as a dose-dependent dysphoria, which includes anxiety, crying spells, fearfulness, irritability, and social withdrawal.

  *Parkinsonian extrapyramidal effects* often occur during the first few days of treatment and are usually mild to moderately severe. Although severe extrapyramidal effects have been reported to occur at relatively low doses, most are dose-related and may decrease in severity or disappear when dosage is reduced.

Incidence less frequent
  *Extrapyramidal effects, dystonic* (difficulty in swallowing; inability to move eyes; muscle spasms, especially of the face, neck, or back; twisting movements of the body); *menstrual changes; tardive dyskinesia* (lip smacking or puckering; puffing of cheeks; rapid or worm-like movements of tongue; uncontrolled chewing movements; uncontrolled movements of arms and legs)

  Note: Risk of developing *tardive dyskinesia* or of developing irreversible tardive dyskinesia may increase with long-term treatment and with total cumulative dose. The symptoms of tardive dyskinesia may be masked during therapy, but may appear after reduction of dose or withdrawal of pimozide. There is no known effective treatment. Careful observation during pimozide therapy for early signs of tardive dyskinesia and reduction of dosage or discontinuation of medication may prevent a more severe manifestation of the syndrome. Tardive dyskinesia is more prevalent among elderly patients, especially females, on high-dose therapy.

Incidence rare
  *Allergic reaction* (skin rash and itching; swelling of face); ***blood dyscrasias*** (sore throat and fever; unusual bleeding or bruising); ***jaundice, obstructive*** (yellow eyes or skin); ***neuroleptic malignant syndrome (NMS)*** (convulsions; difficult or unusually fast breathing; fast heartbeat or irregular pulse; high fever; high or low [irregular] blood pressure; increased sweating; loss of bladder control; severe muscle stiffness); *tardive dystonia* (increased blinking or spasms of eyelid; unusual facial expressions or body positions; uncontrolled twisting movements of neck, trunk, arms, or legs)

  Note: *NMS* is a potentially fatal symptom complex. Additional signs of NMS may include elevated creatine kinase (CK), myoglobinuria (rhabdomyolysis), and acute renal failure. NMS may occur at any time during neuroleptic therapy, but is more commonly seen soon after start of therapy, or after patient has switched from one neuroleptic to another, during combined therapy with another psychotropic medication, or after a dosage increase.

### Those indicating need for medical attention only if they continue or are bothersome
Incidence more frequent
  *Blurred vision or other vision problems; constipation; drowsiness; dryness of mouth; hypotension, orthostatic* (dizziness, lightheadedness, or fainting when getting up from a lying or sitting position); *skin discoloration*

  Note: *Orthostatic hypotension* is most common in elderly and debilitated patients for several hours after administration of pimozide.

Incidence less frequent
  *Asthenia* (tiredness or weakness); *decreased sexual ability; diarrhea; headache; loss of appetite and weight; mental depression; nausea and vomiting*

### Those indicating the need for medical attention if they occur after the medication is discontinued
  *Dyskinesia, withdrawal emergent* (lip smacking or puckering; puffing of cheeks; rapid or worm-like movements of tongue; uncontrolled chewing movements; uncontrolled movements of arms and legs)

## Overdose

For specific information on the agents used in the management of pimozide overdose, see:
- Albumin Human (Systemic) monograph;
- Benztropine in Antidyskinetics (Systemic) monograph;
- Diazepam in Benzodiazepines (Systemic) monograph;
- Diphenhydramine in Antihistamines (Systemic) monograph;
- Magnesium Sulfate (Systemic) monograph; and/or
- Metaraminol, Norepinephrine, and/or Phenylephrine in Sympathomimetic Agents–Cardiovascular Use (Parenteral-Systemic) monograph.

For more information on the management of overdose or unintentional ingestion, **contact a Poison Control Center** (see *Poison Control Center Listing*).

### Clinical effects of overdose
Note: The clinical effects of pimozide overdose are generally an exaggeration of adverse effects seen at therapeutic doses.

The following effects have been selected on the basis of their potential clinical significance (possible signs and symptoms in parentheses where appropriate)—not necessarily inclusive:

Acute
  ***Coma; electrocardiogram (ECG) abnormalities; extrapyramidal reactions*** (muscle trembling, jerking, or stiffness; uncontrolled movements); *hypotension* (dizziness); *respiratory depression* (troubled breathing); *seizures*

### Treatment of overdose
Treatment is essentially symptomatic and supportive.
  To decrease absorption—
    Initiating gastric lavage. Induction of emesis is not advised, because of possible decreased seizure threshold and extrapyramidal reactions.
  Specific treatment—
    Counteracting hypotension and circulatory collapse with use of intravenous fluids, plasma, or concentrated albumin, and vasopressor agents such as norepinephrine, metaraminol, or phenylephrine. Epinephrine should *not* be used since it may cause paradoxical hypotension.
    Administering intravenous diphenhydramine or benztropine to manage dystonias.
    Administering diazepam to manage seizures.
    Using magnesium sulfate followed by pacing and correction of electrolyte abnormalities if *torsades de pointes* develops.
  Monitoring—
    Immediately monitoring ECG and continuing until parameters are within normal range. Continuing monitoring ECG until parameters have remained within normal range for 24 hours in patients who develop *torsades de pointes*.
    Observing patients for at least 4 days because of the long half-life of pimozide.
  Supportive care—
    Establishing a patent airway and mechanically assisting respiration, if necessary.
    Patients in whom intentional overdose is confirmed or suspected should be referred for psychiatric consultation.

## Patient Consultation

As an aid to patient consultation, refer to *Advice for the Patient, Pimozide (Systemic)*.

In providing consultation, consider emphasizing the following selected information (» = major clinical significance):

### Before using this medication
» Conditions affecting use, especially:
    Sensitivity to pimozide or other neuroleptic agents

Pregnancy—Animal studies have shown fewer pregnancies; retarded fetal development; maternal toxicity; mortality; decreased weight gain; embryotoxicity; increased resorptions

Use in children—Not recommended for conditions other than Tourette's syndrome; therapy should be initiated gradually in patients up to 12 years of age; children may be more sensitive to effects of pimozide

Use in the elderly—Elderly patients are more likely to experience extrapyramidal, anticholinergic, hypotensive, and sedative effects; reduced dosage recommended

Dental—Dry mouth may cause caries, candidiasis, periodontal disease, and discomfort; increased motor activity of face, head, and neck may interfere with some dental procedures; pimozide-induced blood dyscrasias may result in infections, delayed healing, and bleeding

Contraindicated medications Azithromycin, clarithromycin, dirithromycin, erythromycin, other QT interval-prolonging medications, or ritonavir

Other medications, especially alcohol, amphetamines, methylphenidate, other anticholinergic medications, other CNS depression-producing medications, other extrapyramidal reaction-producing medications, or pemoline

Other medical problems, especially cardiac arrhythmias, comatose states, congenital or acquired long QT syndrome, history of breast cancer, hypokalemia, severe CNS depression, or tics other than those caused by Tourette's disorder

**Proper use of this medication**
» Importance of not taking more medication than the amount prescribed because of cardiac effects
» Proper dosing
 Missed dose: Skipping the missed dose and returning to regular dosing schedule; not doubling doses
» Proper storage

**Precautions while using this medication**
Regular visits to physician to check progress of therapy
» Not taking azithromycin, clarithromycin, dirithromycin, erythromycin, other QT interval-prolonging medications or ritonavir during pimozide therapy because of possible life-threatening cardiac arrhythmias
» Checking with physician before discontinuing medication; gradual dosage reduction may be needed
» Avoiding use of alcoholic beverages or other CNS depressants during therapy
» Possible drowsiness, blurred vision, or muscle stiffness; caution when driving, using machinery, or doing other things requiring alertness, clear vision, and good muscle control
 Possible dizziness or lightheadedness; avoiding getting up suddenly from a sitting or lying position
» Caution if any kind of surgery, dental treatment, or emergency surgery is required because of additive CNS-depressant effects of pimozide and medications used in these situations
 Possible dryness of mouth; using sugarless gum or candy, ice, or saliva substitute for relief; checking with physician or dentist if dry mouth continues for more than 2 weeks

**Side/adverse effects**
Side effects are more likely in children and elderly or debilitated patients
» Stopping medication and notifying physician immediately if symptoms of neuroleptic malignant syndrome (NMS) appear
» Notifying physician as soon as possible if early symptoms of tardive dyskinesia appear
 Possibility of withdrawal symptoms
 Signs of potential side effects, especially akathisia, ventricular arrhythmias, parkinsonism, mood or behavior changes, swelling or soreness of breasts (less frequent in males), unusual secretion of milk (rare in males), dystonia, menstrual changes, tardive dyskinesia, allergic reaction, blood dyscrasias, obstructive jaundice, NMS, or tardive dystonia

## General Dosing Information

Periodic attempts should be made to reduce the dosage of pimozide gradually to see whether tics persist at the level and extent first identified. In doing so, consideration should be given to the possibility that any increases in tic intensity and frequency may represent a transient withdrawal-related phenomenon rather than a return of disease symptoms. Two to three weeks should elapse before a final conclusion is reached that an increase in tic manifestations is a function of the underlying disease syndrome rather than a response to pimozide withdrawal. Also, spontaneous remission and fluctuating symptoms may occur in many patients, since pimozide's poor absorption and presystemic metabolism profile may result in highly variable absorption from day to day.

When discontinued, pimozide should be withdrawn gradually, over several weeks if possible, to minimize symptoms of withdrawal.

**For treatment of adverse reactions**
Neuroleptic malignant syndrome (NMS)—
 Treatment is essentially symptomatic and supportive and may include the following:
  • *Discontinuing pimozide immediately.*
  • Hyperthermia—Administering antipyretics (aspirin or acetaminophen); using cooling blanket.
  • Dehydration—Restoring fluids and electrolytes.
  • Cardiovascular instability—Monitoring blood pressure and cardiac rhythm closely.
  • Hypoxia—Administering oxygen; consider airway insertion and assisted ventilation.
  • Muscle rigidity—Dantrolene sodium may be administered (100 to 300 mg per day in divided doses; 1.25 to 1.5 mg per kg of body weight [mg/kg], intravenously). Bromocriptine (5 to 7.5 mg every eight hours) has been used to reverse hyperpyrexia and muscle rigidity.

Parkinsonism—
 Many medical authorities advise that the only appropriate treatment of extrapyramidal symptoms is reduction of the antipsychotic dosage, if possible, to the lowest effective dose. Oral antidyskinetic agents, such as trihexyphenidyl (2 mg three times a day) or benztropine, may be effective in treating more severe parkinsonism and acute motor restlessness but are used sparingly, and then usually for no longer than 3 months. Extrapyramidal symptoms may reappear if both pimozide and the antidyskinetic agent are discontinued simultaneously. The antidyskinetic agent may have to be continued after pimozide is discontinued because of the different excretion rates of the medications. Milder effects may be treated by adjusting dosage.

Akathisia—
 Restlessness may be treated with antiparkinsonian medications, or with propranolol (30 to 120 mg a day), nadolol (40 mg a day), pindolol (5 to 60 mg a day), lorazepam (1 or 2 mg two or three times a day), or diazepam (2 mg two or three times a day).

Dystonia—
 Acute dystonic postures or oculogyric crisis may be relieved by parenteral administration of benztropine (2 mg intramuscularly), diphenhydramine (50 mg intramuscularly), or diazepam (5 to 7.5 mg intravenously), to be followed by oral antidyskinetic medication for one or two days to prevent recurrent dystonic episodes. These effects may be controlled by adjustments of pimozide dosage.

Tardive dyskinesia or tardive dystonia—
 There is no known effective treatment. Dosage of pimozide should be lowered or medication discontinued, if clinically feasible, at earliest signs of tardive dyskinesia or tardive dystonia, to prevent irreversible effects.

## Oral Dosage Forms

Note: Bracketed uses in the *Dosage Forms* section refer to categories of use and/or indications that are not included in U.S. product labeling.

### PIMOZIDE TABLETS USP

**Usual adult dose**
Tourette's syndrome[1]—
 Oral, initially, 1 to 2 mg a day in divided doses, the dosage being increased gradually as needed and tolerated.
 Note: Elderly patients usually require a lower initial dosage and a more gradual dosage titration than do younger patients.
[Psychotic disorders]—
 Oral, initially, 2 to 4 mg once a day, preferably in the morning, the dosage being increased as needed and tolerated by 2 to 4 mg a day at weekly intervals.
 Note: The average maintenance dosage is 6 mg a day, with a usual range of 2 to 12 mg a day.
 Elderly patients usually require a lower initial dosage and a more gradual dosage titration than do younger patients.

**Usual adult prescribing limits**
Tourette's syndrome[1]—
 200 mcg (0.2 mg) per kg of body weight a day or 10 mg a day, whichever is less.
[Psychotic disorders]—
 300 mcg (0.3 mg) per kg of body weight a day or 20 mg a day, whichever is less.
Note: Seizures and sudden unexpected deaths have occurred at dosages above 20 mg a day.

## 2330  Pimozide (Systemic)

**Usual pediatric dose**
Tourette's syndrome[1]—
 Children up to 12 years of age: Dosage has not been established.
 Children 12 years of age and over: Oral, initially 50 mcg (0.05 mg) per kg of body weight, preferably as a single dose, the dosage being increased gradually as needed and tolerated.
Note: For children 2 years of age and over, some clinicians use an initial dosage of 1 mg a day, increased by 1 mg a day at intervals of seven to ten days, as needed and tolerated, until a significant decrease in tics is seen.

**Usual pediatric prescribing limits**
200 mcg (0.2 mg) per kg of body weight a day or 10 mg a day, whichever is less.

**Strength(s) usually available**
U.S.—
 2 mg (Rx) [*Orap* (scored; calcium stearate; cellulose; lactose; corn starch)].
Canada—
 1 mg (Rx) [*Orap* (scored)].
 2 mg (Rx) [*Orap* (scored; calcium stearate; lactose; microcrystalline cellulose; corn starch)].
 4 mg (Rx) [*Orap* (scored; calcium stearate; FD&C Blue No. 1; FD&C Yellow No. 5; lactose; microcrystalline cellulose; corn starch; tartrazine)].
 10 mg (Rx) [*Orap* (scored; calcium stearate; FD&C Yellow No. 6; lactose; microcrystalline cellulose; corn starch)].

**Packaging and storage**
Store below 40 °C (104 °F), preferably between 15 and 30 °C (59 and 86 °F), unless otherwise specified by manufacturer. Store in a tight, light-resistant container.

**Auxiliary labeling**
- May cause drowsiness.
- Avoid alcoholic beverages.

[1]Not included in Canadian product labeling.

Revised: 01/26/98

---

**PINDOLOL**—See *Beta-adrenergic Blocking Agents (Systemic)*

---

# PIPECURONIUM Systemic†

VA CLASSIFICATION (Primary): MS300
Commonly used brand name(s): *Arduan*.
Note: For a listing of dosage forms and brand names by country availability, see *Dosage Forms* section(s).

†Not commercially available in Canada.

## Category
Neuromuscular blocking agent.

## Indications

### Accepted
Muscle (skeletal) relaxation, for surgery—Pipecuronium is indicated as an adjunct to anesthesia to induce skeletal muscle relaxation and to facilitate the management of patients undergoing mechanical ventilation. Pipecuronium has a long duration of action and is recommended only for surgical procedures expected to last 90 minutes or longer.

### Unaccepted
Pipecuronium has not been adequately studied, and is not presently recommended, for facilitating prolonged mechanical ventilation in intensive care patients, for administration prior to or following use of other nondepolarizing neuromuscular blocking agents, or for obstetrical use (Cesarean section).

## Pharmacology/Pharmacokinetics
Note: Pharmacokinetic studies on the volume of distribution, distribution and elimination half-lives, and clearance of pipecuronium have been done in a limited number of patients; data presented below must be considered preliminary and subject to interpatient variability.

**Physicochemical characteristics**
Molecular weight—798.74.

**Mechanism of action/Effect**
Pipecuronium is a nondepolarizing neuromuscular blocking agent. Neuromuscular blocking agents produce skeletal muscle paralysis by blocking neural transmission at the myoneural junction. The paralysis is selective initially and usually appears in the following muscles consecutively: levator muscles of eyelids, muscles of mastication, limb muscles, abdominal muscles, muscles of the glottis, and finally, the intercostal muscles and the diaphragm. Neuromuscular blocking agents have no clinically significant effect on consciousness or the pain threshold.
Nondepolarizing neuromuscular blocking agents inhibit neuromuscular transmission by competing with acetylcholine for the cholinergic receptors of the motor end plate, thereby reducing the response of the end plate to acetylcholine. This type of neuromuscular block is usually antagonized by anticholinesterase agents.

**Distribution**
Volume of distribution (steady-state)—
 Normal renal function: 0.25 (range, 0.12–0.37) L per kg of body weight.
 Renal function impairment: 0.37 (range, 0.28–0.51) L per kg of body weight.

**Half-life**
Distribution—
 Normal renal function: 6.22 (range, 1.34–10.66) minutes.
 Renal function impairment: 4.33 (range, 1.69–6.17) minutes.
Elimination—
 Normal renal function: 1.7 (range, 0.9–2.7) hours. The elimination half-life is not altered by hypothermia and bypass.
 Renal function impairment: 4 (range, 2.0–8.2) hours.

**Onset of action**
Intubating conditions are achieved in 2.5 to 3 minutes with doses of 70 to 100 mcg per kg of body weight (mcg/kg). The time to achieve intubating conditions may be somewhat longer when lower doses are administered.

**Time to peak effect**
In adults, maximum (95%) suppression of the twitch response to peripheral nerve stimulation is achieved in about 5.5 to 6 minutes following a dose of 50 mcg/kg and in about 3 to 5 minutes after single doses of 70 to 85 mcg/kg. The peak effect time is not significantly affected by the type of anesthesia administered.

**Duration of action**
Initial dose—
 Adults:
  Long-acting; dependent on dose and on type of anesthesia. With neurolept (nitrous oxide/fentanyl/droperidol) anesthesia, the expected duration of clinical effect (time until the twitch response returns to 25% of the control value as determined using a peripheral nerve stimulator) is about 30 minutes following a dose of 50 mcg/kg. With "balanced" anesthesia (in which a neuromuscular blocking agent may be used together with other medications, such as an induction agent [e.g., an ultrashort-acting barbiturate or propofol], an opioid analgesic, and an inhalation anesthetic [usually nitrous oxide]), doses of 70 to 85 mcg/kg usually provide about 1 to 2 hours of clinical relaxation. Values ranging from 30 to 175 minutes have been reported with 70 mcg/kg and values ranging from 40 to 211 minutes have been reported with 80 to 85 mcg/kg. After the twitch response has recovered to 25% of control, spontaneous recovery to 50% of the control value takes about 24 minutes (range, 8 to 131 minutes) and spontaneous recovery to 75% of the control value takes about 33 minutes.
  When pipecuronium is administered following recovery from succinylcholine-assisted endotracheal intubation, a dose of 50 mcg/kg provides about 45 minutes of clinical relaxation, and a dose of 70 to 85 mcg/kg provides the same clinical duration as without prior administration of succinylcholine.
 Infants and children:
  Intermediate- to long-acting and age-dependent; the expected duration of clinical effect (time until the twitch response returns to 25% of the control value as determined using a peripheral nerve stimulator) provided by an effective dose is about 13 min-

utes in infants < 3 months of age, 10 to 44 minutes in infants 3 months to 1 year of age, and 18 to 52 minutes in children 1 to 14 years of age. After the twitch response has recovered to 25% of control, spontaneous recovery to 75% of the control value takes about 25 to 30 minutes.

Maintenance doses—
  Adults:
    The expected clinical duration of additional doses of 10 to 15 mcg/kg, administered when the twitch response has returned to 25% of the control value, is about 50 (range, 17 to 175) minutes.

Note: The clinical duration of initial and maintenance doses is increased by use of enflurane or isoflurane, and possibly by other potentiating medications, but is not significantly prolonged by halothane.

In patients with renal function impairment, the duration of action is more variable than in patients with normal renal function; accumulation of pipecuronium may lead to a significant prolongation of neuromuscular blockade.

No significant correlation was found between the duration of pipecuronium-induced neuromuscular blockade and the pharmacokinetic variables studied (volume of distribution, distribution and elimination half-lives, and plasma clearance) in a study in patients with normal renal function.

**Elimination**
Renal— In one study in patients undergoing coronary artery bypass surgery who received 200 mcg/kg (double the currently recommended maximum adult dose), 56% of the administered dose was excreted in the urine within 24 hours, 41% of the dose as unchanged pipecuronium and 15% as the active 3-decacetyl metabolite. In animals, this metabolite has about 40 to 50% of the activity of the parent compound.

Clearance—0.12 to 0.15 L per kg of body weight per hour (L/kg/hr) in patients with normal renal function and 0.08 L/kg/hr in patients with renal function impairment.

## Precautions to Consider

### Cross-sensitivity and/or related problems
Patients sensitive to bromides may be sensitive to pipecuronium bromide also.

### Mutagenicity
No evidence of mutagenicity was found in the Ames test or the Sister Chromatid Exchange test.

### Pregnancy/Reproduction
Fertility—Animal studies have not been done.
Pregnancy—Adequate and well-controlled studies have not been done in pregnant women.
Pipecuronium did not cause teratogenicity in rats receiving up to 50 mcg per kg of body weight intravenously. However, the highest dose caused embryotoxicity (increase in early fetal resorptions) secondary to maternal toxicity.
FDA Pregnancy Category C.
Labor and delivery—Pipecuronium is not recommended for use in obstetrics (Cesarean section) because of insufficient information on placental transfer and possible consequent effects on the neonate. Also, pipecuronium's duration of action exceeds the expected duration of Cesarean section.

### Breast-feeding
It is not known whether pipecuronium is distributed into breast milk. However, problems in nursing babies have not been reported.

### Pediatrics
Children 1 to 14 years of age are less sensitive to the effects of pipecuronium than are adults or infants < 1 year of age. The duration of clinical effect (time to recovery of the twitch response to 25% of the control value) is shorter in infants and children than in adults.

### Geriatrics
One study in patients 66 to 79 years of age has shown that response and dosage requirements for pipecuronium are not significantly different in geriatric patients than in younger adults. However, whether the results reported in the relatively few elderly patients studied to date can be applied to the geriatric population in general has not been determined. Also, elderly patients are more likely to have age-related renal function impairment, which requires caution and possibly dosage reduction and/or longer intervals between doses in patients receiving pipecuronium.

### Drug interactions and/or related problems
The following drug interactions and/or related problems have been selected on the basis of their potential clinical significance (possible mechanism in parentheses where appropriate)—not necessarily inclusive (» = major clinical significance):

Note: Combinations containing any of the following medications, depending on the amount present, may also interact with this medication.

Some of the following interactions have not been documented with pipecuronium. However, because they have been reported to occur with other nondepolarizing neuromuscular blocking agents, the possibility of a significant interaction with pipecuronium must be considered.

» Aminoglycosides, possibly including oral neomycin (if significant quantities are absorbed in patients with renal function impairment) or
» Anesthetics, parenteral-local (large doses leading to significant plasma concentrations) or
Bacitracin or
» Capreomycin or
» Citrate-anticoagulated blood (massive transfusions) or
» Clindamycin or
Colistin or
Colistimethate sodium or
Lidocaine (intravenous doses > 5 mg/kg) or
» Lincomycin or
» Polymyxins or
Procaine (intravenous) or
Tetracyclines or
Trimethaphan (large doses)
  (neuromuscular blocking activity of these medications may be additive to that of neuromuscular blocking agents; increased or prolonged respiratory depression or paralysis [apnea] may occur, but is of minor clinical significance while the patient is being mechanically ventilated; however, caution and careful monitoring of the patient are recommended during and following concurrent or sequential use, especially if there is a possibility of incomplete reversal of neuromuscular blockade postoperatively)

Analgesics, opioid (narcotic), especially those commonly used as adjuncts to anesthesia
  (central respiratory depressant effects of opioid analgesics may be additive to the respiratory depressant effects of neuromuscular blocking agents; increased or prolonged respiratory depression or paralysis [apnea] may occur, but is of minor clinical significance while the patient is being mechanically ventilated; however, caution and careful monitoring of the patient are recommended during and following concurrent or sequential use, especially if there is a possibility of incomplete reversal of neuromuscular blockade postoperatively)
  (although specific information for pipecuronium is not available, high doses of sufentanil reduce initial dosage requirements for other nondepolarizing neuromuscular blocking agents; it is recommended that a peripheral nerve stimulator be used to determine dosage)
  (concurrent use of a neuromuscular blocking agent prevents or reverses muscle rigidity induced by sufficiently high doses of most opioid analgesics, especially alfentanil, fentanyl, or sufentanil)
  (pipecuronium has no vagolytic activity and will therefore not decrease the risk of opioid analgesic–induced bradycardia or hypotension; in some patients [especially patients with compromised cardiac function and/or those receiving a beta-adrenergic blocking agent preoperatively], the incidence and/or severity of these effects may be increased)

Anesthetics, hydrocarbon inhalation, such as:
  Chloroform
  Cyclopropane
  Enflurane
  Ether
  Halothane
  Isoflurane
  Methoxyflurane
  Trichloroethylene
  (neuromuscular blocking activity of inhalation hydrocarbon anesthetics, especially enflurane or isoflurane, may be additive to that of nondepolarizing neuromuscular blocking agents; enflurane and isoflurane have been shown to increase pipecuronium's duration of action by about 50% and 12%, respectively, but halothane has not been shown to prolong pipecuronium's effects significantly)

Antimyasthenics or
Edrophonium
  (these agents antagonize the effects of nondepolarizing neuromuscular blocking agents; parenteral neostigmine or pyridostigmine are indicated to reverse neuromuscular blockade following surgery edrophonium in a dose of 0.5 mg per kg of body weight [mg/kg] is not recommended for reversal of pipecuronium because it has

## Pipecuronium (Systemic)

been reported to be less effective than neostigmine [dose of 40 mcg (0.04 mg)/kg]; use of higher doses of edrophonium or of pyridostigmine for reversal of pipecuronium has not been studied)

(neuromuscular blocking agents may antagonize the effects of antimyasthenics on skeletal muscle; temporary dosage adjustment may be required to control symptoms of myasthenia gravis following surgery)

Calcium salts
 (calcium salts may reverse the effects of nondepolarizing neuromuscular blocking agents)

Doxapram
 (the residual effects of neuromuscular blocking agents may be masked temporarily by doxapram when it is used post-anesthesia)

Magnesium salts, parenteral or
» Procainamide or
» Quinidine
 (these medications may enhance the blockade of the neuromuscular blocking agents; increased or prolonged respiratory depression or paralysis [apnea] may occur but is of minor clinical significance while the patient is being mechanically ventilated; however, caution and careful monitoring of the patient are recommended during and following concurrent or sequential use, especially if there is a possibility of incomplete reversal of neuromuscular blockade postoperatively)

Neuromuscular blocking agents, other
 (pipecuronium may be administered following recovery from succinylcholine when the latter has been administered to facilitate endotracheal intubation; administration of pipecuronium prior to succinylcholine, to prevent or attenuate succinylcholine-induced side effects, has not been studied)
 (administration of pipecuronium in conjunction with other nondepolarizing neuromuscular blocking agents has not been studied)

Potassium-depleting medications, such as:
 Adrenocorticoids, glucocorticoid, especially with significant mineralocorticoid activity
 Adrenocorticoids, mineralocorticoid
 Amphotericin B
 Bumetanide
 Carbonic anhydrase inhibitors
 Corticotropin, chronic therapeutic use of
 Ethacrynic acid
 Furosemide
 Indapamide
 Thiazide diuretics
 (serum potassium determinations and correction of serum potassium concentration may be necessary prior to administration of pipecuronium because hypokalemia induced by these medications may enhance the blockade of nondepolarizing neuromuscular blocking agents; increased or prolonged respiratory depression or paralysis [apnea] may occur but is of minor clinical significance while the patient is being mechanically ventilated; however, caution and careful monitoring of the patient are recommended during and following concurrent or sequential use, especially if there is a possibility of incomplete reversal of neuromuscular blockade postoperatively)

**Laboratory value alterations**
The following have been selected on the basis of their potential clinical significance (possible effect in parentheses where appropriate)—not necessarily inclusive (» = major clinical significance):

With physiology/laboratory test values
 Creatinine concentration and
 Potassium concentration
  (may be increased—incidence of each < 1%)
 Glucose concentration, in blood
  (may be increased—incidence < 1%)

**Medical considerations/Contraindications**
The medical considerations/contraindications included have been selected on the basis of their potential clinical significance (reasons given in parentheses where appropriate)—not necessarily inclusive (» = major clinical significance).

*Risk-benefit should be considered when the following medical problems exist:*

Biliary obstruction or
Hepatic function impairment
 (time to onset and maximum effect, pharmacokinetics, and dosage requirements of pipecuronium have not been studied in patients with moderate or severe hepatic function impairment or biliary obstruction)

Carcinoma, bronchogenic
 (duration of action of neuromuscular blocking agents may be prolonged)

Cardiovascular disease leading to slower circulation time or
Edema or
Other conditions associated with increased distribution volume
 (time to onset of action and maximum effect of pipecuronium may be prolonged; a delay in readiness for intubation or surgery should be anticipated and allowed; administration of higher doses of pipecuronium to compensate for a delayed response is not recommended)

Dehydration or
Electrolyte or acid-base imbalance
 (action of neuromuscular blocking agents may be altered; neuromuscular blockade is usually counteracted by alkalosis and enhanced by acidosis, but mixed imbalances may be present, leading to unpredictable responses)

Hypothermia
 (intensity and duration of action of nondepolarizing neuromuscular blocking agents may be increased)

Myasthenia gravis or
Myasthenic syndrome (Eaton-Lambert syndrome)
 (risk of severe and prolonged muscle paralysis or weakness; a neuromuscular blocking agent with a shorter duration of action may be preferable [although caution is required even with shorter-acting agents])

Pulmonary function impairment or
Respiratory depression
 (risk of additive respiratory depression or impairment)

Renal function impairment, mild or moderate or
» Renal function impairment, severe
 (duration of action of pipecuronium may be prolonged or unpredictable; a reduction in dosage may be necessary, but use of a neuromuscular blocking agent with a more predictable duration of action in patients with renal function impairment [e.g., atracurium or vecuronium] may be preferable)

Sensitivity to pipecuronium or to bromides

## Side/Adverse Effects

Note: Unlike gallamine and pancuronium, pipecuronium has no vagolytic activity. Also, unlike several other neuromuscular blocking agents [especially tubocurarine, and, to a somewhat lesser extent, atracurium, metocurine, or succinylcholine], pipecuronium has not been reported to cause histamine release. It therefore causes minimal hemodynamic disturbance, although bradycardia and/or hypotension may occur because pipecuronium does not counteract the bradycardia and/or hypotension induced by other medications (e.g., anesthetics, opioid analgesics) or vagal stimulation.

The following side/adverse effects have been selected on the basis of their potential clinical significance (possible signs and symptoms in parentheses where appropriate)—not necessarily inclusive:

**Those indicating need for medical attention**
Incidence less frequent (1% or higher)
 *Bradycardia, clinically significant*—incidence 1.4%; *hypotension, clinically significant*—incidence 2.5%

Incidence rare (< 1%)
 *Anuria; atelectasis; atrial fibrillation; cerebrovascular accident; CNS depression; dyspnea; hypertension; hypesthesia; laryngismus; muscle atrophy; myocardial ischemia; respiratory depression; skin rash; thrombosis; urticaria; ventricular extrasystole*

## Overdose

For specific information on the agents used in the management of pipecuronium overdose, see:
• *Atropine (Systemic)* in *Anticholinergics/Antispasmodics (Systemic)* monograph; and/or
• *Neostigmine* in *Antimyasthenics (Systemic)* monograph.

For more information on the management of overdose, **contact a Poison Control Center** (see *Poison Control Center Listing*).

**Treatment of overdose**
Specific treatment—
 Administering anticholinesterase agents, such as neostigmine, to antagonize the action of pipecuronium. Edrophonium (0.5 mg/kg) does not sufficiently antagonize the effects of the medication, i.e., it does not increase the twitch response to peripheral nerve stimulation to 70% of the control value or higher, especially when potent hydrocarbon inhalation anesthetics (enflurane or isoflurane) have been

administered. Use of higher doses of edrophonium or of pyridostigmine for antagonism of pipecuronium has not been studied. It is recommended that atropine or another suitable anticholinergic agent be administered prior to or concurrently with the antagonist to counteract its muscarinic side effects. However, use of an antagonist is merely an adjunct to, and not to be substituted for, the institution of measures to ensure adequate ventilation. Ventilatory assistance must be continued until the patient can maintain an adequate ventilatory exchange unassisted.

Monitoring—
Determining the nature and degree of the neuromuscular blockade, using a peripheral nerve stimulator.
Monitoring of vital organ function for the period of paralysis and for an extended period post-recovery.
Monitoring the patient following successful antagonism, because the duration of action of pipecuronium may exceed that of the antagonist.

Supportive care for apnea or prolonged paralysis—
Maintaining an adequate airway and assisting or controlling ventilation. Artificial respiration should be continued until adequate spontaneous ventilation can be maintained.

## General Dosing Information

Neuromuscular blocking agents have no clinically significant effect on consciousness or the pain threshold; therefore, when used as an adjunct to surgery, the neuromuscular blocking agent should always be used with adequate anesthesia.

Since neuromuscular blocking agents may cause respiratory depression, they should be used only by those individuals experienced in the techniques of tracheal intubation, artificial respiration, and the administration of oxygen under positive pressure; facilities for these procedures should be immediately available.

Pipecuronium is intended for intravenous administration only.

The stated doses are intended as a guideline. Actual dosage must be individualized. It is recommended that a peripheral nerve stimulator be used to monitor response, need for additional doses, and reversal.

The $ED_{95}$ (dose of pipecuronium that will produce a 95% suppression of the twitch response to peripheral nerve stimulation) during balanced anesthesia in adults (geriatric patients as well as younger adults) may range from 21 to 77 (average, 41) mcg per kg of body weight. In infants < 1 year of age, the $ED_{95}$ is within the same range as for adults (generally about 33 to 48 mcg/kg). In children 1 to 14 years of age, the $ED_{95}$ may range from 47 to 80 mcg/kg. In patients of all ages, the $ED_{95}$ is significantly reduced with enflurane or isoflurane, but not halothane, anesthesia (as compared with balanced or neurolept anesthesia).

For obese patients (> 30% above ideal body weight for height), dosage of pipecuronium should be calculated on the basis of ideal body weight. Administration of pipecuronium to obese patients in doses based on actual body weight significantly prolongs the medication's effects.

When nondepolarizing neuromuscular blocking agents are administered concurrently with potent general anesthetics such as enflurane, ether, isoflurane, methoxyflurane, or cyclopropane, a reduction in dosage, as determined using a peripheral nerve stimulator, may be required. However, halothane has not been shown to potentiate significantly the effect of pipecuronium.

It is recommended that reversal of pipecuronium-induced neuromuscular blockade with an antagonist (e.g., neostigmine) be attempted only after some spontaneous recovery, as demonstrated using a peripheral nerve stimulator, has first taken place. Recovery will not occur as rapidly if the antagonist is administered earlier.

## Parenteral Dosage Forms

### PIPECURONIUM BROMIDE FOR INJECTION

**Usual adult dose**
Initial:
For intubation: Intravenous, 70 to 85 mcg (0.07 to 0.085 mg) per kg of actual body weight (normal weight patients) or ideal body weight (obese patients). The lowest dose recommended to provide adequate intubation conditions is 50 mcg per kg of body weight, but the onset of action may be delayed with this dose.
For administration following recovery from succinylcholine-facilitated endotracheal intubation: Intravenous, 50 mcg (0.05 mg) per kg of actual body weight (normal weight patients) or ideal body weight (obese patients) to provide about 45 minutes of relaxation, or 70 to 85 mcg (0.07 to 0.085 mg) per kg of body weight to provide about 1 to 2 hours of muscle paralysis.
Maintenance:
Intravenous, after recovery of the twitch response to peripheral nerve stimulation to 25% of control, 10 to 15 mcg (0.01 to 0.015 mg) per kg of body weight. Lower doses may be sufficient for patients receiving inhalation anesthesia.

Note: For patients with renal function impairment, dosage should be based on creatinine clearance as well as body weight. The following initial doses are recommended:

| Creatinine Clearance (mL/min) | Dose (mcg/kg ideal body weight) |
|---|---|
| <40 | 50 |
| 60 | 55 |
| 80 | 70 |
| 100 | 85 |
| >100 | Up to 100 |

**Usual adult prescribing limits**
Intravenous, 100 mcg (0.1 mg) per kg of actual body weight (normal weight patients) or ideal body weight (obese patients).

**Usual pediatric and adolescent dose**
Initial—
Infants up to 3 months of age: Dosage has not been established.
Infants 3 to 12 months of age: Intravenous, 40 mcg (0.04 mg) per kg of body weight (provides about 10 to 44 minutes of clinical relaxation).
Children 1 to 14 years of age: Intravenous, 57 mcg (0.057 mg) per kg of body weight (provides 18 to 52 minutes of clinical relaxation).
Adolescents over 14 years of age: See *Usual adult dose*.
Maintenance—
Dosage has not been established.

**Usual geriatric dose**
See *Usual adult dose*.

**Size(s) usually available**
U.S.—
10 mg (Rx) [*Arduan* (mannitol 380 mg)].
Canada—
Not commercially available.

**Packaging and storage**
Before reconstitution—
Store between 2 and 30 °C (36 and 86 °F), protected from light, unless otherwise specified by manufacturer.
After reconstitution—
Bacteriostatic water for injection as diluent: Store at room temperature (15 to 30 °C [59 to 86 °F]) or in a refrigerator (2 to 8 °C [36 to 46 °F]).
Other injections as diluent: Store in a refrigerator.

**Preparation of dosage form**
Pipecuronium bromide for injection may be reconstituted with 0.9% sodium chloride injection, 5% dextrose in sodium chloride injection, 5% dextrose in water injection, lactated Ringer's injection, sterile water for injection, or bacteriostatic water for injection. Reconstitution using 10 mL of diluent provides a solution containing 10 mg per mL of pipecuronium bromide.
Caution: Use of diluents containing benzyl alcohol (e.g., bacteriostatic water for injection) is not recommended for preparation of medications for use in neonates. A fatal toxic syndrome consisting of metabolic acidosis, CNS depression, respiratory problems, renal failure, hypotension, and possibly seizures and intracranial hemorrhages has been associated with this use.

**Stability**
The vial of pipecuronium bromide is intended for single-dose use only; unused portions of the reconstituted solution should be discarded.
After reconstitution with bacteriostatic water for injection, pipecuronium should be administered within 5 days.
After reconstitution with injections other than bacteriostatic water for injection, pipecuronium should be administered within 24 hours.

## Selected Bibliography

Larijani GE, Bartkowski RR, Azad SS et al. Clinical pharmacology of pipecuronium bromide. Anesth Analg 1989; 68: 734-9.
Foldes FF, Nagashima H, Nguyen HD, Duncalf D, Goldiner PL. Neuromuscular and cardiovascular effects of pipecuronium. Can J Anaesth 1990 Jul; 37: 549-55.
Pittet JF, Tassonyi E, Morel DR et al. Pipecuronium-induced neuromuscular blockade during nitrous oxide–fentanyl, isoflurane, and halothane anesthesia in adults and children. Anesthesiology 1989 71; 210-3.

Revised: 08/13/91

**PIPERACILLIN**—See *Penicillins (Systemic)*

**PIPERAZINE**—The *Piperazine (Systemic)* monograph is not included in this published version of the USP DI database. Copies of the monograph are available on request from Micromedex, Inc. - Reprint Requests, 6200 S. Syracuse Way, Suite 300, Englewood, CO 80111; telephone (303) 486-6400; telefax (303) 486-6464; Email: USPDI@MDX.COM.

**PIPOTIAZINE**—See *Phenothiazines (Systemic)*

**PIRBUTEROL**—See *Bronchodilators, Adrenergic (Inhalation-Local)*

**PIRENZEPINE**—See *Anticholinergics/Antispasmodics (Systemic)*

**PIROXICAM**—See *Anti-inflammatory Drugs, Nonsteroidal (Systemic)*

**PIVAMPICILLIN**—See *Penicillins (Systemic)*

**PIVMECILLINAM**—See *Penicillins (Systemic)*

**PLAGUE VACCINE**—The *Plague Vaccine (Systemic)* monograph is not included in this published version of the USP DI database. Copies of the monograph are available on request from Micromedex, Inc. - Reprint Requests, 6200 S. Syracuse Way, Suite 300, Englewood, CO 80111; telephone (303) 486-6400; telefax (303) 486-6464; Email: USPDI@MDX.COM.

# PLICAMYCIN   Systemic†

VA CLASSIFICATION (Primary/Secondary): AN200/HS305
Commonly used brand name(s): *Mithracin*.
Another commonly used name in the U.S. is mithramycin.
Note:   For a listing of dosage forms and brand names by country availability, see *Dosage Forms* section(s).

†Not commercially available in Canada.

## Category
Antineoplastic; antihypercalcemic; antihypercalciuric; bone resorption inhibitor.

## Indications
Note:   Bracketed information in the *Indications* section refers to uses that are not included in U.S. product labeling.

**Accepted**
Carcinoma, testicular (treatment)—Plicamycin is indicated for treatment of testicular carcinoma, although use has been replaced by that of more effective agents.
Hypercalcemia, associated with neoplasms (treatment) and
Hypercalciuria, associated with neoplasms (treatment)—Plicamycin is indicated in the treatment of hypercalcemia and hypercalciuria associated with neoplasms, although use has generally been replaced by other agents. Some clinicians have found that a single dose of plicamycin is effective and eliminates the possibility of toxicity.
[Paget's disease of bone (treatment)]—Plicamycin is used in the treatment of Paget's disease; however, its use should be reserved for those patients refractory to other agents.

## Pharmacology/Pharmacokinetics

**Physicochemical characteristics**
Molecular weight—1085.16.

**Mechanism of action/Effect**
Antineoplastic—The exact mechanism of action is unknown. However, it has been shown that plicamycin forms a complex with DNA in the presence of magnesium or other divalent cations, thereby inhibiting DNA-dependent or DNA-directed RNA synthesis.
Antihypercalcemic or
Paget's disease—Plicamycin is believed to lower serum calcium concentrations, but the exact mechanism is unknown. It may act by blocking hypercalcemic action of vitamin D or by inhibiting the effect of parathyroid hormone on osteoclasts. Plicamycin's inhibition of DNA-dependent RNA synthesis appears to render osteoclasts unable to fully respond to parathyroid hormone with the biosynthesis necessary for osteolysis.

**Distribution**
Plicamycin is concentrated in the Kupffer cells of the liver, in renal tubular cells, and along formed bone surfaces. It may localize in areas of active bone resorption. Plicamycin also crosses the blood-brain barrier and enters the cerebrospinal fluid (CSF).

**Onset of action**
When used for hypercalcemia, a reduction in plasma calcium usually occurs within 24 to 48 hours following administration.

**Time to peak effect**
72 hours with a single dose.

**Duration of action**
7 to 10 days with a single dose.

**Elimination**
Renal.

## Precautions to Consider
Note:   Although lower doses are used in the treatment of hypercalcemia than in antitumor treatment, the same precautions and contraindications apply.

**Pregnancy/Reproduction**
Fertility—Studies in male rats receiving doses of 0.6 mg and above per kg of body weight per day showed histologic evidence of inhibition of spermatogenesis.
Pregnancy—Plicamycin is not recommended for use during pregnancy. Although studies have not been done and problems have not been documented in humans, risk-benefit must be considered since the use of plicamycin during pregnancy may be toxic to the fetus.
FDA Pregnancy Category X.

**Breast-feeding**
It is not known whether plicamycin is excreted in breast milk.

**Pediatrics**
No information is available on the relationship of age to the effects of plicamycin in pediatric patients.

**Geriatrics**
No information is available on the relationship of age to the effects of plicamycin in geriatric patients.

**Dental**
The leukopenic and thrombocytopenic effects of plicamycin may result in an increased incidence of microbial infection, delayed healing, and gingival bleeding. Dental work, whenever possible, should be completed prior to initiation of therapy or deferred until blood counts have returned to normal. Patients should be instructed in proper oral hygiene during treatment, including caution in use of regular toothbrushes, dental floss, and toothpicks. Plicamycin may also cause stomatitis associated with considerable discomfort.

### Drug interactions and/or related problems
The following drug interactions and/or related problems have been selected on the basis of their potential clinical significance (possible mechanism in parentheses where appropriate)—not necessarily inclusive (» = major clinical significance):

Note: Combinations containing any of the following medications, depending on the amount present, may also interact with this medication.

In addition to the interactions listed below, the possibility should be considered that additive or multiple effects leading to impaired blood clotting and/or increased risk of bleeding may occur if plicamycin is used concurrently with any other medication having a significant potential for inhibiting platelet aggregation or causing hypoprothrombinemia, thrombocytopenia, or gastrointestinal ulceration or hemorrhage.

» Anticoagulants, coumarin- or indandione-derivative or
» Heparin or
» Thrombolytic agents
(plicamycin-induced hypoprothrombinemia may increase the activity of coumarin- and indandione-derivative anticoagulants and may increase the risk of bleeding in patients receiving heparin or thrombolytic agents; concurrent use is not recommended)

(also, inhibition of platelet aggregation may increase the risk of hemorrhage in patients receiving anticoagulant or thrombolytic therapy)

» Anti-inflammatory drugs, nonsteroidal (NSAIDs) or
» Aspirin or
» Dextran or
» Dipyridamole or
» Sulfinpyrazone or
» Valproic acid
(concurrent use with plicamycin may increase the risk of hemorrhage because of additive or multiple actions, which may decrease the blood-clotting ability, i.e., inhibition of platelet aggregation, by these medications and/or plicamycin combined with induction of hypoprothrombinemia by plicamycin and large doses of aspirin; in addition, the gastrointestinal ulcerative or hemorrhagic potential of aspirin, the NSAIDs, or sulfinpyrazone may increase the risk of hemorrhage in plicamycin-treated patients)

» Bone marrow depressants, other (See *Appendix II*) or
» Hepatotoxic medications (See *Appendix II*) or
» Nephrotoxic medications (See *Appendix II*)
(concurrent use with plicamycin may increase the potential for toxicity)

» Calcium-containing preparations or
» Vitamin D, including calcifediol and calcitriol
(concurrent use may antagonize the effect of plicamycin when used as a calcium antagonist)

» Vaccines, live virus
(because normal defense mechanisms are suppressed by plicamycin therapy, the replication of the vaccine virus may be potentiated, the side/adverse effects of the vaccine virus may be increased, and/or the patient's response to the vaccine may be decreased; immunization of these patients should be undertaken only with extreme caution after careful review of the patient's hematologic status and only with the knowledge and consent of the physician managing the plicamycin therapy; immunization is also contraindicated in persons in close contact with the patient, especially family members)

### Medical considerations/Contraindications
The medical considerations/contraindications included have been selected on the basis of their potential clinical significance (reasons given in parentheses where appropriate)—not necessarily inclusive (» = major clinical significance):

***Except under special circumstances, this medication should not be used when the following medical problems exist:***

» Blood dyscrasias, including thrombocytopathy and thrombocytopenia
(condition may be exacerbated)
» Chickenpox, existing or recent, including recent exposure or
» Herpes zoster
(risk of severe generalized disease)
» Coagulation disorders or increased susceptibility to bleeding due to other causes, including ingestion of aspirin or other potent platelet-aggregation inhibitors within the week prior to plicamycin therapy
(increased risk of hemorrhage)

*Risk-benefit should be considered when the following medical problems exist:*

Electrolyte imbalance, especially hypocalcemia, hypokalemia, or hypophosphatemia or
» Hepatic function impairment, severe or
» Renal function impairment, severe
(condition may be exacerbated)
Sensitivity to plicamycin
» Caution should be used also in patients who have had previous cytotoxic drug therapy and radiation therapy, and in cases of general debility.

### Patient monitoring
The following may be especially important in patient monitoring (other tests may be warranted in some patients, depending on condition; » = major clinical significance):

Bleeding time determinations and
Complete blood count and differential and
Platelet count determinations and
Prothrombin time determinations
(recommended before therapy and then at intervals during therapy that depend on frequency of dose and patient status; a significant increase in prothrombin or bleeding times, which may be early signs of impending hemorrhage, or a significant decrease in the platelet count are indications for discontinuing the medication)

Calcium concentrations, serum and
Phosphorus concentrations, serum and
Potassium concentrations, serum
(any electrolyte imbalance should be corrected before initiation of therapy and at intervals during therapy with plicamycin depending on frequency of dose and patient status)

Hepatic function determinations and
Renal function determinations
(recommended before therapy and then at intervals during therapy that depend on frequency of dose and patient status)

## Side/Adverse Effects

The following side/adverse effects have been selected on the basis of their potential clinical significance (possible signs and symptoms in parentheses where appropriate)—not necessarily inclusive:

### Those indicating need for medical attention
Incidence less frequent
*Hypocalcemia* (muscle and abdominal cramps)

### Those indicating need for medical attention only if they continue or are bothersome
Incidence more frequent
*Anorexia* (loss of appetite); *diarrhea; irritation or soreness of mouth; nausea or vomiting*—may occur 1 to 2 hours after initiation of therapy and continue for 12 to 24 hours

Note: Incidence and severity of *gastrointestinal side effects* may increase with too rapid a rate of administration.

Incidence less frequent
*Drowsiness; fever; headache; mental depression; pain, redness, soreness, or swelling at injection site; unusual tiredness or weakness*

### Those indicating possible hematologic abnormalities and the need for medical attention if they occur after medication is discontinued
*Bloody or black, tarry stools; nosebleed; sore throat and fever; unusual bleeding or bruising; vomiting of blood*

## Overdose

For information on the management of overdose, **contact a Poison Control Center** (see *Poison Control Center Listing*).

### Clinical effects of overdose
The following effects have been selected on the basis of their potential clinical significance (possible signs and symptoms in parentheses where appropriate)—not necessarily inclusive:

*Gastrointestinal bleeding* (bloody or black, tarry stools; vomiting of blood); *hepatotoxicity* (yellow eyes or skin); *nosebleed or other bleeding; leukopenia* (sore throat and fever)—incidence about 6%; *petechial bleeding* (small red spots on skin); *thrombocytopenia* (unusual bleeding or bruising); *toxic epidermal necrolysis* (flushing or redness or swelling of face; skin rash)—possible early symptoms

Note: *Hemorrhagic diathesis*—Incidence more frequent with doses of more than 30 mcg (0.03 mg) per kg of body weight a day and/or for more than 10 doses.

## Patient Consultation

As an aid to patient consultation, refer to *Advice for the Patient, Plicamycin (Systemic)*.

In providing consultation, consider emphasizing the following selected information (» = major clinical significance):

**Before receiving this medication**
» Conditions affecting use, especially:
    Sensitivity to plicamycin
    Pregnancy—Use not recommended during pregnancy; possible toxicity to the fetus
    Dental—Blood dyscrasias may result in increased incidence of gingival bleeding, delayed healing, and microbial infection
    Other medications, especially anticoagulants, aspirin, bone marrow depressants, calcium- or vitamin D–containing preparations, dextran, dipyridamole, hepatotoxic medications, nephrotoxic medications, nonsteroidal anti-inflammatory drugs, sulfinpyrazone, thrombolytics, or valproic acid
    Other medical problems, especially blood disorders, chickenpox, herpes zoster, severe hepatic function impairment, or severe renal function impairment

**Proper use of this medication**
    Frequency of nausea and vomiting; importance of continuing treatment
» Proper dosing

**Precautions after receiving this medication**
    Importance of close monitoring by the physician
» Avoiding salicylate-containing products, which may increase risk of hemorrhage
    Possible need to avoid calcium- and vitamin D–containing products
» Avoiding immunizations unless approved by physician; other persons in patient's household should avoid immunizations with oral poliovirus vaccine; avoiding other persons who have taken oral poliovirus vaccine or wearing a protective mask that covers nose and mouth
    Caution if bone marrow depression occurs:
» Avoiding exposure to persons with bacterial infections, especially during periods of low blood counts; checking with physician immediately if fever or chills, cough or hoarseness, lower back or side pain, or painful or difficult urination occurs
» Checking with physician immediately if unusual bleeding or bruising; black, tarry stools; blood in urine or stools; or pinpoint red spots on skin occur
    Caution in use of regular toothbrush, dental floss, or toothpick; physician, dentist, or nurse may suggest alternatives; checking with physician before having dental work done
    Not touching eyes or inside of nose unless hands washed immediately before
    Using caution to avoid accidental cuts with use of sharp objects such as safety razor or fingernail or toenail cutters
    Avoiding contact sports or other situations where bruising or injury could occur

## General Dosing Information

It is recommended that plicamycin be administered by intravenous infusion only to hospitalized patients by or under the supervision of a physician experienced in the use of cancer chemotherapeutic agents because of the possibility of severe reactions.

Before plicamycin therapy is initiated, dehydration or volume depletion should be corrected.

Rapid direct intravenous injection of plicamycin should be avoided since it may be associated with a higher incidence and greater severity of gastrointestinal side effects.

Special precautions are recommended in patients who develop thrombocytopenia as a result of administration of plicamycin. These may include extreme care in performing invasive procedures; regular inspection of intravenous sites, skin (including perirectal area), and mucous membrane surfaces for signs of bleeding or bruising; limiting frequency of venipuncture and avoiding intramuscular injections; testing urine, emesis, stool and secretions for occult blood; care in use of regular toothbrushes, dental floss, toothpicks, safety razors, and fingernail and toenail cutters; avoiding constipation; and using caution to prevent falls and other injuries. Such patients should avoid alcohol and any aspirin intake because of the risk of gastrointestinal bleeding. Platelet transfusions may be required.

Patients who develop leukopenia should be observed carefully for signs of infection. Antibiotic support may be required. In neutropenic patients who develop fever, broad-spectrum antibiotic coverage should be initiated empirically, pending bacterial cultures and appropriate diagnostic tests.

**Safety considerations for handling this medication**

There is limited but increasing evidence and concern that personnel involved in preparation and administration of parenteral antineoplastics may be at some risk because of the potential mutagenicity, teratogenicity, and/or carcinogenicity of these agents, although the actual risk is unknown. USP advisory panels recommend cautious handling both in preparation and disposal of antineoplastic agents. Precautions that have been suggested include:

- Use of a biological containment cabinet during reconstitution and dilution of parenteral medications and wearing of disposable surgical gloves and masks.
- Use of proper technique to prevent contamination of the medication, work area, and operator during transfer between containers (including proper training of personnel in this technique).
- Cautious and proper disposal of needles, syringes, vials, ampuls, and unused medication.

A number of medical centers have developed detailed guidelines for handling of antineoplastic agents.

**For treatment of adverse effects**

Nausea and vomiting—The use of antiemetics prior to and during treatment with plicamycin may help relieve nausea and vomiting, which may begin 1 to 2 hours after initiation of therapy and persist for 12 to 24 hours.

Extravasation—If local irritation or cellulitis occurs at the injection site, immediate application of a cold pack to the site may prevent pain and swelling. If swelling develops, application of moderate heat may help disperse the medication and reduce the discomfort. If cellulitis occurs, the infusion should be discontinued and then reinstituted at another site.

## Parenteral Dosage Forms

### PLICAMYCIN FOR INJECTION USP

**Usual adult dose**
Antineoplastic—
    Intravenous infusion, 25 to 30 mcg (0.025 to 0.03 mg) per kg of body weight a day, administered over a period of four to six hours, for eight to ten days unless significant side effects or toxicity symptoms occur; or 25 to 50 mcg (0.025 to 0.05 mg) per kg of body weight once a day every other day for up to eight doses or until toxicity requires discontinuation of medication. Additional courses of therapy may be administered at one-month intervals.

Note: The same dose may be given by intravenous push over 20 to 30 minutes to reduce the risk of extravasation.

Doses of more than 30 mcg (0.03 mg) per kg of body weight a day and/or a duration of therapy longer than ten days increases the potential of a hemorrhagic diathesis.

The alternate-day dosage schedule has been shown to decrease the toxicity potential.

Delayed toxicity may occur for as long as seventy-two hours after medication has been discontinued following daily administration, but does not occur when the alternate-day dosage schedule is used.

Antihypercalcemic and
Antihypercalcuric—
    Intravenous infusion, initially 15 to 25 mcg (0.015 to 0.025 mg) per kg of body weight a day, to be administered over a period of four to six hours, for three to four days, the dose to be repeated at one-week or more intervals, if necessary, until the desired response is obtained.

Note: The same dose may be given by intravenous push over 20 to 30 minutes to reduce the risk of extravasation.

Alternatively, normal calcium balance may be maintained by administering one to three doses a week, depending upon the patient's response. Some clinicians recommend a single dose of plicamycin with one repeat dose at 48 hours if normalization of calcium levels has not been achieved.

**Usual pediatric dose**
Dosage has not been established.

**Strength(s) usually available**
U.S.—
    2500 mcg (2.5 mg) (Rx) [*Mithracin*].
Canada—
    Not commercially available.

**Packaging and storage**
Prior to reconstitution, store between 2 and 8 °C (36 and 46 °F). Store in a light-resistant container.

### Preparation of dosage form

To prepare initial dilution of 500 mcg (0.5 mg) of plicamycin per mL, add 4.9 mL of sterile water for injection to the 2500-mcg vial and shake to dissolve. After the appropriate dose has been withdrawn from the vial, discard the unused portion.

For intravenous infusion, the daily dose should be further diluted in 1000 mL of 5% dextrose injection or 0.9% sodium chloride injection and administered by infusion over a period of 4 to 6 hours.

### Stability

Reconstituted solution (500 mcg per mL) should be freshly prepared for each dose and used immediately. Infusion solution is stable for 4 to 6 hours at room temperature. Discard any unused portion of either solution.

Revised: 08/05/97

# PNEUMOCOCCAL VACCINE POLYVALENT  Systemic

VA CLASSIFICATION (Primary): IM100

Note: This monograph refers to the 23-valent vaccine licensed in the U.S. in 1983. This vaccine replaces the 14-valent vaccine licensed in the U.S. in 1977.

Commonly used brand name(s): *Pneumovax 23*; *Pnu-Imune 23*.

Note: For a listing of dosage forms and brand names by country availability, see *Dosage Forms* section(s).

## Category

Immunizing agent (active).

## Indications

### Accepted

Pneumococcal disease (prophylaxis)—Pneumococcal vaccine polyvalent is a vaccine consisting of purified bacterial capsular polysaccharides and containing no viable components. It is indicated for immunization against pneumococcal disease caused by any of the 23 pneumococcal types included in the vaccine. These 23 types are responsible for approximately 90% of serious pneumococcal disease. The main objective of pneumococcal immunization is to prevent the severe effects, such as pneumonia, meningitis, bacteremia, and death, that may occur from a pneumococcal infection.

Pneumococcal vaccine polyvalent is recommended for adults and children 2 years of age or older, who are considered to be at increased risk of pneumococcal infection or its complications, particularly:

- Older adults, especially those 50 years of age and older.
- Adults of any age with chronic illnesses, such as cardiovascular disease, pulmonary disease, Hodgkin's disease, multiple myeloma, cirrhosis, alcoholism, renal failure, cerebrospinal fluid leaks, and conditions associated with immunosuppression.
- Adults and children 2 years of age and older with asymptomatic or symptomatic human immunodeficiency virus (HIV) infection.
- Children 2 years of age or older with chronic illnesses, such as nephrotic syndrome, cerebrospinal fluid leaks, and conditions associated with immunosuppression.
- Persons without a spleen or with splenic dysfunction because of sickle cell disease or other causes. Persons scheduled for elective splenectomy should have the vaccine administered at least 2 weeks prior to surgery to receive the full immunizing effect of the vaccine.
- Persons who are to undergo therapy with medications that cause immunosuppression, including candidates for organ transplants and persons with Hodgkin's disease. When possible, the vaccine should be administered at least 10 days, preferably more than 14 days, prior to the immunosuppression-causing medication to achieve the full immunizing effect of the vaccine. Patients with Hodgkin's disease should not receive the vaccine less than 10 days prior to, or during, immunosuppressive therapy, since some patients so immunized have exhibited post-immunization antibody levels below their preimmunization levels. Since response to vaccination is inadequate for the first 6 months following an organ transplant, if the vaccine is not administered before the organ transplant, administration of the vaccine should wait until 6 months following the transplant to elicit a better antibody response. If the vaccine is not administered to persons with Hodgkin's disease before treatment starts, it should be administered 3 months after treatment ends. However, patients with Hodgkin's disease who have received extensive chemotherapy and/or nodal irradiation should not receive the vaccine at all, since immunization of some intensively treated patients has caused depression of pre-existing levels of antibody to some pneumococcal types.
- Persons in residence institutions, such as orphanages and nursing homes.
- Persons at increased risk of pneumococcal infection who will be traveling outside the U.S., since pneumococcal pneumonia is very common in many developing countries and good medical care may not always be readily available.
- Bedridden persons, since persons with limited mobility tend to pool pulmonary secretions and, therefore, are at increased risk for pulmonary infection.
- Selected persons who have been discharged from a hospital within the past 5 years. Studies have shown that approximately two-thirds of all patients with pneumococcal bacteremia have been discharged from a hospital within the past 5 years. Previous hospital care appears to be a dynamic expression of the impact of age and/or medical condition on a person's risk status.

In general, repeat doses of pneumococcal vaccine are not recommended. Increased frequency and severity of side/adverse effects, including Arthus and systemic reactions, are thought to be caused by pre-existing high antibody levels in persons who have previously received a pneumococcal vaccine of any valence. However, when there is doubt or no information on whether an individual at high risk has previously received a pneumococcal vaccine, the vaccine should be administered. In addition, repeat doses of pneumococcal vaccine may be desirable in patients at high risk of severe illness or death from pneumococcal disease, such as children without a spleen or with sickle cell disease, or persons with chronic renal failure whose antibody levels are likely to decline more rapidly than normally, despite the risk of increased side/adverse effects. The optimum interval between revaccinations is not known. However, for adults at highest risk, reimmunization should be considered 6 or more years after the initial dose. For children with nephrotic syndrome, asplenia, or sickle cell anemia, reimmunization should be considered 3 to 5 years after the initial dose, as long as the child will be 10 years of age or less at the time of reimmunization.

### Unaccepted

Pneumococcal vaccine is not indicated for recurrent otitis media, because the vaccine has not shown significant benefit in preventing otitis media in children.

## Pharmacology/Pharmacokinetics

### Physicochemical characteristics

Source—The currently available vaccines in the U.S. (*Pneumovax 23*, MSD, and *Pnu-Imune 23*, Lederle) contain a mixture of purified capsular polysaccharides from the 23 most prevalent pneumococcal types responsible for approximately 90% of serious pneumococcal disease. Each of the pneumococcal polysaccharide types is produced separately. The resultant 23 polysaccharides are separated from the cells, purified, and combined to give 25 mcg of each type per 0.5-mL dose of the final vaccine.

*Pneumovax 23*, MSD (Canada) brand of pneumococcal vaccine polyvalent also contains 23 polysaccharides.

Other characteristics—The U.S. nomenclature for these 23 types is: 1, 2, 3, 4, 5, 26, 51, 8, 9, 68, 34, 43, 12, 14, 54, 17, 56, 57, 19, 20, 22, 23, 70

The Danish nomenclature for these 23 types is: 1, 2, 3, 4, 5, 6B, 7F, 8, 9N, 9V, 10A, 11A, 12F, 14, 15B, 17F, 18C, 19A, 19F, 20, 22F, 23F, 33F

### Mechanism of action/Effect

Pneumococcal bacteria are surrounded by polysaccharide capsules, which make the bacteria resistant to attack by white blood cells. However, human blood serum contains antibodies, which render the bacteria vulnerable to attack. The vaccine, which is composed of the purified polysaccharides from bacterial cells, stimulates production of these antibodies and provides active immunity to the 23 types of pneumococcal bacteria represented in the vaccine.

### Protective effect

The vaccine is about 60 to 80% effective in preventing infection to all 23 types of pneumococcal bacteria represented in the vaccine in persons with normal immune systems, including the elderly. Since the vaccine contains 23 types of antigens, the overall efficacy of the vaccine will be less than the efficacy of each individual type of antigen. In addition, efficacy may be reduced or nonexistent in persons with certain disease states, especially those who are immunocompromised.

Although the 23-valent vaccine contains only 25 mcg of each antigen per dose as compared to the 14-valent vaccine, which contained 50 mcg of antigen per dose, there appear to be comparable levels of antigenicity.

**Time to protective effect**
Approximately 2 to 3 weeks.

**Duration of protective effect**
Antibody levels for most antigen types in healthy adults remain elevated for at least 5 years. In some persons, the levels fall to prevaccination levels within 10 years. A more rapid reduction in antibody levels may occur in children. In addition, in children without spleens, with sickle cell disease, or with nephrotic syndrome, there may be a decline of antibody levels for some antigen types to prevaccination levels within 3 to 5 years.

## Precautions to Consider

### Cross-sensitivity and/or related problems
Patients allergic to thimerosal may be allergic to the pneumococcal vaccine available in the U.S. because it may contain a small amount of thimerosal.

### Pregnancy/Reproduction
Pregnancy—Studies have not been done in humans. However, if the vaccine is administered during pregnancy, it should be given after the first trimester and only to women at high risk of pneumococcal disease.
Studies have not been done in animals.
FDA Pregnancy Category C.

### Breast-feeding
It is not known whether pneumococcal vaccine is distributed into breast milk. However, problems in humans have not been documented.

### Pediatrics
Infants and children younger than 2 years of age—Immunization is not recommended for infants and children younger than 2 years of age, since this age group may not show adequate response to many of the antigens, and antibody levels stimulated by the vaccine may not persist.
Children 2 years of age and older—Response to one of the important pediatric pneumococcal types, type 14, is decreased in children who are less than 5 years of age. Other pediatrics-specific problems that would limit the usefulness of this vaccine in children 2 years of age and older are not expected.

### Geriatrics
Appropriate studies on the relationship of age to the effects of pneumococcal vaccine have not been performed in the geriatric population. However, geriatrics-specific problems that would limit the usefulness of this vaccine in the elderly are not expected.

### Drug interactions and/or related problems
The following drug interactions and/or related problems have been selected on the basis of their potential clinical significance (possible mechanism in parentheses where appropriate)—not necessarily inclusive (» = major clinical significance):

Note: Combinations containing any of the following medications, depending on the amount present, may also interact with this medication.

Immunosuppressive agents or
Radiation therapy
(because normal defense mechanisms are suppressed, the patient's antibody response to the pneumococcal vaccine may be decreased. If possible, persons who are to undergo therapy with medications that cause immunosuppression, including candidates for organ transplants, should receive the vaccine at least 10 days, and preferably more than 14 days, prior to receiving the immunosuppression-causing medication to receive the full immunizing effect of the vaccine. The precaution does not apply to corticosteroids used as replacement therapy, for short-term [less than 2 weeks] systemic therapy, or by other routes of administration that do not cause immunosuppression)

(patients with Hodgkin's disease should not receive the vaccine less than 10 days prior to, or during, immunosuppressive therapy, since some patients so immunized have exhibited post-immunization antibody levels below their preimmunization levels. In addition, patients with Hodgkin's disease who have received extensive chemotherapy and/or nodal irradiation should not receive the vaccine at all, since immunization of some intensively treated patients caused depression of pre-existing levels of antibody to some pneumococcal types)

» Pneumococcal vaccine polyvalent, other
(persons previously immunized with pneumococcal vaccine of any valence generally should not be revaccinated with pneumococcal vaccine polyvalent 23, because of increased frequency and severity of side/adverse effects, including Arthus and systemic reactions. However, it may be desirable to administer subsequent doses of vaccine to patients at high risk of severe illness or death from pneumococcal disease [See *Indications*.])

### Medical considerations/Contraindications
The medical considerations/contraindications included have been selected on the basis of their potential clinical significance (reasons given in parentheses where appropriate)—not necessarily inclusive (» = major clinical significance).

*Risk-benefit should be considered when the following medical problems exist:*

Febrile illness, severe
(to avoid confusing manifestations of illness with possible side/adverse effects of vaccine; minor illnesses, such as upper respiratory infection, do not preclude administration of vaccine)

Sensitivity to pneumococcal vaccine

Thrombocytopenic purpura, idiopathic
(in one report, two stabilized patients experienced a relapse 2 to 14 days after vaccination; this relapse lasted up to 2 weeks)

## Side/Adverse Effects

Note: Neurological disorders, such as paresthesias and acute radiculoneuropathy, including Guillain-Barré syndrome (GBS), have been reported rarely in temporal association with pneumococcal vaccine administration; however, no causal relationship has been established, and the incidence of GBS in vaccinated persons appears to be no greater than the incidence in the general population.

Some persons previously vaccinated with a pneumococcal vaccine of any valence and subsequently revaccinated with the same or a different polyvalent pneumococcal vaccine have experienced increased frequency and severity of side/adverse effects, including Arthus and systemic reactions.

It is recommended that persons who experience neurological symptoms or signs following administration of pneumococcal vaccine should not be reimmunized.

The following side/adverse effects have been selected on the basis of their potential clinical significance (possible signs and symptoms in parentheses where appropriate)—not necessarily inclusive:

### Those indicating need for medical attention
Incidence rare
*Anaphylactic reaction* (difficulty in breathing or swallowing; hives; itching, especially of soles or palms; reddening of skin, especially around ears; swelling of eyes, face, or inside of nose; unusual tiredness or weakness, sudden and severe); *fever over 39 °C (102 °F)*

### Those indicating need for medical attention only if they continue or are bothersome
Incidence more frequent
*Redness, soreness, hard lump, swelling, or pain at injection site*
Incidence less frequent or rare
*Adenitis* (swollen glands); *arthralgia or myalgia* (aches or pain in joints or muscles); *asthenia* (unusual tiredness or weakness); *fever of 38.3 °C (101 °F) or less; malaise* (vague feeling of bodily discomfort); *skin rash*

## Patient Consultation

As an aid to patient consultation, refer to *Advice for the Patient, Pneumococcal Vaccine Polyvalent (Systemic)*.

In providing consultation, consider emphasizing the following selected information (» = major clinical significance):

### Before receiving this vaccine
» Conditions affecting use, especially:
Sensitivity to pneumococcal vaccine or thimerosal
Pregnancy—If needed, administer vaccine following the first trimester and only to women at high risk of pneumococcal disease
Use in children—Not recommended for infants and children younger than 2 years of age
Other medications, especially previous use of any pneumococcal vaccine

### Proper use of this vaccine
» Proper dosing

### Precautions after receiving this vaccine
» Notifying all patient's physicians that patient has received pneumococcal vaccine polyvalent 23 so that the information can be included in patient's medical records; the vaccine is usually administered only once

### Side/adverse effects
Signs of potential side effects, especially anaphylactic reaction or fever over 39 °C (102 °F)

## General Dosing Information
The dosage of pneumococcal vaccine polyvalent is the same for all persons: children and adults.

When sterilizing syringes before vaccination, care should be taken to avoid preservatives, antiseptics, detergents, and disinfectants, since the vaccine is easily inactivated by these substances.

Pneumococcal vaccine polyvalent is administered by subcutaneous or intramuscular injection. It is not recommended for intradermal injection, because it may cause severe local reactions. Also, intravenous administration is not recommended.

Pneumococcal vaccine polyvalent, a polysaccharide vaccine, can be administered concurrently with the following, using separate body sites, separate syringes, and the precautions that apply to each immunizing agent:
- Polysaccharide vaccines, other, such as haemophilus b polysaccharide vaccine, haemophilus b conjugate vaccine, or meningococcal polysaccharide vaccine.
- Influenza vaccine, whole or split virus.
- Diphtheria toxoid, tetanus toxoid, and/or pertussis vaccine.
- Live virus vaccines, such as measles, mumps, and/or rubella vaccines.
- Poliovirus vaccines (oral [OPV], inactivated [IPV], or enhanced-potency inactivated [enhanced-potency IPV]).
- Immune globulin and disease-specific immune globulins.
- Hepatitis B recombinant or plasma-derived vaccine, or other inactivated vaccines, except cholera, typhoid, and plague. It is recommended that cholera, typhoid, and plague vaccines be administered on separate occasions because of these vaccines' propensity to cause side/adverse effects.

Patients who require antibiotic prophylaxis against pneumococcal infection should continue to receive antibiotic therapy after vaccination with pneumococcal vaccine.

### For treatment of adverse effects
Recommended treatment includes
- For mild hypersensitivity reaction—Administering antihistamines, and, if necessary, corticosteroids.
- For severe hypersensitivity or anaphylactic reaction—Administering epinephrine. Antihistamines or corticosteroids may also be administered as required.

## Parenteral Dosage Forms

### PNEUMOCOCCAL VACCINE POLYVALENT INJECTION

#### Usual adult and adolescent dose
Immunizing agent (active)—
Intramuscular or subcutaneous, 0.5 mL, preferably into the outer aspect of the upper arm or into the lateral mid-thigh.

#### Usual pediatric dose
Immunizing agent (active)—
Infants and children up to 2 years of age: Use is not recommended, since this age group may not show adequate response to many of the antigens, and antibody levels stimulated by the vaccine may not persist.
Children 2 years of age and older: See *Usual adult and adolescent dose*.

#### Strength(s) usually available
U.S.—
25 mcg of polysaccharide from each of the 23 capsular types of pneumococci represented in the vaccine in each 0.5 mL dose (Rx) [*Pneumovax 23* (phenol 0.25%); *Pnu-Imune 23* (thimerosal 0.01%)].
Canada—
25 mcg of polysaccharide from each of the 23 capsular types of pneumococci represented in the vaccine in each 0.5 mL dose (Rx) [*Pneumovax 23* (phenol 0.25%)].

#### Packaging and storage
Store manufacturer-supplied filled syringes, unopened vials, and partially used vials of the vaccine between 2 and 8 °C (36 and 46 °F), unless otherwise specified by manufacturer. Protect from freezing.

#### Stability
The vaccine is a clear, colorless solution. It should not be used if it is discolored or contains a precipitate.

#### Incompatibilities
A sterile syringe free of preservatives, antiseptics, disinfectants, and detergents should be used for each injection because these substances may inactivate the vaccine.

#### Auxiliary labeling
- Store in refrigerator.

Revised: 07/12/94

---

# PODOFILOX   Topical—INTRODUCTORY VERSION

BAN: Podophyllotoxin
VA CLASSIFICATION (Primary): DE500
Commonly used brand name(s): *Condylox*.
Another commonly used name is podophyllotoxin.
Note: For a listing of dosage forms and brand names by country availability, see *Dosage Forms* section(s).

## Category
Antimitotic agent (topical).

## Indications

### Accepted
Condyloma acuminatum (treatment)—Podofilox is indicated for the treatment of condyloma acuminatum of the external genital areas; the gel, but not the solution, may be used for perianal warts. Neither the gel nor the solution should be used to treat warts on mucous membranes, including membranous areas of the urethra, rectum, and vagina.

Using a 3-day-on and 4-day-off treatment regimen of 0.5% podofilox solution for 2 to 4 weeks, 50% of patients (35 of 75 patients) showed clearing of up to 79% of their warts (412 of 524 warts); 35% of the warts reappeared in 60% of these patients. In two multicenter clinical studies using a 3-day-on and 4-day-off treatment regimen of 0.5% gel for 4 weeks, 25.6% of 106 patients and 38.4% of 176 patients showed complete clearing of their anogenital warts.

## Pharmacology/Pharmacokinetics

### Physicochemical characteristics
Source—Synthesized and purified from the plant families Coniferae (species of *Juniperus*) and Berberidaceae (species of *Podophyllum*).
Molecular weight—414.41.

### Mechanism of action/Effect
The exact mechanism of action for podofilox is unknown. Podofilox is a potent mitotoxic agent that inhibits cell mitosis; cell division stops, other cellular processes are impaired, necrosis occurs, and the affected tissues gradually erode.

### Absorption
Applying 0.05 mL of 0.5% podofilox solution topically to external genitals does not result in detectable serum concentrations; however, applying 0.1 to 1.5 mL results in systemic absorption. Multiple doses do not accumulate.

### Half-life
Elimination—1 to 4.5 hours.

### Time to peak concentration
Topically, 0.1 to 1.5 mL of 0.05% podofilox solution—1 to 2 hours.

### Peak serum concentration
Topically, 0.1 to 1.5 mL of 0.05% podofilox solution—1 to 17 nanograms per mL.

## Precautions to Consider

### Carcinogenicity
Animal studies have not shown podofilox to be carcinogenic, including one study of podofilox topically administered to mice in doses of 0.04, 0.2, and 1 mg per kg of body weight (mg/kg) a day for 80 weeks.

### Mutagenicity
Podofilox is not mutagenic according to the Ames plate reverse mutation assay (at concentrations up to 5 mg podofilox, with or without metabolic activation) and BALB/3T3 cells (at concentrations up to 0.008 micrograms per mL [mcg/mL] without metabolic activation and 12 mcg/mL with activation). Chromosome damage occurs at higher doses; 25 mg/

kg (75 mg per square meter of body surface area) of podofilox caused disruption and breakage of chromosomes *in vivo* in the mouse micronucleus assay.

### Pregnancy/Reproduction
Fertility—Problems in humans have not been documented.

Podofilox did not impair fertility in two generations of rats given daily topical doses of 0.2 mg/kg of body weight (1.18 mg per square meter of body surface area) (corresponding to the recommended human daily dose) during gametogenesis, mating, gestation, parturition, and lactation.

Pregnancy—Studies have not been done in humans; however, dose-related systemic absorption has occurred.

Podofilox was embryotoxic in rats that were given daily intraperitoneal doses of 5 mg/kg of body weight (29.5 mg per square meter of body surface area; corresponding to 19 times the maximum human recommended dose [MHRD]). It was not teratogenic in rats that were given daily topical doses of 0.21 mg/kg of body weight (2.95 mg per square meter of body surface area; corresponding to two times the MHRD) for 13 days.

FDA Pregnancy Category C.

### Breast-feeding
It is not known if podofilox is distributed into breast milk; however, dose-related systemic absorption has occurred and the potential for serious adverse problems exists.

### Pediatrics
Appropriate studies on the relationship of age to the effects of podofilox have not been performed in the pediatric population. Safety and efficacy have not been established.

### Geriatrics
No information is available on the relationship of age to the effects of podofilox in geriatric patients.

### Medical considerations/Contraindications
The medical considerations/contraindications included have been selected on the basis of their potential clinical significance (reasons given in parentheses where appropriate)—not necessarily inclusive (» = major clinical significance).

*Risk-benefit should be considered when the following medical problem exists:*
Sensitivity to podofilox

## Side/Adverse Effects
The following side/adverse effects have been selected on the basis of their potential clinical significance (possible signs and symptoms in parentheses where appropriate)—not necessarily inclusive:

### Those indicating need for medical attention
Incidence more frequent
*Bleeding of skin, local*—less than 5% for solution, 22.9% for gel; *burning feeling of skin, local; dizziness*—less than 5% for solution only, indicating systemic absorption; *phimosis* (problems with foreskin of penis)—less than 5% for solution only; *headache*—7% for gel only, indicating systemic absorption; *hematuria* (bloody urine)—less than 5% for solution only; *inflammation of skin, local* (redness or swelling of skin); *itching of skin, local; malodor* (bad odor)—less than 5% for solution only; *pain during sexual intercourse*—less than 5% for solution only; *pain of skin, local; scarring of skin*—less than 5% for solution only; *skin erosion, local* (skin ulcers); *vesicle formation* (blistering, crusting, or scabbing of treated skin); *vomiting*—less than 5% for solution only, indicating systemic absorption

Note: Local *burning feeling of skin* (64% in males, 78% in females), *itching of skin* (50% in males, 65% in females), and *pain of skin* (50% in males, 72% in females) occur more frequently in females than in males. Severe reactions occur within the first 2 weeks of beginning treatment and, for the podofilox solution, are more frequent and severe in females than in males. *Inflammation of skin* (71% in males, 63% in females) occurs more frequently in males than females, and *skin ulcers* (67% in males and females) occur equally in both genders.

### Those indicating need for medical attention only if they continue or are bothersome
Incidence more frequent
*Desquamation, local* (peeling of treated skin); *chafing or dryness of skin, local; insomnia* (trouble in sleeping)—less than 5% for solution only; *soreness or tenderness of skin, local; stinging or tingling of skin, local*

Incidence less frequent
*Discoloration of skin, local* (changes in color of treated skin)—for gel only; *skin rash*—for gel only

## Overdose
For more information on the management of overdose or unintentional ingestion, **contact a Poison Control Center** (see *Poison Control Center Listing*).

### Clinical effects of overdose
The following effects have been selected on the basis of their potential clinical significance (possible signs and symptoms in parentheses where appropriate)—not necessarily inclusive:

Signs of systemic absorption of topical administration—in order of appearance
*Nausea; vomiting; diarrhea; bone marrow depression* (chills; fever; sore throat; unusual bleeding or bruising); *oral ulcers*

Note: *Bone marrow depression* occurred following 5 to 10 intravenous doses of 0.5 to 1 mg/kg a day, but was reversible.

### Treatment of overdose
Treatment of systemic toxicity or accidental ingestion is essentially supportive.

To decrease absorption—Wash the skin free of any remaining drug.

Supportive care—Patients in whom intentional overdose is known or suspected should be referred for psychiatric consultation.

## Patient Consultation
As an aid to patient consultation, refer to *Advice for the Patient, Podofilox (Topical)—Introductory Version*.

In providing consultation, consider emphasizing the following selected information (» = major clinical significance):

### Before using this medication
» Conditions affecting use, especially:
Sensitivity to podofilox

### Proper use of this medication
» Carefully reading patient directions that come with medication before using
» Avoiding contact with eyes and mucous membranes, including mucous membranes of vagina, rectum, and urethra; if contact occurs, immediately flushing eyes with water for 15 minutes or thoroughly washing area of mucous membranes with water
» Importance of not using more medication than the amount prescribed or increasing the frequency to greater than 3 times a week or for more than 4 treatment cycles
» Not applying the medication to any other wart without discussing with the physician; not exceeding a total dose of 10 square centimeters
» Proper administration
Proper use of applicators; not reusing
Applying medication to approved wart area only
Washing medication off normal skin
Drying treated area before allowing it contact with normal skin
Washing hands and properly discarding applicator(s) after podofilox application
» Proper dosing
Missed dose: Applying as soon as possible, then returning to regular schedule
» Proper storage

### Precautions while using this medication
Understanding that podofilox may not prevent wart recurrence or stop new warts from appearing
Contains alcohol and may be flammable; not using near heat, open flame, or while smoking

### Side/adverse effects
Signs of potential side effects, especially bleeding of skin, local; burning feeling of skin, local; dizziness (solution only); phimosis (solution only); headache (gel only); hematuria (solution only); inflammation of skin, local; itching of skin, local; malodor (solution only); pain during sexual intercourse (solution only); pain of skin, local; scarring of skin (solution only); skin erosion; vesicle formation; and vomiting (solution only)

## General Dosing Information
On advice of the health care professional, the patient should be able to identify the type of warts podofilox can and cannot be applied to and understand the correct method for applying podofilox. It is particularly important not to apply podofilox to squamous cell carcinomas.

If contact with eyes occurs, patient should wash eyes with a large amount of water and seek professional advice.

Hands should be washed before and after administering podofilox.

Area of treatment with podofilox should be completely dry before allowing treated skin to come in contact with normal skin.

Treatment with podofilox should be discontinued if response of wart to podofilox is unsatisfactory after four treatment cycles. Applying podofilox more frequently than recommended will not increase efficacy but can result in increasing the rate of local adverse effects or cause systemic absorption.

## Topical Dosage Forms

### PODOFILOX GEL

**Usual adult dose**
Condyloma acuminatum—
 Topical, to external genital or perianal warts, two times a day for three consecutive days via applicator tip or finger, then treatment should be discontinued for four consecutive days and cycle repeated until there is no visible wart or for up to four treatment cycles. Treatment should be limited to ten square centimeters or less of wart tissue, and the amount applied should not exceed 0.5 grams of gel per day.

**Usual adult prescribing limits**
Safety and efficacy beyond four treatment cycles have not been established.

**Usual pediatric dose**
Condyloma acuminatum—
 Safety and efficacy have not been established.

**Strength(s) usually available**
U.S.—
 0.5% (Rx) [*Condylox* (alcohol; butylated hydroxytoluene; glycerin; hydroxypropyl cellulose; lactic acid; sodium lactate)].

Note: Packaging includes an applicator tip.

**Packaging and storage**
Store below 40 °C (104 °F), preferably between 15 and 30 °C (59 and 86 °F), unless otherwise specified by manufacturer.

**Auxiliary labeling**
• For external use only.
• Do not freeze.

**Additional information**
Podofilox gel is flammable; keep away from open flame.

### PODOFILOX TOPICAL SOLUTION

**Usual adult dose**
Condyloma acuminatum—
 Topical, to external genital warts, two times a day (every twelve hours) for three consecutive days via applicator tip, then treatment should be discontinued for four consecutive days and cycle repeated until there is no visible wart or for up to four treatment cycles. Treatment should be limited to ten square centimeters or less of wart tissue, and the amount applied should not exceed 0.5 mL of solution per day.

**Usual adult prescribing limits**
Safety and efficacy beyond four treatment cycles have not been established.

**Usual pediatric dose**
Condyloma acuminatum—
 Safety and efficacy have not been established.

**Strength(s) usually available**
U.S.—
 0.5% (Rx) [*Condylox* (alcohol—95%; lactic acid; sodium lactate)].

**Packaging and storage**
Store below 40 °C (104 °F), preferably between 15 and 30 °C (59 and 86 °F), unless otherwise specified by manufacturer.

**Auxiliary labeling**
• For external use only.
• Do not freeze.

**Additional information**
Podofilox is flammable; keep away from open flame.

Developed: 06/27/98

---

# PODOPHYLLUM   Topical†

VA CLASSIFICATION (Primary): DE500

Commonly used brand name(s): *Podocon-25; Podofin*.

Note: For a listing of dosage forms and brand names by country availability, see *Dosage Forms* section(s).

†Not commercially available in Canada.

## Category
Cytotoxic (topical).

## Indications

**General considerations**
Podophyllum contains a number of unidentified ingredients, and its activity may vary widely depending on the source of the material.

**Accepted**
Condyloma acuminatum (treatment)—Podophyllum is indicated for the treatment of condyloma acuminatum (venereal warts).

Epitheliomatosis, multiple superficial (treatment) or
Keratoses, pre-epitheliomatosis (treatment) or
Papilloma, of the larynx, juvenile (treatment)—Podophyllum is used in the treatment of multiple superficial epitheliomatosis, such as multiple superficial or infiltrating basal cell epithelioma, squamous cell epithelioma (prickle cell epithelioma), and basal-squamous cell epithelioma (mixed or transitional cell epithelioma); seborrheic, actinic, and roentgen ray keratoses; and juvenile papilloma of the larynx.

**Unaccepted**
Podophyllum has been used in the treatment of general types of verrucae, such as vulgaris (common warts), filiformis (filiform warts), plana (flat warts), and plantaris (plantar warts); however, it is much less effective in these types of warts than in venereal warts. Also, podophyllum therapy is less effective than other types of treatment for these warts.

## Pharmacology/Pharmacokinetics

**Physicochemical characteristics**
Source—Dried resin from the roots and rhizomes of *Podophyllum peltatum* (mandrake or May apple plant), the North American variety; active constituents are lignans including podophyllotoxin (20%), alpha-peltatin (10%), and beta-peltatin (5%).

**Mechanism of action/Effect**
Podophyllum resin's major active constituent, podophyllotoxin, is a lipid-soluble compound that easily crosses cell membranes. Podophyllotoxin and its derivatives are potent cytotoxic agents that inhibit cell mitosis and deoxyribonucleic acid (DNA) synthesis in a manner similar to that of colchicine. Cell division is arrested, and other cellular processes are impaired, gradually resulting in the disruption of cells and erosion of the tissue.

**Absorption**
Topical podophyllum is systemically absorbed; absorption may be increased if podophyllum is applied to friable, bleeding, or recently biopsied warts.

## Precautions to Consider

**Cross-sensitivity and/or related problems**
Patients sensitive to benzoin may be sensitive to this medication also because some preparations may contain tincture of benzoin.

**Pregnancy/Reproduction**
Pregnancy—Topical podophyllum is absorbed systemically and can cross the placenta. It should not be used during any phase of pregnancy, because of its teratogenic potential. Following oral administration during pregnancy, podophyllum has been reported to cause fetal abnormalities, such as skin tags on the ears and cheeks, limb malformations, and septal heart defects, as well as polyneuritis. Intrauterine death has occurred following topical application to vulval warts during the 32nd week of pregnancy. In one patient, minor fetal anomalies, including preauricular skin tags and a simian crease on the left hand, occurred following topical application during the 23rd, 24th, 25th, 28th, and 29th weeks of pregnancy.

Warts of the vaginal, perianal, or anal areas requiring treatment during pregnancy should be treated by alternative methods, such as electrodesiccation, diathermy, curettage, surgical excision, or cryosurgery with liquid nitrogen or dry ice.

### Breast-feeding
Topical podophyllum is systemically absorbed. However, it is not known whether topical podophyllum is distributed into breast milk. Problems in humans have not been documented.

### Pediatrics
Appropriate studies on the relationship of age to the effects of topical podophyllum have not been performed in the pediatric population. However, no pediatrics-specific problems have been documented to date.

### Geriatrics
Appropriate studies on the relationship of age to the effects of topical podophyllum have not been performed in the geriatric population. However, no geriatrics-specific problems have been documented to date.

### Laboratory value alterations
The following have been selected on the basis of their potential clinical significance (possible effect in parentheses where appropriate)—not necessarily inclusive (» = major clinical significance):

With physiology/laboratory test values
    Alkaline phosphatase and
    Aspartate aminotransferase (AST [SGOT]) and
    Lactate dehydrogenase (LDH)
        (serum values may be increased in association with renal failure and hepatotoxicity)

### Medical considerations/Contraindications
The medical considerations/contraindications included have been selected on the basis of their potential clinical significance (reasons given in parentheses where appropriate)—not necessarily inclusive (» = major clinical significance).

***Risk-benefit should be considered when the following medical problems exist:***
» Friable, bleeding, or recently biopsied warts
   (risk of systemic toxicity may be increased)
  Sensitivity to podophyllum

## Side/Adverse Effects
Note: Podophyllum resin topical solution is highly irritating to the eye and to mucous membranes in general.

Podophyllum can cause severe systemic toxicity, which may result from either topical application or ingestion. The toxic effects are usually reversible but have been fatal. Death can occur with ingestion of podophyllum in amounts as small as 300 mg.

Serious systemic toxicity has occurred following topical application of podophyllum to large areas or in excessive amounts, or when the medication was allowed to remain in contact with the skin or mucous membranes for a prolonged period of time.

The risk of systemic toxicity may be increased when podophyllum is applied to friable, bleeding, or recently biopsied warts, or when the medication is inadvertently applied to normal skin or mucous membranes surrounding the affected area(s).

Renal failure and hepatotoxicity have occurred following topical application of podophyllum.

Adverse effects on the nervous system may occur following topical application of podophyllum; these are usually delayed in onset and prolonged in duration.

Cerebral toxicity (manifested by altered sensorium ranging from mild confusion to coma) may occur following topical application of podophyllum and continue for 7 to 10 days during which the electroencephalogram (EEG) may show generalized slowing.

The following side/adverse effects have been selected on the basis of their potential clinical significance (possible signs and symptoms in parentheses where appropriate)—not necessarily inclusive:

### Those indicating need for medical attention
***Burning, redness, or other irritation of affected area; skin rash or itching***—allergic reaction to benzoin, which may be present in some preparations

## Overdose
For specific information on the agents used in the management of podophyllum overdose, see:
• *Charcoal, Activated (Oral-Local)* monograph.

For more information on the management of overdose or unintentional ingestion, **contact a Poison Control Center** (see *Poison Control Center Listing*).

### Clinical effects of overdose
The following effects have been selected on the basis of their potential clinical significance (possible signs and symptoms in parentheses where appropriate)—not necessarily inclusive:

Initial symptoms of systemic toxicity
   ***Abdominal or stomach pain; clumsiness or unsteadiness; confusion; decreased or loss of reflexes; diarrhea***—sometimes severe and prolonged; ***excitement, irritability, or nervousness; hallucinations; leukopenia*** (sore throat and fever); ***muscle weakness; nausea or vomiting; thrombocytopenia*** (unusual bleeding or bruising)

Delayed symptoms of systemic toxicity
   ***Autonomic neuropathy*** (difficult or painful urination; dizziness or lightheadedness, especially when getting up from a lying or sitting position; fast heartbeat); ***difficulty in breathing; drowsiness; paralytic ileus*** (constipation; nausea and vomiting; pain in upper abdomen or stomach, mild, dull, and continuing); ***peripheral neuropathy*** (numbness, tingling, pain, or weakness in hands or feet); ***seizures***

   Note: If *peripheral neuropathy* occurs, it usually appears about 2 weeks after podophyllum application, may worsen progressively for up to 3 months, and may persist for up to 9 months or longer.

### Treatment of overdose
Treatment of systemic toxicity or accidental ingestion is essentially supportive and may include the following:

To decrease absorption—If podophyllum is accidentally ingested and the patient is conscious, emesis should be immediately induced. If the patient is unconscious, gastric lavage should be performed. Activated charcoal may also be administered.

To enhance elimination—Charcoal hemoperfusion may be beneficial in life-threatening or deteriorating conditions.

Monitoring—Electrolytes, serum calcium, and hemoglobin concentrations should be closely monitored.

Supportive care—Intravenous therapy and respiratory support should be administered if necessary. Patients in whom intentional overdose is known or suspected should be referred for psychiatric consultation.

## Patient Consultation
As an aid to patient consultation, refer to *Advice for the Patient, Podophyllum (Topical)*.
In providing consultation, consider emphasizing the following selected information (» = major clinical significance):

### Before using this medication
» Conditions affecting use, especially:
    Sensitivity to podophyllum or benzoin
    Pregnancy—Podophyllum should not be used during pregnancy, because it is absorbed through the mother's skin
    Breast-feeding—Podophyllum is absorbed through the mother's skin
    Other medical problems, especially friable, bleeding, or recently biopsied warts, because of increased risk of systemic toxicity

### Proper use of this medication
» Importance of keeping away from mouth; medication is poisonous
» Avoiding contact with the eyes and mucous membranes; if contact occurs, immediately flushing eyes with water for 15 minutes, and thoroughly washing skin with soap and water or (if preparation contains tincture of benzoin) swabbing it with rubbing alcohol
» Not using near heat, open flame, or while smoking
» Importance of not using more medication than the amount prescribed
» Not using on moles or birthmarks
» Not using on friable, bleeding, or recently biopsied warts

*Proper administration*
   Preventing dissemination of podophyllum to uninvolved skin—Applying petrolatum around affected areas before applying podophyllum and/or applying talcum powder to treated area immediately after applying podophyllum
   Using a toothpick or a cotton-tipped or glass applicator to apply medication
   Applying one drop at a time, allowing time between drops for drying, until affected area is covered
   Following application of podophyllum, allowing medication to remain on affected area for 1 to 6 hours as directed by physician; removing medication by thoroughly washing affected area with soap and water or, if preparation contains tincture of benzoin, swabbing it with rubbing alcohol
   Washing hands immediately after using medication

» Proper dosing
  Missed dose: Applying as soon as possible
» Proper storage

**Side/adverse effects**
Signs of potential side effects, especially burning, redness, or other irritation of affected area; skin rash or itching; or initial or delayed symptoms of systemic toxicity

## General Dosing Information

Some clinicians recommend that podophyllum be used only under medical supervision because of its potentially serious adverse effects.

Old, discolored, dried, or gritty preparations of podophyllum should not be used.

Podophyllum should not be applied to friable, bleeding, or recently biopsied warts, because systemic absorption of the medication may be increased.

Podophyllum should not be used on moles or birthmarks, since acute inflammation or ulceration may occur.

Podophyllum is most frequently used in a concentration of 25%; however, concentrations of 5 to 10% have been recommended for very large lesions (> 10 to 20 cm$^2$) in order to minimize the risk of toxicity.

Also, to minimize the risk of toxicity, application of podophyllum should be limited to small areas of intact skin.

If podophyllum is to be self-administered, patients should be instructed to use the medication with great caution. It should be applied only to the affected areas, avoiding contact with normal tissue. This medication can cause severe erosive damage to normal skin.

If podophyllum accidentally comes in contact with normal tissue, it should be removed, preferably by thoroughly washing with soap and water, or, if the podophyllum preparation contains tincture of benzoin, swabbing with rubbing alcohol.

Great care should be taken to avoid contact with the eyes because podophyllum can cause corneal damage. If contact does occur, the eyes should be immediately and thoroughly flushed with water for 15 minutes.

To prevent dissemination of the medication to uninvolved skin, petrolatum may be applied to normal skin surrounding the affected areas prior to application of podophyllum and/or talcum powder may be applied to the treated area immediately following application of podophyllum.

A toothpick or a cotton-tipped or glass applicator should be used to apply the topical solution one drop at a time, until the affected area is covered. Sufficient time should be allowed between drops for drying.

**For condyloma acuminatum**
Following application of podophyllum, the medication should be allowed to remain on the affected area for a period of 1 to 6 hours as prescribed by the physician.

At the end of the treatment period, the medication should be removed, preferably by thoroughly washing with soap and water. Some clinicians recommend removing podophyllum preparations that contain tincture of benzoin by swabbing with rubbing alcohol; however, this may be more irritating than washing with soap and water.

A minimum of 7 days should elapse between treatments because of the risk of systemic toxicity. Treatment may be repeated at weekly intervals for up to 6 weeks; however, if a beneficial effect does not occur within 6 weeks, alternative therapy should be considered.

**For multiple superficial epitheliomatosis or pre-epitheliomatosis keratoses**
Before each subsequent application of the medication, the necrotic tissue should be removed by curettage or wiped away with gauze.

In response to treatment, the lesion usually sloughs off leaving a superficial ulcer and a moderate degree of dermatitis of the immediate surrounding tissue. When treatment is discontinued, the lesion may be dressed with a mild antiseptic ointment; healing usually occurs in a few days, except in very large lesions, which may take longer to heal.

## Topical Dosage Forms

### PODOPHYLLUM RESIN TOPICAL SOLUTION USP

**Usual adult and adolescent dose**
Condyloma acuminatum—
  Topical, to the skin, as a 10 to 25% solution for a period of one to six hours; treatment may be repeated at one-week intervals for up to six weeks.
Multiple superficial epitheliomatosis or
Pre-epitheliomatosis keratoses—
  Topical, to the skin, as a 25% solution once a day; treatment should be continued for several days following the initial slough.
Juvenile papilloma of the larynx—
  Topical, to the lesion, as a 12.5% solution once a day. The intervals of treatment can be gradually increased as the lesions become smaller; however, applications at short intervals give the best results.

**Usual pediatric dose**
See *Usual adult and adolescent dose*.

**Strength(s) usually available**
U.S.—
  25% (Rx) [*Podocon-25*; *Podofin*].
Note: Other strengths are currently not commercially available; compounding required for prescriptions.
Canada—
  Podophyllum resin of the North American variety is not commercially available.

**Packaging and storage**
Store below 40 °C (104 °F), preferably between 15 and 30 °C (59 and 86 °F), unless otherwise specified by manufacturer. Store in a tight, light-resistant container. Protect from freezing.

**Preparation of dosage form**
For treatment of juvenile papilloma of the larynx, the 25% solution should be diluted with an equal volume of 95% alcohol to yield the 12.5% solution.

A 25% Podophyllum Resin Topical Solution USP may be prepared extemporaneously by mixing 25 grams of the alcohol-soluble extractive of podophyllum resin in alcohol and 10 grams of the alcohol-soluble extractive of benzoin in alcohol, and diluting with alcohol to make 100 mL.

The solution should be prepared with native North American podophyllum resin, rather than a mixture of North American and Indian resins, because the Indian resin is stronger and more irritating than the North American variety. Also, the resin should be free of guaiacium gum, which may be a sensitizer.

Other vehicles that may be used for preparation of podophyllum resin topical solution include mineral oil or collodion.

**Stability**
Exposure to light, air, and warmth may cause precipitation and darkening of the solution because of evaporation and decomposition; such solutions should be discarded.

**Auxiliary labeling**
- Poison.
- For external use only.
- Shake well.
- Keep container tightly closed.

Revised: 08/15/94
Interim revision: 08/19/97

# POLIOVIRUS VACCINE   Systemic

This monograph includes information on the following: 1) Poliovirus Vaccine Inactivated; 2) Poliovirus Vaccine Inactivated Enhanced Potency; 3) Poliovirus Vaccine Live Oral.

VA CLASSIFICATION (Primary): IM100

Commonly used brand name(s): *Ipol*[2]; *Orimune*[3].

Other commonly used names are: Enhanced-potency IPV [Poliovirus Vaccine Inactivated Enhanced Potency] IPV [Poliovirus Vaccine Inactivated] N-IPV [Poliovirus Vaccine Inactivated Enhanced Potency] OPV [Poliovirus Vaccine Live Oral] Sabin vaccine [Poliovirus Vaccine Live Oral] Salk vaccine [Poliovirus Vaccine Inactivated] TOPV [Poliovirus Vaccine Live Oral]

Note: For a listing of dosage forms and brand names by country availability, see *Dosage Forms* section(s).

## Category
Immunizing agent (active).

# Indications

## Accepted

Poliomyelitis (prophylaxis)—IPV, enhanced-potency IPV, and OPV are indicated for immunization against poliomyelitis caused by poliovirus types 1, 2, and 3 according to the following recommendations.

Unless otherwise contraindicated, all infants from age 6 to 12 weeks, all children, all adolescents up to 18 years of age, and adults at greater risk of exposure to polioviruses than the general population who do not have time to receive IPV immunization should be immunized against poliomyelitis with OPV.

OPV is the vaccine of choice for infants and children up to 18 years of age because the vaccine induces intestinal immunity that provides resistance to reinfection with polioviruses, is easy to administer, is well accepted by parents, results in immunization of some contacts of the vaccinated children, and has a record of having essentially eliminated poliomyelitis associated with wild poliovirus in the U.S.

Immunization with IPV or enhanced-potency IPV is recommended for adults who are at greater risk of exposure to polioviruses than the general population. However, since enhanced-potency IPV is more consistently immunogenic than IPV, it is generally preferred to IPV. IPV or enhanced-potency IPV is the vaccine of choice over OPV, with certain exceptions, for adults 18 years of age and older, especially those with no history of poliovirus vaccination, because the risk of vaccine-associated paralysis following OPV is slightly higher for adults than for children. However, routine primary poliovirus vaccination with IPV or enhanced-potency IPV of adults (18 years of age or older) residing in the U.S. and Canada who have not had a primary series as children is not necessary. Most adults are already immune and also have a very small risk of exposure to polioviruses in the U.S. and Canada.

In addition, the following persons should be immunized against poliomyelitis:

- Persons traveling to countries with endemic or epidemic poliomyelitis, whether or not they have been previously immunized.
- Unimmunized adults at increased risk of exposure to polioviruses.
- Incompletely immunized adults at increased risk of exposure to polioviruses.
- Previously vaccinated adults at increased risk of exposure to polioviruses.
- Personnel in day-care centers and custodial institutions for children.
- Medical personnel and employees in medical facilities should be immunized with IPV or enhanced-potency IPV instead of OPV because virus may be shed after receipt of OPV and inadvertent contact with susceptible immunocompromised patients may occur.
- Persons at risk during a poliomyelitis epidemic. OPV should be administered to all persons within the epidemic area who are over 6 weeks of age and have not been completely immunized or whose immunization status is unknown, with the exception of persons with immunodeficiency considerations. Infants can receive OPV at birth, but because successful immunization is less likely in newborn infants, a complete series of OPV beginning when the infants are 6 weeks of age should also be administered.
- Members of communities or specific population groups with disease caused by wild polioviruses.
- Newborn infants living in tropical endemic areas where the incidence of poliomyelitis is increasing should receive OPV at birth. However, because successful immunization is less likely in newborn infants, a complete series of OPV beginning when the infants are 6 weeks of age should also be administered. There should be a minimum interval of 4 weeks between the neonatal dose and the first dose of the primary series of OPV; in addition, subsequent doses of the primary series should be administered at 4-week intervals. Optimally, the neonate should be immunized with OPV 3 days after birth, and breast-feeding should be withheld for 2 or 3 hours before and after immunization to allow for the establishment of the vaccine viruses in the infant's gut.
- Laboratory workers handling specimens that may contain polioviruses.
- Immunodeficient patients and their household contacts, whether or not the immunodeficient patient had at some earlier time received a poliovirus immunization when his/her immune status was normal. This is because some immunodeficiencies impair the immune response to antigens against which the immune system was previously primed. IPV or enhanced-potency IPV is the poliovirus vaccine of choice. Although patients with immune deficiency diseases may not develop a protective immune response, immunization with IPV or enhanced-potency IPV should be attempted anyway. OPV should not be given to persons residing in the household of an immunocompromised or immunosuppressed person, because live poliovirus is excreted by the recipient of OPV and may be communicable to the immunocompromised or immunosuppressed person. If protection against poliomyelitis is required, IPV or enhanced-potency IPV should be used for immunizing household contacts of immunocompromised or immunosuppressed persons.
- Members of a household in which there is a family history of acquired or hereditary immunodeficiency. IPV or enhanced-potency IPV is the poliovirus vaccine of choice. OPV should not be given to a member of a household in which there is a family history of acquired or hereditary immunodeficiency unless or until the immune status of the family members as well as the patient is known.

Adults who have not been immunized or who are inadequately immunized with either OPV, IPV, or enhanced-potency IPV are at a very small risk (approximately 1 case in 5 million doses of OPV distributed) of developing OPV-associated paralytic poliomyelitis when children in the household are given OPV. These adults should receive IPV or enhanced-potency IPV. However, because of the overriding importance of ensuring timely immunization of children and the extreme rarity of OPV-associated disease in contacts, children should be immunized on schedule with OPV regardless of the poliovirus-vaccine status of adult household contacts. Only if the child's immunization will not be jeopardized or unduly delayed should the adult be immunized before administering OPV to the child. Adults who want to be immunized should receive at least 2 doses of IPV or enhanced-potency IPV a month apart before the children are immunized, and preferably, the full primary series. The children may receive their first dose of OPV at the same time that the adults receive their third dose of IPV or their second dose of enhanced-potency IPV. Adult household contacts who are not adequately immunized prior to the child's receiving OPV should be informed of the small risk involved and of the precautions to be taken, such as hand washing after changing the immunized infant's diaper.

Poliovirus vaccines are not effective in modifying cases of existing poliomyelitis or preventing cases of incubating poliomyelitis.

# Pharmacology/Pharmacokinetics

## Physicochemical characteristics

Source—
  Produced from a mixture of 3 types of attenuated polioviruses that have been propagated in monkey kidney cell culture.
  Poliovirus vaccine inactivated (IPV) and Poliovirus vaccine inactivated enhanced potency (enhanced-potency IPV): The polioviruses are inactivated with formaldehyde.
  Poliovirus vaccine live oral (OPV): Contains the live, attenuated polioviruses.

## Mechanism of action/Effect

Administration of poliovirus vaccine inactivated (IPV), poliovirus vaccine inactivated enhanced potency (enhanced-potency IPV), or poliovirus vaccine live oral (OPV) simulates natural infection by inducing systemic immunity. In addition, OPV induces active mucosal immunity because the live viruses multiply in the intestinal tract. These live viruses persist in the intestinal tract for at least 4 to 6 weeks. The antibodies formed by the administration of a primary series of IPV, enhanced-potency IPV, or OPV protect the person against clinical poliomyelitis infection by any of the 3 types of poliovirus.

## Other actions/effects

Live poliovirus is excreted by persons recently immunized with OPV, especially following the first dose. The vaccine viruses are excreted in the immunized person's feces for at least 6 to 8 weeks and also from the nose or throat for 7 to 10 days.

OPV induces intestinal immunity that provides resistance to reinfection with polioviruses, including the simultaneous infection by wild polioviruses. This is of special value in epidemic-control campaigns. Persons immunized with IPV or enhanced-potency IPV are more likely to be subclinically infected with and excrete in the feces either wild strains or attenuated vaccine virus strains. Immunization with IPV, enhanced-potency IPV, or especially OPV has greatly reduced the circulation of wild polioviruses, and inapparent infection with wild strains no longer contributes significantly to establishing or maintaining immunity; this makes universal vaccination of infants and children even more important.

## Protective effect

A primary vaccination series with 3 doses of OPV, 3 doses of enhanced-potency IPV, or 4 doses of IPV produces immunity to all three poliovirus types in more than 95% of recipients. When OPV is used, many persons are protected after a single dose and most are protected after 2 doses. When enhanced-potency IPV is used, most persons are protected after the second dose. An antibody response to OPV usually occurs within 7 to 10 days after administration and peaks approximately 21 days later.

### Duration of protective effect
With IPV, although vaccine-induced antibodies have persisted for 12 years in some persons, the duration of immunity following primary immunization with the currently available IPV has not been established.

Although conclusive studies are not yet available with enhanced-potency IPV, unpublished studies of an enhanced-potency IPV with a lower antigen content than the U.S. product have shown 100% seropositivity 5 years after the third dose.

With OPV, 95% of children studied 5 years after full immunization had protective antibodies to all 3 types of poliovirus, and some studies show persistence of local intestinal immunity in some persons for more than 6 years; however, the duration of humoral and intestinal immunity following primary immunization with OPV has not been established.

## Precautions to Consider

### Cross-sensitivity and/or related problems
Persons sensitive to one poliovirus vaccine may be sensitive to the other poliovirus vaccines also.

In addition, in the U.S., patients allergic to the following may be allergic to poliovirus vaccines also:
- Neomycin, which may be contained in IPV, enhanced-potency IPV, and OPV.
- Polymyxin B, which may be contained in enhanced-potency IPV.
- Streptomycin, which may be contained in IPV, enhanced-potency IPV, and OPV.

In Canada, patients allergic to the following may be allergic to poliovirus vaccines also:
- Neomycin, which may be contained in IPV, enhanced-potency IPV, and OPV.
- Penicillin, which may be contained in OPV.
- Polymyxin B, which may be contained in OPV.
- Streptomycin, which may be contained in IPV, enhanced-potency IPV, and OPV.

A history of hypersensitivity reactions other than anaphylaxis, such as delayed-type allergic reaction (contact dermatitis), generally does not preclude immunization.

### Carcinogenicity/Mutagenicity
Studies have not been done.

### Pregnancy/Reproduction
Fertility—Studies have not been done.

Pregnancy—Studies have not been done in humans, and problems in humans have not been documented. Although routine immunization of pregnant women is not recommended, if the risk of exposure is or will be high during pregnancy, it is recommended that IPV be administered. However, if time is available before the risk of exposure occurs, some experts recommend that IPV be administered. Enhanced-potency IPV is not recommended for use in pregnant women, because of the lack of data on possible adverse effects.

Although live poliovirus is shed by persons recently immunized with OPV, especially following the first dose, OPV can be administered to children of pregnant women without special risk to the pregnant woman or the fetus.

Studies have not been done in animals.

FDA Pregnancy Category C.

### Breast-feeding
*IPV*—Problems in humans have not been documented.
*Enhanced-potency IPV*—Problems in humans have not been documented.
*OPV*—Although poliovirus antibodies may be distributed into breast milk, mothers who breast-feed can receive OPV without any interruption in the feeding schedule. In addition, breast-feeding does not interfere with the usual immunization of infants with OPV. However, when a neonate is immunized at birth, as may occur in tropical endemic areas or during a poliomyelitis epidemic, breast-feeding should be withheld for 2 or 3 hours before and after immunization with OPV because the colostrum may interfere with the establishment of the vaccine viruses in the neonate's gut.

### Pediatrics
Infants up to 6 weeks of age—Use is not recommended.

Infants and children 6 weeks of age and older—Pediatrics-specific problems that would limit the usefulness of this vaccine in children in this age group are not expected.

### Geriatrics
Appropriate studies on the relationship of age to the effects of poliovirus vaccine have not been performed in the geriatric population. However, geriatrics-specific problems that would limit the usefulness of this vaccine in the elderly are not expected.

### Drug interactions and/or related problems
The following drug interactions and/or related problems have been selected on the basis of their potential clinical significance (possible mechanism in parentheses where appropriate)—not necessarily inclusive (» = major clinical significance):

Note: Combinations containing any of the following medications, depending on the amount present, may also interact with this vaccine.

Blood products, antibody-containing or
Immune globulin (IG)
(do not appear to interfere with the immune response to OPV; OPV may be administered concurrently with immune globulins if necessary. Since IPV and enhanced-potency IPV are inactivated products, there is no reason to suspect interference, and IPV or enhanced-potency IPV can be administered without regard to immune globulins)

» Immunosuppressants or
» Radiation therapy
(because normal defense mechanisms are suppressed, the patient's antibody response to any of the poliovirus vaccines may be decreased; in addition, the use of a live virus vaccine, such as OPV, may potentiate the replication of the vaccine virus, possibly causing poliomyelitis infection secondary to the vaccine; therefore, OPV should not be administered to these patients; IPV or enhanced-potency IPV should be administered instead. The precaution does not apply to corticosteroids used as replacement therapy, for short-term [less than 2 weeks] systemic therapy, or by other routes of administration that do not cause immunosuppression)

(where there is a family history of congenital or hereditary immune deficiency conditions, the patient should not be vaccinated with OPV until his/her immune competence is demonstrated; IPV or enhanced-potency IPV should be administered instead)

Live virus vaccines, other
(although data are lacking on impairment of antibody responses to rubella, measles, mumps, or OPV when these vaccines are administered on different days within 1 month of each other, the chance exists that the immune responses may be impaired when live virus vaccines are administered in this manner; therefore, when feasible, live virus vaccines not administered on the same day should be given at least 1 month apart)

### Medical considerations/Contraindications
The medical considerations/contraindications included have been selected on the basis of their potential clinical significance (reasons given in parentheses where appropriate)—not necessarily inclusive (» = major clinical significance).

Note: A past history of clinical poliomyelitis in otherwise healthy persons does not preclude the administration of IPV, enhanced-potency IPV, or OPV if such administration is otherwise indicated.

Persons who are immunized with OPV should avoid close contact for at least 6 to 8 weeks with persons with altered immune status.

*Except under special circumstances, this vaccine should not be used when the following medical problems exist:*

» Debilitated condition, advanced or
» Illness, moderate or severe, with or without fever
(administration of IPV, enhanced-potency IPV, or OPV should be postponed or avoided; minor illnesses, such as mild upper respiratory infections, do not preclude administration of vaccine)

» Diarrhea, persistent or
» Viral infection or
» Vomiting, persistent
(the presence of other viruses, including poliovirus and other enteroviruses, in the intestinal tract may interfere with the replication of OPV and therefore with final immunity. Alternatives in the presence of the above illnesses include administration of IPV or, in the case of persistent diarrhea, the administration of OPV without it counting as part of the primary series)

» Immune deficiency conditions, congenital or hereditary, family history of or
» Immune deficiency conditions, primary or acquired
(because of reduced or suppressed defense mechanisms, patients who are immunocompromised or immunosuppressed should not receive live virus vaccines, such as OPV; IPV or enhanced-potency IPV should be administered instead)

(persons with leukemia in remission may receive live virus vaccines, such as OPV, if at least 3 months have passed since their last chemotherapy treatment) (persons with asymptomatic or symptomatic human immunodeficiency virus [HIV] infection may receive IPV or enhanced-potency IPV, but not OPV)

(when there is a family history of congenital or hereditary immune deficiency conditions, the patient should not be vaccinated with OPV until his/her immune competence is demonstrated; IPV or enhanced-potency IPV should be administered instead)

Sensitivity to poliovirus vaccine

## Side/Adverse Effects

Note: The risk of developing OPV-associated paralytic poliomyelitis is as follows in unimmunized persons:
- Approximately 1 case in 5 million doses of OPV distributed, in adults living in the same household as children who are given OPV.
- Approximately 1 case in 3.2 million doses of OPV distributed, in all normal vaccine recipients or their close contacts.
- Approximately 1 case in 2.6 million doses of OPV distributed, in all cases (normal as well as immune-deficient recipients and all close contacts).

No paralytic poliomyelitis reactions to poliovirus vaccine inactivated (IPV) have occurred since the 1955 incident in which the vaccine contained live viruses that had escaped inactivation. Although Guillain-Barré syndrome (GBS) has occurred following IPV, no causal relationship has been established. In addition, no other serious side effects of IPV have been documented.

Since there is no evidence that IPV causes serious side effects, poliovirus vaccine inactivated enhanced potency (enhanced-potency IPV) is not expected to cause serious side effects either.

A history of hypersensitivity reactions other than anaphylaxis, such as delayed-type allergic reaction (contact dermatitis), generally does not preclude immunization.

The following side/adverse effects have been selected on the basis of their potential clinical significance (possible signs and symptoms in parentheses where appropriate)—not necessarily inclusive:

**Those indicating need for medical attention**
Incidence rare
*Anaphylactic reaction* (difficulty in breathing or swallowing; hives; itching, especially of soles or palms; reddening of skin, especially around ears; swelling of eyes, face, or inside of nose; unusual tiredness or weakness, sudden and severe)

**Those indicating need for medical attention only if they continue or are bothersome**
Incidence less frequent
*Delayed-type allergic reaction, cell-mediated* (itching or skin rash)—with injection; *fever over 38.5 °C (101.3 °F)*—incidence 5% with injection; *redness, soreness, hard lump, tenderness, or pain at injection site*—with injection

## Patient Consultation

As an aid to patient consultation, refer to *Advice for the Patient, Poliovirus Vaccine (Systemic)*.
In providing consultation, consider emphasizing the following selected information (» = major clinical significance):

**Before using this vaccine**
» Conditions affecting use, especially:
Sensitivity to poliovirus vaccine or allergy to neomycin, penicillin, polymyxin B, or streptomycin
Use in children—Not recommended in infants up to 6 weeks of age
Other medications, especially immunosuppressants or radiation therapy
Other medical problems, especially advanced debilitated condition; moderate or severe illness, with or without fever; persistent diarrhea or vomiting; viral infection; family history of congenital or hereditary immune deficiency conditions; or primary or acquired immune deficiency conditions
Diet—Patients on low-sugar diets should be cautioned that the oral solution form of poliovirus vaccine may be administered on a sugar cube

**Proper use of this vaccine**
» Proper dosing

**Precautions after receiving this vaccine**
Checking with physician before receiving any other live virus vaccines within 1 month of this vaccine

**Side/adverse effects**
In rare instances (approximately 1 case in 3.2 million doses of distributed vaccine), healthy persons who have taken the live oral polio vaccine (OPV) and healthy persons who are close contacts of adults or children who have taken OPV have been infected by the poliovirus and become paralyzed
No paralysis caused by polio infection has occurred with the injected inactivated polio vaccine (IPV) since 1955 when the vaccine contained live viruses that accidentally had not been inactivated
Signs of potential side effects, especially anaphylactic reaction

## General Dosing Information

Poliovirus vaccine inactivated (IPV) and poliovirus vaccine inactivated enhanced potency (enhanced-potency IPV) are administered subcutaneously. The vaccines should not be administered intravenously.

Poliovirus vaccine live oral (OPV) is administered orally. The vaccine should not be administered parenterally.

A primary series of IPV is 4 doses; a primary series of enhanced-potency IPV or of OPV is 3 doses. If a combination of IPV and OPV or a combination of IPV and enhanced-potency IPV is used, a total of 4 doses constitutes a primary series. If a combination of enhanced-potency IPV and OPV is used, a total of 3 doses constitutes a primary series.

The multiple doses of IPV, enhanced-potency IPV, or OPV in the primary series are not administered as boosters, but to ensure that immunity to all three types of poliovirus has been achieved.

For IPV, enhanced-potency IPV, or OPV, time intervals between doses that are longer than those recommended for routine primary immunization do not require additional doses of vaccine.

Although the fourth dose of diphtheria-tetanus-pertussis (DTP) vaccine and the third dose of OPV have traditionally been administered to children 18 months of age, and measles-mumps-rubella (MMR) vaccine has traditionally been administered to children 15 months of age, it is now recommended that DTP, OPV, and MMR be administered concurrently to children 15 months of age. MMR should not be postponed in order to administer these vaccines concurrently at 18 months of age. In addition, the traditional method is still an acceptable alternative.

OPV, a live virus vaccine, can be administered concurrently with the following, using separate body sites, separate syringes, and the precautions that apply to each immunizing agent:
- Polysaccharide vaccines, such as haemophilus b polysaccharide vaccine, haemophilus b conjugate vaccine, meningococcal polysaccharide vaccine, or pneumococcal polyvalent vaccine.
- Influenza vaccine, whole or split virus.
- Diphtheria toxoid, tetanus toxoid, and/or pertussis vaccine.
- Live virus vaccines, other, such as measles, mumps, and/or rubella vaccines, but only if the vaccines are administered on the same day; otherwise they should be administered at least 1 month apart.
- Immune globulin and disease-specific immune globulins.
- Hepatitis B recombinant or plasma-derived vaccine.
- Inactivated vaccines, except cholera, parenteral typhoid, and plague. It is recommended that cholera, parenteral typhoid, and plague vaccines be administered on separate occasions because of these vaccines' propensity to cause side/adverse effects.
- Typhoid vaccine, live, oral. May be administered concurrently with, or at any interval before or after, OPV.

IPV or enhanced-potency IPV, an inactivated vaccine, can be administered concurrently with the following, using separate body sites, separate syringes, and the precautions that apply to each immunizing agent:
- Polysaccharide vaccines, such as haemophilus b polysaccharide vaccine, haemophilus b conjugate vaccine, meningococcal polysaccharide vaccine, or pneumococcal polyvalent vaccine.
- Influenza vaccine, whole or split virus.
- Diphtheria toxoid, tetanus toxoid, and/or pertussis vaccine.
- Live virus vaccines, such as measles, mumps, and/or rubella vaccines.
- Immune globulin and disease-specific immune globulins.
- Hepatitis B recombinant or plasma-derived vaccine.
- Inactivated vaccines, other, except cholera, parenteral typhoid, and plague. It is recommended that cholera, parenteral typhoid, and plague vaccines be administered on separate occasions because of these vaccines' propensity to cause side/adverse effects.

Persons traveling to countries with endemic or epidemic poliomyelitis:
- At a minimum, all travelers should receive a complete primary series of OPV, IPV, or enhanced-potency IPV, depending on age. In addition, travelers, regardless of age, who have previously completed the primary series of OPV, IPV, or enhanced-potency IPV should receive an additional dose of OPV or enhanced-potency IPV.

- If at least 4 weeks remain before departure, inadequately vaccinated adults 18 years of age and older should receive, at intervals of not less than 4 weeks, additional doses of IPV or enhanced-potency IPV up to the total number of doses recommended to complete the primary series.
- Regardless of age, travelers who have not had a primary series and who have less than 4 weeks before beginning their travels should receive one dose of either OPV or enhanced-potency IPV. Such travelers who are under 18 years of age should then complete the primary series of OPV, at the recommended intervals, whether they remain in the foreign country or return to the U.S. or Canada; such travelers 18 years of age and older should complete the primary series of OPV, IPV, or enhanced-potency IPV only if they remain in the foreign country or plan to travel again to a country with endemic or epidemic poliomyelitis.
- If time permits, infants and children under 2 years of age should receive at least 3 doses of OPV before travel. Intervals between doses may be reduced to 4 weeks to maximize immunization status before departure. If the infant is under 6 weeks of age, a dose of OPV should be given before travel, but the dose should not be counted as part of the 3-dose primary series of OPV. Thereafter, if the infant remains in the foreign country or if there are plans to travel again before the primary series is completed, doses of the primary 3-dose series of OPV should be scheduled at 4-week intervals, otherwise the regular immunization schedule may be used.

Unimmunized adults at increased risk of exposure to polioviruses:
- Primary immunization with IPV or enhanced-potency IPV is recommended whenever possible. If time allows and IPV is being administered, 3 doses should be given at intervals of 1 to 2 months with a fourth dose given 6 to 12 months after the third dose. If time allows and enhanced-potency IPV is being administered, 2 doses should be given at intervals of 1 to 2 months with a third dose given 6 to 12 months after the second dose.
- If at least 8 weeks are available before protection is required, 3 doses of enhanced-potency IPV should be given at least 4 weeks apart.
- If less than 8, but at least 4 weeks are available before protection is required, 2 doses of IPV or enhanced-potency IPV should be given at least 4 weeks apart.
- If less than 4 weeks are available before protection is required, a single dose of either OPV or enhanced-potency IPV should be given.
- Generally, if the person remains at increased risk, the remaining doses of IPV, enhanced-potency IPV, or OPV should be given at the usual intervals.

Incompletely immunized adults who are at increased risk of exposure to polioviruses and who have previously received only 1 dose of OPV, fewer than 3 doses of IPV, or a combination of OPV and IPV totaling fewer than 3 doses should receive at least 1 dose of either OPV or enhanced-potency IPV. If time permits, the remaining required doses of OPV, IPV, or enhanced-potency IPV should be administered regardless of the interval since the previously administered dose(s) or the type of vaccine previously received.

Adults who have previously completed a primary course of OPV, IPV, or enhanced-potency IPV and who are at increased risk of exposure to polioviruses should receive an additional dose of OPV, IPV, or enhanced-potency IPV, regardless of which vaccine was previously used. For OPV, IPV, and enhanced-potency IPV, the need for further supplementary doses has not been established. However, if OPV has been used exclusively, further supplementary doses are probably not necessary. If IPV has been used exclusively, further supplementary doses may be given every 5 years (U.S.) or 10 years (Canada).

Pregnant women at increased risk of poliomyelitis:
- Although routine immunization of pregnant women is not recommended, if the risk of exposure is or will be high during pregnancy, it is recommended that OPV be administered. However, if time is available before the risk of exposure occurs, some experts recommend that IPV be administered instead.
- Enhanced-potency IPV is not recommended for use in pregnant women, because of the lack of data on possible adverse effects.
- If OPV is used, 2 doses should be administered at a 6- to 8-week interval with a third dose given at least 6 weeks later (customarily 8 to 12 months later).
- If IPV is used, 3 doses should be administered at intervals of 1 to 2 months with a fourth dose given 6 to 12 months later.
- If there is not time for either of the above schedules and at least 4 weeks are available, 2 doses of IPV should be given 4 weeks apart. If less than 4 weeks are available, a single dose of OPV should be given.
- The remaining required doses of either IPV or OPV should be given at the appropriate intervals only if the woman remains at increased risk.

**For treatment of adverse effects**
Recommended treatment includes:
- For mild hypersensitivity reaction—Administering antihistamines and, if necessary, corticosteroids.
- For severe hypersensitivity or anaphylactic reaction—Administering epinephrine. Antihistamines or corticosteroids may also be administered as required.

---

## POLIOVIRUS VACCINE INACTIVATED

## Parenteral Dosage Forms
### POLIOVIRUS VACCINE INACTIVATED (Injection) USP

**Usual adult dose**
Immunizing agent (active)—
  Subcutaneously, 1 mL:
    First dose:
      At initial visit.
    Second dose:
      Four to eight weeks after the first dose.
    Third dose:
      Four to eight weeks after the second dose.
    Fourth dose:
      Six to twelve months after the third dose.
    Note: If a booster is required following the primary series, either IPV or OPV may be administered.
          If immediate protection is needed against poliomyelitis, OPV or enhanced-potency IPV should be administered.

**Usual pediatric dose**
Immunizing agent (active)—
  Subcutaneously, 1 mL—
    First dose:
      At initial visit, preferably at 6 to 12 weeks of age, commonly with the first DTP inoculation at 2 months of age.
    Second dose:
      Four to eight weeks after the first dose, commonly with the second DTP inoculation at 4 months of age.
    Third dose:
      Four to eight weeks after the second dose, commonly with the third DTP inoculation at 6 months of age.
    Fourth dose:
      Six to twelve months after the third dose, commonly with the MMR and fourth DTP inoculations at 15 months of age.
    First booster dose:
      Children who have completed the primary series of 4 doses of IPV should receive a booster dose of IPV or enhanced-potency IPV or 1 dose of OPV upon entering school, usually between 4 to 6 years of age. However, this booster dose of IPV or enhanced-potency IPV or the OPV dose is not required in children who receive the fourth dose of the primary series of IPV on or after their fourth birthday.
    Additional booster doses:
      In the U.S.: Every five years after the last dose of the primary series or after the first booster dose, whichever occurs last, up until 18 years of age unless a complete primary series of OPV has been administered.
      In Canada: Every ten years after the last dose of the primary series or after the first booster dose, whichever occurs last.
Note: In the U.S. and Canada, OPV is the poliovirus vaccine of choice for infants and children up to 18 years of age.

**Strength(s) usually available**
U.S.—
  The vaccine meets the requirements of the specific monkey potency test by virus-neutralizing antibody production, based on the U.S. Reference Poliovirus Antiserum, such that the ratio of the geometric mean titer of the group of monkey serums representing the vaccine to the mean titer value of the reference serum is not less than 1.29 for Type 1 (Mahoney), 1.13 for Type 2 (M.E.F.1), and 0.72 for Type 3 (Saukett) (Rx) [GENERIC].
Canada—
  The vaccine contains three types of poliovirus: Type 1 (Mahoney), Type 2 (M.E.F.1), and Type 3 (Saukett), grown in monkey kidney cell cultures (Rx) [GENERIC].

**Packaging and storage**
Store between 2 and 8 °C (36 and 46 °F). Do not freeze.

**Auxiliary labeling**
- Shake well.
- Do not freeze.

## POLIOVIRUS VACCINE INACTIVATED ENHANCED POTENCY

### Parenteral Dosage Forms
**POLIOVIRUS VACCINE INACTIVATED ENHANCED POTENCY (Injection)**

**Usual adult dose**
Immunizing agent (active)—
Subcutaneously, 0.5 mL:
First dose:
At initial visit.
Second dose:
Four to eight weeks (preferably eight weeks) after the first dose.
Third dose:
Six to twelve months (preferably closer to twelve months) after the second dose.
Note: If a booster is required following the primary series, either enhanced-potency IPV or OPV may be administered.

If immediate protection is needed against poliomyelitis, OPV or enhanced-potency IPV should be administered.

**Usual pediatric dose**
Immunizing agent (active)—
Subcutaneously, 0.5 mL:
First dose:
At 6 to 8 weeks of age (preferably at 8 weeks of age), commonly with the first DTP inoculation at 2 months of age.
Second dose:
Four to eight weeks (preferably eight weeks) after the first dose, commonly with the second DTP inoculation at 4 months of age.
Third dose:
Six to twelve months (preferably closer to twelve months) after the second dose, commonly with the MMR and fourth DTP inoculations at 15 months of age.
First booster dose:
Children who have completed the primary series of 3 doses of enhanced-potency IPV should receive a booster dose of enhanced-potency IPV or 1 dose of OPV upon entering school, usually between 4 to 6 years of age. However, this booster dose of enhanced-potency IPV or the OPV dose is not required in children who receive the third dose of the primary series of enhanced-potency IPV on or after their fourth birthday.
Additional booster doses:
The need for routinely administered booster doses of enhanced-potency IPV is not known at this time.
Note: In the U.S. and Canada, OPV is the poliovirus vaccine of choice for infants and children up to 18 years of age.

**Strength(s) usually available**
U.S.—
40, 8, and 32 D-Antigen units of types 1, 2, and 3, respectively, determined by comparison to a reference preparation, per 0.5 mL (Rx) [*Ipol*; GENERIC].
Canada—
40, 8, and 32 D-Antigen units of types 1, 2, and 3, respectively, determined by comparison to a reference preparation, per 0.5 mL (Rx) [GENERIC].

**Packaging and storage**
Store between 2 and 8 °C (36 and 46 °F). Do not freeze.

**Auxiliary labeling**
- Shake well.
- Do not freeze.

## POLIOVIRUS VACCINE LIVE ORAL

### Oral Dosage Forms
**POLIOVIRUS VACCINE LIVE ORAL (Oral Solution) USP**

**Usual adult dose**
Immunizing agent (active)—
Oral, 0.5 mL (U.S.) or 0.5 mL or 3 drops (Canada—specific dose depends on manufacturer)
U.S.:
2 doses administered not less than six and preferably eight weeks apart, with the third dose administered six to twelve months following the second dose.
Canada:
2 or 3 doses administered six to twelve weeks apart.
Note: Except in certain circumstances as specified in *General Dosing Information* and *Indications*, in the U.S. and Canada, OPV is not indicated for adults; IPV or enhanced-potency IPV is the poliovirus vaccine of choice in the U.S. and Canada when immunization is indicated for adults. Where OPV *is* indicated for adults, the frequency and number of doses may be different from the *Usual adult dose* above according to the specific circumstances (see *General Dosing Information*).

**Usual pediatric dose**
Immunizing agent (active)—
Oral, 0.5 mL (U.S.) or 0.5 mL or 3 drops (Canada—specific dose depends on manufacturer).
Infants:
First dose—
U.S.—At 6 to 12 weeks of age, commonly with the first DTP inoculation at 2 months of age.
Canada—Not earlier than 2 months of age.
Second dose—
U.S.—Not less than six and preferably eight weeks after the first dose, commonly with the second DTP inoculation at 4 months of age.
Canada—Six to twelve weeks after the first dose.
Third dose—
U.S.—Eight to twelve months after the second dose, commonly with the MMR and fourth DTP inoculations at 15 months of age, but may be administered at any time between 12 and 24 months of age.
Canada—Six to twelve weeks after the second dose.
Booster doses—
U.S.—Upon entering school, usually between 4 to 6 years of age. However, this booster dose is not required in children who receive the third dose of the primary series on or after their fourth birthday.
Canada—Eight to fifteen months after the third dose; during the first school year; and around 15 years of age.
Note: U.S.—An optional additional dose may be administered at 6 months of age (along with the third DTP inoculation) in areas with a high risk of poliovirus exposure.
Children up to age 18 who did not follow the above schedule:
U.S.: The first two doses should be administered not less than six and preferably eight weeks apart, and the third dose should be administered six to twelve months following the second dose.
Canada: 2 doses six to twelve weeks apart, followed by the booster doses above.
Note: When there are time constraints with regard to immunization, the vaccination schedule may be accelerated for infants and children up to 18 years of age so that the first dose may be given at or after 6 weeks of age, the second dose given 6 to 8 weeks later, and the third dose given 6 weeks to 12 months later. Moreover, the second and third doses may be given as close as 4 weeks apart if necessary.

**Strength(s) usually available**
U.S.—
The equivalent of $10^{5.4}$ to $10^{6.4}$ for Type 1, $10^{4.5}$ to $10^{5.5}$ for Type 2, and $10^{5.2}$ to $10^{6.2}$ for Type 3 of the TCID$_{50}$ (quantity of virus estimated to infect 50% of inoculated cultures) of the U.S. Reference Poliovirus, Live, Attenuated, per 0.5 mL (Rx) [*Orimune*].
Canada—
Approximately 1,000,000 infectious particles of Type 1, approximately 100,000 infectious particles of Type 2, and approximately 300,000 infectious particles of Type 3, per 0.5 mL (Rx) [GENERIC (I.A.F.)].
Approximately 1,000,000 infectious particles of Type 1, approximately 100,000 infectious particles of Type 2, and approximately 300,000 infectious particles of Type 3, per 3-drop dose (Rx) [GENERIC (Connaught)].

**Packaging and storage**
Preserve at a temperature that will maintain ice continuously in a solid state. Because of its sorbitol content, this vaccine may remain fluid at temperatures above −14 °C (+7 °F). If frozen, the vaccine must be completely thawed prior to use. Preserve thawed vaccine at a temperature between 2 and 8 °C (36 and 46 °F). Vaccine that has been thawed may be carried through a maximum of 10 freeze-thaw cycles, provided the temperature does not exceed 8 °C (46 °F) during the periods of thaw and provided the total cumulative duration of thaw does not exceed 24 hours. If the 24-hour period is exceeded, the vaccine must be used within 30 days, during which time it must be stored at a temperature between 2 and 8 °C (36 and 46 °F).

### Preparation of dosage form
The vaccine must be completely thawed prior to use.

The vaccine may be administered directly or mixed with distilled water, chlorine-free tap water, Syrup NF, or milk. Alternatively, it may be adsorbed on foods, such as bread, cake, or cube sugar.

### Stability
The vaccine contains phenol red as a pH indicator. The usual color of the vaccine is pink, although some containers of vaccine may exhibit a yellow coloration. The color of the vaccine prior to use (red-pink-yellow) has no effect on the virus or efficacy of the vaccine.

### Auxiliary labeling
- For oral use only.

Revised: 07/12/94

---

**POLIOVIRUS VACCINE INACTIVATED**—See *Poliovirus Vaccine (Systemic)*

---

**POLIOVIRUS VACCINE INACTIVATED ENHANCED POTENCY**—See *Poliovirus Vaccine (Systemic)*

---

**POLIOVIRUS VACCINE LIVE ORAL**—See *Poliovirus Vaccine (Systemic)*

---

**POLOXAMER 188**—See *Laxatives (Local)*

---

**POLYCARBOPHIL**—See *Laxatives (Local)*

---

# POLYETHYLENE GLYCOL AND ELECTROLYTES  Local

VA CLASSIFICATION (Primary): GA209

Note: For a listing of dosage forms and brand names by country availability, see *Dosage Forms* section(s).

## Category
Evacuant (bowel).

## Indications
**Accepted**

Bowel evacuation, preoperative, and

Bowel evacuation, pre-radiography—Polyethylene glycol (PEG) 3350 and electrolytes oral solution is indicated for bowel cleansing prior to gastrointestinal examination (e.g., colonoscopy, barium enema, intravenous pyelography) and colon surgery.

For double contrast barium enema, administration of the PEG-electrolyte solution alone has not been found to be an adequate method of bowel cleansing. PEG-electrolyte solution followed by oral administration of bisacodyl has been reported to achieve better removal of feces and correct degraded mucosal coating.

## Pharmacology/Pharmacokinetics
**Physicochemical characteristics**

Molecular weight—Potassium chloride: 74.55.
Sodium bicarbonate: 84.01.
Sodium chloride: 58.44.
Sodium sulfate: 322.20.
Osmolality—280 mOsmol per kg of water.

**Mechanism of action/Effect**

Evacuant (bowel)—Cleansing of the bowel is achieved by fluid overload with the osmotically balanced PEG-electrolyte solution, which induces a liquid stool within a short period of time. The concentration of electrolytes in the solution causes no net absorption or secretion of ions; thus no significant changes in water or electrolyte balance occur.

**Absorption**

Negligible absorption from gastrointestinal tract.

**Onset of action**

30 to 60 minutes.

**Elimination**

Negligible renal excretion (<0.1%).

## Precautions to Consider
**Carcinogenicity/Mutagenicity**

Studies to evaluate carcinogenic or mutagenic potential have not been performed.

**Pregnancy/Reproduction**

Pregnancy—Studies have not been done in humans.
Studies have not been done in animals.

FDA Pregnancy Category C.

**Breast-feeding**

It is not known whether PEG-electrolyte solution is distributed into breast milk. However, problems in humans have not been documented.

**Pediatrics**

Studies performed in children ranging in age from 6 months to 18 years have not demonstrated pediatrics-specific problems that would limit the usefulness of PEG-electrolyte solution in children.

**Geriatrics**

Appropriate studies performed to date have not demonstrated geriatrics-specific problems that would limit the usefulness of PEG-electrolyte solution in the elderly.

**Drug interactions and/or related problems**

The following drug interactions and/or related problems have been selected on the basis of their potential clinical significance (possible mechanism in parentheses where appropriate)—not necessarily inclusive (» = major clinical significance):

» Oral medications, other
   (other oral medications administered within 1 hour of administration of PEG-electrolyte solution may be flushed from the gastrointestinal tract and not absorbed)

**Laboratory value alterations**

The following have been selected on the basis of their potential clinical significance (possible effect in parentheses where appropriate)—not necessarily inclusive (» = major clinical significance):

With diagnostic test results
   Barium sulfate, rectal
      (administration of PEG-electrolyte solution on the same day as a barium enema [either single or double contrast] may result in retained fluid and thus barium dilution and may prevent barium coating of the intestinal wall)

**Medical considerations/Contraindications**

The medical considerations/contraindications included have been selected on the basis of their potential clinical significance (reasons given in parentheses where appropriate)—not necessarily inclusive (» = major clinical significance).

*Except under special circumstances, this medication should not be used when the following medical problems exist:*

» Intestinal obstruction or
» Paralytic ileus or
» Perforated bowel or
» Toxic colitis or
» Toxic megacolon
   (condition may be aggravated; colonic perforation may occur in patients with intestinal obstruction or toxic colitis)

*Risk-benefit should be considered when the following medical problems exist:*

Aspiration, predisposition to or
Impaired gag reflex or
Regurgitation, predisposition to or

Unconscious or semiconscious state
  (administration via nasogastric tube may increase risk of complications)
Ulcerative colitis, severe
  (condition may be aggravated)

## Side/Adverse Effects

Note: Hypothermia was reported in one patient after ingestion of 5 liters of chilled PEG-electrolyte solution.

One patient experienced cardiac asystole after a large bowel movement following administration of PEG-electrolyte solution. Further studies are needed to establish a causal relationship.

The following side/adverse effects have been selected on the basis of their potential clinical significance (possible signs and symptoms in parentheses where appropriate)—not necessarily inclusive:

### Those indicating need for medical attention
Incidence rare
  *Allergic reaction* (skin rash)

### Those indicating need for medical attention only if they continue or are bothersome
Incidence more frequent
  *Bloating; nausea*
Incidence less frequent
  *Abdominal or stomach cramps; anal irritation; vomiting*

## Patient Consultation

As an aid to patient consultation, refer to *Advice for the Patient, Polyethylene Glycol and Electrolytes (Local)*.
In providing consultation, consider emphasizing the following selected information (» = major clinical significance):

### Before using this medication
» Conditions affecting use, especially:
    Other oral medicines administered within 1 hour of solution
    Other medical problems, especially intestinal obstruction, paralytic ileus, perforated bowel, toxic colitis, or toxic megacolon

### Proper use of this medication
  Special preparatory instructions may be given; patient should inquire in advance
» Taking solution exactly as directed for best test results
» Drinking all the solution for best results, unless otherwise directed by physician
» Fasting for at least 3 hours prior to ingestion of solution; clear liquids are allowed after ingestion of solution
  Directions for the preparation of the powder dosage form
» Proper dosing
» Proper storage

### Side/adverse effects
  Signs of potential side effects, especially allergic reaction

## General Dosing Information

### Diet/Nutrition
Fasting is recommended for at least 3 hours prior to administration of the PEG-electrolyte solution.

The PEG-electrolyte solution may be administered on the morning of the examination, as long as enough time is allowed for the patient to drink the solution (3 hours) and for complete bowel evacuation (1 additional hour). If the patient is having a barium enema examination, the PEG-electrolyte solution should be administered early (e.g., 6 pm) the evening before the examination to permit proper mucosal coating by barium. No foods except clear liquids are allowed after administration of the solution.

Rapid drinking of each portion of the the PEG-electrolyte solution is recommended rather than drinking small amounts continuously.

## Oral Dosage Forms

### POLYETHYLENE GLYCOL 3350 AND ELECTROLYTES ORAL SOLUTION

#### Usual adult and adolescent dose
Bowel evacuant—
  Oral, 240 mL every ten minutes, up to 4 L, or until the fecal discharge is clear and free of solid matter.
  Note: May also be given via nasogastric tube at a rate of 20 to 30 mL per minute (1.2 to 1.8 L per hour).

#### Usual pediatric dose
Bowel evacuant—Oral or by continuous nasogastric drip, 25 to 40 mL per kg of body weight per hour until the fecal discharge is clear and free of solid matter.

#### Usual geriatric dose
See *Usual adult and adolescent dose*.

#### Strength(s) usually available
U.S.—

| Product | Content (mg/100 mL) ||||| 
|---|---|---|---|---|---|
| | PEG 3350 | NaCl | NaHCO$_3$ | Na$_2$SO$_4$ | KCl |
| U.S.— | | | | | |
| *OCL* (Rx) | 6000 | 146 | 168 | 569 | 75 |
| Canada— | | | | | |
| *Peglyte* (OTC) | 5960 | 150 | 170 | 570 | 80 |

#### Packaging and storage
Store between 15 and 30 °C (59 and 86 °F). Store in a tight container.

#### Incompatibilities
The addition of flavoring agents, such as sugar, nutritional supplements, or other sweeteners, is *not* recommended. Such additives may change the osmolality of the solution; sucrose or glucose may cause fluid and electrolyte absorption. Additives may also predispose to colonic bacterial fermentation and formation of combustible gases.

### POLYETHYLENE GLYCOL 3350 AND ELECTROLYTES FOR ORAL SOLUTION USP

#### Usual adult and adolescent dose
See *Polyethylene Glycol 3350 and Electrolytes Oral Solution*.

#### Usual pediatric dose
See *Polyethylene Glycol 3350 and Electrolytes Oral Solution*.

#### Usual geriatric dose
See *Polyethylene Glycol 3350 and Electrolytes Oral Solution*.

#### Size(s) usually available
U.S.—

| Product | Content (mg/100 mL) ||||| 
|---|---|---|---|---|---|
| | PEG 3350 | NaCl | NaHCO$_3$ | Na$_2$SO$_4$ | KCl |
| U.S.— | 6000 | 146 | 168 | 568 | 74.5 |
| *Co-Lav* (Rx) | | | | | |
| *Colovage* (Rx) | | | | | |
| *Colyte* (Rx) | | | | | |
| *Colyte-flavored* (Rx) | | | | | |
| *Go-Evac* (Rx) | | | | | |
| *GoLYTELY* (Rx) | | | | | |
| *NuLYTELY* (Rx) | 10500 | 280 | 143 | — | 37 |
| *NuLYTELY, Cherry Flavor* (Rx) | | | | | |
| Canada— | 6000 | 146 | 168 | 568 | 75 |
| *Colyte* (OTC) | | | | | |
| *GoLYTELY* (OTC) | | | | | |
| *Klean-Prep* (OTC) | | | | | |
| *Peglyte* (OTC) | 6000 | 150 | 170 | 570 | 80 |

#### Packaging and storage
Store below 40 °C (104 °F), preferably between 15 and 30 °C (59 and 86 °F), unless otherwise specified by manufacturer. Store in a tight container.

Note: After reconstitution, solution should be refrigerated to improve palatability.

#### Preparation of dosage form
See manufacturer's package label for complete instructions on reconstitution.
Tap water must be used for reconstitution.
To assure that all ingredients have dissolved, solution must be shaken vigorously.

#### Stability
Reconstituted solution should be used within 48 hours. Unused portion should be discarded.

#### Incompatibilities
The addition of flavoring agents, such as sugar, nutritional supplements, or other sweeteners, is *not* recommended. Such additives may change the

# PORFIMER Systemic—INTRODUCTORY VERSION

VA CLASSIFICATION (Primary): AN900

Commonly used brand name(s): *Photofrin.*

Note: For a listing of dosage forms and brand names by country availability, see *Dosage Forms* section(s).

## Category
Antineoplastic.

## Indications

**Accepted**

Carcinoma, esophageal (treatment)—Porfimer is indicated for the palliative treatment of partial or complete obstruction of the esophagus due to esophageal cancer in patients who cannot be satisfactorily treated with Nd:YAG laser therapy.

Carcinoma, lung, non–small cell (NSCLC) (treatment)—Porfimer is indicated for treatment of microinvasive endobronchial NSCLC in patients for whom surgery and radiotherapy are not indicated.

## Pharmacology/Pharmacokinetics

**Mechanism of action/Effect**

Porfimer, a mixture of oligomers of up to eight porphyrin units, is a photosensitizing agent that, in combination with light, can cause cellular damage and tumor death. Tumor selectivity occurs as a result of selective distribution and retention of porfimer in tumor tissue, and by the selective delivery of light. Illumination of target tissues with 630 nanometer wavelength laser light induces a photochemical reaction that activates porfimer. This light activation initiates a chain reaction, producing singlet oxygen, superoxide, and hydroxyl radicals, which damage mitochondria and intracellular membranes. Porfimer photodynamic therapy causes the release of thromboxane $A_2$, which results in vasoconstriction, activation and aggregation of platelets, and increased clotting. These factors contribute to ischemic necrosis, which leads to tissue and tumor death.

**Distribution**

The average steady-state volume of distribution for porfimer was 0.49 L per kilogram, following a 2 mg per kilogram (mg/kg) dose administered to four male cancer patients.

After intravenous injection, porfimer is distributed throughout a variety of tissues, but is selectively retained in tumors, skin, and organs of the reticuloendothelial system (including liver and spleen).

**Protein binding**

Very high (approximately 90%).

**Half-life**

Elimination—Approximately 250 hours, following a 2 mg/kg dose administered to four male patients.

Note: Porfimer is eliminated more quickly from some tissues (over 40 to 72 hours). However, it is retained longer in tumors; skin; and organs of the reticuloendothelial system, including liver and spleen.

**Peak plasma concentration**

Mean, 15 micrograms per mL (mcg/mL), following a 2 mg/kg dose administered to four male patients.

Note: The mean plasma concentration of porfimer 48 hours after intravenous injection was 2.6 mcg/mL.

**Elimination**

The total plasma clearance of porfimer was 0.051 mL per minute per kilogram of body weight, following a 2 mg/kg dose administered to four male patients.

In dialysis—Not dialyzable.

## Precautions to Consider

**Carcinogenicity**

Studies have not been done.

**Mutagenicity**

Adequate studies to evaluate the mutagenicity of porfimer without light have not been performed. Porfimer photodynamic therapy demonstrated no mutagenic effects in the Ames test, Chinese hamster ovary/HGPRT gene mutation assay, mouse LYR83 cells, or in the mouse micronucleus test. However, when exposed to visible light, porfimer was mutagenic in Chinese hamster ovary cells, causing an increase in sister chromatid exchange. When exposed to near UV light, porfimer caused an increase in Chinese hamster lung fibroblasts. Porfimer photodynamic therapy caused an increase in thymidine kinase mutants and DNA-protein cross-links in mouse L5178Y cells and produced a light-dependent increase in DNA-strand breaks in human cervical carcinoma cells.

**Pregnancy/Reproduction**

Fertility—Studies in rats administered doses of 4 mg per kg of body weight (mg/kg) per day (0.32 times the recommended human dose on a mg per square meter of body surface area [mg/m$^2$] basis) before conception through Day 7 of pregnancy have not shown that porfimer impairs fertility. However, long-term dosing in rats caused testicular hypertrophy, discoloration of ovaries and testes, and decreased parent weight.

Pregnancy—Adequate and well-controlled studies in humans have not been done.

In general, the use of a contraceptive is recommended during porfimer photodynamic therapy.

Studies in rats administered doses of 8 mg/kg per day (0.64 times the recommended human dose on a mg/m$^2$ basis) for 10 days during organogenesis showed that porfimer was toxic to both dam and fetus, causing delayed ossification, increased resorptions, decreased litter size, and decreased fetal body weight. However, porfimer did not cause major malformations or developmental changes at this dose in rats. Studies in rabbits administered doses of 4 mg/kg per day (0.65 times the recommended human dose on a mg/m$^2$ basis) for 13 days during organogenesis showed that porfimer caused no major malformations. However, maternal toxicity that resulted in increased resorptions, decreased litter size, and decreased fetal body weight was observed at this dose in rabbits.

Porfimer, administered to rats at doses of 4 mg/kg per day (0.32 times the recommended human dose on a mg/m$^2$ basis) for at least 42 days late in pregnancy through lactation, produced a reversible decline in the growth of rat offspring.

FDA Pregnancy Category C.

Labor—Porfimer has not been found to affect labor in rats administered doses of 4 mg/kg per day (0.32 times the recommended human dose on a mg/m$^2$ basis).

**Breast-feeding**

It is not known whether porfimer is distributed into breast milk. However, breast-feeding is not recommended because of the risk of serious adverse reactions in the infant.

**Pediatrics**

No information is available on the relationship of age to the effects of porfimer in pediatric patients. Safety and efficacy have not been established.

**Geriatrics**

Almost 80% of the patients in clinical trials with porfimer were older than 60 years of age. There were no apparent differences in efficacy or safety in these patients compared with younger adults. Dosage adjustment is not necessary in geriatric patients.

**Drug interactions and/or related problems**

The following drug interactions and/or related problems have been selected on the basis of their potential clinical significance (possible mechanism in parentheses where appropriate)—not necessarily inclusive (» = major clinical significance):

Note: Combinations containing any of the following medications, depending on the amount present, may also interact with this medication.

Allopurinol
(concurrent use may decrease the efficacy of photodynamic therapy)

---

**POLYTHIAZIDE**—See *Diuretics, Thiazide (Systemic)*

---

osmolality of the solution; sucrose or glucose may cause fluid and electrolyte absorption. Additives may also predispose to colonic bacterial fermentation and formation of combustible gases.

Revised: 08/15/95

Corticosteroids, glucocorticoid
(prior and concurrent use of corticosteroids may inhibit the production of thromboxane $A_2$ and may decrease the efficacy of photodynamic therapy)
Medications that decrease blood clotting, vasoconstriction, or platelet aggregation, such as:
Calcium channel blockers or
Prostaglandin synthesis inhibitors or
Thromboxane $A_2$ inhibitors
(concurrent use may decrease the efficacy of photodynamic therapy)
Medications that decrease active oxygen species or scavenge radicals, such as:
Beta-carotene or
Dimethyl sulfoxide (DMSO) or
Ethanol or
Formate or
Mannitol
(concurrent use may decrease the activity of photodynamic therapy)
Photosensitizing agents, other, including:
Griseofulvin or
Phenothiazines or
Sulfonamides or
Sulfonylurea hypoglycemic agents or
Tetracyclines or
Thiazide diuretics
(concurrent use may increase photosensitivity)

**Laboratory value alterations**
The following have been selected on the basis of their potential clinical significance (possible effect in parentheses where appropriate)—not necessarily inclusive (» = major clinical significance):

With physiology/laboratory test values
Hematocrit or
Hemoglobin
(may be decreased as a result of tumor bleeding induced by photodynamic therapy)

**Medical considerations/Contraindications**
The medical considerations/contraindications included have been selected on the basis of their potential clinical significance (reasons given in parentheses where appropriate)—not necessarily inclusive (» = major clinical significance).

*Except under special circumstances, this medication should not be used when the following medical problems exist:*

*For use in esophageal carcinoma or non–small cell lung carcinoma (NSCLC)*
» Allergic reaction to porphyrins, history of
» Porphyria
» Tumor erosion into a major blood vessel
(risk of potentially fatal hemorrhage after resolution of tumor)
*For use in esophageal carcinoma only*
» Bronchoesophageal fistula
» Tracheoesophageal fistula
» Tumor erosion into the trachea or bronchial tree
(photodynamic therapy is not recommended because of the risk of producing a tracheoesophageal or bronchoesophageal fistula)

*Risk-benefit should be considered when the following medical problems exist:*

*For use in esophageal carcinoma or NSCLC*
» Tissue ischemia at site of therapy
(may interfere with photodynamic therapy)
*For use in esophageal carcinoma only*
» Esophageal varices
(high risk of bleeding if laser light is directed onto variceal areas; extreme caution to avoid such placement is recommended)
*For use in NSCLC only*
» Endobronchial tumor invading deeply into bronchial wall
(possibility of fistula formation after tumor resolution)
» Endobronchial tumor location or configuration that increases the risk of airway obstruction resulting from treatment-induced inflammation
» Obstructing tumor after prior radiotherapy
(substantially higher risk of fatal hemorrhage)

**Patient monitoring**
The following may be especially important in patient monitoring (other tests may be warranted in some patients, depending on condition; » = major clinical significance):

» Respiration
(monitoring for signs of respiratory distress is needed between photodynamic therapy for endobronchial tumors and the follow-up debridement bronchoscopy because treatment-induced inflammation, mucositis, and necrotic debris can result in airway obstruction; if respiratory distress occurs, immediate bronchoscopy to open the airway is recommended)

## Side/Adverse Effects

Note: Most adverse effects are a result of a local inflammatory response and occur in or around the region of illumination.

Some cardiovascular, gastrointestinal, and respiratory side effects may be related to mediastinal inflammation.

Coughing, dysphagia, dyspnea, and photosensitivity reactions affecting the skin and eyes may occur in patients being treated for either esophageal carcinoma or non–small cell lung carcinoma (NSCLC). Most of the other side/adverse effects listed below have been reported only with use of photodynamic therapy for esophageal carcinoma. Adverse effects reported only with treatment for NSCLC are identified as such.

The following side/adverse effects have been selected on the basis of their potential clinical significance (possible signs and symptoms in parentheses where appropriate)—not necessarily inclusive:

**Those indicating need for medical attention**
Incidence more frequent
*Abdominal pain; anemia* (unusual tiredness or weakness); *candidiasis* (white patches inside the mouth); *cardiovascular effects, including atrial fibrillation* (fast or irregular heartbeat); *and heart failure* (shortness of breath; swelling of the feet and lower legs); *chest pain; dyspnea* (troubled breathing); *edema* (swelling of face; swelling of feet or lower legs; unusual weight gain); *endobronchial stricture* (troubled breathing)—reported only with treatment for NSCLC; *esophageal edema* (difficulty in swallowing); *fever; hemoptysis* (spitting blood)—reported only with treatment for NSCLC; *hypertension*—usually asymptomatic; *hypotension* (dizziness; fainting)—usually asymptomatic; *mucositis resulting in edema, exudates, and airway obstruction* (shortness of breath or troubled breathing)—reported only with treatment for NSCLC; *pleural effusion* (chest pain); *pneumonia* (cough; fever; shortness of breath; tightness in chest or wheezing); *urinary tract infection* (difficult, burning, or painful urination; frequent urge to urinate; bloody or cloudy urine)

Note: *Anemia* occurs more frequently, as the result of tumor bleeding caused by photodynamic therapy, when the treated esophageal tumor is > 10 centimeters long and is located in the lower third of the esophagus.

*Cardiovascular effects* occur more frequently with treatment of an esophageal tumor located in the middle third of the esophagus.

*Chest pain* is usually a localized, inflammatory response to photodynamic therapy for an esophageal tumor.

*Esophageal edema* occurs more frequently with treatment of an esophageal tumor located in the upper third of the esophagus.

In patients being treated for NSCLC, bleeding resulting in *hemoptysis* may be fatal, especially in patients who have undergone previous radiation therapy. In controlled studies in patients receiving palliative treatment for obstructing lung carcinoma, fatal hemorrhaging occurred in 21% of the patients who had received prior radiation therapy and in less than 1% of those who had not received such treatment.

Incidence less frequent
*Angina pectoris* (chest pain); *bronchospasm or pulmonary edema* (wheezing; shortness of breath); *coughing; dysphagia* (difficulty in swallowing); *endobronchial ulceration* (painful and/or difficult breathing)—reported only with treatment for NSCLC; *esophageal perforation* (chest pain, severe; troubled breathing; swelling of the neck; vomiting); *gastric ulcer* (severe abdominal or stomach pain); *ileus* (abdominal pain, severe; constipation, severe; vomiting); *jaundice* (yellow eyes or skin); *peritonitis* (abdominal or stomach pain, severe; chills; nausea and vomiting, severe); *respiratory failure* (troubled breathing)

Note: *Esophageal perforations* may occur during photodynamic therapy when endoscopies are performed on patients with complete esophageal obstruction.

**Those indicating need for medical attention only if they continue or are bothersome**
Incidence more frequent
*Asthenia* (weakness); *constipation, mild; diarrhea; insomnia* (trouble in sleeping); *nausea and vomiting, mild; photosensitivity reaction* (blistering, reddening, and/or swelling of skin)—occurs in 20% of patients

Note: Patients are likely to remain at risk of developing photosensitivity reactions for 30 days after porfimer administration.

Incidence less frequent
*Vision-related problems, including abnormal vision; diplopia* (double vision); *ocular discomfort; and photophobia* (eye pain when looking at bright light, including vehicle headlights)

## Overdose

For more information on the management of overdose, **contact a Poison Control Center** (see *Poison Control Center Listing*).

### Clinical effects of overdose

The following effects have been selected on the basis of their potential clinical significance (possible signs and symptoms in parentheses where appropriate)—not necessarily inclusive:

Acute and chronic
*Photosensitivity* (blistering of skin; increased sensitivity of eyes to sunlight or other bright lights, including vehicle headlights; increased sensitivity of skin to sunlight or bright indoor light; ocular discomfort; reddening of skin; swelling of skin)

Note: The effect of overdose on the duration of photosensitivity is unknown.

### Treatment of overdose

If an overdose of porfimer is administered, patients should protect skin and eyes from direct sun or bright indoor light for 30 days and then be tested for residual photosensitivity.

Laser light treatment should not be administered.

Porfimer is not dialyzable.

There is no information on the effects of an overdose of laser light following porfimer.

## Patient Consultation

As an aid to patient consultation, refer to *Advice for the Patient, Porfimer (Systemic—Introductory Version)*.

In providing consultation, consider emphasizing the following selected information (» = major clinical significance):

### Before using this medication
» Conditions affecting use, especially:
  Pregnancy—Use is not recommended because of maternal and fetotoxic effects in animal studies; advisability of using contraception
  Breast-feeding—Not recommended because of potential risks to the infant
  Other medical problems, especially porphyria

### Proper use of this medication
» Proper dosing

### Precautions while using this medication
» Possibility of ocular sensitivity to sunlight or other bright lights, including vehicle headlights; using dark sunglasses as protection
» Avoiding exposure of skin to sunlight and other bright lights (e.g., indoor lamps without shades) for 30 days after administration because of the risk of dermal photosensitivity reactions; sunscreen products will not protect against such reactions
» Not avoiding exposure to ambient indoor light, which helps to clear porfimer from the skin
» After 30 days, testing skin for residual photosensitivity by exposing a small skin area (not facial) to sunlight for 10 minutes; if blistering, reddening, or swelling occurs, continuing to avoid sunlight and bright lights for an additional 2 weeks, then testing again
  Retesting before full exposure to sunlight after traveling to an area with stronger sunlight than at home, even after testing has demonstrated disappearance of residual photosensitivity to usual levels of sunlight

### Side/adverse effects
Signs of dermal or ocular photosensitivity reactions, which may occur at any time within 30 days after treatment
Signs of other potential side effects, especially:
  For esophageal carcinoma patients—Abdominal pain; anemia; candidiasis; cardiovascular effects, including atrial fibrillation and heart failure; chest pain; coughing; dyspnea; edema; esophageal edema; fever; hypertension; hypotension; pleural effusion; pneumonia; urinary tract infection; angina pectoris; bronchospasm or pulmonary edema; esophageal perforation; gastric ulcer; ileus; jaundice; peritonitis; and respiratory failure (depending on location of tumor)
  For lung carcinoma patients—Endobronchial stricture; hemoptysis; mucositis; coughing; dysphagia; and endobronchial ulceration

## General Dosing Information

Patients receiving porfimer should be under the supervision of a physician experienced in photodynamic therapy with porfimer and light delivery devices.

If photodynamic therapy is being used prior to or following radiation therapy, sufficient time should elapse between the two treatments to allow the inflammation induced by the earlier treatment to subside. After completion of photodynamic therapy, radiation therapy may commence after a delay of 2 to 4 weeks. After completion of radiation therapy, a delay of 4 weeks before institution of photodynamic therapy is recommended.

Prior to initiation of a new course of porfimer photodynamic therapy for esophageal carcinoma, the patient should be examined for the presence of either bronchoesophageal or tracheoesophageal fistula.

Care should be taken to avoid extravasation. If extravasation occurs during intravenous administration, the area surrounding the injection site should be protected from light for approximately 30 days.

Porfimer may cause photosensitivity reactions for approximately 30 days after administration; therefore, caution should be exercised to avoid exposure of skin and eyes to direct sunlight and bright indoor light (dental lights, operating room lights, unshaded light bulbs at close proximity). Porfimer is slowly and safely inactivated by ambient indoor light by means of a photobleaching reaction; therefore, patients should avoid spending long periods of time in darkened rooms and should expose themselves to ambient indoor light.

Before exposing any skin to bright lights or direct sunlight, patients should test themselves for residual photosensitivity by exposing a small portion of their skin to sunlight for 10 minutes. If erythema, blistering, or edema of the skin does not occur within 24 hours, patients may slowly increase their exposure to bright lights or sunlight. If a photosensitivity reaction occurs at the test site, patients should continue to avoid bright lights or sunlight exposure for an additional 2 weeks, when skin testing should be repeated. Facial skin should not be used for photosensitivity testing because skin surrounding the eyes may be more sensitive. Patients traveling to geographic locations that have increased sunlight levels should retest their photosensitivity level.

Ultraviolet sunscreens offer no protection against a photosensitivity reaction because porfimer is activated by visible light.

Ocular sensitivity to sunlight or other bright lights (including vehicle headlights) can occur. When outside, patients should wear dark sunglasses that transmit less than 4% of white light for approximately 30 days following intravenous administration of porfimer.

### For treatment of adverse effects

For substernal chest pain in patients being treated for esophageal carcinoma: Short-term treatment with an opioid analgesic may be required.

For airway obstruction in patients being treated for non–small cell lung carcinoma (NSCLC): Mucus plugs may be removed via bronchoscopy, using suction or forceps.

For endobronchial stricture in patients being treated for NSCLC: Stent placement may be required.

### Safety considerations for handling this medication

It is recommended that skin and eye contact be avoided because porfimer may be a skin and eye irritant in the presence of bright light. Exposed personnel should follow the recommendations for the treatment and prevention of photosensitivity reactions.

The use of disposable surgical gloves and eye protection is recommended.

Porfimer spills may be wiped up with a damp cloth. It is recommended that all contaminated materials be disposed of in a polyethylene bag, according to local regulations for handling hazardous materials.

## Parenteral Dosage Forms

### PORFIMER SODIUM FOR INJECTION

**Usual adult dose**
Esophageal carcinoma or
Non–small cell lung carcinoma—
  Intravenous, 2 mg per kg of body weight, injected slowly (over three to five minutes), followed by illumination with laser light and debridement of tumor at appropriate intervals.

Note: Photodynamic treatment with porfimer may be given for a total of three courses of therapy, each separated by at least thirty days.

Administration of a course of porfimer photodynamic therapy occurs in two stages. In the first stage of therapy, porfimer is administered by slow intravenous injection over a period of three to five minutes. The second stage of therapy begins forty to fifty hours later, and consists of the application of a 630 nanometer wavelength laser light to the tumor. Debridement of esophageal tumors should be performed two days later, and debridement of endobronchial tumors should be performed two to three days later. A second application of laser light may be commenced 96 to 120 hours after the first laser light treatment. The tumor should be debrided before the second light treatment, but additional porfimer is not given.

The total light dose determines the extent of the photoactivation of porfimer. For esophageal carcinoma, a dose of 300 joules per centimeter of tumor length, over a period of twelve minutes and thirty seconds, is recommended. For lung carcinoma, a dose of 200 joules per centimeter of tumor length, administered over eight minutes and twenty seconds, is recommended. The laser light is delivered to a tumor by cylindrical fiberoptic diffusers passed through an endoscope.

**Usual pediatric dose**
Safety and efficacy have not been established.

**Usual geriatric dose**
See *Usual adult dose*.

**Strength(s) usually available**
U.S.—
  75 mg (single-dose vial) (Rx) [*Photofrin*].

**Packaging and storage**
Store between 20 and 25 °C (68 and 77 °F).

**Preparation of dosage form**
Porfimer sodium for injection is reconstituted for intravenous administration by adding 31.8 mL of 5% dextrose injection or 0.9% sodium chloride injection to the 75-mg vial, producing a concentration of 2.5 mg per mL.

**Stability**
After reconstitution, porfimer for injection should be protected from bright light and used immediately.

Developed: 04/8/97
Revised: 07/02/98

---

**POTASSIUM ACETATE**—See *Potassium Supplements (Systemic)*

---

**POTASSIUM BICARBONATE**—See *Potassium Supplements (Systemic)*

---

**POTASSIUM BICARBONATE AND POTASSIUM CHLORIDE**—See *Potassium Supplements (Systemic)*

---

**POTASSIUM BICARBONATE AND POTASSIUM CITRATE**—See *Potassium Supplements (Systemic)*

---

**POTASSIUM BITARTRATE AND SODIUM BICARBONATE**—See *Laxatives (Local)*

---

**POTASSIUM CHLORIDE**—See *Potassium Supplements (Systemic)*

---

**POTASSIUM CITRATE**—See *Citrates (Systemic)*

---

**POTASSIUM CITRATE AND CITRIC ACID**—See *Citrates (Systemic)*

---

**POTASSIUM CITRATE AND SODIUM CITRATE**—See *Citrates Systemic*

---

**POTASSIUM GLUCONATE**—See *Potassium Supplements (Systemic)*

---

**POTASSIUM GLUCONATE AND POTASSIUM CHLORIDE**—See *Potassium Supplements (Systemic)*

---

**POTASSIUM GLUCONATE AND POTASSIUM CITRATE**—See *Potassium Supplements (Systemic)*

---

# POTASSIUM IODIDE    Systemic

VA CLASSIFICATION (Primary/Secondary): HS852/AD900; AM700; TN499

Commonly used brand name(s): *Pima; Thyro-Block*.

Other commonly used names are KI and SSKI.

Note: For a listing of dosage forms and brand names by country availability, see *Dosage Forms* section(s).

## Category
Antihyperthyroid agent; radiation protectant (thyroid gland); thyroid inhibitor; antifungal (systemic); iodine replenisher.

## Indications
Note: Bracketed information in the *Indications* section refers to uses that are not included in U.S. product labeling.

**Accepted**

Hyperthyroidism (treatment)[1]—Potassium iodide is indicated in the treatment of hyperthyroidism.

Radiation protection, thyroid gland—Potassium iodide is indicated as a radiation protectant (thyroid gland) prior to and following oral administration or inhalation of radioactive isotopes of iodine or in radiation emergencies.

[Erythema nodosum (treatment)][1]—Potassium iodide is used in the treatment of erythema nodosum.

[Iodine deficiency (treatment)][1]—Potassium iodide is used in the treatment of iodine deficiency.

[Sporotrichosis, cutaneous lymphatic (treatment)][1]—Potassium iodide is used in the treatment of cutaneous lymphatic sporotrichosis.

[Thyroid involution, preoperative][1]—Potassium iodide is used concurrently with an antithyroid agent to induce thyroid involution prior to thyroidectomy.

**Unaccepted**

Potassium iodide has not been shown to have a clinically significant expectorant action.

[1]Not included in Canadian product labeling.

## Pharmacology/Pharmacokinetics

**Physicochemical characteristics**
Molecular weight—166.00.

**Mechanism of action/Effect**
Antihyperthyroid agent—
  In hyperthyroid patients, potassium iodide produces rapid remission of symptoms by inhibiting the release of thyroid hormone into the circulation. The effects of potassium iodide on the thyroid gland

include reduction of vascularity, a firming of the glandular tissue, shrinkage of the size of individual cells, reaccumulation of colloid in the follicles, and increases in bound iodine. These actions may facilitate thyroidectomy when the medication is given prior to surgery.

Radiation protectant—
When administered prior to and following administration of radioactive isotopes and in radiation emergencies involving the release of radioactive iodine, potassium iodide protects the thyroid gland by blocking the thyroidal uptake of radioactive isotopes of iodine.

When potassium iodide is administered simultaneously with radiation exposure, the protectant effect is approximately 97%. Potassium iodide given 12 and 24 hours before exposure yields a 90% and 70% protectant effect, respectively. However, potassium iodide administered 1 and 3 hours after exposure results in an 85% and 50% protectant effect, respectively. Potassium iodide administered more than 6 hours after exposure is thought to have a negligible protectant effect.

## Precautions to Consider

### Pregnancy/Reproduction
Potassium iodide crosses the placenta; use during pregnancy may result in abnormal thyroid function and/or goiter in the infant.

### Breast-feeding
Potassium iodide is distributed into breast milk; use by nursing mothers may cause skin rash and thyroid suppression in the infant.

### Pediatrics
Potassium iodide may cause skin rash and thyroid suppression in infants. Appropriate studies have not been performed for use as a systemic antifungal.

### Geriatrics
Appropriate studies on the relationship of age to the effects of potassium iodide have not been performed in the geriatric population. However, geriatrics-specific problems that would limit the usefulness of this medication in the elderly are not expected.

### Dental
Potassium iodide may cause salivary gland swelling or tenderness, burning of mouth or throat, metallic taste, soreness of teeth and gums, and unusual increase in salivation.

### Drug interactions and/or related problems
The following drug interactions and/or related problems have been selected on the basis of their potential clinical significance (possible mechanism in parentheses where appropriate)—not necessarily inclusive (» = major clinical significance):

Note: Combinations containing any of the following medications, depending on the amount present, may also interact with this medication.

» Antithyroid agents
(concurrent use of these medications with potassium iodide may potentiate the hypothyroid and goitrogenic effects of antithyroid agents or potassium iodide; baseline thyroid status should be determined at periodic intervals to detect changes in the thyroid-pituitary response)

Captopril or
Enalapril or
Lisinopril
(concurrent use of captopril, enalapril, or lisinopril with potassium iodide may result in hyperkalemia; serum potassium concentrations should be monitored)

» Diuretics, potassium-sparing
(concurrent use with potassium iodide may increase the effects of potassium, possibly resulting in hyperkalemia and cardiac arrhythmias or cardiac arrest; serum potassium concentrations should be monitored)

» Lithium
(concurrent use with potassium iodide may potentiate the hypothyroid and goitrogenic effects of either medication; baseline thyroid status should be determined at periodic intervals to detect changes in the thyroid-pituitary response)

Sodium iodide I 131, therapeutic
(potassium iodide may decrease thyroidal uptake of I 131)

### Laboratory value alterations
The following have been selected on the basis of their potential clinical significance (possible effect in parentheses where appropriate)—not necessarily inclusive (» = major clinical significance):

With diagnostic test results
Thyroid function studies
Thyroid imaging, radionuclide and
Thyroid uptake tests
(potassium iodide may decrease thyroidal uptake of I 131, I 123, and sodium pertechnetate Tc 99m)

### Medical considerations/Contraindications
The medical considerations/contraindications included have been selected on the basis of their potential clinical significance (reasons given in parentheses where appropriate)—not necessarily inclusive (» = major clinical significance).

*Risk-benefit should be considered when the following medical problems exist:*

» Hyperkalemia
(condition may be exacerbated)

Hyperthyroidism (for use other than thyroid inhibitor)
(prolonged use of iodine may cause thyroid gland hyperplasia, thyroid adenoma, goiter, or hypothyroidism)

Myotonia congenita
(condition may be exacerbated by potassium)

» Renal function impairment
(may cause excessive serum potassium concentrations)

Sensitivity to potassium iodide

Tuberculosis
(may cause irritation and increase secretions)

### Patient monitoring
The following may be especially important in patient monitoring (other tests may be warranted in some patients, depending on condition; » = major clinical significance):

Serum potassium concentrations
(recommended at periodic intervals during therapy in patients with renal function impairment)

## Side/Adverse Effects

The following side/adverse effects have been selected on the basis of their potential clinical significance (possible signs and symptoms in parentheses where appropriate)—not necessarily inclusive:

### Those indicating need for medical attention
Incidence less frequent
*Allergic reactions, specifically angioedema* (swelling of the arms, face, legs, lips, tongue, and/or throat); *arthralgia* (joint pain); *eosinophilia; swelling of lymph nodes; urticaria* (hives)

With prolonged use
*Iodism* (burning of mouth or throat; gastric irritation; increased watering of mouth; metallic taste; severe headache; skin lesions; soreness of teeth and gums; symptoms of head cold); *potassium toxicity* (confusion; irregular heartbeat; numbness, tingling, pain, or weakness in hands or feet; unusual tiredness; weakness or heaviness of legs)

### Those indicating need for medical attention only if they continue or are bothersome
Incidence less frequent
*Diarrhea; nausea or vomiting; stomach pain*

## Patient Consultation

As an aid to patient consultation, refer to *Advice for the Patient, Potassium Iodide (Systemic)*.

In providing consultation, consider emphasizing the following selected information (» = major clinical significance):

### Before using this medication
» Conditions affecting use, especially:
Sensitivity to iodine or potassium iodide
Pregnancy—May cause thyroid problems or goiter in the newborn infant
Breast-feeding—May cause skin rash and thyroid problems in nursing babies
Use in children—May cause skin rash and thyroid problems in nursing infants
Dental—May cause swelling of salivary glands, burning of mouth or throat, metallic taste, soreness of teeth and gums, or increase in salivation
Other medications, especially antithyroid agents, diuretics (potassium sparing), or lithium
Other medical problems, especially hyperkalemia or renal function impairment

## Potassium Iodide (Systemic)

**Proper use of this medication**
» Taking after meals or with food or milk to minimize gastrointestinal irritation
*Proper administration technique for oral liquids:*
  Taking medication by mouth even if dispensed in a dropper bottle
  Not using if solution turns brownish yellow
  Taking medication in a full glass (240 mL) of water or in fruit juice, milk, or broth to improve taste and lessen gastric upset; drinking full dose
  If crystals form in solution, warming closed container in warm water and gently shaking container
*Proper administration technique for uncoated tablets:*
  Dissolving each tablet in ½ glass (120 mL) of water or milk before taking; drinking full dose
» Compliance with full course of therapy (fungal infections)
» Proper dosing
  Missed dose: Taking as soon as possible; not taking if almost time for next dose; not doubling doses
» Proper storage
*For use as a radiation protectant (thyroid gland)*
  Taking medication only upon instructions from state or local health authorities
» Taking medication daily for 10 days, unless otherwise instructed; not taking more medication or more often than instructed

**Precautions while using this medication**
Regular visits to physician to check progress during therapy
» Caution in patients on potassium-restricted diet

**Side/adverse effects**
Signs of potential side effects, especially allergic reactions, iodism, or potassium toxicity

## General Dosing Information

The potassium content is 6 mEq (234 mg) per gram of potassium iodide.

To minimize stomach upset, the medication may be administered after meals and at bedtime with food or milk.

To protect against possible gastrointestinal injury, which has been associated with the oral ingestion of concentrated potassium salt preparations, it is recommended that the oral solution be administered in a full glass (240 mL) of water, or in fruit juice, milk, or broth. It is also recommended that each regular tablet be dissolved in ½ glass (120 mL) of water or milk before ingestion.

Prolonged use may result in hypothyroidism, parotitis, iodism, and, particularly in postpubescent patients, acneiform skin lesions.

## Oral Dosage Forms

Note: Bracketed uses in the *Dosage Forms* section refer to categories of use and/or indications that are not included in U.S. product labeling.

### POTASSIUM IODIDE ORAL SOLUTION USP

**Usual adult and adolescent dose**
Antihyperthyroid agent[1]—
  Oral, 250 mg three times a day.
Radiation protectant (thyroid gland)—
  Oral, 100 to 150 mg twenty-four hours prior to and once a day for three to ten days following administration of, or exposure to, radioactive isotopes of iodine.
[Antifungal (systemic)][1]—
  Oral, 600 mg three times a day, the dosage being increased by 60 mg at each dose until the maximum tolerated dose is reached.
[Iodine replenisher][1]—
  Oral, 5 to 10 mg per day.
[Thyroid inhibitor—Thyroid involution, preoperative][1]: Prior to thyroidectomy—
  Oral, 5 drops of a 1-gram-per-mL solution (approximately 250 mg) three times a day for ten days before surgery, usually administered concurrently with an antithyroid agent.

**Usual adult prescribing limits**
Up to 12 grams daily.

**Usual pediatric dose**
Radiation protectant (thyroid gland)—
  Infants up to 1 year of age: Oral, 65 mg once a day for ten days following administration of, or exposure to, radioactive isotopes of iodine.
  Infants and children 1 year of age and older: Oral, 130 mg once a day for ten days following administration of, or exposure to, radioactive isotopes of iodine.
[Antifungal (systemic)][1]—
  Dosage has not been established.
[Iodine replenisher][1]—
  Oral, 1 mg per day.
[Thyroid inhibitor—Thyroid involution, preoperative][1]—
  See *Usual adult and adolescent dose.*

**Strength(s) usually available**
U.S.—
  1 gram per mL (Rx) [GENERIC].

**Packaging and storage**
Store below 40 °C (104 °F), preferably between 15 and 30 °C (59 and 86 °F), unless otherwise specified by manufacturer. Store in a tight, light-resistant container. Protect from freezing.

**Stability**
Crystallization may occur under normal conditions of storage, especially if refrigerated; however, on warming and shaking, the crystals will redissolve.

Free iodine may be liberated by oxidation of the potassium iodide, causing the solution to turn brownish yellow in color. If this occurs, the solution should be discarded.

**Auxiliary labeling**
• For oral use only.
• Do not refrigerate.
• Continue medicine for full time of treatment (antifungal).

### POTASSIUM IODIDE SYRUP

**Usual adult and adolescent dose**
Radiation protectant (thyroid gland)—
  Oral, 100 to 150 mg twenty-four hours prior to and once a day for three to ten days following administration of, or exposure to, radioactive isotopes of iodine.
[Antifungal (systemic)][1]—
  Oral, 600 mg three times a day, the dosage being increased by 60 mg at each dose until the maximum tolerated dose is reached.
[Iodine replenisher][1]—
  Oral, 5 to 10 mg per day.
[Thyroid inhibitor—Thyroid involution, preoperative][1]: Prior to thyroidectomy—
  Oral, 4 mL (approximately 260 mg) three times a day for ten days before surgery, usually administered concurrently with an antithyroid agent.

**Usual adult prescribing limits**
Up to 12 grams daily.

**Usual pediatric dose**
Radiation protectant (thyroid gland)—
  Infants up to 1 year of age: Oral, 65 mg once a day for ten days following administration of, or exposure to, radioactive isotopes of iodine.
  Infants and children 1 year of age and older: Oral, 130 mg once a day for ten days following administration of, or exposure to, radioactive isotopes of iodine.
[Antifungal (systemic)][1]—
  Dosage has not been established.
[Iodine replenisher][1]—
  Oral, 1 mg per day.
[Thyroid inhibitor—Thyroid involution, preoperative][1]—
  See *Usual adult and adolescent dose.*

**Strength(s) usually available**
U.S.—
  325 mg per 5 mL (Rx) [*Pima*].

**Packaging and storage**
Store below 40 °C (104 °F), preferably between 15 and 30 °C (59 and 86 °F), in a well-closed container, unless otherwise specified by manufacturer. Protect from freezing.

**Auxiliary labeling**
• For oral use only.
• Continue medicine for full time of treatment (for 3-day uncinariasis treatment).

Note: When dispensing, include a calibrated liquid-measuring device.

### POTASSIUM IODIDE TABLETS USP

**Usual adult and adolescent dose**
Radiation protectant (thyroid gland)—
  Oral, 100 to 150 mg twenty-four hours prior to and once a day for three to ten days following administration of, or exposure to, radioactive isotopes of iodine.
[Antifungal (systemic)][1]—
  Oral, 600 mg three times a day, the dosage being increased by 60 mg at each dose until the maximum tolerated dose is reached.

[Iodine replenisher][1]—
   Oral, 5 to 10 mg per day.
[Thyroid inhibitor—Thyroid involution, preoperative][1]: Prior to thyroidectomy—
   Oral, Dissolve 2 tablets (approximately 260 mg) in 1 glassful of water, three times a day for ten days before surgery, usually administered concurrently with an antithyroid agent.

**Usual adult prescribing limits**
Up to 12 grams daily.

**Usual pediatric dose**
Radiation protectant (thyroid gland)—
   Infants up to 1 year of age: Oral, 65 mg once a day for ten days following administration of, or exposure to, radioactive isotopes of iodine.
   Infants and children 1 year of age and older: Oral, 130 mg once a day for ten days following administration of, or exposure to, radioactive isotopes of iodine.
[Antifungal (systemic)][1]—
   Dosage has not been established.
[Iodine replenisher][1]—
   Oral, 1 mg per day.
[Thyroid inhibitor—Thyroid involution, preoperative][1]—
   See *Usual adult and adolescent dose*.

**Strength(s) usually available**
U.S.—
   Not commercially available; however, potassium iodide tablets are available to government and public health organizations for use in radiation emergencies.
Canada—
   130 mg (Rx) [*Thyro-Block*].

**Packaging and storage**
Store below 40 °C (104 °F), preferably between 15 and 30 °C (59 and 86 °F), unless otherwise specified by manufacturer. Store in a tight container.

**Auxiliary labeling**
• Dissolve in liquid before taking.
• Continue medicine for full time of treatment (for 3-day uncinariasis treatment).

## POTASSIUM IODIDE TABLETS (ENTERIC-COATED) USP

Note: Enteric-coated potassium iodide tablets are not recommended since the administration of this dosage form has been associated with small bowel lesions, which can cause obstruction, hemorrhage, perforation, and possibly death.

**Strength(s) usually available**
U.S.—
   300 mg (Rx) [GENERIC].

[1]Not included in Canadian product labeling.

Revised: 04/14/92
Interim revision: 08/26/94

## POTASSIUM PHOSPHATES—See *Phosphates (Systemic)*

## POTASSIUM AND SODIUM PHOSPHATES—See *Phosphates (Systemic)*

# POTASSIUM SUPPLEMENTS   Systemic

This monograph includes information on the following: 1) Potassium Acetate†; 2) Potassium Bicarbonate; 3) Potassium Bicarbonate and Potassium Chloride; 4) Potassium Bicarbonate and Potassium Citrate†; 5) Potassium Chloride; 6) Potassium Gluconate; 7) Potassium Gluconate and Potassium Chloride†; 8) Potassium Gluconate and Potassium Citrate†; 9) Trikates†.

VA CLASSIFICATION (Primary): TN403

Commonly used brand name(s): *Apo-K*[5]; *Cena-K*[5]; *Effer-K*[4]; *Gen-K*[5]; *Glu-K*[6]; *K+10*[5]; *K+Care*[5]; *K+Care ET*[2]; *K-10*[5]; *K-8*[5]; *K-Dur*[5]; *K-Electrolyte*[2]; *K-G Elixir*[6]; *K-Ide*[2]; *K-Lease*[5]; *K-Long*[5]; *K-Lor*[5]; *K-Lyte*[2]; *K-Lyte DS*[4]; *K-Lyte/Cl*[3]; *K-Lyte/Cl 50*[3]; *K-Lyte/Cl Powder*[5]; *K-Med 900*[5]; *K-Norm*[5]; *K-Sol*[5]; *K-Tab*[5]; *K-Vescent*[2]; *KCL 5%*[5]; *Kalium Durules*[5]; *Kaochlor 10%*[5]; *Kaochlor S-F 10%*[5]; *Kaochlor-10*[5]; *Kaochlor-20*[5]; *Kaon*[6]; *Kaon-Cl*[5]; *Kaon-Cl 20% Liquid*[5]; *Kaon-Cl-10*[5]; *Kato*[5]; *Kay Ciel*[5]; *Kaylixir*[6]; *Klor-Con 10*[5]; *Klor-Con 8*[5]; *Klor-Con Powder*[5]; *Klor-Con/25 Powder*[5]; *Klor-Con/EF*[2]; *Klorvess*[3]; *Klorvess 10% Liquid*[5]; *Klorvess Effervescent Granules*[3]; *Klotrix*[5]; *Kolyum*[7]; *Micro-K*[5]; *Micro-K 10*[5]; *Micro-K LS*[5]; *Neo-K*[3]; *Potasalan*[5]; *Potassium-Rougier*[6]; *Potassium-Sandoz*[3]; *Roychlor-10%*[5]; *Rum-K*[5]; *Slow-K*[5]; *Ten-K*[5]; *Tri-K*[9]; *Twin-K*[8].

Another commonly used name in the U.S. for trikates is potassium triplex.

Note:   For a listing of dosage forms and brand names by country availability, see *Dosage Forms* section(s).

†Not commercially available in Canada.

## Category
Antihypokalemic; electrolyte replenisher.

## Indications

**Accepted**
Hypokalemia (treatment)—Potassium supplements are indicated in patients with hypokalemia, with or without metabolic alkalosis; in chronic digitalis intoxication; and in patients with hypokalemic familial periodic paralysis. Potassium supplementation is indicated in severe hypokalemia in patients receiving potassium-wasting diuretics for uncomplicated essential hypertension, when dosage adjustment of the diuretic is ineffective or unwarranted. Potassium supplementation may be needed in patients receiving antibiotics that cause potassium depletion, either by drug-induced nephrotoxicity (e.g., amphotericin B, polymyxin B, or gentamicin) or by a nonreabsorbable anion effect (e.g., azlocillin, carbenicillin, mezlocillin, penicillin, piperacillin, or ticarcillin). Potassium chloride is usually the salt of choice in the treatment of hypokalemia, since it is better absorbed from the gastrointestinal tract than the non-chloride potassium salts, and the chloride ion may be required to correct hypochloremia, which often occurs with hypokalemia. In rare circumstances (e.g., patients with renal tubular acidosis), potassium depletion may be associated with metabolic acidosis and hyperchloremia. In such patients, potassium replacement should be accomplished with potassium salts other than chloride, such as potassium acetate, potassium bicarbonate, potassium citrate, or potassium gluconate.

Hypokalemia (prophylaxis)—Potassium supplements are indicated to prevent hypokalemia in patients who would be at particular risk if hypokalemia were to develop (e.g., digitalized patients with significant cardiac arrhythmias). Potassium depletion will occur when the rate of loss through renal excretion and/or loss from the gastrointestinal tract exceeds the rate of potassium intake. Potassium supplements may also be indicated in patients who suffer from hepatic cirrhosis with ascites; states of aldosterone excess with normal renal function; certain diarrheal states, including those induced by chronic laxative use; prolonged vomiting; Bartter's syndrome; potassium-losing nephropathy; and in patients, including children, on long-term corticosteroid therapy.

Deficiency of potassium may lead to muscle weakness, irregular heartbeat, mood or mental changes, or nausea or vomiting.

**Acceptance not established**
There are insufficient data to show that potassium supplementation lowers *blood pressure* in hypertensive patients.

**Unaccepted**
Enteric-coated tablets of potassium chloride are no longer recommended for use because of the high incidence of severe injury to adjacent gastrointestinal tissues during tablet dissolution.

## Pharmacology/Pharmacokinetics

**Physicochemical characteristics**
Molecular weight—
   Potassium acetate: 98.14.
   Potassium bicarbonate: 100.12.
   Potassium chloride: 74.55.
   Potassium citrate: 324.41.
   Potassium gluconate: 234.25.

## Mechanism of action/Effect
Potassium is the predominant cation (approximately 150 to 160 mEq per liter) within cells. Intracellular sodium content is relatively low. In extracellular fluid, sodium predominates and the potassium content is low (3.5 to 5 mEq per liter). A membrane-bound enzyme, sodium-potassium–activated adenosinetriphosphatase (Na$^+$K$^+$ ATPase), actively transports or pumps sodium out and potassium into cells to maintain these concentration gradients. The intracellular to extracellular potassium gradients are necessary for the conduction of nerve impulses in such specialized tissues as the heart, brain, and skeletal muscle, and for the maintenance of normal renal function and acid-base balance. High intracellular potassium concentrations are necessary for numerous cellular metabolic processes.

## Elimination
Renal—90%.
Fecal—10%.

# Precautions to Consider

## Carcinogenicity
No data are available on long-term potential for carcinogenicity in animals or humans. Potassium is a normal dietary constituent.

## Pregnancy/Reproduction
Pregnancy—Studies have not been done in humans.
Studies have not been done in animals.
FDA Pregnancy Category C.

## Breast-feeding
Problems in humans have not been documented.

## Pediatrics
Appropriate studies on the relationship of age to the effects of potassium supplements have not been performed in the pediatric population. However, no pediatrics-specific problems have been documented to date.

## Geriatrics
Although appropriate studies on the relationship of age to the effects of potassium supplements have not been performed in the geriatric population, no geriatrics-specific problems have been sufficiently documented to date. However, elderly patients are at greater risk of developing hyperkalemia due to age-related changes in the ability of the kidneys to excrete potassium.

## Drug interactions and/or related problems
The following drug interactions and/or related problems have been selected on the basis of their potential clinical significance (possible mechanism in parentheses where appropriate)—not necessarily inclusive (» = major clinical significance):

Note: Combinations containing any of the following, depending on the amount present, may also interact with this medication.

Amphotericin B or
Corticosteroids, glucocorticoid, especially with significant mineralocorticoid activity or
Corticosteroids, mineralocorticoid or
Corticotropin (ACTH) or
Gentamicin or
Penicillins (including azlocillin, carbenicillin, mezlocillin, piperacillin, ticarcillin) or
Polymyxin B
(potassium requirements may be increased in patients receiving these medications, due to renal potassium wasting; close monitoring of serum potassium is recommended)

» Angiotensin-converting enzyme (ACE) inhibitors or
» Anti-inflammatory drugs, nonsteroidal (NSAIDs) or
» Beta-adrenergic blocking agents or
Blood from blood bank (may contain up to 30 mEq of potassium per liter of plasma or up to 65 mEq per liter of whole blood when stored for more than 10 days) or
Cyclosporine or
» Diuretics, potassium-sparing or
» Heparin or
» Low-salt milk or
Potassium-containing medications, other or
Salt substitutes
(concurrent use with potassium supplements may increase serum potassium concentrations, which may cause severe hyperkalemia and lead to cardiac arrest, especially in renal insufficiency; low-salt milk may contain up to 60 mEq of potassium per liter and most salt substitutes contain substantial amounts of potassium; in addition, use of NSAIDs in combination with potassium supplements may increase the risk of gastrointestinal side effects)

» Anticholinergics or other medications with anticholinergic activity (See *Appendix II*)
(concurrent use with potassium chloride oral supplements, especially solid dosage forms, may increase severity of gastrointestinal lesions produced by potassium chloride alone; if symptoms develop, patients should be carefully monitored endoscopically for evidence of lesions)

Calcium salts, parenteral
(potassium supplements should be used cautiously in patients receiving parenteral calcium salts because of the danger of precipitating cardiac arrhythmias)

» Digitalis glycosides, in the presence of heart block
(potassium supplements are not recommended for concurrent use in digitalized patients with severe or complete heart block; however, if potassium supplements must be used to prevent or correct hypokalemia in digitalized patients, careful monitoring of serum potassium concentrations is extremely important)

» Diuretics, thiazide
(increased risk of hyperkalemia when a potassium-wasting diuretic is discontinued after concurrent use with a potassium supplement)

Exchange resins, sodium cycle, such as sodium polystyrene sulfonate
(whether these medications are administered orally or rectally, serum potassium concentrations are reduced by sodium replacement of the potassium; fluid retention may occur in some patients because of the increased sodium intake)

Insulin or
Sodium bicarbonate
(concurrent use of these medications decreases serum potassium concentration by promoting a shift of potassium ion into the cells)

Laxatives
(chronic use or overuse of laxatives may reduce serum potassium concentrations by promoting excessive potassium loss from the intestinal tract)

## Medical considerations/Contraindications
The medical considerations/contraindications included have been selected on the basis of their potential clinical significance (reasons given in parentheses where appropriate)—not necessarily inclusive (» = major clinical significance).

Except under special circumstances, this medication should not be used when hyperkalemia exists, because further increases in serum potassium may cause cardiac arrest.

*Risk-benefit should be considered when the following medical problems exist:*

*For potassium acetate only*
Alkalosis, metabolic or respiratory
(acetate is a precursor to bicarbonate, which may exacerbate the condition)

*For all potassium supplements*
» Diarrhea, prolonged or severe, resulting in severe dehydration
(the loss of fluid in combination with use of potassium supplements may cause renal toxicity, which may increase the risk of hyperkalemia; if potassium supplements are given in the presence of diarrhea, serum potassium should be monitored)

» Esophageal compression or
» Gastric emptying, delayed or
» Intestinal obstruction or stricture or
» Peptic ulcer
(delayed passage of potassium supplements through the gastrointestinal tract may cause or worsen gastrointestinal irritation, especially with solid dosage forms)

» Familial periodic paralysis or
Myotonia congenita
(potassium supplements may aggravate these conditions, although some patients with familial periodic paralysis may require potassium supplementation)

» Heart block, severe or complete
(increased risk of hyperkalemia, especially in digitalized patients; careful monitoring of serum potassium concentrations is recommended)

» Hyperkalemia, or conditions predisposing to hyperkalemia, such as:
Acidosis, metabolic, acute
Adrenal insufficiency
Dehydration, acute
Diabetes mellitus, uncontrolled
Physical exercise, strenuous, in unconditioned persons
Renal failure, chronic

Tissue breakdown, extensive
(increased serum potassium concentrations possibly leading to cardiac arrest may occur; exercise-induced hyperkalemia is transient and is a problem only in patients with renal insufficiency from dehydration or those taking medications that increase serum potassium)
Sensitivity to potassium

**Patient monitoring**
The following may be especially important in patient monitoring (other tests may be warranted in some patients, depending on condition; » = major clinical significance):

Electrocardiograms (ECG) and
Potassium concentrations, serum and
Renal function determinations, especially serum creatinine and urine output
(monitoring recommended at periodic intervals during oral therapy; recommended concurrently during parenteral therapy)
Magnesium concentrations, serum
(determinations recommended in patients with refractory hypokalemia; coexisting magnesium depletion may need correction to replenish serum potassium and/or cell potassium concentrations)
pH determinations, serum
(used to help determine existence of acidosis or alkalosis and thus allow improved interpretation of serum potassium measurements; utilized more often during parenteral therapy)

## Side/Adverse Effects

The following side/adverse effects have been selected on the basis of their potential clinical significance (possible signs and symptoms in parentheses where appropriate)—not necessarily inclusive:

**Those indicating need for medical attention**
Incidence less frequent
*Hyperkalemia* (confusion; irregular or slow heartbeat; numbness or tingling in hands, feet, or lips; shortness of breath or difficult breathing; unexplained anxiety; unusual tiredness or weakness; weakness or heaviness of legs)
Note: *Hyperkalemia* side effects are considered rare when oral dosage forms of potassium are administered to patients having normal renal function. When hyperkalemia is present, severe muscle weakness and a slow, irregular heartbeat are the most common symptoms. When the medication is administered parenterally, the incidence of irregular heartbeat (arrhythmias) may become more frequent.
Irregular heartbeat is usually the earliest clinical indication of hyperkalemia and is readily detected by ECG.
Incidence rare
*Irritation, contact, of the alimentary tract* (continuing abdominal or stomach pain, cramping, or soreness; chest or throat pain, especially when swallowing; stools containing fresh or digested blood)
Note: *Irritation of the alimentary tract* may occur when potassium is in contact with ulcerous areas, or when there is a high concentration of potassium in one area; the latter has resulted from improper release from oral dosage form, or from delayed passage of the dosage form through the alimentary tract.

**Those indicating need for medical attention only if they continue or are bothersome**
Incidence more frequent
*For oral dosage forms*
**Diarrhea; nausea; stomach pain, discomfort, or gas, mild; vomiting**
Note: These side effects occur more frequently when the medication is not taken with food or is not diluted properly.

## Patient Consultation

As an aid to patient consultation, refer to *Advice for the Patient, Potassium Supplements (Systemic).*
In providing consultation, consider emphasizing the following selected information (» = major clinical significance):

**Description of use**
Description should include function in the body; signs of deficiency

**Importance of diet**
Importance of proper nutrition
Potassium content of selected foods
Recommended daily intake for potassium
Not exceeding recommended amounts of potassium

**Before using this medication**
» Conditions affecting use, especially:
Sensitivity to potassium
Use in the elderly—Risk of developing hyperkalemia due to age-related changes in ability of kidneys to excrete potassium
Other medications, especially beta adrenergic blocking agents, nonsteroidal anti-inflammatory drugs, anticholinergics, potassium-sparing and thiazide diuretics, low-salt milk, other potassium-containing medications, ACE inhibitors, digitalis glycosides, or heparin
Other medical problems, especially delayed gastric emptying, esophageal compression, or intestinal obstruction or stricture, peptic ulcer; heart block; hyperkalemia or conditions predisposing to hyperkalemia for all potassium supplements; metabolic or respiratory acidosis for potassium acetate

**Proper use of this medication**
*Proper administration technique*
Necessary dilution of liquid dosage forms
Taking tablets and capsules with adequate liquids
Complete dissolution of effervescent dosage forms prior to taking
Not using tomato juice for dilution if on a sodium-restricted diet
Not crushing or chewing extended-release dosage forms, unless otherwise directed
Sprinkling contents of some extended-release capsules and some tablets over soft food such as applesauce or mixing with fruit juice, if unable to swallow whole, but only when directed to do so
» Taking each dose immediately after a meal or with food
» Compliance with therapy, especially when taking diuretics and digitalis
» Proper dosing
Missed dose: Taking as soon as possible if remembered within 2 hours; going back to regular dosage schedule; not doubling doses
» Proper storage

**Precautions while using this medication**
Regular visits to physician to check progress of therapy; serum potassium monitoring may be necessary
» Not taking salt substitutes or low-salt milk or food unless approved by physician; importance of carefully reading labels of all low-salt foods to prevent excess intake of potassium
Checking with physician before beginning strenuous physical exercise if out of condition, to prevent possible hyperkalemia
» Checking with physician at once if signs of gastrointestinal bleeding are observed

**Side/adverse effects**
Expended wax matrix from some potassium chloride extended-release tablets may be seen in stool and be alarming to patient, although not necessarily an indication of improper dissolution of tablet or lack of bioavailability of potassium chloride
Signs of potential side effects, especially hyperkalemia or contact irritation of the alimentary tract

## General Dosing Information

Caution must be observed in the attempt to correct hypokalemia in order to avoid overcompensation and a resultant hyperkalemia with accompanying cardiac arrhythmias.

The normal adult concentration of serum potassium is 3.5 to 5.0 millimoles or mEq per liter with 4.5 millimoles or mEq often being used for a reference point. Potassium concentrations exceeding 5.5 mEq per liter are dangerous because of possible initiation of cardiac arrhythmias. Normal potassium concentrations tend to be higher in neonates (7.7 mEq per liter) than in adults.

Serum potassium concentrations do not necessarily indicate the true body potassium content. A rise in plasma pH (alkalosis) and chronic acidosis may decrease plasma potassium concentration by promoting potassium excretion and increase the intracellular potassium concentration. Conversely, a decrease in blood pH (acute acidosis) can cause an increase in serum potassium by inhibiting potassium excretion. However, it is necessary to attempt to restore serum potassium to normal in familial periodic paralysis, even though there is no total body potassium depletion.

Adequate renal function is essential for therapy with potassium supplements, since the kidneys maintain normal potassium balance. A gradual increase in the amount of potassium ingested leads to an increased ability of the kidneys to excrete potassium, thus preventing lethal hyperkalemia. The risk-benefit of potassium supplements should be considered in any patient with a higher-than-normal serum creatinine concentration.

Abrupt discontinuation of supplemental potassium to a patient suffering concurrent potassium losses, and also receiving digitalis preparations, may result in digitalis toxicity.

One gram of potassium acetate provides 10.26 mEq of potassium.
One gram of potassium bicarbonate provides 10 mEq of potassium.
One gram of potassium chloride provides 13.41 mEq of potassium.
One gram of potassium citrate provides 9.26 mEq of potassium.
One gram of potassium gluconate provides 4.27 mEq of potassium.

### For oral dosage forms only
*Because of their ulcerogenic tendency and the incidence of local tissue destruction produced from their dissolution, use of compressed tablets or enteric-coated tablets is not recommended.*

Solid tablet dosage forms should not be used in patients with delayed gastric emptying, esophageal compression, or intestinal obstruction or stricture. The use of potassium tablets in such conditions increases the possibility of tissue destruction by high, local concentrations of potassium released by the tablet.

### For parenteral dosage forms only
Infusion of insulin- or glucose-containing or sodium bicarbonate solutions may decrease serum potassium concentrations because of a shift of potassium into the cells.

Before commencing intravenous administration of potassium chloride for large-dose replacement therapy:
- Serum potassium concentrations should be determined.
- Renal function should be determined. Adequate urine output should be ensured.
- Concentrated potassium chloride injection must be diluted and thoroughly mixed with a larger volume (1000 mL) of fluid suitable for intravenous administration, preferably to a concentration of 40 mEq of potassium per liter, not to exceed 80 mEq per liter.
- When mixing in soft or bag-type containers of large-volume parenteral fluids, extra care must be used to ensure complete mixing and absence of pools of concentrated material.
- In dehydrated patients, a liter of potassium-free hydrating solution such as 0.2 or 0.45% sodium chloride injection is sometimes rapidly infused to ensure hydration and adequate renal function in select patients whose condition will tolerate bolus fluids. In such patients, serum potassium should be measured, and potassium added to the solution if serum potassium levels fall.

During intravenous potassium chloride administration:
- To avoid hyperkalemia, the infusion rate must not be rapid; a rate of 10 mEq of potassium per hour is usually considered to be safe as long as urine output is adequate. As a general rule, the rate should never exceed 1 mEq per minute for adults, or 0.02 mEq per kg of body weight per minute for children.
- Close patient monitoring by clinical observation, frequent electrocardiograms (especially during administration at the higher rates), and serum potassium determinations may be desirable as indicated by the situation.
- If renal dysfunction, especially acute renal failure as evidenced by oliguria and/or rising serum creatinine, should occur during infusion of potassium chloride, the infusion should be stopped at once. Subsequent infusion, if needed, should be administered very cautiously and with close monitoring.

### Diet/Nutrition
Oral potassium supplements should be taken with or immediately after a meal to minimize possible stomach upset or laxative action. Most oral tablets or capsules should be swallowed whole, never crushed or chewed. However, some commercial extended-release products, because of microencapsulation, may be crushed, chewed, or sprinkled on a spoonful of soft food if the patient is unable to swallow the solid dosage form whole. The oral solution, soluble tablet, and powder forms should be completely dissolved in at least one-half glass (120 mL) of cold water or juice, then sipped slowly over a 5- to 10-minute period.

Recommended dietary intakes for potassium are defined differently worldwide.

For U.S.—
The Recommended Dietary Allowances (RDAs) for vitamins and minerals are determined by the Food and Nutrition Board of the National Research Council and are intended to provide adequate nutrition in most healthy persons under usual environmental stresses. In addition, a different designation may be used by the FDA for food and dietary supplement labeling purposes, as with Daily Value (DV). DVs replace the previous labeling terminology United States Recommended Daily Allowances (USRDAs).

For Canada—
Recommended Nutrient Intakes (RNIs) for vitamins, minerals, and protein are determined by Health and Welfare Canada and provide recommended amounts of a specific nutrient while minimizing the risk of chronic diseases.

There is no RDA or RNI established for potassium; 1600 to 2000 mg (40 to 50 mEq) per day is considered adequate for adults.

Low-salt milk and salt substitutes may contain substantial amounts of potassium. These and other low-salt foods, especially breads and canned foods, should be avoided during treatment with potassium supplements, unless otherwise specified by the health care professional. Serum potassium may increase with resulting hyperkalemia, especially in patients with renal insufficiency.

The following table indicates the potassium content of selected foods:

| Food (amount) | Milligrams of potassium | Milliequivalents of potassium |
|---|---|---|
| Acorn squash, cooked (1 cup) | 896 | 23 |
| Potato with skin, baked (1 long) | 844 | 22 |
| Spinach, cooked (1 cup) | 838 | 21 |
| Lentils, cooked (1 cup) | 731 | 19 |
| Kidney beans, cooked (1 cup) | 713 | 18 |
| Split peas, cooked (1 cup) | 710 | 18 |
| White navy beans, cooked (1 cup) | 669 | 17 |
| Butternut squash, cooked (1 cup) | 583 | 15 |
| Watermelon (1/16) | 560 | 14 |
| Raisins (½ cup) | 553 | 14 |
| Yogurt, low-fat, plain (1 cup) | 531 | 14 |
| Orange juice, frozen (1 cup) | 503 | 13 |
| Brussel sprouts, cooked (1 cup) | 494 | 13 |
| Zucchini, cooked, sliced (1 cup) | 456 | 12 |
| Banana (medium) | 451 | 12 |
| Collards, frozen, cooked (1 cup) | 427 | 11 |
| Cantaloupe (¼) | 412 | 11 |
| Milk, low-fat 1% (1 cup) | 348 | 9 |
| Broccoli, frozen, cooked (1 cup) | 332 | 9 |

### For treatment of adverse effects
Treatment of hyperkalemia includes:
- If appropriate, discontinuing blood products, foods and medication that contain potassium, as well as ACE inhibitors, beta blocking agents, nonsteroidal anti-inflammatory drugs (NSAIDs), heparin, cyclosporine, and potassium-sparing diuretics.
- Administering 10% dextrose containing 10 to 20 units of insulin per liter at a rate of 300 to 500 mL of solution per hour. This will facilitate a shift of potassium into the cells.
- Correcting any existing acidosis with 50 mEq intravenous sodium bicarbonate over 5 minutes. The dose may be repeated in 10 to 15 minutes if needed. This will facilitate a shift of potassium into the cells.
- Administering a calcium salt (calcium gluconate, 0.5 to 1 gram, over a 2-minute period) to antagonize the cardiotoxic effects in patients whose electrocardiograms (ECGs) show absent P waves, or a broad QRS complex, and who are not receiving digitalis glycosides. Doses may be repeated after 2-minute intervals.
- Utilizing exchange resins to remove excess potassium from the body by adsorption and/or exchange of potassium. The oral dose of sodium polystyrene sulfonate is 20 to 50 grams of the resin dissolved in 100 to 200 mL of 20% sorbitol. The dose may by given every 4 hours up to four or five daily doses until potassium levels return to normal. It may also be given as a retention enema by mixing 8 grams of sodium polystyrene sulfonate and 50 grams of sorbitol in 200 mL of water. The retention enema exchanges potassium faster than the oral sodium polystyrene sulfonate.
- Utilizing hemodialysis or peritoneal dialysis to reduce serum potassium concentrations. May be necessary in patients with renal function impairment.
- Ascertaining adequate urine output and, if not contraindicated by the clinical condition of the patient, maintaining a high urine output with normal saline solutions and loop diuretics.

Caution must be observed when treating hyperkalemia in digitalized patients, since rapid reduction of serum potassium concentrations may induce digitalis toxicity.

---

## POTASSIUM ACETATE

## Parenteral Dosage Forms

Note: **Injectable potassium products must be diluted prior to intravenous administration. Direct patient injection of potassium concentrate may be instantaneously fatal.**

## POTASSIUM ACETATE INJECTION USP

**Usual adult and adolescent dose**
Electrolyte replenisher or
Hypokalemia (treatment)—
 Intravenous infusion, the dose and rate of infusion to be determined by the individual requirements of each patient, up to 400 mEq of potassium a day (usually not more than 3 mEq per kg of body weight). The response of the patient, as determined by the measurement of serum potassium concentration and the electrocardiogram following the initial 40 to 60 mEq infused, should indicate the subsequent infusion rate required.
 Serum potassium *greater* than 2.5 mEq per liter: Intravenous infusion, up to 200 mEq of potassium a day in a concentration less than 30 mEq per liter and at a rate not exceeding 10 mEq per hour.
 Serum potassium *less* than 2.0 mEq per liter with ECG changes or paralysis (urgent treatment): Intravenous infusion, up to 400 mEq of potassium a day in a suitable concentration and at a rate up to, but usually not exceeding, 20 mEq per hour.
 Note: Some urgent situations may require a dosage and/or rate of administration that temporarily exceeds those stated above.
Hypokalemia (prophylaxis)—
 Intravenous infusion, as part of total parenteral nutrition solutions, the specific amount determined by individual patient need.

**Usual pediatric dose**
Electrolyte replenisher or
Hypokalemia (treatment)—
 Intravenous infusion, up to 3 mEq of potassium per kg of body weight or 40 mEq per square meter of body surface a day. Volume of administered fluids must be adjusted to body size.
Hypokalemia (prophylaxis)—
 Intravenous infusion, as part of total parenteral nutrition solutions, the specific amount determined by individual patient need.

**Strength(s) usually available**
U.S.—
 2 mEq of potassium per mL (Rx) [GENERIC].
 4 mEq of potassium per mL (Rx) [GENERIC].
Canada—
 Not commercially available.

**Packaging and storage**
Store below 40 °C (104 °F), preferably between 15 and 30 °C (59 and 86 °F), unless otherwise specified by manufacturer. Protect from freezing.

---

## POTASSIUM BICARBONATE

## Oral Dosage Forms

### POTASSIUM BICARBONATE EFFERVESCENT TABLETS FOR ORAL SOLUTION USP

**Usual adult and adolescent dose**
Hypokalemia (prophylaxis or treatment)—
 Oral, 25 to 50 mEq of potassium dissolved in one-half to one glass (120 to 240 mL) of cold water one or two times a day, the dosage being adjusted as needed and tolerated.

**Usual adult prescribing limits**
Up to 100 mEq of potassium a day.

**Usual pediatric dose**
Dosage has not been established.

**Strength(s) usually available**
U.S.—
 6.5 mEq of potassium (650 mg) (Rx) [GENERIC].
 20 mEq of potassium (Rx) [*K+ Care ET*].
 25 mEq of potassium (Rx) [*K+ Care ET; K-Electrolyte; K-Ide; Klor-Con/EF; K-Lyte; K-Vescent;* GENERIC].
Canada—
 25 mEq of potassium (Rx) [*K-Lyte*].

**Packaging and storage**
Store below 40 °C (104 °F), preferably between 15 and 30 °C (59 and 86 °F), unless otherwise specified by manufacturer. Store in a tight container or original foil packaging.

**Auxiliary labeling**
- Take dissolved in cold water.
- Take with or immediately after food.

**Note**
Dispense in original foil packaging to help maintain moisture-free condition until use.

---

## POTASSIUM BICARBONATE AND POTASSIUM CHLORIDE

## Oral Dosage Forms

### POTASSIUM BICARBONATE AND POTASSIUM CHLORIDE FOR EFFERVESCENT ORAL SOLUTION USP

**Usual adult and adolescent dose**
Hypokalemia (prophylaxis or treatment)—
 Oral, 20 mEq of potassium dissolved in one-half to one glass (120 to 240 mL) of cold water one or two times a day, the dosage being adjusted as needed and tolerated.

**Usual adult prescribing limits**
Up to 100 mEq of potassium a day.

**Usual pediatric dose**
Dosage has not been established.

**Strength(s) usually available**
U.S.—
 20 mEq of potassium per 2.8-gram packet (Rx) [*Klorvess Effervescent Granules*].
Canada—
 20 mEq of potassium per 2.8-gram packet (Rx) [*Neo-K*].

**Packaging and storage**
Store below 40 °C (104 °F), preferably between 15 and 30 °C (59 and 86 °F), unless otherwise specified by manufacturer. Store in a tight container or original foil packaging.

**Auxiliary labeling**
- Take dissolved in cold water.
- Take with or immediately after food.

**Note**
Dispense in original foil packaging to help maintain moisture-free condition until use.

### POTASSIUM BICARBONATE AND POTASSIUM CHLORIDE EFFERVESCENT TABLETS FOR ORAL SOLUTION USP

**Usual adult and adolescent dose**
Hypokalemia (prophylaxis or treatment)—
 Oral, 20, 25, or 50 mEq of potassium dissolved in one-half to one glass (120 to 240 mL) of cold water one or two times a day, the dosage being adjusted as needed and tolerated.

**Usual adult prescribing limits**
Up to 100 mEq of potassium a day.

**Usual pediatric dose**
Dosage has not been established.

**Strength(s) usually available**
U.S.—
 20 mEq of potassium (Rx) [*Klorvess*].
 25 mEq of potassium (Rx) [*K-Lyte/Cl*].
 50 mEq of potassium (Rx) [*K-Lyte/Cl 50*].
Canada—
 12 mEq of potassium (Rx) [*Potassium-Sandoz*].

**Packaging and storage**
Store below 40 °C (104 °F), preferably between 15 and 30 °C (59 and 86 °F), unless otherwise specified by manufacturer. Store in a tight container or original foil packaging.

**Auxiliary labeling**
- Take dissolved in cold water.
- Take with or immediately after food.

**Note**
Dispense in original foil packaging to help maintain moisture-free condition until use.

## POTASSIUM BICARBONATE AND POTASSIUM CITRATE

## Oral Dosage Forms

### POTASSIUM BICARBONATE AND POTASSIUM CITRATE EFFERVESCENT TABLETS FOR ORAL SOLUTION

**Usual adult and adolescent dose**
Hypokalemia (prophylaxis or treatment)—
    Oral, 25 or 50 mEq of potassium dissolved in one-half to one glass (120 to 240 mL) of cold water one or two times a day, the dosage being adjusted as needed and tolerated.

**Usual adult prescribing limits**
Up to 100 mEq of potassium a day.

**Usual pediatric dose**
Dosage has not been established.

**Strength(s) usually available**
U.S.—
    25 mEq of potassium (Rx) [*Effer-K*].
    50 mEq of potassium (Rx) [*K-Lyte DS*].
Canada—
    Not commercially available.

**Packaging and storage**
Store below 40 °C (104 °F), preferably between 15 and 30 °C (59 and 86 °F), unless otherwise specified by manufacturer. Store in original foil packaging.

**Auxiliary labeling**
• Take dissolved in cold water.
• Take with or immediately after food.

**Note**
Dispense in original foil packaging to help maintain moisture-free condition until use.

## POTASSIUM CHLORIDE

## Oral Dosage Forms

### POTASSIUM CHLORIDE EXTENDED-RELEASE CAPSULES USP

**Usual adult and adolescent dose**
Hypokalemia (prophylaxis)—
    Oral, the equivalent of 16 to 24 mEq of potassium a day, divided into two or three doses, the dosage being adjusted as needed and tolerated.
Hypokalemia (treatment)—
    Oral, 40 to 100 mEq of potassium a day, divided into two or three doses, the dosage being adjusted as needed and tolerated.

**Usual adult prescribing limits**
Up to 100 mEq of potassium a day.

**Usual pediatric dose**
Dosage has not been established.

**Strength(s) usually available**
U.S.—
    8 mEq (600 mg) of potassium (Rx) [*Micro-K*; GENERIC].
    10 mEq (750 mg) of potassium (Rx) [*K-Lease*; *K-Norm*; *Micro-K 10*; GENERIC].
Canada—
    8 mEq (600 mg) of potassium (Rx) [*Micro-K*].
    10 mEq (750 mg) of potassium (Rx) [*Micro-K 10*].

**Packaging and storage**
Store below 30 °C (86 °F). Store in a tight container.

**Auxiliary labeling**
• Swallow capsules whole with a full glass of water.
• Do not chew or crush.
• Take with or immediately after food.

**Note**
Extended release over an 8- to 10-hour period. Polymeric particle coating of one product allows contents of the capsule to be sprinkled over soft food or mixed with juice.

### POTASSIUM CHLORIDE ORAL SOLUTION USP

**Usual adult and adolescent dose**
Hypokalemia (prophylaxis or treatment)—
    Oral, 20 mEq of potassium diluted in one-half glass (120 mL) of cold water or juice one to four times a day, the dosage being adjusted as needed and tolerated.

**Usual adult prescribing limits**
Up to 100 mEq of potassium a day.

**Usual pediatric dose**
Hypokalemia (prophylaxis or treatment)—
    Oral, 15 to 40 mEq of potassium per square meter of body surface or 1 to 3 mEq of potassium per kg of body weight a day administered in divided doses and well diluted in water or juice.

**Strength(s) usually available**
U.S.—
    10 mEq (750 mg) of potassium per 15 mL (Rx) [GENERIC (alcohol 5%)].
    20 mEq (1.5 grams) of potassium per 15 mL (Rx) [*Cena-K*; *Kaochlor 10%* (alcohol 5%; tartrazine); *Kaochlor S-F 10%* (alcohol 5%); *Kay Ciel* (alcohol 4%); *Klorvess 10% Liquid* (alcohol 0.75%); *Potasalan* (alcohol 4%); GENERIC].
    30 mEq (2.25 grams) of potassium per 15 mL (Rx) [*Rum-K*].
    40 mEq (3 grams) of potassium per 15 mL (Rx) [*Cena-K*; *Kaon-Cl 20% Liquid* (alcohol 5%); GENERIC].
Canada—
    10 mEq (750 mg) of potassium per 15 mL (Rx) [*KCL 5%*].
    20 mEq (1.5 grams) of potassium per 15 mL (Rx) [*K-10*; *Kaochlor-10*; *Roychlor-10%*].
    40 mEq (3 grams) of potassium per 15 mL (Rx) [*Kaochlor-20*].

**Packaging and storage**
Store below 40 °C (104 °F), preferably between 15 and 30 °C (59 and 86 °F), unless otherwise specified by manufacturer. Store in a tight container. Protect from freezing.

**Stability**
Some commercial preparations contain coloring agents that fade when exposed to light. Active ingredients are not affected by light.

**Auxiliary labeling**
• Take mixed in cold water or juice.
• Take with or immediately after food.

### POTASSIUM CHLORIDE FOR ORAL SOLUTION USP

**Usual adult and adolescent dose**
Hypokalemia (prophylaxis or treatment)—
    Oral, 15 to 25 mEq of potassium diluted in four to six ounces (180 mL) of cold water two to four times a day, the dosage being adjusted as needed and tolerated.

**Usual adult prescribing limits**
Up to 100 mEq of potassium a day.

**Usual pediatric dose**
Hypokalemia (prophylaxis or treatment)—
    Oral, 15 to 25 mEq of potassium per square meter of body surface, or 1 to 3 mEq of potassium per kg of body weight a day administered in divided doses and well diluted in water or juice.

**Strength(s) usually available**
U.S.—
    10 mEq (745 mg) of potassium per packet (Rx) [GENERIC].
    15 mEq (1.12 grams) of potassium per packet (Rx) [*K+Care*; *K-Lor*].
    20 mEq (1.5 grams) of potassium per packet (Rx) [*Gen-K*; *Kato*; *Kay Ciel*; *K+Care*; *K-Ide*; *K-Lor*; *Klor-Con Powder*; *K-Sol*; GENERIC].
    25 mEq (1.8 grams) of potassium per packet or dose (Rx) [*Gen-K*; *K+Care*; *Klor-Con/25 Powder*; *K-Lyte/Cl Powder* (bulk or packet); GENERIC].
Canada—
    20 mEq (1.5 grams) of potassium per packet (Rx) [*K-Lor*].
    25 mEq (1.8 grams) of potassium per packet (Rx) [*K-Lyte/Cl*].

**Packaging and storage**
Store below 40 °C (104 °F), preferably between 15 and 30 °C (59 and 86 °F), unless otherwise specified by manufacturer. Store in a tight container.

**Auxiliary labeling**
• Take dissolved in cold water or juice.
• Take with or immediately after food.

### POTASSIUM CHLORIDE FOR ORAL SUSPENSION

**Usual adult and adolescent dose**
Hypokalemia (prophylaxis or treatment)—
  Oral, 20 mEq of potassium mixed in two to six ounces (180 mL) of cold water one to five times a day, the dosage being adjusted as needed and tolerated.

**Usual adult prescribing limits**
Up to 100 mEq of potassium a day.

**Usual pediatric dose**
Dosage has not been established.

**Strength(s) usually available**
U.S.—
  20 mEq (1.5 grams) of potassium per packet (Rx) [*Micro-K LS*].
Canada—
  Not commercially available.

**Packaging and storage**
Store below 40 °C (104 °F), preferably between 15 and 30 °C (59 and 86 °F), in a tight container, unless otherwise specified by manufacturer.

**Preparation of dosage form**
Add granules to 2 to 6 ounces of water or juice, and stir for 1 minute before swallowing. The granules may also be added to 2 ounces of orange juice, tomato juice, apple juice, or milk.

**Auxiliary labeling**
• Take dissolved in cold water or juice.
• Take with or immediately after food.

Note: May be sprinkled on food.

### POTASSIUM CHLORIDE EXTENDED-RELEASE TABLETS USP

**Usual adult and adolescent dose**
Hypokalemia (prophylaxis or treatment)—
  Oral, 6.7 to 20 mEq of potassium (approximately 500 to 1.5 grams of potassium chloride, respectively) three times a day.

**Usual adult prescribing limits**
Up to 100 mEq of potassium a day.

**Usual pediatric dose**
Dosage has not been established.

**Strength(s) usually available**
U.S.—
  6.7 mEq (500 mg) of potassium (Rx) [*Kaon-Cl* (tartrazine)].
  8 mEq (600 mg) of potassium (Rx) [*K-8; Klor-Con 8; Slow-K;* GENERIC].
  10 mEq (750 mg) of potassium (Rx) [*K + 10; Kaon-Cl-10* (tartrazine); *K-Dur; Klor-Con 10; Klotrix; K-Tab; Ten-K* (scored); GENERIC].
  20 mEq (1.5 grams) of potassium (Rx) [*K-Dur* (scored)].
Canada—
  6.7 mEq (500 mg) of potassium (Rx) [*K-Long*].
  8 mEq (600 mg) of potassium (Rx) [*Apo-K; Slow-K*].
  10 mEq (750 mg) of potassium (Rx) [*Kalium Durules*].
  12 mEq (900 mg) of potassium (Rx) [*K-Med 900*].
  20 mEq (1500 mg) of potassium (Rx) [*K-Dur* (scored)].

**Packaging and storage**
Store below 30 °C (86 °F). Store in a tight container.

**Auxiliary labeling**
• Swallow tablets whole with a full glass of water.
• Do not chew or crush unless otherwise directed.
• Take with or immediately after food.

**Additional information**
Most extended-release tablets utilize an inert wax matrix from which the drug is slowly leached out as it passes through the gastrointestinal tract. The expended wax matrix may appear intact in the stool.

The extended-release tablets without a wax matrix may be swallowed whole or broken or crushed and sprinkled on food.

## Parenteral Dosage Forms

### POTASSIUM CHLORIDE FOR INJECTION CONCENTRATE USP

Note: **Injectable potassium chloride products in strengths of 1.5 mEq and 2 mEq per mL must be diluted prior to intravenous administration. Direct patient injection of potassium concentrate may be instantaneously fatal. However, injectable potassium chloride products in strengths of 0.1, 0.2, 0.3, and 0.4 mEq per mL are intended for use with a calibrated infusion device and do not require dilution.**

**Usual adult and adolescent dose**
Electrolyte replenisher or
Hypokalemia (treatment)—
  Intravenous infusion, the dose and rate of infusion to be determined by the individual requirements of each patient, up to 400 mEq of potassium a day (usually not more than 3 mEq per kg of body weight). The response of the patient, as determined by the measurement of serum potassium concentration and the electrocardiogram following the initial 40 to 60 mEq infused, should indicate the subsequent infusion rate required.
  Serum potassium *greater* than 2.5 mEq per liter: Intravenous infusion, up to 200 mEq of potassium a day in a concentration less than 30 mEq per liter and at a rate not exceeding 10 mEq per hour.
  Serum potassium *less* than 2.0 mEq per liter with ECG changes or paralysis (urgent treatment): Intravenous infusion, up to 400 mEq of potassium a day in a suitable concentration and at a rate up to, but usually not exceeding, 20 mEq per hour.

Note: Some urgent situations may require a dosage and/or rate of administration that temporarily exceeds those stated above.

Hypokalemia (prophylaxis)—
  Intravenous infusion, as part of total parenteral nutrition solutions, the specific amount determined by individual patient need.

**Usual pediatric dose**
Electrolyte replenisher or
Hypokalemia (treatment)—
  Intravenous infusion, up to 3 mEq of potassium per kg of body weight or 40 mEq per square meter of body surface a day. Volume of administered fluids must be adjusted to body size.
Hypokalemia (prophylaxis)—
  Intravenous infusion, as part of total parenteral nutrition solutions, the specific amount determined by individual patient need.

**Strength(s) usually available**
U.S.—
  0.1 mEq of potassium per mL (Rx) [GENERIC].
  0.2 mEq of potassium per mL (Rx) [GENERIC].
  0.3 mEq of potassium per mL (Rx) [GENERIC].
  0.4 mEq of potassium per mL (Rx) [GENERIC].
  1.5 mEq of potassium per mL (Rx) [GENERIC].
  2 mEq of potassium per mL (Rx) [GENERIC].
  3 mEq of potassium per mL (Rx) [GENERIC].
  10 mEq of potassium per mL (Rx) [GENERIC].

Note: To alert the practitioner to the potential danger of administering potassium chloride not intended for use in a calibration device (e.g., 1.5 or 2 mEq per mL) undiluted, USP requires that Potassium Chloride for Injection Concentrate products in vials be identified with black caps and ferrules. Ampuls must have a black band above the constriction. In addition, the words "Must Be Diluted" must appear on the cap and overseal of the cap, and the product label must bear the boxed warning "Concentrate Must Be Diluted Before Use."

Potassium chloride products in strengths of 0.1, 0.2, 0.3, and 0.4 mEq per mL are intended for use with a calibrated infusion device and do not require dilution.

Canada—
  2 mEq of potassium per mL (Rx) [GENERIC].

**Packaging and storage**
Store below 40 °C (104 °F), preferably between 15 and 30 °C (59 and 86 °F), unless otherwise specified by manufacturer. Protect from freezing.

**Incompatibilities**
Potassium chloride should not be added to mannitol, blood or blood products, or amino acid or lipid-containing solutions because it may precipitate these substances from solution or cause lysis of infused red blood cells.

---

## POTASSIUM GLUCONATE

## Oral Dosage Forms

### POTASSIUM GLUCONATE ELIXIR USP

**Usual adult and adolescent dose**
Hypokalemia (prophylaxis or treatment)—
  Oral, 20 mEq of potassium diluted in one-half glass (120 mL) of cold water or juice two to four times a day, the dosage being adjusted as needed and tolerated.

**Usual adult prescribing limits**
Up to 100 mEq of potassium daily.

## Potassium Supplements (Systemic)

**Usual pediatric dose**
Antihypokalemic—
Oral, 20 to 40 mEq of potassium per square meter of body surface, or 2 to 3 mEq per kg of body weight a day, administered in divided doses and well diluted in water or juice.

**Strength(s) usually available**
U.S.—
20 mEq of potassium (4.68 grams of potassium gluconate) per 15 mL (Rx) [*Kaon* (alcohol 5%); *Kaylixir* (alcohol 5%); *K-G Elixir* (alcohol 5%); GENERIC].
Canada—
20 mEq of potassium (4.68 grams of potassium gluconate) per 15 mL (Rx) [*Kaon; Potassium-Rougier*].

**Packaging and storage**
Store below 40 °C (104 °F), preferably between 15 and 30 °C (59 and 86 °F), unless otherwise specified by manufacturer. Store in a tight, light-resistant container. Protect from freezing.

**Stability**
Some commercial preparations contain coloring agents that fade when exposed to light. Active ingredients are not affected by light.

**Auxiliary labeling**
- Take mixed in cold water or juice.
- Take with or immediately after food.
- Keep container tightly closed.

### POTASSIUM GLUCONATE TABLETS USP

Note: Certain strengths of potassium gluconate may be available over-the-counter in some stores. Unless directed by the physician, use of these products should be discouraged.

**Usual adult and adolescent dose**
Hypokalemia (prophylaxis or treatment)—
Oral, 5 to 10 mEq of potassium two to four times a day.

**Usual adult prescribing limits**
Up to 100 mEq of potassium a day.

**Usual pediatric dose**
Dosage has not been established.

**Strength(s) usually available**
U.S.—
2 mEq of potassium (500 mg of potassium gluconate) [*Glu-K (Rx)*; GENERIC].
2.3 mEq of potassium (550 mg of potassium gluconate) (Rx/OTC) [GENERIC].
2.5 mEq of potassium (595 mg of potassium gluconate) (Rx/OTC) [GENERIC].
Canada—
Not commercially available.

**Packaging and storage**
Store below 40 °C (104 °F), preferably between 15 and 30 °C (59 and 86 °F), unless otherwise specified by manufacturer. Store in a tight container.

**Auxiliary labeling**
- Take with or immediately after food.
- Swallow tablet whole with a full glass of water.
- Do not chew or crush.

---

## *POTASSIUM GLUCONATE AND POTASSIUM CHLORIDE*

## Oral Dosage Forms

### POTASSIUM GLUCONATE AND POTASSIUM CHLORIDE ORAL SOLUTION USP

**Usual adult and adolescent dose**
Hypokalemia (prophylaxis or treatment)—
Oral, 20 mEq of potassium diluted in 30 mL or more of cold water or juice two to four times a day, the dosage being adjusted as needed and tolerated.

**Usual adult prescribing limits**
Up to 100 mEq of potassium a day.

**Usual pediatric dose**
Hypokalemia (prophylaxis or treatment)—
Oral, 20 to 40 mEq of potassium per square meter of body surface or 2 to 3 mEq per kg of body weight a day, administered in divided doses and well diluted in water or juice.

**Strength(s) usually available**
U.S.—
20 mEq of potassium per 15 mL (Rx) [*Kolyum*].
Canada—
Not commercially available.

**Packaging and storage**
Store below 40 °C (104 °F), preferably between 15 and 30 °C (59 and 86 °F), unless otherwise specified by manufacturer. Store in a tight container. Protect from freezing.

**Stability**
Some commercial preparations contain coloring agents that fade when exposed to light. Active ingredients are not affected by light.

**Auxiliary labeling**
- Take mixed in cold water or juice.
- Take with or immediately after food.
- Keep container tightly closed.

### POTASSIUM GLUCONATE AND POTASSIUM CHLORIDE FOR ORAL SOLUTION USP

**Usual adult and adolescent dose**
Hypokalemia (prophylaxis or treatment)—
Oral, 20 mEq of potassium diluted in 30 mL or more of cold water or juice two to four times a day, the dosage being adjusted as needed and tolerated.

**Usual adult prescribing limits**
Up to 100 mEq of potassium a day.

**Usual pediatric dose**
Hypokalemia (prophylaxis or treatment)—
Oral, 20 to 40 mEq of potassium per square meter of body surface or 2 to 3 mEq per kg of body weight a day, administered in divided doses and well diluted in water or juice.

**Strength(s) usually available**
U.S.—
20 mEq of potassium per 5-gram packet (Rx) [*Kolyum*].
Canada—
Not commercially available.

**Packaging and storage**
Store below 40 °C (104 °F), preferably between 15 and 30 °C (59 and 86 °F), unless otherwise specified by manufacturer. Store in a tight container or original package.

**Auxiliary labeling**
- Take mixed in cold water or juice.
- Take with or immediately after food.

**Note**
Dispense in original packet to help maintain moisture-free condition until use.

---

## *POTASSIUM GLUCONATE AND POTASSIUM CITRATE*

## Oral Dosage Forms

### POTASSIUM GLUCONATE AND POTASSIUM CITRATE ORAL SOLUTION USP

**Usual adult and adolescent dose**
Hypokalemia (prophylaxis or treatment)—
Oral, 20 mEq of potassium diluted in one-half glass (120 mL) of cold water or juice two to four times a day, the dosage being adjusted as needed and tolerated.

**Usual adult prescribing limits**
Up to 100 mEq of potassium a day.

**Usual pediatric dose**
Hypokalemia (prophylaxis or treatment)—
Oral, 20 to 40 mEq of potassium per square meter of body surface or 2 to 3 mEq per kg of body weight a day, administered in divided doses and well diluted in water or juice.

**Strength(s) usually available**
U.S.—
20 mEq of potassium per 15 mL (Rx) [*Twin-K*].
Canada—
Not commercially available.

**Packaging and storage**
Store below 40 °C (104 °F), preferably between 15 and 30 °C (59 and 86 °F), unless otherwise specified by manufacturer. Store in a tight container. Protect from freezing.

USP DI

### Stability
Some commercial preparations contain coloring agents that fade when exposed to light. Active ingredients are not affected by light.

### Auxiliary labeling
- Take mixed in cold water or juice.
- Take with or immediately after food.
- Keep container tightly closed.

---
### TRIKATES
---

Note: Trikates consists of potassium acetate, potassium bicarbonate, and potassium citrate.

## Oral Dosage Forms

### TRIKATES ORAL SOLUTION USP

**Usual adult and adolescent dose**
Hypokalemia (prophylaxis or treatment)—
   Oral, 15 mEq of potassium three or four times a day diluted in one-half glass (120 mL) of cold water or juice, the dosage being adjusted as needed and tolerated.

**Usual adult prescribing limits**
Up to 100 mEq of potassium a day.

**Usual pediatric dose**
Hypokalemia (prophylaxis or treatment)—
   Oral, 15 to 30 mEq of potassium per square meter of body surface or 2 to 3 mEq per kg of body weight a day, administered in divided doses and well diluted in water or juice.

### Strength(s) usually available
U.S.—
   15 mEq of potassium per 5 mL (Rx) [*Tri-K*].
Canada—
   Not commercially available.

### Packaging and storage
Store below 40 °C (104 °F), preferably between 15 and 30 °C (59 and 86 °F), unless otherwise specified by manufacturer. Store in a tight, light-resistant container. Protect from freezing.

### Auxiliary labeling
- Take mixed in cold water or juice.
- Take with or immediately after food.

Revised: 07/16/92
Interim revision: 07/11/95

---

**PRALIDOXIME**—The *Pralidoxime (Systemic)* monograph is not included in this published version of the USP DI database. Copies of the monograph are available on request from Micromedex, Inc. - Reprint Requests, 6200 S. Syracuse Way, Suite 300, Englewood, CO 80111; telephone (303) 486-6400; telefax (303) 486-6464; Email: USPDI@MDX.COM.

---

# PRAMIPEXOLE   Systemic—INTRODUCTORY VERSION

VA CLASSIFICATION (Primary): CN500
Commonly used brand name(s): *Mirapex*.
Note: For a listing of dosage forms and brand names by country availability, see *Dosage Forms* section(s).

## Category
Antidyskinetic (dopamine agonist).

## Indications

**Accepted**
Parkinson's disease, idiopathic (treatment)—Pramipexole is indicated for treatment of the symptoms of idiopathic Parkinson's disease. Its efficacy has been demonstrated in patients with early Parkinson's disease, as well as in patients with advanced disease receiving concomitant levodopa therapy.

## Pharmacology/Pharmacokinetics

**Physicochemical characteristics**
Molecular weight—302.27.

**Mechanism of action/Effect**
Pramipexole is a non-ergot dopamine agonist with high relative *in vitro* specificity and full intrinsic activity at the $D_2$ subfamily of dopamine receptors; it binds with higher affinity to $D_3$ than to $D_2$ or $D_4$ receptor subtypes. The relevance of this receptor specificity in Parkinson's disease is not known. Pramipexole's mechanism of action in the treatment of Parkinson's disease is not precisely known, but is believed to be related to its ability to stimulate dopamine receptors in the striatum. This theory is supported by electrophysiologic studies in animals that have demonstrated that pramipexole influences striatal neuronal firing rates via activation of dopamine receptors in the striatum and the substantia nigra, the site of neurons that send projections to the striatum.

**Absorption**
Rapid. Absolute bioavailability is greater than 90%, indicating that pramipexole is well absorbed and undergoes little presystemic metabolism. Food does not affect the extent of absorption.

**Distribution**
Extensive. Volume of distribution ($Vol_D$) is about 500 L. Pramipexole distributes into red blood cells, as indicated by an erythrocyte-to-plasma ratio of approximately 2.

**Protein binding**
Low (15%).

**Biotransformation**
No metabolites have been identified in plasma or urine.

**Half-life**
Elimination—
   About 8 hours in young, healthy volunteers.
   About 12 hours in elderly volunteers.

**Time to peak concentration**
Approximately 2 hours; the time to peak concentration is increased by about an hour if pramipexole is taken with a meal.

**Steady state concentration**
Pramipexole displays linear pharmacokinetics over the clinical dosage range. Steady-state concentrations are achieved within 2 days of dosing.

**Elimination**
Renal, with 90% of a pramipexole dose recovered in urine, almost all as unchanged drug. Nonrenal routes of elimination may contribute to a small extent. Renal clearance of pramipexole is approximately three times higher than the glomerular filtration rate, indicating secretion by the renal tubules, probably by the organic cationic transport system.
Pramipexole clearance is about 30% lower in females than in males. Most of this difference can be accounted for by differences in body weight, as there is no difference in half-life between females and males.
Pramipexole clearance may be reduced by about 30% in Parkinson's disease patients as compared with healthy elderly volunteers. Patients with Parkinson's disease appear to have reduced renal function, which may be related to the poorer general health of these patients. However, the pharmacokinetics of pramipexole are comparable between early and advanced Parkinson's disease patients.
Clearance of pramipexole decreases with age, most likely due to age-related reduction in renal function. Clearance was about 30% lower and half-life about 40% longer in elderly (65 years of age or older) volunteers as compared with that in younger (up to 40 years of age) volunteers.
Clearance of pramipexole was about 60% lower in patients with moderate impairment of renal function, and about 75% lower in patients with severe renal function impairment, as compared with clearance in healthy volunteers. Dosage reductions in these patients are recommended. Pramipexole clearance correlates well with creatinine clearance; thus, creatinine clearance can be used as a predictor of the extent of decrease in pramipexole clearance and can be used to guide dosage reductions. (See *Usual adult dose*.)
In dialysis—
   A negligible amount of pramipexole is removed by dialysis; clearance is extremely low in dialysis patients.

Potassium Supplements (Systemic)  2365

## Precautions to Consider

### Carcinogenicity/Tumorigenicity
Two-year carcinogenicity studies with pramipexole conducted in mice and rats resulted in no significant increases in tumor occurrence.

### Mutagenicity
Pramipexole was not mutagenic or clastogenic in a battery of assays, including the *in vitro* Ames assay, V79 gene mutation assay for HGPRT mutants, chromosomal aberration assay in Chinese hamster ovary cells, and *in vivo* mouse micronucleus assay.

### Pregnancy/Reproduction
Fertility—In rat fertility studies, administration of pramipexole at a dose of 2.5 mg per kg of body weight (mg/kg) per day (5.4 times the highest clinical human dose on a mg per square meter of body surface area [mg/m$^2$] basis), resulted in prolonged estrous cycles and inhibited implantation. These effects were associated with reductions in serum concentrations of prolactin, a hormone necessary for implantation and maintenance of early pregnancy in rats.

Pregnancy—Adequate and well-controlled studies have not been done in humans.

In animal studies, female rats that received pramipexole throughout pregnancy at a dose of 2.5 mg/kg of body weight (5.4 times the highest clinical human dose on a mg/m$^2$ basis) showed evidence of inhibited implantation. Administration of 1.5 mg of pramipexole per kg per day to pregnant rats during the period of organogenesis (gestation days 7 through 16) resulted in a high incidence of total resorption of embryos. These findings are thought to be due to the prolactin-lowering effects of pramipexole, since prolactin is necessary for implantation and maintenance of early pregnancy in rats (but not in rabbits or humans). Because of the pregnancy disruption and early embryonic loss in these studies, the teratogenic potential of pramipexole could not be adequately evaluated. Postnatal growth inhibition occurred in the offspring of rats treated with 0.5 mg pramipexole per kg per day (approximately equivalent to the highest human clinical dose on a mg/m$^2$basis) or greater during the latter part of pregnancy and throughout lactation. In pregnant rabbits receiving up to 10 mg of pramipexole per kg per day during organogenesis, there was no evidence of adverse effects on embryo-fetal development.

FDA Pregnancy Category C.

### Breast-feeding
It is not known whether pramipexole is distributed into breast milk. However, a radiolabeled single-dose study in lactating rats showed that drug-related materials were distributed into milk; concentrations of radioactivity in milk were three to six times greater than concentrations in plasma at equivalent time points.

Other studies have shown that pramipexole therapy has resulted in inhibition of prolactin secretion in humans and rats. Because of the potential for serious adverse reactions in the nursing infant, discontinuation of nursing or discontinuation of pramipexole is recommended.

### Pediatrics
Appropriate studies on the relationship of age to the effects of pramipexole have not been performed in the pediatric population. Safety and efficacy have not been established.

### Geriatrics
Pramipexole clearance was approximately 30% lower in subjects older than 65 years of age as compared with younger subjects because of an age-related reduction in renal function; this resulted in an increase in elimination half-life from approximately 8.5 hours to 12 hours.

In clinical studies, 38.7% of patients were older than 65 years of age. The relative risk of hallucination was increased in elderly patients. There were no other apparent differences in efficacy and safety of pramipexole between older and younger patients.

### Drug interactions and/or related problems
The following drug interactions and/or related problems have been selected on the basis of their potential clinical significance (possible mechanism in parentheses where appropriate)—not necessarily inclusive (» = major clinical significance):

Note: Inhibitors of cytochrome P450 enzymes would not be expected to affect the elimination of pramipexole because pramipexole is not appreciably metabolized by these enzymes *in vivo* or *in vitro*. Pramipexole does not inhibit CYP enzymes CYP1A2, CYP2C9, CYP2C19, CYP2E1, or CYP3A4. Inhibition of CYP2D6 was not observed at pramipexole plasma concentrations following the highest recommended clinical dose (1.5 mg three times a day).

Combinations containing any of the following medications, depending on the amount present, may also interact with this medication.

» Carbidopa and levodopa combination or
» Levodopa
(concomitant administration with pramipexole may cause an increase in peak levodopa plasma concentration by about 40%, and a decrease in time to peak levodopa plasma concentration from 2.5 to 0.5 hours)
(pramipexole may potentiate the dopaminergic side effects of levodopa, causing or exacerbating preexisting dyskinesia; reducing levodopa dosage may ameliorate this effect)

Cimetidine
(by inhibiting renal tubular secretion of organic bases via the cationic transport system, cimetidine caused a 50% increase in the area under the plasma concentration–time curve [AUC] of pramipexole, as well as a 40% increase in the half-life of pramipexole in a small series of patients)

Dopamine antagonists, including:
  Haloperidol
  Metoclopramide
  Phenothiazines
  Thioxanthenes
  (since pramipexole is a dopamine agonist, its actions may be diminished by dopamine antagonists)

Medications excreted by renal secretion, including:
  Diltiazem
  Quinidine
  Quinine
  Ranitidine
  Triamterene
  Verapamil
  (coadministration of agents that are secreted via the cationic transport system decreases the clearance of pramipexole by about 20%; agents secreted via the anionic transport system have little effect on the clearance of pramipexole)

### Medical considerations/Contraindications
The medical considerations/contraindications included have been selected on the basis of their potential clinical significance (reasons given in parentheses where appropriate)—not necessarily inclusive (» = major clinical significance).

*Risk-benefit should be considered when the following medical problems exist:*

Fibrotic complications from ergot-derived dopaminergic agents, history of
  (condition may recur)
» Hallucinations
  (condition may be exacerbated)
» Hypotension or
» Orthostatic hypotension
  (condition may be exacerbated)
» Renal function impairment
  (elimination may be impaired; dosage adjustments are necessary)
Retinal degeneration, or retinal problems
  (studies in albino rats have shown retinal degeneration and loss of photoreceptor cells; although the significance of this effect in humans has not been established, disruption of disk shedding [a mechanism universally present in vertebrates] may be involved)
Sensitivity to pramipexole

### Patient monitoring
The following may be especially important in patient monitoring (other tests may be warranted in some patients, depending on condition; » = major clinical significance):

Monitoring for symptoms of orthostatic hypotension
  (particularly important during dose escalation)

## Side/Adverse Effects

Note: Dopamine agonists appear to impair the systemic regulation of blood pressure, resulting in orthostatic hypotension, especially during dose escalation. In addition, patients with Parkinson's disease appear to have an impaired capacity to respond to an orthostatic challenge. Clear orthostatic effects were demonstrated in normal volunteers who received pramipexole. In clinical trials of pramipexole, however, incidence of clinically significant orthostatic hypotension was no greater in patients receiving the medication than in those patients receiving placebo. The explanation for this unexpected finding is not known; it may reflect a unique property of pramipexole, it may be the result of very careful dose titration, or it may be a factor of the patient selection criteria for the clinical trials, which excluded patients with active cardiovascular disease or significant baseline orthostatic hypotension.

A case of rhabdomyolysis occurred in a 49-year-old male with advanced Parkinson's disease who received pramipexole. Symptoms resolved upon discontinuation of pramipexole.

Pramipexole may cause or exacerbate preexisting dyskinesia. It may also potentiate the dopaminergic side effects of levodopa. Dyskinesia may be ameliorated by reducing the concomitant dose of levodopa.

Pathologic retinal changes consisting of degeneration and loss of photoreceptor cells were observed in albino rats given pramipexole in the premarketing carcinogenicity study. Retinal changes were not observed in albino mice, pigmented rats, monkeys, or minipigs. The potential significance of these effects for humans has not been established; however, this effect cannot be disregarded because it may involve disruption of disk shedding, a mechanism that is universally present in vertebrates.

A symptom complex (characterized by elevated temperature, muscular rigidity, altered consciousness, and autonomic instability) that resembles neuroleptic malignant syndrome and has no other obvious etiology has been reported in association with rapid dose reduction, withdrawal of, or changes in antiparkinsonian therapy. This effect was not observed during premarketing trials of pramipexole, but potentially could occur with the use of this dopaminergic agent.

Fibrotic complications, including retroperitoneal fibrosis, pulmonary infiltrates, pleural effusion, and pleural thickening, have been reported in some patients treated with ergot-derived dopaminergic agents. These complications may resolve upon discontinuation of the medication, but complete resolution does not always occur. Although these effects are believed to be associated with the ergoline structure of these compounds, it is not known if non–ergot-derived dopamine agonists such as pramipexole may produce similar adverse effects.

The following side/adverse effects have been selected on the basis of their potential clinical significance (possible signs and symptoms in parentheses where appropriate)—not necessarily inclusive:

### Those indicating need for medical attention
Incidence more frequent
*Asthenia* (unusual tiredness or weakness); *drowsiness; dyskinesia* (twitching, twisting, or other unusual body movements); *hallucinations* (seeing, hearing, or feeling things that are not there)—higher risk in elderly patients; *insomnia* (trouble in sleeping); *nausea; orthostatic hypotension* (dizziness, lightheadedness, or fainting, especially when standing up)

Note: In the placebo-controlled premarketing trials conducted in patients with early Parkinson's disease, *hallucinations* were observed in 9% of patients receiving pramipexole, as compared with 2.6% of patients receiving placebo. In the placebo-controlled premarketing trials conducted in patients with advanced Parkinson's disease who were concomitantly receiving levodopa, 16.5% of patients reported hallucinations, as compared with 3.8% of patients receiving placebo. Age appears to increase the risk of hallucinations attributable to pramipexole. In the early Parkinson's disease patients in these studies, the incidence of hallucinations was 1.9 times higher in pramipexole patients than in placebo patients younger than 65 years of age, and 6.8 times higher than in placebo patients older than 65 years of age. In the advanced Parkinson's disease patients (who were receiving concomitant levodopa) in these studies, the incidence of hallucinations was 3.5 times higher than in placebo patients younger than 65 years of age, and 5.2 times higher than placebo in patients older than 65 years of age.

Incidence less frequent
*Akathisia* (restlessness or need to keep moving); *amnesia* (memory loss); *confusion; diplopia or other eye or vision changes* (double vision or other changes in vision); *dysphagia* (difficulty in swallowing); *edema; fever; frequent urination; muscle or joint pain; myasthenia* (muscle weakness); *paranoid reaction* (fearfulness, suspiciousness, or other mental changes); *pneumonia* (cough; shortness of breath; troubled breathing; tightness in chest; wheezing)

Incidence rare
*Abnormal thinking; chest pain; delusions* (mood or mental changes); *dizziness; dyspnea* (troubled breathing); *peripheral edema* (swelling of arms or legs); *urinary incontinence* (loss of bladder control); *urinary tract infection* (bloody or cloudy urine; difficult, burning, or painful urination; frequent urge to urinate)

### Those indicating need for medical attention only if they continue or are bothersome
Incidence more frequent
*Constipation; dryness of mouth*

Incidence less frequent
*Abnormal dreams; anorexia* (loss of appetite); *decreased libido or impotence* (decreased sexual drive or ability); *increased sweating; malaise* (general feeling of discomfort or illness); *rhinitis* (runny nose); *skin problems, such as rash; weight loss*

## Overdose
For information on the management of overdose or unintentional ingestion of pramipexole, **contact a Poison Control Center** (see *Poison Control Center Listing*).

### Treatment of overdose
There is no known antidote for overdosage of a dopamine agonist.

To decrease absorption—Gastric lavage may be indicated.

Specific treatment—If signs of central nervous system (CNS) stimulation are present, a phenothiazine or butyrophenone neuroleptic agent may be indicated; however, the efficacy of such medications in reversing the effects of overdosage has not been assessed.

Monitoring—Electrocardiogram (ECG) monitoring may be indicated.

Supportive care—General supportive measures, including administration of intravenous fluids, may be indicated. Patients in whom intentional overdose is confirmed or suspected should be referred for psychiatric consultation.

## Patient Consultation
In providing consultation, consider emphasizing the following selected information (» = major clinical significance):

### Before using this medication
» Conditions affecting use, especially:
   Sensitivity to pramipexole
   Pregnancy—Studies in rats showed evidence of inhibited implantation and a high incidence of total resorption of embryos
   Breast-feeding—Not recommended because of potential for serious adverse effects in the infant
   Use in the elderly—Age-related reductions in renal function may require dosage adjustments; also, increased risk of occurrence of hallucinations
   Other medications, especially carbidopa and/or levodopa
   Other medical problems, especially hallucinations, hypotension, orthostatic hypotension, or renal function impairment

### Proper use of this medication
» Compliance with therapy; not taking more or less medicine than prescribed
» Proper dosing
   Missed dose: Taking as soon as possible; not taking if almost time for next dose; not doubling doses
» Proper storage

### Precautions while using this medication
» Regular visits to physician to check progress of therapy
» Checking with physician before discontinuing medication; gradual dosage reduction may be needed
» Possible drowsiness, dizziness, lightheadedness, vision problems, weakness, or muscular incoordination; caution when driving or doing jobs requiring alertness, clear vision, and coordination
» Caution when getting up suddenly from lying or sitting position
» Possible hallucinations, especially in older patients

### Side/adverse effects
Signs of potential side effects, especially asthenia, drowsiness, dyskinesia, hallucinations, insomnia, nausea, orthostatic hypotension, akathisia, amnesia, confusion, diplopia or other eye or vision changes, dysphagia, edema, fever, frequent urination, muscle or joint pain, myasthenia, paranoid reaction, pneumonia, abnormal thinking, chest pain, delusions, dizziness, dyspnea, peripheral edema, urinary incontinence, and urinary tract infection

## General Dosing Information
Pramipexole doses should be titrated slowly in all patients. Dosage goal should be to achieve maximum therapeutic effect balanced against the principal side effects of dyskinesia, hallucinations, somnolence, and dry mouth.

When pramipexole is used in combination with levodopa, the dosage requirements of levodopa may be reduced. In one controlled study in advanced Parkinson's disease patients, the levodopa dosage was reduced by an average of 27% from baseline.

It is recommended that pramipexole be discontinued gradually over a period of 1 week. However, abrupt discontinuation has been uneventful in some studies.

## Pramipexole (Systemic)

**Diet/Nutrition**
Taking pramipexole with food may reduce the occurrence of nausea.

## Oral Dosage Forms

### PRAMIPEXOLE TABLETS

Note: In clinical studies, dosage was initiated at subtherapeutic doses to avoid intolerable adverse effects and orthostatic hypotension, and then gradually titrated upwards.

**Usual adult dose**
Parkinson's disease, idiopathic—
  In patients with normal renal function:
    Oral, initially 0.375 mg a day, administered in three divided doses. Dosages should be increased gradually at intervals of 5 to 7 days. A suggested schedule for titration follows:

Ascending Dosage Schedule of Pramipexole

| Week | Dosage | Total Daily Dose |
|---|---|---|
| 1 | 0.125 mg three times a day | 0.375 mg |
| 2 | 0.25 mg three times a day | 0.75 mg |
| 3 | 0.5 mg three times a day | 1.5 mg |
| 4 | 0.75 mg three times a day | 2.25 mg |
| 5 | 1 mg three times a day | 3 mg |
| 6 | 1.25 mg three times a day | 3.75 mg |
| 7 | 1.5 mg three times a day | 4.5 mg |

Maintenance: Pramipexole was effective and well tolerated over a dosage range of 1.5 to 4.5 mg a day (administered in divided doses three times a day) with or without concomitant levodopa. In one fixed-dose study in early Parkinson's disease patients, pramipexole doses of 3, 4.5, and 6 mg a day were not shown to provide any significant benefit beyond that achieved at a dose of 1.5 mg a day.

  In patients with impaired renal function:

Pramipexole Dosage in Renal Impairment

| Renal Status | Initial Dose | Maximum Dose |
|---|---|---|
| Normal to mild impairment (creatinine clearance > 60 mL/min) | 0.125 mg three times a day | 1.5 mg three times a day |
| Moderate impairment (creatinine clearance of 35 to 59 mL/min) | 0.125 mg two times a day | 1.5 mg two times a day |
| Severe impairment (creatinine clearance of 15 to 34 mL/min) | 0.125 mg a day | 1.5 mg a day |
| Very severe impairment (creatinine clearance less than 15 mL/min) and hemodialysis patients | Use of pramipexole has not been adequately studied in this patient population | |

**Usual pediatric dose**
Safety and efficacy have not been established.

**Strength(s) usually available**
U.S.—
  0.125 mg (Rx) [*Mirapex* (colloidal silicon dioxide; corn starch; magnesium stearate; mannitol; povidone)].
  0.25 mg (Rx) [*Mirapex* (scored; colloidal silicon dioxide; corn starch; magnesium stearate; mannitol; povidone)].
  1 mg (Rx) [*Mirapex* (scored; colloidal silicon dioxide; corn starch; magnesium stearate; mannitol; povidone)].
  1.5 mg (Rx) [*Mirapex* (scored; colloidal silicon dioxide; corn starch; magnesium stearate; mannitol; povidone)].

**Packaging and storage**
Store between 20 and 25 °C (68 and 77 °F). Protect from light.

**Auxiliary labeling**
• May cause drowsiness.
• May cause dizziness.

Developed: 11/17/97

---

**PRAMOXINE**—See *Anesthetics (Mucosal-Local)*; *Anesthetics (Topical)*

---

**PRAMOXINE AND MENTHOL**—See *Anesthetics (Topical)*

---

**PRAVASTATIN**—See *HMG-CoA Reductase Inhibitors (Systemic)*

---

**PRAZEPAM**—See *Benzodiazepines (Systemic)*

---

# PRAZIQUANTEL  Systemic†

VA CLASSIFICATION (Primary): AP200
Commonly used brand name(s): *Biltricide*.
Note: For a listing of dosage forms and brand names by country availability, see *Dosage Forms* section(s).

†Not commercially available in Canada.

## Category
Anthelmintic (systemic).
Note: Praziquantel is an unusually broad-spectrum anthelmintic.

## Indications
Note: Bracketed information in the *Indications* section refers to uses that are not included in U.S. product labeling.

**Accepted**
Clonorchiasis (treatment)—Praziquantel is indicated in the treatment of clonorchiasis caused by *Clonorchis sinensis* (Chinese or Oriental liver fluke).
Opisthorchiasis (treatment)—Praziquantel is indicated in the treatment of opisthorchiasis caused by *Opisthorchis viverrini* and *O. felineus* (liver flukes).
Schistosomiasis (treatment)—Praziquantel is indicated in the treatment of schistosomiasis caused by *Schistosoma mekongi*, *S. japonicum*, *S. mansoni*, and *S. hematobium*.
[Cysticercosis (treatment)] or
[Neurocysticercosis (treatment)]—Praziquantel is used in the treatment of all types of cysticercosis (except ocular cysticercosis). Concurrent use of corticosteroids may also be necessary in the treatment of neurocysticercosis to control edema and/or other reactions to death of the cysticerci.
[Diphyllobothriasis (treatment)]—Praziquantel is used in the treatment of diphyllobothriasis.
[Dipylidiasis (treatment)]—Praziquantel is used in the treatment of dipylidiasis.
[Hymenolepiasis (treatment)]—Praziquantel is used in the treatment of hymenolepiasis caused by *Hymenolepis nana* (dwarf tapeworm).
[Metagonimiasis (treatment)]—Praziquantel is used in the treatment of metagonimiasis caused by *Metagonimus yokogawai* (intestinal fluke).
[Paragonimiasis (treatment)]—Praziquantel is used in the treatment of paragonimiasis caused by *Paragonimus westermani* (Oriental lung fluke) and other *Paragonimus* species.
[Taeniasis (treatment)]—Praziquantel is used in the treatment of taeniasis caused by *Taenia solium* (pork tapeworm) and *T. saginata* (beef tapeworm).

Not all species or strains of a particular helminth may be susceptible to praziquantel.

**Unaccepted**
Praziquantel is not indicated in the treatment of ocular cysticercosis since destruction of the parasite in the eye may result in irreparable lesions.

Praziquantel is not likely to be effective in the treatment of human echinococcosis caused by *Echinococcus* species or fascioliasis caused by *Fasciola hepatica* (sheep liver fluke).

## Pharmacology/Pharmacokinetics

**Physicochemical characteristics**
Molecular weight—312.41.

**Mechanism of action/Effect**
Vermicidal; precise mechanism of action unknown, but may involve synergy between praziquantel and the host's humoral immune response in *S. mansoni*; praziquantel is rapidly taken up by helminths and also appears to increase permeability of helminth's cell membrane, leading to a loss of intracellular calcium; massive contraction and paralysis of the helminth's musculature rapidly result; after exposure to praziquantel, tegument in neck region of adult helminths develops blebs, which appear to burst and disintegrate; praziquantel also produces intense vacuolization at several sites in tegument of adult schistosomes; in *S. mansoni*, this is followed by phagocytic attachment to parasite and, ultimately, death.

**Absorption**
Helminth—Rapidly taken up by schistosomes, other flukes, and adult tapeworms.
Human—Rapidly absorbed following oral administration, even when taken with meals; however, praziquantel undergoes extensive first-pass metabolism with only a small amount of active drug likely to reach the systemic circulation.

**Distribution**
Helminth—Appears evenly distributed throughout.
Human—Distributed to serum and cerebrospinal fluid (CSF); concentrations in CSF are approximately 15 to 20% of the total amount of free and bound praziquantel in serum. Praziquantel levels in the bile, feces, and breast milk range from less than 10% to 20% of plasma concentrations.

**Protein binding**
High (80 to 85%).

**Biotransformation**
Helminth—Does not appear to be metabolized by cestodes or schistosomes.
Human—Pronounced first-pass effect; rapidly and completely metabolized to inactive mono- and polyhydroxylated derivatives.

**Half-life**
Praziquantel—0.8 to 1.5 hours.
Metabolites—4 to 6 hours.

**Time to peak serum concentration**
1 to 3 hours.

**Peak serum concentration**
Normal liver function—0.2 to 2.0 mcg per mL after therapeutic doses.
Moderate to severe liver function impairment—Plasma concentrations significantly elevated (2 to 4 times) in one study.

**Elimination**
Renal, rapid; metabolites excreted primarily in urine; 72% excreted within 24 hours; approximately 80% excreted within 4 days; small amounts also excreted in feces.

## Precautions to Consider

**Carcinogenicity**
Long-term carcinogenicity studies in rats and golden hamsters have not shown any carcinogenic effects.

**Mutagenicity**
Mutagenicity studies have not shown mutagenic activity in tissue-, host-, and urine-mediated assays with *Salmonella typhimurium;* in dominant lethal and micronucleus tests in mice; and in spermatogonial tests in Chinese hamsters. Also, studies using other species of organisms (e.g., *Schizosaccharomyces, Saccharomyces, Drosophila*) have not shown mutagenic activity. Although mutagenic effects in *Salmonella* tests have been reported by one laboratory, they were not confirmed in the same strain by other laboratories.

**Pregnancy/Reproduction**
Pregnancy—Adequate and well-controlled studies in humans have not been done.

Studies in rats and rabbits given up to 40 times the usual human dose have not shown that praziquantel impairs fertility or is teratogenic. However, praziquantel has been shown to cause an increase in the abortion rate in rats given 3 times the single human dose.
FDA Pregnancy Category B.

**Breast-feeding**
Praziquantel is excreted in breast milk; concentrations are approximately 25% of those found in the maternal serum. Nursing mothers should stop breast-feeding when beginning treatment with praziquantel. Breast-feeding should not be resumed until 72 hours after treatment is completed. During this time, the breast milk should be expressed and discarded.

**Pediatrics**
Appropriate studies on the relationship of age to the effects of praziquantel have not been performed in children up to 4 years of age. However, no pediatrics-specific problems have been documented to date in children 4 years of age and older.

**Geriatrics**
No information is available on the relationship of age to the effects of praziquantel in geriatric patients.

**Drug interactions and/or related problems**
The following drug interactions and/or related problems have been selected on the basis of their potential clinical significance (possible mechanism in parentheses where appropriate)—not necessarily inclusive (» = major clinical significance):

Note: Combinations containing any of the following medications, depending on the amount present, may also interact with this medication.

Carbamazepine or
Phenytoin
 (one small, single-dose, controlled study found that epileptic patients taking carbamazepine or phenytoin had significantly lower plasma concentrations of praziquantel [7.9% and 24% of the control group, respectively]; this effect is thought to be due to induction of the cytochrome P-450 microsomal enzyme system by carbamazepine and phenytoin; patients on carbamazepine or phenytoin may require a larger dose of praziquantel)

Dexamethasone
 (one study found that concurrent administration of dexamethasone with praziquantel reduced praziquantel plasma concentrations by approximately 50%)

**Medical considerations/Contraindications**
The medical considerations/contraindications included have been selected on the basis of their potential clinical significance (reasons given in parentheses where appropriate)—not necessarily inclusive (» = major clinical significance):

*Except under special circumstances, this medication should not be used when the following medical problem exists:*
» Ocular cysticercosis
 (destruction of parasites in the eye may result in irreparable ocular lesions)

*Risk-benefit should be considered when the following medical problems exist:*
Hypersensitivity to praziquantel
Liver disease, moderate to severe
 (peak plasma concentrations were found to be significantly higher in patients with moderate to severe liver disease; higher concentrations were associated with an increased incidence of side effects; the increased bioavailability in patients with hepatosplenic schistosomiasis is presumed to be a result of decreased first-pass metabolism; however, the elimination half-life was not found to be significantly different between patients with and patients without liver disease)

**Patient monitoring**
The following may be especially important in patient monitoring (other tests may be warranted in some patients, depending on condition; » = major clinical significance):

*For Schistosoma hematobium*
» Urine examinations
 (examinations for eggs may be required approximately 1, 3, and 6 months following treatment with praziquantel to determine efficacy or provide proof of cure; no patient should be considered cured unless urine examinations have been negative for several months)

*For tapeworms, flukes, and other Schisotosoma species*
» Stool examinations
 (may be required approximately 1, 3, and 12 months following treat-

ment with praziquantel to determine efficacy or provide proof of cure; where expulsion of the tapeworm[s] is uncertain, stool examinations for the presence of eggs or segments of the worm[s] may be required periodically; no patient should be considered cured unless stool examinations have been negative for 3 months)

## Side/Adverse Effects

The following side/adverse effects have been selected on the basis of their potential clinical significance (possible signs and symptoms in parentheses where appropriate)—not necessarily inclusive:

**Those indicating need for medical attention only if they continue or are bothersome**
Incidence more frequent
*Central nervous system effects* (dizziness; drowsiness; headache; malaise); *fever; gastrointestinal effects* (abdominal cramps or pain; loss of appetite; nausea or vomiting; bloody diarrhea); *increased sweating*
Incidence less frequent
*Skin rash, hives, or itching*

## Patient Consultation

As an aid to patient consultation, refer to *Advice for the Patient, Praziquantel (Systemic)*.
In providing consultation, consider emphasizing the following selected information (» = major clinical significance):

**Before using this medication**
» Conditions affecting use, especially:
   Hypersensitivity to praziquantel
   Breast-feeding—Praziquantel is excreted in breast milk
   Other medical problems, especially ocular cysticercosis

**Proper use of this medication**
No special preparations (e.g., dietary restrictions or fasting, concurrent medications, purging, or cleansing enemas) required before, during, or immediately after therapy
» Not chewing tablets; swallowing tablets whole with small amount of liquid during meals to avoid bitter taste, which may cause gagging and vomiting
» Compliance with therapy
» Proper dosing
   Missed dose: Taking as soon as possible; not taking if almost time for next dose; not doubling doses
» Proper storage

**Precautions while using this medication**
Importance of physician checking progress after treatment
Checking with physician if no improvement after completing course of therapy
» Caution if dizziness or drowsiness occurs; not driving, using machines, or doing other jobs that require alertness while taking praziquantel and for 24 hours after discontinuing it

## General Dosing Information

No special preparations (e.g., dietary restrictions or fasting, concurrent medications, purging, or cleansing enemas) are required before, during, or immediately after treatment with praziquantel.

A bitter taste develops if praziquantel tablets are held in the mouth or chewed; this may result in gagging or vomiting. Therefore, praziquantel tablets, either whole or partial, should be swallowed unchewed with a small amount of liquid during meals.

Patients with severely impaired hepatic function may require a reduction in dose because elevated plasma concentrations have been associated with an increased incidence of side effects.

In the treatment of neurocysticercosis, praziquantel may be most effective in symptomatic patients with viable cysts within the cerebral parenchyma and in the rapidly progressive form of cysticercosis. Patients with intraventricular cysts, meningeal cysts, and old, dead, calcified cysts will probably not benefit from treatment with praziquantel. Also, a single ring-enhancing lesion with surrounding edema likely represents a dying cyst for which praziquantel will not be useful.

## Oral Dosage Forms

Note: Bracketed uses in the *Dosage Forms* section refer to categories of use and/or indications that are not included in U.S. product labeling.

### PRAZIQUANTEL TABLETS USP

**Usual adult and adolescent dose**
Clonorchiasis—
   Oral, 25 mg per kg of body weight three times a day for one day. May be repeated if required.
Schistosomiasis—
   *S. haematobium* and
   *S. mansoni:* Oral, 20 mg per kg of body weight two times a day for one day.
   *S. japonicum* and
   *S. mekongi:* Oral, 20 mg per kg of body weight three times a day for one day.
   Note: Doses should be spaced not less than four and not more than six hours apart.
      40 to 60 mg per kg of body weight as a single dose may also be given.
[Diphyllobothriasis]—
   *D. latum:* Oral, 10 to 20 mg per kg of body weight as a single dose.
   *D. pacificum:* Oral, 10 to 20 mg per kg of body weight as a single dose.
[Dipylidiasis]—
   Oral, 10 to 20 mg per kg of body weight as a single dose.
[Hymenolepiasis]—
   Oral, 25 mg per kg of body weight as a single dose. Heavy infection may require repeated therapy after ten days.
[Metagonimiasis]—
   Oral, 25 mg per kg of body weight three times a day for one day.
[Neurocysticercosis]—
   Oral, 16.7 to 33 mg per kg of body weight three times a day for fourteen to thirty days. May be repeated in two to six months if required.
Opisthorchiasis—
   Oral, 25 mg per kg of body weight three times a day for one day. May be repeated if required.
[Paragonimiasis]—
   Oral, 25 mg per kg of body weight three times a day for two days.
[Taeniasis—*Taenia solium* infections]:
   Oral, 10 mg per kg of body weight as a single dose.

**Usual adult prescribing limits**
Doses up to 75 mg per kg of body weight daily have been tolerated without serious adverse effects.

**Usual pediatric dose**
Children up to 4 years of age—Dosage has not been established.
Children 4 years of age and over—See *Usual adult and adolescent dose*.

**Strength(s) usually available**
U.S.—
   600 mg (Rx) [*Biltricide*].
Canada—
   Not commercially available.
Note: Tablets are triple-scored for dosage adjustment (e.g., pediatric use).

**Packaging and storage**
Store below 30 °C (86 °F), unless otherwise specified by manufacturer.

**Auxiliary labeling**
• May cause dizziness or drowsiness.
• Swallow tablets whole.
• Take with liquid during meals.
• Continue medicine for full time of treatment.

Revised: 03/23/93

---

# PRAZOSIN   Systemic

VA CLASSIFICATION (Primary/Secondary): CV150/CV409; CV900; AD900; GU900

Commonly used brand name(s): *Minipress*.

Note: For a listing of dosage forms and brand names by country availability, see *Dosage Forms* section(s).

## Category

Antihypertensive; vasodilator, congestive heart failure; antidote (to ergot alkaloid poisoning); vasospastic therapy adjunct; benign prostatic hyperplasia therapy agent.

## Indications

Note: Bracketed information in the *Indications* section refers to uses that are not included in U.S. product labeling.

**Accepted**
Hypertension (treatment)—Prazosin is indicated in the treatment of hypertension.

[Congestive heart failure (treatment)][1]—Prazosin may be used as an adjunct to digoxin and diuretics for the treatment of congestive heart failure. However, prazosin has not been shown to improve survival in these patients.

[Toxicity, ergot alkaloid (treatment)][1]—Prazosin is used for treatment of peripheral vasospasm caused by ergot alkaloid overdose.

[Pheochromocytoma (treatment)][1]—Prazosin is used for the management of hypertension associated with pheochromocytoma.

[Raynaud's phenomenon (treatment)][1]—Prazosin is used for treatment of Raynaud's phenomenon.

[Benign prostatic hyperplasia (BPH) (treatment)][1]—Prazosin is used for the treatment of urinary symptoms associated with benign prostatic hyperplasia. Prazosin has been shown to improve urinary flow and symptoms of BPH. However, the long-term effects of prazosin on the incidence of acute urinary obstruction or other complications of BPH or on the need for surgery have not yet been determined.

[1]Not included in Canadian product labeling.

## Pharmacology/Pharmacokinetics

### Physicochemical characteristics
Molecular weight—419.87.
pKa—6.5.

### Mechanism of action/Effect
Prazosin is a selective alpha $_1$-adrenergic blocking agent. The alpha $_1$-adrenergic blocking action is thought to account primarily for its effects.
Hypertension—
  Prazosin produces vasodilation and reduces peripheral resistance but generally has little effect on cardiac output. Antihypertensive effect is usually not accompanied by reflex tachycardia. There is little or no effect on renal blood flow or glomerular filtration rate.
Congestive heart failure—
  Beneficial effects, resulting from vasodilation, are due to decreased systemic resistance, preload and afterload reduction, and resulting improved cardiac output.
Raynaud's phenomenon—
  Therapeutic effect for vasospasm is due to inhibition of vasoconstriction by blocking of postsynaptic alpha$_1$ receptors.
Benign prostatic hyperplasia—
  Relaxation of smooth muscle in the bladder neck, prostate, and prostate capsule produced by alpha$_1$-adrenergic blockade results in a reduction in urethral resistance and pressure, bladder outlet resistance, and urinary symptoms.

### Other actions/effects
Prazosin may affect serum lipids. The most consistent changes observed are a decrease in levels of serum total cholesterol and low density lipoprotein (LDL) cholesterol. However, the implications of these changes are unclear.

### Absorption
Well-absorbed from gastrointestinal tract; bioavailability is variable (50 to 85%).

### Protein binding
Very high (97%; 20% to red blood cells).

### Biotransformation
Primarily hepatic. Several metabolites have been identified in humans and animals (6-O-demethyl, 7-O-demethyl, 2-[1-piperazinyl]-4-amino-6,7-dimethoxyquinazoline, 2,4-diamino-6,7-dimethoxyquinazoline); in dog studies, three of the metabolites were shown to be responsible for approximately 10 to 25% of prazosin's hypotensive activity.

### Half-life
2 to 3 hours; unchanged in renal function impairment, but may increase to more than double (6 to 8 hours) in congestive heart failure.

### Onset of action
Hypertension—Within 30 to 90 minutes after a single dose.
Congestive heart failure—Rapid.

### Time to peak concentration
1 to 3 hours.

### Time to peak effect
Hypertension—
  Single dose: 2 to 4 hours.
  Multiple doses: Up to 3 to 4 weeks of therapy may be required for maximal therapeutic effect.
Congestive heart failure—
  1 hour.

### Duration of action
Hypertension—Single dose: 7 to 10 hours.
Congestive heart failure—6 hours.

### Elimination
Primarily in bile and feces; 6 to 10% in urine. Excreted as unchanged drug (5 to 11%) and metabolites. Elimination of prazosin may be slower in patients with congestive heart failure than in normal subjects.
In dialysis—Not dialyzable.

## Precautions to Consider

### Cross-sensitivity and/or related problems
Patients sensitive to other quinazolines (doxazosin, terazosin) may also be sensitive to prazosin.

### Carcinogenicity
An 18-month study in rats given prazosin at doses of more than 225 times the usual maximum recommended human dose of 20 mg per day did not demonstrate carcinogenic potential.

### Mutagenicity
Prazosin was not mutagenic in in vitro genetic toxicology studies.

### Pregnancy/Reproduction
Fertility—A study in male rats given subcutaneous injections of prazosin (1.4 mg per kg of body weight [mg/kg]) revealed reduced fertility manifested by a suppression of the fertilizing potential of spermatozoa.
A fertility and general reproductive performance study in male and female rats given prazosin at a dose of 75 mg/kg (225 times the usual maximum recommended human dose) demonstrated decreased fertility. However, when rats were given 25 mg/kg (75 times the usual maximum recommended human dose) decreased fertility was not seen.

Pregnancy—Adequate and well-controlled studies in humans have not been done. However, limited uncontrolled use of prazosin and a beta-blocking agent for the control of severe hypertension in 44 pregnant women revealed no drug-related fetal abnormalities or adverse effects. Also, use of prazosin during the last trimester in 8 pregnant women with hypertension produced no prolonged clinical problems. All infants were developing normally 6 to 30 months following delivery.
In rats given doses more than 225 times the usual maximum recommended human dose, prazosin has been shown to be associated with decreased litter weight at birth and at 1, 4, and 21 days of age. There was no evidence, however, of drug-related external, visceral, or skeletal abnormalities.
In pregnant rabbits and pregnant monkeys given doses of more than 225 times and 12 times the usual maximum recommended human dose, respectively, no drug-related external, visceral, or skeletal abnormalities were observed in the fetuses.
FDA Pregnancy Category C.

### Breast-feeding
Prazosin is distributed into breast milk in small amounts.

### Pediatrics
Appropriate studies on the relationship of age to the effects of prazosin have not been performed in the pediatric population. However, no pediatrics-specific problems have been documented to date.

### Geriatrics
Although appropriate studies on the relationship of age to the effects of prazosin have not been performed in the geriatric population, geriatrics-specific problems are not expected to limit the usefulness of prazosin in the elderly. However, elderly patients may be more sensitive to the hypotensive effects and are more likely to have age-related renal function impairment, which may require lower prazosin doses. In addition, the risk of prazosin-induced hypothermia may be increased in elderly patients.

### Drug interactions and/or related problems
The following drug interactions and/or related problems have been selected on the basis of their potential clinical significance (possible mechanism in parentheses where appropriate)—not necessarily inclusive (» = major clinical significance):

Note: Combinations containing any of the following medications, depending on the amount present, may also interact with this medication.

  Anti-inflammatory drugs, nonsteroidal (NSAIDs), especially indomethacin
    (antihypertensive effects of prazosin may be reduced when it is used concurrently with these agents; indomethacin, and possibly other NSAIDs, may antagonize the antihypertensive effect by inhibiting renal prostaglandin synthesis and/or by causing sodium and fluid retention; the patient should be carefully monitored to confirm that the desired effect is being obtained)

Hypotension-producing medications, other (see *Appendix II*)
(antihypertensive effects may be potentiated when these medications are used concurrently with prazosin; although some antihypertensive and/or diuretic combinations are frequently used to therapeutic advantage, dosage adjustments are necessary when these medications are used concurrently)

Sympathomimetics
(antihypertensive effects of prazosin may be reduced when it is used concurrently with these agents; the patient should be carefully monitored to confirm that the desired effect is being obtained)
(concurrent use of prazosin antagonizes the peripheral vasoconstriction produced by high doses of dopamine)
(concurrent use of prazosin may decrease the pressor response to ephedrine)
(concurrent use of prazosin may block the alpha-adrenergic effects of epinephrine, possibly resulting in severe hypotension and tachycardia)
(concurrent use of prazosin usually decreases, but does not reverse or completely block, the pressor effect of metaraminol)
(prior administration of prazosin may decrease the pressor effect and shorten the duration of action of methoxamine and phenylephrine)

**Laboratory value alterations**
The following have been selected on the basis of their potential clinical significance (possible effect in parentheses where appropriate)—not necessarily inclusive (» = major clinical significance):

With diagnostic test results
Vanillylmandelic acid (VMA), urinary
(concentrations may be increased; false positive results may occur in screening tests for pheochromocytoma)

**Medical considerations/Contraindications**
The medical considerations/contraindications included have been selected on the basis of their potential clinical significance (reasons given in parentheses where appropriate)—not necessarily inclusive (» = major clinical significance):

*Risk-benefit should be considered when the following medical problems exist:*

Angina pectoris
(may induce angina or aggravate pre-existing angina)
» Cardiac disease, severe
(prazosin is usually not used alone, although it may improve cardiac performance in some patients with severe refractory congestive heart failure)
Narcolepsy
(may exacerbate cataplexy; however, a clear cause-effect relationship has not been established)
Renal function impairment
(increased sensitivity to prazosin's effects; lower doses may be required)
Sensitivity to prazosin

**Patient monitoring**
The following may be especially important in patient monitoring (other tests may be warranted in some patients, depending on condition; » = major clinical significance):

» Blood pressure measurements
(recommended at periodic intervals in patients being treated for hypertension; selected patients may be trained to perform blood pressure measurements at home and report the results at regular physician visits)

## Side/Adverse Effects

Note: A "first-dose orthostatic hypotensive reaction" sometimes occurs, most frequently 30 to 90 minutes after the initial dose of prazosin, and may be severe. Syncope or other postural symptoms, such as dizziness, may occur. Subsequent occurrence with dosage increases is also possible. Incidence appears to be dose-related; thus, it is important that therapy be initiated with the lowest possible dose. Patients who are volume-depleted or sodium-restricted may be more sensitive to the orthostatic hypotensive effects of prazosin, and the effect may be exaggerated after exercise.

Hypotensive side effects may be more likely to occur in geriatric patients.

The following side/adverse effects have been selected on the basis of their potential clinical significance (possible signs and symptoms in parentheses where appropriate)—not necessarily inclusive:

**Those indicating need for medical attention**
Incidence more frequent
*Dizziness; orthostatic hypotension* (dizziness or lightheadedness when getting up from a lying or sitting position; sudden fainting)
Incidence less frequent
*Edema* (swelling of feet or lower legs); *palpitations* (pounding heartbeat); *urinary incontinence* (loss of bladder control)
Incidence rare
*Angina* (chest pain); *dyspnea* (shortness of breath); *priapism* (painful, inappropriate erection of the penis, continuing)

**Those indicating need for medical attention only if they continue or are bothersome**
Incidence more frequent
*Drowsiness; headache; malaise* (lack of energy)
Incidence less frequent
*Dryness of mouth; fatigue* (unusual tiredness or weakness); *nervousness*
Incidence rare
*Nausea; urinary frequency* (frequent urge to urinate)

## Overdose
For more information on the management of overdose or unintentional ingestion, **contact a Poison Control Center** (see *Poison Control Center Listing*).

**Treatment of overdose**
Recommended treatment for prazosin overdose includes: Treatment of circulatory failure, either by placing the patient in the supine position and elevating the legs or by using additional measures if shock is present, is most important; volume expanders may be used to treat shock, followed, if necessary, by administration of a vasopressor; symptomatic, supportive treatment and monitoring of fluid and electrolyte status.

## Patient Consultation
As an aid to patient consultation, refer to *Advice for the Patient, Prazosin (Systemic)*.
In providing consultation, consider emphasizing the following selected information (» = major clinical significance):

**Before using this medication**
» Conditions affecting use, especially:
Sensitivity to quinazolines
Breast-feeding—Distributed into breast milk in small amounts
Use in the elderly—Increased sensitivity to hypotensive effects and increased risk of prazosin-induced hypothermia
Other medical problems, especially severe cardiac disease

**Proper use of this medication**
Compliance with therapy; taking medication at the same times each day to maintain the therapeutic effect
» Proper dosing
Missed dose: Taking as soon as possible; not taking if almost time for next dose; not doubling doses
» Proper storage
*For use as an antihypertensive*
Possible need for control of weight and diet, especially sodium intake
» Patient may not experience symptoms of hypertension; importance of taking medication even if feeling well
» Does not cure, but helps control hypertension; possible need for lifelong therapy; serious consequences of untreated hypertension
*For use in benign prostatic hyperplasia (BPH)*
Relieves symptoms of BPH but does not change the size of the prostate; may not prevent the need for surgery in the future

**Precautions while using this medication**
Making regular visits to physician to check progress
» Caution if dizziness, lightheadedness, or sudden fainting occurs, especially after initial dose; taking first dose at bedtime
» Caution when getting up suddenly from a lying or sitting position
» Caution in using alcohol, while standing for long periods or exercising, and during hot weather because of enhanced orthostatic hypotensive effects
» Possibility of drowsiness
» Caution when driving or doing anything else requiring alertness because of possible drowsiness, dizziness, or lightheadedness
» Not taking other medications, especially nonprescription sympathomimetics, unless discussed with physician

### Side/adverse effects
Signs of potential side effects, especially dizziness, orthostatic hypotension, edema, palpitations, urinary incontinence, angina, dyspnea, and priapism

## General Dosing Information
Dosage of prazosin should be adjusted to meet the individual requirements of each patient, on the basis of blood pressure response.

Prazosin may be used alone or in combination with a thiazide diuretic or beta-adrenergic blocker, both of which reduce the tendency for sodium and water retention, although they also produce additive hypotension. If combination therapy is indicated, individual titration is required to ensure the lowest possible therapeutic dose of each drug.

In order to minimize the "first-dose orthostatic hypotensive reaction," an initial dose of 1 mg is recommended, with gradual increments as needed. Administration of the initial dose at bedtime is recommended, as well as the initial dose of each increment.

When a diuretic or other antihypertensive agent is added to prazosin therapy, the dose of prazosin should be reduced to 1 or 2 mg three times a day, followed by titration of dosage of the combination. When prazosin is added to existing diuretic or antihypertensive therapy, the dose of the other agent should be reduced and prazosin started at a dose of 0.5 or 1 mg two or three times a day.

Tolerance to the effects of prazosin may occur during treatment of congestive heart failure but usually not during treatment of hypertension. An early, transient (usually within the first few doses) blunting of hemodynamic effect may occur due to reflex activation of the sympathetic nervous system. The hemodynamic effect may spontaneously restore with uninterrupted therapy or the blunted effect may be overcome by temporarily interrupting prazosin therapy. A later apparent tolerance may result from fluid retention, requiring increased doses of diuretics; this effect may be minimized by increasing the dose of prazosin, temporarily interrupting prazosin therapy, or substituting another vasodilator.

## Oral Dosage Forms
Note: Bracketed uses in the *Dosage Forms* section refer to categories of use and/or indications that are not included in U.S. product labeling.

### PRAZOSIN HYDROCHLORIDE CAPSULES USP
Note: The dosing and strengths of the dosage forms available are expressed in terms of prazosin base (not the hydrochloride salt).

**Usual adult dose**
Antihypertensive—
   Initial: Oral, 1 mg (base) two or three times a day.
   Maintenance: Oral, adjusted gradually to meet individual requirements, most commonly 6 to 15 mg (base) a day in two or three divided doses.
[Toxicity, ergot alkaloid]—
   Oral, 1 mg three times a day.
[Vasospastic therapy adjunct—Raynaud's phenomenon]—
   Oral, 1 mg three times a day.
[Benign prostatic hyperplasia]—
   Initial: Oral, 1 mg (base) two times a day.
   Maintenance: Oral, 1 to 5 mg (base) two times a day.
Note: Geriatric patients may be more sensitive to the effects of the usual adult dose.

**Usual adult prescribing limits**
Daily doses higher than 20 mg (base) usually do not have increased efficacy, although some patients respond to up to 40 mg a day.

**Usual pediatric dose**
Antihypertensive—
   Oral, 50 to 400 mcg (0.05 to 0.4 mg) (base) per kg of body weight per day in two or three divided doses. Single doses should not exceed 7 mg, and the total daily dose should not exceed 15 mg per day.

**Strength(s) usually available**
U.S.—
   1 mg (base) (Rx) [*Minipress* (sucrose) [GENERIC (sucrose)].
   2 mg (base) (Rx) [*Minipress* (sucrose) [GENERIC (sucrose)].
   5 mg (base) (Rx) [*Minipress* (sucrose) [GENERIC (sucrose)].
Canada—
   Not commercially available.

**Packaging and storage**
Store below 40 °C (104 °F), preferably between 15 and 30 °C (59 and 86 °F), unless otherwise specified by manufacturer. Store in a well-closed, light-resistant container.

**Auxiliary labeling**
• Do not take other medicines without your doctor's advice.
• May cause dizziness.

**Note**
Check refill frequency to determine compliance in hypertensive patients.

### PRAZOSIN HYDROCHLORIDE TABLETS
Note: The dosing and strengths of the dosage forms available are expressed in terms of prazosin base (not the hydrochloride salt).

**Usual adult dose**
Antihypertensive—
   Initial: Oral, 500 mcg (0.5 mg) two or three times a day for at least 3 days. If tolerated, increase to 1 mg (base) two or three times a day for a further 3 days.
   Maintenance: Oral, adjusted gradually to meet individual requirements, most commonly 6 to 15 mg (base) a day in two or three divided daily doses.
Toxicity, ergot alkaloid[1]—
   Oral, 1 mg three times a day.
Vasospastic therapy adjunct—Raynaud's phenomenon[1]—
   Oral, 1 mg three times a day.
Benign prostatic hyperplasia[1]—
   Initial: Oral, 1 mg (base) two times a day.
   Maintenance: Oral, 1 to 5 mg (base) two times a day.
Note: Geriatric patients may be more sensitive to the effects of the usual adult dose.

**Usual adult prescribing limits**
Daily doses higher than 20 mg (base) usually do not have increased efficacy, although some patients respond to up to 40 mg a day.

**Usual pediatric dose**
Antihypertensive—
   See *Prazosin Hydrochloride Capsules USP*.

**Strength(s) usually available**
U.S.—
   Not commercially available.
Canada—
   1 mg (base) (Rx) [*Minipress* (scored); GENERIC].
   2 mg (base) (Rx) [*Minipress* (scored); GENERIC].
   5 mg (base) (Rx) [*Minipress* (scored); GENERIC].

**Packaging and storage**
Store below 40 °C (104 °F), preferably between 15 and 30 °C (59 and 86 °F), unless otherwise specified by manufacturer. Store in a well-closed, light-resistant container.

**Auxiliary labeling**
• Do not take other medicines without your doctor's advice.
• May cause dizziness.

**Note**
Check refill frequency to determine compliance in hypertensive patients.

[1]Not included in Canadian product labeling.

## Selected Bibliography
The fifth report of the Joint National Committee on Detection, Evaluation, and Treatment of High Blood Pressure. Arch Intern Med 1993; 153: 154-83.

Revised: 08/02/94
Interim revision: 08/19/98

# PRAZOSIN AND POLYTHIAZIDE Systemic

VA CLASSIFICATION (Primary): CV401

**NOTE:** The *Prazosin and Polythiazide (Systemic)* monograph is maintained on the USP DI electronic data base. For a printed copy of the most recent revision of the complete monograph, contact Micromedex, Inc. - Reprint Requests, 6200 S. Syracuse Way, Suite 300, Englewood, CO 80111; telephone (303) 486-6400; telefax (303) 486-6464; Email: USPDI@MDX.COM.

For information on the specific components of this combination, see the *USP DI* monographs for *Diuretics, Thiazide (Systemic)* and *Prazosin (Systemic)*.

The information that follows is selectively abstracted from the complete monograph and is provided to facilitate drug use review and patient counseling.

Note: For a listing of dosage forms and brand names by country availability, see *Dosage Forms* section(s).

## Category
Antihypertensive.

## Indications

**Accepted**

Hypertension (treatment)—Prazosin and polythiazide combination is indicated in the treatment of hypertension.

Fixed-dosage combinations are generally not recommended for initial therapy and are useful for subsequent therapy only when the proportion of the component agents corresponds to the dose of the individual agents, as determined by titration.

## Patient Consultation

As an aid to patient consultation, refer to *Advice for the Patient, Prazosin and Polythiazide (Systemic)*.

In providing consultation, consider emphasizing the following selected information (» = major clinical significance):

**Before using this medication**
» Conditions affecting use, especially:
  Sensitivity to quinazolines, thiazide diuretics, other sulfonamide-type medications, bumetanide, furosemide, or carbonic anhydrase inhibitors
  Pregnancy—Not recommended for routine use; thiazide diuretics may cause jaundice, thrombocytopenia, hypokalemia in infant
  Breast-feeding—Distributed into breast milk; recommended that nursing mothers avoid thiazides diuretics during first month of breast-feeding because of reports of suppression of lactation
  Use in children—Caution if giving to infants with jaundice
  Use in the elderly—Elderly patients may be more sensitive to hypotensive effects; potential for increased risk of prazosin-induced hypothermia and electrolyte effects of polythiazide
  Other medications, especially cholestyramine, colestipol, digitalis glycosides, or lithium
  Other medical problems, especially anuria, severe cardiac disease, severe renal function impairment, or infants with jaundice

**Proper use of this medication**
  Possible need for control of weight and diet, especially sodium intake
» Patient may not experience symptoms of hypertension; importance of taking medication even if feeling well
» Does not cure, but helps control hypertension; possible need for lifelong therapy; serious consequences of untreated hypertension
  Diuretic effects of the medication and timing of doses to minimize inconvenience of diuresis
  Compliance with therapy; taking medication at the same times each day to maintain the therapeutic effect
» Proper dosing
  Missed dose: Taking as soon as possible; not taking if almost time for next dose; not doubling doses
» Proper storage

**Precautions while using this medication**
  Making regular visits to physician to check progress
» Not taking other medications, especially nonprescription sympathomimetics, unless discussed with physician
  Possibility of hypokalemia; possible need for additional potassium in diet; not changing diet without first checking with physician
  To prevent dehydration, checking with physician if severe nausea, vomiting, or diarrhea occurs and continues
  May increase blood sugar levels in diabetics
  Possible photosensitivity; avoiding unprotected exposure to sun; using protective clothing and sun block product; avoiding use of sunlamp, tanning bed, or tanning booth
» Caution if dizziness, lightheadedness, or sudden fainting occurs, especially after initial dose; taking first dose at bedtime
» Caution when getting up suddenly from a lying or sitting position
» Caution in using alcohol, while standing for long periods or exercising, and during hot weather because of enhanced orthostatic hypotensive effects
» Possibility of drowsiness
» Caution when driving or doing anything else requiring alertness because of possible drowsiness, dizziness, or lightheadedness

**Side/adverse effects**

Signs of potential side effects, especially dizziness, edema, urinary incontinence, priapism, electrolyte imbalance, orthostatic hypotension, agranulocytosis, allergic reaction, angina, cholecystitis, pancreatitis, hepatic function impairment, palpitations, shortness of breath, hyperuricemia, gout, and thrombocytopenia

## Oral Dosage Forms

### PRAZOSIN HYDROCHLORIDE AND POLYTHIAZIDE CAPSULES

**Usual adult dose**
Antihypertensive—
  Oral, 1 capsule two or three times a day, as determined by individual titration with the component agents.

Note: Geriatric patients may be more sensitive to the effects of the usual adult dose and may require a lower dose in order to prevent syncope.

**Usual pediatric dose**
Antihypertensive—
  As determined by individual titration with the component agents.

**Strength(s) usually available**
U.S.—
  1 mg of prazosin (base) and 500 mcg (0.5 mg) of polythiazide (Rx) [*Minizide* (sucrose)].
  2 mg of prazosin (base) and 500 mcg (0.5 mg) of polythiazide (Rx) [*Minizide* (sucrose)].
  5 mg of prazosin (base) and 500 mcg (0.5 mg) of polythiazide (Rx) [*Minizide* (sucrose)].

Canada—
  Not commercially available.

**Auxiliary labeling**
• Do not take other medicines without your doctor's advice.

Revised: 07/21/92
Interim revision: 07/20/94; 08/20/98

---

**PREDNISOLONE**—See *Corticosteroids—Glucocorticoid Effects (Systemic); Corticosteroids (Ophthalmic)*

---

**PREDNISONE**—See *Corticosteroids—Glucocorticoid Effects (Systemic)*

---

**PREGNANCY TEST KITS FOR HOME USE**—The *Pregnancy Test Kits for Home Use* monograph is not included in this published version of the USP DI database. Copies of the monograph are available on request from Micromedex, Inc. - Reprint Requests, 6200 S. Syracuse Way, Suite 300, Englewood, CO 80111; telephone (303) 486-6400; telefax (303) 486-6464; Email: USPDI@MDX.COM.

---

**PRILOCAINE**—See *Anesthetics (Parenteral-Local)*

# PRIMAQUINE Systemic

VA CLASSIFICATION (Primary): AP101

Note: For a listing of dosage forms and brand names by country availability, see *Dosage Forms* section(s).

## Category
Antiprotozoal.

## Indications
Note: Bracketed information in the *Indications* section refers to uses that are not included in U.S. product labeling.

### Accepted
Malaria (treatment)—Primaquine is indicated for the prevention of relapses (radical cure) of malaria caused by *Plasmodium vivax* [and *P. ovale*]. Primaquine is also effective against the gametocytes of *P. falciparum*.

[Pneumonia, *Pneumocystis carinii* (treatment)][1]—Primaquine is used in combination with clindamycin in the treatment of *Pneumocystis carinii* pneumonia (PCP) in patients unresponsive or intolerant to standard therapy.

[1]Not included in Canadian product labeling.

## Pharmacology/Pharmacokinetics

### Physicochemical characteristics
Chemical group—8-aminoquinoline.
Molecular weight—455.34.

### Mechanism of action/Effect
The precise mechanism of action has not been determined, but may be based on primaquine's ability to bind to and alter the properties of DNA. Primaquine is highly active against the exoerythrocytic stages of *P. vivax* and *P. ovale* and against the primary exoerythrocytic stages of *P. falciparum*. It is also highly active against the sexual forms (gametocytes) of plasmodia, especially *P. falciparum*, disrupting transmission of the disease by eliminating the reservoir from which the mosquito carrier is infected.

### Absorption
Rapidly absorbed; bioavailability is approximately 96%.

### Distribution
Extensively distributed; unlike the 4-aminoquinoline antimalarials, there is no evidence of accumulation of primaquine or carboxyprimaquine in blood cells; the whole blood to plasma distribution ratio was 0.93 in one study of patients being treated with 15 mg (base) daily for 14 days.
Apparent Vol$_D$=mean 248 L (range, 149 to 303 L).

### Biotransformation
Rapidly converted to carboxyprimaquine, the principal plasma metabolite. It is not known whether this metabolite has antimalarial activity.

### Half-life
Primaquine—Mean, 5.8 hours (range, 3.7 to 7.4 hours).
Carboxyprimaquine—22 to 30 hours.

### Time to peak concentration
Primaquine—Approximately 2 to 3 hours.
Carboxyprimaquine—Approximately 7 hours (range, 2.6 to 8).

### Peak Serum Concentration
Primaquine (steady state)—
   15 mg (base): 50 to 66 nanograms per mL.
   30 mg (base): Approximately 104 nanograms per mL.
Carboxyprimaquine—
   15 mg (base) single dose: 291 to 736 nanograms per mL.
   15 mg (base) daily, on day 14: 432 to 1240 nanograms per mL.

### Elimination
Less than 2% of oral primaquine dose excreted in urine within 24 hours.

## Precautions to Consider

### Cross-sensitivity and/or related problems
Patients hypersensitive to iodoquinol, a chemically related 8-aminoquinoline, may be hypersensitive to this medication also.

### Pregnancy/Reproduction
Pregnancy—Primaquine is not recommended during pregnancy because it may cross the placenta and may cause hemolytic anemia in utero in G6PD-deficient fetuses.

### Breast-feeding
It is not known whether primaquine is excreted in breast milk. However, problems in humans have not been documented.

### Pediatrics
Appropriate studies on the relationship of age to the effects of primaquine have not been performed in the pediatric population. However, no pediatrics-specific problems have been documented to date.

### Geriatrics
No information is available on the relationship of age to the effects of primaquine in geriatric patients.

### Drug interactions and/or related problems
The following drug interactions and/or related problems have been selected on the basis of their potential clinical significance (possible mechanism in parentheses where appropriate)—not necessarily inclusive (» = major clinical significance):

Note: Combinations containing any of the following medications, depending on the amount present, may also interact with this medication.

Bone marrow depressants (See *Appendix II*) or
» Hemolytics, other (See *Appendix II*)
   (concurrent use of primaquine with bone marrow depressants may increase the leukopenic effects; if concurrent use is required, close observation for myelotoxic effects should be considered)
   (concurrent use of primaquine with other hemolytics may increase the potential for toxic side effects)

» Quinacrine
   (concurrent use is not recommended since it may increase the toxic effects of primaquine)

### Medical considerations/Contraindications
The medical considerations/contraindications included have been selected on the basis of their potential clinical significance (reasons given in parentheses where appropriate)—not necessarily inclusive (» = major clinical significance).

*Risk-benefit should be considered when the following medical problems exist:*

Favism or acute hemolytic anemia, history of (family or personal) or
» Glucose-6-phosphate dehydrogenase (G6PD) deficiency
   (primaquine may cause hemolytic anemia, especially in G6PD-deficient patients)

Hypersensitivity to primaquine

Nicotinamide adenine dinucleotide (NADH) methemoglobin reductase deficiency
   (primaquine may cause methemoglobinemia, especially in patients with NADH methemoglobin reductase deficiency)

### Patient monitoring
The following may be especially important in patient monitoring (other tests may be warranted in some patients, depending on condition; » = major clinical significance):

Blood cell counts and
Hemoglobin determinations
   (recommended at weekly intervals during therapy in patients with G6PD deficiency since anemia, methemoglobinemia, and leukopenia have been reported following administration of large doses of primaquine; a mild leukocytosis has also been observed; primaquine should be discontinued immediately if a sudden decrease in hemoglobin concentration, erythrocyte count, or leukocyte count occurs)

» Glucose-6-phosphate dehydrogenase (G6PD) determinations
   (required prior to treatment, especially in Caucasians of Mediterranean origin, Blacks, Asians, and Orientals; if a deficiency is found, primaquine should be given with caution since hemolytic effects may be exaggerated)

## Side/Adverse Effects

The following side/adverse effects have been selected on the basis of their potential clinical significance (possible signs and symptoms in parentheses where appropriate)—not necessarily inclusive:

### Those indicating need for medical attention
Incidence more frequent
   **Hemolytic anemia** (dark urine; back, leg, or stomach pains; loss of appetite; pale skin; unusual tiredness or weakness; fever)—severity of hemolysis in patients with G6PD deficiency is directly related to the degree of deficiency and the dose of primaquine administered

## Primaquine (Systemic)

Incidence less frequent
>*Methemoglobinemia* (cyanosis—bluish fingernails, lips, or skin; dizziness or lightheadedness; difficulty breathing; unusual tiredness or weakness)—especially with high doses or in patients with NADH methemoglobin reductase deficiency

Incidence rare
>*Leukopenia* (sore throat and fever)

**Those indicating need for medical attention only if they continue or are bothersome**
Incidence more frequent
>*Gastrointestinal effects* (abdominal pain or cramps, nausea or vomiting)

## Patient Consultation

As an aid to patient consultation, refer to *Advice for the Patient, Primaquine (Systemic)*.
In providing consultation, consider emphasizing the following selected information (» = major clinical significance):

### Before using this medication
» Conditions affecting use, especially:
    Hypersensitivity to primaquine
    Pregnancy—Use is not recommended
    Other medications, especially other hemolytics and quinacrine
    Other medical problems, especially G6PD deficiency

### Proper use of this medication
» Taking with meals or antacids to minimize gastric irritation
» Compliance with full course of therapy
» Proper dosing
    Missed dose: Taking as soon as possible; not taking if almost time for next dose; not doubling doses
» Proper storage

### Precautions while using this medication
Regular visits to physician to check progress during therapy

### Side/adverse effects
Signs of potential side effects, especially hemolytic anemia, leukopenia, and methemoglobinemia.

## General Dosing Information

Primaquine may be taken with meals or antacids to minimize gastric irritation.

When used to prevent relapses, primaquine may be administered concurrently or consecutively with chloroquine or hydroxychloroquine.

## Oral Dosage Forms

Note: Bracketed uses in the *Dosage Forms* section refer to categories of use and/or indications that are not included in U.S. product labeling.

### PRIMAQUINE PHOSPHATE TABLETS USP

**Usual adult and adolescent dose**
Malaria—
    Oral, 26.3 mg (15 mg base) once a day for fourteen days.
    Note: For some strains of *Plasmodium vivax* (particularly those from Southeast Asia), a dose of 39.4 to 52.6 mg (22.5 to 30 mg base) daily for fourteen days may be required for radical cure of malaria.
    To eliminate gametocytes of *P. falciparum*, a single dose of 78.9 mg (45 mg base) may be administered.
[*Pneumocystis carinii* pneumonia][1]—
    Oral, 26.3 mg to 52.6 mg (15 to 30 mg base) once a day for twenty-one days.

**Usual pediatric dose**
Malaria—
    Oral, 680 mcg (390 mcg base) (0.68 mg [0.39 mg base]) per kg of body weight once a day for fourteen days.

**Strength(s) usually available**
U.S.—
    26.3 mg (15 mg base) (Rx) [GENERIC].
Canada—
    26.3 mg (15 mg base) (Rx) [GENERIC].

**Packaging and storage**
Store below 40 °C (104 °F), preferably between 15 and 30 °C (59 and 86 °F), unless otherwise specified by manufacturer. Store in a well-closed, light-resistant container.

**Auxiliary labeling**
• Continue medicine for full time of treatment.

[1] Not included in Canadian product labeling.

Revised: 01/19/93

---

# PRIMIDONE   Systemic

VA CLASSIFICATION (Primary): CN400
Commonly used brand name(s): *Apo-Primidone; Myidone; Mysoline; PMS Primidone; Sertan*.
Note: For a listing of dosage forms and brand names by country availability, see *Dosage Forms* section(s).

## Category
Anticonvulsant.

## Indications
Note: Bracketed information in the *Indications* section refers to uses that are not included in U.S. product labeling.

### Accepted
Epilepsy (treatment)—Primidone, either alone or used concomitantly with other anticonvulsants, is indicated in the control of generalized tonic-clonic (grand mal), nocturnal myoclonic, complex partial (psychomotor), and simple partial (cortical focal) epileptic seizures.
[Essential tremor (treatment)][1]—Primidone is used in the treatment of essential (familial) tremor. Although propranolol is considered to be the treatment of choice for essential tremor, primidone provides effective treatment for some patients.

[1] Not included in Canadian product labeling.

## Pharmacology/Pharmacokinetics

**Physicochemical characteristics**
Molecular weight—218.25.

**Mechanism of action/Effect**
Unknown, but anticonvulsant effects are thought to be due to the parent compound, primidone, as well as its two active metabolites, phenobarbital and phenylethylmalonamide (PEMA), whose actions may be synergistic.

**Absorption**
Rapid, usually complete with wide individual variation. Bioavailability—90 to 100% (indirect estimates).

**Distribution**
Primidone has a volume of distribution ($V_D$) of 0.64 to 0.86 liters per kg.
Primidone and its metabolites pass into breast milk, reaching a mean concentration of 75% of maternal steady-state serum levels.

**Half-life**
Primidone—3 to 23 hours.
Phenobarbital metabolite—75 to 126 hours.
PEMA metabolite—10 to 25 hours.

**Time to peak concentration**
Average 3 to 4 hours.

**Therapeutic serum concentration**
5 to 12 mcg of primidone per mL(mcg/mL) (23 to 55 mmol/L), which produces phenobarbital serum concentrations of 20 to 40 mcg/mL (86 to 172 mmol/L). Some clinicians have suggested that the optimal mean plasma primidone concentration is 12 mcg/mL with an associated mean derived phenobarbital concentration of 15 mcg/mL resulting in a primidone-to-phenobarbital ratio of 0.8; however, much variation occurs among patients.

|  | Protein Binding (%) | Biotransformation | Elimination (% unchanged) |
|---|---|---|---|
| Primidone | 0–20 | Hepatic; 2 active metabolites: phenobarbital (15–25%) and PEMA. PEMA is the major metabolite and less active than phenobarbital | Renal (64) |
| PEMA (metabolite) | Negligible | No further metabolism | Renal (6.6) |
| Phenobarbital (metabolite) | 50 | Hepatic (therapeutic doses of primidone produce therapeutic blood concentrations of phenobarbital) | Renal (5.1) |

## Precautions to Consider

### Cross-sensitivity and/or related problems
Patients sensitive to barbiturates may be sensitive to this medication also.

### Pregnancy/Reproduction
Pregnancy—Adequate and well-controlled studies in humans have not been done. However, reports have suggested an association between the use of other anticonvulsant drugs and an increased incidence of birth defects (fetal hydantoin syndrome) in newborns. Symptoms similar to fetal hydantoin syndrome, i.e., growth retardation, craniofacial and heart abnormalities, and hypoplasia of the fingernails and distal phalanges, have been shown to occur with primidone also.

Neonatal hemorrhage, with a coagulation defect resembling vitamin K deficiency, has been described in newborns whose mothers were taking primidone and other anticonvulsants. Risk may be reduced by administering water-soluble vitamin K prophylactically to the mother 1 month prior to and during delivery and also to the neonate, intramuscularly or subcutaneously, immediately after birth.

### Breast-feeding
Primidone is distributed into breast milk in substantial amounts, and the use of primidone by nursing mothers may cause unusual drowsiness in the neonate.

### Pediatrics
Some children may react to primidone with paradoxical excitement and restlessness.

### Geriatrics
Unusual restlessness and excitement may sometimes occur as a paradoxical reaction in the elderly.

### Drug interactions and/or related problems
The following drug interactions and/or related problems have been selected on the basis of their potential clinical significance (possible mechanism in parentheses where appropriate)—not necessarily inclusive (» = major clinical significance):

Note: Combinations containing any of the following medications, depending on the amount present, may also interact with this medication.

Although not all of the following interactions have been documented to pertain specifically to primidone, a potential exists for their occurrence because of the barbiturate metabolite of primidone.

Acetaminophen
(when acetaminophen in therapeutic doses is used concurrently in patients receiving chronic primidone therapy, its effects may be decreased because of increased metabolism resulting from induction of hepatic microsomal enzymes by the phenobarbital metabolite; also, risk of hepatotoxicity with single toxic doses or prolonged use of acetaminophen may be increased in chronic alcoholics or in patients regularly using hepatic-enzyme inducing agents)

» Adrenocorticoids, glucocorticoid and mineralocorticoid or
» Anticoagulants, coumarin- or indandione-derivative or
Antidepressants, tricyclic or
Chloramphenicol or
» Contraceptives, oral, estrogen-containing or
» Corticotropin (ACTH) or
Cyclosporine or
Dacarbazine or
Digitalis glycosides, with possible exception of digoxin or
Disopyramide or
Doxycycline or
Levothyroxine or
Metronidazole or
Mexiletine or
Quinidine
(concurrent use with primidone may decrease the effects of these medications because of increased metabolism resulting from induction of hepatic microsomal enzymes by the barbiturate metabolite; dosage increases may be necessary during and after primidone therapy)

(use of a nonhormonal method of birth control or a progestin-only oral contraceptive may be necessary during primidone therapy)

(also, concurrent use of tricyclic antidepressants with primidone may enhance central nervous system [CNS] depression, lower convulsive threshold, and decrease the effects of primidone; dosage adjustments may be necessary to control seizures)

» Alcohol or
» CNS depression–producing medications, other (See *Appendix II*)
(concurrent use may potentiate the CNS and respiratory depressant effects of either these medications or primidone; dosage adjustment of primidone may be necessary)

Amphetamines
(concurrent use may cause a delay in the intestinal absorption of the phenobarbital metabolite)

» Anticonvulsants, other
(concurrent use may cause a change in the pattern of epileptiform seizures because of altered medication metabolism; monitoring of plasma concentrations of both medications is recommended; dosage adjustments may be necessary)

(carbamazepine induces metabolism and decreases effects of primidone; monitoring of plasma concentrations is recommended as a guide to dosage if either medication is added or withdrawn from an existing regimen)

(concurrent use of valproic acid with primidone may cause higher serum concentrations of primidone leading to increased CNS depression and neurological toxicity because of protein binding displacement and reduced metabolism; half-life of valproic acid may be decreased; in addition, primidone may enhance valproic acid hepatotoxicity, presumably through the formation of hepatotoxic valproate metabolites; dosage adjustment of primidone may be necessary)

Carbonic anhydrase inhibitors
(osteopenia induced by primidone may be enhanced; it is recommended that patients receiving concurrent therapy be monitored for early signs of osteopenia and that the carbonic acid anhydrase inhibitor be discontinued and appropriate treatment initiated if necessary)

Cyclophosphamide
(concurrent use with primidone may induce microsomal metabolism to increase the formation of alkylating metabolites of cyclophosphamide, thereby reducing the half-life and increasing the leukopenic activity of cyclophosphamide)

Enflurane or
Halothane or
Methoxyflurane
(chronic use of primidone prior to anesthesia may increase anesthetic metabolism, leading to increased risk of hepatotoxicity)

(also, chronic use of primidone prior to anesthesia with methoxyflurane may increase formation of nephrotoxic metabolites, leading to increased risk of nephrotoxicity)

Fenoprofen
(concurrent use with primidone may decrease the elimination half-life of fenoprofen, possibly because of increased metabolism resulting from induction of hepatic microsomal enzyme activity; fenoprofen dosage adjustment may be required)

Folic acid
(requirements for folic acid may be increased in patients receiving anticonvulsant therapy)

Griseofulvin
(antifungal effects may be decreased when griseofulvin is used concurrently with primidone because of impaired absorption resulting in decreased serum concentrations; although the effect of decreased serum concentrations on therapeutic response has not been established, concurrent use preferably should be avoided)

Guanadrel or
Guanethidine
(concurrent use with primidone may aggravate orthostatic hypotension)

Haloperidol or
Loxapine or
Maprotiline or
Molindone or
Phenothiazines or
Thioxanthenes
(concurrent use may lower the seizure threshold because of altered metabolism; CNS depression may be increased; decreases in primidone dosage may be necessary)
(serum concentrations of neuroleptics may be significantly reduced when these medications are used concurrently with primidone because of increased metabolism)

Leucovorin
(large doses may counteract the anticonvulsant effects of primidone)

Methylphenidate
(concurrent use may increase serum concentrations of primidone because of metabolism inhibition, possibly resulting in toxicity; dosage adjustments may be necessary)

» Monoamine oxidase (MAO) inhibitors, including furazolidone, procarbazine, or selegiline
(concurrent use may prolong the effects of primidone because metabolism of the barbiturate metabolite may be inhibited; changes in the pattern of epileptiform seizures may occur; dosage adjustments of primidone may be necessary)

Phenobarbital
(although concurrent use with primidone is rarely indicated, since primidone is metabolized to phenobarbital, it may cause a change in the pattern of epileptiform seizures because of altered medication metabolism and also increase the sedative effect of either primidone or the barbiturate anticonvulsant; decreases in primidone dosage may be necessary)

Phenylbutazone
(concurrent use may decrease the efficacy of the phenobarbital metabolite of primidone by inducing hepatic microsomal enzymes and increasing its metabolism; also, hepatic enzyme inducers such as barbiturates may increase phenylbutazone metabolism and decrease its half-life)

Posterior pituitary
(concurrent use with primidone may increase the risk of cardiac arrhythmias and coronary insufficiency)

Rifampin
(concurrent use of rifampin with barbiturates may enhance the metabolism of hexobarbital by induction of hepatic microsomal enzymes, resulting in lower serum concentrations; there is conflicting data on rifampin's effect on phenobarbital blood levels; dosage adjustment may be required)

Vitamin D
(effects may be reduced by primidone, because of accelerated metabolism by hepatic microsomal enzyme induction; vitamin D supplementation may be required in patients on long-term primidone therapy to prevent osteomalacia, although rickets is rare)

Xanthines, such as:
Aminophylline
Caffeine
Oxtriphylline
Theophylline
(concurrent use with primidone, because of the barbiturate metabolite, may increase metabolism of the xanthines [except dyphylline] by induction of hepatic microsomal enzymes, resulting in increased theophylline clearance)

### Laboratory value alterations
The following have been selected on the basis of their potential clinical significance (possible effect in parentheses where appropriate)—not necessarily inclusive (» = major clinical significance):

With diagnostic test results
Cyanocobalamin Co 57
(absorption of radioactive cyanocobalamin may be impaired by concurrent use of primidone)

Metyrapone test
(increased metabolism of metyrapone by an hepatic enzyme inducer such as primidone may decrease the response to metyrapone)

Phentolamine test
(primidone may cause a false-positive phentolamine test; it is recommended that all medications be withdrawn at least 24 hours, preferably 48 to 72 hours, prior to a phentolamine test)

With physiology/laboratory test values
Bilirubin concentrations, serum
(may be decreased in patients with congenital nonhemolytic unconjugated hyperbilirubinemia and in epileptics; this effect is presumably due to induction of glucuronyl transferase, the enzyme responsible for the conjugation of bilirubin)

### Medical considerations/Contraindications
The medical considerations/contraindications included have been selected on the basis of their potential clinical significance (reasons given in parentheses where appropriate)—not necessarily inclusive (» = major clinical significance).

*This medication should not be used when the following medical problem exists:*
» Porphyria, acute intermittent or variegate, or history of
(barbiturate metabolite of primidone may aggravate symptoms of porphyria by inducing enzymes responsible for porphyrin synthesis)

*Risk-benefit should be considered when the following medical problems exist:*
Hepatic function impairment
(possible systemic accumulation of barbiturate metabolite)
Hyperkinesia
(may be precipitated or aggravated by primidone)
Renal function impairment
(possible systemic accumulation of barbiturate metabolite)
» Respiratory diseases such as asthma, emphysema, or those involving dyspnea or obstruction
(serious ventilatory depression may occur)
Sensitivity to primidone or barbiturates

### Patient monitoring
The following may be especially important in patient monitoring (other tests may be warranted in some patients, depending on condition; » = major clinical significance):

Blood cell counts, complete and
Blood chemistry profiles
(manufacturer recommends that these tests be completed every 6 months)
Folate concentrations, serum
(determinations recommended periodically because of increased folate requirements of patients on long-term anticonvulsant therapy)
Phenobarbital concentrations, serum, and
Primidone concentrations, serum
(since phenobarbital is a major metabolite of primidone, serum concentrations of both may be required in some patients at periodic intervals to maintain maximum therapeutic efficacy)

## Side/Adverse Effects
The following side/adverse effects have been selected on the basis of their potential clinical significance (possible signs and symptoms in parentheses where appropriate)—not necessarily inclusive:

### Those indicating need for medical attention
Incidence less frequent
*Paradoxical reaction* (unusual excitement or restlessness)—especially in children and the elderly
Incidence rare
*Anemia, megaloblastic* (unusual tiredness or weakness); *skin rash*
Note: *Megaloblastic anemia* may respond to folic acid without discontinuation of anticonvulsant therapy.

Signs of intolerance or overdose
*Confusion; diplopia* (double vision); *nystagmus* (continuous, uncontrolled back-and-forth and/or rolling eye movements); *shortness of breath or troubled breathing*

### Those indicating need for medical attention only if they continue or are bothersome
Incidence more frequent
*Ataxia* (clumsiness or unsteadiness); *dizziness*
Incidence less frequent
*Anorexia* (loss of appetite); *drowsiness; impotence* (decreased sexual ability); *mood or mental changes; nausea or vomiting*—usually decreases or disappears with continued use of medication

## Patient Consultation
As an aid to patient consultation, refer to *Advice for the Patient, Primidone (Systemic)*.
In providing consultation, consider emphasizing the following selected information (» = major clinical significance):

### Before using this medication
» Conditions affecting use, especially:
  Sensitivity to primidone or barbiturates
  Pregnancy—Abnormalities similar to fetal hydantoin syndrome may occur; neonatal hemorrhaging may occur at delivery
  Breast-feeding—Distributed into breast milk, causing drowsiness in the baby
  Use in children—Paradoxical excitement and restlessness may occur
  Use in the elderly—Paradoxical excitement and restlessness may occur
  Other medications, especially adrenocorticoids, anticoagulants, estrogens, estrogen-containing contraceptives, CNS depression–producing medications, other anticonvulsants, or monoamine oxidase inhibitors
  Other medical problems, especially acute intermittent porphyria, or respiratory diseases

### Proper use of this medication
» Compliance with therapy; taking every day in doses spaced as directed
» Proper dosing
  Missed dose: Taking as soon as possible, unless within an hour of next scheduled dose; not doubling doses
» Proper storage

### Precautions while using this medication
Regular visits to physician to check progress of therapy
Checking with physician before discontinuing medication; gradual dosage reduction may be needed
Caution if any kind of surgery, dental treatment, or emergency treatment is required
» Avoiding use of alcoholic beverages; not taking other CNS depressants unless prescribed by physician
» Possible drowsiness; caution when driving or doing other things requiring alertness
» Possible dizziness or lightheadedness; caution when getting up suddenly from a lying or sitting position
Caution if any laboratory tests required; possible interference with results of cyanocobalamin Co 57, metyrapone, or phentolamine tests.

### Side/adverse effects
Signs of potential side effects, especially excitement or restlessness, allergic reaction, or megaloblastic anemia

## General Dosing Information

Because primidone serum concentrations vary greatly among patients after oral administration, it is very important that the dosage be individualized. One of primidone's metabolites, phenobarbital, greatly influences its serum concentration, side effects, and interactions, as well as its therapeutic effect.

When primidone is to be discontinued, dosage should be reduced gradually. Abrupt withdrawal may precipitate status epilepticus.

When used with or to replace other anticonvulsant therapy, the dosage of primidone should be increased gradually while that of the other medication is maintained or decreased gradually in order to maintain seizure control. When therapy with primidone alone is the objective, the transition should not be completed in less than 2 weeks.

Many of the common side effects such as nausea, dizziness, and drowsiness diminish in frequency and intensity with continued use of the medication or reduction of dosage.

### Diet/Nutrition
Patients on long-term anticonvulsant therapy have increased folate requirements. In addition, patients on long-term therapy may require vitamin D supplementation to prevent osteomalacia.

## Oral Dosage Forms
Note: Bracketed uses in the *Dosage Forms* section refer to categories of use and/or indications that are not included in U.S. product labeling.

### PRIMIDONE ORAL SUSPENSION USP

**Usual adult and adolescent dose**
Anticonvulsant—
  Initial—
    Oral, 100 or 125 mg once a day at bedtime for the first three days, the daily dose being increased to 100 or 125 mg two times a day for the fourth, fifth, and sixth days, and then increased to 100 or 125 mg three times a day for the seventh, eighth, and ninth days. On the tenth day a maintenance dosage of 250 mg three times a day may be established and then adjusted according to patient needs and tolerance but not to exceed 2 grams a day.
Note: Initial doses as low as 25 mg twice a day have been used in patients experiencing troublesome nausea and vomiting.
  Maintenance—
    Oral, 250 mg three or four times a day.
[Tremorlytic][1]
    Oral, initially 50 to 62.5 mg a day, the dosage being increased as needed and tolerated up to a maximum of 750 mg a day.

**Usual pediatric dose**
Anticonvulsant—
  Children up to 8 years of age:
    Initial—Oral, 50 mg at bedtime for the first three days, the daily dose being increased to 50 mg two times a day for the fourth, fifth, and sixth days and then increased to 100 mg two times a day for the seventh, eighth, and ninth days.
    Maintenance—Oral, on the tenth day, 125 to 250 mg three times a day (or 10 to 25 mg per kg of body weight a day given in divided doses), the dosage being adjusted according to patient needs and tolerance.
  Children 8 years of age and over:
    See *Usual adult and adolescent dose*.

**Strength(s) usually available**
U.S.—
  250 mg per 5 mL (Rx) [*Mysoline* (ammonia solution [diluted]; citric acid; D&C Yellow No. 10; FD&C Yellow No. 6; magnesium aluminum silicate; methylparaben; propylparaben; saccharin sodium; sodium alginate; sodium citrate; sodium hypochlorite solution; sorbic acid; sorbitan monolaurate; purified water; flavors)].
Canada—
  Not commercially available.

**Packaging and storage**
Store below 40 °C (104 °F), preferably between 15 and 30 °C (59 and 86 °F), unless otherwise specified by manufacturer. Store in a tight, light-resistant container. Protect from freezing.

**Auxiliary labeling**
• Shake well.
• May cause drowsiness.
• Avoid alcoholic beverages.
• Do not freeze.

### PRIMIDONE TABLETS USP

**Usual adult and adolescent dose**
See *Primidone Oral Suspension USP*.

**Usual pediatric dose**
See *Primidone Oral Suspension USP*.

**Strength(s) usually available**
U.S.—
  50 mg (Rx) [*Mysoline* (lactose)].
  250 mg (Rx) [*Myidone*; *Mysoline*; GENERIC].
Canada—
  125 mg (Rx) [*Apo-Primidone*; *PMS Primidone*; *Sertan*].
  250 mg (Rx) [*Apo-Primidone*; *Mysoline* (lactose); *PMS Primidone*; *Sertan*; GENERIC].

**Packaging and storage**
Store below 40 °C (104 °F), preferably between 15 and 30 °C (59 and 86 °F), unless otherwise specified by manufacturer. Store in a well-closed container.

**Auxiliary labeling**
• May cause drowsiness.
• Avoid alcoholic beverages.

### PRIMIDONE CHEWABLE TABLETS

**Usual adult and adolescent dose**
See *Primidone Oral Suspension USP*.

**Usual pediatric dose**
See *Primidone Oral Suspension USP*.

**Strength(s) usually available**
U.S.—
  Not commercially available.
Canada—
  125 mg (Rx) [*Mysoline* (lactose)].

# PROBENECID  Systemic

VA CLASSIFICATION (Primary): MS400
Commonly used brand name(s): *Benemid; Benuryl; Probalan.*
Note: For a listing of dosage forms and brand names by country availability, see *Dosage Forms* section(s).

## Category
Antigout agent; antibiotic therapy adjunct; antihyperuricemic.

## Indications
Note: Bracketed information in the *Indications* section refers to uses that are not included in U.S. product labeling.

**Accepted**
Gouty arthritis, chronic (treatment) or
Hyperuricemia (treatment)—Probenecid is indicated for the long-term management of hyperuricemia associated with chronic gout. It is recommended only for patients whose 24-hour renal excretion of urate is 800 mg (4.8 mmol) or lower (i.e., patients who are hyperuricemic as a result of underexcretion, rather than overproduction, of urate). The aim of probenecid therapy is to reduce the number of acute gout attacks.

Probenecid is not effective in the treatment of acute gout attacks and does not eliminate the need to use colchicine or a nonsteroidal anti-inflammatory drug (NSAID) to relieve an attack. Also, probenecid therapy should not be initiated during an attack, because it may induce fluctuations in urate concentration that may result in prolongation of the attack or initiation of a new attack.

[Probenecid is sometimes used in the treatment of hyperuricemia not associated with gout. However, treatment of asymptomatic hyperuricemia is often unnecessary; the need for such therapy should be determined on an individual basis][1].

Antibiotic therapy, adjunct—Probenecid is indicated as an adjunct to therapy with penicillins [and some of the cephalosporin antibiotics][1]. It is used primarily when high antibiotic plasma and tissue concentrations are required. Adjunctive use of probenecid is included in some of the U.S. Centers for Disease Control (CDC) guidelines for the treatment of sexually transmitted diseases such as gonorrhea, acute pelvic inflammatory disease (outpatient treatment), and neurosyphilis.

**Unaccepted**
Probenecid is not recommended in circumstances in which there is an especially high risk of adverse effects associated with crystallization and deposition of urate in renal tissues, such as formation of renal calculi and uric acid nephropathy. It therefore should not be used for treatment of gout in patients whose 24-hour urate excretion exceeds 800 mg (4.8 mmol) or who have extensive tophi, or for treatment of hyperuricemia associated with neoplastic disease or its treatment (chemotherapy with rapidly cytolytic antineoplastic agents or radiation therapy). Allopurinol, which decreases the quantity of urate that reaches the kidneys in addition to decreasing the concentration of urate in the blood, is recommended in these circumstances.

[1] Not included in Canadian product labeling.

## Pharmacology/Pharmacokinetics

**Physicochemical characteristics**
Molecular weight—285.36.
pKa—3.4.

**Mechanism of action/Effect**
Antigout agent; antihyperuricemic—Probenecid is a uricosuric agent. By competitively inhibiting the active reabsorption of urate at the proximal renal tubule, it increases the urinary excretion of uric acid and lowers serum urate concentrations. By lowering serum concentrations of uric acid below its solubility limits, probenecid may decrease or prevent urate deposition, tophi formation, and chronic joint changes; promote resolution of existing urate deposits; and, after several months of therapy, reduce the frequency of acute attacks of gout. Probenecid has no anti-inflammatory or analgesic activity.

Antibiotic therapy adjunct—Probenecid is a competitive inhibitor of the secretion of weak organic acids, including penicillins and some of the cephalosporin antibiotics, at the proximal and distal renal tubules. It thereby increases blood concentrations of these antibiotics (penicillin concentrations may increase 2- to 4-fold), increases their elimination half-life, and prolongs their duration of action.

**Other actions/effects**
Probenecid also inhibits the renal and/or biliary transport, as well as transport into or out of the cerebrospinal fluid (CSF), of many other endogenous compounds and medications.

**Absorption**
Rapid and complete.

**Protein binding**
High to very high (75 to 95%); primarily to albumin.

**Biotransformation**
Hepatic; rapid and extensive. Metabolites include probenecid monoacyl glucuronide, a carboxylated metabolite, and hydroxylated compounds that have uricosuric activity.

**Half-life**
Dose-dependent; 3 to 8 hours following administration of a 500-mg dose; 6 to 12 hours following administration of larger doses.

**Time to peak concentration**
Adults—2 to 4 hours following a single 1-gram dose; 4 hours following a single 2-gram dose.

**Peak serum concentration**
> 30 mcg per mL (mcg/mL) (105 micromoles/L) following a single 1-gram dose; 150 to 200 mcg/mL (525 to 700 micromoles/L) following a single 2-gram dose.

**Therapeutic plasma concentration**
Uricosuric effect—100 to 200 mcg/mL (350 to 700 micromoles/L).
Suppression of penicillin excretion—40 to 60 mcg/mL (140 to 210 micromoles/L).

**Time to peak effect**
Uricosuric—30 minutes.
Suppression of penicillin excretion—2 hours.

**Duration of action**
The effect on penicillin plasma concentration persists for about 8 hours following a single dose.

**Elimination**
Primarily via hepatic metabolism, followed by renal excretion of metabolites. About 5 to 10% of a dose is excreted unchanged within 24 to 48 hours. Probenecid excretion is dependent upon urinary pH and is increased in alkaline urine; however, the uricosuric activity is not altered.

## Precautions to Consider

**Pregnancy/Reproduction**
Pregnancy—Probenecid crosses the placenta and appears in cord blood. However, the medication has been administered to pregnant women without known adverse effects occurring.

**Breast-feeding**
It is not known whether probenecid is excreted in breast milk. However, problems in humans have not been documented.

**Pediatrics**
Antibiotic therapy adjunct—Studies performed to date have not demonstrated pediatrics-specific problems that would limit the usefulness of probenecid in children 2 to 14 years of age. Use in children younger than 2 years of age is not recommended.

Antigout agent or
Antihyperuricemic—No information is available on the relationship of age to the effects of probenecid as an antigout or antihyperuricemic agent in pediatric patients.

**Geriatrics**
No information is available on the relationship of age to the effects of probenecid in geriatric patients. However, elderly patients are more likely to have age-related renal function impairment, which requires caution in patients receiving probenecid.

**Drug interactions and/or related problems**
The following drug interactions and/or related problems have been selected on the basis of their potential clinical significance (possible mechanism in parentheses where appropriate)—not necessarily inclusive (» = major clinical significance):

See also *Laboratory value alterations*.

Note: Combinations containing any of the following medications, depending on the amount present, may also interact with this medication.

Acyclovir, systemic
(probenecid may decrease renal tubular secretion of acyclovir, resulting in increased and prolonged acyclovir serum and cerebrospinal fluid [CSF] concentrations, prolonged elimination half-life in serum and CSF, and, potentially, increased toxicity)

Alcohol or
Diazoxide or
Mecamylamine or
Pyrazinamide
(these medications may increase serum uric acid concentrations; pyrazinamide may also more directly antagonize probenecid's uricosuric activity; dosage adjustment of probenecid may be necessary to control hyperuricemia and gout)

Allopurinol
(probenecid increases urinary excretion of oxipurinol, the active metabolite of allopurinol; however, the antihyperuricemic effects of the two medications are additive and increased therapeutic benefit has been reported with concurrent use)

Aminosalicylate sodium
(probenecid may decrease renal tubular secretion of aminosalicylate sodium, resulting in increased and prolonged serum concentrations and/or toxicity; however, probenecid is not currently recommended as an adjunct to therapy with this medication; patients should be monitored and dosage adjustments made as necessary during and after concurrent therapy)

Anti-inflammatory drugs, nonsteroidal (NSAIDs), especially:
» Indomethacin and
» Ketoprofen
(probenecid decreases the renal clearance of ketoprofen by approximately 66%, ketoprofen protein binding by 28%, and formation and renal clearance of ketoprofen conjugates, leading to greatly increased ketoprofen plasma concentration and risk of toxicity; concurrent use is not recommended)

(probenecid may decrease renal excretion and biliary clearance of indomethacin, leading to increased plasma concentration, elimination half-life [in one study, the elimination half-life was increased from 10.1 to 17.6 hours], and toxicity, and possibly resulting in increased effectiveness; if concurrent use is required, it is recommended that indomethacin be administered in reduced dosage and that increases in dosage be made slowly and in small increments)

(probenecid has also been shown to increase the plasma concentration of naproxen [by 50%], and meclofenamate, and may also increase the plasma concentration of other NSAIDs, possibly enhancing effectiveness and/or increasing the potential for toxicity; a reduction of NSAID dosage may be required if adverse effects occur)

(probenecid may increase the plasma concentrations of sulindac and its sulfone metabolite and slightly decrease the plasma concentrations of the active sulfide metabolite)

» Antineoplastic agents, rapidly cytolytic
(concurrent use with probenecid is not recommended because of the risk of uric acid nephropathy; allopurinol is the antihyperuricemic agent of choice for reducing risks [gout and/or urate nephropathy] associated with chemotherapy-induced hyperuricemia; also, rapidly cytolytic antineoplastic agents may increase serum uric acid concentrations and interfere with control of pre-existing hyperuricemia and gout)

» Aspirin or other salicylates, including bismuth subsalicylate
(chronic administration of a salicylate with probenecid may interfere with probenecid's uricosuric effect [but not its effect on penicillin excretion]; also, probenecid inhibits the uricosuria induced by high doses of salicylates and may inhibit salicylate excretion, possibly leading to increased salicylate concentrations and toxicity; chronic use of a salicylate, especially in large [antirheumatic] doses, together with probenecid is not recommended)

(occasional use of a salicylate in low to moderate analgesic doses, or chronic administration of 80 mg per day of aspirin as an antithrombotic, is not likely to interfere with probenecid's uricosuric effect)

» Cephalosporins or
» Penicillins
(probenecid decreases renal tubular secretion of penicillins and those cephalosporins excreted by this mechanism, resulting in increased and prolonged antibiotic serum concentrations, prolonged elimination half-life, and increased risk of toxicity; adjunctive use of probenecid provides therapeutic benefit when high and/or prolonged plasma and tissue concentrations of these antibiotics are required; however, probenecid has no effect on the secretion of cefoperazone, ceforanide, ceftazidime, ceftriaxone, or moxalactam)

(probenecid also decreases renal tubular secretion of sulbactam, resulting in increased sulbactam plasma concentrations, but has no effect on renal tubular secretion of clavulanic acid [agents used in combination with some of the beta-lactam antibiotics to protect the antibiotics from enzymatic degradation])

Chlorpropamide and possibly other sulfonylurea antidiabetic agents
(probenecid decreases chlorpropamide elimination, leading to increased plasma concentration and elimination half-life and possibly to an enhanced or prolonged hypoglycemic effect; although an effect of probenecid on the elimination of other sulfonylurea antidiabetic agents has not been determined, the possibility of similar effects should be considered)

Ciprofloxacin or
Norfloxacin
(probenecid decreases renal tubular secretion of ciprofloxacin [by about 50%] and norfloxacin, leading to increased and more prolonged serum concentrations, prolonged elimination half-life, and increased risk of toxicity of the antibacterials)

Clofibrate
(probenecid may decrease renal and metabolic clearances and alter the protein binding of clofibrate, thereby increasing clofibrate's therapeutic and toxic effects)

Dapsone
(concurrent administration with probenecid results in dapsone plasma concentrations being increased by 50% 4 hours after administration and by 25% 8 hours after administration; the patient should be observed for signs of dapsone toxicity and dosage decreased if necessary)

Dyphylline
(probenecid may increase the half-life of dyphylline, possibly permitting less frequent dyphylline dosing)

Furosemide
(probenecid may inhibit renal tubular secretion of furosemide, leading to increased furosemide serum concentrations)

Ganciclovir
(probenecid may decrease the renal clearance of ganciclovir)

» Heparin
(probenecid may increase and prolong the anticoagulant effects of heparin)

Imipenem (available only as imipenem and cilastatin combination)
(since concurrent use with probenecid results in only minimal increase in the serum concentration and half-life of imipenem, such concurrent use to increase imipenem blood concentration is not recommended)

Lorazepam or
Oxazepam or
Temazepam
(probenecid may impair glucuronide conjugation of these benzodiazepines, resulting in increased effects and possibly excessive sedation)

» Methotrexate
(when methotrexate is used as an antineoplastic agent, concurrent use of probenecid is not recommended because of the risk of uric acid nephropathy; allopurinol is the antihyperuricemic agent of choice in this situation)

(probenecid may inhibit renal excretion of methotrexate, possibly leading to toxic plasma concentrations even with the relatively low doses of methotrexate used for noncancerous indications; if used concurrently with probenecid, methotrexate dosage should be de-

» Nitrofurantoin
(probenecid may inhibit renal tubular secretion of nitrofurantoin, resulting in increased serum concentrations and/or toxicity and reduced urinary concentrations and effectiveness as a urinary antiseptic; a reduction of probenecid dosage may be necessary to ensure effectiveness against urinary tract infection)

Riboflavin (vitamin B$_2$)
(probenecid decreases gastrointestinal absorption of riboflavin; requirements for riboflavin may be increased in patients receiving probenecid)

Rifampin
(probenecid may compete with rifampin for hepatic uptake when the two medications are used concurrently, resulting in increased and prolonged rifampin blood concentrations and/or toxicity; however, the effect on rifampin blood concentrations is inconsistent and concurrent use of probenecid to increase rifampin blood concentrations is not recommended)

Sodium benzoate and sodium phenylacetate
(probenecid may interfere with renal elimination of the conjugated products of these agents)

Sulfinpyrazone
(probenecid inhibits the renal secretion of sulfinpyrazone and its active metabolite; however, the uricosuric effects of the medications are additive, and increased therapeutic benefit has been reported with concurrent use)

Sulfonamides
(probenecid decreases renal excretion of sulfonamides, resulting in increased total serum concentrations of these medications, which may increase the risk of toxicity, but concurrent use provides no therapeutic advantage because free serum concentrations of antibacterial sulfonamides are not increased; sulfonamide serum concentrations should be determined at periodic intervals when these medications are used concurrently with probenecid for a prolonged period of time)

Thiopental
(administration of probenecid 3 hours prior to induction of anesthesia with thiopental significantly reduced the required dose of thiopental and prolonged its effects)

» Zidovudine
(probenecid inhibits hepatic glucuronidation and renal tubular secretion of zidovudine, resulting in increased serum concentrations and prolonged elimination half-life; this may increase the risk of toxicity, or possibly permit a reduction in daily zidovudine dosage; however, in 1 small trial, a very high incidence of skin rash occurred in patients receiving the medications concurrently)

**Laboratory value alterations**
The following have been selected on the basis of their potential clinical significance (possible effect in parentheses where appropriate)—not necessarily inclusive (» = major clinical significance):

With diagnostic test results
Aminohippuric acid (PAH) clearance studies and
Phenolsulfonphthalein (PSP) clearance studies
(probenecid decreases renal clearance of PAH and PSP, leading to reduced urine concentrations and misleading test results)

Glucose, urine, determinations
(a reducing substance present in the urine of patients receiving probenecid may cause false-positive test results with copper sulfate urine sugar tests, but not with glucose enzymatic urine sugar tests)

Renal function studies using iodohippurate sodium I 123, iodohippurate sodium I 131, or technetium Tc 99m gluceptate
(probenecid may decrease kidney uptake of these diagnostic aids because of probenecid's inhibitory action on the enzyme transport system in the proximal tubule)

With physiology/laboratory test values
Homovanillic acid (HVA) and
5-Hydroxyindoleacetic acid (5-HIAA)
(probenecid inhibits transport of these substances from the cerebrospinal fluid [CSF] into the blood, resulting in increased CSF concentrations and reduced urine concentrations; however, the changes in HVA and 5-HIAA concentrations are not as great in patients with parkinsonian syndrome and mental depression, respectively, as in healthy individuals)

17-Ketosteroid concentrations, urine
(may be decreased)

Phosphorus
(reabsorption may be increased in hypoparathyroid, but not euparathyroid, individuals)

**Medical considerations/Contraindications**
The medical considerations/contraindications included have been selected on the basis of their potential clinical significance (reasons given in parentheses where appropriate)—not necessarily inclusive (» = major clinical significance).

*Except under special circumstances, this medication should not be used when the following medical conditions exist:*

» Any condition in which there is an increased risk of uric acid renal calculus formation or urate nephropathy, such as:
» Cancer chemotherapy with rapidly cytolytic antineoplastic agents
» Radiation therapy for malignancy
» Renal calculi or history of, especially uric acid calculi
» Urate excretion higher than 800 mg (4.8 mmol) in 24 hours
» Urate nephropathy or history of
(probenecid is likely to induce, or to exacerbate pre-existing, renal calculi and/or urate nephropathy; allopurinol is recommended instead)

» Renal function impairment, moderate to severe
(probenecid's efficacy decreases with increasing degrees of renal function impairment; the medication is completely ineffective when the patient's creatinine clearance is lower than 30 mL per minute)

*Risk-benefit should be considered when the following medical problems exist:*

Allergic reaction to probenecid, history of
» Blood dyscrasias
(may be exacerbated)

Peptic ulcer, history of
(increased risk of gastrointestinal side effects)

» Renal function impairment, mild
(probenecid's efficacy begins to decrease when the creatinine clearance is 80 mL per minute; although higher doses may be effective in patients with gout who have mild renal function impairment, use of probenecid to increase penicillin concentrations is not recommended for these patients)

**Patient monitoring**
The following may be especially important in patient monitoring (other tests may be warranted in some patients, depending on condition; » = major clinical significance):

Acid-base balance determinations
(recommended at periodic intervals if urinary alkalizers are used concurrently with probenecid in uricosuric therapy)

» Serum uric acid concentrations and/or
» Urine uric acid (24-hour) determinations
(monitoring may be required for proper dosing when probenecid is used as an antihyperuricemic; the effect of probenecid may be measured by a reduction of serum uric acid concentration [the upper limit of normal is about 7 mg per 100 mL (420 micromoles/L) for men and postmenopausal women and about 6 mg per 100 mL (360 micromoles/L) for premenopausal women but may vary, depending on the patient and laboratory methodology] or, more directly, by a significant increase in 24-hour uric acid excretion)

## Side/Adverse Effects

The following side/adverse effects have been selected on the basis of their potential clinical significance (possible signs and symptoms in parentheses where appropriate)—not necessarily inclusive:

**Those indicating need for medical attention**
Incidence less frequent
*Renal calculi, urate* (lower back and/or side pain; painful urination, with or without blood in urine); *dermatitis, allergic* (skin rash, hives, and/or itching)

Incidence rare
*Anaphylaxis* (changes in facial skin color; skin rash, hives, and/or itching; fast or irregular breathing; puffiness or swelling of the eyelids or around the eyes; shortness of breath, troubled breathing, tightness in chest, and/or wheezing); *anemia* (unusual tiredness and/or weakness if severe)—often asymptomatic; *aplastic anemia* (shortness of breath, troubled breathing, tightness in chest, and/or wheezing; sores, ulcers, or white spots on lips or in mouth; swollen and/or painful glands; unusual bleeding or bruising; unusual tiredness or weakness); *hemolytic anemia* (troubled breathing, exertional; unusual tiredness or weakness)—may be associated with glucose-6-phosphate dehydrogenase (G6PD) deficiency; *fever, allergic; hepatic necrosis* (yellow eyes or

skin); ***leukopenia*** (rarely, fever or chills; cough or hoarseness; lower back or side pain; painful or difficult urination)—usually asymptomatic; ***nephrotic syndrome*** (cloudy urine; swelling of face); ***pain in back and/or ribs; renal colic*** (pain, severe and/or sharp, in lower back and/or side); ***urate nephropathy*** (symptoms of renal impairment, e.g., increased blood pressure; shortness of breath, troubled breathing, tightness in chest, and/or wheezing; sudden decrease in amount of urine; swelling of face, fingers, feet, and/or lower legs; unusual tiredness or weakness; weight gain)

**Those indicating need for medical attention only if they continue or are bothersome**
Incidence more frequent
***Gouty arthritis, acute attack*** (joint pain; redness; swelling); ***headache; loss of appetite; nausea or vomiting, mild***

Note: An increase in the frequency of *acute attacks of gout* during the first few months of therapy may be anticipated, unless adequate prophylaxis with colchicine (or, if the patient is unable to take colchicine, a nonsteroidal anti-inflammatory drug [NSAID]) is given concurrently with the probenecid. Up to 20% of patients started on treatment with probenecid alone may experience acute attacks within the first few days of treatment.

Incidence less frequent
***Dizziness; flushing or redness of face; frequent urge to urinate; sore gums***

## Overdose

For specific information on the agents in the management of probenecid overdose, see:
- *Acetazolamide* in *Carbonic Anhydrase Inhibitors (Systemic)* monograph;
- *Allopurinol (Systemic)* monograph;
- *Diazepam* in *Benzodiazepines (Systemic)* monograph; and/or
- *Potassium Citrate* in *Citrates (Systemic)* monograph.

For more information on the management of overdose or unintentional ingestion, **contact a Poison Control Center** (see *Poison Control Center Listing*).

**Clinical effects of overdose**
The following effects have been selected on the basis of their potential clinical significance (possible signs and symptoms in parentheses where appropriate)—not necessarily inclusive:

Acute
Note: One case of overdose has been reported, in which an extremely high dose (< 45 grams) produced central nervous system (CNS) stimulation, clonic-tonic seizures, severe vomiting, and respiratory failure.

**Treatment of overdose**
Specific treatment—
For uric acid calculi or urate nephropathy:
Recommended measures include administration of large quantities of fluids and of allopurinol to increase urine flow and reduce uric acid formation, respectively. A urinary pH of 6 to 6.5 should be achieved and maintained by administration of alkali such as potassium citrate. If necessary to maintain the desired urinary pH through the night acetazolamide may also be given at bedtime. Other interventions designed to facilitate removal of renal calculi may also be needed. See the package inserts or *Acetazolamide* in *Carbonic Anhydrase Inhibitors (Systemic)*, *Allopurinol (Systemic)*, or *Potassium Citrate* in *Citrates (Systemic)* for specific dosing guidelines for use of these products.

For convulsions:
Administering appropriate anticonvulsive therapy such as intravenous diazepam. See the package insert or *Diazepam* in *Benzodiazepines (Systemic)* for specific dosing guidelines for use of this product.

Supportive care—General measures, such as monitoring the patient and instituting supportive treatment as needed. Patients in whom intentional overdose is known or suspected should be referred for psychiatric consultation.

## Patient Consultation

As an aid to patient consultation, refer to *Advice for the Patient, Probenecid (Systemic)*.
In providing consultation, consider emphasizing the following selected information (» = major clinical significance):

**Before using this medication**
» Conditions affecting use, especially:
Allergic reaction to probenecid, history of
Pregnancy—Probenecid crosses the placenta

Other medications, especially antibiotics, antivirals, indomethacin, ketoprofen, antineoplastic agents, aspirin or other salicylates, including bismuth subsalicylate (when probenecid used as antihyperuricemic or antigout agent), heparin, methotrexate, nitrofurantoin, or zidovudine

Other medical problems, especially cancer being treated by cytolytic medication or radiation (x-ray) therapy; kidney stones or other kidney problems, especially if caused by uric acid, or history of; renal function impairment; and blood dyscrasias

**Proper use of this medication**
Taking with food or an antacid to minimize gastric irritation
Missed dose: Taking as soon as possible; not taking if almost time for next dose; not doubling doses
» Proper dosing
» Proper storage

*For use as antigout agent*
Several months of continuous therapy may be required for maximum effectiveness
» Medication does not relieve acute attacks but rather helps to prevent them; need to continue taking probenecid with medication prescribed for gout attacks

*For use as antihyperuricemic (including gout therapy)*
Importance of high fluid intake and compliance with therapy for alkalinization of urine, if prescribed

**Precautions while using this medication**
Regular visits to physician to check progress during long-term therapy
Caution if any laboratory tests required; possible interference with test results
Diabetics: May cause false results with copper sulfate urine sugar tests, but not with glucose enzymatic urine sugar tests

*For use as antihyperuricemic (including gout therapy)*
» Aspirin or other salicylates may decrease uricosuric effects of probenecid; checking with physician regarding concurrent use, since effect is dependent on salicylate dose and duration of use
» Possibility that alcohol taken in large amounts may increase blood uric acid concentration and reduce effectiveness of medication

**Side/adverse effects**
Signs and symptoms of potential side effects, especially renal calculi, allergic dermatitis, anaphylaxis, anemia, aplastic anemia, hemolytic anemia, fever, hepatic necrosis, leukopenia, nephrotic syndrome, pain in back and/or ribs, renal colic, and urate nephropathy

## General Dosing Information

Probenecid therapy for gouty arthritis should not be initiated until 2 to 3 weeks after an acute attack has subsided. However, if an acute attack occurs in a patient already receiving probenecid, the medication should be continued at the same dose while full therapeutic doses of colchicine or a nonsteroidal anti-inflammatory drug (NSAID) are given to relieve the attack.

Probenecid may be administered with food or an antacid to minimize gastric irritation. A reduction in the dose may reduce gastrointestinal intolerance.

Determination of serum or 24-hour urine uric acid concentrations may be necessary for proper dosing in uricosuric therapy.

To reduce the risk of urate stone formation in patients with hyperuricemia, a high fluid intake (no less than 2.5 to 3 liters daily) and maintenance of an alkaline urine by administration of sodium bicarbonate (3 to 7.5 grams daily), potassium citrate (7.5 grams daily), or acetazolamide (250 mg daily) are recommended. The risk of urate stone formation is highest during the first few weeks of therapy, when urate excretion is high; after hyperuricemia has been controlled, and urinary excretion of uric acid decreases, the need for these measures is reduced.

Since probenecid may increase the frequency of acute attacks of gout during the early months of therapy, prophylactic doses of colchicine (or, if the patient cannot take colchicine, an NSAID) should be administered concurrently during the first 3 to 6 months of probenecid therapy. However, even with colchicine prophylactic therapy, acute attacks of gout requiring treatment with full therapeutic doses of colchicine or an NSAID may occur.

In gouty arthritis, higher doses may be required for patients with mild renal function impairment. However, it is recommended that dosage be reduced in geriatric patients with possible renal function impairment.

Probenecid is included as an adjunct to antibiotic therapy in some of the U.S. Centers for Disease Control (CDC) recommendations for the treatment of sexually transmitted diseases. The current CDC recommendations may be consulted for a complete description of all of the recommended treatment regimens.

## Oral Dosage Forms

### PROBENECID TABLETS USP

**Usual adult and adolescent dose**
Antigout agent or
Antihyperuricemic—
  Initial: Oral, 250 mg two times a day for one week.
  Maintenance: Oral, 500 mg two times a day. In nongeriatric patients, if this dose does not control symptoms, or if the 24-hour uric acid excretion is not above 700 mg, the daily dose may be increased by 500 mg per day at 4-week intervals, if necessary, up to a maximum of 3 grams per day.
  Note: The initial dose may be eliminated, and treatment started with the usual maintenance dose, when patients previously controlled with other uricosuric therapy are transferred to probenecid.
     When acute attacks of gout have not occurred for at least 6 months, and the serum uric acid concentrations remain within normal limits, the daily dose of probenecid may be reduced by 500 mg every 6 months until the lowest effective maintenance dose is reached.
Antibiotic therapy adjunct—
  Penicillin or cephalosporin therapy (general): Oral, 500 mg four times a day. If the antibiotic is being administered parenterally, the probenecid should be administered at least thirty minutes prior to the antibiotic.
  Treatment of sexually transmitted diseases: Oral, 1 gram as a single dose, administered simultaneously or concurrently with appropriate antibiotic therapy.
  Note: For treatment of neurosyphilis—Oral, 500 mg four times a day, concurrently with one dose of 2.4 million units of penicillin G procaine per day, for ten to fourteen days.

**Usual adult prescribing limits**
Antigout agent or
antihyperuricemic agent—
  Oral, 3 grams per day.

**Usual pediatric dose**
Antihyperuricemic—
  Dosage has not been established.
Antibiotic therapy adjunct—
  Penicillin or cephalosporin therapy (general):
    Children up to 2 years of age—Use is not recommended.
    Children 2 to 14 years of age or
    Children weighing up to 50 kg—Oral, initially 25 mg per kg of body weight or 700 mg per square meter of body surface area, then 10 mg per kg of body weight or 300 mg per square meter of body surface area, four times a day.
    Children weighing over 50 kg—See *Usual adult and adolescent dose*.
  Note: If the antibiotic is being administered parenterally, the probenecid should be administered at least thirty minutes prior to the antibiotic.
  Treatment of gonorrhea:
    Postpubertal children and/or children weighing over 45 kg—Oral, 1 gram as a single dose, administered simultaneously or concurrently with appropriate antibiotic therapy.

**Strength(s) usually available**
U.S.—
  500 mg (Rx) [*Benemid* (scored); *Probalan;* GENERIC].
Canada—
  500 mg (OTC) [*Benemid* (scored); *Benuryl*].

**Packaging and storage**
Store below 40 °C (104 °F), preferably between 15 and 30 °C (59 and 86 °F), unless otherwise specified by manufacturer. Store in a well-closed container.

Revised: 09/01/92

# PROBENECID AND COLCHICINE  Systemic

VA CLASSIFICATION (Primary): MS400

**NOTE:** The *Probenecid and Colchicine (Systemic)* monograph is maintained on the USP DI electronic data base. For a printed copy of the most recent revision of the complete monograph, contact Micromedex, Inc. - Reprint Requests, 6200 S. Syracuse Way, Suite 300, Englewood, CO 80111; telephone (303) 486-6400; telefax (303) 486-6464; Email: USPDI@MDX.COM.

For information on the specific components of this combination, see the *USP DI* monographs for *Colchicine (Systemic)* and *Probenecid (Systemic)*.

The information that follows is selectively abstracted from the complete monograph and is provided to facilitate drug use review and patient counseling.

Note: For a listing of dosage forms and brand names by country availability, see *Dosage Forms* section(s).

## Category
Antigout agent.

## Indications

**Accepted**
Gouty arthritis, chronic (treatment)—Probenecid and colchicine combination is indicated for the treatment of chronic gouty arthritis in patients having frequent, recurrent acute attacks.

Probenecid is used to control hyperuricemia. Therapy with this uricosuric agent is recommended only for patients whose 24-hour renal excretion of urate is 800 mg (4.8 mmol) or lower (i.e., patients who are hyperuricemic as a result of underexcretion, rather than overproduction, of urate). The aim of probenecid therapy is to reduce the number of acute gout attacks. Probenecid therapy should not be initiated during an acute attack because it may produce fluctuations in urate concentration that may result in prolongation of the attack or initiation of a new attack. Even when probenecid therapy is started several weeks after an acute attack, the frequency of acute attacks may be increased during the early months of therapy. Therefore, prophylactic doses of the colchicine in this combination medication are usually administered for the first 3 to 6 months of probenecid therapy.

**Unaccepted**
Probenecid is not recommended in circumstances in which there is an especially high risk of adverse effects associated with crystallization and deposition of urate in renal tissues, such as formation of renal calculi and uric acid nephropathy. It therefore should not be used for treatment of gout in patients whose 24-hour urate excretion exceeds 800 mg (4.8 mmol) or who have extensive tophi. Allopurinol, which decreases the quantity of urate that reaches the kidneys in addition to decreasing the concentration of urate in the blood, is recommended in these circumstances.

## Patient Consultation
As an aid to patient consultation, refer to *Advice for the Patient, Probenecid and Colchicine (Systemic)*.

In providing consultation, consider emphasizing the following selected information (» = major clinical significance):

**Before using this medication**
» Conditions affecting use, especially:
   Allergic reaction to probenecid or sensitivity to colchicine, history of
   Pregnancy—Probenecid crosses the placenta; colchicine reported to be teratogenic in humans
   Use in the elderly—Increased susceptibility to cumulative colchicine toxicity
   Other medications, especially antibiotics, antivirals, bone marrow depressants or blood dyscrasia–causing medications, indomethacin, ketoprofen, antineoplastic agents, aspirin or other salicylates, including bismuth subsalicylate, heparin, methotrexate, nitrofurantoin, or zidovudine
   Other medical problems, especially alcohol abuse, severe cardiac or gastrointestinal disorders; cancer being treated by cytolytic medication or radiation (x-ray) therapy; kidney stones or other kidney problems, especially if caused by uric acid, or history of; renal function impairment; hepatic function impairment; stomach ulcer or other stomach problems, and blood dyscrasias

**Proper use of this medication**
Taking with food or an antacid to minimize gastric irritation
Importance of not taking more medication than the amount prescribed

Several months of continuous therapy may be required for maximum effectiveness
» Medication does not relieve acute attacks of gout but rather helps to prevent them; need to continue taking probenecid and colchicine with medication prescribed for gout attacks
Importance of high fluid intake and compliance with therapy for alkalinization of urine, if prescribed
» Proper dosing
Missed dose: Taking as soon as possible; not taking if almost time for next dose; not doubling doses
» Proper storage

**Precautions while using this medication**
Regular visits to physician to check progress during therapy
Caution if any laboratory tests required; possible interference with test results
Diabetics: May cause false results with copper sulfate urine sugar tests, but not with glucose enzymatic urine sugar tests
» Aspirin or other salicylates may decrease uricosuric effects of probenecid; checking with physician regarding concurrent use, since effect is dependent on salicylate dose and duration of use
» Possibility that alcohol taken in large amounts may increase the risk of colchicine-induced gastrointestinal toxicity; also, may increase uric acid concentrations and thereby reduce effectiveness of medication
» For patients taking high doses (4 tablets a day): Discontinuing at once and notifying physician as soon as possible if symptoms of gastrointestinal toxicity occur

**Side/adverse effects**
Signs and symptoms of potential side effects, especially renal calculi, allergic dermatitis, anaphylaxis, anemia, aplastic anemia, hemolytic anemia, fever, hepatic necrosis, leukopenia, nephrotic syndrome, pain in back and/or ribs, renal colic, urate nephropathy, colchicine-induced gastrointestinal toxicity, and peripheral neuritis

## Oral Dosage Forms

### PROBENECID AND COLCHICINE TABLETS USP

**Usual adult dose**
Antigout agent—
Initial: Oral, 1 tablet a day for one week.
Maintenance: Oral, 1 tablet two times a day. In nongeriatric patients, if this dose does not control symptoms or if the 24-hour uric acid excretion is not above 700 mg, the daily dosage may be increased by 1 tablet every four weeks as tolerated (usually not above 4 tablets per day). If the increase in colchicine dosage is not desired or tolerated, administration of additional probenecid alone may be required.
Note: The initial dose may be eliminated, and treatment started with the usual maintenance dose, when patients previously controlled with other uricosuric therapy are transferred to probenecid.
When acute attacks of gout have not occurred for at least six months, and the serum uric acid concentrations remain within normal limits, the daily dose may be reduced by 1 tablet every six months until the lowest effective maintenance dose is reached. Alternatively, prophylactic use of colchicine may be discontinued and the patient treated with maintenance doses of probenecid alone.

**Usual pediatric dose**
Dosage has not been established.

**Strength(s) usually available**
U.S.—
500 mg of probenecid and 500 mcg (0.5 mg) of colchicine (Rx) [*ColBenemid; Col-Probenecid; Proben-C;* GENERIC].

Revised: 09/09/92
Interim revision: 08/27/94

# PROBUCOL Systemic*

VA CLASSIFICATION (Primary): CV609

Commonly used brand name(s): *Lorelco*.

Note: For a listing of dosage forms and brand names by country availability, see *Dosage Forms* section(s).

*Not commercially available in U.S.

## Category
Antihyperlipidemic.

## Indications

**Accepted**
Hyperlipidemia (treatment)—Probucol is recommended for use as an adjunct to dietary measures in patients with primary hypercholesterolemia(type IIa hyperlipoproteinemia) and a significant risk of coronary artery disease, who have not responded to diet or other measures alone. Probucol reduces plasma cholesterol concentrations, but has a variable effect on serum triglyceride concentrations, and so is not useful in patients with elevated triglyceride concentrations alone. Its use is limited in other types of hyperlipidemia (including type IIb) because it may cause further elevation of triglycerides. Its main advantage over the anion exchange resins is its ease of administration and better acceptance and tolerance by the patient.

For additional information on initial therapeutic guidelines related to the treatment of hyperlipidemia, see *Appendix III*.

## Pharmacology/Pharmacokinetics

**Physicochemical characteristics**
Molecular weight—516.84.

**Mechanism of action/Effect**
Probucol lowers serum cholesterol by increasing the fractional rate of low-density lipoprotein (LDL) catabolism in the final metabolic pathway for cholesterol elimination from the body. Additionally, probucol may inhibit early stages of cholesterol biosynthesis and slightly inhibit dietary cholesterol absorption. Recent information suggests that probucol may inhibit the oxidation and tissue deposition of LDL cholesterol, thereby inhibiting atherogenesis.

**Absorption**
Absorption from the gastrointestinal tract is limited and variable (about 7%).

**Distribution**
Accumulates in fat tissue with prolonged treatment.

**Half-life**
Ranges from 12 hours to more than 500 hours, the longest half-life probably being in adipose tissue.

**Time to peak plasma concentration**
Plasma concentrations increase slowly and reach steady state after 3 to 4 months; they also decline slowly after withdrawal, by 60% after 6 weeks and by 80% after 6 months.

**Time to peak effect**
Maximal reduction in plasma cholesterol concentrations usually occurs within 20 to 50 days after initiation of probucol therapy, although a further decrease may occur gradually over several months. A clinical response usually occurs within 1 to 3 months.

**Elimination**
Biliary (slowly in the feces).
Renal, very little (mainly as unchanged drug).

## Precautions to Consider

**Carcinogenicity**
Two-year studies in rats did not reveal carcinogenicity.

**Mutagenicity**
Mutagenic studies were negative.

**Pregnancy/Reproduction**
Fertility—Studies in rats and rabbits did not reveal adverse effects on fertility.

Pregnancy—Studies in humans have not been done.
Studies in rats and rabbits at doses up to 50 times the human dose have not shown that probucol causes adverse effects on the fetus.

FDA Pregnancy Category B.

**Breast-feeding**
It is not known whether probucol is distributed into human breast milk. However, it is distributed into the milk of animals. Use of probucol while breast-feeding is not recommended, because of potentially serious adverse effects on nursing infants.

#### Pediatrics
Appropriate studies on the relationship of age to the effects of probucol have not been performed in the pediatric population. However, use in children under 2 years of age is not recommended since cholesterol is required for normal development.

#### Geriatrics
No information is available on the relationship of age to the effects of probucol in geriatric patients.

#### Drug interactions and/or related problems
The following drug interactions and/or related problems have been selected on the basis of their potential clinical significance (possible mechanism in parentheses where appropriate)—not necessarily inclusive (» = major clinical significance):

Note: Combinations containing any of the following medications, depending on the amount present, may also interact with this medication.

Antiarrhythmics with QT interval prolongation, such as:
  Amiodarone
  Bretylium
  Disopyramide
  Encainide
  Flecainide
  Lidocaine
  Mexiletine
  Moricizine
  Procainamide
  Propafenone
  Quinidine
  Sotalol
  Tocainide or
Antidepressants, tricyclic or
Phenothiazines
  (additive QT interval prolongation may increase risk of ventricular tachycardia)

Beta-adrenergic blocking agents or
Digoxin
  (the effect of beta-adrenergic blocking agents on the atrial rate and the effect of digoxin on AV block can cause bradycardia; when these medications are given in conjunction with a medication that prolongs the QT interval [i.e. probucol], the risk of ventricular tachycardia may be increased)

Chenodiol or
Ursodiol
  (effect may be decreased when enodiol or ursodiol is used concurrently with antihyperlipidemics since they tend to increase cholesterol saturation of bile)

#### Laboratory value alterations
The following have been selected on the basis of their potential clinical significance (possible effect in parentheses where appropriate)—not necessarily inclusive (» = major clinical significance):

With physiology/laboratory test values
  Alanine aminotransferase (ALT [SGPT]), serum and
  Alkaline phosphatase, serum and
  Aspartate aminotransferase (AST [SGOT]), serum and
  Bilirubin and
  Blood urea nitrogen (BUN) and
  Creatine kinase (CK) and
  Glucose, blood, and
  Uric acid, serum
    (concentrations may be slightly increased)
  Electrocardiogram (ECG)
    (QT interval prolongation may occur)
  Eosinophil concentrations in blood and
  Hematocrit and
  Hemoglobin concentrations
    (may be decreased)

#### Medical considerations/Contraindications
The medical considerations/contraindications included have been selected on the basis of their potential clinical significance (reasons given in parentheses where appropriate)—not necessarily inclusive (» = major clinical significance):

*Except under special circumstances, this medication should not be used when the following medical problems exist:*
» Primary biliary cirrhosis
  (may further raise the cholesterol concentration)
» QT interval prolongation
  (probucol may prolong QT interval)

*Risk-benefit should be considered when the following medical problems exist:*
Bradycardia, intrinsic, severe or
Hypokalemia or
Hypomagnesemia
  (the risk of ventricular tachycardia may be increased because probucol prolongs the QT interval)
» Cardiac arrhythmias or evidence of recent or progressive myocardial damage
  (condition may be exacerbated; probucol should be used only with periodic electrocardiogram [ECG] monitoring)
» Congestive heart failure, unresponsive or
Gallstones
  (conditions may be exacerbated)
Hepatic function impairment
  (higher blood levels of probucol may result)
Sensitivity to probucol

#### Patient monitoring
The following may be especially important in patient monitoring (other tests may be warranted in some patients, depending on condition; » = major clinical significance):

» Cholesterol, serum and
» Triglycerides, serum
  (determinations recommended prior to initiation of therapy and every 3 to 4 months during therapy to confirm efficacy; if an increase in serum triglyceride concentrations occurs, adjustment of the diet is recommended; if the increase persists, it is recommended that probucol therapy be withdrawn)
ECG
  (recommended at periodic intervals in patients with a history of cardiac arrhythmias; probucol therapy should be withdrawn if cardiac arrhythmias or a prolonged QT interval occurs)

## Side/Adverse Effects
Note: Prolongation of QT interval associated with serious arrhythmias has been reported in patients treated with probucol.

The following side/adverse effects have been selected on the basis of their potential clinical significance (possible signs and symptoms in parentheses where appropriate)—not necessarily inclusive:

#### Those indicating need for medical attention
Incidence more frequent
  *Eosinophilia; QT interval prolongation and ventricular arrhythmias* (dizziness or fainting; pounding heartbeat; fast or irregular heartbeat)
Incidence rare
  *Anemia* (unusual tiredness or weakness); *angioneurotic edema* (swellings on face, hands, or feet, or in mouth); *thrombocytopenia* (unusual bleeding or bruising)

#### Those indicating need for medical attention only if they continue or are bothersome
Incidence more frequent
  *Gastrointestinal irritation* (bloating; diarrhea; nausea and vomiting; stomach pain)
  Note: *Gastrointestinal irritation* is usually transient and mild.
Incidence less frequent
  *Dizziness; headache; paresthesia* (numbness or tingling of fingers, toes, or face)

## Patient Consultation
As an aid to patient consultation, refer to *Advice for the Patient, Probucol (Systemic)*.

In providing consultation, consider emphasizing the following selected information (» = major clinical significance):

#### Before using this medication
Diet as preferred therapy; importance of following prescribed diet
» Conditions affecting use, especially:
  Sensitivity to probucol
  Breast-feeding—Use not recommended because of potentially serious adverse effects on nursing infants
  Use in children—Not recommended in children under 2 years of age since cholesterol is required for normal development
  Other medical problems, especially primary biliary cirrhosis, and cardiac abnormalities including congestive heart failure and QT interval prolongation

#### Proper use of this medication
» Importance of not taking more or less medication than the amount prescribed

This medication does not cure the condition but rather helps control it
» Compliance with prescribed diet
  Taking with meals, since medication is more effective with food
» Proper dosing
  Missed dose: Taking as soon as possible; not taking if almost time for next dose; not doubling doses
» Proper storage

**Precautions while using this medication**
» Importance of close monitoring by the physician
» Checking with physician before discontinuing medication; blood lipid concentrations may increase significantly

**Side/adverse effects**
Signs of potential side effects, especially angioneurotic edema, blood dyscrasias, QT interval prolongation, and tachycardia

## General Dosing Information
See also *Patient Monitoring*.

If unexplained or cardiovascular-related syncope occurs, probucol therapy should be withdrawn and ECG monitored.

If response is inadequate after 4 months of treatment, probucol therapy should be re-evaluated and possibly withdrawn, except in the case of xanthoma tuberosum, which may require up to 1 year of treatment as long as reduction in size and/or number of xanthomata occurs.

When probucol is discontinued, an appropriate hypolipidemic diet and monitoring of serum lipids are recommended until the patient stabilizes, since a rise in serum cholesterol concentrations to or above the original base may occur.

**Diet/Nutrition**
It is recommended that probucol be taken with food to maximize absorption.

## Oral Dosage Forms
### PROBUCOL TABLETS
**Usual adult dose**
Antihyperlipidemic—
  Oral, 500 mg two times a day with the morning and evening meals.

**Usual pediatric dose**
Dosage has not been established.

**Strength(s) usually available**
U.S.—
  Not commercially available.
Canada—
  250 mg (Rx) [*Lorelco*].

**Packaging and storage**
Store below 40 °C (104 °F), preferably between 15 and 30 °C (59 and 86 °F), in a well-closed, light-resistant container, unless otherwise specified by manufacturer.

**Auxiliary labeling**
• Take with meals.

## Selected Bibliography
Howard P. Probucol in hypercholesterolemia. Ann Pharmacother 1989; 23: 880-1.

National Cholesterol Education Program. Second Report of the Expert Panel on Detection, Evaluation, and Treatment of High Blood Cholesterol in Adults (Adult Treatment Panel II). Circulation 1994; 89(3): 1329-445.

Knodel LC, Talbert RL. Adverse effects of hypolipidaemic drugs. Med Toxicol 1987; 2: 10-32.

Revised: 04/13/93
Interim revision: 06/28/95; 08/19/97; 08/24/98

---

# PROCAINAMIDE   Systemic

VA CLASSIFICATION (Primary): CV300
Commonly used brand name(s): *Procan SR; Promine; Pronestyl; Pronestyl-SR*.
Note:  For a listing of dosage forms and brand names by country availability, see *Dosage Forms* section(s).

## Category
Antiarrhythmic.

## Indications
Note:  Bracketed information in the *Indications* section refers to uses that are not included in U.S. product labeling.

**Accepted**
Arrhythmias, ventricular (treatment)—Procainamide is indicated in the treatment of life-threatening ventricular arrhythmias, such as sustained ventricular tachycardia. Parenteral procainamide also is indicated for treatment of ventricular extrasystoles and cardiac arrhythmias associated with anesthesia and surgery.

[Arrhythmias, supraventricular (treatment)]—Procainamide is used for the conversion and management of atrial fibrillation and paroxysmal atrial tachycardia.

## Pharmacology/Pharmacokinetics

**Physicochemical characteristics**
Molecular weight—271.79.
pKa—9.23.

**Mechanism of action/Effect**
Direct cardiac effect—Decreases excitability, conduction velocity, automaticity, and membrane responsiveness with prolonged refractory period. No effect on contractility or cardiac output unless myocardial damage present. Larger doses may induce atrioventricular (AV) block. In the Vaughan Williams classification of antiarrhythmics, procainamide is considered to be a Class I antiarrhythmic.

**Other actions/effects**
Relatively weak anticholinergic action diminishes vagal transmission, resulting in increased heart rate, usually with higher dosages. Alpha-adrenergic blockade does not occur. Also causes peripheral vasodilation.

**Absorption**
Oral—Rapid; 75 to 95% complete but may vary.
Intramuscular—Rapid.
Intravenous—Immediate.

**Protein binding**
Low (15 to 20%).

**Biotransformation**
Hepatic; approximately 25% of dose is converted to the active metabolite N-acetylprocainamide (NAPA); up to 40% conversion occurs in patients who are rapid acetylators or those with renal function impairment.

**Half-life**
Procainamide—About 2.5 to 4.5 hours (11 to 20 hours in renal function impairment).
N-acetylprocainamide—About 6 hours.

**Therapeutic serum concentration**
Procainamide—4 to 10 mg per L; higher levels may be needed in some patients such as those with sustained ventricular tachycardia.
NAPA—10 to 30 mg per L.

**Time to peak effect**
Oral—60 to 90 minutes.
Intravenous—Immediately.
Intramuscular—15 to 60 minutes.

**Elimination**
Renal, 50 to 60% unchanged. The cardioactive metabolite, NAPA, has a slower excretion rate than the parent compound. In cases of renal function impairment or congestive heart failure, this metabolite tends to accumulate rapidly in the serum to toxic concentrations, while the serum concentration of procainamide appears to be within acceptable limits.
In dialysis—Procainamide and NAPA are removable by hemodialysis but not by peritoneal dialysis.

## Precautions to Consider

**Cross-sensitivity and/or related problems**
Patients sensitive to procaine or other related agents may be sensitive to procainamide also.

**Carcinogenicity/Mutagenicity**
Long-term studies in animals have not been done.

## Pregnancy/Reproduction

Pregnancy—Procainamide crosses the placenta. Adequate and well-controlled studies have not been done in humans. Some reports of procainamide use in pregnant women seem to indicate that although procainamide and *N*-acetylprocainamide (NAPA) appear in fetal serum, no adverse effects on the fetus or neonate have been noted. However, there is a potential risk of drug accumulation and maternal hypotension leading to uteroplacental insufficiency and ventricular arrhythmias.

FDA Pregnancy Category C.

## Breast-feeding

Procainamide and NAPA are distributed into breast milk.

## Pediatrics

Appropriate studies on the relationship of age to the effects of procainamide have not been performed in the pediatric population. Occasional use in pediatric patients has not demonstrated pediatrics-specific problems that would limit the usefulness of procainamide in these patients. However, dosage requirements to achieve and maintain effective therapeutic concentrations may be higher in some pediatric patients than in adults.

## Geriatrics

Appropriate studies on the relationship of age to the effects of procainamide have not been performed in the geriatric population. However, elderly patients may be more prone to hypotension, especially with parenteral use or when very high doses are given. In addition, elderly patients are more likely to have age-related renal function impairment, which may require lower doses in patients receiving procainamide.

## Dental

The leukopenic and thrombocytopenic effects of procainamide may result in an increased incidence of microbial infection, delayed healing, and gingival bleeding. If leukopenia or thrombocytopenia occurs, dental work should be deferred until blood counts have returned to normal, and patients should be instructed in proper oral hygiene, including caution in use of regular toothbrushes, dental floss, and toothpicks.

The secondary anticholinergic effects of procainamide may decrease or inhibit salivary flow, especially in middle-aged or elderly patients, thus contributing to the development of caries, periodontal disease, oral candidiasis, and discomfort.

## Drug interactions and/or related problems

The following drug interactions and/or related problems have been selected on the basis of their potential clinical significance (possible mechanism in parentheses where appropriate)—not necessarily inclusive (» = major clinical significance):

Note: Combinations containing any of the following medications, depending on the amount present, may also interact with this medication.

» Antiarrhythmics, other
(concurrent use with procainamide may produce additive cardiac effects)

Anticholinergics, especially atropine or related compounds (see *Appendix II* ), or
Antidyskinetics or
Antihistamines
(concurrent use with procainamide may intensify atropine-like side effects because of the secondary anticholinergic activities of procainamide; patients should be advised to report occurrence of gastrointestinal problems promptly since paralytic ileus may occur with concurrent therapy)

» Antihypertensives
(concurrent use with procainamide, especially intravenous procainamide, may produce additive hypotensive effects)

» Antimyasthenics
(neuromuscular blocking action and/or secondary anticholinergic activity of procainamide may antagonize the effect of antimyasthenics on skeletal muscle; dosage adjustments of antimyasthenics may be necessary to control symptoms of myasthenia gravis)

Bethanechol
(concurrent use with procainamide may antagonize the cholinergic effects of bethanechol)

Bone marrow depressants (see *Appendix II* )
(concurrent use of procainamide with these medications may increase the leukopenic and/or thrombocytopenic effects; if concurrent use is required, close observation for toxic effects should be considered)

Bretylium
(concurrent administration may counteract inotropic effect of bretylium and potentiate hypotension)

» Neuromuscular blocking agents
(effects of these medications may be prolonged or enhanced when they are used concurrently with procainamide; careful postoperative monitoring of the patient may be necessary following concurrent or sequential use, especially if there is a possibility of incomplete reversal of neuromuscular blockade)

» Pimozide
(concurrent use with procainamide may potentiate cardiac arrhythmias, which are seen on electrocardiogram [ECG] as prolongation of QT interval)

## Laboratory value alterations

The following have been selected on the basis of their potential clinical significance (possible effect in parentheses where appropriate)—not necessarily inclusive (» = major clinical significance):

With diagnostic test results
Bentiromide
(administration of procainamide during a bentiromide test period will invalidate test results since procainamide is also metabolized to arylamines and will thus increase the percent of para-aminobenzoic acid [PABA] recovered; discontinuation of procainamide at least 3 days prior to the administration of bentiromide is recommended)

Edrophonium tests
(may be altered)

With physiology/laboratory test values
Alanine aminotransferase (ALT [SGPT]), serum and
Alkaline phosphatase, serum and
Aspartate aminotransferase (AST [SGOT]), serum and
Bilirubin, serum and
Lactate dehydrogenase (LDH), serum
(concentrations may be increased)

Antinuclear antibody (ANA) titers
(occur in 60 to 70% of patients after 1 to 2 months of procainamide therapy; may increase with continued therapy)

Direct antiglobulin (Coombs') tests
(may produce positive results)

ECG changes such as:
QRS widening, and less frequently
PR and QT prolongation and
Reduced voltage of QRS and T waves
(may occur with large doses)

Leukocyte counts, including neutrophils and
Platelet counts
(may rarely be decreased)

## Medical considerations/Contraindications

The medical considerations/contraindications included have been selected on the basis of their potential clinical significance (reasons given in parentheses where appropriate)—not necessarily inclusive (» = major clinical significance).

*Except under special circumstances, this medication should not be used when the following medical problems exist:*

» Atrioventricular (AV) block, complete, and also 2nd and 3rd degree AV block unless controlled by electrical pacemaker
(risk of additive cardiac depression)

» Torsades de pointes
(procainamide may aggravate this arrhythmia)

*Risk-benefit should be considered when the following medical problems exist:*

» AV block or
» Bundle branch block or
» Digitalis intoxication, severe
(risk of additive cardiac depression and ventricular asystole or fibrillation)

Bronchial asthma
(possible hypersensitivity)

» Congestive heart failure or
Hepatic function impairment or
» Renal function impairment
(possible accumulation leading to toxicity; lower doses may be required in patients with congestive heart failure or renal function impairment)

» Lupus erythematosus, history of
(procainamide may precipitate active lupus)

» Myasthenia gravis
(procainamide may increase muscle weakness)

Sensitivity to procainamide

» Ventricular tachycardia during an occlusive coronary episode

**Patient monitoring**
The following may be especially important in patient monitoring (other tests may be warranted in some patients, depending on condition; » = major clinical significance):

Antinuclear antibody (ANA) titers
(recommended at periodic intervals during prolonged use of procainamide or if symptoms of a lupus-like reaction occur; procainamide should be withdrawn if a steady increase in ANA titer occurs)

Blood pressure determinations and
» Cardiac function monitoring, including ECG
(recommended at periodic intervals with oral therapy and concurrently with parenteral administration; procainamide should be withdrawn if an excessive blood pressure reduction or QRS widening occurs, and immediately if signs of impending heart block occur)

Complete blood cell counts (especially leukocyte counts)
(recommended every 2 weeks during the first 3 months of therapy, then at longer intervals throughout maintenance, especially in patients taking the extended-release dosage form or after cardiovascular surgery; procainamide should be withdrawn if leukocyte counts fall)

Plasma procainamide and N-acetylprocainamide (NAPA) concentrations
(recommended at periodic intervals to aid in dosage adjustment, especially in patients with congestive heart failure or hepatic or renal function impairment, and when switching from regular oral to extended-release dosage form; risk of toxicity may be increased when the summed concentration of procainamide and NAPA exceeds 25 to 30 mg/L)

## Side/Adverse Effects

Note: Agranulocytosis, bone marrow depression, neutropenia, hypoplastic anemia, and thrombocytopenia have been reported with an incidence of about 0.5% in patients receiving procainamide. Fatalities have been reported, especially in cases of agranulocytosis (20 to 25% mortality in reported cases). Most cases have been noted in the first 12 weeks of therapy.

In the National Heart, Lung, and Blood Institute's Cardiac Arrhythmias Suppression Trial (CAST), treatment with encainide or flecainide was found to be associated with excessive mortality or increased nonfatal cardiac arrest rate, as compared with placebo, in patients with asymptomatic, non–life-threatening arrhythmias who had a recent myocardial infarction. The implications of these results for other patient populations or other antiarrhythmic agents are uncertain.

Tachycardia may occur at high plasma procainamide concentrations as a reflex sympathetic response to the hypotensive effect, due to the anticholinergic effect on the atrioventricular (AV) node, or in response to slowing of the atrial rate in treatment of atrial fibrillation. Tachycardia is especially hazardous in patients with myocardial damage, because of the risk of emboli. Adequate digitalization reduces, but does not abolish, the risk.

Intravenous administration may cause a transient but sometimes severe reduction in blood pressure, especially in conscious patients. Hypotension is less frequent with intramuscular administration and rare with oral use (except with excessive doses).

Ventricular asystole or fibrillation may occur, especially with too-rapid intravenous administration or excessive doses; death has occurred rarely.

The following side/adverse effects have been selected on the basis of their potential clinical significance (possible signs and symptoms in parentheses where appropriate)—not necessarily inclusive:

**Those indicating need for medical attention**
Incidence less frequent
*Allergic reaction or systemic lupus erythematosus (SLE)–like syndrome* (fever and chills; joint pain or swelling; pains with breathing; skin rash or itching)

Note: After extended maintenance therapy nearly 80% of patients treated show an increased titer of antinuclear antibodies (an early sign of developing SLE), often within 1 to 12 months of commencing therapy. Nearly 30% of these patients develop clinical symptoms that resemble SLE. This *SLE-like condition* is usually reversible with discontinuation of procainamide therapy.

Incidence rare
*Central nervous system (CNS) effects* (confusion; hallucinations; mental depression); *Coombs' positive hemolytic anemia* (unusual tiredness or weakness); *leukopenia (neutropenia) and possible agranulocytosis, which may be fatal* (fever, chills, or sore mouth, gums, or throat); *thrombocytopenia* (unusual bleeding or bruising)

Note: *Coombs' positive hemolytic anemia* may be related to the SLE-like syndrome.

*Leukopenia* may be more likely to occur with use of the extended-release dosage form, especially after cardiovascular surgery. Leukopenia usually occurs within the first 3 months of therapy, and counts recover within a few weeks after procainamide is withdrawn. Leukopenia also may occur in association with the SLE-like syndrome.

*Thrombocytopenia* may be related to the SLE-like syndrome.

**Those indicating need for medical attention only if they continue or are bothersome**
Incidence more frequent, especially with daily doses > 4 grams
*Diarrhea; loss of appetite*
Incidence less frequent
*Dizziness or lightheadedness*

## Overdose

For more information on the management of overdose or unintentional ingestion, **contact a Poison Control Center** (see *Poison Control Center Listing*).

**Clinical effects of overdose**
The following effects have been selected on the basis of their potential clinical significance (possible signs and symptoms in parentheses where appropriate)—not necessarily inclusive:

*Confusion; decrease in urination; dizziness, severe, or fainting; drowsiness; fast or irregular heartbeat; nausea and vomiting*

**Treatment of overdose**
Treatment is primarily symptomatic and supportive. Gastric lavage, emesis, hemodialysis, pressor medication, and maintenance of airway are of possible benefit, according to the patient's condition.

## Patient Consultation

As an aid to patient consultation, refer to *Advice for the Patient, Procainamide (Systemic)*.
In providing consultation, consider emphasizing the following selected information (» = major clinical significance):

**Before using this medication**
» Conditions affecting use, especially:
Sensitivity to procaine or other related agents
Pregnancy—Procainamide crosses the placenta
Breast-feeding—Procainamide and NAPA are distributed into breast milk
Use in children—Higher doses may be needed to maintain adequate therapeutic concentrations in some patients
Use in the elderly—May be more susceptible to hypotension
Dental—May be more susceptible to microbial infection, delayed healing, and gingival bleeding because of risk of leukopenia and thrombocytopenia; may cause dryness of mouth
Other medications, especially other antiarrhythmics, antihypertensives, antimyasthenics, neuromuscular blocking agents, and pimozide
Other medical problems, especially atrioventricular block, torsades de pointes, severe digitalis intoxication, congestive heart failure, renal function impairment, lupus erythematosus, myasthenia gravis, or ventricular tachycardia during an occlusive coronary episode

**Proper use of this medication**
» Taking exactly as directed even if feeling well
Taking on empty stomach for faster absorption, or with food or milk to reduce stomach irritation
Proper administration of extended-release tablets: Swallowing tablets whole, without breaking, crushing, or chewing
» Importance of not missing doses and of taking at evenly spaced intervals
» Proper dosing
Missed dose: Taking as soon as possible if remembered within 2 hours (4 hours for extended-release tablets); not taking if remembered later; not doubling doses
» Proper storage

**Precautions while using this medication**
Regular visits to physician to check progress
» Checking with physician before discontinuing medication; gradual dosage reduction may be necessary to avoid worsening of condition
» Caution if any kind of surgery (including dental surgery) or emergency treatment is required
Carrying medical identification card or bracelet

» Possibility of dizziness with high dosage, especially in elderly; caution when driving or doing things requiring alertness
Caution if any laboratory tests required; possible interference with test results

**Side/adverse effects**
Signs of potential side effects, especially allergic reaction, SLE-like syndrome, CNS effects, Coombs' positive hemolytic anemia, leukopenia, and thrombocytopenia
Extended-release tablet matrix may be seen in stool and is to be expected

## General Dosing Information

Dosage must be adjusted to meet the individual requirements of each patient, on the basis of clinical response.

Procainamide therapy should be withdrawn if signs or symptoms of systemic lupus erythematosus (SLE)–like syndrome, leukopenia, or hemolytic anemia occur.

**For treatment of atrial fibrillation**
Patients should be digitalized prior to administration of procainamide to reduce the risk of enhancing atrioventricular (AV) conduction, which may result in ventricular rate acceleration.

**For oral dosage forms only**
A period of 3 to 4 hours should elapse after the last intravenous dose before administration of the first oral dose.

**For parenteral dosage forms only**
Procainamide Hydrochloride Injection USP is always diluted before intravenous administration.

Intravenous administration should be limited to hospitals where monitoring facilities are available.

Intramuscular injection usually is used only when the oral or intravenous routes are not feasible.

Procainamide intravenous injection should be administered at a rate not exceeding 50 mg per minute.

Because hypotension may develop rapidly during intravenous administration, it is highly recommended that blood pressure be monitored continuously, with the patient in a supine position. Phenylephrine and norepinephrine injections should be available to counteract severe hypotension.

**Diet/Nutrition**
Oral procainamide should preferably be taken with a glass of water on an empty stomach (either 1 hour before or 2 hours after meals) for faster absorption; however, it may be taken with meals or immediately after meals to lessen gastrointestinal irritation.

## Oral Dosage Forms

Note: Bracketed information in the *Indications* section refers to uses that are not included in U.S. product labeling.

### PROCAINAMIDE HYDROCHLORIDE CAPSULES USP

**Usual adult dose**
[Atrial arrhythmias]—
   Initial: Oral, 1.25 grams, followed in one to two hours by 750 mg if necessary; then 500 mg to 1 gram every two or three hours as needed and tolerated.
   Maintenance: Oral, 500 mg to 1 gram every four to six hours, the dosage being adjusted as needed and tolerated.
Ventricular arrhythmias—
   Oral, 50 mg per kg of body weight per day in eight divided doses (every three hours), the dosage being adjusted as needed and tolerated.
Note: Geriatric patients may be more sensitive to the hypotensive effects of the usual adult dose.
   Geriatric patients or patients with renal, hepatic, or cardiac insufficiency may require lower doses or longer dosing intervals.

**Usual adult prescribing limits**
Maintenance—Up to 6 grams daily.

**Usual pediatric dose**
Antiarrhythmic—
   Oral, 12.5 mg per kg of body weight or 375 mg per square meter of body surface four times a day.

**Strength(s) usually available**
U.S.—
   250 mg (Rx) [*Promine; Pronestyl* (lactose); GENERIC].
   375 mg (Rx) [*Promine; Pronestyl* (lactose); GENERIC].
   500 mg (Rx) [*Promine; Pronestyl;* GENERIC].
Canada—
   250 mg (Rx) [*Pronestyl*].
   375 mg (Rx) [*Pronestyl*].
   500 mg (Rx) [*Pronestyl;* GENERIC].

**Packaging and storage**
Store below 40 °C (104 °F), preferably between 15 and 30 °C (59 and 86 °F), unless otherwise specified by manufacturer. Store in a tight container.

**Stability**
Procainamide is hygroscopic.

**Auxiliary labeling**
• Keep container tightly closed.
• Do not take other medicines without your doctor's advice.

### PROCAINAMIDE HYDROCHLORIDE TABLETS USP

**Usual adult dose**
See *Procainamide Hydrochloride Capsules USP*.

**Usual pediatric dose**
See *Procainamide Hydrochloride Capsules USP*.

**Strength(s) usually available**
U.S.—
   250 mg (Rx) [*Pronestyl* (tartrazine); GENERIC].
   375 mg (Rx) [*Pronestyl* (tartrazine)].
   500 mg (Rx) [*Pronestyl* (tartrazine)].
Canada—
   Not commercially available.

**Packaging and storage**
Store below 40 °C (104 °F), preferably between 15 and 30 °C (59 and 86 °F), unless otherwise specified by manufacturer. Store in a tight container.

**Stability**
Procainamide is hygroscopic.

**Auxiliary labeling**
• Keep container tightly closed.
• Do not take other medicines without your doctor's advice.

### PROCAINAMIDE HYDROCHLORIDE EXTENDED-RELEASE TABLETS USP

**Usual adult dose**
[Atrial arrhythmias]—
   Maintenance: Oral, 1 gram every six hours, the dosage being adjusted as needed and tolerated.
Ventricular arrhythmias—
   Maintenance: Oral, 50 mg per kg of body weight per day in four divided doses (every six hours), the dosage being adjusted as needed and tolerated.
Note: The extended-release dosage form is intended for maintenance dosage, and not for initial dosage.
   Geriatric patients may be more sensitive to the hypotensive effects of the usual adult dose.

**Usual adult prescribing limits**
Maintenance—Up to 6 grams daily.

**Usual pediatric dose**
Not generally used in children. See instead *Procainamide Hydrochloride Capsules USP*.

**Strength(s) usually available**
U.S.—
   250 mg (Rx) [*Procan SR* (lactose; methylparaben; propylparaben); GENERIC].
   500 mg (Rx) [*Procan SR* (scored; lactose; methylparaben; propylparaben); *Pronestyl-SR;* GENERIC].
   750 mg (Rx) [*Procan SR;* GENERIC].
   1 gram (Rx) [*Procan SR*].
Canada—
   250 mg (Rx) [*Procan SR* (lactose; parabens)].
   500 mg (Rx) [*Procan SR* (parabens); *Pronestyl-SR*].
   750 mg (Rx) [*Procan SR* (scored)].
   1 gram (Rx) [*Procan SR* (scored)].

**Packaging and storage**
Store below 30 °C (86 °F), unless otherwise specified by manufacturer. Store in a tight container.

**Stability**
Procainamide is hygroscopic.

**Auxiliary labeling**
- Keep container tightly closed.
- Do not take other medicines without your doctor's advice.
- Swallow tablets whole.

**Note**
Extended-release tablets utilize a wax matrix, which may be detected in the stool.

## Parenteral Dosage Forms

### PROCAINAMIDE HYDROCHLORIDE INJECTION USP

**Usual adult dose**
Antiarrhythmic—
  Intramuscular—
    50 mg per kg of body weight per day in divided doses given every three to six hours.
  Intravenous—
    Initial:
      Intravenous (direct), 100 mg (diluted in an appropriate volume of 5% dextrose injection to facilitate control of dosage rate) administered slowly (not exceeding 50 mg per minute) and repeated every five minutes until arrhythmia is controlled or up to a maximum total dose of 1 gram, or
      Intravenous infusion, 500 to 600 mg diluted and administered at a constant rate over a period of twenty-five to thirty minutes.
    Maintenance:
      Intravenous infusion, diluted and administered at a rate of 2 to 6 mg per minute to maintain control of arrhythmia.

**Usual pediatric dose**
Dosage has not been established.

**Strength(s) usually available**
U.S.—
  100 mg per mL (Rx) [*Pronestyl* (benzyl alcohol; sodium bisulfite); GENERIC].
  500 mg per mL (Rx) [*Pronestyl* (sodium bisulfite; methylparaben); GENERIC].
Canada—
  100 mg per mL (Rx) [*Pronestyl* (benzyl alcohol; sodium bisulfite)].
  500 mg per mL (Rx) [*Pronestyl* (sodium bisulfite; methylparaben)].

**Packaging and storage**
Store between 15 and 30 °C (59 and 86 °F), unless otherwise specified by manufacturer. Protect from freezing. Protect from light.

**Preparation of dosage form**
For administration by intravenous infusion, dilute 200 mg to 1 gram of Procainamide Hydrochloride Injection USP to a concentration of 2 or 4 mg per mL using a suitable volume of 5% dextrose injection.

**Stability**
A slight yellowing will not alter potency; however, do not use if markedly discolored (darker than light amber) or if a precipitate is present.

Revised: 08/04/93

---

**PROCAINE**—See *Anesthetics (Parenteral-Local)*

---

# PROCARBAZINE   Systemic

VA CLASSIFICATION (Primary): AN900
Commonly used brand name(s): *Matulane; Natulan*.
Note: For a listing of dosage forms and brand names by country availability, see *Dosage Forms* section(s).

## Category
Antineoplastic.

## Indications
Note: Bracketed information in the *Indications* section refers to uses that are not included in U.S. product labeling.

**Accepted**
Lymphomas, Hodgkin's (treatment) or
[Lymphomas, non-Hodgkin's (treatment)][1]—Procarbazine is indicated, in combination with other agents, for treatment of Hodgkin's disease (Stage III and IV) and some non-Hodgkin's lymphomas.
[Tumors, brain, primary (treatment)][1]—Procarbazine is indicated for treatment of primary brain tumors.
[Multiple myeloma (treatment)][1]—Procarbazine is indicated for treatment of multiple myeloma.

[1]Not included in Canadian product labeling.

## Pharmacology/Pharmacokinetics

**Physicochemical characteristics**
Molecular weight—257.76.

**Mechanism of action/Effect**
Procarbazine is an alkylating agent. The exact mechanism of antineoplastic action is unknown but is thought to resemble that of the alkylating agents; procarbazine is cell cycle–specific for the S phase of cell division. Procarbazine is thought to inhibit DNA, RNA, and protein synthesis.

**Other actions/effects**
Procarbazine causes weak inhibition of monoamine oxidase (MAO). MAO inhibitors prevent the inactivation of tyramine by hepatic and gastrointestinal monoamine oxidase. Tyramine in the bloodstream releases norepinephrine from the sympathetic nerve terminals and produces a sudden increase in blood pressure.

**Absorption**
Rapidly and completely absorbed from the gastrointestinal tract.

**Distribution**
Crosses the blood-brain barrier.

**Biotransformation**
Hepatic.

**Half-life**
Approximately 10 minutes.

**Elimination**
Renal—70% (as metabolite).

## Precautions to Consider

**Carcinogenicity/Mutagenicity**
Secondary malignancies are potential delayed effects of many antineoplastic agents, although it is not clear whether the effect is related to their mutagenic or immunosuppressive action. The effect of dose and duration of therapy is also unknown, although risk seems to increase with long-term use. Although information is limited, available data seem to indicate that the carcinogenic risk is greatest with the alkylating agents.
Procarbazine is a potent carcinogen in animals and, because it is an alkylating agent, is also likely to be carcinogenic in humans.

**Pregnancy/Reproduction**
Fertility—Gonadal suppression, resulting in amenorrhea or azoospermia, may occur in patients taking antineoplastic therapy, especially with the alkylating agents. In general, these effects appear to be related to dose and length of therapy and may be irreversible. Prediction of the degree of testicular or ovarian function impairment is complicated by the common use of combinations of several antineoplastics, which makes it difficult to assess the effects of individual agents. Procarbazine affects spermatogenesis in humans.
Pregnancy—Procarbazine is frequently teratogenic in animals and there have been reports of minor malformations or premature births when it is given later in pregnancy in humans.
First trimester: It is usually recommended that use of antineoplastics, especially combination chemotherapy, be avoided whenever possible, especially during the first trimester. Although information is limited because of the relatively few instances of antineoplastic administration during pregnancy, the mutagenic, teratogenic, and carcinogenic potential of these medications must be considered.
Other hazards to the fetus include adverse reactions seen in adults.
In general, use of a contraceptive is recommended during cytotoxic drug therapy.
FDA Pregnancy Category D.

### Breast-feeding
Although very little information is available regarding distribution of antineoplastic agents into breast milk, breast-feeding is not recommended while procarbazine is being administered because of the risks to the infant (adverse effects, mutagenicity, carcinogenicity).

### Pediatrics
Appropriate studies with procarbazine have not been performed in the pediatric population. However, pediatrics-specific problems that would limit the usefulness of this medication in children are not expected.

### Geriatrics
Although appropriate studies with procarbazine have not been performed in the geriatric population, the potential for increased vascular accidents (especially in the event of sudden hypertensive episodes), increased sensitivity to hypotensive effects, and reduced metabolic capacity discourages the first-time use of MAO inhibitors in patients over 60 years of age. When an MAO inhibitor is prescribed for an elderly patient, the patient's history of depression, ability to comply with prescribing instructions, and any potential drug interactions must also be considered. In addition, elderly patients are more likely to have age-related renal function impairment, which may require a lower dosage or, in severe cases, avoidance of use of procarbazine.

### Dental
The bone marrow depressant effects of procarbazine may result in an increased incidence of microbial infection, delayed healing, and gingival bleeding. Dental work, whenever possible, should be completed prior to initiation of therapy or deferred until blood counts have returned to normal. Patients should be instructed in proper oral hygiene during treatment, including caution in use of regular toothbrushes, dental floss, and toothpicks.

Procarbazine may also cause stomatitis that is associated with considerable discomfort.

The secondary anticholinergic effects of procarbazine may decrease or inhibit salivary flow, especially in middle-aged or elderly patients, thus contributing to the development of caries, periodontal disease, oral candidiasis, and discomfort.

### Drug interactions and/or related problems
The following drug interactions and/or related problems have been selected on the basis of their potential clinical significance (possible mechanism in parentheses where appropriate)—not necessarily inclusive (» = major clinical significance):

Note: Combinations containing any of the following medications, depending on the amount present, may also interact with this medication.

Most drug interactions are due to procarbazine's monoamine oxidase–inhibiting activity.

» Alcohol
(concurrent use with procarbazine may result in a disulfiram-like reaction and additive central nervous system (CNS) depression and postural hypotension; also, possible tyramine content in alcoholic beverages, especially beer, wine, or ale, may induce hypertensive reactions)

» Anesthetics, local, with epinephrine or levonordefrin or
» Cocaine
(concurrent use with procarbazine may cause severe hypertension due to sympathomimetic effects)

(cocaine should not be administered during or within 14 days following administration of an MAO inhibitor)

» Anesthetics, spinal
(hypotensive effects may be potentiated when spinal anesthetics are used concurrently with procarbazine; discontinuation of procarbazine at least 10 days before elective surgery if spinal anesthesia is planned may be advisable)

» Anticholinergics or other medications with anticholinergic activity (see *Appendix II*) or
Antidyskinetic agents or
» Antihistamines
(concurrent use with procarbazine may intensify anticholinergic effects because of the secondary anticholinergic activities of MAO inhibitors; also, MAO inhibitors may block detoxification of anticholinergics, thus potentiating their action; patients should be advised to report occurrence of gastrointestinal problems promptly since paralytic ileus may occur with concurrent therapy)

(concurrent use with MAO inhibitors may also prolong and intensify CNS depressant and anticholinergic effects of antihistamines; concurrent use is not recommended)

Anticoagulants, coumarin- and indandione-derivative
(concurrent use may increase anticoagulant activity; although the mechanism of action and clinical significance are unknown, caution is recommended)

Anticonvulsants
(concurrent use of anticonvulsants with procarbazine may lead to increased CNS depressant effects as well as a change in the pattern of epileptiform seizures; dosage adjustment of anticonvulsant may be necessary)

» Antidepressants, tricyclic
(in addition to increased anticholinergic effects, concurrent use with procarbazine may result in hyperpyretic crises, severe convulsions, and death; however, recent studies have shown that some tricyclic antidepressants can be used concurrently with MAO inhibitors with no adverse effects if both medications are initiated simultaneously at lower than usual doses and the doses raised gradually, or if the MAO inhibitor is gradually added to the tricyclic also at low doses; tricyclics should not be added to an established MAO inhibitor regimen; careful monitoring for side effects of either medication is necessary)

» Antidiabetic agents, sulfonylurea or
» Insulin
(procarbazine may enhance hypoglycemic effects; dosage reduction of hypoglycemic medication may be necessary during and after such combined therapy)

Antihypertensives or
Diuretics or
Hypotension-producing medications, other (see *Appendix II*)
(concurrent use with procarbazine may result in an enhanced hypotensive effect; dosage adjustment may be necessary)

(antihypertensives with CNS depressant effects, such as clonidine, guanabenz, methyldopa, or metyrosine, may increase CNS depression)

Beta-adrenergic blocking agents, including ophthalmic beta-blockers absorbed systemically
(possible significant hypertension may theoretically occur up to 14 days following discontinuation of procarbazine; however, sufficient clinical reports are lacking)

Blood dyscrasia–causing medications (see *Appendix II*)
(leukopenic and/or thrombocytopenic effects of procarbazine may be increased with concurrent or recent therapy if these medications cause the same effects; dosage adjustment of procarbazine, if necessary, should be based on blood counts)

» Bone marrow depressants, other (see *Appendix II*) or
Radiation therapy
(additive bone marrow depression may occur; dosage reduction may be required when two or more bone marrow depressants, including radiation, are used concurrently or consecutively)

Bromocriptine
(concurrent use may increase serum prolactin concentrations and interfere with effects of bromocriptine; dosage adjustment of bromocriptine may be necessary)

» Buspirone
(concurrent use with MAO inhibitors is not recommended because elevation of blood pressure may occur)

» Caffeine-containing preparations
(concurrent use of excessive amounts of caffeine, consumed in chocolate, coffee, cola, tea, or "stay awake" products, with procarbazine may produce dangerous cardiac arrhythmias or severe hypertension because of sympathomimetic effects of caffeine)

» Carbamazepine or
» Cyclobenzaprine or
» Maprotiline or
» Monoamine oxidase (MAO) inhibitors, other, including furazolidone and pargyline
(concurrent use with procarbazine is not recommended on an outpatient basis, as hyperpyretic crises, severe seizures, and death could result; prior to initiation of procarbazine therapy, 14 days should elapse after discontinuance of any of these medications)

» CNS depression–producing medications, other (see *Appendix II*)
(CNS depression and postural hypotension may be enhanced; concurrent use with antihistamines is not recommended)

» Dextromethorphan
(concurrent use with procarbazine may cause excitation, hypertension, and hyperpyrexia)

» Doxapram
(concurrent use may increase the pressor effects of either doxapram or procarbazine)

» Fluoxetine
(concurrent use may result in confusion, agitation, restlessness, and gastrointestinal symptoms, or possibly hyperpyretic episodes, severe convulsions, and hypertensive crises. Based on experience with tricyclic antidepressants, at least 14 days should elapse between discontinuation of an MAO inhibitor and initiation of fluoxetine. However, because of the long half-lives of fluoxetine and its active metabolite, at least 5 weeks [approximately 5 half-lives of norfluoxetine] should elapse between discontinuation of fluoxetine and initiation of therapy with an MAO inhibitor. Administration of an MAO inhibitor within 5 weeks of discontinuation of fluoxetine may increase the risk of serious events. While a causal relationship to fluoxetine has not been established, death has been reported following the initiation of an MAO inhibitor shortly after fluoxetine administration was stopped)

» Guanadrel or
» Guanethidine or
» Rauwolfia alkaloids
(administration to patients receiving procarbazine may result in sudden release of accumulated catecholamines and a hypertensive reaction; parenteral administration is not recommended during and for 1 week following procarbazine therapy)

(when an MAO inhibitor is added to existing therapy with a rauwolfia alkaloid, serious potentiation of CNS depressant effects may result; however, if a rauwolfia alkaloid is added to an MAO inhibitor regimen, CNS excitation and hypertension may result from release of excessive amounts of accumulated norepinephrine and serotonin)

Haloperidol or
Loxapine or
Molindone or
Phenothiazines or
Pimozide or
Thioxanthenes
(concurrent use may prolong and intensify the sedative, hypotensive, and anticholinergic effects of either these medications or procarbazine)

» Levodopa
(concurrent use with MAO inhibitors is not recommended, as the combination may result in sudden moderate to severe hypertensive crisis; a period of 2 to 4 weeks is recommended after withdrawal of MAO inhibitors before levodopa is administered)

» Meperidine and possibly other opioid (narcotic) analgesics
(concurrent use with procarbazine may produce immediate excitation, sweating, rigidity, and severe hypertension; in some patients, hypotension, severe respiratory depression, coma, convulsions, hyperpyrexia, vascular collapse, and death may occur; reactions may be due to accumulation of serotonin resulting from MAO inhibition; avoidance of meperidine use within 2 to 3 weeks following procarbazine is recommended; other opioid analgesics, such as morphine, are not likely to cause such severe reactions and may be used cautiously in reduced dosage in patients receiving MAO inhibitors; however, it is recommended that a small test dose [one quarter of the usual dose] or several small incremental test doses over a period of several hours should first be administered to permit observation of any adverse effects)

(caution is also recommended in the use of alfentanil, fentanyl, or sufentanil as an adjunct to anesthesia if the patient has received procarbazine within 14 days; although the risk of a significant interaction has been questioned, the use of a small test dose is advised to detect any possible interaction)

» Methyldopa
(concurrent use with procarbazine may cause hyperexcitability; also headache, severe hypertension, and hallucinations have been reported)

» Methylphenidate
(concurrent use with procarbazine may potentiate the CNS stimulant effects of methylphenidate, possibly resulting in a hypertensive crisis; should not be administered during or within 14 days following the administration of procarbazine)

Metrizamide
(concurrent use with procarbazine may lower the seizure threshold; procarbazine should be discontinued at least 48 hours before myelography and should not be resumed for at least 24 hours after procedure)

Phenylephrine, nasal or ophthalmic
(if significant systemic absorption of nasal or ophthalmic phenylephrine occurs, concurrent use with procarbazine may potentiate pressor effects; these medications should not be administered during or within 14 days following the administration of procarbazine)

» Sympathomimetics
(concurrent use with procarbazine may prolong and intensify cardiac stimulant and vasopressor effects [including headache, cardiac arrhythmias, vomiting, sudden and severe hypertensive and hyperpyretic crises] of these medications because of release of catecholamines that accumulate in intraneuronal storage sites during MAO inhibitor therapy; these medications should not be administered during or within 14 days following the administration of procarbazine)

» Tryptophan
(concurrent use with MAO inhibitors may cause hyperreflexia, shivering, hyperventilation, hyperthermia, mania or hypomania, and disorientation or confusion; when tryptophan is added to an MAOI regimen, it should be started in low dosages and the dose titrated upwards gradually with close monitoring of mental status and blood pressure)

» Tyramine- or other high pressor amine–containing foods and beverages, such as aged cheese; beer; reduced-alcohol and alcohol-free beer and wine; red and white wines; sherry; liqueurs; yeast/protein extracts; fava or broad bean pods; smoked or pickled meats, poultry, or fish; fermented sausage (bologna, pepperoni, salami, summer sausage) or other fermented meat; and any overripe fruit
(concurrent use with procarbazine may cause sudden and severe hypertensive reactions; reactions are usually limited to a few hours and easily treated with phentolamine; severity depends on amount of tyramine ingested, rate of gastric emptying, and length of interval between dose of procarbazine and ingestion of tyramine; when procarbazine is discontinued, dietary restrictions must continue for at least 2 weeks; other tyramine- or high pressor amine–containing foods, such as yogurt, sour cream, cream cheese, cottage cheese, chocolate, and soy sauce, if eaten when fresh and in moderation, are considered unlikely to cause serious problems)

Vaccines, killed virus
(because normal defense mechanisms may be suppressed by procarbazine therapy, the patient's antibody response to the vaccine may be decreased. The interval between discontinuation of medications that cause immunosuppression and restoration of the patient's ability to respond to the vaccine depends on the intensity and type of immunosuppression-causing medication used, the underlying disease, and other factors; estimates vary from 3 months to 1 year)

» Vaccines, live virus
(because normal defense mechanisms may be suppressed by procarbazine therapy, concurrent use with a live virus vaccine may potentiate the replication of the vaccine virus, may increase the side/adverse effects of the vaccine virus, and/or may decrease the patient's antibody response to the vaccine; immunization of these patients should be undertaken only with extreme caution after careful review of the patient's hematologic status and only with the knowledge and consent of the physician managing the procarbazine therapy. The interval between discontinuation of medications that cause immunosuppression and restoration of the patient's ability to respond to the vaccine depends on the intensity and type of immunosuppression-causing medication used, the underlying disease, and other factors; estimates vary from 3 months to 1 year. Immunization with oral poliovirus vaccine should also be postponed in persons in close contact with the patient, especially family members)

**Medical considerations/Contraindications**
The medical considerations/contraindications included have been selected on the basis of their potential clinical significance (reasons given in parentheses where appropriate)—not necessarily inclusive (» = major clinical significance).

*Except under special circumstances, this medication should not be used when the following medical problems exist:*
» Alcoholism, active
» Congestive heart failure
» Hepatic function impairment, severe
(procarbazine may precipitate hepatic precoma in patients with cirrhosis, who are extremely sensitive to its effects)
» Pheochromocytoma
(pressor substances secreted by such tumors may alter blood pressure during therapy with MAO inhibitors)
» Renal function impairment, severe
(cumulative effects of procarbazine may occur because of reduced renal excretion)

*Risk-benefit should be considered when the following medical problems exist:*

» Bone marrow depression
» Cardiac arrhythmias
» Cardiovascular disease or coronary insufficiency
    (ischemia may be aggravated as a result of reduced blood pressure)
  Cerebrovascular disease
    (cerebral ischemia may be aggravated as a result of reduced blood pressure)
» Chickenpox, existing or recent (including recent exposure) or
» Herpes zoster
    (risk of severe generalized disease)
  Diabetes mellitus
    (procarbazine may alter insulin or oral hypoglycemic requirements)
  Epilepsy
    (pattern of epileptiform seizures may be changed)
» Headaches, severe or frequent
    (headache as a first sign of hypertensive reaction during therapy may be masked)
» Hepatic function impairment
    (procarbazine may precipitate hepatic precoma in patients with cirrhosis, who are extremely sensitive to its effects; lower dosage is recommended; use not recommended in severe function impairment)
  Hyperthyroidism
    (sensitivity to pressor amines may be increased)
» Infection
» Paranoid schizophrenia or other hyperexcitable personality states
    (MAO inhibitors may cause excessive stimulation in schizophrenic patients; in manic-depressive states, may effect a swing from depressive to manic phase)
  Parkinsonism
    (may be aggravated)
» Renal function impairment
    (cumulative effects may occur; lower dosage is recommended; use not recommended in severe function impairment)
  Sensitivity to procarbazine
» Caution should be used also in patients who have had previous cytotoxic drug therapy or radiation therapy.
» In addition, caution should be used in patients who have undergone sympathectomy, who may be more sensitive to the hypotensive effects of MAO inhibitors.

**Patient monitoring**
The following may be especially important in patient monitoring (other tests may be warranted in some patients, depending on condition; » = major clinical significance):

» Alanine aminotransferase (ALT [SGPT]) values, serum and
» Aspartate aminotransferase (AST [SGOT]) values, serum and
» Bilirubin concentrations, serum and
» Lactate dehydrogenase (LDH) values, serum
    (determinations recommended prior to initiation of therapy and at periodic intervals during therapy; frequency varies according to clinical state, agent, dose, and other agents being used concurrently)
  Blood urea nitrogen (BUN) concentrations and
  Creatinine concentrations, serum
    (determinations recommended prior to initiation of therapy and at periodic intervals during therapy; frequency varies according to clinical state, agent, dose, and other agents being used concurrently)
» Bone marrow aspiration studies
    (recommended prior to initiation of procarbazine therapy and at time of maximum hematologic response to ensure adequate bone marrow reserve)
» Hematocrit or hemoglobin and
» Platelet count and
» Total and, if appropriate, differential leukocyte count
    (determinations recommended prior to initiation of therapy and at periodic intervals during therapy; frequency varies according to clinical state, agent, dose, and other agents being used concurrently)

## Side/Adverse Effects

Note: Many "side effects" of antineoplastic therapy are unavoidable and represent the medication's pharmacologic action. Some of these (for example, leukopenia and thrombocytopenia) are actually used as parameters to aid in individual dosage titration.

Except for hematologic, pulmonary, and gastrointestinal toxicity, adverse effects of procarbazine resemble those of the MAO inhibitors used in treating psychiatric disorders.

Toxicity is increased in patients with renal or hepatic function impairment or bone marrow depression.

The following side/adverse effects have been selected on the basis of their potential clinical significance (possible signs and symptoms in parentheses where appropriate)—not necessarily inclusive:

**Those indicating need for medical attention**
Incidence more frequent
  *Anemia; CNS stimulation, excessive* (confusion; convulsions; hallucinations); *immunosuppression, infection, or leukopenia* (fever or chills; cough or hoarseness; lower back or side pain; painful or difficult urination)—usually asymptomatic; *thrombocytopenia* (unusual bleeding or bruising; black, tarry stools; blood in urine or stools; pinpoint red spots on skin)—usually asymptomatic; *hemolytic anemia* (continuing tiredness or weakness); *missing menstrual periods; pneumonitis* (cough; shortness of breath; thickening of bronchial secretions)
  Note: With leukopenia and thrombocytopenia, the nadir of the platelet count occurs after about 4 weeks, followed by the leukocyte count, with recovery complete in about 6 weeks.
    Missing menstrual periods occur with high doses.
Incidence less frequent
  *Gastrointestinal toxicity* (diarrhea); *hepatotoxicity* (yellow eyes or skin); *peripheral neuropathy* (tingling or numbness of fingers or toes; unsteadiness or awkwardness); *stomatitis* (sores in mouth and on lips)
Incidence rare
  *Allergic reaction* (skin rash, hives or itching; wheezing); *hypertensive crisis* (severe chest pain; enlarged pupils; fast or slow heartbeat; severe headache; increased sensitivity of eyes to light; increased sweating, possibly with fever or cold, clammy skin; stiff or sore neck); *orthostatic hypotension* (fainting)

**Those indicating need for medical attention only if they continue or are bothersome**
Incidence more frequent
  *CNS stimulation, excessive* (drowsiness; muscle or joint pain; muscle twitching; nervousness; nightmares; trouble in sleeping); *nausea and vomiting; unusual tiredness or weakness*
Incidence less frequent
  *Constipation; darkening of skin; difficulty in swallowing; dry mouth; feeling of warmth and redness in face; headache; loss of appetite; mental depression; orthostatic hypotension* (dizziness or lightheadedness when getting up from a lying or sitting position)

**Those not indicating need for medical attention**
Incidence less frequent
  *Loss of hair*

## Overdose

For more information on the management of overdose or unintentional intestion, **contact a Poison Control Center** (see *Poison Control Center listing*).

**Treatment of overdose**
Note: Symptoms resulting from overdose may be absent or minimal for nearly 12 hours following ingestion, and develop slowly thereafter, reaching a maximum in 24 to 48 hours. Immediate hospitalization and close monitoring of patient are essential during this period.

Treatment may include the following:
  Induction of vomiting or gastric lavage with protected airway followed by instillation of charcoal slurry in early overdose.
  Treatment of signs and symptoms of CNS stimulation with diazepam, administered intravenously and slowly.
  Treatment of hypotension and vascular collapse with intravenous fluids and a dilute pressor agent.
  Support of respiration by management of the airway, and mechanical ventilation with the use of supplemental oxygen, as required.
  Close monitoring of body temperature and vigorous treatment of hyperpyrexia with antipyretics and a cooling blanket. Maintenance of fluid and electrolyte balance is essential.
  Reduction of symptoms of hypermetabolic state (coma, respiratory failure, hyperpyrexia, tachycardia, muscular rigidity, tremor, and hyperreflexia) with intravenous dantrolene sodium at 2.5 mg per kg of body weight (mg/kg) a day in divided doses, with careful monitoring for signs of hepatotoxicity and pleural or pericardial effusions.
  Hemodialysis may be beneficial but is of unproven value.
  Pathophysiologic effects of massive overdose may persist for several days; recovery from mild overdose may take 3 to 4 days.

## Patient Consultation

As an aid to patient consultation, refer to *Advice for the Patient, Procarbazine (Systemic)*.

In providing consultation, consider emphasizing the following selected information (» = major clinical significance):

### Before using this medication

Conditions affecting use, especially:
Sensitivity to procarbazine
Pregnancy—Advisability of using contraception; telling physician immediately if pregnancy is suspected
Breast-feeding—Not recommended because of risk of serious side effects
Use in the elderly—Potential for increased vascular accidents, increased sensitivity to hypotensive effects; first-time use discouraged in patients over 60 years of age
Other medications, especially alcohol, anticholinergics or other medications with anticholinergic activity, antihistamines, buspirone, caffeine-containing preparations, carbamazepine, CNS-depressants, cocaine, cyclobenzaprine, dextromethorphan, doxapram, fluoxetine, furazolidone, guanadrel, guanethidine, insulin, levodopa, local anesthetics with epinephrine or levonordefrin, maprotiline, meperidine and possibly other opioid analgesics, methyldopa, methylphenidate, other bone marrow depressants, other monoamine oxidase inhibitors, pargyline, previous cytotoxic drug or radiation therapy, rauwolfia alkaloids, spinal anesthetics, sulfonylurea antidiabetic agents, sympathomimetics, tricyclic antidepressants, or tryptophan
Other medical problems, especially active alcoholism, bone marrow depression, cardiac arrhythmias, chickenpox or recent exposure, congestive heart failure, coronary insufficiency, severe or frequent headaches, hepatic function impairment, herpes zoster, other infection, paranoid schizophrenia or other hyperexcitable personality states, pheochromocytoma, sympathectomy, or renal function impairment

### Proper use of this medication

» Importance of not taking more or less medication than the amount prescribed
Caution in taking combination chemotherapy; taking each medication at the right time
» Frequency of nausea and vomiting; importance of continuing medication despite stomach upset
Checking with physician if vomiting occurs shortly after dose is taken
» Proper dosing
Missed dose: Taking as soon as remembered if within a few hours; not taking if several hours have passed or if almost time for next dose; not doubling doses
» Proper storage

### Precautions while using this medication

» Importance of close monitoring by the physician
» Checking with hospital emergency room or physician if symptoms of hypertensive crisis develop
» Avoiding use of tyramine-containing foods, alcoholic beverages and large quantities of caffeine-containing beverages, over-the-counter cold and cough medicines, and other medication unless prescribed; having list of such for reference
» Obeying rules of caution during 14 days after discontinuing medication
» Caution in taking alcohol or other CNS depressants
» Caution if drowsiness occurs, especially when driving or doing things requiring alertness
» Avoiding immunizations unless approved by physician; other persons in patient's household should avoid immunizations with oral poliovirus vaccine; avoiding other persons who have taken oral poliovirus vaccine or wearing a protective mask that covers nose and mouth

*Caution if bone marrow depression occurs*
» Avoiding exposure to persons with infections, especially during periods of low blood counts; checking with physician immediately if fever or chills, cough or hoarseness, lower back or side pain, or painful or difficult urination occurs
» Checking with physician immediately if unusual bleeding or bruising; black, tarry stools; blood in urine or stools; or pinpoint red spots on skin occur
Caution in use of regular toothbrush, dental floss, or toothpick; physician, dentist, or nurse may suggest alternatives; checking with physician before having dental work done
Not touching eyes or inside of nose unless hands washed immediately before
Using caution to avoid accidental cuts with use of sharp objects such as safety razor or fingernail or toenail cutters
Avoiding contact sports or other situations where bruising or injury could occur
Diabetics: Checking urine or blood sugar levels
» Caution if any kind of surgery (including dental surgery) or emergency treatment is required
Carrying medical identification card

### Side/adverse effects

May cause adverse effects such as blood problems, loss of hair, hypertensive crisis, and cancer; importance of discussing possible effects with physician
Signs of potential side effects, especially anemia, excessive CNS stimulation, immunosuppression, infection, leukopenia, thrombocytopenia, hemolytic anemia, missing menstrual periods, pneumonitis, gastrointestinal toxicity, hepatotoxicity, peripheral neuropathy, stomatitis, allergic reaction, hypertensive crisis, and orthostatic hypotension
Physician or nurse can help in dealing with side effects

## General Dosing Information

Patients receiving procarbazine should be under supervision of a physician experienced in cancer chemotherapy.

A variety of dosage schedules and regimens of procarbazine, alone or in combination with other antitumor agents, are used. The prescriber may consult medical literature as well as the manufacturer's literature in choosing a specific dosage.

Dosage must be adjusted to meet the individual requirements of each patient, based on clinical response and appearance or severity of toxicity.

Although dosages are based on the patient's actual weight, use of estimated lean body weight is recommended in obese patients or those with weight gain due to edema, ascites, or other abnormal fluid retention.

It is recommended that procarbazine therapy be discontinued promptly if any of the following occur:
Allergic reaction
Central nervous system signs or symptoms, such as paresthesias, neuropathies, or confusion
Diarrhea
Hemorrhage or bleeding tendencies
Leukopenia (< 4000 white blood cells per cubic millimeter)
Stomatitis
Thrombocytopenia (< 100,000 platelets per cubic millimeter)

Therapy may be resumed at a lower dosage when the clinical and laboratory examinations are satisfactory.

Because of the risk of enhanced bone marrow toxicity, an interval of at least 1 month (based on bone marrow studies) is recommended before starting procarbazine therapy after a patient has received radiation or chemotherapy with medications that depress bone marrow function.

After dosage is stopped, monoamine oxidase (MAO) inhibitor effects of this medication may persist for up to 2 weeks after withdrawal (time required for regeneration of enzyme). During this period, food and drug contraindications must be observed.

Special precautions are recommended in patients who develop thrombocytopenia as a result of administration of procarbazine. These may include extreme care in performing invasive procedures; regular inspection of intravenous sites, skin (including perirectal area), and mucous membrane surfaces for signs of bleeding or bruising; limiting frequency of venipuncture and avoiding intramuscular injections; testing urine, emesis, stool, and secretions for occult blood; care in use of regular toothbrushes, dental floss, toothpicks, safety razors, and fingernail and toenail cutters; avoiding constipation; and using caution to prevent falls and other injuries. Such patients should avoid alcohol and any aspirin intake because of the risk of gastrointestinal bleeding. Platelet transfusions may be required.

Patients who develop leukopenia should be observed carefully for signs of infection. Antibiotic support may be required. In neutropenic patients who develop fever, broad-spectrum antibiotic coverage should be initiated empirically, pending bacterial cultures and appropriate diagnostic tests.

## Diet/Nutrition

Foods and beverages containing tyramine or other high pressor amines, such as aged cheese; beer; reduced-alcohol and alcohol-free beer and wine; red and white wines; sherry; liqueurs; yeast/protein extracts; fava or broad bean pods; smoked or pickled meats, poultry, or fish; fermented sausage (bologna, pepperoni, salami, summer sausage) or other fermented meat; and any overripe fruit, when used concurrently with MAO inhibitors, may cause sudden and severe hypertensive reactions. The reactions are usually limited to a few hours and are easily treated with phentolamine. The severity depends on the amount of tyramine ingested, rate of gastric emptying, and length of the interval between

# 2396  Procarbazine (Systemic)

the dose of MAO inhibitor and ingestion of tyramine. When MAO inhibitors are discontinued, dietary restrictions must continue for at least 2 weeks. Other foods, such as yogurt, sour cream, cream cheese, cottage cheese, chocolate, and soy sauce, if eaten when fresh and in moderation, are considered unlikely to cause serious problems.

**For treatment of hypertensive crisis**
Recommended treatment includes:
- Discontinuing MAO inhibitor.
- Lowering blood pressure immediately with intravenous administration of 5 mg of phentolamine, with care being taken to inject slowly, to prevent excessive hypotensive effect.
- Reducing fever by external cooling.

**Combination chemotherapy**
Procarbazine may be used in combination with other agents in various regimens. As a result, incidence and/or severity of side effects may be altered and different dosages (usually reduced) may be used. For example, procarbazine is part of the following chemotherapeutic combinations (some commonly used acronyms are in parentheses):
— carmustine, cyclophosphamide, vinblastine, procarbazine, and prednisone (BCVPP).
— cyclophosphamide, doxorubicin, methotrexate, and procarbazine (CAMP).
— cyclophosphamide, vincristine, procarbazine, and prednisone (COPP).
— mechlorethamine, vincristine, procarbazine, and prednisone (MOPP).

For specific dosages and schedules, consult the literature. For information regarding each agent, consult the individual monographs.

## Oral Dosage Forms

### PROCARBAZINE HYDROCHLORIDE CAPSULES USP

Note: The doses and strength are expressed in terms of procarbazine base, not the hydrochloride salt.

**Usual adult dose**
Lymphomas, Hodgkin's—
Initial: Oral, 2 to 4 mg (base) per kg of body weight (to the nearest 50 mg) a day in single or divided doses for the first week, followed by 4 to 6 mg per kg of body weight a day until leukopenia, thrombocytopenia, or maximum response occurs.

Note: If hematologic toxicity occurs, the medication is withdrawn until the toxicity is resolved, then treatment may be resumed with 1 to 2 mg (base) per kg of body weight a day.
Maintenance: Oral, 1 to 2 mg (base) per kg of body weight a day.

**Usual pediatric dose**
Lymphomas, Hodgkin's—
Initial: Oral, 50 mg (base) per square meter of body surface area a day for the first week, followed by 100 mg per square meter of body surface area a day until leukopenia, thrombocytopenia, or maximum response occurs.

Note: If hematologic toxicity occurs, the medication is withdrawn until the toxicity is resolved, then treatment may be resumed with 50 mg (base) per square meter of body surface area a day.
Maintenance: Oral, 50 mg (base) per square meter of body surface area a day.

Note: This dosage schedule is a guideline only. Undue toxicity in the form of tremors, coma, and seizures has occurred; therefore, dosage must be individualized based on clinical response and appearance of toxicity.

**Strength(s) usually available**
U.S.—
  50 mg (base) (Rx) [*Matulane*].
Canada—
  50 mg (base) (Rx) [*Natulan*].

**Packaging and storage**
Store below 40 °C (104 °F), preferably between 15 and 30 °C (59 and 86 °F), unless otherwise specified by manufacturer. Store in a tight, light-resistant container.

**Auxiliary labeling**
- Avoid alcoholic beverages.
- May cause drowsiness.
- Avoid certain foods as directed.

Revised: 08/90
Interim revision: 08/05/93; 06/30/94; 09/30/97

---

**PROCATEROL**—See *Bronchodilators, Adrenergic (Inhalation-Local)*

---

**PROCHLORPERAZINE**—See *Phenothiazines (Systemic)*

---

**PROCYCLIDINE**—See *Antidyskinetics (Systemic)*

---

**PROGESTERONE**—See *Progestins (Systemic)*

---

# PROGESTERONE INTRAUTERINE DEVICE (IUD)†

VA CLASSIFICATION (Primary): GU400
Commonly used brand name(s): *Progestasert*.
Note: For a listing of dosage forms and brand names by country availability, see *Dosage Forms* section(s).

†Not commercially available in Canada.

## Category
Contraceptive (intrauterine-local).

## Indications

**Accepted**
Pregnancy (prophylaxis)—Progesterone intrauterine devices are recommended as a contraceptive method, primarily for parous women who are in a mutually monogamous relationship and have no history of pelvic inflammatory disease (PID).

An IUD may **not** be an appropriate choice for nulliparous or low parity women whose lifestyle (involvement in multiple relationships or in a nonmonogamous relationship) may expose them to sexually transmitted diseases (STDs) or for women at risk of developing PID because PID, if it develops, potentially may be more severe for these women. The IUD is **not** generally recommended for women whose uterine cavity measures less than 6.5 centimeters (cm).

IUDs do not protect against sexually transmitted diseases including human immunodeficiency virus (HIV) infection or acquired immunodeficiency syndrome (AIDS).

The following table presents the results of studies examining contraceptive failure rates calculated using the life-table method. The first column lists the contraceptive method used. The second column indicates the percentage of women experiencing an accidental pregnancy in the first year of use of a contraceptive method while using the method perfectly under clinical conditions. The range of failure rates in the clinical trials may be explained by interstudy variations in study design or patient population characteristics, such as motivation, fecundity, or socioeconomic factors (including education). The third column indicates contraceptive failure rates in the first year of contraceptive use under clinical conditions for typical couples who start using a method (not necessarily for the first time). Failure rates among adolescents may be higher due to poorer compliance than in other age groups.

| Method used | Failure rate range (over 12 months) in clinical studies (%) | Typical first year failure rate (%) |
|---|---|---|
| None | 78–94 | 85 |
| Spermicides* | 0.3–37 | 21 |
| Periodic abstinence† | 13–35 | 20 |
| Withdrawal | 7–22 | 19 |
| Cervical cap with spermicide | 6–27 | 18 |
| Diaphragm with spermicide | 2–23 | 18 |
| Condom without spermicide | 2–14 | 12 |
| IUD | | |
|   Progesterone-releasing | 1.9–2.0 | 2 |
|   Copper-T 200 | 3.0–3.6 | |
|   Copper-T 200Ag‡ | 0–1.2 | |
|   Copper-T 220C§ | 0.9–1.8 | |
|   Copper-T 380A | 0.5–0.8 | 0.8 |
|   Copper-T 380S | 0.9 | |
| Oral contraceptive | | 3 |
|   Estrogen and progestin | 0–6 | |
|   Progestin only | 1–10 | |
| Medroxyprogesterone injection (90-day) | 0–0.3 | 0.3 |
| Levonorgestrel (implants) | | |
|   Six capsules | 0–0.09 | 0.09 |
|   Two rods | 0–0.2 | 0.3 |
| Sterilization | | |
|   Female# | 0–8 | 0.4 |
|   Male | 0–0.5 | 0.15 |

*Spermicides studied include creams, foams, gels, jellies, and suppositories.

†Methods studied include calendar, ovulation method, and symptothermal (cervical mucus method supplemented by basal body temperature in post-ovulatory phases, post-ovulation phases, post-ovulation).

‡Life-table method rate is unavailable for Copper-T 200Ag and the Pearl method rate at 12 months was reported; these methods at 12 months are considered comparable.

§Copper-T 220C is manufactured with copper sleeves instead of copper wire; often used as a control in clinical studies.

#Methods studied include culdotomy, laparoscopy, minilaparotomy, electrocoagulation, laparotomy, tubal diathermy and/or use of rings or clips.

## Pharmacology/Pharmacokinetics

**Physicochemical characteristics**

Physical description—The ethylene/vinyl coacetate polymer (EVA) T-shaped body has a 36 millimeter tubular vertical stem that contains a reservoir of 38 mg of microcrystallized progesterone (initially) and radiopaque barium sulfate (to monitor location) dispersed in silicone fluid; the horizontal arms measure 32 millimeters. In addition, the T-shaped body contains two blue-black monofilament threads (to monitor placement and aid in IUD removal).

**Mechanism of action/Effect**

Contraceptive, intrauterine-local—

The progesterone intrauterine device prevents pregnancy in 98% of users in the first year of use. The precise mechanism of action has not been fully elucidated; a number of mechanisms may contribute to the contraceptive effect.

Progesterone is thought to enhance an unfavorable uterine environment for implantation by suppressing endometrial proliferation and to inhibit sperm penetration by causing cervical mucus to become thick and scanty. Progesterone also may directly inhibit metabolism, capacitation, and swimming speed of the sperm. Other normal cyclic reproductive function, including ovulation, continues as it does with other IUDs.

In general, IUDs produce cellular reactions that can lead to local superficial ulceration in adjacent uterine cells. This causes a foreign-body inflammatory response leading to biochemical and morphological changes in the endometrial tissue and uterine fluid, including increased infiltration of leukocytes, especially macrophages. This action adds to progesterone's ability to interfere with sperm migration, fertilization and, to a lesser extent, with implantation.

**Other actions/effects**

Progesterone may decrease the endometrial content of prostaglandins and decrease the concentration of blood vessels in the endometrium which may result in fewer complaints of dysmenorrhea and a lower total volume of menstrual blood loss in women using a progesterone IUD.

**Absorption**

Readily absorbed into uterine epithelium; systemic progesterone absorption is low and not considered to be clinically significant. Progesterone IUDs release progesterone continuously into the uterus at an average rate of 65 mcg per day by membrane controlled diffusion from the reservoir. This membrane barrier allows delivery of progesterone but prevents diffusion of silicone fluid and barium sulfate from the reservoir.

**Distribution**

Local, uterine.

**Biotransformation**

Rapid metabolism by endometrium.

**Half-life**

Several minutes.

**Onset of action**

Local contraceptive action begins immediately after insertion.

**Duration of action**

The manufacturer recommends progesterone IUD replacement within 12 months. Local contraceptive action terminates quickly on removal.

## Precautions to Consider

**Carcinogenicity/Tumorigenicity/Mutagenicity**

Studies have not been done in either animals or humans.

**Pregnancy/Reproduction**

Fertility—In most women, fertility resumes on removal of the IUD. Up to 76% of women desiring pregnancy conceive successfully within 12 months after IUD removal, and 49% of women conceive within the first 3 months.

Monogamous women with monogamous partners have little risk of primary tubal infertility attributable to progesterone IUDs unless there are other risk factors, such as endometriosis or past history of surgery on the female reproductive system. IUDs increase the risk of tubal infertility caused by obstruction in or damage to the fallopian tubes, which are problems associated with pelvic inflammatory disease (PID) or an infection in the uterus or fallopian tubes. This risk from the insertion procedure is highest within the first few months after IUD insertion.

Pregnancy—Use of a progesterone IUD is not recommended during pregnancy although there is no clear clinical evidence of adverse effects for infants conceived with an IUD *in situ*. Long-term effects on the offspring if conceived with a progesterone IUD present are not known. A congenital anomaly, bilateral inguinal hernia, has occurred, but causal relationship was not established.

An IUD *in utero* during pregnancy has resulted in maternal sepsis (usually, but not exclusively, in the second trimester, secondary to a septic abortion or chorioamnionitis) and, rarely, death. If pregnancy occurs with an IUD *in situ*, risk-benefit of leaving the IUD *in situ* versus IUD removal must be carefully considered. If an IUD remains *in utero*, possible complications include a 50% risk of spontaneous abortion and an increased risk of premature rupture of membranes, labor, and delivery.

If a pregnancy occurs with a progesterone IUD in place, the IUD should be removed if the string is visible and the removal is easy. However, manipulation of the IUD may stimulate spontaneous abortion. If the string is not visible, removal of the IUD may be attempted under ultrasound guidance, and/or the termination of the pregnancy should be considered.

When a pregnancy occurs with a progesterone IUD *in situ*, the possibility of an ectopic pregnancy should be considered as the IUD protects against intrauterine pregnancy more than it protects against extrauterine pregnancy. Studies indicate that about 1 ectopic pregnancy per 200 users per year occurs with a progesterone IUD *in situ*, a rate similar to that of noncontracepting sexually active women but approximately 6 times higher than that of women using nonmedicated IUDs. Clinical trials also show that the risk of ectopic pregnancy occurring in nulliparous women is twice that of parous women, 1 ectopic pregnancy of 3.6 pregnancies versus 1 ectopic pregnancy in 6.2 pregnancies, respectively.

Diagnosis of ectopic pregnancy may be difficult because early symptoms (enlarged and tender breasts, dizziness, faintness, nausea, unusual tiredness or weakness, lower abdominal pain, cramping or tenderness [possibly severe], vaginal bleeding [possibly heavy and/or unexpected], or absent or delayed menstrual cycle) are nonspecific and variable. Also, 83% of patients continue to have menses, and 53% do not suspect pregnancy.

Delivery—If an intrauterine pregnancy continues with an IUD *in situ*, the risk for premature delivery is increased along with the usual complications of premature infants.

Postpartum—It is recommended that postpartum IUD insertion be performed 8 weeks or more after delivery (interval insertion) or after complete involution of the uterus has occurred, although individual needs and desires should be taken into consideration by the physician. The risk of an IUD expulsion or uterine perforation caused by an IUD is lower for interval insertions than for postplacental insertions (insertions performed within 10 minutes after delivery). Immediate postpartum insertions (insertions performed within 48 hours after delivery) or immediate postabortion insertions may involve a risk of uterine perforation by the IUD similar to that for interval insertions, but the expulsion rate is higher. Higher expulsion rates in postpartum women may be due to the difficulty in placing the IUD sufficiently high in the fundus.

**Breast-feeding**
Problems in humans have not been documented. IUDs are recommended by the World Health Organization (WHO) for use as a contraceptive method because IUDs do not interfere with lactation.

**Adolescents**
Sexually active adolescents may be better served with a contraceptive method that also protects against sexually transmitted diseases (STDs). In general, young age and nulliparity in women appear to be associated with a higher expulsion rate, possibly due to a more reactive myometrium and irregular and heavy menses.

**Drug interactions and/or related problems**
The following drug interactions and/or related problems have been selected on the basis of their potential clinical significance (possible mechanism in parentheses where appropriate)—not necessarily inclusive (» = major clinical significance):

Note: Combinations containing the following medication, depending on the amount present, may also interact with this device.

Anticoagulants
(use of anticoagulants may initially potentiate the risk of abnormal uterine bleeding around the time of the progesterone IUD insertion; risk lessens with use but spotting may persist)

**Laboratory value alterations**
The following have been selected on the basis of their potential clinical significance (possible effect in parentheses where appropriate)—not necessarily inclusive (» = major clinical significance):

With physiology/laboratory test values
Glucose, plasma
(glucose measurements induced by glucose tolerance tests were slightly elevated at 3 hours according to studies in women using progesterone IUDs at 6 and 12 months; fasting and 0.5 hour glucose measurements were unchanged)

Insulin concentration, serum
(measurements induced by glucose tolerance tests in women using progesterone IUDs for 12 months have shown that insulin concentrations taken at fasting, 0.5 hour, and 3 hours increased from 10.3, 69, and 40.5 microunits/mL to 18.1, 118.4, and 68.5 microunits/mL, respectively; insulin concentrations at 1 and 2 hours were not significantly changed)

Triglyceride, plasma, fasting
(although no change was shown at 6 months, a study showed that triglyceride concentrations decreased at 12 months from 76.3 to 61.8 mg/dL for women using progesterone IUDs for 12 months)

**Medical considerations/Contraindications**
The medical considerations/contraindications included have been selected on the basis of their potential clinical significance (reasons given in parentheses where appropriate)—not necessarily inclusive (» = major clinical significance).

*Except under special circumstances, this device should not be used when the following medical problems exist:*

» Acquired immunodeficiency syndrome (AIDS) or
» Autoimmune diseases or
» Malignancy treated with antineoplastic agents and/or radiation or
» Malignancy, uterine or cervical, known or suspected or
» Any other condition associated with or resulting in decreased immunity and/or increased susceptibility to infection
(possible increased risk of infection with an IUD when a patient lacks an intact immune system)

» Bleeding, genital, of unknown etiology
(insertion of a progesterone IUD may initially exacerbate uterine bleeding, then, with continued use, decrease uterine bleeding; this could mask other serious underlying conditions and delay the diagnosis of the condition)

» Ectopic pregnancy, history of
(may increase risk of ectopic pregnancy with contraceptive failure, especially in nulliparous women)

» Infection or inflammation in female reproductive tract, including
Abortion, recent septic
Cervicitis
Endometritis
Genital actinomyces-like infection
PID, acute or history of
Sexually transmitted diseases during last 12 months
Vaginitis, excluding candidiasis but including bacterial vaginosis, until controlled
(use of an IUD, when any of the above conditions is present, may predispose the patient to upper genital tract infections that may range in severity from mild to life-threatening; risk is highest within the first 30 days after IUD insertion)
(women with a history of PID may be at increased risk of developing PID; nulliparous women may be at greater risk than parous women)
(significant risk of infection progressing to PID may be related to acquisition of or exposure to PID-associated sexually transmitted diseases)

» Surgery involving the uterus or fallopian tubes
(women currently using an IUD may have an increased risk of surgical complications; also, in cases of contraception failure, women having had surgery involving the uterus or fallopian tubes may have additional risk for developing an ectopic pregnancy)

» Uterine abnormalities or cavity distortion
(possibility of decreased contraceptive effectiveness; increased risk of IUD expulsion or IUD perforation of the uterus)

*Risk-benefit should be considered when the following medical problems exist:*

Bradycardia, neurovascular, history of or
Syncope, neurovascular, history of
(short-term syncope or bradycardia may occur with IUD insertion; increased risk if these conditions are present)

Cervical stenosis
(may prevent ease of insertion of IUD; excessive force to overcome this resistance is not advised)

» Coagulopathy
(use of a progesterone IUD when increased vascularity and permeability and decreased hemostatic response exists may increase risk of of an IUD expulsion)

Diabetes, insulin-dependent
(IUDs may be a good choice for diabetics; however, complications from infection, if infection occurs, are potentially more likely)

Heart defect, valvular or congenital
(insertion of an IUD may represent a potential source of septic emboli, since these patients are prone to develop subacute bacterial endocarditis)

**Patient monitoring**
The following may be especially important in patient monitoring (other tests may be warranted in some patients, depending on condition; » = major clinical significance):

Papanicolaou (Pap) test
(recommended annually; examination for actinomycosis-like organisms and, if appropriate, gonococcal and chlamydial tests should be performed)

» Physical examination
recommended once during the first 3 months and at 12 months after insertion for removal; special attention should be given to reports of delayed menses and/or pelvic pain because of the possibility of ectopic pregnancies with failed IUD contraception

## Side/Adverse Effects

Note: Cervical laceration, cervical or uterine perforations, and/or abdominal displacement of the IUD may progress to peritonitis, sepsis, pelvic inflammatory disease (PID), abdominal adhesions, intestinal penetration, intestinal obstruction, cystic masses in the pelvis, and local inflammatory reaction with abscess formation, including tuboovarian abscess. Certain of these adverse effects of IUDs, although very rare, can lead to a loss of fertility, require partial or total removal of reproductive organs, and, in extremely rare circumstances, cause death. An IUD must be surgically removed as soon as feasible after IUD displacement has been diagnosed.

Because many of the side effects listed below present with uterine bleeding and pain, these symptoms should always be evaluated even though they may not signify a serious problem. Persistent or recurring abnormal uterine bleeding and/or abdominal pain may lessen with continued progesterone IUD use. Other problems such as cervical or uterine perforation, IUD displacement, ectopic pregnancy, PID, and IUD embedment should be ruled out.

The following side/adverse effects have been selected on the basis of their potential clinical significance (possible signs and symptoms in parentheses where appropriate)—not necessarily inclusive:

**Those indicating need for medical attention**
Incidence more frequent
*Abdominal pain or cramping on insertion, continuing; intermenstrual spotting or uterine bleeding* (uterine bleeding between menstrual periods); *uterine bleeding on insertion, continuing*

Note: *Abdominal pain* or *uterine bleeding* should be investigated if it continues beyond several days after IUD insertion. *Intermenstrual spotting* can be expected for up to 6 months after insertion and *intermenstrual uterine bleeding* may stop within 3 months. The amount of menstrual blood loss usually is less than preinsertion levels.

Incidence rare
*Cervical perforation or laceration; embedment of IUD or perforation of the uterus* (severe abdominal pain or cramping; unexpected, heavy vaginal bleeding, sharp pain on insertion); *fragmentation of device; neurovascular episodes* (dizziness; faintness)—at time of insertion; *PID* (dull or aching abdominal pain, continuing; fever; odorous vaginal discharge; unusual tiredness or weakness; unusual uterine bleeding)— 2 to 3.1%

Note: Increased risk of *PID* occurs within the first 3 months of IUD insertion; ectopic pregnancy should be ruled out before treatment of PID because of similar presenting symptoms. Also, PID and actinomycosis-like infection may be asymptomatic.

## Patient Consultation

As an aid to patient consultation, refer to *Advice for the Patient, Progesterone Intrauterine Device (IUD)*.

In providing consultation, consider emphasizing the following selected information (» = major clinical significance):

**Before using this device**
Note: In the U.S., the health care professional is required by U.S. federal regulation to provide a patient information brochure to the patient regarding the use of IUDs for contraception, discussing it and other methods of contraception.
» Conditions affecting use, especially:
Pregnancy—IUD use is not recommended for women during pregnancy, those planning to become pregnant shortly, or women who have had an ectopic pregnancy. If contraception fails with a progesterone IUD, complications to the mother or infant are possible whether the pregnancy continues with the IUD *in situ* or the device is removed; also, the risk of uterine perforation and expulsion of the IUD may be increased when an IUD is inserted before 8 weeks postpartum
Use in adolescents—Sexually active adolescents may be better served with a contraceptive method that also protects against sexually transmitted diseases (STDs); IUD use in adolescents of young age and nulliparous women appears to be associated with a higher expulsion rate
Other medical problems, especially acquired immunodeficiency syndrome (AIDS), autoimmune diseases, immunosuppressive therapy, malignancy of the cervix or uterus, or any other conditions of decreased immunity or increased risk of infection; coagulopathy; genital bleeding of unknown etiology; history of ectopic pregnancy; infection or inflammation in female reproductive tract; surgery involving the uterus or fallopian tubes; or uterine abnormalities or cavity distortion

**Proper use of this device**
» Reading a copy of the patient information brochure provided by the health care professional helps explain possible side effects, risks, and warning signs of trouble with the IUD
Spermicides are not needed with a properly placed IUD
» Checking for changes in the IUD thread length after the monthly menses, if not more often, as instructed by physician
» Proper dosing, including IUD removal or replacement times

**Precautions while using this device**
» Visiting physician regularly to check progress, especially within the first 3 months, preferably the first month, and at 12 months for removal
» Alerting medical personnel before having diagnostic or therapeutic procedures such as surgery involving the uterus or fallopian tubes
» Notifying physician immediately if a partial or complete expulsion is suspected; using another form of nonhormonal contraception until evaluated by a physician; patient should not try to remove the IUD or re-insert it

» Reporting missed or scanty menses to physician immediately and using other nonhormonal contraceptive methods
» Reporting symptoms of possible pregnancy, including ectopic pregnancy, to physician in the rare case when IUD contraceptive effects fail
» Notifying physician and using other nonhormonal contraceptive methods if any of the following occur:
—Abnormal vaginal bleeding
—Exposure to sexually transmitted diseases
—Feeling the tip of the IUD at the cervix or pain during sexual intercourse
—Change in length of IUD threads or disappearance of IUD threads on periodic observation after menses
—Lifestyle change from a mutually monogamous relationship
—Pelvic/lower abdominal pain or cramping, unusual or severe, possibly with fever
—Vaginal discharge or signs of genital lesions or sores
Progesterone IUDs should not interfere with the proper use of other vaginal products such as tampons or condoms

**Side/adverse effects**
Signs of potential side effects, especially abdominal pain or cramping on insertion (continuing), intermenstrual spotting or uterine bleeding, uterine bleeding on insertion (continuing), cervical perforation or laceration, embedment of IUD, fragmentation of device, perforation of the uterus, neurovascular episodes on insertion, pelvic inflammatory disease (PID)

## General Dosing Information

In the U.S., the health care professional is required by U.S. Federal Regulations (21 CFR 310.502) to give the patient a copy of the Patient Information for an Informed Decision to ensure complete understanding of the risks and benefits, safety, and efficacy of the progesterone IUD.

It is generally believed that perforations occur at the time of insertion, although they may not be detected until later. Adequate training of those health care professionals inserting the device may help prevent cervical or uterine perforation. A number of supervised insertions may be necessary before a solo attempt. The degree of training needed depends on the health care professional's skill and experience with IUD aseptic insertion techniques and uterus manipulation.

The manufacturer's product information should be consulted for specific directions.

The IUD may be inserted at any time during the menstrual cycle. Many physicians prefer insertion at the end of or within 2 days after a menstrual period to reduce the possibility of inserting an IUD in the presence of an undiagnosed pregnancy. However, the optimal time for insertion appears to be the periovulatory period. Caution should be used to avoid inserting a second IUD, as patients may forget about a previously inserted IUD or may assume it to be expelled.

Using aseptic technique and removing the IUD from the sterile packaging no more than 5 minutes before the insertion procedure are recommended. Prophylactic treatment with antibiotics theoretically may reduce the risk of infection, which is 6 times higher within the first 20 days after insertion. Regimens include doxycycline 200 mg orally one hour before insertion, or erythromycin 500 mg orally one hour before insertion and 500 mg orally six hours after insertion. This may be of limited benefit and unnecessary for women at low risk of sexually transmitted disease (STDs).

It is recommended that an IUD be removed for the following medical reasons: pelvic infection, genital actinomycosis, dyspareunia, pregnancy (when able to remove the IUD), endometrial or cervical malignancy, uterine or cervical perforation, or partial expulsion.

If the retrieval threads cannot be seen, they may have retracted into the uterus or have been broken, or the IUD may have been expelled. Pregnancy, both uterine and ectopic, should be considered before attempting to locate the IUD. Although ultrasound is the preferred method of locating a malpositioned IUD, high- or intermediate-strength magnetic resonance imaging (MRI), uterine probe, or x-rays may also be used.

Removing an intraperitoneal progesterone IUD as soon as medically feasible after the diagnosis is recommended because of the possibility of abdominal adhesion formation, intestinal penetration, and local inflammatory reaction with abscess formation and erosion of adjacent viscera, maternal sepsis, or, rarely, death.

The manufacturer's information should be consulted for the recommended removal procedure. If an IUD is difficult to remove, the procedure may need to be done in a hospital or operating room. Another type of contraception should begin immediately after IUD removal if contraception is desired.

## Progesterone Intrauterine Device (IUD)

### For treatment of adverse effects
Recommended treatment consists of the following:
- For pain—Treating with mild analgesics for several hours after IUD insertion.
- For pelvic inflammatory disease (PID)—Removing the progesterone IUD and treating the patient with appropriate broad-spectrum antibiotics; the patient's partner may require treatment with broad-spectrum antibiotics as well.

Note: HIV-infected women with PID who are immunocompromised may be at increased risk of a complicated clinical course and should be hospitalized for intravenous therapy.

## Intrauterine Dosage Form

### PROGESTERONE INTRAUTERINE CONTRACEPTIVE SYSTEM USP

#### Usual adult and adolescent dose
Contraceptive—
Intrauterine, one device; the maximum duration of use is 12 months.

#### Strength(s) usually available
U.S.—
38 mg progesterone (Rx) [*Progestasert*].

Canada—
Not commercially available.

#### Packaging and storage
Store below 40 °C (104 °F), preferably between 15 and 30 °C (59 and 86 °F), unless otherwise specified by manufacturer. Preserve in sealed, single-unit containers.

#### Note
Provide patient with patient package insert (PPI).

### Selected Bibliography
Farley TM, Rosenberg MJ, Rowe PJ, et al. Intrauterine devices and pelvic inflammatory disease: an international perspective. Lancet 1992 Mar 28; 339: 785-8.
Liskin L, Fox G. IUDs: an appropriate contraceptive for many women. Popul Rep B; Intrauterine Devices, (4), Washington, DC, 1982.
Trussell J, Hatcher RA, Cates W Jr, et al. Contraceptive failure in the United States: an update. Stud Fam Plann 1990; 21(1): 51-4.

Developed: 12/04/95

---

# PROGESTINS   Systemic

This monograph includes information on the following: 1) Hydroxyprogesterone†; 2) Levonorgestrel; 3) Medrogestone*; 4) Medroxyprogesterone; 5) Megestrol; 6) Norethindrone; 7) Norgestrel†; 8) Progesterone

Note: For information pertaining to the use of estrogens and progestins oral contraceptives, see *Estrogens and Progestins Oral Contraceptives (Systemic)* and for use of progesterone intrauterine device, see *Progesterone Intrauterine Device (IUD)*.

INN:
  Hydroxyprogesterone caproate—Hydroxyprogesterone
  Medroxyprogesterone acetate—Medroxyprogesterone
  Megestrol acetate—Megestrol
  Norethindrone—Norethisterone

BAN:
  Hydroxyprogesterone caproate—Hydroxyprogesterone
  Medroxyprogesterone acetate—Medroxyprogesterone
  Megestrol acetate—Megestrol
  Norethindrone—Norethisterone

VA CLASSIFICATION (Primary/Secondary):
  Hydroxyprogesterone—HS103
  Levonorgestrel—HS103/HS104
  Medrogestone—HS103
  Medroxyprogesterone—HS103/AN500; HS104
  Megestrol—HS103/AN500
  Norethindrone—HS103/HS104
  Norgestrel—HS103/HS104
  Progesterone—HS103

Commonly used brand name(s): *Alti-MPA*[4]; *Amen*[4]; *Apo-Megestrol*[5]; *Aygestin*[6]; *Colprone*[3]; *Crinone*[8]; *Curretab*[4]; *Cycrin*[4]; *Depo-Provera*[4]; *Depo-Provera Contraceptive Injection*[4]; *Gen-Medroxy*[4]; *Gesterol 50*[8]; *Gesterol LA 250*[1]; *Hy/Gestrone*[1]; *Hylutin*[1]; *Megace*[5]; *Megace OS*[5]; *Micronor*[6]; *NORPLANT System*[2]; *Nor-QD*[6]; *Norlutate*[6]; *Novo-Medrone*[4]; *Ovrette*[7]; *PMS-Progesterone*[8]; *Pro-Span*[1]; *Prodrox*[1]; *Prometrium*[8]; *Provera*[4]; *Provera Pak*[4].

Another commonly used name for norethindrone is norethisterone.

Note: For a listing of dosage forms and brand names by country availability, see *Dosage Forms* section(s).

*Not commercially available in U.S.
†Not commercially available in Canada.

## Category
Progestational agent—Hydroxyprogesterone; Medrogestone; Medroxyprogesterone (oral); Norethindrone; Norgestrel; Progesterone.
Antianoretic—Megestrol.
Anticachectic—Megestrol.
Antineoplastic—Medroxyprogesterone (parenteral); Megestrol.
Contraceptive (systemic)—Levonorgestrel; Medroxyprogesterone (parenteral); Norethindrone (base); Norgestrel.
Diagnostic aid (estrogen production)—Hydroxyprogesterone; Medroxyprogesterone (oral); Progesterone (parenteral).
Infertility therapy adjunct—Progesterone (vaginal).
Ovarian hormone therapy agent adjunct—Medroxyprogesterone (oral); Progesterone (oral).

## Indications
Note: Bracketed information in the *Indications* section refers to uses that are not included in U.S. product labeling.

### Accepted
Amenorrhea, secondary (treatment)
Dysfunctional uterine bleeding (treatment) or
Menses, induction of (treatment)—Hydroxyprogesterone, medrogestone, oral medroxyprogesterone, norethindrone acetate, and parenteral progesterone are indicated in the treatment of menstrual disorders, including secondary amenorrhea and dysfunctional uterine bleeding (DUB) caused by hormonal imbalance in the absence of organic pathology. Progesterone oral capsules[1] and progesterone vaginal gel are indicated in the treatment of secondary amenorrhea. The 8% strength of vaginal gel is used only if the patient fails to respond to treatment with the 4% progesterone vaginal gel. Hydroxyprogesterone is also indicated for the production of a secretory endometrium and desquamation. The uterus must be sufficiently primed with endogenous or exogenous estrogen for the progestins to produce a secretory-like endometrium and endometrial shedding after progestin use ends. Withdrawal bleeding usually occurs 3 to 7 days after discontinuation of the progestin for women with an intact uterus.

Anorexia (treatment)
Cachexia (treatment) or
Weight loss, significant (treatment)—Megestrol suspension is indicated in the treatment of anorexia, cachexia, unexplained significant weight loss (loss of 10% or more of base-line body weight) associated with acquired immunodeficiency syndrome (AIDS). [Megestrol tablets are indicated in the treatment of anorexia, cachexia, and unexplained significant weight loss associated with cancer].

Assisted reproductive technologies, in females or
[Corpus luteum insufficiency (treatment)][1]—Progesterone vaginal gel is indicated to replace the progesterone hormone in female patients whose infertility is due to partial or complete ovarian failure. Progesterone vaginal gel is indicated to supplement endogenous progesterone for luteal phase progesterone deficiency. Extemporaneously prepared [progesterone suppositories][1] have also been used for these indications.

Carcinoma, breast (treatment)—Megestrol and [oral and parenteral medroxyprogesterone] are indicated in the treatment of breast carcinoma; [medroxyprogesterone] is indicated for use in postmenopausal women only. It is used as adjunctive or palliative therapy in the treatment of advanced (inoperable, recurrent, or metastatic) hormonally dependent carcinoma.

Carcinoma, endometrial (treatment)—[Oral] or parenteral medroxyprogesterone, and megestrol are indicated for the treatment of endometrial carcinoma. It is used as adjunctive and/or palliative therapy in the treatment of advanced (recurrent or metastatic) hormonally dependent carcinoma.

Carcinoma, prostate (treatment)—[Megestrol] is indicated in the treatment of hormonally dependent and advanced prostate carcinoma as palliative therapy.

Carcinoma, renal (treatment)—Parenteral medroxyprogesterone is also indicated in the treatment of metastatic renal carcinomaas adjunctive and/or palliative therapy when used in the treatment of advanced (recurrent or metastatic) hormonally dependent carcinoma.

Endometriosis (treatment)—Norethindrone acetate, [parenteral medroxyprogesterone], and [oral medroxyprogesterone][1] are indicated in the treatment of endometriosis.

Estrogen production, endogenous (diagnosis)—Hydroxyprogesterone, [oral medroxyprogesterone], and [parenteral progesterone] are indicated as a test for endogenous estrogen production and can be used to determine whether low levels of estrogen are present if withdrawal bleeding does not occur after a progestin challenge in menopausal women before estrogen-progestin ovarian hormone therapy is considered. However, determination that serum gonadotropins are elevated is the standard way to confirm menopause.

[Hyperplasia, endometrial (treatment)][1] or
Hyperplasia, endometrial, estrogen-induced (prophylaxis)—Megestrol and oral medroxyprogesterone have been used to treat endometrial hyperplasia without atypia, which is usually not a precursor of carcinoma. Complex atypical hyperplasia (previously called adenomatous hyperplasia) is usually best treated surgically, but in some high risk patients or when future pregnancy is desired, high continuous doses of progestins have been used.

For prevention, [oral medroxyprogesterone], [norethindrone][1], medrogestone, and [oral progesterone] can be used to oppose the effects of estrogen on the endometrium in menopausal women who take estrogens for ovarian hormone therapy (OHT), also called hormone replacement therapy (HRT) and estrogen replacement therapy (ERT). All menopausal patients receiving progestins do not have recognized endometrial shedding; there is frequently amenorrhea after several months of treatment with estrogen-progestin regimens. The optimal or recommended length for estrogen replacement after menopause has not been established. Studies have shown that administration of a progestin for a minimum of 10 to 14 days of an estrogen cycle in women with an intact uterus is required for major reduction of endometrial hyperplasia and endometrial carcinoma compared with an estrogen-only cycle. Other dosing regimens for estrogens and progestins, including low continuous daily dosing, are also used. Progestins without estrogens may be used for debilitating menopausal symptoms in patients who have breast cancer and are candidates for progestin therapy but cannot take estrogens.

Pregnancy, prevention of—Levonorgestrel, parenteral medroxyprogesterone, norethindrone (base), and norgestrel are indicated for the prevention of pregnancy. Progestin-only oral contraceptives are also called minipills and progestin-only oral pills (POPs).

The following table presents the results of studies examining contraceptive failure rates calculated using the life-table method. The first column lists the contraceptive method used. The second column indicates the percentage of women experiencing an accidental pregnancy in the first year of use of a contraceptive method while using the method perfectly under clinical conditions. The range of failure rates in the clinical trials may be explained by interstudy variations in study design or patient population characteristics, such as motivation, fecundity, or socioeconomic factors (including education). The third column indicates contraceptive failure rates in the first year of contraceptive use under clinical conditions for typical couples who start using a method (not necessarily for the first time). Failure rates among adolescents may be higher due to poorer compliance than in other age groups.

| Method used | Failure rate range (over 12 months) in clinical studies (%) | Typical first year failure rate (%) |
|---|---|---|
| None | 78–94 | 85 |
| Spermicides* | 0.3–37 | 21 |
| Periodic abstinence† | 13–35 | 20 |
| Withdrawal | 7–22 | 19 |
| Cervical cap with spermicide | 6–27 | 18 |
| Diaphragm with spermicide | 2–23 | 18 |
| Condom without spermicide | 2–14 | 12 |
| IUD | | |
| Progesterone-releasing | 1.9–2 | 2 |
| Copper-T 200 | 3–3.6 | |
| Copper-T 200Ag‡ | 0–1.2 | |
| Copper-T 220C§ | 0.9–1.8 | |
| Copper-T 380A | 0.5–0.8 | 0.8 |
| Copper-T 380S | 0.9 | |

| Method used | Failure rate range (over 12 months) in clinical studies (%) | Typical first year failure rate (%) |
|---|---|---|
| Oral contraceptive | | 3 |
| Estrogen and progestin | 0–6 | |
| Progestin only | 1–10 | 0.5 |
| Progestin injection | | |
| Medroxyprogesterone (90-day) | 0–0.3 | 0.3 |
| Levonorgestrel (subdermal) | | |
| Six implants | 0–0.09 | 0.09 |
| Two rods | 0–0.2 | 0.3 |
| Sterilization | | |
| Female# | 0–8 | 0.4 |
| Male | 0–0.5 | 0.15 |

*Spermicides studied include creams, foams, gels, jellies, and suppositories.

†Methods studied include calendar, ovulation method, symptothermal (cervical mucus method supplemented by basal body temperature post-ovulation).

‡Life table method rate is unavailable for Copper-T 200Ag and the Pearl method rate at 12 months was reported; these methods at 12 months are considered comparable.

§Copper-T 220C is manufactured with copper sleeves instead of copper wire; often used as a control in clinical studies.

#Methods studied include culdotomy laparoscopy, minilaparotomy, electrocoagulation, laparotomy, tubal diathermy and/or use of rings or clips.

[Polycystic ovary syndrome (treatment)][1]—Medroxyprogesterone is used in the treatment of endometrial hyperplasia and its consequences in syndromes, such as polycystic ovary syndrome.

[Puberty, precocious (treatment)][1]—Parenteral medroxyprogesterone is accepted therapy for use in the treatment of precocious puberty but has been replaced by other treatment modalities.

**Unaccepted**

There is no evidence that progesterone is effective in the treatment of premenstrual syndrome.

Progestins are no longer recommended for use as pregnancy tests because of possible teratogenic effects with synthetic progestins; also, other tests available are quicker and easier to perform.

With the exception of progesterone in patients who are progesterone deficient, progestins have no proven value in the treatment of threatened abortion and are no longer recommended for such use.

Unlike oral medroxyprogesterone, parenteral medroxyprogesterone is not recommended by the manufacturer for treatment of secondary amenorrhea or dysfunctional uterine bleeding.

Megestrol is not recommended for prophylactic use to avoid weight loss.

[1]Not included in Canadian product labeling.

## Pharmacology/Pharmacokinetics

See *Table 1*, page 2412.

**Physicochemical characteristics**
Molecular weight—
  Hydroxyprogesterone caproate: 428.62.
  Levonorgestrel: 312.45.
  Medrogestone: 340.51.
  Medroxyprogesterone acetate: 386.53.
  Megestrol acetate: 384.52.
  Norethindrone: 298.43.
  Norethindrone acetate: 340.47.
  Norgestrel: 312.45.
  Progesterone: 314.47.

**Mechanism of action/Effect**

Progestins enter target cells by passive diffusion and bind to cytosolic (soluble) receptors that are loosely bound in the nucleus. The steroid receptor complex initiates transcription, resulting in an increase in protein synthesis.

Progestins are capable of affecting serum concentrations of other hormones, particularly estrogen. Estrogenic effects are modified by the progestins, either by reducing the availability or stability of the hormone receptor complex or by turning off specific hormone-responsive genes by direct interaction with the progestin receptor in the nucleus. In addition, estrogen priming is necessary to increase progestin effects by upregulating the number of progestin receptors and/or increasing progesterone production, causing a negative feedback mechanism that inhibits estrogen receptors.

Depending on the progestin and its dose, progestin may demonstrate varying degrees of progestational effects. Also, other hormonal effects, such as estrogenic-, anabolic-, androgenic-, or glucocorticoid-inducing or suppressing effects are demonstrated to different degrees and depend on the progestin type and dose. For example, an androgenic effect may be expressed by 19-nor derivatives of testosterone but not by other progestins. The androgenic effects of norethindrone are minor to moderate; norethindrone acetate is twice as potent as norethindrone. Norgestrel and levonorgestrel have androgenic effects if unopposed by estrogens. Rare cases of adrenal suppression have been reported in patients using megestrol. While the progestational effects dominate, the other effects can become important when choosing the appropriate progestin or monitoring side effects. Progestins are not used exclusively for other than their progestational effects, as the other effects are highly variable and unreliable.

Progestational agents—Progestins produce significant antiproliferative changes in the endometrium. As progestin levels fall after estrogen priming in the second half of the menstrual cycle, uterine bleeding may occur. Depending on the estrogen-progestin regimen, the progestin dose may be sufficient to cause amenorrhea.

Antianoretic or anticachectic—The mechanism that produces weight gain has not been fully elucidated; however, megestrol appears to have appetite-stimulant and metabolic effects that result in weight gain while causing minimal fluid retention. The underlying cause of wasting should be treated concurrently to optimize management of catabolism.

Antineoplastic—The mechanism has not been fully elucidated; however, several mechanisms may be involved that are dependent on the type and dose of progestin. In certain doses, progestins can produce a diminished response to endogenous hormones in tumor cells by decreasing the number of steroid hormone receptors (estrogen, progesterone, androgen, and glucocorticoid); the degree of variation of response is tissue- and progestin-dependent. The suppression of the growth of hormone-sensitive cells may be due to a direct cytotoxic effect or antiproliferative effects on cell cycle growth and an increased terminal cell differentiation. At higher doses, some progestins compete for the glucocorticoid receptor, resulting in suppressed adrenal production of estradiol and androstenedione. Still-higher progestin doses are able to completely suppress the hypothalamic-pituitary-adrenal axis (HPA axis), an effect that is important in the treatment of estrogen- or testosterone-sensitive tumors.

Contraceptive (systemic)—Inhibition of the secretion of gonadotropins from the anterior pituitary prevents ovulation and follicular maturation and is one of the contraceptive actions of levonorgestrel, parenteral medroxyprogesterone, norethindrone, and norgestrel. These effects do not occur with low-dose oral medroxyprogesterone, which is not used for contraception. In some patients using low-dose progestin-only contraceptives, particularly norethindrone (base) and levonorgestrel subdermal implants, ovulation is not suppressed consistently from cycle to cycle. The contraceptive effect of the progestin is achieved through other mechanisms that result in interference with fertilization and implantation in the luteal cycle, such as thickening of the cervical mucus and changes in the endometrium. In males, medroxyprogesterone suppresses the Leydig cell function.

### Other actions/effects

Progestins increase body temperature, stimulate the respiratory center, and, in some cases, may provide pain relief. The mechanism by which progesterone and medroxyprogesterone mediate thermogenic effects is not clear. It has been suggested that progesterone influences neurotransmitters and neuropeptides in the brain, notably endogenous opioids, interleukin-1, and serotonin, that raise body temperature. Also, medroxyprogesterone may reduce hypercapnia in certain patients by stimulating the respiratory center. Pain relief from high-dose progestins may be due in part to an anti-inflammatory action.

Locally the progestins relax the uterine smooth muscle, sustain pregnancy, decrease the immune response, and, acting with estrogen, stimulate breast tissue growth.

Some progestins cause sodium and water retention. Progesterone doses of 50 to 100 mg may produce a moderate catabolic effect and transient increase in sodium chloride excretion. In addition, use of some progestins may result in dose-related adverse effects on carbohydrate and lipid metabolism.

Progestins influence bone density. When progestins have been used without estrogen, a positive effect has been shown in postmenopausal women and a possible negative effect in premenopausal women; the latter may depend on the degree to which a progestin can reduce ovarian estrogen production, a dose-dependent effect. When progestins have been used sequentially with continuously administered estrogen, a synergistic protective effect on bone density has been shown. Specifically, placebo-controlled studies of postmenopausal women showed that medroxyprogesterone decreased the rate of cortical bone loss but did not protect trabecular areas of the skeleton, such as the spine, equally from bone loss in all studies. A low-dose combination of continuously administered estrogen and sequentially administered progestin therapy showed protective effects against bone loss that were similar to those of higher doses of estrogen therapy alone. This effect may be due to an increase of progestin receptors caused by estrogen, to an antagonistic effect of progestin binding to glucocorticoid receptors, or to a stimulatory effect of progestin acting on progestin receptors within osteoblasts. Additional studies are needed to confirm and fully characterize these results.

Other health benefits of progestational hormone therapy may include less painful menstruation, less menstrual blood loss and anemia, fewer pelvic infections, and lower incidence of uterine cancers.

### Absorption

Progestins—Well absorbed.

Levonorgestrel subdermal implants and parenteral medroxyprogesterone acetate—Well-absorbed during controlled release with wide intra- and intersubject variability. Initial release rate for a set of levonorgestrel subdermal implants is approximately 80 micrograms of levonorgestrel per 24 hours. This rate declines over the first 6 to 18 months to an approximately constant release rate of 30 micrograms of levonorgestrel per 24 hours over the remainder of the 5 years of use.

Progesterone—Micronized progesterone improves surface area contact and absorption compared to nonmicronized progesterone; both types have been used in extemporaneously prepared formulations.

Micronized progesterone, oral—Luteal phase concentrations of progesterone are maintained for approximately 9 to 12 hours after oral administration. Food significantly increases absorption as shown by increases in the area under the plasma concentration–time curve (AUC) and peak concentration, but the time to peak concentration is not affected.

Micronized progesterone, vaginal gel—Since the progesterone is soluble in both the water and oil phases, the vaginal gel (as an oil and water emulsion) provides a prolonged action and an absorption half-life of 25 to 50 hours.

## Precautions to Consider

### Carcinogenicity

The benefit of lowering the incidence of endometrial hyperplasia and endometrial cancer by adding progestin to an estrogen regimen in ovarian hormone therapy to counter estrogen's effect on the uterus is established.

*Medroxyprogesterone*—

Long-term studies in humans using parenteral medroxyprogesterone for contraception have found no increase in the overall risk of ovarian, liver, breast, or cervical cancer and have found a prolonged, protective effect of reducing the risk of endometrial cancer for at least 8 years. The possible protective effect may be lessened with concomitant use of estrogen; however, the lifetime risk for developing endometrial cancer is not increased in women with a uterus who take estrogen plus a progestin for 10 to 20 years. In the short-term, the initial risk of breast cancer with parenteral medroxyprogesterone exposure may be increased in the first 4 years after initial exposure in women under 35 years of age. The risk lessens with duration of use and results in no overall increase of risk for developing breast cancer.

Studies of monkeys administered doses of 3, 30, and 150 mg per kg (mg/kg) of body weight every 90 days for 10 years produced undifferentiated carcinoma of the uterus in a few monkeys dosed at 150 mg/kg. No uterine malignancies were reported in monkeys taking other doses or in the control monkeys; no uterine abnormalities were produced in similar studies of rats after 2 years. The relevance of these findings to humans is not known.

### Tumorigenicity/Mutagenicity

*Hydroxyprogesterone, levonorgestrel, medrogestone, norgestrel, norethindrone, and progesterone*—

Studies have not been done.

*Medroxyprogesterone*—

Studies in humans have not been done.

Mammary nodules, some of which were malignant in the high-dose group, developed in a number of beagles given doses of 3 or 75 mg/kg of medroxyprogesterone every 90 days for 7 years. In studies of monkeys, doses of 3, 30, or 150 mg/kg of medroxyprogesterone given every 90 days for 10 years produced transient mammary nodules in the 3 and 30 mg/kg groups, with none reported in the 150 mg/kg group during the study; hyperplastic nodules had developed in 3 monkeys that had been administered 30 mg/kg of medroxyprogesterone; no breast abnormalities were produced in rats after 2 years. Caution is warranted in applying these results of animal studies of progestins to their use in humans because of the hormonal differences between species. Also, humans and beagles metabolize medroxyprogesterone differently, and beagles are particularly susceptible to this type of breast tumor and develop these tumors spontaneously without progestin use.

There was no mutagenic response in the Ames and micronucleus tests.

*Megestrol—*

Studies in humans have not been done.

Studies of female dogs given megestrol for up to 7 years showed an increased incidence of both benign and malignant tumors; 2-year studies of female rats demonstrated an increased incidence of pituitary tumors. These effects were not found in monkey studies.

**Pregnancy/Reproduction**

Fertility—Progestins cause a decrease in quantity and/or change the quality of cervical mucus and may interfere with sperm function, fertilization, and subsequently, the occurrence of pregnancy. This effect depends on the dose and type of the progestin. High-dose or long-term use of progestins may cause a delayed return to fertility.

*Levonorgestrel subdermal implants—*

After removal, 40% of those women wanting to conceive did so by 3 months; 76% conceived within 1 year, percentages are similar to normal pregnancy rates.

*Medroxyprogesterone—*

It has been reported that of the women who discontinued parenteral medroxyprogesterone to become pregnant, 68% conceived within 12 months, 83% conceived within 15 months, and 93% conceived within 18 months after discontinuation (range, 4 to 31 months; median 10 months). The return of fertility is a function of the uptake and metabolism of parenteral medroxyprogesterone; follicular activity has been reported to return 3 to 37 days after parenteral medroxyprogesterone is nondetectable in serum, whereas, luteal function is delayed by 14 to 102 days.

Animal studies with medroxyprogesterone have reported no impairment of fertility in first- or second-generation studies.

*Megestrol—*

Studies in humans have not been done.

Studies of rats given megestrol in doses of 0.05 to 12.5 mg per kg of body weight (mg/kg), which are lower than the human dose of 13.3 mg/kg, resulted in impaired reproductive capability of male offspring produced from megestrol-treated females; similar results were found in studies of dogs.

*Progesterone—*

Progesterone has been used successfully with assisted reproductive technologies to support embryo implantation and to maintain pregnancy if needed.

Pregnancy—Progestins, in general, should be withheld during pregnancy. Progestins cross the placenta. Although many studies fail to demonstrate an increase in teratogenicity when progestins are given in the first trimester, the possibility that genital abnormalities may appear in male and female fetuses exposed to progestins during that period has been suggested by some studies. The low number of abnormalities reported include an increased risk of hypospadias in male fetuses exposed to intrauterine progesterone and virilization of the female fetus' external genitalia when exposed to ethisterone and norethindrone. There is some controversy about the reliability of these reports. The significant concentration of endogenous natural progesterone produced during pregnancy is devoid of teratogenic effects.

Ectopic pregnancy is possible with contraception failure because some progestin-only contraceptives reduce ectopic pregnancy risk substantially, but prevent ectopic pregnancy less effectively than intrauterine pregnancy. For progestin-only oral contraceptives, the ectopic pregnancy rate reported is 4.1 per 100 pregnancies. The rate of ectopic pregnancy for a set of levonorgestrel subdermal implants is 1.3 per 1000 woman-years. This is lower than those for women not using any contraceptive method (2.7 to 3 ectopic pregnancies per 1000 woman-years). However, the risk may increase with longer duration of use of levonorgestrel subdermal implants and increased weight of the user; risk does not increase in women of normal weight.

*Hydroxyprogesterone and progesterone—*

Use is generally not recommended during pregnancy, unless prescribed in the treatment of female infertility due to progesterone deficiency. Hydroxyprogesterone and progesterone have been used to prevent habitual or threatened abortion within the first few months of pregnancy. There are no adequate and well-controlled studies in humans to document that such use is effective during the first 4 months of pregnancy in preventing miscarriage; use is generally limited to certain cases of hormonal imbalance. Progesterone has been used successfully with assisted reproductive technologies to support embryo implantation and maintain pregnancy. Progesterone may be used to treat corpus luteum deficiency in early pregnancy. Progesterone replacement or supplementation does not appear to be efficacious when a hormone imbalance does not exist. In addition, the progesterone's effects on the uterus may delay the spontaneous miscarriage of a defective ovum.

FDA Pregnancy Category D.

*Levonorgestrel, norethindrone, and norgestrel—*

Use is not recommended during pregnancy. Virilization of the female fetus has been reported with norethindrone in a few cases, but a causal relationship has not been conclusively proven.

FDA Pregnancy Category X.

*Medroxyprogesterone—*

Use is not recommended in pregnancy. Studies in humans have shown that medroxyprogesterone may decrease intrauterine growth. Polysyndactyly in the offspring of women who had used parenteral medroxyprogesterone during pregnancy was reported in a few case-reports; this effect has not been seen in major studies. Furthermore, there has been no evidence of problems associated with growth and development in children exposed *in utero* to medroxyprogesterone and followed to adolescence.

In studies of pregnant beagles given doses of 1, 10, and 30 mg/kg of body weight per day for 6 months, clitoral hypertrophy appeared in the female pups of the high-dose group; no abnormalities were reported in the male pups. No abnormalities were detected in the treated female pups' offspring. Caution is warranted in transferring this information to humans because beagle dogs metabolize medroxyprogesterone differently than do humans.

Medroxyprogesterone, parenteral—FDA Pregnancy Category X.

Note: An FDA pregnancy category has not been assigned for medroxyprogesterone tablets.

*Megestrol—*

Use is not recommended during pregnancy. Risk-benefit must be carefully considered.

Studies in pregnant rats given high doses of megestrol decreased fetal birth weight, produced fewer live births, and resulted in reversible feminization of some male fetuses.

Megestrol suspension—FDA Pregnancy Category X.

Megestrol tablets—FDA Pregnancy Category D.

**Breast-feeding**

Progestins are distributed into breast milk in variable amounts and, depending on the progestin and dose, may increase or decrease quantity or quality or have no effect on breast milk. The effect on the nursing infant has not been determined for many progestins.

No adverse effects on breast milk's quantity or quality have been seen with progestin-only contraceptives, or specifically, when norethindrone or medroxyprogesterone was used for contraception within 5 days postpartum or after the establishment of lactation. Progestin-only contraceptives are recommended in breast-feeding women when oral contraception is desired. The manufacturers and distributors of levonorgestrel subdermal implants and parenteral medroxyprogesterone for contraception recommend that their initial use for contraception begin at 6 weeks postpartum for exclusively breast-feeding mothers. Additionally, no adverse effects have been reported in a study of nursing infants exposed to parenteral medroxyprogesterone and followed through puberty or in another study of 80 nursing infants exposed to levonorgestrel subdermal implants 6 weeks after delivery and followed for 3 years.

Progestins used in very high doses are not recommended for use by nursing mothers.

**Pediatrics**

No information is available on the relationship of age to the effects of progestins in pediatric patients. Safety and efficacy have not been established. Serious adverse effects have not been reported in small children who ingested large doses of oral contraceptives.

**Adolescents**

Safety and efficacy of progestin-only contraceptives are expected to be the same in postpubertal adolescents as they are in adults. However, special counseling for medication compliance and prevention of sexually transmitted diseases (STDs) is needed. Studies have shown that adolescents tend to have a higher failure rate with the use of any type of contraceptive that requires strict compliance, such as oral progestins for contraception, and its use is not generally recommended in this age group. Although parenteral medroxyprogesterone and levonorgestrel subdermal implants do not require daily compliance, readministration of their doses after 3 months (13 weeks) and after 5 years, respectively, is important. Furthermore, none of the progestin contraceptives protect against STDs, which are significant risk-factors for this age group.

**Geriatrics**
No information is available on the relationship of age to the effects of progestins in geriatric patients.

**Dental**
Increased concentrations of progestins increase the normal oral flora growth rate, leading to an increase in inflammation of the gingival tissues and increased bleeding. A strictly enforced program of teeth cleaning by a professional, combined with plaque control by the patient, will minimize severity.

**Drug interactions and/or related problems**
The following drug interactions and/or related problems have been selected on the basis of their potential clinical significance (possible mechanism in parentheses where appropriate)—not necessarily inclusive (» = major clinical significance):

Note: Combinations containing any of the following medications, depending on the amount present, may also interact with this medication.

» Aminoglutethimide
(may significantly lower the serum concentrations of oral and parenteral medroxyprogesterone by an undetermined mechanism; it has been suggested that aminoglutethimide may decrease the intestinal absorption of oral medroxyprogesterone)

» Hepatic enzyme inducing medications, such as
Carbamazepine or
Phenobarbital or
Phenytoin or
Rifabutin or
Rifampin
(decreased efficacy of some progestins, including levonorgestrel subdermal implants, has been suggested to be caused by enhanced metabolism of the progestins by these drugs)

(phenytoin and rifampin increase the serum concentrations of sex hormone–binding globulin [SHBG]; this significantly decreases the serum concentration of free drug for some progestins, which is a special concern in patients using progestins for contraception)

(drug interaction data are not available for rifabutin, but because its structure is similar to that of rifampin, similar precautions with its use with progestins may be warranted. Megestrol has been shown not to affect the pharmacokinetics of rifabutin; whether rifabutin changes megestrol pharmacokinetics has not been studied)

**Laboratory value alterations**
The following have been selected on the basis of their potential clinical significance (possible effect in parentheses where appropriate)—not necessarily inclusive (» = major clinical significance):

With diagnostic test results
Biopsy
(pathologist should be notified of relevant specimens)

Glucose tolerance test
(varies with progestin and dose, glucose tolerance may be increased or decreased)

Metyrapone
(lower response than normally expected)

With laboratory test values
Apolipoprotein A and
High-density lipoproteins (HDL) and
Total cholesterol and
Triglycerides
(serum concentrations may be increased or decreased and may differ depending on type of progestin, dose, dosing, and duration of therapy. In general, all progestins will lower triglyceride and total cholesterol concentrations. Parenteral medroxyprogesterone, in low doses, produces no significant decrease in HDL cholesterol concentrations; oral doses may blunt an estrogen-induced increase of HDL. In contrast, 19-nor-testosterone–derived progestins significantly lower HDL cholesterol as well as total cholesterol)

Apolipoprotein B and
Low-density lipoproteins (LDL)
(serum concentrations may be increased and may differ depending on type of progestin, dose, dosing, and duration of therapy)
(LDL concentrations increased initially in some studies and then returned to normal or below normal baseline levels when progestins were given for a year. Additionally, serum estrogen concentrations seemed to influence the cyclicality and degree to which LDL concentration increased; progestins affected the values to a lesser extent when estrogen levels were normal)

Clotting factors II, VII, VIII, IX, and X and
Prothrombin
(serum concentrations may be increased although studies have not shown consistent results; no change in clotting factors has been reported with parenteral medroxyprogesterone for contraception)

Gonadotropin and
Sex hormone–binding globulin (SHBG)
(serum concentration may be decreased)

Liver function tests
(values may be increased; if abnormal with parenteral medroxyprogesterone use, liver tests may be repeated 4 to 6 months after its discontinuation)

$T_3$-uptake
(values may be decreased because of increase in thyroid-binding globulin [TBG]; free $T_4$ concentration is unaltered)

$T_4$, total
(unaffected by most progestins but concentrations are slightly decreased with levonorgestrel; free $T_4$ concentration is unaltered)

**Medical considerations/Contraindications**
The medical considerations/contraindications included have been selected on the basis of their potential clinical significance (reasons given in parentheses where appropriate)—not necessarily inclusive (» = major clinical significance).

*Except under special circumstances, these medications should not be used when the following medical problems exist:*

» Allergy to peanuts for oral or parenteral progesterone
» Breast malignancies or tumors, known or suspected
(may worsen conditions in some nonresponsive patients; however, some progestins are used for palliative treatment in select patients)
» Hepatic disease, acute, including benign or malignant liver tumors
(metabolism of 19-nor derivatives of testosterone-type progestins may be impaired; also, progestins may worsen the condition)

Hypersensitivity to progestins
» Pregnancy, known or suspected
(use of synthetic progestins during pregnancy may result in virilization of a female fetus and, in a small number of cases, increase the risk of hypospadias in a male fetus)
(use for pregnancy diagnosis is contraindicated)
» Thrombophlebitis or thromboembolic disease, active
(the large doses of progestins used to treat breast and prostate cancer have been associated with a slight risk of thrombogenic conditions; mechanism is unclear and may be due to underlying condition. Problems have not been associated with low doses used for contraception, including parenteral medroxyprogesterone, progestin-only oral contraceptives, and levonorgestrel subdermal implants)
» Urinary tract bleeding, undiagnosed or
» Uterine or genital bleeding, undiagnosed
(use of a progestin may delay diagnosis by masking underlying conditions, including cancer)

*Risk-benefit should be considered when the following medical problems exist:*

Asthma or
Cardiac insufficiency, significant or
Epilepsy or
Hypertension or
Migraine headaches or
Renal dysfunction, significant
(fluid retention may be caused by some progestins, especially in high doses, and may aggravate these conditions)

CNS disorders, such as depression or convulsions, history of
(progestins, such as levonorgestrel, medroxyprogesterone, or norethindrone, may make these conditions worse. Cases of convulsions have been reported with use of parenteral medroxyprogesterone; however, a clear association has not been established. In one small study of 14 women with uncontrolled seizures, medroxyprogesterone reduced their seizure frequency by 30%. However, use of many medications for seizure control reduce the contraceptive efficacy of many contraceptives)

Diabetes mellitus
(high doses of progestins may alter carbohydrate metabolism by an unknown mechanism, producing a mild decrease in glucose tolerance in some patients. New-onset diabetes mellitus and exacerbation of preexisting diabetes mellitus have been reported in patients taking high or chronic doses of megestrol. Progestin-only oral contraceptives do not usually affect carbohydrate metabolism, but may occasionally affect lipid metabolism. No clinical significance on

fasting blood glucose is seen in nondiabetics receiving low doses of oral progestins for contraception)

(levonorgestrel's effects on carbohydrate metabolism appear to be minimal for nondiabetics but are considered inconclusive for prediabetics and diabetics)

(parenteral medroxyprogesterone may decrease glucose tolerance for some patients by an undetermined mechanism; it has been used with caution for contraception in diabetics)

Hepatic disease or dysfunction, history of
(metabolism of progestins, specifically androgenic progestins, may be impaired and contribute to the hepatic condition)

Hyperlipidemia
(some progestins, specifically androgenic progestins, might increase LDL and lower HDL levels and aggravate problems in controlling hyperlipidemia)

Significant risk factors for low bone mineral content
(the overall effect on bone density for progestins has yet to be established and may depend on type of progestin, dose, and gender and age of patient. A retrospective cross-sectional study has reported that women using parenteral medroxyprogesterone for contraception had bone density measurements lower than the control group of premenopausal women but higher than the control group of postmenopausal women. Specifically, medroxyprogesterone may temporarily increase the loss of trabecular bone and additionally increase the risk of osteoporosis. The greatest bone loss is evident in the early years of use, is usually reversible, and possibly reflects other factors, such as hypoestrogenism, when progestin is used alone. A prospective study has reported that the use of oral medroxyprogesterone alone for treatment of menopausal symptoms showed a protective effect against loss of bone; other studies, particularly those in which a progestin was combined with estrogen, have also shown a protective effect)

» Thromboembolic disorders, including cerebrovascular disease, pulmonary embolism, retinal thrombosis, history of or
Thrombophlebitis, history of
(the large doses of progestins used to treat breast and prostate cancer have been associated with a slight risk of thrombogenic conditions; mechanism is unclear and may be due to the underlying condition. Problems have also occurred with megestrol. Problems have not been associated with low doses used for contraception, including parenteral medroxyprogesterone, progestin-only oral contraceptives, or levonorgestrel subdermal implants for patients with a history of thromboembolic disorders or thrombophlebitis)

**Patient monitoring**
The following may be especially important in patient monitoring (other tests may be warranted in some patients, depending on condition; » = major clinical significance):

Breast examinations
(should be performed routinely, especially with prolonged progestin use)

Papanicolaou (Pap) test and
Physical examination
(as determined by physician, with special attention being given to abdomen, breast and pelvic organs; pre- and post-inspection of site of insertion and removal of levonorgestrel subdermal implants with annual inspection of implantation site during use)

## Side/Adverse Effects

The following side/adverse effects have been selected on the basis of their potential clinical significance (possible signs and symptoms in parentheses where appropriate)—not necessarily inclusive:

**Those indicating need for medical attention**
Incidence more frequent
*Amenorrhea* (stopping of menstrual periods); *breakthrough menstrual bleeding or metromenorrhagia* (medium to heavy uterine bleeding between regular monthly periods); *hyperglycemia* (dry mouth; frequent urination; loss of appetite; unusual thirst)—16% with high doses of megestrol; *menorrhagia* (increased amount of menstrual bleeding occurring at regular monthly periods); *spotting* (light uterine bleeding between regular monthly periods)—17% for levonorgestrel subdermal implants or oral progestins for contraception

Note: *For all progestins*, if *abnormal uterine bleeding* is persistent (longer than 10 days at a time) or recurring (heavier than normal menses occurring longer than 10 months after beginning therapy or more often than monthly), malignancy should be considered as a cause of the bleeding.

*For progestins used for cycle control or as part of ovarian hormone therapy:* Breakthrough uterine bleeding is not as prevalent as it is with progestin-only contraceptives; therefore, any unexpected uterine bleeding that persists for 3 to 6 months should be investigated.

*For oral progestins for contraception:* Breakthrough menstrual bleeding or spotting is common.

*For parenteral medroxyprogesterone:* Amenorrhea increases with duration of use (12 months—55% and 24 months—68%). Breakthrough menstrual bleeding occurs in 90% of users.

*For levonorgestrel subdermal implants:* After 1 year of use of levonorgestrel subdermal implants, total uterine blood loss decreases from baseline levels of 31 mL per month to 24 mL per month. Amenorrhea occurs in 9.4 to 15% of users of the subdermal implants and breakthrough menstrual bleeding occurs in 28% of users, persisting throughout treatment.

Incidence less frequent
*Galactorrhea* (unexpected or increased flow of breast milk); ***mental depression; skin rash***

Incidence rare
***Adrenal suppression or insufficiency or hypotension*** (dizziness; nausea or vomiting; unusual tiredness or weakness)—may occur during chronic megestrol treatment or on its withdrawal; ***Cushing's syndrome*** (backache; filling or rounding out of the face; irritability; menstrual irregularities; mental depression; unusual decrease in sexual desire or ability in men; unusual tiredness or weakness)—may occur during chronic megestrol treatment; ***thromboembolism or thrombus formation*** (headache or migraine; loss of or change in speech, coordination, or vision; pain or numbness in chest, arm, or leg; shortness of breath, unexplained)—severe and sudden, with high doses of progestins for noncontraceptive uses

Note: It is not clear if the *thromboembolism or thrombus formation* associated with use of progestins in high doses is due to the treatment or to the underlying condition that is being treated, such as cancer. Thrombophlebitis, pulmonary embolism, and heart failure have occurred with use of megestrol; fatalities occurred in some cases.

**Those indicating need for medical attention only if they continue or are bothersome**
Incidence more frequent
*Abdominal pain or cramping; dizziness; drowsiness*—for progesterone only; *edema* (bloating or swelling of ankles or feet); *headache, mild*—up to 24% with levonorgestrel subdermal implants; *mood changes*—up to 16% for levonorgestrel subdermal implants; *nervousness; ovarian enlargement or ovarian cyst formation* (abdominal pain)—10% for levonorgestrel subdermal implants; *pain, redness, or skin irritation at the site of injection or implantation*—including local skin color change and residual lump; *unusual tiredness or weakness; unusual or rapid weight gain*

Note: For parenteral medroxyprogesterone for contraception: Average *weight gain* is 2.5 to 7.5 kilograms (kg) after 1 to 6 years of use.

*Ovarian enlargement or ovarian cyst formation* occurring with levonorgestrel subdermal implants is almost always transient and rarely requires surgery.

Incidence less frequent
*Acne; breast pain or tenderness; hot flashes; insomnia* (trouble in sleeping); *libido decrease* (loss of sexual desire); *loss or gain of body, facial, or scalp hair; melasma* (brown spots on exposed skin, which may persist after treatment stops); *nausea*—subsides in 3 months for low dose progestins for contraception

**Those indicating need for medical attention if they occur after medication is discontinued**
*Adrenal suppression or insufficiency or hypotension* (dizziness; nausea or vomiting; unusual tiredness or weakness)—may occur on withdrawal of chronic megestrol treatment; *delayed return of fertility in females* (stopping of menstrual periods; unusual menstrual bleeding, continuing)

Note: Progestin-only oral contraceptives and progestins used for ovarian hormone therapy have not been shown to cause *adrenal suppression or insufficiency* or *delayed return of fertility*.

## Patient Consultation

As an aid to patient consultation, refer to *Advice for the Patient, Progestins—For Noncontraceptive Use (Systemic)* or *Progestins—For Contraceptive Use (Systemic)*.

In providing consultation, consider emphasizing the following selected information (» = major clinical significance):

**Before using this medication**
» Conditions affecting use, especially:

Allergy to peanuts, for oral or parenteral progesterone, or history of hypersensitivity to progestins

Carcinogenicity—Studies are ongoing and have not been done with all progestins. Use of progestins with estrogens in ovarian hormone therapy lowers the incidences of endometrial hyperplasia and endometrial cancer. Significantly, a prolonged (8-year) study in women using injectable medroxyprogesterone for contraception has found a protective effect against endometrial cancer. Long-term studies of parenteral medroxyprogesterone have found no increase in overall risk of breast, ovarian, liver, or cervical cancer. Women 35 years of age or younger may have an increased risk of breast cancer during the first four years following initial use

Pregnancy—With the exception of hydroxyprogesterone and progesterone, use is not recommended during pregnancy. When progestins are used in doses for contraception, ectopic pregnancy is possible, although rare. Alternative methods of contraception should be used by fertile and sexually active females when high dose progestins are used for noncontraceptive purposes, such as in treatment of cancer; physician should be told immediately if pregnancy is suspected

Breast-feeding—Progestins are distributed into breast milk in variable amounts; high doses may increase or decrease the quantity or quality of breast milk while low doses have no effect on breast milk and are recommended for use in breast-feeding women needing contraception; adverse effects in the nursing infant have not been reported

Use in adolescents—Adolescents tend to have a greater risk for sexually transmitted diseases (STDs) and have a higher failure rate for oral progestins for contraception because of compliance problems. Adolescents who are at increased risk for STDs or those failing to comply with strict dosing schedule for contraceptives (a strict 24-hour dose regimen for oral medications or replacement doses for contraceptive injection and implants) may be better served with another form of contraception

Dental—May predispose patient to increased bleeding and inflammation of the gingival tissues; teeth cleaning and plaque control should minimize severity

Other medications, especially aminoglutethimide and hepatic enzyme inducers, such as carbamazepine, phenobarbital, phenytoin, rifabutin, or rifampin

Other medical problems, especially active thrombophlebitis or thromboembolic disease; acute hepatic disease, including benign or malignant tumors; history of thromboembolic disease; known or suspected breast malignancy or tumor; known or suspected pregnancy; undiagnosed genital, uterine, or urinary tract bleeding

**Proper use of this medication**
Reading patient directions
» Importance of not taking more or less medication than the amount prescribed
» Proper dosing

Missed dose for noncontraceptive uses of progestins (except for progesterone capsules): Taking as soon as possible; not taking if almost time for next dose; not doubling doses

Missed dose for progesterone capsules: If 200 mg at bedtime is missed, taking 100 mg in the morning, then going back to regular dose schedule. If 300 mg a day is missed, not taking the missed doses, then going back to regular dose schedule

Missed dose for medroxyprogesterone injection for contraceptive use: If next injection is delayed longer than 13 weeks, using a back-up method of contraception and checking with physician about continuing the medication

Missed dose for progestin-only oral contraceptives: If one or more tablets are missed or if dose is delayed by 3 hours or more, taking the missed dose as soon as remembered, continuing your regular dosing schedule, and using a backup method, such as condoms or spermicides, for the next 48 hours if planning to have sexual intercourse. A dose that is 3 hours late is considered a missed dose

» Proper storage

*For contraception use*
Caution that progestins do not protect against sexually transmitted diseases, including human immunodeficiency virus (HIV) infection or acquired immunodeficiency syndrome (AIDS)

*For levonorgestrel subdermal implants*
Insertion procedure by a health care professional takes 15 minutes under local anesthesia
» Caring for insertion site requires removing pressure dressing in 24 hours, leaving steristrips (sterile tape) on incisions for 3 days, keeping covered and dry, taking care not to bump site or to lift heavy objects for 24 hours, and expecting some swelling and bruising at site of insertion
» Full contraceptive protection begins within 24 hours when insertion is done within 7 days of the beginning of the menstrual period; otherwise, another birth control method must be used during the rest of the first menstrual cycle; protection ends immediately after removal
» Removal procedure may be done at any time by a health care professional. After 5 years of use the subdermal implants should be removed and, if desired, a new set of subdermal implants can be inserted at this time; the removal procedure takes 20 minutes or longer under local anesthesia; rarely, some difficult cases may require skin healing after an unsuccessful attempt

*For medroxyprogesterone for contraception*
» Importance of receiving an injection by a health care professional every 3 months (13 weeks)

Stopping use by simply not receiving the injection

Full contraceptive protection begins immediately after initial injection without need for additional birth control methods if given within the first 5 days of a normal menstrual period, within the first 5 days postpartum if not breast-feeding, and, if exclusively breast-feeding, at the sixth postpartum week. Protection continues when an injection is given every 3 months (13 weeks)

*For oral progestins for contraception*
» Compliance with therapy, taking medication at the same time each day at 24-hour intervals

When switching from estrogen and progestin oral contraceptives, the first dose of the progestin-only oral contraceptive should be taken the next day after the last active tablet of the oral estrogen and progestin oral contraceptive is administered. The placebo (inactive) tablets of the 28-day cycle can be discarded

Also, when switching, full protection begins within 48 hours if the dose is taken on the first day of the menstrual period; if treatment is begun at other times, a back-up method should be used for 3 weeks as a conservative approach

A chance of pregnancy is increased for each missed dose

*For noncontraception use*
Caution in taking combination therapy; taking each medication at the right time

**Precautions while using this medication**
» Regular visits to health care professional
» Caution when driving or doing things requiring alertness because the medication may cause dizziness; for progesterone capsules, dizziness or drowsiness may occur 1 to 4 hours after ingestion

Checking with doctor immediately if uterine bleeding (spotting or breakthrough menstrual bleeding) continues longer than 3 months or if menstruation is delayed by 45 days

» Contacting doctor immediately if pregnancy is suspected or a menstrual period is missed

If scheduled for laboratory tests, tell physician if taking progestins; certain blood tests may be affected

Possibility of dental problems, such as tenderness, swelling, or bleeding of gums; checking with dentist if there are questions about care of teeth or gums or if tenderness, swelling, or bleeding of gums occurs; patient should follow good cleaning procedures, such as regular brushing and flossing of teeth, massaging gums, and having dentist clean teeth regularly

*For contraceptive use*
» Using a second method of birth control when taking medications that reduce effectiveness of progestins

If vomiting occurs for any reason shortly after taking the progestin-only oral contraceptive pill, do not take another dose, resume your normal dosing schedule and use an additional backup method for 48 hours

*For noncontraceptive use*
» Advisability of using contraceptive methods while taking progestins for noncontraceptive uses if fertile and sexually active

For progesterone (vaginal) dosage form: Avoiding use of other vaginal products for 6 hours before and for 6 hours after administering progesterone vaginally to ensure its complete absorption

**Side/adverse effects**
Signs of potential side effects, especially amenorrhea; breakthrough menstrual bleeding or metromenorrhagia; hyperglycemia; menorrhagia; spotting; galactorrhea; mental depression; skin rash; adrenal suppression or insufficiency or hypotension (megestrol only); Cush-

ing's syndrome (megestrol only), or thromboembolism or thrombus formation

## General Dosing Information

### For all progestins
The cyclical administration of progestins is based on an assumed menstrual cycle of 28 days.

Onset of the female menopause may be masked by the use of progestins.

Follicular atresia may be delayed, allowing the growth and development of follicles that clinically may appear to be ovarian cysts, especially with levonorgestrel subdermal implants. In most cases, enlarged follicles disappear spontaneously, but, rarely, they may rupture, causing abdominal pain and requiring surgical intervention.

Discontinue medication pending eye examination if there is sudden partial or complete loss of vision or sudden onset of proptosis (exophthalmos or abnormal protrusion of the eyeball), diplopia (seeing double), or migraine. Also, discontinue medication if examination reveals papilledema or if thrombotic disorder occurs or is suspected.

The patient package insert is mandatory for progestational drugs to convey information regarding birth defects to premenopausal women unless childbearing is impossible. However, it is recommended that the patient package insert also be given to patients taking or using progestins for noncontraceptive purposes.

### For contraception use
Although some progestin products protect against pregnancy, none protects against HIV infection or AIDS.

Another contraceptive method should be used and pregnancy should be ruled out before resuming use of hormonal contraceptives if two tablets or an injection is missed.

### For levonorgestrel subdermal implants
Insertion (usually a 15-minute procedure using local anesthesia) should be performed within the first 7 days of a normal menstrual period or immediately postabortion. Insertion is not recommended by the manufacturer in the first 6-weeks postpartum for breast-feeding women.

All 6 implants are inserted subdermally in a fanlike pattern about 15 degrees apart (totaling 75 degrees) in the midportion of the upper arm (8 to 10 centimeters above the crease in the elbow).

Proper insertion technique for insertion or removal of subdermal implants reduces the incidence of hard-to-remove subdermal implants, expulsions, and improper placement of subdermal implants. Bruising and some scarring may occur with insertion or removal procedures. Insertion site complications at 1-year follow-up include 0.8% skin infection, 0.4% expulsion, and 4.7% local skin reaction; in approximately 41% of women with a skin infection, an expulsion of an implant resulted.

When an implant is expelled, a new subdermal implant may be inserted in the same incision, although any infection or unusual wound or incision site problems should heal before a new sterile subdermal implant is inserted. Other contraceptive methods should be used concurrently when fewer than 6 subdermal implants are in place. Also, if removal of all subdermal implants is not successful with the first attempt, the skin should be allowed to heal completely before a second attempt of removal.

Removal of the levonorgestrel implants (usually a 20-minute procedure) may occur on request at any time or at the end of the fifth year of use, and should be considered if prolonged immobilization is anticipated or if persistent infection develops at the implantation site. Used subdermal implants should be disposed of by using the Centers for Disease Control guidelines for biohazardous waste.

### For oral progestins for contraception
When used as oral contraceptives, progestins are administered daily without interruption, regardless of menstrual cycle.

When switching a patient from estrogen and progestin oral contraceptives, a new progestin-only oral contraceptive is begun on the 22nd day; the inactive or placebo tablets of the 28-day cycle should be discarded. Full contraceptive protection begins within 48 hours if the first oral progestin dose is taken on Day 1 of the menstrual cycle. A back-up birth control method should be used for 3 weeks (a conservative approach) if the patient is started at any other time.

### For parenteral medroxyprogesterone
The formulation of parenteral medroxyprogesterone for noncontraceptive use (400 mg/mL) should not be used for contraceptive uses, even if the proper dose (150 mg) is considered. Efficacy issues arose and resulted in discontinuation of a clinical trial conducted by the manufacturer using a lower volume dose than that used in the formulation of medroxyprogesterone for contraception. Dose adjustment is not necessary for body weight but it is reported that plasma concentration and duration decreased by a mean of 3.3 picograms/mL per kg increase of body weight because of its accumulation in fat cells; therefore, return to fertility may be especially prolonged in obese women.

Injecting into the deltoid muscle as opposed to the gluteal muscle is recommended by some clinicians to lessen absorption problems that may occur because of rubbing the injection site while sitting.

### For noncontraceptive uses
For women who are using progestins for other reasons besides contraception, concurrent contraceptive methods should be used if fertile and sexually active.

Response rates are about 15 to 16% in patients using progestins for treating endometrial carcinoma with high-grade resistant tumors and may be significantly better with low-grade malignancy; response rate decreases for tumors of increasing grade and in those tumors negative for both estrogen and progesterone receptors; median survival is approximately 9 to 10 months.

Response rates are approximately 5% and of short duration in patients using progestins for treating renal carcinoma; routine receptor assay is not helpful in predicting appropriate patients.

Response rates of up to about 40% have been reported when high-dose oral medroxyprogesterone has been used to treat breast cancer.

Decisions to treat menopausal symptoms with hormones for a limited time (1 to 5 years) or to use hormones to prevent diseases in postmenopausal women for a longer period of time (10 to 20 years), or a lifetime, should be separate decisions. Counseling asymptomatic postmenopausal women about the benefits and risks of long-term estrogen and progestin ovarian hormone therapy to prevent disease and prolong life is complex. It is dependent on an individual's risk of breast cancer, osteoporosis, and coronary heart disease and whether a uterus is present (progestins are not needed when the uterus is absent). Adding a progestin to estrogen therapy may benefit postmenopausal women at risk for osteoporosis, slightly reduce estrogen's protective effect against coronary heart disease (women at more risk are provided the greatest benefit), and slightly increase the risk of breast cancer over that of non-users. Women should understand that the benefits and risks of preventive ovarian hormone therapy depend on their risk status.

### For medroxyprogesterone
Re-establishment of menstrual cycle may be delayed (up to 18 months or longer) and is difficult to predict following the intramuscular administration of medroxyprogesterone. Because of the prolonged action and the resulting difficulty in predicting the time of withdrawal bleeding following injection, parenteral medroxyprogesterone is not recommended for treatment of secondary amenorrhea or dysfunctional uterine bleeding; oral medroxyprogesterone is the preferred mode of therapy.

### For megestrol
The magnitude and rate of weight gain are highly dependent on megestrol dose and are significantly greater with higher doses. The greatest effect can be maintained at a lower dose of 400 mg a day in the second to fourth months when 800 mg a day is taken in the first month, although some studies have reported further benefit when the dose is not lowered.

Adrenal suppression may occur with normal dosing range; effects on HIV viral replication have not been determined.

### For progesterone
For oral progesterone:
  If only one dose of progesterone capsules is needed, it should be taken at bedtime to minimize the side effect of dizziness or drowsiness experienced by patients within 1 to 4 hours after taking 200 mg progesterone.

  If a progesterone dose is taken in the morning, the patient should take it 2 hours after eating breakfast.

For vaginal progesterone:
  Synthetic progestins are more potent than natural progesterone; i.e., 20 to 25 mg progesterone (intramuscular) has an effect equivalent to 100 mg progesterone (vaginal suppository) or 5 to 10 mg medroxyprogesterone (oral) or 50 mg medroxyprogesterone (intramuscular).

  Use of other vaginal products should be avoided for at least 6 hours before or 6 hours after administering progesterone vaginally to ensure its complete absorption.

### For treatment of adverse effects
For megesterol—
  Reports of adrenal suppression or insufficiency have been reported in patients during treatment and at treatment discontinuation of high or chronic doses of megestrol, whereas Cushing's syndrome has been reported during treatment with high or chronic doses of me-

gestrol. Recommended treatment of adrenal insufficiency consists of the following:
- Laboratory evaluation for adrenal insufficiency.
- Physiologic replacement doses of a rapid-acting glucocorticosteroid.

# HYDROXYPROGESTERONE

## Summary of Differences
Category:
  Progestational agent; diagnostic aid.
Indications:
  Amenorrhea, dysfunctional uterine bleeding, induction of menses, and test for endogenous estrogen production.
Pharmacology/pharmacokinetics:
  More potent than progesterone with longer duration of action.
  Synthetic 17-hydroxy derivative of progesterone with progestogenic, androgenic, and glucocorticoid effects.

## Parenteral Dosage Forms

### HYDROXYPROGESTERONE CAPROATE INJECTION USP

**Usual adult and adolescent dose**
Amenorrhea or
Dysfunctional uterine bleeding—
  Intramuscular, 375 mg.
Estrogen production, endogenous, diagnosis or
Menses, induction of—
  Intramuscular, 125 to 250 mg given on Day 10 of the menstrual cycle, repeated every seven days until suppression is no longer desired.
  Note: Withdrawal bleeding usually occurs within three to seven days after discontinuing therapy.

**Strength(s) usually available**
U.S.—
  125 mg per mL (Rx) [GENERIC].
  250 mg per mL (Rx) [Gesterol LA 250; Hy/Gestrone; Hylutin; Prodrox; Pro-Span; GENERIC].
Canada—
  Not commercially available.

**Packaging and storage**
Store below 40 °C (104 °F), preferably between 15 and 30 °C (59 and 86 °F), unless otherwise specified by manufacturer. Protect from freezing.

**Note**
Castor or sesame oils are commonly used as the vehicle for intramuscular injection.
Include mandatory patient package insert (PPI) when dispensing to premenopausal patient unless reproduction is impossible.

# LEVONORGESTREL

## Summary of Differences
Category:
  Contraceptive.
Indications:
  Pregnancy prophylaxis.
Pharmacology/pharmacokinetics:
  19-nor derivative of testosterone; has progestational and androgenic effects.
Precautions:
  Breast-feeding—Generally recommended for use 6 weeks postpartum in breast-feeding women but has been used 5 days postpartum after establishment of lactation.
  Laboratory value alterations—Serum $T_3$ concentrations may be slightly elevated and $T_4$ concentrations may be decreased; total serum $T_4$ concentrations are unaffected.
  Medical considerations/contraindications—Levonorgestrel subdermal implants have not caused thrombogenic disorders, but caution may be necessary with use in patients with a history of thrombosis. Caution is necessary in patients with a history of CNS disorders, such as depression or history of convulsions.
Side effects:
  Breakthrough menstrual bleeding or spotting, reduced amount of menstrual bleeding, and amenorrhea are predominant side effects. These bleeding irregularities may persist but are less problematic with time. Other side effects include ovarian enlargement or cysts (usually reversible with continued use), acne, headaches, and mood changes.

## Additional Dosing Information
See also *General Dosing Information*.
Special training for insertion, removal, and disposal of levonorgestrel subdermal implants includes knowledge and familiarity of procedures by physician and patient.

## Subdermal Dosage Form

### LEVONORGESTREL IMPLANTS

**Usual adult and adolescent dose**
Pregnancy, prevention of—
  Subdermally, one set of six implants surgically inserted every five years.

**Strength(s) usually available**
U.S.—
  216 mg (Rx) [NORPLANT System].
Canada—
  216 mg (Rx) [NORPLANT System].

**Packaging and storage**
Store below 40 °C (104 °F), preferably between 15 and 30 °C (59 and 86 °F), unless otherwise specified by manufacturer. Store away from excess heat or moisture.

**Note**
Include mandatory patient package insert (PPI) when dispensing progestins to premenopausal patient unless reproduction is impossible.

# MEDROGESTONE

## Summary of Differences
Category:
  Progestational agent.
Indications:
  Secondary amenorrhea, dysfunctional uterine bleeding, induction of menses, and, in conjunction with estrogens, for endometrial shedding in menopausal women.
Pharmacology/pharmacokinetics:
  17-hydroxy derivative of progesterone; highly progestational, devoid of estrogenic, androgenic, glucocorticoid, or anti-androgenic effects.

## Oral Dosage Forms

### MEDROGESTONE TABLETS

**Usual adult and adolescent dose**
Amenorrhea, secondary or
Dysfunctional uterine bleeding or
Hyperplasia, endometrial, estrogen-induced, postmenopausal, prophylaxis or
Menses, induction of—
  Oral, 5 to 10 mg a day on Days 15 through 25 of monthly cycle.
  Note: Withdrawal bleeding usually occurs within three to seven days after discontinuing therapy.
    An optimum secretory transformation of an endometrium that has been adequately primed with either endogenous or exogenous estrogens (Days 5 to 25 of the menstrual cycle) may be reestablished with three or more cycles.

**Strength(s) usually available**
U.S.—
  Not commercially available.
Canada—
  5 mg (Rx) [Colprone (scored)].

**Packaging and storage**
Store below 40 °C (104 °F), preferably between 15 and 30 °C (59 and 86 °F), unless otherwise specified by manufacturer. Store in a well-closed container.

# MEDROXYPROGESTERONE

## Summary of Differences
Category:
  Oral medroxyprogesterone used as a progestational agent, antineoplastic agent, and diagnostic aid (test for endogenous estrogen production). Parenteral medroxyprogesterone used as adjunct in antineo-

plastic therapy and indicated as contraceptive agent in a special parenteral formulation.

Indications:
Oral and parenteral medroxyprogesterone indicated to treat breast carcinoma in postmenopausal women and endometrial hyperplasia in conditions such as polycystic ovary syndrome; however, only parenteral medroxyprogesterone is indicated for adjunct treatment of metastatic renal or endometrial carcinoma and endometriosis. Parenteral medroxyprogesterone is accepted therapy for precocious puberty, but has been replaced by other modalities. Unlike parenteral medroxyprogesterone, oral medroxyprogesterone is indicated for secondary amenorrhea, dysfunctional uterine bleeding, induction of menses, carcinoma, ovarian hormone therapy in menopause, and testing for endogenous estrogen production.

Unlike oral medroxyprogesterone, parenteral medroxyprogesterone is not recommended for treatment of secondary amenorrhea or dysfunctional uterine bleeding.

Pharmacology/pharmacokinetics:
17-hydroxy derivative of progesterone with progestogenic, androgenic, and glucocorticoid effects.

Precautions:
Fertility—Luteal function may be delayed after cessation of parenteral medroxyprogesterone treatment for contraception, especially in obese females of reproductive age.
Pregnancy—Use in pregnancy has produced problems in the fetus and is not recommended. Doses used for contraception have not appeared to produce problems for nursing infants after lactation is established.
Drug interactions—Use of aminoglutethimide may lower serum concentrations of medroxyprogesterone and interfere with intestinal absorption of oral dose.
Medical considerations/contraindications—Low dose parenteral medroxyprogesterone can be used with caution for contraception in women with diabetes mellitus. High doses (but not low doses) have rarely been associated with thromboembolic disorders or thrombophlebitis.

Side/adverse effects:
Bloating or swelling of face, ankles, or feet more likely with higher doses.

## Additional Dosing Information

See also *General Dosing Information*.

Re-establishment of menstrual cycle can be delayed and difficult to predict following the parenteral dose. Also, only the 150 mg/mL formulation and a 150-mg dose should be used for contraception; a special dose adjustment for the obese patient is not needed; however, contraceptive efficacy in patients over 90 kg has not been evaluated.

## Oral Dosage Forms

Note: Bracketed uses in the *Dosage Forms* section refer to categories of use or indications that are not included in U.S. product labeling.

### MEDROXYPROGESTERONE ACETATE TABLETS USP

**Usual adult or adolescent dose**
Amenorrhea, secondary—
Oral, 5 to 10 mg a day for five to ten days, started any time during cycle.
Dysfunctional uterine bleeding—
Oral, 5 to 10 mg a day for five to ten days, commencing on the calculated Day 16 or Day 21 of the menstrual cycle.
Menses, induction of—
Oral, 10 mg daily for ten days starting on Day 16 of the menstrual cycle. If bleeding is controlled satisfactorily, two or more subsequent cycles of the treatment should be given.
[Hyperplasia, endometrial, estrogen-induced, postmenopausal, prophylaxis]—
There are several recommended dosing schedules
Oral, 5 to 10 mg medroxyprogesterone a day for ten or fourteen days beginning on Days 12 or 16 through Day 25, estrogen is taken on Day 1 through Day 25, and neither estrogen nor medroxyprogesterone is taken on the twenty-fifth day through the end of the month.
Oral, 5 to 10 mg medroxyprogesterone a day taken on the first ten to fourteen days along with continuous estrogen dosing.
Oral, 2.5 or 5 mg medroxyprogesterone a day taken continuously with continuous estrogen dosing.

Note: Other regimens may differ but also may be appropriate. Withdrawal bleeding usually occurs within three to seven days after discontinuing therapy.

[Carcinoma, breast, postmenopausal women]—
Oral, 400 mg a day in divided doses.
[Carcinoma, endometrial]—
Initial: Oral, 200 to 400 mg a day for two to three months.
Maintenance: Oral, 200 mg a day.

Note: Improvement may not be evident until eight to ten weeks following initiation of therapy for breast or endometrial carcinoma. However, treatment should be discontinued when there is rapid progression of the disease at any time during therapy.

[Endometriosis][1]—
Oral, 10 to 40 mg a day for six to nine months.
[Estrogen production, endogenous, diagnosis]—
Oral, 10 mg a day for five to ten days. Withdrawal bleeding will occur three to seven days following therapy if the uterus has been sufficiently primed with endogenous estrogen.
[Hyperplasia, endometrial, treatment][1]—
There are several recommended dosing schedules
Oral, 10 mg a day for three to six months.
Oral, 10 mg a day for twenty-one days each month for three months. Then the dose is reduced to 10 mg a day for ten to fourteen days a month.
Oral, 20 mg a day for thirty days every six months.

Note: Other regimens may differ but also may be appropriate.

**Strength(s) usually available**
U.S.—
2.5 mg (Rx) [*Cycrin* (scored); *Provera* (scored); GENERIC].
5 mg (Rx) [*Cycrin* (scored); *Provera* (scored); GENERIC].
10 mg (Rx) [*Amen* (scored); *Curretab* (scored); *Cycrin* (scored); *Provera* (scored); GENERIC].
Canada—
2.5 mg (Rx) [*Alti-MPA*; *Gen-Medroxy* (scored); *Novo-Medrone* (scored); *Provera*].
5 mg (Rx) [*Alti-MPA*; *Gen-Medroxy* (scored); *Novo-Medrone* (scored); *Provera* (scored); *Provera Pak* (scored)].
10 mg (Rx) [*Alti-MPA*; *Gen-Medroxy* (scored); *Novo-Medrone* (scored); *Provera* (scored)].
100 mg (Rx) [*Provera* (scored)].

Note: Brand name *Provera Pak* contains 14 tablets in blister packaging.

**Packaging and storage**
Store below 40 °C (104 °F), preferably between 15 and 30 °C (59 and 86 °F), unless otherwise specified by manufacturer.

**Note**
Include mandatory patient package insert (PPI) when dispensing progestins to premenopausal patient unless reproduction is impossible.

## Parenteral Dosage Forms

Note: Bracketed uses in the *Dosage Forms* section refer to categories of use or indications that are not included in U.S. product labeling.

### MEDROXYPROGESTERONE ACETATE INJECTABLE SUSPENSION USP

Note: Formerly known as Sterile Medroxyprogesterone Acetate Suspension, USP.

**Usual adult or adolescent dose**
Carcinoma, endometrial or
Carcinoma, renal—
Initial: Intramuscular, 400 mg to 1 gram once a week until improvement and stabilization occur.
Maintenance: Intramuscular, 400 mg or more once a month.
[Carcinoma, breast]—
Initial: Intramuscular, 500 mg a day for twenty-eight days.
Maintenance: Intramuscular, 500 mg two times a week.

Note: Improvement may not be evident for eight to ten weeks of therapy for breast or endometrial carcinoma. However, treatment should be discontinued when there is rapid progression of the disease at any time during therapy.

[Endometriosis]—
There are several recommended dosing schedules
Intramuscular, 50 mg once a week for at least six months.
Intramuscular, 100 mg every two weeks for at least six months.
Intramuscular, 150 mg every 3 months for at least six months.
Pregnancy, prevention of—
Intramuscular, 150 mg every three months.

Note: Dosage does not need to be adjusted for body weight in patients weighing less than 90 kg, but dosage has not been studied in patients weighing more than 90 kg. It is recommended that the first injection be given during the first five days after onset of a normal menstrual period; within five days postpartum if not breast-feeding, and if exclusively breast-feeding, at six weeks postpartum. A physician should determine that a patient is not pregnant if more than thirteen weeks will elapse between injections.

**Strength(s) usually available**
U.S.—
   150 mg per mL (Rx) [*Depo-Provera Contraceptive Injection*].
   400 mg per mL (Rx) [*Depo-Provera*].
   Note: Brand name *Depo-Provera Contraceptive Injection* is available in vials or as prefilled syringes.
Canada—
   50 mg per mL (Rx) [*Depo-Provera*].
   150 mg per mL (Rx) [*Depo-Provera*].

**Packaging and storage**
Store below 40 °C (104 °F), preferably between 15 and 30 °C (59 and 86 °F), unless otherwise specified by manufacturer. Protect from freezing.

**Preparation of dosage form**
Should be shaken vigorously before administration.

**Auxiliary labeling**
• Shake well.

**Note**
Include mandatory patient package insert (PPI) when dispensing progestins to premenopausal patient unless reproduction is impossible.

[1]Not included in Canadian product labeling.

## *MEGESTROL*

## Summary of Differences
Category:
   Antianoretic, anticachectic, antineoplastic.
Indications:
   Endometrial or breast carcinoma; anorexia, cachexia and significant weight loss, associated with cancer (tablets) and acquired immunodeficiency syndrome (AIDS) (suspension); and advanced prostate carcinoma. Not recommended for prophylactic avoidance of weight loss.
Pharmacology/pharmacokinetics:
   17-hydroxy derivative of progesterone; progestogenic, glucocorticoid, and anti-estrogenic effects.
Precautions:
   Fertility—Impaired fertility shown in male offspring of megestrol-treated females in studies in rats and dogs.
   Pregnancy—Use is not recommended.

## Additional Dosing Information
See also *General Dosing Information*.

Magnitude and rate of weight gain are dose-related; lower doses of 400 mg are recommended after the first month, although some results have shown weight gain continuing with 800 mg given continuously for 4 months.

## Oral Dosage Forms
Note: Bracketed uses in the *Dosage Forms* section refer to categories of use or indications that are not included in U.S. product labeling.

### MEGESTROL ACETATE SUSPENSION

**Usual adult and adolescent dose**
Anorexia or
Cachexia or
Weight-loss, significant—
   For patients with AIDS: Oral, 800 mg a day the first month, then 400 or 800 mg a day for three more months.

**Strength(s) usually available**
U.S.—
   40 mg per milliliter (mL) (Rx) [*Megace* (alcohol 0.06%; sucrose)].
Canada—
   40 mg per milliliter (mL) (Rx) [*Megace OS* (alcohol 0.06%; sucrose)].

**Packaging and storage**
Store between 15 and 25 °C (59 and 77 °F). Protect from heat. Store in a well-closed container.

**Auxiliary labeling**
• Shake well.

**Note**
Include patient package insert (PPI) when dispensing.

### MEGESTROL ACETATE TABLETS USP

**Usual adult and adolescent dose**
[Anorexia] or
[Cachexia] or
[Weight-loss, significant]—
   For patients with cancer: Oral, 400 to 800 mg a day as a single daily dose.
Carcinoma, breast—
   Oral, 160 mg a day as a single dose or in divided doses.
Carcinoma, endometrial—
   Oral, 40 to 320 mg a day in divided doses.
[Carcinoma, prostate, advanced]—
   Oral, 120 mg once a day with 0.1 mg diethylstilbesterol a day.
Note: At least two months of continuous treatment is considered an adequate period for determining the efficacy of megestrol.
[Hyperplasia, endometrial, treatment][1]—
   Oral, 20 to 40 mg a day for 14 days or longer every month.

**Strength(s) usually available**
U.S.—
   20 mg (Rx) [*Megace* (scored); GENERIC].
   40 mg (Rx) [*Megace* (scored); GENERIC].
Canada—
   40 mg (Rx) [*Apo-Megestrol* (scored); *Megace* (scored)].
   160 mg (Rx) [*Apo-Megestrol* (scored); *Megace*].

**Packaging and storage**
Store below 40 °C (104 °F), preferably between 15 and 30 °C (59 and 86 °F), unless otherwise specified by manufacturer. Store in a well-closed container.

**Note**
Include patient package insert (PPI) when dispensing.

[1]Not included in Canadian product labeling.

## *NORETHINDRONE*

## Summary of Differences
Category:
   Indicated as a progestational agent (norethindrone base and acetate) and contraceptive agent (norethindrone base).
Indication:
   Norethindrone acetate indicated for secondary amenorrhea, dysfunctional uterine bleeding, induction of menses, and endometriosis. Norethindrone base is indicated for contraception while the acetate form is not.

## Oral Dosage Forms

### NORETHINDRONE TABLETS USP

**Usual adult and adolescent dose**
Pregnancy, prevention of—
   Oral, 350 mcg (0.35 mg) a day, starting on Day 1 of the menstrual cycle and continuing uninterrupted at the same time every day of the year, whether or not menstrual bleeding occurs.

**Strength(s) usually available**
U.S.—
   350 mcg (0.35 mg) (Rx) [*Micronor; Nor-QD*].
Canada—
   350 mcg (0.35 mg) (Rx) [*Micronor*].

**Packaging and storage**
Store below 40 °C (104 °F), preferably between 15 and 30 °C (59 and 86 °F), unless otherwise specified by manufacturer. Store in a well-closed container.

**Note**
Include mandatory patient package insert (PPI) when dispensing progestins to premenopausal patient unless reproduction is impossible.

### NORETHINDRONE ACETATE TABLETS USP

**Usual adult and adolescent dose**
Amenorrhea, secondary or
Dysfunctional uterine bleeding—
   Oral, 2.5 to 10 mg a day on Day 5 through Day 25 of the menstrual cycle or for five to ten days during the last half of menstrual cycle.
   Note: Withdrawal bleeding occurs within three to seven days after progestin treatment ends.

Endometriosis—
    Initial: Oral, 5 mg a day for two weeks, increasing by 2.5 mg a day at two-week intervals to reach a total dose of 15 mg a day.
    Maintenance: Oral, 15 mg a day for six to nine months, unless temporarily discontinued because of breakthrough menstrual bleeding.

**Strength(s) usually available**
U.S.—
    5 mg (Rx) [*Aygestin* (scored)].
Canada—
    5 mg (Rx) [*Norlutate*].

**Packaging and storage**
Store below 40 °C (104 °F), preferably between 15 and 30 °C (59 and 86 °F), unless otherwise specified by manufacturer. Store in a well-closed container.

**Note**
Include mandatory patient package insert (PPI) when dispensing progestins to premenopausal patients unless reproduction is impossible.

---

## NORGESTREL

## Summary of Differences
Category:
    Contraceptive agent.
Indication:
    Pregnancy prophylaxis.
Pharmacology/pharmacokinetics:
    19-nor derivative of testosterone; has progestogenic, estrogenic, androgenic, and anti-estrogenic effects.

## Oral Dosage Forms
### NORGESTREL TABLETS USP
**Usual adult and adolescent dose**
Pregnancy, prevention of—
    Oral, 75 mcg (0.075 mg) a day, starting on Day 1 of menstrual cycle and continuing uninterrupted at the same time every day of the year whether or not menstrual bleeding occurs.

**Strength(s) usually available**
U.S.—
    75 mcg (0.075 mg) (Rx) [*Ovrette*].
Canada—
    Not commercially available.

**Packaging and storage**
Store below 40 °C (104 °F), preferably between 15 and 30 °C (59 and 86 °F), unless otherwise specified by manufacturer. Store in a well-closed container.

**Note**
Include mandatory patient package insert (PPI) when dispensing progestins to premenopausal patients unless reproduction is impossible.

---

## PROGESTERONE

## Summary of Differences
Category:
    Progestational agent.
Indications:
    Indicated for secondary amenorrhea and dysfunctional uterine bleeding but is also used for corpus luteum insufficiency.
Pharmacology/pharmacokinetics:
    Natural hormone with progestational, androgenic, and anti-estrogenic effects.
Precautions:
    Pregnancy—Although not proven effective, progesterone has been used during first few months of pregnancy to prevent habitual or threatened abortion due to hormonal imbalance but may also delay expulsion of a defective ovum.

## Additional Dosing Information
See also *General Dosing Information*.
Twenty to 25 mg progesterone (intramuscular) produces an equivalent progestogenic effect compared to 100 mg progesterone (vaginal suppository).

## Oral Dosage Forms
### PROGESTERONE CAPSULES (Micronized)
**Usual adult dose**
Amenorrhea, secondary[1]—
    Oral, 400 mg once a day in the evening for ten days.
[Hyperplasia, endometrial, estrogen-induced, postmenopausal, prophylaxis]—
    Oral, 200 mg once a day at bedtime for fourteen days beginning Day 8 through Day 21 of a twenty-eight–day cycle or beginning Day 12 to Day 25 of a thirty-day cycle. A dose of 300 mg progesterone divided as 100 mg in the morning two hours after breakfast and 200 mg at bedtime may be required for patients taking doses of estrogen 1.25 mg or greater. The progestin dose should be adjusted until desired uterine response is achieved (regular withdrawal uterine bleeding or amenorrhea). In many treatment regimens, the last five to seven days of each month are often left free of hormone use.

**Strength(s) usually available**
U.S.—
    100 mg (Rx) [*Prometrium* (glycerin; lecithin; peanut oil; titanium dioxide)].
Canada—
    100 mg (Rx) [*Prometrium* (glycerin; lecithin; peanut oil; titanium dioxide)].

**Packaging and storage**
Store between 15 and 30 °C (59 and 86 °F), unless otherwise specified by manufacturer. Protect from light.

**Auxiliary labeling**
May cause dizziness or drowsiness.

**Note**
Include patient package insert (PPI) when dispensing progestins to premenopausal patients, unless reproduction is impossible.

## Parenteral Dosage Forms
Note: Bracketed uses in the *Dosage Forms* section refer to categories of use or indications that are not included in U.S. product labeling.

### PROGESTERONE INJECTION USP
**Usual adult and adolescent dose**
Amenorrhea, secondary—
    Intramuscular, 5 to 10 mg a day for six to ten consecutive days or 100 to 150 mg injected intramuscularly as a single dose.
    Note: If there has been sufficient ovarian activity to produce a proliferative endometrium or two weeks of prior estrogen therapy, withdrawal bleeding will occur forty-eight to seventy-two hours after the last injection. The patient should discontinue therapy if menstrual cycle occurs. This may be followed by spontaneous normal cycles. Progesterone should be discontinued if menses occurs during the series of injections.
Dysfunctional uterine bleeding—
    Intramuscular, 5 to 10 mg a day for six consecutive days.
    Note: Bleeding should cease within six days. When estrogen is being given, the administration of progesterone should begin after two weeks of estrogen therapy. Progesterone should be discontinued if menses occurs during the series of injections.
[Corpus luteum insufficiency][1]—
    Intramuscular, 12.5 mg or more a day initiated within several days of ovulation. Treatment duration is usually two weeks, but it may be continued, if necessary, up to eleventh week of gestation.
[Estrogen production, endogenous, diagnosis][1]—
    Intramuscular, 100 mg as a single dose.

**Strength(s) usually available**
U.S.—
    50 mg per mL (Rx) [*Gesterol 50* (in sesame seed oil; benzyl alcohol 10%); GENERIC (in sesame seed or peanut oil)].
Canada—
    50 mg per mL (Rx) [*PMS-Progesterone* (in sesame seed oil; benzyl alcohol 10%)].

**Packaging and storage**
Store below 40 °C (104 °F), preferably between 15 and 30 °C (59 and 86 °F), unless otherwise specified by manufacturer. Protect from freezing.

**Auxiliary labeling**
May cause dizziness or drowsiness.

**Note**
Include mandatory patient package insert (PPI) when dispensing progestins to premenopausal patients unless reproduction is impossible.

## Vaginal Dosage Forms
### PROGESTERONE GEL (Micronized)
Note: Bracketed uses in the *Dosage Forms* section refer to categories of use or indications that are not included in U.S. product labeling.

### Usual adult and adolescent dose
Amenorrhea, secondary—
  Vaginal, 45 mg (one applicatorful of 4% vaginal gel) once every other day for up to six doses. Dose may be increased to 90 mg (one applicatorful of 8% vaginal gel) once every other day for up to six doses.

Note: Increasing the dose to 90 mg by doubling the amount of the 4% vaginal gel used does not increase the amount of medication absorbed, and the 8% vaginal gel should be used instead.

Assisted reproductive technologies, in females or
[Corpus luteum insufficiency][1]—
  For patients needing luteal phase support: Vaginal, 90 mg (one applicatorful of 8% vaginal gel) once a day for progesterone supplementation. For patients undergoing *in vitro* fertilization (IVF), treatment may begin within 24 hours of embryo transfer and continue through Day 30 post-transfer. If pregnancy occurs, treatment can be extended until placental autonomy is achieved, up to ten to twelve weeks.
  For patients with partial or complete ovarian failure: Vaginal, 90 mg (one applicatorful of 8% vaginal gel) two times a day to receive full progesterone replacement doses while undergoing donor oocyte transfer procedure. If pregnancy occurs, treatment can be extended until placental autonomy is achieved, up to ten to twelve weeks.

### Strength(s) usually available
U.S.—
  4% (Rx) [*Crinone*].
  8% (Rx) [*Crinone*].
  Note: Available as single-use prefilled applicators. One applicatorful of 4% or 8% vaginal gel delivers 1.125 grams of gel.
Canada—
  Not commerically available.

### Packaging and storage
Store between 15 and 25 °C (59 and 77 °F), unless otherwise specified by manufacturer.

### Auxiliary labeling
For vaginal use only. May cause dizziness or drowsiness.

## PROGESTERONE SUPPOSITORIES
Note: Because progesterone suppositories are not commercially available in the U.S. or Canada, the bracketed uses and the use of the superscript 1 in this *Dosage Forms* section reflect the lack of labeled (approved) indications for this product in these countries.

### Usual adult and adolescent dose
[Assisted reproductive technologies, in females][1] or
[Corpus luteum insufficiency][1]—
  Vaginal, 25 to 100 mg one to two times a day initiated within several days of ovulation. Treatment duration is usually continued if the patient is pregnant up to about the eleventh week of gestation.

### Strength(s) usually available
U.S.—
  Not commercially available. Compounding required for prescription.
Canada—
  Not commercially available. Compounding required for prescription.

### Packaging and storage
Store between 2 and 8 °C (36 and 46 °F), in a tight container.

### Preparation of dosage form
A formulation that has been used for the extemporaneous compounding of progesterone suppositories is as follows:
- 710 mg (0.71 grams) progesterone powder
- 33.7 grams polyethylene glycol 400
- 22.3 grams polyethylene glycol 6000

Makes 28 suppositories, 25 mg progesterone per suppository.

### Auxiliary labeling
- For vaginal use only.
- Refrigerate. Do not freeze.

[1]Not included in Canadian product labeling.

## Selected Bibliography
### General
Grady D, Rubin SM, Petitti DB, et al. Hormone therapy to prevent disease and prolong life in postmenopausal women. Ann Intern Med 1992 Dec; 117(12): 1016-37.

### General
American College of Physicians. Clinical Guideline. Guidelines for counseling postmenopausal women about preventive hormone therapy. Ann Intern Med 1992 Dec; 117(12): 1038-41.

Revised: 06/29/98

## Table 1. Pharmacokinetics

| Drug | Protein* binding (%) | Biotransformation | Elimination half-life (hrs) | Time to peak concentration (hrs) | Peak serum concentration ng/mL | Peak serum concentration Dose (mg) | Renal elimination (%) | Fecal elimination (%) |
|---|---|---|---|---|---|---|---|---|
| Natural: | | | | | | | | |
| Progesterone† | Very high (90% or more) | Hepatic | Several minutes, after absorption | | | | 50–60 | 10 |
| Oral, micronized | | | | 2–4 | 24.3 | 200 | | |
| IM | | | | 28 | 39.1 | 45 | | |
| IM | | | | 19.6 | 53.8 | 90 | | |
| Vaginal gel, micronized | | | | 55 | 13.2 | 45 | | |
| Vaginal gel, micronized | | | | 34.8 | 14.9 | 45 | | |
| Synthetic 17-hydroxy derivatives: | | | | | | | | |
| Hydroxyprogesterone caproate | Very high (90% or more) | Hepatic | | | | | | |
| Medroxyprogesterone acetate | Very high (90% or more) | Hepatic | | | | | 15–22 | 45–80 |
| Oral | | | 30 | Within 2–4 | 19–35 | 10 | | |
| IM | | No first-pass hepatic effect | 50 days | 3 weeks | 1–7 | 150‡ | | |
| Medrogestone | | | 4 | 1 | | | | |

### Table 1. Pharmacokinetics (continued)

| Drug | Protein* binding (%) | Biotransformation | Elimination half-life (hrs) | Time to peak concentration (hrs) | Peak serum concentration ng/mL | Peak serum concentration Dose (mg) | Renal elimination (%) | Fecal elimination (%) |
|---|---|---|---|---|---|---|---|---|
| Megestrol acetate | Very high (90% or more) | Hepatic | 38 (13–104) | | | | 66 | 20 |
| Oral | | | | 2–3 | 200 | 160 | | |
| Oral | | | | 2–3 | 753 | 600 | | |
| Synthetic 19-nor derivatives: | | | | | | | | |
| Levonorgestrel subdermal implants | Very high§ (90% or more) | No first-pass hepatic effect | 16 (8–30) | 24 | 1.6, within first week | 216** | 45 | 32 |
| 3 months | | | | | 0.4 | | | |
| 12 months | | | | | 0.32 | | | |
| 60 months | | | | | 0.26 | | | |
| Norgestrel | Very high (90% or more) | | 20 | | | | | |
| Norethindrone | Very high# (90% or more) | Hepatic first pass effect | 8 (6–12) | 2 | | | 50 | 20–40 |
| Norethindrone acetate | Very high (90% or more) | Hepatic first pass effect | 8 | | | | | |

*Sex hormone–binding globulin (SHBG) synthesis is stimulated by estrogens and inhibited by androgens; levels are twice as high in women as in men.
†Progesterone binds strongly to cortisol binding globulin (CBG) 17.7%, SHBG 0.6%, and weakly to albumin 79.3%. Absorption is the rate-limiting step for the elimination half-life.
‡Pertains to parenteral medroxyprogesterone for contraception injection formulation (150mg/mL) only given every 3 months.
§Levonorgestrel: Free, 1.1–1.7%; SHBG 92–62%; albumin 37.56%, but suppresses SHBG by 33%.
#Norethindrone: Free 3.5%; SHBG 35.5%; albumin 61%.
**216 mg is the loading dose for 6 levonorgestrel implants; a mean dose of 35 mcg levonorgestrel is released daily.

**PROGUANIL**—The *Proguanil (Systemic)* monograph is not included in this published version of the USP DI database. Copies of the monograph are available on request from Micromedex, Inc. - Reprint Requests, 6200 S. Syracuse Way, Suite 300, Englewood, CO 80111; telephone (303) 486-6400; telefax (303) 486-6464; Email: USPDI@MDX.COM.

**PROMAZINE**—See *Phenothiazines (Systemic)*

**PROMETHAZINE**—See *Antihistamines, Phenothiazine-derivative (Systemic)*

# PROPAFENONE   Systemic

VA CLASSIFICATION (Primary): CV300
Commonly used brand name(s): *Rythmol*.

Note:   For a listing of dosage forms and brand names by country availability, see *Dosage Forms* section(s).

## Category
Antiarrhythmic.

## Indications
Note:   Bracketed information in the *Indications* section refers to uses that are not included in U.S. product labeling.

### Accepted
Arrhythmias, ventricular (treatment)—Propafenone is indicated for suppression of documented life-threatening ventricular arrhythmias, including sustained ventricular tachycardia.

[Arrhythmias, supraventricular (treatment)][1]—Propafenone may be used for the treatment of supraventricular arrhythmias such as, intranodal and extranodal (e.g., Wolff-Parkinson-White Syndrome) reentrant tachycardias. Data for use of propafenone in the treatment of atrial fibrillation/flutter are less convincing, although it may help some patients. Caution is warranted when administering propafenone to patients in atrial fibrillation/flutter and structural heart disease because of the possibility of serious proarrhythmia, including ventricular tachycardia.

### Unaccepted
Use of propafenone is not recommended in the U.S. for treatment of less severe arrhythmias such as nonsustained ventricular tachycardias or frequent premature ventricular contractions, even if patients are symptomatic, because of results of a study in patients following a myocardial infarction that found increased mortality in patients with non–life-threatening ventricular arrhythmias who were treated with encainide and flecainide.

[1]Not included in Canadian product labeling.

## Pharmacology/Pharmacokinetics

### Physicochemical characteristics
Molecular weight—377.91.
pKa—9.

### Mechanism of action/Effect
Reduces the inward sodium current in Purkinje and myocardial cells. Decreases excitability, conduction velocity, and automaticity in atrioventricular (AV) nodal, His-Purkinje, and intraventricular tissue, and causes a slight but significant prolongation of refractory periods in AV nodal tissue. The greatest effect is on the His-Purkinje system. Decreases the rate of rise of the action potential without markedly affecting its duration. Also, prolongs conduction velocity and effective refractory periods in accessory pathways in both directions. Electrophysiologic effects are greater in ischemic than in normal myocardial tissue. In the Vaughan Williams classification of antiarrhythmics, propafenone is considered to be a class IC agent.

### Other actions/effects
Negative inotropic effect. Has approximately one-fortieth the beta-adrenergic blocking activity of propranolol, which may become clinically significant in some patients. Has weak calcium channel blocking properties. Has local anesthetic activity approximately equal to that of procaine.

### Absorption
Rapid and nearly complete, with more than 90% of an oral dose absorbed. Systemic bioavailability ranges from 5 to 50%, reflecting significant first-pass metabolism. Such a wide range in systemic bioavailability is related to two factors. The presence of food increases bioavailability for extensive metabolizers (more than 90% of patients). In addition, bioavailability increases as dosage increases. Absolute bioavailability is 3.4% for a 150-mg tablet compared to 10.6% for a 300-mg tablet.

### Protein binding
Very high (97%).

### Biotransformation
Hepatic; significant first-pass effect. In over 90% of patients, rapidly and extensively metabolized to 2 active metabolites, 5-hydroxypropafenone and N-depropylpropafenone, which have antiarrhythmic activity comparable to propafenone but which are present in concentrations less than 20% of propafenone concentrations. In less than 10% of patients and in patients also receiving quinidine, more slowly metabolized (these patients also have a diminished ability to metabolize debrisoquin, encainide, metoprolol, and dextromethorphan); little, if any, 5-hydroxypropafenone is present in plasma.

### Half-life
In extensive metabolizers (more than 90% of patients)—2 to 10 hours.
In poor metabolizers (less than 10% of patients)—10 to 32 hours.

### Time to peak plasma concentration
1 to 3.5 hours.

### Time to steady-state plasma concentration
Multiple doses—4 to 5 days.

### Steady-state plasma concentrations
Wide interindividual variability. In extensive metabolizers, pharmacokinetics are nonlinear; because of saturable first-pass metabolism, a 3-fold increase in dose may result in a 10-fold increase in steady-state plasma concentrations; however, in poor metabolizers, pharmacokinetics are linear.

### Peak plasma concentration
In poor metabolizers, concentrations are 1.5 to 2 times those of extensive metabolizers at doses of 675 to 900 mg per day.

### Elimination
Renal—38% as metabolites; less than 1% as unchanged drug.
Fecal—53% as metabolites.

## Precautions to Consider

### Carcinogenicity
Studies in rats and mice at oral doses of up to 270 mg per kg of body weight (mg/kg) per day and 360 mg/kg per day, respectively, revealed no evidence of carcinogenicity.

### Mutagenicity
The mouse dominant lethal test, rat bone marrow chromosome analysis, Chinese hamster bone marrow and spermatogonia chromosome analysis, Chinese hamster micronucleus test, and Ames bacterial test were negative.

### Pregnancy/Reproduction
Fertility—A reversible reduction in sperm count (within normal range) occurred after short-term administration in humans, but chronic administration did not have this effect.

Reversible impairment of spermatogenesis occurs in monkeys, dogs, and rabbits after high intravenous doses.

Pregnancy—Adequate and well-controlled studies in humans have not been done.

Studies in rats and rabbits at doses of up to 40 and 10 times the maximum recommended human dose, respectively, have not shown that propafenone causes teratogenicity in the fetus; however, a perinatal and postnatal study in rats at doses of 6 times the maximum recommended human dose or greater found a dose-related increase in maternal and neonatal mortality, decreased maternal and pup body weight gain, and reduced neonatal physiological development.

FDA Pregnancy Category C.

### Breast-feeding
Propafenone and 5-OH-propafenone are excreted in breast milk at concentrations lower than those found in maternal plasma. However, problems in humans have not been documented.

### Pediatrics
Safety and efficacy have not been established. However, limited use of propafenone in neonates, infants, and children seems to indicate that the incidence of side effects in pediatric patients is similar to that reported in adults. Proarrhythmic effects have been reported in the pediatric population, as in the adult population, including an incident of sudden death which may or may not have been related to propafenone. Therefore, propafenone should be used with caution in pediatric patients.

### Geriatrics
Although appropriate studies on the relationship of age to the effects of propafenone have not been performed in the geriatric population, no geriatrics-specific problems have been documented to date. However, elderly patients are more likely to have age-related hepatic and renal function impairment, which may require dosage reduction in patients receiving propafenone.

### Drug interactions and/or related problems
The following drug interactions and/or related problems have been selected on the basis of their potential clinical significance (possible mechanism in parentheses where appropriate)—not necessarily inclusive (» = major clinical significance):

Anesthetics, local
   (concurrent use with propafenone may increase the risk of central nervous system [CNS] side effects)

Antiarrhythmics, other
   (although some antiarrhythmic agents may be used in combination for therapeutic advantage, combined use may sometimes potentiate risk of adverse cardiac effects)

Beta-adrenergic blocking agents
   (concurrent use with propafenone results in significant increases in plasma concentrations and half-life of propranolol and metoprolol, without affecting plasma propafenone concentrations; dosage reduction of the beta-blocker may be necessary)

Cimetidine
   (concurrent use of cimetidine produces a 20% [approximate] increase in plasma concentrations of propafenone; however, because of wide interindividual variability in plasma concentrations and, therefore, lack of direct correlation with clinical effect, effects of propafenone on electrocardiogram parameters are unchanged)

» Digoxin
   (concurrent use with propafenone results in an increase in serum digoxin concentrations ranging from 35 to 85%, which appears to be unrelated to digoxin renal clearance but which may be related to a decrease in volume of distribution and nonrenal clearance; careful monitoring of digoxin concentrations and dosage reduction of digoxin are recommended when propafenone is initiated; subsequent dosage adjustments should be based on plasma digoxin concentrations)

Quinidine
   (small doses completely inhibit hydroxylation of propafenone, effectively making patients poor metabolizers of propafenone; however, dosage adjustment of propafenone is usually not necessary)

» Warfarin
   (concurrent use with propafenone results in a significant increase [approximately 40%] in mean steady-state warfarin plasma concentrations, with a corresponding increase in prothrombin time of approximately 25%; monitoring of prothrombin time and appropriate adjustment of warfarin dosage are recommended during concurrent use)

### Laboratory value alterations
The following have been selected on the basis of their potential clinical significance (possible effect in parentheses where appropriate)—not necessarily inclusive (» = major clinical significance):

With physiology/laboratory test values
   Electrocardiogram (ECG) changes such as:
      QRS widening and
      PR prolongation
         (occur in most patients; dose-related)

Note: ECG changes produced by propafenone do not necessarily indicate efficacy, toxicity, or overdose.

   Antinuclear antibody (ANA) titers, positive
      (may occur rarely; reversible after withdrawal and sometimes during continued propafenone treatment; usually not symptomatic, but one case of lupus erythematosus, which reversed on withdrawal, has been reported)

### Medical considerations/Contraindications
The medical considerations/contraindications included have been selected on the basis of their potential clinical significance (reasons given in parentheses where appropriate)—not necessarily inclusive (» = major clinical significance).

*Except under special circumstances, this medication should not be used when the following medical problems exist:*

» Atrioventricular (AV) block, pre-existing second or third degree without pacemaker, or
» Right bundle branch block associated with a left hemiblock (bifascicular block) without pacemaker
    (risk of complete heart block)

*Risk-benefit should be considered when the following medical problems exist:*

Asthma or
Bronchospasm, nonallergenic (e.g., chronic bronchitis, emphysema)
    (because of its beta-adrenergic blocking effect, propafenone may promote bronchospasm)
» Cardiogenic shock or
» Sinus bradycardia
    (risk of further myocardial depression)
Cardiomyopathy
» Congestive heart failure
    (negative inotropic effect of propafenone; also, risk of further depression of myocardial contractility because of beta-adrenergic blocking activity of propafenone)
Hepatic function impairment
    (reduced first-pass effect results in increased bioavailability, to approximately 70%; increased half-life; dosage of propafenone should be reduced to approximately 20 to 30% of the usual dose, with careful monitoring)
Hypokalemia or hyperkalemia
    (effects of propafenone may be altered; any electrolyte imbalance should be corrected prior to beginning therapy with propafenone)
Hypotension, marked
    (may be aggravated)
Myocardial infarction, history of, especially with associated left ventricular function impairment
Renal function impairment
    (reduced elimination; dosage reduction may be necessary)
Sensitivity to propafenone
» Sick sinus syndrome
    (sinus node recovery time prolonged; sinus bradycardia, sinus pause, or sinus arrest may occur)
Caution is recommended in patients with permanent pacemakers or temporary pacing electrodes; propafenone may increase endocardial pacing thresholds and may suppress ventricular escape rhythms; use is not recommended in patients with existing poor thresholds or nonprogrammable pacemakers unless suitable pacing rescue is available.

**Patient monitoring**
The following may be especially important in patient monitoring (other tests may be warranted in some patients, depending on condition; » = major clinical significance):

» Electrocardiogram (ECG)
    (recommended prior to initiation of therapy and at periodic intervals during therapy to help assess efficacy and detect possible proarrhythmic effects)

## Side/Adverse Effects

Note: In the National Heart, Lung and Blood Institute's Cardiac Arrhythmia Suppression Trial (CAST), encainide and flecainide treatment were found to be associated with excessive mortality or increased nonfatal cardiac arrest rate as compared with placebo in patients with asymptomatic, non–life-threatening arrhythmias who had a recent myocardial infarction. The implications of these results for other patient populations or other antiarrhythmic agents are uncertain.

Adverse cardiac effects reported with propafenone administration include new or exacerbated ventricular arrhythmias in about 4.7% of patients; new or exacerbated congestive heart failure in 1% or less of patients; first, second, or third degree atrioventricular (AV) block in 2.5%, 0.6%, and 0.2% of patients, respectively; sinus bradycardia in 1.5% of patients; and rarely, sinus pause or sinus arrest.

Incidence of cardiac and other effects is at least partially dose-related.

Signs of overdose, usually most severe within 3 hours of ingestion, include hypotension, somnolence, bradycardia, AV dissociation, and intra-atrial and intraventricular conduction disturbances; asystole may develop. Convulsions and high grade ventricular arrhythmias have been reported rarely.

The following side/adverse effects have been selected on the basis of their potential clinical significance (possible signs and symptoms in parentheses where appropriate)—not necessarily inclusive:

**Those indicating need for medical attention**
Incidence more frequent
    *Ventricular tachyarrhythmias* (fast or irregular heartbeat)
Note: Like other antiarrhythmic agents, propafenone may induce new arrhythmias and/or worsen an existing arrhythmia. *Ventricular tachyarrhythmias* are dose-related and potentially fatal; incidence increased in patients with sustained ventricular tachycardia, coronary artery disease, or history of myocardial infarction. Proarrhythmic effects usually occur during the first week of therapy, although effects are also seen later.
Incidence less frequent
    *Angina* (chest pain); *bradycardia* (slow heartbeat); *congestive heart failure* (shortness of breath, swelling of feet or lower legs)
Incidence rare
    *Agranulocytosis* (fever or chills); *conduction abnormalities, including atrioventricular block, bundle branch block; hypotension* (low blood pressure); *joint pain; supraventricular tachyarrhythmias, including atrial flutter, atrial fibrillation; trembling or shaking*

**Those indicating need for medical attention only if they continue or are bothersome**
Incidence more frequent
    *Dizziness; taste disturbance* (change in taste; bitter or metallic taste)
Incidence less frequent
    *Blurred vision; constipation or diarrhea; dryness of mouth; headache; nausea and/or vomiting; skin rash; unusual tiredness or weakness*

## Overdose
For more information on the management of overdose or unintentional ingestion, **contact a Poison Control Center** (see *Poison Control Center Listing*).

**Treatment of overdose**
Treatment is primarily supportive and symptomatic and may include: Defibrillation and infusion of dopamine and isoproterenol to control rhythm and blood pressure; intravenous diazepam for convulsions; mechanical respiratory assistance and external cardiac massage.

## Patient Consultation
As an aid to patient consultation, refer to *Advice for the Patient, Propafenone (Systemic)*.

In providing consultation, consider emphasizing the following selected information (» = major clinical significance):

**Before using this medication**
» Conditions affecting use, especially:
    Sensitivity to propafenone
        Pregnancy—Reduces fertility in monkeys, dogs, and rabbits; in rats, causes increased maternal and neonatal mortality, decreased maternal and infant weight gain, and reduced neonatal development
    Other medications, especially digoxin or warfarin
    Other medical problems, especially second or third degree atrioventricular (AV) block, right bundle branch block associated with a left hemiblock, cardiogenic shock, congestive heart failure, sick sinus syndrome, or sinus bradycardia

**Proper use of this medication**
» Compliance with therapy; taking as directed even if feeling well
» Importance of not missing doses and taking at evenly spaced intervals
    Missed dose: Taking as soon as possible if remembered within 4 hours; not taking if remembered later; not doubling doses
» Proper storage

**Precautions while using this medication**
Regular visits to physician to check progress
Carrying medical identification card or bracelet
» Caution if any kind of surgery (including dental surgery) or emergency treatment is required
Caution when driving or doing things requiring alertness because of possible dizziness

**Side/adverse effects**
Signs of potential side effects, especially ventricular tachyarrhythmias, angina, congestive heart failure, agranulocytosis, bradycardia, conduction abnormalities, hypotension, joint pain, and trembling or shaking

## Propafenone (Systemic)

### General Dosing Information

Because of wide interindividual variability in plasma concentrations, careful titration of dosage is recommended. However, because steady-state concentrations are achieved after the same amount of time in both extensive and poor metabolizers, and because the difference in peak plasma concentrations decreases at high doses and the active 5-hydroxy metabolite is absent in poor metabolizers, the recommended dosage regimen is the same for both groups of patients.

Dosage increments should be made no more frequently than every 3 to 4 days.

It is recommended that treatment be initiated in the hospital because of the increased risk of proarrhythmic effects associated with propafenone administration.

In general, it is recommended that previous antiarrhythmic therapy be withdrawn 2 to 5 half-lives before initiation of propafenone therapy.

In patients with pacemakers, pacing threshold should be monitored and programmed at periodic intervals during propafenone therapy.

### Oral Dosage Forms

#### PROPAFENONE HYDROCHLORIDE TABLETS

**Usual adult dose**
Antiarrhythmic—Ventricular or
[Antiarrhythmic—Supraventricular][1]—
  Oral, initially 150 mg every eight hours, increased, if necessary, after three to four days to 225 mg every eight hours (U.S. labeling) or 300 mg every twelve hours (Canadian labeling); may be further increased after an additional three to four days, if necessary, to 300 mg every eight hours.

**Usual pediatric dose**
Safety and efficacy have not been established.

**Strength(s) usually available**
U.S.—
  150 mg (Rx) [*Rythmol* (scored)].
  225 mg (Rx) [*Rythmol* (scored)].
  300 mg (Rx) [*Rythmol* (scored)].
Canada—
  150 mg (Rx) [*Rythmol*].
  300 mg (Rx) [*Rythmol* (scored)].

**Packaging and storage**
Store between 15 and 30 °C (59 and 86 °F), in a tight, light-resistant container, unless otherwise specified by manufacturer.

[1] Not included in Canadian product labeling.

### Selected Bibliography

Chow MS, Lebsack C, Hilleman D. Propafenone: A new antiarrhythmic agent. Clin Pharm 1988; 7: 869-77.

Harron DW, Brogden RN. Propafenone. A review of its pharmacodynamic and pharmacokinetic properties, and therapeutic use in the treatment of arrhythmias. Drugs 1987; 34: 617-47.

Funck-Brentano C, Kroemer HK, Lee JT, Roden DM. Propafenone. N Engl J Med 1990; 322(8): 518-25.

Revised: 10/07/92
Interim revision: 08/02/93

---

**PROPANTHELINE**—See *Anticholinergics/Antispasmodics (Systemic)*

---

**PROPIOMAZINE**—The *Propiomazine (Systemic)* monograph is not included in this published version of the USP DI database. Copies of the monograph are available on request from Micromedex, Inc. - Reprint Requests, 6200 S. Syracuse Way, Suite 300, Englewood, CO 80111; telephone (303) 486-6400; telefax (303) 486-6464; Email: USPDI@MDX.COM.

---

# PROPOFOL   Systemic

VA CLASSIFICATION (Primary/Secondary): CN203/CN206; CN309
Commonly used brand name(s): *Diprivan*.
Another commonly used name is disoprofol.
Note: For a listing of dosage forms and brand names by country availability, see *Dosage Forms* section(s).

## Category
Anesthetic, general; anesthesia adjunct; sedative-hypnotic.

## Indications

### Accepted
Anesthesia, general or
Anesthesia, general, adjunct—Propofol is indicated for the induction of general anesthesia. It is also indicated for maintenance of anesthesia utilizing balanced techniques with other appropriate agents such as opioids and inhalation anesthetics.

Sedation—Propofol is indicated for sedation in critically ill patients confined to intensive care units.

Propofol is indicated to produce sedation or amnesia as a supplement to local or regional anesthetics, and in diagnostic procedures, such as endoscopy (i.e., Monitored Anesthesia Care [MAC]).

Although cardiovascular, respiratory, and sedative effects must be carefully monitored, propofol provides good control of depth of sedation, and the rapid return of spontaneous ventilation following discontinuation of propofol infusion allows early extubation. Tachyphylaxis, delayed awakening, or cumulative effects have not been reported after prolonged administration of propofol as they have with prolonged infusion of thiopental, diazepam, or midazolam. In addition, propofol does not suppress adrenocortical function as does etomidate.

## Pharmacology/Pharmacokinetics

**Physicochemical characteristics**
Molecular weight—178.28.
pH—Propofol emulsion: 7 to 8.5.

**Mechanism of action/Effect**
Propofol is a short-acting hypnotic. Its mechanism of action has not been well-defined.

**Other actions/effects**
Hemodynamic effects:
  Propofol's hemodynamic effects are generally more pronounced than those of other intravenous anesthetic agents. Arterial hypotension, with readings decreased by as much as 30% or more, has been reported, possibly due to inhibition of sympathetic vasoconstrictor nerve activity. Hypotensive effects are generally proportional to dose and rate of administration of propofol, and may be potentiated by opioid analgesics. Endotracheal intubation and surgical stimulation may increase arterial pressure; increases in heart rate and/or blood pressure to greater than baseline values, which occur frequently with other agents, are not as significant with propofol, possibly due to central sympatholytic and/or vagotonic effects. Propofol may also decrease systemic vascular resistance, myocardial blood flow, and oxygen consumption. The mechanism of these effects may involve direct vasodilation and negative inotropy. Effects such as decreased stroke volume and cardiac output have been demonstrated in some studies.
Respiratory effects:
  Propofol is a respiratory depressant, frequently producing apnea that may persist for longer than 60 seconds, depending on factors such as premedication, rate of administration, dose administered, and presence of hyperventilation or hyperoxia. In addition, propofol may produce significant decreases in respiratory rate, minute volume, tidal volume, mean inspiratory flow rate, and functional residual capacity. These respiratory depressant effects may be the result of depression of the central inspiratory drive as opposed to a change in central timing. The ventilatory depressant effects of propofol may be counteracted by painful surgical stimulation.
Cerebral effects:
  Propofol decreases cerebral blood flow, cerebral metabolic oxygen consumption, and intracranial pressure, and increases cerebrovascular resistance. It does not appear to affect cerebrovascular reactivity to changes in arterial carbon dioxide tension.

Other effects:
  Preliminary findings suggest that in patients with normal intraocular pressure, propofol decreases intraocular pressure by as much as 30 to 50%. This decrease may be associated with a concomitant decrease in systemic vascular resistance.
  Clinical studies have shown that propofol does not cause significant signs of histamine release or significant increases in plasma immunoglobulin or complement $C_3$ levels. Respiratory resistance after tracheal intubation is lower when propofol is used for induction of anesthesia than when thiopental or high-dose etomidate is used for induction of anesthesia.
  Although propofol has the potential for affecting adrenal steroidogenesis, it does not appear to block cortisol and aldosterone secretion in response to surgical stress or adrenocorticotropic hormone (ACTH) in clinical practice. Although transient decreases in plasma cortisol concentrations have occurred, these reductions have not been sustained.
  Propofol appears to have no analgesic activity. In addition, animal studies have demonstrated no significant effect on coagulation profiles.
  Limited experience with propofol in susceptible patients and animal studies has not demonstrated a propensity to induce malignant hyperthermia.
  Propofol has antiemetic properties. Anesthesia with propofol results in less nausea and vomiting than anesthesia with desflurane, enflurane, isoflurane, methohexital, nitrous oxide, or thiopental.

**Distribution**
Propofol is rapidly and extensively distributed in the body. It crosses the blood-brain barrier quickly, and its short duration of action is due to rapid redistribution from the CNS to other tissues, high metabolic clearance, and high lipophilicity.
Volumes of distribution—
  Initial apparent ($Vol_D$): 13 to 76 liters (L).
  Steady-state ($Vol_{DSS}$): 171 to 349 L.
  Elimination ($Vol_D$): 209 to 1008 L.
  Steady-state ($Vol_{DSS}$) in pediatric patients: 9.5 ± 3.71 liters per kg of body weight (L/kg).

**Protein binding**
Very high (95 to 99%).

**Biotransformation**
Hepatic; rapidly undergoes glucuronide conjugation to inactive metabolites. An unidentified route of extrahepatic metabolism may also exist, suggested by the fact that propofol clearance exceeds estimated hepatic blood flow.

**Half-life**
Distribution—
  Two distribution phases:
    Rapid—2 to 4 minutes.
    Slower—30 to 64 minutes.
Elimination—
  Terminal elimination half-life is 3 to 12 hours; prolonged administration of propofol may result in a longer duration.
Note: The long terminal elimination half-life of propofol does not reflect elimination, as more than 70% is eliminated during the first 2 phases. Some investigators believe that the second exponential phase half-life (30 to 64 minutes) best explains the properties of propofol in clinical practice.
Other—
  Blood-brain equilibration half-life: 2.9 minutes.

**Onset of action**
Loss of consciousness occurs rapidly and smoothly, usually within 40 seconds (one arm-brain circulation time) from the start of intravenous injection of propofol. Loss of consciousness is dependent on the dose administered, the rate of administration, and the extent of premedication.

**Plasma concentrations**
Propofol concentrations of 1.5 to 6 mcg per mL (8.42 to 33.66 micromoles per liter [micromoles/L]) will maintain hypnosis, although needs vary with type of surgery and use of other anesthetic agents.

**Duration of action**
Mean duration following a single bolus dose of 2 to 2.5 mg per kg of body weight is 3 to 5 minutes.

**Time to recovery**
Recovery from anesthesia with propofol is rapid, with minimal psychomotor impairment. Emergence following induction (with 2 to 2.5 mg of propofol per kg) and maintenance (with 0.1 to 0.2 mg of propofol per kg per minute) for up to 2 hours occurs in most patients within 8 minutes. If an opioid has been used, recovery may take up to 19 minutes.

Recovery occurs faster than recovery following the use of etomidate, methohexital, midazolam, or thiopental. When anesthesia has included use of an opioid with propofol, recovery has occurred more quickly than with similar use of etomidate, midazolam, or thiopental.
Many investigators have noted clearheadedness in patients emerging from propofol anesthesia, and less residual impairment of performance than in patients who received methohexital has been reported.

**Elimination**
Renal; approximately 70% of a dose is excreted in the urine within 24 hours after administration, and 90% is excreted within 5 days. Clearance of propofol ranges from 1.6 to 3.4 liters per minute in healthy 70 kg patients. As the age of the patient increases, total body clearance of propofol may decrease. Clearance rates ranging from 1.4 to 2.2 liters per minute in patients 18 to 35 years of age have been reported, in contrast to clearance rates of 1 to 1.8 liters per minute in patients 65 to 80 years of age.
Note: Pharmacokinetic parameters of propofol appear to be unaffected by gender, obesity, chronic hepatic cirrhosis, and chronic renal failure.

## Precautions to Consider

**Carcinogenicity**
Studies have not been done.

**Mutagenicity**
The Ames mutation test using *Salmonella* species, gene mutation/gene conversion using *Saccharomyces cerevisiae*, cytogenetic studies in Chinese hamsters, and a mouse micronucleus test have failed to demonstrate mutagenic potential by propofol.

**Pregnancy/Reproduction**
Fertility—Studies in rats given doses up to 6 times the human dose for varying lengths of time have shown no evidence of impaired fertility.
Pregnancy—Propofol crosses the placenta. Adequate and well-controlled studies in humans have not been done.
Studies in animals have shown propofol to cause increased maternal deaths in rats and rabbits and decreased pup survival during the lactating period when the dams received 6 times the recommended human dose.
FDA Pregnancy Category B.
Labor and delivery—A study was conducted in 74 patients comparing the use of propofol with that of thiamylal-isoflurane for induction and maintenance of anesthesia during cesarean section. The study did not show any problems ec the mothers or in the neonates with the use of propofol. There was no difference between the neonates in the two groups in Apgar scores or the neurological and adaptive capacity scores (NACS). However, the manufacturer states that use of propofol is not recommended since data are insufficient to support its use in obstetrics, including cesarean section deliveries.

**Breast-feeding**
Propofol is distributed into breast milk. However, the effects of oral administration of small amounts of propofol are not known.

**Pediatrics**
Appropriate studies with propofol for sedation have not been performed in the pediatric population. There are case reports in the medical literature of pediatric patients developing metabolic acidosis after receiving propofol for sedation in the intensive care unit (ICU). Rarely, deaths have occurred. The role of propofol in these deaths is controversial. Other causes of metabolic acidosis could not be ruled out, and a causal relationship could not be established.
Note: Propofol is approved by the FDA for use in pediatric patients 3 years of age and older for induction and maintenance of anesthesia and as a component of balanced anesthesia.

**Geriatrics**
Dosage requirements are lower in geriatric patients than in younger adult patients, probably due to pharmacokinetic differences rather than pharmacodynamic differences in geriatric patients. Lower induction doses and a slower maintenance infusion rate should be used in geriatric patients, due to reduced total body clearance and volume of distribution in these patients.

**Drug interactions and/or related problems**
The following drug interactions and/or related problems have been selected on the basis of their potential clinical significance (possible mechanism in parentheses where appropriate)—not necessarily inclusive (» = major clinical significance):
Note: Combinations containing any of the following medications, depending on the amount present, may also interact with this medication.

» Alcohol or
» CNS depression–producing medications, other, including those commonly used for preanesthetic medication or induction or supplementation of anesthesia (see *Appendix II*)
   (concurrent administration may increase the CNS-depressant, respiratory-depressant, or hypotensive effects of propofol, as well as decreasing anesthetic requirements and prolonging recovery from anesthesia; dosage adjustments may be required; propofol may also decrease the emetic effects of some opioid drugs)
  Droperidol
   (droperidol may compete with propofol for binding sites in the chemoreceptor trigger zone; concurrent use of propofol and droperidol to control nausea and vomiting is less effective than using propofol alone)

### Medical considerations/Contraindications
The medical considerations/contraindications included have been selected on the basis of their potential clinical significance (reasons given in parentheses where appropriate)—not necessarily inclusive (» = major clinical significance).

*Risk-benefit should be considered when the following medical problems exist:*

Circulatory disorders or
Compromised cardiovascular function
   (may be aggravated by cardiovascular-depressant and hypotensive effects)
Disorders of lipid metabolism, such as primary hyperlipoproteinemia, diabetic hyperlipemia, or pancreatitis
   (may be aggravated by emulsion vehicle of propofol)
Increased intracranial pressure or
Impaired cerebral circulation
   (substantial decreases in mean arterial pressure and cerebral perfusion may occur)
Sensitivity to propofol or its emulsion vehicle
Caution is also recommended in geriatric, debilitated, and/or hypovolemic patients, because they may require lower induction and maintenance doses.

## Side/Adverse Effects
Note: Postoperative infections and subsequent deaths have been reported following the use of propofol that was not administered using strict aseptic technique.
   Rarely, a clinical syndrome including bronchospasm, erythema, and hypotension has occurred shortly after administration of propofol, and sequelae including anoxic brain damage and death have been reported; concurrent use of other agents makes a causal relationship unclear.

The following side/adverse effects have been selected on the basis of their potential clinical significance (possible signs and symptoms in parentheses where appropriate)—not necessarily inclusive:

### Those indicating need for medical attention
Incidence more frequent
   *Apnea; bradycardia; hypotension*

Incidence less frequent or rare
   *Hypertension; perioperative myoclonia, rarely including opisthotonus; pancreatitis* (abdominal pain)—symptoms may not occur until after discharge from medical care following use of propofol

### Those indicating need for medical attention only if they continue or are bothersome
Incidence more frequent
   *Involuntary muscle movements, temporary; nausea and/or vomiting; pain, burning, or stinging at injection site*
   Note: *Excitatory movements* reportedly occur more often than with thiopental but less often than with etomidate or methohexital.
      *Pain* is usually mild and short-lived, and may be decreased by using the larger veins of the forearm or the antecubital fossa or a dedicated intravenous catheter. Pain may be decreased by prior intravenous injection of 10 to 20 mg of lidocaine. Post-injection thrombosis or phlebitis is rare.
Incidence less frequent or rare
   *Abdominal cramping; cough; dizziness; fever; flushing; headache; hiccups; tingling, numbness, or coldness at injection site*

## Overdose
For specific information on the management of a propofol overdose, see:
  • *Atropine* in *Anticholinergics/Antispasmodics* monograph; and/or
  • *Sympathomimetic Agents—Cardiovascular Use (Parenteral-Systemic)* monograph.

For more information on the management of overdose, **contact a Poison Control Center** (see *Poison Control Center Listing*).

### Clinical effects of overdose
The following effects have been selected on the basis of their potential clinical significance (possible signs and symptoms in parentheses where appropriate)—not necessarily inclusive:

Acute
   *Cardiovascular depression; respiratory depression*

### Treatment of overdose
Specific treatment—
   Discontinuation of propofol.
   For respiratory depression: artificial ventilation with oxygen.
   For cardiovascular depression: elevation of legs, increasing flow rate of intravenous fluids, and administration of pressor agents and/or anticholinergic agents.
Monitoring—
   Patients should be continuously monitored for signs of significant hypotension and/or bradycardia.

## Patient Consultation
As an aid to patient consultation, refer to *Advice for the Patient, Anesthetics, General (Systemic)*.
In providing consultation, consider emphasizing the following selected information (» = major clinical significance):

### Before using this medication
» Conditions affecting use, especially:
   Sensitivity to propofol or its emulsion vehicle
   Pregnancy—Propofol crosses the placenta
   Use of propofol is not recommended in labor and delivery because data are insufficient to support its use in obstetrics
   Use in the elderly—Lower induction and maintenance doses are recommended
   Other medications, especially other CNS depressants

### Proper use of this medication
Proper dosing

### Precautions after receiving this medication
Possibility of psychomotor impairment following use of anesthetics; for about 24 hours following anesthesia, using added caution in driving or performing other tasks requiring alertness and coordination
Avoiding use of alcohol or other CNS depressants within 24 hours following anesthesia except as directed by physician or dentist

### Side/adverse effects
Signs of potential side effects, especially pancreatitis

## General Dosing Information
**Propofol should be administered only by individuals qualified in the use of general anesthetics. Appropriate resuscitative and endotracheal intubation equipment, oxygen, and medications for prevention and treatment of anesthetic emergencies must be immediately available. Airway patency must be maintained at all times.**

Propofol emulsion is for intravenous administration only. Although clinical experience and animal studies have shown that inadvertent intra-arterial injection of propofol usually produces minimal tissue reaction, intra-arterial injection of propofol is not recommended.

To minimize the pain, burning, or stinging patients may experience at the site of injection of propofol, a larger vein of the forearm or the antecubital fossa may be used as the infusion site. Pretreatment of the injection site with one mL of 1% lidocaine may also decrease the incidence of this side effect.

Dosage of propofol must be individualized for each patient, with the dose titrated to achieve the desired clinical effect. Lower doses are usually required for elderly, debilitated, or higher risk surgical patients, or those with circulatory disorders. The dosage of intravenously administered propofol should be adjusted according to the type and amount of premedication used.

Rapid intravenous injection of propofol should not be used in elderly, debilitated, hypovolemic, or higher risk surgical patients. Rapid intravenous injection of propofol in these patients may result in cardiopulmonary depression including hypotension, apnea, airway obstruction and/or oxygen desaturation.

When propofol is administered by infusion, it is recommended that drop counters, syringe pumps, or volumetric pumps be utilized to control infusion rates.

When nitrous oxide, oxygen, and propofol are used for maintenance of general anesthesia, supplemental analgesic agents are generally required; neuromuscular blocking agents may also be required. Concurrent use of propofol with neuromuscular blocking agents does not significantly alter the onset, intensity, or duration of action of these agents.

Propofol injection contains 0.005% disodium edetate, but it is not an antimicrobially preserved product under USP standards. The vehicle is capable of supporting the rapid growth of microorganisms, and particulate or bacterial contamination may be difficult to detect because propofol injection is opaque. Rarely, failure to use strict aseptic technique has resulted in sepsis in patients to whom contaminated solution was administered. Therefore, strict aseptic technique must be maintained, and propofol injection should be administered promptly after opening. Unused portions of the injection, as well as reservoirs, intravenous lines, or solutions containing propofol injection, must be discarded at the end of the procedure or within 12 hours (6 hours if propofol was transferred from the original container).

Propofol should not be infused through filters with pore size smaller than 5 microns because infusion through a smaller filter may cause breakdown of the emulsion.

## Parenteral Dosage Forms

### PROPOFOL INJECTION

#### Usual adult and adolescent dose

Dosage must be individualized and titrated to the desired clinical effect; however, as a general guideline—
Anesthesia, general (induction)
Adults up to 55 years of age and/or American Society of Anesthesiologists (ASA) I or II patients:
Intravenous, 2 to 2.5 mg per kg of body weight (approximately 40 mg every ten seconds until onset of induction).
Cardiac patients:
Intravenous, 0.5 to 1.5 mg per kg of body weight (approximately 20 mg every ten seconds until onset of induction).
Elderly, debilitated, hypovolemic, and/or ASA III or IV patients:
Intravenous, 1 to 1.5 mg per kg of body weight (approximately 20 mg every ten seconds until onset of induction).
Neurosurgical patients:
Intravenous, 1 to 2 mg per kg of body weight (approximately 20 mg every ten seconds until onset of induction).
Note: Slow injection of the induction dose of propofol may result in longer induction times and a lower percentage of successful inductions, probably due to rapid redistribution from the CNS; however, slow injection of doses is preferable, in order to diminish some of the cardiovascular effects.

Rapid intravenous injection of propofol should not be used in elderly, debilitated, hypovolemic, or higher-risk surgical patients. Rapid intravenous injection of propofol in these patients may result in cardiopulmonary depression including hypotension, apnea, airway obstruction and/or oxygen desaturation.

Anesthesia, general, adjunct (maintenance)
Adults up to 55 years of age and/or ASA I or II patients:
Intravenous infusion, 100 to 200 mcg (0.1 to 0.2 mg) per kg of body weight per minute (6 to 12 mg per kg of body weight per hour), with 60 to 70% nitrous oxide and oxygen.
Note: During the initial ten to fifteen minutes following induction, higher infusion rates of 150 to 200 mcg (0.15 to 0.2 mg) per kg of body weight per minute are generally required. Infusion rates should subsequently be decreased by 30 to 50% during the first half-hour of maintenance.

Infusion rates should always be titrated downward in the absence of light anesthesia to avoid administration of propofol at rates higher than clinically necessary. In general, rates of 50 to 100 mcg (0.05 to 0.1 mg) per kg of body weight per minute should be achieved during maintenance to optimize recovery times.
Intravenous intermittent injection, 20 to 50 mg increments, administered as needed. Alternatively, some clinicians recommend increments of 500 mcg (0.5 mg) per kg of body weight.
Adults receiving propofol for maintenance of general anesthesia for cardiac surgery:
Intravenous infusion, 50 to 150 mcg (0.05 to 0.15 mg) per kg of body weight per minute (3 to 9 mg per kg of body weight per hour). The use of an opioid as the primary anesthetic will result in a need for dosing of propofol at the lower end of this range, and the use of low-dose opioid as a secondary agent will result in a need for dosing of propofol at the higher end of this range.
Adults receiving propofol for maintenance of general anesthesia for neurosurgery:
Intravenous infusion, 100 to 200 mcg (0.1 to 0.2 mg) per kg of body weight per minute (6 to 12 mg per kg of body weight per hour).
Elderly, debilitated, hypovolemic, and/or ASA III or IV patients:
Intravenous infusion, 50 to 100 mcg (0.05 to 0.1 mg) per kg of body weight per minute (3 to 6 mg per kg of body weight per hour).
Sedation
Intensive care:
Intravenous infusion, 27 mcg (0.027 mg) per kg of body weight per minute (1.62 mg per kg of body weight per hour).
Note: The mean requirement for sedation in the intensive care unit is 27 mcg per kg of body weight per minute, but the requirements vary widely, from 2.8 to 130 mcg per kg of body weight per minute. Lower rates of administration may be sufficient for patients receiving benzodiazepines or opioid analgesics. Older patients (i.e., those 55 years of age and older) require less propofol for sedation than younger patients (i.e., those up to 55 years of age) (20 and 38 mcg per kg of body weight per minute, respectively). In all cases, the infusion should be initiated slowly and titrated to effect.

Monitored Anesthesia Care (MAC):
Initiation: Intravenous infusion, 100 to 150 mcg (0.1 to 0.15 mg) per kg of body weight per minute (6 to 9 mg per kg of body weight per hour) for three to five minutes; or slow intravenous injection over three to five minutes, 0.5 mg per kg of body weight.
Maintenance: Intravenous infusion, 25 to 50 mcg (0.025 to 0.05 mg) per kg of body weight per minute (1.5 to 3 mg per kg of body weight per hour).
Note: During the initial ten to fifteen minutes following induction, higher infusion rates of 25 to 75 mcg (0.025 to 0.075 mg) per kg of body weight per minute (1.5 to 4.5 mg per kg of body weight per hour) may be needed.

In titrating to clinical effect, two minutes should be allowed to observe effects after an adjustment in dose. When propofol is used to provide MAC for elderly, debilitated, or ASA III or IV patients, the rate of administration and dose should be reduced to eighty percent of the usual adult dose.

#### Usual pediatric dose

Anesthesia, general (induction)—
Pediatric patients (ASA I or II) 3 years of age or older: Intravenous, 2.5 to 3.5 mg per kg of body weight.
Note: Propofol is approved for induction of anesthesia in pediatric patients 3 years of age and older. However, propofol has been used in pediatric patients younger than 3 years of age for induction of anesthesia. In one study, infants 1 to 6 months of age required 3 mg per kg of body weight for induction of anesthesia.
Anesthesia, general, adjunct (maintenance)—
Pediatric patients (ASA I or II) 3 years of age or older: Intravenous infusion, 125 to 150 mcg (0.125 to 0.15 mg) per kg of body weight per minute (7.5 to 9 mg per kg of body weight per hour) in most instances.
Note: During the initial one-half hour following induction, higher infusion rates of 200 to 300 mcg (0.2 to 0.3 mg) per kg of body weight per minute (12 to 18 mg per kg of body weight per hour) may be needed. After one-half hour, the dose may be decreased to 125 to 150 mcg (0.125 to 0.15 mg) per kg of body weight per minute (7.5 to 9 mg per kg of body weight per hour) in most cases.

Children 5 years of age and younger may require larger weight-adjusted maintenance doses than older children.

#### Strength(s) usually available

U.S.—
10 mg per mL (Rx) [*Diprivan* (soybean oil 10% w/v; glycerol 2.25% w/v; purified egg phosphatide [lecithin] 1.2% w/v; disodium edetate 0.005%)].
Canada—
10 mg per mL (Rx) [*Diprivan* (soybean oil 10% w/v; glycerol 2.25% w/v; purified egg phosphatide [lecithin] 1.2% w/v; disodium edetate 0.005%)].

## Propofol (Systemic)

**Packaging and storage**
Store between 4 and 22 °C (40 and 72 °F). Refrigeration is not recommended. Protect from light.

**Preparation of dosage form**
Propofol is compatible with 5% dextrose in water, lactated Ringer's solution, lactated Ringer's and 5% dextrose in water, and combinations of 5% dextrose with 0.45% or 0.2% sodium chloride.

If propofol is diluted prior to administration, only 5% Dextrose Injection USP should be used as a diluent, and the final concentration should not be less than 2 mg per mL to preserve the emulsion base. The dilution is more stable in glass than in plastic.

**Stability**
Propofol injection contains 0.005% disodium edetate, but it is not an antimicrobially preserved product under USP standards. The vehicle is capable of supporting the rapid growth of microorganisms, and particulate or bacterial contamination may be difficult to detect because propofol injection is opaque. Therefore, strict aseptic technique must be maintained. Propofol injection should be administered promptly after opening. Unused portions of the injection, as well as reservoirs, IV lines, or solutions containing propofol injection, must be discarded at the end of the procedure or within 12 hours (6 hours if propofol was transferred from the original container).

Propofol should not be used if there is evidence of separation of the emulsion phases.

**Incompatibilities**
The manufacturer states that propofol emulsion should not be mixed with other therapeutic agents prior to administration. In addition, propofol should not be coadministered through the same IV catheter with blood or plasma; although the clinical significance is not known, *in vitro* studies have shown that the globular component of the emulsion vehicle has formed aggregates when in contact with human and animal blood, plasma, and serum.

**Auxiliary labeling**
- Shake well before use.
- Protect from light.

**Selected Bibliography**
Sebel P, Lowdon J. Propofol: a new intravenous anesthetic. Anesthesiology 1989; 71: 260-77.
White PF. Propofol: pharmacokinetics and pharmacodynamics. Seminars in Anesthesia 1988; 7 Suppl 1: 4-20.
Fulton B, Sorkin E. Propofol: an overview of its pharmacology and a review of its clinical efficacy in intensive care sedation. Drugs 1995; 50: 636-57.

Revised: 07/07/98

---

**PROPOXYPHENE** — See *Opioid (Narcotic) Analgesics (Systemic)*

---

**PROPRANOLOL** — See *Beta-adrenergic Blocking Agents (Systemic)*

---

**PROPYLTHIOURACIL** — See *Antithyroid Agents (Systemic)*

---

# PROTAMINE Systemic

BAN: Protamine sulphate
VA CLASSIFICATION (Primary): BL118
Note: For a listing of dosage forms and brand names by country availability, see *Dosage Forms* section(s).

## Category
Antidote (to heparin).

## Indications
Note: Bracketed information in the *Indications* section refers to uses that are not included in U.S. product labeling.

**Accepted**
Toxicity, heparin (treatment) or
[Toxicity, enoxaparin (treatment)][1]—Protamine is indicated in the treatment of severe heparin overdose resulting in hemorrhage; it is also used to neutralize the hemorrhagic effects following overdose of the low molecular weight heparin, enoxaparin. Transfusion of whole blood or fresh frozen plasma may also be required to replace lost volume if hemorrhaging has been severe; this may dilute, but will not neutralize the effects of, heparin.

Protamine is also indicated for administration following cardiac or arterial surgery or dialysis procedures when required to neutralize the effects of heparin administered during extracorporeal circulation.

**Unaccepted**
Protamine is not used in treating minor heparin overdose that may respond to withdrawal of heparin, or in treating hemorrhage not caused by heparin.

[1] Not included in Canadian product labeling.

## Pharmacology/Pharmacokinetics
**Mechanism of action/Effect**
Protamine is a strongly basic substance that combines with the strongly acidic heparin to form a stable complex. Heparin produces its effects indirectly, apparently by forming a complex with and producing a conformational change in the antithrombin III (heparin cofactor) molecule, resulting in potentiation of antithrombin III activity. One study has indicated that by combining with heparin, protamine causes a dissociation of the heparin-antithrombin III complex, resulting in loss of anticoagulant activity.

**Other actions/effects**
Protamine has some anticoagulant activity of its own when administered in the absence of heparin or in doses larger than those required to neutralize heparin, but it is not used as an anticoagulant. This anticoagulant effect may be caused by protamine's antithromboplastin activity, which results in inhibition of thrombin generation.

**Onset of action**
30 seconds to 1 minute.

**Duration of action**
2 hours; dependent on body temperature.

## Precautions to Consider

**Pregnancy/Reproduction**
Pregnancy—Studies have not been done in humans.
Studies have not been done in animals.
FDA Pregnancy Category C.

**Breast-feeding**
It is not known whether protamine is distributed into breast milk. However, problems in humans have not been documented.

**Pediatrics**
Appropriate studies performed to date have not demonstrated pediatrics-specific problems that would limit the usefulness of protamine in children.

**Geriatrics**
Appropriate studies on the relationship of age to the effects of protamine have not been performed in the geriatric population. However, geriatrics-specific problems that would limit the usefulness of this medication in the elderly are not expected.

**Medical considerations/Contraindications**
The medical considerations/contraindications included have been selected on the basis of their potential clinical significance (reasons given in parentheses where appropriate)—not necessarily inclusive (» = major clinical significance).

*Risk-benefit should be considered when the following medical problems exist:*

» Allergic reaction to protamine, history of
  Antibodies to protamine in the sera of infertile or vasectomized men or
  Prior exposure to protamine or other protamine-containing medications, e.g., protamine insulin
    (increased risk of allergic reaction)

**Patient monitoring**
The following may be especially important in patient monitoring (other tests may be warranted in some patients, depending on condition; » = major clinical significance):
Blood coagulation tests
(recommended as a guide to protamine efficacy and dosage; in the operating room, activated clotting time [ACT], either manual or automated, is most often used to monitor neutralization of large doses of heparin)
Blood titration tests with protamine
(may be necessary as a guide to protamine dosage, especially when large doses of heparin have been administered)

## Side/Adverse Effects

The following side/adverse effects have been selected on the basis of their potential clinical significance (possible signs and symptoms in parentheses where appropriate)—not necessarily inclusive:

**Those indicating need for medical attention**
Incidence more frequent—usually caused by too-rapid administration of medication
*Bradycardia; cardiovascular collapse or shock*—may be caused by a direct myocardial effect and/or peripheral vasodilatation; *decrease in blood pressure, sudden*—may reach hypotensive levels; *dyspnea*
Incidence less frequent
*Anaphylactic or anaphylactoid reaction; bleeding*—may be caused by protamine overdose or by a rebound of heparin activity; *hypertension, pulmonary and/or systemic; noncardiogenic pulmonary edema*—reported in patients on cardiopulmonary bypass undergoing cardiovascular surgery
Note: *Anaphylactic or anaphylactoid reactions* may be more likely to occur in patients with a history of allergy to fish (because protamine is prepared from the sperm or mature testes of fish [salmon or related species]), patients who have been previously exposed to protamine, and patients with protamine antibodies; however, a definite relationship between allergy to fish and allergic reactions to protamine sulfate has not been established. In addition, a reaction similar to anaphylaxis may occur when protamine is administered too rapidly.

**Those indicating need for medical attention only if they continue or are bothersome**
Incidence less frequent or rare
*Back pain*—reported rarely in conscious patients undergoing procedures such as cardiac catheterization; *feeling of warmth; feeling of weakness; flushing; nausea or vomiting*

## General Dosing Information

Protamine sulfate is administered by intravenous injection only. A concentration of 10 mg of protamine sulfate per mL is usually used.

Facilities for treating shock and other symptoms of anaphylaxis should be available whenever protamine sulfate is administered.

Prior to administration of protamine, it is recommended that care be taken to assure that the patient's blood volume is adequate. Hypovolemia may increase the risk of peripheral vasodilatation, which may lead to cardiovascular collapse, especially following too-rapid administration of protamine.

The stated doses are intended as a guideline only. It is strongly recommended that blood coagulation tests be used to determine optimum dosage of protamine, especially when neutralizing large doses of heparin given during cardiac or arterial surgery.

Tests used to monitor protamine therapy include activated clotting time (ACT), activated partial thromboplastin time (APTT), thrombin time (TT), and/or direct titration of a sample of the patient's blood with protamine. The tests should be performed at least 5 to 15 minutes following initial administration of protamine and repeated as necessary. Neutralization of heparin used during extracorporeal circulation may be monitored using sequential ACT testing with a dose/response curve that correlates the test results with the quantity of heparin remaining to be neutralized. However, hypothermia may decrease the accuracy of these tests.

APTT and TT may not be useful in monitoring protamine therapy after administration of enoxaparin because enoxaparin, in therapeutic doses, does not alter the value of these tests.

Bleeding may recur if too much protamine, which has anticoagulant activity of its own, is administered or if the effects of heparin persist longer than the effects of protamine. The half-life of heparin is 60 to 360 minutes with an average of 90 minutes. The half-life is dose dependent (the larger the dose, the longer the half-life) and subject to intra- and interpatient variation. It has been proposed that the rebound of heparin effect may be caused by metabolism of protamine with resultant dissociation of the heparin-protamine complex and/or by release of heparin from storage or binding sites. Heparin rebound is especially likely to occur following administration of large doses of heparin, such as those used during cardiopulmonary bypass procedures, and has been reported to occur as late as 18 hours following initial complete neutralization of heparin. Prolonged monitoring of the patient is necessary so that additional doses of protamine may be administered if coagulation test results indicate that they are required.

As time elapses following intravenous administration of heparin, less protamine is required because of rapidly decreasing heparin blood concentrations. For example, 30 minutes after the intravenous administration of heparin, approximately one-half the amount of protamine sulfate is sufficient for neutralization. However, absorption of heparin may be prolonged following subcutaneous administration. For neutralizing heparin given subcutaneously, an initial loading dose of 25 to 50 mg of protamine sulfate, followed by administration of the remainder of the calculated protamine sulfate dose as an intravenous infusion over a period of 8 to 16 hours, has been recommended.

## Parenteral Dosage Forms

Note: Bracketed uses in the *Dosage Forms* section refer to categories of use and/or indications that are not included in U.S. product labeling.

### PROTAMINE SULFATE INJECTION USP

**Usual adult and adolescent dose**
Heparin toxicity—
Intravenous, 1 mg of protamine sulfate for approximately every 100 USP units of heparin to be neutralized, or as determined by blood coagulation test results.
[Enoxaparin toxicity][1]—
Intravenous, 1 mg of protamine sulfate for approximately every 1 mg of enoxaparin to be neutralized.
Note: Protamine sulfate should be administered at a rate of 5 mg per minute, not to exceed 50 mg in any ten-minute period.
Additional doses may be required as indicated by blood coagulation studies.
Since protamine has anticoagulant activity of its own, it is not advisable to administer more than 100 mg of protamine sulfate over a 2-hour period of time (the duration of action of protamine), unless blood coagulation tests indicate a larger requirement.

**Usual pediatric dose**
See *Usual adult and adolescent dose*.

**Strength(s) usually available**
U.S.—
10 mg per mL (Rx) [GENERIC].
Canada—
10 mg per mL (Rx) [GENERIC].

**Packaging and storage**
Store between 2 and 8 °C (36 and 46 °F), or between 15 and 30 °C (59 and 86 °F), as directed by the manufacturer. Protect from freezing.

**Preparation of dosage form**
Protamine sulfate injection is intended for use without further dilution; however, if further dilution is desired, 5% dextrose injection or 0.9% sodium chloride injection may be used.

**Stability**
Contains no preservatives; discard unused portion of opened container. Diluted solutions should not be stored because they contain no preservative.

**Incompatibilities**
Protamine sulfate solutions are incompatible with certain antibiotics, including several of the cephalosporins and penicillins. It is recommended that no other medications be mixed with protamine sulfate unless they are known to be compatible.

### PROTAMINE SULFATE FOR INJECTION USP

**Usual adult and adolescent dose**
See *Protamine Sulfate Injection USP*.

**Usual pediatric dose**
See *Protamine Sulfate Injection USP*.

**Size(s) usually available**
U.S.—
Not commercially available.
Canada—
Not commercially available.

**2422  Protamine (Systemic)**

**Packaging and storage**
Store below 40 °C (104 °F), preferably between 15 and 30 °C (59 and 86 °F), unless otherwise specified by manufacturer.

**Preparation of dosage form**
Five mL of bacteriostatic water for injection containing 0.9% benzyl alcohol should be added to the vial containing 50 mg of protamine sulfate and shaken vigorously to dissolve. Each mL of the resultant solution will contain 10 mg of protamine sulfate.

**Stability**
Reconstituted solutions should be refrigerated and used within 24 hours.

**Incompatibilities**
Protamine sulfate solutions are incompatible with certain antibiotics, including several of the cephalosporins and penicillins. It is recommended that no other medications be mixed with protamine sulfate unless they are known to be compatible.

¹Not included in Canadian product labeling.

Revised: 03/24/94

---

**PROTIRELIN**—The *Protirelin (Systemic)* monograph is not included in this published version of the USP DI database. Copies of the monograph are available on request from Micromedex, Inc. - Reprint Requests, 6200 S. Syracuse Way, Suite 300, Englewood, CO 80111; telephone (303) 486-6400; telefax (303) 486-6464; Email: USPDI@MDX.COM.

---

**PROTRIPTYLINE**—See *Antidepressants, Tricyclic (Systemic)*

---

**PRUSSIAN BLUE**—The *Prussian Blue (Oral-Local)* monograph is not included in this published version of the USP DI database. Copies of the monograph are available on request from Micromedex, Inc. - Reprint Requests, 6200 S. Syracuse Way, Suite 300, Englewood, CO 80111; telephone (303) 486-6400; telefax (303) 486-6464; Email: USPDI@MDX.COM.

---

# PSEUDOEPHEDRINE  Systemic

VA CLASSIFICATION (Primary): RE200

Commonly used brand name(s): *Balminil Decongestant Syrup; Benylin Decongestant; Cenafed; Chlor-Trimeton Non-Drowsy Decongestant 4 Hour; Decofed; Dorcol Children's Decongestant Liquid; Drixoral Non-Drowsy Formula; Efidac/24; Eltor 120; Genaphed; Halofed; Halofed Adult Strength; Maxenal; Myfedrine; Novafed; PediaCare Infants' Oral Decongestant Drops; Pseudo; Pseudogest; Robidrine; Sudafed; Sudafed 12 Hour; Sudafed Liquid, Children's; Sufedrin.*

Note: For a listing of dosage forms and brand names by country availability, see *Dosage Forms* section(s).

## Category
Decongestant, nasal (systemic).

## Indications

**Accepted**
Congestion, nasal (treatment)
Congestion, sinus (treatment) or
Congestion, eustachian tube (treatment)—Pseudoephedrine is indicated for temporary relief of congestion associated with acute coryza, acute eustachian salpingitis, serous otitis media with eustachian tube congestion, vasomotor rhinitis, and aerotitis (barotitis) media. Pseudoephedrine also may be indicated as an adjunct to analgesics, antihistamines, antibiotics, antitussives, or expectorants for optimum results in allergic rhinitis, croup, acute and subacute sinusitis, acute otitis media, and acute tracheobronchitis.

## Pharmacology/Pharmacokinetics

**Physicochemical characteristics**
Molecular weight—Pseudoephedrine hydrochloride: 201.70.
Pseudoephedrine sulfate: 428.54.

**Mechanism of action/Effect**
Pseudoephedrine acts on alpha-adrenergic receptors in the mucosa of the respiratory tract, producing vasoconstriction. The medication shrinks swollen nasal mucous membranes; reduces tissue hyperemia, edema, and nasal congestion; and increases nasal airway patency. Also, drainage of sinus secretions may be increased and obstructed eustachian ostia may be opened.

**Biotransformation**
Pseudoephedrine is incompletely metabolized in the liver.

**Onset of action**
15 to 30 minutes.

**Time to peak effect**
Within 30 to 60 minutes.

**Duration of action**
Tablets, oral solution, and syrup–3 to 4 hours.
Extended-release capsules and tablets–8 to 12 hours.

**Elimination**
Renal. About 55 to 75% of a dose is excreted unchanged. The rate of excretion is accelerated in acidic urine.

## Precautions to Consider

**Cross-sensitivity and/or related problems**
Patients sensitive to other sympathomimetics (for example, albuterol, amphetamines, ephedrine, epinephrine, isoproterenol, metaproterenol, norepinephrine, phenylephrine, phenylpropanolamine, terbutaline) may be sensitive to this medication also.

**Pregnancy/Reproduction**
Pregnancy—Studies in humans have not been done.
Studies in animals have not shown that pseudoephedrine causes teratogenic effects in the fetus. However, pseudoephedrine reduced average weight, length, and rate of skeletal ossification in the animal fetus.
FDA Pregnancy Category B.

**Breast-feeding**
Pseudoephedrine is distributed into breast milk; use by nursing mothers is not recommended, because of the higher than usual risk to infants, especially newborn and premature infants, of side effects from sympathomimetic amines.

**Pediatrics**
Pseudoephedrine should be used with caution in infants, especially newborn and premature infants, because of the higher than usual risk of side/adverse effects.

**Geriatrics**
No information is available on the relationship of age to the effects of pseudoephedrine in geriatric patients. However, elderly patients are more likely to have age-related prostatic hypertrophy, which may require adjustment of dosage in patients receiving pseudoephedrine.

**Drug interactions and/or related problems**
The following drug interactions and/or related problems have been selected on the basis of their potential clinical significance (possible mechanism in parentheses where appropriate)—not necessarily inclusive (» = major clinical significance):

Note: Combinations containing any of the following medications, depending on the amount present, may also interact with this medication.

Anesthetics, hydrocarbon inhalation, such as:
Chloroform
Cyclopropane
Enflurane
Halothane
Isoflurane
Methoxyflurane
Trichloroethylene
(administration of pseudoephedrine prior to or shortly after anesthesia with chloroform, cyclopropane, halothane, or trichloroethylene may increase the risk of severe ventricular arrhythmias, especially in patients with pre-existing heart disease, because these an-

esthetics greatly sensitize the myocardium to the effects of sympathomimetics)
(enflurane, isoflurane, or methoxyflurane may also cause some sensitization of the myocardium to the effects of sympathomimetics; caution is recommended in patients taking pseudoephedrine)

Antihypertensives or
Diuretics used as antihypertensives
(antihypertensive effects may be reduced when these medications are used concurrently with pseudoephedrine; the patient should be carefully monitored to confirm that the desired effect is being obtained)

» Beta-adrenergic blocking agents
(concurrent use with pseudoephedrine may inhibit the therapeutic effect of these medications; beta-blockade may result in unopposed alpha-adrenergic activity of pseudoephedrine with a risk of hypertension and excessive bradycardia and possible heart block)

Central nervous system (CNS) stimulation–producing medications, other (see *Appendix II*)
(concurrent use with pseudoephedrine may result in additive CNS stimulation to excessive levels, which may cause unwanted effects such as nervousness, irritability, insomnia, or possibly convulsions or cardiac arrhythmias; close observation is recommended)

Citrates
(concurrent use may inhibit urinary excretion and prolong the duration of action of pseudoephedrine)

» Cocaine, mucosal-local
(in addition to increasing CNS stimulation, concurrent use with pseudoephedrine may increase the cardiovascular effects of either or both medications and the risk of adverse effects)

Digitalis glycosides
(concurrent use with pseudoephedrine may increase the risk of cardiac arrhythmias; caution and electrocardiographic monitoring are very important if concurrent use is necessary)

Levodopa
(concurrent use with pseudoephedrine may increase the possibility of cardiac arrhythmias; dosage reduction of the sympathomimetic is recommended)

Monoamine oxidase (MAO) inhibitors, including furazolidone, procarbazine, and selegiline
(concurrent use may prolong and intensify the cardiac stimulant and vasopressor effects of pseudoephedrine because of release of catecholamines, which accumulate in intraneuronal storage sites during MAO inhibitor therapy, resulting in headache, cardiac arrhythmias, vomiting, or sudden and severe hypertensive and/or hyperpyretic crises; pseudoephedrine should not be administered during or within 14 days following administration of MAO inhibitors)

Nitrates
(concurrent use with pseudoephedrine may reduce the antianginal effects of these medications)

Rauwolfia alkaloids
(concurrent use may inhibit the action of pseudoephedrine by depleting catecholamine stores)

Sympathomimetics, other
(in addition to possibly increasing CNS stimulation, concurrent use may increase the cardiovascular effects of either other sympathomimetics or pseudoephedrine and the potential for side effects)

Thyroid hormones
(concurrent use may increase the effects of either these medications or pseudoephedrine; thyroid hormones enhance risk of coronary insufficiency when sympathomimetic agents are administered to patients with coronary artery disease; dosage adjustment is recommended, although problem is reduced in euthyroid patients)

**Medical considerations/Contraindications**
The medical considerations/contraindications included have been selected on the basis of their potential clinical significance (reasons given in parentheses where appropriate)—not necessarily inclusive (» = major clinical significance).

*Risk-benefit should be considered when the following medical problems exist:*
Cardiovascular disease, including ischemic heart disease, or
» Coronary artery disease, severe or
Hypertension, mild to moderate or
» Hypertension, severe
(condition may be exacerbated due to drug-induced cardiovascular effects)

Diabetes mellitus
Glaucoma, predisposition to
Hyperthyroidism
Prostatic hypertrophy
Sensitivity to pseudoephedrine or other sympathomimetics

## Side/Adverse Effects
The following side/adverse effects have been selected on the basis of their potential clinical significance (possible signs and symptoms in parentheses where appropriate)—not necessarily inclusive:

**Those indicating need for medical attention**
Incidence rare—more frequent with high doses
*Convulsions; hallucinations; irregular or slow heartbeat; shortness of breath or troubled breathing*

**Those indicating need for medical attention only if they continue or are bothersome**
Incidence more frequent
*Nervousness; restlessness; trouble in sleeping*
Incidence less frequent
*Difficult or painful urination; dizziness or lightheadedness; fast or pounding heartbeat; headache; increased sweating; nausea or vomiting; trembling; troubled breathing; unusual paleness; weakness*

## Overdose
For more information on the management of overdose or unintentional ingestion, **contact a Poison Control Center** (see *Poison Control Center Listing*).

**Clinical effects of overdose**
The following effects have been selected on the basis of their potential clinical significance (possible signs and symptoms in parenthesis where appropriate)–not necessarily inclusive:

Acute and chronic effects
*Convulsions; fast breathing; hallucinations; increase in blood pressure; irregular heartbeat, continuing; shortness of breath or troubled breathing, severe or continuing; slow or fast heartbeat, severe or continuing; unusual nervousness, restlessness, or excitement*

**Treatment of overdose**
To decrease absorption—
Because pseudoephedrine is rapidly absorbed from the gut, emetics and gastric lavage should be instituted within 4 hours of overdosage in order to be effective. Charcoal is useful only if administered within 1 hour. However, if an extended-release preparation was taken, there will be more time for benefit from these measures.
To enhance elimination—
Forced diuresis will increase elimination of pseudoephedrine provided renal function is adequate; however, diuresis is not recommended for severe overdosage.
Specific treatment—
For delirium or convulsions, intravenous diazepam may be administered.
The cardiac state should be monitored and serum electrolytes measured. If there are signs of cardiac toxicity, intravenous propranolol may be indicated.
Hypokalemia may be treated, if necessary, with a slow infusion of a dilute potassium chloride solution; serum potassium concentration should be monitored during and for several hours after administration of potassium chloride.

## Patient Consultation
As an aid to patient consultation, refer to *Advice for the Patient, Pseudoephedrine (Systemic)*.
In providing consultation, consider emphasizing the following selected information (» = major clinical significance):

**Before using this medication**
» Conditions affecting use, especially:
Sensitivity to pseudoephedrine or other sympathomimetics
Pregnancy—In animal studies, pseudoephedrine caused reduced average weight, length, and rate of skeletal ossification in animal fetus
Breast-feeding—Pseudoephedrine distributed into breast milk; use by nursing mothers not recommended because of higher than usual risk of side effects for infants, especially newborn and premature infants
Use in children—Caution should be used in infants, especially newborn and premature infants, because of higher than usual risk of side/adverse effects

Other medications, especially beta-adrenergic blocking agents, mucosal-local cocaine, or monoamine oxidase (MAO) inhibitors
Other medical problems, especially severe coronary artery disease or severe hypertension

**Proper use of this medication**
*Proper administration of extended-release dosage forms*
Swallowing capsules or tablets whole; if capsule too large to swallow, mixing contents with jam or jelly and swallowing without chewing
Not crushing or chewing capsules; not crushing, breaking, or chewing tablets
» Taking the medication a few hours before bedtime to minimize the possibility of insomnia
» Importance of not taking more medication than the amount recommended
» Proper dosing
Missed dose: Taking right away if remembered within an hour or so; not taking if remembered later; not doubling doses
» Proper storage

**Precautions while using this medication**
» Checking with physician if symptoms do not improve within 7 days or if fever is present

**Side/adverse effects**
Signs of potential side effects, especially convulsions, hallucinations, irregular or slow heartbeat, and shortness of breath or troubled breathing

## General Dosing Information

To minimize the possibility of insomnia, the last dose of pseudoephedrine for each day should be administered a few hours before bedtime.

For patients who have difficulty in swallowing the extended-release capsule, the contents of the capsule may be mixed with jam or jelly and taken without chewing.

## Oral Dosage Forms

### PSEUDOEPHEDRINE HYDROCHLORIDE CAPSULES

**Usual adult and adolescent dose**
Decongestant, nasal—
Oral, 60 mg every four to six hours.

**Usual adult prescribing limits**
240 mg in twenty-four hours.

**Usual pediatric dose**
Decongestant, nasal—
Children up to 12 years of age: Use is not recommended.
Children 12 years of age and over: See *Usual adult and adolescent dose*.

**Strength(s) usually available**
U.S.—
Not commercially available.
Canada—
60 mg (OTC) [*Benylin Decongestant*].

**Packaging and storage**
Store below 40 °C (104 °F), preferably between 15 and 30 °C (59 and 86 °F), in a well-closed container, unless otherwise specified by manufacturer.

### PSEUDOEPHEDRINE HYDROCHLORIDE EXTENDED-RELEASE CAPSULES

**Usual adult and adolescent dose**
Decongestant, nasal—
Oral, 120 mg every twelve hours, or 240 mg every twenty-four hours.

**Usual adult prescribing limits**
240 mg in twenty-four hours.

**Usual pediatric dose**
Decongestant, nasal—
Children up to 12 years of age: Use is not recommended.
Children 12 years of age and over: See *Usual adult and adolescent dose*.

**Strength(s) usually available**
U.S.—
120 mg (Rx) [*Novafed*].
Canada—
120 mg (OTC) [*Eltor 120*; GENERIC].

**Packaging and storage**
Store below 40 °C (104 °F), preferably between 15 and 30 °C (59 and 86 °F), in a tight container, unless otherwise specified by manufacturer. Protect from light.

**Auxiliary labeling**
• Swallow capsules whole.

### PSEUDOEPHEDRINE HYDROCHLORIDE ORAL SOLUTION

**Usual adult and adolescent dose**
Decongestant, nasal—
See *Pseudoephedrine Hydrochloride Capsules*.

**Usual adult prescribing limits**
See *Pseudoephedrine Hydrochloride Capsules*.

**Usual pediatric dose**
Decongestant, nasal—
Oral, 4 mg per kg of body weight or 125 mg per square meter of body surface per day, administered in four divided doses; or for
Children up to 2 years of age: Dosage must be individualized.
Children 2 to 6 years of age: Oral, 15 mg every four to six hours, not to exceed 60 mg in twenty-four hours.
Children 6 to 12 years of age: Oral, 30 mg every four to six hours, not to exceed 120 mg in twenty-four hours.
Children 12 years of age and over: See *Pseudoephedrine Hydrochloride Capsules*.

**Strength(s) usually available**
U.S.—
7.5 mg per 0.8 mL (OTC) [*PediaCare Infants' Oral Decongestant Drops*].
15 mg per 5 mL (OTC) [*Dorcol Children's Decongestant Liquid*].
30 mg per 5 mL (OTC) [*Myfedrine; Sudafed Liquid, Children's*].
Canada—
Not commercially available.

**Packaging and storage**
Store below 40 °C (104 °F), preferably between 15 and 30 °C (59 and 86 °F), in a well-closed container, unless otherwise specified by manufacturer. Protect from freezing. Protect from light.

### PSEUDOEPHEDRINE HYDROCHLORIDE SYRUP USP

**Usual adult and adolescent dose**
Decongestant, nasal—
See *Pseudoephedrine Hydrochloride Capsules*.

**Usual adult prescribing limits**
See *Pseudoephedrine Hydrochloride Capsules*.

**Usual pediatric dose**
Decongestant, nasal—
Children up to 12 years of age: See *Pseudoephedrine Hydrochloride Oral Solution*.
Children 12 years of age and over: See *Pseudoephedrine Hydrochloride Capsules*.

**Strength(s) usually available**
U.S.—
30 mg per 5 mL (OTC) [*Cenafed; Decofed; Pseudogest; Sufedrin;* GENERIC].
Canada—
30 mg per 5 mL (OTC) [*Balminil Decongestant Syrup* (alcohol; parabens); *Robidrine* (alcohol 1.4%; sugar); *Sudafed* (methylparaben; sucrose)].

**Packaging and storage**
Store below 40 °C (104 °F), preferably between 15 and 30 °C (59 and 86 °F), unless otherwise specified by manufacturer. Store in a tight, light-resistant container. Protect from freezing.

### PSEUDOEPHEDRINE HYDROCHLORIDE TABLETS USP

**Usual adult and adolescent dose**
Decongestant, nasal—
See *Pseudoephedrine Hydrochloride Capsules*.

**Usual adult prescribing limits**
See *Pseudoephedrine Hydrochloride Capsules*.

**Usual pediatric dose**
Decongestant, nasal—
Children up to 12 years of age: See *Pseudoephedrine Hydrochloride Oral Solution*.
Children 12 years of age and over: See *Pseudoephedrine Hydrochloride Capsules*.

**Strength(s) usually available**
U.S.—
30 mg (OTC) [*Decofed; Genaphed; Halofed; Pseudo; Pseudogest; Sudafed* (povidone; sodium benzoate); GENERIC].

60 mg (OTC) [*Cenafed; Decofed; Halofed Adult Strength; Pseudo; Pseudogest; Sudafed* (sodium starch glycolate; sucrose); *Sufedrin;* GENERIC].

Canada—
 60 mg (OTC) [*Robidrine* (scored); *Sudafed* (scored; lactose)].

**Packaging and storage**
Store below 40 °C (104 °F), preferably between 15 and 30 °C (59 and 86 °F), unless otherwise specified by manufacturer. Store in a tight container.

### PSEUDOEPHEDRINE HYDROCHLORIDE EXTENDED-RELEASE TABLETS

**Usual adult and adolescent dose**
Decongestant, nasal—
 See *Pseudoephedrine Hydrochloride Extended-Release Capsules*.

**Usual adult prescribing limits**
See *Pseudoephedrine Hydrochloride Extended-Release Capsules*.

**Usual pediatric dose**
Decongestant, nasal—
 Children up to 12 years of age: Use is not recommended.
 Children 12 years of age and over: See *Pseudoephedrine Hydrochloride Extended-Release Capsules*.

**Strength(s) usually available**
U.S.—
 120 mg (OTC) [*Sudafed 12 Hour*].
 240 mg (OTC) [*Efidac/24*].
Canada—
 120 mg (OTC) [*Maxenal; Sudafed 12 Hour*].

**Packaging and storage**
Store below 40 °C (104 °F), preferably between 15 and 30 °C (59 and 86 °F), in a tight container, unless otherwise specified by manufacturer. Protect from light.

**Auxiliary labeling**
• Swallow tablets whole.

### PSEUDOEPHEDRINE SULFATE TABLETS

**Usual adult and adolescent dose**
Decongestant, nasal—
 See *Pseudoephedrine Hydrochloride Capsules*.

**Usual adult prescribing limits**
See *Pseudoephedrine Hydrochloride Capsules*.

**Usual pediatric dose**
Decongestant, nasal—
 Children up to 12 years of age: See *Pseudoephedrine Hydrochloride Oral Solution*.
 Children 12 years of age and over: See *Pseudoephedrine Hydrochloride Capsules*.

**Strength(s) usually available**
U.S.—
 60 mg (OTC) [*Chlor-Trimeton Non-Drowsy Decongestant 4 Hour* (scored; lactose; povidone)].

Canada—
 Not commercially available.

**Packaging and storage**
Store between 2 and 30 °C (36 and 86 °F), in a well-closed container, unless otherwise specified by manufacturer. Protect from light.

### PSEUDOEPHEDRINE SULFATE EXTENDED-RELEASE TABLETS

**Usual adult and adolescent dose**
Decongestant, nasal—
 See *Pseudoephedrine Hydrochloride Extended-Release Capsules*.

**Usual adult prescribing limits**
See *Pseudoephedrine Hydrochloride Extended-Release Capsules*.

**Usual pediatric dose**
Decongestant, nasal—
 Children up to 12 years of age: Use is not recommended.
 Children 12 years of age and over: See *Pseudoephedrine Hydrochloride Extended-Release Capsules*.

**Strength(s) usually available**
U.S.—
 120 mg (OTC) [*Drixoral Non-Drowsy Formula* (butylparaben; lactose; povidone; sugar)].
Canada—
 Not commercially available.

**Packaging and storage**
Store between 2 and 30 °C (36 and 86 °F), in a well-closed container, unless otherwise specified by manufacturer. Protect from light.

**Auxiliary labeling**
• Swallow tablets whole.

Revised: 04/19/94

---

**PSYLLIUM** — See *Laxatives (Local)*

---

**PSYLLIUM HYDROPHILIC MUCILLOID** — See *Laxatives (Local)*

---

**PYRANTEL** — The *Pyrantel (Oral-Local)* monograph is not included in this published version of the USP DI database. Copies of the monograph are available on request from Micromedex, Inc. - Reprint Requests, 6200 S. Syracuse Way, Suite 300, Englewood, CO 80111; telephone (303) 486-6400; telefax (303) 486-6464; Email: USPDI@MDX.COM.

---

# PYRAZINAMIDE  Systemic

VA CLASSIFICATION (Primary): AM500

Commonly used brand name(s): *Tebrazid; pms-Pyrazinamide*.

Note: For a listing of dosage forms and brand names by country availability, see *Dosage Forms* section(s).

## Category
Antibacterial (antimycobacterial).

## Indications

**General considerations**
Tuberculosis is a highly infectious life-threatening bacterial disease with 8 million new cases and 3 million deaths reported worldwide each year to the World Health Organization (WHO). The vast majority of these cases are in developing countries; however, tuberculosis also has emerged as an important public health problem in the U.S. in recent years after the decline in number of cases observed between 1950 and 1980.

The resurgence of tuberculosis in the U.S. has been complicated by an increase in the proportion of patients with strains resistant to antituberculosis medications. Outbreaks of multidrug-resistant tuberculosis have been documented in hospitals and prisons. Drug-resistant tuberculosis, particularly that caused by strains resistant to isoniazid and rifampin, is much harder to treat and often is fatal. Among acquired immunodeficiency syndrome (AIDS) patients infected with tuberculosis bacilli resistant to both rifampin and isoniazid, a case-fatality rate of 91% has been reported. Recent investigations of outbreaks of multidrug-resistant tuberculosis have found an extraordinarily high case-fatality rate, with the median time to mortality being reached between 4 and 16 weeks. In almost all instances, these outbreaks have involved patients with severe immunosuppression as a result of infection with the human immunodeficiency virus (HIV).

Acquired drug resistance develops during treatment for drug-sensitive tuberculosis with regimens that are poorly conceived or poorly complied with, allowing the emergence of naturally occurring drug-resistant mutations. Resistant organisms from affected patients may subsequently infect other people who have not been infected with *M. tuberculosis* previously, resulting in primary drug resistance.

Resistance to antituberculosis agents can develop not only in the strain that caused the initial disease, but also as a result of reinfection with a new strain of *M. tuberculosis* strain that is drug-resistant. Reinfection with a new multidrug-resistant *M. tuberculosis* can occur during therapy for the original infection or after completion of therapy. Most recent data suggest that outcomes can be improved if patients promptly begin therapy with two or more drugs that have *in vitro* activity against the multidrug-resistant isolate.

HIV infection is the strongest risk factor yet identified for the development of tuberculosis disease in persons infected with tuberculosis. In addition, persons with HIV infection are at an increased risk of tuberculosis resulting either from newly acquired disease or from reactivation of latent infections. Tuberculosis is a major clinical manifestation of immunodeficiency induced by HIV. In hospital-based retrospective studies, high rates of tuberculosis have been found among patients with AIDS. In communities where tuberculosis and HIV infection are common, the prevalence of HIV seropositivity among patients with tuberculosis is greatly increasing.

WHO has estimated that 5.6 million people worldwide and 80,000 people in the U.S. are infected with both HIV and tuberculosis. Persons dually infected with *M. tuberculosis* and HIV have a high risk of developing clinically active tuberculosis. One study of HIV-positive drug users with positive tuberculin skin test results found a rate of the development of active tuberculosis to be 8 cases per 100 person-years (8% yearly) as compared with the 10% lifetime risk (1 to 3% risk within the first year after skin test conversion) in the general population.

Persons who are known to be HIV-infected and who are contacts of patients with infectious tuberculosis should be carefully evaluated for evidence of tuberculosis. If there are no findings suggestive of current tuberculosis, preventive therapy with isoniazid should be given. Because HIV-infected contacts are not managed in the same way as those who are not HIV-infected, HIV testing is recommended if there are known or suspected risk factors for their acquiring HIV infection.

According to investigators at the National Institute of Allergy and Infectious Diseases (NIAID), levels of HIV in the bloodstream increase 5- to 160-fold in HIV-infected persons who develop active tuberculosis. Clinical and epidemiologic observations have demonstrated that HIV-infected individuals have an estimated 113-times higher risk and AIDS patients have a 170-times higher risk as compared with uninfected persons. Furthermore, the problem of drug resistance may worsen as the HIV epidemic spreads. Immunosuppressed patients with HIV infection who subsequently become infected with *M. tuberculosis* have an extraordinarily high risk of developing active tuberculosis within a short period of time.

In addition to the convincing evidence that HIV infection increases the risk and worsens the course of tuberculosis, there is increasing clinical evidence that coinfection with *M. tuberculosis* accelerates progression of disease caused by HIV infection. Understanding the interaction of these two pathogens is clinically important, given the high prevalence of patients coinfected with HIV and *M. tuberculosis* in both the U.S. and Africa; it is estimated that by the year 2000 about 500,000 deaths per year will occur in coinfected patients worldwide.

Persons with a positive tuberculin skin test and HIV infection, and persons with a positive tuberculin skin test and at risk of acquiring HIV infection with unknown HIV status should be considered for tuberculosis preventive therapy regardless of age. One study showed that isoniazid prophylaxis in HIV-infected, tuberculin-positive individuals not only decreased the incidence of tuberculosis disease, but also delayed the progression to AIDS and death.

Twelve months of preventive therapy is recommended for adults and children with HIV infection and other conditions associated with immunosuppression. Persons with HIV infection should receive at least 6 months of preventive therapy. The American Academy of Pediatrics recommends that children receive 9 months of therapy.

Tuberculosis control programs should ensure that drug susceptibility tests are performed on all initial isolates of *M. tuberculosis* and the results are reported promptly to the primary care provider and the local health department. Tuberculosis control programs should monitor local drug resistance rates to assess the effectiveness of local tuberculosis control efforts and to determine the appropriateness of the currently recommended initial tuberculosis treatment regimen for the area.

Relapse of rifampin-resistant tuberculosis has been reported in HIV-infected patients. Reinfection with new strains of *M. tuberculosis* has also been reported in these patients. Rifampin-resistant tuberculosis is a serious threat because responses to therapy are more difficult to achieve and require long courses of treatment. Therefore, careful follow-up of HIV-infected patients with treated tuberculosis is essential.

Multidrug-resistant tuberculosis also has been transmitted to persons without HIV infection in health care facilities. Together with the lack of effective agents for second-line treatment and methods of prophylaxis, the transmission of multidrug-resistant strains of *M. tuberculosis* may create a substantial reservoir of latently infected people and the potential for clinical multidrug-resistant tuberculosis for many years to come.

Several studies have documented a high prevalence of extrapulmonary disease in HIV-infected patients with clinical tuberculosis disease, particularly in conjunction with pulmonary manifestations. Cutaneous miliary tuberculosis, also known as *tuberculosis cutis miliaris disseminata*, was in the past a rare condition in adults, with only 24 cases reported in nearly a century. However, since the first reported case of cutaneous miliary tuberculosis in 1990 in a patient with AIDS, five additional cases have been reported in HIV-infected patients. Its appearance can be quite nondescript; therefore, a high level of suspicion must be maintained, particularly for patients with CD4+ cell counts of < 200 per cubic millimeter, in order to diagnose the condition and initiate therapy appropriately.

### Accepted
Tuberculosis (treatment)—Pyrazinamide is indicated, in combination with other antimycobacterial drugs, in the treatment of tuberculosis. Pyrazinamide is effective only against mycobacteria.

Not all species or strains of a particular organism may be susceptible to pyrazinamide.

## Pharmacology/Pharmacokinetics

Note: Preliminary data suggest that patients coinfected with the human immunodeficiency virus (HIV) and mycobacteria (*Mycobacterium tuberculosis* or *M. avium*) have altered pharmacokinetic profiles for antimycobacterial agents. In particular, malabsorption of these agents appears to occur frequently, and could seriously affect the efficacy of treatment.

### Physicochemical characteristics
Molecular weight—123.11.

### Mechanism of action/Effect
Unknown; pyrazinamide may be bacteriostatic or bactericidal, depending on its concentration and the susceptibility of the organism. It is active *in vitro* at an acidic pH of 5.6 or less, similar to that found in early, active tubercular inflammatory lesions.

### Absorption
Rapidly and almost completely absorbed from the gastrointestinal tract.

### Distribution
Wide, to most fluids and tissues, including liver, lungs, kidneys, and bile. Pyrazinamide has excellent penetration into the cerebrospinal fluid (CSF), ranging from 87 to 105% of the corresponding serum concentration.

$Vol_D$—0.57 to 0.74 L per kg.

### Protein binding
Pyrazinamide—Low (10 to 20%).
Pyrazinoic acid—Low (approximately 31%).

### Biotransformation
Hepatic; hydrolyzed by a microsomal deamidase to pyrazinoic acid, an active metabolite, and then hydroxylated by xanthine oxidase to 5-hydroxypyrazinoic acid.

### Half-life
Distribution—
    Approximately 1.6 hours.
Elimination—
    Pyrazinamide:
        Normal renal function—Approximately 9.5 hours.
        Chronic renal failure—Approximately 26 hours.
    Pyrazinoic acid:
        Normal renal function—Approximately 12 hours.
        Chronic renal failure—Approximately 22 hours.

### Time to peak serum concentration
Pyrazinamide—1 to 2 hours.
Pyrazinoic acid—4 to 5 hours.

### Peak serum concentration
Pyrazinamide—
    Approximately 19 mcg/mL after a single dose of 14 mg per kg of body weight (mg/kg).
    Approximately 39 mcg/mL after a single dose of 27 mg/kg.
Pyrazinoic acid—
    Approximately 3 mcg/mL after a single dose of 14 mg/kg.
    Approximately 4.5 mcg/mL after a single dose of 27 mg/kg.

### Elimination
Renal; approximately 3% of unchanged pyrazinamide, 33% of pyrazinoic acid, and 36% of remaining identifiable metabolites excreted in urine within 72 hours.

In dialysis—A single 3- to 4-hour hemodialysis session reduced serum pyrazinamide concentrations by approximately 55% and pyrazinoic acid concentrations by 50 to 60%.

## Precautions to Consider

### Cross-sensitivity and/or related problems
Patients hypersensitive to ethionamide, isoniazid, niacin (nicotinic acid), or other chemically related medications may be hypersensitive to this medication also.

### Carcinogenicity
Pyrazinamide was administered in the diets of rats and mice. The estimated daily dose was 2 grams per kg (grams/kg), or 40 times the maximum human dose, for the mouse, and 0.5 gram/kg, or 10 times the maximum human dose, for the rat. Pyrazinamide was not carcinogenic in rats or male mice. No conclusion was possible for female mice due to insufficient numbers of surviving control mice.

### Mutagenicity
Pyrazinamide was not mutagenic in the Ames bacterial test, but it did induce chromosomal aberrations in human lymphocyte cell cultures.

### Pregnancy/Reproduction
Pregnancy—

Note: Pregnant women with tuberculosis should be managed in concert with an expert in the management of tuberculosis. Women who have only pulmonary tuberculosis are not likely to infect the fetus until after delivery, and congenital tuberculosis is extremely rare. *In utero* infections with tubercle bacilli, however, can occur after maternal bacillemia occurs at different stages in the course of tuberculosis. Miliary tuberculosis can seed the placenta and thereby gain access to the fetal circulation. In women with tuberculous endometritis, transmission of infection to the fetus can result from fetal aspiration of bacilli at the time of delivery. A third mode of transmission is through ingestion of infected amniotic fluid *in utero*.

If active disease is diagnosed during pregnancy, a 9-month regimen of isoniazid and rifampin, supplemented by an initial course of ethambutol if drug resistance is suspected, is recommended. Pyrazinamide usually is not given because of inadequate data regarding teratogenesis. Hence, a 9-month course of therapy is necessary for drug-susceptible disease. When isoniazid resistance is a possibility, isoniazid, ethambutol, and rifampin are recommended initially. One of these medications can be discontinued after 1 or 2 months, depending on results of susceptibility tests. If rifampin or isoniazid is discontinued, treatment is continued for a total of 18 months; if ethambutol is discontinued, treatment is continued for a total of 9 months. Prompt initiation of chemotherapy is mandatory to protect both the mother and fetus. If isoniazid or rifampin resistance is documented, an expert in the management of tuberculosis should be consulted.

Asymptomatic pregnant women with positive tuberculin skin tests and normal chest radiographs should receive preventive therapy with isoniazid for 9 months if they are HIV seropositive or have recently been in contact with an infectious person. For these individuals, preventive therapy should begin after the first trimester. In other circumstances in which none of these risk factors is present, although no harmful effects of isoniazid to the fetus have been observed, preventive therapy can be delayed until after delivery.

For all pregnant women receiving isoniazid, pyridoxine should be prescribed. Isoniazid, ethambutol, and rifampin appear to be relatively safe for the fetus. The benefit of ethambutol and rifampin for therapy of active disease in the mother outweighs the risk to the infant. Streptomycin and pyrazinamide should not be used unless they are essential to the control of the disease.

Adequate and well-controlled studies in humans have not been done; the risk for teratogenicity has not been determined.

Animal reproduction studies have not been conducted with pyrazinamide.

FDA Pregnancy Category C.

### Breast-feeding
Pyrazinamide is distributed into breast milk in small amounts.

### Pediatrics
Note: If an infant is suspected of having congenital tuberculosis, a Mantoux tuberculin skin test, chest radiograph, lumbar puncture, and appropriate cultures should be performed promptly. Regardless of the skin test results, treatment of the infant should be initiated promptly with isoniazid, rifampin, pyrazinamide, and streptomycin or kanamycin. In addition, the mother should be evaluated for the presence of pulmonary or extrapulmonary (including uterine) tuberculosis. If the physical examination or chest radiograph support the diagnosis of tuberculosis, the patient should be treated with the same regimen as that used for tuberculous meningitis. The drug susceptibilities of the organism recovered from the mother and/or infant should be determined.

Possible isoniazid resistance should always be considered, particularly in children from population groups in which drug resistance is high, especially in foreign-born children from countries with a high prevalence of drug-resistant tuberculosis. For contacts who are likely to have been infected by an index case with isoniazid-resistant but rifampin-susceptible organisms, and in whom the consequences of the infection are likely to be severe (e.g., children up to 4 years of age), rifampin (10 mg per kg of body weight, maximum 600 mg, given daily in a single dose) should be given in addition to isoniazid (10 mg per kg, maximum 300 mg, given daily in a single dose) until susceptibility test results from the index case are available. If the index case is known or proven to be excreting organisms resistant to isoniazid, then isoniazid should be discontinued and rifampin given for a total of 9 months. Isoniazid alone should be given if no proof of exposure to isoniazid-resistant organisms is found. Optimal therapy for children with tuberculosis infection caused by organisms resistant to isoniazid and rifampin is unknown. In deciding on therapy in this situation, consultation with an expert is advised.

Adjuvant treatment with corticosteroids in treating tuberculosis is controversial. Corticosteroids have been used for therapy in children with tuberculous meningitis to reduce vasculitis, inflammation, and, as a result, intracranial pressure. Data indicate that dexamethasone may lower mortality rates and lessen long-term neurologic impairment. The administration of corticosteroids should be considered in all children with tuberculous meningitis, and also may be considered in children with pleural and pericardial effusions (to hasten reabsorption of fluid), severe miliary disease (to mitigate alveolocapillary block), and endobronchial disease (to relieve obstruction and atelectasis). Corticosteroids should be given only when accompanied by appropriate antituberculosis therapy. Consultation with an expert in the treatment of tuberculosis should be obtained when corticosteroid therapy is considered.

Appropriate studies on the relationship of age to the effects of pyrazinamide have not been performed in the pediatric population. However, no pediatrics-specific problems have been documented to date.

### Geriatrics
Appropriate studies on the relationship of age to the effects of pyrazinamide have not been performed in the geriatric population. However, no geriatrics-specific problems have been documented to date.

### Drug interactions and/or related problems
The following drug interactions and/or related problems have been selected on the basis of their potential clinical significance (possible mechanism in parentheses where appropriate)—not necessarily inclusive (» = major clinical significance):

Note: Combinations containing any of the following medications, depending on the amount present, may also interact with this medication.

Allopurinol or
Colchicine or
Probenecid or
Sulfinpyrazone
(pyrazinamide may increase serum uric acid concentrations and decrease the efficacy of antigout therapy; dosage adjustments of these medications may be necessary to control hyperuricemia and gout when antigout medications are used concurrently with pyrazinamide)

Cyclosporine
(concurrent use with pyrazinamide may decrease the serum concentrations of cyclosporine, possibly leading to inadequate immunosuppression; cyclosporine serum concentrations should be monitored)

### Laboratory value alterations
The following have been selected on the basis of their potential clinical significance (possible effect in parentheses where appropriate)—not necessarily inclusive (» = major clinical significance):

With diagnostic test results
Ketone determinations, urine
(may react with sodium nitroprusside tests, such as *Acetest* or *Chemstrip K;* both pyrazinamide and pyrazinoic acid produce an interfering pink-brown color reaction with nitroprusside)

With physiology/laboratory test values
Alanine aminotransferase (ALT [SGPT]) and
Aspartate aminotransferase (AST [SGOT])
(values may be increased)

Uric acid, serum
(concentration may be increased)

**Medical considerations/Contraindications**
The medical considerations/contraindications included have been selected on the basis of their potential clinical significance (reasons given in parentheses where appropriate)—not necessarily inclusive (» = major clinical significance).

*Risk-benefit should be considered when the following medical problems exist:*

Gout, history of
(pyrazinamide can increase serum uric acid concentrations and precipitate an acute attack of gout)

» Hepatic function impairment, severe
(pyrazinamide is metabolized in the liver and, in high doses, can be hepatotoxic)

» Hypersensitivity to pyrazinamide, ethionamide, isoniazid, niacin (nicotinic acid), or other chemically related medications

**Patient monitoring**
The following may be especially important in patient monitoring (other tests may be warranted in some patients, depending on condition; » = major clinical significance):

Hepatic function determinations
(AST [SGOT] and ALT [SGPT] determinations may be required prior to and every 2 to 4 weeks during treatment; however, elevated serum enzyme values may not be predictive of clinical hepatitis and values may return to normal despite continued treatment; patients with impaired hepatic function should not receive pyrazinamide unless it is crucial to therapy)

Uric acid concentrations, serum
(may be required during treatment since elevated serum uric acid concentrations frequently occur, possibly precipitating acute gout)

## Side/Adverse Effects

The following side/adverse effects have been selected on the basis of their potential clinical significance (possible signs and symptoms in parentheses where appropriate)—not necessarily inclusive:

**Those indicating need for medical attention**
Incidence more frequent
*Arthralgia* (pain in the large and small joints)—related to hyperuricemia; usually mild and self-limiting
Incidence rare
*Gouty arthritis* (pain and swelling of joints, especially big toe, ankle, and knee; tense, hot skin over affected joints); *hepatotoxicity* (loss of appetite; unusual tiredness or weakness; yellow eyes or skin)—related to large doses, i.e., 40 to 50 mg per kg of body weight per day for prolonged periods of time

**Those indicating need for medical attention only if they continue or are bothersome**
Incidence rare
*Itching; skin rash*

## Patient Consultation

As an aid to patient consultation, refer to *Advice for the Patient, Pyrazinamide (Systemic)*.

In providing consultation, consider emphasizing the following selected information (» = major clinical significance):

**Before using this medication**
» Conditions affecting use, especially:
Hypersensitivity to pyrazinamide, ethionamide, isoniazid, niacin (nicotinic acid), or other chemically related medications
Breast-feeding—Pyrazinamide is distributed into breast milk
Other medical problems, especially severe hepatic function impairment

**Proper use of this medication**
» Compliance with full course of therapy, which may take months
» Proper dosing
Missed dose: Taking as soon as possible; not taking if almost time for next dose; not doubling doses
» Proper storage

**Precautions while using this medication**
» Regular visits to physician to check progress
Checking with physician if no improvement within 2 to 3 weeks
» Diabetics: May interfere with urine ketone determinations

**Side/adverse effects**
Signs of side effects, especially arthralgia, gouty arthritis, and hepatotoxicity

## General Dosing Information

Since bacterial resistance may develop rapidly when pyrazinamide is administered alone in the treatment of tuberculosis, it only should be administered concurrently with other antitubercular medications.

The duration of treatment with an antituberculosis regimen is at least 6 months, and may be continued for 2 years. Uncomplicated pulmonary tuberculosis is often successfully treated within 6 to 12 months. Several different treatment regimens are currently recommended.

The duration of antituberculosis therapy is based on the patient's clinical and radiographic responses, smear and culture results, and susceptibility studies of *Mycobacterium tuberculosis* isolates from the patient or the suspect source case. With directly observed therapy (DOT), clinical evaluation is an integral component of each visit for administration of medication. Careful monitoring of the clinical and bacteriologic responses to therapy on a monthly basis in sputum-positive patients is important.

If therapy is interrupted, the treatment schedule should be extended to a later completion date. Although guidelines cannot be provided for every situation, the following factors need to be considered in establishing a new date for completion:
• The length of interruption;
• The time during therapy (early or late) in which interruption occurred; and
• The patient's clinical, radiographic, and bacteriologic status before, during, and after interruption. Consultation with an expert is advised.

Therapy should be administered based on the following guidelines, published by the American Thoracic Society (ATS) and by the Centers for Disease Control and Prevention (CDC), and endorsed by the American Academy of Pediatrics (AAP).
• A 6-month regimen consisting of isoniazid, rifampin, and pyrazinamide given for 2 months followed by isoniazid and rifampin for 4 months is the preferred treatment for patients infected with fully susceptible organisms who adhere to the treatment course.
• Ethambutol (or streptomycin in children too young to be monitored for visual acuity) should be included in the initial regimen until the results of drug susceptibility studies are available, and unless there is little possibility of drug resistance (i.e., there is less than 4% primary resistance to isoniazid in the community, and the patient has had no previous treatment with antituberculosis medications, is not from a country with a high prevalence of drug resistance, and has no known exposure to a drug-resistant case).
• Alternatively, a 9-month regimen of isoniazid and rifampin is acceptable for persons who cannot or should not take pyrazinamide. Ethambutol (or streptomycin in children too young to be monitored for visual acuity) should also be included until the results of drug susceptibility studies are available, unless there is little possibility of drug resistance. If isoniazid resistance is demonstrated, rifampin and ethambutol should be continued for a minimum of 12 months.
• Consideration should be given to treating all patients with DOT. DOT programs have been demonstrated to increase adherence in patients receiving antituberculosis chemotherapy in both rural and urban settings.
• Multidrug-resistant tuberculosis (i.e., resistance to at least isoniazid and rifampin) presents difficult treatment problems. Treatment must be individualized and based on susceptibility studies. In such cases, consultation with an expert in tuberculosis is recommended.
• Children should be managed in essentially the same ways as adults, but doses of the medications must be adjusted appropriately and specific important differences between the management of adults and children addressed. However, optimal therapy of tuberculosis in children with HIV infection has not been established. The Committee on Infectious Diseases of the AAP recommends that therapy always should include at least three drugs initially, and should be continued for a minimum period of 9 months. Isoniazid, rifampin, and pyrazinamide with or without ethambutol or an aminoglycoside should be given for at least the first 2 months. A fourth drug may be needed for disseminated disease and whenever drug-resistant disease is suspected.
• Extrapulmonary tuberculosis should be managed according to the principles and with the drug regimens outlined for pulmonary tuberculosis, except in children who have miliary tuberculosis, bone/joint tuberculosis, or tuberculous meningitis. These children should receive a minimum of 12 months of therapy.
• A 4-month regimen of isoniazid and rifampin is acceptable therapy for adults who have active tuberculosis and who are sputum smear– and culture–negative, if there is little possibility of drug resistance.

ATS, CDC, and AAP recommend preventive treatment of tuberculosis infection in the following patients:

- Preventive therapy with isoniazid given for 6 to 12 months is effective in decreasing the risk of future tuberculosis disease in adults and children with tuberculosis infection demonstrated by a positive tuberculin skin test reaction.
- Persons with a positive skin test and any of the following risk factors should be considered for preventive therapy regardless of age:
    — Persons with HIV infection.
    — Persons at risk for HIV infection with unknown HIV status.
    — Close contacts of sputum-positive persons with newly diagnosed infectious tuberculosis.
    — Newly infected persons (recent skin test convertors).
    — Persons with medical conditions reported to increase the risk of tuberculosis (i.e., diabetes mellitus, corticosteroid therapy and other immunosuppressive therapy, intravenous drug users, hematologic and reticuloendothelial malignancies, end-stage renal disease, and clinical conditions associated with rapid weight loss or chronic malnutrition).

In some circumstances, persons with negative skin tests should be considered for preventive therapy. These include children who are close contacts of infectious tuberculosis cases and anergic HIV-infected adults at increased risk of tuberculosis, tuberculin-positive adults with abnormal chest radiographs showing fibrotic lesions probably representing old healed tuberculosis, adults with silicosis, and persons who are known to be HIV-infected and who are contacts of patients with infectious tuberculosis.

- In the absence of any of the above risk factors, persons up to 35 years of age with a positive skin test who are in the following high-incidence groups should be also considered for preventive therapy:
    — Foreign-born persons from high-prevalence countries.
    — Medically underserved low-income persons from high-prevalence populations (especially blacks, Hispanics, and Native Americans).
    — Residents of facilities for long-term care (e.g., correctional institutions, nursing homes, and mental institutions).
- Twelve months of preventive therapy is recommended for adults and children with HIV infection and other conditions associated with immunosuppression. Persons without HIV infection should receive preventive therapy for at least 6 months.
- In persons younger than 35 years of age, routine monitoring for adverse effects of isoniazid should consist of a monthly symptom review. For persons 35 years of age and older, hepatic enzymes should be measured prior to starting isoniazid and monitored monthly throughout treatment, in addition to monthly symptom reviews.
- Persons who are presumed to be infected with isoniazid-resistant organisms should be treated with rifampin rather than with isoniazid.
- As with the treatment of active tuberculosis, the key to success of preventive treatment is patient adherence to the prescribed regimen. Although not evaluated in clinical studies, directly observed, twice-weekly preventive therapy may be appropriate for adults and children at risk, who cannot or will not reliably self-administer therapy.

Rifampin is an essential component of the currently recommended regimen for treating tuberculosis. This regimen is effective in treating HIV-infected patients with tuberculosis, and consists of isoniazid and rifampin for a minimum period of 6 months, plus pyrazinamide and either ethambutol or streptomycin for the first 2 months.

Because of the common association of tuberculosis with HIV infection, an increasing number of patients probably will be considered candidates for combined therapy with rifampin and protease inhibitors. Prompt initiation of appropriate pharmacologic therapy for patients with HIV infection who acquire tuberculosis is critical because tuberculosis may become rapidly fatal. The management of these patients is complex, requires an individualized approach, and should be undertaken only by or in consultation with an expert. In addition, all HIV-infected patients at risk for tuberculosis infection should be carefully evaluated and administered isoniazid preventive treatment if indicated, regardless of whether they are receiving protease inhibitor therapy.

For HIV-infected patients diagnosed with drug-susceptible tuberculosis and for whom protease inhibitor therapy is being considered but has not been initiated, the suggested management strategy is to complete tuberculosis treatment with a regimen containing rifampin before starting therapy with a protease inhibitor. The duration of antituberculosis regimen is at least 6 months, and therapy should be administered according to the guidelines developed by ATS and CDC, including the recommendation to carefully assess clinical and bacteriologic responses in patients coinfected with HIV and to prolong treatment if response is slow or suboptimal.

Health care or correctional institutions experiencing outbreaks of tuberculosis that are resistant to isoniazid and rifampin, or are resuming therapy for a patient with a prior history of antitubercular therapy, may need to begin five- or six-drug regimens as initial therapy. These regimens should include the four-drug regimen and at least three medications to which the suspected multidrug-resistant strain may be susceptible.

Most infants ≤ 12 months of age with tuberculosis are asymptomatic at the time of diagnosis, and the gastric aspirate cultures in these patients have a high yield for *M. tuberculosis*. When an infant is suspected of having tuberculosis, a thorough household investigation should be undertaken. A 6-month regimen of isoniazid and rifampin supplemented during the first 2 months by pyrazinamide has been found to be well-tolerated and effective in infants with pulmonary tuberculosis. Furthermore, twice-weekly DOT appears to be as effective as daily therapy, and is an essential alternative in patients for whom social issues prevent reliable daily therapy.

Physicians caring for children should be familiar with the clinical forms of the disease in infants to enable them to make an early diagnosis. Any child, especially one in a high-risk group or area, who has unexplained pneumonia, cervical adenitis, bone or joint infections, or aseptic meningitis should have a Mantoux tuberculin skin test performed, and a detailed epidemiologic history for tuberculosis should be obtained.

Management of a newborn infant whose mother, or other household contact, is suspected of having tuberculosis is based on individual considerations. If possible, separation of the mother, or contact, and infant should be minimized. The Committee on Infectious Diseases of the AAP offers the following recommendations in the management of the newborn infant whose mother, or any other household contact, has tuberculosis:

- *Mother, or any other household contact, with a positive tuberculin skin test reaction but no evidence of current disease:* Investigation of other members of the household or extended family to whom the infant may later be exposed is indicated. If no evidence of current disease is found in the mother or in members of the extended family, the infant should be tested with a Mantoux tuberculin skin test at 3 to 4 months of age. When the family members cannot be promptly tested, consideration should be given to administering isoniazid (10 mg per kg of body weight a day) to the infant until skin testing and other evaluation of the family members have excluded contact with a case of active tuberculosis. The infant does not need to be hospitalized during this time if adequate follow-up can be arranged, but adherence to medication administration should be closely monitored. The mother also should be considered for isoniazid therapy.
- *Mother with untreated (newly diagnosed) disease or disease that has been treated for 2 or more weeks and who is judged to be noncontagious at delivery:* Careful investigation of household members and extended family is mandatory. A chest radiograph and Mantoux tuberculin skin test should be performed on the infant at 3 to 4 months and at 6 months of age. Separation of the mother and infant is not necessary if adherence to treatment for the mother and infant is assured. The mother can breast-feed. The infant should receive isoniazid even if the tuberculin skin test and chest radiograph do not suggest clinical tuberculosis, since cell-mediated immunity of a degree sufficient to mount a significant reaction to tuberculin skin testing may develop as late as 6 months of age in an infant infected at birth. Isoniazid can be discontinued if the Mantoux skin test is negative at 3 to 4 months of age, the mother is adherent to treatment and has a satisfactory clinical response, and no other family members have infectious tuberculosis. The infant should be examined carefully at monthly intervals. If nonadherence is documented, the mother has an acid-fast bacillus (AFB)–positive sputum or smear, and supervision is impossible, the infant should be separated from the ill family member and Bacillus Calmette-Guérin (BCG) vaccine may be considered for the infant. However, the response to the vaccine in infants may be delayed and inadequate for prevention of tuberculosis.
- *Mother has current disease and is suspected of having been contagious at the time of delivery:* The mother and infant should be separated until the infant is receiving therapy or the mother is confirmed to be noncontagious. Otherwise, management is the same as when the disease is judged to be noncontagious to the infant at delivery.
- *Mother has hematogenously spread tuberculosis (e.g., meningitis, miliary disease, or bone involvement):* The infant should be evaluated for congenital tuberculosis. If clinical and radiographic findings do not support the diagnosis of congenital tuberculosis, the infant should be separated from the mother until she is judged to be noncontagious. The infant should be given isoniazid until 3 or 4 months of age, at which time the Mantoux skin test should be repeated. If the skin test is positive, isoniazid should be continued for a total of 12 months. If the skin test is negative and the chest radiograph is normal, isoniazid may be discontinued, depending on the status of the mother and whether there are other cases of infectious tuberculosis in the family. The infant should continue to be examined carefully at monthly intervals.

Patients with impaired renal function do not require a reduction in dose; however, patients on hemodialysis should receive the usual dose at the end of each dialysis session.

## Oral Dosage Forms

### PYRAZINAMIDE TABLETS USP

**Usual adult and adolescent dose**
Tuberculosis—
    In combination with other antitubercular drugs: Oral, 15 to 30 mg per kg of body weight once a day; or 50 to 70 mg per kg of body weight two or three times a week, depending on the treatment regimen.

Note: The usual dose of pyrazinamide for persons infected with human immunodeficiency virus (HIV) is 20 to 30 mg per kg of body weight per day for the first two months of therapy.

**Usual adult prescribing limits**
A maximum of 2 grams when taken daily, 3 grams per dose for the three times a week regimen, 4 grams per dose for the two times a week regimen.

**Usual pediatric dose**
See *Usual adult and adolescent dose*.

Note: The usual maximum dose in children is 2 grams when taken daily, 3 grams per dose for the three times a week regimen, 4 grams per dose for the two times a week regimen.

**Strength(s) usually available**
U.S.—
    500 mg (Rx) [GENERIC].
Canada—
    500 mg (Rx) [*pms-Pyrazinamide; Tebrazid*].

**Packaging and storage**
Store below 40 °C (104 °F), preferably between 15 and 30 °C (59 and 86 °F), unless otherwise specified by the manufacturer. Store in a well-closed container.

**Auxiliary labeling**
• Continue medicine for full time of treatment.

## Selected Bibliography

The American Thoracic Society (ATS). Ad Hoc Committee on the Scientific Assembly on Microbiology, Tuberculosis, and Pulmonary Infections. Treatment of tuberculosis and tuberculosis infection in adults and children. Clin Infect Dis 1995; 21: 9-27

Revised: 08/22/97

---

**PYRETHRINS AND PIPERONYL BUTOXIDE**—The *Pyrethrins and Piperonyl Butoxide (Topical)* monograph is not included in this published version of the USP DI database. Copies of the monograph are available on request from Micromedex, Inc. - Reprint Requests, 6200 S. Syracuse Way, Suite 300, Englewood, CO 80111; telephone (303) 486-6400; telefax (303) 486-6464; Email: USPDI@MDX.COM.

---

**PYRIDOSTIGMINE**—See *Antimyasthenics (Systemic)*

---

# PYRIDOXINE Systemic

VA CLASSIFICATION (Primary): VT104

Commonly used brand name(s): *Beesix; Doxine; Nestrex; Pyri; Rodex; Vitabee 6*.

Another commonly used name is vitamin $B_6$.

Note: For a listing of dosage forms and brand names by country availability, see *Dosage Forms* section(s).

## Category

Nutritional supplement (vitamin); antidote (to cycloserine poisoning; to isoniazid poisoning).

Note: Pyridoxine is a water-soluble vitamin.

## Indications

Note: Bracketed information in the *Indications* section refers to uses that are not included in U.S. product labeling.

**Accepted**

Pyridoxine deficiency (prophylaxis and treatment)—Pyridoxine is indicated for prevention and treatment of pyridoxine deficiency states. Pyridoxine deficiency may occur as a result of inadequate nutrition or intestinal malabsorption but does not occur in healthy individuals receiving an adequate balanced diet. Simple nutritional deficiency of individual B vitamins is rare since dietary inadequacy usually results in multiple deficiencies. For prophylaxis of pyridoxine deficiency, dietary improvement, rather than supplementation, is advisable. For treatment of pyridoxine deficiency, supplementation is preferred.

Deficiency of pyridoxine may lead to xanthurenic aciduria, sideroblastic anemia, neurologic problems, seborrheic dermatitis, and cheilosis.

Recommended intakes may be increased and/or supplementation may be necessary in the following conditions or persons (based on documented pyridoxine deficiency):
Alcoholism
Burns
Congenital metabolic dysfunction—cystathioninuria, homocystinuria, hyperoxaluria, xanthurenic aciduria
Congestive heart failure
Fever, chronic
Gastrectomy
Hemodialysis
Hyperthyroidism
Infants receiving unfortified formulas such as evaporated milk
Infection
Intestinal diseases—celiac, diarrhea, regional enteritis, sprue
Malabsorption syndromes associated with hepatic-biliary tract disease such as alcoholism with cirrhosis
Stress, prolonged

Recommended intakes for pyridoxine are related to protein intake.

Some unusual diets (e.g., reducing diets that drastically restrict food selection) may not supply minimum daily requirements of pyridoxine. Supplementation is necessary in patients receiving total parenteral nutrition (TPN) or undergoing rapid weight loss or in those with malnutrition, because of inadequate dietary intake.

Recommended intakes for all vitamins and most minerals are increased during pregnancy. Many physicians recommend that pregnant women receive multivitamin and mineral supplements, especially those pregnant women who do not consume an adequate diet and those in high-risk categories (i.e., women carrying more than one fetus, heavy cigarette smokers, and alcohol and drug abusers). Taking excessive amounts of a multivitamin and mineral supplement may be harmful to the mother and/or fetus and should be avoided.

Recommended intakes for all vitamins and most minerals are increased during breast-feeding.

Recommended intakes may be increased by the following medications: Cycloserine, ethionamide, hydralazine, immunosuppressants, isoniazid, penicillamine, and estrogen-containing oral contraceptives.

Some neonates exhibit a hereditary pyridoxine dependency syndrome and require pyridoxine in the first week of life to prevent anemia and mental retardation; the cause is unknown but signs are hyperirritability and epileptiform seizures.

[Cycloserine toxicity (treatment)] or
[Isoniazid toxicity (treatment)]—Pyridoxine is also used as an antidote in cycloserine poisoning and to terminate seizures and prevent neuropathy associated with isoniazid poisoning.

**Unaccepted**

Pyridoxine has not been proven effective for treatment of acne and other dermatoses, alcohol intoxication, asthma, hemorrhoids, kidney stones, mental disorders, migraine headaches, morning sickness or radiation sickness, premenstrual tension, or for stimulation of lactation or appetite.

## Pharmacology/Pharmacokinetics

**Physicochemical characteristics**
Molecular weight—205.64.

### Mechanism of action/Effect

Nutritional supplement—Pyridoxine is converted in erythrocytes to pyridoxal phosphate and to a lesser extent pyridoxamine phosphate, which act as coenzymes for various metabolic functions affecting protein, carbohydrate, and lipid utilization. Pyridoxine is involved in conversion of tryptophan to niacin or serotonin, breakdown of glycogen to glucose-1-phosphate, conversion of oxalate to glycine, synthesis of gamma aminobutyric acid (GABA) within the CNS, and synthesis of heme.

Antidote—Pyridoxine increases the excretion of certain drugs (e.g., cycloserine and isoniazid) that act as pyridoxine antagonists.

### Absorption

The B vitamins are readily absorbed from the gastrointestinal tract, except in malabsorption syndromes. Pyridoxine is absorbed mainly in the jejunum.

### Protein binding

Pyridoxal phosphate—Totally bound to plasma proteins.
Pyridoxine—Not bound to plasma proteins.

### Storage

Pyridoxine is stored mainly in the liver, with lesser amounts stored in muscle and brain.

### Biotransformation

Hepatic.

### Half-life

15 to 20 days.

### Elimination

Renal (almost entirely as metabolites). Excess beyond daily needs is excreted, largely unchanged, in urine.

In dialysis—Removed by hemodialysis; dialysis patients should receive increased amounts (100 to 300% of USRDA).

## Precautions to Consider

### Pregnancy/Reproduction

Pregnancy—Problems in humans have not been documented with intake of normal daily recommended amounts. However, exposure to large doses of pyridoxine *in utero* may result in a pyridoxine dependency syndrome in the neonate.

FDA Pregnancy Category A (parenteral pyridoxine).

### Breast-feeding

Problems in humans have not been documented with intake of normal daily recommended amounts.

### Pediatrics

Problems in pediatrics have not been documented with intake of normal daily recommended amounts.

### Geriatrics

Problems in geriatrics have not been documented with intake of normal daily recommended amounts.

### Drug interactions and/or related problems

The following drug interactions and/or related problems have been selected on the basis of their potential clinical significance (possible mechanism in parentheses where appropriate)—not necessarily inclusive (» = major clinical significance):

Note: Combinations containing any of the following medications, depending on the amount present, may also interact with pyridoxine.

Cycloserine or
Ethionamide or
Hydralazine or
Immunosuppressants, such as:
  Azathioprine
  Chlorambucil
  Corticosteroids
  Corticotropin (ACTH)
  Cyclophosphamide
  Cyclosporine
  Mercaptopurine, or
Isoniazid or
Penicillamine
  (may cause anemia or peripheral neuritis by acting as pyridoxine antagonists or increasing renal excretion of pyridoxine; recommended intakes for pyridoxine may be increased in patients receiving these medications)

Estrogens or
Contraceptives, estrogen-containing, oral
  (may increase recommended intakes for pyridoxine)

» Levodopa
  (concurrent use with pyridoxine is not recommended since levodopa's antiparkinsonian effects are reversed by as little as 5 mg of pyridoxine orally; this problem does not occur with the carbidopa-levodopa combination)

### Laboratory value alterations

The following have been selected on the basis of their potential clinical significance (possible effect in parentheses where appropriate)—not necessarily inclusive (» = major clinical significance):

With diagnostic test results
  Urobilinogen determinations using Ehrlich's reagent
    (pyridoxine may produce false-positive results)

### Medical considerations/Contraindications

The medical considerations/contraindications included have been selected on the basis of their potential clinical significance (reasons given in parentheses where appropriate)—not necessarily inclusive (» = major clinical significance).

*Risk-benefit should be considered when the following medical problem exists:*

Sensitivity to pyridoxine

## Side/Adverse Effects

Doses of 200 mg per day for over 30 days have been reported to produce a pyridoxine dependency syndrome.

High doses of pyridoxine (2 to 6 grams per day) taken for several months have caused a severe sensory neuropathy, progressing from unstable gait and numb feet to numbness and clumsiness of hands. This condition seems to be reversible on withdrawal of pyridoxine, although some residual weakness has been observed.

## Patient Consultation

As an aid to patient consultation, refer to *Advice for the Patient, Pyridoxine (Vitamin $B_6$) (Systemic)*.

In providing consultation, consider emphasizing the following selected information (» = major clinical significance):

### Description of use

Description should include function in the body, signs of deficiency, and unproven uses

### Importance of diet

Importance of proper nutrition; supplement may be needed because of inadequate dietary intake
Food sources of pyridoxine; effects of processing
Not using vitamins as substitute for balanced diet
Recommended daily intakes for pyridoxine

### Before using this dietary supplement

» Conditions affecting use, especially:
  Sensitivity to pyridoxine
  Pregnancy—Use of large doses in pregnancy may cause pyridoxine dependency syndrome in the neonate
  Other medications, especially levodopa

### Proper use of this dietary supplement

» Proper dosing
Proper administration of extended-release capsule dosage forms: Swallowing whole without crushing, breaking, or chewing; contents of capsule may be mixed with jam or jelly and swallowed without chewing
Proper administration of extended-release tablet dosage forms: Swallowing whole without crushing, breaking, or chewing
Missed dose: No cause for concern because of length of time necessary for depletion; remembering to take as directed
» Proper storage

### Side/adverse effects

Signs of potential side effects, especially sensory neuropathy

## General Dosing Information

Because of the infrequency of single B vitamin deficiencies, combinations are commonly administered. Many commercial combinations of B vitamins are available.

### For parenteral dosage forms only

In most cases, parenteral administration is indicated only when oral administration is not acceptable (for example, in nausea, vomiting, preoperative and postoperative conditions) or possible (for example, in malabsorption syndromes or following gastric resection).

### Diet/Nutrition

Recommended dietary intakes for pyridoxine are defined differently worldwide.

For U.S.—
The Recommended Dietary Allowances (RDAs) for vitamins and minerals are determined by the Food and Nutrition Board of the Na-

tional Research Council and are intended to provide adequate nutrition in most healthy persons under usual environmental stresses. In addition, a different designation may be used by the FDA for food and dietary supplement labeling purposes, as with Daily Value (DV). DVs replace the previous labeling terminology United States Recommended Daily Allowances (USRDAs).

For Canada—
Recommended Nutrient Intakes (RNIs) for vitamins, minerals, and protein are determined by Health and Welfare Canada and provide recommended amounts of a specific nutrient while minimizing the risk of chronic diseases.

Daily recommended intakes for pyridoxine are generally defined as follows:
Infants and children:
  Birth to 3 years of age: 0.3 to 1 mg.
  4 to 6 years of age: 1.1 mg.
  7 to 10 years of age: 1.4 mg.
Adolescent and adult males:
  1.7 to 2 mg.
Adolescent and adult females:
  1.4 to 1.6 mg.
Pregnant females:
  2.2 mg.
Breast-feeding females:
  2.1 mg.

The best dietary sources of pyridoxine include meats, bananas, lima beans, egg yolks, peanuts, and whole-grain cereals. Substantial loss of pyridoxal and pyridoxamine (but not pyridoxine) occurs during cooking.

## Oral Dosage Forms

### PYRIDOXINE HYDROCHLORIDE EXTENDED-RELEASE CAPSULES

**Usual adult and adolescent dose**
Deficiency (prophylaxis)—Oral, amount based on normal daily recommended intakes—
  Adolescent and adult males—1.7 to 2 mg.
  Adolescent and adult females—1.4 to 1.6 mg.
  Pregnant females—2.2 mg.
  Breast-feeding females—2.1 mg.
Deficiency (treatment)—
  Treatment dose is individualized by prescriber based on severity of deficiency.

**Usual pediatric dose**
Dosage form not appropriate for pediatric patients.

**Strength(s) usually available**
U.S.—
  150 mg (OTC) [*Rodex*].
Canada—
  Not commercially available.

Note: The strength of this pyridoxine preparation may exceed the dosage range recommended by USP DI Advisory Panels based on the amount necessary to meet normal nutritional needs.

**Packaging and storage**
Store below 40 °C (104 °F), preferably between 15 and 30 °C (59 and 86 °F), in a well-closed container, unless otherwise specified by manufacturer. Protect from light.

**Auxiliary labeling**
• Swallow capsules whole.

### PYRIDOXINE HYDROCHLORIDE TABLETS USP

**Usual adult and adolescent dose**
See *Pyridoxine Hydrochloride Extended-release Capsules*.

**Usual pediatric dose**
Deficiency (prophylaxis)—Oral, amount based on normal daily recommended intakes—
  Birth to 3 years of age—0.3 to 1 mg.
  4 to 6 years of age—1.1 mg.
  7 to 10 years of age—1.4 mg.
Deficiency (treatment)—
  Treatment dose is individualized by prescriber based on severity of deficiency.

**Strength(s) usually available**
U.S.—
  10 mg (OTC) [GENERIC].
  25 mg (OTC) [*Nestrex*; GENERIC].
  50 mg (OTC) [GENERIC].
  100 mg (OTC) [GENERIC].
  200 mg (OTC) [GENERIC].
  250 mg (OTC) [GENERIC].
  500 mg (OTC) [GENERIC].
Canada—
  25 mg (OTC) [GENERIC].
  50 mg (OTC) [GENERIC].
  100 mg (OTC) [GENERIC].
  250 mg (OTC) [GENERIC].

Note: Some strengths of these pyridoxine preparations may exceed the dosage range recommended by USP DI Advisory Panels based on the amount necessary to meet normal nutritional needs.

**Packaging and storage**
Store below 40 °C (104 °F), preferably between 15 and 30 °C (59 and 86 °F), unless otherwise specified by manufacturer. Store in a well-closed container. Protect from light.

### PYRIDOXINE HYDROCHLORIDE EXTENDED-RELEASE TABLETS

**Usual adult and adolescent dose**
See *Pyridoxine Hydrochloride Extended-release Capsules*.

**Usual pediatric dose**
Dosage form not appropriate for pediatric patients.

**Strength(s) usually available**
U.S.—
  100 mg (OTC) [GENERIC].
  200 mg (OTC) [GENERIC].
  500 mg (OTC) [GENERIC].
Canada—
  Not commercially available.

Note: Some strengths of these pyridoxine preparations may exceed the dosage range recommended by USP DI Advisory Panels based on the amount necessary to meet normal nutritional needs.

## Parenteral Dosage Forms

Note: Bracketed uses in the *Dosage Forms* section refer to categories of use and/or indications that are not included in U.S. product labeling.

### PYRIDOXINE HYDROCHLORIDE INJECTION USP

**Usual adult and adolescent dose**
Deficiency (prophylaxis)—
  Intravenous infusion, as part of total parenteral nutrition solutions, the specific amount determined by individual patient need.
Deficiency (treatment)—
  In patients receiving total parenteral nutrition: The specific amount determined by individual patient need.
  Pyridoxine dependency syndrome: Initial—Intramuscular or intravenous, 30 to 600 mg per day.
  Drug-induced deficiency: Intramuscular or intravenous, 50 to 200 mg per day for three weeks, followed by 25 to 100 mg per day as needed.
[Cycloserine poisoning]—
  Intramuscular or intravenous, 300 mg or more per day.
[Isoniazid poisoning (10 grams or more)]—
  An amount of pyridoxine equal to amount of isoniazid ingested—Intravenous, 4 grams followed by 1 gram intramuscular every 30 minutes.

**Usual pediatric dose**
Deficiency (prophylaxis)—
  Intravenous infusion, as part of total parenteral nutrition solutions, the specific amount determined by individual patient need.
Deficiency (treatment)—
  In patients receiving total parenteral nutrition: The specific amount determined by individual patient need.
  Pyridoxine dependency syndrome in infants (with seizures): Initial—Intramuscular or intravenous, 10 to 100 mg.

**Strength(s) usually available**
U.S.—
  100 mg per mL (Rx) [*Beesix* (1.5% benzyl alcohol); *Doxine; Pyri; Rodex; Vitabee 6;* GENERIC].
Canada—
  100 mg per mL (Rx) [GENERIC].

**Packaging and storage**
Store below 40 °C (104 °F), preferably between 15 and 30 °C (59 and 86 °F), unless otherwise specified by manufacturer. Protect from light. Protect from freezing.

---

Revised: 09/21/92
Interim revision: 08/22/94; 05/01/95

**PYRILAMINE**—See *Antihistamines (Systemic)*

# PYRIMETHAMINE   Systemic

VA CLASSIFICATION (Primary/Secondary): AP101/AP109
Commonly used brand name(s): *Daraprim*.
Note: For a listing of dosage forms and brand names by country availability, see *Dosage Forms* section(s).

## Category
Antiprotozoal.

## Indications
Note: Bracketed information in the *Indications* section refers to uses that are not included in U.S. product labeling.

### Accepted
Malaria (treatment)—Pyrimethamine is indicated in combination with sulfadoxine and quinine in the treatment of chloroquine-resistant *Plasmodium falciparum* malaria. It is also indicated in combination with mefloquine and sulfadoxine, or quinine and sulfadoxine in the treatment of chloroquine-resistant *P. falciparum* malaria acquired in Southeast Asia, Bangladesh, East Africa, or the Amazon basin. Pyrimethamine is indicated in combination with sulfadoxine in the presumptive treatment of chloroquine-resistant *P. falciparum* malaria for self-treatment of febrile illness when medical care is not immediately available.

Toxoplasmosis (treatment)—Pyrimethamine is indicated in combination with a sulfapyrimidine-type sulfonamide in the treatment of toxoplasmosis caused by *Toxoplasma gondii*. [Pyrimethamine is also used with clindamycin in the treatment of toxoplasmosis in patients who are unresponsive to or intolerant of standard therapy.][1]

[Isosporiasis (prophylaxis and treatment)][1]—Pyrimethamine is used with sulfadoxine in the prophylaxis and treatment of isosporiasis caused by *Isospora belli*. It has also been used alone in a limited number of patients in the prophylaxis and treatment of isosporiasis.

[Pneumonia, *Pneumocystis carinii* (treatment)][1]—Pyrimethamine is used in combination with sulfadiazine, sulfadoxine, or dapsone, in the treatment of mild to moderate pneumonia caused by *Pneumocystis carinii* in patients who are unresponsive to or intolerant of standard therapy.

Not all species or strains of a particular organism may be susceptible to pyrimethamine. Resistance to pyrimethamine has been reported in *P. falciparum* and *P. vivax* malaria and may be widespread in certain areas.

### Unaccepted
Pyrimethamine is not indicated alone in the treatment of acute attacks of malaria in nonimmune patients. Fast-acting schizonticides (e.g., 4-aminoquinolines, quinine) are preferred for these patients.

[1]Not included in Canadian product labeling.

## Pharmacology/Pharmacokinetics

### Physicochemical characteristics
Molecular weight—248.71.

### Mechanism of action/Effect
Binds to and reversibly inhibits the protozoal enzyme dihydrofolate reductase, selectively blocking conversion of dihydrofolic acid to its functional form, tetrahydrofolic acid. This depletes folate, an essential cofactor in the biosynthesis of nucleic acids, resulting in interference with protozoal nucleic acid and protein production. Protozoal dihydrofolate reductase is many times more tightly bound by pyrimethamine than the corresponding mammalian enzyme.

Exerts its effect in the folate biosynthesis at a step immediately subsequent to the one at which sulfonamides exert their effect. When administered concurrently with sulfonamides, synergism occurs, which is attributed to inhibition of tetrahydrofolate production at 2 sequential steps in its biosynthesis.

Active against asexual erythrocytic forms and, to a lesser degree, tissue forms of *P. falciparum* malaria. Does not destroy gametocytes, but arrests sporogony in the mosquito. Used alone, pyrimethamine does not produce radical cure in vivax or ovale malaria since it does not kill the latent hepatic stages of these parasites.

### Absorption
Well absorbed following oral administration.

### Distribution
Widely distributed; mainly concentrated in blood cells, kidneys, lungs, liver, and spleen. Crosses into the cerebrospinal fluid (CSF), with concentrations ranging from 13 to 26% of the corresponding serum concentrations. The mean whole blood to plasma concentration ratio was 0.87 in 1 study. Also crosses the placenta and is excreted in breast milk.
$Vol_D$ ranges from 2.3 to 3.1 liters per kg.

### Protein binding
High (87%).

### Biotransformation
Hepatic.

### Half-life
Adults—Range, 80 to 123 hours. However, the half-life of pyrimethamine has been found to be as short as 23 hours in studies in patients with acquired immunodeficiency syndrome (AIDS), suggesting the possibility of a genetic variation in the metabolism of pyrimethamine or altered hepatic function secondary to HIV infection.
Infants (approximately 1 year old)—Approximately 64 hours (range, 52 to 87 hours).

### Time to peak plasma concentration
Approximately 3 hours (range, 2 to 6 hours).

### Peak plasma concentration
Adults—0.13 to 0.31 mcg/mL after a 25 mg dose.
Infants (approximately 1 year old)—1.3 mcg/mL after a dose of 1 mg per kg of body weight (mg/kg) per day; 0.7 mcg/mL 4 hours after a dose when administered at 1 mg/kg every Monday, Wednesday, and Friday.

### Elimination
Renal—Primary route; 20 to 30% excreted unchanged in urine. Urinary excretion may persist for 30 days or longer.
In dialysis—The serum concentration of pyrimethamine fell by approximately 47% after peritoneal dialysis in one patient.

## Precautions to Consider

### Carcinogenicity
Pyrimethamine has been reported to be associated with 2 cases of cancer in humans. Chronic granulocytic leukemia and reticulum cell sarcoma developed in patients receiving long-term pyrimethamine therapy for toxoplasmosis. Pyrimethamine also produced a significant increase in the number of lung tumors in mice given high-dose intraperitoneal pyrimethamine.

### Mutagenicity
An increase in the number of structural and numerical aberrations was found in the chromosomes analyzed from the bone marrow of rats dosed with pyrimethamine. Structural chromosome aberrations were induced by pyrimethamine in human blood lymphoctyes cultured *in vitro*. Pyrimethamine was positive in the L5178Y/TK +/− mouse lymphoma assay without metabolic activation. However, it was found to be nonmutagenic in the Ames point mutation assay, the Rec assay, and the *E. coli* WP2 assay.

### Pregnancy/Reproduction
Fertility—The fertility index of rats treated with pyrimethamine was lowered when high doses were used, suggesting possible toxic effects on the whole organism and/or conceptuses.

Pregnancy—Pyrimethamine crosses the placenta. Studies in humans have not shown that pyrimethamine causes teratogenic effects. Also, use in pregnant women to date has not shown pyrimethamine to be teratogenic. However, use is not generally recommended during the first 14 to 16 weeks of pregnancy since studies in animals have shown that pyrimethamine may cause birth defects in the fetus and may interfere with folic acid metabolism, especially when given in large doses such as those required in the treatment of toxoplasmosis. If pyrimethamine is necessary in the treatment of toxoplasmosis during pregnancy, it is recommended that leucovorin (folinic acid) be given concurrently.

FDA Pregnancy Category C.

### Breast-feeding
Pyrimethamine is excreted in breast milk. It is estimated that a nursing infant would ingest approximately 3 to 4 mg over 48 hours after the ingestion of a single 75 mg dose by the mother. Problems in humans have not been documented. However, pyrimethamine may interfere with folic acid metabolism in nursing infants, especially when given to

nursing women in large doses such as those required in the treatment of toxoplasmosis.

**Pediatrics**
Pyrimethamine has been used in children, and no pediatrics-specific problems have been documented to date.

**Geriatrics**
No information is available on the relationship of age to the effects of pyrimethamine in geriatric patients.

**Dental**
High doses of pyrimethamine not supplemented by leucovorin (folinic acid) may cause a folic acid deficiency, which may be characterized by a change in or loss of taste, or pain, burning, or inflammation of the tongue.

The leukopenic and thrombocytopenic effects of high doses of pyrimethamine may result in an increased incidence of certain microbial infections, delayed healing, and gingival bleeding. If leukopenia or thrombocytopenia occurs, dental work should be deferred until blood counts have returned to normal. Patients should be instructed in proper oral hygiene, including caution in use of regular toothbrushes, dental floss, and toothpicks.

**Drug interactions and/or related problems**
The following drug interactions and/or related problems have been selected on the basis of their potential clinical significance (possible mechanism in parentheses where appropriate)—not necessarily inclusive (» = major clinical significance):

Note: Combinations containing any of the following medications, depending on the amount present, may also interact with this medication.

» Bone marrow depressants (See *Appendix II* )
(concurrent use of pyrimethamine with bone marrow depressants may increase the leukopenic and/or thrombocytopenic effects; if concurrent use is required, the possibility of increased myelotoxic effects should be considered, especially when pyrimethamine is used in large doses such as those required in the treatment of toxoplasmosis)

Folate antagonists, other, (See *Appendix II* )
(concurrent use of other folate antagonists with pyrimethamine or use of pyrimethamine between courses of other folate antagonists is not recommended because of the possible development of megaloblastic anemia)

**Medical considerations/Contraindications**
The medical considerations/contraindications included have been selected on the basis of their potential clinical significance (reasons given in parentheses where appropriate)—not necessarily inclusive (» = major clinical significance):

*Risk-benefit should be considered when the following medical problems exist:*

» Anemia or
» Bone marrow depression
(pyrimethamine may cause folic acid deficiency, resulting in megaloblastic anemia, and blood dyscrasias, including agranulocytosis and thrombocytopenia)

Hepatic function impairment
(pyrimethamine is metabolized in the liver)

Hypersensitivity to pyrimethamine

» Seizure disorders, history of
(pyrimethamine may cause central nervous system [CNS] toxicity when used in high doses, as in the treatment of toxoplasmosis)

**Patient monitoring**
The following may be especially important in patient monitoring (other tests may be warranted in some patients, depending on condition; » = major clinical significance):

» Complete blood counts (CBCs) and
» Platelet counts
(may be required weekly during therapy in patients receiving high dosage, as in the treatment of toxoplasmosis)

## Side/Adverse Effects

Note: When pyrimethamine is used for malaria in usual recommended dosage, side/adverse effects usually are rare; however, with large doses, as for toxoplasmosis, side effects may occur more frequently unless pyrimethamine is given concurrently with folinic acid.

The following side/adverse effects have been selected on the basis of their potential clinical significance (possible signs and symptoms in parentheses where appropriate)—not necessarily inclusive:

**Those indicating need for medical attention**
Incidence more frequent with high doses
*Atrophic glossitis* (pain, burning, or inflammation of the tongue; change in or loss of taste)—due to folic acid deficiency; *blood dyscrasias, specifically agranulocytosis* (fever and sore throat); *megaloblastic anemia* (unusual tiredness or weakness); *or thrombocytopenia* (unusual bleeding or bruising)

Incidence rare
*Hypersensitivity* (skin rash)

**Those indicating need for medical attention only if they continue or are bothersome**
Incidence more frequent with high doses
*Gastrointestinal disturbances* (anorexia; diarrhea; nausea and vomiting)

## Overdose

For specific information on the agents used in the management of pyrimethamine overdose, see:
- *Barbiturates (Systemic)* monograph;
- *Benzodiazepines (Systemic)* monograph; and/or
- *Leucovorin (Systemic)* monograph.

For more information on the management of overdose or unintentional ingestion, **contact a Poison Control Center** (see *Poison Control Center Listing*).

**Clinical effects of overdose**
The following effects have been selected on the basis of their potential clinical significance (possible signs and symptoms in parentheses where appropriate)—not necessarily inclusive:

Acute
In order of occurrence: *Gastrointestinal toxicity* (abdominal pain; severe and repeated vomiting); *neurotoxicity* (hyperexcitability; seizures)—usually occurs within 30 minutes to 2 hours of ingestion; *respiratory depression; circulatory collapse*

**Treatment of overdose**
Recommended treatment for pyrimethamine overdose includes:
To decrease absorption—
Gastric emptying by aspiration and lavage.
Specific treatment—
Control of CNS stimulation, including seizures, by parenteral administration of benzodiazepines or short-acting barbiturates. Administration of leucovorin, 5 to 15 mg (up to 50 mg in cerebral toxoplasmosis) intramuscularly daily for 3 days or longer, to counteract the effects of folic acid antagonism (e.g., reduced white blood cell counts) induced by pyrimethamine.
Monitoring—
Monitoring of hematopoietic status for at least 1 month following overdose.
Supportive care—
Mechanical assistance of respiration, if necessary. Patients in whom intentional overdose is confirmed or suspected should be referred for psychiatric consultation.

## Patient Consultation

As an aid to patient consultation, refer to *Advice for the Patient, Pyrimethamine (Systemic)*.

In providing consultation, consider emphasizing the following selected information (» = major clinical significance):

**Before using this medication**
» Conditions affecting use, especially:
Hypersensitivity to pyrimethamine
Pregnancy—Pyrimethamine crosses the placenta
Breast-feeding—Pyrimethamine is excreted in breast milk
Dental—High doses may cause atrophic glossitis, leukopenia, or thrombocytopenia
Other medications, especially bone marrow depressants
Other medical problems, especially anemia, bone marrow depression, or a history of seizure disorders

**Proper use of this medication**
» Keeping medication out of reach of children; overdose is very dangerous
Taking with meals or a snack if gastric irritation occurs
» Compliance with full course of therapy
» Importance of not missing doses and taking medication on a regular schedule
» Proper dosing
Missed dose: Taking as soon as possible; not taking if almost time for next dose; not doubling doses
» Proper storage

### Precautions while using this medication
» Regular visits to physician to check blood counts, especially during high-dose therapy for toxoplasmosis
Checking with physician if no improvement within a few days
Importance of taking leucovorin concurrently if anemia occurs
Using caution in use of regular toothbrushes, dental floss, and toothpicks; deferring dental work until blood counts have returned to normal; checking with physician or dentist concerning proper oral hygiene

### Side/adverse effects
Signs of potential side effects, especially blood dyscrasias, hypersensitivity, and symptoms of folic acid deficiency

## General Dosing Information
Pyrimethamine may cause gastric irritation, sometimes resulting in vomiting, when given in high doses. To minimize this, pyrimethamine may be taken with meals or a snack or the dosage may be reduced.

Therapy should be discontinued if symptoms of folic acid deficiency occur. However, to prevent folic acid deficiency, leucovorin (folinic acid) may be administered concurrently to restore normal hematopoiesis. Leucovorin does not interfere with the antiprotozoal activity of pyrimethamine. Since malarial parasites are unable to utilize preformed folic acid, the antimalarial effect of pyrimethamine should not be affected. However, folic acid may interfere with the action of pyrimethamine on *T. gondii*, and concurrent use in toxoplasmosis is not recommended. In adults, 5 to 15 mg of leucovorin may be given orally, intramuscularly, or intravenously once a day for 3 days or as required. Alternatively, adults may be given 9 mg of leucovorin 2 or 3 times a week. Doses of up to 50 mg per day of leucovorin have been used with pyrimethamine in AIDS patients. Infants may be given 1 mg of leucovorin once a day.

Patients with impaired renal function receiving pyrimethamine prophylactically do not generally require a reduction in dose. However, patients receiving pyrimethamine more frequently should be monitored closely for signs of toxicity.

### For toxoplasmosis
The dose of pyrimethamine that is required in the treatment of toxoplasmosis is 10 to 20 times greater than the antimalarial dose. Concurrent prophylactic administration of leucovorin in doses up to 50 mg daily with pyrimethamine is recommended to avoid folic acid deficiency.

In patients with seizure disorders, small initial doses of pyrimethamine are recommended in the treatment of toxoplasmosis to avoid potential CNS toxicity.

In patients who also have AIDS, treatment with pyrimethamine and sulfonamides may be required indefinitely. Clindamycin has been used with pyrimethamine in doses of 900 mg to 2.4 grams daily in patients who experienced adverse reactions to sulfonamides.

## Oral Dosage Forms
Note: Bracketed uses in the *Dosage Forms* section refer to categories of use and/or indications that are not included in U.S. product labeling.

### PYRIMETHAMINE TABLETS USP
**Usual adult and adolescent dose**
Malaria—
  Treatment:
    Chloroquine-resistant *P. falciparum* malaria—Oral, 75 mg of pyrimethamine in combination with 1.5 grams of sulfadoxine as a single dose on day three of quinine therapy.
    Chloroquine-resistant *P. falciparum* malaria acquired in Southeast Asia, Bangladesh, East Africa, or the Amazon basin—Oral, 75 mg of pyrimethamine in combination with 750 mg of mefloquine and 1.5 grams of sulfadoxine as a single dose.
  Presumptive treatment:
    Oral, 75 mg of pyrimethamine in combination with 1.5 grams of sulfadoxine as a single dose for self-treatment of febrile illness when medical care is not immediately available.
Toxoplasmosis—
  AIDS patients:
    Loading dose—Oral, 100 to 200 mg of pyrimethamine per day in combination with 500 mg to 1.5 grams of a sulfadiazine every six hours, or 600 mg of clindamycin every six hours, for one to two days.
    Treatment—Oral, 50 to 100 mg of pyrimethamine per day in combination with 500 mg to 1.5 grams of a sulfadiazine every six hours, or 600 mg of clindamycin every six hours, for three to six weeks.
    Maintenance—Oral, 25 to 50 mg of pyrimethamine per day in combination with 250 mg to 1 gram of a sulfadiazine every six hours, or 600 mg of clindamycin every six hours, as life-long therapy.
  Other patients—
    Loading dose—Oral, 50 to 200 mg per day in combination with 250 mg to 1 gram of a sulfapyrimidine-type sulfonamide every six hours, for one to two days.
    Treatment—Oral, 25 to 50 mg per day in combination with 125 to 500 mg of a sulfapyrimidine-type sulfonamide every six hours, for two to four weeks if patient is immunocompetent, and four to six weeks if patient is immunocompromised.
[Isosporiasis][1]—
  Treatment: Oral, 50 to 75 mg of pyrimethamine per day for three to four weeks.
  Prophylaxis: Oral, 25 mg of pyrimethamine in combination with 500 mg of sulfadoxine once a week; or 25 mg of pyrimethamine alone once a day.
  Note: These doses are based on very limited data.

**Usual pediatric dose**
Malaria—
  Treatment:
    Chloroquine-resistant *P. falciparum* malaria—Oral, 1.25 mg per kg of body weight of pyrimethamine in combination with 25 mg per kg of body weight of sulfadoxine as a single dose on day three of quinine therapy.
    Chloroquine-resistant *P. falciparum* malaria acquired in Southeast Asia, Bangladesh, East Africa, or the Amazon basin—Oral, 1 mg per kg of body weight of pyrimethamine in combination with 10 mg per kg of body weight of mefloquine and 20 mg per kg of body weight of sulfadoxine as a single dose.
  Presumptive treatment, for self-treatment of febrile illness when medical care is not immediately available:
    Children 5 to 10 kg of body weight—Oral, 12.5 mg of pyrimethamine and 250 mg of sulfadoxine combination (½ tablet) as a single dose.
    Children 11 to 20 kg of body weight—Oral, 25 mg of pyrimethamine and 500 mg of sulfadoxine combination (1 tablet) as a single dose.
    Children 21 to 30 kg of body weight—Oral, 37.5 mg of pyrimethamine and 750 mg of sulfadoxine combination (1½ tablets) as a single dose.
    Children 31 to 45 kg of body weight—Oral, 50 mg of pyrimethamine and 1 gram of sulfadoxine combination (2 tablets) as a single dose.
    Children greater than 45 kg of body weight—Oral, 75 mg of pyrimethamine and 1.5 grams of sulfadoxine combination (3 tablets) as a single dose.
Toxoplasmosis—
  In combination with the usual pediatric dose of a sulfapyrimidine-type sulfonamide: Oral, 1 mg of pyrimethamine per kg of body weight once a day for one to three days; then 0.5 mg of pyrimethamine per kg of body weight once a day for four to six weeks.
Note: In infants with confirmed congenital toxoplasmosis, treatment should be continued for a minimum of six months if there are no signs of infection, and for one year if there are signs of significant infection.

**Strength(s) usually available**
U.S.—
  25 mg (Rx) [*Daraprim* (scored)].
Canada—
  25 mg (Rx) [*Daraprim* (scored)].

**Packaging and storage**
Store below 40 °C (104 °F), preferably between 15 and 30 °C (59 and 86 °F), unless otherwise specified by manufacturer. Store in a tight, light-resistant container.

**Preparation of dosage form**
For patients who cannot take oral solids—According to the manufacturer, the tablets may be crushed to prepare a 1% solution in normal saline. The solution is stable for 24 hours at room temperature. Cherry Syrup NF or sucrose-containing solutions may also be used as vehicles. However, pyrimethamine prepared in these vehicles should be used immediately after preparation.

**Auxiliary labeling**
• Continue medicine for full time of treatment.
• Keep out of reach of children.

### Pyrimethamine (Systemic)

**Note**
Explain potential danger of accidental overdose.
Consider dispensing in unit-dose packaging in child-resistant containers ("double-barrier" packaging).

[1]Not included in Canadian product labeling.

Revised: 01/19/93

**PYRITHIONE**—The *Pyrithione (Topical)* monograph is not included in this published version of the USP DI database. Copies of the monograph are available on request from Micromedex, Inc. - Reprint Requests, 6200 S. Syracuse Way, Suite 300, Englewood, CO 80111; telephone (303) 486-6400; telefax (303) 486-6464; Email: USPDI@MDX.COM.

**PYRVINIUM**—The *Pyrvinium (Oral-Local)* monograph is not included in this published version of the USP DI database. Copies of the monograph are available on request from Micromedex, Inc. - Reprint Requests, 6200 S. Syracuse Way, Suite 300, Englewood, CO 80111; telephone (303) 486-6400; telefax (303) 486-6464; Email: USPDI@MDX.COM.

**QUAZEPAM**—See *Benzodiazepines (Systemic)*

# QUETIAPINE Systemic—INTRODUCTORY VERSION

VA CLASSIFICATION (Primary): CN709

Note: For a listing of dosage forms and brand names by country availability, see *Dosage Forms* section(s).

## Category
Antipsychotic.

## Indications

**Accepted**

Psychotic disorders (treatment)—Quetiapine is indicated for the treatment of the manifestations of psychotic disorders. The effectiveness of quetiapine for more than 6 weeks has not been evaluated in controlled trials.

## Pharmacology/Pharmacokinetics

**Physicochemical characteristics**
Chemical group—Dibenzothiazepine derivative.
Molecular weight—Quetiapine fumarate: 883.11.
Solubility—Quetiapine fumarate is moderately soluble in water.

**Mechanism of action/Effect**
The exact mechanism by which quetiapine exerts its antipsychotic effect is unknown. However, this effect may be mediated through antagonism of dopamine type 2 ($D_2$) and serotonin type 2 ($5-HT_2$) receptors.

Quetiapine is an antagonist at serotonin $5-HT_{1A}$ and $5-HT_2$, dopamine $D_1$ and $D_2$, histamine $H_1$, and adrenergic $alpha_1$ and $alpha_2$ receptors. Quetiapine has no significant affinity for cholinergic muscarinic or benzodiazepine receptors. Drowsiness and orthostatic hypotension associated with use of quetiapine may be explained by its antagonism of histamine $H_1$ and adrenergic $alpha_1$ receptors, respectively.

**Other actions/effects**
In clinical trials, quetiapine produced a dose-related decrease in total and free thyroxine ($T_4$) concentrations. This decrease was apparent early in treatment with quetiapine, and no further changes occurred during continued therapy. At the high end of the quetiapine therapeutic dosage range, total and free thyroxine concentrations were decreased by about 20%. About 0.4% (10/2386) of patients in clinical trials experienced increases in thyroid-stimulating hormone (TSH) concentrations and six of these patients required thyroid hormone replacement therapy.

Prolactin concentration increases, which were associated with an increased incidence of mammary gland neoplasia, were seen in rat studies with quetiapine. However, prolactin concentration increases were not demonstrated in human clinical trials.

Cataracts developed in the eyes of dogs during chronic quetiapine dosing. Also, changes in the lenses of the eyes have been observed in patients during long-term quetiapine therapy, although a causal relationship to quetiapine has not been established.

**Absorption**
Rapidly and well absorbed. Food increases peak plasma concentration ($C_{max}$) and area under the plasma concentration–time curve (AUC) by 25% and 15%, respectively.

**Distribution**
Extensively distributed throughout the body, with an apparent volume of distribution ($Vol_D$) of $10 \pm 4$ L/kg.

**Protein binding**
High (83%) to plasma proteins; does not alter the binding of warfarin or diazepam to human serum albumin *in vitro* and quetiapine binding is not altered *in vitro* by warfarin or diazepam.

**Biotransformation**
Quetiapine is extensively metabolized in the liver. Less than 1% of an orally administered dose is excreted unchanged. The major metabolic pathways are sulfoxidation, which *in vitro* studies indicate is mediated by the cytochrome P450 3A4 (CYP3A4) isoenzyme, and oxidation. The major metabolites of quetiapine are inactive.

**Half-life**
Elimination—
Mean, about 6 hours.

**Time to peak concentration**
Peak plasma concentration is reached within 1.5 hours of dosing.

**Elimination**
Renal—
Approximately 73% of an orally administered dose is excreted renally.
Fecal—
Approximately 20% of an orally administered dose is excreted in the feces.

## Precautions to Consider

**Carcinogenicity/Tumorigenicity**
Statistically significant increases in the incidence of thyroid gland follicular cell adenomas were seen in male mice receiving quetiapine at daily dosages that were equivalent to 1.5 and 4.5 times the maximum recommended human dose (MRHD) on a mg per square meter of body surface area (mg/m$^2$) basis and in male rats receiving three times the MRHD on a mg/m$^2$ basis, possibly as a result of chronic stimulation of the thyroid gland by thyroid-stimulating hormone (TSH). Although the results were not definitive, quetiapine toxicity studies in rats and mice showed changes in thyroxine concentrations, thyroxine clearance, and TSH concentrations that are consistent with the proposed mechanism of increased thyroxine clearance leading to increased TSH concentrations and increased thyroid gland stimulation.

Statistically significant increases in the incidence of mammary gland adenocarcinomas were seen in female rats receiving quetiapine at daily dosages that were equivalent to 0.3 to 3 times the MRHD on a mg/m$^2$ basis. In a 1-year quetiapine toxicity study, median serum prolactin concentrations were increased a maximum of 32-fold in male rats, and 13-fold in female rats. The mammary gland neoplasms seen in rodents after chronic administration of antipsychotic medications are considered to be prolactin-mediated.

The relevance of these findings to humans is unknown.

**Mutagenicity**
Quetiapine produced a reproducible increase in mutations in one of six strains in *in vitro* bacterial gene mutation assays in the presence of metabolic activation. An *in vitro* chromosomal aberration assay in cultured human lymphocytes and an *in vivo* micronucleus assay in rats found no evidence of clastogenic potential.

**Pregnancy/Reproduction**
Fertility—In male Sprague-Dawley rats, the interval to mate and the number of matings required to produce pregnancy increased at quetiapine doses equivalent to 0.6 and 1.8 times the MRHD on a mg/m$^2$ basis. These effects were still present 2 weeks after discontinuation of quetiapine in the rats that had received 1.8 times the MRHD. No effects on mating or fertility were seen in male rats receiving $\leq 0.3$ times the MRHD on a mg/m$^2$ basis.

In female Sprague-Dawley rats, the interval to mate increased and the number of matings and the number of matings resulting in pregnancy decreased at a quetiapine dose equivalent to 0.6 times the MRHD on a mg/m$^2$ basis. Irregular estrus cycles increased at doses equivalent to 0.1 and 0.6 times the MRHD on a mg/m$^2$ basis. No effects on estrus, mating, or fertility were seen in female rats receiving $\leq 0.01$ times the MRHD on a mg/m$^2$ basis.

Pregnancy—Adequate and well-controlled studies in humans have not been done.

Quetiapine showed no teratogenic potential in rats and rabbits dosed at 0.3 to 2.4 and 0.6 to 2.4 times the MRHD on a mg/m$^2$ basis, respectively, during the period of organogenesis. However, in rats, delays in skeletal ossification were seen in the fetuses at all doses. Also, reduced fetal body weight and reduced maternal weight gain and/or increased maternal deaths were seen at the highest dose used. In rabbits, reduced maternal weight gain and/or increased maternal deaths were seen at all doses, delays in skeletal ossification in the fetuses were seen at doses of 1.2 and 2.4 times the MRHD on a mg/m$^2$ basis, and reduced fetal body weight and an increased incidence of minor soft tissue anomaly in the fetuses were seen at the highest dose used. In a perinatal/postnatal study in rats receiving 0.01 to 0.24 times the MRHD on a mg/m$^2$ basis, no drug-related effects were observed. However, in a preliminary perinatal/postnatal study in rats receiving three times the MRHD on a mg/m$^2$ basis, increases in fetal and pup deaths and decreases in mean litter weight were found.

FDA Pregnancy Category C.

Labor and delivery—The effects of quetiapine on labor and delivery are unknown.

**Breast-feeding**
Quetiapine is distributed into the milk of animals. It is not known whether quetiapine is distributed into breast milk, but breast-feeding while taking quetiapine is not recommended.

**Pediatrics**
No information is available on the relationship of age to the effects of quetiapine in pediatric patients. Safety and efficacy have not been established.

**Geriatrics**
No geriatrics-specific problems that would limit the usefulness of quetiapine in the elderly were seen in studies that included subjects 65 years of age and older. However, the mean plasma clearance of quetiapine in elderly patients was 30 to 50% less than in younger patients. Reduced initial and target dosages, and slower dosage titration may be necessary in elderly patients.

**Drug interactions and/or related problems**
The following drug interactions and/or related problems have been selected on the basis of their potential clinical significance (possible mechanism in parentheses where appropriate)—not necessarily inclusive (» = major clinical significance):

Note: Combinations containing any of the following medications, depending on the amount present, may also interact with this medication.

» Alcohol or
» Central nervous system (CNS) depression–producing medications, other (see *Appendix II*)
  (quetiapine has been shown to potentiate the cognitive and motor effects of alcohol)

Antihypertensive agents
  (hypotensive effects of these medications may be enhanced)

Cimetidine
  (oral clearance of quetiapine was decreased by 20% when coadministered with cimetidine 400 mg three times a day)

» Cytochrome P450 3A (CYP3A) isoenzyme inhibitors, such as:
  Erythromycin
  Fluconazole
  Itraconazole
  Ketoconazole
  (although there is no experience with the combination of quetiapine and a potent CYP3A enzyme inhibitor, caution is advised since quetiapine's major route of metabolism involves CYP3A4)

Dopamine agonists or
Levodopa
  (effects of these medications may be antagonized by quetiapine)

» Enzyme inducers, hepatic, cytochrome P450 (see *Appendix II*)
  (mean oral clearance of quetiapine was increased fivefold in patients receiving phenytoin; higher doses of quetiapine may be required during concomitant therapy with an enzyme-inducing medication; a decrease in quetiapine dosage may be required when enzyme-inducer therapy is discontinued)

Lorazepam
  (mean oral clearance of lorazepam was decreased by 20% when coadministered with quetiapine 250 mg three times a day)

Thioridazine
  (oral clearance of quetiapine was increased by 65% when coadministered with thioridazine 200 mg two times a day)

**Laboratory value alterations**
The following have been selected on the basis of their potential clinical significance (possible effect in parentheses where appropriate)—not necessarily inclusive (» = major clinical significance):

With physiology/laboratory test values
  Alanine aminotransferase (ALT [SGPT]) and
  Aspartate transaminase (AST [SGOT])
    (elevated values have been reported, usually within the first 3 weeks of quetiapine use; approximately 6% of patients in a sample of clinical trials experienced elevations of greater than three times the upper limit of normal; all patients were asymptomatic, and values returned to baseline with continued use of quetiapine)

  Cholesterol, total and
  Triglycerides
    (increases from baseline of 11% and 17%, respectively, which were weakly related to body weight increases, were reported in patients in a sample of clinical trials)

  Thyroid function tests
    (a dose-related decrease in total and free thyroxine [$T_4$] concentrations, which was about 20% at the highest quetiapine doses used, was seen in clinical trials; this decrease was apparent early in treatment with quetiapine, and no further changes occurred with continued therapy; about 0.4% [10/2386] of patients in clinical trials experienced increases in thyroid-stimulating hormone [TSH] concentrations and six of these patients required thyroid hormone replacement therapy)

**Medical considerations/Contraindications**
The medical considerations/contraindications included have been selected on the basis of their potential clinical significance (reasons given in parentheses where appropriate)—not necessarily inclusive (» = major clinical significance).

*Except under special circumstances, this medication should not be used when the following medical problem exists:*
» Hypersensitivity to quetiapine

*Risk-benefit should be considered when the following medical problems exist:*

Alzheimer's dementia
  (dysphagia associated with use of antipsychotic medications may increase risk of aspiration pneumonia)
  (possible increased risk of seizures because of lowered seizure threshold with Alzheimer's dementia)

» Breast cancer, or history of
  (although elevated prolactin concentrations have not been demonstrated in clinical trials of quetiapine, elevations have occurred with use of other antipsychotic medications and in animal studies of quetiapine; studies have found approximately one third of human breast cancers to be prolactin-dependent *in vitro*)

» Cardiovascular disease, including:
  Conduction abnormalities or
  Heart failure or
  Myocardial infarction or ischemia, or history of or
» Cerebrovascular disease or
» Conditions that would predispose to hypotension, including:
  Dehydration or
  Hypovolemia
    (orthostatic hypotension may be exacerbated or may exacerbate pre-existing cardiovascular or cerebrovascular conditions; if hypotension occurs during dosage titration, it is recommended that dosage be returned to the previous level)
    (dehydration may predispose patient to increased core body temperature, and antipsychotic medications may disrupt the body's ability to lower core body temperature, thus increasing the risk of heatstroke)

Drug abuse or dependence, history of
  (patients should be observed closely for signs of misuse or abuse of quetiapine, as with any new CNS medication)

» Hepatic function impairment
  (higher blood concentrations of quetiapine may occur; dosage adjustments may be necessary)

Hypothyroidism
  (decreases in total and free thyroxine ($T_4$) occurred during clinical trials of quetiapine)

Seizures, or history of
  (seizures occurred rarely in premarketing studies of quetiapine; it is recommended that quetiapine be used with caution in patients with a history of seizures or a decreased seizure threshold)

**Patient monitoring**
The following may be especially important in patient monitoring (other tests may be warranted in some patients, depending on condition; » = major clinical significance):

Careful supervision of patients with suicidal tendencies
  (recommended in high-risk patients, since the possibility of suicide attempt is inherent in schizophrenia; prescribing the smallest quantity of medication necessary for good patient management is recommended to prevent overdosing)

» Ophthalmologic exams
  (examination of the lens of the eye by methods adequate to detect cataract formation, such as slit lamp examination, is recommended at baseline and every 6 months during treatment with quetiapine; lens changes have been observed in patients during long-term quetiapine therapy and cataracts developed in dogs during chronic quetiapine dosing)

# Side/Adverse Effects

Note: Disturbances of body temperature regulation have been associated with use of other antipsychotic agents. Caution is advised in administering quetiapine to patients who will be experiencing conditions that may contribute to an elevation in core body temperature, such as strenuous exercise, exposure to extreme heat, dehydration, or concomitant treatment with anticholinergic medications.

The neuroleptic malignant syndrome (NMS) has been associated with the use of antipsychotic agents. Two possible cases were reported during clinical trials with quetiapine. NMS is a potentially fatal symptom complex that may include: hyperpyrexia; muscle rigidity; altered mental status; and autonomic instability seen as irregular pulse or blood pressure, tachycardia, diaphoresis, and cardiac dysrhythmia. Elevated creatine kinase, myoglobinuria (rhabdomyolysis), and acute renal failure also may occur. Differential diagnosis should exclude serious medical illnesses, such as pneumonia or systemic infection, presenting in conjunction with extrapyramidal effects, as well as central anticholinergic toxicity, heatstroke, drug fever, and primary CNS pathology.

Tardive dyskinesia, a syndrome of potentially irreversible, involuntary, dyskinetic movements, has been reported in patients taking other antipsychotic medications. Tardive dyskinesia occurs more frequently in elderly patients, especially women, than in younger patients. The risk of developing the syndrome and of experiencing irreversible effects appears to increase with treatment duration and total cumulative dose, although it may develop at any time during antipsychotic therapy. There is no known treatment for tardive dyskinesia, although partial or complete remission may occur when the antipsychotic medication is withdrawn. Alternatively, the antipsychotic medication may suppress the signs of the syndrome, masking the underlying process. For these reasons, quetiapine should be used only in those patients with chronic illness that is responsive to antipsychotic medication, and for whom potentially less harmful treatments are unavailable or inappropriate. Also, the smallest effective dose of quetiapine should be used and the need for continuing treatment should be assessed periodically.

The following side/adverse effects have been selected on the basis of their potential clinical significance (possible signs and symptoms in parentheses where appropriate)—not necessarily inclusive:

**Those indicating need for medical attention**
Incidence less frequent
*Dysarthria* (trouble in speaking); *dyspnea* (trouble in breathing); *extrapyramidal symptoms, parkinsonian* (trouble in speaking or swallowing; loss of balance control; masklike face; shuffling walk; slowed movements; stiffness of arms or legs; trembling and shaking of hands and fingers); *flu-like symptoms* (fever; chills; muscle aches); *leukopenia* (fever, chills, or sore throat); *peripheral edema* (swelling of feet or lower legs); *skin rash*

Incidence rare
*Changes in lenses of eyes*—usually asymptomatic; *hypothyroidism* (loss of appetite; weight gain; dry, puffy skin; tiredness); *hypotension* (low blood pressure); *menstrual changes; neuroleptic malignant syndrome (NMS)* (difficult or unusually fast breathing; fast heartbeat or irregular pulse; high fever; high or low [irregular] blood pressure; increased sweating; loss of bladder control; severe muscle stiffness; seizures; unusually pale skin; unusual tiredness or weakness); *seizures; unusual secretion of milk*—seen in females

Note: *Changes in the lenses of the eyes* have been observed in patients during long-term quetiapine therapy and cataracts have developed in dogs during chronic quetiapine dosing. Regular ophthalmologic examinations are recommended during quetiapine therapy.

**Those indicating need for medical attention only if they continue or are bothersome**
Incidence more frequent
*Constipation; dizziness; drowsiness; dry mouth; dyspepsia* (indigestion); *increased weight; postural hypotension* (dizziness, lightheadedness, or fainting, especially when getting up from a lying or sitting position)

Note: *Dyspepsia* and *increased weight* are dose-related. In pooled data from 3- to 6-week trials, 23% of patients receiving quetiapine and 6% of patients receiving placebo gained ≥ 7% of their baseline body weight.

Incidence less frequent
*Abdominal pain; abnormal vision; anorexia* (decrease in appetite); *asthenia* (decreased strength and energy); *headache; hypertonia* (increased muscle tone); *increased sweating; palpitation* (feeling of fast or irregular heartbeat); *pharyngitis* (sore throat); *rhinitis* (stuffy or runny nose); *tachycardia* (fast heartbeat)

Note: *Abdominal pain* is dose-related.

## Overdose

For specific information on the agents used in the management of quetiapine overdose, see:
- *Antidyskinetics (Systemic)* monograph;
- *Charcoal, Activated (Oral-Local)* monograph;
- *Laxatives (Local)* monograph; and/or
- *Sympathomimetic Agents–Cardiovascular Use (Parenteral-Systemic)* monograph.

For more information on the management of overdose or unintentional ingestion, **contact a Poison Control Center** (see *Poison Control Center Listing*).

**Clinical effects of overdose**
Note: Effects of overdose may be similar to side effects experienced at therapeutic doses, but may be more severe or several effects may occur together.
The following effects have been selected on the basis of their potential clinical significance (possible signs and symptoms in parentheses where appropriate)—not necessarily inclusive:

Acute
*Drowsiness; heart block* (slow or irregular heartbeat); *hypotension* (low blood pressure); *hypokalemia* (weakness); *tachycardia* (fast heartbeat)

Note: First degree *heart block* and *hypokalemia* were seen in one patient after an estimated overdose of 9600 mg of quetiapine.

**Treatment of overdose**
Treatment is symptomatic and supportive.

To decrease absorption—Gastric lavage, following intubation in unconscious patients, and administration of charcoal with a laxative should be considered. Induction of emesis is not recommended due to risk of aspiration if patient is obtunded or experiencing seizures or dystonic reactions of the head and neck.

Specific treatment—Administering antiarrhythmic therapy, if needed. However, disopyramide, procainamide, and quinidine have the potential to add to the possible QT-interval–prolonging effects of quetiapine overdosage. Also, bretylium may add to the hypotensive effect of quetiapine, due to additive alpha-adrenergic receptor blockade. Hypotension may be treated with intravenous fluids and/or sympathomimetic agents. However, epinephrine and dopamine may exacerbate hypotension through beta-adrenergic stimulation in the presence of quetiapine-induced alpha-adrenergic receptor blockade. Anticholinergic (antidyskinetic) medication should be administered in the presence of severe extrapyramidal symptoms.

Monitoring—Continuous electrocardiographic (ECG) monitoring is recommended to detect possible arrhythmias.

Supportive care—Establish and maintain airway and ensure adequate oxygenation and ventilation. Patients in whom intentional overdose is confirmed or suspected should be referred for psychiatric consultation.

## Patient Consultation

In providing consultation, consider emphasizing the following selected information (» = major clinical significance):

**Before using this medication**
» Conditions affecting use, especially:
Breast-feeding—Distributed into milk of animals; use in nursing mothers not recommended
Other medications, especially alcohol, CYP3A isoenzyme inhibitors, other CNS depression–producing medications, or hepatic enzyme inducers
Other medical problems, especially breast cancer or history of breast cancer, cardiovascular disease, cerebrovascular disease, conditions that would predispose to hypotension, hepatic function impairment, or hypersensitivity to quetiapine

**Proper use of this medication**
Compliance with therapy; not taking more or less medicine than prescribed
Taking with or without food, on a full or empty stomach, as directed by physician
» Proper dosing
Missed dose: Taking as soon as remembered; skipping if almost time for next dose; not doubling doses.
» Proper storage

**Precautions while using this medication**
Possible drowsiness, especially during first 3 to 5 days of therapy; caution when driving, operating machinery, or doing other jobs that require alertness

Possible orthostatic hypotension; rising slowly from a sitting or lying position

Possible impairment of ability to regulate core body temperature; avoiding overheating and dehydration

Avoiding use of alcoholic beverages; not taking other CNS depressants unless prescribed by physician

**Side/adverse effects**
Signs of potential side effects, especially dysarthria, dyspnea, parkinsonian extrapyramidal symptoms, flu-like symptoms, leukopenia, peripheral edema, skin rash, changes in lenses of eyes, hypothyroidism, hypotension, menstrual changes, neuroleptic malignant syndrome (NMS), seizures, and unusual secretion of milk (in females)

## General Dosing Information

Since the possibility of suicide is inherent in schizophrenia, patients should not have access to large quantities of quetiapine. To reduce the risk of overdose, the patient should be supplied with the smallest quantity of medication necessary for satisfactory patient management.

**Diet/Nutrition**
Quetiapine may be administered with or without food, on a full or empty stomach. Food marginally increases quetiapine absorption.

**For treatment of adverse effects**
Neuroleptic malignant syndrome (NMS)—Recommended treatment consists of the following:
- *Discontinuing quetiapine and other medications not essential to current therapy.*
- Providing intensive symptomatic treatment and medical monitoring.
- Treating any concomitant serious medical problems for which specific treatments are available.
- After recovery, giving careful consideration to the reintroduction of antipsychotic drug therapy in patients with severe psychosis requiring treatment, because of possible recurrence of NMS; closely monitoring patients in whom antipsychotic drug therapy is reintroduced after recovery from NMS.

Tardive dyskinesia—There is no known effective treatment. If signs and symptoms of tardive dyskinesia appear, discontinuation of quetiapine treatment should be considered if clinically feasible. To minimize the occurrence of tardive dyskinesia, chronic antipsychotic treatment should be in the smallest effective dose for the shortest duration necessary to produce a satisfactory clinical response.

## Oral Dosage Form

Note: The available dosage form contains quetiapine fumarate, but dosage and strength are expressed in terms of the base.

### QUETIAPINE TABLETS

**Usual adult dose**
Antipsychotic—
Oral, initially 25 mg (base) two times a day, with increases of 25 to 50 mg (base) two or three times a day to a target dosage range of 300 to 400 mg (base) a day, in divided doses given two or three times a day, by the fourth day. Further dosage adjustments may be made in increments or decrements of 25 to 50 mg (base) two times a day at intervals of two days.

Note: A slower rate of dosage titration and a lower target dosage should be considered in geriatric patients and in patients with hepatic impairment, predisposition to hypotension, or other debilitation.

A dose-response study did not find dosages above 300 mg (base) a day to be more efficacious than a dosage of 300 mg (base) a day.

When reinstituting quetiapine therapy in a patient who has discontinued quetiapine for more than one week, the initial titration schedule should be followed. If discontinuation has been for less than one week, quetiapine may be reinstituted at the previous maintenance dosage.

**Usual adult prescribing limits**
800 mg (base) a day.

**Usual pediatric dose**
Antipsychotic—
Safety and efficacy have not been established.

**Strength(s) usually available**
U.S.—
25 mg (base) (Rx) [*Seroquel*].
100 mg (base) (Rx) [*Seroquel*].
200 mg (base) (Rx) [*Seroquel*].

**Packaging and storage**
Store at controlled room temperature, 20 to 25 ºC (68 to 77 ºF), unless otherwise specified by manufacturer.

**Auxiliary labeling**
- Avoid alcoholic beverages.
- May cause dizziness or drowsiness.

Developed: 12/19/97

---

**QUINACRINE**—The *Quinacrine (Systemic)* monograph is not included in this published version of the USP DI database. Copies of the monograph are available on request from Micromedex, Inc. - Reprint Requests, 6200 S. Syracuse Way, Suite 300, Englewood, CO 80111; telephone (303) 486-6400; telefax (303) 486-6464; Email: USPDI@MDX.COM.

---

**QUINAPRIL**—See *Angiotensin-converting Enzyme (ACE) Inhibitors (Systemic)*

---

**QUINESTROL**—See *Estrogens (Systemic)*

---

**QUINETHAZONE**—See *Diuretics, Thiazide (Systemic)*

---

# QUINIDINE  Systemic

VA CLASSIFICATION (Primary/Secondary): CV300/AP101

Commonly used brand name(s): *Apo-Quinidine; Cardioquin; Cin Quin; Cin-Quin; Duraquin; Novoquinidin; Quinaglute Dura-tabs; Quinalan; Quinate; Quinidex Extentabs; Quinora.*

Note: For a listing of dosage forms and brand names by country availability, see *Dosage Forms* section(s).

## Category
Antiarrhythmic; antimalarial.

## Indications

**Accepted**
Cardiac arrhythmias (prophylaxis and treatment)—Treatment and control of:
Atrial fibrillation, established
Atrial flutter
Paroxysmal atrial fibrillation
Paroxysmal atrial tachycardia
Paroxysmal atrioventricular (AV) junctional rhythm
Paroxysmal ventricular tachycardia not associated with complete heart block
Premature contractions, atrial and ventricular
Malaria (treatment)[1]—Intravenous quinidine is indicated in the treatment of life-threatening *Plasmodium falciparum* malaria.

[1]Not included in Canadian product labeling.

## Pharmacology/Pharmacokinetics

**Physicochemical characteristics**
Molecular weight—Quinidine gluconate: 520.58.
Quinidine sulfate: 782.95.

**Mechanism of action/Effect**
Quinidine has both direct and indirect (anticholinergic) effects on cardiac tissue. Automaticity, conduction velocity, and membrane responsive-

ness are decreased, possibly because quinidine inhibits movement of potassium ions across membranes. The effective refractory period is prolonged. The anticholinergic action reduces vagal tone. An alpha-adrenergic blocking action often produces increased beta-adrenergic effects such as peripheral vasodilation. In the Vaughan Williams classification of antiarrhythmics, quinidine is considered to be a Class I antiarrhythmic.

**Protein binding**
High (70 to 80%).

**Biotransformation**
Hepatic; some cardioactive metabolites.

**Half-life**
About 6 hours.

**Time to peak concentration**
Oral:
  Quinidine gluconate: 3 to 4 hours.
  Quinidine sulfate: 1 to 1.5 hours.
Intramuscular:
  1 hour.

**Therapeutic serum concentration**
Usually 3 to 6 mcg per mL; toxic effects commonly occur at concentrations above 8 mcg per mL.

**Duration of action**
Oral—
  Regular tablets or capsules: 6 to 8 hours.
  Extended-release tablets: About 12 hours.

**Elimination**
Renal, about 10 to 50% unchanged. Excretion is increased in acidic urine and decreased in alkaline urine.
In dialysis—Small amounts removed by hemodialysis, none by peritoneal dialysis.

## Precautions to Consider

**Cross-sensitivity and/or related problems**
Patients sensitive to quinine may be sensitive to this medication also.

**Carcinogenicity/Mutagenicity**
Studies have not been done in either animals or humans.

**Pregnancy/Reproduction**
Pregnancy—Studies have not been done in humans. However, quinine, a closely related medication, has produced congenital abnormalities of the central nervous system (CNS) and extremities, has caused ototoxicity in the neonate, and has an oxytocic effect.
Studies have not been done in animals.
FDA Pregnancy Category C.

**Breast-feeding**
Quinidine is distributed into breast milk. However, problems have not been documented.

**Pediatrics**
Appropriate studies on the relationship of age to the effects of quinidine have not been performed in the pediatric population. Use of extended-release dosage forms is not recommended.

**Geriatrics**
Although appropriate studies on the relationship of age to the effects of quinidine have not been performed in the geriatric population, geriatrics-specific problems that would limit the usefulness of this medication in the elderly are not expected. However, elderly patients are more likely to have age-related renal function impairment, which may require dosage adjustment in patients receiving quinidine.

**Dental**
The secondary anticholinergic effects of quinidine may decrease or inhibit salivary flow, especially in middle-aged or elderly patients, thus contributing to the development of caries, periodontal disease, oral candidiasis, and discomfort.

**Drug interactions and/or related problems**
The following drug interactions and/or related problems have been selected on the basis of their potential clinical significance (possible mechanism in parentheses where appropriate)—not necessarily inclusive (» = major clinical significance):

Note: Combinations containing any of the following medications, depending on the amount present, may also interact with this medication.

» Alkalizers, urinary, such as:
    Antacids, calcium- and/or magnesium-containing
    Carbonic anhydrase inhibitors
    Citrates
    Sodium bicarbonate
    (concurrent use may increase the potential for toxic effects of quinidine; serum quinidine concentration is increased by enhanced renal absorption, which is promoted by the higher urinary pH; dosage adjustments may be needed when urinary alkalizer therapy is initiated or discontinued or if the dosage is changed)

» Antiarrhythmics, other or
Phenothiazines or
Rauwolfia alkaloids
    (concurrent use with quinidine may result in additive cardiac effects)

Anticholinergics (see *Appendix II* )
    (concurrent use with quinidine may intensify atropine-like side effects because of the secondary anticholinergic activities of quinidine)

» Anticoagulants, coumarin- or indandione-derivative
    (concurrent use with quinidine may cause additive hypoprothrombinemia as a result of alteration of procoagulant factor synthesis or catabolism and increased receptor affinity for the anticoagulant; dosage adjustments of anticoagulant may be necessary during and after quinidine therapy)

Antimyasthenics
    (neuromuscular blocking and/or secondary anticholinergic actions of quinidine may antagonize the effect of antimyasthenics on skeletal muscle; dosage adjustments of antimyasthenics may be necessary to control symptoms of myasthenia gravis)

Bethanechol
    (concurrent use with quinidine may antagonize the cholinergic effects of bethanechol)

Bretylium
    (concurrent administration with quinidine may counteract inotropic effect of bretylium and potentiate hypotension)

Cimetidine
    (as a result of inhibition of hepatic microsomal enzymes, cimetidine reduces total body clearance and prolongs the half-life of quinidine; dosage adjustment may be necessary)

Digitalis glycosides
    (concurrent use is reported to have increased serum concentrations of digoxin; studies also indicate possible increased serum concentrations of digitoxin when used concurrently with quinidine. Serum concentrations of the glycoside should be monitored and dosage adjusted as indicated)

Hepatic enzyme inducers (see *Appendix II* )
    (concurrent use with quinidine may decrease serum quinidine concentrations because of enhanced hepatic metabolism; adjustments of quinidine dosage may be necessary)

» Neuromuscular blocking agents
    (effects may be potentiated when these medications are used concurrently with quinidine; careful postoperative monitoring of the patient may be necessary following concurrent or sequential use, especially if there is a possibility of incomplete reversal of neuromuscular blockade)

» Pimozide
    (concurrent use with quinidine may potentiate cardiac arrhythmias, which are seen on electrocardiogram [ECG] as prolongation of QT interval)

Potassium-containing medications
    (concurrent use usually enhances quinidine's effects)

Quinine
    (concurrent use with quinidine may increase the possibility of cinchonism)

**Medical considerations/Contraindications**
The medical considerations/contraindications included have been selected on the basis of their potential clinical significance (reasons given in parentheses where appropriate)—not necessarily inclusive (» = major clinical significance).

*Except under special circumstances, this medication should not be used when the following medical problems exist:*

» Atrioventricular (AV) block, complete or
» Digitalis toxicity with AV conduction disorder or
» Intraventricular conduction defects, severe
    (additive cardiac depression)

*Risk-benefit should be considered when the following medical problems exist:*

Asthma or emphysema
    (possible hypersensitivity)

» AV block, incomplete
  (quinidine may produce complete block)
» Digitalis intoxication
  (additive cardiac depression and intracardial conduction inhibition)
» Hepatic function impairment or
» Renal function impairment
  (possible quinidine accumulation; dosage adjustment may be required)
  Hyperthyroidism
  Hypokalemia
  (possible reduced effect of quinidine)
  Infections, acute
» Myasthenia gravis
  (quinidine may increase muscle weakness)
  Psoriasis
  Sensitivity to quinidine
» Thrombocytopenia, or history of

**Patient monitoring**
The following may be especially important in patient monitoring (other tests may be warranted in some patients, depending on condition; » = major clinical significance):
  Blood cell counts and
  Hepatic function determinations and
  Renal function determinations
    (may be required during long-term therapy)
  Blood pressure determinations
    (recommended frequently during intravenous therapy)
  ECG monitoring, continuous and
  Potassium concentrations, serum and
  Quinidine concentrations, serum
    (recommended especially when daily oral dose exceeds 2 grams or during parenteral administration; widening of QRS complex by 50% is evidence of possible quinidine cardiotoxicity)

## Side/Adverse Effects

Note: Quinidine is potentially cardiotoxic, especially at dosages exceeding 2.4 grams per day. Possible cardiovascular effects include QRS widening, cardiac asystole, ventricular ectopic beats, idioventricular rhythms (including ventricular tachycardia and fibrillation), paradoxical tachycardia, and arterial embolism.

The following side/adverse effects have been selected on the basis of their potential clinical significance (possible signs and symptoms in parentheses where appropriate)—not necessarily inclusive:

**Those indicating need for medical attention**
Incidence less frequent
  *Allergic reaction* (fever; skin rash, hives, or itching; wheezing, shortness of breath, or troubled breathing); *cinchonism* (blurred vision or any change in vision; dizziness or lightheadedness, severe; headache; ringing or buzzing in ears or any loss of hearing); *hypotension or extreme CNS effects* (fainting)
  Note: In sensitive patients, *cinchonism* may occur after a single dose.
Incidence rare
  *Anemia* (unusual tiredness or weakness); *tachycardia, paradoxical* (fast heartbeat); *thrombocytopenia* (unusual bleeding or bruising)

**Those indicating need for medical attention only if they continue or are bothersome**
Incidence more frequent
  *Bitter taste; diarrhea; flushing of skin with itching; loss of appetite; nausea or vomiting; stomach pain or cramping*
Incidence less frequent
  *Confusion*

## Overdose

For more information on the management of overdose or unintentional ingestion, **contact a Poison Control Center** (see *Poison Control Center Listing*).

**Treatment of overdose**
Treatment is primarily supportive and symptomatic.
Recent oral ingestion may benefit from emesis and/or gastric lavage.
Oxygen, mechanical respiratory assistance, electronic cardiac pacing, hypertensives, urine acidifiers, and intravenous fluids may be indicated.
Hemodialysis is rarely necessary, although reported to be slightly effective in reducing plasma quinidine concentrations.

## Patient Consultation

As an aid to patient consultation, refer to *Advice for the Patient, Quinidine (Systemic).*
In providing consultation, consider emphasizing the following selected information (» = major clinical significance):

**Before using this medication**
» Conditions affecting use, especially:
    Sensitivity to quinine
    Breast-feeding—Distributed into breast milk
    Use in children—Use of extended-release dosage form not recommended
    Dental—May decrease or inhibit salivary flow
    Other medications, especially antiarrhythmics, anticoagulants, neuromuscular blocking agents, pimozide, and urinary alkalizers
    Other medical problems, especially complete or incomplete atrioventricular block, digitalis toxicity, severe intraventricular conduction defects, hepatic or renal function impairment, myasthenia gravis, or thrombocytopenia

**Proper use of this medication**
  Taking medication with water at least 1 hour before or 2 hours after meals for better absorption; may be taken with food or milk to lessen gastrointestinal irritation
  Proper administration of extended-release tablets: Swallowing tablet whole; not breaking, crushing, or chewing before swallowing
» Compliance with therapy; taking as directed even if feeling well
» Proper dosing
  Missed dose: Taking as soon as possible if remembered within 2 hours; if remembered later, not taking at all; not doubling doses
» Proper storage

**Precautions while using this medication**
  Regular visits to physician to check progress
» Checking with physician before discontinuing medication
» Caution if any kind of surgery (including dental surgery) or emergency treatment is required
  Carrying medical identification card
» Checking with physician if symptoms of quinidine intolerance occur

**Side/adverse effects**
  Signs of potential side effects, especially allergic reaction, cinchonism, hypotension or extreme CNS effects, anemia, paradoxical tachycardia, and thrombocytopenia

## General Dosing Information

Dosage must be adjusted to meet the individual requirements of each patient, on the basis of clinical response.

A test dose of one regular oral tablet may be administered prior to quinidine therapy to check for intolerance.

Higher serum quinidine concentrations are usually required to correct atrial arrhythmias than to correct ventricular arrhythmias.

There is a risk that quinidine may enhance atrioventricular (AV) conduction resulting in ventricular rate acceleration during treatment of atrial fibrillation or flutter. Digitalization prior to quinidine administration may reduce this risk.

**Diet/Nutrition**
This medication is preferably taken with a full glass (240 mL) of water on an empty stomach 1 hour before or 2 hours after meals for better absorption; however, it may be taken with food or milk when necessary to lessen gastrointestinal irritation.

## Oral Dosage Forms

### QUINIDINE GLUCONATE TABLETS

**Usual adult dose**
Antiarrhythmic—
  Oral, 325 to 650 mg every six hours as needed and tolerated.

**Usual pediatric dose**
Dosage has not been established.

**Strength(s) usually available**
U.S.—
  Not commercially available.
Canada—
  325 mg (Rx) [*Quinate*].

**Packaging and storage**
Store below 40 °C (104 °F), preferably between 15 and 30 °C (59 and 86 °F), in a well-closed container, unless otherwise specified by manufacturer. Protect from light.

**Auxiliary labeling**
- Do not take other medicines without advice from your doctor.

### QUINIDINE GLUCONATE EXTENDED-RELEASE TABLETS

**Usual adult dose**
Antiarrhythmic—
Oral, 324 to 660 mg every six to twelve hours as needed and tolerated.

**Usual pediatric dose**
Use is not recommended.

**Strength(s) usually available**
U.S.—
324 mg (equivalent to 243 mg of quinidine sulfate) (Rx) [*Quinaglute Dura-tabs; Quinalan;* GENERIC].
330 mg (equivalent to 248 mg of quinidine sulfate) (Rx) [*Duraquin*].
Canada—
324 mg (Rx) [*Quinaglute Dura-tabs*].

**Packaging and storage**
Store below 40 °C (104 °F), preferably between 15 and 30 °C (59 and 86 °F), in a well-closed container, unless otherwise specified by manufacturer. Protect from light.

**Auxiliary labeling**
- Swallow tablet whole. Do not break or chew.
- Do not take other medicines without advice from your doctor.

### QUINIDINE POLYGALACTURONATE TABLETS

**Usual adult dose**
Antiarrhythmic—
Initial—Oral, 275 to 825 mg every three to four hours for three or four doses with subsequent doses being increased by 137.5 to 275 mg every third or fourth dose until rhythm is restored or toxic effects occur.
Maintenance—Oral, 275 mg two or three times a day as needed and tolerated.

**Usual pediatric dose**
Antiarrhythmic—
Oral, 8.25 mg per kg of body weight or 247.5 mg per square meter of body surface five times a day.

**Strength(s) usually available**
U.S.—
275 mg (equivalent to 200 mg of quinidine sulfate) (Rx) [*Cardioquin*].
Canada—
275 mg (equivalent to 200 mg of quinidine sulfate) (Rx) [*Cardioquin*].

**Packaging and storage**
Store below 40 °C (104 °F), preferably between 15 and 30 °C (59 and 86 °F), in a well-closed container, unless otherwise specified by manufacturer.

**Auxiliary labeling**
- Do not take other medicines without advice from your doctor.

### QUINIDINE SULFATE CAPSULES USP

**Usual adult dose**
Antiarrhythmic—
Initial—
Premature atrial and ventricular contractions—Oral, 200 to 300 mg three or four times per day.
Paroxysmal supraventricular tachycardias—Oral, 400 to 600 mg every two or three hours until the paroxysm is terminated.
Atrial flutter—Oral, by individual titration following digitalization.
Conversion of atrial fibrillation—Oral, 200 mg every two or three hours for five to eight doses, with subsequent daily increases as needed and tolerated.
Maintenance—
Oral, 200 to 300 mg three or four times a day as needed and tolerated.

**Usual adult prescribing limits**
Up to 4 grams daily.

**Usual pediatric dose**
Antiarrhythmic—
Oral, 6 mg per kg of body weight or 180 mg per square meter of body surface five times a day.

**Strength(s) usually available**
U.S.—
200 mg (Rx) [*Cin-Quin;* GENERIC].
300 mg (Rx) [*Cin-Quin*].
Canada—
Not commercially available.

**Packaging and storage**
Store below 40 °C (104 °F), preferably between 15 and 30 °C (59 and 86 °F), unless otherwise specified by manufacturer. Store in a tight, light-resistant container.

**Auxiliary labeling**
- Do not take other medicines without advice from your doctor.

### QUINIDINE SULFATE TABLETS USP

**Usual adult dose**
Antiarrhythmic—See *Quinidine Sulfate Capsules USP*.

**Usual adult prescribing limits**
Up to 4 grams daily.

**Usual pediatric dose**
Antiarrhythmic—See *Quinidine Sulfate Capsules USP*.

**Strength(s) usually available**
U.S.—
100 mg (Rx) [*Cin-Quin*].
200 mg (Rx) [*Cin-Quin; Quinora;* GENERIC].
300 mg (Rx) [*Cin Quin; Quinora*].
Canada—
200 mg (Rx) [*Apo-Quinidine; Novoquinidin;* GENERIC].

**Packaging and storage**
Store below 40 °C (104 °F), preferably between 15 and 30 °C (59 and 86 °F), unless otherwise specified by manufacturer. Store in a well-closed, light-resistant container.

**Auxiliary labeling**
- Do not take other medicines without advice from your doctor.

### QUINIDINE SULFATE EXTENDED-RELEASE TABLETS USP

**Usual adult dose**
Antiarrhythmic—
Oral, 300 or 600 mg every eight to twelve hours as needed and tolerated.

**Usual pediatric dose**
Use is not recommended.

**Strength(s) usually available**
U.S.—
300 mg (Rx) [*Quinidex Extentabs*].
Canada—
300 mg (Rx) [*Quinidex Extentabs*].

**Packaging and storage**
Store between 15 and 30 °C (59 and 86 °F), unless otherwise specified by manufacturer. Store in a well-closed, light-resistant container.

**Auxiliary labeling**
- Swallow tablets whole. Do not break or chew.
- Do not take other medicines without advice from your doctor.

## Parenteral Dosage Forms

### QUINIDINE GLUCONATE INJECTION USP

Note: The dosing and strengths of the dosage form are expressed in terms of the gluconate salt.

**Usual adult dose**
Antiarrhythmic—
Intramuscular, 600 mg (salt) initially; then 400 mg (salt) repeated as often as every two hours if necessary.
Intravenous infusion, 800 mg (salt) in 40 mL of 5% Dextrose Injection USP administered at a rate of 1 mL per minute with electrocardiogram (ECG) and blood pressure monitoring.
Antimalarial[1]—
Intravenous infusion, continuous, initially, 10 mg (salt) per kg of body weight in an appropriate volume of 5% dextrose or 0.9% sodium chloride infused over one to two hours; followed immediately by 20 mcg (0.02 mg) (salt) per kg of body weight per minute until parasitemia decreases to less than one percent or oral therapy can be instituted.
Intravenous infusion, intermittent, initially, 24 mg (salt) per kg of body weight in a volume of 250 mL 5% dextrose or 0.9% sodium chloride infused over four hours; then, eight hours after the beginning of the initial dose, 12 mg (salt) per kg of body weight infused over four hours; this is administered every eight hours until parasitemia decreases to less than one percent or until oral therapy can be instituted.

Note: The intermittent intravenous infusion provides a larger dose of quinidine and may be potentially more toxic than the continuous intravenous infusion.

Standard oral antiplasmodial therapy should be instituted as soon as it is practical. Usually this occurs within 24 to 48 hours of starting quinidine therapy. When the parasite density is ≤ 1% or the patient can tolerate oral therapy, oral quinine may be substituted for intravenous quinidine. The standard duration of combined quinidine/quinine therapy is seventy-two hours when treatment with a second drug (e.g., tetracycline or sulfadoxine/pyrimethamine) is given. However, *Plasmodium falciparum* acquired in Thailand requires seven days of quinidine and/or quinine and seven days of tetracycline.

Continuous ECG and blood pressure monitoring are recommended. Quinidine infusion should be temporarily slowed or discontinued if prolongation of QT interval greater than 0.6 seconds, a QRS interval increase of more than 25% over baseline, or hypotension unresponsive to moderate fluid challenge occurs.

**Usual adult prescribing limits**
Up to 5 grams daily.

**Usual pediatric dose**
Dosage has not been established.

**Strength(s) usually available**
U.S.—
    80 mg per mL (Rx) [GENERIC].
Canada—
    Not commercially available.

**Packaging and storage**
Store below 40 °C (104 °F), preferably between 15 and 30 °C (59 and 86 °F), unless otherwise specified by manufacturer. Protect from freezing. Protect from light.

## QUINIDINE SULFATE INJECTION

**Usual adult dose**
Antiarrhythmic—
    Intramuscular, 190 to 380 mg every two to four hours, up to a total dose of 3 grams a day.
Note: An initial test dose of 95 mg given intramuscularly is recommended.

**Usual adult prescribing limits**
3 grams daily.

**Usual pediatric dose**
Dosage has not been established.

**Strength(s) usually available**
U.S.—
    Not commercially available.
Canada—
    190 mg per mL (Rx) [GENERIC (propylene glycol)].

**Packaging and storage**
Store below 40 °C (104 °F), preferably between 15 and 30 °C (59 and 86 °F), unless otherwise specified by manufacturer. Protect from freezing. Protect from light.

[1]Not included in Canadian product labeling.

Revised: 03/24/94

# QUININE   Systemic

VA CLASSIFICATION (Primary/Secondary): AP101/MS900

Note: For a listing of dosage forms and brand names by country availability, see *Dosage Forms* section(s).

## Category
Antiprotozoal; antimyotonic.

## Indications
Note: Bracketed information in the *Indications* section refers to uses that are not included in U.S. product labeling.

**Accepted**
Malaria (treatment)—Quinine is indicated concurrently with tetracycline, doxycycline, clindamycin, pyrimethamine plus sulfadiazine, or pyrimethamine plus sulfadoxine in the treatment of chloroquine-resistant malaria caused by *Plasmodium falciparum*.

[Leg cramps (prophylaxis and treatment)]—Quinine is indicated in the prophylaxis and treatment of nocturnal recumbency leg muscle cramps, including those associated with arthritis, diabetes, varicose veins, thrombophlebitis, arteriosclerosis, and static foot deformities.

[Babesiosis (treatment)][1]—Quinine is used concurrently with clindamycin in the treatment of severe babesiosis caused by *Babesia microti*.

[1]Not included in Canadian product labeling.

## Pharmacology/Pharmacokinetics

**Physicochemical characteristics**
Molecular weight—782.95.

**Mechanism of action/Effect**
Antiprotozoal—The precise mechanism of action of quinine in malaria has not been determined but may be based on its ability to concentrate in parasitic acid vesicles, causing an elevation of pH in intracellular organelles. This is thought to disrupt the intracellular transport of membrane components and macromolecules, and phospholipase activity. Quinine has a schizonticidal action. Its ability to concentrate in parasitized erythrocytes may account for its selective toxicity against the erythrocytic stages of the 4 malarial parasites, including *P. falciparum* strains resistant to chloroquine. The drug is also gametocidal against *P. vivax* and *P. malariae*.

Antimyotonic—Quinine increases the refractory period of skeletal muscle by direct action on the muscle fiber, and the distribution of calcium within the muscle fiber, thereby diminishing the response to tetanic stimulation. It also decreases the excitability of the motor end-plate region, reducing the responses to repetitive nerve stimulation and to acetylcholine.

**Absorption**
Rapidly and almost completely absorbed. Bioavailability is approximately 80% in healthy subjects.

**Distribution**
Distribution of quinine may vary depending on the degree of illness; the volume of distribution is smaller in patients with cerebral malaria and increases with recovery. Children and pregnant women have a smaller volume of distribution than do nonpregnant adults. Plasma and red blood cell (RBC) concentrations appear to be similar before infection; however, during a malaria attack, plasma concentrations are considerably higher than RBC concentrations. Quinine does not freely cross the blood-brain barrier; the cerebrospinal fluid to plasma ratio is approximately 7%. Quinine crosses the placenta and is distributed into breast milk; peak concentrations are reached in breast milk approximately 90 minutes after oral administration.
    $Vol_D$—
        Adults:
            Cerebral malaria—Approximately 1.2 liters per kg.
            Uncomplicated malaria—Approximately 1.7 liters per kg.
        Children:
            Uncomplicated malaria—Approximately 0.8 liters per kg.

**Protein binding**
Higher (>90%) in patients with cerebral malaria, pregnant women, and children; approximately 85 to 90% in patients with uncomplicated malaria; and approximately 70% in healthy adults.

**Biotransformation**
Hepatic; >80% metabolized by the liver. Metabolites have less activity than the parent drug.

**Half-life**
Adults—
    Cerebral malaria: Approximately 18 hours.
    Uncomplicated malaria: Approximately 16 hours.
    Healthy persons: Approximately 11 hours.
Children—
    Uncomplicated malaria: Approximately 12 hours.
Acute overdose—
    Approximately 26 hours.

**Time to peak serum concentration**
Acute malaria—Approximately 5.9 hours.
Convalescence—Approximately 3.2 hours.

**Mean serum concentration**
Approximately 7 mcg per mL, following chronic administration of total daily doses of 1 gram. Plasma concentrations are higher in patients with cerebral malaria due to reduced clearance and volume of distribution; concentrations decrease as patient recovers.

**Elimination**
Primarily renal, with about 20% excreted as unchanged drug. Excretion of quinine is increased in acidic urine.
Dialysis—Exchange transfusion, hemodialysis, peritoneal dialysis, and hemofiltration have little effect on plasma quinine concentrations.

# Precautions to Consider

### Cross-sensitivity and/or related problems
Patients hypersensitive to quinidine may be hypersensitive to this medication also.

### Carcinogenicity
A study in rats, given quinine sulfate in drinking water at a concentration of 0.1% for up to 20 months, has not shown that quinine is carcinogenic.

### Mutagenicity
Micronucleus tests in male and female mice, given 2 intraperitoneal injections of quinine dihydrochloride 24 hours apart in doses of 0.5 millimole per kg of body weight, have not shown that quinine is mutagenic. Direct *Salmonella typhimurium* tests were also negative. However, when mammalian liver homogenate was added, positive results were obtained.

Sister chromatid exchange (SCE) tests, micronucleus tests, and chromosome aberration tests in Chinese hamsters, given quinine hydrochloride orally in doses of 100 mg per kg of body weight (mg/kg), have not shown that quinine is mutagenic.

Micronucleus tests and chromosome aberration tests in mice, given quinine hydrochloride orally in doses of 100 mg/kg, have not shown that quinine is mutagenic. However, the SCE test showed an increase in SCEs per cell. Tests were repeated in 2 inbred strains of mice, using oral doses of 55, 75, and 110 mg of quinine hydrochloride per kg of body weight. The effects were more pronounced in these mice and the increase in SCEs per cell demonstrated a linear dose relationship. One of the inbred strains of mice showed positive micronucleus test results. The chromosome aberration tests also showed an increase in chromatid breaks. In addition, the Ames test was negative for point mutation.

### Pregnancy/Reproduction
Fertility—No information is available on the effect of quinine on fertility in animals or humans.

Pregnancy—Quinine crosses the placenta; one study found the cord plasma concentration to be approximately one-third the concentration of quinine in maternal plasma. Quinine has been used to treat patients with *P. falciparum* malaria in the third trimester of pregnancy. However, the risk of quinine to the fetus must be balanced against the danger of *P. falciparum* malaria, which is potentially life-threatening, especially during pregnancy. Studies in humans have shown that quinine causes congenital malformations, especially when given in large doses (e.g., up to 30 grams for attempted abortion). These malformations include deafness related to auditory nerve hypoplasia, limb anomalies, visceral defects, and visual changes. In addition, quinine may have an oxytoxic action on the uterus and has been shown to cause abortion when taken in toxic amounts. Stillbirths have also been reported in mothers taking quinine during pregnancy.

Studies in rabbits and guinea pigs have shown that quinine is teratogenic. However, no teratogenic effects were seen in mice, rats, dogs, or monkeys.

FDA Pregnancy Category X.

### Breast-feeding
Quinine is distributed into breast milk in small amounts. One study suggests that a breast-fed infant will receive approximately 1.5 to 3.0 mg per day of quinine base from maternal therapy. Problems in humans have not been documented.

### Pediatrics
Appropriate studies on the relationship of age to the effects of quinine for use as an antimyotonic have not been performed in the pediatric population. Antimalarial studies performed to date have shown that children have a decreased elimination half-life and volume of distribution; however, pediatrics-specific problems that would limit the usefulness of quinine in children have not been documented.

### Geriatrics
No information is available on the relationship of age to the effects of quinine in geriatric patients.

### Drug interactions and/or related problems
The following drug interactions and/or related problems have been selected on the basis of their potential clinical significance (possible mechanism in parentheses where appropriate)—not necessarily inclusive (» = major clinical significance):

Note: Combinations containing any of the following medications, depending on the amount present, may also interact with this medication.

Antacids, aluminum-containing
(concurrent use of aluminum-containing antacids with quinine may decrease or delay the absorption of quinine)

Anticoagulants, coumarin- or indandione-derivative
(hypoprothrombinemic effects may be increased when these agents are used concurrently with quinine because of decreased hepatic synthesis of procoagulant factors; hypoprothrombinemia can be prevented by coadministration of vitamin K; dosage adjustments may be necessary during and after quinine therapy)

Antimyasthenics
(concurrent use of medications with neuromuscular blocking action may antagonize the effect of antimyasthenics on skeletal muscle; temporary dosage adjustments of antimyasthenics may be necessary to control symptoms of myasthenia gravis during and following concurrent use)

Cimetidine
(concurrent use of cimetidine with quinine may reduce the clearance of quinine)

Digitoxin or
Digoxin
(concurrent use of digoxin with quinine may result in increased digoxin serum concentrations and increased digoxin effect by decreasing the nonrenal clearance of digoxin; concurrent use of quinidine with digitoxin has been reported to result in increased digitoxin serum concentrations and increased digitoxin effect as well; because of the similarities of the digitalis glycosides and the similarities of quinine and quinidine, serum digoxin and digitoxin concentrations should be monitored periodically during concurrent therapy with quinine, and dosage adjustments made as indicated)

Hemolytics, other (See *Appendix II* ) or
Neurotoxic medications, other (See *Appendix II* ) or
Ototoxic medications, other, (See *Appendix II* )
(concurrent use of these medications with quinine may increase the potential for toxicity)

» Mefloquine
(concurrent use with quinine may result in an increased incidence of seizures and of electrocardiogram abnormalities, predisposing the patient to arrhythmias; it is recommended that mefloquine be administered at least 12 hours after the last dose of quinine)

(patients taking weekly mefloquine prophylaxis may be found to have mefloquine-resistant malaria that requires treatment with quinine; because mefloquine has a very long half-life [approximately 20 days], it will remain in the body long after the drug has been discontinued. Although there is insufficient information available, it is recommended that if quinine must be given that the patient be hospitalized, if possible, and monitored for QT prolongation and possible rhythm disturbances. Seizure activity may also be potentiated in these patients. In patients considered to be at high risk for a seizure, additional precautions and interventions may be indicated)

Neuromuscular blocking agents
(neuromuscular blockade may be potentiated when these agents are used concurrently with quinine)

Quinidine
(concurrent use with quinine may increase the possibility of QT prolongation or cinchonism)

### Laboratory value alterations
The following have been selected on the basis of their potential clinical significance (possible effect in parentheses where appropriate)—not necessarily inclusive (» = major clinical significance):

With diagnostic test results
17-ketogenic steroid, urinary
(quinine may cause increased values for urinary 17-ketogenic steroids when the metyrapone or Zimmerman method is used)

### Medical considerations/Contraindications
The medical considerations/contraindications included have been selected on the basis of their potential clinical significance (reasons given in parentheses where appropriate)—not necessarily inclusive (» = major clinical significance).

*Risk-benefit should be considered when the following medical problems exist:*

» Blackwater fever, history of
(interrupted or recurrent quinine therapy in patients with *P. falciparum* infections may predispose them to the complications of blackwater fever, including anemia and hemolysis with renal failure)

Cardiac arrhythmias, history of, or QT prolongation
(a prolonged QT interval has been noted in patients being treated for cerebral malaria, without correlation with plasma quinine concentration; patients with a history of cardiac arrhythmias or QT prolongation may be at risk for arrhythmias while taking quinine)

Glucose-6-phosphate dehydrogenase (G6PD) deficiency
(hemolysis or hemolytic anemia may occur in G6PD-deficient patients; however, quinine has been safely given in therapeutic doses to patients with G6PD deficiency)

» Hypersensitivity to quinine or quinidine
» Hypoglycemia
(quinine stimulates release of insulin from the pancreas; hypoglycemia may also be a complication of severe *P. falciparum* malaria, especially in children and during pregnancy)

» Myasthenia gravis
(quinine may exacerbate muscle weakness in myasthenia gravis due to its neuromuscular blocking effects)

» Purpura, thrombocytopenic, or history of
(quinine may cause thrombocytopenic purpura, especially in highly sensitive patients or in patients with a previous history of this reaction to quinine)

## Side/Adverse Effects

The following side/adverse effects have been selected on the basis of their potential clinical significance (possible signs and symptoms in parentheses where appropriate)—not necessarily inclusive:

**Those indicating need for medical attention**
Incidence rare

*Hematologic effects, specifically agranulocytosis* (sore throat and fever); *Coombs' positive hemolytic anemia* (back, leg, or stomach pains; loss of appetite; pale skin; unusual tiredness or weakness; fever); *hypoprothrombinemia* (unusual bleeding or bruising); *or thrombocytopenia* (unusual bleeding or bruising); *hypoglycemia* (anxiety; chills; cold sweats; cool, pale skin; headache; increased hunger; nausea; nervousness; shakiness); *hypersensitivity, specifically fever; hemolytic uremic syndrome* (often presents with abdominal pain, nausea and vomiting, muscle aches, bruising, fever and chills, sweating); *hepatotoxicity* (abdominal pain; nausea; pale stools; yellow skin and eyes); *skin rash; redness; hives; itching; wheezing; shortness of breath; or difficult breathing*

Note: *Hemolytic uremic syndrome* (HUS) is a multi-system disorder that is characterized by hemolytic anemia, thrombocytopenia, disseminated intravascular coagulation (DIC), and acute renal failure. This reaction may occur within hours of a single ingestion of quinine. Several case reports have been published describing patients who have had an acute hypersensitivity reaction to quinine that resulted in adult HUS.

*Hypoprothrombinemia* may be reversed with vitamin K administration.

**Those indicating need for medical attention only if they continue or are bothersome**
Incidence more frequent

*Cinchonism* (blurred vision or change in color vision; headache, severe; nausea or vomiting; ringing or buzzing in ears or transient loss of hearing)—usually develops when plasma concentrations exceed 7 to 10 mcg per mL, but may occur at lower levels; *gastrointestinal disturbances* (abdominal or stomach cramps or pain; diarrhea; nausea or vomiting)

## Overdose

For specific information on the agents used in the management of quinine overdose, see:
- *Charcoal, Activated (Oral-Local)* monograph; and/or
- *Ipecac (Oral-Local)* monograph.

For more information on the management of overdose or unintentional ingestion, **contact a Poison Control Center** (see *Poison Control Center Listing*).

**Clinical effects of overdose**
The following effects have been selected on the basis of their potential clinical significance (possible signs and symptoms in parentheses where appropriate)—not necessarily inclusive:

Acute and chronic
*Cardiovascular toxicity* (cardiac arrest; electromechanical dissociation; hypotension; left bundle branch block; myocardial depression; ventricular arrhythmias); *central nervous system toxicity* (coma; confusion; delirium; respiratory arrest; restlessness; seizures; somnolence); *ocular toxicity* (visual deficits, including peripheral field defects, scotoma, blindness)—some sight is usually recovered

**Treatment of overdose**
Recommended treatment consists of the following:

To decrease absorption—
Using gastric lavage or inducing emesis with ipecac syrup to remove residual quinine from the stomach. Repeated dosing of activated charcoal every 4 hours may be beneficial in shortening the half-life of quinine in an overdose.

To enhance elimination—
Although excretion of quinine is increased in acidic urine, administration of forced acid diuresis has had little impact on quinine elimination by the kidney, which accounts for only 20% of the total body clearance. Peritoneal dialysis, hemodialysis, exchange transfusion, charcoal hemoperfusion, resin hemoperfusion, and plasmapheresis have not been found to be effective in the management of quinine overdose.

Specific treatment—
Stellate ganglionic block has not been shown to be of value in treating quinine-induced blindness and may cause an increase in complications. Caution should be used in administration of antiarrhythmics since quinine has class 1 antiarrhythmic properties that can be potentiated.

Supportive care—
Supportive measures such as maintaining an open airway, respiration, and circulation may be administered. Patients in whom intentional overdose is confirmed or suspected should be referred for psychiatric consultation.

## Patient Consultation

As an aid to patient consultation, refer to *Advice for the Patient, Quinine (Systemic)*.

In providing consultation, consider emphasizing the following selected information (» = major clinical significance):

**Before using this medication**
» Conditions affecting use, especially:
Hypersensitivity to quinine
Pregnancy—Quinine has been found to be teratogenic; it has also caused stillbirths and abortions in pregnant women
Breast-feeding—Quinine is distributed into breast milk
Other medications, especially mefloquine
Other medical problems, especially a history of blackwater fever, hypoglycemia, myasthenia gravis, and a history of thrombocytopenic purpura

**Proper use of this medication**
» Importance of not taking more medication than the amount recommended
» Taking medication with or after meals to minimize possible gastrointestinal irritation
» Compliance with full course of therapy in malaria
» Proper dosing
Missed dose: Taking as soon as possible; not taking if almost time for next dose; not doubling doses
» Proper storage

**Precautions while using this medication**
» Caution if blurred vision or change in color vision occurs

**Side/adverse effects**
Signs of side effects, especially hematologic effects, specifically agranulocytosis, Coombs' positive hemolytic anemia, hypoprothrombinemia, or thrombocytopenia; hypoglycemia; and hypersensitivity, specifically fever, hemolytic uremic syndrome, hepatotoxicity, skin rash, redness, hives, itching, wheezing, shortness of breath, or difficult breathing

## General Dosing Information

This medication should be taken with or after meals to minimize gastrointestinal irritation.

In the treatment of chloroquine-resistant *P. falciparum* malaria, quinine is given concurrently with tetracycline, clindamycin, or pyrimethamine in combination with sulfadiazine or sulfadoxine.

In the treatment of nocturnal recumbency leg cramps, quinine may be discontinued if leg cramps do not occur after several consecutive nights of therapy, to determine if continued therapy is needed.

Plasma concentrations above 10 mg per 100 mL may cause severe symptoms of cinchonism.

### Bioequivalence information
Bioavailability of quinine is extensive and rapid in healthy subjects. Studies using various salts of quinine have indicated no marked difference in the rate and extent of absorption of quinine in the capsule and plain tablet dosage forms.

## Oral Dosage Forms

Note: Bracketed uses in the *Dosage Forms* section refer to categories of use and/or indications that are not included in U.S. product labeling. The dosing and dosage forms available are expressed in terms of quinine sulfate (salt). Bioavailability studies have indicated no marked difference in the rate and extent of absorption of quinine in the capsule and plain tablet dosage forms.

### QUININE SULFATE CAPSULES USP

**Usual adult and adolescent dose**
Malaria: For chloroquine-resistant *Plasmodium falciparum* malaria—
   Oral, 600 to 650 mg every eight hours for at least three days in most areas of the world (seven days in Southeast Asia) with concurrent administration of 250 mg of tetracycline every six hours for seven days; or concurrent administration of 100 mg of doxycycline every twelve hours for seven days; or concurrent administration of 1.5 grams of sulfadoxine and 75 mg of pyrimethamine combination as a single dose; or concurrent administration of 900 mg of clindamycin three times a day for three days.

[Antimyotonic]—
   Nocturnal recumbency leg cramps: Oral, 200 to 300 mg at bedtime; if an additional dose of 200 to 300 mg is needed, it may be taken following the evening meal.

[Babesiosis][1]—
   Oral, 650 mg three or four times a day with concurrent intravenous administration of 300 to 600 mg clindamycin four times a day for seven to ten days.

**Usual pediatric dose**
Malaria: For chloroquine-resistant *Plasmodium falciparum* malaria—
   Oral, 8.3 mg per kg of body weight every eight hours for at least three days in most areas of the world (seven days in Southeast Asia) with concurrent administration of 5 mg per kg of body weight of tetracycline every six hours for seven days in children over 8 years of age; or concurrent administration of 6.7 to 13.3 mg per kg of body weight of clindamycin three times a day for three days; or concurrent administration of 1.25 mg per kg of body weight of pyrimethamine in combination with 25 mg per kg of body weight of sulfadoxine as a single dose.

[Antimyotonic]—
   Dosage has not been established.

[Babesiosis][1]—
   Dosage has not been established; however, based on one case report in an infant, the suggested dose is: Oral, 25 mg per kg of body weight per day with concurrent intravenous or intramuscular administration of 20 mg per kg of body weight per day of clindamycin for seven to ten days.

**Strength(s) usually available**
U.S.—
   200 mg (Rx) [GENERIC].
   300 mg (Rx) [GENERIC].
   325 mg (Rx) [GENERIC].
Canada—
   200 mg (Rx) [GENERIC].
   300 mg (Rx) [GENERIC].

**Packaging and storage**
Store below 40 °C (104 °F), preferably between 15 and 30 °C (59 and 86 °F), unless otherwise specified by manufacturer. Store in a well-closed container.

**Auxiliary labeling**
- May cause vision problems.
- Continue medication for full time of treatment.

### QUININE SULFATE TABLETS USP

**Usual adult and adolescent dose**
See *Quinine Sulfate Capsules USP*.

**Usual pediatric dose**
See *Quinine Sulfate Capsules USP*.

**Strength(s) usually available**
U.S.—
   260 mg (Rx) [GENERIC].
   325 mg (Rx) [GENERIC].
Canada—
   Not commercially available.

**Packaging and storage**
Store below 40 °C (104 °F), preferably between 15 and 30 °C (59 and 86 °F), unless otherwise specified by manufacturer. Store in a well-closed container.

**Auxiliary labeling**
- May cause vision problems.
- Continue medication for full time of treatment.

---

[1]Not included in Canadian product labeling.

Revised: 02/23/93
Interim revision: 06/23/95

# RABIES IMMUNE GLOBULIN Systemic

VA CLASSIFICATION (Primary): IM500

Commonly used brand name(s): *Hyperab; Imogam.*

Other commonly used names are HRIG and RIG.

Note: For a listing of dosage forms and brand names by country availability, see *Dosage Forms* section(s).

## Category

Immunizing agent (passive).

## Indications

### Accepted

Rabies (prophylaxis)—Rabies immune globulin is indicated for post-exposure immunization against rabies infection in persons who have not been previously immunized against rabies with rabies vaccine. Rabies immune globulin is used in conjunction with rabies vaccine.

### Unaccepted

Post-exposure prophylaxis is not recommended for persons inadvertently exposed to modified live rabies virus (MLV) vaccines intended for animals. Although vaccine-induced rabies has occurred in animals administered these vaccines, there have been no reported rabies cases among humans resulting from exposure to needle sticks or sprays with licensed MLV vaccines.

## Pharmacology/Pharmacokinetics

### Physicochemical characteristics

Source—

Rabies immune globulin is an antirabies gamma globulin obtained from the plasma of hyperimmunized human donors. It is concentrated by cold ethanol fractionation. The rabies neutralizing antibody content is usually standardized to contain 150 International Units (IU) per mL. One Canadian product is standardized to contain 300 International Units (IU) per mL. The International Unit of potency is equivalent to the U.S. unit of potency.

### Mechanism of action/Effect

Following intramuscular administration, rabies immune globulin provides immediate passive antibodies for a short period of time. This protects the patient until the patient can produce active antibodies from the rabies vaccine.

### Protective effect

When the post-exposure prophylaxis regimen has included local wound treatment, passive immunization, and active immunization, 100% effectiveness has been shown. However, rabies has occasionally developed in persons when key elements of the rabies post-exposure prophylaxis regimen were omitted or incorrectly administered. This has occurred outside the United States in cases in which patients' wounds were not cleansed with soap and water or other antiviral agents, rabies vaccine was not administered in the deltoid area but rather in the gluteal area, and passive immunization was not administered around the wound site.

### Time to protective effect

An adequate titer of passive antibody is present 24 hours after injection.

### Duration of protective effect

Short; rabies immune globulin has a half-life of approximately 21 days.

## Precautions to Consider

### Cross-sensitivity and/or related problems

Patients sensitive to other human immune globulin products may be sensitive to rabies immune globulin (RIG) also.

### Pregnancy/Reproduction

Pregnancy—Studies have not been done in humans. Because of the potential consequences of rabies virus infection, and because there is no indication that fetal abnormalities have been associated with use of RIG in pregnant women, pregnancy is not considered to be a contraindication to use.

Studies have not been done in animals.

FDA Pregnancy Category C.

### Breast-feeding

Problems in humans have not been documented.

### Pediatrics

Appropriate studies on the relationship of age to the effects of RIG have not been performed in the pediatric population. However, pediatrics-specific problems that would limit the usefulness of this medicine in children are not expected.

### Geriatrics

No information is available on the relationship of age to the effects of RIG in geriatric patients.

### Drug interactions and/or related problems

The following drug interactions and/or related problems have been selected on the basis of their potential clinical significance (possible mechanism in parentheses where appropriate)—not necessarily inclusive (» = major clinical significance):

Note: Combinations containing any of the following medications, depending on the amount present, may also interact with this medication.

Live virus vaccines
(antibodies contained in RIG may interfere with the body's immune response to certain live virus vaccines; live virus vaccines, such as measles, mumps, and rubella, should be administered at least 14 days prior to, or at least 3 months after, administration of RIG)

### Medical considerations/Contraindications

The medical considerations/contraindications included have been selected on the basis of their potential clinical significance (reasons given in parentheses where appropriate)—not necessarily inclusive (» = major clinical significance).

***Risk-benefit should be considered when the following medical problems exist:***

» Immunoglobulin A (IgA) deficiencies, in patients who have known antibody to IgA
(small amounts of IgA may be present in RIG and may cause a severe allergic reaction in patients with antibody to IgA)

Sensitivity to RIG

Sensitivity to thimerosal
(the RIG available in the U.S. and Canada contains thimerosal)

## Side/Adverse Effects

Note: Severe systemic adverse effects to rabies immune globulin (RIG) are rare.

Although not reported with RIG, anaphylaxis, angioneurotic edema, and nephrotic syndrome have been reported rarely with other immune globulin products.

If necessary, physicians should consult with the state public health department, the Centers for Disease Control (CDC), Canadian National Advisory Committee on Immunization (NACI), and/or the World Health Organization (WHO) regarding the management of serious adverse reactions.

There is no evidence that hepatitis B virus (HBV), human immunodeficiency virus (HIV), or other viruses have been transmitted by commercially available RIG in the U.S.

Since RIG is given in conjunction with rabies vaccine, adverse effects generally associated with rabies vaccine have also been temporally associated with RIG.

The following side/adverse effects have been selected on the basis of their potential clinical significance (possible signs and symptoms in parentheses where appropriate)—not necessarily inclusive:

### Those indicating need for medical attention only if they continue or are bothersome

Incidence less frequent

***Fever; pain, soreness, tenderness, or stiffness of the muscles at the place(s) of injection***—may persist for several hours following injection

## Patient Consultation

As an aid to patient consultation, refer to *Advice for the Patient, Rabies Immune Globulin (Systemic).*

In providing consultation, consider emphasizing the following selected information (» = major clinical significance):

### Before using this medication

» Conditions affecting use, especially:

Sensitivity to rabies immune globulin, other human immune globulins, or thimerosal

Other medical problems, especially immunoglobulin A (IgA) deficiencies

### Proper use of this medication

» Proper dosing

## General Dosing Information

The recommended dose of rabies immune globulin (RIG) is 20 International Units (IU) per kg of body weight. Since RIG may partially suppress active production of rabies antibody, it is recommended that no more than the recommended dose be administered.

If anatomically feasible, up to one-half of the dose of RIG should be thoroughly infiltrated into the area(s) around the wound(s) and the rest should be administered intramuscularly in the gluteal area.

Care should be taken to avoid injection of RIG into or near blood vessels or nerves.

All post-exposure therapy should begin with immediate and thorough cleansing of all the patient's wounds with soap and water. Studies have shown that wound cleansing greatly reduces the likelihood of rabies.

Appropriate management of persons who may have been exposed to rabies depends on the assessment of the risk of infection. The incubation period for rabies infection varies with respect to the location and severity of the bite. The incubation period is usually 2 to 6 weeks, but can be longer. For bites to the face or extensive bites elsewhere on the body, the incubation period may be as short as 10 to 17 days. Decisions about management should be made promptly. Persons who have been bitten by animals suspected of being, or proven, rabid should begin therapy within 24 hours. If necessary, physicians should consult with the local or state public health department, the Centers for Disease Control (CDC), the Canadian National Advisory Committee on Immunization (NACI), and/or the World Health Organization (WHO) regarding the need for rabies prophylaxis.

The essential components of the rabies post-exposure prophylaxis regimen are local wound treatment, passive immunization with RIG (unless the patient has been previously immunized against rabies), and active immunization with rabies vaccine. Rabies has occasionally developed in persons when key elements of this regimen were omitted or incorrectly performed. In addition, tetanus prophylaxis and antibacterial medications may be administered as required. Both passive immunization with RIG (except for patients who have been previously immunized against rabies) and active immunization with rabies vaccine are required regardless of the interval between exposure and initiation of therapy. However, RIG should not be administered in the same syringe or into the same body site as the rabies vaccine.

Persons are considered to have been previously immunized against rabies (and as such should not receive RIG as part of the post-exposure therapy) if they have previously received complete regimens of pre- or post-exposure rabies prophylaxis with human diploid cell rabies vaccine (HDCV) or rabies vaccine adsorbed (RVA) or if they have been documented to have had an adequate antibody response to another rabies vaccine, such as duck embryo rabies vaccine. Regardless of the antibody titer that is present before post-exposure therapy occurs, an anamnestic antibody response should occur following the administration of the next dose of rabies vaccine.

RIG, when indicated, is administered only once, usually at the beginning of the post-exposure therapy regimen. RIG provides immediate passive antibodies until the patient can produce active antibodies from the rabies vaccine. If not given on the first day, RIG may be given any time up through the 7th day of the therapy regimen. Beyond the 7th day, RIG is not indicated, since an active antibody response to the rabies vaccine is presumed to have begun, and passive antibody may interfere with the body's active response.

If post-exposure prophylaxis is administered outside the U.S., additional prophylaxis may be desirable when the patient returns to the U.S. Physicians should contact the state public health department or the CDC for specific advice. This is important, since treatment regimens and products vary from country to country.

## Parenteral Dosage Forms

### RABIES IMMUNE GLOBULIN (HUMAN) (RIG) USP

**Usual adult and adolescent dose**
Immunizing agent (passive)—
    Intramuscular: 20 International Units (IU) per kg of body weight. If anatomically feasible, up to one-half of the dose should be thoroughly infiltrated into the area(s) around the wound(s) and the rest should be administered intramuscularly in the gluteal area.

Note: Rabies immune globulin (RIG) is used in conjunction with rabies vaccine and should be administered at the time of the first rabies vaccine dose or no later than the 7th day of rabies vaccine therapy.

**Usual pediatric dose**
See *Usual adult and adolescent dose*.

**Strength(s) usually available**
U.S.—
    150 International Units (IU) per mL (Rx) [*Imogam* (thimerosal); *Hyperab* (thimerosal)].
Canada—
    150 International Units (IU) per mL (Rx) [*Imogam* (thimerosal); *Hyperab* (thimerosal)].
    300 International Units (IU) per mL (Rx) [GENERIC (may contain thimerosal)].

Note: The International Unit of potency is equivalent to the U.S. unit of potency.

**Packaging and storage**
Store between 2 and 8 °C (35 and 46 °F), unless otherwise specified by manufacturer. Do not freeze.

**Stability**
The solution should be discarded if it has been frozen.
The solution should not be used if it is discolored or contains particulate matter.
Rabies immune globulin (RIG) should not be heated. It may be warmed slightly by holding the vial in one's hands, but it should not be placed in warm water or an incubator.

**Incompatibilities**
RIG should not be administered in the same syringe or into the same body site as the rabies vaccine.

**Auxiliary labeling**
- Store in refrigerator.
- Do not freeze.
- Discard if vaccine has been frozen.

## Selected Bibliography

Chabala S, Williams M, Amenta R, et al. Confirmed rabies exposure during pregnancy: treatment with human rabies immune globulin and human diploid cell vaccine. Am J Med 1991 Oct; 91: 423-4.

Centers for Disease Control and Prevention. Rabies prevention-United States, 1991: recommendations of the Immunization Practices Advisory Committee (ACIP). MMWR 1991 Mar 22; 40(RR-3): 1-19.

Frenia ML, Lafin SM, Barone JA. Features and treatment of rabies. Clin Pharm 1992 Jan; 11(1): 37-47.

Developed: 08/31/94

---

# RABIES VACCINE    Systemic

This monograph includes information on the following: 1) Rabies Vaccine Adsorbed†; 2) Rabies Vaccine, Human Diploid Cell.

VA CLASSIFICATION (Primary): IM100

Commonly used brand name(s): *Imovax*[2]; *Imovax I.D*[2].

Other commonly used names are: HDCV [Rabies Vaccine, Human Diploid Cell] RVA [Rabies Vaccine Adsorbed]

Note: For a listing of dosage forms and brand names by country availability, see *Dosage Forms* section(s).

†Not commercially available in Canada.

## Category
Immunizing agent (active).

## Indications

**Accepted**

Rabies (prophylaxis)—Rabies vaccine is indicated for post-exposure immunization against rabies infection. Rabies vaccine is also indicated for pre-exposure immunization of persons with a high risk of rabies infection, such as veterinarians, animal handlers, certain laboratory workers, persons spending more than 1 month in areas of foreign countries where rabies (usually canine) is endemic, and other persons whose activities bring them into frequent contact with rabies virus or potentially rabid animals, such as dogs, cats, skunks, raccoons, and bats. Pre-exposure immunization is also recommended for persons who frequently handle or administer modified live rabies virus (MLV) vaccines intended for animals because of the possibility of exposure via needle sticks or sprays. Pre-exposure immunization is indicated for several reasons. It

**2450    Rabies Vaccine (Systemic)**

may protect persons whose post-exposure therapy may be delayed and it simplifies post-exposure therapy, both of which may be important for persons in areas where immunizing products may not be available or where available products may carry a high risk of adverse reactions. In addition, pre-exposure immunization may protect persons with inapparent exposure to rabies.

### Unaccepted
Post-exposure prophylaxis is not recommended for persons inadvertently exposed to modified live rabies virus (MLV) vaccines intended for animals. Although vaccine-induced rabies has occurred in animals administered these vaccines, there have been no reported rabies cases among humans resulting from exposure to needle sticks or sprays with licensed MLV vaccines.

Rabies vaccine is not intended for use in persons who exhibit clinical manifestation of rabies infection.

## Pharmacology/Pharmacokinetics

### Physicochemical characteristics
Source—
- Human diploid cell vaccine (HDCV): Most HDCV products are prepared from Wistar's Pitman-Moore strain of rabies virus grown in MRC-5 human diploid cell culture. The vaccine virus is concentrated and then inactivated by betapropiolactone. One Canadian product is prepared from the CL-77 strain of rabies virus grown in MRC-5 human diploid cell culture. This vaccine undergoes a unique purification process. It is also inactivated by betapropiolactone.
- Rabies vaccine adsorbed (RVA): RVA is prepared from the CVS Kissling/MDPH strain of rabies virus grown in a diploid cell line derived from fetal rhesus monkey lung cells. The vaccine virus is inactivated by betapropiolactone and concentrated by adsorption to aluminum phosphate.

Description—
- HDCV: Solid, having a creamy white to orange color, and having the characteristic appearance of substances dried from the frozen state. The reconstituted suspension is a pinkish-yellow to red color because of the presence of phenol red.
- RVA: Suspension, having a pink color because of the presence of phenol red.

### Mechanism of action/Effect
Following intradermal or intramuscular administration, rabies vaccine induces the formation of protective antibodies to rabies virus, thereby providing active immunity to rabies virus.

### Protective effect
HDCV and RVA are considered equally effective and safe. When the post-exposure prophylaxis regimen has included local wound treatment, passive immunization, and active immunization, 100% effectiveness has been shown. However, rabies has occasionally developed in persons when key elements of the rabies post-exposure prophylaxis regimen were omitted or incorrectly administered. This has occurred outside the United States in cases in which patients' wounds were not cleansed with soap and water or other antiviral agents, rabies vaccine was not administered in the deltoid area, but rather in the gluteal area, and passive immunization was not administered around the wound site.

The presence of acceptable antibody titers following pre-exposure or post-exposure prophylaxis is demonstrated by complete neutralization of the challenge virus at a 1:25 serum dilution (from serum collected 2 to 4 weeks after therapy) by the rapid fluorescent focus inhibition test (RFFIT). This dilution is approximately equivalent to the minimum titer of 0.5 International Units (IU) recommended by the World Health Organization (WHO).

When considering the administration of booster doses of rabies vaccine, the minimum acceptable antibody titer is demonstrated by complete neutralization of the challenge virus at a 1:5 serum dilution by the RFFIT test.

### Time to protective effect
Induction of active antibody production begins within 7 to 10 days.

### Duration of protective effect
Two or more years. Studies have shown that 2 years after the 3-dose pre-exposure prophylaxis regimen with rabies vaccine, a 1:5 serum dilution failed to neutralize the challenge virus completely by the RFFIT test in 2 to 7% of persons who received the vaccine intramuscularly and 5 to 17% of persons who received the vaccine intradermally.

## Precautions to Consider

### Pregnancy/Reproduction
Pregnancy—Studies have not been done in humans. Because of the potential consequences of rabies virus infection, and because there is no indication that fetal abnormalities have been associated with use of rabies vaccine in pregnant women, pregnancy is not considered to be a contraindication to post-exposure prophylaxis. In addition, if there is a substantial risk of exposure to rabies, pre-exposure prophylaxis may also be administered during pregnancy.

Studies have not been done in animals.

FDA Pregnancy Category C.

### Breast-feeding
Problems in humans have not been documented.

### Pediatrics
*HDCV (intradermal)*—Appropriate studies on the relationship of age to the effects of rabies vaccine have not been performed in the pediatric population. However, pediatrics-specific problems that would limit the usefulness of this vaccine in children are not expected.

*HDCV (intramuscular)*—Appropriate studies performed to date have not demonstrated pediatrics-specific problems that would limit the usefulness of rabies vaccine in children.

*RVA*—Appropriate studies on the relationship of age to the effects of rabies vaccine have not been performed in children up to 6 years of age. However, pediatrics-specific problems that would limit the usefulness of this vaccine in children are not expected.

### Geriatrics
No information is available on the relationship of age to the effects of rabies vaccine in geriatric patients.

### Drug interactions and/or related problems
The following drug interactions and/or related problems have been selected on the basis of their potential clinical significance (possible mechanism in parentheses where appropriate)—not necessarily inclusive (» = major clinical significance):

Note: Combinations containing any of the following medications, depending on the amount present, may also interact with this medication.

» Chloroquine and possibly other related antimalarials, such as mefloquine
(chloroquine, and possibly other related antimalarials, interferes with the antibody response to rabies vaccine. If the intradermal route is used for pre-exposure rabies immunization, rabies prophylaxis should be initiated at least one month prior to travel [i.e., at least 2 weeks before initiation of antimalarial therapy] to allow for the formation of adequate rabies antibodies; if rabies prophylaxis cannot be initiated at least one month prior to travel, the intramuscular route should be used for pre-exposure rabies prophylaxis, since the intramuscular route is considered to have an adequate margin of safety when given within 2 weeks of antimalarial therapy. If post-exposure therapy is required during concurrent use of chloroquine, it is prudent to test for an adequate response to the rabies vaccine)

» Corticosteroids or
» Immunosuppressive agents or
» Radiation therapy
(because normal defense mechanisms are suppressed, concurrent use with rabies vaccine may decrease the patient's antibody response to rabies vaccine. During post-exposure prophylaxis against possible rabies infection, these agents should not be administered unless they are essential for the treatment of other conditions. If these agents must be used concurrently, it is important to test for an adequate response to the rabies vaccine. Pre-exposure prophylaxis for rabies should be postponed if possible. If persons are at risk of rabies exposure and must have pre-exposure prophylaxis, the intramuscular, not the intradermal, agent should be administered and the patient should be tested for an adequate response to the rabies vaccine)

### Medical considerations/Contraindications
The medical considerations/contraindications included have been selected on the basis of their potential clinical significance (reasons given in parentheses where appropriate)—not necessarily inclusive (» = major clinical significance):

*Risk-benefit should be considered when the following medical problems exist:*

» Febrile illness, severe
(to avoid confusing manifestations of illness with possible side/adverse effects of vaccine; minor illnesses, such as upper respiratory infection, do not preclude administration of vaccine. Although pre-exposure prophylaxis may be postponed during severe febrile illness, post-exposure prophylaxis should be initiated on schedule)

» Immune complex–like hypersensitivity reaction to rabies vaccine, history of
(persons who have experienced an immune complex–like hyper-

sensitivity reaction following immunization with either human diploid cell vaccine [HDCV] or rabies vaccine adsorbed [RVA] should not receive further doses of the same type of rabies vaccine; although it is not known whether cross-sensitivity exists between the two types of rabies vaccine, it may be helpful to administer the other type of rabies vaccine if additional treatment is necessary; in addition, one specially purified Canadian HDCV vaccine [Rabies Vaccine Inactivated, Diploid Cell Origin, Dried—Connaught] has not been associated with this reaction [see *Side/Adverse Effects*]; additional doses of the same type of rabies vaccine should be administered only if the other types of rabies vaccine are not available and prophylaxis is essential [e.g., patient requires post-exposure prophylaxis or patient requires pre-exposure prophylaxis because of a high risk of rabies exposure and inadequate antibody titers])

» Immune deficiency conditions, congenital or hereditary, family history of, or
» Immune deficiency conditions, primary or acquired
(because normal defense mechanisms are suppressed or reduced, there may be a decrease in the patient's antibody response to rabies vaccine. Following post-exposure prophylaxis, it is essential to test for an adequate response to the rabies vaccine. Pre-exposure prophylaxis should use the intramuscular, not the intradermal, route of administration and the patient should be tested for an adequate response to the rabies vaccine)

Sensitivity to bovine serum, human albumin, kanamycin, monkey proteins, neomycin, polymyxin B, or thimerosal
(the rabies vaccines available in the U.S. and Canada contain one or more of these ingredients; it may be possible to select a product not having the agent causing sensitivity)

Sensitivity to rabies vaccine

**Patient monitoring**
The following may be especially important in patient monitoring (other tests may be warranted in some patients, depending on condition; » = major clinical significance):

Rabies antibody titer, serum
(may be determined when there is doubt as to whether an adequate antibody response has occurred following pre-exposure or post-exposure prophylaxis; the acceptable antibody titer is demonstrated by complete neutralization of the challenge virus at a 1:25 serum dilution [from serum collected 2 to 4 weeks after therapy] by the rapid fluorescent focus inhibition test [RFFIT]. This dilution is approximately equivalent to the minimum titer of 0.5 International Units [IU] recommended by the World Health Organization (WHO). Determination of the need for a booster dose of rabies vaccine is based on the minimum acceptable antibody titer, which is demonstrated by complete neutralization of the challenge virus at a 1:5 serum dilution by the RFFIT test)

## Side/Adverse Effects

Note: All available methods of systemic prophylaxis against rabies are complicated by occasional adverse effects; however, these adverse effects are rarely severe.

If necessary, physicians should consult with the state public health department, the Centers for Disease Control (CDC), Canadian National Advisory Committee on Immunization (NACI), and/or the World Health Organization (WHO) regarding the management of serious adverse reactions.

In approximately 6% of persons receiving a booster dose of human diploid cell vaccine (HDCV), a non–life-threatening immune complex–like reaction occurs 2 to 21 days later. Patients develop a generalized urticaria or rash, which is sometimes accompanied by arthralgia, arthritis, angioedema, nausea, vomiting, fever, or malaise. The reaction occurs much less frequently among persons receiving a primary immunization series, and rarely, if at all, after the first dose of a primary series. The reaction is thought to be caused by human serum albumin present in the product that has become allergenic by interaction with betapropiolactone. A similar reaction occurs after 7 to 14 days in less than 1% of persons receiving a booster, but not a primary, dose of rabies virus adsorbed (RVA), even though human serum albumin is not used in the production of RVA. However, RVA also is inactivated by betapropiolactone. It is not known whether a person hypersensitive to HDCV is hypersensitive to RVA also, or vice versa. Administration of booster doses of a specially purified HDCV vaccine, currently available in Canada (Rabies Vaccine Inactivated, Diploid Cell Origin, Dried—Connaught), has not been associated with this reaction.

Three cases of neurologic illness resembling Guillain-Barré syndrome that resolved without sequelae in 12 weeks have been reported following administration of rabies vaccine. In addition, a few other subacute central and peripheral nervous system disorders have been temporally associated with the vaccine, but a causal relationship has not been established.

The following side/adverse effects have been selected on the basis of their potential clinical significance (possible signs and symptoms in parentheses where appropriate)—not necessarily inclusive:

**Those indicating need for medical attention**
Incidence rare
*Immune complex–like reaction* (hives or skin rash)—less frequent with booster doses

**Those indicating need for medical attention only if they continue or are bothersome**
Incidence more frequent
*Abdominal pain* (stomach or abdomen pain); *chills; dizziness; fatigue* (tiredness or weakness); *fever; headache; itching, pain, redness, or swelling at the place of injection; malaise* (general feeling of discomfort or illness); *muscle or joint aches; nausea*

## Patient Consultation

As an aid to patient consultation, refer to *Advice for the Patient, Rabies Vaccine (Systemic)*.

In providing consultation, consider emphasizing the following selected information (» = major clinical significance):

**Before using this medication**
» Conditions affecting use, especially:
Sensitivity to rabies vaccine or to bovine serum, human albumin, kanamycin, monkey proteins, neomycin, polymyxin B, or thimerosal, which may also be present in the vaccine
Other medications, especially chloroquine and possibly other related antimalarials, such as mefloquine; corticosteroids; immunosuppressive agents; or radiation therapy
Other medical problems, especially febrile illness, severe; immune complex–like hypersensitivity reaction to rabies vaccine, history of; immune deficiency conditions, congenital or hereditary, family history of; or immune deficiency conditions, primary or acquired

**Proper use of this medication**
» Importance of not missing doses; keeping appointments with physician
» Proper dosing
» Missed dose: Contacting physician as soon as possible

**Precautions while using this medication**
» Caution if dizziness occurs; not driving, using machines, or doing anything else that requires alertness while receiving rabies vaccine

**Side/adverse effects**
Signs of potential side effects, especially immune complex–like reaction

## General Dosing Information

The dosage is the same for all persons, children and adults.

Rabies vaccine is administered either intramuscularly or intradermally, depending on the product and the indication. The products are not interchangable with respect to the route of administration. Care should be taken to avoid injection of the vaccine into or near blood vessels or nerves.

Rabies vaccine should not be administered into the gluteal area (buttocks), since administration into this area of the body results in lower antibody titers.

It is not considered necessary to document seroconversion by testing serum samples from patients completing pre- or post-exposure prophylaxis except under unusual instances, such as when the person is known to be immunosuppressed. Studies at the Centers for Disease Control (CDC) have shown that persons tested 2 to 4 weeks after completion of pre- or post-exposure rabies prophylaxis, administered according to Immunization Practices Advisory Committee (ACIP) guidelines, developed adequate antibody response to rabies. If documentation of seroconversion is required, serum collected 2 to 4 weeks after pre-exposure or post-exposure prophylaxis, and diluted 1:25, should completely neutralize the challenge virus by the rapid fluorescent focus inhibition test (RFFIT). This dilution is approximately equivalent to the minimum titer of 0.5 International Units (IU) recommended by the World Health Organization (WHO).

**For pre-exposure immunization only**
For pre-exposure immunization, either the intradermal or intramuscular product may be used. If the intradermal vaccine is used and is inadvertently injected subcutaneously, another dose of intradermal vaccine should be administered at a different site.

Pre-exposure immunization does not eliminate the need for prompt post-exposure prophylaxis following an exposure. However, pre-exposure immunization eliminates the need for administration of rabies immune globulin and reduces the number of injections of rabies vaccine needed for post-exposure prophylaxis.

Pre-exposure booster immunization is administered to persons who have received the pre-exposure immunization series, who remain at risk of rabies exposure by reasons of occupation or avocation, and whose 1:5 diluted serum does not completely neutralize the challenge virus by the RFFIT test. Depending on the person's degree of risk of rabies exposure, serum testing should be performed every 6 months to 2 years. As an alternative to serum testing for those persons who, based on their degree of risk, would require serum testing every 2 years, a booster can be administered every 2 years.

**For post-exposure immunization only**
All post-exposure therapy should begin with immediate and thorough cleansing of all the patient's wounds with soap and water. Studies have shown that wound cleansing greatly reduces the likelihood of rabies.

For post-exposure immunization, the intramuscular vaccine, not the intradermal vaccine, should be used.

Appropriate management of persons who may have been exposed to rabies depends on the assessment of the risk of infection. The incubation period for rabies infection varies with respect to the location and severity of the bite. For bites to the face or extensive bites elsewhere on the body, the incubation period may be as short as 17 days. Decisions about management should be made promptly. Persons who have been bitten by animals suspected of being, or proven, rabid should begin therapy within 24 hours. If necessary, physicians should consult with the local or state public health department, CDC, the Canadian National Advisory Commitee on Immunization (NACI), and/or WHO regarding the need for rabies prophylaxis.

The essential components of the rabies post-exposure prophylaxis regimen are local wound treatment, passive immunization with rabies immune globulin (RIG) (unless the patient has been previously immunized against rabies), and active immunization with rabies vaccine. Rabies has occasionally developed in persons when key elements of this regimen were omitted or incorrectly performed. In addition, tetanus prophylaxis and antibacterial medications may be administered as required. Both passive immunization with RIG (except for patients who have been previously immunized against rabies) and active immunization with rabies vaccine are required regardless of the interval between exposure and initiation of therapy.

Persons are considered to have been previously immunized against rabies (and as such should not receive RIG as part of the post-exposure therapy) if they have previously received complete regimens of pre- or post-exposure rabies prophylaxis with human diploid cell rabies vaccine (HDCV) or rabies vaccine adsorbed (RVA) or if they have been documented to have had an adequate antibody response to another rabies vaccine, such as duck embryo rabies vaccine. Regardless of the antibody titer that is present before post-exposure therapy occurs, an anamnestic antibody response should occur following the administration of the next dose of rabies vaccine.

RIG, when indicated, is administered only once, usually at the beginning of the post-exposure therapy regimen. RIG provides immediate passive antibodies until the patient can produce active antibodies from the rabies vaccine. If not given on the first day, RIG may be given any time up through the 7th day of the therapy regimen. Beyond the 7th day, RIG is not indicated, since an active antibody response to the rabies vaccine is presumed to have begun. RIG should not be administered in the same syringe or into the same body site as the rabies vaccine. In addition, since RIG may partially suppress active production of rabies antibody, it is recommended that no more than the recommended dose be administered.

WHO recommends a 6-dose series (administered on Days 0, 3, 7, 14, 30, and 90) of HDCV, and probably RVA, for persons not previously immunized with rabies vaccine. The WHO regimen is considered safe and effective. However, studies conducted at CDC have shown that a 5-dose regimen of HDCV or RVA was also safe and effective and induced an adequate antibody response in all recipients tested.

If post-exposure prophylaxis is administered outside the U.S., additional prophylaxis may be desirable when the patient returns to the U.S. Physicians should contact the state public health department or the CDC for specific advice. This is important, since treatment regimens and products vary from country to country.

**For treatment of adverse effects**
Recommended treatment consists of the following:
- Antihistamines may be administered for mild hypersensitivity reactions.
- Anti-inflammatory and antipyretic agents (e.g., aspirin) may be administered for local or mild systemic adverse reactions.
- Epinephrine may be administered to treat severe hypersensitivity or anaphylactic reaction.
- If possible, corticosteroids should not be administered, because when given in immunosuppressive doses, they may reduce the production of rabies antibodies. If corticosteroids are administered, it is important to test for an adequate response to the rabies vaccine, especially during post-exposure prophylaxis.

---

### RABIES VACCINE ADSORBED

## Parenteral Dosage Forms

### RABIES VACCINE ADSORBED SUSPENSION (RVA) USP

**Usual adult and adolescent dose**
Immunizing agent (active)—
 Intramuscular, into the deltoid muscle:
  Pre-exposure immunization:
   1 mL on Days 0, 7, and 21 or 28, for a total of three doses.
  Pre-exposure booster immunization, if required:
   1 mL as a single dose.
   Note: See *General Dosing Information* for the parameters for administering booster doses.
  Post-exposure immunization of persons who have been previously immunized against rabies:
   1 mL on Days 0 and 3, for a total of two doses.
  Post-exposure immunization of persons who have not been previously immunized against rabies:
   1 mL on Days 0, 3, 7, 14, and 28, for a total of five doses.
   Note: For persons who have not been previously immunized against rabies, rabies immune globulin (RIG) should be administered on Day 0 along with the first dose of the vaccine. See *General Dosing Information*.

**Usual pediatric dose**
See *Usual adult and adolescent dose*.
 Note: The vaccine may be administered into the anterolateral aspect of the thigh if the child does not have sufficient deltoid muscle mass.

**Strength(s) usually available**
U.S.—
 Greater than or equal to 2.5 International Units (IU) of rabies antigen per mL (Rx) [GENERIC (no more than 2 mg aluminum phosphate per mL; 0.01% thimerosal)].
Canada—
 Not commercially available.

**Packaging and storage**
Store between 2 and 8 °C (35 and 46 °F), unless otherwise specified by manufacturer. Do not freeze.

**Preparation of dosage form**
The vial should be shaken gently to ensure complete suspension of the aluminum phosphate adjuvant before withdrawing the dose into a syringe.

**Stability**
The suspension should be discarded if it has been frozen.
The suspension should not be used if it is discolored or contains particulate matter.

**Auxiliary labeling**
- Do not freeze.
- Discard if vaccine has been frozen.
- Store in refrigerator

**Note**
The suspension is a light pink color because of the presence of phenol red indicator.

---

### RABIES VACCINE, HUMAN DIPLOID CELL

## Parenteral Dosage Forms

### RABIES VACCINE, HUMAN DIPLOID CELL (FOR INTRADERMAL INJECTION) (HDCV)

**Usual adult and adolescent dose**
Immunizing agent (active)—
 Intradermal, on the deltoid muscle:
  Pre-exposure immunization:
   0.1 mL on Days 0, 7, and 21 or 28, for a total of three doses.

Pre-exposure booster immunization, if required:
  0.1 mL as a single dose.
    Note: See *General Dosing Information* for the parameters for administering booster doses.

**Usual pediatric dose**
See *Usual adult and adolescent dose*.

**Strength(s) usually available**
U.S.—
  Greater than or equal to 2.5 International Units (IU) of rabies antigen per mL of reconstituted suspension (Rx) [*Imovax I.D* (contains no preservatives or stabilizers)].
Canada—
  Not commercially available.

**Packaging and storage**
Store between 2 and 8 °C (35 and 46 °F), unless otherwise specified by manufacturer. Do not freeze.

**Preparation of dosage form**
The freeze-dried vaccine is contained in the single-dose syringe. The plunger of the syringe should be pushed so that the leading edge of the black stopper is even with the broken blue line on the side of the syringe. The needle should be inserted into the diluent bottle in such a way that both syringe and bottle remain upright. The needle should be in the diluent at all times during withdrawal in order to prevent air bubbles. The diluent should be drawn into the syringe until the end of the syringe's black stopper is at the solid blue line on the side of the syringe. The protective rubber cap should be replaced on the needle, and the freeze-dried vaccine should be allowed to completely dissolve. The syringe may be shaken if necessary. The reconstituted vaccine should be used immediately.

**Stability**
The vaccine should be administered immediately following reconstitution, or reconstituted vaccine should be discarded.
The reconstituted vaccine should not be used if it is discolored or contains particulate matter.

**Auxiliary labeling**
• Use reconstituted vaccine immediately.

## RABIES VACCINE, HUMAN DIPLOID CELL (FOR INTRAMUSCULAR INJECTION) (HDCV) USP

**Usual adult and adolescent dose**
Immunizing agent (active)—
  Intramuscular, into the deltoid muscle:
    Pre-exposure immunization:
      1 mL on Days 0, 7, and 21 or 28, for a total of three doses.
    Pre-exposure booster immunization, if required:
      1 mL as a single dose.
        Note: See *General Dosing Information* for the parameters for administering booster doses.
    Post-exposure immunization of persons who have been previously immunized against rabies:
      1 mL on Days 0 and 3, for a total of two doses.
    Post-exposure immunization of persons who have not been previously immunized against rabies:
      1 mL on Days 0, 3, 7, 14, and 28, for a total of five doses.
        Note: For persons who have not been previously immunized against rabies, rabies immune globulin (RIG) should be administered on Day 0 along with the first dose of the vaccine. See *General Dosing Information*.

**Usual pediatric dose**
See *Usual adult and adolescent dose*.
Note: The intramuscular vaccine may be administered into the anterolateral aspect of the thigh if the child does not have sufficient deltoid muscle mass.

**Strength(s) usually available**
U.S.—
  Greater than or equal to 2.5 International Units (IU) of rabies antigen per mL of reconstituted suspension (Rx) [*Imovax* (contains no preservatives or stabilizers)].
Canada—
  Greater than or equal to 2.5 International Units (IU) of rabies antigen per mL of reconstituted suspension (Rx) [GENERIC (diluent may contain 0.01% thimerosal)].

**Packaging and storage**
Store between 2 and 8 °C (35 and 46 °F), unless otherwise specified by manufacturer. Do not freeze.

**Preparation of dosage form**
The freeze-dried vaccine should be reconstituted in its vial by using the 1 mL of diluent supplied in the disposable syringe. The longer of the two needles should be used to introduce the diluent into the vaccine vial. The contents of the vial should be gently swirled until they are completely dissolved. The total amount of dissolved vaccine in the vial should be drawn into the syringe. In order to do this, the vial should be set in an upright position on a table. The needle used for reconstitution should be removed and replaced with the smaller needle that will be used for administration. The reconstituted vaccine should be used immediately.

**Stability**
The vaccine should be administered immediately following reconstitution, or the reconstituted vaccine should be discarded.
The reconstituted vaccine should not be used if it is discolored or contains particulate matter.

**Auxiliary labeling**
• Use reconstituted vaccine immediately.

## Selected Bibliography

Centers for Disease Control and Prevention. Rabies prevention-United States, 1991: recommendations of the Immunization Practices Advisory Committee (ACIP). MMWR 1991 Mar 22; 40(RR-3): 1-19.
Centers for Disease Control and Prevention. Systemic allergic reactions following immunization with human diploid cell rabies vaccine. MMWR 1984 Apr 13; 33(14): 185-7.
Frenia ML, Lafin SM, Barone JA. Features and treatment of rabies. Clin Pharm 1992 Jan; 11(1): 37-47.

Developed: 08/31/94

---

**RABIES VACCINE ADSORBED**—See *Rabies Vaccine (Systemic)*

---

**RABIES VACCINE, HUMAN DIPLOID CELL**—See *Rabies Vaccine (Systemic)*

---

**RACEMETHIONINE**—The *Racemethionine (Systemic)* monograph is not included in this published version of the USP DI database. Copies of the monograph are available on request from Micromedex, Inc. - Reprint Requests, 6200 S. Syracuse Way, Suite 300, Englewood, CO 80111; telephone (303) 486-6400; telefax (303) 486-6464; Email: USPDI@MDX.COM.

---

# RADIOIODINATED ALBUMIN  Systemic

VA CLASSIFICATION (Primary): DX202
Commonly used brand name(s): *IHSA I 125*; *Jeanatope*; *Megatope*.
Note: For a listing of dosage forms and brand names by country availability, see *Dosage Forms* section(s).

## Category
Diagnostic aid, radioactive (fluid and blood loss).

## Indications

**Accepted**
Blood and plasma volumes determinations—Iodinated I 125 and I 131 albumin are indicated for use in determinations of total blood and plasma volumes.

**Unaccepted**
Radioiodinated albumin has been used in determinations of cardiac and pulmonary blood volumes and circulation times and of cardiac output; in protein turnover studies to help determine gastrointestinal loss of

protein. Iodinated I 131 albumin has been used for the delineation of the heart and great vessels; in placenta localization for the detection of placenta previa; and in brain scanning for the localization of cerebral neoplasms. However, these agents generally have been replaced by more effective and/or safer agents for these indications.

## Physical Properties

### Nuclear data

| Radionuclide (half-life) | Decay constant | Mode of decay | Principal emissions (keV) | Mean number of emissions/ disintegration |
|---|---|---|---|---|
| I 125 (60.14 days) | 0.00048 h$^{-1}$ | Gamma and x-ray emissions | Gamma (35.0) x-ray (28.0) | 0.067 1.40 |
| I 131 (8.08 days) | 0.00358 h$^{-1}$ | Beta and gamma emissions | Beta (191.6) Gamma (364.4) | 0.90 0.81 |

## Pharmacology/Pharmacokinetics

### Mechanism of action/Effect
Human serum albumin occurs naturally as the major protein component of blood. When labeled with iodine I 125 or I 131 and given intravenously, it is distributed throughout the body similarly to the patient's serum albumin, and serves as a suitable tracer with which to determine plasma or blood volume. The radioconcentration can be quantitated in blood samples withdrawn at periodic intervals, after injection of the radioiodinated albumin. Although the gamma emissions of I 131 are suitable for external imaging, the biodistribution of iodinated I 131 albumin is seldom evaluated by *in vivo* imaging.

### Distribution
Radioiodinated serum albumin—Within 10 minutes throughout intravascular pool; more slowly into extravascular space. Can also be detected in the lymph and in certain body tissues within 10 minutes after injection; maximum distribution throughout the extravascular space does not occur until 2 to 4 days following injection.

Radioiodine—Small amount of released iodine I 125 or iodine I 131 (resulting from degradation of radioiodinated albumin) is selectively concentrated in thyroid gland; also concentrated in choroid plexus, gastric mucosa, salivary glands, stomach, and lactating breast.

### Radiation dosimetry

**I 125**
**Estimated absorbed radiation dose***

| Organ | mGy/MBq | rad/mCi |
|---|---|---|
| Heart | 0.69 | 2.56 |
| Spleen | 0.59 | 2.19 |
| Lungs | 0.57 | 2.11 |
| Red marrow | 0.37 | 1.37 |
| Kidneys | 0.33 | 1.22 |
| Bone surfaces | 0.32 | 1.19 |
| Adrenals | 0.30 | 1.11 |
| Liver | 0.30 | 1.11 |
| Thyroid | 0.26 | 0.96 |
| Pancreas | 0.23 | 0.85 |
| Stomach wall | 0.21 | 0.78 |
| Small intestine | 0.21 | 0.78 |
| Large intestine (upper) | 0.21 | 0.78 |
| Large intestine (lower) | 0.20 | 0.74 |
| Bladder wall | 0.20 | 0.74 |
| Breast | 0.20 | 0.74 |
| Ovaries | 0.20 | 0.74 |
| Uterus | 0.20 | 0.74 |
| Testes | 0.16 | 0.59 |
| Other tissue | 0.19 | 0.70 |

Effective dose: 0.34 mSv/MBq (1.26 rem/mCi)

*For adults; intravenous injection

**I 131**
**Estimated absorbed radiation dose***

| Organ | mGy/MBq | rad/mCi |
|---|---|---|
| Heart | 1.9 | 7.03 |
| Lungs | 1.5 | 5.55 |
| Spleen | 1.5 | 5.55 |
| Bone surfaces | 0.97 | 3.59 |
| Adrenals | 0.94 | 3.59 |
| Kidneys | 0.88 | 3.26 |
| Liver | 0.72 | 2.66 |
| Thyroid | 0.70 | 2.59 |
| Red marrow | 0.66 | 2.44 |
| Breast | 0.55 | 2.04 |
| Stomach wall | 0.53 | 1.96 |
| Small intestine | 0.52 | 1.92 |
| Large intestine (upper) | 0.52 | 1.92 |
| Uterus | 0.51 | 1.89 |
| Large intestine (lower) | 0.50 | 1.85 |
| Ovaries | 0.49 | 1.81 |
| Bladder wall | 0.49 | 1.81 |
| Testes | 0.46 | 1.70 |
| Other tissue | 0.47 | 1.74 |

Effective dose: 0.86 mSv/MBq (3.18 rem/mCi)

*For adults; intravenous injection

### Half-time
Normal human serum albumin—Approximately 14 days (range, 10 to 20 days); dependent on initial rate of excretion, which is determined by the quality of the labeled albumin.

### Elimination
Primarily renal; about 2% eliminated in feces.

## Precautions to Consider

### Cross-sensitivity and/or related problems
Patients sensitive to human serum albumin–containing products may be sensitive to these products also.

### Pregnancy/Reproduction
Pregnancy—Iodine I 125 and I 131 cross the placenta and may cause severe and irreversible hypothyroidism in the fetus; the fetal thyroid begins to concentrate iodine during approximately the 12th week of gestation. Radioiodinated albumin is usually not recommended for use during pregnancy; however, if used, prior administration of potassium iodide (e.g., Lugol's solution or SSKI) may reduce the risk of fetal thyroid irradiation.

The possibility of pregnancy should be assessed in women of child-bearing potential. Clinical situations exist where the benefit to the patient and fetus, based on information derived from radiopharmaceutical use, outweighs the risks from fetal exposure to radiation. In these situations, the physician should use discretion and reduce the radiopharmaceutical dose to the lowest possible amount.

*Radioiodinated albumin—*
  Studies have not been done in humans with either iodinated I 131 albumin or iodinated I 125 albumin.
  Studies have not been done in animals.

FDA Pregnancy Category C.

### Breast-feeding
Iodine I 125 and I 131 are distributed into breast milk. Because of the potential risk to the infant from radiation exposure, temporary discontinuation of nursing is recommended for a length of time that may be assessed by measuring the activity of breast milk and estimating the radiation exposure to the infant.

### Pediatrics
Although radioiodinated albumin is used in children, there have been no specific studies evaluating its safety and efficacy in children. When this radiopharmaceutical is used in children, the diagnostic benefit should be judged to outweigh the potential risk of radiation.

### Geriatrics
Appropriate studies on the relationship of age to the effects of radioiodinated albumin have not been performed in the geriatric population. However, no geriatrics-specific problems have been documented to date.

### Diagnostic interference

The following have been selected on the basis of their potential clinical significance (possible effect in parentheses where appropriate)—not necessarily inclusive (» = major clinical significance):

With *other* diagnostic test results
  Thyroid function determinations and
  Thyroid imaging
    (potassium iodide [e.g., Lugol's solution] used prior to the administration of radioiodinated albumin may cause a decrease in radioactive iodine or pertechnetate ion uptake for several weeks)

### Medical considerations/Contraindications

The medical considerations/contraindications included have been selected on the basis of their potential clinical significance (reasons given in parentheses where appropriate)—not necessarily inclusive (» = major clinical significance).

*Risk-benefit should be considered when the following medical problem exists:*
» Sensitivity to human serum albumin-containing products

## Side/Adverse Effects

Presently, there are no known side/adverse effects associated with the use of iodinated I 125 or I 131 albumin as a diagnostic aid. However, as with any protein-containing preparation, allergic reactions are possible.

## Patient Consultation

As an aid to patient consultation, refer to *Advice for the Patient, Radiopharmaceuticals (Diagnostic)*.

In providing consultation, consider emphasizing the following selected information (» = major clinical significance):

### Description of use
  Action in the body: Radioactive albumin's distribution in body same as normal albumin
  Dilution of radioactivity in blood pool permits calculation of its volume
  Small amounts of radioactivity used in diagnosis; radiation received is low and considered safe

### Before having this test
» Conditions affecting use, especially:
    Sensitivity to human serum albumin
    Pregnancy—Risk to fetus from radiation exposure as opposed to benefit derived from use should be considered; possibility of hypothyroidism in fetus
    Breast-feeding—Iodine I 125 and I 131 are distributed into breast milk; temporary discontinuation of nursing recommended because of risk to infant from radiation exposure
    Use in children—Risk from radiation exposure as opposed to benefit derived from use should be considered

### Preparation for this test
  Special preparatory instructions may be given; patient should inquire in advance

### Precautions after having this test
Possible interference with future thyroid tests

### Side/adverse effects
No side/adverse effects reported; allergic reactions are possible

## General Dosing Information

Radiopharmaceuticals are to be administered only by or under the supervision of physicians who have had extensive training in the safe use and handling of radioactive materials and who are authorized by the Nuclear Regulatory Commission (NRC) or the appropriate Federal or Agreement State agency, if required or, outside the U.S., the appropriate authority.

Epinephrine, antihistamines, and corticosteroid agents should be available during the administration of radioiodinated albumin because of the possibility of allergic reactions.

To minimize the uptake of radioactive iodine by the thyroid, potassium iodide (e.g., Lugol's solution or SSKI) may be used one to three times daily, beginning at least 24 hours before and continuing for one or two weeks after administration of radioiodinated albumin.

### Safety considerations for handling this radiopharmaceutical

Improper handling of this radiopharmaceutical may cause radioactive contamination. Guidelines for handling radioactive material have been prepared by scientific, professional, state, federal, and international bodies and are available to the specially qualified and authorized users who have access to radiopharmaceuticals.

## Parenteral Dosage Forms

### IODINATED I 125 ALBUMIN INJECTION USP

**Usual adult and adolescent administered activity**
Total blood and plasma volume determinations—
  Intravenous, 0.185 to 1.85 megabecquerels (5 to 50 microcuries).
  Note: For repeat blood volume determinations, the total dosage per week should not exceed 7.4 megabecquerels (200 microcuries).
        See manufacturer's package instructions for preparation of the reference solution and for formula used in the calculation of blood and plasma volumes.

**Usual pediatric administered activity**
Dosage must be individualized by physician.

**Usual geriatric administered activity**
See *Usual adult and adolescent administered activity*.

**Size(s) usually available**
U.S.—
  At time of calibration: Per single-dose syringe
    0.37 megabecquerel (10 microcuries) per 1.5 mL (Rx) [*IHSA I 125*].
  At time of calibration: Per multiple-dose vial
    37 megabecquerels (1 millicurie) (Rx) [*Jeanatope*].
Canada—
  Content information not available at present (Rx) [GENERIC].

**Packaging and storage**
Store between 2 and 8 °C (36 and 46 °F). Protect from freezing.

**Note**
Caution—Radioactive material.

### IODINATED I 131 ALBUMIN INJECTION USP

**Usual adult and adolescent administered activity**
Total blood and plasma volume determinations—
  Intravenous, 0.185 to 1.85 megabecquerels (5 to 50 microcuries).
  Note: For repeat blood volume determinations, the total dosage per week should not exceed 7.4 megabecquerels (200 microcuries).
        See manufacturer's package instructions for preparation of the reference solution and for formula used in the calculation of blood and plasma volumes.

**Usual pediatric administered activity**
Dosage must be individualized by physician.

**Usual geriatric administered activity**
See *Usual adult and adolescent administered activity*.

**Size(s) usually available**
U.S.—
  At time of calibration: Per multiple-dose vial
    37 megabecquerels (1 millicurie) per mL (Rx) [*Megatope*].
Canada—
  At time of calibration: Per multiple-dose vial
    0.185 to 0.555 megabecquerels (5 to 15 microcuries) per mL (Rx) [GENERIC].
    3.7 to 37 megabecquerels (0.1 to 1 millicurie) per mL (Rx) [GENERIC].

**Packaging and storage**
Store between 2 and 8 °C (36 and 46 °F). Protect from freezing.

**Note**
Caution—Radioactive material.

Revised: 07/20/93
Interim revision: 08/02/94

---

# RALOXIFENE   Systemic—INTRODUCTORY VERSION

VA CLASSIFICATION (Primary): HS900
Commonly used brand name(s): *Evista*.
Another commonly used name is keoxifene hydrochloride.

Note: For a listing of dosage forms and brand names by country availability, see *Dosage Forms* section(s).

## Category
Estrogen receptor modulator, selective; osteoporosis prophylactic.

## Indications

### Accepted
**Osteoporosis, postmenopausal (prophylaxis)**—Raloxifene is indicated for the prevention of osteoporosis in postmenopausal women. The effects on risk of fracture are not known. Safety of raloxifene in premenopausal females has not been established and its use is not recommended. Also, use of estrogens as ovarian hormone therapy (OHT) with raloxifene has not been studied and their concurrent use is not recommended. Safety and efficacy of raloxifene have not been studied in men.

### Unaccepted
Raloxifene is not effective in reducing the hot flashes or flushes of estrogen deficiency, such as those occurring during the menopause.

## Pharmacology/Pharmacokinetics

### Physicochemical characteristics
Note: Raloxifene shows high interindividual variability as seen by an approximate 30% coefficient of variation in most pharmacokinetic parameters.
Chemical group—Nonsteroidal, benzothiophene derivative.
Molecular weight—Raloxifene hydrochloride: 510.06.

### Mechanism of action/Effect
**Selective estrogen receptor modulator**—Estrogen receptors regulate gene expression by ligand-, tissue-, or gene-specific pathways or a combination of these. Raloxifene acts as a ligand for the estrogen receptor and, depending on the tissue's subtype of estrogen receptors or available cellular proteins, can cause an estrogenic agonist or antagonist reaction or may not cause any apparent change in a tissue's gene expression.

**Osteoporosis prophylactic**—Raloxifene has estrogen-like effects on bone and increases bone mineral density. It reduces resorption of bone and decreases overall bone turnover, as shown by radiocalcium kinetics studies and by bone turnover markers in the serum and urine. Postmenopausal females who took daily doses of 60 mg raloxifene and 400 to 600 mg of calcium showed a statistically significant increase in bone mineral density (BMD) in the hip, spine, and total body at 12 months that was maintained at 24 months as measured by dual-energy radiography (DXA) compared with women taking a placebo and similar calcium doses. The extent of bone density increase is less with use of raloxifene than with daily doses of 0.625 mg conjugated estrogens. The placebo/calcium females lost 1% of BMD over 24 months. The effects of raloxifene on the forearm have been inconsistent between studies. It is not established whether raloxifene's effect of increasing BMD results in a reduced number of skeletal fractures.

### Other actions/effects
Raloxifene has estrogen-like effects for lowering serum total and low-density lipoprotein (LDL) cholesterol, but it does not affect serum concentrations of total high-density lipoprotein (HDL) cholesterol or triglycerides. Raloxifene has not been associated with other estrogen-like effects, such as endometrial proliferation, breast pain, or breast enlargement.

### Absorption
Raloxifene is rapidly absorbed after oral administration. Absolute raloxifene bioavailability is 2%, approximately 60% of an oral dose is absorbed, and enterohepatic cycling occurs. Although not considered clinically significant, absorption may increase when raloxifene is given with a high-fat meal, as shown by a 28% increase in peak serum concentration ($C_{max}$) and a 16% increase in the area under the plasma concentration–time curve (AUC).

### Distribution
For 30 to 150 mg single doses of raloxifene, the apparent volume of distribution ($Vol_D$) is 2348 L per kg (L/kg) and is not dose-dependent.

### Protein binding
Raloxifene and its glucuronide conjugates are highly bound to plasma proteins albumin and alpha-1-acid glycoprotein, but not to sex hormone–binding globulin.

### Biotransformation
First-pass metabolism to the glucuronide conjugate is extensive; 1% unconjugated raloxifene appears in the plasma as a result of interconversion between conjugated and unconjugated forms.

### Half-life
Elimination—32.5 hours (range 15.8 to 86.6) with multiple dosing.

### Elimination
Primarily fecal, 0.2% renal (unchanged) and 6% renal (glucuronide metabolite).

## Precautions to Consider

### Carcinogenicity/Tumorigenicity
Raloxifene did not increase the risk of endometrial or breast cancer in patients taking raloxifene for up to 39 months when compared with patients taking placebos.

In a 21-month study, there was an increased incidence of benign tumors of granulosal, thecal, or epithelial cell origin in female mice given raloxifene doses of 9 to 242 mg per kg of body weight (mg/kg) (corresponding to 0.3 to 34 times the systemic exposure of that achieved in postmenopausal women taking a 60-mg daily dose). Malignant tumors of granulosal/thecal origin occurred at the higher doses. There was an increased incidence of testicular interstitial cell tumors, prostatic adenomas, and adenocarcinomas in male mice given 41 mg/kg or 210 mg/kg of raloxifene (corresponding to 4.7 to 24 times the systemic exposure in humans); the higher dose showed incidence of prostatic leiomyoblastomas.

In a 2-year study, there was an increased incidence of benign granulosal or thecal cell ovarian tumors in nonovariectomized female rats of reproductive age given doses of 279 mg/kg of raloxifene (corresponding to approximately 400 times the systemic exposure of that achieved in humans).

The clinical relevance of the animal data to humans is not known.

### Mutagenicity
Raloxifene was not found to be mutagenic in the following tests or assays: Ames test, unscheduled DNA synthesis assay in rat hepatocytes, mouse lymphoma assay for mammalian cell mutation, chromosomal aberration assay in Chinese hamster ovary cells, *in vivo* sister chromatid exchanges assay in Chinese hamsters, and *in vivo* micronucleus test in mice.

### Pregnancy/Reproduction
Reproduction studies in rats given raloxifene are consistent with estrogen receptor activity.

Fertility—In rats given at least 5 mg/kg a day of raloxifene (corresponding to 0.8 times or more the human dose based on mg per squared meter [$mg/m^2$] of body surface area), no pregnancies occurred. In male rats, 100 mg/kg of raloxifene a day for 2 weeks (corresponding to 16 times the human dose based on body surface area) did not affect sperm production or quality or reproductive performance. In female rats, 0.1 to 10 mg/kg a day of raloxifene (corresponding to 0.02 to 1.5 times the human dose based on body surface area) reversibly disrupted estrous cycles, inhibited ovulation, and delayed and disrupted embryo implantation, resulting in prolonged gestation and a small litter size.

Pregnancy—Raloxifene is not recommended during pregnancy. Risk-benefit should be considered carefully.

Studies in animals have shown that raloxifene decreased neonatal survival, delayed and disrupted parturition, and caused fetal abortion, ventricular septal defects, hydrocephaly, wavy ribs, kidney cavitation, lymphoid compartment size reduction, growth reduction, and pituitary hormone content changes. Although no ovarian or vaginal pathology resulted, effects in adult offspring included uterine hypoplasia and reduced fertility.

FDA Pregnancy Category X.

### Breast-feeding
It is not known whether raloxifene is distributed into breast milk. However, use of raloxifene during breast-feeding is not recommended.

### Geriatrics
Appropriate studies performed to date have not demonstrated geriatrics-specific problems that would limit the usefulness of raloxifene in the elderly.

### Surgical
Raloxifene should be discontinued for at least 72 hours prior to and during prolonged bed rest or immobilization, such as during postsurgical recovery, because of increased risk of venous thromboembolic events. The medication should be resumed only after the patient is fully ambulatory.

### Drug interactions and/or related problems
The following drug interactions and/or related problems have been selected on the basis of their potential clinical significance (possible mechanism in parentheses where appropriate)—not necessarily inclusive (» = major clinical significance):

Note: Combinations containing any of the following medications, depending on the amount present, may also interact with this medication.

» Cholestyramine
  (reduces the absorption and enterohepatic recycling of raloxifene by 60%; concomitant use is not recommended)

» Estrogens, systemic
  (raloxifene is not recommended for use with estrogens)

Highly protein-bound drugs, such as:
- Clofibrate
- Diazepam
- Diazoxide
- Ibuprofen
- Indomethacin
- Naproxen
  (caution is recommended in using concurrently since raloxifene is highly bound to plasma proteins)

» Warfarin
  (raloxifene alone does not affect the protein-binding of warfarin, but concurrent use has decreased the prothrombin time by 10% in single-dose studies; when given concurrently, prothrombin time should be monitored and the dose of warfarin may need an initial adjustment)

### Laboratory value alterations
The following have been selected on the basis of their potential clinical significance (possible effect in parentheses where appropriate)—not necessarily inclusive (» = major clinical significance):

With physiology/laboratory test values
- Albumin concentration, serum and
- Calcium concentration, total, serum and
- Phosphate concentration, serum and
- Protein concentration, total, serum
  (slightly decreased)
- Cholesterol concentrations, total, serum and
- Lipoproteins concentrations, low-density (LDL), serum
  (compared with the patients' baselines, serum total cholesterol concentrations decreased 5% in 24-month data and 6.6% in a 6-month study; LDL decreased 8% in the 24-month data and 10.9% in a 6-month study)
- Corticosteroid-binding globulin and
- Sex steroid–binding globulin and
- Thyroid-binding globulin
  (may modestly increase serum protein–binding globulins without increasing the free fraction of corresponding hormones)
- Fibrinogen concentration, serum and
- Lipoprotein (a) concentration
  (in a 6-month study, fibrinogen decreased by a median of 12.2% from patients' baselines and lipoprotein (a) decreased by a median of 4.1% from patients' baselines)
- Lipoproteins concentrations, high-density-3 (HDL-3), serum
  (serum HDL-3 concentrations decreased by a median of 2.5% compared with the patients' baselines in a 6-month study; no effect occurred for serum concentrations of triglycerides and serum total high-density lipoprotein [HDL] cholesterol)
- Platelet count
  (slightly decreased)

### Medical considerations/Contraindications
The medical considerations/contraindications included have been selected on the basis of their potential clinical significance (reasons given in parentheses where appropriate)—not necessarily inclusive (» = major clinical significance).

*Except under special circumstances, this medication should not be used when the following medical problem exists:*

» Thromboembolic disorders, active or history of, including deep vein thrombosis, pulmonary embolism, and retinal vein thrombosis (may be exacerbated)

*Risk-benefit should be considered when the following medical problems exist:*

» Congestive heart failure or
» Neoplasia or
» Other conditions of increased thromboembolic risk
  (underlying thromboembolic disorders may be exacerbated)
  Hepatic function impairment
  (may increase plasma concentrations of raloxifene. In patients with cirrhosis classified as Child-Pugh Class A, plasma concentrations of raloxifene were 2.5 times greater than expected, correlating with their total bilirubin concentrations; safety and efficacy in patients with severe hepatic function impairment have not been evaluated)
  Sensitivity to raloxifene

### Patient monitoring
The following may be especially important in patient monitoring (other tests may be warranted in some patients, depending on condition; » = major clinical significance):

Physical examination
  (every year or more frequently as determined by physician, with special attention given to breast and pelvic organs)

## Side/Adverse Effects
The following side/adverse effects have been selected on the basis of their potential clinical significance (possible signs and symptoms in parentheses where appropriate)—not necessarily inclusive:

**Those indicating need for medical attention**
Incidence more frequent
  *Chest pain*—4%; *cystitis or urinary tract infection* (bloody or cloudy urine; difficult, burning, or painful urination; frequent urge to urinate)—3.3 to 4%; *endometrial disorder*—3.1%; *fever*—3.1%; *infection of the body as a whole; influenza-like syndrome; sinusitis; or pharyngitis* (body aches or pain; congestion in throat; cough; dryness or soreness of throat; fever; loss of voice; runny nose)—7 to 15%; *leg cramping*—5.9%; *peripheral edema* (swelling of hands, ankles, or feet)—3.3%; *skin rash*—5.5%; *vaginitis* (vaginal itching)—4.3%

Incidence less frequent
  *Gastroenteritis* (abdominal pain, severe; diarrhea; loss of appetite; nausea; weakness)—2.6%; *laryngitis* (cough; dryness or soreness of throat; hoarseness; trouble in swallowing)—2.2%; *migraine headaches*—2.4%; *pneumonia* (aching body pains; congestion in lungs; difficulty in breathing; fever; sore throat)—2.6%

Incidence rare
  *Thromboembolism or thrombus formation* (coughing blood; headache or migraine headache; loss of or change in speech, coordination, or vision; pain or numbness in chest, arm, or leg; shortness of breath, unexplained)

**Those indicating need for medical attention only if they continue or are bothersome**
Incidence less frequent
  *Arthralgia; arthritis; or myalgia* (joint or muscle pain; swollen joints)—4 to 10.7%; *gastrointestinal disturbances* (nausea; passing of gas; upset stomach; vomiting); *hot flashes* (feelings of warmth; sudden sweating)—24.6%, especially common during the first 6 months of treatment; *insomnia* (trouble in sleeping)—5.5%; *leukorrhea* (increased white vaginal discharge)—3.3%; *mental depression*—6.4%; *sweating*—3.1%; *weight gain, unexplained*—8.8%

## Patient Consultation
As an aid to patient consultation, refer to *Advice for the Patient, Raloxifene (Systemic)—Introductory Version*.
In providing consultation, consider emphasizing the following selected information (» = major clinical significance):

### Before using this medication
» Conditions affecting use, especially:
  Sensitivity to raloxifene or allergies to product's components
  Pregnancy—Not recommended for use during pregnancy. Approved for use in postmenopausal women only. Raloxifene has been associated with fetal abnormalities in animals
  Breast-feeding—Not recommended for use during breast-feeding
  Surgical—Discontinue use 72 hours before surgery, until patient is fully mobilized
  Other medications, especially cholestyramine; estrogens (systemic); or warfarin
  Other medical problems, especially congestive heart failure, neoplasia, or other conditions of increased thromboembolic risk; or thromboembolic disorders, active or history of (deep vein thrombosis, pulmonary embolism, and retinal vein thrombosis)

### Proper use of this medication
» Reading patient directions that come with medication carefully before using
» Not taking more or less of medication than your physician ordered
» Proper dosing
  Missed dose: Skipping missed dose and resuming regular dosing schedule; not doubling dose
» Proper storage

### Precautions while using this medication
» Regular visits to physician, keeping appointments even if feeling well
» Discussing continuing medication with physician before having surgery or periods of immobility, including the inactivity of long trips, because of potential increased risk of thromboembolism
» Stopping medication immediately and checking with physician if pregnancy is suspected; present use is for postmenopausal women only
» Reporting occurrences of vaginal bleeding, breast pain, or swelling of hands or feet

» Importance of weight-bearing exercise and calcium and vitamin D supplements for prevention of osteoporosis

### Side/adverse effects
Signs of potential side effects, especially chest pain; cystitis or urinary tract infection; endometrial disorder; fever; infection of the body as a whole, influenza-like syndrome, sinusitis, or pharyngitis; leg cramping; peripheral edema; skin rash; vaginitis; gastroenteritis; laryngitis; migraine headaches; pneumonia; thromboembolism or thrombus formation

## General Dosing Information

Because of increased risk of venous thromboembolic events, raloxifene should be discontinued for at least 72 hours prior to surgery and during prolonged bed rest or immobilization, such as in postsurgical recovery or during a long trip when mobility is not possible. To prevent thromboembolic events while taking raloxifene, the patient should understand the importance of mobility during a long trip. The medication may be resumed only after the patient is fully ambulatory.

If a pregnancy is possible and is suspected, patient should stop using the medication and contact physician immediately. Present use is for postmenopausal women only.

Since raloxifene does not act like an estrogen to stimulate the uterus or breast, patients should report any occurrences of vaginal bleeding, breast pain or enlargement, or swelling of hands or feet while on raloxifene.

Exercise can be recommended to all patients to prevent development of osteoporosis. Calcium supplementation should be considered as an additional preventive measure if patient's dietary intake is inadequate.

### Diet/Nutrition
Raloxifene may be given without regard to meals.

## Oral Dosage Forms

### RALOXIFENE HYDROCHLORIDE TABLETS
Note: Formerly known as keoxifene hydrochloride.

### Usual adult dose
Osteoporosis prophylactic—
  Oral, 60 mg once a day, without regard to meals.

### Usual adult prescribing limits
Efficacy beyond 2 years for prevention of osteoporosis has not been determined; however, safety data for venous thrombus embolism and breast and uterine cancers are available for up to 39 months.

### Usual geriatric dose
See *Usual adult dose*.

### Strength(s) usually available
U.S.—
  60 mg (Rx) [*Evista* (anhydrous lactose; lactose monohydrate; polyethylene glycol; povidone; propylene glycol)].

### Packaging and storage
Store between 15 and 30 °C (59 and 86 °F), preferably between 20 and 25 °C (68 and 77 °F), unless otherwise specified by manufacturer.

### Caution
The previously available product *E-Vista*, the brand name for hydroxyzine hydrochloride, should not be confused with *Evista*, raloxifene hydrochloride. They are different products with completely different indications.

### Note
Include patient information when dispensing.

Developed: 3/26/98
Interim revision: 8/10/98

---

**RAMIPRIL**—See *Angiotensin-converting Enzyme (ACE) Inhibitors (Systemic)*

---

**RANITIDINE**—See *Histamine H₂-receptor Antagonists (Systemic)*

---

# RANITIDINE BISMUTH CITRATE    Systemic—INTRODUCTORY VERSION

VA CLASSIFICATION (Primary): GA303
Commonly used brand name(s): *Tritec*.
Note: For a listing of dosage forms and brand names by country availability, see *Dosage Forms* section(s).

## Category
Antiulcer agent.

## Indications

### General considerations
Because ranitidine bismuth citrate is intended for use in combination with clarithromycin, some of the information included in this monograph is based on the combined use of both agents. For further information regarding clarithromycin, refer to the *Clarithromycin (Systemic)* monograph.

### Accepted
Ulcer, active duodenal (treatment)—Ranitidine bismuth citrate (RBC), in combination with clarithromycin, is indicated for the treatment of active duodenal ulcer associated with *Helicobacter pylori* infection. Eradication of *H. pylori* has been demonstrated to reduce the risk of duodenal ulcer recurrence. RBC should not be prescribed alone for the treatment of active duodenal ulcer.

Patients in whom *H. pylori* is not eradicated following combination treatment with RBC and clarithromycin should be considered to be infected with an *H. pylori* strain that is resistant to clarithromycin, and should not be re-treated with a regimen containing clarithromycin. No adequate data were collected during clinical trials or *in vitro* studies to indicate that RBC can either decrease or increase emerging resistance of *H. pylori* to clarithromycin.

## Pharmacology/Pharmacokinetics

### Physicochemical characteristics
Note: Ranitidine bismuth citrate (RBC) is a complex of ranitidine, trivalent bismuth, and citrate. Following ingestion, RBC dissociates in intragastric fluid yielding ranitidine and soluble and insoluble forms of bismuth.

Molecular weight—Approximately 651.

### Mechanism of action/Effect
Antisecretory—Ranitidine inhibits both daytime and nocturnal basal gastric acid secretions as well as gastric acid secretion stimulated by food, betazole, and pentagastrin. Ranitidine does not alter plasma pepsinogen I and II concentrations or pepsin activity. Ranitidine has little or no effect on fasting or postprandial serum gastrin.

### Absorption
Bismuth—Variable. Rate and extent of absorption do not increase with ranitidine bismuth citrate doses up to 800 mg; above 800 mg, however, they increase more than proportionally. An oral RBC dose of 800 mg administered 30 minutes after a meal resulted in a 50% decrease in the rate of bismuth absorption and a 25% decrease in the extent of bismuth absorption, as compared with the same dose administered 30 minutes before a meal. Absorption of bismuth following ingestion of an 800-mg dose of RBC is increased when the gastric pH exceeds 6. The absorption and gastrointestinal mucosal penetration of bismuth from RBC are unaffected by the degree of gastritis, the presence of *H. pylori* infection, or the presence of an active ulcer.

Ranitidine—Rate and extent of absorption increase proportionally with increasing doses of up to 1600 mg. Multiple dosing of RBC over a 28-day period showed no evidence of ranitidine accumulation.

### Protein binding
Bismuth—98%.
Ranitidine—Averages 15%.

### Biotransformation
Bismuth—Unknown.
Ranitidine—Metabolized to the N-oxide, S-oxide, and N-desmethyl metabolites, which account for 4%, 1%, and 1% of the dose, respectively.

### Half-life
Bismuth—Terminal half-life of 11 to 28 days.
Ranitidine—Elimination half-life of 2.8 to 3.1 hours.

### Time to peak concentration
Following administration of a single 400-mg oral dose of RBC to healthy volunteers, peak plasma concentrations occurred respectively at:
Bismuth—15 to 60 minutes.
Ranitidine—0.5 to 5 hours.

### Peak plasma concentration
Following administration of a single 400-mg oral dose of RBC to healthy volunteers, mean peak plasma concentrations measured respectively were:
Bismuth—3.3 ($\pm$ 2) nanograms per mL.
Ranitidine—455 ($\pm$ 145.3) nanograms per mL.

### Elimination
Bismuth—Polyexponential. Up to 28% recovered in the feces during a 6-day post-dose period; also undergoes minor excretion in the bile. Less than 1% of bismuth was recovered in the urine following oral administration of RBC.
Ranitidine—Renal, accounting for 30% of an oral dose. Ranitidine has an average renal clearance rate of 530 mL per minute, indicating active tubular secretion.

## Precautions to Consider

### Cross-sensitivity and/or related problems
Patients sensitive to ranitidine bismuth citrate or any of its ingredients may be sensitive to this medication.

### Carcinogenicity
In animal studies, ranitidine bismuth citrate was not shown to be carcinogenic.

### Mutagenicity
Ranitidine bismuth citrate (RBC) was not genotoxic in the Ames test, the mouse lymphoma cell forward mutation test, the *ex vivo* rat gastric mucosal unscheduled DNA synthesis (UDS) test, or the *in vivo* rat micronucleus test. RBC was positive in the *in vitro* human lymphocyte chromosomal aberration assay.

### Pregnancy/Reproduction
Fertility—Ranitidine bismuth citrate had no effect on fertility or reproductive performance in rats given oral doses of 18 times the recommended human dose.
Pregnancy—No adequate and well-controlled studies have been conducted in pregnant women. In premarketing clinical trials, five women became pregnant while taking ranitidine bismuth citrate (RBC) alone at varied doses; of these, three had normal pregnancies and newborns, and the fourth had a voluntary abortion. The fifth woman (a Caucasian with a history of unexplained spontaneous abortions) delivered a baby with postaxial polydactyly after receiving RBC for 7 days prior to conception and for 20 days after conception. The investigator considered the event to be unrelated to RBC administration, and a causal relationship has not been definitively established. In American whites, the incidence rate of postaxial polydactyly ranges from 1:3300 to 1:630 live births.
Studies performed in pregnant rats and rabbits (administered RBC at 18 and 6 times the recommended human dose, respectively) showed no teratogenic effects attributable to RBC.
FDA Pregnancy Category C.

### Breast-feeding
It is not known if ranitidine bismuth citrate is distributed into breast milk. However, in animal studies, ranitidine and bismuth have been found in the milk of rats.

### Pediatrics
Safety and efficacy have not been established.

### Geriatrics
Clinically insignificant increases in ranitidine plasma concentrations were observed in elderly patients, possibly due to decreased renal clearance in this age group. Bismuth plasma concentrations in older patients were equivalent to those seen in the overall population. While dosing adjustments are not usually necessary in elderly patients, ranitidine bismuth citrate should be administered with caution in patients with impaired renal function; RBC is not recommended for patients with a creatinine clearance less than 25 mL per minute.

### Pharmacogenetics
There is no evidence of any racial differences in the pharmacokinetics of bismuth based on trough concentrations observed in clinical studies.

### Drug interactions and/or related problems
Note: Concurrent administration of ranitidine bismuth citrate (RBC) and clarithromycin increases the plasma concentrations of ranitidine by 57% and of bismuth (at trough) by 48%; the plasma concentration of the principal metabolite of clarithromycin, 14-hydroxy-clarithromycin, is increased by 31%.

For additional drug interactions that may be due to either ranitidine or clarithromycin, please refer to the respective monographs.

### Laboratory value alterations
The following have been selected on the basis of their potential clinical significance (possible effect in parentheses where appropriate)—not necessarily inclusive (» = major clinical significance):

With diagnostic test results
Urine protein test
(false-positive reactions may occur with the use of Multistix®; testing with sulfosalicylic acid is recommended)

With physiology/laboratory test values
Alanine aminotransferase (ALT [SGPT]) and
Aspartate aminotransferase (AST [SGOT])
(transient changes in serum values may occur)

### Medical considerations/Contraindications
The medical considerations/contraindications included have been selected on the basis of their potential clinical significance (reasons given in parentheses where appropriate)—not necessarily inclusive (» = major clinical significance).

*Risk-benefit should be considered when the following medical problems exist:*

Acute porphyria, history of
(condition may be exacerbated)
» Renal function impairment
(decreased elimination may lead to increased plasma levels and toxicity of ranitidine and bismuth; use is not recommended in patients with a creatinine clearance less than 25 mL per minute)
Sensitivity to ranitidine bismuth citrate or any of its ingredients

## Side/Adverse Effects
Note: For additional adverse effects that may be due to either ranitidine or clarithromycin, please refer to the respective monographs.

The following side/adverse effects have been selected on the basis of their potential clinical significance (possible signs and symptoms in parentheses where appropriate)—not necessarily inclusive:

### Those indicating need for medical attention
Incidence more frequent
*Diarrhea; headache*

Incidence less frequent
*Dizziness; insomnia* (trouble in sleeping); **nausea; pruritus** (itching); *vomiting*

Incidence rare
*Anaphylaxis* (fast heartbeat; swelling of face; wheezing or troubled breathing); **constipation; skin rash; stomach pain**

### Those not indicating need for medical attention
Incidence more frequent
*Taste disturbances* (change in sense of taste)

Incidence less frequent
*Darkening of tongue and/or stools*

## Overdose
For more information on the management of overdose or unintentional ingestion, **contact a Poison Control Center** (see *Poison Control Center Listing*).

### Clinical effects of overdose
There has been limited experience with overdosage with ranitidine bismuth citrate. Adverse effects were usually reversible, nonspecific, and without adverse sequelae. Bismuth intoxication from prolonged overdosage or deliberate self-poisoning may result in neurotoxicity, nephrotoxicity, and possibly other symptoms seen with the use of soluble bismuth compounds.

### Treatment of overdose
To decrease absorption—Measures should be taken to remove unabsorbed material from the gastrointestinal tract.

Supportive care—Supportive measures should be taken. Patients in whom intentional overdose is confirmed or suspected should be referred for psychiatric consultation.

## Patient Consultation
In providing consultation, consider emphasizing the following selected information (» = major clinical significance):

**Before using this medication**
» Conditions affecting use, especially:
Sensitivity to ranitidine bismuth citrate (RBC) or any of its ingredients
Mutagenicity—RBC had positive results in the *in vitro* human lymphocyte chromosomal aberration assay
Pregnancy—No adequate and well-controlled studies in humans; one of five women who became pregnant while taking RBC delivered a baby with postaxial polydactyly, but a causal relationship has not been definitively established
Breast-feeding—Not known if ranitidine and bismuth are distributed into human breast milk; both have been found in the milk of rats
Other medical problems, especially renal function impairment

**Proper use of this medication**
» Compliance with full course of treatment
» Proper dosing
Missed dose: Taking as soon as remembered. If almost time for the next dose, skip the missed dose and continue on regular dosing schedule until the medication is finished; not doubling doses
» Proper storage

**Precautions while using this medication**
» Caution if dizziness or lightheadedness occurs

**Side/adverse effects**
Signs of potential side effects, especially diarrhea, headache, dizziness, insomnia, nausea, pruritus, vomiting, anaphylaxis, constipation, skin rash, and stomach pain
Darkening of tongue and/or stools caused by bismuth may be alarming to patient, although medically insignificant

## General Dosing Information
Caution should be exercised in the use of ranitidine bismuth citrate (RBC) in patients with impaired renal function; use is not recommended in patients with a creatinine clearance less than 25 mL per minute.

**Diet/Nutrition**
Ranitidine bismuth citrate and clarithromycin may be given without regard to food.

## Oral Dosage Forms

### RANITIDINE BISMUTH CITRATE TABLETS

**Usual adult dose**
Antiulcer—
Oral, 400 mg two times a day for four weeks, in conjunction with clarithromycin 500 mg three times a day for the first two weeks.
Note: Ranitidine bismuth citrate should be used with caution in patients with renal function impairment; use is not recommended in patients with a creatinine clearance less than 25 mL per minute.

**Usual pediatric dose**
Safety and efficacy have not been established.

**Usual geriatric dose**
See *Usual adult dose*.
Note: Ranitidine bismuth citrate and clarithromycin may be taken without regard to meals.

**Strength(s) usually available**
U.S.—
400 mg (Rx) [*Tritec* (film-coated; FD&C Blue No. 2 Aluminum Lake; magnesium stearate; methylhydroxypropylcellulose; microcrystalline cellulose; Povidone K30; anhydrous sodium carbonate; titanium dioxide; triacetin)].
Note: Each 400-mg tablet is approximately equivalent to 162 mg of ranitidine (base), 128 mg of trivalent bismuth, and 110 mg of citrate.

**Packaging and storage**
Store between 2 and 30 °C (36 and 86 °F) in a dry place. Protect from light.

Developed: 11/03/97

---

# RAUWOLFIA ALKALOIDS  Systemic

This monograph includes information on the following: 1) Deserpidine†; 2) Rauwolfia Serpentina†; 3) Reserpine.
VA CLASSIFICATION (Primary): CV409
Commonly used brand name(s): *Harmonyl*[1]; *Novoreserpine*[3]; *Raudixin*[2]; *Rauval*[2]; *Rauverid*[2]; *Reserfia*[3]; *Serpalan*[3]; *Serpasil*[3]; *Wolfina*[2].
Note: For a listing of dosage forms and brand names by country availability, see *Dosage Forms* section(s).

†Not commercially available in Canada.

## Category
Antihypertensive; vasospastic therapy adjunct.

## Indications
Note: Bracketed information in the *Indications* section refers to uses that are not included in U.S. product labeling.

**Accepted**
Hypertension (treatment)—Rauwolfia alkaloids are indicated in the treatment of hypertension.
[Raynaud's phenomenon (treatment)][1]—Reserpine has also been used to treat Raynaud's phenomenon.

**Unaccepted**
Rauwolfia alkaloids have been used for relief of symptoms in agitated psychotic states such as schizophrenia; however, use as antipsychotics and sedatives has been superseded by use of more effective, safer agents.

[1]Not included in Canadian product labeling.

## Pharmacology/Pharmacokinetics
Note: Information (except physicochemical characteristics) available only for reserpine.

**Physicochemical characteristics**
Molecular weight—
Reserpine: 608.69.
pKa—
Deserpidine: 5.67.
Reserpine: 6.6.

**Mechanism of action/Effect**
Acts at postganglionic sympathetic nerve endings; depletes tissue and central nervous system (CNS) stores of catecholamines and serotonin; antihypertensive activity thought to be due to reduced cardiac output and possibly some decrease in peripheral resistance.

**Absorption**
Reserpine is readily absorbed after oral administration.

**Protein binding**
None (bound to sites involved with storage of biogenic amines; may persist in body for several days).

**Biotransformation**
Hepatic.

**Half-life**
Normal—
Initial: 4.5 hours.
Terminal: 45 to 168 hours.
Anuric—
Terminal: 87 to 323 hours.

**Onset of action**
Antihypertensive—Oral: Several days to 3 weeks (multiple doses).
Catecholamine depletion—Within 1 hour (single dose).

**Time to peak effect**
Antihypertensive—Oral: 3 to 6 weeks (multiple doses).
Catecholamine depletion—Within 24 hours (single dose).

**Duration of action**
Antihypertensive—Oral: 1 to 6 weeks.

**Elimination**
Fecal—More than 60%, mainly unchanged, in 4 days.
Renal—8%, less than 1% unchanged, in 4 days.

## Precautions to Consider

### Cross-sensitivity and/or related problems
Patients sensitive to one rauwolfia alkaloid may be sensitive to other rauwolfia alkaloids also.

### Carcinogenicity/Tumorigenicity
The suggestion that long-term use of reserpine (and also, presumably, other rauwolfia alkaloids) may increase the risk of breast cancer in postmenopausal women has been controversial. A few epidemiologic studies have suggested a slightly increased risk of breast cancer in women who have used reserpine. However, other studies have not confirmed this finding.

Studies in rats and mice at 100 to 300 times the usual human dose found an increased incidence of mammary fibroadenomas in females, and malignant tumors of the seminal vesicles and malignant adrenal medullary tumors in males.

### Pregnancy/Reproduction
Fertility—Long-term animal studies have not been done with the rauwolfia alkaloids to determine their effect on fertility in males or females.

Pregnancy—Rauwolfia alkaloids cross the placenta. Adequate and well-controlled studies have not been done in humans. However, possible adverse effects in infants of mothers who received rauwolfia alkaloids include increased respiratory secretions, nasal congestion, cyanosis and anorexia.

Reserpine was found to be teratogenic in rats given parenteral doses of up to 2 mg per kg of body weight (mg/kg) and was embryocidal in guinea pigs given parenteral doses of 0.5 mg per day.

FDA Pregnancy Category C.

### Breast-feeding
Problems in humans have not been documented. However, rauwolfia alkaloids are distributed into breast milk. Possible adverse effects in infants of mothers who received rauwolfia alkaloids include increased respiratory secretions, nasal congestion, cyanosis, and anorexia.

### Pediatrics
Appropriate studies on the relationship of age to the effects of the rauwolfia alkaloids have not been performed in the pediatric population. However, pediatrics-specific problems that would limit the usefulness of these medications in children are not expected.

### Geriatrics
Although appropriate studies on the relationship of age to the effects of the rauwolfia alkaloids have not been performed in the geriatric population, the elderly may be more sensitive to the CNS depressant and hypotensive effects. In addition, elderly patients are more likely to have age-related renal function impairment, which may require caution in patients receiving rauwolfia alkaloids. A lower dose is recommended in the elderly.

### Dental
Use of rauwolfia alkaloids may decrease or inhibit salivary flow, thus contributing to the development of caries, periodontal disease, oral candidiasis, and discomfort.

### Drug interactions and/or related problems
The following drug interactions and/or related problems have been selected on the basis of their potential clinical significance (possible mechanism in parentheses where appropriate)—not necessarily inclusive (» = major clinical significance):

Note: Combinations containing any of the following medications, depending on the amount present, may also interact with this medication.

Alcohol or
CNS depression–producing medications (See *Appendix II*)
(concurrent use may enhance the CNS depressant effects of either these medications or rauwolfia alkaloids)

Anti-inflammatory drugs, nonsteroidal (NSAIDs), especially indomethacin
(antihypertensive effects of rauwolfia alkaloids may be reduced when used concurrently with these agents; indomethacin, and possibly other NSAIDs, may antagonize the antihypertensive effect by inhibiting renal prostaglandin synthesis and/or by causing sodium and fluid retention; the patient should be carefully monitored to confirm that the desired effect is being obtained)

Anticholinergics or other medications with anticholinergic action (See *Appendix II*)
(concurrent use of rauwolfia alkaloids may antagonize the inhibitory action of these medications on gastric acid secretion)

Beta-adrenergic blocking agents, including ophthalmic beta-blockers absorbed systemically
(concurrent administration with beta-blockers may result in additive and possibly excessive beta-adrenergic blockade; although this effect is largely theoretical, close observation is recommended since bradycardia and hypotension may occur)

Bromocriptine
(reserpine may increase serum prolactin concentrations, and interfere with effects of bromocriptine; dosage adjustment of bromocriptine may be necessary)

Digitalis glycosides or
Quinidine
(concurrent use may result in cardiac arrhythmias; although this interaction is controversial and does not appear to be significant with usual doses, caution is recommended, especially when large doses of rauwolfia alkaloids are used in digitalized patients)

Extrapyramidal reaction–causing medications, other (See *Appendix II*)
(concurrent use with rauwolfia alkaloids may potentiate the extrapyramidal effects)

Hypotension-producing medications, other, except MAO inhibitors (See *Appendix II*)
(antihypertensive effects may be potentiated when these medications are used concurrently with rauwolfia alkaloids; although some combinations are frequently used for therapeutic advantage, when used concurrently dosage adjustments may be necessary)
(concurrent use of guanadrel or guanethidine with rauwolfia alkaloids may cause an increased incidence of orthostatic hypotension or bradycardia)

Levodopa
(rauwolfia alkaloids may cause dopamine depletion and parkinsonian effects, decreasing the therapeutic effects of levodopa; dosage adjustments of either or both medications may be necessary)

» Monoamine oxidase (MAO) inhibitors, including furazolidone, procarbazine, and selegiline
(when an MAO inhibitor is added to existing therapy with rauwolfia alkaloids, serious potentiation of CNS depressant effect may result; however, if a rauwolfia alkaloid is added to an MAO inhibitor regimen, excessive stimulation of receptors caused by the sudden release of accumulated norepinephrine and serotonin may result in moderate to sudden and severe hypertension and hyperpyrexia, which can reach crisis levels; administration of rauwolfia alkaloids is not recommended during and for 1 week following MAO inhibitor therapy)

*Sympathomimetics*
(antihypertensive effects of rauwolfia alkaloids may be reduced when used concurrently with these agents; the patient should be carefully monitored to confirm that the desired effect is being obtained)

Indirect-acting amines, such as amphetamines, phenylpropanolamine, pseudoephedrine, and tyramine, or
Direct- and indirect-acting (primarily indirect-acting) amines, such as ephedrine and mephentermine
(rauwolfia alkaloids inhibit the action of indirect-acting sympathomimetics by depleting catecholamine stores)

Direct-acting amines such as epinephrine or norepinephrine (levarterenol) or
Direct- and indirect-acting (primarily direct-acting) amines such as appetite suppressants (except fenfluramine), dobutamine, dopamine, metaraminol, methoxamine, and phenylephrine
(rauwolfia alkaloids may theoretically prolong the action of direct-acting sympathomimetics by preventing uptake into storage granules; a "denervation supersensitivity" response is also possible; although concurrent use with rauwolfia alkaloids is not known to produce severe adverse effects, a significant increase in blood pressure has been documented when phenylephrine ophthalmic drops have been administered to patients taking reserpine, and caution and close observation are recommended; on the other hand, concurrent use with fenfluramine may increase the hypotensive effects of rauwolfia alkaloids)

### Laboratory value alterations
The following have been selected on the basis of their potential clinical significance (possible effect in parentheses where appropriate)—not necessarily inclusive (» = major clinical significance):

With diagnostic test results
Urinary steroid colorimetric determinations by modified Glenn-Nelson technique or Holtorff Koch modification of Zimmerman reaction
(falsely low because rauwolfia alkaloids slightly decrease absorbance)

With physiology/laboratory test values
- Catecholamine excretion, urinary
  (an overall decrease is usually noted with chronic administration of rauwolfia alkaloids)
- Prolactin concentrations, serum
  (may be increased)
- Vanillylmandelic acid (VMA), urinary excretion
  (chronic administration of rauwolfia alkaloids results in an overall decrease)

### Medical considerations/Contraindications
The medical considerations/contraindications included have been selected on the basis of their potential clinical significance (reasons given in parentheses where appropriate)—not necessarily inclusive (» = major clinical significance).

*Risk-benefit should be considered when the following medical problems exist:*
- Cardiac arrhythmias
- Cardiac depression
- Epilepsy
- » Gallstones or
- » Peptic ulcer or
- » Ulcerative colitis
  (rauwolfia alkaloids increase gastrointestinal motility and secretion; may precipitate biliary colic)
- » Mental depression, or history of
- Parkinsonism
- Pheochromocytoma
- Renal function impairment
  (patients with renal insufficiency may adjust poorly to reduced blood pressure levels. However, dosage reduction is not necessary in these patients)
- Respiratory problems
- Sensitivity to the rauwolfia alkaloid prescribed
- » Caution is required also in patients receiving electroconvulsive therapy, as well as in the severely debilitated.

### Patient monitoring
The following may be especially important in patient monitoring (other tests may be warranted in some patients, depending on condition; » = major clinical significance):
- » Blood pressure measurements
  (recommended at periodic intervals in patients being treated for hypertension; selected patients may be trained to perform blood pressure measurements at home and report the results at regular physician visits)

## Side/Adverse Effects
Note: Side effects occur more frequently with high-dose administration.

The following side/adverse effects have been selected on the basis of their potential clinical significance (possible cause in parentheses where appropriate)—not necessarily inclusive:

**Those indicating need for medical attention**
Incidence more frequent
  *Dizziness*
Incidence less frequent
  *Arrhythmias* (irregular heartbeat); *black, tarry stools; bloody vomit, stomach cramps or pain; bradycardia* (slow heartbeat); *chest pain; drowsiness or faintness; headache; impotence or decreased sexual interest; lack of energy or weakness; mental depression or inability to concentrate; nervousness or anxiety; shortness of breath; vivid dreams or nightmares or early-morning sleeplessness*
  Note: CNS effects are dose-related, occurring more frequently with doses exceeding 500 mcg (0.5 mg) per day.
Incidence rare
  *Painful or difficult urination; skin rash or itching; stiffness or trembling and shaking of hands and fingers; thrombocytopenia* (unusual bleeding or bruising)

**Those indicating need for medical attention only if they continue or are bothersome**
Incidence more frequent
  *Anorexia* (loss of appetite); *diarrhea; dryness of mouth; nasal congestion* (stuffy nose); *nausea and vomiting*
Incidence less frequent
  *Edema, peripheral* (swelling of feet and lower legs)

**Those indicating the need for medical attention if they occur after medication is discontinued**
  *Arrhythmias* (irregular heartbeat); *bradycardia* (slow heartbeat); *drowsiness or faintness; impotence or decreased sexual interest; lack of energy or weakness; mental depression or inability to concentrate; nervousness or anxiety; vivid dreams or nightmares or early-morning sleeplessness*
- Note: *Mental depression* may have an insidious onset, may be severe enough to cause suicide, and may persist for several months following withdrawal of this medication.

## Overdose
For more information on the management of overdose or unintentional ingestion, **contact a Poison Control Center** (see *Poison Control Center Listing*).

### Clinical effects of overdose
The following effects have been selected on the basis of their potential clinical significance (possible signs and symptoms in parentheses where appropriate)—not necessarily inclusive:
  *Dizziness or drowsiness, severe; flushing of skin; pinpoint pupils of eyes; slow pulse*

### Treatment of overdose
Immediate evacuation of the stomach and instillation of an activated charcoal slurry.

Supportive, symptomatic treatment.

If treatment with a vasopressor is necessary, one with a direct action on smooth muscle (phenylephrine, norepinephrine, metaraminol) should be used.

The patient should be observed for at least 72 hours.

## Patient Consultation
As an aid to patient consultation, refer to *Advice for the Patient, Rauwolfia Alkaloids (Systemic)*.

In providing consultation, consider emphasizing the following selected information (» = major clinical significance):

**Before using this medication**
- » Conditions affecting use, especially:
  - Sensitivity to any of the rauwolfia alkaloids
  - Pregnancy—Teratogenic in animals
  - Breast-feeding—Distributed into breast milk
  - Use in the elderly—May be more sensitive to the CNS depressant and hypotensive effects
  - Dental—May decrease or inhibit salivary flow
  - Other medications, especially monoamine oxidase (MAO) inhibitors
  - Other medical problems, especially gallstones, peptic ulcer, ulcerative colitis, or mental depression

**Proper use of this medication**
- Possible need for control of weight and diet, especially sodium intake
- » Patient may not experience symptoms of hypertension; importance of taking medication even if feeling well
- » Does not cure but helps control hypertension; possible need for lifelong therapy; serious consequences of untreated hypertension
- Compliance with therapy; taking medication at the same time(s) each day to maintain the therapeutic effect
- Caution in taking combination therapy; taking each medication at the right time
- Taking with meals or milk to reduce gastrointestinal irritation
- » Proper dosing
- Missed dose: Not taking missed dose at all and not doubling doses
- » Proper storage

**Precautions while using this medication**
- Making regular visits to physician to check progress
- » Not taking other medications, especially nonprescription sympathomimetics, unless discussed with physician
- » Caution if any kind of surgery (including dental surgery) or emergency treatment is required
- » Caution if depression or changes in sleep pattern occur
- » Caution in taking alcohol or other CNS depressants
- » Caution when driving or doing things requiring alertness because of possible drowsiness or dizziness
- Possible dryness of mouth; using sugarless candy or gum, ice, or saliva substitute for relief; checking with physician or dentist if dry mouth continues for more than 2 weeks
- Nasal stuffiness may occur; nasal decongestants or other OTC preparations containing sympathomimetics should not be used without first consulting physician or pharmacist

**Side/adverse effects**
Dizziness, arrhythmias, bradycardia, black, tarry stools, bloody vomit, chest pain, drowsiness or faintness, headache, impotence or decreased sexual interest, lack of energy or weakness, mental depression or inability to concentrate, nervousness or anxiety, vivid dreams or nightmares or early-morning sleeplessness, shortness of breath

## General Dosing Information

Dosage must be adjusted to meet the individual requirements of each patient, on the basis of clinical response, with the lowest effective dosage being utilized in order to minimize problems with mental depression, orthostatic hypotension, and other side effects.

Rauwolfia alkaloids are usually used in combination with a diuretic to prevent sodium and water retention.

A lower dose is recommended in the elderly or severely debilitated.

Doses higher than the recommended dose should be used with caution because of the risk of severe mental depression.

Antihypertensive effects of rauwolfia alkaloids may not be observed for a few days to several weeks after oral administration and may persist for 1 to 6 weeks after withdrawal of the medication. It is recommended that adjustments in dosage be made every 7 to 14 days to allow the full effects of the preceding dose to occur.

It is recommended that this medication be withdrawn at the first sign of despondency, early-morning insomnia, loss of appetite, impotence, or self-deprecation.

It is recommended that rauwolfia alkaloids be withdrawn 2 weeks before electroconvulsive therapy is employed.

Recent evidence suggests that withdrawal of catecholamine-depleting antihypertensive therapy prior to surgery is not necessary, but that the anesthesiologist must be aware of such therapy. Administration of atropine prior to induction may prevent excessive bradycardia. If a hypotensive episode occurs, use of a weak direct-acting sympathomimetic agent is recommended.

**Diet/Nutrition**
It is recommended that these medications be taken with food or milk to minimize gastrointestinal upset.

---

### *DESERPIDINE*

## Oral Dosage Forms
**DESERPIDINE TABLETS**

**Usual adult dose**
Antihypertensive—
Oral, 250 to 500 mcg (0.25 to 0.5 mg) a day as a single dose or in two divided daily doses.

Note: Geriatric patients may be more sensitive to the effects of the usual adult dose.

**Usual pediatric dose**
Dosage has not been established.

**Strength(s) usually available**
U.S.—
250 mcg (0.25 mg) (Rx) [*Harmonyl*].
Canada—
Not commercially available.

**Packaging and storage**
Store below 40 °C (104 °F), preferably between 15 and 30 °C (59 and 86 °F). Store in a tight container. Protect from light.

**Auxiliary labeling**
• Take with meals or milk.
• Do not take other medicines without your doctor's advice.

**Note**
Check refill frequency to determine compliance in hypertensive patients.

---

### *RAUWOLFIA SERPENTINA*

## Oral Dosage Forms
**RAUWOLFIA SERPENTINA TABLETS USP**

**Usual adult dose**
Antihypertensive—
Oral, 50 to 200 mg a day as a single dose or in two divided daily doses.

Note: Geriatric patients may be more sensitive to the effects of the usual adult dose.

**Usual pediatric dose**
Dosage has not been established.

**Strength(s) usually available**
U.S.—
50 mg (Rx) [*Raudixin; Rauval; Rauverid;* GENERIC].
100 mg (Rx) [*Raudixin; Rauval; Wolfina;* GENERIC].
Canada—
Not commercially available.

**Packaging and storage**
Store below 40 °C (104 °F), preferably between 15 and 30 °C (59 and 86 °F). Store in a tight, light-resistant container.

**Auxiliary labeling**
• Take with meals or milk.
• Do not take other medicines without your doctor's advice.

**Note**
Check refill frequency to determine compliance in hypertensive patients.

---

### *RESERPINE*

## Oral Dosage Forms

Note: Bracketed uses in the *Dosage Forms* section refer to categories of use and/or indications that are not included in U.S. product labeling.

**RESERPINE TABLETS USP**

**Usual adult dose**
Antihypertensive or
[Vasospastic therapy adjunct—Raynaud's phenomenon][1]—
Oral, 100 to 250 mcg (0.1 to 0.25 mg) a day.

Note: Geriatric patients may be more sensitive to the effects of the usual adult dose.

**Usual pediatric dose**
Antihypertensive—
Oral, 5 to 20 mcg (0.005 to 0.02 mg) per kg of body weight or 150 to 600 mcg (0.15 to 0.6 mg) per square meter of body surface a day in one or two divided daily doses.

**Strength(s) usually available**
U.S.—
100 mcg (0.1 mg) (Rx) [*Serpalan;* GENERIC].
250 mcg (0.25 mg) (Rx) [*Serpalan;* GENERIC].
1 mg (Rx) [GENERIC].
Canada—
250 mcg (0.25 mg) (Rx) [*Novoreserpine; Reserfia; Serpasil;* GENERIC].

**Packaging and storage**
Store below 40 °C (104 °F), preferably between 15 and 30 °C (59 and 86 °F). Store in a tight, light-resistant container.

**Auxiliary labeling**
• Take with meals or milk.
• Do not take other medicines without your doctor's advice.

**Note**
Check refill frequency to determine compliance in hypertensive patients.

[1]Not included in Canadian product labeling.

## Selected Bibliography

The fifth report of the Joint National Committee on Detection, Evaluation, and Treatment of High Blood Pressure (JNC V). Arch Intern Med 1993; 153(2): 154-83.

Revised: 07/28/92
Interim revision: 07/20/94; 08/19/98

---

## RAUWOLFIA ALKALOIDS AND THIAZIDE DIURETICS—The *Rauwolfia Alkaloids and Thiazide Diuretics (Systemic)* monograph is not included in this published version of the USP DI database. Copies of the monograph are available on request from Micromedex, Inc. - Reprint Requests, 6200 S. Syracuse Way, Suite 300, Englewood, CO 80111; telephone (303) 486-6400; telefax (303) 486-6464; Email: USPDI@MDX.COM.

**RAUWOLFIA SERPENTINA**—See *Rauwolfia Alkaloids (Systemic)*

# REMIFENTANIL  Systemic

VA CLASSIFICATION (Primary/Secondary): CN206/CN101

Note: Controlled substance classification
U.S.—Schedule II
Canada—N

Commonly used brand name(s): *Ultiva*.

Note: For a listing of dosage forms and brand names by country availability, see *Dosage Forms* section(s).

## Category
Anesthesia adjunct (opioid analgesic).

## Indications

**Accepted**

Anesthesia adjunct—Remifentanil is indicated as an opioid analgesic adjunct for the induction and maintenance of general anesthesia, and as the analgesic component of anesthetic care in the immediate postoperative period[1]. Remifentanil is also indicated as an analgesic supplement to local or regional anesthesia[1] in a monitored anesthesia setting.

**Unaccepted**

Remifentanil is not a general anesthetic, and should not be used alone for induction of general anesthesia; the use of remifentanil as the sole agent to induce general anesthesia may not provide adequate anesthesia, is associated with a high incidence of apnea, muscle rigidity, and bradycardia/tachycardia, and may be associated with an unacceptable incidence of recall.

Remifentanil should not be used for epidural or intrathecal administration, because glycine in the formulation may cause neurotoxicity.

[1]Not included in Canadian product labeling.

## Pharmacology/Pharmacokinetics

**Physicochemical characteristics**

Chemical group—Piperidine propanoic acid methyl ester, hydrochloride salt.
Molecular weight—412.92.
pH—2.5 to 3.5.
pKa—7.07.

**Mechanism of action/Effect**

Remifentanil exerts its analgesic effect via agonist actions at mu-opioid receptors.

**Other actions/effects**

Remifentanil depresses respiration and cardiac function in a dose-dependent manner.

Remifentanil can cause skeletal muscle rigidity, especially if it is administered in moderate to high doses over a short period of time. Doses greater than 1 mcg per kg of body weight (mcg/kg) administered over 30 to 60 seconds may cause chest wall rigidity and glottic closure. Peripheral muscle rigidity can occur with lower doses.

**Distribution**

Remifentanil has biphasic distribution. The initial volume of distribution of remifentanil is about 100 mL per kg of body weight (mL/kg). Remifentanil is then distributed to peripheral tissues with a steady-state volume of distribution of 350 mL/kg.

**Protein binding**

High (70%), primarily to alpha$_1$-acid glycoprotein.

**Biotransformation**

Hydrolyzed to a carboxylic acid metabolite by nonspecific esterases in the blood and tissues. This metabolite has minimal activity.

**Half-life**

Distribution—
Rapid distribution—1 minute.
Slower distribution—6 minutes.
Elimination—
3 to 10 minutes.

Note: Remifentanil elimination is not dependent on dose. Elimination of remifentanil occurs rapidly, even after prolonged continuous infusion. Context-sensitive half-time (CSHT), the time to a 50% decrease of an effective site concentration after a continuous infusion is stopped, is a more useful parameter than elimination half-life to describe the activity of remifentanil. The CSHT for remifentanil is 3 to 4 minutes, regardless of the duration of the infusion.

**Onset of action**

Within 1 minute.

**Peak serum concentration**

Dependent on dose.

**Time to peak effect**

1 to 2 minutes after a single intravenous injection.

**Duration of action**

5 to 10 minutes following discontinuation of an infusion of remifentanil; the duration of action is shorter following a single intravenous injection of a low or moderate dose of remifentanil.

**Elimination**

After hydrolysis of remifentanil by nonspecific esterases, the carboxylic acid metabolite is excreted by the kidneys; remifentanil is not metabolized by pseudocholinesterase.

In dialysis—
The carboxylic acid metabolite is removed by hemodialysis, with an extraction ratio of about 30%.

## Precautions to Consider

**Cross-sensitivity and/or related problems**

Patients allergic to alfentanil, fentanyl, or sufentanil may be allergic to remifentanil also.

**Carcinogenicity/Tumorigenicity**

Studies have not been done to determine the carcinogenic and tumorigenic potential of remifentanil.

**Mutagenicity**

Mutagenicity was not observed in *in vitro* testing in prokaryotic cells. No clastogenic effect was observed in the cultured Chinese hamster ovary cell test, in the *in vivo* test of unscheduled DNA synthesis in rat hepatocytes, or in the mouse micronucleus assay. Mutagenicity was seen with metabolic activation in the *in vitro* mouse lymphoma assay.

**Pregnancy/Reproduction**

Fertility—Adequate and well-controlled studies have not been done in humans.

Remifentanil reduced the fertility of male rats when administered at doses 40 times greater than the maximum recommended human dose (MRHD) for 70 days. Fertility was not affected in female rats given doses 80 times greater than the MRHD for 15 days prior to mating.

Pregnancy—Remifentanil crosses the placenta. Adequate and well-controlled studies have not been done in humans.

Teratogenic effects were not observed in studies of rats and rabbits given 400 and 125 times the MRHD, respectively.

FDA Pregnancy Category C.

Labor and delivery—Respiratory depression may occur in newborns whose mothers are given remifentanil shortly before delivery. In preapproval clinical studies of labor and delivery, fetal blood concentrations of remifentanil were 50 to nearly 100% of maternal concentrations.

**Breast-feeding**

It is not known whether remifentanil is distributed into breast milk. However, since related drugs are distributed into breast milk, it is expected that remifentanil may be distributed into breast milk. Since remifentanil is eliminated rapidly, problems are not expected when remifentanil is administered to a nursing mother.

**Pediatrics**

Appropriate studies on the relationship of age to the effects of remifentanil have not been performed in children up to 2 years of age. Distribution, clearance, and half-life in children 2 to 13 years of age were similar to those in adult patients.

**Geriatrics**

The clearance of remifentanil is reduced in geriatric patients as compared with that in younger adult patients. In addition, geriatric patients are more sensitive to the effects of remifentanil. Geriatric patients have greater interpatient variability as compared with younger adult patients.

It is recommended that the initial dose of remifentanil be reduced by 50% in geriatric patients.

**Surgical**
Remifentanil is eliminated rapidly. Within 5 to 10 minutes after the discontinuation of a remifentanil infusion, no opioid analgesia is present. Surgical patients may experience a sudden onset of postoperative pain unless other analgesics are administered. Initiation of postoperative pain management should be considered prior to emergence from anesthesia.

**Drug interactions and/or related problems**
The following drug interactions and/or related problems have been selected on the basis of their potential clinical significance (possible mechanism in parentheses where appropriate)—not necessarily inclusive (» = major clinical significance):

Note: Combinations containing any of the following medications, depending on the amount present, may also interact with this medication.

» Anesthetics, barbiturate or
» Anesthetics, inhalation or
» Benzodiazepines or
» Propofol
(the effects of remifentanil are synergistic with barbiturate or inhalation anesthetics, benzodiazepines, and propofol, increasing the risk of hypotension and respiratory depression; the dose of remifentanil or the dose of anesthetic, benzodiazepine, or propofol should be decreased)

Atropine or
Glycopyrrolate
(may reverse bradycardia caused by remifentanil)

Ephedrine or
Epinephrine or
Norepinephrine
(may reverse hypotension caused by remifentanil)

Neuromuscular blocking agents
(attenuates the skeletal muscle rigidity induced by remifentanil)

Opioid antagonists, such as:
» Nalmefene
» Naloxone
» Naltrexone
(opioid antagonists may reverse the hypotension, muscle rigidity, and respiratory depression induced by remifentanil; the analgesic effects of remifentanil may also be reversed, leading to pain and sympathetic hyperactivity)

**Medical considerations/Contraindications**
The medical considerations/contraindications included have been selected on the basis of their potential clinical significance (reasons given in parentheses where appropriate)—not necessarily inclusive (» = major clinical significance).

*Except under special circumstances, this medication should not be used when the following medical problem exists:*
» Allergic reaction to alfentanil, fentanyl, remifentanil, or sufentanil, history of

*Risk-benefit should be considered when the following medical problems exist:*
Cardiac bradyarrhythmias
(may be exacerbated)

Hepatic function impairment
(patients with hepatic function impairment may be more sensitive to the respiratory depressant effects of remifentanil; clearance of remifentanil is unchanged in patients with hepatic function impairment as compared with patients with normal hepatic function)

Obesity
(bradycardia or reduced respiratory drive may occur; it is recommended that dosing for obese patients [patients weighing more than 130% of ideal body weight] be initiated based on ideal body weight [IBW], and then titrated to achieve the desired effect)

Respiratory impairment, pre-existing
(respiratory drive may be further decreased; respiratory support may be required with doses that usually permit spontaneous breathing)

**Patient monitoring**
The following may be especially important in patient monitoring (other tests may be warranted in some patients, depending on condition; » = major clinical significance):

» Blood oxygenation and
» Blood pressure and
» Respiratory status and
» Vital signs, other
(it is recommended that patients be monitored continuously; when remifentanil is used for surgical or diagnostic procedures, it is recommended that the patient be monitored continuously by someone not involved in conducting the surgical or diagnostic procedure, and who is expert in the management of the airway and providing artificial respiration, because rapid changes in patient status may occur)

## Side/Adverse Effects

The following side/adverse effects have been selected on the basis of their potential clinical significance (possible signs and symptoms in parentheses where appropriate)—not necessarily inclusive:

**Those indicating need for medical attention**
Incidence more frequent
*Hypotension; muscle rigidity, including chest wall rigidity* (difficulty breathing)

Incidence less frequent
*Bradycardia*

Incidence rare
*Agitation; apnea* (bluish lips or skin); *hypertension; postoperative pain; pruritus* (itching); *respiratory depression* (slow breathing)

Note: Although *postoperative pain* occurred rarely in preapproval clinical trials, it may not be a rare event in clinical practice. The rapid elimination of remifentanil and the subsequent loss of opioid analgesia may result in postoperative pain unless pain management is initiated prior to emergence from anesthesia.

**Those indicating need for medical attention only if they continue or are bothersome**
Incidence more frequent
*Nausea*

Incidence less frequent
*Headache; shivering; vomiting*

## Overdose

For specific information on the agents used in the management of remifentanil overdose, see:
- Atropine in *Anticholinergics/Antispasmodics (Systemic)* monograph;
- Epinephrine in *Sympathomimetic Agents—Cardiovascular Use (Parenteral-Systemic)* monograph;
- Glycopyrrolate in *Anticholinergics/Antispasmodics (Systemic)* monograph;
- Isoproterenol in *Sympathomimetic Agents—Cardiovascular Use (Parenteral-Systemic)* monograph;
- Naloxone in *Naloxone (Systemic)* monograph; and/or
- Succinylcholine in *Neuromuscular Blocking Agents (Systemic)* monograph.

For more information on the management of overdose, **contact a Poison Control Center** (see *Poison Control Center Listing*).

**Clinical effects of overdose**
Note: The clinical effects of overdose are an extension of the pharmacologic effects of remifentanil.

The following effects have been selected on the basis of their potential clinical significance (possible signs and symptoms in parentheses where appropriate)—not necessarily inclusive:

Acute
*Apnea* (bluish lips or skin); *bradycardia; glottic closure; hypotension; hypoxemia* (bluish lips or skin); *muscle rigidity, including chest wall rigidity*

**Treatment of overdose**
Specific treatment:
Discontinue administration of remifentanil; administer oxygen and support ventilation. Since the context-sensitive half-time (CSHT) of remifentanil is very short, discontinuing the infusion and supporting ventilation may be the only measures required in many cases of overdose.

For bradycardia:
Atropine or glycopyrrolate may be needed to treat bradycardia. Epinephrine or isoproterenol may be needed to treat bradycardia in patients receiving beta-adrenergic blocking agents.

For chest wall rigidity and glottic closure:
Administration of a rapidly acting neuromuscular blocking agent (e.g., rocuronium or succinylcholine) may reverse chest wall rigidity and glottic closure. It may be necessary to treat chest wall rigidity and glottic closure to allow artificial ventilation.

An opioid antagonist (e.g., naloxone) may be used to reverse chest wall rigidity and glottic closure. However, loss of analgesia may result.

Note: Use of naloxone is not the preferred method for treating chest wall rigidity and glottic closure. The preferred method for treating chest wall rigidity and glottic closure is administration of a neuromuscular blocking agent to allow artificial ventilation. This approach avoids the danger of sudden loss of analgesia and sympathetic overactivity. The use of naloxone should be reserved for situations in which treatment of chest wall rigidity and glottic closure with a neuromuscular blocking agent and artificial ventilation is not possible or desirable.

For respiratory depression:
Maintain a patent airway. Initiate assisted or controlled ventilation. Treatment of chest wall rigidity may be required to facilitate assisted ventilation.

If adequate spontaneous ventilation does not return within several minutes of discontinuing remifentanil, other causes of ventilatory depression should be considered. The need for opioid antagonists also should be reconsidered in these circumstances.

Monitoring—
Vital signs and oxygenation should be monitored continuously.

Supportive care—
Support cardiovascular function with fluids and vasopressors as needed.

## Patient Consultation

As an aid to patient consultation, refer to *Advice for the Patient, Narcotic Analgesics—For Surgery and Obstetrics (Systemic)*.

In providing consultation, consider emphasizing the following selected information (» = major clinical significance):

### Before receiving this medication
» Conditions affecting use, especially:
Allergy to alfentanil, fentanyl, remifentanil, or sufentanil
Pregnancy—Remifentanil crosses the placenta; respiratory depression may occur in newborns whose mothers are given remifentanil shortly before delivery
Breast-feeding—Related drugs are distributed into breast milk; since remifentanil is eliminated rapidly, problems are not expected when remifentanil is given to a nursing mother
Use in the elderly—Increased sensitivity and greater interpatient variability to the effects of remifentanil; reduced clearance of remifentanil
Other medications, especially barbiturate anesthetics, benzodiazepines, inhalation anesthetics, nalmefene, naloxone, naltrexone, or propofol

### Side/adverse effects
Signs of potential side effects, especially hypotension, muscle rigidity, bradycardia, agitation, apnea, hypertension, postoperative pain, pruritus, and respiratory depression

## General Dosing Information

Remifentanil should be used only in closely monitored situations by persons trained in the use of anesthetic drugs, airway management, and cardiac and respiratory resuscitation. Equipment for emergency endotracheal intubation and resuscitation, oxygen, and an opioid antagonist must be immediately available while remifentanil is administered. Blood oxygenation and vital signs must be monitored continuously while remifentanil is administered.

Remifentanil should be injected into intravenous tubing close to the site of entry into the patient. When remifentanil is discontinued, remifentanil remaining in the intravenous tubing should be cleared to prevent accidental administration of remifentanil when another medication or fluid is infused through the intravenous line. Accidental administration of remifentanil can result in respiratory depression and chest wall rigidity.

Skeletal muscle rigidity may result from rapid injection of remifentanil or from overdoses of remifentanil. Injection of more than 1 mcg per kg of body weight over 30 to 60 seconds, or infusion of greater than 0.1 mcg per kg of body weight per minute, may result in chest wall rigidity and glottic closure.

The dose of remifentanil for obese patients should be based on ideal body weight, not actual body weight.

Remifentanil should not be infused through the same intravenous line at the same time as blood because esterases in the blood may inactivate the drug.

Remifentanil should not be used for epidural or intrathecal administration, because glycine in the formulation may cause neurotoxicity.

Infusions of remifentanil should be administered only with an infusion device.

Spontaneously breathing patients receiving infusions of remifentanil should not receive additional intermittent injections of remifentanil due to the potential for overdose.

When remifentanil is administered to a patient as an analgesic supplement to local or regional anesthesia, it is recommended that the patient also receive supplemental oxygen.

Because of its extremely short context-sensitive half-time (CSHT), intermittent intravenous injections for analgesia in postoperative patients are not recommended. However, closely monitored continuous infusions may be used in selected patients. Since rapid changes in the status of the patient are possible while receiving remifentanil, it may be advisable to switch the patient to another opioid analgesic while the patient is still in the intraoperative period.

Discontinuation of remifentanil will result in rapid discontinuation of opioid effects, including analgesia. The analgesic needs of the patient should be considered before remifentanil is discontinued. The transition from remifentanil to another analgesic may be accomplished by administering another analgesic intravenously during the intraoperative period or by reducing the dose of remifentanil administered to the patient from anesthetic doses to analgesic doses when surgery has been completed, then gradually switching to another analgesic.

### For treatment of adverse effects
Recommended treatment consists of the following:
- Muscle rigidity occurring during administration of remifentanil can be treated with discontinuation of the drug, reduction of the rate of administration of the drug, or administration of a rapidly acting neuromuscular blocking agent. Simultaneous endotracheal intubation and ventilation may be necessary. Hypnotic induction agents, including inhalational agents, may be used to prevent muscle rigidity.

## Parenteral Dosage Forms

Note: The dosing and strengths of the dosage form available are expressed in terms of remifentanil base (not the hydrochloride salt).

### REMIFENTANIL HYDROCHLORIDE FOR INJECTION

**Usual adult dose**
Induction of general anesthesia, adjunct—
Intravenous infusion, [0.5 to 1 mcg (0.0005 to 0.001 mg) (base) per kg of body weight, administered with an inhalation or intravenous anesthetic.][1]

Note: The FDA-approved dosage of remifentanil as an adjunct in the induction of general anesthesia is 0.5 to 1 mcg (0.0005 to 0.001 mg) (base) per kg of body weight per minute, administered with an inhalation or intravenous anesthetic. However, most USP medical experts believe the approved dosage is unnecessarily high.

Maintenance of nitrous oxide anesthesia (general), adjunct—
Intravenous infusion, [0.05 to 0.2 mcg (0.00005 to 0.0002 mg) (base) per kg of body weight per minute][1]; supplemental doses of 0.5 to 1 mcg (0.0005 to 0.001 mg) per kg of body weight may be administered every two to five minutes if needed because of inadequate anesthesia or transiently increased surgical stress.

Note: The FDA-approved dosage of remifentanil for the maintenance of nitrous oxide anesthesia is 0.4 (range, 0.1 to 2) mcg per kg of body weight per minute. However, most USP medical experts believe the approved dosage is unnecessarily high. Additionally, many USP medical experts believe that any adjustments needed in the dose of remifentanil should be accomplished by adjustments in the rate of the infusion, not by giving additional intermittent injections of remifentanil. Administration of intermittent supplemental doses increases the risks of bradycardia, hypotension, respiratory depression, and chest wall rigidity.

It should be noted that both the FDA-approved and USP-recommended dosages for the maintenance of nitrous oxide anesthesia are incompatible with spontaneous ventilation; patients receiving these dosages require ventilatory support.

Maintenance of isoflurane or propofol anesthesia (general), adjunct—
Intravenous infusion, [0.05 to 0.2 mcg (0.00005 to 0.0002 mg) (base) per kg of body weight per minute][1]; supplemental doses of 0.5 to 1 mcg (0.0005 to 0.001 mg) per kg of body weight may be administered every two to five minutes if needed because of inadequate anesthesia or transiently increased surgical stress.

Note: The FDA-approved dosage of remifentanil for the maintenance of isoflurane or propofol anesthesia is 0.25 (range, 0.05 to 2) mcg per kg of body weight per minute. However, most USP medical experts believe this dosage is unnecessarily high. Additionally, many USP medical experts believe that any adjustments needed in the dose of remifentanil should be accomplished by adjustments in the rate of the infusion, not by giving additional intermittent injections of remifentanil. Administration of intermittent supplemental doses increases the risks of bradycardia, hypotension, respiratory depression, and chest wall rigidity.

It should be noted that both the FDA-approved and USP-recommended dosages for the maintenance of isoflurane or propofol anesthesia are incompatible with spontaneous ventilation; patients receiving these dosages require ventilatory support.

Continuation into the immediate postoperative period[1]—
  Intravenous infusion, 0.1 mcg (0.0001 mg) (base) per kg of body weight per minute initially; the infusion may be adjusted every five minutes in increments of 0.025 mcg (0.000025 mg) per kg of body weight per minute to reach the desired balance of analgesia and adequate respiratory rate.

Note: Remifentanil is intended for use only into the immediate postoperative period; the use of remifentanil for periods longer than sixteen hours postoperatively has not been studied. Continuation of remifentanil into the postoperative period should be reserved for selected patients in whom conversion to another opioid analgesic in the intraoperative period is not advisable, and only when the patient will be closely monitored by personnel trained in use of anesthetic drugs, airway management, and cardiac and respiratory resuscitation. Equipment for emergency endotracheal intubation and resuscitation, oxygen, and an opioid antagonist must be immediately available. Blood oxygenation and vital signs must be monitored continuously while remifentanil is administered.

Analgesic supplement to local or regional anesthesia in a monitored anesthesia setting[1]—
  Intravenous—
    When used with benzodiazepine sedation (i.e., midazolam 2 mg)— 0.5 mcg (0.0005 mg) (base) per kg of body weight, administered over thirty to sixty seconds as a single dose [sixty to][1] ninety seconds before the local anesthetic is administered.
    When used without benzodiazepine sedation—1 mcg (0.001 mg) per kg of body weight administered over thirty to sixty seconds as a single dose [sixty to][1] ninety seconds before the local anesthetic is administered.
  Intravenous infusion—
    When used with benzodiazepine sedation (i.e., midazolam 2 mg)— 0.05 mcg (0.00005 mg) (base) per kg of body weight per minute, beginning five minutes before placement of local or regional block; after placement of the block, the infusion rate should be decreased to 0.025 mcg (0.000025 mg) per kg of body weight per minute. Thereafter, the infusion can be adjusted in increments of 0.025 mcg (0.000025 mg) per kg of body weight per minute at five-minute intervals.
    When used without benzodiazepine sedation—0.1 mcg (0.0001 mg) per kg of body weight per minute beginning five minutes before placement of local or regional block; after placement of the block, the infusion rate should be decreased to 0.05 mcg (0.00005 mg) per kg of body weight per minute. Thereafter, the infusion can be adjusted in increments of 0.025 mcg (0.000025 mg) per kg of body weight per minute at five-minute intervals.

Note: Administration of more than 0.2 mcg per kg of body weight per minute is associated with respiratory depression. This effect should be considered if remifentanil is administered to a patient whose ventilation is not assisted or controlled.

In obese patients, the initial dose of remifentanil should be based on ideal body weight (IBW), then titrated to achieve the desired effect.

**Usual pediatric dose**
Anesthesia adjunct—
  Infants and children up to 2 years of age: Dosage has not been established.
  Children 2 years of age or older[1]: See *Usual adult dose*.

**Usual geriatric dose**
Anesthesia adjunct—
  The initial dose for geriatric patients should be 50% of the usual adult dose. The dose should be titrated to achieve the desired effect.

**Size(s) usually available**
U.S.—
  1 mg (base) (Rx) [*Ultiva* (lyophilized powder; glycine 15 mg; hydrochloric acid)].
  2 mg (base) (Rx) [*Ultiva* (lyophilized powder; glycine 15 mg; hydrochloric acid)].
  5 mg (base) (Rx) [*Ultiva* (lyophilized powder; glycine 15 mg; hydrochloric acid)].
Canada—
  1 mg (base) (Rx) [*Ultiva* (lyophilized powder; glycine 15 mg; hydrochloric acid)].
  2 mg (base) (Rx) [*Ultiva* (lyophilized powder; glycine 15 mg; hydrochloric acid)].
  5 mg (base) (Rx) [*Ultiva* (lyophilized powder; glycine 15 mg; hydrochloric acid)].

**Packaging and storage**
Store between 2 and 25 °C (36 and 77 °F).

**Preparation of dosage form**
One mL of diluent per mg of remifentanil (base) should be added to the vial, resulting in a solution containing 1 mg of remifentanil per mL. Remifentanil should be further diluted as follows before administration to the patient: the 1-mg vial of remifentanil can be diluted with 40 or 20 mL for a final concentration of 25 or 50 mcg (0.025 or 0.05 mg) per mL, respectively; the 2-mg vial of remifentanil can be diluted with 80 or 40 mL for a final concentration of 25 or 50 mcg (0.025 or 0.05 mg) per mL, respectively; and the 5-mg vial of remifentanil can be diluted with 200, 100, or 20 mL for a final concentration of 25, 50, or 250 mcg (0.025, 0.05, or 0.25 mg) per mL, respectively.

Remifentanil may be diluted with sterile water for injection, 5% dextrose injection, 5% dextrose and 0.9% sodium chloride injection, lactated Ringer's injection, lactated Ringer's and 5% dextrose injection, 0.9% sodium chloride injection, or 0.45% sodium chloride injection.

Remifentanil does not contain an antimicrobial preservative. Aseptic technique should be used when diluting remifentanil.

**Stability**
After preparation with sterile water for injection, 5% dextrose injection, 5% dextrose and 0.9% sodium chloride injection, lactated Ringer's and 5% dextrose injection, 0.9% sodium chloride injection, or 0.45% sodium chloride injection, the solution should be used within 24 hours. After preparation with lactated Ringer's injection, the solution should be used within 4 hours. The prepared solution should be inspected for particulate matter and clarity before administration to the patient, and should be discarded if particulate matter is present.

**Incompatibilities**
Remifentanil should not be infused through the same intravenous line at the same time as blood because esterases in the blood may inactivate the drug.

---

[1]Not included in Canadian product labeling.

## Selected Bibliography
Bürkle H, Dunbar S, Aken H. Remifentanil: a novel, short-acting, mu-opioid. Anesth Analg 1996; 83: 646-51.
Glass P. Remifentanil: a new opioid. J Clin Anesth 1995; 7: 558-63.
Egan T. Remifentanil pharmacokinetics and pharmacodynamics: a preliminary appraisal. Clin Pharmacokinet 1995; 29: 80-94.

Developed: 08/13/97

---

# REPAGLINIDE  Systemic—INTRODUCTORY VERSION

VA CLASSIFICATION (Primary): HS509
Commonly used brand name(s): *Prandin*.
Note: For a listing of dosage forms and brand names by country availability, see *Dosage Forms* section(s).

## Category
Antidiabetic agent.

## Indications
**Accepted**
Diabetes, type 2 (treatment)—Repaglinide is indicated as adjunctive therapy to diet and exercise in the management of patients with type 2 diabetes (previously referred to as non–insulin-dependent diabetes mellitus [NIDDM]). It is also indicated in combination with metformin in patients whose hyperglycemia cannot be controlled by diet and exercise or by either metformin or repaglinide alone. In clinical trials, combination therapy with repaglinide and metformin demonstrated a synergistic improvement in glycosylated hemoglobin and fasting plasma glu-

cose concentrations as compared with either medication alone. If adequate glycemic control is not achieved with combination therapy, repaglinide and metformin probably should be discontinued and insulin therapy instituted.

## Pharmacology/Pharmacokinetics

### Physicochemical characteristics
Class—Meglitinide.
Molecular weight—452.6.

### Mechanism of action/Effect
Repaglinide lowers blood glucose concentrations by stimulating the release of insulin from functioning beta cells of pancreatic islet tissue. This is accomplished by a selective ion channel mechanism. Repaglinide inhibits adenosine triphosphate (ATP)-potassium channels on the beta cell membrane and potassium efflux. The resulting depolarization and calcium influx induces insulin secretion.

### Absorption
Rapid and complete following oral administration.

### Distribution
The mean absolute bioavailability is 56%. Volume of distribution at steady-state was 31 L following intravenous administration to healthy volunteers.

### Protein binding
Very high (> 98%).

### Biotransformation
Completely metabolized by oxidative biotransformation and direct conjugation with glucuronic acid. The major metabolites are an oxidized dicarboxylic acid (M2), the aromatic amine (M1), and the acyl glucuronide (M7), none of which contributes to the glucose-lowering effect. The cytochrome P450 3A4 isoenzyme has been shown to be involved in the N-dealkylation of repaglinide to M2 and the further oxidation to M1.

### Half-life
Approximately 1 hour.

### Time to peak concentration
Approximately 1 hour.

### Peak plasma concentration
9.8, 18.3, 26, and 65.8 nanograms per mL following doses of 0.5, 1, 2, and 4 mg, respectively. The peak plasma concentration may be decreased by 20% when repaglinide is administered with food.

### Elimination
Fecal (approximately 90%, 60% as M2 and < 2% as parent compound); renal (approximately 8%, 0.1% as parent compound). Total body clearance was 38 L per hour following intravenous administration to healthy volunteers.
In dialysis—
There is no evidence that repaglinide is dialyzable using hemodialysis.

## Precautions to Consider

### Carcinogenicity/Tumorigenicity
No evidence of carcinogenicity was found in mice or female rats administered repaglinide at doses up to and including 500 mg per kg of body weight (mg/kg) per day or 120 mg/kg per day, respectively, for 104 weeks. These doses represent approximately 125 or 60 times the clinical exposure on a mg per square meter of body surface area (mg/m$^2$) basis. However, in male rats there was an increased incidence of benign adenomas of the thyroid and liver at doses above 30 mg/kg per day for thyroid tumors and above 60 mg/kg per day for liver tumors. These doses represent 15 and 30 times, respectively, the clinical exposure on a mg/m$^2$ basis.

### Mutagenicity
No evidence of mutagenicity was found in a series of *in vitro* and *in vivo* studies including the Ames test, *in vitro* forward cell mutation assay in V79 cells, *in vitro* chromosomal aberration assay in human lymphocytes, unscheduled and replicating DNA synthesis in rat liver, and *in vivo* mouse and rat micronucleus tests.

### Pregnancy/Reproduction
Fertility—Repaglinide had no effect on the fertility of male and female rats administered doses of 300 mg/kg per day and up to 80 mg/kg per day, respectively. These doses represent greater than 40 times the clinical exposure on a mg/m$^2$ basis.
Pregnancy—Studies have not been done in humans.
It is recommended that insulin be used during pregnancy for maintenance of blood glucose concentrations as close to normal as possible. Abnormal maternal blood glucose concentrations have been associated with a higher incidence of congenital anomalies.
No evidence of teratogenicity was found in rats or rabbits administered 40 or 0.8 times, respectively, the clinical exposure on a mg/m$^2$ basis throughout pregnancy. However, rat pups developed skeletal deformities during the postnatal period when the dams were exposed to doses 15 times the clinical exposure on a mg/m$^2$ basis on days 17 to 22 of gestation.
FDA Pregnancy Category C.

### Breast-feeding
It is not known whether repaglinide is distributed into breast milk. However, it is distributed into the milk of lactating rats and has been shown to lower glucose concentrations in the pups. In addition, some pups developed skeletal abnormalities, including shortening, thickening, and bending of the humerus during the postnatal period. Consideration should be given to discontinuing breast-feeding or discontinuing repaglinide and instituting insulin if blood glucose cannot be controlled by diet alone.

### Pediatrics
Appropriate studies on the relationship of age to the effects of repaglinide have not been performed in the pediatric population. Safety and efficacy have not been established.

### Geriatrics
Studies performed in approximately 415 patients 65 years of age or older have not demonstrated geriatrics-specific problems that would limit the usefulness of repaglinide in the elderly. However, hypoglycemia may be difficult to recognize in elderly patients.

### Pharmacogenetics
In a 1-year study in the U.S., the glucose-lowering effect was comparable in black and white patients with type 2 diabetes. In a dose-response study in the U.S., there was no difference in the area under the plasma concentration–time curve (AUC) between Hispanic and white patients.

### Drug interactions and/or related problems
The following drug interactions and/or related problems have been selected on the basis of their potential clinical significance (possible mechanism in parentheses where appropriate)—not necessarily inclusive (» = major clinical significance):

Note: Combinations containing any of the following medications, depending on the amount present, may also interact with this medication.

» Beta-adrenergic blocking agents or
Chloramphenicol or
Highly protein-bound medications, such as:
  Anticoagulants, coumarin-derivative
  Anti-inflammatory drugs, nonsteroidal (NSAIDs)
  Probenecid
  Salicylates or
Monoamine oxidase (MAO) inhibitors or
Sulfonamides
  (these medications enhance the hypoglycemic effect of repaglinide; patients should be observed closely for symptoms of hypoglycemia or loss of glycemic control when repaglinide is added to or withdrawn from a regimen containing these medications)
  (beta-adrenergic blocking agents may blunt some of the symptoms of hypoglycemia, making detection of this condition more difficult)

Erythromycin or
Ketoconazole or
Miconazole
  (these medications may inhibit repaglinide metabolism; however, it is not known whether this effect on metabolism results in an increase in the plasma concentration of repaglinide)

Hyperglycemia-causing medications, such as:
  Calcium channel blocking agents
  Corticosteroids
  Diuretics, especially thiazide diuretics
  Estrogens
  Isoniazid
  Niacin
  Oral contraceptives
  Phenothiazines
  Phenytoin
  Sympathomimetic agents
  Thyroid hormones
    (these medications may cause loss of glycemic control; patients should be observed closely for symptoms of hypoglycemia or loss of glycemic control when repaglinide is added to or withdrawn from a regimen containing these medications)

Other drugs metabolized by cytochrome P450 CYP3A4, such as:
  Barbiturates
  Carbamazepine
  Rifampin
  Troglitazone
    (these medications may increase repaglinide metabolism; however, it is not known if this effect results in a decrease in the plasma concentration of repaglinide)

**Laboratory value alterations**
The following have been selected on the basis of their potential clinical significance (possible effect in parentheses where appropriate)—not necessarily inclusive (» = major clinical significance):

With physiology/laboratory test values
  Electrocardiogram (ECG)
    (rarely, may be abnormal)
  Liver enzymes
    (rarely, may be elevated)

**Medical considerations/Contraindications**
The medical considerations/contraindications included have been selected on the basis of their potential clinical significance (reasons given in parentheses where appropriate)—not necessarily inclusive (» = major clinical significance).

*Except under special circumstances, this medication should not be used when the following medical problems exist:*
» Diabetes, type 1 or
» Diabetic ketoacidosis, with or without coma
    (these conditions should be treated with insulin)

*Risk-benefit should be considered when the following medical problems exist:*
  Adrenal insufficiency or
  Debilitated physical condition or
  Hepatic function impairment or
  Malnutrition or
  Pituitary insufficiency
    (these conditions may cause increased sensitivity to the glucose-lowering effect of repaglinide; caution is recommended)
» Hepatic function impairment
    (AUC and peak plasma concentration [$C_{max}$] may be increased in patients with moderate or severe impairment; caution and longer intervals between dosage adjustments are recommended)
  Infection or
  Surgery or
  Trauma or
  Unusual stress
    (these conditions may cause loss of glycemic control; temporary insulin therapy may be necessary)
» Renal function impairment
    (AUC and $C_{max}$ may be increased; adjustments to the initial dosage usually are not necessary, but subsequent increases in dosage should be made carefully in patients with renal function impairment or renal failure requiring hemodialysis)
  Sensitivity to repaglinide

**Patient monitoring**
The following may be especially important in patient monitoring (other tests may be warranted in some patients, depending on condition; » = major clinical significance):
» Blood glucose determinations
    (recommended periodically to determine the minimum effective dose of repaglinide, to confirm that blood glucose concentration is maintained within acceptable targets, and to detect inadequate lowering of glucose concentration after initial administration [primary failure] or loss of adequate glucose-lowering response after an initial period of efficacy [secondary failure])
» Glycosylated hemoglobin (hemoglobin $A_{1c}$ [$HbA_{1c}$]) determinations
    (recommended every 3 months to assess long-term glycemic control)

## Side/Adverse Effects

Note: It has been suggested, based on a study conducted by the University Group Diabetes Program (UGDP), that certain sulfonylurea antidiabetic agents increase cardiovascular mortality in diabetic patients, a population that already has a greater risk of cardiovascular disease and mortality when blood glucose is not controlled. Despite questions regarding the interpretation of the results and the adequacy of the experimental design, the findings of the UGDP study provide an adequate basis for caution, especially for certain high-risk patients with coronary artery disease, congestive heart failure, or angina pectoris. Given the similarities in the mechanisms of action of sulfonylureas and repaglinide, the patient should be informed of the potential risks and advantages of repaglinide and of alternative modes of therapy.

The following side/adverse effects have been selected on the basis of their potential clinical significance (possible signs and symptoms in parentheses where appropriate)—not necessarily inclusive:

**Those indicating need for medical attention**
Incidence more frequent
  *Bronchitis* (cough; fever; pain in the chest; shortness of breath); *hypoglycemia* (anxiety; behavior change similar to drunkenness; blurred vision; cold sweats; coma; confusion; cool pale skin; difficulty in concentrating; drowsiness; excessive hunger; fast heartbeat; headache; nausea; nervousness; nightmares; restless sleep; seizures; shakiness; slurred speech; unusual tiredness or weakness)—incidence 16% in clinical trials; *sinusitis* (headache; runny nose; sinus congestion with pain); *upper respiratory infection* (cough; fever; runny or stuffy nose; sneezing; sore throat)

  Note: The incidence of *hypoglycemia* is greater in patients who have not previously been treated with oral antidiabetic agents and in patients whose hemoglobin $A_{1c}$ is less than 8%.

Incidence less frequent
  *Allergic reaction* (fever with or without chills; headache; nausea with or without vomiting; runny nose; shortness of breath, tightness in chest, trouble in breathing, or wheezing; skin rash, itching, or hives; tearing of eyes); *angina; chest pain; tooth disorder; urinary tract infection* (bloody or cloudy urine; burning, painful, or difficult urination; frequent urge to urinate)

Incidence rare
  *Cardiovascular effects including arrhythmias; hypertension; and myocardial infarction; leukopenia* (cough or hoarseness; fever or chills; lower back or side pain; painful or difficult urination)—usually asymptomatic; *thrombocytopenia* (black, tarry stools; blood in urine or stools; pinpoint red spots on skin; unusual bleeding or bruising)—usually asymptomatic

**Those indicating need for medical attention only if they continue or are bothersome**
Incidence more frequent
  *Arthralgia* (joint pain); *back pain; diarrhea; headache; nausea; rhinitis* (stuffy nose)

Incidence less frequent
  *Constipation; indigestion; paresthesias* (sensation of burning, numbness, tightness, tingling, warmth, or heat); *vomiting*

## Overdose

For more information on the management of overdose or unintentional ingestion, **contact a Poison Control Center** (see *Poison Control Center Listing*).

**Clinical effects of overdose**
The following effects have been selected on the basis of their potential clinical significance (possible signs and symptoms in parentheses where appropriate)—not necessarily inclusive:

  *Hypoglycemia* (anxiety; behavior change similar to drunkenness; blurred vision; cold sweats; coma; confusion; cool pale skin; difficulty in concentrating; drowsiness; excessive hunger; fast heartbeat; headache; nausea; nervousness; nightmares; restless sleep; seizures; shakiness; slurred speech; unusual tiredness or weakness)

**Treatment of overdose**
Specific treatment—
  Mild hypoglycemia without neurologic symptoms or loss of consciousness should be treated with immediate ingestion of glucose and adjustments to medication dosage and/or meal patterns.
  Severe hypoglycemia including coma, seizures, or other neurologic impairment requires immediate emergency medical assistance. The patient should immediately be given an intravenous injection of a 50% glucose solution followed by a continuous infusion of a 10% glucose solution to maintain a blood glucose concentration above 100 mg per dL.

Monitoring—
  The patient should be monitored for at least 24 to 48 hours.

## Patient Consultation

As an aid to patient consultation, refer to *Advice for the Patient, Repaglinide (Systemic)—Introductory Version*.

In providing consultation, consider emphasizing the following selected information (» = major clinical significance):

### Before using this medication
» Conditions affecting use, especially:
  Sensitivity to repaglinide
  Pregnancy—Use of insulin is recommended during pregnancy for maintenance of blood glucose concentrations as close to normal as possible
  Breast-feeding—Breast-feeding should be discontinued, or repaglinide should be discontinued and insulin given, if blood glucose cannot be controlled by diet alone
  Use in the elderly—Hypoglycemia may be difficult to recognize
  Other medications, especially beta-adrenergic blocking agents
  Other medical problems, especially diabetic ketoacidosis, hepatic function impairment, renal function impairment, or type 1 diabetes

### Proper use of this medication
» Adhering to recommended regimens for diet, exercise, and glucose monitoring
» Taking medication 15 to 30 minutes before each meal
» Proper dosing
  Missed dose: Skipping a dose if a meal is skipped; adding a dose if an extra meal is eaten
» Proper storage

### Precautions while using this medication
» Regular visits to physician to check progress
» *Carefully following special instructions of health care team*
  Discussing use of alcohol
  Not taking other medications unless discussed with physician
  Getting counseling for family members to help the patient with diabetes; also, special counseling for pregnancy planning and contraception
  Making travel plans that include readiness for diabetic emergencies and eating meals at the usual times, even with changing time zones
» Preparing for and understanding what to do in case of diabetic emergency; carrying medical history and current medication list and wearing medical identification
» Recognizing what brings on symptoms of hypoglycemia, such as using other antidiabetic medication; delaying or missing a meal; exercising more than usual; drinking significant amounts of alcohol; or illness, including vomiting or diarrhea
» Recognizing symptoms of hypoglycemia: anxiety; behavior change similar to drunkenness; blurred vision; cold sweats; confusion; cool, pale skin; difficulty in concentrating; drowsiness; excessive hunger; fast heartbeat; headache; nausea; nervousness; nightmares; restless sleep; shakiness; slurred speech; and unusual tiredness or weakness
» Knowing what to do if symptoms of hypoglycemia occur, such as eating glucose tablets or gel, corn syrup, honey, or sugar cubes; drinking fruit juice, nondiet soft drink, or sugar dissolved in water; or getting emergency medical assistance if symptoms are severe
» Recognizing what brings on symptoms of hyperglycemia, such as not taking enough antidiabetic medication, skipping a dose of antidiabetic medication, overeating or not following meal plan, having a fever or infection, or exercising less than usual
» Recognizing symptoms of hyperglycemia and ketoacidosis: blurred vision; drowsiness; dry mouth; flushed, dry skin; fruit-like breath odor; increased urination (frequency and volume); ketones in urine; loss of appetite; stomachache, nausea, or vomiting; tiredness; troubled breathing (rapid and deep); unconsciousness; and unusual thirst
» Knowing what to do if symptoms of hyperglycemia occur, such as checking blood glucose and contacting a member of the health care team

### Side/adverse effects
Signs of potential side effects, especially bronchitis, hypoglycemia, sinusitis, upper respiratory infection, allergic reaction, angina, chest pain, tooth disorder, urinary tract infection, cardiovascular effects, leukopenia, and thrombocytopenia

## General Dosing Information

### Diet/Nutrition
Repaglinide may be taken 15 to 30 minutes before a meal.
Taking repaglinide with meals decreases the risk of hypoglycemia.

## Oral Dosage Forms

### REPAGLINIDE TABLETS

#### Usual adult dose
Antidiabetic agent—
  For patients not previously treated with a blood glucose–lowering medication or whose hemoglobin $A_{1c}$ (Hb$A_{1c}$) is less than 8%: Oral, initially 0.5 mg fifteen to thirty minutes before each meal. The dose may be adjusted up to 4 mg as determined by blood glucose response (usually assessed by fasting concentration).
  For patients previously treated with a blood glucose–lowering medication and whose Hb$A_{1c}$ is greater than or equal to 8%: Oral, initially 1 or 2 mg fifteen to thirty minutes before each meal. The dose may be adjusted up to 4 mg as determined by blood glucose response (usually assessed by fasting concentration).

Note: For both patients not previously treated and those previously treated with blood glucose–lowering medications, at least one week should elapse to assess response after each dose adjustment. However, in patients with hepatic function impairment, the interval between dose adjustments should be increased.

When repaglinide is taken in combination with metformin, the dosing guidelines are the same as for repaglinide monotherapy.

When used to replace therapy with other oral antidiabetic agents, repaglinide may be started on the day after the final dose of previous therapy is given. The patient should be monitored for possible overlapping hypoglycemic effects. Monitoring for up to one week or longer may be required when the patient is transferred from longer half-life agents, such as chlorpropamide.

#### Usual adult prescribing limits
16 mg per day.

#### Usual pediatric dose
Safety and efficacy have not been established.

#### Strength(s) usually available
U.S.—
  0.5 mg (Rx) [*Prandin* (calcium hydrogen phosphate [anhydrous]; microcrystalline cellulose; maize starch; polacrilin potassium; povidone; glycerol 85%; magnesium stearate; meglumine; poloxamer)].
  1 mg (Rx) [*Prandin* (calcium hydrogen phosphate [anhydrous]; microcrystalline cellulose; maize starch; polacrilin potassium; povidone; glycerol 85%; magnesium stearate; meglumine; poloxamer; iron oxide [yellow])].
  2 mg (Rx) [*Prandin* (calcium hydrogen phosphate [anhydrous]; microcrystalline cellulose; maize starch; polacrilin potassium; povidone; glycerol 85%; magnesium stearate; meglumine; poloxamer; iron oxide [red])].

#### Packaging and storage
Store below 25 ºC (77 ºF), in a tight container. Protect from moisture.

Developed: 07/30/98

---

**RESERPINE**—See *Rauwolfia Alkaloids (Systemic)*

---

**RESERPINE HYDRALAZINE AND HYDROCHLOROTHIAZIDE**—The *Reserpine, Hydralazine, and Hydrochlorothiazide (Systemic)* monograph is not included in this published version of the USP DI database. Copies of the monograph are available on request from Micromedex, Inc. - Reprint Requests, 6200 S. Syracuse Way, Suite 300, Englewood, CO 80111; telephone (303) 486-6400; telefax (303) 486-6464; Email: USPDI@MDX.COM.

---

**RESORCINOL**—The *Resorcinol (Topical)* monograph is not included in this published version of the USP DI database. Copies of the monograph are available on request from Micromedex, Inc. - Reprint Requests, 6200 S. Syracuse Way, Suite 300, Englewood, CO 80111; telephone (303) 486-6400; telefax (303) 486-6464; Email: USPDI@MDX.COM.

---

**RESORCINOL AND SULFUR**—The *Resorcinol and Sulfur (Topical)* monograph is not included in this published version of the USP DI database. Copies of the monograph are available on request from Micromedex, Inc. - Reprint Requests, 6200 S. Syracuse Way, Suite 300, Englewood, CO 80111; telephone (303) 486-6400; telefax (303) 486-6464; Email: USPDI@MDX.COM.

# RESPIRATORY SYNCYTIAL VIRUS IMMUNE GLOBULIN INTRAVENOUS  Systemic

VA CLASSIFICATION (Primary): IM500
Commonly used brand name(s): *RespiGam*.
Another commonly used name is RSV-IGIV.

Note: For a listing of dosage forms and brand names by country availability, see *Dosage Forms* section(s).

## Category
Immunizing agent (passive).

## Indications

### General considerations
Respiratory syncytial virus (RSV), a negative-strand enveloped ribonucleic acid (RNA) virus of the paramyxovirus family, is considered to be a major cause of morbidity and mortality in the developing world. In the U.S., RSV causes an estimated 90,000 hospitalizations and 4500 deaths each year from lower respiratory tract infection in both infants and young children.

RSV strains are classified into groups A and B on the basis of the antigenic structure of the G protein. Among hospitalized infants, group A RSV infection results in greater disease severity than does group B infection. Unlike influenza, infection with RSV does not elicit long-term immunity, since RSV contains a single segment of RNA that does not facilitate major antigenic evolution. The mechanism by which group A RSV may cause more severe illness is unknown, but could result from functional differences in the viral genome or protein.

RSV activity in the U.S. is monitored by the National Respiratory and Enteric Virus Surveillance System (NREVSS), a voluntary, laboratory-based system. Outbreaks occur annually throughout the U.S. Onset of disease activity usually occurs in November and continues through April or early May, with peak activity occurring from late January through mid-February.

During the RSV season, health care providers should consider the role of RSV as a cause of acute respiratory disease in both children and adults. RSV is a common, but preventable, cause of nosocomially acquired infection; the risk for nosocomial transmission increases during community outbreaks. Nosocomial outbreaks or transmission of RSV can be controlled with strict attention to contact-isolation procedures.

Individuals at greatest risk for RSV-associated complications include preterm infants, children less than 6 months of age with chronic lung disease (especially those with bronchopulmonary dysplasia [BPD]) or congenital heart disease (CHD), immunocompromised individuals, and geriatric patients.

RSV causes acute respiratory illness in patients of any age. However, in infants and young children, it is the most important cause of bronchiolitis and pneumonia. Most severe manifestations of infection with RSV (e.g., bronchiolitis and pneumonia) occur in infants 2 to 6 months of age. During the first few weeks of life, particularly in preterm infants, respiratory signs can be minimal. Lethargy, irritability, and poor feeding, sometimes accompanied by apneic episodes, may be the major signs. RSV infection in older children and adults usually manifests as an upper respiratory tract illness, occasionally with bronchitis. Exacerbation of asthma or other chronic lung conditions is also common.

Nearly all children are infected by 2 years of age, and 1 to 2% of those infected require hospitalization. Among those admitted to the hospital with no apparent risk factors for severe disease, 4 to 15% are admitted to the intensive care unit (ICU), 1 to 5% require assisted ventilation, and < 1% die. In contrast, among children with underlying heart and lung disease, prematurity (i.e., gestation ≤ 32 weeks), and young age (i.e., ≤ 6 weeks), the corresponding figures for ICU, ventilation, and mortality range from 10 to 40%, 8 to 27%, and up to 10%, respectively.

Although traditionally recognized as the most common cause of lower respiratory tract disease in young children, RSV also has been shown to be a cause of serious illness in elderly adults. RSV is a predictable cause of disease each winter in older persons living in the community, in nursing homes, or attending senior day care programs. Similar to influenza, a well-recognized pathogen in the elderly, peaks of RSV activity in the community are associated with excess rates of mortality in persons over 65 years of age.

Immunity to RSV is incomplete and reinfection throughout life is common. However, although reinfection with RSV occurs throughout life, analysis of immune mechanisms following natural infection suggests that both humoral and mucosal antibodies may contribute to at least partial protection. Illness severity in infants has been related to the level of serum antibody to RSV, and passively administered high-titer RSV immunoglobulin has been demonstrated to protect infants who are at greater risk of acquiring the most severe disease.

Respiratory syncytial virus immune globulin intravenous (RSV-IGIV) has demonstrated efficacy only in the prophylaxis of children at high risk for RSV-related lower respiratory tract infection. One clinical trial has demonstrated that RSV-IGIV treatment is safe, but not efficacious, in the treatment of children with BPD, CHD, or premature gestation who are hospitalized with RSV-related lower respiratory tract infection.

### Accepted
Respiratory syncytial virus infection (prophylaxis)—Respiratory syncytial virus immune globulin intravenous (RSV-IGIV) is indicated for the prevention of serious lower respiratory tract infection caused by RSV in children younger than 24 months of age with bronchopulmonary dysplasia (BPD) or a history of premature birth (gestation ≤ 32 weeks).

## Pharmacology/Pharmacokinetics

### Physicochemical characteristics
Source—Respiratory syncytial virus immune globulin intravenous (RSV-IGIV) is a sterile solution of immune globulin G (IgG) purified from pooled adult human plasma selected for high titers of neutralizing antibody against respiratory syncytial virus (RSV). The product is purified using Cohn-Oncley cold ethanol fractionation and a solvent detergent partitioning method to inactivate blood-borne pathogens.

### Mechanism of action/Effect
RSV-IGIV contains a high concentration of neutralizing and protective antibodies directed against RSV. *In vitro* tests demonstrated that RSV-IGIV can neutralize clinical isolates of RSV.

### Protective effect
Studies in otherwise healthy children have shown that the frequency of primary and recurrent RSV infection is inversely correlated to the titer of RSV-neutralizing antibodies measured before the onset of the RSV season.

A randomized, double-blind, placebo-controlled, clinical trial was conducted at 54 centers in the U.S. (the PREVENT trial) during the 1994 to 1995 RSV season. This study included 510 children with bronchopulmonary dysplasia and/or a history of prematurity. These children were randomized to receive either 750 mg per kg of body weight (mg/kg) RSV-IGIV or placebo (1% albumin). In the study's comparison of treated patients with control patients, the incidence of RSV hospitalization was reduced by 41%, total days of RSV hospitalization were reduced by 53%, total RSV hospital days with increased supplemental oxygen requirements were reduced by 60%, and total RSV hospital days with a moderate or severe lower respiratory tract infection were reduced by 54%. The total days of hospitalization for respiratory illness per 100 randomized children were compared between placebo patients and RSV-IGIV patients. There were 317 days per 100 control children and 170 days per 100 treated children.

One month after the second, third, and fourth monthly infusion of respiratory syncytial virus immune globulin intravenous 750 mg/kg, titers were 1:477 ± 85, 1:490 ± 61, and 1:429 ± 23, respectively. Experts expect that protection against RSV infection is obtained with titers of 1:200 to 1:400.

Studies of adult volunteers have shown that immunity to RSV frequently lasts only a few months. By the next annual RSV epidemic, most of the population is susceptible to reinfection by the same strain of virus.

### Half-life
22 to 28 days.

## Precautions to Consider

### Cross-sensitivity and/or related problems
Respiratory syncytial virus immune globulin intravenous (RSV-IGIV) should be given with caution to patients with a history of prior systemic allergic reactions following the administration of human immunoglobulin preparations.

### Pregnancy/Reproduction
Pregnancy—Studies have not been done in humans.
Studies have not been done in animals.
FDA Pregnancy Category C.

### Breast-feeding
It is not known whether RSV-IGIV is distributed into breast milk. However, problems in humans have not been documented.

### Pediatrics
Infants with underlying pulmonary disease may be sensitive to extra fluid volume. Infusion of RSV-IGIV, particularly in children with bronchopulmonary dysplasia (BPD), may precipitate symptoms of fluid overload. Therefore, RSV-IGIV should be administered with caution to infants with underlying pulmonary disease. Vital signs should be monitored to help indicate fluid overload, and, if indicated, a loop diuretic should be administered.

The safety and efficacy of RSV-IGIV in children with congenital heart disease (CHD) has not been established. In one study, although equivalent proportions of children in RSV-IGIV and control groups had adverse events, a large number of RSV-IGIV recipients had severe or life-threatening adverse reactions. These reactions were most frequently observed in infants with CHD with right to left shunts who underwent cardiac surgery before treatment with RSV-IGIV.

### Geriatrics
No information is available on the relationship of age to the effects of RSV-IGIV in geriatric patients.

### Drug interactions and/or related problems
The following drug interactions and/or related problems have been selected on the basis of their potential clinical significance (possible mechanism in parentheses where appropriate)—not necessarily inclusive (» = major clinical significance):

Note: Combinations containing any of the following medications, depending on the amount present, may also interact with this medication.

Live virus vaccines
(concurrent administration of RSV-IGIV with measles, mumps, rubella, or varicella live virus vaccines may interfere with the patient's immune response to these vaccines; immunization with measles, mumps, rubella, or varicella live virus vaccines should be deferred for 9 months after the last dose of RSV-IGIV; in addition, limited information available from infants who received RSV-IGIV concurrently with one or more doses of their primary immunization series indicates that antibody responses to diphtheria and tetanus toxoids, and pertussis vaccine, and *Haemophilus* b vaccine may be decreased; however, no changes are required to the primary immunization schedule for these agents)

### Medical considerations/Contraindications
The medical considerations/contraindications included have been selected on the basis of their potential clinical significance (reasons given in parentheses where appropriate)—not necessarily inclusive (» = major clinical significance).

*Except under special circumstances, this medication should not be used when the following medical problems exist:*

» Allergic reaction to human immunoglobulins
» Immunoglobulin A (IgA) deficiencies, selective, in patients who are known to have antibodies to IgA
(small amounts of IgA may be present in RSV-IGIV and may cause a severe allergic reaction in patients with antibodies to IgA)

*Risk-benefit should be considered when the following medical problem exists:*

Sensitivity to RSV-IGIV

### Patient monitoring
The following may be especially important in patient monitoring (other tests may be warranted in some patients, depending on condition; » = major clinical significance):

Vital signs
(infants with underlying pulmonary disease who may be sensitive to extra fluid volume may be at risk of developing hypotension, anaphylaxis, or a severe allergic reaction, which may lead to shock; the patient's vital signs should be monitored continuously, and the patient should be observed carefully throughout the infusion)

## Side/Adverse Effects
Note: Severe reactions, such as anaphylaxis or angioneuropathy, have been reported in association with intravenous immunoglobulins, even in patients not known to be sensitive to human immunoglobulins or blood products. In one clinical trial, serious allergic reactions were noted in two patients who received respiratory syncytial virus immune globulin intravenous (RSV-IGIV). These reactions were manifested as an acute episode of cyanosis, mottling, and fever in one patient, and as respiratory distress in the other.

Rare occurrences of aseptic meningitis syndrome (AMS) have been reported in association with immune globulin intravenous (IGIV) treatment. AMS usually begins within several hours to 2 days following IGIV treatment and is characterized by symptoms and signs that include severe headache, drowsiness, fever, photophobia, painful eye movements, muscle rigidity, and nausea and vomiting. Cerebrospinal fluid studies generally demonstrate pleocytosis, predominantly granulocytic, and elevated protein levels. Patients exhibiting such symptoms and signs should be thoroughly evaluated to rule out other causes of meningitis. AMS may occur more frequently in association with high-dose (2 grams per kg of body weight) IGIV treatment. Discontinuation of IGIV treatment has resulted in remission of AMS within several days without sequelae.

Except for hypersensitivity reactions, adverse reactions to IGIV are related to the rate of infusion, and may be relieved by decreasing the rate or temporarily stopping infusion. Loop diuretics should be available for the management of patients who are at risk of fluid overload.

The following side/adverse effects have been selected on the basis of their potential clinical significance (possible signs and symptoms in parentheses where appropriate)—not necessarily inclusive:

**Those indicating need for medical attention**
Incidence rare
*Anaphylactic reaction* (difficulty in breathing and swallowing; hives; itching, especially of feet and hands; reddening of skin, especially around ears; swelling of eyes, face, or inside of nose; unusual tiredness or weakness, sudden and severe); *fever of 39.2 °C (102.6 °F) or more; respiratory distress; tachycardia* (increased heart rate); *vomiting*

## Patient Consultation
As an aid to patient consultation, refer to *Advice for the Patient, Respiratory Syncytial Virus Immune Globulin Intravenous (Systemic).*

In providing consultation, consider emphasizing the following selected information (» = major clinical significance):

**Before using this medication**
» Conditions affecting use, especially:
Sensitivity to respiratory syncytial virus immune globulin intravenous (RSV-IGIV)
Use in children—Using with caution in children with bronchopulmonary dysplasia; safety and efficacy of RSV-IGIV in children with congenital heart disease have not been established
Other medical problems, especially history of allergic reactions to human immunoglobulins, or selective IgA deficiencies

**Proper use of this medication**
» Proper dosing

**Side/adverse effects**
Signs of potential side effects, especially, anaphylactic reaction, fever of 39.2 °C (102.6 °F), respiratory distress, tachycardia, and vomiting

## General Dosing Information
Although systemic reactions to human immunoglobulin preparations are rare, serious allergic reactions were reported following respiratory syncytial virus immune globulin intravenous (RSV-IGIV) administration. Therefore, appropriate precautions should be taken prior to RSV-IGIV infusion to prevent allergic or other unwanted reactions. These precautions should include review of the patient's history regarding possible sensitivity and the ready availability of epinephrine 1:1000 and other appropriate agents used to control immediate allergic reactions.

RSV-IGIV has been approved for use in infants and children younger than 24 months with bronchopulmonary dysplasia (BPD) or a history of premature birth (≤ 32 weeks of gestation). In addition to BPD and prematurity, other factors may influence the decision about the use of RSV-IGIV prophylaxis. These include conditions that predispose to respiratory complications (e.g., neurologic disease in very-low-birth-weight infants), the number of young siblings, child care center attendance, exposure to cigarette smoke in the home, anticipated cardiac surgery, ease of intravenous access, medication- and infusion-related costs, practicality and tolerability of monthly infusions, and the distance to and availability of hospital care for severe respiratory illness. For many infants qualifying for the approved indications, the risk of rehospitalization for serious respiratory illness will be low, and the cost of logistic difficulties associated with RSV-IGIV use may outweigh potential benefits. The effectiveness of RSV-IGIV for children who receive an incomplete single infusion or less than the recommended total monthly infusions has not been assessed.

The Committee on Infectious Diseases and the Committee on Fetus and Newborn of the American Academy of Pediatrics (AAP) offer the following recommendations on the use of RSV-IGIV in infants and children:

• RSV-IGIV prophylaxis should be considered for infants and children younger than 2 years of age with BPD who currently are receiving or have received oxygen therapy within the 6 months before the antici-

pated respiratory syncytial virus (RSV) season. Patients with BPD with more severe underlying lung disease may benefit clinically from prophylaxis for two RSV seasons, whereas those with less severe underlying disease may benefit only for the first season. Decisions regarding individual patients may need additional input from neonatologists, intensive care specialists, or pulmonologists.
- Infants born at 32 weeks or less of gestation without BPD also may benefit from RSV-IGIV prophylaxis. In these infants, major risk factors to consider are gestational age and chronologic age at the start of the RSV season. Infants born at 28 weeks of gestation or less may benefit from prophylaxis up to 12 months of age. Infants born at 29 to 32 weeks of gestation may benefit from prophylaxis up to 6 months of age. Decisions regarding each patient should be individualized. Practitioners may wish to use RSV rehospitalization data from their own region to assist in the decision-making process.
- RSV-IGIV is not approved for patients with congenital heart disease (CHD). Available data indicate that RSV-IGIV should not be used in patients who have cyanotic CHD. However, patients with BPD and/or prematurity who meet the criteria in recommendations mentioned above and who also have asymptomatic acyanotic CHD (e.g., patent ductus arteriosus or ventricular septal defect) may benefit from prophylaxis.
- RSV-IGIV use, either prophylactically or therapeutically, has not been evaluated in randomized trials in immunocompromised pediatric patients. Although specific recommendations for all immunocompromised patients cannot be made, children with severe immunodeficiencies (e.g., severe combined immunodeficiency or severe acquired immunodeficiency syndrome [AIDS]) may benefit from RSV-IGIV. If these infants and children are receiving immune globulin intravenous (IGIV) monthly, providers may consider substituting RSV-IGIV during the RSV season.
- RSV is known to be transmitted in the hospital setting and to cause serious disease in high-risk infants. In high-risk hospitalized infants, the major means to prevent RSV disease is strict observance of infection control practices, including the use of rapid means to identify RSV-infected infants. If an RSV outbreak is documented in a high-risk unit (e.g., pediatric intensive care unit), primary emphasis should be placed on proper infection control practices. The need for, and efficacy of, RSV-IGIV prophylaxis in these situations have not been documented.
- RSV-IGIV prophylaxis should be initiated before the onset of the RSV season and terminated at the end of the RSV season. In most areas of the U.S., the usual time for the beginning of RSV outbreaks is October to December and termination is March to May, but regional differences occur. The onset of RSV occurs earlier in the southern states than in the northern states. Practitioners should check with health departments and/or diagnostic virology laboratories in their geographic areas to determine the optimal schedule.
- In infants and children receiving RSV-IGIV prophylaxis (750 mg per kg of body weight [mg/kg] dose), immunization with measles, mumps, and rubella virus vaccine live and varicella live virus vaccine should be deferred for 9 months after the last dose. There are no data on the use of RSV-IGIV and the response to hepatitis B vaccine, but there is no reason to anticipate any interference because RSV-IGIV does not contain antibodies to hepatitis B surface antigen. RSV-IGIV use should not alter the primary immunization schedule for diphtheria and tetanus toxoids, whole-cell or acellular pertussis vaccine, *Haemophilus* b vaccine, and poliovirus vaccines (inactivated poliovirus vaccine [IPV] or oral poliovirus vaccine [OPV]).
- A critical aspect of RSV prevention in high-risk infants is education of parents and other care givers about the importance of reducing exposure to, and transmission of, RSV. Preventive measures include limiting, where feasible, exposure to cigarette smoke and contagious settings (e.g., child care centers) and emphasis on hand washing in all settings, including the home, especially during periods when contacts of high-risk children have respiratory infections.

**For treatment of adverse effects**
Recommended treatment consists of the following:
- For mild hypersensitivity reaction—Administering antihistamines, and, if necessary, corticosteroids.
- For severe hypersensitivity or anaphylactic reaction—Administering epinephrine. Antihistamines or corticosteroids also may be administered as required.

## Parenteral Dosage Forms

### RESPIRATORY SYNCYTIAL VIRUS IMMUNE GLOBULIN INTRAVENOUS INJECTION

**Usual adult and adolescent dose**
Use is not recommended.

**Usual pediatric dose**
Respiratory syncytial virus infection (prophylaxis)—
   Children younger than 2 years of age: Intravenous infusion, the maximum recommended total dosage is 750 mg per kg of body weight administered as a single monthly infusion beginning in September or October and continuing for a total of five doses.

Note: Respiratory syncytial virus immune globulin intravenous should be administered intravenously at a rate of 1.5 mL per kg of body weight per hour for 15 minutes. If not contraindicated by the patient's clinical condition, the rate can be increased to 3 mL per kg of body weight per hour for 15 minutes, and finally to a maximum rate of 6 mL per kg of body weight per hour. The maximum recommended rate of infusion should not be exceeded. The patient should be monitored closely during and after each rate change. A slower rate of infusion may be indicated in children who are volume sensitive, such as those with bronchopulmonary dysplasia (BPD) or prematurity.
   Children 2 years of age and older: Use is not recommended.

**Strength(s) usually available**
U.S.—
   Each 50-mL vial contains 2500 mg ± 500 mg immunoglobulin, primarily IgG and trace amounts of IgA and IgM (Rx) [*RespiGam*].
Canada—
   Each 50-mL vial contains 2500 mg ± 500 mg immunoglobulin, primarily IgG and trace amounts of IgA and IgM (Rx) [*RespiGam*].

**Packaging and storage**
Store between 2 and 8 °C (36 and 46 °F), unless otherwise specified by the manufacturer. Protect from freezing.

**Stability**
A solution that has been frozen should be discarded.

**Auxiliary labeling**
- Do not freeze.

## Selected Bibliography

American Academy of Pediatrics. Recommendations of the Committee on Infectious Diseases and the Committee on Fetus and Newborn: respiratory syncytial virus immune globulin intravenous—indications for use. Pediatrics 1997; 99(4): 645-50.

Connor E, Top F, Kramer A, et al. The PREVENT Study Group. Reduction of respiratory syncytial virus hospitalization among premature infants and infants with bronchopulmonary dysplasia using respiratory syncytial virus immune globulin prophylaxis. Pediatrics 1997; 99(1): 93-9.

Developed: 07/29/98

---

# RETEPLASE, RECOMBINANT  Systemic—INTRODUCTORY VERSION

VA CLASSIFICATION (Primary): BL115
Commonly used brand name(s): *Retavase*.
Note: For a listing of dosage forms and brand names by country availability, see *Dosage Forms* section(s).

## Category
Thrombolytic.

## Indications

**Accepted**
Thrombosis, coronary arterial, acute (treatment)—Reteplase is indicated for use in the management of acute myocardial infarction (AMI) in adults to improve ventricular function following AMI, reduce the incidence of congestive heart failure, and reduce mortality associated with AMI.

## Pharmacology/Pharmacokinetics

**Physicochemical characteristics**
Source—Reteplase is a nonglycosylated deletion mutein of tissue plasminogen activator produced by recombinant DNA technology in *Escherichia coli*, and purified by chromatographic separation.
Molecular weight—39,571 daltons.

**Mechanism of action/Effect**
Reteplase catalyzes the cleavage of endogenous plasminogen to generate plasmin, which in turn degrades the fibrin matrix of the thrombus, resulting in thrombolysis.

**Half-life**
Elimination, effective, based on the measurement of thrombolytic activity—13 to 16 minutes.

**Time to peak effect**
In a controlled trial, 36 of 56 patients treated for an acute myocardial infarction had a decrease in fibrinogen concentrations to below 100 mg per dL within 2 hours following double-bolus administration of reteplase.

**Duration of action**
After an initial decrease in fibrinogen concentrations following double-bolus administration of reteplase, the mean fibrinogen concentration returned to the baseline value by 48 hours.

**Elimination**
Hepatic and renal.

## Precautions to Consider

**Carcinogenicity**
Long-term studies to evaluate the carcinogenic potential of reteplase have not been done.

**Mutagenicity**
Studies to determine mutagenicity, chromosomal aberrations, gene mutations, and micronuclei induction were negative at all concentrations tested.

**Pregnancy/Reproduction**
Fertility—Studies in rats revealed no effects on fertility at doses up to 15 times the human dose (4.31 units per kg [Units/kg]).

Pregnancy—Studies have not been done in humans.
The most common complication of thrombolytic therapy is bleeding, and certain conditions, including pregnancy, can increase this risk. Reteplase should be used during pregnancy only if the potential benefit justifies the potential risk to the fetus.
Reteplase has been shown to have an abortifacient effect in rabbits when given in doses three times the human dose (0.86 Units/kg). Administration to pregnant rabbits resulted in hemorrhaging in the genital tract leading to abortions in mid-gestation. Studies in rats at doses up to 15 times the human dose (4.31 Units/kg) revealed no evidence of fetal anomalies.
FDA Pregnancy Category C.

**Breast-feeding**
It is not known whether reteplase is distributed into breast milk. However, problems in humans have not been documented.

**Pediatrics**
No information is available on the relationship of age to the effects of reteplase in pediatric patients. Safety and efficacy have not been established.

**Geriatrics**
The risk of intracranial hemorrhage and other types of hemorrhage is increased in patients of advanced age. Patients should be carefully evaluated and the anticipated benefits of reteplase therapy should be weighed against the potential risks.

**Critical/Emergency care**
Standard management of myocardial infarction should be implemented concomitantly with reteplase. Arterial and venous punctures should be minimized. Noncompressible arterial puncture must be avoided and internal jugular and subclavian venous punctures should be avoided to minimize bleeding. Should an arterial puncture be necessary during the administration of reteplase, it is preferable to use an upper extremity vessel that is accessible to manual compression. Pressure should be applied for at least 30 minutes, a pressure dressing applied, and the puncture site checked frequently for evidence of bleeding. Venipunctures should be performed carefully and only as required.

**Drug interactions and/or related problems**
The following drug interactions and/or related problems have been selected on the basis of their potential clinical significance (possible mechanism in parentheses where appropriate)—not necessarily inclusive (» = major clinical significance):

Note: Combinations containing any of the following medications, depending on the amount present, may also interact with this medication.

» Anticoagulants, coumarin- or indandione-derivative or
» Heparin or
» Platelet aggregation inhibitors (See *Appendix II*), such as:
  Abciximab
  Aspirin
  Dipyridamole
  (the risk of bleeding may be increased when these agents are administered prior to or after reteplase therapy; however, heparin and aspirin have been administered concomitantly with and following the administration of reteplase in the management of acute myocardial infarction; careful monitoring for bleeding is recommended, especially at arterial puncture sites)

**Laboratory value alterations**
The following have been selected on the basis of their potential clinical significance (possible effect in parentheses where appropriate)—not necessarily inclusive (» = major clinical significance):

With diagnostic test results
  Coagulation tests and
  Tests for systemic fibrinolysis
    (reteplase, when present in blood in pharmacologic concentrations, remains active under *in vitro* conditions, which can lead to degradation of fibrinogen in blood samples removed for analysis; therefore, results of these tests may be unreliable unless specific precautions are taken to prevent *in vitro* fibrinolytic artifacts)

**Medical considerations/Contraindications**
The medical considerations/contraindications included have been selected on the basis of their potential clinical significance (reasons given in parentheses where appropriate)—not necessarily inclusive (» = major clinical significance).

*Except under special circumstances, this medication should not be used when the following medical problems exist:*

» Aneurysm, intracranial or
» Arteriovenous malformation or
» Bleeding, active or
» Brain tumor or
» Cerebrovascular accident, or history of or
» Hemostatic disorders or
» Neurosurgery, intracranial or intraspinal, recent or
» Trauma to the central nervous system (CNS), recent
    (increased risk of uncontrollable hemorrhage)
» Hypertension, severe uncontrolled
    (increased risk of cerebral hemorrhage)

*Risk-benefit should be considered when the following medical problems exist:*

Any condition in which the risk of bleeding or hemorrhage is present or would be difficult to control because of its location, such as:
  Cerebrovascular disease
» Childbirth, recent
» Coagulation defects, uncontrolled, or other hemostatic defects, including those secondary to severe hepatic or renal disease
» Endocarditis, bacterial, subacute
» Gastrointestinal bleeding, recent
  Genitourinary bleeding, recent
  Hemorrhagic retinopathy, diabetic or other hemorrhagic ophthalmic conditions
  Hepatic function impairment, severe
  Hypertension, moderate, not optimally controlled, i.e., $\geq$ 180 mm Hg systolic and/or $\geq$ 110 mm Hg diastolic
» Organ biopsy, recent
  Pregnancy
  Puncture of noncompressible blood vessel, recent
  Renal function impairment, severe
» Surgery, major, recent
» Trauma, recent
  Infection at or near site of thrombus, obstructed intravenous catheter, or occluded arteriovenous cannula
    (risk of spreading the infection into and via the circulation)
» Mitral stenosis with atrial fibrillation or other indications of probable left heart thrombus
    (risk of new embolic phenomena including those to cerebral vessels)

Pericarditis, acute
(risk of hemopericardium, which may lead to cardiac tamponade)

## Side/Adverse Effects

Note: *Bleeding*, the most common side effect encountered during reteplase therapy, occurs both internally (intracranial, retroperitoneal, gastrointestinal, genitourinary, or respiratory) and superficially (venous cutdowns, arterial punctures, sites of recent surgical intervention). Bleeding may occur from recent puncture sites as fibrin is lysed during therapy with reteplase. The risk of *intracranial hemorrhage* is increased in patients of advanced age or with elevated blood pressure.

*Cardiac arrhythmias* may occur during or following coronary thrombolysis. These are not necessarily direct effects of the medication and may be associated with the myocardial infarction itself, or may be induced by sudden reperfusion. Specific arrhythmias that have been reported include sinus bradycardia, accelerated idioventricular rhythm, ventricular premature depolarizations, supraventricular tachycardia, ventricular tachycardia, and ventricular fibrillation.

The following side/adverse effects have been selected on the basis of their potential clinical significance (possible signs and symptoms in parentheses where appropriate)—not necessarily inclusive:

**Those indicating need for medical attention**
Incidence more frequent
**Bleeding or oozing from cuts, invaded or disturbed sites, wounds, or gums**
Incidence less frequent or rare
**Allergic reaction** (flushing or redness of skin; mild headache; mild muscle pain; nausea; skin rash, hives, or itching; troubled breathing or wheezing); **cholesterol embolism; fever; hypotension; internal bleeding** (abdominal pain or swelling; back pain or backaches; bloody urine; bloody or black, tarry stools; constipation caused by hemorrhage-induced paralytic ileus or intestinal obstruction; coughing up blood; dizziness; headaches, sudden, severe, and/or continuing; joint pain, stiffness, or swelling; muscle pain or stiffness, severe or continuing; nosebleeds; unexpected or unusually heavy bleeding from vagina; vomiting of blood or material that looks like coffee grounds); **stroke, hemorrhagic** (confusion; double vision; impairment of speech; weakness in arms or legs)

**Those indicating need for medical attention only if they continue or are bothersome**
Incidence less frequent
**Nausea and/or vomiting**

## Patient Consultation

As an aid to patient consultation, refer to *Advice for the Patient, Thrombolytic Agents (Systemic)*.

In providing consultation, consider emphasizing the following selected information (» = major clinical significance):

**Before using this medication**
» Conditions affecting use, especially:
  Use in the elderly—Increased risk of hemorrhage
  Other medications, especially anticoagulants, heparin, and platelet aggregation inhibitors
  Other medical problems, especially conditions leading to an increased risk of uncontrollable or cerebral hemorrhage, and mitral stenosis

**Proper use of this medication**
» Proper dosing

**Precautions while using this medication**
» Importance of compliance with strict bed rest or other measures to minimize bleeding

**Side/adverse effects**
Signs of potential side effects, especially bleeding or oozing from cuts, invaded or disturbed sites, wounds, or gums; allergic reaction; cholesterol embolism; fever; hypotension; internal bleeding; and hemorrhagic stroke

## General Dosing Information

The potency of reteplase is expressed in units using a reference standard that is specific for reteplase and is not comparable with units used for other thrombolytic agents.

Intramuscular injections and nonessential handling of the patient should be avoided during treatment with reteplase to minimize bleeding.

Reteplase should be given via an intravenous line in which no other medication is being simultaneously injected or infused.

There is no experience with patients receiving repeat courses of therapy with reteplase. Reteplase did not induce the formation of reteplase-specific antibodies in any of the patients who were tested for antibody formation in clinical trials.

### For treatment of adverse effects

Recommended treatment consists of the following:
- For anaphylactoid reactions—The second bolus of reteplase should not be given, and appropriate therapy should be initiated.
- For serious bleeding (not controllable by local pressure)—Concomitant anticoagulant therapy should be terminated immediately. Heparin effects can be reversed with protamine. In addition, the second bolus of reteplase should not be given if the serious bleeding occurs before it is administered.
- For reperfusion arrhythmias—Standard antiarrhythmic measures should be followed. It is recommended that antiarrhythmic therapy for bradycardia and/or ventricular irritability be available when reteplase is administered.

## Parenteral Dosage Forms

### RETEPLASE, RECOMBINANT FOR INJECTION

Note: Reteplase is administered as a double-bolus injection.

**Usual adult dose**
Thrombosis, coronary arterial, acute—
  Intravenous, 10 units administered over two minutes. The second 10-unit dose is given thirty minutes after initiation of the first injection.

**Usual pediatric dose**
Safety and efficacy have not been established.

**Strength(s) usually available**
U.S.—
  10.8 units (18.8 mg) per single-dose vial (Rx) [*Retavase* (supplied as a kit containing 2 single-dose reteplase vials, 2 single-dose diluent vials for reconstitution [10 mL Sterile Water for Injection USP], 2 sterile 10 mL syringes with 20-gauge needle attached, 2 sterile dispensing pins, 2 sterile 20-gauge needles for dose administration, and 2 alcohol swabs)].

**Packaging and storage**
Store between 2 and 25 °C (36 and 77 °F). Protect from light.

**Preparation of dosage form**
Reteplase should be reconstituted only with Sterile Water for Injection USP (without preservatives). The reconstituted preparation results in a colorless solution containing reteplase 1 unit per mL. Slight foaming may occur during reconstitution; however, large bubbles dissipate when the solution is left undisturbed for a few minutes. The following steps should be taken for reconstitution:
1. Withdraw 10 mL of Sterile Water for Injection USP from the vial using the 10 mL syringe with attached needle.
2. Remove and discard the needle and connect the syringe to the dispensing pin via the Luer-lock port.
3. Insert the spike end of the dispensing pin into the vial of reteplase and transfer the 10 mL of Sterile Water for Injection USP.
4. Swirl the vial gently to dissolve the reteplase, with the dispensing pin and syringe still attached to the vial.
5. Withdraw 10 mL of the reconstituted reteplase solution back into the syringe. A small amount of solution will remain in the vial due to overfill.
6. Detach the syringe from the dispensing pin and attach the sterile 20-gauge needle provided. The 10-mL dose is now ready for administration.

**Stability**
The reconstituted solution should be used within 4 hours when stored between 2 and 30 °C (36 and 86 °F). It should be discarded if not used within this time. However, because reteplase for injection contains no preservatives, it should not be reconstituted until immediately prior to use. Any unused solution must be discarded.

**Incompatibilities**
*Do not add any other medication to the container of reteplase solution or administer other medications through the same intravenous line. Heparin and reteplase are incompatible when combined in solution. If reteplase is to be injected through an intravenous line containing heparin, a 0.9% sodium chloride or 5% dextrose solution should be flushed through the line prior to and following the reteplase injection.*

Developed: 05/14/97

# RH$_O$(D) IMMUNE GLOBULIN Systemic

CVA CLASSIFICATION (Primary): IM 500

Commonly used brand name(s): *Gamulin Rh; HypRho-D Full Dose; HypRho-D Mini-Dose; MICRhoGAM; Mini-Gamulin Rh; RhoGAM; WinRho SD*.

Other commonly used names are anti-D gammaglobulin; anti-D (Rh$_o$) immunoglobulin; anti-Rh immunoglobulin; anti-Rh$_o$(D); D(Rh$_o$) immune globulin; RhD immune globulin; Rh immune globulin; Rh-IG; and Rh$_o$(D) immune human globulin.

Note: For a listing of dosage forms and brand names by country availability, see *Dosage Forms* section(s).

## Category
Immunizing agent (passive).

## Indications

**Accepted**

Sensitization of Rh$_o$(D)–negative females to Rh$_o$(D)–positive blood (prophylaxis) or

Rh hemolytic disease of the newborn (prophylaxis)—Rh$_o$(D) immune globulin is indicated in Rh$_o$(D)–negative females of child-bearing age or younger who have not been previously sensitized to the Rh$_o$(D) erythrocyte factor and who may be exposed to the factor during one or more of the following events: the birth of an Rh$_o$(D)–positive infant; incomplete pregnancy terminating in the delivery of an Rh$_o$(D)–positive fetus (e.g., spontaneous or induced abortion or ruptured tubal pregnancy); amniocentesis, abdominal trauma during pregnancy, or transplacental hemorrhage, while carrying an Rh$_o$(D)–positive fetus; or transfusion involving mismatched Rh$_o$(D)–positive blood. Treating these females prophylactically prevents sensitization to the Rh$_o$(D) erythrocyte factor, which in turn prevents Rh hemolytic disease (erythroblastosis fetalis) in Rh$_o$(D)–positive neonates. See *Mechanism of action/Effect*.

## Pharmacology/Pharmacokinetics

**Physicochemical characteristics**

Source—A sterile, nonpyrogenic solution of immune globulin that contains antibody to the erythrocyte factor Rh$_o$(D). The solution is prepared from large pools of human blood plasma.

**Mechanism of action/Effect**

By providing passive Rh$_o$(D) antibody, Rh$_o$(D) immune globulin suppresses the immune response to Rh$_o$(D)–positive blood in nonsensitized Rh$_o$(D)–negative females. This prevents sensitization to the Rh$_o$(D) erythrocyte factor and the subsequent formation of active Rh$_o$(D) antibody. This in turn prevents the occurrence of Rh hemolytic disease (erythroblastosis fetalis) in Rh$_o$(D)–positive neonates, which results from *in utero* exposure to maternal Rh$_o$(D) antibody.

**Protective effect**

Administration of Rh$_o$(D) immune globulin (full dose) within 72 hours of a delivery of a full-term Rh$_o$(D)–positive infant by an Rh$_o$(D)–negative mother reduces the incidence of Rh immunization from the usual 12 or 13% to 1 or 2%. The 1 or 2% treatment failures are thought to be due to immunization that occurred during the latter part of pregnancy. Studies have shown that 2 doses, the first given at 28 weeks gestation and the second given following delivery, can reduce treatment failures to 0.1%.

Studies have shown that administration of Rh$_o$(D) immune globulin (minidose) within 3 hours following termination of pregnancy prior to 13 weeks of gestation in Rh$_o$(D)–negative females who have not been previously sensitized to the Rh$_o$(D) factor was 100% effective in preventing Rh immunization.

**Duration of protective effect**

The half-life of Rh$_o$(D) immune globulin is 23 to 26 days.

## Precautions to Consider

**Cross-sensitivity and/or related problems**

Patients sensitive to other human immune globulin products may be sensitive to Rh$_o$(D) immune globulin also.

**Pregnancy/Reproduction**

Pregnancy—Adequate and well-controlled studies have not been done in pregnant women. However, use of Rh$_o$(D) immune globulin (full dose) during the third trimester has not produced evidence of hemolysis in the infant.

Studies have not been done in animals.

FDA Pregnancy Category C.

**Breast-feeding**

Problems in humans have not been documented.

**Pediatrics**

No information is available on the relationship of age to the effects of Rh$_o$(D) immune globulin in pediatric patients. Safety and efficacy have not been established.

**Drug interactions and/or related problems**

The following drug interactions and/or related problems have been selected on the basis of their potential clinical significance (possible mechanism in parentheses where appropriate)—not necessarily inclusive (» = major clinical significance):

Note: Combinations containing any of the following medications, depending on the amount present, may also interact with this medication.

Live virus vaccines
(antibodies contained in Rh$_o$(D) immune globulin may interfere with the body's immune response to certain live virus vaccines; live virus vaccines, such as measles, mumps, and rubella, should be administered at least 3 months after administration of Rh$_o$(D) immune globulin)

**Laboratory value alterations**

The following have been selected on the basis of their potential clinical significance (possible effect in parentheses where appropriate)—not necessarily inclusive (» = major clinical significance):

With diagnostic test results
Antibody screening test, maternal
(passively acquired anti-Rh$_o$(D) may be detected in maternal serum if antibody screening tests are performed subsequent to administration of Rh$_o$(D) immune globulin antepartum or postpartum)

Direct antiglobulin test, neonate
(infants born to women administered Rh$_o$(D) immune globulin antepartum may have a weakly positive direct antiglobulin test result at birth)

With physiology/laboratory test values
Bilirubin, serum
(concentrations may be elevated in persons receiving multiple doses of Rh$_o$(D) immune globulin, e.g., following a mismatched transfusion involving Rh$_o$(D)–positive blood. The elevation is believed to be due to a relatively rapid rate of foreign red cell destruction)

**Medical considerations/Contraindications**

The medical considerations/contraindications included have been selected on the basis of their potential clinical significance (reasons given in parentheses where appropriate)—not necessarily inclusive (» = major clinical significance).

*Risk-benefit should be considered when the following medical problems exist:*

» Immunoglobulin A (IgA) deficiencies, selective, in patients who have known antibody to IgA
(small amounts of IgA may be present in Rh$_o$(D) immune globulin and may cause a severe allergic reaction in patients with antibody to IgA)

Sensitivity to Rh$_o$(D) immune globulin

Sensitivity to thimerosal
(the Rh$_o$(D) immune globulin available in the U.S. and Canada may contain thimerosal)

## Side/Adverse Effects

Note: Severe systemic adverse effects to Rh$_o$(D) immune globulin are rare.

The following side/adverse effects have been selected on the basis of their potential clinical significance (possible signs and symptoms in parentheses where appropriate)—not necessarily inclusive:

**Those indicating need for medical attention only if they continue or are bothersome**

Incidence less frequent
*Fever; soreness at the place of injection*

## Patient Consultation

As an aid to patient consultation, refer to *Advice for the Patient, Rh$_o$(D) Immune Globulin (Systemic)*.

In providing consultation, consider emphasizing the following selected information (» = major clinical significance):

**Before using this medication**
» Conditions affecting use, especially:
  Sensitivity to Rh$_o$(D) immune globulin, other human immune globulins, or thimerosal
  Other medical problems, especially immunoglobulin A (IgA) deficiencies

**Proper use of this medication**
» Proper dosing

## General Dosing Information

Rh$_o$(D) immune globulin is *not* for use in neonates.

Rh$_o$(D) immune globulin should be administered only to Rh$_o$(D)–negative females. However, if there is doubt about the mother's Rh type, she should be given Rh$_o$(D) immune globulin. Doubt may arise when a large fetomaternal hemorrhage occurring late in pregnancy or during delivery infuses enough fetal red blood cells into the maternal circulation to cause a weak mixed field positive D$^u$ test result.

Although Rh$_o$(D) immune globulin is not effective in Rh$_o$(D)–negative females who have been already sensitized to the Rh$_o$(D) erythrocyte factor, administration to these females does not increase the risk of adverse effects.

When Rh typing of the fetus or newborn infant is not possible, the fetus or newborn infant should be assumed to be Rh$_o$(D)–positive, unless the father can be determined to be Rh$_o$(D)–negative.

Since 1 full dose of Rh$_o$(D) immune globulin available in the U.S. contains Rh$_o$(D) antibody sufficient to suppress the immunizing potential of approximately 15 mL of Rh$_o$(D)–positive packed red blood cells or 30 mL of Rh$_o$(D)–positive whole blood, the amount of Rh$_o$(D)–positive blood present in the mother's circulation should be carefully determined, since more than 1 dose of Rh$_o$(D) immune globulin may be required. A fetal red blood cell count can be performed on the maternal blood to determine the dosage of Rh$_o$(D) immune globulin required.

For all except one indication, at least 1 full dose of Rh$_o$(D) immune globulin is indicated. If a pregnancy is terminated prior to 13 weeks of gestation, the patient may be administered a mini-dose (approximately 1/6 of the full dose) of Rh$_o$(D) immune globulin instead of a full dose, since it is estimated that the total volume of red blood cells in a fetus at 12 weeks of gestation is less than 2.5 mL. For a pregnancy that is terminated at or beyond 13 weeks of gestation, the patient should receive at least 1 full dose of Rh$_o$(D) immune globulin.

Rh$_o$(D) immune globulin should be administered to the Rh$_o$(D)–negative female within 72 hours after the incompatible event involving Rh$_o$(D)–positive blood. If the event is a mismatched transfusion involving Rh$_o$(D)–positive blood, Rh$_o$(D) immune globulin should be administered within 72 hours, but preferably as soon as possible. If the event is a pregnancy terminated prior to 13 weeks of gestation, and the mini-dose of Rh$_o$(D) immune globulin will be given, the mini-dose should be administered within 72 hours, but preferably within 3 hours.

To maintain protection throughout pregnancy once Rh$_o$(D) immune globulin is administered, the level of passively acquired anti-Rh$_o$(D) should not be allowed to fall below the level required to prevent an immune response to Rh$_o$(D)–positive blood. Additional doses of Rh$_o$(D) immune globulin should be administered during pregnancy at approximately 12-week intervals following the first dose. In all cases, the postpartum dose of Rh$_o$(D) immune globulin should be administered, unless the previous dose was within 3 weeks of delivery and any fetomaternal hemorrhage that occurs during delivery produces less than 15 mL of red blood cells. For example, if an incompatible event involving Rh$_o$(D)–positive blood requires administration of Rh$_o$(D) immune globulin at 13 to 18 weeks of gestation, an additional dose should be administered at 26 to 28 weeks of gestation, followed by the postpartum dose within 72 hours of delivery. If the first dose is administered at 26 to 28 weeks of gestation, the postpartum dose is still required.

Rh$_o$(D) immune globulin should be administered by intramuscular injection. The U.S. products should not be administered intravenously. One Canadian product is indicated for either intravenous or intramuscular use.

## Parenteral Dosage Forms

### RH$_O$(D) IMMUNE GLOBULIN (HUMAN) (FOR INJECTION)

**Usual adult and adolescent dose**
Immunizing agent (passive)—
  Intramuscular, into the deltoid muscle or the anterolateral aspect of the thigh, or intravenous: a sufficient amount of Rh$_o$(D) antibody to suppress the immunizing potential of the amount of Rh$_o$(D)–positive blood calculated or estimated to be present in the female's circulation because of pregnancy or transfusion.

**Usual pediatric dose**
Immunizing agent (passive)—
  Intramuscular, into the deltoid muscle or the anterolateral aspect of the thigh, or intravenous: a sufficient amount of Rh$_o$(D) antibody to suppress the immunizing potential of the amount of Rh$_o$(D)–positive blood calculated or estimated to be present in the female's circulation because of transfusion.

Note: See *General Dosing Information* for the parameters for administering Rh$_o$(D) immune globulin.

If the patient requires administration of more than 1 vial/syringe of Rh$_o$(D) immune globulin, the contents of the vials/syringes may be administered at different sites at the same time or at intervals over time, provided that the entire dose is administered with 72 hours of the event.

**Strength(s) usually available**
U.S.—
  Not commercially available.
Canada—
  Sufficient Rh$_o$(D) antibody to suppress the immunizing potential of approximately 6 mL of Rh$_o$(D)–positive packed red blood cells or 12 mL of Rh$_o$(D)–positive whole blood (Rx) [*WinRho SD* (contains no preservatives)].
  Full dose: Sufficient Rh$_o$(D) antibody to suppress the immunizing potential of approximately 15 mL of Rh$_o$(D)–positive packed red blood cells or 30 mL of Rh$_o$(D)–positive whole blood (Rx) [*WinRho SD* (contains no preservatives)].

Note: Each full dose of Rh$_o$(D) immune globulin contains at least as much anti-Rh$_o$(D) as is contained in 1 mL of the U.S. Reference Rh$_o$(D) immune globulin. A full dose of Rh$_o$(D) immune globulin has traditionally been referred to as a "300 mcg" dose; however, this is *not* the actual anti-Rh$_o$(D) content of the product. Studies have shown that the U.S. Reference contains 820 International Units (IU) of anti-Rh$_o$(D) per mL, which is thought to be equivalent to 164 mcg per mL.

**Packaging and storage**
Store between 2 and 8 °C (36 and 46 °F), unless otherwise specified by manufacturer. Protect from freezing.

**Preparation of dosage form**
A suitable syringe and needle should be used to withdraw the diluent. 1.25 mL of diluent should be used for an intramuscular injection or 2.5 mL of diluent should be used for an intravenous injection. The diluent should be injected slowly into the vial containing the freeze-dried pellet so that the liquid is directed onto the inside glass wall of the vial. The pellet should be wet by gently tilting and inverting the vial. Frothing should be avoided. While the vial is held upright, it should be gently swirled until the pellet is dissolved. This should take less than 10 minutes.

**Stability**
The reconstituted solution may be stored at room temperature for up to 4 hours. It should be discarded if it is not used within 4 hours.
The solution should not be used if it is discolored or contains particulate matter.

**Auxiliary labeling**
• Do not freeze the powder, diluent, or the reconstituted solution.
• Use the reconstituted solution within 4 hours.

### RH$_O$(D) IMMUNE GLOBULIN (HUMAN) (INJECTION) USP

**Usual adult and adolescent dose**
Immunizing agent (passive)—
  Intramuscular, into the deltoid muscle or the anterolateral aspect of the thigh: a sufficient amount of Rh$_o$(D) antibody to suppress the immunizing potential of the amount of Rh$_o$(D)–positive blood calculated or estimated to be present in the female's circulation because of pregnancy or transfusion.

**Usual pediatric dose**
Immunizing agent (passive)—
  Intramuscular, into the deltoid muscle or the anterolateral aspect of the thigh: a sufficient amount of Rh$_o$(D) antibody to suppress the immunizing potential of the amount of Rh$_o$(D)–positive blood calculated or estimated to be present in the female's circulation because of transfusion.

Note: See *General Dosing Information* for the parameters for administering Rh$_o$(D) immune globulin.

If the patient requires administration of more than 1 vial/syringe of $Rh_o(D)$ immune globulin, the contents of the vials/syringes may be administered at different sites at the same time or at intervals over time, provided that the entire dose is administered with 72 hours of the event.

**Strength(s) usually available**

U.S.—
- Mini-dose: Sufficient $Rh_o(D)$ antibody to suppress the immunizing potential of approximately 2.5 mL of $Rh_o(D)$–positive packed red blood cells or 5 mL of $Rh_o(D)$–positive whole blood (Rx) [*HypRho-D Mini-Dose* (thimerosal); *MICRhoGAM* (thimerosal); *Mini-Gamulin Rh* (thimerosal)].
- Full dose: Sufficient $Rh_o(D)$ antibody to suppress the immunizing potential of approximately 15 mL of $Rh_o(D)$–positive packed red blood cells or 30 mL of $Rh_o(D)$–positive whole blood (Rx) [*Gamulin Rh* (thimerosal); *HypRho-D Full Dose* (thimerosal); *RhoGAM* (thimerosal)].

Canada—
- Full dose: Sufficient $Rh_o(D)$ antibody to suppress the immunizing potential of approximately 15 mL of $Rh_o(D)$–positive packed red blood cells or 30 mL of $Rh_o(D)$–positive whole blood (Rx) [*HypRho-D Full Dose* (thimerosal)].

Note: Each full dose of $Rh_o(D)$ immune globulin contains at least as much anti-$Rh_o(D)$ as contained in 1 mL of the U.S. Reference $Rh_o(D)$ immune globulin. A full dose of $Rh_o(D)$ immune globulin has traditionally been referred to as a "300 mcg" dose; however, this is *not* the actual anti-$Rh_o(D)$ content of the product. Studies have shown that the U.S. Reference contains 820 International Units (IU) of anti-$Rh_o(D)$ per mL, which is thought to be equivalent to 164 mcg per mL.

Each mini-dose of $Rh_o(D)$ immune globulin contains not less than one-sixth of the amount of anti-$Rh_o(D)$ that is contained in 1 mL of the U.S. Reference $Rh_o(D)$ immune globulin.

**Packaging and storage**
Store between 2 and 8 °C (36 and 46 °F), unless otherwise specified by manufacturer. Protect from freezing.

**Stability**
The solution should be discarded if it has been frozen. The solution should not be used if it is discolored or contains particulate matter.

**Auxiliary labeling**
- Store in refrigerator.
- Do not freeze.
- Discard if solution has been frozen.

## Selected Bibliography

Bayliss KM, Kueck BD, Johnson ST, et al. Detecting fetomaternal hemorrhage: a comparison of five methods. Transfusion 1991 May; 31(4): 303-7.

Duerbeck NB, Seeds JW. Rhesus immunization in pregnancy: a review. Obstet Gynecol Surv 1993 Dec; 48(12): 801-10.

Developed: 08/31/94
Interim revision: 06/02/95

---

# RIBAVIRIN Systemic

VA CLASSIFICATION (Primary): AM809
Commonly used brand name(s): *Virazole*.
Another commonly used name is tribavirin.
Note: For a listing of dosage forms and brand names by country availability, see *Dosage Forms* section(s).

## Category
Antiviral (systemic).
Note: Ribavirin is a broad-spectrum antiviral active *in vitro* against a wide variety of DNA and RNA viruses.

## Indications
Note: Bracketed information in the *Indications* section refers to uses that are not included in U.S. product labeling.

**Accepted**

Respiratory syncytial virus (RSV) infection, lower respiratory tract (treatment)—Ribavirin inhalation solution is indicated as a primary agent in the treatment of lower respiratory tract disease (including bronchiolitis and pneumonia) caused by respiratory syncytial virus (RSV) in hospitalized infants and young children who are at high risk for severe or complicated RSV infection; this category includes premature infants and infants with structural or physiologic cardiopulmonary disorders, bronchopulmonary dysplasia, immunodeficiency, or imminent respiratory failure. Ribavirin is indicated in the treatment of RSV infections in infants requiring mechanical ventilator assistance.

[Influenza A (treatment)][1] or
[Influenza B (treatment)][1]—Ribavirin inhalation solution is used as a secondary agent in the treatment of influenza A and B in young adults when treatment is started early (e.g., within 24 hours of initial symptoms) in the course of the disease.

[Lassa fever (prophylaxis and treatment)][1] or
[Viral hemorrhagic fever (prophylaxis and treatment)][1]—Oral and intravenous ribavirin are used in the treatment of Lassa fever and as postexposure prophylaxis in contacts at high risk. It may be similarly effective with other viral hemorrhagic fevers, including hemorrhagic fever with renal syndrome, Crimean-Congo hemorrhagic fever, and Rift Valley fever.

**Unaccepted**

Ribavirin is not indicated in children with mild RSV lower respiratory tract involvement who require a shorter hospitalization than that required for completion of a full course of ribavirin treatment (i.e., 3 to 7 days).

[1]Not included in Canadian product labeling.

## Pharmacology/Pharmacokinetics

**Physicochemical characteristics**
Molecular weight—244.21.

**Mechanism of action/Effect**
Virustatic; mechanism not completely understood, but does not alter viral attachment, penetration, or uncoating and does not induce cellular production of interferon; however, reversal of its antiviral action by guanosine and xanthosine suggests that ribavirin may act as a competitive inhibitor of cellular enzymes that act on these metabolites. Ribavirin is rapidly transported into cells and acts within virus-infected cells. Ribavirin is readily phosphorylated intracellularly by adenosine kinase to ribavirin mono-, di-, and triphosphate metabolites. Ribavirin triphosphate (RTP) is a potent competitive inhibitor of inosine monophosphate (IMP) dehydrogenase, influenza virus RNA polymerase, and messenger RNA (mRNA) guanylyltransferase, the latter resulting in inhibition of the capping of mRNA. These diverse effects result in a marked reduction of intracellular guanosine triphosphate (GTP) pools and inhibition of viral RNA and protein synthesis. Ultimately, viral replication and spreading to other cells are prevented or greatly inhibited.

**Other actions/effects**
May have immunologic effects; decreases in neutralizing antibody responses to respiratory syncytial virus (RSV) infection have been reported in ribavirin-treated patients. The clinical significance of this effect is unknown. Ribavirin has also been shown to significantly reduce viral shedding in RSV-infected patients.

**Absorption**
Inhalation—A small amount is systemically absorbed following inhalation.
Oral—Rapidly absorbed from the gastrointestinal tract following oral administration; bioavailability is approximately 45%.

**Distribution**
Distributed to plasma, respiratory tract secretions, and erythrocytes (RBCs). Large amounts of ribavirin triphosphate are sequestered in RBCs, reaching a plateau in approximately 4 days and remaining sequestered for weeks after administration. Significant concentrations (greater than 67%) may be found in the cerebrospinal fluid after prolonged administration.

$Vol_D$ = Approximately 647 to 802 liters.

**Protein binding**
No significant plasma protein binding.

**Biotransformation**
Hepatic (probable); phosphorylated intracellularly to mono-, di-, and triphosphate metabolites, the latter being active; metabolized also to 1,2,4-triazole carboxamide metabolite; secondary metabolic pathway involves amide hydrolysis to tricarboxylic acid, deribosylation, and breakdown of the triazole ring.

## Half-life
**Distribution—**
  Intravenous: Approximately 0.2 hours.
**Elimination—**
  Inhalation: 9.5 hours.
  Intravenous and oral (single dose): 0.5 to 2 hours.
  In erythrocytes: 40 days.
**Terminal—**
  Intravenous and oral:
    Single dose—27 to 36 hours.
    Steady state—Approximately 151 hours.

## Time to peak plasma concentration
Intravenous—End of infusion.
Oral—1 to 1.5 hours.

## Therapeutic plasma concentration
Therapeutically effective concentrations depend primarily on the duration of exposure and patient minute volume. Concentrations in respiratory tract secretions are much higher than corresponding plasma concentrations.

## Mean peak plasma concentration
Inhalation—
  Approximately 0.2 mcg per mL (0.8 micromoles) in pediatric patients receiving ribavirin aerosol by face mask 2.5 hours per day for 3 days.
  Approximately 1.7 mcg per mL (6.8 micromoles) in pediatric patients receiving ribavirin aerosol by face mask or mist tent 20 hours per day for 5 days.
Intravenous—
  Approximately 43 micromoles per liter after a single 600 mg dose.
  Approximately 72 micromoles per liter after a single 1200 mg dose.
Oral—
  Approximately 5 micromoles per liter at the end of the first week of administration of 200 mg every 8 hours.
  Approximately 11 micromoles per liter at the end of the first week of administration of 400 mg every 8 hours.

## Elimination
Inhalation—
  Renal: Approximately 30 to 55% excreted as the 1,2,4-triazole carboxamide metabolite in urine within 72 to 80 hours.
  Fecal: Approximately 15% excreted in feces within 72 hours.
Intravenous—
  Approximately 19% excreted unchanged in 24 hours; approximately 24% excreted unchanged in 48 hours.
Oral—
  Approximately 7% excreted unchanged in 24 hours; approximately 10% excreted unchanged in 48 hours.
In dialysis—
  Significant amounts of ribavirin are not removed by hemodialysis.

# Precautions to Consider

## Carcinogenicity/Tumorigenicity
Studies have shown that ribavirin induces cell transformation in a mammalian system (Balb/C 3T3 cell line). Although carcinogenicity studies are incomplete and inconclusive, results thus far suggest that chronic feeding of ribavirin to rats in doses of 16 to 60 mg per kg of body weight (mg/kg) can induce benign mammary, pancreatic, pituitary, and adrenal gland tumors.

## Mutagenicity
Studies have shown that ribavirin is mutagenic to mammalian cells (L5178Y) in culture. However, microbial mutagenicity assays and dominant lethal assays in mice have not shown that ribavirin is mutagenic.

## Pregnancy/Reproduction
Fertility—Although the effects of lower doses have not been studied, studies have shown that ribavirin causes testicular lesions (tubular atrophy) in adult rats given oral doses as low as 16 mg/kg daily. However, the fertility of ribavirin-treated animals (male or female) has not been adequately investigated.

Pregnancy—Ribavirin is contraindicated during pregnancy. Studies in humans have not been done. Although ribavirin is not indicated for use in adults in the U.S., healthcare workers and visitors who spend time at the patient's bedside may become environmentally exposed to ribavirin. Female healthcare workers and visitors who are pregnant, or may become pregnant, should be advised of the potential risks of exposure.

Studies in primates (e.g., baboons) have not shown that ribavirin causes adverse effects on the fetus; however, ribavirin crosses the placenta and studies in other animals have shown that it is teratogenic and/or embryocidal in nearly all species tested; studies in hamsters given daily oral doses of 2.5 mg/kg and studies in rats given daily oral doses of 10 mg/kg have shown teratogenicity. Malformations of the skull, palate, eye, jaw, skeleton, and gastrointestinal tract have been observed in animal studies, and survival of fetuses and offspring was reduced. Studies in rabbits given daily oral doses as low as 1 mg/kg have shown that ribavirin is embryocidal.

FDA Pregnancy Category X.

## Breast-feeding
It is not known whether ribavirin is excreted in human breast milk. However, ribavirin is excreted in the breast milk of animals and has been shown to be toxic to lactating animals and their offspring. Ribavirin aerosol is not indicated in the treatment of nursing mothers since respiratory syncytial virus (RSV) infection is self-limited in this population.

## Pediatrics
Ribavirin inhalation solution is indicated in the treatment of RSV infection only in children.

## Geriatrics
Ribavirin inhalation solution is not indicated for use in geriatric patients.

## Drug interactions and/or related problems
The following drug interactions and/or related problems have been selected on the basis of their potential clinical significance (possible mechanism in parentheses where appropriate)—not necessarily inclusive (» = major clinical significance):

Note: Combinations containing any of the following medications, depending on the amount present, may also interact with this medication.

Zidovudine
  (*in vitro* studies have shown that when combined, ribavirin and zidovudine are reproducibly antagonistic and should not be used concurrently; ribavirin inhibits the phosphorylation of zidovudine to its active triphosphate form)

## Medical considerations/Contraindications
The medical considerations/contraindications included have been selected on the basis of their potential clinical significance (reasons given in parentheses where appropriate)—not necessarily inclusive (» = major clinical significance).

*Risk-benefit should be considered when the following medical problems exist:*

Anemia, severe
  (intravenous and oral ribavirin may cause anemia that is reversible when the drug is discontinued)
Hypersensitivity to ribavirin

## Patient monitoring
The following may be especially important in patient monitoring (other tests may be warranted in some patients, depending on condition; » = major clinical significance):

Hematocrit
  (hematocrit should be monitored periodically since intravenous and oral ribavirin may cause anemia)

# Side/Adverse Effects
Note: Although the manufacturer's literature includes a number of side effects, most studies indicate that ribavirin inhalation solution causes little or no systemic toxicity.

The following side/adverse effects have been selected on the basis of their potential clinical significance (possible signs and symptoms in parentheses where appropriate)—not necessarily inclusive:

## Those indicating need for medical attention
Incidence more frequent—intravenous and oral only
  *Anemia* (unusual tiredness or weakness)
Note: Anemia is reversible with discontinuation of ribavirin.

## Those indicating need for medical attention only if they continue or are bothersome
Incidence less frequent—intravenous and oral only
  *CNS effects* (fatigue; headache; insomnia)—usually with higher doses; *gastrointestinal effects* (anorexia; nausea)

Incidence rare—inhalation only
  *In patients*
    **Skin irritation due to prolonged drug contact; skin rash**
  *In healthcare worker*
    **Headache; itching, redness, or swelling of eye**

## Patient Consultation

As an aid to patient consultation, refer to *Advice for the Patient, Ribavirin (Systemic)*.

In providing consultation, consider emphasizing the following selected information (» = major clinical significance):

**Before using this medication**
» Conditions affecting use, especially:
  Pregnancy—Ribavirin is contraindicated during pregnancy. Female healthcare workers and visitors who are pregnant or may become pregnant may become environmentally exposed to ribavirin and should be advised of the potential risks of exposure

**Proper use of this medication**
» Importance of receiving medication for full course of therapy and on regular or continuous schedule
» Proper dosing

## General Dosing Information

Before using, become thoroughly familiar with the Viratek Small Particle Aerosol Generator (SPAG) Model SPAG-2 Operator's Manual for operating instructions.

According to the manufacturer, ribavirin inhalation solution should be administered using the Viratek SPAG Model SPAG-2 only. It should not be administered using any other aerosol-generating device. Ribavirin inhalation solution is usually administered using an infant oxygen hood attached to the SPAG-2 aerosol generator. However, administration by face mask may be necessary if an oxygen hood cannot be utilized (see SPAG-2 manual). With use of the recommended concentration (20 mg per mL) of ribavirin in the SPAG reservoir, the average ribavirin inhalation solution concentration over a 12-hour period is approximately 190 micrograms per liter of air.

Use of ribavirin inhalation solution in infants requiring mechanical ventilation should be undertaken only by health care workers familiar with this mode of administration and the specific ventilator being used. The dose for infants requiring mechanical ventilation is the same as for those who do not. Precipitation of ribavirin within the ventilator apparatus, including endotracheal tubes, may cause obstruction, resulting in increased positive end expiratory pressure and increased positive inspiratory pressure. Accumulation of fluid in the tubing ("rain out") has also been observed. To try to avoid this, instructions must be followed carefully. Either a pressure or volume cycle ventilator may be used in conjunction with the SPAG-2. Patients should have their endotracheal tubes suctioned every 1 to 2 hours, and their pulmonary pressures monitored frequently (every 2 to 4 hours). For both pressure and volume ventilators, heated wire connective tubing and bacteria filters in series in the expiratory limb of the system must be used to minimize the risk of ribavirin precipitation in the system and the subsequent risk of ventilator dysfunction. Bacteria filters must be changed frequently, i.e., every 4 hours. Water column pressure release valves should be used in the ventilator circuit for pressure cycled ventilators, and may be utilized with volume cycled ventilators. Refer to the SPAG-2 manual for detailed instructions.

Ribavirin aerosolization, using a small particle aerosol generator, produces particles of 1.2 to 1.6 microns (mass mean diameter) in size. Ribavirin inhalation solution has been administered by this method at the rate of 12.5 liters per minute via an infant oxygen hood or mask, tent, or tubing of a respirator. Using a ribavirin concentration of 20 mg per mL, this method delivers approximately 1.8 mg per kg of body weight (mg/kg) per hour in infants and children up to 6 years of age.

Although ribavirin inhalation solution has been administered using a tent, the volume of distribution and the condensation area are larger and the efficacy of this method has been evaluated in only a small number of patients.

Although ribavirin treatment may be initiated before the results of diagnostic tests are received, treatment should not be continued without laboratory confirmation of respiratory syncytial virus (RSV) infection.

Ribavirin inhalation solution treatment is generally effective when initiated within the first 3 days of RSV pneumonia. Early treatment may be necessary to achieve efficacy and to avoid further damage to the patient's lungs.

## Inhalation Dosage Forms

### RIBAVIRIN FOR INHALATION SOLUTION USP

**Usual adult and adolescent dose**
Respiratory syncytial virus (RSV) infection, lower respiratory tract—
Dosage has not been established.

**Usual pediatric dose**
Respiratory syncytial virus (RSV) infection, lower respiratory tract—
Oral inhalation, via a Viratek Small Particle Aerosol Generator (SPAG) Model SPAG-2 utilizing a 20-mg-per-mL ribavirin concentration in the reservoir, over a twelve- to eighteen-hour period per day for at least three to a maximum of seven days.

Note: Various ribavirin dosage regimens have been utilized in RSV pneumonia and other infections, including virtually continuous aerosolization for three to six days and aerosolization over a four-hour period three times a day for three days.

**Size(s) usually available**
U.S.—
  6 grams (Rx) [*Virazole*].
Canada—
  6 grams (Rx) [*Virazole*].

**Packaging and storage**
Prior to reconstitution, store between 15 and 25 °C (59 and 78 °F), in a dry place.

**Preparation of dosage form**
To prepare initial dilution for oral inhalation, add a measured quantity of sterile water for injection (without antimicrobial agents or other added substances) or sterile water for inhalation, sufficient for dissolution, to each 6-gram vial. Transfer the resulting solution to a clean, sterilized 500-mL wide-mouth Erlenmeyer flask (SPAG-2 reservoir). Further dilute the solution to a final volume of 300 mL with sterile water for injection or sterile water for inhalation to provide a final concentration of 20 mg per mL.

Prior to administration, visually inspect the final solution for particulate matter and discoloration.

When the solution level in the SPAG-2 reservoir is low, discard the remaining solution before adding freshly reconstituted solution to the reservoir.

**Stability**
The stability of ribavirin for inhalation solution (lyophilized powder) is unaffected by temperature, light, and moisture.

After reconstitution, solutions retain their potency at room temperature (20 to 30 °C [68 to 86 °F]) for 24 hours.

Ribavirin solutions are colorless.

**Incompatibilities**
Ribavirin for inhalation solution should not be administered concurrently with other medications administered by aerosolization.

## Oral Dosage Forms

Note: Bracketed uses in the *Dosage Forms* section refer to categories of use and/or indications that are not included in U.S. product labeling.

### RIBAVIRIN FOR ORAL SOLUTION

Note: Ribavirin for Inhalation Solution USP is the dosage form being used because an oral solution is not commercially available.

**Usual adult and adolescent dose**
[Lassa fever (prophylaxis)][1]—
Oral, 500 mg every six hours for seven to ten days.

**Usual pediatric dose**
Children 10 years of age and older—See *Usual adult and adolescent dose*.
Children 6 to 9 years of age—Oral, 400 mg every six hours for seven to ten days.
Children less than 6 years of age—Dosage has not been established.

**Strength(s) usually available**
U.S.—
  Dosage form not commercially available. Compounding required for prescription.
Canada—
  Dosage form not commercially available. Compounding required for prescription.

**Packaging and storage**
Prior to reconstitution, store between 15 and 25 °C (59 and 78 °F), in a dry place.

**Preparation of dosage form**
To prepare initial dilution for oral solution, add a measured quantity of sterile water for injection (without antimicrobial agents or other added substances) or sterile water for inhalation, sufficient for dissolution, to each 6-gram vial. Add dissolved solution to 0.9% sodium chloride or 5% dextrose in water.

**Stability**
The stability of ribavirin for inhalation solution (lyophilized powder) is unaffected by temperature, light, and moisture.

After reconstitution, solutions retain their potency at room temperature (20 to 30 °C [68 to 86 °F]) for 24 hours.
Ribavirin solutions are colorless.

## Parenteral Dosage Forms

Note: Bracketed uses in the *Dosage Forms* section refer to categories of use and/or indications that are not included in U.S. product labeling.

### RIBAVIRIN FOR INJECTION

Note: Ribavirin for Inhalation Solution USP is the dosage form being used because a parenteral solution is not commercially available.

**Usual adult and adolescent dose**
[Lassa fever (treatment)][1]—
Intravenous infusion, 30 mg per kg of body weight loading dose, then 16 mg per kg of body weight every six hours for four days, then 8 mg per kg of body weight every eight hours for six more days. Infuse over 15 to 20 minutes.

**Usual pediatric dose**
Dosage has not been established.

**Strength(s) usually available**
U.S.—
Dosage form not commercially available. Compounding required for prescription.
Canada—
Dosage form not commercially available. Compounding required for prescription.

**Packaging and storage**
Prior to reconstitution, store between 15 and 25 °C (59 and 78 °F), in a dry place.

**Preparation of dosage form**
To prepare initial dilution for parenteral use, add a measured quantity of sterile water for injection (without antimicrobial agents or other added substances) or sterile water for inhalation, sufficient for dissolution, to each 6-gram vial. Add to 0.9% sodium chloride or 5% dextrose in water and infuse over 15 to 20 minutes.

**Stability**
The stability of ribavirin for inhalation solution (lyophilized powder) is unaffected by temperature, light, and moisture.
After reconstitution, solutions retain their potency at room temperature (20 to 30 °C [68 to 86 °F]) for 24 hours.
Ribavirin solutions are colorless.

[1] Not included in Canadian product labeling.

## Selected Bibliography

McCormick JB, et al. Lassa fever-effective therapy with ribavirin. New Engl J Med 1986; 314(1): 20-6.
Frankel LR, Wilson CW, Demers RR, et al. A technique for the administration of ribavirin to mechanically ventilated infants with severe respiratory syncytial virus infection. Crit Care Med 1987; 15: 1051-4.
Outwater KM, Meissner HC, Peterson MB. Ribavirin administration to infants receiving mechanical ventilation. Am J Dis Child 1988; 142: 512-5.
Demers RR, Parker J, Frankel LR, et al. Administration of ribavirin to neonatal and pediatric patients during mechanical ventilation. Respir Care 1986; 31: 1188-96.

Revised: 02/23/93
Interim revision: 06/08/94

---

# RIBOFLAVIN Systemic

VA CLASSIFICATION (Primary): VT106
A commonly used name is vitamin B$_2$.
Note: For a listing of dosage forms and brand names by country availability, see *Dosage Forms* section(s).

## Category

Nutritional supplement (vitamin).
Note: Riboflavin (vitamin B$_2$) is a water-soluble vitamin.

## Indications

### Accepted

Riboflavin deficiency (prophylaxis and treatment)—Riboflavin is indicated for prevention and treatment of riboflavin deficiency states. Riboflavin deficiency may occur as a result of inadequate nutrition or intestinal malabsorption but does not occur in healthy individuals receiving an adequate balanced diet. Simple nutritional deficiency of individual B vitamins is rare since dietary inadequacy usually results in multiple deficiencies. For prophylaxis of riboflavin deficiency, dietary improvement, rather than supplementation, is advisable. For treatment of riboflavin deficiency, supplementation is preferred.

Deficiency of riboflavin (ariboflavinosis) may lead to angular stomatitis, cheilosis, corneal vascularization, and dermatoses. Severe deficiency may cause normocytic, normochromic anemia and neuropathy.

Requirements for riboflavin may be increased and/or supplementation may be necessary in the following persons or conditions (although clinical deficiencies are usually rare):
Burns
Fever, chronic
Gastrectomy
Hepatic-biliary tract disease—alcoholism with cirrhosis, obstructive jaundice
Hyperbilirubinemia in neonates as phototherapy due to photo-decomposition of riboflavin by blue light
Hyperthyroidism
Infection, prolonged
Intestinal disease—celiac, tropical sprue, regional enteritis, persistent diarrhea
Malignancy
Stress, prolonged

Recommended intakes for riboflavin are related to caloric intake.

Some unusual diets (e.g., reducing diets that drastically restrict food selection) may not supply minimum daily requirements of riboflavin. Supplementation is necessary in patients receiving total parenteral nutrition (TPN) or undergoing rapid weight loss or in those with malnutrition, because of inadequate dietary intake.

Recommended intakes for all vitamins and most minerals are increased during pregnancy. Many physicians recommend that pregnant women receive multivitamin and mineral supplements, especially those pregnant women who do not consume an adequate diet and those in high-risk categories (i.e., women carrying more than one fetus, heavy cigarette smokers, and alcohol and drug abusers). Taking excessive amounts of a multivitamin and mineral supplement may be harmful to the mother and/or fetus and should be avoided.

Recommended intakes for all vitamins and most minerals are increased during breast-feeding.

Recommended intakes may be increased by the following medications: Phenothiazines, tricyclic antidepressants, and probenecid.

### Unaccepted

Riboflavin has not been proven effective for treatment of acne, burning foot syndrome, congenital methemoglobinemia, migraine headaches, or muscle cramps.

## Pharmacology/Pharmacokinetics

**Physicochemical characteristics**
Molecular weight—376.37.
pKa—10.2.

**Mechanism of action/Effect**
Riboflavin is converted to 2 coenzymes, flavin mononucleotide (FMN) and flavin adenine dinucleotide (FAD), which are necessary for normal tissue respiration. Riboflavin is also required for activation of pyridoxine, conversion of tryptophan to niacin, and may be involved in maintaining erythrocyte integrity.

**Absorption**
The B vitamins are readily absorbed from the gastrointestinal tract, except in malabsorption syndromes. Riboflavin is absorbed mainly in the duodenum. Alcohol inhibits intestinal absorption of riboflavin.

**Protein binding**
Metabolites (FAD and FMN)—Moderate (60%).

**Storage**
Riboflavin and metabolites are distributed into all body tissues and breast milk. A small amount is stored in the liver, spleen, kidneys, and heart.

**Biotransformation**
Hepatic.

**Half-life**
Oral or intramuscular administration—66 to 84 minutes.

**Elimination**
Renal (almost entirely as metabolites). Excess beyond daily needs is excreted, largely unchanged, in urine. Riboflavin is present in the feces.
In dialysis—Hemodialysis removes riboflavin, but more slowly than normal renal excretion.

## Precautions to Consider

**Pregnancy/Reproduction**
Problems in humans have not been documented with intake of normal daily recommended amounts.

**Breast-feeding**
Problems in humans have not been documented with intake of normal daily recommended amounts.

**Pediatrics**
Problems in pediatrics have not been documented with intake of normal daily recommended amounts.

**Geriatrics**
Problems in geriatrics have not been documented with intake of normal daily recommended amounts.

**Drug interactions and/or related problems**
The following drug interactions and/or related problems have been selected on the basis of their potential clinical significance (possible mechanism in parentheses where appropriate)—not necessarily inclusive (» = major clinical significance):

Note: Combinations containing any of the following medications, depending on the amount present, may also interact with this medication.

Alcohol
(impairs intestinal absorption of riboflavin)

Antidepressants, tricyclic or
Phenothiazines
(requirements for riboflavin may be increased in patients receiving these medications)

Probenecid
(concurrent use decreases gastrointestinal absorption of riboflavin; requirements for riboflavin may be increased in patients receiving probenecid)

**Laboratory value alterations**
The following have been selected on the basis of their potential clinical significance (possible effect in parentheses where appropriate)—not necessarily inclusive (» = major clinical significance):

Note: Usually occurs only with large doses.

With diagnostic test results
Urinary catecholamine concentration measurements by fluorimetric methods
(riboflavin may produce fluorescent substances and falsely elevated results)

Urobilinogen determinations using Ehrlich's reagent
(riboflavin may produce false-positive results)

## Side/Adverse Effects

While toxicity with high doses of riboflavin has not been reported, high doses of other water-soluble vitamins have been known to cause problems.

Large doses of riboflavin may cause yellow discoloration of urine.

## Patient Consultation

As an aid to patient consultation, refer to *Advice for the Patient, Riboflavin (Vitamin B₂) (Systemic)*.

In providing consultation, consider emphasizing the following selected information (» = major clinical significance):

**Description of use**
Description should include function in the body, signs of deficiency, and unproven uses

**Importance of diet**
Importance of proper nutrition; supplement may be needed because of inadequate dietary intake
Food sources of riboflavin; effects of processing
Not using vitamins as substitute for balanced diet
Recommended daily intake for riboflavin

**Proper use of this dietary supplement**
» Proper dosing
Missed dose: No cause for concern because of length of time necessary for depletion; remembering to take as directed
» Proper storage

**Side/adverse effects**
Possible yellow discoloration of urine with large doses; no cause for concern

## General Dosing Information

Because of the infrequency of single B vitamin deficiencies, combinations are commonly administered. Many commercial combinations of B vitamins are available.

**Diet/Nutrition**
Recommended dietary intakes for riboflavin are defined differently worldwide.
For U.S.—
The Recommended Dietary Allowances (RDAs) for vitamins and minerals are determined by the Food and Nutrition Board of the National Research Council and are intended to provide adequate nutrition in most healthy persons under usual environmental stresses. In addition, a different designation may be used by the FDA for food and dietary supplement labeling purposes, as with Daily Value (DV). DVs replace the previous labeling terminology United States Recommended Daily Allowances (USRDAs).
For Canada—
Recommended Nutrient Intakes (RNIs) for vitamins, minerals, and protein are determined by Health and Welfare in Canada and provide recommended amounts of a specific nutrient while minimizing the risk of chronic diseases.

Daily recommended intakes for riboflavin are generally defined as follows:

| Persons | U.S. (mg) | Canada (mg) |
|---|---|---|
| Infants and children | | |
| Birth to 3 years of age | 0.4–0.8 | 0.3–0.7 |
| 4 to 6 years of age | 1.1 | 0.9 |
| 7 to 10 years of age | 1.2 | 1–1.3 |
| Adolescent and adult males | 1.4–1.8 | 1–1.6 |
| Adolescent and adult females | 1.2–1.3 | 1–1.1 |
| Pregnant females | 1.6 | 1.1–1.4 |
| Breast-feeding females | 1.7–1.8 | 1.4–1.5 |

These are ususally provided by adequate diets.

The best dietary sources of riboflavin include milk and dairy products, fish, meats, green leafy vegetables, and whole grain and enriched cereals and bread. There is little loss of riboflavin from foods with ordinary cooking.

## Oral Dosage Forms

### RIBOFLAVIN TABLETS USP

**Usual adult and adolescent dose**
Deficiency (prophylaxis)—
Oral, amount based on normal daily recommended intakes:

| Persons | U.S. (mg) | Canada (mg) |
|---|---|---|
| Adolescent and adult males | 1.4–1.8 | 1–1.6 |
| Adolescent and adult females | 1.2–1.3 | 1–1.1 |
| Pregnant females | 1.6 | 1.1–1.4 |
| Breast-feeding females | 1.7–1.8 | 1.4–1.5 |

Deficiency (treatment)—
Treatment dose is individualized by prescriber based on severity of deficiency.

**Usual pediatric dose**
Deficiency (prophylaxis)—
Oral, amount based on intake of normal daily recommended intakes:

| Persons | U.S. (mg) | Canada (mg) |
|---|---|---|
| Infants and children | | |
| Birth to 3 years of age | 0.4–0.8 | 0.3–0.7 |
| 4 to 6 years of age | 1.1 | 0.9 |
| 7 to 10 years of age | 1.2 | 1–1.3 |

Deficiency (treatment)—
Treatment dose is individualized by prescriber based on severity of deficiency.

**Strength(s) usually available**
U.S.—
  10 mg (OTC) [GENERIC].
  25 mg (OTC) [GENERIC].
  50 mg (OTC) [GENERIC].
  100 mg (OTC) [GENERIC].
  250 mg (OTC) [GENERIC].
Canada—
  5 mg (OTC) [GENERIC].
  100 mg (OTC) [GENERIC].

Note: Some strengths of these riboflavin preparations may exceed the dosage range recommended by USP DI Advisory Panels based on the amount necessary to meet normal nutritional needs.

**Packaging and storage**
Store below 40 °C (104 °F), preferably between 15 and 30 °C (59 and 86 °F), unless otherwise specified by manufacturer. Store in a tight, light-resistant container.

Revised: 08/22/92
Interim revision: 07/29/94; 05/01/95

## RICE SYRUP SOLIDS AND ELECTROLYTES—See
*Carbohydrates and Electrolytes (Systemic)*

# RIFABUTIN  Systemic

VA CLASSIFICATION (Primary): AM900
Commonly used brand name(s): *Mycobutin*.
Note: For a listing of dosage forms and brand names by country availability, see *Dosage Forms* section(s).

## Category
Antibacterial (antimycobacterial).

## Indications
**Accepted**
*Mycobacterium avium* complex (MAC) disease (prophylaxis)—Rifabutin is indicated for the prevention of disseminated MAC disease in patients with advanced human immunodeficiency virus (HIV) infection.

Rifabutin also has *in vitro* activity against many strains of *Mycobacterium tuberculosis*. However, there is no evidence that rifabutin is effective as a prophylactic agent for tuberculosis. Isoniazid and rifabutin may be given concurrently for the prophylaxis of tuberculosis and MAC, respectively. Cross-resistance between rifampin and rifabutin is commonly observed with *M. tuberculosis* and *M. avium* complex isolates that are highly resistant to rifampin.

## Pharmacology/Pharmacokinetics
**Physicochemical characteristics**
Molecular weight—847.02.

**Mechanism of action/Effect**
Rifabutin inhibits DNA-dependent RNA polymerase in susceptible strains of *Escherichia coli* and *Bacillus subtilis*, but not in mammalian cells. Rifabutin does not inhibit this enzyme in resistant strains of *E. coli*. It is not known whether rifabutin inhibits DNA-dependent RNA polymerase in *Mycobacterium avium* or in *M. intracellulare*, which constitute *M. avium* complex (MAC).

**Absorption**
Readily absorbed from the gastrointestinal tract. High-fat meals slow the rate, but not the extent, of absorption. Bioavailability is approximately 20%.

**Distribution**
Highly lipophilic; widely distributed with extensive intracellular tissue uptake. Rifabutin crosses the blood-brain barrier; cerebrospinal fluid (CSF) concentrations are approximately 50% of the corresponding serum concentration.

$Vol_D$ = Approximately 9 liters per kg.

**Protein binding**
High (approximately 85%).

**Biotransformation**
Hepatic; 5 metabolites have been identified.

**Half-life**
Mean terminal—45 hours (range, 16 to 69 hours).

**Time to peak concentration**
2 to 4 hours.

**Peak serum concentration**
375 nanograms per mL after a single oral dose of 300 mg in healthy volunteers.

**Elimination**
30% fecal; 5% unchanged in the urine; 5% unchanged in the bile; 53% in urine as metabolites.
In dialysis—Hemodialysis is not expected to enhance elimination.

## Precautions to Consider
**Cross-sensitivity and/or related problems**
Patients sensitive to other rifamycins (e.g., rifampin) may also be sensitive to rifabutin.

**Carcinogenicity**
Long-term carcinogenicity studies found that rifabutin was not carcinogenic in mice at doses of up to 180 mg per kg of body weight (mg/kg) per day, or approximately 36 times the recommended human daily dose. Rifabutin was not carcinogenic in rats at doses of up to 60 mg/kg per day, or 12 times the recommended human dose.

**Mutagenicity**
Rifabutin was not mutagenic in the Ames test using both rifabutin-susceptible and -resistant strains or in *Schizosaccharomyces pombe* $P_1$ and was not genotoxic in V-79 Chinese hamster cells, human lymphocytes *in vitro*, or mouse bone marrow cells *in vivo*.

**Pregnancy/Reproduction**
Fertility—Fertility was impaired in male rats given 160 mg/kg of rifabutin, or 32 times the recommended human daily dose.

Pregnancy—Adequate and well-controlled studies have not been done in humans.

No teratogenicity was seen in rats and rabbits given rifabutin at doses of up to 200 mg/kg (40 times the recommended human daily dose). There was a decrease in fetal viability in rats given 200 mg/kg per day. At 40 mg/kg per day, rifabutin caused an increase in rat fetal skeletal variants. In rabbits, rifabutin was maternotoxic and there was an increase in fetal skeletal anomalies at 80 mg/kg per day.

FDA Pregnancy Category B.

**Breast-feeding**
It is not known whether rifabutin is distributed into human breast milk.

**Pediatrics**
The safety and efficacy of rifabutin in the prophylaxis of *Mycobacterium avium* complex (MAC) in children have not been established. Limited data are available about the use of rifabutin in children; it was used, along with 2 other antimycobacterials, to treat MAC in 22 HIV-positive children. The mean doses used were 18.5 mg/kg in infants one year of age, 8.6 mg/kg in children 2 to 10 years of age, and 4 mg/kg in adolescents 14 to 16 years of age. Side effects seen in children were similar to those seen in adults.

**Geriatrics**
No information is available on the relationship of age to the effects of rifabutin in geriatric patients.

**Drug interactions and/or related problems**
The following drug interactions and/or related problems have been selected on the basis of their potential clinical significance (possible mechanism in parentheses where appropriate)—not necessarily inclusive (» = major clinical significance):

Note: Didanosine (ddI) and rifabutin coadministration has been studied in AIDS patients; rifabutin does not appear to affect the pharmacokinetics of didanosine and no dosage modifications are necessary.

  Combinations containing any of the following medications, depending on the amount present, may also interact with this medication.

Aminophylline or
Anticoagulants, coumarin- or indandione-derivative or
Antidiabetic agents, oral or
Barbiturates or
Beta-adrenergic blocking agents, systemic or
Chloramphenicol or

Clofibrate or
Contraceptives, estrogen-containing, oral or
Corticosteroids, glucocorticoid and mineralocorticoid or
Cyclosporine or
Dapsone or
Diazepam or
Digitalis glycosides or
Disopyramide or
Estramustine or
Estrogens or
Ketoconazole or
Mexiletine or
Oxtriphylline or
Phenytoin or
Quinidine or
Theophylline or
Tocainide or
Verapamil, oral
    (rifampin is structurally related to rifabutin; rifampin is known to reduce the activity of many drugs [including those listed above] due to its hepatic enzyme–inducing properties; rifabutin appears to be a less potent enzyme inducer of the hepatic cytochrome P-450 system than rifampin. Drug interaction data are unavailable for rifabutin itself; therefore, it is recommended that patients taking rifabutin concurrently with these medications be monitored since the significance of possible drug interactions is not known)

Fluconazole
    (pharmacokinetic studies with fluconazole and rifabutin show that fluconazole appears to increase the serum concentration of rifabutin; however, this is not thought to have clinical significance and rifabutin dosing does not need to be modified in patients receiving fluconazole; in addition, the pharmacokinetics of fluconazole were unchanged)

Methadone
    (concurrent administration with rifabutin has no significant effect on the pharmacokinetics of methadone; however, a few patients may require methadone dosage modification if symptoms of narcotic withdrawal occur)

» Zidovudine
    (steady-state plasma concentrations and the area under the plasma concentration-time curve [AUC] of zidovudine were decreased after repeated rifabutin dosing in healthy volunteers and HIV-positive patients in phase I trials; the mean decreases in peak plasma concentration and AUC were 48% and 32%, respectively. However, a population pharmacokinetic analysis of zidovudine concentration versus time data from two phase III studies showed a nonsignificant trend for rifabutin to increase the apparent clearance of zidovudine. *In vitro* studies have demonstrated that rifabutin does not affect the inhibition of HIV by zidovudine)

### Laboratory value alterations
The following have been selected on the basis of their potential clinical significance (possible effect in parentheses where appropriate)—not necessarily inclusive (» = major clinical significance):

With physiology/laboratory test values
Neutrophil count
    (rifabutin may cause neutropenia)
Platelet count
    (rifabutin may, in rare cases, cause thrombocytopenia)

### Medical considerations/Contraindications
The medical considerations/contraindications included have been selected on the basis of their potential clinical significance (reasons given in parentheses where appropriate)—not necessarily inclusive (» = major clinical significance).

***Except under special circumstances, this medication should not be used when the following medical problems exist:***
» Hypersensitivity to rifabutin or rifampin
» Tuberculosis, active
    (patients with active tuberculosis must be treated with an effective combination of antitubercular agents; administration of single-agent rifabutin for prophylaxis of MAC to patients with active tuberculosis is likely to lead to the development of tuberculosis that is resistant to both rifabutin and rifampin)

### Patient monitoring
The following may be especially important in patient monitoring (other tests may be warranted in some patients, depending on condition; » = major clinical significance):

Platelet count
White blood cell count
    (recommended periodically since rifabutin may cause neutropenia and, rarely, thrombocytopenia)

## Side/Adverse Effects
The following side/adverse effects have been selected on the basis of their potential clinical significance (possible signs and symptoms in parentheses where appropriate)—not necessarily inclusive:

### Those indicating need for medical attention
Incidence more frequent
    *Skin rash*
Incidence rare
    *Arthralgia* (joint pain); *dysgeusia* (change in taste); *myalgia* (muscle pain); *neutropenia* (fever and sore throat); *pseudojaundice* (yellow skin); *uveitis* (eye pain; loss of vision)
    Note: Uveitis is usually associated with doses larger than 1050 mg per day.

### Those indicating need for medical attention only if they continue or are bothersome
Incidence more frequent
    *Nausea; vomiting*

### Those not indicating need for medical attention
Incidence more frequent
    *Reddish orange to reddish brown discoloration of urine, feces, saliva, skin, sputum, sweat, and tears*
    Note: Tears discolored by rifabutin may also discolor soft contact lenses.

## Patient Consultation
As an aid to patient consultation, refer to *Advice for the Patient, Rifabutin (Systemic)*.
In providing consultation, consider emphasizing the following selected information (» = major clinical significance):

### Before using this medication
» Conditions affecting use, especially:
    Hypersensitivity to rifabutin or rifampin
    Other medications, especially zidovudine
    Other medical problems, especially active tuberculosis

### Proper use of this medication
Taking on an empty stomach, or with food if gastrointestinal irritation occurs
» Compliance with full course of therapy, which may take months
» Proper dosing
    Missed dose: Taking as soon as possible; not taking if almost time for next dose; not doubling doses
» Proper storage

### Precautions while using this medication
» Regular visits to physician to check progress
» Medication causes tears to turn reddish orange to reddish brown and may also permanently discolor soft contact lenses; avoiding the use of soft contact lenses during treatment

### Side/adverse effects
Signs of potential side effects, especially skin rash, arthralgia, dysgeusia, myalgia, neutropenia, pseudojaundice, and uveitis
Reddish orange to reddish brown discoloration of urine, stools, saliva, skin, sputum, sweat, and tears may be alarming to patient, although medically insignificant

## General Dosing Information
Rifabutin is absorbed more rapidly if taken on an empty stomach. However, if gastrointestinal irritation occurs, administering rifabutin at doses of 150 mg two times a day with food may help reduce stomach upset.
Contents of rifabutin capsules may be mixed with applesauce for patients who are unable to swallow the capsules.

## Oral Dosage Forms

### RIFABUTIN CAPSULES

#### Usual adult and adolescent dose
*Mycobacterium avium* complex (MAC) disease (prophylaxis)—
    Oral, 300 mg once a day, or 150 mg two times a day.

#### Usual pediatric dose
Dosage has not been established; however, MAC prophylaxis should follow recommendations similar to those for adults and adolescents. Limited data are available about the use of rifabutin in children; it has been used in the treatment of MAC in HIV-positive children. The mean doses

used were 18.5 mg per kg of body weight in infants one year of age, 8.6 mg per kg of body weight in children 2 to 10 years of age, and 4 mg per kg of body weight in adolescents 14 to 16 years of age. Side effects seen in children were similar to those seen in adults.

**Strength(s) usually available**
U.S.—
  150 mg (Rx) [*Mycobutin*].
Canada—
  150 mg (Rx) [*Mycobutin*].

**Packaging and storage**
Store between 15 and 30 °C (59 and 86 °F). Store in a tightly closed container.

**Auxiliary labeling**
- Continue medicine for full time of treatment.
- May discolor body fluids.

Revised: 06/22/94

# RIFAMPIN Systemic

INN: Rifampicin
VA CLASSIFICATION (Primary/Secondary): AM500/AM900
Commonly used brand name(s): *Rifadin; Rifadin IV; Rimactane; Rofact.*
Note: For a listing of dosage forms and brand names by country availability, see *Dosage Forms* section(s).

## Category
Antibacterial (antimycobacterial; antileprosy agent).

## Indications
Note: Bracketed information in the *Indications* section refers to uses that are not included in U.S. product labeling.

**General considerations**

Tuberculosis is a highly infectious life-threatening bacterial disease with 8 million new cases and 3 million deaths reported worldwide each year to the World Health Organization (WHO). The vast majority of these cases are in developing countries; however, tuberculosis also has emerged as an important public health problem in the U.S. in recent years after the decline in number of cases observed between 1950 and 1980.

The resurgence of tuberculosis in the U.S. has been complicated by an increase in the proportion of patients with strains resistant to antituberculosis medications. Outbreaks of multidrug-resistant tuberculosis have been documented in hospitals and prisons. Drug-resistant tuberculosis, particularly that caused by strains resistant to isoniazid and rifampin, is much harder to treat and often is fatal. Among acquired immunodeficiency syndrome (AIDS) patients infected with tuberculosis bacilli resistant to both rifampin and isoniazid, a case-fatality rate of 91% has been reported. Recent investigations of outbreaks of multidrug-resistant tuberculosis have found an extraordinarily high case-fatality rate, with the median time to mortality being reached between 4 and 16 weeks. In almost all instances, these outbreaks have involved patients with severe immunosuppression by infection with the human immunodeficiency virus (HIV).

Acquired drug resistance develops during treatment for drug-sensitive tuberculosis with regimens that are poorly conceived or poorly complied with, allowing the emergence of naturally occurring drug-resistant mutations. Resistant organisms from affected patients may subsequently infect other people who have not been infected with *M. tuberculosis* previously, resulting in primary drug resistance.

Resistance to antituberculosis agents can develop not only in the strain that caused the initial disease, but also as a result of reinfection with a new strain of *M. tuberculosis* that is drug-resistant. Reinfection with a new multidrug-resistant *M. tuberculosis* strain can occur during therapy for the original infection or after completion of therapy. Most recent data suggest that outcomes can be improved if patients promptly begin therapy with two or more drugs that have *in vitro* activity against the multidrug-resistant isolate.

HIV infection is the strongest risk factor yet identified for the development of active tuberculosis disease in persons infected with tuberculosis. In addition, persons with HIV infection are at an increased risk of tuberculosis resulting either from newly acquired disease or from reactivation of latent infections. Tuberculosis is a major clinical manifestation of immunodeficiency induced by HIV. In hospital-based retrospective studies, high rates of tuberculosis have been found among patients with AIDS. In communities where tuberculosis and HIV infection are common, the prevalence of HIV seropositivity among patients with tuberculosis is greatly increasing.

WHO has estimated that 5.6 million people worldwide and 80,000 people in the U.S. are infected with both HIV and tuberculosis. Persons dually infected with *M. tuberculosis* and HIV have a high risk of developing clinically active tuberculosis. One study of HIV-positive drug users with positive tuberculin skin test results found a rate of the development of active tuberculosis to be 8 cases per 100 person-years (8% yearly) as compared with the 10% lifetime risk (1 to 3% risk within the first year after skin test conversion) in the general population.

Persons who are known to be HIV-infected and who are contacts of patients with infectious tuberculosis should be carefully evaluated for evidence of tuberculosis. If there are no findings suggestive of current tuberculosis, preventive therapy with isoniazid should be given. Because HIV-infected contacts are not managed in the same way as those who are not HIV-infected, HIV testing is recommended if there are known or suspected risk factors for their acquiring HIV infection.

According to investigators at the National Institute of Allergy and Infectious Diseases (NIAID), levels of HIV in the bloodstream increase 5- to 160-fold in HIV-infected persons who develop active tuberculosis. Clinical and epidemiologic observations have demonstrated that HIV-infected individuals have an estimated 113-times higher risk and AIDS patients have a 170-times higher risk compared with uninfected persons. Furthermore, the problem of drug resistance may worsen as the HIV epidemic spreads. Immunosuppressed patients with HIV infection who subsequently become infected with *M. tuberculosis* have an extraordinarily high risk of developing active tuberculosis within a short period of time.

In addition to the convincing evidence that HIV infection increases the risk and worsens the course of tuberculosis, there is increasing clinical evidence that coinfection with *M. tuberculosis* accelerates progression of disease caused by HIV infection. Understanding the interaction of these two pathogens is clinically important, given the high prevalence of patients coinfected with HIV and *M. tuberculosis* in both the U.S. and Africa; it is estimated that by the year 2000 about 500,000 deaths per year will occur in coinfected patients worldwide.

Persons with a positive tuberculin skin test and HIV infection, and persons with a positive tuberculin skin test and at risk of acquiring HIV infection with unknown HIV status should be considered for tuberculosis preventive therapy regardless of age. One study showed that isoniazid prophylaxis in HIV-infected, tuberculin-positive individuals not only decreased the incidence of tuberculosis disease, but also delayed the progression to AIDS and death.

Twelve months of preventive therapy is recommended for adults and children with HIV infection and other conditions associated with immunosuppression. Persons with HIV infection should receive at least 6 months of preventive therapy. The American Academy of Pediatrics recommends that children receive 9 months of therapy.

Tuberculosis control programs should ensure that drug susceptibility tests are performed on all initial isolates of *M. tuberculosis* and the results are reported promptly to the primary care provider and the local health department. Tuberculosis control programs should monitor local drug resistance rates to assess the effectiveness of local tuberculosis control efforts and to determine the appropriateness of the currently recommended initial tuberculosis treatment regimen for the area.

Relapse of rifampin-resistant tuberculosis has been reported in HIV-infected patients. Reinfection with new strains of *M. tuberculosis* has also been reported in these patients. Rifampin-resistant tuberculosis is a serious threat because responses to therapy are more difficult to achieve and require long courses of treatment. Therefore, careful follow-up of HIV-infected patients with treated tuberculosis is essential.

Multidrug-resistant tuberculosis also has been transmitted to persons without HIV infection in health care facilities. Together with the lack of effective agents for second-line treatment and methods of prophylaxis, the transmission of multidrug-resistant strains of *M. tuberculosis* may create a substantial reservoir of latently infected people and the potential for clinical multidrug-resistant tuberculosis for many years to come.

Several studies have documented a high prevalence of extrapulmonary disease in HIV-infected patients with clinical tuberculosis disease, particularly in conjunction with pulmonary manifestations. Cutaneous miliary tuberculosis, also known as *tuberculosis cutis miliaris disseminata*, was in the past a rare condition in adults, with only 24 cases reported in nearly a century. However, since the first reported case of cutaneous miliary tuberculosis in 1990 in a patient with AIDS, five additional cases have been reported in HIV-infected patients. Its appearance can be quite nondescript; therefore, a high level of suspicion must be maintained, particularly for patients with CD4+ cell counts of < 200 per cubic millimeter, in order to diagnose the condition and initiate therapy appropriately.

**Accepted**

Tuberculosis (treatment)—Rifampin is indicated in combination with other antituberculosis medications in the treatment of all forms of tuberculosis, including tuberculous meningitis.

Meningococcal infections (prophylaxis)—Rifampin is indicated in the treatment of close contacts of patients with proved or suspected infection caused by *Neisseria meningitidis*. These contacts include other household members, children in nurseries, persons in day care centers, and closed populations, such as military recruits. Health care providers who have intimate exposure (e.g., mouth-to-mouth resuscitation) with index cases also should receive prophylactic therapy.

[*Haemophilus influenzae* type b infection (prophylaxis)][1]—Rifampin is used in the treatment of close contacts of patients with proved or suspected infections caused by *H. influenzae* type b if at least one of the contacts is 4 years of age or younger. A close contact is defined as one who has spent 4 or more hours per day for 5 of the 7 most recent days with the index case.

[Leprosy (treatment)][1]—Rifampin is used in combination with other agents in the treatment of leprosy (Hansen's disease).

[Mycobacterial infections, atypical (treatment)][1]—Rifampin is used in combination with other agents in the treatment of certain atypical (nontuberculous) mycobacterial infections, such as those caused by *Mycobacterium avium* complex (MAC).

[Rifampin, administered concurrently with other antistaphylococcal agents, also may be used in the treatment of serious infections caused by *Staphylococcus* species (including methicillin-resistant and multidrug-resistant strains)][1].

**Unaccepted**

Rifampin is not indicated as a sole agent in the treatment of meningococcal infections because of the possibility of the rapid emergence of resistant organisms.

---

[1]Not included in Canadian product labeling.

## Pharmacology/Pharmacokinetics

Note: Preliminary data suggest that patients coinfected with human immunodeficiency virus (HIV) and mycobacteria (*Mycobacterium tuberculosis* or *M. avium*) have altered pharmacokinetic profiles for antimycobacterial drugs. In particular, malabsorption of these agents appears to occur frequently, and could seriously affect the efficacy of treatment.

**Physicochemical characteristics**
Molecular weight—822.96.

**Mechanism of action/Effect**
Rifampin, a semisynthetic broad-spectrum bactericidal antibiotic, inhibits bacterial RNA synthesis by binding strongly to the beta subunit of DNA-dependent RNA polymerase, preventing attachment of the enzyme to DNA, and thus blocking initiation of RNA transcription.

**Absorption**
Well absorbed from the gastrointestinal tract.

**Distribution**
Diffuses well to most body tissues and fluids, including the cerebrospinal fluid (CSF), where concentrations are increased if the meninges are inflamed; concentrations in the liver, gallbladder, bile, and urine are higher than those found in the blood; therapeutic concentrations are achieved in the saliva, reaching 20% of serum concentrations; crosses the placenta, with fetal serum concentrations at birth found to be approximately 33% of the maternal serum concentration; penetrates into aqueous humor; and is distributed into breast milk. Being lipid-soluble, rifampin may reach and kill susceptible intracellular, as well as extracellular, bacteria including *Mycobacteria* species.

Vol$_D$—1.6 L per kg.

**Protein binding**
High to very high (89%).

**Biotransformation**
Hepatic; rapidly deacetylated by auto-induced microsomal oxidative enzymes to active metabolite (25-*O*-desacetylrifampin). Other identified metabolites include rifampin quinone, desacetyl rifampin quinone, and 3-formylrifampin.

**Half-life**
Absorption half-life—
 Approximately 0.6 hour.
Elimination half-life—
 Initially, 3 to 5 hours; with repeated administration, half-life decreases to 2 to 3 hours.

**Time to peak concentration**
1.5 to 4 hours after oral administration; peak concentration may be decreased and delayed following administration with food.

**Peak plasma concentration**
Oral—
 Adults: 7 to 9 mcg/mL after a dose of 600 mg.
 Children (6 to 58 months old): Approximately 11 mcg/mL after a dose of 10 mg per kg of body weight (mg/kg) mixed in applesauce or simple syrup.
Intravenous—
 Adults: Approximately 17.5 mcg/mL after a 30 minute infusion of 600 mg.
 Children (3 months to 12 years old): Approximately 26 mcg/mL after a 30 minute infusion of 300 mg per square meter.

**Elimination**
Biliary/fecal; enterohepatic recirculation of rifampin, but not of its deacetylated active metabolite; 60 to 65% of dose appears in feces.
Renal: 6 to 15% excreted as unchanged drug, and 15% excreted as active metabolite in urine; 7% excreted as inactive 3-formyl derivative.
Rifampin does not accumulate in patients with impaired renal function; its rate of excretion is increased during the first 6 to 10 days of therapy, probably because of auto-induction of hepatic microsomal oxidative enzymes; after high doses, excretion may be slower because of saturation of its biliary excretory mechanism.
 In dialysis—Rifampin is not removed from the blood by either hemodialysis or peritoneal dialysis.

## Precautions to Consider

**Tumorigenicity**
Studies in female mice of a strain known to be particularly susceptible to the spontaneous development of hepatomas have shown that rifampin, given in doses of 2 to 10 times the maximum human dose for 1 year, causes a significant increase in the development of hepatomas. However, studies in male mice of the same strain, in other strains of male or female mice, or in rats have not shown that rifampin is tumorigenic.

**Pregnancy/Reproduction**
Note: Tuberculosis in pregnancy should be managed in concert with an expert in the management of tuberculosis. Women who have only pulmonary tuberculosis are not likely to infect the fetus until after delivery, and congenital tuberculosis is extremely rare. *In utero* infections with tubercle bacilli, however, can occur after maternal bacillemia occurs at different stages in the course of tuberculosis. Miliary tuberculosis can seed the placenta and thereby gain access to the fetal circulation. In women with tuberculous endometritis, transmission of infection to the fetus can result from fetal aspiration of bacilli at the time of delivery. A third mode of transmission is through ingestion of infected amniotic fluid *in utero*.

If active disease is diagnosed during pregnancy, a 9-month regimen of isoniazid and rifampin, supplemented by an initial course of ethambutol if drug resistance is suspected, is recommended. Pyrazinamide usually is not given because of inadequate data regarding teratogenesis. Hence, a 9-month course of therapy is necessary for drug-susceptible disease. When isoniazid resistance is a possibility, isoniazid, ethambutol, and rifampin are recommended initially. One of these medications can be discontinued after 1 or 2 months, depending on results of susceptibility tests. If rifampin or isoniazid is discontinued, treatment is continued for a total of 18 months; if ethambutol is discontinued, treatment is continued for a total of 9 months. Prompt initiation of chemotherapy is mandatory to protect both the mother and fetus. If isoniazid or rifampin resistance is documented, an expert in the management of tuberculosis should be consulted.

Asymptomatic pregnant women with positive tuberculin skin tests and normal chest radiographs should receive preventive therapy with isoniazid for 9 months if they are HIV seropositive or have recently been in contact with an infectious person. For these individuals, preventive therapy should begin after the first trimester. In other circumstances in which none of these risk factors is present, although no harmful effects of isoniazid to the fetus have been observed, preventive therapy can be delayed until after delivery.

For all pregnant women receiving isoniazid, pyridoxine should be prescribed. Isoniazid, ethambutol, and rifampin appear to be relatively safe for the fetus. The benefit of ethambutol and rifampin for therapy of active disease in the mother outweighs the risk to the infant. Streptomycin and pyrazinamide should not be used unless they are essential to the control of the disease.

Pregnancy—Rifampin crosses the placenta. It has rarely caused postnatal hemorrhages in the mother and infant when administered during the last few weeks of pregnancy; vitamin K may be indicated. Neonates should be carefully observed for evidence of adverse effects.

Imperfect osteogenesis and embryotoxicity were reported in rabbits given up to 20 times the usual daily human dose. Studies in rodents have shown that rifampin given in doses of 150 to 250 mg per kg of body weight (mg/kg) daily causes congenital malformations, primarily cleft palate and spina bifida.

FDA Pregnancy Category C.

### Breast-feeding
Rifampin is distributed into breast milk. Problems in humans have not been documented.

### Pediatrics
Note: If an infant is suspected of having congenital tuberculosis, a Mantoux tuberculin skin test, chest radiograph, lumbar puncture, and appropriate cultures should be performed promptly. Regardless of the skin test results, treatment of the infant should be initiated promptly with isoniazid, rifampin, pyrazinamide, and streptomycin or kanamycin. In addition, the mother should be evaluated for the presence of pulmonary or extrapulmonary (including uterine) tuberculosis. If the physical examination or chest radiograph support the diagnosis of tuberculosis, the patient should be treated with the same regimen as that used for tuberculous meningitis. The drug susceptibilities of the organism recovered from the mother and/or infant should be determined.

Possible isoniazid resistance should always be considered, particularly in children from population groups in which drug resistance is high, especially in foreign-born children from countries with a high prevalence of drug-resistant tuberculosis. For contacts who are likely to have been infected by an index case with isoniazid-resistant but rifampin-susceptible organisms, and in whom the consequences of the infection are likely to be severe (e.g., children up to 4 years of age), rifampin (10 mg per kg of body weight, maximum 600 mg, given daily in a single dose) should be given in addition to isoniazid (10 mg per kg, maximum 300 mg, given daily in a single dose) until susceptibility test results for the isolate from the index case are available. If the index case is known or proven to be excreting organisms resistant to isoniazid, then isoniazid should be discontinued and rifampin given for a total of 9 months. Isoniazid alone should be given if no proof of exposure to isoniazid-resistant organisms is found. Optimal therapy for children with tuberculosis infection caused by organisms resistant to isoniazid and rifampin is unknown. In deciding on therapy in this situation, consultation with an expert is advised.

Adjuvant treatment with corticosteroids in treating tuberculosis is controversial. Corticosteroids have been used for therapy in children with tuberculous meningitis to reduce vasculitis, inflammation, and, as a result, intracranial pressure. Data indicate that dexamethasone may lower mortality rates and lessen long-term neurologic impairment. The administration of corticosteroids should be considered in all children with tuberculous meningitis, and also may be considered in children with pleural and pericardial effusions (to hasten reabsorption of fluid), severe miliary disease (to mitigate alveolocapillary block), and endobronchial disease (to relieve obstruction and atelectasis). Corticosteroids should be given only when accompanied by appropriate antituberculosis therapy. Consultation with an expert in the treatment of tuberculosis should be obtained when corticosteroid therapy is considered.

Appropriate studies performed to date have not demonstrated pediatrics-specific problems that would limit the usefulness of rifampin in children.

### Geriatrics
Appropriate studies on the relationship of age to the effects of rifampin have not been performed in the geriatric population. However, no geriatrics-specific problems have been documented to date.

### Dental
The leukopenic and thrombocytopenic effects of rifampin may result in an increased incidence of certain microbial infections, delayed healing, and gingival bleeding. If leukopenia or thrombocytopenia occurs, dental work should be deferred until blood counts have returned to normal. Patients should be instructed in proper oral hygiene, including caution in use of regular toothbrushes, dental floss, and toothpicks.

Rifampin may cause a hypersensitivity reaction of sore mouth or tongue.

### Drug interactions and/or related problems
The following drug interactions and/or related problems have been selected on the basis of their potential clinical significance (possible mechanism in parentheses where appropriate)—not necessarily inclusive (» = major clinical significance):

Note: Combinations containing any of the following medications, depending on the amount present, may also interact with this medication.

» Alcohol
(concurrent daily consumption of alcohol may increase the risk of rifampin-induced hepatotoxicity and increased metabolism of rifampin; dosage adjustments of rifampin may be necessary, and patients should be monitored closely for signs of hepatotoxicity)

» Aminophylline or
» Oxtriphylline or
» Theophylline
(rifampin may increase metabolism of theophylline, oxtriphylline, and aminophylline by induction of hepatic microsomal enzymes, resulting in increased theophylline clearance)

Anesthetics, hydrocarbon inhalation, except isoflurane
(chronic use of hepatic enzyme–inducing agents prior to anesthesia, except isoflurane, may increase anesthetic metabolism, leading to increased risk of hepatotoxicity)

» Anticoagulants, coumarin- or indandione-derivative
(concurrent use with rifampin may enhance the metabolism of these anticoagulants by induction of hepatic microsomal enzymes, resulting in a considerable decrease in the activity and effectiveness of the anticoagulants; prothrombin time determinations may be required as frequently as once a day; dosage adjustments of anticoagulants may be required before and after rifampin therapy)

» Antidiabetic agents, oral
(concurrent use with rifampin may enhance the metabolism of tolbutamide, chlorpropamide, and glyburide by induction of hepatic microsomal enzymes, resulting in lower serum sulfonylurea concentrations; although not documented, other oral antidiabetic agents may also interact with rifampin; dosage adjustment may be required)

» Azole antifungals
(concurrent use may increase the metabolism of the azole antifungals, lowering their plasma concentrations; depending on the clinical situation, the dose of an azole antifungal may need to be increased during concurrent use with rifampin)

Barbiturates
(concurrent use with rifampin may enhance the metabolism of hexobarbital by induction of hepatic microsomal enzymes, resulting in lower serum concentrations; there are conflicting data on rifampin's effect on phenobarbital; dosage adjustment may be required)

Beta-adrenergic blocking agents, systemic
(concurrent use of metoprolol or propranolol with rifampin has resulted in reduced plasma concentrations of these two beta-adrenergic blocking agents due to enhanced metabolism of hepatic microsomal enzymes by rifampin; although not documented, other beta-adrenergic blocking agents may also interact with rifampin)

Bone marrow depressants (see *Appendix II* )
(concurrent use of bone marrow depressants with rifampin may increase the leukopenic and/or thrombocytopenic effects; if concurrent use is required, close observation for myelotoxic effects should be considered)

» Chloramphenicol
(concurrent use with rifampin may enhance the metabolism of chloramphenicol by induction of hepatic microsomal enzymes, resulting in significantly lower serum chloramphenicol concentrations; dosage adjustment may be necessary)

Clofazimine
(concurrent use with rifampin has resulted in reduced absorption of rifampin, delaying its time to peak concentration, and increasing its half-life)

Clofibrate
(concurrent use with rifampin may enhance the metabolism of clofibrate by induction of hepatic microsomal enzymes, resulting in significantly lower serum clofibrate concentrations)

» Contraceptives, estrogen-containing, oral
(concurrent use with rifampin may decrease the effectiveness of estrogen-containing oral contraceptives because of stimulation of estrogen metabolism or reduction in enterohepatic circulation of estrogens, resulting in menstrual irregularities, intermenstrual

bleeding, and unplanned pregnancies; patients should be advised to use an additional method of contraception throughout the whole cycle while taking rifampin and estrogen-containing oral contraceptives concurrently)

» Corticosteroids, glucocorticoid and mineralocorticoid
(concurrent use with rifampin may enhance the metabolism of corticosteroids by induction of hepatic microsomal enzymes, resulting in a considerable decrease in corticosteroid plasma concentrations; dosage adjustment may be required; rifampin has also counteracted endogenous cortisol and produced acute adrenal insufficiency in patients with Addison's disease)

Cyclosporine
(rifampin may enhance metabolism of cyclosporine by induction of hepatic microsomal enzymes and intestinal cytochrome P450 enzymes; dosage adjustment may be required)

Dapsone
(concurrent use with rifampin may decrease the effect of dapsone because of increased metabolism resulting from stimulation of hepatic microsomal enzyme activity; dapsone concentrations may be decreased by half; dapsone dosage adjustments are not required during concurrent therapy with rifampin for leprosy)

Diazepam
(concurrent use with rifampin may enhance the elimination of diazepam, resulting in decreased plasma concentrations; whether this effect applies to other benzodiazepines has not been determined; dosage adjustment may be necessary)

» Digitalis glycosides
(concurrent use with rifampin may enhance the metabolism of digoxin or digitoxin by induction of hepatic microsomal enzymes, resulting in significantly lower serum digoxin or digitoxin concentrations; dosage adjustment may be necessary)

» Disopyramide or
» Mexiletine or
Propafenone or
» Quinidine or
» Tocainide
(concurrent use with rifampin may enhance the metabolism of these antiarrhythmics by induction of hepatic microsomal enzymes, resulting in significantly lower serum antiarrhythmic concentrations; serum antiarrhythmic concentrations should be monitored and dosage adjustment may be necessary)

» Estramustine or
» Estrogens
(concurrent use of estramustine or estrogens with rifampin may result in significantly reduced estrogenic effect because of stimulation of estrogen metabolism or reduction in enterohepatic circulation of estrogens)

» Hepatotoxic medications, other (see *Appendix II*)
(concurrent use of rifampin and other hepatotoxic medications may increase the potential for hepatotoxicity; patients should be monitored closely for signs of hepatotoxicity)

» Human immunodeficiency virus (HIV) protease inhibitors
(rifampin accelerates the metabolism of protease inhibitors, such as indinavir, nelfinavir, ritonavir, and saquinavir through induction of hepatic P450 cytochrome oxidases, resulting in subtherapeutic levels of the protease inhibitors; in addition, protease inhibitors retard the metabolism of rifampin, resulting in increased serum levels of rifampin and the likelihood of increased toxicity; concurrent use of HIV protease inhibitors with rifampin is not recommended)

» Isoniazid
(concurrent use of isoniazid with rifampin may increase the risk of hepatotoxicity, especially in patients with pre-existing hepatic function impairment and/or in fast acetylators of isoniazid; patients should be monitored closely for signs of hepatotoxicity during the first 3 months of therapy)

» Methadone
(concurrent use with rifampin may decrease the effects of methadone because of stimulation of hepatic microsomal enzyme activity and/or impaired absorption, resulting in symptoms of methadone withdrawal if the patient is dependent on methadone; dosage adjustments may be necessary during and after rifampin therapy)

» Phenytoin
(concurrent use with rifampin may stimulate the hepatic metabolism of phenytoin, increasing its elimination and thus counteracting its anticonvulsant effects; careful monitoring of serum hydantoin concentrations and dosage adjustments may be necessary before and after rifampin therapy)

Probenecid
(may compete with rifampin for hepatic uptake when used concurrently, resulting in increased and more prolonged rifampin serum concentrations and/or toxicity; however, the effect on rifampin serum concentrations is inconsistent, and concurrent use of probenecid to increase rifampin serum concentrations is not recommended)

Trimethoprim
(concurrent use with rifampin may significantly increase the elimination and shorten the elimination half-life of trimethoprim)

» Verapamil, oral
(rifampin has been found to accelerate the metabolism of oral verapamil, resulting in a significant decrease in serum verapamil concentration and reversing its cardiovascular effects; concurrent use of intravenous verapamil with rifampin was found to have only minor effects on verapamil's clearance and no significant effect on cardiovascular effects)

## Laboratory value alterations
The following have been selected on the basis of their potential clinical significance (possible effect in parentheses where appropriate)—not necessarily inclusive (» = major clinical significance):

With diagnostic test results
Coombs' (antiglobulin) tests, direct
(may become positive rarely during rifampin therapy)

Dexamethasone suppression test
(rifampin may prevent the inhibitory action of a standard dexamethasone dose administered for the overnight suppression test, rendering the test abnormal; it is recommended that rifampin therapy be discontinued 15 days before the dexamethasone suppression test is administered)

Folate determinations, serum and
Vitamin $B_{12}$ determinations, serum
(therapeutic concentrations of rifampin may interfere with standard microbiological assays for serum folate and vitamin $B_{12}$; alternative methods must be considered when determining serum folate and vitamin $B_{12}$ concentrations in patients taking rifampin)

Sulfobromophthalein (BSP) uptake and excretion
(hepatic uptake and excretion of BSP in liver function tests may be delayed by rifampin, resulting in BSP retention; the BSP test should be performed prior to the daily dose of rifampin to avoid false-positive test results)

Urinalyses based on spectrometry or color reaction
(rifampin may interfere with urinalyses that are based on spectrometry or color reaction due to rifampin's reddish-orange to reddish-brown discoloration of urine)

With physiology/laboratory test values
Alanine aminotransferase (ALT [SGPT]) and
Alkaline phosphatase and
Aspartate aminotransferase (AST [SGOT])
(values may be increased)

Bilirubin, serum and
Blood urea nitrogen (BUN) and
Uric acid, serum
(concentrations may be increased)

## Medical considerations/Contraindications
The medical considerations/contraindications included have been selected on the basis of their potential clinical significance (reasons given in parentheses where appropriate)—not necessarily inclusive (» = major clinical significance).

*Risk-benefit should be considered when the following medical problems exist:*
» Alcoholism, active or in remission or
» Hepatic function impairment
(rifampin is metabolized in the liver and may also be hepatotoxic)
Hypersensitivity to rifampin

## Patient monitoring
The following may be especially important in patient monitoring (other tests may be warranted in some patients, depending on condition; » = major clinical significance):

» Hepatic function determinations
(ALT [SGPT], AST [SGOT], alkaline phosphatase, and serum bilirubin determinations may be indicated prior to and monthly or more frequently during treatment; however, elevated serum enzyme values may not be predictive of clinical hepatitis and may return to normal despite continued treatment

## Side/Adverse Effects

Note: Intermittent use of rifampin may increase the chance of a patient developing the "flu-like" syndrome, as well as acute hemolysis or renal failure. These reactions are thought to be immunologically mediated and intermittent use should be limited to those conditions, such as leprosy, in which its safety and efficacy have been established.

The following side/adverse effects have been selected on the basis of their potential clinical significance (possible signs and symptoms in parentheses where appropriate)—not necessarily inclusive:

**Those indicating need for medical attention**
Incidence less frequent
*"Flu-like" syndrome* (chills; difficult breathing; dizziness; fever; headache; muscle and bone pain; shivering); *hypersensitivity* (itching; redness; skin rash)
Incidence rare
*Blood dyscrasias* (sore throat; unusual bleeding or bruising); *hepatitis* (yellow eyes or skin); *hepatitis prodromal symptoms* (loss of appetite; nausea or vomiting; unusual tiredness or weakness); *interstitial nephritis* (bloody or cloudy urine, greatly decreased frequency of urination or amount of urine)

**Those indicating need for medical attention only if they continue or are bothersome**
Incidence more frequent
*Gastrointestinal disturbances* (diarrhea; stomach cramps)
Incidence less frequent
*Fungal overgrowth* (sore mouth or tongue)

**Those not indicating need for medical attention**
Incidence more frequent
*Reddish-orange to reddish-brown discoloration of urine, feces, saliva, sputum, sweat, and tears*
Note: Tears discolored by rifampin may also discolor soft contact lenses.

## Overdose

The information below applies to the clinical effects and treatment of rifampin overdose.

**Clinical effects of rifampin overdose**
The following effects have been selected on the basis of their potential clinical significance (possible signs and symptoms in parentheses where appropriate)—not necessarily inclusive:
Acute and chronic effects
*Mental obtundation* (mental changes); *periorbital or facial edema* (swelling around the eyes or the whole face); *pruritus, generalized* (itching over the whole body); *Redman syndrome* (red-orange discoloration of skin, mucous membranes, and sclera)
Note: Fatalities are more likely to occur if there is underlying hepatic disease, frequent use or abuse of alcohol, or concurrent intake of other hepatotoxic medications.

**Treatment of rifampin overdose**
To decrease absorption—
Evacuating stomach contents using ipecac syrup or gastric lavage.
Administering an activated charcoal slurry to help adsorb residual rifampin in the gastrointestinal tract.
Supportive care—
Supportive therapy.

## Patient Consultation

As an aid to patient consultation, refer to *Advice for the Patient, Rifampin (Systemic)*.
In providing consultation, consider emphasizing the following selected information (» = major clinical significance):

**Before using this medication**
» Conditions affecting use, especially:
Hypersensitivity to rifampin
Pregnancy—Rifampin crosses the placenta and has rarely caused post-natal hemorrhages in the mother and infant when administered during the last few weeks of pregnancy
Breast-feeding—Rifampin is distributed into breast milk
Dental—Patients who develop blood dyscrasias may be at increased risk of microbial infections, delayed healing, and gingival bleeding
Other medications, especially aminophylline, azole antifungals, corticosteroids, coumarin- or indandione-derivative anticoagulants, oral antidiabetic agents, chloramphenicol, estrogen-containing oral contraceptives, digitalis glycosides, disopyramide, estramustine, estrogens, hepatotoxic medications, HIV protease inhibitors, isoniazid, methadone, mexiletine, oxtriphylline, phenytoin, quinidine, tocainide, theophylline, or oral verapamil
Other medical problems, especially alcoholism, active or in remission, or impairment of hepatic function

**Proper use of this medication**
Taking with a full glass (240 mL) of water on an empty stomach, 1 hour before or 2 hours after a meal, or with food if gastrointestinal irritation occurs
Proper administration technique for patients unable to swallow capsules
» Compliance with full course of therapy, which may take months or years to complete
» Proper dosing
Missed dose: Taking as soon as possible; not taking if almost time for next dose; not doubling doses; intermittent dosing may result in more frequent and/or severe side effects
» Proper storage

**Precautions while using this medication**
» Regular visits to physician to check progress
Checking with physician if no improvement within 2 to 3 weeks
» Using an alternative method of contraception if taking estrogen-containing oral contraceptives concurrently
» Avoiding alcoholic beverages concurrently with this medication
» Need to report prodromal signs of hepatotoxicity to physician
» Medication causes urine, feces, saliva, sputum, sweat, and tears to turn reddish-orange to reddish-brown and may also permanently discolor soft contact lenses; avoiding the wearing of soft contact lenses
Using caution in use of regular toothbrushes, dental floss, and toothpicks; deferring dental work until blood counts have returned to normal; checking with physician or dentist concerning proper oral hygiene
Possible interference with laboratory values

**Side/adverse effects**
Reddish-orange to reddish-brown discoloration of urine, stools, saliva, sputum, sweat, and tears may be alarming to patient, although medically insignificant; however, tears discolored by rifampin may also discolor soft contact lenses
Signs of potential side effects, especially "flu-like" syndrome, hypersensitivity, blood dyscrasias, hepatitis, hepatitis prodromal symptoms, and interstitial nephritis

## General Dosing Information

Rifampin preferably should be taken with a full glass (240 mL) of water on an empty stomach (either 1 hour before or 2 hours after a meal) to obtain optimum absorption. However, it may be taken with food if gastrointestinal irritation occurs.

Contents of rifampin capsules may be mixed with applesauce or jelly for patients who are unable to swallow the capsules.

Since bacterial resistance may develop rapidly when rifampin is administered alone in the treatment of tuberculosis, it should be administered only concurrently with other antituberculosis medications.

The duration of treatment with an antituberculosis regimen is at least 6 months and may be continued for to 2 years. Uncomplicated pulmonary tuberculosis is often successfully treated within 6 to 12 months. Several different treatment regimens are currently recommended.

The duration of antituberculosis therapy is based on the patient's clinical and radiographic responses, smear and culture results, and susceptibility studies of *Mycobacterium tuberculosis* isolates from the patient or the suspect source case. With directly observed therapy (DOT), clinical evaluation is an integral component of each visit for administration of medication. Careful monitoring of the clinical and bacteriologic responses to therapy on a monthly basis in sputum-positive patients is important.

If therapy is interrupted, the treatment schedule should be extended to a later completion date. Although guidelines cannot be provided for every situation, the following factors need to be considered in establishing a new date for completion:
• The length of interruption;
• The time during therapy (early or late) in which interruption occurred; and
• The patient's clinical, radiographic, and bacteriologic status before, during, and after interruption. Consultation with an expert is advised.

Therapy should be administered based on the following guidelines, published by the American Thoracic Society (ATS) and by the Centers for Disease Control and Prevention (CDC), and endorsed by the American Academy of Pediatrics (AAP).
• A 6-month regimen consisting of isoniazid, rifampin, and pyrazinamide given for 2 months followed by isoniazid and rifampin for 4

months is the preferred treatment for patients infected with fully susceptible organisms who adhere to the treatment course.
- Ethambutol (or streptomycin in children too young to be monitored for visual acuity) should be included in the initial regimen until the results of drug susceptibility studies are available, and unless there is little possibility of drug resistance (i.e., there is less than 4% primary resistance to isoniazid in the community, and the patient has had no previous treatment with antituberculosis medications, is not from a country with a high prevalence of drug resistance, and has no known exposure to a drug-resistant case).
- Alternatively, a 9-month regimen of isoniazid and rifampin is acceptable for persons who cannot or should not take pyrazinamide. Ethambutol (or streptomycin in children too young to be monitored for visual acuity) should also be included until the results of drug susceptibility studies are available, unless there is little possibility of drug resistance. If isoniazid resistance is demonstrated, rifampin and ethambutol should be continued for a minimum of 12 months.
- Consideration should be given to treating all patients with DOT. DOT programs have been demonstrated to increase adherence in patients receiving antituberculosis chemotherapy in both rural and urban settings.
- Multidrug-resistant tuberculosis (i.e., resistance to at least isoniazid and rifampin) presents difficult treatment problems. Treatment must be individualized and based on susceptibility studies. In such cases, consultation with an expert in tuberculosis is recommended.
- Children should be managed in essentially the same ways as adults, but doses of the medications must be adjusted appropriately and specific important differences between the management of adults and children addressed. However, optimal therapy of tuberculosis in children with HIV infection has not been established. The Committee on Infectious Diseases of the AAP recommends that therapy always should include at least three drugs initially, and should be continued for a minimum period of 9 months. Isoniazid, rifampin, and pyrazinamide with or without ethambutol or an aminoglycoside should be given for at least the first 2 months. A fourth drug may be needed for disseminated disease and whenever drug-resistant disease is suspected.
- Extrapulmonary tuberculosis should be managed according to the principles and with the drug regimens outlined for pulmonary tuberculosis, except in children who have miliary tuberculosis, bone/joint tuberculosis, or tuberculous meningitis. These children should receive a minimum of 12 months of therapy.
- A 4-month regimen of isoniazid and rifampin is acceptable therapy for adults who have active tuberculosis and who are sputum smear– and culture–negative, if there is little possibility of drug resistance.

ATS, CDC, and AAP recommend preventive treatment of tuberculosis infection in the following patients:
- Preventive therapy with isoniazid given for 6 to 12 months is effective in decreasing the risk of future tuberculosis disease in adults and children with tuberculosis infection demonstrated by a positive tuberculin skin test reaction.
- Persons with a positive skin test and any of the following risk factors should be considered for preventive therapy regardless of age:
  —Persons with HIV infection.
  —Persons at risk for HIV infection with unknown HIV status.
  —Close contacts of sputum-positive persons with newly diagnosed infectious tuberculosis.
  —Newly infected persons (recent skin test convertors).
  —Persons with medical conditions reported to increase the risk of tuberculosis (i.e., diabetes mellitus, corticosteroid therapy and other immunosuppressive therapy, intravenous drug users, hematologic and reticuloendothelial malignancies, end-stage renal disease, and clinical conditions associated with rapid weight loss or chronic malnutrition).

In some circumstances, persons with negative skin tests should be considered for preventive therapy. These include children who are close contacts of infectious tuberculosis cases and anergic HIV-infected adults at increased risk of tuberculosis, tuberculin-positive adults with abnormal chest radiographs showing fibrotic lesions probably representing old healed tuberculosis, adults with silicosis, and persons who are known to be HIV-infected and who are contacts of patients with infectious tuberculosis.
- In the absence of any of the above risk factors, persons up to 35 years of age with a positive skin test who are in the following high-incidence groups should be also considered for preventive therapy:
  —Foreign-born persons from high-prevalence countries.
  —Medically underserved low-income persons from high-prevalence populations (especially blacks, Hispanics, and Native Americans).
  —Residents of facilities for long-term care (e.g., correctional institutions, nursing homes, and mental institutions).

- Twelve months of preventive therapy is recommended for adults and children with HIV infection and other conditions associated with immunosuppression. Persons without HIV infection should receive preventive therapy for at least 6 months.
- In persons younger than 35 years of age, routine monitoring for adverse effects of isoniazid should consist of a monthly symptom review. For persons 35 years of age and older, hepatic enzymes should be measured prior to starting isoniazid and monitored monthly throughout treatment, in addition to monthly symptom reviews.
- Persons who are presumed to be infected with isoniazid-resistant organisms should be treated with rifampin rather than with isoniazid.
- As with the treatment of active tuberculosis, the key to success of preventive treatment is patient adherence to the prescribed regimen. Although not evaluated in clinical studies, directly observed, twice-weekly preventive therapy may be appropriate for adults and children at risk, who cannot or will not reliably self-administer therapy.

Protease inhibitors interact with rifamycin derivatives, such as rifampin and rifabutin, which are used to treat and prevent the mycobacterial infections commonly observed in HIV-infected patients. Rifamycins accelerate the metabolism of protease inhibitors through induction of hepatic cytochrome P450 oxidases, resulting in subtherapeutic levels of the protease inhibitors. In addition, protease inhibitors retard the metabolism of rifamycins, resulting in increased serum levels of rifamycins and the likelihood of increased drug toxicity.

Rifampin is an essential component of the currently recommended regimen for treating tuberculosis. This regimen is effective in treating HIV-infected patients with tuberculosis, and consists of isoniazid and rifampin for a minimum period of 6 months, plus pyrazinamide and either ethambutol or streptomycin for the first 2 months. Therefore, information concerning the pharmacokinetic interactions between protease inhibitors and rifampin is important for health care workers involved in tuberculosis control and the care of patients coinfected with tuberculosis and HIV, because clinicians may decrease or restrict the use of rifampin in the treatment of patients who are candidates for therapy with both protease inhibitors and rifampin.

Because of the common association of tuberculosis with HIV infection, an increasing number of patients probably will be considered candidates for combined therapy with rifampin and protease inhibitors. Prompt initiation of appropriate pharmacologic therapy for patients with HIV infection who acquire tuberculosis is critical because tuberculosis may become rapidly fatal. The management of these patients is complex, requires an individualized approach, and should be undertaken only by or in consultation with an expert. In addition, all HIV-infected patients at risk for tuberculosis infection should be carefully evaluated and administered isoniazid preventive treatment if indicated, regardless of whether they are receiving protease inhibitor therapy.

For HIV-infected patients diagnosed with drug-susceptible tuberculosis and for whom protease inhibitor therapy is being considered but has not been initiated, the suggested management strategy is to complete tuberculosis treatment with a regimen containing rifampin before starting therapy with a protease inhibitor. The duration of antituberculosis regimen is at least 6 months, and therapy should be administered according to the guidelines developed by ATS and CDC, including the recommendation to carefully assess clinical and bacteriologic responses in patients coinfected with HIV and to prolong treatment if response is slow or suboptimal.

There are three options for managing HIV-infected patients with tuberculosis who are undergoing protease inhibitor therapy when tuberculosis is diagnosed. Option I is discontinuation of therapy with the protease inhibitor while a tuberculosis treatment regimen that includes rifampin is followed. However, because that interruption in the administration of the prescribed protease inhibitor can induce HIV resistance to the protease inhibitor and possibly to other medications within the protease inhibitor class, and because discontinuation of the protease inhibitor therapy may be detrimental to the patient's clinical status, some clinicians may be reluctant to discontinue protease inhibitor therapy for the duration of tuberculosis treatment. In such cases, option II and option III may be considered. Because the risks and benefits of all of these options are unknown, clinicians should make management decisions on a case-by-case basis to provide optimal patient care.
- Option I. This option involves discontinuing therapy with the protease inhibitor and completing a short (minimum 6 months) course of tuberculosis treatment with a regimen containing rifampin. The anti-tuberculosis regimen should be administered according to the guidelines developed by ATS and CDC, and the duration of therapy should be prolonged in patients with slow or suboptimal responses. Protease inhibitor therapy may be resumed when treatment with rifampin is discontinued. Antiretroviral agents other than protease inhibitors may be used concurrently with rifampin. Although the risks associated with complete discontinuation of protease inhibitor therapy during tuberculosis treat-

ment are unclear, they may be serious; however, the risks and complications associated with tuberculosis treatment regimens that do not include rifampin are known. Potential consequences include prolonged duration of therapy to at least 18 to 24 months, increased likelihood of treatment failure and mortality, slower conversion of sputum culture to negative with patients remaining infectious for longer periods of time, and the adverse effect of tuberculous disease on the progression of HIV infection. Therefore, antituberculosis treatment regimens without rifampin are not recommended for the treatment of rifampin-susceptible tuberculosis.

• Option II. To minimize the interruption of protease inhibitor therapy, one option is to use a four-drug tuberculosis treatment regimen that includes rifampin (i.e., daily isoniazid, pyrazinamide, rifampin, and ethambutol or streptomycin) for a minimum of 2 months, and until bacteriologic response is achieved (i.e., sputum conversion to culture-negative status) and the results from the susceptibility testing are available. After bacteriologic response and drug susceptibility have been documented (usually 3 months), treatment may be modified to a 16-month continuation-phase regimen consisting of isoniazid (15 mg per kg of body weight) and ethambutol (50 mg per kg of body weight) two times per week. This regimen allows the reintroduction of protease inhibitor therapy. Some experts recommend adding a third agent, such as streptomycin, during this continuation phase if the infecting organism is not resistant to the agent. Option II cannot be recommended for patients with proven isoniazid-resistant tuberculosis.

• Option III. Another management option is to continue protease inhibitor therapy with indinavir (800 mg every 8 hours) and administer a four-drug, 9-month tuberculosis treatment regimen containing daily rifabutin (150 mg a day) instead of rifampin. When this option is used for tuberculosis management, clinicians should conduct careful monitoring, possibly including measurement of serum concentrations of rifabutin. This alternative tuberculosis therapy is recommended based on the pharmacokinetic characteristics of rifabutin and limited data from clinical trials. Rifabutin is a rifamycin derivative with comparable antituberculosis activity *in vitro*, but with less hepatic cytochrome P450 enzyme–inducing effect than rifampin. An international multicenter study indicated that a 6-month regimen containing rifabutin at a daily dose of either 150 or 300 mg is as effective in treating tuberculosis as a similar regimen containing rifampin. In a small clinical trial, a rifabutin-containing regimen was effective in treating tuberculosis in patients coinfected with HIV. In addition, limited data from pharmacokinetic studies suggest that the combination of rifabutin 150 mg a day and indinavir resulted in acceptable levels of both agents. Option III cannot be recommended for patients undergoing therapy with ritonavir or saquinavir. For these patients, the decision to change the prescribed protease inhibitor to indinavir and to prescribe rifabutin for tuberculosis therapy should be made in consultation with an expert in the use of protease inhibitors to manage HIV infection.

Neither option II nor option III has been studied in large clinical trials of HIV-infected patients or patients undergoing protease inhibitor therapy during tuberculosis treatment. For these reasons, if either of these options is selected for managing patients with tuberculosis, CDC recommends the following interim guidelines until additional data are available and formal guidelines are issued:

• On initiation of therapy, frequent bacteriologic evaluations should be performed to document sputum conversion to culture-negative status, and after culture conversion, to detect any possible treatment failures.
• The duration of therapy should be extended to at least 18 months for option II or 9 months for option III.
• Only indinavir should be used with option III.
• Monitoring for drug toxicity should be performed carefully.
• DOT should be used throughout treatment.
• During the first 2 years after completion of therapy, periodic evaluation should be performed (including an assessment of bacteriologic status at 6 months), and patients should be instructed to report symptoms indicating relapse of tuberculous disease promptly.

HIV-infected patients diagnosed with drug-resistant tuberculosis or diagnosed clinically with tuberculosis but without culture and susceptibility test results should be evaluated on a case-by-case basis and managed in consultation with a tuberculosis expert.

Most infants ≤ 12 months of age with tuberculosis are asymptomatic at the time of diagnosis, and the gastric aspirate cultures in these patients have a high yield for *M. tuberculosis*. When an infant is suspected of having tuberculosis, a thorough household investigation should be undertaken. A 6-month regimen of isoniazid and rifampin supplemented during the first 2 months by pyrazinamide has been found to be well-tolerated and effective in infants with pulmonary tuberculosis. Furthermore, twice-weekly DOT appears to be as effective as daily therapy, and is an essential alternative in patients for whom social issues prevent reliable daily therapy.

Physicians caring for children should be familiar with the clinical forms of the disease in infants to enable them to make an early diagnosis. Any child, especially one in a high-risk group or area, who has unexplained pneumonia, cervical adenitis, bone or joint infections, or aseptic meningitis should have a Mantoux tuberculin skin test performed, and a detailed epidemiologic history for tuberculosis should be obtained.

Management of a newborn infant whose mother, or other household contact, is suspected of having tuberculosis is based on individual considerations. If possible, separation of the mother, or contact, and infant should be minimized. The Committee on Infectious Diseases of the AAP offers the following recommendations in the management of the newborn infant whose mother, or any other household contact, has tuberculosis:

• *Mother, or any other household contact, with a positive tuberculin skin test reaction but no evidence of current disease:* Investigation of other members of the household or extended family to whom the infant may later be exposed is indicated. If no evidence of current disease is found in the mother or in members of the extended family, the infant should be tested with a Mantoux tuberculin skin test at 3 to 4 months of age. When the family members cannot be promptly tested, consideration should be given to administering isoniazid (10 mg per kg of body weight a day) to the infant until skin testing and other evaluation of the family members have excluded contact with a case of active tuberculosis. The infant does not need to be hospitalized during this time if adequate follow-up can be arranged, but adherence to medication administration should be closely monitored. The mother also should be considered for isoniazid therapy.

• *Mother with untreated (newly diagnosed) disease or disease that has been treated for 2 or more weeks and who is judged to be noncontagious at delivery:* Careful investigation of household members and extended family is mandatory. A chest radiograph and Mantoux tuberculin skin test should be performed on the infant at 3 to 4 months and at 6 months of age. Separation of the mother and infant is not necessary if adherence to treatment for the mother and infant is assured. The mother can breast-feed. The infant should receive isoniazid even if the tuberculin skin test and chest radiograph do not suggest clinical tuberculosis, since cell-mediated immunity of a degree sufficient to mount a significant reaction to tuberculin skin testing may develop as late as 6 months of age in an infant infected at birth. Isoniazid can be discontinued if the Mantoux skin test is negative at 3 to 4 months of age, the mother is adherent to treatment and has a satisfactory clinical response, and no other family members have infectious tuberculosis. The infant should be examined carefully at monthly intervals. If nonadherence is documented, the mother has an acid-fast bacillus (AFB)–positive sputum or smear, and supervision is impossible, the infant should be separated from the ill family member and Bacillus Calmette-Guérin (BCG) vaccine may be considered for the infant. However, the response to the vaccine in infants may be delayed and inadequate for prevention of tuberculosis.

• *Mother has current disease and is suspected of having been contagious at the time of delivery:* The mother and infant should be separated until the infant is receiving therapy or the mother is confirmed to be noncontagious. Otherwise, management is the same as when the disease is judged to be noncontagious to the infant at delivery.

• *Mother has hematogenously spread tuberculosis (e.g., meningitis, miliary disease, or bone involvement):* The infant should be evaluated for congenital tuberculosis. If clinical and radiographic findings do not support the diagnosis of congenital tuberculosis, the infant should be separated from the mother until she is judged to be noncontagious. The infant should be given isoniazid until 3 or 4 months of age, at which time the Mantoux skin test should be repeated. If the skin test is positive, isoniazid should be continued for a total of 12 months. If the skin test is negative and the chest radiograph is normal, isoniazid may be discontinued, depending on the status of the mother and whether there are other cases of infectious tuberculosis in the family. The infant should continue to be examined carefully at monthly intervals.

Health care or correctional institutions experiencing outbreaks of tuberculosis that are resistant to isoniazid and rifampin, or that are resuming therapy for a patient with a prior history of antitubercular therapy, may need to begin five- or six-drug regimens as initial therapy. These regimens should include the four-drug regimen and at least three medications to which the suspected multi-drug-resistant strain may be susceptible.

Side effects may be more frequent and/or severe with intermittent administration (600 mg once or twice weekly).

Patients with severe hepatic function impairment usually require a 50% reduction in dose of rifampin.

Patients with renal function impairment do not require a reduction in dose. In addition, rifampin plasma concentrations are not significantly altered in patients with decreased glomerular filtration rates (GFR) or in anuric patients.

## Oral Dosage Forms

Note: Bracketed uses in the *Dosage Forms* section refer to categories of use and/or indications that are not included in U.S. product labeling.

### RIFAMPIN CAPSULES USP

**Usual adult and adolescent dose**
Tuberculosis—
    In combination with other antituberculosis medications: Oral, 600 mg once a day for the entire treatment period; or 10 mg per kg of body weight, up to 600 mg, two or three times a week, depending on the treatment regimen.
Meningococcal infection (prophylaxis)—
    Oral, 600 mg once a day for four days.
[*Haemophilus influenzae* infection (prophylaxis)][1]—
    Oral, 600 mg once a day for four days.
[Leprosy][1]—
    In combination with other antileprosy agents:
    For multibacillary leprosy—Oral, 600 mg once a month for a minimum of two years or until smear is negative, whichever is longer.
    For paucilbacillary leprosy—Oral, 600 mg once a month for a minimum of six months.
Note: Debilitated patients—Oral, 10 mg per kg of body weight once a day.

**Usual adult prescribing limits**
600 mg daily.

**Usual pediatric dose**
Infants up to 1 month of age—
    Tuberculosis: In combination with other antituberculosis medications—Oral, 10 to 20 mg per kg of body weight once a day; or 10 to 20 mg per kg of body weight, two or three times a week, depending on the treatment regimen.
    Meningococcal infection (prophylaxis)—
    Oral, 5 mg per kg of body weight every twelve hours for two days.
    [*Haemophilus influenzae* infection (prophylaxis)][1]—
    Oral, 10 mg per kg of body weight once a day for four days.
Children 1 month of age and over—
    Tuberculosis: In combination with other antituberculosis medications—Oral, 10 to 20 mg per kg of body weight, up to 600 mg, once a day; or 10 to 20 mg per kg of body weight, up to 600 mg, two or three times a week, depending on the treatment regimen.
    Meningococcal infection (prophylaxis): Oral, 10 mg per kg of body weight every twelve hours for two days.
    [*Haemophilus influenzae* infection (prophylaxis)][1]—
    Oral, 20 mg per kg of body weight once a day for four days.
Note: The maximum daily dose should not exceed 600 mg.

**Usual geriatric dose**
Tuberculosis—
    Oral, 10 mg per kg of body weight once a day.

**Strength(s) usually available**
U.S.—
    150 mg (Rx) [*Rifadin*].
    300 mg (Rx) [*Rifadin; Rimactane;* GENERIC].
Canada—
    150 mg (Rx) [*Rifadin; Rimactane; Rofact*].
    300 mg (Rx) [*Rifadin; Rimactane; Rofact*].

**Packaging and storage**
Store below 40 °C (104 °F). Store in a tight, light-resistant container.

**Auxiliary labeling**
• Continue medicine for full time of treatment.
• Avoid alcoholic beverages.
• May discolor body fluids.

**Note**
Contents of the capsules may also be mixed with applesauce or jelly.

### RIFAMPIN ORAL SUSPENSION USP

**Usual adult and adolescent dose**
See *Rifampin Capsules USP*.

**Usual adult prescribing limits**
600 mg daily.

**Usual pediatric dose**
See *Rifampin Capsules USP*.
Note: The maximum daily dose should not exceed 600 mg.

**Usual geriatric dose**
See *Rifampin Capsules USP*.

**Strength(s) usually available**
U.S.—
    Not commercially available. Compounding required for prescription.
Canada—
    Not commercially available. Compounding required for prescription.

**Packaging and storage**
Preserve in a tight, light-resistant glass or plastic prescription bottle, with a child-resistant closure. Store at controlled room temperature.

**Preparation of dosage form**
Rifampin oral suspension is compounded as follows:
    Rifampin .................................................... 1.2 grams
    Syrup, a sufficient quantity to make ............................ 120 mL
Transfer 1.2 grams of rifampin, or the contents of rifampin capsules, into a mortar. If necessary, gently crush the capsule contents with a pestle to produce a fine powder. Add about 2 mL of syrup to the mortar, and triturate until a smooth paste is formed. Add about 10 mL of syrup, and triturate to form a suspension. Continue to add syrup, until about 80 mL has been added. Transfer this suspension to a 120-mL precalibrated light-resistant glass or plastic prescription bottle. Rinse the mortar and pestle with successive small portions of syrup, and add the rinses to the bottle. Shake vigorously. If necessary, add citric acid or sodium citrate to adjust to a pH of 5. Add a suitable flavor if desired. Add sufficient syrup to make the product measure 120 mL, and shake vigorously.

**Stability**
Rifampin suspension compounded for oral use should be discarded 30 days after the day on which it was compounded.

**Auxiliary labeling**
• Continue medicine for full time of treatment.
• Avoid alcoholic beverages.
• May discolor body fluids.
• Shake well before using.

## Parenteral Dosage Forms

Note: Bracketed uses in the *Dosage Forms* section refer to categories of use and/or indications that are not included in U.S. product labeling.

### RIFAMPIN FOR INJECTION USP

**Usual adult and adolescent dose**
Tuberculosis—
    In combination with other antituberculosis medications: Intravenous, 600 mg once a day for the entire treatment period; or 10 mg per kg of body weight, up to 600 mg, two or three times a week, depending on the treatment regimen.
Meningococcal infection (prophylaxis)—
    Intravenous, 600 mg two times a day for two days.
[Leprosy]—
    In combination with other antileprosy agents: Intravenous, 600 mg once a month for a minimum of two years or until smear is negative, whichever is longer.
Note: Debilitated patients—Intravenous, 10 mg per kg of body weight once a day.

**Usual adult prescribing limits**
600 mg daily.

**Usual pediatric dose**
Infants up to 1 month of age—
    Tuberculosis: In combination with other antituberculosis medications—Intravenous, 10 to 20 mg per kg of body weight once a day; or 10 to 20 mg per kg of body weight two or three times a week, depending on the treatment regimen.
    Meningococcal infection (prophylaxis): Intravenous, 5 mg per kg of body weight every twelve hours for two days.
Children 1 month of age and over—
    Tuberculosis: In combination with other antituberculosis medications—Intravenous, 10 to 20 mg per kg of body weight, up to 600 mg, once a day; or 10 to 20 mg per kg of body weight, up to 600 mg, two or three times a week, depending on the treatment regimen.
    Meningococcal infection (prophylaxis): Intravenous, 10 mg per kg of body weight every twelve hours for two days.
Note: The maximum daily dose should not exceed 600 mg.

**Usual geriatric dose**
Tuberculosis: Intravenous, 10 mg per kg of body weight once a day.

**Strength(s) usually available**
U.S.—
    600 mg (Rx) [*Rifadin IV*].
Canada—
    Not commercially available.

**Packaging and storage**
Store below 40 °C (104 °F). Store in a tight, light-resistant container.

### Preparation of dosage form
To prepare for initial dilution for intravenous use, 10 mL of sterile water for injection should be added to each 600-mg vial. Vial should be gently swirled to completely dissolve the rifampin.

For intermittent infusion, the calculated amount of reconstituted rifampin to be administered should be added to 500 mL of 5% dextrose in water and infused over 3 hours. In some cases, the calculated amount of rifampin may be added to 100 mL of 5% dextrose in water and infused over 30 minutes.

### Stability
5% dextrose in water is the recommended infusion medium. Sterile saline may be used; however, this slightly reduces the stability of rifampin. Other solutions are not recommended.

After reconstitution, the solution of 60 mg per mL is stable at room temperature for 24 hours. After dilution in 100 or 500 mL, solutions are also stable at room temperature for 24 hours.

[1]Not included in Canadian product labeling.

## Selected Bibliography
The American Thoracic Society (ATS). Ad Hoc Committee on the Scientific Assembly on Microbology, Tuberculosis, and Pulmonary Infections. Treatment of tuberculosis and tuberculosis infection in adults and children. Clin Infect Dis 1995; 21: 9-27

Revised: 08/22/97
Interim revision: 08/12/98

# RIFAMPIN AND ISONIAZID  Systemic

INN: Rifampin—Rifampicin
VA CLASSIFICATION (Primary): AM500
NOTE: The *Rifampin and Isoniazid (Systemic)* monograph is maintained on the USP DI electronic data base. For a printed copy of the most recent revision of the complete monograph, contact Micromedex, Inc. - Reprint Requests, 6200 S. Syracuse Way, Suite 300, Englewood, CO 80111; telephone (303) 486-6400; telefax (303) 486-6464; Email: USPDI@MDX.COM.

For information on the specific components of this combination, see the *USP DI* monographs for *Isoniazid (Systemic)* and *Rifampin (Systemic)*.

The information that follows is selectively abstracted from the complete monograph and is provided to facilitate drug use review and patient counseling.

Note: For a listing of dosage forms and brand names by country availability, see *Dosage Forms* section(s).

## Category
Antibacterial (antimycobacterial).

## Indications

### General considerations
Tuberculosis is a highly infectious life-threatening bacterial disease with 8 million new cases and 3 million deaths reported worldwide each year to the World Health Organization (WHO). The vast majority of these cases are in developing countries; however, tuberculosis also has emerged as an important public health problem in the U.S. in recent years after the decline in number of cases observed between 1950 and 1980.

The resurgence of tuberculosis in the U.S. has been complicated by an increase in the proportion of patients with strains resistant to antituberculosis medications. Outbreaks of multidrug-resistant tuberculosis have been documented in hospitals and prisons. Drug-resistant tuberculosis, particularly that caused by strains resistant to isoniazid and rifampin, is much harder to treat and often is fatal. Among acquired immunodeficiency syndrome (AIDS) patients infected with tuberculosis bacilli resistant to both rifampin and isoniazid, a case-fatality rate of 91% has been reported. Recent investigations of outbreaks of multidrug-resistant tuberculosis have found an extraordinarily high case-fatality rate, with the median time to mortality being reached between 4 and 16 weeks. In almost all instances, these outbreaks have involved patients with severe immunosuppression by infection with the human immunodeficiency virus (HIV).

Acquired drug resistance develops during treatment for drug-sensitive tuberculosis with regimens that are poorly conceived or poorly complied with, allowing the emergence of naturally occurring drug-resistant mutations. Resistant organisms from affected patients may subsequently infect other people who have not been infected with *M. tuberculosis* previously, resulting in primary drug resistance.

Resistance to antituberculosis agents can develop not only in the strain that caused the initial disease, but also as a result of reinfection with a new strain of *M. tuberculosis* that is drug-resistant. Reinfection with a new multidrug-resistant *M. tuberculosis* strain can occur during therapy for the original infection or after completion of therapy. Most recent data suggest that outcomes can be improved if patients promptly begin therapy with two or more drugs that have *in vitro* activity against the multidrug-resistant isolate.

HIV infection is the strongest risk factor yet identified for the development of active tuberculosis disease in persons infected with tuberculosis. In addition, persons with HIV infection are at an increased risk of tuberculosis resulting either from newly acquired disease or from reactivation of latent infections. Tuberculosis is a major clinical manifestation of immunodeficiency induced by HIV. In hospital-based retrospective studies, high rates of tuberculosis have been found among patients with AIDS. In communities where tuberculosis and HIV infection are common, the prevalence of HIV seropositivity among patients with tuberculosis is greatly increasing.

WHO has estimated that 5.6 million people worldwide and 80,000 people in the U.S. are infected with both HIV and tuberculosis. Persons dually infected with *M. tuberculosis* and HIV have a high risk of developing clinically active tuberculosis. One study of HIV-positive drug users with positive tuberculin skin test results found a rate of the development of active tuberculosis to be 8 cases per 100 person-years (8% yearly) as compared with the 10% lifetime risk (1 to 3% risk within the first year after skin test conversion) in the general population.

Persons who are known to be HIV-infected and who are contacts of patients with infectious tuberculosis should be carefully evaluated for evidence of tuberculosis. If there are no findings suggestive of current tuberculosis, preventive therapy with isoniazid should be given. Because HIV-infected contacts are not managed in the same way as those who are not HIV-infected, HIV testing is recommended if there are known or suspected risk factors for their acquiring HIV infection.

According to investigators at the National Institute of Allergy and Infectious Diseases (NIAID), levels of HIV in the bloodstream increase 5- to 160-fold in HIV-infected persons who develop active tuberculosis. Clinical and epidemiologic observations have demonstrated that HIV-infected individuals have an estimated 113-times higher risk and AIDS patients have a 170-times higher risk as compared with uninfected persons. Furthermore, the problem of drug resistance may worsen as the HIV epidemic spreads. Immunosuppressed patients with HIV infection who subsequently become infected with *M. tuberculosis* have an extraordinarily high risk of developing active tuberculosis within a short period of time.

In addition to the convincing evidence that HIV infection increases the risk and worsens the course of tuberculosis, there is increasing clinical evidence that coinfection with *M. tuberculosis* accelerates progression of disease caused by HIV infection. Understanding the interaction of these two pathogens is clinically important, given the high prevalence of patients coinfected with HIV and *M. tuberculosis* in both the U.S. and Africa; it is estimated that by the year 2000 about 500,000 deaths per year will occur in coinfected patients worldwide.

Persons with a positive tuberculin skin test and HIV infection, and persons with a positive tuberculin skin test and at risk of acquiring HIV infection with unknown HIV status should be considered for tuberculosis preventive therapy regardless of age. One study showed that isoniazid prophylaxis in HIV-infected, tuberculin-positive individuals not only decreased the incidence of tuberculosis disease, but also delayed the progression to AIDS and death.

Twelve months of preventive therapy is recommended for adults and children with HIV infection and other conditions associated with immunosuppression. Persons with HIV infection should receive at least 6 months of preventive therapy. The American Academy of Pediatrics recommends that children receive 9 months of therapy.

Tuberculosis control programs should ensure that drug susceptibility tests are performed on all initial isolates of *M. tuberculosis* and the results are reported promptly to the primary care provider and the local health department. Tuberculosis control programs should monitor local drug resistance rates to assess the effectiveness of local tuberculosis control efforts and to determine the appropriateness of the currently recommended initial tuberculosis treatment regimen for the area.

Relapse of rifampin-resistant tuberculosis has been reported in HIV-infected patients. Reinfection with new strains of *M. tuberculosis* has also been reported in these patients. Rifampin-resistant tuberculosis is a serious threat because responses to therapy are more difficult to achieve and require long courses of treatment. Therefore, careful follow-up of HIV-infected patients with treated tuberculosis is essential.

Multidrug-resistant tuberculosis also has been transmitted to persons without HIV infection in health care facilities. Together with the lack of effective agents for second-line treatment and methods of prophylaxis, the transmission of multidrug-resistant strains of *M. tuberculosis* may create a substantial reservoir of latently infected people and the potential for clinical multidrug-resistant tuberculosis for many years to come.

Several studies have documented a high prevalence of extrapulmonary disease in HIV-infected patients with clinical tuberculosis disease, particularly in conjunction with pulmonary manifestations. Cutaneous miliary tuberculosis, also known as *tuberculosis cutis miliaris disseminata*, was in the past a rare condition in adults, with only 24 cases reported in nearly a century. However, since the first reported case of cutaneous miliary tuberculosis in 1990 in a patient with AIDS, five additional cases have been reported in HIV-infected patients. Its appearance can be quite nondescript; therefore, a high level of suspicion must be maintained, particularly for patients with CD4+ cell counts of < 200 per cubic millimeter, in order to diagnose the condition and initiate therapy appropriately.

**Accepted**
Tuberculosis (treatment)—Rifampin and isoniazid combination is indicated in the treatment of pulmonary tuberculosis when the patient has been titrated on the individual components and the efficacy of the combination has been established.

**Unaccepted**
Rifampin and isoniazid combination is not indicated for initial treatment or prophylaxis of pulmonary tuberculosis, for meningococcal infections, or in the treatment of asymptomatic meningococcal carriers to eliminate *Neisseria meningitidis* from the nasopharynx.

## Patient Consultation

As an aid to patient consultation, refer to *Advice for the Patient, Rifampin and Isoniazid (Systemic)*.
In providing consultation, consider emphasizing the following selected information (» = major clinical significance):

**Before using this medication**
» Conditions affecting use, especially:
  Hypersensitivity to rifampin, isoniazid, ethionamide, pyrazinamide, niacin (nicotinic acid), or other chemically related medications
  Pregnancy—Isoniazid and rifampin cross the placenta. It is recommended that isoniazid and rifampin be used to treat pregnant women with tuberculosis; however, rifampin has rarely caused postnatal hemorrhage in the mother and infant when administered during the last few weeks of pregnancy
  Breast-feeding—Isoniazid and rifampin are distributed into breast milk
  Use in children—Use of the fixed-dose combination is not recommended in pediatric patients
  Use in the elderly—Patients over the age of 50 have the highest incidence of hepatitis
  Dental—Patients who develop blood dyscrasias may be at increased risk of microbial infections, delayed healing, and gingival bleeding
  Other medicines, especially daily alcohol use, alfentanil, aminophylline, coumarin- or indandione-derivative anticoagulants, oral antidiabetic agents, azole antifungals, carbamazepine, chloramphenicol, corticosteroids, digitalis glycosides, disopyramide, disulfiram, estramustine, estrogens, ketoconazole, other hepatotoxic medications, methadone, mexiletine, oral estrogen-containing contraceptives, oxtriphylline, phenytoin, quinidine, theophylline, tocainide, or verapamil
  Other medical problems, especially alcoholism, active or in remission, or hepatic function impairment

**Proper use of this medication**
  Taking this medication with food or antacids, but not within 1 hour of aluminum-containing antacids, if gastrointestinal irritation occurs
» Compliance with full course of therapy, which may take months or years
» Taking pyridoxine concurrently to prevent or minimize symptoms of peripheral neuritis
» Proper dosing
  Missed dose: Taking as soon as possible; not taking if almost time for next dose; not doubling doses; intermittent dosing may result in more frequent and/or severe side effects
» Proper storage

**Precautions while using this medication**
» Regular visits to physician to check progress, as well as ophthalmologic examinations if signs of optic neuritis occur
  Checking with physician if no improvement within 2 to 3 weeks
» Using an alternate method of contraception if taking estrogen-containing oral contraceptives concurrently
» Avoiding alcoholic beverages concurrently with this medication
  Checking with physician if vascular reactions occur following concurrent ingestion of cheese or fish with isoniazid-containing medications
» Medication causes urine, feces, saliva, sputum, sweat, and tears to turn reddish-orange to reddish-brown and may also permanently discolor soft contact lenses; avoiding the wearing of soft contact lenses
» Need to report to physician promptly prodromal signs of hepatitis or peripheral neuritis
  Caution in use of regular toothbrushes, dental floss, and toothpicks; deferring dental work until blood counts have returned to normal; checking with physician or dentist concerning proper oral hygiene
  Possible interference with diagnostic tests

**Side/adverse effects**
  Signs of potential side effects, especially blood dyscrasias, hepatitis, hepatitis prodromal symptoms, hypersensitivity, neurotoxicity, optic neuritis, peripheral neuritis, "flu-like" syndrome, and interstitial nephritis
  Hepatitis may be more likely to occur in patients over 50 years of age
  Reddish-orange to reddish-brown discoloration of urine, stools, saliva, sputum, sweat, and tears may be alarming to patient, although medically insignificant; however, tears discolored by rifampin may also discolor soft contact lenses

## Oral Dosage Forms

### RIFAMPIN AND ISONIAZID CAPSULES USP

**Usual adult and adolescent dose**
Tuberculosis—
  Oral, 600 mg of rifampin and 300 mg of isoniazid once a day for the entire treatment period.

**Usual pediatric dose**
Use of the fixed-dose combination is not recommended in pediatric patients.

Note: See individual components for dosage recommendations.

**Strength(s) usually available**
U.S.—
  300 mg of rifampin and 150 mg of isoniazid (Rx) [*Rifamate*].
Canada—
  Not commercially available.

**Auxiliary labeling**
• Continue medicine for full time of treatment.
• Avoid alcoholic beverages.
• May discolor body fluids.

Revised: 08/29/97

---

# RIFAMPIN, ISONIAZID, AND PYRAZINAMIDE    Systemic

**VA CLASSIFICATION (Primary):** AM500

**NOTE:** The *Rifampin, Isoniazid, and Pyrazinamide (Systemic)* monograph is maintained on the USP DI electronic data base. For a printed copy of the most recent revision of the complete monograph, contact Micromedex, Inc. - Reprint Requests, 6200 S. Syracuse Way, Suite 300, Englewood, CO 80111; telephone (303) 486-6400; telefax (303) 486-6464; Email: USPDI@MDX.COM.

For information on the specific components of this combination, see the *USP DI* monographs for *Isoniazid (Systemic)*, *Pyrazinamide (Systemic)*, and *Rifampin (Systemic)*.

The information that follows is selectively abstracted from the complete monograph and is provided to facilitate drug use review and patient counseling.

Note: For a listing of dosage forms and brand names by country availability, see *Dosage Forms* section(s).

## Category

Antibacterial (antimycobacterial).

## Indications

### General considerations

Tuberculosis is a highly infectious life-threatening bacterial disease with 8 million new cases and 3 million deaths reported worldwide each year to the World Health Organization (WHO). The vast majority of these cases are in developing countries; however, tuberculosis also has emerged as an important public health problem in the U.S. in recent years after the decline in number of cases observed between 1950 and 1980.

The resurgence of tuberculosis in the U.S. has been complicated by an increase in the proportion of patients with strains resistant to antituberculosis medications. Outbreaks of multidrug-resistant tuberculosis have been documented in hospitals and prisons. Drug-resistant tuberculosis, particularly that caused by strains resistant to isoniazid and rifampin, is much harder to treat and often is fatal. Among acquired immunodeficiency syndrome (AIDS) patients infected with tuberculosis bacilli resistant to both rifampin and isoniazid, a case-fatality rate of 91% has been reported. Recent investigations of outbreaks of multidrug-resistant tuberculosis have found an extraordinarily high case-fatality rate, with the median time to mortality being reached between 4 and 16 weeks. In almost all instances, these outbreaks have involved patients with severe immunosuppression by infection with the human immunodeficiency virus (HIV).

Acquired drug resistance develops during treatment for drug-sensitive tuberculosis with regimens that are poorly conceived or poorly complied with, allowing the emergence of naturally occurring drug-resistant mutations. Resistant organisms from affected patients may subsequently infect other people who have not been infected with *M. tuberculosis* previously, resulting in primary drug resistance.

Resistance to antituberculosis agents can develop not only in the strain that caused the initial disease, but also as a result of reinfection with a new strain of *M. tuberculosis* that is drug-resistant. Reinfection with a new multidrug-resistant *M. tuberculosis* strain can occur during therapy for the original infection or after completion of therapy. Most recent data suggest that outcomes can be improved if patients promptly begin therapy with two or more drugs that have *in vitro* activity against the multidrug-resistant isolate.

HIV infection is the strongest risk factor yet identified for the development of active tuberculosis disease in persons infected with tuberculosis. In addition, persons with HIV infection are at an increased risk of tuberculosis resulting either from newly acquired disease or from reactivation of latent infections. Tuberculosis is a major clinical manifestation of immunodeficiency induced by HIV. In hospital-based retrospective studies, high rates of tuberculosis have been found among patients with AIDS. In communities where tuberculosis and HIV infection are common, the prevalence of HIV seropositivity among patients with tuberculosis is greatly increasing.

WHO has estimated that 5.6 million people worldwide and 80,000 people in the U.S. are infected with both HIV and tuberculosis. Persons dually infected with *M. tuberculosis* and HIV have a high risk of developing clinically active tuberculosis. One study of HIV-positive drug users with positive tuberculin skin test results found a rate of the development of active tuberculosis to be 8 cases per 100 person-years (8% yearly) as compared with the 10% lifetime risk (1 to 3% risk within the first year after skin test conversion) in the general population.

Persons who are known to be HIV-infected and who are contacts of patients with infectious tuberculosis should be carefully evaluated for evidence of tuberculosis. If there are no findings suggestive of current tuberculosis, preventive therapy with isoniazid should be given. Because HIV-infected contacts are not managed in the same way as those who are not HIV-infected, HIV testing is recommended if there are known or suspected risk factors for their acquiring HIV infection.

According to investigators at the National Institute of Allergy and Infectious Diseases (NIAID), levels of HIV in the bloodstream increase 5- to 160-fold in HIV-infected persons who develop active tuberculosis. Clinical and epidemiologic observations have demonstrated that HIV-infected individuals have an estimated 113-times higher risk and AIDS patients have a 170-times higher risk compared with uninfected persons. Furthermore, the problem of drug resistance may worsen as the HIV epidemic spreads. Immunosuppressed patients with HIV infection who subsequently become infected with *M. tuberculosis* have an extraordinarily high risk of developing active tuberculosis within a short period of time.

In addition to the convincing evidence that HIV infection increases the risk and worsens the course of tuberculosis, there is increasing clinical evidence that coinfection with *M. tuberculosis* accelerates progression of disease caused by HIV infection. Understanding the interaction of these two pathogens is clinically important, given the high prevalence of patients coinfected with HIV and *M. tuberculosis* in both the U.S. and Africa; it is estimated that by the year 2000 about 500,000 deaths per year will occur in coinfected patients worldwide.

Persons with a positive tuberculin skin test and HIV infection, and persons with a positive tuberculin skin test and at risk of acquiring HIV infection with unknown HIV status should be considered for tuberculosis preventive therapy regardless of age. One study showed that isoniazid prophylaxis in HIV-infected, tuberculin-positive individuals not only decreased the incidence of tuberculosis disease, but also delayed the progression to AIDS and death.

Twelve months of preventive therapy is recommended for adults and children with HIV infection and other conditions associated with immunosuppression. Persons with HIV infection should receive at least 6 months of preventive therapy. The American Academy of Pediatrics recommends that children receive 9 months of therapy.

Tuberculosis control programs should ensure that drug susceptibility tests are performed on all initial isolates of *M. tuberculosis* and the results are reported promptly to the primary care provider and the local health department. Tuberculosis control programs should monitor local drug resistance rates to assess the effectiveness of local tuberculosis control efforts and to determine the appropriateness of the currently recommended initial tuberculosis treatment regimen for the area.

Relapse of rifampin-resistant tuberculosis has been reported in HIV-infected patients. Reinfection with new strains of *M. tuberculosis* has also been reported in these patients. Rifampin-resistant tuberculosis is a serious threat because responses to therapy are more difficult to achieve and require long courses of treatment. Therefore, careful follow-up of HIV-infected patients with treated tuberculosis is essential.

Multidrug-resistant tuberculosis also has been transmitted to persons without HIV infection in health care facilities. Together with the lack of effective agents for second-line treatment and methods of prophylaxis, the transmission of multidrug-resistant strains of *M. tuberculosis* may create a substantial reservoir of latently infected people and the potential for clinical multidrug-resistant tuberculosis for many years to come.

Several studies have documented a high prevalence of extrapulmonary disease in HIV-infected patients with clinical tuberculosis disease, particularly in conjunction with pulmonary manifestations. Cutaneous miliary tuberculosis, also known as *tuberculosis cutis miliaris disseminata*, was in the past a rare condition in adults, with only 24 cases reported in nearly a century. However, since the first reported case of cutaneous miliary tuberculosis in 1990 in a patient with AIDS, five additional cases have been reported in HIV-infected patients. Its appearance can be quite nondescript; therefore, a high level of suspicion must be maintained, particularly for patients with CD4+ cell counts of < 200 per cubic millimeter, in order to diagnose the condition and initiate therapy appropriately.

### Accepted

Tuberculosis (treatment)—Rifampin, isoniazid, and pyrazinamide combination is indicated in the initial phase of the short-course treatment of all forms of tuberculosis. During this phase, usually lasting 2 months, rifampin, isoniazid, and pyrazinamide combination should be administered on a daily, continuous basis. Additional medications are indicated if multidrug-resistant tuberculosis is suspected.

## Patient Consultation

As an aid to patient consultation, refer to *Advice for the Patient, Rifampin, Isoniazid, and Pyrazinamide (Systemic)*.

In providing consultation, consider emphasizing the following selected information (» = major clinical significance):

### Before using this medication

» Conditions affecting use, especially:
    Hypersensitivity to rifampin, isoniazid, pyrazinamide, ethionamide, niacin (nicotinic acid), rifabutin, or other chemically related medications
    Pregnancy—Isoniazid and rifampin cross the placenta
    Breast-feeding—Isoniazid, pyrazinamide, and rifampin are distributed into breast milk
    Use in children—Use of the fixed-dose combination is not recommended in pediatric patients up to 15 years of age

**2496  Rifampin, Isoniazid, and Pyrazinamide (Systemic)**

Use in the elderly—Patients 50 years of age and older have the highest incidence of hepatitis with use of isoniazid

Other medications, especially daily alcohol consumption, alfentanil, aminophylline, coumarin- or indanedione-derivative anticoagulants, oral antidiabetic agents, azole antifungals, carbamazepine, chloramphenicol, oral estrogen-containing contraceptives, corticosteroids, digitalis glycosides, disopyramide, disulfiram, estramustine, estrogens, other hepatotoxic medications, HIV protease inhibitors, ketoconazole, methadone, mexiletine, oxtriphylline, phenytoin, quinidine, theophylline, tocainide, or oral verapamil

Other medical problems, especially alcoholism, active or in remission, or hepatic function impairment

### Proper use of this medication
Taking this medication with food or antacids, but not within 1 hour of aluminum-containing antacids, if gastrointestinal irritation occurs
» Compliance with full course of therapy, which may take months or years
» Taking pyridoxine concurrently to prevent or minimize symptoms of peripheral neuritis
» Proper dosing
Missed dose: Taking as soon as possible; not taking if almost time for next dose; not doubling doses; intermittent dosing may result in more frequent and/or severe side effects
» Proper storage

### Precautions while using this medication
» Regular visits to physician to check progress, as well as ophthalmologic examinations if signs of optic neuritis occur
Checking with physician if no improvement within 2 to 3 weeks
» Using an alternate method of contraception if taking estrogen-containing oral contraceptives concurrently
» Avoiding alcoholic beverages while taking this medication
» Checking with physician if vascular reactions occur following concurrent ingestion of cheese or fish with isoniazid-containing medication
» Medication causes urine, feces, saliva, sputum, sweat, and tears to turn reddish-orange to reddish-brown and may also permanently discolor soft contact lenses; avoiding the wearing of soft contact lenses
» Need to report to physician promptly prodromal signs of hepatitis or peripheral neuritis
Using caution in use of regular toothbrushes, dental floss, and toothpicks; deferring dental work until blood counts have returned to normal; checking with physician or dentist concerning proper oral hygiene

Possible interference with diagnostic tests
» Diabetics: May interfere with urine ketone determinations

### Side/adverse effects
Hepatitis caused by isoniazid is more likely to occur in patients 50 years of age and older
Reddish-orange to reddish-brown discoloration of urine, stools, saliva, sputum, sweat, and tears may be alarming to patient, although medically insignificant; however, tears discolored by rifampin may also discolor soft contact lenses
Signs of potential side effects, especially arthralgia, hepatitis, hepatitis prodromal symptoms, peripheral neuritis, "flu-like" syndrome, hypersensitivity, blood dyscrasias, interstitial nephritis, neurotoxicity, and optic neuritis

## Oral Dosage Forms

### RIFAMPIN, ISONIAZID AND PYRAZINAMIDE TABLETS

**Usual adult dose**
Tuberculosis—
Patients weighing 44 kg or less: Oral, 4 tablets once a day.
Patients weighing between 45 and 54 kg: Oral, 5 tablets once a day.
Patients weighing 55 kg or more: Oral, 6 tablets once a day.

**Usual pediatric dose**
Tuberculosis—
Children and adolescents up to 15 years of age: Use of the fixed-dose combination is not recommended.
Adolescents 15 years of age and older: See *Usual adult dose*.

Note: See individual components for dosage recommendations.

**Strength(s) usually available**
U.S.—
  120 mg rifampin, 50 mg isoniazid, and 300 mg pyrazinamide (Rx) [*Rifater*].
Canada—
  Not commercially available.

**Auxiliary labeling**
• Continue taking the medicine for full time of treatment.
• Avoid alcoholic beverages.
• May discolor body fluids.

Revised: 08/29/97

---

# RIFAPENTINE    Systemic—INTRODUCTORY VERSION

VA CLASSIFICATION (Primary): AM500
Commonly used brand name(s): *Priftin*.
Note: For a listing of dosage forms and brand names by country availability, see *Dosage Forms* section(s).

## Category
Antibacterial (antimycobacterial).

## Indications

### Accepted
Tuberculosis, pulmonary (treatment)—Rifapentine is indicated in combination with other antituberculosis medications in the treatment of pulmonary tuberculosis.

### Unaccepted
Rifapentine is not indicated as a sole agent in the treatment of pulmonary tuberculosis because of the possibility of the rapid emergence of resistant organisms.

## Pharmacology/Pharmacokinetics

### Physicochemical characteristics
Molecular weight—877.04.

### Mechanism of action/Effect
Rifapentine, a cyclopentyl rifamycin, inhibits DNA-dependent RNA polymerase in susceptible strains of *Mycobacterium tuberculosis* but not in mammalian cells. At therapeutic levels, rifapentine exhibits bactericidal activity against both intracellular and extracellular *M. tuberculosis* organisms. Both rifapentine and the 25-desacetyl metabolite accumulate in human monocyte–derived macrophages with intracellular/extracellular ratios approximately 24:1 and 7:1, respectively.

### Absorption
The relative bioavailability of rifapentine after a single 600 mg dose to healthy adult volunteers was 70%. The absolute bioavailability of rifapentine has not been determined.

### Protein binding
In healthy volunteers, rifapentine and the 25-desacetyl metabolite were 97.7% and 93.2% bound to plasma proteins respectively. Rifapentine was mainly bound to albumin.

### Time to peak concentration
5 to 6 hours after a single 600 mg dose.

### Elimination
Fecal—70%.
Renal—17%.
  In dialysis—Rifapentine is not removed from the blood by hemodialysis.

## Precautions to Consider

### Cross-sensitivity and/or related problems
Patients sensitive to other rifamycins (e.g., rifabutin and rifampin) may also be sensitive to rifapentine.

### Carcinogenicity
Carcinogenicity studies with rifapentine have not been completed.

### Mutagenicity
Rifapentine was negative in the following genotoxicity tests:
  • *In vitro* gene mutation assay in bacteria (Ames test).
  • *In vitro* point mutation test in *Aspergillus nidulans*.
  • *In vitro* gene conversion assay in *Saccharomyces cerevisiae*.
  • *In vitro* host-mediated (mouse) gene conversion assay with *Saccharomyces cerevisiae*.

- *In vitro* Chinese hamster ovary cell/hypoxanthine-guanine phosphoribosyl transferase (CHO/HGPRT) forward mutation assay.
- *In vitro* chromosomal aberration assay utilizing rat lymphocytes.
- *In vivo* mouse bone marrow micronucleus assay.

**Pregnancy/Reproduction**
Fertility—Fertility and reproductive performance were not affected by oral administration of rifapentine to male and female rats at doses of up to one third of the human dose (based on body surface area conversions).

Pregnancy—There have been no adequate and well-controlled studies in pregnant women; however, rifapentine should be used during pregnancy only if the potential benefit justifies the potential risk to the fetus. In one clinical study, 6 patients randomized to rifapentine became pregnant; two had normal deliveries, two had first trimester spontaneous abortions, one had an elective abortion, and one patient was lost to follow-up. Of the two patients who spontaneously aborted, co-morbid conditions of alcohol abuse in one and HIV infection in the other were noted.

Rifapentine is chemically related to rifampin. When administered during the last few weeks of pregnancy, rifampin can cause postnatal hemorrhages in the mother and infant for which treatment with vitamin K may be indicated. Therefore, patients who receive rifapentine during the last few weeks of pregnancy and their newborn infants should have appropriate clotting parameters evaluated.

Rifapentine has been shown to be teratogenic in rats and rabbits. In rats, when given in doses 0.6 times the human dose (based on body surface area comparisons) during the period of organogenesis, pups showed cleft palates, right aortic arch, increased incidence of delayed ossification, and increased number of ribs. Rabbits treated with rifapentine at doses between 0.3 and 1.3 times the human dose (based on body surface area comparisons) displayed major malformations including ovarian agenesis, per varus, arhinia, microphthalmia and irregularities of the ossified facial tissues.

FDA Pregnancy Category C.

**Breast-feeding**
It is not known whether rifapentine is distributed into breast milk. Because many drugs are excreted in human milk and because of the potential for serious adverse reactions in nursing infants, a decision should be made whether to discontinue nursing or discontinue the drug, taking into account the importance of the drug to the mother.

**Pediatrics**
Infants and children up to 12 years of age—Safety and efficacy have not been established.

Children 12 years of age and older—Pediatrics-specific problems that would limit the usefulness of rifapentine in this age group are not expected.

**Geriatrics**
Following oral administration of a single 600-mg dose of rifapentine to 14 elderly (≥ 65 years) healthy male volunteers, the pharmacokinetics of rifapentine and its 25-desacetyl metabolite were similar to that observed for young (18 to 45 years) healthy male volunteers. Therefore, geriatrics-specific problems that would limit the usefulness of rifapentine in the elderly are not expected.

**Dental**
The leukopenic and thrombocytopenic effects of rifapentine may result in an increased incidence of certain microbial infections, delayed healing, and gingival bleeding. If leukopenia or thrombocytopenia occurs, dental work should be deferred until blood counts have returned to normal. Patients should be instructed in proper oral hygiene, including caution in use of regular toothbrushes, dental floss, and toothpicks.

**Drug interactions and/or related problems**
The following drug interactions and/or related problems have been selected on the basis of their potential clinical significance (possible mechanism in parentheses where appropriate)—not necessarily inclusive (» = major clinical significance):

Note: Combinations containing any of the following medications, depending on the amount present, may also interact with this medication.

» Alcohol
(concurrent daily consumption of alcohol may increase the risk of rifapentine-induced hepatotoxicity and increased metabolism of rifapentine; dosage adjustment of rifapentine may be necessary, and patients should be monitored closely for signs of hepatotoxicity)

Amitriptyline
Nortriptyline
(concurrent use with rifapentine may enhance the metabolism of amitriptyline and nortriptyline by induction of hepatic microsomal enzymes, resulting in lower serum concentrations; dosage adjustment may be required)

» Antidiabetic agents, oral
(concurrent use with rifapentine may enhance the metabolism of sulfonylureas by induction of hepatic microsomal enzymes, resulting in lower serum sulfonylurea concentrations; dosage adjustment may be required)

» Azole antifungals
(concurrent use with rifapentine may increase the metabolism of azole antifungals, lowering their plasma concentrations; depending on the clinical situation, the dose of an azole antifungal may need to be increased)

Barbiturates
(concurrent use with rifapentine may enhance the metabolism of barbiturates by induction of hepatic microsomal enzymes, resulting in lower serum concentrations; dosage adjustment may be required)

» Chloramphenicol or
» Ciprofloxacin or
» Clarithromycin or
» Doxycycline
(concurrent use with rifapentine may enhance the metabolism of these antibiotics by induction of hepatic microsomal enzymes, resulting in significantly lower serum antibiotic concentrations; dosage adjustment may be required)

Clofibrate
(concurrent use with rifapentine may enhance the metabolism of clofibrate by induction of hepatic microsomal enzymes, resulting in significantly lower clofibrate serum concentrations; dosage adjustment may be necessary)

» Contraceptives, estrogen-containing, oral
(concurrent use with rifapentine may decrease the effectiveness of estrogen-containing oral contraceptives because of stimulation of estrogen metabolism or reduction in enterohepatic circulation of estrogens, resulting in menstrual irregularities, intermenstrual bleeding, and unplanned pregnancies; patients should be advised to change to nonhormonal methods of birth control)

» Corticosteroids, glucocorticoid and mineralocorticoid
(concurrent use with rifapentine may enhance the metabolism of corticosteroids by induction of hepatic microsomal enzymes, resulting in a considerable decrease in corticosteroid plasma concentrations; dosage adjustment may be required)

Cyclosporine
Tacrolimus
(rifapentine may enhance the metabolism of cyclosporine and tacrolimus by induction of hepatic microsomal enzymes and intestinal cytochrome P450 enzymes; dosage adjustment may be required)

Dapsone
(concurrent use with rifapentine may decrease the effect of dapsone because of increased metabolism resulting from stimulation of hepatic microsomal enzyme activity; dapsone concentrations may be decreased)

» Delavirdine
» Zidovudine
(concurrent use with rifapentine may enhance the metabolism of delavirdine and zidovudine by induction of hepatic microsomal enzymes, resulting in lower serum concentrations; dosage adjustment may be required)

Diazepam
(concurrent use with rifapentine may enhance the metabolism of diazepam, resulting in decreased plasma concentrations; dosage adjustment may be required)

» Digitalis glycosides
(concurrent use with rifapentine may enhance the metabolism of digoxin or digitoxin by induction of hepatic microsomal enzymes, resulting in significantly lower serum digoxin or digitoxin concentrations; dosage adjustment may be required)

» Diltiazem or
» Nifedipine or
» Verapamil
(rifapentine may accelerate the metabolism of these calcium channel blocking agents, resulting in a significant decrease in serum calcium channel blocking agent concentration and reversing their cardiovascular effects; dosage adjustment may be required)

» Disopyramide or
» Mexiletine or
» Quinidine or
» Tocainide
(concurrent use with rifapentine may enhance the metabolism of these antiarrhythmics by induction of hepatic microsomal enzymes, resulting in significantly lower serum antiarrhythmic concentra-

tions; serum antiarrhythmic should be monitored and dosage adjustment may be required)

Haloperidol
(concurrent use with rifapentine may enhance the metabolism of haloperidol by induction of hepatic microsomal enzymes, resulting in lower serum concentrations; dosage adjustment may be required)

» Human immunodeficiency virus (HIV) protease inhibitors
(rifapentine accelerates the metabolism of protease inhibitors such as indinavir, nelfinavir, ritonavir, and saquinavir through induction of hepatic P450 cytochrome oxidases, resulting in subtherapeutic levels of protease inhibitors; concurrent use of HIV protease inhibitors with rifapentine is not recommended)

Levothyroxine
(concurrent use with rifapentine may enhance the metabolism of levothyroxine by induction of hepatic microsomal enzymes, resulting in lower serum concentrations; dosage adjustment may be required)

» Methadone
(concurrent use with rifapentine may decrease the effects of methadone because of stimulation of hepatic microsomal enzyme activity and/or impaired absorption, resulting in symptoms of methadone withdrawal if the patient is dependent on methadone; dosage adjustments may be necessary during and after rifapentine therapy)

» Phenytoin
(concurrent use with rifapentine may stimulate the hepatic metabolism of phenytoin, increasing its elimination and thus counteracting its anticonvulsant effects; careful monitoring of serum hydantoin concentrations and adjustments may be necessary before and after rifapentine therapy)

Quinine
(concurrent use with rifapentine may enhance the metabolism of quinine by induction of hepatic microsomal enzymes, resulting in lower serum concentrations; dosage adjustment may be required)

Sildenafil
(concurrent use with rifapentine may enhance the metabolism of sildenafil by induction of hepatic microsomal enzymes, resulting in lower serum concentrations; dosage adjustment may be required)

» Theophylline
(rifapentine may increase the metabolism of theophylline by induction of hepatic microsomal enzymes, resulting in increased theophylline clearance; dosage adjustments may be necessary during and after rifapentine therapy)

» Warfarin
(concurrent use with rifapentine may enhance the metabolism of warfarin by induction of hepatic microsomal enzymes, resulting in a considerable decrease in the activity and effectiveness of warfarin; prothrombin time determinations may be required as frequently as once a day; dosage adjustments of warfarin may be required before and after rifapentine therapy)

## Laboratory value alterations
The following have been selected on the basis of their potential clinical significance (possible effect in parentheses where appropriate)—not necessarily inclusive (» = major clinical significance):

With diagnostic test results
Folate determinations, serum and
Vitamin $B_{12}$ determinations, serum
(therapeutic concentrations of rifapentine may interfere with standard microbiological assays for serum folate and vitamin $B_{12}$; alternative methods must be considered when determining serum folate and vitamin $B_{12}$ concentrations in patients taking rifapentine)

Urinalyses based on spectrometry or color reaction
(rifapentine may interfere with urinalyses that are based on spectrometry or color reaction due to rifapentine's reddish-orange to reddish-brown discoloration of urine)

Note: Hyperbilirubinemia resulting from competition for excretory pathways between rifapentine and bilirubin cannot be excluded since competition between the related drug rifampin and bilirubin can occur. An isolated report showing a moderate rise in bilirubin and/or transaminase level is not in itself an indication for interrupting treatment; rather the decision should be made after repeating the tests, noting trends in the levels, and considering them in conjunction with the patient's clinical condition.

With physiology/laboratory test values
Alanine aminotransferase (ALT [SGPT]) and
Alkaline phosphatase and
Aspartate aminotransferase (AST [SGOT])
(values may be increased)

Bilirubin, serum and
Blood urea nitrogen (BUN) and
Uric acid, serum
(concentrations may be increased)

## Medical considerations/Contraindications
The medical considerations/contraindications included have been selected on the basis of their potential clinical significance (reasons given in parentheses where appropriate)—not necessarily inclusive (» = major clinical significance).

*Risk-benefit should be considered when the following medical problems exist:*

» Alcoholism, active or in remission or
» Hepatic function impairment
(multidrug antituberculosis treatments, including the rifamycin class, are associated with serious hepatic adverse effects; patients with abnormal liver test results and/or liver disease should be given rifapentine only in cases of necessity and then with caution and under strict medical supervision; in these patients, careful monitoring of liver tests [especially serum transaminases] should be carried out prior to therapy and then every 2 to 4 weeks during therapy; if signs of liver disease occur or worsen, rifapentine should be discontinued)

» Hypersensitivity to rifabutin, rifampin, or rifapentine

## Patient monitoring
The following may be especially important in patient monitoring (other tests may be warranted in some patients, depending on condition; » = major clinical significance):

Alanine aminotransferase (ALT [SGPT]) and
Alkaline phosphatase and
Aspartate aminotransferase (AST [SGOT]) and
Bilirubin, serum
(recommended prior to treatment and monthly or more frequently during treatment)

Complete blood counts (CBCs)
(monitoring of CBC recommended to detect rifapentine-induced blood dyscrasias)

# Side/Adverse Effects

The following side/adverse effects have been selected on the basis of their potential clinical significance (possible signs and symptoms in parentheses where appropriate)—not necessarily inclusive:

### Those indicating need for medical attention
Incidence more frequent
**Hematuria, pyuria, or proteinuria** (blood in urine); **hyperuricemia** (joint pain; lower back or side pain; swelling of feet or lower legs)

Note: In the tuberculosis treatment clinical trial known as Study 008, *hyperuricemia* was the most frequently reported adverse effect that was assessed as treatment-related. However, hyperuricemia most likely was related to the pyrazinamide in the treatment regimen, since no case was reported in the continuation phase when pyrazinamide was no longer included in the treatment regimen.

Incidence less frequent
**Anemia** (unusual tiredness or weakness); **arthralgia** (joint pain); **leukopenia or neutropenia** (sore throat and fever); **mood or behavior changes** (aggressive reaction); **hepatitis** (yellow eyes or skin); **pancreatitis** (nausea; severe abdominal or stomach pain; vomiting); **thrombocytopenia** (black, tarry stools; blood in urine or stools; pinpoint red spots on skin; unusual bleeding or bruising)

Incidence rare
**Diarrhea, nausea and/or vomiting; hypertension** (dizziness; severe or continuing headaches; increase in blood pressure)

Note: Pseudomembranous colitis has been reported to occur with various antibiotics, including other rifamycins. *Diarrhea*, particularly if severe and/or persistent, occurring during treatment or in the initial weeks following treatment, may be symptomatic of *Clostridium difficile*–associated disease, the most severe form of which is pseudomembranous colitis. If pseudomembranous colitis is suspected, rifapentine should be stopped immediately and the patient should be treated with supportive and specific treatment without delay (e.g., oral vancomycin). Products inhibiting peristalsis are contraindicated in this clinical situation.

### Those indicating need for medical attention only if they continue or are bothersome
Incidence less frequent
*Acne; anorexia* (loss of appetite); *constipation; fatigue* (unusual tiredness)

### Those not indicating need for medical attention
Incidence more frequent
*Reddish-orange to reddish-brown discoloration of urine, feces, saliva, sputum, sweat, and tears*
Note: Tears discolored by rifapentine may also discolor soft contact lenses.

## Overdose

For more information on the management of overdose or unintentional ingestion, **contact a Poison Control Center** (see *Poison Control Center Listing*).

### Clinical effects of overdose
Note: Experience with rifapentine overdose is very limited. In reported cases, only very few adverse effects occurred.

### Treatment of overdose
Note: There is no experience with the treatment of acute overdose with rifapentine at doses exceeding 1200 mg per dose.

While there is no experience with the treatment of acute overdose with rifapentine, clinical experience with rifamycins suggests that gastric lavage to evacuate gastric contents (within a few hours of overdose), followed by instillation of an activated charcoal slurry into the stomach, may help adsorb any remaining drug from the gastrointestinal tract.

Forced diuresis and hemodialysis are of no benefit in the treatment of rifapentine overdose.

## Patient Consultation

As an aid to patient consultation, refer to *Advice for the Patient, Rifapentine (Systemic)—Introductory Version*.
In providing consultation, consider emphasizing the following selected information (» = major clinical significance):

### Before using this medication
» Conditions affecting use, especially:
  Hypersensitivity to rifabutin, rifampin, or rifapentine
  Pregnancy—Rifapentine may cause postnatal hemorrhages in the mother and the infant when administered during the last few weeks of pregnancy
  Other medications, especially alcohol, azole antifungals, ciprofloxacin, chloramphenicol, clarithromycin, corticosteroids, delavirdine, digitalis glycosides, diltiazem, disopyramide, doxycycline, estrogen-containing oral contraceptives, human immunodeficiency virus (HIV) protease inhibitors, methadone, mexiletine, nifedipine, oral antidiabetic agents, phenytoin, quinidine, theophylline, tocainide, verapamil, warfarin, or zidovudine
  Other medical problems, especially alcoholism, active or in remission, or impairment of hepatic function

### Proper use of this medication
» Compliance with full course of therapy, which may take months or years to complete
» Proper dosing
  Missed dose: Taking as soon as possible; not taking if almost time for next dose; not doubling doses
» Proper storage

### Precautions while using this medication
» Regular visits to physician to check progress
  Checking with physician if no improvement within 2 to 3 weeks, or if symptoms become worse
  Stopping taking this medication and checking with physician immediately if this medication causes very tired or very weak feeling, a loss of appetite, nausea, or vomiting
» Using an alternative method of contraception if taking estrogen-containing oral contraceptives concurrently
» Avoiding alcoholic beverages concurrently with this medication
» Medication causes urine, stools, saliva, sputum, sweat, and tears to turn reddish-orange to reddish-brown and may also permanently discolor soft contact lenses; avoiding the wearing of soft contact lenses
  Using caution in use of regular toothbrushes, dental floss, and toothpicks; deferring dental work until blood counts have returned to normal; checking with physician or dentist concerning proper oral hygiene
  Possible interference with laboratory values

### Side/adverse effects
Signs of potential side effects, especially hematuria, pyuria, proteinuria, hyperuricemia, anemia, arthralgia, leukopenia or neutropenia, mood or behavior changes, hepatitis, pancreatitis, thrombocytopenia, diarrhea, nausea, vomiting, and hypertension
Reddish-orange to reddish-brown discoloration of urine, stools, saliva, sputum, sweat, tears may be alarming to patient, although medically insignificant; however, tears discolored by rifapentine may also discolor soft contact lenses

## General Dosing Information

For patients with propensity to nausea, vomiting, or gastrointestinal upset, administration of rifapentine with food may be useful.

In the intensive phase of short-course therapy, which is to continue for 2 months, 600 mg of rifapentine should be given twice a week with an interval of not less than 3 days (72 hours) between doses.

Rifapentine should be administered only concurrently with other antituberculosis medications. It should not be used alone in initial treatment or re-treatment of pulmonary tuberculosis.

Compliance with all drugs in the intensive phase (i.e., rifapentine, isoniazid, pyrazinamide, ethambutol, or streptomycin), especially on days when rifapentine is not administered, is imperative to assure early sputum conversion and protection against relapse.

The American Thoracic Society (ATS) and the Centers for Disease Control and Prevention (CDC) also recommend that either streptomycin or ethambutol be added to the regimen unless the likelihood of isoniazid resistance is very low. The need for streptomycin or ethambutol should be reassessed when the results of susceptibility testing are known.

An initial tuberculosis treatment regimen with less than four drugs may be considered if the following criteria are met:
• If primary resistance to isoniazid is less than 4% in the community.
• If the patient has had no previous treatment with antituberculosis medications.
• If the patient is not from a country with a high prevalence of drug resistance.
• If the patient has had no known exposure to a drug-resistant case.

Following the intensive phase, treatment should be continued with rifapentine once weekly for 4 months in combination with isoniazid or an appropriate agent for susceptible organisms.

Concomitant administration of pyridoxine (vitamin $B_6$) is recommended in the malnourished, in those predisposed to neuropathy (e.g., alcoholics and diabetics), and in adolescents.

Experience in human immunodeficiency virus (HIV)–infected patients is limited. In an ongoing CDC tuberculosis trial, five out of 30 HIV-infected patients randomized to once-weekly rifapentine and isoniazid in the continuation phase who completed treatment relapsed. Four of these patients developed rifampin mono-resistant (RMR) tuberculosis. Each RMR patient had late-stage HIV infection, low CD4 counts, and extrapulmonary disease, and documented concomitant administration of antifungal azoles. As with other antituberculosis treatments, when rifapentine is used in HIV-infected patients, a more aggressive regimen should be employed (e.g., more frequent dosing). Once-weekly rifapentine dosing in HIV-infected patients during the continuation phase of treatment is not recommended.

## Oral Dosage Forms

### RIFAPENTINE TABLETS

#### Usual adult and adolescent dose
Tuberculosis, pulmonary (treatment)—
  In combination with other antituberculosis medications: Oral, 600 mg twice a week with an interval of not less than three days (seventy-two hours) between doses.

#### Usual pediatric dose
Infants and children up to 12 years of age—
  Safety and efficacy have not been established.
Children 12 years of age and older—
  See *Usual adult and adolescent dose*.

#### Strength(s) usually available
U.S.—
  150 mg (Rx) [*Priftin*].

### Packaging and storage
Store below 40 °C (104 °F), preferably between 15 and 30 °C (59 and 86 °F), unless otherwise specified by manufacturer. Protect from excessive heat and humidity.

### Auxiliary labeling
- Continue medicine for full time of treatment.
- Avoid alcoholic beverages.
- May discolor body fluids.

Developed: 08/03/98

# RILUZOLE  Systemic†

VA CLASSIFICATION (Primary): CN900
Commonly used brand name(s): *Rilutek*.
Note: For a listing of dosage forms and brand names by country availability, see *Dosage Forms* section(s).

†Not commercially available in Canada.

## Category
Amyotrophic lateral sclerosis (ALS) therapy agent.

## Indications

### Accepted
Amyotrophic lateral sclerosis (ALS) (treatment)—Riluzole is indicated in the treatment of ALS; it may slow the progression of ALS by extending the survival and/or time to tracheostomy.

In two placebo-controlled studies, riluzole was shown to improve survival early in the trials; however, muscle strength and neurological functioning were not improved. Also, no statistically significant difference in mortality was seen at the conclusion of these studies.

## Pharmacology/Pharmacokinetics

### Physicochemical characteristics
Chemical group—Benzothiazole.
Molecular weight—234.20.

### Mechanism of action/Effect
Riluzole presynaptically inhibits glutamate release in the central nervous system (CNS) and postsynaptically interferes with the effects of excitatory amino acids. Although the etiology of ALS is unknown, current hypotheses suggest that glutamic acid may play a secondary role in mediating the neurodegenerative processes in the disease. Another pharmacological property of riluzole that may be related to its effect is inactivation of voltage-dependent sodium channels.

### Other actions/effects
In animal models, riluzole has demonstrated anticonvulsant effects at doses twice the recommended human daily dose, and myorelaxant and sedative properties at doses twenty times the recommended human daily dose. Anti-ischemic properties have also been reported.

### Absorption
Riluzole is well absorbed (approximately 90%), and has an absolute bioavailability of about 60%. Administration with a high fat meal decreases absorption, decreasing the area under the plasma concentration–time curve (AUC) by about 20% and decreasing peak blood levels by about 45%.

### Distribution
Riluzole penetrates the brain very readily.

### Protein binding
Very high (96%); bound mainly to albumin and lipoproteins.

### Biotransformation
Riluzole is extensively metabolized to six major and a number of minor metabolites, which have not all been identified to date. Metabolism is mostly hepatic, consisting of cytochrome P450–dependent hydroxylation and glucuronidation. P450 1A2 is the primary isozyme involved in N-hydroxylation; CYP 2D6, CYP 2C19, CYP 3A4, and CYP 2E1 are considered unlikely to contribute significantly to riluzole metabolism in humans.

### Half-life
Elimination—Approximately 12 hours after multiple dosing.

### Time to steady-state concentration
Steady-state is reached in less than 5 days. The pharmacokinetics of riluzole are linear over the dose range of 25 to 100 mg administered every 12 hours.

### Elimination
There is marked interindividual variability in the clearance of riluzole, most likely due to variability of activity of the CYP 1A2 isoenzyme involved in the N-hydroxylation of the parent compound.
Renal: 90% of a single 150-mg radiolabeled dose administered to healthy males was recovered in the urine over 7 days, of which only 2% was unchanged riluzole. More than 85% of the metabolites recovered in the urine were glucuronide metabolites.
Fecal: 5% of a single 150-mg radiolabeled dose administered to healthy males was recovered in the feces over 7 days.

## Precautions to Consider

### Carcinogenicity
Long-term studies to determine the carcinogenic potential of riluzole have not been completed to date.

### Mutagenicity
There was no evidence of mutagenic or clastogenic potential in the Ames test, the mouse lymphoma assay, or the *in vivo* assays in the mouse and rat. There was an equivocal clastogenic response in the *in vitro* lymphocyte chromosomal aberration assay.

### Pregnancy/Reproduction
Fertility—Riluzole impaired fertility when administered to male and female rats prior to and during mating at a dose of 15 mg per kg of body weight (mg/kg) or 1.5 times the maximum daily dose on a mg per square meter of body surface area basis.
Pregnancy—Adequate and well-controlled studies in humans have not been done.
Embryotoxicity and maternal toxicity were observed when riluzole was administered to pregnant rats and rabbits during the period of organogenesis at doses of 27 mg/kg and 60 mg/kg, respectively (2.6 and 11.5 times the maximum human recommended dose [MHRD], respectively). Administration of riluzole to rats during gestation and lactation at doses of 15 mg/kg (or 1.5 times the MHRD) produced adverse effects such as a decrease in implantations and an increase in intrauterine deaths. Viability and growth of the offspring also were adversely affected.
FDA Pregnancy Category C.

### Breast-feeding
It is not known whether riluzole is distributed into human milk. However, it is distributed into maternal milk in rats. Because of the potential for serious adverse effects, it is recommended that women receiving riluzole not breast-feed.

### Pediatrics
No information is available on the relationship of age to the effects of riluzole in pediatric patients. Safety and efficacy have not been established.

### Geriatrics
Although appropriate studies on the relationship of age to the effects of riluzole have not been performed in the geriatric population, no geriatrics-specific problems have been documented to date. However, elderly patients are more likely to have age-related renal function impairment, which may cause decreased clearance of riluzole. About 30% of the patients included in controlled clinical trials were over 65 years of age; no differences in adverse effects between the younger and older patients were observed.

### Pharmacogenetics
Riluzole clearance in Japanese subjects native to Japan has been shown to be 50% lower than riluzole clearance in Caucasians after adjusting for body weight. Although it is not clear if this effect is due to genetic or environmental factors, alcohol intake, coffee intake, other dietary preferences, or smoking, Japanese subjects may possess a lower capacity (oxidative and/or conjugative) for metabolizing riluzole.
Female subjects may possess lower metabolic capacity to eliminate riluzole as compared to males, due to lower activity of the CYP 1A2 isozyme. This gender effect may result in increased blood concentration of riluzole and its metabolites. However, in controlled trials, no gender effect on favorable or adverse effects of riluzole was noted.

### Drug interactions and/or related problems
The following drug interactions and/or related problems have been selected on the basis of their potential clinical significance (possible mechanism in parentheses where appropriate)—not necessarily inclusive (» = major clinical significance):

Note: Clinical studies designed to evaluate the interaction of riluzole with other drugs have not been conducted.

Combinations containing any of the following medications, depending on the amount present, may also interact with this medication.

Alcohol
(it is not known if alcohol increases the risk of serious hepatotoxicity with riluzole; patients should be discouraged from drinking excessive amounts of alcohol)

Allopurinol or
Hepatotoxic agents or
Methyldopa or
Sulfasalazine
(because of the potential for additive hepatotoxic effects, caution should be exercised in prescribing these medications to a patient receiving riluzole)

Amitriptyline or
Caffeine or
Phenacetin or
Quinolones or
Tacrine or
Theophylline or
Other agents that potentially inhibit CYP 1A2
(inhibitors of CYP 1A2 may decrease the rate of elimination of riluzole)

(potential interactions may occur when riluzole is administered concomitantly with other agents that are also metabolized by CYP 1A2)

Charbroiled food or
Cigarette smoke or
Omeprazole or
Rifampicin
(inducers of CYP 1A2 may increase the rate of elimination of riluzole)

### Laboratory value alterations
The following have been selected on the basis of their potential clinical significance (possible effect in parentheses where appropriate)—not necessarily inclusive (» = major clinical significance):

With diagnostic test results
Coombs' (antiglobulin) test, direct
(positive results may occur)

With physiology/laboratory test values
Alkaline phosphataseor
Gamma glutamyl transferase (GGT) or
Lactic dehydrogenase
(values may be increased)

» Aminotransferases, serum
(elevated values occur in many patients, even those with no prior history of liver disease; experience in nearly 800 ALS patients predicts that about 50% of riluzole-treated patients will experience at least one alanine aminotransferase [ALT (SGPT)] level above the upper limit of normal (ULN), about 8% will have elevations > 3 times the ULN, and about 2% will have elevations > 5 times the ULN)

(in clinical trials, maximum increases in serum ALT usually occurred within 3 months after initiation of therapy with riluzole; patients were continued on riluzole if ALT values were < 5 times the ULN, and levels usually decreased to < 2 times the ULN within 2 to 6 months; if ALT values exceeded 5 times the ULN, riluzole was discontinued, so there is no clinical experience to date with continuing riluzole treatment in ALS patients with ALT values > 5 times the ULN)

Erythrocyte counts or
Hematocrit values or
Hemoglobin values
(levels may fall below the lower limit of normal; in clinical trials the changes were mostly mild and transient, and appeared to show a dose-response relationship)

Gamma globulins
(values may be increased)

### Medical considerations/Contraindications
The medical considerations/contraindications included have been selected on the basis of their potential clinical significance (reasons given in parentheses where appropriate)—not necessarily inclusive (» = major clinical significance).

*Except under special circumstances, this medication should not be used when the following medical problem exists:*

» Severe hepatic function impairment
(increased risk of liver toxicity)

*Risk-benefit should be considered when the following medical problems exist:*

Hepatic function impairment
(metabolism of riluzole and its metabolites may be decreased, leading to higher plasma levels)

Renal function impairment
(excretion of riluzole and its metabolites may be decreased, leading to higher plasma levels)

Sensitivity to riluzole

### Patient monitoring
The following may be especially important in patient monitoring (other tests may be warranted in some patients, depending on condition; » = major clinical significance):

Hepatic function tests including:
Alanine aminotransferase (ALT [SGPT]) and
Aspartate aminotransferase (AST [SGOT]) and
Bilirubin and
Gamma glutamyl transferase (GGT)
(serum values of aminotransferases should be measured prior to and during riluzole treatment; serum ALT values should be monitored every month for the first 3 months of treatment, every 3 months during the remainder of the first year, and periodically thereafter)

(if riluzole therapy is continued in patients with ALT values > 5 times the upper limit of normal [ULN], frequent [at least weekly] monitoring of complete liver function is recommended; treatment should be discontinued if ALT values exceed 10 times the ULN or if clinical jaundice develops)

White blood cell counts
(because of the occurrence of rare but marked neutropenia [absolute neutrophil count less than 500 per cubic millimeter], patients reporting febrile illness should have white cell counts checked)

## Side/Adverse Effects
Note: Adverse effects can worsen the quality of life of ALS patients receiving riluzole; however, in one study, adverse reactions to the drug reportedly did not outweigh its therapeutic effect on survival.

The following side/adverse effects have been selected on the basis of their potential clinical significance (possible signs and symptoms in parentheses where appropriate)—not necessarily inclusive:

### Those indicating need for medical attention
Incidence more frequent
*Aggravation reaction* (worsening of symptoms of ALS); *including worsening of asthenia* (unusual tiredness or weakness); *and spasticity; diarrhea; nausea; vomiting*

Note: *Diarrhea, nausea,* and *worsening of asthenia* may be dose-related.

Incidence less frequent
*Respiratory disorders, including decreased lung function* (difficulty in breathing); *increased cough, and pneumonia*

Incidence rare
*Angioedema* (swelling of the eyelids, mouth, lips, tongue, and/or throat); *dysphagia* (trouble in swallowing); *exfoliative dermatitis* (redness, scaling, or peeling of the skin); *facial edema* (swelling of face); *hypertension, mild to moderate* (high blood pressure); *hypokalemia* (increased thirst; irregular heartbeat; mood or mental changes; muscle cramps, pain, or weakness); *hyponatremia* (lack of energy); *incoordination* (lack of coordination); *jaundice* (yellow eyes or skin); *mental depression; neutropenia* (fever; chills; continuing sores in mouth); *phlebitis* (pain, tenderness, bluish color, or swelling of foot or leg); *seizures; tachycardia* (fast or pounding heartbeat); *urinary tract problems, including infections* (bloody or cloudy urine; frequent urge to urinate); *and dysuria* (painful or difficult urination)

### Those indicating need for medical attention only if they continue or are bothersome
Incidence more frequent
*Abdominal pain or gas; anorexia* (loss of appetite); *circumoral paresthesia* (numbness or tingling around the mouth); *dizziness; somnolence* (drowsiness); *vertigo*

# Riluzole (Systemic)

Note: *Anorexia, circumoral paresthesia, dizziness, somnolence,* and *vertigo* may be dose-related. *Dizziness* may occur more commonly in females than in males.

Incidence less frequent
*Back or muscle pain or stiffness; constipation; dermatological problems, including alopecia* (hair loss); *eczema* (skin rash); *and pruritus* (itching); *headache; insomnia* (trouble in sleeping); *malaise* (general feeling of discomfort or illness); *peripheral edema* (swelling of feet or legs); *rhinitis* (runny nose); *stomatitis* (irritation or soreness of mouth)

## Overdose

For more information on the management of overdose or unintentional ingestion, **contact a Poison Control Center** (see *Poison Control Center Listing*).

### Clinical effects of overdose
No cases of overdose with riluzole have been reported to date.

### Treatment of overdose
No specific antidote or information on treatment is available.

If an overdose occurs, riluzole should be discontinued immediately.

Supportive care—Treatment should be directed toward alleviating symptoms of overdose. Patients in whom intentional overdose is confirmed or suspected should be referred for psychiatric consultation.

## Patient Consultation

As an aid to patient consultation, refer to *Advice for the Patient, Riluzole (Systemic)*.

In providing consultation, consider emphasizing the following selected information (» = major clinical significance):

### Before using this medication
» Conditions affecting use, especially:
  Sensitivity to riluzole
  Pregnancy—Studies have shown adverse effects in animals receiving doses greater than recommended maximum human daily doses
  Breast-feeding—Not recommended because of risk of serious side effects
  Other medical problems, especially severe hepatic function impairment

### Proper use of this medication
Taking on a regular basis and at the same time of the day (e.g., morning and evening)
Taking on an empty stomach
Missed dose: skipping missed dose; starting again with next scheduled dose
» Proper storage

### Precautions while using this medication
Reporting any febrile illnesses promptly to physician
» Caution when driving or doing jobs requiring alertness, because of the potential for drowsiness, dizziness, or vertigo
Avoiding excessive alcohol intake

### Side/adverse effects
Aggravation reaction; asthenia; spasticity; diarrhea; nausea; vomiting; respiratory disorders, including decreased lung function, increased cough, and pneumonia; angioedema; dysphagia; exfoliative dermatitis; facial edema; hypertension; hypokalemia; hyponatremia; incoordination; jaundice; mental depression; neutropenia; phlebitis; seizures; tachycardia; and urinary tract problems including infections and dysuria

## General Dosing Information

Riluzole should be taken on a regular basis and at the same time of day (e.g., morning and evening). To avoid food-related decreases in bioavailability, riluzole should be given on an empty stomach, one hour before or two hours after meals.

## Oral Dosage Forms

### RILUZOLE TABLETS

**Usual adult dose**
Amyotrophic lateral sclerosis—Oral, 50 mg every twelve hours, taken on an empty stomach.

Note: Higher daily doses result in no increased benefit, but increased incidence of adverse effects.

**Usual adult prescribing limits**
100 mg a day.

**Usual pediatric dose**
Safety and efficacy have not been established.

**Usual geriatric dose**
See *Usual adult dose*.

**Strength(s) usually available**
U.S.—
  50 mg (Rx) [*Rilutek*].
Canada—
  Not commercially available.

**Packaging and storage**
Store between 20 and 25 °C (68 and 77 °F). Protect from bright light.

**Auxiliary labeling**
- May cause drowsiness.
- Take on an empty stomach.
- Avoid alcoholic beverages.

Developed: 07/30/96

---

# RIMANTADINE  Systemic†

VA CLASSIFICATION (Primary): AM809

Commonly used brand name(s): *Flumadine*.

Note: For a listing of dosage forms and brand names by country availability, see *Dosage Forms* section(s).

†Not commercially available in Canada.

## Category
Antiviral (systemic).

## Indications

### Accepted
Influenza A (prophylaxis and treatment)—Rimantadine is indicated for the prophylaxis of respiratory tract infections caused by influenza A virus in adults and children, and the treatment of respiratory tract infections caused by influenza A virus in adults.

Influenza A virus strains that are resistant to amantadine or rimantadine are cross-resistant to the other medication.

Although rimantadine is structurally similar to amantadine, differing only in the 10-carbon ring side chain, rimantadine, unlike amantadine, is not effective in the control of Parkinson's disease.

## Pharmacology/Pharmacokinetics

### Physicochemical characteristics
Molecular weight—215.77.

### Mechanism of action/Effect
Rimantadine is thought to exert its inhibitory effect early in the viral replicative cycle, possibly by blocking or greatly reducing the uncoating of viral RNA within host cells. Genetic studies suggest that a single amino acid change on the transmembrane portion of the M2 protein can completely eliminate influenza A virus' susceptibility to rimantadine.

### Absorption
Well absorbed; tablets and syrup are absorbed equally well after oral administration.

### Distribution
Vol$_D$—
  Adults: 17 to 25 L/kg.
  Children: Mean of 289 L.
Concentrations in the nasal mucus average 50% higher than those in plasma.

### Protein binding
Moderate (approximately 40%).

### Biotransformation
Extensively metabolized in the liver; glucuronidation and hydroxylation are the major metabolic pathways.

### Half-life
Young adults (22 to 44 years old)—25 to 30 hours.
Older adults (71 to 79 years old) and patients with chronic liver disease—
  Approximately 32 hours.
Children (4 to 8 years old)—13 to 38 hours.

### Time to peak concentration
1 to 4 hours.

### Peak serum concentration
Steady state—
  100 mg once a day: Approximately 181 nanograms per mL.
  100 mg twice a day: Approximately 416 nanograms per mL.
Rimantadine concentrations in elderly nursing home patients were found to be nearly 3 times those of younger adults.

### Elimination
Renal; > 90% recovered in the urine within 72 hours, mostly as metabolites. Less than 25% excreted in urine as unchanged drug.
In dialysis—Hemodialysis has a negligible effect on the clearance of rimantadine.

## Precautions to Consider

### Cross-sensitivity and/or related problems
Patients who are hypersensitive to amantadine may also be hypersensitive to rimantadine.

### Carcinogenicity
Carcinogenicity studies in animals have not been performed.

### Mutagenicity
No mutagenic effects were seen when rimantadine was evaluated in several standard mutagenicity assays.

### Pregnancy/Reproduction
Fertility—A study in male and female rats given doses of up to 60 mg per kg of body weight (mg/kg) per day (3 times the maximum human dose based on body surface area comparisons) showed no impairment of fertility.

Pregnancy—Adequate and well-controlled studies in humans have not been done.

Rimantadine crosses the placenta in mice. It has been shown to be embryotoxic in rats when given at a dose of 200 mg/kg per day (11 times the maximum human dose based on body surface area comparisons), and has caused fetal resorption. Maternal toxicity included ataxia, tremors, seizures, and significantly reduced weight gain. Rimantadine was not embryotoxic when given to rabbits in doses of up to 50 mg/kg per day (5 times the maximum human dose based on body surface area comparisons). However, there was evidence of a change in the ratio of fetuses with 12 ribs to fetuses with 13 ribs; normally the ratio is 50:50 in a litter, but the ratio was 80:20 after rimantadine treatment.

FDA Pregnancy Category C.

### Breast-feeding
It is not known whether rimantadine is distributed into breast milk. However, it is distributed into the milk of rats. Rimantadine concentrations in the milk of rats were twice those found in serum 2 to 3 hours after administration.

### Pediatrics
Appropriate studies on the relationship of age to the effects of rimantadine have not been performed in neonates and infants up to one year of age. However, use of rimantadine in children older than 1 year of age has not been shown to cause any pediatrics-specific problems that would limit its usefulness in children.

### Geriatrics
Elderly patients, particularly those in chronic care facilities, are more likely than younger adults or children to experience adverse effects associated with rimantadine, primarily central nervous system (CNS) and gastrointestinal side effects.

### Drug interactions and/or related problems
The following drug interactions and/or related problems have been selected on the basis of their potential clinical significance (possible mechanism in parentheses where appropriate)—not necessarily inclusive (» = major clinical significance):

Note: Combinations containing any of the following medications, depending on the amount present, may also interact with this medication.

Acetaminophen or
Aspirin
  (concurrent use of acetaminophen or aspirin with rimantadine reduces the peak serum concentration of rimantadine by approximately 11%; the clinical significance is thought to be minimal at this time)
Cimetidine
  (concurrent use of a single dose of rimantadine with cimetidine reduces rimantadine clearance by 18% in healthy adults; the clinical significance is thought to be minimal at this time)

### Medical considerations/Contraindications
The medical considerations/contraindications included have been selected on the basis of their potential clinical significance (reasons given in parentheses where appropriate)—not necessarily inclusive (» = major clinical significance).

*Risk-benefit should be considered when the following medical problems exist:*
» Epilepsy, history of, or other seizure disorders
  (amantadine increases the risk of seizures; seizures have also been reported with rimantadine in 2 patients with a history of seizures who had previously been withdrawn from their anticonvulsants)
» Hepatic function impairment
  (a single-dose study done in patients with severe liver dysfunction showed a reduction in rimantadine clearance by 50% compared to healthy subjects)
Hypersensitivity to amantadine or rimantadine
» Renal function impairment, severe
  (a single-dose study done in patients with end-stage renal failure showed a reduction in rimantadine clearance by 40%, and an increase in elimination half-life by 60%, compared to healthy subjects; a dosage reduction is recommended in patients with a creatinine clearance of ≤ 10 mL/min [0.17 mL/second])

## Side/Adverse Effects

Note: Rimantadine has fewer CNS side effects than does amantadine. Elderly patients have a higher incidence of side effects, primarily CNS and gastrointestinal side effects, than do younger patients at conventional doses.

The following side/adverse effects have been selected on the basis of their potential clinical significance (possible signs and symptoms in parentheses where appropriate)—not necessarily inclusive:

**Those indicating need for medical attention only if they continue or are bothersome**
Incidence less frequent
  *CNS effects* (difficulty in concentrating; difficulty in sleeping; dizziness; headache; nervousness; unusual tiredness); *gastrointestinal disturbances* (dryness of mouth; loss of appetite; nausea; stomach pain; vomiting)

## Patient Consultation

As an aid to patient consultation, refer to *Advice for the Patient, Rimantadine (Systemic)*.
In providing consultation, consider emphasizing the following selected information (» = major clinical significance):

### Before using this medication
» Conditions affecting use, especially:
    Hypersensitivity to amantadine or rimantadine
    Pregnancy—High doses were embryotoxic and maternotoxic in rats
    Other medical problems, especially epilepsy or a history of seizures, liver function impairment and renal function impairment

### Proper use of this medication
» Receiving a flu shot if recommended by your doctor
» Taking before exposure or as soon as possible after exposure
» Compliance with full course of therapy
» Importance of not missing doses and taking at evenly spaced times
  Proper administration technique for oral liquid

## Rimantadine (Systemic)

» Proper dosing
  Missed dose: Taking as soon as possible; not taking if almost time for next dose; not doubling doses
» Proper storage

**Precautions while using this medication**
  Caution if dizziness occurs
  Checking with physician if no improvement within a few days

## General Dosing Information

Chemoprophylactic administration should be started in anticipation of contact with, or as soon as possible after exposure to, persons having influenza A virus infections. Administration should be continued for at least 10 days following exposure. During an influenza epidemic, rimantadine should be given daily, usually for 6 to 8 weeks in most communities or until active immunity can be expected from administration of inactivated influenza A virus vaccine. Rimantadine has been reported to be effective for post-exposure prophylaxis of household contacts, but appeared to be less effective when used prophylactically in members of households in which index cases were being treated concurrently for influenza A. Failure was apparently due to transmission of drug-resistant strains of the virus.

If administered concurrently with inactivated influenza A virus vaccine until protective antibodies develop, rimantadine should be continued chemoprophylactically for 2 to 3 weeks after the vaccine has been administered. However, since the vaccine is only 70 to 80% effective, continued administration of rimantadine may be beneficial in elderly or high-risk patients. If the vaccine is unavailable or contraindicated, rimantadine should be administered for up to 90 days in cases of possible repeated or unknown exposure.

Treatment of influenza A virus infection with rimantadine should be started within 24 to 48 hours after the onset of symptoms and should be continued for 5 to 7 days. Optimal duration of therapy has not been established.

## Oral Dosage Forms

### RIMANTADINE HYDROCHLORIDE SYRUP

**Usual adult and adolescent dose**
Antiviral—
  Prophylaxis: Oral, 100 mg two times a day.
  Treatment: Oral, 100 mg two times a day for approximately five to seven days from the inital onset of symptoms.

Note: In adults with impaired renal function (creatinine clearance ≤ 10 mL/minute [0.17 mL/second]) or severe hepatic dysfunction, and in elderly nursing home patients, a dose of 100 mg once a day is recommended.

Although the manufacturer recommends twice-a-day dosing, once-a-day dosing has been well-tolerated and as effective because of the long elimination half-life of rimantadine.

**Usual pediatric dose**
Antiviral—Prophylaxis:
  Children up to 10 years of age: Oral, 5 mg per kg of body weight once a day. Maximum daily dose should not exceed 150 mg.
  Children 10 years of age and over: See *Usual adult and adolescent dose*.

**Strength(s) usually available**
U.S.—
  50 mg per 5 mL (Rx) [*Flumadine* (methylparaben; propylparaben; sodium saccharin)].
Canada—
  Not commercially available.

**Packaging and storage**
Store below 40 °C (104 °F), preferably between 15 and 30 °C (59 and 86 °F), unless otherwise specified by manufacturer.

**Auxiliary labeling**
• Continue medicine for full time of treatment.

### RIMANTADINE HYDROCHLORIDE TABLETS

**Usual adult and adolescent dose**
See *Rimantadine Hydrochloride Syrup*.

**Usual pediatric dose**
See *Rimantadine Hydrochloride Syrup*.

**Strength(s) usually available**
U.S.—
  100 mg (Rx) [*Flumadine*].
Canada—
  Not commercially available.

**Packaging and storage**
Store below 40 °C (104 °F), preferably between 15 and 30 °C (59 and 86 °F), unless otherwise specified by manufacturer.

**Auxiliary labeling**
• Continue medicine for full time of treatment.

Developed: 03/29/94

---

# RIMEXOLONE Ophthalmic—INTRODUCTORY VERSION

VA CLASSIFICATION (Primary): OP301
Commonly used brand name(s): *Vexol*.
Note: For a listing of dosage forms and brand names by country availability, see *Dosage Forms* section(s).

## Category

Corticosteroid (ophthalmic); anti-inflammatory (steroidal), ophthalmic.

## Indications

**Accepted**
Inflammation, postoperative (treatment)—Rimexolone is indicated for the treatment of postoperative inflammation following ocular surgery.

Uveitis, anterior (treatment)—Rimexolone is indicated for the treatment of anterior uveitis.

## Pharmacology/Pharmacokinetics

**Physicochemical characteristics**
Molecular weight—370.53.
pH—Ophthalmic suspension—6 to 8.
Tonicity—260 to 320 mOsmol per kg.

**Mechanism of action/Effect**
Corticosteroids suppress the inflammatory response to a variety of inciting agents of a mechanical, chemical, or immunological nature. They inhibit edema, cellular infiltration, capillary dilatation, fibroblastic proliferation, deposition of collagen, and scar formation that are associated with inflammation.

**Absorption**
Rimexolone is systemically absorbed. Rimexolone 1% administered hourly in each eye during waking hours for 1 week produced serum concentrations of less than 80 to 470 picograms per mL. The mean serum concentration was approximately 130 picograms per mL. In the same study, during the second week, the frequency of administration was decreased to every 2 hours while awake, producing a mean serum concentration of approximately 100 picograms per mL.

**Biotransformation**
Rimexolone undergoes extensive metabolism. Following intravenous administration of radiolabeled rimexolone in rats, more than 80% of the dose was excreted in the feces as rimexolone and metabolites. Metabolites have been shown to be either less active than rimexolone or inactive in human glucocorticoid receptor binding assays.

**Half-life**
Not reliably estimated, because a large number of samples were below the quantitation limit of the assay (80 picograms per mL). However, based on the time required to reach steady state, the half-life appears to be short (1 to 2 hours).

**Peak serum concentration**
Rimexolone 1% produced serum concentrations that were at, or near, steady state after hourly administration of five to seven doses.

**Elimination**
Feces; 80% as rimexolone and metabolites.

## Precautions to Consider

**Carcinogenicity**
Long-term studies have not been done.

### Mutagenicity
Rimexolone was shown to be nonmutagenic in a battery of *in vitro* and *in vivo* mutagenicity assays.

### Pregnancy/Reproduction
Fertility—In one study, fertility and reproductive capability were not impaired in rats that had plasma levels of 42 nanograms per mL of rimexolone, which is approximately 200 times the levels obtained in clinical studies of ophthalmic rimexolone (less than 0.2 nanogram per mL in humans).

Pregnancy—Adequate and well-controlled studies have not been done in pregnant women. Rimexolone should be used in pregnant women only if the benefits to the mother outweigh the potential risk to the fetus.

Corticosteroids are recognized to cause fetal resorption and malformations in animals. Rimexolone was shown to be teratogenic and embryotoxic in rabbits administered 0.5 mg per kg of body weight a day subcutaneously, which was the lowest dose tested and approximately two times the recommended human ophthalmic dose.

FDA Pregnancy Category C.

### Breast-feeding
It is not known whether ophthalmic corticosteroids could result in sufficient systemic absorption to produce detectable quantities in human breast milk. Caution should be exercised when ophthalmic corticosteroids are administered to breast-feeding women.

### Pediatrics
Appropriate studies on the relationship of age to the effects of ophthalmic rimexolone have not been performed in children. Safety and efficacy have not been established.

### Geriatrics
No information is available on the relationship of age to the effects of ophthalmic rimexolone in geriatric patients.

### Medical considerations/Contraindications
The medical considerations/contraindications included have been selected on the basis of their potential clinical significance (reasons given in parentheses where appropriate)—not necessarily inclusive (» = major clinical significance).

*Except under special circumstances, this medication should not be used when the following medical problems exist:*
» Fungal diseases, ocular or
» Herpes simplex keratitis, epithelial (dendritic keratitis) or
» Infections of the eye, other, including acute, purulent infections or
» Mycobacterial infection, ocular or
» Viral diseases, such as vaccinia, varicella, and other viral diseases of the cornea and conjunctiva
  (corticosteroids decrease resistance to bacterial, fungal, and viral infections; application may mask or exacerbate existing infections and encourage the development of new or secondary infections)
» Sensitivity to rimexolone

*Risk-benefit should be considered when the following medical problems exist:*
» Diseases causing thinning of the cornea or sclera
  (use may result in perforation)

### Patient monitoring
The following may be especially important in patient monitoring (other tests may be warranted in some patients, depending on condition; » = major clinical significance):

Ophthalmologic examinations, including tonometry and slit-lamp examinations
  (intraocular pressure should be checked frequently; if rimexolone is administered in the presence of herpes simplex infection, great caution and frequent slit-lamp examinations are required)

## Side/Adverse Effects
Note: Prolonged use of rimexolone may result in glaucoma or ocular hypertension, damage to the optic nerve, defects in visual acuity and visual fields, and posterior subcapsular cataract formation.

Prolonged use may also result in secondary ocular infections, including herpes simplex, due to suppression of host response.

Fungal infections of the cornea are prone to develop during long-term corticosteroid treatment. Fungal invasion should be considered in any persistent corneal ulceration where a corticosteroid is, or was, in use.

The following side/adverse effects have been selected on the basis of their potential clinical significance (possible signs and symptoms in parentheses where appropriate)—not necessarily inclusive.

**Those indicating need for medical attention**
Incidence less frequent or rare
  *Blurred vision; conjunctival edema* (swelling of the lining of the eyelids); *corneal edema, erosion, staining, or ulcer* (blurred vision or other change in vision); *eye discharge, discomfort, dryness, irritation, pain, or tearing; foreign body sensation* (feeling of something in the eye); *hyperemia* (eye redness); *increased fibrin; increased intraocular pressure; infiltrate* (eye redness, irritation, or pain); *keratitis* (eye redness, irritation, or pain); *pharyngitis* (sore throat); *pruritus* (itching); *rhinitis* (stuffy or runny nose)

**Those indicating need for medical attention only if they continue or are bothersome**
Incidence less frequent or rare
  *Browache; headache; hypotension* (unusual tiredness or weakness; dizziness, lightheadness, or faintness); *lid margin crusting* (crusting in corner of eye); *photophobia* (increased sensitivity of eyes to light); *sticky sensation of eyelids; taste perversion* (change in taste)

## Patient Consultation
As an aid to patient consultation, refer to *Advice for the Patient, Rimexolone (Ophthalmic)—Introductory Version.*

In providing consultation, consider emphasizing the following selected information (» = major clinical significance):

**Before using this medication**
» Conditions affecting use, especially:
    Sensitivity to rimexolone or other corticosteroids
    Pregnancy—Rimexolone administered subcutaneously was teratogenic and embryotoxic in studies in rabbits
    Other medical problems, especially diseases causing thinning of the cornea or sclera; fungal diseases, ocular; herpes simplex keratitis, epithelial (dendritic keratitis); infections of the eye, other, including acute, purulent infections; mycobacterial infection, ocular; or viral diseases, such as vaccinia, varicella, and other viral diseases of the cornea and conjunctiva

**Proper use of this medication**
Shaking suspension well before applying
» Proper administration technique; preventing contamination; not touching applicator tip to any surface
» Proper dosing
   Missed dose: Using missed dose as soon as possible; if almost time for next dose, skipping missed dose and going back to regular dosing schedule
» Proper storage

**Precautions while using this medication**
Need for ophthalmologic examinations during prolonged therapy

**Side/adverse effects**
Signs of potential side effects, especially blurred vision; conjunctival edema; corneal edema, erosion, staining, or ulcer; eye discharge, discomfort, dryness, irritation, pain, or tearing; foreign body sensation; hyperemia; increased fibrin; increased intraocular pressure; infiltrate; keratitis; pharyngitis; pruritus; and rhinitis

## General Dosing Information
Rimexolone is not for injection.

## Ophthalmic Dosage Forms
### RIMEXOLONE OPHTHALMIC SUSPENSION

**Usual adult and adolescent dose**
Postoperative inflammation—
  Topical, to the conjunctiva, 1 or 2 drops in the affected eye four times a day beginning twenty-four hours after surgery and continuing throughout the first two weeks of the postoperative period.
Anterior uveitis—
  Topical, to the conjunctiva, 1 or 2 drops in the affected eye every hour during waking hours for the first week, 1 drop every two hours during waking hours of the second week, and then tapering the frequency until uveitis is resolved.

**Usual pediatric dose**
Safety and efficacy have not been established.

**Strength(s) usually available**
U.S.—
  1% (Rx) [*Vexol* (benzalkonium chloride 0.01%; mannitol; carbomer 934P; polysorbate 80; sodium chloride; edetate disodium; sodium hydroxide; hydrochloric acid)].

**Packaging and storage**
Store between 4 and 30 °C (39 and 86 °F).

**Auxiliary labeling**
- For the eye.
- Shake well.
- Store container upright.

Developed: 09/20/95
Revised: 08/13/98

# RISEDRONATE Systemic—INTRODUCTORY VERSION

VA CLASSIFICATION (Primary): HS303
Commonly used brand name(s): *Actonel*.
Note: For a listing of dosage forms and brand names by country availability, see *Dosage Forms* section(s).

## Category
Bone resorption inhibitor.

## Indications
**Accepted**
Paget's disease of bone (treatment)—Risedronate is indicated for the treatment of Paget's disease of bone (osteitis deformans) in patients with alkaline phosphatase concentrations that are at least two times the upper limit of normal, those who are symptomatic, or those at risk for future complications from the disease. Signs and symptoms of Paget's disease may include bone pain, deformity, and/or fractures; increased concentrations of *N*-telopeptide of type I collagen, serum alkaline phosphatase, and/or urinary hydroxyproline; neurologic disorders associated with skull lesions and spinal deformities; and elevated cardiac output and other vascular disorders associated with increased vascularity of bones.

## Pharmacology/Pharmacokinetics
**Physicochemical characteristics**
Chemical group—A pyridinyl bisphosphonate.
Molecular weight—Anhydrous: 305.1.
Hemi-pentahydrate: 350.13.
Solubility—Soluble in water and in aqueous solutions, and essentially insoluble in common organic solvents.

**Mechanism of action/Effect**
Risedronate binds to bone hydroxyapatite and, at the cellular level, inhibits osteoclasts. Although the osteoclasts adhere normally to the bone surface, they show evidence of reduced active resorption (e.g., lack of ruffled border). Evidence from studies in rats and dogs indicates that risedronate treatment reduces bone turnover (activation frequency, i.e., the number of sites at which bone is remodeled) and bone resorption at remodeling sites.

**Absorption**
Rapid and independent of dose, occurring throughout the upper gastrointestinal tract. Mean oral bioavailability is 0.63% and is decreased when administered with food. Administration either 0.5 hour before breakfast or 2 hours after dinner reduces the extent of absorption by 55% compared to the fasting state (no food or drink for 10 hours before or 4 hours after administration). Administration 1 hour before breakfast reduces the extent of absorption by 30% compared with the fasting state.

**Distribution**
Studies in rats and dogs with intravenously administered single doses of radiolabeled risedronate showed that approximately 60% of the dose was distributed to bone.
The mean steady-state volume of distribution is 6.3 liters per kg of body weight in humans.

**Protein binding**
Plasma—Low (about 24%).

**Biotransformation**
There is no evidence that risedronate is metabolized in humans or animals.

**Half-life**
Initial—
 Approximately 1.5 hours.
Terminal exponential—
 220 hours (which may represent the dissociation of risedronate from the surface of bone).

**Time to peak concentration**
1 hour.

**Time to peak effect**
3 months in one study.

**Duration of action**
At least 16 months in one study.

**Elimination**
Fecal, unabsorbed drug (unchanged).
Renal, unchanged, approximately 50% of the absorbed dose within 24 hours, 85% over 28 days. Mean renal clearance is 105 mL per minute (mL/min) and mean total clearance is 122 mL/min, the difference primarily reflecting nonrenal clearance or clearance due to adsorption to bone.
Note: Renal clearance is not concentration-dependent and there is a linear relationship between renal clearance and creatinine clearance.

## Precautions to Consider
**Carcinogenicity**
Long-term studies to determine the carcinogenic potential of residronate have not been done in humans or animals.

**Mutagenicity**
Risedronate was not found to be mutagenic in a number of assays, including *in vitro* bacterial mutagenesis in *Salmonella* and *Escherichia coli* (Ames assay), mammalian cell mutagenesis in CHO/HGPRT assay, unscheduled DNA synthesis in rat hepatocytes, and an assessment of chromosomal aberrations *in vivo* in rat bone marrow. Positive results were obtained in a chromosomal aberration assay in CHO cells at highly cytotoxic concentrations (>675 mcg per mL, survival of 6% to 7%); however, when the assay was repeated at doses exhibiting appropriate cell survival (29%), there was no evidence of chromosomal damage.

**Pregnancy/Reproduction**
Fertility—Studies in female rats at oral doses of 16 mg per kg of body weight (mg/kg) per day (approximately five times the human 30-mg dose on a mg per square meter of body surface area [mg/m$^2$] basis) found inhibition of ovulation. At doses of 7 and 16 mg/kg per day (two and five times the human 30-mg dose on a mg/m$^2$ basis), decreased implantation was noted. Studies in male rats at doses of 40 mg/kg per day (13 times the human 30-mg dose on a mg/m$^2$ basis) found testicular and epididymal atrophy and inflammation. Studies in male dogs at a dose of 8 mg/kg per day (approximately eight times the human 30-mg dose on a mg/m$^2$ basis) found moderate to severe spermatid maturation block after 13 weeks. Studies in male rats at doses of 16 mg/kg per day (five times the human 30-mg dose on a mg/m$^2$ basis) found testicular atrophy after 13 weeks. Findings tended to show an increased severity with increased dose and exposure time.

Pregnancy—Adequate and well-controlled studies in humans have not been done.
Studies in rats at doses of 16 and 80 mg/kg per day (5 and 27 times the human 30-mg dose on a mg/m$^2$ basis) during gestation found decreased survival of neonates. Body weight was increased in neonates from dams treated with 7.1 and 16 mg/kg (two and five times the human 30-mg dose on a mg/m$^2$ basis), but decreased in neonates from dams treated with 80 mg/kg (27 times the human 30-mg dose based on a mg/m$^2$ basis). In rats treated during gestation, the number of fetuses exhibiting incomplete ossification of sternebrae or skull was statistically significantly decreased at 3.2 mg/kg per day, but increased at 7.1 mg/kg per day (one and two times the human 30-mg dose on a mg/m$^2$ basis). Statistically significant decreases in the number of fetuses exhibiting unossified fetal sternebrae occurred at these same doses. In rats treated with 16 and 80 mg/kg per day (5 and 27 times the human 30-mg dose on a mg/m$^2$ basis), both incomplete ossification and the number of unossified sternebrae were increased. When female rats were treated with 3.2 and 7.1 mg/kg per day (one and two times the human 30-mg dose on a mg/m$^2$ basis), a low incidence of cleft palate was observed in fetuses. Studies in rabbits at doses of up to 10 mg/kg per day during gestation (seven times the human 30-mg dose on a mg/m$^2$ basis) found no significant fetal ossification effects. However, in rabbits treated with

10 mg/kg per day, 1 of 14 litters was aborted and 1 of 14 litters was delivered prematurely.

Like other bisphosphonates, risedronate in doses as low as 3.2 mg/kg per day (equal to the human 30-mg dose on a mg/m² basis) during mating and gestation has resulted in periparturient hypocalcemia and mortality in pregnant rats allowed to deliver.

FDA Pregnancy Category C.

**Breast-feeding**
It is not known whether risedronate passes into human breast milk. However, a small degree of lacteal transfer has been detected in lactating rats for a 24-hour period postdosing. Risk-benefit should be considered before breast-feeding during risedronate treatment.

**Pediatrics**
Studies on the relationship of age to the effects of risedronate in pediatric patients (younger than 18 years of age) have not been done. Safety and efficacy have not been established.

**Geriatrics**
Studies indicate that bioavailability and disposition of risedronate are similar in patients older than 60 years of age to those in younger adults. No dosage adjustment is necessary.

**Drug interactions and/or related problems**
The following drug interactions and/or related problems have been selected on the basis of their potential clinical significance (possible mechanism in parentheses where appropriate)—not necessarily inclusive (» = major clinical significance):

Note: Combinations containing any of the following medications, depending on the amount present, may also interact with this medication.

» Antacids containing calcium or
» Calcium-containing preparations
　(simultaneous use may interfere with the absorption of risedronate)
　Anti-inflammatory agents, nonsteroidal or
　Aspirin
　　(concurrent use may result in increased gastrointestinal irritation)

**Laboratory value alterations**
The following have been selected on the basis of their potential clinical significance (possible effect in parentheses where appropriate)—not necessarily inclusive (» = major clinical significance):

With diagnostic test results
　Bone imaging
　　(bisphosphonates are known to interfere with the use of bone imaging agents)

With physiology/laboratory test values
　Calcium and
　Phosphorus
　　(small, asymptomatic decreases in serum concentrations have occurred in some patients)

**Medical considerations/Contraindications**
The medical considerations/contraindications included have been selected on the basis of their potential clinical significance (reasons given in parentheses where appropriate)—not necessarily inclusive (» = major clinical significance).

*Risk-benefit should be considered when the following medical problems exist:*
　Gastrointestinal disorders, upper
　　(bisphosphonates may cause upper gastrointestinal disorders such as dysphagia, esophagitis, esophageal ulcer, and gastric ulcer; caution is recommended with use of risedronate in these conditions)
» Renal function impairment
　　(renal clearance is significantly decreased [by about 70%] in patients with creatinine clearance of approximately 30 mL per minute [mL/min]; use is not recommended in patients with creatinine clearance less than 30 mL/min; no dosage adjustment is necessary when creatinine clearance is 30 mL/min or higher)
» Sensitivity to risedronate

**Patient monitoring**
The following may be especially important in patient monitoring (other tests may be warranted in some patients, depending on condition; » = major clinical significance):

» Alkaline phosphatase, serum values
　(determinations recommended to confirm effectiveness of risedronate therapy)

## Side/Adverse Effects

The following side/adverse effects have been selected on the basis of their potential clinical significance (possible signs and symptoms in parentheses where appropriate)—not necessarily inclusive:

**Those indicating need for medical attention**
Incidence more frequent (incidence 11.5%)
　*Abdominal or stomach pain; skin rash*
　Note: *Abdominal or stomach pain* may be associated with dysphagia, esophagitis, esophageal ulcers, or gastric ulcer.
Incidence less frequent (incidence 3 to 5%)
　*Belching; bone pain; colitis* (abdominal or stomach pain, severe; cramping)
　Note: *Belching* may be a symptom of esophagitis.
Incidence rare
　*Iritis, acute* (red, sore eyes)

**Those indicating need for medical attention only if they continue or are bothersome**
Incidence more frequent (incidence 18 to 33%)
　*Arthralgia* (joint pain); *diarrhea; headache*
Incidence less frequent (incidence 3 to 10%)
　*Amblyopia* (blurred vision or a change in vision); *asthenia* (weakness); *bronchitis* (cough); *chest pain; constipation; dizziness; dry eyes; flu-like syndrome* (fever; general feeling of discomfort or illness); *leg cramps; myasthenia* (weakness); *nausea; peripheral edema* (swelling of feet or lower legs); *sinusitis* (headache); *tinnitus* (ringing in the ears)

## Overdose

For more specific information on the agents used in the management of risedronate overdose, see:
• *Calcium Supplements (Systemic)* monograph.

For more information on the management of overdose or unintentional ingestion, **contact a Poison Control Center** (see *Poison Control Center Listing*).

**Clinical effects of overdose**
Although overdose with risedronate has not been reported, decreases in serum calcium (including signs and symptoms of hypocalcemia) would be expected to occur with substantial overdose in some patients.

**Treatment of overdose**
To decrease absorption—Gastric lavage may remove unabsorbed drug. Administration of milk or antacids to chelate risedronate may be helpful.
Specific treatment—Standard procedures for treatment of hypocalcemia, including administration of intravenous calcium, would be expected to restore physiologic amounts of ionized calcium and to relieve signs and symptoms of hypocalcemia.

## Patient Consultation

As an aid to patient consultation, refer to *Advice for the Patient, Risedronate (Systemic)—Introductory Version*.

In providing consultation, consider emphasizing the following selected information (» = major clinical significance):

**Before using this medication**
» Conditions affecting use, especially:
　Sensitivity to risedronate
　Pregnancy—Studies in animals showed decreased weight gain, incomplete fetal ossification, and decreased survival of the fetus
　Breast-feeding—Distributed into milk in lactating rats; risk-benefit should be considered
　Other medications, especially calcium-containing antacids or other calcium-containing preparations
　Other medical problems, especially renal function impairment

**Proper use of this medication**
» Taking with 6 to 8 ounces of plain water on empty stomach, at least 30 minutes before first food, beverage, or medication of the day
» Not lying down for at least 30 minutes after taking risedronate
　Possible need for calcium and vitamin D supplementation
» Proper dosing
　Missed dose: Not taking later in the day; continuing usual schedule the next morning
» Proper storage

**Precautions while using this medication**
　Importance of close monitoring by physician

**Side/adverse effects**
　Signs of potential side effects, especially abdominal or stomach pain, skin rash, belching, bone pain, colitis, or acute iritis

## General Dosing Information

To facilitate delivery of risedronate to the stomach and reduce esophageal irritation, patients should not lie down for at least 30 minutes after taking risedronate.

Hypocalcemia and other disturbances of bone and mineral metabolism should be treated effectively before risedronate therapy is initiated.

### Diet/Nutrition

Risedronate should be taken with 6 to 8 ounces of plain water. Absorption of risedronate is best when it is taken in the morning, at least 30 minutes before the first food, beverage, or medication of the day. Waiting longer than 30 minutes will improve the absorption of risedronate.

A well-balanced diet with adequate intake of calcium and vitamin D should be maintained. Calcium and vitamin D supplements may be prescribed if necessary.

## Oral Dosage Forms

### RISEDRONATE SODIUM TABLETS

**Usual adult dose**
Paget's disease of bone (treatment)—
  30 mg once a day for two months. Re-treatment may be considered, after a posttreatment observation period of at least two months, if relapse occurs, or if treatment fails to normalize serum alkaline phosphatase values. For retreatment, the dose and duration of therapy are the same as for initial treatment.

**Usual pediatric dose**
Safety and efficacy in children younger than 18 years of age have not been established.

**Strength(s) usually available**
U.S.—
  30 mg (Rx) [*Actonel* (lactose monohydrate)].

**Packaging and storage**
Store between 20 and 25 °C (68 and 77 °F).

**Auxiliary labeling**
• Take on an empty stomach.

Developed: 08/12/98

---

# RISPERIDONE   Systemic

VA CLASSIFICATION (Primary): CN709
Commonly used brand name(s): *Risperdal*.
Note:  For a listing of dosage forms and brand names by country availability, see *Dosage Forms* section(s).

## Category

Antipsychotic.
Note:  Risperidone is considered by some experts to be an atypical antipsychotic. Universal acceptance of the exact parameters that define an antipsychotic as an atypical agent has not been established. Differences in binding affinities and activity at various receptor sites may explain the differing profiles of the newer antipsychotics.

## Indications

### Accepted

Psychotic disorders (treatment)—Risperidone is used to treat the manifestations of psychotic disorders. It appears to produce a significant improvement in both the positive and negative symptoms of schizophrenia.

## Pharmacology/Pharmacokinetics

### Physicochemical characteristics

Chemical group—A benzisoxazole derivative.
Molecular weight—410.49.
$pKa_1$—8.24.
$pKa_2$—3.11.

### Mechanism of action/Effect

The mechanism by which risperidone exerts its antipsychotic effect is unknown. Risperidone is a selective monoaminergic antagonist with a strong affinity for serotonin type 2 (5-$HT_2$) receptors and a slightly weaker affinity for dopamine type 2 ($D_2$) receptors. The antipsychotic activity of risperidone may be mediated through antagonism at a combination of these receptor sites, particularly through blockade of cortical serotonin receptors and limbic dopamine systems.

Risperidone also has moderate affinity for the $alpha_1$-adrenergic, $alpha_2$-adrenergic, and $H_1$-histaminergic receptors. The affinity of risperidone for the serotonin 5-$HT_{1A}$, 5-$HT_{1C}$, and 5-$HT_{1D}$ receptors is low to moderate, while its affinity for dopamine $D_1$ receptors and the haloperidol-sensitive sigma site is weak.

Risperidone has negligible affinity for cholinergic-muscarinic, beta-adrenergic, and serotonin 5-$HT_{1B}$ and 5-$HT_3$ receptors.

### Other actions/effects

Cardiovascular effects reflect the vascular alpha-adrenergic antagonistic activity of risperidone, as evidenced by such dose-related effects as hypotension and reflex tachycardia. The potential for proarrhythmic effects exists, due to risperidone's ability to prolong the QT interval in some patients.

Risperidone changes sleep architecture by promoting deep slow-wave sleep, thereby improving sleep patterns. This effect is most likely due to risperidone's blockade of serotonin receptors.

Substantial and sustained elevations in serum prolactin levels are induced by risperidone. It appears that tolerance to hyperprolactinemia does not occur, but the condition is reversible upon withdrawal of risperidone. Increases in prolactin concentrations are likely due to risperidone's blockade of dopamine receptors.

Preliminary reports suggest that risperidone may suppress pre-existing dyskinesias and may exhibit a low propensity for inducing extrapyramidal symptoms or tardive dyskinesia. However, some clinicians believe that risperidone is likely to cause tardive movement disorders because of its relatively potent blockade of $D_2$ receptors. Additional data from long-term studies are needed to resolve these issues.

Risperidone exerts an antiemetic effect in animals that may also occur in humans, potentially masking signs and symptoms of other medical problems.

Disturbances of body temperature regulation have been reported with the use of other antipsychotics; both hypothermia and hyperthermia have been reported with the use of risperidone.

### Absorption

Rapid and extensive. Food does not significantly affect the extent of absorption; therefore, risperidone may be given without respect to meals.

The relative bioavailability of risperidone from a tablet is 94% when compared with a solution. The absolute oral bioavailability of risperidone is 70%; the absolute bioavailability of the active moiety (risperidone plus 9-hydroxy-risperidone) approaches 100%, irrespective of the route of administration or the metabolic phenotype status of the patient.

### Distribution

Rapid and extensive. The volume of distribution ($Vol_D$) at steady state is about 1.1 L per kg. In animals, risperidone and 9-hydroxy-risperidone are distributed into milk, reaching concentrations comparable to plasma concentrations.

### Protein binding

Risperidone—Very high (90%).
9-hydroxy-risperidone—High (77%).
Note:  In plasma, risperidone is predominantly bound to albumin and $alpha_1$-acid glycoprotein (AGP). Although the pharmacokinetics of risperidone in patients with hepatic function impairment are similar to those in healthy young controls, the mean free fraction of risperidone in plasma is increased by about 35% due to decreased concentrations of albumin and AGP.

### Biotransformation

Risperidone is extensively metabolized in the liver by the cytochrome P450 2D6 (CYP2D6) isoenzyme. The main metabolic pathway, hydroxylation, yields the major active metabolite 9-hydroxy-risperidone. The pharmacologic activity, potency, and safety of this metabolite are comparable to those of its parent compound.

### Half-life
Elimination—
- Overall mean elimination half-life of the active moiety (risperidone plus 9-hydroxy-risperidone) ranges from 20 to 24 hours.
- In patients with renal function impairment, increased elimination half-lives have been reported. Dosage reductions for patients with renal function impairment are recommended.

### Time to peak concentration
Mean peak risperidone plasma concentrations occur within 1 to 2 hours following oral administration.

### Time to steady-state plasma concentrations
Steady-state concentrations of the active moiety (risperidone plus 9-hydroxy-risperidone) are achieved within 5 to 6 days.

### Peak plasma concentration
In one study in healthy volunteers, peak plasma concentrations of the active moiety (risperidone plus 9-hydroxy-risperidone) ranging from 9 to 16 nanograms/mL were reported following oral administration of 1 mg of risperidone. However, no correlation between plasma concentrations and therapeutic effect has been definitively established.

### Plasma concentrations
Although interindividual plasma concentrations vary considerably, plasma concentrations of risperidone, 9-hydroxy-risperidone, and the active moiety (risperidone plus 9-hydroxy-risperidone) are dose-proportional and linear over the therapeutic dosing range.

### Elimination
Renal—
- In patients with normal renal function: Approximately 70% of administered oral dose.
- In patients with moderate to severe renal function impairment: Renal clearance of the active moiety (risperidone plus 9-hydroxy-risperidone) may be decreased by 60 to 80%.

Fecal—
- Approximately 15% of administered oral dose.

## Precautions to Consider

### Carcinogenicity/Tumorigenicity
Significant increases in the incidence of mammary gland adenocarcinomas and pituitary adenomas occurred in female Swiss albino mice that received risperidone for 18 months at doses of 2.4 and 9.4 times, respectively, the maximum recommended human dose (MRHD) on a mg per kg of body weight (mg/kg) basis (0.2 and 0.75 times, respectively, the MRHD on a mg per square meter of body surface area [mg/m$^2$] basis). In Wistar rats that received risperidone for 25 months, males dosed at 9.4 times the MRHD on a mg/kg basis (1.5 times the MHRD on a mg/m$^2$ basis) exhibited increased incidences of endocrine pancreas adenomas and mammary gland neoplasms; also, mammary gland adenocarcinomas were reported in males dosed at 37.5 times the MRHD on a mg/kg basis (6 times the MRHD on a mg/m$^2$ basis) and in females dosed at 2.4 times the MRHD on a mg/kg basis (0.4 times the MRHD on a mg/m$^2$ basis).

Risperidone, like other agents that antagonize dopamine D$_2$ receptors, elevates prolactin concentrations; the elevation persists during chronic administration. Tissue culture experiments indicate that approximately one-third of human breast cancers are prolactin-dependent *in vitro*, a factor of potential importance if use of this medication is contemplated in a patient with a previously detected breast cancer. Although disturbances such as galactorrhea, amenorrhea, gynecomastia, and impotence have been reported, the clinical significance of elevated serum prolactin concentrations is unknown for most patients. An increase in pituitary gland, mammary gland, and pancreatic islet cell hyperplasia and/or neoplasia has been found in rodents after chronic administration of medications (including risperidone) that increase prolactin release. However, neither clinical studies nor epidemiologic studies conducted to date have shown an association between chronic administration of these medications and tumorigenesis in humans; the available evidence is considered too limited to be conclusive at this time.

### Mutagenicity
Risperidone demonstrated no mutagenic potential in the following tests: Ames reverse mutation test, mouse lymphoma assay, *in vitro* rat hepatocyte DNA-repair assay, *in vivo* micronucleus test in mice, the sex-linked recessive lethal test in *Drosophila*, and the chromosomal aberration test in human lymphocytes or Chinese hamster cells.

### Pregnancy/Reproduction
Fertility—In three reproductive studies, risperidone was shown to impair mating but not fertility in Wistar rats that received 0.1 to 3 times the MRHD on a mg/m$^2$ basis; this effect apparently occurred only in female rats. In a study in beagle dogs, sperm motility and concentration were decreased at risperidone doses of 0.6 to 10 times the MRHD on a mg/m$^2$ basis. Dose-related decreases in serum testosterone were also noted. Serum testosterone and sperm parameters partially recovered but remained decreased after discontinuation of risperidone.

Pregnancy—Adequate and well-controlled studies in humans have not been done.

Agenesis of the corpus callosum in an infant exposed to risperidone *in utero* has been reported. However, a causal relationship to risperidone therapy has not been established.

In three teratogenicity studies conducted in rats and rabbits that received 0.4 to 6 times the MRHD of risperidone on a mg/m$^2$ basis, the incidence of malformations was not increased as compared with controls. In three reproductive studies in rats, there was an increase in pup deaths during the first 4 days of lactation at doses of 0.1 to 3 times the MRHD on a mg/m$^2$ basis; it is not known whether these deaths were due to a direct effect on the fetuses or pups, or to effects on the dams. In another study in rats receiving risperidone doses of 1.5 times the MRHD on a mg/m$^2$ basis, there was an increase in the number of stillborn pups.

FDA Pregnancy Category C.

Labor and delivery—The effect of risperidone on labor and delivery is not known.

### Breast-feeding
Risperidone and 9-hydroxy-risperidone are distributed into the milk of animals in concentrations greater than or equal to plasma concentrations. It is not known if these substances are distributed into human breast milk.

### Pediatrics
No information is available on the relationship of age to the effects of risperidone in pediatric patients. Safety and efficacy in children up to 18 years of age have not been established.

### Geriatrics
There is limited experience in the use of risperidone in the elderly. In healthy elderly patients, decreases in renal clearance and increases in the elimination half-life of the active moiety (risperidone plus 9-hydroxy-risperidone) have been reported. Also, geriatric patients generally have decreased renal function, decreased hepatic function, decreased cardiac function, and an increased tendency to postural hypotension. Therefore, reduced risperidone doses are recommended.

### Pharmacogenetics
Hydroxylation of risperidone via the cytochrome P450 2D6 (CYP2D6) isoenzyme is subject to genetic polymorphism. About 6 to 8% of Caucasians and a low percentage of Asians have little or no CYP2D6 activity and are considered poor metabolizers. Patients taking risperidone who have normal CYP2D6 activity (considered extensive metabolizers) have lower plasma concentrations of risperidone and higher concentrations of 9-hydroxy-risperidone than do patients who are poor metabolizers. Although blood levels of risperidone and 9-hydroxy-risperidone can differ by up to sevenfold, there is no difference in the area under the plasma concentration–time curve (AUC) for the combination, and clinical data do not indicate that the ratio affects either therapeutics or incidence of adverse effects. Overall, the pharmacokinetic parameters of the active moiety (risperidone plus 9-hydroxy-risperidone) are similar in all metabolizers. Therefore, the metabolic phenotype status of patients is not considered to have clinically significant effects on risperidone therapy.

### Drug interactions and/or related problems
The following drug interactions and/or related problems have been selected on the basis of their potential clinical significance (possible mechanism in parentheses where appropriate)—not necessarily inclusive (» = major clinical significance):

Note: Medications that inhibit the cytochrome P450 2D6 (CYP2D6) isoenzyme potentially could inhibit the metabolism of risperidone. However, since only the relative amounts of risperidone and 9-hydroxy-risperidone and not the total concentration of active moiety (risperidone plus 9-hydroxy-risperidone) would be affected, no marked changes in activity should occur. *In vitro*, medications metabolized by other P450 isoenzymes (including CYP1A1, CYP1A2, CYP2C9, CYP2C19, and CYP3A4) are only weak inhibitors of risperidone metabolism.

Similarly, risperidone potentially could interfere with the metabolism of other medications metabolized via CYP2D6; however, risperidone is bound relatively weakly to the enzyme, so these effects seem unlikely to be clinically significant.

*In vitro* studies have shown no significant interactions caused by other highly protein-bound agents displacing or being displaced by risperidone.

Combinations containing any of the following medications, depending on the amount present, may also interact with this medication.

» Alcohol or
» Central nervous system (CNS) depression–producing medications, other (see *Appendix II*)
(additive CNS depressant effects may occur)
» Antihypertensive medications
(potential hypotensive effects of these medications can enhance hypotensive effects of risperidone)
» Bromocriptine or
» Levodopa or
» Pergolide
(risperidone may antagonize the effects of levodopa and dopamine agonists)
» Carbamazepine
(chronic administration of carbamazepine may increase the clearance of risperidone)
» Clozapine
(chronic administration of clozapine may decrease the clearance of risperidone)

### Laboratory value alterations
The following have been selected on the basis of their potential clinical significance (possible effect in parentheses where appropriate)—not necessarily inclusive (» = major clinical significance):

With physiology/laboratory test values
Electrocardiogram
(prolongation of the QT interval has occurred in some patients)
Prolactin concentrations, serum
(sustained elevations occur during therapy with risperidone)

### Medical considerations/Contraindications
The medical considerations/contraindications included have been selected on the basis of their potential clinical significance (reasons given in parentheses where appropriate)—not necessarily inclusive (» = major clinical significance).

*Risk-benefit should be considered when the following medical problems exist:*

Brain tumor or
Intestinal obstruction or
Medication overdose or
Reye's syndrome
(risperidone's antiemetic effect may mask signs and symptoms of these conditions)
» Breast cancer
(prolactin-dependent cancer may be exacerbated)
» Cardiovascular disease, including heart failure, conduction abnormalities, or history of myocardial infarction or
» Cerebrovascular disease
(condition may be exacerbated by risperidone-induced hypotension)
» Dehydration or
» Hypovolemia
(these conditions may increase likelihood or severity of risperidone-induced hypotension)
Drug abuse or dependence, history of
(although no evidence of drug-seeking behavior was seen in clinical trials, patients with a history of drug abuse should be observed closely for any signs of misuse of risperidone, as with any new CNS medication)
» Hepatic function impairment, severe
(metabolism and protein binding of risperidone may be decreased; reduced dosage is recommended)
» Parkinson's disease
(may be exacerbated)
» Renal function impairment, severe
(excretion of the active moieties of risperidone may be decreased; reduced dosage is recommended)
» Risk factors for *torsades de pointes*, including bradycardia, electrolyte imbalance, or concomitant intake of other medications that prolong the QT interval
(risk of *torsades de pointes* may be increased)
» Seizures, history of
(seizure threshold may be lowered)
Sensitivity to risperidone

### Patient monitoring
The following may be especially important in patient monitoring (other tests may be warranted in some patients, depending on condition; » = major clinical significance):

Abnormal-movement determinations
(recommended at periodic intervals to detect extrapyramidal symptoms)
Careful observation for early signs of tardive dyskinesia
(recommended at periodic intervals; since there is no known effective treatment if the syndrome develops, risperidone should be discontinued, if clinically feasible, at the earliest signs, usually fine, worm-like movements of the tongue, to stop further development)

## Side/Adverse Effects
The following side/adverse effects have been selected on the basis of their potential clinical significance (possible signs and symptoms in parentheses where appropriate)—not necessarily inclusive:

### Those indicating need for medical attention
Incidence more frequent
*Akathisia* (restlessness or need to keep moving); **anxiety or nervousness; changes in vision, including disturbances of accommodation and blurred vision; sexual dysfunction or decreased libido** (decreased sexual performance or desire); **dizziness; dysmenorrhea or menorrhagia** (menstrual changes); **extrapyramidal effects, dystonic** (muscle spasms of face, neck and back; tic-like or twitching movements; twisting movements of body; inability to move eyes; weakness of arms and legs); **extrapyramidal effects, parkinsonian** (difficulty in speaking or swallowing; loss of balance control; mask-like face; shuffling walk; stiffness of arms or legs; trembling and shaking of hands and fingers); **insomnia** (trouble in sleeping); **micturition disturbances or polyuria** (problems in urination or increase in amount of urine); **mood or mental changes, including aggressive behavior, agitation, difficulty in concentration, and memory problems; skin rash or itching**

Note: *Extrapyramidal symptoms* are dose-related; *sexual dysfunction* and *decreased libido*, or *vision changes* may be dose-related.
*Menorrhagia* may be associated with increased prolactin concentrations.

Incidence less frequent
*Amenorrhea* (menstrual changes); **back pain; cardiovascular effects, including orthostatic hypotension** (dizziness or lightheadedness)—especially when getting up from a lying or sitting position; **orthostatic dizziness; hypotension; palpitation** (fast or irregular heartbeat); **chest pain, and reflex tachycardia or tachycardia** (fast heartbeat); **dyspnea** (trouble in breathing); **galactorrhea** (unusual secretion of milk); **seborrhea** (skin condition caused by excess release of oil—may be accompanied by dandruff and oily skin)

Note: *Amenorrhea* and *galactorrhea* are associated with increased prolactin concentrations. *Orthostatic dizziness*, *palpitation*, and *tachycardia* may be dose-related.

Incidence rare
*Anorexia* (loss of appetite); **hyperthermia** (dizziness; fast, shallow breathing; fast, weak heartbeat; headache; muscle cramps; pale, clammy skin; thirst); **or hypothermia** (confusion; drowsiness; poor coordination; shivering); **mania or hypomania** (talking, feeling, and acting with excitement and activity that cannot be controlled); **neuroleptic malignant syndrome (NMS)** (difficult or unusually fast breathing; fast heartbeat or irregular pulse; high fever; high or low [irregular] blood pressure; increased sweating; loss of bladder control; severe muscle stiffness; seizures; unusually pale skin; unusual tiredness or weakness); **polydipsia** (extreme thirst); **priapism** (prolonged, painful, inappropriate erection of the penis); **seizures** (convulsions); **tardive dyskinesia** (lip smacking or puckering; puffing of cheeks; rapid or worm-like movements of tongue; uncontrolled chewing movements; uncontrolled movements of arms and legs); **tardive dystonia** (increased blinking or spasms of eyelid; unusual facial expressions or body positions; uncontrolled twisting movements of neck, trunk, arms, or legs); **thrombocytopenic purpura** (unusual bleeding or bruising)

### Those indicating need for medical attention only if they continue or are bothersome
Incidence more frequent
*Asthenia, fatigue, or lassitude* (unusual tiredness or weakness); **constipation; cough; decreased salivation or dryness of mouth; diarrhea; drowsiness; dyspepsia** (heartburn); **headache; increased dream activity; increased duration of sleep; nausea; pharyngitis** (sore throat); **rhinitis** (stuffy or runny nose); **weight gain**

Note: *Asthenia, lassitude, or fatigue, drowsiness, increased duration of sleep*, and *weight gain* may be dose-related. *Rhinitis* is most likely due to alpha-adrenoceptor–mediated nasal congestion.

Incidence less frequent
*Abdominal pain; arthralgia* (joint pain); **dry skin; increased pigmentation** (darkening of skin color); **increased salivation** (increased water-

ing of mouth); *increased sweating; photosensitivity* (increased sensitivity of the skin to sun); *vomiting; weight loss*

Note: *Increased pigmentation* may be dose-related.

**Those indicating the need for medical attention if they occur after the medication is discontinued**

*Withdrawal emergent dyskinesia* (lip smacking or puckering; puffing of cheeks; rapid or worm-like movements of tongue; uncontrolled chewing movements; uncontrolled movements of arms and legs)

## Overdose

For specific information on the agents used in the management of risperidone overdose, see *Charcoal, Activated (Oral-Local)* monograph.

For more information on the management of overdose or unintentional ingestion, **contact a Poison Control Center** (see *Poison Control Center Listing*).

**Clinical effects of overdose**

The following effects have been selected on the basis of their potential clinical significance (possible signs and symptoms in parentheses where appropriate)—not necessarily inclusive:

Acute and chronic effects

*Drowsiness; extrapyramidal symptoms; electrocardiogram (ECG) abnormalities, especially prolonged QT interval; electrolyte disturbances; hypotension; seizures; tachycardia*

**Treatment of overdose**

There is no specific antidote for risperidone. Treatment is essentially symptomatic and supportive.

To decrease absorption—
Gastric lavage should be considered. Activated charcoal may be administered with a laxative. The risk of aspiration with induced emesis is increased if the patient is obtunded, seizing, or experiencing dystonic movements of the head and neck.

Specific treatment—
For treatment of severe extrapyramidal symptoms: Administration of anticholinergic agents may be indicated.
For treatment of arrhythmias caused by risperidone toxicity: Selection of an appropriate antiarrhythmic agent—Use of disopyramide, procainamide, or quinidine may add to risperidone toxicity by prolonging the QT interval. Also, the alpha-adrenergic blocking properties of bretylium may add to risperidone's effects, producing problematic hypotension.
For treatment of hypotension or circulatory collapse: Selection of an appropriate sympathomimetic—Beta-adrenergic stimulation properties of epinephrine or dopamine may worsen the hypotension induced by risperidone's alpha-adrenergic blockade.

Monitoring—
Cardiovascular monitoring should be initiated immediately to detect arrhythmias. Serum electrolytes should also be monitored.

Supportive care—
Supportive measures such as establishing intravenous lines, hydration, correction of electrolyte imbalance, oxygenation, and support of ventilatory function are essential for maintaining the vital functions of the patient. Patients in whom intentional overdose is confirmed or suspected should be referred for psychiatric consultation.

## Patient Consultation

As an aid to patient consultation, refer to *Advice for the Patient, Risperidone (Systemic)*.

In providing consultation, consider emphasizing the following selected information (» = major clinical significance):

**Before using this medication**
» Conditions affecting use, especially:
Sensitivity to risperidone
Pregnancy—Agenesis of the corpus callosum reported in one infant, but causal relationship not established
Breast-feeding—Risperidone appears in animal milk at levels approximating plasma concentrations
Use in the elderly—Older patients may be at increased risk for adverse effects; reduced dosage recommended
Other medications, especially antihypertensives, bromocriptine, carbamazepine, clozapine, CNS depressants, levodopa, or pergolide
Other medical problems, especially breast cancer, cardiovascular disease, cerebrovascular disease, dehydration, hepatic function impairment, history of seizures, hypovolemia, Parkinson's disease, renal function impairment, or risk factors for *torsades de pointes*

**Proper use of this medication**
» Compliance with therapy; not taking more or less medicine than prescribed
» Proper dosing
Stirring measured dose of oral solution into water, coffee, orange juice, or low-fat milk prior to use; not mixing with cola or tea
Missed dose: Taking as soon as possible; if almost time for next dose, skipping missed dose; not doubling doses
» Proper storage

**Precautions while using this medication**
» Regular visits to physician to check progress of therapy
» Checking with physician before discontinuing medication; gradual dosage reduction may be needed
» Avoiding use of alcoholic beverages; not taking other CNS depressants unless prescribed by physician
» Caution if any kind of surgery, dental treatment, or emergency treatment is required; telling physician or dentist in charge about treatment with risperidone because of possible drug interactions or adverse effects
» Possible blurred vision, dizziness, or drowsiness; caution when driving or doing jobs requiring alertness or clear vision
» Possible dizziness or lightheadedness; caution when getting up suddenly from a lying or sitting position
» Possible skin photosensitivity; avoiding unprotected exposure to sun; wearing protective clothing; using a sun block product that includes protection against both UVA-caused photosensitivity reactions and UVB-caused sunburn reactions; avoiding use of sunlamp, tanning bed, or tanning booth
Possible heatstroke or hypothermia; caution during exercise, hot baths, or exposure to extreme temperatures

**Side/adverse effects**
Akathisia; anxiety or nervousness; changes in vision; sexual dysfunction or decreased libido; dizziness; dysmenorrhea or menorrhagia; extrapyramidal effects; insomnia; micturition disturbances or polyuria; mood or mental changes; skin rash or itching; amenorrhea; back pain; cardiovascular effects; dyspnea; galactorrhea; seborrhea; anorexia; hyperthermia or hypothermia; mania or hypomania; neuroleptic malignant syndrome; polydipsia; priapism; seizures; tardive dyskinesia; tardive dystonia; thrombocytopenic purpura

## General Dosing Information

Risperidone dosage must be individualized by cautious titration from the lower dosage range, to avoid orthostatic hypotension. The need for risperidone should be reassessed periodically, and the patient maintained at the lowest possible dosage level.

Since the possibility of suicide is inherent in schizophrenia, patients should not have access to large quantities of this medication. To reduce the risk of overdose, some clinicians recommend that the patient be supplied with the smallest quantity of medication necessary for satisfactory patient management.

There is a significant curvilinear dose-response relationship over the range of 1 to 16 mg of risperidone a day. This represents an "optimal dose" curve, along which maximum activity of risperidone occurs at doses of 4 to 8 mg a day. In trials using two-times-a-day dosing, daily doses greater than 6 mg of risperidone were not proven to be more efficacious than lower risperidone doses and were associated with increased adverse effects. In a trial using once-a-day dosing, the 8-mg dose was generally more effective than the 4-mg dose.

**Diet/Nutrition**
Risperidone may be given without regard to food.

**Bioequivalenence information**
The oral solution and 1-mg tablet forms of risperidone are bioequivalent.

**For treatment of adverse effects**
Neuroleptic malignant syndrome (NMS)—Treatment is essentially symptomatic and supportive and may include the following:
• *Discontinuing risperidone immediately.*
• Hyperthermia—Administering antipyretics (aspirin or acetaminophen); using cooling blanket.
• Dehydration—Restoring fluids and electrolytes.
• Cardiovascular instability—Monitoring blood pressure and cardiac rhythm closely; use of sodium nitroprusside may allow vasodilation with subsequent heat loss from the skin in patients with less dominant muscle rigidity.
• Hypoxia—Administering oxygen; considering airway insertion and assisted ventilation.
• Muscle rigidity—Administering dantrolene sodium (100 to 300 mg per day in divided doses, or 1.25 to 1.5 mg per kg of body weight, intravenously) for muscle relaxation; or amantadine (100 mg two times

a day) or bromocriptine (5 mg three times a day) to restore central balance of dopamine and acetylcholine at the receptor site.
- If neuroleptics must be continued because of severe psychosis, initial treatment may consist of:
    —At least 5 days of neuroleptic abstinence before rechallenge.
    —Use of a neuroleptic of a different class from the one causing NMS.
    —Use of a low dose.
    —Using the neuroleptic only for controlling the psychosis.

Tardive dyskinesia or tardive dystonia—No known effective treatment. Dosage of risperidone should be lowered or medication discontinued, if clinically feasible, at earliest signs of tardive dyskinesia or tardive dystonia to prevent possible irreversible effects.

## Oral Dosage Forms

### RISPERIDONE ORAL SOLUTION

Note: The oral solution and 1-mg tablet forms of risperidone are bioequivalent.

**Usual adult dose**
Antipsychotic—
Oral, 1 mg two times a day on the first day; the dose may be increased to 2 mg two times a day on the second day, and further increased to 3 mg two times a day on the third day. However, although this regimen was employed in early trials of risperidone, many patients reportedly have been unable to tolerate such rapid titration. Slower titration may be necessary in many patients. Further dosage adjustments should be made as needed and tolerated in increments or decrements of 1 to 2 mg a day at intervals of no less than one week, thus enabling steady-state plasma concentrations to be reached before further dosage changes are instituted. Total daily doses of up to 8 mg may be administered in a single dose or in two divided doses.

Note: Dosing regimens for risperidone are somewhat controversial. Some clinicians advocate an initial dosing schedule of 0.5 to 1 mg two times a day, with the dosage being increased as needed and tolerated at intervals of three to five days, until a total daily dose of 4 to 8 mg is reached; that dosage level usually is maintained for one to two weeks prior to any further changes in dose.

Debilitated patients, as well as those who have severe hepatic or renal function impairment, and those who are predisposed to hypotension or for whom hypotension would pose a risk, should receive reduced doses, following the regimen described in the *Usual geriatric dose* section.

If risperidone treatment is to be reinitiated in a patient who previously was receiving risperidone therapy, the initial titration schedule should be followed.

When switching from other antipsychotics to risperidone, immediate discontinuation of the previous treatment may be acceptable for some patients, while more gradual discontinuation may be most appropriate for other patients. In all cases, the period of overlapping antipsychotic administration should be minimized. When switching patients from depot antipsychotics, risperidone may be instituted in place of the next scheduled depot injection, if medically appropriate. The need for continuing administration of medication to control extrapyramidal symptoms should be re-evaluated periodically.

**Usual adult prescribing limits**
16 mg per day.

Note: In adults with severe hepatic function impairment, the usual prescribing limit is 4 mg per day.

**Usual pediatric dose**
Safety and efficacy in children younger than 18 years of age have not been established.

**Usual geriatric dose**
Antipsychotic—
Oral, initially 0.5 mg two times a day. The dose may be increased as needed and tolerated in increments of 0.5 mg two times a day. Increases to dosages above 1.5 mg two times a day generally should occur at intervals of at least one week. It is recommended that titration to the target dosage be accomplished on a two-times-a-day regimen. Once-a-day dosing may be instituted after at least two to three days at the target dosage.

Note: There is potential for accumulation of risperidone in the elderly.

**Usual geriatric prescribing limits**
3 mg per day.

**Strength(s) usually available**
U.S.—
  1 mg per mL (Rx) [*Risperdal* (benzoic acid; purified water; sodium hydroxide; tartaric acid)].
Canada—
  1 mg per mL (Rx) [*Risperdal*].

**Packaging and storage**
Store at controlled room temperature, between 15 and 25 °C (59 and 77 °F), unless otherwise specified by manufacturer. Protect from light and freezing.

**Preparation of dosage form**
Measure the dose with the pipette provided and thoroughly stir the dose into about 100 mL (3 to 4 ounces) of a compatible beverage. Compatible beverages include water, coffee, orange juice, and low-fat milk.

**Incompatibilities**
Risperidone oral solution is not compatible with cola or tea.

**Auxiliary labeling**
- Avoid alcoholic beverages.
- Dilute dose before taking.
- May cause drowsiness.

**Note**
When dispensing, include the manufacturer-provided calibrated dispensing pipette.

### RISPERIDONE TABLETS

Note: The oral solution and 1-mg tablet forms of risperidone are bioequivalent.

**Usual adult dose**
See *Risperidone Oral Solution*.

**Usual adult prescribing limits**
See *Risperidone Oral Solution*.

**Usual pediatric dose**
See *Risperidone Oral Solution*.

**Usual geriatric dose**
See *Risperidone Oral Solution*.

**Usual geriatric prescribing limits**
See *Risperidone Oral Solution*.

**Strength(s) usually available**
U.S.—
  1 mg (Rx) [*Risperdal* (scored; colloidal silicon dioxide; corn starch; hydroxypropyl methylcellulose; lactose; magnesium stearate; microcrystalline cellulose; propylene glycol; sodium lauryl sulfate)].
  2 mg (Rx) [*Risperdal* (colloidal silicon dioxide; corn starch; FD&C Yellow No. 6 Aluminum Lake; hydroxypropyl methylcellulose; lactose; magnesium stearate; microcrystalline cellulose; propylene glycol; sodium lauryl sulfate; talc; titanium dioxide)].
  3 mg (Rx) [*Risperdal* (colloidal silicon dioxide; corn starch; D&C Yellow No. 10; hydroxypropyl methylcellulose; lactose; magnesium stearate; microcrystalline cellulose; propylene glycol; sodium lauryl sulfate; talc; titanium dioxide)].
  4 mg (Rx) [*Risperdal* (colloidal silicon dioxide; corn starch; D&C Yellow No. 10; FD&C Blue No. 2 Aluminum Lake; hydroxypropyl methylcellulose; lactose; magnesium stearate; microcrystalline cellulose; propylene glycol; sodium lauryl sulfate; talc; titanium dioxide)].
Canada—
  1 mg (Rx) [*Risperdal* (scored; lactose)].
  2 mg (Rx) [*Risperdal* (lactose)].
  3 mg (Rx) [*Risperdal* (lactose)].
  4 mg (Rx) [*Risperdal* (lactose)].

**Packaging and storage**
Store at controlled room temperature, between 15 and 25 °C (59 and 77 °F), unless otherwise specified by manufacturer. Protect from light and moisture.

**Auxiliary labeling**
- Avoid alcoholic beverages.
- May cause drowsiness.

## Selected Bibliography

Grant S, Fitton A. Risperidone. A review of its pharmacology and therapeutic potential in the treatment of schizophrenia. Drugs 1994; 48(2): 253-73.

Cohen LJ. Risperidone. Pharmacotherapy 1994; 14(3): 253-65.

Developed: 09/12/95
Interim revision: 11/17/97; 08/07/98

# RITODRINE Systemic

VA CLASSIFICATION (Primary/Secondary): AU100/GU900
Commonly used brand name(s): *Yutopar; Yutopar S.R.*
Note: For a listing of dosage forms and brand names by country availability, see *Dosage Forms* section(s).

## Category
Tocolytic.

## Indications

**Accepted**

Premature labor (prophylaxis and treatment)—Intravenous ritodrine is indicated in the treatment of preterm labor in patients with a pregnancy of 20 or more weeks' gestation. Preterm labor is defined as rhythmic uterine contractions less than 10 minutes apart accompanied by progressive cervical effacement and/or dilation before the end of the 37th week of gestation. By prolonging gestation, ritodrine may reduce the incidence of neonatal mortality and respiratory distress syndrome by allowing time for the fetus to age and the fetal lung to mature or time for corticosteroids to be administered to the mother to enhance lung maturity in the fetus. Suitable patients must have intact amniotic membranes, cervical dilation usually but not always less than 4 centimeters (cm), and cervical effacement less than 80%. Use is not recommended prior to the 20th week of pregnancy.

For intravenous ritodrine to be most effective, it is recommended that therapy begin as soon as the diagnosis of preterm labor is confirmed. Due to the potential risks for the patient and fetus, a physician experienced in the use of intravenous ritodrine should be present to intervene in case of an emergency.

Intravenous ritodrine is less likely to inhibit labor when labor is advanced (cervical dilation more than 4 cm or effacement more than 80%) or when patient is close to term; its use, according to one study, may be best in pregnancies of less than 28 weeks. Risk-benefit should be cautiously assessed for those women in advanced labor or whose amniotic membranes have ruptured as safety and efficacy have not been established for these patients; use of ritodrine is not recommended. Risk of intrauterine infection when amniotic membranes are ruptured must be considered.

Although oral ritodrine is indicated in the treatment of preterm labor in Canada, it is the opinion of the USP Obstetrics and Gynecology Advisory Panel that oral ritodrine cannot be recommended because its efficacy has not been established to be more effective than a placebo and alternative therapies may be more beneficial. Bed rest at home and early admission may be better alternatives than using oral ritodrine in treatment of preterm labor, including retreatment of recurrent preterm labor.

## Pharmacology/Pharmacokinetics

**Physicochemical characteristics**
Molecular weight—323.82.

**Mechanism of action/Effect**
Ritodrine, a beta-2–adrenergic agonist, relaxes the uterus by stimulating the beta-2–adrenergic receptors of the uterine muscle, which causes a decrease in the intensity and frequency of uterine contractions. Specifically, ritodrine decreases uterine myometrial contractility by increasing cellular cyclic adenosine monophosphate (cAMP) and increasing cell membrane cytokines that increase and sequester intracellular calcium. Without intracellular calcium, the activation of contractile protein of smooth muscle is prevented and the uterus relaxes.

**Other actions/effects**
In addition to stimulating the beta-2–adrenergic receptors of the uterine smooth muscle, ritodrine stimulates beta-adrenergic receptors of bronchial and vascular smooth muscles. The cardiostimulatory effects, including increased cardiac output, increased maternal and fetal heart rates, and widening of the maternal pulse pressure, are probably due to relaxation of vascular smooth muscle. Relaxation of vascular smooth muscle stimulates the beta-1–adrenergic receptors and the reflex response to blood pressure. Also, during intravenous administration, ritodrine transiently increases maternal and fetal blood glucose and maternal plasma insulin concentrations. Other metabolic changes include increased cAMP, lactic acid, and free fatty acids, and decreased serum potassium concentration.

**Distribution**
Ritodrine and its conjugates transfer via placenta into the fetal circulation; fetal and maternal concencentrations may be equal.

**Protein binding**
Low (almost exclusively to albumin).

**Biotransformation**
Hepatic (inactive metabolites); metabolized to conjugates by both the mother and the fetus.

**Half-life**
Intravenous—Nonpregnant females—
  Distribution: 6 to 9 minutes.
  Elimination: 1.7 to 2.6 hours.

**Onset of action**
Intravenous—5 minutes (at effective dose).

**Peak serum concentration**
Intravenous—32 to 52 nanograms per mL after infusion of 9 mg over 60 minutes in nonpregnant females.

**Elimination**
Renal (71 to 93%; conjugated metabolites; with 90% of dose eliminated within 24 hours).
In dialysis—Removable by dialysis.

## Precautions to Consider

**Cross-sensitivity and/or related problems**
Patients sensitive to sulfites may be sensitive to intravenous ritodrine because of the sulfite preservative present.

**Carcinogenicity/Tumorigenicity**
Studies in rats receiving ritodrine orally found no increased risk of carcinogenicity or tumorigenicity.

**Pregnancy/Reproduction**
Pregnancy—Adequate and well-controlled studies in humans have not been done in women with a pregnancy of less than 20 weeks' gestation. A small number of children 7 to 9 years of age who had been exposed to ritodrine prenatally were studied for up to 2 years and did not show increased risk of abnormalities. Risk-benefit to the fetus must be considered since ritodrine crosses the placenta. Neonatal hypoglycemia, tachycardia, and ileus have been reported; ketoacidosis has resulted in fetal death. Neonatal hypocalcemia and hypotension have occurred with other beta-adrenergic stimulants, although they have not been reported with ritodrine.
Studies in animals have not shown that ritodrine causes adverse effects on the fetus.
FDA Pregnancy Category B.

**Drug interactions and/or related problems**
The following drug interactions and/or related problems have been selected on the basis of their potential clinical significance (possible mechanism in parentheses where appropriate)—not necessarily inclusive (» = major clinical significance):

Note: Combinations containing any of the following medications, depending on the amount present, may also interact with this medication.

  Anesthetics, potent, general or
  Diazoxide, parenteral or
  Magnesium sulfate or
  Meperidine
    (may potentiate cardiovascular effects of intravenous ritodrine, especially cardiac arrhythmias or hypotension)

» Beta-adrenergic agonists, other or
  Parasympatholytic agents, such as atropine or
  Sympathomimetics
    (concurrent use may cause an additive sympathomimetic effect and greatly increase the likelihood of developing side effects, including hypertension from a parasympatholytic agent or cardiac problems from another tocolytic agent. A sufficient time interval should elapse prior to administering another sympathomimetic agent [90% of an intravenous dose is eliminated within 24 hours])

» Beta-adrenergic blocking agents
    (these agents antagonize the effects of ritodrine, and although agents with greater beta-1–adrenergic selectivity may be less antagonistic, concurrent use is not recommended)

» Corticosteroids, long-acting
    (corticosteroids are often used concurrently to enhance fetal lung maturity; however, intravenous ritodrine and, to a lesser extent, cor-

ticosteroids each expand plasma volume by causing sodium retention. Intravenous ritodrine further increases plasma volume and may cause overhydration. One possible result of overhydration is maternal pulmonary edema, which has occurred with or without corticosteroid administration. Restricting and monitoring fluids helps prevent maternal pulmonary edema; however, on occurrence, discontinuance of ritodrine should be considered. Maternal ketoacidosis has also been reported with concurrent use of high doses of corticosteroids)

**Laboratory value alterations**
The following have been selected on the basis of their potential clinical significance (possible effect in parentheses where appropriate)—not necessarily inclusive (» = major clinical significance):

With physiology/laboratory test values
  Alanine aminotransferase (ALT [SGPT]) or
  Aspartate aminotransferase (AST [SGOT])
    (increased serum concentrations have been reported in less than 1% of patients receiving ritodrine and other beta-adrenergic agonists)
  Blood pressure, maternal and
  Cardiac output, maternal and
  Heart rate, fetal and maternal
    (increased maternal heart rate, increased maternal systolic blood pressure, and decreased maternal diastolic blood pressure occur in 80 to 100% of patients treated with intravenous ritodrine; oral ritodrine frequently causes small increases in maternal heart rate but usually does not affect fetal heart rate or maternal blood pressure)
  Free fatty acid, serum and
  Glucose, blood and
  Insulin, serum
    (concentrations may be transiently increased during intravenous infusion but usually return to pretreatment concentrations within 48 to 72 hours, even with continued infusion)
  Potassium
    (serum concentration may be decreased during intravenous infusion; related to changes in glucose and insulin; maximum effect occurs within 2 hours after infusion is started and concentrations return to normal 30 minutes to 48 hours after withdrawal)

**Medical considerations/Contraindications**
The medical considerations/contraindications included have been selected on the basis of their potential clinical significance (reasons given in parentheses where appropriate)—not necessarily inclusive (» = major clinical significance).

*Except under special circumstances, this medication should not be used when the following medical problems exist:*
» Cardiovascular diseases, maternal, especially those associated with arrhythmias or
» Hyperthyroidism, uncontrolled or
» Hypovolemia or
» Pheochromocytoma
    (ritodrine may precipitate arrhythmias or heart failure; occult cardiac disease may be unmasked)
» Chorioamnionitis or
» Intrauterine fetal death or
» Nonreassuring fetal status
    (premature labor should not be suppressed for these problems or conditions)
» Eclampsia and severe preeclampsia or
» Hypertension, uncontrolled or
» Pulmonary hypertension
    (ritodrine may aggravate these conditions and, if these conditions cannot be controlled, preterm labor should not be suppressed)

*Risk-benefit should be considered when the following medical problems exist:*
» Abruptio placentae or
» Hemorrhage, maternal or
» Placenta previa or
» Preeclampsia, mild to moderate
    (ritodrine may aggravate these conditions and, if they cannot be controlled, premature labor should not be suppressed)
  Allergy or sensitivity to ritodrine or sulfites
» Diabetes mellitus
    (may be aggravated; maternal ketoacidosis has also been reported, especially in patients with poorly controlled diabetes; insulin dose may need to be increased; neonatal glucose should be checked after delivery)
  Hypertension or
  Migraine headaches, or history of
    (these conditions may be aggravated; also, transient cerebral ischemia has been reported with the use of other beta-adrenergic agonist therapy in patients who had migraines during ritodrine administration)

**Patient monitoring**
The following may be especially important in patient monitoring (other tests may be warranted in some patients, depending on condition; » = major clinical significance):

  Assessment of gestational age and fetal maturity
    (to diagnose preterm labor)
» Blood count determinations
    (patients using ritodrine long-term, especially intravenous use for 2 or 3 weeks, should be monitored for development of leukopenia or agranulocytosis)
» Blood glucose, maternal and neonatal and
» Fluid and electrolyte status, maternal and neonatal
    (should be monitored carefully during prolonged intravenous administration, especially in diabetic patients or those receiving corticosteroids, potassium-depleting diuretics, or digitalis glycosides; neonatal blood glucose should be determined promptly after delivery)
  Cardiac function monitoring, maternal, such as electrocardiogram (ECG) and/or
  Pulmonary function monitoring, maternal
    (baseline ECG should be done to rule out occult maternal cardiac disease; pulmonary function monitoring and an ECG should also be done immediately in patients complaining of chest pain or tightness during ritodrine therapy and ritodrine should be temporarily discontinued until ECG is assessed; a persistent high tachycardia [over 140 beats per minute] may be related to impending pulmonary edema)
  Heart rate, fetal and
  Heart rate and blood pressure, maternal and
  Uterine activity
    (should be monitored frequently during intravenous administration)

## Side/Adverse Effects

Note: Most adverse effects of ritodrine are related to its beta-adrenergic stimulating activity and are usually dose-related.
  Maternal ketoacidosis has been reported, especially in patients also receiving high doses of corticosteroids or in patients with poorly controlled diabetes mellitus.

The following side/adverse effects have been selected on the basis of their potential clinical significance (possible signs and symptoms in parentheses where appropriate)—not necessarily inclusive:

**Those indicating need for medical attention**
Incidence more frequent
  *Angina or cardiac disease, previously undiagnosed* (chest pain or tightness)—15% with intravenous use; *diastolic blood pressure reduction, maternal* (lightheadedness or dizziness)—80 to 100% with intravenous use; *hyperglycemia, maternal* (blurred vision; drowsiness; dry mouth; flushed, dry skin; fruit-like breath odor; increased frequency and volume of urination; ketones in urine; loss of appetite; somnolence; stomachache, nausea, or vomiting; tiredness; troubled breathing, rapid and deep; unconsciousness; unusual thirst)—80 to 100% with intravenous use, transient for 48 to 72 hours; *pulmonary edema* (shortness of breath)—15% with intravenous use; *tachycardia or other cardiac arrhythmias, maternal and fetal* (fast or irregular heartbeat)—1% with oral use and 80 to 100% with intravenous use

Note: Increased cardiac output resulting from the use of beta-adrenergic agonists may result in *cardiac arrhythmias* or *angina* (with or without ECG changes) that has usually been associated with unrecognized cardiopulmonary disease, which may lead to myocardial ischemia, myocardial infarction, and possibly death.

At the recommended intravenous infusion rate in one study, the *maternal and fetal heartbeat* averaged 130 (range, 60 to 180) and 164 (range, 130 to 200) beats per minute, respectively. The maternal systolic and diastolic blood pressure measurements averaged 128 mm Hg (range, 96 to 162 mm Hg) and 48 mm Hg (range, 0 to 76 mm Hg), respectively. Only 1% of patients with persistent *tachycardia* or *severely decreased diastolic blood pressure* required withdrawal from the medication; these severe effects were managed successfully by dose reduction. Oral administration was associated with only a small increase in maternal heart rate and little or no effect on maternal blood pressure or fetal heart rate.

*Maternal hyperglycemia* may cause fetal or neonatal hypoglycemia.

Serious maternal *pulmonary edema* has occurred during intravenous administration of ritodrine or other beta-adrenergic agonists for premature labor or after delivery. Although the exact cause is unknown, it appears to be related to circulatory fluid overload with subsequent pulmonary edema, and has occurred more frequently with concurrent corticosteroid administration; maternal death has been reported with or without concomitantly administered corticosteroids. Other contributing factors may include hypokalemia, twin gestations, sustained tachycardia (> 140 beats per minute), undiagnosed cardiopulmonary disease, and catecholamine-induced cardiac injury. If pulmonary edema develops during administration, ritodrine should be discontinued.

Incidence rare
*Agranulocytosis or leukopenia* (sore throat or fever)—with intravenous use for 2 to 3 weeks, reversible on discontinuation; *hepatic function impairment or hepatitis* (yellow eyes or skin)—reported in less than 1% of patients using ritodrine and other beta-adrenergic agonists

**Those indicating need for medical attention only if they continue or are bothersome**
Incidence more frequent
*Erythema* (reddened skin)—10 to 50% with intravenous use; *headache*—10 to 50% with intravenous use; *nausea*—5 to 8% with oral use and 10 to 50% with intravenous use; *palpitations* (pounding or racing heartbeat)—10 to 15% with oral use and 33% with intravenous use; *trembling*—10 to 15% with oral use and 10 to 50% with intravenous use; *vomiting*—5 to 8% with oral use and 10 to 50% with intravenous use

Incidence less frequent or rare
*Psychological symptoms* (anxiety, emotional upset, jitteriness, nervousness, restlessness)—5 to 8% with oral or intravenous use; *skin rash*—3 to 4% with oral use and rare with intravenous use

**Those indicating possible maternal pulmonary edema and need for medical attention if they occur after medication is discontinued**
*Shortness of breath*

## Overdose

For specific information on the agents used in the management of ritodrine overdose, see:
- *Beta-adrenergic Blocking Agents (Systemic)* monograph;
- *Charcoal, Activated (Oral-Local)* monograph; and/or
- *Furosemide (Systemic)* in the *Diuretics, Loop* monograph.

For more information on the management of overdose or unintentional ingestion, **contact a Poison Control Center** (see *Poison Control Center Listing*).

**Clinical effects of overdose**
The following effects have been selected on the basis of their potential clinical significance (possible signs and symptoms in parentheses where appropriate)—not necessarily inclusive:
*Nausea or vomiting, severe; nervousness or trembling, severe; pulmonary edema* (shortness of breath, severe); *tachycardia* (fast or irregular heartbeat, severe)

Note: The dose required to produce overdose symptoms varies by individual.

**Treatment of overdose**
Discontinuation of ritodrine is often all that is required if symptoms are not severe.

To enhance elimination—Renal dialysis for all dosage forms, if needed. Overdose of oral ritodrine may require induction of emesis, followed by administration of activated charcoal.

Specific treatment—Beta-adrenergic blocking agents are used to antagonize the actions of ritodrine and to treat arrhythmias. Loop diuretics are indicated as adjuncts to treat maternal pulmonary edema.

Supportive care—Supportive measures such as establishing intravenous lines, correction of hydration or electrolyte balance, especially potassium or calcium, oxygenation, and support of ventilatory function are essential for maintaining the vital functions of the patient.

## Patient Consultation

As an aid to patient consultation, refer to *Advice for the Patient, Ritodrine (Systemic)*.

In providing consultation, consider emphasizing the following selected information (» = major clinical significance):

**Before using this medication**
» Conditions affecting use, especially:
Sensitivity to ritodrine or sulfite preservative
Other medications, especially beta-adrenergic agonists (other), beta-adrenergic blocking agents, or long-acting corticosteroids
Other medical problems, especially abruptio placentae, cardiovascular disease (maternal), chorioamnionitis, diabetes mellitus, eclampsia, hemorrhage (maternal), hypertension (uncontrolled), hyperthyroidism (uncontrolled), hypovolemia, intrauterine fetal death, nonreassuring fetal status, pheochromocytoma, placenta previa, preeclampsia, or pulmonary hypertension

**Proper use of this medication**
» Proper dosing
Missed dose: Taking if remembered within an hour or so; not taking if remembered later; not doubling doses
» Proper storage

**Precautions while using this medication**
» Checking with physician immediately if contractions begin again or in case of ruptured membranes
» Not taking other medications, especially OTC sympathomimetics, unless discussed with physician

**Side/adverse effects**
Signs of potential side effects, especially angina or cardiac disease (previously undiagnosed)(maternal), diastolic blood pressure reduction (maternal), hyperglycemia (maternal), tachycardia or other cardiac arrhythmias (maternal or fetal), agranulocytosis or leukopenia, hepatic function impairment or hepatitis, or pulmonary edema

## General Dosing Information

Side effects, including tachycardia (maternal heart rate of greater than 120 or fetal heart rate of greater than 170 to 180), may be reduced without reducing ritodrine's effectiveness by slowing the rate of infusion or decreasing the dose.

If labor persists despite administration of the maximum dose, it is recommended that ritodrine therapy be withdrawn; however, in cases of recurrence of unwanted preterm labor, ritodrine treatment may be repeated.

Ritodrine should be discontinued as soon as labor is irreversible in order to allow for metabolic recovery (reversal of maternal hyperglycemia or fetal hypoglycemia or hypocalcemia) before delivery.

**For parenteral dosage forms only**
For better dose titration, it is recommended that ritodrine intravenous infusion be administered by means of a controlled infusion device, such as electronic volumetric controller, volumetric intravenous infusion pump, or intravenous microdrip chamber able to measure 60 drops per mL. The patient should be placed in the left lateral position to minimize hypotension. Fluids should be closely monitored to prevent circulatory fluid overload.

Concurrent administration of excessive intravenous fluids or saline intravenous solutions with ritodrine therapy may cause circulatory fluid overload and maternal pulmonary edema. Use of saline solutions, such as Sodium Chloride Injection USP, Ringer's Injection USP, or Hartmann's solution, should be avoided.

Ambulation may be resumed gradually after 36 to 48 hours if contractions do not recur and patient is clinically stable.

## Oral Dosage Forms

### RITODRINE HYDROCHLORIDE EXTENDED-RELEASE CAPSULES

**Usual adult dose**
Tocolytic—
Initial: Oral, 40 mg thirty minutes before the intravenous infusion is discontinued, then 40 mg every eight hours for twenty-four hours.
Maintenance: Oral, 40 mg every eight to twelve hours until term (or until the 37th week of gestation) or as medical judgment dictates.

**Usual adult prescribing limits**
Up to 120 mg a day.

**Strength(s) usually available**
U.S.—
Not commercially available.
Canada—
40 mg (Rx) [*Yutopar S.R*].

**Packaging and storage**
Store between 15 and 40 °C (59 and 104 °F), preferably below 30 °C (86 °F), unless otherwise specified by manufacturer. Store in a tight container.

### RITODRINE HYDROCHLORIDE TABLETS USP

**Usual adult dose**
Tocolytic—
Initial: Oral, 10 mg thirty minutes before the intravenous infusion is discontinued, then 10 mg every two hours for twenty-four hours.
Maintenance: Oral, 10 to 20 mg every four to six hours until term (or until the 37th week of gestation) or as medical judgment dictates.

**Usual adult prescribing limits**
Up to 120 mg a day.

**Strength(s) usually available**
U.S.—
Not commercially available.
Canada—
10 mg (Rx) [*Yutopar*].

**Packaging and storage**
Store between 15 and 40 °C (59 and 104 °F), preferably below 30 °C (86 °F). Store in a tight container.

## Parenteral Dosage Forms

### RITODRINE HYDROCHLORIDE INJECTION USP

**Usual adult dose**
Tocolytic—
Initial: Intravenous, 50 to 100 mcg (0.05 to 0.1 mg) per minute, increased every ten minutes as necessary in increments of 50 mcg (0.05 mg) to the effective dose that balances uterine response and unwanted effects (increased maternal heart rate and decreased blood pressure and increased fetal heart rate), or until the maternal heart rate reaches 130 beats per minute.
Maintenance: Intravenous, 150 to 350 mcg (0.15 to 0.35 mg) per minute at the lowest dose that maintains a relaxed uterus; however, as soon as labor is irreversible or the maximum dose of 350 mcg (0.35 mg) per minute is reached, ritodrine should be discontinued.
Note: Injection must be diluted before use unless premixed solution is used. Intravenous infusion should be continued for twelve to forty-eight hours after uterine contractions stop. Ritodrine should be administered in a separate intravenous line. Other medications of any type should not be administered via the same tubing.

**Usual adult prescribing limits**
Intravenous, up to 350 mcg (0.35 mg) per minute.

**Strength(s) usually available**
U.S.—
10 mg per mL (Rx) [*Yutopar*; GENERIC].
15 mg per mL (Rx) [*Yutopar*; GENERIC].
Canada—
10 mg per mL (Rx) [*Yutopar*].

**Packaging and storage**
Store between 15 and 40°C (59 and 104 °F), preferably below 30 °C (86 °F).

**Preparation of dosage form**
Ritodrine Hydrochloride Injection USP may be prepared for intravenous infusion by dilution of 150 mg in 500 mL of 5% Dextrose Injection USP to produce a solution containing 300 mcg (0.3 mg) of ritodrine hydrochloride per mL. More concentrated solutions may be prepared in cases where fluid restriction is necessary. In general, use of saline diluents, such as Sodium Chloride Injection USP, Ringer's Injection USP, or Hartmann's solution as the infusion solution should be avoided because of the risk of pulmonary edema.

**Stability**
Ritodrine hydrochloride is stable for up to 48 hours following preparation of intravenous infusion containing 300 mcg (0.3 mg) per mL. Ritodrine Hydrochloride Injection USP should not be used if the solution is discolored or contains particulate matter.

### RITODRINE HYDROCHLORIDE IN 5% DEXTROSE INJECTION

**Usual adult dose**
Tocolytic—See *Ritodrine Hydrochloride Injection USP*.
Note: Intravenous infusion should be continued for twelve to forty-eight hours after uterine contractions stop. Ritodrine should be administered in a separate intravenous line. Other medications of any type should not be administered via the same tubing.

**Usual adult prescribing limits**
See *Ritodrine Hydrochloride Injection USP*.

**Strength(s) usually available**
U.S.—
150 mg per 500 mL of 5% Dextrose Injection USP (premix) (Rx) [GENERIC].
Canada—
Not commercially available.

**Packaging and storage**
Store below 40 °C (104 °F), preferably between 15 and 30 °C (59 and 86 °F), unless otherwise specified by manufacturer. Protect from freezing.
Note: If more concentrated solutions are needed when fluid restriction is necessary, ritodrine hydrochloride injection should be used to prepare the solution.

**Stability**
Ritodrine Hydrochloride in 5% Dextrose Injection USP should not be used if the solution is discolored or contains particulate matter.

## Selected Bibliography
Wischnik A. Risk-benefit assessment of tocolytic drugs. Drug Safety 1991 6(5): 371-80.

Revised: 06/28/96

---

# RITONAVIR   Systemic—INTRODUCTORY VERSION

VA CLASSIFICATION (Primary): AM803
Commonly used brand name(s): *Norvir*.
Note: For a listing of dosage forms and brand names by country availability, see *Dosage Forms* section(s).

## Category
Antiviral (systemic).

## Indications

**General considerations**
Cross-resistance between ritonavir (a protease inhibitor) and reverse transcriptase inhibitors is thought to be unlikely because each affects a different part of human immunodeficiency virus (HIV) replication. However, it is unknown whether there is cross-resistance between ritonavir and other protease inhibitors.

**Accepted**
Human immunodeficiency virus (HIV) infection (treatment) or
Immunodeficiency syndrome, acquired (AIDS) (treatment)—Ritonavir is indicated in combination with nucleoside analogs or as monotherapy for the treatment of HIV infection or AIDS.

## Pharmacology/Pharmacokinetics

**Physicochemical characteristics**
Molecular weight—720.95.

**Mechanism of action/Effect**
Ritonavir is a protease inhibitor. It inhibits both human immunodeficiency virus proteases (HIV-1 and HIV-2), which leaves these enzymes incapable of processing the gag-pol polyprotein precursor. This leads to the production of noninfectious immature HIV particles.

**Absorption**
In one study, when ritonavir oral solution was administered with food, the peak plasma concentration was decreased by 23% and the extent of absorption was decreased by 7% as compared with administration under fasting conditions. However, administration of the oral solution with chocolate milk, Advera®, or Ensure® did not significantly affect the extent and rate of absorption. When administered with food, 600 mg of ritonavir capsules and oral solution yielded comparable areas under the plasma concentration–time curve in two studies. The extent of absorption of ritonavir from the capsules was 15% higher when administered with a meal than under fasting conditions.

**Protein binding**
Very high (98 to 99%).

### Biotransformation
Hepatic; five metabolites have been identified in the urine and feces. Isopropylthiazole oxidation metabolite (M-2) is the major metabolite and has antiviral activity similar to that of ritonavir; however, plasma concentrations of M-2 are low. The cytochrome P450 enzymes CYP3A and CYP2D6 are primarily involved in ritonavir metabolism.

### Half-life
3 to 5 hours.

### Time to peak concentration
Two hours after administration of 600 mg of oral solution under fasting conditions.
Four hours after administration of 600 mg of oral solution with food.

### Peak serum concentration
Approximately 11 micrograms per mL after administration of 600 mg every 12 hours.

### Elimination
Fecal; approximately 86% of the dose was excreted in the feces, with approximately 34% excreted as unchanged drug.
Renal; approximately 11% of the administered dose was excreted into the urine, with approximately 4% excreted as unchanged drug.

## Precautions to Consider

### Carcinogenicity
Long-term carcinogenicity studies in animals have not been completed.

### Mutagenicity
Ritonavir was not found to be mutagenic in a series of *in vitro* and *in vivo* assays, including bacterial reverse mutation (Ames test) using *Salmonella typhimurium* and *Escherichia coli*, mouse lymphoma, mouse micronucleus, and human lymphocyte chromosome aberration assays.

### Pregnancy/Reproduction
Fertility—There was no effect on the fertility of rats receiving ritonavir exposures approximately 40% (male) and 60% (female) of those achieved with the recommended human therapeutic dose. Use of higher doses was not feasible due to hepatic toxicity.

Pregnancy—Adequate and well-controlled studies have not been done in humans.

When ritonavir was administered to pregnant rats and rabbits, no treatment-related malformations were observed. Early resorptions, decreased fetal body weight, ossification delays, and developmental variations occurred in rats at a maternally toxic dosage, equivalent to approximately 30% of the recommended therapeutic dose. There was a slight increase in cryptorchidism in rats exposed to approximately 22% of the recommended therapeutic dose. Resorptions, decreased litter size, and decreased fetal weights also occurred in rabbits administered a maternally toxic dosage equivalent to 1.8 times the recommended therapeutic dose on a mg per square meter of body surface area basis.

FDA Pregnancy Category B.

### Breast-feeding
It is not known whether ritonavir is distributed into breast milk.

### Pediatrics
The adverse event profile seen in HIV-infected patients 2 to 16 years of age receiving ritonavir was similar to that of adults. Evaluation of the antiviral efficacy in pediatric patients is ongoing.

### Geriatrics
No information is available on the relationship of age to the effects of ritonavir in geriatric patients. Pharmacokinetic studies have not been done in older patients.

### Drug interactions and/or related problems
The following drug interactions and/or related problems have been selected on the basis of their potential clinical significance (possible mechanism in parentheses where appropriate)—not necessarily inclusive (» = major clinical significance):

Note: Combinations containing any of the following medications, depending on the amount present, may also interact with this medication.

Ritonavir clearance may be increased by the use of other medications that increase the activity of the cytochrome P450 enzyme CYP3A, resulting in decreased ritonavir plasma concentrations. Also, ritonavir may produce a large increase in the plasma concentration of certain highly metabolized medications due to ritonavir's high affinity for several cytochrome P450 enzyme isoforms. The affinity for the isoforms is in the following rank order: CYP3A > CYP2D6 > CYP2C9, CYP2C19 >> CYP2A6, CYP1A2, CYP2E1.

» Amiodarone or
» Astemizole or
» Bepridil or
» Bupropion or
» Cisapride or
» Clozapine or
» Dihydroergotamine or
» Encainide or
» Ergotamine or
» Flecainide or
» Meperidine or
» Pimozide or
» Piroxicam or
» Propafenone or
» Propoxyphene or
» Quinidine or
» Rifabutin or
» Terfenadine
(these medications should not be administered concurrently with ritonavir; concurrent administration with ritonavir is likely to produce a large increase in the plasma concentrations of these medications, which may increase the risk of arrhythmias, hematologic abnormalities, seizures, or other potentially serious adverse effects)

» Clarithromycin
(in one study, concurrent administration increased the area under the plasma concentration–time curve [AUC] of clarithromycin by 77% and the peak plasma concentration [$C_{max}$] by 31%; dosing does not need to be adjusted in patients with normal renal function; however, for patients with a creatinine clearance of 30 to 60 mL/minute [0.5 to 1 mL/second], the dose of clarithromycin should be reduced by 50%, and for patients with a creatinine clearance of less than 30 mL/minute [0.5 mL/second], the dose of clarithromycin should be reduced by 75%)

» Clorazepate or
» Diazepam or
» Estazolam or
» Flurazepam or
» Midazolam or
» Triazolam or
» Zolpidem
(these medications should not be administered concurrently with ritonavir; concurrent administration with ritonavir is likely to produce a large increase in the plasma concentrations of these medications, which may produce extreme sedation and respiratory depression)

» Contraceptives, estrogen-containing, oral
(in one study, concurrent administration decreased the AUC of ethinyl estradiol by 40%; an oral contraceptive with a higher estrogen content or an alternative method of contraception should be considered)

Desipramine
(in one study, concurrent administration increased the AUC of desipramine by 145% and the $C_{max}$ of desipramine by 22%; dosage reduction of desipramine should be considered)

Disulfiram or
Metronidazole
(ritonavir capsules and oral solution contain alcohol, which can produce a disulfiram-alcohol reaction when concurrently administered with disulfiram or metronidazole)

Saquinavir
(concurrent administration extensively inhibits the metabolism of saquinavir, resulting in greatly increased saquinavir levels; safety has not been established)

» Theophylline
(in one study, concurrent administration reduced the AUC of theophylline by 43% and the $C_{max}$ by 32%; theophylline concentrations should be monitored and the dosage of theophylline may need to be adjusted)

### Laboratory value alterations
The following have been selected on the basis of their potential clinical significance (possible effect in parentheses where appropriate)—not necessarily inclusive (» = major clinical significance):

With physiology/laboratory test values
Alanine aminotransferase (ALT [SGPT]), serum and
Aspartate aminotransferase (AST [SGOT]), serum and
Creatine kinase (CK) and
Gamma-glutamyltransferase (GGT)
(values may be increased)

Glucose, plasma and
Triglycerides, serum and
Uric acid, serum
(concentrations may be increased)

### Medical considerations/Contraindications
The medical considerations/contraindications included have been selected on the basis of their potential clinical significance (reasons given in parentheses where appropriate)—not necessarily inclusive (» = major clinical significance).

*Except under special circumstances, this medication should not be used when the following medical problem exists:*
» Hypersensitivity to ritonavir

*Risk-benefit should be considered when the following medical problems exist:*
Hemophilia
(increased bleeding, including spontaneous skin hematomas and hemarthrosis, has been reported in patients with hemophilia types A and B who are receiving protease inhibitor therapy; a causal relationship has not been established)
Hepatic function impairment
(because ritonavir is primarily metabolized by the liver, it should be used with caution in patients with hepatic function impairment)

### Patient monitoring
The following may be especially important in patient monitoring (other tests may be warranted in some patients, depending on condition; » = major clinical significance):
Blood glucose determinations
(recommended to monitor closely patient's plasma glucose concentrations; development of hyperglycemia or diabetes may be associated with the use of protease inhibitors)

## Side/Adverse Effects
The following side/adverse effects have been selected on the basis of their potential clinical significance (possible signs and symptoms in parentheses where appropriate)—not necessarily inclusive:

### Those indicating need for medical attention
Incidence less frequent
*Circumoral paresthesia* (numbness or tingling feeling around the mouth); *peripheral paresthesia* (numbness or tingling feeling in the hands or feet)
Incidence rare
*Diabetes or hyperglycemia* (dry or itchy skin; fatigue; hunger, increased; thirst, increased; unexplained weight loss; urination, increased); *ketoacidosis* (confusion; dehydration; mouth odor, fruity; nausea; vomiting; weight loss)

### Those indicating need for medical attention only if they continue or are bothersome
Incidence more frequent
*Asthenia* (generalized weakness); *gastrointestinal disturbances* (diarrhea; loss of appetite; nausea; stomach pain; vomiting); *taste perversion* (change in sense of taste)
Incidence less frequent
*Dizziness; headache; somnolence* (sleepiness)

## Overdose
Information on ritonavir overdose in humans is limited. There is one report of a patient who took 1500 mg a day of ritonavir for two days. The patient experienced paresthesias, which resolved after the dose was decreased. One case of renal failure with eosinophilia has also been reported with ritonavir overdose. The approximate lethal dose was found to be more than 20 times the recommended human dose in rats and 10 times the recommended human dose in mice.

For more information on the management of overdose or unintentional ingestion, **contact a Poison Control Center** (see *Poison Control Center Listing*).

### Treatment of overdose
To decrease absorption—Induction of emesis or performing gastric lavage.
To enhance elimination—Administration of activated charcoal.
Monitoring—Monitoring of vital signs and observation of the clinical status of the patient.
Supportive care—Patients in whom intentional overdose is known or suspected should be referred for psychiatric consultation.

## Patient Consultation
As an aid to patient consultation, refer to *Advice for the Patient, Ritonavir (Systemic)—Introductory Version.*
In providing consultation, consider emphasizing the following selected information (» = major clinical significance):

### Before using this medication
» Conditions affecting use, especially:
Hypersensitivity to ritonavir
Use in children—Safety and effectiveness have not been established in children up to 2 years of age
Other medications, especially amiodarone, astemizole, bepridil, bupropion, cisapride, clarithromycin, clorazepate, clozapine, diazepam, dihydroergotamine, encainide, ergotamine, estazolam, flecainide, flurazepam, meperidine, midazolam, oral estrogen-containing contraceptives, pimozide, piroxicam, propafenone, propoxyphene, quinidine, rifabutin, terfenadine, theophylline, triazolam, or zolpidem

### Proper use of this medication
» Importance of taking ritonavir with food
» Importance of not taking more medication than prescribed; importance of not discontinuing ritonavir without checking with physician
» Compliance with full course of therapy
» Importance of not missing doses and of taking at evenly spaced times
Not sharing medication with others
» Proper dosing
Missed dose: Taking as soon as possible; not taking if almost time for next dose; not doubling doses
» Proper storage

### Precautions while using this medication
» Because ritonavir may interact with other medications, not taking any other medications (prescription or nonprescription) without first checking with physician
» Regular visits to physician for blood tests and monitoring of blood glucose concentrations
» Using an additional method of contraception if taking estrogen-containing oral contraceptives concurrently

### Side/adverse effects
Signs of potential side effects, especially circumoral paresthesia, peripheral paresthesia, diabetes or hyperglycemia, or ketoacidosis

## General Dosing Information
If an adult or adolescent patient experiences nausea or other adverse events upon initiation of 600 mg two times a day, the following dose escalation may be beneficial: 300 mg two times a day, then increasing the dose by 100 mg two times a day up to 600 mg two times a day.

If a pediatric patient cannot tolerate a dose of 400 mg per square meter of body surface area two times a day due to adverse events, the highest tolerated dose should be used for maintenance therapy in combination with other antiretroviral agents.

Patients who are initiating both ritonavir and nucleoside analogs may improve gastrointestinal tolerance by initiating ritonavir alone and then adding the nucleoside analog within 2 weeks.

The taste of ritonavir oral solution may be improved by mixing with chocolate milk, *Ensure®*, or *Advera®* within one hour of dosing.

## Oral Dosage Forms

### RITONAVIR CAPSULES

**Usual adult and adolescent dose**
Antiviral—
Oral, 600 mg two times a day with food.

**Usual pediatric dose**
This dosage form usually is not used in children. See *Ritonavir Oral Solution.*

**Strength(s) usually available**
U.S.—
100 mg (Rx) [*Norvir* (ethanol)].

**Packaging and storage**
Store in the refrigerator between 2 and 8 °C (36 and 46 °F). Protect from light.

**Auxiliary labeling**
• Take with food.
• Continue medicine for full time of treatment.
• Refrigerate.
• Do not take other medications without physician's advice.

### RITONAVIR ORAL SOLUTION

**Usual adult and adolescent dose**
This dosage form usually is not used in adults or adolescents. See *Ritonavir Capsules.*

**Usual pediatric dose**
Infants and children up to 2 years of age: Safety and efficacy have not been established.

Children 2 years of age and older: Oral, 250 mg per square meter [mg/m²] of body surface area two times a day, increasing by 50 mg/m² of body surface area two times a day in two- to three-day intervals, up to a total dosage of 400 mg/m² of body surface area two times a day, according to the following table:

| Body Surface Area (m²) | 250 mg/m² (given two times a day) | 300 mg/m² (given two times a day) | 350 mg/m² (given two times a day) | 400 mg/m² (given two times a day) |
|---|---|---|---|---|
| 0.25 | 0.8 mL (62.5 mg) | 0.9 mL (75 mg) | 1.1 mL (87.5 mg) | 1.25 mL (100 mg) |
| 0.5 | 1.6 mL (125 mg) | 1.9 mL (150 mg) | 2.2 mL (175 mg) | 2.5 mL (200 mg) |
| 1 | 3.1 mL (250 mg) | 3.75 mL (300 mg) | 4.4 mL (350 mg) | 5 mL (400 mg) |
| 1.25 | 3.9 mL (312.5 mg) | 4.7 mL (375 mg) | 5.5 mL (437.5 mg) | 6.25 mL (500 mg) |
| 1.5 | 4.7 mL (375 mg) | 5.6 mL (450 mg) | 6.6 mL (525 mg) | 7.5 mL (600 mg) |

Body surface area (m²) = $\sqrt{([\text{height (cm)}] \times \text{weight (kg)}]/3600)}$

**Usual pediatric prescribing limits**
1200 mg per day.

**Strength(s) usually available**
U.S.—
   80 mg per mL (Rx) [*Norvir* (ethanol; saccharin sodium)].

**Packaging and storage**
Store at room temperature between 20 and 25 °C (68 and 77 °F); it should not be refrigerated. The oral solution should be stored in the original container.

**Auxiliary labeling**
- Shake well.
- Take with food.
- Continue medicine for full time of treatment.
- Do not take other medications without physician's advice.

Developed: 01/27/97
Interim revision: 09/09/97; 08/24/98

# RITUXIMAB    Systemic—INTRODUCTORY VERSION

VA CLASSIFICATION (Primary): AN900
Commonly used brand name(s): *Rituxan*.
   Note:  For a listing of dosage forms and brand names by country availability, see *Dosage Forms* section(s).

## Category
Monoclonal antibody; antineoplastic.

## Indications
**Accepted**
Lymphomas, non-Hodgkin's (treatment)—Rituximab is indicated for treatment of relapsed or refractory low-grade or follicular CD20-positive, B-cell non-Hodgkin's lymphoma.

## Pharmacology/Pharmacokinetics
**Physicochemical characteristics**
Source—Synthetic (genetically engineered) chimeric murine/human monoclonal antibody, an IgG1-kappa immunoglobulin containing murine light- and heavy-chain variable region sequences and human constant region sequences. It is composed of two heavy chains of 451 amino acids and two light chains of 213 amino acids (based on cDNA analysis). The chimeric anti-CD20 antibody is produced by mammalian cell (Chinese hamster ovary) suspension culture in a nutrient medium containing gentamicin (although gentamicin does not appear in the final product). Purification procedure includes affinity and ion exchange chromatography, as well as specific viral inactivation and removal procedures.
Molecular weight— 145 kilodaltons.
pH—6.5.
Binding affinity—For CD20 antigen: Approximately 8 nanomolar.

**Mechanism of action/Effect**
Rituximab, a murine/human monoclonal antibody, binds to the antigen CD20 (human B-lymphocyte–restricted differentiation antigen, Bp35). This antigen is a hydrophobic transmembrane protein, with a molecular weight of approximately 35,000 daltons, that is located on pre-B and mature B lymphocytes. It is also expressed on more than 90% of B-cell non-Hodgkin's lymphomas but not expressed on hematopoietic stem cells, pro-B cells, normal plasma cells, or other normal tissues. CD20 regulates an early step or steps in the activation process for cell cycle initiation and differentiation and may also function as a calcium ion channel. It is not shed from the cell surface and does not internalize upon antibody binding. No free CD20 antigen is found in the circulation.
The mechanism of antineoplastic action may involve mediation of B cell lysis (seen *in vitro*) by means of binding of the Fab domain of rituximab to the CD20 antigen on B lymphocytes and by recruitment of immune effector functions by the Fc domain. Cell lysis may be the result of complement-dependent cytotoxicity (CDC) and antibody-dependent cellular cytotoxicity (ADCC). In addition, the antibody has been shown to induce apoptosis in the DHL-4 human B-cell lymphoma line.
Rituximab binds to lymphoid cells in the thymus, the white pulp of the spleen, and a majority of B lymphocytes in peripheral blood and lymph nodes. However, there appears to be little or no binding to non-lymphoid tissues.

**Half-life**
Intravenous infusion (for four doses)—
   After the first dose: Mean, 59.8 hours (range, 11.1 to 104.6 hours).
   After the fourth dose: Mean, 174 hours (range, 26 to 442 hours).
Note:  The wide range may be related to variable tumor burden among patients, as well as the changes that were seen in CD20-positive (normal and malignant) B-cell populations with repeated administration.
   No difference has been found in the rate of elimination of rituximab, as measured by serum half-life, in responders versus nonresponders.
   Rituximab has been found to be detectable in serum for 3 to 6 months after completion of treatment.

**Onset of action**
Depletion of circulating B cells (measured as CD19-positive cells)— Within the first three doses.
Depletion of tissue-based B cells (measured in lymph node biopsies)— Fourteen days after a single dose.
Note:  Rituximab treatment results in depletion of both circulating and tissue-based B cells.

**Peak serum concentration**
Inversely correlated with baseline values for the number of circulating CD20-positive B cells and measures of disease burden.
Note:  Trough serum concentrations also are inversely correlated with baseline values for the number of circulating CD20-positive B cells and measures of disease burden.
   Median steady-state serum concentrations have been found to be higher in responders than in nonresponders.
   Serum concentrations have been found to be higher in patients with International Working Formulation (IWF) subtypes B, C, and D as compared to those with subtype A.

**Duration of action**
Depletion of circulating B cells (measured as CD19-positive cells)—Up to 6 to 9 months after treatment, with median B-cell levels returning to normal by 12 months following completion of treatment.
Note:  Sustained and statistically significant reductions in IgG and IgM serum concentrations occurred from the fifth through the eleventh month after administration, but only 14% of patients experienced reductions in IgG and/or IgM serum concentrations to values below the normal range.

## Precautions to Consider
**Cross-sensitivity and/or related problems**
Patients sensitive to murine proteins may also be sensitive to rituximab.
**Carcinogenicity**
Long-term studies in animals have not been done.

**Mutagenicity**
Long-term studies in animals have not been done.

**Pregnancy/Reproduction**
Fertility—Studies in animals have not been done.

Pregnancy—Studies in humans have not been done.

Studies in animals have not been done.

Immunoglobulin G (IgG) is known to cross the placenta and therefore could cause fetal B cell depletion.

It is recommended that women of childbearing potential use effective contraception during treatment and for up to 12 months following treatment with rituximab. Risk-benefit should be considered before use of rituximab during pregnancy.

FDA Pregnancy Category C.

**Breast-feeding**
It is not known whether rituximab is distributed into human breast milk. However, human IgG is distributed into human milk, although the potential for absorption and consequent immunosuppression in the infant is unknown. It is recommended that women treated with rituximab not breast-feed until circulating drug levels are no longer detectable.

**Pediatrics**
Safety and efficacy have not been established.

**Drug interactions and/or related problems**
The following drug interactions and/or related problems have been selected on the basis of their potential clinical significance (possible mechanism in parentheses where appropriate)—not necessarily inclusive (» = major clinical significance):

Antihypertensive medications
   (withholding of antihypertensive medications for 12 hours prior to rituximab administration should be considered because rituximab may cause hypotension)

Vaccines, killed virus or
Vaccines, live virus
   (rituximab theoretically may inhibit the generation of an anamnestic or humoral response to any vaccine)

**Laboratory value alterations**
The following have been selected on the basis of their potential clinical significance (possible effect in parentheses where appropriate)—not necessarily inclusive (» = major clinical significance):

With physiology/laboratory test values
   B-cell counts and
   Immunoglobulin concentrations
      (may be decreased: B cell depletion is associated with a decrease in serum immunoglobulin concentrations in a minority of patients; however, incidence of infection does not appear to be increased)
   Blood pressure
      (may be increased or decreased)
   Calcium, serum
      (decreases in concentrations have been reported infrequently)
   Glucose, serum
      (increases in concentrations [hyperglycemia] have been reported infrequently)
   Hemoglobin concentrations and
   Hematocrit
      (may be decreased)
   Lactate dehydrogenase (LDH), serum
      (increases in values have been reported infrequently)
   Neutrophil counts and
   Platelet counts
      (may be decreased)

**Medical considerations/Contraindications**
The medical considerations/contraindications included have been selected on the basis of their potential clinical significance (reasons given in parentheses where appropriate)—not necessarily inclusive (» = major clinical significance).

*Except under special circumstances, this medication should not be used when the following medical problems exist:*
» Sensitivity (type I) or previous anaphylactic reaction to rituximab
» Sensitivity (type I) or previous anaphylactic reaction to murine proteins

*Risk-benefit should be considered when the following medical problems exist:*
   Cardiac conditions (history of), including
      Angina
      Arrhythmias
         (recurrences have been reported during rituximab therapy; monitoring throughout the infusion and immediately postinfusion is recommended)

**Patient monitoring**
The following may be especially important in patient monitoring (other tests may be warranted in some patients, depending on condition; » = major clinical significance):

Blood counts, complete and
Platelet counts
   (recommended at periodic intervals during therapy, more frequently in patients who develop cytopenias)

Electrocardiogram (ECG)
   (continuous monitoring recommended during administration of rituximab and during the immediate post-infusion period in patients with pre-existing cardiac conditions, including angina and arrhythmias; for patients who develop clinically significant arrhythmias during rituximab administration, continuous monitoring is recommended during subsequent administrations)

## Side/Adverse Effects

Note: Patients treated with rituximab were evaluated for the presence of human antimurine antibody (HAMA) and human antichimeric antibody (HACA); development of these titers is associated with allergic or hypersensitivity reactions in patients treated with murine or chimeric monoclonal antibodies. No HAMA was detected and HACA was detected in less than 1% of patients.

Severe and life-threatening (grades 3 and 4) reactions have occurred in a total of 10% of patients. These included (in some cases, only in one patient) abdominal pain, anemia, angioedema, arthralgia, arrhythmia, asthenia, asthma, bronchiolitis obliterans, bronchospasm, chills, coagulation disorder, dyspnea, headache, hypertension, hypotension, hypoxia, increased cough, leukopenia, nausea, neutropenia, pruritus, rhinitis, skin rash, thrombocytopenia, urticaria, and vomiting.

In most cases, incidence of side/adverse effects is the same for one course or several courses of treatment. However, side/adverse effects seen more frequently in re-treated subjects have included anemia, anorexia, asthenia, dizziness, flushing, leukopenia, mental depression, night sweats, peripheral edema, pruritus, respiratory symptoms, tachycardia, throat irritation, and thrombocytopenia.

The incidence of any side/adverse effect in patients with bulky disease versus those with lesions less than 10 centimeters in diameter was similar. However, incidence of specific side/adverse effects (dizziness, neutropenia, thrombocytopenia, myalgia, anemia, chest pain) was higher in patients with lesions greater than 10 centimeters in diameter. In addition, the incidence of any grade 3 or 4 event was higher (31% versus 13%) and the incidence of grade 3 or 4 neutropenia, anemia, hypotension, and dyspnea was higher in patients with bulky disease versus those with lesions less than 10 centimeters in diameter.

Although rituximab depletes B cells in 70 to 80% of patients, with an associated decrease in serum immunoglobulins in a minority of patients, the incidence of infection does not appear to be increased. Most infections that occur are not serious. Serious (grade 3) bacterial events reported in clinical trials included sepsis due to listeria, staphylococcal bacteremia, and polymicrobial sepsis; in the post-treatment period (30 days to 11 months after the last dose), bacterial infections reported included sepsis, and significant viral infections reported included herpes simplex infections and herpes zoster.

The following side/adverse effects have been selected on the basis of their potential clinical significance (possible signs and symptoms in parentheses where appropriate)—not necessarily inclusive:

### Those indicating need for medical attention
Incidence more frequent
   ***Infusion-related reaction; including angioedema*** (feeling of swelling of tongue or throat); ***bronchospasm or dyspnea*** (shortness of breath); ***fatigue*** (unusual tiredness); ***fever and chills; flushing of face; headache; hypotension*** (dizziness); ***nausea; pruritus*** (itching); ***rhinitis*** (runny nose); ***urticaria*** (skin rash); ***and vomiting***

Note: *Fever and chills* occur in a majority of patients during the first rituximab infusion. *Infusion-related reactions* usually occur within 30 minutes to 2 hours of the beginning of the first infusion and can be resolved by slowing or interrupting the infusion and administering supportive care (intravenous saline, diphenhydramine, and acetaminophen). The incidence of these reactions is decreased with subsequent infusions.

Mild to moderate *hypotension* may require interruption of the infusion, with or without administration of intravenous saline (sodium chloride).

Isolated cases of a severe *infusion-related reaction* requiring administration of epinephrine have been reported with use of rituximab for indications other than the labeled indication.

Approximately 25% of patients who experienced *bronchospasm* have required treatment with bronchodilators.

Incidence less frequent
*Anemia* (unusual tiredness or weakness)—usually asymptomatic; *conjunctivitis* (red, itchy lining of eye); *hypertension*—asymptomatic; *neutropenia* (fever or chills; cough or hoarseness; lower back or side pain; painful or difficult urination)—usually asymptomatic; *pain at site of injection; peripheral edema* (swelling of feet or lower legs); *thrombocytopenia* (unusual bleeding or bruising; black, tarry stools; blood in urine or stools; pinpoint red spots on skin)

Note: During the treatment period, and for up to 30 days following the last dose, severe *anemia, neutropenia,* or *thrombocytopenia* has been reported in 1%, 1.9%, and 1.3% of patients, respectively.

Incidence rare
*Angina* (chest pain); *cardiac arrhythmias, including ventricular tachycardia, supraventricular tachycardia, trigeminy, and irregular pulse* (irregular heartbeat)

Note: Bradycardia also has been reported.

**Those indicating need for medical attention only if they continue or are bothersome**
Incidence less frequent—1 to 5%
*Abdominal or stomach pain; agitation or anxiety; arthralgia* (joint pain); *asthenia or hypotonia* (feeling of weakness); *back pain; change in taste; diarrhea; dyspepsia* (heartburn); *hypesthesia or paresthesia* (numbness or tingling of hands or feet); *increased cough; insomnia* (trouble in sleeping); *lacrimation disorder* (dry eyes); *loss of appetite; malaise* (general feeling of discomfort or illness); *myalgia* (muscle pain); *nervousness; sore throat; swelling of stomach*

**Those indicating the need for medical attention if they occur after medication is discontinued**
*Anemia* (unusual tiredness or weakness)—usually asymptomatic; *neutropenia* (fever or chills; cough or hoarseness; lower back or side pain; painful or difficult urination)—usually asymptomatic; *thrombocytopenia* (unusual bleeding or bruising; black, tarry stools; blood in urine or stools; pinpoint red spots on skin)

Note: During the treatment period, and for up to 30 days following the last dose, severe *anemia, neutropenia,* or *thrombocytopenia* has been reported in 1%, 1.9%, and 1.3% of patients, respectively.

## Patient Consultation

In providing consultation, consider emphasizing the following selected information (» = major clinical significance):

**Before using this medication**
» Conditions affecting use, especially:
Type I sensitivity or previous anaphylactic reaction to rituximab or to murine proteins
Pregnancy—Use of contraception recommended in women of child-bearing potential; risk-benefit should be considered during pregnancy
Breast-feeding—Not recommended as long as rituximab is detectable in the blood because of the risk of absorption and consequent immunosuppression in the infant

**Proper use of this medication**
» Proper dosing

**Side/adverse effects**
Signs of potential side effects, especially infusion-related reaction (angioedema, bronchospasm or dyspnea, fatigue, fever and chills,

flushing of face, headache, hypotension, nausea, pruritus, rhinitis, urticaria, vomiting), conjunctivitis, pain at site of injection, peripheral edema, thrombocytopenia, angina, and cardiac arrhythmias
Asymptomatic side effects, including anemia, hypertension, and neutropenia.

## General Dosing Information

Rituximab is recommended for administration by intravenous infusion only. Rapid intravenous (push or bolus) administration is not recommended.

It is recommended that medications for hypersensitivity reactions (e.g., epinephrine, antihistamines, corticosteroids) be available for each administration of rituximab.

Premedication with acetaminophen and diphenhydramine may attenuate the hypersensitivity reaction and should be considered before each dose of rituximab.

If a severe infusion-related reaction occurs, it is recommended that the infusion be discontinued. The infusion may be resumed at a 50% reduction in rate (e.g., from 100 mg/hr to 50 mg/hr) when symptoms have completely resolved. Treatment of symptoms with diphenhydramine and acetaminophen is recommended, along with bronchodilators or intravenous sodium chloride if indicated. In most cases, the occurrence of non–life-threatening reactions has not prevented completion of the full course of therapy.

If a serious or life-threatening cardiac arrhythmia occurs, it is recommended that the infusion be discontinued. Cardiac monitoring during and following subsequent infusions is recommended in patients who develop clinically significant arrhythmias.

## Parenteral Dosage Forms

### RITUXIMAB CONCENTRATE FOR INJECTION

**Usual adult dose**
Lymphomas, non-Hodgkin's (treatment)—
Intravenous infusion, 375 mg per square meter of body surface area once a week for four doses (on days 1, 8, 15, and 22).

Note: An initial intravenous infusion rate of 50 mg per hour (mg/hr) is recommended. If hypersensitivity or other infusion-related events do not occur, the infusion rate may be increased in 50 mg/hr increments every thirty minutes up to a maximum rate of 400 mg/hr. For subsequent infusions, an initial rate of 100 mg/hr may be used, increased in 100 mg/hr increments at thirty-minute intervals up to a maximum rate of 400 mg/hr.

**Usual pediatric dose**
Safety and efficacy have not been established.

**Strength(s) usually available**
U.S.—
10 mg per mL (Rx) [*Rituxan* (sodium chloride; sodium citrate dihydrate; polysorbate 80)].

**Packaging and storage**
Store between 2 and 8 °C (36 and 46 °F). Protect from direct sunlight.

**Preparation of dosage form**
Rituximab concentrate for injection is prepared for administration by intravenous infusion by withdrawing the necessary amount of drug and diluting it, in an infusion bag, to a final concentration of 1 to 4 mg per mL (mg/mL) with 0.9% sodium chloride injection or 5% dextrose injection. The bag is then gently inverted to mix the solution.

**Stability**
Contains no preservative; any unused portion of a vial should be discarded. Rituximab solutions prepared for intravenous infusion are stable for 24 hours at 2 to 8 °C (36 to 46 °F) and for an additional 12 hours at room temperature. Incompatibilities between rituximab and polyvinyl chloride or polyethylene infusion bags have not been observed.

Developed: 03/23/98

# ROCURONIUM Systemic

VA CLASSIFICATION (Primary): MS300
Commonly used brand name(s): *Zemuron*.
Note: For a listing of dosage forms and brand names by country availability, see *Dosage Forms* section(s).

## Category

Neuromuscular blocking agent.

## Indications

### Accepted
Muscle (skeletal) relaxation, for surgery—Rocuronium is indicated as an adjunct to general anesthesia to facilitate rapid-sequence or routine tracheal intubation and to induce skeletal muscle relaxation during surgery or mechanical ventilation.

### Acceptance not established
Rocuronium has not been studied for long-term use in the intensive care unit (ICU). Prolonged paralysis and/or skeletal muscle weakness may occur with chronic use in the ICU.

## Pharmacology/Pharmacokinetics

### Physicochemical characteristics
Chemical group—Aminosteroid compound.
Molecular weight—609.69.

### Mechanism of action/Effect
Rocuronium is a nondepolarizing neuromuscular blocking agent with a rapid to intermediate onset of action depending on dose and with an intermediate duration of action. Rocuronium produces neuromuscular blockade by competing with acetylcholine for cholinergic receptors at the motor end plate.

### Other actions/effects
Rocuronium causes increases in heart rate of over 30% of baseline in some patients. While the etiology of the tachycardia is believed to be multi-factorial, vagal blockade may contribute to tachycardia. Rocuronium is more likely than vecuronium but less likely than pancuronium to cause tachycardia.

Rocuronium may cause histamine release. In a study of histamine release, 1 of 88 (1.1%) patients receiving rocuronium had clinically significant concentrations of histamine. In pre-marketing clinical trials, rocuronium administration was accompanied by clinical signs of histamine release (e.g., flushing, rash, or bronchospasm) in 9 of 1137 (0.8%) patients. No clinical evidence of histamine release was observed in one study of 45 patients designed to provoke histamine release by the rapid injection of rocuronium.

### Distribution
Approximately 80% of the initial rocuronium dose is redistributed. As administration of rocuronium continues, tissue compartments fill. Within 4 to 8 hours, less rocuronium is redistributed away from the site of action, and the dosage requirement to maintain neuromuscular blockade via continuous infusion falls to about 20% of the initial infusion rate.
Volume of distribution—
    Adults with normal hepatic and renal function: 0.26 L per kg of body weight (L/kg).
    Adults with hepatic function impairment: 0.53 L/kg.
    Renal transplant patients (adults): 0.34 L/kg.
    Geriatric patients (>65 years of age): 0.22 L/kg.
    Infants 3 to 12 months of age: 0.3 L/kg.
    Children 1 to 3 years of age: 0.26 L/kg.
    Children 3 to 8 years of age: 0.21 L/kg.

### Protein binding
Low (30%).

### Biotransformation
Deacetylated in the liver to 17-desacetyl-rocuronium, a metabolite believed to have little neuromuscular blocking activity.

### Half-life
Distribution—
    Rocuronium has a biphasic distribution. The rapid distribution half-life is 1 to 2 minutes, and the slower distribution half-life is 14 to 18 minutes.
Elimination—
    Adult and geriatric patients with normal hepatic function: 1.4 to 2.4 hours.
    Adult and geriatric patients with hepatic function impairment: 4.3 hours.
    Renal transplant patients (adults): 2.4 hours.
    Infants 3 to 12 months of age: 1.3 hours.
    Children 1 to 3 years of age: 1.1 hours.
    Children 3 to 8 years of age: 0.8 hour.

### Onset of action
With doses of 0.6 mg rocuronium per kg of body weight administered over 5 seconds, effective intubating conditions are achieved within 60 to 70 seconds.
Note: Onset of action of rocuronium may be delayed in patients with conditions, such as cardiovascular disease and advanced age, associated with slowed circulation.

### Time to peak effect
The time to peak effect is dependent on dosage, the age of the patient, and the anesthetic administered concurrently. The median times to maximum block are given below.
Adults 18 to 64 years of age under opioid/nitrous oxide/oxygen anesthesia—
    0.45 mg per kg of body weight (mg/kg): 3 (range, 1.3–8.2) minutes.
    0.6 mg/kg: 1.8 (range, 0.6–13) minutes.
    0.9 mg/kg: 1.4 (range, 0.8–6.2) minutes.
    1.2 mg/kg: 1 (range, 0.6–4.7) minute.
Geriatric patients 65 years of age and older under opioid/nitrous oxide/oxygen anesthesia—
    0.6 mg/kg: 3.7 (range, 1.3–11.3) minutes.
    0.9 mg/kg: 2.5 (range, 1.2–5) minutes.
    1.2 mg/kg: 1.3 (range, 1.2–4.7) minutes.
Infants 3 months to 1 year of age under halothane anesthesia—
    0.6 mg/kg: 0.8 (range, 0.3–3) minute.
    0.8 mg/kg: 0.7 (range, 0.5–0.8) minute.
Children 1 to 12 years of age under halothane anesthesia—
    0.6 mg/kg: 1 (range, 0.5–3.3) minute.
    0.8 mg/kg: 0.5 (range, 0.3–1) minute.

### Duration of action
Duration of clinical effect (the time until spontaneous return of the twitch response to 25% of control value as determined using a peripheral nerve stimulator) is dependent on dosage
Adults 18 to 64 years of age:
    0.45 mg/kg—22 (range, 12–31) minutes.
    0.6 mg/kg—31 (range, 15–85) minutes.
    0.9 mg/kg—58 (range, 27–111) minutes.
    1.2 mg/kg—67 (range, 38–160) minutes.
Geriatric patients 65 years of age and older:
    0.6 mg/kg—46 (range, 22–73) minutes.
    0.9 mg/kg—62 (range, 49–75) minutes.
    1.2 mg/kg—94 (range, 64–138) minutes.
Infants 3 months to 1 year of age:
    0.6 mg/kg—41 (range, 24–68) minutes.
    0.8 mg/kg—40 (range, 27–70) minutes.
Children 1 to 12 years of age:
    0.6 mg/kg—26 (range, 17–39) minutes.
    0.8 mg/kg—30 (range, 17–56) minutes.
Median time to spontaneous recovery from 25 to 75% of the control value is 13 minutes in adults.

### Elimination
Biliary and renal.

## Precautions to Consider

### Carcinogenicity/Tumorigenicity
Studies have not been done to evaluate the carcinogenic or tumorigenic potential of rocuronium.

### Mutagenicity
No mutagenic effect was observed with the Ames test. No chromosomal abnormalities were induced in cultured mammalian cells. The micronucleus test did not suggest mutagenic potential.

### Pregnancy/Reproduction
Fertility—Studies have not been done.

Pregnancy—Rocuronium crosses the placenta. Adequate and well-controlled studies in humans have not been done.

No teratogenic effects were seen in a teratogenicity study in rats at dosages of 0.3 mg per kg of body weight (mg/kg).

FDA Pregnancy Category B.

Delivery—Rocuronium was administered in doses of 0.6 mg/kg to 55 patients for rapid-sequence induction of anesthesia for cesarean section. Patients were also given thiopental at doses of 4 to 6 mg/kg. Anesthesia was maintained with isoflurane, and nitrous oxide in oxygen. No neonate had an Apgar score below seven at 5 minutes after birth. Neonatal blood (umbilical venous) concentrations of rocuronium were 18% of maternal levels. Intubating conditions were poor or inadequate at 1 minute in four patients receiving 4 mg/kg of thiopental. Increasing the thiopental dose to 6 mg/kg improved intubating conditions; however, increasing the thiopental dose to improve intubating conditions is controversial and is not recommended due to an increased chance of central nervous system (CNS) depression in the neonate. Rocuronium is not recommended for rapid-sequence induction in cesarean section patients.

### Breast-feeding
It is not known if rocuronium is distributed into breast milk. However, problems in humans have not been documented.

### Pediatrics

Appropriate studies on the relationship of age to the effects of rocuronium have not been performed in infants less than 3 months of age. Rocuronium was studied in 228 pediatric patients 3 months to 12 years of age in pre-approval clinical trials. When halothane anesthesia was used without atropine pretreatment, a high incidence of tachycardia (exceeding 30% over baseline) was observed in patients given 0.6 to 0.8 mg/kg of rocuronium. A smaller, transient increase in heart rate was observed in another study of pediatric patients.

As compared to adults, children have increased clearance of rocuronium. As compared to children, infants have a longer duration of paralysis after an intubating dose of rocuronium.

Some pediatric patients have experienced tachycardia, increased blood pressure, and resistance to neuromuscular blockade when phenylephrine nose drops were administered after rocuronium.

### Geriatrics

Appropriate studies performed to date have not demonstrated geriatrics-specific problems that would limit the usefulness of rocuronium in the elderly. However, geriatric patients may have a delayed onset of effect as compared to other adult patients.

Geriatric patients have a slightly prolonged duration of clinical effect as compared to other adult patients, perhaps due to age-related changes in renal and hepatic perfusion. The rate of spontaneous recovery (25 to 75%) in geriatric patients is not different from that in other adults.

### Drug interactions and/or related problems

The following drug interactions and/or related problems have been selected on the basis of their potential clinical significance (possible mechanism in parentheses where appropriate)—not necessarily inclusive (» = major clinical significance):

Note: Combinations containing any of the following medications, depending on the amount present, may also interact with this medication.

» Aminoglycosides or
» Bacitracin or
» Colistin or
» Polymyxins or
» Sodium colistimethate or
Tetracyclines or
» Vancomycin
(neuromuscular blocking activity of these medications may be additive to that of rocuronium; prolongation of neuromuscular blocking activity is possible when these medications and rocuronium are used concurrently)

Aminophylline or
Theophylline
(resistance to neuromuscular blockade may occur; higher doses of rocuronium may be needed)

» Anesthetics, inhalation, especially enflurane and isoflurane
(the neuromuscular blocking activity of inhalation anesthetics may be additive to that of rocuronium; median spontaneous recovery time is prolonged by enflurane and isoflurane, but not by halothane; the infusion rate of rocuronium should be reduced by 40% when it is used concurrently with enflurane or isoflurane; the use of rocuronium with other inhalation anesthetics has not been fully studied)

Atropine or
Hyoscyamine
(vagolytic activity of atropine and hyoscyamine may be additive or synergistic with the vagolytic activity of rocuronium; tachycardia has been observed when atropine or hyoscyamine was administered to patients with rocuronium-induced neuromuscular blockade; increased tachycardia also may occur with other anticholinergic drugs)

» Magnesium salts
(magnesium in large doses [e.g., for management of toxemia of pregnancy] may cause enhancement of blockade)

Neuromuscular blocking agents, nondepolarizing, other
(the use of rocuronium with other nondepolarizing neuromuscular blocking agents has not been fully studied; interactions have been reported when other nondepolarizing neuromuscular blocking agents were used in succession)
(the use of rocuronium with mivacurium results in synergistic activity)
(the use of rocuronium before succinylcholine to reduce side effects of succinylcholine has not been studied; if rocuronium is used following use of succinylcholine, it should not be given until recovery from succinylcholine has been observed)

Phenylephrine
(resistance to neuromuscular blockade may occur, perhaps due to changes in perfusion of the muscle tissue; some pediatric patients receiving phenylephrine nose drops in conjunction with rocuronium experienced tachycardia)

Phenytoin
(resistance to neuromuscular blockade may occur with chronic phenytoin therapy, perhaps due to receptor up-regulation; diminished magnitude of blockade and shortened duration of blockade may occur)

» Quinidine
(injection of quinidine during recovery from other neuromuscular blocking agents can cause recurrent paralysis; the same interaction is possible with rocuronium)

### Medical considerations/Contraindications

The medical considerations/contraindications included have been selected on the basis of their potential clinical significance (reasons given in parentheses where appropriate)—not necessarily inclusive (» = major clinical significance).

*Except under special circumstances, this medication should not be used when the following medical problem exists:*

» Hypersensitivity to rocuronium bromide

*Risk-benefit should be considered when the following medical problems exist:*

Acid-base or electrolyte imbalance
(action of rocuronium may be altered; resistance or enhanced effects may occur)

Burns
(resistance to neuromuscular blocking agents may occur)

» Cachexia or debilitation
(profound neuromuscular block may occur)

Cardiovascular disease
(onset of action of rocuronium may be delayed in patients with conditions, such as cardiovascular disease, in which circulation is slowed)

Hepatic function impairment
(duration of action may be prolonged as compared to patients with normal hepatic function; greater interpatient variability may be observed in patients with hepatic function impairment, necessitating close monitoring of twitch response)

» Neuromuscular diseases, such as myasthenia gravis or myasthenic syndrome
(profound effects may occur with small doses of rocuronium)

Pulmonary hypertension or valvular heart disease
(rocuronium may be associated with increased pulmonary vascular resistance)

Renal function impairment
(duration of action may be prolonged as compared to patients with normal renal function; greater interpatient variability is observed in patients with renal function impairment, necessitating close monitoring of twitch response)

### Patient monitoring

The following may be especially important in patient monitoring (other tests may be warranted in some patients, depending on condition; » = major clinical significance):

Degree of neuromuscular blockade
(a peripheral nerve stimulator may be used to determine the adequacy of spontaneous recovery or antagonism; recovery from neuromuscular blockade also should be evaluated clinically by assessment of 5-second head lift, phonation, ventilation, and ability to protect upper airway)

## Side/Adverse Effects

Note: It is not known whether rocuronium can precipitate malignant hyperthermia in susceptible humans, although it is believed to be unlikely. Malignant hyperthermia has not been reported with administration of rocuronium, nor did rocuronium precipitate malignant hyperthermia when tested in susceptible swine. However, clinicians using rocuronium should be familiar with the signs, symptoms, and treatment of malignant hyperthermia.

The following side/adverse effects have been selected on the basis of their potential clinical significance—not necessarily inclusive:

### Those indicating need for medical attention
Incidence less frequent
*Hypertension; hypotension*

Incidence rare
*Arrhythmia; bronchospasm; pruritus; rhonchi; skin rash; swelling at injection site; tachycardia; wheezing*

**Those indicating need for medical attention only if they continue or are bothersome**
Incidence more frequent
*Pain on injection*
Incidence rare
*Hiccups; nausea; vomiting*

## Overdose

Note: No cases of overdose with rocuronium have been reported. Management of rocuronium overdose is the same as management of overdose of the other neuromuscular blocking agents.

For specific information on the agents used in the management of rocuronium overdose, see:
- *Atropine* in *Anticholinergics/Antispasmodics (Systemic)* monograph;
- *Edrophonium (Systemic)* monograph;
- *Glycopyrrolate* in *Anticholinergics/Antispasmodics (Systemic)* monograph;
- *Neostigmine* in *Antimyasthenics (Systemic)* monograph; and/or
- *Pyridostigmine* in *Antimyasthenics (Systemic)* monograph.

For more information on the management of overdose, **contact a Poison Control Center** (see *Poison Control Center Listing*).

**Clinical effects of overdose**
The following effects have been selected on the basis of their potential clinical significance—not necessarily inclusive:

Acute effects
*Apnea; prolonged paralysis*

**Treatment of overdose**
The primary treatment consists of maintenance of a patent airway and controlled ventilation until recovery of neuromuscular function. After evidence of spontaneous recovery, further recovery may be facilitated by administration of an anticholinesterase agent (e.g., edrophonium, neostigmine, pyridostigmine) and an anticholinergic agent (e.g., atropine or glycopyrrolate). Use of a peripheral nerve stimulator to monitor recovery from paralysis is recommended.

## General Dosing Information

Rocuronium should be administered under the direct supervision of an experienced clinician familiar with the actions and potential complications of neuromuscular blocking agents. Equipment and materials for endotracheal intubation, assisted or controlled ventilation, and oxygen therapy, and an agent for reversal should be immediately available.

Rocuronium has no effect on consciousness or pain threshold. Therefore, when rocuronium is used, adequate analgesia and sedation should also be administered.

Doses must be individualized. The stated doses are to be used as a guideline. The degree of neuromuscular blockade should be monitored clinically and with a peripheral nerve stimulator. While the use of a peripheral nerve stimulator can help monitor neuromuscular function, studies comparing the action of rocuronium at the vocal cords and at the adductor pollicis show that onset is quicker at the vocal cords, but maximum block achieved with a given dose is less intense at the vocal cords as compared to the adductor pollicis. The diaphragm is more resistant to rocuronium than is the adductor pollicis. Differences in the action of rocuronium at these locations should be considered when using a peripheral nerve stimulator to monitor drug effect. Relaxation of the vocal cords and diaphragm is more likely to determine intubating conditions than is the degree of block achieved at the adductor pollicis, the site measured with a peripheral nerve stimulator.

Onset of action of rocuronium may be delayed in patients with conditions, such as cardiovascular disease and advanced age, associated with slowed circulation. More time should be allowed for onset of effect in these patients. Higher doses to facilitate more rapid onset should not be used since such doses will result in longer duration of action.

In most clinical trials, the dose for obese patients was determined using actual body weight (ABW). In one study in which the dose for obese patients was determined by ideal body weight (IBW), the patients experienced longer time to maximum block, shorter clinical duration, and unsatisfactory intubating conditions. In obese patients, it is recommended that the dose be determined according to ABW.

Extravasation of rocuronium may result in local irritation. If extravasation occurs, the injection or infusion should be terminated immediately and restarted in another vein.

Injection of rocuronium prior to loss of consciousness is associated with severe, burning pain at the site of injection when administered through a peripheral vein. Although some healthcare practitioners administer lidocaine prior to intravenous injection of rocuronium to attenuate this effect, this technique has not been tested by a controlled trial. Generally, rocuronium should not be administered until loss of consciousness.

Rocuronium is recommended for intravenous administration only.

Reversal of rocuronium blockade should not be attempted until demonstration of some spontaneous recovery from neuromuscular blockade. Reversal of rocuronium can be accomplished more rapidly with edrophonium as compared to neostigmine at a return to 25% of control. At a return to 10% of control, reversal of neuromuscular blockade is accomplished more completely and rapidly with neostigmine as compared to edrophonium.

## Parenteral Dosage Forms

### ROCURONIUM BROMIDE FOR INJECTION

**Usual adult dose**
Neuromuscular blocking agent—
Initial:
For rapid sequence intubation:
Intravenous, 0.6–1.2 mg per kg of body weight.
For tracheal intubation:
Intravenous, 0.6 mg per kg of body weight.

Note: This dose results in blockade sufficient for intubation in one (range, 0.4–6) minute, allows intubation to be completed within two minutes, and achieves maximum blockade within three minutes. A lower dose of 0.45 mg per kg of body weight may be used with a small prolongation of time to blockade sufficient for intubation (1.3 minutes) and of time to achievement of maximum blockade (within 4 minutes). With a dose of 0.45 mg per kg of body weight, intubation can still be accomplished in most patients within two minutes. Doses of 0.9 and 1.2 mg per kg of body weight have been administered during surgery under opioid/nitrous oxide/oxygen anesthesia without adverse cardiovascular effects.

The use of a priming dose (i.e., administration of 10% of the dose of rocuronium, followed three minutes later by the remaining 90% of the intubating dose) significantly shortened the onset time in one study. However, the peripheral intravenous injection of priming doses into patients who are conscious can be expected to be associated with burning pain on injection. Patients may experience sensations of weakness and difficulty breathing after receiving a priming dose.

Maintenance:
Intravenous:
Doses of 0.1, 0.15, and 0.2 mg per kg of body weight given when twitch response returns to 25% of the control value provide a median of twelve (range, 2–31), seventeen (range, 6–50), and twenty-four (range, 7–69) minutes, respectively, of clinical relaxation under opioid/nitrous oxide/oxygen anesthesia. Additional maintenance doses should be guided by recovery of neuromuscular function following the initial dose and should not be administered until recovery of neuromuscular function is evident.

Intravenous infusion:
0.01 to 0.012 mg per kg of body weight per minute after evidence of recovery from the intubating dose. Additional doses may be needed until steady-state has been achieved. The rate of the maintenance infusion must be individualized for each patient and should be guided by the patient's twitch response to peripheral stimulation. In clinical trials, satisfactory blockade was obtained with maintenance infusion rates of 0.004 to 0.016 mg/kg per minute.

**Usual pediatric dose**
Neuromuscular blocking agent—
Initial:
Infants up to 3 months of age—Dosage has not been established.
Infants and children 3 months to 12 years of age—Intubation: Intravenous, 0.6 mg per kg of body weight.

Note: The median time to maximum blockade in pediatric patients is one (range, 0.5–3.3) minute. The intubating dose provides a median time of clinical relaxation of forty-one (range, 24–68) minutes in infants 3 months to 1 year of age and twenty-seven (range, 17–41) minutes in children 1 to 12 years of age.

Maintenance:
   Intravenous—Doses of 0.075 to 0.125 mg per kg of body weight administered when twitch response returns to 25% of the control value to provide an additional seven to ten minutes of clinical relaxation.
   Intravenous infusion—0.012 mg per kg per minute administered when twitch response returns to 10% of the control value. The rate should be adjusted based on twitch response to peripheral nerve stimulation.

### Usual geriatric dose
See *Usual adult dose*.

Note: Onset of action may be delayed in some geriatric patients. Geriatric patients exhibit a slightly prolonged duration of clinical effect.

### Strength(s) usually available
U.S.—
   10 mg/mL (Rx) [*Zemuron*].
Canada—
   10 mg/mL (Rx) [*Zemuron*].

### Packaging and storage
Store between 2 and 8 °C (36 and 46 °F). Protect from freezing.

### Preparation of dosage form
Rocuronium may be prepared with 0.9% sodium chloride injection, 5% dextrose in sodium chloride injection, 5% dextrose in water injection, lactated Ringers injection, or sterile water for injection.

### Stability
After reconstitution with one of the diluents listed above, rocuronium should be used within 24 hours. The prepared solution should be inspected for particulate matter and clarity before being administered to the patient, and should be discarded if particulate matter is present. Prior to reconstitution, rocuronium should be used within 30 days after removal from refrigeration.

### Incompatibilities
Rocuronium is incompatible with alkaline solutions (e.g., barbiturate solutions). The immediate formation of a precipitate after sequential injection of thiopental and rocuronium through the same intravenous line has been reported, even with flushing of the line between injections.

### Selected Bibliography
Magorian T, Flannery KB, Miller RD. Comparison of rocuronium, succinylcholine, and vecuronium for rapid-sequence induction of anesthesia in adult patients. Anesthesiology 1993; 79: 913-8.
Bevan DR, Fiset P, Balendran P, et al. Pharmacodynamic behaviour of rocuronium in the elderly. Can J Anaesth 1993; 40: 127-32.
Hunter JM. New neuromuscular blocking drugs. N Engl J Med 1995; 332: 1691-9.

Developed: 06/28/96

---

# ROPINIROLE  Systemic—INTRODUCTORY VERSION

VA CLASSIFICATION (Primary): CN500
Commonly used brand name(s): *Requip*.
Note: For a listing of dosage forms and brand names by country availability, see *Dosage Forms* section(s).

## Category
Antidyskinetic (dopamine agonist).

## Indications
### Accepted
Parkinson's disease, idiopathic (treatment)—Ropinirole is used to treat the symptoms of idiopathic Parkinson's disease. Its efficacy has been demonstrated in patients with early Parkinson's disease, as well as in patients with advanced disease receiving concomitant levodopa therapy.

## Pharmacology/Pharmacokinetics
### Physicochemical characteristics
Molecular weight—
   Ropinirole: 260.38.
   Ropinirole hydrochloride: 296.84.

### Mechanism of action/Effect
Ropinirole is a non-ergoline dopamine agonist with a high relative *in vitro* specificity and full intrinsic activity at the $D_2$ and $D_3$ dopamine receptor subtypes; it binds with higher affinity to $D_3$ than to $D_2$ or $D_4$ receptor subtypes. The relevance of this binding specificity in Parkinson's disease is not known. Ropinirole's mechanism of action in the treatment of Parkinson's disease is not precisely known, but is believed to be due to the stimulation of post-synaptic dopamine $D_2$-type receptors within the caudate-putamen in the brain. This conclusion is supported by studies in various animal models of Parkinson's disease that show that ropinirole improves motor function. In particular, ropinirole attenuates the motor deficits induced by lesioning the ascending striatonigral dopaminergic pathway with the neurotoxin 1-methyl-4-phenyl-1,2,3,6-tetrahydropyridine (MPTP) in primates.

### Other actions/effects
Ropinirole has moderate *in vitro* affinity for opioid receptors. Ropinirole and its metabolites have negligible *in vitro* affinity for dopamine $D_1$, 5-$HT_1$, 5-$HT_2$, benzodiazepine, GABA, muscarinic, $alpha_1$, $alpha_2$, and beta adrenoreceptors.

### Absorption
Ropinirole is rapidly and fully absorbed. Absolute bioavailability is 55%, indicating a first pass effect. Relative bioavailability from a tablet compared with an oral solution is 85%. Food does not affect the extent of absorption.

### Distribution
Ropinirole is widely distributed throughout the body, with an apparent volume of distribution ($Vol_D$) of 7.5 L per kg. Studies in rats have shown that ropinirole and/or its metabolites cross the placenta and are distributed into breast milk.

### Protein binding
Up to 40%. Ropinirole has a blood-to-plasma ratio of 1:1.

### Biotransformation
Hepatic. Ropinirole is extensively metabolized to inactive metabolites via N-despropylation and hydroxylation pathways. *In vitro* studies indicate that the major cytochrome P450 isoenzyme involved in the metabolism of ropinirole is CYP1A2.

### Half-life
Elimination—Approximately 6 hours.

### Time to peak concentration
Median time to peak concentration ($T_{max}$) is approximately 1.5 hours. $T_{max}$ is increased by 2.5 hours when ropinirole is taken with a meal.

### Peak serum concentration
Approximate dose-normalized mean peak serum concentration ($C_{max}$) is 2 nanograms per mL per mg ([nanograms/mL]/mg). The $C_{max}$ of ropinirole is decreased by an average of 25% when the medication is taken with a meal.

### Time to steady-state concentration
Steady-state concentrations are expected to be achieved within 2 days of dosing. Single dosing predicts that accumulation will occur with multiple dosing. Ropinirole displays linear kinetics over the therapeutic dosing range of 1 to 8 mg three times a day.

### Elimination
Renal. Over 88% of a radiolabeled dose is recovered in urine; less than 10% of an administered dose is excreted as unchanged drug.
   In dialysis—
      Although the effect of hemodialysis on ropinirole removal is not known, removal is unlikely because of the relatively high apparent volume of distribution of the medication.

## Precautions to Consider
### Carcinogenicity/Tumorigenicity
Two-year carcinogenicity studies were conducted in Charles River CD-1 mice at doses of 5, 15, and 50 mg per kg of body weight (mg/kg) per day and in Sprague-Dawley rats at doses of 1.5, 15, and 50 mg/kg per day (top doses equivalent to 10 times and 20 times, respectively, the maximum recommended human dose [MRHD] of 24 mg per day on a mg per square meter of body surface area [mg/m$^2$] basis). In the male rat, there was a significant increase in testicular Leydig cell adenomas at all doses tested, i.e., ≥ 1.5 mg/kg (0.6 times the MRHD on a mg/m$^2$ basis). This finding is of questionable significance because the endocrine mechanisms believed to be involved in the production of Leydig cell hyperplasia and adenomas in rats are not relevant to humans. In the

female mouse, there was an increase in benign uterine endometrial polyps at a dose of 50 mg/kg per day (10 times the MRHD on a mg/m$^2$ basis).

**Mutagenicity**
Ropinirole was not mutagenic or clastogenic in the *in vitro* Ames test, the *in vitro* chromosome aberration test in human lymphocytes, the *in vitro* mouse lymphoma (L1578Y cells) assay, and the *in vivo* mouse micronucleus test.

**Pregnancy/Reproduction**
Fertility—When administered to female rats prior to and during mating and throughout pregnancy, ropinirole caused disruption of implantation at doses of 20 mg/kg per day (8 times the MRHD on a mg/m$^2$ basis) or greater. This effect is thought to be due to the prolactin-lowering effect of ropinirole. In humans, chorionic gonadotropin, not prolactin, is essential for implantation. In rat studies, low doses of ropinirole (5 mg/kg) given during the prolactin-dependent phase of early pregnancy (gestation days 0 to 8) did not affect female fertility at dosages of up to 100 mg/kg per day (40 times the MRHD on a mg/m$^2$ basis). No effect on male fertility was observed in rats at dosages of up to 125 mg/kg per day (50 times the MRHD on a mg/m$^2$ basis).

Pregnancy—Adequate and well-controlled studies have not been done in humans. Ropinirole should be used during pregnancy only if the potential benefit outweighs the potential risk to the fetus.

In animal reproduction studies, ropinirole has been shown to have adverse effects on embryo-fetal development, including teratogenic effects. Ropinirole given to pregnant rats during organogenesis (20 mg/kg on gestation days 6 and 7, followed by 20, 60, 90, 120, or 150 mg/kg on gestation days 8 through 15) resulted in decreased fetal body weight at 60 mg/kg per day, increased fetal death at 90 mg/kg per day, and digital malformations at 150 mg/kg per day (24, 36, and 60 times the maximum recommended clinical dose on a mg/m$^2$ basis, respectively). The combined administration of ropinirole (10 mg/kg per day [8 times the MRHD on a mg/m$^2$ basis]) and levodopa (250 mg/kg per day) to pregnant rabbits during organogenesis produced a greater incidence and severity of fetal malformations (primarily digit defects) than were seen in the offspring of rabbits treated with levodopa alone. No indication of an effect on development of the conceptus was observed in rabbits when a maternally toxic dose of ropinirole was administered alone (20 mg/kg per day [16 times the MRHD on a mg/m$^2$ basis]). In a perinatal-postnatal study in rats, 10 mg/kg per day (4 times the MRHD on a mg/m$^2$ basis) of ropinirole impaired growth and development of nursing offspring and altered neurological development of female offspring.

FDA Pregnancy Category C.

**Breast-feeding**
Studies in rats have shown that ropinirole and/or its metabolites are distributed into breast milk. Dopamine agonist activity is a possibility in the nursing infant.

**Pediatrics**
Appropriate studies on the relationship of age to the effects of ropinirole have not been performed in the pediatric population. Safety and efficacy have not been established.

**Geriatrics**
Ropinirole clearance is reduced by 30% in patients older than 65 years of age as compared with that in younger patients. Dosage adjustments are not necessary because dose titration is based on individual clinical response.

The incidence of hallucinations appears to be greater in the elderly.

**Pharmacogenetics**
The influence of race on the pharmacokinetics of ropinirole has not been evaluated.

**Drug interactions and/or related problems**
The following drug interactions and/or related problems have been selected on the basis of their potential clinical significance (possible mechanism in parentheses where appropriate)—not necessarily inclusive (» = major clinical significance):

Note: Since *in vitro* metabolism studies have shown that CYP1A2 is the major enzyme responsible for the metabolism of ropinirole, substrates or inhibitors of this enzyme, when coadministered with ropinirole, have the potential to alter its clearance. Therefore, if a potent inhibitor of CYP1A2 is initiated or discontinued during ropinirole therapy, dosage adjustments may be necessary.

Combinations containing any of the following medications, depending on the amount present, may also interact with this medication.

» Carbidopa and levodopa combination and
» Levodopa
(administration of 2 mg of ropinirole three times a day increased the mean steady-state concentration of levodopa by 20%; however, the area under the plasma concentration–time curve [AUC] was unaffected; when ropinirole is administered concomitantly, the dose of levodopa may be gradually reduced as needed and tolerated)
(ropinirole may potentiate the dopaminergic side effects of levodopa and may cause or exacerbate preexisting dyskinesia; reducing the dosage of levodopa may ameliorate this effect)

Ciprofloxacin
(coadministration of ciprofloxacin with ropinirole increased the AUC of ropinirole by 84% on average, and the peak plasma concentration by 60% through inhibition of the metabolism of ropinirole via the hepatic isoenzyme CYP1A2)

Dopamine antagonists, including:
  Haloperidol
  Metoclopramide
  Phenothiazines
  Thioxanthenes
(since ropinirole is a dopamine agonist, its actions may be diminished by dopamine antagonists)

Estrogens
(population pharmacokinetic analysis revealed that estrogens [mainly ethinyl estradiol, with an intake of 0.6 to 3 mg over a 4-month to 23-year period] reduced the oral clearance of ropinirole by 36% in 16 patients; with careful clinical titration, dosage adjustments of ropinirole may not be needed unless estrogen therapy is initiated or discontinued during ropinirole treatment)

Tobacco, smoking
(increased clearance of ropinirole is expected, since smoking induces the CYP1A2 isoenzyme)

**Laboratory value alterations**
The following have been selected on the basis of their potential clinical significance (possible effect in parentheses where appropriate)—not necessarily inclusive (» = major clinical significance):

With physiology/laboratory test values
Alkaline phosphatase
(values may be increased)

Prolactin concentrations
(prolactin secretion in healthy male volunteers is suppressed by ropinirole at doses as low as 0.2 mg)

**Medical considerations/Contraindications**
The medical considerations/contraindications included have been selected on the basis of their potential clinical significance (reasons given in parentheses where appropriate)—not necessarily inclusive (» = major clinical significance).

*Risk-benefit should be considered when the following medical problems exist:*

Fibrotic complications from ergot-derived dopaminergic agents, history of
(condition may recur)

» Hallucinations
(condition may be exacerbated)

Hepatic function impairment
(the pharmacokinetics of ropinirole have not been studied in patients with impaired hepatic function; however, these patients may have higher plasma concentrations and lower clearance than do patients with normal hepatic function; doses should be titrated with caution in this patient population)

» Hypotension or
» Orthostatic hypotension
(condition may be exacerbated)

Retinal degeneration, or retinal problems
(studies in albino rats have shown retinal degeneration; the potential significance of this effect in humans has not been established; however, disruption of disk shedding [a mechanism universally present in vertebrates] may be involved)

Sensitivity to ropinirole

**Patient monitoring**
The following may be especially important in patient monitoring (other tests may be warranted in some patients, depending on condition; » = major clinical significance):

Monitoring for symptoms of orthostatic hypotension
(particularly important during dose escalation)

# Side/Adverse Effects

Note: Dopamine agonists appear to impair the systemic regulation of blood pressure, with resulting orthostatic hypotension, especially during dose escalation. In addition, patients with Parkinson's disease appear to have an impaired capacity to respond to an orthostatic challenge.

Retinal degeneration was observed in albino rats that received ropinirole in the premarketing carcinogenicity study. This effect was not noted in albino mice, pigmented rats, or monkeys. The potential significance for humans has not been established; however, this effect cannot be disregarded because it may involve disruption of disk shedding, a mechanism that is universally present in vertebrates.

A symptom complex (characterized by elevated temperature, muscular rigidity, altered consciousness, and autonomic instability) that resembles neuroleptic malignant syndrome and has no other obvious etiology has been reported in association with rapid dose reduction, withdrawal of, or changes in antiparkinsonian therapy. This effect was not observed during premarketing trials of ropinirole, but potentially could occur with the use of this dopaminergic agent.

Fibrotic complications, including retroperitoneal fibrosis, pulmonary infiltrates, pleural effusion, and pleural thickening, have been reported in some patients treated with ergot-derived dopaminergic agents. These complications may resolve upon discontinuation of the medication, but complete resolution does not always occur. Although these effects are believed to be associated with the ergoline structure of these compounds, it is not known if non–ergot-derived dopamine agonists such as ropinirole may produce similar adverse effects.

The following side/adverse effects have been selected on the basis of their potential clinical significance (possible signs and symptoms in parentheses where appropriate)—not necessarily inclusive:

**Those indicating need for medical attention**
Incidence more frequent
*Asthenia* (unusual tiredness or weakness); ***confusion; dependent edema*** (swelling of legs); ***dizziness; dyskinesia*** (twisting, twitching, or other unusual body movements)—may be dose-related; ***falling; hallucinations*** (seeing, hearing, or feeling things that are not there)—may be dose-related; ***nausea; orthostatic hypotension*** (dizziness, lightheadedness, or fainting, especially when standing up); ***somnolence*** (drowsiness); ***syncope*** (fainting); ***viral infection; worsening of parkinsonism***

Note: In placebo-controlled premarketing trials conducted in patients with early Parkinson's disease, *hallucinations* were observed in 5.2% of patients receiving ropinirole, as compared with 1.4% of patients receiving placebo. Among those patients with advanced Parkinson's disease who were concomitantly receiving levodopa, 10.1% of patients receiving ropinirole experienced hallucinations, as compared with 4.2% of patients receiving placebo. The incidence of hallucinations appears to be higher in elderly patients.

*Syncope*, sometimes associated with bradycardia, was observed in placebo-controlled trials in patients receiving ropinirole alone or in combination with levodopa. In patients with early Parkinson's disease who were receiving ropinirole, 11.5% experienced syncope, as compared with 1.4% of patients who were receiving placebo. In patients with advanced Parkinson's disease, 2.9% of those receiving ropinirole plus levodopa reported syncope, as compared with 1.7% of those receiving placebo plus levodopa.

Incidence less frequent
***Abdominal pain; amnesia*** (loss of memory); ***bronchitis*** (cough; shortness of breath; tightness in chest; wheezing); ***cardiac arrhythmias*** (irregular or pounding heartbeat); ***chest pain; difficulty in concentrating; diplopia, xerophthalmia, or other eye or vision problems; dyspnea*** (troubled breathing); ***hematuria*** (blood in urine); ***hypertension; hypotension; mental depression; pain; pain in arms or legs; paresthesia*** (tingling, numbness, or prickly feelings); ***pharyngitis*** (sore throat); ***tachycardia*** (fast heartbeat); ***urinary tract infection*** (burning, pain, or difficulty in urinating); ***vomiting***

Incidence rare
***Anxiety or nervousness; chills; dysphagia*** (trouble in swallowing); ***fever; joint pain; muscle cramps, pain, or spasms; sinus infection*** (fever; headache; nasal congestion); ***tinnitus*** (buzzing or ringing in ears); ***upper respiratory infection*** (cough; fever; runny nose; sneezing); ***urinary incontinence*** (loss of bladder control)

**Those indicating need for medical attention only if they continue or are bothersome**
Incidence less frequent
*Abnormal dreams; anorexia* (loss of appetite); *constipation; diarrhea; dryness of mouth; flushing; headache; heartburn or gas; hot flashes; impotence* (decrease in sexual desire or performance); *increased sweating; malaise* (general feeling of discomfort or illness); ***tremor; weight loss; yawning***

## Overdose

For information on the management of ropinirole overdose or unintentional ingestion, **contact a Poison Control Center** (see *Poison Control Center Listing*).

**Clinical effects of overdose**
Symptoms of ropinirole overdose will most likely be related to its dopaminergic activity.

The following effects have been selected on the basis of their potential clinical significance (possible signs and symptoms in parentheses where appropriate)—not necessarily inclusive:

*Agitation; chest pain; confusion; grogginess; increased dyskinesia, including mild oro-facial dyskinesia; nausea; orthostatic hypotension; sedation; vomiting*

**Treatment of overdose**
To decrease absorption—Gastric lavage may be indicated.

Supportive care—General supportive measures are recommended. Vital signs should be maintained. Patients in whom intentional overdose is confirmed or suspected should be referred for psychiatric consultation.

## Patient Consultation

In providing consultation, consider emphasizing the following selected information (» = major clinical significance):

**Before using this medication**
» Conditions affecting use, especially:
  Sensitivity to ropinirole
  Pregnancy—Animal studies have shown adverse effects on embryo-fetal development, including teratogenicity
  Breast-feeding—Potential for serious adverse effects in nursing infant
  Use in the elderly—Age-related reductions in renal function may require dosage adjustments; also, increased risk of occurrence of hallucinations
  Other medications, especially carbidopa and/or levodopa
  Other medical problems, especially hallucinations, hypotension, or orthostatic hypotension

**Proper use of this medication**
» Compliance with therapy; not taking more or less medication than prescribed
» Proper dosing
  Missed dose: Taking dose as soon as possible; not taking if almost time for next dose; not doubling doses
» Proper storage

**Precautions while using this medication**
» Regular visits to physician to check progress of therapy
» Checking with physician before discontinuing medication; gradual dosage reduction may be needed
» Possible drowsiness, dizziness, lightheadedness, vision problems, weakness, or muscular incoordination; caution when driving or doing jobs requiring alertness, clear vision, and coordination
» Caution when getting up suddenly from lying or sitting position
» Possible occurrence of hallucinations

**Side/adverse effects**
Signs of potential side effects, especially asthenia; confusion; dependent edema; dizziness; dyskinesia; falling; hallucinations; nausea; orthostatic hypotension; somnolence; syncope; viral infection; worsening of parkinsonism; abdominal pain; amnesia; bronchitis; cardiac arrhythmias; chest pain; difficulty in concentrating; diplopia, xerophthalmia, or other eye or vision problems; dyspnea; hematuria; hypertension; hypotension; mental depression; pain; pain in arms or legs; paresthesia; pharyngitis; tachycardia; urinary tract infection; vomiting; anxiety or nervousness; chills; dysphagia; fever; joint pain; muscle cramps, pain, or spasms; sinus infection; tinnitus; upper respiratory infection; and urinary incontinence

## General Dosing Information

Ropinirole doses should be titrated slowly in all patients. Dosage goal should be to achieve maximum therapeutic effect balanced against the principal side effects of nausea, dizziness, somnolence, and dyskinesia.

When ropinirole is used in combination with levodopa, the required dosage of levodopa may be reduced. In clinical trials, the levodopa dose was reduced on average by 31% from baseline.

It is recommended that ropinirole be discontinued gradually over a 7-day period. The frequency of administration should be reduced to two times a day for 4 days, then to once a day for the remaining 3 days before complete withdrawal of ropinirole.

**Diet/Nutrition**
Ropinirole may be taken with or without food. Taking this medication with food possibly may reduce the occurrence of nausea.

## Oral Dosage Forms

### ROPINIROLE HYDROCHLORIDE TABLETS

Note: In clinical studies, dosage was initiated at subtherapeutic levels and gradually titrated to therapeutic response.

**Usual adult dose**
Parkinson's disease, idiopathic—
Oral, initially 0.25 mg three times a day. Based on patient response, dosage should be increased at weekly intervals. A suggested schedule for titration follows:

| \multicolumn{3}{c}{Ascending Dosage Schedule of Ropinirole} |
| Week | Dosage | Total Daily Dose |
|---|---|---|
| 1 | 0.25 mg three times a day | 0.75 mg |
| 2 | 0.5 mg three times a day | 1.5 mg |
| 3 | 0.75 mg three times a day | 2.25 mg |
| 4 | 1 mg three times a day | 3 mg |

**Usual adult prescribing limits**
24 mg a day.

**Usual pediatric dose**
Safety and efficacy have not been established.

**Strength(s) usually available**
U.S.—
0.25 mg (Rx) [*Requip* (croscarmellose sodium; hydrous lactose; magnesium stearate; microcrystalline cellulose; Aluminum Lake; FD&C Blue No. 2; hydroxypropyl methylcellulose; iron oxides; polyethylene glycol; polysorbate 80; talc; titanium dioxide)].
0.5 mg (Rx) [*Requip* (croscarmellose sodium; hydrous lactose; magnesium stearate; microcrystalline cellulose; Aluminum Lake; FD&C Blue No. 2; hydroxypropyl methylcellulose; iron oxides; polyethylene glycol; polysorbate 80; talc; titanium dioxide)].
1 mg (Rx) [*Requip* (croscarmellose sodium; hydrous lactose; magnesium stearate; microcrystalline cellulose; Aluminum Lake; FD&C Blue No. 2; hydroxypropyl methylcellulose; iron oxides; polyethylene glycol; polysorbate 80; talc; titanium dioxide)].
2 mg (Rx) [*Requip* (croscarmellose sodium; hydrous lactose; magnesium stearate; microcrystalline cellulose; Aluminum Lake; FD&C Blue No. 2; hydroxypropyl methylcellulose; iron oxides; polyethylene glycol; polysorbate 80; talc; titanium dioxide)].
5 mg (Rx) [*Requip* (croscarmellose sodium; hydrous lactose; magnesium stearate; microcrystalline cellulose; Aluminum Lake; FD&C Blue No. 2; hydroxypropyl methylcellulose; iron oxides; polyethylene glycol; polysorbate 80; talc; titanium dioxide)].

**Packaging and storage**
Store at controlled room temperature between 20 and 25 °C (68 and 77 °F). Protect from light.

**Auxiliary labeling**
- May cause drowsiness.
- May cause dizziness.

Developed: 11/17/97

---

**ROPIVACAINE**—The *Ropivacaine (Parenteral-Local)* monograph is not included in this published version of the USP DI database. Copies of the monograph are available on request from Micromedex, Inc. - Reprint Requests, 6200 S. Syracuse Way, Suite 300, Englewood, CO 80111; telephone (303) 486-6400; telefax (303) 486-6464; Email: USPDI@MDX.COM.

---

# RUBELLA AND MUMPS VIRUS VACCINE LIVE   Systemic†

VA CLASSIFICATION (Primary): IM100

Note: This monograph is specific for the Wistar RA 27/3 strain of live attenuated rubella virus grown in human diploid cell (WI-38) culture, and the Jeryl Lynn (B level) strain of mumps virus grown in cell cultures of chick embryos.

Commonly used brand name(s): *BIAVAX II*.

Note: For a listing of dosage forms and brand names by country availability, see *Dosage Forms* section(s).

†Not commercially available in Canada.

## Category
Immunizing agent (active).

## Indications

**General considerations**
Persons generally can be considered immune to rubella and/or mumps if they have documentation of adequate immunization with rubella and mumps vaccine on or after their first birthdays, if they have laboratory evidence of rubella and/or mumps immunity, or if they have a physician's diagnosis of previous mumps infection. Since the clinical diagnosis of rubella infection is unreliable, it should not be considered in assessing immune status to rubella.

Although serologic tests may be conducted to determine the susceptibility of persons of unknown immunity, studies have indicated there is no evidence of increased risk of adverse reactions due to vaccination with live rubella and/or mumps virus vaccine in persons already immune to rubella and/or mumps.

Previously nonimmunized children of susceptible pregnant women should receive live attenuated rubella vaccine, because an immunized child is less likely to acquire natural rubella and introduce the virus into the household.

Measles, mumps, and rubella virus vaccine live should be used for vaccinating individuals who are likely to be susceptible to more than one of these viruses, unless otherwise contraindicated.

Vaccines containing measles antigen should be administered routinely to persons 12 to 15 months of age or older. Most individuals born before 1957 generally can be considered immune to measles and mumps because of probable previous infection, even though, in the case of mumps, they may not have had clinically recognizable disease. However, birth before 1957 provides only presumptive evidence of immunity; mumps can occur in some persons born before 1957.

Children vaccinated with rubella and mumps virus vaccine live when younger than 12 months of age should be revaccinated. Based on available evidence, there is no reason to routinely revaccinate persons who were vaccinated originally when 12 months of age or older. However, persons should be revaccinated if there is evidence to suggest that the initial immunization was ineffective.

**Accepted**
Rubella and mumps (prophylaxis)—Rubella and mumps virus vaccine live is indicated for simultaneous immunization against rubella (German measles) and mumps in persons 12 to 15 months of age or older who already have evidence of immunity to measles.

The main objectives of rubella and mumps immunization are:
- To prevent intrauterine infection of the fetuses of women exposed to rubella, which can result in miscarriage, abortion, stillbirth, or in congenital rubella syndrome in the neonate.
- To prevent complications, such as orchitis, which may occur in up to 20% of postpubescent and adult men infected with the mumps virus; and meningoencephalitis, which may occur in up to 15% of persons infected with the mumps virus. In addition, mumps infection during the first trimester of pregnancy may increase the rate of spontaneous abortion.

Unless otherwise contraindicated, all susceptible persons 12 months of age or older should be immunized against rubella and mumps, including:
- Women of childbearing potential, if they are not pregnant and if they are counseled not to become pregnant for 3 months following vaccination. Since there is an increased risk of acquiring rubella while traveling outside the U.S., females of childbearing age should be immunized before leaving the country.
- Postpartum women, preferably before discharge from the hospital. Breast-feeding is not a contraindication to vaccination. Although rubella vaccine virus can be distributed into breast milk, breast-fed newborns generally remain asymptomatic.
- Household contacts of susceptible pregnant women or of other persons with medical contraindications to mumps vaccination, to reduce the risk

to persons unable to receive rubella and mumps vaccine. Vaccinated persons do not transmit rubella and mumps vaccine virus.

- Persons who have been exposed to rubella and/or mumps, since a single exposure may not cause infection and postexposure vaccination provides future protection. There is no evidence to suggest that vaccinating an individual incubating rubella or mumps is harmful, but neither will it prevent illness.
- Persons traveling outside the U.S. These persons should receive either a single antigen vaccine or a combined antigen vaccine, as appropriate, prior to international travel. However, measles, mumps, and rubella virus vaccine live is preferred for persons likely to be susceptible to mumps and rubella; and if a single-antigen measles vaccine is not readily available, travelers should receive measles, mumps, and rubella virus vaccine live regardless of their immune status to mumps or rubella.
- Children 12 months of age and older, including school-aged children.

## Pharmacology/Pharmacokinetics

### Physicochemical characteristics

Source—Rubella and mumps virus vaccine live contains a sterile, lyophilized preparation of live attenuated Wistar RA 27/3 strain of rubella virus grown in human diploid (WI-38) cell culture and Jeryl Lynn (B level) strain of mumps virus grown in cell cultures of chick embryos. The vaccine viruses are the same as those used in the manufacture of rubella virus vaccine live and mumps virus vaccine live. The two viruses are mixed before they are lyophilized.

### Mechanism of action/Effect

Following subcutaneous injection, rubella and mumps vaccine produces a modified, noncommunicable rubella and mumps infection and provides active immunity to rubella and mumps.

### Protective effect

Clinical studies of 73 double seronegative children 12 months to 2 years of age demonstrated that rubella and mumps virus vaccine is highly immunogenic and generally well tolerated. In these studies, a single injection of the vaccine induced rubella hemagglutination-inhibition (HI) antibodies in 100%, and mumps neutralizing antibodies in 97%, of susceptible vaccinated individuals.

The RA 27/3 rubella strain in rubella and mumps virus vaccine elicits higher immediate postvaccination HI, complement-fixing, and neutralizing antibody levels than other strains of rubella vaccine and has been shown to induce a broader profile of circulating antibodies, including anti-theta and anti-iota precipitating antibodies. The RA 27/3 rubella strain immunologically simulates natural infection more closely than other rubella vaccine viruses. The increased levels and broader profile of antibodies produced by the RA 27/3 strain of rubella virus vaccine appear to correlate with greater resistance to subclinical reinfection with the wild virus, and provide greater confidence for lasting immunity.

### Duration of protective effect

The immunity conferred by the vaccine appears to be long-lasting. Vaccine-induced antibody levels following the administration of rubella and mumps vaccine have been shown to persist for at least 2 years without substantial decline. Antibody levels after immunization with a rubella and mumps vaccine containing the HPV-77 strain of rubella have persisted for 10.5 years without substantial decline. Protective antibodies have been observed 18 years after rubella vaccination. If the present pattern continues, it will provide a basis for the expectation that immunity following vaccination will be permanent. However, continued surveillance will be required to demonstrate this point. Continuous serosurveillance is also important to monitor the immunity status in the population and especially to ensure that the immunity is sufficient during childbearing years.

## Precautions to Consider

### Cross-sensitivity and/or related problems

Patients allergic to systemic or topical neomycin may be allergic to rubella and mumps virus vaccine live because each 0.5-mL dose contains approximately 25 mcg of neomycin, which is used in the production of the vaccine to prevent bacterial overgrowth in the viral culture.

A history of hypersensitivity reactions (such as delayed-type allergic reaction contact dermatitis) to neomycin generally does not preclude immunization. Anaphylaxis due to topically or systemically administered neomycin precludes immunization.

Patients allergic to gelatin also may be allergic to the rubella and mumps virus vaccine live, since gelatin is used as a stabilizer in the production of the vaccine.

Patients allergic to eggs may be allergic to the rubella and mumps virus vaccine live, since mumps virus vaccine is produced in chick embryo cell cultures. However, the vaccine may be administered to egg-allergic children without prior skin testing or the use of protocols requiring gradually increasing doses of vaccine. There is no evidence to indicate that persons with allergies to chicken or chicken feathers are at increased risk of reaction to the vaccine.

### Pregnancy/Reproduction

Pregnancy—Although adequate studies have not been done in humans, use in pregnant women is not recommended.

Rubella vaccine virus crosses the placenta and has been recovered from the products of conception of some aborted fetuses of women who received the vaccine just prior to or during pregnancy. However, from 1971 through 1988, the Centers for Disease Control and Prevention (CDC) monitored 210 susceptible pregnant women who had received the RA 27/3 strain of rubella virus vaccine within 3 months before or after conception and who carried their pregnancies to term. Although some neonates had serologic evidence of rubella virus infection, none had malformations associated with congenital rubella syndrome. Therefore, vaccination of a pregnant woman should not in itself indicate the need for abortion, although the final decision rests with the woman and her physician. The risk of congenital rubella syndrome associated with maternal infection with the wild virus during the first trimester of pregnancy is at least 20%. Since the risk of teratogenicity is not known, and appears to be minimal, there is still a theoretical risk of fetal abnormality caused by the vaccine virus.

Although mumps vaccine virus has not been isolated from electively aborted fetuses of women who were vaccinated during pregnancy, the vaccine virus may infect the placenta. In addition, natural mumps infection can infect the placenta and fetus, but there is no evidence that natural mumps infection during pregnancy causes congenital malformations. Therefore, there is no reason to suspect, or evidence to indicate, that mumps vaccine would cause congenital malformations.

It is recommended that pregnancy be avoided for 3 months following vaccination.

Studies have not been done in animals.

FDA Pregnancy Category C.

### Breast-feeding

It is not known whether mumps vaccine is distributed into breast milk. Although rubella vaccine may be distributed into breast milk and infants may subsequently show serologic evidence of rubella infection or mild clinical illness typical of acquired rubella, studies have not shown that these effects cause serious clinical problems.

### Pediatrics

Immunization is not recommended for infants up to 12 months of age, since maternal rubella- and mumps-neutralizing antibodies may interfere with the immune response. Therefore, children vaccinated when younger than 12 months of age should be revaccinated.

When rubella and mumps vaccines are part of a combination vaccination that includes measles vaccine, the minimum age for vaccination is 12 to 15 months in order to maximize measles seroconversion. Children who received the monovalent measles vaccine rather than the combination measles, mumps, and rubella virus vaccine live on or after their first birthdays also should receive a primary dose of mumps and rubella vaccines. Children who were vaccinated when younger than 12 months of age should be revaccinated at 15 months of age.

Children with end-stage renal disease receiving maintenance hemodialysis have a degree of immunosuppression that reduces their response to vaccination. One small trial showed that 80% of these vaccinated children developed antibodies to rubella, while only 50% developed mumps antibodies. Therefore, it may be necessary to monitor postvaccination antibody levels in children with end-stage renal disease, and to revaccinate those children who have failed to demonstrate seroconversion.

### Drug interactions and/or related problems

The following drug interactions and/or related problems have been selected on the basis of their potential clinical significance (possible mechanism in parentheses where appropriate)—not necessarily inclusive (» = major clinical significance):

Note: Combinations containing any of the following medications, depending on the amount present, may also interact with this medication.

Blood products or
Immune globulins
  (concurrent administration with rubella and mumps virus vaccine live may interfere with the patient's immune response to the vaccine because of the possibility of antibodies to rubella and mumps viruses in these products; rubella and mumps virus vaccine live should be administered at least 14 days before, or 3 months after, administration of blood products or immune globulins; the effect of immune globulin preparations on the immune globulin response to mumps virus vaccine is unknown)

» Immunosuppressive agents or
» Radiation therapy
  (because normal defense mechanisms are suppressed, concurrent

use with rubella and mumps virus vaccine live may potentiate the replication of the vaccine virus, increase the side/adverse effects of the vaccine virus, and/or may decrease the patient's antibody response to rubella and mumps virus vaccine live. The reaction may be severe enough to cause death. The interval between discontinuing medications that cause immunosuppression and regaining the ability to respond to rubella and mumps virus vaccine live depends on the intensity and type of immunosuppressive medication being used, the underlying disease, and other factors; estimates vary from 3 months to 1 year. Patients with leukemia that is in remission should not receive rubella and mumps virus vaccine live until at least 3 months after the last dose of chemotherapy. The precaution does not apply to corticosteroids used as replacement therapy, for short-term [less than 2 weeks] systemic therapy, or for other routes of administration that do not cause immunosuppression)

Live virus vaccines, other
(data are lacking on impairment of antibody responses to rubella, measles, mumps, or oral poliovirus vaccine [OPV] when these vaccines are administered on different days within 1 month of each other; however, OPV and measles, mumps, and rubella virus vaccine [or its component vaccines] can be administered at any time before, with, or after each other, if indicated)

## Laboratory value alterations
The following have been selected on the basis of their potential clinical significance (possible effect in parentheses where appropriate)—not necessarily inclusive (» = major clinical significance):

With diagnostic test results
» Tuberculin skin test
(short-term suppression of tuberculin skin test results lasting several weeks may occur and may result in false-negative tests; if required, tuberculin skin tests should be done before, simultaneously with, or at least 4 to 6 weeks after administration of rubella and mumps virus vaccine live)

With physiology/laboratory test values
Platelets, blood
(counts may be decreased)

## Medical considerations/Contraindications
The medical considerations/contraindications included have been selected on the basis of their potential clinical significance (reasons given in parentheses where appropriate)—not necessarily inclusive (» = major clinical significance).

*Except under special circumstances, this medication should not be used when the following medical problems exist:*

» Febrile illness, severe
(manifestations of illness may be confused with possible side/adverse effects of vaccine; however, minor illnesses, such as upper respiratory infection, do not preclude administration of vaccine)
» Immune deficiency conditions, congenital or hereditary, family history of, or
» Immune deficiency conditions, primary or acquired
(because of reduced or suppressed defense mechanisms, the use of live virus vaccines, including rubella and mumps virus vaccine live, may potentiate the replication of the vaccine virus, and/or may decrease the patient's antibody response to rubella and mumps)
(persons with leukemia that is in remission may receive live virus vaccines if at least 3 months have passed since the last chemotherapy treatment)
(persons infected with human immunodeficiency virus [HIV] may receive rubella and mumps virus vaccine live if they are not severely lymphopenic)
(when there is a family history of congenital or hereditary immune deficiency conditions, the patient should not be vaccinated until immunocompetence is demonstrated)

*Risk-benefit should be considered when the following medical problems exist:*

Allergy to eggs or
Allergy to neomycin
(A history of hypersensitivity reactions to neomycin, such as delayed-type allergic reaction or contact dermatitis, generally does not preclude immunization. Anaphylaxis due to topically or systemically administered neomycin precludes immunization. The vaccine may be administered to egg-allergic children without prior skin testing or the use of protocols requiring gradually increasing doses of vaccine. In addition, no allergy to rubella and mumps virus vaccine has been found in patients allergic to chicken feathers or chicken)

Allergy to gelatin
(patients allergic to gelatin also may be allergic to rubella and mumps virus vaccine live, since gelatin is used as a stabilizer in the production of the vaccine)
Sensitivity to rubella and mumps virus vaccine live
Thrombocytopenia or history of vaccine-associated thrombocytopenia
(persons who experienced thrombocytopenia with the first dose of vaccine may develop thrombocytopenia with additional doses. These persons should have serologic testing performed in order to determine the need for additional doses of vaccine. The risk-benefit ratio should be evaluated before considering vaccination in such cases)

**Patient monitoring**
The following may be especially important in patient monitoring (other tests may be warranted in some patients, depending on condition; » = major clinical significance):

Seroconversion test
(may be performed 6 to 8 weeks following vaccination in patients for whom immunity is considered crucial [e.g., persons traveling outside the U.S. or women in high-risk areas who intend to become pregnant], since vaccination with rubella and mumps virus vaccine live may not result in seroconversion in all susceptible patients)

## Side/Adverse Effects
Note: The side/adverse effects associated with the use of rubella and mumps virus vaccine live are the same as those expected to follow administration of the monovalent vaccines given separately. However, it is very important to differentiate between vaccine-induced side/adverse effects and natural infection.

Revaccination of prior vaccinees appears to be associated with relatively low side/adverse effect rates.

The incidence of side/adverse effects increases with age and is generally higher in females.

A history of hypersensitivity reactions other than anaphylaxis, such as delayed-type allergic reaction (contact dermatitis), generally does not preclude immunization.

Encephalitis and other central nervous system (CNS) reactions have been temporally related to mumps virus vaccine administration; however, no causal relationship has been established. The incidence of these disorders in patients vaccinated with mumps virus vaccine is no more frequent than the incidence found in the general population.

Isolated incidents of Guillain-Barré syndrome (GBS) have been reported after immunization with rubella-containing vaccines.

Persons who are immune to rubella and/or mumps virus because of past vaccination or infection usually do not experience side/adverse effects from the vaccine.

Excretion of small amounts of the live attenuated rubella virus from the nose or throat has occurred in the majority of susceptible individuals 7 to 28 days after vaccination. However, there is no confirmed evidence to indicate that the vaccine virus is transmitted to susceptible persons who are in contact with the vaccinated individuals.

The following side/adverse effects have been selected on the basis of their potential clinical significance (possible signs and symptoms in parentheses where appropriate)—not necessarily inclusive:

### Those indicating need for medical attention
Incidence less frequent
*Optic neuritis* (pain or tenderness of eyes)—may occur from 1 to 4 weeks after immunization, lasting less than 1 week

Incidence rare
*Anaphylactic reaction* (difficulty in breathing or swallowing; hives; itching, especially of feet or hands; reddening of skin, especially around ears; swelling of eyes, face, or inside of nose; unusual tiredness or weakness, sudden and severe); *encephalitis or meningoencephalitis* (confusion; headache, severe or continuing; irritability; stiff neck; vomiting); *fever over 39.4 ºC (103 ºF); orchitis in postpubescent and adult males* (pain, tenderness, or swelling in testicles and scrotum); *peripheral neuropathy, polyneuritis, or polyneuropathy* (pain, numbness, or tingling of hands, arms, legs, or feet)—may occur from 1 to 4 weeks after immunization, lasting less than 1 week; *thrombocytopenic purpura* (bruising or purple spots on skin)

### Those indicating need for medical attention only if they continue or are bothersome
Incidence more frequent
*Lymphadenopathy or parotitis* (swelling of glands in neck)—may occur from 1 to 4 weeks after immunization, lasting less than 1 week;

*reaction to acid pH of vaccine* (burning or stinging at injection site); *skin rash*

Incidence less frequent

*Allergic reaction, delayed-type, cell-mediated* (itching, swelling, redness, tenderness, or hard lump at place of injection); *arthralgia or arthritis* (aches or pain in joints)—may occur from 1 to 10 weeks after immunization, lasting less than 1 week; *malaise* (vague feeling of bodily discomfort)—may occur from 1 to 4 weeks after immunization, lasting less than 1 week; *mild headache, sore throat, or runny nose*—may occur from 1 to 4 weeks after immunization, lasting less than 1 week; *nausea*

Note: One study showed that the RA 27/3 strain of rubella virus vaccine live administered to susceptible adult women is not associated with clinically important acute or chronic joint disease. Therefore, rubella vaccination should continue to be used to protect susceptible adult women from rubella in order to advance the goal of eliminating the congenital rubella syndrome. The incidence of *arthralgia or arthritis* is increased greatly in women of childbearing age. Generally the older the woman, the greater the incidence, severity, and duration of arthralgia or arthritis. However, even in older women, the symptoms generally are well tolerated and rarely interfere with normal activities. No persistent joint disorders have been reported.

## Patient Consultation

As an aid to patient consultation, refer to *Advice for the Patient, Rubella and Mumps Virus Vaccine Live (Systemic)*.

In providing consultation, consider emphasizing the following selected information (» = major clinical significance):

**Before receiving this vaccine**
» Conditions affecting use, especially:
Sensitivity to rubella and mumps virus vaccine live, or allergy to gelatin or neomycin
Pregnancy—Use of rubella and mumps virus vaccine live during pregnancy or pregnancy within 3 months of immunization is not recommended
Use in children—Use is not recommended for infants younger than 12 months of age
Other medications, especially immunosuppressive agents or radiation therapy
Other medical problems, especially severe febrile illness, family history of congenital or hereditary immune deficiency conditions, or primary or acquired immune deficiency conditions

**Proper use of this medication**
Waiting at least 14 days after receiving vaccine before receiving blood products or immune globulins
Waiting at least 3 months after administration of blood products or immune globulins before receiving vaccine; however, the effect of immune globulin preparations on the response to mumps virus vaccine is unknown
» Proper dosing

**Precautions after receiving this vaccine**
» Not becoming pregnant for 3 months without first checking with physician, because of theoretical possibility of birth defects
Checking with physician before receiving tuberculin skin test within 4 to 6 weeks of this vaccine, since the results of the test may be affected by the vaccine

**Side/adverse effects**
Signs of potential side effects, especially optic neuritis; anaphylactic reaction; encephalitis or meningoencephalitis; fever over 39.4 °C (103 °F); orchitis in postpubescent and adult males; peripheral neuropathy; polyneuritis; or polyneuropathy; and thrombocytopenic purpura

## General Dosing Information

The dosage of rubella and mumps virus vaccine live is the same for both children and adults.

Rubella and mumps virus vaccine live is administered subcutaneously. It should not be injected intravenously.

When sterilizing syringes and skin before vaccination, care should be taken to avoid preservatives, antiseptics, detergents, and disinfectants, because the vaccine virus is easily inactivated by these substances.

To prevent inactivation of the vaccine, it is recommended that only the diluent provided by the manufacturer be used.

A 25-gauge, 5/8th-inch needle is recommended for administration of the vaccine.

Although rubella and mumps vaccines are available as a combination vaccine (rubella and mumps virus vaccine live) and, as such, are administered as a single injection, the commercially available individual vaccines should not be mixed in the same syringe or administered at the same body site.

Although the fourth dose of diphtheria, tetanus, and pertussis (DTP) vaccine and the third dose of oral poliovirus vaccine (OPV) traditionally have been administered to children 18 months of age, and measles, mumps, and rubella virus vaccine live has traditionally been administered to children 12 to 15 months of age, it is now recommended that DTP, OPV, and measles, mumps, and rubella virus vaccine live be administered concurrently to children 12 to 15 months of age. Measles, mumps, and rubella virus vaccine live should not be postponed in order to administer these vaccines concurrently at 18 months of age.

Rubella and mumps virus vaccine, a live virus vaccine, may be administered concurrently with the following, using separate body sites, separate syringes, and the precautions that apply to each immunizing agent:
- Polysaccharide vaccines, such as Haemophilus b conjugate vaccine, Haemophilus b polysaccharide vaccine, meningococcal polysaccharide vaccine, or pneumococcal polyvalent vaccine.
- Influenza vaccine, whole or split virus.
- Diphtheria toxoid, tetanus toxoid, and/or pertussis vaccine.
- Live virus vaccines, other, such as measles, mumps, OPV, and varicella. OPV and measles, mumps, and rubella virus vaccine (or its component vaccines) can be administered at any time before, with, or after each other, if indicated.
- Inactivated poliovirus vaccine (IPV) or enhanced-potency inactivated poliovirus vaccine (enhanced-potency IPV).
- Hepatitis B recombinant or plasma-derived vaccine.
- Inactivated vaccines, other, except cholera, plague, and typhoid. It is recommended that cholera, plague, and typhoid vaccines be administered on separate occasions because of these vaccines' propensity to cause side/adverse effects.

**For treatment of adverse effects**
Recommended treatment consists of the following:
- For mild hypersensitivity reaction—Administering antihistamines, and, if necessary, corticosteroids.
- For severe hypersensitivity or anaphylactic reaction—Administering epinephrine. Antihistamines or corticosteroids also may be administered as required.

## Parenteral Dosage Forms

### RUBELLA AND MUMPS VIRUS VACCINE LIVE (FOR INJECTION) USP

**Usual adult and adolescent dose**
Immunizing agent (active)—
Subcutaneous, 0.5 mL, preferably into the outer aspect of the upper arm.

**Usual pediatric dose**
Immunizing agent (active)—
Infants up to 12 months of age: Use is not recommended.
Infants and children 12 months of age and older: See *Usual adult and adolescent dose*.

Note: Administration of measles, mumps, and rubella virus vaccine live yields results similar to those from administration of individual measles, mumps, and rubella vaccines at different sites. Therefore, there is no medical basis for administering these vaccines separately for routine vaccination instead of the preferred measles, mumps, and rubella combined vaccine. Measles, mumps, and rubella virus vaccine live should be used for vaccinating individuals who are likely to be susceptible to more than one of these viruses, unless otherwise contraindicated. The Committee on Infectious Diseases of the American Academy of Pediatrics (AAP) and the Advisory Committee on Immunization Practices (ACIP) recommend that all children receive a second dose of measles-containing vaccine. The second dose of measles, mumps, and rubella virus vaccine live is routinely recommended at 4 to 6 years of age, but may be administered at any visit provided at least 1 month has elapsed since receipt of the first dose. The preadolescent health visit at 11 to 12 years of age can serve as a catch-up opportunity to verify vaccination status and administer the vaccine to those children who have not yet received two doses of a measles-containing vaccine.

**Strength(s) usually available**
U.S.—
Not less than the equivalent of 1000 median tissue culture infective dose [$TCID_{50}$] of the U.S. Reference Rubella Virus and not less than the equivalent of 20,000 $TCID_{50}$ of the U.S. Reference Mumps

Virus in each 0.5-mL dose. (Rx) [*BIAVAX II* (neomycin approximately 25 mcg)].

Canada—
Not commercially available.

**Packaging and storage**
Store the lyophilized form of the vaccine, the diluent, and the reconstituted form of the vaccine between 2 and 8 °C (36 and 46 °F), unless otherwise specified by manufacturer.
Alternatively, the diluent for the single-dose vials may be stored between 15 and 30 °C (59 and 86 °F).
Protect both the lyophilized form and the reconstituted form of the vaccine from light.

**Preparation of dosage form**
To reconstitute, use only the diluent provided by the manufacturer, since it is free of preservatives and other substances that might inactivate the vaccine.
Single-dose vial—The entire volume of diluent (approximately 0.5 mL) should be withdrawn into the syringe. All the diluent in the syringe should be injected into the vial of lyophilized vaccine and agitated to mix thoroughly. The entire contents of the vial should be withdrawn into the syringe and the total volume of restored vaccine injected subcutaneously.

**Stability**
Both the lyophilized and the reconstituted vaccine should be stored between 2 and 8 °C (36 and 46 °F) and protected from light. Improper storage and protection may inactivate the vaccine.
The reconstituted vaccine should be used as soon as possible. Unused reconstituted vaccine should be discarded after 8 hours.
The reconstituted vaccine is clear yellow. It should not be used if it is discolored.

**Incompatibilities**
Preservatives or other substances may inactivate the vaccine; therefore, only the diluent supplied by the manufacturer should be used for reconstitution.
A sterile syringe free of preservatives, antiseptics, disinfectants, and detergents should be used for each injection and/or reconstitution of the vaccine. These substances may inactivate the live virus vaccine.

**Auxiliary labeling**
• Protect from light.
• Store in refrigerator.
• Discard reconstituted vaccine if not used within 8 hours.

**Note**
The date and the time of reconstitution should be indicated on the vial if the reconstituted vaccine is not used at once.

Developed: 04/29/97

# RUBELLA VIRUS VACCINE LIVE  Systemic

VA CLASSIFICATION (Primary): IM100

Note: This monograph is specific to the sterile, lyophilized preparation of the Wistar RA 27/3 strain of live attenuated rubella virus grown in human diploid cell (WI-38) culture.

Commonly used brand name(s): *Meruvax II*.

Note: For a listing of dosage forms and brand names by country availability, see *Dosage Forms* section(s).

## Category
Immunizing agent (active).

## Indications

**General considerations**
Persons generally can be considered immune to rubella if they have documentation of adequate immunization with rubella vaccine on or after their first birthdays, or if they have laboratory evidence of rubella immunity. Since the clinical diagnosis of rubella infection is unreliable, it should not be considered in assessing immune status to rubella.

Although serologic tests may be conducted to determine the susceptibility of persons of unknown immunity, studies have indicated that there is no evidence of increased risk of adverse reactions from live rubella virus vaccination in persons already immune to rubella.

Previously nonimmunized children of susceptible pregnant women should receive live attenuated rubella virus vaccine because an immunized child is less likely to acquire natural rubella infection and thus introduce the virus into the household.

Measles, mumps, and rubella virus vaccine live should be used for vaccinating individuals who are likely to be susceptible to more than one of these viruses, unless otherwise contraindicated.

Children vaccinated with rubella virus vaccine live at less than 12 months of age should be revaccinated. Based on available evidence, there is no reason to routinely revaccinate persons who were vaccinated originally when 12 months of age or older. However, persons should be revaccinated if there is evidence to suggest that the initial immunization was ineffective.

**Accepted**
Rubella (prophylaxis)—Rubella virus vaccine live is indicated for immunization against rubella (German measles) in persons 12 months of age or older.

The main objective of rubella immunization is to prevent intrauterine infection of the fetus, which can result in miscarriage, abortion, stillbirth, or in congenital rubella syndrome in the neonate.

Unless otherwise contraindicated, all susceptible persons 12 months of age or older should be immunized against rubella, including:

• All children 12 months of age and older. All children 12 months of age and older should receive rubella virus vaccine live, preferably as the combined measles, mumps, and rubella virus vaccine live, as part of the routine childhood immunization schedule. Infants less than 12 months of age may retain maternal rubella-neutralizing antibodies that may interfere with the development of an immune response to rubella virus vaccine live. Therefore, children vaccinated when less than 12 months of age should be revaccinated. Older children who have not received rubella virus vaccine live should be vaccinated promptly. Because a history of rubella illness is not a reliable indicator of immunity, all children should be vaccinated unless the vaccine is contraindicated.

• Adolescent and adult females who are not pregnant. The routine serologic testing of all women of childbearing age to determine susceptibility to rubella can be effective, but is expensive. Accordingly, rubella vaccination of a woman who is not known to be pregnant and has no history of vaccination is justifiable without serologic testing. Vaccinated women should be counseled to avoid becoming pregnant for a 3-month period following vaccination.

• Postpartum women. Prenatal screening should be carried out on all pregnant women not known to be immune. Women who have just delivered infants should be vaccinated before discharge from the hospital, unless they are known to be immune. Although such women are unlikely to become pregnant, counseling to avoid conception for 3 months following vaccination is still necessary. It is estimated that postpartum vaccination of all women not known to be immune could have prevented approximately 40% of recent congenital rubella syndrome cases. Breast-feeding is not a contraindication to vaccination. Although women can excrete rubella vaccine virus in breast milk, their newborns generally remain asymptomatic.

• Women attending any medical setting. Vaccination of susceptible women of childbearing age should be part of routine general medical and gynecologic outpatient care, should take place in all family-planning settings, and should become routine before discharge from a hospital for any reason, if there are no contraindications. Vaccination should be offered to adults, especially women of childbearing age, any time they make contact with the health-care system, including when their children undergo routine examinations or immunizations.

• International travelers. Persons without evidence of rubella immunity who travel abroad should be vaccinated against rubella because rubella is endemic and even epidemic in many countries throughout the world. No immunization or record of immunization is required for entry into the U.S. However, international travelers should have immunity to rubella (i.e., laboratory evidence of rubella antibodies or verified rubella vaccination on or after the first birthday). Protection is especially important for susceptible women of childbearing age, particularly those planning to remain out of the country for a prolonged period. These persons should receive either a single-antigen vaccine or a combined antigen vaccine as appropriate, prior to international travel. However, measles, mumps, and rubella virus vaccine live is preferred for persons likely to be susceptible to more than one of these viruses; if a single-antigen rubella virus vaccine is not readily available, travelers should receive measles, mumps, and rubella virus vaccine live regardless of their immune status to measles and mumps.

• Medical personnel. Medical personnel, both male and female (e.g., volunteers, trainees, nurses, physicians), who might transmit rubella to pregnant patients or other personnel, should have immunity against rubella. Consideration should be given to making rubella immunity a condition of employment. All medical personnel who have patient contact and who are beginning employment should have proof of rubella immunity or prior vaccination.

• Adolescent and adult males. Vaccination of adolescent and adult males may be a useful procedure in preventing or controlling outbreaks of rubella in circumscribed population groups (e.g., military bases and schools). Ascertainment of rubella immune status and availability of rubella immunization for males should be components of the health care program in places employing women of childbearing age (e.g., day-care centers, schools, colleges, prisons, companies, government offices, and industrial sites).

## Pharmacology/Pharmacokinetics

### Physicochemical characteristics
Source—Rubella virus vaccine live is a sterile, lyophilized preparation of the Wistar RA 27/3 strain of live attenuated rubella virus grown in human diploid cell (WI-38) culture.

### Mechanism of action/Effect
Following subcutaneous injection, rubella virus vaccine live produces a modified, noncommunicable rubella infection and provides active immunity to rubella.

### Protective effect
Extensive clinical trials of rubella virus vaccines, prepared using the Wistar RA 27/3 strain of rubella virus, have been carried out in more than 28,000 human subjects in the U.S. and, in more than 20 other countries. A single injection of the vaccine has been shown to induce rubella hemagglutinin-inhibiting (HI) antibodies in 97% or more of susceptible persons. The Wistar RA 27/3 rubella strain elicits higher immediate postvaccination HI, complement-fixing, and neutralizing antibody levels than other strains of rubella vaccine and has been shown to induce a broader profile of circulating antibodies including anti-theta and anti-iota precipitating antibodies. The Wistar RA 27/3 rubella strain immunologically simulates natural infection more closely than other rubella vaccine virus strains. The increased levels and broader profile of antibodies produced by the Wistar RA 27/3 strain of rubella virus vaccine appear to correlate with greater resistance to subclinical reinfection with the wild virus, and provide greater confidence for lasting immunity.

### Duration of protective effect
Vaccine-induced antibody levels have been shown to persist for at least 10 years without substantial decline. If the present pattern continues, it will provide a basis for the expectation that immunity following vaccination will be permanent. However, continued surveillance will be required to demonstrate this point.

## Precautions to Consider

### Pregnancy/Reproduction
Pregnancy—In a 10-year survey involving over 700 pregnant women who received rubella virus vaccine live (of whom 189 received the Wistar RA 27/3 strain) within 3 months before or after conception, none of the newborns had abnormalities compatible with congenital rubella syndrome. However, there is evidence suggesting transmission of rubella vaccine viruses to products of conception.

The possible effects of the vaccine on fetal development are unknown at this time. If vaccination of postpubertal females is undertaken, pregnancy should be avoided for three months following vaccination.

Studies have not been done in animals.

FDA Pregnancy Category C.

### Breast-feeding
Although women can excrete rubella vaccine virus in breast milk, their newborn generally remain asymptomatic. Therefore, breast-feeding is not a contraindication to vaccination.

### Pediatrics
Infants up to 12 months of age may retain maternal rubella-neutralizing antibodies that may interfere with the immune response to rubella virus vaccine live. Therefore, children vaccinated at less than 12 months of age should be revaccinated. Based on available evidence, there is no reason to routinely revaccinate persons who were vaccinated originally when 12 months of age or older. However, persons should be revaccinated if there is evidence to suggest that the initial immunization was ineffective.

Children with end-stage renal disease receiving maintenance hemodialysis have a degree of immunosuppression that reduces their response to vaccination. One small trial showed that only 80% of these vaccinated children developed antibodies to rubella. Therefore, it may be necessary to monitor postvaccination antibody levels in children with end-stage renal disease, and to revaccinate those children who have failed to demonstrate seroconversion.

Children with human immunodeficiency virus (HIV) infection without overt clinical manifestations of immunosuppression may be vaccinated. However, it may be necessary to monitor postvaccination antibody levels in these children because immunization may be less effective in HIV-infected persons than in uninfected persons.

### Drug interactions and/or related problems
The following drug interactions and/or related problems have been selected on the basis of their potential clinical significance (possible mechanism in parentheses where appropriate)—not necessarily inclusive (» = major clinical significance):

Note: Combinations containing any of the following medications, depending on the amount present, may also interact with this medication.

Blood products or
Immune globulins
(concurrent administration with rubella virus vaccine live may interfere with the patient's immune response to the vaccine because of the possibility of antibodies to rubella virus in these products; rubella virus vaccine live should be administered at least 14 days before, or 3 months after, administration of blood products or immune globulins)

» Immunosuppressive agents or
» Radiation therapy
(because normal defense mechanisms are suppressed, concurrent use with rubella virus vaccine live may potentiate the replication of the vaccine virus, may increase the side/adverse effects of the vaccine, and/or may decrease the patient's antibody response to rubella vaccine. The interval between discontinuation of medications that cause immunosuppression and restoration of the patient's ability to respond to rubella virus vaccine live depends on the intensity and type of immunosuppressive medication used, the underlying disease, and other factors; estimates vary from 3 months to 1 year. Patients with leukemia in remission should not receive rubella virus vaccine live until at least 3 months after their last chemotherapy. This precaution does not apply to corticosteroids used as replacement therapy, for short-term [less than 2 weeks] systemic therapy, or by other routes of administration that do not cause immunosuppression)

Live virus vaccines, other
(data are lacking on impairment of antibody responses to measles, mumps, or oral poliovirus vaccine [OPV] when these vaccines are administered on different days within 1 month of each other; however, OPV and measles, mumps, and rubella virus vaccine live [or its component vaccines] can be administered at any time before, with, or after each other, if indicated)

### Laboratory value alterations
The following have been selected on the basis of their potential clinical significance (possible effect in parentheses where appropriate)—not necessarily inclusive (» = major clinical significance):

With diagnostic test results
Tuberculin skin test
(short-term suppression of response to tuberculin skin test lasting several weeks may occur and may result in false-negative test results; if required, tuberculin skin tests should be done before, simultaneously with, or 4 to 6 weeks after administration of rubella vaccine)

With physiology/laboratory test values
Blood platelets
(counts may be decreased)

### Medical considerations/Contraindications
The medical considerations/contraindications included have been selected on the basis of their potential clinical significance (reasons given in parentheses where appropriate)—not necessarily inclusive (» = major clinical significance).

*Except under special circumstances, this vaccine should not be used when the following medical problems exist:*

» Febrile illness, severe
(the decision to administer or delay vaccination because of current or recent febrile illness depends largely on the cause of the illness and the severity of symptoms; minor illnesses, such as upper res-

piratory infection, do not preclude administration of vaccine; for persons whose compliance with medical care cannot be ensured, every opportunity should be taken to provide appropriate vaccination)

(children with moderate or severe febrile illnesses can be vaccinated as soon as they have recovered from the acute phase of the illness; this waiting period avoids superimposing adverse effects of vaccination on the underlying illness or mistakenly attributing a manifestation of the underlying illness to the vaccine; performing routine physical examinations or measuring temperatures are not prerequisites for vaccinating infants and children who appear to be in good health; asking the parent or guardian if the child is ill, postponing vaccination for children with moderate or severe febrile illnesses, and vaccinating those without contraindications are appropriate procedures in childhood immunization programs)

» Immune deficiency conditions, congenital or hereditary, family history of, or
» Immune deficiency conditions, primary or acquired

(replication of vaccine viruses can be enhanced in persons with immune deficiency diseases and in persons with immunosuppression, as occurs with leukemia, lymphoma, generalized malignancy, or therapy with alkylating agents, antimetabolites, radiation, or large doses of corticosteroids)

(patients with leukemia in remission who have not received chemotherapy for at least 3 months may receive live virus vaccines)

(the exact amount of systemically absorbed corticosteroids and the duration of administration needed to suppress the immune system of an otherwise healthy child are not well defined; most experts agree that corticosteroid therapy usually does not contraindicate administration of live virus vaccines when therapy is short term [i.e., less than 2 weeks], low to moderate dose, long-term alternate-day treatment with short-acting preparations, maintenance physiologic doses [replacement therapy], or administered topically [skin or eyes], by aerosol, or by intra-articular, bursal, or tendon injection; although of recent theoretical concern, no evidence of increased severe reactions to live virus vaccines has been reported among persons receiving corticosteroid therapy by aerosol, and such therapy is not in itself a reason to delay vaccination)

(the immunosuppressive effects of steroid treatment vary, but many clinicians consider a dose equivalent to 2 mg per kg of body weight (mg/kg) or a total of 20 mg per day of prednisone as sufficiently immunosuppressive to raise a concern about the safety of vaccination with live virus vaccines; corticosteroids used in greater-than-physiologic doses also can reduce the immune response to vaccines; physicians should wait at least 3 months after discontinuation of therapy before administering a live virus vaccine to patients who have received high systemically absorbed doses of corticosteroids for ≥ 2 weeks)

***Risk-benefit should be considered when the following medical problems exist:***

Allergy to neomycin
(patients allergic to systemic or topical neomycin may be allergic to rubella virus vaccine live because each 0.5-mL dose contains approximately 25 mcg of neomycin, which is used in the production of the vaccine to prevent bacterial overgrowth in the viral culture. A history of hypersensitivity reactions, such as delayed-type allergic reaction (contact dermatitis), to neomycin generally does not preclude immunization. However, a history of anaphylaxis due to topically or systemically administered neomycin precludes immunization)

Allergy to gelatin
(patients allergic to gelatin also may be allergic to rubella virus vaccine live, since gelatin is used as a stabilizer in the production of the vaccine)

Thrombocytopenia or vaccine-associated thrombocytopenia
(persons who experienced thrombocytopenia with the first dose of vaccine may also develop thrombocytopenia with additional doses. These persons should have serologic testing performed in order to determine the need for additional doses of vaccine. The risk-benefit ratio should be evaluated before considering vaccination in such cases)

Sensitivity to rubella virus vaccine live

**Patient monitoring**
The following may be especially important in patient monitoring (other tests may be warranted in some patients, depending on condition; » = major clinical significance):

Seroconversion test
(may be performed 6 to 8 weeks following vaccination in patients in whom immunity is considered crucial [e.g., women in high-risk areas who intend to become pregnant], since vaccination with rubella virus vaccine live may not result in seroconversion in all susceptible patients)

## Side/Adverse Effects

Note: Surveillance of adverse reactions in the U.S. and other countries indicates that measles, mumps, and rubella virus vaccine live (or its component vaccines) can, in rare circumstances, cause clinically apparent thrombocytopenia within two months following vaccination. In prospective studies, the reported incidence of clinically apparent thrombocytopenia after measles, mumps, and rubella virus vaccine live vaccination ranged from one case per 30,000 vaccinated children in Finland and Great Britain to one case per 40,000 in Sweden, with a temporal clustering of cases occurring 2 to 3 weeks after vaccination. With passive surveillance, the reported incidence was approximately one case per 100,000 vaccine doses distributed in Canada and France, and approximately one case per 1 million doses distributed in the U.S. The clinical course of these cases was usually transient and benign, although hemorrhage occurred rarely. Furthermore, the risk of thrombocytopenia during rubella or measles infection is much greater than the risk after vaccination. According to some reports, the risk of thrombocytopenia may be higher for persons who previously had idiopathic thrombocytopenic purpura, particularly for those who had thrombocytopenic purpura after an earlier dose of measles, mumps, and rubella virus vaccine live.

The following side/adverse effects have been selected on the basis of their potential clinical significance (possible signs and symptoms in parentheses where appropriate)—not necessarily inclusive:

**Those indicating need for medical attention**
Incidence less frequent
*Optic neuritis* (pain or tenderness of eyes)—may occur from 1 to 4 weeks after immunization, lasting less than 1 week

Incidence rare
*Anaphylactic reaction* (difficulty in breathing or swallowing; hives; itching, especially of feet or hands; reddening of skin, especially around ears; swelling of eyes, face, or inside of nose; unusual tiredness or weakness, sudden and severe); *encephalitis or meningoencephalitis* (confusion, convulsions, severe or continuing headache, stiff neck, unusual irritability, or vomiting); *peripheral neuropathy, polyneuritis, or polyneuropathy* (pain, numbness, or tingling of hands, arms, legs, or feet)—may occur from 1 to 4 weeks after immunization, lasting less than 1 week; *thrombocytopenic purpura* (bruising or purple spots on skin)

**Those indicating need for medical attention only if they continue or are bothersome**
Incidence more frequent
*Lymphadenopathy or parotitis*—incidence rare for parotitis (swelling of glands in neck)—may occur from 1 to 4 weeks after immunization, lasting less than 1 week; *reaction due to acid pH of vaccine* (burning or stinging at place of injection); *skin rash*

Incidence less frequent
*Arthralgia or arthritis* (aches or pain in joints)—may occur from 1 to 10 weeks after immunization, lasting less than 1 week; *delayed-type cell-mediated allergic reaction* (itching, swelling, redness, tenderness, or hard lump at place of injection); *malaise* (vague feeling of bodily discomfort)—may occur from 1 to 4 weeks after immunization, lasting less than 1 week; *mild headache, sore throat, runny nose, or fever*—may occur from 1 to 4 weeks after immunization, lasting less than 1 week; *nausea*

Note: Following vaccination with rubella virus vaccine live, *arthralgia* and transient *arthritis* occur more frequently in susceptible adults than in children, and more frequently in susceptible postpubertal females than in susceptible males. Arthralgia or arthritis is rare following vaccination of children with the Wistar RA 27/3 strain of rubella virus vaccine live. However, by contrast, approximately 25% of susceptible postpubertal females develop arthralgia, and approximately 10% have been reported to have arthritis-like signs and symptoms following vaccination with the Wistar RA 27/3 strain of rubella virus vaccine live. Transient peripheral neuritic complaints, such as paresthesias and pain in the arms and legs have occurred rarely.

One study showed that the Wistar RA 27/3 strain of rubella virus vaccine live administered to susceptible adult women is not associated with clinically important acute or chronic joint disease. Therefore, rubella vaccination should continue to be used to protect susceptible adult women from rubella infection with the aim of eliminating congenital rubella syndrome.

## Patient Consultation

As an aid to patient consultation, refer to *Advice for the Patient, Rubella Virus Vaccine Live (Systemic)*.

In providing consultation, consider emphasizing the following selected information (» = major clinical significance):

### Before using this vaccine
Conditions affecting use, especially:
Sensitivity to rubella vaccine or allergy to gelatin or neomycin
Pregnancy—Use of rubella virus vaccine live during pregnancy or pregnancy within 3 months of immunization is not recommended
Use in children—Not recommended for infants less than 12 months of age, since maternal antibodies may interfere with the infant's immune response
Other medications, especially immunosuppressive agents or radiation therapy
Other medical problems, especially severe febrile illness, family history of congenital or hereditary immune deficiency conditions, or primary or acquired immune deficiency conditions

### Proper use of this vaccine
» Proper dosing

### Precautions after receiving this vaccine
Not becoming pregnant for 3 months without first checking with physician, because of theoretical possibility of birth defects
Checking with physician before receiving tuberculin skin test within 4 to 6 weeks of this vaccine, since the results of the test may be affected by rubella vaccine
Waiting at least 14 days after receiving vaccine before receiving blood products or immune globulins
Waiting at least 3 months after administration of blood products or immune globulins before receiving vaccine

### Side/adverse effects
The incidence of side/adverse effects, especially arthralgia and arthritis, increases with age and is generally higher in females
Some side/adverse effects, such as fever, headache, runny nose, or sore throat; peripheral neuropathy, polyneuritis, or polyneuropathy; optic neuritis; lymphadenopathy or parotitis; and malaise may occur from 1 to 4 weeks after immunization (arthralgia or arthritis may occur from 1 to 10 weeks after immunization) and usually last less than 1 week
Signs of potential side effects, especially anaphylactic reaction, encephalitis, meningoencephalitis, optic neuritis, peripheral neuropathy, polyneuritis, polyneuropathy, and thrombocytopenic purpura

## General Dosing Information

The American Academy of Pediatrics (AAP) and the Advisory Committee on Immunization Practices (ACIP) recommend that all children 12 to 15 months of age receive two doses of measles, mumps, and rubella virus vaccine live. Children who received the monovalent rubella vaccine rather than the measles, mumps, and rubella virus vaccine live on or after their first birthdays also should receive a primary dose of measles and mumps vaccines, and doses of measles, mumps, and rubella virus vaccine live or other measles-containing vaccines should be separated by at least one month.

The dosage of rubella virus vaccine live is the same for both children and adults.

When sterilizing syringes and skin before vaccination, care should be taken to avoid contact of the vaccine with preservatives, antiseptics, detergents, and disinfectants, since the vaccine virus is easily inactivated by these substances.

To prevent inactivation of the vaccine, it is recommended that only the diluent provided by the manufacturer be used.

A 25-gauge, 5/8th-inch needle is recommended for administration of the vaccine.

Rubella virus vaccine live is administered subcutaneously. It should not be injected intravenously.

Although measles, mumps, and rubella vaccines are commercially available as a combination vaccine (measles, mumps, and rubella virus vaccine live) and, as such, are administered as a single injection, the commercially available individual vaccines should not be mixed in the same syringe or administered at the same body site.

In general, simultaneous administration of the most widely used live and inactivated vaccines does not impair antibody responses or increase rates of adverse effects. Vaccines recommended for administration at 12 to 15 months of age can be administered at either one or two visits. There are equivalent antibody responses and no clinically significant increases in the frequency of adverse events when diphtheria toxoid, tetanus toxoid, and pertussis vaccine (DTP); measles, mumps, and rubella virus vaccine live; oral poliovirus vaccine (OPV) or inactivated poliovirus vaccine (IPV); and *Haemophilus influenzae* type b conjugate vaccine (HbCV; Hib vaccine) are administered either simultaneously at different sites or at separate times. If a child might not be brought back for future vaccinations, all vaccines (including DTP [or DTaP]; measles, mumps, and rubella virus vaccine live; OPV [or IPV]; varicella; HbCV [Hib]; and hepatitis B vaccines may be administered simultaneously, as appropriate to the child's age and previous vaccination status.

### For treatment of adverse effects
Recommended treatment includes:
- For mild hypersensitivity reaction—Administering antihistamines and, if necessary, corticosteroids.
- For severe hypersensitivity or anaphylactic reaction—Administering epinephrine. Antihistamines or corticosteroids also may be administered as required.

## Parenteral Dosage Forms

### RUBELLA VIRUS VACCINE LIVE (FOR INJECTION) USP

#### Usual adult and adolescent dose
Immunizing agent (active)—
Subcutaneous, 0.5 mL, preferably into the outer aspect of the upper arm.

#### Usual pediatric dose
Infants up to 12 months of age—
Use is not recommended.
Infants and children 12 months of age and older—See *Usual adult and adolescent dose*.

#### Strength(s) usually available
U.S.—
Not less than the equivalent of 1000 median tissue culture infective doses [TCID$_{50}$] of the U.S. Reference Rubella Virus Live in each 0.5-mL dose (Rx) [*Meruvax II*].
Canada—
Not less than the equivalent of 1000 median tissue culture infective doses [TCID$_{50}$] of a reference rubella virus live in each 0.5-mL dose (Rx) [*Meruvax II*; GENERIC].

#### Packaging and storage
Store the lyophilized form of the vaccine, the diluent, and the reconstituted form of the vaccine between 2 and 8 °C (36 and 46 °F), unless otherwise specified by the manufacturer.
Alternatively, the diluent for the single-dose vials only may be stored between 15 and 30 °C (59 and 86 °F).
Protect both the lyophilized form and the reconstituted form of the vaccine from light.

#### Preparation of dosage form
To reconstitute, use only the diluent provided by the manufacturer, since it is free of preservatives or other substances that might inactivate the vaccine.
Single-dose vial—Withdraw the entire volume of diluent (approximately 0.5 mL) into the syringe. Inject all the diluent in the syringe into the vial of lyophilized vaccine and agitate to mix thoroughly. Withdraw the entire contents into the syringe and inject the total volume of restored vaccine subcutaneously.
10-dose vial (in U.S., available only to government agencies/institutions)—Withdraw the entire contents (7 mL) of the diluent vial into the syringe to be used for reconstitution. Inject all of the diluent in the syringe into the 10-dose vial of lyophilized vaccine and agitate to mix thoroughly. The 10-dose container can be used with either syringes or a jet injector. Since the vaccine and diluent do not contain preservatives, special care should be taken to prevent contamination of the multiple-dose vial of vaccine. In addition, the vial should be stored properly until the reconstituted vaccine is used. Discard unused vaccine after 8 hours.
50-dose vial (in U.S., available only to government agencies/institutions)—Withdraw the entire contents (30 mL) of the diluent vial into the syringe to be used for reconstitution. Inject all of the diluent in the syringe into the 50-dose vial of lyophilized vaccine and agitate to mix thoroughly. The 50-dose container is designed to be used only with a jet injector. Since the vaccine and diluent do not contain preservatives, special care should be taken to prevent contamination of the multiple-dose vial of vaccine. In addition, the vial should be stored properly until the reconstituted vaccine is used. Discard unused vaccine after 8 hours.

#### Stability
Both the lyophilized and reconstituted vaccine should be protected from light, which may inactivate the virus.
Use the reconstituted vaccine as soon as possible. Unused reconstituted vaccine should be discarded after 8 hours.

The reconstituted vaccine is clear yellow. It should not be used if it is discolored.

**Incompatibilities**

Preservatives or other substances may inactivate the vaccine; therefore, only the diluent supplied by the manufacturer should be used for reconstitution.

A sterile syringe free of preservatives, antiseptics, disinfectants, and detergents should be used for each injection and/or reconstitution of the vaccine because these substances may inactivate the live virus vaccine.

**Auxiliary labeling**
- Protect from light.
- Store in refrigerator.
- Discard reconstituted vaccine if not used within 8 hours.

**Note**

The date and time of reconstitution should be indicated on the vial if the reconstituted vaccine is not used at once.

Revised: 07/23/97

# RUBIDIUM Rb 82   Systemic†

VA CLASSIFICATION (Primary): DX201

Commonly used brand name(s): *CardioGen-82*.

Note: For a listing of dosage forms and brand names by country availability, see *Dosage Forms* section(s).

†Not commercially available in Canada.

## Category

Diagnostic aid, radioactive (cardiac disease).

## Indications

Note: Bracketed information in the *Indications* section refers to uses that are not included in U.S. product labeling.

**Accepted**

Cardiac imaging, positron emission tomographic

Myocardial perfusion imaging, positron emission tomographic or

Myocardial infarction (diagnosis)—Positron emission tomography using rubidium Rb 82 ($^{82}$Rb-PET) is used to distinguish normal from abnormal regions of myocardial perfusion (blood flow) in patients with suspected myocardial infarction.

[Ischemia, myocardial (diagnosis)]—$^{82}$Rb-PET is used in studies of myocardial perfusion under resting conditions and after pharmacologic coronary vasodilation with dipyridamole or adenosine to detect myocardium with abnormal perfusion reserve secondary to coronary artery disease.

[Coronary artery disease (diagnosis)]—$^{82}$Rb-PET is used in studies of myocardial perfusion before and after physiologic or pharmacologic stress (either exercise or dipyridamole or adenosine infusion) to detect coronary artery disease and characterize its extent and severity.

## Physical Properties

**Nuclear data**

| Radionuclide (half-life) | Mode of decay | Principal photon emissions (keV) | Mean number of emissions/ disintegration |
|---|---|---|---|
| Rb 82 (75 sec) | Positron decay | Gamma (511 each)* | 1.91 |

*Following positron emission, at the moment of annihilation two gamma rays are released, which are used for imaging purposes. Detection device used is a positron emission tomography (PET) unit.

## Pharmacology/Pharmacokinetics

**Mechanism of action/Effect**

Rubidium Rb 82 appears to accumulate, as a function of blood flow, in cells of myocardium and other tissues in a manner analogous to potassium. Compared with normal myocardium, areas of ischemia or infarction exhibit low Rb 82 uptake because of diminished blood flow and/or viability. Imaging equipment can record regional differences in rubidium Rb 82 uptake.

**Distribution**

Rapidly cleared from blood after intravenous administration. Myocardial activity noted within the first minute after injection. Also taken up to a variable degree by all other organs and tissues (with little uptake by normal brain because Rb 82 has limited ability to cross an intact blood-brain barrier).

**Time to radioactivity visualization**

2 to 7 minutes after injection.

**Radiation dosimetry**

Estimated absorbed radiation dose*

| Organ | mGy/MBq | rad/mCi |
|---|---|---|
| Thyroid | 0.038 | 0.14 |
| Adrenals | 0.020 | 0.074 |
| Kidneys | 0.018 | 0.067 |
| Spleen | 0.0050 | 0.018 |
| Pancreas | 0.0045 | 0.017 |
| Small intestine | 0.0039 | 0.014 |
| Large intestine wall (upper) | 0.0039 | 0.014 |
| Large intestine wall (lower) | 0.0039 | 0.014 |
| Stomach wall | 0.0038 | 0.014 |
| Heart | 0.0033 | 0.012 |
| Lungs | 0.0024 | 0.0089 |
| Red marrow | 0.00099 | 0.0037 |
| Liver | 0.00097 | 0.0036 |
| Bone surfaces | 0.00067 | 0.0025 |
| Ovaries | 0.00024 | 0.00089 |
| Uterus | 0.00021 | 0.00078 |
| Breast | 0.00019 | 0.00070 |
| Other tissue | 0.00023 | 0.00085 |

Effective dose: 0.0048 mSv/MBq (0.018 rem/mCi)

*For adults; intravenous injection. Data based on the International Commission on Radiological Protection (ICRP) Publication 53—Radiation dose to patients from radiopharmaceuticals.

**Elimination**

Renal.

## Precautions to Consider

**Carcinogenicity/Mutagenicity**

Long-term animal studies to evaluate carcinogenic or mutagenic potential of rubidium Rb 82 have not been performed.

**Pregnancy/Reproduction**

Pregnancy—Adequate and well-controlled studies have not been done in humans. The possibility of pregnancy should be assessed in women of child-bearing potential. Clinical situations exist where the benefit to the patient and fetus, based on information derived from radiopharmaceutical use, outweighs the risks from fetal exposure to radiation. In this situation, the physician should use discretion and reduce the radiopharmaceutical dose to the lowest possible amount. However, exposure of the embryo or fetus to radiation with the use of rubidium Rb 82 is very low due to the rapid clearance of rubidium Rb 82 from the blood and its short physical half-life.

Studies have not been done in animals.

FDA Pregnancy Category C.

**Breast-feeding**

It is not known whether rubidium Rb 82 is distributed into breast milk; however, due to rubidium Rb 82's short physical half-life, excretion of the agent during lactation is unlikely to result in significant radiation exposure to the breast-feeding infant.

It is not known whether Sr 82 and Sr 85 contaminants are distributed into breast milk; however, due to the small amounts of these contaminants present, excretion during lactation is unlikely to result in significant exposure of the breast-feeding infant to radiation.

**Pediatrics**

No information is available on the relationship of age to the effects of rubidium Rb 82 in pediatric patients. When rubidium Rb 82 is used in children, the diagnostic benefit should be judged to outweigh the potential risk of radiation.

**Geriatrics**

Diagnostic studies performed to date using rubidium Rb 82 have not demonstrated geriatrics-specific problems that would limit its usefulness in the elderly.

**Drug interactions and/or related problems**

There are no known drug interactions and/or related problems associated with the use of rubidium Rb 82.

**Diagnostic interference**

The following have been selected on the basis of their potential clinical significance (possible effect in parentheses where appropriate)—not necessarily inclusive (» = major clinical significance):

With results of this test
   *Due to medical problems or conditions*
      Diabetes mellitus
         (marked alterations in blood glucose, insulin, or pH may affect transport of rubidium Rb 82, possibly affecting quality of images)

**Medical considerations/Contraindications**

The medical considerations/contraindications included have been selected on the basis of their potential clinical significance (reasons given in parentheses where appropriate)—not necessarily inclusive (» = major clinical significance).
See also *Diagnostic interference*.

*Risk-benefit should be considered when the following medical problem exists:*
   Congestive heart failure
      (hemodynamic disturbances may occur due to transitory increase in circulatory volume load)

## Side/Adverse Effects

There are no known side/adverse effects associated with the use of rubidium Rb 82.

## Patient Consultation

As an aid to patient consultation, refer to *Advice for the Patient, Radiopharmaceuticals (Diagnostic)*.
In providing consultation, consider emphasizing the following selected information (» = major clinical significance):

**Description of use**
   Action in the body: Concentration of radioactivity in heart allows images to be obtained
   Small amounts of radioactivity used in diagnosis; radiation exposure is low and considered safe

**Before having this test**
» Conditions affecting use, especially:
   Pregnancy—Risk to fetus from radiation exposure as opposed to benefit derived from use should be considered
   Use in children—Risk of radiation exposure as opposed to benefit derived from use should be considered

**Preparation for this test**
   Special preparatory instructions may be given; patient should inquire in advance

## General Dosing Information

Radiopharmaceuticals are to be administered only by or under the supervision of physicians who have had extensive training in the safe use and handling of radioactive materials and who are authorized by the appropriate Federal or state regulatory agency, if required, or, outside the U.S., the appropriate authority.

**Safety considerations for handling this radiopharmaceutical**

Improper handling of this radiopharmaceutical may cause radioactive contamination. Guidelines for handling radioactive material have been prepared by scientific, professional, state, federal, and international bodies and are available to the specially qualified and authorized users who have access to radiopharmaceuticals.

## Parenteral Dosage Forms

**RUBIDIUM CHLORIDE Rb 82 INJECTION**

**Usual adult and adolescent administered activity**

Cardiac imaging—
   Intravenous, 1480 megabecquerels (40 millicuries) (range, 1110 to 2220 megabecquerels [30 to 60 millicuries]), administered at a rate of 50 mL per minute not to exceed a cumulative volume of 200 mL.

**Usual adult prescribing limits**

Up to 2220 megabecquerels (60 millicuries), as a single dose. Limit for multiple injection series is 4440 megabecquerels (120 millicuries).

**Usual pediatric administered activity**

Dosage must be individualized by physician.

**Usual geriatric administered activity**

See *Usual adult and adolescent administered activity*.

**Strength(s) usually available**

U.S.—
   The activity in megabecquerels (millicuries) of rubidium Rb 82 obtained in each elution depends on potency of generator (Rx) [*CardioGen-82*].

Note: Rubidium Rb 82 generator is supplied in the form of strontium Sr 82 adsorbed on a hydrous stannic oxide column with an activity of 3330 to 5550 megabecquerels (90 to 150 millicuries) of Sr 82 at calibration time.

Canada—
   Not commercially available.

**Packaging and storage**

Store below 40 °C (104 °F), preferably between 15 and 30 °C (59 and 86 °F). Protect from freezing.

**Preparation of dosage form**

At least 10 minutes should be allowed between elutions for regeneration of Rb 82.
Additive-free sodium chloride injection must be used as the diluent.
The first 50 mL eluate should be discarded each day the generator is eluted.
For full preparation instructions, the rubidium Rb 82 generator package insert and the Rb 82 infusion system operator's manual should be consulted.

**Stability**

Almost all of the radioactivity in the eluate decays within 15 minutes after the end of elution.

**Note**

Caution—Radioactive material.

## Selected Bibliography

Williams KA, Ryan JW, Resnekov L, et al. Planar positron imaging of rubidium-82 for myocardial infarction: a comparison with thallium-201 and regional wall motion. Am Heart J 1989; 118(3): 601-10.

Schwaiger M, Muzik O. Assessment of myocardial perfusion by positron emission tomography. Am J Cardiol 1991; 67: 35D-43D.

Gould KL. Clinical cardiac PET using generator-produced Rb 82: a review. Cardiovasc Intervent Radiol 1989; 12(5): 245-51.

Revised: 06/14/93
Interim revision: 08/02/94

# SALICYLATES Systemic

This monograph includes information on the following: 1) Aspirin‡; 2) Aspirin, Buffered‡; 3) Choline Salicylate†; 4) Choline and Magnesium Salicylates; 5) Magnesium Salicylate; 6) Salsalate; 7) Sodium Salicylate.

VA CLASSIFICATION (Primary/Secondary):
Aspirin
    Tablets—CN103/CN104; CN850; MS101; BL170
    Chewable Tablets—CN103/CN104; CN850; MS101; BL170
    Chewing Gum Tablets—CN103
    Delayed-release Tablets—CN103/CN104; CN850; MS101; BL170
    Extended-release Tablets—CN103/CN104; CN850; MS101
    Suppositories—CN103/CN104; CN850; MS101
Aspirin and Caffeine—CN103/CN104; CN850; MS101
Aspirin, Buffered—CN103/CN104; CN850; MS101; BL170
Aspirin and Caffeine, Buffered—CN103/CN104; CN850; MS101; BL170
Choline Salicylate—CN103/CN104; CN850; MS101
Choline and Magnesium Salicylates—CN103/CN104; CN850; MS101
Magnesium Salicylate—CN103/CN104; CN850; MS101
Salsalate—MS101/CN103; CN104; CN850
Sodium Salicylate—CN103/CN104; CN850; MS101

Note: For information on a buffered aspirin product that is used for its antacid as well as its analgesic and antithrombotic effects, see *Aspirin, Sodium Bicarbonate, and Citric Acid (Systemic)*.

Commonly used brand name(s): *217*[1]; *217 Strong*[1]; *Acuprin 81*[1]; *Amigesic*[6]; *Anacin*[1]; *Anacin Caplets*[1]; *Anacin Extra Strength*[1]; *Anacin Maximum Strength*[1]; *Anacin Tablets*[1]; *Anaflex 750*[6]; *Antidol*[1]; *Apo-ASA*[1]; *Apo-ASEN*[1]; *Arco Pain Tablet*[1]; *Arthrisin*[1]; *Arthritis Pain Ascriptin*[2]; *Arthritis Pain Formula*[2]; *Arthritis Strength Bufferin*[2]; *Arthropan*[3]; *Artria S.R*[1]; *Aspergum*[1]; *Aspir-Low*[1]; *Aspirin Caplets*[1]; *Aspirin Children's Tablets*[1]; *Aspirin Plus Stomach Guard Extra Strength*[2]; *Aspirin Plus Stomach Guard Regular Strength*[2]; *Aspirin Regimen Bayer Adult Low Dose*[1]; *Aspirin Regimen Bayer Regular Strength Caplets*[1]; *Aspirin Tablets*[1]; *Aspirin, Coated*[1]; *Aspirtab*[1]; *Aspirtab-Max*[1]; *Astone*[1]; *Astrin*[1]; *Backache Caplets*[5]; *Bayer Children's Aspirin*[1]; *Bayer Select Maximum Strength Backache Pain Relief Formula*[5]; *Bufferin Caplets*[2]; *Bufferin Extra Strength Caplets*[2]; *Bufferin Tablets*[2]; *Buffex*[2]; *Buffinol*[2]; *Buffinol Extra*[2]; *C2*[1]; *C2 Buffered*[2]; *CMT*[4]; *Calmine*[1]; *Cama Arthritis Pain Reliever*[2]; *Cope*[2]; *Coryphen*[1]; *Disalcid*[6]; *Doan's Backache Pills*[5]; *Doan's Regular Strength Tablets*[5]; *Dodd's Extra Strength*[7]; *Dodd's Pills*[7]; *Dolomine*[1]; *Easprin*[1]; *Ecotrin Caplets*[1]; *Ecotrin Tablets*[1]; *Empirin*[1]; *Entrophen 10 Super Strength Caplets*[1]; *Entrophen 15 Maximum Strength Tablets*[1]; *Entrophen Caplets*[1]; *Entrophen Extra Strength*[1]; *Entrophen Tablets*[1]; *Extended-release Bayer 8-Hour*[1]; *Extra Strength Bayer Arthritis Pain Formula Caplets*[1]; *Extra Strength Bayer Aspirin Caplets*[1]; *Extra Strength Bayer Aspirin Tablets*[1]; *Extra Strength Bayer Plus Caplets*[2]; *Gensan*[1]; *Genuine Bayer Aspirin Caplets*[1]; *Genuine Bayer Aspirin Tablets*[1]; *Gin Pain Pills*[7]; *Halfprin*[1]; *Headache Tablet*[1]; *Healthprin Adult Low Strength*[1]; *Healthprin Full Strength*[1]; *Healthprin Half-Dose*[1]; *Herbopyrine*[1]; *Instantine*[1]; *Kalmex*[1]; *Magan*[5]; *Magnaprin*[2]; *Marthritic*[6]; *Maximum Strength Arthritis Foundation Safety Coated Aspirin*[1]; *Maximum Strength Ascriptin*[2]; *Maximum Strength Doan's Analgesic Caplets*[5]; *Mobidin*[5]; *Mono-Gesic*[6]; *Nervine*[1]; *Norwich Aspirin*[1]; *Norwich Aspirin*[1]; *Novasen*[1]; *Novasen Sp.C*[1]; *P-A-C Revised Formula*[1]; *PMS-ASA*[1]; *Pain Aid*[1]; *Regular Strength Ascriptin*[2]; *Salflex*[6]; *Salsitab*[6]; *Sero-Gesic*[5]; *Sloprin*[1]; *St. Joseph Adult Chewable Aspirin*[1]; *Tri-Buffered ASA*[2]; *Tricosal*[4]; *Trilisate*[4]; *Trilisate*[4]; *ZORprin*[1].

Other commonly used names are Acetylsalicylic Acid [Aspirin‡] ASA [Aspirin‡] Choline Magnesium Trisalicylate [Choline and Magnesium Salicylates] Salicylsalicylic Acid [Salsalate]

Note: For a listing of dosage forms and brand names by country availability, see *Dosage Forms* section(s).

†Not commercially available in Canada.

‡*Aspirin* is a brand name in Canada; acetylsalicylic acid is the generic name. ASA, a commonly used designation for aspirin (or acetylsalicylic acid) in both the U.S. and Canada, is the term used in Canadian product labeling.

## Category

Note: All of the salicylates have analgesic, anti-inflammatory, and antipyretic actions; however, clinical uses among specific agents or dosage formulations may vary because of actual pharmacokinetic differences, lack of specific testing, and/or lack of clinical-use data.

Analgesic—Aspirin; Aspirin, Buffered; Choline Salicylate; Choline and Magnesium Salicylates; Magnesium Salicylate; [Salsalate]; Sodium Salicylate.
Anti-inflammatory (nonsteroidal)—Aspirin; Aspirin, Buffered; Choline Salicylate; Choline and Magnesium Salicylates; Magnesium Salicylate; [Salsalate]; Sodium Salicylate.
Antipyretic—Aspirin; Aspirin, Buffered; Choline Salicylate; Choline and Magnesium Salicylates; [Magnesium Salicylate]; [Salsalate]; Sodium Salicylate.
Antirheumatic (nonsteroidal anti-inflammatory)—Aspirin; Aspirin, Buffered; Choline Salicylate; Choline and Magnesium Salicylates; Magnesium Salicylate; Salsalate; Sodium Salicylate.
Platelet aggregation inhibitor—Aspirin Tablets; Aspirin Tablets (Chewable); Aspirin Delayed-release Tablets; Aspirin, Buffered.
Antithrombotic—Aspirin Tablets; Aspirin Tablets (Chewable); Aspirin Delayed-release Tablets; Aspirin, Buffered.
Myocardial infarction prophylactic—Aspirin Tablets; Aspirin Tablets (Chewable); Aspirin Delayed-release Tablets; Aspirin, Buffered.
Myocardial reinfarction prophylactic—Aspirin Tablets; Aspirin Tablets (Chewable); Aspirin Delayed-release Tablets; Aspirin, Buffered.

## Indications

Note: Bracketed information in the *Indications* section refers to uses that are not included in U.S. product labeling.

**Accepted**

Pain (treatment) or
Fever (treatment)—Salicylates are indicated to relieve mild to moderate pain such as headache, toothache, and menstrual cramps and to reduce fever. These medications provide only symptomatic relief; additional therapy to treat the cause of the pain or fever should be instituted when necessary. However, the presence of an illness that may predispose toward Reye's syndrome (i.e., an acute febrile illness, especially influenza or varicella) should be ruled out before salicylate therapy is initiated in a pediatric or adolescent patient.

Salicylates are recommended for relief of mild to moderate bone pain caused by metastatic neoplastic disease. However, careful patient selection is necessary, especially in patients receiving chemotherapy, because of the platelet aggregation–inhibiting effect of aspirin and because salicylates may cause hypoprothrombinemia or gastrointestinal or renal toxicity.

Delayed-release formulations containing aspirin or sodium salicylate may not be as useful as immediate-release formulations for single-dose administration for analgesia or antipyresis because the delayed absorption prolongs the onset of action.

Note: The FDA has proposed that caffeine (present as an analgesic adjuvant in some aspirin products) be classified as a Category III ingredient (i.e., lacking documentation of efficacy) in OTC analgesic/antipyretic medications.

Inflammation, nonrheumatic (treatment)—Salicylates are indicated to relieve myalgia, musculoskeletal pain, and other symptoms of nonrheumatic inflammatory conditions such as athletic injuries, bursitis, capsulitis, tendinitis, and nonspecific acute tenosynovitis.

Arthritis, rheumatoid (treatment)
Arthritis, juvenile (treatment) or
Osteoarthritis (treatment)—Salicylates are indicated for the symptomatic relief of acute and chronic rheumatoid arthritis, juvenile arthritis, osteoarthritis, and related rheumatic diseases. Aspirin is usually the first agent to be used and may be the drug of choice in patients able to tolerate prolonged therapy with high doses. These agents do not affect the progressive course of rheumatoid arthritis.

Concurrent treatment with a glucocorticoid or a disease-modifying antirheumatic agent may be needed, depending on the condition being treated and patient response.

[Salicylates are also used to reduce arthritic complications associated with systemic lupus erythematosus.]

Rheumatic fever (treatment)—Salicylates are indicated to reduce fever and inflammation in rheumatic fever. However, they do not prevent cardiac or other complications associated with this condition. Sodium salicylate should be avoided in rheumatic fever if congestive cardiac complications are present because of its sodium content. Also, large doses of any salicylate should be avoided in rheumatic fever if severe carditis is present because of possible adverse cardiovascular effects.

Platelet aggregation (prophylaxis)—Aspirin (tablets, chewable tablets, delayed-release capsules or tablets, and buffered formulations) is indicated as a platelet aggregation inhibitor in the following:

Ischemic attacks, transient, in males (prophylaxis)
Thromboembolism, cerebral (prophylaxis) or
[Thromboembolism, cerebral, recurrence (prophylaxis)][1]—Aspirin is indicated in the treatment of men who have had transient brain ischemia due to fibrin platelet emboli to reduce the recurrence of transient ischemic attacks (TIAs) and the risk of stroke and death.

[Aspirin is also used in the treatment of women with transient brain ischemia due to fibrin platelet emboli. However, its efficacy in preventing stroke and death in female patients has not been established.][1]

[Aspirin is also indicated in the treatment of patients with documented, unexplained TIAs associated with mitral valve prolapse. However, if TIAs continue to occur after an adequate trial of aspirin therapy, aspirin should be discontinued and an oral anticoagulant administered instead.][1]

[Aspirin is also indicated to prevent initial or recurrent cerebrovascular embolism, TIAs, and stroke following carotid endarterectomy.]

[Aspirin is indicated in the treatment of patients who have had a completed thrombotic stroke, to prevent a recurrence.][1]

Myocardial infarction (prophylaxis) or
Myocardial reinfarction (prophylaxis)—Aspirin is indicated to prevent myocardial infarction in patients with unstable angina pectoris and to prevent recurrence of myocardial infarction in patients with a history of myocardial infarction.

In one study, aspirin significantly reduced the rate of reocclusion, reinfarction, stroke, and death when a single dose was administered within a few hours after the onset of symptoms of acute myocardial infarction and daily thereafter. The benefit of early treatment with aspirin was additive to that of streptokinase. Therefore, it is recommended that aspirin therapy be initiated as soon as possible after the onset of symptoms, even if the patient is receiving thrombolytic therapy.

[One study has shown that aspirin may also prevent myocardial infarction in individuals 50 years of age and older who have no history of unstable angina pectoris or myocardial infarction. However, the incidence of hemorrhagic stroke (but not the total number of hemorrhagic plus thrombotic strokes) was slightly increased in subjects receiving aspirin. Also, the incidence of myocardial infarction, although higher in the placebo group than in the aspirin group, was low in both groups. Therefore, aspirin's benefit in apparently healthy individuals has not been established. However, aspirin may be indicated for prevention of an initial myocardial infarction in selected patients, especially those who may be at risk because of the presence of chronic stable coronary artery disease (as shown by exertional or episodic angina pectoris, abnormal coronary arteriogram, or positive stress test) and/or other risk factors.][1]

[Thromboembolism (prophylaxis)]—Aspirin is used in low doses to decrease the risk of thromboembolism following orthopedic (hip) surgery (especially total hip replacement) and in patients with arteriovenous shunts.

Platelet aggregation inhibitors, although not as consistently effective as an anticoagulant or an anticoagulant plus dipyridamole, may provide some protection against the development of thromboembolic complications in patients with mechanical prosthetic heart valves. Therefore, administration of aspirin, alone or in combination with dipyridamole, may be considered if anticoagulant therapy is contraindicated for these patients. Patients with bioprosthetic cardiac valves who are in normal sinus rhythm generally do not require prolonged antithrombotic therapy, but long-term aspirin administration may be considered on an individual basis.[1]

Aspirin is also indicated, alone[1] or in combination with dipyridamole, to reduce the risk of thrombosis and/or reocclusion of saphenous vein aortocoronary bypass grafts following coronary bypass surgery.

Aspirin is also indicated, alone or in combination with dipyridamole, to reduce the risk of thrombosis and/or reocclusion of prosthetic or saphenous vein femoral popliteal bypass grafts.[1]

Because the patient may be at risk for thromboembolic complications, including myocardial infarction and stroke, long-term aspirin therapy may also be indicated for maintaining patency following coronary or peripheral vascular angioplasty and for treating patients with peripheral vascular insufficiency caused by arteriosclerosis.[1]

Prolonged antithrombotic therapy is generally not needed to maintain vessel patency following vascular reconstruction procedures in high-flow, low-resistance arteries larger than 6 mm in diameter. However, long-term aspirin therapy may be indicated, because patients requiring such procedures may be at risk for other thrombotic complications.[1]

[Kawasaki disease (treatment)][1]—Aspirin is indicated for its anti-inflammatory, antipyretic, and antithrombotic effects in the treatment of Kawasaki disease (Kawasaki syndrome, mucocutaneous lymph node syndrome) in children. It reduces fever, relieves inflammation (e.g., lymphadenitis, mucositis, conjunctivitis, serositis), and may reduce the occurrence of cardiovascular complications. However, the combination of high-dose intravenous gamma globulin and aspirin has been shown to be more effective than aspirin alone in reducing the formation of coronary artery abnormalities.

---

[1]Not included in Canadian product labeling.

## Pharmacology/Pharmacokinetics

### Physicochemical characteristics

Note: Aspirin is an acetylated salicylate; the other salicylates are nonacetylated.

Molecular weight—
  Aspirin: 180.16.
  Choline salicylate: 241.29.
  Magnesium salicylate: 370.60 (tetrahydrate); 298.53 (anhydrous).
  Salsalate: 258.23.
  Sodium salicylate: 160.11.

pKa—
  Aspirin: 3.5.
  Note: The other salicylates are also acidic.

### Mechanism of action/Effect

The analgesic, antipyretic, and anti-inflammatory effects of aspirin are due to actions by both the acetyl and the salicylate portions of the intact molecule as well as by the active salicylate metabolite. The actions of other salicylates are due only to the salicylate portion of the molecule. Aspirin directly inhibits the activity of the enzyme cyclo-oxygenase to decrease the formation of precursors of prostaglandins and thromboxanes from arachidonic acid. Salicylate may competitively inhibit prostaglandin formation. Although many of the therapeutic and adverse effects of these medications may result from inhibition of prostaglandin synthesis (and consequent reduction of prostaglandin activity) in various tissues, other actions may also contribute significantly to the therapeutic effects.

Analgesic—
  Salicylates: Produce analgesia through a peripheral action by blocking pain impulse generation and via a central action, possibly in the hypothalamus. The peripheral action may predominate and probably involves inhibition of the synthesis of prostaglandins, and possibly inhibition of the synthesis and/or actions of other substances, which sensitize pain receptors to mechanical or chemical stimulation.
  Caffeine: A mild central nervous system (CNS) stimulant. Caffeine-induced constriction of cerebral blood vessels, which leads to a decrease in cerebral blood flow and in the oxygen tension of the brain, may contribute to relief of some types of headache. It has been suggested that the addition of caffeine to aspirin may provide a more rapid onset of action and/or enhanced pain relief with lower doses of analgesic. However, the FDA has determined that studies performed to date have not demonstrated that caffeine is an effective analgesic adjuvant or that it does not interfere with aspirin's efficacy as an antipyretic.

Anti-inflammatory (nonsteroidal)—
  Exact mechanisms have not been determined. Salicylates may act peripherally in inflamed tissue, probably by inhibiting the synthesis of prostaglandins and possibly by inhibiting the synthesis and/or actions of other mediators of the inflammatory response. Inhibition of leukocyte migration, inhibition of the release and/or actions of lysosomal enzymes, and actions on other cellular and immunological processes in mesenchymal and connective tissues may be involved.

Antipyretic—
  May produce antipyresis by acting centrally on the hypothalamic heat-regulating center to produce peripheral vasodilation resulting in increased cutaneous blood flow, sweating, and heat loss. The central action may involve inhibition of prostaglandin synthesis in the hypothalamus; however, there is some evidence that fevers caused by endogenous pyrogens that do not act via a prostaglandin mechanism may also respond to salicylate therapy.

Antirheumatic (nonsteroidal anti-inflammatory)—
  Act via analgesic and anti-inflammatory mechanisms; the therapeutic effects are not due to pituitary-adrenal stimulation.

Platelet aggregation inhibitor—
  The platelet aggregation–inhibiting effect of aspirin specifically involves the compound's ability to act as an acetyl donor to the platelet membrane; the nonacetylated salicylates have no clinically significant effect on platelet aggregation. Aspirin affects platelet function by inhibiting the enzyme prostaglandin cyclooxygenase in platelets, thereby preventing the formation of the aggregating agent thromboxane $A_2$. This action is irreversible; the effects persist for the life of the platelets exposed. Aspirin may also inhibit formation

of the platelet aggregation inhibitor prostacyclin (prostaglandin I$_2$) in blood vessels; however, this action is reversible. These actions may be dose-dependent. Although there is some evidence that doses lower than 100 mg per day may not inhibit prostacyclin synthesis, optimum dosage that will suppress thromboxane A$_2$ formation without suppressing prostacyclin generation has not been determined.

**Other actions/effects**

It is proposed that the gastrointestinal toxicity of salicylates, especially aspirin, may be caused primarily by reduction of the activity of prostaglandins (which exert a protective effect on the gastrointestinal mucosa) because upper gastrointestinal toxicity has been reported following rectal or parenteral administration of nonsteroidal anti-inflammatory drugs. However, when administered orally, these acidic medications (unless administered in an enteric-coated formulation) probably also exert a direct irritant or erosive effect on the mucosa.

**Absorption**

Salicylates—
  Absorption is generally rapid and complete following oral administration but may vary according to specific salicylate used, dosage form, and other factors such as tablet dissolution rate and gastric or intraluminal pH.
  Food decreases the rate, but not the extent, of absorption.
  Absorption from enteric-coated formulations is generally delayed.
  Absorption of aspirin from the chewing gum tablet is incomplete as compared with absorption from the oral tablet.
  Following rectal administration of aspirin, absorption is delayed and incomplete as compared with absorption following oral administration of equal doses.
  Absorption of aspirin is impaired during the early febrile stage of Kawasaki disease, then increases toward normal in the convalescent stage.
Caffeine—
  Well absorbed from the gastrointestinal tract.

**Distribution**

In breast milk—
  Aspirin: Peak salicylate concentrations of 173 to 483 mcg per mL have been measured 5 to 8 hours after maternal ingestion of a single 650-mg dose.
  Sodium salicylate: A total of 3 to 4 mg of salicylate is excreted following maternal ingestion of a single dose of 20 mg per kg of body weight (mg/kg).

**Protein binding**

Salicylate—High (to albumin); decreases as plasma salicylate concentration increases, with reduced plasma albumin concentration or renal dysfunction, and during pregnancy.
Caffeine—Low.

**Biotransformation**

Salicylate compounds are largely hydrolyzed in the gastrointestinal tract, liver, and blood to salicylate, which is further metabolized primarily in the liver.
Caffeine—Hepatic.

**Half-life**

Aspirin—
  15 to 20 minutes (for intact molecule); rapidly hydrolyzed to salicylate.
  In breast milk (as salicylate)—3.8 to 12.5 hours (average 7.1 hours) following a single 650-mg dose of aspirin.
Salicylate—
  Dependent on dose and on urinary pH; about 2 to 3 hours with low or single doses and 20 hours or longer with very high doses; with repeated dosing using antirheumatic doses, may range from 5 to 18 hours.
Caffeine—
  3 to 4 hours.

**Time to peak plasma concentration**

Generally 1 to 2 hours with single doses; may be more rapid with liquid dosage forms; may be delayed with salsalate (as compared with aspirin) or with delayed-release tablet or capsule formulations.

**Time to steady-state plasma concentration**

Increases as daily dosage and plasma concentrations are increased; with large (antirheumatic) doses of aspirin, may require up to 7 days.

**Therapeutic plasma concentration**

Salicylate—
  Analgesic and antipyretic: 25 to 50 mcg per mL (2.5 to 5 mg per 100 mL); these concentrations are generally reached with single analgesic/antipyretic doses.
  Anti-inflammatory/antirheumatic: 150 to 300 mcg per mL (15 to 30 mg per 100 mL). Steady-state plasma concentrations within this range are usually reached with therapeutic antirheumatic doses. However, because of interindividual differences in salicylate kinetics, wide variations in steady-state plasma concentrations may be produced in different patients by the same dose. Also, with large or repeated doses, major metabolic pathways become saturated; small changes in dosage may result in large changes in plasma concentration.

**Time to peak effect**

Antirheumatic—May require 2 to 3 weeks or more of continuous therapy.

**Elimination**

Aspirin and salicylate salts—
  Renal; primarily as free salicylic acid and conjugated metabolites.
Salsalate—
  About 13% of a dose excreted as conjugated salsalate; small amounts also excreted unchanged. The remainder of the dose is excreted as free or conjugated salicylate.
Note: Total salicylate excretion does not increase proportionately with dose, but excretion of unmetabolized salicylic acid is increased with higher doses; also, there are large interindividual differences in elimination kinetics. In addition, the rate of excretion of total salicylate and the quantity of free salicylic acid eliminated are increased in alkaline urine and decreased in acidic urine.
In dialysis—Salicylate—
  Hemodialysis—Clearances of 35 to 100 mL per minute have been reported.
  Peritoneal dialysis—Removed more slowly than with hemodialysis; clearances of 45 to 90 mL per hour have been reported in infants.
Caffeine—Renal; primarily as metabolites. About 1 to 2% of a dose is excreted unchanged.

## Precautions to Consider

**Cross-sensitivity and/or related problems**

Patients sensitive to one salicylate, including methyl salicylate (oil of wintergreen), or to other nonsteroidal anti-inflammatory drugs (NSAIDs) may be sensitive to other salicylates also.
Patients sensitive to aspirin may not necessarily be sensitive to nonacetylated salicylates.
Patients sensitive to tartrazine dye may be sensitive to aspirin also, and vice versa.
Cross-sensitivity between aspirin and other NSAIDs that results in bronchospastic or cutaneous reactions may be eliminated if the patient undergoes a desensitization procedure (See *General Dosing Information*).
Patients sensitive to other xanthines (aminophylline, dyphylline, oxtriphylline, theobromine, theophylline) may be sensitive to caffeine also.

**Pregnancy/Reproduction**

Fertility—Salicylates have caused increased numbers of fetal resorptions in animal studies.
Pregnancy—
  *First trimester*
    For salicylates—Salicylates readily cross the placenta. Although it has been reported that salicylate use during pregnancy may increase the risk of birth defects in humans, controlled studies using aspirin have not shown proof of teratogenicity. Studies in humans with other salicylates have not been done. Studies in animals have shown that salicylates cause birth defects including fissure of the spine and skull; facial clefts; eye defects; and malformations of the CNS, viscera, and skeleton (especially the vertebrae and ribs). (Aspirin extended-release tablets: FDA Pregnancy Category D; Magnesium salicylate and salsalate: FDA Pregnancy Category C.)
    For caffeine—Caffeine crosses the placenta and achieves blood and tissue concentrations similar to maternal concentrations. Studies in humans have not shown that caffeine causes birth defects. However, studies in animals have shown that caffeine causes skeletal abnormalities in the digits and phalanges (when given in doses equivalent to the caffeine content of 12 to 24 cups of coffee daily throughout pregnancy or when given in very large single doses, i.e., 50 to 100 mg per kg of body weight [mg/kg]) and retarded skeletal development (when given in lower doses).
  *Third trimester*
    Chronic, high-dose salicylate therapy may result in prolonged gestation, increased risk of postmaturity syndrome (fetal damage or death due to decreased placental function if pregnancy is greatly prolonged), and increased risk of maternal antenatal hemorrhage. Also, ingestion of salicylates, especially aspirin, during the last 2 weeks of pregnancy may increase the risk of fetal or neonatal hemorrhage. The possibility that regular use late in pregnancy may result in constriction or premature closure of the fetal ductus arteriosus, possibly leading to persistent pulmonary hypertension and heart failure in the neonate, must also be considered. Overuse or abuse of aspirin late in pregnancy has been

reported to increase the risk of stillbirth or neonatal death, possibly because of antenatal hemorrhage or premature ductus arteriosus closure, and to decrease birthweight; however, studies using therapeutic doses of aspirin have not shown these adverse effects. Pregnant women should be advised not to take aspirin during the last trimester of pregnancy unless such therapy is prescribed and monitored by a physician.

Labor and delivery—Chronic, high-dose salicylate therapy late in pregnancy may result in prolonged labor, complicated deliveries, and increased risk of maternal or fetal hemorrhage.

### Breast-feeding
*For salicylates*—
Problems in humans with usual analgesic doses have not been documented. However, salicylate is distributed into breast milk; with chronic, high-dose use, intake by the infant may be high enough to cause adverse effects.

In one study, peak salicylate concentrations of 173 to 483 mcg per mL were measured in breast milk 5 to 8 hours after maternal ingestion of a single dose of 650 mg of aspirin. The half-life in breast milk was 3.8 to 12.5 hours (average 7.1 hours).

Following maternal ingestion of 20 mg/kg of sodium salicylate, a total of 3 to 4 mg of salicylate is distributed into breast milk.

*For caffeine*—
Caffeine is distributed into breast milk in very small amounts; at recommended dosages, concentration in the infant is considered to be insignificant.

### Pediatrics
*For salicylates*—
Aspirin use may be associated with the development of Reye's syndrome in children and teenagers with acute febrile illnesses, especially influenza and varicella. It is recommended that salicylate therapy not be initiated in febrile pediatric or adolescent patients until after the presence of such an illness has been ruled out. Also, it is recommended that chronic salicylate therapy in these patients be discontinued if a fever occurs, and not resumed until it has been determined that an illness that may predispose to Reye's syndrome is not present or has run its course. Other forms of salicylate toxicity may also be more prevalent in pediatric patients, especially children who have a fever or are dehydrated.

Especially careful monitoring of the serum salicylate concentration is recommended in pediatric patients with Kawasaki disease. Absorption of aspirin is impaired during the early febrile stage of the disease; therapeutic anti-inflammatory plasma salicylate concentrations may be extremely difficult to achieve. Also, as the febrile stage passes, absorption is improved; salicylate toxicity may occur if dosage is not readjusted.

*For caffeine*—
Pediatric patients are especially susceptible to overdose of caffeine and its adverse CNS effects.

### Geriatrics
Geriatric patients may be more susceptible to the toxic effects of salicylates, possibly because of decreased renal function. Lower doses than those usually recommended for adults, especially for long-term use or for use of long-acting salicylates (such as choline and magnesium salicylates and salsalate), may be required.

### Drug interactions and/or related problems
The following drug interactions and/or related problems have been selected on the basis of their potential clinical significance (possible mechanism in parentheses where appropriate)—not necessarily inclusive (» = major clinical significance):

Note: Combinations containing any of the following medications, depending on the amount present, may also interact with this medication.

In addition to the interactions listed below, the possibility should be considered that additive or multiple effects leading to impaired blood clotting and/or increased risk of bleeding may occur if a salicylate, especially aspirin, is used concurrently with any medication having a significant potential for causing hypoprothrombinemia, thrombocytopenia, or gastrointestinal ulceration or hemorrhage.

*For all salicylates*
Acetaminophen
(prolonged concurrent use of acetaminophen with a salicylate is not recommended because chronic, high-dose administration of the combined analgesics [1.35 grams daily, or cumulative ingestion of 1 kg annually, for 3 years or longer] significantly increases the risk of analgesic nephropathy, renal papillary necrosis, end-stage renal disease, and cancer of the kidney or urinary bladder; also, it is recommended that for short-term use the combined dose of acetaminophen plus a salicylate not exceed that recommended for acetaminophen or a salicylate given individually)

Acidifiers, urinary, such as:
Ammonium chloride
Ascorbic acid (Vitamin C)
Potassium or sodium phosphates
(acidification of the urine by these medications decreases salicylate excretion, leading to increased salicylate plasma concentrations; initiation of therapy with these medications in patients stabilized on a salicylate may lead to toxic salicylate concentrations)

(aspirin may increase urinary excretion of ascorbic acid; clinical significance is unclear, but some clinicians recommend ascorbic acid supplementation in patients receiving prolonged high-dose aspirin therapy)

Alcohol or
» Nonsteroidal anti-inflammatory drugs (NSAIDs), other
(concurrent use of these medications with a salicylate may increase the risk of gastrointestinal side effects, including ulceration and gastrointestinal blood loss; also, concurrent use of a salicylate with an NSAID may increase the risk of severe gastrointestinal side effects without providing additional symptomatic relief and is therefore not recommended)

(aspirin may decrease the bioavailability of many NSAIDs, including diflunisal, fenoprofen, indomethacin, meclofenamate, piroxicam [to 80% of the usual plasma concentration], and the active sulfide metabolite of sulindac; aspirin has also been shown to decrease the protein binding and increase the plasma clearance of ketoprofen, and to decrease the formation and excretion of ketoprofen conjugates)

(concurrent use of other NSAIDs with aspirin may also increase the risk of bleeding at sites other than the gastrointestinal tract because of additive inhibition of platelet aggregation)

» Alkalizers, urinary, such as:
Carbonic anhydrase inhibitors
Citrates
Sodium bicarbonate or
Antacids, chronic high-dose use, especially calcium- and/or magnesium-containing
(alkalinization of the urine by these medications increases salicylate excretion, leading to decreased salicylate plasma concentrations, reduced effectiveness, and shortened duration of action; also, withdrawal of a urinary alkalizer from a patient stabilized on a salicylate may increase the plasma salicylate concentration to a toxic level; however, the antacids present in buffered aspirin formulations may not be present in sufficient quantity to alkalinize the urine)

(metabolic acidosis induced by carbonic anhydrase inhibitors may increase penetration of salicylate into the brain and increase the risk of salicylate toxicity in patients taking large [antirheumatic] doses of salicylate; if acetazolamide is used to produce forced alkaline diuresis in the treatment of salicylate poisoning, the increased risk of severe metabolic acidosis and increased salicylate toxicity must be considered and an alkaline intravenous solution given concurrently)

» Anticoagulants, coumarin- or indandione-derivative or
» Heparin or
» Thrombolytic agents, such as:
Alteplase
Anistreplase
Streptokinase
Urokinase
(salicylates may displace a coumarin- or indandione-derivative anticoagulant from its protein-binding sites, and, in high doses, may cause hypoprothrombinemia, leading to increased anticoagulation and risk of bleeding)

(the potential occurrence of gastrointestinal ulceration or hemorrhage during salicylate, especially aspirin, therapy may cause increased risk to patients receiving anticoagulant or thrombolytic therapy)

(because aspirin-induced inhibition of platelet function may lead to prolonged bleeding time and increased risk of hemorrhage, concurrent use of aspirin with an anticoagulant or a thrombolytic agent is recommended only within a carefully monitored antithrombotic regimen; although a recent study has shown that initiation of therapy with 160 mg of aspirin a day concurrently with short-term [1-hour] intravenous infusion of streptokinase in patients with acute coronary arterial occlusion significantly decreases the risk of reocclusion, reinfarction, stroke, and death without increasing the risk of adverse effects [as compared with streptokinase alone], other studies using higher doses of aspirin and/or more prolonged administration of a thrombolytic agent have demonstrated an increased risk of bleeding)

Anticonvulsants, hydantoin
(salicylates may decrease hydantoin metabolism, leading to increases in hydantoin plasma concentrations, efficacy, and/or toxicity; adjustment of hydantoin dosage may be required when chronic salicylate therapy is initiated or discontinued)

» Antidiabetic agents, oral or
Insulin
(effects of these medications may be increased by large doses of salicylates; dosage adjustments may be necessary; potentiation of oral antidiabetic agents may be caused partially by displacement from serum proteins; glipizide and glyburide, because of their nonionic binding characteristics, may not be affected as much as the other oral agents; however, caution in concurrent use is recommended)

Antiemetics, including antihistamines and phenothiazines
(antiemetics may mask the symptoms of salicylate-induced ototoxicity, such as dizziness, vertigo, and tinnitus)

Bismuth subsalicylate
(ingestion of large repeated doses as for traveler's diarrhea may produce substantial plasma salicylate concentrations; concurrent use with large doses of analgesic salicylates may increase the risk of salicylate toxicity)

» Cefamandole or
» Cefoperazone or
» Cefotetan or
» Plicamycin or
» Valproic acid
(these medications may cause hypoprothrombinemia; in addition, plicamycin or valproic acid may inhibit platelet aggregation; concurrent use with aspirin may increase the risk of bleeding because of additive interferences with blood clotting)

(hypoprothrombinemia induced by large doses of salicylates, and the potential occurrence of gastrointestinal ulceration or hemorrhage during salicylate, especially aspirin, therapy, may increase the risk of bleeding complications in patients receiving these medications)

(concurrent use of aspirin with valproic acid has also been reported to increase the plasma concentration of valproic acid and induce valproic acid toxicity)

Corticosteroids or
Corticotropin (ACTH), chronic therapeutic use of
(corticosteroids or corticotropin may increase salicylate excretion, resulting in lower plasma concentrations and increased salicylate dosage requirements; salicylism may result when corticosteroids or corticotropin dosage is subsequently decreased or discontinued, especially in patients receiving large [antirheumatic] doses of salicylate; also, the risk of gastrointestinal side effects, including ulceration and gastrointestinal blood loss, may be increased; however, concurrent use in the treatment of arthritis may provide additive therapeutic benefit and permit reduction of corticosteroid or corticotropin dosage)

(because corticosteroids and corticotropin may cause sodium and fluid retention, caution in concurrent use with large doses of sodium salicylate is recommended)

Furosemide
(in addition to increasing the risk of ototoxicity, concurrent use of furosemide with high doses of salicylate may lead to salicylate toxicity because of competition for renal excretory sites)

Laxatives, cellulose-containing
(concurrent use may reduce the salicylate effect because of physical binding or other absorptive hindrance; medications should be administered 2 hours apart)

» Methotrexate
(salicylates may displace methotrexate from its binding sites and decrease its renal clearance, leading to toxic methotrexate plasma concentrations; if they are used concurrently, methotrexate dosage should be decreased, the patient observed for signs of toxicity, and/or methotrexate plasma concentration monitored; also, it is recommended that salicylate therapy be discontinued 24 to 48 hours prior to administration of a high-dose methotrexate infusion, and not resumed until the plasma methotrexate concentration has decreased to a nontoxic level [usually at least 12 hours postinfusion])

Ototoxic medications, other (See *Appendix II*), especially
» Vancomycin
(concurrent or sequential administration of these medications with a salicylate should be avoided because the potential for ototoxicity may be increased; hearing loss may occur and may progress to deafness even after discontinuation of the medication; these effects may be reversible, but usually are permanent)

» Platelet aggregation inhibitors (See *Appendix II*)
(concurrent use with aspirin is not recommended, except in a monitored antithrombotic regimen, because the risk of bleeding may be increased)

(the potential occurrence of gastrointestinal ulceration or hemorrhage during salicylate therapy, and the hypoprothrombinemic effect of large doses of salicylate, may cause increased risk to patients receiving a platelet aggregation inhibitor)

» Probenecid or
» Sulfinpyrazone
(concurrent use of a salicylate is not recommended when these medications are used to treat hyperuricemia or gout, because the uricosuric effect of these medications may be decreased by doses of salicylates that produce serum salicylate concentrations above 5 mg per 100 mL; also, these medications may inhibit the uricosuric effect achieved when serum salicylate concentrations are above 10 to 15 mg per 100 mL)

(probenecid may decrease renal clearance and increase plasma concentrations and toxicity of salicylates)

(sulfinpyrazone may decrease salicylate excretion and/or displace salicylate from its protein binding sites, possibly leading to increased salicylate concentrations and toxicity)

(although low doses of sulfinpyrazone and aspirin have been used concurrently to provide additive inhibition of platelet aggregation, the efficacy of the combination has not been established and the increased risk of bleeding must be considered; also, concurrent use of sulfinpyrazone with aspirin may increase the risk of gastrointestinal ulceration or hemorrhage)

Salicylic acid or other salicylates, topical
(concurrent use with systemic salicylates may increase the risk of salicylate toxicity if significant quantities are absorbed)

Vitamin K
(requirements for this vitamin may be increased in patients receiving high doses of salicylate)

Zidovudine
(in theory, aspirin may competitively inhibit the hepatic glucuronidation and decrease the clearance of zidovudine, leading to potentiation of zidovudine toxicity; the possibility must be considered that aspirin toxicity may also be increased)

*For buffered aspirin formulations, choline and magnesium salicylates, and magnesium salicylate (in addition to those interactions listed above as applying to all salicylates)*

» Ciprofloxacin or
» Enoxacin or
» Itraconazole or
» Ketoconazole or
» Lomefloxacin or
» Norfloxacin or
» Ofloxacin or
» Tetracyclines, oral
(antacids present in buffered aspirin formulations, and the magnesium in choline and magnesium salicylates or magnesium salicylate, interfere with absorption of these medications; if used concurrently, the interacting salicylate should be taken at least 6 hours before or 2 hours after ciprofloxacin or lomefloxacin, 8 hours before or 2 hours after enoxacin, 2 hours after itraconazole, 3 hours before or after ketoconazole, 2 hours before or after norfloxacin or ofloxacin, and 3 to 4 hours before or after a tetracycline)

*For enteric-coated formulations (in addition to those interactions listed above as applying to all salicylates)*
Antacids or
Histamine $H_2$-receptor antagonists
(concurrent administration of these medications, which increase intragastric pH, with an enteric-coated medication may cause premature dissolution, and loss of the protective effect, of the enteric coating)

*For formulations containing caffeine (in addition to those interactions listed above as applying to all salicylates)*
CNS stimulation–producing medications, other (See *Appendix II*)
(concurrent use with caffeine may result in excessive CNS stimulation, which may cause unwanted effects such as nervousness, irritability, insomnia, or possibly convulsions or cardiac arrhythmias; close observation is recommended)

Lithium
(caffeine increases urinary excretion of lithium, thereby possibly reducing its therapeutic effect)

Monoamine oxidase (MAO) inhibitors, including furazolidone, pargyline, and procarbazine
  (concurrent use of large amounts of caffeine with MAO inhibitors may produce dangerous cardiac arrhythmias or severe hypertension because of the sympathomimetic side effects of caffeine)

**Laboratory value alterations**
The following have been selected on the basis of their potential clinical significance (possible effect in parentheses where appropriate)—not necessarily inclusive (» = major clinical significance):

With diagnostic test results
*For all salicylates*
  Copper sulfate urine sugar tests
    (false-positive test results may occur with chronic use of salicylates in doses equivalent in salicylate content to 2.4 grams or more of aspirin a day, i.e., 3.2 grams of choline salicylate, 2.4 grams of choline and magnesium salicylates, 2 grams of magnesium salicylate, 1.8 grams of salsalate, or 2.4 grams of sodium salicylate a day)
  Gerhardt test for urine aceto-acetic acid
    (interference may occur because reaction with ferric chloride produces a reddish color that persists after boiling)
  Glucose enzymatic urine sugar tests
    (false-negative test results may occur with chronic use of salicylates in doses equivalent in salicylate content to 2.4 grams or more of aspirin a day, i.e., 3.2 grams of choline salicylate, 2.4 grams of choline and magnesium salicylates, 2 grams of magnesium salicylate, 1.8 grams of salsalate, or 2.4 grams of sodium salicylate a day)
  Renal function test using phenolsulfonphthalein (PSP)
    (salicylate may competitively inhibit renal tubular secretion of PSP, thereby decreasing urinary PSP concentration and invalidating test results)
  Serum uric acid determinations
    (falsely increased values may occur with colorimetric assay methods when plasma salicylate concentrations exceed 13 mg per 100 mL; the uricase assay method is not affected)
  Thyroid imaging, radionuclide
    (chronic salicylate administration may depress thyroid function; salicylate therapy should be discontinued at least 1 week prior to administration of the radiopharmaceutical; however, a rebound effect may occur following discontinuation of salicylate therapy, resulting in a period of 3 to 10 days of increased thyroidal uptake)
  Urine vanillylmandelic acid (VMA) determinations
    (values may be falsely increased or decreased, depending on method used)

*For aspirin only (in addition to those interferences listed above for all salicylates)*
  Protirelin-induced thyroid-stimulating hormone (TSH) release determinations
    (TSH response to protirelin may be decreased by 2 to 3.6 grams of aspirin daily; peak TSH concentrations occur at the same time after administration, but are reduced)
  Urine 5-hydroxyindoleacetic acid (5-HIAA) determinations
    (aspirin may alter results when fluorescent method is used)

*For caffeine-containing formulations (in addition to the diagnostic interferences listed above)*
  Myocardial perfusion imaging, radionuclide, when adenosine or dipyridamole is used as an adjunct to the radiopharmaceutical
    (caffeine may reverse the effects of adenosine or dipyridamole on myocardial blood flow, thereby interfering with test results; patients should be advised to avoid caffeine for at least 8 to 12 hours prior to the test)

With physiology/laboratory test values
*For all salicylates*
  Liver function tests, including:
    Serum alanine aminotransferase (ALT [SGPT]) and
    Serum alkaline phosphatase and
    Serum aspartate aminotransferase (AST [SGOT])
    (abnormalities may occur, especially in patients with juvenile rheumatoid arthritis, systemic lupus erythematosus, or pre-existing history of liver disease, or when plasma salicylate concentrations exceed 25 mg per 100 mL; liver function test values may return to normal despite continued use or when dosage is decreased; however, if severe abnormalities occur, or if there is evidence of active liver disease, the medication should be discontinued and used with caution in the future)
  Prothrombin time
    (may be prolonged with large doses of salicylates, especially if plasma concentrations exceed 30 mg per 100 mL)
  Serum cholesterol concentrations
    (may be decreased by chronic use of salicylates in doses equivalent in salicylate content to 5 grams or more of aspirin per day, i.e., 6.7 grams of choline salicylate, 5 grams of choline and magnesium salicylates, 4.1 grams of magnesium salicylate, 3.8 grams of salsalate, or 5 grams of sodium salicylate a day)
  Serum potassium concentrations
    (may be decreased because of increased potassium excretion caused by direct effect on renal tubules)
  Serum thyroxine ($T_4$) concentrations and
  Serum triiodothyronine ($T_3$) concentrations
    (may be decreased when determined by radioimmunoassay—with large doses of salicylates)
  Serum uric acid concentrations
    (may be increased or decreased, depending on salicylate dosage; plasma salicylate concentrations below 10 to 15 mg per 100 mL increase serum uric acid concentrations and higher plasma salicylate concentrations decrease uric acid concentrations)
  $T_3$ resin uptake
    (may be increased with large doses of salicylates)

*For aspirin only (in addition to the interferences listed above)*
  Bleeding time
    (may be prolonged by aspirin for 4 to 7 days because of suppressed platelet aggregation; as little as 40 mg of aspirin affects platelet function for at least 96 hours following administration; however, clinical bleeding problems have not been reported with small doses [150 mg or less])

**Medical considerations/Contraindications**
The medical considerations/contraindications included have been selected on the basis of their potential clinical significance (reasons given in parentheses where appropriate)—not necessarily inclusive (» = major clinical significance).

*Except under special circumstances, this medication should not be used when the following medical problems exist:*
*For all salicylates*
» Bleeding ulcers or
» Hemorrhagic states, other active
    (may be exacerbated, especially by aspirin)
» Hemophilia or other bleeding problems, including coagulation or platelet function disorders
    (increased risk of hemorrhage, especially with aspirin)

*For aspirin only (in addition to the contraindications listed above for all salicylates)*
» Angioedema, anaphylaxis, or other severe sensitivity reaction induced by aspirin or other NSAIDs, history of or
» Nasal polyps associated with asthma, induced or exacerbated by aspirin
    (high risk of severe sensitivity reaction to aspirin)
» Thrombocytopenia
    (increased risk of bleeding because aspirin inhibits platelet aggregation)

*For choline and magnesium salicylates and for magnesium salicylate only (in addition to the contraindications listed above for all salicylates)*
» Renal insufficiency, chronic advanced
    (risk of hypermagnesemic toxicity)

*Risk-benefit should be considered when the following medical problems exist:*
*For all salicylates*
  Anemia
    (may be exacerbated by gastrointestinal blood loss during salicylate, especially aspirin, therapy; also, salicylate-induced peripheral vasodilation may lead to pseudoanemia)
  Conditions predisposing to fluid retention, such as:
    Compromised cardiac function or
    Hypertension
    (in patients with carditis, high doses of salicylates may precipitate congestive heart failure or pulmonary edema)
    (patients with congestive heart disease may be more susceptible to adverse renal effects)
    (sodium content of sodium salicylate may be detrimental to these patients when large doses are administered chronically)
» Gastritis, erosive or
» Peptic ulcer
    (may be exacerbated because of ulcerogenic effects, especially with aspirin; risk of gastrointestinal bleeding is increased)

Gout
(salicylates may increase serum uric acid concentrations and may interfere with efficacy of uricosuric agents)

Hepatic function impairment
(salicylates metabolized hepatically; also, patients with decompensated hepatic cirrhosis may be more susceptible to adverse renal effects)
(in severe hepatic impairment, inhibition of platelet function by aspirin may increase the risk of hemorrhage)

Hypoprothrombinemia or
Vitamin K deficiency
(increased risk of bleeding because of antiplatelet action of aspirin and the hypoprothrombinemic effect of high doses of salicylates)

Renal function impairment
(salicylate elimination may be reduced; also, the risk of renal adverse effects may be increased)
(choline and magnesium salicylates or magnesium salicylate should be used with caution in patients with mild or moderate renal impairment because of the risk of hypermagnesemic toxicity; however, as stated above, these medications should *not* be used if chronic advanced renal insufficiency is present)

Sensitivity reaction, mild, to aspirin or other NSAIDs, history of
(risk of sensitivity reaction, especially with aspirin)

Symptoms of nasal polyps associated with bronchospasm, or angioedema, anaphylaxis, or other severe allergic reactions induced by aspirin or other NSAIDs
(although cross-sensitivity leading to severe reactions occurs very rarely with the nonacetylated salicylates, caution is recommended; however, as indicated above, aspirin should *not* be used)

Thyrotoxicosis
(may be exacerbated by large doses)

*For aspirin only (in addition to those listed above for all salicylates)*
» Asthma
(increased risk of bronchospastic sensitivity reaction)

Glucose-6-phosphate dehydrogenase (G6PD) deficiency
(rarely, aspirin has caused hemolytic anemia in these patients)

*For formulations containing caffeine*
Cardiac disease, severe
(high doses of caffeine may increase risk of tachycardia or extrasystoles, which may lead to heart failure)

Sensitivity to caffeine, history of
(risk of allergic reaction)

## Patient monitoring
The following may be especially important in patient monitoring (other tests may be warranted in some patients, depending on condition; » = major clinical significance):

*For all salicylates*
Hematocrit determinations
(may be required at periodic intervals during prolonged high-dose therapy because of the possibility of gastrointestinal blood loss, especially with aspirin)

Hepatic function determinations
(may be required prior to initiation of antirheumatic therapy and if symptoms of hepatotoxicity occur during therapy; salicylate-induced hepatotoxicity may be especially likely to occur in patients, especially children, with rheumatic fever, systemic lupus erythematosus, juvenile arthritis, or pre-existing hepatic disease)

Serum salicylate concentrations
(monitoring required at periodic intervals during prolonged high-dose therapy as a guide to dosage, safety, and efficacy, especially in children; because aspirin absorption in children with Kawasaki disease is erratic and varies at different stages of the disease, monitoring of plasma salicylate concentration in these patients is critical)

*For choline and magnesium salicylates and magnesium salicylate only (in addition to those listed above for all salicylates)*
Serum magnesium concentration
(monitoring recommended during therapy with large doses in patients with renal insufficiency because of the possibility of hypermagnesemic toxicity)

## Side/Adverse Effects
Note: Salicylates may decrease renal function, especially when serum salicylate concentrations reach 250 mcg per mL (25 mg per 100 mL). However, the risk of complications due to this action appears minimal in patients with normal renal function.

Aspirin-induced bronchospasm is most likely to occur in patients with the triad of asthma, allergies, and nasal polyps induced by aspirin. Nonacetylated salicylates may rarely cause bronchospastic reactions in susceptible people when very large doses are given.

Angioedema or urticaria may be more likely to occur in patients with a history of recurrent idiopathic angioedema or urticaria.

Gastrointestinal side effects are more likely to occur with aspirin than with other salicylates; also, they may be more likely to occur with chronic, high-dose administration than with occasional use. Use of enteric-coated formulations may reduce the potential for gastrointestinal side effects.

Adverse effects are more likely to occur at serum salicylate concentrations of 300 mcg per mL (30 mg per 100 mL) or above; however, they may also occur at lower serum concentrations, especially in patients 60 years of age or older. Serum concentrations at which adverse or toxic effects have been reported during chronic therapy include:

| Salicylate Concentration (mcg per mL/ mg per 100 mL) | Effect |
|---|---|
| 195–210/ 19.5–21 | Mild toxicity (tinnitus, decreased hearing) |
| 250/25 | Hepatotoxicity (abnormal liver function tests) |
| 250/25 | Decreased renal function |
| 300/30 | Decreased prothrombin time |
| 310/31 | Deafness |
| 350/35 | Hyperventilation |
| > 400/40 | Metabolic acidosis, other signs of severe toxicity |

The following side/adverse effects have been selected on the basis of their potential clinical significance (possible signs and symptoms in parentheses where appropriate)—not necessarily inclusive:

**Those indicating need for medical attention**
Incidence less frequent or rare
*Anaphylactoid reaction* (bluish discoloration or flushing or redness of skin; coughing; difficulty in swallowing; dizziness or feeling faint, severe; skin rash, hives [may include giant urticaria], and/or itching; stuffy nose; swelling of eyelids, face, or lips; tightness in chest, troubled breathing, and/or wheezing, especially in asthmatic patients); *anemia* (unusual tiredness or weakness)—for aspirin or buffered aspirin only; may occur secondary to gastrointestinal microbleeding; *anemia, hemolytic* (troubled breathing, exertional; unusual tiredness or weakness)—reported with aspirin only, almost always in patients with glucose-6-phosphate (G6PD) deficiency; *bronchospastic allergic reaction* (shortness of breath, troubled breathing, tightness in chest, and/or wheezing); *dermatitis, allergic* (skin rash, hives, or itching); *gastrointestinal ulceration, possibly with bleeding* (bloody or black, tarry stools; stomach pain, severe; vomiting of blood or material that looks like coffee grounds)

Incidence unknown
*Rectal irritation*—for aspirin suppository dosage form

**Those indicating need for medical attention only if they continue or are bothersome**
Incidence more frequent with aspirin; less frequent with enteric-coated or buffered formulations and with other salicylates
*Gastrointestinal irritation* (mild stomach pain; heartburn or indigestion; nausea with or without vomiting)

Incidence less frequent
*For caffeine-containing formulations*
*CNS stimulation* (trouble in sleeping, nervousness, or jitters)

## Overdose
For specific information on the agents used in the management of salicylate overdose, see:
- Vitamin K$_1$—Phytonadione in *Vitamin K (Systemic)* monograph.

For more information on the management of overdose or unintentional ingestion, **contact a Poison Control Center** (see *Poison Control Center Listing*).

**Clinical effects of overdose**
The following effects have been selected on the basis of their potential clinical significance (possible signs and symptoms in parentheses where appropriate)—not necessarily inclusive:

Acute and chronic
*Mild overdose*
**Salicylism** (Continuing ringing or buzzing in ears or hearing loss; confusion; severe or continuing diarrhea, stomach pain, and or headache; dizziness or lightheadedness; severe drowsiness; fast or deep breathing; continuing nausea and/or vomiting; uncontrollable flapping movements of the hands, especially in elderly patients; increased thirst; vision problems)—tinnitus and/or headache may be the earliest symptoms of salicylism

*Severe overdose*
***Bloody urine; convulsions; hallucinations; severe nervousness, excitement, or confusion; shortness of breath or troubled breathing; unexplained fever***
> Note: In young children, the only signs of an overdose may be changes in behavior, severe drowsiness or tiredness, and/or fast or deep breathing.
>
> Laboratory findings in overdose may indicate encephalographic abnormalities, alterations in acid-base balance (especially respiratory alkalosis and metabolic acidosis), hyperglycemia or hypoglycemia (especially in children), ketonuria, hyponatremia, hypokalemia, and proteinuria.

**Treatment of overdose**
To decrease absorption—Emptying the stomach via induction of emesis (taking care to guard against aspiration) or gastric lavage.

Administering activated charcoal.

To enhance elimination—Inducing forced alkaline diuresis to increase salicylate excretion. However, bicarbonate should not be administered orally for this purpose because salicylate absorption may be increased. Also, if acetazolamide is used, the increased risk of severe metabolic acidosis and salicylate toxicity (caused by increased penetration of salicylate into the brain because of metabolic acidosis) must be considered. Some emergency care practitioners recommend that acetazolamide not be used at all in the treatment of salicylate overdose. Others state that acetazolamide may be used, provided that precautions are taken to prevent systemic metabolic acidosis, such as concurrent administration of an alkaline intravenous solution, e.g., one that contains sodium bicarbonate or sodium lactate.

Institution of exchange transfusion, hemodialysis, peritoneal dialysis, or hemoperfusion as needed in severe overdose.

Specific treatment—Administering blood or vitamin $K_1$ if necessary to treat hemorrhaging.

Monitoring—Monitoring for pulmonary edema and convulsions and instituting appropriate therapy if required.

Monitoring serum salicylate concentration until it is apparent that the concentration is decreasing to the nontoxic range. When a large single dose of an immediate-release formulation has been ingested, salicylate concentrations of 500 mcg per mL (50 mg per 100 mL; 3.62 mmol/L) 2 hours after ingestion indicate serious toxicity; salicylate concentrations above 800 mcg per mL (80 mg per 100 mL; 5.79 mmol/L) 2 hours after ingestion indicate possible fatality. In addition, prolonged monitoring may be necessary in massive overdosage because absorption may be delayed; if a determination performed prior to 6 hours after ingestion fails to show a toxic salicylate concentration, the determination should be repeated. Although the following values are not reliable for predicting the severity of toxicity after chronic or repeated ingestions, or after ingestion of a large single dose of a delayed-release (enteric-coated) or extended-release formulation, salicylate concentrations considered indicative of varying degrees of toxicity are as follows:

| Time After Ingestion | Salicylate Concentration | | |
|---|---|---|---|
| | mcg/mL | mg/100 mL | mmol/L |
| Mild toxicity | | | |
| 6 hr | 450–650 | 45–65 | 3.26–4.71 |
| 12 hr | 350–550 | 35–55 | 2.53–3.98 |
| Moderate toxicity | | | |
| 6 hr | 650–900 | 65–90 | 4.71–6.52 |
| 12 hr | 550–750 | 55–75 | 3.98–5.43 |
| Severe toxicity | | | |
| 6 hr | > 900 | > 90 | > 6.52 |
| 12 hr | > 750 | > 75 | > 5.43 |

Supportive care—Monitoring and supporting vital functions. Correcting hyperthermia; fluid, electrolyte, and acid-base imbalances; ketosis; and plasma glucose concentration as needed. Patients in whom intentional overdose is known or suspected should be referrred for psychiatric consultation.

## Patient Consultation
As an aid to patient consultation, refer to *Advice for the Patient, Salicylates (Systemic).*

In providing consultation, consider emphasizing the following selected information (» = major clinical significance):

### Before using this medication
» Conditions affecting use, especially:
>  Sensitivity to any of the salicylates, including methyl salicylate, or nonsteroidal anti-inflammatory drugs (NSAIDs), history of
>
>  Pregnancy—Salicylates and caffeine (present in some formulations) cross the placenta; high-dose chronic use or abuse of aspirin in the third trimester may be hazardous to the mother as well as the fetus and/or neonate, causing heart problems in fetus or neonate and/or bleeding in mother, fetus, or neonate; high-dose chronic use or abuse of any salicylate late in pregnancy may also prolong and complicate labor and delivery; not taking aspirin during the third trimester unless prescribed by physician
>
>  Breast-feeding—Salicylates and caffeine (present in some formulations) are excreted in breast milk
>
>  Use in children and teenagers—Checking with physician before giving to children or teenagers with symptoms of acute febrile illness, especially influenza or varicella, because of the risk of Reye's syndrome; determining ahead of time what physician wants done if a child receiving chronic therapy develops fever or other symptoms of acute illness that may predispose to Reye's syndrome; also, increased susceptibility to salicylate toxicity in children, especially with fever and dehydration
>
>  Use in the elderly—Increased susceptibility to salicylate toxicity
>
>  Other medications, especially anticoagulants, antidiabetic agents (oral), those cephalosporins that may cause hypoprothrombinemia, plicamycin, valproic acid, methotrexate, NSAIDs, platelet aggregation inhibitors, probenecid, sulfinpyrazone, urinary alkalizers, and vancomycin; also, for buffered aspirin, choline and magnesium salicylates, and magnesium salicylate: fluoroquinolone antibiotics, itraconazole, ketoconazole, and oral tetracyclines
>
>  Other medical problems, especially coagulation or platelet function disorders, gastrointestinal problems such as ulceration or erosive gastritis (especially a bleeding ulcer), thyrotoxicosis, and (for choline and magnesium salicylates and for magnesium salicylate) chronic advanced renal insufficiency
>
>  Diet—Sodium content of sodium salicylate must be considered for patients on a sodium-restricted diet, especially with chronic use of antirheumatic doses

### Proper use of this medication
» Taking nonenteric-coated oral dosage forms after meals or with food to minimize stomach irritation

» Taking all tablet or capsule dosage forms with a full glass of water and not lying down for 15 to 30 minutes after taking

» Not taking aspirin or buffered aspirin if it has a strong vinegar-like odor

Not chewing aspirin or buffered aspirin dosage forms within 7 days after tonsillectomy, tooth extraction, or other oral surgery

Not placing aspirin or buffered aspirin tablet directly on tooth or gum surface, to prevent tissue damage

*Proper administration of*
  *Aspirin*
>  Chewable tablets—May be chewed, dissolved in liquid, crushed, or swallowed whole
>
>  Delayed-release tablets—Must be swallowed whole
>
>  Extended-release tablets—May be broken or crumbled (but not ground up) if necessary, unless specified by manufacturer to be swallowed whole; see manufacturer's prescribing information
>
>  Suppository—Proper administration technique

  *Choline and magnesium salicylates oral solution*
>  Liquid may be mixed with fruit juice just prior to taking, if desired

  *Sodium salicylate delayed-release tablets*
>  Tablets must be swallowed whole

Importance of not taking more medication than prescribed by physician or dentist or recommended on package label

Unless otherwise directed by physician, children not taking more often than 5 times daily

Compliance with therapy (for arthritis); may take 2 to 3 weeks or longer for maximum effectiveness

» Proper dosing
Missed dose: If on scheduled dosing regimen—taking as soon as possible; not taking if almost time for next dose; not doubling doses

» Proper storage

**Precautions while using this medication**
» Possibility of overdose if other medications containing aspirin or other salicylates (possibly including topical products) are used
» Regular visits to physician to check progress if long-term or high-dose therapy is prescribed

*Checking with physician if*
  Taking for pain or fever, and pain persists for longer than 10 days for adults or 5 days for children, fever persists for longer than 3 days, condition becomes worse, new symptoms occur, or redness or swelling is present
  Taking for sore throat, and sore throat is severe, persists for longer than 2 days, or occurs together with or is followed by fever, headache, rash, nausea, or vomiting
  Symptoms of ringing or buzzing in ears or headache occur during long-term therapy

*Patients taking aspirin as a platelet aggregation inhibitor*
» Taking only the amount of aspirin prescribed; checking with prescribing physician about proper medication to use for relief of pain, fever, or arthritis
» Not discontinuing treatment for any reason without first consulting prescribing physician
» Not taking acetaminophen, ibuprofen, or other NSAIDs concurrently with salicylates for longer than a few days, unless specifically prescribed by physician or dentist, especially if using salicylates on a long-term and/or high-dose basis

*Diabetics: Possibility of false urine sugar test results with prolonged use (per day) of—*
  8 or more 325-mg (5-grain), 4 or more 500-mg or 650-mg (10-grain), 3 or more 800-mg or 975-mg (15-grain) doses of aspirin
  8 or more 325-mg (5-grain) or 4 or more 500-mg or 650-mg (10-grain) doses of buffered aspirin or sodium salicylate
  4 or more 870-mg doses of choline salicylate
  5 or more 500-mg, 4 or more 750-mg, or 2 or more 1000-mg, doses of choline and magnesium salicylates
  7 or more regular strength, or 4 or more extra-strength, tablets of magnesium salicylate
  4 or more 500-mg, or 3 or more 750-mg, doses of salsalate
  Checking with physician, nurse, or pharmacist if unsure of daily dose being taken, if changes in urine sugar test results occur, or if any other questions, especially if diabetes not well-controlled
  Caution if any kind of surgery is required; not taking aspirin for 5 days prior to surgery unless otherwise directed by physician or dentist because of risk of bleeding
  Checking with health care professional before using buffered aspirin, choline and magnesium salicylates, or magnesium salicylate concurrently with a fluoroquinolone antibiotic, itraconazole, ketoconazole, or an oral tetracycline; these salicylate formulations may interfere with absorption of the anti-infective agent
  Not taking a cellulose-containing laxative within 2 hours of a salicylate
  Alcohol consumption may increase probability of stomach problems (for oral dosage forms only)
  Checking with physician if rectal irritation occurs with aspirin suppositories
  Caution if any laboratory tests required; possible interference with some test results by salicylates; possible interference with dipyridamole-assisted myocardial imaging by formulations containing caffeine
» Suspected overdose: Getting emergency help immediately

**Side/adverse effects**
  Signs of potential side effects, especially allergic reactions, anemia, and gastrointestinal toxicity and, with aspirin suppositories, rectal irritation

## General Dosing Information

A reduction in initial dosage is recommended for geriatric patients, especially those receiving long-acting salicylates (e.g., choline and magnesium salicylates, salsalate) or prolonged therapy. These patients may be more susceptible to salicylate toxicity, especially if accumulation occurs because of impaired renal function. If the reduced dosage is not effective, dosage may gradually be increased as tolerated.

For treatment of arthritis, dosage is usually increased gradually until symptoms are relieved, therapeutic plasma concentrations are achieved, or signs of toxicity, such as tinnitus or headache, occur. If these signs should appear, dosage should be reduced. However, tinnitus is not a reliable index of maximum salicylate tolerance, especially in very young or geriatric patients or those with impaired hearing.

For treatment of arthritis, dosage adjustments should not be made more frequently than once weekly, unless a reduction in dosage is required because of side effects, because up to 7 days may be required to achieve steady-state plasma concentrations.

The risk of Reye's syndrome must be considered when salicylates are administered to children and teenagers. It is recommended that salicylates be withheld from pediatric and adolescent patients with a fever or other symptoms of an illness that may predispose to Reye's syndrome until it has been determined that such an illness is not present or has run its course.

Dosage should be reduced if fever or illness causes fluid depletion, especially in children.

In general, it is recommended that aspirin therapy be discontinued 5 days before surgery to prevent possible occurrence of bleeding problems.

Patients who experience bronchospastic or cutaneous allergic reactions to aspirin may be desensitized to these effects by administration of initially small and gradually increasing doses of aspirin. *Desensitization must be carried out only by clinicians who are familiar with the technique, and only in a facility having trained personnel, medications, and equipment immediately available for treating any adverse reaction to the medication (especially anaphylaxis or severe bronchospasm).* This procedure also desensitizes the patient to other nonsteroidal anti-inflammatory drugs (NSAIDs). However, unless aspirin or another NSAID is then administered on a daily basis, sensitivity to these medications re-develops within a few days.

**For oral dosage forms only**
These medications (except enteric-coated formulations) should be administered after meals or with food to lessen gastric irritation.

It is recommended that tablet and capsule dosage forms of these medications always be administered with a full glass (240 mL) of water and that the patient remain in an upright position for 15 to 30 minutes after administration. These measures may reduce the risk of the medication becoming lodged in the esophagus, which has been reported to cause prolonged esophageal irritation and difficulty in swallowing in some patients receiving NSAIDs.

It is recommended that aspirin or buffered aspirin products not be chewed before swallowing for at least 7 days following tonsillectomy or oral surgery because of possible injury to oral tissues from prolonged contact with aspirin.

Aspirin or buffered aspirin tablets should not be placed directly on a tooth or gum surface because of possible injury to tissues.

Concurrent use of an antacid and/or a histamine ($H_2$)-receptor antagonist (cimetidine, famotidine, or ranitidine) may protect against salicylate-induced gastric irritation or ulceration. However, the fact that chronic, high-dose antacid use may alkalinize the urine and increase salicylate excretion must be considered. Also, because these medications may cause premature dissolution, and loss of the protective effect, of enteric coatings, they will not provide additive protection against gastric irritation when administered concurrently with enteric-coated dosage forms.

---

## ASPIRIN

## Summary of Differences

Category/indications:
  Aspirin (tablets, chewable tablets, and delayed-release tablets) also indicated as a platelet aggregation inhibitor.
Pharmacology/pharmacokinetics:
  Aspirin irreversibly inhibits platelet aggregation.
Precautions:
  Cross-sensitivity and/or related problems—
    Risk of cross-sensitivity with other nonsteroidal anti-inflammatory drugs (NSAIDs) significantly greater than with other salicylates.
  Drug interactions and/or related problems—
    May increase ascorbic acid requirement (prolonged high-dose use).
    Theoretically, may decrease zidovudine clearance.
    Higher risk of bleeding (compared with other salicylates) when used concurrently with other medications that may inhibit blood clotting or cause gastrointestinal ulceration or bleeding.
  Laboratory value alterations—
    Interferes with urine 5-hydroxyindoleacetic acid determinations.
    Interferes with protirelin-induced thyroid-stimulating hormone release determinations.
    Prolongs bleeding time.
  Medical considerations/contraindications—
    Should not be used in patients with a history of severe sensitivity reactions to aspirin, other NSAIDs, nasal polyps and asthma, or thrombocytopenia
    Should be used with caution in patients with asthma or glucose-6-phosphate dehydrogenase (G6PD) deficiency.

Side/adverse effects:
- More ulcerogenic than other salicylates.
- Rarely, causes hemolytic anemia (in patients with G6PD deficiency).
- Suppository dosage form may cause rectal bleeding.

## Additional Dosing Information

See also *General Dosing Information*.

Salicylate toxicity requiring treatment generally occurs with doses of 200 mg per kg of body weight (mg/kg), especially in children.

The general doses for aspirin products other than aspirin chewing gum tablets are based on the FDA's dosing recommendations for aspirin. The dosage unit of 80 mg (1.23 grains) is used for pediatric doses; the dosage unit of 325 mg (5 grains) is used for adult doses. The conversion factor of 1 grain equal to 65 mg is used. Strengths of specific products may vary, depending on the manufacturer.

The extended-release tablet, the suppository, and the chewing gum tablet dosage forms may give incomplete or unreliable absorption.

Chewable aspirin tablets may be chewed, dissolved in liquid, or swallowed whole.

The delayed-release tablets must be swallowed whole.

Some extended-release tablets may be broken or crumbled but must not be ground up before swallowing. Others must be swallowed whole. Consult manufacturers' prescribing information for individual products.

## Oral Dosage Forms

Note: Bracketed uses in the *Dosage Forms* section refer to categories of use and/or indications that are not included in U.S. product labeling.

### ASPIRIN TABLETS USP

**Usual adult and adolescent dose**

Analgesic/antipyretic—
  Oral, 325 to 500 mg every three hours, 325 to 650 mg every four hours, or 650 mg to 1000 mg every six hours as needed, while symptoms persist.
  Note: For patient self-medication, it is recommended that the total daily dose not exceed 4 grams, and that a physician be consulted if pain is not relieved within ten days, fever within three days, or sore throat within two days.

Antirheumatic (nonsteroidal anti-inflammatory)—
  Oral, 3.6 to 5.4 grams a day in divided doses.
  Note: In acute rheumatic fever, up to 7.8 grams a day in divided doses may be given.

Platelet aggregation inhibitor—
  Oral, 80 to 325 mg a day, with the following exceptions
  Ischemic attacks, transient, in males or
  [Thromboembolism, cerebral, recurrence][1]—
    Oral, 1 gram a day. Dosage may be reduced to 325 mg a day if the patient is unable to tolerate the higher dose.
  [Ischemic attacks, transient, occurring in association with mitral valve prolapse][1]—
    Oral, 325 mg to 1 gram a day.
  [Prevention of thrombosis or occlusion of coronary bypass graft]—
    Oral, 325 mg seven hours postoperatively (via a nasogastric tube), then 325 mg three times daily, concurrently with 75 mg of dipyridamole. Dipyridamole may be discontinued one week postoperatively, but aspirin should be continued indefinitely.
    Platelet aggregation inhibitor therapy is most effective when it is initiated two days prior to scheduled surgery. However, preoperative administration of aspirin has been shown to increase perisurgical bleeding and is not recommended. Therapy is therefore initiated with dipyridamole (recommended dosage 100 mg four times a day for two days prior to surgery and 100 mg one hour postoperatively [via a nasogastric tube]). Dipyridamole therapy is continued postoperatively (recommended dosage 75 mg seven hours postoperatively, via a nasogastric tube, then 75 mg three times a day, concurrently with aspirin) for at least one week.

Note: Although the doses recommended above for use of aspirin as a platelet aggregation inhibitor have been found effective in clinical studies, optimum dosage has not been established. For indications other than prevention of transient ischemic attacks or recurrence of cerebral thromboembolism, lower doses are often used. A few studies have shown that 160 mg of aspirin every twenty-four hours, or 325 mg every forty-eight hours, may effectively inhibit platelet aggregation while minimizing the risk of aspirin-induced side effects. Other studies have shown that single doses of 40 to 80 mg also inhibit platelet aggregation.

**Usual pediatric dose**

Analgesic/antipyretic—
  Oral, 1.5 grams per square meter of body surface a day in four to six divided doses; or for
  Children up to 2 years of age: Dosage must be individualized by physician.
  Children 2 to 4 years of age: Oral, 160 mg every four hours as needed, while symptoms persist.
  Children 4 to 6 years of age: Oral, 240 mg every four hours as needed, while symptoms persist.
  Children 6 to 9 years of age: Oral, 320 to 325 mg every four hours as needed, while symptoms persist.
  Children 9 to 11 years of age: Oral, 320 to 400 mg every four hours as needed, while symptoms persist.
  Children 11 to 12 years of age: Oral, 320 to 480 mg every four hours as needed, while symptoms persist.
  Note: It is recommended that children up to 12 years of age receive no more than five doses in each twenty-four-hour period, unless otherwise directed by a physician, and that a physician be consulted if pain is not relieved within five days, fever within three days, or sore throat within two days.

Antirheumatic (nonsteroidal anti-inflammatory)—
  Oral, 80 to 100 mg per kg of body weight a day in divided doses.
  Note: If an adequate response is not achieved within one or two weeks, dosage adjustment should be based on measurement of plasma salicylate concentration. Up to 130 mg per kg of body weight per day may be required in some patients.

[Kawasaki disease][1]—
  During the early febrile stage: Oral, 80 to 120 mg (average 100 mg) per kg of body weight a day in four divided doses for fourteen days or until inflammation has subsided. However, absorption may be impaired or erratic during this stage of the illness, and considerably higher doses may be required. It is recommended that dosage be adjusted to achieve and maintain a plasma salicylate concentration of 20 to 30 mg per 100 mL.
  During the convalescent stage: Oral, 3 to 5 mg per kg of body weight a day as a single dose. If no coronary artery abnormalities occur, treatment is usually continued for a minimum of eight weeks. If coronary artery abnormalities occur, it is recommended that treatment be continued for at least one year, even if the abnormalities regress, and longer if abnormalities persist.

**Strength(s) usually available**

U.S.—
  81 mg (OTC) [*Aspir-Low; Healthprin Adult Low Strength* (scored); GENERIC].
  162.5 mg (OTC) [*Healthprin Half-Dose* (scored)].
  325 mg (OTC) [*Aspirtab; Empirin; Genuine Bayer Aspirin Caplets; Genuine Bayer Aspirin Tablets; Healthprin Full Strength* (scored); *Norwich Aspirin;* GENERIC].
  500 mg (OTC) [*Aspirtab-Max; Extra Strength Bayer Aspirin Caplets; Extra Strength Bayer Aspirin Tablets; Norwich Aspirin;* GENERIC].
  650 mg (OTC) [GENERIC].
Canada—
  300 mg of ASA (OTC) [*Headache Tablet*].
  325 mg of ASA (OTC) [*Apo-ASA; Aspirin Caplets; Aspirin Tablets; PMS-ASA;* GENERIC].
  500 mg of ASA (OTC) [*Aspirin Caplets; Aspirin Tablets*].
Note: Strengths of specific products labeled in grains may vary, depending on the manufacturer.

**Packaging and storage**
Store below 40 °C (104 °F), preferably between 15 and 30 °C (59 and 86 °F), unless otherwise specified by manufacturer. Store in a tight container.

**Auxiliary labeling**
• Take with food and a full glass of water.

### ASPIRIN TABLETS (CHEWABLE) USP

**Usual adult and adolescent dose**
See *Aspirin Tablets USP*.

**Usual pediatric dose**
See *Aspirin Tablets USP*.

**Strength(s) usually available**
U.S.—
  81 mg (OTC) [*Bayer Children's Aspirin; St. Joseph Adult Chewable Aspirin;* GENERIC].
Canada—
  80 mg of ASA (OTC) [*Aspirin Children's Tablets*].

**Packaging and storage**
Store below 40 °C (104 °F), preferably between 15 and 30 °C (59 and 86 °F), unless otherwise specified by manufacturer. Store in a tight container.

**Auxiliary labeling**
- May be chewed.
- Take with food and a full glass of water.

### ASPIRIN CHEWING GUM TABLETS

**Usual adult and adolescent dose**
Analgesic—
   Oral, 454 to 650 mg. May be repeated every four hours as needed.
Note: For patient self-medication, it is recommended that a physician be consulted if pain is not relieved within ten days or sore throat within two days.

**Usual pediatric dose**
Analgesic—
   Children up to 3 years of age: Dosage must be individualized by physician.
   Children 3 to 6 years of age: Oral, 227 mg. May be repeated up to three times a day.
   Children 6 to 12 years of age: Oral, 227 to 454 mg. May be repeated up to four times a day.
Note: It is recommended that children up to 12 years of age receive no more than five doses in each twenty-four-hour period, unless otherwise directed by a physician, and that a physician be consulted if pain is not relieved within five days or sore throat within two days.

**Strength(s) usually available**
U.S.—
   227 mg (OTC) [*Aspergum*].
Canada—
   325 mg of ASA (OTC) [*Aspergum*].

**Packaging and storage**
Store below 40 °C (104 °F), preferably between 15 and 30 °C (59 and 86 °F), unless otherwise specified by manufacturer.

**Auxiliary labeling**
- To be chewed.
- Take with food.
- Drink a full glass of water after chewing.

### ASPIRIN DELAYED-RELEASE TABLETS USP

**Usual adult and adolescent dose**
See *Aspirin Tablets USP*.

**Usual pediatric dose**
See *Aspirin Tablets USP*.

**Strength(s) usually available**
U.S.—
   81 mg (OTC) [*Acuprin 81; Aspirin Regimen Bayer Adult Low Dose; Ecotrin Caplets; Ecotrin Tablets; Halfprin;* GENERIC].
   162 mg (OTC) [*Halfprin*].
   325 mg (OTC) [*Aspirin Regimen Bayer Regular Strength Caplets; Ecotrin Caplets; Ecotrin Tablets; Norwich Aspirin;* GENERIC].
   500 mg (OTC) [*Ecotrin Caplets; Ecotrin Tablets; Extra Strength Bayer Arthritis Pain Formula Caplets; Maximum Strength Arthritis Foundation Safety Coated Aspirin; Norwich Aspirin;* GENERIC].
   650 mg (OTC) [GENERIC].
   975 mg (Rx) [*Easprin;* GENERIC].
Canada—
   325 mg of ASA (OTC) [*Apo-ASEN; Aspirin, Coated; Astrin; Coryphen; Entrophen Caplets; Entrophen Tablets; Novasen; Novasen Sp.C;* GENERIC].
   500 mg of ASA (OTC) [*Aspirin, Coated; Entrophen Extra Strength*].
   650 mg of ASA (OTC) [*Apo-ASEN; Coryphen; Entrophen 10 Super Strength Caplets; Novasen; Novasen Sp.C;* GENERIC].
   975 mg of ASA (OTC) [*Entrophen 15 Maximum Strength Tablets;* GENERIC].

**Packaging and storage**
Store below 40 °C (104 °F), preferably between 15 and 30 °C (59 and 86 °F), unless otherwise specified by manufacturer. Store in a tight container.

**Auxiliary labeling**
- Swallow tablets whole.
- Take with a full glass of water.

### ASPIRIN EXTENDED-RELEASE TABLETS USP

**Usual adult and adolescent dose**
Analgesic—
   Oral, 650 mg to 1.3 grams as 650-mg tablets every eight hours, or 1.6 grams as 800-mg tablets twice a day.
Note: The extended-release tablets have not been recommended by FDA for use as a platelet aggregation inhibitor.
   For treatment of arthritis, the recommended analgesic dose may be administered initially, then adjusted according to patient requirements and response.

**Usual pediatric dose**
Pediatric strength not available.

**Strength(s) usually available**
U.S.—
   650 mg (OTC) [*Extended-release Bayer 8-Hour* (scored)].
   800 mg (Rx) [*Sloprin; ZORprin;* GENERIC].
   975 mg (Rx) [GENERIC].
Canada—
   325 mg of ASA (OTC) [*Arthrisin*].
   650 mg of ASA (OTC) [*Arthrisin; Artria S.R*].

**Packaging and storage**
Store below 40 °C (104 °F), preferably between 15 and 30 °C (59 and 86 °F), unless otherwise specified by manufacturer. Store in a tight container.

**Auxiliary labeling**
- Take with food and a full glass of water.
- Swallow tablets whole (if specified by manufacturer).

### ASPIRIN AND CAFFEINE CAPSULES

**Usual adult and adolescent dose**
See *Aspirin Tablets USP*. Dosage is based only on the aspirin component.

**Usual pediatric dose**
Analgesic/Antipyretic—
   Children up to 6 years of age: Product of suitable strength not available.
   Children 6 years of age and older: Oral, 325 mg every four hours as needed, while symptoms persist.
Note: It is recommended that children up to 12 years of age receive no more than five doses in each twenty-four-hour period, unless otherwise directed by a physician, and that a physician be consulted if pain is not relieved within five days, fever within three days, or sore throat within two days.
Antirheumatic (nonsteroidal anti-inflammatory)—
   Oral, 80 to 100 mg per kg of body weight a day in divided doses.
Note: If an adequate response is not achieved within one or two weeks, dosage adjustment should be based on measurement of plasma salicylate concentration. Up to 130 mg per kg of body weight per day may be required in some patients.

**Strength(s) usually available**
U.S.—
   Not commercially available.
Canada—
   325 mg of ASA and 55 mg of caffeine (OTC) [*Astone*].

**Packaging and storage**
Store below 40 °C (104 °F), preferably between 15 and 30 °C (59 and 86 °F), in a well-closed container, unless otherwise specified by manufacturer.

**Auxiliary labeling**
- Take with food and a full glass of water.

### ASPIRIN AND CAFFEINE TABLETS

**Usual adult and adolescent dose**
See *Aspirin Tablets USP*. Dosage is based only on the aspirin component.

**Usual pediatric dose**
Analgesic/Antipyretic—
   Children up to 9 years of age: Product of suitable strength not available.
   Children 9 years of age and older: Oral, 325 to 400 mg every four hours as needed, while symptoms persist.
Note: It is recommended that children up to 12 years of age receive no more than five doses in each twenty-four-hour period, unless otherwise directed by a physician, and that a physician be consulted if pain is not relieved within five days, fever within three days, or sore throat within two days.
Antirheumatic (nonsteroidal anti-inflammatory)—
   Oral, 80 to 100 mg per kg of body weight a day in divided doses.
Note: If an adequate response is not achieved within one or two weeks, dosage adjustment should be based on measurement of plasma

salicylate concentration. Up to 130 mg per kg of body weight per day may be required in some patients.

**Strength(s) usually available**
U.S.—
- 400 mg of aspirin and 32 mg of caffeine (OTC) [*Anacin Caplets; Anacin Tablets; Gensan; P-A-C Revised Formula*].
- 500 mg of aspirin and 32 mg of caffeine (OTC) [*Anacin Maximum Strength*].

Canada—
- 325 mg of ASA and 4 mg of caffeine [*Kalmex*].
- 325 mg of ASA and 15 mg of caffeine (OTC) [*C2* (double-scored)].
- 325 mg of ASA and 30 mg of caffeine citrate equivalent to 15 mg of caffeine base (OTC) [*Herbopyrine; 217* (scored)].
- 325 mg of ASA and 30 mg of caffeine (OTC) [*Nervine*].
- 325 mg of ASA and 32 mg of caffeine (OTC) [*Anacin*].
- 325 mg of ASA and 32.4 mg of caffeine (OTC) [*Antidol*].
- 325 mg of ASA and 33 mg of caffeine (OTC) [*Calmine; Dolomine*].
- 325 mg of ASA and 65 mg of caffeine (OTC) [*Instantine*].
- 375 mg of ASA and 30 mg of caffeine citrate equivalent to 15 mg of caffeine base [*Arco Pain Tablet*].
- 500 mg of ASA and 30 mg of caffeine citrate equivalent to 15 mg of caffeine base (OTC) [*217 Strong*].
- 500 mg of ASA and 32 mg of caffeine (OTC) [*Anacin Extra Strength; Pain Aid*].

**Packaging and storage**
Store below 40 °C (104 °F), preferably between 15 and 30 °C (59 and 86 °F), in a well-closed container, unless otherwise specified by manufacturer.

**Auxiliary labeling**
- Take with food and a full glass of water.

## Rectal Dosage Forms

Note: Bracketed uses in the *Dosage Forms* section refer to categories of use and/or indications that are not included in U.S. product labeling.

### ASPIRIN SUPPOSITORIES USP

**Usual adult and adolescent dose**
Analgesic/antipyretic—
  Rectal, 325 to 650 mg every four hours as needed, while symptoms persist.
  Note: For patient self-medication, it is recommended that the total daily dose not exceed 4 grams, and that a physician be consulted if pain is not relieved within ten days, fever within three days, or sore throat within two days.
Antirheumatic (nonsteroidal anti-inflammatory)—
  Rectal, 3.6 to 5.4 grams a day in divided doses.
  Note: In acute rheumatic fever, up to 7.8 grams a day in divided doses may be given.
Platelet aggregation inhibitor—
  The suppositories have not been recommended by FDA for use as a platelet aggregation inhibitor.

**Usual pediatric dose**
Analgesic/antipyretic—
  Rectal, 1.5 grams per square meter of body surface a day in four to six divided doses; or for
  Children up to 2 years of age—Dosage must be individualized by physician.
  Children 2 to 4 years of age—Rectal, 160 mg every four hours as needed, while symptoms persist.
  Children 4 to 6 years of age—Rectal, 240 mg every four hours as needed, while symptoms persist.
  Children 6 to 9 years of age—Rectal, 325 mg every four hours as needed, while symptoms persist.
  Children 9 to 11 years of age—Rectal, 325 to 400 mg every four hours as needed, while symptoms persist.
  Children 11 to 12 years of age—Rectal, 325 to 480 mg every four hours as needed, while symptoms persist.
  Note: Do not exceed 2.5 grams per square meter of body surface per day. It is recommended that children up to 12 years of age receive no more than five doses in each twenty-four-hour period, unless otherwise directed by a physician, and that a physician be consulted if pain is not relieved within five days, fever within three days, or sore throat within two days.
Antirheumatic (nonsteroidal anti-inflammatory)—
  Rectal, 80 to 100 mg per kg of body weight a day in divided doses.
  Note: If an adequate response is not achieved within one or two weeks, dosage adjustment should be based on measurement of plasma salicylate concentration. Up to 130 mg per kg of body weight per day may be required in some patients.

[Kawasaki disease][1]—
  During the early febrile stage: Rectal, 80 to 120 mg (average 100 mg) per kg of body weight a day in four divided doses for fourteen days or until inflammation has subsided. However, absorption may be impaired or erratic during this stage of the illness, and considerably higher doses may be required. It is recommended that dosage be adjusted to achieve and maintain a plasma salicylate concentration of 20 to 30 mg per 100 mL.
  During the convalescent stage: Rectal, 3 to 5 mg per kg of body weight a day as a single dose. If no coronary artery abnormalities occur, treatment is usually continued for a minimum of eight weeks. If coronary artery abnormalities occur, it is recommended that treatment be continued for at least one year, even if the abnormalities regress, and longer if abnormalities persist.

**Strength(s) usually available**
U.S.—
- 60 mg (OTC) [GENERIC].
- 120 mg (OTC) [GENERIC].
- 125 mg (OTC) [GENERIC].
- 200 mg (OTC) [GENERIC].
- 300 mg (OTC) [GENERIC].
- 325 mg (OTC) [GENERIC].
- 600 mg (OTC) [GENERIC].
- 650 mg (OTC) [GENERIC].
- 1.2 grams (OTC) [GENERIC].

Canada—
- 150 mg of ASA (OTC) [*PMS-ASA;* GENERIC].
- 650 mg of ASA (OTC) [*PMS-ASA;* GENERIC].

Note: The strengths of the specific products may not conform to the recommended pediatric doses. Also, the strengths of some products labeled in grains may vary, depending on the manufacturer.

**Packaging and storage**
Store between 8 and 15 °C (46 and 59 °F), unless otherwise specified by manufacturer. Store in a well-closed container, in a cool place.

**Auxiliary labeling**
- Store in a cool place. May be refrigerated.
- For rectal use only.

[1]Not included in Canadian product labeling.

---

## ASPIRIN, BUFFERED

## Summary of Differences

Category/indications:
  Aspirin, buffered, also indicated as a platelet aggregation inhibitor.
Pharmacology/pharmacokinetics:
  Aspirin irreversibly inhibits platelet aggregation.
Precautions:
  Cross-sensitivity and/or related problems—
    Risk of cross-sensitivity with other nonsteroidal anti-inflammatory drugs (NSAIDs) significantly greater with aspirin than with other salicylates.
  Drug interactions and/or related problems—
    Aspirin may increase ascorbic acid requirement (prolonged high-dose use).
    Theoretically, aspirin may decrease zidovudine clearance.
    Higher risk of bleeding (compared with other salicylates) when aspirin is used concurrently with other medications that may inhibit blood clotting or cause gastrointestinal ulceration or bleeding.
    Antacids present as buffering agents may decrease absorption of fluoroquinolone antibiotics, itraconazole, ketoconazole, and oral tetracyclines.
  Laboratory value alterations—
    Aspirin interferes with urine 5-hydroxyindoleacetic acid determinations.
    Aspirin interferes with protirelin-induced thyroid stimulating hormone release determinations.
    Aspirin prolongs bleeding time.
  Medical considerations/contraindications—
    Aspirin should not be used in patients with a history of severe sensitivity reactions to aspirin, other NSAIDs, nasal polyps and asthma, or thrombocytopenia.
    Aspirin should be used with caution in patients with asthma or glucose-6-phosphate dehydrogenase (G6PD) deficiency.

Side/adverse effects:
- Aspirin is more ulcerogenic than other salicylates.
- Rarely, aspirin causes hemolytic anemia (in patients with G6PD deficiency).

## Additional Dosing Information

See also *General Dosing Information*.

The doses for buffered aspirin formulations are based on the FDA's dosing recommendations for aspirin. The dosage unit of 325 mg (5 grains) is used. The conversion factor of 1 grain equal to 65 mg is used. Strengths of specific products may vary, depending on the manufacturer.

The amount and type of buffering may vary among products.

## Oral Dosage Forms

Note: Bracketed uses in the *Dosage Forms* section refer to categories of use and/or indications that are not included in U.S. product labeling.

### ASPIRIN, ALUMINA, AND MAGNESIA TABLETS USP

**Usual adult and adolescent dose**

Analgesic/antipyretic—
  Oral, 500 mg every three or four hours or 1000 mg every six hours as needed, while symptoms persist.
  Note: For patient self-medication, it is recommended that the total daily dose not exceed 4 grams, and that a physician be consulted if pain is not relieved within ten days, fever within three days, or sore throat within two days.

Antirheumatic (nonsteroidal anti-inflammatory)—
  Oral, 3.6 to 5.4 grams a day in divided doses.
  Note: In acute rheumatic fever, up to 7.8 grams a day in divided doses may be given.

Platelet aggregation inhibitor—
  Oral, 325 mg a day, with the following exceptions:
  Ischemic attacks, transient, in males or—
  [Thromboembolism, cerebral, recurrence][1]—
    Oral, 1 gram a day. Dosage may be reduced to 325 mg a day if the patient is unable to tolerate the higher dose.
  [Ischemic attacks, transient, occurring in association with mitral valve prolapse][1]—
    Oral, 325 mg to 1 gram a day.
  [Prevention of thrombosis or occlusion of coronary bypass graft]—
    Oral, 325 mg seven hours postoperatively (via a nasogastric tube), then 325 mg three times daily, concurrently with 75 mg of dipyridamole. Dipyridamole may be discontinued one week postoperatively, but aspirin should be continued indefinitely.
    Platelet aggregation inhibitor therapy is most effective when it is initiated two days prior to scheduled surgery. However, preoperative administration of aspirin has been shown to increase perisurgical bleeding and is not recommended. Therapy is therefore initiated with dipyridamole (recommended dosage 100 mg four times a day for two days prior to surgery and 100 mg one hour postoperatively [via a nasogastric tube]). Dipyridamole therapy is continued postoperatively (recommended dosage 75 mg seven hours postoperatively, via a nasogastric tube, then 75 mg three times a day, concurrently with aspirin) for at least one week.
  Note: Although the doses recommended above for use of aspirin as a platelet aggregation inhibitor have been found effective in clinical studies, optimum dosage has not been established. For indications other than prevention of transient ischemic attacks or recurrence of cerebral thromboembolism, lower doses are often used. A few studies have shown that 160 mg of aspirin every twenty-four hours, or 325 mg every forty-eight hours, may effectively inhibit platelet aggregation while minimizing the risk of aspirin-induced side effects.

  For most antithrombotic indications, lower doses than can be achieved with the aspirin, alumina, and magnesia formulation are used. However, this formulation may be used when 500-mg or 1-gram doses are appropriate.

**Usual pediatric dose**

Analgesic/antipyretic—
  Product of suitable strength not available.
Antirheumatic (nonsteroidal anti-inflammatory)—
  Oral, 80 to 100 mg per kg of body weight a day in divided doses.
  Note: If an adequate response is not achieved within one or two weeks, dosage adjustment should be based on measurement of plasma salicylate concentration. Up to 130 mg per kg of body weight per day may be required in some patients.

[Kawasaki disease][1]—
  During the early febrile stage: Oral, 80 to 120 mg (average 100 mg) per kg of body weight a day in four divided doses for fourteen days or until inflammation has subsided. However, absorption may be impaired or erratic during this stage of the illness, and considerably higher doses may be required. It is recommended that dosage be adjusted to achieve and maintain a plasma salicylate concentration of 20 to 30 mg per 100 mL.
  During the convalescent stage: Oral, 3 to 5 mg per kg of body weight a day as a single dose. If no coronary artery abnormalities occur, treatment is usually continued for a minimum of eight weeks. If coronary artery abnormalities occur, it is recommended that treatment be continued for at least one year, even if the abnormalities regress, and longer if abnormalities persist.

**Strength(s) usually available**

U.S.—
  500 mg of aspirin, with 27 mg of aluminum hydroxide and 100 mg of magnesium hydroxide (OTC) [*Arthritis Pain Formula*].
Canada—
  Not commercially available.

**Packaging and storage**
Store below 40 °C (104 °F), preferably between 15 and 30 °C (59 and 86 °F), unless otherwise specified by manufacturer. Store in a tight container.

**Auxiliary labeling**
- Take with food and a full glass of water.

### ASPIRIN, ALUMINA, AND MAGNESIUM OXIDE TABLETS USP

**Usual adult and adolescent dose**

Analgesic/antipyretic or
Antirheumatic (nonsteroidal anti-inflammatory)—
  See *Aspirin, Alumina, and Magnesia Tablets USP*. Dosage is based only on the aspirin component.
Platelet aggregation inhibitor—
  See *Aspirin, Alumina, and Magnesia Tablets USP*. Dosage is based only on the aspirin component. For most antithrombotic indications, lower doses than can be achieved with the aspirin, alumina, and magnesium oxide formulation are used. However, this formulation may be used when 500-mg or 1-gram doses are appropriate.

**Usual pediatric dose**
See *Aspirin, Alumina, and Magnesia Tablets USP*. Dosage is based only on the aspirin component.

**Strength(s) usually available**

U.S.—
  500 mg of aspirin, with dried aluminum hydroxide gel equivalent to 125 mg of aluminum hydroxide and 150 mg of magnesium oxide (OTC) [*Cama Arthritis Pain Reliever*].
Canada—
  Not commercially available.

**Packaging and storage**
Store below 40 °C (104 °F), preferably between 15 and 30 °C (59 and 86 °F), unless otherwise specified by manufacturer. Store in a tight container.

**Auxiliary labeling**
- Take with food and a full glass of water.

### BUFFERED ASPIRIN TABLETS USP

**Usual adult and adolescent dose**

Analgesic/antipyretic—
  Oral, 325 to 500 mg every three hours, 325 to 650 mg every four hours, or 650 mg to 1000 mg every six hours as needed, while symptoms persist.
  Note: For patient self-medication, it is recommended that the total daily dose not exceed 4 grams, and that a physician be consulted if pain is not relieved within ten days, fever within three days, or sore throat within two days.

Platelet aggregation inhibitor—
  See *Aspirin, Alumina, and Magnesia Tablets USP*.

**Usual pediatric dose**

Analgesic/antipyretic—
  Oral, 1.5 grams of aspirin per square meter of body surface a day in four to six divided doses; or for
  Children up to 2 years of age: Dosage must be individualized by physician.
  Children 2 to 4 years of age: Oral, ½ of a 325-mg tablet every four hours as needed, while symptoms persist.

Children 4 to 6 years of age: Oral, ¾ of a 325-mg tablet every four hours as needed, while symptoms persist.
Children 6 to 9 years of age: Oral, 1 tablet (325 mg) every four hours as needed, while symptoms persist.
Children 9 to 11 years of age: Oral, 1 to 1¼ tablets (325 mg each) every four hours as needed, while symptoms persist.
Children 11 to 12 years of age: Oral, 1 to 1½ tablets (325 mg each) every four hours as needed, while symptoms persist.
Note: It is recommended that children up to 12 years of age receive no more than five doses in each twenty-four-hour period, unless otherwise directed by a physician, and that a physician be consulted if pain is not relieved within five days, fever within three days, or sore throat within two days.

Antirheumatic (nonsteroidal anti-inflammatory)—
Oral, 80 to 100 mg of aspirin per kg of body weight a day in divided doses.
Note: If an adequate response is not achieved within one or two weeks, dosage adjustment should be based on measurement of plasma salicylate concentration. Up to 130 mg per kg of body weight of aspirin per day may be required in some patients.

[Kawasaki disease][1]—
During the early febrile stage: Oral, 80 to 120 mg (average 100 mg) per kg of body weight a day in four divided doses for fourteen days or until inflammation has subsided. However, absorption may be impaired or erratic during this stage of the illness, and considerably higher doses may be required. It is recommended that dosage be adjusted to achieve and maintain a plasma salicylate concentration of 20 to 30 mg per 100 mL.
During the convalescent stage: Oral, 3 to 5 mg per kg of body weight a day as a single dose. If no coronary artery abnormalities occur, treatment is usually continued for a minimum of eight weeks. If coronary artery abnormalities occur, it is recommended that treatment be continued for at least one year, even if the abnormalities regress, and longer if abnormalities persist.

**Strength(s) usually available**
U.S.—
325 mg of aspirin (OTC) [*Arthritis Pain Ascriptin; Bufferin Caplets; Bufferin Tablets; Buffex; Buffinol; Magnaprin; Regular Strength Ascriptin;* GENERIC].
500 mg of aspirin (OTC) [*Arthritis Strength Bufferin; Buffinol Extra; Extra Strength Bayer Plus Caplets; Maximum Strength Ascriptin*].
Canada—
325 mg of ASA (OTC) [*Aspirin Plus Stomach Guard Regular Strength; Bufferin Caplets; Tri-Buffered ASA;* GENERIC].
500 mg of ASA (OTC) [*Aspirin Plus Stomach Guard Extra Strength; Bufferin Extra Strength Caplets;* GENERIC].
Note: See individual product label for buffering agent(s).
The strengths of the specific products may not conform to the recommended pediatric doses.

**Packaging and storage**
Store below 40 °C (104 °F), preferably between 15 and 30 °C (59 and 86 °F), unless otherwise specified by manufacturer. Store in a tight container.

**Auxiliary labeling**
- Take with food and a full glass of water.

## BUFFERED ASPIRIN AND CAFFEINE TABLETS

**Usual adult and adolescent dose**
See *Buffered Aspirin Tablets USP*. Dosage is based only on the aspirin component.

**Usual pediatric dose**
Analgesic/antipyretic—
Oral, 1.5 grams of aspirin per square meter of body surface a day in four to six divided doses; or for
Children up to 2 years of age: Dosage must be individualized by physician.
Children 2 to 4 years of age: Oral, ½ of a 325-mg tablet every four hours as needed, while symptoms persist.
Children 4 to 6 years of age: Oral, ¾ of a 325-mg tablet every four hours as needed, while symptoms persist.
Children 6 to 9 years of age: Oral, 1 tablet (325 mg) every four hours as needed, while symptoms persist.
Children 9 to 11 years of age: Oral, 1 to 1¼ tablets (325 mg each) every four hours as needed, while symptoms persist.
Children 11 to 12 years of age: Oral, 1 to 1½ tablets (325 mg each) or 1 tablet (421 mg) every four hours as needed, while symptoms persist.

Note: It is recommended that children up to 12 years of age receive no more than five doses in each twenty-four-hour period, unless otherwise directed by a physician, and that a physician be consulted if pain is not relieved within five days, fever within three days, or sore throat within two days.

Antirheumatic (nonsteroidal anti-inflammatory)—
Oral, 80 to 100 mg of aspirin per kg of body weight a day in divided doses.
Note: If an adequate response is not achieved within one or two weeks, dosage adjustment should be based on measurement of plasma salicylate concentration. Up to 130 mg per kg of body weight of aspirin per day may be required in some patients.

**Strength(s) usually available**
U.S.—
421 mg of aspirin and 32 mg of caffeine (OTC) [*Cope*].
Canada—
325 mg of ASA and 15 mg of caffeine (OTC) [*C2 Buffered* (scored)].
Note: See individual product label for buffering agent(s).
The strengths of the specific products may not conform to the recommended pediatric doses.

**Packaging and storage**
Store below 40 °C (104 °F), preferably between 15 and 30 °C (59 and 86 °F), unless otherwise specified by manufacturer. Store in a tight container.

**Auxiliary labeling**
- Take with food and a full glass of water.

[1]Not included in Canadian product labeling.

---

## CHOLINE SALICYLATE

## Summary of Differences
Pharmacology/pharmacokinetics:
Choline salicylate does not have a clinically significant effect on platelet aggregation.
Precautions:
Cross-sensitivity and/or related problems—Lower risk than with aspirin of cross-sensitivity to nonsteroidal anti-inflammatory drugs (NSAIDs).
Drug interactions and/or related problems—Lower risk of bleeding (compared with aspirin) when used concurrently with other medications that may inhibit blood clotting or cause gastrointestinal ulceration or bleeding.
Medical considerations/contraindications—May be used in patients with a history of severe sensitivity reactions to aspirin or other NSAIDs, although caution is advised.
Side/adverse effects:
Less ulcerogenic than aspirin.

## Additional Dosing Information
See also *General Dosing Information*.

The nonarthritic doses are based on the FDA's dosing recommendations for aspirin.

A 435-mg dose of choline salicylate is equivalent in salicylate content to 325 mg of aspirin.

## Oral Dosage Forms
### CHOLINE SALICYLATE ORAL SOLUTION

**Usual adult and adolescent dose**
Analgesic/antipyretic—
Oral, 435 to 669 mg (equivalent in salicylate content to 325 to 500 mg of aspirin) every three hours, 435 to 870 mg (equivalent in salicylate content to 325 to 650 mg of aspirin) every four hours, or 870 to 1338 mg (equivalent in salicylate content to 650 to 1000 mg of aspirin) every six hours as needed, while symptoms persist.
Note: For patient self-medication, it is recommended that the total daily dose not exceed 5352 mg, and that a physician be consulted if pain is not relieved within ten days, fever within three days, or sore throat within two days.

Antirheumatic (nonsteroidal anti-inflammatory)—
Oral, 4.8 to 7.2 grams (equivalent in salicylate content to 3.6 to 5.4 grams of aspirin) a day in divided doses.

## Salicylates (Systemic)

**Usual pediatric dose**

Analgesic/antipyretic—
  Oral, 2 grams (equivalent in salicylate content to 1.5 grams of aspirin) per square meter of body surface a day in four to six divided doses; or for
  Children up to 2 years of age: Dosage must be individualized by physician.
  Children 2 to 4 years of age: Oral, 217.5 mg (equivalent in salicylate content to 162.5 mg of aspirin) every four hours as needed, while symptoms persist.
  Children 4 to 6 years of age: Oral, 326.5 mg (equivalent in salicylate content to 243.8 mg of aspirin) every four hours as needed, while symptoms persist.
  Children 6 to 9 years of age: Oral, 435 mg (equivalent in salicylate content to 325 mg of aspirin) every four hours as needed, while symptoms persist.
  Children 9 to 11 years of age: Oral, 435 to 543.8 mg (equivalent in salicylate content to 325 to 406.3 mg of aspirin) every four hours as needed, while symptoms persist.
  Children 11 to 12 years of age: Oral, 435 to 652.5 mg (equivalent in salicylate content to 325 to 487.5 mg of aspirin) every four hours as needed, while symptoms persist.
  Note: It is recommended that children up to 12 years of age receive no more than five doses in each twenty-four-hour period, unless otherwise directed by a physician, and that a physician be consulted if pain is not relieved within five days, fever within three days, or sore throat within two days.

Antirheumatic (nonsteroidal anti-inflammatory)—
  Oral, 107 to 133 mg (equivalent in salicylate content to 80 to 100 mg of aspirin) per kg of body weight a day in divided doses.
  Note: If an adequate response is not achieved within one or two weeks, dosage adjustment should be based on measurement of plasma salicylate concentration. Up to 174 mg (equivalent in salicylate content to 130 mg of aspirin) per kg of body weight per day may be required in some patients.

**Strength(s) usually available**

U.S.—
  870 mg (equivalent in salicylate content to 650 mg of aspirin) per 5 mL (OTC) [*Arthropan*].
Canada—
  Not commercially available.

**Packaging and storage**
Store below 40 °C (104 °F), preferably between 15 and 30 °C (59 and 86 °F), in a well-closed container, unless otherwise specified by manufacturer. Protect from freezing.

**Auxiliary labeling**
• Take with food or a full glass of water.

---

### CHOLINE AND MAGNESIUM SALICYLATES

## Summary of Differences

Pharmacology/pharmacokinetics:
  This medication does not have a clinically significant effect on platelet aggregation.
Precautions:
  Cross-sensitivity and/or related problems—
    Lower risk than with aspirin of cross-sensitivity to nonsteroidal anti-inflammatory drugs (NSAIDs).
  Drug interactions and/or related problems—
    Lower risk of bleeding (compared with aspirin) when used concurrently with other medications that may inhibit blood clotting or cause gastrointestinal ulceration or bleeding.
    Magnesium may decrease absorption of fluoroquinolone antibiotics, itraconazole, ketoconazole, and oral tetracyclines.
  Medical considerations/contraindications—
    Should not be used in patients with chronic advanced renal impairment because of risk of hypermagnesemic toxicity.
    May be used in patients with a history of severe sensitivity reactions to aspirin or other NSAIDs, although caution is advised.
  Patient monitoring—
    Monitoring of serum magnesium concentration recommended if large doses administered to patients with renal insufficiency.
Side/adverse effects:
  Less ulcerogenic than aspirin.

## Additional Dosing Information

See also *General Dosing Information*.
Choline and magnesium salicylates oral solution may be mixed with fruit juices just prior to administration.

## Oral Dosage Forms

### CHOLINE AND MAGNESIUM SALICYLATES ORAL SOLUTION

**Usual adult and adolescent dose**
Analgesic or
Antipyretic—
  Oral, 2 to 3 grams of salicylate a day in two or three divided doses.
Anti-inflammatory (nonsteroidal) or
Antirheumatic—
  Oral, 3 grams of salicylate a day in a single dose at bedtime, or in two or three divided doses, initially. Dosage must then be adjusted according to the requirements and response of the individual patient.

**Usual pediatric dose**
Analgesic
Antipyretic or
Anti-inflammatory (nonsteroidal)—
  Children weighing up to 37 kg: Oral, 50 mg of salicylate per kg of body weight per day in two divided doses.
  Children weighing more than 37 kg: Oral, 2.2 grams of salicylate a day in two divided doses.

**Strength(s) usually available**
U.S.—
  500 mg of salicylate (contains 293 mg of choline salicylate and 362 mg of magnesium salicylate) per 5 mL (Rx) [*Trilisate*].
Note: Each 5-mL dose of this medication is equivalent in salicylate content to 650 mg of aspirin.
Canada—
  Not commercially available.

**Packaging and storage**
Store below 40 °C (104 °F), preferably between 15 and 30 °C (59 and 86 °F), unless otherwise specified by manufacturer. Protect from freezing.

**Auxiliary labeling**
• Take with food or a full glass of water.

### CHOLINE AND MAGNESIUM SALICYLATES TABLETS

**Usual adult and adolescent dose**
See *Choline and Magnesium Salicylates Oral Solution*.

**Usual pediatric dose**
See *Choline and Magnesium Salicylates Oral Solution*.

**Strength(s) usually available**
U.S.—
  500 mg of salicylate (contains 293 mg of choline salicylate and 362 mg of magnesium salicylate) (Rx) [*CMT*; *Tricosal*; *Trilisate* (scored); GENERIC].
  750 mg of salicylate (contains 440 mg of choline salicylate and 544 mg of magnesium salicylate) (Rx) [*CMT*; *Tricosal*; *Trilisate* (scored); GENERIC].
  1000 mg of salicylate (contains 587 mg of choline salicylate and 725 mg of magnesium salicylate) (Rx) [*CMT*; *Tricosal*; *Trilisate* (scored); GENERIC].
Canada—
  500 mg of salicylate (contains 293 mg of choline salicylate and 362 mg of magnesium salicylate) (Rx) [*Trilisate* (scored)].
Note: Each 500-mg tablet is equivalent in salicylate content to 650 mg of aspirin. Each 750-mg tablet is equivalent in salicylate content to 975 mg of aspirin. Each 1000-mg tablet is equivalent in salicylate content to 1.3 grams of aspirin.

**Packaging and storage**
Store below 40 °C (104 °F), preferably between 15 and 30 °C (59 and 86 °F), in a well-closed container, unless otherwise specified by manufacturer.

**Auxiliary labeling**
• Take with food and a full glass of water.

## MAGNESIUM SALICYLATE

### Summary of Differences
Pharmacology/pharmacokinetics:
    Magnesium salicylate does not have a clinically significant effect on platelet aggregation.
Precautions:
    Cross-sensitivity and/or related problems—
        Lower risk than with aspirin of cross-sensitivity to nonsteroidal anti-inflammatory drugs (NSAIDs).
    Drug interactions and/or related problems—
        Lower risk of bleeding (compared with aspirin) when used concurrently with other medications that may inhibit blood clotting or cause gastrointestinal ulceration or bleeding.
        Magnesium may decrease absorption of fluoroquinolone antibiotics, itraconazole, ketoconazole, and oral tetracyclines.
    Medical considerations/contraindications—
        Should not be used in patients with chronic advanced renal impairment.
        May be used in patients with a history of severe sensitivity reactions to aspirin or other NSAIDs, although caution is advised.
    Patient monitoring—
        Monitoring of serum magnesium concentration recommended if large doses are administered to patients with renal insufficiency.
Side/adverse effects:
    Less ulcerogenic than aspirin.

### Additional Dosing Information
See also *General Dosing Information*.

A 545-mg dose of magnesium salicylate is equivalent in salicylate content to 650 mg of aspirin.

### Oral Dosage Forms

#### MAGNESIUM SALICYLATE TABLETS USP
**Usual adult and adolescent dose**
Analgesic/antipyretic
Antirheumatic (nonsteroidal anti-inflammatory)—
    Oral, 2 regular-strength tablets (containing the equivalent of 303.7 mg of anhydrous magnesium salicylate per tablet) every four hours as needed, up to a maximum of 12 tablets a day, or
    Oral, 2 extra-strength tablets (containing the equivalent of 467 mg of anhydrous magnesium salicylate, or more, per tablet) every six hours as needed, up to a maximum of 8 tablets a day.
Note: For patient self-medication, it is recommended that a physician be consulted if pain is not relieved within ten days, fever within three days, or sore throat within two days.

**Usual pediatric dose**
Dosage has not been established.

**Strength(s) usually available**
U.S.—
    377 mg of magnesium salicylate tetrahydrate equivalent to 303.7 mg of anhydrous magnesium salicylate (OTC) [*Doan's Regular Strength Tablets*].
    545 mg (Rx) [*Magan*].
    580 mg of magnesium salicylate tetrahydrate equivalent to 467 mg of anhydrous magnesium salicylate (OTC) [*Backache Caplets; Bayer Select Maximum Strength Backache Pain Relief Formula; Maximum Strength Doan's Analgesic Caplets*].
    600 mg (Rx) [*Mobidin* (scored)].
Canada—
    325 mg (OTC) [*Doan's Backache Pills*].
    650 mg (OTC) [*Sero-Gesic*].

**Packaging and storage**
Store below 40 °C (104 °F), preferably between 15 and 30 °C (59 and 86 °F), unless otherwise specified by manufacturer. Store in a tight container.

**Auxiliary labeling**
• Take with food and a full glass of water.

## SALSALATE

### Summary of Differences
Pharmacology/pharmacokinetics:
    Salsalate does not have a clinically significant effect on platelet aggregation.
Precautions:
    Cross-sensitivity and/or related problems—Lower risk than with aspirin of cross-sensitivity to nonsteroidal anti-inflammatory drugs (NSAIDs).
    Drug interactions and/or related problems—Lower risk of bleeding (compared with aspirin) when used concurrently with other medications that may inhibit blood clotting or cause gastrointestinal ulceration or bleeding.
    Medical considerations/contraindications—May be used in patients with a history of severe sensitivity reactions to aspirin or other NSAIDs, although caution is advised.
Side/adverse effects:
    Less ulcerogenic than aspirin.

### Additional Dosing Information
**Bioequivalenence information**
Bioavailability or bioequivalence problems among different brands of Salsalate Tablets USP have not been documented.

### Oral Dosage Forms

#### SALSALATE CAPSULES USP
**Usual adult and adolescent dose**
Antirheumatic—
    Oral, 1 gram three times a day initially. Dosage may then be titrated according to patient response.

**Usual pediatric dose**
Dosage has not been established.

**Strength(s) usually available**
U.S.—
    500 mg (Rx) [*Disalcid;* GENERIC].
    750 mg (Rx) [GENERIC].
Canada—
    Not commercially available.

**Packaging and storage**
Store between 15 and 30 °C (59 and 86 °F), in a light-resistant container, unless otherwise specified by manufacturer. Store in a tight container.

**Auxiliary labeling**
• Take with food and a full glass of water.

#### SALSALATE TABLETS USP
Note: Bioavailability or bioequivalence problems among different brands of Salsalate Tablets USP have not been documented.

**Usual adult and adolescent dose**
Analgesic/antipyretic or
Antirheumatic—
    Oral, 500 mg to 1 gram two or three times a day initially. Dosage may then be titrated according to patient response.

**Usual pediatric dose**
Dosage has not been established.

**Strength(s) usually available**
U.S.—
    500 mg (Rx) [*Amigesic; Disalcid* (scored); *Mono-Gesic; Salflex; Salsitab;* GENERIC].
    750 mg (Rx) [*Amigesic* (scored); *Anaflex 750; Disalcid* (scored); *Marthritic; Mono-Gesic* (scored); *Salflex* (scored); *Salsitab* (scored); GENERIC].
Canada—
    500 mg (Rx) [*Disalcid* (scored)].
    750 mg (Rx) [*Disalcid* (scored)].

**Packaging and storage**
Store between 15 and 30 °C (59 and 86 °F), in a light-resistant container, unless otherwise specified by manufacturer. Store in a tight container.

**Auxiliary labeling**
• Take with food and a full glass of water.

## SODIUM SALICYLATE

### Summary of Differences
Pharmacology/pharmacokinetics:
    Sodium salicylate does not have a clinically significant effect on platelet aggregation.
Precautions:
    Cross-sensitivity and/or related problems—
        Lower risk than with aspirin of cross-sensitivity to nonsteroidal anti-inflammatory drugs (NSAIDs).

**Salicylates (Systemic)**

Drug interactions and/or related problems—
Caution required when large doses administered concurrently with sodium-retaining medications.
Lower risk of bleeding (compared with aspirin) when used concurrently with other medications that may inhibit blood clotting or cause gastrointestinal ulceration or bleeding.
Medical considerations/contraindications—
Caution required in hypertensive patients or those on a sodium-restricted diet because of sodium content.
May be used in patients with a history of severe sensitivity reactions to aspirin or other NSAIDs, although caution is advised.
Side/adverse effects:
Less ulcerogenic than aspirin.

## Additional Dosing Information

See also *General Dosing Information*.

The nonarthritic doses are based on the FDA's dosing recommendations for sodium salicylate. The dosage unit of 325 mg (5 grains) is used for adult doses. The conversion factor of 65 mg equal to 1 grain is used. Strengths of specific products may vary, depending on the manufacturer.

The uncoated tablet form of sodium salicylate should be administered with food or a full glass (240 mL) of water to lessen gastric irritation.

Each 325-mg tablet of sodium salicylate contains 2 mEq (46 mg) of sodium.

## Oral Dosage Forms
### SODIUM SALICYLATE TABLETS USP
**Usual adult and adolescent dose**
Analgesic/antipyretic—
Oral, 325 to 650 mg every four hours as needed, while symptoms persist.

Note: For patient self-medication, it is recommended that the total daily dose not exceed 4 grams, and that a physician be consulted if pain is not relieved within ten days, fever within three days, or sore throat within two days.

Antirheumatic (nonsteroidal anti-inflammatory)—
Oral, 3.6 to 5.4 grams a day in divided doses.

**Usual pediatric dose**
Analgesic/antipyretic—
Oral, 1.5 grams per square meter of body surface a day in four to six divided doses; or for
Children up to 6 years of age: Product of suitable strength not available.
Children 6 years of age and older: Oral, 325 mg every four hours as needed, while symptoms persist.

Note: It is recommended that children up to 12 years of age receive no more than five doses in each twenty-four-hour period, unless otherwise directed by a physician, and that a physician be consulted if pain is not relieved within five days, fever within three days, or sore throat within two days.

Antirheumatic (nonsteroidal anti-inflammatory)—
Oral, 80 to 100 mg per kg of body weight a day in divided doses.

Note: If an adequate response is not achieved within one or two weeks, dosage adjustment should be based on measurement of plasma salicylate concentration. Up to 130 mg per kg of body weight per day may be required in some patients.

**Strength(s) usually available**
U.S.—
Not commercially available.
Canada—
325 mg (OTC) [*Dodd's Pills; Gin Pain Pills*].
500 mg [*Dodd's Extra Strength*].

Note: The strengths of the specific products may not conform to the recommended pediatric dose. Also, the strengths of individual products labeled in grains may vary, depending on the manufacturer.

**Packaging and storage**
Store below 40 °C (104 °F), preferably between 15 and 30 °C (59 and 86 °F), unless otherwise specified by manufacturer. Store in a well-closed container.

**Auxiliary labeling**
• Take with food and a full glass of water.

### SODIUM SALICYLATE DELAYED-RELEASE TABLETS
**Usual adult and adolescent dose**
See *Sodium Salicylate Tablets USP*.
**Usual pediatric dose**
See *Sodium Salicylate Tablets USP*.
**Strength(s) usually available**
U.S.—
325 mg (OTC) [GENERIC].
650 mg (OTC) [GENERIC].
Canada—
Not commercially available.

Note: Strengths of individual products labeled in grains may vary, depending on the manufacturer.

**Packaging and storage**
Store between 15 and 30 °C (59 and 86 °F), in a well-closed container, unless otherwise specified by manufacturer.

**Auxiliary labeling**
• Swallow tablets whole.
• Take with a full glass of water.

Revised: August 1990
Interim revision: 07/25/95

---

**SALICYLIC ACID**—The *Salicylic Acid (Topical)* monograph is not included in this published version of the USP DI database. Copies of the monograph are available on request from Micromedex, Inc. - Reprint Requests, 6200 S. Syracuse Way, Suite 300, Englewood, CO 80111; telephone (303) 486-6400; telefax (303) 486-6464; Email: USPDI@MDX.COM.

---

**SALICYLIC ACID AND SULFUR**—The *Salicylic Acid and Sulfur (Topical)* monograph is not included in this published version of the USP DI database. Copies of the monograph are available on request from Micromedex, Inc. - Reprint Requests, 6200 S. Syracuse Way, Suite 300, Englewood, CO 80111; telephone (303) 486-6400; telefax (303) 486-6464; Email: USPDI@MDX.COM.

---

**SALICYLIC ACID, SULFUR, AND COAL TAR**—The *Salicylic Acid, Sulfur, and Coal Tar (Topical)* monograph is not included in this published version of the USP DI database. Copies of the monograph are available on request from Micromedex, Inc. - Reprint Requests, 6200 S. Syracuse Way, Suite 300, Englewood, CO 80111; telephone (303) 486-6400; telefax (303) 486-6464; Email: USPDI@MDX.COM.

---

**SALMETEROL**—See *Bronchodilators, Adrenergic (Inhalation-Local)*.

---

**SALSALATE**—See *Salicylates (Systemic)*.

---

# SAQUINAVIR Systemic—INTRODUCTORY VERSION

VA CLASSIFICATION (Primary): AM803
Commonly used brand name(s): *Fortovase; Invirase*.

Note: For a listing of dosage forms and brand names by country availability, see *Dosage Forms* section(s).

## Category
Antiviral (systemic).

# Indications

## General considerations
Saquinavir is a human immunodeficiency virus (HIV) protease inhibitor. Cross-resistance between saquinavir (following prolonged [24 to 127 weeks] treatment with saquinavir mesylate capsules) and other HIV protease inhibitors, such as indinavir, nelfinavir, and ritonavir, has been observed in clinical isolates. However, cross-resistance between saquinavir and reverse transcriptase inhibitors is thought to be unlikely because they affect different parts of HIV replication.

The key mutations conferring viral resistance to saquinavir are at codons L90M and G48V. In clinical isolates from patients treated with either saquinavir mesylate capsules or saquinavir soft gelatin capsules, the L90M mutation predominated. Although the mutations in HIV protease characterizing resistance to saquinavir differ from those seen in patients treated with indinavir, nelfinavir, or ritonavir, additional mutations may occur during long-term treatment. The mutations may lead to resistance to other protease inhibitors.

## Accepted
Human immunodeficiency virus (HIV) infection (treatment) or
Immunodeficiency syndrome, acquired (AIDS) (treatment)—Saquinavir, in combination with other antiretroviral agents, is indicated in the treatment of HIV infection or AIDS. Saquinavir soft gelatin capsule (*Fortovase*) is the preferred dosage form, according to the Food and Drug Administration.

# Pharmacology/Pharmacokinetics

Note: Two capsule formulations of saquinavir currently are available: saquinavir mesylate capsules (*Invirase*) and saquinavir soft gelatin capsules (*Fortovase*). Unless otherwise indicated, the information provided in this monograph refers to both capsule formulations of saquinavir. Saquinavir is the active ingredient in both products.

## Physicochemical characteristics
Molecular weight—Saquinavir base: 670.86.
Saquinavir mesylate: 766.96.

## Mechanism of action/Effect
Saquinavir inhibits the activity of human immunodeficiency virus (HIV) protease. HIV protease cleaves viral polyprotein precursors in HIV-infected cells to generate functional proteins that are essential for maturation of the virus. Inhibition of HIV protease results in the production of immature, noninfectious virus particles.

## Absorption
Saquinavir mesylate capsules (*Invirase*):
Absolute bioavailability averaged 4% (range, 1 to 9%) in healthy volunteers who received a single 600-mg dose following a high-fat meal; low bioavailability was thought to be due to incomplete absorption and extensive first-pass metabolism. The area under the plasma concentration–time curve (AUC) and peak plasma concentration ($C_{max}$) values were 2.5 times higher in HIV-infected patients following multiple dosing than after a single dose. HIV-infected patients had AUC and $C_{max}$ values that were approximately twice those of healthy volunteers when both groups were administered the same treatment regimen.

Administration of saquinavir with a high-fat meal increased the AUC and $C_{max}$ to approximately twice the concentrations seen following administration with a low-calorie, lower-fat meal. The effect of food persisted for up to 2 hours.

Saquinavir soft gelatin capsules (*Fortovase*):
The bioavailability of the soft gelatin capsule formulation was estimated to be 331% of that of the original saquinavir mesylate capsule formulation. In healthy volunteers receiving single doses of saquinavir soft gelatin capsules (300 to 1200 mg), or in HIV-infected patients receiving multiple doses (400 to 1200 mg three times a day), a greater than dose-proportional increase in the plasma concentration of saquinavir was observed.

## Distribution
In two patients, distribution into the cerebrospinal fluid was minimal when compared with concentrations from corresponding plasma samples.
$Vol_D$—Approximately 700 liters (mean) at steady state.

## Protein binding
Very high (98%).

## Biotransformation
Hepatic; over 90% of saquinavir is metabolized by the cytochrome P450 isoenzyme CYP3A4. Saquinavir is thought to undergo extensive first-pass metabolism and is rapidly metabolized to a variety of inactive mono- and di-hydroxylated compounds.

## Elimination
Fecal—Approximately 88% of orally administered saquinavir is eliminated fecally as unchanged saquinavir and metabolites within 48 hours of dosing.
Renal—Approximately 1% of orally administered saquinavir is eliminated unchanged in the urine within 48 hours of dosing.

# Precautions to Consider

## Carcinogenicity
Carcinogenicity studies in rats and mice have not been completed.

## Mutagenicity
Mutagenicity and genotoxicity studies, with and without metabolic activation where appropriate, have not shown saquinavir to be mutagenic *in vitro* in the Ames test or the Chinese hamster lung V79/HPRT test. Saquinavir does not induce chromosomal damage *in vivo* in the mouse micronucleus assay or *in vitro* in human peripheral blood lymphocytes, and does not induce primary DNA damage *in vitro* in the unscheduled DNA synthesis test.

## Pregnancy/Reproduction
Fertility—Fertility and reproduction were not affected in rats given saquinavir at plasma exposures (area under the plasma concentration–time curve [AUC] values) of up to five times those achieved in humans at the recommended dose for saquinavir mesylate capsules (or approximately 50% of AUC values achieved in humans at the recommended dose for saquinavir soft gelatin capsules).

Pregnancy—Adequate and well-controlled studies have not been done in humans.

Embryotoxicity and teratogenicity were not seen in rats given saquinavir at plasma exposures (AUC values) of up to five times those achieved in humans at the recommended dose for saquinavir mesylate capsules (1800 mg per day) (or approximately 50% of AUC values achieved in humans at the recommended dose for saquinavir soft gelatin capsules), or in rabbits at plasma exposures of four times those achieved at the recommended clinical dose for saquinavir mesylate capsules (or approximately 40% of AUC values achieved in humans at the recommended dose for saquinavir soft gelatin capsules). Studies in rats administered saquinavir from late pregnancy through lactation at plasma concentrations (AUC values) of up to five times those achieved in humans at the recommended dose for saquinavir mesylate capsules (or approximately 50% of AUC values achieved in humans at the recommended dose for saquinavir soft gelatin capsules) showed that saquinavir had no effect on survival, growth, and development of offspring to the time of weaning.

FDA Pregnancy Category B.

## Breast-feeding
It is not known whether saquinavir is distributed into breast milk. The U.S. Public Health Services Centers for Disease Control and Prevention advises human immunodeficiency virus (HIV)–infected women not to breast-feed, to avoid potential postnatal transmission of HIV to a child who may not be infected.

## Pediatrics
No information is available on the relationship of age to the effects of saquinavir in pediatric patients. Safety, efficacy, and pharmacokinetics of saquinavir in HIV-infected children up to 16 years of age have not been established.

## Geriatrics
No information is available on the relationship of age to the effects of saquinavir in geriatric patients. Safety, efficacy, and pharmacokinetics of saquinavir have not been studied in HIV-infected patients older than 65 years of age.

## Drug interactions and/or related problems
The following drug interactions and/or related problems have been selected on the basis of their potential clinical significance (possible mechanism in parentheses where appropriate)—not necessarily inclusive (» = major clinical significance):

Note: Combinations containing any of the following medications, depending on the amount present, may also interact with this medication.

» Astemizole or
» Cisapride or
» Ergot derivatives or
» Midazolam or
» Terfenadine or
» Triazolam
(concurrent use of saquinavir with terfenadine has resulted in an increase in the plasma concentrations of terfenadine; competition for the cytochrome P450 enzyme CYP3A by saquinavir may also

inhibit the metabolism of astemizole, cisapride, ergot derivatives, midazolam, or triazolam; due to the potential for serious and/or life-threatening cardiac arrhythmias or prolonged sedation, concurrent use of any of these medications with saquinavir soft gelatin capsules is not recommended)

» Calcium channel blocking agents or
Clindamycin or
Dapsone or
» Quinidine
(concurrent administration of saquinavir mesylate capsules with these medications, which are substrates of the CYP3A4 isoenzyme of the cytochrome P450 enzyme system, may result in elevated plasma concentrations of these medications; patients should be monitored for toxicities associated with these medications)

» Carbamazepine or
» Dexamethasone or
» Phenobarbital or
» Phenytoin or
» Rifabutin or
» Rifampin or
» Other medications that are metabolic inducers of the cytochrome P450 enzyme system (see *Appendix II*)
(concurrent administration of rifabutin or rifampin with saquinavir mesylate capsules has resulted in a decrease in the steady-state AUC and peak plasma concentration [$C_{max}$] of saquinavir by approximately 80% and 40%, respectively; carbamazepine, dexamethasone, phenobarbital, phenytoin, or other medications that induce CYP3A4 may also reduce saquinavir plasma concentrations; use of alternative medications should be considered if patients are taking either formulation of saquinavir)

Clarithromycin
(concurrent use of saquinavir soft gelatin capsules with clarithromycin has resulted in a 177% increase in the AUC for saquinavir, a 45% increase in the AUC for clarithromycin, and a 24% decrease in the AUC for the active metabolite 14-hydroxyclarithromycin)

» Delavirdine
(concurrent use has resulted in a fivefold increase in the AUC for saquinavir mesylate capsules; in one small, preliminary study, hepatic enzyme activities were elevated in 13% of subjects during the first several weeks of dual therapy with delavirdine and saquinavir mesylate capsules; hepatic function should be monitored if these medications are administered concurrently)

Indinavir or
Nelfinavir or
» Ritonavir
(concurrent administration of saquinavir mesylate capsules or saquinavir soft gelatin capsules with indinavir has resulted in a 364% increase in the AUC for saquinavir; concurrent administration of saquinavir mesylate capsules or saquinavir soft gelatin capsules with nelfinavir has resulted in a 392% increase in the AUC for saquinavir and an 18% increase in the AUC for nelfinavir; there are currently no safety and efficacy data from the use of these combinations)
(in HIV-infected patients, concurrent administration of saquinavir mesylate capsules [400 or 600 mg two times a day] with ritonavir [400 or 600 mg two times a day] has resulted in AUC values for saquinavir that were at least 17-fold greater than historical AUC values in patients receiving saquinavir 600 mg three times a day without ritonavir; when used in combination therapy for up to 24 weeks, doses greater than 400 mg two times a day of either ritonavir or saquinavir mesylate capsules were associated with an increase in adverse events; plasma exposures achieved with saquinavir mesylate capsules [400 mg two times a day] and ritonavir [400 mg two times a day] are similar to those achieved with saquinavir soft gelatin capsules [400 mg two times a day] and ritonavir [400 mg two times a day])

Ketoconazole
(concurrent use of ketoconazole with saquinavir has resulted in steady-state AUC and $C_{max}$ values for saquinavir that were three times those seen with saquinavir alone; no dosage adjustment is necessary when these two medications are administered together; the pharmacokinetics of ketoconazole are unaffected)

Zalcitabine or
Zidovudine
(concurrent administration of saquinavir with zalcitabine and zidovudine as triple therapy resulted in no change in absorption, metabolism, or elimination for any of these medications)

**Laboratory value alterations**
The following have been selected on the basis of their potential clinical significance (possible effect in parentheses where appropriate)—not necessarily inclusive (» = major clinical significance):

With physiology/laboratory test values
Alanine aminotransferase (ALT [SGPT]), serum or
Amylase, serum or
Aspartate aminotransferase (AST [SGOT]), serum or
Creatine kinase (CK) or
Gamma-glutamyltransferase
(values may be increased)
Bilirubin or
Potassium
(concentrations may be increased)
Glucose, plasma
(concentrations may be decreased or increased)

**Medical considerations/Contraindications**
The medical considerations/contraindications included have been selected on the basis of their potential clinical significance (reasons given in parentheses where appropriate)—not necessarily inclusive (» = major clinical significance).

*Except under special circumstances, this medication should not be used when the following medical problem exists:*
» Hypersensitivity to saquinavir

*Risk-benefit should be considered when the following medical problems exist:*
Hemophilia
(increased bleeding, including spontaneous skin hematomas and hemarthrosis, has been reported in patients with hemophilia types A and B who are receiving protease inhibitor therapy; a causal relationship has not been established)
Hepatic function impairment
(saquinavir is metabolized primarily by the liver; in patients with underlying hepatitis B or C, cirrhosis, or other hepatic abnormalities, there have been reports of exacerbation of chronic hepatic dysfunction, including portal hypertension, with saquinavir therapy; although a causal relationship has not been established, caution should be used when administering saquinavir to patients with hepatic function impairment)

**Patient monitoring**
The following may be especially important in patient monitoring (other tests may be warranted in some patients, depending on condition; » = major clinical significance):
» Blood glucose determinations
(close monitoring of patient's plasma glucose concentrations is recommended; development of hyperglycemia or diabetes may be associated with the use of protease inhibitors)

## Side/Adverse Effects
Note: Saquinavir is indicated in combination with other antiretroviral agents. Saquinavir was not found to alter the pattern, frequency, or severity of toxicities associated with nucleoside analog reverse transcriptase inhibitors. Most side effects were considered to be mild. However, ketoacidosis has been reported in rare cases for patients receiving protease inhibitor therapy.

If a serious or severe toxicity occurs during treatment with saquinavir, saquinavir therapy should be interrupted until the cause of the event is identified or the toxicity resolves. At that time, resumption of treatment with full-dose saquinavir may be considered.

The following side/adverse effects have been selected on the basis of their potential clinical significance (possible signs and symptoms in parentheses where appropriate)–not necessarily inclusive:

**Those indicating need for medical attention**
Incidence rare
*Diabetes or hyperglycemia* (dry or itchy skin; fatigue; hunger, increased; thirst, increased; unexplained weight loss; urination, increased); *ketoacidosis* (confusion; dehydration; mouth odor, fruity; nausea; vomiting; weight loss); *paresthesia* (burning or prickling sensation); *skin rash*

**Those indicating need for medical attention only if they continue or are bothersome**
Incidence less frequent
*Asthenia* (weakness); *gastrointestinal disturbances* (abdominal pain; diarrhea; mouth ulcers; nausea)

Incidence rare
*Headache*

## Overdose

No acute toxicities were seen in one patient who ingested a single dose of 8 grams of saquinavir mesylate capsules; emesis was induced within 2 to 4 hours after ingestion. No serious toxicities were reported in patients taking 7200 mg per day for 25 weeks in a phase II study.

For more information on the management of overdose or unintentional ingestion, **contact a Poison Control Center** (see *Poison Control Center Listing*).

## Patient Consultation

As an aid to patient consultation, refer to *Advice for the Patient, Saquinavir (Systemic)—Introductory Version*.

In providing consultation, consider emphasizing the following selected information (» = major clinical significance)

**Before taking this medication**
- » Conditions affecting use, especially:
    - Hypersensitivity to saquinavir
    - Breast-feeding—It is recommended that HIV-infected mothers do not breast-feed to avoid potential postnatal transmission of HIV to an uninfected infant
    - Use in children—Saquinavir has not been studied in children up to 16 years of age
    - Other medications, especially astemizole, calcium channel blocking agents, carbamazepine, cisapride, delavirdine, dexamethasone, ergot derivatives, midazolam, phenobarbital, phenytoin, quinidine, rifabutin, rifampin, ritonavir, terfenadine, triazolam, or other medications that are metabolic inducers of the cytochrome P450 enzyme system

**Proper use of this medication**
- » Importance of taking saquinavir with a meal or within 2 hours after a meal
- » Importance of not taking more medication than prescribed; importance of not discontinuing saquinavir or other antiretroviral agents without checking with physician
- » Compliance with full course of therapy
- » Importance of not missing doses and of taking at evenly spaced times
- Not sharing medication with others
- » Proper dosing
- Missed dose: Taking as soon as possible; not taking if almost time for next dose; not doubling doses
- » Proper storage

**Precautions while using this medication**
- » Because saquinavir may interact with other medications, not taking any other medications (prescription or nonprescription) without first consulting your physician
- » Regular visits to physician for blood tests and monitoring of blood glucose concentrations

**Side/adverse effects**
Signs of potential side effects, especially diabetes or hyperglycemia, ketoacidosis, paresthesia, and skin rash

## General Dosing Information

Saquinavir should be taken with a meal or within 2 hours after a meal.

## Oral Dosage Forms

Note: The dosing and strength of the dosage forms available are expressed in terms of saquinavir base.

### SAQUINAVIR SOFT GELATIN CAPSULES

**Usual adult dose**
Human immunodeficiency virus (HIV) infection—
    Oral, 1200 mg three times a day with a meal or within two hours of eating a meal, in combination with other appropriate antiretroviral agents.

**Usual pediatric dose**
Children up to 16 years of age—Safety and efficacy have not been established.

**Strength(s) usually available**
U.S.—
    200 mg (Rx) [*Fortovase*].

**Packaging and storage**
Store in a refrigerator between 2 and 8 °C (36 and 46 °F) in a tight container.

**Stability**
Capsules stored in the refrigerator remain stable until the expiration date printed on the label. Capsules that are brought to room temperature (25 °C [77 °F]) are stable for up to 3 months.

**Auxiliary labeling**
- Refrigerate.
- Continue for full time of treatment.
- Take with food.
- Do not take other medications without physician's advice.

### SAQUINAVIR MESYLATE CAPSULES

**Usual adult dose**
Human immunodeficiency virus (HIV) infection—
    Oral, 600 mg (base) three times a day within two hours after a meal, in combination with other appropriate antiretroviral agents.

**Usual pediatric dose**
Children up to 16 years of age—Safety and efficacy have not been established.

**Strength(s) usually available**
U.S.—
    200 mg (base) (Rx) [*Invirase* (lactose)].

**Packaging and storage**
Store between 15 and 30 °C (59 and 86 °F) in a tight container.

**Auxiliary labeling**
- Continue for full time of treatment.
- Take with food.
- Do not take other medications without physician's advice.

Developed: 01/27/97
Interim revision: 09/11/97; 03/30/98; 08/05/98

---

**SARGRAMOSTIM**—See *Colony Stimulating Factors (Systemic)*

---

**SCOPOLAMINE**—See *Anticholinergics/Antispasmodics (Systemic); Scopolamine (Ophthalmic)*

---

# SCOPOLAMINE Ophthalmic†

VA CLASSIFICATION (Primary): OP600
Commonly used brand name(s): *Isopto Hyoscine*.
Another commonly used name is hyoscine.

Note: For a listing of dosage forms and brand names by country availability, see *Dosage Forms* section(s).

†Not commercially available in Canada.

## Category

Cycloplegic; mydriatic.

## Indications

Note: Bracketed information in the *Indications* section refers to uses that are not included in U.S. product labeling.

**Accepted**
Refraction, cycloplegic—Scopolamine is indicated for measurement of refractive errors. Scopolamine is not useful for refraction in adults, because of its long duration of action.

Uveitis (treatment)—Scopolamine is indicated for pupil dilation and ciliary muscle relaxation, which are desirable in acute and sub-acute inflammatory conditions of the iris and uveal tract.

## Scopolamine (Ophthalmic)

[Synechiae, posterior (prophylaxis)] or
Synechiae, posterior (treatment)—Scopolamine may be indicated for pupil dilation to break posterior synechiae. In addition, scopolamine is used in the prophylaxis of posterior synechiae.

Mydriasis, postoperative—Scopolamine may be indicated for postoperative mydriasis.

Iridocyclitis, postoperative (treatment) or
Iridocyclitis, preoperative (treatment)—Scopolamine is indicated in certain preoperative and postoperative conditions when a medication having mydriatic and cycloplegic properties is required in the treatment of iridocyclitis.

[Iridocyclitis (treatment)]—Scopolamine is also used in the treatment of iridocyclitis at times other than postoperative or preoperative conditions.

Mydriasis, in diagnostic procedures—Scopolamine is indicated in diagnostic procedures to produce mydriasis.

Note: Scopolamine may be useful in patients who are allergic to atropine.

## Pharmacology/Pharmacokinetics

### Mechanism of action/Effect
Scopolamine (a belladonna alkaloid) is an anticholinergic agent that blocks the responses of the sphincter muscle of the iris and the accommodative muscle of the ciliary body to stimulation by acetylcholine. Dilation of the pupil (mydriasis) and paralysis of accommodation (cycloplegia) result.

### Duration of action
Has shorter duration of action than atropine.
Residual cycloplegia and mydriasis may persist for approximately 3 to 7 days following instillation of medication.

## Precautions to Consider

### Cross-sensitivity and/or related problems
Patients sensitive to any of the other belladonna alkaloids may be sensitive to scopolamine also.

### Pregnancy/Reproduction
Pregnancy—Problems in humans have not been documented; however, ophthalmic scopolamine may be systemically absorbed.

### Breast-feeding
Problems in humans have not been documented; however, ophthalmic scopolamine may be systemically absorbed.

### Pediatrics
An increased susceptibility to scopolamine and similar drugs (such as atropine) has been reported in infants and young children and in children with blond hair, blue eyes, Down's syndrome, spastic paralysis, or brain damage; therefore, scopolamine should be used with great caution in these patients.

### Geriatrics
Geriatric patients are more susceptible to the effects of scopolamine and similar drugs (such as atropine), thus increasing the potential for systemic side effects.

### Drug interactions and/or related problems
The following drug interactions and/or related problems have been selected on the basis of their potential clinical significance (possible mechanism in parentheses where appropriate)—not necessarily inclusive (» = major clinical significance):

Note: Combinations containing any of the following medications, depending on the amount present, may also interact with this medication.

Anticholinergics or medications with anticholinergic activity, other (See *Appendix II*)
(if significant systemic absorption of ophthalmic scopolamine occurs, concurrent use of other anticholinergics or medications with anticholinergic activity may result in potentiated anticholinergic effects)

Antiglaucoma agents, cholinergic, long-acting, ophthalmic
(concurrent use with scopolamine may antagonize the antiglaucoma and miotic actions of ophthalmic long-acting cholinergic antiglaucoma agents, such as demecarium, echothiophate, and isoflurophate; concurrent use with scopolamine may also antagonize the antiaccommodative convergence effects of these medications when they are used for the treatment of strabismus)

Antimyasthenics or
Potassium citrate or
Potassium supplements
(if significant systemic absorption of ophthalmic scopolamine occurs, concurrent use may increase the chance of toxicity and/or side effects of these systemic medications because of the anticholinergic-induced slowing of gastrointestinal motility)

Carbachol or
Physostigmine or
Pilocarpine
(concurrent use with scopolamine may interfere with the antiglaucoma action of carbachol, physostigmine, or pilocarpine. Also, concurrent use may counteract the mydriatic effect of scopolamine; this counteraction may be used to therapeutic advantage)

CNS depression–producing medications (See *Appendix II*)
(if significant systemic absorption of ophthalmic scopolamine occurs, concurrent use of medications having CNS effects, such as antiemetic agents, phenothiazines, or barbiturates, may result in opisthotonos, convulsions, coma, and extrapyramidal symptoms)

### Medical considerations/Contraindications
The medical considerations/contraindications included have been selected on the basis of their potential clinical significance (reasons given in parentheses where appropriate)—not necessarily inclusive (» = major clinical significance).

*Risk-benefit should be considered when the following medical problems exist:*

Brain damage, in children
Down's syndrome (mongolism), in children and adults
» Glaucoma, primary, or predisposition to angle closure
Keratoconus
(scopolamine may produce fixed dilated pupil)
Sensitivity to scopolamine
Spastic paralysis, in children
Synechiae between the iris and lens

## Side/Adverse Effects

Note: An increased susceptibility to scopolamine and similar drugs (such as atropine) has been reported in infants, young children, children with blond hair or blue eyes, adults and children with Down's syndrome, children with brain damage or spastic paralysis, and the elderly. This susceptibility increases the potential for systemic side effects.

Prolonged use of scopolamine may produce local irritation, resulting in follicular conjunctivitis, vascular congestion, edema, exudate, contact dermatitis, or an eczematoid dermatitis.

The following side/adverse effects have been selected on the basis of their potential clinical significance (possible signs and symptoms in parentheses where appropriate)—not necessarily inclusive:

### Those indicating need for medical attention
Symptoms of systemic absorption
*Clumsiness or unsteadiness; confusion or unusual behavior; dryness of skin; fever; flushing or redness of face; hallucinations; skin rash; slurred speech; swollen stomach in infants; tachycardia (fast or irregular heartbeat); unusual drowsiness; tiredness or weakness; xerostomia (thirst or dryness of mouth)*

### Those indicating need for medical attention only if they continue or are bothersome
*Blurred vision; eye irritation not present before therapy; increased sensitivity of eyes to light; swelling of the eyelids*

## Overdose

For specific information on the agents used in the management of ophthalmic scopolamine overdose, see:
- *Atropine* in *Anticholinergics/Antispasmodics (Systemic)* monograph;
- *Diazepam* in *Benzodiazepines (Systemic)* monograph;
- *Physostigmine (Systemic)* monograph.

For more information on the management of overdose or unintentional ingestion, **contact a Poison Control Center** (see *Poison Control Center Listing*).

### Treatment of overdose
For accidental ingestion, emesis or gastric lavage with 4% tannic acid solution is recommended.

For systemic effects, 0.2 to 1 mg (0.2 mg in children) physostigmine should be administered intravenously as a dilution containing 1 mg in 5 mL of normal saline. The solution should be injected over a period of not less than 2 minutes. Dosage may be repeated every 5 minutes up to a total dose of 2 mg in children and 6 mg in adults in each 30-minute period.

Physostigmine is contraindicated in hypotensive reactions.

ECG monitoring is recommended during physostigmine administration.

Excitement may be controlled by diazepam or a short-acting barbiturate.

It is recommended that 1 mg of atropine be available for immediate injection if the physostigmine causes bradycardia, convulsion, or bronchoconstriction.

Supportive therapy may require oxygen and assisted respiration; cool water baths for fever, especially in children; and catheterization for urinary retention. In infants and small children, the body surface should be kept moist.

## Patient Consultation

As an aid to patient consultation, refer to *Advice for the Patient, Atropine/Homatropine/Scopolamine (Ophthalmic)*.

In providing consultation, consider emphasizing the following selected information (» = major clinical significance):

**Before using this medication**
» Conditions affecting use, especially:
   Sensitivity to atropine, homatropine, or scopolamine
   Use in children—Infants and young children and children with blond hair or blue eyes may be especially sensitive to the effects of scopolamine; this may increase the chance of side effects during treatment
   Use in the elderly—Geriatric patients are more susceptible to the effects of scopolamine and similar drugs (such as atropine), thus increasing the potential for systemic side effects
   Other medical problems, especially primary glaucoma or predisposition to angle closure

**Proper use of this medication**
Proper administration technique
   Washing hands immediately after application to remove any medication that may be on them; if applying medication to infants or children, washing their hands immediately afterwards also, and not letting any medication get into their mouths; wiping off any medication that may have accidentally gotten on the infant or child, including his or her face and eyelids
   Preventing contamination: Not touching applicator tip to any surface; keeping container tightly closed
» Importance of not using more medication than the amount prescribed
» Proper dosing
   Missed dose: If dosing schedule is—
      Once a day: Applying as soon as possible if remembered same day; if remembered later, skipping missed dose and going back to regular dosing schedule; not doubling doses
      More than once a day: Applying as soon as possible; if almost time for next dose, skipping missed dose and going back to regular dosing schedule; not doubling doses
» Proper storage

**Precautions while using this medication**
» Medication causes blurred vision and increased sensitivity of the eyes to light; checking with physician if these effects continue longer than 7 days after discontinuation of scopolamine

**Side/adverse effects**
   Signs of potential side effects, especially symptoms of systemic absorption

## General Dosing Information

Scopolamine has a cycloplegic effect comparable to that of atropine.

Although some manufacturers recommend a dose of 2 drops of an ophthalmic solution at appropriate intervals, the conjunctival sac will usually hold only 1 drop.

More frequent instillation or use of a stronger concentration may be required to produce adequate cycloplegia in eyes with brown or hazel irides than in eyes with blue irides.

To avoid excessive systemic absorption, patient should press finger to the lacrimal sac during, and for 2 or 3 minutes following, instillation of the solution.

## Ophthalmic Dosage Forms

Note: Bracketed uses in the *Dosage Forms* section refer to categories of use and/or indications that are not included in U.S. product labeling.

## SCOPOLAMINE HYDROBROMIDE OPHTHALMIC SOLUTION USP

**Usual adult and adolescent dose**
Cycloplegic refraction—
   Topical, to the conjunctiva, 1 drop of a 0.25% solution one hour prior to refraction.
Uveitis—
   Topical, to the conjunctiva, 1 drop of a 0.25% solution up to four times a day, depending on the severity of the condition.
Posterior synechiae (treatment)—
   Topical, to the conjunctiva, 1 drop of a 0.25% solution every ten minutes for three applications.
   Note: To enhance the mydriatic effect of scopolamine, 1 drop of a 2.5 or 10% phenylephrine solution may be instilled every ten minutes for three applications. Extreme caution should be used if 10% phenylephrine is administered.
[Posterior synechiae (prophylaxis)]—
   Topical, to the conjunctiva, 1 drop of a 0.25% solution one or two times a day as needed to maintain mydriasis.
Postoperative mydriasis—
   Topical, to the conjunctiva, 1 drop of a 0.25% solution once a day. Administration two or three times a day may be necessary for patients with dark brown irides.
[Iridocyclitis (other than preoperative or postoperative)] or
Postoperative iridocyclitis or
Preoperative iridocyclitis—
   Topical, to the conjunctiva, 1 drop of a 0.25% solution one to four times a day as needed to maintain mydriasis, the dose being decreased as the severity of the inflammation decreases.
Mydriasis in diagnostic procedures—
   Topical, to the conjunctiva, 1 drop of a 0.25% solution as needed to maintain mydriasis.

**Usual pediatric dose**
Cycloplegic refraction—
   Topical, to the conjunctiva, 1 drop of a 0.25% solution two times a day for two days prior to refraction.
Uveitis—
   Topical, to the conjunctiva, 1 drop of a 0.25% solution up to four times a day, depending on the severity of the condition and the size and weight of the child.
[Posterior synechiae (prophylaxis)]—
   See *Usual adult and adolescent dose*.
[Iridocyclitis (other than preoperative or postoperative)] or
Postoperative iridocyclitis or
Preoperative iridocyclitis—
   See *Usual adult and adolescent dose*.
   Note: The pediatric dose should be individualized based on the age and weight of the child as well as the severity of the inflammation.
Mydriasis in diagnostic procedures—
   See *Usual adult and adolescent dose*.

**Strength(s) usually available**
U.S.—
   0.25% (Rx) [*Isopto Hyoscine* (benzalkonium chloride 0.01%)].
Canada—
   Not commercially available.

**Packaging and storage**
Store below 40 °C (104 °F), preferably between 15 and 30 °C (59 and 86 °F), unless otherwise specified by manufacturer. Store in a tight container. Protect from freezing. Protect from light.

**Auxiliary labeling**
• For the eye.
• Keep container tightly closed.

Revised: 06/21/94

## SECOBARBITAL—See *Barbiturates (Systemic)*

# SELEGILINE Systemic

VA CLASSIFICATION (Primary): CN500

Commonly used brand name(s): *Apo-Selegiline; Carbex; Eldepryl; Gen-Selegiline; Novo-Selegiline; Nu-Selegiline; SD Deprenyl; Selegiline-5.*

Other commonly used names are deprenil and deprenyl.

Note: For a listing of dosage forms and brand names by country availability, see *Dosage Forms* section(s).

## Category
Antidyskinetic.

## Indications

Note: Bracketed information in the *Indications* section refers to uses that are not included in U.S. product labeling.

**Accepted**

Parkinsonism (treatment adjunct)—Selegiline is indicated for use with levodopa or levodopa and carbidopa combination in the treatment of idiopathic Parkinson's disease (paralysis agitans).

[Some studies have suggested that the initial use of selegiline may delay the need for addition of levodopa to the treatment regimen; in addition, these studies have shown that selegiline alone or in combination with levodopa may slow the progression of Parkinson's disease, possibly by preventing selective destruction of dopaminergic neurons in the substantia nigra. One retrospective study showed selegiline to possibly prolong the life span of patients with idiopathic Parkinson's disease.]

[The addition of selegiline to levodopa in patients experiencing fluctuating responses ("wearing off" effect or "on-off" phenomenon) may be of moderate benefit. However, the initial response to selegiline may not be sustained, with the degree of improvement declining over 6 months to 4 years. Selegiline is ineffective in advanced disease with extreme fluctuations. Motor control fluctuations may be due to factors other than the central pharmacokinetics of dopamine; hence prolongation of dopamine effects may fail in some cases to improve this problem.]

Note: Preliminary studies have demonstrated that selegiline may be useful as an antidepressant, usually when given in doses greater than those used for its antidyskinetic effect. However, there are *insufficient data* to definitively establish effectiveness of selegiline and criteria for its use in mental depression.

## Pharmacology/Pharmacokinetics

**Physicochemical characteristics**
Molecular weight—223.75.

**Mechanism of action/Effect**

The action of selegiline is thought to be related to its irreversible inhibition of monoamine oxidase type B (MAO B), the major form of the enzyme in the human brain. MAO B, which is involved in the oxidative deamination of dopamine in the brain, is inhibited when selegiline binds covalently and stoichiometrically to the isoalloxazine flavin adenine dinucleotide (FAD) at its active center. Administration of 10 mg of selegiline a day produces almost complete inhibition of MAO B in the brain. Selegiline becomes a nonselective inhibitor of all monoamine oxidase (MAO) at higher doses, possibly at 20 to 40 mg a day. At these doses, tyramine-mediated hypertensive reactions from MAO A blockade ("cheese reactions") may occur.

Selegiline (or its metabolites) may also act through other mechanisms to increase dopaminergic activity, including interfering with dopamine re-uptake at the synapse.

**Absorption**
Rapidly absorbed from the gastrointestinal tract.

**Distribution**
Crosses the blood-brain barrier.

**Biotransformation**
Rapidly and completely metabolized to *N*-desmethyldeprenyl, l-methamphetamine, and l-amphetamine.

**Half-life**
The mean half-lives of the 3 active metabolites that were found in serum and urine following a single dose of selegiline are as follows—
  *N*-desmethyldeprenyl: 2 hours.
  l-amphetamine: 17.7 hours.
  l-methamphetamine: 20.5 hours.
Elimination—
  Selegiline: 39 (range, 16 to 69) hours.

**Time to peak plasma concentration**
0.5 to 2 hours.

**Duration of action**
Duration of clinical action depends on the regeneration time of MAO B.

**Elimination**
Renal; slow. 45% of a 10 mg dose appears in the urine as metabolites (*N*-desmethyldeprenyl, l-amphetamine, and l-methamphetamine) within 48 hours of ingestion.

## Precautions to Consider

**Carcinogenicity**
Long-term animal studies have revealed no evidence of carcinogenic effects.

**Pregnancy/Reproduction**
Pregnancy—Studies in humans have not been done.
Studies in animals have not shown that selegiline causes adverse effects on the fetus. Reproduction studies in rats and rabbits given approximately 250 and 350 times the comparable human dose, respectively, have revealed no evidence of teratogenic effects.
FDA Pregnancy Category C.

**Breast-feeding**
It is not known whether selegiline is excreted in breast milk.

**Pediatrics**
No published pediatrics-specific information is available. Safety and efficacy have not been established.

**Geriatrics**
No geriatrics-related problems have been documented in studies done to date that included elderly patients.

**Dental**
Selegiline may decrease or inhibit salivary flow, thus contributing to the development of caries, periodontal disease, oral candidiasis, and discomfort.

**Drug interactions and/or related problems**
The following drug interactions and/or related problems have been selected on the basis of their potential clinical significance (possible mechanism in parentheses where appropriate)—not necessarily inclusive (» = major clinical significance):

Note: Combinations containing any of the following medications, depending on the amount present, may also interact with this medication.

*For all doses of selegiline*
» Antidepressants, tricyclic
  (asystole, diaphoresis, hypertension, syncope, changes in behavior and mental status, impaired consciousness, hyperpyrexia, seizures, muscular rigidity, and tremors have occurred with concurrent use of selegiline and tricyclic antidepressants. Concurrent use is not recommended; at least 14 days should elapse between discontinuation of selegiline and initiation of a tricyclic antidepressant)

» Fluoxetine or
» Fluvoxamine or
» Nefazodone or
» Paroxetine or
» Sertraline or
» Venlafaxine
  (a reaction resembling the serotonin syndrome has been reported rarely following concurrent use of selegiline with selective serotonin re-uptake inhibitors (SSRIs). [The serotonin syndrome may occur as the result of combining a serotonergic agent with an MAO inhibitor. The syndrome may be manifest by mental status changes (confusion, hypomania), restlessness, myoclonus, hyperreflexia, diaphoresis, shivering, tremor, diarrhea, incoordination, and/or fever. If recognized early, the syndrome usually resolves quickly upon withdrawal of the offending agents.] Concurrent use of selegiline with SSRIs is not recommended because of the potential for autonomic instability, muscular rigidity, severe agitation, or delirium. At least 14 days should elapse between discontinuation of an MAO inhibitor and initiation of an SSRI. However, because of the long half-lives of fluoxetine and its active metabolite, at least 5 weeks [approximately 5 half-lives] should elapse between discontinuation of fluoxetine and initiation of therapy with an MAO inhibitor. Also, based on the half-life of venlafaxine, at least 7 days should elapse between discontinuation of venlafaxine and initiation of therapy with an MAO inhibitor.)

Levodopa
(although selegiline is used in conjunction with levodopa, it may enhance levodopa-induced dyskinesias, nausea, orthostatic hypotension, confusion, and hallucinations; reduction of levodopa dosage may be necessary within 2 to 3 days after the initiation of selegiline therapy)

» Meperidine, and possibly other opioid (narcotic) analgesics
(at least one interaction of meperidine with selegiline has been reported; concurrent use of meperidine with nonselective monoamine oxidase inhibitors [MAOIs] may produce immediate excitation, sweating, rigidity, and severe hypertension; in some patients, hypotension, severe respiratory depression, coma, convulsions, hyperpyrexia, vascular collapse, and death may occur; avoidance of meperidine use within 2 to 3 weeks following MAO inhibition is recommended; other opioid analgesics such as morphine are not likely to cause such severe reactions and may be used cautiously in reduced dosage in patients receiving MAOIs; however, it is recommended that a small test dose [one quarter of the usual dose] or several small incremental test doses over a period of several hours should first be administered to permit observation of any adverse effects; caution is also recommended in the use of alfentanil, fentanyl, or sufentanil as an adjunct to anesthesia if the patient has received an MAOI within 14 days; because the risk of a significant interaction has been questioned, the use of a small test dose is advised to detect any possible interaction)

*For doses of 20 mg or more of selegiline per day*
» Tyramine- or other high pressor amine–containing foods and beverages, such as aged cheese; fava or broad bean pods; yeast/protein extracts; smoked or pickled meats, poultry, or fish; fermented sausage (bologna, pepperoni, salami, summer sausage) or other fermented meat; sauerkraut; any overripe fruit; beer; reduced-alcohol and alcohol-free beer and wine; red and white wines; sherry; and liqueurs
(concurrent use with MAOIs, including selegiline in doses of 20 mg a day or greater, may cause sudden and severe hypertensive reactions; reactions are usually limited to a few hours and are easily treated with rapidly acting hypotensive agents [such as labetalol, nifedipine, or, if necessary in severe cases refractory to other agents, phentolamine]; severity of reaction depends on amount of tyramine ingested, rate of gastric emptying, and length of interval between dose of MAOI and ingestion of tyramine; when MAOIs are discontinued, dietary restrictions must continue for at least 2 weeks; other tyramine- or high pressor amine–containing foods, such as yogurt, sour cream, cream cheese, cottage cheese, chocolate, and soy sauce, if eaten when fresh and in moderation, are considered unlikely to cause serious problems)

### Medical considerations/Contraindications
The medical considerations/contraindications included have been selected on the basis of their potential clinical significance (reasons given in parentheses where appropriate)—not necessarily inclusive (» = major clinical significance).

*Risk-benefit should be considered when the following medical problems exist:*

Dementia, profound or
Psychosis, severe or
Tardive dyskinesia or
Tremor, excessive
(condition may be exacerbated)

» Peptic ulcer disease, history of
(activation of pre-existing ulcers may occur, probably due to stimulation of the H₂receptors in the stomach or inhibition of MAO-mediated gastric histamine catabolism)

Sensitivity to selegiline

### Side/Adverse Effects
Note: Selegiline enhances the dose-related side effects of levodopa, but few side effects are attributable to selegiline itself. When selegiline is used as an adjunct to levodopa or levodopa and carbidopa combination, adverse effects can usually be ameliorated by reducing the dose of levodopa or levodopa and carbidopa.

In addition, selegiline may cause elevation of liver enzymes.

The following side/adverse effects have been selected on the basis of their potential clinical significance (possible signs and symptoms in parentheses where appropriate)—not necessarily inclusive:

### Those indicating need for medical attention
Incidence more frequent
*Dyskinesias* (increase in unusual movements of body); *mood or other mental changes*

Incidence less frequent or rare
*Angina pectoris, new or increased* (chest pain); *arrhythmias* (irregular heartbeat); *asthma* (wheezing, difficulty in breathing, or tightness in chest); *bradycardia, sinus* (slow heartbeat); *edema, peripheral* (swelling of feet or lower legs); *motor/coordination/extrapyramidal effects* (difficulty in speaking; loss of balance control; uncontrolled movements, especially of face, neck, and back; restlessness or desire to keep moving; twisting movements of body); *gastrointestinal bleeding* (bloody or black, tarry stools; severe stomach pain; vomiting of blood or material that looks like coffee grounds); *hallucinations; headache, severe; hypertension, severe; orthostatic hypotension* (dizziness or lightheadedness, especially when getting up from a lying or sitting position); *prostatic hypertrophy* (difficult or frequent urination); *tardive dyskinesia* (lip smacking or puckering; puffing of cheeks; rapid or worm-like movements of tongue; uncontrolled chewing movements; uncontrolled movements of arms and legs)

Symptoms of hypertensive crisis
*Chest pain, severe; enlarged pupils; fast or slow heartbeat; headache, severe; increased sensitivity of eyes to light; increased sweating, possibly with fever or cold, clammy skin; nausea or vomiting, severe; stiff or sore neck*

### Those indicating need for medical attention only if they continue or are bothersome
Incidence more frequent
*Abdominal or stomach pain; dizziness or feeling faint; dryness of mouth; insomnia* (trouble in sleeping); *nausea or vomiting*

Incidence less frequent or rare
*Anxiety, nervousness, or restlessness; apraxia, increased* (inability to move); *blepharospasm* (sudden closing of eyelids); *blurred or double vision; body ache or back or leg pain; bradykinesia, increased* (slowed movements); *chills; constipation or diarrhea; diaphoresis* (increased sweating); *drowsiness; headache; heartburn; hypertension or hypotension* (high or low blood pressure); *impaired memory*—more frequent with doses greater than 10 mg a day; *slow or difficult urination; frequent urge to urinate; irritability, temporary; loss of appetite or weight loss; muscle cramps or numbness of fingers or toes; palpitations or tachycardia* (pounding or fast heartbeat); *paresthesias, circumoral* (burning of lips or mouth); *or burning of throat; photosensitivity* (increased sensitivity of skin and eyes to sunlight); *skin rash; tinnitus* (ringing or buzzing in ears); *taste changes; unusual feeling of well-being; unusual tiredness or weakness*

With doses greater than 10 mg a day
*Bruxism* (clenching, gnashing, or grinding teeth); *muscle twitches or myoclonic jerks* (sudden jerky movements of body)

Note: *Bruxism* and *myoclonic jerks* may be considered to be adverse effects only if not previously present and beginning shortly after the start of therapy with selegiline.

## Overdose
For specific information in the agents used in the management of selegiline overdose, see:
• *Charcoal, Activated (Oral-Local)* monograph.

For more information on the management of overdose of unintentional ingestion, **contact a Poison Control Center** (see *Poison Control Center Listing*).

### Clinical effects of overdose
No specific information is available regarding overdoses with selegiline. Since overdose is likely to cause significant inhibition of both MAO type A and type B, symptoms of overdose may resemble those of nonselective MAO inhibitors.

Symptoms of MAOI overdose
*Agitation or irritability; chest pain; convulsions; cool, clammy skin; diaphoresis* (increased sweating); *dizziness, severe, or fainting; fast or irregular pulse, continuing; high or low blood pressure; hyperpyrexia* (high fever); *opisthotonus* (severe spasm where the head and heels are bent backward and the body arched forward); *respiratory depression* (troubled breathing); *trismus* (difficulty opening the mouth; lockjaw)

Note: Symptoms resulting from overdose may be absent or minimal for nearly 12 hours after ingestion, and develop slowly thereafter, reaching a maximum in 24 to 48 hours. Death has resulted. Immediate hospitalization and close monitoring of patient is essential during this period.

### Treatment of overdose
Treatment may include the following:
To decrease absorption—
Induction of emesis or gastric lavage with protected airway followed by instillation of charcoal slurry in early overdose.

**Specific treatment—**
  Treatment of signs and symptoms of central nervous system (CNS) stimulation with diazepam, administered intravenously and slowly. Phenothiazine derivatives should be avoided.
  Treatment of hypotension and vascular collapse with intravenous fluids and, if necessary, a dilute pressor agent. Adrenergic agents may produce a markedly increased pressor response.
  Vigorous treatment of hyperpyrexia with antipyretics and a cooling blanket.
**Monitoring—**
  Close monitoring of body temperature.
**Supportive care—**
  Maintenance of fluid and electrolyte balance.
  Support of respiration by management of the airway, and mechanical ventilation with the use of supplemental oxygen, as required.
  Patients in whom intentional overdose is confirmed or suspected should be referred for psychiatric consultation.

## Patient Consultation

As an aid to patient consultation, refer to *Advice for the Patient, Selegiline (Systemic)*.

In providing consultation, consider emphasizing the following selected information (» = major clinical significance):

**Before using this medication**
» Conditions affecting use, especially:
  Sensitivity to selegiline
  Other medications, especially fluoxetine, fluvoxamine, meperidine and possibly other narcotic (opioid) analgesics, nefazodone, paroxetine, sertraline, tricyclic antidepressants, or venlafaxine
  Other medical problems, especially a history of peptic ulcer disease

**Proper use of this medication**
» Importance of not taking more medication than the amount prescribed; to do so may increase the risk of side effects
  Missed dose: Taking as soon as possible; not taking in the late afternoon or evening; not taking if almost time for next dose; not doubling doses.
» Proper storage

**Precautions while using this medication**
» If taking 20 mg or more of selegiline a day, avoiding tyramine-containing foods, alcoholic beverages, and large quantities of caffeine-containing beverages, over-the-counter cold and cough medicines, and other medications, unless prescribed
» Checking with hospital emergency room or physician if symptoms of hypertensive crisis develop
» Possibility of orthostatic hypotension; caution when getting up suddenly from a lying or sitting position
  Possible dryness of mouth; using sugarless candy or gum, ice, or saliva substitute for relief; checking with physician or dentist if dryness of mouth continues for more than 2 weeks

**Side/adverse effects**
Signs of potential side effects, especially dyskinesias, mood or mental changes, angina pectoris, arrhythmias, asthma, bradycardia, peripheral edema, extrapyramidal effects, hallucinations, severe headache, severe hypertension, gastrointestinal bleeding, orthostatic hypotension, prostatic hypertrophy, and tardive dyskinesia

## General Dosing Information

Selegiline should not be used in the treatment of Parkinson's disease at doses exceeding 10 mg a day because of the risks associated with non-selective inhibition of monoamine oxidase (MAO). A tyramine-mediated hypertensive reaction has been reported when selegiline was administered at a dose of 20 mg a day. In addition, selegiline in doses greater than 10 mg a day has not demonstrated increased effectiveness in the treatment of Parkinson's disease.

When selegiline is used as an adjunct to levodopa or levodopa and carbidopa combination, adverse effects such as involuntary movements or hallucinations may result, and doses of levodopa may need to be reduced. If necessary, doses of levodopa should be reduced after 2 to 3 days by 10 to 30%, and possibly by as much as 50% with continued therapy.

Because selegiline may produce insomnia, it should not be administered in the late afternoon or evening.

**Diet/Nutrition**
Selegiline should be administered with breakfast and lunch to minimize possible nausea and insomnia.

When monoamine oxidase inhibitors, including selegiline at doses of 20 mg a day or greater, are used concurrently with foods and beverages containing tyramine or other high pressor amines, sudden and severe hypertensive reactions may result. These reactions are usually limited to a few hours and are easily treated with rapidly acting hypotensive agents (such as labetalol, nifedipine, or, if necessary in severe cases refractory to other agents, phentolamine). The severity of the reaction depends on the amount of tyramine ingested, the rate of gastric emptying, and the length of the interval between the dose of MAO inhibitor and ingestion of tyramine. When MAO inhibitors are discontinued, dietary restrictions must continue for at least 2 weeks. Foods and beverages containing tyramine or other high pressor amines include aged cheese; fava or broad bean pods; yeast/protein extracts; smoked or pickled meats, poultry, or fish; fermented sausage (bologna, pepperoni, salami, summer sausage) or other fermented meat; sauerkraut; any over-ripe fruit; beer; reduced-alcohol and alcohol-free beer and wine; red and white wines; sherry; and liqueurs. Other foods, such as yogurt, sour cream, cream cheese, cottage cheese, chocolate, and soy sauce, if eaten when fresh and in moderation, are considered unlikely to cause serious problems.

## Oral Dosage Forms

### SELEGILINE HYDROCHLORIDE CAPSULES

**Usual adult dose**
Parkinsonism—
  Oral, 5 mg two times a day, at breakfast and lunch.
Note: In some cases, some clinicians recommend that the total daily dose be divided (2.5 mg four times a day) to decrease the side effects induced by concomitant administration of levodopa.

**Usual pediatric dose**
Safety and efficacy have not been established.

**Usual geriatric dose**
See *Usual adult dose*.

**Strength(s) usually available**
U.S.—
  5 mg (Rx) [*Eldepryl*].
Canada—
  Not commercially available.

**Packaging and storage**
Store below 40 °C (104 °F), preferably between 15 and 30 °C (59 and 86 °F), in a well-closed container, unless otherwise specified by manufacturer.

**Auxiliary labeling**
• Avoid alcoholic beverages.

### SELEGILINE HYDROCHLORIDE TABLETS USP

**Usual adult dose**
See *Selegiline Hydrochloride Capsules*.

**Usual pediatric dose**
See *Selegiline Hydrochloride Capsules*.

**Usual geriatric dose**
See *Selegiline Hydrochloride Capsules*.

**Strength(s) usually available**
U.S.—
  5 mg (Rx) [*Carbex*; GENERIC].
Canada—
  5 mg (Rx) [*Apo-Selegiline; Eldepryl; Gen-Selegiline; Novo-Selegiline; Nu-Selegiline; SD Deprenyl; Selegiline-5*].

**Packaging and storage**
Store below 40 °C (104 °F), preferably between 15 and 30 °C (59 and 86 °F), in a well-closed container, unless otherwise specified by manufacturer.

**Auxiliary labeling**
• Avoid alcoholic beverages.

## Selected Bibliography

Yahr MD. R-(—)-Deprenyl and parkinsonism. J Neural Transm 1987; 25(Suppl): 5-12.
Golbe LI. Deprenyl as symptomatic therapy in Parkinson's disease. Clin Neuropharmacol 1988 Oct; 11(5): 387-400.

Revised: 09/30/92
Interim revision: 08/20/96; 01/21/98

---

**SELENIOUS ACID**—See *Selenium Supplements (Systemic)*

USP DI                                                                                                                                    Selenium    2563

**SELENIUM**—See *Selenium Supplements (Systemic)*

**SELENIUM SULFIDE**—The *Selenium Sulfide (Topical)* monograph is not included in this published version of the USP DI database. Copies of the monograph are available on request from Micromedex, Inc. - Reprint Requests, 6200 S. Syracuse Way, Suite 300, Englewood, CO 80111; telephone (303) 486-6400; telefax (303) 486-6464; Email: USPDI@MDX.COM.

# SELENIUM SUPPLEMENTS   Systemic

This monograph includes information on the following: 1) Selenious Acid†; 2) Selenium.

VA CLASSIFICATION (Primary): TN499

Commonly used brand name(s): Sele-Pak[1]; Selepen[1].

Note:   For a listing of dosage forms and brand names by country availability, see *Dosage Forms* section(s).

†Not commercially available in Canada.

## Category
Nutritional supplement (mineral).

## Indications
**Accepted**

Selenium deficiency (prophylaxis and treatment)—Selenium supplements are indicated in the prevention and treatment of selenium deficiency, which may result from inadequate nutrition or intestinal malabsorption, but does not occur in healthy individuals receiving an adequate balanced diet. For prophylaxis of selenium deficiency, dietary improvement, rather than supplementation, is advisable. For treatment of selenium deficiency, supplementation is preferred.

Deficiency of selenium may lead to lightening in color of the fingernail beds, muscle discomfort or weakness, and cardiomyopathy.

Clinical deficiencies of selenium in the U.S. are rare. Selenium supplements may be necessary in Keshan disease, a form of selenium deficiency that has been reported in areas of the world in which the soil is poor in selenium.

Some unusual diets (e.g., reducing diets that drastically restrict food selection) may not supply minimum daily requirements of selenium. Supplementation may be necessary in patients receiving total parenteral nutrition (TPN) or undergoing rapid weight loss or in those with malnutrition, because of inadequate dietary intake.

Recommended intakes for all vitamins and most minerals are increased during pregnancy. Many physicians recommend that pregnant women receive multivitamin and mineral supplements, especially those pregnant women who do not consume an adequate diet and those in high-risk categories (i.e., women carrying more than one fetus, heavy cigarette smokers, and alcohol and drug abusers). However, taking excessive amounts of multivitamin and mineral supplements may be harmful to the mother and/or fetus and should be avoided.

Recommended intakes for most vitamins and minerals are increased during breast-feeding.

**Acceptance not established**

There are insufficient data to show that selenium may reduce the occurrence of certain types of *cancer*.

## Pharmacology/Pharmacokinetics

**Physicochemical characteristics**
Molecular weight—
   Elemental selenium: 78.96.
   Selenious acid: 128.97.

**Mechanism of action/Effect**
Selenium is necessary for the enzyme glutathione peroxidase, which facilitates the lowering of tissue peroxide levels in the body by destroying hydrogen peroxide. There is an overlap in action of selenium and vitamin E in that both are responsible for lowering tissue peroxide levels.

**Absorption**
Readily absorbed.

**Storage**
Selenium is stored primarily in red cells, liver, spleen, heart, nails, and tooth enamel, but also in testes and sperm.

**Elimination**
Primarily in urine; to a lesser extent in the feces.

## Precautions to Consider

**Pregnancy/Reproduction**

Pregnancy—Adequate and well controlled studies in humans have not been done and problems in humans have not been documented with intake of normal daily recommended amounts.

High doses of selenium (15 to 30 micrograms per egg) have been found to cause adverse embryological effects in chickens.

FDA Pregnancy Category C (parenteral selenium).

**Breast-feeding**
Problems in humans have not been documented with intake of normal daily recommended amounts.

**Pediatrics**
Problems in pediatrics have not been documented with intake of normal daily recommended amounts.

Selenium injection that contains benzyl alcohol as a preservative should not be used in newborn and immature infants. The use of benzyl alcohol in neonates has been associated with a fatal toxic syndrome consisting of metabolic acidosis and central nervous system (CNS), respiratory, circulatory, and renal function impairment.

**Geriatrics**
Problems in geriatrics have not been documented with intake of normal daily recommended amounts.

**Medical considerations/Contraindications**
The medical considerations/contraindications included have been selected on the basis of their potential clinical significance (reasons given in parentheses where appropriate)—not necessarily inclusive (» = major clinical significance).

*Risk-benefit should be considered when the following medical problems exist:*
   Gastrointestinal disease and
   Renal function impairment
      (may cause high levels of selenium; reduction of dosage may be necessary)

**Patient monitoring**
The following may be especially important in patient monitoring (other tests may be warranted in some patients, depending on condition; » = major clinical significance):
   Selenium, plasma
      (weekly plasma selenium monitoring may be recommended by some clinicians for patients receiving short-term total parenteral nutrition [TPN]; monthly monitoring may be recommended with long-term use.)

## Overdose
For more information on the management of overdose or unintentional ingestion, **contact a Poison Control Center** (see *Poison Control Center Listing*).

**Clinical effects of overdose**
Symptoms of overdose
   *Dermatitis* (itching of skin); *diarrhea; fingernail weakening; garlic odor of breath and sweat; hair loss; irritability; metallic taste; nausea and vomiting; unusual tiredness and weakness*

## Patient Consultation
As an aid to patient consultation, refer to *Advice for the Patient, Selenium Supplements (Systemic)*.

In providing consultation, consider emphasizing the following selected information (» = major clinical significance):

**Description of use**
   Description should include function in the body, signs of deficiency, conditions that may cause deficiency of selenium

**Importance of diet**
- Importance of proper nutrition; supplement may be needed because of inadequate dietary intake
- Food sources of selenium
- Recommended daily intake for selenium

**Proper use of this dietary supplement**
» Proper dosing
- Missed dose: No cause for concern because of length of time necessary for depletion; remembering to take as directed
» Proper storage

## General Dosing Information

Because of the infrequency of selenium deficiency alone, combinations of selenium with several vitamins and/or minerals are commonly administered. Many commercial vitamin-mineral complexes are available.

**For parenteral dosage forms only**
In most cases, parenteral administration is indicated only when oral administration is not acceptable (for example, in nausea, vomiting, preoperative and postoperative conditions) or possible (for example, in malabsorption syndromes or following gastric resection).

**Diet/Nutrition**
Recommended dietary intakes for selenium are defined differently worldwide.
For U.S.—
  The Recommended Dietary Allowances (RDAs) for vitamins and minerals are determined by the Food and Nutrition Board of the National Research Council and are intended to provide adequate nutrition in most healthy persons under usual environmental stresses. In addition, a different designation may be used by the FDA for food and dietary supplement labeling purposes, as with Daily Value (DV). DV replaces the previous labeling terminology United States Recommended Daily Allowances (USRDAs).
For Canada—
  Recommended Nutrient Intakes (RNIs) for vitamins, minerals, and protein are determined by Health and Welfare Canada and provide recommended amounts of a specific nutrient while minimizing the risk of chronic diseases.
  Daily recommended intakes for selenium are generally defined as follows:
    Infants and children—
      Birth to 3 years: 10 to 20 mcg.
      4 to 6 years: 20 mcg.
      7 to 10 years: 30 mcg.
    Adolescent and adult males—
      40 to 70 mcg.
    Adolescent and adult females—
      45 to 55 mcg.
    Pregnant females—
      65 mcg.
    Lactating females—
      75 mcg.
The best sources of selenium include grains (depending on selenium content of soil), seafood, liver, and lean red meat.

---

### SELENIOUS ACID

## Parenteral Dosage Forms
### SELENIOUS ACID INJECTION USP

**Usual adult and adolescent dose**
Deficiency (treatment)—
  Intravenous, 100 mcg a day of elemental selenium for 24 to 31 days, added to total parenteral nutrition (TPN).
Deficiency (prophylaxis)—
  Intravenous, 20 to 40 mcg of elemental selenium a day, added to total parenteral nutrition (TPN).

**Usual pediatric dose**
Deficiency (prophylaxis and treatment)—
  Intravenous, 3 mcg of elemental selenium per kilogram of body weight a day, added to total parenteral nutrition (TPN).

Note: Selenium injection that contains benzyl alcohol as a preservative should not be used in newborn and immature infants. The use of benzyl alcohol in neonates has been associated with a fatal toxic syndrome consisting of metabolic acidosis and CNS, respiratory, circulatory, and renal function impairment.

**Strength(s) usually available**
U.S.—
  40 mcg elemental selenium per mL (Rx) [*Sele-Pak* (0.9% benzyl alcohol); *Selepen* (0.9% benzyl alcohol); GENERIC].
Canada—
  Not commercially available.

**Packaging and storage**
Store below 40 °C (104 °F), preferably between 15 and 30 °C (59 and 86 °F), unless otherwise specified by manufacturer.

**Preparation of dosage form**
Selenious acid is compatible with amino acids, dextrose, electrolytes, and other trace elements usually used for total parenteral nutrition (TPN).

---

### SELENIUM

## Oral Dosage Forms
### SELENIUM TABLETS

**Usual adult and adolescent dose**
Deficiency (prophylaxis)—Oral, amount based on normal daily recommended intakes—
  Adolescent and adult males—40 to 70 mcg.
  Adolescent and adult females—45 to 55 mcg.
  Pregnant females—65 mcg.
  Lactating females—75 mcg.
Deficiency (treatment)—
  Treatment dose is individualized by prescriber based on severity of deficiency.

**Usual pediatric dose**
Deficiency (prophylaxis)—Oral, amount based on normal daily recommended intakes—
  Birth to 3 years of age—10 to 20 mcg.
  4 to 6 years of age—20 mcg.
  7 to 10 years of age—30 mcg.
Deficiency (treatment)—
  Treatment dose is individualized by prescriber based on severity of deficiency.

**Strength(s) usually available**
U.S.—
  50 mcg elemental selenium (OTC) [GENERIC (yeast)].
  100 mcg elemental selenium (OTC) [GENERIC].
  200 mcg elemental selenium (OTC) [GENERIC].
Canada—
  50 mcg elemental selenium (OTC) [GENERIC (yeast)].
  100 mcg elemental selenium (OTC) [GENERIC (yeast)].
  Note: Some strengths of these selenium preparations may exceed the dosage range recommended by USP DI Advisory Panels based on the amount necessary to meet normal nutritional needs.

**Packaging and storage**
Store below 40 °C (104 °F), preferably between 15 and 30 °C (59 and 86 °F), unless otherwise specified by manufacturer.

Revised: 04/16/92
Interim revision: 06/06/92; 08/15/94; 05/01/95

---

**SENNA**—See *Laxatives (Local)*

---

**SENNOSIDES**—See *Laxatives (Local)*

# SERMORELIN Systemic—INTRODUCTORY VERSION

VA CLASSIFICATION (Primary): HS900
Commonly used brand name(s): *Geref.*

Note: For a listing of dosage forms and brand names by country availability, see *Dosage Forms* section(s).

## Category

Growth hormone–releasing hormone.

## Indications

**Accepted**

Growth hormone deficiency (treatment)—Sermorelin is indicated for treatment of idiopathic growth hormone deficiency in prepubertal children with growth failure. These patients are expected to retain pituitary responsiveness to growth hormone–releasing hormone. Treatment should be initiated at a bone age of 7.5 years or less in females and 8 years or less in males.

Note: The effect of treatment with sermorelin on final adult height has not been determined.

Sermorelin has not been studied in, and therefore is not recommended for treatment of, patients with growth hormone deficiency secondary to an intracranial lesion.

## Pharmacology/Pharmacokinetics

**Physicochemical characteristics**

Source—Synthetic. Sermorelin acetate is the acetate salt of an amidated synthetic 29–amino acid peptide (GRF 1-29 NH$_2$) that corresponds to the amino-terminal segment of the naturally occurring human growth hormone–releasing hormone (GHRH or GRF) that consists of 44 amino acid residues.

Molecular weight—Sermorelin: 3358 daltons.

pH—5 to 5.5 (after reconstitution with sodium chloride injection).

**Mechanism of action/Effect**

Like naturally occurring GHRH, sermorelin stimulates the pituitary gland to release growth hormone, resulting in an increase in the concentration of growth hormone in the plasma.

**Absorption**

The mean absolute bioavailability was approximately 6% following a subcutaneous dose of 2 mg administered to healthy volunteers.

**Distribution**

The mean volume of distribution ranged from 23.7 to 25.8 L following intravenous doses of 0.25 to 1 mg administered to healthy volunteers.

**Half-life**

11 to 12 minutes following intravenous or subcutaneous administration.

**Time to peak concentration**

5 to 20 minutes following a subcutaneous dose of 2 mg to healthy volunteers.

**Elimination**

Rapidly cleared from the circulation at a rate of 2.4 to 2.8 L per minute in adults.

## Precautions to Consider

**Carcinogenicity**

Long-term animal studies to determine the carcinogenic potential of sermorelin have not been done.

**Mutagenicity**

No evidence of mutagenicity has been found in studies done to date.

**Pregnancy/Reproduction**

Pregnancy—Adequate and well-controlled studies have not been done in humans.

Studies in rats and rabbits at doses of 0.5 mg per kg of body weight per day (three and six times the daily human dose based on body surface area, respectively) produced minor variations in the fetuses.

FDA Pregnancy Category C.

**Breast-feeding**

It is not known whether sermorelin is distributed into breast milk.

**Drug interactions and/or related problems**

The following drug interactions and/or related problems have been selected on the basis of their potential clinical significance (possible mechanism in parentheses where appropriate)—not necessarily inclusive (» = major clinical significance):

Note: Combinations containing any of the following medications, depending on the amount present, may also interact with this medication.

» Corticosteroids, glucocorticoid
(concurrent use may inhibit the response to sermorelin)

**Laboratory value alterations**

The following have been selected on the basis of their potential clinical significance (possible effect in parentheses where appropriate)—not necessarily inclusive (» = major clinical significance):

With physiology/laboratory test values
  Alkaline phosphatase
    (values may be increased)
  Insulin-like growth factor 1 (IGF-1) and
  Phosphorus, inorganic
    (concentrations may be increased)

**Medical considerations/Contraindications**

The medical considerations/contraindications included have been selected on the basis of their potential clinical significance (reasons given in parentheses where appropriate)—not necessarily inclusive (» = major clinical significance):

*Risk-benefit should be considered when the following medical problems exist:*

» Hypothyroidism
  (untreated hypothyroidism can impair the response to sermorelin)
Sensitivity to sermorelin

**Patient monitoring**

The following may be especially important in patient monitoring (other tests may be warranted in some patients, depending on condition; » = major clinical significance):

» Bone age
  (determinations recommended periodically during treatment, especially in patients who have reached puberty and/or are receiving concomitant thyroid replacement therapy; in these patients, epiphyseal maturation may progress rapidly)
» Height
  (determinations recommended at least every 6 months during treatment)
» Thyroid function
  (determinations recommended prior to, and periodically during, treatment because untreated hypothyroidism can impair the response to sermorelin)

## Side/Adverse Effects

Note: Many patients develop antibodies to growth hormone–releasing hormone at least once during treatment with sermorelin. However, the significance of these antibodies is not known. Their presence does not appear to affect growth, nor do they cause specific side effects. In addition, a positive test for antibodies at one growth assessment may become negative by the next assessment.

No generalized allergic reactions have been reported with sermorelin therapy.

Intravenous administration for diagnostic purposes has been associated with flushing of the face; headache; injection site pain, redness, and/or swelling; nausea; pallor; parageusia; tightness in the chest; and vomiting.

The following side/adverse effects have been selected on the basis of their potential clinical significance (possible signs and symptoms in parentheses where appropriate)—not necessarily inclusive:

**Those indicating need for medical attention**
Incidence more frequent
  *Injection site reaction* (pain; redness; swelling)—incidence 17%
Incidence rare—less than 1%
  *Trouble in swallowing; urticaria* (itching)

**Those indicating need for medical attention only if they continue or are bothersome**
Incidence rare—less than 1%
  *Dizziness; flushing; headache; hyperactivity* (trouble sitting still); *somnolence* (sleepiness)

## Patient Consultation

As an aid to patient consultation, refer to *Advice for the Patient, Sermorelin (Systemic)—Introductory Version.*

## Sermorelin (Systemic)—Introductory Version

In providing consultation, consider emphasizing the following selected information (» = major clinical significance):

**Before using this medication**
» Conditions affecting use, especially:
    Sensitivity to sermorelin
    Other medications, especially glucocorticoid corticosteroids
    Other medical problems, especially hypothyroidism

**Proper use of this medication**
» Compliance with therapy
» Reading patient directions carefully with regard to:
    —Preparation of the injection
    —Use of disposable syringes and needles; safe handling and disposal of syringes and needles
    —Proper administration technique
    —Stability of the injection
» Carefully selecting and rotating injection sites, following physician's recommendations
» Proper dosing
» Proper storage

**Precautions while using this medication**
» Importance of regular visits to physician

**Side/adverse effects**
Signs of potential side effects, especially injection site reaction, trouble in swallowing, and urticaria

## General Dosing Information

Sermorelin is to be administered only by or under the supervision of a physician who is experienced in the diagnosis and treatment of growth disorders.

Prior to initiation of treatment, a sermorelin growth hormone stimulation test is recommended in all patients. Treatment should be excluded if the resulting peak growth hormone concentration is 2 nanograms per mL or less.

Subcutaneous injection sites should be rotated.

Care should be taken to ensure that the child receiving sermorelin continues to grow at a rate consistent with the child's age and stage of development. Growth hormone therapy should be considered for children whose response to sermorelin is poor or waning.

The efficacy of sermorelin when used for longer than 1 year and its effect on final adult height have not been determined.

## Parenteral Dosage Forms

### SERMORELIN ACETATE FOR INJECTION

**Usual pediatric dose**
Growth hormone deficiency—
    Subcutaneous, 0.03 mg per kg of body weight once a day at bedtime.
Note: Initially, treatment should continue for a period of six months.
    Treatment should be discontinued once the epiphyses are fused.

**Size(s) usually available**
U.S.—
    0.5 mg (Rx) [*Geref* (mannitol 5 mg; dibasic sodium phosphate; monobasic sodium phosphate)].
    1 mg (Rx) [*Geref* (mannitol 5 mg; dibasic sodium phosphate; monobasic sodium phosphate)].

**Packaging and storage**
Store between 2 and 8 °C (36 and 46 °F).

**Preparation of dosage form**
Sermorelin acetate for injection is reconstituted for subcutaneous administration by adding 0.5 to 1 mL of sodium chloride injection to the vial. The diluent should be aimed against the vial wall and the vial swirled gently with a rotary motion until the contents have dissolved completely.

**Stability**
Sermorelin should be administered immediately following reconstitution. Any unused portion of a vial should be discarded.

Developed: 06/17/98

---

# SERTRALINE Systemic

VA CLASSIFICATION (Primary/Secondary): CN603/CN900
Commonly used brand name(s): *Zoloft*.
Note: For a listing of dosage forms and brand names by country availability, see *Dosage Forms* section(s).

## Category

Antidepressant; antiobsessional agent; antipanic agent.

## Indications

### Accepted

Depressive disorder, major (treatment)—Sertraline is indicated for the treatment of major depressive disorder. Treatment of acute depressive episodes typically requires 6 to 12 months of antidepressant therapy. Patients with recurrent or chronic depression may require long-term treatment. Sertraline showed effective maintenance of antidepressant response for up to 52 weeks of treatment in a placebo-controlled trial.

Obsessive-compulsive disorder (treatment)—Sertraline is indicated for the treatment of obsessions and compulsions in adults and children[1] 6 years of age and older with obsessive-compulsive disorder.

Panic disorder (treatment)—Sertraline is indicated for the treatment of panic disorder with or without agoraphobia.

[1]Not included in Canadian product labeling.

## Pharmacology/Pharmacokinetics

**Physicochemical characteristics**
Chemical group—Naphthylamine derivative. Chemically unrelated to tricyclic or tetracyclic antidepressants.
Molecular weight—Sertraline hydrochloride: 342.7.
Solubility—Sertraline hydrochloride is slightly soluble in water and sparingly soluble in ethyl alcohol.

**Mechanism of action/Effect**
Sertraline is a potent and selective inhibitor of neuronal uptake of serotonin (5-hydroxytryptamine [5-HT]). It has only weak effects on neuronal uptake of norepinephrine and dopamine. Chronic administration of sertraline in animals has resulted in down-regulation of postsynaptic beta-adrenergic receptors. Sertraline's inhibition of serotonin reuptake enhances serotonergic transmission, which results in subsequent inhibition of adrenergic activity in the locus ceruleus. Specifically, sertraline depresses the firing of the raphe serotonin neurons; this, in turn, increases the activity of the locus ceruleus, with consequent desensitization of the postsynaptic beta-receptors and presynaptic alpha$_2$-receptors.

Sertraline lacks affinity for adrenergic (alpha$_1$, alpha$_2$, or beta) receptors, muscarinic-cholinergic receptors, gamma aminobutyric acid (GABA) receptors, dopaminergic receptors, histaminergic receptors, serotonergic (5-HT$_{1A}$, 5-HT$_{1B}$, 5-HT$_2$) receptors, and benzodiazepine receptors. Sertraline does not inhibit monoamine oxidase.

**Other actions/effects**
Sertraline inhibits the isoenzyme cytochrome P450 2D6 (CYP2D6). When used in low clinical doses, sertraline probably inhibits CYP2D6 less than other selective serotonin reuptake inhibitors.

Sertraline blocks the uptake of serotonin into human platelets as well as into neurons. There have been rare reports of altered platelet function and of abnormal bleeding or purpura in patients taking sertraline.

Sertraline has anorectic effects.

**Absorption**
Slow but consistent. Bioavailability and absorption rate are increased if sertraline is taken with food.

**Distribution**
Both sertraline and its metabolites are extensively distributed into tissues. In animal studies, the volume of distribution (Vol$_D$) exceeded 20 liters/kilogram (L/kg).

**Protein binding**
Very high (98%). However, at concentrations up to and greater than those achieved during therapeutic dosing of sertraline, neither sertraline nor its major metabolite, *N*-desmethylsertraline, altered plasma protein binding of warfarin or propranolol *in vitro*.

**Biotransformation**
Undergoes extensive first-pass metabolism in the liver. The primary initial pathway is *N*-demethylation to form *N*-desmethylsertraline, which is substantially less active than the parent compound, exhibiting only about 1/8 of its activity. Animal testing has shown that *N*-desmethyl-

sertraline does not contribute appreciably to the pharmacologic activity or toxicity of the parent compound. Both sertraline and N-desmethylsertraline undergo oxidative deamination and subsequent reduction, hydroxylation, and glucuronide conjugation.

**Half-life**
Elimination—
  Sertraline: 24 to 26 hours.
  N-desmethylsertraline: 62 to 104 hours.

**Onset of action**
Antidepressant and antipanic effects—2 to 4 weeks.
Antiobsessional effects may take longer to achieve.

**Time to peak concentration**
Time to reach mean peak plasma concentration ($T_{max}$) following administration of 50 to 200 mg of sertraline once daily for 14 days ranged from 4.5 to 8.4 hours. When sertraline was administered with food, $T_{max}$ fell from 8 hours to 5.5 hours post-dosing.

**Time to steady-state concentration**
After once-daily dosing of sertraline in adult subjects, steady-state plasma concentrations were reached in about 7 days. Based on a 14-day kinetics study, steady state should be reached after 2 to 3 weeks in older patients.

**Peak plasma concentration**
Mean peak plasma concentration ($C_{max}$) and area under the plasma concentration–time curve (AUC) after a single dose of sertraline were proportional to dose over the range of 50 to 200 mg, demonstrating linear pharmacokinetics. When sertraline was administered with food, $C_{max}$ increased by 25% and AUC increased slightly.

**Elimination**
Renal—
  In two healthy male subjects, about 40 to 45% of an administered radioactive dose was recovered in the urine within 9 days, with less than 0.2% recovered unchanged.
Fecal—
  In two healthy male subjects, about 40 to 45% of an administered radioactive dose was recovered in feces within 9 days, including 12 to 14% unchanged sertraline.
In dialysis—
  Due to large volume of distribution, dialysis is not believed to be effective.

## Precautions to Consider

**Carcinogenicity**
In lifetime carcinogenicity studies, there was a dose-related increase in the incidence of liver adenomas in male CD-1 mice receiving sertraline at doses of 10 to 40 mg per kg of body weight (mg/kg) per day (less than and equal to the maximum recommended human dose [MRHD] on a mg per square meter of body surface area [mg/m$^2$] basis). However, liver adenomas have a variable rate of spontaneous occurrence in the CD-1 mouse, and the significance of this finding to use in humans is unknown. No increase in liver adenomas was seen in Long-Evans rats or in female CD-1 mice receiving doses of up to 40 mg/kg. No increase in the incidence of hepatocellular carcinomas was seen in the studies. Female rats receiving 40 mg/kg (two times the MRHD on a mg/m$^2$ basis) had an increase in follicular adenomas of the thyroid, unaccompanied by thyroid hyperplasia. Rats receiving 10 to 40 mg/kg (0.5 to 2 times the MRHD on a mg/m$^2$ basis) showed an increase in uterine adenocarcinomas compared with placebo controls, but this effect was not clearly drug-related.

**Mutagenicity**
Sertraline had no genotoxic effects, with or without metabolic activation, based on the bacterial mutation assay, mouse lymphoma mutation assay, or tests for cytogenic aberrations in vivo in mouse bone marrow and in vitro in human lymphocytes.

**Pregnancy/Reproduction**
Fertility—A decrease in fertility was seen in one of two studies in rats that received 80 mg/kg of sertraline per day (four times the MRHD on a mg/m$^2$ basis).
Pregnancy—A prospective study compared birth outcomes of 267 pregnancies that were exposed to the selective serotonin reuptake inhibitors (SSRIs) sertraline (50 mg/day, range 25 to 250 mg/day), paroxetine (30 mg/day, range 10 to 60 mg/day), or fluvoxamine (50 mg/day, range 25 to 200 mg/day) with those of 267 pregnancies that were exposed to medications or medical treatments that are known to be nonteratogenic. Sertraline was taken at some time during 147 of the SSRI-exposed pregnancies. Based on interviews with the mothers 6 to 9 months after the births, no differences in the infants' gestational ages or mean birth weights, or in the rates of major malformations, spontaneous or elective abortions, or stillbirths were found between the two groups. Also, no differences were found between infants exposed to SSRIs during the first trimester only and infants exposed to SSRIs throughout gestation. The behavioral effects of in utero sertraline exposure were not examined.
No teratogenic effects were demonstrated in studies in rats and rabbits receiving approximately four times the MRHD on a mg/m$^2$ basis. However, delayed ossification occurred in fetuses of rats and rabbits given sertraline dosages of 10 mg/kg per day (one half the MRHD on a mg/m$^2$ basis) and 40 mg/kg per day (four times the MRHD on a mg/m$^2$ basis), respectively, during the period of organogenesis. Also, an increase in pup stillbirths and pup deaths during the first 4 days of life and a decrease in pup weights were seen in rats when dams were given a sertraline dose of 20 mg/kg per day (equal to the MRHD on a mg/m$^2$ basis) through the last one third of gestation and through lactation. There was no effect on pup mortality at doses ≤ 10 mg/kg per day (one half the MRHD on a mg/m$^2$ basis). The decrease in pup survival was due to in utero exposure to sertraline. The clinical significance of these effects is unknown.
FDA Pregnancy Category C.
Labor and delivery—The effect of sertraline on labor and delivery is not known.

**Breast-feeding**
Sertraline is distributed into breast milk. Very low levels of sertraline and/or N-desmethylsertraline (< 2 nanograms/mL) were detected in the plasma of breast-fed infants of mothers who were receiving sertraline. However, no adverse effects in the infants were seen during the short-term (< 2 years) follow-up.

**Pediatrics**
Sertraline has been tested in children 6 to 17 years of age and, in effective doses, has not been shown to cause different side effects or problems than it does in adults. However, the effects of long-term use of sertraline on the growth, development, and maturation of children and adolescents are unknown. Because of the anorectic effect of sertraline, body weight and growth should be monitored in children receiving long-term treatment.

**Geriatrics**
No geriatrics-specific problems have been documented in studies done to date that included elderly patients. However, in one study, clearance of sertraline in 16 elderly patients was about 40% lower than clearance in a group of younger subjects, indicating that steady-state will take 2 to 3 weeks to achieve in elderly patients. A reduced initial dosage is recommended in elderly patients.

**Drug interactions and/or related problems**
The following drug interactions and/or related problems have been selected on the basis of their potential clinical significance (possible mechanism in parentheses where appropriate)—not necessarily inclusive (» = major clinical significance):

Note:  Sertraline inhibits cytochrome P450 2D6 (CYP2D6) and a potential exists for clinically significant interactions with medications that are metabolized by this isoenzyme, particularly medications having a narrow therapeutic index, such as tricyclic antidepressants and the type 1C antiarrhythmics propafenone and flecainide. A lower dosage of these medications may be needed when they are used concomitantly with sertraline, and an increase in dosage may be necessary after discontinuation of sertraline following concomitant use.

  Combinations containing any of the following medications, depending on the amount present, may also interact with this medication.

  Alcohol
    (although sertraline has not been shown to alter alcohol metabolism and does not appear to potentiate cognitive and psychomotor effects of alcohol in normal subjects, concomitant use is not recommended)

» Antidepressants, tricyclic (TCAs)
    (sertraline may inhibit the metabolism of TCAs; in a pharmacokinetic study in 18 healthy males, 50 mg per day of sertraline increased the mean area under the plasma concentration–time curve [AUC] and mean maximum plasma concentration [$C_{max}$] of desipramine by 23% and 31%, respectively; in 12 healthy males, 150 mg per day of sertraline increased the AUC and $C_{max}$ of desipramine by 54% and 22%, respectively, when desipramine was administered, and increased the AUC and $C_{max}$ of desipramine [a metabolite of imipramine] by 129% and 55%, respectively, when imipramine was administered; imipramine AUC and $C_{max}$ were increased by 68% and 39%, respectively, in the second study; TCA plasma concentration monitoring and dosage adjustments of the TCA and/or sertraline may be necessary)

» Astemizole or
» Terfenadine
(because sertraline inhibits cytochrome P450 enzymes and may increase plasma concentrations of these medications, thereby increasing the risk of cardiac arrhythmias, concurrent use is not recommended)

Cimetidine
(AUC, $C_{max}$, and mean half-life of sertraline were increased by 50%, 24%, and 26%, respectively, compared with placebo values, when a single dose of 100 mg of sertraline was administered on the second day of administration of 800 mg per day of cimetidine)

Diazepam
(after 21 days of dosing with sertraline or placebo, clearance of diazepam following a single intravenous dose was decreased from baseline by 32% in subjects administered sertraline and by 19% in subjects administered placebo; however, the clinical significance of this interaction is unknown)

» Highly protein-bound medications, especially:
Digitoxin
Warfarin
(caution in concurrent use with sertraline is recommended because of possible displacement of either medication from protein-binding sites, leading to increased plasma concentrations of the free [unbound] medications and increased risk of adverse effects; however, sertraline did not alter plasma protein binding of warfarin or propranolol *in vitro*)
(after single oral doses of warfarin in six healthy males, the prothrombin time was increased and the protein binding of warfarin was decreased compared with both baseline and the placebo group values after 21 days of sertraline dosing that was escalated from 50 mg per day to 200 mg per day; changes were small but statistically significant; prothrombin time should be carefully monitored when sertraline therapy is initiated or stopped in patients taking warfarin)

Lithium
(although a placebo-controlled clinical trial in normal volunteers demonstrated no alteration in steady-state lithium levels or renal clearance of lithium, close monitoring of lithium concentrations is recommended; also, concurrent use may lead to an increased incidence of serotonin-associated side effects)

» Moclobemide
(because of the potentially fatal effects of concomitant use of sertraline and nonselective, irreversible monoamine oxidase [MAO] inhibitors, and the increased risk of development of the serotonin syndrome with concomitant use of sertraline and the selective, reversible MAO-A inhibitor moclobemide, concurrent use is not recommended; allowing a washout period of 3 to 7 days is advised between discontinuing moclobemide and initiating sertraline therapy, and allowing a washout period of 2 weeks is advised between discontinuing sertraline and initiating moclobemide therapy)

» Monoamine oxidase (MAO) inhibitors, including furazolidone, procarbazine, and selegiline
(concurrent use of MAO inhibitors with sertraline may result in hyperpyretic episodes, severe convulsions, hypertensive crises, or the serotonin syndrome; fatalities have occurred. Concomitant use of MAO inhibitors with sertraline is **contraindicated**. A wash-out period of at least 14 days should elapse between discontinuation of either medication [the MAO inhibitor or sertraline] and initiation of the other)

» Serotonergics or other medications or substances with serotonergic activity (see *Appendix II*)
(increased risk of developing the serotonin syndrome, a rare but potentially fatal hyperserotonergic state; symptoms typically occur shortly [hours to days] after the addition of a serotonergic agent to a regimen that includes other serotonin-enhancing drugs, such as sertraline, or an increase in dosage of a serotonergic agent; symptoms include agitation, diaphoresis, diarrhea, fever, hyperreflexia, incoordination, mental status changes [confusion, hypomania], myoclonus, shivering, or tremor; the syndrome usually resolves shortly after the discontinuation of the serotonergic agents)

Tolbutamide
(in a placebo-controlled study in 25 healthy male volunteers, clearance of tolbutamide following a single intravenous dose was decreased by 16% from baseline after 22 days of sertraline dosing that was escalated from 50 mg per day to 200 mg per day; blood glucose should be monitored, and the dosage of tolbutamide reduced if hypoglycemia occurs)

**Laboratory value alterations**
The following have been selected on the basis of their potential clinical significance (possible effect in parentheses where appropriate)—not necessarily inclusive (» = major clinical significance):

With physiology/laboratory test values
Alanine aminotransferase (ALT [SGPT]) or
Aspartate aminotransferase (AST [SGOT])
(values increased to ≥ 3 times the upper limit of normal have been reported infrequently; increases usually occur within 1 to 9 weeks of initiation of therapy, with values generally normalizing after sertraline is discontinued)

Total cholesterol or
Triglycerides
(mean increases of 3% and 5%, respectively, have been reported)

Uric acid, serum
(mean decreases of approximately 7% have been reported)

**Medical considerations/Contraindications**
The medical considerations/contraindications included have been selected on the basis of their potential clinical significance (reasons given in parentheses where appropriate)—not necessarily inclusive (» = major clinical significance).

*Risk-benefit should be considered when the following medical problems exist:*

» Hepatic function impairment
(in a single-dose study, mean elimination half-life of sertraline was prolonged from 22 hours in healthy subjects to 52 hours in patients with mild, stable cirrhosis; peak concentrations and AUC were increased 1.7 and 4.4 times, respectively, in patients with hepatic impairment; decreased dosage or less frequent dosing is recommended)

Mania, history of
(activation of mania or hypomania was reported in approximately 0.4% of patients during premarketing testing of sertraline, and occurs most frequently in patients with bipolar disorder)

Neurological impairment, including developmental delay
(risk of seizures may be increased)

Renal function impairment
(results of an open-label study showed no difference between pharmacokinetic parameters of sertraline in patients with renal impairment ranging from mild to severe [but not requiring regular hemodialysis] and those of a matched healthy group with no renal impairment; however, since clinical experience with long-term sertraline treatment in patients with renal impairment is lacking, caution is recommended)

Seizure disorders
(seizures occurred in approximately 0.2% of subjects in clinical trials of sertraline for obsessive-compulsive disorder, with most cases occurring in patients with a pre-existing seizure disorder or a family history of seizure disorder; as with other antidepressants, sertraline should be introduced with care)

Sensitivity to sertraline
Weight loss
(although the weight loss associated with sertraline use is usually about one to two pounds [0.4 to 0.9 kg], there have been rare reports of significant weight loss; significant weight loss may be undesirable in some patients)

**Patient monitoring**
The following may be especially important in patient monitoring (other tests may be warranted in some patients, depending on condition; » = major clinical significance):

Careful supervision of patients with suicidal tendencies
(recommended especially during early treatment phase before peak effectiveness of sertraline is achieved; although sertraline has a wide margin of safety when taken in overdose, limiting the total amount of medication in the patient's possession is recommended)

## Side/Adverse Effects

Note: Side effects may be dose-related and time-related. Severity of side effects appears to lessen with decreased doses or after administration for longer than 2 weeks.

The following side/adverse effects have been selected on the basis of their potential clinical significance (possible signs and symptoms in parentheses where appropriate)—not necessarily inclusive:

**Those indicating need for medical attention**
Incidence more frequent
*Sexual dysfunction* (decreased sexual desire or ability)

Note: *Sexual dysfunction* may include decreased libido, impotence, delayed ejaculation, or anorgasmia. Delayed ejaculation is the most commonly seen form of sexual dysfunction associated with sertraline use.

Incidence less frequent or rare
*Abnormal bleeding* (red or purple spots on skin; nose bleeds); *akathisia* (inability to sit still; restlessness); *breast tenderness or enlargement; or galactorrhea* (unusual secretion of milk)—in females; *extrapyramidal effects, dystonic* (unusual or sudden body or facial movements or postures); *fever; hyponatremia* (confusion; drowsiness; dryness of mouth; increased thirst; lack of energy; seizures); *mania or hypomania* (fast talking and excited feelings or actions that are out of control)—may be more frequent in patients with bipolar disorder; *palpitation* (fast or irregular heartbeat); *serotonin syndrome* (diarrhea; fever; increased sweating; mood or behavior changes; overactive reflexes; racing heartbeat; restlessness; shivering or shaking); *skin rash, hives, or itching*

Note: *Hyponatremia* is probably the result of the syndrome of inappropriate antidiuretic hormone secretion (SIADH). Most cases have been in elderly patients or in volume-depleted patients, such as patients taking diuretics.

The *serotonin syndrome* is most likely to occur shortly (within hours to days) after an increase in sertraline dosage or the addition of another serotonergic agent to the patient's regimen. The syndrome may include cardiac arrhythmias, coma, disseminated intravascular coagulation, hypertension or hypotension, renal failure, respiratory failure, seizures, or severe hyperthermia.

**Those indicating need for medical attention only if they continue or are bothersome**
Incidence more frequent
*Dizziness; drowsiness; gastrointestinal effects; including anorexia* (decrease in appetite); *diarrhea or loose stools; dryness of mouth; nausea; stomach or abdominal cramps, gas, or pain; or weight loss; headache; increased sweating; insomnia* (trouble in sleeping); *tiredness or weakness; tremor* (trembling or shaking)

Note: *Weight loss* in patients in controlled trials was usually about one to two pounds [0.4 to 0.9 kg]. Significant weight loss was reported rarely.

Incidence less frequent
*Anxiety, agitation, or nervousness; changes in vision, including blurred vision; constipation; flushing or redness of skin, with feeling of warmth or heat; increased appetite; vomiting; yawning*

**Those indicating the need for medical attention if they occur after medication is discontinued**
*Agitation; anxiety; dizziness; gait instability* (trouble in walking); *headache; increased sweating; insomnia* (trouble in sleeping); *nausea; tremor* (trembling or shaking); *unusual tiredness; vertigo* (feeling of constant movement of self or surroundings)

Note: Discontinuation symptoms are usually mild, and are often mistaken for influenza.

## Overdose
For specific information on the agents used in the management of sertraline overdose, see *Charcoal, Activated (Oral-Local)* monograph.

For more information on the management of overdose or unintentional ingestion, **contact a Poison Control Center** (see *Poison Control Center Listing*).

**Clinical effects of overdose**
Note: Sertraline has a wide margin of safety in overdose. However, deaths have occurred in overdoses involving sertraline in combination with other drugs and/or alcohol.

Symptoms of overdose resemble the side/adverse effects occurring with therapeutic doses, but may be more intense or several symptoms may occur together.

The following effects have been selected on the basis of their potential clinical significance (possible signs and symptoms in parentheses where appropriate)—not necessarily inclusive:

Acute
*Anxiety; drowsiness; electrocardiogram (ECG) changes; mydriasis* (unusually large pupils); *nausea; tachycardia* (unusually fast heartbeat); *vomiting*

Note: Some patients may develop the serotonin syndrome, a potentially fatal symptom complex, in response to acute overdose with sertraline. The serotonin syndrome may be manifested by mental status changes, restlessness, myoclonus, hyperreflexia, diaphoresis, shivering, tremor, diarrhea, incoordination, and/or fever.

**Treatment of overdose**
There is no specific antidote for sertraline. Treatment is essentially symptomatic and supportive.

To decrease absorption—Administering activated charcoal, which may be used with sorbitol, may be as effective as or more effective than emesis or gastric lavage.

Monitoring—Monitoring cardiac function and vital signs.

Supportive care—Establishing and maintaining airway. Patients in whom intentional overdose is confirmed or suspected should be referred for psychiatric consultation.

Note: Dialysis, forced diuresis, hemoperfusion, and exchange transfusions are unlikely to be of benefit due to sertraline's large volume of distribution and high degree of protein binding.

## Patient Consultation
As an aid to patient consultation, refer to *Advice for the Patient, Sertraline (Systemic)*.

In providing consultation, consider emphasizing the following selected information (» = major clinical significance):

**Before using this medication**
» Conditions affecting use, especially:
   Sensitivity to sertraline
   Pregnancy—No difference in birth outcome was found between 267 SSRI-exposed pregnancies (147 to sertraline) and 267 pregnancies exposed to known nonteratogenic medications or procedures; behavioral effects were not studied
   Breast-feeding—Distributed into breast milk; the long-term effects on nursing infants are unknown
   Use in children—Body weight and growth should be monitored during long-term treatment because of anorectic effect
   Use in the elderly—Clearance is reduced; reduced initial dosage is recommended
   Contraindicated medications—MAO inhibitors
   Other medications, especially astemizole, digitoxin, moclobemide, serotonergics or other medications or substances with serotonergic activity, terfenadine, tricyclic antidepressants, and warfarin
   Other medical problems, especially hepatic dysfunction

**Proper use of this medication**
» Compliance with therapy; not taking more or less medicine than prescribed
   Taking with or without food, as directed by physician
» Four weeks or more of therapy may be required before antidepressant or antipanic effects are achieved; antiobsessional effects may take longer to achieve
» Proper dosing
   Missed dose: Discussing with physician what to do about any missed doses since some patients take sertraline in the morning and other patients take sertraline in the evening
» Proper storage

**Precautions while using this medication**
Regular visits to physician to check progress of therapy
» Not taking sertraline with or within 14 days of taking an MAO inhibitor; not taking an MAO inhibitor within 14 days of taking sertraline
   Avoiding use of alcoholic beverages
» Possible drowsiness, impairment of judgment, thinking, or motor skills; caution when driving or doing jobs requiring alertness or coordination until effects of medication are known
» Checking with physician before discontinuing sertraline; dosage tapering may be required

**Side/adverse effects**
Sexual dysfunction; abnormal bleeding; akathisia; breast tenderness or enlargement, or galactorrhea (in females); extrapyramidal effects, dystonic; fever; hyponatremia; mania or hypomania; serotonin syndrome; skin rash, hives, or itching
Possible discontinuation symptoms, including agitation, anxiety, dizziness, gait instability, headache, increased sweating, insomnia, nausea, tremor, unusual tiredness, or vertigo

## General Dosing Information
Potentially suicidal patients, particularly those who may use alcohol excessively, should not have access to large quantities of this medication since they may continue to exhibit suicidal tendencies until significant improvement occurs. Some clinicians recommend that the patient be supplied with the least amount of medication necessary for satisfactory patient management.

Activation of hypomania or mania has been reported in patients treated with sertraline. Risk is greatest in patients with a history of bipolar disorder.

When discontinued, sertraline should be withdrawn gradually to help avoid the occurrence of discontinuation symptoms, including agitation, anxiety, dizziness, gait instability, headache, increased sweating, insomnia, nausea, tremor, unusual tiredness, or vertigo. Discontinuation symptoms are usually mild and are often mistaken for influenza.

**Diet/Nutrition**
Sertraline may be taken with or without food. Some clinicians advise their patients to take this medication with food to lessen gastrointestinal side effects.

**For treatment of adverse effects**
Serotonin syndrome—The serotonin syndrome usually resolves shortly after discontinuation of serotonergic medications. Treatment is essentially symptomatic and supportive. However, the nonspecific serotonergic receptor antagonists cyproheptadine and methysergide have been reported to be of some use in shortening the duration of the serotonin syndrome.

## Oral Dosage Forms

Note: The dosing and strengths of the dosage forms available are expressed in terms of sertraline base.

### SERTRALINE HYDROCHLORIDE CAPSULES

**Usual adult dose**
Depression or
Obsessive-compulsive disorder—
  Oral, initially 50 mg (base) a day as a single morning or evening dose. The dosage may be increased after several weeks in increments of 50 mg, with increases made at intervals of at least one week, as needed and tolerated.
Note: Some clinicians recommend an initial dosage of 25 mg a day for one to two days.
Panic disorder—
  Oral, initially 25 mg (base) a day, as a single morning or evening dose. After one week, the dosage should be increased to 50 mg (base) a day, as a single dose. Further dosage increases may be made in increments of 50 mg, at intervals of at least one week, as needed and tolerated.
Note: Patients with hepatic function impairment should receive a lower dosage or less frequent dosing than patients with normal hepatic function.

**Usual adult prescribing limits**
200 mg (base) a day.

**Usual pediatric dose**
Depression or
Panic disorder—
  Safety and efficacy have not been established.
Obsessive-compulsive disorder[1]—
  Children 6 to 13 years of age: Oral, initially 25 mg (base) a day as a single morning or evening dose. Dosage may be increased at intervals of at least one week, as needed and tolerated.
  Children 13 to 17 years of age: Oral, initially 50 mg (base) a day as a single morning or evening dose. Dosage may be increased at intervals of at least one week, as needed and tolerated.
Note: To avoid excessive dosing when the dosage is being increased, consideration should be given to the generally lower body weights of children as compared with adult body weights.

**Usual pediatric prescribing limits**
See *Usual adult prescribing limits*.

**Usual geriatric dose**
Depression or
Obsessive-compulsive disorder or
Panic disorder—
  Oral, initially 25 mg (base) a day, as a single morning or evening dose; dosage may be increased gradually as needed and tolerated.

**Strength(s) usually available**
U.S.—
  Not commercially available.
Canada—
  25 mg (base) (Rx) [*Zoloft* (anhydrous lactose; corn starch; magnesium stearate; sodium lauryl sulfate)].
  50 mg (base) (Rx) [*Zoloft* (anhydrous lactose; corn starch; magnesium stearate; sodium lauryl sulfate)].
  100 mg (base) (Rx) [*Zoloft* (anhydrous lactose; corn starch; magnesium stearate; sodium lauryl sulfate)].
  150 mg (base) (Rx) [*Zoloft* (anhydrous lactose; corn starch; magnesium stearate; sodium lauryl sulfate)].
  200 mg (base) (Rx) [*Zoloft* (anhydrous lactose; corn starch; magnesium stearate; sodium lauryl sulfate)].

**Packaging and storage**
Store below 40 °C (104 °F), preferably between 15 and 30 °C (59 and 86 °F), unless otherwise specified by manufacturer.

**Auxiliary labeling**
- May cause dizziness or drowsiness.
- Avoid alcoholic beverages.

### SERTRALINE HYDROCHLORIDE TABLETS

**Usual adult dose**
See *Sertraline Hydrochloride Capsules*.

**Usual adult prescribing limits**
See *Sertraline Hydrochloride Capsules*.

**Usual pediatric dose**
See *Sertraline Hydrochloride Capsules*.

**Usual pediatric prescribing limits**
See *Sertraline Hydrochloride Capsules*.

**Usual geriatric dose**
Depression or
Obsessive-compulsive disorder or
Panic disorder—
  Oral, initially 12.5 to 25 mg (base) a day, as a single morning or evening dose; dosage may be increased gradually as needed and tolerated.

**Strength(s) usually available**
U.S.—
  25 mg (base) (Rx) [*Zoloft* (scored; dibasic calcium phosphate dihydrate; D&C Yellow #10 aluminum lake; FD&C Blue #1 aluminum lake; FD&C Red #40 aluminum lake; hydroxypropyl cellulose; hydroxypropyl methylcellulose; magnesium stearate; microcrystalline cellulose; polyethylene glycol; polysorbate 80; sodium starch glycolate; titanium dioxide)].
  50 mg (base) (Rx) [*Zoloft* (scored; dibasic calcium phosphate dihydrate; FD&C Blue #2 aluminum lake; hydroxypropyl cellulose; hydroxypropyl methylcellulose; magnesium stearate; microcrystalline cellulose; polyethylene glycol; polysorbate 80; sodium starch glycolate; titanium dioxide)].
  100 mg (base) (Rx) [*Zoloft* (scored; dibasic calcium phosphate dihydrate; hydroxypropyl cellulose; hydroxypropyl methylcellulose; magnesium stearate; microcrystalline cellulose; polyethylene glycol; polysorbate 80; sodium starch glycolate; synthetic yellow iron oxide; titanium dioxide)].
Canada—
  Not commercially available.

**Packaging and storage**
Store below 40 °C (104 °F), preferably between 15 and 30 °C (59 and 86 °F), unless otherwise specified by manufacturer.

**Auxiliary labeling**
- May cause dizziness or drowsiness.
- Avoid alcoholic beverages.

---

[1]Not included in Canadian product labeling.

Revised: 08/07/98

---

**SEVOFLURANE**—The *Sevoflurane (Inhalation-Systemic)* monograph is not included in this published version of the USP DI database. Copies of the monograph are available on request from Micromedex, Inc. - Reprint Requests, 6200 S. Syracuse Way, Suite 300, Englewood, CO 80111; telephone (303) 486-6400; telefax (303) 486-6464; Email: USPDI@MDX.COM.

# SIBUTRAMINE  Systemic—INTRODUCTORY VERSION

VA CLASSIFICATION (Primary): GA751
Note: Controlled substance in the U.S.—Schedule IV
Commonly used brand name(s): *Meridia*.
Note: For a listing of dosage forms and brand names by country availability, see *Dosage Forms* section(s).

## Category
Appetite suppressant.

## Indications

### General considerations
Cardiac valve dysfunction and primary pulmonary hypertension have been associated with the use of centrally acting appetite suppressants that cause the release of serotonin (5-hydroxytryptamine, 5-HT) from nerve terminals while inhibiting the reuptake of 5-HT. Sibutramine acts in part by inhibiting the reuptake of 5-HT, but has no effect on 5-HT release. A comparison of echocardiograms performed on 132 patients who had received 15 mg per day of sibutramine and 77 patients who had received placebo for 0.5 to 16 months (mean 7.6 months) found no difference in the incidence of valvular heart disease between the two groups. A second study in 25 patients comparing echocardiograms administered at baseline to those administered after 3 months of treatment with 5 to 30 mg per day of sibutramine detected no cases of valvular heart disease. Similarly, no cases of primary pulmonary hypertension were reported during premarketing clinical studies of sibutramine.

In two 12-month studies of sibutramine in obese subjects, maximum weight loss was achieved by 6 months and statistically significant weight loss was maintained over 12 months.

### Accepted
Obesity, exogenous (treatment)—Sibutramine is indicated for the management of obesity, including weight loss and maintenance of weight loss, in patients on a reduced-calorie diet. Sibutramine should be used only in obese patients with an initial body mass index $\geq$ 30 kg of body weight per square meter of height (kg/m$^2$) or with an initial body mass index $\geq$ 27 kg/m$^2$ in the presence of other risk factors, such as hypertension, diabetes, and dyslipidemia. Safety and efficacy of sibutramine use for more than 1 year have not been evaluated in controlled trials.

## Pharmacology/Pharmacokinetics

### Physicochemical characteristics
Chemical group—Cyclobutanemethanamine.
Molecular weight—Sibutramine hydrochloride monohydrate: 334.33.
Solubility—In water at pH 5.2: 2.9 mg/mL.
Partition coefficient—Octanol:water at pH 5: 30.9.

### Mechanism of action/Effect
*In vivo* studies have shown that sibutramine and its primary and secondary amine metabolites potently inhibit the reuptake of norepinephrine and serotonin (5-hydroxytryptamine, 5-HT). These metabolites also inhibit the reuptake of dopamine *in vitro*, but at a potency that is threefold less than that with which they inhibit norepinephrine and 5-HT reuptake. *In vitro* testing found sibutramine to be much less potent than its active metabolites in inhibiting monoamine reuptake. Therefore, the pharmacological actions of sibutramine are thought to be due predominantly to its active metabolites. Neither sibutramine nor its active metabolites causes the release of monoamines or inhibits monoamine oxidase. Also, all active moieties have low affinity for serotonin (5-HT$_1$, 5-HT$_{1A}$, 5-HT$_{1B}$, 5-HT$_{2A}$, 5-HT$_{2C}$), norepinephrine (beta, beta$_1$, beta$_3$, alpha$_1$, alpha$_2$), dopamine (D$_1$, D$_2$), benzodiazepine, and glutamate (NMDA) receptors, and they show no evidence of anticholinergic or antihistaminergic actions.

### Other actions/effects
Inhibits 5-HT uptake by platelets as well as by neurons, which may affect platelet functioning.

### Absorption
Rapidly absorbed following oral administration; undergoes extensive first-pass metabolism in the liver to form mono- and di-desmethyl active metabolites. Absolute bioavailability is unknown, but mass balance studies indicate that at least 77% of a single oral dose is absorbed.

Food increases the time to peak plasma concentration and decreases the peak plasma concentrations of the desmethyl metabolites by about 3 hours and 30%, respectively, but does not affect the area under the plasma concentration–time curves (AUC) of the desmethyl metabolites.

### Distribution
Rapidly and extensively distributed into tissues.

### Protein binding
Sibutramine—Very high (97%); to human plasma proteins.
Mono-desmethylsibutramine—Very high (94%); to human plasma proteins.
Di-desmethylsibutramine—Very high (94%); to human plasma proteins.
Although protein binding is very high, interactions with other highly protein-bound medications are not anticipated because of the low therapeutic concentrations and basic characteristics of sibutramine and its active metabolites.

### Biotransformation
Hepatic. Sibutramine is metabolized principally by the cytochrome P450 3A4 (CYP3A4) isoenzyme to two active desmethyl metabolites, mono-desmethylsibutramine and di-desmethylsibutramine, which are hydroxylated and conjugated to inactive metabolites.

### Half-life
Elimination—
Sibutramine: 1.1 hours.
Mono-desmethylsibutramine: 14 hours.
Di-desmethylsibutramine: 16 hours.

### Time to peak concentration
Sibutramine—1.2 hours.
Desmethyl metabolites—3 to 4 hours.
Steady-state plasma concentrations of the desmethyl metabolites are reached within 4 days of dosing and are approximately twofold higher than single-dose plasma concentrations.

### Peak plasma concentration
In 18 obese subjects, after a single 15-mg dose of sibutramine, the mean peak plasma concentration of mono-desmethylsibutramine was 4 nanograms/mL (range 3.2 to 4.8 nanograms/mL) and of di-desmethylsibutramine was 6.4 nanograms/mL (range 5.6 to 7.2 nanograms/mL).

### Elimination
Primarily renal, as inactive metabolites.

## Precautions to Consider

### Carcinogenicity/tumorigenicity
Two-year studies in rats and mice, given sibutramine in daily doses that resulted in combined area under the plasma concentration–time curves (AUCs) of the two active metabolites that were 0.5 to 21 times those seen in patients taking the maximum recommended human dose (MRHD), showed an increased incidence of benign tumors of the testicular interstitial cells in male rats. These tumors are commonly seen in rats, and the clinical significance of this finding is unknown. No evidence of carcinogenicity was seen in mice or in female rats.

### Mutagenicity
The two active metabolites of sibutramine had equivocal bacterial mutagenic activity in the Ames test. However, neither sibutramine nor its active metabolites showed evidence of mutagenicity in a number of other appropriate tests.

### Pregnancy/Reproduction
Fertility—Studies in rats showed no evidence of impairment of fertility with sibutramine administration.

Pregnancy—Adequate and well-controlled studies in humans have not been done.

No evidence of teratogenicity was seen in studies in which rats were given daily doses of sibutramine that produced an AUC of the active metabolites that was approximately 43 times that produced in humans receiving the MRHD. However, maternal toxicity and impaired nest-building behavior, which led to decreased pup survival, were seen. Maternal toxicity and increased incidences of broad short snout, short rounded pinnae, short tail, and short thickened long bones in the limbs of offspring were seen in Dutch Belted rabbits given daily doses of sibutramine that produced an AUC of the active metabolites greater than five times that produced in humans receiving the MRHD. Using comparable doses, two studies in New Zealand White rabbits yielded conflicting results. One study found an increased incidence and the other a decreased incidence of cardiovascular anomalies in the offspring of rabbits given sibutramine compared with the offspring of control rabbits.

FDA Pregnancy Category C.

### Breast-feeding
It is not known whether sibutramine or its metabolites are distributed into breast milk.

## Sibutramine (Systemic)—Introductory Version

### Pediatrics
Appropriate studies on the relationship of age to the effects of sibutramine have not been performed in the pediatric population. Safety and efficacy in children up to 16 years of age have not been established.

### Geriatrics
Appropriate studies on the relationship of age to the effects of sibutramine have not been performed in the geriatric population. However, no geriatrics-specific problems have been documented to date and plasma concentrations of sibutramine's active metabolites were similar between subjects 61 to 77 years of age and subjects 19 to 30 years of age after a single 15-mg dose.

### Pharmacogenetics
Although pharmacokinetic data indicate that mean maximum plasma concentration and area under the plasma concentration–time curve are slightly higher in females than in males, this difference is not likely to be clinically significant, and no dosage adjustments based on gender are recommended.

### Dental
Use of sibutramine may decrease or inhibit salivary flow, thus contributing to the development of dental caries, periodontal disease, oral candidiasis, and discomfort.

### Drug interactions and/or related problems
The following drug interactions and/or related problems have been selected on the basis of their potential clinical significance (possible mechanism in parentheses where appropriate)—not necessarily inclusive (» = major clinical significance):

Note: In a study of 12 healthy female volunteers, sibutramine did not interfere with the efficacy of oral contraceptives.

Combinations containing any of the following medications, depending on the amount present, may also interact with this medication.

Alcohol
(a single-dose study found no clinically significant psychomotor effects with concomitant use; however, use of excess alcohol with sibutramine is not recommended)

» Appetite suppressants, other
(sibutramine has not been studied and should not be used in combination with other centrally acting appetite suppressants)

Medications that may increase blood pressure and/or heart rate, other, such as:
Ephedrine or
Phenylpropanolamine or
Pseudoephedrine or
Cough, cold, and allergy products that contain such agents
(sibutramine may increase blood pressure and/or heart rate; concurrent use has not been evaluated)

Medications that inhibit cytochrome P450 3A4 (CYP3A4), such as:
Erythromycin or
Ketoconazole
(CYP3A4 is involved in sibutramine metabolism and the potential exists for a decrease in sibutramine clearance; in small clinical drug interaction studies with erythromycin and ketoconazole, the effects on sibutramine clearance were small to moderate)

» Monoamine oxidase (MAO) inhibitors, including furazolidone, procarbazine, and selegiline
(there have been reports of serious, sometimes fatal, reactions in patients taking MAO inhibitors in combination with other serotonergic agents; concurrent use is **contraindicated** and at least 2 weeks should elapse between discontinuing one medication [MAO inhibitor or sibutramine] and beginning the other)

» Serotonergics or medications or substances with serotonergic activity (see *Appendix II*)
(increased risk of development of the serotonin syndrome, a rare but potentially fatal hyperserotonergic state that may occur in patients receiving serotonergic medications, usually in combination; symptoms typically occur shortly [hours to days] after the addition of a serotonergic agent to a regimen that includes serotonin-enhancing drugs or an increase in dosage of a serotonergic agent; symptoms include agitation, diaphoresis, diarrhea, fever, hyperreflexia, incoordination, mental status changes [confusion, hypomania], myoclonus, shivering, or tremor; cardiac arrhythmias, coma, disseminated intravascular coagulation, hypertension or hypotension, renal failure, respiratory failure, seizures, and severe hyperthermia also have been reported; the syndrome usually resolves shortly after discontinuation of serotonergic medications; treatment is essentially symptomatic and supportive)

### Laboratory value alterations
The following have been selected on the basis of their potential clinical significance (possible effect in parentheses where appropriate)—not necessarily inclusive (» = major clinical significance):

With physiology/laboratory test values
» Blood pressure determinations and
» Heart rate
(mean increases of 1 to 3 mm Hg in systolic and diastolic blood pressure and four to five beats per minute in heart rate occurred during clinical trials of sibutramine; if a sustained increase in blood pressure or heart rate occurs, a reduction in sibutramine dosage or discontinuation of sibutramine therapy should be considered)

Lipids, serum and
Uric acid, serum
(weight loss induced by sibutramine has been accompanied by increases in serum high-density lipoprotein cholesterol concentrations and by decreases in serum triglyceride, total cholesterol, low-density lipoprotein cholesterol, and uric acid concentrations)

Liver function tests
(increases in serum concentrations of aspartate aminotransferase [AST (SGOT)], alanine aminotransferase [ALT (SGPT)], gamma-glutamyltransferase [GGT], lactate dehydrogenase [LDH], alkaline phosphate, and bilirubin were reported in 1.6% of sibutramine-treated obese patients and 0.8% of placebo-control patients in clinical trials; clinically significant elevations were rare; abnormal values were sporadic, did not show a clear dose-response relationship, and often diminished with continued treatment)

### Medical considerations/Contraindications
The medical considerations/contraindications included have been selected on the basis of their potential clinical significance (reasons given in parentheses where appropriate)—not necessarily inclusive (» = major clinical significance).

*Except under special circumstances, this medication should not be used when the following medical problems exist:*
» Anorexia nervosa or
» Hypertension, uncontrolled or poorly controlled
(may be exacerbated)

*Risk-benefit should be considered when the following medical problems exist:*
» Cardiac arrhythmia, or history of or
» Congestive heart failure, or history of or
» Coronary artery disease, or history of or
» Stroke, or history of
(sibutramine is not recommended for use in these patients because of its association with increases in blood pressure and heart rate)

» Drug abuse or dependence, history of
(patients must be carefully observed for signs of misuse of sibutramine, such as development of tolerance, increasing dosage, and drug-seeking behavior)

Gallstones, or history of
(weight loss may precipitate or exacerbate gallstone formation)

Glaucoma, narrow angle
(sibutramine can cause mydriasis and should be used with caution in these patients)

» Hepatic function impairment, severe or
» Renal function impairment, severe
(pharmacokinetic studies indicate that no dosage adjustment is needed in patients with mild to moderate hepatic function impairment, and sibutramine's extensive metabolism to inactive metabolites suggests that no dosage adjustment will be needed in patients with mild to moderate renal function impairment; however, sibutramine has not been studied in patients with severe hepatic or renal function impairment and use is not recommended in these patients)

» Hypertension, well-controlled or
» Hypertension, history of
(may be exacerbated; sibutramine should be used with caution in these patients and should not be used in patients with uncontrolled or poorly controlled hypertension)

Seizures, history of
(increased risk of having seizures; seizures were reported in < 0.1% of patients in premarketing studies of sibutramine)

Sensitivity to sibutramine

### Patient monitoring
The following may be especially important in patient monitoring (other tests may be warranted in some patients, depending on condition; » = major clinical significance):

» Blood pressure and
» Heart rate
(recommended in all patients before starting therapy with sibutramine and at regular intervals during treatment; if sustained elevations occur, a decrease in sibutramine dosage or discontinuation of sibutramine therapy should be considered)

## Side/Adverse Effects

Note: Cardiac valve dysfunction and primary pulmonary hypertension have been associated with the use of other centrally acting appetite suppressants. The mechanism of action of sibutramine does not include the promotion of serotonin (5-HT) release from nerve terminals as did the mechanism of the appetite suppressants that were associated with these adverse events. A comparison of echocardiograms performed on 132 patients receiving 15 mg per day of sibutramine with those performed on 77 patients receiving placebo for 0.5 to 16 months (mean 7.6 months) found no difference in the incidence of valvular heart disease between the two groups. A second study in 25 patients comparing echocardiograms administered at baseline to those administered after 3 months of treatment with 5 to 30 mg per day of sibutramine detected no cases of valvular heart disease. Similarly, no cases of pulmonary hypertension were reported during premarketing clinical studies of sibutramine.

Mean increases of 1 to 3 mm Hg in systolic and diastolic blood pressure and four to five beats per minute in heart rate occurred during clinical trials of sibutramine. However, some patients experienced substantial increases in blood pressure, leading to discontinuation of sibutramine in 0.4% of patients. Tachycardia also led to discontinuation of sibutramine in 0.4% of patients. Placebo discontinuation rates for hypertension and tachycardia were 0.4% and 0.1%, respectively.

The following side/adverse effects have been selected on the basis of their potential clinical significance (possible signs and symptoms in parentheses where appropriate)—not necessarily inclusive:

**Those indicating need for medical attention**
Incidence less frequent
*Dysmenorrhea* (painful menstruation); *edema* (swelling of body or of feet and ankles); *influenza-like symptoms* (chills; achiness); *hypertension* (increased blood pressure); *mental depression; tachycardia* (fast heartbeat)

Incidence rare
*Abnormal bleeding* (bruising or red spots or patches on skin; excessive bleeding following injury); *acute interstitial nephritis* (swelling of body or of feet and ankles; unusual weight gain); *emotional lability* (rapidly changing mood); *migraine* (severe headache); *seizures; skin rash*

Note: *Abnormal bleeding* may be related to inhibition of serotonin uptake into platelets caused by sibutramine and its metabolites.

A single case of biopsy-confirmed *acute interstitial nephritis* was reported during premarketing studies. The patient fully recovered after discontinuing sibutramine and receiving dialysis and oral corticosteroids.

*Seizures* were reported in < 0.1% of patients in premarketing studies of sibutramine. Some of these patients had predisposing factors, including prior history of epilepsy and brain tumor. If seizures develop, sibutramine should be discontinued.

**Those indicating need for medical attention only if they continue or are bothersome**
Incidence more frequent
*Constipation; diarrhea; dizziness; dryness of mouth; headache; insomnia* (trouble in sleeping); *rhinitis* (stuffy or runny nose)

Incidence less frequent
*Abdominal pain; anxiety; back pain; drowsiness; dyspepsia* (indigestion); *increased appetite; increased sweating; increased thirst; nausea; nervousness; paresthesia* (burning, itching, prickling, or tingling of skin); *taste perversion* (change in sense of taste); *vasodilation* (unusual warmth or flushing of skin)

## Overdose

For specific information on the agents used in the management of sibutramine overdose, see *Beta-adrenergic Blocking Agents (Systemic)* monograph.

For more information on the management of overdose or unintentional ingestion, **contact a Poison Control Center** (see *Poison Control Center Listing*).

**Clinical effects of overdose**
Note: Experience with sibutramine overdose is very limited. In reported cases, few adverse effects and no apparent sequelae occurred. Increased heart rate (120 beats per minute) was reported in a 45-year-old male who ingested 400 mg of sibutramine.

**Treatment of overdose**
Treatment of sibutramine overdose is symptomatic and supportive.

Specific treatment—Beta-adrenergic blocking agents may be used cautiously to control elevated blood pressure or tachycardia.

Monitoring—Cardiac and vital signs should be monitored.

Supportive care—Establish and maintain patent airway. Patients in whom intentional overdose is confirmed or suspected should be referred for psychiatric consultation.

Note: Forced diuresis and hemodialysis are of unknown benefit in treatment of sibutramine overdose.

## Patient Consultation

As an aid to patient consultation, refer to *Advice for the Patient, Sibutramine (Systemic)—Introductory Version.*

In providing consultation, consider emphasizing the following selected information (» = major clinical significance):

**Before using this medication**
» Conditions affecting use, especially:
Use in children—Safety and efficacy not established in children up to 16 years of age
Dental—Decreased salivary flow may contribute to caries, periodontal disease, oral candidiasis, and discomfort
Contraindicated medications—Monoamine oxidase (MAO) inhibitors
Other medications, especially appetite suppressants, other; or serotonergics or medications or substances with serotonergic activity
Other medical problems, especially anorexia nervosa; cardiac arrhythmia, or history of; congestive heart failure, or history of; coronary artery disease, or history of; drug abuse or dependence, history of; hepatic or renal function impairment, severe; hypertension, or history of; or stroke, or history of

**Proper use of this medication**
» Taking as directed; not increasing dose, not taking more frequently, and not taking for a longer time than directed by physician because of potential cardiovascular adverse effects
Following reduced-calorie diet, as directed by physician
Taking with or without food, on a full or empty stomach, as directed by physician
» Proper dosing
Missed dose: Taking as soon as possible if remembered the same day; not taking if remembered the next day; returning to regular dosing schedule; not doubling doses
» Proper storage

**Precautions while using this medication**
» Importance of regular visits to physician to check progress of therapy and monitor blood pressure and heart rate
» Not increasing dosage if tolerance develops; checking with physician
» Not taking an MAO inhibitor within 2 weeks of sibutramine; not taking sibutramine within 2 weeks of an MAO inhibitor
Limiting alcohol consumption
» Notifying physician as soon as possible if skin rash, hives, or other allergic reactions occur
» Possible dizziness, drowsiness, or impaired judgment; caution in driving or doing other things that require alertness and sound judgment until effects are known
Possible dryness of mouth; using sugarless candy or gum, ice, or saliva substitute for relief; checking with physician or dentist if dry mouth continues for more than 2 weeks

**Side/adverse effects**
Signs of potential side effects, especially dysmenorrhea, edema, influenza-like symptoms, hypertension, mental depression, tachycardia, abnormal bleeding, acute interstitial nephritis, emotional lability, migraine, seizures, and skin rash

## General Dosing Information

Sibutramine should not be prescribed until organic causes for obesity, such as untreated hypothyroidism, have been ruled out.

In sibutramine obesity trials of 6 months or longer, the patients who lost at least 1.8 kg (4 pounds) of body weight during the first 4 weeks of treatment were much more likely than the patients who lost less than this to subsequently lose at least 5% of their initial body weight at a given dose. If a patient does not lose at least 1.8 kg (4 pounds) in the first 4 weeks of sibutramine treatment, therapy should be re-evaluated and sibutramine dosage should be increased, or sibutramine use should be discontinued.

## Sibutramine (Systemic)—Introductory Version

**Diet/Nutrition**
Sibutramine may be taken with or without food.
A reduced-calorie diet should be followed during sibutramine therapy.

## Oral Dosage Form

### SIBUTRAMINE HYDROCHLORIDE MONOHYDRATE CAPSULES

**Usual adult dose**
Obesity, exogenous—
  Oral, initially 10 mg once a day, usually in the morning. If weight loss is inadequate after four weeks of therapy, dosage may be increased to 15 mg once a day, taking into consideration effects on heart rate and blood pressure.
Note: Patients who do not tolerate the 10-mg dose may benefit from a 5-mg dose.

**Usual adult prescribing limits**
15 mg per day.

**Usual pediatric dose**
Safety and efficacy in children up to 16 years of age have not been established.

**Usual geriatric dose**
See *Usual adult dose*.
Note: Dosing in elderly patients should be approached cautiously because of the high incidence of concomitant disease states and medication use in this population.

**Strength(s) usually available**
U.S.—
  5 mg (Rx) [*Meridia* (colloidal silicon dioxide; D&C Yellow No. 10; FD&C Blue No. 2; gelatin; lactose monohydrate; microcrystalline cellulose; magnesium stearate; titanium dioxide)].
  10 mg (Rx) [*Meridia* (colloidal silicon dioxide; FD&C Blue No. 2; gelatin; lactose monohydrate; microcrystalline cellulose; magnesium stearate; titanium dioxide)].
  15 mg (Rx) [*Meridia* (colloidal silicon dioxide; D&C Yellow No. 10; gelatin; lactose monohydrate; microcrystalline cellulose; magnesium stearate; titanium dioxide)].

**Packaging and storage**
Store at 25 ºC (77 ºF), with excursions between 15 and 30 ºC (59 and 86 ºF) permitted, in a tight, light-resistant container, unless otherwise specified by manufacturer. Protect from heat and moisture.

**Auxiliary labeling**
• May cause dizziness or drowsiness

**Note**
Sibutramine is a controlled substance in the U.S.

Developed: 04/16/98

---

# SILDENAFIL  Systemic—INTRODUCTORY VERSION

VA CLASSIFICATION (Primary): GU900
Note: For a listing of dosage forms and brand names by country availability, see *Dosage Forms* section(s).

## Category
Impotence therapy agent (systemic).

## Indications

**General considerations**
Erectile dysfunction that is medication-induced or caused by endocrine problems, such as hypogonadism or hypothyroidism or hyperthyroidism, should be evaluated and appropriately treated before sildenafil treatment is considered.
Cardiac risk associated with sexual activity should be individually assessed prior to initiating any treatment for erectile dysfunction.

**Accepted**
Erectile dysfunction (treatment)—Sildenafil is indicated to facilitate erections in men with erectile dysfunction.
  Sildenafil has been evaluated in 3000 patients (19 to 87 years of age) in twenty-one studies of up to 6 months. Compared with patients taking a placebo, patients taking sildenafil demonstrated statistically significant improvement in treatment of erectile dysfunction of organic, psychogenic, or mixed etiologies (mean onset of 5 years). Sildenafil was effective in a broad range of patients, including those with a history of coronary artery disease, hypertension, other cardiac disease, peripheral vascular disease, diabetes mellitus, depression, coronary artery bypass graft (CABG), radical prostatectomy, transurethral resection of the prostate (TURP), and spinal cord injury. Sildenafil was also effective in patients taking antidepressant, antipsychotic, antihypertensive, or diuretic medications.

## Pharmacology/Pharmacokinetics

**Physicochemical characteristics**
Molecular weight—666.7.

**Mechanism of action/Effect**
Impotence therapy agent—Sildenafil is a selective inhibitor of phosphodiesterase type 5 (PDE5), an enzyme responsible for degrading cyclic guanosine monophosphate (cGMP) in the corpus cavernosum. By diminishing the effect of PDE5, sildenafil facilitates the effect of nitric oxide during sexual stimulation: cGMP levels increase, smooth muscle relaxes, and blood flows into the corpus cavernosum, producing an erection. Without sexual stimulation, sildenafil has no effect on erections.

*In vitro* studies show that sildenafil's potency for action on phosphodiesterases differs. Sildenafil's action is greater for PDE5 than for the following phosphodiesterases: PDE1 ( 80 times); PDE2 and PDE4 ( 1000 times); PDE3 (about 4000 times), and PDE6 (about 10 times). PDE3 controls cardiac contractility and PDE6, an enzyme found in the retina, may be involved in color vision abnormalities reported for the higher dose of sildenafil. The active metabolite of sildenafil has approximately 50% potency for PDE5, and contributes approximately 20% of sildenafil's effect.

**Absorption**
Rapidly absorbed; absolute bioavailability is approximately 40%. A high-fat meal reduces absorption as shown by reducing the maximum plasma concentration ($C_{max}$) by 29% and delaying time to peak concentration ($T_{max}$) by 60 minutes.

**Distribution**
The mean steady state volume of distribution ($Vol_{ss}$) is 105 liters. Less than 0.001% of sildenafil remained in the semen of healthy volunteers at 90 minutes.

**Protein binding**
Very high (96% bound to plasma proteins).

**Biotransformation**
Hepatic metabolism, via cytochrome P450 (CYP) 3A4 (major route) and CYP2C9 (minor route). Sildenafil is converted by N-desmethylation to an active metabolite with properties similar to those of the parent, sildenafil. Parent and active metabolite are metabolized further.

**Half-life**
4 hours (terminal half-life for parent and major metabolite).

**Onset of action**
Within 0.5 hour after administration.

**Time to peak concentration**
30 to 120 minutes under fasting conditions; sildenafil is delayed by 60 minutes when given with a high-fat meal.

**Peak serum concentration**
Sildenafil—Not listed in the manufacturer's labeling; major metabolite has 40% of the serum concentration of sildenafil.

**Duration of action**
Up to 4 hours, but with less response than that seen at 2 hours.

**Elimination**
Feces (80% of the administered dose as metabolites); urine (13% of the administered dose as metabolites).

## Precautions to Consider

### Carcinogenicity
In 24-month animal studies, sildenafil was not found to be carcinogenic in male rats given 29 times the maximum recommended human dose (MRHD) or in female rats given 42 times the MRHD. In 18- to 21-month studies, sildenafil was not carcinogenic in mice given 10 mg per kg of body weight (mg/kg) a day, corresponding to 0.6 times the MRHD (based on a mg per square meter of body surface area).

### Mutagenicity
Sildenafil was not found to be mutagenic for *in vivo* mouse micronucleus assay or *in vitro* human lymphocytes assay and bacterial or Chinese hamster ovary cell assays.

### Pregnancy/Reproduction
Fertility—Single doses of 100 mg sildenafil given to males did not impair sperm motility or morphology.

In animal studies, sildenafil did not impair fertility in rats given sildenafil in doses of 60 mg/kg a day for 36 days in females and for 102 days in males, corresponding to an area under the plasma concentration–time curve (AUC) that was greater than 25 times that produced in humans.

Pregnancy—Adequate and well-controlled studies in humans have not been done. Sildenafil is not indicated for use in females.

In animal studies, sildenafil was not teratogenic, embryotoxic, or fetotoxic in rats and rabbits given up to 200 mg/kg a day during organogenesis, corresponding to 20 to 40 times the MRHD as calculated per body surface area of a 50-kg person.

FDA Pregnancy Category B.

### Breast-feeding
Problems in humans have not been documented; sildenafil is not indicated for use in females.

### Geriatrics
Healthy volunteers 65 years of age and over cleared sildenafil less effectively from the plasma than did healthy younger volunteers 18 to 45 years of age as shown by a 40% increase of AUC in older adults. Using an initial lower dose of 25 mg is recommended for patients 65 years of age and over.

### Drug interactions and/or related problems
The following drug interactions and/or related problems have been selected on the basis of their potential clinical significance (possible mechanism in parentheses where appropriate)—not necessarily inclusive (» = major clinical significance):

Note: Combinations containing any of the following medications, depending on the amount present, may also interact with this medication.

The safety and efficacy of combining sildenafil treatment with other impotence therapy agents have not been studied.

There is no difference in the side effect profiles of patients taking sildenafil with antihypertensive medications compared with those of patients taking sildenafil without antihypertensive medications.

» Enzyme inhibitors, hepatic, cytochrome P450 (CYP) 3A4 including:
    Cimetidine
    Erythromycin
    Itraconazole
    Ketoconazole
    Mibefradil
(an increase in sildenafil plasma concentrations is likely to occur with CYP3A4 inhibitors because they reduce the metabolism and clearance of sildenafil; using a lower dose of 25 mg is recommended for patients taking these medications. Plasma concentrations of sildenafil increased 56% when a 50-mg dose of sildenafil was administered with cimetidine; AUC of sildenafil increased 182% when a single 100-mg dose of sildenafil was administered after steady-state concentrations of erythromycin were achieved at 5 days; similar reactions are expected with stronger CYP3A4 inhibitors, such as ketoconazole, itraconazole, and mibefradil)

Enzyme inducers, hepatic, cytochrome P450 (CYP) 3A4, including rifampin
(a decrease in sildenafil plasma concentrations is likely to occur with CYP3A4 inducers because they increase the metabolism and clearance of sildenafil)

» Nitrates, including nitroglycerin
(sildenafil potentiates the hypotensive effect of nitrates; concomitant use is not recommended)

### Medical considerations/Contraindications
The medical considerations/contraindications included have been selected on the basis of their potential clinical significance (reasons given in parentheses where appropriate)—not necessarily inclusive (» = major clinical significance).

*Risk-benefit should be considered when the following medical problems exist:*

Abnormalities of the penis, such as:
    Anatomical deformity
    Angulation of the penis
    Cavernosal fibrosis
    Hypospadia, severe
    Peyronie's disease
(patients who have an anatomical deformity, angulation of the penis, cavernosal fibrosis, or Peyronie's disease are at increased risk of developing problems when using impotence therapy agents, including sildenafil)

Bleeding disorders, including peptic ulcer, active or
Coagulation defects, severe
(risk of bleeding may be increased since sildenafil may inhibit platelet aggregation as shown in *in vitro* studies; further study is needed. Safety information is not available for use of sildenafil in these patients)

Cardiovascular disease
(cardiac risk associated with sexual activity should be individually assessed prior to initiating any treatment for erectile dysfunction)

» Cirrhosis or
» Hepatic function impairment, severe
(sildenafil clearance was reduced in volunteers with hepatic cirrhosis [Child-Pugh A and B], resulting in an increase of AUC by 84% and of $C_{max}$ by 47% when compared with data of age-matched volunteers who had no hepatic impairment; using a lower initial dose of 25 mg of sildenafil is recommended for these patients)

Leukemia or
Myeloma, multiple or
Polycythemia or
Priapism, history of or
Sickle cell disease or
Thrombocythemia
(although priapism was not reported in clinical trials of sildenafil, patients with these predisposing conditions have an increased risk of priapism)

» Renal function impairment, severe
(creatinine clearance of less than 30 mL/min [severe renal insufficiency] significantly reduced sildenafil clearance, approximately doubling AUC and $C_{max}$ compared with those of age-matched volunteers who had no renal impairment; using a lower initial dose of 25 mg of sildenafil is recommended for these patients. Creatinine clearance of 30 to 80 mL/min [mild to moderate renal insufficiency] did not alter pharmacokinetics of 50 mg sildenafil as a single dose)

Retinitis pigmentosa
(a minority of patients with this condition also experience genetic disorders of retinal phosphodiesterases; safety information is not available for use of sildenafil in these patients)

Sensitivity to sildenafil

## Side/Adverse Effects

Note: In clinical studies, priapism was not reported.

The following side/adverse effects have been selected on the basis of their potential clinical significance (possible signs and symptoms in parentheses where appropriate)—not necessarily inclusive:

### Those indicating need for medical attention
Incidence less frequent—2 to 3%
*Abnormal vision, including blurred vision; color change perception* (seeing shades of colors differently than before); *or sensitivity to light*—may be mild and transient; *dizziness; urinary tract infection or cystitis* (bladder pain; cloudy or bloody urine; increased frequency of urination; pain on urination)

Note: In fixed-dose studies, *abnormal vision* was more common at the 100-mg dose (incidence of 11%) than at lower doses.

Incidence rare—Less than 2%

Note: The following side/adverse effects reported in clinical trials of sildenafil have not been established as being caused by sildenafil.

*Allergic reaction* (skin rash; hives; itching of skin); *anemia or asthenia* (unusual tiredness or weakness); *arthrosis; arthritis; gout or hyperuricemia; synovitis or tenosynovitis; tendon rupture* (bone pain; lower back or side pain; painful, swollen joints); *breast enlargement; cardiovascular effects, such as angina pectoris* (chest pain); *AV block* (fainting; trouble in breathing; unusual weakness); *cardiac arrest* (heart failure); ***cerebral thrombosis*** (confusion; numbness of hands); ***hypotension, including orthostatic hypotension*** (dizziness or lightheadedness, especially when getting up from a lying or sitting position; low blood pressure); ***migraine headache; myocardial ischemia*** (chest pain; shortness of breath); ***palpitation*** (pounding heartbeat); ***syncope*** (fainting); ***and tachycardia*** (fast heartbeat); ***chills; deafness; edema*** (swelling of face, hands, feet, or lower legs); ***hyperglycemia*** (faintness; nausea; paleness of skin; sweating); ***or hypoglycemia reaction*** (anxiety; behavior change similar to drunkenness; blurred vision; cold sweats; confusion; cool, pale skin; difficulty in concentrating; drowsiness; excessive hunger; fast heartbeat; headache; nausea; nervousness; nightmares; restless sleep; shakiness; slurred speech; unusual tiredness or weakness)—especially for patients with diabetes mellitus; ***hypernatremia*** (confusion; convulsions; decrease in amount of urine or in frequency of urination; dizziness; fast heartbeat; headache; increased thirst; swelling of feet or lower legs; twitching of muscles; unusual tiredness or weakness); ***leukopenia*** (sore throat and fever or chills); ***myasthenia*** (weakness of muscles); ***ophthalmic effects, such as cataracts; conjunctivitis*** (feeling of something in the eye; redness, itching, or tearing of eyes); ***dry eyes; eye hemorrhage*** (eye pain); ***and mydriasis*** (increase in size of pupil); ***shock*** (fainting); ***skin effects, such as contact dermatitis; pruritus; or urticaria*** (hives; itching; redness of skin); ***exfoliative dermatitis*** (dryness, redness, scaling, or peeling of the skin); ***herpes simplex*** (groups of skin lesions with swelling; unusual feeling of burning or stinging of skin); ***and skin ulcers***

**Those indicating need for medical attention only if they continue or are bothersome**
Incidence more frequent
 *Dyspepsia* (stomach discomfort following meals)—7%; *flushing*—10%; *headache*—16%; *nasal congestion*—4%
 Note: In fixed-dose studies, *dyspepsia* was more common at the 100-mg dose (incidence of 17%) than at lower doses.

Incidence less frequent
 *Diarrhea*

Incidence rare—Less than 2%
 Note: The following side/adverse effects reported in clinical trials of sildenafil have not been established as being caused by sildenafil.
 ***Abdominal pain; CNS symptoms, such as abnormal dreams; ataxia*** (clumsiness or unsteadiness); ***decreased reflexes*** (lack of coordination); ***hypertonia*** (tense muscles); ***hypesthesia*** (increased skin sensitivity); ***insomnia*** (trouble in sleeping); ***mental depression; neuralgia; neuropathy; paresthesia; or tremor*** (aches, pains, or weakness of muscles; numbness or tingling of hands, legs, or feet; trembling and shaking; unusual feeling of burning or stinging of skin); ***somnolence*** (sleepiness); ***and vertigo*** (sensation of motion, usually whirling, either of one's self or of one's surroundings); ***ear pain; gastrointestinal effects, such as colitis*** (severe diarrhea or stomach cramps); ***dry mouth, esophagitis, gastritis, and stomatitis*** (difficulty in swallowing; redness or irritation of the tongue; sores in mouth and on lips); ***gastroenteritis*** (abdominal pain; diarrhea, severe; nausea); ***gingivitis*** (redness, soreness, swelling, or bleeding of gums); ***rectal bleeding; and vomiting; increased amount of saliva; increased sweating or thirst; myalgia*** (aches or pains in muscles); ***respiratory effects, such as asthma; bronchitis; dyspnea; laryngitis; pharyngitis; and sinusitis*** (cough; shortness of breath or troubled breathing; tightness of chest or wheezing); ***tinnitus*** (ringing or buzzing in ears); ***urogenital effects, such as abnormal ejaculation or anorgasmia*** (failure to experience a sexual orgasm; sexual problems in men, continuing); ***nocturia*** (waking to urinate at night); ***urinary frequency, and urinary incontinence*** (loss of bladder control)

## Overdose
For more information on the management of overdose or unintentional ingestion, **contact a Poison Control Center** (see *Poison Control Center Listing*).

**Clinical effects of overdose**
In studies with healthy volunteers taking single doses of up to 800 mg, adverse events were similar to those seen at lower doses but incidence rates were increased.

**Treatment of overdose**
To enhance elimination—Renal dialysis is not expected to accelerate clearance of sildenafil; sildenafil is highly bound to plasma proteins and is not eliminated in the urine.

Supportive care—Supportive treatment should be adopted as required. Patients in whom intentional overdose is confirmed or suspected should be referred for psychiatric consultation.

## Patient Consultation
As an aid to patient consultation, refer to *Advice for the Patient, Sildenafil (Systemic)—Introductory Version*.
In providing consultation, consider emphasizing the following selected information (» = major clinical significance):

**Before using this medication**
» Conditions affecting use, especially:
 Sensitivity to sildenafil
 Use in the elderly—Patients 65 years of age and older should be started at 25 mg of sildenafil because of their slower metabolism and clearance and should be monitored more often for side/adverse effects
 Other medications, especially enzyme inhibitors, hepatic, cytochrome P450 3A4, including cimetidine, erythromycin, itraconazole, ketoconazole, and mibefradil; or nitrates, including nitroglycerin
 Other medical problems, especially cirrhosis or severe hepatic or renal function impairment

**Proper use of this medication**
» Reading patient package insert
 Knowing that medication begins to work within 30 minutes after taking it and effect continues for up to 4 hours, lessening after 2 hours
» Proper dosing
» Proper storage

**Precautions while using this medication**
» Concurrent use of other impotence therapy agents is not presently recommended
» Complying with therapy dose recommendations; importance of not exceeding prescribed dosage and frequency of use

**Side/adverse effects**
 Signs of potential side effects, especially abnormal vision, including blurred vision, color change perception, and sensitivity to light; dizziness; urinary tract infection or cystitis
 Signs of potential side effects (although not proven to be caused by sildenafil, but reported in clinical trials), especially allergic reaction; anemia or asthenia; arthrosis, arthritis, gout or hyperuricemia, synovitis (including tenosynovitis), tendon rupture; breast enlargement; cardiovascular effects, such as angina pectoris, AV block, cardiac arrest, cerebral thrombosis, migraine headache, palpitation, tachycardia, hypotension (including orthostatic hypotension), myocardial ischemia, and syncope; chills; deafness; edema; hyperglycemia or hypoglycemia—especially for patients with diabetes mellitus; hypernatremia; leukopenia; myasthenia; ophthalmic effects, such as cataracts, conjunctivitis, dry eyes, eye hemorrhage, mydriasis; shock; or skin effects, such as contact dermatitis, exfoliative dermatitis, herpes simplex, pruritus, skin ulcer, and urticaria

## General Dosing Information
For treatment of untreated erectile dysfunction—Sildenafil improved frequency, firmness, and maintenance of erections; frequency of orgasm; frequency and level of desire; frequency, satisfaction, and enjoyment of intercourse; and overall relationship satisfaction.

For treatment of erectile dysfunction due to a radical prostatectomy–Across all trials, sildenafil improved the erections of 43% of patients compared with improvement in 15% of the patients taking a placebo.

For treatment of erectile dysfunction due to complications of diabetes mellitus—Sildenafil improved frequency of successful penetration during sexual activity and maintenance of erections after penetration, compared to patients taking a placebo. Fifty-seven percent of patients taking sildenafil reported improved erections compared with 10% of patients taking a placebo.

For treatment of erectile dysfunction due to a spinal cord injury—Sildenafil improved frequency of successful penetration during sexual activity and maintenance of erections after penetration. Eighty-three percent of patients taking sildenafil reported improved erections compared with 12% of patients taking a placebo.

For treatment of erectile dysfunction due to psychogenic etiology—Sildenafil improved frequency of successful penetration during sexual activity and maintenance of erections after penetration. Eighty-four percent of patients taking sildenafil reported improved erections compared with 26% of patients taking a placebo.

## Oral Dosage Forms

### SILDENAFIL CITRATE

**Usual adult dose**
Erectile dysfunction—
   Oral, 50 mg (base) one hour (range, one half to four hours) before sexual intercourse once a day if needed. As tolerated, subsequent doses may be increased to 100 mg or decreased to 25 mg once a day.

**Usual adult prescribing limits**
100 mg once a day.

**Usual geriatric dose**
Erectile dysfunction—
   Oral, 25 mg (base) one hour (range, one half to four hours) before sexual intercourse once a day if needed. As tolerated, subsequent doses may be increased.

**Strength(s) usually available**
U.S.—
   25 mg (base) (Rx) [*Viagra* (croscarmellose sodium; lactose; magnesium stearate)].
   50 mg (base) (Rx) [*Viagra* (croscarmellose sodium; lactose; magnesium stearate)].
   100 mg (base) (Rx) [*Viagra* (croscarmellose sodium; lactose; magnesium stearate)].

**Packaging and storage**
Store below 40 °C (104 °F), preferably between 15 and 30 °C (59 and 86 °F).

**Note**
Include patient information insert (PPI) when dispensing.

Developed: 05/28/98

---

**SILICONE OIL 5000 CENTISTOKES**—The *Silicone Oil 500 Centistokes (Parenteral-Local)* monograph is not included in this published version of the USP DI database. Copies of the monograph are available on request from Micromedex, Inc. - Reprint Requests, 6200 S. Syracuse Way, Suite 300, Englewood, CO 80111; telephone (303) 486-6400; telefax (303) 486-6464; Email: USPDI@MDX.COM.

---

**SILVER SULFADIAZINE**—The *Silver Sulfadiazine (Topical)* monograph is not included in this published version of the USP DI database. Copies of the monograph are available on request from Micromedex, Inc. - Reprint Requests, 6200 S. Syracuse Way, Suite 300, Englewood, CO 80111; telephone (303) 486-6400; telefax (303) 486-6464; Email: USPDI@MDX.COM.

---

**SIMETHICONE**—The *Simethicone (Oral-Local)* monograph is not included in this published version of the USP DI database. Copies of the monograph are available on request from Micromedex, Inc. - Reprint Requests, 6200 S. Syracuse Way, Suite 300, Englewood, CO 80111; telephone (303) 486-6400; telefax (303) 486-6464; Email: USPDI@MDX.COM.

---

**SIMVASTATIN**—See *HMG-CoA Reductase Inhibitors (Systemic)*

---

**SINCALIDE**—The *Sincalide (Systemic)* monograph is not included in this published version of the USP DI database. Copies of the monograph are available on request from Micromedex, Inc. - Reprint Requests, 6200 S. Syracuse Way, Suite 300, Englewood, CO 80111; telephone (303) 486-6400; telefax (303) 486-6464; Email: USPDI@MDX.COM.

---

# SKELETAL MUSCLE RELAXANTS   Systemic

This monograph includes information on the following: 1) Carisoprodol; 2) Chlorphenesin[†]; 3) Chlorzoxazone[†]; 4) Metaxalone[†]; 5) Methocarbamol; 6) Orphenadrine.

VA CLASSIFICATION (Primary/Secondary):
   Carisoprodol—MS200
   Chlorphenesin—MS200
   Chlorzoxazone—MS200
   Metaxalone—MS200
   Methocarbamol—MS200
   Orphenadrine Citrate—MS200
   Orphenadrine Hydrochloride—AU350

Commonly used brand name(s): *Antiflex*[6]; *Banflex*[6]; *Carbacot*[5]; *Disipal*[6]; *EZE-DS*[3]; *Flexoject*[6]; *Maolate*[2]; *Mio-Rel*[6]; *Myolin*[6]; *Myotrol*[6]; *Norflex*[6]; *Orfro*[6]; *Orphenate*[6]; *Paraflex*[3]; *Parafon Forte DSC*[3]; *Relaxazone*[3]; *Remular*[3]; *Remular-S*[3]; *Robaxin*[5]; *Robaxin-750*[5]; *Skelaxin*[4]; *Skelex*[5]; *Soma*[1]; *Strifon Forte DSC*[3]; *Vanadom*[1].

Note:   For a listing of dosage forms and brand names by country availability, see *Dosage Forms* section(s).

[†]Not commercially available in Canada.

## Category

Skeletal muscle relaxant—Carisoprodol; Chlorphenesin; Chlorzoxazone; Metaxalone; Methocarbamol; Orphenadrine Citrate.
Parkinsonism therapy adjunct—Orphenadrine Hydrochloride.

## Indications

**Accepted**
Spasm, skeletal muscle (treatment)—Skeletal muscle relaxants are indicated as adjuncts to other measures, such as rest and physical therapy, for the relief of muscle spasm associated with acute, painful musculoskeletal conditions.

Parkinsonism (treatment adjunct)—Orphenadrine hydrochloride is indicated (but is rarely used) as an adjunct to physical therapy and other medications in the treatment of postencephalic, arteriosclerotic, or idiopathic parkinsonism. It produces symptomatic relief of tremor. The medication may be used concurrently with reduced dosages of more potent medications in treating patients who cannot tolerate effective doses of the other medications.

**Unaccepted**
Methocarbamol is also FDA-approved for control of the neuromuscular manifestations of tetanus. However, it has largely been replaced in the treatment of tetanus by diazepam, or, in severe cases, a neuromuscular blocking agent such as pancuronium. Such therapy is used as an adjunct to other measures, such as debridement, tetanus antitoxin, penicillin, tracheotomy, fluid and electrolyte replacement, and supportive treatment.

## Pharmacology/Pharmacokinetics

See *Table 1*, page 2582.
See *Table 2*, page 2583.

**Physicochemical characteristics**
Molecular weight—
   Carisoprodol: 260.34.
   Chlorphenesin carbamate: 245.66.
   Chlorzoxazone: 169.57.
   Metaxalone: 221.26.
   Methocarbamol: 241.25.
   Orphenadrine citrate: 461.51.
   Orphenadrine hydrochloride: 305.85.

**Mechanism of action/Effect**
Skeletal muscle relaxant—Precise mechanism of action has not been determined. These agents act in the central nervous system (CNS) rather than directly on skeletal muscle. Several of these medications have been shown to depress polysynaptic reflexes preferentially. The muscle relaxant effects of most of these agents may be related to their CNS

depressant (sedative) effects. Carisoprodol blocks interneuronal activity in the descending reticular formation and in the spinal cord. Chlorzoxazone acts primarily at the spinal cord level and at subcortical areas of the brain. Orphenadrine has analgesic activity, which may contribute to its skeletal muscle relaxant properties.

Parkinsonism therapy adjunct—Orphenadrine has mild anticholinergic actions, which produce its beneficial effect in parkinsonism.

**Other actions/effects**
Orphenadrine also has anticholinergic properties.

## Precautions to Consider

### Cross-sensitivity and/or related problems
Patients sensitive to other carbamate derivatives (for example, carbromal, meprobamate, mebutamate, or tybamate) may be sensitive to carisoprodol also.

### Pregnancy/Reproduction
Pregnancy—
  *Carisoprodol, chlorzoxazone, and methocarbamol*—
    Problems in humans have not been documented.
  *Chlorphenesin*—
    Studies have not been done in either animals or humans.
  *Metaxalone*—
    Although studies in humans have not been done, studies in rats have not shown that metaxalone causes adverse effects in the fetus.
  *Orphenadrine*—
    Problems in humans have not been documented.
    Studies in animals have not been done.
    Orphenadrine citrate—FDA Pregnancy Category C.

### Breast-feeding
*Carisoprodol*—
  Carisoprodol is distributed into breast milk in concentrations that may reach 2 to 4 times the maternal plasma concentrations; use by nursing mothers may cause sedation and gastrointestinal upset in the infant.
*Chlorphenesin, chlorzoxazone, metaxalone, methocarbamol, and orphenadrine*—
  It is not known whether these medications are distributed into breast milk. However, problems in humans have not been documented.

### Pediatrics
*Carisoprodol*—
  Although appropriate studies with carisoprodol have not been performed in the pediatric population, the medication has been used in children. Pediatrics-specific problems that would limit the use of carisoprodol in these patients have not been documented.
*Chlorphenesin, metaxalone, methocarbamol, and orphenadrine*—
  No information is available on the relationship of age to the effects of these medications in pediatric patients. Safety and efficacy have not been established.
*Chlorzoxazone*—
  This medication has been used in children. Pediatrics-specific problems that would limit use of chlorzoxazone in these patients have not been documented.

### Geriatrics
No information is available on the relationship of age to the effects of skeletal muscle relaxants in geriatric patients. However, elderly males are more likely to have age-related prostatic hypertrophy and may therefore be adversely affected by orphenadrine's anticholinergic activity. Also, elderly patients are more likely to have age-related renal function impairment, which may require that parenteral methocarbamol not be used at all and that other skeletal muscle relaxants be used with caution.

### Dental
*Orphenadrine*—
  The peripheral anticholinergic effects of orphenadrine may decrease or inhibit salivary flow, thus contributing to the development of caries, periodontal disease, oral candidiasis, and discomfort.

### Drug interactions and/or related problems
The following drug interactions and/or related problems have been selected on the basis of their potential clinical significance (possible mechanism in parentheses where appropriate)—not necessarily inclusive (» = major clinical significance):

Note: Combinations containing any of the following medications, depending on the amount present, may also interact with this medication.

*For all skeletal muscle relaxants*
» Alcohol or
» CNS depression–producing medications, other (See *Appendix II* )

(concurrent use with a skeletal muscle relaxant may result in additive CNS depressant effects; caution is recommended and dosage of one or both agents should be reduced )

*For orphenadrine (in addition to the interaction listed above)*
  Anticholinergics or other medications with anticholinergic action (See *Appendix II* )
    (anticholinergic effects may be intensified when these medications are used concurrently with orphenadrine because of orphenadrine's secondary anticholinergic activity)

### Laboratory value alterations
The following have been selected on the basis of their potential clinical significance (possible effect in parentheses where appropriate)—not necessarily inclusive (» = major clinical significance):

With diagnostic test results
*For metaxalone*
  Copper sulfate urine sugar tests
    (false-positive test results may occur, possibly because of the presence of an unknown reducing substance; results of tests using glucose oxidase are not affected)

*For methocarbamol*
  5-Hydroxyindoleacetic acid (5-HIAA), in urine, determinations
    (values may be falsely increased when the nitrosonaphthol reagent is used)
  Vanillylmandelic acid (VMA), in urine, determinations
    (values may be falsely increased when the Gitlow screening method is used; no error occurs when the quantitative procedure of Sunderman is used)

With physiology/laboratory test values
*For metaxalone*
  Cephalin flocculation tests
    (elevations may occur without concurrent changes in other liver function tests)

### Medical considerations/Contraindications
The medical considerations/contraindications included have been selected on the basis of their potential clinical significance (reasons given in parentheses where appropriate)—not necessarily inclusive (» = major clinical significance).

See *Table 3,* page 2583.

### Patient monitoring
The following may be especially important in patient monitoring (other tests may be warranted in some patients, depending on condition; » = major clinical significance):

*For metaxalone*
  Liver function tests
    (recommended periodically during prolonged metaxalone therapy, especially if the patient has pre-existing hepatic function impairment or disease)

*For methocarbamol*
  Renal function determinations
    (recommended if parenteral therapy lasts 3 days or more because the polyethylene glycol 300 vehicle may be nephrotoxic)

*For orphenadrine*
  Blood count and
  Liver function tests and
  Renal function tests
    (recommended during prolonged therapy since the safety of continuous long-term use has not been established)

## Side/Adverse Effects

See *Table 4,* page 2584.

Note: Rarely, an idiosyncratic reaction to carisoprodol may occur within minutes or hours following the first dose of the medication. Reported symptoms include agitation, ataxia, confusion, disorientation, dizziness, euphoria, extreme weakness, speech disturbances, temporary loss of vision or other vision disturbances, and transient quadriplegia. Symptoms usually subside within several hours, but in some cases, supportive and symptomatic therapy, including hospitalization, may be necessary.

Psychological dependence and abuse have occurred very rarely with carisoprodol. Signs of abstinence have not been reported with clinical usage; however, in one study abrupt withdrawal of 100 mg per kg of body weight (mg/kg) per day of carisoprodol (5 times the recommended daily dose) produced withdrawal symptoms including abdominal cramps, insomnia, chills, headache, and nausea.

USP DI

## Oral Dosage Forms

### SILDENAFIL CITRATE

**Usual adult dose**
Erectile dysfunction—
  Oral, 50 mg (base) one hour (range, one half to four hours) before sexual intercourse once a day if needed. As tolerated, subsequent doses may be increased to 100 mg or decreased to 25 mg once a day.

**Usual adult prescribing limits**
100 mg once a day.

**Usual geriatric dose**
Erectile dysfunction—
  Oral, 25 mg (base) one hour (range, one half to four hours) before sexual intercourse once a day if needed. As tolerated, subsequent doses may be increased.

**Strength(s) usually available**
U.S.—
  25 mg (base) (Rx) [*Viagra* (croscarmellose sodium; lactose; magnesium stearate)].
  50 mg (base) (Rx) [*Viagra* (croscarmellose sodium; lactose; magnesium stearate)].
  100 mg (base) (Rx) [*Viagra* (croscarmellose sodium; lactose; magnesium stearate)].

**Packaging and storage**
Store below 40 °C (104 °F), preferably between 15 and 30 °C (59 and 86 °F).

**Note**
Include patient information insert (PPI) when dispensing.

Developed: 05/28/98

---

**SILICONE OIL 5000 CENTISTOKES**—The *Silicone Oil 500 Centistokes (Parenteral-Local)* monograph is not included in this published version of the USP DI database. Copies of the monograph are available on request from Micromedex, Inc. - Reprint Requests, 6200 S. Syracuse Way, Suite 300, Englewood, CO 80111; telephone (303) 486-6400; telefax (303) 486-6464; Email: USPDI@MDX.COM.

**SILVER SULFADIAZINE**—The *Silver Sulfadiazine (Topical)* monograph is not included in this published version of the USP DI database. Copies of the monograph are available on request from Micromedex, Inc. - Reprint Requests, 6200 S. Syracuse Way, Suite 300, Englewood, CO 80111; telephone (303) 486-6400; telefax (303) 486-6464; Email: USPDI@MDX.COM.

**SIMETHICONE**—The *Simethicone (Oral-Local)* monograph is not included in this published version of the USP DI database. Copies of the monograph are available on request from Micromedex, Inc. - Reprint Requests, 6200 S. Syracuse Way, Suite 300, Englewood, CO 80111; telephone (303) 486-6400; telefax (303) 486-6464; Email: USPDI@MDX.COM.

**SIMVASTATIN**—See *HMG-CoA Reductase Inhibitors (Systemic)*

**SINCALIDE**—The *Sincalide (Systemic)* monograph is not included in this published version of the USP DI database. Copies of the monograph are available on request from Micromedex, Inc. - Reprint Requests, 6200 S. Syracuse Way, Suite 300, Englewood, CO 80111; telephone (303) 486-6400; telefax (303) 486-6464; Email: USPDI@MDX.COM.

---

# SKELETAL MUSCLE RELAXANTS   Systemic

This monograph includes information on the following: 1) Carisoprodol; 2) Chlorphenesin†; 3) Chlorzoxazone†; 4) Metaxalone†; 5) Methocarbamol; 6) Orphenadrine.

VA CLASSIFICATION (Primary/Secondary):
  Carisoprodol—MS200
  Chlorphenesin—MS200
  Chlorzoxazone—MS200
  Metaxalone—MS200
  Methocarbamol—MS200
  Orphenadrine Citrate—MS200
  Orphenadrine Hydrochloride—AU350

Commonly used brand name(s): *Antiflex*[6]; *Banflex*[6]; *Carbacot*[5]; *Disipal*[6]; *EZE-DS*[3]; *Flexoject*[6]; *Maolate*[2]; *Mio-Rel*[6]; *Myolin*[6]; *Myotrol*[6]; *Norflex*[6]; *Orfro*[6]; *Orphenate*[6]; *Paraflex*[3]; *Parafon Forte DSC*[3]; *Relaxazone*[3]; *Remular*[3]; *Remular-S*[3]; *Robaxin*[5]; *Robaxin-750*[5]; *Skelaxin*[4]; *Skelex*[5]; *Soma*[1]; *Strifon Forte DSC*[3]; *Vanadom*[1].

Note: For a listing of dosage forms and brand names by country availability, see *Dosage Forms* section(s).

†Not commercially available in Canada.

## Category

Skeletal muscle relaxant—Carisoprodol; Chlorphenesin; Chlorzoxazone; Metaxalone; Methocarbamol; Orphenadrine Citrate.
Parkinsonism therapy adjunct—Orphenadrine Hydrochloride.

## Indications

**Accepted**

Spasm, skeletal muscle (treatment)—Skeletal muscle relaxants are indicated as adjuncts to other measures, such as rest and physical therapy, for the relief of muscle spasm associated with acute, painful musculoskeletal conditions.

Parkinsonism (treatment adjunct)—Orphenadrine hydrochloride is indicated (but is rarely used) as an adjunct to physical therapy and other medications in the treatment of postencephalic, arteriosclerotic, or idiopathic parkinsonism. It produces symptomatic relief of tremor. The medication may be used concurrently with reduced dosages of more potent medications in treating patients who cannot tolerate effective doses of the other medications.

**Unaccepted**

Methocarbamol is also FDA-approved for control of the neuromuscular manifestations of tetanus. However, it has largely been replaced in the treatment of tetanus by diazepam, or, in severe cases, a neuromuscular blocking agent such as pancuronium. Such therapy is used as an adjunct to other measures, such as debridement, tetanus antitoxin, penicillin, tracheotomy, fluid and electrolyte replacement, and supportive treatment.

## Pharmacology/Pharmacokinetics

See *Table 1*, page 2582.
See *Table 2*, page 2583.

**Physicochemical characteristics**
Molecular weight—
  Carisoprodol: 260.34.
  Chlorphenesin carbamate: 245.66.
  Chlorzoxazone: 169.57.
  Metaxalone: 221.26.
  Methocarbamol: 241.25.
  Orphenadrine citrate: 461.51.
  Orphenadrine hydrochloride: 305.85.

**Mechanism of action/Effect**
Skeletal muscle relaxant—Precise mechanism of action has not been determined. These agents act in the central nervous system (CNS) rather than directly on skeletal muscle. Several of these medications have been shown to depress polysynaptic reflexes preferentially. The muscle relaxant effects of most of these agents may be related to their CNS

depressant (sedative) effects. Carisoprodol blocks interneuronal activity in the descending reticular formation and in the spinal cord. Chlorzoxazone acts primarily at the spinal cord level and at subcortical areas of the brain. Orphenadrine has analgesic activity, which may contribute to its skeletal muscle relaxant properties.

Parkinsonism therapy adjunct—Orphenadrine has mild anticholinergic actions, which produce its beneficial effect in parkinsonism.

**Other actions/effects**
Orphenadrine also has anticholinergic properties.

## Precautions to Consider

### Cross-sensitivity and/or related problems
Patients sensitive to other carbamate derivatives (for example, carbromal, meprobamate, mebutamate, or tybamate) may be sensitive to carisoprodol also.

### Pregnancy/Reproduction
Pregnancy—
*Carisoprodol, chlorzoxazone, and methocarbamol*—
Problems in humans have not been documented.
*Chlorphenesin*—
Studies have not been done in either animals or humans.
*Metaxalone*—
Although studies in humans have not been done, studies in rats have not shown that metaxalone causes adverse effects in the fetus.
*Orphenadrine*—
Problems in humans have not been documented.
Studies in animals have not been done.
Orphenadrine citrate—FDA Pregnancy Category C.

### Breast-feeding
*Carisoprodol*—
Carisoprodol is distributed into breast milk in concentrations that may reach 2 to 4 times the maternal plasma concentrations; use by nursing mothers may cause sedation and gastrointestinal upset in the infant.
*Chlorphenesin, chlorzoxazone, metaxalone, methocarbamol, and orphenadrine*—
It is not known whether these medications are distributed into breast milk. However, problems in humans have not been documented.

### Pediatrics
*Carisoprodol*—
Although appropriate studies with carisoprodol have not been performed in the pediatric population, the medication has been used in children. Pediatrics-specific problems that would limit the use of carisoprodol in these patients have not been documented.
*Chlorphenesin, metaxalone, methocarbamol, and orphenadrine*—
No information is available on the relationship of age to the effects of these medications in pediatric patients. Safety and efficacy have not been established.
*Chlorzoxazone*—
This medication has been used in children. Pediatrics-specific problems that would limit use of chlorzoxazone in these patients have not been documented.

### Geriatrics
No information is available on the relationship of age to the effects of skeletal muscle relaxants in geriatric patients. However, elderly males are more likely to have age-related prostatic hypertrophy and may therefore be adversely affected by orphenadrine's anticholinergic activity. Also, elderly patients are more likely to have age-related renal function impairment, which may require that parenteral methocarbamol not be used at all and that other skeletal muscle relaxants be used with caution.

### Dental
*Orphenadrine*—
The peripheral anticholinergic effects of orphenadrine may decrease or inhibit salivary flow, thus contributing to the development of caries, periodontal disease, oral candidiasis, and discomfort.

### Drug interactions and/or related problems
The following drug interactions and/or related problems have been selected on the basis of their potential clinical significance (possible mechanism in parentheses where appropriate)—not necessarily inclusive (» = major clinical significance):

Note: Combinations containing any of the following medications, depending on the amount present, may also interact with this medication.

*For all skeletal muscle relaxants*
» Alcohol or
» CNS depression–producing medications, other (See *Appendix II* )
(concurrent use with a skeletal muscle relaxant may result in additive CNS depressant effects; caution is recommended and dosage of one or both agents should be reduced )

*For orphenadrine (in addition to the interaction listed above)*
Anticholinergics or other medications with anticholinergic action (See *Appendix II* )
(anticholinergic effects may be intensified when these medications are used concurrently with orphenadrine because of orphenadrine's secondary anticholinergic activity)

### Laboratory value alterations
The following have been selected on the basis of their potential clinical significance (possible effect in parentheses where appropriate)—not necessarily inclusive (» = major clinical significance):

With diagnostic test results
*For metaxalone*
Copper sulfate urine sugar tests
(false-positive test results may occur, possibly because of the presence of an unknown reducing substance; results of tests using glucose oxidase are not affected)
*For methocarbamol*
5-Hydroxyindoleacetic acid (5-HIAA), in urine, determinations
(values may be falsely increased when the nitrosonaphthol reagent is used)
Vanillylmandelic acid (VMA), in urine, determinations
(values may be falsely increased when the Gitlow screening method is used; no error occurs when the quantitative procedure of Sunderman is used)

With physiology/laboratory test values
*For metaxalone*
Cephalin flocculation tests
(elevations may occur without concurrent changes in other liver function tests)

### Medical considerations/Contraindications
The medical considerations/contraindications included have been selected on the basis of their potential clinical significance (reasons given in parentheses where appropriate)—not necessarily inclusive (» = major clinical significance).

See *Table 3*, page 2583.

### Patient monitoring
The following may be especially important in patient monitoring (other tests may be warranted in some patients, depending on condition; » = major clinical significance):

*For metaxalone*
Liver function tests
(recommended periodically during prolonged metaxalone therapy, especially if the patient has pre-existing hepatic function impairment or disease)

*For methocarbamol*
Renal function determinations
(recommended if parenteral therapy lasts 3 days or more because the polyethylene glycol 300 vehicle may be nephrotoxic)

*For orphenadrine*
Blood count and
Liver function tests and
Renal function tests
(recommended during prolonged therapy since the safety of continuous long-term use has not been established)

## Side/Adverse Effects

See *Table 4*, page 2584.

Note: Rarely, an idiosyncratic reaction to carisoprodol may occur within minutes or hours following the first dose of the medication. Reported symptoms include agitation, ataxia, confusion, disorientation, dizziness, euphoria, extreme weakness, speech disturbances, temporary loss of vision or other vision disturbances, and transient quadriplegia. Symptoms usually subside within several hours, but in some cases, supportive and symptomatic therapy, including hospitalization, may be necessary.

Psychological dependence and abuse have occurred very rarely with carisoprodol. Signs of abstinence have not been reported with clinical usage; however, in one study abrupt withdrawal of 100 mg per kg of body weight (mg/kg) per day of carisoprodol (5 times the recommended daily dose) produced withdrawal symptoms including abdominal cramps, insomnia, chills, headache, and nausea.

## Overdose

For more information on the management of overdose or unintentional ingestion, **contact a Poison Control Center** (see *Poison Control Center Listing*).

**Carisoprodol**

To decrease absorption—Emptying the stomach via induction of emesis or gastric lavage.

Specific treatment—Administering respiratory assistance, CNS stimulants, and pressor agents cautiously, if necessary.

To enhance elimination—Removing carisoprodol from the body via induction of diuresis, osmotic (mannitol) diuresis, peritoneal dialysis, or hemodialysis.

Monitoring—Monitoring urinary output.

Taking care to prevent overhydration.

Monitoring the patient for relapse due to incomplete gastric emptying and delayed absorption, and administering additional treatment as required.

Supportive care—Administering supportive treatment of observed symptoms.

Chlorphenesin—
- To decrease absorption—Emptying the stomach via institution of saline catharsis or gastric lavage.
- Supportive care—Administering supportive therapy of observed symptoms.

Chlorzoxazone—
- To decrease absorption—Emptying the stomach via induction of emesis or gastric lavage.
- Specific treatment—Administering oxygen and artificial respiration for respiratory depression and plasma volume expanders or vasopressors for hypotension.
- Supportive care—Administering supportive treatment of observed symptoms.

Note: Cholinergic medications and analeptic medications are of no value in chlorzoxazone overdose and should not be used.

Metaxalone—
- Experience with overdose causing major toxicity is extremely limited.
- To decrease absorption—Emptying the stomach via induction of emesis or gastric lavage.
- Supportive care—Administering supportive treatment of observed symptoms.

Methocarbamol—
- To decrease absorption—Emptying the stomach via induction of emesis or gastric lavage (if administered orally).
- To enhance elimination—The usefulness of forced diuresis or hemodialysis in treating overdose has not been determined.
- Supportive care—Administering supportive treatment of observed symptoms.

Orphenadrine—
- To decrease absorption—Emptying the stomach via induction of emesis or gastric lavage (if administered orally).
- To enhance elimination—Maintaining a high-volume urinary output. Institution of hemodialysis or peritoneal dialysis may be of some benefit if the serum concentration exceeds 4 mcg per mL.
- Supportive care—Administering intravenous fluids and circulatory support as required. Administering supportive treatment of observed symptoms.

Note: Patients in whom intentional overdose is known or suspected should be referred for psychiatric consultation.

## Patient Consultation

See *Table 5*, page 2585.

---

### CARISOPRODOL

## Summary of Differences

Pharmacology/pharmacokinetics:
- Physicochemical characteristics—Molecular weight: 260.34.
- Biotransformation—Hepatic; one metabolite is meprobamate.
- Half-life—8 hours
- Onset of action—0.5 hour.
- Time to peak concentration—4 hours (350-mg single dose).
- Peak serum concentration—4–7 mcg per mL.
- Duration of action—4–6 hours.
- Elimination—Renal, <1% as unchanged carisoprodol. Carisoprodol is dialyzable.

Precautions:
- Cross-sensitivity and/or related problems—May occur with other carbamate derivatives.

Breast-feeding—Distributed into breast milk in significant quantities; may cause sedation and gastrointestinal upset in the nursing infant.

Medical considerations/contraindications—
- Should not be used in patients with known or suspected acute intermittent porphyria.
- Caution also recommended in patients with a history of drug abuse or dependence.

Side/adverse effects:
- Idiosyncratic reactions may occur shortly after first dose.
- Psychological dependence and abuse reported very rarely.
- Also may cause orthostatic hypotension, fast heartbeat, mental depression, clumsiness or unsteadiness, fever (allergic), stinging or burning of eyes, angioedema, bronchospastic allergic reaction, blurred vision, and flushing.

## Oral Dosage Forms

### CARISOPRODOL TABLETS USP

**Usual adult and adolescent dose**
Skeletal muscle relaxant—
Oral, 350 mg four times a day.

**Usual pediatric dose**
Skeletal muscle relaxant—
Children up to 5 years of age: Dosage has not been established.
Children 5 to 12 years of age: Oral, 6.25 mg per kg of body weight four times a day.

**Strength(s) usually available**
U.S.—
350 mg (Rx) [*Soma; Vanadom;* GENERIC].
Canada—
350 mg (Rx) [*Soma*].

**Packaging and storage**
Store below 40 °C (104 °F), preferably between 15 and 30 °C (59 and 86 °F), unless otherwise specified by manufacturer. Store in a well-closed container.

**Auxiliary labeling**
- May cause drowsiness.
- Avoid alcoholic beverages.

---

### CHLORPHENESIN

## Summary of Differences

Pharmacology/pharmacokinetics:
- Physicochemical characteristics—Molecular weight: 245.66.
- Absorption—Rapid; complete.
- Biotransformation—Hepatic; at least partially metabolized.
- Half-life—2.3–5 hours
- Time to peak concentration—1–3 hours.
- Peak serum concentration—3.8–17 mcg per mL (800-mg single dose).
- Elimination—Renal; 85% of a dose excreted within 24 hours as the glucuronide metabolite.

Side/adverse effects:
- Gastrointestinal bleeding reported, but causal relationship not established.
- Also may cause fever (allergic), agranulocytosis, leukopenia, or thrombocytopenia.

## Additional Dosing Information

The safety of administering chlorphenesin for longer than 8 weeks has not been established.

## Oral Dosage Forms

### CHLORPHENESIN CARBAMATE TABLETS

**Usual adult and adolescent dose**
Skeletal muscle relaxant—
Oral, 800 mg three times a day initially; may be decreased to 400 mg four times a day or less, as required to maintain the desired response.

**Usual pediatric dose**
Safety and efficacy have not been established.

**Strength(s) usually available**
U.S.—
400 mg (Rx) [*Maolate*].
Canada—
Not commercially available.

## CHLORZOXAZONE

### Summary of Differences
Pharmacology/pharmacokinetics:
  Physicochemical characteristics—Molecular weight: 169.57.
  Absorption—Rapid; complete.
  Biotransformation—Hepatic.
  Half-life—1.1 hours.
  Onset of action—Within 1 hour.
  Time to peak concentration—1–2 hours.
  Peak serum concentration—10–30 mcg per mL (750-mg single dose).
  Duration of action—3–4 hours.
  Elimination—Renal; <1% as unchanged chlorzoxazone.
Precautions:
  Medical considerations/contraindications: Also should be used with caution in patients with allergies (or history of).
Side/adverse effects:
  Also may cause agranulocytosis, gastrointesinal bleeding, angioedema, anemia, diarrhea, heartburn, and constipation.
  Hepatotoxicity reported, but causal association not established.

### Additional Dosing Information
Discontinuation of chlorzoxazone therapy is recommended if symptoms of hepatotoxicity or sensitivity (e.g., skin rash, hives, or itching) occur.

### Oral Dosage Forms
**CHLORZOXAZONE TABLETS USP**

**Usual adult and adolescent dose**
Skeletal muscle relaxant—
  Oral, 250 to 750 mg three or four times a day; usually 500 mg three or four times a day initially and increased or decreased as determined by patient response.

**Usual pediatric dose**
Skeletal muscle relaxant—
  Oral, 20 mg per kg of body weight or 600 mg per square meter of body surface, in three or four divided doses; or 125 to 500 mg three or four times a day, according to the child's age and weight.

**Strength(s) usually available**
U.S.—
  250 mg (Rx) [*Paraflex; Remular-S;* GENERIC].
  500 mg (Rx) [*EZE-DS; Parafon Forte DSC* (scored); *Relaxazone; Remular; Strifon Forte DSC;* GENERIC].
Canada—
  Not commercially available.

**Packaging and storage**
Store between 15 and 30 °C (59 and 86 °F), unless otherwise specified by manufacturer. Store in a tight container.

**Preparation of dosage form**
*Single dose*—Tablets may be crushed and mixed with food or liquid for ease of administration.

**Auxiliary labeling**
- May cause drowsiness.
- Avoid alcoholic beverages.

## METAXALONE

### Summary of Differences
Pharmacology/pharmacokinetics:
  Physicochemical characteristics—Molecular weight: 221.26.
  Biotransformation—Hepatic.
  Half-life—2–3 hours
  Onset of action—1 hour.
  Time to peak concentration—2 hours (800-mg single dose).
  Peak serum concentration—295 mcg per mL (800-mg single dose).
  Elimination—Renal.
Precautions:
  Laboratory value alterations—
    May interfere with copper sulfate urine sugar test results.
    May cause liver function test abnormalities.
  Medical considerations/contraindications—Also should not be used in patients with hemolytic anemia or a history of hemolytic anemia, especially if drug-induced.
  Patient monitoring—Liver function tests recommended during prolonged therapy.
Side/adverse effects:
  Also may cause hemolytic anemia and hepatotoxicity.

### Additional Dosing Information
Discontinuation of metaxalone therapy is recommended if signs of hepatotoxicity occur.

### Oral Dosage Forms
**METAXALONE TABLETS**

**Usual adult and adolescent dose**
Skeletal muscle relaxant—
  Oral, 800 mg three or four times a day.

**Usual pediatric dose**
Safety and efficacy have not been established.

**Strength(s) usually available**
U.S.—
  400 mg (Rx) [*Skelaxin* (scored)].
Canada—
  Not commercially available.

**Packaging and storage**
Store below 40 °C (104 °F), preferably between 15 and 30 °C (59 and 86 °F), in a well-closed container, unless otherwise specified by manufacturer.

**Auxiliary labeling**
- May cause drowsiness.
- Avoid alcoholic beverages.

## METHOCARBAMOL

### Summary of Differences
Pharmacology/pharmacokinetics:
  Physicochemical characteristics—Molecular weight: 241.25.
  Absorption—Rapid.
  Biotransformation—Probably hepatic.
  Half-life (elimination)—0.9–2.2 hours.
    Onset of action—
      Oral: Within 0.5 hour.
      Intravenous: Immediate.
    Time to peak concentration—
      Oral: 2 hours (2-gram single dose).
      Intravenous: Almost immediate.
    Peak serum concentration—
      Oral: 16 mcg per mL (2-gram single dose).
      Intravenous: 19 mcg per mL (1-gram single dose).
    Elimination—
      Renal and fecal.
Precautions:
  Laboratory value alterations—Urinary 5-Hydroxyindoleacetic acid (5-HIAA) values may be falsely increased (with nitrosonaphthol reagent).
  Urinary vanillylmandelic acid (VMA) values may be falsely increased (with the Gitlow screening method).
  Medical considerations/contraindications—
    Parenteral dosage form should not be used in patients with renal function impairment or disease because the polyethylene glycol 300 vehicle is nephrotoxic.
    Parenteral dosage form also should be used with caution in patients with epilepsy.
  Patient monitoring—Renal function determinations recommended if parenteral therapy lasts 3 days or more.
Side/adverse effects:
  Parenteral dosage form also reported to cause convulsions, fainting, slow heartbeat, muscle weakness, nystagmus, and facial flushing, especially when given too rapidly.
  Parenteral dosage form may also cause pain or peeling of skin at injection site and thrombophlebitis.
  Also may cause fever (allergic), conjunctivitis and nasal congestion, and leukopenia.

May be more likely than other muscle relaxants to cause blurred or double vision.

### Additional Dosing Information

**For parenteral dosage forms only**
The injection may be given intravenously or intramuscularly. Subcutaneous administration is not recommended.
The polyethylene glycol 300 vehicle in the parenteral dosage form may be nephrotoxic.
The medication may be administered intravenously undiluted at a rate not to exceed 3 mL (300 mg) per minute. It may also be given as an intravenous infusion in sodium chloride injection or 5% dextrose injection.
The patient should lie down during and for at least 10 to 15 minutes following intravenous administration.
Extravasation should be avoided, since the injection is hypertonic and may cause thrombophlebitis.
The manufacturer's labeling should be consulted for special directions for use in tetanus.
Not more than 5 mL (500 mg) should be given intramuscularly into each gluteal region at one time. The injections may be repeated at 8-hour intervals, if necessary.

## Oral Dosage Forms

### METHOCARBAMOL TABLETS USP

**Usual adult and adolescent dose**
Skeletal muscle relaxant—
  Initial: Oral, 1.5 grams four times a day for the first forty-eight to seventy-two hours of therapy. For severe conditions, 8 grams a day may be administered initially.
  Maintenance: Oral, 750 mg every four hours; 1 gram four times a day; or 1.5 grams three times a day.
Note: If used as adjunctive therapy in the treatment of tetanus—Via nasogastric tube, up to 24 grams a day depending on patient response.

**Usual pediatric dose**
Safety and efficacy have not been established.

**Strength(s) usually available**
U.S.—
  500 mg (Rx) [*Carbacot; Robaxin;* GENERIC].
  750 mg (Rx) [*Carbacot; Robaxin-750;* GENERIC].
Canada—
  500 mg (OTC) [*Robaxin* (scored)].
  750 mg (OTC) [*Robaxin-750* (scored)].

**Packaging and storage**
Store below 40 °C (104 °F), preferably between 15 and 30 °C (59 and 86 °F), unless otherwise specified by manufacturer. Store in a tight container.

**Preparation of dosage form**
For administration via nasogastric tube—Crush tablets and suspend in water or saline solution.

**Auxiliary labeling**
- May cause drowsiness.
- Avoid alcoholic beverages.

## Parenteral Dosage Forms

### METHOCARBAMOL INJECTION USP

**Usual adult and adolescent dose**
Skeletal muscle relaxant—
  Intramuscular or intravenous, 1 to 3 grams a day for three days. Following a drug-free interval of forty-eight hours, the course may be repeated if necessary.
Note: If used as adjunctive therapy in the treatment of tetanus—Intravenous, 1 or 2 grams by direct intravenous injection. An additional 1 or 2 grams may be administered by intravenous infusion, so that a total initial dose of up to 3 grams is administered. This regimen should be repeated every six hours until therapy via a nasogastric tube can be instituted.

**Usual adult prescribing limits**
Total adult dosage should not exceed 3 grams per day. Also, the medication should not be administered for more than three consecutive days except in the treatment of tetanus.

**Usual pediatric dose**
Skeletal muscle relaxant—
  Safety and efficacy in children up to 12 years of age have not been established for conditions other than tetanus.

Note: If used as adjunctive therapy in the treatment of tetanus—Intravenous, 15 mg per kg of body weight every six hours.

**Strength(s) usually available**
U.S.—
  100 mg per mL (1 gram per 10-mL single-dose ampul or vial) (Rx) [*Carbacot; Robaxin; Skelex;* GENERIC].
Canada—
  100 mg per mL (1 gram per 10-mL single-dose vial) (OTC) [*Robaxin*].

**Packaging and storage**
Store below 40 °C (104 °F), preferably between 15 and 30 °C (59 and 86 °F), unless otherwise specified by manufacturer. Protect from freezing.

**Preparation of dosage form**
For intravenous infusion—Dilute with sodium chloride injection or 5% dextrose injection; 10 mL (1 gram) of medication should be diluted to not more than 250 mL of infusion. After dilution, the injection should not be refrigerated.

---

## ORPHENADRINE

## Summary of Differences

Category:
  Hydrochloride salt indicated to relieve tremor in parkinsonism.
Pharmacology/pharmacokinetics—
  Physicochemical characteristics: Molecular weight—
    Orphenadrine citrate—461.51.
    Orphenadrine hydrochloride—305.85.
  Mechanism of action (parkinsonism therapy adjunct)—
    Has anticholinergic activity.
  Protein binding—
    Low.
  Biotransformation—
    Hepatic.
  Half-life—
    14 hours (parent compound; half-life of metabolites may range from 2 to 25 hours).
  Onset of action:
    Orphenadrine citrate—
      Oral (extended-release tablets)—Within 1 hour.
      Intramuscular—5 minutes.
      Intravenous—Immediate.
    Orphenadrine hydrochloride—
      Oral—Within 1 hour.
  Time to peak concentration:
    Orphenadrine citrate—
      Oral (extended-release tablets)—6–8 hours (100-mg single dose).
      Intramuscular—0.5 hour (60-mg single dose).
      Intravenous—Immediate.
    Orphenadrine hydrochloride—
      Oral—3 hours (50-mg single dose).
  Peak serum concentration:
    Orphenadrine citrate—
      Oral (extended-release tablets)—60–120 nanograms per mL (100-mg single dose).
    Orphenadrine hydrochloride: Oral—110–210 nanograms per mL (100-mg single dose).
  Elimination—
    Renal and fecal.
Precautions:
  Dental—May cause dryness of mouth.
  Medical considerations/contraindications—
    Also should not be used in patients with medical conditions in which anticholinergic actions are detrimental.
    Also should be used with caution in patients with cardiac disease or arrhythmias, especially tachycardia.
  Patient monitoring—Blood count and hepatic and renal function tests recommended during prolonged therapy.
Side/adverse effects:
  Also may cause side effects typical of anticholinergics and aplastic anemia.
  Also may cause hallucinations, syncope, confusion (especially in the elderly), and blurred or double vision; anticholinergic as well as CNS actions may contribute to these effects.

## Additional Dosing Information

The safety of continuous long-term administration of orphenadrine has not been established.

## Oral Dosage Forms

### ORPHENADRINE CITRATE EXTENDED-RELEASE TABLETS

**Usual adult and adolescent dose**
Skeletal muscle relaxant—
  Oral, 100 mg two times a day, in the morning and evening.

**Usual pediatric dose**
Safety and efficacy have not been established.

**Strength(s) usually available**
U.S.—
  100 mg (Rx) [*Norflex*; GENERIC].
Canada—
  100 mg (OTC) [*Norflex*].

**Packaging and storage**
Store below 40 °C (104 °F), preferably between 15 and 30 °C (59 and 86 °F), in a tight, light-resistant container, unless otherwise specified by manufacturer.

**Auxiliary labeling**
• May cause drowsiness.
• Avoid alcoholic beverages.

### ORPHENADRINE HYDROCHLORIDE TABLETS

**Usual adult and adolescent dose**
Skeletal muscle relaxant
and Parkinsonism therapy adjunct—
  Oral, 50 mg three times a day.

Note: Smaller doses may suffice if other antiparkinson medications are being administered concurrently.

**Usual adult prescribing limits**
Up to 250 mg a day.

**Usual pediatric dose**
Dosage has not been established.

**Strength(s) usually available**
U.S.—
  Not commercially available.
Canada—
  50 mg (OTC) [*Disipal*].

**Packaging and storage**
Store below 40 °C (104 °F), preferably between 15 and 30 °C (59 and 86 °F), in a tight container, unless otherwise specified by manufacturer.

**Auxiliary labeling**
• May cause drowsiness.
• Avoid alcoholic beverages.

## Parenteral Dosage Forms

### ORPHENADRINE CITRATE INJECTION USP

**Usual adult and adolescent dose**
Skeletal muscle relaxant—
  Intramuscular or intravenous, 60 mg every twelve hours as needed.

**Usual pediatric dose**
Safety and efficacy have not been established.

**Strength(s) usually available**
U.S.—
  30 mg per mL (Rx) [*Antiflex*; *Banflex*; *Flexoject*; *Mio-Rel*; *Myolin*; *Myotrol*; *Norflex*; *Orfro*; *Orphenate*; GENERIC].
Canada—
  30 mg per mL (OTC) [*Norflex* (sodium bisulfite)].

**Packaging and storage**
Store below 40 °C (104 °F), preferably between 15 and 30 °C (59 and 86 °F), unless otherwise specified by manufacturer. Protect from light. Protect from freezing.

## Selected Bibliography

Elenbaas JK. Central acting oral skeletal muscle relaxants. Am J Hosp Pharm 1980; 37: 1313-23.
Waldman HJ. Centrally acting skeletal muscle relaxants and associated drugs. J Pain Symptom Manage 1994; 9: 434-41.

Revised: 08/11/95

## Table 1. Pharmacology/Pharmacokinetics

| Drug | Absorption | Protein Binding (%) | Biotransformation | Half-life (hr) | Elimination Primary (% Excreted Unchanged)/ Secondary |
|---|---|---|---|---|---|
| Carisoprodol | | | Hepatic* | 8 | Renal (<1)† |
| Chlorphenesin | Rapid; complete | | Hepatic‡ | 2.3–5 | Renal§ |
| Chlorzoxazone | Rapid; complete | | Hepatic | 1.1 | Renal (<1) |
| Metaxalone | | | Hepatic | 2–3 | Renal |
| Methocarbamol | Rapid | | Probably hepatic | 0.9–2.2 | Renal/fecal |
| Orphenadrine | | Low | Hepatic | 14# | Renal/fecal |

*One of the metabolites is meprobamate.
†Distributed into breast milk; concentration may reach 2 to 4 times the maternal plasma concentration. Also, may be removed from the circulation via hemodialysis and peritoneal dialysis.
‡At least partially metabolized.
§85% of a dose excreted within 24 hours as the glucuronide metabolite.
#For the parent compound; half-life of metabolites may range from 2 to 25 hours.

## Table 2. Pharmacology/Pharmacokinetics

| Drug | Onset of Action | Time to Peak Concentration (hr) (single dose) | Peak Serum Concentration (single dose) | Duration of Action (hr) |
|---|---|---|---|---|
| Carisoprodol | 0.5 hr | 4 (350 mg) | 4–7 mcg/mL | 4–6 |
| Chlorphenesin | | 1–3 | 3.8–17 mcg/mL (800 mg) | |
| Chlorzoxazone | Within 1 hr | 1–2 | 10–30 mcg/mL (750 mg) | 3–4 |
| Metaxalone | 1 hr | 2 (800 mg) | 295 mcg/mL (800 mg) | |
| Methocarbamol | | | | |
|   Oral | Within 0.5 hr | 2 (2 grams) | 16 mcg/mL (2 grams) | |
|   IV (300 mg/min) | Immediate | Almost immediate | 19 mcg/mL (1 gram) | |
| Orphenadrine citrate* | | | | |
|   Oral (extended-release tablets) | Within 1 hr | 6 to 8 (100 mg) | 60–120 nanograms/mL (100 mg) | 12 |
|   IM | 5 min | 0.5 (60 mg) | | |
|   IV | Immediate | Immediate | | |
| Orphenadrine hydrochloride† | Within 1 hr | 3 (50 mg) | 110–210 nanograms/mL (100 mg) | 8 |

*Relief of muscle spasm.
†In parkinsonism.

## Table 3. Medical Considerations/Contraindications

The medical considerations/contraindications included have been selected on the basis of their potential clinical significance (reasons given in parentheses where appropriate)—not necessarily inclusive (» = major clinical significance).

Legend:
I = Carisoprodol
II = Chlorphenesin
III = Chlorzoxazone
IV = Metaxalone
V = Methocarbamol
VI = Orphenadrine

| | I | II | III | IV | V | VI |
|---|---|---|---|---|---|---|
| ***Except under special circumstances, these medications should not be used when the following medical problems exist:*** | | | | | | |
| » Achalasia or | | | | | | ✔ |
| » Bladder neck obstruction or | | | | | | ✔ |
| » Glaucoma, or predisposition to, or | | | | | | ✔ |
| » Myasthenia gravis or | | | | | | ✔ |
| » Peptic ulcer, stenosing, or | | | | | | ✔ |
| » Prostatic hypertrophy or | | | | | | ✔ |
| » Pyloric or duodenal obstruction (anticholinergic actions detrimental in these conditions) | | | | | | ✔ |
| » Hemolytic anemia, or history of, especially if drug-induced (may be induced by metaxalone) | | | | ✔ | | |
| » Porphyria, acute intermittent, known or suspected | ✔ | | | | | |
| » Renal function impairment or disease (for parenteral dosage form only—polyethylene glycol 300 vehicle is nephrotoxic and may cause increased urea retention and acidosis in these patients) | | | | | ✔ | |
| ***Risk-benefit should be considered when the following medical problems exist:*** | | | | | | |
| Allergic reaction to the medication considered for use, history of | ✔ | ✔ | ✔ | ✔ | ✔ | ✔ |
| Allergies or history of | | | | ✔ | | |
| Cardiac disease or arrhythmias or Tachycardia (orphenadrine may cause tachycardia) | | | | | | ✔ ✔ |
| CNS depression (may be exacerbated) | ✔ | ✔ | ✔ | ✔ | ✔ | ✔ |
| Drug abuse or dependence, history of (psychological dependence and abuse reported rarely) | ✔ | | | | | |
| Epilepsy (for parenteral dosage form only—may increase risk of seizures) | | | | | ✔ | |
| Hepatic function impairment (metabolized in liver) | ✔ | ✔ | | | ✔ | ✔ |

## Table 3. Medical Considerations/Contraindications *(continued)*

The medical considerations/contraindications included have been selected on the basis of their potential clinical significance (reasons given in parentheses where appropriate)— not necessarily inclusive (» = major clinical significance).

Legend:
**I**=Carisoprodol
**II**=Chlorphenesin
**III**=Chlorzoxazone
**IV**=Metaxalone
**V**=Methocarbamol
**VI**=Orphenadrine

| | I | II | III | IV | V | VI |
|---|---|---|---|---|---|---|
| » Hepatic function impairment or disease (metabolized in liver; also, potentially hepatotoxic) | | | ✔ | ✔ | | |
| Renal function impairment (excreted via kidneys) | ✔ | ✔ | ✔ | ✔ | ✔ | ✔ |
| » Renal function impairment, severe (excreted via kidneys) | | | | ✔ | | |

## Table 4. Side/Adverse Effects*

The following side/adverse effects have been selected on the basis of their potential clinical significance (possible signs and symptoms in parentheses where appropriate)—not necessarily inclusive:

Legend:
**I**=Carisoprodol
**II**=Chlorphenesin
**III**=Chlorzoxazone
**IV**=Metaxalone
**V**=Methocarbamol
**VI**=Orphenadrine

| | I | II | III | IV | V | VI |
|---|---|---|---|---|---|---|
| **Medical attention needed** | | | | | | |
| *Anticholinergic effects, specifically:* | | | | | | |
|   *Decreased urination* | — | — | — | — | — | L |
|   *Increased intraocular pressure* (eye pain) | — | — | — | — | — | L |
| *Cardiovascular effects, specifically:* | | | | | | |
|   *Fast heartbeat*—with orphenadrine, anticholinergic activity may contribute to this effect | L | U | U | U | U | L |
|   *Pounding heartbeat* | U | U | U | U | U | L |
|   *Slow heartbeat*—with parenteral dosage form only | — | — | — | — | L‡ | U |
|   *Thrombophlebitis* (local pain, tenderness, heat, redness, swelling at site of affected vein)—with parenteral administration only | — | — | — | — | R | U |
| *Central nervous system effects, specifically:* | | | | | | |
|   *Convulsions* | U | U | U | U | R‡ | U |
|   *Fainting*—with carisoprodol, may also be caused by orthostatic hypotension | L | U | U | U | R‡ | L |
|   *Hallucinations*—orphenadrine's anticholinergic activity may contribute to this effect | U | U | U | U | U | R |
|   *Mental depression* | L | U | U | U | U | U |
| *Gastrointestinal bleeding* (bloody or black, tarry stools; vomiting of blood or material that looks like coffee grounds) | U | R† | R | U | U | U |
| *Hematologic effects, specifically:* | | | | | | |
|   *Agranulocytosis* (fever with or without chills; sores, ulcers, or white spots on lips or in mouth; sore throat) | U | R | R | U | U | U |
|   *Anemia* (unusual tiredness or weakness) | U | U | R | U | U | U |
|   *Anemia, aplastic [pancytopenia]* (shortness of breath, troubled breathing, tightness in chest, and/or wheezing; sores, ulcers, or white spots on lips or in mouth; swollen and/or painful glands; unusual bleeding or bruising; unusual tiredness or weakness) | R† | U | U | U | U | R |
|   *Anemia, hemolytic* (troubled breathing, exertional; unusual tiredness or weakness) | U | U | U | R | U | U |
|   *Leukopenia* (usually asymptomatic; rarely, fever or chills, cough or hoarseness, lower back or side pain, painful or difficult urination) | R† | R | U | R | R | U |
|   *Thrombocytopenia* (usually asymptomatic; rarely, unusual bleeding or bruising; black, tarry stools; blood in urine or stools; pinpoint red spots on skin) | U | R | U | U | U | U |
| *Hepatotoxicity* (yellow eyes or skin) | U | U | R† | R | U | U |
| *Hypersensitivity reactions, specifically:* | | | | | | |
|   *Anaphylactic or anaphylactoid reaction* (changes in facial skin color; skin rash, hives, and/or itching; fast or irregular breathing; puffiness or swelling of the eyelids or around the eyes; shortness of breath, troubled breathing, tightness in chest, and/or wheezing)—with carisoprodol, anaphylactic shock with sudden, severe decrease in blood pressure and collapse has also occurred | R | R | R | R | U | U |
|   *Angioedema* (hive-like swellings, large, on face, eyelids, mouth, lips, and/or tongue) | L | U | R | U | U | U |
|   *Bronchospastic allergic reaction* (shortness of breath, troubled breathing, tightness in chest, and/or wheezing) | L | U | U | U | U | U |
|   *Conjunctivitis and nasal congestion* (stuffy nose and red or bloodshot eyes) | U | U | U | U | L | U |
|   *Dermatitis, allergic* (skin rash, hives, itching, and/or redness)—with carisoprodol, fixed drug eruptions with cross-sensitivity to meprobamate have also been reported; with chlorzoxazone, petechial rashes and ecchymoses have also been reported | L | R | R | R | L | U |
|   *Eosinophilia* | R | U | U | U | U | U |

## Table 4. Side/Adverse Effects* *(continued)*

| The following side/adverse effects have been selected on the basis of their potential clinical significance (possible signs and symptoms in parentheses where appropriate)—not necessarily inclusive: | Legend: I=Carisoprodol II=Chlorphenesin III=Chlorzoxazone |  |  | IV=Metaxalone V=Methocarbamol VI=Orphenadrine |  |  |
|---|---|---|---|---|---|---|
|  | I | II | III | IV | V | VI |
| *Erythema multiforme* (fever with or without chills; muscle cramps or pain; skin rash; sores, ulcers, or white spots on lips or in mouth) | R | U | U | U | U | U |
| *Fever, allergic* | L | R | U | U | L | U |
| *Stinging or burning of eyes* | L | U | U | U | U | U |
| **Medical attention needed only if continuing or bothersome** |  |  |  |  |  |  |
| *Anticholinergic effects* (dryness of mouth [more frequent], confusion, difficult urination, constipation, unusually large pupils, blurred or double vision, weakness) | — | — | — | — | — | L |
| *Central nervous system effects, specifically:* |  |  |  |  |  |  |
| *Blurred or double vision or any change in vision*—with orphenadrine, anticholinergic activity may also contribute to this effect | R | U | U | U | M | L |
| *Clumsiness or unsteadiness* | R | U | U | U | U | U |
| *Confusion*—with orphenadrine, anticholinergic activity may also contribute to this effect, especially in elderly patients | U | L | U | U | U | L |
| *Dizziness or lightheadedness*—with carisoprodol, orthostatic hypotension may also contribute to this effect | L | L | M | M | M | L |
| *Drowsiness* | M | L | M | M | M | L |
| *Headache* | L | R | L | M | L | L |
| *Muscle weakness* | U | R | U | U | L‡ | R |
| *Nystagmus* (uncontrolled movements of eyes) | U | U | U | U | L‡ | U |
| *Stimulation, paradoxical* (excitement, nervousness, restlessness, irritability, trouble in sleeping) | L | R | L | M | U | L |
| *Trembling* | L | U | U | U | U | L |
| *Flushing or redness of face* | L | U | U | U | L‡ | U |
| *Gastrointestinal irritation, specifically:* |  |  |  |  |  |  |
| *Abdominal or stomach cramps or pain* | L | R | L | M | U | L |
| *Constipation*—with orphenadrine, anticholinergic activity may contribute to this effect | U | U | L | U | U | L |
| *Diarrhea* | U | U | L | U | U | U |
| *Heartburn* | U | U | L | U | U | U |
| *Hiccups* | L | U | U | U | U | U |
| *Nausea or vomiting* | L | R | L | M | L | L |
| *Pain or peeling at place of injection* | — | — | — | — | L‡ | U |

*Differences in frequency of occurrence may reflect either lack of clinical-use data or actual pharmacologic distinctions among agents (although their pharmacologic similarity suggests that side effects occurring with one may occur with the others, except for those caused by anticholinergic activity, which is specific for orphenadrine). M = more frequent; L = less frequent; R = rare; U = unknown.
†A causal association has not been established.
‡Usually reported with too-rapid intravenous administration.

## Table 5. Patient Consultation

| As an aid to patient consultation, refer to *Advice for the Patient, Skeletal Muscle Relaxants (Systemic)* or *Orphenadrine (Systemic)*. In providing consultation, consider emphasizing the following selected information (» = major clinical significance): | Legend: I=Carisoprodol II=Chlorphenesin III=Chlorzoxazone |  |  | IV=Metaxalone V=Methocarbamol VI=Orphenadrine |  |  |
|---|---|---|---|---|---|---|
|  | I | II | III | IV | V | VI |
| **Before using this medication** |  |  |  |  |  |  |
| » Conditions affecting use, especially: |  |  |  |  |  |  |
| Sensitivity to the muscle relaxant considered for use, history of, and, for carisoprodol, sensitivity to other carbamate derivatives | ✓ | ✓ | ✓ | ✓ | ✓ | ✓ |
| Breast-feeding—Carisoprodol distributed into breast milk and may cause sedation and gastrointestinal upset in the infant; problems in nursing infants have not been reported with other skeletal muscle relaxants | ✓ |  |  |  |  |  |
| Other medications, especially other CNS depression–producing medications | ✓ | ✓ | ✓ | ✓ | ✓ | ✓ |
| Other medical problems, especially: |  |  |  |  |  |  |
| Acute intermittent porphyria (known or suspected) | ✓ |  |  |  |  |  |
| Conditions that may be adversely affected by anticholinergic activity |  |  |  |  |  | ✓ |
| Hemolytic anemia, or history of |  |  |  | ✓ |  |  |
| Hepatic function impairment or disease | ✓ | ✓ | ✓ | ✓ | ✓ | ✓ |
| Renal function impairment or disease | ✓ | ✓ | ✓ | ✓ | ✓ | ✓ |

*For parenteral administration only.

## Table 5. Patient Consultation (continued)

As an aid to patient consultation, refer to *Advice for the Patient, Skeletal Muscle Relaxants (Systemic)* or *Orphenadrine (Systemic)*.

In providing consultation, consider emphasizing the following selected information (» = major clinical significance):

Legend:
I = Carisoprodol
II = Chlorphenesin
III = Chlorzoxazone
IV = Metaxalone
V = Methocarbamol
VI = Orphenadrine

| | I | II | III | IV | V | VI |
|---|---|---|---|---|---|---|
| **Proper use of this medication** | | | | | | |
| Tablets may be crushed and mixed with food or liquid for ease of administration | | | | ✔ | ✔ | ✔ |
| » Proper dosing | ✔ | ✔ | ✔ | ✔ | ✔ | ✔ |
| Missed dose: Taking if remembered within an hour or so; not taking if remembered later; not doubling doses | ✔ | ✔ | ✔ | ✔ | ✔ | |
| » Proper storage | ✔ | ✔ | ✔ | ✔ | ✔ | ✔ |
| **Precautions while using this medication** | | | | | | |
| Regular visits to physician to check progress during prolonged therapy | ✔ | ✔ | ✔ | ✔ | ✔ | ✔ |
| » Avoiding use of alcohol or other CNS depressants during therapy unless prescribed or otherwise approved by physician | ✔ | ✔ | ✔ | ✔ | ✔ | ✔ |
| » Caution if any of the following occur: | | | | | | |
| Blurred vision or other vision problems | ✔ | | | | ✔ | ✔ |
| Clumsiness or unsteadiness | ✔ | | | | | |
| Dizziness or lightheadedness | ✔ | ✔ | ✔ | ✔ | ✔ | ✔ |
| Drowsiness | ✔ | ✔ | ✔ | ✔ | ✔ | ✔ |
| Faintness | ✔ | | | | ✔ | ✔ |
| Muscle weakness | | | | | | ✔ |
| Possible dryness of mouth; using sugarless gum or candy, ice, or saliva substitute for relief; checking with dentist if dry mouth continues for more than 2 weeks | | | | | | ✔ |
| Diabetics: May cause false-positive urine sugar tests | | | | ✔ | | |
| **Side/adverse effects** | | | | | | |
| Signs and symptoms of potential side effects, especially: | | | | | | |
| Allergic reactions | ✔ | ✔ | ✔ | ✔ | ✔ | ✔ |
| Anticholinergic effects | | | | | | ✔ |
| Blood dyscrasias | | ✔ | | ✔ | ✔ | |
| Convulsions | | | | | ✔* | |
| Fainting | ✔ | | | | ✔* | ✔ |
| Fast heartbeat | ✔ | | | | | ✔ |
| Gastrointestinal bleeding | | | | ✔ | | |
| Hallucinations | | | | | | ✔ |
| Hepatotoxicity | | | | ✔ | | |
| Mental depression | ✔ | | | | | |
| Pounding heartbeat | | | | | | ✔ |
| Slow heartbeat | | | | | ✔* | |
| Medication may color urine orange or reddish purple | | | ✔ | | | |
| Medication may color urine black, brown, or green, especially if allowed to stand | | | | | | ✔ |

*For parenteral administration only.

---

**SODIUM ASCORBATE**—See *Ascorbic Acid (Systemic)*

**SODIUM BENZOATE AND SODIUM PHENYLACETATE**—The *Sodium Benzoate and Sodium Phenylacetate (Systemic)* monograph is not included in this published version of the USP DI database. Copies of the monograph are available on request from Micromedex, Inc. - Reprint Requests, 6200 S. Syracuse Way, Suite 300, Englewood, CO 80111; telephone (303) 486-6400; telefax (303) 486-6464; Email: USPDI@MDX.COM.

---

# SODIUM BICARBONATE Systemic

VA CLASSIFICATION (Primary/Secondary): GA110/TN409
Commonly used brand name(s): *Arm and Hammer Pure Baking Soda; Bellans; Citrocarbonate; Soda Mint*.
Note: For a listing of dosage forms and brand names by country availability, see *Dosage Forms* section(s).

## Category

Alkalizer (systemic; urinary)—Sodium Bicarbonate Injection USP; Sodium Bicarbonate Oral Powder USP; Sodium Bicarbonate Tablets USP.
Antacid—Effervescent Sodium Bicarbonate; Sodium Bicarbonate Oral Powder USP; Sodium Bicarbonate Tablets USP.
Electrolyte replenisher—Sodium Bicarbonate Injection USP.

## Indications

Note: Bracketed information in the *Indications* section refers to uses that are not included in U.S. product labeling.

**Accepted**
Metabolic acidosis (treatment)—
Acute mild to moderate
In renal tubular disorders
In severe renal disease (renal tubular acidosis)
In circulatory insufficiency, due to shock or severe dehydration
In cardiac arrest
In extracorporeal circulation of blood and
In primary lactic acidosis, severe—Oral sodium bicarbonate is indicated in the treatment of metabolic acidosis. It is preferred over parenteral therapy in acute mild to moderate acidosis. Oral sodium bicarbonate is

also indicated to correct acidosis in renal tubular disorders. Parenteral sodium bicarbonate is indicated to minimize risks of metabolic acidosis in severe renal disease, circulatory insufficiency due to shock or severe dehydration, extracorporeal circulation of blood, cardiac arrest, and severe primary lactic acidosis.

Intravenous sodium bicarbonate has been used to minimize the risks of metabolic acidosis in uncontrolled diabetes; however, it generally has been replaced by low-dose insulin therapy and saline, potassium, and fluid replacement. With low-dose insulin therapy there is less risk of developing serious hypoglycemia and/or hypokalemia.

Renal calculi, uric acid (prophylaxis)—Oral sodium bicarbonate is indicated to reduce uric acid crystallization as an adjuvant to uricosuric medication in gout.

Hyperacidity (treatment)—Also indicated orally to provide symptomatic relief of upset stomach associated with hyperacidity. It may also be used in the treatment of the symptoms of peptic ulcer disease.

Diarrhea (treatment adjunct)—Parenteral sodium bicarbonate is indicated in severe diarrhea in which the loss of bicarbonate is significant.

Toxicity, nonspecific (treatment)—Parenteral sodium bicarbonate is indicated in the treatment of certain drug intoxications, including barbiturates, and in poisoning by salicylates or methyl alcohol.

Sodium bicarbonate is not recommended for use as an antidote following the ingestion of strong mineral acids, since the formation of carbon dioxide may distend the weakened stomach and lead to gastric rupture.

Sodium bicarbonate has been used as a urinary alkalizer to increase sulfonamide solubility and prevent crystallization that may lead to renal calculi or nephrotoxicity; however, poorly soluble sulfonamides are rarely used now.

[Sodium bicarbonate has been used in the treatment of sickle cell anemia; however, it generally has been replaced by more effective agents.]

## Pharmacology/Pharmacokinetics

### Physicochemical characteristics
Molecular weight—84.01.

### Mechanism of action/Effect
Alkalizer, systemic—Increases the plasma bicarbonate, buffers excess hydrogen ion concentration, and raises blood pH, thereby reversing the clinical manifestations of acidosis.

Alkalizer, urinary—Increases the excretion of free bicarbonate ions in the urine, thus effectively raising the urinary pH. By maintaining an alkaline urine, the actual dissolution of uric acid stones may be accomplished.

Antacid—Reacts chemically to neutralize or buffer existing quantities of stomach acid but has no direct effect on its output. This action results in increased pH value of stomach contents, thus providing relief of hyperacidity symptoms.

### Elimination
Renal; $CO_2$ formed is eliminated via lungs.

## Precautions to Consider

### Pregnancy/Reproduction
Pregnancy—Problems in humans have not been documented; however, risk-benefit must be considered, since sodium bicarbonate is absorbed systemically. Chronic use may lead to systemic alkalosis. The sodium load that is absorbed can also cause edema and weight gain.

For parenteral dosage form: Studies have not been done in humans.

Studies have not been done in animals.

FDA Pregnancy Category C.

### Breast-feeding
It is not known whether sodium bicarbonate is distributed into breast milk. However, problems in humans have not been documented.

### Pediatrics
Antacids should not be given to young children (up to 6 years of age) unless prescribed by a physician. Since children are not usually able to describe their symptoms precisely, proper diagnosis should precede the use of an antacid. This will avoid the complication of an existing condition (e.g., appendicitis) or the appearance of more severe adverse effects.

### Geriatrics
No information is available on the relationship of age to the effects of sodium bicarbonate in geriatric patients. However, elderly patients are more likely to have age-related renal function impairment, which may require caution in patients receiving sodium bicarbonate.

### Drug interactions and/or related problems
The following drug interactions and/or related problems have been selected on the basis of their potential clinical significance (possible mechanism in parentheses where appropriate)—not necessarily inclusive (» = major clinical significance):

Note: Not all interactions between sodium bicarbonate and other oral medications have been identified in this monograph. Because concurrent use may increase or reduce the rate and/or extent of absorption of other oral medications, patients should be advised not to take any other oral medications within 1 to 2 hours of sodium bicarbonate.

Combinations containing any of the following medications, depending on the amount present, may also interact with this medication.

Acidifiers, urinary, such as:
  Ammonium chloride
  Ascorbic acid
  Potassium or sodium phosphates
    (antacids may alkalinize the urine and counteract the effect of urinary acidifiers; frequent use of antacids, especially in high doses, is best avoided by patients receiving therapy to acidify the urine)

Amphetamines or
Quinidine
  (urinary excretion may be inhibited when these medications are used concurrently with sodium bicarbonate, possibly resulting in toxicity; dosage adjustment may be needed when sodium bicarbonate therapy is initiated or discontinued or if dosage is changed)

Anticholinergics or other medications with anticholinergic action (See Appendix II )
  (concurrent use with sodium bicarbonate may decrease absorption, reducing the effectiveness of the anticholinergic; doses of these medications should be spaced 1 hour apart from doses of sodium bicarbonate; also, urinary excretion may be delayed by alkalinization of the urine, thus potentiating the side effects of the anticholinergic)

Calcium-containing preparations or
Milk or milk products
  (concurrent and prolonged use with sodium bicarbonate may result in the milk-alkali syndrome)

Ciprofloxacin or
Norfloxacin or
Ofloxacin
  (alkalinization of the urine may reduce the solubility of ciprofloxacin, norfloxacin, or ofloxacin in the urine; patients should be observed for signs of crystalluria and nephrotoxicity)

Citrates
  (concurrent use with antacids containing sodium bicarbonate may result in systemic alkalosis)

  (concurrent use with sodium bicarbonate may promote the development of calcium stones in patients with uric acid stones, due to sodium ion opposition to the hypocalciuric effect of the alkaline load; may also cause hypernatremia)

Enteric-coated medications, such as bisacodyl
  (concurrent administration of antacids with enteric-coated tablets may cause the enteric coating to dissolve too rapidly, resulting in gastric or duodenal irritation)

Ephedrine
  (urine alkalinization induced by sodium bicarbonate may increase the half-life of ephedrine and prolong its duration of action, especially if the urine remains alkaline for several days or longer; dosage adjustment of ephedrine may be necessary)

Histamine $H_2$-receptor antagonists, such as
  Cimetidine
  Famotidine
  Nizatidine
  Ranitidine
  (concurrent use with sodium bicarbonate may be indicated in the treatment of peptic ulcer to relieve pain; however, simultaneous administration of antacids of medium to high potency [80 mmol to 150 mmol HCl] is not recommended since absorption of these medications may be decreased; patients should be advised not to take any antacids within one-half to 1 hour of histamine $H_2$-receptor antagonists)

Iron supplements or preparations, oral
  (absorption may be decreased when these preparations are used concurrently with antacids containing carbonate; because of the formation of less soluble complexes, iron supplements should not be taken within 1 hour before or 2 hours after sodium bicarbonate)

» Ketoconazole
  (sodium bicarbonate may cause increased gastrointestinal pH; concurrent administration with sodium bicarbonate may result in a

marked reduction in absorption of ketoconazole; patients should take sodium bicarbonate at least 2 hours after ketoconazole)

Lithium
(sodium bicarbonate enhances lithium excretion, possibly resulting in decreased efficacy; this may be partly due to the sodium content)

» Mecamylamine
(alkalinization of the urine caused by sodium bicarbonate slows excretion and prolongs the effects of mecamylamine; concurrent use is not recommended)

» Methenamine
(alkalinization of the urine caused by sodium bicarbonate may reduce the effectiveness of methenamine by inhibiting its conversion to formaldehyde; concurrent use is not recommended)

Mexiletine
(marked alkalinization of the urine caused by sodium bicarbonate may retard renal excretion of mexiletine)

Potassium supplements
(concurrent use of sodium bicarbonate infusion decreases serum potassium concentration by promoting a shift of potassium ion into the cells)

Salicylates
(alkalinization of the urine may increase renal salicylate excretion and lower serum salicylate concentrations; dosage adjustments of salicylates may be necessary when chronic high-dose antacid therapy with sodium bicarbonate is started or stopped, especially in patients receiving large doses of the salicylate, such as those with rheumatoid arthritis and rheumatic fever)

Sucralfate
(concurrent use with sodium bicarbonate may be indicated in the treatment of duodenal ulcer to relieve pain; however, simultaneous administration is not recommended since antacids, such as sodium bicarbonate, may interfere with binding of sucralfate to the mucosa; patients should be advised not to take sodium bicarbonate within one-half hour before or 1 hour after sucralfate)

» Tetracyclines, oral
(absorption may be decreased when oral tetracyclines are used concurrently with sodium bicarbonate because of increase in intragastric pH; patients should be advised not to take sodium bicarbonate within 1 to 2 hours of tetracyclines)

**Laboratory value alterations**
The following have been selected on the basis of their potential clinical significance (possible effect in parentheses where appropriate)—not necessarily inclusive (» = major clinical significance):

With diagnostic test results
» Gastric acid secretion test
(concurrent use of sodium bicarbonate may antagonize the effect of pentagastrin or histamine in the evaluation of gastric acid secretory function; administration of sodium bicarbonate is not recommended on the morning of the test)

With physiology/laboratory test values
pH, systemic and urinary
(may be increased)

**Medical considerations/Contraindications**
The medical considerations/contraindications included have been selected on the basis of their potential clinical significance (reasons given in parentheses where appropriate)—not necessarily inclusive (» = major clinical significance).

*Except under special circumstances, this medication should not be used when the following medical problems exist:*

For parenteral dosage form
» Alkalosis, metabolic or respiratory
(may be exacerbated)

» Chloride loss due to vomiting or continuous gastrointestinal suction
(increased risk of severe alkalosis)

» Hypocalcemia
(increased risk of alkalosis producing tetany)

*Risk-benefit should be considered when the following medical problems exist:*

» Anuria or oliguria
(increased risk of excessive sodium retention)

» Edematous sodium-retaining conditions such as:
Cirrhosis of liver
Congestive heart failure
Renal function impairment
Toxemia of pregnancy

» Hypertension
(may be exacerbated)

For antacid use
» Appendicitis or symptoms of
(sodium bicarbonate may complicate existing condition)
» Bleeding, gastrointestinal or rectal, undiagnosed

**Patient monitoring**
The following may be especially important in patient monitoring (other tests may be warranted in some patients, depending on condition; » = major clinical significance):

Arterial blood pH determinations and
Bicarbonate concentrations, serum
(periodic monitoring during parenteral administration is recommended to avoid overdosage and alkalosis)

pH determinations, urinary
(monitoring is recommended for dosage adjustment when sodium bicarbonate is used as a urinary alkalizer)

Renal function determinations
(recommended at periodic intervals with long-term use of frequent, repeated dosage)

## Side/Adverse Effects

The following side/adverse effects have been selected on the basis of their potential clinical significance (possible signs and symptoms in parentheses where appropriate)—not necessarily inclusive:

**Those indicating need for medical attention**
With excessive parenteral administration
*Hypokalemia* (dryness of mouth; increased thirst; irregular heartbeat; mood or mental changes; muscle cramps or pain; weak pulse)

With large doses
*Swelling of feet or lower legs*

**Those indicating need for medical attention only if they continue or are bothersome**
Incidence less frequent
*Increased thirst; stomach cramps*

## Overdose

For specific information on the agents used in the management of sodium bicarbonate overdose, see
• *Potassium Chloride* in *Potassium Supplements* monograph and/or
• *Calcium Gluconate* in *Calcium Supplements* monograph.

For information on the management of overdose or unintentional ingestion, **contact a Poison Control Center** (see *Poison Control Center Listing*).

**Clinical effects of overdose**
With large doses or in renal insufficiency
*Metabolic alkalosis* (mood or mental changes; muscle pain or twitching; nervousness or restlessness; slow breathing; unpleasant taste; unusual tiredness or weakness)

With long-term use
*Hypercalcemia associated with milk-alkali syndrome* (frequent urge to urinate; continuing headache; continuing loss of appetite; nausea or vomiting; unusual tiredness or weakness)

**Treatment of overdose**
Stop administration of sodium bicarbonate and all other alkali.
Supportive care—
Hydration with sodium chloride 0.9% intravenous injection.
Specific treatment—
Parenteral administration of potassium chloride if hypokalemia present.
Parenteral administration of calcium gluconate if hypocalcemia is present, for severe alkalosis.
Parenteral administration of ammonium chloride or hydrochloric acid, for severe alkalosis.
Hemodialysis for severe alkalosis.

## Patient Consultation

As an aid to patient consultation, refer to *Advice for the Patient, Sodium Bicarbonate (Systemic)*.
In providing consultation, consider emphasizing the following selected information (» = major clinical significance):

**Before using this medication**
» Conditions affecting use, especially:
Pregnancy—Chronic use may lead to systemic alkalosis; sodium may cause edema and weight gain
Use in children—Not recommended, because serious side effects may result

Other medications, especially ketoconazole, mecamylamine, methenamine, or oral tetracyclines

Other medical problems, especially anuria or oliguria, appendicitis, bleeding of gastrointestinal tract or rectum, chloride loss, edema, hypertension, hypocalcemia, or metabolic or respiratory alkalosis

**Proper use of this medication**
Following physician's or manufacturer's instructions
» Proper dosing
Missed dose: If on regular dosing schedule—Taking as soon as possible; not taking if almost time for next dose; not doubling doses
» Proper storage
*For antacid use*
» Compliance with therapy, especially for ulcer patients
Taking 1 and 3 hours after meals and at bedtime for maximum effectiveness (for ulcer patients)

**Precautions while using this medication**
Regular visits to physician to check progress during long-term therapy
» Not taking:
—within 1 to 2 hours of other oral medication
—for a prolonged period of time because of increased possibility of side effects
Caution for sodium restriction
*For antacid use*
» Not taking:
—if symptoms of appendicitis are present; checking with physician for proper diagnosis
—concurrently with large amounts of milk or milk products
—for more than 2 weeks or if problem is recurring, unless otherwise directed by physician

**Side/adverse effects**
Signs of potential side effects, especially hypokalemia

## General Dosing Information

Prolonged sodium bicarbonate therapy is not recommended because of the high risk of causing metabolic alkalosis or sodium overload.

In acute mild to moderate acidosis, oral treatment is preferred to intravenous therapy. In severe acute acidosis, sodium bicarbonate may be given intravenously.

**For oral dosage forms only**
Sodium bicarbonate is a fast-acting antacid, but has a short duration of effect. It has a high neutralizing capacity.

The maximum daily dosage of sodium is 200 mEq (16.6 grams of sodium bicarbonate) in patients younger than 60 years of age and 100 mEq (8.3 grams of sodium bicarbonate) in patients 60 years of age or older.

When sodium bicarbonate is used as an antacid, the maximum dosage allowed should not be taken for more than 2 weeks except with the advice or under the supervision of a physician.

In the treatment of peptic ulcer disease, sodium bicarbonate may be administered 1 and 3 hours after meals and at bedtime. Additional doses of antacids may be administered to relieve the pain that may occur between the regularly scheduled doses.

**For parenteral dosage forms only**
Commercially available parenteral solutions are generally hypertonic and require dilution.

Sodium bicarbonate solution may be administered intravenously or, following dilution to isotonicity (1.5%), subcutaneously.

For intravenous administration, suitable concentrations range from 1.5% (isotonic) to 8.4% (undiluted), depending on the clinical condition and requirements of the patient.

For subcutaneous administration, an isotonic solution (1.5%) of sodium bicarbonate may be prepared by diluting 1 mL of 8.4% sodium bicarbonate solution with 4.6 mL of sterile water for injection. However, it should be noted that absorption from subcutaneous administration is unpredictable. This route of administration is not generally recommended except in those cases where the intravenous route is not available.

Bicarbonate therapy should always be planned in a careful, controlled way, since the degree of response to a given dose is not precisely predictable. Ideally, sodium bicarbonate should always be given according to the results of measurement of arterial blood pH, carbon dioxide content of the plasma, and calculation of base deficit.

Excessive administration may induce hypokalemia and may predispose the patient to cardiac arrhythmias.

Too rapid administration of sodium bicarbonate may produce severe alkalosis, which may be accompanied by hyperirritability or tetany.

Overdosage and alkalosis may be avoided by giving repeated small doses. Periodic monitoring is recommended.

Rapid injection (10 mL per minute) of hypertonic sodium bicarbonate solutions may produce hypernatremia, a decrease in cerebrospinal fluid pressure, and possible intracranial hemorrhage, especially in neonates and children under 2 years of age. No more than 8 mEq per kg of body weight per day of a 4.2% solution should be administered.

In cardiac arrest emergencies, the risk of rapid infusion may be necessary because of the fatality risk due to acidosis.

Adequate alveolar ventilation must be ensured following sodium bicarbonate administration during cardiac arrest, to allow for the continued excretion of the carbon dioxide released. This is important for the control of arterial pH.

## Oral Dosage Forms

### EFFERVESCENT SODIUM BICARBONATE

**Usual adult and adolescent dose**
Antacid—
Oral, 3.9 to 10 grams in a glass of cold water after meals.
Note: Patients 60 years of age and over—Oral, 1.9 to 3.9 grams after meals.

**Usual adult and adolescent prescribing limits**
Oral, 19.5 grams per day.

**Usual pediatric dose**
Antacid—
Children up to 6 years of age: Dosage must be individualized by physician.
Children 6 to 12 years of age: Oral, 1 to 1.9 grams in a glass of cold water after meals.

**Strength(s) usually available**
U.S.—
780 mg of sodium bicarbonate and 1.82 grams of sodium citrate per teaspoonful (3.9 grams) (OTC) [*Citrocarbonate*].
Canada—
780 mg of sodium bicarbonate and 1.82 grams of sodium citrate per teaspoonful (3.9 grams) (OTC) [*Citrocarbonate*].

**Packaging and storage**
Store below 40 °C (104 °F), preferably between 15 and 30 °C (59 and 86 °F), in a tight container, unless otherwise specified by manufacturer.

**Note**
Alert patients on sodium-restricted diet. Product contains 30.46 mEq (700.6 mg) of sodium per 3.9 grams.

### SODIUM BICARBONATE ORAL POWDER USP

**Usual adult and adolescent dose**
Antacid—
Oral, ½ teaspoonful in a glass of water every two hours, the dose being adjusted as needed.
Urinary alkalizer—
Oral, 1 teaspoonful in a glass of water every four hours, the dose being adjusted as needed.

**Usual adult prescribing limits**
Up to 60 years of age—Up to 4 teaspoonfuls daily.

**Usual pediatric dose**
Dosage has not been established.

**Size(s) usually available**
U.S.—
120 grams (OTC) [*Arm and Hammer Pure Baking Soda;* GENERIC].
240 grams (OTC) [*Arm and Hammer Pure Baking Soda;* GENERIC].
480 grams (OTC) [*Arm and Hammer Pure Baking Soda;* GENERIC].
2400 grams (OTC) [*Arm and Hammer Pure Baking Soda;* GENERIC].
Canada—
Information not available [GENERIC].

Note: Each ½ teaspoonful contains 20.9 mEq (476 mg) of sodium.

**Packaging and storage**
Store below 40 °C (104 °F), preferably between 15 and 30 °C (59 and 86 °F), unless otherwise specified by manufacturer. Store in a well-closed container.

**Note**
Alert patients on sodium-restricted diet. Products contain 41.8 mEq (952 mg) of sodium per teaspoonful.

### SODIUM BICARBONATE TABLETS USP

**Usual adult and adolescent dose**
Antacid—
Oral, 325 mg to 2 grams one to four times a day.

## Sodium Bicarbonate (Systemic)

Urinary alkalizer—
  Oral, 4 grams initially, then 1 to 2 grams every four hours.

**Usual adult prescribing limits**
Up to 16 grams daily.

**Usual pediatric dose**
Antacid—
  Children up to 6 years of age: Dosage has not been established.
  Children 6 to 12 years of age: Oral, 520 mg; may be repeated once in thirty minutes.
Urinary alkalizer—
  Oral, 1 to 10 mEq (23 to 230 mg) per kg of body weight per day, the dose being adjusted as needed.

**Strength(s) usually available**
U.S.—
  325 mg (OTC) [*Soda Mint;* GENERIC].
  520 mg (OTC) [*Bellans*].
  650 mg (OTC) [GENERIC].
Canada—
  500 mg (OTC) [GENERIC].

**Packaging and storage**
Store below 40 °C (104 °F), preferably between 15 and 30 °C (59 and 86 °F), unless otherwise specified by manufacturer. Store in a well-closed container.

**Note**
Alert patients on sodium-restricted diet. Products contain sodium as follows: 325 mg tablets (3.9 mEq), 520 mg tablets (6.2 mEq), and 650 mg tablets (7.7 mEq).

## Parenteral Dosage Forms

### SODIUM BICARBONATE INJECTION USP

**Usual adult and adolescent dose**
Systemic alkalizer—
  In cardiac arrest: Intravenous, initially 1 mEq per kg of body weight; 0.5 mEq per kg of body weight may be repeated every ten minutes of continued arrest.
  In less urgent forms of metabolic acidosis: Intravenous infusion, 2 to 5 mEq per kg of body weight, administered over a period of four to eight hours.
  Note: Frequency of administration and the size of the dose may be reduced after severe symptoms have abated.
Urinary alkalizer—
  Intravenous, 2 to 5 mEq per kg of body weight, administered over a period of four to eight hours.

**Usual pediatric dose**
Systemic alkalizer—
  In cardiac arrest: Intravenous, 1 mEq per kg of body weight initially, then 0.5 mEq per kg of body weight every ten minutes of continued arrest.
  In less urgent forms of metabolic acidosis: Older children— See *Usual adult and adolescent dose.*
Urinary alkalizer—
  See *Usual adult and adolescent dose.*

**Strength(s) usually available**
U.S.—
  4.2% (Rx) [GENERIC].
  5% (Rx) [GENERIC].
  7.5% (Rx) [GENERIC].
  8.4% (Rx) [GENERIC].
Canada—
  4.2% (Rx) [GENERIC].
  7.5% (Rx) [GENERIC].
  8.4% (Rx) [GENERIC].

Note:

| Concentration per mL of Aqueous Solution | Sodium Content (mg/mL) |
|---|---|
| 4% (0.48 mEq) | 11 |
| 4.2% (0.5 mEq) | 11.5 |
| 5% (0.595 mEq) | 13.8 |
| 7.5% (0.892 mEq) | 20.5 |
| 8.4% (1 mEq) | 23 |

**Packaging and storage**
Store below 40 °C (104 °F), preferably between 15 and 30 °C (59 and 86 °F), unless otherwise specified by manufacturer. Protect from freezing.

**Preparation of dosage form**
Sterile water for injection, sodium chloride injection, dextrose injection (5%), or other standard electrolyte solutions may be used as diluents.
For dilution and preparation of injection, see manufacturer's package insert.

**Stability**
A sterile 7.5% solution of sodium bicarbonate in polypropylene syringes may remain stable for up to 100 days if refrigerated (2 to 8 °C), or up to 45 days at room temperature.
Stability may be increased by refrigerating the sodium bicarbonate injection and the syringes before preparation, rinsing the syringes twice with refrigerated sterile water for injection, minimizing the contact of the solution with air by expelling the air from the syringes, and taping the plunger in place to minimize its movement caused by escaping carbon dioxide.
Solutions of sodium bicarbonate should not be boiled or heated. When heated, it may decompose and be converted to the carbonate.
Haze formation or precipitation may result when sodium bicarbonate is added to infusion solution containing calcium.
Do not use the injection if it contains a precipitate.

**Incompatibilities**
Sodium bicarbonate is incompatible with acids, acidic salts, many alkaloidal salts, aspirin, atropine, bismuth salicylate, calcium-containing solutions, dobutamine, dopamine hydrochloride, epinephrine, isoproterenol hydrochloride, morphine sulfate, norepinephrine bitartrate, regular insulin, and tubocurarine chloride.

Revised: 02/03/92
Interim revision: 08/10/94

---

**SODIUM CHLORIDE**—The *Sodium Chloride (Parenteral-Local)* monograph is not included in this published version of the USP DI database. Copies of the monograph are available on request from Micromedex, Inc. - Reprint Requests, 6200 S. Syracuse Way, Suite 300, Englewood, CO 80111; telephone (303) 486-6400; telefax (303) 486-6464; Email: USPDI@MDX.COM.

---

# SODIUM CHROMATE Cr 51   Systemic

INN:  Sodium Chromate ($^{51}$Cr)
VA CLASSIFICATION (Primary): DX201
Commonly used brand name(s): *Chromitope.*
Note:  For a listing of dosage forms and brand names by country availability, see *Dosage Forms* section(s).

## Category
Diagnostic aid, radioactive (red blood cell disease; gastrointestinal bleeding; platelet survival).

## Indications
Note:  Bracketed information in the *Indications* section refers to uses that are not included in U.S. product labeling.

Accepted
Red blood cells, labeling of—
  Sodium chromate Cr 51 is indicated for *in vitro* labeling of autologous red blood cells. Cr 51–labeled red blood cells are indicated for the following diagnostic studies:
    Red blood cell volume or mass determinations: To determine and evaluate red blood cell volume or mass in the differential diagnosis and follow-up of patients with polycythemia.
    Red blood cell survival time determinations and
    Red blood cell sequestration studies: To study the rate of disappearance of red blood cells from the circulation in cases of splenic sequestration accompanying such diseases as hereditary spherocytosis, acquired hemolytic anemia, or hemolytic anemia secondary to lymphoma or leukemia. These data may be helpful in deciding the need for splenectomy.

Bleeding, gastrointestinal (diagnosis): To evaluate patients suspected of gastrointestinal bleeding, to quantify the amount of blood loss.

[Platelets, labeling of]—
Sodium chromate Cr 51 is used for the labeling of autologous platelets to be used for the following study:
[Platelet survival studies]: To determine platelet survival time and sites of platelet destruction and/or sequestration in the evaluation of patients with thrombocytopenia.

## Physical Properties

### Nuclear Data

| Radionuclide (half-life) | Mode of decay | Principal photon emissions (keV) | Mean number of emissions/ disintegration |
|---|---|---|---|
| Cr 51 (27.7 days) | Electron capture | Gamma (320) | 0.1 |

## Pharmacology/Pharmacokinetics

### Mechanism of action/Effect

*In vitro*, the hexavalent radioactive chromium Cr 51 readily penetrates the erythrocyte and binds to hemoglobin. Unbound chromium Cr 51 is reduced to the trivalent state by the addition of a reducing agent, such as ascorbic acid, so no further binding occurs *in vivo*. Unbound chromium Cr 51 can be removed by cell washing with isotonic saline. When the chromium Cr 51–labeled cells are injected, the Cr 51 is slowly eluted from the cells in the circulation at a rate of 1% per day. The labeled cells eventually undergo destruction in the reticuloendothelial tissues mainly in the spleen, from which the deposited radioactivity is again slowly eluted. After intravenous injection of the labeled red blood cells, the trivalent state of chromium Cr 51 is maintained until the labeled red blood cells are sequestered by the spleen, at which time the chromium Cr 51 is released to the plasma. Samples of the patient's blood are obtained and measured in a scintillation well counter for red blood cell volume and survival time determinations. External counting with scintillation probes is used to evaluate relative splenic and hepatic sequestration. To determine actual gastrointestinal bleeding, stool is collected and measurements of the amount of radioactivity in the stool are performed.

### Half-life

Normal labeled red blood cells survival half-time—25 to 35 days.

Note: The apparent short survival time, as compared to the 120-day true life span of red blood cells, is due to the elution of chromium from the cells and to cell damage that probably occurs during blood withdrawal and labeling.

### Radiation dosimetry

| Organ | Estimated absorbed radiation dose* |||||
|---|---|---|---|---|
| | Cr 51-labeled red blood cells || Cr 51-labeled platelets ||
| | mGy/MBq | rad/mCi | mGy/MBq | rad/mCi |
| Spleen | 1.6 | 5.92 | 2.6 | 9.63 |
| Heart | 0.51 | 1.89 | 0.096 | 0.36 |
| Lungs | 0.32 | 1.18 | 0.072 | 0.27 |
| Liver | 0.24 | 0.89 | 0.3 | 1.11 |
| Kidneys | 0.22 | 0.81 | 0.11 | 0.41 |
| Adrenals | 0.22 | 0.81 | 0.11 | 0.41 |
| Pancreas | 0.19 | 0.70 | 0.18 | 0.67 |
| Red marrow | 0.14 | 0.52 | 0.19 | 0.7 |
| Stomach wall | 0.14 | 0.52 | 0.096 | 0.36 |
| Thyroid | 0.12 | 0.44 | 0.022 | 0.081 |
| Bone surfaces | 0.11 | 0.41 | 0.09 | 0.33 |
| Breast | 0.099 | 0.37 | 0.03 | 0.11 |
| Small intestine | 0.095 | 0.35 | 0.044 | 0.16 |
| Large intestine (upper) | 0.094 | 0.35 | 0.045 | 0.17 |
| Uterus | 0.085 | 0.31 | 0.028 | 0.1 |
| Bladder wall | 0.075 | 0.28 | 0.018 | 0.067 |
| Ovaries | 0.082 | 0.30 | 0.032 | 0.12 |
| Large intestine (lower) | 0.081 | 0.30 | 0.032 | 0.12 |
| Testes | 0.063 | 0.23 | 0.013 | 0.048 |
| Other tissues | 0.085 | 0.31 | 0.034 | 0.13 |

| Radionuclide | Effective dose* ||||
|---|---|---|---|---|
| | Cr 51-labeled red blood cells || Cr 51-labeled platelets ||
| | mSv/MBq | rem/mCi | mSv/MBq | rem/mCi |
| Cr 51 | 0.26 | 0.96 | 0.24 | 0.89 |

*For adults; intravenous injection. Data based on the International Commission on Radiological Protection (ICRP) Publication 53—Radiation dose to patients from radiopharmaceuticals.

### Elimination

Renal (unbound/released trivalent chromium Cr 51) and fecal (less than 1% eliminated in the feces of normal patients).

## Precautions to Consider

### Carcinogenicity/Mutagenicity

Long-term animal studies to evaluate carcinogenic or mutagenic potential of sodium chromate Cr 51 have not been performed.

### Pregnancy/Reproduction

Pregnancy—Studies have not been done in humans with sodium chromate Cr 51. The possibility of pregnancy should be assessed in women of child-bearing potential. Clinical situations exist where the benefit to the patient and fetus, based on information derived from radiopharmaceutical use, outweighs the risks from radiation exposure to the fetus. In these situations, the physician should use discretion and reduce the radiopharmaceutical dose to the lowest possible amount.

Studies have not been done in animals.

FDA Pregnancy Category C.

### Breast-feeding

Sodium chromate Cr 51 is distributed into breast milk. Because of the potential risk to the infant from radiation exposure, temporary discontinuation of nursing is recommended for a length of time that may be assessed by measuring the activity in breast milk and estimating the radiation exposure to the infant.

### Pediatrics

Although sodium chromate Cr 51 is used in children, there have been no specific studies evaluating safety and efficacy of sodium chromate Cr 51 in children. When this radiopharmaceutical is used in children, the diagnostic benefit should be judged to outweigh the potential risk of radiation.

### Geriatrics

Appropriate studies on the relationship of age to the effects of sodium chromate Cr 51 have not been performed in the geriatric population. However, no geriatrics-specific problems have been documented to date.

### Drug interactions and/or related problems

See *Diagnostic interference*.

### Diagnostic interference

The following have been selected on the basis of their potential clinical significance (possible effect in parentheses where appropriate)—not necessarily inclusive (» = major clinical significance):

With results of *this* test
Stannous pyrophosphate
(red blood cell labeling may be inhibited in double tracer red blood cell survival studies by the presence of stannous pyrophosphate used in the labeling of Tc 99m; washing red blood cells before labeling with chromium Cr 51 is recommended to avoid this effect)

## Side/Adverse Effects

Currently, there are no known side/adverse effects associated with the use of sodium chromate Cr 51 as a diagnostic aid.

## Patient Consultation

As an aid to patient consultation, refer to *Advice for the Patient, Radiopharmaceuticals (Diagnostic)*.

In providing consultation, consider emphasizing the following selected information (» = major clinical significance):

### Description of use

Action in the body: Distribution in body of injected radioactive red blood cells same as that of normal red blood cells
Radioactivity in blood or stool samples is measured
Small amounts of radioactivity used in diagnosis; radiation exposure is low and considered safe

### Before having this test
» Conditions affecting use, especially:
　Pregnancy—Risk to fetus from radiation exposure as opposed to benefit derived from use should be considered
　Breast-feeding—Distributed into breast milk; temporary discontinuation of nursing recommended because of risk to infant from radiation exposure
　Use in children—Risk of radiation exposure as opposed to benefit derived from use should be considered

### Preparation for this test
Special preparatory instructions may apply; patient should inquire in advance

### Precautions after having this test
No special precautions

## General Dosing Information
Radiopharmaceuticals are to be administered only by or under the supervision of physicians who have had extensive training in the safe use and handling of radioactive materials and who are authorized by the Nuclear Regulatory Commission (NRC) or the appropriate Agreement State agency, if required, or, outside the U.S., the appropriate authority.

The possibility of contamination of labeled red blood cells necessitates the use of sterile techniques for the collection, labeling, rinsing, suspending, and injection of labeled red blood cells.

Extreme care must be taken in blood withdrawal and labeling procedures to ensure that red blood cells are not damaged. Damaged labeled red blood cells will be rapidly sequestered by reticuloendothelial cells of spleen and liver, resulting in erroneous red cell volume and survival determinations.

Manufacturer's package insert or other appropriate literature should be consulted for specific method of labeling red blood cells.

### Safety considerations for handling this radiopharmaceutical
Improper handling of this radiopharmaceutical may cause radioactive contamination. Guidelines for handling radioactive material have been prepared by scientific, professional, state, federal, and international bodies and are available to the specially qualified and authorized users who have access to radiopharmaceuticals.

## Parenteral Dosage Forms
Note: Bracketed uses in the *Dosage Forms* section refer to categories of use and/or indications that are not included in U.S. product labeling.

### SODIUM CHROMATE Cr 51 INJECTION USP
#### Usual adult and adolescent administered activity
Red blood cell dynamics—
　Volume or mass determinations—
　　Intravenous, 0.37 to 1.11 megabecquerels (0.01 to 0.03 millicurie).
　Survival time determinations—
　　Intravenous, 5.55 megabecquerels (0.15 millicurie).
　Gastrointestinal blood loss—
　　Intravenous, 7.4 megabecquerels (0.2 millicurie).
[Platelet survival studies]—
　Intravenous, 0.185 to 0.555 megabecquerel (5 to 15 microcuries).

#### Usual pediatric administered activity
Dosage must be individualized by physician.

#### Usual geriatric administered activity
See *Usual adult and adolescent administered activity*.

#### Strength(s) usually available
U.S.—
　3.7 megabecquerels (0.1 millicurie) per mL at time of calibration, having a specific activity of no less than 370 megabecquerels (10 millicuries) per mg of sodium chromate at time of use (Rx) [GENERIC].
　9.25 megabecquerels (0.25 millicurie) per 1.25-mL vial at time of calibration, having a specific activity of no less than 370 megabecquerels (10 millicuries) per mg of sodium chromate at time of use (Rx) [*Chromitope*].
　37 megabecquerels (1 millicurie) per 5-mL vial at time of calibration, having a specific activity of no less than 370 megabecquerels (10 millicuries) per mg of sodium chromate at time of use (Rx) [*Chromitope*].
Canada—
　1.85 to 74 megabecquerels (0.05 to 2 millicuries) per mL (Rx) [GENERIC].

#### Packaging and storage
Store below 30 °C (86 °F), preferably between 15 and 30 °C (59 and 86 °F), unless otherwise specified by manufacturer.

#### Note
Caution—Radioactive material.

## Selected Bibliography
International Committee for Standardization in Haematology. Recommended methods for measurement of red-cell and plasma volumes. J Nucl Med 1980; 21: 793-800.

Sisson JC. Red blood cell survival including red blood cell sequestration. In: Carey JE, Kline RC, Keyes JW, editors. Manual of nuclear medicine procedures. 4th ed. Boca Raton, FL: CRC Press, 1983: 134-6.

Revised: 04/30/96

---

**SODIUM CITRATE AND CITRIC ACID**—See *Citrates (Systemic)*

---

# SODIUM FLUORIDE   Systemic

VA CLASSIFICATION (Primary): TN407

Commonly used brand name(s): *Flozenges; Fluor-A-Day; Fluoritab; Fluoritabs; Fluorodex; Fluorosol; Flura; Flura-Drops; Flura-Loz; Karidium; Luride; Luride Lozi-Tabs; Luride-SF Lozi-Tabs; PDF; Pedi-Dent; Pediaflor; Pharmaflur; Pharmaflur 1.1; Pharmaflur df; Phos-Flur; Solu-Flur*.

Note: For a listing of dosage forms and brand names by country availability, see *Dosage Forms* section(s).

## Category
Dental caries prophylactic; nutritional supplement (mineral).

## Indications
### Accepted
Dental caries (prophylaxis)—Sodium fluoride is indicated as a dietary supplement for prevention of dental caries in children in those areas where the level of naturally occurring fluoride in the drinking water is inadequate. In optimally fluoridated communities, sodium fluoride supplementation may be necessary in infants that are totally breast-fed or receive ready-to-use formulas or in children consuming nonfluoridated bottled water rather than tap water. Sodium fluoride supplementation may also be indicated in those situations where home water filtration systems remove fluoride. This usually occurs with reverse osmosis or distillation units, but not with carbon charcoal filters.

Evidence that oral systemic fluoride supplements reduce dental caries in adults is lacking.

Note: Sodium fluoride has been used to treat osteoporosis and otospongiosis in adults; however, its use is controversial and further studies are needed. The doses used in osteoporosis and otospongiosis have potential for toxicity, including skeletal fluorosis, osteomalacia, widening of unmineralized osteoid seams, and upper gastrointestinal ulceration.

## Pharmacology/Pharmacokinetics
### Physicochemical characteristics
Molecular weight—41.99.

### Mechanism of action/Effect
Fluoride ion becomes incorporated into and stabilizes the apatite crystal of bone and teeth. Fluoride acts primarily to promote remineralization of decalcified enamel and may interfere with growth and development of dental plaque bacteria. Deposition of fluoride ion in the enamel surface of teeth increases resistance to acid and to development of caries.

### Absorption
Fluorides in solution or in the form of rapidly soluble salts are readily and almost completely absorbed from the gastrointestinal tract.

### Storage
In bone and developing teeth.

**Time to peak serum concentration**
30 to 60 minutes.

**Elimination**
Primarily renal (approximately 50%), with small amounts in feces and sweat.

## Precautions to Consider

### Carcinogenicity
Fluoride in the concentrations shown to be effective against tooth decay has not been shown to cause cancer in individuals who receive fluoride over prolonged periods.

### Pregnancy/Reproduction
Problems in humans have not been documented with intake of normal daily recommended amounts. Fluoride readily crosses the placenta.

There is conflicting evidence as to whether administration of fluoride supplements to women during pregnancy will help prevent caries in the child.

### Breast-feeding
Problems in humans have not been documented with intake of normal daily recommended amounts. Trace amounts of fluoride are distributed into breast milk, although the concentration is not high enough to provide benefits to the infant.

### Pediatrics
Problems in pediatrics have not been documented with intake of normal daily recommended amounts. Chronic overdose may cause fluorosis of the teeth (if given during the period of tooth-enamel formation) and osseous changes.

### Geriatrics
Problems in geriatrics have not been documented with intake of normal daily recommended amounts. Elderly patients are more likely to have age-related renal failure, which may require caution if patients are receiving large doses for osteoporosis or otospongiosis. The elderly are also more likely to develop stress fractures, gastrointestinal ulceration, and arthralgia from large doses of sodium fluoride.

### Dental
Excessive doses of sodium fluoride may result in fluorosis of teeth if taken during tooth formation years.

### Drug interactions and/or related problems
The following drug interactions and/or related problems have been selected on the basis of their potential clinical significance (possible mechanism in parentheses where appropriate)—not necessarily inclusive (» = major clinical significance):

Note: Combinations containing any of the following, depending on the amount present, may also interact with this medication.

Aluminum hydroxide
(may decrease absorption and increase fecal excretion of fluoride; aluminium hydroxide–containing medications should be taken 2 hours before or after sodium fluoride)

Calcium supplements
(concurrent use with sodium fluoride may cause the calcium ions to complex with fluoride and inhibit absorption of both fluoride and calcium; if sodium fluoride is used with calcium supplements to treat osteoporosis, a 1- to 2-hour interval should elapse between doses of the two)

### Laboratory value alterations
The following have been selected on the basis of their potential clinical significance (possible effect in parentheses where appropriate)—not necessarily inclusive (» = major clinical significance):

With diagnostic test results
Alkaline phosphatase concentrations, serum
(results may be elevated)

Aspartate aminotransferase (AST [SGOT]) concentrations, serum
(may be falsely increased)

### Medical considerations/Contraindications
The medical considerations/contraindications included have been selected on the basis of their potential clinical significance (reasons given in parentheses where appropriate)—not necessarily inclusive (» = major clinical significance).

*Except under special circumstances, this medication should not be used when the following medical conditions exist:*

Arthralgia or
Gastrointestinal ulceration
(conditions may be exacerbated, especially with high doses)
Renal insufficiency, severe
(condition may be exacerbated; may lead to higher blood levels of fluoride due to a decrease in excretion of fluoride; dosage reduction may be necessary)

*Risk-benefit should be considered when the following medical problems exist:*

High dental fluorosis, or prevalence in other members of the immediate community

### Patient monitoring
The following may be especially important in patient monitoring (other tests may be warranted in some patients, depending on condition; » = major clinical significance):

Dental examination
(recommended once or twice a year in most patients, and more frequently in those highly prone to developing caries)

## Side/Adverse Effects

The following side/adverse effects have been selected on the basis of their potential clinical significance (possible signs and symptoms in parentheses where appropriate)—not necessarily inclusive:

### Those indicating need for medical attention
Incidence rare
*Ulceration of oral mucous membranes* (sores in mouth and on lips)

## Overdose

For specific information on the agents used in the management of fluoride overdose, see
- *Calcium Supplements (Systemic)* monograph.

For more information on the management of overdose or unintentional ingestion **contact a Poison Control Center** (see *Poison Control Center Listing*).

### Clinical effects of overdose

Note: Stomach upset may occur with ingestion of 5 to 20 mg of sodium fluoride. The lethal dose is not known, but has been estimated as 5 to 10 grams of sodium fluoride in untreated adults and 5 mg of fluoride ion per kilogram of body weight in children.

Severe acute fluoride overdose can cause hypocalcemia and tetany and bone pain, especially in the feet and ankles, of uncertain cause; electrolyte disturbances and cardiac arrhythmias have been reported, progressing to cardiac failure or respiratory arrest in some cases.

Osseous changes, including skeletal fluorosis, osteomalacia, and osteosclerosis, may also result from excessive, chronic doses.

The following effects have been selected on the basis of their potential clinical significance (possible signs and symptoms in parentheses where appropriate)—not necessarily inclusive

Chronic effects (fluorosis and osteosclerosis)
*Pain and aching of bones, stiffness, or white, brown, or black discoloration of teeth*—occur only during periods of tooth development in children

Acute effects
*Black, tarry stools; bloody vomit; diarrhea; drowsiness; faintness; increased watering of mouth; nausea or vomiting; shallow breathing; stomach cramps or pain; tremors; unusual excitement; watery eyes; weakness*

### For treatment of acute overdose
Specific treatment—
Administration of intravenous dextrose.
Gastric lavage with calcium chloride or calcium hydroxide solution to precipitate fluoride.
Intravenous calcium gluconate if hypocalcemia occurs.
Monitoring—
Monitor respiration, blood pressure, and ECG.
Supportive care—
Maintenance of high urine output.
Patients in whom intentional overdose is confirmed or suspected should be referred for psychiatric consultation.

## Patient Consultation

As an aid to patient consultation, refer to *Advice for the Patient, Sodium Fluoride (Systemic)*.

In providing consultation, consider emphasizing the following selected information (» = major clinical significance):

### Importance of diet
Importance of proper nutrition; fluoride may be needed because of inadequate dietary intake
Dietary sources of fluoride; effects of processing

Recommended daily intake for fluoride
Remembering not to take more than recommended

**Before using this medication**
» Conditions affecting use, especially:
Pregnancy—Fluoride crosses the placenta
Breast-feeding—Trace amount distributed into breast milk
Use in children—Chronic overdose may cause dental fluorosis and osseous changes
Use in the elderly—High doses used for osteoporosis or otospongiosis not recommended in elderly patients with arthralgia, gastrointestinal ulceration, or renal insufficiency
Dental—Excessive doses taken during tooth formation years may result in tooth fluorosis

**Proper use of this medication**
» Importance of not using more medication than the amount prescribed
» Proper dosing
Missed dose: Taking as soon as possible; not taking if almost time for next dose; not doubling doses
*For individuals taking the chewable tablet dosage form*
Chewing or crushing tablets before swallowing
Advisability of taking at bedtime after brushing teeth; not eating or drinking for at least 15 minutes after taking
*For individuals taking the oral solution dosage form*
Proper use of the dropper bottle
» Avoiding use of glass with fluoride-containing solutions since fluoride etches glass
May be dropped directly into the mouth or mixed with cereal, fruit juice, or other food (except calcium-containing foods or beverages)
» Proper storage

**Precautions while using this medication**
Checking with health care professional as soon as possible after moving to another geographic area to see if continued treatment at the same dosage is necessary, since fluoride levels of community drinking water vary; also checking if changing infant feeding habits, drinking water, or filtration
Not taking calcium supplements or aluminum hydroxide-containing products and sodium fluoride at the same time; use should be separated by 2 hours
» Informing health care professional if teeth show signs of mottling

**Side/adverse effects**
Signs of potential side effects especially oral mucous membrane ulceration

## General Dosing Information

Optimal benefit of fluorides must be established on an individual basis, taking into consideration the fluoride content of the water supply when determining the dose. Some studies have found that systemic fluoride ingestion from toothpaste use in young children is significant.

The amount of fluoride from all sources should be taken into account when determining the therapeutic dose. For example, infant formulas made with fluoridated water provide a significant amount. Also, some schools in communities without water fluoridation have added up to 4.5 times the optimal fluoride level to the school's water supply to ensure that children receive adequate fluoride.

Use of fluoride supplements is generally not recommended when community drinking water contains more than 0.6 parts per million (ppm) of fluoride.

A fluoride level of approximately 1 ppm (0.6 to 1.2 ppm) in water is generally considered optimal for development of decay-resistant teeth without causing fluorosis, the actual value depending on the annual mean maximum daily temperature of the geographic area.

2.2 mg of sodium fluoride is equivalent to 1 mg of fluoride ion.

Since therapy with oral, systemic fluoride supplements is most effective on unerupted teeth, it is recommended that children receive oral fluoride supplementation until the age of 13 (or when the second molars have erupted) to provide maximum benefit to both deciduous and permanent teeth. Subsequent periodic topical application of fluoride for life may be advisable to prolong the cariostatic benefits, since beneficial effects, particularly in caries-prone individuals, appear to be lost a year or two after topical use is discontinued.

The recommended dose should not be exceeded, since prolonged overdosage may cause dental fluorosis in children and osseous changes in children and adults.

Mottling of tooth enamel (dental fluorosis) occurs with excessive ingestion of fluoride (e.g., continual use of drinking water containing greater than 2 ppm of fluoride) during the period of tooth development in children.

Stiffness (skeletal fluorosis) occurs with chronic ingestion of water containing 4 to 14 ppm of fluoride.

Generalized effects (renal damage, albuminuria, goiter) occur only after chronic ingestion of large amounts of fluoride over 10 to 20 years.

It is recommended that fluoride preparations (especially the chewable tablets) taken on a once-a-day basis be taken at bedtime after the teeth have been thoroughly brushed (to also provide some topical benefit from the fluoride).

Sodium fluoride (25 to 60 mg a day) may stabilize the progression of hearing loss in some patients with otospongiosis.

**Diet/Nutrition**
Nausea (although rare with doses of fluoride taken for dental caries) may be reduced by taking sodium fluoride with or just after meals, provided that the foods do not contain calcium, since calcium may interfere with fluoride absorption.

The oral solution may be administered undiluted or mixed with cereal, fluids, or other food. However, absorption of sodium fluoride may be reduced when taken with calcium-rich foods or beverages.

Recommended dietary intakes for fluoride are defined differently worldwide.
For U.S.—
The Recommended Dietary Allowances (RDAs) for vitamins and minerals are determined by the Food and Nutrition Board of the National Research Council and are intended to provide adequate nutrition in most healthy persons under usual environmental stresses. In addition, a different designation may be used by the FDA for food and dietary supplement labeling purposes, as with Daily Value (DV). DVs replace the previous labeling terminology United States Recommended Daily Allowances (USRDAs).
For Canada—
Recommended Nutrient Intakes (RNIs) for vitamins, minerals, and protein are determined by Health and Welfare Canada and provide recommended amounts of a specific nutrient while minimizing the risk of chronic diseases.

There is no RDA or RNI established for fluoride. Daily recommended intakes for fluoride are generally defined as follows
Infants and children:
Birth to 3 years: 0.1 to 1.5 mg.
4 to 6 years: 1 to 2.5 mg.
7 to 10 years: 1.5 to 2.5 mg.
Adolescents and adults:
1.5 to 4 mg.

Sources of fluoride other than fluoridated drinking water include fish that are consumed with their bones and tea. Cooking foods in fluorinated water can increase their fluoride content as can cooking with Teflon- (a fluoride-containing polymer) coated utensils and pans. However, cooking foods in utensils and pans with an aluminum surface can decrease their fluoride content.

## Oral Dosage Forms

### SODIUM FLUORIDE LOZENGES
**Usual pediatric dose**
Dental caries prophylactic or
Nutritional supplement—
Dosage of fluoride recommended by the American Dental Association, the American Academy of Pediatrics, and the American Academy of Pediatric Dentistry for communities where the level of fluoride in drinking water is 0.6 ppm or less

| Water Fluoride (ppm) | Age (yr) | Dose of Fluoride Ion (mg per day) |
|---|---|---|
| <0.3 | Birth to 0.5 | 0 |
|  | 0.5 to 3 | 0.25 |
|  | 3 to 6 | 0.5 |
|  | 6 to 16 | 1 |
| 0.3–0.6 | Birth to 3 | 0 |
|  | 3 to 6 | 0.25 |
|  | 6 to 16 | 0.5 |
| >0.6 | Birth to 16 | 0 |

Note: In Canada a different dosing schedule may be used. The Canadian Dental Association recommendations differ from that of the American Dental Association.

**Strength(s) usually available**
U.S.—
2.2 mg (1 mg of fluoride ion) (Rx) [*Flura-Loz*].

Canada—
- 1.1 mg (OTC) [*Flozenges*].
- 2.2 mg (OTC) [*Flozenges*].

**Packaging and storage**
Store below 40 °C (104 °F), preferably between 15 and 30 °C (59 and 86 °F), unless otherwise specified by manufacturer. Store in a tight container.

## SODIUM FLUORIDE ORAL SOLUTION USP

**Usual pediatric dose**
See *Sodium Fluoride Lozenges*.

**Strength(s) usually available**
U.S.—
- 0.275 mg (0.125 mg of fluoride ion) per drop (Rx) [*Karidium; Luride;* GENERIC].
- 0.44 mg (0.2 mg of fluoride ion) per mL (Rx) [*Phos-Flur*].
- 0.55 mg (0.25 mg of fluoride ion) per drop (Rx) [*Fluoritab; Flura-Drops*].
- 1.1 mg (0.5 mg of fluoride ion) per mL (Rx) [*Pediaflor* (alcohol less than 0.5%)].

Canada—
- 2 mg (0.905 mg of fluoride ion) per mL (OTC) [*PDF*].
- 2.2 mg (1 mg of fluoride ion) per 4 drops (Rx) [*Solu-Flur*].
- 2.21 mg (1 mg of fluoride ion) per 8 drops (0.5 mL) (OTC) [*Karidium*].
- 5.56 mg (1 mg of fluoride ion) per mL (OTC) [*Fluor-A-Day*].
- 6.9 mg (3.12 mg of fluoride ion) per mL (OTC) [*Fluorosol; Pedi-Dent;* GENERIC].

**Packaging and storage**
Store below 40 °C (104 °F), preferably between 15 and 30 °C (59 and 86 °F), unless otherwise specified by manufacturer. Store in a tight, plastic container. Protect from freezing.

**Auxiliary labeling**
- Keep out of reach of children.

**Note**
To reduce the risk associated with accidental ingestion and overdosage, it is recommended that no more than 264 mg of sodium fluoride be dispensed at one time. The American Dental Association Council on Dental Therapeutics considers a limit of 300 mg acceptable when sodium fluoride is dispensed to children in prepackaged containers.
Since size of drop dispensed and strength vary among commercial preparations, always dispense the same brand for refills on a prescription.

## SODIUM FLUORIDE TABLETS USP

**Usual pediatric dose**
See *Sodium Fluoride Lozenges*.

**Strength(s) usually available**
U.S.—
- 1.1 mg (0.5 mg of fluoride ion) (Rx) [GENERIC].
- 2.2 mg (1 mg of fluoride ion) (Rx) [*Flura; Karidium;* GENERIC].

Canada—
- 2.2 mg (1 mg fluoride ion) (OTC) [*Fluorosol; Karidium;* GENERIC].

**Packaging and storage**
Store below 40 °C (104 °F), preferably between 15 and 30 °C (59 and 86 °F), unless otherwise specified by manufacturer. Store in a tight container.

**Auxiliary labeling**
- Keep out of reach of children.

**Note**
To reduce the risk associated with accidental ingestion and overdosage, it is recommended that no more than 264 mg of sodium fluoride be dispensed at one time. The American Dental Association Council on Dental Therapeutics considers a limit of 300 mg acceptable when sodium fluoride is dispensed to children in prepackaged containers.

## SODIUM FLUORIDE CHEWABLE TABLETS USP

**Usual pediatric dose**
See *Sodium Fluoride Lozenges*.

**Strength(s) usually available**
U.S.—
- 0.55 mg (0.25 mg of fluoride ion) (Rx) [*Luride Lozi-Tabs*].
- 1.1 mg (0.5 mg of fluoride ion) (Rx) [*Fluoritab* (scored); *Fluorodex; Luride Lozi-Tabs; Pharmaflur 1.1;* GENERIC].
- 2.2 mg (1 mg of fluoride ion) (Rx) [*Fluoritab; Fluorodex; Karidium; Luride Lozi-Tabs; Luride-SF Lozi-Tabs; Pharmaflur; Pharmaflur df;* GENERIC].

Canada—
- 2.2 mg (1 mg of fluoride ion) (OTC) [*Fluor-A-Day; Fluoritabs; Pedi-Dent; Solu-Flur;* GENERIC].

**Packaging and storage**
Store below 40 °C (104 °F), preferably between 15 and 30 °C (59 and 86 °F), unless otherwise specified by manufacturer. Store in a tight container.

**Auxiliary labeling**
- Keep out of reach of children.

**Note**
To reduce the risk associated with accidental ingestion and overdosage, it is recommended that no more than 264 mg of sodium fluoride be dispensed at one time. The American Dental Association Council on Dental Therapeutics considers a limit of 300 mg acceptable when sodium fluoride is dispensed to children in prepackaged containers.

Revised: 07/17/92
Interim revision: 08/07/95

# SODIUM FLUORIDE F 18  Systemic*†

VA CLASSIFICATION (Primary): DX201

Note: For a listing of dosage forms and brand names by country availability, see *Dosage Forms* section(s).

*Not commercially available in the U.S.
†Not commercially available in Canada.

## Category
Diagnostic aid, radioactive (bone disease).

## Indications

Note: Because sodium fluoride F 18 is no longer commercially available in the U.S. and is not available in Canada, the bracketed information and the use of superscript 1 in this monograph reflect the lack of labeled (approved) indications for this product.

**Accepted**
[Skeletal imaging, positron emission tomographic][1]—Sodium fluoride F 18 is used as a skeletal imaging agent to delineate areas of abnormal osteogenesis, such as those occurring with metastatic bone disease, Paget's disease, arthritic disease, osteomyelitis, and fractures. Also, it is used to assess changes in bone metabolism and to identify extraosseous sites of bone formation or calcification. It is useful in demonstrating increased blood flow and osteoblastic activity in onlay bone grafts and regions of osteosynthesis. It has been used in patients with osteogenic sarcoma to study their response to radiotherapy and for the early detection of recurrence of disease. In addition, it has been used as an adjunct to other imaging procedures (e.g., bone marrow imaging or whole body imaging with fludeoxyglucose F 18) in order to delineate the skeleton.

[1]Not included in Canadian product labeling.

## Physical Properties

**Nuclear Data**

| Radionu-clide (half-life) | Decay constant | Mode of decay | Principal photon emissions (keV) | Mean number of emissions/ disintegration |
|---|---|---|---|---|
| F 18 (110 min) | 0.0063 min$^{-1}$ | Positron decay | Gamma* (511) | 1.94 |

*The two gamma rays emitted in opposite directions at the moment of positron annihilation are used for imaging purposes.

## Pharmacology/Pharmacokinetics

**Physicochemical characteristics**
Source—Produced in an accelerator with $H_2O^{18}$ targets; may be produced in a reactor.

## Mechanism of action/Effect
The fluoride ion becomes incorporated into bone as a result of an ion exchange (with hydroxyl ions) at the surface of the hydroxyapatite crystal. The passage of the fluoride ion from the plasma through the extracellular fluid space into the hydration shell surrounding each bone crystal occurs within minutes. Blood flow and/or blood concentration are the most important factors in the delivery of the agent to sites of uptake. Fluoride F 18 is taken up in bone in proportion to blood flow and bone metabolic activity. Thus, visualization of osseous lesions is possible since skeletal uptake of fluoride F 18 is altered in areas of abnormal osteogenesis.

## Distribution
Following intravenous administration, about half of the fluoride ions are rapidly taken up by the skeleton where they remain during the time period of their radioactive decay. The remainder are distributed into the extracellular fluid and eliminated by renal excretion within a few hours. The fluoride ions normally accumulate in the skeleton in a symmetrical way, and with greater deposition in the axial skeleton and in the bones around joints than in the appendicular skeleton and in the shafts of long bones. Increased deposition occurs around fracture sites, and in bones affected by osteomyelitis, fibrous dysplasia, spondylitis tuberculosis, Paget's disease, hyperostosis frontalis interna, myositis ossificans, tumors, and in rapidly growing epiphyses.

## Time to radioactivity visualization
Imaging may begin 1 hour after administration.

## Radiation dosimetry

| Organ | Estimated absorbed radiation dose* | |
|---|---|---|
| | mGy/MBq | mrad/mCi |
| Bladder wall | 0.22 | 815 |
| Bone surfaces | 0.04 | 148 |
| Kidneys | 0.02 | 74 |
| Uterus | 0.019 | 70 |
| Large intestine (lower) | 0.013 | 48 |
| Ovaries | 0.013 | 48 |
| Testes | 0.011 | 40 |
| Adrenals | 0.010 | 37 |
| Small intestine | 0.0094 | 34 |
| Large intestine (upper) | 0.0089 | 32 |
| Spleen | 0.0074 | 27 |
| Pancreas | 0.0073 | 27 |
| Liver | 0.0069 | 25 |
| Lungs | 0.0068 | 25 |
| Thyroid | 0.0068 | 25 |
| Stomach wall | 0.0067 | 25 |
| Breast | 0.0061 | 23 |
| Other tissue | 0.0084 | 31 |

Effective dose: 0.027 mSv/MBq (0.1 rem/mCi)

*For adults; intravenous injection. Data based on the International Commission on Radiological Protection (ICRP) Publication 53—Radiation dose to patients from radiopharmaceuticals.

## Elimination
Primarily renal (approximately 20% within the first 2 hours after administration).

Note: When imaging the pelvis, spine, and the limbs, background interference may result from accumulation of the radiopharmaceutical in the bladder.

## Precautions to Consider

### Pregnancy/Reproduction
Pregnancy—Fluoride is known to readily cross the placenta.

### Breast-feeding
Trace amounts of fluoride are distributed into breast milk. Temporary discontinuation of nursing may need to be considered.

### Pediatrics
Although sodium fluoride F 18 is used in children, there have been no specific studies evaluating safety and efficacy in children.

### Geriatrics
Diagnostic studies performed to date have not demonstrated geriatrics-specific problems that would limit the usefulness of sodium fluoride F 18 in the elderly.

## Side/Adverse Effects
There are no known side/adverse effects associated with the use of sodium fluoride F 18.

## Patient Consultation
As an aid to patient consultation, refer to *Advice for the Patient, Radiopharmaceuticals (Diagnostic)*.

In providing consultation, consider emphasizing the following selected information (» = major clinical significance):

### Description of use
Action in the body: Concentration of radioactivity in bone allows images to be obtained

Small amounts of radioactivity used in diagnosis; radiation received is low and considered safe

### Before having this test
» Conditions affecting use, especially:
Breast-feeding—Fluoride is distributed into breast milk; temporary discontinuation of nursing may be recommended

### Preparation for this test
Special preparatory instructions may be given; patient should inquire in advance

Increasing intake of fluids and voiding before test begins for best imaging results

### Precautions after having this test
No special precautions

## General Dosing Information
Radiopharmaceuticals are to be administered only by or under the supervision of physicians who have had extensive training in the safe use and handling of radioactive materials and who are authorized by the appropriate federal or state regulatory agency, if required, or, outside the U.S., the appropriate authority.

The patient should increase intake of fluids following the administration of sodium fluoride F 18 injection and void prior to imaging procedures to optimize image quality.

### Safety considerations for handling this radiopharmaceutical
Guidelines for the receipt, storage, handling, dispensing, and disposal of radioactive materials are available from scientific, professional, state, federal, and international bodies. Handling of this radiopharmaceutical should be limited to those individuals who are appropriately qualified and authorized.

## Parenteral Dosage Forms

### SODIUM FLUORIDE F 18 INJECTION USP

#### Usual adult and adolescent administered activity
Skeletal imaging—
Intravenous, 370 megabecquerels (10 millicuries).

#### Usual pediatric administered activity
Skeletal imaging—
Dosage must be individualized by physician.

#### Usual geriatric administered activity
Skeletal imaging—
See *Usual adult and adolescent administered activity*.

#### Strength(s) usually available
U.S.—
Prepared on-site at various clinical facilities and at centralized nuclear pharmacies.
Canada—
Not commercially available.

#### Packaging and storage
For immediate use.

#### Note
Caution—Radioactive material.

Developed: 08/20/98

# SODIUM IODIDE  Systemic†

VA CLASSIFICATION (Primary/Secondary): TN499/HS852
Commonly used brand name(s): *Iodopen*.
Note: For a listing of dosage forms and brand names by country availability, see *Dosage Forms* section(s).

†Not commercially available in Canada.

## Category
Nutritional supplement (mineral); antihyperthyroid agent.

## Indications
Note: Bracketed information in the *Indications* section refers to uses that are not included in U.S. product labeling.

### Accepted
Iodine deficiency (prophylaxis and treatment)—Sodium iodide is indicated in the prevention and treatment of iodine deficiency, which may result from inadequate nutrition or intestinal malabsorption, but does not occur in healthy individuals receiving an adequate balanced diet. For prophylaxis of iodine deficiency, dietary improvement, rather than supplementation, is advisable. For treatment of iodine deficiency, supplementation is preferred. Due to the introduction of iodized salt, iodine deficiency in the U.S. is rare; however, it continues to be a problem worldwide.

Deficiency of iodine may lead to thyroid dysfunction, goiter, mental deficiency, hearing loss, and cretinism.

Some diets (e.g., reducing diets that drastically restrict food selection) may not supply minimum daily requirements of iodine. Supplementation may be necessary in patients receiving long-term total parenteral nutrition (TPN) or undergoing rapid weight loss or in those with malnutrition, because of inadequate dietary intake.

Recommended intakes for all vitamins and most minerals are increased during pregnancy. Many physicians recommend that pregnant women receive multivitamin and mineral supplements, especially those pregnant women who do not consume an adequate diet and those in high-risk categories (i.e., women carrying more than one fetus, heavy cigarette smokers, and alcohol and drug abusers). However, taking excessive amounts of multivitamin and mineral supplements may be harmful to the mother and/or fetus and should be avoided.

Maternal iodine deficiency before or during early pregnancy may lead to neurological damage and fetal hypothyroidism or cretinism in later pregnancy.

Recommended intakes for all vitamins and most minerals are increased during breast-feeding.

[Thyrotoxicosis crisis (treatment adjunct)]—Intravenous sodium iodide may be used as a treatment adjunct for thyrotoxicosis crisis.

## Pharmacology/Pharmacokinetics

### Physicochemical characteristics
Molecular weight—Elemental iodine: 126.9.
Sodium iodide: 149.89.

### Mechanism of action/Effect
Antihyperthyroid agent—In thyrotoxicosis crisis, sodium iodide produces rapid remission of symptoms by inhibiting the release of thyroid hormone into the circulation.

Nutritional supplement—Sodium iodide is oxidized to iodine, which is an essential component of the thyroid hormones, triiodothyronine ($T_3$) and thyroxin ($T_4$). These hormones are among the factors that regulate energy transformation, growth, reproduction, neuromuscular function, and cellular metabolism.

### Absorption
Oral iodine is rapidly and completely absorbed from the gastrointestinal tract. It is also absorbed from the skin and lungs. Iodine is recycled from inactive iodothyronines.

### Protein binding
Totally protein bound.

### Storage
Iodine is stored primarily in the thyroid gland and muscle, but also in the skin, skeleton, mammary glands, and hair.

### Elimination
Iodine is eliminated via the kidneys, liver, skin, lungs, and intestine.

## Precautions to Consider

### Pregnancy/Reproduction
Pregnancy—Problems in humans have not been documented with intake of normal daily recommended amounts. Sodium iodide crosses the placenta; use of high doses during pregnancy may result in abnormal thyroid function and/or goiter in the infant.

### Breast-feeding
Problems in humans have not been documented with intake of normal daily recommended amounts. Sodium iodide is distributed into breast milk; excessive iodide use by nursing mothers may cause skin rash and thyroid suppression in the infant.

### Pediatrics
Problems in pediatrics have not been documented with intake of normal daily recommended amounts. Iodides may cause skin rash and thyroid suppression in infants.

### Geriatrics
Problems in geriatrics have not been documented with intake of normal daily recommended amounts.

### Dental
Oral and intravenous iodine may cause salivary gland swelling or tenderness, burning of mouth or throat, metallic taste, soreness of teeth and gums, and unusual increase in salivation.

### Drug interactions and/or related problems
The following drug interactions and/or related problems have been selected on the basis of their potential clinical significance (possible mechanism in parentheses where appropriate)—not necessarily inclusive (» = major clinical significance):

Note: Combinations containing any of the following, depending on the amount present, may also interact with sodium iodide supplements.

» Antithyroid agents
(antithyroid agents block the oxidation of iodide to iodine in the thyroid gland)

Iodine-containing compounds used for cleansing or
» Iodine-containing preparations, other
(concurrent use with other iodine products may increase serum iodine concentrations; iodine-containing cleansers are more likely to cause a problem in infants)

» Lithium
(concurrent use with sodium iodide may potentiate the hypothyroid and goitrogenic effects of either medication; baseline thyroid status should be determined at periodic intervals to detect changes in the thyroid-pituitary response)

Sodium iodide I 131, therapeutic
(sodium iodide may decrease thyroid uptake of I 131)

### Laboratory value alterations
The following have been selected on the basis of their potential clinical significance (possible effect in parentheses where appropriate)—not necessarily inclusive (» = major clinical significance):

With diagnostic test results
Thyroid function studies and
Thyroid imaging, radionuclide, and
Thyroid uptake tests
(sodium iodide may decrease thyroidal uptake of I 131, I 123, and sodium pertechnetate Tc 99m)

### Medical considerations/Contraindications
The medical considerations/Contraindications included have been selected on the basis of their potential clinical significance (reasons given in parentheses where appropriate)—not necessarily inclusive (» = major clinical significance).

*Risk-benefit should be considered when the following medical problems exist:*

Hyperthyroidism
(prolonged use of iodine may cause thyroid gland hyperplasia, thyroid adenoma, goiter, or hypothyroidism)

Renal function impairment
(may cause excessive serum iodine concentrations)

Sensitivity to iodine or sodium iodide

Tuberculosis
(use may cause irritation and increase secretions)

## Patient monitoring

The following may be especially important in patient monitoring (other tests may be warranted in some patients, depending on condition; » = major clinical significance):

Thyroid function
(periodic monitoring is recommended as a guideline for adjusting dosage)

## Side/Adverse Effects

The following side/adverse effects have been selected on the basis of their potential clinical significance (possible signs and symptoms in parentheses where appropriate)—not necessarily inclusive:

**Those indicating need for medical attention**
Incidence less frequent
*Allergic reaction, specifically angioedemia* (swelling of the arms, face, legs, lips, tongue, and/or throat); *arthralgia* (joint pain); *eosinophilia; swelling of lymph nodes*

With prolonged use
*Iodism* (burning of mouth or throat; gastric irritation; increased watering of mouth; metallic taste; severe headache; skin lesions; soreness of teeth and gums)

## Patient Consultation

As an aid to patient consultation, refer to *Advice for the Patient, Sodium Iodide (Systemic)*.
In providing consultation, consider emphasizing the following selected information (»= major clinical significance):

**Description of use**
*For use as a nutritional supplement*
Description should include function in the body, signs of deficiency, conditions that may cause iodine deficiency

**Importance of diet**
*For use as a nutritional supplement*
Importance of proper nutrition; supplement may be needed because of inadequate dietary intake
Food sources of iodine
Recommended daily intake for iodine

**Before using this medication**
» Conditions affecting use, especially:
Sensitivity to iodine or sodium iodide
Pregnancy—High doses may cause thyroid problems or goiter in the newborn infant
Breast-feeding—High doses may cause skin rash and thyroid problems in nursing babies
Use in children—High doses may cause skin rash and thyroid problems in infants
Dental—May cause swelling of salivary glands, burning of mouth or throat, metallic taste, soreness of teeth and gums, or increase in salivation
Other medications, especially antithyroid agents, lithium, or other iodine-containing medications
Other medical problems, especially renal function impairment, thyroid disease, or tuberculosis

**Proper use of this medication**
*For use as a nutritional supplement*
» Proper dosing
Missed dose: No cause for concern because of length of time necessary for depletion; remembering to take as directed
» Proper storage

**Precautions while using this medication**
*For use as a nutritional supplement*
Other products contain iodine; making sure not to get too much, especially for infants and small children

**Side/adverse effects**
» Signs of potential side effects, especially allergic reactions or iodism

## General Dosing Information

**For use as a nutritional supplement**
Because of the infrequency of iodine deficiency alone, combinations of several vitamins and/or minerals are commonly administered. In the oral form, iodine is available only as a vitamin/mineral complex.

**For parenteral dosage forms only**
For use as a nutritional supplement:
In most cases, parenteral administration is indicated only when oral administration is not acceptable (for example, in nausea, vomiting, and preoperative and postoperative conditions) or possible (for example, in malabsorption syndromes or following gastric resection).

**Diet/Nutrition**
Recommended dietary intakes for iodine are defined differently worldwide.
For U.S—
The Recommended Dietary Allowances (RDAs) for vitamins and minerals are determined by the Food and Nutrition Board of the National Research Council and are intended to provide adequate nutrition in most healthy persons under usual environmental stresses. In addition, a different designation may be used by the FDA for food and dietary supplement labeling purposes, as with Daily Value (DV). DVs replace the previous labeling terminology United States Recommended Daily Allowances (USRDAs).
For Canada—
Recommended Nutrient Intakes (RNIs) for vitamins, minerals, and protein are determined by Health and Welfare Canada and provide recommended amounts of a specific nutrient while minimizing the risk of chronic diseases.
Daily recommended intakes for iodine are generally defined as follows:

| Persons | U.S. (mcg) | Canada (mcg) |
| --- | --- | --- |
| Infants and children | | |
| Birth to 3 years of age | 40–70 | 30–65 |
| 4 to 6 years of age | 90 | 85 |
| 7 to 10 years of age | 120 | 95–125 |
| Adolescent and adult males | 150 | 125–160 |
| Adolescent and adult females | 150 | 110–160 |
| Pregnant females | 175 | 135–185 |
| Breast-feeding females | 200 | 160–210 |

These are usually provided by adequate diets.
The best sources of iodine include seafood, iodized salt (in moderation), and vegetables grown in iodine-rich soils. Iodine-containing mist from the ocean is also an important source. Iodized salt provides 76 mcg of iodine per gram of salt.

## Parenteral Dosage Forms

### SODIUM IODIDE INJECTION

**Usual adult dose**
Deficiency (prophylaxis or treatment)—
Intravenous infusion, 1 to 2 mcg elemental iodide per kg of body weight a day added to total parenteral nutrition (TPN).
Note: For pregnant and lactating women, the recommended dosage is 2 to 3 mcg elemental iodide per kg of body weight a day added to TPN.
[Hyperthyroidism]—
Intravenous infusion, 0.5 to 1 gram every 12 hours until stable, the first dose being given at least one hour after the initial dose of antithyroid agent.

**Usual pediatric dose**
Deficiency (prophylaxis or treatment)—
Intravenous infusion, 2 to 3 mcg elemental iodide per kg of body weight a day added to TPN.

**Strength(s) usually available**
U.S.—
100 mcg elemental iodide (118 mcg sodium iodide) per mL (Rx) [*Iodopen;* GENERIC].
Canada—
Not commercially available.

**Packaging and storage**
Store below 40 °C (104 °F), preferably between 15 and 30 °C (59 and 86 °F), unless otherwise specified by manufacturer.

**Preparation of dosage form**
The manufacturer states that sodium iodide can be added to total parenteral nutrition (TPN) solutions, and is physically compatible with amino acid solutions, dextrose solutions, electrolytes, and other trace elements.

Revised: 02/26/92
Interim revision: 08/19/94; 06/19/95

# SODIUM IODIDE I 123 Systemic

VA CLASSIFICATION (Primary): DX201

Note: For a listing of dosage forms and brand names by country availability, see *Dosage Forms* section(s).

## Category
Diagnostic aid, radioactive (thyroid disorders).

## Indications

### Accepted
Thyroid function studies or

Thyroid uptake tests—Sodium iodide I 123 is indicated in thyroid uptake tests, in which thyroid function is evaluated by determining the fraction of administered radioiodine activity taken up by the thyroid gland. The thyroid uptake test is used in the diagnosis and confirmation of suspected hyperthyroidism and in calculating the activity to be administered for radioactive iodine therapy.

Thyroid imaging, radionuclide—Sodium iodide I 123 is indicated in thyroid imaging for the evaluation of thyroid function and size; thyroid nodules; carcinoma; and masses in the lingual region, neck, and mediastinum.

Sodium iodide I 123 is generally preferable to sodium iodide I 131 because of its lower patient radiation doses and better imaging properties. It also may be the radiopharmaceutical of choice in children who require diagnosis of thyroid function and imaging of the thyroid.

## Physical Properties

### Nuclear data

| Radionuclide (half-life*) | Decay constant | Mode of decay | Principal photon emissions (keV) | Mean number of emissions/ disintegration |
|---|---|---|---|---|
| I 123 (13.2 hr) | 0.0533 h$^{-1}$ | Electron capture | Gamma (159) | 0.83 |

*In the euthyroid patient, 5 to 30% of the administered sodium iodide I 123 is concentrated in the thyroid gland at 24 hours and has an effective half-life of 13 hours. The remaining administered activity is distributed within the extracellular fluid and has an effective half-life of 8 hours.

## Pharmacology/Pharmacokinetics

### Mechanism of action/Effect
The action of radioiodide is based on one of the normal functions of the thyroid gland, which is the accumulation and retention of iodine as required in the synthesis of thyroid hormones. Thyroid retention of radioiodide permits quantification of organ uptake and imaging of anatomical distribution in thyroid tissue. Sodium iodide I 123 is also concentrated in functioning papillary, follicular, or mixed papillary/follicular thyroid cancer and metastases, although to a lesser extent than in normal thyroid tissue.

### Absorption
Readily absorbed from upper gastrointestinal tract.

### Distribution
Selectively concentrated and bound to tyrosyl residues of thyroglobulin in the thyroid gland; also concentrated, but not bound, in the choroid plexus, gastric mucosa, salivary glands, nasal mucosa, stomach, and lactating breast tissue, with the remainder being distributed within the extracellular fluid.

### Half-life
Biological (for thyroid compartment)—
  Euthyroid: 80 days.
  Hyperthyroid: 5 to 40 days.

### Time to radioactivity visualization
4 to 24 hours.

### Radiation dosimetry
See *Table 1*, page 2601.

### Elimination
Renal—Primary, 50 to 75% of administered activity eliminated in the urine of euthyroid patients with normal renal function within 48 hours.
Fecal and salivary—Secondary (less than 2% of administered activity).

## Precautions to Consider

### Carcinogenicity/Mutagenicity
No long-term animal studies have been performed to evaluate carcinogenic or mutagenic potential of sodium iodide I 123.

### Pregnancy/Reproduction
Pregnancy—Well-controlled studies have not been done in humans. However, investigational studies performed in retrospect have not shown sodium iodide I 123 to cause adverse effects in the fetus.

The possibility of pregnancy should be assessed in women of child-bearing potential. Clinical situations exist where the benefit to the patient and fetus, based on information derived from radiopharmaceutical use, outweighs the risks from fetal exposure to radiation. In these situations, the physician should use discretion and reduce the radiopharmaceutical dose to the lowest possible amount.

Studies have not been done in animals.

FDA Pregnancy Category C.

### Breast-feeding
Iodide I 123 is distributed into breast milk and may reach concentrations equal to or greater than concentrations in maternal plasma. It has been recommended that breast-feeding may be resumed when the radiation dose to the infant's thyroid does not exceed 150 mrad. A method to calculate the radiation dose to the infant's thyroid has been proposed based on the effective half-life of the radionuclide, the activity administered to the mother, the fraction of administered activity ingested by the infant, and the radiation dose to the infant's thyroid per unit of activity ingested. It has been estimated that the time required before nursing may be resumed after administration of 1.11 megabecquerels (30 microcuries) of sodium iodide I 123 is 16 days for a product contaminated with 4.9% of I 124 and 91 days for a product contaminated with 1.9% of I 125. Because of the difficulty of maintaining the maternal milk supply for such an extended period of time, complete cessation of nursing is usually recommended.

### Pediatrics
Although sodium iodide I 123 is used in children, there have been no specific studies evaluating its safety and efficacy in pediatric patients.

### Geriatrics
Although appropriate studies on the relationship of age to the effects of sodium iodide I 123 have not been performed in the geriatric population, no geriatrics-specific problems have been documented to date.

### Drug interactions and/or related problems
See *Diagnostic interference*.

### Diagnostic interference
The following have been selected on the basis of their potential clinical significance (possible effect in parentheses where appropriate)—not necessarily inclusive (» = major clinical significance):

With results of *this* test
*Due to other medications*
  Amiodarone or
  Antithyroid preparations—thioamide derivatives or aromatic preparations or
  Benzodiazepines or
  Contrast media, iodinated or
  Corticosteroids or
  Goitrogenic foods (e.g., cabbage, turnips) or
  Iodine-containing foods or
  Iodine-containing preparations or
  Iodine-contaminated bromides or
  Iodine, stable or
  Monovalent anions (e.g., perchlorate, thiocyanate) or
  Pyrazolone derivatives, such as phenylbutazone or
  Salicylates or
  Salt, iodized, excessive intake of or
  Thiopental or
  Thyroid blocking agents, such as strong iodine solution, potassium iodide, or potassium perchlorate or
  Thyroid preparations, natural or synthetic
    (may decrease thyroidal uptake of iodide I 123; it is recommended that these medications be withheld for the following periods of time prior to administration of sodium iodide I 123: several months for amiodarone; 1 week for corticosteroids; 4 weeks for benzodiazepines; 2 to 4 weeks for intravascular iodinated contrast media and more than 4 weeks for cholecystographic agents; 2 to 4 weeks for iodine-containing preparations, such as vitamins, expectorants, antitussives, and topical medications; 1 to 2 weeks for pyrazolone

derivatives; 1 week for thiopental; 4 to 6 weeks for thyroxine and 2 to 3 weeks for triiodothyronine)
(a rebound effect may occur following the sudden withdrawal of antithyroid preparations, resulting in a period of up to 5 days of very high thyroidal uptake; it is recommended that antithyroid medications be discontinued 1 week prior to administration of sodium iodide I 123 ; however, for early uptake studies [i.e., 15 to 30 minutes] to determine iodide trapping [not organification] the treatment with thioamide drugs does not need to be interrupted)
(chronic salicylate administration may cause a depression of thyroid function; salicylate therapy should be discontinued at least 1 to 2 week prior to sodium iodide I 123 administration; however, a rebound effect may also occur following discontinuation of salicylate therapy, resulting in a period of 3 to 10 days of increased thyroidal uptake)

*Due to medical problems or conditions*

Iodine deficiency or
Low serum chlorides or
Nephrosis
(may increase thyroidal uptake of I 123)

Renal function impairment
(lack of normal excretion of iodine may cause an increase or decrease in the body iodide pool, resulting in false high or low uptake determinations)

**Medical considerations/Contraindications**
The medical considerations/contraindications included have been selected on the basis of their potential clinical significance (reasons given in parentheses where appropriate)—not necessarily inclusive (» = major clinical significance).
See also *Diagnostic interference*.
Sensitivity to the radiopharmaceutical preparation

## Side/Adverse Effects

The following side/adverse effects have been selected on the basis of their potential clinical significance (possible signs and symptoms in parentheses where appropriate)—not necessarily inclusive:

**Those indicating need for medical attention only if they continue or are bothersome**
Incidence rare
*Headache; nausea or vomiting; skin rash, hives, or itching*

## Patient Consultation

As an aid to patient consultation, refer to *Advice for the Patient, Radiopharmaceuticals (Diagnostic)*.
In providing consultation, consider emphasizing the following selected information (»= major clinical significance):

**Description of use**
*Action in the body*
Iodide I 123 uptake by the thyroid same as uptake of nonradioactive iodine
Localization of iodide I 123 in thyroid allows thyroid uptake quantification and visualization of thyroid tissue
Small amounts of radioactivity used in diagnosis; radiation exposure is relatively low and considered safe

**Before having this test**
» Conditions affecting use, especially:
Pregnancy—Sodium iodide I 123 crosses placenta; risk to fetus from radiation exposure as opposed to benefit derived from use should be considered
Breast-feeding—Iodide I 123 is distributed into breast milk; complete cessation of nursing recommended for this infant because of risk to infant from radiation exposure (present administration of I 123 will not affect breast-feeding of future infants)

**Preparation for this test**
Special preparatory instructions may apply; patient should inquire in advance

**Precautions after having this test**
To decrease radiation exposure to the urinary bladder: Increasing intake of fluids to promote more frequent voiding to help eliminate radioactive iodine

## General Dosing Information

Radiopharmaceuticals are to be administered only by or under the supervision of physicians who have had extensive training in the safe use and handling of radioactive materials and who are authorized by the appropriate Federal or state agency, if required, or, outside the U.S., the appropriate authority.

Uptake measurements are generally made at 4 and/or 24 hours, and thyroid imaging is usually performed 18 to 24 hours after sodium iodide I 123 administration. However, it has been demonstrated that a 4- to 5-hour interval after administration of sodium iodide I 123 may be adequate for thyroid imaging, especially in hyperthyroid patients with high percentage uptakes.

Since sodium iodide I 123 may contain small amounts of longer-lived isotopes of iodine (e.g., I 124, I 125), it should be used as soon as possible on the day of calibration. The use of this radiopharmaceutical beyond the day of calibration results in an increased ratio of these isotopes to I 123 and, therefore, in unnecessary patient radiation from the relatively greater quantities of these contaminants.

**Safety considerations for handling this radiopharmaceutical**
Improper handling of this radiopharmaceutical may cause radioactive contamination. Guidelines for handling radioactive material have been prepared by scientific, professional, state, federal, and international bodies and are available to the specially qualified and authorized users who have access to radiopharmaceuticals.

## Oral Dosage Forms

### SODIUM IODIDE I 123 CAPSULES USP

**Usual adult and adolescent administered activity**
Diagnostic aid—
Oral, 3.7 to 14.8 megabecquerels (100 to 400 microcuries).
Note: For uptake studies only, dosages in the lower end of the range (e.g., 3.7 megabecquerels) are recommended.
For thyroid imaging, higher dosages (e.g., 14.8 megabecquerels) are generally used.

**Usual pediatric administered activity**
Diagnostic aid—
Dosage must be individualized by physician. A minimum dosage of 0.37 megabecquerels (10 microcuries) is required for uptake studies and 1.85 megabecquerels (50 microcuries) for thyroid imaging.
Note: The available strength of the capsule does not conform to the recommended pediatric dosages. For this reason, in actual practice, the administered activity is usually 3.7 megabecquerels (100 microcuries). If smaller dosage is required, the capsule must be dissolved and an aliquot taken.

**Usual geriatric administered activity**
See *Usual adult and adolescent administered activity*.

**Strength(s) usually available**
U.S.—
3.7 megabecquerels (100 microcuries) of I 123 at time of calibration (Rx) [GENERIC].
7.4 megabecquerels (200 microcuries) of I 123 at time of calibration (Rx) [GENERIC].
Canada—
Not commercially available.

**Packaging and storage**
Store below 40 °C (104 °F), preferably between 15 and 30 °C (59 and 86 °F), unless otherwise specified by manufacturer. Store in a well-closed container.

**Stability**
Capsules should be administered within 24 hours after calibration, unless otherwise stated by manufacturer. Sodium iodide I 123 preparations may contain small amounts of longer-lived isotopes of iodine (e.g., I 124, I 125). The use of this radiopharmaceutical beyond the day of calibration results in an increased ratio of these isotopes to I 123 and, therefore, in unnecessary patient radiation from the relatively greater quantities of these contaminants.

**Note**
Caution—Radioactive material.

### SODIUM IODIDE I 123 SOLUTION USP

**Usual adult and adolescent administered activity**
Diagnostic aid—
See *Sodium Iodide I 123 Capsules USP*.

**Usual pediatric administered activity**
Diagnostic aid—
See *Sodium Iodide I 123 Capsules USP*.

**Usual geriatric administered activity**
See *Usual adult and adolescent administered activity*.

**Strength(s) usually available**
U.S.—
Not commercially available.

Canada—
Content information not available at present (Rx) [GENERIC].

**Packaging and storage**
Store below 40 °C (104 °F), preferably between 15 and 30 °C (59 and 86 °F), unless otherwise specified by manufacturer.

**Stability**
Solution should be used within 24 hours after calibration, unless otherwise stated by manufacturer. Sodium iodide I 123 preparations may contain small amounts of longer-lived isotopes of iodine (e.g., I 124, I 125). The use of this radiopharmaceutical beyond the day of calibration results in an increased ratio of these isotopes to I 123 and, therefore, in unnecessary patient radiation from the relatively greater quantities of these contaminants.

**Note**
Caution—Radioactive material.

**Additional information**
Radioiodide stock solutions and any dilutions thereof must be maintained at a pH of 7.5 to 9.0 in order to minimize oxidation of iodide to volatile forms of iodine. Additionally, 0.2% sodium thiosulfate may be incorporated into these solutions if an antioxidant is desired.

## Selected Bibliography

Braverman LE, Utiger RD, editors. Werner and Ingbar's the thyroid: a fundamental and clinical text. 6th ed. Philadelphia: J.B. Lippincott Company, 1991: 437-45.

Ryo UY, Vaidya PV, Schneider AB, et al. Thyroid imaging agents: a comparison of I 123 and Tc 99m pertechnetate. Radiology 1983; 148: 819-22.

Revised: 08/25/94

## Table 1. Radiation dosimetry

| Organ | Maximum thyroid uptake (%) | I 123 mGy/MBq | I 123 rad/mCi | I 124‡ mGy/MBq | I 124‡ rad/mCi | I 125‡ MGy/MGq | I 125‡ rad/mCi |
|---|---|---|---|---|---|---|---|
| Bladder wall | 0 | 0.090 | 0.33 | 0.78 | 2.9 | 0.1 | 0.37 |
| | 5 | 0.085 | 0.31 | 0.74 | 2.7 | 0.095 | 0.35 |
| | 15 | 0.076 | 0.28 | 0.67 | 2.5 | 0.085 | 0.31 |
| | 25 | 0.069 | 0.26 | 0.6 | 2.2 | 0.076 | 0.28 |
| | 55 | 0.043 | 0.16 | 0.38 | 1.4 | 0.047 | 0.17 |
| Uterus | 0 | 0.014 | 0.052 | 0.11 | 0.41 | 0.0095 | 0.035 |
| | 5 | 0.016 | 0.059 | 0.12 | 0.44 | 0.0093 | 0.034 |
| | 15 | 0.015 | 0.056 | 0.11 | 0.41 | 0.0092 | 0.034 |
| | 25 | 0.014 | 0.052 | 0.11 | 0.41 | 0.0088 | 0.033 |
| | 55 | 0.012 | 0.044 | 0.097 | 0.36 | 0.0075 | 0.028 |
| Kidneys | 0 | 0.011 | 0.041 | 0.1 | 0.37 | 0.01 | 0.037 |
| | 5 | 0.012 | 0.044 | 0.1 | 0.37 | 0.0092 | 0.034 |
| | 15 | 0.010 | 0.037 | 0.094 | 0.35 | 0.0086 | 0.032 |
| | 25 | 0.011 | 0.041 | 0.097 | 0.36 | 0.0081 | 0.03 |
| | 55 | 0.0091 | 0.034 | 0.075 | 0.28 | 0.0064 | 0.024 |
| Ovaries | 0 | 0.0098 | 0.036 | 0.079 | 0.29 | 0.0064 | 0.024 |
| | 5 | 0.012 | 0.044 | 0.091 | 0.34 | 0.007 | 0.026 |
| | 15 | 0.012 | 0.044 | 0.089 | 0.33 | 0.0069 | 0.026 |
| | 25 | 0.011 | 0.041 | 0.088 | 0.33 | 0.0069 | 0.026 |
| | 55 | 0.011 | 0.041 | 0.084 | 0.31 | 0.0066 | 0.024 |
| Large intestine wall (lower) | 0 | 0.0097 | 0.036 | 0.087 | 0.32 | 0.0067 | 0.025 |
| | 5 | 0.011 | 0.041 | 0.093 | 0.34 | 0.0076 | 0.028 |
| | 15 | 0.011 | 0.041 | 0.092 | 0.34 | 0.0075 | 0.028 |
| | 25 | 0.011 | 0.041 | 0.090 | 0.33 | 0.0074 | 0.027 |
| | 55 | 0.0098 | 0.036 | 0.084 | 0.31 | 0.007 | 0.026 |
| Red marrow | 0 | 0.0094 | 0.035 | 0.059 | 0.21 | 0.0083 | 0.031 |
| | 5 | 0.0092 | 0.034 | 0.065 | 0.24 | 0.01 | 0.037 |
| | 15 | 0.0093 | 0.034 | 0.086 | 0.32 | 0.017 | 0.063 |
| | 25 | 0.0098 | 0.036 | 0.11 | 0.41 | 0.023 | 0.085 |
| | 55 | 0.011 | 0.041 | 0.17 | 0.63 | 0.043 | 0.16 |
| Small intestine | 0 | 0.0085 | 0.031 | 0.071 | 0.26 | 0.0058 | 0.021 |
| | 5 | 0.043 | 0.16 | 0.37 | 1.37 | 0.042 | 0.16 |
| | 15 | 0.043 | 0.16 | 0.37 | 1.37 | 0.042 | 0.16 |
| | 25 | 0.043 | 0.16 | 0.37 | 1.37 | 0.042 | 0.16 |
| | 55 | 0.042 | 0.16 | 0.37 | 1.37 | 0.042 | 0.16 |
| Bone surfaces | 0 | 0.0097 | 0.036 | 0.053 | 0.2 | 0.0074 | 0.027 |
| | 5 | 0.0068 | 0.025 | 0.053 | 0.2 | 0.0092 | 0.034 |
| | 15 | 0.0071 | 0.026 | 0.072 | 0.27 | 0.016 | 0.06 |
| | 25 | 0.0075 | 0.028 | 0.092 | 0.34 | 0.024 | 0.089 |
| | 55 | 0.0086 | 0.032 | 0.15 | 0.56 | 0.045 | 0.17 |

*Data based on the International Commission on Radiological Protection (ICRP) Publication 53—Radiation Dose to Patients from Radiopharmaceuticals.

†Estimates based on intravenous administration. With oral administration there is a radiation dose to the stomach in addition to that due to iodide in gastric and salivary secretions. Assuming a mean residence time in the stomach of one-half hour, the absorbed dose to the stomach wall is increased by approximately 40% for I 123 with oral administration, while the dose to organs and tissues other than the stomach wall is decreased by 3% for I 123.

‡Levels of I 124 and I 125 contamination in sodium iodide I 123 preparations vary with the manufacturing source/production method. The ratio of the concentration of I 123, I 124, and I 125 changes with time.

§With thyroid blocking, thyroid uptakes ranging from 0.5% to 2.0% will still occur. Under these circumstances the effective dose to the adult will range from 0.016 to 0.025 mSv/MBq (0.059 to 0.092 rem/mCi) for I 123.

#The effective dose is virtually identical after oral or intravenous administration.

## Table 1. Radiation dosimetry (continued)

| Organ | Maximum thyroid uptake (%) | Estimated absorbed radiation dose*† |||||| 
|---|---|---|---|---|---|---|---|
| | | I 123 || I 124‡ || I 125‡ ||
| | | mGy/MBq | rad/mCi | mGy/MBq | rad/mCi | MGy/MGq | rad/mCi |
| Large intestine wall (upper) | 0 | 0.0080 | 0.030 | 0.068 | 0.25 | 0.0058 | 0.021 |
| | 5 | 0.019 | 0.070 | 0.13 | 0.48 | 0.016 | 0.06 |
| | 15 | 0.018 | 0.067 | 0.13 | 0.48 | 0.016 | 0.06 |
| | 25 | 0.018 | 0.067 | 0.13 | 0.48 | 0.016 | 0.06 |
| | 55 | 0.018 | 0.067 | 0.13 | 0.48 | 0.016 | 0.06 |
| Pancreas | 0 | 0.0076 | 0.028 | 0.061 | 0.23 | 0.0056 | 0.021 |
| | 5 | 0.014 | 0.052 | 0.11 | 0.41 | 0.0092 | 0.034 |
| | 15 | 0.014 | 0.052 | 0.11 | 0.41 | 0.0092 | 0.034 |
| | 25 | 0.014 | 0.052 | 0.12 | 0.44 | 0.0092 | 0.034 |
| | 55 | 0.014 | 0.052 | 0.13 | 0.48 | 0.0092 | 0.034 |
| Spleen | 0 | 0.0070 | 0.026 | 0.058 | 0.21 | 0.0056 | 0.021 |
| | 5 | 0.0096 | 0.036 | 0.079 | 0.29 | 0.0058 | 0.021 |
| | 15 | 0.0095 | 0.035 | 0.083 | 0.31 | 0.0058 | 0.021 |
| | 25 | 0.0096 | 0.036 | 0.087 | 0.32 | 0.0059 | 0.022 |
| | 55 | 0.0097 | 0.036 | 0.098 | 0.36 | 0.0058 | 0.021 |
| Adrenals | 0 | 0.0070 | 0.026 | 0.072 | 0.27 | 0.0048 | 0.018 |
| | 5 | 0.0064 | 0.024 | 0.066 | 0.24 | 0.0036 | 0.013 |
| | 15 | 0.0063 | 0.023 | 0.072 | 0.27 | 0.0036 | 0.013 |
| | 25 | 0.0064 | 0.024 | 0.078 | 0.29 | 0.0036 | 0.013 |
| | 55 | 0.0065 | 0.024 | 0.093 | 0.34 | 0.0036 | 0.013 |
| Testes | 0 | 0.0069 | 0.026 | 0.074 | 0.27 | 0.0053 | 0.02 |
| | 5 | 0.0055 | 0.020 | 0.058 | 0.21 | 0.0037 | 0.014 |
| | 15 | 0.0053 | 0.020 | 0.057 | 0.21 | 0.0036 | 0.013 |
| | 25 | 0.0052 | 0.019 | 0.056 | 0.21 | 0.0036 | 0.013 |
| | 55 | 0.0046 | 0.017 | 0.051 | 0.19 | 0.0034 | 0.013 |
| Stomach wall | 0 | 0.0069 | 0.026 | 0.057 | 0.21 | 0.0053 | 0.02 |
| | 5 | 0.068 | 0.25 | 0.58 | 2.15 | 0.071 | 0.26 |
| | 15 | 0.068 | 0.25 | 0.58 | 2.15 | 0.071 | 0.26 |
| | 25 | 0.068 | 0.25 | 0.58 | 2.15 | 0.071 | 0.26 |
| | 55 | 0.068 | 0.25 | 0.6 | 2.2 | 0.071 | 0.26 |
| Liver | 0 | 0.0067 | 0.025 | 0.058 | 0.21 | 0.0054 | 0.02 |
| | 5 | 0.0062 | 0.023 | 0.056 | 0.21 | 0.0042 | 0.016 |
| | 15 | 0.0062 | 0.023 | 0.061 | 0.23 | 0.0042 | 0.016 |
| | 25 | 0.0063 | 0.023 | 0.066 | 0.24 | 0.0042 | 0.016 |
| | 55 | 0.0064 | 0.024 | 0.081 | 0.3 | 0.0042 | 0.016 |
| Lungs | 0 | 0.0061 | 0.023 | 0.051 | 0.19 | 0.0055 | 0.02 |
| | 5 | 0.0054 | 0.020 | 0.057 | 0.21 | 0.0057 | 0.021 |
| | 15 | 0.0057 | 0.021 | 0.086 | 0.32 | 0.0087 | 0.032 |
| | 25 | 0.0061 | 0.023 | 0.11 | 0.41 | 0.012 | 0.044 |
| | 55 | 0.0072 | 0.027 | 0.2 | 0.74 | 0.021 | 0.078 |
| Breast | 0 | 0.0056 | 0.021 | 0.052 | 0.19 | 0.0051 | 0.019 |
| | 5 | 0.0046 | 0.017 | 0.052 | 0.19 | 0.004 | 0.015 |
| | 15 | 0.0047 | 0.017 | 0.073 | 0.27 | 0.0046 | 0.017 |
| | 25 | 0.0050 | 0.019 | 0.093 | 0.34 | 0.0053 | 0.02 |
| | 55 | 0.0056 | 0.021 | 0.15 | 0.56 | 0.0073 | 0.027 |
| Thyroid | 0 | 0.0051 | 0.019 | 0.05 | 0.19 | 0.0047 | 0.017 |
| | 5 | 0.63 | 2.33 | 42.0 | 155.56 | 47.0 | 174.07 |
| | 15 | 1.9 | 7.03 | 130.0 | 481.48 | 140.0 | 518.52 |
| | 25 | 3.2 | 11.84 | 210.0 | 777.78 | 240.0 | 888.89 |
| | 55 | 7.0 | 25.9 | 470.0 | 1740.74 | 520.0 | 1925.93 |
| Other tissue | 0 | 0.0064 | 0.024 | 0.056 | 0.21 | 0.0052 | 0.019 |
| | 5 | 0.0063 | 0.023 | 0.069 | 0.25 | 0.021 | 0.078 |
| | 15 | 0.0068 | 0.025 | 0.11 | 0.41 | 0.053 | 0.2 |
| | 25 | 0.0074 | 0.027 | 0.14 | 0.52 | 0.086 | 0.32 |
| | 55 | 0.0092 | 0.034 | 0.25 | 0.93 | 0.18 | 0.67 |

|  | Effective dose# | | | | | | | | | | | | | | |
|---|---|---|---|---|---|---|---|---|---|---|---|---|---|---|---|
|  | I 123 Maximum thyroid uptake (%)§ | | | | | I 124 Maximum thyroid uptake (%) | | | | | I 125 Maximum thyroid uptake (%) | | | | |
|  | 0 | 5 | 15 | 25 | 55 | 0 | 5 | 15 | 25 | 55 | 0 | 5 | 15 | 25 | 55 |
| mSv/MBq | 0.013 | 0.038 | 0.075 | 0.11 | 0.23 | 0.11 | 1.4 | 4.0 | 6.5 | 14 | 0.012 | 1.4 | 4.3 | 7.1 | 16 |
| rem/mCi | 0.048 | 0.14 | 0.28 | 0.41 | 0.85 | 0.41 | 5.18 | 14.8 | 24.05 | 51.8 | 0.044 | 5.18 | 15.91 | 26.27 | 59.2 |

*Data based on the International Commission on Radiological Protection (ICRP) Publication 53—Radiation Dose to Patients from Radiopharmaceuticals.

†Estimates based on intravenous administration. With oral administration there is a radiation dose to the stomach in addition to that due to iodide in gastric and salivary secretions. Assuming a mean residence time in the stomach of one-half hour, the absorbed dose to the stomach wall is increased by approximately 40% for I 123 with oral administration, while the dose to organs and tissues other than the stomach wall is decreased by 3% for I 123.

‡Levels of I 124 and I 125 contamination in sodium iodide I 123 preparations vary with the manufacturing source/production method. The ratio of the concentration of I 123, I 124, and I 125 changes with time.

§With thyroid blocking, thyroid uptakes ranging from 0.5% to 2.0% will still occur. Under these circumstances the effective dose to the adult will range from 0.016 to 0.025 mSv/MBq (0.059 to 0.092 rem/mCi) for I 123.

#The effective dose is virtually identical after oral or intravenous administration.

# SODIUM IODIDE I 131 Systemic—Diagnostic

VA CLASSIFICATION (Primary): DX201

Note: For a listing of dosage forms and brand names by country availability, see *Dosage Forms* section(s).

## Category

Diagnostic aid, radioactive (thyroid disorders).

## Indications

### Accepted

Thyroid function studies or

Thyroid uptake tests—Sodium iodide I 131 is indicated in thyroid uptake tests, in which thyroid function is evaluated by determining the fraction of administered radioiodine activity taken up by the thyroid gland. The thyroid uptake test is used in the diagnosis and confirmation of suspected hyperthyroidism and in calculating the activity to be administered for radioactive iodine therapy.

Thyroid imaging, radionuclide—Sodium iodide I 131 is indicated in thyroid imaging for the evaluation of thyroid function and size; thyroid nodules; carcinoma; masses in the lingual region, neck and mediastinum; and in the localization of functioning metastatic thyroid tumor. It is useful in the pre- and post-operative evaluation of patients with thyroid carcinoma. It is also used to assess the effects of therapy on these patients.

Sodium iodide I 123 or sodium pertechnetate Tc 99m (for thyroid imaging) may be preferable to sodium iodide I 131 because of their lower patient radiation doses and better imaging properties. Sodium iodide I 123 may also be the radiopharmaceutical of choice in children who require diagnosis of thyroid function and imaging of the thyroid.

## Physical Properties

### Nuclear data

| Radionuclide (half-life*) | Decay constant | Mode of decay | Principal emissions (keV) | Mean number of emissions/ disintegration |
|---|---|---|---|---|
| I 131 (8.08 days) | 0.00358 h$^{-1}$ | Beta | Beta (191.6) | 0.90 |
|  |  |  | Gamma (364.5) | 0.81 |

*For diagnostic use: In the euthyroid patient, 5 to 30% of the administered sodium iodide I 131 is concentrated in the thyroid gland at 24 hours and has an effective half-life of approximately 7.6 days. The remainder is distributed within the extracellular fluid and has an effective half-life of approximately 0.34 day.

## Pharmacology/Pharmacokinetics

### Mechanism of action/Effect

The action of radioiodide is based on one of the normal functions of the thyroid gland, which is the accumulation and retention of iodine as required for the synthesis of thyroid hormones. Thyroid retention of sodium iodide I 131 permits quantification of organ uptake and imaging of anatomical distribution in thyroid tissue. Radioiodide is also concentrated in functioning papillary, follicular, or mixed papillary/follicular thyroid cancer and metastases, although to a lesser extent than in normal thyroid tissue.

### Absorption

Readily absorbed from gastrointestinal tract.

### Distribution

Selectively concentrated and bound to tyrosyl residues of thyroglobulin in the thyroid gland; also concentrated, but not bound, in the choroid plexus, gastric mucosa, salivary glands, nasal mucosa, and lactating breast tissue with the remainder being distributed within the extracellular fluid.

### Half-life

Biological (for thyroid compartment)—
  Euthyroid: 80 days.
  Hyperthyroid: 5 to 40 days.

### Time to radioactivity visualization

18 to 24 hours.

Note: Imaging of functional thyroid metastases is generally performed at 24 to 96 hours to allow maximal uptake and minimal blood-pool retention.

## Radiation dosimetry

| Organ | Maximum thyroid uptake (%) | mGy/MBq | rad/mCi |
|---|---|---|---|
| Bladder wall | 0 | 0.61 | 2.26 |
|  | 5 | 0.58 | 2.15 |
|  | 15 | 0.52 | 1.93 |
|  | 25 | 0.46 | 1.70 |
|  | 55 | 0.29 | 1.07 |
| Uterus | 0 | 0.054 | 0.20 |
|  | 5 | 0.055 | 0.20 |
|  | 15 | 0.054 | 0.20 |
|  | 25 | 0.052 | 0.19 |
|  | 55 | 0.046 | 0.17 |
| Kidneys | 0 | 0.065 | 0.24 |
|  | 5 | 0.063 | 0.24 |
|  | 15 | 0.060 | 0.22 |
|  | 25 | 0.058 | 0.21 |
|  | 55 | 0.051 | 0.19 |
| Ovaries | 0 | 0.042 | 0.16 |
|  | 5 | 0.044 | 0.16 |
|  | 15 | 0.043 | 0.16 |
|  | 25 | 0.043 | 0.16 |
|  | 55 | 0.041 | 0.15 |
| Large intestine wall (lower) | 0 | 0.043 | 0.16 |
|  | 5 | 0.043 | 0.16 |
|  | 15 | 0.042 | 0.16 |
|  | 25 | 0.041 | 0.15 |
|  | 55 | 0.040 | 0.15 |
| Red marrow | 0 | 0.035 | 0.13 |
|  | 5 | 0.038 | 0.14 |
|  | 15 | 0.054 | 0.20 |
|  | 25 | 0.070 | 0.26 |
|  | 55 | 0.12 | 0.44 |
| Small intestine | 0 | 0.038 | 0.14 |
|  | 5 | 0.28 | 1.04 |
|  | 15 | 0.28 | 1.04 |
|  | 25 | 0.28 | 1.04 |
|  | 55 | 0.28 | 1.04 |
| Bone surfaces | 0 | 0.032 | 0.12 |
|  | 5 | 0.032 | 0.12 |
|  | 15 | 0.047 | 0.17 |
|  | 25 | 0.061 | 0.23 |
|  | 55 | 0.11 | 0.41 |
| Large intestine wall (upper) | 0 | 0.037 | 0.14 |
|  | 5 | 0.059 | 0.22 |
|  | 15 | 0.059 | 0.22 |
|  | 25 | 0.059 | 0.22 |
|  | 55 | 0.058 | 0.21 |
| Pancreas | 0 | 0.035 | 0.13 |
|  | 5 | 0.050 | 0.19 |
|  | 15 | 0.052 | 0.19 |
|  | 25 | 0.053 | 0.20 |
|  | 55 | 0.058 | 0.21 |
| Spleen | 0 | 0.034 | 0.13 |
|  | 5 | 0.039 | 0.14 |
|  | 15 | 0.042 | 0.16 |
|  | 25 | 0.044 | 0.16 |
|  | 55 | 0.051 | 0.19 |
| Adrenals | 0 | 0.037 | 0.14 |
|  | 5 | 0.032 | 0.12 |
|  | 15 | 0.036 | 0.13 |
|  | 25 | 0.039 | 0.14 |
|  | 55 | 0.049 | 0.18 |
| Testes | 0 | 0.037 | 0.14 |
|  | 5 | 0.029 | 0.11 |
|  | 15 | 0.028 | 0.10 |
|  | 25 | 0.027 | 0.10 |
|  | 55 | 0.026 | 0.10 |
| Stomach wall | 0 | 0.034 | 0.13 |
|  | 5 | 0.45 | 1.67 |
|  | 15 | 0.46 | 1.67 |
|  | 25 | 0.46 | 1.67 |
|  | 55 | 0.46 | 1.67 |
| Liver | 0 | 0.033 | 0.12 |
|  | 5 | 0.030 | 0.11 |
|  | 15 | 0.032 | 0.12 |
|  | 25 | 0.035 | 0.13 |
|  | 55 | 0.043 | 0.16 |
| Lungs | 0 | 0.031 | 0.11 |
|  | 5 | 0.034 | 0.13 |
|  | 15 | 0.053 | 0.20 |
|  | 25 | 0.072 | 0.27 |
|  | 55 | 0.13 | 0.48 |
| Breast | 0 | 0.033 | 0.12 |
|  | 5 | 0.031 | 0.11 |
|  | 15 | 0.043 | 0.16 |
|  | 25 | 0.055 | 0.20 |
|  | 55 | 0.091 | 0.34 |
| Thyroid | 0 | 0.029 | 0.11 |
|  | 5 | 72.00 | 266.67 |
|  | 15 | 210.00 | 777.78 |
|  | 25 | 360.00 | 1333.33 |
|  | 55 | 790.00 | 2925.93 |
| Other tissue | 0 | 0.032 | 0.12 |
|  | 5 | 0.040 | 0.15 |
|  | 15 | 0.065 | 0.24 |
|  | 25 | 0.090 | 0.33 |
|  | 55 | 0.16 | 0.59 |

Effective dose§

| | Maximum thyroid uptake (%)‡ | | | | |
|---|---|---|---|---|---|
| | 0 | 5 | 15 | 25 | 55 |
| mSv/MBq | 0.072 | 2.30 | 6.60 | 11.00 | 24.00 |
| rem/mCi | 0.27 | 8.51 | 24.42 | 40.70 | 88.80 |

*Data based on the International Commission on Radiological Protection (ICRP) Publication 53—Radiation Dose to Patients from Radiopharmaceuticals.

†Estimates based on intravenous administration. With oral administration there is a radiation dose to the stomach in addition to that due to iodide in gastric and salivary secretions. Assuming a mean residence time in the stomach is half an hour, the absorbed dose to the stomach wall is increased by approximately 30% with oral administration, while the dose to organs and tissues other than the stomach wall is decreased by less than 3%.

‡With thyroid blocking, thyroid uptakes ranging from 0.5 to 2.0% will still occur. Under these circumstances the effective dose to the adult will range from 0.30 to 0.97 mSv/MBq (1.11 to 3.59 rem/mCi).

§The effective dose is virtually identical after oral or intravenous administration.

### Elimination
Renal: Primary, 50 to 75% of the administered activity eliminated in the urine of euthyroid patients with normal renal function within 48 hours.
Fecal and salivary: Secondary (less than 2% of the administered activity).
Breast milk: Up to 20% of administered activity appears in the milk within 24 hours.

## Precautions to Consider

### Carcinogenicity
Experiments in animals with sodium iodide I 131 have demonstrated that radioiodide administration can induce thyroid adenomas and carcinomas.

### Pregnancy/Reproduction
Pregnancy—Risk-benefit must be considered since radioiodides cross the placenta and may cause severe and irreversible hypothyroidism in the neonate.

The possibility of pregnancy should be assessed in women of child-bearing potential. Clinical situations exist in which the benefit to the patient and fetus, based on information derived from radiopharmaceutical use, outweighs the risks from fetal exposure to radiation. In these situations, the physician should use discretion and reduce the radiopharmaceutical dose to the lowest possible amount.

Studies have not been done in animals.

FDA Pregnancy Category C.

**Breast-feeding**

Iodide I 131 is distributed into breast milk and may reach concentrations equal to or greater than concentrations in maternal plasma. It has been recommended that nursing can be resumed, after administration of a radiopharmaceutical, when the likelihood of the infant's ingested effective dose equivalent (EDE) is below 1 mSv (100 mrem). A method to calculate the EDE has been proposed based on the effective half-life of the radionuclide, the activity administered to the mother, the fraction of administered activity ingested by the infant, and the total body effective dose equivalent to the newborn infant per unit of activity ingested. According to this method, it has been estimated that, for sodium iodide I 131, the time to reduce the EDE to the infant to below 1 mSv (100 mrem) is approximately 10 weeks after administration of 40 megabecquerels (1.08 millicuries) (maximum administered activity) to the mother. Because of the difficulty of maintaining the maternal milk supply for such an extended period of time, complete cessation of nursing is usually recommended for large administered activities of sodium iodide I 131.

**Pediatrics**

Sodium iodide I 123 or sodium pertechnetate Tc 99m, because of its lower patient radiation dose, may be the radiopharmaceutical of choice in children and growing adolescents who require diagnosis of thyroid function and imaging of the thyroid.

**Geriatrics**

Although appropriate studies on the relationship of age to the effects of radiodiodide have not been performed in the geriatric population, no geriatrics-specific problems have been documented to date.

**Drug interactions and/or related problems**

See *Diagnostic interference*.

**Diagnostic interference**

The following have been selected on the basis of their potential clinical significance (possible effect in parentheses where appropriate)—not necessarily inclusive (» = major clinical significance):

With results of *this* test
*Due to other medications*
   Amiodarone or
   Antithyroid preparations—thioamide derivatives or aromatic preparations or
   Benzodiazepines or
   Contrast media, iodinated or
   Corticosteroids or
   Goitrogenic foods (e.g., cabbage, turnips) or
   Iodine-containing foods or
   Iodine-containing preparations or
   Iodine-contaminated bromides or
   Iodine, stable or
   Monovalent anions (e.g., perchlorate, thiocyanate) or
   Pyrazolone derivatives, such as phenylbutazone or
   Salicylates, chronic administration of or
   Salt, iodized, excessive intake of or
   Thiopental or
   Thyroid blocking agents, such as strong iodine solution, potassium iodide, or potassium perchlorate or
   Thyroid preparations, natural or synthetic
      (may decrease thyroidal uptake of iodide I 131; it is recommended that these medications be withheld for the following periods of time prior to administration of sodium iodide I 131: several months for amiodarone; 1 week for corticosteroids; 4 weeks for benzodiazepines; 2 to 4 weeks for intravascular iodinated contrast media and more than 4 weeks for cholecystographic agents; 2 to 4 weeks for iodine-containing preparations, such as vitamins, expectorants, antitussives, and topical medications; 1 to 2 weeks for pyrazolone derivatives; 1 week for thiopental; 4 to 6 weeks for thyroxine and 2 to 3 weeks for triiodothyronine)
      (a rebound effect may occur following the sudden withdrawal of antithyroid preparations, resulting in a period of up to 5 days of very high thyroidal uptake; it is recommended that antithyroid medications be discontinued 3 to 4 days prior to administration of sodium iodide I 131; however, for early uptake studies [i.e., 15 to 30 minutes] to determine iodide trapping [not organification] the treatment with thioamide drugs does not need to be interrupted)
      (chronic salicylate administration may cause a depression of thyroid function; salicylate therapy should be discontinued at least 1 to 2 weeks prior to sodium iodide I 131 administration; however, a rebound effect may also occur following discontinuation of salicylate therapy, resulting in a period of 3 to 10 days of increased thyroidal uptake)

*Due to medical problems or conditions*
   Iodine deficiency or
   Low serum chlorides or
   Nephrosis
      (may increase thyroidal uptake of I 131)
   Renal function impairment
      (lack of normal excretion of iodine may cause an increase or decrease in the body iodide pool, resulting in falsely high or low uptake determinations)

**Medical considerations/Contraindications**

The medical considerations/contraindications included have been selected on the basis of their potential clinical significance (reasons given in parentheses where appropriate)—not necessarily inclusive (» = major clinical significance).

See also *Diagnostic interference*.

***Risk-benefit should be considered when the following medical problem exists:***

Sensitivity to the radiopharmaceutical preparation

## Side/Adverse Effects

The following side/adverse effects have been selected on the basis of their potential clinical significance (possible signs and symptoms in parentheses where appropriate)—not necessarily inclusive:

**Those indicating need for medical attention only if they continue or are bothersome**

Incidence rare
   *Headache; nausea or vomiting; skin rash, hives, or itching*

## Patient Consultation

As an aid to patient consultation, refer to *Advice for the Patient, Radiopharmaceuticals (Diagnostic)*.

In providing consultation, consider emphasizing the following selected information (» = major clinical significance):

**Description of use**
   Action in the body: Iodide I 131 uptake by the thyroid and functioning thyroid cancer metastases same as uptake of nonradioactive iodine
   Localization of iodide I 131 in thyroid allows thyroid uptake quantification and visualization of thyroid tissue; localization of iodide I 131 in functioning thyroid cancer metastases allows their detection, evaluation, and response to therapy
   Small amounts of radioactivity used in diagnosis; radiation exposure is relatively low and considered safe

**Before having this test**
» Conditions affecting use, especially:
   Pregnancy—Radioiodide crosses placenta; risk to fetus from radiation exposure as opposed to benefit derived from use should be considered
   Breast-feeding—Iodide I 131 is distributed into breast milk; complete cessation of nursing recommended for this infant when activity administered is large because of risk to infant from radiation exposure (present administration of I 131 will not affect breast-feeding of future infants)
   Use in children—Diagnostic benefit should be judged to outweigh potential risk of radiation

**Preparation for this test**
   Special preparatory instructions may apply; patient should inquire in advance

## General Dosing Information

Radiopharmaceuticals are to be administered only by or under the supervision of physicians who have had extensive training in the safe use and handling of radioactive materials and who are authorized by the appropriate Federal or state agency, if required, or, outside the U.S., the appropriate authority.

The estimated absorbed radiation dose to the thyroid is dependent on thyroidal uptake of radioiodine and the thyroid mass.

Adequate hydration of the patient is recommended before and after administration of sodium iodide I 131 to assure rapid elimination of the iodide that is not incorporated into the gland.

Uptake measurements are generally made at 4 and/or 24 hours, and thyroid imaging is usually performed 18 to 24 hours after sodium iodide I 131 administration. For imaging functioning metastatic thyroid tumor, imaging is usually performed 24 to 96 hours after sodium iodide I 131 administration.

## Safety considerations for handling this medication
Improper handling of this radiopharmaceutical may cause radioactive contamination. Guidelines for handling radioactive material have been prepared by scientific, professional, state, federal, and international bodies and are available to the specially qualified and authorized users who have access to radiopharmaceuticals.

## Oral Dosage Forms

### SODIUM IODIDE I 131 CAPSULES USP

**Usual adult administered activity**
Diagnostic aid—
  Thyroid uptake—
    Oral, 0.185 to 0.55 megabecquerel (5 to 15 microcuries).
    Note: Most uptake dosages of iodine I 131 are currently 0.55 megabecquerel (15 microcuries) or less. Only patients in whom hyperthyroidism is strongly suspected or in whom substernal thyroid nodules are likely would receive a dosage as high as 3.7 megabecquerels (100 microcuries).
  Thyroid imaging—
    Oral, 1.85 to 3.7 megabecquerels (50 to 100 microcuries).
      Localization of thyroid tumor metastases—
        Oral, 37 to 370 megabecquerels (1 to 10 millicuries).

**Usual pediatric administered activity**
Diagnostic aid—
  Dosage must be individualized by physician.
  For uptake studies, a minimum dosage of 0.037 megabecquerel (1 microcurie) and a maximum dosage of 0.55 megabecquerel (15 microcuries) have been used.
  For thyroid imaging, a minimum dosage of 0.185 megabecquerel (5 microcuries) and a maximum of 1.3 megabecquerels (35 microcuries) for lingular thyroid have been used. For mediastinal mass, a minimum dosage of 0.55 megabecquerel (15 microcuries) and a maximum of 3.7 megabecquerels (100 microcuries) have been used.
  Note: Sodium iodide I 123 or sodium pertechnetate Tc 99m (for thyroid imaging) may be preferable to sodium iodide I 131 because of its lower patient radiation doses. Sodium iodide I 123 may also be the radiopharmaceutical of choice in children who require diagnosis of thyroid function and imaging of the thyroid.

**Usual geriatric administered activity**
See *Usual adult administered activity.*

**Strength(s) usually available**
U.S.—
  0.3, 0.5, 1.1, 2, and 3.7 megabecquerels (8, 15, 30, 50, and 100 microcuries, respectively) per capsule at time of calibration (Rx) [GENERIC].

Canada—
  0.33, 0.61, 1.11, 2.03, and 3.70 megabecquerels (9, 16.5, 30, 55, and 100 microcuries, respectively) per capsule at time of calibration (Rx) [GENERIC].

**Packaging and storage**
Store below 40 °C (104 °F), preferably between 15 and 30 °C (59 and 86 °F), unless otherwise specified by manufacturer. Store in a well-closed container.

**Note**
Caution—Radioactive material.

### SODIUM IODIDE I 131 SOLUTION USP

**Usual adult administered activity**
Diagnostic aid—
  See *Sodium Iodide I 131 Capsules USP.*

**Usual pediatric administered activity**
See *Sodium Iodide I 131 Capsules USP.*

**Usual geriatric administered activity**
See *Usual adult administered activity.*

**Strength(s) usually available**
U.S.—
  Available in the U.S. for therapeutic use only.
Canada—
  925 megabecquerels (25 millicuries) per 10-mL vial, at time of calibration (Rx) [GENERIC].

**Packaging and storage**
Store below 40 °C (104 °F), preferably between 15 and 30 °C (59 and 86 °F), unless otherwise specified by manufacturer.

**Note**
Caution—Radioactive material.

**Additional information**
Radioiodide stock solutions and any dilutions thereof must be maintained at a pH of 7.5 to 9.0 in order to minimize oxidation of iodide to volatile forms of iodine. In addition, 0.2% sodium thiosulfate may be incorporated into these solutions if an antioxidant is desired.

## Selected Bibliography
Ross DS. Evaluation of the thyroid nodule. J Nucl Med 1991; 32(11): 2181-92.

Revised: 09/02/94

---

# SODIUM IODIDE I 131    Systemic—Therapeutic

VA CLASSIFICATION (Primary): AN600
Commonly used brand name(s): *Iodotope.*
Note: For a listing of dosage forms and brand names by country availability, see *Dosage Forms* section(s).

## Category
Antihyperthyroid agent; Antineoplastic.

## Indications

**Accepted**
Hyperthyroidism (treatment)—Sodium iodide I 131 is indicated for the treatment of diffuse toxic goiter (Graves' disease), single or multiple toxic nodular goiter, and recurrent hyperthyroidism following surgical or medical treatment. Sodium iodide I 131 may be used in patients of any age if medically appropriate.
Carcinoma, thyroid (treatment)—Sodium iodide I 131 is indicated for the treatment of functioning metastatic papillary or follicular carcinoma of the thyroid. The amount of sodium iodide I 131 used for the treatment of thyroid carcinoma is variable and depends upon the amount of normal thyroid tissue remaining and the extent of thyroid metastases and the degree to which they accumulate sodium iodide I 131.

## Physical Properties

**Nuclear data**

| Radionuclide (half-life*) | Decay constant | Mode of decay | Principal emissions (keV) | Mean number of emissions/ disintegration |
|---|---|---|---|---|
| I 131 (8.08 days) | 0.00358 h$^{-1}$ | Beta | Beta (191.6) | 0.90 |
|  |  |  | Gamma (364.5) | 0.81 |

*For therapeutic use: In the hyperthyroid patient, a percent of the administered dose equal to the fractional radioiodide uptake (usually between 35 and 90%) of the administered sodium iodide I 131 is concentrated in the thyroid gland and has an effective half-life of approximately 4 to 6 days. The non-thyroidal sodium iodide I 131 is distributed within the extracellular fluid and has an effective half-life of approximately 0.34 day.

## Pharmacology/Pharmacokinetics

**Mechanism of action/Effect**
The action of therapeutic radioiodide is based on one of the normal functions of the thyroid gland, which is the accumulation and retention of iodine as required for the synthesis of thyroid hormones. Radioiodide may also be concentrated in papillary, follicular, or mixed papillary/follicular thyroid cancer and metastases, although to a lesser extent than in normal thyroid tissue. When large doses of sodium iodide I 131 are given orally, it is possible to selectively damage or destroy thyroidal

tissue as required in the treatment of hyperthyroidism or thyroid carcinoma.

**Absorption**
Readily absorbed from gastrointestinal tract.

**Distribution**
Selectively concentrated and bound to tyrosyl residues of thyroglobulin in the thyroid gland; also concentrated, but not protein-bound, in the choroid plexus, gastric mucosa, salivary glands, nasal mucosa, and lactating breast tissue, with the remainder being distributed within the extracellular fluid.

**Half-life**
Biological (for thyroid compartment)—
  Euthyroid: 80 days.
  Hyperthyroid: 5 to 40 days.

**Onset of therapeutic action**
Approximately 2 to 4 weeks.

**Time to peak therapeutic effect**
Approximately 2 to 4 months.

**Radiation dosimetry**

| Organ | I 131 Estimated absorbed radiation dose*† |||
|---|---|---|---|
| | Maximum thyroid uptake (%) | mGy/MBq | rad/mCi |
| Bladder wall | 0 | 0.61 | 2.26 |
| | 5 | 0.58 | 2.15 |
| | 15 | 0.52 | 1.93 |
| | 25 | 0.46 | 1.70 |
| | 55 | 0.29 | 1.07 |
| Uterus | 0 | 0.054 | 0.20 |
| | 5 | 0.055 | 0.20 |
| | 15 | 0.054 | 0.20 |
| | 25 | 0.052 | 0.19 |
| | 55 | 0.046 | 0.17 |
| Kidneys | 0 | 0.065 | 0.24 |
| | 5 | 0.063 | 0.24 |
| | 15 | 0.060 | 0.22 |
| | 25 | 0.058 | 0.21 |
| | 55 | 0.051 | 0.19 |
| Ovaries | 0 | 0.042 | 0.16 |
| | 5 | 0.044 | 0.16 |
| | 15 | 0.043 | 0.16 |
| | 25 | 0.043 | 0.16 |
| | 55 | 0.041 | 0.15 |
| Large intestine wall (lower) | 0 | 0.043 | 0.16 |
| | 5 | 0.043 | 0.16 |
| | 15 | 0.042 | 0.16 |
| | 25 | 0.041 | 0.15 |
| | 55 | 0.040 | 0.15 |
| Red marrow | 0 | 0.035 | 0.13 |
| | 5 | 0.038 | 0.14 |
| | 15 | 0.054 | 0.20 |
| | 25 | 0.070 | 0.26 |
| | 55 | 0.12 | 0.44 |
| Small intestine | 0 | 0.038 | 0.14 |
| | 5 | 0.28 | 1.04 |
| | 15 | 0.28 | 1.04 |
| | 25 | 0.28 | 1.04 |
| | 55 | 0.28 | 1.04 |
| Bone surfaces | 0 | 0.032 | 0.12 |
| | 5 | 0.032 | 0.12 |
| | 15 | 0.047 | 0.17 |
| | 25 | 0.061 | 0.23 |
| | 55 | 0.11 | 0.41 |
| Large intestine wall (upper) | 0 | 0.037 | 0.14 |
| | 5 | 0.059 | 0.22 |
| | 15 | 0.059 | 0.22 |
| | 25 | 0.059 | 0.22 |
| | 55 | 0.058 | 0.21 |
| Pancreas | 0 | 0.035 | 0.13 |
| | 5 | 0.050 | 0.19 |
| | 15 | 0.052 | 0.19 |
| | 25 | 0.053 | 0.20 |
| | 55 | 0.058 | 0.21 |

| Organ | I 131 Estimated absorbed radiation dose*† |||
|---|---|---|---|
| | Maximum thyroid uptake (%) | mGy/MBq | rad/mCi |
| Spleen | 0 | 0.034 | 0.13 |
| | 5 | 0.039 | 0.14 |
| | 15 | 0.042 | 0.16 |
| | 25 | 0.044 | 0.16 |
| | 55 | 0.051 | 0.19 |
| Adrenals | 0 | 0.037 | 0.14 |
| | 5 | 0.032 | 0.12 |
| | 15 | 0.036 | 0.13 |
| | 25 | 0.039 | 0.14 |
| | 55 | 0.049 | 0.18 |
| Testes | 0 | 0.037 | 0.14 |
| | 5 | 0.029 | 0.11 |
| | 15 | 0.028 | 0.10 |
| | 25 | 0.027 | 0.10 |
| | 55 | 0.026 | 0.10 |
| Stomach wall | 0 | 0.034 | 0.13 |
| | 5 | 0.45 | 1.67 |
| | 15 | 0.46 | 1.67 |
| | 25 | 0.46 | 1.67 |
| | 55 | 0.46 | 1.67 |
| Liver | 0 | 0.033 | 0.12 |
| | 5 | 0.030 | 0.11 |
| | 15 | 0.032 | 0.12 |
| | 25 | 0.035 | 0.13 |
| | 55 | 0.043 | 0.16 |
| Lungs | 0 | 0.031 | 0.11 |
| | 5 | 0.034 | 0.13 |
| | 15 | 0.053 | 0.20 |
| | 25 | 0.072 | 0.27 |
| | 55 | 0.13 | 0.48 |
| Breast | 0 | 0.033 | 0.12 |
| | 5 | 0.031 | 0.11 |
| | 15 | 0.043 | 0.16 |
| | 25 | 0.055 | 0.20 |
| | 55 | 0.091 | 0.34 |
| Thyroid | 0 | 0.029 | 0.11 |
| | 5 | 72.00 | 266.67 |
| | 15 | 210.00 | 777.78 |
| | 25 | 360.00 | 1333.33 |
| | 55 | 790.00 | 2925.93 |
| Other tissue | 0 | 0.032 | 0.12 |
| | 5 | 0.040 | 0.15 |
| | 15 | 0.065 | 0.24 |
| | 25 | 0.090 | 0.33 |
| | 55 | 0.16 | 0.59 |

| | Effective dose§ |||||
|---|---|---|---|---|---|
| | Maximum Thyroid Uptake (%)‡ |||||
| | 0 | 5 | 15 | 25 | 55 |
| mSv/MBq | 0.072 | 2.3 | 6.6 | 11 | 24 |
| rem/mCi | 0.27 | 8.51 | 24.42 | 40.7 | 88.8 |

  *Data based on the International Commission on Radiological Protection (ICRP) Publication 53—Radiation Dose to Patients from Radiopharmaceuticals.
  †Estimates based on intravenous administration. With oral administration there is a radiation dose to the stomach in addition to that due to iodide in gastric and salivary secretions. Assuming a mean residence time in the stomach of 30 minutes, the absorbed dose to the stomach wall is increased by approximately 30% with oral administration, while the dose to organs and tissues other than the stomach wall is not significantly changed.
  ‡With thyroid blocking, thyroid uptakes ranging from 0.5 to 2.0% will still occur. Under these circumstances, the effective dose to the adult will range from 0.30 to 0.97 mSv/MBq (1.11 to 3.59 rem/mCi) for I 131.
  §The effective dose is virtually identical after oral or intravenous administration.

**Elimination**
Renal—Primary, 50 to 75% of the administered activity eliminated in the urine of euthyroid patients with normal renal function within 48 hours.
Fecal and salivary—Secondary.

Breast milk—Up to 20% of administered activity appears in the milk within 24 hours.

## Precautions to Consider

### Carcinogenicity
Experiments in animals with sodium iodide I 131 have demonstrated that radioiodide administration can induce thyroid adenomas and carcinomas. However, studies in humans have shown no conclusive evidence of thyroid carcinoma in hyperthyroid patients treated with sodium iodide I 131.

Also, studies with sodium iodide I 131 have not demonstrated that leukemia occurs more frequently in patients treated with this medication than in other hyperthyroid patients.

### Mutagenicity
Mutagenic effects have not been clearly established in clinical studies of patients treated with sodium iodide I 131. However, chromosomal changes have been reported in laboratory studies.

### Pregnancy/Reproduction
Fertility—A follow-up study of 627 women treated for differentiated thyroid carcinoma with sodium iodide I 131 revealed no evidence of fertility impairment.

Pregnancy—Iodide I 131 crosses the placenta and may cause severe and irreversible hypothyroidism in the neonate; the fetal thyroid begins to concentrate iodine during approximately the 12th week of gestation. Sodium iodide I 131 is contraindicated for the treatment of disease during pregnancy.

To avoid the possibility of fetal exposure to radiation, in those circumstances where the patient's pregnancy status is uncertain a pregnancy test should be performed and will help to prevent inadvertent administration of this preparation during pregnancy.

Studies have not been done in animals.

FDA Pregnancy Category X.

### Breast-feeding
Radioiodide is distributed into breast milk and may reach concentrations equal to or greater than concentrations in maternal plasma. It has been recommended that nursing be resumed after administration of a radiopharmaceutical, when the likelihood of the infant's ingested effective dose equivalent (EDE) is below 1 mSv (100 mrem). A method to calculate the EDE has been proposed based on the effective half-life of the radionuclide, the activity administered to the mother, the fraction of administered activity ingested by the infant, and the total body effective dose equivalent to the newborn infant per unit of activity ingested. According to this method, it has been estimated that the time to reduce the EDE to the infant to below 1 mSv (100 mrem) is approximately 10 weeks after administration of 40 megabecquerels (1.08 millicuries) of sodium iodide I 131 to the mother. Because of the difficulty of maintaining the maternal milk supply for such an extended period of time, complete cessation of nursing is usually recommended. Also, to minimize the absorbed radiation dose to the breast tissue and to ensure that mammary secretory activity has ceased, breast-feeding should be discontinued several weeks before starting treatment with sodium iodide I 131.

### Pediatrics
There is no conclusive evidence linking carcinogenicity, leukemogenicity, and mutagenicity to radioiodide therapy in children and growing adolescents.

Retrospective studies in children and adolescents treated with sodium iodide I 131 for hyperthyroidism have shown that sodium iodide I 131 is effective for both the initial treatment of hyperthyroidism and in cases in which other treatment modalities have failed. However, the occurrence of vomiting in the early post-treatment period may present management problems in some pediatric patients.

### Geriatrics
Geriatric patients with severe thyrotoxic cardiac disease should be given antithyroid agents and/or beta-blockers, such as propranolol, for 4 to 6 weeks prior to treatment with radioiodide to help reduce possible aggravation of the condition by radiation thyroiditis. Antithyroid drugs must be discontinued at least 3 to 4 days prior to treatment and should not be readministered until 1 week after treatment. However, a beta-blocker may be used throughout the treatment period if needed.

### Drug interactions and/or related problems
The following drug interactions and/or related problems have been selected on the basis of their potential clinical significance (possible mechanism in parentheses where appropriate)—not necessarily inclusive (» = major clinical significance):

Amiodarone or
Antithyroid preparations—thioamide derivatives or aromatic preparations or
Benzodiazepines or
Contrast media, iodinated or
Corticosteroids or
Goitrogenic foods (e.g., cabbage, turnips) or
Iodine-containing foods or
Iodine-containing preparations or
Iodine-contaminated bromides or
Iodine, stable or
Monovalent anions (e.g., perchlorate, thiocyanate) or
Pyrazolone derivatives, such as phenylbutazone or
Salicylates, chronic administration of or
Salt, iodized, excessive intake of or
Thiopental or
Thyroid blocking agents, such as strong iodine solution, potassium iodide, or potassium perchlorate or
Thyroid preparations, natural or synthetic
(may decrease thyroidal uptake of iodide I 131; it is recommended that these medications or preparations be withheld for the following periods of time prior to administration of sodium iodide I 131: 1 week for corticosteroids; 4 weeks for benzodiazepines; 2 to 4 weeks for intravascular iodinated contrast media and more than 4 weeks for cholecystographic agents; 2 to 4 weeks for iodine-containing preparations, such as vitamins, expectorants, antitussives, and topical medications; 1 to 2 weeks for pyrazolone derivatives; 1 week for thiopental; 4 to 6 weeks for thyroxine and 2 to 3 weeks for triiodothyronine)

(a rebound effect may occur following the sudden withdrawal of antithyroid preparations, resulting in a period of up to 5 days of very high thyroidal uptake; it is recommended that antithyroid medications be discontinued 3 to 4 days prior to administration of sodium iodide I 131)

(chronic salicylate administration may cause a depression of thyroid function; salicylate therapy should be discontinued at least 1 to 2 weeks prior to sodium iodide I 131 administration; however, a rebound effect may also occur following discontinuation of salicylate therapy, resulting in a period of 3 to 10 days of increased thyroidal uptake)

Bone marrow depressants, other (See *Appendix II*)
(concurrent use may rarely increase the bone marrow depressant effects of these medications and radiation therapy; dosage reduction of other bone marrow depressant medications may be required)

### Medical considerations/Contraindications
The medical considerations/contraindications included have been selected on the basis of their potential clinical significance (reasons given in parentheses where appropriate)—not necessarily inclusive (» = major clinical significance).

*Risk-benefit should be considered when the following medical problems exist:*

Diarrhea or
Vomiting
(radiation exposure and loss of therapeutic dose may result)

Low serum chlorides or
Nephrosis
(may increase thyroidal uptake of iodide I 131)

Renal function impairment
(may decrease excretion of radioiodide, resulting in increased radiation exposure)

Sensitivity to the radiopharmaceutical preparation

Thyrotoxic cardiac disease, severe, especially in the elderly
(hyperthyroidism may be aggravated by radiation thyroiditis if antithyroid agents and/or beta-blockers, such as propranolol, are not given prior to and after treatment)

### Patient monitoring
The following may be especially important in patient monitoring (other tests may be warranted in some patients, depending on condition; » = major clinical significance):

Thyroid hormones, serum
(determinations of serum concentrations are recommended every 2 to 3 months during the first year after treatment of hyperthyroidism, and annually thereafter, since hypothyroidism may occur several years after treatment)

## Side/Adverse Effects

Note: The incidence of hypothyroidism following the treatment of Graves' disease is approximately 15 to 25% in the first post-treatment year and increases approximately 2 to 3% per year thereafter. The greater the life expectancy of the patient following treatment, the greater the risk of developing hypothyroidism.

The following side/adverse effects have been selected on the basis of their potential clinical significance (possible signs and symptoms in parentheses where appropriate)—not necessarily inclusive:

**Those indicating need for medical attention**
>> *Hypothyroidism* (changes in menstrual periods; clumsiness; coldness; drowsiness; dry, puffy skin; headache; listlessness; muscle aches; temporary thinning of hair [may occur 2 to 3 months after treatment]; unusual tiredness or weakness; weight gain)—dose-dependent
Note: *Hypothyroidism* may occur several years following successful treatment of hyperthyroidism; therefore, annual blood tests for thyroid hormone concentration are recommended.

Incidence rare
*Following treatment of hyperthyroidism*
**Exaggerated hyperthyroid state** (excessive sweating, fast heartbeat, fever, palpitations, unusual irritability or unusual tiredness)—due to radiation thyroiditis

*Following treatment of thyroid carcinoma*
**Leukopenia** (cough or hoarseness, fever or chills, lower back or side pain, painful or difficult urination); **thrombocytopenia** (unusual bleeding or bruising; black, tarry stools; blood in urine or stools; pinpoint red spots on skin)

**Those indicating need for medical attention only if they continue or are bothersome**
Incidence less frequent
*Following treatment of hyperthyroidism or thyroid carcinoma*
**Radiation thyroiditis** (neck tenderness or swelling or sore throat)

*Following treatment of thyroid carcinoma*
**Temporary loss of taste; radiation gastritis** (temporary nausea and vomiting); **radiation sialadenitis** (tenderness of salivary glands)

## Patient Consultation
As an aid to patient consultation, refer to *Advice for the Patient, Sodium Iodide I 131 (Therapeutic).*
In providing consultation, consider emphasizing the following selected information (>> = major clinical significance):

**Description of use**
Action in the body: Radioiodide uptake by the thyroid and functioning thyroid cancer metastases same as uptake of nonradioactive iodine
Large doses are used therapeutically to damage or destroy thyroidal tissue in management of hyperthyroidism or thyroid carcinoma

**Before using this medication**
>> Conditions affecting use, especially:
Pregnancy—Radioiodide crosses placenta; risk to fetus from radiation exposure; use contraindicated because of possibility of causing hypothyroidism in newborn
Breast-feeding—Distributed into breast milk; complete cessation of nursing recommended because of risk to infant from radiation exposure; possibility of causing hypothyroidism in newborn
Use in children—Vomiting may present management problems in some children

**Proper use of this medication**
Special preparatory instructions may apply; patient should inquire in advance

**Precautions after using this medication**
*Following treatment of hyperthyroidism or thyroid carcinoma*
To prevent radiation contamination of other persons or environment: For 48 to 96 hours after receiving radioiodide—
>> Not kissing anyone and not handling or using another person's eating or drinking utensils, toothbrush, or bathroom glass
>> Not engaging in sexual activities
Avoiding close and prolonged contact with others, especially children and pregnant women
Sleeping alone
>> Washing sink and tub after use (including brushing teeth)
>> Washing hands after using or cleaning toilet
Using separate towels and washcloths
Laundering clothes and linens separately
>> Double-flushing toilet
To decrease radiation exposure to the urinary bladder: Increasing intake of fluids to promote more frequent voiding to help eliminate radioactive iodine

*Following treatment of hyperthyroidism*
Periodic blood tests to check thyroid hormone concentration

**Side/adverse effects**
Signs of potential side effects, especially hypothyroidism or hyperthyroid state (following treatment of hyperthyroidism); leukopenia and thrombocytopenia (following treatment of thyroid carcinoma)

## General Dosing Information
Radiopharmaceuticals are to be administered only by or under the supervision of physicians who have had extensive training in the safe use and handling of radioactive materials and who are authorized by the Nuclear Regulatory Commission (NRC) or appropriate state agency, or, outside the U.S., the appropriate authority.

Adequate hydration of the patient is recommended before and after administration of radioiodide to assure rapid elimination of the iodide that is not incorporated into the gland.

The radiation dose to the thyroid gland from sodium iodide I 131 is dependent upon the uptake as well as the size of the gland and the amount of radioiodide administered. Thyroidal uptake and size should be determined by the physician prior to treatment and may be useful in calculating the therapeutic dose.

**Safety considerations for handling this medication**
Guidelines for the receipt, storage, handling, dispensing, and disposal of radioactive materials are available from scientific, professional, state, federal, and international bodies. Handling of this radiopharmaceutical should be limited to those individuals who are appropriately qualified and authorized.

Safety considerations for patients after treatment—
Large amount of radioactivity may be excreted in the urine, feces, perspiration, saliva, and on the skin of patients treated with radioiodide. This may present a contamination hazard during hospitalization and after discharge (current Nuclear Regulatory Commission [NRC] regulations require a hospital stay until the retained radioactivity is less than 1.1 gigabecquerels [30 millicuries] or until the measured dose rate from the patient is less than 0.05 millisieverts [mSv] [5 millirems (mrem)] per hour at a distance of one meter). For this reason
• Patients need to be instructed at time of discharge in techniques to prevent transfer of radioactivity to family members and the environment after release from the hospital.
• For most radioiodide thyroid carcinoma therapy patients, close contact with other persons may be resumed 2 to 4 days after release from the hospital; the time period may be longer for hyperthyroid therapy patients since the excretion of radioiodide in these patients is not as rapid as in the thyroid carcinoma patients.

## Oral Dosage Forms

### SODIUM IODIDE I 131 CAPSULES USP
**Usual adult and adolescent administered activity**
Disease therapy—
Antihyperthyroid agent—
Oral, 148 to 370 megabecquerels (4 to 10 millicuries).
Note: The administered activity is usually individualized based on the estimated weight of the patient's thyroid gland and measurement of the 24-hour radioiodide uptake.
Toxic nodular goiter and other serious thyroid conditions may require larger dosages (e.g., 555 to 1110 megabecquerels [15 to 30 millicuries]).
Antineoplastic:
Ablation of normal thyroid tissue—
Oral, 1.85 gigabecquerels (50 millicuries), with a range of 1.1 to 3.7 gigabecquerels (30 to 100 millicuries).
Subsequent therapy for metastases—
Oral, 3.7 to 7.4 gigabecquerels (100 to 200 millicuries).

**Usual pediatric administered activity**
Dosage must be individualized by physician.

**Usual geriatric administered activity**
See *Usual adult and adolescent administered activity.*

**Strength(s) usually available**
U.S.—
28 megabecquerels to 3.7 gigabecquerels (0.75 to 100 millicuries) per capsule at time of calibration (Rx) [GENERIC].
37 megabecquerels to 1.85 gigabecquerels (1 to 50 millicuries) per capsule at time of calibration (Rx) [*Iodotope*].
37 megabecquerels to 4.81 gigabecquerels (1 to 130 millicuries) per capsule at time of calibration (Rx) [*Iodotope*].

Canada—
Each gelatin capsule contains an individually dispensed dose of sodium iodide I 131 as prescribed (Rx) [GENERIC].

**Packaging and storage**
Store between 15 and 30 °C (59 and 86 °F), unless otherwise specified by manufacturer. Store in a well-closed container.

**Note**
Caution—Radioactive material.

### SODIUM IODIDE I 131 SOLUTION USP

**Usual adult and adolescent administered activity**
See *Sodium Iodide I 131 Capsules USP*.

**Usual pediatric administered activity**
See *Sodium Iodide I 131 Capsules USP*.

**Usual geriatric administered activity**
See *Usual adult and adolescent administered activity*.

**Strength(s) usually available**
U.S.—
129.5 megabecquerels to 5.5 gigabecquerels (3.5 to 150 millicuries) per vial at time of calibration (Rx) [GENERIC (sodium bisulfite 0.1%, edetate disodium 0.2%)].
259 megabecquerels to 3.93 gigabecquerels (7 to 106 millicuries) per vial at time of calibration (Rx) [*Iodotope* (edetate disodium 1 mg per mL)].
Canada—
Each vial contains an individually dispensed dose of sodium iodide I 131 as prescribed (Rx) [GENERIC].

**Packaging and storage**
Store between 15 and 30 °C (59 and 86 °F), unless otherwise specified by manufacturer.

**Note**
Caution—Radioactive material.

**Additional information**
Radioiodide stock solutions and any dilutions thereof must be maintained at a pH of 7.5 to 9.0 in order to minimize oxidation of iodide to volatile forms of iodine. Additionally, 0.2% sodium thiosulfate may be incorporated into these solutions if an antioxidant is desired.

### Selected Bibliography

Sugrue D, McEvoy M, Feely J, et al. Hyperthyroidism in the land of Graves', results of treatment by surgery, radioiodine, and carbimazole in 837 patients. Q J Med 1980; 49: 51-61.

Levetan C, Wartofsky L. A clinical guide to the management of Graves' disease with radioactive iodine. Endocr Pract 1995; 1: 205-12.

Revised: 07/15/96

**SODIUM NITRITE**—The *Sodium Nitrite (Systemic)* monograph is not included in this published version of the USP DI database. Copies of the monograph are available on request from Micromedex, Inc. - Reprint Requests, 6200 S. Syracuse Way, Suite 300, Englewood, CO 80111; telephone (303) 486-6400; telefax (303) 486-6464; Email: USPDI@MDX.COM.

# SODIUM PERTECHNETATE Tc 99m     Mucosal-Local

VA CLASSIFICATION (Primary): DX201

Note: For information on sodium pertechnetate Tc 99m injection for intravenous administration, see *Sodium Pertechnetate Tc 99m (Systemic)*.
For information on sodium pertechnetate Tc 99m injection for ophthalmic administration, see *Sodium Pertechnetate Tc 99m (Ophthalmic)*.

Note: For a listing of dosage forms and brand names by country availability, see *Dosage Forms* section(s).

## Category
Diagnostic aid, radioactive (urinary bladder disorders).

## Indications

**Accepted**
Urinary bladder imaging, radionuclide—Sodium pertechnetate Tc 99m is indicated in direct isotopic cystography for the detection of vesicoureteral reflux.

## Physical Properties

**Nuclear data**

| Radionuclide (half-life) | Decay constant | Mode of decay | Principal photon emissions (keV) | Mean number of emissions/ disintegration ($\geq 0.01$) |
|---|---|---|---|---|
| Tc 99m (6.0 hr) | 0.1151 hr$^{-1}$ | Isomeric transition to Tc 99 | Gamma (18) Gamma (140.5) | 0.062 0.891 |

## Pharmacology/Pharmacokinetics

**Mechanism of action/Effect**
Urinary bladder imaging—Sodium pertechnetate Tc 99m is confined within the urinary tract after direct instillation via catheter into the bladder. The dynamic sequence of filling and voiding is recorded on film and/or digital device; reflux activity into the ureters and/or renal collecting system during filling and voiding can thus be detected.

**Elimination**
Direct intraurethral instillation—Almost total with normal micturition.

## Precautions to Consider

**Pregnancy/Reproduction**

Pregnancy—Although systemic absorption of sodium pertechnetate is minimal with intraurethral administration, fetal exposure to radiation may result from radioactivity localized in the bladder. Adequate and well-controlled studies with sodium pertechnetate Tc 99m have not been done in humans. The possibility of pregnancy should be assessed in women of child-bearing potential. Clinical situations exist in which the benefit to the patient and fetus derived from information from radiopharmaceutical use outweighs the risks from fetal exposure to radiation. In these situations, the physician should use discretion and reduce the administered activity of the radiopharmaceutical to the lowest possible amount.

Studies have not been done in animals.

FDA Pregnancy Category C.

**Breast-feeding**
Although Tc 99m is known to be distributed into breast milk, discontinuation of breast-feeding is generally not required because systemic absorption of sodium pertechnetate Tc 99m after intraurethral administration is minimal. Also, the activity administered for this procedure is much less than that used for other procedures.

**Pediatrics**
Diagnostic studies performed to date using sodium pertechnetate Tc 99m have not demonstrated pediatrics-specific problems that would limit its usefulness in children. Risk of radiation exposure as opposed to benefit derived from use should be considered.

**Geriatrics**
Although appropriate studies on the relationship of age to the effects of sodium pertechnetate Tc 99m have not been performed in the geriatric population, no geriatrics-specific problems have been documented to date.

**Medical considerations/Contraindications**
The medical considerations/contraindications included have been selected on the basis of their potential clinical significance (reasons given in parentheses where appropriate)—not necessarily inclusive (» = major clinical significance).

*Except under special circumstances, this medication should not be used when the following medical problems exist:*

» Obstruction to urethral catheterization, such as in extensive urinary tuberculosis, bladder tumors, urethral obstructions, and prostate enlargement

» Urinary tract infection, upper, acute
(procedure may increase risk of complications)

### Side/Adverse Effects
There are no known side/adverse effects associated with the intraurethral use of sodium pertechnetate Tc 99m as a diagnostic aid.

### Patient Consultation
As an aid to patient consultation, refer to *Advice for the Patient, Radiopharmaceuticals (Diagnostic)*.
In providing consultation, consider emphasizing the following selected information (» = major clinical significance):

**Description of use**
*Actions in the body*
Direct instillation into bladder allows recording of dynamic sequence of filling and voiding to detect vesico-ureteral reflux
Small amounts of radioactivity used in diagnosis; radiation exposure is low and considered safe

**Before having this test**
» Conditions affecting use, especially:
Pregnancy—Risk to fetus from radiation exposure as opposed to benefit derived from use should be considered
Use in children—Risk of radiation exposure as opposed to benefit derived from use should be considered
Other medical problems, especially obstruction or acute upper urinary tract infection

**Preparation for this test**
Special preparatory instructions may be given; patient should inquire in advance

### General Dosing Information
Radiopharmaceuticals are to be administered only by or under the supervision of physicians who have had extensive training in the safe use and handling of radioactive materials and who are authorized by the Nuclear Regulatory Commission (NRC) or the appropriate Agreement State agency or, outside the U.S., the appropriate authority.
Manufacturer's package insert or other appropriate literature should be consulted for optimal times when imaging should be performed.

**Safety considerations for handling this medication**
Improper handling of this radiopharmaceutical may cause radioactive contamination. Guidelines for handling radioactive material have been prepared by scientific, professional, state, federal, and international bodies and are available to the specially qualified and authorized users who have access to radiopharmaceuticals.

## Mucosal-Local Dosage Forms

### SODIUM PERTECHNETATE Tc 99m INJECTION USP

**Usual adult and adolescent administered activity**
Urinary bladder imaging—
Intraurethral instillation via catheter, 18.5 to 37 megabecquerels (0.5 to 1 millicurie).

**Usual pediatric administered activity**
See *Usual adult and adolescent administered activity*.

**Usual geriatric administered activity**
See *Usual adult and adolescent administered activity*.

**Strength(s) usually available**
U.S.—
740 megabecquerels to 3.7 gigabecquerels (20 to 100 millicuries) per mL at time of calibration.
Note: Sodium pertechnetate Tc 99m injection is supplied as a molybdenum Mo 99/technetium Tc 99m generator in sizes of Mo 99 ranging from 30.7 to 614.2 gigabecquerels (830 to 16,600 millicuries); 9.25 to 111 gigabecquerels (250 to 3000 millicuries) [*Ultra-TechneKow FM*]; or 8.3 to 100 gigabecquerels (225 to 2700 millicuries) [*TechneLite*]. Each eluate of the generator should not contain more than the USP limit of 0.15 kilobecquerel of molybdenum Mo 99 per megabecquerel of technetium Tc 99m (0.15 microcurie Mo 99 per millicurie Tc 99m) per administered activity at the time of administration.
Canada—
Sodium pertechnetate Tc 99m injection is supplied as a molybdenum Mo 99/technetium Tc 99m generator in sizes of Mo 99 ranging from 8.3 to 100 gigabecquerels (225 to 2700 millicuries). Each eluate of the generator should not contain more than the Canadian Regulatory limit of 1.1 kilobecquerels of molybdenum Mo 99 per 37 megabecquerels of technetium Tc 99m (0.03 microcurie Mo 99 per millicurie Tc 99m) per administered activity at the time of administration.

**Packaging and storage**
Store below 40 °C (104 °F), preferably between 15 and 30 °C (59 and 86 °F), unless otherwise specified by manufacturer. Protect from freezing.

**Stability**
Generator eluate does not contain an antimicrobial agent, and thus should be used within 12 hours from the time of generator elution.

**Note**
Caution—Radioactive material.

Developed: 08/30/94

# SODIUM PERTECHNETATE Tc 99m Ophthalmic

VA CLASSIFICATION (Primary): DX201
Note: For information on sodium pertechnetate Tc 99m injection for oral or parenteral administration see *Sodium Pertechnetate Tc 99m (Systemic)*.
For information on sodium pertechnetate Tc 99m injection for intraurethral administration, see *Sodium Pertechnetate Tc 99m (Mucosal-Local)*.

Note: For a listing of dosage forms and brand names by country availability, see *Dosage Forms* section(s).

## Category
Diagnostic aid, radioactive (nasolacrimal disorders).

## Indications
**Accepted**
*Dacryoscintigraphy*—Sodium pertechnetate Tc 99m is indicated for imaging the nasolacrimal drainage system in adults.

## Physical Properties

### Nuclear data

| Radionuclide (half-life) | Decay constant | Mode of decay | Principal photon emissions (keV) | Mean number of emissions/ disintegration (≥0.01) |
|---|---|---|---|---|
| Tc 99m (6.0 hr) | 0.1151 h$^{-1}$ | Isomeric transition to Tc 99 | Gamma 18 | 0.062 |
| | | | Gamma 140.5 | 0.889 |

## Pharmacology/Pharmacokinetics

**Mechanism of action/Effect**
Sodium pertechnetate Tc 99m, when administered as eye drops, mixes with tears within the conjunctival space and follows the same path as tears through the nasolacrimal drainage system. Thus, any anatomical or functional blockage of the draining system will be visualized.

**Absorption**
Minimal transconjunctival absorption after instillation in eye.

**Distribution**
Distributed within conjunctival space; passes into the inferior meatus of the nose through the nasolacrimal drainage system.

**Radiation dosimetry**
Following ophthalmic administration of sodium pertechnetate Tc 99m, the estimated absorbed radiation doses to an adult are:

Eye lens—
- If lacrimal fluid turnover is 16% per minute: 0.04 mGy/megabecquerel (0.14 mrad/microcurie).
- If lacrimal fluid turnover is 100% per minute: 0.006 mGy/megabecquerel (0.02 mrad/microcurie).
- If drainage system is blocked: 1.09 mGy/megabecquerel (4.04 mrads/microcurie).

Ovaries (no blockage of drainage system)—0.008 mGy/megabecquerel (0.03 mrad/microcurie).
Testes (no blockage of drainage system)—0.002 mGy/megabecquerel (0.009 mrad/microcurie).
Thyroid (no blockage of drainage system)—0.04 mGy/megabecquerel (0.13 mrad/microcurie).

**Elimination**
Most of Tc 99m escapes within a few minutes of normal drainage and tearing.

## Precautions to Consider

**Pregnancy/Reproduction**
Pregnancy—Transconjunctival absorption of sodium pertechnetate Tc 99m is minimal. However, studies have not been done in humans.
Studies have not been done in animals.
FDA Pregnancy Category C.

**Breast-feeding**
Although transconjunctival absorption of sodium pertechnetate Tc 99m is minimal, risk-benefit must be considered since Tc 99m is known to be distributed into breast milk.

**Pediatrics**
Appropriate studies on the relationship of age to the effects of sodium pertechnetate Tc 99m have not been performed in children.

**Geriatrics**
Appropriate studies on the relationship of age to the effects of sodium pertechnetate Tc 99m have not been performed in the geriatric population. However, no geriatrics-specific problems have been documented to date.

## Side/Adverse Effects
There are no known side/adverse effects associated with the ophthalmic use of sodium pertechnetate Tc 99m as a diagnostic aid.

## Patient Consultation
As an aid to patient consultation, refer to *Advice for the Patient, Radiopharmaceuticals (Diagnostic)*.
In providing consultation, consider emphasizing the following selected information (» = major clinical significance):

**Description of use**
Action in the body: Transit through nasolacrimal drainage system allows visualization to detect blockage within
Small amounts of radioactivity used in diagnosis; radiation exposure is low and considered safe

**Before having this test**
» Conditions affecting use, especially:
Breast-feeding—Tc 99m distributed into breast milk

**Preparation for this test**
Special preparatory instructions may be given; patient should inquire in advance

**Precautions after having this test**
Blowing nose and rinsing eyes to minimize radiation exposure

## General Dosing Information
Radiopharmaceuticals are to be administered only by or under the supervision of physicians who have had extensive training in the safe use and handling of radionuclides and who are licensed by the Nuclear Regulatory Commission (NRC) or the appropriate Agreement State agency or, outside the U.S., the appropriate authority.

Sodium pertechnetate Tc 99m should be instilled into the eye by using a micropipette or a similar method of administration that ensures the accuracy of the dose.

Blowing the nose and rinsing the eyes with sterile distilled water or an isotonic sodium chloride solution is recommended after the nasolacrimal imaging procedures to minimize the absorbed radiation dose.

**Safety considerations for handling this radiopharmaceutical**
Improper handling of this radiopharmaceutical may cause radioactive contamination. Guidelines for handling radioactive material have been prepared by scientific, professional, state, federal, and international bodies and are available to the specially qualified and authorized users who have access to radiopharmaceuticals.

## Ophthalmic Dosage Forms

### SODIUM PERTECHNETATE Tc 99m INJECTION USP

**Usual adult and adolescent administered activity**
Topical, to the conjunctiva, 3.7 megabecquerels (100 microcuries).

**Usual geriatric administered activity**
See *Usual adult and adolescent administered activity*.

**Strength(s) usually available**
U.S.—
740 megabecquerels to 3.7 gigabecquerels (20 to 100 millicuries) per mL at time of calibration (Rx).
Sodium pertechnetate Tc 99m injection is supplied as a Molybdenum Mo 99/Technetium Tc 99m generator in sizes of Mo 99 ranging from 30.7 to 614.2 gigabecquerels (830 to 16,600 millicuries); or 9.25 to 111 gigabecquerels (250 to 3000 millicuries) [*UltraTechneKow FM*]; or 8.3 to 100 gigabecquerels (225 to 2700 millicuries) [*TechneLite*]. Each eluate of the generator should not contain more than the USP limit of 0.15 kilobecquerel of molybdenum Mo 99 per megabecquerel of technetium Tc 99m (0.15 microcurie Mo 99 per millicurie Tc 99m) per administered dose at the time of administration.

Canada—
740 megabecquerels to 3.7 gigabecquerels (20 to 100 millicuries) per mL at time of calibration (Rx).
Sodium pertechnetate Tc 99m injection is supplied as a Molybdenum Mo 99/Technetium Tc 99m generator in sizes of Mo 99 ranging from 8.3 to 100 gigabecquerels (225 to 2700 millicuries). Each eluate of the generator should not contain more than the Canadian Regulatory limit of 1.1 kilobecquerels of molybdenum Mo 99 per 37 megabecquerels of techentium Tc 99m (0.03 microcurie Mo 99 per millicurie Tc 99m) per administered dose at the time of administration.

**Packaging and storage**
Store below 40 °C (104 °F), preferably between 15 and 30 °C (59 and 86 °F), unless otherwise specified by manufacturer. Protect from freezing.

**Stability**
Generator eluate does not contain an antimicrobial agent, and thus, should be used within 12 hours from the time of generator elution.

**Note**
Caution—Radioactive material.

Revised: 06/23/94

---

# SODIUM PERTECHNETATE Tc 99m Systemic

VA CLASSIFICATION (Primary): DX201

Note: For information on sodium pertechnetate Tc 99m injection for intraurethral administration, see *Sodium Pertechnetate Tc 99m (Mucosal-Local)*.
For information on sodium pertechnetate Tc 99m injection for ophthalmic administration, see *Sodium Pertechnetate Tc 99m (Ophthalmic)*.
Note: For a listing of dosage forms and brand names by country availability, see *Dosage Forms* section(s).

## Category
Diagnostic aid, radioactive (vascular disorders; brain disorders; thyroid disorders; salivary gland disorders; cardiac disorders; gastrointestinal disorders).

## Indications
Note: Bracketed information in the *Indications* section refers to uses that are not included in U.S. product labeling.

**Accepted**

Blood pool imaging, radionuclide—Sodium pertechnetate Tc 99m is indicated for blood pool imaging, especially radionuclide angiography.

Brain imaging, radionuclide and

Angiography, cerebral, radionuclide—Sodium pertechnetate Tc 99m is indicated for brain imaging, including cerebral radionuclide angiography. It is used to screen patients for primary brain tumors, to detect cerebral metastases, to evaluate patients with cerebrovascular disease, to localize arteriovenous malformations, to detect intracranial injury due to trauma, to localize intracranial abscesses, and to monitor patients with intracranial diseases. However, this procedure has been almost entirely replaced by other imaging procedures, including computed tomography (CT) and magnetic resonance imaging (MRI).

Thyroid imaging, radionuclide—Sodium pertechnetate Tc 99m is indicated for thyroid imaging in the evaluation of thyroid nodules; carcinoma; and masses in the lingual region, neck, and mediastinum; and to study thyroid size, position, and function. Sodium pertechnetate Tc 99m may be preferred over the radioiodine study in thyroid scanning in cases in which the radioiodine is unsuccessful because of poor uptake, in children to reduce radiation exposure, and when results of the procedure are needed as soon as possible. However, sodium iodide I 131 or I 123 may be preferred over sodium pertechnetate Tc 99m for characterizing the function of thyroid nodules or for detecting substernal or lingual thyroids.

Salivary gland imaging, radionuclide—Sodium pertechnetate Tc 99m is indicated in adult patients for salivary gland imaging as an adjunct in the evaluation of space-occupying lesions and in the evaluation of the size, position, and function of the gland.

Placenta localization—Sodium pertechnetate Tc 99m is indicated for placenta localization. However, this procedure has generally been replaced by ultrasound procedures.

[Gastric mucosa imaging, radionuclide][1]—Sodium pertechnetate Tc 99m is used to localize Meckel's diverticula.

[Red blood cells, labeling of][1]—Sodium pertechnetate Tc 99m is used for in vitro or in vivo labeling of red blood cells (which have been pretreated with stannous ion). Red blood cells labeled with sodium pertechnetate Tc 99m are used for the following diagnostic studies:

Cardiac blood pool imaging, radionuclide—To evaluate cardiac function, including measurement of cardiac output, ejection fraction, and wall motion.

Bleeding, gastrointestinal (diagnosis)—To evaluate patients suspected of having gastrointestinal bleeding, to detect the site of bleeding and help establish the amount of bleeding.

[1]Not included in Canadian product labeling.

## Physical Properties

### Nuclear data

| Radionuclide (half-life) | Decay constant | Mode of decay | Principal photon emissions (keV) | Mean number of emissions/ disintegration (≥0.01) |
|---|---|---|---|---|
| Tc 99m (6.0 hr) | 0.1151 hr$^{-1}$ | Isomeric transition to Tc 99 | Gamma (18) | 0.062 |
| | | | Gamma (140.5) | 0.891 |

## Pharmacology/Pharmacokinetics

### Mechanism of action/Effect

Vascular disorders—Pertechnetate Tc 99m remains in the intravascular space long enough to allow external detection for the evaluation of blood flow patterns in brain or in other regions of the body, or to allow the depiction of the large blood pool in the heart or major vessels.

Brain disorders—The mechanism by which pertechnetate Tc 99m accumulates in the abnormal areas of the brain is not precisely known but is most likely related to a change in the blood-brain barrier permeability.

Thyroid disorders—Pertechnetate Tc 99m is handled by the body in a way similar to the iodide ion. Pertechnetate Tc 99m is trapped by the thyroid (but not organified) and remains in the gland long enough for images to be obtained.

Salivary gland disorders—Exact mechanism of action is unknown. However, pertechnetate Tc 99m is handled by the body in a way similar to the iodide ion and, since radioiodine is known to concentrate in the duct cells of the salivary glands, this is also probably true for pertechnetate Tc 99m. The accumulation in the glands is sufficient to allow images to be obtained.

Gastrointestinal disorders—Meckel's diverticula: Following intravenous injection, sodium pertechnetate Tc 99m binds to albumin in the serum. It is then handled by the body in a way similar to that for chloride ions by the gastric mucosa, which concentrates and secretes sodium pertechnetate Tc 99m.

Red blood cells, labeling of—When used for cardiac blood pool imaging or detection of gastrointestinal bleeding, pretreatment of red blood cells with stannous ions causes Tc 99m (as sodium pertechnetate Tc 99m) to bind to the red blood cells in vivo with about 70 to 80% of the injected radioactivity remaining in the blood pool long enough to provide images of the cardiac chambers or sites of active (rapid) or cumulative (intermittent) gastrointestinal bleeding. A modified in vivo/in vitro method of labeling red blood cells usually results in a greater percentage of the injected radioactivity remaining in the blood pool.

Placenta localization—The large pool of maternal blood in the placenta accumulates more radionuclide than the surrounding less vascular structures (i.e., fetus and uterus). The accumulation is sufficient to allow images to be obtained.

### Absorption

Oral—Usually well absorbed from gastrointestinal tract; may be incomplete in some patients.

### Distribution

Intravenous or oral—Selectively concentrated in intracranial lesions with altered blood-brain barrier, thyroid gland, salivary glands, stomach and intestines, and choroid plexus; remainder distributed within circulatory system and extracellular spaces.

### Protein binding

High (75% of plasma radioactivity is loosely bound).

### Half-life

Elimination$_1$—
 Blood: 10 minutes.
 Cerebrospinal fluid (CSF): < 1 hour.
Elimination$_2$—
 Blood: 6 hours.
 CSF: 11 to 12 hours.

### Time to peak concentration

Oral—
 Blood: 1 to 3 hours.
Intravenous—
 CSF: 3½ hours.
 Thyroid (euthyroid patients): 15 minutes to 2 hours.

### Radiation dosimetry

| | Estimated absorbed radiation dose* | | | |
|---|---|---|---|---|
| | Without blocking agent | | With blocking agent | |
| Organ | mGy/MBq | rad/mCi | mGy/MBq | rad/mCi |
| Large intestine wall (upper) | 0.062 | 0.23 | 0.0032 | 0.012 |
| Thyroid | 0.023 | 0.085 | 0.021 | 0.078 |
| Stomach wall | 0.029 | 0.11 | 0.0032 | 0.012 |
| Large intestine wall (lower) | 0.022 | 0.08 | 0.0045 | 0.017 |
| Bladder wall | 0.019 | 0.07 | 0.032 | 0.12 |
| Small intestine | 0.018 | 0.067 | 0.0041 | 0.015 |
| Ovaries | 0.01 | 0.037 | 0.0047 | 0.017 |
| Salivary glands | 0.0093 | 0.034 | | |
| Uterus | 0.0081 | 0.03 | 0.0066 | 0.024 |
| Red marrow | 0.0061 | 0.023 | 0.0045 | 0.017 |
| Pancreas | 0.0059 | 0.022 | 0.0035 | 0.013 |
| Kidneys | 0.005 | 0.019 | 0.0047 | 0.017 |
| Spleen | 0.0044 | 0.016 | 0.0032 | 0.012 |
| Liver | 0.0039 | 0.014 | 0.0031 | 0.011 |
| Bone surfaces | 0.0039 | 0.014 | 0.0038 | 0.014 |
| Adrenals | 0.0036 | 0.013 | 0.0033 | 0.012 |
| Lungs | 0.0027 | 0.01 | 0.0028 | 0.01 |
| Testes | 0.0027 | 0.01 | 0.0032 | 0.012 |
| Breast | 0.0023 | 0.0085 | 0.0025 | 0.0093 |
| Other tissue | 0.0034 | 0.013 | 0.0029 | 0.011 |

## Sodium Pertechnetate Tc 99m (Systemic)

| Radionuclide | Effective dose* Without blocking agent mSv/MBq | rem/mCi | Effective dose* With blocking agent mSv/MBq | rem/mCi |
|---|---|---|---|---|
| Tc 99m | 0.013 | 0.048 | 0.0053 | 0.020 |

*For adults; intravenous injection of sodium pertechnetate Tc 99m. Data based on the International Commission on Radiological Protection (ICRP) Publication 53—Radiation dose to patients from radiopharmaceuticals.

**Elimination**
Oral or intravenous—
  Renal: Primary, 15 to 50% of administered Tc 99m is eliminated within 24 hours.
  Fecal: Secondary, 10 to 55% of administered Tc 99m is eliminated in the feces within 3 days.

## Precautions to Consider

### Pregnancy/Reproduction
Pregnancy—Tc 99m as sodium pertechnetate crosses the placenta. The possibility of pregnancy should be assessed in women of child-bearing potential. Clinical situations exist in which the benefit to the patient and fetus derived from information from radiopharmaceutical use outweighs the risks from fetal exposure to radiation. In these situations, the physician should use discretion and reduce the radiopharmaceutical dose to the lowest possible amount.
Studies have not been done in animals.
FDA Pregnancy Category C.

### Breast-feeding
Tc 99m as sodium pertechnetate is distributed into breast milk. It has been estimated that after a 24-hour discontinuation of breast-feeding, the breast-fed infant's exposure to radiation will be less than 20 mrems after a 20-millicurie dose of sodium pertechnetate Tc 99m. Accordingly, discontinuation of breast-feeding for 24 hours is generally recommended for this radiopharmaceutical. If the patient wishes further guidance concerning her individual circumstances, the activity in breast milk can be measured and the radiation dose to the infant estimated to determine how long discontinuation of breast-feeding is appropriate.

### Pediatrics
Diagnostic studies performed to date using sodium pertechnetate Tc 99m have not demonstrated pediatrics-specific problems that would limit its usefulness in children. When this radiopharmaceutical is used in children, as with other groups of patients, the diagnostic benefit should be judged to outweigh the potential risk of radiation.
For brain or blood pool imaging, potassium perchlorate should be administered prior to sodium pertechnetate Tc 99m, in order to minimize thyroidal uptake.

### Geriatrics
Appropriate studies on the relationship of age to the effects of sodium pertechnetate Tc 99m have not been performed in the geriatric population. However, no geriatrics-specific problems have been documented to date.

### Drug interactions and/or related problems
See *Diagnostic interference*.

### Diagnostic interference
The following have been selected on the basis of their potential clinical significance (possible effect in parentheses where appropriate)—not necessarily inclusive (» = major clinical significance):
With results of *brain imaging*
  Due to other medications
    Antacids, aluminum-containing
      (prior administration of aluminum-containing antacids may decrease uptake of sodium pertechnetate Tc 99m in brain lesions)
    Antineoplastics, especially intrathecally-administered
      (chemotherapeutic neurotoxicity may result in patchy increased brain uptake or localization in ventricles or meninges)
    Corticosteroids, glucocorticoid
      (concurrent use may decrease brain tumor or abscess uptake of sodium pertechnetate Tc 99m because of reduced peritumor edema caused by large doses of the steroid)
    Technetium Tc 99m pyrophosphate
      (brain scan may give either false-positive or false-negative results when performed after a bone scan using technetium Tc 99m pyrophosphate that contains stannous ions; to avoid false results, brain scan may be performed prior to bone scan or with a brain imaging agent other than sodium pertechnetate Tc 99m)

With results of *thyroid uptake tests* and *thyroid imaging*
  Due to other medications
    Antacids, aluminum-containing or
    Amiodarone or
    Antithyroid agents—thioamide derivatives or aromatic preparations or
    Contrast media, iodinated or
    Corticosteroids or
    Goitrogenic foods (e.g., cabbage, turnips) or
    Iodine-containing foods or
    Iodine-containing preparations or
    Iodine-contaminated bromides or
    Iodine, stable or
    Monovalent anions (e.g., perchlorate, thiocyanate) or
    Pyrazolone derivatives, such as oxyphenbutazone and phenylbutazone or
    Salicylates, chronic administration of, or
    Salt, iodized, excessive intake of or
    Thiopental or
    Thyroid blocking agents, such as strong iodine solution, potassium iodide, or potassium perchlorate or
    Thyroid preparations, natural or synthetic
      (may decrease thyroidal uptake of pertechnetate ion)
      (a rebound effect may occur following the sudden withdrawal of antithyroid preparations, resulting in a period of up to 5 days of very high thyroidal uptake)
      (a rebound effect may also occur when discontinuing salicylate therapy, resulting in a period of 3 to 10 days of increased thyroidal uptake)
With results of *salivary gland imaging*
  Due to other medications
    Perchlorate or
    Sodium iodide I 131, therapeutic
      (may decrease salivary uptake of pertechnetate ion)
With results of *gastric mucosa imaging*
  Due to other medications
    Antacids, aluminum-containing
      (prior administration of aluminum-containing antacids may decrease stomach uptake and urinary excretion of sodium pertechnetate Tc 99m and thus interfere with Meckel's diverticula evaluation)
    Perchlorate
      (may decrease gastric uptake of sodium pertechnetate Tc 99m if given prior to imaging of Meckel's diverticulum)
With results of *cardiac blood pool imaging* and *diagnosis of gastrointestinal bleeding* using Tc 99m-labeled red blood cells
  Due to other medications
    Digoxin or
    Doxorubicin or
    Heparin sodium or
    Hydralazine or
    Methyldopa or
    Prazosin or
    Propranolol or
    Quinidine or
    Radiopaque agents, water-soluble organic iodides, with intravascular administration
      (these medications may impair blood pool imaging by decreasing the labeling efficiency of red blood cells)
  Due to medical problems or conditions
    Goiter, toxic diffuse or
    Hyperthyroidism
      (thyroid uptake may be increased)
    Lupus erythematosus
      (labeling of red blood cells may be decreased)
    Transfusion-induced reaction
      (labeling efficiency may be decreased because of red blood cell antibody formation)

### Medical considerations/Contraindications
The medical considerations/contraindications included have been selected on the basis of their potential clinical significance (reasons given in parentheses where appropriate)—not necessarily inclusive (» = major clinical significance).
See also *Diagnostic interference*.

*Risk-benefit should be considered when the following medical problem exists:*
  Sensitivity to the radiopharmaceutical preparation

## Side/Adverse Effects
The following side/adverse effects have been selected on the basis of their potential clinical significance (possible signs and symptoms in parentheses where appropriate)—not necessarily inclusive:

**Those indicating need for medical attention**
Incidence less frequent or rare
 *Allergic reaction* (skin rash, hives, or itching)

## Patient Consultation
As an aid to patient consultation, refer to *Advice for the Patient, Radiopharmaceuticals (Diagnostic)*.
In providing consultation, consider emphasizing the following selected information (» = major clinical significance):

**Description of use**
Actions in the body
 Concentration of pertechnetate Tc 99m in intravascular spaces, in abnormal areas of brain, in thyroid, salivary glands, and stomach tissue allows visualization of these areas
 Distribution in body of injected radioactive red blood cells same as normal red blood cells
 Small amounts of radioactivity used in diagnosis; radiation exposure is low and considered safe

**Before having this test**
» Conditions affecting use, especially:
 Sensitivity to the radiopharmaceutical preparation
 Pregnancy—Sodium pertechnetate Tc 99m crosses placenta; risk to fetus from radiation exposure as opposed to benefit derived from use should be considered
 Breast-feeding—Tc 99m as sodium pertechnetate distributed into breast milk; discontinuation of nursing for 24 hours recommended to decrease possibility of risk to infant from radiation exposure
 Use in children—Possible risk of radiation exposure as opposed to benefit derived from use should be considered

**Preparation for this test**
Special preparatory instructions may be given; patient should inquire in advance
Fasting for 6 hours before administration (oral only)
Fasting for 8 to 12 hours before Meckel's diverticulum imaging

**Precautions after having this test**
Fasting for 2 hours after administration (oral only)

**Side/adverse effects**
Signs of potential side effects, especially allergic reaction

## General Dosing Information
Radiopharmaceuticals are to be administered only by or under the supervision of physicians who have had extensive training in the safe use and handling of radioactive materials and who are authorized by the Nuclear Regulatory Commission (NRC) or the appropriate Agreement State agency, if required, or, outside the U.S., the appropriate authority.

Sodium pertechnetate Tc 99m is usually administered intravenously but may be given orally, except for cystography in which it is instilled into the bladder (see *Sodium Pertechnetate Tc 99m, Mucosal-Local*) and for lacrimal drainage studies in which it is placed on the eye (see *Sodium Pertechnetate Tc 99m, Ophthalmic*).

When sodium pertechnetate Tc 99m is given orally, fasting is recommended for at least 6 hours before and 2 hours after administration.

Prior to the administration of sodium pertechnetate Tc 99m for brain or blood pool imaging, up to 1 gram of pharmaceutical grade potassium perchlorate may be given orally to help block the uptake of Tc 99m into the thyroid gland, salivary glands, choroid plexus, and gastric mucosa. This is especially important in children receiving sodium pertechnetate Tc 99m for brain or blood pool imaging in order to reduce the absorbed radiation dose to the thyroid gland.

Manufacturer's package insert or other appropriate literature should be consulted for optimal times when imaging should be performed.

**Safety considerations for handling this medication**
Improper handling of this radiopharmaceutical may cause radioactive contamination. Guidelines for handling radioactive material have been prepared by scientific, professional, state, federal, and international bodies and are available to the specially qualified and authorized users who have access to radiopharmaceuticals.

## Oral or Parenteral Dosage Forms
Note: Bracketed uses in the *Dosage Forms* section refer to categories of use and/or indications that are not included in U.S. product labeling.

## SODIUM PERTECHNETATE Tc 99m INJECTION USP
**Usual adult and adolescent administered activity**
Vascular disorders or —
 Intravenous, 370 to 1110 megabecquerels (10 to 30 millicuries).
Brain disorders—
 Intravenous or oral, 370 to 740 megabecquerels (10 to 20 millicuries).
Thyroid disorders—
 Intravenous or oral, 37 to 370 megabecquerels (1 to 10 millicuries).
Salivary gland disorders—
 Intravenous, 37 to 185 megabecquerels (1 to 5 millicuries).
Placenta localization—
 Intravenous, 37 to 111 megabecquerels (1 to 3 millicuries).
[Gastrointestinal disorders (Meckel's diverticula)][1]—
 Intravenous, 185 to 555 megabecquerels (5 to 15 millicuries).
 Note: Some investigators have used cimetidine prior to Meckel's imaging to produce a more intense and prolonged uptake of sodium pertechnetate Tc 99m by the gastric mucosa in both the stomach and in Meckel's diverticulum. Cimetidine is thought to work by blocking acid secretion from the mucosa, leading to an increased accumulation of sodium pertechnetate Tc 99m.
 Also, some investigators have used glucagon, with or without pentagastrin, to inhibit intestinal peristalsis and allow pooling of secreted sodium pertechnetate Tc 99m.
[Cardiac disorders][1]—
 Intravenous, 555 to 1295 megabecquerels (15 to 35 millicuries) of Tc 99m-labeled red blood cells.
 Note: For cardiac blood pool imaging, the injection of 0.5 to 2.1 mg of stannous ion 15 to 60 minutes before the administration of sodium pertechnetate Tc 99m injection is necessary to promote the labeling of Tc 99m to red blood cells.
[Gastrointestinal bleeding][1]—
 Intravenous, 740 to 1110 megabecquerels (20 to 30 millicuries) of Tc 99m-labeled red blood cells.

**Usual pediatric administered activity**
Vascular disorders or
Brain disorders—
 Intravenous or oral, 5 to 10 megabecquerels (140 to 280 microcuries) per kg of body weight.
 Note: For radionuclide angiography performed as part of the brain imaging or blood pool procedures, a minimum of 111 to 185 megabecquerels (3 to 5 millicuries) should be used.
Thyroid disorders—
 Intravenous or oral, 2 to 3 megabecquerels (60 to 80 microcuries) per kg of body weight.
[Gastrointestinal disorders (Meckel's diverticula)][1]—
 Intravenous, 1.85 to 3.7 megabecquerels (50 to 100 microcuries) per kg of body weight.

**Usual geriatric administered activity**
See *Usual adult and adolescent administered activity*.

**Strength(s) usually available**
U.S.—
 740 megabecquerels to 3.7 gigabecquerels (20 to 100 millicuries) per mL at time of calibration.
Note: Sodium pertechnetate Tc 99m injection is supplied as a molybdenum Mo 99/technetium Tc 99m generator in sizes of Mo 99 ranging from 30.7 to 614.2 gigabecquerels (830 to 16,600 millicuries); 9.25 to 111 gigabecquerels (250 to 3000 millicuries) [*Ultra-TechneKow FM*]; or 8.3 to 100 gigabecquerels (225 to 2700 millicuries) [*TechneLite*]. Each eluate of the generator should not contain more than the USP limit of 0.15 kilobecquerel of molybdenum Mo 99 per megabecquerel of technetium Tc 99m (0.15 microcurie Mo 99 per millicurie Tc 99m) per administered dose at the time of administration.
Canada—
 Sodium pertechnetate Tc 99m injection is supplied as a molybdenum Mo 99/technetium Tc 99m generator in sizes of Mo 99 ranging from 8.3 to 100 gigabecquerels (225 to 2700 millicuries). Each eluate of the generator should not contain more than the Canadian Regulatory limit of 1.1 kilobecquerels of molybdenum Mo 99 per 37 megabecquerels of technetium Tc 99m (0.03 microcurie Mo 99 per millicurie Tc 99m) per administered dose at the time of administration.

**Packaging and storage**
Store below 40 °C (104 °F), preferably between 15 and 30 °C (59 and 86 °F), unless otherwise specified by manufacturer. Protect from freezing.

**Stability**
Generator eluate does not contain an antimicrobial agent, and thus, should be used within 12 hours from the time of generator elution.

## Note
Caution—Radioactive material.

[1]Not included in Canadian product labeling.

## Selected Bibliography
Campbell CM, Khafagi FA. Insensitivity of Tc 99m pertechnetate for detecting metastases of differentiated thyroid carcinoma. Clin Nucl Med 1990; 15(1): 1–4.

Gupta SM, Luna E, Kingsley S, et al. Detection of gastrointestinal bleeding by radionuclide scintigraphy. Am J Gastroenterol 1984; 79: 26-31.

Revised: 08/19/94

---

**SODIUM PHENYLBUTYRATE**—The *Sodium Phenylbutyrate (Systemic)* monograph is not included in this published version of the USP DI database. Copies of the monograph are available on request from Micromedex, Inc. - Reprint Requests, 6200 S. Syracuse Way, Suite 300, Englewood, CO 80111; telephone (303) 486-6400; telefax (303) 486-6464; Email: USPDI@MDX.COM.

**SODIUM PHOSPHATE**—See *Laxatives (Local)*

---

# SODIUM PHOSPHATE P 32    Systemic

VA CLASSIFICATION (Primary): AN600

Note: For a listing of dosage forms and brand names by country availability, see *Dosage Forms* section(s).

## Category
Antineoplastic.

## Indications
Note: Bracketed information in the *Indications* section refers to uses that are not included in U.S. product labeling.

**Accepted**

Polycythemia rubra vera (treatment)
Leukemia, chronic myelocytic (treatment)
Leukemia, chronic lymphocytic (treatment) and
[Thrombocythemia, essential (treatment)][1]—Sodium phosphate P 32 is indicated for the treatment of polycythemia rubra vera, chronic myelocytic leukemia, chronic lymphocytic leukemia, and essential thrombocythemia. In the treatment of polycythemia vera, sodium phosphate P 32 should be used with adjunctive phlebotomy.

Bone lesions, metastatic (treatment)—Sodium phosphate P 32 is indicated in the palliative treatment of bone pain in selected patients with multiple areas of skeletal metastases from carcinomas of the prostate, lung, and breast.

[1]Not included in Canadian product labeling.

## Physical Properties
**Nuclear Data**

| Radionuclide (half-life) | Mode of decay | Mean energy (keV) | Mean number of emissions/ disintegration |
|---|---|---|---|
| P 32 (14.3 days) | Beta emission | 695 | 1 |

## Pharmacology/Pharmacokinetics
**Mechanism of action/Effect**

Antineoplastic—

Polycythemia vera: Phosphorus (as phosphate) incorporates into the deoxyribonucleic acid (DNA), and is therefore concentrated to a very high degree in rapidly proliferating hematopoietic cells. Subsequent radiation damage to these cells halts their reproduction.

Metastatic bone lesions: Sodium phosphate P 32 concentrates in areas of rapid bone formation associated with metastatic tumor localized to bone. The beta emissions of sodium phosphate P 32 result in localized therapeutic radiation and destruction of tumor cells localized to the bone matrix.

**Distribution**

Diffuses rapidly from circulating blood into extra- and intracellular fluids following intravenous administration; concentrates mostly in bone marrow, liver, and spleen.

**Half-life**

Biological half-life—Whole body: 39 days (mean).

**Radiation dosimetry**

| | Estimated absorbed radiation dose* ||
|---|---|---|
| Organ | mGy/MBq | rad/mCi |
| Red marrow | 11.00 | 40.74 |
| Bone surfaces | 11.00 | 40.74 |
| Breast | 0.92 | 3.41 |
| Adrenals | 0.74 | 2.74 |
| Bladder wall | 0.74 | 2.74 |
| Kidneys | 0.74 | 2.74 |
| Large intestine wall (upper) | 0.74 | 2.74 |
| Large intestine wall (lower) | 0.74 | 2.74 |
| Liver | 0.74 | 2.74 |
| Lungs | 0.74 | 2.74 |
| Ovaries | 0.74 | 2.74 |
| Pancreas | 0.74 | 2.74 |
| Spleen | 0.74 | 2.74 |
| Small intestine | 0.74 | 2.74 |
| Stomach wall | 0.74 | 2.74 |
| Testes | 0.74 | 2.74 |
| Thyroid | 0.74 | 2.74 |
| Uterus | 0.74 | 2.74 |
| Other tissue | 0.74 | 2.74 |

Effective dose: 2.2 mSv/MBq (8.14 rem/mCi)

*For adults; intravenous injection. Data based on the International Commission on Radiological Protection (ICRP) Publication 53—Radiation dose to patients from radiopharmaceuticals.

**Elimination**

Primarily renal; a very small percentage in the feces. In normal patients, 5 to 10% eliminated in the urine within 24 hours and about 20% eliminated within a week.

Note: Fecal excretion increases if sodium phosphate P 32 is administered orally.

## Precautions to Consider
**Carcinogenicity/Mutagenicity**

Long-term animal studies to evaluate carcinogenic or mutagenic potential of sodium phosphate P 32 have not been performed.

**Pregnancy/Reproduction**

Pregnancy—Studies have not been done with sodium phosphate P 32 in humans. Radiopharmaceuticals are generally not recommended for therapeutic use during pregnancy because of the risk to the fetus from radiation exposure.

To avoid the possibility of fetal exposure to radiation, in those circumstances where the patient's pregnancy status is uncertain, a pregnancy test will help to prevent inadvertent administration of this preparation during pregnancy.

Studies have not been done in animals.

FDA Pregnancy Category C.

**Breast-feeding**

Sodium phosphate P 32 may be distributed into breast milk. Because of the potential risk to the infant from radiation exposure, breast-feeding should be discontinued.

**Pediatrics**

Although sodium phosphate P 32 is used in children, there have been no specific studies evaluating its safety and efficacy in children. When this radiopharmaceutical is used in children, the therapeutic benefit should be judged to outweigh the potential risk of radiation.

**Geriatrics**
Geriatric patients may be more sensitive to the effects of radiation; smaller doses and longer intervals between doses are recommended.

**Drug interactions and/or related problems**
The following drug interactions and/or related problems have been selected on the basis of their potential clinical significance (possible mechanism in parentheses where appropriate)—not necessarily inclusive (» = major clinical significance):

Bone marrow depressants, other (See *Appendix II*)
(concurrent use may increase the bone marrow depressant effects of these medications and radiation therapy; dosage reduction of other bone marrow depressant medication may be required)

**Laboratory value alterations**
The following have been selected on the basis of their potential clinical significance (possible effect in parentheses where appropriate)—not necessarily inclusive (» = major clinical significance):

With physiology/laboratory test values
Blood urea nitrogen (BUN)
Calcium, serum
(concentrations may be increased)

**Medical considerations/Contraindications**
The medical considerations/contraindications included have been selected on the basis of their potential clinical significance (reasons given in parentheses where appropriate)—not necessarily inclusive (» = major clinical significance).

*Except under special circumstances, this medication should not be used when the following medical problems exist:*

» Bone metastases with leukocyte count less than 5,000 per microliter and platelet count less than 100,000 per microliter
» Myelocytic leukemia, chronic, with leukocyte count less than 20,000 per microliter

*Risk-benefit must be considered when the following medical problem exists:*

Sensitivity to the radiopharmaceutical preparation

**Patient monitoring**
The following may be especially important in patient monitoring (other tests may be warranted in some patients, depending on condition; » = major clinical significance):

Blood studies, including hemoglobin determinations and leukocyte, erythrocyte, and platelet counts, and
Bone marrow studies
(recommended prior to therapy and at regular intervals during and after therapy)

## Side/Adverse Effects

Note: Leukopenia, thrombocytopenia, and anemia may occur following administration of large therapeutic doses. Also, at present, about 15% of patients with polycythemia vera may develop acute leukemia following therapy with sodium phosphate P 32.

In patients pretreated with testosterone, a transient increase in bone pain has been reported.

**Those indicating need for medical attention**
Incidence more frequent
*Following treatment of bone pain*
**Pancytopenia** (diarrhea; fever; nausea; vomiting)

## Patient Consultation

As an aid to patient consultation, refer to *Advice for the Patient, Sodium Phosphate P 32 (Therapeutic)*.
In providing consultation, consider emphasizing the following selected information (» = major clinical significance):

**Description of use**
*Action in the body*
Incorporation of phosphate P 32 into red cells of bone marrow causing reduction in their proliferation
Incorporation of phosphate P 32 into rapidly forming bone matrix associated with metastatic tumors localized to bone; beta emissions result in tumor cell destruction

**Before using this medication**
» Conditions affecting use, especially:
Sensitivity to the radiopharmaceutical preparation
Pregnancy—Risk to fetus from radiation exposure
Breast-feeding—Distributed into breast milk; cessation of nursing recommended because of risk to infant from radiation exposure
Use in children—Risk from radiation exposure as opposed to benefit derived from use should be considered

**Proper use of this medication**
Special preparatory instructions may apply; patient should inquire in advance

**Side/adverse effects**
Signs of potential side effects, especially pancytopenia; and leukopenia, thrombocytopenia, and anemia (with large therapeutic doses)

## General Dosing Information

Radiopharmaceuticals are to be administered only by or under the supervision of physicians who have had extensive training in the safe use and handling of radioactive materials and who are authorized by the Nuclear Regulatory Commission (NRC) or the appropriate Agreement State agency, if required, or, outside the U.S., the appropriate authority.

Sodium phosphate P 32 solution should not be used for intracavitary therapy (e.g., intraperitoneal treatment of metastasis of ovarian carcinoma).

Visual inspection of the injection is recommended to avoid the accidental intravenous administration of chromic phosphate P 32. Sodium phosphate P 32 is a clear, colorless solution, whereas chromic phosphate P 32 is a green, cloudy liquid intended for intracavitary therapy.

The dosage of sodium phosphate P 32 in the treatment of polycythemia vera is dependent on the stage of the disease, the patient's surface area or body weight, and the erythrocyte, leukocyte, and platelet counts.

The initial dose of sodium phosphate P 32 in the treatment of chronic leukemia is calculated on the basis of the leukocyte count. Subsequent doses are based upon the response of the patient.

A phlebotomy should be performed in patients with polycythemia vera before or after the administration of sodium phosphate P 32 to maintain the hematocrit at normal levels during the induction period.

**Safety considerations for handling this radiopharmaceutical**
Improper handling of this radiopharmaceutical may cause radioactive contamination. Guidelines for handling radioactive material have been prepared by scientific, professional, state, federal, and international bodies and are available to the specially qualified and authorized users who have access to radiopharmaceuticals.

## Parenteral Dosage Forms

### SODIUM PHOSPHATE P 32 SOLUTION USP

**Usual adult and adolescent administered activity**
Antineoplastic—
Polycythemia rubra vera—
Intravenous, 111 to 185 megabecquerels (3 to 5 millicuries); may be repeated in twelve weeks if needed.
Note: An initial dose of 85.1 megabecquerels (2.3 millicuries) per square meter of body surface is usually recommended (not to exceed 185 megabecquerels [5 millicuries]). Subsequent doses are based on patient response.
Chronic leukemia—
Intravenous, 37 to 111 megabecquerels (1 to 3 millicuries).
Metastatic bone lesions—
One type of regimen used is as follows—Intravenous, 370 to 777 megabecquerels (10 to 21 millicuries) given over a three- to four-week period (e.g., 111 megabecquerels [3 millicuries] given the first day, followed by two 74-megabecquerel [2-millicurie] doses given every other day during the first week; two 74-megabecquerel [2-millicurie] doses given during the second and third week; thereafter, 37 megabecquerels [1 millicurie] given two times a week until a total of 777 megabecquerels [21 millicuries] is administered).

**Usual pediatric administered activity**
Dosage has not been established.

**Usual geriatric administered activity**
See *Usual adult and adolescent administered activity*.
Note: Geriatric patients should receive smaller doses with longer intervals between doses.

**Strength(s) usually available**
U.S.—
25 megabecquerels (0.67 millicurie) per mL at time of calibration (Rx) [GENERIC].
Canada—
Provided in various concentrations in multiple-dose vial (Rx) [GENERIC].

## Sodium Phosphate P 32 (Systemic)

**Packaging and storage**
Store below 40 °C (104 °F), preferably between 15 and 30 °C (59 and 86 °F), unless otherwise specified by manufacturer. Protect from freezing.

**Note**
Caution—Radioactive material.
Not for intracavitary use.

Revised: 07/16/93
Interim revision: 08/02/94

**SODIUM PHOSPHATES**—See *Laxatives (Local)*; *Phosphates (Systemic)*

# SODIUM POLYSTYRENE SULFONATE  Local

VA CLASSIFICATION (Primary): AD400
Commonly used brand name(s): *K-Exit*; *Kayexalate*; *Kionex*; *PMS-Sodium Polystyrene Sulfonate*; *SPS Suspension*.

Note: For a listing of dosage forms and brand names by country availability, see *Dosage Forms* section(s).

## Category
Antihyperkalemic.

## Indications
**Accepted**
Hyperkalemia (treatment)—Sodium polystyrene sulfonate is indicated in the treatment of hyperkalemia associated with oliguria or anuria due to acute renal failure.

## Pharmacology/Pharmacokinetics
**Mechanism of action/Effect**
Antihyperkalemic—In the intestine (mostly the large intestine), sodium ions are released and are replaced by potassium and other cations before the resin is passed from the body.

**Other actions/effects**
Sodium polystyrene sulfonate also exchanges small amounts of other cations such as magnesium and calcium.

**Absorption**
Not absorbed from gastrointestinal tract; exchanges sodium for potassium and is excreted from the intestine.

**Onset of action**
Hours to days; therefore, other measures such as dialysis may be necessary in emergency situations.

## Precautions to Consider
**Carcinogenicity/Mutagenicity**
Studies have not been done to evaluate the carcinogenic or mutagenic potential of sodium polystyrene sulfonate.

**Pregnancy/Reproduction**
Pregnancy—Studies have not been done in humans.
Studies have not been done in animals.
FDA Pregnancy Category C.

**Breast-feeding**
It is not known whether sodium polystyrene sulfonate is distributed into breast milk.

**Pediatrics**
Appropriate studies on the relationship of age to the effects of sodium polystyrene sulfonate have not been performed in the pediatric population. However, pediatrics-specific problems that would limit the usefulness of this medication in children are not expected.

**Geriatrics**
Although appropriate studies on the relationship of age to the effects of sodium polysytrene sulfonate have not been performed in the geriatric population, the elderly may be more likely to develop fecal impaction.

**Drug interactions and/or related problems**
The following drug interactions and/or related problems have been selected on the basis of their potential clinical significance (possible mechanism in parentheses where appropriate)—not necessarily inclusive (» = major clinical significance):

Note: Combinations containing any of the following medications, depending on the amount present, may also interact with this medication.

» Antacids or
» Laxatives
   (sodium polystyrene sulfonate may bind with magnesium or calcium found in nonsystemic antacids and laxatives, preventing neutralization of bicarbonate ions and leading to systemic alkalosis that may be severe; concurrent use is not recommended, although the risk may be less with rectal administration of the resin)

Diuretics, potassium-sparing or
Potassium supplements
   (sodium polystyrene sulfonate reduces serum potassium concentrations by replacing potassium with sodium; fluid retention may occur in some patients because of the increased sodium intake)

**Laboratory value alterations**
The following have been selected on the basis of their potential clinical significance (possible effect in parentheses where appropriate)—not necessarily inclusive (» = major clinical significance):

With physiology/laboratory test values
Calcium and
Magnesium
   (serum concentrations may be decreased since sodium polystyrene sulfonate exchanges for cations in addition to potassium)

**Medical considerations/Contraindications**
The medical considerations/contraindications included have been selected on the basis of their potential clinical significance (reasons given in parentheses where appropriate)—not necessarily inclusive (» = major clinical significance).

*Risk-benefit should be considered when the following medical problems exist:*

Edematous conditions, such as:
   Congestive heart failure, severe or
   Hypertension, severe
      (may require compensatory restriction of sodium intake from other sources or use of dialysis instead of sodium polystyrene sulfonate)

Sensitivity to sodium polystyrene sulfonate

**Patient monitoring**
The following may be especially important in patient monitoring (other tests may be warranted in some patients, depending on condition; » = major clinical significance):

Bicarbonate concentrations, serum
   (determinations recommended once a week during chronic therapy, especially if patient is also receiving antacids or laxatives)

Calcium concentrations, serum or
Magnesium concentrations, serum
   (determinations recommended in patients receiving sodium polystyrene sulfonate for longer than 3 days)

Electrocardiogram (ECG)
   (may be useful in some patients)

» Potassium concentrations, serum
   (determinations recommended at least once a day or as necessary to monitor effectiveness of treatment)

## Side/Adverse Effects
Note: Cases of colonic necrosis have been reported and may have occurred because cleansing enemas were not administered before and after treatment with sodium polystyrene sulfonate enemas. However, some clinicians think that colonic necrosis may be caused by using sorbitol as a vehicle for sodium polystyrene sulfonate.

The following side/adverse effects have been selected on the basis of their potential clinical significance (possible signs and symptoms in parentheses where appropriate)—not necessarily inclusive:

**Those indicating need for medical attention**
Incidence less frequent—dose-related
  *Fecal impaction* (severe stomach pain with nausea and vomiting); *hypocalcemia* (abdominal and muscle cramps); *hypokalemia* (confusion with irritability; delayed thought processes; irregular heartbeat; severe muscle weakness); *sodium retention* (decrease in urination; swelling of hands, feet, or lower legs; weight gain)

**Those indicating need for medical attention only if they continue or are bothersome**
Incidence more frequent—especially with large doses
  *Constipation; loss of appetite; nausea or vomiting*

## General Dosing Information

Exchange efficiency of sodium polystyrene sulfonate resin is approximately 33%; although each gram contains about 4.1 mEq (mmol) of sodium, 15 grams of resin bind about 46.5 mEq (mmol) of potassium in exchange for the release of an equal amount of sodium. However, these values are variable and electrolyte balance must be monitored to determine dosage and duration of therapy.

Treatment with sodium polystyrene sulfonate may be discontinued when the serum potassium concentrations have been reduced to 4 to 5 mEq (mmol) per liter.

**For oral use**
Sodium Polystyrene Sulfonate USP is usually mixed with sorbitol. However, to improve palatability, Sodium Polystyrene Sulfonate USP may be mixed with food or a beverage, with the sorbitol given in addition. Alternate vehicles for mixing include warm water, 1% methylcellulose, or 5 to 10% dextrose in water.

To prevent constipation, patients should be treated with oral 70% sorbitol syrup, 10 to 20 mL every 2 hours as needed to produce one or two watery stools a day, or a mild laxative. This will also hasten elimination of potassium and help prevent fecal impaction.

**For rectal use**
The rectal route is recommended when the patient is vomiting or is restricted from taking anything by mouth (NPO), or when there are upper gastrointestinal tract problems.

After a cleansing enema, the resin suspension is introduced into the rectum via a Foley catheter, and is gently agitated during administration to keep the particles in suspension; administration is followed by flushing with 50 to 100 mL of fluid. The enema is retained as long as possible (anywhere from 30 to 45 minutes to 4 to 10 hours) and is followed by a non–sodium-containing cleansing enema. To prevent back leakage, elevation of the hips on pillows or a knee-chest position may be necessary. In a child, the buttocks may be taped together.

Note: Cases of colonic necrosis have been reported and may have occurred because cleansing enemas were not administered before and after treatment with sodium polystyrene sulfonate enemas. However, some clinicians think that colonic necrosis may be caused by using sorbitol as a vehicle for sodium polystyrene sulfonate.

## Oral/Rectal Dosage Forms

### SODIUM POLYSTYRENE SULFONATE SUSPENSION USP

**Usual adult dose**
Antihyperkalemic—
  Oral, 15 grams one to four times a day, up to 40 grams four times a day.
  Note: A dose of 15 grams is approximately equivalent to 4 *level* tablespoonfuls.
  Rectal, 25 to 100 grams as needed, administered as a retention enema or inserted into the rectum in a dialysis bag to facilitate recovery. Sodium polystyrene sulfonate is less effective with rectal administration than by the oral route.

**Usual pediatric dose**
Antihyperkalemic—
  Oral, usually 1 gram per kg of body weight per dose as needed to correct hyperkalemia.
  Rectal, 1 gram per kg of body weight per dose, administered as a retention enema or inserted into the rectum in a dialysis bag to facilitate recovery. Sodium polystyrene sulfonate is less effective with rectal administration than by the oral route.

**Strength(s) usually available**
U.S.—
  250 mg per mL (Rx) [*SPS Suspension* [GENERIC (Roxane—sorbitol 235 mg)].
Canada—
  250 mg per mL (Rx) [*PMS-Sodium Polystyrene Sulfonate* (sorbitol 235 mg)].

**Packaging and storage**
Store below 40 °C (104 °F), preferably between 15 and 30 °C (59 and 86 °F), unless otherwise specified by manufacturer. Store in a well-closed container. Protect from freezing.

**Stability**
Heating may alter the exchange properties of the resin.

**Auxiliary labeling**
• Shake well before using.

### SODIUM POLYSTYRENE SULFONATE (FOR SUSPENSION) USP

**Usual adult dose**
Antihyperkalemic—
  Oral, 15 grams one to four times a day, up to 40 grams four times a day.
  Note: A dose of 15 grams is approximately equivalent to 4 *level* teaspoonfuls.
  Rectal, 25 to 100 grams as needed, administered as a retention enema or inserted into the rectum in a dialysis bag to facilitate recovery. Sodium polystyrene sulfonate is less effective with rectal administration than by the oral route.

**Usual pediatric dose**
See *Sodium Polystyrene Sulfonate Suspension USP*.

**Strength(s) usually available**
U.S.—
  3.5 grams per level teaspoonful (Rx) [*Kayexalate; Kionex* [GENERIC].
Canada—
  3.5 grams per level teaspoonful (Rx) [*Kayexalate; K-Exit; PMS-Sodium Polystyrene Sulfonate*].

**Packaging and storage**
Store below 40 °C (104 °F), preferably between 15 and 30 °C (59 and 86 °F), unless otherwise specified by manufacturer. Store in a well-closed container.

**Preparation of dosage form**
To facilitate and hasten action and prevent constipation, Sodium Polystyrene Sulfonate USP should be suspended in 3 to 4 mL of 70% sorbitol syrup (which acts as an osmotic cathartic) per gram of resin. The resin also may be mixed with water or a diet appropriate for a patient with renal failure and administered orally through a plastic tube.

For rectal administration, Sodium Polystyrene Sulfonate USP is suspended in 100 to 200 mL of an aqueous vehicle (for example, 25% sorbitol, 1% methylcellulose, or 10% dextrose). Care should be taken that the paste is not too thick because it will be less effective.

**Stability**
The suspension should be freshly prepared and used within 24 hours. Heating may alter the exchange properties of the resin.

**Auxiliary labeling**
• Shake well before using.

Revised: 08/15/95

## SODIUM SALICYLATE—See *Salicylates (Systemic)*

## SODIUM THIOSULFATE

The *Sodium Thiosulfate (Systemic)* monograph is not included in this published version of the USP DI database. Copies of the monograph are available on request from Micromedex, Inc. - Reprint Requests, 6200 S. Syracuse Way, Suite 300, Englewood, CO 80111; telephone (303) 486-6400; telefax (303) 486-6464; Email: USPDI@MDX.COM.

## SOMATREM—See *Growth Hormone (Systemic)*

## SOMATROPIN RECOMBINANT—See *Growth Hormone (Systemic)*

**SOTALOL**—See *Beta-adrenergic Blocking Agents (Systemic)*

# SPARFLOXACIN Systemic—INTRODUCTORY VERSION

VA CLASSIFICATION (Primary): AM402
Commonly used brand name(s): *Zagam*.
Note: For a listing of dosage forms and brand names by country availability, see *Dosage Forms* section(s).

## Category
Antibacterial (systemic).

## Indications

**Accepted**

Bronchitis, bacterial exacerbations (treatment)—Sparfloxacin is indicated in the treatment of bacterial exacerbations of bronchitis caused by *Chlamydia pneumoniae*, *Enterobacter cloacae*, *Haemophilus influenzae*, *Haemophilus parainfluenzae*, *Klebsiella pneumoniae*, *Moraxella catarrhalis*, *Staphylococcus aureus*, or *Streptococcus pneumoniae*.

Pneumonia, community-acquired (treatment)—Sparfloxacin is indicated in the treatment of community-acquired pneumonia caused by *C. pneumoniae*, *H. influenzae*, *H. parainfluenzae*, *M. catarrhalis*, *Mycoplasma pneumoniae*, or *S. pneumoniae*.

## Pharmacology/Pharmacokinetics

**Physicochemical characteristics**
Chemical group—Fluoroquinolone.
Molecular weight—392.41.

**Mechanism of action/Effect**
Bactericidal; sparfloxacin acts intracellularly by inhibiting DNA gyrase. DNA gyrase is an essential bacterial enzyme that controls DNA topology and assists in DNA replication, repair, deactivation, and transcription.

**Absorption**
Well absorbed after oral administration. Bioavailability is approximately 92%.

**Distribution**
Widely distributed into body fluids and tissues. Concentrations in lower respiratory tract tissues and fluids are three to six times higher than the corresponding plasma concentrations.
$Vol_D$—Approximately 3.9 liters per kg.

**Protein binding**
Moderate (approximately 45%).

**Biotransformation**
Hepatic; metabolized primarily by phase II glucuronidation to form a glucuronide conjugate. Metabolism does not utilize or interfere with the cytochrome P450 enzyme system.

**Half-life**
Elimination—Mean, approximately 20 hours (range, 16 to 30 hours).

**Time to peak concentration**
Approximately 4 hours (range, 3 to 6 hours).

**Peak serum concentration**
Approximately 1.3 mcg per mL (mcg/mL) after an initial 400-mg loading dose.
Approximately 1.1 mcg/mL at steady-state after administration of 200 mg every 24 hours.

**Elimination**
Fecal—50%.
Renal—50%; approximately 10% of an orally administered dose is excreted in the urine unchanged.
In dialysis—It is not known whether sparfloxacin is removed by dialysis.

## Precautions to Consider

**Cross-sensitivity and/or related problems**
Patients allergic to one fluoroquinolone or other chemically related quinolone derivatives (e.g., cinoxacin, nalidixic acid) may be allergic to other fluoroquinolones also.

**Carcinogenicity**
Sparfloxacin was not carcinogenic in mice or rats that were administered 3.5 and 6.2 times, respectively, the maximum human dose (400 mg per day) based on a mg per square meter of body surface area basis (mg/m$^2$) for 104 weeks. These doses correspond to plasma concentrations approximately equal to (in mice) and 2.2 times greater than (in rats) maximum human plasma concentrations.

**Mutagenicity**
Sparfloxacin was not mutagenic in *Salmonella typhimurium* TA98, TA100, TA1535, or TA1537, in *Escherichia coli* strain WP2 uvrA, or in Chinese hamster lung cells. Sparfloxacin and other fluoroquinolones have been shown to be mutagenic in *S. typhimurium* strain TA102 and to induce DNA repair in *E. coli*, possibly due to the inhibition of bacterial DNA gyrase. Sparfloxacin induced chromosomal aberrations in Chinese hamster lung cells *in vitro* at cytotoxic concentrations; however, no increase in chromosomal aberrations or micronuclei in bone marrow cells was observed after sparfloxacin was administered orally to mice.

**Pregnancy/Reproduction**
Fertility—Sparfloxacin had no effect on the fertility or reproductive performance of male or female rats at oral doses up to 15.4 times the maximum recommended human dose (400 mg), on a mg/m$^2$ basis.

Pregnancy—Adequate and well-controlled studies in humans have not been done. Since sparfloxacin has been shown to cause arthropathy in immature animals, use is recommended in pregnancy only if the potential benefit to the mother outweighs the potential risk to the fetus.

Reproduction studies performed in rats, rabbits, and monkeys at oral doses 6.2, 4.4, and 2.6 times higher than the maximum recommended human dose, respectively, on a mg/m$^2$ basis, did not show evidence of teratogenic effects. At these doses, sparfloxacin produced clear evidence of maternal toxicity in rabbits and in monkeys, and slight evidence of maternal toxicity in rats. When administered to pregnant rats at clearly defined maternally toxic doses, sparfloxacin induced a dose-dependent increase in the incidence of ventricular septal defects in fetuses. Among the three species tested, this effect was specific to the rat.

FDA Pregnancy Category C.

**Breast-feeding**
Sparfloxacin is distributed into breast milk. Because of the potential for serious adverse effects in nursing infants, a decision should be made whether to avoid nursing or to discontinue taking sparfloxacin.

**Pediatrics**
Safety and efficacy have not been established in patients up to 18 years of age. Fluoroquinolones have been shown to cause arthropathy and osteochondrosis in immature animals of several species.

**Geriatrics**
Appropriate studies performed to date have not demonstrated geriatrics-specific problems that would limit the usefulness of sparfloxacin in the elderly. However, elderly patients are more likely to have age-related renal function impairment, which may require adjustment of dosage in patients receiving sparfloxacin.

**Drug interactions and/or related problems**
The following drug interactions and/or related problems have been selected on the basis of their potential clinical significance (possible mechanism in parentheses where appropriate)—not necessarily inclusive (» = major clinical significance):

Note: Unlike other fluoroquinolones, sparfloxacin does not alter the pharmacokinetics of cimetidine, digoxin, probenecid, theophylline or other methylxanthines, or warfarin.

Combinations containing any of the following medications, depending on the amount present, may also interact with this medication.

» Amiodarone or
» Astemizole or
» Cisapride or
» Disopyramide or
» Erythromycin or
» Pentamidine or
» Phenothiazines or
» Terfenadine or
» Tricyclic antidepressants or
» Other medications reported to prolong the QTc interval
(concurrent use of sparfloxacin with amiodarone and disopyramide has resulted in torsades de pointes; concurrent use of sparfloxacin with amiodarone, astemizole, cisapride, disopyramide, erythromycin, pentamidine, phenothiazines, terfenadine, tricyclic antidepres-

sants, or any other QTc-prolonging medication reported to cause torsades de pointes is contraindicated)
- » Antacids, aluminum-, calcium-, and/or magnesium-containing or
- » Ferrous sulfate or
- » Sucralfate or
  Zinc
    (antacids, ferrous sulfate, sucralfate, and zinc may reduce absorption of sparfloxacin by chelation, resulting in lower serum and urine concentrations; therefore, concurrent use is not recommended; it is recommended that sparfloxacin be taken at least 4 hours after any of these medications)

**Laboratory value alterations**
The following have been selected on the basis of their potential clinical significance (possible effect in parentheses where appropriate)—not necessarily inclusive (» = major clinical significance):
With diagnostic test results
  *Mycobacterium tuberculosis* culture
    (sparfloxacin may produce a false-negative culture result for *M. tuberculosis* by suppressing mycobacterial growth)

With physiology/laboratory test values
  Alanine aminotransferase (ALT [SGPT]) and
  Alkaline phosphatase and
  Aspartate aminotransferase (AST [SGOT])
    (serum values may be increased)
  White blood cells
    (count may be increased)

**Medical considerations/Contraindications**
The medical considerations/contraindications included have been selected on the basis of their potential clinical significance (reasons given in parentheses where appropriate)—not necessarily inclusive (» = major clinical significance).

*Except under special circumstances, this medication should not be used when the following medical problems exist:*
- » Photosensitivity, history of
    (moderate to severe phototoxic reactions have occurred in patients exposed to direct or indirect sunlight or to artificial ultraviolet light during or following sparfloxacin treatment; these reactions also have occurred in patients exposed to shaded or diffuse light, including exposure through glass or during cloudy weather; sparfloxacin should not be used in patients with a history of photosensitivity or whose lifestyle or employment will not permit compliance with the required safety precautions)
- » Previous allergic reaction to fluoroquinolones or other chemically related quinolone derivatives
- » QTc prolongation
    (sparfloxacin has been found to increase the QTc interval, predisposing patients with QTc prolongation to the development of torsades de pointes)

*Risk-benefit should be considered when the following medical problems exist:*
- » Cardiovascular conditions predisposing the patient to proarrhythmic conditions
    (sparfloxacin is not recommended in patients with cardiovascular conditions predisposing the patient to proarrhythmic conditions, such as hypokalemia, significant bradycardia, congestive heart failure, myocardial ischemia, and atrial fibrillation)
  Central nervous system (CNS) disorders, including cerebral arteriosclerosis or epilepsy
    (sparfloxacin may cause CNS stimulation or toxicity, increasing the risk of seizures in patients with these conditions)
- » Renal function impairment
    (sparfloxacin is excreted renally; it is recommended that patients with a creatinine clearance of less than 50 mL per minute receive a reduced dose of sparfloxacin)

## Side/Adverse Effects

Note: Sparfloxacin has been found to increase the QTc interval in healthy volunteers. After a single 400-mg loading dose, a mean increase in the QTc interval of 11 milliseconds in 2.9% of subjects was observed; at steady state, the mean increase was 7 milliseconds in 1.9% of subjects. In clinical trials with 1489 patients, the mean prolongation was 10 milliseconds in 2.5% of patients; 0.7% had a QTc interval greater than 500 milliseconds; however, no arrhythmias were observed. The magnitude of this prolongation does not increase with repeated administration, and the QTc interval returns to baseline within 48 hours of the last dose.

Moderate to severe phototoxic reactions have occurred in patients exposed to direct or indirect sunlight, or to artificial ultraviolet light, during or following sparfloxacin treatment; these reactions also have occurred in patients exposed to shaded or diffuse light, including exposure through glass or during cloudy weather. Phototoxic reactions have occurred with and without the use of sunscreens or sunblocks and have occurred after a single dose of sparfloxacin. Some sunscreen products that block UVA spectrum wavelengths (those containing the active ingredients octocrylene or Parsol® 1789) can moderate the phototoxic effects; however, many over-the-counter sunscreens do not provide adequate UVA protection. The overall incidence of phototoxicity was 7.9% in clinical trials, with 4.1% of the reactions defined as mild, 3.3% as moderate, and 0.6% as severe. In rare cases, reactions recurred up to several weeks after stopping sparfloxacin therapy. Patients should discontinue sparfloxacin at the first sign or symptom of phototoxicity. Sparfloxacin should not be used in patients with a history of photosensitivity or whose lifestyle or employment will not permit compliance with the required safety precautions.

There have been reports of ruptures of the tendons in the shoulder or hand, or of the Achilles tendon, requiring surgical repair or resulting in prolonged disability, in patients taking sparfloxacin and other fluoroquinolones. Patients should discontinue sparfloxacin if they experience pain, inflammation, or rupture of a tendon. They should rest and refrain from exercise until the diagnosis of tendinitis or tendon rupture has been excluded. Tendon rupture can occur at any time during or after sparfloxacin therapy.

The following side/adverse effects have been selected on the basis of their potential clinical significance (possible signs and symptoms in parentheses where appropriate)—not necessarily inclusive:

**Those indicating need for medical attention**
Incidence more frequent
  *Phototoxicity* (blisters; itching; rash; redness; sensation of skin burning; swelling)
Incidence less frequent
  *QTc prolongation*
Incidence rare
  *CNS stimulation* (acute psychosis; agitation; confusion; hallucinations; tremors); **hypersensitivity reactions** (skin rash, itching, or redness); **pseudomembranous colitis** (abdominal or stomach cramps and pain, severe; abdominal tenderness; diarrhea, watery and severe, which may also be bloody; fever); *tendinitis or tendon rupture* (pain, inflammation, or swelling in calves, shoulders, or hands)

**Those indicating need for medical attention only if they continue or are bothersome**
Incidence less frequent
  *CNS effects* (dizziness; drowsiness; headache; lightheadedness; nervousness; trouble in sleeping); **gastrointestinal effects** (abdominal or stomach pain or discomfort; diarrhea; nausea; vomiting); *taste perversion* (changes in sense of taste); *vaginal candidiasis* (vaginal itching and discharge)

**Those indicating possible pseudomembranous colitis and the need for medical attention if they occur after medication is discontinued**
  *Abdominal or stomach cramps and pain, severe; abdominal tenderness; diarrhea, watery and severe, which may also be bloody; fever*

## Overdose

There is no known antidote for sparfloxacin overdose. It is not known whether sparfloxacin is removed by dialysis.

No deaths occurred within a 14-day observation period after administration of up to 5000 mg per kg of body weight (mg/kg) in mice and rats, or up to 600 mg/kg in dogs. Clinical signs observed included inactivity in mice and dogs; diarrhea in mice and rats; and vomiting, salivation, and tremors in dogs.

For more information on the management of overdose or unintentional ingestion, **contact a Poison Control Center** (see *Poison Control Center Listing*).

**Treatment of overdose**
Monitoring—Electrocardiogram (ECG) monitoring is recommended due to possible QTc prolongation.

Supportive care—The patient should avoid sun exposure for 5 days. Patients in whom intentional overdose is confirmed or suspected should be referred for psychiatric consultation.

## Patient Consultation

As an aid to patient consultation, refer to *Advice for the Patient, Sparfloxacin (Systemic)—Introductory Version*.

## 2622  Sparfloxacin (Systemic)—Introductory Version

In providing consultation, consider emphasizing the following selected information (» = major clinical significance):

**Before using this medication**
» Conditions affecting use, especially:
  Allergy to fluoroquinolones or other quinolone derivatives
  Pregnancy—Sparfloxacin is recommended for use during pregnancy only if the potential benefit to the mother outweighs the potential risk to the fetus because sparfloxacin has been shown to cause arthropathy in immature animals
  Breast-feeding—Sparfloxacin is distributed into breast milk; caution should be exercised in making the decision whether to breast-feed, since sparfloxacin has been shown to cause arthropathy in immature animals
  Use in children—Safety and efficacy have not been established in children up to 18 years of age because sparfloxacin has been shown to cause arthropathy in immature animals
  Other medications, especially amiodarone; aluminum-, calcium-, and/or magnesium-containing antacids; astemizole; cisapride; disopyramide; erythromycin; ferrous sulfate; other medications that prolong the QTc interval; pentamidine; phenothiazines; sucralfate; terfenadine; or tricyclic antidepressants
  Other medical problems, especially cardiovascular conditions that predispose the patient to proarrhythmic conditions, photosensitivity reactions (history of), QTc prolongation, or renal function impairment

**Proper use of this medication**
» Sparfloxacin may be taken with food, milk, or caffeine-containing products
  Importance of maintaining adequate fluid intake
» Importance of not missing doses, and taking at evenly spaced times
» Proper dosing
  Missed dose: Taking as soon as possible; not taking if almost time for next dose; not doubling doses
» Proper storage

**Precautions while using this medication**
  Checking with physician if no improvement within a few days
» Avoiding concurrent use of antacids, ferrous sulfate, sucralfate, or zinc and sparfloxacin; taking these products at least 4 hours after administration of sparfloxacin
*Possible phototoxicity reactions*
» Avoiding exposure to direct or indirect sunlight and to artificial ultraviolet light (e.g., sunlamps) during treatment, and for 5 days after therapy
» Discontinuing sparfloxacin at the first sign or symptom of phototoxicity, such as blistering, itching, rash, redness, sensation of skin burning, or swelling
» If phototoxicity has occurred, avoiding further sunlight and artificial light until the phototoxicity reaction has been resolved, or for 5 days, whichever is longer
» Discontinuing sparfloxacin at the first sign of skin rash or other allergic reaction
» Caution when driving or doing anything else requiring alertness because of possible dizziness, drowsiness, or lightheadedness
» Discontinuing sparfloxacin and notifying physician if pain, inflammation, or rupture of a tendon is experienced; resting and refraining from exercise until the diagnosis of tendinitis or tendon rupture has been excluded

**Side/adverse effects**
  Signs of potential side effects, especially phototoxicity, QTc prolongation, CNS stimulation, hypersensitivity reactions, pseudomembranous colitis, and tendinitis or tendon rupture

## General Dosing Information

**Diet/Nutrition**
Sparfloxacin may be taken with food, milk, or caffeine-containing products.

**For treatment of adverse effects**
For antibiotic-associated pseudomembranous colitis (AAPMC)
  • Some patients may develop antibiotic-associated pseudomembranous colitis (AAPMC), caused by *Clostridium difficile* toxin, during or following administration of sparfloxacin. Mild cases may respond to discontinuation of the drug alone. Moderate to severe cases may require fluid, electrolyte, and protein replacement.
  • In cases not responding to the above measures or in more severe cases, oral doses of an antibacterial medication effective against *C. difficile* should be administered.
  • In addition, antibiotic-associated pseudomembranous colitis may result in severe watery diarrhea, which may occur during therapy or up to several weeks after therapy is discontinued. If diarrhea occurs, administration of antiperistaltic antidiarrheals (e.g., diphenoxylate and atropine combination, loperamide, opiates) is not recommended since they may delay the removal of toxins from the colon, thereby prolonging and/or worsening the condition.

## Oral Dosage Forms

### SPARFLOXACIN TABLETS

**Usual adult dose**
Antibacterial—
  Oral, 400 mg on the first day, then 200 mg every twenty-four hours for a total of ten days of therapy.

Note: The recommended dose for patients with renal function impairment (creatinine clearance less than 50 mL per minute) is 400 mg on the first day, then 200 mg every forty-eight hours for a total of nine days of therapy.

**Usual adult prescribing limits**
400 mg.

**Usual pediatric dose**
Appropriate studies on the relationship of age to the effects of sparfloxacin have not been performed in patients up to 18 years of age. Safety and efficacy have not been established.

**Strength(s) usually available**
U.S.—
  200 mg (Rx) [*Zagam*].

**Packaging and storage**
Store below 40 °C (104 °F), preferably between 15 and 30 °C (59 and 86 °F), unless otherwise specified by the manufacturer.

**Auxiliary labeling**
• Continue medicine for full time of treatment.
• Avoid too much sun or use of sunlamp.

Developed: 07/31/97
Interim revision: 08/10/98

# SPECTINOMYCIN   Systemic

VA CLASSIFICATION (Primary): AM900
Commonly used brand name(s): *Trobicin*.
Note: For a listing of dosage forms and brand names by country availability, see *Dosage Forms* section(s).

## Category
Antibacterial (systemic).

## Indications
Note: Bracketed information in the *Indications* section refer to uses that are not included in U.S. product labeling.

**Accepted**
Gonorrhea, endocervical (treatment)
Gonorrhea, rectal (treatment) or
Gonorrhea, urethral (treatment)—Spectinomycin is indicated as a secondary agent in the treatment of endocervical, rectal, and urethral gonorrhea caused by nonresistant, penicillinase-producing (PPNG), or chromosomally mediated resistant *Neisseria gonorrhoeae* (CMRNG).

Spectinomycin is also indicated in the treatment of recent sexual partners of patients known to have gonorrhea.[1]

Because many patients with gonorrhea have coexisting infections with *Chlamydia trachomatis*, a 7-day course of tetracycline, doxycycline, or erythromycin should follow spectinomycin treatment as presumptive treatment for chlamydial infections.

[Gonorrhea, disseminated (treatment)][1]—Spectinomycin is also used in the treatment of disseminated gonococcal infection in patients who are allergic to beta-lactam antibiotics.

Not all species or strains of a particular organism may be susceptible to spectinomycin.

**Unaccepted**
Spectinomycin is not effective in the treatment of pharyngeal gonorrhea, syphilis, *C. trachomatis*, or nongonococcal urethritis.

[1]Not included in Canadian product labeling.

## Pharmacology/Pharmacokinetics

**Physicochemical characteristics**
Molecular weight—495.35.

**Mechanism of action/Effect**
Bacteriostatic; inhibits protein synthesis by interacting with the 30S ribosomal subunit of bacterial cells.

**Absorption**
Rapidly and almost completely absorbed following intramuscular administration.

**Distribution**
Concentrates in the urine; does not distribute well into the saliva.
Vol$_D$=Approximately 0.33 liters per kg.

**Protein binding**
Not significantly bound to plasma proteins.

**Half-life**
Normal renal function—1 to 3 hours.
Renal function impairment (creatinine clearance < 20 mL per minute [0.33 mL per second])—10 to 30 hours.

**Time to peak concentration**
1 hour following a single 2-gram intramuscular dose.
2 hours following a single 4-gram intramuscular dose.

**Peak serum concentration**
Approximately 100 mcg per mL 1 hour following a single, intramuscular dose of 2 grams.
Approximately 160 mcg per mL 2 hours following a single, intramuscular dose of 4 grams.

**Elimination**
Up to 100% of a 4-gram dose excreted in urine within 48 hours in biologically active form.
In dialysis—Hemodialysis decreases serum spectinomycin concentrations by approximately 50%.

## Precautions to Consider

**Pregnancy/Reproduction**
Pregnancy—Adequate and well-controlled studies in humans have not been done. However, spectinomycin has been recommended in the treatment of gonococcal infections in pregnant patients who are allergic to penicillins, cephalosporins, or probenecid.
Studies in animals have not shown that spectinomycin causes adverse effects on the fetus.

**Breast-feeding**
It is not known whether spectinomycin is excreted in breast milk. Problems in humans have not been documented.

**Pediatrics**
Spectinomycin has been recommended in the treatment of gonococcal infections in pediatric patients who are allergic to penicillins or cephalosporins. However, the diluent recommended for reconstitution of spectinomycin contains 0.945% benzyl alcohol, which has been associated with a fatal gasping syndrome in infants. Because of this toxicity concern, use of spectinomycin is not recommended in infants.

**Geriatrics**
No information is available on the relationship of age to the effects of spectinomycin in geriatric patients.

**Medical considerations/Contraindications**
The medical considerations/contraindications included have been selected on the basis of their potential clinical significance (reasons given in parentheses where appropriate)—not necessarily inclusive (» = major clinical significance).

*Risk-benefit should be considered when the following medical problem exists:*
Hypersensitivity to spectinomycin

## Side/Adverse Effects

The following side/adverse effects have been selected on the basis of their potential clinical significance (possible signs and symptoms in parentheses where appropriate)—not necessarily inclusive:

**Those indicating need for medical attention**
Incidence rare
*Hypersensitivity* (chills or fever; itching or redness of the skin)

**Those indicating need for medical attention only if they continue or are bothersome**
Incidence rare
*Dizziness; gastrointestinal disturbance* (abdominal cramps; nausea and vomiting); *pain at site of injection*

## Patient Consultation

As an aid to patient consultation, refer to *Advice for the Patient, Spectinomycin (Systemic)*.
In providing consultation, consider emphasizing the following selected information (» = major clinical significance):

**Before receiving this medication**
» Conditions affecting use, especially:
  Hypersensitivity to spectinomycin
  Use in children—Use is not recommended in infants; benzyl alcohol, contained in the recommended diluent, has been associated with a fatal gasping syndrome in infants

**Proper use of this medication**
Giving one dose of spectinomycin intramuscularly; second dose may be required in some infections
Use of condom by male sexual partner to prevent infection; possible need for concurrent treatment of partner to prevent reinfection
» Proper dosing

**Precautions after receiving this medication**
Checking with physician if no improvement within a few days
» Caution if dizziness occurs

## General Dosing Information

Spectinomycin must be administered by intramuscular injection only, deep into the upper, outer quadrant of the gluteal muscle. Intramuscular injections should not exceed 2 grams (5 mL) in each site.

**For treatment of adverse effects**
Recommended treatment consists of the following:
• Epinephrine, corticosteroids, and/or antihistamines for serious allergic reactions.
• Airway support and oxygen for severe anaphylactic reactions.

## Parenteral Dosage Forms

Note: Bracketed uses in the *Dosage Forms* section refer to categories of use and/or indications that are not included in U.S. product labeling.

### STERILE SPECTINOMYCIN HYDROCHLORIDE FOR SUSPENSION USP

**Usual adult and adolescent dose**
Endocervical, rectal, or urethral gonorrhea—
  Intramuscular, 2 grams as a single dose.
[Disseminated gonorrhea][1]—
  Intramuscular, 2 grams every twelve hours for three days.

Note: Dosage may be repeated if reinfection occurs or is strongly suspected.

**Usual adult prescribing limits**
Up to 4 grams as a single dose, divided and administered in two separate sites, have been used in geographic areas in which antibiotic-resistant organisms are prevalent.

**Usual pediatric dose**
Endocervical, rectal, or urethral gonorrhea—
  Infants: Use is not recommended.
  Children up to 45 kg of body weight: Intramuscular, 40 mg per kg of body weight as a single dose.
  Children 45 kg of body weight and over: Intramuscular, 2 grams as a single dose.

**Size(s) usually available**
U.S.—
  2 grams (Rx) [*Trobicin* (diluent contains benzyl alcohol 0.945%)].
  4 grams (Rx) [*Trobicin* (diluent contains benzyl alcohol 0.945%)].
Canada—
  2 grams (Rx) [*Trobicin*].

**Packaging and storage**
Prior to reconstitution, store below 40 °C (104 °F), preferably between 15 and 30 °C (59 and 86 °F), unless otherwise specified by manufacturer. Protect diluent from freezing.

Note: Store reconstituted sterile spectinomycin hydrochloride suspension between 15 and 30 °C (59 and 86 °F).

## Preparation of dosage form
To prepare initial dilution for intramuscular use, add 3.2 mL of bacteriostatic water for injection (with benzyl alcohol 0.945%) to each 2-gram vial and 6.2 mL of diluent to each 4-gram vial to provide a concentration of 400 mg per mL.

Shake the vial vigorously immediately after addition of the diluent and before withdrawing each dose. Inject spectinomycin suspension using a 20-gauge needle.

## Stability
After reconstitution for intramuscular use with bacteriostatic water for injection (preserved with benzyl alcohol 0.945%), suspensions retain their potency for 24 hours at 15 to 30 °C (59 to 86 °F).

[1]Not included in Canadian product labeling.

Revised: 02/23/93

---

**SPERMICIDES**—The *Spermicides (Vaginal)* monograph is not included in this published version of the USP DI database. Copies of the monograph are available on request from Micromedex, Inc. - Reprint Requests, 6200 S. Syracuse Way, Suite 300, Englewood, CO 80111; telephone (303) 486-6400; telefax (303) 486-6464; Email: USPDI@MDX.COM.

---

# SPIRAMYCIN Systemic*

JAN: Spiramycin—Acetylspiramycin
VA CLASSIFICATION (Primary/Secondary): AM200/AP900
Commonly used brand name(s): *Provamicina; Rovamicina; Rovamycine; Rovamycine 250; Rovamycine 500; Rovamycine-250; Rovamycine-500; Spiramycine Coquelusédal*.

Note: For a listing of dosage forms and brand names by country availability, see *Dosage Forms* section(s).

*Not commercially available in U.S.

## Category
Antibacterial (systemic); antiprotozoal.

## Indications

### General considerations
Spiramycin is a macrolide antimicrobial agent with activity against gram-positive organisms, including *Streptococcus pyogenes* (group A beta-hemolytic streptococci), *S. viridans*, *Corynebacterium diphtheriae*, and methicillin-sensitive *Staphylococcus aureus*. Increasing resistance has left spiramycin with inconsistent activity against *S. pneumoniae* and enterococcus. Spiramycin also has activity against some gram-negative bacteria, such as *Neisseria meningitidis*, *Bordetella pertussis*, and *Campylobacter*. *Neisseria gonorrhoeae* is inconsistently sensitive, and approximately 50% of *Haemophilus influenzae* strains are sensitive to spiramycin. *Clostridium* species are sensitive; however, Enterobacteraceae, *Pseudomonas* species, as well as *Bacteroides fragilis*, and most other gram-negative bacteria are resistant. Spiramycin also has activity against other organisms, including *Mycoplasma pneumoniae*, *Chlamydia trachomatis*, *Toxoplasma gondii*, *Legionella pneumophila*, and spirochetes.

Cross-resistance between spiramycin and erythromycin has been reported.

### Accepted
Toxoplasmosis (treatment)[1]—Spiramycin is used as an alternative agent in the treatment of toxoplasmosis during pregnancy. Pyrimethamine and sulfadiazine combination is considered to be more effective than spiramycin. However, because spiramycin has not been found to be teratogenic and has been found to be safe in the pregnant woman, fetus, and newborn, it is often used to treat toxoplasmosis during pregnancy and congenital toxoplasmosis. Spiramycin reduces the transmission of toxoplasmosis from the pregnant woman to the fetus; however, it will not affect the severity of disease in an already infected fetus.

Although spiramycin is effective in the treatment of some bacterial infections, spiramycin is considered to be a secondary agent and other medications are generally used in place of spiramycin.

### Acceptance not established
Spiramycin has not been shown to be clearly effective in the treatment of *cryptosporidiosis* in immunocompromised patients. Data are mixed and relapse often occurs after spiramycin is discontinued. *Cryptosporidiosis* is usually self-limiting in non-immunocompromised patients.

### Unaccepted
Because spiramycin does not reach adequate concentrations in the cerebrospinal fluid, spiramycin is not accepted in the treatment of *meningitis* or in preventing *toxoplasma encephalitis*.

[1]Not included in Canadian product labeling.

## Pharmacology/Pharmacokinetics

### Physicochemical characteristics
Chemical group—A 16-membered ring macrolide antibiotic.
Molecular weight—843.1.
pKa—7.9.

### Mechanism of action/Effect
The mechanism of action of spiramycin is not clear; however, it is thought to reversibly bind to the 50 S subunit of bacterial ribosomes, resulting in blockage of the transpeptidation or translocation reactions, inhibiting protein synthesis and subsequent cell growth. It is primarily bacteriostatic, but may be bactericidal against more sensitive strains when used in high concentrations. Spiramycin also accumulates in high concentrations in the bacterial cell. Unlike erythromycin, spiramycin does not produce gastrointestinal motility stimulation.

### Absorption
The absorption of spiramycin is incomplete, with an oral bioavailability of 33 to 39% (range, 10 to 69%). The rate of absorption is slower than that of erythromycin and is thought to be due to the high pKa (7.9) of spiramycin, suggesting a high degree of ionization in the acidic stomach. Studies have shown that administration with food reduces bioavailability by approximately 50% and delays the time to peak serum concentration.

### Distribution
Spiramycin is highly concentrated in tissues, such as the lungs, bronchi, tonsils, sinuses, and female pelvic tissues. These high tissue concentrations persist long after serum concentrations have fallen to low levels. Peak concentrations in the saliva are 1.3 to 4.8 times greater than those found in the serum. Spiramycin crosses the placenta and is distributed into breast milk; however, fetal blood concentrations are only 50% of the maternal serum concentrations. Concentrations in the placenta are up to 5 times higher than the corresponding serum concentration. High concentrations are also found in the bile, polymorphonuclear leukocytes, and macrophages. Biliary concentrations are 15 to 40 times higher than the serum concentration. Spiramycin does not cross the blood-brain barrier.

$Vol_D$ is large and variable (383 to 660 L).

### Protein binding
Low (10 to 25%).

### Biotransformation
Spiramycin metabolism has not been well studied; however, spiramycin is thought to be metabolized in the liver to active metabolites.

### Half-life
Intravenous—
  Young persons (18 to 32 years of age): Approximately 4.5 to 6.2 hours.
  Elderly persons (73 to 85 years of age): Approximately 9.8 to 13.5 hours.
Oral—
  5.5 to 8 hours.
Rectal (in children)—
  Approximately 8 hours.

### Time to peak concentration
Intravenous—End of infusion.
Oral—3 to 4 hours.
Rectal (in children)—1.5 to 3 hours.

### Peak serum concentration
Intravenous—
  2.3 mcg per mL (mcg/mL) after a 500-mg dose.

Oral—
    Approximately 1 mcg/mL after a 1-gram dose.
    1.6 to 3.1 mcg/mL after a 2-gram dose.
Rectal (in children)—
    Approximately 1.6 mcg per mL after a 1.3 million IU dose.

**Elimination**
Fecal—Biliary elimination is substantial, with over 80% of an administered dose excreted in the bile; enterohepatic recycling may occur.
Renal—Urinary excretion accounts for only 4 to 14% of an administered dose.

## Precautions to Consider

**Cross-sensitivity and/or related problems**
Patients with hypersensitivity reactions to other macrolides (e.g., erythromycin, azithromycin, clarithromycin, troleandomycin, dirithromycin, josamycin) may also have hypersensitivity to spiramycin.

**Pregnancy/Reproduction**
Pregnancy—Spiramycin crosses the placenta and reaches concentrations in the placenta up to five times higher than that in the corresponding serum. Spiramycin is used in pregnant women to decrease the risk of toxoplasmosis transmission to the fetus. It is reported to decrease the transmission from 25 to 8% in the first trimester, from 54 to 19% in the second trimester, and from 65 to 44% in the third trimester. However, spiramycin will not affect the severity of disease in an already infected fetus. Fetal blood concentrations are only 50% of the maternal serum concentrations. Spiramycin has not been found to be teratogenic, and has been found to be safe in the pregnant woman, fetus, and newborn.

**Breast-feeding**
Spiramycin is distributed into breast milk.

**Pediatrics**
Studies performed in infants and children have not demonstrated pediatrics-specific problems that would limit the usefulness of spiramycin in children.

**Geriatrics**
No information is available on the relationship of age to the effects of spiramycin in geriatric patients. However, one small pharmacokinetic study showed that elderly patients (73 to 85 years of age) had an elimination half-life that was twice as long as that in younger patients.

**Drug interactions and/or related problems**
The following drug interactions and/or related problems have been selected on the basis of their potential clinical significance (possible mechanism in parentheses where appropriate)—not necessarily inclusive (» = major clinical significance):

Note: Unlike erythromycin, a related macrolide, spiramycin does not bind to hepatic cytochrome P-450 isoenzymes and has not been shown to interact with cyclosporine or theophylline.

Combinations containing either of the following medications, depending on the amount present, may interact with this medication.

Levodopa and carbidopa combination
    (concurrent use of spiramycin with levodopa and carbidopa combination has resulted in an increase in the elimination half-life of levodopa; this is thought to be due to the inhibition of carbidopa absorption by spiramycin secondary to modified gastrointestinal motility)

**Laboratory value alterations**
The following have been selected on the basis of their potential clinical significance (possible effect in parentheses where appropriate)—not necessarily inclusive (» = major clinical significance):

With physiology/laboratory test values
Alanine aminotransferase (ALT [SGPT]) and
Alkaline phosphatase, serum
    (values may be increased rarely)

**Medical considerations/Contraindications**
The medical considerations/contraindications included have been selected on the basis of their potential clinical significance (reasons given in parentheses where appropriate)—not necessarily inclusive (» = major clinical significance).

*Risk-benefit should be considered when the following medical problems exist:*

Biliary obstruction or
Hepatic function impairment
    (biliary obstruction or hepatic function impairment may decrease the elimination of spiramycin, which may increase the risk of side effects)
Hypersensitivity to spiramycin or another macrolide

**Patient monitoring**
The following may be especially important in patient monitoring (other tests may be warranted in some patients, depending on condition; » = major clinical significance):

Hepatic function determinations
    (may be required in patients with hepatic function impairment receiving high-dose spiramycin; spiramycin has also been reported to cause cholestatic hepatitis)

## Side/Adverse Effects

Note: Severe adverse reactions due to spiramycin are rare. Hypersensitivity reactions and gastrointestinal disturbances occur most frequently. Thrombocytopenia, QT prolongation in an infant, cholestatic hepatitis, acute colitis, and ulcerated esophagitis have each only been reported as single case reports in the literature; there were two case reports of intestinal mucosal injury.

Thrombocytopenia, reported in a patient infected with human immunodeficiency virus (HIV), was thought to be induced by spiramycin-IgG immune complexes adsorbed onto the surface of platelets.

The two cases of intestinal mucosal injury occurred with high doses of spiramycin. Endoscopic examination revealed erosions of the small bowel wall with loss of the small intestinal folds, marked damage to the large and small bowel with flattened epithelial cells, multifocal apoptosis, and regenerative epithelial changes.

The following side/adverse effects have been selected on the basis of their potential clinical significance (possible signs and symptoms in parentheses where appropriate)—not necessarily inclusive:

**Those indicating need for medical attention**
Incidence less frequent
    *Hypersensitivity reactions, specifically skin rash and itching; thrombocytopenia* (unusual bleeding or bruising)
Incidence rare
    *Cardiac toxicity, specifically QT prolongation* (irregular heartbeat; recurrent fainting); *cholestatic hepatitis* (abdominal pain; nausea; vomiting; yellow eyes or skin); *gastrointestinal toxicity, specifically acute colitis* (abdominal pain and tenderness; bloody stools; fever); *intestinal injury* (abdominal pain and tenderness); *ulcerated esophagitis* (chest pain; heartburn); *pain at site of injection*

**Those indicating need for medical attention only if they continue or are bothersome**
Incidence less frequent
    *Gastrointestinal disturbances* (diarrhea; nausea; stomach pain; vomiting)

## Patient Consultation

As an aid to patient consultation, refer to *Advice for the Patient, Spiramycin (Systemic)*.

In providing consultation, consider emphasizing the following selected information (» = major clinical significance):

**Before using this medication**
» Conditions affecting use, especially:
    Hypersensitivity to spiramycin or other macrolides
    Breast-feeding—Spiramycin is distributed into breast milk

**Proper use of this medication**
» Taking on an empty stomach
» Compliance with full course of therapy
» Importance of taking medication on regular schedule and not missing doses
» Proper administration of spiramycin suppositories
» Proper dosing
    Missed dose: taking as soon as possible; not taking if almost time for next dose; not doubling dose
» Proper storage

**Precautions while using this medication**
Checking with physician if no improvement within a few days

**Side/adverse effects**
Signs of potential side effects, especially hypersensitivity reactions, cardiac toxicity, cholestatic hepatitis, gastrointestinal toxicity, or pain at site of injection

## General Dosing Information

**For oral dosage form only**
Administration of spiramycin with food reduces bioavailability by approximately 50% and delays the time to peak serum concentration. Spiramycin should be taken on an empty stomach.

**For rectal dosage form only**
Before rectal administration of spiramycin suppositories, the suppository should be dipped in cold water, then introduced quickly and deeply into the rectum.

## Oral Dosage Forms

### SPIRAMYCIN CAPSULES

Note: Dosing of spiramycin may be expressed as either milligrams (mg) or International Units (IU). One mg of spiramycin is equivalent to approximately 3000 IU.

**Usual adult and adolescent dose**
Antibacterial—
    Oral, 1 to 2 grams (3,000,000 to 6,000,000 IU) two times a day; or 500 mg to 1 gram (1,500,000 to 3,000,000 IU) three times a day. For severe infections, the dose may be increased to 2 to 2.5 grams (6,000,000 to 7,500,000 IU) two times a day.

Note: Toxoplasmosis in pregnant women[1]
    First trimester: Oral, 3 grams (9,000,000 IU) per day, divided into three or four doses.
    Second and third trimesters: Oral, 25 to 50 mg of pyrimethamine per day in combination with 2 to 3 grams of sulfadiazine per day and folinic acid 5 mg per day for three weeks, alternating with 3 grams (9,000,000 IU) of spiramycin, divided into three or four doses, for three weeks.

**Usual pediatric dose**
Antibacterial—
    Children 20 kg of body weight and over: Oral, 25 mg (75,000 IU) per kg of body weight two times a day, or 16.7 mg (50,000 IU) per kg of body weight three times a day.

Note: Toxoplasmosis[1]
    Subclinical congenital infection: Oral, 0.5 to 1 mg per kg of body weight per day of pyrimethamine in combination with 50 to 100 mg per kg of body weight per day of sulfadiazine for four weeks, alternating with 50 to 100 mg (150,000 to 300,000 IU) per kg of body weight of spiramycin for six weeks; these dosing courses are repeated for one year.
    Overt congenital infection: Oral, 0.5 to 1 mg per kg of body weight per day of pyrimethamine in combination with 50 to 100 mg per kg of body weight per day of sulfadiazine and folinic acid 5 mg every three days for six months, alternating with 50 to 100 mg (150,000 to 300,000 IU) per kg of body weight of spiramycin in combination with pyrimethamine and sulfadiazine for four weeks; these dosing courses are repeated until 18 months of age.

**Strength(s) usually available**
U.S.—
    Not commercially available. However, physicians who wish to use spiramycin should contact the FDA's Division of Anti-Infective Drug Products (301-443-4310).
Canada—
    250 mg (750,000 IU) (Rx) [*Rovamycine 250*].
    500 mg (1,500,000 IU) (Rx) [*Rovamycine 500*].

**Packaging and storage**
Store below 40 °C (104 °F), preferably between 15 and 30 °C (59 and 86 °F), unless otherwise specified by manufacturer.

**Auxiliary labeling**
• Continue medicine for full time of treatment.
• Take on an empty stomach.

### SPIRAMYCIN TABLETS

Note: Dosing of spiramycin may be expressed as either milligrams (mg) or International Units (IU). One mg of spiramycin is equivalent to approximately 3000 IU.

**Usual adult and adolescent dose**
See *Spiramycin Capsules*.

**Usual pediatric dose**
See *Spiramycin Capsules*.

**Strength(s) usually available**
U.S.—
    Not commercially available. However, physicians who wish to use spiramycin should contact the FDA's Division of Anti-Infective Drug Products (301-443-4310).
Canada—
    Not commercially available.
France—
    500 mg (1,500,000 IU) (Rx) [*Rovamycine*].
    1 gram (3,000,000 IU) (Rx) [*Rovamycine*].
Germany—
    250 mg (750,000 IU) (Rx) [*Rovamycine-250*].
    500 mg (1,500,000 IU) (Rx) [*Rovamycine-500*].
Italy—
    1 gram (3,000,000 IU) (Rx) [*Rovamicina*].
Mexico—
    500 mg (1,500,000 IU) (Rx) [*Provamicina*].
Spain—
    500 mg (1,500,000 IU) (Rx) [*Rovamycine*].

**Packaging and storage**
Store below 40 °C (104 °F), preferably between 15 and 30 °C (59 and 86 °F), unless otherwise specified by manufacturer.

**Auxiliary labeling**
• Continue medicine for full time of treatment.
• Take on an empty stomach.

## Parenteral Dosage Forms

### SPIRAMYCIN ADIPATE INJECTION

Note: Dosing of spiramycin may be expressed as either milligrams (mg) or International Units (IU). One mg of spiramycin is equivalent to approximately 3000 IU.
    The dosing and strengths of spiramycin adipate injection are expressed in terms of the base (not the adipate salt).

**Usual adult and adolescent dose**
Antibacterial—
    Intravenous infusion, 500 mg (1,500,000 IU) (base), by slow intravenous infusion, every eight hours. For severe infections, the dose may be doubled to 1 gram (3,000,000 IU) every eight hours.

**Usual pediatric dose**
Dosage has not been established.

**Strength(s) usually available**
U.S.—
    Not commercially available.
Canada—
    Not commercially available.
France—
    500 mg (1,500,000 IU) (base) (Rx) [*Rovamycine*].

**Packaging and storage**
Store below 40 °C (104 °F), preferably between 15 and 30 °C (59 and 86 °F), unless otherwise specified by manufacturer.

**Preparation of dosage form**
For initial dilution, 4 mL of sterile water for injection should be added to each 500-mg (1,500,000 IU) (base) vial.
After initial dilution, the solution may be further diluted in a minimum of 100 mL of 5% dextrose injection solution and administered by slow intravenous infusion.

**Stability**
After reconstitution, the solution retains its potency for 12 hours.

**Incompatibilities**
It is recommended that spiramycin injection not be mixed with any other medications.

## Rectal Dosage Forms

### SPIRAMYCIN ADIPATE SUPPOSITORIES

Note: Dosing of spiramycin may be expressed as either milligrams (mg) or International Units (IU). One mg of spiramycin is equivalent to approximately 3000 IU.
    The dosing and strengths of spiramycin adipate suppositories are expressed in terms of the adipate salt (not the base).

**Usual adult and adolescent dose**
Antibacterial—
    Rectal, two to three 750 mg (1,950,000 IU) suppositories every 24 hours.

**Usual pediatric dose**
Antibacterial—
    Newborns: Rectal, one 250 mg (650,000 IU) suppository per 5 kg of body weight every 24 hours.
    Children up to 12 years of age: Rectal, two to three 500 mg (1,300,000 IU) suppositories every 24 hours.
    Children 12 years of age and over: See *Usual adult and adolescent dose*.

**Strength(s) usually available**
U.S.—
    Not commercially available.

USP DI

Canada—
  Not commercially available.
France—
  250 mg (650,000 IU) (Rx) [*Spiramycine Coquelusédal*].
  500 mg (1,300,000 IU) (Rx) [*Spiramycine Coquelusédal*].
  750 mg (1,950,000 IU) (Rx) [*Spiramycine Coquelusédal*].

**Packaging and storage**
Store below 40 °C (104 °F), preferably between 15 and 30 °C (59 and 86 °F), unless otherwise specified by manufacturer.

**Auxiliary labeling**
• For rectal use only.

¹Not included in Canadian product labeling.

Developed: 05/28/96

**SPIRONOLACTONE**—See *Diuretics, Potassium-sparing (Systemic)*

**STANOZOLOL**—See *Anabolic Steroids (Systemic)*

# STAVUDINE  Systemic

VA CLASSIFICATION (Primary): AM809
Commonly used brand name(s): *Zerit*.
Another commonly used name is d4T.
Note: For a listing of dosage forms and brand names by country availability, see *Dosage Forms* section(s).

## Category
Antiviral (systemic).

## Indications
**Accepted**
Human immunodeficiency virus (HIV) infection (treatment)—Stavudine is indicated for the treatment of patients with HIV infection who have received prolonged previous treatment with zidovudine.
  The duration of clinical benefit from antiretroviral therapy may be limited. If disease progression occurs during stavudine treatment, an alternative antiretroviral therapy is recommended.

## Pharmacology/Pharmacokinetics
**Physicochemical characteristics**
Molecular weight—224.22.

**Mechanism of action/Effect**
Stavudine, a nucleoside analog of thymidine, is rapidly phosphorylated by cellular enzymes to its active moiety, stavudine triphosphate. Stavudine triphosphate inhibits human immunodeficiency virus (HIV) replication by competing with the natural substrate, deoxythymidine triphosphate, and by inhibiting viral DNA synthesis by acting as a terminator of chain elongation. In addition, stavudine triphosphate inhibits cellular DNA polymerases beta and gamma, and markedly reduces the synthesis of mitochondrial DNA.
A concentration of 0.009 mg/mL of stavudine is required to inhibit HIV replication by 50% *in vitro*. The *in vitro* potency of stavudine against HIV is similar to that of zidovudine.

**Absorption**
Stavudine is rapidly absorbed with an oral bioavailability of 78 to 86%. Stavudine may be taken with food or on an empty stomach. Administration with food results in a decrease in peak plasma concentration ($C_{max}$) of approximately 45%; however, the systemic availability, as measured by the area under the plasma concentration–time curve (AUC), remains unchanged.

**Distribution**
Crosses the blood-brain barrier and distributes into the cerebrospinal fluid (CSF); the mean CSF to plasma concentration ratio was 55% (range, 16 to 97%) when measured in 6 children. Also, stavudine distributes equally between red blood cells and plasma.
$Vol_D$—
  Adults: 0.8 to 1.1 L per kg (L/kg).
  Children: Approximately 0.68 L/kg.

**Protein binding**
Negligible.

**Biotransformation**
Phosphorylated intracellularly to stavudine triphosphate, the active substrate for HIV-reverse transcriptase.

**Half-life**
Normal renal function—
  Adults: 1 to 1.6 hours.
  Children: 0.9 to 1.1 hours.
Renal function impairment (creatinine clearance < 25 mL/min [< 0.42 mL/sec])—
  Approximately 4.8 hours.
Intracellular half-life of stavudine triphosphate—
  Approximately 3.5 hours.

**Time to peak concentration**
0.5 to 1.5 hour.

**Peak serum concentration**
Approximately 1.4 micrograms/mL (6.2 micromoles/L) after a single oral dose of 70 mg.

**Elimination**
Renal (glomerular filtration and tubular secretion); approximately 40% is excreted unchanged in the urine in 6 to 24 hours.
Approximately 50% of an administered dose undergoes nonrenal elimination. Although the exact metabolic fate is unknown, stavudine may be cleaved to thymine, and the subsequent degradation and/or utilization of thymine may account for the unrecovered stavudine.
In dialysis—It is not known whether stavudine is removed by hemodialysis or peritoneal dialysis.

## Precautions to Consider
**Carcinogenicity**
Long-term carcinogenicity studies of stavudine have not been completed in animals.

**Mutagenicity**
No evidence of mutagenicity was found in the Ames test, *Escherichia coli* reverse mutation assay, or the CHO/HGPRT mammalian cell forward gene mutation assay, with and without metabolic activation. Positive results were produced in the *in vitro* human lymphocyte clastogenesis and mouse fibroblast assays, and in the *in vivo* mouse micronucleus test. In the *in vitro* assays, stavudine produced an increased frequency of chromosome abberations in human lymphoctyes at concentrations of 25 to 250 mcg per mL (mcg/mL), without metabolic activation, and increased the frequency of transformed foci in mouse fibroblast cells at concentrations of 25 to 2500 mcg/mL, with and without metabolic activation. In the *in vivo* micronucleus assay, stavudine was clastogenic in bone marrow cells of mice following administration of oral doses of 600 to 2000 mg per kg of body weight (mg/kg) per day for 3 days.

**Pregnancy/Reproduction**
Fertility—No evidence of impaired fertility was seen in rats given stavudine at doses that resulted in peak serum concentrations that were up to 216 times those observed in humans who received a clinical dosage of 1 mg/kg per day.

Pregnancy—Adequate and well-controlled studies have not been done in humans. It is not known whether stavudine crosses the placenta in humans. Also, it is not known whether stavudine reduces perinatal transmission of HIV infection, as does zidovudine. Stavudine should be used during pregnancy only if clearly needed.
Stavudine crosses the placenta in rats. Reproduction studies done in rats and rabbits exposed to levels of stavudine up to 399 and 183 times, respectively, those seen at a clinical dosage in humans of 1 mg/kg per day, based on peak serum concentrations, revealed no evidence of teratogenicity. The incidence of common skeletal variation, unossified or incomplete ossification of sternebra, in fetuses was increased in rats at 399 times the human exposure, but not at 216 times the human exposure. A slight postimplantation loss was seen at 216 times the human exposure, but no effect was seen at approximately 135 times the human exposure. An increase in rat neonatal mortality occurred at 399 times

the human exposure, while survival was unaffected at approximately 135 times the human exposure. The concentration of stavudine in rat fetal tissue was approximately one-half the concentration of that in maternal plasma.

FDA Pregnancy Category C.

**Breast-feeding**
It is not known whether stavudine is distributed into human breast milk. However, it has been found to pass readily into the milk of lactating rats.

There have been case reports of HIV being transmitted from an infected mother to her nursing infant through breast milk. Therefore, breast-feeding is not recommended in HIV-infected mothers, to avoid potential postnatal transmission of HIV to the nursing infant.

**Pediatrics**
A pharmacokinetic study has been done in a small number of children 5 weeks to 15 years of age. The pharmacokinetic and side effect profiles of stavudine in children were similar to those in adults.

**Geriatrics**
No information is available on the relationship of age to the effects of stavudine in geriatric patients. However, elderly patients are more likely to have an age-related decrease in renal function, which may require a reduction in dose.

**Drug interactions and/or related problems**
The following drug interactions and/or related problems have been selected on the basis of their potential clinical significance (possible mechanism in parentheses where appropriate)—not necessarily inclusive (» = major clinical significance):

Note: Combinations containing any of the following medications, depending on the amount present, may also interact with this medication.

Medications that may cause peripheral neuropathy, such as:
» Chloramphenicol or
» Cisplatin or
» Dapsone or
» Didanosine or
» Ethambutol or
» Ethionamide or
» Hydralazine or
» Isoniazid or
» Lithium or
» Metronidazole or
» Nitrofurantoin or
» Phenytoin or
» Vincristine or
» Zalcitabine
(since stavudine has been shown to cause peripheral neuropathy, other medications associated with the development of neuropathy should be avoided during stavudine therapy or, if concurrent use is necessary, used with caution)

Zidovudine
(*in vitro* studies detected an antagonistic antiviral effect between stavudine and zidovudine at a molar ratio of 20 to 1, respectively; concurrent use is not recommended until *in vivo* studies demonstrate that these medications are not antagonistic in their anti-HIV activity)

**Laboratory value alterations**
The following have been selected on the basis of their potential clinical significance (possible effect in parentheses where appropriate)—not necessarily inclusive (» = major clinical significance):

With physiology/laboratory test values
» Alanine aminotransferase (ALT [SGPT]) and
  Alkaline phosphatase and
» Aspartate aminotransferase (AST [SGOT])
  (serum values have increased to greater than 5 times the upper normal limit, but returned to baseline when therapy was discontinued)

Mean corpuscular volume (MCV)
  (may be increased)

**Medical considerations/Contraindications**
The medical considerations/contraindications included have been selected on the basis of their potential clinical significance (reasons given in parentheses where appropriate)—not necessarily inclusive (» = major clinical significance).

*Risk-benefit should be considered when the following medical problems exist:*

Alcoholism, active or a history of, or
Hepatic function impairment
  (stavudine may exacerbate hepatic dysfunction in patients with pre-existing liver disease or a history of alcohol abuse)

» Peripheral neuropathy
  (stavudine may cause peripheral neuropathy; if symptoms of peripheral neuropathy develop, stavudine therapy should be interrupted; if symptoms resolve completely, reinstatement of therapy at a lower dose may be considered)

» Renal function impairment
  (patients with renal function impairment may be at increased risk of toxicity due to decreased clearance of stavudine; patients with a creatinine clearance of < 50 mL/min [0.83 mL/sec] may require a reduction in dose)

**Patient monitoring**
The following may be especially important in patient monitoring (other tests may be warranted in some patients, depending on condition; » = major clinical significance):

» Alanine aminotransferase (ALT [SGPT]) and
  Alkaline phosphatase and
» Aspartate aminotransferase (AST [SGOT])
  (serum values may be increased to greater than 5 times the upper normal limit)

Amylase, serum and
Lipase, serum
  (values may be increased)

## Side/Adverse Effects

The following side/adverse effects have been selected on the basis of their potential clinical significance (possible signs and symptoms in parentheses where appropriate)—not necessarily inclusive:

**Those indicating need for medical attention**
Incidence more frequent
  *Peripheral neuropathy* (tingling, burning, numbness, or pain in the hands or feet)
  
  Note: *Sensory peripheral neuropathy*, which is the major side effect of stavudine, may also be seen with severe HIV disease. Therefore, differentiation between this side effect of stavudine and the complications of HIV disease may be difficult. *Peripheral neuropathy* occurred in 19 to 24% of adult patients with advanced HIV infection who were treated with stavudine, compared with 13% of adult patients with less advanced HIV infection who were treated with stavudine. It may resolve if stavudine therapy is stopped promptly. Symptoms may become worse temporarily after discontinuation of therapy. If symptoms resolve completely, resumption of treatment at a lower dose may be considered.

Incidence less frequent
  *Arthralgia* (joint pain); *hypersensitivity* (fever; skin rash); *myalgia* (muscle pain)

Incidence rare
  *Anemia* (unusual tiredness or weakness); *pancreatitis* (nausea, vomiting, severe abdominal pain)
  
  Note: *Pancreatitis* was reported in 1% of patients enrolled in clinical trials.

**Those indicating need for medical attention only if they continue or are bothersome**
Incidence more frequent
  *Chills and fever*

Incidence less frequent
  *Asthenia* (lack of strength or energy; weakness); *gastrointestinal disturbances* (abdominal pain; diarrhea; loss of appetite; nausea or vomiting); *headache; insomnia* (difficulty in sleeping)

## Overdose

For more information on the management of overdose or unintentional ingestion, **contact a Poison Control Center** (see *Poison Control Center Listing*).

**Clinical effects of overdose**
The following effects have been selected on the basis of their potential clinical significance (possible signs and symptoms in parentheses where appropriate)—not necessarily inclusive:

Acute
Adults treated with 12 to 24 times the recommended daily dose of stavudine showed no acute toxicity.

Chronic
  *Hepatotoxicity* (dark or amber urine; loss of appetite; pale stools; stomach pain; unusual tiredness or weakness; yellow eyes or skin); *peripheral neuropathy* (tingling, burning, numbness, or pain in the hands or feet)

## Treatment of overdose
Supportive care—Patients in whom intentional overdose is confirmed or suspected should be referred for psychiatric consultation.

## Patient Consultation
As an aid to patient consultation, refer to *Advice for the Patient, Stavudine (Systemic)*.

In providing consultation, consider emphasizing the following selected information (» = major clinical significance):

**Before using this medication**
- » Conditions affecting use, especially:
  - Pregnancy—Stavudine should be used during pregnancy only if clearly needed
  - Breast-feeding—Breast-feeding is not recommended, because of potential postnatal transmission of HIV to the nursing infant
  - Use in children—Stavudine has been studied in a small number of children; the side effect profile is similar to that for adults
  - Other medications, especially those associated with peripheral neuropathy
  - Other medical problems, especially peripheral neuropathy and renal function impairment

**Proper use of this medication**
- » Importance of not taking more medication than prescribed; importance of not discontinuing medication without checking with physician
- » Compliance with full course of therapy
- » Importance of not missing doses and of taking at evenly spaced times
- Not sharing medication with others
- » Proper dosing
  - Missed dose: Taking as soon as possible; not taking if almost time for next dose; not doubling doses
- » Proper storage

**Precautions while using this medication**
- » Regular visits to physician for blood tests
- » Importance of not taking other medications concurrently without checking with physician
- » Taking steps to avoid spreading HIV infection

**Side/adverse effects**
Signs of potential side effects, especially peripheral neuropathy, arthralgia, hypersensitivity, myalgia, anemia, and pancreatitis

## General Dosing Information
Patients with symptoms of peripheral neuropathy or clinically significant elevations in serum concentrations of hepatic transaminases should discontinue taking stavudine. If symptoms or serum enzyme elevations resolve completely, stavudine may be reintroduced at 50% of the regular dose.

Stavudine may be taken on a full or empty stomach.

## Oral Dosage Forms

### STAVUDINE CAPSULES

**Usual adult and adolescent dose**
Human immunodeficiency virus (HIV) infection—
  Adults and adolescents 60 kg of body weight or greater: Oral, 40 mg every twelve hours.
  Adults and adolescents less than 60 kg of body weight: Oral, 30 mg every twelve hours.

Note: Patients with renal function impairment may require a reduction in dose as follows:

| Creatinine clearance (mL/min)/(mL/sec) | Recommended dose based on patient's body weight ≥ 60 kg | < 60 kg |
|---|---|---|
| > 50/0.83 | See *Usual adult and adolescent dose* | See *Usual adult and adolescent dose* |
| 26-50/0.43-0.83 | 20 mg every 12 hours | 15 mg every 12 hours |
| 10-25/0.17-0.42 | 20 mg every 24 hours | 15 mg every 24 hours |

Data are insufficient to recommend a dose for patients with creatinine clearance < 10 mL per minute (0.17 mL per second) or for patients undergoing hemodialysis.

**Usual pediatric dose**
This dosage form is usually not used for children. See *Stavudine for Oral Solution*.

**Strength(s) usually available**
U.S.—
  15 mg (Rx) [*Zerit* (lactose; methylparaben; propylparaben)].
  20 mg (Rx) [*Zerit* (lactose; methylparaben; propylparaben)].
  30 mg (Rx) [*Zerit* (lactose; methylparaben; propylparaben)].
  40 mg (Rx) [*Zerit* (lactose; methylparaben; propylparaben)].
Canada—
  5 mg (Rx) [*Zerit* (lactose)].
  15 mg (Rx) [*Zerit* (lactose)].
  20 mg (Rx) [*Zerit* (lactose)].
  30 mg (Rx) [*Zerit* (lactose)].
  40 mg (Rx) [*Zerit* (lactose)].

**Packaging and storage**
Store at controlled room temperature, preferably between 15 and 30 °C (59 and 86 °F), in a tight container.

**Auxiliary labeling**
• Continue medicine for full time of treatment.

### STAVUDINE FOR ORAL SOLUTION

**Usual adult and adolescent dose**
See *Stavudine Capsules*.

**Usual pediatric dose**
Human immunodeficiency virus (HIV) infection—
  Infants and children 30 kg of body weight or greater: Oral, 30 mg every twelve hours.
  Infants and children up to 30 kg of body weight: Oral, 1 mg per kg of body weight every twelve hours.

**Strength(s) usually available**
U.S.—
  1 mg per mL (when reconstituted according to manufacturer's instructions) (available in 200-mL bottles) (Rx) [*Zerit* (methylparaben; propylparaben; sucrose)].
Canada—
  Not commercially available.

**Packaging and storage**
Prior to reconstitution, store at controlled room temperature, preferably between 15 and 30 °C (59 and 86 °F), in a tight container. Protect from excessive moisture.
After reconstitution, store in a refrigerator (2 to 8 °C [36 to 46 °F]).

**Preparation of dosage form**
To prepare stavudine for oral solution, add 202 mL of purified water to each bottle and shake vigorously to dissolve. This will provide 200 mL of dispensible solution. The solution may appear slightly hazy.

**Stability**
Reconstituted solutions are stable for up to 30 days when refrigerated.

**Auxiliary labeling**
• Shake prior to use.
• Continue medicine for full time of treatment.

Developed: 11/28/94
Interim revision: 04/20/98

---

**STREPTOKINASE**—See *Thrombolytic Agents (Systemic)*

---

**STREPTOMYCIN**—See *Aminoglycosides (Systemic)*

---

# STREPTOZOCIN   Systemic

VA CLASSIFICATION (Primary): AN200

Commonly used brand name(s): *Zanosar*.

Note: For a listing of dosage forms and brand names by country availability, see *Dosage Forms* section(s).

## Category
Antineoplastic.

# Indications

Note: Bracketed information in the *Indications* section refers to uses that are not included in U.S. product labeling.

### Accepted
Carcinoma, islet cell (treatment) or

Carcinoma, pancreatic (treatment)—Streptozocin is indicated for treatment of symptomatic or progressive metastatic islet cell carcinoma of the pancreas (both functional and nonfunctional). It is also indicated for treatment of metastatic [non–islet cell carcinoma of the pancreas][1].

[Tumors, gastrointestinal carcinoid (treatment)][1]—Streptozocin also is indicated for treatment of malignant metastatic gastrointestinal carcinoid tumors.

---
[1]Not included in Canadian product labeling.

# Pharmacology/Pharmacokinetics

### Physicochemical characteristics
Molecular weight—265.22.

### Mechanism of action/Effect
Streptozocin is an alkylating agent of the nitrosourea type.

Streptozocin is considered cell cycle–phase nonspecific, although it particularly inhibits progression out of the $G_2$ phase of cell division.

The mechanism of streptozocin's antineoplastic action is not completely understood, but activity appears to occur as a result of formation of methylcarbonium ions, which alkylate or bind with many intracellular molecular structures including nucleic acids. Its cytotoxic action is probably due to cross-linking of strands of DNA, resulting in inhibition of DNA synthesis. Streptozocin has little effect on RNA or protein synthesis. Its alkylating activity is weak compared to that of other nitrosoureas.

### Other actions/effects
Streptozocin also has a diabetogenic or hyperglycemic effect as a result of selective uptake into and toxicity to pancreatic islet beta cells involving lowering of beta cell nicotinamide adenine dinucleotide (NAD). Irreversible damage to the cell results in degranulation and loss of insulin secretion.

### Distribution
Very little streptozocin crosses the blood-brain barrier, but metabolites do; 2 hours after administration, cerebrospinal fluid (CSF) concentrations are approximately equal to plasma concentrations.

### Biotransformation
Hepatic.

### Half-life
Initial—
  Unchanged drug: 5 to 15 minutes.
  Metabolites: 6 minutes.
Intermediate—
  Metabolites: 3.5 hours.
Terminal—
  Unchanged drug: 35 minutes.
  Metabolites: 40 hours.

### Elimination
Renal (as unchanged drug and at least 3 identified metabolites, including methylnitrosoureas).
Fecal (less than 1%).
Significant respiratory excretion also occurs.

# Precautions to Consider

### Carcinogenicity/Mutagenicity/Tumorigenicity
Streptozocin administration has reportedly been followed by development of acute myelocytic leukemia in one patient. Streptozocin is mutagenic in bacteria, plants, and mammalian cells and has been shown to be tumorigenic (renal, hepatic, stomach, and pancreatic tumors) in animals and carcinogenic in mice. Topical exposure in rats has resulted in development of benign tumors at the site.

### Pregnancy/Reproduction
Fertility—Gonadal suppression, resulting in amenorrhea or azoospermia, may occur in patients receiving antineoplastic therapy, especially with the alkylating agents. In general, these effects appear to be related to dose and length of therapy and may be irreversible. Prediction of the degree of testicular or ovarian function impairment is complicated by the common use of combinations of several antineoplastics, which makes it difficult to assess the effects of individual agents.

Streptozocin adversely affects fertility in male and female rats.

Pregnancy—Streptozocin crosses the placenta. Studies in humans have not been done.

First trimester: It is usually recommended that use of antineoplastics, especially combination chemotherapy, be avoided whenever possible, especially during the first trimester. Although information is limited because of the relatively few instances of antineoplastic administration during pregnancy, the mutagenic, teratogenic, and carcinogenic potential of these medications must be considered.

Other hazards to the fetus include adverse reactions seen in adults.

In general, use of a contraceptive is recommended during cytotoxic drug therapy.

Studies in animals have shown that streptozocin causes teratogenicity in rats and is abortifacient in rabbits.

FDA Pregnancy Category C.

### Breast-feeding
It is not known whether streptozocin is distributed into breast milk. Although very little information is available regarding distribution of antineoplastic agents in breast milk, breast-feeding is not recommended during chemotherapy because of the risks to the infant (adverse effects, mutagenicity, carcinogenicity).

### Pediatrics
Appropriate studies on the relationship of age to the effects of streptozocin have not been performed in the pediatric population.

### Geriatrics
No information is available on the relationship of age to the effects of streptozocin in geriatric patients. However, elderly patients are more likely to have age-related renal function impairment, which may require caution in patients receiving streptozocin.

### Dental
The bone marrow depressant effects of streptozocin may result in an increased incidence of microbial infection, delayed healing, and gingival bleeding. If leukopenia and/or thrombocytopenia occur, dental work should be deferred until blood counts have returned to normal and patients should be instructed in proper oral hygiene including caution in use of regular toothbrushes, dental floss, and toothpicks.

### Drug interactions and/or related problems
The following drug interactions and/or related problems have been selected on the basis of their potential clinical significance (possible mechanism in parentheses where appropriate)—not necessarily inclusive (» = major clinical significance):

Note: Combinations containing any of the following medications, depending on the amount present, may also interact with this medication.

Blood dyscrasia–causing medications (see *Appendix II*)
  (leukopenic and/or thrombocytopenic effects of streptozocin may be increased with concurrent or recent therapy if these medications cause the same effects; dosage adjustment of streptozocin, if necessary, should be based on blood counts)

Bone marrow depressants, other (see *Appendix II*) or
Radiation therapy
  (additive bone marrow depression may occur, although myelosuppressive effects of streptozocin are rare; dosage reduction may be required when two or more bone marrow depressants, including radiation, are used concurrently or consecutively)

  (streptozocin may prolong the half-life of doxorubicin when used concurrently; dosage reduction of doxorubicin is recommended)

Corticosteroids, glucocorticoid or
Corticotropin (ACTH)
  (concurrent use may increase the hyperglycemic effect of streptozocin)

» Nephrotoxic medications (see *Appendix II*)
  (concurrent use may result in enhanced nephrotoxicity and is not recommended)

Nicotinamide
  (concurrent use may reduce the diabetogenic effect of streptozocin but does not appear to alter the antitumor effect)

» Phenytoin
  (may protect pancreatic beta cells from the toxic effects of streptozocin, thus reducing its therapeutic effects; concurrent use is not recommended)

Vaccines, killed virus
  (because normal defense mechanisms may be suppressed by streptozocin therapy, the patient's antibody response to the vaccine may be decreased. The interval between discontinuation of medications that cause immunosuppression and restoration of the patient's ability to respond to the vaccine depends on the intensity and type of immunosuppression-causing medication used, the underlying disease, and other factors; estimates vary from 3 months to 1 year)

» Vaccines, live virus
  (because normal defense mechanisms may be suppressed by streptozocin therapy, concurrent use with a live virus vaccine may po-

tentiate the replication of the vaccine virus, may increase the side/adverse effects of the vaccine virus, and/or may decrease the patient's antibody response to the vaccine; immunization of these patients should be undertaken only with extreme caution after careful review of the patient's hematologic status and only with the knowledge and consent of the physician managing the streptozocin therapy. The interval between discontinuation of medications that cause immunosuppression and restoration of the patient's ability to respond to the vaccine depends on the intensity and type of immunosuppression-causing medication used, the underlying disease, and other factors; estimates vary from 3 months to 1 year. Immunization with oral poliovirus vaccine should also be postponed in persons in close contact with the patient, especially family members)

**Laboratory value alterations**
The following have been selected on the basis of their potential clinical significance (possible effect in parentheses where appropriate)—not necessarily inclusive (» = major clinical significance):

With physiology/laboratory test values
   Alanine aminotransferase (ALT [SGPT]) and
   Alkaline phosphatase and
   Aspartate aminotransferase (AST [SGOT]) and
   Bilirubin and
   Lactate dehydrogenase (LDH)
      (serum values may be increased, indicating hepatotoxicity)
   Albumin concentrations in blood
      (may be decreased, indicating hepatotoxicity)
   Blood urea nitrogen (BUN) concentrations and
   Creatinine concentrations, plasma and
   Protein concentrations, urinary
      (may be increased, indicating renal toxicity; usually transient, but permanent damage may occur)
   Glucose
      (blood concentrations may be initially decreased because of sudden release of insulin)
   Hematocrit
      (may rarely be mildly increased; reduction in hematocrit is generally more common than leukopenia or thrombocytopenia)
   Phosphate
      (blood concentrations may be decreased, as an early indication of renal toxicity)

**Medical considerations/Contraindications**
The medical considerations/contraindications included have been selected on the basis of their potential clinical significance (reasons given in parentheses where appropriate)—not necessarily inclusive (» = major clinical significance).

*Risk-benefit should be considered when the following medical problems exist:*
   Bone marrow depression or
   Infection
      (possible hematological toxicity, although this is rare)
» Chickenpox, existing or recent (including recent exposure) or
» Herpes zoster
      (risk of severe generalized disease)
   Diabetes mellitus
      (streptozocin causes hypoglycemia)
» Hepatic function impairment
      (reduced biotransformation and possible increased toxicity of streptozocin; streptozocin can have hepatotoxic effects)
» Renal function impairment
      (streptozocin causes severe renal toxicity)
   Sensitivity to streptozocin
   Caution should be used also in patients who have had previous cytotoxic drug therapy or radiation therapy.

**Patient monitoring**
The following may be especially important in patient monitoring (other tests may be warranted in some patients, depending on condition; » = major clinical significance):

   Alanine aminotransferase (ALT [SGPT]) values, serum and
   Aspartate aminotransferase (AST [SGOT]) values, serum and
   Bilirubin concentrations, serum and
   Lactate dehydrogenase (LDH) values, serum
      (determinations recommended prior to initiation of therapy and at periodic intervals during therapy; frequency varies according to clinical state, agent, and other agents being used concurrently)
» Blood urea nitrogen (BUN) concentrations and
» Creatinine clearance determinations and
» Creatinine concentrations, plasma and
» Electrolyte concentrations, serum and
» Urinalysis, serial, to detect proteinuria
      (recommended prior to, at least weekly during, and for 4 weeks following each course of therapy, to monitor for renal toxicity)
» Glucose concentrations, blood
      (recommended at periodic intervals)
   Hematocrit or hemoglobin and
   Leukocyte count, total and, if appropriate, differential and
   Platelet count
      (determinations recommended prior to initiation of therapy and at periodic intervals during therapy; frequency varies according to clinical state, agent, and other agents being used concurrently)
   Insulin concentrations, fasting
      (in patients with functional pancreatic tumors, serial monitoring allows a determination of biochemical response to therapy)
   Uric acid concentrations, serum
      (recommended prior to initiation of therapy and at periodic intervals during therapy; frequency varies according to clinical state, agent, and other agents being used concurrently)

## Side/Adverse Effects

Note: Many "side effects" of antineoplastic therapy are unavoidable and represent the medication's pharmacologic action. Some of these (for example, leukopenia and thrombocytopenia) are actually used as parameters to aid in individual dosage titration.

The following side/adverse effects have been selected on the basis of their potential clinical significance (possible signs and symptoms in parentheses where appropriate)—not necessarily inclusive:

**Those indicating need for medical attention**
Incidence more frequent— 28 to 73%
   *Renal toxicity and failure* (swelling of feet or lower legs; unusual decrease in urination)
   Note: *Renal toxicity* (proteinuria, glycosuria, hypophosphatemia, azotemia, renal tubular acidosis) occurs frequently. Mild proteinuria is one of the first signs of renal toxicity. Toxicity is dose-related and cumulative and may be fatal in some cases.

Incidence less frequent
   *Hypoglycemia* (anxiety, nervousness, or shakiness; chills, cold sweats, or cool, pale skin; drowsiness or unusual tiredness or weakness; fast pulse; headache; unusual hunger)—occurring shortly after injection; *pain or redness at site of injection*—caused by rapid intravenous injection or extravasation
   Note: Although streptozocin is diabetogenic, a sudden release of insulin may occur initially. Mild to moderate glucose tolerance abnormalities have been reported; they are usually reversible, although insulin shock with hypoglycemia has occurred.

Incidence rare
   *Hepatotoxicity*—usually not symptomatic; *leukopenia or infection* (fever or chills; cough or hoarseness; lower back or side pain; painful or difficult urination)—usually asymptomatic; *thrombocytopenia* (unusual bleeding or bruising; black, tarry stools; blood in urine or stools; pinpoint red spots on skin)—usually asymptomatic
   Note: Hematological toxicity is rare but has been fatal in some cases.

**Those indicating need for medical attention only if they continue or are bothersome**
Incidence more frequent
   *Nausea and vomiting*
   Note: *Nausea and vomiting* occur in most patients, usually within 2 to 4 hours after a dose and may be severe; usually become progressively worse over a course of therapy; antiemetics have little effect.

Incidence less frequent
   *Diarrhea*

**Those indicating the need for medical attention if they occur after medication is discontinued**
   *Renal toxicity* (decrease in urination; swelling of feet or lower legs)

## Patient Consultation

As an aid to patient consultation, refer to *Advice for the Patient, Streptozocin (Systemic)*.
In providing consultation, consider emphasizing the following selected information (» = major clinical significance):

**Before using this medication**
» Conditions affecting use, especially:
      Sensitivity to streptozocin

**2632   Streptozocin (Systemic)**

Pregnancy—Use not recommended because of mutagenic, teratogenic, and carcinogenic potential, advisability of using contraception; telling physician immediately if pregnancy is suspected

Breast-feeding—Not recommended because of risk of serious side effects

Other medications, especially nephrotoxic medications or phenytoin

Other medical problems, especially chickenpox, herpes zoster, hepatic function impairment, or renal function impairment

### Proper use of this medication
Importance of ample fluid intake and subsequent increase in urine output to aid excretion and reduce renal toxicity

Frequency of nausea and vomiting; importance of continuing medication despite stomach upset

» Proper dosing

### Precautions while using this medication
» Importance of close monitoring by physician
» Avoiding immunizations unless approved by physician; other persons in patient's household should avoid immunizations with oral poliovirus vaccine; avoiding other persons who have taken oral poliovirus vaccine or wearing a protective mask that covers nose and mouth
» Possibility of local tissue injury and scarring if infiltration of intravenous solution occurs; telling doctor or nurse right away about redness, pain, or swelling at injection site

### Side/adverse effects
Signs of potential side effects, especially renal toxicity and failure, hypoglycemia, pain or redness at site of injection caused by rapid intravenous injection or extravasation, hepatotoxicity, leukopenia, infection, and thrombocytopenia

Physician or nurse can help in dealing with side effects

## General Dosing Information

Patients receiving streptozocin should be under supervision of a physician experienced in cancer chemotherapy.

A variety of dosage schedules and regimens of streptozocin, alone or in combination with other antitumor agents, are used. The prescriber may consult the medical literature as well as the manufacturer's literature in choosing a specific dosage.

Dosage must be adjusted to meet the individual requirements of each patient, on the basis of clinical response and appearance or severity of toxicity.

Streptozocin may be administered by rapid intravenous injection or as a short (over a 10- to 15-minute period) or long (over a 6-hour period) intravenous infusion.

Streptozocin has also been administered as a continuous, 5-day intravenous infusion. Although incidence of renal toxicity and nausea and vomiting appeared to be reduced, other side effects including lethargy, confusion, and depression were reported.

Care must be taken to avoid extravasation during administration because of the risk of severe ulceration and necrosis.

If extravasation of streptozocin occurs during intravenous administration, as indicated by local burning or stinging, the injection or infusion should be stopped immediately and resumed, completing the dose, in another vein.

Although the manufacturer does not recommend intra-arterial administration because of the possibility that renal toxicity may occur more rapidly, streptozocin has been administered intra-arterially by a number of investigators, for example, in patients with hepatic metastases.

It is recommended that intravenous dextrose be immediately available, especially when the first dose of streptozocin is administered, because of the risk of hypoglycemia due to a sudden release of insulin.

It is recommended that each course of streptozocin therapy be followed by a 4- to 6-week observation period in order to detect any renal toxicity.

It is recommended that dosage of streptozocin be reduced or treatment withdrawn if significant renal toxicity occurs. Subsequent doses should not be given until renal function returns to normal.

Concomitant hydration with each dose may reduce renal toxicity by promoting rapid excretion in a dilute urine.

### Safety considerations for handling this medication
There is limited but increasing evidence and concern that personnel involved in preparation and administration of parenteral antineoplastics may be at some risk because of the potential mutagenicity, teratogenicity, and/or carcinogenicity of these agents, although the actual risk is unknown. USP advisory panels recommend cautious handling both in preparation and disposal of antineoplastic agents. Precautions that have been suggested include:
• Use of a biological containment cabinet during reconstitution and dilution of parenteral medications and wearing of disposable surgical gloves and masks.
• Use of proper technique to prevent contamination of the medication, work area, and operator during transfer between containers (including proper training of personnel in this technique).
• Cautious and proper disposal of needles, syringes, vials, ampuls, and unused medication.

A number of medical centers have developed detailed guidelines for handling of antineoplastic agents.

## Parenteral Dosage Forms

### STREPTOZOCIN FOR INJECTION

**Usual adult dose**
Carcinoma, islet cell—
  Intravenous, 500 mg per square meter of body surface area per day for five consecutive days every six weeks or
  Intravenous, 1 gram per square meter of body surface area once a week for two weeks, increased thereafter if necessary, up to a maximum dose of 1.5 grams per square meter of body surface area.

  Note: A single course usually consists of four to six once-a-week doses, but may be longer.

**Usual adult prescribing limits**
Up to 1.5 grams per square meter of body surface area as a single dose (because of the risk of azotemia).

**Usual pediatric dose**
Dosage has not been established.

**Size(s) usually available**
U.S.—
  1 gram (Rx) [Zanosar (citric acid anhydrous 220 mg)].
Canada—
  1 gram (Rx) [Zanosar].

**Packaging and storage**
Store between 2 and 8 °C (36 and 46 °F), unless otherwise specified by manufacturer. Protect from light.

**Preparation of dosage form**
Streptozocin for injection is reconstituted for intravenous use by adding 9.5 mL of 5% dextrose injection or 0.9% sodium chloride injection to the vial, producing a clear, pale-gold solution containing 100 mg of streptozocin and 22 mg of citric acid per mL.

Reconstituted solutions may be further diluted with 5% dextrose injection or 0.9% sodium chloride injection for administration by intravenous infusion. Addition of the 100 mg of streptozocin per mL solution to 10 to 200 mL of 5% dextrose injection followed by administration over a 15-minute period by infusion may prevent local pain and phlebitis.

**Stability**
Reconstituted solutions should be used within 12 hours if kept at room temperature.

Because the product contains no preservatives, the vial should not be used for more than one dose.

A change in color from pale gold to dark brown indicates decomposition.

**Note**
If accidental contact with skin or mucous membranes occurs, immediately wash the affected area with soap and water.

Revised: 08/26/92
Interim revision: 06/30/94; 09/30/97

---

# STRONTIUM CHLORIDE SR 89   Systemic

VA CLASSIFICATION (Primary): AN600
Commonly used brand name(s): *Metastron*.
Note: For a listing of dosage forms and brand names by country availability, see *Dosage Forms* section(s).

## Category
Antineoplastic.

# Indications

## Accepted
Bone lesions, metastatic (treatment)—Strontium chloride Sr 89 is indicated in the palliative treatment of bone pain in selected patients with multiple areas of skeletal metastases from carcinomas of the prostate, breast, and possibly, from other carcinomas.

# Physical Properties

## Nuclear data

| Radionuclide (half-life) | Mode of decay | Maximum energy (MeV) | Mean number of emissions/ disintegration |
|---|---|---|---|
| Sr 89 (50.5 days) | Beta | 1.463 | 1 |

# Pharmacology/Pharmacokinetics

## Mechanism of action/Effect
Antineoplastic—Metastatic bone lesions: Strontium chloride Sr 89, a calcium analog, follows the same biochemical pathways as calcium does *in vivo* and concentrates in areas of increased osteogenesis (i.e., increased mineral turnover), not in marrow cells. Thus, reactive osteoid being formed at sites of primary bone tumors and metastases accumulate strontium to a much higher level than does surrounding normal bone. The retained strontium can deliver a radiation dose sufficiently large to produce a palliative effect. Due to the short range of the beta particles, the cells close to regions containing strontium will be preferentially irradiated.

## Distribution
Distribution similar to calcium analogs with fairly rapid clearance from the blood and selective localization in bone hydroxyapatite.

## Onset of action
Pain relief may begin between 7 and 21 days following administration of strontium chloride Sr 89, with maximum relief by 6 weeks.

## Duration of action
Duration of pain relief averages 6 months, with a range of 4 to 12 months.

## Radiation dosimetry

| | Estimated absorbed radiation dose*† | |
|---|---|---|
| Organ | mGy/MBq | rad/mCi |
| Bone surfaces | 17.0 | 62.96 |
| Red marrow | 11.0 | 40.74 |
| Large intestine wall (lower) | 4.7 | 17.41 |
| Large intestine wall (upper) | 1.8 | 6.67 |
| Bladder wall | 1.3 | 4.81 |
| Breast | 0.96 | 3.55 |
| Adrenals | 0.78 | 2.89 |
| Stomach wall | 0.78 | 2.89 |
| Kidneys | 0.78 | 2.89 |
| Liver | 0.78 | 2.89 |
| Lungs | 0.78 | 2.89 |
| Ovaries | 0.78 | 2.89 |
| Pancreas | 0.78 | 2.89 |
| Spleen | 0.78 | 2.89 |
| Testes | 0.78 | 2.89 |
| Thyroid | 0.78 | 2.89 |
| Uterus | 0.78 | 2.89 |
| Small intestine | 0.023 | 0.085 |
| Other tissue | 0.78 | 2.89 |
| Effective dose: 2.9 mSv/MBq (10.73 rem/mCi) | | |

*For adults; intravenous injection. Data based on the International Commission on Radiological Protection (ICRP) Publication 53—Radiation dose to patients from radiopharmaceuticals.

†The absorbed dose to individual metastatic sites ranges from 60 to 610 mGy/MBq (220 to 2260 rad/mCi) with a mean dose of 230 mGy/MBq (850 rad/mCi).

## Elimination
Renal, by glomerular filtration (two-thirds of excreted activity), and fecal (one-third) in patients with bone metastases. Renal excretion is greatest in the first 2 days after treatment. Strontium 89 is lost from normal bone with an initial biological half-life of 14 days, but retained much longer in metastatic bone lesions. Patients with extensive metastases may retain 50 to 100% of the administered activity in bone and may excrete less than do persons without bone lesions. Whole body retention of strontium varies according to individual urinary plasma clearance and metastatic load in the skeleton; between 12 and 90% of the administered activity is retained 3 months after administration of strontium chloride Sr 89.

# Precautions to Consider

## Carcinogenicity/Mutagenicity
Thirty-three out of 40 rats receiving 10 consecutive monthly doses of either 250 or 350 microcuries per kg of body weight of strontium chloride Sr 89 developed malignant bone tumors after a latency period of approximately 9 months.

## Pregnancy/Reproduction
Pregnancy—Adequate and well-controlled studies with strontium chloride Sr 89 have not been done in humans. Radiopharmaceuticals are generally not recommended for therapeutic use during pregnancy because of the risk to the fetus from radiation exposure. Strontium chloride Sr 89 would be expected to cause adverse effects, such as bone marrow toxicity, in the fetus.

To avoid the possibility of fetal exposure to radiation, in those circumstances in which the patient's pregnancy status is uncertain, a pregnancy test will help to prevent inadvertent administration of this preparation during pregnancy.

Studies have not been done in animals.

FDA Pregnancy Category D.

## Breast-feeding
Strontium chloride Sr 89 acts as a calcium analog and is expected to be distributed into breast milk. Because of the potential risk to the infant from radiation exposure, complete cessation of nursing is recommended after strontium chloride Sr 89 has been administered.

## Pediatrics
There have been no specific studies evaluating the safety and efficacy of strontium chloride Sr 89 in children.

## Geriatrics
Appropriate studies on the relationship of age to the effects of strontium chloride Sr 89 have not been performed in the geriatric population. However, no geriatrics-specific problems have been documented to date.

## Drug interactions and/or related problems
The following drug interactions and/or related problems have been selected on the basis of their potential clinical significance (possible mechanism in parentheses where appropriate)—not necessarily inclusive (» = major clinical significance):

» Blood-dyscrasia–causing medications (See *Appendix II*)
(leukopenic and/or thrombocytopenic effects of strontium chloride Sr 89 may be increased)

» Calcium-containing medications
(saturation of bone-binding sites by calcium may cause decreased bone uptake of strontium chloride Sr 89; calcium-containing medications should be discontinued at least 2 weeks before therapy with strontium chloride Sr 89; calcium-containing medication may be resumed approximately 2 weeks after strontium chloride Sr 89 therapy)

## Laboratory value alterations
The following have been selected on the basis of their potential clinical significance (possible effect in parentheses where appropriate)—not necessarily inclusive (» = major clinical significance):

With physiology/laboratory test values
Alkaline phosphatase
(serum values may be decreased, reflecting tumoricidal effect)

Serum tumor markers, such as prostatic specific antigen (PSA) and prostate acid phosphatase (PAP)
(concentration may be decreased, reflecting tumoricidal effect)

## Medical considerations/Contraindications
The medical considerations/contraindications included have been selected on the basis of their potential clinical significance (reasons given in parentheses where appropriate)—not necessarily inclusive (» = major clinical significance).

*Except under special circumstances, this medication should not be used when the following medical problem exists:*

» Bone marrow depression, with platelet count less than 60,000 per microliter and white cell count less than 2,400 per microliter, especially with previous or concomitant chemotherapy or radiotherapy administration
(increased risk of toxicity due to compromised bone marrow)

# Strontium Chloride Sr 89 (Systemic)

*Risk-benefit must be considered when the following medical problems exist:*

Sensitivity to the radiopharmaceutical preparation

Urinary incontinence
(increased risk of radiation contamination of environment; therefore, urinary catheterization is recommended)

Very short life-expectancy
(use not warranted since onset of pain relief may not occur for 10 to 20 days)

**Patient monitoring**

The following may be especially important in patient monitoring (other tests may be warranted in some patients, depending on condition; » = major clinical significance):

» Blood studies, including leukocyte and platelet counts
(recommended prior to therapy and at least once every other week for 3 to 4 months after therapy)

## Side/Adverse Effects

Note: A single case of fatal septicemia following leukopenia has been reported during clinical trials.

**Those indicating need for medical attention**
Incidence rare
*Bone marrow depression leading to thrombocytopenia* (unusual bleeding or bruising; black, tarry stools; blood in urine or stools; pinpoint red spots on skin); *and leukopenia* (cough or hoarseness; fever or chills; lower back or side pain; painful or difficult urination)

Note: On the average, platelet concentrations may fall by 30% of pretreatment levels (i.e., fall to 70% of baseline); however, this effect is generally reversible, and the majority of patients maintain platelet counts that are within normal limits. The nadir of platelet depression occurs in most patients about 6 weeks after administration of strontium chloride Sr 89.

Bone marrow toxicity may be difficult to evaluate because marrow suppression is common in patients with prostate cancer and extensive bone metastases.

**Those indicating need for medical attention only if they continue or are bothersome**
Incidence more frequent
*Flare reaction* (increase in bone pain, transient); *flushing*—with rapid administration

## Patient Consultation

As an aid to patient consultation, refer to *Advice for the Patient, Strontium Chloride Sr 89 (Therapeutic)*.

In providing consultation, consider emphasizing the following selected information (» = major clinical significance):

**Description of use**
Action in the body: Active incorporation of strontium 89 into bone mineral, especially in areas of tumor involvement; localized radiation exposure to these sites provides reduction in bone pain

**Before using this medication**
» Conditions affecting use, especially:
Sensitivity to the radiopharmaceutical preparation
Pregnancy—Use not recommended; risk to fetus from radiation exposure
Breast-feeding—May be distributed into breast milk; cessation of nursing is recommended because of risk to infant from radiation exposure
Other medications, especially blood dyscrasia–causing and calcium-containing

**Proper use of this medication**
Special preparatory instructions may apply; patient should inquire in advance
Notifying physician prior to administration if having an incontinence problem; catheterization may be required to prevent radiation contamination

**Precautions after using this medication**
» Importance of close monitoring by the physician
*To prevent radiation contamination of other persons or environment:*
For the first week—
» Using a normal toilet instead of a urinal
» Double-flushing toilet
» Wiping any spilled urine with a tissue and flushing it away
» Washing hands after using or cleaning toilet
» Immediately laundering clothes and linens soiled with urine or blood; washing them separately from other clothes
» Washing away any spilled blood

» Caution if significant bone marrow depression occurs
*Abnormally low white blood cell counts—*
Avoiding exposure to persons with bacterial infections, especially during periods of low blood counts; checking with physician immediately if fever or chills, cough or hoarseness, lower back or side pain, or painful or difficult urination occurs
Caution in use of regular toothbrush, dental floss, or toothpick; physician, dentist, or nurse may suggest alternatives; checking with physician before having dental work done
Not touching eyes or inside of nose unless hands washed immediately before

*Abnormally low platelet counts—*
Using caution to avoid accidental cuts with use of sharp objects such as safety razor or fingernail or toenail cutters
Avoiding contact sports or other situations where bruising or injury could occur

**Side/adverse effects**
Signs of potential side effects, especially bone marrow depression

## General Dosing Information

Radiopharmaceuticals are to be administered only by or under the supervision of physicians who have had extensive training in the safe use and handling of radioactive materials and who are authorized by the Nuclear Regulatory Commission (NRC) or the appropriate Agreement State agency, if required, or, outside the U.S., the appropriate authority.

The presence of bone metastases must be confirmed (e.g., by skeletal imaging with a technetium Tc 99m–labeled phosphate or phosphonate radiopharmaceutical) prior to therapy with strontium chloride Sr 89.

Treatment may be repeated at intervals of 3 months or more if pain recurs. However, previous hematologic response, current platelet level, and other signs of bone marrow depression should be carefully evaluated before therapy with strontium chloride Sr 89 is repeated.

**Safety considerations for handling this medication**
Improper handling of this radiopharmaceutical may cause radioactive contamination. Guidelines for handling radioactive material have been prepared by scientific, professional, state, federal, and international bodies and are available to the specially qualified and authorized users who have access to radiopharmaceuticals

## Parenteral Dosage Forms

### STRONTIUM CHLORIDE Sr 89 INJECTION USP

**Usual adult administered activity**
Antineoplastic—
Metastatic bone lesions: Intravenous, 1.5 to 2.2 megabecquerels (40 to 60 microcuries) per kg of body weight, or a total administered activity of 148 megabecquerels (4 millicuries) given slowly (one to two minutes) as a single dose.

Note: Repeated administration at intervals of less than ninety days is generally not recommended.

**Usual pediatric administered activity**
Children up to 18 years of age: Minimum dosage has not been established.

**Usual geriatric administered activity**
See *Usual adult administered activity*.

**Strength(s) usually available**
U.S.—
148 megabecquerels (4 millicuries) in 4-mL volume per 10-mL vial, containing 10.9 to 22.6 mg of strontium chloride per mL, and a specific activity of 2.96 to 6.17 megabecquerels (80 to 167 microcuries) per mg of strontium, at time of calibration (Rx) [*Metastron*].
Canada—
150 megabecquerels (4.05 millicuries) in 4-mL volume per 10-mL vial, containing 13.4 to 20.1 mg of strontium chloride per mL, and a specific activity of 3.33 to 5 megabecquerels (90 to 135 microcuries) per mg of strontium, at time of calibration (Rx) [*Metastron*].

**Packaging and storage**
Store between 15 and 25 °C (59 and 77 °F), unless otherwise specified by manufacturer. Protect from freezing.

**Stability**
Product should not be used beyond 4 weeks after calibration.

**Note**
Caution—Radioactive material.

## Selected Bibliography

Hansen DV, Holmes ER, Catton G, et al. Strontium 89 therapy for painful osseous metastatic prostate and breast cancer. Am Fam Physician 1993; 47(8): 1795-800.

Laing AH, Ackery DM, Bayly RJ, et al. Strontium 89 chloride for pain palliation in prostatic skeletal malignancy. Br J Radiol 1991; 64(765): 816-22.

Porter AT, McEwan AJ, Powe JE, et al. Results of a randomized phase-III trial to evaluate the efficacy of strontium 89 adjuvant to local field external beam irradiation in the management of endocrine resistant metastatic prostate cancer. Int J Radiat Oncol Biol Phys 1993; 25(5): 805-13.

Robinson RG, Preston DF, Baxter KG, et al. Clinical experience with strontium 89 in prostatic and breast cancer patients. Semin Oncol 1993; 20(3 Suppl 2): 44-8.

Robinson RG, Preston DF, Spicer JA, et al. Radionuclide therapy of intractable bone pain: emphasis on strontium 89. Semin Nucl Med 1992; 22(1): 28-32.

Revised: 06/23/94
Interim revision: 05/18/95

**SUCCIMER**—The *Succimer (Systemic)* monograph is not included in this published version of the USP DI database. Copies of the monograph are available on request from Micromedex, Inc. - Reprint Requests, 6200 S. Syracuse Way, Suite 300, Englewood, CO 80111; telephone (303) 486-6400; telefax (303) 486-6464; Email: USPDI@MDX.COM.

**SUCCINYLCHOLINE CHLORIDE**—See *Neuromuscular Blocking Agents (Systemic)*

# SUCRALFATE   Oral-Local

VA CLASSIFICATION (Primary): GA302

Commonly used brand name(s): *Apo-sucralfate; Carafate; Sulcrate; Sulcrate Suspension Plus.*

Note:   For a listing of dosage forms and brand names by country availability, see *Dosage Forms* section(s).

## Category
Antiulcer agent; gastric mucosa protectant.

## Indications
Note:   Bracketed information in the *Indications* section refers to uses that are not included in U.S. product labeling.

**Accepted**

Ulcer, duodenal (treatment)—Sucralfate is indicated in the short-term (up to 8 weeks) treatment of duodenal ulcer.

Ulcer, duodenal (prophylaxis)—Sucralfate is used in the prevention of duodenal ulcer recurrence.

[Ulcer, gastric (treatment)]—Sucralfate is used for the short-term treatment of benign gastric ulcer.

[Arthritis, rheumatoid (treatment adjunct)][1]—Sucralfate is used for the relief of gastrointestinal symptoms associated with the use of nonsteroidal anti-inflammatory drugs in the treatment of rheumatoid arthritis.

[Stress-related mucosal damage (prophylaxis and treatment)]—Sucralfate is used to prevent and treat gastrointestinal, stress-induced ulceration and bleeding, especially in intensive care patients.

[Reflux, gastroesophageal (treatment)]—Sucralfate is used in the treatment of gastroesophageal reflux disease.

[1]Not included in Canadian product labeling.

## Pharmacology/Pharmacokinetics

**Physicochemical characteristics**
Sucralfate is an aluminum salt of a sulfated disaccharide.

**Mechanism of action/Effect**
Exact mechanism of action is not known; however, sucralfate is thought to form an ulcer-adherent complex with proteinaceous exudate, such as albumin and fibrinogen, at the ulcer site, protecting it against further acid attack. To a lesser extent, sucralfate forms a viscous, adhesive barrier on the surface of intact mucosa of the stomach and duodenum. Sucralfate also inhibits pepsin activity and has been found to bind bile salts *in vitro*. Recent information suggests that sucralfate may increase the production of prostaglandin $E_2$ and gastric mucus.

**Absorption**
Up to 5% of the disaccharide component and less than 0.02% of aluminum is absorbed from the gastrointestinal tract following an oral sucralfate dose.

**Elimination**
Mostly fecal; small amounts of sulfate disaccharide are eliminated in the urine.

## Precautions to Consider

**Pregnancy/Reproduction**

Pregnancy—Studies in humans have not been done.
Studies in animals have not shown that sucralfate causes adverse effects on the fetus.

FDA Pregnancy Category B.

**Breast-feeding**
Problems in humans have not been documented.

**Pediatrics**
Appropriate studies to date have not demonstrated pediatrics-specific problems that would limit the usefulness of sucralfate in children.

**Geriatrics**
Although adequate and well-controlled studies on the relationship of age to the effects of sucralfate have not been performed in the geriatric population, no geriatrics-specific problems have been documented to date.

**Drug interactions and/or related problems**
The following drug interactions and/or related problems have been selected on the basis of their potential clinical significance (possible mechanism in parentheses where appropriate)—not necessarily inclusive (» = major clinical significance):

Note:   Combinations containing any of the following medications, depending on the amount present, may also interact with this medication.

  Aluminum-containing medications, such as:
   Antacids
   Antidiarrheals
   Aspirin, buffered with aluminum
   Vaginal douches
    (concurrent use with sucralfate in patients with renal failure may cause aluminum toxicity)

  Antacids
    (concurrent use with antacids in the treatment of duodenal ulcer may be indicated for the relief of pain; however, simultaneous administration is not recommended since antacids may interfere with binding of sucralfate to the mucosa; patient should be advised not to take antacids within ½ hour before or after sucralfate)

  Cimetidine or
  Ranitidine
    (concurrent use with sucralfate may decrease the absorption of cimetidine or ranitidine; patients should be advised to take cimetidine or ranitidine 2 hours before sucralfate)

» Ciprofloxacin or
» Norfloxacin or
» Ofloxacin
    (concurrent use with sucralfate may decrease the absorption of ciprofloxacin, norfloxacin, or ofloxacin by chelation, resulting in lower serum and urine concentrations of these 3 medicines; patients should be advised to take ciprofloxacin, norfloxacin, or ofloxacin 2 to 3 hours before sucralfate)

» Digoxin or
» Theophylline
    (concurrent use with sucralfate may decrease the absorption of digoxin or theophylline; patients should be advised not to take sucralfate within 2 hours of digoxin or theophylline)

» Phenytoin
(concurrent use with sucralfate may decrease the absorption of phenytoin enough to reduce the steady-state blood concentrations of phenytoin with a resultant loss of seizure control; patients should be advised not to take sucralfate within 2 hours of phenytoin)

Tetracyclines, oral
(absorption may be decreased when oral tetracyclines are used concurrently with sucralfate, since sucralfate is an aluminum salt and may form nonabsorbable complexes with tetracycline; patients should be advised not to take sucralfate within 2 hours of tetracyclines)

### Medical considerations/Contraindications
The medical considerations/contraindications included have been selected on the basis of their potential clinical significance (reasons given in parentheses where appropriate)—not necessarily inclusive (» = major clinical significance).

*Risk-benefits should be considered when the following medical problems exist:*
Dysphagia or
Gastrointestinal tract obstruction disease
(patients with these conditions may be at risk of bezoar formation because of the protein-binding properties of sucralfate)
Renal failure
(absorption of the aluminum in sucralfate in patients with renal failure may cause aluminum toxicity, especially with long-term use)
Sensitivity to sucralfate

### Patient monitoring
The following may be especially important in patient monitoring (other tests may be warranted in some patients, depending on condition; » = major clinical significance):

Serum aluminum concentrations
(determinations may be increased in patients with renal failure)

## Side/Adverse Effects
Note: Occurrence of drowsiness progressing to seizures in patients with renal failure may indicate aluminum toxicity.

The following side/adverse effects have been selected on the basis of their potential clinical significance (possible signs and symptoms in parentheses where appropriate)—not necessarily inclusive:

### Those indicating need for medical attention only if they continue or are bothersome
Incidence more frequent
  *Constipation*
Incidence less frequent or rare
  *Backache; diarrhea; dizziness or lightheadedness; drowsiness; dryness of mouth; indigestion; nausea; skin rash, hives, or itching; stomach cramps or pain*

## Patient Consultation
As an aid to patient consultation, refer to *Advice for the Patient, Sucralfate (Oral)*.
In providing consultation, consider emphasizing the following selected information (» = major clinical significance):

### Before using this medication
» Conditions affecting use, especially:
  Sensitivity to sucralfate
  Other medications, especially ciprofloxacin, digoxin, norfloxacin, ofloxacin, phenytoin, and theophylline

### Proper use of this medication
Taking on empty stomach 1 hour before meals and at bedtime
Compliance with full course of therapy and keeping appointments for check-ups
» Proper dosing
  Missed dose: Taking as soon as possible; not taking if almost time for next dose; not doubling doses
» Proper storage

### Precautions while using this medication
» Not taking antacids within ½ hour before or after sucralfate

### Side/adverse effects
Signs of potential side effects, especially aluminum toxicity

## General Dosing Information
Sucralfate should be taken with water on an empty stomach, 1 hour before each meal and at bedtime, for maximum effectiveness.

Short-term treatment with sucralfate may result in complete healing of the ulcer but it may not alter the posthealing frequency or severity of duodenal ulceration.

If required, antacids may be administered ½ hour before or after sucralfate for the relief of pain.

Even though the symptoms of duodenal ulcers may subside, unless healing has been documented by x-ray or endoscopic examination, therapy should continue for at least 4 to 8 weeks.

Use of sucralfate in a nasogastric feeding tube has resulted in bezoar formation with other medications or enteral feedings, due to the protein-binding properties of sucralfate.

## Oral Dosage Forms
Note: Bracketed uses in the *Dosage Forms* section refer to categories of use and/or indications that are not included in U.S. product labeling.

### SUCRALFATE ORAL SUSPENSION
**Usual adult and adolescent dose**
Duodenal ulcer (treatment)—
  Oral, 1 gram four times a day one hour before each meal and at bedtime; or 2 grams two times a day on waking and at bedtime on an empty stomach.
[Gastroesophageal reflux]—
  Oral, 1 gram four times a day one hour before each meal and at bedtime.
[Stress-related mucosal damage (prophylaxis)]—
  Oral, 1 gram four to six times a day.
  Note: Duration of treatment for prophylaxis of stress ulceration must be individually determined and should be continued for as long as risk factors are present; usually, treatment does not continue longer than fourteen days.

**Usual pediatric dose**
Duodenal ulcer (treatment)—
  Dosage has not been established.
[Gastroesophageal reflux]—
  Oral, 500 mg to 1 gram four times a day one hour before each meal and at bedtime.

**Strength(s) usually available**
U.S.—
  500 mg per 5 mL (Rx) [*Carafate*].
Canada—
  500 mg per 5 mL (Rx) [*Sulcrate*].
  1 gram per 5 mL (Rx) [*Sulcrate Suspension Plus* (caramel-flavored)].

**Packaging and storage**
Store below 40 °C (104 °F), preferably between 15 and 30 °C (59 and 86 °F), in a tight container, unless otherwise specified by manufacturer. Protect from freezing.

**Auxiliary labeling**
• Shake well.

### SUCRALFATE TABLETS USP
**Usual adult and adolescent dose**
Duodenal ulcer (treatment)—
  Oral, 1 gram four times a day one hour before each meal and at bedtime.
Duodenal ulcer (prophylaxis)—
  Oral, 1 gram two times a day on an empty stomach.
[Gastric ulcer (treatment)] or
[Gastroesophageal reflux]—
  Oral, 1 gram four times a day one hour before each meal and at bedtime.

**Usual pediatric dose**
Duodenal ulcer (treatment)—
  Dosage has not been established.
[Gastroesophageal reflux]—
  Oral, 500 mg four times a day one hour before each meal and at bedtime.

**Strength(s) usually available**
U.S.—
  1 gram (Rx) [*Carafate*; GENERIC].
Canada—
  1 gram (Rx) [*Apo-sucralfate*; *Sulcrate*].

**Packaging and storage**
Store below 40 °C (104 °F), preferably between 15 and 30 °C (59 and 86 °F), in a tight container, unless otherwise specified by manufacturer.

**Auxiliary labeling**
- Continue medicine for full time of treatment.

Revised: 03/24/92
Interim revision: 08/17/94; 07/26/96; 01/07/98; 02/23/98

---

**SUFENTANIL**—See *Fentanyl Derivatives (Systemic)*

---

**SULCONAZOLE**—The *Sulconazole (Topical)* monograph is not included in this published version of the USP DI database. Copies of the monograph are available on request from Micromedex, Inc. - Reprint Requests, 6200 S. Syracuse Way, Suite 300, Englewood, CO 80111; telephone (303) 486-6400; telefax (303) 486-6464; Email: USPDI@MDX.COM.

---

**SULFACETAMIDE**—See *Sulfonamides (Ophthalmic)*

---

**SULFADIAZINE**—See *Sulfonamides (Systemic)*

---

# SULFADOXINE AND PYRIMETHAMINE Systemic

VA CLASSIFICATION (Primary): AP101
Commonly used brand name(s): *Fansidar*.
Note: For a listing of dosage forms and brand names by country availability, see *Dosage Forms* section(s).

## Category
Antiprotozoal.

## Indications
Note: Bracketed information in the *Indications* section refers to uses that are not included in U.S. product labeling.

**Accepted**
Malaria (prophylaxis)—Sulfadoxine and pyrimethamine combination is indicated as a secondary agent in the prophylaxis of chloroquine-resistant *Plasmodium falciparum* malaria. However, because of its potentially life-threatening toxicity, it is not recommended for weekly use in the prophylaxis of chloroquine-resistant *P. falciparum* malaria in travelers to areas where chloroquine-resistant malaria is endemic. It is indicated **only** in persons at high risk of chloroquine-resistant malaria in remote areas who are unable to take alternative medication.

Malaria (treatment)—Sulfadoxine and pyrimethamine combination is indicated in combination with quinine as a primary agent in the treatment of chloroquine-resistant *P. falciparum* malaria. It is also indicated in the presumptive treatment of chloroquine-resistant *P. falciparum* malaria for self-treatment of febrile illness when medical care is not immediately available (within 24 hours).

[Isosporiasis (prophylaxis)][1]—Sulfadoxine is used with pyrimethamine in the prophylaxis of isosporiasis caused by *Isospora belli* in patients with acquired immunodeficiency disease.

Some strains of *P. falciparum* have developed resistance to sulfadoxine and pyrimethamine combination.

[1]Not included in Canadian product labeling.

## Pharmacology/Pharmacokinetics

**Physicochemical characteristics**
Molecular weight—Sulfadoxine: 310.33.
Pyrimethamine: 248.71.

**Mechanism of action/Effect**
Sulfadoxine—
  Bacteriostatic; Structural analog of aminobenzoic acid (PABA); competitively inhibits a bacterial enzyme, dihydropteroate synthetase, which is responsible for incorporation of PABA into dihydrofolic acid. This blocks the synthesis of dihydrofolic acid and decreases the amount of metabolically active tetrahydrofolic acid, a cofactor for the synthesis of purines, thymidine, and DNA.
  Susceptible bacteria are those that must synthesize folic acid. The action of sulfonamides is antagonized by PABA and its derivatives (e.g., procaine and tetracaine) and by the presence of pus or tissue breakdown products, which provide the necessary components for bacterial growth.
Pyrimethamine—
  Binds to and reversibly inhibits the protozoal enzyme dihydrofolate reductase, selectively blocking conversion of dihydrofolic acid to its functional form, tetrahydrofolic acid. This depletes folate, an essential cofactor in the biosynthesis of nucleic acids, resulting in interference with protozoal nucleic acid and protein production.
  Protozoal dihydrofolate reductase is many times more tightly bound by pyrimethamine than is the corresponding mammalian enzyme.
  Pyrimethamine exerts its effect in the folate biosynthesis at a step immediately subsequent to the one at which sulfonamides exert their effect. When pyrimethamine is administered concurrently with sulfonamides, synergism occurs, which is attributed to inhibition of tetrahydrofolate production at two sequential steps in its biosynthesis.
  Pyrimethamine is active against asexual erythrocytic forms and, to a lesser degree, tissue forms of *P. falciparum* malaria. It does not destroy gametocytes, but arrests sporogony in the mosquito.

**Absorption**
Well absorbed following oral administration.

**Distribution**
Pyrimethamine—Widely distributed; mainly concentrated in red and white blood cells, kidneys, lungs, liver, and spleen. Crosses into the cerebrospinal fluid (CSF), with concentrations ranging from 13 to 26% of the corresponding serum concentrations.
Sulfadoxine and pyrimethamine both cross the placenta and are excreted in breast milk.

**Protein binding**
Pyrimethamine—High (87%).
Sulfadoxine—High (> 90%).

**Biotransformation**
Pyrimethamine—Hepatic.

**Half-life**
Elimination—
  Sulfadoxine: Approximately 100 to 230 hours (mean, approximately 169 hours).
  Pyrimethamine: Approximately 54 to 148 hours (mean, approximately 111 hours).

**Time to peak plasma concentration**
Sulfadoxine—2.5 to 6 hours.
Pyrimethamine—Approximately 3 hours (range, 2 to 6 hours).

**Peak plasma concentration**
Sulfadoxine—Approximately 50 to 75 mcg per mL, 2.5 to 6 hours following a single oral dose of 500 mg of sulfadoxine and 25 mg of pyrimethamine.
Pyrimethamine—Approximately 0.13 to 0.4 mcg per mL, 1.5 to 8 hours following a single oral dose of 500 mg of sulfadoxine and 25 mg of pyrimethamine.

**Elimination**
Sulfadoxine—
  Renal: Excreted primarily unchanged by the kidneys.
Pyrimethamine—
  Renal: Primary route; 20 to 30% excreted unchanged in urine. Urinary excretion may persist for 30 days or longer.
  In dialysis: The serum concentration of pyrimethamine was decreased by approximately 47% after peritoneal dialysis in one patient.

## Precautions to Consider

**Cross-sensitivity and/or related problems**
For sulfadoxine—Patients allergic to one sulfonamide may be allergic to other sulfonamides also. Patients allergic to furosemide, thiazide diuretics, sulfonylureas, or carbonic anhydrase inhibitors may be allergic to sulfonamides also.

## Carcinogenicity/Tumorigenicity
For sulfadoxine—Long-term administration of sulfonamides in rats has been shown to result in thyroid malignancies.

For pyrimethamine—Pyrimethamine has not been shown to be carcinogenic in female mice or in male or female rats.

## Mutagenicity
For pyrimethamine—Pyrimethamine has been shown to be mutagenic in laboratory animals and in human bone marrow following 3 or 4 consecutive daily doses totaling 200 to 300 mg. However, pyrimethamine has not been shown to be mutagenic in the Ames test.

## Pregnancy/Reproduction
Fertility—Studies in rats given sulfadoxine and pyrimethamine combination in doses of 105 mg per kg of body weight (mg/kg) daily or pyrimethamine alone in doses of 15 mg/kg daily have shown that both regimens cause testicular changes.

The fertility of male rats and the ability of male or female rats to mate has not been shown to be adversely affected when sulfadoxine and pyrimethamine combination was given in doses of up to 210 mg/kg daily.

The pregnancy rate of female rats was significantly reduced when the rats were given doses of 31.5 mg/kg daily (approximately 30 times the weekly prophylactic dose) or higher, but was not adversely affected at doses of 10.5 mg/kg daily.

Pregnancy—Sulfonamides and pyrimethamine cross the placenta. Adequate and well-controlled studies in humans have not been done. Sulfadoxine and pyrimethamine combination may interfere with folic acid metabolism in the fetus and is generally not recommended for use during pregnancy. However, malaria in pregnant women may be more severe than in nonpregnant women and may result in maternal death. The risk of adverse pregnancy outcomes, including premature births, stillbirths, and abortion, may be increased. These risks should be weighed against the risks and benefits of sulfadoxine and pyrimethamine combination use during pregnancy. Women of child-bearing potential who travel to areas where chloroquine-resistant malaria is endemic should be warned not to become pregnant.

Studies in rats given weekly doses approximately 12 times the weekly prophylactic dose have shown that sulfadoxine and pyrimethamine combination is teratogenic. Studies in rats given sulfadoxine and pyrimethamine (20:1) have shown that the minimum oral teratogenic dose is approximately 18 mg of sulfadoxine and 0.9 mg of pyrimethamine per kg of body weight. However, studies in rabbits given doses as high as 400 mg of sulfadoxine and 20 mg of pyrimethamine per kg of body weight have not shown that sulfadoxine and pyrimethamine combination is teratogenic.

FDA Pregnancy Category C.

## Breast-feeding
Sulfadoxine and pyrimethamine are excreted in breast milk. Use is not recommended in nursing women since sulfonamides may cause kernicterus in nursing infants. In addition, pyrimethamine may interfere with folic acid metabolism in nursing infants, especially when given in large doses to nursing women.

## Pediatrics
Sulfadoxine and pyrimethamine combination is contraindicated in infants under 2 months of age since sulfonamides may cause kernicterus in neonates.

## Geriatrics
No information is available on the relationship of age to the effects of sulfadoxine and pyrimethamine combination in geriatric patients.

## Dental
Sulfadoxine and pyrimethamine combination may cause a change in or loss of taste; soreness, redness, swelling, burning, or stinging of the tongue; sore throat or difficulty in swallowing; and ulcers, sores, or white spots in the mouth.

The leukopenic and thrombocytopenic effects of sulfadoxine and pyrimethamine combination may result in an increased incidence of certain microbial infections, delayed healing, and gingival bleeding. If leukopenia or thrombocytopenia occurs, dental work should be deferred until blood counts have returned to normal. Patients should be instructed in proper oral hygiene, including caution in use of regular toothbrushes, dental floss, and toothpicks.

## Drug interactions and/or related problems
The following drug interactions and/or related problems have been selected on the basis of their potential clinical significance (possible mechanism in parentheses where appropriate)—not necessarily inclusive (» = major clinical significance):

Note: Combinations containing any of the following medications, depending on the amount present, may also interact with this medication.

Anticoagulants, coumarin- or indandione-derivative or
Anticonvulsants, hydantoin or
Antidiabetic agents, oral
(these medications may be displaced from protein-binding sites and/or their metabolism may be inhibited by some sulfonamides, resulting in increased or prolonged effects and/or toxicity; dosage adjustments may be necessary during and after sulfonamide therapy)

» Bone marrow depressants (See *Appendix II* )
(concurrent use of these medications with sulfadoxine and pyrimethamine combination may increase the leukopenic and/or thrombocytopenic effects; if concurrent use is required, close observation for myelotoxic effects should be considered, especially when sulfadoxine and pyrimethamine combination is used in high doses)

Folate antagonists, other (See *Appendix II* )
(concurrent use of other folate antagonists with pyrimethamine or use of pyrimethamine between courses of other folate antagonists is not recommended because of the possibility of megaloblastic anemia)

» Hemolytics, other (See *Appendix II* )
(concurrent use with sulfonamides may increase the potential for toxic side effects)

» Hepatotoxic medications, other (See *Appendix II* )
(concurrent use with sulfonamides may result in an increased incidence of hepatotoxicity; patients, especially those on prolonged administration or those with a history of liver disease, should be carefully monitored)

Methotrexate or
Phenylbutazone or
Sulfinpyrazone
(the effects of these medications may be potentiated during concurrent use with some sulfonamides because of displacement from plasma protein-binding sites)

## Medical considerations/Contraindications
The medical considerations/contraindications included have been selected on the basis of their potential clinical significance (reasons given in parentheses where appropriate)—not necessarily inclusive (» = major clinical significance).

*Except under special circumstances, this medication should not be used when the following medical problem exists:*

» Allergy to sulfonamides, pyrimethamine, furosemide, thiazide diuretics, sulfonylureas, or carbonic anhydrase inhibitors

*Risk-benefit should be considered when the following medical problems exist:*

» Anemia or
» Bone marrow depression
(pyrimethamine may cause folic acid deficiency, resulting in megaloblastic anemia; sulfonamides and pyrimethamine may cause blood dyscrasias, including agranulocytosis and thrombocytopenia)

Hepatic function impairment
(sulfonamides and pyrimethamine are metabolized in the liver; may cause fulminant hepatic necrosis)

» Porphyria
(sulfonamides may precipitate an acute attack of porphyria)

» Renal function impairment
(pyrimethamine and sulfadoxine are eliminated primarily through the kidneys)

Seizure disorders
(pyrimethamine may cause central nervous system [CNS] toxicity when used in high doses)

## Patient monitoring
The following may be especially important in patient monitoring (other tests may be warranted in some patients, depending on condition; » = major clinical significance):

» Complete blood counts (CBCs)
(may be required prior to and monthly or less frequently during treatment to detect blood dyscrasias in patients on prolonged therapy; therapy should be discontinued if a significant decrease in the count of any formed blood elements occurs)

Urinalyses
(may be required prior to and periodically during treatment to detect crystalluria and/or urinary calculi formation in patients on long-term or high-dose therapy and in patients with impaired renal function)

## Side/Adverse Effects

Note: **Fatalities have occurred, although rarely, due to severe reactions such as Stevens-Johnson syndrome, toxic epidermal necrolysis, fulminant hepatic necrosis, agranulocytosis, aplastic anemia, and other blood dyscrasias.** These toxicities were associated with multiple dosing regimens. Therapy should be discontinued at the first appearance of skin rash or if symptoms of folic acid deficiency occur.

The following side/adverse effects have been selected on the basis of their potential clinical significance (possible signs and symptoms in parentheses where appropriate)—not necessarily inclusive:

### Those indicating need for medical attention
Incidence more frequent
*Atrophic glossitis* (pain, burning, or inflammation of the tongue; change in or loss of taste)—due to folic acid deficiency with high doses; *blood dyscrasias, specifically agranulocytosis* (fever and sore throat); *megaloblastic anemia* (unusual tiredness or weakness); *or thrombocytopenia* (unusual bleeding or bruising); *hypersensitivity* (skin rash; fever); *photosensitivity* (increased sensitivity of skin to sunlight)

Incidence less frequent
*Hepatitis* (yellow eyes and skin); *Stevens-Johnson syndrome* (aching of joints and muscles; redness, blistering, peeling, or loosening of skin; unusual tiredness or weakness)

Incidence rare
*Crystalluria or hematuria;* (blood in urine; lower back pain; pain or burning while urinating); *goiter or thyroid function disturbance* (swelling of front part of neck)

### Those indicating need for medical attention only if they continue or are bothersome
Incidence more frequent
*CNS effects* (anxiety; drowsiness; fatigue; headache; nervousness); *gastrointestinal disturbances* (abdominal pain; diarrhea; nausea or vomiting)

## Overdose

For specific information on the agents used in the management of sulfadoxine and pyrimethamine overdose, see:
- *Barbiturates (Systemic)* monograph;
- *Benzodiazepines (Systemic)* monograph; and/or
- *Leucovorin (Systemic)* monograph.

For more information on the management of overdose or unintentional ingestion, **contact a Poison Control Center** (see *Poison Control Center Listing*).

### Clinical effects of overdose
The following effects have been selected on the basis of their potential clinical significance (possible signs and symptoms in parentheses where appropriate)—not necessarily inclusive:

Acute—In order of occurrence:
*Gastrointestinal toxicity* (anorexia; severe vomiting); *central nervous system (CNS) toxicity* (ataxia; trembling; seizures); *blood dyscrasias, specifically leukopenia* (fever and sore throat); *megaloblastic anemia* (unusual tiredness or weakness); *or thrombocytopenia* (unusual bleeding or bruising)

### Treatment of overdose
Recommended treatment includes:
To decrease absorption—
  Gastric emptying by emesis or lavage.
Specific treatment—
  Control of CNS stimulation, including seizures, by parenteral administration of benzodiazepines or short-acting barbiturates.
  Administration of leucovorin, 5 to 15 mg a day intramuscularly for 3 days or longer, to counteract the effects of folic acid antagonism (e.g., reduced white blood cell counts) induced by the pyrimethamine component.
  Adequate hydration to prevent renal damage.
Monitoring—
  Monitoring of renal and hematopoietic status for at least 1 month following overdose.
Supportive care—
  Mechanical assistance of respiration, if necessary. Patients in whom intentional overdose is confirmed or suspected should be referred for psychiatric consultation.

## Patient Consultation

As an aid to patient consultation, refer to *Advice for the Patient, Sulfadoxine and Pyrimethamine (Systemic)*.
In providing consultation, consider emphasizing the following selected information (» = major clinical significance):

### Before using this medication
» Conditions affecting use, especially:
  Allergy to sulfonamides, furosemide, thiazide diuretics, sulfonylureas, carbonic anhydrase inhibitors, or pyrimethamine
  Pregnancy—Pyrimethamine and sulfadoxine cross the placenta. Use not recommended because of possible interference with folic acid metabolism in fetus
  Breast-feeding—Pyrimethamine and sulfadoxine are excreted in breast milk. Use not recommended because of possible kernicterus in the infant
  Use in children—Use is not recommended in children under 2 months of age because of possible kernicterus
  Dental—High doses may cause atrophic glossitis, leukopenia, or thrombocytopenia
  Other medications, especially bone marrow depressants, other hemolytics, or other hepatotoxic medications
  Other medical problems, especially anemia, bone marrow depression, porphyria, or renal function impairment

### Proper use of this medication
» Not giving to infants under 2 months of age; keeping medication out of reach of children
» Maintaining adequate fluid intake; taking with meals or a snack if gastric irritation occurs
» Proper storage
*For prevention of malaria*
  Starting medication 1 to 2 weeks before entering malarious area to ascertain patient response and allow time to substitute another medication if reactions occur
» Continuing medication while staying in area and for 4 weeks after leaving area; checking with physician immediately if fever develops while traveling or within 2 months after departure from endemic area
» Importance of not missing doses and taking medication on a regular schedule
» Proper dosing
  Missed dose: Taking as soon as possible; not taking if almost time for next dose; not doubling doses
*For treatment of malaria*
» Compliance with therapy
*For self-treatment of presumptive malaria*
» After taking this medication, continuing to take an alternative effective malaria medication once a week

### Precautions while using this medication
» Stopping medication immediately and reporting promptly to physician signs of skin rash, itching, redness, mouth or genital lesions, or sore throat
*Mosquito-control measures to reduce the chance of getting malaria*
  Sleeping under mosquito netting
  Wearing long-sleeved shirts or blouses and long trousers to protect arms and legs when mosquitoes are out
  Applying mosquito repellant to uncovered areas of skin when mosquitoes are out
*For prevention of malaria*
» Regular visits to physician to check blood counts
  Importance of taking leucovorin concurrently if anemia occurs
  Using caution in use of regular toothbrushes, dental floss, and toothpicks; deferring dental work until blood counts have returned to normal; checking with physician or dentist concerning proper oral hygiene
» Possible photosensitivity reactions
*For self-treatment of presumptive malaria*
  Checking with physician as soon as possible, especially if no improvement within 48 hours

### Side/adverse effects
Signs of potential side effects, especially atrophic glossitis; blood dyscrasias, specifically agranulocytosis, megaloblastic anemia, or thrombocytopenia; hypersensitivity; photosensitivity; hepatitis; Stevens-Johnson syndrome; crystalluria or hematuria; and goiter or thyroid function disturbance

## General Dosing Information

Sulfadoxine and pyrimethamine combination may be administered alone for the presumptive treatment, or sequentially with quinine in the treatment of acute attacks, of documented falciparum malaria.

Fluid intake should be sufficient to maintain urine output of at least 1200 to 1500 mL per day in adults.

Sulfadoxine and pyrimethamine combination may cause gastric irritation, sometimes resulting in vomiting, when given in high doses. If this occurs, the medication may be taken with meals or a snack or the dosage may be reduced.

**Therapy with sulfadoxine and pyrimethamine combination should be discontinued if skin rash or symptoms of folic acid deficiency occur.** However, to prevent folic acid deficiency, leucovorin (folinic acid) may be administered to restore normal hematopoiesis. Leucovorin does not interfere with the antiprotozoal activity of the pyrimethamine component. In addition, since malarial parasites are unable to utilize preformed folic acid, the antimalarial effect of pyrimethamine should not be affected. In adults, 5 to 15 mg of leucovorin may be given orally, intramuscularly, or intravenously once a day for 3 days or as required. Alternatively, adults may be given 9 mg of leucovorin 2 or 3 times a week. Infants may be given 1 mg of leucovorin once a day.

Because of its potentially life-threatening toxicity, sulfadoxine and pyrimethamine combination is no longer recommended for weekly use as a prophylactic agent **except** in persons at high risk of chloroquine-resistant malaria, in remote areas, who are unable to take alternative medications. If this combination is used, prophylaxis should be started 1 week before the patient enters a malarious area and should be continued for 4 weeks after the patient leaves the area. Starting the medication before the patient enters the malarious area will help to determine the patient's tolerance to the medication and allow time to substitute other antimalarials if the patient develops allergies to the medication or experiences other adverse effects.

## Oral Dosage Forms

Note: Bracketed uses in the *Dosage Forms* section refer to categories of use and/or indications that are not included in U.S. product labeling.

### SULFADOXINE AND PYRIMETHAMINE TABLETS USP

**Usual adult and adolescent dose**
Malaria—
  Treatment: Chloroquine-resistant *P. falciparum* malaria—Oral, 3 tablets as a single dose on day three of quinine therapy.
  Presumptive treatment: Oral, 3 tablets as a single dose for self-treatment of febrile illness when medical care is not immediately available.
  Chemoprophylaxis: Oral, 1 tablet once every seven days; or 2 tablets once every fourteen days.
[Isosporiasis (prophylaxis)][1]—
  Oral, 1 tablet once every seven days.

**Usual pediatric dose**
Malaria—
  Treatment:
    Chloroquine-resistant *P. falciparum* malaria
    Children up to 2 months of age:
      Use is contraindicated since sulfonamides may cause kernicterus in neonates.
    Children 2 months of age and over:
      Oral, 1.25 mg per kg of body weight of pyrimethamine in combination with 25 mg per kg of body weight of sulfadoxine as a single dose on day three of quinine therapy.
  Presumptive treatment, for self-treatment of febrile illness when medical care is not immediately available:
    Children up to 2 months of age:
      Use is contraindicated since sulfonamides may cause kernicterus in neonates.
    Children 2 months of age and over:
      Children 5 to 10 kg of body weight: Oral, ½ tablet as a single dose.
      Children 11 to 20 kg of body weight: Oral, 1 tablet as a single dose.
      Children 21 to 30 kg of body weight: Oral, 1½ tablets as a single dose.
      Children 31 to 45 kg of body weight: Oral, 2 tablets as a single dose.
      Children greater than 45 kg of body weight: Oral, 3 tablets as a single dose.
  Chemoprophylaxis:
    Infants up to 2 months of age:
      Use is contraindicated since sulfonamides may cause kernicterus in neonates.
    Infants and children 2 months to 4 years of age:
      Oral, ¼ tablet once every seven days; or ½ tablet once every fourteen days.
    Children 4 to 8 years of age:
      Oral, ½ tablet once every seven days; or 1 tablet once every fourteen days.
    Children 9 to 14 years of age:
      Oral, ¾ tablet once every seven days; or 1½ tablets once every fourteen days.
    Children over 14 years of age:
      See *Usual adult and adolescent dose*.

**Strength(s) usually available**
U.S.—
  500 mg of sulfadoxine and 25 mg of pyrimethamine (Rx) [*Fansidar*].
Canada—
  500 mg of sulfadoxine and 25 mg of pyrimethamine (Rx) [*Fansidar*].

**Packaging and storage**
Store below 40 °C (104 °F), preferably between 15 and 30 °C (59 and 86 °F), unless otherwise specified by manufacturer. Store in a well-closed, light-resistant container.

**Auxiliary labeling**
- Take with a full glass of water.
- Avoid too much sun or use of sunlamp or tanning bed or booth.
- Continue medicine for full time of treatment (chemoprophylaxis).
- Keep out of reach of children.

**Note**
Explain potential danger of accidental overdose in children.
Consider dispensing in unit-dose packaging in child-resistant containers ("double-barrier" packaging).

[1]Not included in Canadian product labeling.

Revised: 02/23/93

---

## SULFAMETHIZOLE — See *Sulfonamides (Systemic)*

## SULFAMETHOXAZOLE — See *Sulfonamides (Systemic)*

## SULFANILAMIDE — See *Sulfonamides (Vaginal)*

---

# SULFAPYRIDINE   Systemic

VA CLASSIFICATION (Primary): DE890
Commonly used brand name(s): *Dagenan*.
Note: For a listing of dosage forms and brand names by country availability, see *Dosage Forms* section(s).

## Category
Dermatitis herpetiformis suppressant.

## Indications
Note: Bracketed information in the *Indications* section refers to uses that are not included in U.S. product labeling.

**Accepted**
Dermatitis herpetiformis (treatment)—Sulfapyridine is indicated as a secondary agent in the treatment of dermatitis herpetiformis (Duhring's disease).

[Dermatosis, subcorneal pustular (treatment)][1]—Sulfapyridine is used as a secondary agent in the treatment of subcorneal pustular dermatosis (Sneddon-Wilkinson disease).

[Pemphigoid (treatment)][1]—Sulfapyridine is used as a secondary agent in the treatment of bullous pemphigoid.

[Pyoderma gangrenosum (treatment)][1]—Sulfapyridine is used as secondary agent in the treatment of pyoderma gangrenosum.

[1]Not included in Canadian product labeling.

## Pharmacology/Pharmacokinetics

**Physicochemical characteristics**
Molecular weight—249.29.

**Mechanism of action/Effect**
Dermatitis herpetiformis—Unknown.

**Absorption**
Absorption from gastrointestinal tract is slow and incomplete (approximately 60–80%).

**Distribution**
Sulfonamides readily cross the placenta; sulfapyridine also crosses into the cerebrospinal fluid.
Vol$_D$=0.4 to 1.2 L per kg.

**Protein binding**
Variable (approximately 50%); acetylated metabolites are more highly protein bound than the free drug. Sulfonamides compete with bilirubin for binding to albumin. Kernicterus may develop in premature infants or neonates. Binding is decreased in patients with severely impaired renal function.

**Biotransformation**
Hepatic; sulfapyridine is metabolized by acetylation and hydroxylation, followed by conjugation with glucuronic acid. Sulfapyridine is metabolized to inactive metabolites, which retain the toxicity of the parent compound. Metabolism is increased with renal function impairment and decreased with hepatic failure.

**Half-life**
6 to 14 hours.

**Time to peak concentration**
4 to 6 hours following administration of a single dose.

**Duration of action**
Intermediate-acting sulfonamide.

**Elimination**
Sulfapyridine and metabolites excreted primarily in urine; up to 80% of sulfapyridine may be reabsorbed by the renal tubules.

## Precautions to Consider

**Cross-sensitivity and/or related problems**
Patients allergic to other sulfonamides may be allergic to this medication also.
Patients allergic to furosemide, thiazide diuretics, sulfonylureas, or carbonic anhydrase inhibitors may be allergic to this medication also.

**Carcinogenicity/Tumorigenicity**
Long-term administration of sulfonamides in rats has been shown to result in thyroid malignancies. However, rats appear to be more susceptible to the goitrogenic effects of sulfonamides than do other animal species.

**Pregnancy/Reproduction**
Fertility—Sulfapyridine has been shown to cause oligospermia and infertility in men.
Pregnancy—Sulfapyridine crosses the placenta. Adequate and well-controlled studies in humans have not been done. However, sulfonamides may cause kernicterus in the neonate. Therefore, use is not recommended during pregnancy.
Studies in rats and mice, given 7 to 25 times the human therapeutic dose orally, have shown that certain sulfonamides cause a significant increase in the incidence of cleft palate and other bony abnormalities.

**Breast-feeding**
Sulfapyridine is excreted in breast milk in concentrations that are 30 to 60% of those in the maternal serum. Use is not recommended in nursing women since sulfonamides may cause kernicterus in nursing infants.
Sulfonamides may cause hemolytic anemia in glucose-6-phosphate dehydrogenase (G6PD)–deficient neonates.

**Pediatrics**
Use is not recommended in pediatric patients since they do not usually develop dermatitis herpetiformis.

**Geriatrics**
No information is available on the relationship of age to the effects of sulfapyridine in geriatric patients.

**Dental**
The leukopenic and thrombocytopenic effects of sulfapyridine may result in an increased incidence of certain microbial infections, delayed healing, and gingival bleeding. If leukopenia or thrombocytopenia occurs, dental work should be deferred until blood counts have returned to normal. Patients should be instructed in proper oral hygiene, including caution in use of regular toothbrushes, dental floss, and toothpicks.

**Drug interactions and/or related problems**
The following drug interactions and/or related problems have been selected on the basis of their potential clinical significance (possible mechanism in parentheses where appropriate)—not necessarily inclusive (» = major clinical significance):

Note: Combinations containing any of the following medications, depending on the amount present, may also interact with this medication.

» Anticoagulants, coumarin- or indandione-derivative or
» Anticonvulsants, hydantoin or
» Antidiabetic agents, oral
  (may be displaced from protein-binding sites and/or metabolism may be inhibited by sulfonamides, resulting in increased or prolonged effects and/or toxicity; dosage adjustments may be necessary during and after sulfonamide therapy)

Bone marrow depressants (See *Appendix II* )
  (concurrent use of sulfapyridine with bone marrow depressants may increase the leukopenic and/or thrombocytopenic effects of these medications; if concurrent use is required, close observation for myelotoxic effects should be considered)

» Hemolytics, other (See *Appendix II* )
  (concurrent use with sulfapyridine may increase the potential for toxic side effects)

» Hepatotoxic medications, other (See *Appendix II* )
  (concurrent use with sulfonamides may result in an increased incidence of hepatotoxicity; patients, especially those on prolonged administration or those with a history of liver disease, should be carefully monitored)

» Methotrexate or
Phenylbutazone or
Sulfinpyrazone
  (the effects of these medications may be potentiated during concurrent use with sulfonamides because of displacement from plasma protein-binding sites; phenylbutazone has also been reported to potentiate the effects of sulfonamides)

**Laboratory value alterations**
The following have been selected on the basis of their potential clinical significance (possible effect in parentheses where appropriate)—not necessarily inclusive (» = major clinical significance):

With diagnostic test results
Bentiromide
  (administration of sulfonamides during a bentiromide test period will invalidate test results since sulfonamides are also metabolized to arylamines and will thus increase the percent of PABA recovered; discontinuation of sulfonamides at least 3 days prior to the administration of bentiromide is recommended)

**Medical considerations/Contraindications**
The medical considerations/contraindications included have been selected on the basis of their potential clinical significance (reasons given in parentheses where appropriate)—not necessarily inclusive (» = major clinical significance).

*Risk-benefit should be considered when the following medical problems exist:*

Allergy to sulfapyridine, other sulfonamides, furosemide, thiazide diuretics, sulfonylureas, or carbonic anhydrase inhibitors

» Blood dyscrasias
  (sulfapyridine may cause agranulocytosis, aplastic anemia, or other blood dyscrasias)

» Glucose-6-phosphate dehydrogenase (G6PD) deficiency
  (sulfapyridine may cause hemolytic anemia in G6PD-deficient patients)

» Hepatic function impairment
  (sulfonamides are metabolized in the liver and may cause hepatitis)

» Porphyria
  (sulfonamides may precipitate an acute attack of porphyria)

» Renal function impairment
  (sulfapyridine is excreted primarily through the kidneys)

**Patient monitoring**
The following may be especially important in patient monitoring (other tests may be warranted in some patients, depending on condition; » = major clinical significance):

» Complete blood counts (CBCs)
  (may be required prior to and monthly during treatment to detect blood dyscrasias in patients on prolonged therapy; therapy should

be discontinued if a significant decrease in the count of any formed blood elements occurs)
- » Glucose-6-phosphate dehydrogenase (G6PD) determinations
  (are recommended prior to treatment in Caucasians of Mediterranean origin, Orientals, and blacks; if a deficiency is found, sulfapyridine should be given with caution since hemolytic effects may be exacerbated in these patients; dosage adjustments and/or discontinuation of the medication may be required)
- Urinalyses
  (may be required prior to and periodically during treatment to detect crystalluria and/or urinary calculi formation in patients on long-term or high-dose therapy and in patients with impaired renal function)

## Side/Adverse Effects

Note: Fatalities have occurred, although rarely, due to severe reactions such as Stevens-Johnson syndrome, toxic epidermal necrolysis, fulminant hepatic necrosis, agranulocytosis, aplastic anemia, other blood dyscrasias, and hypersensitivity reactions. Therapy should be discontinued at the first appearance of skin rash or any serious side/adverse effects.

Sulfapyridine has been shown to cause oligospermia and infertility in men.

The following side/adverse effects have been selected on the basis of their potential clinical significance (possible signs and symptoms in parentheses where appropriate)—not necessarily inclusive:

**Those indicating need for medical attention**
Incidence more frequent
  *Headache, continuing; hypersensitivity* (itching; skin rash; fever); *photosensitivity* (increased sensitivity of skin to sunlight)

Incidence less frequent
  *Blood dyscrasias* (pale skin; sore throat; unusual bleeding or bruising; unusual tiredness or weakness); *hepatitis* (yellow eyes or skin); *Lyell's syndrome or Stevens-Johnson syndrome* (aching of joints and muscles; difficulty in swallowing; redness, blistering, peeling, or loosening of skin; unusual tiredness or weakness)

Incidence rare
  *Crystalluria or hematuria* (blood in urine; lower back pain; pain or burning while urinating); *goiter or thyroid function disturbance* (swelling of front part of neck)

**Those indicating need for medical attention only if they continue or are bothersome**
Incidence more frequent
  *Gastrointestinal disturbances* (diarrhea; anorexia; nausea or vomiting)

## Patient Consultation

As an aid to patient consultation, refer to *Advice for the Patient, Sulfapyridine (Systemic)*.
In providing consultation, consider emphasizing the following selected information (» = major clinical significance):

**Before using this medication**
- » Conditions affecting use, especially:
  - Allergies to other sulfonamides, furosemide, thiazide diuretics, sulfonylureas, or carbonic anhydrase inhibitors
  - Pregnancy—Crosses the placenta; not recommended during pregnancy since sulfonamides may cause kernicterus in the neonate
  - Breast-feeding—Excreted in breast milk; not recommended in nursing women since sulfonamides may cause kernicterus in nursing infants
  - Use in children—Not recommended since pediatric patients do not usually develop dermatitis herpetiformis
  - Other medications, especially anticoagulants (coumarin- or indandione-derivative), anticonvulsants (hydantoin), antidiabetic agents (oral), hemolytics, hepatotoxic medications, and methotrexate
  - Other medical problems, especially blood dyscrasias, G6PD deficiency, hepatic function impairment, porphyria, and renal function impairment

**Proper use of this medication**
- » Maintaining adequate fluid intake to help prevent crystalluria and urinary calculi formation

*For dermatitis herpetiformis*
  Possible need for a strict, gluten-free diet in the treatment of dermatitis herpetiformis

Using for 6 to 12 months may be required before reducing the dose or discontinuing medication
- » Proper dosing
  Missed dose: Taking as soon as possible if symptoms return or worsen; not taking if symptoms do not return or worsen
- » Proper storage

**Precautions while using this medication**
- » Regular visits to physician to check blood counts in patients on long-term therapy
  Checking with physician if no improvement within a few days
  Using caution in use of regular toothbrushes, dental floss, and toothpicks; deferring dental work until blood counts have returned to normal; checking with doctor or dentist concerning proper oral hygiene
- » Possible photosensitivity reactions; using sunscreen lotion or avoiding unprotected exposure to sun or use of sunlamp
  Possible interference with bentiromide diagnostic test for pancreatic function

**Side/adverse effects**
  Signs of potential side effects, especially blood dyscrasias, crystalluria or hematuria, goiter or thyroid function disturbance, headache (continuing), hepatitis, hypersensitivity, Lyell's syndrome or Stevens-Johnson syndrome, or photosensitivity

## General Dosing Information

Fluid intake should be sufficient to maintain a urine output of at least 1200 to 1500 mL per day in adults, to prevent crystalluria and urinary calculi formation.

If dermatitis herpetiformis recurs, increased dosage may be required. The maintenance dose should not exceed the minimum effective dose.

In the treatment of dermatitis herpetiformis, use of a strict, gluten-free diet for 6 to 12 months may allow a reduction in dose or discontinuation of sulfapyridine.

## Oral Dosage Forms

Note: Bracketed uses in the *Dosage Forms* section refer to categories of use and/or indications that are not included in U.S. product labeling.

### SULFAPYRIDINE TABLETS USP

**Usual adult and adolescent dose**
Dermatitis herpetiformis—
  Oral, initially 250 mg to 1 gram four times a day until improvement occurs. Daily dosage should then be reduced by 250- to 500-mg decrements every three days until a symptom-free maintenance dose is achieved.

  Note: Sulfapyridine may also be given two times a day in evenly divided doses.

[Dermatosis, subcorneal pustular][1]—
  Oral, 500 mg two times a day to 750 mg four times a day.
[Pemphigoid][1]—
  Oral, 1 gram three times a day.

**Usual adult prescribing limits**
Dermatitis herpetiformis—Up to 6 grams daily.

**Usual pediatric dose**
Use is not recommended in pediatric patients since they do not usually develop dermatitis herpetiformis.

**Strength(s) usually available**
U.S.—
  500 mg (Rx) [GENERIC].
Canada—
  500 mg (Rx) [*Dagenan;* GENERIC].

**Packaging and storage**
Store below 40 °C (104 °F), preferably between 15 and 30 °C (59 and 86 °F), unless otherwise specified by manufacturer. Store in a well-closed, light-resistant container.

**Auxiliary labeling**
- Take with a full glass of water.
- Avoid too much sun or use of sunlamp.

---

[1]Not included in Canadian product labeling.

Revised: 02/01/93

# SULFASALAZINE Systemic

BAN: Sulphasalazine.
JAN: Salazosulfapyridine.

VA CLASSIFICATION (Primary/Secondary): GA400/MS109

Commonly used brand name(s): *Alti-Sulfasalazine; Alti-Sulfasalazine (Enteric-Coated); Azulfidine; Azulfidine EN-Tabs; PMS-Sulfasalazine; PMS-Sulfasalazine E.C.; S.A.S. Enteric-500; S.A.S.-500; Salazopyrin; Salazopyrin EN-Tabs.*

Another commonly used name is salicylazosulfapyridine.

Note: For a listing of dosage forms and brand names by country availability, see *Dosage Forms* section(s).

## Category
Bowel disease (inflammatory) suppressant; antirheumatic (disease-modifying).

## Indications
Note: Bracketed information in the *Indications* section refers to uses that are not included in U.S. product labeling.

### Accepted
Bowel disease, inflammatory (prophylaxis and treatment)—Sulfasalazine is indicated to treat and to maintain remission of inflammatory bowel disease (e.g., ulcerative colitis or Crohn's disease affecting the colon). It is indicated in the treatment of mild to moderate ulcerative colitis and as adjunctive treatment of severe ulcerative colitis.

Arthritis, rheumatoid (treatment)—Sulfasalazine is indicated for the treatment of rheumatoid arthritis in patients who have responded inadequately to, or who are intolerant of, analgesics or other nonsteroidal anti-inflammatory drugs (NSAIDs).

[Ankylosing spondylitis (treatment)][1]—Sulfasalazine is used in the treatment of ankylosing spondylitis.

[1]Not included in Canadian product labeling.

## Pharmacology/Pharmacokinetics

**Physicochemical characteristics**
Molecular weight—398.39.

**Mechanism of action/Effect**
Bowel disease (inflammatory) suppressant—Uncertain; may be related to sulfasalazine's immunosuppressant effects, which have been observed in animals, its affinity for connective tissue, and/or its relatively high concentrations in serous fluids, the liver, and intestinal wall. Sulfasalazine is considered a vehicle for carrying its principal metabolites to the colon. Unabsorbed sulfasalazine is cleaved in the colon by intestinal bacteria to form sulfapyridine and mesalamine (5-aminosalicylic acid; 5-ASA), both of which may act locally within the gut. Mesalamine, which is different from aminosalicylates used to treat tuberculosis, is thought to be the major active moiety. Mucosal production of arachidonic acid metabolites, both through the cyclooxygenase and the lipoxygenase pathways, is increased in patients with inflammatory bowel disease. Mesalamine appears to diminish inflammation by inhibiting cyclooxygenase and lipoxygenase, thereby decreasing the production of prostaglandins, and leukotrienes and hydroxyeicosatetraenoic acids (HETEs), respectively. It is also believed that mesalamine acts as a scavenger of oxygen-derived free radicals, which are produced in greater numbers in patients with inflammatory bowel disease.

Antirheumatic (disease-modifying)—Uncertain; sulfapyridine moiety may suppress the activity of natural killer cells and impair lymphocyte transformation.

**Absorption**
Sulfasalazine—Poorly absorbed; approximately 20% of ingested sulfasalazine dose reaches the systemic circulation. The remaining ingested dose is split by colonic bacteria into its components, sulfapyridine and mesalamine.

Sulfapyridine—Most of the sulfapyridine metabolized from sulfasalazine (60–80%) is absorbed in the colon following oral administration.

Mesalamine (5-ASA)—Approximately 25% of the mesalamine metabolized from sulfasalazine is absorbed in the colon following oral administration.

**Distribution**
Distributed to serum, connective tissue, serous fluids, liver, and intestinal wall. The apparent volume of distribution (Vol$_D$) of sulfasalazine in 8 healthy volunteers was 64 L. The Vol$_D$ of sulfapyridine was found to be 0.4 to 1.2 L per kg.

**Protein binding**
Sulfasalazine—Very high (Approximately 99%).
Sulfapyridine—Moderate (Approximately 50%).
Mesalamine (5-ASA)—Moderate (Approximately 43%).

**Biotransformation**
Sulfasalazine (unabsorbed)—Cleaved in the colon by intestinal bacteria to form sulfapyridine and mesalamine.
Sulfapyridine (absorbed)—Acetylated and hydroxylated in the liver, followed by conjugation with glucuronic acid.
Mesalamine (5-ASA) (absorbed)—Acetylated in the intestinal mucosal wall and the liver.

**Half-life**
Sulfasalazine—5 to 10 hours.
Sulfapyridine—6 to 14 hours, depending on acetylator status.
Mesalamine (5-ASA)—0.6 to 1.4 hours.

**Time to peak serum concentration**
Sulfasalazine oral suspension:
    Sulfasalazine: Approximately 1.5 to 6 hours.
    Sulfapyridine: Approximately 9 to 24 hours.
Sulfasalazine tablets:
    Sulfasalazine: Approximately 1.5 to 6 hours.
    Sulfapyridine: Approximately 6 to 24 hours.
Sulfasalazine enteric-coated tablets:
    Sulfasalazine: Approximately 3 to 12 hours.
    Sulfapyridine: Approximately 12 to 24 hours.

**Mean peak serum concentration**
Sulfasalazine oral suspension—
    Sulfasalazine: Approximately 20 mcg per mL 3 hours following a single oral 2-gram dose.
    Sulfapyridine: Approximately 19 mcg per mL 12 hours following a single oral 2-gram dose.
    Mesalamine (5-ASA): Approximately 4 mcg per mL following a single oral 2-gram dose.
Sulfasalazine tablets—
    Sulfasalazine: Approximately 14 mcg per mL 3 hours following a single oral 2-gram dose.
    Sulfapyridine: Approximately 21 mcg per mL 12 hours following a single oral 2-gram dose.
    Mesalamine (5-ASA): Approximately 4 mcg per mL following a single oral 2-gram dose.
Sulfasalazine enteric-coated tablets—
    Sulfasalazine: Approximately 6 mcg per mL 6 hours following a single oral 2-gram dose.
    Sulfapyridine: Approximately 13 mcg per mL 12 hours following a single oral 2-gram dose.
    Mesalamine (5-ASA): Approximately 4 mcg per mL following a single oral 2-gram dose.

**Elimination**
Fecal—Trace amounts of sulfasalazine, approximately 5% of sulfapyridine, and approximately 67% of mesalamine are found in feces.
Renal—Approximately 75 to 91% of sulfasalazine and sulfapyridine metabolites excreted in urine within 3 days, depending on the dosage form used. Mesalamine is excreted in urine mostly in acetylated form.

## Precautions to Consider

**Cross-sensitivity and/or related problems**
Patients allergic to one sulfonamide may be allergic to other sulfonamides also.
Patients allergic to salicylates, furosemide, thiazide diuretics, sulfonylureas, or carbonic anhydrase inhibitors may be allergic to this medication also.

**Carcinogenicity/Tumorigenicity**
Long-term studies have not been done to evaluate the carcinogenic potential of sulfasalazine. However, long-term administration of sulfonamides to rats has been shown to result in thyroid malignancies. In addition, rats appear to be especially susceptible to the goitrogenic effects of sulfonamides.

**Mutagenicity**
No evidence of mutagenicity was observed in *in vitro* tests for point mutations and chromosome aberrations.

**Pregnancy/Reproduction**
Fertility—Studies in rats and rabbits given doses of up to 6 times the human dose have not shown that sulfasalazine impairs female fertility. However, these studies have shown that sulfasalazine does impair male fer-

tility. In addition, oligospermia and infertility, reported to be reversible upon discontinuation of sulfasalazine, have been reported in men.

Pregnancy—Sulfasalazine and sulfapyridine cross the placenta. Adequate and well-controlled studies in humans have not been done. However, a national survey of 186 women with inflammatory bowel disease (IBD) who took sulfasalazine, alone or concurrently with corticosteroids, showed an incidence of adverse effects in the fetus comparable to that in 245 untreated IBD pregnancies. Another study of 1445 pregnancies in which sulfonamides, including sulfasalazine, were taken did not show that sulfasalazine causes fetal malformations.

Appropriate studies have not been performed on the effect of sulfasalazine on growth, development, and functional maturation of children whose mothers received sulfasalazine during pregnancy.

Studies in rats and rabbits given doses of up to 6 times the human dose have not shown that sulfasalazine causes adverse effects in the fetus.

FDA Pregnancy Category B.

### Breast-feeding
Uncleaved sulfasalazine is distributed into breast milk in small amounts. Sulfapyridine is distributed into breast milk in concentrations that are 30 to 60% of those in the maternal serum. Although sulfonamides may displace bilirubin from protein-binding sites in the fetal plasma, hyperbilirubinemia has occurred rarely.

Sulfonamides may cause hemolytic anemia in glucose-6-phosphate dehydrogenase (G6PD)–deficient neonates.

### Pediatrics
Use is contraindicated in infants and children up to 2 years of age because sulfonamides may cause kernicterus.

### Geriatrics
Appropriate studies performed to date have not demonstrated geriatrics-specific problems that would limit the usefulness of sulfasalazine in the elderly.

### Pharmacogenetics
Mean serum concentrations of sulfapyridine and its metabolites may be significantly increased in patients who are slow acetylators. Eskimo, Oriental, and American Indian populations have the lowest prevalence of slow acetylators, while Egyptian, Israeli, Scandinavian, other Caucasian, and black populations have the highest prevalence of slow acetylators.

### Dental
The leukopenic and thrombocytopenic effects of sulfasalazine may result in an increased incidence of certain microbial infections, delayed healing, and gingival bleeding. If leukopenia or thrombocytopenia occurs, dental work should be deferred until blood counts have returned to normal. Patients should be instructed in proper oral hygiene, including caution in use of regular toothbrushes, dental floss, and toothpicks.

### Drug interactions and/or related problems
The following drug interactions and/or related problems have been selected on the basis of their potential clinical significance (possible mechanism in parentheses where appropriate)—not necessarily inclusive (» = major clinical significance):

Note: Combinations containing any of the following medications, depending on the amount present, may also interact with this medication.

» Anticoagulants, coumarin- or indandione-derivative or
» Anticonvulsants, hydantoin or
» Antidiabetic agents, oral
(may be displaced from protein binding sites and/or metabolism may be inhibited by sulfonamides, resulting in increased or prolonged effects and/or toxicity; dosage adjustments may be necessary during and after sulfonamide therapy)

Bone marrow depressants (see *Appendix II* )
(concurrent use of sulfasalazine with bone marrow depressants may increase the leukopenic and/or thrombocytopenic effects; if concurrent use is required, close observation for myelotoxic effects should be considered)

Digitalis glycosides or
Folic acid
(sulfasalazine may inhibit absorption and lower the serum concentrations of these medications; folic acid requirements may be increased in patients receiving sulfasalazine; patients taking digitalis glycosides should be monitored closely for evidence of altered digitalis effect)

» Hemolytics, other (see *Appendix II* )
(concurrent use with sulfasalazine may increase the potential for toxic side effects)

» Hepatotoxic medications, other (see *Appendix II* )
(concurrent use with sulfonamides may result in an increased incidence of hepatotoxicity; patients, especially those on prolonged administration or those with a history of liver disease, should be carefully monitored)

» Methotrexate or
Phenylbutazone or
Sulfinpyrazone
(the effects of these medications may be potentiated during concurrent use with sulfonamides because of displacement from plasma protein binding sites; phenylbutazone and sulfinpyrazone have also been reported to potentiate the effects of sulfonamides)

### Laboratory value alterations
The following have been selected on the basis of their potential clinical significance (possible effect in parentheses where appropriate)—not necessarily inclusive (» = major clinical significance):

With diagnostic test results
Bentiromide
(administration of sulfonamides during a bentiromide test period will invalidate test results because sulfonamides are also metabolized to arylamines and will thus increase the percent of *p*-aminobenzoic acid (PABA) recovered; discontinuation of sulfonamides at least 3 days prior to the administration of bentiromide is recommended)

### Medical considerations/Contraindications
The medical considerations/contraindications included have been selected on the basis of their potential clinical significance (reasons given in parentheses where appropriate)—not necessarily inclusive (» = major clinical significance).

*Except under special circumstances, this medication should not be used when the following medical problem exists:*

» Intestinal obstruction or
» Urinary obstruction
» Previous allergic reaction to sulfasalazine, sulfonamides, salicylates, furosemide, thiazide diuretics, sulfonylureas, or carbonic anhydrase inhibitors

*Risk-benefit should be considered when the following medical problems exist:*

» Allergy, severe or
» Asthma, bronchial
(risk of hypersensitivity reaction to sulfasalazine may be increased with use of sulfasalazine)
» Blood dyscrasias
(sulfasalazine may cause agranulocytosis, aplastic anemia, or other blood dyscrasias)
» Glucose-6-phosphate dehydrogenase (G6PD) deficiency
(sulfasalazine may cause hemolytic anemia in G6PD-deficient patients)
» Hepatic function impairment
(sulfonamides are metabolized in the liver and may cause hepatitis)
» Porphyria
(sulfonamides may precipitate an acute attack of porphyria)
» Renal function impairment
(the metabolite, sulfapyridine, is excreted primarily through the kidneys)

### Patient monitoring
The following may be especially important in patient monitoring (other tests may be warranted in some patients, depending on condition; » = major clinical significance):

» Complete blood counts (CBCs)
(recommended prior to, and every 2 to 3 weeks for the first 2 to 3 months of treatment, then every 3 to 6 months during treatment to detect blood dyscrasias in patients on prolonged therapy; therapy should be discontinued if a significant decrease in the count of any formed blood elements occurs)

» Liver function tests
(recommended prior to, and every 2 weeks for the first 3 months of treatment, then monthly during the second 3 months of treatment, and thereafter once every 3 months and as clinically indicated during treatment to detect hepatotoxicity)

Proctoscopy and
Sigmoidoscopy
(may be required periodically during treatment to determine patient response and dosage adjustments)

Sulfapyridine concentrations, serum
(determinations may be useful since concentrations greater than 50

mcg/mL appear to be associated with an increased incidence of adverse reactions)

Urinalyses
(may be required prior to and periodically during treatment)

## Side/Adverse Effects

Note: Deaths have been reported from hypersensitivity reactions, agranulocytosis, aplastic anemia, other blood dyscrasias, renal and hepatic damage, irreversible neuromuscular and central nervous system (CNS) changes, and fibrosing alveolitis in patients taking sulfasalazine. If toxic or hypersensitivity reactions occur, sulfasalazine should be discontinued immediately.

Oligospermia and infertility, reported to be reversible upon discontinuation of sulfasalazine, have been reported in males taking this medication.

Daily doses of 4 grams or more and total sulfapyridine serum concentrations > 50 mcg per mL may be associated with an increased incidence of side/adverse effects.

The following side/adverse effects have been selected on the basis of their potential clinical significance (possible signs and symptoms in parentheses where appropriate)—not necessarily inclusive:

**Those indicating need for medical attention**
Incidence more frequent
*Headache, continuing; hypersensitivity reaction* (aching of joints; fever; itching; skin rash); *photosensitivity* (increased sensitivity of skin to sunlight)

Incidence less frequent or rare
*Blood dyscrasias, including agranulocytosis or neutropenia* (fever and sore throat); *aplastic anemia* (fever, chills, or sore throat; unusual bleeding or bruising; unusual tiredness or weakness); *Heinz body or hemolytic anemia* (back, leg, or stomach pains; loss of appetite; pale skin; unusual tiredness or weakness; fever); *leukopenia* (fever, chills, or sore throat); *or thrombocytopenia* (unusual bleeding or bruising); *cyanosis* (bluish fingernails, lips, or skin); *exacerbation of ulcerative colitis* (bloody diarrhea; fever; rash); *hepatitis* (yellow eyes or skin); *interstitial pneumonitis* (cough; difficult breathing; fever); *Stevens-Johnson syndrome* (aching of joints and muscles; redness, blistering, peeling, or loosening of skin; unusual tiredness or weakness); *systemic lupus erythematosus (SLE)–like syndrome* (blisters on skin; chest pain; general feeling of discomfort or illness; skin rash, hives, and/or itching); *toxic epidermal necrolysis* (difficulty in swallowing; redness, blistering, peeling, or loosening of skin)

**Those indicating need for medical attention only if they continue or are bothersome**
Incidence more frequent
*Gastrointestinal disturbances* (abdominal or stomach pain or upset; diarrhea; loss of appetite; nausea or vomiting)

**Those not indicating need for medical attention**
Incidence more frequent
*Orange-yellow discoloration of urine or skin*

## Overdose

For specific information on the agents used in the management of sulfasalazine overdose, see *Ipecac (Oral-Local)* monograph.

For more information on the management of overdose or unintentional ingestion, **contact a Poison Control Center** (see *Poison Control Center Listing*).

The severity of sulfasalazine toxicity is directly related to the total serum sulfapyridine concentration. Daily doses of 4 grams or more and total sulfapyridine serum concentrations > 50 mcg per mL may be associated with an increased incidence of side/adverse effects.

**Clinical effects of overdose**
The following effects have been selected on the basis of their potential clinical significance (possible signs and symptoms in parentheses where appropriate)—not necessarily inclusive:

*Anuria, crystalluria, or hematuria* (blood in urine; lack of urination; lower back pain; pain or burning while urinating); *drowsiness; gastrointestinal disturbances* (abdominal or stomach pain or upset; diarrhea; loss of appetite; nausea or vomiting); *seizures*

**Treatment of overdose**
To decrease absorption—the stomach may be emptied by inducing emesis with ipecac syrup (taking care to guard against aspiration) or by gastric lavage.

To enhance elimination—The urine may be alkalinized and, if kidney function is normal, fluids forced. If anuria is present, fluids and salt should be restricted. Catheterization of the ureters may be indicated when there is complete renal blockage by crystals. The low molecular weight of sulfasalazine and its metabolites may facilitate removal by dialysis.

Monitoring—Serum sulfapyridine concentrations may be monitored so that the progress of recovery can be followed.

Supportive care—Patients in whom intentional overdose is confirmed or suspected should be referred for psychiatric consultation.

## Patient Consultation

As an aid to patient consultation, refer to *Advice for the Patient, Sulfasalazine (Systemic)*.

In providing consultation, consider emphasizing the following selected information (» = major clinical significance):

**Before using this medication**
» Conditions affecting use, especially:
Allergies to sulfasalazine, sulfonamides, salicylates, furosemide, thiazide diuretics, sulfonylureas, carbonic anhydrase inhibitors
Pregnancy—Sulfasalazine and sulfapyridine cross the placenta
Breast-feeding—Sulfasalazine and sulfapyridine are distributed into breast milk
Use in children—Use is contraindicated in infants and children up to 2 years of age because sulfonamides may cause kernicterus
Other medications, especially coumarin- or indandione-derivative anticoagulants, hemolytics, hepatotoxic medications, hydantoin anticonvulsants, methotrexate, and oral antidiabetic agents
Other medical problems, especially intestinal obstruction, urinary obstruction, severe allergies, bronchial asthma, blood dyscrasias, G6PD deficiency, hepatic function impairment, porphyria, and renal function impairment

**Proper use of this medication**
» Not giving to infants up to 2 years of age; sulfasalazine may cause kernicterus
Taking after meals or with food to lessen gastrointestinal irritation
» Maintaining adequate fluid intake
Proper administration technique for enteric-coated tablets
» Compliance with full course of therapy
» Proper dosing
Missed dose: Taking as soon as possible; not taking if almost time for next dose; not doubling doses
» Proper storage

**Precautions while using this medication**
» Regular visits to physician to check blood counts in patients on long-term therapy
Checking with physician if no improvement within 1 or 2 months
Using caution in use of regular toothbrushes, dental floss, and toothpicks; deferring dental work until blood counts have returned to normal; checking with physician or dentist concerning proper oral hygiene
» Possible photosensitivity reactions
» Caution if dizziness occurs
Possible interference with bentiromide diagnostic test for pancreatic function

**Side/adverse effects**
Signs of potential side effects, especially headache (continuing), hypersensitivity reaction, photosensitivity, blood dyscrasias, cyanosis, exacerbation of ulcerative colitis, hepatitis, interstitial pneumonitis, Stevens-Johnson syndrome, systemic lupus erythematosus (SLE)–like syndrome, and toxic epidermal necrolysis
Orange-yellow discoloration of alkaline urine or skin may be alarming to patient although medically insignificant

## General Dosing Information

Fluid intake should be sufficient to maintain urine output of at least 1200 to 1500 mL per day in adults.

Sulfasalazine should preferably be taken immediately after meals or with food. Also, when sulfasalazine is being taken for inflammatory bowel disease, the total daily dose may be spread evenly over a 24-hour period. In some patients it may be necessary to initiate therapy with smaller doses (e.g., 1 to 2 grams daily) to lessen gastrointestinal irritation.

When endoscopic examination confirms satisfactory improvement, dosage may be reduced to maintenance level. If diarrhea recurs, dosage should be increased to previously effective level.

Patients with impaired renal function may require a reduction in dose.

Adverse reactions tend to increase with total daily doses of 4 grams or more or with serum concentrations greater than the equivalent of 50 mcg of sulfapyridine per mL.

Patients experiencing mild hypersensitivity reactions may be "desensitized" to allow continued treatment with sulfasalazine. Desensitization in-

## Sulfasalazine (Systemic)

volves withdrawal of the medication followed by reinstitution, beginning with a lower dose and increasing it slowly over at least 23 days. Desensitization should not be attempted in patients with a history of agranulocytosis. Some medical experts believe that with the availability of mesalamine preparations, desensitization may no longer be indicated.

### Diet/Nutrition
Folic acid requirements may be increased in patients on sulfasalazine therapy, because sulfasalazine inhibits the absorption of folic acid.

### For treatment of adverse effects
Recommended treatment consists of the following:
- Discontinuing the drug immediately if agranulocytosis or hypersensitivity reactions occur.
- Controlling hypersensitivity reactions with antihistamines and/or corticosteroids.

## Oral Dosage Forms

### SULFASALAZINE TABLETS USP

**Usual adult and adolescent dose**
Bowel disease (inflammatory) suppressant—
   Initial: Oral, 1 gram every six to eight hours. An initial dose of 500 mg every six to twelve hours may be recommended to lessen gastrointestinal side effects.
   Maintenance: Oral, 500 mg every six hours, adjusted according to patient response and tolerance.
Antirheumatic (disease-modifying)—
   Oral, 500 mg to 1 gram daily for the first week, with the daily dose being increased by 500 mg each week, up to a maintenance dose of 2 grams daily. The dose may be administered two times a day. If no response is seen after two months, the dose may be increased to 3 grams daily.

**Usual adult prescribing limits**
Total daily doses of greater than 4 grams may increase the risk of side effects and toxicity.

**Usual pediatric dose**
Bowel disease (inflammatory) suppressant—
   Infants and children up to 2 years of age:
      Use is contraindicated because sulfonamides may cause kernicterus.
   Children 2 years of age and older:
      Initial—Oral, 6.7 to 10 mg per kg of body weight every four hours; 10 to 15 mg per kg of body weight every six hours; or 13.3 to 20 mg per kg of body weight every eight hours.
      Maintenance—Oral, 7.5 mg per kg of body weight every six hours.
Antirheumatic (disease-modifying)—
   Safety and efficacy have not been established.

**Usual geriatric dose**
See *Usual adult and adolescent dose*.

**Strength(s) usually available**
U.S.—
   500 mg (Rx) [*Azulfidine*; GENERIC].
Canada—
   500 mg (Rx) [*Alti-Sulfasalazine* (scored); *PMS-Sulfasalazine* (scored); *Salazopyrin* (scored); *S.A.S.-500* (scored); GENERIC].

**Packaging and storage**
Store below 40 °C (104 °F), preferably between 15 and 30 °C (59 and 86 °F), unless otherwise specified by manufacturer. Store in a well-closed container.

**Auxiliary labeling**
- Take with a full glass of water.
- Avoid use of sunlamp and unprotected exposure to sun.
- Continue medicine for full time of treatment.
- May discolor urine.

### SULFASALAZINE TABLETS (ENTERIC-COATED) USP

**Usual adult and adolescent dose**
See *Sulfasalazine Tablets USP*.

**Usual adult prescribing limits**
See *Sulfasalazine Tablets USP*.

**Usual pediatric dose**
See *Sulfasalazine Tablets USP*.

**Usual geriatric dose**
See *Sulfasalazine Tablets USP*.

**Strength(s) usually available**
U.S.—
   500 mg (Rx) [*Azulfidine EN-Tabs*; GENERIC].
Canada—
   500 mg (Rx) [*Alti-Sulfasalazine (Enteric-Coated)*; *PMS-Sulfasalazine E.C.*; *Salazopyrin EN-Tabs*; *S.A.S. Enteric-500*; GENERIC].

**Packaging and storage**
Store below 40 °C (104 °F), preferably between 15 and 30 °C (59 and 86 °F), unless otherwise specified by manufacturer. Store in a well-closed container.

**Auxiliary labeling**
- Take with a full glass of water.
- Avoid use of sunlamp and unprotected exposure to sun.
- Continue medicine for full time of treatment.
- May discolor urine.
- Swallow tablets whole.

**Note**
Dissolution of enteric-coated tablets is much more variable and unreliable than that of nonenteric-coated tablets.

## Rectal Dosage Forms

### SULFASALAZINE RECTAL SUSPENSION

**Usual adult and adolescent dose**
Bowel disease (inflammatory) suppressant—
   Rectal, 3 grams each night at bedtime.

**Usual pediatric dose**
Bowel disease (inflammatory) suppressant—
   Infants and children up to 2 years of age: Use is contraindicated because sulfonamides cause kernicterus.
   Children 2 years of age and older: Dosage has not been established.

**Usual geriatric dose**
See *Usual adult and adolescent dose*.

**Strength(s) usually available**
U.S.—
   Not commercially available.
Canada—
   3 grams per 100-mL unit (Rx) [*Salazopyrin*].

**Packaging and storage**
Store below 40 °C (104 °F), preferably between 15 and 30 °C (59 and 86 °F), unless otherwise specified by manufacturer.

**Auxiliary labeling**
- For rectal use.
- Shake well.
- Continue medicine for full time of treatment.

## Selected Bibliography
Allgayer H. Sulfasalazine and 5-ASA compounds. Gastrointest Pharmacol 1992; 21: 643-57.

Revised: 08/11/98

---

# SULFINPYRAZONE   Systemic

VA CLASSIFICATION (Primary): MS400
Commonly used brand name(s): *Anturan*; *Anturane*; *Apo-Sulfinpyrazone*; *Novopyrazone*.

Note: For a listing of dosage forms and brand names by country availability, see *Dosage Forms* section(s).

## Category
Antigout agent; antihyperuricemic.

## Indications
Note: Bracketed information in the *Indications* section refers to uses that are not included in U.S. product labeling.

### Accepted
Gouty arthritis, chronic (treatment) or
Hyperuricemia (treatment)—Sulfinpyrazone is indicated for the long-term management of hyperuricemia associated with chronic gout. It is recommended only for patients whose 24-hour renal excretion of urate is 800 mg (4.8 mmol) or lower (i.e., patients who are hyperuricemic as a

result of underexcretion, rather than overproduction, of urate). The aim of sulfinpyrazone therapy is to reduce the number of acute gout attacks.

Sulfinpyrazone is not effective in the treatment of acute gout attacks and does not eliminate the need to use colchicine or a nonsteroidal anti-inflammatory drug (NSAID) to relieve an attack. Also, sulfinpyrazone therapy should not be initiated during an attack, because it may induce fluctuations in urate concentration that may result in prolongation of the attack or initiation of a new attack.

[Sulfinpyrazone is sometimes used in the treatment of hyperuricemia not associated with gout. However, treatment of asymptomatic hyperuricemia is often unnecessary; the need for such therapy should be determined on an individual basis.][1]

Although a few studies have shown that sulfinpyrazone may reduce the risk of reinfarction and/or sudden cardiac death during the first 7 months after an initial myocardial infarction, the results of these studies have been questioned on methodological grounds. Aspirin is the drug of choice for preventing reinfarction, because its efficacy is more clearly established. However, sulfinpyrazone may be a suitable alternative for patients unable to take aspirin for this indication.

**Unaccepted**
Sulfinpyrazone is not recommended in circumstances in which there is an especially high risk of adverse effects associated with crystallization and deposition of urate in renal tissues, such as formation of renal calculi and uric acid nephropathy. It therefore should not be used for treatment of gout in patients whose 24-hour urate excretion exceeds 800 mg (4.8 mmol) or who have extensive tophi, or for treatment of hyperuricemia associated with neoplastic disease or its treatment (chemotherapy with rapidly cytolytic antineoplastic agents or radiation therapy). Allopurinol, which decreases the quantity of urate that reaches the kidneys in addition to decreasing the concentration of urate in the blood, is recommended in these circumstances.

Sulfinpyrazone has also been used to prevent the occurrence or reoccurrence of venous thrombosis or embolism and thrombotic complications associated with rheumatic mitral stenosis, unstable angina pectoris, and transient cerebral ischemic attacks. Also, sulfinpyrazone has been used to prevent occlusion (by clotted blood) of aortocoronary bypass grafts, arteriovenous shunts, and prosthetic mitral valves. However, sulfinpyrazone's efficacy has not been established and further study has been recommended. Aspirin is the agent of choice for these indications. Dipyridamole is also effective in protecting against thrombotic complications associated with prosthetic valves or other foreign surfaces.

---
[1] Not included in Canadian product labeling.

## Pharmacology/Pharmacokinetics

**Physicochemical characteristics**
Chemical group—A pyrazole compound chemically related to phenylbutazone.
Molecular weight—404.48.
pKa—2.8.

**Mechanism of action/Effect**
Antigout agent; antihyperuricemic—Sulfinpyrazone is a uricosuric agent. By competitively inhibiting the active reabsorption of urate at the proximal renal tubule, it increases the urinary excretion of uric acid and lowers serum urate concentrations. By lowering serum concentrations of uric acid below its solubility limits, sulfinpyrazone may decrease or prevent urate deposition, tophi formation, and chronic joint changes; promote resolution of existing urate deposits; and, after several months of therapy, reduce the frequency of acute attacks of gout. Sulfinpyrazone does not have clinically useful anti-inflammatory or analgesic activity.

Antithrombotic; myocardial infarction prophylactic—Sulfinpyrazone restores toward normal the shortened platelet survival time often associated with thromboembolic disorders. It decreases platelet adhesiveness to subendothelial cells and possibly to prosthetic surfaces. Although sulfinpyrazone also inhibits the activity of the enzyme cyclo-oxygenase, resulting in decreased synthesis of thromboxane $A_2$ (a prostaglandin in platelets that promotes aggregation) and the platelet release reaction (an essential step in platelet aggregation and subsequent thrombus formation), it is a relatively weak inhibitor of platelet aggregation. Whether inhibition of platelet aggregation contributes significantly to the medication's antithrombotic activity has therefore been questioned. Sulfinpyrazone's effects on platelets are due primarily to an active sulfide metabolite.

**Other actions/effects**
Although sulfinpyrazone lacks clinically useful anti-inflammatory or analgesic activity, it inhibits prostaglandin synthesis and shares some of the risks associated with phenylbutazone (to which it is chemically related) and other nonsteroidal anti-inflammatory drugs (NSAIDs), including the potential for causing gastrointestinal, renal, or hematologic toxicity.

There is some evidence that sulfinpyrazone induces the activity of hepatic microsomal enzymes and, with chronic use, enhances its own metabolism. Although sulfinpyrazone has been shown to increase antipyrine clearance, the possibility that it may induce the metabolism of other medications has not been fully investigated. However, sulfinpyrazone has been shown to inhibit (rather than increase) metabolism of several medications, including warfarin, tolbutamide, and phenytoin, that are metabolized via the hepatic P-450 microsomal enzyme system.

**Absorption**
Rapid and complete.

**Protein binding**
Very high (98 to 99%).

**Biotransformation**
Hepatic and intestinal. The sulfide metabolite is formed primarily by intestinal microflora following enterohepatic circulation of sulfinpyrazone. The number and quantity of metabolites formed, especially the quantity of the sulfide metabolite, are subject to considerable interpatient variation.

At least 4 of the known metabolites are active. p-Hydroxy-sulfinpyrazone has about 33 to 50% of the uricosuric activity of the parent compound. The sulfide derivative, but not the sulfone or p-hydroxysulfide derivative, also has slight uricosuric activity. The sulfide, sulfone, and p-hydroxysulfide metabolites are approximately 10, 5, and 2 times as potent, respectively, and the p-hydroxy-sulfinpyrazone metabolite is about half as potent, as sulfinpyrazone itself in altering platelet function. However, only the sulfide metabolite is considered to contribute significantly toward the medication's antithrombotic activity.

**Half-life**
Elimination—
  Sulfinpyrazone:
    Approximately 4 to 6 hours. Single-dose studies have provided some evidence for the existence of an early elimination half-life of approximately 2 to 3 hours and a late elimination half-life (beginning approximately 20 hours after administration) of approximately 6 hours.
  p-Hydroxy-sulfinpyrazone:
    200-mg single dose—Approximately 1 hour.
    400-mg single dose and
    Steady-state, following administration of 400 mg twice a day for 23 days—Approximately 2.6 hours.
  Sulfide metabolite:
    Single doses—Approximately 11 to 12 hours, although one study reported a mean value of 20.9 hours after a single 400-mg dose.
    Steady-state—Approximately 14 hours, following administration of 200 mg 4 times a day for 6 days or 400 mg twice a day for 23 days.

**Onset of action**
Antithrombotic effect—Approximately 4 days.

**Time to peak concentration**
Sulfinpyrazone—Approximately 1 to 2 hours. Values at steady-state (after administration of 200 mg 4 times a day for 6 days or 400 mg twice a day for 23 days) are not significantly different from those found with single 400-mg oral doses.

p-Hydroxy-sulfinpyrazone—Approximately 2.5 hours, after administration of a single 400-mg dose and at steady-state (following administration of 400 mg twice a day for 23 days).

Sulfide metabolite—Generally 11 to 12 hours after administration of a single dose, although one study reported a mean value of 19 hours after a single 400-mg dose. Mean values under steady-state conditions (after administration of 200 mg 4 times a day for 6 days or administration of 400 mg twice a day for 23 days) are lower by about 4 to 5 hours than those determined after single doses.

**Peak serum concentration**
Sulfinpyrazone—
  Single 200-mg dose: Approximately 13 mcg per mL (mcg/mL) (32.1 micromoles/L).
  Single 400-mg dose: Approximately 26 to 30 mcg/mL (64.2 to 74.1 micromoles/L).
  Chronic administration of 600 to 800 mg a day: Two studies, one in which values were determined in patients who had been treated continuously for 2.5 years and another in which values were determined after administration of 200 mg 4 times a day for 6 days, reported maximum values of approximately 16 to 21 mcg/mL (39.5 to 51.9 micromoles/L). In a third study, maximum concentrations of 13.5 mcg/mL (33.3 micromoles/L) were measured after administration of 400 mg twice a day for 23 days; this value is approxi-

mately half of that found in the same study after administration of a single 400-mg dose.

*p*-Hydroxy-sulfinpyrazone—
  Single 200-mg dose: Less than 0.5 mcg/mL.
  Single 400-mg dose: Approximately 0.7 mcg/mL.
  Chronic administration of 800 mg a day: Approximately 0.2 mcg/mL.

Sulfide metabolite—
  Single 200-mg dose: Approximately 2.6 mcg/mL.
  Single 400-mg dose: Approximately 1 mcg/mL in 1 study and 3.5 mcg/mL in another.
  Chronic administration of 600 to 800 mg a day: Maximum values of approximately 14 mcg/mL were reported in one study after administration of 200 mg 4 times a day for 6 days. However, lower values (approximately 2.5 to 5 mcg/mL) were reported in other studies in which sulfinpyrazone was administered for a longer time (23 days in 1 study and at least 2.5 years in the other).

**Time to peak effect**
Antithrombotic effect—Approximately 1 to 2 weeks after initiation of treatment with 200 mg 4 times a day.

**Duration of action**
Single dose—The uricosuric action usually lasts for 4 to 6 hours, but may persist for up to 10 hours in some patients.

**Elimination**
95% renal; 5% fecal. Approximately 25% of a dose is excreted in the urine as free sulfinpyrazone and another 25% as sulfinpyrazone glucuronide. Up to 45% of a dose is excreted in the urine as metabolites, mostly as their glucuronide conjugates.

## Precautions to Consider

### Cross-sensitivity and/or related problems
Patients sensitive to aspirin, oxyphenbutazone, or phenylbutazone may be sensitive to this medication also. In challenge tests, sulfinpyrazone caused dyspnea, wheezing, and/or a fall in peak expiratory flow rate in 4 of 11 patients with aspirin-induced asthma but no reaction in individuals with documented sensitivity (history of anaphylaxis and positive skin tests) to dipyrone.

The possibility of cross-sensitivity between sulfinpyrazone and other nonsteroidal anti-inflammatory drugs (NSAIDs) should be considered, especially for patients in whom cross-sensitivity between aspirin and other NSAIDs has been reported.

### Carcinogenicity
No evidence of carcinogenicity was found in a 2-year study in rats receiving up to 500 mg per kg of body weight per day.

### Pregnancy/Reproduction
Pregnancy—Problems in humans have not been documented.
Studies in animals on the teratogenic potential of sulfinpyrazone have yielded inconclusive results.

### Breast-feeding
It is not known whether sulfinpyrazone is excreted in breast milk.

### Pediatrics
No published information is available on the relationship of age to the effects of sulfinpyrazone in pediatric patients.

### Geriatrics
No published information is available on the relationship of age to the effects of sulfinpyrazone in geriatric patients. However, elderly patients are more likely to have age-related renal function impairment, which may decrease the efficacy of uricosuric agents and/or increase the risk of adverse effects in patients receiving sulfinpyrazone.

### Drug interactions and/or related problems
The following drug interactions and/or related problems have been selected on the basis of their potential clinical significance (possible mechanism in parentheses where appropriate)—not necessarily inclusive (» = major clinical significance):

Note: Combinations containing any of the following medications, depending on the amount present, may also interact with this medication.

In addition to the interactions listed below, the possibility should be considered that additive or multiple effects leading to impaired blood clotting and/or increased risk of bleeding may occur if sulfinpyrazone is administered concurrently with any medication having a significant potential for causing hypoprothrombinemia, thrombocytopenia, or gastrointestinal ulceration or hemorrhage.

Alcohol or
Diazoxide or
Mecamylamine or
Pyrazinamide
  (these medications may increase serum uric acid concentrations; dosage adjustment of sulfinpyrazone may be necessary to control hyperuricemia)

Aminosalicylate sodium
  (sulfinpyrazone may decrease renal tubular secretion of aminosalicylate sodium, resulting in increased and more prolonged serum concentrations and/or toxicity; patient should be monitored and dosage adjusted as necessary)

» Anticoagulants, coumarin- or indandione-derivative or
» Heparin or
» Thrombolytic agents, such as:
  Alteplase (tissue-type plasminogen activator, recombinant)
  Anistreplase (anisoylated plasminogen-streptokinase activator complex, APSAC)
  Streptokinase
  Urokinase
  (prolongation of the prothrombin time and severe gastrointestinal or renal bleeding have resulted from concurrent use of sulfinpyrazone with acenocoumarol [nicoumalone] or warfarin; studies have demonstrated that sulfinpyrazone has stereoselective effects on warfarin kinetics, i.e., it displaces from protein-binding sites and increases clearance of the (R)-enantiomer of warfarin, but inhibits metabolism of the substantially more potent (S)-enantiomer by the hepatic P-450 enzyme system, resulting in a net increase in warfarin activity; careful monitoring of the prothrombin time is recommended when sulfinpyrazone therapy is initiated or discontinued so that anticoagulant dosage can be adjusted as needed)
  (although sulfinpyrazone has also been shown to inhibit enzymatic metabolism of phenprocoumon, concurrent use of the 2 medications does not lead to a significant increase in the prothrombin time, possibly because a comparatively small quantity of phenprocoumon is eliminated via this mechanism; however, inhibition of platelet function by sulfinpyrazone, and its potential for causing gastrointestinal ulceration or hemorrhage, may increase the risk of hemorrhage in patients receiving any anticoagulant or thrombolytic agent)

Antidiabetic agents, oral
  (sulfinpyrazone may decrease the metabolism of an oral antidiabetic agent, leading to prolonged half-life and increased hypoglycemic effect; dosage adjustments may be necessary during and following sulfinpyrazone therapy)

Anti-inflammatory drugs, nonsteroidal (NSAIDs) or
» Platelet aggregation–inhibiting medications (See *Appendix II*)
  (concurrent use with sulfinpyrazone may increase the risk of bleeding because of additive inhibition of platelet function and sulfinpyrazone's potential for causing gastrointestinal ulceration or hemorrhage; concurrent use with NSAIDs may also increase the risk of gastrointestinal ulceration or hemorrhage)

Antimicrobial agents
  (antimicrobial therapy may suppress formation by intestinal microflora of the active sulfide metabolite of sulfinpyrazone, which is responsible for sulfinpyrazone's antithrombotic activity)

» Antineoplastic agents, rapidly cytolytic
  (concurrent use with sulfinpyrazone is not recommended because of the risk of uric acid nephropathy; allopurinol is the antihyperuricemic agent of choice for reducing risks [gout and/or urate nephropathy] associated with chemotherapy-induced hyperuricemia; also, rapidly cytolytic antineoplastic agents may increase serum uric acid concentrations and interfere with control of pre-existing hyperuricemia and gout)

» Aspirin or other salicylates, including bismuth subsalicylate
  (salicylates inhibit sulfinpyrazone's uricosuric action; although occasional use of a salicylate in low to moderate analgesic doses, or chronic administration of 80 mg per day of aspirin as an antithrombotic, is not likely to interfere with sulfinpyrazone's uricosuric effect, chronic use of analgesic or antirheumatic doses of a salicylate together with sulfinpyrazone is not recommended; sulfinpyrazone also inhibits the uricosuria induced by high doses of salicylates; in addition, sulfinpyrazone may decrease excretion of salicylate and/or displace salicylate from its plasma protein-binding sites, possibly leading to increased salicylate concentrations and toxicity)
  (low doses of sulfinpyrazone and aspirin have been used together as an antithrombotic regimen in a few studies; however, whether the combination is more effective than aspirin alone has not been established, and the increased risk of bleeding must be considered)

» Cefamandole or
» Cefoperazone or
» Cefotetan or
» Moxalactam or
» Plicamycin or

» Valproic acid
(these medications may cause hypoprothrombinemia; in addition, plicamycin or valproic acid may inhibit platelet aggregation, and moxalactam may also cause irreversible platelet damage; inhibition of platelet function by sulfinpyrazone, as well as its potential for causing gastrointestinal ulceration or hemorrhage, may increase the risk of severe hemorrhage when these medications are used concurrently)

» Nitrofurantoin
(sulfinpyrazone may increase serum concentrations of nitrofurantoin by decreasing its renal clearance, possibly increasing the potential for toxic reactions and reducing nitrofurantoin's effectiveness as a urinary tract anti-infective; concurrent use should be avoided)

Phenytoin and possibly other hydantoin anticonvulsants
(sulfinpyrazone may displace these medications from plasma protein-binding sites and decrease their metabolism, possibly leading to increased plasma concentration and elimination half-life; although hydantoin plasma concentration is not consistently increased, it is recommended that patients be monitored for signs of hydantoin toxicity during concurrent use)

Probenecid
(probenecid inhibits the renal tubular secretion of sulfinpyrazone and its active para-hydroxy metabolite; however, the uricosuric effects of the medications are additive, and increased therapeutic benefit has been reported during concurrent use)

**Laboratory value alterations**
The following have been selected on the basis of their potential clinical significance (possible effect in parentheses where appropriate)—not necessarily inclusive (» = major clinical significance):

With diagnostic test results
» Aminohippuric acid (PAH) clearance studies and Phenolsulfonphthalein (PSP) clearance studies
(sulfinpyrazone decreases renal clearance of PAH and PSP, leading to reduced urine concentrations and misleading test results)

**Medical considerations/Contraindications**
The medical considerations/contraindications included have been selected on the basis of their potential clinical significance (reasons given in parentheses where appropriate)—not necessarily inclusive (» = major clinical significance).

*Except under special circumstances, this medication should not be used when the following medical conditions exist:*

» Any condition in which there is an increased risk of uric acid renal calculus formation or urate nephropathy, such as:
» Cancer chemotherapy with rapidly cytolytic antineoplastic agents
» Radiation therapy for malignancy
» Renal calculi or history of, especially uric acid calculi
» Urate excretion higher than 800 mg (4.8 mmol) in 24 hours
» Urate nephropathy or history of
(sulfinpyrazone is likely to induce, or exacerbate pre-existing, renal calculi and/or urate nephropathy; allopurinol is the antihyperuricemic agent recommended in these circumstances)

» Blood dyscrasias
(may be exacerbated)
» Peptic ulcer, active
(may be exacerbated)
» Renal function impairment, moderate to severe
(may be exacerbated; also, sulfinpyrazone's efficacy as a uricosuric agent decreases with increasing degrees of renal function impairment, and the medication may be completely ineffective when the patient's creatinine clearance is lower than 30 mL per minute [0.5 mL per second])

*Risk-benefit should be considered when the following medical problems exist:*

Bronchospastic reaction to aspirin, history of or
Sensitivity to sulfinpyrazone or to NSAIDs, especially oxyphenbutazone or phenylbutazone, history of
(risk of cross-sensitivity)
Blood dyscrasias, history of
(increased risk of sulfinpyrazone-induced blood dyscrasias)
» Gastrointestinal inflammation or ulceration, active or history of or
» Peptic ulcer, history of
(may be exacerbated or reactivated; if sulfinpyrazone is used for patients with these conditions, concurrent use of an appropriate treatment or prophylactic regimen for gastrointestinal ulceration should be considered)

» Renal function impairment, mild
(may be exacerbated; also, sulfinpyrazone's efficacy as a uricosuric agent begins to decrease when the creatinine clearance is 80 mL per minute [1.33 mL per second])

**Patient monitoring**
The following may be especially important in patient monitoring (other tests may be warranted in some patients, depending on condition; » = major clinical significance):

Blood counts
(recommended at periodic intervals during therapy)
Renal function determinations
(recommended at periodic intervals during therapy for patients with renal function impairment)
» Uric acid determinations
(monitoring of uric acid concentrations may be required for proper dosing in uricosuric therapy; the effect of sulfinpyrazone may be measured by a reduction of serum uric acid concentration [the upper limit of normal is about 7 mg per 100 mL (420 micromoles/L) for men and postmenopausal women and about 6 mg per 100 mL (360 micromoles/L) for premenopausal women but may vary, depending on the patient and laboratory methodology] or, more directly, by a significant increase in 24-hour urinary uric acid excretion)

## Side/Adverse Effects

The following side/adverse effects have been selected on the basis of their potential clinical significance (possible signs and symptoms in parentheses where appropriate)—not necessarily inclusive:

**Those indicating need for medical attention**
Incidence more frequent
*Renal calculi, urate* (lower back and/or side pain, painful urination, with or without blood in urine)—may occur in up to 10% of patients early in sulfinpyrazone treatment
Incidence less frequent
*Dermatitis, allergic* (skin rash)
Incidence rare
*Agranulocytosis* (fever with or without chills; sores, ulcers, or white spots on lips or in mouth; sore throat); *anemia* (unusual tiredness or weakness); *aplastic anemia; [pancytopenia]* (shortness of breath, troubled breathing, tightness in chest, and/or wheezing; sores, ulcers, or white spots on lips or in mouth; swollen and/or painful glands; unusual bleeding or bruising; unusual tiredness or weakness); *fever, allergic; gastrointestinal bleeding* (bloody or black, tarry stools; vomiting of blood or material that looks like coffee grounds); *leukopenia* (fever with or without chills; sore throat; unusual tiredness or weakness); *renal failure, possibly associated with urate nephropathy* (increased blood pressure; shortness of breath, troubled breathing, tightness in chest, and/or wheezing; sudden decrease in amount of urine; swelling of face, fingers, feet, and/or lower legs; unusual tiredness or weakness; weight gain); *thrombocytopenia* (rarely, unusual bleeding or bruising; black, tarry stools; blood in urine or stools; pinpoint red spots on skin)—usually asymptomatic

Note: *Renal failure not associated with urate nephropathy* has been reported, rarely, during sulfinpyrazone therapy, but a direct causal relationship has not always been clearly established. Sulfinpyrazone has caused *acute interstitial nephritis* (including cases documented as being hypersensitivity-mediated) and *acute renal tubular necrosis* in a few patients. Also, *transient renal function impairment* (which improved despite continued administration) has occurred in postmyocardial infarction patients and postaortocoronary bypass patients receiving sulfinpyrazone. It has been proposed that sulfinpyrazone may cause transient renal ischemia by temporarily inhibiting the synthesis of renal vasodilator prostaglandins and/or kinins, and that the presence of congestive heart failure may be a predisposing factor in the development of sulfinpyrazone-induced renal complications.

**Those indicating need for medical attention only if they continue or are bothersome**
Incidence more frequent
*Gouty arthritis, acute attack* (joint pain; redness; swelling); *nausea or vomiting; stomach pain*
Note: An increase in the frequency of *acute attacks of gout* during the first few months of therapy may be anticipated, unless adequate prophylaxis with colchicine (or, if the patient is unable to take colchicine, a nonsteroidal anti-inflammatory drug [NSAID]) is given concurrently with the sulfinpyrazone. Up to 20% of patients started on treatment with a uricosuric agent alone may experience acute attacks within the first few days of treatment.

## Overdose

For specific information on the agents used in the management of sulfinpyrazone overdose, see:
- *Acetazolamide* in *Carbonic Anhydrase Inhibitors (Systemic)* monograph;
- *Allopurinol (Systemic)* monograph; and/or
- *Potassium citrate* in *Citrates (Systemic)* monograph.

For more information on the management of overdose or unintentional ingestion, **contact a Poison Control Center** (see *Poison Control Center Listing* ).

### Clinical effects of overdose
The following effects have been selected on the basis of their clinical significance (possible signs and symptoms in parentheses where appropriate)—not necessarily inclusive:

Acute and chronic
*Clumsiness or unsteadiness; convulsions; diarrhea; nausea or vomiting, severe or continuing; stomach pain, severe or continuing; difficulty in breathing*

### Treatment of overdose
To decrease absorption—Emptying the stomach by induction of emesis or performing gastric lavage.

Specific treatment—If severe renal function impairment occurs, hemodialysis may be needed.

For uric acid calculi or urate nephropathy:

Recommended measures include administration of large quantities of fluids and of allopurinol to increase urine flow and reduce uric acid formation, respectively. A urinary pH of 6 to 6.5 should be achieved and maintained by administration of alkali such as potassium citrate. If necessary to maintain the desired urinary pH through the night, acetazolamide may also be given at bedtime. Other interventions designed to facilitate removal of renal calculi may also be needed.

Supportive care—Monitoring the patient and instituting supportive treatment as needed. Patients in whom intentional overdose is known or suspected should be referred for psychiatric consultation.

## Patient Consultation

As an aid to patient consultation, refer to *Advice for the Patient, Sulfinpyrazone (Systemic)*.

In providing consultation, consider emphasizing the following selected information (» = major clinical significance):

### Before using this medication
» Conditions affecting use, especially:
Sensitivity to sulfinpyrazone or NSAIDs, especially aspirin, oxyphenbutazone, or phenylbutazone, history of
Other medications, especially anticoagulants, rapidly cytolytic antineoplastic agents, aspirin or other salicylates, hypoprothrombinemia-inducing cephalosporins, moxalactam, nitrofurantoin, platelet aggregation inhibitors, plicamycin, and valproic acid
Other medical problems, especially cancer treated with rapidly cytolytic antineoplastic agents or radiation therapy, renal calculi or history of (especially uric acid calculi), renal function impairment, blood dyscrasias, gastrointestinal inflammation or ulceration, and active peptic ulcer

### Proper use of this medication
» Taking with food or an antacid to minimize gastrointestinal irritation
» Compliance with therapy
Importance of high fluid intake and compliance with therapy for alkalinization of urine, if prescribed, to minimize kidney stone formation
» Proper dosing
Missed dose: Taking as soon as possible; not taking if almost time for next dose; not doubling doses
» Proper storage
*For use as antigout agent*
Several months of continuous therapy may be required for maximum effectiveness
» Medication does not relieve acute gout attacks but rather helps to prevent them; need to continue taking sulfinpyrazone with medication prescribed for gout attacks

### Precautions while using this medication
Regular visits to physician to check progress during therapy
Caution if any laboratory tests required; possible interference with test results
*For use as antihyperuricemic (including gout therapy)*
» Aspirin or other salicylates may decrease the uricosuric effects of sulfinpyrazone; checking with physician regarding concurrent use, since effect is dependent on salicylate dose and duration of use
» Possibility that alcohol taken in large amounts may increase blood uric acid concentration and reduce effectiveness of medication

### Side/adverse effects
Signs and symptoms of potential side effects, especially renal calculi, dermatitis, blood dyscrasias, fever, gastrointestinal bleeding, and renal failure

## General Dosing Information

Sulfinpyrazone therapy for gouty arthritis should not be initiated until 2 to 3 weeks after an acute attack has subsided. However, if an acute attack occurs in a patient already receiving sulfinpyrazone, the medication should be continued at the same dose while therapeutic doses of colchicine or a nonsteroidal anti-inflammatory drug (NSAID) are given to relieve the attack.

Sulfinpyrazone may be administered with food or an antacid to reduce gastrointestinal irritation.

Because sulfinpyrazone may increase the frequency of acute attacks of gout during the early months of therapy, prophylactic doses of colchicine (or, if the patient is unable to take colchicine, an NSAID) should be administered concurrently during the first 3 to 6 months of sulfinpyrazone therapy. However, even with prophylactic therapy, acute attacks of gout requiring treatment with full therapeutic doses of colchicine or an NSAID may occur.

To reduce the risk of urate stone formation, especially in patients with hyperuricemia, it is recommended that sulfinpyrazone therapy be initiated with a low dose, followed by a gradual increase in dosage. Also, a high fluid intake (no less than 2.5 to 3 liters daily) and maintenance of an alkaline urine by administration of sodium bicarbonate (3 to 7.5 grams daily), potassium citrate (7.5 grams daily), or acetazolamide (250 mg daily) are recommended. The risk of urate stone formation is highest during the first few weeks of therapy, when urate excretion is high; after hyperuricemia has been controlled and urinary excretion of uric acid decreases, the need for these measures is reduced.

Sulfinpyrazone may be given concurrently with allopurinol for treatment of gout; the antihyperuricemic effects of the 2 medications are additive.

Determination of serum or urine (24-hour) uric acid concentrations may be necessary for proper dosing in uricosuric therapy.

## Oral Dosage Forms

Note: Bracketed uses in the *Dosage Forms* section refer to categories of use and/or indications that are not included in U.S. product labeling.

### SULFINPYRAZONE CAPSULES USP

**Usual adult dose**
Antigout agent—
Initial—
Oral, 100 to 200 mg two times a day, the dose being increased by 200 mg a day at two-day intervals, if necessary, up to a maximum of 800 mg per day.

Note: Some clinicians recommend initiating treatment with a lower dose of 50 mg two times a day and increasing the dose more gradually (e.g., at three- to four-day intervals).

Patients who were previously controlled with other uricosuric therapy may be transferred to sulfinpyrazone at full maintenance dosage.

Maintenance—
Oral, dosage to be adjusted to the lowest dose that maintains the serum uric acid concentration at the desired level, usually 200 to 400 mg per day. However, some patients may require maintenance doses of up to 800 mg a day.

Note: The initial dose recommended for treatment of gout is also appropriate if sulfinpyrazone is used as an antithrombotic. However, it is recommended that myocardial reinfarction prophylaxis with sulfinpyrazone not be initiated until at least fourteen days after the acute event. Delaying treatment may decrease the risk of renal function impairment in patients receiving sulfinpyrazone for this purpose.

For preventing myocardial reinfarction, the usual maintenance dose is 800 mg per day, in four divided doses. For other antithrombotic indications, the usual maintenance dose is 600 to 800 mg per day, in three or four divided doses.

**Usual pediatric dose**
Dosage has not been established.

**Strength(s) usually available**
U.S.—
200 mg (Rx) [*Anturane*; GENERIC].
Canada—
Not commercially available.

**Packaging and storage**
Store below 40 °C (104 °F), preferably between 15 and 30 °C (59 and 86 °F), unless otherwise specified by manufacturer. Store in a well-closed container.

### SULFINPYRAZONE TABLETS USP
**Usual adult dose**
See *Sulfinpyrazone Capsules USP*.

**Usual pediatric dose**
Dosage has not been established.

**Strength(s) usually available**
U.S.—
 100 mg (Rx) [*Anturane*; GENERIC].

Canada—
 100 mg (Rx) [*Anturan; Apo-Sulfinpyrazone; Novopyrazone*].
 200 mg (Rx) [*Anturan; Apo-Sulfinpyrazone; Novopyrazone*].

**Packaging and storage**
Store below 40 °C (104 °F), preferably between 15 and 30 °C (59 and 86 °F), unless otherwise specified by manufacturer. Store in a well-closed container.

Revised: 01/19/93

**SULFISOXAZOLE**—See *Sulfonamides (Ophthalmic); Sulfonamides (Systemic)*

# SULFONAMIDES  Ophthalmic

This monograph includes information on the following: 1) Sulfacetamide; 2) Sulfisoxazole.

INN:
 Sulfisoxazole—Sulfafurazole

BAN:
 Sulfacetamide—Sulphacetamide
 Sulfisoxazole—Sulphafurazole

VA CLASSIFICATION (Primary): OP201

Commonly used brand name(s): *Ak-Sulf*[1]; *Bleph-10*[1]; *Cetamide*[1]; *Gantrisin*[2]; *I-Sulfacet*[1]; *Isopto-Cetamide*[1]; *Ocu-Sul-10*[1]; *Ocu-Sul-15*[1]; *Ocu-Sul-30*[1]; *Ocusulf-10*[1]; *Ophthacet*[1]; *Sodium Sulamyd*[1]; *Spectro-Sulf*[1]; *Steri-Units Sulfacetamide*[1]; *Sulf-10*[1]; *Sulfair*[1]; *Sulfair 10*[1]; *Sulfair 15*[1]; *Sulfair Forte*[1]; *Sulfamide*[1]; *Sulfex*[1]; *Sulten-10*[1].

Note: For a listing of dosage forms and brand names by country availability, see *Dosage Forms* section(s).

## Category
Antibacterial (ophthalmic).

## Indications
Note: Bracketed information in the *Indications* section refers to uses that are not included in U.S. product labeling.

**Accepted**
Conjunctivitis, bacterial (treatment) or
Ocular infections, other (treatment)—Ophthalmic sulfonamides are indicated in the treatment of conjunctivitis and other superficial ocular infections caused by susceptible organisms.

Trachoma (treatment) or
Chlamydial infections, other (treatment)—Ophthalmic sulfonamides are indicated concurrently with systemic sulfonamides in the treatment of trachoma and other chlamydial infections.

[Blepharitis, bacterial (treatment)]—Ophthalmic sulfonamides are used in the treatment of bacterial blepharitis.

[Blepharoconjunctivitis (treatment)]—Ophthalmic sulfonamides are used in the treatment of blepharoconjunctivitis.

[Keratitis, bacterial (treatment)]—Ophthalmic sulfonamides are used in the treatment of bacterial keratitis.

[Keratoconjunctivitis, bacterial (treatment)]—Ophthalmic sulfonamides are used in the treatment of bacterial keratoconjunctivitis.

Note: Not all species or strains of a particular organism may be susceptible to a specific sulfonamide.

## Pharmacology/Pharmacokinetics
**Physicochemical characteristics**
Molecular weight—
 Sulfacetamide sodium: 254.24.
 Sulfisoxazole diolamine: 372.44.

**Mechanism of action/Effect**
Sulfonamides are broad-spectrum, bacteriostatic anti-infectives. They are structural analogs of aminobenzoic acid (PABA) and competitively inhibit a bacterial enzyme, dihydropteroate synthetase, that is responsible for incorporation of PABA into dihydrofolic acid. This blocks the synthesis of dihydrofolic acid and decreases the amount of metabolically active tetrahydrofolic acid, a cofactor for the synthesis of purines, thymidine, and DNA.

Susceptible bacteria are those that must synthesize folic acid. The action of sulfonamides is antagonized by PABA and its derivatives (e.g., procaine and tetracaine) and by the presence of pus or tissue breakdown products, which provide the necessary components for bacterial growth.

**Absorption**
Following topical application of sulfacetamide (30% solution) to the eye, small amounts may be absorbed into the cornea.

## Precautions to Consider
**Cross-sensitivity and/or related problems**
Patients sensitive to one sulfonamide may be sensitive to other sulfonamides also.

Patients sensitive to furosemide, thiazide diuretics, sulfonylureas, or carbonic anhydrase inhibitors may be sensitive to sulfonamides also.

**Pregnancy/Reproduction**
Problems in humans have not been documented.

**Breast-feeding**
Problems in humans have not been documented.

**Pediatrics**
Appropriate studies on the relationship of age to the effects of sulfonamides have not been performed in the pediatric population.

**Geriatrics**
Appropriate studies on the relationship of age to the effects of sulfonamides have not been performed in the geriatric population. However, no geriatrics-specific problems have been documented to date.

**Drug interactions and/or related problems**
The following drug interactions and/or related problems have been selected on the basis of their potential clinical significance (possible mechanism in parentheses where appropriate)—not necessarily inclusive (» = major clinical significance):

Note: Combinations containing any of the following medications, depending on the amount present, may also interact with this medication.

» Silver preparations, such as silver nitrate, mild silver protein
 (topical sulfonamides are incompatible with silver salts; concurrent use is not recommended)

**Medical considerations/Contraindications**
The medical considerations/contraindications included have been selected on the basis of their potential clinical significance (reasons given in parentheses where appropriate)—not necessarily inclusive (» = major clinical significance).

*Risk-benefit should be considered when the following medical problem exists:*
Sensitivity to sulfonamides

## Side/Adverse Effects
The following side/adverse effects have been selected on the basis of their potential clinical significance (possible signs and symptoms in parentheses where appropriate)—not necessarily inclusive:

**Those indicating need for medical attention**
Incidence more frequent
 *Hypersensitivity* (itching, redness, swelling, or other sign of irritation not present before therapy)

## Patient Consultation

As an aid to patient consultation, refer to *Advice for the Patient, Sulfonamides (Ophthalmic)*.

In providing consultation, consider emphasizing the following selected information (» = major clinical significance):

**Before using this medication**
» Conditions affecting use, especially:
   Sensitivity to sulfonamides, furosemide, thiazide diuretics, sulfonylureas, or carbonic anhydrase inhibitors
   Other medications, especially silver preparations, such as silver nitrate or mild silver protein

**Proper use of this medication**
   Proper administration technique for ophthalmic solution and ophthalmic ointment
» Compliance with full course of therapy
» Proper dosing
   Missed dose: Applying as soon as possible; not applying if almost time for next dose
» Proper storage

**Precautions while using this medication**
   Blurred vision after application of ophthalmic ointments
   Possibility of stinging or burning after application
   Checking with physician if no improvement within a few days

**Side/adverse effects**
   Signs of potential side effects, especially hypersensitivity

## General Dosing Information

At night the ophthalmic ointment may be used as an adjunct to the ophthalmic solution to provide prolonged contact with the medication.

Although some manufacturers recommend a dose of 2 drops of an ophthalmic solution at appropriate intervals, the conjunctival sac will usually hold only 1 drop.

---
### SULFACETAMIDE
---

## Ophthalmic Dosage Forms

### SULFACETAMIDE SODIUM OPHTHALMIC OINTMENT USP

**Usual adult and adolescent dose**
Ophthalmic antibacterial—
   Topical, to the conjunctiva, a thin strip (approximately 1.25 to 2.5 cm) of ointment four times a day and at bedtime.

**Usual pediatric dose**
Dosage has not been established.

**Strength(s) usually available**
U.S.—
   10% (Rx) [*Ak-Sulf; Bleph-10; Cetamide; Ocu-Sul-10; Sodium Sulamyd; Sulfair 10;* GENERIC].
Canada—
   10% (Rx) [*Cetamide; Sodium Sulamyd*].

**Packaging and storage**
Store below 40 °C (104 °F), preferably between 15 and 30 °C (59 and 86 °F), unless otherwise specified by manufacturer. Protect from freezing.

**Auxiliary labeling**
• For the eye.
• Continue medicine for full time of treatment.

### SULFACETAMIDE SODIUM OPHTHALMIC SOLUTION USP

**Usual adult and adolescent dose**
Ophthalmic antibacterial—
   Topical, to the conjunctiva, 1 drop every one to three hours during the day and less frequently during the night.

**Usual pediatric dose**
Dosage has not been established.

**Strength(s) usually available**
U.S.—
   10% (Rx) [*Ak-Sulf; Bleph-10; I-Sulfacet; Ocu-Sul-10; Ocusulf-10; Ophthacet; Sodium Sulamyd; Spectro-Sulf; Sulf-10; Sulfair; Sulfair 10; Sulfamide; Sulten-10;* GENERIC].
   15% (Rx) [*Isopto-Cetamide; I-Sulfacet; Ocu-Sul-15; Spectro-Sulf; Steri-Units Sulfacetamide; Sulfair; Sulfair 15;* GENERIC].
   30% (Rx) [*I-Sulfacet; Ocu-Sul-30; Sodium Sulamyd; Spectro-Sulf; Sulfair; Sulfair Forte;* GENERIC].
Canada—
   10% (Rx) [*Ak-Sulf; Bleph-10; Isopto-Cetamide; Sodium Sulamyd; Sulfex*].
   30% (Rx) [*Sodium Sulamyd*].

**Packaging and storage**
Store between 8 and 15 °C (46 and 59 °F). Store in a tight, light-resistant container.

**Stability**
Sulfonamide solutions become dark brown with time. When this occurs, solutions should be discarded.

**Auxiliary labeling**
• For the eye.
• Keep in a cool place.
• Continue medicine for full time of treatment.
• Discard if dark brown.

**Note**
Dispense in original unopened container.

---
### SULFISOXAZOLE
---

## Ophthalmic Dosage Forms

Note: The dosing and strengths of the dosage forms available are expressed in terms of sulfisoxazole base.

### SULFISOXAZOLE DIOLAMINE OPHTHALMIC OINTMENT USP

**Usual adult and adolescent dose**
Ophthalmic antibacterial—
   Topical, to the conjunctiva, a thin strip (approximately 1.25 to 2.5 cm) of ointment one to three times a day and at bedtime.

**Usual pediatric dose**
See *Usual adult and adolescent dose*.

**Strength(s) usually available**
U.S.—
   4% (base) (each gram of ophthalmic ointment contains 55.6 mg of sulfisoxazole diolamine, equivalent to approximately 40 mg of sulfisoxazole) (Rx) [*Gantrisin* (phenylmercuric nitrate 1:50,000)].

**Packaging and storage**
Store below 40 °C (104 °F), preferably between 15 and 30 °C (59 and 86 °F), unless otherwise specified by manufacturer. Protect from freezing.

**Auxiliary labeling**
• For the eye.
• Continue medicine for full time of treatment.

### SULFISOXAZOLE DIOLAMINE OPHTHALMIC SOLUTION USP

**Usual adult and adolescent dose**
Ophthalmic antibacterial—
   Topical, to the conjunctiva, 1 drop three or more times a day.

**Usual pediatric dose**
Ophthalmic antibacterial—
   Infants up to 2 months of age: Use is not recommended.
   Infants and children over 2 months of age: See *Usual adult and adolescent dose*.

**Strength(s) usually available**
U.S.—
   4% (base) (each mL of ophthalmic solution contains 55.6 mg of sulfisoxazole diolamine, equivalent to approximately 40 mg of sulfisoxazole) (Rx) [*Gantrisin* (phenylmercuric nitrate 1:100,000)].

**Packaging and storage**
Store below 40 °C (104 °F), preferably between 15 and 30 °C (59 and 86 °F), unless otherwise specified by manufacturer. Store in a tight, light-resistant container. Protect from freezing.

**Auxiliary labeling**
• For the eye.
• Continue medicine for full time of treatment.

**Note**
Dispense in original unopened container.

Revised: 07/01/93

# SULFONAMIDES Systemic

This monograph includes information on the following: 1) Sulfadiazine; 2) Sulfamethizole†; 3) Sulfamethoxazole; 4) Sulfisoxazole.

INN:
   Sulfisoxazole—Sulfafurazole

BAN:
   Sulfadiazine—Sulphadiazine
   Sulfamethizole†—Sulphamethizole
   Sulfamethoxazole—Sulphamethoxazole
   Sulfisoxazole—Sulphafurazole

JAN:
   Sulfamethoxazole—Acetylsulfamethoxazole
   Sulfamethoxazole—Sulfamethoxazole sodium

VA CLASSIFICATION (Primary): AM650

Commonly used brand name(s): *Apo-Sulfamethoxazole*[3]; *Apo-Sulfisoxazole*[4]; *Gantanol*[3]; *Gantrisin*[4]; *Novo-Soxazole*[4]; *Sulfizole*[4]; *Thiosulfil Forte*[2]; *Urobak*[3].

Note: For a listing of dosage forms and brand names by country availability, see *Dosage Forms* section(s).

†Not commercially available in Canada.

## Category
Antibacterial (urinary)—Sulfamethizole.
Antibacterial (systemic)—Sulfadiazine; Sulfamethoxazole; Sulfisoxazole.
Antiprotozoal—Sulfadiazine; Sulfamethoxazole; Sulfisoxazole.

## Indications
Note: Bracketed information in the *Indications* section refers to uses that are not included in U.S. product labeling.

**General considerations**
Sulfonamides are active *in vitro* against a broad spectrum of gram-positive and gram-negative bacteria. They also have activity *in vitro* against *Actinomyces*, *Chlamydia trachomatis*, *Nocardia asteroides*, *Plasmodium falciparum*, and *Toxoplasma gondii*. Susceptibility of an organism to sulfonamides is variable; many bacteria have become resistant to sulfonamides, with resistance occurring in more than 20% of community and nosocomial bacterial isolates. Resistance has developed in strains of staphylococci, *Neisseria gonorrhoeae*, *N. meningitidis*, Enterbacteriaceae, and *Pseudomonas* species.

**Accepted**
Chancroid (treatment)—Sulfonamides are indicated in the treatment of chancroid caused by *Haemophilus ducreyi*. However, other agents, such as erythromycin and ceftriaxone, are considered to be first line agents.

Chlamydial infections, endocervical and urethral (treatment)[1]—Sulfonamides are indicated in the treatment of endocervical and urethral infections caused by *Chlamydia trachomatis*. However, other agents, such as doxycycline and azithromycin, are considered to be first line agents.

Conjunctivitis, inclusion (treatment)—Sulfonamides are indicated in the treatment of neonatal inclusion conjunctivitis caused by *Chlamydia trachomatis*. However, other agents, such as erythromycin, are considered to be first line agents.

Malaria (treatment)—Sulfonamides are indicated as adjunctive therapy in the treatment of chloroquine-resistant *Plasmodium falciparum*.

Meningitis (prophylaxis)[1]—Sulfonamides are indicated in the prophylaxis of meningitis caused by susceptible strains of *Neisseria meningitidis*. However, other agents, such as rifampin, are considered to be first line agents.

Nocardiosis (treatment)—Sulfonamides are indicated in the treatment of nocardiosis caused by *Nocardia asteroides*.

Otitis media (treatment)[1]—Sulfonamides are indicated in combination with other antibacterials in the treatment of otitis media caused by susceptible strains of *H. influenzae*, streptococci, and pneumococci.

Rheumatic fever (prophylaxis)[1]—Sulfadiazine, [sulfamethoxazole], and [sulfisoxazole] are indicated in the prophylaxis of rheumatic fever associated with group A beta-hemolytic streptococcal infections. However, other agents, such as penicillin, are considered to be first line agents.

Toxoplasmosis (treatment)[1]—Sulfonamides are indicated in combination with pyrimethamine in the treatment of toxoplasmosis caused by *Toxoplasma gondii*.

Trachoma (treatment)—Sulfonamides are indicated in the treatment of ocular trachoma caused by *Chlamydia trachomatis*. However, other agents, such as doxycycline and azithromycin, are considered to be first line agents.

Urinary tract infections, bacterial (treatment)—Sulfonamides are indicated in the treatment of acute, uncomplicated urinary tract infections caused by susceptible bacteria. Because sulfamethizole produces low plasma levels and is rapidly eliminated, it is recommended only for use in urinary tract infections, not systemic infections. Sulfadiazine is not recommended for the treatment of urinary tract infections because of its relatively lower urine solubility and the increased chance of crystalluria; other, more soluble agents, such as sulfisoxazole, are generally preferred.

[Lymphogranuloma venereum (treatment)][1]—Sulfonamides are used in the treatment of lymphogranuloma venereum caused by *Chlamydia* species. However, other agents, such as doxycycline and erythromycin, are considered to be first line agents.

[Paracoccidioidomycosis (treatment)][1]—Sulfadiazine is used in the treatment of paracoccidioidomycosis caused *Paracoccidioides brasiliensis*.

Not all species or strains of a particular organism may be susceptible to a specific sulfonamide.

**Unaccepted**
Sulfonamides should not be used in the treatment of Group A beta-hemolytic streptococcal tonsillopharyngitis since they may not eradicate streptococci and therefore may not prevent sequelae such as rheumatic fever.

Sulfonamides are also not effective in treating rickettsial, viral, tuberculous, actinomycotic, fungal, or mycoplasmal infections. They are also not effective in the treatment of shigellosis.

[1]Not included in Canadian product labeling.

## Pharmacology/Pharmacokinetics

**Physicochemical characteristics**
Molecular weight—
   Sulfadiazine: 250.28.
   Sulfamethizole: 270.34.
   Sulfamethoxazole: 253.28.
   Sulfisoxazole: 267.31.
   Sulfisoxazole acetyl: 309.35.

**Mechanism of action/Effect**
Sulfonamides are broad-spectrum, bacteriostatic anti-infectives. They are structural analogs of para-aminobenzoic acid (PABA) and competitively inhibit a bacterial enzyme, dihydropteroate synthetase, that is responsible for incorporation of PABA into dihydrofolic acid, the immediate precursor of folic acid. This blocks the synthesis of dihydrofolic acid and decreases the amount of metabolically active tetrahydrofolic acid, a cofactor for the synthesis of purines, thymidine, and DNA.
Susceptible bacteria are those that must synthesize folic acid. Mammalian cells require preformed folic acid and cannot synthesize it. The action of sulfonamides is antagonized by PABA and its derivatives (e.g., procaine and tetracaine) and by the presence of pus or tissue breakdown products, which provide the necessary components for bacterial growth.

**Absorption**
All sulfonamides are rapidly and well absorbed (70–100%).

**Distribution**
Widely distributed throughout body tissues and fluids, including pleural, peritoneal, synovial, and ocular fluids, as well as the vagina and middle ear. Sulfadiazine is distributed throughout total body water, while sulfisoxazole is distributed primarily to extracellular fluid (ECF). Sulfadiazine, sulfamethoxazole, and sulfisoxazole penetrate into the cerebrospinal fluid (CSF); sulfadiazine reaches 32 to 65%, sulfamethoxazole reaches 14 to 30%, and sulfisoxazole reaches 30 to 50% of corresponding blood concentrations. Sulfonamides may be detected in the urine in approximately 30 minutes. They readily cross the placenta and are distributed into breast milk, also.

Urine solubility—
   Sulfadiazine: Less soluble in urine; increased risk of crystalluria.
   Sulfamethizole: Highly soluble in urine.
   Sulfamethoxazole: Acetylated metabolite less soluble in urine; increased risk of crystalluria.
   Sulfisoxazole: Highly soluble in urine.

Vol_D—
  Sulfamethoxazole: Approximately 0.15 L per kg of body weight (L/kg).
  Sulfisoxazole: Approximately 0.21 L/kg.

**Protein binding**
Variable; acetylated metabolites are more highly protein bound than the free drug. Sulfonamides compete with bilirubin for binding to albumin. Kernicterus may develop in premature infants or neonates. Binding is decreased in patients with severely impaired renal function. Only free, unbound drug has antibacterial activity.
Sulfadiazine—38 to 48%.
Sulfamethizole—Approximately 90%.
Sulfamethoxazole—60 to 70%.
Sulfisoxazole—85 to 90%.

**Biotransformation**
Hepatic; primarily by acetylation to inactive metabolites, which retain the toxicity of the parent compound. Some hepatic glucuronide conjugation may occur. Metabolism is increased with renal function impairment and decreased with hepatic failure.

**Half-life**
Sulfadiazine—
  Normal renal function: Approximately 10 hours.
  Renal failure: Approximately 34 hours.
Sulfamethizole—
  Normal renal function: Approximately 1.5 hours.
Sulfamethoxazole—
  Normal renal function: 6 to 12 hours.
  Renal failure: 20 to 50 hours.
Sulfisoxazole—
  Normal renal function: 3 to 7 hours.
  Renal failure: 6 to 12 hours.

**Time to peak concentration**
Sulfadiazine—3 to 6 hours.
Sulfamethoxazole—2 to 4 hours.
Sulfisoxazole—2 to 4 hours.

**Peak serum concentration**
Free unbound sulfonamide—
  Sulfadiazine: Single 2-gram dose—Approximately 30 to 60 mcg/mL.
  Sulfamethoxazole: Single 2-gram dose—Approximately 80 to 100 mcg/mL.
  Sulfisoxazole: Single 2-gram dose—40 to 50 mcg/mL.

**Duration of action**
Sulfadiazine—Short-acting sulfonamide.
Sulfamethizole—Short-acting sulfonamide.
Sulfamethoxazole—Intermediate-acting sulfonamide.
Sulfisoxazole—Short-acting sulfonamide.

**Elimination**
Renal, by glomerular filtration, with some tubular secretion and reabsorption of both active medication and metabolites. Excretion is increased in alkaline urine; small amounts are excreted in the feces, bile, and other body secretions.
  Percent of medication unchanged in the urine—
    Sulfadiazine: 60 to 85% in 48 to 72 hours.
    Sulfamethizole: Approximately 95%.
    Sulfamethoxazole: 20 to 40%.
    Sulfisoxazole: Approximately 52% in 48 hours.
    Sulfisoxazole acetyl: Approximately 58% in 72 hours.
In dialysis—
  Peritoneal dialysis is not effective and hemodialysis is only moderately effective in removing sulfonamides.

## Precautions to Consider

**Cross-sensitivity and/or related problems**
Patients allergic to one sulfonamide may be allergic to other sulfonamides also.
Patients allergic to furosemide, thiazide diuretics, sulfonylureas, or carbonic anhydrase inhibitors may be allergic to sulfonamides also.

**Carcinogenicity**
Sulfamethoxazole—
  Long-term studies to evaluate the carcinogenic potential of sulfamethoxazole have not been done.
Sulfisoxazole—
  Studies in mice given daily oral doses of up to 18 times the highest recommended human daily dose for 103 weeks, and rats given 4 times the highest recommended human daily dose have not shown that sulfisoxazole is carcinogenic in either male or female mice or rats.

**Mutagenicity**
Sulfamethizole—
  No long-term mutagenicity studies have been done in animals or humans.
Sulfamethoxazole—
  Bacterial mutagenicity studies with sulfamethoxazole have not been done. Studies in human leukocytes cultured *in vitro* with sulfamethoxazole using concentrations that exceeded therapeutic serum concentrations have not shown that sulfamethoxazole causes chromosomal damage.
Sulfisoxazole—
  Bacterial mutagenicity studies with sulfisoxazole have not been done. However, sulfisoxazole has not been shown to be mutagenic when tested in *Escherichia coli* Sd-4-73 strains in the absence of a metabolic activating system.

**Pregnancy/Reproduction**
Fertility—
  Sulfamethizole—
    No long-term fertility studies have been done in animals or humans.
  Sulfamethoxazole—
    Studies in rats, given oral doses of 350 mg of sulfamethoxazole per kg of body weight daily, have not shown that it causes any adverse effects on fertility or general reproductive performance.
  Sulfisoxazole—
    Studies in rats given daily doses of 7 times the highest recommended daily dose have not shown that sulfisoxazole causes adverse effects on mating behavior, conception rate, or fertility index (percent of animals pregnant).
Pregnancy—
  Sulfadiazine—
    FDA Pregnancy Category C.
  Sulfamethizole—
    FDA Pregnancy Category C.
  Sulfamethoxazole—
    Sulfamethoxazole crosses the placenta. Large, adequate, and well-controlled studies in humans have not been done.
    Studies in rats given oral doses of 533 mg of sulfamethoxazole per kg of body weight have shown that it causes teratogenic effects (primarily cleft palates). However, doses of 512 mg of sulfamethoxazole per kg of body weight did not cause cleft palates in rats.
    Studies in rabbits given doses of 150 to 350 mg of sulfamethoxazole per kg of body weight daily have shown that sulfamethoxazole causes increased maternal mortality but has no adverse effects on the fetus.
    FDA Pregnancy Category C.
  Sulfisoxazole—
    Sulfisoxazole crosses the placenta and enters the fetal circulation. Adequate and well-controlled studies in humans have not been done.
    Studies in rats and rabbits given daily doses of 7 times the highest recommended human daily dose have not shown that sulfisoxazole is teratogenic. However, in studies in rats and mice given doses of 9 times the highest recommended human daily dose, sulfisoxazole caused cleft palates in both mice and rats and skeletal defects in rats.
    FDA Pregnancy Category C.
Labor and delivery—Sulfonamides are not recommended at term since sulfonamides may cause kernicterus in the newborn.

**Breast-feeding**
Sulfonamides are distributed into breast milk. Use is not recommended in nursing women since sulfonamides may cause kernicterus in nursing infants. Also, sulfonamides may cause hemolytic anemia in glucose-6-phosphate dehydrogenase (G6PD)–deficient infants.

**Pediatrics**
Except as concurrent adjunctive therapy with pyrimethamine in the treatment of congenital toxoplasmosis, use of sulfonamides is contraindicated in infants up to 2 months of age. Sulfonamides compete for bilirubin binding sites on plasma albumin, increasing the risk of kernicterus in the newborn. Also, because the acetyltransferase system is not fully developed in the newborn, increased blood concentrations of the free sulfonamide can further increase the risk of kernicterus.

**Geriatrics**
Elderly patients may be at increased risk of severe side/adverse effects. Severe skin reactions, generalized bone marrow depression, and decreased platelet count (with or without purpura) are the most frequently reported severe side/adverse effects in the elderly. An increased incidence of thrombocytopenia with purpura has been reported in elderly

patients who are receiving diuretics, primarily thiazides, concurrently with sulfamethoxazole. The potential for these problems should also be considered for elderly patients taking other sulfonamide medications.

**Pharmacogenetics**
Sulfonamides are metabolized primarily by acetylation. Patients can be divided into 2 groups, slow and fast acetylators. Slow acetylators have a higher incidence of severe sulfonamide reactions, although a slow acetylator phenotype is not thought to be the sole reason for sulfonamide toxicity. The incidence of the slow acetylator phenotype is approximately 50% in North American blacks and whites. Approximately 30% of the Hispanic population and 10% of the Asian population are slow acetylators. Also, acquired immunodeficiency syndrome (AIDS) patients with acute illness, but not AIDS patients who are stable or human immunodeficiency virus (HIV)–infected patients without AIDS, have an increased incidence of slow acetylation.

**Dental**
The leukopenic and thrombocytopenic effects of sulfonamides may result in an increased incidence of certain microbial infections, delayed healing, and gingival bleeding. If leukopenia or thrombocytopenia occurs, dental work should be deferred until blood counts have returned to normal. Patients should be instructed in proper oral hygiene, including caution in use of regular toothbrushes, dental floss, and toothpicks.

**Drug interactions and/or related problems**
The following drug interactions and/or related problems have been selected on the basis of their potential clinical significance (possible mechanism in parentheses where appropriate)—not necessarily inclusive (» = major clinical significance):

Note: Combinations containing any of the following medications, depending on the amount present, may also interact with this medication.

» Anticoagulants, coumarin- or indandione-derivative or
» Anticonvulsants, hydantoin or
» Antidiabetic agents, oral
(these medications may be displaced from protein binding sites and/or their metabolism may be inhibited by some sulfonamides, resulting in increased or prolonged effects and/or toxicity; dosage adjustments may be necessary during and after sulfonamide therapy)

Bone marrow depressants (See *Appendix II*)
(concurrent use of bone marrow depressants with sulfonamides may increase the leukopenic and/or thrombocytopenic effects; if concurrent use is required, close observation for myelotoxic effects should be considered)

Contraceptives, estrogen-containing, oral
(concurrent long-term use of sulfonamides may result in increased incidence of breakthrough bleeding and pregnancy)

Cyclosporine
(concurrent use with sulfonamides may increase the metabolism of cyclosporine, resulting in decreased plasma concentrations and potential transplant rejection, and additive nephrotoxicity; plasma cyclosporine concentrations and renal function should be monitored)

» Hemolytics, other (See *Appendix II*)
(concurrent use with sulfonamides may increase the potential for toxic side effects)

» Hepatotoxic medications, other (See *Appendix II*)
(concurrent use with sulfonamides may result in an increased incidence of hepatotoxicity; patients, especially those on prolonged administration or those with a history of liver disease, should be carefully monitored)

» Methenamine
(in acid urine, methenamine breaks down into formaldehyde, which may form an insoluble precipitate with certain sulfonamides, especially those that are less soluble in urine, and may also increase the danger of crystalluria; concurrent use is not recommended)

» Methotrexate or
Phenylbutazone or
Sulfinpyrazone
(the effects of methotrexate may be potentiated during concurrent use with sulfonamides because of displacement from plasma protein binding sites; phenylbutazone and sulfinpyrazone may displace sulfonamides from plasma protein binding sites, increasing sulfonamide concentrations)

Penicillins
(since bacteriostatic drugs may interfere with the bactericidal effect of penicillins in the treatment of meningitis or in other situations where a rapid bactericidal effect is necessary, it is best to avoid concurrent therapy)

**Laboratory value alterations**
The following have been selected on the basis of their potential clinical significance (possible effect in parentheses where appropriate)—not necessarily inclusive (» = major clinical significance):

With diagnostic test results
Benedict's test
(sulfonamides may produce a false-positive Benedict's test for urine glucose)
Jaffé alkaline picrate reaction assay
(sulfamethoxazole may interfere with the Jaffé alkaline picrate reaction assay for creatinine, resulting in overestimations of approximately 10% in the normal values for creatinine)
Sulfosalicylic acid test
(sulfonamides may produce a false-positive sulfosalicylic acid test for urine protein)
Urine urobilinogen test strip (e.g., Urobilistix)
(sulfonamides may interfere with the urine urobilinogen [Urobilistix] test for urinary urobilinogen)

With physiology/laboratory test values
Alanine aminotransferase (ALT [SGPT]), serum and
Aspartate aminotransferase (AST [SGOT]), serum and
Bilirubin, serum
(values may be increased)
Blood urea nitrogen (BUN) and
Creatinine, serum
(concentrations may be increased)

**Medical considerations/Contraindications**
The medical considerations/contraindications included have been selected on the basis of their potential clinical significance (reasons given in parentheses where appropriate)—not necessarily inclusive (» = major clinical significance).

*Except under special circumstances, this medication should not be used when the following medical problems exist:*

Allergy to sulfonamides, furosemide, thiazide diuretics, sulfonylureas, or carbonic anhydrase inhibitors

*Risk-benefit should be considered when the following medical problems exist:*

» Blood dyscrasias or
» Megaloblastic anemia due to folate deficiency
(sulfonamides may cause blood dyscrasias)
» Glucose-6-phosphate dehydrogenase (G6PD) deficiency
(hemolysis may occur)
» Hepatic function impairment
(sulfonamides are metabolized in the liver; delayed metabolism may increase the risk of toxicity; also, sulfonamides may cause fulminant hepatic necrosis)
» Porphyria
(sulfonamides may precipitate an acute attack of porphyria)
» Renal function impairment
(sulfonamides are renally excreted; delayed elimination may increase the risk of toxicity; also, sulfonamides may cause tubular necrosis or interstitial nephritis)

**Patient monitoring**
The following may be especially important in patient monitoring (other tests may be warranted in some patients, depending on condition; » = major clinical significance):

Complete blood counts (CBCs)
(may be required prior to and monthly during treatment to detect blood dyscrasias in patients on prolonged therapy; therapy should be discontinued if a significant decrease in the count of any formed blood elements occurs)
Urinalyses
(may be required prior to and periodically during treatment to detect crystalluria and/or urinary calculi formation in patients on long-term or high-dose therapy and in patients with impaired renal function)

## Side/Adverse Effects

Note: Fatalities have occurred, although rarely, due to severe reactions such as Stevens-Johnson syndrome, toxic epidermal necrolysis, fulminant hepatic necrosis, agranulocytosis, aplastic anemia, and other blood dyscrasias. Therapy should be discontinued at the first appearance of skin rash or any serious side/adverse effects.

Patients with acquired immunodeficiency syndrome (AIDS) may have a greater incidence of side/adverse effects, especially rash, fever, and leukopenia, than do non-AIDS patients.

The multiorgan toxicity of sulfonamides is thought to be the result of the way sulfonamides are metabolized in certain patients. It is probably due to the inability of the body to detoxify reactive metabolites. Sulfonamides are metabolized primarily by acetylation. Patients can be divided into slow and fast acetylators. Slow acetylation of sulfonamides makes more of the medication available for metabolism by the oxidative pathways of the cytochrome P-450 system. These pathways produce reactive toxic metabolites, such as hydroxylamine and nitroso compounds. The metabolites are normally detoxified by scavengers, such as glutathione. However, some populations, such as human immunodeficiency virus (HIV)–infected patients, have low concentrations of glutathione and these metabolites accumulate, producing toxicity. Patients who are slow acetylators have a higher incidence of sulfonamide hypersensitivity reactions, although severe toxicity has also been seen in fast acetylators. Acetylation status alone cannot fully explain sulfonamide toxicity since approximately 50% of North American blacks and whites are slow acetylators and severe reactions occur in less than 1% of patients treated with sulfonamides. However, decreased acetylation may increase the amount of sulfonamide metabolized to toxic metabolites.

Crytalluria is more likely to occur with a less soluble sulfonamide, such as sulfadiazine. It occurs most often with the administration of high doses, and can be minimized by maintaining a high urine flow and alkalinizing the urine.

The following side/adverse effects have been selected on the basis of their potential clinical significance (possible signs and symptoms in parentheses where appropriate)—not necessarily inclusive:

### Those indicating need for medical attention
Incidence more frequent
*Hypersensitivity* (fever; itching; skin rash); *photosensitivity* (increased sensitivity of skin to sunlight)

Incidence less frequent
*Blood dyscrasias* (fever and sore throat; pale skin; unusual bleeding or bruising; unusual tiredness or weakness); *hepatitis* (yellow eyes or skin); *Lyell's syndrome* (difficulty in swallowing; redness, blistering, peeling, or loosening of skin); *Stevens-Johnson syndrome* (aching joints and muscles; redness, blistering, peeling, or loosening of skin; unusual tiredness or weakness)

Incidence rare
*Central nervous system toxicity* (confusion; disorientation; euphoria; hallucination; mental depression); *Clostridium difficile* colitis (severe abdominal or stomach cramps and pain; abdominal tenderness; watery and severe diarrhea, which may also be bloody; fever); *crystalluria or hematuria* (blood in urine; lower back pain; pain or burning while urinating); *goiter or thyroid function disturbance* (swelling of front part of neck); *interstitial nephritis or tubular necrosis* (greatly increased or decreased frequency of urination or amount of urine; increased thirst; loss of appetite; nausea; vomiting)

Note: *C. difficile colitis* may occur up to several weeks after discontinuation of these medications.

### Those indicating need for medical attention only if they continue or are bothersome
Incidence more frequent
*Central nervous system effects* (dizziness; headache; lethargy); *gastrointestinal disturbances* (diarrhea; loss of appetite; nausea or vomiting)

## Patient Consultation
As an aid to patient consultation, refer to *Advice for the Patient, Sulfonamides (Systemic)*.

In providing consultation, consider emphasizing the following selected information (» = major clinical significance):

### Before using this medication
» Conditions affecting use, especially:
  Allergy to sulfonamides, furosemide, thiazide diuretics, sulfonylureas, carbonic anhydrase inhibitors
  Pregnancy—Sulfonamides cross the placenta; not recommended at term since sulfonamides may cause kernicterus in newborn
  Breast-feeding—Sulfonamides are distributed into breast milk; may cause kernicterus in nursing infants
  Use in children—Sulfonamides are contraindicated in infants up to 2 months of age since sulfonamides may cause kernicterus in neonates
  Use in the elderly—Elderly patients may be at increased risk of severe side/adverse effects
  Other medications, especially coumarin- or indandione-derivative anticoagulants, hydantoin anticonvulsants, oral antidiabetic agents, other hemolytics, other hepatotoxic medications, methenamine, or methotrexate
  Other medical problems, especially blood dyscrasias, G6PD deficiency, hepatic function impairment, megaloblastic anemia, porphyria, and renal function impairment

### Proper use of this medication
» Not giving to infants under 2 months of age
» Maintaining adequate fluid intake
   Proper administration technique for oral liquids
» Compliance with full course of therapy
» Importance of not missing doses and taking at evenly spaced times
» Proper dosing
   Missed dose: Taking as soon as possible; not taking if almost time for next dose; not doubling doses
» Proper storage

### Precautions while using this medication
» Regular visits to physician to check blood counts
   Checking with physician if no improvement within a few days
   Using caution in use of regular toothbrushes, dental floss, and toothpicks; deferring dental work until blood counts have returned to normal; checking with physician or dentist concerning proper oral hygiene
» Possible photosensitivity reactions
» Caution if dizziness occurs

### Side/adverse effects
Severe skin problems and blood problems may be more likely to occur in the elderly who are taking sulfamethoxazole, especially if taking diuretics concurrently

Signs of potential side effects, especially hypersensitivity, photosensitivity, blood dyscrasias, hepatitis, Lyell's syndrome, Stevens-Johnson syndrome, central nervous system toxicity, *C. difficile* colitis, crystalluria or hematuria, goiter or thyroid function disturbance, and interstitial nephritis or tubular necrosis

## General Dosing Information
Fluid intake should be sufficient to maintain urine output of at least 1200 mL per day in adults.

---

## SULFADIAZINE

## Summary of Differences
Indications: Because of its relatively low urine solubility and the increased chance of crystalluria, sulfadiazine is not recommended for the treatment of urinary tract infections. Sulfadiazine is used for the prophylaxis of rheumatic fever and, in combination with pyrimethamine, for the treatment of toxoplasmosis and malaria caused by chloroquine-resistant *P. falciparum*.

## Additional Dosing Information
Fluid intake should be sufficient to maintain urine output of at least 1200 mL per day in adults.

Patients with impaired renal function may require a reduction in dose.

## Oral Dosage Forms
### SULFADIAZINE TABLETS USP
Usual adult and adolescent dose
Antibacterial (systemic) or
Antiprotozoal—
   Oral, 2 to 4 grams initially, then 1 gram every four to six hours.
   Meningitis (prophylaxis):
      Oral, 1 gram every twelve hours for two days.
   Rheumatic fever (prophylaxis):
      Oral, 1 gram once a day.
   Toxoplasmosis:
      AIDS patients: Oral, 1 to 2 grams of sulfadiazine every 6 hours with 50 to 100 mg of pyrimethamine per day and 10 to 25 mg of leucovorin per day.
      Pregnant women: Oral, 1 gram of sulfadiazine every 6 hours with 25 mg of pyrimethamine per day after week 16 of the pregnancy. With this regimen, 5 to 15 mg of leucovorin per day is administered.

**Usual pediatric dose**
Antibacterial (systemic) or
Antiprotozoal—
  Infants up to 2 months of age: Use is not recommended.
  Infants 2 months of age and over: Oral, 75 mg per kg of body weight initially, then 37.5 mg per kg of body weight every six hours or 25 mg per kg of body weight every four hours.
  Toxoplasmosis: Oral, 50 mg of sulfadiazine per kg of body weight two times a day, administered concurrently with 2 mg of pyrimethamine per kg of body weight per day for two days, then 1 mg of pyrimethamine per kg of body weight per day for two to six months, then of 1 mg pyrimethamine per kg of body weight per day three times per week. With this regimen, 5 mg of leucovorin is administered three times a week. The three medications should be given for a total of twelve months.

Note:  The maximum dose for children should not exceed 6 grams daily.

**Strength(s) usually available**
U.S.—
  500 mg (Rx) [GENERIC].
Canada—
  500 mg (Rx) [GENERIC].

**Packaging and storage**
Store below 30 °C (86 °F), unless otherwise specified by manufacturer. Store in a tight container. Protect from light.

**Auxiliary labeling**
- Take with a full glass of water.
- Avoid too much sun or use of sunlamp.
- May cause dizziness.
- Continue medicine for full time of treatment.

---

## SULFAMETHIZOLE

## Summary of Differences
Indications: Sulfamethizole is recommended for use only in the treatment of urinary tract infections, not systemic infections.

## Additional Dosing Information
Fluid intake should be sufficient to maintain urine output of at least 1200 mL per day in adults.

Patients with impaired renal function may require a reduction in dose.

## Oral Dosage Forms
### SULFAMETHIZOLE TABLETS USP

**Usual adult and adolescent dose**
Antibacterial—
  Oral, 500 mg to 1 gram every six to eight hours.

**Usual pediatric dose**
Antibacterial—
  Infants up to 2 months of age: Use is not recommended.
  Infants 2 months of age and over: Oral, 7.5 to 11.25 mg per kg of body weight every six hours.

**Strength(s) usually available**
U.S.—
  500 mg (Rx) [*Thiosulfil Forte*].
Canada—
  Not commercially available.

**Packaging and storage**
Store below 30 °C (86 °F), unless otherwise specified by manufacturer. Store in a tight container.

**Auxiliary labeling**
- Take with a full glass of water.
- Avoid too much sun or use of sunlamp.
- May cause dizziness.
- Continue medicine for full time of treatment.

---

## SULFAMETHOXAZOLE

## Additional Dosing Information
Fluid intake should be sufficient to maintain urine output of at least 1200 mL per day in adults.

Although sulfamethoxazole has a greater tendency to cause crystalluria than sulfisoxazole because of slower absorption and excretion, alkalinization of the urine is usually unnecessary.

Therapy should be continued for at least 7 to 10 days in urinary tract infections.

Patients with impaired renal function may require a reduction in dose.

## Oral Dosage Forms
### SULFAMETHOXAZOLE TABLETS USP

**Usual adult and adolescent dose**
Antibacterial (systemic) or
Antiprotozoal—
  Mild to moderate infections: Oral, 2 grams initially, then 1 gram every eight to twelve hours.
  Severe infections: Oral, 4 grams initially, then 2 grams every eight to twelve hours.

**Usual pediatric dose**
Antibacterial (systemic) or
Antiprotozoal—
  Infants up to 2 months of age: Except as concurrent adjunctive therapy with pyrimethamine in the treatment of congenital toxoplasmosis, use is contraindicated since sulfonamides may cause kernicterus in neonates.
  Infants and children 2 months of age and over: Oral, 50 to 60 mg per kg of body weight (maximum—2 grams) initially, then 25 to 30 mg per kg of body weight every twelve hours.

Note:  The maximum dose for children should not exceed 75 mg per kg of body weight per day.

**Strength(s) usually available**
U.S.—
  500 mg (Rx) [*Gantanol; Urobak*].
Canada—
  500 mg (Rx) [*Apo-Sulfamethoxazole* (scored); GENERIC].

**Packaging and storage**
Store below 40 °C (104 °F), preferably between 15 and 30 °C (59 and 86 °F), unless otherwise specified by manufacturer. Store in a well-closed, light-resistant container.

**Auxiliary labeling**
- Take with a full glass of water.
- May cause dizziness.
- Avoid too much sun or use of sunlamp.
- Continue medicine for full time of treatment.

---

## SULFISOXAZOLE

## Additional Dosing Information
Fluid intake should be sufficient to maintain urine output of at least 1200 mL per day in adults.

Because of its relatively high solubility even in acid urine, the risk of crystalluria with sulfisoxazole is low and alkalinization of the urine is usually unnecessary.

Therapy should be continued for at least 7 to 10 days in urinary tract infections.

Patients with impaired renal function may require a reduction in dose.

## Oral Dosage Forms
### SULFISOXAZOLE TABLETS USP

**Usual adult and adolescent dose**
Antibacterial (systemic) or
Antiprotozoal—
  Oral, 2 to 4 grams initially, then 750 mg to 1.5 grams every four hours; or 1 to 2 grams every six hours.

**Usual adult prescribing limits**
Up to 8 grams daily.

**Usual pediatric dose**
Antibacterial (systemic) or
Antiprotozoal—
  Infants up to 2 months of age: Except as concurrent adjunctive therapy with pyrimethamine in the treatment of congenital toxoplasmosis, use is contraindicated since sulfonamides may cause kernicterus in neonates.
  Infants and children 2 months of age and over: Oral, 75 mg per kg of body weight or 2 grams per square meter of body surface initially, then 25 mg per kg of body weight or 667 mg per square meter of body surface every four hours; or 37.5 mg per kg of body weight or 1 gram per square meter of body surface every six hours.

Note:  The maximum dose for children should not exceed 6 grams daily.

## Sulfonamides (Systemic)

**Strength(s) usually available**
U.S.—
500 mg (Rx) [*Gantrisin* (scored); GENERIC].
Canada—
500 mg (Rx) [*Apo-Sulfisoxazole; Novo-Soxazole; Sulfizole*].

**Packaging and storage**
Store below 40 °C (104 °F), preferably between 15 and 30 °C (59 and 86 °F), unless otherwise specified by manufacturer. Store in a well-closed, light-resistant container.

**Auxiliary labeling**
- Take with a full glass of water.
- May cause dizziness.
- Avoid too much sun or use of sunlamp.
- Continue medicine for full time of treatment.

### SULFISOXAZOLE ACETYL ORAL SUSPENSION USP

**Usual adult and adolescent dose**
See *Sulfisoxazole Tablets USP*.

**Usual adult prescribing limits**
See *Sulfisoxazole Tablets USP*.

**Usual pediatric dose**
See *Sulfisoxazole Tablets USP*.

**Strength(s) usually available**
U.S.—
500 mg per 5 mL (Rx) [*Gantrisin* (alcohol 0.3%; parabens; sucrose); GENERIC].
Canada—
Not commercially available.

**Packaging and storage**
Store below 40 °C (104 °F), preferably between 15 and 30 °C (59 and 86 °F), unless otherwise specified by manufacturer. Store in a tight, light-resistant container. Protect from freezing.

**Auxiliary labeling**
- Shake well.
- Take with a full glass of water.
- May cause dizziness.
- Avoid too much sun or use of sunlamp.
- Continue medicine for full time of treatment.

**Note**
When dispensing, include a calibrated liquid-measuring device.

### SULFISOXAZOLE ACETYL ORAL SYRUP

**Usual adult and adolescent dose**
See *Sulfisoxazole Tablets USP*.

**Usual adult prescribing limits**
See *Sulfisoxazole Tablets USP*.

**Usual pediatric dose**
See *Sulfisoxazole Tablets USP*.

**Strength(s) usually available**
U.S.—
500 mg per 5 mL (Rx) [*Gantrisin*].
Canada—
Not commercially available.

**Packaging and storage**
Store below 40 °C (104 °F), preferably between 15 and 30 °C (59 and 86 °F), unless otherwise specified by manufacturer. Store in a tight, light-resistant container. Protect from freezing.

**Auxiliary labeling**
- Take with a full glass of water.
- May cause dizziness.
- Avoid too much sun or use of sunlamp.
- Continue medicine for full time of treatment.

**Note**
When dispensing, include a calibrated liquid-measuring device.

Revised: 08/25/95

---

# SULFONAMIDES Vaginal

This monograph includes information on the following: 1) Sulfanilamide; 2) Triple Sulfa.

VA CLASSIFICATION (Primary): GU301

Commonly used brand name(s): *AVC*[1]; *Sultrin*[2]; *Trysul*[2].

Another commonly used name for triple sulfa is sulfathiazole, sulfacetamide, and sulfabenzamide.

Note: For a listing of dosage forms and brand names by country availability, see *Dosage Forms* section(s).

## Category
Anti-infective (vaginal).

## Indications

### Unaccepted
The U.S. Food and Drug Administration (FDA) announced on May 31, 1979, that its Anti-infective and Topical Drugs Advisory Committee and Fertility and Maternal Health Advisory Committee, as well as other studies, had concluded there was no adequate evidence that the then-available vaginal sulfonamides formulations were effective either for the treatment of vulvovaginitis caused by *Candida albicans*, *Trichomonas vaginalis*, or *Gardnerella vaginalis (Haemophilus vaginalis)* or for relief of the symptoms of these conditions.

In addition, in the opinion of USP medical experts, triple sulfa vaginal preparations are not effective for any indication, including vulvovaginitis caused by *Gardnerella vaginalis* and use as a deodorant in saprophytic infections following radiation therapy. Also, USP medical experts do not recommend the use of vaginal sulfonamides, including the reformulated single-entity preparations, for the treatment of fungal infections of the vagina.

## Pharmacology/Pharmacokinetics

### Physicochemical characteristics
Molecular weight—
Sulfabenzamide: 276.32.
Sulfacetamide: 214.25.
Sulfanilamide: 172.21.
Sulfathiazole: 255.32.
Sulfisoxazole: 267.31.

**Mechanism of action/Effect**
Sulfonamides— See *Sulfonamides (Systemic)*.

**Absorption**
Sulfonamides are absorbed through the vaginal mucosa.

## Precautions to Consider

### Cross-sensitivity and/or related problems
Patients sensitive to one sulfonamide may be sensitive to other sulfonamides also.

Patients sensitive to furosemide, thiazide diuretics, sulfonylureas, or carbonic anhydrase inhibitors may be sensitive to sulfonamides also.

Use of topical sulfonamides may lead to sensitization, resulting in hypersensitivity reactions with subsequent topical or systemic use of the medication.

### Carcinogenicity/Tumorigenicity
Studies in rats have shown that long-term administration of sulfonamides may cause thyroid malignancy. However, rats appear to be especially susceptible to the goitrogenic effects of sulfonamides.

### Pregnancy/Reproduction
Pregnancy—Safe use of vaginal sulfonamides during pregnancy has not been established. Sulfonamides are absorbed from the vaginal mucosa, readily cross the placenta, and appear in the fetal circulation. Fetal serum concentrations are approximately 50 to 90% of maternal serum concentrations. Adequate and well-controlled studies of most sulfonamides have not been done in either animals or humans. However, studies in rats and mice given high oral doses (7 to 25 times the human therapeutic dose) have shown that certain short-, intermediate-, and long-acting sulfonamides cause a significant increase in the incidence of cleft palate and other bony abnormalities in the fetus.

FDA Pregnancy Category C.

### Breast-feeding
Sulfonamides are absorbed from the vaginal mucosa and are distributed into breast milk. Use is not recommended in nursing mothers since sulfonamides may cause hyperbilirubinemia in the infant. In addition,

sulfonamides may cause hemolytic anemia in glucose-6-phosphate dehydrogenase (G6PD)–deficient neonates.

**Pediatrics**
No information is available on the relationship of age to the effects of sulfonamides in pediatric patients.

**Geriatrics**
No information is available on the relationship of age to the effects of sulfonamides in geriatric patients.

**Medical considerations/Contraindications**
The medical considerations/contraindications included have been selected on the basis of their potential clinical significance (reasons given in parentheses where appropriate)—not necessarily inclusive (» = major clinical significance).

*Risk-benefit should be considered when the following medical problems exist:*

Glucose-6-phosphate dehydrogenase (G6PD) deficiency
   (hemolytic anemia may occur in G6PD-deficient patients)
Hepatic function impairment
   (sulfonamides are metabolized in the liver; may cause hyperbilirubinemia in nursing infants)
Porphyria
   (sulfonamides may precipitate an acute attack of porphyria)
Renal function impairment
Sensitivity to sulfonamides, furosemide, thiazide diuretics, sulfonylureas, or carbonic anhydrase inhibitors or, depending on product, to peanut oil, lanolin, or parabens

## Side/Adverse Effects

Note: Treatment should be discontinued if local or systemic toxicity or hypersensitivity occurs. One case of agranulocytosis has occurred on use of vaginal triple sulfa cream, and Stevens-Johnson syndrome has occurred rarely and can be fatal.

The following side/adverse effects have been selected on the basis of their potential clinical significance (possible signs and symptoms in parentheses where appropriate)—not necessarily inclusive:

**Those indicating need for medical attention**
Incidence less frequent
   *Hypersensitivity* (itching, burning, skin rash, redness, swelling, or other sign of irritation not present before therapy)
Incidence rare
   *Skin reaction, local* (burning at site of application)

**Those indicating need for medical attention only if they continue or are bothersome**
Incidence less frequent or rare
   *Rash or irritation of penis of sexual partner*

## Patient Consultation

As an aid to patient consultation, refer to *Advice for the Patient, Sulfonamides (Vaginal)*.

In providing consultation, consider emphasizing the following selected information (» = major clinical significance):

**Before using this medication**
» Conditions affecting use, especially:
   Sensitivity to sulfonamides, furosemide, thiazide diuretics, sulfonylureas, or carbonic anhydrase inhibitors, or, depending on product, to peanut oil, lanolin, or parabens
   Pregnancy—Sulfonamides are absorbed from vaginal mucosa and appear in fetal circulation
   Breast-feeding—Distributed into breast milk; not recommended for use in nursing mothers

**Proper use of this medication**
Reading patient instructions before using
Proper administration technique; checking with physician before using applicator if pregnant
» Compliance with full course of therapy, even if menstruation begins
» Proper dosing
   Missed dose: Inserting as soon as possible; not inserting if almost time for next dose
» Proper storage

**Precautions while using this medication**
Checking with physician if no improvement within a few days
Protecting clothing because of possible soiling with vaginal sulfonamides; avoiding the use of tampons
*Using hygienic measures to cure infection and prevent reinfection*
   Wearing cotton panties instead of synthetic underclothes
   Wearing only freshly washed underclothes
» Use of condom by partner to prevent reinfection; possible need for concurrent treatment of male partner; continuing medication if intercourse occurs during treatment
» Use of douche for hygienic purposes, if advised by doctor, prior to next dose; not overfilling vagina with douche solution; avoiding use of a douche during pregnancy

**Side/adverse effects**
Sulfonamides may cause thyroid malignancy with long-term administration in rats; however, rats may be more susceptible to goitrogenic effects of sulfonamides
Signs of potential side effects, especially hypersensitivity or local skin reaction

## General Dosing Information

Treatment should be continued for 30 days or through one complete menstrual cycle, unless otherwise directed by physician.

---

### SULFANILAMIDE

## Vaginal Dosage Forms

### SULFANILAMIDE VAGINAL CREAM

**Usual adult and adolescent dose**
Intravaginal, 1 applicatorful (approximately 6 grams) one or two times a day for thirty days.

**Usual pediatric dose**
Use and dose have not been established.

**Strength(s) usually available**
U.S.—
   15% (Rx) [*AVC* (methylparaben; propylene glycol; propylparaben); GENERIC].
Canada—
   15% (Rx) [*AVC* (methylparaben; propylene glycol; propylparaben)].

**Packaging and storage**
Store between 15 and 30 °C (59 and 86 °F), in a well-closed container, unless otherwise specified by manufacturer. Protect from freezing.

**Stability**
Sulfanilamide vaginal cream darkens with age. However, this does not affect potency.

**Auxiliary labeling**
• For the vagina.
• Continue medicine for full time of treatment.

**Note**
When dispensing, include patient instructions and brochure.

### SULFANILAMIDE VAGINAL SUPPOSITORIES

**Usual adult and adolescent dose**
Intravaginal, 1 suppository one or two times a day for thirty days.

**Usual pediatric dose**
Use and dose have not been established.

**Strength(s) usually available**
U.S.—
   1.05 grams (Rx) [*AVC* (methylparaben; propylparaben)].
Canada—
   Not commercially available.

**Packaging and storage**
Store below 30 °C (86 °F), in a well-closed container, unless otherwise specified by manufacturer. Protect from freezing and moisture.

**Auxiliary labeling**
• For the vagina.
• Continue medicine for full time of treatment.

**Note**
When dispensing, include patient instructions and brochure.

## TRIPLE SULFA

### Vaginal Dosage Forms
#### TRIPLE SULFA VAGINAL CREAM USP
**Usual adult and adolescent dose**
Intravaginal, 1 applicatorful (approximately 4 to 5 grams) two times a day for four to six days. The dose may then be reduced to one-half or one-fourth applicatorful two times a day.

**Usual pediatric dose**
Use and dose have not been established.

**Strength(s) usually available**
U.S.—
3.42% of sulfathiazole, 2.86% of sulfacetamide, and 3.7% of sulfabenzamide (Rx) [*Sultrin* (methylparaben; peanut oil; propylparaben; propylene glycol); *Trysul* (methylparaben; peanut oil; propylparaben); GENERIC].
Canada—
3.42% of sulfathiazole, 2.86% of sulfacetamide, and 3.7% of sulfabenzamide (Rx) [*Sultrin* (lanolin; methylparaben; peanut oil; propylparaben; propylene glycol)].

**Packaging and storage**
Store between 15 and 30 °C (59 and 86 °F), unless otherwise specified by manufacturer. Store in a well-closed, light-resistant container or in a collapsible tube. Protect from freezing.

**Auxiliary labeling**
- For the vagina.
- Continue medicine for full time of treatment.

**Note**
When dispensing, include patient instructions and brochure.

#### TRIPLE SULFA VAGINAL TABLETS USP
**Usual adult and adolescent dose**
Intravaginal, 1 tablet two times a day for ten days. May be repeated if necessary.

**Usual pediatric dose**
Use and dose have not been established.

**Strength(s) usually available**
U.S.—
172.5 mg of sulfathiazole, 143.75 mg of sulfacetamide, and 184 mg of sulfabenzamide (Rx) [*Sultrin*; GENERIC].
Canada—
Not commercially available.

**Packaging and storage**
Store between 15 and 30 °C (59 and 86 °F), unless otherwise specified by manufacturer. Store in a well-closed, light-resistant container.

**Auxiliary labeling**
- For the vagina.
- Continue medicine for full time of treatment.

**Note**
When dispensing, include patient instructions and brochure.

Revised: 08/13/98

# SULFONAMIDES AND PHENAZOPYRIDINE  Systemic

This monograph includes information on the following: 1) Sulfamethoxazole and Phenazopyridine; 2) Sulfisoxazole and Phenazopyridine.

VA CLASSIFICATION (Primary): AM650

**NOTE:** The *Sulfonamides and Phenazopyridine (Systemic)* monograph is maintained on the USP DI electronic data base. For a printed copy of the most recent revision of the complete monograph, contact Micromedex, Inc. - Reprint Requests, 6200 S. Syracuse Way, Suite 300, Englewood, CO 80111; telephone (303) 486-6400; telefax (303) 486-6464; Email: USPDI@MDX.COM.

For information on the specific components of this combination, see the *USP DI* monographs for *Phenazopyridine (Systemic)* and *Sulfonamides (Systemic)*.

The information that follows is selectively abstracted from the complete monograph and is provided to facilitate drug use review and patient counseling.

Note: For a listing of dosage forms and brand names by country availability, see *Dosage Forms* section(s).

## Category
Antibacterial-analgesic (urinary tract).

## Indications
**Accepted**
Urinary tract infections, bacterial (treatment)—Sulfonamide and phenazopyridine combinations are indicated in the treatment of the acute, painful phase of uncomplicated urinary tract infections caused by *Escherichia coli*, *Klebsiella* species, *Enterobacter* species, *Proteus mirabilis*, *P. vulgaris*, and *Staphylococcus aureus*. After relief of pain has been obtained, treatment should be continued with either sulfamethoxazole or sulfisoxazole alone.

Not all species or strains of a particular organism may be susceptible to a specific sulfonamide.

## Patient Consultation
As an aid to patient consultation, refer to *Advice for the Patient, Sulfonamides and Phenazopyridine (Systemic)*.

In providing consultation, consider emphasizing the following selected information (» = major clinical significance):

**Before using this medication**
» Conditions affecting use, especially:
  Allergies to sulfonamides, furosemide, thiazide diuretics, sulfonylureas, carbonic anhydrase inhibitors, or phenazopyridine
  Pregnancy—Sulfonamides cross the placenta; use is contraindicated at term since sulfonamides may cause kernicterus
  Breast-feeding—Sulfonamides are excreted in breast milk; may cause kernicterus in the nursing infant
  Use in children—Use is contraindicated in children up to 12 years of age
  Other medications, especially coumarin- or indandione-derivative anticoagulants, hydantoin anticonvulsants, oral antidiabetic agents, hemolytics, hepatotoxic medications, methenamine, and methotrexate
  Other medical problems, especially blood dyscrasias, G6PD deficiency, hepatic function impairment, hepatitis, megaloblastic anemia due to folate deficiency, porphyria, and renal function impairment

**Proper use of this medication**
» Maintaining adequate fluid intake; taking with or following meals if gastrointestinal irritation occurs
» Compliance with full course of therapy
» Importance of not missing doses and taking at evenly spaced times
» Proper dosing; not giving to infants and children up to 12 years of age
  Missed dose: Taking as soon as possible; not taking if almost time for next dose; not doubling doses
» Proper storage

**Precautions while using this medication**
  Checking with physician if no improvement within a few days or if symptoms become worse
  Using caution with regular toothbrushes, dental floss, and toothpicks; deferring dental work until blood counts have returned to normal; checking with physician or dentist concerning proper oral hygiene
» Possible photosensitivity reactions
» Caution if dizziness occurs
» Medication causes urine to turn reddish orange and may stain clothing
» Diabetics: May cause false urine sugar and urine ketone test results

**Side/adverse effects**
  Reddish orange discoloration of urine may be alarming to patient although medically insignificant
  Signs of potential side effects, especially blood dyscrasias, crystalluria, goiter, headache, hematuria, hemolytic anemia, hepatitis, hypersensitivity, interstitial nephritis, Lyell's syndrome, methemoglobinemia, photosensitivity, Stevens-Johnson syndrome, thyroid function disturbance, and tubular necrosis

## SULFAMETHOXAZOLE AND PHENAZOPYRIDINE

### Oral Dosage Forms

**SULFAMETHOXAZOLE AND PHENAZOPYRIDINE HYDROCHLORIDE TABLETS**

**Usual adult and adolescent dose**
Urinary tract infections, bacterial—
　Oral, 2 grams of sulfamethoxazole and 400 mg of phenazopyridine hydrochloride initially, then 1 gram of sulfamethoxazole and 200 mg of phenazopyridine hydrochloride every twelve hours for up to two days.

**Usual pediatric dose**
Urinary tract infections, bacterial—
　Infants and children up to 12 years of age: Use is contraindicated.
　Children 12 years of age and over: See *Usual adult and adolescent dose*.

**Strength(s) usually available**
U.S.—
　500 mg of sulfamethoxazole and 100 mg of phenazopyridine hydrochloride (Rx) [*Azo Gantanol; Azo-Sulfamethoxazole;* GENERIC].
Canada—
　Not commercially available.

**Auxiliary labeling**
- Take with a full glass of water.
- Avoid too much sun or use of sunlamp.
- May cause dizziness.
- Continue medicine for full time of treatment.
- May discolor urine.

## SULFISOXAZOLE AND PHENAZOPYRIDINE

### Oral Dosage Forms

**SULFISOXAZOLE AND PHENAZOPYRIDINE HYDROCHLORIDE TABLETS**

**Usual adult and adolescent dose**
Urinary tract infections, bacterial—
　Oral, 2 to 3 grams of sulfisoxazole and 200 to 300 mg of phenazopyridine hydrochloride initially, then 1 gram of sulfisoxazole and 100 mg of phenazopyridine hydrochloride every six hours for up to two days.

**Usual pediatric dose**
Urinary tract infections, bacterial—
　Infants and children up to 12 years of age: Use is contraindicated.
　Children 12 years of age and over: See *Usual adult and adolescent dose*.

**Strength(s) usually available**
U.S.—
　500 mg of sulfisoxazole and 50 mg of phenazopyridine hydrochloride (Rx) [*Azo Gantrisin; Azo-Sulfisoxazole; Azo-Truxazole; Sul-Azo;* GENERIC].
Canada—
　500 mg of sulfisoxazole and 50 mg of phenazopyridine hydrochloride (Rx) [*Azo Gantrisin*].

**Auxiliary labeling**
- Take with a full glass of water.
- Avoid too much sun or use of sunlamp.
- May cause dizziness.
- Continue medicine for full time of treatment.
- May discolor urine.

Revised: 02/01/93

# SULFONAMIDES AND TRIMETHOPRIM　Systemic

This monograph includes information on the following: 1) Sulfadiazine and Trimethoprim*; 2) Sulfamethoxazole and Trimethoprim

BAN:
　Sulfadiazine—Sulphadiazine
　Sulfamethoxazole—Sulphamethoxazole

JAN:
　Sulfamethoxazole—Acetylsulfamethoxazole
　Sulfamethoxazole—Sulfamethoxazole sodium

VA CLASSIFICATION (Primary): AM650

NOTE:　The *Sulfonamides and Trimethoprim (Systemic)* monograph is maintained on the USP DI electronic data base. For a printed copy of the most recent revision of the complete monograph, contact Micromedex, Inc. - Reprint Requests, 6200 S. Syracuse Way, Suite 300, Englewood, CO 80111; telephone (303) 486-6400; telefax (303) 486-6464; Email: USPDI@MDX.COM.

For information on the specific components of this combination, see the *USP DI* monographs for *Sulfonamides (Systemic)* and *Trimethoprim (Systemic)*.

The information that follows is selectively abstracted from the complete monograph and is provided to facilitate drug use review and patient counseling.

Note:　For a listing of dosage forms and brand names by country availability, see *Dosage Forms* section(s).

*Not commercially available in U.S.

## Category

Antibacterial (systemic)—Sulfadiazine and Trimethoprim; Sulfamethoxazole and Trimethoprim.
Antiprotozoal—Sulfamethoxazole and Trimethoprim.

## Indications

Note:　Bracketed information in the *Indications* section refers to uses that are not included in U.S. product labeling.

**General considerations**
Sulfonamides, such as sulfadiazine and sulfamethoxazole, used together with trimethoprim, produce synergistic antibacterial activity. Sulfadiazine and sulfamethoxazole have equal antibacterial properties, covering the same spectrum of activity. These sulfonamides, in combination with trimethoprim, are active *in vitro* against many gram-positive and gram-negative aerobic organisms. They have minimal activity against anaerobic bacteria. Susceptible gram-positive organisms include many *Staphylococcus aureus*, including some methicillin-resistant strains, *S. saprophyticus*, some group A beta-hemolytic streptococci, *Streptococcus agalactiae*, and most but not all strains of *S. pneumoniae*. Gram-negative organisms that are susceptible include *Escherichia coli*, many *Klebsiella* species, *Citrobacter diversus* and *C. fruendii*, *Enterobacter*-species, *Salmonella* species, *Shigella* species, *Haemophilus influenzae*, including some ampicillin-resistant strains, *H. ducreyi*, *Morganella morganii*, *Proteus vulgaris* and *P. mirabilis*, and some *Serratia* species. Sulfonamide and trimethoprim combinations also have activity against *Acinetobacter* species, *Providencia rettgeri*, *P. stuarti*, *Aeromonas*, *Brucella*, and *Yersinia* species. They are also usually active against *Neisseria meningitidis*, *Branhamella (Moraxella) catarrhalis*, and some, but not all, *N. gonorrhoeae*. *Pseudomonas aeruginosa* is usually resistant, but *P. cepacia* and *P. maltophilia* may be sensitive.

The major difference between sulfadiazine and sulfamethoxazole exists in their respective pharmacokinetics. The primary distinction is that sulfadiazine is metabolized to a much lesser extent than is sulfamethoxazole. This allows for a higher urinary concentration of unchanged sulfadiazine, as well as an increased risk of crystalluria when it is administered in high doses; the antibacterial urinary concentration of sulfadiazine is maintained over a 24-hour interval, allowing for once-a-day dosing in adults. Also, sulfadiazine achieves higher concentrations in the bile and cerebrospinal fluid.

**Accepted**
Bronchitis (treatment)—Oral sulfamethoxazole and trimethoprim combination is indicated in adults in the treatment of acute exacerbations of chronic bronchitis caused by susceptible organisms.

Enterocolitis, *Shigella* species (treatment)—Oral and parenteral sulfamethoxazole and trimethoprim combinations are indicated in the treatment of enterocolitis caused by susceptible strains of *Shigella flexneri* and *S. sonnei*.

Otitis media, acute (treatment)—Oral sulfamethoxazole and trimethoprim combination is indicated in the treatment of acute otitis media caused by susceptible organisms in children.

Pneumonia, *Pneumocystis carinii* (prophylaxis)[1]—Oral sulfamethoxazole and trimethoprim combination is indicated in the prophylaxis of *Pneumocystis carinii* pneumonia (PCP) in patients who are immunocompromised and considered to be at increased risk of developing PCP, including patients with acquired immunodeficiency syndrome (AIDS). It is considered to be the treatment of choice for this indication. Sulfamethoxazole and trimethoprim combination is indicated in both secondary prophylaxis (patients who have already had at least one episode of PCP), and primary prophylaxis (HIV-infected adults with a CD4 lymphocyte count less than or equal to 200 cells per cubic millimeter and/or less than 20% of total lymphocytes; all children born to HIV-infected mothers, beginning at 4 to 6 weeks of age, and subsequent prophylaxis given as determined on the basis of age-specific CD4 lymphocyte count) of PCP.

Pneumonia, *Pneumocystis carinii* (treatment)—Oral and parenteral sulfamethoxazole and trimethoprim combinations are indicated as primary agents in the treatment of *Pneumocystis carinii* pneumonia (PCP) in immunocompromised patients, including patients with acquired immunodeficiency syndrome (AIDS). Pentamidine is considered an alternative agent for PCP.

Traveler's diarrhea (treatment)—Oral sulfamethoxazole and trimethoprim combination is indicated in the treatment of traveler's diarrhea caused by susceptible strains of enterotoxigenic *Escherichia coli* and *Shigella* species.

Urinary tract infections, bacterial (treatment)—Sulfadiazine and trimethoprim combination and oral and parenteral sulfamethoxazole and trimethoprim combinations are indicated in the treatment of urinary tract infections caused by susceptible organisms.

[Biliary tract infections (treatment)]—Sulfamethoxazole and trimethoprim combination is used in the treatment of biliary tract infections caused by susceptible organisms.

[Bone and joint infections (treatment)]—Sulfamethoxazole and trimethoprim combination is used in the treatment of bone and joint infections caused by susceptible organisms.

[Chancroid (treatment)][1]—Sulfamethoxazole and trimethoprim combination is used as an alternative agent in the treatment of chancroid.

[Chlamydial infections (treatment)][1]—Sulfamethoxazole and trimethoprim combination is used as an alternative agent in the treatment of chlamydial infections.

[Cyclospora infections (treatment)][1]—Sulfamethoxazole and trimethoprim combination is used in the treatment of diarrhea caused by *Cyclospora cayetanensis*, but may not completely eradicate the organism.

[Endocarditis, bacterial (treatment)][1]—Sulfamethoxazole and trimethoprim combination is used as an alternative agent in the treatment of bacterial endocarditis caused by susceptible organisms.

[Gonorrhea, endocervical and urethral, uncomplicated (treatment)]—Sulfamethoxazole and trimethoprim combination is used as an alternative agent in the treatment of gonorrhea caused by susceptible organisms.

[Granuloma inguinale (treatment)][1]—Sulfamethoxazole and trimethoprim combination is used as an alternative agent in the treatment of granuloma inguinale.

[Isosporiasis (prophylaxis and treatment)][1]—Sulfamethoxazole and trimethoprim combination is used in the prophylaxis and treatment of isosporiasis caused by *Isospora belli*.

[Lymphogranuloma venereum (treatment)][1]—Sulfamethoxazole and trimethoprim combination is used in the treatment of lymphogranuloma venereum.

[Meningitis (treatment)]—Sulfamethoxazole and trimethoprim combination is used as an alternative agent in the treatment of meningitis caused by susceptible organisms.

[Nocardiosis (treatment)]—Sulfamethoxazole and trimethoprim combination is used in the treatment of nocardiosis.

[Paracoccidioidomycosis (treatment)][1]—Sulfamethoxazole and trimethoprim combination is used in the treatment of paracoccidioidomycosis.

[Paratyphoid fever (treatment)] or
[Typhoid fever (treatment)]—Sulfamethoxazole and trimethoprim combination is used as an alternative agent in the treatment of paratyphoid and typhoid fevers caused by susceptible strains.

[Septicemia, bacterial (treatment)]—Sulfamethoxazole and trimethoprim combination is used as an alternative agent in the treatment of bacterial septicemia caused by susceptible organisms.

[Sinusitis (treatment)][1]—Sulfamethoxazole and trimethoprim combination is used in the treatment of sinusitis caused by susceptible organisms.

[Skin and soft tissue infections (treatment)]—Sulfamethoxazole and trimethoprim combination is used in the treatment of skin and soft tissue infections, including burn wound infections caused by susceptible organisms.

[Toxoplasmosis (prophylaxis)][1]—Sulfamethoxazole and trimethoprim combination is used in the primary prophylaxis of toxoplasmosis in patients with AIDS.

[Urinary tract infections, bacterial (prophylaxis)][1]—Sulfamethoxazole and trimethoprim combination is used in the prophylaxis of bacterial urinary tract infections.

[Whipple's disease (treatment)][1]—Sulfamethoxazole and trimethoprim combination is used in the treatment of Whipple's disease.

Not all strains of a particular organism may be susceptible to sulfonamide and trimethoprim combinations.

**Unaccepted**

Sulfamethoxazole and trimethoprim combination is not indicated for prophylaxis or prolonged therapy in otitis media. Sulfamethoxazole and trimethoprim combination is not effective in the treatment of syphilis and *Ureaplasm urealyticum*.

Sulfamethoxazole and trimethoprim combination should not be used in the treatment of group A beta-hemolytic streptococcal tonsillopharyngitis since it may not eradicate streptococci and therefore may not prevent sequelae such as rheumatic fever.

---

[1]Not included in Canadian product labeling.

## Patient Consultation

As an aid to patient consultation, refer to *Advice for the Patient, Sulfonamides and Trimethoprim (Systemic)*.

In providing consultation, consider emphasizing the following selected information (» = major clinical significance):

### Before using this medication
» Conditions affecting use, especially:
  Allergy to sulfonamides, furosemide, thiazide diuretics, sulfonylureas, carbonic anhydrase inhibitors, sulfites, or trimethoprim
  Pregnancy—Sulfonamides and trimethoprim cross the placenta; trimethoprim may interfere with folic acid metabolism; use is not recommended at term since sulfonamides may cause jaundice, hemolytic anemia, and kernicterus in neonates
  Breast-feeding—Sulfonamides and trimethoprim are distributed into breast milk; sulfonamides may cause kernicterus in nursing infants; trimethoprim may interfere with folic acid metabolism
  Use in children—Sulfadiazine and trimethoprim combination is contraindicated in infants up to 3 months of age and sulfamethoxazole and trimethoprim combination is contraindicated in infants up to 2 months of age for most indications since sulfonamides may cause kernicterus in neonates; however, sulfamethoxazole and trimethoprim combination is indicated in all infants born to human immunodeficiency virus (HIV)–infected mothers, starting at 4 to 6 weeks
  Use in the elderly—Elderly patients, especially those also taking diuretics, may be at increased risk of severe side/adverse effects
  Other medications, especially coumarin- or indandione-derivative anticoagulants, hydantoin anticonvulsants, oral antidiabetic agents, other hemolytics, other hepatotoxic medications, methenamine, or methotrexate
  Other medical problems, especially blood dyscrasias, G6PD deficiency, hepatic function impairment, megaloblastic anemia due to folic acid deficiency, porphyria, and renal function impairment

### Proper use of this medication
» Not giving sulfadiazine and trimethoprim combination to infants under 3 months of age, or sulfamethoxazole and trimethoprim combination to infants under 2 months of age, except under special circumstances
» Maintaining adequate fluid intake
  Proper administration technique for oral liquids
» Compliance with full course of therapy
» Importance of not missing doses and taking at evenly spaced times
» Proper dosing
  Missed dose: Taking as soon as possible; not taking if almost time for next dose; not doubling doses
» Proper storage

### Precautions while using this medication
» Regular visits to physician to check blood counts
  Checking with physician if no improvement within a few days
  Caution in use of regular toothbrushes, dental floss, and toothpicks; deferring dental work until blood counts have returned to normal; checking with physician or dentist concerning proper oral hygiene

- » Possible skin photosensitivity
- » Caution if dizziness occurs

**Side/adverse effects**

Severe skin problems and blood problems may be more likely to occur in elderly patients who are taking sulfamethoxazole and trimethoprim combination, especially if diuretics are being taken concurrently

Signs of potential side effects, especially hypersensitivity, photosensitivity, blood dyscrasias, cholestatic hepatitis, Stevens-Johnson syndrome, toxic epidermal necrolysis, aseptic meningitis, central nervous system toxicity, *Clostridium difficile* colitis, crystalluria, hematuria, goiter, thyroid function disturbance, interstitial nephritis, tubular necrosis, methemoglobinemia, and thrombophlebitis

---

### SULFADIAZINE AND TRIMETHOPRIM

## Oral Dosage Forms

### SULFADIAZINE AND TRIMETHOPRIM ORAL SUSPENSION

**Usual adult and adolescent dose**
Antibacterial—
  Oral, 820 mg of sulfadiazine and 180 mg of trimethoprim once a day.

**Usual pediatric dose**
Antibacterial—
  Infants up to 3 months of age: Use is not recommended.
  Children 3 months to 12 years of age: Oral, 7 mg of sulfadiazine and 1.5 mg of trimethoprim per kg of body weight every twelve hours.
  Children over 12 years of age: See *Usual adult and adolescent dose*.

**Strength(s) usually available**
U.S.—
  Not commercially available.
Canada—
  205 mg of sulfadiazine and 45 mg of trimethoprim per 5 mL (Rx) [*Coptin*].

**Auxiliary labeling**
- Shake well.
- Take with a full glass of water.
- May cause dizziness.
- Avoid too much sun or use of sunlamp.
- Continue medicine for full time of treatment.

### SULFADIAZINE AND TRIMETHOPRIM TABLETS

**Usual adult and adolescent dose**
See *Sulfadiazine and Trimethoprim Oral Suspension*.

**Usual pediatric dose**
See *Sulfadiazine and Trimethoprim Oral Suspension*.

**Strength(s) usually available**
U.S.—
  Not commercially available.
Canada—
  410 mg of sulfadiazine and 90 mg of trimethoprim (Rx) [*Coptin*].
  820 mg of sulfadiazine and 180 mg of trimethoprim (Rx) [*Coptin 1*].

**Auxiliary labeling**
- Take with a full glass of water.
- May cause dizziness.
- Avoid too much sun or use of sunlamp.
- Continue medicine for full time of treatment.

---

### SULFAMETHOXAZOLE AND TRIMETHOPRIM

## Oral Dosage Forms

Note: Bracketed uses in the *Dosage Forms* section refer to categories of use and/or indications that are not included in U.S. product labeling.

### SULFAMETHOXAZOLE AND TRIMETHOPRIM ORAL SUSPENSION USP

**Usual adult and adolescent dose**
Antibacterial (systemic)—
  Oral, 800 mg of sulfamethoxazole and 160 mg of trimethoprim every twelve hours.
Antiprotozoal—
  Pneumocystis carinii pneumonia:
    Treatment:
      Oral, 18.75 to 25 mg of sulfamethoxazole and 3.75 to 5 mg of trimethoprim per kg of body weight every six hours for fourteen to twenty-one days.
    Prophylaxis[1]:
      Oral, 800 mg of sulfamethoxazole and 160 mg of trimethoprim once a day.
      Acceptable alternative dosing schedules include—
        Oral, 800 mg of sulfamethoxazole and 160 mg of trimethoprim three times a week (e.g., Monday, Wednesday, Friday).
        Oral, 400 mg of sulfamethoxazole and 80 mg of trimethoprim once a day.
[Toxoplasmosis (prophylaxis)][1]:
  Oral, 800 mg of sulfamethoxazole and 160 mg of trimethoprim once a day.
  Acceptable alternative dosing schedules include:
    Oral, 800 mg of sulfamethoxazole and 160 mg of trimethoprim three times a week (e.g., Monday, Wednesday, Friday).
    Oral, 400 mg of sulfamethoxazole and 80 mg of trimethoprim once a day.

**Usual pediatric dose**
Antibacterial (systemic)—
  Infants up to 2 months of age:
    Use is not recommended since sulfonamides may cause kernicterus in neonates.
  Infants 2 months of age and over:
    Infants and children up to 40 kg of body weight—Oral, 20 to 30 mg of sulfamethoxazole and 4 to 6 mg of trimethoprim per kg of body weight every twelve hours.
  Children 40 kg of body weight and over—See *Usual adult and adolescent dose*.
Antiprotozoal—
  Pneumocystis carinii pneumonia (PCP):
    Treatment—
      Oral, 18.75 to 25 mg of sulfamethoxazole and 3.75 to 5 mg of trimethoprim per kg of body weight every six hours for fourteen to twenty-one days.
    Prophylaxis[1]—
      Children 4 weeks of age and over—
        Oral, 375 mg of sulfamethoxazole per square meter and 75 mg of trimethoprim per square meter of body surface two times a day, three times a week on consecutive days (e.g., Monday, Tuesday, Wednesday).
      Acceptable alternative dosing schedules include—
        Oral, 750 mg of sulfamethoxazole per square meter and 150 mg of trimethoprim per square meter of body surface as a single daily dose three times a week on consecutive days (e.g., Monday, Tuesday, Wednesday).
        Oral, 375 mg of sulfamethoxazole per square meter and 75 mg of trimethoprim per square meter of body surface two times a day seven days a week.
        Oral, 375 mg of sulfamethoxazole per square meter and 75 mg of trimethoprim per square meter of body surface two times a day, three times a week on alternate days (e.g., Monday, Wednesday, Friday).
    Note: PCP prophylaxis is recommended for all infants born to HIV-infected mothers starting at 4 weeks of age, regardless of their CD4 lymphocyte counts. However, if the infant is receiving zidovudine during the first 6 weeks of life for the prevention of perinatal HIV transmission, sulfamethoxazole and trimethoprim combination prophylaxis should be delayed until zidovudine is discontinued at 6 weeks of age, to reduce the chance of anemia that may occur if these two medications are given concurrently.
[Toxoplasmosis (prophylaxis)][1]:
  Oral, 375 mg of sulfamethoxazole per square meter and 75 mg of trimethoprim per square meter of body surface two times a day, three times a week on consecutive days (e.g., Monday, Tuesday, Wednesday).
  Acceptable alternative dosing schedules include—
    Oral, 750 mg of sulfamethoxazole per square meter and 150 mg of trimethoprim per square meter of body surface as a single daily dose three times a week on consecutive days (e.g., Monday, Tuesday, Wednesday).
    Oral, 375 mg of sulfamethoxazole per square meter and 75 mg of trimethoprim per square meter of body surface two times a day seven days a week.

Oral, 375 mg of sulfamethoxazole per square meter and 75 mg of trimethoprim per square meter of body surface two times a day, three times a week on alternate days (e.g., Monday, Wednesday, Friday).

**Strength(s) usually available**
U.S.—
   200 mg of sulfamethoxazole and 40 mg of trimethoprim per 5 mL (Rx) [*Bactrim Pediatric; Cotrim Pediatric; Septra Pediatric; Sulfatrim Pediatric; Sulfatrim Suspension;* GENERIC].
Canada—
   200 mg of sulfamethoxazole and 40 mg of trimethoprim per 5 mL (Rx) [*Apo-Sulfatrim; Bactrim; Novo-Trimel; Nu-Cotrimox; Septra*].

**Auxiliary labeling**
- Shake well.
- Take with a full glass of water.
- May cause dizziness.
- Avoid too much sun or use of sunlamp.
- Continue medicine for full time of treatment.

### SULFAMETHOXAZOLE AND TRIMETHOPRIM TABLETS USP

**Usual adult and adolescent dose**
See *Sulfamethoxazole and Trimethoprim Oral Suspension USP*.

**Usual adult prescribing limits**
See *Sulfamethoxazole and Trimethoprim Oral Suspension USP*.

**Usual pediatric dose**
See *Sulfamethoxazole and Trimethoprim Oral Suspension USP*.

**Strength(s) usually available**
U.S.—
   400 mg of sulfamethoxazole and 80 mg of trimethoprim (Rx) [*Bactrim; Cotrim; Septra; Sulfatrim; Sulfatrim S/S;* GENERIC].
   800 mg of sulfamethoxazole and 160 mg of trimethoprim (Rx) [*Bactrim DS; Cofatrim Forte; Cotrim DS; Septra DS; Sulfatrim-DS;* GENERIC].
Canada—
   100 mg of sulfamethoxazole and 20 mg of trimethoprim (Rx) [*Apo-Sulfatrim*].
   400 mg of sulfamethoxazole and 80 mg of trimethoprim (Rx) [*Apo-Sulfatrim* (scored); *Bactrim; Novo-Trimel* (scored); *Nu-Cotrimox; Septra*].
   800 mg of sulfamethoxazole and 160 mg of trimethoprim (Rx) [*Apo-Sulfatrim DS; Bactrim DS* (scored); *Novo-Trimel D.S.* (scored); *Nu-Cotrimox DS; Roubac; Septra DS*].

**Auxiliary labeling**
- Take with a full glass of water.
- May cause dizziness.
- Avoid too much sun or use of sunlamp.
- Continue medicine for full time of treatment.

## Parenteral Dosage Forms

### SULFAMETHOXAZOLE AND TRIMETHOPRIM FOR INJECTION CONCENTRATE USP

**Usual adult and adolescent dose**
Antibacterial (systemic)—
   Intravenous infusion, 10 to 12.5 mg of sulfamethoxazole and 2 to 2.5 mg of trimethoprim per kg of body weight every six hours; 13.3 to 16.7 mg of sulfamethoxazole and 2.7 to 3.3 mg of trimethoprim per kg of body weight every eight hours; or 20 to 25 mg of sulfamethoxazole and 4 to 5 mg of trimethoprim per kg of body weight every twelve hours.

Antiprotozoal—
   *Pneumocystis carinii* pneumonia: Intravenous infusion, 18.75 to 25 mg of sulfamethoxazole and 3.75 to 5 mg of trimethoprim per kg of body weight every six hours; or 25 to 33.3 mg of sulfamethoxazole and 5.0 to 6.7 mg of trimethoprim per kg of body weight every eight hours for fourteen days.

**Usual pediatric dose**
Infants up to 2 months of age—Use is not recommended since sulfonamides may cause kernicterus in neonates.
Infants 2 months of age and over—See *Usual adult and adolescent dose*.

**Strength(s) usually available**
U.S.—
   400 mg of sulfamethoxazole and 80 mg of trimethoprim per 5 mL (Rx) [*Bactrim I.V.; Septra I.V.;* GENERIC].
Canada—
   400 mg of sulfamethoxazole and 80 mg of trimethoprim per 5 mL (Rx) [*Bactrim; Septra*].

**Preparation of dosage form**
The contents of each vial (5 mL) must be diluted to 75 to 125 mL of 5% dextrose injection prior to administration by intravenous infusion. The resulting solution should be administered by intravenous infusion over a 60- to 90-minute period.
Caution: Use of products containing benzyl alcohol is not recommended for use in neonates. A fatal toxic syndrome consisting of metabolic acidosis, CNS depression, respiratory problems, renal failure, hypotension, and possibly seizures and intracranial hemorrhages has been associated with this use.

**Stability**
After initial dilution with 75 or 125 mL of 5% dextrose injection, infusion should be administered within 2 or 6 hours, respectively.
Do not use if solution is cloudy or contains a precipitate. Do not mix with other medications or solutions.
After initial entry of a needle into the vial, the remaining contents should be used within 48 hours.
Sulfamethoxazole and trimethoprim combination is very unstable when mixed with other medications and diluents other than 5% dextrose injection.

[1]Not included in Canadian product labeling.

Revised: 03/01/96

---

**SULFUR**—The *Sulfur (Topical)* monograph is not included in this published version of the USP DI database. Copies of the monograph are available on request from Micromedex, Inc. - Reprint Requests, 6200 S. Syracuse Way, Suite 300, Englewood, CO 80111; telephone (303) 486-6400; telefax (303) 486-6464; Email: USPDI@MDX.COM.

---

**SULFURATED LIME**—The *Sulfurated Lime (Topical)* monograph is not included in this published version of the USP DI database. Copies of the monograph are available on request from Micromedex, Inc. - Reprint Requests, 6200 S. Syracuse Way, Suite 300, Englewood, CO 80111; telephone (303) 486-6400; telefax (303) 486-6464; Email: USPDI@MDX.COM.

---

**SULINDAC**—See *Anti-inflammatory Drugs, Nonsteroidal (Systemic)*

---

# SUMATRIPTAN   Systemic

VA CLASSIFICATION (Primary): CN105
Commonly used brand name(s): *Imitrex*.
Note: For a listing of dosage forms and brand names by country availability, see *Dosage Forms* section(s).

## Category
Antimigraine agent.

## Indications

**General considerations**
Sumatriptan should not be prescribed for a patient who has not previously been diagnosed as a migraineur, or administered to a migraineur with atypical symptoms, until it has been determined that the patient's headache is not occurring secondary to an evolving potentially serious neurological condition (e.g., cerebrovascular accident or subarachnoid hemorrhage).

## Accepted

Headache, migraine (treatment)—Sumatriptan is indicated to relieve (abort) acute migraine headaches (with or without aura) in patients who do not obtain sufficient relief with analgesics, such as acetaminophen, aspirin, or nonsteroidal anti-inflammatory drugs (NSAIDs). Sumatriptan also relieves the nausea, vomiting, photophobia, and phonophobia that frequently occur in association with migraine headaches.

When incapacitating migraines occur more frequently than twice a month, prophylactic treatment is recommended to reduce the severity and duration, as well as the number, of headaches. Sumatriptan is not used for this purpose. Beta-adrenergic blocking agents, calcium channel blocking agents, tricyclic antidepressants, monoamine oxidase inhibitors, methysergide, pizotyline (pizotifen [not commercially available in the U.S.]), and sometimes cyproheptadine (especially in children) are used for prophylaxis. Other measures that may reduce the need for medication in migraineurs include identification and avoidance of headache precipitants and relaxation and/or biofeedback techniques.

Headache, cluster (treatment)—Sumatriptan injection is indicated for the relief of acute cluster headache episodes. Cluster headaches may occur daily, often more than once a day, for several months (a cluster period), followed by a headache-free interval.

## Unaccepted

Sumatriptan is not recommended for long-term migraine prophylaxis.

Sumatriptan is not recommended for treatment of basilar artery migraine or hemiplegic migraine. Efficacy and safety in these conditions have not been established.

## Pharmacology/Pharmacokinetics

**Physicochemical characteristics**
Source—Synthetic. Sumatriptan is structurally related to serotonin (5-hydroxytryptamine, 5-HT).
Molecular weight—Sumatriptan succinate: 413.5.
pKa—Sumatriptan succinate—
  $pKa_1$ (succinic acid)—4.21 and 5.67
  $pKa_2$ (tertiary amine group)—9.63
  $pKa_3$ (sulfonamide group)— > 12
Sumatriptan succinate: Readily soluble in water and in 0.9% sodium chloride solution.

**Mechanism of action/Effect**
Although sumatriptan's mechanism of action has not been established, suppression of migraine headaches may result from sumatriptan-induced decreases in the firing of serotonergic (5-hydroxytryptaminergic, 5-HT) neurons. Specifically, it is thought that agonist activity at the $5\text{-HT}_{1D}$ receptor subtype provides relief of acute headache. Sumatriptan is a highly selective agonist at this receptor subtype; it has no significant activity at other 5-HT receptor subtypes or at adrenergic, dopaminergic, muscarinic, or benzodiazepine receptors.

It has been proposed that constriction of cerebral blood vessels resulting from $5\text{-HT}_{1D}$ receptor stimulation reduces the pulsation that may be responsible for the pain of vascular headaches. Studies in humans have shown that blood flow velocity in the middle cerebral arteries is significantly reduced during a migraine on the side of the headache, that relief of the headache by sumatriptan is accompanied by return of the blood flow velocity in these vessels to normal, and that sumatriptan treatment does not induce other changes in cerebral hemispheric blood flow. However, other studies have not consistently shown a significant correlation between dilatation of cerebral blood vessels and pain or other symptoms of migraine headaches, or between medication-induced vasoconstriction and relief of these headaches.

It has also been proposed that neurogenic inflammation in areas innervated by the trigeminal nerve may contribute to the development of migraine headaches. Although the cause of the inflammation has not been established, there is some evidence that serotonergic mechanisms may be involved. Sumatriptan may also relieve migraines by decreasing release of neuropeptides and other mediators of inflammation and by reducing extravasation of plasma proteins. A study in humans has demonstrated that concentrations of calcitonin gene-related peptide, a substance that increases vascular permeability and promotes plasma protein extravasation, are elevated during a migraine and return to normal as the headache is relieved by sumatriptan.

**Absorption**
Nasal—Rapid; bioavailability is low (approximately 17%), primarily because of presystemic hepatic metabolism and incomplete absorption.
Oral—Rapid. However, bioavailability is low (approximately 15% of a dose), primarily because of presystemic hepatic metabolism and, to a lesser extent, because of incomplete absorption. The rate and extent of absorption are not affected to a clinically significant extent by administration with food or by the gastric stasis that may accompany migraine headaches.
Subcutaneous—Rapid; bioavailability is approximately 97% of that achieved with an intravenous injection.

**Distribution**
Sumatriptan is rapidly and extensively distributed to tissues but passage across the blood-brain barrier is limited.

**Protein binding**
In plasma—Low (14 to 21%).

**Biotransformation**
Hepatic and extensive; approximately 80% of a dose is metabolized. The major metabolite is an inactive indole acetic acid derivative.
*In vitro* studies with human hepatic microsomes indicate that sumatriptan is metabolized by monoamine oxidase (MAO), primarily the A isoenzyme (MAO-A).

**Half-life**
Distribution—Subcutaneous administration: Approximately 15 minutes.
Elimination—Subcutaneous or oral administration: Approximately 2.5 hours. One study reported a terminal half-life of approximately 7 hours that became apparent about 12 hours after administration of multiple oral doses, but did not contribute substantially to the overall disposition of the medication.
Nasal administration: Approximately 2 hours.

**Onset of action**
Nasal:
  Within 15 minutes.
Oral:
  Within 30 minutes.
Subcutaneous:
  Relief of headache pain: Within 10 minutes.
  Relief of migraine-associated nausea, vomiting, photophobia, phonophobia: Within 20 minutes.

**Time to peak serum concentration:**
Nasal (single 5-mg, 10-mg, or 20-mg dose): Between 1 and 1.5 hours.
Oral (single 100-mg dose): Approximately 2 hours (range, 0.5 to 5 hours). The wide interindividual variability found in pharmacokinetic studies may be related to the appearance of multiple peaks in the concentration over time. Approximately 80% of the maximum value is achieved within 45 minutes.
Subcutaneous (single 6-mg dose): Approximately 12 minutes (range, 5 to 20 minutes).

**Peak serum concentration**
Nasal (5-mg and 20-mg dose): Approximately 5 nanograms per mL (0.012 micromoles/L) and 16 nanograms/mL (0.039 micromoles/L), respectively.
Oral (single 100-mg dose): Approximately 54 nanograms per mL (0.13 micromoles/L) (range, 26.7 to 137 nanograms per mL [0.06 to 0.33 micromoles/L]).
Subcutaneous (single 6-mg dose): Approximately 72 to 74 nanograms per mL; (0.17 to 0.18 micromoles/L) (range, 54.9 to 108.4 nanograms per mL [0.13 to 0.26 micromoles/L]).

**Time to peak effect**
Relief of headache (i.e., moderate or severe pain being reduced to mild or no pain)—
  Oral (single 100-mg dose): Within 2 hours in 50 to 75%, and within 4 hours in an additional 15 to 25%, of patients.
  Subcutaneous (single 6-mg dose): Within 1 hour in 70%, and within 2 hours in an additional 12%, of patients.
Relief of associated symptoms (nausea, vomiting, photophobia, phonophobia)—
  Oral (single 100-mg dose): Within 2 hours.
  Subcutaneous (single 6-mg dose): Within 1 hour in 68%, and within 2 hours in an additional 13%, of patients.

**Duration of action**
Return of migraine headache occurs within 24 to 48 hours in approximately 40% of patients who initially obtain a beneficial response to sumatriptan, i.e., after moderate or severe headache pain has been reduced to mild or no pain. Whether this represents development of a new migraine or breakthrough of a prolonged migraine after the effects of sumatriptan have worn off has not been established.

**Elimination**
Renal, via active renal tubular secretion, following hepatic metabolism. Approximately 80% of a dose is eliminated as metabolites. After nasal administration, approximately 3% of the dose is eliminated as unchanged sumatriptan and 35% as the indole acetic acid metabolite. After oral administration, approximately 57% of a dose is eliminated in the urine (3% of the dose as unchanged sumatriptan, 35% as the indole acetic acid metabolite, and 8% as the glucuronide conjugate of the in-

dole acetic acid metabolite) and another 38% of the dose is eliminated in the feces (9% as unchanged sumatriptan and 11% as the indole acetic acid metabolite). After subcutaneous administration, approximately 22% of a dose is eliminated in the urine as unchanged sumatriptan and another 38% as the indole acetic acid metabolite. Only 0.6% and 3.3% of a dose are eliminated in the feces as unchanged sumatriptan and the indole acetic acid metabolite, respectively.

The effects of renal function impairment on clearance of sumatriptan have not been studied. Approximately 80% of the total clearance is via hepatic biotransformation; therefore, hepatic function impairment may produce clinically significant elevations in the bioavailability of orally administered sumatriptan. However, the elevation in the bioavailability of intranasal sumatriptan is not clinically significant.

## Precautions to Consider

### Tumorigenicity
No evidence of tumorigenicity was found in a 104-week study in rats given sumatriptan by oral gavage in quantities sufficient to achieve peak concentrations up to > 100 times higher than are achieved in humans with a 6-mg subcutaneous dose. Also, although no evidence of tumorigenicity was found in a 78-week study in mice given sumatriptan continuously in drinking water, this study did not use the maximum tolerated dose and is therefore considered inadequate for evaluating potential tumorigenicity in the mouse.

### Mutagenicity
No evidence of mutagenicity was found in a variety of *in vitro* and *in vivo* studies.

### Pregnancy/Reproduction
Fertility—No adverse effects on fertility were found in reproduction studies in rats given up to 60 mg per kg of body weight (mg/kg) per day subcutaneously or up to 500 mg/kg per day orally.

Pregnancy—Adequate and well-controlled studies have not been done in pregnant women.

Studies in rats receiving daily subcutaneous injections of sumatriptan prior to and during pregnancy showed no evidence of teratogenicity or embryolethality. Also, embryolethality did not occur in studies in rats receiving sumatriptan intravenously throughout organogenesis in doses producing plasma concentrations > 50 times higher than those produced by the recommended human subcutaneous dose. However, maternal toxicity and embryotoxicity occurred in rats given oral doses of 1000 mg/kg per day, but not those given 500 mg/kg per day, during organogenesis. Also, term fetuses from Dutch Stride rabbits treated during organogenesis with oral sumatriptan exhibited an increased incidence of cervicothoracic vascular defects and minor skeletal abnormalities. The functional significance of these abnormalities is not known. In other studies, daily administration of sumatriptan to pregnant rabbits throughout the period of organogenesis using oral doses of 100 mg/kg per day or intravenous doses sufficient to produce peak concentrations 3 times those produced in humans after a 6-mg subcutaneous dose resulted in maternal toxicity and/or embryolethality.

FDA Pregnancy Category C.

### Breast-feeding
Sumatriptan is distributed into human breast milk. However, problems in humans have not been documented.

### Pediatrics and adolescents
Appropriate studies on the relationship of age to the effects of sumatriptan have not been done in patients up to 18 years of age. Safety and efficacy have not been established.

### Geriatrics
Information on the relationship of age to the effects of sumatriptan in geriatric patients is extremely limited. No unusual adverse, age-related phenomena occurred in patients older than 60 years of age who participated in clinical trials. However, most published studies report excluding patients older than 65 years of age. Studies in a limited number of healthy subjects 65 to 86 years of age found no differences in pharmacokinetic parameters between these older individuals and younger subjects.

### Drug interactions and/or related problems
The following drug interactions and/or related problems have been selected on the basis of their potential clinical significance (possible mechanism in parentheses where appropriate)—not necessarily inclusive (» = major clinical significance):

Note: Combinations containing any of the following medications, depending on the amount present, may also interact with this medication.

Antidepressants, selective 5-hydroxytryptamine uptake inhibitor or
Lithium or
» Monoamine oxidase (MAO) inhibitors, including furazolidone, procarbazine, and selegiline
(concurrent use of any of these agents with sumatriptan may lead to a potentially dangerous hyperserotonergic state or other adverse effects; sumatriptan should be used with caution in patients receiving these medications)

(sumatriptan is metabolized by the MAO-A isoenzyme; pretreatment of human subjects with an MAO-A inhibitor has been shown to decrease sumatriptan clearance, resulting in substantial increases in the area under the sumatriptan plasma concentration-time curve and the sumatriptan half-life. MAOIs that inhibit the MAO-A isoenzyme include furazolidone, isocarboxazid, moclobemide, phenelzine, toloxatone, and tranylcypromine. MAOIs that inhibit only the MAO-B isoenzyme, such as selegiline, did not produce these effects)

(oral and intranasal sumatriptan should not be used during or within 14 days following administration of an MAO inhibitor; concurrent use of sumatriptan injection with MAO inhibitors is not generally recommended; however, concurrent use would require a dosage adjustment of sumatriptan injection)

Dihydroergotamine or
Ergotamine or
Methysergide
(a delay of 24 hours between administration of dihydroergotamine, ergotamine, or methysergide and sumatriptan is recommended because of the possibility of additive and/or prolonged vasoconstriction)

Selective serotonin reuptake inhibitors, such as:
Fluoxetine
Fluvoxamine
Paroxetine
Sertraline
(concurrent use may result in weakness, hyperreflexia, and incoordination; careful monitoring is recommended)

### Laboratory value alterations
The following have been selected on the basis of their potential clinical significance (possible effect in parentheses where appropriate)—not necessarily inclusive (» = major clinical significance):

With physiology/laboratory test values
Blood pressure and
Peripheral vascular resistance
(may be increased, although increases are generally mild and transient; in clinical studies, clinically significant blood pressure elevations [increase in systolic pressure by 20 mm Hg or to 180 mm Hg; increase in diastolic pressure by 15 mm Hg or to 105 mm Hg] occurred in fewer than 1% of the patients; blood pressure changes after oral administration are smaller and occur more slowly than after subcutaneous administration)

### Medical considerations/Contraindications
The medical considerations/contraindications included have been selected on the basis of their potential clinical significance (reasons given in parentheses where appropriate)—not necessarily inclusive (» = major clinical significance).

*Except under special circumstances, this medication should not be used when the following medical problems exist:*

» Coronary artery disease, especially:
Angina pectoris
Myocardial infarction, history of
Myocardial ischemia, silent documented
Prinzmetal's angina or
» Other conditions in which coronary vasoconstriction would be detrimental
(although sumatriptan has only a slight vasoconstrictive effect on coronary arteries, sumatriptan-induced myocardial ischemia has been documented, primarily in patients with a history of coronary artery disease or susceptibility to coronary artery vasospasm)

» Hypertension, uncontrolled
(may be exacerbated)

*Risk-benefit should be considered when the following medical problems exist:*

Cardiac arrhythmias, especially:
» Tachycardia or
» Cerebrovascular accident, history of
(sumatriptan may cause cerebral hemorrhage, subarachnoid hemorrhage, or stroke; caution should be used when administering in patients at risk for cerebrovascular events)

» Coronary artery disease, predisposition to
    (sumatriptan has rarely caused serious coronary adverse effects; patients in whom coronary artery disease is a possibility on the basis of age or the presence of other risk factors, such as diabetes, hypercholesterolemia, obesity, a strong family history of coronary artery disease, or tobacco smoking should be evaluated for the presence of cardiovascular disease before sumatriptan is prescribed; even after a satisfactory evaluation, the advisability of administering the patient's first dose under medical supervision should be considered)
» Hepatic function impairment or
  Renal function impairment
    (caution is recommended because clearance of sumatriptan may be impaired; because about 80% of the total clearance is via hepatic biotransformation, hepatic function impairment should be more likely than renal function impairment to produce clinically significant increases in sumatriptan concentration; dosage adjustment is recommended in patients with hepatic impairment)
  Hypertension, controlled
    (elevations of systolic and diastolic blood pressure may occur, especially after subcutaneous administration, although these effects are generally mild and transient in hypertensive patients whose blood pressure is adequately controlled by medication; in clinical studies, patients with controlled hypertension experienced mean peak increases of 6 mm Hg, which usually started within 30 minutes after subcutaneous administration and persisted for less than an hour)
» Sensitivity to sumatriptan

## Side/Adverse Effects

Note: Most of the adverse effects reported with sumatriptan are mild and transient (lasting less than 1 hour after subcutaneous injection and 2 hours or less after oral administration) and resolve without treatment. Although several deaths have been reported after administration of sumatriptan, a direct causal relationship could not be established in most cases. Most of the fatalities occurred 3 hours or more after administration and probably were spontaneous events or were caused by underlying disease. Some of the deaths were attributed to strokes, cerebral hemorrhages, or other cerebrovascular events. However, migraineurs are known to be at increased risk of cerebrovascular accidents or transient ischemic attacks; in many of these cases a cerebrovascular event, rather than a migraine, may have been causing the symptoms that led to sumatriptan administration.

Some of the adverse events reported after administration of sumatriptan (e.g., nausea, vomiting, malaise, fatigue, dizziness, vertigo, weakness, drowsiness, sedation) often occur during and/or following a migraine headache; whether sumatriptan contributes to their occurrence has not been established.

Although a causal relationship to sumatriptan has not been established, the following adverse events have also been reported in open, uncontrolled studies (incidences < 1%) and/or postmarketing: cardiac arrhythmias (atrial fibrillation, ventricular fibrillation, ventricular tachycardia, sinus arrhythmia), other transient changes in the electrocardiogram (ST segment elevations, other ST or T-wave changes, prolongation of PR or QTc intervals, nonsustained ventricular premature beats, isolated junctional ectopic beats, atrial ectopic beats, delayed activation of the right ventricle), hypotension, bradycardia, syncope, Prinzmetal's angina, vasodilatation, Raynaud's disease, acute renal failure, seizures, cerebrovascular accident, dysphagia, subarachnoid hemorrhage, polydipsia, dehydration, gastrointestinal reflux, dyspnea, erythema, pruritus, skin rashes, peptic ulceration, gallstones, swelling of extremities, transient hemiplegia, hysteria, globus hystericus, intoxication, mental depression, myoclonia, monoplegia or diplegia, dystonia, dysuria, urinary frequency, renal calculus, photosensitivity, and exacerbation of sunburn.

The following side/adverse effects have been selected on the basis of their potential clinical significance (possible signs and symptoms in parentheses where appropriate)—not necessarily inclusive:

### Those indicating need for medical attention
Incidence less frequent (1 to 3%) with subcutaneous administration; less frequent or rare (< 1%) with oral or nasal administration
  *Chest pain, severe; difficulty in swallowing; heaviness, tightness, or pressure in chest and/or neck*
    Note: Although *chest pain* and *heaviness, tightness, or pressure in the chest and neck* are suggestive of angina pectoris, monitoring of the electrocardiogram (ECG) during such symptoms in clinical studies failed to detect evidence of myocardial ischemia. Conversely, ECG monitoring detected new T-wave abnormalities in a small number of patients, most of whom had abnormal pretreatment ECGs, who were not experiencing relevant symptoms. However, sumatriptan-induced coronary artery vasospasm resulting in symptomatic myocardial ischemia and myocardial infarction have been documented in a few patients, primarily patients with a history of coronary artery disease or susceptibility to coronary artery vasospasm. Several fatalities associated with such complications have been reported following administration of sumatriptan, but in most cases a causal relationship has not been established.

Incidence rare
  *Anaphylactic or anaphylactoid reaction* (changes in facial skin color; skin rash, hives, and/or itching; fast or irregular breathing; puffiness or swelling of the eyelids or around the eyes, face, or lips; shortness of breath, troubled breathing, tightness in chest, and/or wheezing); *dermatitis, allergic* (skin rash, hives, and/or itching); *seizures*

### Those indicating need for medical attention only if they continue or are bothersome
Incidence more frequent
  *Injection site reaction* (burning, pain, or redness); *irritation in the nose* (burning; discharge; pain; or soreness)—occurs with nasal spray only; *nausea or vomiting*; *taste perversion* (change in sense of taste)—occurs with nasal spray only
    Note: *Nausea* and *vomiting* often occur in conjunction with migraine headaches; they are not necessarily caused by (and may actually be relieved by) sumatriptan. However, these effects occurred more frequently after oral than after subcutaneous administration of sumatriptan in clinical trials, possibly because of the unpleasant taste of the dispersible tablet used in the studies.

Incidence up to 13.5% with subcutaneous administration; less frequent (1 to 3%) or rare (< 1%) with nasal or oral administration
  *Atypical sensations* (sensation of burning, warmth, heat, numbness, tightness, or tingling; feeling cold; "strange" feeling); *discomfort in jaw, mouth, throat, tongue, nasal cavity, or sinuses; dizziness; drowsiness; flushing; lightheadedness; muscle aches, cramps, or stiffness; weakness*
    Note: *Flushing* and sensations of *burning, warmth,* or *heat* generally disappear within 10 to 30 minutes after administration of a subcutaneous dose.

Incidence less frequent (1 to 3%) with subcutaneous administration; less frequent or rare (< 1%) with oral and nasal administration
  *Anxiety; general feeling of illness or tiredness; vision changes*

## Overdose
For specific information on the agents used in the management of sumatriptan overdose, see:
  • *Nitroglycerin* in *Nitrates (Systemic)*.

For more information on the management of overdose or unintentional ingestion **contact a Poison Control Center** (see *Poison Control Center Listing*).

### Clinical effects of overdose
Overdose has not been reported in humans. Signs and symptoms that might be anticipated, based on animal studies, include ataxia, convulsions, cyanosis, erythema of extremities, inactivity, injection site reactions (desquamation, hair loss, scab formation), mydriasis, paralysis, reduced respiratory rate, and tremor.

### Treatment of overdose
Although there is no experience with overdose of sumatriptan, treatment may involve:
To decrease absorption—Emptying the stomach by induction of emesis or performing gastric lavage (if ingested orally).
Monitoring—For continuing chest pain or other symptoms consistent with angina pectoris: Monitoring the electrocardiogram for evidence of ischemia and administering appropriate treatment (e.g., nitroglycerin or other coronary artery vasodilators) as needed. Some patients may require further evaluation to determine whether previously undiagnosed coronary artery disease is present. See the package insert or *Nitroglycerin* in *Nitrates (Systemic)* for specific dosing guidelines for use of this product.
Monitoring of patients who have received an overdose of sumatriptan nasal spray should continue for at least 10 hours or while signs or symptoms persist.
Supportive care—Monitoring the patient and instituting supportive treatment as needed. Patients in whom intentional overdose is confirmed or suspected should be referred for psychiatric consultation.

## Patient Consultation

As an aid to patient consultation, refer to *Advice for the Patient, Sumatriptan (Systemic)*.

In providing consultation, consider emphasizing the following selected information (» = major clinical significance):

### Before using this medication
» Conditions affecting use, especially:
  Sensitivity to sumatriptan
  Other medications, especially monoamine oxidase inhibitors
  Other medical problems, especially cerebrovascular accident (history of); coronary artery disease, predisposition to coronary artery disease, or other conditions that may be adversely affected by coronary artery constriction; hepatic function impairment; hypertension (uncontrolled); and tachycardia

### Proper use of this medication
» Not administering if atypical headache symptoms are present; checking with physician instead
  Administering after onset of headache pain
  Additional benefit may be obtained if the patient lies down in a quiet, dark room after administering medication
» Not using additional doses if a first dose does not provide substantial relief; additional sumatriptan is not likely to be effective in these circumstances; taking alternate medication as previously advised by physician, then checking with physician as soon as possible
» Taking additional doses, if needed, for return of migraine after initial relief was obtained, provided that prescribed limits (quantity used and frequency of administration) are not exceeded
» Compliance with prophylactic therapy, if prescribed

*Proper administration of*
  Tablets—Swallowing whole; not breaking, crushing or chewing before taking; taking with full glass of water
  Injection—
    Reading patient instructions provided with medication
    Proper injection technique
    Discarding used cartridge as directed in patient instructions, using container provided; not discarding autoinjector unit because refill cartridges are available
  Nasal—Reading patient instructions provided with medication
» Proper dosing
» Proper storage

### Precautions while using this medication
Checking with physician if usual dose fails to relieve three consecutive headaches, or frequency and/or severity of headaches increases
Avoiding alcohol, which aggravates headache
» Caution if drowsiness or dizziness occurs

### Side/adverse effects
Contacting physician immediately if severe chest pain or signs and symptoms of anaphylactoid reaction occur
Contacting physician at once if mild pain or tightness in chest or throat occurs and persists for more than 1 hour; even if symptoms are of shorter duration, not using medication again without first consulting physician
Signs and symptoms of other potential side effects, including dysphagia, palpitation, and skin rash or eruptions

## General Dosing Information

Clinical studies have not shown a correlation between the duration of a migraine prior to administration of sumatriptan and its ability to abort an acute attack. Because a recent study has shown that administration of sumatriptan during a preheadache aura may neither prevent nor significantly delay the onset of the headache, it is recommended that sumatriptan not be administered prior to the appearance of headache pain.

Lying down and relaxing in a quiet, darkened room after administering a dose of antimigraine medication may contribute to relief of migraines.

Additional doses of sumatriptan should not be administered to patients who do not obtain substantial relief (reduction of initially moderate or severe headache pain to mild or no pain) within 1 or 2 hours after the initial dose. Several clinical trials have failed to demonstrate that a second dose benefits these patients. It is recommended that an analgesic be used as "rescue" medication in the event of an unsatisfactory response to sumatriptan; use of dihydroergotamine, ergotamine, or methysergide is not recommended because of the possibility of additive or prolonged vasoconstriction. Also, the prescriber should be contacted as soon as possible if sumatriptan is ineffective because of the possibility that the patient's symptoms are being caused by a cerebrovascular event. However, patients who do not respond to sumatriptan during one migraine attack may obtain a satisfactory response during subsequent attacks.

Return of migraine headache occurs within 24 to 48 hours in about 40% of patients who initially obtain a beneficial response to sumatriptan. Whether this represents development of a new migraine or breakthrough of a prolonged migraine after the effects of sumatriptan have worn off has not been established. Recurrences following an initial beneficial response may be treated with additional sumatriptan.

Tolerance to the effects of sumatriptan did not occur when the medication was used intermittently to relieve acute migraines for longer than 6 months.

The possibility that overuse of sumatriptan by migraineurs may lead to dependence on the medication and to the development of withdrawal (rebound) or chronic, intractable headaches (as has been documented with too-frequent use of ergotamine and/or analgesics by these patients) has not been evaluated. Some headache specialists recommend that, until more definitive information about the risk of cumulative toxicity and/or dependence is available, courses of sumatriptan treatment should not be administered more often than every five to seven days.

### For oral dosage form only
Sumatriptan tablets are to be swallowed whole (i.e., with the film coating intact) because the unpleasant taste of the contents may cause taste disturbances and/or an increased risk of nausea and vomiting.

### For parenteral dosage form only
Sumatriptan is not to be given intravenously. Clinical trials have shown that intravenous administration is associated with a higher incidence of adverse effects than subcutaneous administration. Specifically, the risk of coronary artery vasospasm and angina may be increased. Long-term users with risk factors of coronary artery disease should receive periodic cardiovascular evaluations.

## Oral Dosage Forms

Note: Sumatriptan tablets contain sumatriptan succinate. However, dosage and strength are expressed in terms of sumatriptan base.

### SUMATRIPTAN TABLETS

**Usual adult dose**
Antimigraine agent—
  Oral, 25 to 100 mg (base) as a single dose. If necessary, additional doses up to 100 mg may be taken at intervals of at least two hours, up to a maximum of 300 mg a day.
  For relief of migraine headache that returns after an initial treatment with sumatriptan injection, additional single oral doses of up to 50 mg may be given at intervals of at least two hours, up to a maximum of 200 mg a day.
  The maximum single dose for patients with hepatic impairment should not exceed 50 mg.

Note: There is no evidence that an initial dose of 100 mg provides substantially greater relief than a dose of 25 mg.

**Usual adult prescribing limits**
Antimigraine agent—
  Oral, not more than 300-mg (base) in twenty-four hours.

**Usual pediatric dose**
Safety and efficacy in patients up to 18 years of age have not been established.

**Strength(s) usually available**
U.S.—
  25 mg (base) (Rx) [*Imitrex* (lactose)].
  50 mg (base) (Rx) [*Imitrex* (lactose)].
Canada—
  50 mg (base [as the succinate salt]) (Rx) [*Imitrex* (lactose)].
  100 mg (base [as the succinate salt]) (Rx) [*Imitrex* (lactose)].

**Packaging and storage**
Store between 2 and 30 °C (36 and 86 °F), unless otherwise specified by manufacturer.

**Auxiliary labeling**
• Swallow tablets whole.
• Take with a full glass of water.

## Nasal Dosage Forms

### SUMATRIPTAN NASAL SOLUTION

**Usual adult dose**
Antimigraine agent—
  Intranasal, 5 mg or 10 mg (1 or 2 sprays) in each nostril, respectively, or 20 mg (1 spray) into one nostril as a single dose.
  Additional doses should not be administered for the same migraine attack. However, a dose may be administered for subsequent attacks provided a minimum of two hours has elapsed since the last dose.

**Usual adult prescribing limits**
Antimigraine agent—
Nasal, not more than 40 mg in twenty-four hours.

**Usual pediatric dose**
Safety and efficacy in patients up to 18 years of age have not been established.

**Strength(s) usually available**
U.S.—
5 mg (base [as the hemisulphate salt]) (Rx) [*Imitrex* (monobasic potassium phosphate; anhydrous dibasic sodium phosphate; sulfuric acid; sodium hydroxide; purified water)].
20 mg (base [as the hemisulphate salt]) (Rx) [*Imitrex* (monobasic potassium phosphate; anhydrous dibasic sodium phosphate; sulfuric acid; sodium hydroxide; purified water)].
Canada—
5 mg (base [as the hemisulphate salt]) (Rx) [*Imitrex* (monobasic potassium phosphate; anhydrous dibasic sodium phosphate; sulfuric acid; sodium hydroxide; purified water)].
20 mg (base [as the hemisulphate salt]) (Rx) [*Imitrex* (monobasic potassium phosphate; anhydrous dibasic sodium phosphate; sulfuric acid; sodium hydroxide; purified water)].

**Packaging and storage**
Store between 2 and 30 °C (36 and 86 °F), protected from light and from freezing, unless otherwise specified by manufacturer.

## Parenteral Dosage Forms

Note: Sumatriptan injection contains sumatriptan succinate. However, dosage and strength are expressed in terms of sumatriptan base.

### SUMATRIPTAN INJECTION

**Usual adult dose**
Antimigraine agent—
Subcutaneous, injected into the outer thigh or the outer upper arm, 6 mg (base). If a beneficial response to this dose is obtained within one or two hours, an additional 6-mg dose may be administered, at least one hour after the first dose, if headache pain returns or increases in severity.

Note: Lower doses may be administered if the patient does not tolerate the usual dose. The auto-injector should not be used for this purpose; doses should be withdrawn from the single-dose vial, using a separate syringe.

One study compared the effects of 6-mg and 8-mg subcutaneous doses of sumatriptan (base) in migraineurs. The 8-mg dose was not significantly more effective than the 6-mg dose; therefore, doses higher than 6 mg are not recommended.

**Usual adult prescribing limits**
Antimigraine agent—
Single subcutaneous doses should not exceed 6 mg (base). No more than two 6-mg doses should be administered within twenty-four hours.

Note: Some clinicians recommend administering no more than two 6-mg doses within forty-eight hours.

**Usual pediatric dose**
Safety and efficacy in patients up to 18 years of age have not been established.

**Strength(s) usually available**
U.S.—
6 mg (base [as the succinate salt]) per 0.5 mL (Rx) [*Imitrex* (sodium chloride 3.5 mg per 0.5 mL)].
Canada—
6 mg (base [as the succinate salt]) per 0.5 mL (Rx) [*Imitrex*].

**Packaging and storage**
Store between 2 and 30 °C (36 and 86 °F), protected from light and from freezing, unless otherwise specified by manufacturer.

### Selected Bibliography

Cady RK, Wendt JK, Kirchner JR, et al. Treatment of acute migraine with subcutaneous sumatriptan. JAMA 1991; 265: 2831-5.
Subcutaneous Sumatriptan International Study Group. Treatment of migraine attacks with sumatriptan. N Engl J Med 1991; 325: 316-21.
Brown EG, Endersby CA, Smith RM, et al. The safety and tolerability of sumatriptan: an overview. Eur Neurol 1991; 31: 339-44.

Revised: 03/27/97
Interim revision: 03/30/98

---

**SUNSCREEN AGENTS**—The *Sunscreen Agents (Topical)* monograph is not included in this published version of the USP DI database. Copies of the monograph are available on request from Micromedex, Inc. - Reprint Requests, 6200 S. Syracuse Way, Suite 300, Englewood, CO 80111; telephone (303) 486-6400; telefax (303) 486-6464; Email: USPDI@MDX.COM.

---

**SUPROFEN**—See *Anti-inflammatory Drugs, Nonsteroidal (Ophthalmic)*.

---

**SURAMIN**—The *Suramin (Systemic)* monograph is not included in this published version of the USP DI database. Copies of the monograph are available on request from Micromedex, Inc. - Reprint Requests, 6200 S. Syracuse Way, Suite 300, Englewood, CO 80111; telephone (303) 486-6400; telefax (303) 486-6464; Email: USPDI@MDX.COM.

---

# SYMPATHOMIMETIC AGENTS—Cardiovascular Use    Parenteral-Systemic

This monograph includes information on the following: 1) Dobutamine; 2) Dopamine; 3) Ephedrine; 4) Epinephrine; 5) Isoproterenol; 6) Mephentermine†; 7) Metaraminol†; 8) Methoxamine; 9) Norepinephrine; 10) Phenylephrine.

INN:
Norepinephrine—Levarterenol
BAN:
Norepinephrine—Noradrenaline
VA CLASSIFICATION (Primary/Secondary):
Dobutamine—AU100/CV900
Dopamine—AU100/CV900
Ephedrine—AU100/CV900
Epinephrine—AU100/CV900
Isoproterenol—AU100/CV300
Mephentermine—AU100/CV900
Metaraminol—AU100/CV900
Methoxamine—AU100/CV900
Norepinephrine—AU100/CV900
Phenylephrine—AU100/CV900; CV300

Commonly used brand name(s): *Adrenalin*[4]; *Aramine*[7]; *Dobutrex*[1]; *Intropin*[2]; *Isuprel*[5]; *Levophed*[9]; *Neo-Synephrine*[10]; *Revimine*[2]; *Vasoxyl*[8]; *Wyamine*[6].

Note: For a listing of dosage forms and brand names by country availability, see *Dosage Forms* section(s).

†Not commercially available in Canada.

## Category

Antiarrhythmic—Isoproterenol; Phenylephrine.
Cardiac stimulant—Dobutamine; Dopamine; Epinephrine.
Vasopressor—Dopamine; Ephedrine; Epinephrine; Mephentermine; Metaraminol; Methoxamine; Norepinephrine; Phenylephrine.

## Indications

**Accepted**
Bradycardia (treatment)—Isoproterenol is indicated for the temporary control of hemodynamically significant bradycardia, such as bradycardia associated with a denervated transplanted heart or third degree heart block due to conduction system disease. Electrical pacing is the pre-

ferred treatment for maintenance of an adequate ventricular rate and isoproterenol is used only for temporary support when electrical pacing is unavailable. Isoproterenol may also be used in long QT-related arrhythmias where underlying bradycardia is common.

Hypotension, acute (prophylaxis and treatment) or
Shock (treatment)—The sympathomimetic agents (except isoproterenol) are indicated for the correction of hypotension, unresponsive to adequate fluid volume replacement, as part of shock syndrome caused by myocardial infarction, trauma, bacteremia, open-heart surgery, renal failure, chronic cardiac decompensation, drug overdose, or other major systemic illness.

The specific choice of drug must be determined by clinical assessment. This assessment may include hemodynamic status, mental status, urine output, and other measures of tissue perfusion. In refractory cases, the use of multiple drug therapy may be necessary for blood pressure support.

In septic shock, low-dose dopamine may be used in conjunction with norepinephrine to maintain renal blood flow.

In hypovolemic shock, the sympathomimetic agents should be used only as adjuncts to energetic fluid volume replacement to provide temporary support for maintaining coronary and cerebral artery perfusion until volume replacement therapy is completed. These medications must not be used as the sole therapy in hypovolemic patients.

In acute hypotension associated with myocardial infarction, sympathomimetic agent-induced increases in myocardial oxygen demand and the work of the heart may outweigh the beneficial effect of the medication. Also, cardiac arrhythmias induced by the sympathomimetic agents may be more likely to occur in patients with myocardial infarction.

Although norepinephrine is indicated in the treatment of acute hypotension occurring during spinal anesthesia, vasopressors that have a longer duration of action (e.g., metaraminol or phenylephrine) are also useful.

Ephedrine is indicated for the correction of hypotension secondary to spinal or other types of nontypical conduction anesthesia. It is also used in hypotensive states following sympathectomy, or following overdose with ganglionic blocking agents, antiadrenergic agents, or other medications that lower blood pressure in the treatment of hypertension.

Metaraminol is indicated for the prevention and treatment of acute hypotension occurring with spinal anesthesia and in the adjunctive treatment of hypotension resulting from hemorrhage, reactions to medications, surgical complications, and shock associated with brain damage due to trauma or tumor. However, metaraminol is not indicated as the sole treatment for hypotension secondary to decreased plasma volume.

Mephentermine is indicated in the treatment of hypotension secondary to ganglionic blockade and hypotension occurring with spinal anesthesia.

Methoxamine is indicated for supporting, restoring, or maintaining blood pressure during general anesthesia with agents that sensitize the myocardium to arrhythmias, such as halothane.

Dobutamine is not recommended for the adjunctive treatment of hypovolemic shock.

Cardiac output, low (treatment) or
Congestive heart failure (treatment)—Dobutamine is indicated to improve cardiac function during cardiac decompensation in congestive heart failure or depressed contractility from cardiac or major vascular surgery.

If a vasopressor is also needed, norepinephrine or dopamine is useful for short-term management. However, stimulation of alpha-1 adrenergic receptors produces vasoconstriction, which is undesirable in most patients with severe heart failure. In certain circumstances, a vasodilating agent such as nitroprusside or nitroglycerin may be used as an adjunct to dobutamine to decrease afterload and pulmonary pressures.

Cardiac arrest (treatment)—Epinephrine is indicated during resuscitation of cardiac standstill or cardiac arrest. Epinephrine is used as an adjunct to restore cardiac rhythm in the treatment of cardiac arrest due to various causes. It also has beneficial hemodynamic effects in the setting of cardiopulmonary resuscitation (CPR), improving myocardial and cerebral blood flow. Epinephrine injection may be used for resuscitation in cardiac arrest following anesthetic accidents; however, it should be used with great caution in patients receiving halogenated hydrocarbon anesthetics, especially halothane, because these anesthetics sensitize the myocardium and cardiac arrhythmias may be induced.

In acute attacks of ventricular standstill, physical measures should be used prior to administration of epinephrine. However, if external cardiac compression and attempts to restore circulation by electrical defibrillation or use of a pacemaker fail, intravenous injection of epinephrine into a major vein may be effective.

Shock, anaphylactic (treatment)—Epinephrine injection is indicated in the emergency treatment of anaphylactic shock.

Tachycardia, supraventricular, paroxysmal (treatment)—Phenylephrine is indicated in the termination of some episodes of paroxysmal supraventricular tachycardia (PSVT).

**Unaccepted**
Isoproterenol is no longer routinely recommended as an inotropic agent. It has been replaced in most clincial settings by newer agents that are less prone to induce ischemia, arrhythmias, or a hypotensive response.

Mephentermine is not recommended in the treatment of hypotension induced by chlorpromazine because it may potentiate, rather than correct, the hypotension secondary to the adrenolytic effects of chlorpromazine.

## Pharmacology/Pharmacokinetics

**Physicochemical characteristics**
Molecular weight—
  Dobutamine: 337.85.
  Dopamine hydrochloride: 189.64.
  Ephedrine sulfate: 428.54.
  Epinephrine: 183.21.
  Isoproterenol hydrochloride: 247.72.
  Mephentermine sulfate: 424.60.
  Metaraminol bitartrate: 317.29.
  Methoxamine hydrochloride: 247.72.
  Norepinephrine bitartrate: 337.28.
  Phenylephrine hydrochloride: 203.67.
Other characteristics—
  pH—
    Dobutamine—9.4
    Dopamine Hydrochloride Injection, USP—2.5 to 5

**Mechanism of action/Effect**
Dobutamine—
  A direct-acting inotropic agent. Dobutamine acts primarily on beta-1 adrenergic receptors, with little effect on beta-2 or alpha receptors. Dobutamine directly stimulates beta-1 receptors of the heart to increase myocardial contractility and stroke volume, resulting in increased cardiac output. Coronary blood flow and myocardial oxygen consumption are usually increased because of increased myocardial contractility. Dobutamine has little effect on systemic vascular resistance, and systolic blood pressure and pulse pressure may remain unchanged or be increased because of increased cardiac output. However, in septic patients with decreased systemic vascular resistance, dobutamine may lower blood pressure without increasing cardiac output. Dobutamine reduces elevated ventricular filling pressure (preload reduction) and facilitates atrioventricular (AV) node conduction. At appropriate doses, an increase in heart rate does not usually occur, but excessive doses have a chronotropic effect. Renal blood flow and urine output may be improved as a result of increased cardiac output rather than as a dopaminergic effect.

Dopamine—
  Dopamine stimulates postsynaptic beta-1 receptors in the myocardium, mediating its positive inotropic and chronotropic effects. Dopamine causes vascular relaxation and promotes sodium excretion through its stimulation of postsynaptic dopamine-1 receptors on vascular smooth muscle and on the kidney. In addition, dopamine stimulates both alpha-1 and alpha-2 receptors, which mediate smooth muscle vasoconstriction. These pharmacologic effects are dose-related, requiring various infusion rates of dopamine to activate different receptors.

  In low doses (0.5 to 3 mcg per kg of body weight [mcg/kg] per minute), dopamine acts predominantly on dopaminergic receptors to cause vasodilation in the renal, mesenteric, coronary, and intracerebral vascular beds. Renal vasodilation results in increased renal blood flow, glomerular filtration rate, urine flow (usually), and sodium excretion.

In low to moderate doses (2 to 10 mcg/kg per minute), beta-1 receptors are stimulated, resulting in a positive inotropic effect on the myocardium and an increase in cardiac output. Systolic blood pressure and pulse pressure may be increased with either no change or a slight increase in diastolic blood pressure. Total peripheral resistance is usually unchanged. Coronary blood flow and myocardial oxygen consumption are usually increased.

In higher doses (10 mcg/kg per minute or above), alpha-adrenergic receptor stimulation predominates, resulting in increased peripheral vascular resistance and renal vasoconstriction (this vasoconstriction may decrease previously increased renal blood flow and urine output). Both systolic and diastolic blood pressures are increased as a result of increased cardiac output and increased peripheral resistance.

Ephedrine—
Ephedrine stimulates both alpha and beta adrenergic receptors and enhances the release of endogenous norepinephrine from sympathetic neurons, resulting in increased systolic and diastolic blood pressure and increased cardiac output. Ephedrine also stimulates the central nervous system (CNS), although to a lesser extent than does amphetamine.

Epinephrine—
Epinephrine predominantly stimulates alpha and beta-1 adrenergic receptors, and has moderate activity at beta-2 adrenergic receptors. At very low doses, (less than 0.01 mcg/kg per minute), epinephrine may decrease blood pressure through dilatation of skeletal muscle vasculature. At doses of 0.04 to 0.1 mcg/kg per minute, stimulation of beta-receptors predominates, increasing heart rate, cardiac output, and stroke volume and decreasing peripheral vascular resistance. At doses exceeding 0.2 mcg/kg per minute, stimulation of alpha adrenergic receptors produces vasoconstriction and increased total peripheral resistance. Doses exceeding 0.3 mcg/kg per minute decrease renal blood flow, gastrointestinal motility, pyloric tone, and splanchnic vascular bed perfusion.

Epinephrine also increases conduction velocity in the myocardium and increases ectopic pacemaker activity. Myocardial oxygen demand is also increased.

Isoproterenol—
Isoproterenol is a pure beta receptor agonist. It is a potent inotrope and chronotrope, increasing cardiac output despite a reduction in mean blood pressure due to peripheral vasodilation.

Mephentermine—
Mephentermine is an alpha adrenergic receptor agonist, but also acts indirectly by releasing endogenous norepinephrine. Cardiac output and systolic and diastolic pressures are usually increased. A change in heart rate is variable, depending on the degree of vagal tone. Sometimes the net vascular effect may be vasodilation. Large doses may depress the myocardium or produce central nervous system (CNS) effects.

Metaraminol—
Metaraminol acts directly on peripheral alpha adrenergic receptors, as well as, indirectly through release of endogenous norepinephrine. Metaraminol produces a positive inotropic effect on the heart and peripheral vasoconstriction.

Methoxamine—
Methoxamine is a relatively selective alpha-1 adrenergic receptor agonist, producing an increase in peripheral vascular resistance. At high doses beta adrenergic receptors may be stimulated, resulting in increased blood pressure. A reflex sinus bradycardia may occur.

Norepinephrine—
Norepinephrine stimulates alpha and beta-1 adrenergic receptors in a dose-related fashion. At lower doses (less than 2 mcg per minute), stimulation of beta-1 receptors results in a positive inotropic and chronotropic effect. At higher doses (greater than 4 mcg per minute), the alpha adrenergic effect predominates, resulting in elevated total peripheral resistance. Chronotropy diminishes as a result of baroreceptor-mediated vagal stimulation.

Norepinephrine may produce vasoconstriction in the mesenteric vascular bed, which can induce splanchnic ischemia and facilitate bacterial translocation from the gut. Norepinephrine also increases renal vascular resistance. However, renal perfusion may actually increase in hypotensive patients through norepinephrine's effect of increasing blood pressure.

Phenylephrine—
Phenylephrine is primarily an alpha-1 adrenergic agonist, which causes marked vasoconstriction.

The following table represents relative receptor agonist activity of the sympathomimetic agents—

|  | RECEPTOR TYPE ||||| 
|---|---|---|---|---|---|
|  | Alpha-1 | Alpha-2 | Beta-1 | Beta-2 | Dopamine |
| Norepinephrine | +++ | +++ | ++ | None | None |
| Epinephrine low dose |  |  | ++ | +++ | None |
| moderate dose | + |  | +++ | +++ |  |
| high dose | +++ | +++ | +++ | +++ |  |
| Dobutamine | + | None | +++ | + | None |
| Dopamine low dose |  | None |  | None |  |
| moderate dose |  |  | +++ |  | +++ |
| high dose | +++ |  |  |  |  |
| Isoproterenol | None | None | +++ | +++ | None |
| Ephedrine (indirect effects via norepinephrine release) | +++ | +++ | ++ | None | None |
| Mephentermine | +++ | None | None | None | None |
| Metaraminol (indirect effects via norepinephrine release) | +++ | +++ | ++ | None | None |
| Methoxamine | +++ | None | None | None | None |
| Phenylephrine | +++ | None | None | None | None |

**Distribution**
Dopamine—
  Adults: Widely distributed in the body; does not extensively cross the blood-brain barrier. About 25% of a dose is taken up into specialized neurosecretory vesicles where hydroxylation occurs, forming norepinephrine.
  Neonates: Apparent volume of distribution—1.8 L per kg.

**Biotransformation**
Dobutamine—Hepatic, to inactive compounds.
Dopamine—Metabolized in the liver, kidney, and plasma by monoamine oxidase (MAO) and catechol-O-methyltransferase (COMT) to inactive metabolites.
Ephedrine—Small amounts in the liver.
Epinephrine—Metabolized by monoamine oxidase (MAO) and catechol-O-methyltransferase (COMT).
Isoproterenol—Metabolism in liver, lungs, and other tissues.
Mephentermine—Hepatic, by N-demethylation and then p-hydroxylation.
Metaraminol—Hepatic.
Methoxamine—Hepatic.
Norepinephrine—Metabolized in the liver, kidney, and plasma by monoamine oxidase (MAO) and catechol-O-methyltransferase (COMT) to inactive metabolites.
Phenylephrine—Hepatic and gastrointestinal.

**Half-life**
Dobutamine—
  About 2 minutes.
Dopamine—
  Adults:
    Plasma—About 2 minutes.
    Elimination—About 9 minutes.
  Neonates:
    Elimination—6.9 minutes (range 5 to 11 minutes).
Epinephrine—
  1 minute.
Ephedrine—
  3 to 6 hours.
Mephentermine—
  17 to 18 hours.
Norepinephrine—
  1 minute.

**Onset of action**
Dobutamine—
  1 to 2 minutes; however, up to 10 minutes may be required when infusion rate is slow.
Dopamine—
  Within 5 minutes.
Epinephrine—
  Rapid.
Isoproterenol—
  Less than 5 minutes.

Mephentermine—
    Intravenous: Very rapid.
    Intramuscular: 5 to 15 minutes.
Metaraminol—
    Intravenous: 1 to 2 minutes.
    Intramuscular: About 10 minutes.
Methoxamine—
    0.5 to 2 minutes.
Norepinephrine—
    Rapid.
Phenylephrine—
    Very rapid.

**Duration of action**
Dobutamine—
    Less than 5 minutes.
Dopamine—
    Less than 10 minutes.
Ephedrine—
    1 hour.
Epinephrine—
    1 to 2 minutes.
Isoproterenol—
    10 minutes.
Mephentermine—
    Intravenous: 15 to 30 minutes.
    Intramuscular: 1 to 4 hours.
Metaraminol—
    20 to 60 minutes.
Methoxamine—
    5 to 15 minutes.
Norepinephrine—
    1 to 2 minutes.
Phenylephrine—
    5 to 20 minutes.

**Elimination**
Dobutamine—Renal; as metabolites.
Dopamine—Renal; 80% of a dose excreted within 24 hours, primarily as metabolites. A very small fraction of a dose is excreted unchanged.
Ephedrine—Renal; mostly as unchanged drug.
Mephentermine—Renal.
Methoxamine—Renal.
Norepinephrine—Renal; primarily as metabolites.

## Precautions to Consider

### Cross-sensitivity and/or related problems
Dobutamine, dopamine, epinephrine, isoproterenol, metaraminol, methoxamine, norepinephrine, and phenylephrine preparations contain sulfites.

### Carcinogenicity/Mutagenicity
Long-term studies have not been done.

### Pregnancy/Reproduction
Fertility—*Dobutamine:* Studies in rats and rabbits have revealed no evidence of fertility impairment.
*Dopamine:* Long-term studies have not been done.
*Isoproterenol:* Studies have not been done.
*Mephentermine:* Long-term studies have not been done.
*Metaraminol:* Long-term studies have not been done.
*Methoxamine:* Long-term studies have not been done.
*Norepinephrine:* Studies have not been done.
*Phenylephrine:* Long-term studies have not been done.

Pregnancy—
    *Dobutamine*—
        Adequate and well-controlled studies in humans have not been done.
        Reproduction studies in rats and rabbits found no evidence of teratogenicity or harm to the fetus.
    *Dopamine*—
        Adequate and well-controlled studies in humans have not been done.
        Studies in animals have not revealed evidence of teratogenic effects. However, administration of dopamine to pregnant rats resulted in a decreased survival rate of the newborn and a potential for the development of cataracts in survivors.
        FDA Pregnancy Category C.
    *Ephedrine*—
        Adequate and well-controlled studies have not be done in humans.
        Studies have not been done in animals.
        FDA Pregnancy Category C.
    *Epinephrine*—
        Adequate and well-controlled studies in humans have not been done.
        Studies in rats given epinephrine at doses 25 times the human dose have revealed teratogenic effects.
        FDA Pregnancy Category C.
    *Isoproterenol*—
        Adequate and well-controlled studies have not been done in humans.
        Studies have not been done in animals.
        FDA Pregnancy Category C.
    *Mephentermine*—
        It is not known whether mephenterine crosses the placenta. However, mephentermine may increase uterine contractions in pregnant women, especially during the third trimester.
        Studies have not been done in animals.
        FDA Pregnancy Category C.
    *Metaraminol*—
        Adequate and well-controlled studies have not been done in humans.
        Metaraminol given to pregnant ewes at a dose of 0.025 mg per kg of body weight (mg/kg) decreased uterine blood flow.
        FDA Pregnancy Category C.
    *Methoxamine*—
        Adequate and well-controlled studies in humans have not been done. However, a fetal death has been reported when the mother received methoxamine concomitantly with other medications. A direct causal relationship has not been established.
        Methoxamine administered to pregnant ewes and monkeys at doses comparable to those used in humans decreased uterine blood flow and heart rate, and adversely affected fetal acid-base status, as evidenced by hypoxia, hypercarbia, and metabolic acidosis. In pregnant ewes, an inverse relationship between pressor response to methoxamine and uteroplacental blood flow was shown at doses ranging from 0.025 to 0.2 mg/kg. A study in baboons given methoxamine at a dose of 1.3 mg/kg over 57 minutes revealed a decrease in uterine blood flow and a possible association with fetal asphyxia.
        FDA Pregnancy Category C.
    *Norepinephrine*—
        Adequate and well-controlled studies have not been done in humans.
        Studies have not been done in animals.
        FDA Pregnancy Category C.
    *Phenylephrine*—
        Adequate and well-controlled studies have not been done in humans.
        Studies have not been done in animals.
        FDA Pregnancy Category C.

Labor and delivery—If vasopressor medications are used to correct hypotension or added to the local anesthetic solution during labor and delivery, some oxytocic medications (e.g., vasopressin, ergotamine, ergonovine, methylergonovine) may cause severe persistent hypertension, and rupture of a cerebral blood vessel may occur during the postpartum period.
*Ephedrine:* Ephedrine, when used to maintain blood pressure during low or other spinal anesthesia for delivery, may accelerate fetal heart rate. Use is not recommended when maternal blood pressure exceeds 130/80 mm Hg.
*Epinephrine:* Use during labor is not recommended because epinephrine may delay the second stage of labor.
*Mephentermine:* Mephentermine may cause a decrease in uterine blood flow, which may result in fetal hypoxia. Transient fetal hypertension has also been reported in animals.

### Breast-feeding
It is not known whether these medications are distributed into breast milk.

### Pediatrics
*Dobutamine*—Dobutamine has been studied in a limited number of pediatric patients up to 18 years of age. There do not appear to be pediatric-specific problems that would limit the usefulness of dobutamine in pediatric patients.
*Dopamine*—Dopamine has been studied in a limited number of pediatric patients up to 18 years of age. Close hemodynamic monitoring is recommended since there is a lack of controlled studies investigating age-dependent dosages and the maximum dosage at which therapeutic response occurs without causing toxicity. In addition, cardiac arrhythmias and gangrene due to extravasation have been reported in pediatric patients.

*Epinephrine*—Epinephrine has been used in pediatric patients during cardiac arrest and there do not appear to be pediatrics-specific problems that would limit its usefulness in this setting. However, caution is recommended to avoid errors in concentration selection and dosing, since two different dilutions of epinephrine are necessary for the dosing regimen.

**Geriatrics**

*Isoproterenol*—Data seem to indicate that elderly patients may exhibit a decreased chronotropic and peripheral vascular response to isoproterenol.

*Norepinephrine*—The pressor response to norepinephrine does not appear to be altered with aging.

*Phenylephrine*—The baroreceptor reflex response to phenylephrine appears to decrease with age.

**Drug interactions and/or related problems**

The following drug interactions and/or related problems have been selected on the basis of their potential clinical significance (possible mechanism in parentheses where appropriate)—not necessarily inclusive (» = major clinical significance):

Note: Combinations containing any of the following medications, depending on the amount present, may also interact with this medication.

Alpha-adrenergic blocking agents, such as:
 Doxazosin
 Labetalol
 Phenoxybenzamine
 Phentolamine
 Prazosin
 Terazosin
 Tolazoline, or
Other medications with alpha-adrenergic blocking action, such as:
 Haloperidol
 Loxapine
 Phenothiazines
 Thioxanthenes
 (concurrent use may antagonize the peripheral vasoconstriction of sympathomimetic agents; however, phentolamine may be used for therapeutic benefit)

» Anesthetics, hydrocarbon inhalation, such as:
 Chloroform
 Enflurane
» Halothane
 Isoflurane
 Methoxyflurane
 (concurrent use of these medications with the sympathomimetic agents may increase the risk of severe atrial and ventricular arrhythmias because these anesthetics greatly sensitize the myocardium; sympathomimetic agents should be used with caution and in substantially reduced doses in patients receiving these anesthetics)

 (enflurane, isoflurane, or methoxyflurane may also sensitize the myocardium to the effects of sympathomimetics; caution is recommended during concurrent use)

» Antidepressants, tricyclic or
» Maprotiline
 (concurrent use may potentiate the cardiovascular and pressor effects of sympathomimetic agents, possibly resulting in arrhythmias, tachycardia, or severe hypertension or hyperpyrexia)

Antihypertensives or
Diuretics used as antihypertensives
 (antihypertensive effects may be reduced when these medications are used concurrently; the patient should be carefully monitored to confirm that the desired effect is being obtained)

Beta-adrenergic blocking agents, ophthalmic or
» Beta-adrenergic blocking agents, systemic
 (concurrent use with sympathomimetic agents may result in mutual inhibition of therapeutic effects; beta-blockade may antagonize the beta-1 adrenergic cardiac effects of sympathomimetic agents)

» Cocaine, mucosal-local
 (concurrent use with sympathomimetic agents may increase the cardiovascular effects of either or both medications and the risk of adverse effects)

» Digitalis glycosides
 (concurrent use with sympathomimetic agents possessing beta-1 adrenergic agonist activity may increase the risk of cardiac arrhythmias; in addition, concurrent use may produce additive inotropic effects though these medications may be used with digitalis glycosides for therapeutic advantage, caution and close electrocardiographic monitoring are recommended during concurrent use)

Diuretics
 (concurrent use may increase the diuretic effect of the diuretic medications or dopamine as a result of dopamine's direct action on dopaminergic receptors to produce vasodilation of renal vasculature and increase renal blood flow; dopamine also has a direct natriuretic effect)

» Doxapram
 (concurrent use may increase the pressor effects of either the sympathomimetic agents or doxapram)

Ergonovine or
» Ergotamine or
Methylergonovine or
Methysergide or
Oxytocin
 (concurrent use of ergonovine, methylergonovine, or methysergide with a sympathomimetic agent may result in enhanced vasoconstriction; dosage adjustments may be necessary)

 (concurrent use of ergotamine with these medications may produce peripheral vascular ischemia and gangrene and is not recommended)

 (concurrent use of ergonovine, ergotamine, methylergonovine, or oxytocin may potentiate the pressor effect of these medications with possible severe hypertension and rupture of cerebral blood vessels)

Guanadrel or
Guanethidine
 (in addition to possibly decreasing the hypotensive effect of guanadrel or guanethidine, concurrent use may potentiate the pressor response to the sympathomimetic agents; these actions are a result of inhibition of sympathomimetic uptake by adrenergic neurons and may lead to hypertension and cardiac arrhythmias)

Levodopa
 (concurrent use with dopamine may increase the possibility of cardiac arrhythmias; dosage reduction of the sympathomimetic is recommended)

Mecamylamine or
Methyldopa
 (in addition to possibly decreasing the hypotensive effects of these medications, concurrent use may enhance the pressor response to sympathomimetic agents)

Methylphenidate
 (concurrent use may potentiate the pressor effect of sympathomimetic agents)

» Monoamine oxidase (MAO) inhibitors, including furazolidone, procarbazine, and selegiline
 (concurrent use may prolong and intensify cardiac stimulation and vasopressor effects because of the release of catecholamines, which accumulate in intraneuronal storage sites during MAO inhibitor therapy; this may result in headache, cardiac arrhythmias, vomiting, or sudden and severe hypertensive and/or hyperpyretic crises; for patients who have been receiving MAO inhibitors 2 to 3 weeks prior to administration of sympathomimetic agents, the initial dosage should be reduced to no more than one-tenth of the usual dose)

Nitrates
 (concurrent use with sympathomimetic agents may reduce the antianginal effects of these medications; also, nitrates may counteract the pressor effect of sympathomimetic agents, possibly resulting in hypotension; however, nitrates and sympathomimetic agents may be used concurrently for therapeutic advantage)

Phenoxybenzamine
 (in addition to phenoxybenzamine antagonizing the peripheral vasoconstriction of the sympathomimetic agents, concurrent use of phenoxybenzamine may produce an exaggerated hypotensive response and tachycardia)

Phenytoin, and possibly other hydantoins
 (concurrent use with dopamine may result in sudden hypotension and bradycardia; this reaction is considered to be dose-rate dependent; if anticonvulsant therapy is necessary during administration of dopamine, an alternative to phenytoin should be considered; caution is also advised with concurrent use of other hydantoins)

Rauwolfia alkaloids
 (in addition to possibly decreasing the hypotensive effects of rauwolfia alkaloids, concurrent use may theoretically prolong the action of direct-acting sympathomimetics, such as dopamine, by preventing uptake into storage granules; a "denervation supersensitivity" response is also possible; although concurrent use is not known to produce severe adverse effects, a significant increase in blood pressure has been documented when phenylephrine ophthalmic drops were administered to patients taking reserpine, and caution and close observation are recommended)

Sympathomimetics, other
(concurrent use may increase the cardiovascular effects and the potential for side effects)

Thyroid hormones
(concurrent use may increase the effects of either these medications or the sympathomimetic agents; thyroid hormones enhance risk of coronary insufficiency when sympathomimetic agents are administered to patients with coronary artery disease; dosage adjustment is recommended, although the problem is reduced in euthyroid patients)

## Medical considerations/Contraindications

The medical considerations/contraindications included have been selected on the basis of their potential clinical significance (reasons given in parentheses where appropriate)—not necessarily inclusive (» = major clinical significance).

*Except under special circumstances, this medication should not be used when the following medical problems exist:*

» Asymmetric septal hypertrophy (idiopathic hypertrophic subaortic stenosis)
(obstruction may increase as myocardial contractility improves with sympathomimetic agents possessing beta-1 adrenergic agonist activity)

» Pheochromocytoma
(severe hypertension may occur)

» Tachyarrhythmias or
Ventricular fibrillation
(exacerbation of arrhythmia may occur; however, epinephrine may be used as an adjunct in the treatment of ventricular fibrillation)

*Risk-benefit should be considered when the following medical problems exist:*

Acidosis, metabolic or
Hypercapnia or
Hypoxia
(may reduce effectiveness and/or increase incidence of side/adverse effects of the sympathomimetic agents; should be corrected prior to or concurrently with administration of sympathomimetic agents)

Atrial fibrillation
(rapid ventricular response may occur since dobutamine facilitates atrioventricular conduction; in patients who have atrial fibrillation with rapid ventricular response, a digitalis preparation should be used prior to institution of therapy with dobutamine)

Glaucoma, narrow angle
(condition may be exacerbated with sympathomimetic agents possessing alpha-1 adrenergic agonist activity)

Hypertension, pulmonary
(condition may be exacerbated due to pulmonary vasoconstriction)

» Hypovolemia
(prior to initiation of sympathomimetic therapy, hypovolemia should be corrected with appropriate volume expanders; volume should be maintained throughout treatment)

Mechanical obstruction, severe, such as severe valvular aortic stenosis
(these agents may be ineffective)

» Myocardial infarction
(excessive doses of sympathomimetic agents possessing beta-1 adrenergic agonist activity may intensify ischemia by increasing myocardial oxygen demands)

Occlusive vascular disease, history of, including:
Arterial embolism
Atherosclerosis
Buerger's disease
Cold injury, e.g., frostbite
Diabetic endarteritis
Raynaud's disease
(possible risk of necrosis and gangrene with sympathomimetic agents possessing alpha-1 adrenergic agonist activity; patients should be closely monitored for decreased circulation to extremities; if decreased circulation occurs, rate of infusion should be reduced or the infusion discontinued)

Sensitivity to other sympathomimetics

» Tachyarrhythmias or ventricular arrhythmias
(condition may be exacerbated)

*For dopamine and dextrose injection only*
Diabetes mellitus, subclinical or overt
(condition may be exacerbated)

## Patient monitoring

The following may be especially important in patient monitoring (other tests may be warranted in some patients, depending on condition; » = major clinical significance):

» Blood pressure, preferably intra-arterial and
» Electrocardiogram (ECG) and
» Urine flow
(continuous monitoring is recommended during therapy with sympathomimetic agents)

» Cardiac output and
» Central venous pressure and
» Pulmonary artery pressure and
» Pulmonary capillary wedge pressure
(recommended during therapy with sympathomimetic agents; however, therapy with low-dose dopamine may not require such intensive monitoring)

*For dobutamine and epinephrine, in addition to the above*
Potassium, serum
(monitoring may be considered due to risk of hypokalemia)

## Side/Adverse Effects

Note: *Peripheral vasoconstriction*, possibly leading to necrosis or gangrene, may occur with prolonged use of sympathomimetic agents with alpha-1 adrenergic agonist activity in high doses or low doses in the presence of peripheral vascular disease.

*Allergic reaction* may occur in preparations containing sulfites.

The following side/adverse effects have been selected on the basis of their potential clinical significance (possible signs and symptoms in parentheses where appropriate)—not necessarily inclusive:

### Those indicating need for medical attention

Incidence less frequent
*Angina; bradycardia; dyspnea; hypertension; hypotension; palpitations; tachycardia; ventricular arrhythmias*—especially with high doses

Note: *Angina, dyspnea, palpitations, tachycardia, and ventricular arrhythmias* are associated with agents possessing beta-adrenergic agonist activity. They may also occur with agents possessing alpha-adrenergic agonist activity if marked degrees of hypertension are induced.

Incidence rare—for dobutamine and epinephrine
*Hypokalemia*

Incidence rare—for dopamine
*Polyuria*

Note: *Polyuria* has been reported in patients receiving dopamine at nonrenal doses.

### Those indicating need for medical attention only if they continue or are bothersome

Incidence more frequent
*Headache; nausea or vomiting*

Incidence less frequent
*Nervousness or restlessness*

## Overdose

For more information on the management of overdose or unintentional ingestion, **contact a Poison Control Center** (see *Poison Control Center Listing*).

### Clinical effects of overdose

The following effects have been selected on the basis of their potential clinical significance (possible signs and symptoms in parentheses where appropriate)—not necessarily inclusive:

*Hypertension, severe*

### Treatment of overdose

For excessive hypertensive effect—The rate of administration should be reduced or the medication temporarily discontinued until blood pressure is decreased. Additional measures are usually not necessary because the duration of action of these agents is short. However, if reduction in the rate of administration or discontinuation of therapy fails to lower the blood pressure, a short-acting alpha-adrenergic blocking agent may be administered.

## General Dosing Information

Patients receiving sympathomimetic agent therapy should be closely monitored. See *Patient monitoring*.

Sympathomimetic agent therapy is not a substitute for replacement of blood, plasma, fluids, and/or electrolytes.

Prior to initiation of therapy, hypovolemia should be fully corrected, if possible, with either whole blood or a plasma volume expander as indicated.

An infusion pump or other suitable metering device should be used to control the rate of infusion in order to avoid unintentional administration of bolus doses.

Dosage must be adjusted to meet the individual requirements of each patient, on the basis of clinical response. Some patients may need higher than usually recommended doses for a time.

Infusions of sympathomimetic agents should be given into a large vein, or preferably, directly into the central circulation.

Caution is recommended to avoid extravasation, which may cause tissue necrosis and sloughing of surrounding tissues.

When discontinuing therapy, the dosage should be reduced gradually, since sudden cessation of therapy may result in severe hypotension. Intravascular fluid should be repleted if necessary to avoid hypotension.

**For treatment of adverse effects**

For extravasation ischemia—To prevent necrosis and sloughing of tissue in areas where extravasation has occurred, the site should be infiltrated promptly with 10 to 15 mL of 0.9% sodium chloride injection containing 5 to 10 mg of phentolamine. A syringe with a fine hypodermic needle should be used and the solution infiltrated liberally throughout the affected area. If the area is infiltrated within 12 hours, the sympathetic blockade with phentolamine produces immediate and noticeable local hyperemic changes. This treatment should be proportionally reduced for pediatric patients.

---
## DOBUTAMINE
---

## Summary of Differences

Indications:
  Indicated for congestive heart failure and low cardiac output.
Pharmacology/pharmacokinetics:
  Mechanism of action/effect—Primarily beta-1 adrenergic agonist; mild alpha-1 and beta-2 agonist.
Precautions to consider:
  Patient monitoring—Serum potassium.
Side/adverse effects:
  Hypokalemia.

## Additional Dosing Information

The concentration of solution administered depends on the dosage and fluid requirements of the patient, but should not exceed 5 mg of dobutamine per mL.

## Parenteral Dosage Forms

Note: The dosing and strengths of the dosage forms available are expressed in terms of dobutamine base (not the hydrochloride salt).

### DOBUTAMINE HYDROCHLORIDE INJECTION

**Usual adult dose**
Cardiac stimulant—
  Intravenous infusion, administered at a rate of 2.5 to 10 mcg (0.0025 to 0.01 mg) (base) per kg of body weight per minute.
  Rates of infusion for concentrations of 250, 500, and 1000 mcg per mL:

| Drug delivery rate (mcg/kg/min) | 250 mcg/mL* (mL/kg/min) | Infusion delivery rate 500 mcg/mL† (mL/kg/min) | 1000 mcg/mL‡ (mL/kg/min) |
|---|---|---|---|
| 2.5 | 0.01 | 0.005 | 0.0025 |
| 5 | 0.02 | 0.01 | 0.005 |
| 7.5 | 0.03 | 0.015 | 0.0075 |
| 10 | 0.04 | 0.02 | 0.01 |
| 12.5 | 0.05 | 0.025 | 0.0125 |
| 15 | 0.06 | 0.03 | 0.015 |

*250 mg per L of diluent.
†500 mg per L or 250 mg/500 mL of diluent.
‡1000 mg per L or 250 mg/250 mL of diluent.

**Usual pediatric dose**
Cardiac stimulant—
  Intravenous infusion, 5 to 20 mcg per kg of body weight per minute.

**Size(s) usually available**
U.S.—
  12.5 mg (base) per mL (Rx) [*Dobutrex* (sodium bisulfite 0.24 mg per mL)].

Canada—
  12.5 mg (base) per mL (Rx) [*Dobutrex* (sodium bisulfite 0.245 mg per mL)].

**Packaging and storage**
Prior to dilution, store between 15 and 30 °C (59 and 86 °F), unless otherwise specified by manufacturer.

**Preparation of dosage form**
The solution must be further diluted to at least 50 mL prior to administration in 5% dextrose injection, 5% dextrose and 0.45% sodium chloride injection, 5% dextrose and 0.9% sodium chloride injection, 10% dextrose injection, lactated Ringer's injection, 5% dextrose in lactated Ringer's injection, 0.9% sodium chloride injection, or sodium lactate injection.

**Stability**
Solutions diluted for intravenous infusion should be used within 24 hours. Freezing may cause crystallization and should be avoided.
Pink discoloration of dobutamine solution indicates slight oxidation of the medication, but there is no significant loss of potency if administered within the recommended time periods.

**Incompatibilities**
Dobutamine is incompatible with alkaline solutions and should not be mixed with solutions such as 5% sodium bicarbonate injection.
Dobutamine injection should not be used in conjunction with other agents or diluents containing both sodium bisulfite and ethanol.
It is recommended that dobutamine injection not be mixed in the same solution with other medications.
Mixture or administration of dobutamine through the same intravenous line as heparin, hydrocortisone sodium succinate, cefazolin, cefamandole, neutral cephalothin, penicillin, or sodium ethacrynate is not recommended.

---
## DOPAMINE
---

## Summary of Differences

Pharmacology/pharmacokinetics:
  Mechanism of action/effect—Dose-related alpha, beta, and dopamine receptor agonist.
  Biotransformation—Metabolized by monoamine oxidase (MAO) and catechol-O-methyltransferase (COMT).
Precautions to consider:
  Drug interactions—Levodopa, phenytoin.
  Pediatrics—Cardiac arrhythmias and gangrene reported.
Side/adverse effects:
  Polyuria reported at nonrenal doses.

## Additional Dosing Information

Dopamine hydrochloride injection must be diluted prior to administration.

When dopamine hydrochloride and dextrose injection is used, the less concentrated 800 mcg (0.8 mg) per mL solution may be preferred when fluid expansion is not a problem. The more concentrated 1.6 or 3.2 mg per mL solutions may be preferred in patients who are fluid restricted or when a slower rate of infusion is desired.

## Parenteral Dosage Forms

### DOPAMINE HYDROCHLORIDE INJECTION USP

**Usual adult dose**
Vasopressor or
Cardiac stimulant—
  Dopaminergic (renal) effects: Intravenous infusion, 0.5 to 3 mcg per kg of body weight per minute.
  Beta-1 adrenergic effects: Intravenous infusion, 2 to 10 mcg per kg of body weight per minute.
  Alpha adrenergic effects: Intravenous infusion, 10 mcg per kg of body weight per minute. The dose may be increased gradually as clinically indicated.

**Usual pediatric dose**
Vasopressor or
Cardiac stimulant—
  Intravenous infusion, 5 to 20 mcg per kg of body weight per minute.

Note: Renal doses of dopamine (0.5 to 3 mcg per kg of body weight per minute) appear to be effective in increasing renal blood flow in pediatric patients, even in premature infants.

Close hemodynamic monitoring is recommended since only limited studies have been conducted in pediatric patients and there is a lack of data evaluating age-dependent doses.

**Strength(s) usually available**
U.S.—
  40 mg per mL (Rx) [*Intropin* (sodium metabisulfite 1%); GENERIC].
  80 mg per mL (Rx) [*Intropin* (sodium metabisulfite 1%); GENERIC].
  160 mg per mL (Rx) [*Intropin* (sodium metabisulfite 1%); GENERIC].
Canada—
  40 mg per mL (Rx) [*Intropin* (sodium bisulfite 1%); *Revimine* (sodium metabisulfite 1%)].

**Packaging and storage**
Store below 40 °C (104 °F), preferably between 15 and 30 °C (59 and 86 °F), unless otherwise specified by manufacturer. Protect from freezing.

**Preparation of dosage form**
Diluents used for preparation of intravenous infusion solutions of dopamine include 0.9% sodium chloride injection, 5% dextrose injection, 5% dextrose and 0.9% sodium chloride injection, 5% dextrose in 0.45% sodium chloride solution, 5% dextrose in lactated Ringer's solution, sodium lactate injection (1/6 molar), and lactated Ringer's injection.
Sodium bicarbonate or other alkaline intravenous solutions should not be used as diluents because dopamine is inactivated in alkaline solutions.
To prepare an intravenous infusion of dopamine hydrochloride, 400 to 800 mg of dopamine should be added to 250 mL of an appropriate diluent solution. The resultant solution contains 1600 or 3200 mcg of dopamine per mL.

**Stability**
Injection should be diluted immediately prior to administration.
After dilution in appropriate intravenous solution for infusion, dopamine is stable for at least 24 hours.
Dopamine injection should not be used if it is darker than slightly yellow or discolored.

**Incompatibilities**
Dopamine is inactivated in alkaline solution (solution becomes pink to violet); therefore, it should not be added to 5% sodium bicarbonate or other alkaline diluent solution. Dopamine is also sensitive to oxidizing agents and iron salts.

## DOPAMINE HYDROCHLORIDE AND DEXTROSE INJECTION USP

**Usual adult dose**
See *Dopamine Hydrochloride Injection USP*.

**Usual pediatric dose**
See *Dopamine Hydrochloride Injection USP*.

**Strength(s) usually available**
U.S.—
  800 mcg (0.8 mg) of dopamine hydrochloride per mL and 5% dextrose (Rx) [GENERIC].
  1.6 mg of dopamine hydrochloride per mL and 5% dextrose (Rx) [GENERIC].
  3.2 mg of dopamine hydrochloride per mL and 5% dextrose (Rx) [GENERIC].
Canada—
  800 mcg (0.8 mg) of dopamine hydrochloride per mL and 5% dextrose (Rx) [GENERIC].
  1.6 mg of dopamine hydrochloride per mL and 5% dextrose (Rx) [GENERIC].

**Packaging and storage**
Store below 40 °C (104 °F), preferably between 15 and 30 °C (59 and 86 °F), unless otherwise specified by manufacturer. Protect from freezing.

**Stability**
Solution should not be administered unless it is clear.
Discard unused portion.

**Incompatibilities**
Dopamine is inactivated in alkaline solution (solution becomes pink to violet); therefore, it should not be added to 5% sodium bicarbonate or other alkaline diluent solution. Dopamine is also sensitive to oxidizing agents and iron salts.
Dextrose solutions without electrolytes should not be administered simultaneously with blood through the same infusion set because of possible pseudoagglutination of red cells.
Additive medications should not be delivered via dopamine in dextrose injection because of possible incompatibilities.

---

## EPHEDRINE

## Summary of Differences
Pharmacology/pharmacokinetics:
  Mechanism of action/effect—Alpha and beta-1 adrenergic agonist; indirect effects via norepinephrine release.

## Additional Dosing Information
When ephedrine is administered intravenously, the injection should be given slowly.

## Parenteral Dosage Forms
### EPHEDRINE SULFATE INJECTION USP

**Usual adult dose**
Vasopressor—
  Intramuscular or subcutaneous, 25 to 50 mg. Dose may be repeated based on blood pressure response.
Note: The intravenous route of administration may be used if an immediate effect is needed.

**Usual pediatric dose**
Vasopressor—
  Intravenous or subcutaneous, 750 mcg per kg of body weight or 25 mg per square meter of body surface area four times a day as needed according to patient response.

**Strength(s) usually available**
U.S.—
  25 mg per mL (Rx) [GENERIC].
  50 mg per mL (Rx) [GENERIC].
Canada—
  50 mg per mL (Rx) [GENERIC].

**Packaging and storage**
Store below 40 °C (104 °F), preferably between 15 and 30 °C (59 and 86 °F), unless otherwise specified by manufacturer. Protect from light.

**Stability**
Should not use if solution is not clear.
Unused portion should be discarded.

---

## EPINEPHRINE

## Summary of Differences
Indications:
  Indicated for anaphylactic shock and cardiac arrest.
Pharmacology/pharmacokinetics:
  Mechanism of action/effect—Has alpha and beta adrenergic receptor action.
  Biotransformation—Metabolized by monoamine oxidase (MAO) and catechol-O-methyltransferase (COMT).
Precautions to consider:
  Patient monitoring—Serum potassium.
Side/adverse effects:
  Hypokalemia.

## Additional Dosing Information
The 1:1000 (1 mg/mL) concentration of epinephrine injection must be diluted before administering intravenously.
Intra-arterial administration of epinephrine injection is not recommended since marked vasoconstriction may result in gangrene.

## Parenteral Dosage Forms
### EPINEPHRINE HYDROCHLORIDE INJECTION

**Usual adult dose**
Vasopressor—
  Intravenous infusion, 1 mcg per minute. The dose may be titrated up to 2 to 10 mcg per minute for desired hemodynamic response.
Cardiac arrest—
  Intravenous, 1 mg every three to five minutes during resuscitation.
Note: Epinephrine may be given by the endotracheal route. However, the optimal dose for this route of administration is not known. A dose that is at least two to two and a half times the peripheral intravenous dose may be needed.

**Usual pediatric dose**
Cardiac arrest—
  Neonates:
    Intravenous, 10 to 30 mcg (0.01 to 0.03 mg) per kg of body weight every three to five minutes.
  Note: Endotracheal administration may be used. However, this may result in low plasma concentrations.
  Children:
    Intravenous, 10 mcg (0.01 mg) per kg of body weight. Subsequent doses of 100 mcg (0.1 mg) per kg of body weight every three to five minutes may be given if needed. In refractory situations, following at least two standard doses, a higher dose may be

used. Subsequent doses of 200 mcg (0.2 mg) per kg of body weight every five minutes may be given.

Note: Two different dilutions of epinephrine are necessary for this dosing regimen. **Caution** is recommended to avoid errors in concentration selection and dosing.

Endotracheal administration may be used. However, absorption and resulting plasma concentrations may be unpredictable.

**Strength(s) usually available**
U.S.—
0.1 mg (100 mcg) per mL (1:10,000) (Rx/OTC) [GENERIC].
1 mg per mL (1:1000) (Rx) [*Adrenalin* (benzyl alcohol; chlorobutanol 0.5%; sodium bisulfite < 0.1% in ampuls and < 0.15% in vials); GENERIC].
Canada—
1 mg per mL (1:1000) (Rx) [GENERIC].

**Packaging and storage**
Store below 40 °C (104 °F), preferably between 15 and 30 °C (59 and 86 °F), unless otherwise specified by manufacturer. Protect from light. Protect from freezing.

**Preparation of dosage form**
Epinephrine 1:1000 should be diluted.

**Stability**
Epinephrine is readily destroyed by alkalies and oxidizing agents (for example, oxygen, chlorine, bromine, iodine, permanganates, chromates, nitrites, and salts of easily reducible metals, especially iron). Do not use if solution is pinkish or brownish in color or contains a precipitate. Discard unused portion.

---

### *ISOPROTERENOL*

## Summary of Differences
Indications:
 Indicated for bradycardia only.
Pharmacology/pharmacokinetics:
 Mechanism of action/effect—Pure beta-adrenergic agonist.

## Parenteral Dosage Forms
**ISOPROTERENOL HYDROCHLORIDE INJECTION USP**

**Usual adult dose**
Bradycardia—
 Intravenous infusion, initially, 2 mcg per minute, the dosage being gradually titrated according to heart rate up to 10 mcg per minute if needed.

**Usual pediatric dose**
Dosage has not been established.

**Strength(s) usually available**
U.S.—
 20 mcg (0.02 mg) per mL (Rx) [GENERIC].
 200 mcg (0.2 mg) per mL (Rx) [*Isuprel* (sodium chloride; sodium lactate; sodium metabisulfite; lactic acid); GENERIC].
Canada—
 200 mcg (0.2 mg) per mL (Rx) [*Isuprel* (sodium lactate; sodium metabisulfite); GENERIC].

**Packaging and storage**
Store below 40 °C (104 °F), preferably between 15 and 30 °C (59 and 86 °F), unless otherwise specified by manufacturer. Protect from light. Protect from freezing.

**Preparation of dosage form**
For preparation of solutions for injection, see manufacturer's package insert.

**Stability**
When exposed to air, alkalies, or metals, isoproterenol may turn pinkish to brownish in color because of oxidation. Do not use if solution is pinkish to brownish in color or contains a precipitate.

---

### *MEPHENTERMINE*

## Summary of Differences
Pharmacology/pharmacokinetics:
 Mechanism of action/effect—Alpha-adrenergic agonist.

## Additional Dosing Information
Mephentermine can be administered intramuscularly.

## Parenteral Dosage Forms
**MEPHENTERMINE SULFATE**

**Usual adult dose**
Vasopressor—
 Hypotension, secondary to spinal anesthesia (prophylaxis):
  Intramuscular, 30 to 45 mg, administered ten to twenty minutes prior to anesthesia, operation, or termination of operative procedure.
 Hypotension, secondary to spinal anesthesia (treatment):
  Intravenous, 30 to 45 mg given as a single dose. Doses of 30 mg may be repeated as needed to maintain the desired level of blood pressure.
  Intravenous infusion (continuous), administered as a 0.1% (1 mg per mL) solution in 5% dextrose in water, the rate of administration and duration of therapy being adjusted according to patient response.
 In obstetrical patients—Intravenous, 15 mg initially, the dose being repeated if needed.

**Usual pediatric dose**
Safety and efficacy have not been established.

**Strength(s) usually available**
U.S.—
 15 mg per mL (Rx) [*Wyamine* (methylparaben 1.8 mg; propylparaben 0.2 mg; sodium acetate)].
 30 mg per mL (Rx) [*Wyamine* (methylparaben 1.8 mg; propylparaben 0.2 mg; sodium acetate)].
Canada—
 Not commercially available.

**Packaging and storage**
Store below 40 °C (104 °F), preferably between 15 and 30 °C (59 and 86 °F), unless otherwise specified by manufacturer. Protect from freezing.

**Preparation of dosage form**
To prepare a 0.1% (1 mg per mL) solution of mephentermine for continuous intravenous infusion, 600 mg of mephentermine should be added to 500 mL of 5% dextrose in water.

**Stability**
Do not use if solution is discolored or contains a precipitate.

---

### *METARAMINOL*

## Summary of Differences
Pharmacology/pharmacokinetics:
 Mechanism of action/effect—Alpha and beta-1 receptor agonist; indirect effects via norepinephrine release.

## Additional Dosing Information
Metaraminol may be given intramuscularly, subcutaneously, or intravenously.

The site for intramuscular or subcutaneous injection should be carefully selected, since use of areas with poor circulation may produce poor patient response and increase the possibility of tissue necrosis, sloughing of tissue, or abscess formation.

Patient's response to initial dose should be observed for at least 10 minutes before increasing dose since the maximum effect is not immediately evident.

## Parenteral Dosage Forms
Note: The dosing and strengths of the dosage forms available are expressed in terms of metaraminol base (not the bitartrate salt).

**METARAMINOL BITARTRATE INJECTION USP**

**Usual adult dose**
Hypotension (prophylaxis)—
 Intramuscular or subcutaneous, 2 to 10 mg (base).
Hypotension (treatment)—
 Intravenous infusion, 15 to 100 mg (base) in 500 mL of 0.9% sodium chloride injection or 5% dextrose injection, administered at a rate adjusted to maintain the desired blood pressure.
Shock, severe—
 Intravenous, 500 mcg (0.5 mg) to 5 mg (base), followed by an intravenous infusion of metaraminol for control of blood pressure.

**Usual adult prescribing limits**
Intravenous infusion, up to 500 mg (base) in 500 mL of infusion fluid (with caution).

**Usual pediatric dose**
Dosage has not been established.

**Strength(s) usually available**
U.S.—
   10 mg (base) per mL (Rx) [*Aramine* (sodium chloride 4.4 mg per mL; methylparaben 0.15%; propylparaben 0.02%; sodium bisulfite 0.2%); GENERIC].
Canada—
   Not commercially available.

**Packaging and storage**
Store below 40 °C (104 °F), preferably between 15 and 30 °C (59 and 86 °F), unless otherwise specified by manufacturer. Protect from light. Protect from freezing.

**Preparation of dosage form**
Metaraminol bitartrate 1% must be diluted prior to use.
The preferred solutions for dilution of metaraminol bitartrate are 0.9% sodium chloride injection and 5% dextrose injection. However, other diluents that may be used include Ringer's injection and lactated Ringer's injection.

**Stability**
After metaraminol and infusion solutions are mixed, they should be used within 24 hours because of the absence of preservatives.

**Incompatibilities**
Metaraminol bitartrate tends to be physically incompatible with other medications of poor solubility in acidic media, such as sodium salts of barbiturates, penicillins, and phenytoin.

## *METHOXAMINE*

## Summary of Differences
Pharmacology/pharmacokinetics:
   Mechanism of action/effect—Selective alpha-1 adrenergic agonist.

## Additional Dosing Information
If methoxamine is administered prophylactically to prevent hypotension during spinal anesthesia, it should be administered by intramuscular injection shortly before or at the time of spinal anesthesia administration. Those patients suffering from hypertension are more likely to experience a greater reduction in blood pressure during spinal anesthesia than patients with blood pressure in a normal range. Higher levels of anesthesia will usually cause a greater drop in blood pressure, which in turn will require an increased dose of methoxamine for control.

Although it is sometimes necessary to repeat intramuscular doses of methoxamine, it is very important to allow adequate time (about 15 minutes) for the previous intramuscular dose to elicit its effect before administration of additional doses.

Methoxamine is administered by slow, intravenous injection when the systolic blood pressure falls to 60 mm of mercury (Hg) or less, or when an emergency situation occurs.

When methoxamine is administered intravenously during emergencies, supplemental doses may be given intramuscularly to provide a prolonged effect.

Rapid administration of methoxamine should be avoided because it would produce added stress on the myocardium from markedly increased peripheral resistance during a reduction in stroke volume and cardiac output.

## Parenteral Dosage Forms
### METHOXAMINE HYDROCHLORIDE INJECTION USP
**Usual adult dose**
Vasopressor—
   Intramuscular, 10 to 15 mg. In cases of moderate hypotension, 5- to 10-mg doses may be adequate. If used during spinal anesthesia, a 10-mg dose may be adequate at low spinal anesthesia levels; however, a 15- to 20-mg dose may be required at high spinal anesthesia levels.
   Intravenous, 3 to 5 mg administered slowly.

**Usual pediatric dose**
Dosage has not been established.

**Strength(s) usually available**
U.S.—
   20 mg per mL (Rx) [*Vasoxyl* (citric acid 0.3%; potassium metabisulfite 0.1%; sodium citrate 0.3%)].
Canada—
   20 mg per mL (Rx) [*Vasoxyl* (bisulfites)].

**Packaging and storage**
Store below 40 °C (104 °F), preferably between 15 and 30 °C (59 and 86 °F), unless otherwise specified by manufacturer. Protect from light. Protect from freezing.

## *NOREPINEPHRINE*

## Summary of Differences
Pharmacology/pharmacokinetics:
   Mechanism of action/effect—Alpha and beta-1 adrenergic agonist.
   Biotransformation—Metabolized by monoamine oxidase (MAO) and catechol-O-methyltransferase (COMT).

## Additional Dosing Information
Prior to administration, norepinephrine injection must be diluted with 5% dextrose in distilled water or 5% dextrose in sodium chloride solution because the dextrose in these fluids protects against significant loss of potency due to oxidation. Administration of norepinephrine in sodium chloride solution alone is not recommended.

When norepinephrine is used as an emergency measure, it can be administered before or concurrently with blood volume replacement, but intraaortic pressure should be maintained to prevent cerebral or coronary artery ischemia.

If whole blood or plasma is indicated to increase blood volume, it should be administered separately (e.g., use of a Y-tube and individual flasks if given simultaneously).

Norepinephrine is administered only by intravenous infusion. Subcutaneous or intramuscular administration is not recommended because of the potent vasoconstrictor effect of norepinephrine.

## Parenteral Dosage Forms
Note: The dosing and strengths of the dosage forms available are expressed in terms of norepinephrine base (not the bitartrate salt).

### NOREPINEPHRINE BITARTRATE INJECTION USP
**Usual adult dose**
Vasopressor—
   Initial: Intravenous infusion, 0.5 to 1 mcg (base) per minute; the dosage being adjusted gradually to achieve desired blood pressure.
   Maintenance: Intravenous infusion, 2 to 12 mcg (base) per minute.
   Note: Patients with refractory shock may require dose up to 30 mcg (base) per minute.

**Usual pediatric dose**
Vasopressor—
   Intravenous infusion, 0.1 mcg (base) per kg of body weight per minute; the dosage being adjusted gradually to achieve desired blood pressure, up to 1 mcg per kg of body weight per minute.

**Strength(s) usually available**
U.S.—
   1 mg (base) per mL (Rx) [*Levophed* (sodium chloride; sodium metabisulfite not more than 2 mg per mL)].
Canada—
   1 mg (base) per mL (Rx) [*Levophed* (sodium bisulfite not more than 2 mg per mL; sodium chloride)].

**Packaging and storage**
Store below 40 °C (104 °F), preferably between 15 and 30 °C (59 and 86 °F), unless otherwise specified by manufacturer. Store in a light-resistant container. Protect from freezing.

**Preparation of dosage form**
Diluents used for preparation of infusion solutions of norepinephrine are 5% dextrose in distilled water or 5% dextrose in sodium chloride solution because the dextrose in these fluids protects against significant loss of potency due to oxidation. Sodium chloride solution alone is not recommended as a diluent.

To prepare an intravenous infusion solution of norepinephrine, add 4 mg of norepinephrine (base) to 250 mL of 5% dextrose solution. The resultant solution contains 16 mcg of norepinephrine base per mL.

**Stability**
Do not use discolored (pink, yellow, or brown) solutions or those containing a precipitate; they should be discarded.
Discard unused portion of norepinephrine solution.

**Incompatibilities**
Norepinephrine is incompatible with iron salts, alkalies, and oxidizing agents; contact should be avoided.

## PHENYLEPHRINE

### Summary of Differences
Indications:
    Also indicated as an antiarrhythmic.
Pharmacology/pharmacokinetics:
    Mechanism of action/effect—Alpha-1 adrenergic agonist.

## Parenteral Dosage Forms
### PHENYLEPHRINE HYDROCHLORIDE INJECTION USP
**Usual adult dose**
Vasopressor—
    Mild or moderate hypotension:
        Intramuscular or subcutaneous, 2 to 5 mg, repeated not more often than every ten to fifteen minutes.
        Intravenous, 200 mcg (0.2 mg), repeated not more often than every ten to fifteen minutes.
        Note: The initial intramuscular or subcutaneous dose should not exceed 5 mg; the initial intravenous dose should not exceed 500 mcg (0.5 mg).
    Severe hypotension and shock:
        Intravenous infusion, 10 mg in 500 mL of 5% dextrose injection USP or 0.9% sodium chloride injection USP, administered initially at a rate of about 100 to 180 mcg (0.1 to 0.18 mg) per minute until blood pressure is stabilized; then at a rate of 40 to 60 mcg (0.04 to 0.06 mg) per minute. If necessary, additional doses in increments of 10 mg or more may be added to the infusion solution and the rate of flow adjusted until the desired blood pressure level is obtained.
    Hypotension during spinal anesthesia:
        Prophylaxis—Intramuscular or subcutaneous, 2 to 3 mg three to four minutes prior to injection of spinal anesthetic.
        Hypotensive emergencies—Intravenous, initially 200 mcg (0.2 mg), the dosage being increased by not more than 200 mcg (0.2 mg) for each subsequent dose, up to a maximum of 500 mcg (0.5 mg) per dose.

Antiarrhythmic—
    Intravenous (rapid), initial dose not exceeding 500 mcg (0.5 mg). Additional doses should not exceed the preceding dose by more than 100 to 200 mcg (0.1 to 0.2 mg).

**Usual pediatric dose**
Hypotension during spinal anesthesia—
    Intramuscular or subcutaneous, 500 mcg (0.5 mg) to 1 mg per twenty-five pounds of body weight.

**Strength(s) usually available**
U.S.—
    10 mg per mL (Rx) [*Neo-Synephrine* (sodium chloride 3.5 mg; sodium citrate 4 mg; citric acid monohydrate 1 mg; sodium metabisulfite not more than 2 mg)].
Canada—
    10 mg per mL (Rx) [*Neo-Synephrine* (sodium chloride 3.5 mg; sodium citrate 4 mg; citric acid monohydrate 1 mg; sodium metabisulfite not more than 2 mg)].

**Packaging and storage**
Store below 40 °C (104 °F), preferably between 15 and 30 °C (59 and 86 °F), unless otherwise specified by manufacturer. Protect from light. Protect from freezing.

**Preparation of dosage form**
To prepare a solution of phenylephrine for direct intravenous injection, 10 mg (1 mL) of phenylephrine hydrochloride injection should be diluted with 9 mL of sterile water for injection USP to provide a solution containing 1 mg of phenylephrine per mL.

## Selected Bibliography
Chernow B, Roth BL. Pharmacologic manipulation of the peripheral vasculature in shock: clinical and experimental approaches. Circ Shock 1986; 18: 141-55.

Kulka PJ, Tryba M. Inotropic support of the critically ill patient. Drugs 1993; 45(5): 654-67.

MacLeod CM. Drugs used in the acutely ill patient. Dis Mon 1993; 39(6): 370-81.

Developed: 10/20/94

# TACRINE  Systemic†

VA CLASSIFICATION (Primary): CN900

Commonly used brand name(s): *Cognex*.

Other commonly used names are tetrahydroaminoacridine and THA.

Note: For a listing of dosage forms and brand names by country availability, see *Dosage Forms* section(s).

†Not commercially available in Canada.

## Category
Dementia symptoms treatment adjunct.

## Indications
**Accepted**

Dementia of the Alzheimer's type, mild to moderate (treatment)—Tacrine is indicated for the symptomatic treatment of mild to moderate dementia of the Alzheimer's type. Clinical trials have found tacrine to be of limited efficacy in the treatment of this condition.

In one high-dose, 30-week clinical trial of tacrine, approximately 43% of the 663 patients enrolled dropped out due to adverse medication effects, primarily elevated transaminase values and gastrointestinal effects, and only 28% of patients randomized to the 160 mg per day (mg/day) treatment group were able to complete the study. Of those patients who achieved the maximum tacrine dosage of 160 mg/day, and completed the 30-week study, 42% showed improvement in the Clinician Interview–Based Impression (CIBI), a global evaluation of change; 42% showed improvement in the Final Comprehensive Consensus Assessment (FCCA), which was similar to the CIBI but included caregivers' impressions; and 40% showed at least a 4 point improvement on the Alzheimer's Disease Assessment Scale—Cognitive subscale (ADAS-Cog), an objective 70-point evaluation of cognitive function. The only significant improvement seen in the lower dosage treatment groups was on the FCCA in the 120 mg/day patients. Among patients who received placebo, 18% showed improvement in the CIBI, 16% showed improvement in the FCCA, and 25% improved on the ADAS-Cog by at least 4 points. The improvements seen in clinical trials of tacrine were comparable in magnitude to the decline that would be expected to occur over a six-month period in a patient with Alzheimer's disease.

## Pharmacology/Pharmacokinetics

**Physicochemical characteristics**

Chemical group—Acridines.
Molecular weight—Tacrine hydrochloride monohydrate: 252.74.
pKa—9.85.

**Mechanism of action/Effect**

While many neuronal systems are affected in Alzheimer's disease, the decline in central cholinergic activity is one of the most pronounced neurotransmitter deficits. This deficit occurs early in the disease process and correlates with decreased scores on dementia ratings scales. Tacrine's primary effect is the reversible inhibition of cholinesterase, butyrylcholinesterase more than acetylcholinesterase. This inhibition is thought to increase the level of acetylcholine available in the central nervous system. In fact, increased levels of acetylcholine have been detected in the cerebrospinal fluid of patients receiving tacrine.

Tacrine may also block potassium channels, increasing the duration of the action potential and augmenting acetylcholine release from cholinergic neurons.

In addition, tacrine may moderate cholinergic activity by acting as a partial agonist or antagonist through direct binding to nicotinic and, with greater affinity, to muscarinic receptors.

Additionally, tacrine inhibits monoamine oxidase (MAO), MAO-A to a greater extent than MAO-B. Tacrine may also inhibit the reuptake of norepinephrine, serotonin, and dopamine.

There is no evidence that tacrine alters the underlying dementing process, and its effect may be expected to lessen as the disease progresses.

**Other actions/effects**

Because of its cholinomimetic action, tacrine may have vagotonic effects on the heart, including bradycardia, and may increase the activity of the gastrointestinal and urinary tracts.

**Absorption**

Tacrine is rapidly absorbed. Probably due to a very high first-pass metabolism, absolute bioavailability is about $17 \pm 13\%$. Bioavailability increases with increasing dose in a nonlinear manner, and large interindividual variations are seen. Food decreases bioavailability by 30 to 40%.

**Distribution**

Volume of distribution ($Vol_D$) is $349 \pm 193$ L.

In rats, tacrine readily penetrates the blood-brain barrier resulting in brain concentrations approximately 10 times those of plasma.

**Protein binding**

Moderate (55%).

**Biotransformation**

Metabolized by the hepaticcytochrome P-450 system. Cytochrome P-450 1A2 is the principal isozyme involved in tacrine metabolism. The major metabolite, 1-hydroxy-tacrine, or velnacrine, has central cholinergic activity.

**Half-life**

Elimination—
  Tacrine: 1.5 to 4 hours.
  1-hydroxy-tacrine (velnacrine): 2.5 to 3.1 hours.

**Time to peak concentration**

0.5 to 3 hours.

**Peak serum concentration**

Peak serum concentration shows wide interindividual variation and is significantly higher in females than in males. In addition, peak serum concentration increases nonlinearly with dose. Because the enzyme system responsible for first-pass metabolism can be saturated at relatively low doses, a larger fraction of a high dose than of a low dose will reach the circulation.

**Elimination**

Negligible amount excreted in urine. In a mass balance study, 336 hours after a single radiolabeled dose was administered, approximately 25% of the radiolabel remained unrecovered, suggesting the possibility that tacrine and/or one or more of its metabolites may be retained.

## Precautions to Consider

**Cross-sensitivity and/or related problems**

Patients hypersensitive to other acridine derivatives, such as the topical antiseptics 9-aminoacridine (e.g., Akrinol, Monacrin), acriflavine (e.g., Panflavin), or proflavine, may be hypersensitive to tacrine.

**Carcinogenicity**

Since some members of its chemical class (acridines) are known to be animal carcinogens, tacrine may be carcinogenic.

**Mutagenicity**

Tacrine was mutagenic in bacteria in the Ames test, but was not mutagenic in an *in vitro* mammalian mutation test. Tacrine induced unscheduled DNA synthesis in rat and mouse hepatocytes *in vitro*.

**Pregnancy/Reproduction**

Fertility—Studies of effects of tacrine on fertility have not been performed.

Pregnancy—Studies have not been done in humans.
Studies have not been done in animals.

FDA Pregnancy Category C.

**Breast-feeding**

Problems in humans have not been documented. It is not known whether tacrine is distributed into breast milk. However, use of tacrine is not recommended in nursing mothers.

**Geriatrics**

Clinical trials of tacrine have included Alzheimer's disease patients 40 years of age and older with no other significant disease; information available on the effects of tacrine is based upon this population. Comparisons with younger age groups have not been performed. However, elderly patients are more likely to have age-related prostate problems, which may require caution in patients receiving tacrine, especially if urinary tract obstruction is present.

**Surgical**

If possible, tacrine should be discontinued on a tapered schedule, under medical supervision, three days before any surgery involving general anesthesia. Possible interactions between tacrine and surgical adjuncts have not been fully characterized. However, tacrine may prolong or exaggerate the effects of neuromuscular blocking agents that are metabolized by plasma cholinesterase.

**Drug interactions and/or related problems**

The following drug interactions and/or related problems have been selected on the basis of their potential clinical significance (possible mechanism in parentheses where appropriate)—not necessarily inclusive (» = major clinical significance):

Note: Possible interactions with hepatic enzyme inducers, hepatic enzyme inhibitors, and medications that are metabolized by the hepatic P-450 enzyme system, other than those listed below, have not been studied, but the possibility of a significant interaction should be considered and the patient should be carefully monitored during and following concurrent use.

Combinations containing any of the following medications, depending on the amount present, may also interact with this medication.

Anticholinergics (See *Appendix II*)
(concurrent use may decrease the effects of either these medications or tacrine)

Cholinomimetics (e.g., bethanechol) and cholinesterase inhibitors (e.g., neostigmine)
(concurrent use may increase the effects of either these medications or tacrine and increase the potential for toxicity)

» Cimetidine
(concurrent use increases peak plasma concentrations and area under the concentration-time curve [AUC] of tacrine, which may increase the potential for toxicity)

» Neuromuscular blocking agents metabolized by plasma cholinesterase (e.g., succinylcholine, mivacurium)
(tacrine inhibits cholinesterase and may prolong or exaggerate muscle relaxation)

» Nonsteroidal anti-inflammatory drugs (NSAIDs)
(tacrine may increase gastric acid secretion, which may contribute to gastrointestinal irritation; patient should be monitored for occult gastrointestinal bleeding)

» Smoking tobacco
(mean plasma concentration of tacrine is 67% lower in current smokers than in nonsmokers; the effectiveness of tacrine in smokers may be decreased)

» Theophylline
(concurrent use increases mean plasma concentration and half-life of theophylline to approximately twice normal values, increasing the potential for toxicity; theophylline plasma concentration should be monitored, and dosage reduced as indicated)

### Medical considerations/Contraindications
The medical considerations/contraindications included have been selected on the basis of their potential clinical significance (reasons given in parentheses where appropriate)—not necessarily inclusive (» = major clinical significance).

***This medication should not be used when the following medical problems exist:***

» Jaundice, tacrine treatment–associated, confirmed by elevated total bilirubin greater than 3 mg per dL (mg/dL), or history of
(condition may be exacerbated or reactivated)

» Known hypersensitivity to tacrine or other acridine derivatives

***Risk-benefit should be considered when the following medical problems exist:***

» Asthma, bronchial, active or latent
(asthma attack may be precipitated)

» Cardiovascular conditions, such as:
Bradycardia
Hypotension
Sick sinus syndrome
(vagotonic effect on heart may exacerbate pre-existing conditions)

» Epilepsy or history of seizures or
» Head injury with loss of consciousness or
» Increased intracranial pressure, preexisting or
» Intracranial lesions or
» Metabolic disorders, unstable
(seizures may occur)

» Gastrointestinal obstruction or
» Urinary tract obstruction
(increased activity of gastrointestinal tract or urinary bladder may be harmful)

» Hepatic function impairment, current or history of
(condition may be exacerbated or reactivated)

» Parkinson's disease
(increased cholinergic activity in the central nervous system may exacerbate condition)

» Peptic ulcer, active or history of
(increased gastric acid secretion may exacerbate or reactivate condition)

### Patient monitoring
The following may be especially important in patient monitoring (other tests may be warranted in some patients, depending on condition; » = major clinical significance):

» Cognitive function
(periodic objective assessment of cognitive status is recommended to determine effectiveness of tacrine treatment)

» Alanine aminotransferase (ALT [SGPT]) serum values
(monitoring every other week is required for the first 16 weeks following initiation of therapy, and for the first 16 weeks following reinstitution of tacrine after a suspension of therapy of more than 4 weeks. Testing frequency may then be reduced to monthly for 2 months, then once every 3 months in the absence of ALT [SGPT] serum value elevations. However, weekly testing should be performed if ALT [SGPT] serum values are greater than twice the upper limit of normal [ULN]. For serum values up to 3 times the ULN, recommended dosage titration may be continued; for serum values greater than 3, and up to 5 times the ULN, the dosage should be reduced by 40 mg per day; dosage titration and monitoring every other week may be resumed when ALT [SGPT] serum values return to within normal limits; for serum values greater than 5 times the ULN, tacrine should be discontinued and the patient should be closely monitored for signs and symptoms of hepatitis; rechallenge may be considered when ALT [SGPT] serum values return to within normal limits)

Note: Experience rechallenging patients who have had ALT (SGPT) serum values greater than 10 times the ULN is limited; risk versus demonstrated benefit should be considered. Patients who have experienced tacrine treatment–related jaundice confirmed by elevated total bilirubin greater than 3 mg per dL (mg/dL) and patients exhibiting clinical signs of hypersensitivity, such as rash or fever, in association with ALT (SGPT) serum value elevations *should permanently discontinue and not be rechallenged* with tacrine.

## Side/Adverse Effects
The following side/adverse effects have been selected on the basis of their potential clinical significance (possible signs and symptoms in parentheses where appropriate)—not necessarily inclusive:

### Those indicating need for medical attention
Incidence more frequent
*Ataxia* (clumsiness or unsteadiness); ***gastrointestinal toxicity, specifically anorexia*** (loss of appetite); ***diarrhea, nausea, or vomiting; hepatotoxicity (50%)*** (change in stool color [rare]; fever [infrequent]; yellow eyes or skin [rare])

Note: Approximately 50% of all patients started on tacrine will develop elevated transaminase serum values, usually within 12 weeks of initiation of therapy. Approximately 25% of all patients started on tacrine will develop transaminase serum values more than 3 times the upper limit of normal (ULN) and will require dosage reduction or discontinuation of tacrine. Females are at greater risk than males for developing transaminase elevation. Rarely, clinical signs of hepatotoxicity emerge, such as jaundice and fever. Liver biopsies in these patients have revealed granulomatous changes and hepatocellular necrosis. In cases of hepatotoxicity reported to date, liver function tests have returned to normal, usually within six weeks of dosage reduction or discontinuation of tacrine.

Incidence less frequent
***Cardiovascular effects, specifically bradycardia*** (slow heartbeat); ***hypertension*** (high blood pressure); ***hypotension*** (low blood pressure); ***or palpitation*** (fast or pounding heartbeat); ***skin rash; syncope*** (fainting)

Incidence rare
***Asthma*** (cough; tightness in chest; trouble in breathing; wheezing); ***convulsions*** (seizures)—associated with cholinergic effects, particularly diarrhea; ***mood or mental changes, specifically aggression, irritability, or nervousness; parkinsonian extrapyramidal effects*** (stiffness of arms or legs; slow movement; trembling and shaking of hands and fingers); ***tachycardia*** (fast heartbeat); ***urinary obstruction*** (trouble in urinating)

### Those indicating need for medical attention only if they continue or are bothersome
Incidence more frequent
***Dizziness; gastrointestinal effects, specifically abdominal pain or cramping, or dyspepsia*** (indigestion); ***headache; myalgia*** (muscle pain)

Incidence less frequent
> *Belching; flushing of skin; hyperventilation* (fast breathing); *insomnia* (trouble in sleeping); *lacrimation, increased* (watering of eyes); *malaise* (general feeling of discomfort or illness); *peripheral edema* (swelling of feet or lower legs); *polyuria* (frequent urination or increased volume of urine); *rhinitis* (runny nose); *salivation, increased* (watering of mouth); *sweating, increased*

## Overdose
For specific information on the agents used in the management of tacrine overdose, see:
- *Atropine sulfate* in *Anticholinergics/Antispasmodics (Systemic)* monograph.

For more information on the management of overdose or unintentional ingestion, **contact a Poison Control Center** (see *Poison Control Center Listing*).

### Clinical effects of overdose
The following effects have been selected on the basis of their potential clinical significance (possible signs and symptoms in parentheses where appropriate)—not necessarily inclusive:
> *Cardiovascular effects, specifically bradycardia* (slow heartbeat); *hypotension* (low blood pressure); *or shock* (fast weak pulse; irregular breathing; large pupils); *convulsions* (seizures); *muscular weakness, increasing*—may lead to death if respiratory muscles are involved; *nausea, severe; salivation, excessive* (watering of mouth); *sweating, excessive; vomiting, severe*

### Treatment of overdose
Specific treatment—Administering intravenous atropine sulfate, initial dose 1 to 2 mg, with subsequent doses based on clinical response.

Supportive care—Providing supportive therapy. Patients in whom intentional overdose is confirmed or suspected should be referred for psychiatric consultation.

## Patient Consultation
As an aid to patient consultation, refer to *Advice for the Patient, Tacrine (Systemic)*.

In providing consultation, consider emphasizing the following selected information (» = major clinical significance):

### Before using this medication
» Conditions affecting use, especially:
  Hypersensitivity to tacrine or other acridine derivatives
  Other medications, especially cimetidine, neuromuscular blocking agents, NSAIDs, smoking tobacco, and theophylline
  Other medical problems, especially asthma, cardiovascular conditions (such as bradycardia, hypotension, or sick sinus syndrome), epilepsy or history of seizures, gastrointestinal or urinary tract obstruction, head injury with loss of consciousness, hepatic function impairment, increased intracranial pressure, intracranial lesions, Parkinson's disease, peptic ulcer, and unstable metabolic disorders

### Proper use of this medication
» Not taking more medication than the amount prescribed because of increased risk of adverse effects
  Taking tacrine on empty stomach if tolerated
  Taking doses at regular intervals for maximum efficacy
» Proper dosing
  Missed dose: taking as soon as possible; not taking if within 2 hours of time for next dose; not doubling doses
» Proper storage

### Precautions while using this medication
» Importance of complying with monitoring schedule and keeping appointments with physician and/or laboratory
  Informing physician when new symptoms arise or when previously noted symptoms increase in severity
  Caution if any kind of surgery or emergency treatment is required; informing physician or dentist in charge that tacrine is being taken
  Caution if dizziness, clumsiness, or unsteadiness occurs
» Not decreasing dose or discontinuing treatment without consulting physician because of possible decline in cognitive function and behavioral disturbances
» Suspected overdose: Getting emergency help at once

### Side/adverse effects
Ataxia; gastrointestinal toxicity, specifically anorexia, diarrhea, nausea, or vomiting; hepatotoxicity; cardiovascular effects, specifically bradycardia, hypertension, hypotension, or palpitation; convulsions; skin rash; syncope; asthma; mood or mental changes, specifically aggression, irritability, or nervousness; parkinsonian extrapyramidal effects; tachycardia; urinary obstruction

## General Dosing Information
Tacrine should be taken on an empty stomach (either 1 hour before meals or 2 hours after meals) for more complete absorption. However, if stomach upset occurs, tacrine may be taken with food.

Tacrine should be taken at regular intervals for best effect.

The rate of dosage escalation may be slowed in patients who are having difficulty tolerating the recommended dosage escalation schedule. However, *dosage escalation should not be accelerated*, or the incidence of serious adverse effects may be increased.

The first dosage increase should not be made earlier than 6 weeks after initiation of tacrine therapy because of the possibility of delayed transaminase elevation.

The patient should be carefully observed for side effects following initiation of therapy and following every dosage increase.

Abrupt discontinuation of tacrine or a decrease of 80 mg or greater in daily tacrine dose has caused decreased cognitive function and behavioral disturbances.

## Oral Dosage Forms
Note: The available dosage form contains tacrine hydrochloride, but dosage and strength are expressed in terms of the base.

### TACRINE CAPSULES

**Usual adult dose**
Alzheimer's dementia—
  Oral, initially 10 mg (base) four times a day. After at least six weeks, if there are no significant transaminase elevations and the patient is tolerating treatment, the dose may be increased to 20 mg four times a day. Further increases to 30 mg four times a day, and then to 40 mg four times a day may be instituted at intervals of at least six weeks, based on patient tolerance.

If elevations of serum transaminase occur, tacrine dosage should be modified. Recommended modifications are:

| Transaminase Serum Value (times Upper Limit of Normal [ULN]) | Treatment Regimen Modification |
|---|---|
| ≤ 3 | No modification. |
| > 3 to ≤ 5 | Reduce the daily dose of tacrine by 40 mg per day. Resume dose titration when transaminase serum values return to within normal limits. |
| > 5 | Stop tacrine treatment. Monitor transaminase serum values until within normal limits. Consider rechallenge with tacrine. |
| > 10 | Rechallenge experience is limited with these patients. Risk versus demonstrated benefit should be considered. |

Note: For rechallenge: Dose titration schedule is the same as that for new patients. However, ALT (SGPT) serum values should be monitored weekly for the first 16 weeks following re-initiation of tacrine therapy. If unacceptable elevations in ALT (SGPT) serum values do not recur, monitoring frequency may be decreased to monthly for 2 months and every 3 months thereafter.

Patients who have experienced tacrine treatment–related jaundice confirmed by elevated total bilirubin greater than 3 mg per dL (mg/dL) and patients exhibiting clinical signs of hypersensitivity, such as rash or fever, in association with ALT (SGPT) serum value elevations *should permanently discontinue and not be rechallenged* with tacrine.

**Usual adult prescribing limits**
Up to 160 mg a day.

**Usual pediatric dose**
Safety and efficacy have not been established.

**Usual geriatric dose**
See *Usual adult dose*.

**Strength(s) usually available**
U.S.—
  10 mg (base) (Rx) [*Cognex* (hydrous lactose; magnesium stearate; microcrystalline cellulose; gelatin NF; silicon dioxide NF; sodium lauryl sulfate NF; D&C Yellow #10; FD&C Green #3; titanium dioxide)].
  20 mg (base) (Rx) [*Cognex* (hydrous lactose; magnesium stearate; microcrystalline cellulose; gelatin NF; silicon dioxide NF; sodium lau-

ryl sulfate NF; D&C Yellow #10; FD&C Blue #1; titanium dioxide)].

30 mg (base) (Rx) [*Cognex* (hydrous lactose; magnesium stearate; microcrystalline cellulose; gelatin NF; silicon dioxide NF; sodium lauryl sulfate NF; D&C Yellow #10; FD&C Blue #1; FD&C Red #40; titanium dioxide)].

40 mg (base) (Rx) [*Cognex* (hydrous lactose; magnesium stearate; microcrystalline cellulose; gelatin NF; silicon dioxide NF; sodium lauryl sulfate NF; D&C Yellow #10; FD&C Blue #1; FD&C Red #40; D&C Red #28; titanium dioxide)].

Canada—
Not commercially available.
Note: Tacrine may be available from the manufacturer through a compassionate use program.

**Packaging and storage**
Store below 40 °C (104 °F), preferably between 15 and 30 °C (59 and 86 °F), in a well-closed container, away from moisture, unless otherwise specified by manufacturer.

**Preparation of dosage form**
For patients who cannot take oral solids—Tacrine capsules may be dissolved in any aqueous solution. However, orange juice will best mask the bitter taste of the medication. The capsule should be placed in the liquid intact to avoid loss of medication through spillage. Some excipients may remain undissolved. Prepare each dose as needed; do not store solution for later use.

**Auxiliary labeling**
- Take on empty stomach.
- May cause dizziness.
- Take exactly as directed.

**Selected Bibliography**
Freeman SE, Dawson RM. Tacrine: A pharmacological review. Prog Neurobiol 1991; 36: 257-77.
Knapp MJ, Knopman DS, Solomon PR, et al. A 30-week randomized controlled trial of high-dose tacrine in patients with Alzheimer's Disease. JAMA 1994 Apr 6; 271(13): 985-91.

Developed: 08/05/94
Interim revision: 08/24/95

# TACROLIMUS Systemic

JAN: Tacrolimus Hydrate.
VA CLASSIFICATION (Primary): IM600
Commonly used brand name(s): *Prograf.*
Another commonly used name is FK 506.
Note: For a listing of dosage forms and brand names by country availability, see *Dosage Forms* section(s).

## Category
Immunosuppressant.

## Indications
Note: Bracketed information in the *Indications* section refers to uses that are not included in U.S. product labeling.

**Accepted**
Transplant rejection, solid organ (prophylaxis)—Tacrolimus is useful for the prevention of rejection of transplanted [heart][1], kidney[1], liver, [lung][1], [pancreas][1], and [small bowel][1] allografts.

[Transplant rejection, solid organ (treatment)]—Tacrolimus is useful for the treatment of rejection of transplanted heart[1], kidney[1], liver, lung[1], pancreas[1], and small bowel[1] allografts.

[Graft-versus-host disease (prophylaxis)][1] or
[Graft-versus-host disease (treatment)][1]—Tacrolimus is useful for the prevention and treatment of graft-versus-host disease in patients receiving bone marrow transplants.

[Uveitis, severe, refractory (treatment)][1]—Tacrolimus is useful for the treatment of severe, refractory uveitis.

**Acceptance not established**
Tacrolimus has been studied for the treatment of *atopic dermatitis*, *nephrotic syndrome*, *pediatric autoimmune enteropathy*, *primary sclerosing cholangitis*, *psoriasis*, *psoriatic arthritis*, and *pyoderma gangrenosum*. More data are needed to assess the place in therapy of tacrolimus for these indications.

There have been additional reports of the use of tacrolimus for other conditions, including:
- *alopecia universalis*;
- *autoimmune chronic active hepatitis*;
- *inflammatory bowel disease*;
- *multiple sclerosis*;
- *primary biliary cirrhosis*; and
- *scleroderma*.

The use of tacrolimus for these conditions cannot be assessed at this time.

[1]Not included in Canadian product labeling.

## Pharmacology/Pharmacokinetics

**Physicochemical characteristics**
Source—
Tacrolimus is a macrolide immunosuppressant produced by *Streptomyces tsukubaensis*.
Molecular weight—822.05.

Solubility—Freely soluble in ethanol; very soluble in chloroform and methanol; practically insoluble in water

**Mechanism of action/Effect**
Tacrolimus inhibits T-lymphocyte activation. This may occur through formation of a complex with FK 506-binding proteins (FKBPs). The complex inhibits calcineurin phosphatase. This is believed to inhibit interleukin-2 (IL-2) gene expression in T-helper lymphocytes.
Tacrolimus also binds to the steroid receptor–associated heat-shock protein 56. This ultimately results in inhibition of transcription of proinflammatory cytokines such as granulocyte–macrophage colony-stimulating factor (GM-CSF), interleukin-1 (IL-1), interleukin-3 (IL-3), interleukin-4 (IL-4), interleukin-5 (IL-5), interleukin-6 (IL-6), interleukin-8 (IL-8), and tumor necrosis factor alpha (TNF alpha).

**Absorption**
Rapid, variable, and incomplete from the gastrointestinal tract; the mean bioavailability of the oral dosage form is 27%, range 5 to 65%; rate of absorption is decreased in the presence of food, but the extent of absorption may or may not be affected, depending on the type of food ingested.
Pediatric patients may have decreased bioavailability as compared to adult patients.

**Distribution**
The volume of distribution (Vol$_D$) when based on plasma obtained from blood samples at 37 °C (98.6 °F) is 5 to 65 L per kg of body weight (L/kg). The Vol$_D$ based on plasma concentration is much higher than the Vol$_D$ based on whole blood concentrations, the difference reflecting the binding of tacrolimus to the red blood cells. The mean Vol$_D$ for patients with liver allografts when measured in whole blood is 0.9 L/kg.

**Protein binding**
High to very high (75 to 99%), primarily to albumin and alpha$_1$-acid glycoprotein.

**Biotransformation**
Hepatic, extensive, primarily by the cytochrome P450 3A enzymes.

**Half-life**
Distribution—
0.9 hour.
Elimination—
Biphasic, variable: Terminal—11.3 hours (range, 3.5 to 40.5 hours).

**Time to peak concentration**
0.5 to 4 hours after oral administration.
Note: The rate of absorption is reduced when tacrolimus is given with food.

**Peak serum concentration**
Plasma or blood—Whole blood concentrations may be 12 to 67 times the plasma concentrations.

**Elimination**
Tacrolimus is eliminated by metabolism. Less than 1% of the dose is eliminated unchanged in urine.
Pediatric patients may have increased clearance as compared with adult patients.

## Tacrolimus (Systemic)

In dialysis—
Tacrolimus is not removed by dialysis.

## Precautions to Consider

### Cross-sensitivity and/or related problems
Patients allergic to castor oil derivatives may be allergic to the injectable dosage form of tacrolimus also, since the injection contains a polyoxyl 60 hydrogenated castor oil vehicle.

### Carcinogenicity
Tacrolimus is associated with an increased risk of malignancy, especially lymphomas and skin malignancies. The increased risk is attributed to the intensity and duration of immunosuppression. The incidence of lymphomas is comparable to that observed with cyclosporine-based immunosuppressive regimens.

### Tumorigenicity
Studies in mice and rats did not show a relationship between the dose of tacrolimus and the incidence of tumors.

### Mutagenicity
Mutagenicity was not observed in bacterial or Chinese hamster cell *in vitro* testing, or *in vivo* tests performed in mice or rat hepatocytes.

### Pregnancy/Reproduction
Fertility—Adequate and well-controlled studies have not been done in humans.

Pregnancy—Tacrolimus crosses the placenta. Pregnancy in patients treated with tacrolimus is possible, with low incidences of hypertension and pre-eclampsia. The use of tacrolimus during pregnancy is associated with premature birth, and hyperkalemia and reversible renal function impairment in neonates. One case of intrauterine growth retardation has been reported. In one series, 27 pregnancies in 21 liver transplant recipients managed with tacrolimus did not result in the loss of any allografts. Prenatal growth and postnatal infant growth for postpartum age were normal. Two of the 27 infants died after being delivered at 23 and 24 weeks gestation. The unsuccessful pregnancies were conceived a few weeks and 11.7 months following the liver transplantations.

Studies in rats showed that tacrolimus use during organogenesis was associated with an increase in late fetal resorptions and a decrease in the number of live births.

FDA Pregnancy Category C.

### Breast-feeding
Tacrolimus is distributed into breast milk. Breast-feeding should be avoided during tacrolimus therapy.

### Pediatrics
Pediatric patients require higher doses of tacrolimus per kg of body weight to maintain trough concentrations similar to those of adult patients. Pediatric patients may have decreased bioavailability and increased clearance as compared with adult patients.

Post-transplant lymphoproliferative disorder (PTLD) may be more common in pediatric patients than in adult patients, especially in pediatric patients up to 3 years of age.

### Geriatrics
No information is available on the relationship of age to the effects of tacrolimus in geriatric patients. Tacrolimus has been used in geriatric patients undergoing transplantation; however, information has not been published on the age-related effects of tacrolimus in these patients. Elderly patients are more likely to have age-related renal function impairment, which may require adjustment of dosage.

### Dental
The immunosuppressive effects of tacrolimus may result in an increased incidence of certain microbial infections and delayed healing. Dental work, whenever possible, should be completed prior to initiation of therapy and undertaken with caution during therapy. Patients should be instructed in proper oral hygiene.

### Drug interactions and/or related problems
The following drug interactions and/or related problems have been selected on the basis of their potential clinical significance (possible mechanism in parentheses where appropriate)—not necessarily inclusive (» = major clinical significance):

Note: Combinations containing any of the following medications, depending on the amount present, may also interact with this medication.

The drug interactions between tacrolimus and clarithromycin, clotrimazole, danazol, erythromycin, fluconazole, hyperkalemia-causing medications, nephrotoxic medications, and rifampin have been observed clinically in patients. The drug interactions between tacrolimus and aluminum hydroxide gel, bromocriptine, cimetidine, cyclosporine, dexamethasone, diltiazem, ethinyl estradiol, itraconazole, ketoconazole, magnesium oxide, nifedipine, omeprazole, sodium bicarbonate, and verapamil have been demonstrated *in vitro* or in experimental animal models.

The extent of induction or inhibition of cytochrome P450 enzymes may depend on the dose of the inducer or inhibitor.

Aluminum hydroxide gel
(adsorbs tacrolimus; may lead to reduced blood concentrations of tacrolimus)

Bromocriptine or
Cimetidine or
Clarithromycin or
Clotrimazole or
» Danazol or
Diltiazem or
Ethinyl estradiol or
» Erythromycin or
» Fluconazole or
» Itraconazole or
» Ketoconazole or
Nifedipine or
Omeprazole or
Verapamil
(may inhibit the metabolism of tacrolimus, leading to increased tacrolimus blood concentrations and toxicity; some agents inhibiting the metabolism of tacrolimus [e.g., azole antifungal agents and calcium channel blocking agents] may be used therapeutically so that lower doses of tacrolimus can be used)

Note: No interaction between fluconazole and tacrolimus was noted in one study in which the medications were administered intravenously to patients receiving bone marrow transplantation. The mechanism of this interaction may be inhibition of metabolism of tacrolimus in the gut, leading to increased absorption. This interaction may not occur to the same extent when tacrolimus is given intravenously as when it is given orally.

Dexamethasone or
» Rifampin
(may induce cytochrome P450 3A enzymes, leading to increased metabolism of tacrolimus and lower blood concentrations)

» Cyclosporine
(increased immunosuppression; tacrolimus may increase the bioavailability of cyclosporine, or may inhibit the metabolism of cyclosporine, leading to increased cyclosporine blood concentrations and toxicity; increased risk of nephrotoxicity with concurrent use)

Hyperkalemia-causing medications (see *Appendix II*), especially:
» Diuretics, potassium-sparing
(concurrent use with tacrolimus may result in hyperkalemia)

Magnesium oxide or
Sodium bicarbonate
(tacrolimus is degraded by an alkaline environment, resulting in decreased bioavailability of tacrolimus; the same interaction may occur with other antacids; a single-dose study examining the effect of magnesium oxide did not show decreased bioavailability)

Muromonab-CD3
(increased incidence of post-transplant lymphoproliferative disorder [PTLD] with concurrent use)

Nephrotoxic medications (see *Appendix II*), such as:
Aminoglycosides or
Amphotericin B or
Anti-inflammatory drugs, nonsteroidal or
Vancomycin
(may be additive or synergistic impairment of renal function)

Vaccines, killed virus
(immune response to vaccines may be decreased)

» Vaccines, live virus
(the immunosuppressive effect of tacrolimus may potentiate the replication of the vaccine virus, may increase the side/adverse effect of the vaccine, and/or may decrease the immune response to the vaccine)

### Laboratory value alterations
The following have been selected on the basis of their potential clinical significance (possible effect in parentheses where appropriate)—not necessarily inclusive (» = major clinical significance):

With physiology/laboratory test values
Alanine aminotransferase (ALT [SGPT]) and
Alkaline phosphatase and
Aspartate aminotransferase (AST [SGOT])
(values may be increased; may indicate hepatotoxicity)

Bilirubin, serum
(concentrations may be increased; may indicate hepatotoxicity)
Blood urea nitrogen (BUN) and
» Creatinine, serum
(concentrations may be increased; may indicate nephrotoxicity)
Calcium and
» Magnesium, serum
(concentrations may be decreased)
Cholesterol, serum
(values may be increased)
» Glucose, blood and
Triglycerides, serum
(concentrations may be increased)
Hematocrit value and
Hemoglobin concentration
(may be decreased)
Leukocytes (neutrophils [WBC])
(blood counts may be increased or decreased)
Platelets
(blood counts may be decreased)
Phosphate and
» Potassium
(serum concentrations may be increased)

**Medical considerations/Contraindications**
The medical considerations/contraindications included have been selected on the basis of their potential clinical significance (reasons given in parentheses where appropriate)—not necessarily inclusive (» = major clinical significance).

*Except under special circumstances, this medication should not be used when the following medical problems exist:*
» Allergy to polyoxyl 60 hydrogenated castor oil
(patients with an allergy to castor oil derivatives may be allergic to tacrolimus injection also, since tacrolimus injection has a castor oil vehicle; intravenous administration of castor oil derivatives has been associated with anaphylactic reactions; the use of tacrolimus injection in patients with an allergy to castor oil derivatives is contraindicated)
» Allergy to tacrolimus, history of
» Malignancy, current
(Tacrolimus use is associated with an increased susceptibility to malignancies)

*Risk-benefit should be considered when the following medical problems exist:*
» Chickenpox, existing or recent (including recent exposure) or
» Herpes zoster
risk of severe generalized disease
Diabetes mellitus
(risk of loss of glucose control)
Hepatic function impairment or
Hepatitis B or C infection, chronic or
» Renal function impairment
(dosage reduction may be required; patients with post-transplant hepatic function impairment may have an increased risk of renal toxicity when taking tacrolimus)
Hyperkalemia
(tacrolimus may exacerbate hyperkalemia)
» Infection
(immunosuppression may exacerbate infections)
Neurologic function impairment
(dosage reduction may be required)

**Patient monitoring**
The following may be especially important in patient monitoring (other tests may be warranted in some patients, depending on condition; » = major clinical significance):
Note: Monitoring intervals may need to be altered based on the condition of the patient.
Alanine aminotransferase (ALT [SGPT]) and
Alkaline phosphatase and
Aspartate aminotransferase (AST [SGOT]) and
Bilirubin, serum
(recommended periodically to monitor hepatic function; more frequent monitoring required in the early post-transplant period)
Blood urea nitrogen (BUN) and
» Creatinine, serum
(recommended to monitor for nephrotoxicity; nephrotoxicity occurs most often in the early post-transplant period, especially if intravenous tacrolimus is administered)
» Blood pressure measurements
(frequent measurements recommended)
Calcium and
» Magnesium and
Phosphate and
» Potassium
(frequent monitoring recommended in the early post-transplant period; periodic monitoring recommended thereafter)
Cholesterol, serum and
Triglycerides, serum
(periodic monitoring recommended)
Complete blood counts (CBCs)
(monitoring of CBC recommended to detect tacrolimus-induced blood dyscrasias; changes in the neutrophil count may also indicate infection)
» Glucose, blood
(frequent monitoring recommended in the early post-transplant period; periodic monitoring recommended thereafter)
» Tacrolimus concentrations, whole blood, trough
(target blood concentrations vary depending on the indication and the transplant center protocol; trough whole blood concentrations of 10 to 20 mcg per mL [mcg/mL] [12.2 to 24.4 micromoles per L (micromoles/L)] are used by some centers in the first month following transplantation; for the subsequent 2 months, lower blood concentrations [i.e., 5 to 15 mcg/mL (6.1 to 18.3 micromoles/L)] are often recommended; after 3 months some centers lower the target blood concentrations to 5 to 10 mcg/mL [6.1 to 12.2 micromoles/L]; higher concentrations are used in intestinal transplantation)
(target blood concentrations vary for pediatric patients, depending on indication and transplant center; for liver transplantation, a consortium of transplant centers recommends trough concentrations of 12 to 15 mcg/L [14.6 to 18.3 micromoles/L] in the first month following transplantation, 10 to 12 mcg/L [12.2 to 14.6 micromoles/L] for the subsequent 2 months, and 5 to 10 mcg/L [6.1 to 12.2 micromoles/L] thereafter; for renal transplantation, one transplant center recommends trough blood concentrations of 20 to 25 mcg/L [24.4 to 30.5 micromoles/L] in the first 2 weeks following transplantation, 15 to 20 mcg/mL [18.3 to 24.4 micromoles/L] for the second 2 weeks following transplantation, 10 to 15 mcg/L [12.2 to 18.3 micromoles/L] for the following 3 months, and 5 to 9 mcg/L [6.1 to 11 micromoles/L] thereafter)
(trough blood concentrations should be measured frequently in the early post-transplant period; tacrolimus blood concentrations often are measured daily until good graft function and good renal function are achieved, and then every other day during the early post-transplant hospitalization; concentrations should be measured after adjustment in the tacrolimus dose, and after the addition or removal of medications that may alter tacrolimus absorption or clearance)
(high tacrolimus blood concentrations are correlated with toxicity; low tacrolimus blood concentrations are not as well-correlated with episodes of rejection; tacrolimus blood concentrations should always be considered in conjunction with the patient's clinical condition when assessing the adequacy of the tacrolimus dose)

## Side/Adverse Effects

Note: Hyperglycemia, nephrotoxicity, and neurotoxicity are the most significant adverse effects resulting from the use of tacrolimus. Other adverse effects (e.g., infection, post-transplant lymphoproliferative disorder [PTLD]) result from the degree of immunosuppression, not specifically from the use of tacrolimus.

The following side/adverse effects have been selected on the basis of their potential clinical significance (possible signs and symptoms in parentheses where appropriate)—not necessarily inclusive:

**Those indicating need for medical attention**
Incidence more frequent
*Asthenia* (loss of energy or weakness); *blood dyscrasias including red cell aplasia* (fever and sore throat; pale skin; unusual bleeding or bruising; unusual tiredness or weakness); *gastrointestinal disturbance, including abdominal pain; diarrhea; loss of appetite; nausea; vomiting; hyperglycemia* (frequent urination); *hyperkalemia* (abdominal pain; nausea or vomiting; weakness); *hypomagnesemia* (muscle trembling or twitching); *infection* (fever or chills); *nephrotoxicity; neurotoxicity, including abnormal dreams; agitation; anxiety; confusion; depression; dizziness; hallucinations* (seeing or hearing things that are not there); *headache; insomnia* (trouble in sleeping); *nervousness; sei-*

zures; *tremor* (trembling and shaking of hands); *paresthesia* (tingling); *peripheral edema* (swelling of ankles, feet, or lower legs); *pleural effusion* (shortness of breath); *pruritus* (itching); *skin rash*

Incidence less frequent
*Cardiovascular effects, including cardiomyopathy* (shortness of breath); *chest pain; hyperlipidemia; hypertension; hyperesthesia* (increased sensitivity to pain); *muscle cramps; neuropathy* (numbness or pain in legs); *osteoporosis; sweating; tinnitus* (ringing in ears); *visual disturbance* (blurred vision)

Incidence rare
*Anaphylaxis* (flushing of face or neck; shortness of breath; wheezing)—with parenteral use; *hepatotoxicity* (flu-like symptoms); *PTLD* (fever; general feeling of discomfort and illness; weight loss)

Note: PTLD may be more common in pediatric patients than in adult patients, especially in pediatric patients up to 3 years of age.

## Overdose

For more information on the management of overdose or unintentional ingestion, **contact a Poison Control Center** (see *Poison Control Center Listing*).

**Clinical effects of overdose**
Early clinical trials used doses of tacrolimus that were later determined to be overdoses. The patients experienced the same side effects as patients receiving lower doses, but the incidence of these effects was greater in patients receiving higher doses of tacrolimus. The patients receiving the overdoses of tacrolimus experienced more new-onset diabetes, nephrotoxicity, and neurotoxicity as compared to patients receiving lower doses.

There is limited literature on the effects of massive overdoses of tacrolimus in humans. Overdoses of up to 7 mg per kg of body weight (mg/kg) have been reported. Most patients did not develop symptoms associated with the overdose.

In toxicity studies in rats, mortalities first occurred at intravenous doses 16 times the recommended human dose.

**Treatment of overdose**
Treatment is symptomatic and supportive. Clearance of tacrolimus cannot be enhanced by dialysis because tacrolimus is extensively bound to erythrocytes and plasma proteins.

Patients in whom intentional overdose is confirmed or suspected should be referred for psychiatric consultation.

## Patient Consultation

As an aid to patient consultation, refer to *Advice for the Patient, Tacrolimus (Systemic)*.

In providing consultation, consider emphasizing the following selected information (» = major clinical significance):

**Before using this medication**
» Conditions affecting use, especially:
  Allergy to tacrolimus or castor oil derivatives
  Carcinogenicity—Use of tacrolimus is associated with an increased incidence of malignancy
  Pregnancy—Tacrolimus crosses the placenta; transplant patients should not conceive shortly after transplantation or while being treated for transplant-related complications
  Breast-feeding—Tacrolimus is distributed into breast milk; breast-feeding should be avoided
  Dental—Dental work should be completed prior to initiation of therapy whenever possible
  Other medications, especially cyclosporine, danazol, erythromycin, fluconazole, itraconazole, ketoconazole, potassium-sparing diuretics, or rifampin
  Other medical problems, especially allergy to polyoxyl 60 hydrogenated castor oil, chickenpox, current malignancy, herpes zoster infection, or renal function impairment

**Proper use of this medication**
» Importance of not using more or less medication than the amount prescribed
  Getting into the habit of taking at the same time each day and in a consistent relationship to the type and timing of the intake of food to help increase compliance and maintain steady blood concentrations
» Checking with physician before discontinuing or changing medication; possible need for lifelong therapy
» Proper dosing
  Missed dose: Taking as soon as possible if remembered within 12 hours; not taking if almost time for next dose; not doubling doses
» Proper storage

**Precautions while using this medication**
» Importance of close monitoring by physician
  Maintaining good dental hygiene and seeing dentist frequently for teeth cleaning
» Not eating raw oysters or other shellfish; making sure they are fully cooked before eating
» Continuing recommended vaccination schedule (except for live vaccines)
» Avoiding exposure to chickenpox, measles, mumps, and rubella; if exposed, seeing physician for prophylactic therapy
  Not traveling to another country without making sure a supply of tacrolimus will be available
  Not eating grapefruit or drinking grapefruit juice

**Side/adverse effects**
Signs of potential side effects, especially asthenia, blood dyscrasias, abdominal pain, diarrhea, loss of appetite, nausea, vomiting, hyperglycemia, hyperkalemia, hypomagnesemia, infection, nephrotoxicity, abnormal dreams, agitation, anxiety, confusion, depression, dizziness, hallucinations, headache, insomnia, nervousness, seizures, tremor, paresthesia, peripheral edema, pleural effusion, pruritus, skin rash, cardiomyopathy, chest pain, hyperlipidemia, hypertension, hyperesthesia, muscle cramps, neuropathy, osteoporosis, sweating, tinnitus, visual disturbance, anaphylaxis, hepatotoxicity, and post-transplant lymphoproliferative disorder

## General Dosing Information

Dosage regimens for tacrolimus vary among transplant centers. Dosage of tacrolimus should be adjusted based on the clinical response of each patient. Whole blood trough concentrations can be used as a guide to appropriate dosing. High whole blood trough concentrations are associated with an increase in toxicity.

Tacrolimus usually is used in conjunction with other immunosuppressants (e.g., corticosteroids and azathioprine). Corticosteroids typically are tapered following transplantation to target doses of prednisone for adult patients of 2.5 to 5 mg per day six months after transplantation. In some cases, it may be possible to wean the patient from other immunosuppressants and maintain the patient on tacrolimus monotherapy.

When converting from cyclosporine to tacrolimus, it is recommended that cyclosporine be discontinued 24 hours before initiating tacrolimus therapy. In some transplant centers, cyclosporine whole blood concentrations are measured, and tacrolimus therapy started if cyclosporine concentrations are less than 100 micrograms per liter (mcg/L).

Patients receiving lower-quality hepatic allografts or with poor early hepatic graft function should receive lower doses of tacrolimus initially. Liver transplant patients with poor hepatic graft function have increased risk for developing renal function impairment.

Antiviral prophylaxis, i.e., with acyclovir, ganciclovir, and immune globulins, may be advisable for some patients receiving tacrolimus, especially cytomegalovirus (CMV) prophylaxis in patients who have not been exposed to CMV prior to transplantation who receive a CMV-positive graft.

Vaccination schedules should be continued, except for live vaccines. Vaccinations against hepatitis A and B are recommended. Inactivated poliovirus vaccine should be used instead of oral poliovirus vaccine for both the patient and for people living in the same household as the patient. Vaccines given to immunosuppressed patients may not result in a protective antibody response. Protective antibody concentrations should be checked after the vaccine has been administered.

If a patient is exposed to measles, mumps, rubella, or varicella for the first time while receiving tacrolimus, the patient should receive prophylactic therapy with immune globulin, i.e., pooled human immune globulin or varicella immune globulin.

**For parenteral dosage forms only**
Because parenteral tacrolimus is associated with the development of more adverse effects, including anaphylaxis and renal function impairment, than is oral tacrolimus, parenteral tacrolimus should be used only in patients unable to take tacrolimus orally. When receiving parenteral tacrolimus, patients should be monitored closely for anaphylaxis, especially during the first 30 minutes of the infusion. Patients receiving tacrolimus parenterally should be switched to oral tacrolimus as soon as it can be tolerated.

**Diet/Nutrition**
The rate of absorption of oral tacrolimus is decreased in the presence of food, but the extent of absorption may or may not be affected, depending on the type of food ingested. Tacrolimus should be given consistently with relation to food.

Bioavailability of tacrolimus may be increased by ingestion of grapefruit or grapefruit juice, resulting in toxic blood concentrations of tacrolimus.

Raw oysters or other shellfish may contain bacteria that can cause serious illness, and possibly death. Even eating oysters from "clean" water or good restaurants does not guarantee that the oysters do not contain the bacteria. Symptoms of this infection include sudden chills, fever, nausea, vomiting, blood poisoning, and sometimes death. Eating raw shellfish is not a problem for most healthy people; however, patients with the following conditions may be at greater risk: cancer, immune disorders, immunosuppression following organ transplantation, long-term corticosteroid use (as for asthma, arthritis, or prevention of graft rejection in organ transplantation), liver disease (including viral hepatitis), excessive alcohol intake (two to three drinks or more per day), diabetes, stomach problems (including previous stomach surgery and low stomach acid), and hemochromatosis.

### For treatment of adverse effects
Recommended treatment consists of the following:
• Many adverse effects (e.g., cardiomyopathy, gastrointestinal toxicity, hyperglycemia, hyperkalemia, hypomagnesemia, nephrotoxicity, neurotoxicity, pruritus, rash) may respond to a reduction in dose. If adverse effects do not respond to a reduction in dose, it may be advisable to convert the patient to a cyclosporine-based immunosuppressant regimen.

## Oral Dosage Forms
Note: Bracketed uses in the *Dosage Forms* section refer to categories of use and/or indications that are not included in U.S. product labeling.

### TACROLIMUS CAPSULES

#### Usual adult and adolescent dose
Transplant rejection, liver (prophylaxis) or
Transplant rejection, kidney (prophylaxis)[1] or
[Transplant rejection, solid organ, other (prophylaxis)][1] or
[Transplant rejection, liver (treatment)] or
[Transplant rejection, solid organ, other (treatment)][1]—
  Oral, 0.1 to 0.15 mg per kg of body weight per day, in two divided doses, initially. The dose should be adjusted based on trough blood concentrations.
[Graft-versus-host disease (prophylaxis)][1]—
  Oral, 0.12 mg per kg of body weight per day in two divided doses, starting when the patient can tolerate oral medications. The dose should be adjusted based on trough blood concentrations.
[Graft-versus-host disease (treatment)][1]—
  Oral, 0.3 mg per kg of body weight per day in two divided doses, starting when the patient can tolerate oral medications. The dose should be adjusted based on trough blood concentrations.
  Tacrolimus is used as part of a regimen to treat graft-versus-host disease. Other agents used to treat graft-versus-host disease may include methotrexate and/or corticosteroids.
[Uveitis, severe, refractory (treatment)][1]—
  Oral, 0.1 to 0.15 mg per kg of body weight per day in two divided doses.

#### Usual pediatric dose
Transplant rejection, liver (prophylaxis) or
Transplant rejection, kidney (prophylaxis)[1] or
[Transplant rejection, solid organ, other (prophylaxis)][1] or
[Transplant rejection, liver (treatment)] or
[Transplant rejection, solid organ, other (treatment)][1]—
  Oral, 0.1 to 0.3 mg per kg of body weight per day, in two divided doses, initially. The dose should be adjusted based on trough blood concentrations.
[Graft-versus-host disease (prophylaxis)][1]—
  See *Usual adult and adolescent dose*. Pediatric patients may require higher doses to attain therapeutic blood trough concentrations.
[Graft-versus-host disease (treatment)][1]—
  See *Usual adult and adolescent dose*. Pediatric patients may require higher doses to attain therapeutic blood trough concentrations.

#### Usual geriatric dose
See *Usual adult and adolescent dose*.

#### Strength(s) usually available
U.S.—
  1 mg (Rx) [*Prograf* (anhydrous; croscarmellose sodium; gelatin; hydroxypropyl methylcellulose; lactose; magnesium stearate; titanium dioxide)].
  5 mg (Rx) [*Prograf* (anhydrous; croscarmellose sodium; ferric oxide; gelatin; hydroxypropyl methylcellulose; lactose; magnesium stearate; titanium dioxide)].
Canada—
  1 mg (Rx) [*Prograf* (anhydrous; croscarmellose sodium; gelatin; hydroxypropyl methylcellulose; lactose; magnesium stearate; titanium dioxide)].
  5 mg (Rx) [*Prograf* (anhydrous; croscarmellose sodium; ferric oxide; gelatin; hydroxypropyl methylcellulose; lactose; magnesium stearate; titanium dioxide)].

#### Packaging and storage
Store between 15 and 30 °C (59 and 86 °F).

Note: Tacrolimus suspension has been extemporaneously compounded by mixing the contents of 5-mg capsules with equal amounts of Ora-Plus™, a suspending vehicle for oral extemporaneous preparations, and Simple Syrup NF, to a final concentration of 0.5 mg per mL (mg/mL). The extemporaneously prepared tacrolimus suspension was found to be stable for at least 56 days in glass and plastic amber bottles stored between 24 and 26 °C (75.2 and 78.8 °F). Bioavailability testing has not been performed using the extemporaneously compounded suspension.

## Parenteral Dosage Forms
Note: Bracketed uses in the *Dosage Forms* section refer to categories of use and/or indications that are not included in U.S. product labeling.

### TACROLIMUS FOR INJECTION
Note: Tacrolimus injection is intended for intravenous infusion only.
  Parenteral tacrolimus should be used only in patients unable to take tacrolimus orally. Patients receiving tacrolimus parenterally should be switched to oral tacrolimus as soon as it can be tolerated.

#### Usual adult and adolescent dose
Transplant rejection, liver (prophylaxis), in patients unable to take oral medications or
Transplant rejection, kidney (prophylaxis), in patients unable to take oral medications[1] or
[Transplant rejection, solid organ, other (prophylaxis), in patients unable to take oral medications][1] or
[Transplant rejection, liver (treatment), in patients unable to take oral medications] or
[Transplant rejection, solid organ, other (treatment), in patients unable to take oral medications][1]—
  Continuous intravenous infusion, 0.01 to 0.05 mg per kg of body weight per day, beginning no sooner than six hours after transplantation. The dose should be adjusted based on trough blood concentrations.
[Graft-versus-host disease (prophylaxis)][1]—
  Intravenous infusion, 0.04 mg per kg of body weight per day as a continuous infusion started the day prior to bone marrow transplantation. The dose should be adjusted based on trough blood concentrations.
[Graft-versus-host disease (treatment)][1]—
  Intravenous infusion, 0.1 mg per kg of body weight per day in two divided doses administered over four hours for each infusion. The dose should be adjusted based on trough blood concentrations.

#### Usual pediatric dose
Transplant rejection, liver (prophylaxis), in patients unable to take oral medications or
Transplant rejection, kidney (prophylaxis), in patients unable to take oral medications[1] or
[Transplant rejection, solid organ, other (prophylaxis), in patients unable to take oral medications][1] or
[Transplant rejection, liver (treatment), in patients unable to take oral medications] or
[Transplant rejection, solid organ, other (treatment), in patients unable to take oral medications][1]—
  See *Usual adult and adolescent dose*.
[Graft-versus-host disease (prophylaxis)][1]—
  See *Usual adult and adolescent dose*. Pediatric patients may require higher doses to attain therapeutic blood trough concentrations.
[Graft-versus-host disease (treatment)][1]—
  Intravenous infusion, 0.1 mg per kg of body weight per day as a continuous infusion.

#### Usual geriatric dose
See *Usual adult and adolescent dose*.

#### Strength(s) usually available
U.S.—
  5 mg per mL (Rx) [*Prograf* (anhydrous; alcohol 80% v/v; polyoxyl 60 hydrogenated castor oil 200 mg per mL)].
Canada—
  5 mg per mL (Rx) [*Prograf* (anhydrous; alcohol 80% v/v; polyoxyl 60 hydrogenated castor oil 200 mg per mL)].

**Packaging and storage**
Store between 5 and 25 °C (41 and 77 °F).

**Preparation of dosage form**
Tacrolimus should be diluted with 5% dextrose injection or 0.9% sodium chloride injection to a concentration between 0.004 and 0.02 mg per mL (mg/mL).

**Stability**
Diluted tacrolimus for injection should be used within 24 hours. The prepared solution should be inspected for particulate matter and clarity before administration to the patient, and should be discarded if particulate matter is present.

**Incompatibilities**
Tacrolimus for injection should not be stored in polyvinyl chloride (PVC) containers because the solution may be adsorbed by PVC containers, and leaching of phthalates in the PVC container may occur.

[1]Not included in Canadian product labeling.

## Selected Bibliography

The US Multicenter FK506 Liver Study Group. A comparison of tacrolimus (FK 506) and cyclosporine for immunosuppression in liver transplantation. N Engl J Med 1994; 331: 1110-5.

Venkataramanan R, Swaminathan A, Prasad T, et al. Clinical pharmacokinetics of tacrolimus. Clin Pharmacokinet 1995; 404-30.
Peters D, Fitton A, Plosker G. Tacrolimus. A review of its pharmacology and therapeutic potential in hepatic and renal transplantation. Drugs 1993; 46: 746-94
Starzl T, Todo S, Fung J, et al. FK 506 for liver, kidney, and pancreas transplantation. Lancet 1989; 2: 1000-4.

Developed: 08/14/97

---

**TALC, STERILE**—The *Talc, Sterile (Intrapleural-Local)—Introductory Version* monograph is not included in this published version of the USP DI database. Copies of the monograph are available on request from Micromedex, Inc. - Reprint Requests, 6200 S. Syracuse Way, Suite 300, Englewood, CO 80111; telephone (303) 486-6400; telefax (303) 486-6464; Email: USPDI@MDX.COM.

---

# TAMOXIFEN Systemic

VA CLASSIFICATION (Primary): AN500

Commonly used brand name(s): *Apo-Tamox; Gen-Tamoxifen; Nolvadex; Nolvadex-D; Novo-Tamoxifen; Tamofen; Tamone; Tamoplex*.

Note: For a listing of dosage forms and brand names by country availability, see *Dosage Forms* section(s).

## Category
Antineoplastic.

## Indications

Note: Bracketed information in the *Indications* section refers to uses that are not included in U.S. product labeling.

**Accepted**
Carcinoma, breast (treatment)—
Node-negative: Tamoxifen is indicated for adjuvant treatment of axillary node-negative breast cancer in women following total mastectomy or segmental mastectomy, axillary dissection, and breast irradiation. Data are insufficient to predict which women are most likely to benefit and to determine if tamoxifen provides any benefit in women with tumors of less than 1 cm.

Node-positive: Tamoxifen is indicated for adjuvant treatment of axillary node-positive breast cancer in postmenopausal women following total mastectomy or segmental mastectomy, axillary dissection, and breast irradiation. In some tamoxifen adjuvant studies, most of the benefit to date has been in the subgroup with 4 or more positive axillary nodes.

Note: The estrogen and progesterone receptor values may help to predict whether adjuvant tamoxifen therapy is likely to be beneficial in node-negative or node-positive breast cancer.

Advanced disease: Tamoxifen is indicated in the treatment of metastatic breast cancer in men and women.

The labeling states that tamoxifen is effective in premenopausal women as an alternative to oophorectomy or ovarian irradiation. Available evidence indicates that women whose tumors are estrogen receptor–positive are more likely to benefit from tamoxifen therapy.

[Melanoma, malignant (treatment)][1]—Tamoxifen is indicated, in combination with other agents, in the treatment of malignant melanoma.

[1]Not included in Canadian product labeling.

## Pharmacology/Pharmacokinetics

Note: Pharmacokinetic studies have been done in women only.

**Physicochemical characteristics**
Molecular weight—563.65.
pKa—8.85.

**Mechanism of action/Effect**
Tamoxifen is a nonsteroidal antiestrogen agent that also has weak estrogenic effects. The exact mechanism of antineoplastic action is unknown, but may be related to its antiestrogen effects; tamoxifen blocks uptake of estradiol.

**Other actions/effects**
Tamoxifen may induce ovulation in anovulatory women, stimulating release of gonadotropin-releasing hormone from the hypothalamus, which in turn stimulates release of pituitary gonadotropins. In oligospermic males, tamoxifen increases serum concentrations of luteinizing hormone (LH), follicle-stimulating hormone (FSH), testosterone, and estrogen. Tamoxifen and some of its metabolites (*N*-desmethyltamoxifen, 4-hydroxytamoxifen) are potent inhibitors of hepatic cytochrome P450 mixed function oxidases; however, the clinical significance of these effects has not been determined.

**Biotransformation**
Hepatic. Enterohepatic circulation is believed to account for prolongation of blood concentrations and fecal excretion.

**Half-life**
Distribution—7 to 14 hours; secondary peaks at 4 or more days may be due to enterohepatic circulation.
Elimination—May exceed 7 days.

**Onset of action**
An objective response usually occurs within 4 to 10 weeks of therapy, but may take several months in patients with bone metastases.

**Duration of action**
Estrogen antagonism may persist for several weeks following a single dose.

**Elimination**
Primary route—Biliary/fecal, mostly as metabolites.
Secondary route—Renal (only small amounts).

## Precautions to Consider

Note: Unless otherwise noted, information in this section is based on reports in women treated with tamoxifen.

**Carcinogenicity**
An increased incidence of endometrial cancer has been associated with tamoxifen treatment in humans. A large randomized study in Sweden found a significantly increased incidence of uterine cancer in women who took tamoxifen as compared with those who received placebo. In the ongoing NSABP B-14 study, an increased incidence of uterine cancer has also been noted; deaths have been reported.

Hepatic carcinogenicity of tamoxifen in rats is well established. Studies in rats at doses of 5, 20, and 35 mg per kg of body weight (mg/kg) per day for up to 2 years found an increased incidence of hepatocellular carcinoma at all doses; the incidence was highest at doses of 20 or 35 mg/kg per day. In a 13-month study of endocrine changes in immature and mature mice, granulosa cell ovarian tumors and interstitial cell testicular tumors were found in tamoxifen-treated mice but not in controls.

**Mutagenicity**
No genotoxic potential was found in a conventional battery of *in vivo* and *in vitro* tests with pro- and eukaryotic test systems with drug metabolizing systems present. However, increased levels of DNA adducts have been found in the livers of rats exposed to tamoxifen. Tamoxifen has also been found to increase levels of micronucleus formation *in vitro* in human lymphoblastoid cell line (MCL-5).

## Pregnancy/Reproduction
Fertility—Tamoxifen may induce ovulation in women.
Tamoxifen affects reproductive function in rats at doses somewhat higher than the human dose.

Pregnancy—Although adequate and well-controlled studies have not been done in humans, spontaneous abortions, birth defects, fetal deaths, and vaginal bleeding have been reported. Because of tamoxofen's estrogenic effect, the possibility of a diethylstilbestrol (DES)-like syndrome in females whose mothers took tamoxifen during pregnancy should be kept in mind. In rodent models of fetal reproductive tract development, at doses of 0.3 to 2.4 times the maximum recommended human dose (MRHD), tamoxifen caused changes in both sexes that are similar to those caused by estradiol, ethynylestradiol, and DES; some of these changes, especially vaginal adenosis, are similar to those found in young women who were exposed *in utero* to DES and who have a 1 in 1000 risk of developing clear-cell adenocarcinoma of the vagina or cervix. Duration of follow-up of the few women exposed to tamoxifen *in utero* to date has not been long enough to confirm or disprove this risk with its use in humans.

In general, use of a barrier or nonhormonal contraceptive is recommended during (and for about 2 months after) tamoxifen therapy in sexually active women.

At dose levels at or below the human dose, reversible nonteratogenic developmental skeletal changes occurred in rats, and a lower incidence of embryo implantation and higher incidence of fetal death or retarded *in utero* growth occurred in rats and rabbits, as well as impaired learning behavior in some rat pups.

FDA Pregnancy Category D.

## Breast-feeding
It is not known whether tamoxifen is distributed into breast milk. Although very little information is available regarding distribution of antineoplastic agents into breast milk, breast-feeding is not recommended during chemotherapy because of the risks to the infant (adverse effects, mutagenicity, carcinogenicity).

## Geriatrics
Appropriate studies on the relationship of age to the effects of tamoxifen have not been performed in the geriatric population. However, this medication is commonly used in elderly patients and geriatrics-specific problems that would limit the usefulness of this medication in the elderly have not been reported and are not expected.

## Drug interactions and/or related problems
The following drug interactions and/or related problems have been selected on the basis of their potential clinical significance (possible mechanism in parentheses where appropriate)—not necessarily inclusive (» = major clinical significance):

Note: Combinations containing any of the following medications, depending on the amount present, may also interact with this medication.

Estrogens
(may interfere with tamoxifen's therapeutic effect)

## Laboratory value alterations
The following have been selected on the basis of their potential clinical significance (possible effect in parentheses where appropriate)—not necessarily inclusive (» = major clinical significance):

With physiology/laboratory test values
Calcium concentrations, serum
(may be increased infrequently, usually in patients with bone metastases; the effect appears to be transient)
Cholesterol and
Triglycerides
(increases in serum concentrations have been seen infrequently)
Hepatic enzymes
(serum values may be increased; rarely, more severe abnormalities, including fatty liver, cholestasis, and hepatitis, have occurred; fatalities have been reported)
Karyopyknotic index on vaginal smears
(variations have been seen infrequently in postmenopausal women treated with tamoxifen)
Papanicolaou (Pap) test
(various degrees of estrogen effect have been seen infrequently in postmenopausal women treated with tamoxifen)
Thyroxine ($T_4$)
(increases in serum concentrations have been reported in a few patients, possibly as a result of increases in thyroid-binding globulin; however, clinical hyperthyroidism has not been reported)

## Medical considerations/Contraindications
The medical considerations/contraindications included have been selected on the basis of their potential clinical significance (reasons given in parentheses where appropriate)—not necessarily inclusive (» = major clinical significance).

*Risk-benefit should be considered when the following medical problems exist:*

Cataracts or vision disturbances
(visual disturbances, including corneal changes, cataracts, and retinopathy, have been reported in patients receiving tamoxifen)
Hyperlipidemia
(increased serum lipid concentrations have been reported infrequently)
Leukopenia
(leukopenia has been reported occasionally in patients receiving tamoxifen)
» Sensitivity to tamoxifen
Thrombocytopenia
(thrombocytopenia has been reported occasionally in patients receiving tamoxifen, although platelet counts recovered even with continued therapy)

## Patient monitoring
The following may be especially important in patient monitoring (other tests may be warranted in some patients, depending on condition; » = major clinical significance):

» Calcium concentrations, serum
(recommended at periodic intervals in patients with bone metastases during initial period of therapy)
Cholesterol concentrations, serum and
Triglyceride concentrations, serum
(may be recommended at periodic intervals in patients with pre-existing hyperlipidemias)
Complete blood count
(may be appropriate at periodic intervals, although leukopenia and thrombocytopenia have not been definitely attributed to tamoxifen)
» Gynecologic examinations
(recommended at regular intervals in women taking tamoxifen, to detect possible endometrial cancers)
Hepatic function tests
(recommended at periodic intervals during therapy)
Ophthalmologic examinations
(recommended prior to initiation of therapy and at periodic intervals during therapy)

# Side/Adverse Effects
Note: Side/adverse effects are usually relatively mild.
Although information is limited, the side effect profile in men seems to be similar to that in women.
A transient, sometimes severe, increase in bone or tumor pain may occur shortly after initiation of therapy but usually subsides with continued tamoxifen treatment. Analgesics may be required during this time.
Tamoxifen induces ovulation, which puts women at risk for becoming pregnant.
Ovarian cysts have been reported in a small number of premenopausal women treated with tamoxifen for advanced breast carcinoma.

The following side/adverse effects have been selected on the basis of their potential clinical significance (possible signs and symptoms in parentheses where appropriate)—not necessarily inclusive:

## Those indicating need for medical attention
Incidence less frequent or rare
*In both females and males*
**Confusion; hepatotoxicity** (yellow eyes or skin)—usually asymptomatic; **ocular toxicity, including retinopathy, keratopathy, cataracts, and optic neuritis** (blurred vision)—may be asymptomatic initially; **pulmonary embolus** (shortness of breath); **thrombosis** (pain or swelling in legs); **weakness or sleepiness**

Note: *Hepatotoxicity* usually consists of elevated hepatic enzyme values. However, more serious liver abnormalities, including fatty liver, cholestasis, and hepatitis, have occurred; fatalities have been reported.

*Ocular toxicity* was previously thought to occur only after high (240 to 320 mg per day), prolonged (17 months or more) tamoxifen dosage. However, there are reports of retinopathy or keratopathy occurring at lower doses (10 to 40 mg per day) and after only a few weeks of tamoxifen therapy, although they are still most commonly associated with several months' therapy. Ocular toxicity may or may not be reversible following withdrawal of tamoxifen. A number of reports included recommendations for baseline and periodic ocular examinations during tamoxifen therapy to detect subclinical toxicity and permit withdrawal of tamoxifen at early stages of toxicity.

*In females only*
**Endometrial hyperplasia, endometrial polyps, or endometrial carcinoma** (change in vaginal discharge; pain or feeling of pressure in pelvis; vaginal bleeding)

**Those indicating need for medical attention only if they continue or are bothersome**
Incidence more frequent— 10 to 20%
*In females only*
**Hot flashes; weight gain**
Note: *Weight gain* is an estrogen effect.
Incidence less frequent
*In both females and males*
**Headache; nausea and/or vomiting, mild; skin rash or dryness; transient local disease flare** (bone pain)
Note: Incidence of *nausea and/or vomiting* is higher with higher doses.
*Transient local disease flare* may also consist of hypercalcemia and/or spinal cord compression, as well as a sudden increase in the size of pre-existing lesions in patients with soft tissue disease, sometimes associated with marked erythema within and surrounding the lesions and/or the development of new lesions. Bone pain or other disease flare usually occurs shortly after initiation of therapy and subsides within 1 to 2 weeks.

*In females only*
**Changes in menstrual period; itching in genital area; vaginal discharge**
*In males only*
**Impotence or decrease in sexual interest**

## Patient Consultation
As an aid to patient consultation, refer to *Advice for the Patient, Tamoxifen (Systemic)*.
In providing consultation, consider emphasizing the following selected information (» = major clinical significance):

**Before using this medication**
» Conditions affecting use, especially:
Sensitivity to tamoxifen
Pregnancy—Use not recommended because of risk of miscarriage, death of the fetus, birth defects, and vaginal bleeding; advisability of using nonhormonal contraception during (and for about 2 months following) therapy; telling physician immediately if pregnancy is suspected
Breast-feeding—Not recommended because of risk of serious side effects

**Proper use of this medication**
» Importance of not taking more or less medication than the amount prescribed

» Frequency of nausea and vomiting; importance of continuing medication despite stomach upset
Checking with physician if vomiting occurs shortly after dose is taken
» Proper dosing
Missed dose: Not taking at all; not doubling doses
» Proper storage

**Precautions while using this medication**
» Importance of close monitoring by the physician
For women: May increase fertility; advisability of using nonhormonal contraception during therapy; telling physician immediately if pregnancy is suspected

**Side/adverse effects**
For women: Increased risk of endometrial carcinoma
Signs of potential side effects, especially confusion, hepatotoxicity, retinopathy, keratopathy, cataracts, optic neuritis, pulmonary embolus, thrombosis, weakness or sleepiness, endometrial hyperplasia, endometrial polyps, and endometrial carcinoma
Physician or nurse can help in dealing with side effects

## General Dosing Information
Patients receiving tamoxifen should be under supervision of a physician experienced in cancer chemotherapy.
If side effects are severe, dosage may sometimes be reduced without loss of control of the disease.
If severe hypercalcemia occurs, tamoxifen should be discontinued.
Ophthalmologic examination is recommended if visual disturbances occur, and withdrawal of tamoxifen should be considered if retinopathy or keratopathy is detected.

## Oral Dosage Forms

### TAMOXIFEN CITRATE TABLETS USP
Note: The dosing and strengths available are expressed in terms of tamoxifen base.

**Usual adult dose**
Breast carcinoma—
Node-negative or node-positive: In women—Oral, 10 mg (base) two times a day (in the morning and evening).
Metastatic: In men and women—Oral, 10 to 20 mg (base) two times a day (in the morning and evening).

**Strength(s) usually available**
U.S.—
10 mg (base) (Rx) [*Nolvadex* (carboxymethylcellulose calcium; magnesium stearate; mannitol; starch); GENERIC].
20 mg (base) (Rx) [*Nolvadex* (carboxymethylcellulose calcium; magnesium stearate; mannitol; starch); GENERIC].
Canada—
10 mg (base) (Rx) [*Apo-Tamox; Gen-Tamoxifen; Nolvadex; Novo-Tamoxifen; Tamofen; Tamone; Tamoplex*].
20 mg (base) (Rx) [*Apo-Tamox; Gen-Tamoxifen; Nolvadex-D; Novo-Tamoxifen; Tamofen; Tamone; Tamoplex*].

**Packaging and storage**
Store between 20 and 25 °C (68 and 77 °F), unless otherwise specified by manufacturer. Store in a well-closed, light-resistant container.

Revised: 08/12/94
Interim revision: 09/30/97

---

# TAMSULOSIN Systemic—INTRODUCTORY VERSION

VA CLASSIFICATION (Primary): GU700
Commonly used brand name(s): *Flomax*.
Note: For a listing of dosage forms and brand names by country availability, see *Dosage Forms* section(s).

## Category
Benign prostatic hyperplasia therapy agent.

## Indications

**Accepted**
Benign prostatic hyperplasia (treatment)—Tamsulosin is indicated in the treatment of symptomatic benign prostatic hyperplasia (BPH). It has been shown to improve urinary flow and the symptoms of BPH.

**Unaccepted**
Tamsulosin is not intended for use as an antihypertensive agent.

## Pharmacology/Pharmacokinetics

**Physicochemical characteristics**
Molecular weight—444.98.

**Mechanism of action/Effect**
Tamsulosin is an alpha$_1$-adrenergic blocking agent exhibiting selectivity for alpha$_1$ receptors in the human prostate. Relaxation of smooth muscle in the bladder neck and prostate produced by alpha$_1$-adrenergic blockade results in improvement in urine flow rate and a reduction in symptoms of BPH.

### Absorption
Absorption is > 90% following oral administration of a 0.4-mg dose under fasting conditions. Bioavailability is increased by 30% and peak concentration is increased by 40 to 70% when tamsulosin is taken in the fasting state compared to the nonfasting state.

### Distribution
Animal studies have found that tamsulosin is widely distributed to most tissues, including aorta, brown fat, gallbladder, heart, kidney, liver, and prostate; it is minimally distributed into the brain, spinal cord, and testes.

### Protein binding
Very high (94 to 99%) to plasma proteins, primarily to alpha-1 glycoprotein; binding is linear over a wide concentration range (20 to 600 nanograms per mL).

### Biotransformation
Tamsulosin is extensively metabolized by cytochrome P450 enzymes in the liver, with < 10% of the dose excreted in the urine unchanged. The metabolites undergo extensive conjugation to glucuronide or sulfate prior to renal excretion.

### Half-life
Healthy individuals (fasting state)—9 to 13 hours.
Target population—14 to 15 hours.
Elimination—5 to 7 hours in plasma following intravenous or oral administration of an immediate-release formulation of tamsulosin.

### Time to peak concentration
4 to 5 hours under fasting conditions and 6 to 7 hours when administered with food.

### Peak serum concentration
Peak plasma concentrations achieved with a 0.4-mg once-daily dose are $10.1 \pm 4.8$ nanograms per mL after a light breakfast and $17.1 \pm 17.1$ nanograms per mL in the fasting state; peak plasma concentrations after administration of a 0.8-mg dose are $29.8 \pm 10.3$ nanograms per mL after a light breakfast, $29.1 \pm 11$ nanograms per mL after a high-fat breakfast, and $41.6 \pm 15.6$ nanograms per mL in the fasting state.

### Elimination
After administration of a radiolabeled dose of tamsulosin, 76% of the dose is recovered in the urine and 21% is recovered in the feces over 168 hours.
  In dialysis—Tamsulosin is unlikely to be removed because of its high protein binding (94 to 99%).

## Precautions to Consider

### Carcinogenicity
Male rats given doses of up to 43 mg per kg of body weight (mg/kg) a day and female rats given doses of 52 mg/kg a day had no increase in tumor incidence, with the exception of a modest increase in the frequency of mammary gland fibroadenomas in female rats receiving doses ≥ 5.4 mg/kg. There were no significant tumor findings in male mice receiving doses of up to 127 mg/kg a day. However, female mice treated for 2 years had statistically significant increases in the incidence of mammary gland fibroadenomas and adenocarcinomas with the highest doses given (45 and 158 mg/kg a day). The highest dose concentrations of tamsulosin evaluated in the rat and mice carcinogenicity studies produced systemic exposures (area under the plasma concentration–time curve [AUC]) in rats and mice eight times the exposures in men receiving 0.8 mg of tamsulosin a day. The increased incidences of mammary gland neoplasms in female rats and mice were considered secondary to tamsulosin-induced hyperprolactinemia. It is not known if tamsulosin elevates prolactin secretion in humans.

### Mutagenicity
Tamsulosin was found nonmutagenic *in vitro* in the Ames reverse mutation test, the mouse lymphoma thymidine kinase assay, the unscheduled DNA repair synthesis assay, and the chromosomal aberration assays in Chinese hamster ovary cells or human lymphocytes. There were no mutagenic effects in the *in vivo* sister chromatid exchange and mouse micronucleus assay.

### Pregnancy/Reproduction
Fertility—Studies in rats receiving tamsulosin in single or multiple daily doses of 300 mg/kg a day (AUC exposure in rats approximately 50 times the maximum human exposure using the maximum therapeutic dose) found a significant reduction in fertility in males. This reduction is thought to be due to an effect of the compound on the vaginal plug formation in female rats, possibly due to changes of semen content or impairment of ejaculation. These effects were reversible, showing improvement by 3 days after a single dose and by 4 weeks after multiple dosing; the effects were completely reversed 9 weeks after discontinuation of multiple dosing. Multiple doses of 10 and 100 mg/kg a day (1/5 and 16 times the anticipated human AUC exposure, respectively) produced no significant effects on fertility in male rats. Studies in female rats found a significant reduction in fertility after single or multiple dosing using 300 mg/kg a day of the R-isomer or a racemic mixture of tamsulosin, respectively. In female rats, the reductions in fertility after single doses of tamsulosin were considered to be associated with impairments in fertilization. Multiple dosing with 10 or 100 mg/kg a day of the racemic mixture of tamsulosin did not significantly alter fertility in female rats.

Pregnancy—Tamsulosin is not indicated for use in women.
Administration of tamsulosin to pregnant female rats at doses of up to 300 mg/kg a day (approximately 50 times the human therapeutic AUC exposure) and to pregnant rabbits at doses of up to 50 mg/kg a day produced no evidence of fetal harm.

FDA Pregnancy Category B.

### Breast-feeding
Tamsulosin is not indicated for use in women.

### Pediatrics
Tamsulosin is not indicated for use in children.

### Geriatrics
The pharmacokinetic disposition of tamsulosin may be slightly prolonged, resulting in a 40% higher exposure (AUC) in older males compared to that of young, healthy males.

### Drug interactions and/or related problems
The following drug interactions and/or related problems have been selected on the basis of their potential clinical significance (possible mechanism in parentheses where appropriate)—not necessarily inclusive (» = major clinical significance):

Note: Combinations containing any of the following medications, depending on the amount present, may also interact with this medication.
  Tamsulosin is extensively metabolized by cytochrome P450 enzymes in the liver. Potential interactions with other cytochrome P450–metabolized compounds have not been determined.

» Alpha$_1$-adrenergic blocking agents, other, such as doxazosin, phentolamine, prazosin, and terazosin
  (concurrent administration may produce an additive effect)

Cimetidine
  (concurrent administration resulted in a 26% decrease in the clearance of tamsulosin and a 44% increase in tamsulosin AUC; tamsulosin should be used with caution in combination with cimetidine, particularly at daily doses higher than 0.4 mg)

» Warfarin
  (caution should be exercised with concurrent administration because of inconclusive results from *in vitro* and *in vivo* studies)

### Medical considerations/Contraindications
The medical considerations/contraindications included have been selected on the basis of their potential clinical significance (reasons given in parentheses where appropriate)—not necessarily inclusive (» = major clinical significance).

*Risk-benefit should be considered when the following medical problem exists:*
Sensitivity to tamsulosin or any component

## Side/Adverse Effects
The following side/adverse effects have been selected on the basis of their potential clinical significance (possible signs and symptoms in parentheses where appropriate)—not necessarily inclusive:

### Those indicating need for medical attention only if they continue or are bothersome
Incidence more frequent (5 to 21%, except as indicated)
  *Abnormal ejaculation; asthenia* (unusual weakness); *back pain; diarrhea*—incidence 4.3% with 0.8-mg dose; *dizziness; headache; rhinitis* (stuffy or runny nose)

  Note: Incidence of *abnormal ejaculation* is 8.4% with the 0.4-mg dose and 18% with the 0.8-mg dose.

Incidence less frequent (< 5%)
  *Chest pain; decreased libido; drowsiness; insomnia* (difficulty in sleeping); *nausea; orthostatic hypotension* (dizziness, fainting, or lightheadedness, especially when getting up from a lying or sitting position)

## Overdose

For more information on the management of overdose or unintentional ingestion, **contact a Poison Control Center** (see *Poison Control Center Listing*).

**Clinical effects of overdose**
The following effects have been selected on the basis of their potential clinical significance (possible signs and symptoms in parentheses where appropriate)—not necessarily inclusive:

**Treatment of overdose**
Specific treatment—Intravenous fluids and vasopressors should be administered if needed.

Monitoring—Renal function should be monitored.

Supportive care—Cardiovascular system must be maintained; to restore blood pressure and normalize the heart rate, patient should be kept in the supine position. Patients in whom intentional overdose is confirmed or suspected should be referred for psychiatric consultation.

## Patient Consultation

As an aid to patient consultation, refer to *Advice for the Patient, Tamsulosin (Systemic)—Introductory Version*.

In providing consultation, consider emphasizing the following selected information (» = major clinical significance):

**Before using this medication**
» Conditions affecting use, especially:
   Sensitivity to tamsulosin or any component
   Other medications, especially alpha$_1$-adrenergic blocking agents or warfarin

**Proper use of this medication**
Taking at the same time each day to help increase compliance
Not crushing, chewing, or opening capsules, unless otherwise directed by a physician
» Proper dosing
Missed dose: Taking as soon as possible; not taking if almost time for next dose; not doubling doses
» Proper storage

**Precautions while using this medication**
Regular visits to physician to check progress
» Caution when getting up suddenly from a lying or sitting position
» Possible dizziness; caution when driving or doing things requiring alertness

**Side/adverse effects**
Signs of potential side effects, especially abnormal ejaculation, decreased libido, or orthostatic hypotension

## General Dosing Information

**Diet/Nutrition**
Tamsulosin should be taken once a day one-half hour after the same meal each day.

## Oral Dosage Forms

### TAMSULOSIN HYDROCHLORIDE CAPSULES

**Usual adult dose**
Benign prostatic hyperplasia—
   Oral, 0.4 mg once a day, approximately one-half hour after the same meal each day. If there is no response after two to four weeks, the dose may be increased to 0.8 mg once a day.
Note: If tamsulosin administration is discontinued or interrupted for several days at either dose, therapy should be restarted with the 0.4-mg dose.

**Usual geriatric dose**
See *Usual adult dose*.

**Strength(s) usually available**
U.S.—
   0.4 mg (Rx) [*Flomax*].

**Packaging and storage**
Store at 20 to 25 °C (68 to 77 °F).

**Auxiliary labeling**
• Do not crush, chew, or open capsules.

Developed: 10/15/97

---

# TAZAROTENE   Topical—INTRODUCTORY VERSION

VA CLASSIFICATION (Primary/Secondary): DE802/DE752
Commonly used brand name(s): *Tazorac*.
Note: For a listing of dosage forms and brand names by country availability, see *Dosage Forms* section(s).

## Category

Antiacne agent (topical); antipsoriatic (topical).

## Indications

**Accepted**
Acne vulgaris (treatment)—Tazarotene, as the 0.1% gel, is indicated in the treatment of mild to moderate facial acne vulgaris. It is not known if tazarotene is effective in treatment of acne vulgaris resistant to antibiotics or for acne treated previously with other retinoid medications.

One study of patients treated with tazarotene or with a vehicle gel for 12 weeks showed that 68% of patients treated with tazarotene gel and 40% of patients using the vehicle gel had more than a 50% reduction in their total number of inflammatory and noninflammatory acne lesions. Another study showed that 48% of patients treated with tazarotene gel and 29% of patients using the vehicle gel had more than a 50% reduction in their total number of inflammatory and noninflammatory acne lesions.

Psoriasis (treatment)—Tazarotene, as the 0.05% and 0.1% gel, is indicated for the treatment of stable plaque psoriasis involving up to 20% of the body surface area.

In two studies of patients treated with 0.05% or 0.1% tazarotene gel or with the vehicle gel for 12 weeks, the 0.1% gel was more effective than the 0.05% gel or vehicle gel in the overall improvement of psoriasis. In these studies, 42% and 52% of patients treated with 0.05% tazarotene gel and 52% and 65% of patients treated with 0.1% tazarotene gel showed more than a 50% global improvement from baseline of psoriasis when evaluated for plaque elevation, scaling, and erythema. In the same study, a 50% global improvement over baseline was seen in 23% and 33% of patients treated with the vehicle gel.

## Pharmacology/Pharmacokinetics

**Physicochemical characteristics**
Chemical group—Tazarotene is a prodrug that is converted to an acetylenic retinoid, tazarotenic acid.
Molecular weight—351.47.

**Mechanism of action/Effect**
Although tazarotene binds to all three members of the retinoic acid receptor family (alpha, beta, and gamma receptors), it binds selectively to beta and gamma receptors and probably modifies gene expression.
   Antiacne agent—The mechanism of action of tazarotene in the treatment of acne vulgaris is not known, but studies suggest that it inhibits corneocyte accumulation in rhino mouse skin and cross-linked envelope formation in human keratocyte cultures.
   Antipsoriatic—The mechanism of action of tazarotene in the treatment of psoriasis is not known. Skin studies done with tazarotene in animals and human cell cultures suggest that it has anti-inflammatory and antiproliferative actions in the skin through gene expression. Tazarotene, by directly reducing the keratinocyte's rate of proliferation, helps to normalize cell differentiation and inhibits the formation of a cornified envelope. Also, tazarotene may modify gene transcription or bind to transcription factors to reduce the erythema common in psoriasis.

**Absorption**
Minimal systemic absorption of tazarotene occurs because of its rapid metabolism in the skin to the active metabolite, tazarotenic acid, which can be systemically absorbed and further metabolized. The use of a nonradiolabeled dose in one study comparing 0.05% to 0.1% tazarotene showed its area under the plasma concentration–time curve (AUC) as 40% higher for 0.1% gel compared to 0.05% gel.

The percentage of tazarotenic acid absorbed from a dose of 0.1% tazarotene (2 mg per square centimeter [2 mg/cm$^2$]) and left on the skin for 10 to 12 hours without occlusion is as follows—

Once a day for 7 days to normal skin (involving 20% of body surface area): 0.91% ± 0.67% tazarotenic acid.

Once a day for 14 days to psoriatic skin (measurement was extrapolated to 20% of involved area from data using 8 to 18% of body surface area): 14.8% tazarotenic acid.

### Distribution
An *in vitro* percutaneous absorption study indicated that 4 to 5% of the applied dose remained in the stratum corneum and 2 to 4% remained in the viable epidermis-dermis layer 24 hours after topical application. Tazarotenic acid is hydrophilic and is quickly metabolized systemically, causing no apparent accumulation within body tissues.

### Protein binding
Tazarotenic acid is highly bound to plasma proteins (> 99%).

### Biotransformation
The prodrug tazarotene undergoes esterase hydrolysis in skin to form its active metabolite, tazarotenic acid. Tazarotenic acid is further metabolized in skin and, after systemic absorption, hepatically metabolized to sulfoxides, sulfones, and other polar products for elimination.

### Half-life
Approximately 18 hours for tazarotenic acid in both normal and psoriatic patients.

### Time to peak concentration
For 0.1% tazarotene—

Dose of 2 mg/cm$^2$ once a day for 7 days to normal skin (involving 20% of body surface area): 9 hours for tazarotenic acid.

Dose of 2 mg/cm$^2$ once a day for 14 days to psoriatic skin (measurement was extrapolated to 20% of involved area from data using 8 to 18% of body surface area): 6 hours for tazarotenic acid.

### Peak serum concentration
For 0.1% tazarotene—

Dose of 2 mg/cm$^2$ once a day for 7 days to normal skin (involving 20% of body surface area): 0.72 ± 5.8 nanogram per mL of tazarotenic acid.

Dose of 2 mg/cm$^2$ once a day for 14 days to psoriatic skin (measurement was extrapolated to 20% of involved area from data using 8 to 18% of body surface area): 18.9 ± 10.6 nanogram per mL of tazarotenic acid.

### Elimination
Tazarotenic acid—Systemically absorbed dose is eliminated by fecal and renal pathways.

## Precautions to Consider

### Cross-sensitivity and/or related problems
Patients sensitive to vitamin A or retinoid derivatives, such as acitretin, etretinate, isotretinoin, or tretinoin may be sensitive to this medication.

### Carcinogenicity
An 88-week topical application study in mice showed that doses of 0.05, 0.125, 0.25, and 1 mg per kg of body weight (mg/kg) a day produced no carcinogenic effect; a dosage reduction from 1 mg to 0.5 mg/kg a day for male mice after 41 weeks occurred due to severe dermal irritation.

### Tumorigenicity
Hairless mice administered topical tazarotene at 0.001%, 0.005%, and 0.01% and exposed to intercurrent ultraviolet radiation for up to 40 weeks developed the expected tumors faster; the clinical relevance to humans is not known.

### Mutagenicity
Tazarotene was not found to be mutagenic in a series of tests or assays, including the Ames test, CHO/HPRT mammalian cell forward gene mutation assay, human lymphocyte assay, and the mouse micronucleus test.

### Pregnancy/Reproduction
Pregnancy—Although adequate and well-controlled studies in humans have not been done, tazarotene is not recommended for use during pregnancy because retinoids may cause fetal harm. Apparently healthy babies have been delivered by mothers who were exposed inadvertently to topical tazarotene during early pregnancy; however, tazarotene treatment should be discontinued and the patient advised about potential risks to the fetus if pregnancy occurs. Teratogenic systemic concentrations of the medication may be produced in humans when tazarotene is applied to 20% of body surface area. This may be a concern in treating psoriasis; systemic absorption from treatment of facial acne vulgaris would be less because of the limited area of application.

It is recommended that a pregnancy test, having a sensitivity of 50 milli-International Units (mIU) per mL for human chorionic gonadotropin, be obtained within 2 weeks prior to initiation of treatment with topical tazarotene, and that tazarotene treatment begin during a normal menstrual period. Women of childbearing age also should be counseled about potential risks to the fetus and about available contraceptive options that may be used during tazarotene therapy.

Studies of rats showed lower than expected body weights and reduced skeletal ossification in fetuses when 0.05% tazarotene was used topically during gestation (Days 6 through 17) at a dose of 0.25 mg/kg per day (corresponding to 1.5 mg/m$^2$ per day). Rabbits that were given topical tazarotene at doses of 0.25 mg/kg per day (corresponding to 2.75 mg/m$^2$ total body surface area per day) during gestation (Days 6 through 18) showed single incidences of known retinoid malformations, including spina bifida, hydrocephaly, and heart anomalies.

In studies of animals given tazarotene orally, developmental delays were seen in rabbits, and teratogenic effects and postimplantation fetal losses were seen in rats and rabbits at doses that produced serum concentrations between 0.7 and 13 times those produced in humans using topical tazarotene over 20% of the total body surface area.

FDA Pregnancy Category X.

### Breast-feeding
It is not known if tazarotene is distributed into breast milk in humans; however, animal studies show that single topical doses of radiolabeled tazarotene are detected in maternal milk. Risk-benefit should be carefully considered.

### Pediatrics
No information is available on the relationship of age to the effects of tazarotene in pediatric patients up to 12 years of age. Safety and efficacy have not been established.

### Drug interactions and/or related problems
The following drug interactions and/or related problems have been selected on the basis of their potential clinical significance (possible mechanism in parentheses where appropriate)—not necessarily inclusive (» = major clinical significance):

Note: Combinations containing any of the following medications, depending on the amount present, may also interact with this medication.

Acne products, topical, or topical products containing a peeling agent, such as
  Antibiotics, topical, such as clindamycin and erythromycin
  Benzoyl peroxide
  Resorcinol
  Salicylic acid
  Sulfur or
Alcohol-containing products, topical, such as
  After-shave lotions
  Astringents
  Cosmetics or soaps with a strong drying effect
  Shaving creams or lotions or
Hair products, skin-irritating, such as hair permanents or hair removal products or
Products containing lime or spices, topical or
Soaps or cleansers, abrasive
  (concurrent use with tazarotene may cause a cumulative irritant or drying effect, especially with the application of peeling, desquamating, or abrasive agents, resulting in excessive irritation of the skin. If irritation results, the strength or dose of tazarotene may need to be reduced or temporarily discontinued until the skin is less sensitive)

Photosensitizing medications, such as
  Fluoroquinolones
  Phenothiazines
  Sulfonamides
  Tetracyclines
  Thiazide diuretics
  (although tazarotene did not induce contact sensitization, phototoxicity, or photoallergy in human dermal safety studies in patients using tazarotene in the treatment of acne vulgaris, concurrent use with these medications may increase the risk of developing photosensitivity, partly due to tazarotene-induced dryness, peeling, and scaling. These effects are more likely to occur during treatment of psoriasis and may occur anytime during treatment. If skin becomes sunburned or irritated, the strength or dose of tazarotene may need to be reduced or temporarily discontinued until the skin is less sensitive)

### Medical considerations/Contraindications
The medical considerations/contraindications included have been selected on the basis of their potential clinical significance (reasons given in parentheses where appropriate)—not necessarily inclusive (» = major clinical significance).

*Risk-benefit should be considered when the following medical problems exist:*
» Eczema
    (tazarotene may cause skin irritation and may worsen this condition)
  Sensitivity to tazarotene, oral vitamin A, or retinoid derivatives, such as acitretin, etretinate, isotretinoin, or tretinoin

## Side/Adverse Effects
Note: A retinoid reaction (erythema, peeling of skin, and stinging or burning sensation of skin) usually occurs with normal use of tazarotene and may be mild. If the retinoid reaction is severe, tazarotene should be discontinued for 1 to 3 days until the symptoms subside and the skin recovers. Symptoms may be less severe for the weaker strength of tazarotene.

The following side/adverse effects have been selected on the basis of their potential clinical significance (possible signs and symptoms in parentheses where appropriate)—not necessarily inclusive:

### Those indicating need for medical attention
Incidence more frequent
  *Burning or stinging sensation of the skin, severe; desquamation, severe* (severe peeling of skin; severe dryness of skin); *erythema, severe* (severe redness of skin); *fissuring of skin* (deep grooves or lines in skin); *localized edema* (pain or swelling of treated skin); *pruritus, severe* (severe itching of skin); *skin discoloration* (change in color of treated skin)

*For patients with psoriasis only*
  *Irritant contact dermatitis* (skin rash)—incidence of 1 to 10%

### Those indicating need for medical attention only if they continue or are bothersome
Incidence more frequent—can indicate therapeutic effect
  *Burning or stinging sensation of the skin, mild*—on application; *desquamation, mild* (mild peeling of skin; mild dryness of skin); *erythema, mild* (mild redness of skin); *pruritus, mild* (mild itching of skin)

## Patient Consultation
As an aid to patient consultation, refer to *Advice for the Patient, Tazarotene (Topical)—Introductory Version*.
In providing consultation, consider emphasizing the following selected information (» = major clinical significance):

### Before using this medication
» Conditions affecting use, especially:
    Sensitivity to tazarotene, oral vitamin A, or retinoid derivatives
    Tumorigenicity—The development rate of expected skin tumors induced by ultraviolet light in mice treated with topical tazarotene was faster than in light-exposed mice not treated with tazarotene; clinical relevance to humans is not known
    Pregnancy—Not recommended for use during pregnancy; initiation of treatment is recommended during menses after a pregnancy test, and contraception should be considered during treatment
    Breast-feeding—Although it is not known if medication is distributed into breast milk, use is not recommended while breast-feeding
    Other medical problems, especially eczema

### Proper use of this medication
» Importance of not using more medication than the amount prescribed
  Reading patient directions carefully before use
*Proper administration*
  *For treatment of acne vulgaris*
    Before applying tazarotene, washing skin with mild or nonallergenic soap or cleanser and warm water; gently patting dry; waiting at least 20 to 30 minutes before applying medication
  *For treatment of acne vulgaris or psoriasis*
» Avoiding contact with the eyes, mouth, and nose; spreading away from these areas when applying medication
» Not applying medication to windburned or sunburned skin or to open wounds
» Waiting for 20 to 30 minutes to allow complete drying of skin if recently washed; applying to wet skin can cause skin irritation
    Applying very sparingly to affected areas only and rubbing in gently but well; washing medication off areas not intended to be treated
    Washing hands immediately after administration

» Proper dosing
  Missed dose: Applying next dose at regularly scheduled time; not doubling doses
» Proper storage

### Precautions while using this medication
» Discontinuing medication and contacting physician if pregnancy is suspected
  For treatment of acne vulgaris—Condition may appear to worsen during the first 3 weeks of therapy; checking with health care professional if acne does not improve within 8 to 12 weeks
  For treatment of psoriasis—Condition may worsen at any time during treatment; checking with health care professional if this occurs
  Not covering treated area with a bandage
  Either checking with health care professional before using or avoiding use of other topical acne or skin products containing a peeling agent (e.g., benzoyl peroxide, resorcinol, salicylic acid, or sulfur), irritating hair products (permanents or hair removal products), sun-sensitizing skin products (including products containing limes or spices), alcohol-containing skin products, or drying or abrasive skin products (some cosmetics or soaps or skin cleansers)
  Avoiding use of vitamin A supplements while using tazarotene, unless otherwise directed by health care professional
  Minimizing exposure of treated areas to sunlight, wind, and cold temperatures to lessen the possibility of sunburn, dryness, or irritation. Also, avoiding use of artificial sunlight (sunlamps).
  Using sunscreen preparations (minimum sun protection factor [SPF] of 15) or wearing protective clothing over treated areas when skin exposure cannot be avoided

### Side/adverse effects
Signs of potential side effects, especially burning or stinging sensation of the skin (severe), desquamation (severe), erythema (severe), fissuring of skin, irritant contact dermatitis—for treatment of psoriasis only, localized edema, pruritus (severe), or skin discoloration
Skin usually becomes irritated with normal use and administration; checking with doctor at any time skin becomes too dry or irritated

## General Dosing Information
Use of adequate birth control in women of reproductive age who are using tazarotene should be discussed, especially during treatment of psoriasis involving 20% of total body surface area.

If tazarotene causes too much skin irritation or peeling, it should not be applied until the skin is healed or less irritated. Tazarotene should not be applied to mucous membranes; administration near the eyes, lips, or nose should be avoided.

Patients should be counseled on the importance of protecting the skin from the sun, wind, cold temperatures, and excessive dryness by using sunscreens of at least SPF 15, moisturizers, and protective clothing. Artificial sunlight, such as sunlamps, should be avoided.

Topical products or medications should not be applied simultaneously with tazarotene; occlusive bandages should not be applied to treated areas.

Using the fingertips when washing the skin helps clean the skin and remove resulting scales and peeling of skin; harsh scrubbing of skin with sponges or washcloths should be avoided.

Tazarotene should be applied to dry skin (20 to 30 minutes should be allowed after washing) to reduce possible skin irritation that worsens or occurs more often if tazarotene is applied any earlier to nondry skin.

### For the treatment of acne
The areas to be treated for acne should be cleansed thoroughly before the medication is applied.

Within the first few weeks, acne can worsen because of exacerbation of deep, previously unseen lesions.

Therapeutic results with use of tazarotene may be noticeable after 4 weeks of therapy; clinical investigations beyond 12 weeks have not been done.

### For the treatment of psoriasis
Therapeutic results on psoriatic lesions and scales may be noticeable after 1 to 4 weeks of therapy, but improvement of the skin redness may take longer. Clinical investigations beyond 1 year have not been done.

During a 1-year study, psoriasis worsened for some patients throughout the treatment period; worsening of the condition should be reported to physician.

The patient should apply tazarotene carefully only to affected skin to minimize the amount of skin irritation.

The safety of using tazarotene over more than 20% of total body surface area has not been established, and systemic absorption would be expected.

## Topical Dosage Forms

### TAZAROTENE GEL

**Usual adult dose**
Acne vulgaris—
  Topical, (as the 0.1% gel) to clean, dry affected areas of facial skin, once a day, usually in the evening or at bedtime.
Psoriasis—
  Topical, (as the 0.05 or 0.1% gel) to affected areas of skin, once a day at bedtime. Treated area should not exceed 20% of total body surface area.

**Usual pediatric dose**
Safety and efficacy have not been established.

**Strength(s) usually available**
U.S.—
  0.05% (Rx) [*Tazorac* (ascorbic acid; benzoyl alcohol 1% w/w; butylated hydroxyanisole; butylated hydroxytoluene; carbomer 934P; edetate disodium; hexylene glycol; poloxamer 407; polyethylene glycol 400; polysorbate 40; purified water; tromethamine)].
  0.1% (Rx) [*Tazorac* (ascorbic acid; benzoyl alcohol 1% w/w; butylated hydroxyanisole; butylated hydroxytoluene; carbomer 934P; edetate disodium; hexylene glycol; poloxamer 407; polyethylene glycol 400; polysorbate 40; purified water; tromethamine)].

**Packaging and storage**
Store below 25 °C (77 °F), preferably between 15 and 30 °C (59 and 86 °F), in a tight container.

**Auxiliary labeling**
• For external use only.
• Avoid prolonged or excessive exposure to direct and/or artificial sunlight while using this medication.

**Note**
Include patient instructions when dispensing.

Developed: 11/14/97
Interim revision: 03/31/98

# TECHNETIUM Tc 99m ALBUMIN  Systemic

VA CLASSIFICATION (Primary): DX201
Commonly used brand name(s): *Frosstimage Albumin*; *Technetium Tc 99m HSA*.
Note: For a listing of dosage forms and brand names by country availability, see *Dosage Forms* section(s).

## Category
Diagnostic aid, radioactive (cardiac disease).

## Indications

**Accepted**
Cardiac blood pool imaging, radionuclide—Technetium Tc 99m albumin by intravenous administration is indicated as a cardiac blood pool imaging agent and as an adjunct in the diagnosis of pericardial effusion and ventricular aneurysm.
  Although technetium Tc 99m albumin is an acceptable agent for cardiac blood pool imaging, it is not as widely used as technetium Tc 99m–labeled red blood cells for this indication.

**Unaccepted**
Technetium Tc 99m albumin has been used in placenta localization and may be used in blood volume determinations. However, for placenta localization, it has generally been replaced by the ultrasound technique. In general, blood volume determinations are performed with Cr 51– or technetium Tc 99m–labeled red blood cells (RBC) for RBC volume determinations, and with radioiodinated serum albumin for plasma volume determinations.
Technetium Tc 99m albumin has been used in lymphoscintigraphy to evaluate lymphatic drainage patterns of malignant melanoma.

## Physical Properties

**Nuclear Data**

| Radionuclide (half-life) | Decay constant | Mode of decay | Principal photon emissions (keV) | Mean number of emissions/ disintegration ($\geq 0.01$) |
|---|---|---|---|---|
| Tc 99m (6 h) | 0.1151 h$^{-1}$ | Isomeric transition to Tc 99 | Gamma (18) | 0.062 |
|  |  |  | Gamma (140.5) | 0.891 |

## Pharmacology/Pharmacokinetics

**Mechanism of action/Effect**
Human albumin occurs naturally as the major protein component of blood. When labeled with technetium Tc 99m and given intravenously, it is distributed throughout the body in much the same way as the patient's serum albumin, and serves as a suitable tracer with which to transiently image the vascular compartment.

**Distribution**
Vascular system; no significant accumulation in organs, except the kidneys, liver, and bladder.

**Half-life**
Biological (normal human serum albumin)—Elimination: 10 to 16 hours.

**Radiation dosimetry**

| | Estimated absorbed radiation dose* ||
|---|---|---|
| Organ | mGy/MBq | rad/mCi |
| Heart | 0.20 | 0.74 |
| Spleen | 0.14 | 0.52 |
| Lungs | 0.13 | 0.48 |
| Bone surfaces | 0.0089 | 0.033 |
| Adrenals | 0.0083 | 0.031 |
| Kidneys | 0.0081 | 0.030 |
| Red marrow | 0.0075 | 0.028 |
| Liver | 0.0073 | 0.027 |
| Pancreas | 0.0064 | 0.024 |
| Stomach wall | 0.0051 | 0.019 |
| Thyroid | 0.0049 | 0.018 |
| Uterus | 0.0048 | 0.018 |
| Small intestine | 0.0048 | 0.018 |
| Large intestine wall (upper) | 0.0047 | 0.017 |
| Breast | 0.0046 | 0.017 |
| Ovaries | 0.0044 | 0.016 |
| Large intestine wall (lower) | 0.0042 | 0.016 |
| Bladder wall | 0.0040 | 0.015 |
| Testes | 0.0029 | 0.011 |
| Other tissue | 0.0040 | 0.015 |

Effective dose: 0.079 mSv/MBq (0.29 rem/mCi)

*For adults; intravenous injection. Data based on the International Commission on Radiological Protection (ICRP) Publication 53—Radiation dose to patients from radiopharmaceuticals.

**Elimination**
Renal, about 39% eliminated within 24 hours.

## Precautions to Consider

**Cross-sensitivity and/or related problems**
Patients sensitive to human albumin products may be sensitive to this product also.

**Pregnancy/Reproduction**
Pregnancy—Tc 99m (as free pertechnetate) crosses the placenta. However, studies have not been done with technetium Tc 99m albumin in humans.
The possibility of pregnancy should be assessed in women of child-bearing potential. Clinical situations exist where the benefit to the patient and fetus, based on information derived from radiopharmaceutical use, outweighs the risks from fetal exposure to radiation. In these situations, the physician should use discretion and reduce the radiopharmaceutical dose to the lowest possible amount.
Studies have not been done in animals.
FDA Pregnancy Category C.

**Breast-feeding**
Although it is not known whether technetium Tc 99m albumin is excreted in breast milk, it is known that Tc 99m as free pertechnetate is excreted in breast milk. Based on the assumption that the Tc 99m in breast milk is in the form of pertechnetate and based on the effective half-life of the radionuclide in breast milk, the daily volume of milk, a dose factor relating the radionuclide to its critical organ (thyroid) in the nursing infant, and the maximum permissible dose to that organ, a guideline has been proposed. According to this guideline, it has been calculated that nursing can be safely resumed when the concentration in breast milk reaches $30.3 \times 10^{-4}$ megabecquerels ($8.2 \times 10^{-2}$ microcuries) per mL. This level of activity is probably reached, in the majority of patients, within 24 hours after administration of technetium Tc 99m–labeled radiopharmaceuticals.

**Pediatrics**
There have been no specific studies evaluating the safety and efficacy of technetium Tc 99m albumin in children. When this radiopharmaceutical is used in children, the diagnostic benefit should be judged to outweigh the potential risk of radiation.

**Geriatrics**
Appropriate studies on the relationship of age to the effects of technetium Tc 99m albumin have not been performed in the geriatric population. However, no geriatrics-specific problems have been documented to date.

**Medical considerations/Contraindications**
The medical considerations/contraindications included have been selected on the basis of their potential clinical significance (reasons given in parentheses where appropriate)—not necessarily inclusive (» = major clinical significance).

*Risk-benefit must be considered when the following medical problem exists:*
>   Sensitivity to human albumin products or to the radiopharmaceutical preparation

## Side/Adverse Effects
The following side/adverse effects have been selected on the basis of their potential clinical significance (possible signs and symptoms in parentheses where appropriate)—not necessarily inclusive:

**Those indicating need for medical attention**
Incidence less frequent
   *Allergic reaction* (shortness of breath; skin rash)

## Patient Consultation
As an aid to patient consultation, refer to *Advice for the Patient, Radiopharmaceuticals (Diagnostic)*.
In providing consultation, consider emphasizing the following selected information (» = major clinical significance):

**Description of use**
   Action in the body: Distribution in body of injected radioactive albumin
   Visualization of radioactivity in blood pool
   Small amounts of radioactivity used in diagnosis; radiation received is low and considered safe

**Before having this test**
» Conditions affecting use, especially:
   Sensitivity to albumin products or to the radiopharmaceutical preparation
   Pregnancy—Technetium Tc 99m (as free pertechnetate) crosses placenta; risk to fetus from radiation exposure as opposed to benefit derived from use should be considered
   Breast-feeding—Not known if technetium Tc 99m albumin is excreted in breast milk, but Tc 99m as free pertechnetate is excreted in breast milk; temporary discontinuation of nursing may be recommended because of risk to infant from radiation exposure
   Use in children—Risk from radiation exposure as opposed to benefit derived from use should be considered

**Preparation for this test**
   Special preparatory instructions may be given; patient should inquire in advance

**Precautions after having this test**
   No special precautions

**Side/adverse effects**
   Signs of potential side effects, especially allergic reaction

## General Dosing Information
Radiopharmaceuticals are to be administered only by or under the supervision of physicians who have had extensive training in the safe use and handling of radioactive materials and who are authorized by the Nuclear Regulatory Commission (NRC) or the appropriate Agreement State agency, if required, or, outside the U.S., the appropriate authority.

Epinephrine, antihistamines, and corticosteroid agents should be available during the administration of technetium Tc 99m albumin because of the possibility of allergic reactions.

Manufacturer's package insert or other appropriate literature should be consulted for optimal times when imaging should be performed.

**Safety considerations for handling this radiopharmaceutical**
Improper handling of this radiopharmaceutical may cause radioactive contamination. Guidelines for handling radioactive material have been prepared by scientific, professional, state, federal, and international bodies and are available to the specially qualified and authorized users who have access to radiopharmaceuticals.

## Parenteral Dosage Forms

### TECHNETIUM Tc 99m ALBUMIN INJECTION USP
**Usual adult administered activity**
Cardiac blood pool imaging—
   Intravenous, 111 to 185 megabecquerels (3 to 5 millicuries).

**Usual pediatric administered activity**
Safety and efficacy have not been established in children under 18 years of age.

**Usual geriatric administered activity**
See *Usual adult administered activity*.

**Strength(s) usually available**
U.S.—
   Reaction vial:
      7 mg of albumin human and 80 mcg (0.08 mg) of stannous tartrate (lyophilized mixture, under nitrogen atmosphere), per 5-mL unit dose vial (Rx) [*Technetium Tc 99m HSA*].
      21 mg of albumin human and 230 mcg (0.23 mg) of stannous tartrate (lyophilized mixture, under nitrogen atmosphere), per 10-mL multidose vial (Rx) [*Technetium Tc 99m HSA*].
Canada—
   Reaction vial: 50 mg of albumin human, 200 mcg (0.2 mg) of stannous chloride dihydrate, and 2 mg potassium biphthalate (lyophilized mixture, under nitrogen atmosphere) (Rx) [*Frosstimage Albumin*].

**Packaging and storage**
Before and after reconstitution—Store between 2 and 8 °C (36 and 46 °F). Protect from freezing.

**Preparation of dosage form**
To prepare injection, an oxidant-free sodium pertechnetate Tc 99m solution is used. See manufacturer's package insert for instructions.

**Stability**
Injection should be administered within 6 hours after preparation.

**Incompatibilities**
If oxidants such as peroxides and hypochlorites are present in the sodium pertechnetate Tc 99m used for labeling, the final preparation may be adversely affected and should be discarded.

**Note**
Caution—Radioactive material.

## Selected Bibliography
Atkins HL, Klopper JF, Ansari AN, et al. A comparison of Tc 99m–labeled human serum albumin and *in vitro* labeled red blood cells for blood pool studies. Clin Nucl Med 1980; 5: 166-9.

Thrall JH, Freitas JE, Swanson D, et al. Clinical comparison of cardiac blood pool visualization with technetium 99m red blood cells labeled *in vivo* and with technetium 99m human serum albumin. J Nucl Med 1978; 19: 796-803.

Revised: 04/05/93
Interim revision: 08/02/94

# TECHNETIUM Tc 99m ALBUMIN AGGREGATED  Systemic

VA CLASSIFICATION (Primary): DX201

Commonly used brand name(s): *AN-MAA; Frosstimage MAA; MPI MAA; Macrotec; Pulmolite; TechneScan MAA*.

Note: For a listing of dosage forms and brand names by country availability, see *Dosage Forms* section(s).

## Category

Diagnostic aid, radioactive (pulmonary disease; vascular disorders); Chemotherapy adjunct.

## Indications

Note: Bracketed information in the *Indications* section refers to uses that are not included in U.S. product labeling.

**Accepted**

Lung imaging, radionuclide—Technetium Tc 99m albumin aggregated is indicated in adult and pediatric patients as a lung imaging agent to be used as an adjunct in the assessment of regional lung perfusion, primarily to screen for pulmonary emboli. It is also useful in the evaluation of the status of pulmonary circulation in such conditions as pulmonary neoplasm, pulmonary tuberculosis, and emphysema.

Venography, radionuclide—Technetium Tc 99m albumin aggregated is indicated to visualize specific regions of the vascular system and the blood flow in such areas, primarily to localize deep venous thrombosis in the lower extremities. Combined radionuclide venography of the lower extremities and pulmonary perfusion imaging may be performed with technetium Tc 99m albumin aggregated.

LeVeen peritoneovenous shunt patency assessment[1]—Intraperitoneal technetium Tc 99m albumin aggregated is indicated in adults to determine the patency of a peritoneovenous shunt in patients with ascites. The appearance of lung activity is used as the criterion for shunt patency.

[Chemotherapy, intra-arterial, infusion adjunct][1]—Technetium Tc 99m albumin aggregated is used as an adjunct to intra-arterial chemotherapy infusion for neoplasms (e.g., hepatic tumors) to assess blood flow, to evaluate catheter placement and tumor perfusion, and to visualize the area of distribution of the infused chemotherapeutic agent.

[1]Not included in Canadian product labeling.

## Physical Properties

**Nuclear Data**

| Radionuclide (half-life) | Decay constant | Mode of decay | Principal photon emissions (keV) | Mean number of emissions/ disintegration ($\geq 0.01$) |
|---|---|---|---|---|
| Tc 99m (6.0 hr) | 0.1151 h$^{-1}$ | Isomeric transition to Tc 99 | Gamma (18) | 0.062 |
| | | | Gamma (140.5) | 0.891 |

## Pharmacology/Pharmacokinetics

**Mechanism of action/Effect**

Diagnostic aid (pulmonary disease)—The intravenously injected albumin particles labeled with technetium Tc 99m are temporarily trapped by the capillary bed of the lungs, making it possible to obtain an image of patent blood flow distribution within lungs.

Diagnostic aid (vascular disorders)—After injection into the dorsal pedal veins, technetium Tc 99m–labeled albumin particles are transported by the blood flow to the lungs where they are trapped in the capillary bed. However, if lower extremity venous thrombosis or obstruction is present, the albumin particles show retention and/or abnormal movement (delayed or collateral flow) in the peripheral veins.

LeVeen peritoneovenous shunt patency assessment—After intraperitoneal injection, clearance of technetium Tc 99m albumin aggregated from the peritoneal cavity may be insignificant, which occurs with peritoneovenous shunt blockage, or it may be very rapid, as with subsequent transfer into the systemic circulation when the shunt is patent. Visualization of radioactivity in lungs indicates shunt patency.

Intra-arterial chemotherapy, infusion adjunct—Albumin particles labeled with technetium Tc 99m infused through an intra-arterial catheter directly into the arterial supply of a neoplasm (or of the organ containing the neoplasm), at the same rate at which the chemotherapeutic agent is to be delivered, are trapped in the capillary bed allowing visualization of the perfusion pattern.

**Absorption**

80 to 90% of the technetium Tc 99m albumin aggregated particles are trapped in the arterioles and capillaries of the lung during the first circulatory transit through the lungs after intravenous injection.

**Distribution**

Dependent on particle size—Particles > 10 to 15 microns: Trapped in pulmonary arterioles and capillaries.

Distribution of particles in the lungs is dependent on regional pulmonary blood flow.

**Half-life**

Biological elimination (from lungs)—Approximately 1 to 10 hours.

**Radiation dosimetry**

| Estimated absorbed radiation dose* |||
|---|---|---|
| Organ | mGy/MBq | rad/mCi |
| Lungs | 0.067 | 0.25 |
| Liver | 0.016 | 0.059 |
| Bladder wall | 0.010 | 0.037 |
| Adrenals | 0.0058 | 0.021 |
| Pancreas | 0.0058 | 0.021 |
| Breast | 0.0056 | 0.021 |
| Red marrow | 0.0044 | 0.016 |
| Spleen | 0.0044 | 0.016 |
| Stomach wall | 0.0040 | 0.015 |
| Kidneys | 0.0037 | 0.014 |
| Bone surfaces | 0.0035 | 0.013 |
| Uterus | 0.0024 | 0.0089 |
| Large intestine wall (upper) | 0.0022 | 0.0081 |
| Small intestine | 0.0021 | 0.0078 |
| Thyroid | 0.0020 | 0.0074 |
| Ovaries | 0.0018 | 0.0067 |
| Large intestine wall (lower) | 0.0016 | 0.0059 |
| Testes | 0.0011 | 0.0041 |
| Other tissue | 0.0029 | 0.011 |

Effective dose: 0.012 mSv/MBq (0.044 rem/mCi)

*For adults; intravenous injection. Data based on the International Commission on Radiological Protection (ICRP) Publication 53— Radiation dose to patients from radiopharmaceuticals.

**Elimination**

Renal, 40 to 75% of injected technetium Tc 99m eliminated within 24 hours.

## Precautions to Consider

**Cross-sensitivity and/or related problems**

Patients sensitive to human serum albumin products may be sensitive to this radiopharmaceutical also.

**Carcinogenicity/Mutagenicity**

Long-term animal studies to evaluate carcinogenic or mutagenic potential of technetium Tc 99m albumin aggregated have not been performed.

**Pregnancy/Reproduction**

Pregnancy—Tc 99m (as free pertechnetate) crosses the placenta. Studies have not been done in humans with technetium Tc 99m albumin aggregated.

The possibility of pregnancy should be assessed in women of child-bearing potential. Clinical situations exist where the benefit to the patient and fetus, based on information derived from radiopharmaceutical use, outweighs the risks from fetal exposure to radiation. In these situations, the physician should use discretion and reduce the radiopharmaceutical dose to the lowest possible amount.

Studies have not been done in animals.

FDA Pregnancy Category C.

**Breast-feeding**

Although it is not known whether technetium Tc 99m albumin aggregated is distributed into breast milk, it is known that Tc 99m as free pertechnetate is distributed into breast milk. It has been estimated that, without discontinuation of breast-feeding, the radiation dose to the breast-fed infant will be less than 20 mrems after the mother receives a 4-millicurie dose of technetium Tc 99m albumin aggregated, assuming that all of the radioactive dose is in the form of Tc 99m pertechnetate. Because of the potential risk to the infant from radiation exposure, temporary discontinuation of nursing is recommended for 6 to 12 hours.

### Pediatrics
Although appropriate studies have not been performed in the pediatric population, the number of particles administered should be reduced to the lowest possible level (≤ 50,000 particles for newborns, ≤ 165,000 particles for 1 year-old infants) in these patients since the pulmonary capillary beds in children do not develop fully for several years after birth.

### Medical considerations/Contraindications
The medical considerations/contraindications included have been selected on the basis of their potential clinical significance (reasons given in parentheses where appropriate)—not necessarily inclusive (» = major clinical significance).

*Except under special circumstances, this medication should not be used when the following medical problem exists:*
- » Pulmonary hypertension, severe
  (deaths associated with administration of aggregated albumin have been reported)

*Risk-benefit should be considered when the following medical problems exist:*
- Cardiac shunt, right-to-left
  (may increase risk because of rapid entry of aggregated albumin into the systemic circulation; it is recommended that the number of particles administered be reduced to 60,000 to 125,000 particles)
- Cor pulmonale, acute or
- Other states of severely impaired pulmonary blood flow
  (aggregated albumin may cause further impairment of blood flow; it is recommended that the number of particles administered be reduced to 125,000 particles or less)
- » Sensitivity to human serum albumin or to the radiopharmaceutical preparation

## Side/Adverse Effects
Note: There are reports of hemodynamic or idiosyncratic reactions associated with the administration of technetium Tc 99m albumin aggregated.

As with any protein-containing preparation, allergic reactions are possible with the use of technetium Tc 99m albumin aggregated.

The following side/adverse effects have been selected on the basis of their potential clinical significance and/or frequency of occurrence (possible signs and symptoms in parentheses where appropriate)—not necessarily inclusive:

**Those indicating need for medical attention**
Incidence less frequent or rare
  *Cyanosis* (bluish discoloration of skin); *wheezing, tightness in chest, or troubled breathing*

Note: *Wheezing, tightness in chest, or troubled breathing* may be initial manifestations of more severe respiratory distress.

**Those indicating need for medical attention only if they continue or are bothersome**
Incidence more frequent
  *Flushing or redness of face*
Incidence less frequent
  *Increased sweating; nausea*

## Patient Consultation
As an aid to patient consultation, refer to *Advice for the Patient, Radiopharmaceuticals (Diagnostic)*.

In providing consultation, consider emphasizing the following selected information (» = major clinical significance):

**Description of use**
  Action in the body: Radioactive albumin particles temporarily trapped in capillaries of lungs
  Tracing of radioactivity demonstrates the distribution of blood flow in lungs
  Small amounts of radioactivity used in diagnosis; radiation received is low and considered safe

**Before having this test**
- » Conditions affecting use, especially:
  Sensitivity to albumin products or to the radiopharmaceutical preparation

  Pregnancy—Technetium Tc 99m (as free pertechnetate) crosses placenta; risk to fetus from radiation exposure as opposed to benefit derived from use should be considered
  Breast-feeding—Not known if distributed into breast milk; temporary discontinuation of nursing may be recommended because of risk to infant from radiation exposure
  Use in children—Risk from radiation exposure as opposed to benefit derived from use should be considered

**Preparation for this test**
  Special preparatory instructions may be given; patient should inquire in advance

**Precautions after having this test**
  No special precautions

**Side/adverse effects**
  Signs of potential side effects, especially allergic reaction or respiratory distress

## General Dosing Information
Radiopharmaceuticals are to be administered only by or under the supervision of physicians who have had extensive training in the safe use and handling of radioactive materials and who are authorized by the Nuclear Regulatory Commission (NRC) or the appropriate Agreement State agency if required, or, outside the U.S., the appropriate authority.

Technetium Tc 99m albumin aggregated should be administered by slow intravenous injection with the patient in a recumbent position. During injection, the aspiration of blood into the syringe should be avoided since this can cause the formation of blood clots (containing the radioactive material) in the syringe, which may result in focal areas of increased radioactivity later on during lung imaging.

125,000 to 2,000,000 particles of aggregated albumin should be administered to adults per dosage.

Pediatric dosages must contain significantly fewer particles than adult dosages since the pulmonary capillary beds in pediatric patients are not as developed. It has been suggested that if 500,000 particles are considered safe in an adult, a newborn should not receive more than 50,000 particles, and a one-year-old no more than 165,000 particles.

Epinephrine, antihistamines, and corticosteroid agents should be available during the administration of technetium Tc 99m albumin aggregated because of the possibility of allergic reactions.

For lung imaging, it is recommended that the patient be positioned under the imaging apparatus before administration of technetium Tc 99m albumin aggregated and that imaging begin immediately after injection.

**Safety considerations for handling this radiopharmaceutical**
Improper handling of this radiopharmaceutical may cause radioactive contamination. Guidelines for handling radioactive material have been prepared by scientific, professional, state, federal, and international bodies and are available to the specially qualified and authorized users who have access to radiopharmaceuticals.

## Parenteral Dosage Forms

### TECHNETIUM Tc 99m ALBUMIN AGGREGATED INJECTION USP

**Usual adult and adolescent administered activity**
Lung imaging—
  Intravenous, 37 to 148 megabecquerels (1 to 4 millicuries).
Venography—
  Intravenous, 74 to 148 megabecquerels (2 to 4 millicuries) per extremity.
LeVeen shunt patency[1]—
  Intraperitoneal, 37 to 111 megabecquerels (1 to 3 millicuries).
  Percutaneous transtubal, 12 to 37 megabecquerels (0.3 to 1 millicurie) in a volume not to exceed 0.5 mL.

Note: The lowest possible number of particles per dosage (60,000 to 125,000) should be administered to patients with right-to-left cardiac shunt or with states of severely impaired pulmonary blood flow.

**Usual pediatric administered activity**
Lung imaging—
  Intravenous, 0.925 to 1.85 megabecquerels (25 to 50 microcuries) per kg of body weight.

Note: In newborns, the total dosage should be at least 7.4 megabecquerels (200 microcuries).

**Usual geriatric administered activity**
See *Usual adult and adolescent administered activity*.

**Strength(s) usually available**

U.S.—
- 0.11 mg albumin aggregated, 0.09 mg stannous tartrate, and 0.3 mL isotonic saline, per reaction vial (Rx) [GENERIC].
- 1.0 mg albumin aggregated, 10.0 mg albumin human, 0.02 mg stannous chloride, 0.12 mg total tin, 10 mg sodium chloride, with 3.6 to 6.5 $\times 10^6$ particles, per 10-mL reaction vial (Rx) [*Pulmolite*].
- 1.5 mg albumin aggregated, 10.0 mg albumin human, 0.07 mg stannous chloride, 0.19 mg total tin, 1.8 mg sodium chloride, with 1.0 to 8.0 $\times 10^6$ particles, per 5-mL reaction vial (Rx) [*Macrotec*].
- 2.0 mg albumin aggregated, 0.5 mg albumin human, 0.12 mg stannous chloride, 80 mg lactose, 24 mg succinic acid, and 1.4 mg sodium acetate, with $8\pm4 \times 10^6$ particles, per 10-mL reaction vial (Rx) [*TechneScan MAA*].
- 2.0 mg albumin aggregated, 0.16 mg stannous chloride, and 17 mg sodium chloride, with $6.8\pm0.8 \times 10^6$ particles, per reaction vial (Rx) [*AN-MAA*].
- 2.5 mg albumin aggregated, 5.0 mg albumin human, 0.06 mg stannous chloride, and 1.2 mg sodium chloride, with 4.0 to 8.0 $\times 10^6$ particles, per 10-mL reaction vial (Rx) [*MPI MAA*; GENERIC].

Canada—
- 2.5 mg albumin aggregated, 5.0 mg albumin human, 0.1 mg stannous chloride (dihydrate), and 1.2 mg sodium chloride, with 4.0 to 8.0 $\times 10^6$ particles, per 10-mL reaction vial (Rx) [*Frosstimage MAA*].

**Packaging and storage**

Store between 2 and 8 °C (36 and 46 °F). Protect from freezing.

**Preparation of dosage form**

To prepare injection, an oxidant-free sodium pertechnetate Tc 99m solution is used. See manufacturer's package insert for instructions.

**Stability**

Preparations in which clumping or foaming of contents are observed should not be used.

Injection should be administered within 3, 6, or 8 hours after preparation, depending on product used.

**Incompatibilities**

If oxidants such as peroxides and hypochlorites are present in the sodium pertechnetate Tc 99m used for labeling, the final preparation may be adversely affected and should be discarded.

**Note**

Caution—Radioactive material.
Agitate gently before using.

[1]Not included in Canadian product labeling.

**Selected Bibliography**

Algeo JH, Powell M, Couacaud J. LeVeen shunt visualization without function using technetium 99m macroaggregated albumin. Clin Nucl Med 1987; 12(9): 741-3.

Revised: 06/14/93
Interim revision: 08/02/94

# TECHNETIUM Tc 99m ALBUMIN COLLOID  Systemic[†]

VA CLASSIFICATION (Primary): DX201

Commonly used brand name(s): *Microlite*.

Note: For a listing of dosage forms and brand names by country availability, see *Dosage Forms* section(s).

[†]Not commercially available in Canada.

## Category

Diagnostic aid, radioactive (hepatic disease; hematologic disease; splenic disease).

## Indications

**Accepted**

Liver imaging, radionuclide—Technetium Tc 99m albumin colloid, administered intravenously, is indicated for imaging the functioning reticuloendothelial cells of the liver in the evaluation of metastatic disease, primary liver tumors, abscesses, and other focal hepatic lesions. It is also indicated in the evaluation of patients with cirrhosis, hepatitis, and other hepatic disorders.

Spleen imaging, radionuclide—Technetium Tc 99m albumin colloid, administered intravenously, is indicated for imaging the functioning reticuloendothelial cells of the spleen, thus serving to demonstrate clinically significant splenomegaly, and for evaluating splenic infarct or splenic rupture.

Bone marrow imaging, radionuclide—Technetium Tc 99m albumin colloid, administered intravenously, is indicated for imaging the functioning reticuloendothelial cells of the bone marrow to complement other hematological studies for the evaluation of hematopoiesis in hematological diseases, such as leukemia, polycythemia, anemias, and myelofibrosis. Also, imaging with technetium Tc 99m albumin colloid helps localize sites for bone marrow biopsy and helps demonstrate or define areas of marrow invasion by metastatic disease and areas of decreased marrow function secondary to radiation therapy.

## Physical Properties

**Nuclear data**

| Radionuclide (half-life) | Decay constant | Mode of decay | Principal photon emissions (keV) | Mean number of emissions/ disintegration ($\geq 0.01$) |
|---|---|---|---|---|
| Tc 99m (6.0 hr) | 0.1151 h$^{-1}$ | Isomeric transition to Tc 99 | Gamma (18) | 0.062 |
|  |  |  | Gamma (140.5) | 0.891 |

## Pharmacology/Pharmacokinetics

**Mechanism of action/Effect**

Diagnostic aid (hepatic disease; hematologic disease; splenic disease)—Radioactive colloids are phagocytized by the reticuloendothelial system of the liver, spleen, and bone marrow, and remain there long enough for scintillation scans of their distribution to be obtained.

**Distribution**

The colloid particles are rapidly phagocytized by the reticuloendothelial system after intravenous administration. Distribution is dependent upon blood flow rates and the functional capacity of the phagocytic cells. In the average normal patient, 80 to 90% of the administered activity localizes in the liver, 5 to 10% in the spleen, and the remainder in bone marrow. Levels of activity in the liver and spleen remain constant for at least 4 hours.

Uptake in the lungs and other soft tissues is possible in the presence of a wide variety of disorders, usually inflammatory or neoplastic.

Note: In progressively severe hepatic dysfunction (e.g., hepatic cirrhosis), greater amounts of the colloid appear in the spleen, bone marrow, and sometimes, in the lungs.

**Half-life**

Elimination from the blood pool—2 to 3 minutes.

**Time to radioactivity visualization**

Liver and spleen imaging—10 to 15 minutes.

Note: In patients with severe hepatic disease, onset of visualization may be delayed because of slower blood clearance of the colloid.

Bone marrow imaging—15 minutes.

## Radiation dosimetry

| | Estimated absorbed radiation dose* | | | |
|---|---|---|---|---|
| | With normal hepatic function | | With parenchymal liver disease (intermediate/advanced) | |
| Organ | mGy/MBq | rad/mCi | mGy/MBq | rad/mCi |
| Spleen | 0.077 | 0.29 | 0.14 | 0.52 |
| Liver | 0.074 | 0.27 | 0.042 | 0.16 |
| Pancreas | 0.012 | 0.044 | 0.018 | 0.066 |
| Red marrow | 0.011 | 0.041 | 0.023 | 0.085 |
| Adrenals | 0.01 | 0.037 | 0.0098 | 0.036 |
| Kidneys | 0.0097 | 0.036 | 0.011 | 0.041 |
| Bone surfaces | 0.0064 | 0.024 | 0.012 | 0.044 |
| Stomach wall | 0.0062 | 0.023 | 0.0098 | 0.036 |
| Large intestine wall (upper) | 0.0056 | 0.021 | 0.0049 | 0.018 |
| Lungs | 0.0055 | 0.20 | 0.0048 | 0.018 |
| Small intestine | 0.0043 | 0.016 | 0.0046 | 0.017 |
| Breast | 0.0027 | 0.01 | 0.0024 | 0.0089 |
| Ovaries | 0.0022 | 0.0081 | 0.0033 | 0.012 |
| Uterus | 0.0019 | 0.0070 | 0.0028 | 0.01 |
| Large intestine wall (lower) | 0.0018 | 0.0067 | 0.0031 | 0.011 |
| Bladder wall | 0.0011 | 0.0041 | 0.0016 | 0.0059 |
| Thyroid | 0.00079 | 0.0029 | 0.0011 | 0.0041 |
| Testes | 0.00062 | 0.0023 | 0.00095 | 0.0035 |
| Other tissue | 0.0028 | 0.01 | 0.0031 | 0.011 |

| | Effective dose* | | | |
|---|---|---|---|---|
| | With normal hepatic function | | With parenchymal liver disease (intermediate/advanced) | |
| Radionuclide | mSv/MBq | rem/mCi | mSv/MBq | rem/mCi |
| Tc 99m | 0.014 | 0.052 | 0.017 | 0.063 |

*For adults; intravenous injection of technetium Tc 99m–labeled large colloids. Data based on the International Commission on Radiological Protection (ICRP) Publication 53—Radiation dose to patients from radiopharmaceuticals.

### Elimination
Renal, 4 to 30% of the administered activity is eliminated by 24 hours after injection.

## Precautions to Consider

### Cross-sensitivity and/or related problems
Patients sensitive to human serum albumin products may be sensitive to this radiopharmaceutical also.

### Carcinogenicity/Mutagenicity
Long-term animal studies to evaluate carcinogenic or mutagenic potential of technetium Tc 99m albumin colloid have not been performed.

### Pregnancy/Reproduction
Pregnancy—Tc 99m (as free pertechnetate) crosses the placenta. Studies with technetium Tc 99m albumin colloid have not been done in humans.
The possibility of pregnancy should be assessed in women of child-bearing potential. Clinical situations exist in which the benefit to the patient and fetus, based on information derived from radiopharmaceutical use, outweighs the risks from fetal exposure to radiation. In these situations, the physician should use discretion and reduce the radiopharmaceutical dose to the lowest possible amount.
Studies have not been done in animals.
FDA Pregnancy Category C.

### Breast-feeding
Although it is not known whether technetium Tc 99m albumin colloid is distributed into breast milk, it is known that Tc 99m as free pertechnetate is distributed into breast milk. Based on the assumption that the Tc 99m in breast milk is in the form of pertechnetate and based on the effective half-life of the radionuclide in breast milk, the daily volume of milk, a dose factor relating the radionuclide to its critical organ (thyroid) in the nursing infant, and the maximum permissible dose to that organ, a guideline has been proposed. According to this guideline, it has been calculated that nursing can be safely resumed when the concentration in breast milk reaches $30.3 \times 10^{-4}$ megabecquerels ($8.2 \times 10^{-2}$ microcuries) per mL. This level of activity is probably reached, in the majority of patients, within 12 to 24 hours after administration of technetium Tc 99m–labeled radiopharmaceuticals.

### Pediatrics
Diagnostic studies performed to date using technetium Tc 99 albumin colloid have not demonstrated pediatrics-specific problems that would limit the usefulness of technetium Tc 99m albumin colloid in children. However, when this radiopharmaceutical is used in children, the diagnostic benefit should be judged to outweigh the potential risk of radiation.

### Geriatrics
Appropriate studies on the relationship of age to the effects of technetium Tc 99m albumin colloid have not been performed in the geriatric population. However, no geriatrics-specific problems have been documented to date.

### Drug interactions and/or related problems
See *Diagnostic interference*.

### Diagnostic interference
The following have been selected on the basis of their potential clinical significance (possible effect in parentheses where appropriate)—not necessarily inclusive (» = major clinical significance):

With results of this test
*Due to other medications*
  Anesthetics, inhalation, such as halothane
    (recent administration of general anesthetics may increase splenic uptake of technetium Tc 99m albumin colloid, probably because the reduced hepatic flow and hepatotoxicity associated with general anesthetics may alter the hepatic radiocolloid extraction efficiency, resulting in an alteration of the normal liver-spleen colloid distribution pattern)
  Chemotherapy, especially with nitrosoureas
    (use of technetium Tc 99m albumin colloid in patients who are undergoing or have recently undergone chemotherapy may result in nonhomogeneous or irregular hepatic uptake, shift of activity from the liver to the bone marrow and spleen, and hepatomegaly; irregular hepatic distribution of radiopharmaceutical may be misinterpreted as malignancy; thus, it is recommended that liver and/or spleen imaging be done prior to initiating chemotherapy with these agents or several weeks after discontinuing therapy)
  Reticuloendothelial system stimulators, such as:
    Dextrose
    Heparin
    Steroid hormones (including estrogen)
    Thyroid hormones
    Vitamin $B_{12}$
    (use of technetium Tc 99m albumin colloid in patients using these medications may result in lung uptake of technetium Tc 99m albumin colloid, probably due to a drug-induced increase in number of free intravascular macrophages, which may migrate to the pulmonary capillary bed and phagocytize colloidal particles there)

*Due to medical problems or conditions*
  Viral infections
    (decreased function of the reticuloendothelial system caused by the viral infection may result in prolonged appearance of the technetium Tc 99m albumin colloid in the blood)

### Medical considerations/Contraindications
The medical considerations/contraindications included have been selected on the basis of their potential clinical significance (reasons given in parentheses where appropriate)—not necessarily inclusive (» = major clinical significance).
See also *Diagnostic interference*.

*Risk-benefit should be considered when the following medical problem exists:*
» Sensitivity to human serum albumin or to the radiopharmaceutical preparation

## Side/Adverse Effects
The following side/adverse effects have been selected on the basis of their potential clinical significance and/or frequency of occurrence (possible signs and symptoms in parentheses where appropriate)—not necessarily inclusive:

### Those indicating need for medical attention
Incidence less frequent or rare
  *Allergic reaction* (coughing or choking; flushing or redness of face; skin rash, hives, or itching; swelling of throat, hands, or feet; wheezing, tightness in chest, or troubled breathing)

  Note: The *allergic reaction* may be the initial manifestation of a more severe anaphylactic reaction.

Those indicating need for medical attention only if they continue or are bothersome
Incidence less frequent
*Abdominal pain; dizziness; fever; flushing of skin; increased sweating; nausea*

## Patient Consultation

As an aid to patient consultation, refer to *Advice for the Patient, Radiopharmaceuticals (Diagnostic).*
In providing consultation, consider emphasizing the following selected information (» = major clinical significance):

**Description of use**
Action in the body: Accumulation of radioactive colloid particles in liver, spleen, and bone marrow
Retention of radioactivity in these organs allows visualization
Small amounts of radioactivity used in diagnosis; radiation received is low and considered safe

**Before having this test**
» Conditions affecting use, especially:
Sensitivity to albumin products or to the radiopharmaceutical preparation
Pregnancy—Technetium Tc 99m (as free pertechnetate) crosses placenta; risk to fetus from radiation exposure as opposed to benefit derived from use should be considered
Breast-feeding—Not known if technetium Tc 99m albumin colloid is distributed into breast milk, but Tc 99m as free pertechnetate is distributed into breast milk; temporary discontinuation of nursing may be recommended because of risk to infant from radiation exposure
Use in children—Risk from radiation exposure as opposed to benefit derived from use should be considered

**Preparation for this test**
Special preparatory instructions may be given; patient should inquire in advance

**Precautions after having this test**
No special precautions

**Side/adverse effects**
Signs of potential side effects, especially allergic reaction

## General Dosing Information

Radiopharmaceuticals are to be administered only by or under the supervision of physicians who have had extensive training in the safe use and handling of radioactive materials and who are authorized by the Nuclear Regulatory Commission (NRC) or the appropriate Agreement State agency if required, or, outside the U.S., the appropriate authority.

Technetium Tc 99m albumin colloid should be administered by intravenous injection and, preferably, with the patient in a recumbent position (in the erect position the liver may appear larger). During injection, the aspiration of blood into the syringe should be avoided since this can cause the formation of blood clots (containing the radioactive material) in the syringe, which may result in focal areas of increased radioactivity during lung imaging.

Epinephrine, antihistamines, and corticosteroids should be available during the administration of technetium Tc 99m albumin colloid because of the possibility of allergic reactions.

**Safety considerations for handling this radiopharmaceutical**
Improper handling of this radiopharmaceutical may cause radioactive contamination. Guidelines for handling radioactive material have been prepared by scientific, professional, state, federal, and international bodies and are available to the specially qualified and authorized users who have access to radiopharmaceuticals.

## Parenteral Dosage Forms

### TECHNETIUM Tc 99m ALBUMIN COLLOID INJECTION

**Usual adult and adolescent administered activity**
Liver, spleen, and/or bone marrow imaging—
Intravenous, 37 to 296 megabecquerels (1 to 8 millicuries).
Note: For bone marrow imaging, 370 to 444 megabecquerels (10 to 12 millicuries) are usually required.

**Usual pediatric administered activity**
Dosage must be individualized by physician.
Liver and spleen imaging—
Activity administered has ranged between 0.55 and 2.75 megabecquerels (15 to 75 microcuries) per kg of body weight, with a usual administered activity of 1.8 megabecquerels (50 microcuries) per kg of body weight.
Note: In newborns, the total minimum administered activity recommended for liver and spleen imaging is 11.1 to 18.5 megabecquerels (300 to 500 microcuries).
Bone marrow imaging—
A dosage of 5.18 megabecquerels (140 microcuries) per kg of body weight is recommended.

**Usual geriatric administered activity**
See *Usual adult and adolescent administered activity.*

**Strength(s) usually available**
U.S.—
1 mg albumin colloid, 10 mg normal human serum albumin, 0.0054 mg stannous chloride (minimum), 0.17 mg total tin (maximum), 1.1 mg poloxamer 188, 0.12 mg medronate disodium, and 10 mg sodium phosphate (anhydrous), per reaction vial (Rx) [*Microlite*].
Canada—
Not commercially available.

**Packaging and storage**
Store between 2 and 8 °C (36 and 46 °F). Protect from freezing. Protect from light.

**Preparation of dosage form**
To prepare injection, an oxidant-free sodium pertechnetate Tc 99m solution is used. See manufacturer's package insert for instructions.

**Stability**
Preparations in which clumping of contents are observed should not be used.
Injection should be administered within 6 hours after preparation.

**Incompatibilities**
If oxidants such as peroxides and hypochlorites are present in the sodium pertechnetate Tc 99m used for labeling, the final preparation may be adversely affected and should be discarded.

**Note**
Caution—Radioactive material.
Agitate gently before using.

## Selected Bibliography

Klingensmith WC, Spitzer VM, Fritzberg AR, et al. Normal appearance and reproducibility of liver-spleen studies with Tc 99m sulfur colloid and Tc 99m microalbumin colloid. J Nucl Med 1983; 24: 8-13.

Saha GB, Feiglin DHI, O'Donnell JK, et al. Experience with technetium Tc 99m albumin colloid kit for reticuloendothelial system imaging. J Nucl Med Technol 1986; 14: 149-51.

Developed: 08/17/94

---

# TECHNETIUM Tc 99m ARCITUMOMAB   Systemic

VA CLASSIFICATION (Primary): DX201
Note: For a listing of brand names for the articles in this monograph, refer to the *General Index.*
Commonly used brand name(s): *CEA-Scan.*
Note: For a listing of dosage forms and brand names by country availability, see *Dosage Forms* section(s).

## Category

Diagnostic aid, radioactive (colorectal disease).

## Indications

Note: Bracketed information in the *Indications* section refers to uses that are not included in U.S. product labeling.

**Accepted**
Carcinoma, colorectal (diagnosis adjunct)—Technetium Tc 99m arcitumomab, in conjunction with standard diagnostic modalities (e.g., computed tomography [CT]), is indicated to detect, locate, and determine the extent of recurrent and/or metastatic colorectal carcinoma involving the liver and the extrahepatic abdominal and pelvic regions in patients with a histologically confirmed diagnosis of colorectal carcinoma. Imaging with technetium Tc 99m arcitumomab provides additional infor-

mation in patients suspected of tumor recurrence or metastasis who have elevated or rising serum carcinoembryonic antigen (CEA) but no evidence of disease by standard diagnostic methods (e.g., abdominal and pelvic CT, chest radiograph, colonoscopy, barium enema).

**Acceptance not established**
Technetium Tc 99m arcitumomab may have a role as an adjunct to mammography in the diagnosis of primary, recurrent, or metastatic mammary cancer, particularly in patients without palpable abnormalities who have indeterminate mammograms. However, at present, there are insufficient data to confirm the usefulness of technetium Tc 99m arcitumomab for this indication.

## Physical Properties
### Nuclear Data

| Radionuclide (half-life) | Mode of decay | Principal photon emissions (keV) | Mean number of emissions/ disintegration |
|---|---|---|---|
| Tc 99m (6 hr) | Isomeric transition to Tc 99 | Gamma (18) Gamma (140.5) | 0.062 0.891 |

## Pharmacology/Pharmacokinetics
### Physicochemical characteristics
Source—Arcitumomab, the Fab' fragment, is derived from purified IMMU-4 by enzymatic digestion with pepsin, which produces F(ab')2 fragments, and by subsequent reduction, the Fab' fragments.
Molecular weight—Arcitumomab: approximately 50,000 daltons.

### Mechanism of action/Effect
Arcitumomab, a Fab' fragment of the murine monoclonal antibody IMMU-4 of the IgG1 subclass, is directed against a 200,000-dalton carcinoembryonic antigen (CEA) that is expressed on the cell surface of numerous tumors, particularly of the gastrointestinal tract (including fetal gastrointestinal tissues) and in certain inflammatory states (e.g., Crohn's disease). The Fab' fragment is used rather than the whole monoclonal antibody because of its more favorable pharmacokinetics (faster blood clearance and minimal liver metabolism) also, it minimizes the frequency of human anti-mouse antibody response. Less than 50% antigen complexation with technetium Tc 99m arcitumomab occurs with plasma CEA levels of up to 2000 nanograms per mL, and antigen complexation is not detectable at serum CEA levels below 250 nanograms per mL. The distribution of radioactivity is recorded by planar scintigraphy and single photon emission computed tomography (SPECT).

### Distribution
After intravenous administration of technetium Tc 99m arcitumomab, there is moderately rapid clearance from the circulation. Blood levels at 1, 5, and 24 hours after technetium Tc 99m arcitumomab injection have been reported as 63%, 23%, and 7% of the administered activity, respectively. Technetium Tc 99m arcitumomab localizes at sites of increased CEA expression, particularly primary and/or metastatic colorectal lesions. Also, accumulation of radioactivity, leading to potential false-positive readings especially with planar imaging, may occur in nontumor areas, such as in major blood pool organs (e.g., heart, major vessels), near the sites of antibody fragment excretion (e.g., kidneys and urinary bladder, and in the gallbladder and intestines).

### Half-life
Elimination—
Initial: Approximately 1 hour.
Terminal: 13 ± 4 hours.

### Time to radioactivity visualization
For optimal target tissue visualization—Planar scintigraphy and SPECT are generally performed 2 to 5 hours after technetium Tc 99m arcitumomab administration. Selected additional views may be obtained for up to 24 hours after administration.

Note: If late imaging is performed (up to 24 hours postinjection), intestinal and gallbladder activity may interfere with true tumor imaging. Late images should be compared to earlier ones (2 to 5 hours) and interpreted cautiously.

### Radiation dosimetry:

| | Estimated absorbed radiation dose* | |
|---|---|---|
| Organ | mGy/MBq (mean) | rad/mCi |
| Kidney | 0.1 | 0.4 |
| Bladder | 0.02 | 0.06 |
| Spleen | 0.02 | 0.06 |
| Liver | 0.01 | 0.04 |
| Red marrow | 0.01 | 0.04 |
| Ovaries | 0.008 | 0.03 |
| Lungs | 0.008 | 0.03 |
| Testes | 0.005 | 0.02 |
| Total body | 0.005 | 0.02 |

Effective dose: 0.009 mSv/MBq (0.03 rem/mCi)

* For adults; intravenous injection.

### Elimination
Renal (primary). Approximately 28% of the administered activity is excreted within the first 24 hours.

## Precautions to Consider
### Cross-sensitivity and/or related problems
Patients sensitive to murine antibody–based products may be sensitive to technetium Tc 99m arcitumomab also.

### Carcinogenicity/ Mutagenicity
Long-term animal studies to evaluate carcinogenic or mutagenic potential of technetium Tc 99m arcitumomab have not been performed.

### Pregnancy/Reproduction
Pregnancy—Tc 99m (as free pertechnetate) crosses the placenta. However, studies to assess transplacental transfer of technetium Tc 99m arcitumomab have not been done in humans.
To avoid the possibility of fetal exposure to radiation, in those circumstances in which the patient's pregnancy status is uncertain, a pregnancy test will help to prevent inadvertent administration of this preparation during pregnancy.
Studies have not been done in animals.
FDA Pregnancy Category C.

### Breast-feeding
Although it is not known whether technetium Tc 99m arcitumomab is distributed into breast milk, it is known that Tc 99m as free pertechnetate is distributed into breast milk. To avoid radiation exposure to the infant, discontinuation of nursing for a period of 24 hours is recommended after administration of technetium Tc 99m–labeled radiopharmaceuticals.

### Pediatrics
Studies on the relationship of age to the effects of technetium Tc 99m arcitumomab have not been performed in the pediatric population. However, pediatrics-specific problems that would limit the usefulness of technetium Tc 99m arcitumomab in children are not expected.

### Geriatrics
Appropriate studies on the relationship of age to the effects of technetium Tc 99m arcitumomab have not been performed in the geriatric population. However, clinical trials and studies that included older patients were conducted, and geriatrics-specific problems that would limit the usefulness of this agent in the elderly are not expected.

### Laboratory value alterations
The following have been selected on the basis of their potential clinical significance (possible effect in parentheses where appropriate)—not necessarily inclusive (» = major clinical significance):

With diagnostic test results
Immunoassays, murine antibody–based
(human anti-murine antibody [HAMA] production may be induced by the administration of murine monoclonal antibodies; although the use of the Fab' fragment almost always eliminates induction of HAMAs, HAMAs in serum may interfere with murine antibody–based immunoassays and with *in vitro* or *in vivo* diagnostic murine antibody–based agents, and may increase the risk of adverse reactions)

### Diagnostic interference
The following have been selected on the basis of their potential clinical significance (possible effect in parentheses where appropriate)—not necessarily inclusive (» = major clinical significance):

With results of this test
*Due to other medical problems or conditions*
Inflammatory lesions, local or
Surgical areas, recent
(localization of technetium Tc 99m arcitumomab may occur at these sites)

**Medical considerations/Contraindications**
The medical considerations/contraindications included have been selected on the basis of their potential clinical significance (reasons given in parentheses where appropriate)—not necessarily inclusive (» = major clinical significance).

*Risk-benefit should be considered when the following medical problems exist:*
Sensitivity to murine antibody–based products or to the radiopharmaceutical preparation

## Side/Adverse Effects

Note: Allergic reactions, including anaphylaxis, can occur in patients receiving murine antibody–based products. Although serious allergic reactions have not been reported during clinical trials with technetium Tc 99m arcitumomab, the possibility must be considered and proper treatment measures should be readily available.

The following side/adverse effects have been selected on the basis of their potential clinical significance (possible signs and symptoms in parentheses where appropriate)—not necessarily inclusive:

**Those indicating need for medical attention only if they continue or are bothersome**
Incidence rare
*Allergic reaction, mild, transient* (itching; skin rash); *bursitis* (pain and inflammation at the joints); *eosinophilia, transient; fever; headache; nausea*

## Patient Consultation

As an aid to patient consultation, refer to *Advice for the Patient, Radiopharmaceuticals (Diagnostic)*.
In providing consultation, consider emphasizing the following selected information (» = major clinical significance):

**Description of use**
Action in the body: Localization of radiolabeled monoclonal antibodies in tumor sites; uptake of radioactivity may be visualized by external imaging
Small amounts of radioactivity used in diagnosis; radiation received is low and considered safe

**Before using this test**
» Conditions affecting use, especially:
Sensitivity to murine antibody–based products or to the radiopharmaceutical preparation
Pregnancy—Technetium Tc 99m (as free pertechnetate) crosses the placenta; risk to fetus from radiation exposure as opposed to benefit derived from study should be considered
Breast-feeding—Not known if technetium Tc 99m arcitumomab is distributed into breast milk, but Tc 99m (as free pertechnetate) is distributed into breast milk; temporary discontinuation of nursing is recommended after administration of this agent to avoid any unnecessary absorbed radiation dose to the infant

**Preparation for this test**
Special preparatory instructions may apply; patient should inquire in advance
Voiding prior to imaging of the pelvis to minimize bladder activity, which may interfere with image interpretation

## General Dosing Information

Radiopharmaceuticals are to be administered only by or under the supervision of physicians who have had extensive training in the safe use and handling of radioactive materials and who are licensed by the Nuclear Regulatory Commission (NRC) or the appropriate Agreement State agency, if required, or, outside the U.S., the appropriate authority.

The patient should void prior to imaging of the pelvis to minimize bladder activity, which may interfere with image interpretation.

Guidelines for the receipt, storage, handling, dispensing, and disposal of radioactive materials are available from scientific, professional, state, federal, and international bodies. Handling of this radiopharmaceutical should be limited to those individuals who are appropriately qualified and authorized.

**For treatment of adverse effects**
Epinephrine and antihistamines should be available during the administration of technetium Tc 99m arcitumomab because of the possibility of allergic reactions.

## Parenteral Dosage Forms

**TECHNETIUM Tc 99m ARCITUMOMAB INJECTION**

**Usual adult administered activity**
Diagnosis of colorectal carcinoma—
Intravenous, 1 mg of arcitumomab radiolabeled with 740 to 1110 megabecquerels (20 to 30 millicuries) of technetium Tc 99m, administered over five to twenty minutes.

**Usual pediatric administered activity**
Minimum dosage has not been established.

**Usual geriatric administered activity**
See *Usual adult administered activity*.

**Strength(s) usually available**
U.S.—
1.25 mg of arcitumomab and 0.29 mg of stannous chloride, per single-use vial (Rx) [*CEA-Scan* (potassium sodium tartrate tetrahydrate; sodium acetate trihydrate; sodium chloride; glacial acetic acid; hydrochloric acid; sucrose)].
Canada—
1.25 mg of arcitumomab and 0.29 mg of stannous chloride, per single-use vial (Rx) [*CEA-Scan* (potassium sodium tartrate tetrahydrate; sodium acetate trihydrate; sodium chloride; glacial acetic acid; hydrochloric acid; sucrose)].

**Packaging and storage**
Before radiolabeling, store between 2 and 8 °C (36 and 46 °F), unless otherwise specified by manufacturer. Protect from freezing.
Note: After radiolabeling, the technetium Tc 99m arcitumomab injection can be kept at room temperature.

**Preparation of dosage form**
To radiolabel the arcitumomab, 1110 megabecquerels (30 millicuries) of a sterile, pyrogen- and oxidant-free sodium pertechnetate Tc 99m in 0.9% sodium chloride solution is used. See the manufacturer's package insert for instructions.

**Stability**
The package insert states that the injection can be administered 5 minutes after radiolabeling. Administration should occur within 4 hours after radiolabeling.

**Caution**
Radioactive material.

## Selected Bibliography

Moffat FL Jr, Vargas-Cuba RD, Serafini AN, et al. Radioimmunodetection of colorectal carcinoma using technetium-99m-labeled Fab' fragments of the IMMU-4 anti-carcinoembryonic antigen monoclonal antibody. Cancer 1994 Feb; 73(3 Suppl): 836-45.
Sirisriro R, Podoloff DA, Patt YZ, et al. 99mTc-IMMU-4 imaging in recurrent colorectal cancer: efficacy and impact on surgical management. Nucl Med Commun 1996 Jul; 17(7): 568-76.

Developed: 08/26/98

# TECHNETIUM Tc 99m BICISATE Systemic

VA CLASSIFICATION (Primary): DX201
Commonly used brand name(s): *Neurolite*.
Another commonly used name for bicisate is ethyl cysteinate dimer (ECD).
Note: For a listing of dosage forms and brand names by country availability, see *Dosage Forms* section(s).

## Category

Diagnostic aid, radioactive (cerebrovascular disease).

## Indications

Note: Bracketed information in the *Indications* section refers to uses that are not included in U.S. product labeling.

## Accepted

Brain imaging, radionuclide—Single-photon emission computed tomography (SPECT) using technetium Tc 99m bicisate is indicated as an adjunct to conventional computed tomography (CT) or magnetic resonance imaging (MRI) in the localization of stroke in patients in whom stroke has already been diagnosed. However, [technetium Tc 99m bicisate is also used in the evaluation and localization of altered regional cerebral perfusion associated with functional impairment in patients with neurological disorders not limited to stroke, but including such disorders as dementia, head trauma, and epilepsy].

## Physical Properties

### Nuclear data

| Radionuclide (half-life) | Decay constant | Mode of decay | Principal photon emissions (keV) | Mean number of emissions/ disintegration ($\geq 0.01$) |
|---|---|---|---|---|
| Tc 99m (6.0 hr) | 0.1151 h$^{-1}$ | Isomeric transition to Tc 99 | Gamma (18) | 0.062 |
|  |  |  | Gamma (140.5) | 0.891 |

## Pharmacology/Pharmacokinetics

### Mechanism of action/Effect

Brain imaging—Technetium Tc 99m bicisate is a lipophilic complex with high first-pass extraction fraction and deposition and retention in the brain in proportion to cerebral blood flow (perfusion). Its radionuclide emissions permit external imaging of the cerebral distribution of the agent, thus allowing the detection of altered regional cerebral perfusion. The retention in the brain of technetium Tc 99m bicisate results from *in vivo* metabolism (deesterification) of the primary complex to polar, less diffusable compounds (mono- and di-acids).

### Distribution

High initial cerebral uptake with rapid blood clearance after intravenous injection (less than 10% of the administered activity remains in the blood after 5 minutes). Approximately 5 to 8% of administered activity localizes in the brain within 5 minutes after injection and exhibits little change for one hour after injection. Brain washout is approximately 20% between 5 and 60 minutes after injection and approximately 10% per hour thereafter.

### Time to radioactivity visualization

10 minutes to 6 hours after injection. Optimal images may be obtained 30 to 60 minutes after administration to allow washout from facial muscles and salivary glands and thereby increase brain-to-soft-tissue ratios.

### Radiation dosimetry

| | Estimated absorbed radiation dose* | | | |
|---|---|---|---|---|
| | With 2-hour void | | With 4.8-hour void | |
| Organ | mGy/ MBq | rad/ mCi | mGy/ MBq | rad/ mCi |
| Urinary bladder wall | 0.03 | 0.11 | 0.073 | 0.27 |
| Gallbladder wall | 0.025 | 0.091 | 0.025 | 0.091 |
| Large intestine wall, upper | 0.016 | 0.061 | 0.017 | 0.063 |
| Large intestine wall, lower | 0.013 | 0.047 | 0.015 | 0.055 |
| Small intestine | 0.0094 | 0.035 | 0.01 | 0.038 |
| Kidneys | 0.0073 | 0.027 | 0.0074 | 0.027 |
| Uterus | 0.0063 | 0.023 | 0.011 | 0.041 |
| Brain | 0.0055 | 0.02 | 0.0055 | 0.02 |
| Ovaries | 0.0054 | 0.022 | 0.008 | 0.03 |
| Liver | 0.0053 | 0.02 | 0.0054 | 0.02 |
| Thyroid | 0.0035 | 0.013 | 0.0035 | 0.013 |
| Bone surfaces | 0.0034 | 0.013 | 0.0038 | 0.014 |
| Adrenals | 0.0025 | 0.009 | 0.0025 | 0.009 |
| Pancreas | 0.003 | 0.011 | 0.003 | 0.011 |
| Red marrow | 0.0024 | 0.009 | 0.0027 | 0.01 |
| Stomach | 0.0024 | 0.009 | 0.0025 | 0.0093 |
| Testes | 0.0022 | 0.008 | 0.0036 | 0.013 |
| Muscle | 0.002 | 0.007 | 0.0024 | 0.009 |

| | Estimated absorbed radiation dose* | | | |
|---|---|---|---|---|
| | With 2-hour void | | With 4.8-hour void | |
| Organ | mGy/ MBq | rad/ mCi | mGy/ MBq | rad/ mCi |
| Spleen | 0.002 | 0.0073 | 0.002 | 0.0073 |
| Lungs | 0.002 | 0.008 | 0.002 | 0.008 |
| Heart wall | 0.0018 | 0.0067 | 0.0018 | 0.0067 |
| Skin | 0.001 | 0.0037 | 0.0012 | 0.0043 |
| Thymus | 0.0013 | 0.0047 | 0.0013 | 0.0047 |
| Breast | 0.00094 | 0.0037 | 0.00094 | 0.0037 |
| Total body | 0.0024 | 0.009 | 0.0029 | 0.011 |

| | Effective dose† | | | |
|---|---|---|---|---|
| | With 2-hour void | | With 4.8-hour void | |
| Radionuclide | mSv/ MBq | rem/ mCi | mSv/ MBq | rem/ mCi |
| Tc 99m | 0.0095 | 0.035 | 0.013 | 0.048 |

*For adults; intravenous injection. Data based on information from the Oak Ridge Associated Universities, Radiopharmaceutical Internal Dose Information Center.

†Calculated according to the method of the International Commission on Radiological Protection (ICRP) publication 60.

### Elimination

Renal—About 50% of the administered activity is excreted as metabolites within 2 hours, and about 74% within 24 hours.

Fecal—About 12% of the administered activity is excreted after 48 hours.

## Precautions to Consider

### Carcinogenicity

Long-term animal studies to evaluate carcinogenic potential of technetium Tc 99m bicisate have not been performed.

### Pregnancy/Reproduction

Pregnancy—Tc 99m (as free pertechnetate) crosses the placenta. Although studies have not been done with technetium Tc 99m bicisate in humans, the estimated absorbed radiation dose to the uterus is 6.99 mGy/1110 MBq (0.69 rad/30 mCi) for a 2-hour void, and 12.2 mGy/1110 MBq (1.23 rad/30 mCi) for a 4.8-hour void. There is no evidence demonstrating embryonic or fetal harm at these doses.

Nevertheless, the possibility of pregnancy should be assessed in women of child-bearing potential. In these situations, the physician should use discretion and reduce the administered activity of the radiopharmaceutical to the lowest possible amount.

Studies have not been done in animals.

FDA Pregnancy Category C.

### Breast-feeding

Although it is not known whether technetium Tc 99m bicisate is distributed into breast milk, it is known that Tc 99m as free pertechnetate is distributed into breast milk. Based on the assumption that the Tc 99m in breast milk is in the form of pertechnetate, and based on the effective half-life of the radionuclide in breast milk, the daily volume of milk, a dose factor relating the radionuclide to its critical organ (thyroid) in the nursing infant, and the maximum permissible dose to that organ, a guideline has been proposed. According to this guideline, it has been calculated that nursing can be safely resumed when the concentration in breast milk reaches $30.3 \times 10^{-4}$ megabecquerels ($8.2 \times 10^{-2}$ microcuries) per mL. This level of activity is probably reached, in the majority of patients, within 24 hours after administration of 740 megabecquerels (20 millicuries) of technetium Tc 99m–labeled radiopharmaceuticals.

### Pediatrics

There have been no specific studies evaluating the safety and efficacy of technetium Tc 99m bicisate in pediatric patients. However, no pediatrics-specific problems have been documented to date.

### Geriatrics

Diagnostic studies performed to date using technetium Tc 99m bicisate have not demonstrated geriatrics-specific problems that would limit the usefulness of technetium Tc 99m bicisate in the elderly.

### Medical considerations/Contraindications

The medical considerations/contraindications included have been selected on the basis of their potential clinical significance (reasons given in parentheses where appropriate)—not necessarily inclusive (» = major clinical significance).

*Risk-benefit should be considered when the following medical problem exists:*
Sensitivity to the radiopharmaceutical preparation

## Side/Adverse Effects

The following side/adverse effects have been selected on the basis of their potential clinical significance (possible signs and symptoms in parentheses where appropriate)—not necessarily inclusive:

**Those indicating need for medical attention**
Incidence rare
*Angina* (chest pain); *difficulty breathing; hallucinations; hypertension; seizures; skin rash*

**Those indicating need for medical attention only if they continue or are bothersome**
Incidence rare
*Agitation or anxiety; dizziness; drowsiness; headache; nausea; parosmia* (transient, mild, pleasant aromatic odor)

## Patient Consultation

As an aid to patient consultation, refer to *Advice for the Patient, Radiopharmaceuticals (Diagnostic)*.
In providing consultation, consider emphasizing the following selected information (» = major clinical significance):

**Description of use**
Action in the body: Concentration of radioactive bicisate in brain
Retention of radioactivity in brain allows visualization
Small amount of radioactivity used in diagnosis; radiation received is low and considered safe

**Before having this test**
» Conditions affecting use, especially:
Sensitivity to the radiopharmaceutical preparation
Pregnancy—Technetium Tc 99m (as free pertechnetate) crosses placenta; reducing administered activity should be considered
Breast-feeding—Not known if technetium Tc 99m bicisate is distributed into breast milk, but Tc 99m as free pertechnetate is distributed into breast milk; temporary discontinuation of nursing may be recommended to avoid any unnecessary absorbed radiation dose to the infant

**Preparation for this test**
Special preparatory instructions may be given; patient should inquire in advance

**Precautions after having this test**
Adequate intake of fluids before and after administration of technetium Tc 99m bicisate; voiding frequently for 2 to 6 hours after administration to promote urine flow and to minimize absorbed radiation dose to bladder

**Side/adverse effects**
Signs of rare, but possible, side effects, especially angina, difficulty breathing, hallucinations, hypertension, seizures, and skin rash

## General Dosing Information

Radiopharmaceuticals are to be administered only by or under the supervision of physicians who have had extensive training in the safe use and handling of radioactive materials and who are authorized by the Nuclear Regulatory Commission (NRC) or the appropriate Agreement State agency, if required, or, outside the U.S., the appropriate authority.

Adequate hydration of the patient is recommended before and after administration of technetium Tc 99m bicisate to promote urinary flow and blood pool clearance. Also, urination is recommended as often as possible for 2 to 6 hours after the examination to promote urine flow, thereby minimizing absorbed radiation dose to the bladder.

**Safety considerations for handling this radiopharmaceutical**
Improper handling of this radiopharmaceutical may cause radioactive contamination. Guidelines for handling radioactive material have been prepared by scientific, professional, state, federal, and international bodies and are available to the specially qualified and authorized users who have access to radiopharmaceuticals.

## Parenteral Dosage Forms

### TECHNETIUM Tc 99m BICISATE INJECTION

**Usual adult and adolescent administered activity**
Brain imaging—
Intravenous, 370 to 1110 megabecquerels (10 to 30 millicuries).

**Usual pediatric administered activity**
Safety and dosage have not been established.

**Usual geriatric administered activity**
See *Usual adult and adolescent administered activity*.

**Strength(s) usually available**
U.S.—
0.9 mg bicisate dihydrochloride, 0.36 mg edetate disodium (dihydrate), 72 mcg (0.072 mg) stannous chloride dihydrate (theoretical), 12 mcg (0.012 mg) stannous chloride dihydrate (minimum), 83 mcg (0.083 mg) total tin (dihydrate) and 24 mg mannitol, in lyophilized form under nitrogen atmosphere, per reaction vial A; and 4.1 mg sodium phosphate dibasic heptahydrate, 0.46 mg sodium phosphate monobasic monohydrate, and enough water for injection to produce 1 mL, per reaction vial B (Rx) [*Neurolite*].
Canada—
0.9 mg bicisate dihydrochloride, 0.36 mg edetate disodium (dihydrate), 72 mcg (0.072 mg) stannous chloride dihydrate (theoretical), 12 mcg (0.012 mg) stannous chloride dihydrate (minimum), 83 mcg (0.083 mg) total tin (dihydrate) and 24 mg mannitol, in lyophilized form under nitrogen atmosphere, per reaction vial A; and 4.1 mg sodium phosphate dibasic heptahydrate, 0.46 mg sodium phosphate monobasic monohydrate, and enough water for injection to produce 1 mL, per reaction vial B (Rx) [*Neurolite*].

**Packaging and storage**
Store between 15 and 30 °C (59 and 86 °F), unless otherwise specified by manufacturer. Protect from light.
Note: Prior to labeling, kit can be stored between 15 and 25 °C (59 and 77 °F).

**Preparation of dosage form**
To prepare injection, an oxidant-free sodium pertechnetate Tc 99m solution is used. See manufacturer's package insert for instructions.

**Stability**
Technetium Tc 99m bicisate is stable at room temperature for a period of at least 8 hours after reconstitution. However, the manufacturer's package insert recommends that the product be used within 6 hours after preparation.

**Incompatibilities**
If oxidants such as peroxides and hypochlorites are present in the sodium pertechnetate Tc 99m used for labeling, the final preparation may be adversely affected and should be discarded.

**Note**
Caution—Radioactive material.

## Selected Bibliography

Holman BL, Hellman RS, Goldsmith SJ, et al. Biodistribution, dosimetry, and clinical evaluation of technetium-99m ethyl cysteinate dimer in normal subjects and in patients with chronic cerebral infarction. J Nucl Med 1989 Jun; 30(6): 1018-24.

Léveillé J, Demonceau G, Walovitch RC. Intrasubject comparison between technetium-99m-ECD and technetium-99m-HMPAO in healthy human subjects. J Nucl Med 1992 Apr; 33: 480-4.

Brass LM, Walovitch RC, Joseph JL, et al. The role of single photon emission computed tomography brain imaging with Tc-99m-bicisate in the localization and definition of mechanism of ischemic stroke. J Cereb Blood Flow Metab 1994; 14(Suppl 1): S91-S98.

Developed: 06/29/95

---

# TECHNETIUM Tc 99m DISOFENIN  Systemic†

VA CLASSIFICATION (Primary): DX201
Commonly used brand name(s): *Hepatolite*.
Another commonly used name is technetium Tc 99m DISIDA.

Note: For a listing of dosage forms and brand names by country availability, see *Dosage Forms* section(s).

†Not commercially available in Canada.

# Technetium Tc 99m Disofenin (Systemic)

## Category
Diagnostic aid, radioactive (hepatobiliary disorders).

## Indications

**Accepted**

*Hepatobiliary imaging, radionuclide*—Technetium Tc 99m disofenin is indicated as a hepatobiliary imaging agent for the evaluation of hepatobiliary tract patency to differentiate jaundice resulting from hepatocellular causes from jaundice resulting from partial or complete biliary obstruction; to differentiate extrahepatic biliary atresia from neonatal hepatitis; to detect cystic duct obstruction associated with acute cholecystitis; and to detect bile leaks.

Also, technetium Tc 99m disofenin may be useful to detect intrahepatic cholestasis and to distinguish it from other hepatobiliary diseases that involve hepatocyte damage.

## Physical Properties

### Nuclear data

| Radionuclide (half-life) | Decay constant | Mode of decay | Principal photon emissions (keV) | Mean number of emissions/disintegration ($\geq 0.01$) |
|---|---|---|---|---|
| Tc 99m (6.0 hr) | 0.1151 h$^{-1}$ | Isomeric transition to Tc 99 | Gamma (18) | 0.062 |
| | | | Gamma (140.5) | 0.891 |

## Pharmacology/Pharmacokinetics

**Physicochemical characteristics**
Molecular weight—Disofenin: 350.41.

**Mechanism of action/Effect**
Based on the clearance of most of the administered activity through the hepatobiliary system. Following intravenous administration, technetium Tc 99m–labeled IDA derivatives, such as disofenin, become bound to plasma proteins (mainly albumin). In the liver, in the space of Disse, technetium Tc 99m disofenin becomes dissociated from the proteins and enters the hepatocyte by a mechanism similar to that of serum bilirubin. Technetium Tc 99m disofenin traverses the hepatocyte unmetabolized and enters the bile canaliculi. Flow beyond the canaliculi is influenced to a large extent by the tone of the sphincter of Oddi and the patency of the bile ducts. Clear visualization of the gallbladder and intestines with technetium Tc 99m disofenin demonstrates hepatobiliary tract patency.

**Distribution**
In circulatory system, with rapid clearance; however, a percentage of the radiopharmaceutical (about 8%) remains in circulation 30 minutes after injection. It is cleared from blood by normal hepatic cells within 10 to 20 minutes. Excreted into bile and stored in gallbladder. The radiopharmaceutical is excreted through the hepatobiliary tract into the intestine. A fraction of the radiopharmaceutical is excreted into the urine. The fraction excreted into the urine is dependent on the extent of biliary disease.

**Time to radioactivity visualization**
In patients with normal hepatobiliary function (fasting state)—
 Gallbladder: 10 to 20 minutes.
 Intestines: 30 to 60 minutes.

Note: Delayed visualization or nonvisualization may occur during the period immediately following a meal or after prolonged fasting.

**Radiation dosimetry**

| | Estimated absorbed radiation dose* | | | |
|---|---|---|---|---|
| | With normal hepatobiliary function | | With parenchymal liver disease | |
| Organ | mGy/MBq | rad/mCi | mGy/MBq | rad/mCi |
| Gallbladder wall | 0.11 | 0.41 | 0.035 | 0.13 |
| Large intestine wall (upper) | 0.092 | 0.34 | 0.033 | 0.12 |
| Large intestine wall (lower) | 0.062 | 0.23 | 0.024 | 0.089 |
| Small intestine | 0.052 | 0.19 | 0.019 | 0.070 |
| Bladder wall | 0.023 | 0.085 | 0.069 | 0.26 |
| Ovaries | 0.020 | 0.074 | 0.0099 | 0.037 |
| Liver | 0.015 | 0.056 | 0.010 | 0.037 |
| Uterus | 0.013 | 0.048 | 0.011 | 0.041 |
| Red marrow | 0.0070 | 0.026 | 0.0038 | 0.014 |
| Kidneys | 0.0063 | 0.023 | 0.0066 | 0.024 |
| Stomach wall | 0.0061 | 0.023 | 0.0027 | 0.010 |
| Pancreas | 0.0057 | 0.021 | 0.0028 | 0.010 |
| Adrenals | 0.0032 | 0.012 | 0.0021 | 0.0078 |
| Bone surfaces | 0.0026 | 0.0096 | 0.0017 | 0.0063 |
| Spleen | 0.0026 | 0.0096 | 0.0015 | 0.0056 |
| Testes | 0.0015 | 0.0056 | 0.0025 | 0.0093 |
| Breast | 0.00061 | 0.0023 | 0.00056 | 0.0021 |
| Thyroid | 0.00012 | 0.00044 | 0.00023 | 0.00085 |
| Other tissue | 0.0030 | 0.011 | 0.0021 | 0.0078 |

| | Effective dose* | | | |
|---|---|---|---|---|
| | With normal hepatobiliary function | | With parenchymal liver disease | |
| Radionuclide | mSv/MBq | rem/mCi | mSv/MBq | rem/mCi |
| Tc 99m | 0.024 | 0.089 | 0.013 | 0.048 |

*For adults; intravenous injection of technetium Tc 99m–labeled iminodiacetic acid (IDA) derivatives. Data based on the International Commission on Radiological Protection (ICRP) Publication 53—Radiation dose to patients from radiopharmaceuticals.

**Elimination**
Primarily fecal; about 9% eliminated in the urine within 2 hours.

Note: In patients with hepatocellular disease or biliary obstruction, elimination through the urinary tract may be greatly increased.

## Precautions to Consider

**Cross-sensitivity and/or related problems**
Patients sensitive to amide-type local anesthetics may be sensitive to technetium Tc 99m disofenin also.

**Carcinogenicity/Mutagenicity**
Long-term animal studies to evaluate carcinogenic or mutagenic potential of technetium Tc 99m disofenin have not been performed.

**Pregnancy/Reproduction**
*Pregnancy*—Tc 99m (as free pertechnetate) crosses the placenta. Studies have not been done with technetium Tc 99m disofenin in humans.

The possibility of pregnancy should be assessed in women of child-bearing potential. Clinical situations exist where the benefit to the patient and fetus, based on information derived from radiopharmaceutical use, outweighs the risks from fetal exposure to radiation. In these situations, the physician should use discretion and reduce the radiopharmaceutical administered activity to the lowest possible amount.

Studies have not been done in animals.

FDA Pregnancy Category C.

**Breast-feeding**
Although it is not known whether technetium Tc 99m disofenin is distributed into breast milk, it is known that Tc 99m as free pertechnetate is distributed into breast milk. Based on the assumption that the Tc 99m in breast milk is in the form of pertechnetate and based on the effective half-life of the radionuclide in breast milk, the daily volume of milk, a dose factor relating the radionuclide to its critical organ (thyroid) in the nursing infant, and the maximum permissible dose to that organ, a guideline has been proposed. According to this guideline, it has been calculated that nursing can be safely resumed when the concentration in breast milk reaches $30.3 \times 10^{-4}$ megabecquerels ($8.2 \times 10^{-2}$ microcuries) per mL. This level of activity is probably reached, in the majority of patients, within 12 to 24 hours after administration of technetium Tc 99m–labeled radiopharmaceuticals.

**Pediatrics**
Diagnostic studies performed to date using technetium Tc 99m disofenin have not demonstrated pediatrics-specific problems that would limit its usefulness in children. However, there have been no specific studies evaluating the safety and efficacy of technetium Tc 99m disofenin in pediatric patients. When this radiopharmaceutical is used in children,

the diagnostic benefit should be judged to outweigh the potential risk of radiation.

### Geriatrics
Appropriate studies on the relationship of age to the effects of technetium Tc 99m disofenin have not been performed in the geriatric population. However, no geriatrics-specific problems have been documented to date.

### Drug interactions and/or related problems
See *Diagnostic interference*.

### Diagnostic interference
The following have been selected on the basis of their potential clinical significance (possible effect in parentheses where appropriate)—not necessarily inclusive (» = major clinical significance):

With results of this test
*Due to other medications*
Alcohol or
Anticholinergics or other medications with anticholinergic action (See *Appendix II* ) or
Bethanechol or
Somatostatin
(may decrease gallbladder emptying thus delaying gallbladder clearance of technetium Tc 99m disofenin)

Erythromycin
(nonvisualization of gallbladder may occur due to erthromycin-induced hepatotoxicity)

Nicotinic acid
(chronic, high-dose nicotinic acid therapy may result in poor extraction and elimination of the radiopharmaceutical, mimicking intrinsic hepatocellular disease)

Opioid (narcotic) analgesics, especially butorphanol, morphine, and meperidine
(delivery of technetium Tc 99m disofenin to the small bowel may be prevented by the opioid analgesics because of constriction of the sphincter of Oddi and increased biliary tract pressure caused by these medications; these actions result in delayed intestinal visualization, which resembles that caused by obstruction of the common bile duct; however, the use of intravenous morphine has been shown to help in the diagnosis of acute cholecystitis when conditions that delay or prevent gallbladder visualization are present)

Parenteral alimentation
(may give false-positive diagnosis of cystic duct obstruction due to stasis of bile in the gallbladder)

*Due to medical problems or conditions*
Fasting, prolonged or
Pancreatitis, acute
(may give false-positive results [nonvisualization or delayed visualization of gallbladder] of cystic duct obstruction due to stasis of bile in gallbladder)

Hepatocellular disease
(nonvisualization or delayed visualization of gallbladder may occur)

Post-prandial state, especially with ingestion of fatty meals
(ingestion of a fatty meal immediately before test may give false-positive results [nonvisualization of gallbladder] of cystic duct obstruction due to gallbladder contraction stimulated by meal ingestion)

### Medical considerations/Contraindications
The medical considerations/contraindications included have been selected on the basis of their potential clinical significance (reasons given in parentheses where appropriate)—not necessarily inclusive (» = major clinical significance).
See also *Diagnostic interference*.

*Risk-benefit should be considered when the following medical problem exists:*
Sensitivity to amide-type local anesthetics or to the radiopharmaceutical preparation

## Side/Adverse Effects
There are no known side/adverse effects associated with the use of technetium Tc 99m disofenin.

## Patient Consultation
As an aid to patient consultation, refer to *Advice for the Patient, Radiopharmaceuticals (Diagnostic)*.
In providing consultation, consider emphasizing the following selected information (» = major clinical significance):

### Description of use
Action in the body: Clearance of radioactive disofenin from blood through hepatobiliary tract
Visualization of radioactivity in intestinal tract and gallbladder shows absence of obstruction of bile ducts
Small amounts of radioactivity used in diagnosis; radiation received is low and considered safe

### Before having this test
» Conditions affecting use, especially:
Sensitivity to amide-type local anesthetics or to the radiopharmaceutical preparation
Pregnancy—Technetium Tc 99m (as free pertechnetate) crosses placenta; risk to fetus from radiation exposure as opposed to benefit derived from use should be considered
Breast-feeding—Not known if technetium Tc 99m disofenin distributed into breast milk, but Tc 99m as free pertechnetate is distributed into breast milk; temporary discontinuation of nursing may be recommended because of risk to infant from radiation exposure
Use in children—Risk from radiation exposure as opposed to benefit derived from use should be considered

### Preparation for this test
Fasting for at least 2, and preferably 4 hours before test to prevent gallbladder nonvisualization

### Precautions after having this test
No special precautions

## General Dosing Information
Radiopharmaceuticals are to be administered only by or under the supervision of physicians who have had extensive training in the safe use and handling of radioactive materials and who are authorized by the Nuclear Regulatory Commission (NRC) or the appropriate Agreement State agency, if required, or, outside the U.S., the appropriate authority.

Administration of phenobarbital (5 mg per kg of body weight [mg/kg] in 2 fractions) for at least 5 days prior to hepatobiliary imaging may enhance and accelerate biliary uptake and excretion of the radiopharmaceutical in the differential diagnosis of extrahepatic atresia from neonatal hepatitis. This will enable determination of the status of the extrahepatic biliary tract in the jaundiced neonate within 24 hours.

Fasting is recommended for at least 2, and preferably 4 hours before the examination since nonvisualization of the gallbladder may result if gallbladder contraction has been stimulated by the ingestion of food.

Prolonged fasting (e.g., more than 24 hours) may result in a false-positive hepatobiliary scan (i.e., nonvisualization of the gallbladder despite a patent cystic duct) due to the development of increased intraluminal gallbladder pressure (biliary stasis or sludge), which reduces radiotracer flow to the gallbladder. To avoid this, prior administration of a cholecystokinetic agent, such as sincalide or cholecystokinin (CCK-8), to induce contraction of the gallbladder is recommended for pre-emptying the gallbladder before the injection of technetium Tc 99m disofenin. Whenever there is doubt about the dietary history of the patient, especially in emergency situations, a cholecystokinetic agent should be administered.

In patients receiving parenteral alimentation, the relative inactivity of the gallbladder results in bile stasis and the formation of thick viscous bile (sludge), which reduces the flow of the radiotracer into the gallbladder. Pretreatment with a cholecystokinetic agent (e.g., intravenous sincalide 0.02 to 0.04 mcg per kg of body weight [mcg/kg]) may be useful to empty stored bile from the gallbladder, and thus may prevent a false-positive hepatobiliary scan.

In patients demonstrating technetium Tc 99m disofenin localization in the gallbladder, a cholecystokinetic agent (e.g., intravenous sincalide 0.02 to 0.04 mcg/kg of body weight) may be useful to stimulate gallbladder contraction and thereby evaluate the contractile function of the gallbladder. Quantitation of gallbladder emptying yields the ejection fraction ($\geq$ 35% is usually considered normal).

Imaging is performed immediately following technetium Tc 99m disofenin administration, and is usually completed in 60 to 90 minutes. Imaging for up to 4 hours or longer may be necessary if no gallbladder or intestinal activity is seen at the earlier times.

When there is no visualization of the gallbladder within an hour of administration of technetium Tc 99m disofenin, but the radiotracer is seen within the small bowel in patients suspected of having acute cholecystitis, morphine sulfate (0.04 mg/kg diluted in 10 mL saline) may be injected intravenously to help confirm the diagnosis. The diagnosis of acute cholecystitis is confirmed if nonvisualization of the gallbladder persists after morphine is administered. Although morphine-augmented cholescintigraphy may cause false-positive and false-negative results in some patients (e.g., acalculous cholecystitis), it may be useful in critically ill patients or patients who have been on prolonged fasting or who are receiving parenteral alimentation.

**Safety considerations for handling this radiopharmaceutical**
Improper handling of this radiopharmaceutical may cause radioactive contamination. Guidelines for handling radioactive material have been prepared by scientific, professional, state, federal, and international bodies and are available to the specially qualified and authorized users who have access to radiopharmaceuticals.

## Parenteral Dosage Forms

### TECHNETIUM Tc 99m DISOFENIN INJECTION USP

**Usual adult and adolescent administered activity**
Hepatobiliary imaging—
　Nonjaundiced patients: Intravenous, 37 to 185 megabecquerels (1 to 5 millicuries) by slow injection.
　Patients with serum bilirubin concentration > 0.08 mmol per L (5 mg per dL): Intravenous, 111 to 296 megabecquerels (3 to 8 millicuries) by slow injection.

**Usual pediatric administered activity**
Hepatobiliary imaging—
　Dosage must be individualized by physician. The minimum recommended administered activity is 37 megabecquerels (1 millicurie), intravenously.

**Usual geriatric administered activity**
See *Usual adult and adolescent administered activity*.

**Strength(s) usually available**
U.S.—
　20 mg disofenin, 0.24 mg (minimum) stannous chloride, and 0.6 mg total tin (maximum tin as stannous chloride) in lyophilized form under nitrogen atmosphere, per reaction vial (Rx) [*Hepatolite*].
Canada—
　Not commercially available.

**Packaging and storage**
Store below 40 °C (104 °F), preferably between 15 and 30 °C (59 and 86 °F), unless otherwise specified by manufacturer. Protect from freezing.

**Preparation of dosage form**
To prepare injection, an oxidant-free sodium pertechnetate Tc 99m solution is used. See manufacturer's package insert for instructions.

**Stability**
Injection should be administered within 6 hours after preparation.

**Note**
Caution—Radioactive material.

### Selected Bibliography
Fink-Bennett D, Balon H, Robbins T, et al. Morphine-augmented cholescintigraphy: its efficacy in detecting acute cholecystitis. J Nucl Med 1991; 32: 1231-3.
Krishnamurthy GT, Turner FE. Pharmacokinetics and clinical application of technetium 99m-labeled hepatobiliary agents. Semin Nucl Med 1990; 20(2): 130-49.
Cherver LR, Nunn AD, Loberg MD. Radiopharmaceuticals for hepatobiliary imaging. Semin Nucl Med 1982; 12(1): 5-17.

Revised: 06/14/93
Interim revision: 08/02/94

---

# TECHNETIUM Tc 99m EXAMETAZIME  Systemic

VA CLASSIFICATION (Primary): DX201
Commonly used brand name(s): *Ceretec*.
Another commonly used name for exametazime is hexamethylpropyleneamine oxime (HM-PAO).
Note:　For a listing of dosage forms and brand names by country availability, see *Dosage Forms* section(s).

## Category
Diagnostic aid, radioactive (cerebrovascular disease; inflammatory disease).

## Indications
Note:　Bracketed information in the *Indications* section refers to uses that are not included in U.S. product labeling.

**Accepted**
Brain imaging, radionuclide—Technetium Tc 99m exametazime is indicated as a brain imaging agent in the detection of altered regional cerebral perfusion in stroke.
Leukocytes, labeling of—Technetium Tc 99m exametazime is indicated for the labeling of autologous leukocytes. Technetium Tc 99m exametazime–labeled leukocytes are used for the following diagnostic studies:
Inflammatory lesions, intra-abdominal (diagnosis)[1];
Bowel disease, inflammatory (diagnosis)—Indicated in scintigraphy to help locate intra-abdominal infection or inflammation and inflammatory bowel disease.
[Dementia, Alzheimer-type (diagnosis)][1]—Technetium Tc 99m exametazime is used as a brain imaging agent to help identify patients with Alzheimer's disease.
[Epilepsy (diagnosis)][1]—Technetium Tc 99m exametazime is used in the evaluation of epilepsy to help find the location of the epileptic focus.
[Brain death (diagnosis)][1]—Technetium Tc 99m exametazime is used to help confirm the diagnosis of brain death.

[1]Not included in Canadian product labeling.

## Physical Properties
**Nuclear data**

| Radionuclide (half-life) | Decay constant | Mode of decay | Principal photon emissions (keV) | Mean number of emissions/ disintegration ($\geq 0.01$) |
|---|---|---|---|---|
| Tc 99m (6.0 hr) | 0.1151 h$^{-1}$ | Isomeric transition to Tc 99 | Gamma (18) | 0.062 |
|  |  |  | Gamma (140.5) | 0.891 |

## Pharmacology/Pharmacokinetics

**Physicochemical characteristics**
Molecular weight—Exametazime: 272.39.

**Mechanism of action/Effect**
Brain imaging—Technetium Tc 99m exametazime is a lipophilic complex able to cross the blood-brain barrier as well as penetrate cell membranes. The agent localizes in the brain as a function of regional cerebral perfusion. Its radionuclide emissions while localized in cerebral tissue permit external imaging of the cerebral distribution of the agent thus helping detect altered regional cerebral perfusion. Technetium Tc 99m exametazime is primarily extracted and trapped by cerebral gray matter and the basal ganglia during the first pass through the brain. It has been proposed that the retention in the brain of technetium Tc 99m exametazime results from *in vivo* conversion of the primary complex to a less lipophilic complex, which is unable to cross the blood-brain barrier.
Labeling of leukocytes—When incubated with leukocytes, which have been isolated from whole blood, the technetium Tc 99m exametazime complex, being lipid-soluble, penetrates the cell membrane of the leukocytes by passive diffusion. The lipophilic complex is then converted to a hydrophilic species, in a process possibly involving intracellular glutathione, thus trapping the technetium Tc 99m label within the cells (mostly neutrophils). The radioactive autologous leukocytes are subsequently reinjected to permit the detection of inflammatory lesions based on the normal physiological accumulation of leukocytes at such sites.

## Distribution

**Brain imaging**—Rapidly cleared from blood after intravenous injection; a maximum of 3.5 to 7% of administered activity localizes in the brain within one minute of injection. Up to 15% of this localized activity is eliminated from the brain within the next 2 minutes after injection, with little or no further loss of activity for the following 24 hours, except by physical decay of technetium Tc 99m. The activity that is not localized in the brain is widely distributed throughout the body, particularly in muscle and soft tissue.

**Diagnosis of inflammatory lesions**—Technetium Tc 99m exametazime–labeled leukocytes tend to concentrate at sites of inflammation. However, there is an initial accumulation of radioactivity in the lungs, liver, spleen, blood pool, bone marrow, and the bladder. Activity is seen in the urine, occasionally in the gallbladder, and consistently in the colon from 4 hours on. Significant colonic activity remains 24 hours after injection. Also, normal areas visualized in earlier scans remain visible.

## Time to radioactivity visualization

**Brain imaging**—Dynamic imaging may be performed within the first 10 minutes post-injection. Static imaging may be performed 15 minutes after injection for up to 6 hours.

**Diagnosis of inflammatory lesions**—Although some inflammatory lesions have been detected at 2 minutes post-injection, images taken at 30 minutes and/or 2 hours are recommended. Optimal planar images are obtained between 2 and 4 hours following administration.

## Radiation dosimetry

Estimated absorbed radiation dose for Technetium Tc 99m Exametazime*

| Organ | mGy/MBq | rad/mCi |
|---|---|---|
| Lacrimal glands | 0.070 | 0.26 |
| Gallbladder wall | 0.051 | 0.19 |
| Kidney | 0.035 | 0.13 |
| Thyroid | 0.027 | 0.10 |
| Upper large intestine wall | 0.021 | 0.079 |
| Liver | 0.015 | 0.054 |
| Lower large intestine wall | 0.015 | 0.054 |
| Bladder wall | | |
| 2 hr void | 0.013 | 0.047 |
| 4 hr void | 0.019 | 0.070 |
| Small intestine wall | 0.012 | 0.044 |
| Brain | 0.0069 | 0.026 |
| Eyes | 0.0069 | 0.026 |
| Ovaries | 0.0063 | 0.023 |
| Bone surfaces | 0.0048 | 0.018 |
| Red marrow | 0.0034 | 0.013 |
| Testes | 0.0018 | 0.007 |
| Total body | 0.0036 | 0.013 |

Effective dose: 0.0092 mSv/MBq (0.034 rem/mCi)†.

Estimated absorbed radiation dose for Technetium Tc 99m Exametazime–labeled leukocytes†‡

| Organ | mGy/MBq | rad/mCi |
|---|---|---|
| Spleen | 0.15 | 0.56 |
| Red marrow | 0.022 | 0.082 |
| Liver | 0.02 | 0.074 |
| Pancreas | 0.014 | 0.052 |
| Ovaries | 0.0042 | 0.016 |
| Uterus | 0.0038 | 0.014 |
| Testes | 0.0017 | 0.0064 |

Effective dose: 0.017 mSv/MBq (0.063 rem/mCi)†.

*For adults; intravenous injection. Data based on information from the Oak Ridge Associated Universities, Radiopharmaceutical Internal Dose Information Center.

†Data based on the International Commission on Radiological Protection (ICRP) Publication 53—Radiation dose to patients from radiopharmaceuticals.

‡Data based on bladder voiding every 3.5 hours.

## Elimination

For technetium Tc 99m exametazime—
  Within 48 hours:
    Fecal (about 50% of the administered activity via hepatobiliary excretion).
    Renal (about 40% of the injected administered activity).

For technetium Tc 99m exametazime–labeled leukocytes—
  Renal (about 15 to 30% of the injected administered activity in 24 hours).
  Fecal (about 6% of the administered activity in 48 hours).

# Precautions to Consider

## Carcinogenicity
Long-term animal studies to evaluate carcinogenic potential of technetium Tc 99m exametazime have not been performed.

## Mutagenicity
Studies in rats have not demonstrated mutagenic potential following intraperitoneal administration at doses of 70, 140, and 280 mg of exametazime per kg of body weight.

## Pregnancy/Reproduction
Pregnancy—Tc 99m (as free pertechnetate) crosses the placenta. However, studies have not been done with technetium Tc 99m exametazime in humans.

The possibility of pregnancy should be assessed in women of child-bearing potential. Clinical situations exist in which the benefit to the patient and fetus, based on information derived from radiopharmaceutical use, outweighs the risks from fetal exposure to radiation. In these situations, the physician should use discretion and reduce the administered activity of the radiopharmaceutical to the lowest possible amount.

Studies have not been done in animals.

FDA Pregnancy Category C.

## Breast-feeding
Although it is not known whether technetium Tc 99m exametazime is distributed into breast milk, it is known that Tc 99m as free pertechnetate is distributed into breast milk. Based on the assumption that the Tc 99m in breast milk is in the form of pertechnetate, and based on the effective half-life of the radionuclide in breast milk, the daily volume of milk, a dose factor relating the radionuclide to its critical organ (thyroid) in the nursing infant, and the maximum permissible dose to that organ, a guideline has been proposed. According to this guideline, it has been calculated that nursing can be safely resumed when the concentration in breast milk reaches $30.3 \times 10^{-4}$ megabecquerels ($8.2 \times 10^{-2}$ microcuries) per mL. This level of activity is probably reached, in the majority of patients, within 24 hours after administration of 740 megabecquerels (20 millicuries) of technetium Tc 99m–labeled radiopharmaceuticals. However, the manufacturer recommends that formula feedings be substituted for breast-feeding for 60 hours.

## Pediatrics
Diagnostic studies performed to date in patients up to 18 years of age have not demonstrated pediatrics-specific problems that would limit the usefulness of technetium Tc 99m exametazime in children. However, there have been no specific studies evaluating the safety and efficacy of technetium Tc 99m exametazime in pediatric patients. When this radiopharmaceutical is used in children, the diagnostic benefit should be judged to outweigh the potential risk of radiation.

For technetium Tc 99m exametazime–labeled leukocytes—Technetium Tc 99m exametazime–labeled leukocytes may be preferred for use in children to indium In 111 oxyquinoline–labeled leukocytes or gallium citrate Ga 67 because of its lower radiation dose.

## Geriatrics
Appropriate studies on the relationship of age to the effects of technetium Tc 99m exametazime have not been performed in the geriatric population. However, no geriatrics-specific problems have been documented to date.

## Drug interactions and/or related problems
See *Diagnostic interference*.

## Diagnostic interference
The following have been selected on the basis of their potential clinical significance (possible effect in parentheses where appropriate)—not necessarily inclusive (» = major clinical significance):

With results of *technetium Tc 99m–labeled leukocyte* studies
  *Due to other medications*
    Antibiotics
      (long-term intravenous antibiotic therapy may result in a false-negative study)

## Medical considerations/Contraindications
The medical considerations/contraindications included have been selected on the basis of their potential clinical significance (reasons given in parentheses where appropriate)—not necessarily inclusive (» = major clinical significance).

**Risk-benefit should be considered when the following medical problem exists:**
Sensitivity to the radiopharmaceutical preparation

## Side/Adverse Effects
The following side/adverse effects have been selected on the basis of their potential clinical significance (possible signs and symptoms in parentheses where appropriate)—not necessarily inclusive:

**Those indicating need for medical attention**
Incidence less frequent or rare
*Allergic reaction* (fever; skin rash; swelling of face); *transient increase in blood pressure*

## Patient Consultation
As an aid to patient consultation, refer to *Advice for the Patient, Radiopharmaceuticals (Diagnostic)*.
In providing consultation, consider emphasizing the following selected information (» = major clinical significance):

**Description of use**
Action in the body: Concentration of radioactive exametazime in brain; concentration of technetium Tc 99m–labeled leukocytes at sites of infection
Retention of radioactivity in brain and sites of infection allows visualization
Small amount of radioactivity used in diagnosis; radiation received is low and considered safe

**Before having this test**
» Conditions affecting use, especially:
   Sensitivity to the radiopharmaceutical preparation
   Pregnancy—Technetium Tc 99m (as free pertechnetate) crosses placenta; risk to fetus from radiation exposure as opposed to benefit derived from use should be considered
   Breast-feeding—Not known if technetium Tc 99m exametazime is distributed into breast milk, but Tc 99m as free pertechnetate is distributed into breast milk; temporary discontinuation of nursing may be recommended to avoid any unnecessary absorbed radiation dose to the infant
   Use in children—For brain imaging: Risk from radiation exposure as opposed to benefit derived from use should be considered

**Preparation for this test**
Special preparatory instructions may be given; patient should inquire in advance

**Precautions after having this test**
Increasing intake of fluids and voiding as often as possible after examination to minimize bladder exposure to radiation

**Side/adverse effects**
Signs of possible side effects, especially allergic reaction and transient increase in blood pressure

## General Dosing Information
Radiopharmaceuticals are to be administered only by or under the supervision of physicians who have had extensive training in the safe use and handling of radioactive materials and who are authorized by the Nuclear Regulatory Commission (NRC) or the appropriate Agreement State agency, if required, or, outside the U.S., the appropriate authority.

Adequate hydration of the patient is recommended before and after examination to promote urinary excretion of radioactivity. Also, urination is recommended as often as possible after the examination to reduce bladder exposure to radiation.

**For brain perfusion imaging**
Dynamic imaging may be performed within the first 10 minutes after injection. Static imaging may be performed from 15 minutes up to 6 hours after injection.

**For labeling of leukocytes**
White blood cells may be damaged by mechanical shearing forces; therefore, it is important to minimize the use of needles when transferring cells. If a syringe cannot be used by itself, wide-bore (19 gauge) needles should be used. When separating the mixed leukocytes from other blood cells, excessive centrifuge speed may damage the cells and increase platelet contamination. However, an adequate centrifuge speed will provide a compact button (pellet).
The manufacturer's package insert or other appropriate literature should be consulted for the specific method of labeling leukocytes.

**Safety considerations for handling this radiopharmaceutical**
Improper handling of this radiopharmaceutical may cause radioactive contamination. Guidelines for handling radioactive material have been prepared by scientific, professional, state, federal, and international bodies and are available to the specially qualified and authorized users who have access to radiopharmaceuticals.

## Parenteral Dosage Forms

### TECHNETIUM Tc 99m EXAMETAZIME INJECTION USP

**Usual adult and adolescent administered activity**
Brain imaging—
   Intravenous, 370 to 740 megabecquerels (10 to 20 millicuries).
Diagnosis of inflammatory lesions—
   Intravenous, 0.259 to 0.925 gigabecquerels (7 to 25 millicuries) of technetium Tc 99m exametazime–labeled leukocytes.

**Usual pediatric administered activity**
Brain imaging—
   Intravenous, 5 to 10 megabecquerels (0.14 to 0.28 millicuries) per kg of body weight with a minimum total dosage of 185 megabecquerels (5 millicuries).
Diagnosis of inflammatory lesions—
   Dosage must be individualized by physician.

**Usual geriatric administered activity**
See *Usual adult and adolescent administered activity*.

**Strength(s) usually available**
U.S.—
   0.5 mg exametazime, 7.6 mcg (0.0076 mg) stannous chloride dihydrate, and 4.5 mg sodium chloride, in lyophilized form under nitrogen atmosphere, per single-dose reaction vial (Rx) [*Ceretec*].
   Note: In addition, the kit contains 1-mL vials of 1% methylene blue injection and 4.5-mL vials of 0.003 M monobasic sodium phosphate and dibasic sodium phosphate in 0.9% sodium chloride injection.
Canada—
   0.5 mg exametazime, 7.6 mcg (0.0076 mg) stannous chloride dihydrate, and 4.5 mg sodium chloride, in lyophilized form under nitrogen atmosphere, per single-dose reaction vial (Rx) [*Ceretec*].

**Packaging and storage**
Store between 20 and 25 °C (68 and 77 °F), unless otherwise specified by manufacturer. Protect from freezing.
Note: Prior to labeling, kit must be stored between 15 and 25 °C (59 and 77 °F).

**Preparation of dosage form**
To prepare injection, an oxidant-free sodium pertechnetate Tc 99m solution is used. Freshly eluted technetium Tc 99m generator eluate must be used for reconstitution to assure the highest radiochemical purity. It is recommended that only eluate from a technetium Tc 99m generator that was previously eluted within 24 hours should be used. Generator eluate more than 2 hours old should not be used. Preservative-free, nonbacteriostatic sodium chloride injection must be used as the diluent for sodium pertechnetate Tc 99m. Bacteriostatic sodium chloride should not be used because it will increase the oxidation products and adversely affect the biological distribution of technetium Tc 99m exametazime. Methylene blue injection may be used to form a stabilizing solution. See manufacturer's package insert for full preparation instructions.
Note: Methylene blue *must not* be used as a stabilizer in the preparation of the technetium Tc 99m exametazime injection to be used for labeling leukocytes.

**Stability**
Without methylene blue stabilizer—Injection must be administered within 30 minutes after preparation since progressive conversion to a less lipophilic complex unable to cross the blood-brain barrier may exceed acceptable limits after this time period.
With methylene blue stabilizer—Injection may be administered within 4 hours after time of reconstitution.

**Incompatibilities**
If oxidants such as peroxides and hypochlorites are present in the sodium pertechnetate Tc 99m used for labeling, the final preparation may be adversely affected and should be discarded.

**Note**
Caution—Radioactive material.

## Selected Bibliography
Roddie ME, Peters AM, Danpure HJ, et al. Inflammation: imaging with Tc 99m HMPAO-labeled leukocytes. Radiology 1988 Mar; 166(3): 767-72.

ered.
Leonard JP, Nowotnik DP, Neirinckx RD. Technetium 99m, 1-HM-PAO: a new radiopharmaceutical for imaging regional brain perfusion using SPECT—a comparison with iodine 123 HIPDM. J Nucl Med 1986; 27(12): 1819-23.

Testa HJ, Snowden JS, Neary D, et al. The use of Tc 99m HM-PAO in the diagnosis of primary degenerative dementia. J Cereb Blood Flow Metab 1988; 8(6): S123-S126.

Revised: 01/11/96

# TECHNETIUM Tc 99m GLUCEPTATE Systemic

VA CLASSIFICATION (Primary): DX201

Commonly used brand name(s): *Frosstimage Gluceptate; Frosstimage Gluco; Glucoscan; TechneScan Gluceptate.*

Another commonly used name is technetium Tc 99m glucoheptonate.

Note: For a listing of dosage forms and brand names by country availability, see *Dosage Forms* section(s).

## Category

Diagnostic aid, radioactive (intracranial lesions; cerebral disorders; renal disorders).

## Indications

**Accepted**

Brain imaging, radionuclide—Technetium Tc 99m gluceptate is indicated as a brain imaging agent to detect and evaluate intracranial lesions, including brain tumors.

Renal imaging, radionuclide—Technetium Tc 99m gluceptate is indicated as a renal imaging agent to evaluate kidney size, shape, and position, especially in parenchymal disorders.

Brain perfusion studies or
Renal perfusion studies—Technetium Tc 99m gluceptate is indicated in dynamic brain and renal perfusion studies.

## Physical Properties

**Nuclear data**

| Radionuclide (half-life) | Decay constant | Mode of decay | Principal photon emissions (keV) | Mean number of emissions/ disintegration ($\geq 0.01$) |
|---|---|---|---|---|
| Tc 99m (6.0 hr) | 0.1151 h$^{-1}$ | Isomeric transition to Tc 99 | Gamma (18) | 0.062 |
| | | | Gamma (140.5) | 0.891 |

## Pharmacology/Pharmacokinetics

**Mechanism of action/Effect**

Diagnostic aid (intracranial lesions; cerebral disorders)—
Technetium Tc 99m gluceptate accumulates, by passive diffusion, in intracranial lesions with an altered blood-brain barrier. The radionuclide emissions may then be detected to determine the presence and localization of the lesion.

Diagnostic aid (renal disorders)—
Based on its rapid clearance through the urinary tract. Urinary clearance of technetium Tc 99m gluceptate occurs by both glomerular filtration and tubular secretion; however, a sufficient amount is retained by the renal cortex to allow delayed static images to be performed for evaluation of cortical morphology.

**Distribution**

Rapidly distributed in and cleared from plasma; up to 15% of dose localizes in the tubules of the renal cortex by 3 hours.

**Radiation dosimetry**

| Estimated absorbed radiation dose* |||
|---|---|---|
| Organ | mGy/MBq | rad/mCi |
| Bladder wall | 0.056 | 0.21 |
| Kidneys | 0.049 | 0.18 |
| Uterus | 0.0077 | 0.029 |
| Adrenals | 0.0046 | 0.017 |
| Ovaries | 0.0046 | 0.017 |
| Large intestine wall (lower) | 0.0044 | 0.016 |
| Red marrow | 0.0039 | 0.014 |
| Spleen | 0.0039 | 0.014 |
| Small intestine | 0.0037 | 0.014 |
| Pancreas | 0.0036 | 0.013 |
| Large intestine wall (upper) | 0.0033 | 0.012 |
| Testes | 0.0029 | 0.011 |
| Stomach wall | 0.0027 | 0.010 |
| Liver | 0.0027 | 0.010 |
| Bone surfaces | 0.0026 | 0.0096 |
| Lungs | 0.0017 | 0.0063 |
| Breast | 0.0014 | 0.0052 |
| Thyroid | 0.0011 | 0.0041 |
| Other tissue | 0.0023 | 0.0085 |

Effective dose: 0.0090 mSv/MBq (0.033 rem/mCi)

*In adults; intravenous administration. Data based on the International Commission on Radiological Protection (ICRP) Publication 53—Radiation dose to patients from radiopharmaceuticals.

**Elimination**

Renal (by both glomerular filtration and renal tubular secretion)—
Normal renal function: about 40% of the administered activity eliminated in 1 hour; about 70% of the administered activity eliminated within 24 hours.
Renal function impairment: Urinary elimination is delayed. Hepatobiliary elimination may occur.

## Precautions to Consider

**Carcinogenicity/Mutagenicity**

Long-term animal studies to evaluate carcinogenic or mutagenic potential of technetium Tc 99m gluceptate have not been performed.

**Pregnancy/Reproduction**

Pregnancy—Tc 99m (as free pertechnetate) crosses the placenta. However, studies have not been done with technetium Tc 99m gluceptate in humans.

The possibility of pregnancy should be assessed in women of child-bearing potential. Clinical situations exist where the benefit to the patient and fetus, based on information derived from radiopharmaceutical use, outweighs the risks from fetal exposure to radiation. In these situations, the physician should use discretion and reduce the radiopharmaceutical dose to the lowest possible amount.

Studies have not been done in animals.

FDA Pregnancy Category C.

**Breast-feeding**

Although it is not known whether technetium Tc 99m gluceptate is distributed into breast milk, it is known that Tc 99m as free pertechnetate is distributed into breast milk. Based on the assumption that the Tc 99m in breast milk is in the form of pertechnetate and based on the effective half-life of the radionuclide in breast milk, the daily volume of milk, a dose factor relating the radionuclide to its critical organ (thyroid) in the nursing infant, and the maximum permissible dose to that organ, a guideline has been proposed. According to this guideline, it has been calculated that nursing can be safely resumed when the concentration in breast milk reaches $30.3 \times 10^{-4}$ megabecquerels ($8.2 \times 10^{-2}$ microcuries) per mL. This level of activity is probably reached, in the majority of patients, within 24 hours after administration of 740 megabecquerels (20 millicuries) of technetium Tc 99m–labeled radiopharmaceuticals.

## Technetium Tc 99m Gluceptate (Systemic)

**Pediatrics**
Diagnostic studies performed in children have not demonstrated pediatrics-specific problems that would limit the usefulness of technetium Tc 99m gluceptate in children. However, when this radiopharmaceutical is used in children, the diagnostic benefit should be judged to outweigh the potential risk of radiation.

**Geriatrics**
Appropriate studies on the relationship of age to the effects of technetium Tc 99m gluceptate have not been performed in the geriatric population. However, no geriatrics-specific problems have been documented to date.

**Drug interactions and/or related problems**
See *Diagnostic interference*.

**Diagnostic interference**
The following have been selected on the basis of their potential clinical significance (possible effect in parentheses where appropriate)—not necessarily inclusive (» = major clinical significance):
With results of *brain imaging*
*Due to other medications*

Corticosteroids, glucocorticoid
(uptake of technetium Tc 99m gluceptate in cerebral tumor or abscess may be decreased because of reduced peritumor edema caused by the corticosteroids)

*Due to medical problems or conditions*

Neurotoxicity, induced by such drugs as:
Cyclophosphamide or
Dactinomycin or
Doxorubicin or
Vincristine
(brain images may show increased activity due to chemotherapeutic neurotoxicity following therapy with these medications)

With results of *renal imaging*
*Due to other medications*

Penicillamine
(concurrent penicillamine therapy may cause transchelation of technetium Tc 99m gluceptate to a compound excreted through the hepatobiliary system, thus resulting in gallbladder visualization; gallbladder visualization may mimic abnormal kidney localization on posterior views of renal images)

Probenecid
(concurrent use may decrease kidney uptake of technetium Tc 99m gluceptate due to a direct inhibition of the enzyme transport system in the proximal tubule by probenecid)

*Due to medical problems or conditions*

Dehydration
(decreased urinary flow may result in poor renal images)

**Medical considerations/Contraindications**
The medical considerations/contraindications included have been selected on the basis of their potential clinical significance (reasons given in parentheses where appropriate)—not necessarily inclusive (» = major clinical significance).
See also *Diagnostic interference*.

Risk benefit must be considered when the following medical problem exists:
Sensitivity to the radiopharmaceutical preparation

## Side/Adverse Effects

The following side/adverse effects have been selected on the basis of their potential clinical significance (possible signs and symptoms in parentheses where appropriate)—not necessarily inclusive:

**Those indicating need for medical attention**
Incidence less frequent or rare
*Allergic reaction* (skin rash, hives, or itching)

## Patient Consultation

As an aid to patient consultation, refer to *Advice for the Patient, Radiopharmaceuticals (Diagnostic)*.
In providing consultation, consider emphasizing the following selected information (» = major clinical significance):

**Description of use**
Action in the body: Concentration of radioactive gluceptate in brain lesions and kidneys
Retention of radioactivity in brain lesions and kidneys allows visualization

Small amount of radioactivity used in diagnosis; radiation received is low and considered safe

**Before having this test**
» Conditions affecting use, especially:
Sensitivity to the radiopharmaceutical preparation
Pregnancy—Technetium Tc 99m (as free pertechnetate) crosses placenta; risk to fetus from radiation exposure as opposed to benefit derived from use should be considered
Breast-feeding—Not known if technetium Tc 99m gluceptate is distributed into breast milk, but Tc 99m as free pertechnetate is distributed into breast milk; temporary discontinuation of nursing may be recommended because of risk to infant from radiation exposure
Use in children—Risk from radiation exposure as opposed to benefit derived from use should be considered

**Preparation for this test**
Special preparatory instructions may be given; patient should inquire in advance

**Precautions after having this test**
Increasing intake of fluids and voiding as often as possible for 4 to 6 hours after examination to minimize radiation dose to bladder

**Side/adverse effects**
Signs of potential side effects, especially allergic reaction

## General Dosing Information

Radiopharmaceuticals are to be administered only by or under the supervision of physicians who have had extensive training in the safe use and handling of radioactive materials and who are authorized by the Nuclear Regulatory Commission (NRC) or the appropriate Agreement State agency, if required, or, outside the U.S., the appropriate authority.

Adequate hydration of the patient is recommended before and after examination to promote urinary flow. Also, urination is recommended as often as possible for 4 to 6 hours after the examination to reduce radiation dose to the bladder.

Manufacturer's package insert or other appropriate literature should be consulted for optimal times when imaging should be performed.

**Safety considerations for handling this radiopharmaceutical**
Improper handling of this radiopharmaceutical may cause radioactive contamination. Guidelines for handling radioactive material have been prepared by scientific, professional, state, federal, and international bodies and are available to the specially qualified and authorized users who have access to radiopharmaceuticals.

## Parenteral Dosage Forms

### TECHNETIUM Tc 99m GLUCEPTATE INJECTION USP

**Usual adult and adolescent administered activity**
Brain imaging or
Brain perfusion studies—
Intravenous, 555 to 740 megabecquerels (15 to 20 millicuries).
Renal imaging or
Renal perfusion studies—
Intravenous, 370 to 555 megabecquerels (10 to 15 millicuries).

**Usual pediatric administered activity**
Brain imaging—
Intravenous, 7.9 to 10.6 megabecquerels (0.21 to 0.28 millicuries) per kg of body weight, with a minimum total dosage of at least 74 megabecquerels (2 millicuries) and a maximum total dosage of 740 megabecquerels (20 millicuries).
Renal imaging—
Intravenous, 5.3 to 10.6 megabecquerels (0.14 to 0.28 millicuries) per kg of body weight, with a minimum total dosage of at least 37 megabecquerels (1 millicurie) and a maximum total dosage of 370 megabecquerels (10 millicuries).

**Usual geriatric administered activity**
See *Usual adult and adolescent administered activity*.

**Strength(s) usually available**
U.S.—
50 mg gluceptate calcium, 0.7 mg minimum stannous tin as stannous chloride dihydrate, and 1.1 mg maximum total tin as stannous chloride dihydrate (in a lyophilized form and under a nitrogen atmosphere), per 10-mL reaction vial (Rx) [*TechneScan Gluceptate*].
200 mg gluceptate sodium, 0.06 mg minimum stannous tin as stannous chloride, and 0.07 mg maximum tin (in a lyophilized form and under a nitrogen atmosphere), per reaction vial (Rx) [*Glucoscan*].

Canada—
- 25 mg gluceptate calcium, 3 mg stannous chloride dihydrate (in lyophilized form under nitrogen atmosphere), per 10-mL reaction vial (Rx) [*Frosstimage Gluceptate*].
- 50 mg gluceptate calcium, 0.7 mg minimum stannous chloride dihydrate, and 1.1 mg maximum total tin expressed as stannous chloride dihydrate (in lyophilized form under nitrogen atmosphere), per 10-mL reaction vial (Rx) [*Frosstimage Gluco*].

**Packaging and storage**
Store between 2 and 8 °C (36 and 46 °F). Protect from freezing.
Note: Prior to labeling, kit can be stored at room temperature.

**Preparation of dosage form**
To prepare injection, an oxidant-free sodium pertechnetate Tc 99m solution is used. See manufacturer's package insert for instructions.

**Stability**
Injection should be administered within 6 hours after preparation.

**Incompatibilities**
If oxidants such as peroxides and hypochlorites are present in the sodium pertechnetate Tc 99m used for labeling, the final preparation may be adversely affected and should be discarded.

**Note**
Caution—Radioactive material.

## Selected Bibliography
Blaufox MD. Procedures of choice in renal nuclear medicine. J Nucl Med 1991; 32: 1301-9.

Revised: 07/26/93
Interim revision: 08/02/94

# TECHNETIUM Tc 99m LIDOFENIN  Systemic

VA CLASSIFICATION (Primary): DX201
Commonly used brand name(s): *Frosstimage HIDA; TechneScan HIDA*.
Note: For a listing of dosage forms and brand names by country availability, see *Dosage Forms* section(s).

## Category
Diagnostic aid, radioactive (hepatobiliary disorders).

## Indications
**Accepted**
Hepatobiliary imaging, radionuclide—Technetium Tc 99m lidofenin is indicated as a hepatobiliary imaging agent for the evaluation of hepatobiliary tract patency to differentiate jaundice resulting from hepatocellular causes from jaundice resulting from partial or complete biliary obstruction; to differentiate extrahepatic biliary atresia from neonatal hepatitis; to detect cystic duct obstruction associated with acute cholecystitis; and to detect bile leaks.

Also, technetium Tc 99m lidofenin may be useful to detect intrahepatic cholestasis and to distinguish it from other hepatobiliary diseases, which involve hepatocyte damage.

## Physical Properties
**Nuclear data**

| Radionuclide (half-life) | Decay constant | Mode of decay | Principal photon emissions (keV) | Mean number of emissions/ disintegration ($\geq 0.01$) |
|---|---|---|---|---|
| Tc 99m (6.0 hr) | 0.1151 h$^{-1}$ | Isomeric transition to Tc 99 | Gamma 18 | 0.062 |
|  |  |  | Gamma 140.5 | 0.891 |

## Pharmacology/Pharmacokinetics
**Physicochemical characteristics**
Molecular weight—Lidofenin: 294.31.

**Mechanism of action/Effect**
Based on the clearance of most of the administered activity through the hepatobiliary system. Following intravenous administration, technetium Tc 99m–labeled IDA derivatives, such as lidofenin, become bound to plasma proteins (mainly albumin). In the liver, in the space of Disse, technetium Tc 99m lidofenin becomes dissociated from the proteins and enters the hepatocyte by a mechanism similar to that of serum bilirubin. Technetium Tc 99m lidofenin traverses through the hepatocyte unmetabolized and enters the bile canaliculi. Flow beyond the canaliculi is influenced to a large extent by the tone of the sphincter of Oddi and the patency of the bile ducts. Clear visualization of the gallbladder and intestines, usually within 15 to 30 minutes of administration, demonstrates hepatobiliary tract patency.

**Distribution**
In circulatory system, with rapid blood clearance (about 5 minutes after injection); however, a percentage of the administered activity (about 10% in patients with normal liver function and in excess of 20% in patients with obstructive jaundice) clears the circulation more slowly. Cleared from blood by normal hepatic cells within 10 to 20 minutes. Excreted into bile and stored in gallbladder. Excreted through hepatobiliary tract into the intestine. A fraction of the administered activity excreted into the urine. The fraction excreted into the urine is dependent on the extent of biliary disease.

**Protein binding**
Low (18% of radioactivity).

**Half-life**
Elimination from blood (with suspected gallbladder disease)—
89% of dose: 3.1 minutes.
7.3% of dose: 26.1 minutes.
3.9% of dose: 14.1 hours.

**Time to radioactivity visualization**
With normal hepatobiliary function—
Liver: 5 minutes; maximum liver uptake by 10 to 15 minutes.
Hepatic duct and gallbladder: 20 to 30 minutes.
Intestines: 15 to 30 minutes.
Note: Delayed visualization or nonvisualization of gallbladder may occur during the period immediately following a meal or after prolonged fasting.
With hepatocellular disease or biliary obstruction—
Delayed visualization or nonvisualization. With serum bilirubin values over 7 to 8 mg per dL (0.12 to 1.37 mmol per L), the biliary system is not well visualized, but liver and intestinal radioactivity may still be observed with levels up to 10 to 13 mg/dL (0.17 to 2.22 mmol/L).

**Radiation dosimetry**

| Organ | With normal hepatobiliary function mGy/MBq | With normal hepatobiliary function rad/mCi | With parenchymal liver disease mGy/MBq | With parenchymal liver disease rad/mCi |
|---|---|---|---|---|
| Gall bladder wall | 0.11 | 0.41 | 0.035 | 0.13 |
| Large intestine wall (upper) | 0.092 | 0.34 | 0.033 | 0.12 |
| Large intestine wall (lower) | 0.062 | 0.23 | 0.024 | 0.089 |
| Small intestine | 0.052 | 0.19 | 0.019 | 0.070 |
| Bladder wall | 0.023 | 0.085 | 0.069 | 0.26 |
| Ovaries | 0.020 | 0.074 | 0.0099 | 0.037 |
| Liver | 0.015 | 0.056 | 0.010 | 0.037 |
| Uterus | 0.013 | 0.048 | 0.011 | 0.041 |
| Red marrow | 0.0070 | 0.026 | 0.0038 | 0.014 |
| Kidneys | 0.0063 | 0.023 | 0.0066 | 0.024 |
| Stomach wall | 0.0061 | 0.023 | 0.0027 | 0.010 |
| Pancreas | 0.0057 | 0.021 | 0.0028 | 0.010 |
| Adrenals | 0.0032 | 0.012 | 0.0021 | 0.0078 |
| Bone surfaces | 0.0026 | 0.0096 | 0.0017 | 0.0063 |
| Spleen | 0.0026 | 0.0096 | 0.0015 | 0.0056 |
| Testes | 0.0015 | 0.0056 | 0.0025 | 0.0093 |
| Breast | 0.00061 | 0.0023 | 0.00056 | 0.0021 |
| Thyroid | 0.00012 | 0.00044 | 0.00023 | 0.00085 |
| Other tissue | 0.0030 | 0.011 | 0.0021 | 0.0078 |

*Estimated absorbed radiation dose

| Radionuclide | Effective dose* | | | |
|---|---|---|---|---|
| | With normal hepatobiliary function | | With parenchymal liver disease | |
| | mSv/MBq | rem/mCi | mSv/MBq | rem/mCi |
| Tc 99m | 0.024 | 0.089 | 0.013 | 0.048 |

*For adults; intravenous injection of technetium Tc 99m–labeled iminodiacetic acid (IDA) derivatives. Data based on the International Commission on Radiological Protection (ICRP) Publication 53—Radiation dose to patients from radiopharmaceuticals.

**Elimination**
Primarily fecal.

Note: In patients with normal liver function, approximately 14% of the administered activity is present in the urinary bladder within 90 minutes after administration. In patients with hepatocellular disease or biliary obstruction, elimination through the urinary tract may be greatly increased. In jaundiced patients, approximately 22% of the administered activity is present in the urine within 90 minutes, and 53% in 18 to 24 hours.

## Precautions to Consider

**Cross-sensitivity and/or related problems**
Patients sensitive to amide-type local anesthetics may be sensitive to technetium Tc 99m lidofenin also.

**Carcinogenicity/Mutagenicity**
Long-term animal studies to evaluate carcinogenic or mutagenic potential of technetium Tc 99m lidofenin have not been performed.

**Pregnancy/Reproduction**
Pregnancy—Tc 99m (as free pertechnetate) crosses the placenta. Studies have not been done with technetium Tc 99m lidofenin in humans.

The possibility of pregnancy should be assessed in women of child-bearing potential. Clinical situations exist where the benefit to the patient and fetus, based on information derived from radiopharmaceutical use, outweighs the risks from fetal exposure to radiation. In these situations, the physician should use discretion and reduce the administered activity of the radiopharmaceutical to the lowest possible amount.

Studies have not been done in animals.

FDA Pregnancy Category C.

**Breast-feeding**
Although it is not known whether technetium Tc 99m lidofenin is distributed into breast milk, it is known that Tc 99m as free pertechnetate is distributed into breast milk. Based on the assumption that the Tc 99m in breast milk is in the form of pertechnetate and based on the effective half-life of the radionuclide in breast milk, the daily volume of milk, a dose factor relating the radionuclide to its critical organ (thyroid) in the nursing infant, and the maximum permissible dose to that organ, a guideline has been proposed. According to this guideline, it has been calculated that nursing can be safely resumed when the concentration in breast milk reaches $30.3 \times 10^{-4}$ megabecquerels ($8.2 \times 10^{-2}$ microcuries) per mL. This level of activity is probably reached, in the majority of patients, within 12 to 24 hours after administration of technetium Tc 99m–labeled radiopharmaceuticals.

**Pediatrics**
Diagnostic studies performed to date using technetium Tc 99m lidofenin have not demonstrated pediatrics-specific problems that would limit its usefulness in children. However, there have been no specific studies evaluating the safety and efficacy of technetium Tc 99m lidofenin in pediatric patients. When this radiopharmaceutical is used in children, the diagnostic benefit should be judged to outweigh the potential risk of radiation.

**Geriatrics**
Appropriate studies on the relationship of age to the effects of technetium Tc 99m lidofenin have not been performed in the geriatric population. However, no geriatrics-specific problems have been documented to date.

**Drug interactions and/or related problems**
See *Diagnostic interference*.

**Diagnostic interference**
The following have been selected on the basis of their potential clinical significance (possible effect in parentheses where appropriate)—not necessarily inclusive (» = major clinical significance):

With results of *this* test
*Due to other medications*
Alcohol or
Anticholinergics or other medications with anticholinergic activity (See *Appendix II* ) or
Bethanechol or
Somatostatin
(may decrease gallbladder emptying, thus delaying gallbladder clearance of technetium Tc 99m lidofenin)
Erythromycin
(nonvisualization of gallbladder may occur due to erthromycin-induced hepatotoxicity)
Nicotinic acid
(chronic, high-dose nicotinic acid therapy may result in poor extraction and elimination of the radiopharmaceutical, mimicking intrinsic hepatocellular disease)
Opioid (narcotic) analgesics, especially butorphanol, morphine, and meperidine
(delivery of technetium Tc 99m lidofenin to the small bowel may be prevented by opioid analgesics because of the constriction of the sphincter of Oddi and the increased biliary tract pressure caused by these medications; these actions result in delayed intestinal visualization, which resembles the delay caused by obstruction of the common bile duct; however, the use of intravenous morphine has been shown to help in the diagnosis of acute cholecystitis when conditions that delay or prevent gallbladder visualization are present)
Parenteral alimentation
(may give false-positive diagnosis of cystic duct obstruction due to stasis of bile in the gallbladder)
*Due to medical problems or conditions*
Fasting, prolonged or
Pancreatitis, acute
(may give false-positive results [nonvisualization or delayed visualization of gallbladder] of cystic duct obstruction due to stasis of bile in gallbladder)
Hepatocellular disease
(nonvisualization or delayed visualization of gallbladder may occur)
Post-prandial state, especially with ingestion of fatty meals
(ingestion of a fatty meal immediately before test may give false-positive results [nonvisualization of gallbladder] of cystic duct obstruction due to gallbladder contraction stimulated by meal ingestion)

**Medical considerations/Contraindications**
The medical considerations/contraindications included have been selected on the basis of their potential clinical significance (reasons given in parentheses where appropriate)—not necessarily inclusive (» = major clinical significance).
See also *Diagnostic interference*.

*Risk-benefit should be considered when the following medical problem exists:*
Sensitivity to amide-type local anesthetics or to the radiopharmaceutical preparation

## Side/Adverse Effects

The following side/adverse effects have been selected on the basis of their potential clinical significance and/or frequency of occurrence (possible signs and symptoms in parentheses where appropriate)—not necessarily inclusive:

**Those indicating need for medical attention only if they continue or are bothersome**
Incidence less frequent or rare
*Chills; nausea; skin rash*

## Patient Consultation

As an aid to patient consultation, refer to *Advice for the Patient, Radiopharmaceuticals (Diagnostic)*.

In providing consultation, consider emphasizing the following selected information (» = major clinical significance):

**Description of use**
Action in the body: Clearance of radioactive lidofenin from blood through hepatobiliary tract
Visualization of radioactivity in intestinal tract and gallbladder shows absence of obstruction of bile ducts
Small amounts of radioactivity used in diagnosis; radiation received is low and considered safe

**Before having this test**
» Conditions affecting use, especially:
   Sensitivity to the radiopharmaceutical preparation or to local anesthetics (amide-type)
   Pregnancy—Technetium Tc 99m (as free pertechnetate) crosses placenta; risk to fetus from radiation exposure as opposed to benefit derived from use should be considered
   Breast-feeding—Not known if technetium Tc 99m lidofenin distributed into breast milk, but Tc 99m as free pertechnetate is distributed into breast milk; temporary discontinuation of nursing may be recommended because of risk to infant from radiation exposure
   Use in children—Risk from radiation exposure as opposed to benefit derived from use should be considered
   Other medical problems, especially prolonged fasting and acute pancreatitis

**Preparation for this test**
Fasting for at least 2 and preferably 4 hours before test to prevent gallbladder nonvisualization

**Precautions after having this test**
No special precautions

## General Dosing Information

Radiopharmaceuticals are to be administered only by or under the supervision of physicians who have had extensive training in the safe use and handling of radioactive materials and who are authorized by the Nuclear Regulatory Commission (NRC) or the appropriate Agreement State agency, if required, or, outside the U.S., the appropriate authority.

Administration of phenobarbital (5 mg per kg of body weight [mg/kg] in 2 divided doses) for at least 5 days prior to hepatobiliary imaging may enhance and accelerate biliary uptake and excretion of the radiopharmaceutical in the differential diagnosis of extrahepatic atresia from neonatal hepatitis. This will enable determination of the status of the extrahepatic biliary tract in the jaundiced neonate within 24 hours.

Fasting is recommended for at least 2 and preferably 4 hours before the examination is recommended since nonvisualization of the gallbladder may result if gallbladder contraction has been stimulated by the ingestion of food.

Prolonged fasting (e.g., more than 24 hours) may result in a false-positive hepatobiliary scan (e.g., nonvisualization of the gallbladder despite a patent cystic duct) due to the development of increased intraluminal gallbladder pressure (biliary stasis or sludge), which reduces radiotracer flow to the gallbladder. To avoid this, prior administration of a cholecystokinetic agent, such as sincalide or cholecystokinin (CCK-8) to induce contraction of the gallbladder, is recommended for pre-emptying the gallbladder before the injection of technetium Tc 99m lidofenin. Whenever there is doubt about the dietary history of the patient, especially in emergency situations, a cholecystokinetic agent should be administered.

In patients receiving parenteral alimentation, the relative inactivity of the gallbladder results in bile stasis and the formation of thick viscous bile (sludge), which reduces the flow of the radiotracer into the gallbladder. Pretreatment with a cholecystokinetic agent (e.g., intravenous sincalide 0.02 to 0.04 microgram per kilogram of body weight) may be useful to empty stored bile from the gallbladder, and thus, may prevent a false-positive hepatobiliary scan.

In patients demonstrating technetium Tc 99m lidofenin localization in the gallbladder, a cholecystokinetic agent (e.g., intravenous sincalide 0.02 to 0.04 microgram per kilogram of body weight) may be useful to stimulate gallbladder contraction and thereby evaluate the contractile function of the gallbladder. Quantitation of gallbladder emptying yields the ejection fraction ($\geq$ 35% is usually considered normal).

Imaging is performed immediately following technetium Tc 99m lidofenin administration, and is usually completed in 60 to 90 minutes. Imaging for up to 4 hours or longer may be necessary if there is no gallbladder or intestinal activity.

When there is no visualization of the gallbladder within an hour of administration of technetium Tc 99m lidofenin, but the radiotracer is seen within the small bowel in patients suspected of having acute cholecystitis, morphine sulfate (0.04 mg/kg diluted in 10 mL saline) may be injected intravenously to help confirm the diagnosis. The diagnosis of acute cholecystitis is confirmed if nonvisualization of the gallbladder persists after morphine is administered. Although morphine-augmented cholescintigraphy may cause false-positive and false-negative results in some patients (e.g., acalculous cholecystitis), it may be useful in critically ill patients or patients who have been on a prolonged fasting or are receiving parenteral alimentation.

**Safety considerations for handling this radiopharmaceutical**
Improper handling of this radiopharmaceutical may cause radioactive contamination. Guidelines for handling radioactive material have been prepared by scientific, professional, state, federal, and international bodies and are available to the specially qualified and authorized users who have access to radiopharmaceuticals.

## Parenteral Dosage Forms

### TECHNETIUM Tc 99m LIDOFENIN INJECTION USP

**Usual adult and adolescent administered activity**
Hepatobiliary imaging—
   Intravenous, 185 megabecquerels (5 millicuries).
Note: Dosage is usually adjusted depending on bilirubin levels.
      A period of 24 hours should elapse before a second dose is administered.

**Usual adult prescribing limits**
370 megabecquerels (10 millicuries).

**Usual pediatric administered activity**
Hepatobiliary imaging—
   With bilirubin levels less than 5 mg per dL (0.08 mmol per L): Intravenous, 2.6 megabecquerels (70 microcuries) per kg of body weight. Minimum total administered activity is 18.5 megabecquerels (500 microcuries).
   With bilirubin levels higher than 5 mg per dL (0.08 mmol per L): Intravenous, 5.18 megabecquerels (140 microcuries) per kg of body weight. Minimum total administered activity is 37 megabecquerels (1 millicurie).

**Usual geriatric administered activity**
See *Usual adult and adolescent administered activity*.

**Strength(s) usually available**
U.S.—
   10 mg lidofenin complexed with 0.8 mg (minimum) stannous chloride dihydrate (maximum tin as stannous chloride dihydrate 1.1 mg) in lyophilized form under nitrogen atmosphere, per 10-mL reaction vial (Rx) [*TechneScan HIDA*].
Canada—
   10 mg lidofenin complexed with 0.8 mg (minimum) stannous chloride dihydrate (maximum tin as stannous chloride dihydrate 1.1 mg) in lyophilized form under nitrogen atmosphere, per 10-mL reaction vial (Rx) [*TechneScan HIDA*].
   10 mg lidofenin complexed with 1 mg stannous chloride dihydrate in lyophilized form under nitrogen atmosphere, per 10-mL reaction vial (Rx) [*Frosstimage HIDA*].

**Packaging and storage**
Store between 2 and 8 °C (36 and 46 °F), unless otherwise specified by manufacturer. Protect from freezing.

**Preparation of dosage form**
To prepare injection, an oxidant-free sodium pertechnetate Tc 99m solution is used. See manufacturer's package insert for instructions.

**Stability**
Injection should be administered within 6 hours after preparation.

**Note**
Caution—Radioactive material.

## Selected Bibliography

Fink-Bennett D, Balon H, Robbins T, et al. Morphine-augmented cholescintigraphy: its efficacy in detecting acute cholecystitis. J Nucl Med 1991; 32: 1231-3.

Krishnamurthy GT, Turner FE. Pharmacokinetics and clinical application of technetium 99m-labeled hepatobiliary agents. Semin Nucl Med 1990; 20(2): 130-49.

Weissman HS, Badia J, Sugarman LA, et al. Spectrum of 99m-Tc-IDA cholescintigraphic patterns in acute cholecystitis. Radiology 1981; 138: 167-75.

Revised: 06/14/93
Interim revision: 08/02/94

# TECHNETIUM Tc 99m MEBROFENIN Systemic

VA CLASSIFICATION (Primary): DX201

Commonly used brand name(s): *Choletec*.

Another commonly used name is technetium Tc 99m BrIDA.

Note: For a listing of dosage forms and brand names by country availability, see *Dosage Forms* section(s).

## Category

Diagnostic aid, radioactive (hepatobiliary disorders).

## Indications

### Accepted

Hepatobiliary imaging, radionuclide—Technetium Tc 99m mebrofenin is indicated as a hepatobiliary imaging agent for the evaluation of hepatobiliary tract patency to differentiate jaundice resulting from hepatocellular causes from jaundice resulting from partial or complete biliary obstruction; to differentiate extrahepatic biliary atresia from neonatal hepatitis; to detect cystic duct obstruction associated with acute cholecystitis; and to detect bile leaks.

Also, technetium Tc 99m mebrofenin may be useful to detect intrahepatic cholestasis and to distinguish it from other hepatobiliary diseases, which involve hepatocyte damage.

## Physical Properties

### Nuclear data

| Radionuclide (half-life) | Decay constant | Mode of decay | Principal photon emissions (keV) | Mean number of emissions/ disintegration ($\geq 0.01$) |
|---|---|---|---|---|
| Tc 99m (6.0 hr) | 0.1151 h$^{-1}$ | Isomeric transition to Tc 99 | Gamma (18) | 0.062 |
| | | | Gamma (140.5) | 0.891 |

## Pharmacology/Pharmacokinetics

### Physicochemical characteristics

Molecular weight—Mebrofenin: 387.23.

### Mechanism of action/Effect

Based on the clearance of most of the administered activity through the hepatobiliary system. Following intravenous administration, technetium Tc 99m–labeled iminodiacetic acid (IDA) derivatives, such as mebrofenin, bind to plasma proteins (mainly albumin). In the liver, in the space of Disse, technetium Tc 99m mebrofenin dissociates from the proteins and enters the hepatocyte by a mechanism similar to that of serum bilirubin. Technetium Tc 99m mebrofenin traverses through the hepatocyte unmetabolized and enters the bile canaliculi. Flow beyond the canaliculi is influenced to a large extent by the tone of the sphincter of Oddi and the patency of the bile ducts. Clear visualization of the gallbladder and intestines, usually within 15 to 30 minutes of administration, demonstrates hepatobiliary tract patency.

### Distribution

In circulatory system, with rapid blood clearance; however, about 17% of the administered activity (twice as much in patients with obstructive jaundice) remains in circulation 10 minutes after injection. Cleared from blood by normal hepatic cells within 10 to 20 minutes. Excreted into bile and stored in gallbladder. Excreted through hepatobiliary tract into the intestine. A small fraction of the administered activity excreted into the urine. The fraction excreted into the urine is dependent on the extent of biliary disease.

### Time to radioactivity visualization

With normal hepatobiliary function—Liver: 5 minutes; maximum liver uptake by 11 minutes.
Hepatic duct and gallbladder: 10 to 15 minutes.
Intestines: 30 to 60 minutes.

Note: Delayed visualization or nonvisualization of the gallbladder may occur during the period immediately following a meal or after prolonged fasting.

### Radiation dosimetry

| Organ | Estimated absorbed radiation dose* |||| 
|---|---|---|---|---|
| | With normal hepatobiliary function || With parenchymal liver disease ||
| | mGy/MBq | rad/mCi | mGy/MBq | rad/mCi |
| Gall bladder wall | 0.11 | 0.41 | 0.035 | 0.13 |
| Large intestine wall (upper) | 0.092 | 0.34 | 0.033 | 0.12 |
| Large intestine wall (lower) | 0.062 | 0.23 | 0.024 | 0.089 |
| Small intestine | 0.052 | 0.19 | 0.019 | 0.070 |
| Bladder wall | 0.023 | 0.085 | 0.069 | 0.26 |
| Ovaries | 0.020 | 0.074 | 0.0099 | 0.037 |
| Liver | 0.015 | 0.056 | 0.010 | 0.037 |
| Uterus | 0.013 | 0.048 | 0.011 | 0.041 |
| Red marrow | 0.0070 | 0.026 | 0.0038 | 0.014 |
| Kidneys | 0.0063 | 0.023 | 0.0066 | 0.024 |
| Stomach wall | 0.0061 | 0.023 | 0.0027 | 0.010 |
| Pancreas | 0.0057 | 0.021 | 0.0028 | 0.010 |
| Adrenals | 0.0032 | 0.012 | 0.0021 | 0.0078 |
| Bone surfaces | 0.0026 | 0.0096 | 0.0017 | 0.0063 |
| Spleen | 0.0026 | 0.0096 | 0.0015 | 0.0056 |
| Testes | 0.0015 | 0.0056 | 0.0025 | 0.0093 |
| Breast | 0.00061 | 0.0023 | 0.00056 | 0.0021 |
| Thyroid | 0.00012 | 0.00044 | 0.00023 | 0.00085 |
| Other tissue | 0.0030 | 0.011 | 0.0021 | 0.0078 |

| Radionuclide | Effective dose* ||||
|---|---|---|---|---|
| | With normal hepatobiliary function || With parenchymal liver disease ||
| | mSv/MBq | rem/mCi | mSv/MBq | rem/mCi |
| Tc 99m | 0.024 | 0.089 | 0.013 | 0.048 |

*For adults; intravenous injection of technetium Tc 99m–labeled iminodiacetic acid (IDA) derivatives. Data based on the International Commission on Radiological Protection (ICRP) Publication 53—Radiation dose to patients from radiopharmaceuticals.

### Elimination

Primarily fecal.

Note: In patients with normal liver function, 1% (mean) of the administered activity is present in the urinary bladder within 3 hours after administration. In patients with hepatocellular disease or biliary obstruction, elimination through the urinary tract may be greatly increased. With mean elevated serum bilirubin levels of 9.8 mg per dL (791.73 micromole per L), 3% (mean) of the administered activity is excreted in the urine within 3 hours and 14.9% (mean) of the administered activity is excreted during 3 to 24 hours.

## Precautions to Consider

### Cross-sensitivity and/or related problems

Patients sensitive to amide-type local anesthetics may be sensitive to technetium Tc 99m mebrofenin also.

### Carcinogenicity/Mutagenicity

Long-term animal studies to evaluate carcinogenic or mutagenic potential of technetium Tc 99m mebrofenin have not been performed.

### Pregnancy/Reproduction

Pregnancy—Tc 99m (as free pertechnetate) crosses the placenta. Studies have not been done with technetium Tc 99m mebrofenin in humans.

The possibility of pregnancy should be assessed in women of child-bearing potential. Clinical situations exist where the benefit to the patient and fetus, based on information derived from radiopharmaceutical use, outweighs the risks from fetal exposure to radiation. In these situations, the physician should use discretion and reduce the administered activity of the radiopharmaceutical to the lowest possible amount.

Studies have not been done in animals.

FDA Pregnancy Category C.

### Breast-feeding

Although it is not known whether technetium Tc 99m mebrofenin is distributed into breast milk, it is known that Tc 99m as free pertechnetate is distributed into breast milk. Based on the assumption that the Tc 99m in breast milk is in the form of pertechnetate and based on the effective half-life of the radionuclide in breast milk, the daily volume of milk, a dose factor relating the radionuclide to its critical organ (thyroid) in the nursing infant, and the maximum permissible dose to that organ, a guideline has been proposed. According to this guideline, it has been calculated that nursing can be safely resumed when the concentration in breast milk reaches $30.3 \times 10^{-4}$ megabecquerels ($8.2 \times 10^{-2}$ microcuries) per mL. This level of activity is probably reached, in the majority of patients, within 12 to 24 hours after administration of technetium Tc 99m–labeled radiopharmaceuticals.

### Pediatrics
Diagnostic studies performed to date using technetium Tc 99m mebrofenin have not demonstrated pediatrics-specific problems that would limit its usefulness in children. However, there have been no specific studies evaluating the safety and efficacy of technetium Tc 99m mebrofenin in pediatric patients. When this radiopharmaceutical is used in children, the diagnostic benefit should be judged to outweigh the potential risk of radiation.

### Geriatrics
Appropriate studies on the relationship of age to the effects of technetium Tc 99m mebrofenin have not been performed in the geriatric population. However, no geriatrics-specific problems have been documented to date.

### Drug interactions and/or related problems
See *Diagnostic interference*.

### Diagnostic interference
The following have been selected on the basis of their potential clinical significance (possible effect in parentheses where appropriate)—not necessarily inclusive (» = major clinical significance):

With results of *this* test
*Due to other medications*
  Alcohol or
  Anticholinergics or other medications with anticholinergic activity (See *Appendix II*) or
  Bethanechol or
  Somatostatin
    (may decrease gallbladder emptying, thus delaying gallbladder clearance of technetium Tc 99m mebrofenin)
  Erythromycin
    (nonvisualization of gallbladder may occur due to erythromycin-induced hepatotoxicity)
  Nicotinic acid
    (chronic, high-dose nicotinic acid therapy may result in poor extraction and elimination of the radiopharmaceutical, mimicking intrinsic hepatocellular disease)
  Opioid (narcotic) analgesics, especially butorphanol, morphine, and meperidine
    (delivery of technetium Tc 99m mebrofenin to the small bowel may be prevented by opioid analgesics because of the constriction of the sphincter of Oddi and the increased biliary tract pressure caused by these medications; these actions result in delayed intestinal visualization, which resembles the delay caused by obstruction of the common bile duct; however, the use of intravenous morphine has been shown to help in the diagnosis of acute cholecystitis when conditions that delay or prevent gallbladder visualization are present)
  Parenteral alimentation
    (may give false-positive diagnosis of cystic duct obstruction because of stasis of bile in the gallbladder)

*Due to medical problems or conditions*
  Fasting, prolonged or
  Pancreatitis, acute
    (may give false-positive results [nonvisualization or delayed visualization of gallbladder] of cystic duct obstruction due to stasis of bile in gallbladder)
  Hepatocellular disease
    (nonvisualization or delayed visualization of gallbladder may occur)
  Postprandial state, especially with ingestion of fatty meals
    (ingestion of a fatty meal immediately prior to study may give false-positive results [nonvisualization of gallbladder] of cystic duct obstruction due to gallbladder contraction stimulated by meal ingestion)

### Medical considerations/Contraindications
The medical considerations/contraindications included have been selected on the basis of their potential clinical significance (reasons given in parentheses where appropriate)—not necessarily inclusive (» = major clinical significance).

See also *Diagnostic interference*.

*Risk-benefit should be considered when the following medical problem exists:*
  Sensitivity to amide-type local anesthetics or to the radiopharmaceutical preparation

## Side/Adverse Effects
There are no known side/adverse effects associated with the use of technetium Tc 99m mebrofenin. However, chills, nausea, and skin rash have been reported with other iminodiacetic acid (IDA) derivatives.

## Patient Consultation
As an aid to patient consultation, refer to *Advice for the Patient, Radiopharmaceuticals (Diagnostic)*.

In providing consultation, consider emphasizing the following selected information (» = major clinical significance):

### Description of use
Action in the body: Clearance of radioactive mebrofenin from blood through hepatobiliary tract

Visualization of radioactivity in intestinal tract and gallbladder shows absence of obstruction of bile ducts

Small amounts of radioactivity used in diagnosis; radiation received is low and considered safe

### Before having this test
» Conditions affecting use, especially:
  Sensitivity to the radiopharmaceutical preparation or to local anesthetics (amide-type)
  Pregnancy—Technetium Tc 99m (as free pertechnetate) crosses placenta; risk to fetus from radiation exposure as opposed to benefit derived from use should be considered
  Breast-feeding—Not known if technetium Tc 99m mebrofenin is distributed into breast milk, but Tc 99m as free pertechnetate is distributed into breast milk; temporary discontinuation of nursing may be recommended because of risk to infant from radiation exposure
  Use in children—Risk from radiation exposure as opposed to benefit derived from use should be considered
  Other medical problems, especially prolonged fasting and acute pancreatitis

### Preparation for this test
Fasting for at least 2 and preferably 4 hours before test to prevent gallbladder nonvisualization

### Precautions after having this test
No special precautions

## General Dosing Information
Radiopharmaceuticals are to be administered only by or under the supervision of physicians who have had extensive training in the safe use and handling of radioactive materials and who are authorized by the Nuclear Regulatory Commission (NRC) or the appropriate Agreement State agency, if required, or, outside the U.S., the appropriate authority.

Administration of phenobarbital (5 mg per kg of body weight [mg/kg] in 2 divided doses) for at least 5 days prior to hepatobiliary imaging may enhance and accelerate biliary uptake and excretion of the radiopharmaceutical in the differential diagnosis of extrahepatic atresia from neonatal hepatitis. This will enable determination of the status of the extrahepatic biliary tract in the jaundiced neonate within 24 hours.

Fasting is recommended for at least 2 and preferably 4 hours before the examination since nonvisualization of the gallbladder may result if gallbladder contraction has been stimulated by the ingestion of food.

Prolonged fasting (e.g., more than 24 hours) may result in a false-positive hepatobiliary scan (e.g., nonvisualization of the gallbladder despite a patent cystic duct) due to the development of increased intraluminal gallbladder pressure (biliary stasis or sludge), which reduces radiotracer flow to the gallbladder. To avoid this, prior administration of a cholecystokinetic agent, such as sincalide or cholecystokinin (CCK-8) to induce contraction of the gallbladder, is recommended for pre-emptying the gallbladder before the injection of technetium Tc 99m mebrofenin. Whenever there is doubt about the dietary history of the patient, especially in emergency situations, a cholecystokinetic agent should be administered.

In patients receiving parenteral alimentation, the relative inactivity of the gallbladder results in bile stasis and the formation of thick viscous bile (sludge), which reduces the flow of the radiotracer into the gallbladder. Pretreatment with a cholecystokinetic agent (e.g., intravenous sincalide 0.02 to 0.04 microgram per kilogram of body weight) may be useful to empty stored bile from the gallbladder, which may prevent a false-positive hepatobiliary scan.

In patients demonstrating technetium Tc 99m mebrofenin localization in the gallbladder, a cholecystokinetic agent (e.g., intravenous sincalide 0.02 to 0.04 microgram per kilogram of body weight) may be useful to stimulate gallbladder contraction and thereby evaluate the contractile function of the gallbladder. Quantitation of gallbladder emptying yields the ejection fraction ($\geq$ 35% is usually considered normal).

Imaging is performed immediately following technetium Tc 99m mebrofenin administration, and is usually completed in 60 to 90 minutes. Imaging for up to 4 hours or longer may be necessary if there is no gallbladder or intestinal activity.

When there is no visualization of the gallbladder within an hour of administration of technetium Tc 99m mebrofenin, but the radiotracer is seen within the small bowel in patients suspected of having acute cholecystitis, morphine sulfate (0.04 mg/kg diluted in 10 mL saline) may be injected intravenously to help confirm the diagnosis. The diagnosis of acute cholecystitis is confirmed if nonvisualization of the gallbladder persists after morphine is administered. Although morphine-augmented cholescintigraphy may cause false-positive and false-negative results in some patients (e.g., acalculous cholecystitis), it may be useful in critically ill patients or patients who have been on prolonged fasting or who are receiving parenteral alimentation.

### Safety considerations for handling this radiopharmaceutical
Improper handling of this radiopharmaceutical may cause radioactive contamination. Guidelines for handling radioactive material have been prepared by scientific, professional, state, federal, and international bodies and are available to the specially qualified and authorized users who have access to radiopharmaceuticals.

## Parenteral Dosage Forms

### TECHNETIUM Tc 99m MEBROFENIN INJECTION

**Usual adult and adolescent administered activity**
Hepatobiliary imaging—
  Nonjaundiced patients: Intravenous, 74 to 185 megabecquerels (2 to 5 millicuries).
  Patients with serum bilirubin concentration > 25.65 micromole per L (1.5 mg per dL): Intravenous, 111 to 370 megabecquerels (3 to 10 millicuries).
  Note: A period of 24 hours should elapse before a second dose is administered.

**Usual pediatric administered activity**
Hepatobiliary imaging—
  Intravenous, 37 megabecquerels (1 millicurie).

**Usual geriatric administered activity**
See *Usual adult and adolescent administered activity*.

**Strength(s) usually available**
U.S.—
  45 mg mebrofenin, 0.54 mg (minimum) stannous fluoride dihydrate, 1.03 mg total tin (maximum as stannous fluoride dihydrate), not more than 5.2 mg methylparaben, and 0.58 mg propylparaben (in a lyophilized form and under nitrogen atmosphere), per multidose reaction vial (Rx) [*Choletec*].
Canada—
  45 mg mebrofenin, 0.73 mg stannous fluoride, 4.5 mg methylparaben, and 0.5 mg propylparaben (in a lyophilized form and under nitrogen atmosphere), per multidose reaction vial (Rx) [*Choletec*].

**Packaging and storage**
Store between 15 and 30 °C (59 and 86 °F), unless otherwise specified by manufacturer. Protect from freezing.

**Preparation of dosage form**
To prepare injection, an oxidant-free sodium pertechnetate Tc 99m solution is used for labeling. See manufacturer's package insert for instructions.

**Stability**
Injection should be administered within 18 hours after preparation.

**Note**
Caution—Radioactive material.

### Selected Bibliography
Fink-Bennett D, Balon H, Robbins T, et al. Morphine-augmented cholescintigraphy: its efficacy in detecting acute cholecystitis. J Nucl Med 1991; 32: 1231-3.

Krishnamurthy GT, Turner FE. Pharmacokinetics and clinical application of technetium 99m–labeled hepatobiliary agents. Semin Nucl Med 1990; 20(2): 130-49.

Weissman HS, Badia J, Sugarman LA, et al. Spectrum of 99m-Tc-IDA cholescintigraphic patterns in acute cholecystitis. Radiology 1981; 138: 167-75.

Revised: 07/26/93
Interim revision: 08/02/94

---

# TECHNETIUM Tc 99m MEDRONATE   Systemic

VA CLASSIFICATION (Primary/): DX201

Commonly used brand name(s): *AN-MDP; Frosstimage MDP; MDP-Squibb; MPI MDP; Osteolite; TechneScan MDP*.

Note: For a listing of dosage forms and brand names by country availability, see *Dosage Forms* section(s).

## Category
Diagnostic aid, radioactive (bone disease).

## Indications
**Accepted**
Skeletal imaging, radionuclide—Technetium Tc 99m medronate is indicated as a skeletal imaging agent to delineate areas of abnormal osteogenesis, such as those that occur with metastatic bone disease, Paget's disease, arthritic disease, osteomyelitis, and fractures.

## Physical Properties
**Nuclear data**

| Radionuclide (half-life) | Decay constant | Mode of decay | Principal photons emissions (keV) | Mean number of emissions/ disintegration ($\geq$0.01) |
|---|---|---|---|---|
| Tc 99m (6.0 hr) | 0.1151 h$^{-1}$ | Isomeric transition to Tc 99 | Gamma (18) | 0.062 |
|  |  |  | Gamma (140.5) | 0.891 |

## Pharmacology/Pharmacokinetics

**Mechanism of action/Effect**
Exact mechanism is not known. It is generally accepted that technetium Tc 99m medronate localizes on the surface of hydroxyapatite crystals by a process termed chemisorption, with blood flow and/or blood concentration being most important in the delivery of the agent to sites of uptake. Visualization of osseous lesions is possible since skeletal uptake of technetium Tc 99m medronate is altered in areas of abnormal osteogenesis.

**Distribution**
Rapidly distributed in and cleared from blood after intravenous administration, with about half the administered activity normally accumulating in the skeleton within 3 to 4 hours after intravenous administration. May also locate within infarcted myocardial cells or other regions of soft tissue necrosis or calcification. Minimal uptake by soft tissue organs, except calcified cartilage, blood vessels, and kidneys.

**Time to radioactivity visualization**
1 to 4 hours (optimal imaging).

**Radiation dosimetry**

| Estimated absorbed radiation dose* |||
|---|---|---|
| Organ | mGy/MBq | rad/mCi |
| Bone surfaces | 0.063 | 0.23 |
| Bladder wall | 0.050 | 0.19 |
| Red marrow | 0.0096 | 0.036 |
| Kidneys | 0.0073 | 0.027 |
| Uterus | 0.0061 | 0.023 |
| Large intestine wall (lower) | 0.0038 | 0.014 |

| Estimated absorbed radiation dose* |||
| Organ | mGy/MBq | rad/mCi |
|---|---|---|
| Ovaries | 0.0035 | 0.013 |
| Testes | 0.0024 | 0.0089 |
| Small intestine | 0.0023 | 0.0085 |
| Large intestine wall (upper) | 0.0020 | 0.0074 |
| Adrenals | 0.0019 | 0.0070 |
| Pancreas | 0.0016 | 0.0059 |
| Spleen | 0.0014 | 0.0052 |
| Liver | 0.0013 | 0.0048 |
| Lungs | 0.0013 | 0.0048 |
| Stomach wall | 0.0012 | 0.0044 |
| Thyroid | 0.0010 | 0.0037 |
| Breast | 0.00088 | 0.0033 |
| Other tissue | 0.0019 | 0.0070 |

Effective dose: 0.008 mSv/MBq (0.030 rem/mCi)

*For adults; intravenous injection of technetium Tc 99m–labeled phosphates and phosphonates. Data based on the International Commission on Radiological Protection (ICRP) Publication 53—Radiation dose to patients from radiopharmaceuticals.

**Elimination**
Renal; 50% (not localized in bone) eliminated within 24 hours.

## Precautions to Consider

**Carcinogenicity/Mutagenicity**
Long-term animal studies to evaluate carcinogenic or mutagenic potential of technetium Tc 99m medronate have not been performed.

**Pregnancy/Reproduction**
Pregnancy—Tc 99m (as free pertechnetate) crosses the placenta. Studies have not been done in humans with technetium Tc 99m medronate.

The possibility of pregnancy should be assessed in women of child-bearing potential. Clinical situations exist where the benefit to the patient and fetus, based on information derived from radiopharmaceutical use, outweighs the risks from fetal exposure to radiation. In these situations, the physician should use discretion and reduce the radiopharmaceutical dose to the lowest possible amount.

Studies have not been done in animals.

FDA Pregnancy Category C.

**Breast-feeding**
Although it is not known whether technetium Tc 99m medronate is distributed into breast milk, it is known that Tc 99m as free pertechnetate is distributed into breast milk. Based on the assumption that the Tc 99m in breast milk is in the form of pertechnetate and based on the effective half-life of the radionuclide in breast milk, the daily volume of milk, a dose factor relating the radionuclide to its critical organ (thyroid) in the nursing infant, and the maximum permissible dose to that organ, a guideline has been proposed. According to this guideline, it has been calculated that nursing can be safely resumed when the concentration in breast milk reaches $30.3 \times 10^{-4}$ megabecquerels ($8.2 \times 10^{-2}$ microcuries) per mL. This level of activity is probably reached, in the majority of patients, within 12 to 24 hours after administration of technetium Tc 99m–labeled radiopharmaceuticals.

**Pediatrics**
Diagnostic studies performed to date using technetium Tc 99m medronate have not demonstrated pediatrics-specific problems that would limit its usefulness in children. However, there have been no specific studies evaluating the safety and efficacy of technetium Tc 99m medronate in pediatric patients. When this radiopharmaceutical is used in children, the diagnostic benefit should be judged to outweigh the potential risk of radiation.

**Geriatrics**
Appropriate studies on the relationship of age to the effects of technetium Tc 99m medronate have not been performed in the geriatric population. However, no geriatrics-specific problems have been documented to date.

**Drug interactions and/or related problems**
See *Diagnostic interference*.

**Diagnostic interference**
The following have been selected on the basis of their potential clinical significance (possible effect in parentheses where appropriate)—not necessarily inclusive (» = major clinical significance):

With results of *this* test
*Due to other medications*
  Antacids, aluminum-containing
    (high blood concentrations of aluminum ion, which may occur in patients with gastrointestinal obstruction or impaired renal function, may cause localization of technetium Tc 99m medronate in the liver)
  Diatrizoate sodium
    (possible renal and hepatic uptake of technetium Tc 99m medronate if diatrizoate sodium is administered intravenously immediately after technetium Tc 99m medronate)
  Etidronate
    (etidronate may interfere with bone uptake of technetium Tc 99m medronate; a 2-week period after discontinuation of etidronate therapy is recommended before performance of a bone scan with technetium Tc 99m medronate)
  Heparin calcium, subcutaneous or
  Iron dextran, intramuscular or
  Meperidine, intramuscular
    (possible accumulation of technetium Tc 99m medronate at site[s] of injection of these medications)
  Iron supplements or preparations
    (iron overload may cause a decrease in bone uptake of technetium Tc 99m medronate)
  Potassium phosphates or
  Potassium and sodium phosphates or
  Sodium phosphates
    (saturation of bone binding sites by phosphorus ions in these medications may cause decreased bone uptake of technetium Tc 99m medronate)

*Due to medical problems or conditions*
  Bone demineralization, glucocorticoid-induced
    (long-term therapy with these medications may induce bone mineral depletion thus causing decreased bone uptake of technetium Tc 99m medronate)
  Gynecomastia, estrogen-induced
    (possible localization of technetium Tc 99m medronate in breast)
  Nephrotoxicity, drug-induced
    (increased retention of technetium Tc 99m medronate in kidneys)
  Obesity
    (attenuation of photons coming from bone may decrease visualization)
  Osteoporosis
    (reduced mineral deposit in bone may result in images with lower target to non-target ratio)
  Renal function impairment
    (decreased clearance of technetium Tc 99m medronate from blood and soft tissues may decrease visualization because of a lower bone to background ratio resulting from the increased circulating activity; also, chronic renal function impairment may cause metastatic calcification and altered biodistribution of technetium Tc 99m medronate)

With results of *other* tests
  Brain imaging
    (brain scans using sodium pertechnetate Tc 99m may result in high blood background activity when performed after a bone scan using technetium Tc 99m medronate, which contains stannous ions; to avoid this potential diagnostic interference, brain scan may be performed prior to bone scan or with a brain imaging agent other than sodium pertechnetate Tc 99m [e.g., technetium Tc 99m pentetate])

**Medical considerations/Contraindications**
The medical considerations/contraindications included have been selected on the basis of their potential clinical significance (reasons given in parentheses where appropriate)—not necessarily inclusive (» = major clinical significance).

See also *Diagnostic interference*.

*Risk-benefit should be considered when the following medical problem exists:*
  Sensitivity to the radiopharmaceutical preparation

## Side/Adverse Effects

The following side/adverse effects have been selected on the basis of their potential clinical significance (possible signs and symptoms in parentheses where appropriate)—not necessarily inclusive:

## Those indicating need for medical attention
Incidence less frequent or rare
   *Allergic reaction* (skin rash, hives, or itching)

## Patient Consultation
As an aid to patient consultation, refer to *Advice for the Patient, Radiopharmaceuticals (Diagnostic)*.

In providing consultation, consider emphasizing the following selected information (» = major clinical significance):

### Description of use
Action in the body: Accumulation of radioactivity in bone

Retention of radioactivity in bone allows visualization of lesions

Small amounts of radioactivity used in diagnosis; radiation received is low and considered safe

### Before having this test
» Conditions affecting use, especially:
   Sensitivity to the radiopharmaceutical preparation
   Pregnancy—Technetium Tc 99m (as free pertechnetate) crosses placenta; risk to fetus from radiation exposure as opposed to benefit derived from use should be considered
   Breast-feeding—Not known if technetium Tc 99m medronate is distributed into breast milk, but Tc 99m as free pertechnetate is distributed into breast milk; temporary discontinuation of nursing may be recommended because of risk to infant from radiation exposure
   Use in children—Risk from radiation exposure as opposed to benefit derived from use should be considered

### Preparation for this test
Special preparatory instructions may be given; patient should inquire in advance

Increasing intake of fluids and voiding frequently after injection and before test begins in order to minimize radiation dose to bladder

Voiding just prior to imaging for best test results

### Precautions after having this test
Increasing intake of fluids and voiding frequently for 4 to 6 hours after test to minimize radiation dose to bladder

### Side/adverse effects
Signs of potential side effects, especially allergic reaction

## General Dosing Information
Radiopharmaceuticals are to be administered only by or under the supervision of physicians who have had extensive training in the safe use and handling of radioactive materials and who are authorized by the Nuclear Regulatory Commission (NRC) or the appropriate Agreement State agency, if required, or, outside the U.S., the appropriate authority.

The patient should increase intake of fluids and void frequently following the administration of technetium Tc 99m medronate injection, and for 4 to 6 hours after the imaging procedures are completed, to minimize radiation dose to the bladder.

Voiding is also recommended immediately prior to imaging procedures to reduce background interference that may result because of the accumulation of the agent in the bladder.

Manufacturer's package insert or other appropriate literature should be consulted for optimal times when imaging should be performed.

### Safety considerations for handling this radiopharmaceutical
Improper handling of this radiopharmaceutical may cause radioactive contamination. Guidelines for handling radioactive material have been prepared by scientific, professional, state, federal, and international bodies and are available to the specially qualified and authorized users who have access to radiopharmaceuticals.

## Parenteral Dosage Forms

### TECHNETIUM Tc 99m MEDRONATE INJECTION USP

**Usual adult and adolescent administered activity**
Skeletal imaging—
   Intravenous, 7.4 megabecquerels (200 microcuries) per kg of body weight, or a total dose of 370 to 740 megabecquerels (10 to 20 millicuries), administered slowly over a period of 30 seconds.

**Usual pediatric administered activity**
Intravenous, 10.4 megabecquerels (0.28 millicuries) per kg of body weight, administered slowly.

Note: The recommended minimum total pediatric administered activity is 37 megabecquerels (1 millicurie); the maximum total pediatric administered activity is 740 megabecquerels (20 millicuries).

**Usual geriatric administered activity**
See *Usual adult and adolescent administered activity*.

**Strength(s) usually available**
U.S.—
   10 mg medronic acid, 0.17 mg (minimum) stannous chloride, and 2 mg ascorbic acid, in a lyophilized form and under nitrogen atmosphere, per 10-mL reaction vial (Rx) [*MPI MDP*].
   10 mg medronic acid and not less than 0.60 mg stannous chloride dihydrate (maximum total tin expressed as stannous chloride dihydrate 1.10 mg), in a lyophilized form and under nitrogen atmosphere, per 10-mL reaction vial (Rx) [*TechneScan MDP*].
   10 mg medronic acid and not less than 0.60 mg stannous chloride dihydrate (maximum total tin expressed as stannous chloride dihydrate 1.10 mg), in a lyophilized form and under nitrogen atmosphere, per 10-mL reaction vial (Rx) [*AN-MDP*].
   10 mg medronate disodium and 0.85 mg stannous chloride dihydrate, in a lyophilized form and under nitrogen atmosphere, per reaction vial (Rx) [*Osteolite*].
   20 mg medronic acid, 11 mg sodium hydroxide, 1 mg ascorbic acid, and 0.33 mg stannous fluoride, in a lyophilized form and under nitrogen atmosphere, per 10-mL reaction vial (Rx) [*MDP-Squibb*].
Canada—
   10 mg medronic acid and not less than 0.8 mg stannous chloride dihydrate (maximum total tin expressed as stannous chloride dihydrate 1.21 mg), in a lyophilized form and under nitrogen atmosphere, per 10-mL reaction vial (Rx) [*Frosstimage MDP*].

**Packaging and storage**
Store between 2 and 8 °C (36 and 46 °F). Protect from freezing.

Note: Before radiolabeling, the kit may be stored at or below room temperature.

**Preparation of dosage form**
To prepare injection, an oxidant-free sodium pertechnetate Tc 99m solution is used. See manufacturer's package insert for instructions.

**Stability**
Injection should be administered within 6 hours after preparation.

**Incompatibilities**
If oxidants such as peroxides and hypochlorites are present in the sodium pertechnetate Tc 99m used for labeling, the final preparation may be adversely affected and should be discarded.

**Note**
Caution—Radioactive material.

## Selected Bibliography
Holder LE. Clinical radionuclide bone imaging. Radiology 1990; 176: 607-14.

Revised: 06/14/93
Interim revision: 08/02/94

# TECHNETIUM Tc 99m MERTIATIDE Systemic

VA CLASSIFICATION (Primary): DX201

Commonly used brand name(s): *TechneScan MAG3*.

Other names commonly used are technetium Tc 99m mercaptoacetyltriglycine and MAG3.

Note: For a listing of dosage forms and brand names by country availability, see *Dosage Forms* section(s).

## Category
Diagnostic aid, radioactive (renal disorders).

## Indications
Note: Bracketed information in the *Indications* section refers to uses that are not included in U.S. product labeling.

## Accepted

Renal imaging, radionuclide or
Renal function studies—Technetium Tc 99m mertiatide is indicated as a renal imaging agent to assess renal perfusion, size, position, configuration, function (including differential renal function), upper urinary tract obstruction, and [active urinoma]. Technetium Tc 99m mertiatide scintigraphy provides renal images and renogram curves for the whole kidney and renal cortex.

In renal transplant patients, technetium Tc 99m mertiatide scintigraphy helps in the follow-up evaluation by providing anatomical information as well as functional analysis of the kidney. In diuretic radionuclide renography, technetium Tc 99m mertiatide provides useful information in the evaluation of obstructive uropathy. Also, angiotensin-converting enzyme (ACE) inhibitors–augmented renography using technetium Tc 99m mertiatide allows the detection of physiologically significant renal artery stenosis and helps in the differential diagnosis of renovascular hypertension.

Technetium Tc 99m mertiatide is used as an indirect measurement of effective renal plasma flow.

[Cystography, voiding, indirect, radionuclide] or
[Urinary bladder imaging, radionuclide]—Technetium Tc 99m mertiatide can be used following renal imaging for assessment of vesico-ureteral reflux.

## Physical Properties

### Nuclear data

| Radionuclide (half-life) | Decay constant | Mode of decay | Principal photon emissions (keV) | Mean number of emissions/ disintegration ($\geq 0.01$) |
|---|---|---|---|---|
| Tc 99m (6.0 hr) | 0.1151 h$^{-1}$ | Isomeric transition to Tc 99 | Gamma (18) | 0.061 |
| | | | Gamma (140.5) | 0.891 |

## Pharmacology/Pharmacokinetics

### Mechanism of action/Effect
The use of technetium Tc 99m mertiatide as a renal imaging agent is based on its clearance through the urinary tract predominantly via active tubular secretion (almost exclusively by the proximal renal tubules) and to a small extent by glomerular filtration. The rate of appearance and excretion and the concentration of technetium Tc 99m mertiatide in the kidney can be monitored to assess renal function.

### Distribution
Rapidly distributed in and cleared from plasma. However, when compared to iodohippurate sodium I 131 (OIH[131]), another renal imaging agent, technetium Tc 99m mertiatide has a significantly slower plasma clearance (50 to 65% of the clearance of OIH[131]).

### Protein binding
High (70 to 90%), but reversible.

### Radiation dosimetry

| Organ | Estimated absorbed radiation dose*† |||||
|---|---|---|---|---|
| | With normal renal function || With impaired renal function ||
| | mGy/ MBq | rad/ mCi | mGy/ MBq | rad/ mCi |
| Uterus | 0.012 | 0.044 | 0.01 | 0.037 |
| Large intestine (lower) | 0.0057 | 0.021 | 0.0051 | 0.019 |
| Ovaries | 0.0054 | 0.02 | 0.0049 | 0.018 |
| Testes | 0.0037 | 0.014 | 0.0034 | 0.013 |
| Kidneys | 0.0034 | 0.013 | 0.014 | 0.052 |
| Small intestine | 0.0023 | 0.0085 | 0.0027 | 0.01 |
| Large intestine (upper) | 0.0017 | 0.0063 | 0.0022 | 0.0081 |
| Muscles | 0.0014 | 0.0052 | 0.0017 | 0.0063 |
| Bone surfaces | 0.0013 | 0.0048 | 0.0022 | 0.0081 |
| Red marrow | 0.00093 | 0.0034 | 0.0015 | 0.0056 |
| Gall bladder | 0.00057 | 0.0021 | 0.0016 | 0.0059 |
| Skin | 0.00046 | 0.0017 | 0.00078 | 0.0029 |
| Pancreas | 0.0004 | 0.0015 | 0.0015 | 0.0056 |
| Stomach | 0.00039 | 0.0014 | 0.0027 | 0.01 |
| Adrenals | 0.00039 | 0.0014 | 0.0016 | 0.0059 |
| Spleen | 0.00036 | 0.0013 | 0.0015 | 0.0056 |
| Liver | 0.00031 | 0.0011 | 0.0014 | 0.0052 |
| Heart | 0.00018 | 0.00067 | 0.00091 | 0.0034 |
| Lungs | 0.00015 | 0.00056 | 0.00079 | 0.0029 |
| Esophagus | 0.00013 | 0.00048 | 0.00074 | 0.0027 |
| Thymus | 0.00013 | 0.00048 | 0.00074 | 0.0027 |
| Thyroid | 0.00013 | 0.00048 | 0.00073 | 0.0027 |
| Bladder | 0.00011 | 0.00041 | 0.083 | 0.031 |
| Brain | 0.0001 | 0.00037 | 0.00061 | 0.0023 |
| Breast | 0.0001 | 0.00037 | 0.00054 | 0.002 |
| Remaining organs | 0.0013 | 0.0048 | 0.0017 | 0.0063 |
| Effective dose | 0.0073 | 0.027 | 0.0063 | 0.023 |
| | mSv/MBq | rem/mCi | mSv/MBq | rem/mCi |

*For adults; intravenous administration.
†Data based on the International Commission on Radiological Protection (ICRP) Publication 53—Radiation dose to patients from radiopharmaceuticals.

### Elimination
Renal (70% of the administered activity in the first 30 minutes, and about 90% of the administered activity in 3 hours). Minimal hepatobiliary elimination (approximately 3% of the administered activity) in normal patients. Hepatobiliary elimination may be increased (approximately 10% of the administered activity) in patients with severe renal function impairment.

Note: The relatively higher extraction fraction (40 to 50%) of technetium Tc 99m mertiatide often provides superior images in patients with impaired renal function compared to technetium Tc 99m pentetate, another renal imaging agent, which has a lower extraction fraction (20%).

## Precautions to Consider

### Pregnancy/Reproduction
Pregnancy—Tc 99m (as free pertechnetate) crosses the placenta. Studies to assess transplacental transfer of technetium Tc 99m mertiatide have not been done in humans.

The possibility of pregnancy should be assessed in women of child-bearing potential. Clinical situations exist in which the benefit to the patient and fetus from information derived from radiopharmaceutical use outweigh the risks from radiation exposure to the fetus. In this situation, the physician should use discretion and reduce the radiopharmaceutical dose to the lowest possible amount consistent with image quality needs.

The patient should be maximally hydrated, and encouraged to urinate frequently.

Studies have not been done in animals.

FDA Pregnancy Category C.

### Breast-feeding
Although it is not known whether technetium Tc 99m mertiatide is distributed into breast milk, it is known that Tc 99m as free pertechnetate is distributed into breast milk. To avoid unnecessary irradiation of the infant, discontinuation of nursing for a period of 24 hours is recommended after administration of technetium Tc 99m–labeled radiopharmaceuticals.

### Pediatrics
Safety and efficacy have not been established in children up to 30 days of age. However, appropriate studies performed to date in older children have not demonstrated pediatrics-specific problems that would limit the usefulness of technetium Tc 99m mertiatide in children.

### Geriatrics
Appropriate studies performed to date have demonstrated a significant decrease in renal clearance of technetium Tc 99m mertiatide in geriatric patients when compared to younger adults.

### Diagnostic interference
The following have been selected on the basis of their potential clinical significance (possible effect in parentheses where appropriate)—not necessarily inclusive (» = major clinical significance):

With results of *this* test
Due to medical problems or conditions
  Dehydration
    (decreased urinary flow may result in a pattern that mimics decreased urine production and/or obstruction)

### Medical considerations/Contraindications
The medical considerations/contraindications included have been selected on the basis of their potential clinical significance (reasons given in parentheses where appropriate)—not necessarily inclusive (» = major clinical significance).
See also *Diagnostic interference*.

*Risk-benefit should be considered when the following medical problem exists:*
  Sensitivity to the radiopharmaceutical preparation

## Side/Adverse Effects
The following side/adverse effects have been selected on the basis of their potential clinical significance (possible signs and symptoms in parentheses where appropriate)—not necessarily inclusive:

### Incidence less frequent or rare
  *Allergic reaction* (skin rash or itching, wheezing or troubled breathing); *increased blood pressure; seizures* (convulsions); *tachycardia* (fast or pounding heartbeat)

### Those indicating need for medical attention only if they continue or are bothersome
Incidence less frequent or rare
  *Chills; fever; nausea; vomiting*

## Patient Consultation
As an aid to patient consultation, refer to *Advice for the Patient, Radiopharmaceuticals (Diagnostic)*.
In providing consultation, consider emphasizing the following selected information (» = major clinical significance):

### Description of use
  Action in the body: Concentration of radioactive mertiatide in kidneys
  Excretion of radioactivity in urine allows visualization and evaluation of renal function
  Small amounts of radioactivity used in diagnosis; radiation received is low and considered safe

### Before having this test
» Conditions affecting use, especially:
    Sensitivity to the radiopharmaceutical preparation
    Pregnancy—Technetium Tc 99m (as free pertechnetate) crosses placenta; risk to fetus from radiation exposure as opposed to benefit derived from study should be considered
    Breast-feeding—Not known if distributed into breast milk; temporary discontinuation of nursing may be recommended because of risk to infant from radiation exposure
    Use in children—Safety and efficacy have not been established in children up to 30 days of age

### Preparation for this test
  Special preparatory instructions may be given; patient should inquire in advance

### Precautions after having this test
  Adequate intake of fluids and voiding as often as possible for 4 to 6 hours after examination to minimize bladder exposure to radiation

## General Dosing Information
Radiopharmaceuticals are to be administered only by or under the supervision of physicians who have had extensive training in the safe use and handling of radionuclides and who are licensed by the Nuclear Regulatory Commission (NRC) or the appropriate Agreement State agency or, outside the U.S., the appropriate authority.

Adequate hydration of the patient is recommended before and after examination to promote urinary flow. Also, urination is recommended as often as possible for 4 to 6 hours after the examination to reduce bladder exposure to radiation.

Manufacturer's package insert or other appropriate literature should be consulted for optimal times when imaging should be performed.

### Safety considerations for handling this radiopharmaceutical
Guidelines for the receipt, storage, handling, dispensing, and disposal of radioactive materials are available from scientific, professional, state, federal, and international bodies. Handling of this radiopharmaceutical should be limited to those individuals who are appropriately qualified and authorized.

## Parenteral Dosage Forms

### TECHNETIUM Tc 99m MERTIATIDE INJECTION USP

**Usual adult and adolescent administered activity**
Renal imaging or
Renal function studies—
  Intravenous, 185 to 370 megabecquerels (5 to 10 millicuries).

**Usual pediatric administered activity**
Renal imaging or
Renal function studies—
  Children up to 30 days of age: Safety and efficacy have not been established.
  Children 30 days of age and over: Intravenous, 2.6 to 5.2 megabecquerels (70 to 140 microcuries) per kilogram of body weight, with a minimum administered activity of 37 megabecquerels (1 millicurie).

**Usual geriatric administered activity**
See *Usual adult and adolescent administered activity*.

**Strength(s) usually available**
U.S.—
  1 mg betiatide (precursor to mertiatide, thiobenzoic acid, *S*-ester with mercaptoacetyltriglycine), 0.05 mg (minimum) stannous chloride dihydrate, and 0.2 mg (maximum) total tin expressed as stannous chloride dihydrate, 40 mg sodium tartrate dihydrate, and 20 mg lactose monohydrate in lyophilized form under argon atmosphere, per 10-mL reaction vial (Rx) [*TechneScan MAG3*].
Canada—
  1 mg betiatide (precursor to mertiatide, thiobenzoic acid, *S*-ester with mercaptoacetyltriglycine), 0.05 mg (minimum) stannous chloride dihydrate, and 0.2 mg (maximum) total tin expressed as stannous chloride dihydrate, 40 mg sodium tartrate dihydrate, and 20 mg lactose monohydrate in lyophilized form under argon atmosphere, per 10-mL reaction vial (Rx) [*TechneScan MAG3*].

**Packaging and storage**
Store between 15 and 30 °C (59 and 86 °F). Protect from freezing.
Note: Before reconstitution, protect kit from light.

**Preparation of dosage form**
To prepare injection, an oxidant-free sodium pertechnetate Tc 99m solution is used. See manufacturer's package insert for instructions.

**Stability**
Product is stable; package insert states that injection must be used within 6 hours after preparation.

**Incompatibilities**
If oxidants such as peroxides and hypochlorites are present in the sodium pertechnetate Tc 99m used for labeling, the final preparation may be adversely affected and should be discarded.

**Note**
Caution—Radioactive material.

## Selected Bibliography
Bubeck B, Brandau W, Weber E, et al. Pharmacokinetics of technetium-99m-MAG3 in humans. J Nucl Med 1990; 31(8): 1285-93.
Eshima D, Taylor A Jr. Technetium-99m mercaptoacetyltriglycine: update on the new Tc 99m renal tubular function agent. Semin Nucl Med 1992; 22(2): 61-73

Revised: 07/23/96

# TECHNETIUM Tc 99 m NOFETUMOMAB MERPENTAN  Systemic†

VA CLASSIFICATION (Primary): DX201
Note: For a listing of brand names for the articles in this monograph, refer to the General Index.

Note: For a listing of dosage forms and brand names by country availability, see *Dosage Forms* section(s).

†Not commercially available in Canada.

## Category
Diagnostic aid, radioactive (pulmonary disease).

## Indications
### Accepted
Carcinoma, lung, primary and metastatic (diagnosis adjunct)—Technetium Tc 99m nofetumomab merpentan is indicated to determine the extent of disease in patients diagnosed with small cell lung cancer (SCLC). It is indicated for the detection of extensive stage disease in patients with biopsy-confirmed SCLC, but who have not yet received treatment. If imaging with technetium Tc 99m nofetumomab merpentan shows limited stage disease, additional diagnostic tests (e.g., bone scintigraphy; computed tomographic [CT] examinations of the head, chest, and abdomen; x-ray of the chest; and/or bone marrow aspirate/biopsy) should be performed to exclude extensive stage disease.

## Physical Properties
### Nuclear Data

| Radionuclide (half-life) | Mode of decay | Principal photon emissions (keV) | Mean number of emissions/ disintegration |
|---|---|---|---|
| Tc 99m (6 hr) | Isomeric transition to Tc 99 | Gamma (18) Gamma (140.5) | 0.062 0.891 |

## Pharmacology/Pharmacokinetics
### Physicochemical characteristics
Source—Mouse spleen cells that have been genetically engineered (by in vitro fermentation) to make monoclonal antibodies (NR-LU-10) of the type that react with the protein on various tumors, including small cell lung cancer (SCLC). Nofetumomab, the Fab fragment, is derived from the enzymatic digestion of purified NR-LU-10 antibody with papain. The radionuclide Tc 99m is attached to the antibody through a diamine dithiolate (N2S2) ligand.

### Mechanism of action/Effect
Nofetumomab, a Fab fragment of the murine monoclonal antibody NR-LU-10 of the IgG2b subclass, is directed against a 40-kilodalton (Kd) glycoprotein antigen expressed on the surface of numerous tumors, including lung (small cell and non–small cell), colon, breast, ovary, pancreas, kidney, and prostate. The distribution of radioactivity is recorded by planar or single photon emission computed tomography [SPECT].

### Distribution
After intravenous administration of technetium Tc 99m nofetumomab merpentan there is an initial rapid extravascular distribution followed by a slower clearance from the circulation. Technetium Tc 99m nofetumomab merpentan localizes to primary and/or metastatic small cell and non–small cell lung cancer, and adenocarcinomas of the breast, ovary, colorectum, and prostate. Also, accumulation of radioactivity may occur in non-tumor areas (e.g., gallbladder, intestine, kidneys, and urinary bladder as a result of excretion), in areas of marked vascularity (e.g., testes, midline nasal area, liver, spleen), or in areas of antigen cross-reactivity (e.g., pituitary gland, salivary gland, thyroid). In addition, radioactivity may accumulate in regions of inflammation, increased vascular pool, or recent surgical areas.

### Half-life
Distribution—1.5 hours (mean).
Elimination— 10.5 hours (mean).

### Time to radioactivity visualization
Total body imaging is generally performed 14 to 17 hours after technetium Tc 99m nofetumomab merpentan administration.

### Radiation dosimetry

| | Estimated absorbed radiation dose* | |
|---|---|---|
| Organ | mGy/MBq | rad/mCi |
| Gallbladder wall | 0.05 | 0.19 |
| Kidney | 0.034 | 0.13 |
| Large intestine wall (upper) | 0.024 | 0.09 |
| Large intestine wall (lower) | 0.017 | 0.067 |
| Small intestine wall | 0.014 | 0.053 |
| Liver | 0.012 | 0.043 |
| Ovaries | 0.0084 | 0.037 |
| Thyroid | 0.0081 | 0.03 |
| Uterus | 0.0077 | 0.029 |
| Lungs | 0.0066 | 0.025 |
| Spleen | 0.005 | 0.019 |
| Red marrow | 0.0042 | 0.016 |
| Testes | 0.004 | 0.015 |
| Total body | 0.0042 | 0.016 |

Effective dose: 0.008 mSv/MBq (0.03 rem/mCi)

*For adults; intravenous injection.

### Elimination
Renal (primary). Approximately 64% of the administered activity is excreted within the first 22 hours.
Note: The primary route of excretion, the kidneys, and the secondary routes of excretion, the hepatobiliary system and the gastrointestinal tract, lead to accumulation of radioactivity in the kidneys, urinary bladder, gallbladder, and intestines, which may interfere with image interpretation.

## Precautions to Consider
### Cross-sensitivity and/or related problems
Patients sensitive to murine antibody–based products may be sensitive to technetium Tc 99m nofetumomab merpentan also.

### Carcinogenicity/Mutagenicity
Long-term animal studies to evaluate carcinogenic or mutagenic potential of technetium Tc 99m nofetumomab merpentan have not been performed.

### Pregnancy/Reproduction
Pregnancy—Tc 99m (as free pertechnetate) crosses the placenta. However, studies to assess transplacental transfer of technetium Tc 99m nofetumomab merpentan have not been done in humans.
To avoid the possibility of fetal exposure to radiation, in those circumstances in which the patient's pregnancy status is uncertain, a pregnancy test will help to prevent inadvertent administration of this preparation during pregnancy. Studies have not been done in animals.
FDA Pregnancy Category C.

### Breast-feeding
Although it is not known whether technetium Tc 99m nofetumomab merpentan is distributed into breast milk, it is known that Tc 99m as free pertechnetate is distributed into breast milk. Because of the potential risk to the infant from radiation exposure, breast-feeding should be discontinued and formula feedings used instead for at least 60 hours after administration of technetium Tc 99m nofetumomab merpentan.

### Pediatrics
Appropriate studies on the relationship of age to the effects of technetium Tc 99m nofetumomab merpentan have not been performed in the pediatric population. Safety and efficacy have not been established.

### Geriatrics
Appropriate studies on the relationship of age to the effects of technetium Tc 99m nofetumomab merpentan have not been performed in the geriatric population. However, clinical trials and studies that included older patients were conducted, and geriatrics-specific problems that would limit the usefulness of this agent in the elderly are not expected.

### Laboratory value alterations
The following have been selected on the basis of their potential clinical significance (possible effect in parentheses where appropriate)—not necessarily inclusive (» = major clinical significance):

With other diagnostic test results
　Immunoassays, murine antibody–based
　　(human anti-murine antibody [HAMA] production may be induced by the administration of murine monoclonal antibodies; HAMA in serum may interfere with murine antibody–based immunoassays and with in vitro or in vivo diagnostic or therapeutic murine antibody–based agents, and may increase the risk of adverse reactions)

## Diagnostic interference

The following have been selected on the basis of their potential clinical significance (possible effect in parentheses where appropriate)—not necessarily inclusive (» = major clinical significance):

With results of *this* test
*Due to medical problems or conditions*

Inflammatory lesions, local or
Surgical areas, recent
(localization of technetium Tc 99m nofetumomab merpentan may occur at these sites)

## Medical considerations/Contraindications

The medical considerations/contraindications included have been selected on the basis of their potential clinical significance (reasons given in parentheses where appropriate)—not necessarily inclusive (» = major clinical significance).

*Risk-benefit should be considered when the following medical problems exist:*

Sensitivity to murine antibody–based products or to the radiopharmaceutical preparation

## Side/Adverse Effects

The following side/adverse effects have been selected on the basis of their potential clinical significance (possible signs and symptoms in parentheses where appropriate)—not necessarily inclusive:

**Those indicating need for medical attention only if they continue or are bothersome**
*Incidence less frequent or rare*

***Allergic reaction, mild, transient*** (skin rash); ***fever***

## Patient Consultation

As an aid to patient consultation, refer to *Advice for the Patient, Radiopharmaceuticals (Diagnostic)*.

In providing consultation, consider emphasizing the following selected information (» = major clinical significance):

**Description of use**
Action in the body: Localization of radiolabeled monoclonal antibodies in tumor sites; uptake of radioactivity may be visualized by external imaging
Small amounts of radioactivity used in diagnosis; radiation received is low and considered safe

**Before using this medication**
» Conditions affecting use, especially:
Sensitivity to murine antibody–based products or to the radiopharmaceutical preparation
Pregnancy—Technetium Tc 99m (as free pertechnetate) crosses the placenta; risk to fetus from radiation exposure as opposed to benefit derived from study should be considered
Breast-feeding—Not known if technetium Tc 99m nofetumomab merpentan is distributed into breast milk, but Tc 99m (as free pertechnetate) is distributed into breast milk; formula feedings should be used for at least 60 hours after administration of this agent to avoid any unnecessary absorbed radiation dose to the infant

**Preparation for this test**
Special preparatory instructions may apply; patient should inquire in advance
Administration of an oral cathartic before imaging to minimize imaging interference due to radioactivity localization in bowel

**Precautions after having this test**
Adequate intake of fluids and frequent voiding for 12 to 14 hours after administration of agent to minimize radiation exposure to the bladder

## General Dosing Information

Radiopharmaceuticals are to be administered only by or under the supervision of physicians who have had extensive training in the safe use and handling of radioactive materials and who are licensed by the Nuclear Regulatory Commission (NRC) or the appropriate Agreement State agency, if required, or, outside the U.S., the appropriate authority.

The patient should increase intake of fluids and void frequently for 12 to 14 hours following the administration of technetium Tc 99m nofetumomab merpentan to minimize radiation dose to the bladder.

Oral administration of a cathartic is recommended after the injection of technetium Tc 99m nofetumomab merpentan, and prior to imaging, to minimize radioactivity in bowel, which may interfere with image interpretation.

**Safety considerations for handling this radiopharmaceutical**
Guidelines for the receipt, storage, handling, dispensing, and disposal of radioactive materials are available from scientific, professional, state, federal, and international bodies. Handling of this radiopharmaceutical should be limited to those individuals who are appropriately qualified and authorized.

**For treatment of adverse effects**
Epinephrine and antihistamines should be available during the administration of technetium Tc 99m nofetumomab merpentan because of the possibility of allergic reactions.

## Parenteral Dosage Forms

### TECHNETIUM Tc 99m NOFETUMOMAB MERPENTAN INJECTION

**Usual adult and administered activity**
*Diagnosis of extent of lung carcinoma*—
Intravenous, 5 to 10 mg of nofetumomab merpentan radiolabeled with 555 to 1110 megabecquerels (15 to 30 millicuries) of technetium Tc 99m, administered over three to five minutes.

Note: At least 555 megabecquerels (15 millicuries) of the final preparation should be administered to ensure an adequate dose of radiolabeled antibody is used to obtain satisfactory images.

**Usual pediatric administered activity**
Safety and efficacy have not been established.

**Usual geriatric administered activity**
See *Usual adult administered activity*.

**Strength(s) usually available**
U.S.—
10 mg of nofetumomab merpentan per 1-mL vial of sodium phosphate–buffered saline solution (Rx) [*Verluma*; GENERIC].
Canada—
Not commercially available.

**Packaging and storage**
Before radiolabeling, store between 2 and 8 °C (36 and 46 °F), unless otherwise specified by manufacturer. Protect from freezing and shaking.

Note: After radiolabeling, the technetium Tc 99m nofetumomab merpentan injection should be kept at room temperature.

**Preparation of dosage form**
To radiolabel the nofetumomab merpentan, a sterile, pyrogen- and oxidant-free sodium pertechnetate Tc 99m in 0.9% sodium chloride solution is used. See the manufacturer's package insert for instructions.

**Stability**
The package insert states that the injection should be administered within 6 hours after radiolabeling, since it does not contain a preservative.

**Caution**
Radioactive material.

## Selected Bibliography

Balaban EP, Walker BS, Cox JV, et al. Radionuclide imaging of bone marrow metastases with a Tc-99m labeled monoclonal antibody to small cell lung carcinoma. Clin Nucl Med 1991 Oct; 16(10): 732-6.

Vansant JP, Johnson DH, O'Donnell, et al. Staging lung carcinoma with a Tc-99m labeled monoclonal antibody. Clin Nucl Med 1992 June; 17(6): 431-8.

Developed: 08/24/98

---

# TECHNETIUM Tc 99m OXIDRONATE  Systemic†

VA CLASSIFICATION (Primary): DX201
Commonly used brand name(s): *Osteoscan-HDP*.

Note: For a listing of dosage forms and brand names by country availability, see *Dosage Forms* section(s).

†Not commercially available in Canada.

## Category
Diagnostic aid, radioactive (bone disease).

## Indications
Note: Bracketed information in the *Indications* section refers to uses that are not included in U.S. product labeling.

### Accepted
Skeletal imaging, radionuclide—Technetium Tc 99m oxidronate is indicated as a skeletal imaging agent in adults and children to delineate areas of abnormal osteogenesis, such as those that occur with metastatic bone disease, Paget's disease, arthritic disease, osteomyelitis, and fractures.

## Physical Properties
### Nuclear data

| Radionuclide (half-life) | Decay constant | Mode of decay | Principal photons emissions (keV) | Mean number of emissions/ disintegration ($\geq 0.01$) |
|---|---|---|---|---|
| Tc 99m (6.0 hr) | 0.1151 h$^{-1}$ | Isomeric transition to Tc 99 | Gamma (18) | 0.062 |
| | | | Gamma (140.5) | 0.891 |

## Pharmacology/Pharmacokinetics
### Mechanism of action/Effect
Exact mechanism is not known. It is generally accepted that technetium Tc 99m oxidronate localizes on the surface of hydroxyapatite crystals by a process termed chemisorption, with blood flow and/or blood concentration being most important in the delivery of the agent to sites of uptake. Visualization of osseous lesions is possible since skeletal uptake of technetium Tc 99m oxidronate is altered in areas of abnormal osteogenesis.

### Distribution
Rapidly distributed in and cleared from blood after intravenous administration, with about half the dose normally accumulating in the skeleton within 3 to 4 hours after injection. May also locate within infarcted myocardial cells or other regions of soft tissue necrosis or calcification. Minimal uptake by soft-tissue organs, except calcified cartilage, blood vessels, and kidneys.

### Time to radioactivity visualization
1 to 4 hours (optimal imaging).

### Radiation dosimetry

| Estimated absorbed radiation dose* |||
|---|---|---|
| Organ | mGy/MBq | rad/mCi |
| Bone surfaces | 0.063 | 0.23 |
| Bladder wall | 0.050 | 0.19 |
| Red marrow | 0.0096 | 0.036 |
| Kidneys | 0.0073 | 0.027 |
| Uterus | 0.0061 | 0.023 |
| Large intestine wall (lower) | 0.0038 | 0.014 |
| Ovaries | 0.0035 | 0.013 |
| Testes | 0.0024 | 0.0089 |
| Small intestine | 0.0023 | 0.0085 |
| Large intestine wall (upper) | 0.0020 | 0.0074 |
| Adrenals | 0.0019 | 0.0070 |
| Pancreas | 0.0016 | 0.0059 |
| Spleen | 0.0014 | 0.0052 |
| Liver | 0.0013 | 0.0048 |
| Lungs | 0.0013 | 0.0048 |
| Stomach wall | 0.0012 | 0.0044 |
| Thyroid | 0.0010 | 0.0037 |
| Breast | 0.00088 | 0.0033 |
| Other tissue | 0.0019 | 0.0070 |

Effective dose: 0.008 mSv/MBq (0.030 rem/mCi)

*For adults; intravenous injection of technetium Tc 99m–labeled phosphates and phosphonates. Data based on the International Commission on Radiological Protection (ICRP) Publication 53—Radiation dose to patients from radiopharmaceuticals.

## Elimination
Renal.

## Precautions to Consider
### Carcinogenicity/Mutagenicity
Long-term animal studies to evaluate carcinogenic or mutagenic potential of technetium Tc 99m oxidronate have not been performed.

### Pregnancy/Reproduction
Pregnancy—Tc 99m (as free pertechnetate) crosses the placenta. Studies with technetium Tc 99m oxidronate have not been done in humans.

The possibility of pregnancy should be assessed in women of child-bearing potential. Clinical situations exist where the benefit to the patient and fetus, based on information derived from radiopharmaceutical use, outweighs the risks from fetal exposure to radiation. In these situations, the physician should use discretion and reduce the radiopharmaceutical dose to the lowest possible amount.

Studies have not been done in animals.

FDA Pregnancy Category C.

### Breast-feeding
Although it is not known whether technetium Tc 99m oxidronate is distributed into breast milk, it is known that Tc 99m as free pertechnetate is distributed into breast milk. Based on the assumption that the Tc 99m in breast milk is in the form of pertechnetate and based on the effective half-life of the radionuclide in breast milk, the daily volume of milk, a dose factor relating the radionuclide to its critical organ (thyroid) in the nursing infant, and the maximum permissible dose to that organ, a guideline has been proposed. According to this guideline, it has been calculated that nursing can be safely resumed when the concentration in breast milk reaches $30.3 \times 10^{-4}$ megabecquerels ($8.2 \times 10^{-2}$ microcuries) per mL. This level of activity is probably reached, in the majority of patients, within 12 to 24 hours after administration of technetium Tc 99m–labeled radiopharmaceuticals.

### Pediatrics
Diagnostic studies performed to date using technetium Tc 99m oxidronate have not demonstrated pediatrics-specific problems that would limit its usefulness in children. However, there have been no specific studies evaluating the safety and efficacy of technetium Tc 99m oxidronate in pediatric patients. When this radiopharmaceutical is used in children, the diagnostic benefit should be judged to outweigh the potential risk of radiation.

### Geriatrics
Appropriate studies on the relationship of age to the effects of technetium Tc 99m oxidronate have not been performed in the geriatric population. However, no geriatrics-specific problems have been documented to date.

### Drug interactions and/or related problems
See *Diagnostic interference*.

### Diagnostic interference
The following have been selected on the basis of their potential clinical significance (possible effect in parentheses where appropriate)—not necessarily inclusive (» = major clinical significance):

With results of *this* test
*Due to other medications*
  Antacids, aluminum-containing
    (high blood concentrations of aluminum ion, which may occur in patients with gastrointestinal obstruction or impaired renal function, may cause localization of technetium Tc 99m oxidronate in the liver)
  Diatrizoate sodium
    (possible renal and hepatic uptake if diatrizoate sodium is administered intravenously immediately after technetium Tc 99m oxidronate)
  Etidronate
    (etidronate may interfere with bone uptake of technetium Tc 99m oxidronate; discontinuation of etidronate therapy before performance of a bone scan with technetium Tc 99m oxidronate is recommended for a 2-week period)
  Heparin calcium, subcutaneous or
  Iron dextran, intramuscular or
  Meperidine, intramuscular
    (possible accumulation of technetium Tc 99m oxidronate at site[s] of injection of these medications)
  Iron supplements or preparations
    (iron overload may cause a decrease in bone uptake of technetium Tc 99m oxidronate)
  Potassium phosphates or
  Potassium and sodium phosphates or

# Technetium Tc 99m Oxidronate (Systemic)

Sodium phosphates
(saturation of bone binding sites by phosphorus ions in these medications may cause decreased bone uptake of technetium Tc 99m oxidronate)

*Due to medical problems or conditions*

Bone demineralization, glucocorticoid-induced
(long-term therapy with glucocorticoids may induce bone mineral depletion, thus causing decreased bone uptake of technetium Tc 99m oxidronate)

Gynecomastia, estrogen-induced
(possible localization of technetium Tc 99m oxidronate in breast)

Nephrotoxicity, drug-induced
(increased retention of technetium Tc 99m oxidronate in kidneys)

Obesity
(decreased visualization may result due to attenuation of photons coming from bone)

Osteoporosis
(reduced mineral deposit in bone may result in images with lower target to non-target ratio)

Renal function impairment
(decreased clearance of technetium Tc 99m oxidronate from blood and soft tissues may impair visualization because of a lower bone to background ratio resulting from the increased circulating activity; also, chronic renal function impairment may cause metastatic calcification and altered biodistribution of technetium Tc 99m oxidronate)

With results of *other* tests

Brain imaging
(brain scans using sodium pertechnetate Tc 99m may result in high blood background activity when performed after a bone scan using technetium Tc 99m oxidronate, which contains stannous ions; to avoid this potential diagnostic interference, brain scan may be performed prior to bone scan or with a brain imaging agent other than sodium pertechnetate Tc 99m [e.g., technetium Tc 99m pentetate])

### Medical considerations/Contraindications

The medical considerations/contraindications included have been selected on the basis of their potential clinical significance (reasons given in parentheses where appropriate)—not necessarily inclusive (» = major clinical significance).

See also *Diagnostic interference*.

*Risk-benefit should be considered when the following medical problem exists:*

Sensitivity to the radiopharmaceutical preparation

## Side/Adverse Effects

The following side/adverse effects have been selected on the basis of their potential clinical significance (possible signs and symptoms in parentheses where appropriate)—not necessarily inclusive:

### Those indicating need for medical attention
Incidence less frequent or rare
*Allergic reaction* (flushing or redness of skin)

### Those indicating need for medical attention if they continue or are bothersome
Incidence less frequent or rare
*Nausea and vomiting*

## Patient Consultation

As an aid to patient consultation, refer to *Advice for the Patient, Radiopharmaceuticals (Diagnostic)*.

In providing consultation, consider emphasizing the following selected information (» = major clinical significance):

### Description of use
Action in the body: Accumulation of radioactivity in bone
Retention of radioactivity in bone allows visualization of lesions
Small amounts of radioactivity used in diagnosis; radiation received is low and considered safe

### Before having this test
» Conditions affecting use, especially:
Sensitivity to the radiopharmaceutical preparation
Pregnancy—Technetium Tc 99m (as free pertechnetate) crosses placenta; risk to fetus from radiation exposure as opposed to benefit derived from use should be considered
Breast-feeding—Not known if technetium Tc 99m oxidronate is distributed into breast milk, but Tc 99m as free pertechnetate is distributed into breast milk; temporary discontinuation of nursing may be recommended because of risk to infant from radiation exposure
Use in children—Risk from radiation exposure as opposed to benefit derived from use should be considered

### Preparation for this test
Special preparatory instructions may be given; patient should inquire in advance
Increasing intake of fluids and voiding frequently after injection and before test begins in order to minimize radiation dose to bladder
Voiding again just prior to imaging for best test results

### Precautions after having this test
Increasing intake of fluids and voiding frequently for 4 to 6 hours after test to minimize radiation dose to bladder

### Side/adverse effects
Signs of potential side effects, especially allergic reaction

## General Dosing Information

Radiopharmaceuticals are to be administered only by or under the supervision of physicians who have had extensive training in the safe use and handling of radioactive materials and who are authorized by the Nuclear Regulatory Commission (NRC) or the appropriate Agreement State agency, if required, or, outside the U.S., the appropriate authority.

The patient should increase intake of fluids and void frequently following the administration of technetium Tc 99m oxidronate injection, and for 4 to 6 hours after the imaging procedures are completed, to minimize radiation dose to the bladder.

Voiding is also recommended immediately prior to imaging procedures to reduce background interference that may result from accumulation of the agent in the bladder.

### Safety considerations for handling this radiopharmaceutical
Improper handling of this radiopharmaceutical may cause radioactive contamination. Guidelines for handling radioactive material have been prepared by scientific, professional, state, federal, and international bodies and are available to the specially qualified and authorized users who have access to radiopharmaceuticals.

## Parenteral Dosage Forms

### TECHNETIUM Tc 99m OXIDRONATE INJECTION USP

**Usual adult and adolescent administered activity**
Skeletal imaging—
Intravenous, 370 to 740 megabecquerels (10 to 20 millicuries), administered slowly.

**Usual adult prescribing limits**
Up to 740 megabecquerels (20 millicuries).

**Usual pediatric administered activity**
Skeletal imaging—
Intravenous, 7.4 to 13 megabecquerels (0.20 to 0.35 millicurie) per kg of body weight, administered slowly.

Note: The recommended minimum total pediatric administered activity is 37 megabecquerels (1 millicurie); the maximum total pediatric administered activity is 740 megabecquerels (20 millicuries).

**Usual geriatric administered activity**
See *Usual adult and adolescent administered activity*.

**Strength(s) usually available**
U.S.—
2.0 mg oxidronate sodium and 0.16 mg stannous chloride, per vial (Rx) [*Osteoscan-HDP*].
Canada—
Not commercially available.

**Packaging and storage**
Store below 40 °C (104 °F), preferably between 15 and 30 °C (59 and 86 °F), unless otherwise specified by manufacturer. Protect from freezing.

Note: Both prior to and following radiolabeling, this product may be stored at or below room temperature.

**Preparation of dosage form**
To prepare injection, an oxidant-free sodium pertechnetate Tc 99m solution is used. See manufacturer's package insert for instructions.

**Stability**
Injection should be administered within 8 hours after preparation.

**Incompatibilities**
If oxidants such as peroxides and hypochlorites are present in the sodium pertechnetate Tc 99m used for labeling, the final preparation may be adversely affected and should be discarded.

Note
Caution—Radioactive material.

## Selected Bibliography
Holder LE. Clinical radionuclide bone imaging. Radiology 1990; 176: 607-14.

Delaloye B, Delaloye-Bischof A, Koppenhagen K, et al. Clinical comparison of Tc 99m-HMDP and Tc 99m-MDP. A multicenter study. Eur J Nucl Med 1985; 11(5): 182-5.

Revised: 07/20/93
Interim revision: 08/02/94

# TECHNETIUM Tc 99m PENTETATE   Systemic

VA CLASSIFICATION (Primary): DX201

Commonly used brand name(s): *AN-DTPA; DTPA (Chelate) Multidose; Frosstimage DTPA; TechneScan DTPA; Techneplex.*

Note: For a listing of dosage forms and brand names by country availability, see *Dosage Forms* section(s).

## Category
Diagnostic aid, radioactive (renal disorders; intracranial lesions; cerebrospinal fluid disorders; pulmonary disease).

## Indications
Note: Bracketed information in the *Indications* section refers to uses that are not included in U.S. product labeling.

**Accepted**

Renal imaging, radionuclide—Technetium Tc 99m pentetate is indicated as a renal imaging agent to evaluate kidney size, position, configuration, and function, especially in parenchymal disorders.

Renal perfusion studies—Technetium Tc 99m pentetate is indicated to assess renal perfusion.

Glomerular filtration rate determination—Technetium Tc 99m pentetate is indicated in excretion studies to estimate glomerular filtration rate (GFR).

Brain imaging, radionuclide—Technetium Tc 99m pentetate is indicated as a brain imaging agent to detect and evaluate intracranial lesions. Although technetium Tc 99m pentetate is an acceptable brain imaging agent, it is being replaced by computed tomography (CT) and magnetic resonance imaging (MRI).

[Cisternography, radionuclide][1]—Technetium Tc 99m pentetate is used to evaluate cerebrospinal fluid (CSF) flow through ventriculoperitoneal and lumboperitoneal shunts.

[Lung imaging, radionuclide][1]—Technetium Tc 99m pentetate administered by inhalation as an aerosol is used to assess airway patency, especially in conjunction with perfusion lung imaging to evaluate pulmonary embolism.

[1]Not included in Canadian product labeling.

## Physical Properties
**Nuclear Data**

| Radionuclide (half-life) | Decay constant | Mode of decay | Principal photon emissions (keV) | Mean number of emissions/ disintegration ($\geq 0.01$) |
|---|---|---|---|---|
| Tc 99m (6.0 hr) | 0.1151 h$^{-1}$ | Isomeric transition to Tc 99 | Gamma (18) | 0.062 |
|  |  |  | Gamma (140.5) | 0.891 |

## Pharmacology/Pharmacokinetics
**Mechanism of action/Effect**

Diagnostic aid (renal function)—The use of technetium Tc 99m pentetate as a renal imaging agent is based on its clearance through the urinary tract by glomerular filtration.

Diagnostic aid (intracranial lesions)—Technetium Tc 99m pentetate normally is prevented by the blood-brain barrier from entering the brain; however, it accumulates by passive diffusion in intracranial lesions that have altered blood-brain barrier.

Diagnostic aid (CSF flow disorders)—Technetium Tc 99m pentetate, when injected intrathecally or intraventricularly mixes and flows with the CSF.

Diagnostic aid (pulmonary disease)—Aerosolized droplets of technetium Tc 99m pentetate, when inhaled, distribute and accumulate in patent airways.

**Distribution**

Rapidly distributed in and cleared from plasma following intravenous administration.

**Protein binding**

Very low (variable, 3.7 to 10% if continuously infused).

**Radiation dosimetry**

| Organ | Estimated absorbed radiation dose* With intravenous injection ||||
|---|---|---|---|---|
|  | Normal renal function || Impaired renal function ||
|  | mGy/ MBq | rad/ mCi | mGy/ MBq | rad/ mCi |
| Bladder wall | 0.065 | 0.24 | 0.022 | 0.081 |
| Uterus | 0.0079 | 0.029 | 0.0063 | 0.023 |
| Kidneys | 0.0044 | 0.016 | 0.0079 | 0.029 |
| Ovaries | 0.0043 | 0.016 | 0.0049 | 0.018 |
| Large intestine wall (lower) | 0.0042 | 0.016 | 0.0047 | 0.017 |
| Testes | 0.0028 | 0.010 | 0.0033 | 0.012 |
| Small intestine | 0.0026 | 0.0096 | 0.0047 | 0.017 |
| Red marrow | 0.0025 | 0.0093 | 0.0052 | 0.019 |
| Large intestine wall (upper) | 0.0022 | 0.0081 | 0.0044 | 0.016 |
| Bone surfaces | 0.0017 | 0.0063 | 0.0044 | 0.016 |
| Pancreas | 0.0015 | 0.0056 | 0.0043 | 0.016 |
| Spleen | 0.0014 | 0.0052 | 0.0040 | 0.015 |
| Adrenals | 0.0014 | 0.0052 | 0.0041 | 0.015 |
| Stomach wall | 0.0013 | 0.0048 | 0.0038 | 0.019 |
| Liver | 0.0013 | 0.0048 | 0.0038 | 0.019 |
| Lungs | 0.0010 | 0.0037 | 0.0033 | 0.012 |
| Breast | 0.00094 | 0.0035 | 0.0030 | 0.011 |
| Thyroid | 0.00079 | 0.0029 | 0.0025 | 0.0093 |
| Other tissue | 0.0017 | 0.0063 | 0.0033 | 0.012 |

| Radionuclide | Effective dose* ||||
|---|---|---|---|---|
|  | Normal renal function || Impaired renal function ||
|  | mSv/ MBq | rem/ mCi | mSv/ MBq | rem/ mCi |
| Tc 99m | 0.0063 | 0.034 | 0.0053 | 0.020 |

| Organ | Estimated absorbed radiation dose* With intrathecal injection ||||
|---|---|---|---|---|
|  | Lumbar injection || Cisternal injection ||
|  | mGy/ MBq | rad/ mCi | mGy/ MBq | rad/ mCi |
| Spinal cord | 0.046 | 0.17 | 0.013 | 0.048 |
| Red marrow | 0.029 | 0.11 | 0.0085 | 0.031 |
| Bladder wall | 0.017 | 0.063 | 0.010 | 0.037 |
| Kidneys | 0.017 | 0.063 | 0.0019 | 0.0070 |
| Adrenals | 0.011 | 0.041 | 0.0018 | 0.0067 |
| Pancreas | 0.0093 | 0.034 | 0.0012 | 0.0044 |
| Small intestine | 0.0081 | 0.030 | 0.00088 | 0.0033 |
| Bone surfaces | 0.0064 | 0.024 | 0.0059 | 0.022 |
| Large intestine wall (upper) | 0.0062 | 0.023 | 0.00071 | 0.0026 |
| Ovaries | 0.0048 | 0.018 | 0.00089 | 0.0033 |
| Spleen | 0.0046 | 0.017 | 0.00066 | 0.0024 |
| Uterus | 0.0045 | 0.017 | 0.0014 | 0.0052 |
| Stomach wall | 0.0042 | 0.016 | 0.00076 | 0.0028 |
| Liver | 0.0038 | 0.014 | 0.00060 | 0.0022 |

| Organ | Estimated absorbed radiation dose* With intrathecal injection |||| 
| | Lumbar injection || Cisternal injection ||
| | mGy/MBq | rad/mCi | mGy/MBq | rad/mCi |
|---|---|---|---|---|
| Brain | 0.0032 | 0.012 | 0.055 | 0.20 |
| Large intestine wall (lower) | 0.0026 | 0.0096 | 0.00075 | 0.0028 |
| Lungs | 0.0024 | 0.0089 | 0.00086 | 0.0032 |
| Thyroid | 0.0013 | 0.0048 | 0.0030 | 0.011 |
| Testes | 0.00089 | 0.0033 | 0.00044 | 0.0016 |
| Breast | 0.00065 | 0.0024 | 0.00054 | 0.0020 |
| Other tissue | 0.0025 | 0.0093 | 0.00086 | 0.0032 |

| Radionuclide | Effective dose* ||||
| | Lumbar injection || Cisternal injection ||
| | mSv/MBq | rem/mCi | mSv/MBq | rem/mCi |
|---|---|---|---|---|
| Tc 99m | 0.011 | 0.041 | 0.0066 | 0.024 |

| Organ | Estimated absorbed radiation dose* With aerosol administration ||
| | mGy/MBq | rad/mCi |
|---|---|---|
| Bladder wall | 0.047 | 0.17 |
| Lungs | 0.017 | 0.063 |
| Uterus | 0.0059 | 0.022 |
| Kidneys | 0.0041 | 0.015 |
| Ovaries | 0.0033 | 0.012 |
| Large intestine wall (lower) | 0.0032 | 0.012 |
| Red marrow | 0.0027 | 0.010 |
| Adrenals | 0.0021 | 0.0078 |
| Small intestine | 0.0021 | 0.0078 |
| Pancreas | 0.0021 | 0.0078 |
| Testes | 0.0021 | 0.0078 |
| Bone surfaces | 0.0019 | 0.0070 |
| Breast | 0.0019 | 0.0070 |
| Large intestine wall (upper) | 0.0019 | 0.0070 |
| Liver | 0.0019 | 0.0070 |
| Spleen | 0.0019 | 0.0070 |
| Stomach wall | 0.0017 | 0.0063 |
| Thyroid | 0.00099 | 0.0037 |
| Other tissue | 0.0018 | 0.0067 |

Effective dose: 0.0070 mSv/MBq (0.026 rem/mCi)*

*In adults. Data based on the International Commission on Radiological Protection (ICRP) Publication 53—Radiation dose to patients from radiopharmaceuticals.

### Elimination
Renal; about 50% of the intravenously administered activity eliminated in 2 hours and about 95% of the administered activity eliminated within 24 hours.

## Precautions to Consider

### Carcinogenicity/Mutagenicity
Long-term animal studies to evaluate carcinogenic or mutagenic potential of technetium Tc 99m pentetate have not been performed.

### Pregnancy/Reproduction
Pregnancy—Tc 99m (as free pertechnetate) crosses the placenta. However, studies have not been done with technetium Tc 99m pentetate in humans.
The possibility of pregnancy should be assessed in women of child-bearing potential. Clinical situations exist where the benefit to the patient and fetus, based on information derived from radiopharmaceutical use, outweighs the risks from fetal exposure to radiation. In these situations, the physician should use discretion and reduce the radiopharmaceutical dose to the lowest possible amount.
Studies have not been done in animals.
FDA Pregnancy Category C.

### Breast-feeding
Although it is not known whether technetium Tc 99m pentetate is distributed into breast milk, it is known that Tc 99m as free pertechnetate is distributed into breast milk. Based on the assumption that the Tc 99m in breast milk is in the form of pertechnetate and based on the effective half-life of the radionuclide in breast milk, the daily volume of milk, a dose factor relating the radionuclide to its critical organ (thyroid) in the nursing infant, and the maximum permissible dose to that organ, a guideline has been proposed. According to this guideline, it has been calculated that nursing can be safely resumed when the concentration in breast milk reaches $30.3 \times 10^{-4}$ megabecquerels ($8.2 \times 10^{-2}$ microcuries) per mL. This level of activity is probably reached, in the majority of patients, within 24 hours after administration of 740 megabecquerels (20 millicuries) of technetium Tc 99m–labeled radiopharmaceuticals.

### Pediatrics
Renal studies performed in children from 1 week to 18 years of age have not demonstrated pediatrics-specific problems that would limit the usefulness of technetium Tc 99m pentetate in children. However, there have been no specific studies evaluating the safety and efficacy of technetium Tc 99m pentetate in pediatric patients. When this radiopharmaceutical is used in children, the diagnostic benefit should be judged to outweigh the potential risk of radiation.

### Geriatrics
Appropriate studies on the relationship of age to the effects of technetium Tc 99m pentetate have not been performed in the geriatric population. However, no geriatrics-specific problems have been documented to date.

### Drug interactions and/or related problems
See *Diagnostic interference*.

### Diagnostic interference
The following have been selected on the basis of their potential clinical significance (possible effect in parentheses where appropriate)—not necessarily inclusive (» = major clinical significance):

With results of *brain imaging*
  Due to other medications
    Corticosteroids, glucocorticoid
      (uptake of technetium Tc 99m pentetate in cerebral tumors may be decreased because of reduced peritumor edema caused by the corticosteroids)

With results of *renal imaging*
  Due to other medications
    Captopril or
    Enalapril or
    Lisinopril
      (in patients with renal artery stenosis, use of angiotensin-converting enzyme inhibitors may result in decreased uptake of technetium Tc 99m pentetate by the affected kidney because of a loss of effective trans-membrane filtration pressure; in the diagnosis of renal artery stenosis, this effect has been used to improve the diagnostic accuracy of renal scintigraphy by exaggerating the asymmetry of function between the ischemic and the contralateral kidneys)

  Due to medical problems or conditions
    Dehydration
      (decreased urinary flow may result in poor renal images and/or decreased glomerular filtration rate [GFR])

### Medical considerations/Contraindications
The medical considerations/contraindications included have been selected on the basis of their potential clinical significance (reasons given in parentheses where appropriate)—not necessarily inclusive (» = major clinical significance).
See also *Diagnostic interference*.

***Risk-benefit must be considered when the following medical problem exists:***
  Sensitivity to the radiopharmaceutical preparation

## Side/Adverse Effects
The following side/adverse effects have been selected on the basis of their potential clinical significance (possible signs and symptoms in parentheses where appropriate)—not necessarily inclusive:

### Incidence less frequent or rare
*Allergic reaction* (skin rash, hives, or itching)

## Patient Consultation
As an aid to patient consultation, refer to *Advice for the Patient, Radiopharmaceuticals (Diagnostic)*.
In providing consultation, consider emphasizing the following selected information (» = major clinical significance):

## Description of use
**Action in the body**
- Accumulation of radioactive pentetate in intracranial lesions, cerebrospinal fluid (CSF), and in airways (with aerosolized administration)
- Elimination by kidneys via glomerular filtration

Retention of radioactivity in intracranial lesions, CSF, and lungs (when inhaled) and excretion through kidneys allows visualization

Small amounts of radioactivity used in diagnosis; radiation received is low and considered safe

## Before having this test
» Conditions affecting use, especially:
Sensitivity to the radiopharmaceutical preparation
Pregnancy—Technetium Tc 99m (as free pertechnetate) crosses placenta; risk to fetus from radiation exposure as opposed to benefit derived from use should be considered
Breast-feeding—Not known if technetium Tc 99m pentetate is distributed into breast milk, but Tc 99m as free pertechnetate is distributed into breast milk; temporary discontinuation of nursing may be recommended because of risk to infant from radiation exposure
Use in children—Risk from radiation exposure as opposed to benefit derived from use should be considered

## Preparation for this test
Special preparatory instructions may be given; patient should inquire in advance

## Precautions after having this test
Adequate intake of fluids and voiding as often as possible for 4 to 6 hours after examination to minimize radiation exposure to bladder

## Side/adverse effects
Signs of potential side effects, especially allergic reaction

# General Dosing Information
Radiopharmaceuticals are to be administered only by or under the supervision of physicians who have had extensive training in the safe use and handling of radioactive materials and who are authorized by the Nuclear Regulatory Commission (NRC) or the appropriate Agreement State agency, if required, or, outside the U.S., the appropriate authority.

Adequate hydration of the patient is recommended before and after examination to promote urinary flow. Also, urination is recommended as often as possible for 4 to 6 hours after the examination to reduce bladder exposure to radiation.

Manufacturer's package insert or other appropriate literature should be consulted for optimal times when imaging should be performed.

### Safety considerations for handling this radiopharmaceutical
Improper handling of this radiopharmaceutical may cause radioactive contamination. Guidelines for handling radioactive material have been prepared by scientific, professional, state, federal, and international bodies and are available to the specially qualified and authorized users who have access to radiopharmaceuticals.

# Parenteral Dosage Forms
Note: Bracketed uses in the *Dosage Forms* section refer to categories of use and/or indications that are not included in U.S. product labeling.

## TECHNETIUM Tc 99m PENTETATE INJECTION USP

**Usual adult and adolescent administered activity**
Renal imaging or
Glomerular filtration rate determination—
 Intravenous, 111 to 185 megabecquerels (3 to 5 millicuries).
Brain imaging or
Renal perfusion studies—
 Intravenous, 370 to 740 megabecquerels (10 to 20 millicuries).
[Cisternography—CSF imaging, ventriculoperitoneal shunt][1]—
 Intraventricular, 37 megabecquerels (1 millicurie) injected into the reservoir of the shunt system.
[Lung imaging][1]—
 Inhalation, 18.5 to 37 megabecquerels (0.5 to 1 millicurie).

**Usual pediatric administered activity**
Renal imaging or
Glomerular filtration rate determination—
 Intravenous, 37 to 185 megabecquerels (1 to 5 millicuries).
[Cisternography][1]—
 [CFS imaging, ventriculoperitoneal shunt][1]: Intraventricular, 7.4 to 37 megabecquerels (0.2 to 1 millicurie) injected into the reservoir of the shunt system.
 [CSF imaging, shunt][1]—Lumbar subarachnoid injection, 11.1 to 37 megabecquerels (0.3 to 1 millicurie).

**Usual geriatric administered activity**
See *Usual adult and adolescent administered activity.*

**Strength(s) usually available**
U.S.—
 5 mg pentetate pentasodium and 0.17 mg (minimum) stannous chloride (in a lyophilized form and under a nitrogen atmosphere), per 10-mL multidose reaction vial (Rx) [*DTPA (Chelate) Multidose; Techneplex*].
 20.6 mg pentetate calcium trisodium, 0.15 mg minimum stannous tin as stannous chloride dihydrate, and 0.30 mg maximum total tin as stannous chloride dihydrate (in a lyophilized form and under a nitrogen atmosphere), per 10-mL multidose reaction vial (Rx) [*AN-DTPA*].
 25 mg pentetate calcium trisodium, 0.25 mg minimum stannous tin as stannous chloride dihydrate, and 0.385 mg maximum total tin as stannous chloride dihydrate (in a lyophilized form and under a nitrogen atmosphere), per 10-mL multidose reaction vial (Rx) [*TechneScan DTPA*].
Canada—
 25 mg pentetate calcium trisodium, 0.25 mg minimum stannous tin as stannous chloride dihydrate, and 0.385 mg maximum total tin as stannous chloride dihydrate (in a lyophilized form and under a nitrogen atmosphere), per 10-mL multidose reaction vial (Rx) [*Frosstimage DTPA*].

**Packaging and storage**
Store between 2 and 8 °C (36 and 46 °F). Protect from freezing.
Note: Before reconstitution, kit may be stored at room temperature.

**Preparation of dosage form**
To prepare injection, an oxidant-free sodium pertechnetate Tc 99m solution is used. See manufacturer's package insert for instructions.

**Stability**
For brain and renal imaging—Injection should be administered within 6 hours after preparation.
For glomerular filtration rate determination—Injection should be administered within 1 hour after preparation.

**Incompatibilities**
If oxidants such as peroxides and hypochlorites are present in the sodium pertechnetate Tc 99m used for labeling, the final preparation may be adversely affected and should be discarded.

**Note**
Caution—Radioactive material.

---

[1]Not included in Canadian product labeling.

## Selected Bibliography
Blaufox MD. Procedures of choice in renal nuclear medicine. J Nucl Med 1991; 32: 1301-9.

Revised: 04/30/96

---

# TECHNETIUM Tc 99m PYROPHOSPHATE   Systemic†

VA CLASSIFICATION (Primary): DX201
Commonly used brand name(s): *MPI Pyrophosphate; Phosphotec; TechneScan PYP*.
Note: For a listing of dosage forms and brand names by country availability, see *Dosage Forms* section(s).

†Not commercially available in Canada.

## Category
Diagnostic aid, radioactive (bone disease; cardiac disease; gastrointestinal bleeding [without Tc 99m label]).

## Indications

### Accepted

For *technetium Tc 99m pyrophosphate*

Skeletal imaging, radionuclide—Technetium Tc 99m pyrophosphate is indicated as a skeletal imaging agent to delineate areas of altered osteogenesis, such as those that occur with metastatic bone disease, Paget's disease, arthritic disease, osteomyelitis, and fractures.

Cardiac imaging, radionuclide—Technetium Tc 99m pyrophosphate is indicated as a cardiac imaging agent to aid in the diagnosis of acute myocardial infarction.

For *sodium pyrophosphate without Tc 99m label*

Red blood cells, labeling of—Intravenous injection of the unlabeled sodium pyrophosphate and stannous chloride complex, when followed by the injection of sodium pertechnetate Tc 99m, is indicated for *in vivo* or modified *in vitro/in vivo* labeling of red blood cells. Red blood cells labeled with sodium pertechnetate Tc 99m are used for blood pool imaging in the following diagnostic study:

Cardiac blood pool imaging, radionuclide—To detect pericardial effusion, intracardiac abnormalities, or ventricular aneurysms.

Bleeding, gastrointestinal (diagnosis)—To detect the site of bleeding in patients suspected of gastrointestinal bleeding.

## Physical Properties

### Nuclear data

| Radionuclide (half-life) | Decay constant | Mode of decay | Principal photons emissions (keV) | Mean number of emissions/ disintegration (≥0.01) |
|---|---|---|---|---|
| Tc 99m (6.0 hr) | 0.1151 h$^{-1}$ | Isomeric transition to Tc 99 | Gamma (18) | 0.062 |
|  |  |  | Gamma (140.5) | 0.891 |

## Pharmacology/Pharmacokinetics

### Physicochemical characteristics
Molecular weight—Sodium pyrophosphate: 265.90.
Stannous chloride: 225.63.

### Mechanism of action/Effect

Skeletal and cardiac imaging—Exact mechanism is not known. It is generally accepted that technetium Tc 99m pyrophosphate localizes on the surface of hydroxyapatite crystals, found in bone and within infarcted myocardial cells, by a process termed chemisorption, with blood flow and/or blood concentration being most important in the delivery of the agent to sites of uptake. Visualization of osseous lesions is possible since skeletal uptake of technetium Tc 99m pyrophosphate is altered in areas of abnormal osteogenesis.

Red blood cells, labeling of—When used for cardiac blood pool imaging or to detect gastrointestinal bleeding, pretreatment with the stannous ion-containing phosphate complex causes the technetium Tc 99m (as sodium pertechnetate Tc 99m) to bind to the red blood cells *in vivo*, with about 76% of the injected radioactivity remaining in the blood pool long enough to provide images of the cardiac chambers or sites of active (rapid) or cumulative (intermittent) gastrointestinal bleeding. Modified *in vitro/in vivo* method of labeling red blood cells usually results in a greater percent of the injected radioactivity remaining in the blood pool.

### Distribution
Selectively concentrated in areas of altered osteogenesis and injured myocardium with minimal uptake by soft-tissue organs.

### Radiation dosimetry

Estimated absorbed radiation dose for Technetium Tc 99m Pyrophosphate*‡

| Organ | mGy/MBq | rad/mCi |
|---|---|---|
| Bone surfaces | 0.063 | 0.23 |
| Bladder wall | 0.050 | 0.19 |
| Red marrow | 0.0096 | 0.036 |
| Kidneys | 0.0073 | 0.027 |
| Uterus | 0.0061 | 0.023 |
| Large intestine wall (lower) | 0.0038 | 0.014 |
| Ovaries | 0.0035 | 0.013 |

Estimated absorbed radiation dose for Technetium Tc 99m Pyrophosphate*‡

| Organ | mGy/MBq | rad/mCi |
|---|---|---|
| Testes | 0.0024 | 0.0089 |
| Small intestine | 0.0023 | 0.0085 |
| Large intestine wall (upper) | 0.0020 | 0.0074 |
| Adrenals | 0.0019 | 0.0070 |
| Pancreas | 0.0016 | 0.0059 |
| Spleen | 0.0014 | 0.0052 |
| Liver | 0.0013 | 0.0048 |
| Lungs | 0.0013 | 0.0048 |
| Stomach wall | 0.0012 | 0.0044 |
| Thyroid | 0.0010 | 0.0037 |
| Breast | 0.00088 | 0.0033 |
| Other tissue | 0.0019 | 0.0070 |

Effective dose: 0.008 mSv/MBq (0.030 rem/mCi)

Estimated absorbed radiation dose for Sodium Pertechnetate Tc 99m†‡

| Organ | mGy/MBq | rad/mCi |
|---|---|---|
| Stomach wall | 0.029 | 0.11 |
| Thyroid | 0.023 | 0.085 |
| Bladder wall | 0.019 | 0.070 |
| Small intestine | 0.018 | 0.067 |
| Ovaries | 0.010 | 0.037 |
| Salivary glands | 0.0093 | 0.034 |
| Uterus | 0.0081 | 0.030 |
| Large intestine wall (upper) | 0.062 | 0.23 |
| Large intestine wall (lower) | 0.062 | 0.23 |
| Red marrow | 0.0061 | 0.022 |
| Pancreas | 0.0059 | 0.022 |
| Kidneys | 0.0050 | 0.019 |
| Spleen | 0.0044 | 0.016 |
| Bone surfaces | 0.0039 | 0.014 |
| Liver | 0.0039 | 0.014 |
| Adrenals | 0.0036 | 0.013 |
| Lungs | 0.0027 | 0.010 |
| Testes | 0.0027 | 0.010 |
| Breast | 0.0023 | 0.0085 |
| Other tissue | 0.0034 | 0.013 |

Effective dose: 0.013 mSv/MBq (0.048 rem/mCi)

*For adults. Intravenous injection of technetium Tc 99m–labeled phosphates and phosphonates for skeletal and cardiac imaging.

†For adults. Intravenous injection of sodium pertechnetate Tc 99m preceded by intravenous administration of unlabeled sodium pyrophosphate for cardiac blood pool imaging. Without blocking agent.

‡Data based on the International Commission on Radiological Protection (ICRP) Publication 53—Radiation dose to patients from radiopharmaceuticals.

### Elimination
Renal, 40% of the administered activity of technetium Tc 99m pyrophosphate eliminated within 24 hours.

## Precautions to Consider

### Carcinogenicity/Mutagenicity
Long-term animal studies to evaluate carcinogenic or mutagenic potential of technetium Tc 99m pyrophosphate have not been performed.

### Pregnancy/Reproduction
Pregnancy—Tc 99m (as free pertechnetate) crosses the placenta. Studies with technetium Tc 99m pyrophosphate have not been done in humans. The possibility of pregnancy should be assessed in women of child-bearing potential. Clinical situations exist where the benefit to the patient and fetus, based on information derived from radiopharmaceutical use, outweighs the risks from fetal exposure to radiation. In these situations, the physician should use discretion and reduce the radiopharmaceutical dose to the lowest possible amount.

Studies have not been done in animals.

FDA Pregnancy Category C.

### Breast-feeding
Although it is not known whether technetium Tc 99m pyrophosphate is distributed into breast milk, it is known that Tc 99m as free pertechnetate is distributed into breast milk. Based on the assumption that the Tc 99m in breast milk is in the form of pertechnetate and based on the

effective half-life of the radionuclide in breast milk, the daily volume of milk, a dose factor relating the radionuclide to its critical organ (thyroid) in the nursing infant, and the maximum permissible dose to that organ, a guideline has been proposed. According to this guideline, it has been calculated that nursing can be safely resumed when the concentration in breast milk reaches $30.3 \times 10^{-4}$ megabecquerels ($8.2 \times 10^{-2}$ microcuries) per mL. This level of activity is probably reached, in the majority of patients, within 12 to 24 hours after administration of technetium Tc 99m–labeled radiopharmaceuticals.

## Pediatrics
Diagnostic studies performed to date using technetium Tc 99m–labeled red blood cells have not demonstrated pediatrics-specific problems that would limit the usefulness of technetium Tc 99m pyrophosphate in children. However, there have been no specific studies evaluating the safety and efficacy of technetium Tc 99m pyrophosphate in pediatric patients. When this radiopharmaceutical is used in children, the diagnostic benefit should be judged to outweigh the potential risk of radiation.

## Geriatrics
Diagnostic studies performed to date using technetium Tc 99m pyrophosphate have not demonstrated geriatrics-specific problems that would limit the usefulness of technetium Tc 99m pyrophosphate in the elderly.

## Drug interactions and/or related problems
See *Diagnostic interference*.

## Diagnostic interference
The following have been selected on the basis of their potential clinical significance (possible effect in parentheses where appropriate)—not necessarily inclusive (» = major clinical significance):

With results of *skeletal imaging*
  Due to other medications
    Amphotericin B or
    Antineoplastics
      (biodistribution of technetium Tc 99m pyrophosphate may be altered with concurrent administration of these medications)
    Antacids, aluminum-containing
      (high blood concentrations of aluminum ion, which may occur in patients with gastrointestinal obstruction or impaired renal function, may cause localization of technetium Tc 99m pyrophosphate in the liver and spleen)
    Diatrizoate sodium
      (possible renal and hepatic uptake if diatrizoate sodium is administered intravenously immediately after technetium Tc 99m pyrophosphate)
    Etidronate
      (etidronate may interfere with bone uptake of technetium Tc 99m pyrophosphate; discontinuation of etidronate therapy for a 2-week period before performance of a bone scan with technetium Tc 99m pyrophosphate is recommended)
    Heparin calcium, subcutaneous or
    Radiation therapy
      (concurrent administration may result in extraosseous accumulation of technetium Tc 99m pyrophosphate)
    Iron dextran, intramuscular or
    Meperidine, intramuscular
      (possible accumulation of technetium Tc 99m pyrophosphate at site of injection of these medications)
    Iron supplements or preparations
      (iron overload may cause a decrease in bone uptake of technetium Tc 99m pyrophosphate)
    Potassium phosphates or
    Potassium and sodium phosphates or
    Sodium phosphates
      (saturation of bone binding sites by phosphorous ions in these medications may cause decreased bone uptake of technetium Tc 99m pyrophosphate)

  Due to medical problems or conditions
    Amyloidosis or
    Carcinomas or
    Cirrhosis or
    Diabetes mellitus or
    Hypercalcemia
      (biodistribution of technetium Tc 99m pyrophosphate may be altered, resulting in an increased uptake by other organs)
    Blood transfusions, repeated
      (may cause a decrease in bone uptake)

    Bone demineralization, glucocorticoid-induced
      (long-term therapy with glucocorticoids may induce bone mineral depletion, thus causing decreased bone uptake of technetium Tc 99m pyrophosphate)
    Gynecomastia, estrogen-induced or
    Lactation
      (possible localization of technetium Tc 99m pyrophosphate in breast)
    Obesity
      (attenuation of photons coming from bone may decrease visualization)
    Osteoporosis
      (reduced mineral deposit in bone may result in images with lower target to non-target ratio)
    Renal function impairment
      (decreased drug clearance from blood and soft tissues may decrease visualization because of a lower bone to background ratio resulting from the increased circulating activity; also, chronic renal function impairment may cause metastatic calcification and altered biodistribution of technetium Tc 99m pyrophosphate)

With results of *cardiac imaging*
  Due to other medications
    Antacids, aluminum-containing
      (high blood concentrations of aluminum ion, which may occur in patients with gastrointestinal obstruction or impaired renal function, may cause localization of technetium Tc 99m pyrophosphate in the liver and spleen)
    Estrogens
      (possible localization of technetium Tc 99m pyrophosphate in breast)
    Heparin sodium
      (diffuse uptake of technetium Tc 99m pyrophosphate into the myocardium, with signs of diminished uptake into the infarct)
    Methylprednisolone
      (methylprednisolone may increase glomerular filtration rate and excretion of technetium Tc 99m pyrophosphate, which results in faster blood clearance of the radiotracer, thus decreasing myocardial uptake of the radiotracer)
    Radiation therapy
      (diffuse myocardial uptake of technetium Tc 99m pyrophosphate)
    Verapamil
      (patchy liver uptake of technetium Tc 99m pyrophosphate may result due to hepatocellular damage caused by verapamil toxicity)

  Due to medical problems or conditions
    Amyloidosis or
    Hyperphosphatemia or
    Sarcoidosis, myocardial
      (diffuse cardiac uptake may occur)
    Angina pectoris, unstable or
    Cardiac contusions or
    Coronary bypass surgery, recent or
    Myocardial infarcts, previous
      (false-positive cardiac images may occur)
    Gynecomastia, estrogen-induced or
    Lactation
      (possible localization of technetium Tc 99m pyrophosphate in breast)
    Myocardial infarcts, time of
      (false-negative cardiac images may occur in the diagnosis of acute myocardial infarction if test is performed too early in the evolutionary phase or too late in the resolution phase of the infarct)

With results of *blood pool imaging (cardiac blood pool imaging and diagnosis of gastrointestinal bleeding)*
  Due to other medications
    Digoxin or
    Doxorubicin or
    Heparin sodium or
    Hydralazine or
    Methyldopa or
    Prazosin or
    Propranolol or
    Quinidine or
    Radiopaque agents, water-soluble organic iodides, with intravascular administration
      (concurrent use with these medications may impair blood pool images by decreasing the labeling efficiency of red blood cells)

## Technetium Tc 99m Pyrophosphate (Systemic)

*Due to medical problems or conditions*
- Goiter, toxic diffuse or
- Hyperthyroidism
  (thyroid uptake may be increased)
- Lupus erythematosus
  (labeling of red blood cells may be decreased)
- Transfusion-induced reaction
  (labeling efficiency may be decreased because of red blood cell antibody formation)

With *other* diagnostic test results
- Brain scan using sodium pertechnetate Tc 99m
  (may give either false-positive or false-negative results when performed after a bone scan using technetium Tc 99m pyrophosphate that contains stannous ions; to avoid false results, brain scan should be performed prior to bone scan or with a brain imaging agent other than sodium pertechnetate Tc 99m)

### Medical considerations/Contraindications
The medical considerations/contraindications included have been selected on the basis of their potential clinical significance (reasons given in parentheses where appropriate)—not necessarily inclusive (» = major clinical significance).
See also *Diagnostic interference*.

*Risk-benefit should be considered when the following medical problem exists:*
Sensitivity to the radiopharmaceutical preparation

### Side/Adverse Effects
The following side/adverse effects have been selected on the basis of their potential clinical significance (possible signs and symptoms in parentheses where appropriate)—not necessarily inclusive:

**Those indicating need for medical attention**
Incidence less frequent or rare
*Allergic reaction* (skin rash, hives, or itching)

## Patient Consultation
As an aid to patient consultation, refer to *Advice for the Patient, Radiopharmaceuticals (Diagnostic)*.
In providing consultation, consider emphasizing the following selected information (» = major clinical significance):

**Description of use**
Action in the body: Accumulation of radioactivity in bone and cardiac tissues and in labeled red blood cells
Retention of radioactivity allows visualization of skeletal or cardiac lesions, or visualization of blood pool
Small amounts of radioactivity used in diagnosis; radiation received is low and considered safe

**Before having this test**
» Conditions affecting use, especially:
Sensitivity to the radiopharmaceutical preparation
Pregnancy—Technetium Tc 99m (as free pertechnetate) crosses placenta; risk to fetus from radiation exposure as opposed to benefit derived from use should be considered
Breast-feeding—Not known if technetium Tc 99m pyrophosphate is distributed into breast milk, but Tc 99m as free pertechnetate is distributed into breast milk; temporary discontinuation of nursing may be recommended because of risk to infant from radiation exposure
Use in children—Risk from radiation exposure as opposed to benefit derived from use should be considered

**Preparation for this test**
Special preparatory instructions may be given; patient should inquire in advance
For cardiac and skeletal imaging: Increasing intake of fluids and voiding frequently after injection and before test begins to minimize radiation dose to bladder; voiding again just prior to imaging for best test results

**Precautions after having this test**
For cardiac and skeletal imaging: Increasing intake of fluids and voiding frequently for 4 to 6 hours after test to minimize radiation dose to bladder

**Side/adverse effects**
Signs of potential side effects, especially allergic reaction

## General Dosing Information
Radiopharmaceuticals are to be administered only by or under the supervision of physicians who have had extensive training in the safe use and handling of radioactive materials and who are authorized by the Nuclear Regulatory Commission (NRC) or the appropriate Agreement State agency, if required, or, outside the U.S., the appropriate authority.
Manufacturer's package insert or other appropriate literature should be consulted for optimal times when imaging should be performed.

**For cardiac and skeletal imaging**
Unless cardiac status indicates otherwise, the patient should increase intake of fluids and void frequently following the administration of technetium Tc 99m pyrophosphate injection, and for 4 to 6 hours after the imaging procedures are completed, to minimize radiation dose to the bladder.
Voiding is also recommended immediately prior to imaging procedures to reduce background interference that may result from accumulation of the agent in the bladder.

**For blood pool imaging (cardiac blood pool imaging and diagnosis of gastrointestinal bleeding)**
Stannous pyrophosphate should be injected by direct venipuncture. Heparinized catheter systems are not recommended.

**Safety considerations for handling this radiopharmaceutical**
Improper handling of this radiopharmaceutical may cause radioactive contamination. Guidelines for handling radioactive material have been prepared by scientific, professional, state, federal, and international bodies and are available to the specially qualified and authorized users who have access to radiopharmaceuticals.

## Parenteral Dosage Forms

### TECHNETIUM Tc 99m PYROPHOSPHATE INJECTION USP

**Usual adult and adolescent administered activity**
For technetium Tc 99m pyrophosphate:
Skeletal imaging or
Cardiac imaging—Intravenous, 555 to 740 megabecquerels (15 to 20 millicuries), administered over a period of ten to twenty seconds.
For sodium pyrophosphate without Tc 99m label:
Blood pool imaging—Intravenous, 5 to 15.4 mg of stannous pyrophosphate (unlabeled) followed, fifteen to sixty minutes later, by the intravenous administration of 740 megabecquerels (20 millicuries) of sodium pertechnetate Tc 99m.

**Usual pediatric administered activity**
Dosage must be individualized by physician.

**Usual geriatric administered activity**
See *Usual adult and adolescent administered activity*.

**Strength(s) usually available**
U.S.—
12 mg of sodium pyrophosphate and 3.4 mg of stannous chloride (anhydrous) per 10-mL reaction vial (Rx) [*TechneScan PYP*].
40 mg sodium pyrophosphate, 0.4 mg stannous fluoride (minimum), and 0.9 mg total tin (maximum) as stannous fluoride, per 5-mL reaction vial (Rx) [*MPI Pyrophosphate; Phosphotec*].
Canada—
Not commercially available.

**Packaging and storage**
Store between 15 and 30 °C (59 and 86 °F), unless otherwise specified by manufacturer. Protect from freezing.
Note: Before reconstitution, store between 2 and 8 °C (36 and 46 °F).

**Preparation of dosage form**
To prepare technetium Tc 99m pyrophosphate injection, an oxidant-free sodium pertechnetate Tc 99m solution is used. See manufacturer's package insert for instructions.
To prepare sodium pyrophosphate injection (unlabeled), stannous pyrophosphate is reconstituted with sodium chloride injection. See manufacturer's package insert for complete instructions.

**Stability**
Injection should be administered within 6 hours after preparation.

**Incompatibilities**
If oxidants such as peroxides and hypochlorites are present in the sodium pertechnetate Tc 99m used for labeling, the final preparation may be adversely affected and should be discarded.

**Note**
Caution—Radioactive material.

Revised: 8/18/93
Interim revision: 08/02/94

# TECHNETIUM Tc 99m (PYRO- AND TRIMETA-) PHOSPHATES Systemic

VA CLASSIFICATION (Primary): DX201
Commonly used brand name(s): *Pyrolite*.

Note: This monograph includes information that applies to both technetium Tc 99m (pyro- and trimeta-) phosphates and to sodium (pyro- and trimeta-) phosphates without Tc 99m label.

Note: For a listing of dosage forms and brand names by country availability, see *Dosage Forms* section(s).

## Category
Diagnostic aid, radioactive (bone disease; cardiac disease; gastrointestinal bleeding [without Tc 99m label]).

## Indications
### Accepted
For technetium Tc 99m (pyro- and trimeta-) phosphates:
Skeletal imaging, radionuclide—Technetium Tc 99m (pyro- and trimeta-) phosphates injection is indicated as a skeletal imaging agent to delineate areas of altered osteogenesis, such as those that occur with metastatic bone disease, Paget's disease, arthritic disease, osteomyelitis, and fractures.
Cardiac imaging, radionuclide—Technetium Tc 99m (pyro- and trimeta-) phosphates injection is indicated as a cardiac imaging agent to aid in the diagnosis of acute myocardial infarction.

For sodium (pyro- and trimeta-) phosphates without Tc 99m label:
Red blood cells, labeling of—Intravenous injection of the unlabeled sodium (pyro- and trimeta-) phosphates component of the kit, when followed by the injection of sodium pertechnetate Tc 99m, is indicated for *in vivo* or modified *in vitro/in vivo* labeling of red blood cells. Red blood cells labeled with sodium pertechnetate Tc 99m are used for blood pool imaging in the following diagnostic studies:
Cardiac blood pool imaging, radionuclide: To detect pericardial effusion, intracardiac abnormalities, or ventricular aneurysms.
Bleeding, gastrointestinal (diagnosis): To evaluate patients suspected of gastrointestinal bleeding, to detect the site of bleeding.

## Physical Properties
### Nuclear data

| Radionuclide (half-life) | Decay constant | Mode of decay | Principal photons (keV) | Mean number of photons/disintegration ($\geq 0.01$) |
|---|---|---|---|---|
| Tc 99m (6.0 hr) | 0.1151 h$^{-1}$ | Isomeric transition to Tc 99 | 18 | 0.062 |
|  |  |  | 140.5 | 0.891 |

## Pharmacology/Pharmacokinetics
### Physicochemical characteristics
Molecular weight—Sodium pyrophosphate: 265.90.
Sodium trimetaphosphate: 305.89.
Stannous chloride: 225.63.

### Mechanism of action/Effect
Skeletal and cardiac imaging—
Exact mechanism is unknown. Technetium Tc 99m (pyro- and trimeta-) phosphates' affinity for hydroxyapatite crystals, found in bone and within infarcted myocardial cells, may be responsible for its skeletal and myocardial uptake, with blood flow and/or blood concentration being most important in the delivery of the phosphate complex for uptake. Since normal myocardial tissue does not appreciably accumulate the phosphate complex, an area of acute damage will appear as a focus of increased activity. Visualization of osseous lesions also is possible since skeletal uptake of technetium Tc 99m (pyro- and trimeta-) phosphates is altered in areas of abnormal osteogenesis.

Red blood cells, labeling of—
When used for cardiac blood pool imaging or to detect gastrointestinal bleeding, pretreatment with the stannous ion–containing phosphate complex causes the technetium Tc 99m (as sodium pertechnetate Tc 99m) to bind to the red blood cells in vivo, with about 75–85% of the injected radioactivity remaining in the blood pool long enough to provide images of the cardiac chambers or sites of active (rapid) or cumulative (intermittent) gastrointestinal bleeding. Modified *in vitro/in vivo* method of labeling red blood cells usually results in a greater percent of the injected radioactivity remaining in the blood pool.

### Distribution
Technetium Tc 99m (pyro- and trimeta-) phosphates is selectively concentrated in areas of altered osteogenesis and injured myocardium with minimal uptake by soft-tissue organs, with the exception of the kidneys.

### Radiation dosimetry

| Mode of administration | Radiation source (% administered activity) | Target organ | mGy/MBq | rad/mCi |
|---|---|---|---|---|
| Intravenous Technetium Tc 99m (Pyro- and trimeta-) Phosphates* | Skeleton (50%) Urinary bladder (50%) | Bladder 2 hr void | 0.026 | 0.097 |
| | | 4.8 hr void | 0.062 | 0.230 |
| | | Skeleton | 0.014 | 0.054 |
| | | Kidneys | 0.013 | 0.047 |
| | | Bone marrow | 0.010 | 0.038 |
| | | Testes 2 hr void | 0.003 | 0.010 |
| | | 4.8 hr void | 0.004 | 0.015 |
| | | Heart Normal | 0.002 | 0.009 |
| | | Impaired | 0.004 | 0.015 |
| | | Ovaries 2 hr void | 0.002 | 0.009 |
| | | 4.8 hr void | 0.004 | 0.015 |
| | | Red marrow | 0.006 | 0.022 |
| | | Total body | 0.004 | 0.015 |
| Intravenous Sodium Pertechnetate Tc 99m† | | Bladder wall | 0.032 | 0.120 |
| | | Blood | 0.014 | 0.052 |
| | | Ovaries | 0.006 | 0.023 |
| | | Spleen | 0.005 | 0.018 |
| | | Testes | 0.003 | 0.012 |
| | | Total body | 0.004 | 0.015 |

*For skeletal and cardiac imaging.
†For blood pool imaging. Preceded by intravenous administration of unlabeled sodium (pyro- and trimeta-) phosphates.

### Elimination
Renal; up to 50% of the dose of technetium Tc 99m (pyro- and trimeta-) phosphates eliminated within the first 3 to 6 hours.

## Precautions to Consider
### Carcinogenicity/Mutagenicity
Long-term animal studies to evaluate carcinogenic or mutagenic potential of technetium Tc 99m (pyro- and trimeta-) phosphates have not been performed.

### Pregnancy/Reproduction
Pregnancy—Tc 99m (as free pertechnetate) crosses the placenta. However, studies have not been done in either animals or humans with technetium Tc 99m (pyro- and trimeta-) phosphates.
Radiopharmaceuticals are usually not recommended during pregnancy because of the risk to the fetus from radiation exposure.
To avoid the possibility of fetal exposure to radiation, in those circumstances where the patient's pregnancy status is uncertain, a pregnancy test will help to prevent inadvertent administration of this preparation during pregnancy.
FDA Pregnancy Category C.

### Breast-feeding
Although it is not known whether technetium Tc 99m (pyro- and trimeta-) phosphates is excreted in breast milk, it is known that Tc 99m as free pertechnetate is excreted in breast milk. Based on the assumption that the Tc 99m in breast milk is in the form of pertechnetate and based on the effective half-life of the radionuclide in breast milk, the daily volume of milk, a dose factor relating the radionuclide to its critical organ (thyroid) in the nursing infant, and the maximum permissible dose to that organ, a guideline has been proposed. According to this guideline,

it has been calculated that nursing can be safely resumed when the concentration in breast milk reaches $30.3 \times 10^{-4}$ megabecquerels ($8.2 \times 10^{-2}$ microcuries) per mL. This level of activity is probably reached, in the majority of patients, within 24 hours after administration of 740 megabecquerels (20 millicuries) of technetium Tc 99m.

### Pediatrics
Diagnostic studies performed to date using technetium Tc 99m–labeled red blood cells have not demonstrated pediatrics-specific problems that would limit the usefulness of technetium Tc 99m (pyro- and trimeta-) phosphates in children. However, because of the potential risk of radiation exposure, risk-benefit must be considered.

### Geriatrics
Although appropriate studies have not been performed in the geriatric population, no geriatrics-specific problems have been documented to date.

### Drug interactions and/or related problems
See *Diagnostic interference*.

### Diagnostic interference
The following have been selected on the basis of their potential clinical significance (possible effect in parentheses where appropriate)—not necessarily inclusive (» = major clinical significance):

With results of *blood pool imaging (cardiac blood pool imaging and diagnosis of gastrointestinal bleeding)*
  *Due to other medications*
    Digoxin or
    Doxorubicin or
    Heparin sodium or
    Hydralazine or
    Methyldopa or
    Prazosin or
    Propranolol or
    Quinidine or
    Radiopaques, water-soluble organic iodides, with intravascular administration
      (concurrent use with these medications may impair blood pool images because of a decrease in labeling of red blood cells)
  *Due to medical problems or conditions*
    Goiter, toxic diffuse or
    Hyperthyroidism
      (thyroid uptake may be increased)
    Lupus erythematosus
      (labeling of red blood cells may be decreased)
    Transfusion-induced reaction
      (labeling efficiency may be decreased because of red blood cell antibody formation)

With results of *cardiac imaging*
  *Due to other medications*
    Antacids, aluminum-containing
      (high blood concentrations of aluminum ion, which may occur in patients with gastrointestinal obstruction or impaired renal function, may cause localization of technetium Tc 99m [pyro- and trimeta-] phosphates in the liver and spleen)
    Estrogens
      (possible localization of technetium Tc 99m [pyro- and trimeta-] phosphates in breast)
    Heparin sodium
      (diffuse uptake of technetium Tc 99m [pyro- and trimeta-] phosphates into the myocardium, with signs of diminished uptake into the infarct)
    Methylprednisolone
      (methylprednisolone may increase glomerular filtration rate and excretion of technetium Tc 99m [pyro- and trimeta-] phosphates, resulting in faster blood clearance of the radiotracer, and thus decreasing myocardial uptake of the radiotracer)
    Radiation therapy
      (diffuse myocardial uptake of technetium Tc 99m [pyro- and trimeta-] phosphates)
    Verapamil
      (patchy liver uptake of technetium Tc 99m [pyro- and trimeta-] phosphates may result due to hepatocellular damage caused by verapamil toxicity)
  *Due to medical problems or conditions*
    Amyloidosis or
    Hyperphosphatemia or
    Sarcoidosis, myocardial
      (diffuse cardiac uptake may occur)
    Angina pectoris, unstable or
    Cardiac contusions or
    Coronary bypass surgery, recent or
    Myocardial infarcts, previous
      (false-positive cardiac images may occur)
    Gynecomastia, estrogen-induced or
    Lactation
      (possible localization of technetium Tc 99m [pyro- and trimeta-] phosphates in breast)
    Hepatic necrosis, massive
      (possible liver uptake of technetium Tc 99m [pyro- and trimeta-] phosphates)
    Myocardial infarcts, time of
      (false-negative cardiac images may occur in the diagnosis of acute myocardial infarction if test is performed too early in the evolutionary phase or too late in the resolution phase of the infarct)

With results of *skeletal imaging*
  *Due to other medications*
    Antacids, aluminum-containing
      (high blood concentrations of aluminum ion, which may occur in patients with gastrointestinal obstruction or impaired renal function, may cause localization of technetium Tc 99m [pyro- and trimeta-] phosphates in the liver)
    Amphotericin B or
    Antineoplastics
      (biodistribution of technetium Tc 99m [pyro- and trimeta-] phosphates may be altered with concurrent administration of these medications)
    Diatrizoate sodium
      (possible renal and hepatic uptake of technetium Tc 99m [pyro- and trimeta-] phosphates if diatrizoate sodium is administered intravenously immediately after technetium Tc 99m [pyro- and trimeta-] phosphates)
    Etidronate
      (etidronate may theoretically interfere with bone uptake of technetium Tc 99m [pyro- and trimeta-] phosphates; clinical significance is unknown)
    Heparin calcium, subcutaneous or
    Radiation therapy
      (concurrent administration may result in extraosseous accumulation of technetium Tc 99m [pyro- and trimeta-] phosphates)
    Iron dextran, intramuscular or
    Meperidine, intramuscular
      (possible accumulation of technetium Tc 99m [pyro- and trimeta-] phosphates at site of injection)
    Iron supplements or preparations
      (iron overload may cause a decrease in bone uptake)
    Potassium phosphates or
    Potassium and sodium phosphates or
    Sodium phosphates
      (saturation of bone binding sites by phosphorous ions in these medications may cause decreased bone uptake)
  *Due to medical problems or conditions*
    Amyloidosis or
    Carcinomas or
    Cirrhosis or
    Diabetes mellitus or
    Hypercalcemia
      (biodistribution of technetium Tc 99m [pyro- and trimeta-] phosphates may be altered, resulting in an increased uptake by other organs)
    Blood transfusions, repeated
      (may cause a decrease in bone uptake)
    Bone demineralization, adrenocorticoid (glucocorticoid)-induced
      (long-term therapy with these medications may induce bone mineral depletion, thus causing decreased bone uptake of technetium Tc 99m [pyro- and trimeta-] phosphates)
    Gynecomastia, estrogen-induced or
    Lactation
      (possible localization of technetium Tc 99m [pyro- and trimeta-] phosphates in breast)
    Obesity
      (attenuation of photons coming from bone may decrease visualization)
    Osteoporosis
      (reduced mineral deposits in bone may result in images with lower target to non-target ratio)

Renal function impairment
(decreased drug clearance from blood and soft tissues may decrease visualization because of a lower bone-to-background ratio resulting from the increased circulating activity; also, chronic renal function impairment may cause metastatic calcification and altered biodistribution of technetium Tc 99m [pyro- and trimeta-] phosphates)

With *other* diagnostic test results
Brain scan using sodium pertechnetate Tc 99m
(may give either false-positive or false-negative results when performed after a bone scan using technetium Tc 99m [pyro- and trimeta-] phosphates because of its stannous ion content; to avoid false results, brain scan should be performed prior to bone scan or with a brain imaging agent other than sodium pertechnetate Tc 99m)

**Medical considerations/Contraindications**
The medical considerations/contraindications included have been selected on the basis of their potential clinical significance (reasons given in parentheses where appropriate)—not necessarily inclusive (» = major clinical significance).
See also *Diagnostic interference*.

*Risk-benefit should be considered when the following medical problem exists:*
Sensitivity to the radiopharmaceutical preparation

## Side/Adverse Effects

The following side/adverse effects have been selected on the basis of their potential clinical significance (possible signs and symptoms in parentheses where appropriate)—not necessarily inclusive:

**Those indicating need for medical attention**
Incidence less frequent or rare
*Allergic reaction* (skin rash, hives, or itching)

## Patient Consultation

As an aid to patient consultation, refer to *Advice for the Patient, Radiopharmaceuticals (Diagnostic)*.
In providing consultation, consider emphasizing the following selected information (» = major clinical significance):

**Description of use**
Action in the body: Accumulation of radioactivity in bone and cardiac tissues and in labeled red blood cells
Retention of radioactivity allows visualization of skeletal or cardiac lesions, or visualization of blood pool
Small amounts of radioactivity used in diagnosis; radiation received is low and considered safe

**Before having this test**
» Conditions affecting use, especially:
Sensitivity to the radiopharmaceutical preparation
Pregnancy—Technetium Tc 99m (as free pertechnetate) crosses placenta; risk to fetus from radiation exposure
Breast-feeding—Not known if excreted in breast milk; temporary discontinuation of nursing may be recommended because of risk to infant from radiation exposure
Use in children—Risk of radiation exposure

**Preparation for this test**
Special preparatory instructions may be given; patient should inquire in advance
For cardiac and skeletal imaging: Increasing intake of fluids and voiding frequently after injection and before test begins to minimize radiation exposure to bladder; voiding again just prior to imaging for best test results

**Precautions after having this test**
For cardiac and skeletal imaging: Increasing intake of fluids and voiding frequently for 4 to 6 hours after test to minimize radiation exposure to bladder

**Side/adverse effects**
Signs of potential side effects, especially allergic reaction

## General Dosing Information

Radiopharmaceuticals are to be administered only by or under the supervision of physicians who have had extensive training in the safe use and handling of radionuclides and who are licensed by the Nuclear Regulatory Commission (NRC) or the appropriate Agreement State agency or, outside the U.S., the appropriate authority.

Manufacturer's package insert or other appropriate literature should be consulted for optimal times when imaging should be performed.

**For cardiac and skeletal imaging**
Unless cardiac status indicates otherwise, the patient should increase intake of fluids and void frequently following the administration of technetium Tc 99m (pyro- and trimeta-) phosphates injection, and for 4 to 6 hours after the imaging procedures are completed, to minimize radiation exposure to the bladder.
Voiding is also recommended immediately prior to imaging procedures to reduce background interference that may result from accumulation of the agent in the bladder.

**For blood pool imaging (cardiac blood pool imaging and diagnosis of gastrointestinal bleeding)**
Unlabeled sodium (pyro- and trimeta-) phosphates should be injected by direct venipuncture. Heparinized catheter systems should not be used.

**Safety considerations for handling this radiopharmaceutical**
Improper handling of this radiopharmaceutical may cause radioactive contamination. Guidelines for handling radioactive material have been prepared by scientific, professional, state, federal, and international bodies and are available to the specially qualified and authorized users who have access to radiopharmaceuticals.

## Parenteral Dosage Forms

### TECHNETIUM Tc 99m (PYRO- AND TRIMETA-) PHOSPHATES INJECTION USP

**Usual adult and adolescent administered activity**
For technetium Tc 99m (pyro- and trimeta-) phosphates:
Skeletal imaging—Intravenous, 555 to 925 megabecquerels (15 to 25 millicuries).
Cardiac imaging—Intravenous, 740 to 1295 megabecquerels (20 to 35 millicuries).
For sodium (pyro- and trimeta-) phosphates without Tc 99m label:
Blood pool imaging—Intravenous, 14 to 42 mg of sodium (pyro- and trimeta-) phosphates (unlabeled) followed by the intravenous administration of 185 to 740 megabecquerels (5 to 20 millicuries) of sodium pertechnetate Tc 99m five to thirty minutes later.

**Usual pediatric administered activity**
Dosage must be individualized by physician.

**Usual geriatric administered activity**
See *Usual adult and adolescent administered activity*.

**Strength(s) usually available**
U.S.—
10 mg of sodium pyrophosphate, 30 mg of sodium trimetaphosphate, 0.95 mg (minimum) of stannous chloride, and 1.8 mg (maximum) total tin, per reaction vial (Rx) [*Pyrolite*].
Canada—
10 mg of sodium pyrophosphate, 30 mg of sodium trimetaphosphate, 0.95 mg (minimum) of stannous chloride, and 1.8 mg (maximum) total tin, per reaction vial (Rx) [*Pyrolite*].

**Packaging and storage**
Store below 40 °C (104 °F), preferably between 15 and 30 °C (59 and 86 °F), unless otherwise specified by manufacturer. Protect from freezing.

**Preparation of dosage form**
To prepare technetium Tc 99m (pyro- and trimeta-) phosphates injection, an oxidant-free sodium pertechnetate Tc 99m solution is used. See manufacturer's package insert for complete instructions.
To prepare sodium (pyro- and trimeta-) phosphates injection (unlabeled), 3 to 4 mL of sterile sodium chloride injection is used. See manufacturer's package insert for complete instructions.

**Stability**
Technetium Tc 99m (pyro- and trimeta-) phosphates injection should be administered within 6 hours after preparation.
Sodium (pyro- and trimeta-) phosphates injection (unlabeled) should be administered within 6 hours after preparation.

**Incompatibilities**
If oxidants such as peroxides and hypochlorites are present in the sodium pertechnetate Tc 99m used for labeling, the final preparation of Technetium Tc 99m (pyro- and trimeta-) phosphates injection may be adversely affected and should be discarded.

**Note**
Caution—Radioactive material.

Revised: October 1990
Interim revision: 08/02/94

# TECHNETIUM Tc 99m SESTAMIBI Systemic

VA CLASSIFICATION (Primary): DX201
Commonly used brand name(s): *Cardiolite*.
Other commonly used names are technetium Tc 99m methoxyisobutylisonitrile and technetium Tc 99m MIBI.

Note: For a listing of dosage forms and brand names by country availability, see *Dosage Forms* section(s).

## Category
Diagnostic aid, radioactive (cardiac disease).

## Indications
Note: Bracketed information in the *Indications* section refers to uses that are not included in U.S. product labeling.

**Accepted**
Cardiac imaging, radionuclide
Myocardial infarction (diagnosis) and
Myocardial perfusion imaging, radionuclide—Technetium Tc 99m sestamibi is indicated in myocardial perfusion imaging to assess the severity and localization of the myocardial infarction. It also helps to demonstrate whether thrombolytic therapy has improved perfusion.

Ischemia, myocardial (diagnosis)[1]—Technetium Tc 99m sestamibi is indicated in patients with known or suspected coronary artery disease to aid in the diagnosis of myocardial ischemia, orient investigative procedures, and guide treatment. In patients with unstable angina, technetium Tc 99m sestamibi is injected at the time of spontaneous chest pain to confirm diagnosis.

Cardiac ventricular function assessment[1] and
[Cardiac wall-motion abnormalities assessment][1]—Technetium Tc 99m sestamibi is indicated for use in the determination of right and/or left ventricular ejection fraction by first-pass radionuclide angiocardiography; it is also used to assess regional wall motion.

[Stress electrocardiography adjunct][1]—Technetium Tc 99m sestamibi is used as an adjunct to stress electrocardiography in the diagnosis of coronary artery disease, allowing simultaneous evaluation of myocardial perfusion and ventricular function.

[Parathyroid imaging, radionuclide][1]—Technetium Tc 99m sestamibi is used for the detection and localization of enlarged parathyroid glands in patients with hyperparathyroidism.

[Thyroid imaging, radionuclide][1]—Technetium Tc 99m sestamibi is used for the detection and localization of various thyroid carcinomas (e.g., medullary, lymphoma, Hurthle cell).

[1] Not included in Canadian product labeling.

## Physical Properties

**Nuclear Data**

| Radionuclide (half-life) | Decay constant | Mode of decay | Principal photon emissions (keV) | Mean number of emissions/ disintegration ($\geq 0.01$) |
|---|---|---|---|---|
| Tc 99m (6.0 hr) | 0.1151 h$^{-1}$ | Isomeric transition to Tc 99 | Gamma (18) | 0.062 |
|  |  |  | Gamma (140.5) | 0.891 |

## Pharmacology/Pharmacokinetics

**Mechanism of action/Effect**
Cardiac imaging—The myocardial uptake of technetium Tc 99m sestamibi appears to occur by a passive diffusion process. The rate of passive uptake is determined by the membrane permeability of the drug and the surface area of the vascular beds to which it is exposed; thus myocardial uptake is related to myocardial blood flow. While the mechanism of myocardial retention is not completely understood, its distribution in myocardium appears to be analogous to that of thallous chloride Tl 201. When injected at rest, technetium Tc 99m sestamibi appears to accumulate in viable myocardial tissue; infarcts are thus delineated as areas of lack of accumulation. When injected at stress (either exercise or pharmacologic vasodilation), technetium Tc 99m sestamibi accumulates in myocardial tissue in relation to myocardial blood flow; thus ischemic areas (e.g., those supplied by stenotic vessels) are detected as areas of less accumulation.

Parathyroid imaging and
Thyroid imaging—Although the precise mechanism of tumor localization is unclear, it has been suggested that technetium Tc 99m sestamibi passively crosses cell membranes and is concentrated primarily within cytoplasm and mitochondria. It has been proposed that malignant cells, because of their increased metabolic rate, maintain greater negative mitochondrial and transmembrane potentials, thus enhancing intracellular accumulation of technetium Tc 99m sestamibi. In thyroid glands with hyperthyroidism, blood flow and the number of mitochondria are increased, which may explain the uptake of technetium Tc 99m sestamibi in hyperthyroid glands. Localization of technetium Tc 99m sestamibi appears to be dependent on blood flow to the tissue, the concentration of technetium Tc 99m sestamibi presented to the tissue, and the size of the gland.

**Distribution**
High volume of distribution, with minimal cardiac redistribution. Rapidly cleared from blood after intravenous administration, accumulating in normal myocardium in relation to blood flow. The fast clearing component clears from the blood with a half-life of 4.3 minutes (at rest). At 5 minutes after injection, about 8% of the administered activity remains in circulation. Lung uptake is generally low, but there is considerable hepatic uptake. Technetium Tc 99m sestamibi is cleared through the biliary system into the intestine.

**Protein binding**
Very low (<1%).

**Half-life**
Elimination—
  Biological:
    Myocardium—6 hours (after rest injection).
    Liver—30 minutes (after rest injection).
  Effective (includes biological half-life and radionuclide decay after rest injection):
    Myocardium—3 hours.
    Liver—28 minutes.

**Radiation dosimetry**

| Organ | At rest Estimated absorbed radiation dose* | | | |
|---|---|---|---|---|
|  | With 2-hour void | | With 4.8-hour void | |
|  | mGy/MBq | rad/mCi | mGy/MBq | rad/mCi |
| Large intestine wall (upper) | 0.049 | 0.18 | 0.049 | 0.18 |
| Large intestine wall (lower) | 0.035 | 0.13 | 0.038 | 0.14 |
| Small intestine | 0.027 | 0.10 | 0.027 | 0.10 |
| Gallbladder wall | 0.018 | 0.067 | 0.018 | 0.067 |
| Kidneys | 0.018 | 0.067 | 0.018 | 0.067 |
| Bladder wall | 0.018 | 0.067 | 0.038 | 0.14 |
| Ovaries | 0.014 | 0.050 | 0.014 | 0.053 |
| Bone surfaces | 0.0063 | 0.023 | 0.0063 | 0.023 |
| Thyroid | 0.0063 | 0.023 | 0.0063 | 0.023 |
| Liver | 0.0054 | 0.02 | 0.0054 | 0.02 |
| Stomach wall | 0.0054 | 0.02 | 0.0054 | 0.02 |
| Red marrow | 0.0046 | 0.017 | 0.0046 | 0.017 |
| Heart wall | 0.0046 | 0.017 | 0.0046 | 0.017 |
| Testes | 0.0027 | 0.010 | 0.0035 | 0.013 |
| Breast | 0.0018 | 0.0067 | 0.0018 | 0.0067 |
| Total body | 0.0045 | 0.017 | 0.0045 | 0.017 |

| Radionuclide | Effective dose | | | |
|---|---|---|---|---|
|  | With 2-hour void | | With 4.8-hour void | |
|  | mSv/MBq | rem/mCi | mSv/MBq | rem/mCi |
| Tc 99m | 0.014 | 0.052 | 0.015 | 0.057 |

| Organ | At stress Estimated absorbed radiation dose* |||| 
|---|---|---|---|---|
| | With 2-hour void || With 4.8-hour void ||
| | mGy/MBq | rad/mCi | mGy/MBq | rad/mCi |
| Large intestine wall (upper) | 0.041 | 0.15 | 0.041 | 0.15 |
| Large intestine wall (lower) | 0.030 | 0.11 | 0.030 | 0.11 |
| Gallbladder wall | 0.025 | 0.093 | 0.025 | 0.093 |
| Small intestine | 0.022 | 0.08 | 0.022 | 0.08 |
| Kidneys | 0.015 | 0.057 | 0.015 | 0.057 |
| Bladder wall | 0.014 | 0.050 | 0.027 | 0.10 |
| Ovaries | 0.011 | 0.040 | 0.012 | 0.043 |
| Bone surfaces | 0.0054 | 0.02 | 0.0054 | 0.02 |
| Stomach wall | 0.0045 | 0.017 | 0.0045 | 0.017 |
| Heart wall | 0.0045 | 0.017 | 0.0045 | 0.017 |
| Red marrow | 0.0045 | 0.017 | 0.0045 | 0.017 |
| Liver | 0.0036 | 0.013 | 0.0036 | 0.013 |
| Lungs | 0.0027 | 0.010 | 0.0018 | 0.0067 |
| Thyroid | 0.0027 | 0.010 | 0.0018 | 0.0067 |
| Testes | 0.0027 | 0.010 | 0.0027 | 0.010 |
| Breast | 0.0018 | 0.0067 | 0.0018 | 0.0067 |
| Total body | 0.0036 | 0.013 | 0.0036 | 0.013 |

| Radionuclide | Effective dose ||||
|---|---|---|---|---|
| | With 2-hour void || With 4.8-hour void ||
| | mSv/MBq | rem/mCi | mSv/MBq | rem/mCi |
| Tc 99m | 0.013 | 0.045 | 0.013 | 0.048 |

*For adults; intravenous injection. Data based on the Radiopharmaceutical Internal Dose Information Center, July 1990. Oak Ridge Associated Universities.

**Elimination**
Within 48 hours—
Renal, 27% of the administered activity.
Fecal, 33% of the administered activity.

## Precautions to Consider

### Pregnancy/Reproduction
Pregnancy—Tc 99m (as free pertechnetate) crosses the placenta. Studies have not been done in humans.
The possibility of pregnancy should be assessed in women of child-bearing potential. Clinical situations exist in which the benefit to the patient and fetus, based on information derived from radiopharmaceutical use, outweighs the risks from radiation exposure to the fetus. In this situation, the physician should use discretion and reduce the administered activity of the radiopharmaceutical to the lowest possible amount.
Studies have not been done in animals.
FDA Pregnancy Category C.

### Breast-feeding
The percentage of the injected dose of technetium Tc 99m sestamibi distributed into milk has been found to be very low (0.0084% during the first 24 hours), and should not necessitate interruption of breast-feeding. However, since Tc 99m as free pertechnetate is distributed into breast milk, discontinuation of nursing for a period of 24 hours is generally recommended after administration of technetium Tc 99m–labeled radiopharmaceuticals.

### Pediatrics
Although used in children, there have been no specific studies evaluating safety and efficacy. When used in children the diagnostic benefit should be judged to outweigh the potential risk of radiation.

### Geriatrics
Appropriate studies on the relationship of age to the effects of technetium Tc 99m sestamibi have not been performed in the geriatric population. However, clinical trials and studies including older patients were conducted and geriatrics-specific problems that would limit the usefulness of this agent in the elderly are not expected.

### Diagnostic interference
The following have been selected on the basis of their potential clinical significance (possible effect in parentheses where appropriate)—not necessarily inclusive (» = major clinical significance):

With results of *this* test
Radiotherapy
(radiation may affect binding of technetium Tc 99m sestamibi to intracellular proteins, thus decreasing its uptake in myocardial cells)

### Medical considerations/Contraindications
The medical considerations/Contraindications included have been selected on the basis of their potential clinical significance (reasons given in parentheses where appropriate)—not necessarily inclusive (» = major clinical significance).

*Risk-benefit should be considered when the following medical problem exists:*
Sensitivity to the radiopharmaceutical preparation

## Side/Adverse Effects

Note: One case has been reported of severe hypersensitivity, which was characterized by dyspnea, hypotension, bradycardia, asthenia, and vomiting within 2 hours after a second injection of technetium Tc 99m sestamibi.

The following side/adverse effects have been selected on the basis of their potential clinical significance (possible signs and symptoms in parentheses where appropriate)—not necessarily inclusive:

**Those indicating need for medical attention only if they continue or are bothersome**
Incidence more frequent
*Metallic or bitter taste*
Incidence less frequent or rare
*Flushing of skin; headache; skin rash*

## Patient Consultation

As an aid to patient consultation, refer to *Advice for the Patient, Radiopharmaceuticals (Diagnostic)*.
In providing consultation, consider emphasizing the following selected information (» = major clinical significance):

**Description of use**
Action in the body: Accumulation of radioactivity in myocardial cells as a function of relative blood flow
Differences in uptake of radioactivity can be visualized
Small amounts of radioactivity used in diagnosis; radiation received is low and considered safe

**Before having this test**
» Conditions affecting use, especially:
Sensitivity to the radiopharmaceutical preparation
Pregnancy—Technetium Tc 99m (as free pertechnetate) crosses placenta; risk to fetus from radiation exposure as opposed to benefit derived from study should be considered
Breast-feeding—Very small amount distributed into breast milk; temporary discontinuation of nursing may be recommended to avoid any unnecessary absorbed radiation dose to the infant
Use in children—Risk from radiation exposure as opposed to benefit derived from use should be considered

**Preparation for this test**
Special preparatory instructions may be given; patient should inquire in advance

## General Dosing Information

Radiopharmaceuticals are to be administered only by or under the supervision of physicians who have had extensive training in the safe use and handling of radioactive materials and who are authorized by the Nuclear Regulatory Commission (NRC) or the appropriate Agreement State agency, if required, or, outside the U.S., the appropriate authority.

Imaging with technetium Tc 99m sestamibi to assess the distribution of myocardial perfusion at the time of the infarct in patients who have received the agent prior to, or at the initiation of, thrombolytic therapy (< 4 hours), is possible up to 6 hours after the intravenous injection of this agent, due to the absence of significant redistribution in the myocardium. Thus, the assessment of the amount of hypoperfused myocardium (e.g., the area at risk) is possible without having to delay the administration of thrombolytic therapy.

In conjunction with exercise or pharmacologic stress testing, technetium Tc 99m sestamibi should be administered at the inception of a period of maximum stress that lasts for approximately 1 to 3 minutes after injection.

After intravenous injection, redistribution of technetium Tc 99m sestamibi in the myocardium is minimal or non-existent. For this reason, separate stress and rest injections are required to distinguish reversible stress-induced ischemia from irreversible perfusion defects.

Technical factors such as tomographic reconstruction artifacts, patient movement, diaphragmatic attenuation, and breast attenuation in female patients may cause false-positive results (false perfusion defects).

High liver extraction of technetium Tc 99m sestamibi may interfere with visualization of the inferior wall of the heart. Delaying imaging for at least 1 hour should facilitate tracer clearance from the liver.

When used to examine myocardial perfusion, the optimal time interval for imaging is approximately 1 to 4 hours after administration of technetium Tc 99m sestamibi.

**Safety considerations for handling this radiopharmaceutical**
Improper handling of this radiopharmaceutical may cause radioactive contamination. Guidelines for handling radioactive material have been prepared by scientific, professional, state, federal, and international bodies and are available to the specially qualified and authorized users who have access to radiopharmaceuticals.

## Parenteral Dosage Forms

Note: Bracketed uses in the *Dosage Forms* section refer to categories of use and/or indications that are not included in U.S. product labeling.

### TECHNETIUM Tc 99m SESTAMIBI INJECTION USP

**Usual adult and adolescent administered activity**
Cardiac imaging—
 Intravenous, 370 to 1110 megabecquerels (10 to 30 millicuries).
 Note: For same-day rest-stress studies, to differentiate ischemia from scar, administration of a low dose (7 millicuries) at rest followed 2 hours later by a higher dose (25 millicuries) at stress has been found to be useful and to give results similar to the 2-day protocol.
[Parathyroid imaging][1]—
 Intravenous, 370 to 740 megabecquerels (10 to 20 millicuries).
[Thyroid imaging][1]—
 Intravenous, 370 to 740 megabecquerels (10 to 20 millicuries).

**Usual pediatric administered activity**
Minimum dosage has not been established.

**Usual geriatric administered activity**
See *Usual adult and adolescent administered activity*.

**Strength(s) usually available**
U.S.—
 1.0 mg of tetrakis (2-methoxy isobutyl isonitrile) Copper (I) tetrafluoroborate, 2.6 mg sodium citrate dihydrate, 1.0 mg L-cysteine hydrochloride monohydrate, 20 mg mannitol, 0.025 mg dihydrate stannous chloride (minimum), 0.075 mg dihydrate stannous chloride, 0.086 mg dihydrate tin chloride (stannous and stannic, maximum), per 5-mL reaction vial (Rx) [*Cardiolite*].

Canada—
 1.0 mg of tetrakis (2-methoxy isobutyl isonitrile) Copper (I) tetrafluoroborate, 2.6 mg sodium citrate dihydrate, 1.0 mg L-cysteine hydrochloride monohydrate, 20 mg mannitol, 0.025 mg dihydrate stannous chloride (minimum), 0.075 mg dihydrate stannous chloride, 0.086 mg dihydrate tin chloride (stannous and stannic, maximum), per 5-mL reaction vial (Rx) [*Cardiolite*].

**Packaging and storage**
Store between 15 and 25 °C (59 and 77 °F), unless otherwise specified by manufacturer. Protect from freezing.

**Preparation of dosage form**
To prepare technetium Tc 99m sestamibi injection, an oxidant-free sodium pertechnetate Tc 99m solution is used. See manufacturer's package insert for instructions.

**Stability**
Product is stable; package insert states that injection must be used within 6 hours after preparation.

**Incompatibilities**
If oxidants such as peroxides and hypochlorites are present in the sodium pertechnetate Tc 99m used for labeling, the final preparation may be adversely affected and should be discarded.

**Note**
Caution—Radioactive material.

[1]Not included in Canadian product labeling.

## Selected Bibliography

Beller GA, Sinusas AJ. Experimental studies of the physiologic properties of technetium-99m isonitriles. Am J Cardiol 1990; 66(13): 5E-8E.

Grégoire J, Théroux P. Detection and assessment of unstable angina using myocardial perfusion imaging: comparison between technetium-99m sestamibi SPECT and 12-lead electrocardiogram. Am J Cardiol 1990; 66(13): 42E-46E.

Isakandrian A, Heo J, Kong B, et al. Use of technetium-99m isonitrile (RP-30A) in assessing left ventricular perfusion and function at rest and during exercise in coronary artery disease and comparison with coronary arteriography and exercise thallium-201 SPECT imaging. Am J Cardiol 1989; 64: 270-5.

Leppo JA, DePuey EG, Johnson LL. A review of cardiac imaging with sestamibi and teboroxime. J Nucl Med 1991; 32: 2012-22.

Revised: 07/20/93
Interim revision: 08/02/94; 04/25/95

# TECHNETIUM Tc 99m SUCCIMER Systemic†

VA CLASSIFICATION (Primary): DX201
Commonly used brand name(s): *MPI DMSA Kidney Reagent*.
Note: For a listing of dosage forms and brand names by country availability, see *Dosage Forms* section(s).

†Not commercially available in Canada.

## Category

Diagnostic aid, radioactive (renal disorders).

## Indications

**Accepted**
Renal imaging, radionuclide—Technetium Tc 99m succimer is indicated as a renal imaging agent to evaluate renal parenchymal disorders.

## Physical Properties

### Nuclear Data

| Radionuclide (half-life) | Decay constant | Mode of decay | Principal photon emissions (keV) | Mean number of emissions/ disintegration (≥0.01) |
|---|---|---|---|---|
| Tc 99m (6.0 hr) | 0.1151 h$^{-1}$ | Isomeric transition to Tc 99 | Gamma (18) | 0.062 |
|  |  |  | Gamma (140.5) | 0.891 |

## Pharmacology/Pharmacokinetics

**Mechanism of action/Effect**
Based on its clearance through the urinary tract. A significant amount is retained in the proximal tubular cells of the renal cortex long enough to allow external detection by means of a scintillation camera.

**Distribution**
Distributed in the plasma, loosely bound to proteins. Cleared from the plasma with a half-time of about 60 minutes, then concentrating in the tubular cells of the renal cortex. After one hour, about 25% of the administered activity is concentrated in the kidneys, increasing to 40% after six hours.

### Radiation dosimetry

| Organ | Estimated absorbed radiation dose*† | |
|---|---|---|
| | mGy/MBq | rad/mCi |
| Kidneys | 0.17 | 0.63 |
| Bladder wall | 0.019 | 0.070 |
| Adrenals | 0.013 | 0.048 |
| Spleen | 0.013 | 0.048 |
| Liver | 0.0097 | 0.036 |
| Pancreas | 0.0090 | 0.033 |
| Red marrow | 0.0063 | 0.023 |
| Stomach wall | 0.0055 | 0.020 |
| Small intestine | 0.0052 | 0.019 |
| Large intestine wall (upper) | 0.0051 | 0.019 |
| Uterus | 0.0046 | 0.017 |
| Ovaries | 0.0037 | 0.014 |
| Bone surfaces | 0.0035 | 0.013 |
| Large intestine wall (lower) | 0.0032 | 0.012 |
| Lungs | 0.0025 | 0.0093 |
| Breast | 0.0018 | 0.0067 |
| Testes | 0.0018 | 0.0067 |
| Thyroid | 0.0011 | 0.0041 |
| Other tissue | 0.0030 | 0.011 |

Effective dose: 0.016 mSv/MBq (0.059 rem/mCi)

*For adults; intravenous injection.
†Data based on the International Commission on Radiological Protection (ICRP) Publication 53—Radiation dose to patients from radiopharmaceuticals.

**Elimination**
Renal (about 16% of the administered activity in 2 hours).

## Precautions to Consider

### Pregnancy/Reproduction
Pregnancy—Tc 99m (as free pertechnetate) crosses the placenta. However, studies have not been done with technetium Tc 99m succimer in humans.

The possibility of pregnancy should be assessed in women of child-bearing potential. Clinical situations exist where the benefit to the patient and fetus, based on information derived from radiopharmaceutical use, outweighs the risks from fetal exposure to radiation. In these situations, the physician should use discretion and reduce the radiopharmaceutical dose to the lowest possible amount.

Studies have not been done in animals.

FDA Pregnancy Category C.

### Breast-feeding
Although it is not known whether technetium Tc 99m succimer is distributed into breast milk, it is known that Tc 99m as free pertechnetate is distributed into breast milk. Based on the assumption that the Tc 99m in breast milk is in the form of pertechnetate and based on the effective half-life of the radionuclide in breast milk, the daily volume of milk, a dose factor relating the radionuclide to its critical organ (thyroid) in the nursing infant, and the maximum permissible dose to that organ, a guideline has been proposed. According to this guideline, it has been calculated that nursing can be safely resumed when the concentration in breast milk reaches $30.3 \times 10^{-4}$ megabecquerels ($8.2 \times 10^{-2}$ microcuries) per mL. This level of activity is probably reached, in the majority of patients, within 12 to 24 hours after administration of technetium Tc 99m–labeled radiopharmaceuticals.

### Pediatrics
Studies performed in children have not demonstrated pediatrics-specific problems that would limit the usefulness of technetium Tc 99m succimer in children. However, because of the potential risk of radiation exposure, risk-benefit must be considered.

### Geriatrics
Appropriate studies on the relationship of age to the effects of technetium Tc 99m succimer have not been performed in the geriatric population. However, no geriatrics-specific problems have been documented to date.

### Diagnostic interference
The following have been selected on the basis of their potential clinical significance (possible effect in parentheses where appropriate)—not necessarily inclusive (» = major clinical significance):

With results of *this* test
*Due to other medications*
   Captopril or
   Enalapril or
   Lisinopril
     (in patients with unilateral renal artery stenosis, use of angiotensin-converting enzyme inhibitors may result in decreased uptake of technetium Tc 99m succimer by the affected kidney because of a loss of effective trans-membrane filtration pressure)
*Due to medical problems or conditions*
   Dehydration
     (decreased urinary flow may result in poor renal images)

### Medical considerations/Contraindications
The medical considerations/contraindications included have been selected on the basis of their potential clinical significance (reasons given in parentheses where appropriate)—not necessarily inclusive (» = major clinical significance).

See also *Diagnostic interference*.

*Risk-benefit should be considered when the following medical problem exists:*
   Sensitivity to the radiopharmaceutical preparation

## Side/Adverse Effects
The following side/adverse effects have been selected on the basis of their potential clinical significance (possible signs and symptoms in parentheses where appropriate)—not necessarily inclusive:

**Those indicating need for medical attention only if they continue or are bothersome**
Incidence rare
   *Fever; flushing or redness of skin; nausea; skin rash; stomach pain; syncope* (fainting)

## Patient Consultation
As an aid to patient consultation, refer to *Advice for the Patient, Radiopharmaceuticals (Diagnostic)*.

In providing consultation, consider emphasizing the following selected information (» = major clinical significance):

### Description of use
   Action in the body: Concentration of radioactive succimer in kidneys
   Retention of radioactivity in kidneys allows visualization
   Small amounts of radioactivity used in diagnosis; radiation received is low and considered safe

### Before having this test
» Conditions affecting use, especially:
   Sensitivity to the radiopharmaceutical preparation
   Pregnancy—Technetium Tc 99m (as free pertechnetate) crosses placenta; risk to fetus from radiation exposure as opposed to benefit derived from use should be considered
   Breast-feeding—Not known if technetium Tc 99m succimer is distributed into breast milk, but Tc 99m as free pertechnetate is distributed into breast milk; temporary discontinuation of nursing may be recommended because of risk to infant from radiation exposure
   Use in children—Risk from radiation exposure as opposed to benefit derived from use should be considered

### Preparation for this test
   Special preparatory instructions may be given; patient should inquire in advance

### Precautions after having this test
   Adequate intake of fluids and voiding as often as possible for 4 to 6 hours after examination to minimize radiation dose to bladder

## General Dosing Information
Radiopharmaceuticals are to be administered only by or under the supervision of physicians who have had extensive training in the safe use and handling of radioactive materials and who are authorized by the Nuclear Regulatory Commission (NRC) or the appropriate Agreement State agency, if required, or, outside the U.S., the appropriate authority.

Adequate hydration of the patient is recommended before and after examination to promote urinary flow. Also, urination is recommended as often as possible for 4 to 6 hours after the examination to reduce radiation exposure to the bladder.

Manufacturer's package insert or other appropriate literature should be consulted for optimal times when imaging should be performed.

## Safety considerations for handling this radiopharmaceutical
Improper handling of this radiopharmaceutical may cause radioactive contamination. Guidelines for handling radioactive material have been prepared by scientific, professional, state, federal, and international bodies and are available to the specially qualified and authorized users who have access to radiopharmaceuticals.

## Parenteral Dosage Forms

### TECHNETIUM Tc 99m SUCCIMER INJECTION USP

**Usual adult and adolescent administered activity**
Renal imaging—
   Intravenous, 74 to 222 megabecquerels (2 to 6 millicuries), administered slowly.

**Usual pediatric administered activity**
Renal imaging—
   Dosage must be individualized by physician. The minimum recommended total dosage is 55 megabecquerels (1.5 millicuries), with a maximum total dosage of 185 megabecquerels (5 millicuries), intravenously.

**Usual geriatric administered activity**
See *Usual adult and adolescent administered activity*.

**Strength(s) usually available**
U.S.—
   1.2 mg succimer and 0.42 mg anhydrous stannous chloride, per 2.2-mL reagent ampule (Rx) [*MPI DMSA Kidney Reagent*].
Canada—
   Not commercially available.

**Packaging and storage**
Store between 15 and 30 °C (59 and 86 °F), in a light-resistant container. Protect from freezing.

**Preparation of dosage form**
To prepare injection, an oxidant-free sodium pertechnetate Tc 99m solution is used. After reconstitution with sodium pertechnetate Tc 99m, the newly formed complex should be allowed to incubate for 10 minutes, at room temperature, to permit the formation of a more desirable succimer complex. See manufacturer's package insert for complete instructions.

**Stability**
Injection should be administered within 30 minutes after preparation.

**Incompatibilities**
If oxidants such as peroxides and hypochlorites are present in the sodium pertechnetate Tc 99m used for labeling, the final preparation may be adversely affected and should be discarded.

**Note**
Caution—Radioactive material.

## Selected Bibliography
Blaufox MD. Procedures of choice in renal nuclear medicine. J Nucl Med 1991; 32: 1301-9.

Revised: 08/18/93
Interim revision: 08/02/94

---

# TECHNETIUM Tc 99m SULFUR COLLOID   Systemic

VA CLASSIFICATION (Primary): DX201
Commonly used brand name(s): *AN-Sulfur Colloid; Frosstimage Sulfur Colloid; TSC; TechneColl; TechneScan Sulfur Colloid*.
Note: For a listing of dosage forms and brand names by country availability, see *Dosage Forms* section(s).

## Category
Diagnostic aid, radioactive (hepatic disease; hematological disease; spleen disease; gastroesophageal disorders; gastrointestinal disorders).

## Indications
Note: Bracketed information in the *Indications* section refers to uses that are not included in U.S. product labeling.

**Accepted**
Liver imaging, radionuclide—Technetium Tc 99m sulfur colloid, administered intravenously, is indicated for imaging the functioning reticuloendothelial cells of the liver in the evaluation of metastatic disease, primary liver tumors, abscesses, and other focal hepatic lesions; and in the evaluation of patients with cirrhosis, hepatitis, and other hepatic disorders.
Spleen imaging, radionuclide—Technetium Tc 99m sulfur colloid, administered intravenously, is indicated for imaging the functioning reticuloendothelial cells of the spleen, thus serving to demonstrate clinically significant splenomegaly, and in the evaluation of splenic infarct, other local splenic lesions, or splenic rupture.
Bone marrow imaging, radionuclide—Technetium Tc 99m sulfur colloid, administered intravenously, is indicated for imaging the functioning reticuloendothelial cells of the bone marrow to complement other hematological studies for the evaluation of hematopoiesis in hematological diseases, such as leukemia, polycythemia, anemias, and myelofibrosis.
Esophageal imaging, radionuclide[1]—Technetium Tc 99m sulfur colloid, administered orally, is indicated in adults and children for esophageal transit studies, gastroesophageal reflux scintigraphy, and the detection of pulmonary aspiration of gastric contents.
LeVeen peritoneovenous shunt patency assessment[1]—Intraperitoneal technetium Tc 99m sulfur colloid is indicated in adults to determine the patency of a peritoneovenous shunt in patients with ascites.
[Bleeding, gastrointestinal (diagnosis)][1]—Technetium Tc 99m sulfur colloid, administered intravenously, is used to detect and locate the site of bleeding in the gastrointestinal tract.
[Gastric emptying studies][1]—Technetium Tc 99m sulfur colloid is used orally in studies to evaluate gastric function in patients with suspected anatomical or functional obstruction, or hypomotility (e.g., gastroparesis).

[1]Not included in Canadian product labeling.

## Physical Properties

**Nuclear data**

| Radionuclide (half-life) | Decay constant | Mode of decay | Principal photon emissions (keV) | Mean number of emissions/ disintegration ($\geq 0.01$) |
|---|---|---|---|---|
| Tc 99m (6.0 hr) | 0.1151 h$^{-1}$ | Isomeric transition to Tc 99 | 18 | 0.062 |
|  |  |  | 140.5 | 0.891 |

## Pharmacology/Pharmacokinetics

**Mechanism of action/Effect**
Diagnostic aid (hepatic disease; hematological disease; spleen disease)—
   Radioactive colloids are phagocytized by the reticuloendothelial system of the liver, spleen, and bone marrow, and remain there long enough for scintillation scans of their distribution to be obtained.
Diagnostic aid (gastroesophageal disorders)—Esophageal transit of technetium Tc 99m sulfur colloid after oral administration is depicted scintigraphically and quantified by computer assistance.
Diagnostic aid (gastrointestinal disorders)—Gastrointestinal bleeding: After intravenous injection, technetium Tc 99m sulfur colloid circulates in the blood until it is cleared by the cells of the reticuloendothelial system. If active gastrointestinal bleeding is occurring during this period, there will be accumulation of the tracer in the lumen of the gastrointestinal tract at the site of bleeding, thus permitting scintigraphic detection and localization.

**Absorption**
Rapidly phagocytized by the reticuloendothelial system after intravenous administration.

**Distribution**
Parenteral—
   Distribution dependent on relative blood flow and functional capacity of phagocytic cells; technetium Tc 99m sulfur colloid is selectively concentrated in reticuloendothelial system of the liver, spleen, and bone marrow. About 80 to 90% of the injected colloidal particles are phagocytized by the Kupffer cells of the liver, 5 to 10% by the spleen, and the balance by the bone marrow.

Uptake may be decreased in the liver and increased in the spleen and bone marrow of patients with impaired portal circulation or Kupffer cell dysfunction.

Several cases of uptake in the lungs and other soft tissues have been reported in the presence of a wide variety of disorders, usually inflammatory or neoplastic.

**Half-life**
Elimination from the blood pool—2.5 minutes.

**Time to radioactivity visualization**
With intravenous administration—
Liver and spleen imaging: 10 to 15 minutes.
Note: Onset of hepatic visualization may be delayed in patients with severe hepatic disease because of slower blood clearance of the radiopharmaceutical, with an overall result of decreased liver uptake and increased spleen and marrow uptake.
Bone marrow imaging: 15 minutes.
With oral administration—
Esophageal imaging: Immediate; usually as the patient swallows, in a single swallow, the water containing technetium Tc 99m sulfur colloid.

**Radiation dosimetry**

| | Estimated absorbed radiation dose* | | | |
|---|---|---|---|---|
| | With normal hepatic function | | With parenchymal liver disease (intermediate/advanced) | |
| Organ | mGy/MBq | rad/mCi | mGy/MBq | rad/mCi |
| Spleen | 0.077 | 0.29 | 0.14 | 0.52 |
| Liver | 0.074 | 0.27 | 0.042 | 0.16 |
| Pancreas | 0.012 | 0.044 | 0.018 | 0.066 |
| Red marrow | 0.011 | 0.041 | 0.023 | 0.085 |
| Adrenals | 0.010 | 0.037 | 0.0098 | 0.036 |
| Kidneys | 0.0097 | 0.036 | 0.011 | 0.041 |
| Bone surfaces | 0.0064 | 0.024 | 0.012 | 0.044 |
| Stomach wall | 0.0062 | 0.023 | 0.0098 | 0.036 |
| Large intestine wall (upper) | 0.0056 | 0.021 | 0.0049 | 0.018 |
| Lungs | 0.0055 | 0.20 | 0.0048 | 0.018 |
| Small intestine | 0.0043 | 0.016 | 0.0046 | 0.017 |
| Breast | 0.0027 | 0.010 | 0.0024 | 0.0089 |
| Ovaries | 0.0022 | 0.0081 | 0.0033 | 0.012 |
| Uterus | 0.0019 | 0.0070 | 0.0028 | 0.010 |
| Large intestine wall (lower) | 0.0018 | 0.0067 | 0.0031 | 0.011 |
| Bladder wall | 0.0011 | 0.0041 | 0.0016 | 0.0059 |
| Thyroid | 0.00079 | 0.0029 | 0.0011 | 0.0041 |
| Testes | 0.00062 | 0.0023 | 0.00095 | 0.0035 |
| Other tissue | 0.0028 | 0.010 | 0.0031 | 0.011 |

| | Effective dose* | | | |
|---|---|---|---|---|
| | With normal hepatic function | | With parenchymal liver disease (intermediate/advanced) | |
| Radionuclide | mSv/MBq | rem/mCi | mSv/MBq | rem/mCi |
| Tc 99m | 0.014 | 0.052 | 0.017 | 0.063 |

*For adults; intravenous injection of technetium Tc 99m–labeled large colloids. Data based on the International Commission on Radiological Protection (ICRP) Publication 53—Radiation dose to patients from radiopharmaceuticals.

**Elimination**
Renal, about 3% of the administered activity eliminated within 48 hours after intravenous administration.

## Precautions to Consider

**Carcinogenicity/Mutagenicity**
Long-term animal studies to evaluate carcinogenic or mutagenic potential of technetium Tc 99m sulfur colloid have not been performed.

**Pregnancy/Reproduction**
Pregnancy—Tc 99m (as free pertechnetate) crosses the placenta. However, studies with technetium Tc 99m sulfur colloid have not been done in humans.
The possibility of pregnancy should be assessed in women of child-bearing potential. Clinical situations exist where the benefit to the patient and fetus, based on information derived from radiopharmaceutical use, outweighs the risks from fetal exposure to radiation. In these situations, the physician should use discretion and reduce the radiopharmaceutical dose to the lowest possible amount.
Studies have not been done in animals.
FDA Pregnancy Category C.

**Breast-feeding**
Although it is not known whether technetium Tc 99m sulfur colloid is distributed into breast milk, it is known that Tc 99m as free pertechnetate is distributed into breast milk. Based on the assumption that the Tc 99m in breast milk is in the form of pertechnetate and based on the effective half-life of the radionuclide in breast milk, the daily volume of milk, a dose factor relating the radionuclide to its critical organ (thyroid) in the nursing infant, and the maximum permissible dose to that organ, a guideline has been proposed. According to this guideline, it has been calculated that nursing can be safely resumed when the concentration in breast milk reaches $30.3 \times 10^{-4}$ megabecquerels ($8.2 \times 10^{-2}$ microcuries) per mL. This level of activity is probably reached, in the majority of patients, within 12 to 24 hours after administration of technetium Tc 99m–labeled radiopharmaceuticals.

**Pediatrics**
Diagnostic studies performed to date using technetium Tc 99 sulfur colloid have not demonstrated pediatrics-specific problems that would limit the usefulness of technetium Tc 99m sulfur colloid in children. However, when this radiopharmaceutical is used in children, the diagnostic benefit should be judged to outweigh the potential risk of radiation.

**Geriatrics**
Appropriate studies on the relationship of age to the effects of technetium Tc 99m sulfur colloid have not been performed in the geriatric population. However, no geriatrics-specific problems have been documented to date.

**Drug interactions and/or related problems**
See *Diagnostic interference*.

**Diagnostic interference**
The following have been selected on the basis of their potential clinical significance (possible effect in parentheses where appropriate)—not necessarily inclusive (» = major clinical significance):

With results of *this* test
*Due to other medications*
Anesthetics, inhalation, such as halothane
(recent administration of general anesthetics may increase splenic uptake of technetium Tc 99m sulfur colloid, probably because the reduced hepatic flow and hepatotoxicity associated with general anesthetics may alter the hepatic radiocolloid extraction efficiency, resulting in a reversal of the normal liver-spleen colloid distribution pattern)

Antacids, aluminum-containing, high doses or long-term use or
Magnesium sulfate, parenteral or
Polyvalent cations
(reticuloendothelial cell imaging may be impaired by polyvalent cations, which cause agglomeration of the individual colloidal particles leading to trapping by the pulmonary capillary bed rather than the reticuloendothelial cells of the liver, spleen, and bone marrow)

Chemotherapy, especially with nitrosoureas
(use of technetium Tc 99m sulfur colloid in patients who are undergoing or have recently undergone chemotherapy, may result in inhomogeneous or irregular hepatic uptake, shift of activity from the liver to the bone marrow and spleen, and hepatomegaly; irregular hepatic distribution of radiopharmaceutical may be misinterpreted as malignancy; thus, it is recommended that liver and/or spleen imaging be done prior to initiating chemotherapy with these agents or several weeks after discontinuing therapy)

Reticuloendothelial system stimulators, such as:
Dextrose
Heparin
Steroid hormones (including estrogen)
Thyroid hormones
Vitamin B$_{12}$
(use of technetium Tc 99m sulfur colloid in patients receiving these medicines may result in lung uptake of technetium Tc 99m sulfur colloid, probably due to a drug-induced increase in number of free intravascular macrophages, which may migrate to pulmonary capillary bed and phagocytize colloidal particles there)

*Due to medical problems or conditions*
Malaria
(diffuse lung uptake of technetium Tc 99m sulfur colloid may occur, probably related to increased reticuloendothelial system activity due to malaria-induced increase in the pulmonary macrophages)

## Medical considerations/Contraindications
The medical considerations/contraindications included have been selected on the basis of their potential clinical significance (reasons given in parentheses where appropriate)—not necessarily inclusive (» = major clinical significance).

*Risk-benefit should be considered when the following medical problem exists:*
Sensitivity to the radiopharmaceutical preparation, especially gelatin-containing preparations

## Side/Adverse Effects
Note: Cardiopulmonary arrest has been reported rarely with the administration of technetium Tc 99m sulfur colloid.

The following side/adverse effects have been selected on the basis of their potential clinical significance (possible signs and symptoms in parentheses where appropriate)—not necessarily inclusive:

**Those indicating need for medical attention**
Incidence rare
*Allergic reaction* (coughing or choking; flushing or redness of face; skin rash, hives, or itching; swelling of throat, hands, or feet; wheezing, tightness in chest, or troubled breathing); *bronchospasm with or without pulmonary edema* (severe wheezing or troubled breathing); *fever; hypotension* (severe tiredness or weakness); *pain or burning sensation at injection site; seizures; slow or irregular heartbeat*

Note: The *allergic reaction* may be the initial manifestation of a more severe anaphylactic reaction.

*Allergic reactions* and *fever* may be caused by the colloid stabilizer (i.e., gelatin) used in the preparation.

**Those indicating need for medical attention only if they continue or are bothersome**
Incidence less frequent or rare
*Dizziness; nausea or vomiting*

## Patient Consultation
As an aid to patient consultation, refer to *Advice for the Patient, Radiopharmaceuticals (Diagnostic).*

In providing consultation, consider emphasizing the following selected information (» = major clinical significance):

**Description of use**
*Action in the body*
Accumulation of radioactive colloid particles in liver, spleen, and bone marrow
Esophageal and gastric transit of radiocolloid
Retention of radioactivity in these organs allows visualization; or transit of radioactivity through mouth/esophagus/stomach allows visualization
Small amounts of radioactivity used in diagnosis; radiation received is low and considered safe

**Before having this test**
» Conditions affecting use, especially:
Sensitivity to radiopharmaceutical preparation
Pregnancy—Technetium Tc 99m (as free pertechnetate) crosses placenta; risk to fetus from radiation exposure as opposed to benefit derived from use should be considered
Breast-feeding—Not known if technetium Tc 99m sulfur colloid is distributed into breast milk, but Tc 99m as free pertechnetate is distributed into breast milk; temporary discontinuation of nursing may be recommended because of risk to infant from radiation exposure
Use in children—Risk of radiation exposure as opposed to benefit derived from use should be considered

**Preparation for this test**
Special preparatory instructions may be given; patient should inquire in advance (fasting required for esophageal imaging and gastric emptying studies)

**Precautions after having this test**
No special precautions

**Side/adverse effects**
Signs of potential side effects, especially allergic reaction, fever, hypotension, pain or burning sensation at injection site, seizures, slow or irregular heartbeat, or respiratory distress

## General Dosing Information
Radiopharmaceuticals are to be administered only by or under the supervision of physicians who have had extensive training in the safe use and handling of radioactive materials and who are authorized by the Nuclear Regulatory Commission (NRC) or the appropriate Agreement State agency, if required, or, outside the U.S., the appropriate authority.

Epinephrine, antihistamines, and corticosteroids should be available during the administration of technetium Tc 99m sulfur colloid because of the possibility of allergic reactions.

**Safety considerations for handling this radiopharmaceutical**
Improper handling of this radiopharmaceutical may cause radioactive contamination. Guidelines for handling radioactive material have been prepared by scientific, professional, state, federal, and international bodies and are available to the specially qualified and authorized users who have access to radiopharmaceuticals.

## Parenteral Dosage Forms
Note: Bracketed uses in the *Dosage Forms* section refer to categories of use and/or indications that are not included in U.S. product labeling.

**TECHNETIUM Tc 99m SULFUR COLLOID INJECTION USP**

**Usual adult and adolescent administered activity**
Liver and/or spleen imaging—
Intravenous, 37 to 296 megabecquerels (1 to 8 millicuries).
Bone marrow imaging—
Intravenous, 111 to 444 megabecquerels (3 to 12 millicuries).
Esophageal imaging[1]—
Gastroesophageal studies: Oral, 5.55 to 11.1 megabecquerels (150 to 300 microcuries).
Pulmonary aspiration studies: Oral, 11.1 to 18.5 megabecquerels (300 to 500 microcuries).
LeVeen shunt patency[1]—
Intraperitoneal, 37 to 111 megabecquerels (1 to 3 millicuries).
Percutaneous transtubal, 12 to 37 megabecquerels (0.3 to 1 millicurie) in a volume not to exceed 0.5 mL.
[Diagnosis of gastrointestinal bleeding][1]—
Intravenous or intra-arterial, 370 megabecquerels (10 millicuries).
[Gastric emptying studies][1]—
Oral, 9.2 to 37 megabecquerels (0.25 to 1 millicurie).
Note: For gastric emptying studies, the dosage may be given in a liquid or incorporated into food such as scrambled eggs.

**Usual pediatric administered activity**
Liver and/or spleen imaging—
Intravenous, 0.55 to 2.75 megabecquerels (15 to 75 microcuries) per kg of body weight.
Note: In newborns the total administered activity should be 7.4 to 18.5 megabecquerels (200 to 500 microcuries), since a minimum administered activity of 7.4 megabecquerels (200 microcuries) is required for this procedure.
Bone marrow imaging—
Intravenous, 1.11 to 5.55 megabecquerels (30 to 150 microcuries) per kg of body weight.
Note: In newborns a maximum total administered activity of 22.2 megabecquerels (600 microcuries) is recommended, since this is the minimum administered activity required for this procedure.
Esophageal imaging[1]—
Gastroesophageal and pulmonary aspiration studies: Oral, 3.7 to 11.1 megabecquerels (100 to 300 microcuries).
Note: Oral dosage may be incorporated into milk feeding. However, to avoid preliminary contamination of the esophagus, the oral dosage may be instilled directly into the stomach by intubation, followed by a dextrose or milk meal.

**Usual geriatric administered activity**
See *Usual adult and adolescent administered activity*.

**Strength(s) usually available**
U.S.—
2 mg sodium thiosulfate anhydrous, 2.3 mg edetate disodium, and 18.1 mg gelatin, per 10-mL multidose reaction vial; 1.5 mL of 0.148 *N* hydrochloric acid solution per syringe A; and 1.5 mL aqueous solution of 38.8 mg sodium biphosphate anhydrous and 11.1 mg sodium hydroxide, per syringe B (Rx) [*AN-Sulfur Colloid; Techne-Scan Sulfur Colloid*].
50 mg phosphoric acid per mL or reaction mixture vial; 12 mg gelatin and 9 mg sodium chloride per mL in one compartment, and 12 mg sodium thiosulfate per mL in the other compartment of syringe I; 36 mg gelatin and 9 mg sodium chloride per mL in one compart-

ment, and 544 mg sodium acetate and 4 mg edetate disodium per mL in the other compartment of syringe II (Rx) [*TechneColl*].

0.5 mL of 1.0 N hydrochloric acid per reaction vial; and two syringes, one containing a 1.1 mL aqueous solution of 1.9 mg sodium thiosulfate anhydrous and the other containing 5.3 mg gelatin in 2.1 mL of an aqueous buffer solution containing 177 mg sodium acetate (Rx) [*TSC*].

Canada—

3 mg sodium thiosulfate, 4.25 mg gelatin, 0.65 mg potassium perrhenate, per mL of reaction vial A; 1 N hydrochloric acid solution per vial B; alkaline buffer solution per vial C (Rx) [*Frosstimage Sulfur Colloid*].

**Packaging and storage**

Store below 40 °C (104 °F), preferably between 15 and 30 °C (59 and 86 °F), unless otherwise specified by manufacturer. Protect from freezing.

**Preparation of dosage form**

To prepare injection, an oxidant-free sodium pertechnetate Tc 99m solution is used. See manufacturer's package insert for instructions.

**Stability**

Preparations containing a flocculent precipitate should not be used.

Injection should be administered within 6 hours after preparation, since particles tend to agglomerate with aging.

**Incompatibilities**

Polyvalent cations may decrease the stability of the colloidal preparation. Solutions of sodium pertechnetate Tc 99m containing more than 10 mcg per mL of aluminum ion should not be used since a flocculent precipitate may form. These larger particles may become lodged in the pulmonary capillary bed rather than in the reticuloendothelial system.

If oxidants such as peroxides and hypochlorites are present in the sodium pertechnetate Tc 99m used for labeling, the final preparation may be adversely affected and it should be discarded.

**Note**

Caution—Radioactive material.
Shake well.

[1]Not included in Canadian product labeling.

## Selected Bibliography

Malmud LS, Fisher RS, Knight LC, et al. Scintigraphic evaluation of gastric emptying. Semin Nucl Med 1982; 12(2): 116-25.

Malmud LS, Fisher RS. Radionuclide studies of esophageal transit and gastrophageal reflux. Semin Nucl Med 1982; 12(2): 104-15.

Alavi A. Detection of gastrointestinal bleeding with Tc 99m sulfur colloid. Semin Nucl Med 1982; 12(2): 126-38.

Revised: 06/23/94

# TECHNETIUM Tc 99m TEBOROXIME Systemic†

VA CLASSIFICATION (Primary): DX201

Commonly used brand name(s): *CardioTec*.

Note: For a listing of dosage forms and brand names by country availability, see *Dosage Forms* section(s).

†Not commercially available in Canada.

## Category

Diagnostic aid, radioactive (cardiac disease).

## Indications

**Accepted**

Cardiac imaging, radionuclide
Myocardial infarction (diagnosis) and
Myocardial perfusion imaging, radionuclide—Technetium Tc 99m teboroxime is indicated in myocardial perfusion imaging to distinguish normal from abnormal myocardium in patients with suspected coronary artery disease (CAD) using rest and stress techniques.

## Physical Properties

**Nuclear data**

| Radionuclide (half-life) | Decay constant | Mode of decay | Principal photon emissions (keV) | Mean number of photons/ disintegration (≥0.01) |
|---|---|---|---|---|
| Tc 99m (6.0 hr) | 0.1151 h$^{-1}$ | Isomeric transition to Tc 99 | Gamma 18 | 0.062 |
| | | | Gamma 140.5 | 0.891 |

## Pharmacology/Pharmacokinetics

**Mechanism of action/Effect**

The mechanisms for uptake and retention of technetium Tc 99m teboroxime by myocardial tissue are not well established. Unlike cationic thallous chloride Tl 201 and technetium Tc 99m sestamibi, technetium Tc 99m teboroxime has a neutral charge. Because of its neutral charge and high lipophilicity, the myocardial uptake of technetium Tc 99m teboroxime appears to occur by a passive diffusion process. The rate of passive uptake is determined by the membrane permeability of the drug, the surface area of the vascular beds to which it is exposed, the vascular and extravascular concentrations of the drug, and the rate of delivery of the drug. While technetium Tc 99m teboroxime's mechanism of myocardial retention is less efficient than that of thallous chloride Tl 201 or technetium Tc 99m sestamibi, its myocardial extraction is higher.

Its rapid myocardial washout allows early repeat studies following the application of a pharmacologic or physical intervention.

**Distribution**

Technetium Tc 99m teboroxime is rapidly cleared from blood after intravenous administration, with high myocardial extraction in proportion to myocardial perfusion even at extremely high flow rates. Myocardial uptake is apparent scintigraphically at 1 minute after injection. A significant amount of the initial myocardial activity is cleared by 20 to 30 minutes after administration.

Liver uptake of technetium Tc 99m teboroxime becomes significant by 5 to 10 minutes after injection and has a slow clearance (half-life approximately 1.5 hours) that can impair visualization of the inferior left ventricular wall.

There is marked first-pass uptake of technetium Tc 99m teboroxime in the lungs with rapid subsequent clearance within the first 2 minutes after injection. This initial lung uptake may complicate first-pass radionuclide angiography image interpretation, since it results in lower ejection fractions, higher pulmonary transit times, higher calculated pulmonary blood volume indices, and poorer left ventricular border definition.

**Protein binding**

Very low (<10%).

**Half-life**

Elimination (myocardium)—10 to 15 minutes.

Note: A biexponential pattern of myocardial washout has been demonstrated in animals and man. About two-thirds of myocardial activity demonstrates an effective half-life of 5.2 minutes; the remaining one-third demonstrates an effective half-life of 3.8 hours. At 10 minutes after injection, approximately 10.4±4.4% (mean) of the injected dose remains in the circulation.

**Radiation dosimetry**

| Mode of administration | Estimated absorbed radiation dose* | | |
|---|---|---|---|
| | Target organ | mGy/MBq | rad/mCi |
| Intravenous | Large intestine, upper | 0.033 | 0.12 |
| | Gallbladder wall | 0.026 | 0.097 |
| | Large intestine, lower | 0.023 | 0.087 |
| | Small intestine | 0.018 | 0.067 |
| | Liver | 0.017 | 0.062 |
| | Ovaries | 0.0098 | 0.036 |
| | Lungs | 0.0076 | 0.028 |
| | Urinary bladder wall | 0.0074 | 0.027 |
| | Heart wall | 0.0055 | 0.020 |
| | Kidneys | 0.0055 | 0.020 |
| | Red marrow | 0.0045 | 0.017 |

**2744 Technetium Tc 99m Teboroxime (Systemic)**

| Mode of administration | Estimated absorbed radiation dose* | | |
|---|---|---|---|
| | Target organ | mGy/MBq | rad/mCi |
| | Spleen | 0.0040 | 0.015 |
| | Brain | 0.0034 | 0.012 |
| | Thyroid | 0.0029 | 0.011 |
| | Testes | 0.0028 | 0.010 |
| | Total body | 0.0045 | 0.017 |

Effective dose: 0.013 mSv/MBq (0.048 rem/mCi)

*Assuming 6-hour gallbladder emptying; 2-hour urinary bladder void.

**Elimination**
Hepatobiliary, mainly. Renal, 22±13% in 24 hours.

## Precautions to Consider

**Carcinogenicity**
Long-term animal studies to evaluate carcinogenic potential of technetium Tc 99m teboroxime have not been performed.

**Mutagenicity**
Decayed technetium Tc 99m teboroxime has not been shown to be mutagenic in a reversion test with bacteria, a chromosomal aberration assay, and an *in vivo* mouse micronucleus assay.

At high concentrations that were toxic to the cells and reduced growth to 33% or less relative to vehicle controls, technetium Tc 99m teboroxime was weakly positive for inducing forward mutations at the TK locus in L5178Y mouse lymphoma cells without metabolic activation. In the presence of metabolic activation, technetium Tc 99m teboroxime gave negative results in this assay.

**Pregnancy/Reproduction**
Pregnancy—Tc 99m (as free pertechnetate) crosses the placenta. However, studies with technetium Tc 99m teboroxime have not been done in humans.

The possibility of pregnancy should be assessed in women of child-bearing potential. Clinical situations exist in which the benefit to the patient and fetus from information derived from radiopharmaceutical use outweighs the risks from fetal exposure to radiation. In these situations, the physician should use discretion and reduce the administered activity of the radiopharmaceutical to the lowest possible amount.

Studies have not been done in animals.

FDA Pregnancy Category C.

**Breast-feeding**
Although it is not known whether technetium Tc 99m teboroxime is distributed into breast milk, it is known that Tc 99m as free pertechnetate is distributed into breast milk. Because of the potential risk to the infant from radiation exposure, discontinuation of nursing for a period of 24 hours is recommended after administration of technetium Tc 99m–labeled radiopharmaceuticals.

**Pediatrics**
Although technetium Tc 99m teboroxime is used in children, there have been no specific studies evaluating safety and efficacy. When used in children, the diagnostic benefit should be judged to outweigh the potential risk of radiation.

**Geriatrics**
Appropriate studies on the relationship of age to the effects of technetium Tc 99m teboroxime have not been performed in the geriatric population. However, clinical trials and studies were conducted including older patients and geriatrics-specific problems that would limit the usefulness of this agent in the elderly are not expected.

**Medical considerations/Contraindications**
The medical considerations/contraindications included have been selected on the basis of their potential clinical significance (reasons given in parentheses where appropriate)—not necessarily inclusive (» = major clinical significance).

*Risk-benefit should be considered when the following medical problem exists:*
Sensitivity to the radiopharmaceutical preparation

## Side/Adverse Effects

The following side/adverse effects have been selected on the basis of their potential clinical significance (possible signs and symptoms in parentheses where appropriate)—not necessarily inclusive:

Those indicating need for medical attention only if they continue or are bothersome
Incidence less frequent or rare
*Burning sensation at injection site; hypotension; metallic taste; nausea; numbness of hand and arm; swelling of face*

## Patient Consultation

As an aid to patient consultation, refer to *Advice for the Patient, Radiopharmaceuticals (Diagnostic)*.
In providing consultation, consider emphasizing the following selected information (» = major clinical significance):

**Description of use**
Action in the body: Accumulation of radioactivity in myocardial cells as a function of relative blood flow
Differences in uptake of radioactivity can be visualized
Small amounts of radioactivity used in diagnosis; radiation dose received is relatively low and considered safe

**Before having this test**
» Conditions affecting use, especially:
Sensitivity to the radiopharmaceutical preparation
Pregnancy—Technetium Tc 99m (as free pertechnetate) crosses placenta; risk to fetus from radiation exposure as opposed to benefit derived from study should be considered
Breast-feeding—Not known if technetium Tc 99m teboroxime is distributed into breast milk, but Tc 99m as free pertechnetate is distributed into breast milk; temporary discontinuation of nursing is recommended to avoid any unnecessary absorbed radiation dose to the infant

**Preparation for this test**
Fasting for 4 to 8 hours before the stress/rest test
Other special preparatory instructions may also be given; patient should inquire in advance

## General Dosing Information

Radiopharmaceuticals are to be administered only by or under the supervision of physicians who have had extensive training in the safe use and handling of radioactive materials and who are licensed by the Nuclear Regulatory Commission (NRC) or the appropriate Agreement State agency, if required, or, outside the U.S., the appropriate authority.

Fasting is usually recommended for 4 to 8 hours before the stress/rest test.

Technical factors such as tomographic reconstruction artifacts, patient movement, diaphragmatic attenuation, and breast attenuation in female patients may cause false-positive results (false perfusion defects).

In conjunction with exercise or pharmacologic vasodilatation stress testing, technetium Tc 99m teboroxime should be administered at the inception of a period of maximum stress that is continued for approximately 30 to 60 seconds after injection.

High liver extraction of technetium Tc 99m teboroxime may interfere with visualization of the inferior wall of the heart. Positioning the patient upright during image acquisition is helpful in minimizing the contribution of liver activity, since in the upright position the liver tends to drop downward, allowing better separation of the cardiac and hepatic activities.

For either rest or stress studies, imaging must begin within 2 to 5 minutes after injection of technetium Tc 99m teboroxime and must be completed within 5 to 10 minutes. After 5 minutes, differential washout of technetium Tc 99m teboroxime begins to introduce artifacts. If image acquisition takes too long, perfusion defects can become less apparent before acquisition is complete, resulting in an underestimation of the number and severity of ischemic segments. A significant amount of the initial myocardial activity is cleared by 20 to 30 minutes after administration.

Rapid myocardial washout and early hepatic uptake necessitates use of rapid imaging protocols, and may require a multiple-headed single-photon emission computed tomography (SPECT) camera to complete image acquisition in 3 to 4 minutes.

**For studies performed in conjunction with pharmacologic stress testing**
Pharmacologic stress, induced by intravenous adenosine or dipyridamole, may be preferred for stress/rest studies using technetium Tc 99m teboroxime since the patient can be infused while in position under the camera, thus eliminating delays between tracer injection and the start of image acquisition.

Technetium Tc 99m teboroxime is usually administered during the third minute of the 4- to 5-minute infusion of adenosine, or 2 minutes after the 4-minute dipyridamole infusion.

## Parenteral Dosage Forms

### TECHNETIUM Tc 99m TEBOROXIME INJECTION

**Usual adult and adolescent administered activity**
Cardiac imaging—
Intravenous, 555 to 1110 megabecquerels (15 to 30 millicuries).

Note: Due to the short residence time of technetium Tc 99m teboroxime in the myocardium, two separate injections are needed for a stress/rest perfusion study.

When a stress study is to be performed prior to a rest study, it is recommended that an interval of 1½ hours be allowed for the effects of exercise to dissipate.

For same-day rest/stress studies, a combined dose of 1295 to 1850 megabecquerels (35 to 50 millicuries) is used.

When a rest study is to be performed prior to a stress study, it is only necessary to wait until the residual myocardial activity clears. In most cases, the stress study may be performed in one hour.

**Usual pediatric administered activity**
Minimum dosage has not been established.

**Usual geriatric administered activity**
See *Usual adult and adolescent administered activity*.

**Strength(s) usually available**
U.S.—
2 mg of cyclohexanedione dioxime, 2 mg of methyl boronic acid, 2 mg pentetic acid, 9 mg citric acid (anhydrous), 100 mg sodium chloride, 50 mg gamma cyclodextrin, and 50 mcg stannous chloride (anhydrous) in lyophilized form under nitrogen atmosphere, per 5-mL reaction vial (Rx) [*CardioTec*].

Note: Technetium Tc 99m teboroxime is a boronic acid technetium dioxime (BATO) derivative.

Canada—
Not commercially available.

**Safety considerations for handling this radiopharmaceutical**
Improper handling of this radiopharmaceutical may cause radioactive contamination. Guidelines for handling radioactive material have been prepared by scientific, professional, state, federal, and international bodies and are available to the specially qualified and authorized users who have access to radiopharmaceuticals.

**Packaging and storage**
Store between 15 and 30 °C (59 and 86 °F), unless otherwise specified by manufacturer. Protect from freezing.

Note: Before radiolabeling, the kit is also stored at room temperature.

**Preparation of dosage form**
To prepare technetium Tc 99m teboroxime injection, an oxidant-free sodium pertechnetate Tc 99m solution is used.

During reconstitution, it is important that air is not added to the nitrogen atmosphere of the vial, since air will cause oxidation, thus decreasing the radiochemical purity of the compound.

See manufacturer's package insert for complete instructions.

**Stability**
Product is stable (24-month shelf life before radiolabeling); U.S. package insert states that injection should be administered within 6 hours after preparation since it does not contain a preservative.

**Incompatibilities**
If oxidants such as peroxides and hypochlorites are present in the sodium pertechnetate Tc 99m used for labeling, the final preparation may be adversely affected and should be discarded. Final preparation should appear clear to slightly opalescent and free of particulate matter and discoloration.

**Note**
Caution—Radioactive material.

### Selected Bibliography

Meerdink DJ, Leppo JA. Experimental studies of the physiologic properties of technetium-99m agents: myocardial transport of perfusion imaging agents. Am J Cardiol 1990; 66(13): 9E-15E.

Berman DS, Kiat H, Van Train KF, et al. Comparison of SPECT using technetium-99m agents and thallium-201 and PET for the assessment of myocardial perfusion and viability. Am J Cardiol 1990; 66(13): 72E-79E.

Johnson LL, Seldin DW. Clinical experience with technetium-99m teboroxime, a neutral, lipophilic myocardial perfusion imaging agent. Am J Cardiol 1990; 66: 63E-67E.

Revised: 05/18/95

---

# TECHNETIUM TC 99M TETROFOSMIN  Systemic†

VA CLASSIFICATION (Primary): DX201

Commonly used brand name(s): *Myoview*.

Note: For a listing of dosage forms and brand names by country availability, see *Dosage Forms* section(s).

†Not commercially available in Canada.

## Category
Diagnostic aid, radioactive (cardiac disease).

## Indications

**Accepted**
Cardiac imaging, radionuclide
Myocardial infarction (diagnosis) or
Myocardial perfusion imaging, radionuclide—Technetium Tc 99m tetrofosmin is indicated in myocardial perfusion imaging to distinguish regions of reversible myocardial ischemia in the presence or absence of infarcted myocardium, following separate administration under stress and rest conditions.

## Physical Properties

**Nuclear Data**

| Radionuclide (half-life) | Decay constant | Mode of decay | Principal photon emissions (keV) | Mean number of photons/ disintegration (≥0.01) |
|---|---|---|---|---|
| Tc 99m (6 hr) | 0.1151 h$^{-1}$ | Isomeric transition to Tc 99 | Gamma (18) | 0.062 |
| | | | Gamma (140.5) | 0.891 |

## Pharmacology/Pharmacokinetics

**Mechanism of action/Effect**
The mechanisms for uptake and retention of technetium Tc 99m tetrofosmin by myocardial tissue are not well established. Technetium Tc 99m tetrofosmin is a lipophilic cationic agent (diphosphine group). The myocardial uptake of technetium Tc 99m tetrofosmin appears to occur by a passive diffusion process. When injected at rest, technetium Tc 99m tetrofosmin appears to accumulate in viable myocardial tissue; infarcts are thus delineated as areas that lack accumulation. When injected at stress, technetium Tc 99m tetrofosmin accumulates in viable myocardial tissue in relation to myocardial blood flow; thus, ischemic areas (e.g., those supplied by stenotic vessels) are detectable as areas of less accumulation.

**Distribution**
Technetium Tc 99m tetrofosmin is rapidly cleared from the blood after intravenous administration (< 5% of administered activity remains in blood by 10 minutes postinjection), accumulating in myocardium, skeletal muscle, liver, spleen, and kidneys in proportion to the regional perfusion. Uptake in myocardium is approximately 1.2% of the administered activity 5 minutes after injection, and approximately 1% at 2 hours. Once technetium Tc 99m tetrofosmin is taken up by the myocardium, there is no, or minimal, redistribution over the following 3 to 4 hours. Washout from the myocardium is slow (4% of myocardial activity per hour postexercise).

Following injection at peak exercise, activity in the liver is lower than that in the heart as early as 5 minutes postinjection, with further decline over time (< 4.5% by 60 minutes). The gallbladder shows slightly higher activity than the heart in the first 15 minutes.

Sequestration of activity by skeletal muscle is enhanced during exercise (probably due to a relative increase in the blood flow to skeletal tissue), but significantly reduced in all other organ systems.

**Time to radioactivity visualization**
Imaging is generally performed at 15 minutes after injection during stress, and at 30 to 60 minutes after injection during rest (delay allows for

hepatic clearance). Imaging is possible for up to 4 hours due to the slow washout of technetium Tc 99m tetrofosmin from myocardium.

Note: Heart-to-liver activity ratios may be dependent on the applied stress condition (e.g., exercise vs. dipyridamole injection). Higher heart-to-liver ratios occur with exercise than with dipyridamole stress.

### Radiation dosimetry

| Organ | Estimated absorbed radiation dose* | | | |
|---|---|---|---|---|
| | With exercise | | At rest | |
| | mGy/MBq | rad/mCi | mGy/MBq | rad/mCi |
| Gallbladder wall | 0.027 | 0.1 | 0.036 | 0.13 |
| Large intestine (upper) | 0.02 | 0.075 | 0.027 | 0.1 |
| Large intestine (lower) | 0.015 | 0.057 | 0.02 | 0.075 |
| Bladder wall | 0.014 | 0.052 | 0.017 | 0.063 |
| Small intestine | 0.012 | 0.045 | 0.015 | 0.057 |
| Ovaries | 0.0077 | 0.029 | 0.0088 | 0.033 |
| Uterus | 0.0071 | 0.026 | 0.0078 | 0.029 |
| Bone surfaces | 0.0062 | 0.023 | 0.0056 | 0.021 |
| Heart wall | 0.0051 | 0.019 | 0.0046 | 0.017 |
| Pancreas | 0.0047 | 0.017 | 0.0045 | 0.017 |
| Thyroid | 0.0047 | 0.017 | 0.0055 | 0.02 |
| Stomach | 0.0044 | 0.016 | 0.0044 | 0.016 |
| Kidneys | 0.0042 | 0.016 | 0.0041 | 0.015 |
| Adrenal glands | 0.004 | 0.015 | 0.0037 | 0.014 |
| Red bone marrow | 0.0038 | 0.014 | 0.0036 | 0.013 |
| Spleen | 0.0038 | 0.014 | 0.0034 | 0.013 |
| Muscle | 0.0034 | 0.013 | 0.0032 | 0.012 |
| Testes | 0.0033 | 0.012 | 0.003 | 0.011 |
| Thymus | 0.0032 | 0.012 | 0.0027 | 0.01 |
| Liver | 0.0031 | 0.012 | 0.0037 | 0.014 |
| Lungs | 0.0032 | 0.012 | 0.0027 | 0.01 |
| Brain | 0.0027 | 0.01 | 0.0022 | 0.008 |
| Breasts | 0.0023 | 0.008 | 0.0019 | 0.007 |
| Skin | 0.0022 | 0.008 | 0.0019 | 0.007 |
| Total body | 0.0037 | 0.014 | 0.0036 | 0.013 |

| Radionuclide | Effective dose* | | | |
|---|---|---|---|---|
| | With exercise | | At rest | |
| | mSv/MBq | rem/mCi | mSv/MBq | rem/mCi |
| Tc 99m | 0.0071 | 0.026 | 0.0082 | 0.03 |

*For adults; intravenous injection. Data based on the Radiopharmaceutical Internal Dose Information Center, August 1996. Oak Ridge Institute for Science and Education.

### Elimination
Within 48 hours—
Renal, approximately 40% of the administered activity under both rest and exercise conditions.
Fecal, approximately 26 to 41% (mean, 34%) of the administered activity at rest, and approximately 17 to 34% (mean, 25%) after exercise.

## Precautions to Consider

### Carcinogenicity
Long-term animal studies to evaluate carcinogenic potential of technetium Tc 99m tetrofosmin have not been performed.

### Mutagenicity
Tetrofosmin has not been shown to be mutagenic *in vitro* in the Ames test, mouse lymphoma and human lymphocyte tests, and in *in vivo* mouse micronucleus assay.

### Pregnancy/Reproduction
Pregnancy—Tc 99m (as free pertechnetate) crosses the placenta. However, studies to assess transplacental transfer of technetium Tc 99m tetrofosmin have not been done in humans.
The possibility of pregnancy should be assessed in women of child-bearing potential. Clinical situations exist in which the benefit to the patient and fetus from information derived from radiopharmaceutical use outweighs the risks from fetal exposure to radiation. In these situations, the physician should use discretion and reduce the administered activity of the radiopharmaceutical to the lowest practical amount.
Studies have not been done in animals.
FDA Pregnancy Category C.

### Breast-feeding
Although it is not known whether technetium Tc 99m tetrofosmin is distributed into breast milk, it is known that Tc 99m as free pertechnetate is distributed into breast milk. To avoid radiation exposure to the infant, discontinuation of nursing for a period of 24 hours is recommended after administration of technetium Tc 99m–labeled radiopharmaceuticals.

### Pediatrics
Although technetium Tc 99m tetrofosmin is used in children, there have been no specific studies evaluating safety and efficacy.

### Geriatrics
Appropriate studies on the relationship of age to the effects of technetium Tc 99m tetrofosmin have not been performed in the geriatric population. However, clinical trials and studies that included older patients were conducted, and geriatrics-specific problems that would limit the usefulness of this agent in the elderly are not expected.

### Medical considerations/Contraindications
The medical considerations/contraindications included have been selected on the basis of their potential clinical significance (reasons given in parentheses where appropriate)—not necessarily inclusive (» = major clinical significance).

*Risk-benefit should be considered when the following medical problem exists:*
Sensitivity to the radiopharmaceutical preparation

## Side/Adverse Effects
The following side/adverse effects have been selected on the basis of their potential clinical significance (possible signs and symptoms in parentheses where appropriate)—not necessarily inclusive:

**Those indicating need for medical attention**
Incidence rare
*Allergic reaction* (skin rash; troubled breathing); **angina** (chest pain); **hypertension**

**Those indicating need for medical attention only if they continue or are bothersome**
Incidence less frequent or rare
*Burning sensation in hard palate; gastrointestinal symptoms* (abdominal or stomach discomfort; vomiting); **hypotension** (lightheadedness; dizziness); *metallic taste; unusual smell*

## Patient Consultation
As an aid to patient consultation, refer to *Advice for the Patient, Radiopharmaceuticals (Diagnostic).*
In providing consultation, consider emphasizing the following selected information (» = major clinical significance):

**Description of use**
Action in the body: Accumulation of radioactivity in myocardial cells as a function of relative blood flow
Differences in uptake of radioactivity can be visualized
Small amounts of radioactivity used in diagnosis; radiation received is low and considered safe

**Before having this test**
» Conditions affecting use, especially:
Sensitivity to the radiopharmaceutical preparation
Pregnancy—Technetium Tc 99m (as free pertechnetate) crosses placenta; risk to fetus from radiation exposure as opposed to benefit derived from study should be considered
Breast-feeding—Not known if technetium Tc 99m tetrofosmin is distributed into breast milk, but Tc 99m as free pertechnetate is distributed into breast milk; temporary discontinuation of nursing is recommended to avoid any unnecessary absorbed radiation dose to the infant

**Preparation for this test**
Fasting for at least 2 hours before the exercise test
Other special preparatory instructions may also be given; patient should inquire in advance

**Precautions after having this test**
Adequate intake of fluids and voiding as often as possible after examination to minimize radiation exposure to bladder

**Side/adverse effects**
Signs of potential side effects, especially allergic reaction, angina, and hypertension

## General Dosing Information
Radiopharmaceuticals are to be administered only by or under the supervision of physicians who have had extensive training in the safe use

and handling of radioactive materials and who are licensed by the Nuclear Regulatory Commission (NRC) or the appropriate Agreement State agency, if required, or, outside the U.S., the appropriate authority.

Fasting is usually recommended, or at least 2 hours should elapse after a light breakfast, before the exercise test.

Adequate hydration of the patient is recommended before and after examination to promote urinary flow. Also, urination is recommended as often as possible after the examination to reduce bladder exposure to radiation.

For exercise studies, imaging may be started as early as 5 minutes after injection of technetium Tc 99m tetrofosmin, with imaging generally performed at 15 minutes. For rest imaging, a delay of 30 minutes is needed in most patients after the administration of technetium Tc 99m tetrofosmin to allow clearance of the tracer from the liver.

**Safety considerations for handling this radiopharmaceutical**
Guidelines for the receipt, storage, handling, dispensing, and disposal of radioactive materials are available from scientific, professional, state, federal, and international bodies. Handling of this radiopharmaceutical should be limited to those individuals who are appropriately qualified and authorized.

## Parenteral Dosage Forms

### TECHNETIUM Tc 99m TETROFOSMIN INJECTION

**Usual adult and adolescent administered activity**
Cardiac imaging—
  Intravenous, 185 to 296 megabecquerels (5 to 8 millicuries) administered at peak exercise; then 555 to 888 megabecquerels (15 to 24 millicuries) administered 4 hours later, at rest.

Note: A two-day protocol has been found to increase image quality. According to this protocol, the rest and stress imaging studies are performed on two separate days; patients receive 500 megabecquerels (14 millicuries) of technetium Tc 99m tetrofosmin on each day.

Also, a combined myocardial imaging protocol involving thallous chloride Tl 201 scintigraphy at rest followed by technetium Tc 99m tetrofosmin imaging after stress is being used. It involves the intravenous administration at rest of 74 megabecquerels (2 millicuries) of thallous chloride Tl 201, with imaging performed 20 minutes postinjection, followed by the administration of 370 megabecquerels (10 millicuries) of technetium Tc 99m tetrofosmin at 4 minutes of exercise, with imaging performed 20 minutes after the completion of the stress test. This combined thallium/tetrofosmin protocol requires a total time of 90 minutes.

**Usual pediatric administered activity**
Minimum dosage has not been established.

**Usual geriatric administered activity**
See *Usual adult and adolescent administered activity*.

**Strength(s) usually available**
U.S.—
  0.23 mg tetrofosmin, 0.03 mg stannous chloride dihydrate, 0.32 mg disodium sulfosalicylate, 1 mg sodium D-gluconate, and 1.8 mg sodium hydrogen carbonate in lyophilized form under nitrogen atmosphere, per vial (Rx) [*Myoview*].
Canada—
  Not commercially available.

**Packaging and storage**
Store between 2 and 25 °C (36 and 77 °F), unless otherwise specified by manufacturer. Protect from freezing.

Note: Before radiolabeling, the kit must be stored between 2 and 8 °C (36 and 46 °F), and protected from light.

**Preparation of dosage form**
To prepare technetium Tc 99m tetrofosmin injection, an oxidant-free sodium pertechnetate Tc 99m solution is used.
Preparation of technetium Tc 99m tetrofosmin injection does not require heating. Instead, a 15-minute incubation period at room temperature is sufficient after radiolabeling.
See manufacturer's package insert for complete instructions.

**Stability**
Product is stable ( 90% radiochemical purity is maintained for 8 hours after reconstitution). Package insert states that injection should be administered within 8 hours after preparation since it does not contain a preservative.

**Incompatibilities**
If oxidants such as peroxides and hypochlorites are present in the sodium pertechnetate Tc 99m used for labeling, the final preparation may be adversely affected and should be discarded. Final preparation should appear clear and free of particulate matter.

**Note**
Caution—Radioactive material.

Developed: 12/04/96

---

**TEMAZEPAM**—See *Benzodiazepines (Systemic)*

---

**TENOXICAM**—See *Anti-inflammatory Drugs, Nonsteroidal (Systemic)*

---

# TENIPOSIDE   Systemic—INTRODUCTORY VERSION

VA CLASSIFICATION (Primary): AN900
Commonly used brand name(s): *Vumon*.
Another commonly used name is VM-26.
Note: For a listing of dosage forms and brand names by country availability, see *Dosage Forms* section(s).

## Category
Antineoplastic.

## Indications

**Accepted**
Leukemia, acute lymphocytic (treatment)—Teniposide is indicated, in combination with other approved anticancer agents, for induction therapy of refractory childhood acute lymphocytic (lymphoblastic) leukemia.

## Pharmacology/Pharmacokinetics

**Physicochemical characteristics**
Source—Semisynthetic derivative of podophyllotoxin.
Chemical group—Podophyllotoxin.
Molecular weight—656.66.
pH—Approximately 5 (adjusted with maleic acid).
Other characteristics—Lipophilic.
Solubility—Insoluble in water and ether; slightly soluble in methanol and very soluble in acetone and dimethylformamide.
Partition coefficient—Octanol/water: Approximately 100.

**Mechanism of action/Effect**
Teniposide is a topoisomerase II inhibitor. It acts at the premitotic stage of cell division to prevent cells from entering mitosis by causing dose-dependent single- and double-stranded breaks in DNA and DNA-protein cross-links. It does not intercalate into or bind strongly to DNA. It is cell phase–specific, acting in the late S or early $G_2$ phase of cell division.

**Distribution**
Limited, probably because of very high plasma protein binding. Mean steady-state volumes of distribution range from 8 to 44 liters per square meter of body surface area ($L/m^2$) in adults and 3 to 11 $L/m^2$ in children. The steady-state volume of distribution is inversely related to plasma albumin concentrations. Teniposide crosses the blood-brain barrier to only a limited extent, although one study found higher concentrations of teniposide in the cerebrospinal fluid (CSF) of patients with brain tumors than in the CSF of patients who did not have brain tumors. Concentrations in saliva, CSF, and malignant ascites fluid are low compared to simultaneous plasma concentrations.

**Protein binding**
Very high (greater than 99%).

**Half-life**
Terminal—
  5 hours.

**Teniposide (Systemic)—Introductory Version**

Note: Plasma teniposide concentrations decline biexponentially following intravenous infusion.

**Peak plasma concentration**
Greater than 40 micrograms per mL (mcg/mL) after intravenous infusions of 137 to 203 mg per square meter of body surface area over a period of 1 to 2 hours in pediatric patients. Concentrations generally declined to less than 2 mcg/mL by 20 to 24 hours after the infusion.

**Elimination**
Renal, 4 to 12% of a dose as unchanged teniposide. In a study of tritium-labeled teniposide in adults, 44% of the radiolabel (parent compound and metabolites) was recovered in urine within 120 hours after dosing.
Fecal, 0 to 10% of a dose.

## Precautions to Consider

### Carcinogenicity
Children with acute lymphocytic leukemia (ALL) in remission who were given maintenance therapy with teniposide once or twice a week (in combination with other antineoplastics) were found to have an approximately twelvefold increase in relative risk of developing secondary acute nonlymphocytic leukemia (ANLL), compared to patients treated with less intensive schedules.

No association was found between a short course of teniposide for induction of remission or consolidation and an increased risk of secondary ANLL, but the number of patients studied was small.

Studies in animals have not been done.

### Mutagenicity
Teniposide has been found to be mutagenic in bacterial and mammalian tests including Ames/*Salmonella* and *B. subtilis* bacterial mutagenicity assays. It caused gene mutations in both Chinese hamster ovary cells and mouse lymphoma cells and DNA damage (as measured by alkaline elution) in human lung carcinoma–derived cell lines. Teniposide also caused aberrations in chromosome structure in primary cultures of human lymphocytes *in vitro* and in L5178y/TK +/− mouse lymphoma cells *in vitro*. Chromosome aberrations were observed *in vivo* in the embryonic tissue of pregnant Swiss albino mice. Teniposide also caused a dose-related increase in sister chromatid exchanges in Chinese hamster ovary cells.

### Pregnancy/Reproduction
Pregnancy—Adequate and well-controlled studies in humans have not been done.

In general, it is recommended that women of childbearing age be advised to avoid becoming pregnant during therapy with teniposide. If a woman becomes pregnant during treatment with teniposide, it is recommended that she be informed of the potential risk to the fetus.

Intravenous administration of teniposide to pregnant rats in doses between 1 and 3 mg per kg of body weight (mg/kg) per day on alternate days from day 6 to day 16 postcoitum (during organogenesis) caused retarded embryonic development, prenatal mortality, and teratogenicity (including spinal and rib defects, deformed extremities, anophthalmia, and celosomia).

FDA Pregnancy Category D.

### Breast-feeding
It is not known whether teniposide is distributed into breast milk. However, it is recommended that any decision regarding breast-feeding during teniposide therapy should take into account the potential risk to the infant.

### Pediatrics
Children with Down syndrome may be more sensitive to the effects of this medicine compared to other children.

### Geriatrics
One case of sudden death attributed to probable arrhythmia and intractable hypotension has been reported in an elderly patient treated with teniposide for a nonleukemic malignancy.

### Drug interactions and/or related problems
The following drug interactions and/or related problems have been selected on the basis of their potential clinical significance (possible mechanism in parentheses where appropriate)—not necessarily inclusive (» = major clinical significance):

Note: Combinations containing any of the following medications, depending on the amount present, may also interact with this medication.

Antiemetics
(the risk of acute central nervous system depression and hypotension may be increased during concurrent use, especially with higher-than-recommended doses of teniposide, probably because of the depressant effects of both the antiemetic and the alcohol present in the teniposide injection)

Methotrexate
(concurrent use with teniposide may slightly increase the plasma clearance of methotrexate; an increase in intracellular concentrations of methotrexate has been observed in the presence of teniposide *in vitro*)

» Sodium salicylate or
» Sulfamethizole or
» Tolbutamide
(therapeutic concentrations of sodium salicylate, sulfamethizole, or tolbutamide have been shown to cause small but significant displacement of teniposide from plasma protein binding sites, which could lead to substantial increases in free plasma teniposide concentrations and, possibly, increased toxicity)

### Medical considerations/Contraindications
The medical considerations/contraindications included have been selected on the basis of their potential clinical significance (reasons given in parentheses where appropriate)—not necessarily inclusive (» = major clinical significance).

*Risk-benefit should be considered when the following medical problems exist:*

» Down syndrome
(patients may be especially sensitive to the myelosuppressive effects of teniposide; a 50% reduction in initial dosage is recommended)

Hepatic function impairment or
Renal function impairment
(caution is recommended, since increases in serum alkaline phosphatase or gamma-glutamyl transpeptidase have been associated with a decrease in the plasma clearance of teniposide and approximately 10% of a dose is eliminated unchanged in the urine; dosage adjustment may be necessary in patients with significant hepatic or renal function impairment)

» Hypoalbuminemia
(the steady-state volume of distribution of teniposide increases with a decrease in plasma albumin concentrations; careful monitoring is recommended)

» Sensitivity to teniposide or to castor oil
hypersensitivity reactions to teniposide injection may be caused by the medication itself or by the polyoxyethylated castor oil present in the injection; patients who are known to be sensitive to castor oil, or who have experienced a previous hypersensitivity reaction to teniposide, should be treated with teniposide only if the benefit clearly outweighs the risk of a probable hypersensitivity reaction

### Patient monitoring
The following may be especially important in patient monitoring (other tests may be warranted in some patients, depending on condition; » = major clinical significance):

» Hemoglobin concentration and
» Leukocyte count, total and, if appropriate, differential and
» Platelet count
(determinations recommended prior to initiation of therapy and at periodic intervals during therapy)

Hepatic function and
Renal function
(determinations recommended prior to initiation of therapy and at periodic intervals during therapy)

» Vital signs
(continuous monitoring recommended for at least the first 60 minutes after the start of a teniposide infusion and at periodic intervals thereafter, to detect possible signs of a hypersensitivity reaction, including anaphylaxis)

## Side/Adverse Effects

The following side/adverse effects have been selected on the basis of their potential clinical significance (possible signs and symptoms in parentheses where appropriate)—not necessarily inclusive:

### Those indicating need for medical attention
Incidence more frequent
*Anemia* (unusual tiredness)—usually asymptomatic; *hypersensitivity reaction* (chills; fever; flushing of the face; hives; hypertension or hypotension; rapid heartbeat; shortness of breath, troubled breathing, tightness in chest, or wheezing); *leukopenia or neutropenia* (fever or chills; cough or hoarseness; lower back or side pain; painful or difficult urination)—symptomatic only if neutropenic fever occurs; *mucositis* (sores in mouth and on lips); *thrombocytopenia* (unusual bleeding or bruising; black, tarry stools; blood in urine or stools; pinpoint red spots on skin)—usually asymptomatic

Note: Bone marrow depression (*leukopenia* or *thrombocytopenia*) may be severe. It is characterized by an early onset and delayed recovery. Bone marrow hypoplasia is a desired end point of therapy in refractory acute lymphocytic leukemia.

The occurrence of *hypersensitivity reactions* appears to be increased in patients with brain tumors or neuroblastoma. Hypersensitivity reactions, including anaphylaxis-like symptoms, may occur on initial or after repeated exposure to teniposide, and may be life-threatening if not treated promptly.

Incidence less frequent
*Hypotension*—usually asymptomatic; *skin rash*

Note: Transient *hypotension* has been reported following rapid intravenous administration.

Incidence rare
*Hepatic function impairment* (yellow eyes or skin)—usually asymptomatic; *neurotoxicity; renal function impairment* (decreased urination; swelling of face, fingers, feet, or lower legs)

**Those indicating need for medical attention only if they continue or are bothersome**
Incidence more frequent
*Nausea or vomiting*—usually mild to moderate; *diarrhea*

**Those not indicating need for medical attention**
Incidence more frequent
*Loss of hair*

Note: *Alopecia*, sometimes progressing to total baldness, is usually reversible.

## Overdose

For more information on the management of overdose or unintentional ingestion, **contact a Poison Control Center** (see *Poison Control Center Listing*).

**Clinical effects of overdose**
The following effects have been selected on the basis of their potential clinical significance (possible signs and symptoms in parentheses where appropriate)—not necessarily inclusive:

Acute and chronic
**Bone marrow suppression** (fever; chills; cough or hoarseness; lower back or side pain; painful or difficult urination; unusual bleeding or bruising; black, tarry stools; blood in urine or stools; pinpoint red spots on skin)

**Treatment of overdose**
Supportive blood product and antibiotic therapy, as indicated, is recommended. There is no known antidote.

## Patient Consultation

As an aid to patient consultation, refer to *Advice for the Patient, Teniposide (Systemic)—Introductory Version*.
In providing consultation, consider emphasizing the following selected information (» = major clinical significance):

**Before using this medication**
» Conditions affecting use, especially:
Sensitivity to teniposide or castor oil
Carcinogenicity—Secondary acute nonlymphocytic leukemia (ANLL) reported
Pregnancy—Use not recommended because of embryotoxic and teratogenic effects in animal studies; notifying physician immediately if pregnancy is suspected
Breast-feeding—Potential risks to the infant should be considered
Other medications, especially sodium salicylate, sulfamethizole, or tolbutamide
Other medical problems, especially Down syndrome or hypoalbuminemia

**Proper use of this medication**
Importance of continuing treatment even if nausea or vomiting occurs
» Proper dosing

**Precautions while using this medication**
» Importance of close monitoring by the physician
Possibility of local tissue injury and scarring if infiltration occurs; telling physician or nurse right away if redness, pain, swelling, or lump under the skin occurs at injection site
» Avoiding immunizations unless approved by physician
Avoiding exposure to persons with bacterial infections, especially during periods of low blood counts

Caution in use of regular toothbrush, dental floss, or toothpick
Not touching eyes or inside of nose unless hands washed immediately before
Caution in activities that may result in cuts, bruises, or injuries

**Side/adverse effects**
Informing physician or nurse immediately if symptoms of a hypersensitivity reaction occur during an injection
Signs of other potential side effects, especially anemia, leukopenia or neutropenia, mucositis, thrombocytopenia, skin rash, hepatic function impairment, neurotoxicity, and renal function impairment
Possibility of hair loss

## General Dosing Information

Patients receiving teniposide should be under the supervision of a physician experienced in cancer chemotherapy.

Teniposide injection must be diluted prior to use. It should be administered by slow intravenous infusion over a period of at least 30 to 60 minutes to prevent hypotension.

Care must be taken to avoid extravasation during intravenous administration, which can result in tissue necrosis and/or thrombophlebitis.

Equipment and medications (including epinephrine and oxygen) necessary for treatment of a possible anaphylactic reaction should be immediately available during each administration of teniposide.

If treatment is reinstituted in a patient who has previously had a hypersensitivity reaction to teniposide, pretreatment with corticosteroids and antihistamines, along with careful clinical observation during and after the infusion, are recommended.

Since occlusion of central venous access devices has occurred during 24-hour teniposide infusions in concentrations of 0.1 to 0.2 mg per mL, frequent observation is recommended to minimize the risk.

**Safety considerations for handling this medication**
The procedure for the preparation, handling, and disposal of teniposide should be the same as that used with other antineoplastic agents.
Direct contact of skin or mucosa with teniposide requires immediate washing with soap and water or thoroughly flushing with water, respectively.
The use of disposable surgical gloves is recommended.

**Combination chemotherapy**
Teniposide may be used in combination with other agents in various regimens. As a result, the incidence and/or severity of side effects may be altered and different dosages (usually reduced) may be used. For example, teniposide is part of the following chemotherapeutic combinations:
—teniposide and cytarabine.
—teniposide and vincristine and prednisone.
For specific dosages and schedules, consult the literature. For information regarding each agent, consult the individual monographs.

**For treatment of adverse effects**
It is recommended that the teniposide infusion be discontinued if significant hypotension develops, and administration of fluids or other supportive therapy be instituted as appropriate. Blood pressure usually returns to normal within hours. If the infusion is then re-started, the administration rate should be reduced and the patient carefully monitored.

It is recommended that anaphylaxis be treated by stopping the infusion immediately and administering antihistamines, corticosteroids, epinephrine, intravenous fluids, and other supportive measures as indicated.

## Parenteral Dosage Forms

### TENIPOSIDE INJECTION

**Usual pediatric dose**
Leukemia, acute lymphocytic—
Intravenous infusion (over at least 30 to 60 minutes), 165 mg per square meter of body surface area two times per week for eight or nine doses, given in combination with intravenous cytarabine (300 mg per square meter of body surface area two times a week for eight or nine doses), or
Intravenous infusion (over at least 30 to 60 minutes), 250 mg per square meter of body surface area once a week for four to eight weeks, given in combination with intravenous vincristine (1.5 mg per square meter of body surface area once a week for four to eight weeks) and oral prednisone (40 mg per square meter of body surface area per day for twenty-eight days).

Note: It is recommended that the first course of teniposide in patients with Down syndrome be given at one half the usual dose. Subsequent courses may utilize higher doses, depending on the degree of myelosuppression and mucositis occurring in previous courses.

## Teniposide (Systemic)—Introductory Version

**Strength(s) usually available**
U.S.—
 10 mg per mL (50 mg per 5-ml ampul) (Rx) [*Vumon* (benzyl alcohol; N,N-dimethylacetamide; polyoxyethylated castor oil; dehydrated alcohol; maleic acid)].

**Packaging and storage**
Store between 2 and 8 °C (36 and 46 °F). The injection is not adversely affected by freezing.

**Preparation of dosage form**
Teniposide injection is prepared for intravenous infusion by dilution with 5% dextrose injection or 0.9% sodium chloride injection to produce a final concentration of 100, 200, or 400 mcg (0.1, 0.2, or 0.3 mg, respectively) or 1 mg of teniposide per mL.

Use of polyvinyl chloride (PVC) containers is not recommended, because of possible leaching of diethylhexylphthalate (DEHP) from PVC bags into the medication. Use of non–DEHP-containing containers, such as glass or polyolefin plastic bags or containers, is recommended instead. Also, non–DEHP intravenous administrations sets, such as lipid administration sets or low DEHP-containing nitroglycerin sets, are recommended. Contact of undiluted (but not diluted) teniposide injection with plastic equipment or devices used to prepare an infusion may result in softening or cracking and possible product leakage.

Caution—Use of products containing benzyl alcohol is generally not recommended for preparation of medications for use in neonates. A fatal toxic syndrome consisting of metabolic acidosis, central nervous system depression, respiratory problems, renal failure, hypotension, and possibly seizures and intracranial hemorrhages has been associated with this use.

**Stability**
It is recommended that teniposide infusions containing 1 mg per mL be administered within 4 hours of preparation to reduce the possibility of precipitation. Teniposide injections that have been diluted to concentrations of 0.1 to 1 mg per mL are chemically stable for up to 24 hours at ambient room temperature and lighting conditions. After dilution, the injection should not be refrigerated. The type of container in which the medication is kept (glass or plastic) does not affect stability.

Precipitation has been reported during 24-hour intravenous infusions of teniposide in concentrations of 0.1 to 0.2 mg per mL, leading to occlusion of central venous access catheters. Precipitation may also occur if the diluted solution is subjected to excessive agitation during preparation. Storage time prior to administration should be kept to a minimum.

**Incompatibilities**
Heparin can cause precipitation of teniposide; therefore, the administration set should be flushed thoroughly with 5% dextrose injection or 0.9% sodium chloride injection before and after administration of teniposide.

Developed: 09/30/97
Interim revision: 08/14/98

# TERAZOSIN   Systemic

VA CLASSIFICATION (Primary/Secondary): CV150/CV409; GU900
Commonly used brand name(s): *Hytrin*.
Note: For a listing of dosage forms and brand names by country availability, see *Dosage Forms* section(s).

## Category
Antihypertensive; benign prostatic hyperplasia therapy agent.

## Indications

**Accepted**
Hypertension (treatment)—Terazosin is indicated in the treatment of hypertension.

Benign prostatic hyperplasia[1]—Terazosin is indicated in the treatment of symptomatic benign prostatic hyperplasia (BPH). It has been shown to improve urinary flow and symptoms of BPH. However, the long-term effects of terazosin on the incidence of surgery, acute urinary obstruction, or other complications of BPH have not yet been determined.

[1]Not included in Canadian product labeling.

## Pharmacology/Pharmacokinetics

**Physicochemical characteristics**
Molecular weight—459.93.
pKa—7.04.

**Mechanism of action/Effect**
Terazosin has a peripheral post-synaptic alpha$_1$-adrenergic blocking action, which is thought to account primarily for its effects.
Hypertension—
 Terazosin produces vasodilation and reduces peripheral resistance but generally has little effect on cardiac output. Antihypertensive effect with chronic dosing is usually not accompanied by reflex tachycardia. There is little or no effect on renal blood flow or glomerular filtration rate.
Benign prostatic hyperplasia—
 Relaxation of smooth muscle in the bladder neck, prostate, and prostate capsule produced by alpha$_1$-adrenergic blockade results in a reduction in urethral resistance and pressure, bladder outlet resistance, and urinary symptoms.

**Other actions/effects**
Terazosin may affect serum lipids. The most consistent changes observed are a decrease in levels of serum total cholesterol and low density lipoprotein (LDL) cholesterol plus very low density lipoprotein (VLDL) cholesterol fraction. However, the implications of these changes are unclear.

**Absorption**
Rapid and nearly complete; not affected by food; minimal first-pass metabolism; bioavailability approximately 90%.

**Protein binding**
Very high (90 to 94%).

**Biotransformation**
Hepatic; four metabolites have been identified, one of which (the piperazine derivative of terazosin) has antihypertensive activity.

**Half-life**
Approximately 12 hours; does not appear to be significantly influenced by renal insufficiency.

**Onset of action**
Single dose—15 minutes.

**Time to peak plasma concentration**
Approximately 1 hour.

**Time to peak effect**
Single dose—2 to 3 hours.
Multiple doses—Up to 6 to 8 weeks.

**Duration of action**
Single dose—24 hours.

**Elimination**
Fecal (biliary)—40%.
Fecal (unchanged)—20%.
Renal—40% (10% unchanged).

## Precautions to Consider

**Carcinogenicity**
Studies in rats for two years at doses of 250 mg per kg of body weight (mg/kg) per day (695 times the maximum recommended human dose [MRHD]) found an increase in benign adrenal medullary tumors in male, but not in female, rats. Studies in mice for two years at a maximum tolerated dose of 32 mg/kg per day found no oncogenic effect.

**Mutagenicity**
Both *in vivo* and *in vitro* tests (Ames test, *in vivo* cytogenetics, dominant lethal test in mice, *in vivo* Chinese hamster chromosome aberration test, V$_{79}$ forward mutation assay) found no evidence of mutagenicity.

**Pregnancy/Reproduction**
Fertility—Testicular atrophy occurred in rats given 40 and 250 mg/kg per day for 1 to 2 years, but not in those given 8 mg/kg per day. Testicular atrophy also occurred in dogs given 300 mg/kg per day (more than 800 times the MRHD) for 3 months, but not in those given 20 mg/kg per day for 1 year.

Pregnancy—Adequate and well-controlled studies in humans have not been done.
Studies in rats given oral doses of 480 mg/kg per day (approximately 1330 times the MRHD) found an increased incidence of fetal resorptions. In offspring of rabbits given 165 times the MRHD, there were increased fetal resorptions, decreased fetal weight, and an increased number of supernumerary ribs. No teratogenicity occurred in either rats or rabbits in these studies.

In peri- and postnatal development studies with rats given 120 mg/kg per day (approximately 300 times the MRHD), postpartum death of pups was increased.

FDA Pregnancy Category C.

**Breast-feeding**
It is not known whether terazosin is distributed into breast milk. However, problems in humans have not been documented.

**Pediatrics**
Appropriate studies on the relationship of age to the effects of terazosin have not been performed in the pediatric population. Safety and efficacy have not been established.

**Geriatrics**
Although appropriate studies on the relationship of age to the effects of terazosin have not been performed in the geriatric population, clinical trials have included patients over 65 years of age and have not demonstrated geriatrics-specific problems that would limit the usefulness of terazosin in the elderly. However, the elderly may be more sensitive to the hypotensive effects of terazosin.

**Drug interactions and/or related problems**
The following drug interactions and/or related problems have been selected on the basis of their potential clinical significance (possible mechanism in parentheses where appropriate)—not necessarily inclusive (» = major clinical significance):

Note: Combinations containing any of the following medications, depending on the amount present, may also interact with this medication.

Anti-inflammatory drugs, nonsteroidal (NSAIDs), especially indomethacin
   (indomethacin, and probably other NSAIDs, may antagonize the antihypertensive effect of terazosin by inhibiting renal prostaglandin synthesis and/or by causing sodium and fluid retention; the patient should be carefully monitored to confirm that the desired effect is being obtained)

Hypotension-producing medications, other (See *Appendix II*)
   (antihypertensive effects may be potentiated when these medications are used concurrently with terazosin; although some antihypertensive and/or diuretic combinations are frequently used to therapeutic advantage, when used concurrently dosage adjustments are necessary)

Sympathomimetics
   (antihypertensive effects of terazosin may be reduced when it is used concurrently with these agents; the patient should be carefully monitored to confirm that the desired effect is being obtained)
   (concurrent use of terazosin antagonizes the peripheral vasoconstriction produced by high doses of dopamine)
   (concurrent use of terazosin may decrease the pressor response to ephedrine)
   (concurrent use of terazosin may block the alpha-adrenergic effects of epinephrine, possibly resulting in severe hypotension and tachycardia)
   (concurrent use of terazosin usually decreases, but does not reverse or completely block, the pressor effect of metaraminol)
   (prior administration of terazosin may decrease the pressor effect and shorten the duration of action of methoxamine and phenylephrine)

**Laboratory value alterations**
The following have been selected on the basis of their potential clinical significance (possible effect in parentheses where appropriate)—not necessarily inclusive (» = major clinical significance):

With physiology/laboratory test values
  Albumin and
  Total protein
    (serum concentrations may be decreased)
  Hemoglobin and hematocrit and
  White blood cells
    (serum concentrations may be decreased)

**Medical considerations/Contraindications**
The medical considerations/contraindications included have been selected on the basis of their potential clinical significance (reasons given in parentheses where appropriate)—not necessarily inclusive (» = major clinical significance).

*Risk-benefit should be considered when the following medical problems exist:*
Angina or
Cardiac disease, severe
   (may induce angina or aggravate pre-existing angina)
Hepatic function impairment
   (although studies in patients with impaired hepatic function have not been done, terazosin undergoes hepatic metabolism, and, therefore, increased sensitivity or prolonged terazosin effect may occur)
Renal function impairment
   (approximately 40% of terazosin dose is eliminated by the kidneys as parent drug or metabolites; therefore, prolonged hypotensive effects may occur)
Sensitivity to terazosin

**Patient monitoring**
The following may be especially important in patient monitoring (other tests may be warranted in some patients, depending on condition; » = major clinical significance):

» Blood pressure measurements
   (recommended at periodic intervals in patients being treated for hypertension; selected patients may be trained to perform blood pressure measurements at home and report the results at regular physician visits)

## Side/Adverse Effects

Note: A "first-dose orthostatic hypotensive reaction" sometimes occurs, most frequently 30 minutes to 2 hours after the initial dose of terazosin, and may be severe. Syncope or other postural symptoms, such as dizziness, may occur. Subsequent occurrence with dosage increases is also possible. Incidence appears to be dose-related; thus, it is important that therapy be initiated with a 1-mg dose given at bedtime. Patients who are volume-depleted or sodium-restricted may be more sensitive to the orthostatic hypotensive effects of terazosin, and the effect may be exaggerated after exercise.

The following side/adverse effects have been selected on the basis of their potential clinical significance (possible signs and symptoms in parentheses where appropriate)—not necessarily inclusive:

**Those indicating need for medical attention**
Incidence more frequent
  *Dizziness*
Incidence less frequent
  *Angina* (chest pain); *dyspnea* (shortness of breath); *edema, peripheral* (swelling of feet or lower legs); *orthostatic hypotension* (dizziness or lightheadedness, when getting up from a lying or sitting position; sudden fainting); *palpitations* (pounding heartbeat); *tachycardia* (fast or irregular heartbeat)

Note: Rarely, weight gain (usually 1 kg [2 lb] or less) may occur with *peripheral edema*.

**Those indicating need for medical attention only if they continue or are bothersome**
Incidence more frequent
  *Asthenia* (unusual tiredness or weakness); *headache*
Incidence less frequent
  *Back or joint pain; blurred vision; nasal congestion* (stuffy nose); *nausea or vomiting; somnolence* (drowsiness)

## Overdose

For more information on the management of overdose or unintentional ingestion, **contact a Poison Control Center** (see *Poison Control Center Listing*).

**Treatment of overdose**
Recommended treatment for terazosin overdose includes: Treatment of circulatory failure, either by placing the patient in the supine position and elevating the legs or by using additional measures if shock is present, is most important; volume expanders may be used to treat shock, followed, if necessary, by administration of a vasopressor; symptomatic, supportive treatment and monitoring of fluid and electrolyte status.

## Patient Consultation

As an aid to patient consultation, refer to *Advice for the Patient, Terazosin (Systemic)*.

In providing consultation, consider emphasizing the following selected information (» = major clinical significance):

**Before using this medication**
» Conditions affecting use, especially:
   Sensitivity to quinazolines

Use in the elderly—Increased sensitivity to hypotensive effects
Other medical problems, especially angina, severe cardiac disease, hepatic function impairment, or renal function impairment

**Proper use of this medication**
Compliance with therapy; taking medication at the same time each day to maintain the therapeutic effect
» Proper dosing
Missed dose: Taking as soon as possible the same day; not taking if not remembered until next day; not doubling doses
» Proper storage
*For use as an antihypertensive*
Possible need for control of weight and diet, especially sodium intake
» Patient may not experience symptoms of hypertension; importance of taking medication even if feeling well
» Does not cure, but helps control hypertension; possible need for lifelong therapy; serious consequences of untreated hypertension
*For use in benign prostatic hyperplasia (BPH)*
Relieves symptoms of BPH but does not change the size of the prostate; may not prevent the need for surgery in the future
May require 2 to 6 weeks of therapy before patient experiences improvement of symptoms

**Precautions while using this medication**
Making regular visits to physician to check progress
» Caution if dizziness, lightheadedness, or sudden fainting occurs, especially after initial dose; taking first dose at bedtime
» Caution when getting up suddenly from a lying or sitting position
» Caution in using alcohol, while standing for long periods or exercising, and during hot weather because of enhanced orthostatic hypotensive effects
» Possibility of drowsiness
» Caution when driving or doing anything else requiring alertness because of possible drowsiness, dizziness, or lightheadedness
» Not taking other medication, especially nonprescription sympathomimetics, unless discussed with physician

**Side/adverse effects**
Signs of potential side effects, especially angina, dizziness, dyspnea, orthostatic hypotension, palpitations, peripheral edema, and tachycardia

## General Dosing Information

In order to minimize the "first-dose orthostatic hypotensive reaction," an initial dose of 1 mg is recommended, with gradual increments as needed. Administration of the initial dose at bedtime is recommended, as well as for the initial dose at each increment.

**For use as an antihypertensive**
Dosage of terazosin should be adjusted to meet the individual requirements of each patient, on the basis of blood pressure response.

Terazosin may be used alone or in combination with a thiazide diuretic or beta-adrenergic blocker, both of which reduce the tendency for sodium and water retention, although they also produce additive hypotension. If combination therapy is indicated, individual titration is required to ensure the lowest possible therapeutic dose of each drug.

When a diuretic or other antihypertensive agent is added to terazosin therapy, the dose of terazosin should be reduced, followed by titration of dosage of the combination. When terazosin is added to existing diuretic or antihypertensive therapy, the dose of the other agent should be reduced and terazosin started at a dose of 1 mg once a day.

**For use in benign prostatic hyperplasia**
Prior to initiation of terazosin therapy, the presence of prostate carcinoma should be ruled out, since prostate carcinoma can present with symptoms similar to those associated with BPH.

## Oral Dosage Forms

### TERAZOSIN HYDROCHLORIDE CAPSULES

Note: The dosing and strengths of the dosage forms available are expressed in terms of terazosin base (not the hydrochloride salt).

**Usual adult dose**
Antihypertensive—
Initial: Oral, 1 mg (base) once a day, at bedtime.
Maintenance: Oral, adjusted gradually to meet individual requirements, usually 1 to 5 mg (base) once a day.
Note: If the antihypertensive effect is not maintained for a full 24 hours, twice daily dosing may be more effective.
Geriatric patients may be more sensitive to the effects of the usual adult dose.
Benign prostatic hyperplasia[1]—
Initial: Oral, 1 mg (base), at bedtime.
Maintenance: Oral, adjusted gradually up to 5 to 10 mg (base) once a day. Doses of 10 mg once a day are generally required for an adequate response.

**Usual adult prescribing limits**
Daily doses higher than 20 mg (base) usually do not have increased efficacy.

**Usual pediatric dose**
Safety and efficacy have not been established.

**Strength(s) usually available**
U.S.—
  1 mg (base) (Rx) [*Hytrin*].
  2 mg (base) (Rx) [*Hytrin*].
  5 mg (base) (Rx) [*Hytrin*].
  10 mg (base) (Rx) [*Hytrin*].
Canada—
  1 mg (base) (Rx) [*Hytrin*].
  2 mg (base) (Rx) [*Hytrin*].
  5 mg (base) (Rx) [*Hytrin*].
  10 mg (base) (Rx) [*Hytrin*].

**Packaging and storage**
Store below 40 °C (104 °F), preferably between 15 and 30 °C (59 and 86 °F), unless otherwise specified by manufacturer.

**Auxiliary labeling**
• Do not take other medicines without your doctor's advice.
• May cause dizziness.

**Note**
Check refill frequency to determine compliance in hypertensive patients.

---

[1]Not included in Canadian product labeling.

## Selected Bibliography

The fifth report of the Joint National Committee on Detection, Evaluation, and Treatment of High Blood Pressure (JNC V). Arch Intern Med 1993; 153(2): 154-83.

Revised: 06/26/92
Interim revision: 07/08/94; 08/19/98

---

# TERBINAFINE Systemic*

VA CLASSIFICATION (Primary): AM700
Commonly used brand name(s): *Lamisil*.
Note: For a listing of dosage forms and brand names by country availability, see *Dosage Forms* section(s).

*Not commercially available in U.S.

## Category

Antifungal (systemic).

## Indications

**General considerations**
Terbinafine has *in vitro* activity against yeasts and a wide range of dermatophyte, filamentous, dimorphic, and dematiaceous fungi. It is fungicidal against dermatophytes, such as *Trichophyton* species, *Microsporum* species, and *Epidermophyton floccosum*, as well as against *Aspergillus* species, *Scopulariopsis brevicaulis*, *Blastomyces dermatitidis*, *Cryptococcus neoformans*, *Sporothrix schenckii*, *Histoplasma capsulatum*, *Candida parapsilosis*, and *Pityrosporum* yeasts. Terbinafine has also been shown to be active *in vitro* against the protozoal organisms *Trypanosoma cruzi* and *Leishmania mexicana mexicana*. However, clinical efficacy has not been demonstrated in the treatment of infections caused by *B. dermatitidis*, *H. capsulatum*, *S. schenckii*, *C. neo-*

*formans*, *T. cruzi*, and *L. mexicana mexicana*. Also, terbinafine is only fungistatic against *Candida albicans*. Clinical studies have found terbinafine to be only moderately effective against skin infections caused by *Candida* species, with a mycological cure of only 65% after 2 to 4 weeks of treatment.

**Accepted**
Onychomycosis (treatment)—Terbinafine is indicated in the treatment of onychomycosis (fungal infection of the nails) caused by dermatophyte fungi.

Tinea capitis (treatment)[1]—Limited data suggest that terbinafine may be used in the treatment of tinea capitis (ringworm of the scalp).

Tinea corporis (treatment)—Terbinafine is indicated in the treatment of tinea corporis (ringworm of the body).

Tinea cruris (treatment)—Terbinafine is indicated in the treatment of tinea cruris (ringworm of the groin; jock itch).

Tinea pedis (treatment)—Terbinafine is indicated in the treatment of interdigital or plantar tinea pedis (ringworm of the foot; athlete's foot).

**Unaccepted**
Terbinafine is not effective in the treatment of pityriasis versicolor because concentrations of oral terbinafine reached in the stratum corneum are not high enough to treat this condition adequately.

---

[1] Not included in Canadian product labeling.

## Pharmacology/Pharmacokinetics

**Physicochemical characteristics**
Chemical group—Allylamine class.
Molecular weight—Terbinafine hydrochloride: 327.90.

**Mechanism of action/Effect**
Terbinafine interferes with fungal ergosterol biosynthesis by inhibiting squalene epoxidase in the fungal cell membrane. This leads to a deficiency of ergosterol and an intracellular accumulation of squalene, thus disrupting fungal membrane function and cell wall synthesis, and resulting in fungal cell death.

**Other actions/effects**
Unlike azole antifungal agents, terbinafine does not inhibit cytochrome P-450 activity and is only weakly bound to hepatic cytochrome P-450, resulting in a low propensity for interference with cytochrome P-450 enzymes involved in drug metabolism and synthesis of steroid hormones and prostaglandins. Terbinafine also has no effect on 14 alpha-demethylation.

Terbinafine's mechanism of action against protozoal organisms is thought to involve inhibition of sterol synthesis.

**Absorption**
Readily absorbed from gastrointestinal tract. Bioavailability is 70 to 80% and is not affected by the presence of food.

**Distribution**
Terbinafine is lipophilic and extensively distributed. It rapidly diffuses from the vascular system, passes through the dermis and epidermis, and concentrates in the lipophilic stratum corneum. It is also distributed via the sebum to hair follicles and sebum-rich skin, resulting in high concentrations in hair follicles, hair, sebum-rich skin, and the nail plate within the first few weeks of therapy. It is also highly distributed to adipose tissue. After 12 days of treatment, concentrations in the stratum corneum exceed those in plasma by a factor of 75 and concentrations in the epidermis and dermis exceed those in plasma by a factor of 25. Blood cells contain approximately 8% of administered terbinafine. Terbinafine is not detected in sweat.

Vol$_D$ at steady state is approximately 948 L.

**Protein binding**
Very high (99%), with binding evenly distributed among all plasma fractions.

**Biotransformation**
Terbinafine undergoes first pass metabolism. It is extensively metabolized in the liver by N-demethylation of the central nitrogen atom, alkyl side-chain oxidation (alkyl oxidation), and arene oxide formation followed by hydrolysis to the corresponding dihydrodiol. Metabolism involves only a small fraction (< 5%) of total hepatic cytochrome P-450 capacity. Fifteen metabolites have been identified, but none are active.

**Half-life**
Absorption—
  Approximately 0.8 hour.
Distribution—
  Approximately 4.6 hours.
Elimination—
  Plasma: 11 to 17 hours.
  Sebum: 3 to 5 days.
  Stratum corneum: 3 to 5 days.
Terminal—
  Sebum: 18 days.
  Plasma: 22 days, due to accumulation in adipose tissue and gradual release after discontinuation of treatment.
  Stratum corneum: 22 days.
  Hair and nails: 24 days.
  Dermis and epidermis: 28 days.

**Time to peak concentration**
Plasma—Approximately 2 hours. Steady state is reached in 10 to 14 days.
Stratum corneum—Maximum concentrations in the stratum corneum were found on Day 12 of treatment. However, terbinafine was detected in lower levels of the stratum corneum 24 hours after a single oral dose, and fungicidal concentrations were found across the whole of the stratum corneum within 7 days.
Nails—Detected in distal nail clippings as early as 3 weeks after the beginning of therapy. Fungicidal levels in nails were maintained for several weeks after discontinuation of therapy.

**Peak serum concentration**
Serum—0.8 to 1.5 mg per L (2.4 to 4.6 micromoles per L).
Nails—250 to 550 nanograms per mg, detected in toenails 3 to 18 weeks after starting therapy, with no progressive increase thereafter during the 48 weeks of therapy.

**Elimination**
Renal—Approximately 80% of an administered dose is excreted in the urine as metabolites.
Fecal—Approximately 20% is eliminated in feces.

## Precautions to Consider

**Carcinogenicity**
An increase in liver tumors was observed in male rats at the highest dose level (69 mg per kg of body weight [mg/kg] per day) during a 123-week carcinogenicity study. Other changes included increased enzyme activity, peroxisome proliferation, and altered triglyceride metabolism. These changes were not seen in mice or monkeys.

**Mutagenicity**
*In vitro* and *in vivo* mutagenicity testing of terbinafine revealed no specific mutagenic or genotoxic properties. *In vitro* tests of cell transformation to malignancy were negative.

**Pregnancy/Reproduction**
Fertility—Fertility studies in animals suggest no adverse effects.
Pregnancy—Adequate and well-controlled studies in humans have not been done.
Fetal toxicity studies in animals suggest no adverse effects.

**Breast-feeding**
Terbinafine is distributed into breast milk. In 2 women, totals of 0.2 and 0.7 mg of terbinafine were detected in the breast milk after a single oral 500-mg dose in the ablactation period.

**Pediatrics**
No information is available on the relationship of age to the effects of terbinafine in pediatric patients. Safety and efficacy have not been established. However, terbinafine has been used to treat tinea capitis in a small number of children 3 to 16 years of age and was generally well tolerated.

**Geriatrics**
No information is available on the relationship of age to the effects of terbinafine in geriatric patients. However, elderly patients are more likely to have age-related renal function impairment, which may require an adjustment of dosage in patients receiving terbinafine.

**Drug interactions and/or related problems**
The following drug interactions and/or related problems have been selected on the basis of their potential clinical significance (possible mechanism in parentheses where appropriate)—not necessarily inclusive (» = major clinical significance):

Note: Combinations containing any of the following medications, depending on the amount present, may also interact with this medication.

» Alcohol or
» Hepatotoxic medications, other (See *Appendix II*)
  (severe hepatitis has been reported rarely with terbinafine; concurrent use of other hepatotoxic medications may increase the risk of hepatotoxicity)

  Caffeine
  (terbinafine was found to decrease the clearance of caffeine by 20%)

- » Enzyme inducers, hepatic, cytochrome P-450 (See *Appendix II*)
    (because terbinafine is hepatically metabolized, medications, such as rifampin, that induce the cytochrome P-450 system may increase the clearance of terbinafine)
- » Enzyme inhibitors, hepatic, cytochrome P-450
    (because terbinafine is hepatically metabolized, medications, such as cimetidine, that inhibit the cytochrome P-450 system may decrease the clearance of terbinafine)

**Laboratory value alterations**
The following have been selected on the basis of their potential clinical significance (possible effect in parentheses where appropriate)—not necessarily inclusive (» = major clinical significance):

With physiology/laboratory test values
   Alanine aminotransferase (ALT [SGPT]) and
   Aspartate aminotransferase (AST [SGOT])
       (values may rarely be transiently increased)

**Medical considerations/Contraindications**
The medical considerations/contraindications included have been selected on the basis of their potential clinical significance (reasons given in parentheses where appropriate)—not necessarily inclusive (» = major clinical significance).

*Risk-benefit should be considered when the following medical problems exist:*
- » Alcoholism, active or in remission or
- » Hepatic function impairment
    (severe hepatitis has been reported with terbinafine on rare occasion; patients with alcoholism or hepatic function impairment may be at increased risk of severe hepatotoxicity; hepatic function impairment was found to reduce the clearance of terbinafine by approximately 30%; it is recommended that patients with pre-existing stable chronic liver function impairment receive a 50% reduction in dose)
- » Hypersensitivity to terbinafine
- » Renal function impairment
    (terbinafine elimination was found to be reduced in patients with renal function impairment; the elimination half-life was increased from 16 to 24 hours; it is recommended that patients with impaired renal function [creatinine clearance < 50 mL per min (0.83 mL per sec) or serum creatinine greater than 3.4 mg per dL (300 micromoles per L)] receive a 50% reduction in dose)

**Patient monitoring**
The following may be especially important in patient monitoring (other tests may be warranted in some patients, depending on condition; » = major clinical significance):

Clinical assessment
    (a follow-up clinical assessment is recommended after terbinafine therapy has ended, to determine whether relapse has occurred; the timing of this assessment depends on the condition being treated; for tinea corporis, tinea cruris, and tinea pedis, it is recommended that the assessment be performed at 6 to 8 weeks following cessation of treatment, for onychomycosis of the fingernails, it is recommended that the assessment be at 4 to 6 months, and for onychomycosis of the toenails, it is recommended that the assessment be at 6 to 9 months following cessation of treatment)

Hepatic function determinations
    (liver function tests are recommended before therapy, and periodically during terbinafine treatment, in patients with hepatic function impairment, alcoholic patients, or patients taking hepatotoxic medications concurrently)

## Side/Adverse Effects

Note: Loss of taste has been reported rarely during terbinafine treatment, with the onset occurring 5 to 8 weeks after the start of therapy. This effect is reversible upon discontinuation of terbinafine, but recovery may take 2 to 6 weeks. There also has been one case of tongue discoloration associated with terbinafine.

The following side/adverse effects have been selected on the basis of their potential clinical significance (possible signs and symptoms in parentheses where appropriate)—not necessarily inclusive:

**Those indicating need for medical attention**
Incidence less frequent
   *Hypersensitivity* (skin rash or itching)
Incidence rare
   *Hepatitis* (dark urine; fatigue; loss of appetite; pale stools; yellow eyes or skin); *neutropenia* (fever, chills, or sore throat); *pancytopenia* (fever, chills, or sore throat; pale skin; unusual bleeding or bruising; unusual tiredness or weakness); *Stevens-Johnson syndrome* (aching joints and muscles; redness, blistering, peeling, or loosening of skin; unusual tiredness or weakness); *toxic epidermal necrolysis* (difficulty in swallowing; redness, blistering, peeling, or loosening of skin)

**Those indicating need for medical attention only if they continue or are bothersome**
Incidence more frequent
   *Gastrointestinal disturbances* (diarrhea; loss of appetite; nausea and vomiting; stomach pain, mild)
Incidence less frequent
   *Change of taste or loss of taste*

## Patient Consultation

As an aid to patient consultation, refer to *Advice for the Patient, Terbinafine (Systemic)*.

In providing consultation, consider emphasizing the following selected information (» = major clinical significance):

**Before using this medication**
- » Conditions affecting use, especially:
    Hypersensitivity to terbinafine
    Breast-feeding—Terbinafine is distributed into breast milk
    Other medications, especially alcohol, cytochrome P-450 enzyme inducers and inhibitors, and other hepatotoxic medications
    Other medical problems, especially alcoholism, hepatic function impairment, and renal function impairment

**Proper use of this medication**
   May be taken with or without food
- » Compliance with full course of therapy
- » Importance of not missing doses and taking at evenly spaced times
- » Proper dosing
    Missed dose: Taking as soon as possible; not taking if almost time for next dose; not doubling doses
- » Proper storage

**Precautions while using this medication**
   Regular visits to physician to check progress during therapy
   Checking with physician if no improvement within a few weeks (or months for onychomycosis)
   Caution in drinking alcoholic beverages during terbinafine therapy

**Side/adverse effects**
   Signs of potential side effects, especially hypersensitivity, hepatitis, neutropenia, pancytopenia, Stevens-Johnson syndrome, and toxic epidermal necrolysis

## General Dosing Information

Terbinafine may be taken with or without food.

To prevent relapse, therapy should be continued until the infecting organism is completely eradicated as determined by clinical or laboratory examination. Representative treatment periods are: onychomycosis, 6 weeks to 3 months; tinea corporis and tinea cruris, 2 to 4 weeks; and tinea pedis, 2 to 6 weeks.

Patients with pre-existing, stable chronic liver dysfunction or impaired renal function (creatinine clearance < 50 mL per min [0.83 mL per sec] or serum creatinine greater than 3.4 mg per dL [300 micromoles per L]) should receive a 50% reduction of the regular dose.

## Oral Dosage Forms

### TERBINAFINE HYDROCHLORIDE TABLETS

**Usual adult and adolescent dose**
Antifungal—
   Onychomycosis: Oral, 125 mg two times a day, or 250 mg once a day, for 6 weeks to 3 months. Some toenail infections may require longer therapy, depending on the extent of the infection.
   Tinea capitis[1]: Oral, 125 mg two times a day, or 250 mg once a day, for 4 to 6 weeks.
   Tinea corporis: Oral, 125 mg two times a day, or 250 mg once a day, for 2 to 4 weeks.
   Tinea cruris: Oral, 125 mg two times a day, or 250 mg once a day, for 2 to 4 weeks.
   Tinea pedis (interdigital or plantar): Oral, 125 mg two times a day, or 250 mg once a day, for 2 to 6 weeks.

**Usual pediatric dose**
Dosage has not been established. However, in one study the following doses were used in the treatment of tinea capitis in children 3 to 16 years of age—
   Children 12.5 to 18.5 kg of body weight: Oral, 62.5 mg once a day.
   Children 18.5 to 25 kg of body weight: Oral, 125 mg once a day.
   Children more than 25 kg of body weight: Oral, 250 mg once a day.

## Strength(s) usually available
U.S.—
  Not commercially available.
Canada—
  125 mg (Rx) [*Lamisil*].
  250 mg (Rx) [*Lamisil*].

## Packaging and storage
Store below 40 °C (104 °F), preferably between 15 and 30 °C (59 and 86 °F), unless otherwise specified by manufacturer.

## Auxiliary labeling
• Continue medicine for full time of treatment.

[1]Not included in Canadian product labeling.

## Selected Bibliography
Balfour JA, Faulds D. Terbinafine. A review of its pharmacodynamic and pharmacokinetic properties, and therapeutic potential in superficial mycoses. Drugs 1992; 43(2): 259-84.

Developed: 06/22/95

---

# TERBINAFINE  Topical†

VA CLASSIFICATION (Primary): DE102
Commonly used brand name(s): *Lamisil*.
Note: For a listing of dosage forms and brand names by country availability, see *Dosage Forms* section(s).

†Not commercially available in Canada.

## Category
Antifungal (topical).

## Indications
**Accepted**
Tinea corporis (treatment) or
Tinea cruris (treatment) or
Tinea pedis, interdigital (treatment) or
Tinea pedis, plantar (treatment)—Terbinafine is indicated as a primary agent in the topical treatment of tinea corporis (ringworm of the body), tinea cruris (ringworm of the groin; jock itch), interdigital tinea pedis (ringworm of the foot; athlete's foot) caused by *Trichophyton rubrum*, *T. mentagrophytes*, or *Epidermophyton floccosum (Acrothesium floccosum)*, and plantar tinea pedis (moccasin-type) caused by *T. mentagrophytes* or *T. rubrum*.

## Pharmacology/Pharmacokinetics
**Physicochemical characteristics**
Source—A synthetic allylamine derivative.
Molecular weight—Terbinafine hydrochloride: 327.90.

**Mechanism of action/Effect**
Fungicidal; inhibits squalene epoxidase (a key enzyme in sterol biosynthesis in fungi), which results in a deficiency in ergosterol and a corresponding increase in squalene within the fungal cell, causing fungal cell death. Also fungistatic; interferes with membrane synthesis and growth.

**Absorption**
Limited absorption may occur.

**Elimination**
Approximately 75% of topically absorbed terbinafine is eliminated in the urine, mostly as metabolites.

## Precautions to Consider
**Cross-sensitivity and/or related problems**
Patients sensitive to the oral form of terbinafine may be sensitive to the topical form also.

**Carcinogenicity/Tumorigenicity**
A 2-year carcinogenicity study in mice showed a 4% incidence of splenic hemangiosarcomas and a 6% incidence of leiomyosarcoma-like tumors of the seminal vesicles in males administered terbinafine orally in doses of 156 mg per kg of body weight (mg/kg) per day. A carcinogenicity study in rats showed a 6% incidence of liver tumors, which were associated with peroxisomal proliferation, and skin lipomas in males administered terbinafine orally in doses of 69 mg/kg per day.

**Mutagenicity**
*In vitro* and *in vivo* genotoxicity tests, including Ames assay, mutagenicity evaluation in Chinese hamster ovarian cells, chromosome aberration test, sister chromatid exchanges, and mouse micronucleus test, revealed no evidence of mutagenic or clastogenic potential for terbinafine.

**Pregnancy/Reproduction**
Fertility—Reproductive studies in rats administered terbinafine orally in doses of up to 300 mg/kg per day did not show any adverse effects on fertility. In addition, terbinafine in doses of 150 mg per day administered intravaginally to pregnant rabbits did not increase the incidence of abortions or premature deliveries and did not affect fetal parameters.

Pregnancy—Adequate and well-controlled studies in humans have not been done.

Terbinafine was not teratogenic when it was administered orally at doses of up to 300 mg/kg per day during organogenesis in rats and rabbits, administered subcutaneously at doses of up to 100 mg/kg per day in rats, or administered percutaneously at doses of up to 150 mg/kg per day in rabbits.

FDA Pregnancy Category B.

**Breast-feeding**
Terbinafine is distributed into breast milk after oral administration. However, it is not known whether terbinafine is distributed into breast milk after topical administration. Breast-feeding women should avoid applying topical terbinafine to the breasts.

Terbinafine was administered orally in single 500-mg doses to two breast-feeding women. The total amounts of terbinafine recovered during the following 72-hour period were 0.65 mg and 0.15 mg. This corresponded to 0.13 and 0.03% of the administered dose, respectively.

**Pediatrics**
No information is available on the relationship of age to the effects of terbinafine in pediatric patients. Safety and efficacy have not been established in infants and children up to 12 years of age.

**Geriatrics**
No information is available on the relationship of age to the effects of terbinafine in geriatric patients.

**Medical considerations/Contraindications**
The medical considerations/contraindications included have been selected on the basis of their potential clinical significance (reasons given in parentheses where appropriate)—not necessarily inclusive (» = major clinical significance).

*Risk-benefit should be considered when the following medical problem exists:*
  Onychomycosis
    (patients with onychomycosis may be less likely to have a favorable response to terbinafine therapy)

## Side/Adverse Effects
The following side/adverse effects have been selected on the basis of their potential clinical significance (possible signs and symptoms in parentheses where appropriate)—not necessarily inclusive:

**Those indicating need for medical attention**
Incidence rare
  *Hypersensitivity* (redness, itching, burning, blistering, swelling, oozing, or other signs of skin irritation not present before use of this medicine)

## Overdose
For more information on the management of overdose or unintentional ingestion, **contact a Poison Control Center** (see *Poison Control Center Listing*).

**Treatment of overdose**
Acute overdosage with topical application of terbinafine hydrochloride is unlikely due to the limited absorption of the topically applied drug and would not be expected to lead to a life-threatening situation.

## Patient Consultation
As an aid to patient consultation, refer to *Advice for the Patient, Terbinafine (Topical)*.

In providing consultation, consider emphasizing the following selected information (» = major clinical significance):

**Before using this medication**
» Conditions affecting use, especially:
  Sensitivity to terbinafine

**Proper use of this medication**
  Applying sufficient medication to cover affected and surrounding areas, and rubbing in gently
» Avoiding contact with the eyes, nose, mouth, and other mucous membranes
» Not applying occlusive dressing over this medication unless directed to do so by physician
» Proper dosing
» Compliance with full course of therapy; fungal infections may require prolonged therapy
  Missed dose: Applying as soon as possible; not applying if almost time for next dose
» Proper storage

**Precautions while using this medication**
  Checking with physician if no improvement within 4 weeks
» Using hygienic measures to help cure infection and prevent reinfection
*For tinea corporis*
  Carefully drying the body after bathing
  Avoiding excess heat and humidity if possible; keeping moisture from accumulating on affected areas of the body
  Wearing well-ventilated, loose-fitting clothing
  Using a bland, absorbent powder once or twice daily; using the powder after the cream has been applied and has disappeared into the skin
*For tinea cruris*
  Avoiding underwear that is tight-fitting or made from synthetic materials; wearing loose-fitting cotton underwear instead
  Using a bland, absorbent powder on the skin; using the powder between administration times for terbinafine
*For tinea pedis*
  Carefully drying feet, especially between toes, after bathing
  Avoiding socks made from wool or synthetic materials; wearing clean, cotton socks and changing them daily or more often if feet perspire excessively
  Wearing sandals or well-ventilated shoes
  Using a bland, absorbent powder between toes, on feet, and in socks and shoes liberally once or twice daily; using the powder between administration times for terbinafine

**Side/adverse effects**
  Signs of potential side effects, especially hypersensitivity

## Topical Dosage Forms

### TERBINAFINE HYDROCHLORIDE CREAM

**Usual adult and adolescent dose**
Tinea corporis or
Tinea cruris—
  Topical, to the skin and surrounding areas, one or two times a day.
Tinea pedis, interdigital—
  Topical, to the skin and surrounding areas, two times a day.

Note: Treatment should be continued for at least one week *and* until there is significant improvement in the clinical signs and symptoms of the disease. Treatment should not exceed four weeks.

Tinea pedis, plantar—
  Topical, to the skin and surrounding areas, two times a day.

Note: Treatment should be continued for two weeks. Treatment may be affected by the presence of onychomycosis. Patients with a toenail infection may be less likely to have a favorable response to terbinafine therapy.

**Usual pediatric dose**
Tinea corporis or
Tinea cruris or
Tinea pedis—
  Infants and children up to 12 years of age: Safety and efficacy have not been established.
  Children 12 years of age and over: See *Usual adult and adolescent dose*.

**Strength(s) usually available**
U.S.—
  1% (Rx) [*Lamisil*].
Canada—
  Not commercially available.

**Packaging and storage**
Store between 5 and 30 °C (41 and 86 °F), unless otherwise specified by manufacturer.

**Auxiliary labeling**
• For external use only.
• Continue medicine for full time of treatment.

## Selected Bibliography
Berman B, et al. Efficacy of a 1-week twice-daily regimen of terbinafine 1% cream in the treatment of interdigital tinea pedis. J Am Acad Derm 1992 Jun; 26(6): 956-60.

Revised: 07/29/93
Interim revision: 08/19/97

---

**TERBUTALINE**—See *Bronchodilators, Adrenergic (Inhalation-Local)*; *Bronchodilators, Adrenergic (Systemic)*

---

**TERCONAZOLE**—See *Antifungals, Azole (Vaginal)*

---

**TERIPARATIDE**—The *Teriparatide (Systemic)* monograph is not included in this published version of the USP DI database. Copies of the monograph are available on request from Micromedex, Inc. - Reprint Requests, 6200 S. Syracuse Way, Suite 300, Englewood, CO 80111; telephone (303) 486-6400; telefax (303) 486-6464; Email: USPDI@MDX.COM.

---

# TESTOLACTONE Systemic†

VA CLASSIFICATION (Primary): AN500
Commonly used brand name(s): *Teslac*.
Note: For a listing of dosage forms and brand names by country availability, see *Dosage Forms* section(s).

†Not commercially available in Canada.

## Category
Antineoplastic.

## Indications

**Accepted**
Testolactone has been used as adjunctive therapy in the palliative treatment of advanced or disseminated breast cancer in postmenopausal women when hormone therapy is indicated; however testolactone generally *has been replaced* by more effective agents.

Testolactone is not recommended for treatment of breast cancer in males.

## Pharmacology/Pharmacokinetics

**Physicochemical characteristics**
Molecular weight—300.40.

**Mechanism of action/Effect**
Testolactone is structurally similar to androgens but is not known to cause virilization. The mechanism of its antineoplastic activity is unknown, although it is reported to inhibit steroid aromatase activity (the effect may be noncompetitive and irreversible) and reduce estrone synthesis from adrenal androstenedione (the major source of estrogen in postmenopausal women).

**Absorption**
Well absorbed from the gastrointestinal tract.

**Biotransformation**
Hepatic.

**Onset of action**
Clinical effects may not be apparent for 6 to 12 weeks.

**Elimination**
Renal.

## Precautions to Consider

### Carcinogenicity/Mutagenicity
Studies have not been done in either animals or humans.

### Pregnancy/Reproduction
Pregnancy—Adequate and well-controlled studies in humans have not been done.

Studies in rats at doses 5 to 15 times the recommended human dose have found that testolactone causes increased fetal mortality, increased abnormal fetal development, and increased mortality in growing pups. It did not cause teratogenicity in rabbits given 2.5 to 7.5 times the recommended human dose.

FDA Pregnancy Category C.

### Breast-feeding
It is not known whether testolactone is distributed into breast milk. However, problems in humans have not been documented.

### Geriatrics
No information is available on the relationship of age to the effects of testolactone in geriatric patients.

### Drug interactions and/or related problems
The following drug interactions and/or related problems have been selected on the basis of their potential clinical significance (possible mechanism in parentheses where appropriate)—not necessarily inclusive (» = major clinical significance):

Anticoagulants, coumarin- or indandione-type
 (effects may be increased by concurrent use of testolactone; dosage adjustment of oral anticoagulants may be necessary)

### Laboratory value alterations
The following have been selected on the basis of their potential clinical significance (possible effect in parentheses where appropriate)—not necessarily inclusive (» = major clinical significance):

With physiology/laboratory test values
 Calcium concentrations, serum
  (may be increased; immobilized patients are especially likely to develop hypercalcemia)
 Creatinine and
 17-Ketosteroid
  (urinary concentrations may be increased)
 Estradiol measured by radioimmunoassay
  (concentrations may be decreased)

### Medical considerations/Contraindications
The medical considerations/contraindications included have been selected on the basis of their potential clinical significance (reasons given in parentheses where appropriate)—not necessarily inclusive (» = major clinical significance).

*Risk-benefit should be considered when the following medical problems exist:*
» Cardiorenal disease
» Hypercalcemia
» Sensitivity to testolactone

### Patient monitoring
The following are especially important in patient monitoring (other tests may be warranted in some patients, depending on condition; » = major clinical significance):

» Calcium concentrations, serum
 (recommended at periodic intervals, especially in patients with active remission of bone metastases)

## Side/Adverse Effects

The following side/adverse effects have been selected on the basis of their potential clinical significance (possible signs and symptoms in parentheses where appropriate)—not necessarily inclusive:

**Those indicating need for medical attention**
Incidence less frequent
 *Peripheral neuropathies* (numbness or tingling of fingers, toes, or face)

**Those indicating need for medical attention only if they continue or are bothersome**
Incidence less frequent
 *Diarrhea; loss of appetite; nausea or vomiting; pain or swelling in feet or lower legs; swelling or redness of tongue*

## Patient Consultation

As an aid to patient consultation, refer to *Advice for the Patient, Testolactone (Systemic)*.

In providing consultation, consider emphasizing the following selected information (» = major clinical significance):

**Before using this medication**
» Conditions affecting use, especially:
 Sensitivity to testolactone
  Pregnancy—Causes increased fetal and pup mortality and abnormal fetal development in rats
  Other medical problems, especially cardiorenal disease

**Proper use of this medication**
» Importance of not taking more or less medication than the amount prescribed
» Possible nausea and vomiting; importance of continuing medication despite stomach upset
 Checking with physician if vomiting occurs shortly after dose is taken
» Proper dosing
 Missed dose: Taking as soon as possible, not taking if almost time for next dose; not doubling doses; checking with physician if two or more doses in a row are missed
» Proper storage

**Precautions while using this medication**
» Importance of close monitoring by the physician

**Side/adverse effects**
 Signs of potential side effects, especially peripheral neuropathies
 Physician or nurse can help in dealing with side effects

## General Dosing Information

Patients receiving testolactone should be under supervision of a physician experienced in cancer chemotherapy.

If hypercalcemia occurs, therapy with testolactone should be withdrawn and the patient treated with large volumes of fluid.

Testolactone should be given for at least 3 months before it is considered ineffective, unless active progression of the disease occurs.

## Oral Dosage Forms

### TESTOLACTONE TABLETS USP

**Usual adult dose**
Breast carcinoma—
 Oral, 250 mg four times a day.

**Strength(s) usually available**
U.S.—
 50 mg (Rx) [*Teslac*].
Canada—
 Not commercially available.

**Packaging and storage**
Store below 40 °C (104 °F), preferably between 15 and 30 °C (59 and 86 °F), unless otherwise specified by manufacturer. Store in a tight container.

Revised: 08/04/92
Interim revision: 09/30/97

---

**TESTOSTERONE**—See *Androgens (Systemic)*

---

**TETANUS ANTITOXIN**—The *Tetanus Antitoxin (Systemic)* monograph is not included in this published version of the USP DI database. Copies of the monograph are available on request from Micromedex, Inc. - Reprint Requests, 6200 S. Syracuse Way, Suite 300, Englewood, CO 80111; telephone (303) 486-6400; telefax (303) 486-6464; Email: USPDI@MDX.COM.

**TETANUS AND DIPHTHERIA TOXOIDS TD**—See *Diphtheria and Tetanus Toxoids (Systemic)*

# TETANUS IMMUNE GLOBULIN HUMAN   Systemic

VA CLASSIFICATION (Primary/Secondary): IM500

Note: This monograph is specific to the sterile solution of tetanus immune globulin prepared from large pools of plasma obtained from individuals immunized with tetanus toxoid.

Commonly used brand name(s): *BayTet*.

Another commonly used name is TIG.

Note: For a listing of dosage forms and brand names by country availability, see *Dosage Forms* section(s).

## Category
Immunizing agent (passive).

## Indications

**General considerations**

Tetanus (lockjaw) is a neurologic disease charcterized by severe muscular spasms. It is caused by the neurotoxin produced by the anaerobic bacterium *Clostridium tetani* in a contaminated wound. Onset is gradual, occurring over 1 to 7 days, and progresses to severe generalized muscle spasms (severe enough to cause spinal fractures), which frequently are aggravated by any external stimulus. Severe spasms persist for 1 week or more and subside in a period of weeks in those who recover. Neonatal tetanus, a common cause of neonatal mortality in developing countries but rare in the U.S., is caused by contamination of the umbilical stump. Local tetanus is manifested by local muscle spasms in areas contiguous to a wound infected with *Clostridium tetani*.

Wound cleaning, debridement when indicated, and proper immunization are important in the prevention and management of tetanus. The need for tetanus toxoid (active immunization), with or without tetanus immune globulin (passive immunization), depends on both the condition of the wound and the patient's vaccination history.

Determining whether the wound is clean or dirty is extremely important in categorizing patients. A wound is considered to be dirty if it is more than 6 hours old, if there is debris in the wound, if the wound is penetrating or deep, if the instrument that caused the wound is contaminated, if the wound is infected, if the wound is caused by a deep partial- or full-thickness burn, or if it is a crush injury.

A thorough attempt must be made to determine whether a patient has completed primary vaccination. Patients with unknown or uncertain previous vaccination histories should be considered to have had no previous tetanus toxoid doses. Patients who have not completed a primary series may require tetanus toxoid and passive immunization with tetanus immune globulin at the time of wound cleaning and debridement.

Tetanus immune globulin provides protection for a longer time than does antitoxin of animal origin, and causes fewer adverse reactions. Therefore, if passive immunization is needed, tetanus immune globulin is the product of choice.

A recent U.S. serologic survey of tetanus immunity indicated that in the majority of the population, tetanus immunity decreases with time after the recipient's most recent vaccination. If a contraindication to using tetanus toxoid–containing preparations exists for a person who has not completed a primary series of tetanus toxoid immunizations and that person has a wound that is neither clean nor minor, only passive immunization should be given, using tetanus immune globulin.

In the U.S., tetanus is primarily a disease of older adults. Of the 99 tetanus patients with complete information reported to the Centers for Disease Control and Prevention (CDC) during 1987 and 1988, 68% were 50 years of age or older. The age distribution of recent cases and the results of serosurveys indicate that many U.S. adults are not protected against tetanus.

**Accepted**

*Clostridium tetani* infection (prophylaxis)—Tetanus immune globulin is indicated for prophylaxis against *C. tetani* infection, and the severe complications that arise from the toxins produced by *C. tetani*, following injury in patients whose immune status against tetanus is uncertain or incomplete.

## Pharmacology/Pharmacokinetics

**Physicochemical characteristics**

Source—
Tetanus immune globulin is a sterile solution of tetanus hyperimmune immunoglobulin, primarily immunoglobulin G (IgG), containing 15 to 18% protein, of which not less than 90% is gamma globulin. Tetanus immune globulin is prepared from large pools of plasma obtained from individuals immunized with tetanus toxoid. Tetanus immune globulin is stabilized with 0.21 to 0.32 molar glycine and contains no preservative. Tetanus immune globulin is standardized against the U.S. standard antitoxin and the U.S. control tetanus toxin and contains not less than 250 tetanus antitoxin units per vial.

pH—
Adjusted to between 6.4 and 7.2 with sodium carbonate or acetic acid.

**Mechanism of action/Effect**

Following intramuscular injection, tetanus immune globulin provides immunity to those individuals who have low or no immunity to the toxin produced by the tetanus organism, *Clostridium tetani*. The antibodies act to neutralize the free form of the powerful exotoxin, tetanospasmin, produced by this bacterium.

**Protective effect**

Therapeutic passive immunization with tetanus immune globulin decreases fatalities in humans. While the therapeutic dose of tetanus immune globulin does not prevent the effects of toxin already bound to the nerve tissue, it should be given promptly because it may modify the course of toxin that has not yet been bound and later may cause symptoms.

**Time to protective effect**

Peak blood concentrations of immunoglobulin G (IgG) are obtained approximately 2 days after intramuscular injection.

**Duration of protective effect**

Short; the half-life of IgG in the circulation of individuals with normal IgG concentrations is approximately 23 days.

## Precautions to Consider

**Pregnancy/Reproduction**

Pregnancy—Studies have not been done in humans. However, there is no evidence to suspect that tetanus immune globulin causes problems in pregnant women.

Studies have not been done in animals.

FDA Pregnancy Category C.

**Breast-feeding**

It is not known whether tetanus immune globulin is distributed into breast milk. However, problems in humans have not been documented.

**Pediatrics**

Appropriate studies on the relationship of age to the effects of tetanus immune globulin have not been performed in the pediatric population. However, pediatrics-specific problems that would limit the usefulness of tetanus immune globulin in children are not expected.

**Geriatrics**

No information is available on the relationship of age to the effects of tetanus immune globulin in geriatric patients. However, there is no evidence that increasing age enhances the risk or diminishes the efficacy of tetanus immune globulin, or that its effects differ from those in younger persons.

**Drug interactions and/or related problems**

The following drug interactions and/or related problems have been selected on the basis of their potential clinical significance (possible mechanism in parentheses where appropriate)—not necessarily inclusive (» = major clinical significance):

Note: Combinations containing any of the following medications, depending on the amount present, may also interact with this medication.

Live virus vaccines
(antibodies in immunoglobulin preparations may interfere with the response to live virus vaccines such as measles, oral poliovirus, and rubella; use of live virus vaccines should be deferred until approximately 3 months after tetanus immune globulin administration; the

effect of immune globulin preparations on the response to mumps and varicella vaccines is unknown, but commercial immune globulin preparations contain antibodies to these viruses)

### Medical considerations/Contraindications

The medical considerations/contraindications included have been selected on the basis of their potential clinical significance (reasons given in parentheses where appropriate)—not necessarily inclusive (» = major clinical significance).

*Risk-benefit should be considered when the following medical problem exists:*

Sensitivity to tetanus immune globulin

## Side/Adverse Effects

Note: Sensitization to repeated injections of human immunoglobulin preparations is extremely rare, even though slight soreness at the site of injection and slight temperature elevation may be noted at times.

In the course of routine injections of large numbers of persons with immunoglobulin preparations, there have been a few isolated occurrences of angioneuropathic edema, nephrotic syndrome, and anaphylactic shock after injection.

The following side/adverse effects have been selected on the basis of their potential clinical significance (possible signs and symptoms in parentheses where appropriate)—not necessarily inclusive:

**Those indicating need for medical attention**
Incidence rare
*Anaphylactic reaction* (difficulty in breathing or swallowing; hives; itching, especially of soles or palms; reddening of skin, especially around ears; swelling of eyes, face, or inside of nose; unusual tiredness or weakness, sudden and severe)

## Patient Consultation

As an aid to patient consultation, refer to *Advice for the Patient, Tetanus Immune Globulin (Systemic)*.

In providing consultation, consider emphasizing the following selected information (» = major clinical significance):

**Before receiving this medication**
» Conditions affecting use, especially:
    Sensitivity to tetanus immune globulin

**Proper use of this medication**
» Proper dosing

**Side/adverse effects**
Signs of potential side effects, especially anaphylactic reaction

## General Dosing Information

Skin tests for allergy should not be performed prior to administration of tetanus immune globulin. The intradermal injection of concentrated immunoglobulin G (IgG) solution often causes localized inflammation due to tissue irritation, which can be misinterpreted as a positive allergic reaction. True allergic responses to human IgG are rare.

Although systemic reactions to human immunoglobulin preparations are rare, appropriate precautions should be taken prior to tetanus immune globulin injection to prevent allergic or other unwanted reactions. These should include review of the patient's history regarding possible sensitivity and the ready availability of epinephrine 1:1000 and other appropriate agents used to control immediate allergic reactions.

Tetanus immune globulin is administered intramuscularly. The preferred sites for intramuscular injections are the anterolateral aspect of the upper thigh and the deltoid muscle of the upper arm. It should not be injected intravenously. Intravenous injection of immune globulin intended for intramuscular use can, on occasion, cause a rapid fall in blood pressure. Therefore, injections should only be made intramuscularly; care should be taken to draw back on the plunger of the syringe before injection in order to be certain that the needle is not in a blood vessel.

It is important to convey immediate passive protection against tetanus, and at the same time begin formation of tetanus antibodies in the injured individual in order to preclude future need for antitoxin. Passive immunization with tetanus immune globulin may be undertaken simultaneously with active immunization using tetanus toxoid in those persons who must receive an immediate injection of tetanus immune globulin and in whom it is desirable to begin or continue (for those patients who have had only one dose of tetanus toxoid) the process of active immunization.

Since tetanus is actually a local infection, proper initial wound care is of paramount importance. The use of tetanus immune globulin is an adjunct to treatment of the wound. However, in approximately 10% of recent tetanus cases, no wound or other break in the skin or mucous membranes could be implicated. Current recommendations for wound management of patients definitely known to have completed a full tetanus toxoid series indicate only a booster dose of tetanus toxoid if more than 5 to 10 years have elapsed since the last dose of toxoid.

Tetanus immune globulin does not interfere with the immune response to tetanus toxoid. However, the two injections should not be given in the same syringe or injected at the same site, since neutralization of the toxoid may occur.

The optimum therapeutic dose for the treatment of tetanus infection has not been established. However, the Committee on Infectious Diseases of the American Academy of Pediatrics (AAP) recommends a single dose of 3000 to 6000 units of tetanus immune globulin for the treatment of tetanus infection.

Antibodies in immune globulin preparations may interfere with the response to live virus vaccines such as oral poliovirus, and rubella. Therefore, use of live virus vaccines should be deferred until approximately 3 months after tetanus immune globulin administration. The concurrent administration of tetanus immune globulin should not interfere with the immune response to oral typhoid vaccine.

Recent evidence suggests high doses of immune globulin can inhibit the immune response to measles vaccine for more than 3 months after administration. Administration of immune globulin can also inhibit the response to rubella vaccine. The effect of immune globulin preparations on the response to mumps and varicella vaccines is unknown, but commercial immune globulin preparations contain antibodies to these viruses.

Blood-containing products, such as immune globulins, can diminish the immune response to measles, mumps, and rubella virus vaccine live or its individual component vaccines. Therefore, after an immune globulin preparation is received, these vaccines should not be administered before the recommended interval. However, the postpartum vaccination of rubella-susceptible women with rubella virus vaccine live or measles, mumps, and rubella virus vaccine live should not be delayed because immune globulin was received during the last trimester of pregnancy or at delivery. These women should be vaccinated immediately after delivery and, if possible, tested at least 3 months later to ensure immunity to rubella and, if necessary, to measles.

If administration of an immune globulin preparation becomes necessary because of imminent exposure to disease, measles, mumps, and rubella virus vaccine live or its individual component vaccines can be administered simultaneously with the immune globulin preparation, although vaccine-induced immunity could be compromised. The vaccine should be administered at an injection site remote from that chosen for the immune globulin inoculation. Unless serologic testing indicates that specific antibodies have been produced, vaccination should be repeated after the recommended interval.

If administration of an immune globulin preparation becomes necessary after measles, mumps, and rubella virus vaccine live or its individual component vaccines have been administered, interference can occur. Usually, vaccine virus replication and stimulation of immunity will occur 1 to 2 weeks after vaccination. Thus, if the interval between administration of any of these vaccines and subsequent administration of an immune globulin preparation is less than 14 days, vaccination should be repeated after the recommended interval, unless serologic testing indicates that antibodies were produced.

Immune globulin preparations interact less with inactivated vaccines and toxoids than with live virus vaccines. Therefore, administration of inactivated vaccines and toxoids either simultaneously with, or at any interval before or after, receipt of immune globulins should not substantially impair the development of a protective antibody response. The vaccine or toxoid and the immune globulin preparation should be administered at different injection sites using the standard recommended dose of vaccine. Increasing the vaccine dose or number of vaccinations for inactivated vaccines or toxoids is not indicated or recommended.

Immunocompromised persons, including those infected with human immunodeficiency virus (HIV), should receive tetanus immune globulin for the same indications and in the same doses as immunocompetent persons.

For emergency tetanus prophylaxis of wounds—
• If uncertain of number or less than three primary doses of tetanus toxoid have been administered: For clean, minor wounds, tetanus and diphtheria toxoids should be administered as soon as possible. For children younger than 7 years of age, diphtheria and tetanus toxoids adsorbed (for pediatric use), diphtheria and tetanus toxoids and pertussis vaccine adsorbed (DTP), or a combination DTP and poliovirus vaccine should be given as part of the routine childhood immunization. For all other wounds, tetanus immune globulin also should be administered.

- If three or more doses of tetanus toxoid have been administered alone or in combination with other vaccines such as DTP: For clean, minor wounds, if more than 10 years have passed since the last dose of tetanus toxoid, tetanus and diphtheria toxoids should be administered as soon as possible. For other, more severe tetanus-prone wounds, if more than 5 years have passed since the last dose of tetanus toxoid, tetanus and diphtheria toxoids should be administered as soon as possible. Generally, tetanus immune globulin is not required in either case.

### For treatment of adverse effects
Recommended treatment consists of the following:
- For mild hypersensitivity reaction—Administering antihistamines, and, if necessary, corticosteroids.
- For severe hypersensitivity or anaphylactic reaction—Administering epinephrine. Antihistamines or corticosteroids also may be administered as required.

## Parenteral Dosage Forms

### TETANUS IMMUNE GLOBULIN INJECTION USP

**Usual adult and adolescent dose**
Immunizing agent (passive)—
  Deep intramuscular injection, 250 units.

Note: In cases of severe or highly contaminated wounds, or when treatment is delayed for more than twenty-four hours, a dose of 500 units may be required. If the threat of tetanus infection persists, repeat doses of tetanus immune globulin can be given at four-week intervals.

**Usual pediatric dose**
Immunizing agent (passive)—
  See *Usual adult and adolescent dose*.

Note: The pediatric dose is the same as for adults. Alternatively, in children younger than 7 years of age, tetanus immune globulin can be given in doses of 4 units per kilogram of body weight.

**Strength(s) usually available**
U.S.—
  Not less than 250 units in each prefilled disposable syringe (Rx) [*BayTet*].
Canada—
  Not less than 250 units in each prefilled disposable syringe (Rx) [GENERIC].

**Packaging and storage**
Store between 2 and 8 °C (36 and 46 °F), unless otherwise specified by manufacturer.

**Stability**
Tetanus immune globulin should not be used if exposed to freezing temperatures.

**Incompatibilities**
Do not administer in the same syringe or at the same body site as tetanus toxoid.

**Auxiliary labeling**
- Do not freeze.

Developed: 06/20/97

# TETANUS TOXOID  Systemic

VA CLASSIFICATION (Primary): IM200

Note: For a listing of dosage forms and brand names by country availability, see *Dosage Forms* section(s).

## Category
Immunizing agent (active).

## Indications

### Accepted
Tetanus (prophylaxis)—Tetanus toxoid is indicated for immunization against tetanus. The main objectives of tetanus immunization are to prevent tetanus infection and the severe complications, including death, that arise from the toxins produced by *Clostridium tetani*. Although the spores of tetanus are ubiquitous, naturally acquired immunity to tetanus does not occur in the U.S., and primary immunization and booster injections are essential to protect persons in all age groups.

Unless otherwise contraindicated, all infants 6 to 8 weeks of age and older, all children, and all adults should be immunized against tetanus with the primary series of tetanus toxoid and a booster injection every 10 years throughout their lives, including:
- Adults, especially those 50 years of age and older. In recent years, approximately two-thirds of persons contracting tetanus have been in this age group.
- Persons with uncertain histories of a complete primary series with tetanus toxoid or immunizing agents containing tetanus toxoid.
- Travelers.
- Persons at increased risk of receiving lacerations and abrasions through their occupation or recreation.
- Persons with known sensitivity to horse serum or with asthma or other allergies. This is to minimize the possible need for passive immunization with tetanus antitoxin (TAT) of animal origin (usually horse) if a wound is received. Although human tetanus immune globulin (TIG) is usually used for passive immunization, TAT of animal origin still may be used in certain areas of the world and has the potential of causing adverse reactions in hypersensitive patients.
- Pregnant women who are unimmunized or inadequately immunized and who may deliver their infants under unhygienic conditions, thereby exposing their infants to neonatal tetanus.
- Those recovering from tetanus. Since a tetanus infection does not confer immunity, especially in the U.S., immunization with tetanus toxoid should be initiated or continued at the time of recovery from the illness.

In addition, persons who are injured may require emergency tetanus prophylaxis depending on the number of primary immunizations, the timing of any boosters, and/or the type of wound received.

It is recommended that infants and children 6 weeks up to 7 years of age receive tetanus toxoid as part of Diphtheria and Tetanus Toxoids and Pertussis Vaccine Adsorbed (DTP) immunization according to the DTP immunization schedule. In those cases where the pertussis vaccine is contraindicated, it is recommended that Diphtheria and Tetanus Toxoids for pediatric use (DT) be administered instead, according to the DT immunization schedule.

It is recommended that children 7 years of age and older and all adults receive tetanus toxoid as part of Tetanus and Diphtheria Toxoids for adult use (Td) both for the primary series and for the booster doses every 10 years.

When the single-entity vaccine is used, tetanus toxoid adsorbed is the vaccine of choice for primary immunization because greater antigenic stimulation and longer lasting immunity are achieved than with the tetanus toxoid (fluid). Most experts feel that tetanus toxoid adsorbed should be used for booster doses as well; others feel that either tetanus toxoid adsorbed or tetanus toxoid (fluid) may be used for booster doses with equal results. Either tetanus toxoid adsorbed or tetanus toxoid (fluid) may be used for emergency tetanus prophylaxis for wounds.

## Pharmacology/Pharmacokinetics

### Physicochemical characteristics
Source—Tetanus toxoid adsorbed and fluid are prepared by growing the tetanus bacilli *Clostridium tetani* on a protein-free, semi-synthetic medium. The tetanus toxin produced by these bacilli is detoxified by using formaldehyde and forms the tetanus toxoid. Thimerosal is added as a preservative. In addition, for tetanus toxoid adsorbed, aluminum phosphate or aluminum potassium sulfate is used as a mineral adjuvant to adsorb the tetanus antigens. This prolongs and enhances the antigenic properties by retarding the rate of absorption of the injected toxoid into the body.

### Mechanism of action/Effect
Following intramuscular injection of tetanus toxoid adsorbed or either intramuscular or subcutaneous injection of tetanus toxoid (fluid), an antigenic response is induced in the immunized patient, causing the formation of tetanus antibodies.

### Protective effect
Tetanus toxoid adsorbed—Most persons possess protective levels of antitoxin to tetanus after two doses. The remaining persons usually obtain protective levels following the third dose of the primary series, which is given approximately one year later.

Tetanus toxoid (fluid)—Does not produce as great an antigenic stimulation as does tetanus toxoid adsorbed, but does provide protective levels.

**Duration of protective effect**
Duration of immunity is unknown, but is generally believed to persist for 10 or more years following a primary series or a booster dose of tetanus toxoid. Tetanus toxoid adsorbed causes greater antigenic stimulation and longer lasting immunity than does the tetanus toxoid (fluid).

## Precautions to Consider

**Cross-sensitivity and/or related problems**
Patients allergic to thimerosal may be allergic to the tetanus toxoid available in the U.S. and Canada because it may contain a small amount of thimerosal.

**Pregnancy/Reproduction**
Pregnancy—Studies have not been done in humans; however, problems in humans have not been documented.
Immune pregnant women confer protection to their infants through transplacental maternal antibody. Pregnant women who are inadequately immunized or unimmunized and who may deliver their infants under unhygienic conditions may expose their infants to neonatal tetanus. For inadequately immunized or unimmunized pregnant women, it is recommended that immunization with tetanus toxoid be initiated or continued during the last two trimesters. Unimmunized women should receive the first two doses of the primary series before childbirth.
Studies have not been done in animals.
FDA Pregnancy Category C.

**Breast-feeding**
Problems in humans have not been documented.

**Pediatrics**
Infants up to 6 weeks of age—Use is not recommended.
Infants and children 6 weeks of age and older—Pediatrics-specific problems that would limit the usefulness of this vaccine in children in this age group are not expected.

**Geriatrics**
Although appropriate studies on the relationship of age to the effects of tetanus toxoid have not been performed in the geriatric population, geriatrics-specific problems are not expected to limit the usefulness of tetanus toxoid in the elderly. However, the immune response in the elderly may be slightly diminished.

**Drug interactions and/or related problems**
The following drug interactions and/or related problems have been selected on the basis of their potential clinical significance (possible mechanism in parentheses where appropriate)—not necessarily inclusive (» = major clinical significance):
Note: Combinations containing any of the following medications, depending on the amount present, may also interact with this medication.

Immunosuppressants or
Radiation therapy
(because normal defense mechanisms are suppressed, the patient's antibody response to tetanus toxoid may be decreased. The precaution does not apply to corticosteroids used as replacement therapy, for short-term [less than 2 weeks] systemic therapy, or by other routes of administration that do not cause immunosuppression. Where possible, immunosuppressive therapy should be interrupted when immunization is required because of a tetanus-prone wound)

**Medical considerations/Contraindications**
The medical considerations/contraindications included have been selected on the basis of their potential clinical significance (reasons given in parentheses where appropriate)—not necessarily inclusive (» = major clinical significance).

*Except under special circumstances, this medication should not be used when the following medical problems exist:*
» Febrile illness, severe or
» Respiratory disease, acute
(routine primary or booster immunization should not be administered until the acute symptoms of the patient's illness have abated; however, emergency tetanus prophylaxis for wounds should be administered as usual. Minor illnesses, such as upper respiratory infection, do not preclude administration of tetanus toxoid)
» Tetanus infection
(tetanus toxoid should not be used to treat a tetanus infection; tetanus antitoxin, preferably tetanus immune globulin (TIG), should be used instead; after recovery, tetanus toxoid should be initiated or continued, since a tetanus infection does not confer immunity)

*Risk-benefit should be considered when the following medical problem exists:*
Sensitivity to tetanus vaccine

## Side/Adverse Effects

Note: If an arthus-type hypersensitivity reaction or a fever greater than 39.4 °C (103 °F) occurs following a dose of tetanus toxoid, the patient usually has very high serum tetanus antitoxin levels and no additional doses of tetanus toxoid should be given for any reason, including wounds, more frequently than every 10 years.
If a systemic allergic or neurologic reaction occurs following a dose of tetanus toxoid, the person should not be further immunized using tetanus toxoid; instead, passive immunization using tetanus immune globulin (TIG) should be used when other than a clean, minor wound is sustained. Neurological reactions, such as peripheral neuropathies, have been temporally related to tetanus toxoid administration; however, no causal relationship has been established.
Booster doses of tetanus toxoid administered more frequently than every 10 years have been reported to result in an increased occurrence and severity of adverse reactions.
Generally, a history of hypersensitivity reactions other than anaphylaxis, such as delayed-type, cell-mediated allergic reaction (contact dermatitis), does not preclude immunization.

The following side/adverse effects have been selected on the basis of their potential clinical significance (possible signs and symptoms in parentheses where appropriate)—not necessarily inclusive:

**Those indicating need for medical attention**
Incidence rare
*Anaphylactic reaction* (difficulty in breathing or swallowing; hives; itching, especially of soles or palms; reddening of skin, especially around ears; swelling of eyes, face, or inside of nose; sudden and severe unusual tiredness or weakness); *neurologic reaction* (confusion; fever over 39.4 °C [103 °F]; severe or continuing headache; seizures; excessive sleepiness; unusual irritability; severe or continuing vomiting)

**Additional side/adverse effects that may occur because of very high serum tetanus antitoxin levels and indicating need for medical attention**
Incidence rare
*Fever over 39.4 °C* (103 °F); *lymphadenopathy* (swelling of glands in armpit); *swelling, blistering, or pain at injection site, which may be severe and extensive*

**Those indicating need for medical attention only if they continue or are bothersome**
Incidence more frequent
*Redness or hard lump at injection site*—may persist for a few days
Incidence less frequent
*Allergic reaction, delayed-type, cell-mediated* (pain, tenderness, itching, or swelling at injection site); *chills, fever, irritability, or unusual tiredness; nodule or sterile abscess at injection site*—probably from the aluminum content of tetanus toxoid adsorbed; may persist for a few weeks; *skin rash*

## Patient Consultation

As an aid to patient consultation, refer to *Advice for the Patient, Tetanus Toxoid (Systemic)*.
In providing consultation, consider emphasizing the following selected information (» = major clinical significance):

**Before using this vaccine**
» Conditions affecting use, especially:
Use in children—Not recommended for infants up to 6 weeks of age
Other medical problems, especially severe febrile illness, acute respiratory disease, or tetanus infection

**Proper use of this vaccine**
» Proper dosing

**Side/adverse effects**
Signs of potential side effects, especially anaphylactic reaction; neurologic reaction; fever over 39.4 °C (103 °F); lymphadenopathy; or swelling, blistering, or pain at injection site

## General Dosing Information

It is recommended that infants and children 6 weeks up to 7 years of age receive tetanus toxoid as part of Diphtheria and Tetanus Toxoids and Pertussis Vaccine Adsorbed (DTP) immunization according to the DTP immunization schedule. In those cases where the pertussis vaccine is contraindicated, it is recommended that Diphtheria and Tetanus Toxoids for pediatric use (DT) be administered instead, according to the DT immunization schedule.

It is recommended that children 7 years of age and older and all adults receive tetanus toxoid as part of Tetanus and Diphtheria Toxoids for adult use (Td), both for the primary series and for the booster doses every 10 years.

The dosage of tetanus toxoid is the same for all persons: infants, children, and adults.

A primary series of tetanus toxoid adsorbed consists of 3 doses; a primary series of tetanus toxoid (fluid) consists of 4 doses. If a combination of tetanus toxoid adsorbed and tetanus toxoid (fluid) is used, a total of 4 doses constitutes a primary series. These primary series include a reinforcing dose administered 6 to 12 months after the first 2 doses of tetanus toxoid adsorbed or after the first 3 doses of tetanus toxoid (fluid) or a combination of both. Basic immunization cannot be considered complete until all of these doses are administered.

Prolonging the interval between the primary immunizing doses probably does not interfere with the final immunity. Any dose of tetanus toxoid, including an emergency prophylactic dose, a person has received during the last 10 years may be counted as one of his immunizing injections.

Persons infected with human immunodeficiency virus (HIV) may receive tetanus toxoid whether they have asymptomatic or symptomatic HIV infection.

Tetanus toxoid can be administered concurrently with the following, using separate body sites, separate syringes, and the precautions that apply to each immunizing agent:
- Tetanus immune globulin (human) or tetanus antitoxin (animal).
- Polysaccharide vaccines, such as haemophilus b polysaccharide vaccine, haemophilus b conjugate vaccine, meningococcal polysaccharide vaccine, or pneumococcal polyvalent vaccine.
- Influenza vaccine, whole or split virus.
- Diphtheria toxoid and/or pertussis vaccine.
- Live virus vaccines, such as measles, mumps, and/or rubella vaccines.
- Poliovirus vaccines (oral [OPV], inactivated [IPV], or enhanced-potency inactivated [enhanced-potency IPV]).
- Immune globulin and disease-specific immune globulins.
- Hepatitis B recombinant or plasma-derived vaccine, or other inactivated vaccines, except cholera, typhoid, and plague. It is recommended that cholera, typhoid, and plague vaccines be administered on separate occasions because of these vaccines' propensity to cause side/adverse effects.

### For tetanus toxoid (fluid) only
Tetanus toxoid (fluid) is administered subcutaneously or intramuscularly into the area of the midlateral muscles (vastus lateralis) of the thigh or into the deltoid. The vaccine should not be injected intravenously.

### For tetanus toxoid adsorbed only
Tetanus toxoid adsorbed is administered intramuscularly into the area of the midlateral muscles (vastus lateralis) of the thigh or into the deltoid. The same muscle site should not be used more than once during the course of the primary immunization. The vaccine should not be injected intravenously.

### Emergency tetanus prophylaxis of wounds
Examples of wounds that are not clean, minor wounds are: wounds contaminated with dirt, feces, soil, or saliva; puncture wounds; wounds caused by tearing; and wounds resulting from missiles, crushing, burns, or frostbite.

Patients who were unimmunized or inadequately immunized prior to injury should complete their primary immunization schedule as soon as possible.

If only tetanus toxoid adsorbed has been used for the primary doses—Patients who receive an emergency prophylactic dose of tetanus toxoid adsorbed after their second primary dose should count the prophylactic dose as their third (last) primary dose if the prophylactic dose is administered at least 6 months after the second primary dose.

If either tetanus toxoid (fluid) or a combination of both toxoids has been used for the primary doses—Patients who receive an emergency prophylactic dose of either tetanus toxoid (fluid) or tetanus toxoid adsorbed after their third primary dose should count the prophylactic dose as their fourth (last) primary dose if the prophylactic dose is administered at least 6 months after the third primary dose.

The decision to administer concomitant passive immunization by using tetanus immune globulin (human) or tetanus antitoxin (animal) depends on such factors as location, type, and severity of the wound; degree and kind of contamination; and the time elapsed since the injury. Some experts feel that tetanus toxoid adsorbed should be used with the selected antitoxin; others feel that either tetanus toxoid adsorbed or tetanus toxoid (fluid) may be used.

### For treatment of adverse effects
Recommended treatment includes
- For mild hypersensitivity reaction—Administering antihistamines and, if necessary, corticosteroids.
- For severe hypersensitivity or anaphylactic reaction—Administering epinephrine. Antihistamines or corticosteroids may also be administered as required.

## Parenteral Dosage Forms

### TETANUS TOXOID (FLUID) INJECTION USP

**Usual adult and adolescent dose**
Tetanus (prophylaxis)—Intramuscular or subcutaneous, 0.5 mL (U.S.) or 1 mL (Canada—Connaught):—
First dose—
  At initial visit.
Second dose—
  4 to 8 weeks after the first dose.
Third dose—
  4 to 8 weeks after the second dose.
Fourth dose—
  6 to 12 months after the third dose.
Booster doses—
  Every 10 years.
Emergency tetanus prophylaxis of wounds:
  U.S.—
    If less than the 4 primary doses have been administered—As soon as possible following any wound. For other than clean, minor wounds, tetanus immune globulin (human) (preferred) or tetanus antitoxin (animal) should also be administered.
    If 4 or more doses have been administered—For a clean, minor wound, as soon as possible if more than 10 years have passed since the last dose. For all other wounds, as soon as possible if more than 5 years have passed since the last dose. No tetanus immune globulin (human) or tetanus antitoxin (animal) is required in either case.
  Canada—
    If less than 2 primary doses have been administered—As soon as possible following any wound. For other than clean, minor wounds, tetanus immune globulin (human) (preferred) or tetanus antitoxin (animal) should also be administered.
    If 2 primary doses have been administered—As soon as possible following any wound. For other than clean, minor wounds, tetanus immune globulin (human) (preferred) or tetanus antitoxin (animal) should also be administered if more than 24 hours have elapsed since the injury.
    If 3 or more doses have been administered—For a clean, minor wound, as soon as possible if more than 10 years have passed since the last dose. For all other wounds, as soon as possible if more than 5 years have passed since the last dose. No tetanus immune globulin (human) or tetanus antitoxin (animal) is required in either case.

**Usual pediatric dose**
See *Usual adult and adolescent dose*.

Note: For infants, the first dose is usually administered at 6 to 8 weeks of age.

**Usual geriatric dose**
See *Usual adult and adolescent dose*.

**Strength(s) usually available**
U.S.—
  4 Lf per 0.5 mL (Rx) [GENERIC (may contain thimerosal)].
Canada—
  10 Lf per 1 mL (Rx) [GENERIC (may contain thimerosal)].
Note: Lf is the quantity of toxoid as assessed by flocculation.

**Packaging and storage**
Store between 2 and 8 °C (36 and 46 °F). Do not freeze.

**Stability**
The vaccine should not be used if exposed to freezing or if cloudy or turbid.

**Auxiliary labeling**
- Shake well.
- Do not freeze.

### TETANUS TOXOID ADSORBED (INJECTION) USP

**Usual adult and adolescent dose**
Tetanus (prophylaxis)—Intramuscular, 0.5 mL:—
First dose—
  At initial visit.

Second dose—
  4 to 8 weeks after the first dose.
Third dose—
  6 to 12 months after the second dose.
Booster doses—
  Every 10 years.
Emergency tetanus prophylaxis of wounds:
  U.S.—
    If less than the 3 primary doses have been administered—As soon as possible following any wound. For other than clean, minor wounds, tetanus immune globulin (human) (preferred) or tetanus antitoxin (animal) should also be administered.
    If 3 or more doses have been administered—For a clean, minor wound, as soon as possible if more than 10 years have passed since the last dose. For all other wounds, as soon as possible if more than 5 years have passed since the last dose. Generally, no tetanus immune globulin (human) or tetanus antitoxin (animal) is required in either case.
  Canada—
    If less than 2 primary doses have been administered—As soon as possible following any wound. For other than clean, minor wounds, tetanus immune globulin (human) (preferred) or tetanus antitoxin (animal) should also be administered.
    If 2 primary doses have been administered—As soon as possible following any wound. For other than clean, minor wounds, tetanus immune globulin (human) (preferred) or tetanus antitoxin (animal) should also be administered if more than 24 hours have elapsed since the injury.
    If 3 or more doses have been administered—For a clean, minor wound, as soon as possible if more than 10 years have passed since the last dose. For all other wounds, as soon as possible if more than 5 years have passed since the last dose. No tetanus immune globulin (human) or tetanus antitoxin (animal) is required in either case.

**Usual pediatric dose**
See *Usual adult and adolescent dose*.
Note:  For infants, the first dose is usually administered at 6 to 8 weeks of age.

**Usual geriatric dose**
See *Usual adult and adolescent dose*.

**Strength(s) usually available**
U.S.—
  5 Lf per 0.5 mL (Rx) [GENERIC (may contain thimerosal)].
  10 Lf per 0.5 mL (Rx) [GENERIC (may contain thimerosal)].
Canada—
  5 Lf per 0.5 mL (Rx) [GENERIC (may contain thimerosal)].
Note:  Lf is the quantity of toxoid as assessed by flocculation.

**Packaging and storage**
Store between 2 and 8 °C (36 and 46 °F). Do not freeze.

**Stability**
The vaccine should not be used if exposed to freezing.

**Auxiliary labeling**
• Shake well.
• Do not freeze.

Revised: 07/12/94

---

## TETRACAINE—See *Anesthetics (Mucosal-Local); Anesthetics (Parenteral-Local); Anesthetics (Topical)*

---

## TETRACAINE AND MENTHOL—See *Anesthetics (Topical)*

---

## TETRACYCLINE—See *Tetracycline Periodontal Fibers (Mucosal-Local); Tetracyclines (Ophthalmic); Tetracyclines (Systemic); Tetracyclines (Topical)*

---

## TETRACYCLINE PERIODONTAL FIBERS—The *Tetracycline Periodontal Fibers (Mucosal-Local)* monograph is not included in this published version of the USP DI database. Copies of the monograph are available on request from Micromedex, Inc. - Reprint Requests, 6200 S. Syracuse Way, Suite 300, Englewood, CO 80111; telephone (303) 486-6400; telefax (303) 486-6464; Email: USPDI@MDX.COM.

---

# TETRACYCLINES  Ophthalmic

This monograph includes information on the following: 1) Chlortetracycline; 2) Tetracycline.
VA CLASSIFICATION (Primary): OP201
Commonly used brand name(s): *Achromycin*[2]; *Aureomycin*[1].
Note:  For a listing of dosage forms and brand names by country availability, see *Dosage Forms* section(s).

## Category
Antibacterial (ophthalmic).

## Indications
Note:  Bracketed information in the *Indications* section refers to uses that are not included in U.S. product labeling.

**Accepted**
Ocular infections (treatment)—Ophthalmic chlortetracycline is indicated in the treatment of superficial ocular infections caused by *Staphylococcus aureus*, *Streptococcus epidemicus (Streptococcus pyogenes)*, *Neisseria gonorrhoeae*, *S. pneumoniae (Diplococcus pneumoniae)*, *Haemophilus influenzae*, *H. ducreyi*, *Klebsiella pneumoniae*, *Francisella tularensis (Pasteurella tularensis)*, *Yersinia pestis (Pasteurella pestis)*, *Escherichia coli*, *Bacillus anthracis*, and *Lymphogranuloma venereum*.
Ophthalmic tetracycline is indicated in the treatment of superficial ocular infections caused by *Staphylococcus aureus*, streptococci including *Streptococcus epidemicus (Streptococcus pyogenes)* and *S. pneumoniae (Diplococcus pneumoniae)*, *Neisseria gonorrhoeae*, and *Escherichia coli*.
Ophthalmia neonatorum (prophylaxis)—Ophthalmic [chlortetracycline] and tetracycline are indicated in the prophylaxis of ophthalmia neonatorum caused by *N. gonorrhoeae* and *Chlamydia trachomatis*.
Trachoma (treatment)—Ophthalmic chlortetracycline and tetracycline are indicated in the treatment of trachoma caused by *Chlamydia trachomatis*. They should be used concurrently with oral tetracyclines.
[Blepharitis, bacterial (treatment)]
[Blepharoconjunctivitis (treatment)]
[Conjunctivitis, bacterial (treatment)]
[Keratitis, bacterial (treatment)]
[Keratoconjunctivitis, bacterial (treatment)] or
[Meibomianitis (treatment)]—Ophthalmic chlortetracycline and tetracycline are used in the treatment of bacterial blepharitis, blepharoconjunctivitis, bacterial conjunctivitis, bacterial keratitis, bacterial keratoconjunctivitis, and meibomianitis.
[Chlamydial infections (treatment)] or
[Rosacea, ocular (treatment)]—Ophthalmic tetracycline is used in the treatment of chlamydial infections and ocular rosacea.
Note:  Not all species or strains of a particular organism may be susceptible to a specific tetracycline.

**Unaccepted**
Tetracycline is not effective against *Haemophilus influenzae*, *Klebsiella* species, *Enterobacter (Aerobacter)* species, *Pseudomonas aeruginosa*, or *Serratia marcescens*.

## Pharmacology/Pharmacokinetics

### Physicochemical characteristics
Molecular weight—
  Chlortetracycline hydrochloride: 515.35.
  Tetracycline hydrochloride: 480.90.

### Mechanism of action/Effect
Tetracyclines are broad-spectrum bacteriostatic agents and act by inhibiting protein synthesis by blocking the binding of aminoacyl tRNA (transfer RNA) to the mRNA (messenger RNA) ribosome complex. Reversible binding occurs primarily at the 30 S ribosomal subunit of susceptible organisms. Bacterial cell wall synthesis is not inhibited.

## Precautions to Consider

### Cross-sensitivity and/or related problems
Patients sensitive to one tetracycline, tetracycline combination, or tetracycline derivative may be sensitive to other tetracyclines also.

### Pregnancy/Reproduction
Pregnancy—Problems in humans have not been documented.

### Breast-feeding
Problems in humans have not been documented.

### Pediatrics
Appropriate studies on the relationship of age to the effects of ophthalmic tetracyclines have not been performed in the pediatric population. However, no pediatrics-specific problems have been documented to date.

### Geriatrics
Appropriate studies on the relationship of age to the effects of tetracyclines have not been performed in the geriatric population. However, no geriatrics-specific problems have been documented to date.

### Medical considerations/Contraindications
The medical considerations/contraindications included have been selected on the basis of their potential clinical significance (reasons given in parentheses where appropriate)—not necessarily inclusive (» = major clinical significance).

*Risk-benefit should be considered when the following medical problem exists:*
  Sensitivity to tetracyclines

## Patient Consultation
As an aid to patient consultation, refer to *Advice for the Patient, Tetracyclines (Ophthalmic)*.
In providing consultation, consider emphasizing the following selected information (» = major clinical significance):

### Before using this medication
» Conditions affecting use, especially:
    Sensitivity to tetracycline, chlortetracycline, or any related antibiotic, such as demeclocycline, doxycycline, methacycline, minocycline, or oxytetracycline

### Proper use of this medication
  Proper administration technique for ophthalmic suspension and ophthalmic ointment
» Compliance with full course of therapy
» Proper dosing
  Missed dose: Applying as soon as possible; not applying if almost time for next dose
» Proper storage

### Precautions while using this medication
  Blurred vision after application of ophthalmic ointments and ophthalmic suspensions in oil (tetracycline)
  Checking with physician if no improvement within a few days

## General Dosing Information
Blurred vision after application of ophthalmic suspensions in oil or ophthalmic ointments is to be expected.

Therapy should be continued for 1 to 2 months or longer in acute and chronic trachoma. Severe infections may also require concurrent oral therapy for trachoma.

In term infants born to mothers with clinically apparent gonorrhea, a single intramuscular or intravenous dose of 50,000 Units of penicillin G potassium is administered concurrently with ophthalmic tetracycline. In low-birth-weight infants, the dose is 20,000 Units.

At night, the ophthalmic ointment may be used as an adjunct to the ophthalmic suspension to provide prolonged contact with the medication.

Although some manufacturers recommend a dose of 2 drops of an ophthalmic solution at appropriate intervals, the conjunctival sac usually will hold only 1 drop.

---
### CHLORTETRACYCLINE
---

## Ophthalmic Dosage Forms

### CHLORTETRACYCLINE HYDROCHLORIDE OPHTHALMIC OINTMENT USP

**Usual adult and adolescent dose**
Ocular infections—
  Topical, to the conjunctiva, a thin strip (approximately 1 cm) of ointment every two to four hours or more frequently.

**Usual pediatric dose**
See *Usual adult and adolescent dose*.

**Strength(s) usually available**
U.S.—
  1% (Rx) [*Aureomycin*].
Canada—
  1% (Rx) [*Aureomycin*].

**Packaging and storage**
Store below 40 °C (104 °F), preferably between 15 and 30 °C (59 and 86 °F), unless otherwise specified by manufacturer. Store in a collapsible ophthalmic ointment tube. Protect from freezing.

**Auxiliary labeling**
• For the eye.
• Continue medicine for full time of treatment.

---
### TETRACYCLINE
---

## Ophthalmic Dosage Forms

### TETRACYCLINE HYDROCHLORIDE OPHTHALMIC OINTMENT USP

**Usual adult and adolescent dose**
Ocular infections—
  Topical, to the conjunctiva, a thin strip (approximately 1 cm) of ointment every two to four hours or more frequently.
Ophthalmia neonatorum—
  Topical, to the conjunctiva, a thin strip (approximately 1 cm) of ointment as a single dose.

**Usual pediatric dose**
See *Usual adult and adolescent dose*.

**Strength(s) usually available**
U.S.—
  1% (Rx) [*Achromycin*].
Canada—
  1% (Rx) [*Achromycin*].

**Packaging and storage**
Store below 40 °C (104 °F), preferably between 15 and 30 °C (59 and 86 °F), unless otherwise specified by manufacturer. Store in a collapsible ophthalmic ointment tube. Protect from freezing.

**Auxiliary labeling**
• For the eye.
• Continue medicine for full time of treatment.

### TETRACYCLINE HYDROCHLORIDE OPHTHALMIC SUSPENSION USP

**Usual adult and adolescent dose**
Ocular infections—
  Topical, to the conjunctiva, 1 drop every six to twelve hours or more frequently.
Ophthalmia neonatorum—
  Topical, to the conjunctiva, 1 drop as a single dose.

**Usual pediatric dose**
See *Usual adult and adolescent dose*.

**Strength(s) usually available**
U.S.—
  1% (Rx) [*Achromycin*].
Canada—
  Not commercially available.

USP DI  Tetracyclines (Ophthalmic) 2765

**Packaging and storage**
Store below 40 °C (104 °F), preferably between 15 and 30 °C (59 and 86° F), unless otherwise specified by manufacturer. Store in a tight, light-resistant glass or plastic container. Protect from freezing.

**Auxiliary labeling**
- Shake well.
- For the eye.
- Continue medicine for full time of treatment.

**Note**
Dispense in original unopened container.

The ophthalmic suspension is available in a base containing light mineral oil and other ingredients that may briefly cause blurred vision after application.

Revised: 07/01/93

# TETRACYCLINES Systemic

This monograph includes information on the following: 1) Demeclocycline; 2) Doxycycline; 3) Minocycline; 4) Oxytetracycline†; 5) Tetracycline.

VA CLASSIFICATION (Primary/Secondary):
  Demeclocycline—AM250/AP109
  Doxycycline—AM250/AP109
  Minocycline—AM250/AP109; DE751; MS109
  Oxytetracycline—AM250/AP109
  Tetracycline—AM250/AP109; DE751

Commonly used brand name(s): *Achromycin*[5]; *Achromycin V*[5]; *Apo-Doxy*[2]; *Apo-Tetra*[5]; *Declomycin*[1]; *Doryx*[2]; *Doxi Film*[2]; *Doxy*[2]; *Doxy-Caps*[2]; *Doxycin*[2]; *Dynacin*[3]; *Minocin*[3]; *Monodox*[2]; *Novodoxylin*[2]; *Novotetra*[5]; *Nu-Tetra*[5]; *Panmycin*[5]; *Robitet*[5]; *Sumycin*[5]; *Terramycin*[4]; *Tetracyn*[5]; *Tija*[4]; *Vibra-Tabs*[2]; *Vibramycin*[2].

Note: For a listing of dosage forms and brand names by country availability, see *Dosage Forms* section(s).

†Not commercially available in Canada.

## Category

Antibacterial (systemic); antiprotozoal—Demeclocycline; Doxycycline; Minocycline; Oxytetracycline; Tetracycline.
Antiacne agent (systemic)—Minocycline (oral); tetracycline (oral).
Antirheumatic (systemic)—Minocycline (oral).
Diuretic (syndrome of inappropriate antidiuretic hormone)—Demeclocycline.

## Indications

Note:  Bracketed information in the *Indications* section refers to uses that are not included in U.S. product labeling.

**Accepted**

Acne vulgaris (treatment)—Although all tetracyclines may be indicated as adjunctive treatment, they are generally no more effective in the initial treatment of acne and are more expensive than tetracycline. However, oral minocycline may be more effective in severe or resistant acne and may be effective in acne unresponsive to oral tetracycline.

Actinomycosis (treatment)—Systemic tetracyclines are indicated in the treatment of actinomycosis caused by *Actinomyces israelii*.

Anthrax (treatment)—Systemic tetracyclines are indicated in the treatment of anthrax caused by *Bacillus anthracis*.

Bronchitis (treatment)
Brucellosis (treatment)
Conjunctivitis, inclusion (treatment) or
Trachoma (treatment)—Systemic tetracyclines are indicated in the treatment of bronchitis, brucellosis, inclusion conjunctivitis, and trachoma.

Genitourinary tract infections (treatment)—Systemic tetracyclines are indicated in the treatment of genitourinary tract infections (including acute epididymo-orchitis) caused by *Neisseria gonorrhoeae*.

Doxycycline is indicated in the treatment of genitourinary tract infections (including acute epididymo-orchitis) caused by *Chlamydia trachomatis*.

Doxycycline, minocycline, oxytetracycline, and tetracycline are indicated in the treatment of uncomplicated genitourinary tract infections (including endocervical infections) caused by *C. trachomatis*.

Minocycline is indicated in the treatment of uncomplicated genitourinary tract infections (including endocervical infections) caused by *Ureaplasma urealyticum*.

Gingivostomatitis, necrotizing ulcerative (treatment)—Systemic tetracyclines are indicated in the treatment of necrotizing ulcerative gingivostomatitis (Vincent's infection) caused by *Fusobacterium fusiformisans* (*Fusiformis fusiformisans*).

Granuloma inguinale (treatment)—Systemic tetracyclines are indicated in the treatment of granuloma inguinale caused by *Calymmatobacterium granulomatis*.

Lymphogranuloma venereum (treatment)—Systemic tetracyclines are indicated in the treatment of lymphogranuloma venereum caused by *Chlamydia* species.

Malaria (prophylaxis)—Doxycycline is indicated in the prophylaxis of malaria due to *Plasmodium falciparum* in short-term travelers (< 4 months) going to areas with chloroquine- and/or pyrimethamine-sulfadoxine–resistant strains.

Meningococcal carriers (treatment)—Oral minocycline is indicated in the treatment of asymptomatic meningococcal carriers to eliminate *Neisseria meningitidis* from the nasopharynx.

Otitis media, acute (treatment)
Pharyngitis, bacterial (treatment)
Pneumonia, *Haemophilus influenzae* (treatment)
Pneumonia, *Klebsiella* species (treatment) or
Sinusitis (treatment)—Systemic tetracyclines are indicated in the treatment of acute otitis media, pharyngitis, pneumonia, and sinusitis caused by *H. influenzae* and *Klebsiella* species.

Doxycycline is indicated in the treatment of the above-listed infections caused by *Staphylococcus aureus*. However, some USP medical experts do not recommend the use of tetracyclines for infections caused by *S. aureus*.

Psittacosis (treatment)—Systemic tetracyclines are indicated in the treatment of psittacosis caused by *Chlamydia psittaci*.

Q fever (treatment)
Rickettsial pox (treatment)
Rocky Mountain spotted fever (treatment) or
Typhus infections (treatment)—Systemic tetracyclines are indicated in the treatment of Q fever, rickettsial pox, Rocky Mountain spotted fever (including tick fevers), and typhus infections caused by Rickettsiae.

Relapsing fever (treatment)—Systemic tetracyclines are indicated in the treatment of relapsing fever caused by *Borrelia recurrentis*.

Skin and soft tissue infections (treatment)—Systemic tetracyclines are indicated in the treatment of skin and soft tissue infections, including burn wound infections, caused by *S. aureus*. However, some USP medical experts do not recommend the use of tetracyclines for infections caused by *S. aureus*.

Syphilis (treatment)—Systemic tetracyclines are indicated in the treatment of syphilis caused by *Treponema pallidum*.

Urethritis, nongonococcal (treatment)—Doxycycline is indicated in the treatment of nongonococcal urethritis caused by *C. trachomatis* and *U. urealyticum*.

Urinary tract infections, bacterial (treatment)—Systemic tetracyclines are indicated in the treatment of urinary tract infections caused by [susceptible organisms, including *Escherichia coli* and] *Klebsiella* species.

Yaws (treatment)—Systemic tetracyclines are indicated in the treatment of yaws caused by *T. pertenue*.

Doxycycline, minocycline, oxytetracycline, and tetracycline are indicated in the treatment of uncomplicated rectal infections caused by *C. trachomatis*. Minocycline is indicated in the treatment of uncomplicated rectal infections caused by *U. urealyticum*.

[Amebiasis, extraintestinal (treatment)]—Tetracycline, a lumenal amebicide, is indicated concurrently or sequentially with metronidazole in the treatment of extraintestinal amebiasis caused by *Entamoeba histolytica*.

[Arthritis, gonococcal (treatment)]
[Bejel (treatment)]
[Biliary tract infections (treatment)]
[Enterocolitis, *Shigella* species (treatment)]
[Intra-abdominal infections (treatment)]
[Pinta (treatment)]
[Plague (treatment)]
[Pneumonia, mycoplasmal (treatment)]
[Septicemia, bacterial (treatment)]
[Tularemia (treatment)] or

[Urethritis, gonococcal (treatment)]—Systemic tetracyclines are indicated in the treatment of the above-listed infections.

[Arthritis, rheumatoid (treatment)][1]—Systemic minocycline is indicated in the treatment of early (< 2 years), mild rheumatoid arthritis *(Evidence rating: I)*,.

[Chlamydial infections (treatment)] or

[Rosacea, ocular (treatment)]—Systemic tetracycline is indicated in the treatment of chlamydial infections and ocular rosacea.

[Gonorrhea (treatment)] or

[Malaria (treatment)]—Systemic doxycycline and tetracycline are indicated in the treatment of gonorrhea and malaria.

[Lyme disease (treatment)]—Doxycycline and tetracycline are indicated in the treatment of early Lyme disease, caused by *Borrelia burgdorferi*.

[Malignant effusions, pleural (treatment)]—Doxycycline is indicated in the treatment of malignant pleural effusions by instillation into the pleural cavity.

[Mycobacterial infections, atypical (treatment)]—Systemic doxycycline and minocycline are indicated in the treatment of atypical mycobacterial infections.

[Nocardiosis (treatment)]—Systemic minocycline is indicated in the treatment of nocardiosis.

[Syndrome of inappropriate antidiuretic hormone (SIADH) (treatment)]—Demeclocycline is indicated in the treatment of syndrome of inappropriate (excess) antidiuretic hormone (SIADH).

[Traveler's diarrhea (prophylaxis and treatment)]—Doxycycline is indicated in the prophylaxis and treatment of traveler's diarrhea caused by enterotoxigenic *Escherichia coli*, *Salmonella* species, and *Shigella* species in high-risk patients in whom diarrhea and dehydration may result in serious consequences because of chronic underlying health problems.

Tetracyclines are also indicated in the treatment of infections caused by *Mycobacterium marinum* (oral minocycline), *Mycoplasma pneumoniae*, *Yersinia pestis*, *Francisella tularensis*, *Bartonella bacilliformis*, *Bacteroides* species, *Vibrio cholerae*, *Campylobacter fetus*, *Brucella* species (concurrently with streptomycin), *E. coli*, *Enterobacter aerogenes*, *Shigella* species, *Acinetobacter* species, streptococci, *Streptococcus pneumoniae*, *N. gonorrhoeae*, *N. meningitidis* (parenteral doxycycline, minocycline, and tetracycline), *Listeria monocytogenes*, *Clostridium* species, and *Actinomyces* species.

Not all species or strains of a particular organism may be susceptible to a specific tetracycline.

**Unaccepted**
Oral minocycline is no longer recommended by the Centers for Disease Control (CDC) for the treatment of meningococcal carriers because of vestibular toxicity. Oral minocycline is not indicated in the treatment of meningococcal infections.

[1]Not included in Canadian product labeling.

## Pharmacology/Pharmacokinetics

**Physicochemical characteristics**
Molecular weight—
  Demeclocycline hydrochloride: 501.32.
  Doxycycline: 462.46.
  Doxycycline hyclate: 1025.89.
  Minocycline hydrochloride: 493.95.
  Oxytetracycline: 496.47.
  Oxytetracycline hydrochloride: 496.9.
  Tetracycline: 444.44.
  Tetracycline hydrochloride: 480.9.

**Mechanism of action/Effect**
Antibacterial (systemic); antiprotozoal—Tetracyclines are broad-spectrum bacteriostatic agents and act by inhibiting protein synthesis by blocking the binding of aminoacyl-tRNA (transfer RNA) to the mRNA (messenger RNA)-ribosome complex. Reversible binding occurs primarily at the 30 S ribosomal subunit of susceptible organisms. Bacterial cell wall synthesis is not inhibited.

Diuretic (Syndrome of inappropriate diuretic hormone [SIADH])—In the treatment of the SIADH, demeclocycline acts by inhibiting ADH-induced water reabsorption in the distal portion of the convoluted tubules and collecting ducts of the kidneys, thereby causing water diuresis.

**Absorption**

| Drug | Absorbed orally (%) | Effect of food on absorption |
| --- | --- | --- |
| Demeclocycline | 66 | Decreased |
| Doxycycline | 90–100 | Insignificant |
| Minocycline | 90–100 | Insignificant |
| Oxytetracycline | 58 | Decreased |
| Tetracycline | 75–77 | Decreased |

**Distribution**
Doxycycline—Achieves therapeutic concentrations in the eye; prostatic concentrations are approximately 60% of serum concentrations.
Minocycline—Achieves high concentrations in saliva, sputum, and tears.
All tetracyclines—Readily distributed to most body fluids, including bile, sinus secretions, and synovial, pleural, ascitic, and gingival crevicular fluids. Cerebrospinal fluid (CSF) concentrations vary and may achieve 10 to 25% of plasma concentrations following parenteral administration. Concentrations in gingival crevicular fluid may be 3 to 7 times serum concentrations. Tetracyclines tend to localize in bone, liver, spleen, tumors, and teeth; also cross the placenta and distribute into breast milk.

**Biotransformation**
Doxycycline and minocycline are partially inactivated by hepatic metabolism.

**Half-life**

| Drug | Half-life Normal (hr) | Half-life Anuric (hr) |
| --- | --- | --- |
| Demeclocycline | 10–17 | 40–60 |
| Doxycycline | 12–22 | 12–22 |
| Minocycline | 11–23 | 11–23 |
| Oxytetracycline | 6–10 | 47–66 |
| Tetracycline | 6–11 | 57–108 |

**Onset of action**
SIADH syndrome (demeclocycline)—24 to 48 hours.

**Time to peak concentration**
Tetracycline—Two to three days may be necessary to achieve therapeutic concentrations of tetracycline.
Other tetracyclines—2 to 4 hours (oral).

**Elimination**
Renal; unchanged, via glomerular filtration.
Fecal; unchanged, via biliary secretion, gastrointestinal secretion, or poor absorption.
Dialysis—Tetracyclines are slowly removed by hemodialysis; although, doxycycline is not removed by hemodialysis. Peritoneal dialysis does not effectively remove tetracyclines.

  Note: Gastrointestinal secretion is an important route of excretion when doxycycline is administered to patients with impaired renal function or azotemia.

| Drug | Distribution* (Vol$_D$—L/kg) | Excretion routes[†] (primary/secondary—% excreted unchanged) | Protein binding |
| --- | --- | --- | --- |
| Demeclocycline | 1.79 | Renal/biliary (42) | High (91%) |
| Doxycycline | 0.7 | Biliary/renal (35) | High (93%) |
| Minocycline | 0.14–0.7 | Biliary/renal (5–10) | Moderate (76%) |
| Oxytetracycline | 0.9–1.9 | Renal/biliary (70) | Low (35%) |
| Tetracycline | 1.3–1.6 | Renal/biliary (60) | Moderate (65%) |

*Diffuses readily into most body tissues, fluids, and/or cavities.
[†]Biliary route involves concentration by the liver and excretion via the bile into the intestine from which partial reabsorption occurs.

## Precautions to Consider

**Cross-sensitivity and/or related problems**
Patients hypersensitive to one tetracycline may be hypersensitive to other tetracyclines also.

Patients hypersensitive to lidocaine, procaine, or other "caine-type" local anesthetics may also be hypersensitive to the lidocaine component of oxytetracycline injection or to the procaine component of tetracycline hydrochloride for intramuscular injection.

### Pregnancy/Reproduction
Pregnancy—Tetracyclines cross the placenta; use is not recommended during the last half of pregnancy since tetracyclines may cause permanent discoloration of teeth, enamel hypoplasia, and inhibition of skeletal growth in the fetus. In addition, fatty infiltration of the liver may occur in pregnant women, especially with high intravenous doses.

FDA Pregnancy Category D.

### Breast-feeding
Tetracyclines are distributed into breast milk; although tetracyclines may form nonabsorbable complexes with breast-milk calcium, use is not recommended because of the possibility of their causing permanent staining of teeth, enamel hypoplasia, inhibition of linear skeletal growth, photosensitivity reactions, and oral and vaginal thrush in infants. In addition, vestibular disturbances may occur with minocycline.

### Pediatrics
In infants and children up to 8 years of age, tetracyclines may cause permanent staining of teeth, enamel hypoplasia, and a decrease in linear skeletal growth rate. Therefore, use is not recommended in patients in these age groups unless other antibacterials are unlikely to be effective or are contraindicated.

Bulging fontanels have been reported in young infants who received full therapeutic doses of tetracyclines. This side effect disappeared rapidly upon discontinuation of the drug.

### Geriatrics
No information is available on the relationship of age to the effects of tetracyclines in geriatric patients.

### Dental
Use of systemic tetracyclines during pregnancy or in infants and children up to 8 years of age may cause permanent discoloration of teeth and enamel hypoplasia. Therefore, use is not recommended unless other antibacterials are unlikely to be effective or are contraindicated. Vital bleaching or aesthetic restoration may be required if staining is objectionable.

Systemic tetracyclines may also contribute to the development of oral candidiasis.

### Drug interactions and/or related problems
The following drug interactions and/or related problems have been selected on the basis of their potential clinical significance (possible mechanism in parentheses where appropriate)—not necessarily inclusive (» = major clinical significance):

Note: Combinations containing any of the following medications, depending on the amount present, may also interact with this medication.

» Antacids or
» Calcium supplements such as calcium carbonate or
» Choline and magnesium salicylates or
» Iron supplements or
» Magnesium salicylate or
» Magnesium-containing laxatives
  Sodium bicarbonate
   (concurrent use may result in formation of nonabsorbable complexes; also, concurrent use with antacids or sodium bicarbonate may result in decreased absorption of oral tetracyclines because of increased intragastric pH; patients should be advised not to take these medications within 1 to 3 hours of oral tetracyclines)

Barbiturates or
Carbamazepine or
Phenytoin
   (concurrent use with doxycycline may result in decreased doxycycline serum concentrations due to induction of microsomal enzyme activity; adjustment of doxycycline dosage or substitution of another tetracycline may be necessary)

» Cholestyramine or
» Colestipol
   (concurrent use with cholestyramine or colestipol may result in binding of oral tetracyclines, thus impairing their absorption; an interval of several hours between administration of cholestyramine or colestipol and oral tetracyclines is recommended)

» Contraceptives, estrogen-containing, oral
   (concurrent long-term use with tetracyclines may result in reduced contraceptive reliability and increased incidence of breakthrough bleeding)

Digoxin
   (although no cases of clinical toxicity have been reported, concurrent use of oral antibiotics may increase serum digoxin concentrations in some individuals; in these individuals, alteration of the gut flora by antibiotics may diminish digoxin conversion to inactive metabolites, resulting in increased serum digoxin concentrations; although limited data are available, this interaction has been reported with oral use of erythromycins, neomycin, and tetracyclines)

Methoxyflurane
   (concurrent use with tetracyclines may increase the potential for nephrotoxicity)

Penicillins
   (since bacteriostatic drugs may interfere with the bactericidal effect of penicillins in the treatment of meningitis or in other situations where a rapid bactericidal effect is necessary, it is best to avoid concurrent therapy)

Vitamin A
   (concurrent use with tetracycline has been reported to cause benign intracranial hypertension)

### Laboratory value alterations
The following have been selected on the basis of their potential clinical significance (possible effect in parentheses where appropriate)—not necessarily inclusive (» = major clinical significance):

With diagnostic test results
  Catecholamine determinations, urine
   (may produce false elevations of urinary catecholamines because of interfering fluorescence in the Hingerty method)

With physiology/laboratory test values
  Alanine aminotransferase (ALT [SGPT]) and
  Alkaline phosphatase and
  Amylase and
  Aspartate aminotransferase (AST [SGOT]) and
  Bilirubin
   (serum concentrations may be increased)
  Blood urea nitrogen (BUN)
   (antianabolic effect of tetracyclines [except doxycycline] may increase BUN concentrations; in patients with significantly impaired renal function, increased serum concentrations of tetracyclines may lead to azotemia, hyperphosphatemia, and acidosis)

### Medical considerations/Contraindications
The medical considerations/contraindications included have been selected on the basis of their potential clinical significance (reasons given in parentheses where appropriate)—not necessarily inclusive (» = major clinical significance).

*Risk-benefit should be considered when the following medical problems exist:*

» Diabetes insipidus, nephrogenic
   (demeclocycline induces a reversible nephrogenic diabetes insipidus)
  Hepatic function impairment
   (doxycycline and minocycline are partially metabolized in the liver; hepatic function impairment may prolong the elimination half-life)
  Hypersensitivity to tetracyclines, or "caine-type" local anesthetics (e.g., lidocaine, procaine)
» Renal function impairment
   (the half-life of tetracyclines, except doxycycline or minocycline, is prolonged in patients with renal function impairment)

## Side/Adverse Effects
Note: Tetracycline-induced hepatotoxicity is usually seen as a fatty degeneration of the liver. It is more likely to occur in pregnant women, in patients receiving high-dose intravenous therapy, and in patients with renal function impairment. However, hepatotoxicity has also occurred in patients without these predisposing conditions. Tetracycline-induced pancreatitis has also been described in association with hepatotoxicity, and without associated liver disease.

The following side/adverse effects have been selected on the basis of their potential clinical significance (possible signs and symptoms in parentheses where appropriate)—not necessarily inclusive:

### Those indicating need for medical attention
Incidence more frequent
  *Staining of infants' or children's teeth; photosensitivity* (increased sensitivity of skin to sunlight)

Incidence less frequent
  *Nephrogenic diabetes insipidus* (greatly increased frequency of urination or amount of urine; increased thirst; unusual tiredness or weak-

ness)—with demeclocycline; *pigmentation of skin and mucous membranes*—primarily with minocycline

Incidence rare
*Benign intracranial hypertension* (anorexia; headache; vomiting; papilledema; visual changes; bulging fontanel in infants); *hepatotoxicity* (abdominal pain; nausea and vomiting; yellowing skin); *pancreatitis* (abdominal pain; nausea and vomiting)

**Those indicating need for medical attention only if they continue or are bothersome**
Incidence more frequent
*CNS toxicity* (dizziness; lightheadedness; unsteadiness); *gastrointestinal disturbances* (cramps or burning of the stomach; diarrhea; nausea or vomiting); *photosensitivity* (increased sensitivity of skin to sunlight)

Incidence less frequent
*Fungal overgrowth* (itching of the rectal or genital areas; sore mouth or tongue); *hypertrophy of the papilla* (darkened or discolored tongue)

## Patient Consultation
As an aid to patient consultation, refer to *Advice for the Patient, Tetracyclines (Systemic)*.

In providing consultation, consider emphasizing the following selected information (» = major clinical significance):

**Before using this medication**
» Conditions affecting use, especially:
  Sensitivity to tetracyclines
  Pregnancy—Tetracyclines cross the placenta; use is not recommended during the last half of pregnancy since tetracyclines may cause permanent staining of teeth, enamel hypoplasia, and inhibition of skeletal growth in the fetus; also, fatty infiltration of the liver may occur in pregnant women, especially with high intravenous doses
  Breast-feeding—Tetracyclines distributed into breast milk; although tetracyclines may form nonabsorbable complexes with breast-milk calcium, use is not recommended because of the possibility of their causing permanent staining of teeth, enamel hypoplasia, inhibition of linear skeletal growth, photosensitivity reactions, and oral and vaginal thrush in infants
  Use in children—In infants and children up to 8 years of age, tetracyclines may cause permanent discoloration of teeth, enamel hypoplasia, and a decrease in linear skeletal growth rate
  Other medications, especially antacids, calcium supplements, cholestyramine, choline and magnesium salicylates, colestipol, estrogen-containing oral contraceptives, iron supplements, magnesium salicylate, or magnesium-containing laxatives
  Other medical problems, especially nephrogenic diabetes insipidus or renal function impairment

**Proper use of this medication**
» Not giving to children up to 8 years of age
  Taking with at least a full glass of water while in an upright position to avoid esophageal ulceration or to decrease gastrointestinal irritation
» Avoiding concurrent use of milk or other dairy products when taking oral demeclocycline, oxytetracycline, and tetracycline; if gastrointestinal irritation still occurs, these medicines may be taken with food
  Oral doxycycline and minocycline may be taken with food or milk if gastric irritation occurs
» Discarding outdated or decomposed tetracyclines (decomposed products may be toxic)
» Compliance with full course of therapy
» Importance of not missing doses and taking at evenly spaced times
» Proper dosing
  Missed dose: Taking as soon as possible; not taking if almost time for next dose; not doubling doses
» Proper storage

**Precautions while using this medication**
Checking with physician if no improvement within a few days (or a few weeks or months for acne patients)
» Avoiding antacids, calcium supplements, choline and magnesium salicylates, iron supplements, magnesium salicylate, magnesium-containing laxatives, sodium bicarbonate within 1 to 3 hours of oral tetracyclines
» Use of an alternate or additional method of contraception if concurrently taking estrogen-containing oral contraceptives
  Caution if surgery with general anesthesia is required
» Possible photosensitivity reactions
» Caution if dizziness, lightheadedness, or unsteadiness occurs

**Side/adverse effects**
Signs of potential side effects such as discoloration of infant's or children's teeth, nephrogenic diabetes insipidus—with demeclocycline, pigmentation of skin and mucous membranes—with minocycline, benign intracranial hypertension, hepatotoxicity, pancreatitis, and photosensitivity

## General Dosing Information
Use of tetracyclines (except doxycycline and minocycline) in patients with impaired renal function is not recommended.

**For oral dosage forms only**
All tetracyclines should be taken with a full glass (240 mL) of water to avoid esophageal ulceration and to decrease gastrointestinal irritation. In addition, most tetracyclines (except doxycycline and minocycline) should preferably be taken on an empty stomach (either 1 hour before or 2 hours after meals) to obtain optimum serum concentrations.

---

### DEMECLOCYCLINE

## Summary of Differences
Indications:
  Also used as a diuretic (syndrome of inappropriate diuretic hormone [SIADH]).
Pharmacology/pharmacokinetics:
  Different mechanism of action in SIADH.
Precautions:
  Drug interactions and/or related problems—Also interacts with desmopressin.
  Medical considerations/contraindications—Caution also needed in nephrogenic diabetes insipidus.
Side/adverse effects:
  May also cause greatly increased frequency of urination or amount of urine, increased thirst, or unusual tiredness or weakness (nephrogenic diabetes insipidus).

## Oral Dosage Forms
Note: Bracketed uses in the *Dosage Forms* section refer to categories of use and/or indications that are not included in U.S. product labeling.

Note: The dosing and dosage forms available are expressed in terms of demeclocycline hydrochloride.

### DEMECLOCYCLINE HYDROCHLORIDE CAPSULES USP

**Usual adult and adolescent dose**
Antibacterial (systemic); antiprotozoal—
  Oral, 150 mg every six hours; or 300 mg every twelve hours.
  Note: Gonorrhea—Oral, 300 mg every twelve hours for four days, up to a total dose of 3 grams.
[Diuretic (SIADH)]—
  Oral, 3.25 to 3.75 mg per kg of body weight every six hours.

**Usual adult prescribing limits**
Antibacterial (systemic); antiprotozoal—
  Up to 2.4 grams daily.
[Diuretic (SIADH)]—
  300 mg to 1.2 grams daily.

**Usual pediatric dose**
Children 8 years of age and over—Antibacterial (systemic); antiprotozoal—
  Oral, 1.65 to 3.3 mg per kg of body weight every six hours; or 3.3 to 6.6 mg per kg of body weight every twelve hours.
Note: Infants and children up to 8 years of age—All tetracyclines form a stable calcium complex in any bone-forming tissue. Accordingly, tetracyclines may cause permanent yellow-gray-brown staining of the teeth, as well as enamel hypoplasia. Also, a decrease in linear skeletal growth rate may occur in premature infants. Therefore, tetracyclines are not recommended in these age groups unless other drugs are unlikely to be effective or are contraindicated.

**Strength(s) usually available**
U.S.—
  150 mg (Rx) [*Declomycin*].
Canada—
  Not commercially available.

**Packaging and storage**
Store below 40 °C (104 °F), preferably between 15 and 30 °C (59 and 86 °F), unless otherwise specified by manufacturer. Store in a tight, light-resistant container.

USP DI

**Auxiliary labeling**
- Continue medicine for full time of treatment.
- Do not take within 1 to 3 hours of other medicines, milk, or other dairy products.
- Avoid too much sun or use of sunlamp.
- Keep container tightly closed in a dry place.

### DEMECLOCYCLINE HYDROCHLORIDE TABLETS USP

**Usual adult and adolescent dose**
See *Demeclocycline Hydrochloride Capsules USP*.

**Usual adult prescribing limits**
See *Demeclocycline Hydrochloride Capsules USP*.

**Usual pediatric dose**
See *Demeclocycline Hydrochloride Capsules USP*.

**Strength(s) usually available**
U.S.—
   150 mg (Rx) [*Declomycin*].
   300 mg (Rx) [*Declomycin*].
Canada—
   150 mg (Rx) [*Declomycin*].
   300 mg (Rx) [*Declomycin*].

**Packaging and storage**
Store below 40 °C (104 °F), preferably between 15 and 30 °C (59 and 86 °F), unless otherwise specified by manufacturer. Store in a tight, light-resistant container.

**Auxiliary labeling**
- Continue medicine for full time of treatment.
- Do not take within 1 to 3 hours of other medicines, milk, or other dairy products.
- Avoid too much sun or use of sunlamp.
- Keep container tightly closed in a dry place.

---
### DOXYCYCLINE
---

## Summary of Differences
Indications:
   Also indicated for the prevention of malaria.
Precautions:
   Drug interactions and/or related problems—
      Also interacts with barbiturates, carbamazepine, and phenytoin.
      No interaction with methoxyflurane.
   Laboratory value alterations—
      No increase in BUN concentrations.
   Medical considerations/contraindications—
      Caution not needed in renal impairment.
General dosing information:
   No dosage reduction in renal impairment.
   May be taken with food, milk, or carbonated beverages.

## Additional Dosing Information
Even though approximately 40% of a dose of doxycycline may be eliminated through the kidneys in patients with normal renal function, patients with impaired renal function do not generally require a reduction in dose since doxycycline alternatively may be eliminated through the liver, biliary tract, and gastrointestinal tract and does not have the antianabolic effect of other tetracyclines.

For oral dosage forms only:
- Doxycycline may be taken with food or milk if gastrointestinal irritation occurs.

## Oral Dosage Forms
Note: Bracketed uses in the *Dosage Forms* section refer to categories of use and/or indications that are not included in U.S. product labeling.

### DOXYCYCLINE FOR ORAL SUSPENSION USP

**Usual adult and adolescent dose**
Antibacterial (systemic); antiprotozoal—
   Oral, 100 mg (base) every twelve hours the first day, then 100 to 200 mg once a day; or 50 to 100 mg every twelve hours.
   Note: Gonococcal infections, uncomplicated (except anorectal infections in men)—Oral, 100 mg (base) every twelve hours for seven days; or 300 mg initially, then 300 mg one hour later.
      Malaria prophylaxis—Oral, 100 mg (base) once a day. Prophylaxis should begin one or two days before travel to the malarious area, be continued daily during travel, and for four weeks after the traveler leaves the malarious area.
      Nongonococcal urethritis caused by *Chlamydia trachomatis* or *Ureaplasma urealyticum*, and
      Uncomplicated urethral, endocervical, or rectal infection caused by *Chlamydia trachomatis*—Oral, 100 mg (base) two times a day for at least seven days.
      Syphilis (primary and secondary)—Oral, 150 mg (base) every twelve hours for at least ten days.
      [Traveler's diarrhea (prophylaxis)]—Oral, 100 mg (base) once a day for three weeks.
      [Lyme disease (treatment)]—Oral, 100 mg (base) two times a day.

**Usual adult prescribing limits**
Up to 300 mg (base) daily; or up to 600 mg daily for five days in acute gonococcal infections.

**Usual pediatric dose**
Antibacterial (systemic); antiprotozoal—
   Children 45 kg of body weight and under: Oral, 2.2 mg (base) per kg of body weight every twelve hours the first day, then 2.2 to 4.4 mg per kg of body weight once a day; or 1.1 to 2.2 mg per kg of body weight every twelve hours.
   Children over 45 kg of body weight: See *Usual adult and adolescent dose*.
   Note: Malaria prophylaxis
      Children over 8 years of age—Oral, 2 mg per kg of body weight, up to 100 mg, once a day. Prophylaxis should begin one or two days before travel to the malarious area, be continued daily during travel, and for four weeks after the traveler leaves the malarious area.
      [Lyme disease (treatment)]—Children over 8 years of age: Oral, 1 to 2 mg per kg of body weight two times a day.
      Infants and children up to 8 years of age—All tetracyclines form a stable calcium complex in any bone-forming tissue. Accordingly, tetracyclines may cause permanent yellow-gray-brown staining of the teeth, as well as enamel hypoplasia. Also, a decrease in linear skeletal growth rate may occur in premature infants. Therefore, tetracyclines are not recommended in these age groups unless other drugs are unlikely to be effective or are contraindicated.

**Strength(s) usually available**
U.S.—
   25 mg per 5 mL, when reconstituted according to manufacturer's instructions (base) (Rx) [*Vibramycin*].
Canada—
   Not commercially available.

**Packaging and storage**
Prior to reconstitution, store below 40 °C (104 °F), preferably between 15 and 30 °C (59 and 86 °F), unless otherwise specified by manufacturer. Store in a tight, light-resistant container.

**Stability**
After reconstitution, suspensions retain their potency for 14 days at room temperature.

**Auxiliary labeling**
- Shake well.
- Continue medicine for full time of treatment.
- Do not take within 1 to 3 hours of other medicines.
- Avoid too much sun or use of sunlamp.
- Beyond-use date.

**Note**
When dispensing, include a calibrated liquid-measuring device.

### DOXYCYCLINE CALCIUM ORAL SUSPENSION USP

**Usual adult and adolescent dose**
See *Doxycycline for Oral Suspension USP*.

**Usual adult prescribing limits**
See *Doxycycline for Oral Suspension USP*.

**Usual pediatric dose**
See *Doxycycline for Oral Suspension USP*.

**Strength(s) usually available**
U.S.—
   50 mg per 5 mL (base) (Rx) [*Vibramycin*].
Canada—
   Not commercially available.

**Packaging and storage**
Store below 40 °C (104 °F), preferably between 15 and 30 °C (59 and 86 °F), unless otherwise specified by manufacturer. Store in a tight, light-resistant container. Protect from freezing.

## Auxiliary labeling
- Shake well.
- Continue medicine for full time of treatment.
- Do not take within 1 to 3 hours of other medicines.
- Avoid too much sun or use of sunlamp.

## Note
When dispensing, include a calibrated liquid-measuring device.

## DOXYCYCLINE HYCLATE CAPSULES USP

### Usual adult and adolescent dose
See *Doxycycline for Oral Suspension USP*.

### Usual adult prescribing limits
See *Doxycycline for Oral Suspension USP*.

### Usual pediatric dose
See *Doxycycline for Oral Suspension USP*.

### Strength(s) usually available
U.S.—
- 50 mg (base) (Rx) [*Monodox; Vibramycin;* GENERIC].
- 100 mg (base) (Rx) [*Doxy-Caps; Monodox; Vibramycin;* GENERIC].

Canada—
- 100 mg (base) (Rx) [*Apo-Doxy; Doxycin; Novodoxylin; Vibramycin*].

### Packaging and storage
Store below 40 °C (104 °F), preferably between 15 and 30 °C (59 and 86 °F), unless otherwise specified by manufacturer. Store in a tight, light-resistant container.

### Auxiliary labeling
- Continue medicine for full time of treatment.
- Do not take within 1 to 3 hours of other medicines.
- Avoid too much sun or use of sunlamp.
- Keep container tightly closed in a dry place.

## DOXYCYCLINE HYCLATE DELAYED-RELEASE CAPSULES USP

### Usual adult and adolescent dose
See *Doxycycline for Oral Suspension USP*.

### Usual adult prescribing limits
See *Doxycycline for Oral Suspension USP*.

### Usual pediatric dose
See *Doxycycline for Oral Suspension USP*.

### Strength(s) usually available
U.S.—
- 100 mg (base) (Rx) [*Doryx;* GENERIC].

Canada—
- 100 mg (base) (Rx) [*Doryx*].

### Packaging and storage
Store below 40 °C (104 °F), preferably between 15 and 30 °C (59 and 86 °F), unless otherwise specified by manufacturer. Store in a tight, light-resistant container.

### Auxiliary labeling
- Continue medicine for full time of treatment.
- Do not take within 1 to 3 hours of other medicines.
- Avoid too much sun or use of sunlamp.
- Keep container tightly closed in a dry place.
- Swallow capsules whole.

### Note
Doxycycline Delayed-release Capsules USP contain enteric-coated pellets.

## DOXYCYCLINE HYCLATE TABLETS USP

### Usual adult and adolescent dose
See *Doxycycline for Oral Suspension USP*.

### Usual adult prescribing limits
See *Doxycycline for Oral Suspension USP*.

### Usual pediatric dose
See *Doxycycline for Oral Suspension USP*.

### Strength(s) usually available
U.S.—
- 100 mg (base) (Rx) [*Doxi Film; Vibra-Tabs;* GENERIC].

Canada—
- 100 mg (base) (Rx) [*Doxycin; Vibra-Tabs*].

### Packaging and storage
Store below 40 °C (104 °F), preferably between 15 and 30 °C (59 and 86 °F), unless otherwise specified by manufacturer. Store in a tight, light-resistant container.

### Auxiliary labeling
- Continue medicine for full time of treatment.
- Do not take within 1 to 3 hours of other medicines.
- Avoid too much sun or use of sunlamp.
- Keep container tightly closed in a dry place.

# Parenteral Dosage Forms

## DOXYCYCLINE HYCLATE FOR INJECTION USP

### Usual adult and adolescent dose
Antibacterial (systemic); antiprotozoal—
- Intravenous infusion, 200 mg (base) once a day or 100 mg every twelve hours the first day, then 100 to 200 mg once a day; or 50 to 100 mg every twelve hours.

Note: Syphilis (primary and secondary)—Intravenous infusion, 150 mg (base) every twelve hours for at least ten days.

### Usual adult prescribing limits
Up to 300 mg (base) daily.

### Usual pediatric dose
Antibacterial (systemic); antiprotozoal—
- Children 45 kg of body weight and under: Intravenous infusion, 4.4 mg (base) per kg of body weight once a day or 2.2 mg per kg of body weight every twelve hours the first day; then 2.2 to 4.4 mg per kg of body weight once a day or 1.1 to 2.2 mg per kg of body weight every twelve hours.
- Children over 45 kg of body weight: See *Usual adult and adolescent dose*.

Note: Infants and children up to 8 years of age—All tetracyclines form a stable calcium complex in any bone-forming tissue. Accordingly, tetracyclines may cause permanent yellow-gray-brown staining of the teeth, as well as enamel hypoplasia. Also, a decrease in linear skeletal growth rate may occur in premature infants. Therefore, tetracyclines are not recommended in these age groups unless other drugs are unlikely to be effective or are contraindicated.

### Size(s) usually available
U.S.—
- 100 mg (base) (Rx) [*Doxy; Vibramycin;* GENERIC].
- 200 mg (base) (Rx) [*Doxy; Vibramycin;* GENERIC].

Canada—
- 100 mg (base) (Rx) [*Vibramycin*].

### Packaging and storage
Prior to reconstitution, store below 40 °C (104 °F), preferably between 15 and 30 °C (59 and 86 °F), unless otherwise specified by manufacturer. Protect from light.

### Preparation of dosage form
To prepare initial dilution for intravenous use, add 10 mL of sterile water for injection or other suitable diluents (see manufacturer's package insert) to each 100-mg vial or 20 mL of diluent to each 200-mg vial. The resulting solution containing the equivalent of 100 to 200 mg of doxycycline may be further diluted in 100 to 1000 mL or in 200 to 2000 mL of suitable diluent, respectively.

### Stability
After reconstitution, intravenous infusions of doxycycline hyclate retain their potency for 12 hours at room temperature or for 72 hours if refrigerated at concentrations of 100 mcg (0.1 mg) to 1 mg per mL in suitable fluids (see manufacturer's package insert). Intravenous infusions of doxycycline hyclate retain their potency for 6 hours at room temperature at concentrations of 100 mcg (0.1 mg) to 1 mg per mL in lactated Ringer's injection or 5% dextrose and lactated Ringer's injection. Infusions must be protected from direct sunlight during administration.

If frozen immediately after reconstitution with sterile water for injection, solutions at concentrations of 10 mg per mL retain their potency up to 8 weeks at −20 °C (−4 °F). Once thawed, solutions should not be refrozen.

### Additional information
Concentrations less than 100 mcg (0.1 mg) per mL or greater than 1 mg per mL are not recommended.

Infusions may be administered over a 1- to 4-hour period. Avoid rapid administration.

Do not administer intramuscularly or subcutaneously.

## MINOCYCLINE

### Summary of Differences
Precautions:
  Laboratory value alterations—No increase in BUN concentrations.
  Medical considerations/contraindications—Caution not needed in renal impairment.
Side/adverse effects:
  May also cause dizziness, lightheadedness, or unsteadiness (central nervous system [CNS] toxicity); and pigmentation of skin and mucous membranes.
General dosing information:
  No dosage reduction in renal impairment.
  May be taken with food or milk.

### Additional Dosing Information
For oral dosage forms only:
- Minocycline may be taken with food or milk if gastrointestinal irritation occurs.

### Oral Dosage Forms

#### MINOCYCLINE HYDROCHLORIDE CAPSULES USP

**Usual adult and adolescent dose**
Antibacterial (systemic); antiprotozoal—
  Oral, 200 mg (base) initially, then 100 mg every twelve hours; or 100 to 200 mg initially, then 50 mg every six hours.
Note: Gonorrhea—Oral, 100 mg (base) every twelve hours for at least four days.
  *Mycobacterium marinum* infections—Oral, 100 mg (base) every twelve hours for six to eight weeks.
  *Neisseria meningitidis* carriers (asymptomatic)—Oral, 100 mg (base) every twelve hours for five days.
  [Rheumatoid arthritis][1]—Oral, 100 mg (base) two times a day.
  Uncomplicated urethral, endocervical, or rectal infection caused by *Chlamydia trachomatis*—Oral, 100 mg (base) two times a day for at least seven days.

**Usual adult prescribing limits**
Up to 350 mg (base) the first day; then up to 200 mg a day.

**Usual pediatric dose**
Antibacterial (systemic); antiprotozoal—
  Children 8 years of age and over: Oral, 4 mg (base) per kg of body weight initially, then 2 mg per kg of body weight every twelve hours.
Note: Infants and children up to 8 years of age—All tetracyclines form a stable calcium complex in any bone-forming tissue. Accordingly, tetracyclines may cause permanent yellow-gray-brown staining of the teeth, as well as enamel hypoplasia. Also, a decrease in linear skeletal growth rate may occur in premature infants. Therefore, tetracyclines are not recommended in these age groups unless other drugs are unlikely to be effective or are contraindicated.

**Strength(s) usually available**
U.S.—
  50 mg (base) (Rx) [*Dynacin*; *Minocin*; GENERIC].
  100 mg (base) (Rx) [*Dynacin*; *Minocin*; GENERIC].
Canada—
  50 mg (base) (Rx) [*Minocin*].
  100 mg (base) (Rx) [*Minocin*].

**Packaging and storage**
Store below 40 °C (104 °F), preferably between 15 and 30 °C (59 and 86 °F), unless otherwise specified by manufacturer. Store in a tight, light-resistant container.

**Auxiliary labeling**
- Continue medicine for full time of treatment.
- Do not take within 1 to 3 hours of other medicines.
- Avoid too much sun or use of sunlamp.
- Keep container tightly closed in a dry place.
- May cause dizziness.

#### MINOCYCLINE HYDROCHLORIDE ORAL SUSPENSION USP

**Usual adult and adolescent dose**
See *Minocycline Hydrochloride Capsules*.

**Usual adult prescribing limits**
See *Minocycline Hydrochloride Capsules USP*.

**Usual pediatric dose**
See *Minocycline Hydrochloride Capsules USP*.

**Strength(s) usually available**
U.S.—
  50 mg (base) (Rx) [*Minocin*].
Canada—
  Not commercially available.

**Packaging and storage**
Store below 40 °C (104 °F), preferably between 15 and 30 °C (59 and 86 °F), unless otherwise specified by manufacturer. Store in a tight, light-resistant container. Protect from freezing.

**Auxiliary labeling**
- Shake well.
- Continue medicine for full time of treatment.
- Do not take within 1 to 3 hours of other medicines.
- Avoid too much sun or use of sunlamp.
- May cause dizziness.

**Note**
When dispensing, include a calibrated liquid-measuring device.

#### MINOCYCLINE HYDROCHLORIDE TABLETS

**Usual adult and adolescent dose**
See *Minocycline Hydrochloride Capsules USP*.

**Usual adult prescribing limits**
See *Minocycline Hydrochloride Capsules USP*.

**Usual pediatric dose**
See *Minocycline Hydrochloride Capsules USP*.

**Strength(s) usually available**
U.S.—
  50 mg (base) (Rx) [GENERIC].
  100 mg (base) (Rx) [GENERIC].
Canada—
  Not commercially available.

**Packaging and storage**
Store below 40 °C (104 °F), preferably between 15 and 30 °C (59 and 86 °F), unless otherwise specified by manufacturer. Store in a tight, light-resistant container. Protect from freezing.

**Auxiliary labeling**
- Continue medicine for full time of treatment.
- Do not take within 1 to 3 hours of other medicines.
- Avoid too much sun or use of sunlamp.
- May cause dizziness.
- Keep container tightly closed and in a dry place.

### Parenteral Dosage Forms

#### STERILE MINOCYCLINE HYDROCHLORIDE USP

**Usual adult and adolescent dose**
Intravenous infusion, 200 mg (base) initially, then 100 mg every twelve hours.

**Usual adult prescribing limits**
Up to 400 mg (base) daily.

**Usual pediatric dose**
Children 8 years of age and over—Intravenous infusion, 4 mg (base) per kg of body weight initially, then 2 mg per kg of body weight every twelve hours.
Note: Infants and children up to 8 years of age—All tetracyclines form a stable calcium complex in any bone-forming tissue. Accordingly, tetracyclines may cause permanent yellow-gray-brown staining of the teeth, as well as enamel hypoplasia. Also, a decrease in linear skeletal growth rate may occur in premature infants. Therefore, tetracyclines are not recommended in these age groups unless other drugs are unlikely to be effective or are contraindicated.

**Size(s) usually available**
U.S.—
  100 mg (base) (Rx) [*Minocin*].
Canada—
  Not commercially available.

**Packaging and storage**
Prior to reconstitution, store below 40 °C (104 °F), preferably between 15 and 30 °C (59 and 86 °F), unless otherwise specified by manufacturer. Protect from light.

**Preparation of dosage form**
To prepare initial dilution for intravenous use, add 5 to 10 mL of sterile water for injection to each 100-mg vial.

The resulting solution may be further diluted in 500 to 1000 mL of 0.9% sodium chloride injection, dextrose injection, dextrose and sodium chloride injection, Ringer's injection, or lactated Ringer's injection, but not in other calcium-containing solutions since a precipitate may form. Administration should be started immediately, but avoid rapid administration.

**Stability**
After reconstitution, solutions retain their potency for 24 hours at room temperature.

---

[1]Not included in Canadian product labeling.

## OXYTETRACYCLINE

## Additional Dosing Information
For parenteral dosage forms only:
- Serum concentrations should not exceed 15 mcg per mL, especially in pregnant or postpartum patients with pyelonephritis.

## Oral Dosage Forms

### OXYTETRACYCLINE HYDROCHLORIDE CAPSULES USP

**Usual adult and adolescent dose**
Antibacterial (systemic); antiprotozoal—
　Oral, 250 to 500 mg (base) every six hours.

Note: Brucellosis—Oral, 500 mg (base) every six hours for three weeks, given concurrently with 1 gram of streptomycin intramuscularly every twelve hours the first week and once a day the second week.
　Gonorrhea, uncomplicated—Oral, 500 mg (base) every six hours, up to a total dose of 9 grams.
　Syphilis—Oral, 500 mg (base) every six hours for fifteen days (early syphilis) or for thirty days (late syphilis).

**Usual adult prescribing limits**
Up to 4 grams (base) daily.

**Usual pediatric dose**
Antibacterial (systemic); antiprotozoal—
　Children 8 years of age and over: Oral, 6.25 to 12.5 mg (base) per kg of body weight every six hours.

Note: Infants and children up to 8 years of age—All tetracyclines form a stable calcium complex in any bone-forming tissue. Accordingly, tetracyclines may cause permanent yellow-gray-brown staining of the teeth, as well as enamel hypoplasia. Also, a decrease in linear skeletal growth rate may occur in premature infants. Therefore, tetracyclines are not recommended in these age groups unless other drugs are unlikely to be effective or are contraindicated.

**Strength(s) usually available**
U.S.—
　250 mg (base) (Rx) [*Terramycin; Tija;* GENERIC].
Canada—
　Not commercially available.

**Packaging and storage**
Store below 40 °C (104 °F), preferably between 15 and 30 °C (59 and 86 °F), unless otherwise specified by manufacturer. Store in a tight, light-resistant container.

**Auxiliary labeling**
- Continue medicine for full time of treatment.
- Do not take within 1 to 3 hours of other medicines, milk, or other dairy products.
- Avoid too much sun or use of sunlamp.
- Keep container tightly closed in a dry place.

## Parenteral Dosage Forms

### OXYTETRACYCLINE INJECTION USP

**Usual adult and adolescent dose**
Antibacterial (systemic); antiprotozoal—
　Intramuscular, 100 mg (base) every eight hours; 150 mg every twelve hours; or 250 mg once a day.

**Usual adult prescribing limits**
Up to 500 mg (base) daily.

**Usual pediatric dose**
Antibacterial (systemic); antiprotozoal—
　Children 8 years of age and over: Intramuscular, 5 to 8.3 mg (base) per kg of body weight every eight hours; or 7.5 to 12.5 mg per kg of body weight every twelve hours. Maximum daily dose should not exceed 250 mg.

Note: Infants and children up to 8 years of age—All tetracyclines form a stable calcium complex in any bone-forming tissue. Accordingly, tetracyclines may cause permanent yellow-gray-brown staining of the teeth, as well as enamel hypoplasia. Also, a decrease in linear skeletal growth rate may occur in premature infants. Therefore, tetracyclines are not recommended in these age groups unless other drugs are unlikely to be effective or are contraindicated.

**Strength(s) usually available**
U.S.—
　50 mg per mL (base) (Rx) [*Terramycin*].
　125 mg per mL (base) (Rx) [*Terramycin*].
　Note: Injection contains 2% of lidocaine.
Canada—
　Not commercially available.

**Packaging and storage**
Store below 40 °C (104 °F), preferably between 15 and 30 °C (59 and 86 °F), unless otherwise specified by manufacturer. Protect from light. Protect from freezing.

**Additional information**
Cross-sensitivity with other "caine-type" local anesthetics may also occur.
For deep intramuscular use only. Do not administer intravenously.
May cause intense pain and local irritation at the site of intramuscular injections.
Since intramuscular administration of oxytetracycline produces lower serum concentrations than oral administration in recommended doses, patients should be changed to an oral dosage form as soon as feasible.
When rapid, high serum concentrations are required, an intravenous form (oxytetracycline hydrochloride) should be used.

### OXYTETRACYCLINE HYDROCHLORIDE FOR INJECTION USP

**Usual adult and adolescent dose**
Antibacterial (systemic); antiprotozoal—
　Intravenous infusion, 250 to 500 mg (base) every twelve hours.

**Usual adult prescribing limits**
Up to 2 grams (base) daily.

**Usual pediatric dose**
Children 8 years of age and over—Antibacterial (systemic); antiprotozoal—
　Intravenous infusion, 5 to 10 mg (base) per kg of body weight every twelve hours.

Note: Infants and children up to 8 years of age—All tetracyclines form a stable calcium complex in any bone-forming tissue. Accordingly, tetracyclines may cause permanent yellow-gray-brown staining of the teeth, as well as enamel hypoplasia. Also, a decrease in linear skeletal growth rate may occur in premature infants. Therefore, tetracyclines are not recommended in these age groups unless other drugs are unlikely to be effective or are contraindicated.

**Size(s) usually available**
U.S.—
　500 mg (base) (Rx) [*Terramycin*].
Canada—
　Not commercially available.

**Packaging and storage**
Prior to reconstitution, store below 40 °C (104 °F), preferably between 15 and 30 °C (59 and 86 °F), unless otherwise specified by manufacturer. Protect from light.

**Preparation of dosage form**
To prepare initial dilution for intravenous use, add 10 mL of sterile water for injection or 5% dextrose injection to each 250- or 500-mg vial.
The resulting solution should be further diluted in at least 100 mL of 5% dextrose injection, 0.9% sodium chloride injection, or Ringer's injection.

**Stability**
After reconstitution, solutions retain their potency for 48 hours if refrigerated.

**Additional information**
Avoid rapid administration. If patient complains of vein irritation, decrease the rate of administration or increase the volume of diluent.
Do not administer intramuscularly or subcutaneously.

## TETRACYCLINE

### Additional Dosing Information
For parenteral dosage forms only:
- Serum concentrations should not exceed 15 mcg per mL, especially in pregnant or postpartum patients with pyelonephritis.

## Oral Dosage Forms

Note: The dosing and dosage forms available are expressed in terms of tetracycline hydrochloride.

### TETRACYCLINE ORAL SUSPENSION USP

**Usual adult and adolescent dose**
Antibacterial (systemic); antiprotozoal—
    Oral, 250 to 500 mg every six hours; or 500 mg to 1 gram every twelve hours.
Antiacne agent (systemic)—
    Oral, 500 mg to 2 grams daily in divided doses initially in moderate to severe cases as adjunctive therapy. When improvement is noted (usually after 3 weeks), dosage should be reduced gradually to a maintenance dose of 125 to 1000 mg daily. Adequate remission of lesions may also be possible with alternate-day or intermittent therapy.
Note: Brucellosis—Oral, 500 mg every six hours for three weeks, given concurrently with 1 gram of streptomycin intramuscularly every twelve hours the first week and once a day the second week.
    Gonorrhea—Oral, 500 mg every six hours for five days.
    Syphilis—Oral, 500 mg every six hours for fifteen days (early syphilis) or for thirty days (late syphilis).
    Uncomplicated urethral, endocervical, or rectal infection caused by *Chlamydia trachomatis*—Oral, 500 mg four times a day for at least seven days.
    [Lyme disease (treatment)]—Oral, 250 to 500 mg four times a day.

**Usual adult prescribing limits**
Up to 4 grams daily.

**Usual pediatric dose**
Antibacterial (systemic); antiprotozoal—
    Children 8 years of age and over: Oral, 6.25 to 12.5 mg per kg of body weight every six hours; or 12.5 to 25 mg per kg of body weight every twelve hours.
Note: [Lyme disease (treatment)]—Children over 8 years of age: Oral, 6.25 to 12.5 mg per kg of body weight four times a day.
    Infants and children up to 8 years of age—All tetracyclines form a stable calcium complex in any bone-forming tissue. Accordingly, tetracyclines may cause permanent yellow-gray-brown staining of the teeth, as well as enamel hypoplasia. Also, a decrease in linear skeletal growth rate may occur in premature infants. Therefore, tetracyclines are not recommended in these age groups unless other drugs are unlikely to be effective or are contraindicated.

**Strength(s) usually available**
U.S.—
    125 mg per 5 mL (Rx) [*Achromycin V; Sumycin;* GENERIC].
Canada—
    125 mg per 5 mL (Rx) [*Novotetra*].

**Packaging and storage**
Store below 40 °C (104 °F), preferably between 15 and 30 °C (59 and 86 °F), unless otherwise specified by manufacturer. Store in a tight, light-resistant container. Protect from freezing.

**Auxiliary labeling**
- Shake well.
- Continue medicine for full time of treatment.
- Do not take within 1 to 3 hours of other medicines, milk or other dairy products.
- Avoid too much sun or use of sunlamp.

**Note**
When dispensing, include a calibrated liquid-measuring device.

### TETRACYCLINE HYDROCHLORIDE CAPSULES USP

**Usual adult and adolescent dose**
See *Tetracycline Oral Suspension USP*.

**Usual adult prescribing limits**
See *Tetracycline Oral Suspension USP*.

**Usual pediatric dose**
See *Tetracycline Oral Suspension USP*.

**Strength(s) usually available**
U.S.—
    250 mg (Rx) [*Achromycin V; Panmycin; Robitet; Sumycin; Tetracyn;* GENERIC].
    500 mg (Rx) [*Achromycin V; Robitet; Sumycin; Tetracyn;* GENERIC].
Canada—
    250 mg (Rx) [*Achromycin V; Apo-Tetra; Novotetra; Nu-Tetra; Tetracyn*].

**Packaging and storage**
Store below 40 °C (104 °F), preferably between 15 and 30 °C (59 and 86 °F), unless otherwise specified by manufacturer. Store in a tight, light-resistant container.

**Auxiliary labeling**
- Continue medicine for full time of treatment.
- Do not take within 1 to 3 hours of other medicines, milk or other dairy products.
- Avoid too much sun or use of sunlamp.
- Keep container tightly closed in a dry place.

### TETRACYCLINE HYDROCHLORIDE TABLETS USP

**Usual adult and adolescent dose**
See *Tetracycline Oral Suspension USP*.

**Usual adult prescribing limits**
See *Tetracycline Oral Suspension USP*.

**Usual pediatric dose**
See *Tetracycline Oral Suspension USP*.

**Strength(s) usually available**
U.S.—
    250 mg (Rx) [*Sumycin*].
    500 mg (Rx) [*Sumycin*].
Canada—
    250 mg (Rx) [*Novotetra*].

**Packaging and storage**
Store below 40 °C (104 °F), preferably between 15 and 30 °C (59 and 86 °F), unless otherwise specified by manufacturer. Store in a tight, light-resistant container.

**Auxiliary labeling**
- Continue medicine for full time of treatment.
- Do not take within 1 to 3 hours of other medicines, milk, or other dairy products.
- Avoid too much sun or use of sunlamp.
- Keep container tightly closed in a dry place.

## Parenteral Dosage Forms

Note: The dosing and dosage forms available are expressed in terms of tetracycline hydrochloride.

### TETRACYCLINE HYDROCHLORIDE FOR INJECTION (INTRAMUSCULAR) USP

**Usual adult and adolescent dose**
Antibacterial (systemic); antiprotozoal—
    Intramuscular, 100 mg every eight hours; 150 mg every twelve hours; or 250 mg once daily.

**Usual adult prescribing limits**
Up to 1 gram daily.

**Usual pediatric dose**
Antibacterial (systemic); antiprotozoal—
    Children 8 years of age and over—Intramuscular, 5 to 8.3 mg per kg of body weight every eight hours; or 7.5 to 12.5 mg per kg of body weight every twelve hours. Maximum daily dose should not exceed 250 mg.
Note: Infants and children up to 8 years of age—All tetracyclines form a stable calcium complex in any bone-forming tissue. Accordingly, tetracyclines may cause permanent yellow-gray-brown staining of the teeth, as well as enamel hypoplasia. Also, a decrease in linear skeletal growth rate may occur in premature infants. Therefore, tetracyclines are not recommended in these age groups unless other drugs are unlikely to be effective or are contraindicated.

**Size(s) usually available**
U.S.—
    250 mg (Rx) [*Achromycin*].
Canada—
    250 mg (Rx) [*Achromycin*].
Note: Contains 2% or 40 mg of procaine hydrochloride per vial (either strength), depending on manufacturer.

## Tetracyclines (Systemic)

**Packaging and storage**
Prior to reconstitution, store below 40 °C (104 °F), preferably between 15 and 30 °C (59 and 86 °F), unless otherwise specified by manufacturer. Protect from light.

**Preparation of dosage form**
To prepare initial dilution for intramuscular use, depending on the manufacturer, add 2 mL of sterile water for injection or 0.9% sodium chloride injection to each 100-mg vial, and 1.8 to 2 mL of diluent to each 250-mg vial.

**Stability**
After reconstitution, solutions retain their potency for 6 to 24 hours at room temperature or for 24 hours if refrigerated, depending on the manufacturer.

**Additional information**
Cross-sensitivity with other "caine-type" local anesthetics may also occur.
For deep intramuscular use only. Do not administer intravenously, subcutaneously, or into fat layers of the skin.
May cause intense pain and local irritation at the site of injection.
Intramuscular injections should not exceed 2 mL in each site. Injection sites should be alternated.
Since intramuscular administration of tetracycline hydrochloride produces lower serum concentrations than oral administration in recommended doses, patients should be changed to an oral dosage form as soon as feasible.
When rapid, high serum concentrations are required, an intravenous form of tetracycline hydrochloride should be used.

Revised: 08/30/92
Interim revision: 03/18/94; 05/26/94; 04/19/95; 08/14/97; 08/03/98

---

# TETRACYCLINES   Topical

This monograph includes information on the following: 1) Chlortetracycline; 2) Meclocycline†; 3) Tetracycline.
VA CLASSIFICATION (Primary/Secondary):
  Chlortetracycline—DE101
  Meclocycline—DE752
  Tetracycline—DE752/DE101
Commonly used brand name(s): *Achromycin*[3]; *Aureomycin*[1]; *Meclan*[2]; *Topicycline*[3].
Note:  For a listing of dosage forms and brand names by country availability, see *Dosage Forms* section(s).

†Not commercially available in Canada.

## Category

Antiacne agent (topical)—Meclocycline; Tetracycline Hydrochloride for Topical Solution.
Antibacterial (topical)—Chlortetracycline; Tetracycline Hydrochloride Ointment.

## Indications

Note: Bracketed information in the *Indications* section refers to uses that are not included in U.S. product labeling.

**Accepted**
Acne vulgaris (treatment)—Meclocycline sulfosalicylate cream and tetracycline hydrochloride for topical solution are indicated for the topical treatment of acne vulgaris. They may be effective in grades II and III acne, which are characterized by inflammatory lesions such as papules and pustules.
Skin infections, bacterial, minor (treatment)—Chlortetracycline hydrochloride ointment and tetracycline hydrochloride ointment are indicated in the topical treatment of minor skin infections caused by streptococci, staphylococci, and other susceptible organisms.
[Skin infections, bacterial, minor (prophylaxis)] or
[Ulcer, dermal (treatment)]—Topical chlortetracycline and tetracycline hydrochloride ointment are used in the prophylaxis of minor bacterial skin infections and in the treatment of dermal ulcer.

Not all species or strains of a particular organism may be susceptible to tetracyclines.

**Unaccepted**
Topical tetracyclines are not effective in deep cystic lesions or in noninflammatory lesions. In addition, topical antibacterials are not generally considered to be as effective as systemic antibacterials in the treatment of acne, especially severe inflammatory acne.

## Pharmacology/Pharmacokinetics

**Physicochemical characteristics**
Molecular weight—
  Chlortetracycline hydrochloride: 515.35.
  Meclocycline sulfosalicylate: 695.05.
  Tetracycline hydrochloride: 480.90.

**Mechanism of action/Effect**
Antiacne agent (topical)—Probably due to their antibacterial activity. Topical tetracyclines are thought to suppress the growth of *Propionibacterium acnes (Corynebacterium acnes)*, an anaerobe found in sebaceous glands and follicles. *P. acnes* produces proteases, hyaluronidases, lipases, and chemotactic factors, all of which can produce inflammatory components or inflammation directly.
Antibacterial (topical)—Tetracyclines are broad-spectrum bacteriostatic agents and act by inhibiting protein synthesis by blocking the binding of aminoacyl tRNA (transfer RNA) to the mRNA (messenger RNA) ribosome complex. Reversible binding occurs primarily at the 30 S ribosomal subunit of susceptible organisms. Bacterial cell wall synthesis is not inhibited.

**Absorption**
Meclocycline—Virtually no absorption following topical application to intact skin.
Tetracycline—Vehicle containing *n*-decyl dimethyl sulfoxide used for topical solution claimed to enhance cutaneous penetration of tetracycline.

**Peak serum concentration**
Up to 0.1 mcg per mL following continuous twice-daily application of tetracycline hydrochloride topical solution to skin.

## Precautions to Consider

**Cross-sensitivity and/or related problems**
Patients sensitive to one tetracycline, tetracycline combination, or tetracycline derivative may be sensitive to other tetracyclines also.

Tetracycline hydrochloride for topical solution—
  A two-year dermal study in mice has not shown that tetracycline hydrochloride for topical solution is carcinogenic.

**Pregnancy/Reproduction**
Fertility—
  *Meclocycline*—
    Adequate and well-controlled studies in humans have not been done. Studies in rats and rabbits, given oral doses of up to 1000 times the human dose (i.e., 1 gram of cream daily), have not shown that meclocycline causes impaired fertility.
  *Tetracycline hydrochloride for topical solution*—
    Adequate and well-controlled studies in humans have not been done. Studies in rats and rabbits, given doses of up to 246 times the human dose (i.e., 0.0325 mL per kg of body weight daily), have not shown that tetracycline hydrochloride for topical solution causes impaired fertility.

Pregnancy—
  *Meclocycline*—
    Adequate and well-controlled studies in humans have not been done.
    Studies in rabbits have shown that meclocycline, applied topically, causes a slight delay in ossification. However, studies in rats and rabbits, given oral doses of up to 1000 times the human dose (i.e., 1 gram of cream daily), have not shown that meclocycline causes other adverse effects on the fetus.
    FDA Pregnancy Category B.
  *Tetracycline hydrochloride for topical solution*—
    Adequate and well-controlled studies in humans have not been done.
    Studies in rats and rabbits, given doses of up to 246 times the human dose (i.e., 0.0325 mL per kg of body weight daily), have not shown that tetracycline hydrochloride for topical solution causes adverse effects on the fetus.
    FDA Pregnancy Category B.

*Tetracyclines, other—*
  Problems in humans have not been documented.

**Breast-feeding**
It is not known whether topical tetracyclines are distributed into breast milk. However, tetracyclines are unlikely to be distributed into breast milk in significant amounts following topical administration, since the total daily dose is small (e.g., less than 5 mg for tetracycline hydrochloride for topical solution) and serum concentrations following topical administration are undetectable or very low (up to 0.1 mcg per mL).

**Pediatrics**
*Tetracycline hydrochloride for topical solution—*
  Appropriate studies have not been performed in children up to 11 years of age. However, no pediatrics-specific problems have been documented to date in children 11 years of age or older.

**Geriatrics**
No information is available on the relationship of age to the effects of topical tetracyclines in geriatric patients.

**Drug interactions and/or related problems**
The following drug interactions and/or related problems have been selected on the basis of their potential clinical significance (possible mechanism in parentheses where appropriate)—not necessarily inclusive (» = major clinical significance):

Note: Combinations containing any of the following medications, depending on the amount present, may also interact with this medication.

*For tetracycline hydrochloride for topical solution*
  Abrasive or medicated soaps or cleansers or
  Acne preparations, topical, other or
  Alcohol-containing preparations, topical, such as after-shave lotions, astringents, perfumed toiletries, or shaving creams or lotions or
  Cosmetics or soaps with a strong drying effect or
  Isotretinoin or
  Medicated cosmetics or "cover-ups" or
  Preparations containing peeling agents, topical, such as benzoyl peroxide, resorcinol, salicylic acid, or sulfur
    (concurrent use with tetracycline hydrochloride for topical solution may cause a cumulative irritant or drying effect, especially with the application of peeling, desquamating, or abrasive agents, resulting in excessive irritation of the skin)

**Medical considerations/Contraindications**
The medical considerations/contraindications included have been selected on the basis of their potential clinical significance (reasons given in parentheses where appropriate)—not necessarily inclusive (» = major clinical significance).

*Risk-benefit should be considered when the following medical problem exists:*
  Sensitivity to tetracyclines

## Side/Adverse Effects

The following side/adverse effects have been selected on the basis of their potential clinical significance (possible signs and symptoms in parentheses where appropriate)—not necessarily inclusive:

**Those indicating need for medical attention**
Incidence less frequent
  *Pain, redness, swelling, or other sign of irritation not present before therapy*

**Those indicating need for medical attention only if they continue or are bothersome**
Incidence more frequent
  *For topical solution*
    *Dry or scaly skin; stinging or burning feeling*
  *For cream and topical solution*
    *Faint yellowing of the skin, especially around hair roots*

## Patient Consultation

As an aid to patient consultation, refer to *Advice for the Patient, Tetracyclines (Topical)*.
In providing consultation, consider emphasizing the following selected information (» = major clinical significance):

**Before using this medication**
» Conditions affecting use, especially:
    Sensitivity to tetracycline or to any related antibiotics, such as chlortetracycline, demeclocycline, doxycycline, methacycline, minocycline, or oxytetracycline; allergy to formaldehyde (contained in meclocycline cream)

**Proper use of this medication**
*For all dosage forms*
» Compliance with full course of therapy, which may take months or longer
  Proper administration technique
  May stain clothing
» Proper dosing
  Missed dose: Applying as soon as possible; not applying if almost time for next dose
» Proper storage
*For cream and topical solution only*
» Importance of applying medication to entire affected area
» Not using in eyes, nose, mouth, or on other mucous membranes
*For topical solution only*
» Not using near heat, open flame, or while smoking
  Not using after expiration date
» Explanation of presence of floating plastic plug
  Not using medication more often than prescribed
  Avoiding too frequent washing of affected areas
*For topical ointment only*
  Not using on deep or puncture wounds or serious burns unless directed by physician
  Not for ophthalmic use

**Precautions while using this medication**
*For cream and topical solution only*
  Checking with physician if no improvement in acne within 6 to 8 weeks
  Waiting at least 1 hour before applying any other topical medication for acne
  May cause slight yellowing of skin
  Fluorescence of treated skin under "black" light
  Proper use of cosmetics
*For topical solution only*
  Checking with physician if treated skin becomes excessively dry
*For topical ointment only*
  Checking with physician if no improvement within 2 weeks

**Side/adverse effects**
  Signs of potential side effects, especially pain, redness, swelling, or other signs of irritation not present before therapy

## General Dosing Information

The treated area(s) may be covered with a gauze dressing if desired (ointment only).

Use of topical antibacterials may lead to skin sensitization, resulting in hypersensitivity reactions with subsequent topical or systemic use of the medication.

In the treatment of acne with meclocycline sulfosalicylate cream or tetracycline hydrochloride for topical solution, noticeable improvement may be seen in 4 to 6 weeks. However, in some patients it may require up to 6 to 8 weeks of treatment before noticeable improvement is seen and up to 8 to 12 weeks before maximum benefit is seen.

---

### CHLORTETRACYCLINE

## Summary of Differences

Indications: Indicated as a topical antibacterial.

## Topical Dosage Forms

**CHLORTETRACYCLINE HYDROCHLORIDE OINTMENT USP**

**Usual adult and adolescent dose**
Antibacterial (topical)—
  Topical, to the skin, one or two times a day.

**Usual pediatric dose**
See *Usual adult and adolescent dose*.

**Strength(s) usually available**
U.S.—
  3% (OTC) [*Aureomycin*].
Canada—
  3% (OTC) [*Aureomycin*].

**Packaging and storage**
Store below 40 °C (104 °F), preferably between 15 and 30 °C (59 and 86 °F), unless otherwise specified by manufacturer. Store in a collapsible tube or in a well-closed, light-resistant container. Protect from freezing.

# Tetracyclines (Topical)

**Auxiliary labeling**
- For external use only.
- Continue medicine for full time of treatment.

## MECLOCYCLINE

### Summary of Differences
Indications: Indicated in the topical treatment of acne vulgaris.
Side/adverse effects: Faint yellowing of the skin, especially around hair roots.

### Additional Dosing Information
See also *General Dosing Information*.

Meclocycline sulfosalicylate cream may also be effective when applied less frequently (e.g., once a day). However, some reports indicate it is much less effective and improvement may be delayed.

### Topical Dosage Forms
**MECLOCYCLINE SULFOSALICYLATE CREAM USP**

**Usual adult and adolescent dose**
Antiacne agent (topical)—
   Topical, to the skin, two times a day, morning and evening.

**Usual pediatric dose**
See *Usual adult and adolescent dose*.

**Strength(s) usually available**
U.S.—
   1% (base) (Rx) [*Meclan* (sodium formaldehyde sulfoxylate)].
Canada—
   Not commercially available.

**Packaging and storage**
Store below 40 °C (104 °F), preferably between 15 and 30 °C (59 and 86 °F), unless otherwise specified by manufacturer. Store in a tight container. Protect from light. Protect from freezing.

**Auxiliary labeling**
- For external use only.
- Continue medicine for full time of treatment.

**Note**
Explain administration technique.

**Additional information**
The cream is compatible with both oil- and water-base systems.

## TETRACYCLINE

### Summary of Differences
Indications: Indicated as a topical antibacterial (ointment) and in the topical treatment of acne vulgaris (topical solution).
Side/adverse effects: For topical solution—Dry or scaly skin; faint yellowing of the skin, especially around hair roots; stinging or burning feeling.

### Additional Dosing Information
See also *General Dosing Information*.

Twice-daily use of tetracycline hydrochloride for topical solution on the face and neck for acne delivers an average daily dose of 2.9 mg of tetracycline to the skin. When used twice daily on the face and neck as well as other acne-affected areas, the average daily dose delivered to the skin is 4.8 mg.

### Topical Dosage Forms
**TETRACYCLINE HYDROCHLORIDE OINTMENT USP**

**Usual adult and adolescent dose**
Antibacterial (topical)—
   Topical, to the skin, one or two times a day.

**Usual pediatric dose**
See *Usual adult and adolescent dose*.

**Strength(s) usually available**
U.S.—
   3% (OTC) [*Achromycin*].
Canada—
   3% (OTC) [*Achromycin*].

**Packaging and storage**
Store preferably between 15 and 30 °C (59 and 86 °F). Store in a well-closed container. Protect from freezing.

**Auxiliary labeling**
- For external use only.
- Continue medicine for full time of treatment.

**TETRACYCLINE HYDROCHLORIDE FOR TOPICAL SOLUTION USP**

**Usual adult and adolescent dose**
Antiacne agent (topical)—Topical, to the skin, two times a day, morning and evening.

**Usual pediatric dose**
Infants and children up to 11 years of age—Dosage has not been established.

**Strength(s) usually available**
U.S.—
   2.2 mg per mL, when reconstituted according to manufacturer's instructions (Rx) [*Topicycline* (sodium bisulfite; 40% ethanol in diluent)].
Canada—
   Not commercially available.

**Packaging and storage**
Prior to reconstitution, store below 40 °C (104 °F), preferably between 15 and 30 °C (59 and 86 °F), unless otherwise specified by manufacturer. Store in a tight, light-resistant container. Protect diluent from freezing.

**Stability**
After reconstitution, solutions retain their potency for 2 months at controlled room temperature (15 to 30 °C [59 to 86 °F]).

**Auxiliary labeling**
- For external use only.
- Continue medicine for full time of treatment.
- Beyond-use date.
- Keep container tightly closed.
- Flammable—Keep from heat and flame.

**Note**
When dispensing, include patient instructions.
Explain the presence of floating plastic plug in the bottle.
Explain administration technique.

**Additional information**
The vehicle is a solution of *n*-decyl methyl sulfoxide and sucrose esters in 40% alcohol.
To maintain an effective concentration of tetracycline hydrochloride, a sufficient amount of 4-epitetracycline hydrochloride is present, which maintains equilibrium between the two.

Revised: 10/27/93

---

# THALIDOMIDE  Systemic†

VA CLASSIFICATION (Primary/Secondary): IM900/MS102
Note: For a listing of dosage forms and brand names by country availability, see *Dosage Forms* section(s).

†Not commercially available in Canada.

## Category
Immunomodulator; anti-inflammatory.

## Indications
Note: Bracketed information in the *Indications* section refers to uses that are not included in U.S. product labeling.

**General considerations**
Thalidomide was first synthesized in 1954. It produced marked sedation in laboratory animals. Dose-escalation studies in rodents failed to show lethality even when thalidomide was given in excess of 10 grams per kilogram of body weight, suggesting that thalidomide was a safe drug. Although the studies were limited in scope, thalidomide was tested in over 1000 adults and children: it was well tolerated, had minimal ad-

dictive potential, and appeared to be an effective alternative to barbiturates. Thus, thalidomide was marketed in Europe in the late 1950s as a sedative/hypnotic (thalidomide was not approved for sale in the U.S.). However, in the early 1960s it became evident that the incidences of a relatively rare birth defect, phocomelia, and of other severe malformations of internal organs were increasing. These specific birth defects soon reached epidemic proportions (more than 10,000 children with birth defects were reported), and retrospective epidemiological research firmly established the causative agent to be thalidomide taken early in the course of pregnancy. Because of its established teratogenicity, thalidomide was withdrawn from the market worldwide.

Due to the attention given to thalidomide's dramatic, previously unknown side effects, lines of research into thalidomide's other properties were abandoned. Research into the anti-inflammatory properties that had been suggested by animal and human studies, including follow-up of surgical patients, was not pursued. Ironically, it was the sedative properties of thalidomide that resulted in its eventual acceptance as an immunomodulatory agent. In 1964, a patient with severe erythema nodosum leprosum (ENL), or type II leprosy reaction, was given thalidomide for sedation (the patient's pain had been so severe that he could not sleep). The patient's ENL lesions had regressed after a few doses of thalidomide, and this response was reversed when treatment was stopped temporarily. Thus, investigation into thalidomide's immunologic activities began, and in 1998 the Food and Drug Administration (FDA) approved the use of thalidomide for the treatment and suppression of ENL.

Due to thalidomide's toxicity, and in an effort to make the chance of fetal exposure to thalidomide as negligible as possible, thalidomide has been approved for marketing in the U.S. only under a special restricted distribution program approved by the FDA. This program is called the System for Thalidomide Education and Prescribing Safety (STEPS). Registration is available to all health care providers who agree to comply with the STEPS program. Under this restricted distribution program, only prescribers and pharmacists registered with the program are allowed to prescribe and dispense thalidomide. In addition, patients must be advised of, agree to, and comply with the requirements of the STEPS program to receive the product.

**Any suspected fetal exposure to thalidomide must be reported immediately** to the FDA via the MedWATCH number at 1-800-FDA-1088 and also to Celgene Corporation (1-888-668-2528). The patient should be referred to an obstetrician/gynecologist experienced in reproductive toxicity for further evaluation and counseling.

**Accepted**
Note: **FOR WOMEN WITH CHILDBEARING POTENTIAL, SEE THE PREGNANCY/REPRODUCTION SECTION OF *PRECAUTIONS TO CONSIDER* FOR RESTRICTIONS ON THE USE OF THALIDOMIDE.**

Erythema nodosum leprosum (ENL) (treatment)[1]—Thalidomide is indicated for the treatment of the cutaneous manifestations of moderate to severe ENL. Thalidomide is not indicated as monotherapy for such ENL treatment in the presence of moderate to severe neuritis.

Erythema nodosum leprosum (ENL), recurrent (suppression)[1]—Thalidomide is indicated as maintenance therapy for prevention and suppression of the cutaneous manifestations of ENL recurrence.

[Behçet's syndrome (treatment)][1]—Thalidomide is indicated for the treatment of the mucocutaneous lesions associated with Behçet's syndrome (*Evidence rating: I*).

[Human immunodeficiency virus (HIV)–associated wasting syndrome (treatment)][1]—Thalidomide is indicated for the treatment of HIV-associated wasting syndrome (*Evidence rating: I*).

[Stomatitis, aphthous (treatment)][1] or
[Stomatitis, aphthous, immunodeficiency-associated (treatment)][1]—Thalidomide is indicated in the treatment of aphthous stomatitis in immunocompetent and HIV-infected patients who do not respond to colchicine, dapsone, or corticosteroid treatment (*Evidence rating: I*). An infectious cause of the lesion should be excluded before thalidomide therapy is considered.

**Acceptance not established**
The use of thalidomide for the treatment of the cutaneous lesions associated with *lupus erythematosus* refractory to other therapies has been studied (*Evidence rating: III*). Although thalidomide appeared to be effective in the small number of patients reported thus far, comparative clinical studies need to be done to determine the role of thalidomide in this indication.

Thalidomide also has been used in the treatment of *graft-versus-host disease* (GVHD) (*Evidence rating: III*). There is currently not enough medical literature or clinical experience to recommend the use of thalidomide for this indication.

**Unaccepted**
Thalidomide is no longer accepted for use as a sedative/hypnotic.
Thalidomide has no antibacterial or antimycotic activity.

[1]Not included in Canadian product labeling.

## Pharmacology/Pharmacokinetics

**Physicochemical characteristics**
Chemical class—Glutamic acid derivative; chemically related to glutethimide and chlorthalidone.
Molecular weight—258.23.

**Mechanism of action/Effect**
Thalidomide is a racemic mixture of two optical isomers in equal amounts. The R-configuration and the S-configuration are more toxic individually than the racemic mixture; the dose at which 50% of animals would be killed (lethal dose [$LD$]$_{50}$) could not be established in mice for racemic thalidomide, whereas $LD_{50}$ values for the R and S configurations are reported to be 0.4 to 0.7 grams per kilogram of body weight (grams/kg) and 0.5 to 1.5 grams/kg, respectively. However, it should be noted that chirally pure thalidomide converts to the racemic mixture when administered. Early studies suggested that the R-configuration is responsible for the sleep-inducing effects of thalidomide, while the S-configuration confers its teratogenicity. More recent studies suggest that the S-configuration may be selectively responsible for all of the sedative, teratogenic, and immunomodulatory properties of thalidomide. It is not clear whether the configuration of the thalidomide molecule determines its neurotoxicity.

The mechanism(s) responsible for the clinical activity of thalidomide are as yet unknown. Although thalidomide was first recognized as a sedating agent, little information is available to ascertain a potential mechanism underlying this effect, and thalidomide is no longer used for this purpose. The teratogenic effects of thalidomide currently are explained by three leading hypotheses: disruption of neural crest development; inhibition of angiogenesis; and down-regulation of adhesion receptors on early limb-bud cells and on cells of the heart in embryos. It has been well established that thalidomide has no antibacterial or antimycotic activity. Thus, the clinical usefulness of thalidomide appears to reside in its anti-inflammatory and/or immunomodulatory properties.

Although the underlying mechanisms of these activities have not yet been defined, detailed pharmacological analyses indicate that the clinical effects result from the thalidomide molecule itself and not from any of its metabolites. Results from *in vitro* and *in vivo* studies demonstrate that thalidomide inhibits the production of tumor necrosis factor–alpha (TNF-alpha) in monocytes, ostensibly by accelerating the degradation of TNF-alpha ribonucleic acid (RNA) transcripts. Other studies suggest that thalidomide may induce the down-regulation of integrin receptors and other surface adhesion proteins, reduce IgM production, alter CD4/CD8 T-cell ratios, and/or inhibit angiogenesis. However, lymphocyte proliferation does not appear to be affected by thalidomide.

Thalidomide has been used successfully to treat various inflammatory conditions characterized by tissue infiltration with polymorphonuclear leukocytes (PMNLs), e.g., erythema nodosum leprosum (ENL) and recurrent mucocutaneous aphthous ulceration. Therapeutic benefit has been attributed to depression of PMNL chemotaxis and, possibly, PMNL phagocytosis. However, thalidomide has been reported also to be effective in other inflammatory processes with predominantly mononuclear cell accumulation, including discoid lupus erythematosus. Thalidomide was found to reduce both monocyte phagocytosis and chemiluminescence, indicating that thalidomide may decrease tissue inflammation and injury by suppressing production of oxygen-derived free radicals and other mediators involved in inflammatory responses.

Erythema nodosum leprosum (ENL)—Thalidomide has been found to reduce circulating TNF-alpha in patients with ENL; this action may be related to thalidomide's ability to reduce the local and systemic symptoms of ENL, and reduce the number of neutrophils and CD4 T-cells in the ENL lesions.

Human immunodeficiency virus (HIV) infection—Thalidomide may suppress viral replication, decrease viral burden, and enhance patient well-being by reducing TNF-alpha–induced fever, malaise, muscle weakness, and cachexia in the immunodepressed host. *In vitro* studies suggest that thalidomide selectively inhibits TNF-alpha production by monocytes. Additionally, *in vitro* experiments in primary macrophages suggest that thalidomide works through the nuclear factor kappa-B (NF-kappa-B) pathway to inhibit HIV-1 viral replication. However, *in vitro* inhibition of HIV-1 by thalidomide cannot be reproduced consistently, and this inhibition has not been shown *in vivo* or in HIV-infected patients. Contrarily, there is some *in vivo* evidence that HIV RNA levels are increased in HIV-infected patients treated with thalidomide (compared with HIV-infected patients treated with placebo).

**Graft-versus-host disease (GVHD)**—Thalidomide has been found to bind less avidly to helper T-lymphocytes than to suppressor and cytotoxic T-lymphocytes. This binding pattern suppresses the activity of helper T-lymphocytes while allowing the development of the cytotoxic and suppressor T-lymphocytes; these latter cells play a critical role in keeping GVHD in check and in promoting transplant tolerance.

### Other actions/effects
Results from human and animal studies suggest that thalidomide also has an effect on the endocrine system. Hyperthyroid states improved in some patients who were receiving thalidomide. Iodine uptake by the thyroid gland was decreased slightly, and myxedema was seen occasionally. An increase in the urinary secretion of 17-hydroxycorticosteroids associated with hypoglycemia also has been reported.

### Absorption
Half-life—Approximately 1.7 hours.

### Distribution
Approximately 121 liters in healthy subjects and 78 liters in HIV-infected patients.

In animal studies, high concentrations of thalidomide were found in the gastrointestinal tract, liver, and kidney; and lower concentrations were found in the muscle, brain, and adipose tissue. Thalidomide crosses the placenta. It is not known whether thalidomide is present in the ejaculate of males.

Patients with Hansen's disease may have an increased bioavailability of thalidomide compared with healthy subjects.

### Protein binding
Highly bound to plasma proteins.

### Biotransformation
Studies on thalidomide metabolism in humans have not been done. In animals, nonenzymatic hydrolytic cleavage appears to be the main pathway of degradation, producing seven major and at least five minor hydrolysis products. Thalidomide may be metabolized hepatically by enzymes of the cytochrome P450 enzyme system. Thalidomide does not appear to induce or inhibit its own metabolism. However, it may interfere with enzyme induction caused by other compounds.

The end product of metabolism, phthalic acid, is excreted as a glycine conjugate.

### Half-life
Elimination—
In healthy subjects, following a single dose of:
  50 mg—5.52 hours.
  200 mg—5.53 hours.
  400 mg—7.29 hours.
In HIV-positive patients, following a single dose of:100 mg—6.5 ± 3.4 hours.
  300 mg—5.7 ± 0.6 hours.
In patients with Hansen's disease, following a single dose of:400 mg—6.86 hours.

### Time to peak concentration
In healthy subjects, following a single dose of—
  50 mg: 2.9 hours.
  200 mg: 3.5 to 4.4 hours.
  400 mg: 4.3 hours.
Taking thalidomide with a high-fat meal increases the time to peak concentration to 6 hours.
In HIV-positive patients, following a single dose of—
  100 mg: 3.4 ± 1.8 hours.
  300 mg: 3.4 ± 1.5 hours.
In patients with Hansen's disease, following a single dose of—
  400 mg: 5.7 hours.

### Peak plasma concentration
In healthy subjects, following a single dose of—
  50 mg: 0.62 microgram per milliliter (mcg/mL).
  200 mg: 1.15 to 1.76 mcg/mL.
  400 mg: 2.82 mcg/mL.
In HIV-positive patients, following a single dose of—
  100 mg: 1.17 ± 0.21 mcg/mL.
  300 mg: 3.47 ± 1.14 mcg/mL.
In patients with Hansen's disease, following a single dose of—
  400 mg: 3.44 mcg/mL.
Taking thalidomide with a high-fat meal does not significantly alter peak plasma concentration values (< 10% change).

### Elimination
Thalidomide has a renal clearance of 1.15 mL per minute; less than 0.7% of the total dose is excreted unchanged.

Thalidomide appears to be well tolerated in patients with severe liver and kidney disease.

## Precautions to Consider

### Mutagenicity
Thalidomide was not mutagenic in *Salmonella typhimurium* or *Escherichia coli* gene mutation assays, in L5178YTK$^{+/-}$ mouse lymphoma cell assays, or in AS52/XPRT mammalian cell forward gene mutation assays, with or without metabolic activation. It was not clastogenic in chromosomal aberration assays using Chinese hamster ovary cells, human lymphocytes, grasshopper neuroblasts (although some unusual chromosome morphology was observed), or *Drosophila melanogaster* somatic cells; in human lymphocyte micronucleus assays; or in bone marrow micronucleus assays using male and female mice and female rabbits.

Note: The unusual chromosome morphologies observed in the grasshopper cytogenetic studies indicate a potential for thalidomide to interact with chromosomal proteins. However, this potential was not evident in the human lymphocyte micronucleus assays, and thalidomide was apparently not reactive to the proteins of mouse skin, as it gave negative results in a mouse local lymph node assay for skin sensitizing agents.

### Pregnancy/Reproduction
Fertility—Studies on the effects of thalidomide on fertility in humans or in animals have not been performed. It is not known whether thalidomide is present in the ejaculate of males.

Pregnancy—**Thalidomide is teratogenic in humans**. The window of embryopathy is small (thought to be from day 21 to day 56 after conception); however, during that time, one dose, producing a serum concentration of as little as 0.9 mcg per mL, can cause birth defects. Malformations include amelia and phocomelia; polydactyly; syndactyly; facial capillary hemangiomas; hydrocephalus; intestinal, cardiovascular, and renal anomalies; and eye, ear, and cranial nerve defects. Other malformations include facial and oculomotor paresthesias; other ocular defects; anal stenoses; vaginal and uterine defects; and heart malformations, which are generally fatal. Mortality at or shortly after birth has been reported at about 40%.

**Thalidomide is contraindicated in women with childbearing potential, unless all of the following criteria have been met (women who have undergone hysterectomy or 24 consecutive months of menopause are not considered to have childbearing potential):**
• Patient is reliable in understanding and carrying out instructions.
• Patient is capable of complying with the mandatory contraceptive measures, pregnancy testing, patient registration, and patient survey as described by the STEPS program.
• Patient has received both oral and written warnings of the risk of possible contraception failure; and of the need to continuously abstain from reproductive heterosexual sexual intercourse, or to use simultaneously two reliable forms of contraception, for at least 1 month before thalidomide therapy, during therapy, and for 1 month following discontinuation of therapy. The two reliable forms of contraception include at least one highly effective method (e.g., intrauterine device [IUD], hormonal contraception, tubal ligation, partner's vasectomy) and one additional effective method (e.g., latex condom, diaphragm, cervical cap). If hormonal or IUD contraception is medically contraindicated, two other effective or highly effective methods may be used.
• Patient acknowledges, in writing, her understanding of these warnings and of the need for using two reliable methods of contraception for 1 month before starting thalidomide therapy, during therapy, and for 1 month following discontinuation of therapy.
• Pregnancy has been definitely excluded through a negative pregnancy test with a sensitivity of at least 50 mIU per mL and appropriate history and physical examination. The pregnancy test should be performed within the 24 hours before beginning thalidomide therapy, weekly during the first month of therapy, and monthly thereafter in women with regular menstrual cycles or every 2 weeks in women with irregular menstrual cycles.
• If the patient is between 12 and 18 years of age, her parent or legal guardian must have read this material and agreed to ensure compliance with the above.

**Thalidomide is contraindicated in sexually mature males, unless all of the following criteria have been met:**
• Patient can reliably understand and carry out instructions.
• Patient is capable of complying with the mandatory contraceptive measures that are appropriate for men, the patient registration, and the patient survey as described by the STEPS program.
• Patient has received both oral and written warnings of the hazards of taking thalidomide and exposing a fetus to this medicine.
• Patient has received both oral and written warnings of the risk of possible contraception failure and of the need to use barrier contracep-

tion (latex condom) when having sexual intercourse with women with childbearing potential, even if he has undergone successful vasectomy.
• Patient acknowledges, in writing, his understanding of these warnings and of the need for using barrier contraception (latex condom), even if he has undergone successful vasectomy, when having sexual intercourse with women with childbearing potential.
• If the patient is between 12 and 18 years of age, his parent or legal guardian must have read this material and agreed to ensure compliance with the above.

FDA Pregnancy Category X.

### Breast-feeding
It is not known whether thalidomide is distributed into breast milk. Thalidomide was given to nursing mothers in the late 1950s. Although the mothers awakened easily to nurse their babies, no information was provided about the effects thalidomide had on the nursing infants. Because of the potential for serious adverse reactions from thalidomide in nursing infants, a decision should be made whether to discontinue nursing or to discontinue taking thalidomide, taking into account the importance of the medication to the mother.

### Pediatrics
No information is available on the pharmacokinetic parameters of thalidomide in patients younger than 18 years of age. Thalidomide has been used to treat approximately 20 patients from 11 to 17 years of age, and the response rates and safety profiles were the same as those for adult patients. In another study, 14 patients from 2 to 19 years of age were treated with thalidomide for chronic graft-versus-host disease, and no pediatrics-specific problems were reported. However, because of thalidomide's toxicity, it should be used with caution, and only after less toxic alternatives have been considered and/or found to be ineffective.

### Geriatrics
Appropriate studies on the relationship of age to the effects of thalidomide have not been performed in the geriatric population. However, thalidomide has been used in clinical trials in patients up to 90 years of age, and no geriatrics-specific problems have been documented to date.

### Drug interactions and/or related problems
The following drug interactions and/or related problems have been selected on the basis of their potential clinical significance (possible mechanism in parentheses where appropriate)—not necessarily inclusive (» = major clinical significance):

Note: The pharmacokinetic profiles of the hormonal contraceptive agents norethindrone (1 mg) and ethinyl estradiol (75 grams) are not changed significantly when coadministered with thalidomide (200 mg per day, to steady-state levels).

Combinations containing any of the following medications, depending on the amount present, may also interact with this medication.

» Alcohol or
» Barbiturates or
» Chlorpromazine or
» CNS depression–producing medications, other (see *Appendix II*) or
» Reserpine
(because thalidomide is a strong sedative, concurrent use may increase the CNS depressant effects of these medications; caution is recommended; the dosage of thalidomide or the other CNS depressant may need to be reduced)

» Chloramphenicol or
» Cisplatin or
» Dapsone or
» Didanosine or
» Ethambutol or
» Ethionamide or
» Hydralazine or
» Isoniazid or
» Lithium or
» Metronidazole or
» Nitrofurantoin or
» Nitrous oxide or
» Phenytoin or
» Stavudine or
» Vincristine or
» Zalcitabine or
» Other medications associated with peripheral neuropathy
(since thalidomide has been shown to cause peripheral neuropathy, which may be irreversible, other medications associated with the development of neuropathy should be used with caution during thalidomide therapy; if concurrent use is necessary, the patient should be monitored closely)

» Carbamazepine or
» Griseofulvin or
» Human immunodeficiency virus (HIV)–protease inhibitors or
» Rifabutin or
» Rifampin
(use of these medications with hormonal contraceptive agents may reduce the effectiveness of the contraception; women requiring treatment with one or more of these medications must abstain from heterosexual sexual intercourse or use two *other* effective or highly effective methods of contraception)

### Medical considerations/Contraindications
The medical considerations/contraindications included have been selected on the basis of their potential clinical significance (reasons given in parentheses where appropriate)—not necessarily inclusive (» = major clinical significance).

*Except under special circumstances, this medication should not be used when the following medical problems exist:*

» Hypersensitivity to thalidomide—more common in HIV-infected patients
» Neutropenia
(decreased white blood cell counts, including neutropenia, have been reported in association with the clinical use of thalidomide; thalidomide treatment should not be initiated with an absolute neutrophil count [ANC] of < 750 per cubic millimeter)
» Peripheral neuropathy
(thalidomide may cause peripheral neuropathy, which may be irreversible; because nerve damage can occur before the patient has any symptoms, thalidomide should not be used in any patient with pre-existing neuropathy or encephalopathy; neuropathy secondary to thalidomide is uncommon in leprosy patients, possibly because high doses are used only for 1 or 2 weeks)

### Patient monitoring
The following may be especially important in patient monitoring (other tests may be warranted in some patients, depending on condition; » = major clinical significance):

» Clinical neurological examinations and
» Nerve conduction studies
(thalidomide may cause peripheral neuropathy, which may be irreversible; although peripheral neuropathy generally occurs over a period of months following long-term use of thalidomide, reports following relatively short-term use also exist; patients should be examined at monthly intervals for the first 3 months of thalidomide therapy for detection of early signs of neuropathy, including numbness, tingling, or pain in the hands and feet; patients should be evaluated periodically thereafter during treatment, and counseled, questioned, and evaluated regularly for signs or symptoms of peripheral neuropathy; electrophysiological testing, consisting of measurement of sensory nerve action potential [SNAP] amplitudes at baseline and every 6 months thereafter, may be considered; the variability in SNAP amplitudes may be limited by having the same examiner perform the baseline and follow-up tests, and by measuring several SNAPs on each occasion; if symptoms of medication-induced neuropathy develop, thalidomide should be *discontinued immediately* to limit further damage; treatment with thalidomide should be reinitiated only if the neuropathy returns to baseline status)

» HIV-viral load
(plasma HIV ribonucleic acid [RNA] levels were found to increase in HIV-positive patients treated with thalidomide compared with HIV-positive patients treated with placebo; it is recommended that HIV-viral load be measured in HIV-positive patients after the first and third months of thalidomide treatment and every 3 months thereafter)

## Side/Adverse Effects

Note: Thalidomide may cause **peripheral neuropathy**, characterized by axonal degeneration without demyelination, affecting mainly sensory fibers in the lower limbs. Neuropathy is manifested initially by paresthesia of the feet, then the hands, followed by burning sensations in the extremities and by muscle cramps. Distribution is generally in a stocking-glove pattern.

Thalidomide does not cause major motor disability, although distal weakness in the feet and depression of the ankle deep tendon reflexes do occur late in the course of the neuropathy; on discontinuation, motor signs revert more readily and completely than sensory symptoms. Patients with mild, new onset, or progressive symptoms of peripheral neuropathy should discontinue thalidomide treatment. Thalidomide-induced neuropathy progresses gradually, over a period of weeks to months; neuropathy generally is reversible if thalidomide treatment is stopped in the early stages of neuropathy. However, symptoms may occur some time after thalidomide treatment has been stopped. Although some researchers have suggested a relationship between the total dose given and the neuropathy, others found no statistically significant correlation between the severity of this effect and total dose. However, the risk of developing polyneuropathy may be 10% or higher in chronically treated patients who do not have Hansen's disease. Results from one clinical study have suggested that smoking may have a protective effect against the development of peripheral neuropathy.

Electrophysiological abnormalities detected before the onset of subjective symptoms have been reported. The most prominent electrophysiological alteration was a decreased sensory nerve action potential (SNAP) amplitude, but decreased sensory and motor conduction velocities, as well as alterations in latencies, were also observed. The number of patients found to have developed neuropathy was consistently higher if electrophysiological tests, rather than clinical symptoms alone, were used for diagnosis. The reduced or absent sensitivity in the extremities was frequently irreversible or was only partially reversible over a long period. The incidence of peripheral neuropathy has ranged widely, from 0.5 to 50%. In human immunodeficiency virus (HIV)–infected patients, the incidence reportedly varies from 15 to 50%. Patients with pre-existing neuropathies may be more sensitive to the development of thalidomide-induced neuropathy. However, neuropathy may also be seen in HIV disease itself. The side effects of thalidomide appear to be more severe and more poorly tolerated in HIV-infected patients.

Detecting thalidomide-induced neuropathy in erythema nodosum leprosum (ENL) patients may be difficult because of the similarity of clinical symptoms and changes in electrophysiological measurements that result from the underlying ENL disease. The incidence of peripheral neuropathy due to thalidomide appears to be low in patients being treated for ENL; this may be because peripheral nerves are consistently affected in lepromatous leprosy and thalidomide improves the neuritis of ENL by reducing inflammation. Gradual dose escalation may be efficacious in avoiding adverse reactions.

The following side/adverse effects have been selected on the basis of their potential clinical significance (possible signs and symptoms in parentheses where appropriate)—not necessarily inclusive:

**Those indicating need for medical attention**
Incidence more frequent
*Peripheral neuropathy* (tingling, burning, numbness, or pain in the hands, arms, feet, or legs; muscle weakness)
Note: If symptoms of thalidomide-induced neuropathy develop, thalidomide should be discontinued *immediately* to limit further damage. Usually, treatment with thalidomide should be reinitiated only if the neuropathy returns to baseline status.

Patients should undergo a baseline neurological exam before beginning thalidomide treatment.

Incidence rare
*Fever; irregular heartbeat; low blood pressure; neutropenia* (fever, chills, or sore throat); *renal failure* (blood in urine; decreased urination); *skin rash*—seen more frequently in HIV-infected patients; may be moderate to severe

**Those indicating need for medical attention only if they continue or are bothersome**
Incidence more frequent
*Dizziness; drowsiness; gastrointestinal intolerance* (constipation; diarrhea; nausea; stomach pain)
Incidence less frequent
*Dryness of mouth; dry skin; headache; increased appetite; mood alterations; swelling in the legs*

## Overdose

For more information on the management of overdose or unintentional ingestion, **contact a Poison Control Center** (see *Poison Control Center Listing*).

**Clinical effects of overdose**
The toxicity of thalidomide is so low that a dose at which 50% of animals would be killed (LD$_{50}$) could not be established. Patients who have attempted suicide or have accidentally overdosed have survived without detectable sequelae. Overdoses of up to 14 grams of thalidomide taken with alcohol have resulted only in somnolence. No respiratory or circulatory problems have been reported.

**Treatment of overdose**
Supportive care—Patients in whom intentional overdose is confirmed or suspected should be referred for psychiatric consultation.

## Patient Consultation

As an aid to patient consultation, refer to *Advice for the Patient, Thalidomide (Systemic)*.
In providing consultation, consider emphasizing the following selected information (» = major clinical significance):

**Before using this medication**
» Conditions affecting use, especially:
   Hypersensitivity to thalidomide
   Pregnancy—Thalidomide is **contraindicated** during pregnancy; it is a known teratogen to the human fetus; women with childbearing potential should have a pregnancy test within 24 hours before starting thalidomide treatment, weekly during the first month of treatment, and every 2 to 4 weeks thereafter; two effective methods of contraception should be used simultaneously for at least 1 month before starting thalidomide treatment, during treatment, and for at least 1 month following discontinuation of treatment
   Other medications, especially alcohol, barbiturates, carbamazepine, chloramphenicol, chlorpromazine, cisplatin, dapsone, didanosine, ethambutol, ethionamide, griseofulvin, HIV–protease inhibitors, hydralazine, isoniazid, lithium, metronidazole, nitrofurantoin, nitrous oxide, phenytoin, reserpine, rifabutin, rifampin, stavudine, vincristine, zalcitabine, other CNS depressants, and other medications associated with peripheral neuropathy
   Other medical problems, especially neutropenia and peripheral neuropathy

**Proper use of this medication**
» Importance of not taking more medication than prescribed; not discontinuing medication without checking with physician
» Not sharing this medicine with others
» Proper dosing
   Missed dose: Taking as soon as possible; not taking if almost time for next dose; not doubling doses
» Proper storage

**Precautions while using this medication**
» Avoiding the use of alcoholic beverages and other medicines that cause drowsiness
» Having a pregnancy test done within 24 hours before starting thalidomide treatment, weekly during the first month of treatment, and every 2 to 4 weeks thereafter in women with childbearing potential
» Abstaining from heterosexual sexual intercourse, or using two effective methods of contraception simultaneously for at least 1 month before starting thalidomide, during treatment, and for at least 1 month following discontinuation of treatment, for women with childbearing potential
» Discontinuing thalidomide and calling physician immediately if mild, new onset, or progressive symptoms of peripheral neuropathy occur

**Side/adverse effects**
Signs of potential side effects, especially peripheral neuropathy, fever, irregular heartbeat, low blood pressure, neutropenia, renal failure, and skin rash

## General Dosing Information

Thalidomide should be taken with water, at least 1 hour after meals. Thalidomide may be taken at bedtime to minimize the impact of its sedative effect, which occurs in nearly all patients when therapy is started. Many patients rapidly adjust to this effect and are able to resume their normal daily activities.

Dosing of thalidomide for erythema nodosum leprosum (ENL) generally should continue until signs and symptoms of active reaction have subsided, usually a period of at least 2 weeks. Patients may then be tapered off thalidomide in 50-mg decrements every 2 to 4 weeks. However, ENL recurrence is very common, often necessitating prolonged (up to several years) suppressive therapy.

Some patients (26% from one clinical study) receiving thalidomide for recurrent aphthous stomatitis have been able to discontinue thalidomide treatment after approximately 27 months of therapy, and a further 43% of patients remained in remission with continued low doses of thalidomide.

## Oral Dosage Forms

Note: Bracketed uses in the *Dosage Forms* section refer to categories of use and/or indications that are not included in U.S. product labeling.

## THALIDOMIDE CAPSULES

### Usual adult and adolescent dose
Erythema nodosum leprosum (ENL)[1]—
  Cutaneous ENL, treatment: Oral, 100 to 300 mg once a day with water, taken at bedtime or at least one hour after the evening meal. Patients weighing less than 50 kilograms should be started at the low end of the dosing range.
  Severe cutaneous ENL, treatment: Oral, up to 400 mg once a day at bedtime or in divided doses with water, at least one hour after meals.
  Note: In patients with moderate to severe neuritis associated with a severe ENL reaction, corticosteroids may be started concomitantly with thalidomide. Corticosteroid use can be tapered and discontinued when the neuritis has ameliorated.
  Recurrent ENL, suppression: Patients who have a documented history of requiring prolonged maintenance treatment to prevent the recurrence of cutaneous ENL or who flare during tapering should be maintained on the minimum dose necessary to control the reaction. Tapering the dosage of thalidomide should be attempted every three to six months, in decrements of 50 mg every two to four weeks.
[Behçet's syndrome][1]—
  Oral, 100 to 300 mg a day with water, at bedtime or at least one hour after meals.
[Human immunodeficiency virus (HIV)–associated wasting syndrome][1]—
  Oral, 100 or 200 mg once a day with water, at bedtime or at least one hour after the evening meal; or 100 mg two times a day with water, at least one hour after meals.
[Stomatitis, aphthous][1]—
  Oral, 50 to 200 mg once a day with water, at bedtime or at least one hour after the evening meal, for four weeks. A maintenance dose of 50 mg four times a day may be required for some patients.

### Usual pediatric dose
Dosing has not been clearly established. Thalidomide was administered to infants and children when it was originally approved as a sedative. Almost all of the more recent case reports and studies have been done in adults.

### Strength(s) usually available
U.S.—
  50 mg (Rx) [*THALOMID* (anhydrous lactose)].
Canada—
  Not commercially available.
Note: In the U.S., thalidomide has orphan drug status for the treatment and maintenance of reactional lepromatous leprosy (Sponsor: Pediatric Pharmaceuticals, Westfield, NJ); for the treatment and prevention of graft-versus-host disease (GVHD) in patients receiving bone marrow transplantation (Sponsors: Andrulis Research Corporation, Bethesda, MD, and Pediatric Pharmaceuticals, Westfield, NJ); for the treatment of the clinical manifestations of mycobacterial infection caused by *Mycobacterium tuberculosis* and nontuberculous mycobacteria (Sponsor: Celgene Corporation, Warren, NJ); for the treatment and prevention of recurrent aphthous ulcers in severely, terminally immunocompromised patients (Sponsors: Celgene Corporation, Warren, NJ, and Andrulis Research Corporation, Bethesda, MD); and for the treatment of human immunodeficiency virus (HIV)–associated wasting syndrome (Sponsor: Celgene Corporation, Warren, NJ).
Canada revoked the total ban on thalidomide in 1984; thalidomide is now available on a limited basis, upon specific authorization, for emergency purposes only.

### Packaging and storage
Store between 15 and 30 °C (59 and 86 °F). Protect from light.

### Auxiliary labeling
- Take with water.
- May cause drowsiness.
- Continue medicine for full time of treatment.

### Note
Thalidomide must be dispensed only as a 1-month or less supply and only upon presentation of a new prescription written within the previous 7 days. Specific informed consent (copy attached as part of the package insert) and compliance with the mandatory patient registry and survey are required for all patients (male and female) prior to dispensing by the pharmacist.

[1]Not included in Canadian product labeling.

### Selected Bibliography
McCarty MF. Thalidomide may impede cell migration in primates by down-regulating integrin beta-chains: potential therapeutic utility in solid malignancies, proliferative retinopathy, inflammatory disorders, neointimal hyperplasia, and osteoporosis. Med Hypotheses 1997; 49: 123-31.

Zwingenberger K, Wnendt S. Immunomodulation by thalidomide: systematic review of the literature and of unpublished observations. J Inflamm 1996; 46: 177-211.

Revised: 08/31/98

---

# THALLOUS CHLORIDE Tl 201   Systemic

VA CLASSIFICATION (Primary): DX201

Note: For a listing of dosage forms and brand names by country availability, see *Dosage Forms* section(s).

## Category
Diagnostic aid, radioactive (myocardial infarction; ischemic heart disease; parathyroid disorders; neoplastic disease).

## Indications
Note: Bracketed information in the *Indications* section refers to uses that are not included in U.S. product labeling.

### Accepted
Cardiac imaging, radionuclide
Myocardial infarction (diagnosis) and
Myocardial perfusion imaging, radionuclide—Thallous chloride Tl 201 is indicated in myocardial perfusion imaging for the diagnosis and localization of myocardial infarction.

Coronary artery disease (diagnosis)—Thallous chloride Tl 201 is indicated in studies of myocardial perfusion done under resting conditions and after physiologic or pharmacologic stress (either exercise or after infusion of dipyridamole, [adenosine][1], or [dobutamine][1]) to detect myocardium with abnormal perfusion reserve secondary to coronary artery disease. Intravenous dipyridamole, [adenosine][1], and [dobutamine][1] are used primarily as substitutes for exercise in patients who are unable to exercise sufficiently to provide the required level of myocardial blood flow augmentation or when exercise is otherwise not feasible.

Parathyroid imaging, radionuclide[1]—Thallous chloride Tl 201 is indicated for the detection and localization of parathyroid tissue in patients with documented hyperparathyroidism. Thallous chloride Tl 201 also may be useful in preoperative screening to localize extrathyroidal and mediastinal sites of parathyroid tissue and for postsurgical reexamination. However, the use of thallous chloride Tl 201 as a parathyroid imaging agent generally has been replaced by technetium Tc 99m sestamibi.

[Tumor imaging, radionuclide][1]—Thallous chloride Tl 201 is used for the detection and localization of various tumors, including thyroid carcinomas, malignant brain neoplasms, lymphomas, and mediastinal tumors, especially for postoperative detection of residual and recurrent tumors and differentiation of these from post-therapy fibrosis or necrosis.

[1]Not included in Canadian product labeling.

## Physical Properties

### Nuclear Data

| Radionuclide (half-life) | Mode of decay | Principal photon emissions (keV) | Mean number of emissions/disintegration |
|---|---|---|---|
| Tl 201 (73.1 hr) | Electron capture | Gamma-4 (135.3) | 0.03 |
| | | Gamma-6 (167.4) | 0.1 |
| | | Mercury x-rays (68.9–80.3) | 0.95 |

## Pharmacology/Pharmacokinetics

### Mechanism of action/Effect

Cardiac imaging—Thallous chloride Tl 201 appears to accumulate in cells of myocardium and other tissues in a manner analogous to that of potassium. The initial biodistribution of thallous chloride Tl 201 in most tissues is primarily related to regional blood flow. Ischemic myocardial cells take up less thallium-201 than nonischemic cells, in proportion to the relative change in blood flow, especially during maximal stress (or pharmacologically induced vasodilation) when the differential in perfusion is most marked between regions supplied by normal coronary arteries and those supplied by stenotic vessels. Imaging equipment can record regional differences in thallium-201 uptake, and thus in myocardial perfusion, confirming the presence or absence of coronary disease.

Parathyroid imaging—Localizes in parathyroid adenomas, parathyroid hyperplasia, and other abnormal tissues, generally in proportion to organ blood flow at the time of injection.

### Distribution

Rapidly cleared from blood after intravenous administration, with the following accumulation—
  Cardiac: 4% within 10 minutes of injection.
  Hepatic: 15%.
  Intracellular: 72%.
  Renal: 3%.
  Testicular: 0.15%.

### Half-life

Biological (approximate)—
  Intracellular: 36 hours.
  Liver, heart, and kidneys: 35.6 hours.
  Testes: 20 hours.

### Time to peak concentration

Myocardium—10 minutes.

### Radiation dosimetry

Estimated absorbed radiation dose*

| Organ | mGy/MBq | rad/mCi |
|---|---|---|
| Testes | 0.56 | 2.1 |
| Kidneys | 0.54 | 2 |
| Large intestine wall (lower) | 0.36 | 1.3 |
| Bone surfaces | 0.34 | 1.3 |
| Thyroid | 0.25 | 0.93 |
| Heart | 0.23 | 0.85 |
| Large intestine wall (upper) | 0.19 | 0.7 |
| Red marrow | 0.18 | 0.67 |
| Liver | 0.18 | 0.67 |
| Small intestine | 0.16 | 0.59 |
| Spleen | 0.14 | 0.52 |
| Stomach wall | 0.12 | 0.44 |
| Lungs | 0.12 | 0.44 |
| Ovaries | 0.12 | 0.44 |
| Pancreas | 0.054 | 0.20 |
| Adrenals | 0.051 | 0.19 |
| Uterus | 0.05 | 0.19 |
| Bladder wall | 0.036 | 0.13 |
| Breast | 0.028 | 0.1 |
| Other tissue | 0.056 | 0.21 |

Effective dose*

| Radionuclide and impurities | mSv/MBq† | rem/mCi† |
|---|---|---|
| Tl 201 | 0.23 | 0.85 |
| Tl 200 | 0.31 | 1.15 |
| Tl 202 | 0.8 | 2.96 |

*In adults. Intravenous administration at rest; uptake in muscles increases two- to threefold during exercise with a corresponding reduction in other tissues. Data based on the International Commission on Radiological Protection (ICRP) Publication 53—Radiation dose to patients from radiopharmaceuticals.

†Effective doses for the radionuclide and its contaminants are expressed per individual unit of activity of each.

### Elimination

Renal and fecal; 4 to 8% of the administered activity eliminated in the urine within 24 hours.

## Precautions to Consider

### Carcinogenicity/Mutagenicity

Long-term animal studies to evaluate carcinogenic or mutagenic potential of thallous chloride Tl 201 have not been performed.

### Pregnancy/Reproduction

Pregnancy—Studies to assess transplacental transfer of thallous chloride Tl 201 have not been done in humans.

The possibility of pregnancy should be assessed in women of child-bearing potential. Clinical situations exist in which the benefit to the patient and fetus, based on information derived from radiopharmaceutical use, outweighs the risks from fetal exposure to radiation. In these situations, the physician should use discretion and reduce the radiopharmaceutical dose to the lowest possible amount consistent with image quality needs.

Studies have not been done in animals.

FDA Pregnancy Category C.

### Breast-feeding

Thallous chloride Tl 201 is distributed into breast milk. To avoid unnecessary irradiation of the infant, temporary discontinuation of nursing is recommended for a length of time that may be assessed by measuring the activity of breast milk and estimating the radiation exposure to the infant.

### Pediatrics

Diagnostic studies performed in children have not demonstrated pediatrics-specific problems that would limit the usefulness of thallous chloride Tl 201 in children.

### Geriatrics

Diagnostic studies performed to date using thallous chloride Tl 201 have not demonstrated geriatrics-specific problems that would limit the usefulness of this agent in the elderly.

### Drug interactions and/or related problems

See *Diagnostic interference*.

### Diagnostic interference

The following have been selected on the basis of their potential clinical significance (possible effect in parentheses where appropriate)—not necessarily inclusive (» = major clinical significance):

With results of *this* test
  *Due to other medications*
    Dexamethasone or
    Furosemide, chronic therapy without potassium replacement or
    Isoproterenol or
    Sodium bicarbonate, intravenous
      (in animal studies, concurrent use increased myocardial uptake of thallous chloride Tl 201; human data are not available)
    Digitalis glycosides or
    Propranolol, intravenous
      (in animal studies, concurrent use decreased myocardial uptake of thallous chloride Tl 201; human data are not available)
  *Due to medical problems or conditions*
    Diabetes mellitus
      (transport of thallium may be affected by alterations in blood glucose, insulin, or pH)
    Postprandial state
      (increased accumulation of thallium in the abdominal viscera [postprandial stomach, liver, spleen, intestines] may interfere with myocardial visualization during the resting, exercise, or pharmacologic stress thallium test)

With results of *adenosine/thallium* or *dipyridamole/thallium* test
  *Due to other medications*
    Caffeine or
    Xanthine-derivative medications
      (these agents antagonize the effects of adenosine or dipyridamole on myocardial blood flow; xanthine-derivative medication should be withheld for 24 to 36 hours prior to test; also, patients should be instructed to avoid ingesting caffeine [from a dietary or medicinal source] for 8 to 12 hours prior to test)

### Medical considerations/Contraindications

The medical considerations/contraindications included have been selected on the basis of their potential clinical significance (reasons given in parentheses where appropriate)—not necessarily inclusive (» = major clinical significance).

*Risk-benefit should be considered when the following medical problems exist:*

» Hypotension
  (increased risk of severe hypotension with either adenosine/thallium or dipyridamole/thallium stress test)

» Pulmonary disease, bronchospastic, history of
    (increased risk of bronchospasm with either adenosine/thallium or dipyridamole/thallium stress test)
  Sensitivity to the radiopharmaceutical preparation
*For adenosine/thallium stress test*
» Atrioventricular (AV) block, pre-existing second or third degree or
» Angina, unstable, history of or
» Congestive heart failure, severe or
» Ischemic cardiomyopathy, severe or
» Myocardial infarction, recent
    (increased risk of severe myocardial ischemia and/or arrhythmia with adenosine/thallium stress test)
*For dipyridamole/thallium stress test*
» Angina, unstable, history of
    (increased risk of severe myocardial ischemia with dipyridamole/thallium stress test)
» Asthma, current or history of
    (increased risk of bronchospasm with dipyridamole/thallium stress test)

## Side/Adverse Effects

The following side/adverse effects have been selected on the basis of their potential clinical significance (possible signs and symptoms in parentheses where appropriate)—not necessarily inclusive:

**Those indicating need for medical attention**
Incidence less frequent or rare
  *Allergic reaction* (skin rash, hives, or itching); *blurred vision; hypotension*

**Those indicating need for medical attention only if they continue or are bothersome**
Incidence less frequent or rare
  *Nausea; sweating*

## Patient Consultation

As an aid to patient consultation, refer to *Advice for the Patient, Radiopharmaceuticals (Diagnostic)*.
In providing consultation, consider emphasizing the following selected information (» = major clinical significance):

**Description of use**
  Action in the body: Accumulation of radioactivity in myocardial cells and parathyroid, thyroid, and tumor tissues
  Differences in uptake of radioactivity can be visualized
  Small amounts of radioactivity used in diagnosis; radiation received is low and considered safe

**Before having this test**
» Conditions affecting use, especially:
    Sensitivity to the radiopharmaceutical preparation
    Pregnancy—Risk to fetus from radiation exposure as opposed to benefit derived from use should be considered
    Breast-feeding—Thallous chloride Tl 201 is distributed into breast milk; temporary discontinuation of nursing recommended to avoid unnecessary irradiation of infant
    Other medical problems, especially current or history of asthma, history of unstable angina, hypotension, pulmonary disease, recent myocardial infarction, severe congestive heart failure

**Preparation for this test**
  Fasting the morning of the resting or exercise thallium test to minimize localization in splanchnic organs and improve myocardial visualization
  Avoiding caffeine ingestion for 8 to 12 hours before adenosine/thallium or dipyridamole/thallium test
  Special preparatory instructions may be given; patient should inquire in advance

**Precautions after having this test**
  No special precautions

**Side/adverse effects**
  Signs of potential side effects, especially allergic reaction, blurred vision, and hypotension

## General Dosing Information

Radiopharmaceuticals are to be administered only by or under the supervision of physicians who have had extensive training in the safe use and handling of radioactive materials and who are authorized by the Nuclear Regulatory Commission (NRC) or the appropriate Agreement State agency, if required, or, outside the U.S., the appropriate authority.

For resting thallium studies, myocardial-to-background ratios are improved when patients are injected while upright and in the fasting state; the upright position reduces the hepatic and gastric concentration of thallium-201. Imaging should begin 10 to 20 minutes after injection of thallous chloride Tl 201.

For thallium studies performed in conjunction with exercise stress testing, thallous chloride Tl 201 should be administered at the inception of a period of maximum stress that lasts for approximately 30 to 60 seconds after injection. To obtain maximum target-to-background ratios, imaging should begin within 10 minutes after administration of thallous chloride Tl 201.

For thallium studies performed in conjunction with pharmacologic stress testing, thallous chloride Tl 201 should be administered 4 to 5 minutes after the 4-minute infusion of dipyridamole, or during the third to fourth minute of the 6-minute infusion of adenosine.

For parathyroid hyperactivity imaging, thallous chloride Tl 201 should be administered before, with, or after a minimal dose of a thyroid imaging agent, such as sodium pertechnetate Tc 99m or sodium iodide I 123, to enable thyroid subtraction imaging.

**Safety considerations for handling this radiopharmaceutical**
Guidelines for the receipt, storage, handling, dispensing, and disposal of radioactive materials are available from scientific, professional, state, federal, and international bodies. Handling of this radiopharmaceutical should be limited to those individuals who are appropriately qualified and authorized.

## Parenteral Dosage Forms

Note: Bracketed uses in the *Dosage Forms* section refer to categories of use and/or indications that are not included in U.S. product labeling.

### THALLOUS CHLORIDE Tl 201 INJECTION USP

**Usual adult and adolescent administered activity**
Cardiac imaging—
  Planar imaging: Intravenous, 37 to 74 megabecquerels (1 to 2 millicuries).
  SPECT imaging: 74 to 148 megabecquerels (2 to 4 millicuries).
Parathyroid imaging[1]—
  Intravenous, 75 megabecquerels (2 millicuries).
[Tumor imaging][1]—
  Intravenous, 55.5 to 111 megabecquerels (1.5 to 3 millicuries).

**Usual pediatric administered activity**
Cardiac imaging and
Parathyroid imaging[1]—
  Dosage must be individualized by physician. The recommended dosage is 1.11 megabecquerels (30 microcuries) per kg of body weight administered intravenously, with a minimum total dosage of 27.75 megabecquerels (750 microcuries) and a maximum total dosage of 111 megabecquerels (3 millicuries).

**Usual geriatric administered activity**
See *Usual adult and adolescent administered activity*.

**Strength(s) usually available**
U.S.—
  37 megabecquerels (1 millicurie) per mL at time of calibration (Rx) [GENERIC].
Canada—
  Content information not available (Rx) [GENERIC].

**Packaging and storage**
Store between 15 and 30 °C (59 and 86 °F), unless otherwise specified by manufacturer. Protect from freezing.

**Stability**
Do not use if contents are turbid.
Injection should be administered within 4 to 6 days after the calibration date, depending on the product used.

**Note**
Caution—Radioactive material.

---
[1]Not included in Canadian product labeling.

## Selected Bibliography

Waxman AD. Thallium-201 in nuclear oncology. Nucl Med Ann 1991; 193-209.
Verani MS. Thallium-201 single-photon emission computed tomography (SPECT) in the assessment of coronary artery disease. Am J Cardiol 1992; 70: 3E-9E.
Wackers FJT. Comparison of thallium-201 and technetium-99m methoxyisobutyl isonitrile. Am J Cardiol 1992; 70: 30E-34E.

Revised: 07/03/96

**THEOPHYLLINE**—See *Bronchodilators, Theophylline (Systemic)*

**THEOPHYLLINE, EPHEDRINE, GUAIFENESIN, AND PHENOBARBITAL**—The *Theophylline, Ephedrine, Guaifenesin, and Phenobarbital (Systemic)* monograph is not included in this published version of the USP DI database. Copies of the monograph are available on request from Micromedex, Inc. - Reprint Requests, 6200 S. Syracuse Way, Suite 300, Englewood, CO 80111; telephone (303) 486-6400; telefax (303) 486-6464; Email: USPDI@MDX.COM.

**THEOPHYLLINE, EPHEDRINE, AND HYDROXYZINE**—The *Theophylline, Ephedrine, and Hydroxyzine (Systemic)* monograph is not included in this published version of the USP DI database. Copies of the monograph are available on request from Micromedex, Inc. - Reprint Requests, 6200 S. Syracuse Way, Suite 300, Englewood, CO 80111; telephone (303) 486-6400; telefax (303) 486-6464; Email: USPDI@MDX.COM.

**THEOPHYLLINE, EPHEDRINE, AND PHENOBARBITAL**—The *Theophylline, Ephedrine, and Phenobarbital (Systemic)* monograph is not included in this published version of the USP DI database. Copies of the monograph are available on request from Micromedex, Inc. - Reprint Requests, 6200 S. Syracuse Way, Suite 300, Englewood, CO 80111; telephone (303) 486-6400; telefax (303) 486-6464; Email: USPDI@MDX.COM.

**THEOPHYLLINE AND GUAIFENESIN**—The *Theophylline and Guaifenesin (Systemic)* monograph is not included in this published version of the USP DI database. Copies of the monograph are available on request from Micromedex, Inc. - Reprint Requests, 6200 S. Syracuse Way, Suite 300, Englewood, CO 80111; telephone (303) 486-6400; telefax (303) 486-6464; Email: USPDI@MDX.COM.

# THIABENDAZOLE  Systemic†

VA CLASSIFICATION (Primary): AP200
Commonly used brand name(s): *Mintezol*.
Note: For a listing of dosage forms and brand names by country availability, see *Dosage Forms* section(s).

†Not commercially available in Canada.

## Category
Anthelmintic (systemic).
Note: Thiabendazole is a broad-spectrum anthelmintic, which has a spectrum similar to that of mebendazole.

## Indications
Note: Bracketed information in the *Indications* section refers to uses that are not included in U.S. product labeling.

### Accepted
Larva migrans, cutaneous (treatment)—Thiabendazole is indicated in the treatment of cutaneous larva migrans (creeping eruption) caused by *Ancylostoma braziliense* (dog and cat hookworm) and *Ancylostoma caninum*.

Larva migrans, visceral (treatment)—Thiabendazole is indicated in the treatment of visceral larva migrans (toxocariasis) caused by *Toxocara canis* and *T. cati* (dog and cat roundworm).

Strongyloidiasis (treatment)—Thiabendazole is indicated in the treatment of strongyloidiasis, including hyperinfection syndrome caused by *Strongyloides stercoralis* (threadworm) in immunosuppressed and non-immunosuppressed patients.

Trichinosis (treatment)—Thiabendazole is indicated in the treatment of trichinosis caused by *Trichinella spiralis* (pork worm) if the patient is known to have ingested trichinous pork within the previous 24 hours. It has little effect on muscle larvae and has not been shown to alter the course of the disease in established infections. However, it does have an effect on the adult worms, and thereby decreases the number of new larvae. Systemic corticosteroids may be used in critically ill patients to minimize inflammatory reactions to *Trichinella* larvae. However, their effectiveness has not been proven.

[Capillariasis (treatment)]—Thiabendazole is used in the treatment of capillariasis caused by *Capillaria philippinensis*.

[Dracunculiasis (treatment)]—Thiabendazole is used in the treatment of dracunculiasis (guinea worm infection) caused by *Dracunculus medinensis*. It has no effect on the worms themselves, but reduces inflammation to permit easier removal of the worm.

[Trichostrongyliasis (treatment)]—Thiabendazole is used in the treatment of trichostrongyliasis caused by *Trichostrongylus* species.

Not all species or strains of a particular helminth may be susceptible to thiabendazole.

### Unaccepted
In the treatment of ascariasis, enterobiasis, trichuriasis, hookworm infection, and multiple helminth infections, thiabendazole generally has been replaced by more effective and less toxic agents, such as mebendazole or pyrantel.

Thiabendazole is not indicated in the prophylaxis of helminth infections.

## Pharmacology/Pharmacokinetics

### Physicochemical characteristics
Molecular weight—201.25.

### Mechanism of action/Effect
Unknown; however, thiabendazole has been shown to inhibit helminth-specific enzyme fumarate reductase; vermicidal; although thiabendazole may also be ovicidal and larvicidal, it has no effect on muscle-encysted *Trichinella spiralis* larvae.

### Other actions/effects
Also has anti-inflammatory, analgesic, antipyretic, and mild antifungal and scabicidal actions.

### Absorption
Rapidly and well absorbed from gastrointestinal tract.

### Distribution
Therapeutic concentrations of thiabendazole were found in the cerebrospinal fluid of one patient with disseminated strongyloidiasis.

### Biotransformation
Hepatic; rapidly and almost completely metabolized to inactive 5-hydroxythiabendazole, which is further metabolized to glucuronide and sulfate conjugates.

### Half-life
Thiabendazole—Normal and anephric: 1.2 hours (range, 0.9 to 2 hours).
5-hydroxythiabendazole—1.7 hours (range, 1.4 to 2 hours).

### Time to peak serum concentration
Thiabendazole—1 to 2 hours.
5-hydroxythiabendazole—2 to 4 hours.

### Peak serum concentration
Thiabendazole—4.5 to 5.0 mcg/mL after a single 25 mg per kg of body weight (mg/kg) dose.
5-hydroxythiabendazole—4 to 10 mcg/mL after a single 25 mg/kg dose.

### Elimination
Renal—Up to 90% or more excreted as inactive metabolites in urine within 48 hours (most during the first 24 hours); <1% excreted unchanged in urine; 5-hydroxythiabendazole excreted in urine as glucuronide and sulfate conjugates.
Fecal—Approximately 5% excreted in feces within 48 hours.
In dialysis—Hemodialysis does not remove significant amounts of thiabendazole or its metabolites from the blood.

## Precautions to Consider

### Carcinogenicity
Numerous short- and long-term studies in animals given doses of up to 15 times the usual human dose have not shown that thiabendazole is carcinogenic.

**Mutagenicity**
*In vitro* microbial mutagen tests, micronucleus tests, and *in vivo* host-mediated assays have not shown that thiabendazole is mutagenic.

**Pregnancy/Reproduction**
Fertility—Studies in mice given doses of thiabendazole 2½ times the usual human dose and studies in rats given doses equivalent to the usual human dose have not shown that thiabendazole adversely affects fertility.
Pregnancy—Adequate and well-controlled studies in humans have not been done.
Studies in rabbits given doses of up to 15 times the usual human dose and studies in rats given doses equivalent to the usual human dose have not shown that thiabendazole causes adverse effects on the fetus. Similarly, studies in mice given doses of up to 2½ times the usual human dose have not shown any adverse effects on the fetus. However, another study in mice given doses of 10 times the usual human dose in olive oil (but not in aqueous suspension) has shown that thiabendazole causes cleft palate and axial skeletal defects.
FDA Pregnancy Category C.

**Breast-feeding**
It is not known whether thiabendazole is excreted in human breast milk. Problems in humans have not been documented; however, because of the potential for serious adverse effects in the nursing infant, breast-feeding may need to be discontinued.

**Pediatrics**
Appropriate studies on the relationship of age to the effects of thiabendazole have not been performed in children up to 13.6 kg of body weight.

**Geriatrics**
No information is available on the relationship of age to the effects of thiabendazole in geriatric patients.

**Drug interactions and/or related problems**
The following drug interactions and/or related problems have been selected on the basis of their potential clinical significance (possible mechanism in parentheses where appropriate)—not necessarily inclusive (» = major clinical significance):
Note: Combinations containing any of the following medications, depending on the amount present, may also interact with this medication.
» Theophylline
(concurrent use of thiabendazole with theophylline may reduce the clearance of theophylline by greater than 50%, possibly resulting in toxic concentrations; theophylline concentrations should be monitored)

**Laboratory value alterations**
The following have been selected on the basis of their potential clinical significance (possible effect in parentheses where appropriate)—not necessarily inclusive (» = major clinical significance):
With physiology/laboratory test values
Aspartate aminotransferase (AST [SGOT]), serum
(rarely, concentration may be transiently increased)

**Medical considerations/Contraindications**
The medical considerations/contraindications included have been selected on the basis of their potential clinical significance (reasons given in parentheses where appropriate)—not necessarily inclusive (» = major clinical significance):

*Risk-benefit should be considered when the following medical problems exist:*
» Hepatic function impairment
(thiabendazole metabolized primarily in liver; may also be hepatotoxic)
Hypersensitivity to thiabendazole
Renal function impairment
(high concentrations of the parent compound may accumulate in renal failure, resulting in neurotoxicity)

**Patient monitoring**
The following may be especially important in patient monitoring (other tests may be warranted in some patients, depending on condition; » = major clinical significance):
*For strongyloidiasis*
» Sputum examinations
(in the diagnosis of strongyloidiasis, sputum examinations may be required when pulmonary signs or symptoms are present, when the possibility of a hyperinfection syndrome exists, or when the patient is immunosuppressed or will be undergoing immunosuppression)

» Stool examinations
(required prior to and approximately 2 to 3 weeks following treatment with thiabendazole to determine efficacy of the medication or establish proof of cure [i.e., absence of eggs, larvae, or worms in the stool]; because of colonic mixing, eggs may persist in the stool for up to 1 week following cure; more frequent stool examinations may be required in the treatment of strongyloidiasis hyperinfection syndrome, especially in immunocompromised patients; follow-up stool examinations are generally not useful in toxocariasis since *Toxocara* species rarely develop into egg-producing adults in humans)

## Side/Adverse Effects
Note: Some patients may excrete a metabolite that imparts an asparagus-like or other unusual odor to the urine.
Thiabendazole may cause severe cases of Stevens-Johnson syndrome, in which fatalities have occurred.

The following side/adverse effects have been selected on the basis of their potential clinical significance (possible signs and symptoms in parentheses where appropriate)—not necessarily inclusive:

**Those indicating need for medical attention**
Incidence more frequent
*Central nervous system (CNS) toxicity* (numbness or tingling in the hands or feet); *gastrointestinal disturbance, severe* (anorexia; diarrhea; nausea and vomiting); *neuropsychiatric toxicity* (delirium; disorientation; hallucinations; irritability)
Incidence less frequent
*Hypersensitivity* (skin rash or itching)
Incidence rare
*Crystalluria* (lower back pain; pain or burning while urinating); *intrahepatic cholestasis* (malaise; nausea and vomiting; dark urine; pale stools; yellow eyes and skin); *ocular symptoms* (blurred or yellow vision; unusual feeling in the eyes); *seizures; Stevens-Johnson syndrome* (aching of joints and muscles; fever and chills; redness, blistering, peeling, or loosening of skin)

**Those indicating need for medical attention only if they continue or are bothersome**
Incidence more frequent
*CNS toxicity* (dizziness; drowsiness; headache; tinnitus); *drying of mucous membranes, especially eyes and mouth*

## Overdose
For more information on the management of overdose or unintentional ingestion, **contact a Poison Control Center** (see *Poison Control Center Listing*).

**Treatment of overdose**
Since there is no specific antidote, treatment of thiabendazole overdose should consist of the following:
To decrease absorption—
Inducing emesis or performing gastric lavage.
Specific treatment—
Symptomatic treatment may be given.
Supportive care—
Supportive measures such as maintaining an open airway, respiration, and circulation may be necessary. Patients in whom intentional overdose is confirmed or suspected should be referred for psychiatric consultation.

## Patient Consultation
As an aid to patient consultation, refer to *Advice for the Patient, Thiabendazole (Systemic)*.
In providing consultation, consider emphasizing the following selected information (» = major clinical significance):

**Before using this medication**
» Conditions affecting use, especially:
Hypersensitivity to thiabendazole
Other medications, especially theophylline
Other medical problems, especially liver function impairment

**Proper use of this medication**
No special preparations (e.g., dietary restrictions or fasting, concurrent medications, purging, or cleansing enemas) required before, during, or immediately after therapy
Taking after meals to minimize common side effects such as nausea, vomiting, dizziness, or loss of appetite

**2786 Thiabendazole (Systemic)**

**Proper administration**
*For oral suspension dosage form*
  Using a calibrated liquid-measuring device to measure each dose accurately
*For chewable tablet dosage form*
  Chewing or crushing tablets before swallowing
» Compliance with full course of therapy; second course may be required in some infections
» Proper dosing
  Missed dose: Taking as soon as possible; not taking if almost time for next dose; not doubling doses
» Proper storage
*For trichinosis*
  Possibly taking systemic corticosteroids concurrently with thiabendazole, especially in patients with severe symptoms, to reduce inflammatory reactions to *Trichinella* larvae

**Precautions while using this medication**
  Regular visits to physician to check progress
» Caution if dizziness, drowsiness, blurred vision, or yellow vision occurs

**Using hygienic measures to prevent reinfection**
*For creeping eruption or visceral larva migrans*
  Keeping dogs and cats off beaches and bathing areas
  Deworming household pets regularly
  Covering children's sandboxes when not in use
*For trichinosis*
  Cooking all pork, pork-containing products, and wild animals thoroughly (at not less than 60 °C until well done) before eating

**Side/adverse effects**
  Asparagus-like or other unusual odor of urine may be alarming to patient although medically insignificant
  Signs of potential side effects, especially CNS toxicity, severe gastrointestinal disturbance, neuropsychiatric toxicity, hypersensitivity, crystalluria, intrahepatic cholestasis, ocular symptoms, seizures, and Stevens-Johnson syndrome

## General Dosing Information

No special preparations (e.g., dietary restrictions or fasting, concurrent medications, purging, or cleansing enemas) are required before, during, or immediately after treatment with thiabendazole.

Thiabendazole should preferably be taken after meals (breakfast and evening meal) to minimize common side effects such as nausea, vomiting, dizziness, or loss of appetite.

Patients who are heavily infected with helminths may require more prolonged treatment.

Patients with impaired hepatic function may require a reduction in dose, also.

**For trichinosis**
Systemic corticosteroids may be given in the treatment of trichinosis to critically ill patients to minimize inflammatory reactions to *Trichinella* larvae. However, their effectiveness has not been proven.

## Oral Dosage Forms

Note: Bracketed uses in the *Dosage Forms* section refer to categories of use and/or indications that are not included in U.S. product labeling.

### THIABENDAZOLE ORAL SUSPENSION USP

**Usual adult and adolescent dose**
Larva migrans, cutaneous—
  Oral, 25 mg per kg of body weight two times a day for two days. May be repeated two days after completion of treatment if active lesions are still present.
Larva migrans, visceral—
  Oral, 25 mg per kg of body weight two times a day for five to seven days. May be repeated in four weeks if required.
Strongyloidiasis—
  Uncomplicated infections: Oral, 25 mg per kg of body weight two times a day for two days.
  [Hyperinfection syndrome]: Oral, 25 mg per kg of body weight two times a day for five to seven days. May be repeated if required.
Trichinosis—
  Oral, 25 mg per kg of body weight two times a day for two to four days, based on patient's response.
[Capillariasis]—
  Oral, 25 mg per kg of body weight once a day for thirty days.
[Dracunculiasis]—
  Oral, 25 mg per kg of body weight two times a day for two days.
[Trichostrongyliasis]—
  Oral, 25 mg per kg of body weight two times a day for two days.
Note: Patients up to 68 kg of body weight—25 mg per kg of body weight two times a day may be given.
  Patients 68 kg of body weight and over—1.5 grams two times a day may be given.

**Usual adult prescribing limits**
Up to 3 grams daily.

**Usual pediatric dose**
Infants and children up to 13.6 kg of body weight—Dosage has not been established in the treatment of strongyloidiasis and trichinosis.
Children 13.6 kg of body weight and over—See *Usual adult and adolescent dose*.

**Strength(s) usually available**
U.S.—
  500 mg per 5 mL (Rx) [*Mintezol*].
Canada—
  Not commercially available.

**Packaging and storage**
Store below 40 °C (104 °F), preferably between 15 and 30 °C (59 and 86 °F), unless otherwise specified by manufacturer. Store in a tight container. Protect from freezing.

**Auxiliary labeling**
• Shake well.
• Take after meals.
• May cause dizziness, drowsiness, blurred vision, or yellow vision.
• Continue medicine for full time of treatment.

**Note**
When dispensing, include a calibrated liquid-measuring device.

### THIABENDAZOLE TABLETS (CHEWABLE) USP

**Usual adult and adolescent dose**
See *Thiabendazole Oral Suspension USP*.

**Usual adult prescribing limits**
See *Thiabendazole Oral Suspension USP*.

**Usual pediatric dose**
See *Thiabendazole Oral Suspension USP*.

**Strength(s) usually available**
U.S.—
  500 mg (Rx) [*Mintezol*].
Canada—
  Not commercially available.

**Packaging and storage**
Store below 40 °C (104 °F), preferably between 15 and 30 °C (59 and 86 °F), unless otherwise specified by manufacturer. Store in a tight container.

**Auxiliary labeling**
• Chew or crush tablets before swallowing.
• Take after meals.
• May cause dizziness, drowsiness, blurred vision, or yellow vision.
• Continue medicine for full time of treatment.

Revised: 02/01/93

---

# THIABENDAZOLE Topical*†

VA CLASSIFICATION (Primary): AP200
Note: For a listing of dosage forms and brand names by country availability, see *Dosage Forms* section(s).

*Not commercially available in the U.S.
†Not commercially available in Canada.

## Category
Anthelmintic (topical).

## Indications
Note: Because topical thiabendazole is not commercially available in the U.S. or Canada, the bracketed information and the use of the su-

perscript 1 in this monograph reflect the lack of labeled (approved) indications for this medication.

### Accepted
[Larva migrans, cutaneous (treatment)][1]—Topical thiabendazole is used in the treatment of cutaneous larva migrans (creeping eruption) caused by *Ancylostoma braziliense* (dog and cat hookworm). Recent reports and some medical experts have suggested the use of systemic ivermectin or albendazole as alternative treatment for cutaneous larva migrans if topical therapy with thiabendazole proves ineffective since its use for this indication is becoming obsolete.

Not all species or strains of a particular helminth may be susceptible to topical thiabendazole.

[1]Not included in Canadian product labeling.

## Pharmacology/Pharmacokinetics
### Physicochemical characteristics
Molecular weight—201.25.

### Mechanism of action/Effect
Unknown; however, thiabendazole has been shown to inhibit helminth-specific enzyme fumarate reductase; vermicidal.

### Absorption
Some systemic absorption may occur from topical preparations applied to the skin.

## Precautions to Consider
### Pregnancy/Reproduction
Pregnancy—Topical thiabendazole may be systemically absorbed. However, problems in humans have not been documented.

### Breast-feeding
Topical thiabendazole may be systemically absorbed. However, problems in humans have not been documented.

### Pediatrics
Appropriate studies on the relationship of age to the effects of topical thiabendazole have not been performed in the pediatric population. However, pediatrics-specific problems that would limit the usefulness of this medication in children are not expected.

### Geriatrics
Appropriate studies on the relationship of age to the effects of topical thiabendazole have not been performed in the geriatric population. However, no geriatrics-specific problems have been documented to date.

### Medical considerations/Contraindications
The medical considerations/contraindications included have been selected on the basis of their potential clinical significance (reasons given in parentheses where appropriate)—not necessarily inclusive (» = major clinical significance).

*Risk-benefit should be considered when the following medical problem exists:*
Sensitivity to thiabendazole

## Patient Consultation
As an aid to patient consultation, refer to *Advice for the Patient, Thiabendazole (Topical).*

In providing consultation, consider emphasizing the following selected information (» = major clinical significance):

### Before using this medication
» Conditions affecting use, especially:
Sensitivity to thiabendazole

### Proper use of this medication
Applying directly to and approximately 5 to 7.5 cm around the slowly advancing end of each burrow or tunnel in the skin
» Compliance with full course of therapy
» Proper dosing
Missed dose: Applying as soon as possible; not applying if almost time for next dose
» Proper storage

### Precautions while using this medication
Checking with physician if no improvement within a few days or if burrow or tunnel continues to advance

## General Dosing Information
Thiabendazole topical suspension should be applied directly to the slowly advancing end of the larval burrow or tunnel in the skin. Since the larvae may have advanced beyond the site of inflammation in the skin, topical thiabendazole should also be applied approximately 5 to 7.5 cm around the presumed end of the burrow or tunnel.

Thiabendazole may also be applied topically as a cream in concentrations up to 15% in a water-soluble base.

## Topical Dosage Forms
### THIABENDAZOLE TOPICAL SUSPENSION
Note: Thiabendazole topical suspension is not commercially available in the U.S. or Canada; thiabendazole oral suspension is being used for topical application. The bracketed information and the use of superscript 1 in the *Dosage Forms* section reflect the lack of labeled (approved) indications for this product.

### Usual adult and adolescent dose
[Cutaneous larva migrans (treatment)][1]—
Topical, to and around the advancing end of each larva burrow in the skin, two to four times a day for two to seven days.

Note: Concentrations of 10 to 15% have been recommended.

### Usual adult prescribing limits
Up to six times a day.

### Usual pediatric dose
[Cutaneous larva migrans (treatment)][1]—
See *Usual adult and adolescent dose.*

### Strength(s) usually available
U.S.—
Dosage form not commercially available. Thiabendazole oral suspension (500 mg per 5 mL) (Rx) [*Mintezol*] is the dosage form used when 10% thiabendazole topical suspension is prescribed. Higher concentrations require compounding.
Canada—
Dosage form not commercially available. Compounding required.

### Packaging and storage
Store below 40 °C (104 °F), preferably between 15 and 30 °C (59 and 86 °F), unless otherwise specified by manufacturer. Protect from freezing.

### Auxiliary labeling
- Shake well.
- For external use only.
- Continue medicine for full time of treatment.

[1]Not included in Canadian product labeling.

Revised: 09/28/93
Interim revision: 05/31/94

# THIAMINE   Systemic

VA CLASSIFICATION (Primary): VT105
Commonly used brand name(s): *Betaxin; Bewon; Biamine.*
Another commonly used name is vitamin $B_1$.
Note: For a listing of dosage forms and brand names by country availability, see *Dosage Forms* section(s).

## Category
Nutritional supplement (vitamin).
Note: Thiamine (vitamin $B_1$) is a water-soluble vitamin.

## Indications
Note: Bracketed information in the *Indications* section refers to uses that are not included in U.S. product labeling.

### Accepted
Thiamine deficiency (prophylaxis and treatment)—Thiamine is indicated for prevention and treatment of thiamine deficiency states. Thiamine deficiency may occur as a result of inadequate nutrition or intestinal malabsorption but does not occur in healthy individuals receiving an adequate balanced diet. Simple nutritional deficiency of individual B vitamins is rare since dietary inadequacy usually results in multiple deficiencies. For prophylaxis of thiamine deficiency, dietary improve-

ment, rather than supplementation, is advisable. For treatment of thiamine deficiency, supplementation is preferred.

Deficiency of thiamine may lead to beriberi (dry or wet) or Wernicke's encephalopathy.

Requirements may be increased and/or supplementation may be necessary in the following persons or conditions (based on documented thiamine deficiency):
Alcoholism
Burns
Fever, chronic
Gastrectomy
Hemodialysis, chronic
Hepatic-biliary tract disease—alcoholism with cirrhosis, hepatic function impairment
Hyperthyroidism
Infection, prolonged
Intestinal disease—celiac, ileal resection, tropical sprue, regional enteritis, persistent diarrhea
Manual labor, heavy, for long periods of time
Stress, prolonged

Recommended intakes for thiamine are related to caloric intake.

Some unusual diets (e.g., reducing diets that drastically restrict food selection) may not supply minimum daily requirements for thiamine. Supplementation is necessary in patients receiving total parenteral nutrition (TPN) or undergoing rapid weight loss or in those with malnutrition, because of inadequate dietary intake.

Recommended intakes for all vitamins and most minerals are increased during pregnancy. Many physicians recommend that pregnant women receive multivitamin and mineral supplements, especially those pregnant women who do not consume an adequate diet and those in high-risk categories (i.e., women carrying more than one fetus, heavy cigarette smokers, and alcohol and drug abusers). Taking excessive amounts of a multivitamin and mineral supplement may be harmful to the mother and/or fetus and should be avoided.

Recommended intakes for all vitamins and most minerals are increased during breast-feeding.

[Encephalomyelopathy, subacute necrotizing (treatment)]
[Maple syrup urine disease (treatment)]
[Pyruvate carboxylase deficiency (treatment)] or
[Hyperalaninemia (treatment)]—Thiamine has been found to be useful for temporary metabolic correction of genetic enzyme deficiency diseases such as subacute necrotizing encephalomyelopathy (SNE, Leigh's disease), maple syrup urine disease (branched-chain aminoacidopathy), and lactic acidosis associated with pyruvate carboxylase deficiency and hyperalaninemia.

**Unaccepted**
Thiamine has not been proven effective for appetite stimulation, treatment of cerebellar syndrome, dermatitis, chronic diarrhea, fatigue, mental disorders, multiple sclerosis, neuritis, or ulcerative colitis, or for use as an insect repellant.

## Pharmacology/Pharmacokinetics

**Physicochemical characteristics**
Molecular weight—337.27.
pKa—4.8 and 9.

**Mechanism of action/Effect**
Thiamine combines with adenosine triphosphate (ATP) to form a coenzyme, thiamine pyrophosphate (thiamine diphosphate, cocarboxylase), which is necessary for carbohydrate metabolism.

**Absorption**
The B vitamins are readily absorbed from the gastrointestinal tract, except in malabsorption syndromes. Thiamine is absorbed mainly in the duodenum. Alcohol inhibits absorption of thiamine.
In individuals with normal gastrointestinal absorption, total maximum daily oral absorption of thiamine is 5 to 15 mg (increased when given in divided daily doses with food).

**Biotransformation**
Hepatic.

**Elimination**
Renal (almost entirely as metabolites). Excess beyond daily needs is excreted as unchanged drug and metabolites in urine.

## Precautions to Consider

**Pregnancy/Reproduction**
Pregnancy—Problems in humans have not been documented with intake of normal daily recommended amounts.

FDA Pregnancy Category A (parenteral thiamine).

**Breast-feeding**
Problems in humans have not been documented with intake of normal daily recommended amounts.

**Pediatrics**
Problems in pediatrics have not been documented with intake of normal daily recommended amounts.

**Geriatrics**
Problems in geriatrics have not been documented with intake of normal daily recommended amounts. Studies have shown that the elderly may have impaired thiamine status, thereby requiring thiamine supplementation.

**Laboratory value alterations**
The following have been selected on the basis of their potential clinical significance (possible effect in parentheses where appropriate)—not necessarily inclusive (» = major clinical significance):

With diagnostic test results
Theophylline concentration determinations, serum, by Schack and Waxler spectrophotometric method
(thiamine may interfere with results)
Uric acid concentration determinations by phototungstate method or
Urobilinogen determinations using Ehrlich's reagent
(thiamine may produce false-positive results)
Note: Usually occurs only with large doses.

**Medical considerations/Contraindications**
The medical considerations/contraindications included have been selected on the basis of their potential clinical significance (reasons given in parentheses where appropriate)—not necessarily inclusive (» = major clinical significance).

*Risk-benefit should be considered when the following medical problems exist:*
Sensitivity to thiamine
Wernicke's encephalopathy
(intravenous glucose loading may precipitate or worsen this condition in thiamine-deficient patients; thiamine should be administered prior to glucose)

## Side/Adverse Effects

The following side/adverse effects have been selected on the basis of their potential clinical significance (possible signs and symptoms in parentheses where appropriate)—not necessarily inclusive:

**Those indicating need for medical attention**
Incidence rare
*Anaphylactic reaction* (coughing; difficulty in swallowing; hives; itching of skin; swelling of face, lips, or eyelids; wheezing or difficulty in breathing)—usually after a large intravenous dose

## Patient Consultation

As an aid to patient consultation, refer to *Advice for the Patient, Thiamine (Vitamin $B_1$) (Systemic)*.

In providing consultation, consider emphasizing the following selected information (» = major clinical significance):

**Description of use**
Description should include function in the body, signs of deficiency, and unproven uses

**Importance of diet**
Importance of proper nutrition; supplement may be needed because of inadequate dietary intake
Food sources of thiamine; effects of processing
Not using vitamins as substitute for balanced diet
Recommended daily intake for thiamine

**Before using this dietary supplement**
» Conditions affecting use, especially:
Sensitivity to thiamine
Use in the elderly—May have impaired thiamine status

**Proper use of this dietary supplement**
» Proper dosing
Missed dose: No cause for concern because of length of time necessary for depletion; remembering to take as directed
» Proper storage

**Side/adverse effects**
Signs of potential side effects, especially anaphylactic reaction

## General Dosing Information

Because of the infrequency of single B vitamin deficiencies, combinations are commonly administered. Many commercial combinations of B vitamins are available.

### For parenteral dosage forms only

In most cases, parenteral administration is indicated only when oral administration is not acceptable (for example, in nausea, vomiting, preoperative and postoperative conditions), or possible (for example, in malabsorption syndromes or following gastric resection).

### Diet/Nutrition

Recommended dietary intakes for thiamine are defined differently worldwide.

For U.S.—
 The Recommended Dietary Allowances (RDAs) for vitamins and minerals are determined by the Food and Nutrition Board of the National Research Council and are intended to provide adequate nutrition in most healthy persons under usual environmental stresses. In addition, a different designation may be used by the FDA for food and dietary supplement labeling purposes, as with Daily Value (DV). DVs replace the previous labeling terminology United States Recommended Daily Allowances (USRDAs).

For Canada—
 Recommended Nutrient Intakes (RNIs) for vitamins, minerals, and protein are determined by Health and Welfare in Canada and provide recommended amounts of a specific nutrient while minimizing the risk of chronic diseases.

Daily recommended intakes for thiamine are generally defined as follows:

| Persons | U.S. (mg) | Canada (mg) |
|---|---|---|
| Infants and children | | |
|   Birth to 3 years of age | 0.3–0.7 | 0.3–0.6 |
|   4 to 6 years of age | 0.9 | 0.7 |
|   7 to 10 years of age | 1 | 0.8–1 |
| Adolescent and adult males | 1.2–1.5 | 0.8–1.3 |
| Adolescent and adult females | 1–1.1 | 0.8–0.9 |
| Pregnant females | 1.5 | 0.9–1 |
| Breast-feeding females | 1.6 | 1–1.2 |

These are usually provided by adequate diets.

The best dietary sources of thiamine include cereals (whole-grain and enriched), meats (especially pork and beef), peas, beans, and nuts. Loss is variable during cooking and may be as high as 50%.

## Oral Dosage Forms

Note: Bracketed uses in the *Dosage Forms* section refer to categories of use and/or indications that are not included in U.S. product labeling.

### THIAMINE HYDROCHLORIDE ELIXIR USP

**Usual adult and adolescent dose**
Deficiency (prophylaxis)—
 Oral, amount based on normal daily recommended intakes:

| Persons | U.S. (mg) | Canada (mg) |
|---|---|---|
| Adolescent and adult males | 1.2–1.5 | 0.8–1.3 |
| Adolescent and adult females | 1–1.1 | 0.8–0.9 |
| Pregnant females | 1.5 | 0.9–1 |
| Breast-feeding females | 1.6 | 1–1.2 |

Deficiency (treatment)—
 Treatment dose is individualized by prescriber based on severity of deficiency. The following dosage has been established: Beriberi (initial in mild or maintenance following severe)—Oral, 5 to 10 mg three times a day.

[Genetic enzyme deficiency diseases]—
 Oral, 10 to 20 mg per day as a single dose (dosage of up to 4 grams per day in divided doses has been used).

**Usual pediatric dose**
Deficiency (prophylaxis)—
 Oral, amount based on intake of normal daily recommended intakes:

| Persons | U.S. (mg) | Canada (mg) |
|---|---|---|
| Infants and children | | |
|   Birth to 3 years of age | 0.3–0.7 | 0.3–0.6 |
|   4 to 6 years of age | 0.9 | 0.7 |
|   7 to 10 years of age | 1 | 0.8–1 |

Deficiency (treatment)—
 Treatment dose is individualized by prescriber based on severity of deficiency. The following dosage has been established: Beriberi (mild)—Oral, 10 per day.

**Strength(s) usually available**
U.S.—
 Not commercially available.
Canada—
 250 mcg (0.25 mg) per 5 mL (OTC) [*Bewon* (16% alcohol; bisulfites)].
 Note: The strength of this thiamine preparation may exceed the dosage range recommended by USP DI Advisory Panels based on the amount necessary to meet normal nutritional needs.

**Packaging and storage**
Store below 40 °C (104 °F), preferably between 15 and 30 °C (59 and 86 °F), unless otherwise specified by manufacturer. Store in a tight, light-resistant container. Protect from freezing.

### THIAMINE HYDROCHLORIDE TABLETS USP

**Usual adult and adolescent dose**
See *Thiamine Hydrochloride Elixir USP*.

**Usual pediatric dose**
See *Thiamine Hydrochloride Elixir USP*.

**Strength(s) usually available**
U.S.—
 5 mg (OTC) [GENERIC].
 10 mg (OTC) [GENERIC].
 25 mg (OTC) [GENERIC].
 50 mg (OTC) [GENERIC].
 100 mg (OTC) [GENERIC].
 250 mg (OTC) [GENERIC].
 500 mg (OTC) [GENERIC].
Canada—
 10 mg (OTC) [GENERIC].
 25 mg (OTC) [GENERIC].
 50 mg (OTC) [GENERIC].
 100 mg (OTC) [GENERIC].
 500 mg (OTC) [GENERIC].
 Note: Some strengths of these thiamine preparations may exceed the dosage range recommended by USP DI Advisory Panels based on the amount necessary to meet normal nutritional needs.

**Packaging and storage**
Store below 40 °C (104 °F), preferably between 15 and 30 °C (59 and 86 °F), unless otherwise specified by manufacturer. Store in a tight, light-resistant container.

## Parenteral Dosage Forms

### THIAMINE HYDROCHLORIDE INJECTION USP

**Usual adult dose**
Deficiency (prophylaxis)—
 Intravenous infusion, as part of total parenteral nutrition solutions, the specific amount determined by individual patient need.
Deficiency (treatment)—
 Intramuscular or intravenous infusion (slow): 5 to 100 mg three times a day followed by maintenance oral administration.

**Usual pediatric dose**
Deficiency (prophylaxis)—
 Intravenous infusion, as part of total parenteral nutrition solutions, the specific amount determined by individual patient need.
Deficiency (treatment)—
 Intramuscular or intravenous infusion (slow), 10 to 25 mg a day.

**Strength(s) usually available**
U.S.—
 100 mg per mL (Rx) [*Biamine* (0.5% chlorobutanol); GENERIC].
Canada—
 100 mg per mL (Rx) [*Betaxin* (0.5% chlorobutanol; 0.5% monothioglycerol); GENERIC].

**Packaging and storage**
Store below 40 °C (104 °F), preferably between 15 and 30 °C (59 and 86 °F), unless otherwise specified by manufacturer. Protect from light. Protect from freezing.

**Incompatibilities**
Thiamine is unstable in neutral or alkaline solutions; therefore, administration with carbonates, citrates, barbiturates, or copper ions is not recommended. In addition, stability is poor in intravenous solutions containing sodium bisulfite as an antioxidant or preservative; if these so-

lutions must be used, they should be used immediately after addition of thiamine.

Revised: 06/24/92
Interim revision: 07/29/94; 05/26/95

**THIETHYLPERAZINE** — The *Thiethylperazine (Systemic)* monograph is not included in this published version of the USP DI database. Copies of the monograph are available on request from Micromedex, Inc. - Reprint Requests, 6200 S. Syracuse Way, Suite 300, Englewood, CO 80111; telephone (303) 486-6400; telefax (303) 486-6464; Email: USPDI@MDX.COM.

**THIOGUANINE** — The *Thioguanine (Systemic)* monograph is not included in this published version of the USP DI database. Copies of the monograph are available on request from Micromedex, Inc. - Reprint Requests, 6200 S. Syracuse Way, Suite 300, Englewood, CO 80111; telephone (303) 486-6400; telefax (303) 486-6464; Email: USPDI@MDX.COM.

**THIOPENTAL** — See *Anesthetics, Barbiturate (Systemic)*

**THIOPROPAZATE** — See *Phenothiazines (Systemic)*

**THIOPROPERAZINE** — See *Phenothiazines (Systemic)*

**THIORIDAZINE** — See *Phenothiazines (Systemic)*

# THIOTEPA  Systemic

VA CLASSIFICATION (Primary): AN100
Note: For a listing of dosage forms and brand names by country availability, see *Dosage Forms* section(s).

## Category
Antineoplastic.

## Indications
Note: Bracketed information in the *Indications* section refers to uses that are not included in U.S. product labeling.

**Accepted**
Carcinoma, breast (treatment)
Carcinoma, ovarian, epithelial (treatment)
Carcinoma, bladder (treatment)[1] or
[Carcinoma, bladder (prophylaxis)][1] — Thiotepa is indicated for treatment of adenocarcinoma of the breast or ovary. It is also indicated for topical treatment of superficial papillary carcinoma of the urinary bladder. Thiotepa also is indicated for prophylaxis of bladder carcinoma.
Lymphomas, Hodgkin's (treatment) — Thiotepa is indicated for treatment of Hodgkin's disease, although its use has been replaced largely by that of other agents.
Malignant effusions, pericardial (treatment) or
Malignant effusions, pleural (treatment) — Thiotepa is indicated by intracavitary administration for controlling effusions secondary to diffuse or localized neoplastic disease of various serosal cavities.

[1]Not included in Canadian product labeling.

## Pharmacology/Pharmacokinetics

**Physicochemical characteristics**
Molecular weight — 189.21.

**Mechanism of action/Effect**
Thiotepa is an alkylating agent of the nitrogen mustard type. Thiotepa is a trifunctional alkylating agent, and is cell cycle–phase nonspecific. Activity occurs as a result of formation of an unstable ethylenimmonium ion, which alkylates or binds with many intracellular molecular structures, including nucleic acids. Its cytotoxic action is primarily due to cross-linking of strands of DNA and RNA, as well as inhibition of protein synthesis.

**Absorption**
Some degree of systemic absorption occurs after local administration. Absorption through bladder mucosa varies from 10% to almost 100% of a dose (related to drug concentration and time of drug contact with the urothelium, and increased by extensive tumor infiltration, mucosal inflammation, endoscopic surgical procedures or radiation therapy, and the presence of vesicoureteral reflux).

**Elimination**
Renal, 85% (largely as metabolites).

## Precautions to Consider

**Carcinogenicity/Mutagenicity**
Secondary malignancies are potential delayed effects of many antineoplastic agents, although it is not clear whether the effect is related to their mutagenic or immunosuppressive action. The effect of dose and duration of therapy is also unknown, although risk seems to increase with long-term use. Although information is limited, available data seem to indicate that the carcinogenic risk is greatest with the alkylating agents.
Thiotepa is carcinogenic and mutagenic in both animals and humans.

**Pregnancy/Reproduction**
Fertility — Gonadal suppression, resulting in amenorrhea or azoospermia, may occur in patients taking antineoplastic therapy, especially with the alkylating agents. In general, these effects appear to be related to dose and length of therapy and may be irreversible. Prediction of the degree of testicular or ovarian function impairment is complicated by the common use of combinations of several antineoplastics, which makes it difficult to assess the effects of individual agents.

Pregnancy — Thiotepa is generally teratogenic in humans, although normal births have been reported.
First trimester: It is usually recommended that use of antineoplastics, especially combination chemotherapy, be avoided whenever possible, especially during the first trimester. Although information is limited because of the relatively few instances of antineoplastic administration during pregnancy, the mutagenic, teratogenic, and carcinogenic potential of these medications must be considered.
Other hazards to the fetus include adverse reactions seen in adults.
In general, use of a contraceptive is recommended during cytotoxic drug therapy.

**Breast-feeding**
Although very little information is available regarding distribution of antineoplastic agents into breast milk, breast-feeding is not recommended while thiotepa is being administered because of the risks to the infant (adverse effects, mutagenicity, carcinogenicity). It is not known whether thiotepa or its metabolites are distributed into breast milk.

**Pediatrics**
Appropriate studies have not been performed in the pediatric population.

**Geriatrics**
No geriatrics-specific information is available on the use of thiotepa in geriatric patients. However, elderly patients are more likely to have age-related renal function impairment, which may require lower dosage and careful monitoring in patients receiving thiotepa.

**Dental**
The bone marrow depressant effects of thiotepa may result in an increased incidence of microbial infection, delayed healing, and gingival bleeding. Dental work, whenever possible, should be completed prior to initiation of therapy or deferred until blood counts have returned to normal. Patients should be instructed in proper oral hygiene during treatment, including caution in use of regular toothbrushes, dental floss, and toothpicks.
Thiotepa may also rarely cause stomatitis associated with considerable discomfort.

### Drug interactions and/or related problems
The following drug interactions and/or related problems have been selected on the basis of their potential clinical significance (possible mechanism in parentheses where appropriate)—not necessarily inclusive (» = major clinical significance):

Note: Combinations containing any of the following medications, depending on the amount present, may also interact with this medication.

Allopurinol or
Colchicine or
» Probenecid or
» Sulfinpyrazone
(thiotepa may raise the concentration of blood uric acid; dosage adjustment of antigout agents may be necessary to control hyperuricemia and gout; allopurinol may be preferred to prevent or reverse thiotepa-induced hyperuricemia because of risk of uric acid nephropathy with uricosuric antigout agents)

Blood dyscrasia–causing medications (see *Appendix II*)
(leukopenic and/or thrombocytopenic effects of thiotepa may be increased with concurrent or recent therapy if these medications cause the same effects; dosage adjustment of thiotepa, if necessary, should be based on blood counts)

» Bone marrow depressants, other (see *Appendix II*) or
» Radiation therapy
(additive bone marrow depression may occur; administration of thiotepa with immunosuppressive medications is not recommended and modification of dosage may be required when thiotepa is administered with radiation therapy)

Succinylcholine
(thiotepa may decrease plasma levels of pseudocholinesterase, the enzyme that metabolizes succinylcholine, thereby enhancing the neuromuscular blockade of succinylcholine; determination of plasma pseudocholinesterase concentrations is recommended prior to use of succinylcholine in patients receiving thiotepa. Increased or prolonged respiratory depression or paralysis (apnea) may occur but is of minor clinical significance while the patient is being mechanically ventilated; however, careful postoperative monitoring of the patient may be necessary following concurrent or sequential use, especially if there is a possibility of incomplete reversal of neuromuscular blockade)

Urokinase
(may increase the efficacy of thiotepa in the treatment of bladder cancer by acting as a plasminogen activator and increasing the amount of medication in tumor tissue)

Vaccines, killed virus
(because normal defense mechanisms may be suppressed by thiotepa therapy, the patient's antibody response to the vaccine may be decreased. The interval between discontinuation of medications that cause immunosuppression and restoration of the patient's ability to respond to the vaccine depends on the intensity and type of immunosuppression-causing medication used, the underlying disease, and other factors; estimates vary from 3 months to 1 year)

» Vaccines, live virus
(because normal defense mechanisms may be suppressed by thiotepa therapy, concurrent use with a live virus vaccine may potentiate the replication of the vaccine virus, may increase the side/adverse effects of the vaccine virus, and/or may decrease the patient's antibody response to the vaccine; immunization of these patients should be undertaken only with extreme caution after careful review of the patient's hematologic status and only with the knowledge and consent of the physician managing the thiotepa therapy. The interval between discontinuation of medications that cause immunosuppression and restoration of the patient's ability to respond to the vaccine depends on the intensity and type of immunosuppression-causing medication used, the underlying disease, and other factors; estimates vary from 3 months to 1 year. Immunization with oral polio virus vaccine should also be postponed in persons in close contact with the patient, especially family members)

### Laboratory value alterations
The following have been selected on the basis of their potential clinical significance (possible effect in parentheses where appropriate)—not necessarily inclusive (» = major clinical significance):

With physiology/laboratory test values
Pseudocholinesterase concentrations in the plasma
(may be decreased very slightly)

Uric acid concentrations in blood and urine
(may be increased)

### Medical considerations/Contraindications
The medical considerations/contraindications included have been selected on the basis of their potential clinical significance (reasons given in parentheses where appropriate)—not necessarily inclusive (» = major clinical significance).

*Risk-benefit should be considered when the following medical problems exist:*
» Bone marrow depression
(lower dosage and careful monitoring recommended)
» Chickenpox, existing or recent (including recent exposure) or
» Herpes zoster
(risk of severe generalized disease)
Gout, history of or
Urate renal stones, history of
(risk of hyperuricemia)
» Hepatic function impairment
(reduced biotransformation; lower dosage and careful monitoring recommended)
» Infection
» Renal function impairment
(reduced elimination; lower dosage and careful monitoring recommended)
Sensitivity to thiotepa
» Tumor cell infiltration of bone marrow
(lower dosage and careful monitoring recommended)
» Caution should be used also in patients who have had previous cytotoxic drug therapy or radiation therapy.

### Patient monitoring
The following may be especially important in patient monitoring (other tests may be warranted in some patients, depending on condition; » = major clinical significance):

Alanine aminotransferase (ALT [SGPT]) concentrations, serum and
Aspartate aminotransferase (AST [SGOT]) concentrations, serum and
Bilirubin concentrations, serum and
Lactate dehydrogenase (LDH) concentrations, serum
(determinations recommended prior to initiation of therapy and at periodic intervals during therapy; frequency varies according to clinical state, agent, dose, and other agents being used concurrently)

Blood urea nitrogen (BUN) concentrations and
Creatinine concentrations, serum
(recommended prior to initiation of therapy and at periodic intervals during therapy; frequency varies according to clinical state, agent, dose, and other agents being used concurrently)

» Hematocrit or hemoglobin and
» Platelet count and
» Total and, if appropriate, differential leukocyte count
(determinations recommended prior to initiation of therapy and at periodic intervals during therapy; frequency varies according to clinical state, agent, dose, and other agents being used concurrently)

Uric acid concentrations, serum
(recommended prior to initiation of therapy and at periodic intervals during therapy; frequency varies according to clinical state, agent, dose, and other agents being used concurrently)

## Side/Adverse Effects
Note: Many "side effects" of antineoplastic therapy are unavoidable and represent the medication's pharmacologic action. Some of these (for example, leukopenia and thrombocytopenia) are actually used as parameters to aid in individual dosage titration.

Side effects (especially bone marrow depression) may also occur after intracavitary administration and may be severe.

The following side/adverse effects have been selected on the basis of their potential clinical significance (possible signs and symptoms in parentheses where appropriate)—not necessarily inclusive:

### Those indicating need for medical attention
Incidence more frequent
***Leukopenia or infection*** (fever or chills; cough or hoarseness; lower back or side pain; painful or difficult urination)—usually asymptomatic; ***thrombocytopenia*** (unusual bleeding or bruising; black, tarry stools; blood in urine; pinpoint red spots on skin)—usually asymptomatic

Note: *Bone marrow depression* may occur up to 1 month after thiotepa is administered.

## Thiotepa (Systemic)

Incidence less frequent
*Hyperuricemia or uric acid nephropathy* (joint pain; lower back or side pain; swelling of feet or lower legs); *pain at site of injection or instillation*
  Note: *Hyperuricemia or uric acid nephropathy* occurs most commonly during initial treatment of patients with lymphoma, as a result of rapid cell breakdown, which leads to elevated serum uric acid concentrations.

Incidence rare
*Anaphylaxis* (skin rash; tightness of throat; wheezing); *renal toxicity after local vesical application* (painful or difficult urination); *stomatitis* (sores in mouth and on lips)

**Those indicating need for medical attention only if they continue or are bothersome**
Incidence less frequent
*Dizziness; hives; loss of appetite; missing menstrual periods; nausea and vomiting*

**Those not indicating need for medical attention**
Incidence less frequent
*Loss of hair*

**Those indicating the need for medical attention if they occur after medication is discontinued**
*Bone marrow depression* (black, tarry stools; blood in urine or stools; cough or hoarseness; fever or chills; lower back or side pain; painful or difficult urination; pinpoint red spots on skin; unusual bleeding or bruising)

## Patient Consultation

As an aid to patient consultation, refer to *Advice for the Patient, Thiotepa (Systemic)*.

In providing consultation, consider emphasizing the following selected information (» = major clinical significance):

**Before using this medication**
  Conditions affecting use, especially:
    Sensitivity to thiotepa
    Pregnancy—Advisability of using contraception; telling physician immediately if pregnancy is suspected
    Breast-feeding—Not recommended because of risk of serious side effects
    Other medications, especially previous cytotoxic medication or radiation therapy, probenecid, or sulfinpyrazone
    Other medical problems, especially bone marrow depression, chickenpox or recent exposure, hepatic function impairment, herpes zoster, other infection, renal function impairment, or tumor cell infiltration of bone marrow

**Proper use of this medication**
  Importance of ample fluid intake and subsequent increase in urine output to aid in excretion of uric acid
  Possible nausea and vomiting; importance of continuing medication despite stomach upset
» Proper dosing

**Precautions while using this medication**
» Importance of close monitoring by physician
  Caution if surgery with general anesthesia is required
» Avoiding immunizations unless approved by physician; other persons in patient's household should avoid immunizations with oral poliovirus vaccine; avoiding other persons who have taken oral poliovirus vaccine or wearing a protective mask that covers nose and mouth

*Caution if bone marrow depression occurs*
» Avoiding exposure to persons with infections, especially during periods of low blood counts; checking with physician immediately if fever or chills, cough or hoarseness, lower back or side pain, or painful or difficult urination occurs
» Checking with physician immediately if unusual bleeding or bruising; black, tarry stools; blood in urine or stools; or pinpoint red spots on skin occur
  Caution in use of regular toothbrush, dental floss, or toothpick; physician, dentist, or nurse may suggest alternatives; checking with physician before having dental work done
  Not touching eyes or inside of nose unless hands washed immediately before
  Using caution to avoid accidental cuts with use of sharp objects such as safety razor or fingernail or toenail cutters
  Avoiding contact sports or other situations where bruising or injury could occur

**Side/adverse effects**
  May cause adverse effects such as blood problems, loss of hair, and cancer; importance of discussing possible effects with physician
  Signs of potential side effects, especially leukopenia, infection, thrombocytopenia, hyperuricemia, uric acid nephropathy, pain at site of injection or instillation, anaphylaxis, renal toxicity after local vesical instillation, and stomatitis
  Physician or nurse can help in dealing with side effects
  Possibility of hair loss; growth should return after treatment has ended

## General Dosing Information

Patients receiving thiotepa should be under supervision of a physician experienced in cancer chemotherapy.

Dosage must be adjusted to meet the individual requirements of each patient, based on clinical response and appearance or severity of toxicity.

It is recommended that thiotepa be administered no more frequently than every 7 days, the risk of cumulative bone marrow toxicity being kept in mind, to allow the full effect of each dose on the leukocyte count to be seen (nadir occurs 5 to 30 days after each dose).

Maintenance therapy at 1- to 4-week intervals is recommended to continue optimal effect once it is obtained.

Initiation of thiotepa therapy in patients who have recently received cytotoxic drug or radiation therapy is not recommended until leukocyte and platelet counts depressed by the previous therapy begin to recover. Leukocyte counts above 2000 per cubic millimeter and platelet counts above 50,000 per cubic millimeter are considered acceptable.

Development of uric acid nephropathy in patients with lymphoma may be prevented by adequate oral hydration, and, in some cases, administration of allopurinol. Alkalinization of urine may be necessary if serum uric acid concentrations are elevated.

Thiotepa may be administered by intravenous, intrapleural, intraperitoneal, intrapericardial, or intratumor injection or by intravesical instillation to the bladder.

It is recommended that thiotepa therapy be discontinued or dosage reduced at the first sign of a sudden large decrease in leukocyte (particularly granulocyte) or platelet count to prevent irreversible bone marrow depression. Therapy may be resumed when leukocyte and platelet counts return to acceptable levels.

Special precautions are recommended in patients who develop thrombocytopenia as a result of administration of thiotepa. These may include extreme care in performing invasive procedures; regular inspection of intravenous sites, skin (including perirectal area), and mucous membrane surfaces for signs of bleeding or bruising; limiting frequency of venipuncture and avoiding intramuscular injections; testing urine, emesis, stool, and secretions for occult blood; care in use of regular toothbrushes, dental floss, toothpicks, safety razors, and fingernail and toenail cutters; avoiding constipation; and using caution to prevent falls and other injuries. Such patients should avoid alcohol and any aspirin intake because of the risk of gastrointestinal bleeding. Platelet transfusions may be required.

Patients who develop leukopenia should be observed carefully for signs of infection. Antibiotic support may be required. In neutropenic patients who develop fever, broad-spectrum antibiotic coverage should be initiated empirically, pending bacterial cultures and appropriate diagnostic tests.

**Safety considerations for handling this medication**

There is limited but increasing evidence and concern that personnel involved in preparation and administration of parenteral antineoplastics may be at some risk because of the potential mutagenicity, teratogenicity, and/or carcinogenicity of these agents, although the actual risk is unknown. USP advisory panels recommend cautious handling both in preparation and disposal of antineoplastic agents. Precautions that have been suggested include:
  • Use of a biological containment cabinet during reconstitution and dilution of parenteral medications and wearing of disposable surgical gloves and masks.
  • Use of proper technique to prevent contamination of the medication, work area, and operator during transfer between containers (including proper training of personnel in this technique).
  • Cautious and proper disposal of needles, syringes, vials, ampuls, and unused medication.

A number of medical centers have developed detailed guidelines for handling of antineoplastic agents.

## Parenteral Dosage Forms

Note: Bracketed uses in the *Dosage Forms* section refer to categories of use and/or indications that are not included in U.S. product labeling.

## THIOTEPA FOR INJECTION USP

**Usual adult and adolescent dose**
Carcinoma, breast or
Carcinoma, ovarian, epithelial or
Malignant effusions, pericardial or
Malignant effusions, pleural—
　Intracavitary or intratumor, 600 to 800 mcg (0.6 to 0.8 mg) per kg of body weight every one to four weeks, with a maintenance dose of 70 to 800 mcg (0.07 to 0.8 mg) per kg of body weight. The dose is reduced in cases of marked debility or weakness, chronic cardiovascular or renal disease, or surgical shock. Maintenance dose is adjusted on the basis of blood counts and given every one to four weeks.
Carcinoma, breast or
Carcinoma, ovarian, epithelial or
Lymphomas, Hodgkin's—
　Intravenous, 300 to 400 mcg (0.3 to 0.4 mg) per kg of body weight every one to four weeks, or 200 mcg (0.2 mg) per kg of body weight for four to five days every two to four weeks. Maintenance dose is adjusted on the basis of blood counts.
Carcinoma, bladder[1]—
　Topical, to the bladder, 30 to 60 mg in 30 to 60 mL of distilled water instilled into the bladder by catheter once a week for four weeks; the course may be repeated monthly if necessary. The patient is dehydrated for eight to twelve hours prior to each dose and should try to retain the volume for two hours. The patient's position may be changed every fifteen minutes to ensure maximum area contact.

**Usual pediatric dose**
Children up to 12 years of age: Dosage has not been established.
Children 12 years of age and over: See *Usual adult and adolescent dose*.

**Size(s) usually available**
U.S.—
　15 mg (Rx) [*Thioplex*; GENERIC].
Canada—
　15 mg (Rx) [GENERIC].

**Packaging and storage**
Store between 2 and 8 °C (36 and 46 °F). Protect from light.

**Preparation of dosage form**
Thiotepa for Injection USP is reconstituted for use by adding 1.5 mL of sterile water for injection (other diluents are not recommended because they would produce a hypertonic solution, which would cause discomfort with injection) to the vial to produce an isotonic solution containing 10 mg of thiotepa per mL.
Reconstituted solutions may be further diluted with 0.9% sodium chloride injection, 5% dextrose injection, 5% dextrose and 0.9% sodium chloride injection, Ringer's injection, or lactated Ringer's injection for intracavitary use, intravenous drip, or perfusion therapy.
Thiotepa may be mixed with 2% Procaine Hydrochloride Injection USP and/or epinephrine hydrochloride 1:1000 for local use into single or multiple sites.

**Stability**
Reconstituted solutions of thiotepa may be stored for 5 days between 2 and 8 °C without significant loss of potency. Reconstituted solutions may be clear to slightly opaque; solutions that are grossly opaque or precipitated should not be used.

[1]Not included in Canadian product labeling.

Revised: 09/90
Interim revision: 08/11/93; 07/05/94; 09/29/97

---

**THIOTHIXENE**—See *Thioxanthenes (Systemic)*

---

# THIOXANTHENES  Systemic

This monograph includes information on the following: 1) Chlorprothixene[†]; 2) Flupenthixol[*]; 3) Thiothixene.
INN: Flupenthixol[*]—Flupentixol
VA CLASSIFICATION (Primary): CN709
Commonly used brand name(s): *Fluanxol*[2]; *Fluanxol Depot*[2]; *Navane*[3]; *Taractan*[1]; *Thiothixene HCl Intensol*[3].
Another commonly used name is flupentixol.

　[*]Not commercially available in U.S.
　[†]Not commercially available in Canada.

## Category
Antipsychotic.

## Indications

**Accepted**
Psychotic disorders (treatment)—Indicated for management of primary and secondary symptoms of psychotic disorders.
　The long-acting flupenthixol decanoate injection may be used in the management of nonagitated, chronic, schizophrenic patients who have been stabilized with short-acting neuroleptics.

**Unaccepted**
Flupenthixol is *not* indicated for the management of severely agitated psychotic patients, psychoneurotic patients, or geriatric patients with confusion and/or agitation.

## Pharmacology/Pharmacokinetics

**Physicochemical characteristics**
Molecular weight—
　Chlorprothixene: 315.86.
　Flupenthixol decanoate: 588.82.
　Flupenthixol dihydrochloride: 507.4.
　Thiothixene: 443.62.
　Thiothixene hydrochloride: 552.57.
Other characteristics
　Structurally and pharmacologically similar to the piperazine phenothiazines, which include acetophenazine, fluphenazine, perphenazine, prochlorperazine, and trifluoperazine.

**Mechanism of action/Effect**
Antipsychotic—Thioxanthenes are thought to benefit psychotic conditions by blocking postsynaptic dopamine receptors in the brain. They also produce an alpha-adrenergic blocking effect and depress the release of most hypothalamic and hypophyseal hormones. However, the concentration of prolactin is increased due to blockade of prolactin inhibitory factor (PIF), which inhibits the release of prolactin from the pituitary gland.

**Other actions/effects**
Antiemetic—Chlorprothixene also inhibits the medullary chemoreceptor trigger zone to produce an antiemetic effect.
Sedative—Chlorprothixene is also thought to cause an indirect reduction of stimuli to the brain stem reticular system to produce a sedative effect.

**Absorption**
Flupenthixol decanoate—Slowly, from the site of injection, and gradually released from the vehicle into the bloodstream, where it is rapidly hydrolyzed to flupenthixol.
Flupenthixol dihydrochloride—Rapid, from gastrointestinal tract.
Thiothixene—Rapid.

**Biotransformation**
Hepatic.

**Half-life**
Elimination—
　Thiothixene:
　　Initial phase—3.4 hours.
　　Late phase—Approximately 34 hours.

**Time to peak concentrations**
Flupenthixol dihydrochloride—3 to 8 hours.
Flupenthixol decanoate—4 to 7 days.
Thiothixene—1 to 3 hours.

**Duration of action**
Chlorprothixene—Intramuscular, up to 12 hours.
Flupenthixol decanoate—3 weeks.

**Elimination**
Chlorprothixene and thiothixene—Primarily renal.
Flupenthixol—Primarily fecal; some renal.

## Precautions to Consider

### Cross-sensitivity and/or related problems
Patients sensitive to one thioxanthene may be sensitive to the others also, and possibly to the phenothiazines.

### Carcinogenicity/Tumorigenicity
Most neuroleptic medications have been found to cause increased serum prolactin concentrations. Although the clinical significance of this increase is not known for most patients, *in vitro* studies have shown approximately one-third of human breast cancers to be prolactin dependent. Additionally, an increase in mammary neoplasms has been found in rodents after chronic administration of neuroleptics. However, a definite association between the chronic administration of these medications and mammary tumorigenesis has not been established.

### Pregnancy/Reproduction
Fertility—Studies with thiothixene in rats and rabbits showed a decrease in fertility.

Pregnancy—Studies in humans have not been done.

Animal studies have shown no birth defects caused by thioxanthenes. However, there have been reports of hyperreflexia in the neonate when phenothiazines were used during pregnancy. Also, studies with thiothixene in rats and rabbits showed an increase in resorption rate. No teratogenic effects were seen after repeated oral administration of thiothixene to rats, rabbits, and monkeys before and during gestation.

### Breast-feeding
It is not known if thioxanthenes are distributed into breast milk. Caution is advised since pharmacologically related phenothiazines are distributed into breast milk, causing an increased risk of tardive dyskinesia and possible drowsiness in the nursing infant.

### Pediatrics
Children appear to be prone to develop neuromuscular or extrapyramidal reactions, especially dystonias, while receiving therapeutic doses of pharmacologically related phenothiazines and should be closely monitored. Adolescents should be monitored very carefully during parenteral therapy with thioxanthenes because they tend to experience a higher incidence of hypotensive and extrapyramidal reactions than do adults.

### Geriatrics
Geriatric patients tend to develop higher plasma concentrations of neuroleptics because of changes in distribution due to decreases in lean body mass, total body water, and albumin, and often an increase in total body fat composition. These patients usually require a lower initial dosage and a more gradual titration of dose.

Elderly patients appear to be more prone to orthostatic hypotension, and exhibit an increased sensitivity to the anticholinergic and sedative effects of neuroleptics. They are also more prone to develop extrapyramidal side effects, such as tardive dyskinesia and parkinsonism. The signs of tardive dyskinesia are persistent, difficult to control, and, in some patients, appear to be irreversible. There is no known effective treatment. Careful observation during treatment for early signs of tardive dyskinesia and dosage adjustment of the thioxanthene may prevent a more severe manifestation of the syndrome.

### Dental
The peripheral anticholinergic effects of thioxanthenes may decrease or inhibit salivary flow, especially in middle-aged or elderly patients, thus contributing to the development of caries, periodontal disease, oral candidiasis, and discomfort.

Extrapyramidal reactions induced by thioxanthenes will result in increased motor activity of the head, face, and neck. Occlusal adjustments, bite registrations, and treatment for bruxism may be made less reliable.

The leukopenic and thrombocytopenic effects of thioxanthenes may result in an increased incidence of microbial infection, delayed healing, and gingival bleeding. If leukopenia or thrombocytopenia occurs, dental work should be deferred until blood counts have returned to normal, and patients should be instructed in proper oral hygiene, including caution in use of regular toothbrushes, dental floss, and toothpicks.

### Drug interactions and/or related problems
The following drug interactions and/or related problems have been selected on the basis of their potential clinical significance (possible mechanism in parentheses where appropriate)—not necessarily inclusive (» = major clinical significance):

Note: Combinations containing any of the following medications, depending on the amount present, may also interact with this medication.

Although not all of the following interactions have been documented specifically for thioxanthenes, a potential exists for their occurrence because of the close similarity of the pharmacological effects of thioxanthenes with those of phenothiazine medications.

» Alcohol or
» Central nervous system (CNS) depression–producing medications, other, especially anesthetics, barbiturates, and opioid (narcotic) analgesics(See *Appendix II*)
(concurrent use may potentiate and prolong the CNS depressant effects of either these medications or the thioxanthenes; dosage adjustments may be necessary)

Amphetamines
(concurrent use with thioxanthenes may inhibit the CNS-stimulating effects of amphetamines due to alpha-adrenergic blockade by the thioxanthenes; also, the antipsychotic effects of thioxanthenes may be reduced when they are used concurrently with amphetamines)

Antacids or
Antidiarrheals, adsorbent
(concurrent use may inhibit the absorption of an orally administered thioxanthene)

Anticholinergics or other medications with anticholinergic action (See *Appendix II*) or
Antidyskinetic agents or
Antihistamines
(anticholinergic effects, especially confusion, hallucinations, nightmares, and increased intraocular pressure, may be potentiated when these medications are used concurrently with thioxanthenes, because of secondary anticholinergic action of thioxanthenes)

Anticonvulsants
(thioxanthenes may lower the seizure threshold; dosage adjustment of anticonvulsant medications may be necessary; potentiation of anticonvulsant effects does not occur)

Antidepressants, tricyclic or
Maprotiline or
Monoamine oxidase (MAO) inhibitors, including furazolidone, procarbazine, or selegiline or
Trazodone
(concurrent use with thioxanthenes may prolong and intensify the sedative and anticholinergic effects of either these medications or the thioxanthenes)

Bromocriptine
(concurrent use with thioxanthenes may increase serum prolactin concentrations and interfere with effects of bromocriptine; dosage adjustment of bromocriptine may be necessary)

Dopamine
(concurrent use may antagonize peripheral vasoconstriction produced by high doses of dopamine, because of the alpha-adrenergic blocking action of thioxanthenes)

Ephedrine
(alpha-adrenergic blocking action of thioxanthenes may decrease the pressor response to ephedrine when it is used concurrently with thioxanthenes)

» Epinephrine
(alpha-adrenergic effects of epinephrine may be blocked when it is used concurrently with thioxanthenes, possibly resulting in severe hypotension and tachycardia)

» Extrapyramidal reaction–causing medications, other (See *Appendix II*)
(concurrent use with thioxanthenes may increase the severity and frequency of extrapyramidal effects)

Guanadrel or
Guanethidine
(concurrent use with thioxanthenes may decrease the hypotensive effects of these medications because of their displacement from and inhibition of uptake by adrenergic neurons)

» Levodopa
(concurrent use with thioxanthenes may inhibit the antiparkinsonian effects of levodopa because thioxanthenes block dopamine receptors in the brain)

Metaraminol
(concurrent use usually decreases, but does not reverse or completely block, the pressor response to metaraminol, because of the alpha-adrenergic blocking action of thioxanthenes)

Methoxamine
(prior administration of thioxanthenes may decrease the pressor effect and duration of action of methoxamine because of the alpha-adrenergic blocking action of thioxanthenes)

Ototoxic medications, especially ototoxic antibiotics (See *Appendix II*)
(concurrent use with thioxanthenes may mask the symptoms of ototoxicity such as tinnitus, dizziness, or vertigo)

Phenylephrine
(prior administration of thioxanthenes may decrease the pressor response to phenylephrine because of the alpha-adrenergic blocking action of thioxanthenes)

Photosensitizing medications, other
(concurrent use with thioxanthenes may cause additive photosensitizing effects)

» Quinidine
(concurrent use with thioxanthenes may result in additive cardiac effects)

**Laboratory value alterations**
The following have been selected on the basis of their potential clinical significance (possible effect in parentheses where appropriate)—not necessarily inclusive (» = major clinical significance):

With diagnostic test results
*For chlorprothixene*
Bilirubin tests, urine
(false-positive results may occur)

Electrocardiogram (ECG) readings
(Q- and T-wave changes may occur)

Immunologic urine pregnancy tests
(depending on the test used, false-positive or false-negative results may occur)

With physiology/laboratory test values
Uric acid
(serum concentrations may be decreased with use of neuroleptics)

**Medical considerations/Contraindications**
The medical considerations/contraindications included have been selected on the basis of their potential clinical significance (reasons given in parentheses where appropriate)—not necessarily inclusive (» = major clinical significance).

*Except under special circumstances, this medication should not be used when the following medical problems exist:*
» Blood dyscrasias or
» Bone marrow depression or
» Circulatory collapse or
» CNS depression or
» Comatose states, drug-induced
(may be exacerbated)

*Risk-benefit should be considered when the following medical problems exist:*
» Alcoholism
(CNS depression may be potentiated)
» Cardiovascular disease
(increased risk of transient hypotension)
Glaucoma, or predisposition to or
Peptic ulcer or
Respiratory disorders due to acute infections, asthma, or emphysema or
Urinary retention
(may be exacerbated)
» Hepatic function impairment
(metabolism may be altered)
Parkinson's disease
(potentiation of extrapyramidal effects)
Prostatic hypertrophy, symptomatic
(increased risk of urinary retention)
» Reye's syndrome
(increased risk of hepatotoxicity in children and adolescents with signs and symptoms suggesting Reye's syndrome)
Seizure disorders
(seizures may be precipitated because of lowered seizure threshold)
Sensitivity to thioxanthenes or phenothiazines

**Patient monitoring**
The following may be especially important in patient monitoring (other tests may be warranted in some patients, depending on condition; » = major clinical significance):

Blood cell counts and differential, especially in patients with sore throat and fever
(may be required at periodic intervals during high-dose or prolonged therapy; agranulocytosis is more likely to occur between the 4th and 10th weeks of therapy; if significant cellular depression occurs, medication should be discontinued and appropriate therapy initiated)

Careful observation for early symptoms of tardive dyskinesia
(recommended at periodic intervals, especially during high-dose or prolonged therapy and in the elderly; since there is no known effective treatment if syndrome should develop, thioxanthenes should be discontinued, if clinically feasible, at the earliest signs, usually fine, worm-like movements of the tongue)

Careful observation for early symptoms of tardive dystonia
(recommended at periodic intervals; since there is no known effective treatment if syndrome should develop, thioxanthenes should be discontinued, if clinically feasible, at the earliest signs)

Liver function tests and
Urine tests for bilirubin and bile
(may be required if jaundice or grippe-like symptoms occur; these side effects are more likely to occur between the 2nd and 4th weeks of therapy)

Ophthalmologic examinations
(may be required at periodic intervals during high-dose or prolonged therapy since deposition of particulate matter in the lens and cornea has occurred)

## Side/Adverse Effects

Note: A few cases of sudden death have been reported in patients who were receiving phenothiazine derivatives. However, there is no definite evidence that the phenothiazines are causative agents.

Although not all of these side effects have been attributed specifically to each thioxanthene or its phenothiazine analog, a potential exists for their occurrence during the use of any thioxanthene or its analog.

The following side/adverse effects have been selected on the basis of their potential clinical significance (possible signs and symptoms in parentheses where appropriate)—not necessarily inclusive:

**Those indicating need for medical attention**
Incidence more frequent
*Akathisia* (severe restlessness or need to keep moving)—may appear within first 6 hours after dose; *dystonic reactions* (difficulty in swallowing; inability to move eyes; muscle spasms, especially of neck and back; unusual twisting movements of body); *extrapyramidal effects, parkinsonian* (difficulty in talking; loss of balance control; mask-like face; shuffling walk; stiffness of arms and legs; trembling and shaking of fingers and hands); *tardive dyskinesia, persistent* (lip smacking or puckering; puffing of cheeks; rapid or worm-like movements of tongue; uncontrolled chewing movements; uncontrolled movements of arms and legs)

Note: *Dystonic reactions* appear most often in children and young adults; usually appear early in treatment and may subside within 24 to 48 hours after medication has been discontinued.

*Parkinsonian extrapyramidal effects* may be seen in the first few days of treatment, but frequency usually increases with increase of dosage; may be more frequent in elderly patients and older children.

*Tardive dyskinesia* is initially dose related, but may increase with long-term treatment and total cumulative dose; may persist after discontinuation of thioxanthenes.

Incidence less frequent
*Allergic reaction* (skin rash); *anticholinergic effect* (difficult urination); *deposition of opaque substances in lens and cornea or retinopathy* (blurred vision or other eye problems); *hypotension* (fainting); *skin discoloration*—more frequent in females on high-dose and prolonged therapy

Incidence rare
*Agranulocytosis or other blood dyscrasias* (sore throat and fever; unusual bleeding or bruising); *heat stroke* (hot, dry skin or lack of sweating; muscle weakness); *jaundice, obstructive* (yellow eyes or skin); *neuroleptic malignant syndrome (NMS)* (convulsions; difficulty in breathing; fast heartbeat; high fever; high or low blood pressure; increased sweating; loss of bladder control; severe muscle stiffness; unusually pale skin; tiredness); *tardive dystonia* (increased blinking or spasms of eyelid; unusual facial expressions or body positions; uncontrolled twisting movements of neck, trunk, arms, or legs)

Note: *Heat stroke* may occur in environmental conditions of high heat and high humidity. Adequate interior temperature control (air-conditioning) must be maintained for institutionalized patients during hot weather because of the increased risk of heat stroke and neuroleptic malignant syndrome (NMS).

*NMS* may occur at any time during neuroleptic therapy, but is more commonly seen soon after start of therapy, after patient has switched from one neuroleptic to another, during combined therapy with another psychotropic medication, or after a dosage increase. Along with the overt signs of skeletal muscle rigidity, hyperthermia, autonomic dysfunction, and altered consciousness, differential diagnosis may reveal leukocytosis (9500 to 26,000 cells per cubic millimeter), elevated liver enzymes, and elevated creatine phosphokinase (CPK).

**Those indicating need for medical attention only if they continue or are bothersome**
Incidence more frequent
*Constipation; decreased sweating; drowsiness, mild; dryness of mouth; increased appetite and weight; increased sensitivity of skin to sunlight; nasal congestion* (stuffy nose); *orthostatic hypotension* (dizziness, lightheadedness, or fainting)

Incidence less frequent
*Changes in menstrual period; decreased sexual ability; swelling of breasts*—in males and females; *unusual secretion of milk*

**Those indicating need for medical attention if they occur after medication is discontinued**
*Dyskinesia, withdrawal emergent* (dizziness; nausea and vomiting; stomach pain; trembling of fingers and hands; uncontrolled, repetitive movements of mouth, tongue, or jaw)

## Overdose
For specific information on the agents used in the management of thioxanthene overdose, see:
- *Amphetamine* or *dextroamphetamine* in *Amphetamines (Systemic)* monograph;
- *Benztropine* in *Antidyskinetics (Systemic)* monograph;
- *Charcoal, Activated (Oral-Local)* monograph;
- *Diazepam* in *Benzodiazepines (Systemic)* monograph;
- *Digitalis Glycosides (Systemic)* monograph;
- *Diphenhydramine* in *Antihistamines (Systemic)* monograph;
- *Norepinephrine* or *phenylephrine* in *Sympathomimetic Agents—Cardiovascular Use (Parenteral-Systemic)* monograph; and/or
- *Phenytoin* in *Anticonvulsants, Hydantoin (Systemic)* monograph.

For more information on the management of overdose or unintentional ingestion, **contact a Poison Control Center** (see *Poison Control Center Listing*).

**Clinical effects of overdose**
The following effects have been selected on the basis of their potential clinical significance (possible signs and symptoms in parentheses where appropriate)—not necessarily inclusive:
*Convulsions; difficulty in breathing, severe; drowsiness, severe, or coma; fast heartbeat; fever; hypotension* (dizziness, severe); *muscle trembling, jerking, stiffness, or uncontrolled movements, severe; small pupils; unusual excitement; unusual tiredness or weakness, severe*

**Treatment of overdose**
Treatment is essentially symptomatic and supportive and may consist of the following:
To decrease absorption—
  Early gastric lavage is often helpful.
  Not attempting to induce emesis because a dystonic reaction of the head and neck may develop that could result in aspiration of vomitus.
  Administering activated charcoal slurry.
  Administering saline cathartic.
Specific treatment—
  Controlling cardiac arrhythmias with intravenous phenytoin, 9 to 11 mg per kg of body weight (mg/kg).
  Digitalizing for cardiac failure.
  Administering a vasopressor, such as norepinephrine or phenylephrine, for hypotension (not using epinephrine, which may cause paradoxical hypotension).
  Controlling convulsions with diazepam followed by phenytoin, 15 mg/kg, administered at a rate no faster than 50 mg per minute.
  Benztropine or diphenhydramine may be administered to manage acute parkinsonian symptoms.
  Severe CNS depression may require administration of a stimulant such as amphetamine or dextroamphetamine (picrotoxin or pentylenetetrazol should be avoided as it may induce convulsions).
Monitoring—
  Monitoring cardiovascular function(for not less than 5 days).
Supportive care—
  Maintaining respiratory function and body temperature.
  Patients in whom intentional overdose is known or suspected should be referred for psychiatric consultation.

Note: Dialysis of thioxanthenes has not been successful.

## Patient Consultation
As an aid to patient consultation, refer to *Advice for the Patient, Thioxanthenes (Systemic)*.
In providing consultation, consider emphasizing the following selected information (» = major clinical significance):

**Before using this medication**
» Conditions affecting use, especially:
  Sensitivity to thioxanthenes or phenothiazines
  Pregnancy—Reports of hyperreflexia in neonates when pharmacologically related phenothiazines were used during pregnancy; animal studies have shown an increase in resorption rates and decreased fertility with phenothiazines
  Breast-feeding—Pharmacologically related phenothiazines are distributed into breast milk causing tardive dyskinesia and possible drowsiness in nursing baby
  Use in children—Children are more prone to extrapyramidal symptoms
  Use in the elderly—Elderly patients are more likely to develop extrapyramidal, anticholinergic, hypotensive, and sedative effects; reduced dosage recommended
  Dental—Thioxanthene-induced blood dyscrasias may result in infections, delayed healing, and bleeding; dry mouth may cause caries and candidiasis; increased motor activity of face, head, and neck may interfere with some dental procedures
  Other medications, especially alcohol or other CNS depression–producing medications, epinephrine, other extrapyramidal reaction–causing medications, levodopa, or quinidine
  Other medical problems, especially blood dyscrasias, bone marrow depression, circulatory collapse, CNS depression, alcoholism, cardiovascular disease, hepatic function impairment, or Reye's syndrome

**Proper use of this medication**
  Taking with food or milk to reduce gastrointestinal irritation
» Diluting thiothixene oral solution with recommended beverages prior to use
» Compliance with therapy; not taking more medication or more often than directed
» May require several weeks of therapy to obtain desired effects
» Proper dosing
  Missed dose: Taking as soon as possible; not taking if within 2 hours of next scheduled dose; continuing on regular schedule; not doubling doses
» Proper storage

**Precautions while using this medication**
  Regular visits to physician to check progress of therapy
  Checking with physician before discontinuing medication; gradual dosage reduction may be needed
» Avoiding use of alcoholic beverages or other CNS depressants during therapy
  Avoiding use of antacids or medicine for diarrhea within 2 hours of taking thioxanthenes
» Caution if any kind of surgery, dental treatment, or emergency treatment is required
» Possible drowsiness; caution when driving, using machines, or doing other things requiring alertness
» Possible dizziness or lightheadedness; caution when getting up suddenly from a lying or sitting position
» Possible heatstroke: caution during exercise or hot weather, or when taking hot baths
» Possible skin photosensitivity; avoiding unprotected exposure to sun; using protective clothing; using a sun block product that includes protection against both UVA-caused photosensitivity reactions and UVB-caused sunburn reactions; avoiding use of sunlamp, tanning bed, or tanning booth
  Possible dryness of mouth; using sugarless gum or candy, ice, or saliva substitute for relief; checking with physician or dentist if dry mouth continues for more than 2 weeks
» Avoiding spilling liquid medication on skin or clothing; may cause contact dermatitis
  Observing precautions for long-acting parenteral form for up to 3 weeks

**Side/adverse effects**
» Stopping medication and notifying physician immediately if symptoms of neuroleptic malignant syndrome (NMS) appear
» Notifying physician as soon as possible if early signs of tardive dyskinesia appear
  Possibility of withdrawal symptoms
  Signs of potential side effects, especially akathisia, dystonias, parkinsonian effects, tardive dyskinesia or dystonia, allergic reactions, anticholinergic effects, deposition of opaque substances in lens and

cornea or retinopathy, hypotension, skin discoloration, blood dyscrasias, heat stroke, obstructive jaundice, and NMS

## General Dosing Information

Dosage must be individualized by titration from the lower dose range. After a favorable psychiatric response is noted (within several days to several months), that dosage should be continued for about 2 weeks, then gradually decreased to the lowest level that will maintain an adequate clinical response.

When extended therapy is discontinued, a gradual reduction in thioxanthene dosage over several weeks is recommended. Abrupt withdrawal may cause some patients on high or long-term dosage to experience transient dyskinetic signs, nausea, vomiting, gastritis, trembling, and dizziness.

The antiemetic effect of thioxanthenes may mask signs of drug toxicity or may obscure diagnosis of conditions whose primary symptom is nausea.

Avoid skin contact with liquid forms of this medication; contact dermatitis has resulted with use of similar medications.

### For parenteral dosage forms only

Because hypotension is a common side effect of thioxanthenes, parenteral administration should be used only for patients who are bedfast or for appropriate acute, ambulatory patients who can be closely monitored. A possible exception may be those patients who are dose-stabilized on the extended-action injectable form.

Intramuscular injections should be administered slowly and deeply into the upper outer quadrant of the buttock or midlateral thigh. Patient should remain lying down for at least half an hour after injection to avoid possible hypotensive effects.

Effects of the extended-action injectable form may last for up to 3 weeks. The precautions and side effects information applies during this period of time.

Geriatric patients and children should be monitored very carefully during parenteral therapy because of a higher incidence of hypotensive and extrapyramidal reactions.

The changeover from other neuroleptic medication to long-acting flupenthixol should be done gradually and under close supervision to prevent overdosage or insufficient suppression of psychotic symptoms before the next injection.

### Diet/Nutrition

This medication may be taken with food or a full glass (240 mL) of water or milk, if necessary, to lessen stomach irritation.

### For treatment of adverse effects

Neuroleptic malignant syndrome (NMS)
Treatment is essentially symptomatic and supportive and may include:
- *Discontinuing thioxanthene immediately.*
- Hyperthermia—Administering antipyretics (aspirin or acetaminophen); using cooling blanket.
- Dehydration—Restoring fluid and electrolytes.
- Cardiovascular instability—Monitoring blood pressure and cardiac rhythm closely.
- Hypoxia—Administering oxygen; considering airway insertion and assisted ventilation.
- Muscle rigidity—Dantrolene sodium may be administered (100 to 300 mg per day in divided doses; 1.25 to 1.5 mg per kg of body weight, intravenously). Bromocriptine (5 to 7.5 mg every eight hours) has been used to reverse hyperpyrexia and muscle rigidity.

Parkinsonism, severe—
Many authorities advise that the only appropriate treatment of extrapyramidal symptoms is reduction of the antipsychotic dosage, if possible. Oral antidyskinetic agents such as trihexyphenidyl (2 mg three times a day), or benztropine, may be effective in treating more severe parkinsonism and acute motor restlessness but should be used sparingly, and then usually for no longer than 3 months. Milder effects may be treated by adjusting dosage. However, in the elderly patient, the use of amantadine (100 to 200 mg) at bedtime minimizes the severe anticholinergic effects that may occur with other antidyskinetics.

Akathisia—
May be treated with antidyskinetic agents, or with propranolol (30 to 120 mg a day); nadolol (40 mg a day); pindolol (5 to 60 mg a day); lorazepam (1 or 2 mg two or three times a day): or diazepam (2 mg two or three times a day).

Dystonia—
Acute dystonic postures or oculogyric crisis may be relieved by parenteral administration of benztropine (2 mg intramuscularly), or diphenhydramine (50 mg intravenously or intramuscularly), or diazepam (5 to 7.5 mg intravenously), to be followed by oral antidyskinetic medication for one or two days to prevent recurrent dystonic episodes. Dosage adjustments of the thioxanthene may control these effects, and discontinuation may reverse severe symptoms.

Tardive dyskinesia or tardive dystonia—
No known effective treatment. Dosage of thioxanthene should be lowered or medication discontinued, if clinically feasible, at earliest signs of tardive dyskinesia or tardive dystonia, to prevent possible irreversible effects.

---

### CHLORPROTHIXENE*

## Summary of Differences

Pharmacology/pharmacokinetics:
Other actions/effects—Antiemetic and sedative effects are more prominent than those of thiothixene.
Duration of action—Intramuscular dosage may produce effects lasting up to 12 hours.

Precautions:
Laboratory value alterations—
More likely to cause Q-T wave changes on ECG readings than is thiothixene.
May produce false-positive results on immunologic urine pregnancy test.
May produce false-positive results on urine bilirubin test.

## Oral Dosage Forms

### CHLORPROTHIXENE ORAL SUSPENSION USP

**Usual adult and adolescent dose**
Antipsychotic—
Oral, 25 to 50 mg three or four times a day.

Note: Geriatric or debilitated patients usually require a lower initial dose, the dosage being increased gradually as needed and tolerated.

**Usual adult prescribing limits**
Up to 600 mg a day.

**Usual pediatric dose**
Antipsychotic—
Children up to 6 years of age: Safety and efficacy have not been established.
Children 6 to 12 years of age: Oral, 10 to 25 mg three or four times a day.

**Strength(s) usually available**
U.S.—
100 mg per 5 mL (Rx) [*Taractan* (benzoic acid; edetate disodium; glycerin; hydrochloric acid; lactic acid; magnesium aluminum silicate; parabens [methyl and propyl]; polyoxyethylene [8] stearate; silicon emulsion; sodium hydroxide; sorbitol; sucrose; FD&C Red No. 40; FD&C Blue No. 1; FD&C Yellow No. 6; flavors; water)].
Canada—
Not commercially available.

**Packaging and storage**
Store below 40 °C (104 °F), preferably between 15 and 30 °C (59 and 86 °F), unless otherwise specified by manufacturer. Store in a tight, light-resistant container. Protect from freezing.

**Auxiliary labeling**
- Shake well.
- May cause drowsiness.
- Avoid alcoholic beverages.
- Do not spill on skin or clothing.

**Note**
Avoid skin contact with liquid forms of this medication; contact dermatitis has resulted.

### CHLORPROTHIXENE TABLETS USP

**Usual adult and adolescent dose**
Antipsychotic—
Oral, 25 to 50 mg three or four times a day.

Note: Geriatric or debilitated patients usually require a lower initial dose, the dosage being increased gradually as needed and tolerated.

**Usual adult prescribing limits**
Up to 600 mg a day.

**Usual pediatric dose**
Antipsychotic—
Children up to 6 years of age: Safety and efficacy have not been established.
Children 6 to 12 years of age: Oral, 10 to 25 mg three or four times a day.

## Strength(s) usually available

U.S.—
- 10 mg (Rx) [*Taractan* (tartrazine)].
- 25 mg (Rx) [*Taractan* (tartrazine)].
- 50 mg (Rx) [*Taractan* (tartrazine)].
- 100 mg (Rx) [*Taractan* (tartrazine)].

Canada—
- Not commercially available.

## Packaging and storage
Store below 40 °C (104 °F), preferably between 15 and 30 °C (59 and 86 °F), unless otherwise specified by manufacturer. Store in a well-closed, light-resistant container.

## Auxiliary labeling
- May cause drowsiness.
- Avoid alcoholic beverages.

# Parenteral Dosage Forms

## CHLORPROTHIXENE INJECTION USP

### Usual adult and adolescent dose
Antipsychotic—
  Intramuscular, 25 to 50 mg three or four times a day.

Note: Geriatric or debilitated patients and adolescents usually require a lower initial dose, the dosage being increased gradually as needed and tolerated.

### Usual pediatric dose
Antipsychotic—
  Children up to 12 years of age: Safety and efficacy have not been established.
  Children 12 years of age and over: See *Usual adult and adolescent dose*.

### Strength(s) usually available
U.S.—
  12.5 mg per mL (Rx) [*Taractan* (parabens [methyl and propyl] 0.2%)].

Canada—
  Not commercially available.

### Packaging and storage
Store below 40 °C (104 °F), preferably between 15 and 30 °C (59 and 86 °F), unless otherwise specified by manufacturer. Protect from light. Protect from freezing.

### Note
Avoid skin contact with liquid forms of this medication; contact dermatitis has resulted with similar medications.

---

## FLUPENTHIXOL

## Additional Dosing Information
See also *General Dosing Information*.

### For parenteral dosage form only
Flupenthixol is for intramuscular injection only. It is *not* for intravenous use.

As with all oily injections, aspiration before injection ensures that inadvertent intravascular injection has not occurred.

Administration is by deep intramuscular injection into the gluteal region.

Patients not previously treated with a long-acting depot neuroleptic should be given a test dose of 5 to 20 mg of flupenthixol decanoate. The 5-mg test dose is usually recommended for elderly or debilitated patients, or for patients who may have a predisposition to extrapyramidal effects.

During the 5 to 10 days following the test dose, the patient should be carefully monitored for therapeutic response and appearance of extrapyramidal side effects. Any oral neuroleptic dosage should be reduced in this period.

A single injection may last for two to three weeks. However, when higher doses are used, a single injection may last for four weeks or more. Since higher doses also increase the incidence of adverse effects, dose increases should be made in increments not to exceed 20 mg.

# Oral Dosage Forms

## FLUPENTHIXOL DIHYDROCHLORIDE TABLETS

### Usual adult dose
Antipsychotic—
  Initial: Oral, 1 mg three times a day, the dosage being increased by 1 mg every two to three days as needed and tolerated.
  Maintenance: Oral, 3 to 6 mg a day in divided doses, up to 12 mg a day or more.

Note: Geriatric or debilitated patients usually require a lower initial dose, the dosage being increased gradually as needed and tolerated.

### Usual pediatric dose
Antipsychotic—
  Safety and efficacy have not been established.

### Strength(s) usually available
U.S.—
  Not commercially available.

Canada—
  0.5 mg (Rx) [*Fluanxol* (sucrose)].
  3 mg (Rx) [*Fluanxol* (sucrose)].

### Packaging and storage
Store below 40 °C (104 °F), preferably between 15 and 30 °C (59 and 86 °F), in a well-closed container, unless otherwise specified by manufacturer. Protect from light.

### Auxiliary labeling
- May cause drowsiness.
- Avoid alcoholic beverages.

# Parenteral Dosage Forms

## FLUPENTHIXOL DECANOATE INJECTION

### Usual adult dose
Antipsychotic—
  Intramuscular, initially 20 to 40 mg, the dose being repeated in four to ten days. Dosage may be increased in increments of not more than 20 mg.

Note: Most patients require 20 to 40 mg every two to three weeks.
  Doses greater than 80 mg are rarely necessary, although higher doses may be used in some patients.

### Usual pediatric dose
Antipsychotic—
  Safety and efficacy have not been established.

### Strength(s) usually available
U.S.—
  Not commercially available.

Canada—
  20 mg per mL (Rx) [*Fluanxol Depot*].
  100 mg per mL (Rx) [*Fluanxol Depot*].

### Packaging and storage
Store below 40 °C (104 °F), preferably between 15 and 30 °C (59 and 86 °F), unless otherwise specified by manufacturer. Protect from light. Protect from freezing.

### Additional information
Vehicle is a thin vegetable oil.

---

## THIOTHIXENE

## Summary of Differences
Precautions: Laboratory value alterations—With physiology/laboratory test values: Serum uric acid may be decreased.

# Oral Dosage Forms

## THIOTHIXENE CAPSULES USP

### Usual adult and adolescent dose
Antipsychotic—
  Oral, initially 2 mg three times a day for milder conditions, or 5 mg two times a day for more severe conditions, the dosage being adjusted gradually as needed and tolerated, usually up to 60 mg a day.

Note: Dosages over 60 mg a day rarely increase the beneficial effect.
  Geriatric or debilitated patients usually require a lower initial dose, the dosage being increased gradually as needed and tolerated.

### Usual pediatric dose
Antipsychotic—
  Children up to 12 years of age: Safety and efficacy have not been established.
  Children 12 years of age and over: See *Usual adult and adolescent dose*.

### Strength(s) usually available
U.S.—
  1 mg (Rx) [*Navane*; GENERIC].
  2 mg (Rx) [*Navane*; GENERIC].
  5 mg (Rx) [*Navane*; GENERIC].

10 mg (Rx) [*Navane;* GENERIC].
20 mg (Rx) [*Navane;* GENERIC].

Canada—
- 2 mg (Rx) [*Navane* (sodium lauryl sulfate; corn starch [gluten]; lactose; magnesium stearate; gelatin; sodium metabisulfite; titanium dioxide; FD&C Red No. 3)].
- 5 mg (Rx) [*Navane* (sodium lauryl sulfate; corn starch [gluten]; lactose; magnesium stearate; gelatin; sodium metabisulfite; titanium dioxide; FD&C Red No. 3; FD&C Yellow No. 6)].
- 10 mg (Rx) [*Navane* (sodium lauryl sulfate; corn starch [gluten]; lactose; magnesium stearate; gelatin; sodium metabisulfite; titanium dioxide; FD&C Red No. 3; FD&C Yellow No. 6)].

**Packaging and storage**
Store below 40 °C (104 °F), preferably between 15 and 30 °C (59 and 86 °F), unless otherwise specified by manufacturer. Store in a well-closed, light-resistant container.

**Auxiliary labeling**
- May cause drowsiness.
- Avoid alcoholic beverages.

### THIOTHIXENE HYDROCHLORIDE ORAL SOLUTION USP

Note: The dosing and strengths of Thiothixene Oral Solution are expressed in terms of thiothixene base (not the hydrochloride salt).

**Usual adult and adolescent dose**
Antipsychotic—
Oral, initially, 2 mg (base) three times a day for milder conditions, or 5 mg two times a day for severe conditions, the dosage being adjusted gradually as needed and tolerated, up to 60 mg a day.

Note: Dosages over 60 mg a day rarely increase the beneficial effect.
Geriatric or debilitated patients usually require a lower initial dose, the dosage being increased gradually as needed and tolerated.

**Usual pediatric dose**
Antipsychotic—
Children up to 12 years of age: Safety and efficacy have not been established.
Children 12 years of age and over: See *Usual adult and adolescent dose.*

**Strength(s) usually available**
U.S.—
5 mg (base) per mL (Rx) [*Navane* (alcohol 7%); *Thiothixene HCl Intensol;* GENERIC].
Canada—
Not commercially available.

**Packaging and storage**
Store below 25 °C (77 °F), unless otherwise specified by manufacturer. Store in a tight, light-resistant container. Protect from freezing.

**Auxiliary labeling**
- May cause drowsiness.
- Avoid alcoholic beverages.
- Do not spill on skin or clothing.
- Must be diluted before use.

**Note**
Avoid skin contact with liquid forms of this medication; contact dermatitis has resulted with similar medications.

Each dose must be diluted just before administration by adding it to a cupful of milk, tomato or fruit juice, water, soup, or carbonated beverage.

Provide a specially marked dosage dropper and explain dilution and dosage measurement to patient if medication is self-administered.

## Parenteral Dosage Forms

Note: The dosing and strengths of the dosage forms available are expressed in terms of thiothixene base (not the hydrochloride salt).

### THIOTHIXENE HYDROCHLORIDE INJECTION USP

**Usual adult and adolescent dose**
Antipsychotic—
Intramuscular, 4 mg (base) two to four times a day, the dosage being adjusted gradually as needed and tolerated, but not to exceed a total of 30 mg a day.

Note: Geriatric or debilitated patients usually require a lower initial dose, the dosage being increased gradually as needed and tolerated.

**Usual pediatric dose**
Antipsychotic—
Children up to 12 years of age: Safety and efficacy have not been established.
Children 12 years of age and over: See *Usual adult and adolescent dose.*

**Strength(s) usually available**
U.S.—
2 mg (base) per mL (Rx) [*Navane* (dextrose 5% w/v; benzyl alcohol 0.9% w/v; propyl gallate 0.02% w/v)].
Canada—
Not commercially available.

**Packaging and storage**
Store between 2 and 8 °C (36 and 46 °F), unless otherwise specified by manufacturer. Protect from light. Protect from freezing.

**Note**
Avoid skin contact with liquid forms of this medication; contact dermatitis has resulted from use of similar medications.

### THIOTHIXENE HYDROCHLORIDE FOR INJECTION USP

**Usual adult and adolescent dose**
Antipsychotic—
Intramuscular, 4 mg (base) two to four times a day, the dosage being adjusted gradually as needed and tolerated, but not to exceed a total of 30 mg a day.

Note: Geriatric or debilitated patients usually require a lower initial dose, the dosage being increased gradually as needed and tolerated.

**Usual pediatric dose**
Antipsychotic—
Children up to 12 years of age: Safety and efficacy have not been established.

**Strength(s) usually available**
U.S.—
5 mg (base) per mL (Rx) [*Navane* (mannitol)].
Canada—
Not commercially available.

**Packaging and storage**
Store between 2 and 8 °C (36 and 46 °F), unless otherwise specified by manufacturer. Store in a light-resistant container. Protect from freezing.

**Preparation of dosage form**
Reconstitute thiothixene hydrochloride for injection with 2.2 mL of sterile water for injection.

**Stability**
Reconstituted product may be stored at room temperature for up to 48 hours before discarding.

**Note**
Avoid skin contact with liquid forms of this medication; contact dermatitis has resulted with similar medications.

Revised: 06/17/93

# THROMBOLYTIC AGENTS  Systemic

This monograph includes information on the following: 1) Alteplase, Recombinant; 2) Anistreplase; 3) Streptokinase; 4) Urokinase.

**VA CLASSIFICATION (Primary):** BL115

Commonly used brand name(s): *Abbokinase*[4]*; Abbokinase Open-Cath*[4]*; Activase*[1]*; Activase rt-PA*[1]*; Eminase*[2]*; Kabikinase*[3]*; Streptase*[3].

Other commonly used names for [Anistreplase] are anisoylated plasminogen-streptokinase activator complex and APSAC; and, for [Alteplase, Recombinant], tissue-type plasminogen activator (recombinant), t-PA, and rt-PA.

Note: For a listing of dosage forms and brand names by country availability, see *Dosage Forms* section(s).

## Category
Thrombolytic.

## Indications
Note: Bracketed information in the *Indications* section refers to uses that are not included in U.S. product labeling.

The selection of thrombolytic therapy must be evaluated individually for each patient based on confirmation of thrombotic disease and assessment of patient condition and history. Some of the indications for thrombolytic therapy are identical to those for heparin or coumarin- or indandione-derivative anticoagulants. However, the goals of thrombolytic therapy and anticoagulant therapy are different. Thrombolytic agents are used primarily to lyse obstructive thrombi and restore blood flow in a recently occluded blood vessel, whereas anticoagulants are used primarily to prevent thrombus formation and extension of existing thrombi. The potential benefit of thrombolytic therapy must be weighed against the risk of bleeding because the risk of hemorrhage may be greater with thrombolytic agents than with heparin or coumarin- or indandione-derivative anticoagulants.

### Accepted
Thrombosis, coronary arterial, acute (treatment)—Alteplase, anistreplase, streptokinase, and [urokinase][1] are indicated for use via intravenous infusion to lyse acute coronary arterial thrombi associated with evolving transmural myocardial infarction. Streptokinase and urokinase are also indicated for use via injection directly into the affected coronary artery. Various studies with intracoronary arterial injection have reported recanalization rates of 72 to 96%. However, intracoronary arterial administration requires prior identification of the site of the thrombus by coronary angiography. Intravenous infusion does not require coronary angiography and is the preferred route of administration because therapy can be instituted more rapidly and can be initiated in locations that lack facilities for cardiac catheterization.

Thrombolytic therapy may relieve chest pain, reduce the incidence of congestive heart failure, improve left ventricular function, limit cardiac damage (i.e., infarct size), and decrease the risk of early death if coronary arterial blood flow is restored before irreversible cardiac damage occurs. The reperfusion rate is dependent on the interval between the onset of symptoms and the initiation of therapy. Higher reperfusion rates are achieved when thrombolytic therapy is started within 4 hours after symptoms of ischemia first appear. However, reductions in mortality can be achieved if thrombolytic therapy is started up to 24 to 36 hours after the onset of symptoms.

Thrombolytic therapy is not a substitute for other measures that may be required to treat acute myocardial infarction or prevent reinfarction. Restoration of coronary arterial blood flow via thrombolysis does not correct underlying conditions that may promote thrombus formation. Recurrent ischemia, with or without reocclusion or overt reinfarction, may occur following initially successful thrombolysis. The risk of reocclusion may depend on the extent of residual stenosis in the affected vessel. Following successful thrombolytic therapy, long-term anticoagulation, platelet aggregation inhibitor therapy, percutaneous transluminal coronary angioplasty (PTCA), or coronary artery bypass graft (CABG) surgery may be required to provide long-lasting protection against reocclusion. However, initial thrombolytic therapy may permit a revascularization procedure to be performed on a delayed or elective, rather than on an emergency, basis.

Stroke, acute ischemic (treatment)—Alteplase[1] is indicated for the management of acute ischemic stroke in adults; it is used to improve neurologic recovery and reduce the incidence of disability. However, the safety and efficacy of alteplase therapy in patients with minor neurologic deficit, or with rapidly improving symptoms prior to the initiation of treatment, have not been evaluated.

Thromboembolism, pulmonary, acute (treatment)—Alteplase[1], streptokinase, and urokinase are indicated, and may be the therapy of choice in selected patients, for the lysis of acute, massive pulmonary emboli producing obstruction or significant filling defects involving two or more lobar pulmonary arteries or an equivalent degree of obstruction in other pulmonary vessels. These agents are also indicated for lysing pulmonary emboli accompanied by unstable hemodynamics, i.e., failure to maintain blood pressure without supportive measures. Heparin is recommended for the treatment of subacute or small emboli; however, some clinicians recommend thrombolytic therapy for comparatively small emboli in patients with limited cardiopulmonary reserve caused by significant cardiac or pulmonary disease. Prior to administration of a thrombolytic agent, the diagnosis should be confirmed by objective means such as pulmonary angiography via an upper extremity vein (preferred) or ventilation-perfusion lung scanning.

Thrombosis, deep venous (treatment)—Streptokinase and [urokinase][1] are indicated for the lysis of acute, extensive deep venous thrombi in the popliteal or more proximal vessels. Thrombolytic therapy may be the treatment of choice for deep venous thrombosis in selected patients. [These agents are also used for the lysis of acute, extensive thrombi in the axillary subclavian veins and vena cavae in selected patients.] However, anticoagulants are recommended for treatment of calf-vein thrombi. Prior to administration of a thrombolytic agent, the diagnosis should be confirmed, preferably by ascending venography or by Doppler ultrasound.

Thromboembolism, arterial, acute (treatment) and
Thrombosis, arterial, acute (treatment)—Streptokinase and [urokinase] are indicated for use via intravenous infusion for the lysis of acute arterial thrombi or emboli. [These agents are also administered locally (via a catheter positioned adjacent to or inserted into the substance of the thrombus as shown by arteriogram) to lyse arterial thrombi or emboli.] Studies have shown that thrombolytic therapy alone may be ineffective for treating chronic arterial occlusion. Angioplasty or distal bypass may be required following initial thrombolytic therapy in order to salvage the affected limb.

Cannula, arteriovenous, clearance—Streptokinase and [urokinase][1] are indicated to clear totally or partially occluded arteriovenous cannulae, as an alternative to surgical revision, when acceptable flow cannot be achieved by conventional mechanical measures.

Catheter, intravenous, clearance—[Streptokinase][1] and urokinase are indicated to restore patency to intravenous catheters, including central venous catheters, obstructed by clotted blood or fibrin deposits.

[Thrombolytic agents are also used to treat renal artery thrombosis, retinal blood vessel occlusions, hemolytic uremic syndrome, and impending renal cortical necrosis. However, controlled studies are required to establish the safety and effectiveness of such therapy in these conditions.][1]

### Unaccepted
Thrombolytic agents should *not* be used to treat superficial thrombophlebitis.

Alteplase has not been sufficiently studied, and is currently not recommended, for treatment of deep venous thrombosis or arterial thrombosis not associated with evolving acute myocardial infarction or for clearing occluded arteriovenous cannulae or obstructed intravenous catheters.

Alteplase and streptokinase are not recommended for treatment of arterial emboli originating in the left side of the heart (e.g., mitral stenosis accompanied by atrial fibrillation) because of the risk of cerebral embolism.

---

[1]Not included in Canadian product labeling.

## Pharmacology/Pharmacokinetics
### Physicochemical characteristics
Molecular weight—
  Alteplase: About 68,000 daltons.
  Anistreplase: About 131,000 daltons.
  Streptokinase: About 46,000 daltons.
  Urokinase: About 33,000 daltons.

### Mechanism of action/Effect
Thrombolytic agents activate the endogenous fibrinolytic system by cleaving the arginine$_{560}$–valine$_{561}$ bond in plasminogen to produce plasmin, an enzyme that degrades fibrin clots, fibrinogen, and other plasma proteins, including the procoagulant factors V and VIII. Alteplase and urokinase cleave the peptide bond directly. Anistreplase and streptokinase act indirectly; they combine with plasminogen to form streptokinase-plasminogen complexes that are converted to streptokinase-plasmin complexes. These activator complexes, rather than streptokinase itself, convert residual plasminogen to plasmin.

Conversion of plasminogen to plasmin occurs within the thrombus or embolus as well as on its surface and in circulating blood. Thrombolytic agents lyse fibrin deposits wherever they exist and can be reached by the plasmin generated; therefore, thrombolytic agents also promote lysis of fibrin deposits responsible for hemostasis.

Alteplase is more clot-selective than the other thrombolytic agents, binding more readily to the fibrin-plasminogen complex within a clot than to circulating (free) plasminogen. However, systemic fibrinolysis does occur with usual therapeutic doses.

### Other actions/effects
Fibrinogenolysis and fibrinolysis induced by thrombolytic agents increase the concentration of fibrinogen- and fibrin-degradation products (FDP/fdp) in the blood. The FDP/fdp exert an anticoagulant effect, probably by impairing fibrin polymerization and possibly by decreasing thrombin generation and/or interfering with platelet function. Alteplase usually reduces the circulating fibrinogen concentration and increases FDP/fdp

concentrations to a lesser extent than does streptokinase, but to about the same extent that urokinase does. However, studies have not shown a significantly lower incidence of bleeding with alteplase than has been reported with the other thrombolytic agents, probably because factors other than the concentrations of fibrinogen and/or FDP/fdp also significantly influence the risk of bleeding (see *Side/Adverse Effects*). Specifically, the risk of bleeding complications associated with thrombolytic therapy may be more dependent on the presence of vascular injury than on the extent of systemic fibrinolysis induced by a specific agent.

Anistreplase has potent proteolytic activity in the systemic circulation. In addition to decreasing plasma concentrations of fibrinogen, the medication lowers plasma concentrations of plasminogen, procoagulant factors V and VIII, and the fibrinolysis inhibitor alpha-2-antiplasmin.

Anistreplase, streptokinase, and urokinase have also been reported to decrease plasma viscosity and erythrocyte aggregation, probably as a result of reduced fibrinogen concentration.

Streptokinase and the streptokinase component of anistreplase are antigenic and induce the formation of antibodies. Elevation of the antistreptokinase antibody titer usually occurs about 5 to 7 days following administration, reaches a peak after 2 to 3 weeks, and may persist for 1 year or longer. The antibodies may cause resistance to subsequent streptokinase or anistreplase therapy, and possibly an increased risk of anaphylaxis or other severe allergic reactions.

**Biotransformation**
Alteplase—Hepatic; rapid.
Urokinase—Hepatic; rapid.

**Half-life**
Alteplase—
Distribution: Approximately 4 minutes.
Elimination: Approximately 35 minutes.
Anistreplase—
The half-life of anistreplase's fibrinolytic activity is 70 to 120 minutes (average about 90 minutes). The deacylation half-life of the complex is about 105 to 120 minutes. The plasma clearance and duration of fibrinolytic activity of the medication are probably controlled primarily by its deacylation rate.
Streptokinase—
Following intravenous administration of 1.5 million International Units (IU) over a 1-hour period: the half-life of the activator complexes (streptokinase-plasminogen and/or streptokinase-plasmin) is 23 minutes.
Urokinase—
Up to 20 minutes. The half-life may be prolonged in patients with hepatic function impairment.

**Time to peak effect**
Reperfusion of the myocardium generally occurs 20 minutes to 2 hours (average 45 minutes) following initiation of intravenous therapy.

**Duration of action**
Thrombolysis may continue for approximately 4 hours following administration of alteplase, streptokinase, or urokinase; the hyperfibrinolytic effect disappears within a few hours following discontinuation of administration. Following administration of anistreplase, thrombolysis may continue for approximately 6 hours, and a systemic hyperfibrinolytic state, as demonstrated by euglobulin clot lysis time determinations, may persist for more than 2 days. For all thrombolytic agents, the prothrombin time may rarely be prolonged for 12 to 24 hours following cessation of therapy because of the decreased plasma concentration of fibrinogen, decreased plasma concentration of factor V and possibly other coagulant factors, and/or the anticoagulant effects of FDP/fdp. However, prolonged, high FDP/fdp concentrations may potentiate bleeding for a longer period of time, especially after administration of non–clot-selective thrombolytic agents.

**Elimination**
Alteplase—Renal; approximately 80% of a dose is excreted in the urine, as metabolites, within 18 hours.
Urokinase—Small quantities are eliminated via the renal and biliary routes.

# Precautions to Consider

### Cross-sensitivity and/or related problems
Patients allergic to streptokinase will be allergic to anistreplase also, and vice versa.

### Carcinogenicity
*Alteplase, anistreplase,* and *urokinase*—Long-term studies to determine whether alteplase, anistreplase, and urokinase have carcinogenic potential have not been done.

### Mutagenicity
*Alteplase*—No mutagenicity was demonstrated in the Ames test or in chromosomal aberration assays in human lymphocytes.

*Anistreplase*—No mutagenicity was demonstrated in chromosomal aberration assays in human lymphocytes.

### Pregnancy/Reproduction
Fertility—*Alteplase*: Studies have not been done in animals.
*Anistreplase*: Studies have not been done in humans.
Studies have not been done in animals.
*Urokinase*: Studies in mice and rats have not shown that urokinase causes impaired fertility.

Pregnancy—It has been suggested that administration of a thrombolytic agent during the first 18 weeks of pregnancy may increase the risk of premature separation of the placenta because fetal attachments to the uterus during this time are composed primarily of fibrin. However, this problem has not been reported following administration of streptokinase or urokinase to patients during the first 2 trimesters of pregnancy.
*Alteplase and anistreplase—*
Studies have not been done in humans.
Studies have not been done in animals.
FDA Pregnancy Category C.
*Streptokinase—*
Streptokinase apparently crosses the human placenta minimally if at all. However, antibodies to streptokinase do cross the placenta. Studies in pregnant women (treated mostly during the second and third trimesters) have not shown evidence of abnormalities or induction of fibrinolysis in the fetus.
Studies have not been done in animals.
FDA Pregnancy Category C.
*Urokinase—*
Adequate and well-controlled studies have not been done in humans.
Studies in mice and rats have not shown that urokinase causes fetal harm when administered in doses up to 1000 times the human dose.
FDA Pregnancy Category B.

Postpartum—Thrombolytic agents should be administered with great caution during the first 10 days postpartum because of the increased risk of hemorrhage.

### Breast-feeding
It is not known whether thrombolytic agents are distributed into breast milk. However, problems in humans have not been documented.

### Pediatrics
Appropriate studies performed to date have not demonstrated pediatrics-specific problems that would limit the usefulness of thrombolytic agents in children.

### Geriatrics
Geriatric patients generally have a poorer prognosis than younger adults following an acute myocardial infarction. They may also be more likely than younger adults to have pre-existing conditions that tend to increase the risk of intracranial bleeding or other hemorrhagic complications. Because the risks of thrombolytic therapy, as well as its potential benefits, are increased in older patients, careful patient selection and monitoring are recommended.

### Drug interactions and/or related problems
The following drug interactions and/or related problems have been selected on the basis of their potential clinical significance (possible mechanism in parentheses where appropriate)—not necessarily inclusive (» = major clinical significance):

Note: Combinations containing any of the following medications, depending on the amount present, may also interact with this medication.

In addition to the interactions listed below, the possibility should be considered that multiple effects leading to further impairment of blood clotting and/or increased risk of hemorrhage may occur if a thrombolytic agent is administered to a patient receiving any medication having a significant potential for causing hypoprothrombinemia, thrombocytopenia, or gastrointestinal ulceration or hemorrhage.

» Anticoagulants, coumarin- or indandione-derivative or
» Enoxaparin or
» Heparin
(concurrent use with antithrombotic or thrombolytic agents increases the risk of hemorrhage; however, heparin is often administered concurrently with intravenous thrombolytic therapy for treatment of acute coronary arterial occlusion or with low doses of thrombolytic agents given intra-arterially; also, thrombolytic therapy may be administered following initial anticoagulant therapy)
(anticoagulants are recommended to prevent additional thrombus formation following thrombolytic therapy for most indications;

however, following intravenous thrombolytic therapy for acute coronary arterial occlusion, the need for anticoagulant administration should be determined on an individual basis; if an anticoagulant is administered under these circumstances, careful monitoring of the patient is recommended because studies have shown that heparin, when administered after intravenous streptokinase for this indication, increases the risk of hemorrhage)

» Antifibrinolytic agents, such as:
  Aminocaproic acid
  Aprotinin
  Tranexamic acid
    (the actions of antifibrinolytic agents and of thrombolytic agents are mutually antagonistic; although antifibrinolytic agents may be effective in treating severe hemorrhage caused by thrombolytic agents, controlled studies to verify their efficacy and safety have not been done)

Antihypertensive agents or
Other hypotension-producing medications
  (the risk of severe hypotension may be increased, especially when streptokinase is administered rapidly for treatment of coronary arterial occlusion)

» Cefamandole or
» Cefoperazone or
» Cefotetan or
» Plicamycin or
» Valproic acid
  (these medications may cause hypoprothrombinemia; in addition, plicamycin or valproic acid may inhibit platelet aggregation; concurrent use with a thrombolytic agent may increase the risk of severe hemorrhage and is not recommended)

Corticosteroids, glucocorticoids or
Corticotropin, chronic therapeutic use or
Ethacrynic acid or
Salicylates, nonacetylated
  (gastrointestinal ulceration or hemorrhage may occur during therapy with these medications and cause increased risk of severe hemorrhage in patients receiving thrombolytic therapy)

» Nonsteroidal anti-inflammatory drugs (NSAIDs), especially:
  Aspirin
  Indomethacin
  Phenylbutazone or
» Other platelet aggregation inhibitors (see *Appendix II*), especially:
  Sulfinpyrazone
  Ticlopidine
    (concurrent use of a platelet aggregation inhibitor and a thrombolytic agent may increase the risk of bleeding and is generally not recommended [except when aspirin therapy for acute myocardial infarction is initiated concurrently with thrombolytic therapy])
    (initiation of aspirin therapy [160 mg per day] before or during intravenous administration of alteplase, anistreplase, or streptokinase for treatment of acute coronary arterial occlusion may reduce significantly the risk of reocclusion, reinfarction, stroke, and death without increasing the risk of adverse effects [as compared to the thrombolytic agent or aspirin alone]; however, larger doses of aspirin have been shown to increase the risk of bleeding in patients receiving thrombolytic agents for other indications; the possibility of hemorrhage should be considered and the patient carefully monitored)
    (the potential occurrence of gastrointestinal ulceration and/or hemorrhage during therapy with NSAIDs [including analgesic or antirheumatic doses of aspirin] or sulfinpyrazone may also cause increased risk to patients receiving thrombolytic therapy)

Thiotepa
  (urokinase may increase the efficacy of thiotepa in the treatment of bladder cancer by acting as a plasminogen activator and increasing the amount of thiotepa in tumor tissue)

## Laboratory value alterations
The following have been selected on the basis of their potential clinical significance (possible effect in parentheses where appropriate)—not necessarily inclusive (» = major clinical significance):

With diagnostic test results
  Coagulation tests and
  Tests for systemic fibrinolysis
    (the fibrinolytic activity of thrombolytic agents persists *in vitro*; unless the patient is extremely resistant to thrombolytic therapy, degradation of fibrinogen in blood samples will lead to unreliable test results [when specific measurements of fibrinogen, rather than a general indication that fibrinolysis is occurring, are required]; the addition of a fibrinolysis inhibitor, e.g., aprotinin [150 to 200 Kallikrein Inhibitor Units per mL of blood] or aminocaproic acid may reduce this effect)

With physiology/laboratory test values
  Activated partial thromboplastin time (APTT) and
  Prothrombin time (PT) and
  Thrombin time (TT)
    (values will be increased unless the patient is extremely resistant to thrombolytic therapy)
  Alpha$_2$-antiplasmin activity and
  Factor V activity and
  Factor VIII activity and
  Fibrinogen activity and
  Plasminogen activity
    (will be decreased unless the patient is extremely resistant to thrombolytic therapy; significant recovery of fibrinogen activity may occur within 18 to 36 hours after discontinuation of thrombolytic therapy, but return of fibrinogen activity to pretreatment values may require up to 48 hours after discontinuation of thrombolytic therapy; recovery of plasminogen activity may also require more than 30 hours)
  Blood pressure
    (may be decreased, especially when a thrombolytic agent is administered rapidly for treatment of acute coronary arterial occlusion; a decrease in blood pressure [not secondary to anaphylaxis or bleeding], which may be severe, has also been reported in about 10% of anistreplase-treated patients)
  Fibrinogen- and fibrin-degradation products (FDP/fdp) concentrations
    (will be increased unless the patient is extremely resistant to thrombolytic therapy; return to pretreatment values may require up to 48 hours after discontinuation of thrombolytic therapy)
  Hematocrit values and
  Hemoglobin concentrations
    (moderate reduction not related to clinical bleeding has been reported in 20% of patients receiving thrombolytic therapy)

## Medical considerations/Contraindications
The medical considerations/contraindications included have been selected on the basis of their potential clinical significance (reasons given in parentheses where appropriate)—not necessarily inclusive (» = major clinical significance).

*Except under special circumstances, this medication should not be used when the following medical problems exist:*

For all thrombolytic agents
» Aneurysm, dissecting and/or intracranial, confirmed or suspected or
» Arteriovenous malformation or
» Bleeding, active or
» Brain tumor, primary, or neoplasm metastatic to the central nervous system (CNS) from other primary sites or
» Cerebrovascular accident, or history of or
» Neurosurgery, intracranial or intraspinal, within past 2 months or
» Surgery, thoracic, recent or
» Trauma to the CNS, recent
    (increased risk of uncontrollable hemorrhage)
» Hypertension, severe, uncontrolled, i.e., ≥ 200 mm Hg systolic and/or ≥ 120 mm Hg diastolic
    (increased risk of cerebral hemorrhage)

*For alteplase used to treat acute ischemic stroke (in addition to medical problems listed above)*
» Bleeding diathesis, such as
    Heparin therapy within 48 hours preceding the onset of stroke along with an elevated APTT at presentation
    Oral anticoagulant therapy with a PT > 15 seconds
    Platelet count < 100,000 per mm$^3$ or
» Hemorrhage, intracranial, evidence of on pretreatment evaluation, or history of or
» Hemorrhage, subarachnoid, suspected or
» Hypertension, severe, uncontrolled, i.e., > 185 mm Hg systolic or > 110 mm Hg diastolic or
» Seizure at the onset of stroke or
» Stroke, recent
    (increased risk of bleeding, which could result in significant disability or death)

*For anistreplase and streptokinase (in addition to medical problems listed above)*
» Anaphylaxis or other severe allergic reaction to streptokinase or anistreplase, history of
    (increased risk of anaphylaxis)

***Risk-benefit should be considered when the following medical problems exist:***

*For all thrombolytic agents*
    Allergic reaction, mild, to the thrombolytic agent considered for use, history of
    Any condition in which the risk of bleeding or hemorrhage is present or would be difficult to control because of its location, such as:
        Cardiopulmonary resuscitation with possibility of internal injury, recent
        Cerebrovascular disease
»   Childbirth within past 10 days
»   Coagulation defects, uncontrolled, or other hemostatic defects, including those secondary to severe hepatic or renal disease
»   Endocarditis, bacterial, subacute
»   Gastrointestinal bleeding, severe, within past 10 days
        Gastrointestinal lesion or ulcer, active or history of
        Genitourinary bleeding within past 10 days
        Hemorrhagic retinopathy, diabetic, or other hemorrhagic ophthalmic conditions
        Hepatic function impairment, severe
        Hypertension, moderate, not optimally controlled, i.e., 180 to 200 mm Hg systolic and/or 110 to 120 mm Hg diastolic
        Invasive procedure, such as lumbar puncture, paracentesis, or thoracentesis, recent
        Knitted dacron graft
»   Neurosurgical procedure more than 2 months previously
»   Organ biopsy within past 10 days
        Pregnancy
»   Puncture of noncompressible blood vessel within past 10 days
»   Surgery, major, other than neurosurgery or thoracic surgery, within past 10 days
        Trauma, minor, recent, other than to the CNS
»   Trauma, severe, recent, other than to the CNS
        Tuberculosis, active, with cavitation of recent onset
    Infection at or near site of thrombus, obstructed intravenous catheter, or occluded arteriovenous cannula
        (risk of spreading the infection into and via the circulation)
    Mitral stenosis with atrial fibrillation or other indications of probable left heart thrombus
        (risk of new embolic phenomena including those to cerebral vessels)
    Pericarditis, acute
        (risk of hemopericardium, which may lead to cardiac tamponade)

*For alteplase used to treat acute ischemic stroke (in addition to medical problems listed above)*
»   Infarct signs, major, on cranial computed tomographic scan, e.g., substantial edema, mass effect, or midline shift or
»   Neurologic deficit, severe, i.e., National Institues of Health Stroke Scale score > 22 at presentation
        (increased risk of intracranial hemorrhage)

*For anistreplase and streptokinase (in addition to medical problems listed above)*
»   Anistreplase or streptokinase therapy within past 5 days to 1 year or Streptococcal infection, recent
        (antistreptococcal antibodies are likely to be present in the circulation; these antibodies may cause a temporary resistance to the therapeutic effects of anistreplase or streptokinase and/or an increased risk of severe allergic reactions to the medication; although resistance may be overcome by increasing the dosage, use of an alternate thrombolytic agent [alteplase or urokinase] is advisable if thrombolytic therapy is needed within 1 year after anistreplase or streptokinase therapy or streptococcal infection)

**Patient monitoring**
The following may be especially important in patient monitoring (other tests may be warranted in some patients, depending on condition; » = major clinical significance):

*Prior to initiation of therapy*
Note:   Initiation of therapy for acute coronary arterial occlusion must **not** be delayed until the results of the tests recommended below are available. However, blood may be drawn prior to initiation of therapy so that appropriate tests can be performed to determine the hemostatic status of the patient, especially if a potential bleeding problem exists or is suspected, and/or to establish baseline values.

»   Coagulation tests, such as: Activated partial thromboplastin time (APTT)
    Fibrin/fibrinogen degradation product (FDP/fdp) titer
    Fibrinogen concentration
    Prothrombin time (PT)
    Thrombin time (TT) and
»   Hematocrit values and
»   Hemoglobin concentrations and
»   Platelet count
        (recommended prior to initiation of therapy to determine the hemostatic status of the patient and/or to establish baseline values so that the presence of fibrinolysis can be confirmed during therapy; heparin therapy should be discontinued before thrombolytic therapy is instituted unless the heparin is being given in conjunction with urokinase for intracoronary administration; also the APTT or TT should be less than 2 times the control value before thrombolytic therapy is instituted)
»   Electrocardiogram (ECG)
        (recommended when acute coronary arterial thrombosis is suspected, to confirm diagnosis and to aid in selecting patients in whom thrombolytic therapy is likely to be most beneficial)

*During and/or following therapy*
    Coagulation tests, such as APTT, PT, or TT and/or
    Tests of fibrinolytic activity, such as fibrinogen concentration, FDP/fdp titer, reptilase clotting time, and/or whole blood euglobulin lysis time
        (recommended 3 to 4 hours following initiation of intravenous therapy for indications other than acute coronary arterial thrombosis; these tests may be repeated every 12 hours for the duration of therapy, if necessary, to determine that a fibrinolytic state exists; however, such tests do not reliably predict either efficacy of medication or risk of bleeding and are not currently recommended for determining maintenance dosage; a TT value equal to or greater than 1.5 times the control value in seconds, or a decrease of fibrinogen concentration to 50% or less of the control value [with alteplase or anistreplase, a reduction to 75% of the control value may be sufficient], indicates that fibrinolysis is occurring)

Note:   Confirmation of fibrinolysis does **not** require that all of the tests listed above be used for each patient. The selection of a particular test for monitoring thrombolytic therapy depends upon physician preference and available laboratory facilities.

    Because heparin also prolongs APTT, PT, and TT, the results of these determinations may be misleading if heparin has been or is being administered; tests that more directly measure fibrinolytic activity may be more reliable.

    Computed tomography and/or
    Impedance plethysmography and/or
    Quantitative Doppler effect determination and/or
    Visualization of affected vessel via angiography or venography
        (may be useful in assessing restoration of blood flow; also, may aid in determining optimum duration of therapy; however, repeated venograms are not recommended)
    Coronary angiography and/or
    Myocardial scanning, radionuclide
        (may be useful for monitoring effectiveness of therapy for coronary arterial thrombosis in evolving transmural myocardial infarction; coronary angiography and myocardial scanning may also be useful for assessing the patency of the coronary vasculature and for determining whether further treatment to prevent reocclusion is needed; however, coronary angiography increases the risk of adverse effects, including severe bleeding, when performed within several days after thrombolytic therapy; it is recommended that the procedure be performed only when necessary [as determined by signs and symptoms of persistent ischemia], preferably after a delay of 7 to 10 days following thrombolytic therapy)
    Creatine kinase activity or other cardiac enzyme determination
        (may be useful for monitoring effectiveness of therapy for acute coronary arterial thrombosis)
»   Electrocardiogram (ECG)
        (monitoring during and following administration for treatment of acute coronary arterial thrombosis is recommended to detect reperfusion atrial or ventricular arrhythmias; also, may be useful as a means of determining effectiveness of treatment because reversal of some abnormalities may occur with recanalization)
    Hematocrit values
        (monitoring recommended to detect possible blood loss during and following thrombolytic therapy)
»   Mental status and
»   Neurologic status
        (monitoring recommended because altered sensorium or neurologic changes may be indicative of intracranial bleeding)
    Stool tests for occult blood loss and
    Urine tests for hematuria
        (recommended periodically during therapy)

» Vital signs, such as blood pressure, pulse, respiratory rate, and temperature
  (continuous monitoring recommended during therapy for acute coronary arterial occlusion to detect adverse effects such as bradycardia, hypotension, and allergic reactions; a reduction in the infusion rate is usually sufficient to correct hypotension)
  (monitoring recommended at least every 4 hours during therapy for other indications; however, a lower extremity should **not** be used for blood pressure determinations when there is a risk of dislodging deep vein thrombi that may be present)

## Side/Adverse Effects

Note: Rarely, thrombolysis causes clot fragmentation with migration of the fragments resulting in additional embolic complications. Patients should be monitored for new embolic phenomena.

Bleeding, the most common side effect encountered during thrombolytic therapy, occurs most frequently at invaded sites (e.g., sites of arterial punctures, venous cutdowns, recent surgery) because thrombolytic agents promote lysis of the fibrin deposits that are needed to maintain hemostasis at these sites. The risk of bleeding at invaded sites is not reduced by administration of a relatively clot-selective agent such as alteplase. Studies comparing alteplase with streptokinase have shown a similar incidence of internal bleeding with both agents. However, most patients in these studies also received heparin or other potentially hemorrhagic medications concurrently with and/or immediately following the thrombolytic agent. Therefore, the frequency of hemorrhage attributable solely to the thrombolytic agent has not been determined. In some patients, bleeding may be severe enough to result in anemia or shock.

Chest pain or cardiac arrhythmias may occur during or following thrombolytic therapy for acute coronary arterial thrombosis. These are not direct effects of the medication. Chest pain may indicate treatment failure or reocclusion. Cardiac arrhythmias may be associated with the myocardial infarction itself, or may be induced by sudden reperfusion. Specific arrhythmias that have been reported include sinus bradycardia, accelerated idioventricular rhythm, ventricular premature depolarizations, ventricular tachycardia, second- and third-degree atrioventricular block, atrial fibrillation, and (especially in patients with coronary instrumentation) ventricular fibrillation. Hypotension may occur in association with reperfusion bradyarrhythmias.

Nausea and vomiting have also been reported during thrombolytic therapy. However, a causal relationship to the medication has not been established because these symptoms occur frequently during acute myocardial infarction.

The lys-plasminogen used in manufacturing anistreplase is obtained from human plasma. To reduce the risk of the patient's contracting viral infections that may be transmitted via human blood–derived products, the material is tested for viral antigens or particles and heat-treated to inactivate viral particles. Hepatitis has not been reported to date.

The following effects have been selected on the basis of their potential clinical significance (possible signs and symptoms in parentheses where appropriate)—not necessarily inclusive:

**Those indicating need for medical attention**
Incidence more frequent
  ***Bleeding or oozing from cuts, invaded or disturbed sites, wounds, or gums; decreased blood pressure, not secondary to bleeding or to streptokinase-induced anaphylaxis***—may be severe, especially when a thrombolytic agent is given rapidly and/or when other medications having hypotensive actions, such as vasodilators or morphine, are used concurrently

Incidence more frequent with anistreplase and streptokinase; less frequent with urokinase
  ***Fever***
  Note: Elevations of body temperature by about 1.5 °F occur in up to 33%, and body temperature as high as 104 °F has been reported in about 3.5%, of patients receiving streptokinase. Approximately 2 to 3% of patients receiving urokinase develop a febrile reaction to the medication. *Fever* has also been reported with alteplase, but a causal relationship has not been established.

Incidence less frequent or rare
  ***Allergic reaction*** (flushing or redness of skin; mild headache; mild muscle pain; nausea; skin rash, hives, or itching; troubled breathing or wheezing)—less frequent with streptokinase and rare with alteplase or urokinase; ***bleeding into subcutaneous tissues*** (bruising); ***cholesterol embolism***—with alteplase, anistreplase, and streptokinase; ***internal bleeding*** (abdominal pain or swelling; back pain or backaches; bloody urine; bloody or black, tarry stools; constipation caused by hemorrhage-induced paralytic ileus or intestinal obstruction; coughing up blood; dizziness; headaches, sudden, severe, and/or continuing; joint pain, stiffness, or swelling; muscle pain or stiffness, severe or continuing; nosebleeds; unexpected or unusually heavy bleeding from vagina; vomiting of blood or material that looks like coffee grounds); ***stroke, hemorrhagic or thromboembolic*** (confusion; double vision; impairment of speech; weakness in arms or legs)—more frequent with alteplase

  Note: Individual symptoms of *internal bleeding* depend on the site of bleeding and have not necessarily been reported with all of the thrombolytic agents; internal bleeding has been reported following intracoronary arterial administration as well as following intravenous administration; with alteplase, the incidences of gastrointestinal, genitourinary, and retroperitoneal bleeding are 5%, 4%, and < 1%, respectively; the incidence of intracranial hemorrhage (ICH) in patients with acute myocardial infarction treated with alteplase is 0.4% with total doses of 100 mg or 1 to 1.4 mg per kg of body weight (mg/kg) and 1.3% with a total dose of 150 mg; the incidence of ICH in patients treated with alteplase for acute ischemic stroke was found to be 15.4% in trials.

Incidence rare—for anistreplase, streptokinase, and urokinase
  ***Allergic reaction, severe, or anaphylaxis*** (changes in facial skin color; fast or irregular breathing; large, hive-like swellings on eyelids, face, mouth, lips, or tongue; puffiness or swelling of the eyelids or around the eyes; shortness of breath, troubled breathing, tightness in chest, and/or wheezing; skin rash, hives, and/or itching)—may also include anaphylactic shock with sudden, severe decrease in blood pressure

  Note: An *anaphylactic reaction* has been reported in a patient following a second course of streptokinase given 1 month after the first course for clearance of an occluded arteriovenous shunt. Therefore, the probability of systemic absorption of streptokinase following use for this purpose must be considered.

**Those not indicating need for medical attention**
Incidence rare
  *Skin lesions*—with streptokinase

## Patient Consultation

As an aid to patient consultation, refer to *Advice for the Patient, Thrombolytic Agents (Systemic)*.

In providing consultation, consider emphasizing the following selected information (» = major clinical significance):

**Before receiving this medication**
» Conditions affecting use, especially:
    Allergic reaction to the thrombolytic agent considered for use, history of, especially a severe allergic reaction to anistreplase or streptokinase
    Use in the elderly—Increased risk of hemorrhage
    Other medications, especially anticoagulants, antifibrinolytic agents, enoxaparin, heparin, hypoprothrombinemia-inducing cephalosporins, nonsteroidal anti-inflammatory drugs, platelet aggregation inhibitors, plicamycin, and valproic acid
    Other medical problems, especially conditions leading to an increased risk of uncontrollable or cerebral hemorrhage, and, for anistreplase and streptokinase, prior treatment with either agent (within past 12 months)

**Proper use of this medication**
» Proper dosing

**Precautions after receiving this medication**
» Importance of compliance with strict bed rest or other measures to minimize bleeding

**Side/adverse effects**
Signs of potential side effects, especially bleeding or oozing from cuts, invaded or disturbed sites, wounds, or gums; decreased blood pressure, not secondary to bleeding or streptokinase-induced anaphylaxis; fever; allergic reaction; bleeding into subcutaneous tissues; cholesterol embolism; internal bleeding; hemorrhagic or thromboembolic stroke; and severe allergic reaction or anaphylaxis

## General Dosing Information

The activity and doses of alteplase are expressed in milligrams, the activity and doses of anistreplase are expressed in units, and the activity and doses of streptokinase and urokinase are expressed in International Units (IU). However, in some countries, individual products may be labeled in other units. Different tests and standards are used to determine activity of each thrombolytic agent.

Thrombolytic therapy for indications other than acute coronary arterial thrombosis and catheter clearance should be performed only in a hospital with the facilities and trained personnel necessary for performance of the recommended diagnostic and monitoring techniques.

Thrombolytic therapy should be instituted as soon as possible following the onset of clinical symptoms because resistance to lysis increases with the age of the thrombus. For coronary arterial thrombosis or occlusion in evolving transmural myocardial infarction, rapid initiation of treatment is critical. However, patients receiving treatment within 6 to 12 hours following the onset of symptoms may also benefit from thrombolytic therapy. In patients who experience intermittent symptoms resulting from alternating coronary artery occlusion and spontaneous recanalization, thrombolytic therapy may limit the extent of myocardial damage even if given late. In addition, late thrombolytic therapy may limit myocardial damage by providing collateral flow in the event of subsequent coronary artery occlusion. For other indications, treatment should preferably be started within:
- Pulmonary embolism—5 to 7 days.
- Deep venous thrombosis—3 to 4 days, although treatment started later may be somewhat successful.
- Arterial thrombosis or thromboembolism (noncoronary)—3 days, although treatment started later may be successful.

Factors that may affect the success of thrombolytic therapy include the age, size, and location of the thrombus, and the extent of pretreatment perfusion, with most failures occurring when no blood is flowing past the thrombus (grade 0 flow as defined in the Thrombolysis in Myocardial Infarction [TIMI] trials). Factors that decrease the efficiency or activation potential of the fibrinolytic system include extremes in body temperature, elevated concentration of endogenous inhibitors, the presence of abnormal proteins or dysfunctional components of the fibrinolytic system, and the presence of high titers of antistreptokinase antibodies.

Prior to initiation of intravenous thrombolytic therapy for indications other than acute coronary arterial thrombosis, heparin (if being given) should be discontinued and the patient's thrombin time (TT) or activated partial thromboplastin time (APTT) should be less than twice the control value.

Thrombolytic agents should be administered via a constant infusion pump. A separate intravenous line, which should be established prior to initiation of thrombolytic therapy to reduce the need for venipuncture during treatment, should be used for administration of other medications, if required.

To minimize the risk of bleeding during thrombolytic therapy, the patient should be kept on strict bed rest and pressure dressings applied to recently invaded sites. *Nonessential handling or moving of the patient, invasive procedures (biopsy, etc.), and intramuscular injections must be avoided. Only essential procedures or diagnostic tests should be performed.* Cutdowns should be performed only if unavoidable. Venipunctures should be performed as carefully and infrequently as possible, preferably only in arm vessels, using a 23-gauge (or smaller) needle. If an arterial puncture is necessary, an upper extremity distal vessel should be used. Manual pressure should be applied for 30 minutes after the arterial puncture, followed by application of a pressure dressing. The puncture site should be checked frequently for signs of bleeding. Profuse bleeding may persist for a prolonged period of time.

*Therapy should be discontinued immediately if bleeding not controllable by local pressure occurs.* Some clinicians recommend that thrombolytic therapy be discontinued permanently if such bleeding occurs. However, other clinicians suggest that reinstitution of therapy using one half the original maintenance dose may be considered if the results of blood coagulation tests performed shortly after the bleeding episode show values higher than the normal therapeutic range. These clinicians further suggest that therapy not be reinstituted until the results of blood coagulation tests have returned to within the normal therapeutic range, and, if bleeding recurs, that therapy be discontinued permanently.

Anticoagulation with heparin (preferably by continuous intravenous infusion) followed, if necessary, by a coumarin or indandione derivative is recommended following thrombolytic therapy for deep venous thrombosis or pulmonary embolism to prevent further thrombus formation. It is usually recommended that heparin be administered only after the patient's TT or APTT returns to less than twice the normal control value. This usually occurs within 2 hours after cessation of thrombolytic therapy. However, heparin therapy may be instituted earlier, depending on clinical circumstances. A loading dose of heparin is generally not recommended, but may be required in some circumstances, especially if the TT or APTT has fallen to substantially less than twice the control value. Administration of a coumarin- or indandione-derivative anticoagulant, if necessary, should be started at least 5 days prior to discontinuation of heparin.

Angioplasty, coronary bypass surgery, or another revascularization procedure may be necessary to provide long-lasting protection against reocclusion, especially if extensive stenosis (> 80%) persists in the affected artery. Performance of these procedures within several days after thrombolytic therapy increases the risk of adverse effects, including hemorrhage, and should therefore be delayed if possible. If such a procedure cannot be postponed, replacement of fibrinogen to 50% of normal activity by administration of cryoprecipitate may reduce the risk of bleeding complications. If systemic fibrinolysis induced by the thrombolytic agent has not yet ceased, administration of an antifibrinolytic agent (e.g., aminocaproic acid, tranexamic acid) will be necessary to prevent immediate lysis of the infused fibrinogen, but the risks of administering an antifibrinolytic agent to a patient undergoing a revascularization procedure must be carefully considered.

### For treatment of acute coronary arterial thrombosis

A suitable antiarrhythmic agent may be administered prior to or concurrently with the thrombolytic agent to prevent reperfusion arrhythmias.

It has been shown that aspirin, administered in conjunction with streptokinase for treatment of coronary arterial thrombosis, significantly decreases the occurrence of reocclusion, reinfarction, stroke, and death, as compared to aspirin or streptokinase administered alone. Although the benefit of aspirin administered with alteplase or anistreplase has not been studied, it is widely held that the combination of aspirin and any thrombolytic agent is likely to have benefit similar to that of aspirin and streptokinase. It is therefore recommended that at least 160 mg of aspirin be administered as soon as possible after myocardial infarction is suspected. It is also recommended that the aspirin be chewed so that it reaches the bloodstream rapidly.

Heparin (in dosage sufficient to prolong the APTT to 1.5 to 2 times the control value) has been administered in conjunction with thrombolytic therapy for acute coronary arterial occlusion. However, recent studies have found that the addition of heparin to a regimen of aspirin and thrombolysis does not significantly improve survival, but does increase the risk of major bleeding and cerebral hemorrhage. In addition, there are little data to show that heparin contributes to sustained coronary artery patency when administered with aspirin and streptokinase or with aspirin and anistreplase. When administered with aspirin and alteplase, intravenous heparin seems to improve coronary artery patency slightly, but the benefit must be weighed against the risk of hemorrhage associated with the use of intravenous heparin.

### For arteriovenous cannula occlusion clearance

First, the cannula should be cleared by careful syringe technique, using heparinized saline solution. If this procedure is unsuccessful, a thrombolytic agent may be used after the effects of prior anticoagulation have been allowed to diminish. After the thrombolytic agent has been instilled in the cannula, the affected cannula limb(s) should be clamped for 2 hours and the patient closely observed for possible adverse effects. After treatment, the contents of the affected cannula limb(s) should be aspirated, and the cannula flushed with saline solution and reconnected.

### For intravenous catheter obstruction clearance

The manufacturer's product information for urokinase should be consulted for a complete description of the recommended procedure.

Excessive pressure should be avoided when instilling a thrombolytic agent into the catheter in order to avoid rupture of the catheter or expulsion of the clot into the circulation.

To prevent air from entering an open central venous catheter, the patient should be instructed to exhale and hold his or her breath any time the catheter is not connected to intravenous tubing or to a syringe.

Intravenous catheters may be obstructed by substances not responsive to thrombolysis (i.e., substances other than clotted blood or fibrin). The possibility that such a precipitate may be forced into the circulation must be considered.

### For treatment of adverse effects

Recommended treatment includes
- For minor bleeding—Applying local measures, such as pressure at the site of bleeding. Although efficacy has not been proved, topical application of an antifibrinolytic agent such as aminocaproic acid may help to stop stubborn minor bleeding. Thrombolytic therapy need not be discontinued unless such measures are unsuccessful and it is determined that the risk to the patient outweighs the benefit of continuing treatment.
- For uncontrollable or internal bleeding—Discontinuing thrombolytic therapy. If necessary, replacement of lost blood and reversal of the bleeding tendency can be accomplished by administration of fresh whole blood, packed red blood cells, cryoprecipitate or fresh frozen plasma, platelets, and/or desmopressin. Plasma volume expanders may be administered; however, dextrans should **not** be used because of their platelet aggregation–inhibiting activity. Heparin, if being given, should be discontinued and consideration given to administration of the heparin antagonist protamine. Also, an antifibrinolytic agent such as aminoca-

proic acid (5 grams initially or over a period of 1 hour, followed by 1 gram per hour for approximately 4 to 8 hours or until the desired response has been obtained), or tranexamic acid may be administered intravenously (preferably by continuous infusion) or orally. However, the efficacy of aminocaproic acid or other antifibrinolytic agents in the treatment of thrombolytic agent–induced hemorrhage has not been documented by controlled studies in humans. Also, the risk of reocclusion or other thrombotic complications must be considered.

- For bradycardia—If necessary, atropine may be administered.
- For reperfusion arrhythmias—Administering a suitable antiarrhythmic agent, such as lidocaine or procainamide. Electrical cardioversion may be needed for ventricular tachycardia or fibrillation.
- For mild hypersensitivity reaction—Administering antihistamines and, if necessary, glucocorticoids.
- For severe hypersensitivity or anaphylactic reaction—Discontinuing thrombolytic therapy and administering epinephrine. Antihistamines and/or glucocorticoids may also be administered as required.
- For sudden hypotension—If sudden hypotension occurs during rapid, high-dose administration, reducing the infusion rate. If sudden hypotension occurs in other circumstances or does not respond to a reduction in the infusion rate, placing the patient in the Trendelenburg position and/or administering volume expanders (other than dextrans), atropine, and/or a vasopressor, e.g., dopamine, as clinical circumstances permit.
- For fever—Administering acetaminophen if treatment is required. Administration of multiple antipyretic doses of aspirin is not recommended.

---

## ALTEPLASE, RECOMBINANT

## Summary of Differences
Indications:
 Indicated in the treatment of acute coronary arterial thrombosis, acute ischemic stroke, and acute pulmonary thromboembolism.
Pharmacology/pharmacokinetics:
 Mechanism of action/effect—
  Acts directly to convert plasminogen to plasmin.
  May be more clot-selective than anistreplase, streptokinase, or urokinase.
 Half-life—
  Biphasic; about 4 minutes for distribution phase and 35 minutes for elimination phase.
Side/adverse effects:
 Incidence of stroke and cerebral hemorrhage greater than with other thrombolytic agents. Incidence and severity of allergic reactions lower than with anistreplase or streptokinase.

## Additional Dosing Information
Alteplase is not antigenic (as are anistreplase and streptokinase) and does not promote antibody formation. Therefore, a second course of alteplase therapy can be administered, if reocclusion occurs, without resistance having developed to the effects of alteplase and without risk of precipitating an anaphylactic reaction. In one study, a second course of alteplase therapy was shown to be effective, without producing significant bleeding complications, in patients exhibiting signs and symptoms of reocclusion following initial thrombolytic therapy for treatment of acute myocardial infarction. However, it must still be considered that a second course of therapy, if initiated before systemic effects of the first dose have subsided, may increase the risk of severe hemorrhage.

A large multi-center study has shown that alteplase, administered in an accelerated or front-loaded dosing regimen within 6 hours of the onset of symptoms of myocardial infarction, may achieve earlier and more complete patency of the infarct-affected artery than does streptokinase in combination with intravenous or subcutaneous heparin, or a combination of alteplase, streptokinase, and intravenous heparin. Twenty-four-hour and 30-day mortality was also lower with the accelerated or front-loaded alteplase regimen than with these combinations.

### For treatment of acute ischemic stroke
The treatment of acute ischemic stroke with alteplase should be limited to facilities that can provide appropriate evaluation and management of intracranial hemorrhage.

*Treatment should only be initiated within 3 hours after the onset of stroke symptoms, and after exclusion of intracranial hemorrhage by a cranial computed tomographic scan or other diagnostic imaging method sensitive to the presence of hemorrhage.*

In patients who have not recently been treated with oral anticoagulants or heparin, alteplase may be given prior to the availability of coagulation study results. However, treatment should be stopped if either a pretreatment prothrombin time > 15 seconds or an elevated APTT is identified.

Blood pressure should be monitored frequently and controlled with appropriate medication during and following alteplase administration.

The safety and efficacy of concomitant administration of heparin and aspirin during the first 24 hours after symptom onset have not been investigated.

## Parenteral Dosage Forms
### ALTEPLASE, RECOMBINANT, FOR INJECTION
**Usual adult dose**
Thrombosis, coronary arterial, acute—
 Standard regimen:
  For patients weighing less than 65 kg—Intravenous, 1.25 mg per kg of body weight administered over a period of three hours, as follows:
   First hour—60% of the total dose. Initially, 6 to 10% of the total dose is given by direct intravenous injection within the first one or two minutes. The next 50 to 54% of the total dose is given via intravenous infusion during the remainder of the hour.
   Second hour—20% of the total dose, via intravenous infusion.
   Third hour—20% of the total dose, via intravenous infusion.
  For patients weighing 65 kg or more—Intravenous, 100 mg, administered over a period of three hours, as follows:
   First hour—60 mg. Initially, 6 to 10 mg is given by direct intravenous injection within the first one or two minutes. The next 50 to 54 mg is given via intravenous infusion during the remainder of the hour.
   Second hour—20 mg, via intravenous infusion.
   Third hour—20 mg, via intravenous infusion.
 Accelerated regimen:
  For patients weighing less than or equal to 67 kg—Intravenous, initially 15 mg followed by an infusion of 0.75 mg per kg of body weight, up to 50 mg, administered over a period of thirty minutes. The infusion should continue for an additional sixty minutes at a dose of 0.5 mg per kg of body weight, up to 35 mg.
  For patients weighing 67 kg or more—Intravenous, initially 15 mg by direct intravenous injection, followed by 50 mg infused over the next thirty minutes, and then 35 mg infused over the next sixty minutes.
 Note: It is recommended that intravenous heparin be administered in conjunction with accelerated-dose alteplase at an initial dose of 5000 USP Heparin Units, followed by 1000 USP Heparin Units per hour (1200 USP Heparin Units per hour for patients weighing more than 80 kg), with the dose adjusted to raise the activated partial thromboplastin time to between 60 and 85 seconds.
Stroke, acute ischemic[1]—
 Intravenous, 0.9 mg per kg of body weight (up to a maximum of 90 mg) infused over sixty minutes, with 10% of the total dose administered by direct intravenous injection over the first minute.
Thromboembolism, pulmonary, acute[1]—
 Intravenous infusion, 100 mg, administered over a period of two hours.
 Note: It is recommended that heparin be used in conjunction with alteplase for treatment of acute pulmonary embolism. Heparin should be administered only if the patient's activated partial thromboplastin time or thrombin time value is no higher than twice the control value, near the end of or immediately following the alteplase infusion.

**Usual pediatric dose**
Dosage has not been established.

**Size(s) usually available**
U.S.—
 50 mg (Rx) [*Activase* (vials contain a vacuum)].
 100 mg (Rx) [*Activase* (vials do *not* contain a vacuum)].
Canada—
 50 mg (Rx) [*Activase rt-PA* (vials contain a vacuum)].
 100 mg (Rx) [*Activase rt-PA* (vials do *not* contain a vacuum)].

**Packaging and storage**
Store between 2 and 30 °C (36 and 86 °F), unless otherwise specified by manufacturer. Protect from excessive exposure to light.

**Preparation of dosage form**
Alteplase should be reconstituted using the diluent provided (sterile water for injection). Bacteriostatic water for injection must not be used. A large-bore (18-gauge) needle (for use with the 50-mg vials), or the

transfer device (for use with the 100-mg vials) should be used to direct the stream of diluent directly into the lyophilized material.

If a vacuum is not present in the 50-mg vial, it should not be used.

When reconstituting the 100-mg vials using the transfer device, the vial of sterile water for injection, with the transfer device inserted, is held upright while the vial of alteplase is held upside down and pushed down onto the piercing pin of the transfer device. The vials are then inverted to allow the sterile water for injection to flow into the alteplase vial. The resulting colorless to pale yellow, transparent solution will contain 1 mg of alteplase per mL. This solution may be used without further dilution or it may be diluted to a concentration of 0.5 mg per mL using an equal volume of 0.9% sodium chloride injection or 5% dextrose injection. Other infusion solutions or preservative-containing solutions should not be used when further diluting the reconstituted solution. The solution may be mixed with gentle swirling and/or slow inversion; excessive agitation should be avoided. Slight foaming may occur during reconstitution; however, large bubbles dissipate when the solution is left undisturbed for a few minutes.

**Stability**

The reconstituted solution should be used within 8 hours when stored between 2 and 30 °C (36 and 86 °F). It should be discarded if not used within this time. However, because alteplase for injection contains no preservatives, it should not be reconstituted until immediately prior to use. Any unused solution must be discarded.

**Incompatibilities**

*Do not add any other medication to the container of alteplase solution or administer other medications through the same intravenous line.*

---

[1]Not included in Canadian product labeling.

---

## *ANISTREPLASE*

## Summary of Differences

Indications:
   Indicated in the treatment of acute coronary arterial thrombosis.
Pharmacology/pharmacokinetics:
   Mechanism of action/effect—Acts indirectly to promote conversion of plasminogen to plasmin.
   Other actions/effects—Antigenic; promotes antibody formation.
   Half-life—70 to 120 minutes (average about 90 minutes). The deacylation half-life of the complex is about 105 to 120 minutes.
Precautions:
   Medical considerations/contraindications—Caution is required in patients who have had a severe hypersensitivity reaction to prior anistreplase or streptokinase therapy or a prior course of anistreplase or streptokinase therapy within the past 12 months.
Side/adverse effects:
   Incidence of mild hypersensitivity and febrile reactions greater than with alteplase or urokinase.
   May cause severe hypersensitivity reactions including anaphylaxis.

## Additional Dosing Information

It is recommended that equipment and medications (such as epinephrine, glucocorticoids, and antihistamines) for treating anaphylaxis be immediately available whenever anistreplase is administered. Some investigators have administered a glucocorticoid (e.g., 100 mg of hydrocortisone or methylprednisolone, intravenously) and/or an antihistamine (e.g., 50 mg of diphenhydramine, intravenously) prior to anistreplase administration, to decrease the risk of severe hypersensitivity and febrile reactions. However, the prophylactic efficacy of these medications has not been established.

Resistance to anistreplase therapy may occur because of the presence of high titers of antibodies following a prior course of anistreplase or streptokinase therapy. A significant titer of these antibodies generally occurs 5 to 7 days following administration of anistreplase or streptokinase and may persist for 1 year (up to 4 years in some patients). Alteplase or urokinase may be administered if thrombolytic therapy is indicated during this time. A recent streptococcal infection may also result in high titers of antibodies and resistance to anistreplase.

## Parenteral Dosage Forms

### ANISTREPLASE FOR INJECTION

**Usual adult dose**
Thrombosis, coronary arterial, acute—
   Intravenous, 30 units, administered over two to five minutes.

**Usual pediatric dose**
Safety and efficacy have not been established.

**Size(s) usually available**
U.S.—
   30 Units per single-dose vial (Rx) [*Eminase* (human albumin 30 mg)].
Canada—
   30 Units per single-dose vial (Rx) [*Eminase* (human albumin 30 mg)].

**Packaging and storage**
Store between 2 and 8 °C (36 and 46 °F), unless otherwise specified by manufacturer.

**Preparation of dosage form**
Five mL of sterile water for injection should be slowly added to the vial containing anistreplase for injection; the stream of water should be directed against the side of the vial. The vial should then be gently rolled (not shaken), to mix the powder with the liquid. Other measures to minimize foaming should also be used.

**Stability**
The reconstituted solution is to be administered within 30 minutes after reconstitution.

The medication contains no preservative. Each vial is intended to provide a single dose only; any unused solution should be discarded.

**Incompatibilities**
*Do not add any other medication to the container of anistreplase solution or administer other medications through the same intravenous line.*

---

## *STREPTOKINASE*

## Summary of Differences

Indications:
   Indicated in the treatment of acute coronary arterial thrombosis, acute pulmonary thromboembolism, deep venous thrombosis, and acute arterial thromboembolism and thrombosis. Also indicated to clear totally or partially occluded arteriovenous cannulae.
Pharmacology/pharmacokinetics:
   Mechanism of action/effect—Acts indirectly to promote conversion of plasminogen to plasmin.
   Other actions/effects—Antigenic; promotes antibody formation.
   Half-life—Following rapid, high-dose administration: 23 minutes (as active activator complex activity).
Precautions:
   Medical considerations/contraindications—Caution required in patients who have had a severe hypersensitivity reaction to prior streptokinase therapy or a prior course of streptokinase therapy within the past 12 months.
Side/adverse effects:
   Incidence of mild hypersensitivity and febrile reactions greater than with urokinase or alteplase.
   May cause severe hypersensitivity reactions including anaphylaxis or, rarely, skin lesions.

## Additional Dosing Information

It is recommended that equipment and medications (such as epinephrine, glucocorticoids, and antihistamines) for treating anaphylaxis be immediately available whenever streptokinase is administered. Some investigators have administered a glucocorticoid (e.g., 100 mg of hydrocortisone or methylprednisolone, intravenously) and/or an antihistamine (e.g., 50 mg of diphenhydramine, intravenously) prior to streptokinase administration, to decrease the risk of severe hypersensitivity and febrile reactions. However, the prophylactic efficacy of these medications has not been established.

Resistance to streptokinase therapy may occur because of the presence of high titers of antibodies to streptokinase following a prior course of streptokinase or anistreplase therapy. A significant titer of these antibodies generally occurs 5 to 7 days following administration of anistreplase or streptokinase and may persist for 1 year (up to 4 years in some patients). Alteplase or urokinase may be administered if thrombolytic therapy is indicated during this time. A recent streptococcal infection may also result in high titers of antibodies and resistance to streptokinase.

For intravenous administration of streptokinase (for indications other than acute coronary arterial thrombosis), a loading dose of 250,000 International Units (IU) is recommended to overcome mild resistance caused by exposure (without recent active infection) to streptococci. Since this loading dose successfully overcomes resistance in 85 to 90% of patients, many clinicians state that a previously recommended resistance test is now considered unnecessary. However, if a thrombin time (TT) determination or other test of fibrinolysis performed after 4 hours of therapy indicates minimal or no fibrinolytic activity, and no clinical improvement is apparent, the possibility of excessive resistance to streptokinase should be considered. Streptokinase should be discontinued and an alternate thrombolytic agent (alteplase or urokinase, but not anistreplase) administered instead.

A previously recommended regimen of variable maintenance dosage with frequent laboratory monitoring has not been shown to increase the efficacy or safety of streptokinase therapy. Therefore, this regimen is not currently recommended and has been replaced by a fixed maintenance dosage schedule.

The dosage and duration of intravenous therapy vary with the condition being treated. The recommended duration of therapy is 24 hours for acute pulmonary embolism (but up to 72 hours if concurrent deep vein thrombosis is suspected); 24 to 72 hours for arterial thrombosis or thromboembolism; and up to 72 hours for deep vein thrombosis. For the individual patient, tests to determine restoration of blood flow, such as angiography or venography of the affected blood vessel, computed tomography, impedance plethysmography, or quantitative Doppler effect, may be useful in determining the optimum duration of administration.

## Parenteral Dosage Forms

### STREPTOKINASE FOR INJECTION

**Usual adult dose**
Thrombosis, coronary arterial, acute—
  Intravenous, 1,500,000 IU, administered within one hour.
  Intra-arterial (via a coronary artery catheter placed via the Judkins or Sones technique), 20,000 IU initially, followed by 2000 IU per minute for one hour.
  Note: Recanalization may occur in less than one hour; however, treatment should be continued following recanalization, to ensure complete lysis of all thrombotic material.
Thromboembolism, pulmonary, acute or
Thrombosis, deep venous or
Thromboembolism or thrombosis, arterial, acute—
  Intravenous, 250,000 IU as an initial loading dose over thirty minutes, followed by 100,000 IU per hour as a continuous infusion.
Cannula, arteriovenous, clearance—
  100,000 to 250,000 IU, instilled slowly into each occluded cannula limb.

**Usual pediatric dose**
Dosage has not been established.

**Size(s) usually available**
U.S.—
  250,000 IU (Rx) [*Kabikinase; Streptase*].
  750,000 IU (Rx) [*Kabikinase; Streptase*].
  1,500,000 IU (Rx) [*Kabikinase; Streptase*].
Canada—
  250,000 IU (Rx) [*Kabikinase; Streptase*].
  750,000 IU (Rx) [*Kabikinase; Streptase*].
  1,500,000 IU (Rx) [*Kabikinase; Streptase*].

**Packaging and storage**
Store between 15 and 30 °C (59 and 86 °F), unless otherwise specified by manufacturer.

**Preparation of dosage form**
For intracoronary artery or intravenous administration—Manufacturer's prescribing information should be consulted for recommendations for reconstituting and further diluting the individual product.
For arteriovenous cannula obstruction clearance—Two mL of sodium chloride injection or 5% dextrose injection should be added to each 250,000-IU vial of streptokinase.

**Stability**
Streptokinase for injection should be reconstituted immediately prior to use. If not administered shortly following reconstitution, the solution should be stored at 2 to 8 °C (36 to 46 °F). If not used within 8 hours after reconstitution, the solution should be discarded.
One manufacturer states that slight flocculation (described as thin translucent fibers) may occur after reconstitution. Shaking the solution during reconstitution may increase flocculation or cause foaming, and should be avoided. The solution may be administered if slight flocculation is present but should be discarded if flocculation is extensive.

**Incompatibilities**
*Do not add any other medication to the container of streptokinase solution or administer other medications through the same intravenous line.*

---

## UROKINASE

### Summary of Differences
Indications:
  Indicated in the treatment of acute coronary arterial thrombosis, acute pulmonary embolism, and to restore patency to intravenous catheters.
Pharmacology/pharmacokinetics:
  Mechanism of action/effect—Acts directly to convert plasminogen to plasmin.
  Half-life—Up to 20 minutes; may be prolonged in patients with hepatic function impairment.
Side/adverse effects:
  Incidence and severity of allergic or febrile reactions lower than with anistreplase or streptokinase.

### Additional Dosing Information

The dosage and duration of urokinase therapy may vary with the condition being treated. For the individual patient, tests to determine restoration of blood flow, such as angiography or venography of the affected blood vessel, computed tomography, impedance plethysmography, or quantitative Doppler effect, may be useful in determining the optimum duration of administration.

**For lysis of coronary artery thrombi**
Prior to intracoronary arterial administration of urokinase, it is recommended that 2500 to 10,000 USP Heparin Units be administered via direct intravenous injection. Prior heparin administration should be considered when calculating heparin dosage.

## Parenteral Dosage Forms

### UROKINASE FOR INJECTION

**Usual adult dose**
Thrombosis, coronary arterial, acute—
  Intra-arterial (via a coronary artery catheter), 6000 IU (4 mL of a solution containing approximately 1500 IU per mL) per minute.
  Note: The average total dose of urokinase required for lysis of coronary artery thrombi is 500,000 IU.
    Urokinase administration should be continued until the artery is maximally opened, usually 15 to 30 minutes after initial opening. The medication has been administered for periods up to 2 hours.
Thromboembolism, pulmonary, acute—
  Intravenous, 4400 IU per kg of body weight initially over a ten minute period, followed by 4400 IU per kg of body weight per hour for approximately 12 hours.
  Note: Manufacturer's product information should be consulted for recommendations concerning the rate of infusion, based on recommended dilution volume of the product.
Catheter, intravenous, clearance—
  After the intravenous tubing has been disconnected and catheter occlusion confirmed, the catheter should be filled with a solution containing 5000 IU per mL of urokinase.

**Usual pediatric dose**
Catheter, intravenous, clearance—
  After the intravenous tubing has been disconnected and catheter occlusion confirmed, the catheter should be filled with a solution containing 5000 IU per mL of urokinase. Alternatively, an intravenous infusion of 150 IU per kg of body weight per hour may be administered over eight hours.

**Size(s) usually available**
U.S.—
  5000 IU (Rx) [*Abbokinase Open-Cath*].
  9000 IU (Rx) [*Abbokinase Open-Cath*].
  250,000 IU (Rx) [*Abbokinase*].
Canada—
  5000 IU (Rx) [*Abbokinase Open-Cath*].
  250,000 IU (Rx) [*Abbokinase*].

Note: The 5000-IU and 9000-IU sizes are intended for intravenous catheter clearance only. Premeasured diluent is included. After reconstitution, the solution prepared from either size contains 5000 IU per mL.

**Packaging and storage**
Store between 2 and 8 °C (36 and 46 °F), unless otherwise specified by manufacturer. Store *Abbokinase Open-Cath* below 25 °C (77 °F). Protect from freezing.

### Preparation of dosage form
For intravenous administration—Manufacturer's prescribing information should be consulted for recommendations for reconstituting and further diluting the product.

For intracoronary arterial administration—Five mL of sterile water for injection *without preservatives* should be added to each of three 250,000-IU vials of urokinase. The vial should be rolled and tilted (not shaken) to facilitate reconstitution. The contents of the three vials should be added to 500 mL of 5% dextrose injection to make a solution containing approximately 1500 IU per mL.

For intravenous catheter clearance (for the 250,000-IU size only)—Five mL of sterile water for injection *without preservatives* should be added to the vial. The vial should be rolled and tilted (not shaken) to facilitate reconstitution. Then, 1 mL of the reconstituted solution should be added to 9 mL of sterile water for injection to make a solution containing 5000 IU per mL.

### Stability
Because urokinase for injection contains no preservatives, it should not be reconstituted until immediately prior to use. Also, any unused solution must be discarded.

Filaments may form in the solution during reconstitution, especially if the vial is shaken. Shaking the vial should be avoided. If necessary, the solution may be filtered through a 0.45-micron or smaller cellulose membrane filter.

### Incompatibilities
*Do not add any other medication to the container of urokinase solution or administer other medications through the same intravenous line.*

### Selected Bibliography
Anderson HV, Willerson JT. Thrombolysis in acute myocardial infarction. N Engl J Med 1993; 329: 703-9.

Revised: 09/01/94
Interim revision: 08/18/97

---

## THYROGLOBULIN — See *Thyroid Hormones (Systemic)*

## THYROID — See *Thyroid Hormones (Systemic)*

---

# THYROID HORMONES  Systemic

This monograph includes information on the following: 1) Levothyroxine; 2) Liothyronine; 3) Liotrix†; 4) Thyroglobulin*†; 5) Thyroid.

VA CLASSIFICATION (Primary/Secondary):
Levothyroxine—HS851/AN500; DX900
Liothyronine—HS851/AN500; DX900
Liotrix—HS851/AN500
Thyroglobulin—HS851/AN500
Thyroid—HS851/AN500

Commonly used brand name(s): *Armour Thyroid*[5]; *Cytomel*[2]; *Eltroxin*[1]; *Levo-T*[1]; *Levothroid*[1]; *Levoxyl*[1]; *PMS-Levothyroxine Sodium*[1]; *Synthroid*[1]; *Thyrar*[5]; *Thyroid Strong*[5]; *Westhroid*[5].

Another commonly used name for Levothyroxine is L-Thyroxine.

Note: For a listing of dosage forms and brand names by country availability, see *Dosage Forms* section(s).

*Not commercially available in the U.S.
†Not commercially available in Canada.

## Category
Thyroid hormone—Levothyroxine; Liothyronine; Liotrix; Thyroglobulin; Thyroid.
Antineoplastic—Levothyroxine; Liothyronine; Liotrix; Thyroglobulin; Thyroid.
Diagnostic aid (thyroid function)—Levothyroxine; Liothyronine.

## Indications
### Accepted
Hypothyroidism (diagnosis and treatment)—Thyroid hormones are indicated as replacement therapy in the treatment of thyroid hormone deficiency (hypothyroidism) of any etiology (except transient hypothyroidism during the recovery phase of subacute thyroiditis), as well as for simple (nonendemic) goiter and chronic lymphocytic (Hashimoto's) thyroiditis[1].

In general, levothyroxine is the preferred thyroid hormone for use in the treatment of hypothyroidism because of the absence of variability and the ease of monitoring of plasma concentrations; it is the drug of choice in the treatment of congenital hypothyroidism. Liothyronine is recommended by some clinicians because of its short half-life and readily reversible effects for initial therapy in myxedema and myxedema coma, as well as for hypothyroid patients who also have heart disease, although there are significant risks associated with the latter use. Liothyronine may also be preferred during preparation for radioisotope scanning procedures or when gastrointestinal absorption processes are impaired. Disadvantages of thyroid extract and thyroglobulin tablets are their variable potencies and the fact that triiodothyronine ($T_3$) and thyroxine ($T_4$) concentrations fluctuate and cannot be used to regulate dosage. Liotrix is no longer considered advantageous because of the natural conversion of $T_4$ to $T_3$ in the tissues.

Goiter (prophylaxis[1] and treatment)—Thyroid hormones are indicated to suppress the growth of some adenomatous goiters, and to prevent the goitrogenic effects of other medications such as lithium, aminosalicylic acid, and some sulfonamide compounds.

Carcinoma, thyroid (prophylaxis and treatment)[1]—Thyroid hormones are indicated in the treatment of thyrotropin-dependent thyroid gland carcinoma. Some clinicians believe that prophylactic administration of thyroid hormones after neck irradiation will prevent development of thyroid gland carcinoma.

Thyroid function studies—Levothyroxine[1] and liothyronine are indicated as diagnostic aids (for example, the $T_3$ suppression test), although this use has generally been replaced by other tests.

### Unaccepted
Use of thyroid hormones to treat vague symptoms such as dry skin, fatigue, constipation, abnormalities of reproductive function, growth retardation, or obesity without laboratory confirmation of contributing hypothyroidism is inappropriate and may cause hyperthyroidism in euthyroid individuals.

[1]Not included in Canadian product labeling.

## Pharmacology/Pharmacokinetics
### Physicochemical characteristics
Source—
  Natural products include thyroglobulin and thyroid.
  Synthetic products include levothyroxine, liothyronine, and liotrix.
Composition—
  Levothyroxine: $T_4$ (thyroxine), with approximately 30% being converted to $T_3$ in peripheral tissues.
  Liothyronine: $T_3$ (triiodothyronine).
  Liotrix, thyroglobulin, and thyroid: $T_3$ and $T_4$.
Molecular weight—
  Levothyroxine sodium: 798.86 (anhydrous).
  Liothyronine sodium: 672.96.
Equivalent strength (approximate), based on clinical response—
  Levothyroxine: 100 mcg (0.1 mg) or less.
  Liothyronine: 25 mcg (0.025 mg).
  Liotrix—
    Levothyroxine and liothyronine: 60 mcg (0.06 mg) and 15 mcg (0.015 mg), or 50 mcg (0.05 mg) and 12.5 mcg (0.0125 mg), respectively.
  Thyroglobulin: 60 mg.
  Thyroid USP: 60 mg.
Note: Because of the difficulty in measuring actual hormonal content of thyroglobulin and Thyroid USP, the measurable amounts of levothyroxine and liothyronine in these preparations may be less than the clinical equivalent. However, for purposes of dosage adjustment, the above equivalent strengths are appropriate.

### Mechanism of action/Effect
The action of thyroid hormones is not completely understood, but they have both catabolic (calorigenic) and anabolic effects and are therefore involved in normal metabolism, growth, and development, especially the development of the central nervous system (CNS) of infants. A feed-

back system involving the hypothalamus, anterior pituitary, and thyroid normally regulates circulating thyroid hormone concentrations.

### Absorption
Oral—
- Levothyroxine: Incomplete and variable, especially when taken with food; average 50 to 75%.
- Liothyronine: Approximately 95%.

Note: Absorption may be reduced in patients with congestive heart failure, malabsorption syndromes, or diarrhea.

### Protein binding
Very high (more than 99%), but not firmly bound.

### Biotransformation
As for endogenous thyroid hormone; levothyroxine (approximately 30%) is deiodinated in peripheral tissues; small amounts are metabolized in the liver and excreted in bile.

### Half-life
Levothyroxine—
- Euthyroid: 6 to 7 days.
- Hypothyroid: 9 to 10 days.
- Hyperthyroid: 3 to 4 days.

Liothyronine—
- Euthyroid: 1 day.
- Hypothyroid: 1.4 days.
- Hyperthyroid: 0.6 day.

Note: Because thyroid and thyroglobulin contain varying amounts of thyroxine and triiodothyronine, their half-lives will vary but will be somewhere between that for $T_4$ and $T_3$.

### Time to peak therapeutic effect
With chronic stable oral dosing—
- Levothyroxine, thyroglobulin, thyroid: 3 to 4 weeks.
- Liothyronine: 48 to 72 hours.

### Duration of therapeutic action
After withdrawal of chronic therapy—
- Levothyroxine, thyroglobulin, thyroid: 1 to 3 weeks.
- Liothyronine: Up to 72 hours.

## Precautions to Consider

Note: The following precautions apply to patients with *abnormal thyroid status* (hypothyroidism or, in some cases, hyperthyroidism). Patients in stable euthyroid condition as a result of continuing thyroid hormone therapy may be expected to respond in the same way as individuals with normal thyroid function and, therefore, the following precautions (except for *Patient monitoring*) do not usually apply in those circumstances.

### Carcinogenicity/Mutagenicity
Studies have not been done in animals. A reported association with breast cancer has not been confirmed and does not justify withholding thyroid hormone treatment.

### Pregnancy/Reproduction
Pregnancy—Thyroid hormones cross the placenta, but only to a limited extent. However, clinical experience in humans has not shown that appropriate use of thyroid hormones causes adverse effects in the fetus. Monitoring of maternal dose is important as maternal dose requirements may change during pregnancy. Intra-amniotic levothyroxine has been used to treat fetal hypothyroidism.

FDA Pregnancy Category A.

### Breast-feeding
Problems in humans have not been documented with appropriate use of thyroid hormones in women who are breast-feeding. Minimal amounts of exogenous thyroid hormones are distributed into breast milk.

### Pediatrics
Studies performed to date have not demonstrated pediatrics-specific problems that would limit the usefulness of thyroid hormones in children. However, caution is necessary in interpreting results of thyroid function tests in neonates, because serum $T_4$ concentrations are transiently elevated and serum $T_3$ concentrations are transiently low, and the infant pituitary is relatively insensitive to the negative feedback effect of thyroid hormones.

### Geriatrics
The elderly may be more sensitive to the effects of thyroid hormones. Thyroid hormone replacement requirements are about 25% lower in some patients over the age of 60 years than in younger adults; therefore, individualization of dose is recommended.

### Drug interactions and/or related problems
The following drug interactions and/or related problems have been selected on the basis of their potential clinical significance (possible mechanism in parentheses where appropriate)—not necessarily inclusive (» = major clinical significance):

Note: Combinations containing any of the following medications, depending on the amount present, may also interact with this medication.

In most cases, relative need for thyroid hormone dosage adjustment will depend on the thyroid state of the patient and the dosages of all medications involved. Dosage adjustment should be based on results of thyroid function tests and clinical status.

» Anticoagulants, coumarin- or indandione-derivative
(the effects of the oral anticoagulant may be altered, depending on the thyroid status of the patient; an increase in dosage of thyroid hormone may necessitate a decrease in oral anticoagulant dosage; adjustment of oral anticoagulant dosage on the basis of prothrombin time is recommended)

Antidepressants, tricyclic
(concurrent use with thyroid hormones may increase the therapeutic and toxic effects of both drugs, possibly due to increased receptor sensitivity to catecholamines; toxic effects include cardiac arrhythmias and CNS stimulation; also the onset of action of tricyclics may be accelerated)

Antidiabetic agents, sulfonylurea or
Insulin
(thyroid hormones may increase insulin or antidiabetic agent requirements; careful monitoring of diabetic control is recommended, especially when thyroid therapy is started, changed, or discontinued)

Beta-adrenergic blocking agents
(may decrease peripheral conversion of $T_4$ [thyroxine] to $T_3$ [triiodothyronine])

» Cholestyramine or
» Colestipol
(concurrent use may decrease the effects of thyroid hormones by binding and delaying or preventing absorption; an interval of 4 to 5 hours between administration of the two medications and regular monitoring of thyroid function tests are recommended)

Corticosteroids, glucocorticoid with mineralocorticoid activity or
Corticosteroids, mineralocorticoid or
Corticotropin (ACTH)
(changes in the thyroid status of the patient that may occur as a result of administration, changes in dosage, or discontinuation of thyroid hormones may necessitate adjustment of corticosteroid dosage because metabolic clearance of corticosteroids is decreased in hypothyroid patients and increased in hyperthyroid patients)

Estrogens
(increase serum thyroxine-binding globulin; in patients with a nonfunctioning thyroid gland, thyroid hormone requirements may be increased)

Hepatic enzyme inducers (See *Appendix II*)
(increase hepatic degradation of levothyroxine, which may result in increased requirements; dosage adjustment may be necessary)
(phenytoin also reduces serum protein binding of levothyroxine, and reduces total and free serum $T_4$ by 15 to 25%; despite this, most patients remain euthyroid and dosage of thyroid hormone does not need to be adjusted)

Ketamine
(concurrent use may produce marked hypertension and tachycardia; cautious administration to patients receiving thyroid hormone therapy is recommended)

Maprotiline
(concurrent use with thyroid hormones may enhance the possibility of cardiac arrhythmias; dosage adjustment may be necessary)

Sodium iodide I 123 or
Sodium iodide I 131 or
Sodium pertechnetate Tc 99m
(thyroid hormones may decrease the normal thyroidal uptake of I 123, I 131, or pertechnetate ion)

Somatrem or
Somatropin
(concurrent excessive use of thyroid hormones with somatrem or somatropin may accelerate epiphyseal closure. However, untreated hypothyroidism may interfere with growth response to somatrem or somatropin; prior and/or concurrent thyroid hormone replacement is recommended)

» Sympathomimetics
(concurrent use may increase the effects of these medications or thyroid hormone; thyroid hormones enhance risk of coronary in-

sufficiency when sympathomimetic agents are administered to patients with coronary artery disease)

**Medical considerations/Contraindications**

The medical considerations/contraindications included have been selected on the basis of their potential clinical significance (reasons given in parentheses where appropriate)—not necessarily inclusive (» = major clinical significance).

*Risk-benefit should be considered when the following medical problems exist:*

» Adrenocortical insufficiency
(must be corrected while thyroid replacement therapy is being given, to prevent precipitation of acute adrenocortical insufficiency)

» Cardiovascular disease, including angina pectoris, arteriosclerosis, coronary artery disease, hypertension, myocardial infarction
(because of the risks associated with overly rapid thyroid hormone replacement and increased metabolic demands; mobilization of myxedema fluid may produce pitting edema 1 to 3 or more weeks after a change in dosage)

Diabetes mellitus
(possible reduced glucose tolerance and increased insulin or oral antidiabetic agent requirements)

» Hyperthyroidism, history of
(residual autonomous thyroid function may be present after therapy for hyperthyroidism, necessitating lower than typical doses)

Malabsorption states, such as celiac disease
(absorption, especially of levothyroxine, is reduced; dosage adjustment may be necessary)

» Pituitary insufficiency
(associated adrenocortical insufficiency must be corrected before thyroid replacement therapy is initiated, to prevent precipitation of acute adrenocortical insufficiency)

Sensitivity to thyroid hormone

» Thyrotoxicosis being treated with antithyroid medication

» Caution is required also in patients with long-standing hypothyroidism or myxedema, who may be more sensitive to effects of thyroid hormones.

**Patient monitoring**

The following may be especially important in patient monitoring (other tests may be warranted in some patients, depending on condition; » = major clinical significance):

Note: In patients receiving levothyroxine, liotrix, or thyroid extract for primary hypothyroidism, serum free $T_4$ index (total serum $T_4$ and $T_3$ resin uptake) or serum free $T_4$ together with a serum thyroid-stimulating hormone (TSH) are the most useful tests for monitoring replacement therapy. Serum TSH measurements are not useful in hypothyroidism secondary to pituitary insufficiency. In the rare patient receiving liothyronine replacement, serum $T_4$ concentrations will remain low and normalization of serum TSH indicates that treatment is adequate. Overdosage with liothyronine can best be recognized by clinical symptoms of hyperthyroidism and/or by a decrease in serum TSH to subnormal levels.

Many medications affect the results of thyroid function tests and may produce false results.

Caution is necessary in interpreting results of thyroid function tests in neonates, because serum $T_4$ concentrations are transiently elevated and serum $T_3$ concentrations are transiently low, and the infant pituitary is relatively insensitive to the negative feedback effect of thyroid hormones.

The following have been found to be the most useful in general and may be especially important in patient monitoring (other tests may be warranted in some patients, depending on condition; » = major clinical significance):

» Free $T_4$ (thyroxine) index determinations or
Free (unbound) $T_4$ determinations
(recommended at periodic intervals in most patients)

Measurement of bone age and
» Measurement of growth and
» Measurement of psychomotor development
(recommended at periodic intervals in children with congenital hypothyroidism)

» Observation for signs of ischemia or tachyarrhythmias
(recommended in hypothyroid patients with cardiovascular disease to aid in adjustment of dosage and to prevent overdosage or overly rapid increase in dosage)

» TSH (thyroid-stimulating hormone) determinations and
» $T_3$ (triiodothyronine) or $T_4$ resin uptake determinations and

» Total serum $T_4$ determinations, by radioimmunoassay and
» Total serum $T_3$ determinations, by radioimmunoassay
(which thyroid function tests are most useful for a particular patient depends on the agent, condition being treated, other agents used concomitantly, and existing conditions that are capable of altering test results by altering serum thyroxine-binding globulin [TBG] concentrations)

## Side/Adverse Effects

Note: Side/adverse effects are dose-related and the dose at which they occur varies with each patient; incidence may be reduced by slowly increasing the initial dose to the minimum effective dose.

Side/adverse effects may occur more rapidly with liothyronine than with levothyroxine or thyroid because of its rapid onset of action.

In infants, excessive doses may result in craniosynostosis.

Partial loss of hair may occur in children during the first few months of treatment; normal hair growth usually returns, even with continued treatment.

The following side/adverse effects have been selected on the basis of their potential clinical significance (possible signs and symptoms in parentheses where appropriate)—not necessarily inclusive:

**Those indicating need for medical attention**

Incidence rare
*Allergic reaction* (skin rash or hives); *hyperthyroidism or overdosage* (changes in appetite; changes in menstrual periods; chest pain; diarrhea; fast or irregular heartbeat; fever; hand tremors; headache; irritability; leg cramps; nervousness; sensitivity to heat; shortness of breath; sweating; trouble in sleeping; vomiting; weight loss); *pseudotumor cerebri, in children* (severe headache)

**Those indicating need for medical attention only if they continue or are bothersome**

*Hypothyroidism or underdosage* (changes in menstrual periods; clumsiness; coldness; constipation; dry, puffy skin; headache; listlessness; muscle aches; sleepiness; tiredness; weakness; weight gain)

## Overdose

For specific information on the agents used in the management of thyroid hormones overdose, see:
- *Beta-adrenergic Blocking Agents (Systemic)* monograph;
- *Charcoal, Activated (Oral-Local)* monograph;
- *Hydrocortisone* in *Corticosteroids—Glucocorticoid Effects (Systemic)* monograph; and/or
- *Digitalis Glycosides (Systemic)* monograph.

For more information on the management of overdose or unintentional ingestion, **contact a Poison Control Center** (see *Poison Control Center Listing*).

**Treatment of overdose**

If symptoms of hyperthyroidism occur, it is recommended that thyroid hormone therapy be withdrawn for 2 to 6 days (1 to 2 days for liothyronine), then resumed at a lower dose.

To decrease absorption—
Acute massive overdose is treated by reducing gastrointestinal absorption, if possible, by means of vomiting, followed by emptying of the stomach and/or use of a charcoal instillation, which may be useful up to 3 to 4 hours after oral ingestion of toxic doses of thyroid hormones.

Specific treatment—
Cardiac glycosides if congestive heart failure develops.
Antiadrenergic agents such as propranolol for treatment of increased sympathetic activity.
Intravenous hydrocortisone to partially inhibit conversion of $T_4$ to $T_3$.

Supportive care—
Administration of oxygen. Implementation of measures to control fever, hypoglycemia, or fluid loss. Patients in whom intentional overdose is confirmed or suspected should be referred for psychiatric consultation.

## Patient Consultation

As an aid to patient consultation, refer to *Advice for the Patient, Thyroid Hormones (Systemic)*.

In providing consultation, consider emphasizing the following selected information (» = major clinical significance):

**Before using this medication**

» Conditions affecting use, especially:
Allergy to thyroid hormones

Pregnancy—Crosses the placenta to a limited extent and has not caused problems in the fetus with appropriate doses; regular monitoring is necessary as maternal dose requirements may change during pregnancy

Breast-feeding—Small amounts are distributed into breast milk

Use in the elderly—Sensitivity to thyroid effects is greater in the elderly than in younger age groups and dose adjustment may be necessary

Other medications, especially cholestyramine, colestipol, coumarin- or indandione-derivative anticoagulants, or sympathomimetics

Other medical problems, especially adrenocortical insufficiency, cardiovascular disease, history of hyperthyroidism, pituitary insufficiency, thyroid sensitivity with long-standing hypothyroidism or myxedema, or thyrotoxicosis

**Proper use of this medication**
» Importance of not taking more or less medication than the amount prescribed; taking medication at the same time every day for consistent effect
» Possible need for lifelong therapy; checking with physician before discontinuing medication
» Proper dosing
  Missed dose: Taking as soon as possible; not taking if almost time for next dose and not doubling doses; notifying physician if two or more doses in a row are missed
» Proper storage

**Precautions while using this medication**
» Importance of close monitoring by the physician
  Caution with angina or coronary artery disease; heavy exercise or exertion may precipitate angina
» Caution if any kind of surgery (including dental surgery) or emergency treatment is required
  Avoiding other medications unless prescribed by physician because of possible interference with effects of thyroid hormone

**Side/adverse effects**
Signs of potential side effects, especially allergic reaction, hyperthyroidism, and pseudotumor cerebri

## General Dosing Information

**Dosage must be adjusted to meet the individual requirements of each patient, on the basis of clinical response and results of thyroid function tests.**

Levothyroxine is the preferred form of thyroid replacement therapy.

Patients who are more than mildly hypothyroid initially should be treated with less than a full replacement dose, with doses then being increased gradually over a period of weeks. Otherwise, nervousness and rapid heart rate may occur.

Thyroid hormone replacement therapy for congenital hypothyroidism should be initiated as soon as possible after birth to minimize impaired mental and physical development. Treatment after about 3 months of age may reverse many of the physical effects but not all of the mental effects of hypothyroidism. Treatment should be continued for life, unless transient hypothyroidism is suspected, in which case therapy may be withdrawn for 2 to 8 weeks after 3 years of age; if thyroid-stimulating hormone (TSH) and thyroxine ($T_4$) concentrations remain normal throughout the withdrawal period, treatment is no longer necessary.

Suppression of TSH to normal levels must not be used as the sole criterion of adequacy of dose in congenital hypothyroidism, since TSH concentrations may remain elevated despite adequate or even excessive doses of thyroid hormone. Maintenance of appropriate $T_4$ concentrations for age is a more accurate guideline during infancy and childhood.

In general, thyroid hormone therapy is begun at a low dose, which is increased gradually to obtain a euthyroid state, followed by the dose required to maintain the response. However, this is not necessary in neonates, in whom rapid replacement is important, and who may be started at the full replacement dose. Adverse effects such as hyperactivity in the older child may be lessened by utilizing a starting dose of one-fourth the full replacement dose, and increasing the dose by one-fourth weekly until the full replacement dose is reached.

Rapid replacement of thyroid hormone is associated with less risk in younger adults than in older ones.

In hypothyroid patients with adrenocortical insufficiency or panhypopituitarism, replacement therapy with thyroid hormones must be preceded by adequate amounts of corticosteroids to prevent precipitation of acute adrenocortical insufficiency by the increase in metabolism. Supplemental corticosteroids may also be necessary for patients with prolonged or severe hypothyroidism, including myxedema.

In hypothyroid patients with myxedema or cardiovascular disease, the initial dosage of thyroid hormones should be very small and must be increased very gradually to prevent precipitation of angina, coronary occlusion, or stroke. If cardiovascular reactions occur, a reduction in thyroid hormone dosage may be required. Although some clinicians prefer to use liothyronine in these patients because its effects disappear more rapidly after withdrawal, regulation of dosage is more difficult and its rapid onset of action may also produce adverse cardiac effects as a result of abrupt changes in metabolic demands.

If, after prolonged therapy (2 to 6 months), no response occurs with physiologic doses or a response occurs only with large doses of thyroid hormone, it is recommended that the diagnosis be reevaluated.

---
### LEVOTHYROXINE
---

## Summary of Differences
Indications: Usual drug of choice. Advantage over thyroid and thyroglobulin is a predictable effect because of standard hormonal content.
Pharmacology/pharmacokinetics: Absorption after oral administration is incomplete and variable, especially when taken with food.
Precautions: Medical problems/contraindications—Absorption may be significantly reduced in patients with malabsorption states.

## Oral Dosage Forms
### LEVOTHYROXINE SODIUM TABLETS USP
**Usual adult dose**
Mild hypothyroidism—
  Initial: Oral, 50 mcg (0.05 mg) as a single daily dose, with increments of 25 to 50 mcg (0.025 to 0.05 mg) at two- to three-week intervals until the desired result is obtained.
  Maintenance: Oral, 75 to 125 mcg (0.075 to 0.125 mg) per day (or 1.5 mcg per kg of body weight per day) as a single daily dose. A higher maintenance dose (up to 200 mcg per day) may be necessary in some patients (e.g., those with malabsorption).
Severe hypothyroidism—
  Initial: Oral, 12.5 to 25 mcg (0.0125 to 0.025 mg) as a single daily dose, with increments of 25 mcg (0.025 mg) at two- to three-week intervals until the desired result is obtained.
  Maintenance: Oral, 75 to 125 mcg (0.075 to 0.125 mg) per day (or 1.5 mcg per kg of body weight per day) as a single daily dose. A higher maintenance dose (up to 200 mcg per day) may be necessary in some patients (e.g., those with malabsorption).
Note: In the elderly and in patients with long-standing hypothyroidism, myxedematous infiltration, or cardiovascular dysfunction, the initial dose is usually 12.5 to 25 mcg (0.0125 to 0.025 mg) a day, and dosage is incremented at three- to four-week intervals. In the elderly, the maintenance dose is usually about 75 mcg (0.075 mg) per day.

**Usual adult prescribing limits**
Failure to respond to a daily dose of 150 mcg (0.15 mg) or more may indicate erroneous diagnosis of hypothyroidism, malabsorption, or poor compliance.

**Usual pediatric dose**
Children less than 6 months of age—Oral, 5 to 6 mcg (0.005 to 0.006 mg) per kg of body weight per day or 25 to 50 mcg (0.025 to 0.05 mg) per day as a single daily dose.
Children 6 to 12 months of age—Oral, 5 to 6 mcg (0.005 to 0.006 mg) per kg of body weight per day or 50 to 75 mcg (0.05 to 0.075 mg) per day as a single daily dose.
Children 1 to 5 years of age—Oral, 3 to 5 mcg (0.003 to 0.005 mg) per kg of body weight per day or 75 to 100 mcg (0.075 to 0.1 mg) per day as a single daily dose.
Children 6 to 10 years of age—Oral, 4 to 5 mcg (0.004 to 0.005 mg) per kg of body weight per day or 100 to 150 mcg (0.1 to 0.15 mg) per day as a single daily dose.
Children over 10 years of age—Oral, 2 to 3 mcg (0.002 to 0.003 mg) per kg of body weight per day as a single daily dose until the adult dose is reached (usually 150 mcg [0.15 mg] per day) up to 200 mcg (0.2 mg) per day.
Note: Premature infants weighing less than 2000 grams, or infants at risk for cardiac failure receive a starting dose of 25 mcg (0.025 mg) a day which may be increased to 50 mcg (0.05 mg) a day in four to six weeks.

**Usual geriatric dose**
See *Usual adult dose*.

**Strength(s) usually available**
U.S.—
  25 mcg (0.025 mg) (Rx) [*Levo-T* (scored); *Levothroid*; *Levoxyl*; *Synthroid* (scored); GENERIC].

50 mcg (0.05 mg) (Rx) [*Levo-T* (scored); *Levothroid; Levoxyl; Synthroid* (scored); GENERIC].
75 mcg (0.075 mg) (Rx) [*Levo-T* (scored); *Levothroid; Levoxyl; Synthroid* (scored); GENERIC].
88 mcg (0.088 mg) (Rx) [*Levothroid; Levoxyl; Synthroid* (scored)].
100 mcg (0.1 mg) (Rx) [*Levo-T* (scored); *Levothroid; Levoxyl; Synthroid* (scored); GENERIC].
112 mcg (0.112 mg) (Rx) [*Levothroid; Levoxyl; Synthroid* (scored)].
125 mcg (0.125 mg) (Rx) [*Levo-T* (scored); *Levothroid; Levoxyl; Synthroid* (scored); GENERIC].
137 mcg (0.137 mg) (Rx) [*Levothroid; Levoxyl*].
150 mcg (0.15 mg) (Rx) [*Levo-T* (scored); *Levothroid; Levoxyl; Synthroid* (scored); GENERIC].
175 mcg (0.175 mg) (Rx) [*Levothroid; Levoxyl; Synthroid* (scored)].
200 mcg (0.2 mg) (Rx) [*Levo-T* (scored); *Levothroid; Levoxyl; Synthroid* (scored); GENERIC].
300 mcg (0.3 mg) (Rx) [*Levo-T* (scored); *Levothroid; Levoxyl; Synthroid* (scored); GENERIC].

Canada—
25 mcg (0.025 mg) (Rx) [*PMS-Levothyroxine Sodium* (scored); *Synthroid* (scored)].
50 mcg (0.05 mg) (Rx) [*Eltroxin; PMS-Levothyroxine Sodium* (scored); *Synthroid* (scored)].
75 mcg (0.075 mg) (Rx) [*PMS-Levothyroxine Sodium* (scored); *Synthroid* (scored)].
88 mcg (0.088 mg) (Rx) [*Synthroid* (scored)].
100 mcg (0.1 mg) (Rx) [*Eltroxin; PMS-Levothyroxine Sodium* (scored); *Synthroid* (scored)].
112 mcg (0.112 mg) (Rx) [*Synthroid* (scored)].
125 mcg (0.125 mg) (Rx) [*PMS-Levothyroxine Sodium* (scored); *Synthroid* (scored)].
150 mcg (0.15 mg) (Rx) [*Eltroxin; PMS-Levothyroxine Sodium* (scored); *Synthroid* (scored)].
175 mcg (0.175 mg) (Rx) [*Synthroid* (scored)].
200 mcg (0.2 mg) (Rx) [*Eltroxin; PMS-Levothyroxine Sodium* (scored); *Synthroid* (scored)].
300 mcg (0.3 mg) (Rx) [*Eltroxin; PMS-Levothyroxine Sodium* (scored); *Synthroid* (scored)].

**Packaging and storage**
Store below 40 °C (104 °F), preferably between 15 and 30 °C (59 and 86 °F), unless otherwise specified by manufacturer. Store in a tight, light-resistant container.

**Auxiliary labeling**
• Take on empty stomach.
• Do not take other medicines without your doctor's advice.

**Note**
Caution is recommended when changing products because of the potential difference in actual levothyroxine content between brands.

## Parenteral Dosage Forms

### LEVOTHYROXINE SODIUM INJECTION

**Usual adult dose**
Hypothyroidism—
Intravenous or intramuscular, 50 to 100 mcg (0.05 to 0.1 mg) as a single daily dose.
Myxedema coma or stupor—
Initial: Intravenous, 200 to 500 mcg (0.2 to 0.5 mg), even in the elderly; an additional 100 to 300 mcg (0.1 to 0.3 mg) may be given on the second day if improvement has not occurred, followed by continuous daily administration of smaller doses, until the patient can tolerate oral administration.
Note: Smaller doses may be required in patients with concomitant cardiovascular disease.

**Usual pediatric dose**
Hypothyroidism—
Intravenous or intramuscular, daily dose equal to 75% of the usual oral pediatric dose.

**Usual geriatric dose**
See *Usual adult dose*.

**Strength(s) usually available**
U.S.—
Not commercially available.
Canada—
Not commercially available.

**Packaging and storage**
Store below 40 °C (104 °F), preferably between 15 and 30 °C (59 and 86 °F), unless otherwise specified by manufacturer.

### LEVOTHYROXINE SODIUM FOR INJECTION

**Usual adult dose**
See *Levothyroxine Sodium Injection*.

**Usual pediatric dose**
See *Levothyroxine Sodium Injection*.

**Usual geriatric dose**
See *Levothyroxine Sodium Injection*.

**Size(s) usually available**
U.S.—
200 mcg (0.2 mg) (Rx) [*Levothroid; Synthroid;* GENERIC].
500 mcg (0.5 mg) (Rx) [*Levothroid; Synthroid;* GENERIC].
Canada—
500 mcg (0.5 mg) (Rx) [*Synthroid*].

**Packaging and storage**
Store below 40 °C (104 °F), preferably between 15 and 30 °C (59 and 86 °F), unless otherwise specified by manufacturer. Protect from light.

**Preparation of dosage form**
Levothyroxine sodium for injection may be reconstituted for parenteral use by adding 0.5, 2, or 5 mL of Sodium Chloride Injection USP (without preservative) to the 50-, 200-, or 500-mcg vial, respectively, and shaking to dissolve, producing a solution containing 100 mcg (0.1 mg) per mL.

**Stability**
Solution should be freshly reconstituted immediately prior to each dose. Any unused portion should be discarded.

---

## LIOTHYRONINE

## Summary of Differences
Indications:
Advantage over thyroid and thyroglobulin is a predictable effect because of standard hormonal content. May be preferred over levothyroxine when a rapid effect or rapidly reversible effect is desired, or when gastrointestinal absorption processes or peripheral conversion of $T_4$ (thyroxine) to $T_3$ (triiodothyronine) is impaired; however, regulation of dosage is more difficult and rapid onset of action may also produce adverse cardiac effects as a result of abrupt changes in metabolic demands.
Pharmacology/pharmacokinetics:
Maximal effects with continued use occur within 48 to 72 hours and persist for up to 72 hours after withdrawal.
Side/adverse effects:
May occur more rapidly with liothyronine than with levothyroxine or thyroid.
General dosing information:
Rapid action and abrupt increase in metabolic demands may produce adverse cardiac effects.
If symptoms of hyperthyroidism occur, withdrawal for 2 to 3 days is recommended before resumption at a lower dose.

## Additional Dosing Information
See also *General Dosing Information*.

When a patient is transferred to liothyronine from other thyroid therapy, the other therapy is discontinued and liothyronine is initiated at a low dosage, increased gradually on the basis of patient response. Keep in mind that the effects of liothyronine occur rapidly, while the effects of other thyroid hormones may persist for several weeks.

Liothyronine may be given in divided daily doses to minimize fluctuations in $T_3$ concentrations.

## Oral Dosage Forms

### LIOTHYRONINE SODIUM TABLETS USP

**Usual adult dose**
Mild hypothyroidism—
Initial: Oral, 25 mcg (0.025 mg) a day, with increments of 12.5 or 25 mcg (0.0125 or 0.025 mg) every one or two weeks until the desired result is obtained.
Maintenance: Oral, 25 to 50 mcg (0.025 to 0.05 mg) a day.
Myxedema—
Initial: Oral, 2.5 to 5 mcg (0.0025 to 0.005 mg) a day, with increments of 5 to 10 mcg (0.005 to 0.01 mg) every one or two weeks. When 25 mcg (0.025 mg) a day is reached, increments may sometimes be by 12.5 to 25 mcg (0.0125 to 0.025 mg) every one or two weeks.
Maintenance: Oral, 25 to 50 mcg (0.025 to 0.05 mg) a day.

**Simple (nontoxic) goiter**—
  Initial: Oral, 5 mcg (0.005 mg) a day, with increments of 5 to 10 mcg (0.005 to 0.01 mg) every one or two weeks. When 25 mcg (0.025 mg) a day is reached, increments may be by 12.5 or 25 mcg (0.0125 or 0.025 mg) every week.
  Maintenance: Oral, 50 to 100 mcg (0.05 to 0.1 mg) a day.
Note: In patients with cardiovascular disease, the initial dose is 5 mcg (0.005 mg) a day, with increments of no more than 5 mcg every two weeks. In the elderly also, the initial dose is 5 mcg a day, with increments of no more than 5 mcg at the recommended intervals.

### Usual pediatric dose
Cretinism—
  USP Advisory Panels do not recommend use for cretinism in children because of significant question about $T_3$ crossing the blood-brain barrier.

### Usual geriatric dose
See *Usual adult dose*.

### Strength(s) usually available
U.S.—
  5 mcg (0.005 mg) (Rx) [*Cytomel*].
  25 mcg (0.025 mg) (Rx) [*Cytomel* (scored); GENERIC].
  50 mcg (0.05 mg) (Rx) [*Cytomel* (scored)].
Canada—
  5 mcg (0.005 mg) (base) (Rx) [*Cytomel*].
  25 mcg (0.025 mg) (base) (Rx) [*Cytomel* (scored)].

### Packaging and storage
Store below 40 °C (104 °F), preferably between 15 and 30 °C (59 and 86 °F), unless otherwise specified by manufacturer. Store in a tight container.

### Auxiliary labeling
• Do not take other medicines without your doctor's advice.

---

## LIOTRIX

## Summary of Differences
Indications: Advantage over thyroid and thyroglobulin is a predictable effect because of standard hormonal content; provision of a product containing $T_3$ (triiodothyronine) no longer considered an advantage because of natural conversion of $T_4$ (thyroxine) to $T_3$ in the tissues.

## Oral Dosage Forms
### LIOTRIX TABLETS USP

#### Usual adult and adolescent dose
Hypothyroidism without myxedema—
  Initial: Oral, 50 mcg (0.05 mg) of levothyroxine and 12.5 mcg (0.0125 mg) of liothyronine a day, with increments of a like amount at monthly intervals until the desired result is obtained.
  Maintenance: Oral, 50 to 100 mcg (0.05 to 0.1 mg) of levothyroxine and 12.5 to 25 mcg (0.0125 to 0.025 mg) of liothyronine a day.
Myxedema or hypothyroidism with cardiovascular disease—
  Initial: Oral, 12.5 mcg (0.0125 mg) of levothyroxine and 3.1 mcg (0.0031 mg) of liothyronine a day, with increments of a like amount at two- to three-week intervals until the desired result is obtained.
  Maintenance: Oral, 50 to 100 mcg (0.05 to 0.1 mg) of levothyroxine and 12.5 to 25 mcg (0.0125 to 0.025 mg) of liothyronine a day.
Note: In the elderly, the initial dose is one-fourth to one-half the usual adult dose, doubled at six- to eight-week intervals until the desired result is obtained.

#### Usual pediatric dose
Cretinism or severe hypothyroidism—
  See *Usual adult and adolescent dose* for myxedema.
Hypothyroidism—
  See *Usual adult and adolescent dose* for hypothyroidism without myxedema.
Note: Increments in dosage are made at two-week intervals in children.
  Dosage should always be based on results of thyroid function tests.

#### Usual geriatric dose
See *Usual adult and adolescent dose*.

#### Strength(s) usually available
U.S.—

| Levothyroxine sodium (mcg) | Liothyronine sodium (mcg) | Brand name |
|---|---|---|
| 12.5 | 3.1 | *Thyrolar* (Rx) |
| 25 | 6.25 | *Thyrolar* (Rx) |
| 50 | 12.5 | *Thyrolar* (Rx) |
| 100 | 25 | *Thyrolar* (Rx) |
| 150 | 37.5 | *Thyrolar* (Rx) |

Canada—
  Not commercially available.

#### Packaging and storage
Store below 40 °C (104 °F), preferably between 15 and 30 °C (59 and 86 °F), unless otherwise specified by manufacturer. Store in a tight container.

#### Auxiliary labeling
• Do not take other medicines without your doctor's advice.

#### Note
Be very careful always to dispense the same brand of liotrix that a patient has received previously.

---

## THYROGLOBULIN

## Summary of Differences
Indications: Disadvantages include variable hormonal content of commercial preparations and fluctuation of $T_3$ (triiodothyronine) and $T_4$ (thyroxine) concentrations produced.

## Oral Dosage Forms
### THYROGLOBULIN TABLETS USP

#### Usual adult and adolescent dose
Hypothyroidism without myxedema—
  Initial: Oral, 32 mg a day, with increments every one or two weeks until the desired result is obtained.
  Maintenance: Oral, 65 to 160 mg a day.
Myxedema or hypothyroidism with cardiovascular disease—
  Initial: Oral, 16 to 32 mg a day, with increments of a like amount every two weeks until the desired result is obtained.
  Maintenance: 65 to 160 mg a day.

#### Usual pediatric dose
Cretinism or severe hypothyroidism—
  See *Usual adult and adolescent dose* for myxedema.
Hypothyroidism—
  See *Usual adult and adolescent dose* for hypothyroidism without myxedema.
Note: Dosage should always be based on results of thyroid function tests.
  Levothyroxine is considered the drug of choice in the treatment of congenital hypothyroidism.

#### Strength(s) usually available
U.S.—
  Not commercially available.
Canada—
  Not commercially available.

#### Packaging and storage
Store below 40 °C (104 °F), preferably between 15 and 30 °C (59 and 86 °F), unless otherwise specified by manufacturer. Store in a tight container.

#### Auxiliary labeling
• Do not take other medicines without your doctor's advice.

---

## THYROID

## Summary of Differences
Indications: Disadvantages include variable hormonal content of commercial preparations and fluctuation of $T_3$ (triiodothyronine) and $T_4$ (thyroxine) concentrations produced.

## Oral Dosage Forms
### THYROID TABLETS USP

**Usual adult and adolescent dose**
Hypothyroidism without myxedema—
  Initial: Oral, 60 mg a day, with increments of 30 mg at monthly intervals until the desired result is obtained.
  Maintenance: Oral, 60 to 120 mg a day.
Myxedema or hypothyroidism with cardiovascular disease—
  Initial: Oral, 15 mg a day, increased to 30 mg a day after two weeks, and to 60 mg a day after a further two weeks. Careful clinical assessment is recommended after one month and two months of treatment at 60 mg a day. If necessary, dosage may then be increased to 120 mg a day. If necessary, further increases of 30 or 60 mg may be made.
  Maintenance: Oral, 60 to 120 mg a day.
Note: An initial dose of 7.5 to 15 mg a day is recommended in the elderly; this dose may be doubled every six to eight weeks until the desired result is obtained.

**Usual pediatric dose**
Cretinism or severe hypothyroidism—
  See *Usual adult and adolescent dose* for myxedema.
Hypothyroidism—
  See *Usual adult and adolescent dose* for hypothyroidism without myxedema.
Note: Dosage should always be based on results of thyroid function tests. Levothyroxine is considered the drug of choice in the treatment of congenital hypothyroidism.

**Usual geriatric dose**
See *Usual adult and adolescent dose*.

**Strength(s) usually available**
U.S.—
  Regular
    15 mg (Rx) [*Armour Thyroid*; GENERIC].
    30 mg (Rx) [*Armour Thyroid*; *Westhroid*; GENERIC].
    60 mg (Rx) [*Armour Thyroid*; *Westhroid*; GENERIC].
    90 mg (Rx) [*Armour Thyroid*].
    120 mg (Rx) [*Armour Thyroid*; *Westhroid*; GENERIC].
    180 mg (Rx) [*Armour Thyroid*; *Westhroid*; GENERIC].
    240 mg (Rx) [*Armour Thyroid*; *Westhroid*].
    300 mg (Rx) [*Armour Thyroid*; *Westhroid*; GENERIC].
  Bovine
    30 mg (Rx) [*Thyrar*].
    60 mg (Rx) [*Thyrar*].
    120 mg (Rx) [*Thyrar*].
  Strong (contains iodine 0.3%)
    30 mg (Rx) [*Thyroid Strong*].
    60 mg (Rx) [*Thyroid Strong*].
    120 mg (Rx) [*Thyroid Strong*].
    180 mg (Rx) [*Thyroid Strong*].
Canada—
  Regular
    30 mg (Rx) [GENERIC].
    60 mg (Rx) [GENERIC].
    125 mg (Rx) [GENERIC].
Note: Administration of strengths above 120 mg may result in thyrotoxic symptoms.

**Packaging and storage**
Store below 40 °C (104 °F), preferably between 15 and 30 °C (59 and 86 °F), unless otherwise specified by manufacturer. Store in a tight container.

**Auxiliary labeling**
• Do not take other medicines without your doctor's advice.

Revised: 05/22/92
Interim revision: 07/25/94; 01/08/95; 06/26/96

---

**THYROTROPIN**—The *Thyrotropin (Systemic)* monograph is not included in this published version of the USP DI database. Copies of the monograph are available on request from Micromedex, Inc. - Reprint Requests, 6200 S. Syracuse Way, Suite 300, Englewood, CO 80111; telephone (303) 486-6400; telefax (303) 486-6464; Email: USPDI@MDX.COM.

---

# TIAGABINE Systemic—INTRODUCTORY VERSION

VA CLASSIFICATION (Primary): CN400
Commonly used brand name(s): *Gabitril*.
Note: For a listing of dosage forms and brand names by country availability, see *Dosage Forms* section(s).

## Category
Anticonvulsant.

## Indications
**Accepted**
Epilepsy (treatment adjunct)—Tiagabine is indicated as an adjunct to other anticonvulsant medications in the treatment of partial seizures in adults and children 12 years of age and older.

## Pharmacology/Pharmacokinetics

**Physicochemical characteristics**
Molecular weight—Tiagabine hydrochloride: 412.

**Mechanism of action/Effect**
The precise mechanism of tiagabine's antiseizure effects is unknown. *In vitro* experiments have documented tiagabine's ability to enhance the activity of gamma-aminobutyric acid (GABA), the major inhibitory neurotransmitter in the central nervous system (CNS). These experiments have shown that tiagabine binds to recognition sites associated with the GABA uptake carrier. It is thought that this binding enables tiagabine to block GABA uptake into presynaptic neurons, permitting more GABA to be available for receptor binding on the surfaces of post-synaptic cells. Inhibition of GABA uptake has been shown for synaptosomes, neuronal cell cultures, and glial cell cultures.
*In vitro* binding studies have shown that tiagabine does not significantly inhibit the uptake of dopamine, norepinephrine, serotonin, glutamate, or choline, and shows little or no binding to dopamine $D_1$ and $D_2$; muscarinic; serotonin $5HT_{1A}$, $5HT_2$, and $5HT_3$; beta$_1$- and beta$_2$-adrenergic; alpha$_1$- and alpha$_2$-adrenergic; histamine $H_2$ and $H_3$; adenosine $A_1$ and $A_2$; opiate mu and $K_1$; *N*-methyl-*D*-aspartate (NMDA) glutamate; and GABA$_A$ receptors. Tiagabine also lacks significant affinity for sodium or calcium channels. At concentrations 20 to 400 times those inhibiting the uptake of GABA, tiagabine binds to histamine $H_1$, serotonin $5HT_{1B}$, benzodiazepine, and chloride channel receptors.

**Absorption**
Tiagabine is rapidly and nearly completely absorbed (> 95%), with an absolute bioavailability of about 90%. Food slows the rate but not the extent of absorption.

**Protein binding**
Very high (96%), mainly to serum albumin and alpha-1–acid glycoprotein.

**Biotransformation**
Hepatic; not fully elucidated. At least two metabolic pathways have been identified: thiophene ring oxidation, leading to an inactive metabolite, and glucuronidation. Tiagabine is most likely metabolized primarily by the 3A isoform subfamily of hepatic cytochrome P450 (CYP3A); contributions to the metabolism of tiagabine from isoenzymes CYP1A2, CYP2D6, or CYP2C19 have not been excluded.
In patients with moderate hepatic impairment (Child-Pugh Class B), clearance of unbound tiagabine was reduced by about 60%. Patients with impaired liver function may require lower initial and maintenance doses of tiagabine and/or longer dosing intervals than patients with normal hepatic function.

**Half-life**
Elimination—
  Normal volunteers: 7 to 9 hours.
  Epileptic patients taking hepatic enzyme-inducing drugs: 4 to 7 hours.
Note: In clinical trials, most patients were induced.

**Time to peak concentration**
Approximately 45 minutes following an oral dose administered in the fasting state. The presence of food (i.e., a high fat meal) may prolong the time to reach maximum concentration to 2.5 hours.

### Other pharmacokinetic parameters
A diurnal effect was observed on the pharmacokinetics of tiagabine. Mean steady-state minimum plasma concentration ($C_{min}$) values were 40% lower in the evening than in the morning. The area under the plasma concentration–time curve (AUC) values at steady-state were 15% lower following the evening dose as compared to the AUC values following the morning dose.

### Elimination
Approximately 2% of an oral dose of tiagabine is excreted unchanged. Of the remaining dose, 25% and 63% are excreted into the urine and feces, respectively, primarily as metabolites.

## Precautions to Consider

### Carcinogenicity/Tumorigenicity
A carcinogenicity study in rats receiving 200 mg of tiagabine per kg of body weight (mg/kg) a day (36 to 100 times the maximum recommended human dosage [MRHD] of 56 mg a day) for 2 years resulted in small but statistically significant increases in the incidences of hepatocellular adenomas in female rats and Leydig cell tumors of the testis in male rats. The significance of these findings relative to the use of tiagabine in humans is not known. The no effect dosage for induction of tumors in this study was 100 mg/kg a day (17 to 50 times the MRHD). No statistically significant increases in tumor formation were noted in mice at dosages of up to 250 mg/kg a day (20 times the MRHD on a mg per square meter of body surface area [mg/m$^2$] basis).

### Mutagenicity
Tiagabine produced an increase in structural chromosome aberration frequency in human lymphocytes *in vitro* in the absence of metabolic activation; no increase in chromosomal aberration frequencies was demonstrated in this assay in the presence of metabolic activation. No evidence of genetic toxicity was found in the *in vitro* bacterial gene mutation assays, the *in vitro* HGPRT forward mutation assay in Chinese hamster lung cells, the *in vivo* mouse micronucleus test, or an unscheduled DNA synthesis assay.

### Pregnancy/Reproduction
Fertility—Studies in male and female rats receiving tiagabine prior to and during mating, gestation, and lactation have shown no impairment of fertility at doses of up to 100 mg/kg a day (approximately 16 times the MRHD on a mg/m$^2$ basis). Lowered maternal weight gain and decreased viability and growth in the rat pups did occur at this dose.

Pregnancy—Adequate and well-controlled studies in humans have not been done.

Tiagabine has been shown to have adverse effects on embryo-fetal development, including teratogenic effects, when administered to pregnant rats and rabbits at doses greater than the human therapeutic dose.

An increased incidence of malformed fetuses (various craniofacial, appendicular, and visceral defects) and decreased fetal weights were observed following oral administration of 100 mg/kg a day to pregnant rats during the period of organogenesis. This dose is approximately 16 times the MRHD on a mg/m$^2$ basis. Maternal toxicity (transient weight loss and reduced maternal weight gain during gestation) was associated with this dose, but there was no evidence to suggest that the teratogenic effects were secondary to the maternal effects. No adverse maternal or embryo-fetal effects were seen at a dose of 20 mg/kg a day (3 times the MRHD on a mg/m$^2$ basis).

Decreased maternal weight gain, increased resorption of embryos, and increased incidence of fetal variations, but not malformations, were observed when pregnant rabbits were administered 25 mg of tiagabine per kg a day (8 times the MRHD on a mg/m$^2$ basis) during organogenesis. The no effect level for maternal and embryo-fetal toxicity in rabbits was 5 mg/kg a day (equivalent to the MRHD on a mg/m$^2$ basis).

Decreased maternal weight gain during gestation, an increase in stillbirths, and decreased postnatal offspring viability and growth were observed in female rats that received tiagabine 100 mg/kg a day during late gestation and throughout parturition and lactation.

FDA Pregnancy Category C.

### Breast-feeding
It is not known whether tiagabine and/or its metabolites are distributed into human milk or what effects it may have on the nursing infant. Animal studies have shown that tiagabine and/or its metabolites appear in the milk of rats. Risk-benefit must be considered.

### Pediatrics
Adequate and well-controlled studies have not been conducted in children up to 12 years of age. However, pharmacokinetic studies in a small number of children 3 to 10 years of age showed that apparent clearance (per unit of body surface area) and volume of distribution (per kg) of tiagabine were similar to those in adults when both groups were receiving enzyme-inducing anticonvulsants (e.g., carbamazepine or phenytoin). In children taking a non–enzyme-inducing anticonvulsant (e.g., valproate), the clearance of tiagabine based upon body weight and body surface area was 2- and 1.5-fold higher, respectively, than in un-induced adults with epilepsy. Safety and efficacy in children up to 12 years of age have not been established.

### Geriatrics
The pharmacokinetic profile of tiagabine in healthy elderly adults was similar to that in healthy young adults. However, only a small number of patients over 65 years of age were exposed to tiagabine during clinical evaluation; therefore, safety and efficacy in this age group have not been established.

### Pharmacogenetics
Population pharmacokinetic analyses indicated that tiagabine clearance values were not significantly different in white, black, or Hispanic patients with epilepsy.

### Drug interactions and/or related problems
The following drug interactions and/or related problems have been selected on the basis of their potential clinical significance (possible mechanism in parentheses where appropriate)—not necessarily inclusive (» = major clinical significance):

Note: Administration of hepatic enzyme-inducing medications will increase the clearance of tiagabine.

Combinations containing any of the following medications, depending on the amount present, may also interact with this medication.

Alcohol or
Central nervous system (CNS) depression–producing medications, other (see *Appendix II*)
(increased CNS depression may occur)

» Carbamazepine
(tiagabine clearance is increased by 60% in patients taking carbamazepine)

» Phenobarbital
(tiagabine clearance is increased by 60% in patients taking phenobarbital)

» Phenytoin
(tiagabine clearance is increased by 60% in patients taking phenytoin)

» Primidone
(tiagabine clearance is increased by 60% in patients taking primidone)

Valproic acid
(tiagabine causes a slight decrease [about 10%] in steady-state valproate concentrations; *in vitro* studies have shown that valproate decreased the protein binding of tiagabine from 96.3 to 94.8%, resulting in an increase of approximately 40% in the free tiagabine concentration; clinical relevance of this finding is unknown)

### Medical considerations/Contraindications
The medical considerations/contraindications included have been selected on the basis of their potential clinical significance (reasons given in parentheses where appropriate)—not necessarily inclusive (» = major clinical significance).

*Risk-benefit should be considered when the following medical problems exist:*

Electroencephalogram (EEG) abnormalities
(patients with a history of spike and wave discharges on EEG have been reported to have exacerbations of EEG abnormalities associated with cognitive/neuropsychiatric events; these clinical events may, in some cases, be a manifestation of underlying seizure activity; dosage adjustments may be required)

Hepatic function impairment
(dosage reductions or longer dosing intervals may be required)

Sensitivity to tiagabine

Status epilepticus, history of
(condition may be precipitated)

### Patient monitoring
The following may be especially important in patient monitoring (other tests may be warranted in some patients, depending on condition; » = major clinical significance):

Therapeutic monitoring of plasma concentrations
(a therapeutic range for tiagabine plasma concentrations has not been established; in controlled trials, trough plasma concentrations observed in patients randomized to tiagabine doses that were statistically significantly more effective than placebo ranged from < 1 nanogram/mL to 234 nanograms/mL; because of the potential for interactions between tiagabine and drugs that induce or inhibit he-

patic metabolizing enzymes, obtaining tiagabine plasma concentrations before and after changes are made in the patient's medication regimen may be useful)

## Side/Adverse Effects

Note: In studies in dogs receiving a single dose of radiolabeled tiagabine, residual binding in the retina and uvea after 3 weeks was apparent. Binding to melanin is likely. The ability of available tests to detect potentially adverse consequences of the binding of tiagabine to melanin-containing tissue is unknown, and no systematic monitoring for relevant ophthalmologic changes during the clinical development of tiagabine was conducted. However, long-term (up to 1 year) toxicological studies of tiagabine in dogs showed no treatment-related ophthalmoscopic changes, and macro- and microscopic examinations of the eye were unremarkable. Although there are no specific recommendations for periodic ophthalmologic monitoring, the possibility of long-term ophthalmologic effects exists.

The following side/adverse effects have been selected on the basis of their potential clinical significance (possible signs and symptoms in parentheses where appropriate)—not necessarily inclusive:

### Those indicating need for medical attention
Incidence more frequent
*Difficulty in concentrating or paying attention*—may be dose-related; *ecchymosis* (blue or purple spots on skin)

Incidence less frequent
*Ataxia* (clumsiness or unsteadiness); *confusion; mental depression; paresthesias* (burning, numbness, or tingling sensations); *pruritus* (itching); *speech and/or language problems*

Incidence rare
*Abnormal gait* (walking in unusual manner); *agitation; emotional lability* (quick to react or overreact emotionally); *generalized weakness; hostility; memory problems; nystagmus* (uncontrolled back-and-forth and/or rolling eye movements); *rash; urinary tract infection* (bloody or cloudy urine; burning, pain, or difficulty in urinating; frequent urge to urinate)

Note: Moderately severe to incapacitating *generalized weakness* has been reported in about 1% of patients with epilepsy following administration of tiagabine. Weakness resolved in all cases following a reduction in dose or discontinuation of tiagabine.

Four patients treated with tiagabine during premarketing clinical testing developed serious *rashes*; two cases were described as maculopapular, one case was described as vesiculobullous, and one case was diagnosed as Stevens-Johnson syndrome. A causal relationship to tiagabine has not been established. However, drug-associated rash can, if extensive and serious, cause irreversible morbidity, even death.

### Those indicating need for medical attention only if they continue or are bothersome
Incidence more frequent
*Asthenia* (unusual tiredness or weakness)—may be dose-related; *diarrhea; dizziness; influenza-like syndrome* (chills; fever; headache; muscle aches or pain); *nervousness; pharyngitis* (sore throat); *somnolence* (drowsiness); *tremor*—may be dose-related; *vomiting*

Incidence less frequent
*Abdominal pain; amblyopia* (impaired vision); *cough, increased; increased appetite; insomnia* (trouble in sleeping); *mouth ulcers; muscle weakness; myalgia* (muscle ache or pain); *nausea; pain (unspecified); vasodilation* (flushing)

## Overdose

For information on the management of overdose or unintentional ingestion of tiagabine, **contact a Poison Control Center** (see *Poison Control Center Listing*).

### Clinical effects of overdose
The following effects have been selected on the basis of their potential clinical significance (possible signs and symptoms in parentheses where appropriate)—not necessarily inclusive:

Acute
*Agitation, severe; ataxia, severe* (clumsiness or unsteadiness); *confusion, severe; hostility; impaired consciousness* (coma); *lethargy* (sluggishness); *mental depression; myoclonus* (severe muscle twitching or jerking); *precipitation of a tonic-clonic seizure* (increase in seizures); *somnolence, severe* (drowsiness); *speech problems, severe; weakness*

### Treatment of overdose
There is no specific antidote for overdose with tiagabine.
To decrease absorption—Elimination of unabsorbed drug by inducing emesis or by gastric lavage, if indicated; usual precautions to maintain the airway should be taken.
To enhance elimination—Since tiagabine is primarily metabolized by the liver and highly protein-bound, dialysis is not likely to be beneficial.
Monitoring—Monitoring of vital signs.
Supportive care—General supportive care, including observation of clinical status. Patients in whom intentional overdose is confirmed or suspected should be referred for psychiatric consultation.

## Patient Consultation

As an aid to patient consultation, refer to Advice for the Patient, Tiagabine (Systemic).
In providing consultation, consider emphasizing the following selected information (» = major clinical significance):

### Before using this medication
» Conditions affecting use, especially:
  Sensitivity to tiagabine
  Pregnancy—Teratogenicity and maternal toxicity have been demonstrated in animal studies
  Other medications, especially carbamazepine, phenobarbital, phenytoin, or primidone

### Proper use of this medication
» Compliance with therapy; not taking more or less medicine than prescribed
  Taking with food
» Proper dosing
  Missed dose: Taking as soon as possible; if almost time for next dose, skipping missed dose and returning to regular dosing schedule; not doubling doses
» Proper storage

### Precautions while using this medication
» Possible dizziness, drowsiness, impairment of thinking or motor skills; caution when driving or doing jobs requiring alertness or coordination
  Discussing alcohol use or use of other CNS depressants with physician
» Not discontinuing tiagabine abruptly; consulting physician about gradually reducing dosage

### Side/adverse effects
Signs of potential side effects, especially difficulty in concentrating or paying attention, ecchymosis, ataxia, confusion, mental depression, paresthesias, pruritus, speech and/or language problems, abnormal gait, agitation, emotional lability, generalized weakness, hostility, memory problems, nystagmus, rash, and urinary tract infection

## General Dosing Information

Anticonvulsants should not be abruptly discontinued because of the possibility of increasing seizure frequency. Unless safety concerns require a more rapid withdrawal, tiagabine should be withdrawn gradually.

### Diet/Nutrition
Tiagabine should be taken with food.

## Oral Dosage Forms

### TIAGABINE HYDROCHLORIDE TABLETS

Note: Clinical trials of adjunctive use of tiagabine were conducted in patients taking enzyme-inducing anticonvulsants (e.g., barbiturates, carbamazepine, phenytoin). Patients taking only non–enzyme-inducing anticonvulsants (e.g., gabapentin, lamotrigine, valproate) may require a lower dose or slower titration of tiagabine. Patients taking a combination of inducing and non-inducing anticonvulsants should be considered to be induced.

#### Usual adult dose
Anticonvulsant—
  Oral, initially 4 mg once a day. The total daily dose may be increased by 4 to 8 mg at weekly intervals until clinical response is achieved or a dose of 56 mg a day is reached. The total daily dose should be given in divided doses two to four times a day.

Note: Dosage modification of concomitant anticonvulsants is not necessary, unless clinically indicated.

## Tiagabine (Systemic)—Introductory Version

A typical dosing titration regimen for patients taking enzyme-inducing anticonvulsants follows:

| Week | Initiation and titration schedule | Total daily dose |
|---|---|---|
| 1 | Initiate at 4 mg once a day | 4 mg/day |
| 2 | Increase total daily dose by 4 mg | 8 mg/day (in two divided doses) |
| 3 | Increase total daily dose by 4 mg | 12 mg/day (in three divided doses) |
| 4 | Increase total daily dose by 4 mg | 16 mg/day (in two to four divided doses) |
| 5 | Increase total daily dose by 4 to 8 mg | 20 to 24 mg/day (in two to four divided doses) |
| 6 | Increase total daily dose by 4 to 8 mg | 24 to 32 mg/day (in two to four divided doses) |
| Usual adult maintenance dose | | 32 to 56 mg/day in two to four divided doses |

Note: Dosage reduction may be necessary in patients with liver disease due to reduced clearance of tiagabine.

**Usual adult prescribing limits**
56 mg a day.

Note: Doses above 56 mg a day have not been evaluated in adequate and well-controlled studies.

**Usual pediatric dose**
Anticonvulsant—
Children 12 to 18 years of age—Oral, initially 4 mg once a day. The total daily dose may be increased by 4 mg at the beginning of the second week of therapy. Thereafter, the total daily dose may be further increased by 4 to 8 mg at weekly intervals until clinical response is achieved or a dose of 32 mg a day is reached. The total daily dose should be given in divided doses two to four times a day.

Note: Dosage modification of concomitant anticonvulsants is not necessary, unless clinically indicated.
Children up to 12 years of age—Safety and efficacy have not been established.

**Usual adolescent prescribing limits**
32 mg a day.

Note: Doses above 32 mg a day have been tolerated in a small number of adolescent patients for a relatively short time.

**Usual geriatric dose**
See *Usual adult dose*.

U.S.—
4 mg (Rx) [*Gabitril* (film-sealed; ascorbic acid; colloidal silicon dioxide; crospovidone; hydrogenated vegetable oil wax; hydroxypropyl cellulose; hydroxypropyl methylcellulose; lactose; magnesium stearate; microcrystalline cellulose; pregelatinized starch; stearic acid; titanium dioxide; D&C Yellow No. 10)].
12 mg (Rx) [*Gabitril* (film-sealed; ascorbic acid; colloidal silicon dioxide; crospovidone; hydrogenated vegetable oil wax; hydroxypropyl cellulose; hydroxypropyl methylcellulose; lactose; magnesium stearate; microcrystalline cellulose; pregelatinized starch; stearic acid; titanium dioxide; D&C Yellow No. 10; FD&C Blue No. 1)].
16 mg (Rx) [*Gabitril* (film-sealed; ascorbic acid; colloidal silicon dioxide; crospovidone; hydrogenated vegetable oil wax; hydroxypropyl cellulose; hydroxypropyl methylcellulose; lactose; magnesium stearate; microcrystalline cellulose; pregelatinized starch; stearic acid; titanium dioxide; D&C Blue No. 2)].
20 mg (Rx) [*Gabitril* (film-sealed; ascorbic acid; colloidal silicon dioxide; crospovidone; hydrogenated vegetable oil wax; hydroxypropyl cellulose; hydroxypropyl methylcellulose; lactose; magnesium stearate; microcrystalline cellulose; pregelatinized starch; stearic acid; titanium dioxide; D&C Red No. 30)].

**Packaging and storage**
Store between 20 and 25 ºC (68 and 77 ºF). Protect from light and moisture.

**Auxiliary labeling**
- Take with food.
- May cause drowsiness.
- May cause dizziness.

Developed: 02/26/98

---

**TIAPROFENIC ACID**—See *Anti-inflammatory Drugs, Nonsteroidal (Systemic)*

---

**TICARCILLIN**—See *Penicillins (Systemic)*

---

# TICLOPIDINE  Systemic

VA CLASSIFICATION (Primary): BL117
Commonly used brand name(s): *Ticlid*.

Note: For a listing of dosage forms and brand names by country availability, see *Dosage Forms* section(s).

## Category
Antithrombotic; platelet aggregation inhibitor.

## Indications

**Accepted**
Stroke, thromboembolic, initial or recurrent (prophylaxis)—Ticlopidine is indicated to reduce the risk of a recurrent thromboembolic stroke in patients who have had a completed thrombotic stroke. It is also indicated to reduce the risk of an initial completed thromboembolic stroke in patients who have experienced stroke precursors, such as transient ischemic attack, transient monocular blindness (amaurosis fugax), reversible ischemic neurological deficit (RIND), or minor stroke. In one study in patients who had experienced an ischemic stroke, ticlopidine produced slight but significant neurologic improvement.

Although ticlopidine was somewhat more effective than aspirin in preventing initial strokes in patients with stroke precursors in a major study, it caused significantly more adverse effects than aspirin. Also, ticlopidine may cause neutropenia and agranulocytosis. It is therefore recommended that ticlopidine therapy be reserved for patients unable to take aspirin for stroke prophylaxis and patients who develop strokes despite aspirin therapy, and only when close hematologic monitoring is possible.

## Pharmacology/Pharmacokinetics

**Physicochemical characteristics**
Chemical group—Thienopyridine derivative.
Molecular weight—300.25.

**Mechanism of action/Effect**
Ticlopidine is an inhibitor of platelet aggregation; doses of 250, 375, and 500 mg a day inhibit platelet aggregation by 20 to 50%, 30 to 60%, and 50 to 70%, respectively. Doses higher than 500 mg per day do not produce a significant additional increase in the extent of inhibition.

The mechanism by which ticlopidine inhibits platelet aggregation has not been fully characterized. Ticlopidine inhibits adenosine diphosphate (ADP)-induced binding of fibrinogen to the platelet membrane at a specific receptor site (the glycoprotein IIb-IIIa complex). Release of platelet granule constituents, platelet-platelet interactions, and platelet adhesion to the endothelium and to atheromatous plaque are inhibited. Ticlopidine has no significant inhibitory effect on other endogenous substances known to promote platelet aggregation; it does not interfere with the synthesis or activity of cyclo-oxygenase, phosphodiesterase, or platelet cyclic adenosine monophosphate (cAMP), or with adenosine uptake. Also, ticlopidine does not alter mobilization or influx of calcium ions.

There is a lag time of several days for ticlopidine to exert its maximum effect on platelet function, probably by acting on platelet membranes during megakaryocytopoietic development rather than on already circulating platelets. Ticlopidine-induced inhibition of platelet aggregation persists for the life of the platelet.

Ticlopidine prolongs the template bleeding time, but has no effect in usual assays of coagulation or fibrinolysis.

Ticlopidine also reduces fibrinogen concentrations and blood viscosity, and increases the filterability rates of both whole blood and red cells, which may contribute to the beneficial effects in patients with vascular disease.

**Absorption**
Rapid; 80% or more of a dose is absorbed. Absorption is increased when the medication is taken after a meal.

**Protein binding**
Very high (98%), primarily to serum albumin and lipoproteins, and, to a lesser extent (15% or less), to alpha-1-acid glycoprotein. Protein binding of metabolites is about 40 to 50%.

**Biotransformation**
Hepatic; extensive. At least 20 metabolites have been identified. It has been proposed that 1 or more active metabolites may account for ticlopidine's activity, because the intact agent is an extremely weak platelet aggregation inhibitor *in vitro* at the concentrations achieved *in vivo*. However, no active metabolite has been identified.

Biotransformation of ticlopidine may be saturable; plasma concentrations achieved after a single dose increase disproportionately to the dose. Also, steady-state plasma concentrations are approximately twice as high as those achieved after administration of a single dose. In addition, the percentage of unmetabolized ticlopidine present in the circulation is 5% after a single dose and 15% at steady-state.

**Half-life**
Elimination—
  Single 250-mg dose: About 7.9 hours in subjects 20 to 43 years of age; about 12.6 hours in subjects 65 to 76 years of age.
  Repeated dosing with 250 mg twice a day: About 4 days in subjects 20 to 43 years of age; about 5 days in subjects 65 to 76 years of age.

**Onset of action**
Repeated dosing with 250 mg twice a day—Inhibition of platelet aggregation is detectable within 2 days; clinically significant inhibition (more than 50%) occurs within 4 days.

**Time to peak concentration**
Single 250-mg dose—About 2 hours.

**Peak concentration**
Single 250-mg dose—0.4 to 0.6 mcg per mL (mcg/mL) (1.33 to 1.99 micromoles/L); subject to substantial inter- and intrasubject variation. Values obtained when the medication is taken with meals are about 20% higher than those obtained when the medication is taken on an empty stomach. Values obtained when the medication is taken following an aluminum- and magnesium-containing antacid are about 18% lower than those obtained when the medication is not taken after an antacid.

Plasma concentrations may be increased slightly in patients with hepatic function impairment (advanced cirrhosis) and significantly increased in patients with renal function impairment. The area under the curve is increased by about 28% in patients with mild renal function impairment (creatinine clearances of 50 to 80 mL per minute) and by about 60% in patients with moderate renal function impairment (creatinine clearances of 20 to 50 mL per minute).

**Time to steady-state concentration**
Repeated administration of 250 mg twice a day—14 to 21 days.

**Steady-state concentration**
Repeated administration of 250 mg twice a day—About 1 to 2 mcg/mL (3.33 to 6.66 micromoles/L); may be increased in elderly patients. The area under the curve in elderly subjects receiving 250 mg twice a day for 21 days is 2 to 3 times as high as in younger subjects.

**Time to peak effect**
Repeated dosing with 250 mg twice a day: Maximal inhibition of platelet aggregation (60 to 70%) is achieved in 8 to 11 days.

**Duration of action**
After discontinuation of treatment, recovery of platelet function occurs as exposed platelets are replaced. In the majority of patients, bleeding time and other platelet function tests return to pretreatment levels within 1 to 2 weeks.

**Elimination**
Renal (about 60% of a dose) and biliary/fecal (about 23% of a dose). Unchanged ticlopidine accounts for trace amounts of the quantity eliminated in the urine and about 33% of the quantity eliminated in the feces.

The plasma clearance rate after administration of 250 mg twice a day for 21 days is about 1.52 L per minute in young subjects (average age 29 years) and about 0.56 L per minute in elderly subjects (average age 70 years). The plasma clearance rate is decreased by about 37% in patients with mild renal function impairment (creatinine clearances 50 to 80 mL per minute) and by about 52% in patients with moderate renal function impairment (creatinine clearances 20 to 50 mL per minute).

## Precautions to Consider

**Carcinogenicity/Tumorigenicity**
No evidence of carcinogenicity or tumorigenicity was found in a 2-year study in rats receiving oral doses of up to 100 mg per kg of body weight (mg/kg) per day (610 mg per square meter of body surface area [mg/m$^2$] per day). These doses are equivalent to up to 14 times the human clinical dose on an mg/kg basis and 2 times the clinical dose on an mg/m$^2$ basis (based on a human weighing 70 kg and having a body surface area of 1.73 m$^2$). Also, no evidence of tumorigenicity or carcinogenicity was found in a 78-week study in mice receiving oral doses of up to 275 mg/kg per day (1180 mg/m$^2$ per day). These doses are equivalent to up to 40 times the clinical dose on a mg/kg basis and 4 times the clinical dose on an mg/m$^2$ basis.

**Mutagenicity**
No evidence of mutagenic activity was found in the Ames test, rat hepatocyte DNA-repair assay, Chinese hamster fibroblast chromosomal aberration test (all *in vitro*) or in the mouse spermatozoid morphology test, Chinese hamster micronucleus test, and Chinese hamster bone marrow cell sister chromatid exchange test (all *in vivo*).

**Pregnancy/Reproduction**
Fertility—Ticlopidine had no effect on fertility in male or female rats in doses of up to 400 mg/kg per day.

Pregnancy—Adequate and well-controlled studies have not been performed in pregnant women.

No evidence of teratogenicity was found in studies in mice receiving up to 200 mg/kg per day, rats receiving up to 400 mg/kg per day, or rabbits receiving up to 200 g/kg per day. However, maternal toxicity (decreased food intake and weight gain) and fetotoxicity occurred in mice receiving 200 mg/kg per day, rats receiving 400 mg/kg per day, and rabbits receiving 100 g/kg per day.

FDA Pregnancy Category B.

**Breast-feeding**
It is not known whether ticlopidine is distributed into human breast milk. However, problems in humans have not been documented.

**Pediatrics**
No information is available on the relationship of age to the effects of ticlopidine in pediatric patients. Safety and efficacy have not been established.

**Geriatrics**
Appropriate studies performed to date have not demonstrated geriatrics-specific problems that would limit the usefulness of ticlopidine in the elderly. In major clinical trials, approximately 45% of the patients were 65 years of age or older; 12% were more than 75 years of age. Although clearance of ticlopidine is lower in elderly patients than in younger adults, and plasma concentrations are higher than in younger adults, elderly individuals in these studies did not receive lower doses. No overall differences in efficacy or safety were observed.

**Dental**
Because of the risk of increased blood loss, it is recommended that ticlopidine be discontinued 10 to 14 days prior to dental surgery.

Ticlopidine may cause neutropenia, which may result in an increased incidence of microbial infection, delayed healing, and gingival bleeding. If severe neutropenia occurs, dental work should be deferred until blood counts have returned to normal. Also, patients should be instructed in proper oral hygiene, including caution in use of regular toothbrushes, dental floss, and toothpicks.

**Surgical**
Because of the risk of increased surgical blood loss, it is recommended that ticlopidine be discontinued 10 to 14 days prior to elective surgery. In emergency situations, transfusion of fresh platelets may improve hemostasis. Although intravenous administration of 20 mg of methylprednisolone to ticlopidine-treated patients has been shown to return the bleeding time to normal within 2 hours, the effect of such treatment on perisurgical hemostasis has not been established.

**Drug interactions and/or related problems**
The following drug interactions and/or related problems have been selected on the basis of their potential clinical significance (possible mechanism in parentheses where appropriate)—not necessarily inclusive (» = major clinical significance):

Note:  Combinations containing any of the following medications, depending on the amount present, may also interact with this medication.

In addition to the interactions listed below, the possibility should be considered that additive or multiple effects leading to an increased risk of bleeding may occur if ticlopidine is administered concurrently with any other medication that has significant platelet aggregation-inhibiting activity or a significant potential for causing hypoprothrombinemia, thrombocytopenia, or gastrointestinal ulceration or hemorrhage.

Antacids, aluminum- and magnesium-containing
(plasma concentrations of ticlopidine are decreased by about 18% when it is administered after an aluminum- and magnesium-containing antacid; information about the effects of single-ingredient antacids on ticlopidine concentrations is not available, but the possibility of a similar effect should be considered; it is recommended that ticlopidine and an antacid be administered at least 1 to 2 hours apart)

» Anticoagulants, coumarin- or indandione-derivative or
» Heparin or
» Thrombolytic agents, such as:
   Alteplase
   Anistreplase
   Streptokinase
   Urokinase
   (the possibility of additive effects on blood clotting mechanisms leading to an increased risk of bleeding cannot be discounted; particularly careful clinical monitoring of the patient is recommended if concurrent use is necessary)

   (in one study, concurrent administration of warfarin and ticlopidine was associated with an increased risk of medication-induced hepatitis)

» Aspirin or
» Nonsteroidal anti-inflammatory drugs (NSAIDs) or
» Platelet aggregation inhibitors, other (see *Appendix II*)
   (concurrent use of ticlopidine with these agents may increase the risk of bleeding because of additive inhibition of platelet aggregation; also, the potential for aspirin- or NSAID-induced gastrointestinal ulceration or hemorrhage exists)

   (concurrent use of ticlopidine and aspirin is not recommended; in one study, the risk of bleeding was higher, and bleeding episodes occurred earlier, in patients receiving combined therapy with low doses of aspirin and ticlopidine [81 mg and 100 mg per day, respectively] than in patients receiving larger doses of either agent alone; studies have also shown that the combination of medications prolongs bleeding time to a greater extent than either agent alone; these effects are probably due to potentiation by ticlopidine of aspirin-mediated inhibition of platelet aggregation, since studies have shown that inhibition of collagen-induced platelet aggregation [an effect of aspirin], but not of adenosine diphosphate [ADP]-induced platelet aggregation [an effect of ticlopidine] is increased in the presence of both agents)

Phenytoin
(several cases of elevated phenytoin plasma concentrations with associated somnolence and lethargy have been reported following ticlopidine administration)

Xanthines, such as:
   Aminophylline
   Oxtriphylline
   Theophylline
   (theophylline elimination half-life may be increased by about 40%, and total plasma clearance of theophylline decreased by about 35%, when a xanthine is administered to a patient receiving ticlopidine)

**Laboratory value alterations**
The following have been selected on the basis of their potential clinical significance (possible effect in parentheses where appropriate)—not necessarily inclusive (» = major clinical significance):

With physiology/laboratory test values
   Alkaline phosphatase and
   Bilirubin and
   Transaminases
   (values may be elevated; in clinical studies, the incidence of elevations to more than twice the upper limit of normal was 7.6% for alkaline phosphatase and 3.1% for aspartate aminotransferase [AST (SGOT)]; increases generally occurred within 1 to 4 months after initiation of therapy; although no progressive increases were reported, treatment was discontinued in most patients)

» Bleeding time
   (prolongation to 2 to 5 times the pretreatment value is expected during ticlopidine treatment, although maximal effects on bleeding time may be delayed for some time after platelet aggregation tests indicate maximal inhibition; ticlopidine-induced prolongation of bleeding time may be reduced in patients receiving chronic glucocorticoid treatment, although ticlopidine's effect on ADP-induced platelet aggregation is not altered; also, prolongation of bleeding time may be reversed by a single intravenous dose of 20 mg of methylprednisolone)

Cholesterol, total and
Triglycerides
(serum concentrations may be elevated; in clinical studies, total serum cholesterol was increased by 8 to 10% after about 1 month of ticlopidine treatment, but further increases did not occur thereafter; also, the ratios of lipoprotein subfractions were not altered)

» Neutrophil count and
Platelet count
(may be decreased; in clinical trials, the overall incidence of neutropenia [absolute neutrophil count (ANC) < 1200 neutrophils/mm³] was 2.4%, and that of severe neutropenia [ANC < 450 neutrophils/mm³] about 0.8%; neutropenia generally occurs between 3 and 12 weeks after initiation of treatment, is associated with inhibition of granulocyte cell line maturation, and is generally reversed within a few weeks after discontinuation of treatment)

(thrombocytopenia may occur in conjunction with, or independently of, neutropenia, generally between 3 and 12 weeks after initiation of treatment; in clinical trials, the incidence of thrombocytopenia was 0.4%; recovery generally occurs after discontinuation)

**Medical considerations/Contraindications**
The medical considerations/contraindications included have been selected on the basis of their potential clinical significance (reasons given in parentheses where appropriate)—not necessarily inclusive (» = major clinical significance).

*Except under special circumstances, this medication should not be used when the following medical problems exist:*

» Bleeding, active and
» Hemophilia or other coagulation defects or hemostatic disorders
   (risk of severe bleeding)
» Hematopoietic disorders such as:
   Neutropenia
   Thrombocytopenia
      (may be exacerbated)
» Hepatic function impairment, severe
   (increased risk of bleeding because severe hepatic function impairment may result in decreased synthesis of clotting factor precursors)

*Risk-benefit should be considered when the following medical problems exist:*

» Any condition in which there is a significant risk of bleeding, such as:
   Gastrointestinal ulceration
   Surgery
   Trauma
» Renal function impairment, severe
   (clearance of ticlopidine decreases, and concentrations increase, with increasing degrees of renal function impairment; although ticlopidine is well tolerated by patients with mild or moderate degrees of renal function impairment, caution and close monitoring are recommended in patients with severe renal disease because experience in such patients is limited; a reduction in dosage may be needed, but studies with reduced doses of ticlopidine have not been done)

Sensitivity to ticlopidine

**Patient monitoring**
The following may be especially important in patient monitoring (other tests may be warranted in some patients, depending on condition; » = major clinical significance):

Bleeding time and
Platelet count
(determinations may be needed to assess the risk of bleeding complications when procedures that have a significant risk of bleeding, such as surgery or dental work, are needed during or shortly following ticlopidine therapy)

» Complete blood count and
» Platelet count and
» White blood cell differentials
(because of the risk of neutropenia and/or thrombocytopenia, these checks should be performed every 2 weeks, starting at baseline before treatment is begun, for the first 3 months of treatment; more frequent monitoring may be needed for patients whose absolute neutrophil counts are declining or are 30% below the baseline count, since severe neutropenia may develop rapidly [over a few days]. Treatment should be discontinued if clinical evaluation and repeat laboratory testing confirm the presence of neutropenia or thrombocytopenia [neutrophil count reduced to 1200 per cubic millimeter or lower; platelet count reduced to 80,000 per cubic millimeter or lower]. If treatment is discontinued for any reason within the first

3 months, continued monitoring for at least another 2 weeks following discontinuation is recommended because of ticlopidine's long plasma half-life. Because the risk of these complications decreases substantially after the first 3 months of therapy [although cases have been reported after several months or even years of treatment], further testing is needed only if signs and symptoms suggestive of severe neutropenia or thrombocytopenia occur)

## Side/Adverse Effects

Note: Most of the side/adverse effects reported with ticlopidine, including *neutropenia or agranulocytosis, thrombocytopenia, gastrointestinal disturbances,* and *skin rash,* appear within the first 3 months of treatment, although some may occur or recur several months later. Rarely, *neutropenia, thrombocytopenia, or thrombotic thrombocytopenic purpura* has occurred after years of treatment. Fatalities associated with *severe neutropenia, agranulocytosis, pancytopenia, aplastic anemia, immune thrombocytopenia,* or *thrombotic thrombocytopenic purpura* have been reported.

Ticlopidine-induced *gastrointestinal disturbances* may occur in up to 40% of the patients receiving the medication. They are generally mild and usually disappear within 1 or 2 weeks without discontinuation of treatment; however, about 13% of the patients withdrew from clinical studies because of them. In some cases of severe or bloody diarrhea, colitis was later diagnosed.

In addition to the side/adverse effects listed below, rare cases of the following have been reported in postmarketing surveillance programs: *pancytopenia, hemolytic anemia with reticulocytosis, allergic pneumonitis, systemic lupus erythematosus, peripheral neuropathy, vasculitis, serum sickness, arthropathy, nephrotic syndrome, myositis, hyponatremia, immune thrombocytopenia, thrombotic thrombocytopenic purpura, eosinophilia, bone marrow depression, aplastic anemia, hepatocellular jaundice, hepatic necrosis, peptic ulcer, renal failure, sepsis,* and *angioedema.* A causal relationship has not always been established.

The following side/adverse effects have been selected on the basis of their potential clinical significance (possible signs and symptoms in parentheses where appropriate)—not necessarily inclusive:

**Those indicating need for medical attention**
Incidence more frequent
*Skin rash*—incidence 5.1%
Note: Usually disappears within several days after treatment is discontinued, and may not recur upon reinstitution of treatment. However, there have been rare reports of severe rashes including Stevens-Johnson syndrome, erythema multiforme, and exfoliative dermatitis.

Incidence less frequent
*Bleeding complications* (abdominal pain [severe] or swelling; back pain; blood in eyes; blood in urine; bloody or black, tarry stools; bruising or purple areas on skin; coughing up blood; decreased alertness; dizziness; headache, severe or continuing; joint pain or swelling; nosebleeds; paralysis or problems with coordination; stammering or other difficulty in speaking; unusually heavy bleeding or oozing from cuts or wounds; unusually heavy or unexpected menstrual bleeding; vomiting of blood or material that looks like coffee grounds)—depending on the site of bleeding; in clinical studies the incidence of intracerebral bleeding was 0.5% and that of epistaxis was 0.5 to 1%; *itching of skin*—incidence 1.3%; *neutropenia, including agranulocytosis* (fever, chills, sore throat, other signs of infection; ulcers, sores, or white spots in mouth)—incidence 2.4% overall, 0.8% severe [absolute neutrophil count (ANC) < 450 neutrophils/mm$^3$]; *purpura* (red or purple spots on skin, varying in size from pinpoint to large bruises)—incidence 2.2%

Incidence rare
*Hepatitis or cholestatic jaundice* (yellow eyes or skin); *hives*—incidence 0.5 to 1%; *ringing or buzzing in ears*—incidence 0.5 to 1%; *skin rash, severe, including erythema multiforme* (fever; malaise; red skin lesions, often with a purple center); *or Stevens-Johnson syndrome* (blistering, peeling, or loosening of skin and mucous membranes; fever; malaise); *or exfoliative dermatitis* (fever; malaise; red, thickened, or scaly skin); *thrombocytopenia* (unusual bleeding or bruising; black, tarry stools; blood in urine or stools; pinpoint red spots on skin)—usually asymptomatic; incidence 0.4%
Note: Bulla formation involving the eyes or other organ systems may occur with *Stevens-Johnson syndrome.*
*Thrombocytopenia* may occur independently of, or in conjunction with, neutropenia.

**Those indicating need for medical attention only if they continue or are bothersome**
Incidence more frequent
*Abdominal pain*—incidence 3.7%; *diarrhea*—incidence 12.5%; *indigestion*—incidence 7%; *nausea*—incidence 7%
Incidence less frequent
*Bloating or gas*—incidence 1.5%; *dizziness*—incidence 1.1%; *vomiting*—incidence 1.9%

## Overdose

Only one case of overdose has been reported, in which a single 6000-mg dose was ingested by a 38-year-old male. The patient's bleeding time was prolonged and the alanine aminotransferase (ALT [SGPT]) value was increased. There were no other abnormalities or symptoms, and the patient recovered without treatment.

For more information on the management of overdose or unintentional ingestion, **contact a Poison Control Center** (see *Poison Control Center Listing*).

## Patient Consultation

As an aid to patient consultation, refer to *Advice for the Patient, Ticlopidine (Systemic).*

In providing consultation, consider emphasizing the following selected information (» = major clinical significance):

**Before using this medication**
» Conditions affecting use, especially:
   Sensitivity to ticlopidine
   Dental—Risk of increased blood loss during dental procedures
   Other medications, especially anticoagulants or platelet aggregation inhibitors
   Other medical problems, especially bleeding (active), medical problems in which there is a significant risk of bleeding, hematopoietic disorders, severe hepatic function impairment, and severe renal function impairment
   Surgical—Risk of increased blood loss during surgical procedures

**Proper use of this medication**
Taking medication with food to increase absorption and to reduce the risk of gastrointestinal irritation
Compliance with prescribed treatment regimen
» Proper dosing
Missed dose: Taking as soon as possible; not taking if almost time for next dose; not doubling doses
» Proper storage

**Precautions while using this medication**
» Importance of regular blood tests to detect potential adverse effects during the first 3 months of treatment
» Need to inform all health care providers of use of medication; medication should be discontinued 10 to 14 days prior to elective procedures with a risk of bleeding
» Because of risk of bleeding, obtaining physician's opinion before participating in activities with substantial risk of injury and contacting physician immediately if injury occurs
» Notifying physician immediately if signs and symptoms of bleeding, infection, or thrombocytopenia occur
Possibility that risk of bleeding may continue for 1 to 2 weeks after treatment is discontinued

**Side/adverse effects**
Signs of potential side effects, especially skin rash, bleeding complications, itching of skin, neutropenia, agranulocytosis, purpura, hepatitis or cholestatic jaundice, hives, ringing or buzzing in the ears, erythema multiforme, Stevens-Johnson syndrome, exfoliative dermatitis, and thrombocytopenia

## General Dosing Information

Ticlopidine should be taken with meals to achieve maximum absorption and reduce the risk of gastrointestinal side effects.

It is recommended that ticlopidine therapy be discontinued temporarily if an injury that results in a substantial risk of bleeding occurs.

It is recommended that ticlopidine therapy be discontinued 10 to 14 days prior to elective surgery, including dental extraction, because of the risk of increased blood loss.

**Diet/Nutrition**
Absorption of ticlopidine is increased when the medication is taken after a meal.

### For treatment of adverse effects
Recommended treatment consists of the following
- In general—Monitoring the patient and instituting supportive measures as needed.
- For bleeding complications—Although administration of methylprednisolone (20 mg, intravenously) returns the bleeding time to normal in ticlopidine-treated patients, clinical experience indicating that such treatment improves hemostasis is lacking. Platelet transfusions may be helpful, although they are usually not indicated for thrombotic thrombocytopenic purpura occuring in patients taking ticlopidine. In addition, other measures to control bleeding in specific areas must be employed as needed.

## Oral Dosage Forms

### TICLOPIDINE HYDROCHLORIDE TABLETS

**Usual adult dose**
Antithrombotic—
  Oral, 250 mg twice a day, taken with food.

**Usual pediatric and adolescent dose**
Safety and efficacy in patients up to 18 years of age have not been established.

**Usual geriatric dose**
See *Usual adult dose*.

**Strength(s) usually available**
U.S.—
  250 mg (Rx) [*Ticlid* (citric acid; magnesium stearate; microcrystalline cellulose; povidone; starch; stearic acid)].
Canada—
  250 mg (Rx) [*Ticlid* (citric acid; magnesium stearate; microcrystalline cellulose; povidone; corn starch; stearic acid); GENERIC].

**Packaging and storage**
Store below 40 °C (104 °F), preferably between 15 and 30 °C (59 and 86 °F), unless otherwise specified by manufacturer.

**Auxiliary labeling**
- Take with food.

## Selected Bibliography
Gent M, Blakely JA, Easton JD, et al. The Canadian American ticlopidine study (CATS) in thromboembolic stroke. Lancet 1989; 333: 1215-20.
Hass WK, Easton D, Adams HP Jr, et al. A randomized trial comparing ticlopidine hydrochloride with aspirin for the prevention of stroke in high-risk patients. N Engl J Med 1989; 321: 501-7.

Revised: 08/06/96
Interim revision: 08/15/97

---

# TILUDRONATE   Systemic—INTRODUCTORY VERSION

VA CLASSIFICATION (Primary): HS303
Commonly used brand name(s): *Skelid*.
Note:  For a listing of dosage forms and brand names by country availability, see *Dosage Forms* section(s).

## Category
Bone resorption inhibitor.

## Indications

**Accepted**
Paget's disease of bone (treatment)—Tiludronate is indicated for the treatment of Paget's disease (osteitis deformans) in patients with alkaline phosphatase concentrations at least two times the upper limit of normal, those who are symptomatic, or those at risk for future complications from the disease. Signs and symptoms of Paget's disease may include bone pain, deformity, and/or fractures; increased concentrations of serum alkaline and/or urinary hydroxyproline; and neurologic disorders.

## Pharmacology/Pharmacokinetics

**Physicochemical characteristics**
Molecular weight—380.6.

**Mechanism of action/Effect**
Tiludronate reduces toward normal the rate of bone turnover in pagetic patients. *In vitro* studies have shown that tiludronate inhibits osteoclasts by inhibiting the osteoclastic proton pump and by disrupting the cytoskeletal ring structure (possibly by inhibition of protein-tyrosine-phosphatase), which leads to detachment of osteoclasts from the bone surface. This causes a reduction in the enzymatic and transport processes that lead to resorption of the mineralized matrix.

**Absorption**
Studies in healthy males showed that the mean oral bioavailability was 6 ± 2% after a single dose equivalent to 400 mg tiludronic acid was administered after an overnight fast and 4 hours before a standard breakfast. Oral bioavailability was reduced by 90% when a single dose equivalent to 400 mg tiludronic acid was administered with, or 2 hours after, a standard breakfast. In clinical studies, efficacy was demonstrated when tiludronate was administered at least 2 hours before or after meals.

**Distribution**
Studies in rats showed that tiludronate is distributed to bone and soft tissues.

**Protein binding**
High (approximately 90%) to human serum protein, primarily albumin, at plasma concentrations of tiludronic acid between 1 and 10 mg per L (mg/L).

**Biotransformation**
There is little to no evidence that tiludronate is metabolized in humans or animals. *In vitro* studies have shown that tiludronic acid is not metabolized in human liver microsomes or hepatocytes.

**Half-life**
Distribution—
  30 days in the bone of rats, depending on the status of bone turnover.
Elimination—
  In healthy subjects: 50 hours from plasma after administration of a single, oral dose equivalent to 400 mg tiludronic acid.
  In pagetic patients: Approximately 150 hours from plasma after administration of oral doses equivalent to 400 mg tiludronic acid a day for 12 days.
  In patients with renal insufficiency (creatinine clearance between 11 and 18 mL per minute [mL/min]): 205 hours from plasma after administration of a single, oral dose equivalent to 400 mg tiludronic acid.

**Time to peak concentration**
1.5 ± 0.9 hours in the plasma of healthy males after administration of a single, oral dose equivalent to 400 mg tiludronic acid, taken 4 hours before the first meal of the day.

**Peak serum concentration**
In healthy males—2.66 ± 1.22 mg/L in the plasma after administration of a single, oral dose equivalent to 400 mg tiludronic acid, taken 4 hours before the first meal of the day.
In patients with renal insufficiency (creatinine clearance between 11 and 18 mL/min)—Approximately 3 mg/L in the plasma after administration of a single, oral dose equivalent to 400 mg tiludronic acid.

**Elimination**
Renal; approximately 60% of an intravenous dose is excreted in the urine as tiludronic acid within 13 days. In healthy subjects, the renal clearance was 0.54 ± 0.14 L per hour (L/hr) after intravenous administration of a 20-mg dose.

## Precautions to Consider

**Carcinogenicity**
Studies to determine the carcinogenic potential of tiludronate have not been done in humans or animals.

**Mutagenicity**
Tiludronate was not genotoxic in the *in vitro* microbial mutagenesis assay with and without metabolic activation, in the human lymphocyte assay, in a yeast cell assay for forward mutation and mitotic crossing over, and in the *in vivo* mouse micronucleus test.

**Pregnancy/Reproduction**
Fertility—Studies in male and female rats given tiludronate at doses of 75 mg per kg of body weight (mg/kg) a day (up to 2 times the human dose of 400 mg a day based on body surface area) found no effect on fertility.
Pregnancy—Adequate and well-controlled studies in humans have not been done.
Studies in rabbits given tiludronate doses of 42 mg/kg a day and 130 mg/kg a day (2 and 5 times the human dose of 400 mg, respectively, a day based on body surface area) on days 6 through 18 of gestation found dose-related scoliosis. Studies in mice given tiludronic acid doses of

375 mg/kg a day (7 times the human dose of 400 mg a day based on body surface area) on days 6 through 15 of gestation found a slightly decreased maternal body weight gain, increased postimplantation loss, and a decreased number of fetuses per dam; in addition, malformations of the paw were noted in six fetuses from the same litter. Teratology studies in rats given tiludronic acid at doses of 375 mg/kg a day (ten times the human dose of 400 mg a day based on body surface area) on days 6 through 18 of gestation found decreased maternal body weight, a reduced percent of implantations, increased postimplantation loss, and increased intrauterine deaths; there were no teratogenic effects in the fetuses.

Protracted parturition and maternal death, possibly due to maternal hypocalcemia, occurred in rats receiving tiludronic acid at doses of 75 mg/kg a day (2 times the human dose of 400 mg a day based on body surface area) on day 15 of gestation through day 25 postpartum.

FDA Pregnancy Category C.

**Breast-feeding**
It is not known whether tiludronate is distributed into human breast milk.

**Pediatrics**
No information is available on the relationship of age to the effects of tiludronate in pediatric patients. Safety and efficacy have not been established.

**Geriatrics**
Appropriate studies performed to date have not demonstrated geriatrics-specific problems that would limit the usefulness of tiludronate in the elderly.

**Drug interactions and/or related problems**
The following drug interactions and/or related problems have been selected on the basis of their potential clinical significance (possible mechanism in parentheses where appropriate)—not necessarily inclusive (» = major clinical significance):

Note: Combinations containing any of the following, depending on the amount present, may also interact with this medication.

Food and beverages or
» Medications, oral (including aluminum- or magnesium-containing antacids) or
» Mineral supplements (including calcium) or
» Salicylates or salicylate-containing compounds
(simultaneous use may interfere with the absorption of tiludronate; the bioavailability of tiludronate is decreased by 60% when aluminum- or magnesium-containing antacids are administered 1 hour before tiludronate, by 80% when tiludronate is administered with calcium preparations, and by 50% when salicylates are taken 2 hours after tiludronate; aluminum- or magnesium-containing antacid preparations should be taken at least 2 hours after taking tiludronate; beverages, food, mineral supplements [including calcium], or salicylates should not be taken within 2 hours before or after taking tiludronate)

Indomethacin
(concurrent use may increase the bioavailability of tiludronate two- to four-fold; indomethacin should not be taken within 2 hours before or 2 hours after taking tiludronate)

**Medical considerations/Contraindications**
The medical considerations/contraindications included have been selected on the basis of their potential clinical significance (reasons given in parentheses where appropriate)—not necessarily inclusive (» = major clinical significance):

*Except under special circumstances, this medication should not be used when the following medical problems exist:*
» Gastrointestinal diseases such as dysphagia, esophagitis, esophageal ulcer, or gastric ulcer
(bisphosphonates, including tiludronate may exacerbate these conditions)
» Renal function impairment when creatinine clearance is < 30 mL per minute
(use is not recommended due to lack of experience; elimination of tiludronate may be reduced)

*Risk-benefit should be considered when the following medical problems exist:*
Hyperparathyroidism or
Hypocalcemia or
Vitamin D deficiency
(bisphosphonates, including tiludronate may exacerbate these conditions)

Sensitivity to tiludronate

**Patient monitoring**
The following may be especially important in patient monitoring (other tests may be warranted in some patients, depending on condition; » = major clinical significance):

Alkaline phosphatase, serum or
Hydroxyproline, urinary
(determinations recommended periodically to assess effectiveness of therapy; values should decrease with treatment)

## Side/Adverse Effects

The following side/adverse effects have been selected on the basis of their potential clinical significance (possible signs and symptoms in parentheses where appropriate)—not necessarily inclusive:

**Those indicating need for medical attention**
Incidence more frequent (5 to 10%)
*Respiratory tract infection, upper* (cough; fever; head congestion; hoarseness or other voice changes; nasal congestion; runny nose; sneezing; sore throat)

Incidence less frequent (< 5%)
*Cataract* (blurred or decreased vision); *chest pain; edema* (swelling of face; swelling of feet or lower legs; unusual weight gain); *glaucoma* (blurred vision; eye pain; headache)

**Those indicating need for medical attention only if they continue or are bothersome**
Incidence more frequent (5 to 10% or as indicated)
*Back pain; body pain, general*—incidence 21%; *gastrointestinal symptoms, such as diarrhea; dyspepsia* (upset stomach); *nausea; headache*

Incidence less frequent (< 5%)
*Arthralgia* (joint pain); *conjunctivitis* (red or irritated eyes); *cough; dizziness; flatulence* (gas); *flu-like syndrome* (fever; joint pain; muscle pain); *pharyngitis* (pain in throat); *rhinitis* (runny nose); *skin rash; vomiting*

## Overdose

For information on the management of overdose or unintentional ingestion, **contact a Poison Control Center** (see *Poison Control Center Listing*).

**Treatment of overdose**
Specific treatment—Patients should be treated for signs of renal insufficiency and hypocalcemia.

Supportive care—Patients in whom intentional overdose is confirmed or suspected should be referred for psychiatric consultation.

## Patient Consultation

As an aid to patient consultation, refer to *Advice for the Patient, Tiludronate (Systemic)—Introductory Version*.

In providing consultation, consider emphasizing the following selected information (» = major clinical significance)

**Before using this medication**
» Conditions affecting use, especially:
Sensitivity to tiludronate
Pregnancy—Studies in animals showed scoliosis, decreased maternal weight gain, increased postimplantation loss, decreased number of fetuses per dam, fetal paw malformations, reduced percent of implantations, and increased intrauterine deaths
Other medications, especially salicylates or compounds that contain salicylates, medications (including aluminum- or magnesium-containing antacids) or mineral supplements (including calcium)
Other medical problems, especially gastrointestinal diseases or renal function impairment

**Proper use of this medication**
» Taking with 6 to 8 ounces of plain water on empty stomach
Possible need for calcium and vitamin D supplements
» Proper dosing
Missed dose: Taking as soon as possible; not taking if almost time for next dose; not doubling doses
» Proper storage

**Side/adverse effects**
Signs of potential side effects, especially upper respiratory tract infection; cataract; chest pain; edema; and glaucoma

## General Dosing Information

**Diet/Nutrition**
Tiludronate should be taken with 6 to 8 ounces of plain water. Tiludronate should not be taken within 2 hours of taking beverages (including mineral water), food, medications, or mineral supplements.

Some patients may be instructed to take calcium or vitamin D supplements if their diet is inadequate. These supplements should be taken 2 hours before or 2 hours after taking tiludronate.

## Oral Dosage Forms

Note: The dosing and strengths of the dosage forms available are expressed in terms of tiludronic acid (not the disodium salt).

### TILUDRONATE DISODIUM TABLETS

**Usual adult and adolescent dose**
Paget's disease of bone—
  Oral, 400 mg tiludronic acid a day at least two hours before or after taking beverages, food, medications, or mineral supplements. Treatment should continue for three months. The dose should be taken with six to eight ounces of plain water. Retreatment may be considered for some patients following a three-month post-treatment evaluation period.

**Usual pediatric dose**
Safety and efficacy have not been established.

**Usual geriatric dose**
See *Usual adult and adolescent dose*.

**Size(s) usually available**
U.S.—
  200 mg (tiludronic acid) (equivalent to 240 mg tiludronate disodium) (Rx) [*Skelid* (lactose)].

**Packaging and storage**
Store between 15 and 30 °C (59 and 86 °F), unless otherwise specified by the manufacturer.

**Auxiliary labeling**
• Take on empty stomach.

Developed: 08/15/97

---

**TIMOLOL**—See *Beta-adrenergic Blocking Agents (Ophthalmic)*; *Beta-adrenergic Blocking Agents (Systemic)*

---

**TIOCONAZOLE**—See *Antifungals, Azole (Vaginal)*

---

# TIOPRONIN  Systemic†

VA CLASSIFICATION (Primary): GU900
Commonly used brand name(s): *Thiola*.
Note: For a listing of dosage forms and brand names by country availability, see *Dosage Forms* section(s).

†Not commercially available in Canada.

## Category
Antiurolithic (cystine calculi).

## Indications

**Accepted**
Cystinuria (treatment) or
Renal calculi, cystine (prophylaxis)—Tiopronin is indicated for the prevention of cystine kidney stones in patients with severe homozygous cystinuria who have a urinary cystine concentration greater than 500 mg a day; are resistant to treatment with high fluid intake, alkali, and diet modification; or have had adverse reactions to penicillamine.

## Pharmacology/Pharmacokinetics

**Physicochemical characteristics**
Molecular weight—163.19.

**Mechanism of action/Effect**
Tiopronin is an active reducing agent that undergoes thiol-disulfide exchange with cystine (cysteine-cysteine disulfide) to form tiopronin-cystine disulfide, which is more water-soluble than cystine and is readily excreted. As a result, urinary cystine calculi are prevented.

**Distribution**
Up to 48% of a dose appears in the urine during the first 4 hours and 78% by 72 hours.

**Onset of action**
Rapid.

**Duration of action**
Very short; effect of tiopronin shown to disappear within 8 to 10 hours after administration.

**Elimination**
Renal.

## Precautions to Consider

**Cross-sensitivity and/or related problems**
Patients sensitive to penicillamine may be sensitive to this medication also.

**Carcinogenicity**
Long-term carcinogenicity studies in animals have not been performed.

**Pregnancy/Reproduction**
Pregnancy—Adequate and well-controlled studies in humans have not been done.

Since penicillamine has been shown to cause skeletal defects, cleft palates, and an increased number of resorptions when administered to rats at 10 times the recommended human dose, a similar teratogenic effect might be expected for tiopronin. Also, high doses of tiopronin in animals have been shown to interfere with maintenance of pregnancy and viability of the fetus.
FDA Pregnancy Category C.

**Breast-feeding**
Tiopronin may be distributed into breast milk. It is recommended that mothers taking tiopronin not breast-feed because of potentially serious adverse effects on nursing infants.

**Pediatrics**
Appropriate studies on the relationship of age to the effects of tiopronin have not been performed in the pediatric population. However, no pediatrics-specific problems have been documented to date.

**Geriatrics**
Although appropriate studies on the relationship of age to the effects of tiopronin have not been performed in the geriatric population, no geriatrics-specific problems have been documented to date. However, elderly patients are more likely to have age-related renal function impairment, which may require adjustment of dosage or dosing interval in patients receiving tiopronin.

**Drug interactions and/or related problems**
The following drug interactions and/or related problems have been selected on the basis of their potential clinical significance (possible mechanism in parentheses where appropriate)—not necessarily inclusive (» = major clinical significance):

Note: Combinations containing any of the following medications, depending on the amount present, may also interact with this medication.

Bone marrow depressants (See *Appendix II*)
  (concurrent use of these medications with tiopronin may increase the leukopenic and/or thrombocytopenic effects; if concurrent use is required, close observation for toxic effects should be considered)

Hepatotoxic medications (See *Appendix II*)
  (concurrent use of these medications with tiopronin may increase the hepatotoxic effects of either medication)

Nephrotoxic medications (See *Appendix II*)
  (concurrent use of these medications with tiopronin may increase the nephrotoxic effects of either medication)

**Medical considerations/Contraindications**
The medical considerations/contraindications included have been selected on the basis of their potential clinical significance (reasons given in parentheses where appropriate)—not necessarily inclusive (» = major clinical significance).

*Risk-benefit should be considered when the following medical problems exist:*

» Agranulocytosis, aplastic anemia or thrombocytopenia, history of
  (risk of recurrence)

Hepatic function impairment
  (condition may be exacerbated)
Renal function impairment, current or history of
  (cumulative effects of tiopronin may occur)
Sensitivity to tiopronin or penicillamine

**Patient monitoring**
The following may be especially important in patient monitoring (other tests may be warranted in some patients, depending on condition; » = major clinical significance):

Abdominal roentgenogram (KUB)
  (recommended on a yearly basis to monitor the size and appearance/disappearance of stone[s])
Albumin concentrations, serum and
Hemoglobin determinations and
Urinary protein determinations, 24-hour
  (recommended at frequent intervals)
Blood cell counts, white and
» Platelet counts, direct
  (therapy should be discontinued when peripheral white count is below 3500 per cubic mm and platelet count is below 100,000 cubic mm)
Hepatic function determinations
  (recommended at 2, 4, and 6 weeks of therapy)
Urinalysis, routine
  (recommended every 3 to 6 months during treatment; proteinuria may develop from membranous glomerulopathy and may be severe enough to cause nephrotic syndrome)
Urinary cystine concentrations
Urinary pH, 24-hour, determinations with pH electrode
  (determinations recommended after the first and third months of therapy and every 6 months thereafter to determine effectiveness of tiopronin in treatment of cystinuria)

## Side/Adverse Effects

The following side/adverse effects have been selected on the basis of their potential clinical significance (possible signs and symptoms in parentheses where appropriate)—not necessarily inclusive:

**Those indicating need for medical attention**
Incidence more frequent
*Dermatologic effects specifically ecchymosis* (pain, swelling, tenderness of subcutaneous tissue in affected area); *elastosis perforans serpiginosa; or pemphigus* (itching of skin); *skin rash or itching; ulcers or sores in mouth; urticaria* (hives); *jaundice* (yellow skin or eyes)
  Note: If *pemphigus-type reaction* develops, tiopronin therapy should be stopped. Steroid treatment may be necessary.
    *Skin rash* may appear during the first few months of treatment, but may be controlled with antihistamine therapy. Less commonly, rash may appear late in the course of treatment (after more than 6 months); this rash is usually located on the trunk and is associated with intense pruritus. The early rash recedes when tiopronin therapy is discontinued and seldom recurs when treatment is restarted at a lower dosage. The later rash recedes slowly after discontinuation of tiopronin and usually recurs when treatment is restarted.

Incidence less frequent
*Allergic reactions, specifically adenopathy* (tenderness of glands); *arthralgia* (pain in joints); *or chills; dyspnea or respiratory distress* (difficulty in breathing); *fever; increased bleeding; laryngeal edema* (difficulty in breathing; difficulty in swallowing; hoarseness); *myalgia* (muscle pain); *weakness; hematologic abnormalities, specifically anemia* (unusual tiredness or weakness); *eosinophilia; leukopenia* (sore throat and fever); *or thrombocytopenia* (unusual bleeding or bruising); *renal effects, specifically edema* (swelling of feet or lower legs); *hematuria* (bloody urine); *nephrotic syndrome* (cloudy or bloody urine; high blood pressure; swelling of feet or lower legs); *or proteinuria* (cloudy urine)
  Note: Drug-induced *fever* may develop during the first month of therapy. This will recede when tiopronin is discontinued; therapy can then be reinstated at smaller doses and increased until desired levels are achieved.
    *Leukopenia* of granulocytic series may develop without eosinophilia. *Thrombocytopenia* may be immunologic in origin or occur on an idiosyncratic basis. The reduction in peripheral white blood cell count to less than 3500 per cubic mm or in platelet count to below 100,000 per cubic mm mandates cessation of therapy.

Incidence rare
*Goodpasture's syndrome* (difficulty in breathing, spitting up blood, unusual tiredness or weakness); *myasthenia gravis syndrome* (difficulty in breathing, chewing, talking, or swallowing; double vision; muscle weakness); *pulmonary effects, specifically bronchiolitis* (cough; difficulty in breathing; fever); *dyspnea* (difficulty in breathing); *hemoptysis* (coughing up blood); *pharyngitis* (hoarseness; sore throat); *or pulmonary infiltrates* (cough; chest pain; unusual tiredness or weakness); *systemic lupus erythematosus (SLE)–like syndrome* (fever, general feeling of discomfort, illness, or weakness; joint pain; skin rash, blisters, hives or itching; swelling of lymph glands)
  Note: With abnormal urinary findings of *hemoptysis* and *pulmonary infiltrates*, tiopronin treatment should be stopped.
    Appearance of *myasthenia gravis syndrome* requires cessation of tiopronin therapy.
    *SLE-like syndrome* may be associated with a positive antinuclear antibody test, but not necessarily nephropathy. It may require discontinuance of tiopronin treatment.

**Those indicating need for medical attention only if they continue or are bothersome**
Incidence more frequent
*Gastrointestinal disturbances, specifically abdominal pain; anorexia* (loss of appetite); *bloating or gas; diarrhea or soft stools; or nausea and vomiting; warts; wrinkling, peeling, or unusually dry skin*

Incidence less frequent
*Changes in taste or smell*

## Patient Consultation

As an aid to patient consultation, refer to *Advice for the Patient, Tiopronin (Systemic)*.
In providing consultation, consider emphasizing the following selected information (» = major clinical significance):

**Before using this medication**
» Conditions affecting use, especially:
    Sensitivity to tiopronin or penicillamine
    Breast-feeding—May be distributed into breast milk; may cause potentially serious adverse effects in nursing infants
    Other medical problems, especially agranulocytosis, aplastic anemia, or thrombocytopenia (history of)

**Proper use of this medication**
Taking medication on empty stomach
Importance of high fluid intake, especially at night
Possible need for low-methionine diet
Compliance with therapy; checking with physician before discontinuing medication since interruption of therapy may cause sensitivity reactions when therapy is reinstituted
» Proper dosing
    Missed dose: Taking as soon as possible; not taking if almost time for next dose; not doubling doses
» Proper storage

**Precautions while using this medication**
Regular visits to physician to check progress during therapy

**Side/adverse effects**
Signs of potential side effects, especially dermatologic effects, allergic reactions, hematologic abnormalities, jaundice, renal effects, Goodpasture's syndrome, myasthenia gravis syndrome, pulmonary effects, and systemic lupus erythematosus (SLE)–like syndrome

## General Dosing Information

Tiopronin therapy should be added to a treatment regimen only when the patient continues to form cystine stones on a high fluid intake (3 liters per day) and alkali therapy to maintain a urinary pH at a high normal range (6.5 to 7.0). Calcium phosphate nephrolithiasis may result if urinary alkalinization (pH is increased above 7.0) is continued without aggressively maintaining a high fluid intake.

To help prevent the formation of cystine stones, a high fluid intake is recommended. The patient should drink 2 full glasses (8 ounces each) of water with each meal and at bedtime. The patient should drink another 2 glasses (8 ounces each) during the night when the urine is more concentrated and more acidic than during the day.

For patients who have developed toxicity to penicillamine, tiopronin therapy may be initiated at lower doses.

Dosage of tiopronin should be based on the amount required to keep the urinary cystine concentration below the solubility limit (generally < 250 mg per L). The extent of cystine excretion is generally dependent on tiopronin dosage.

## Tiopronin (Systemic)

### Diet/Nutrition
A diet low in methionine may be necessary to minimize cystine production (methionine is a precursor to cystine and is found in animal proteins such as milk, eggs, cheese, and fish). This diet is not recommended in growing children or during pregnancy because of its low protein content.

Tiopronin should be taken on an empty stomach (either 30 minutes before meals or 2 hours after meals) for faster absorption.

## Oral Dosage Forms

### TIOPRONIN TABLETS

**Usual adult dose**
Oral, initially, 800 mg a day in three divided doses, adjusted according to urinary cystine concentrations.

**Usual pediatric dose**
Children up to 9 years of age—Dosage has not been established.
Children 9 years of age and older—Oral, initially 15 mg per kg of body weight a day in three divided doses, adjusted according to urinary cystine concentrations.

**Strength(s) usually available**
U.S.—
  100 mg (Rx) [*Thiola* (sugar-coated)].
Canada—
  Not commercially available.

**Packaging and storage**
Store between 15 and 30 °C (59 and 86 °F), in a tight container, unless otherwise specified by manufacturer.

**Auxiliary labeling**
- Take on an empty stomach.

Revised: 05/19/92
Interim revision: 08/09/94

---

# TIROFIBAN  Systemic—INTRODUCTORY VERSION

VA CLASSIFICATION (Primary): BL117
Commonly used brand name(s): *Aggrastat*.
Note: For a listing of dosage forms and brand names by country availability, see *Dosage Forms* section(s).

## Category
Platelet aggregation inhibitor.

## Indications

**Accepted**
Thrombosis, acute coronary syndrome–related (prophylaxis)—Tirofiban is indicated, in combination with heparin, for the prevention of acute cardiac ischemic complications in patients with acute coronary syndrome (unstable angina or non–Q-wave myocardial infarction). These patients are at high risk for myocardial infarction and sudden death due to progression of total coronary artery occlusion, whether managed medically or with percutaneous coronary intervention (PCI).

Note: Acute coronary syndrome is defined as prolonged ($\geq 10$ minutes) or repetitive symptoms of cardiac ischemia occurring at rest or with minimal exertion, associated with either ST-T wave changes on electrocardiogram or elevated cardiac enzymes. This definition includes unstable angina and non–Q-wave myocardial infarction but excludes myocardial infarction that is associated with Q waves or nontransient ST-segment elevation.

Tirofiban has been studied in settings that included the use of aspirin and heparin.

## Pharmacology/Pharmacokinetics

**Physicochemical characteristics**
Molecular weight—495.08.
pH—Tirofiban hydrochloride injection or premixed injection: 5.5 to 6.5.

**Mechanism of action/Effect**
Tirofiban inhibits platelet aggregation by reversibly binding to the platelet receptor glycoprotein (GP) IIb/IIIa of human platelets, thus preventing the binding of fibrinogen. Inhibition of platelet aggregation occurs in a dose- and concentration-dependent manner.

**Distribution**
The steady-state volume of distribution ranges from 22 to 42 liters.

**Protein binding**
Not highly bound to plasma proteins; protein binding is concentration-independent over the range of 0.01 to 25 mcg per mL. Unbound fraction in human plasma is 35%.

**Biotransformation**
Metabolism appears to be limited.

**Half-life**
Elimination—
  Approximately 2 hours.

**Time to peak effect**
> 90% platelet inhibition by the end of the 30-minute intravenous infusion.

**Elimination**
Renal, 65% (largely unchanged).
Fecal, 25% (largely unchanged).
  In dialysis—
    Removable by hemodialysis.

Note: Plasma clearance in healthy subjects has been found to be 213 to 314 mL per minute (mL/min), with renal clearance accounting for 39 to 69% of plasma clearance. In patients with coronary artery disease, plasma clearance ranges from 152 to 267 mL/min, with renal clearance accounting for 39% of plasma clearance.

## Precautions to Consider

**Carcinogenicity**
No studies have been done.

**Mutagenicity**
Tirofiban was not found to be mutagenic in vitro in the microbial mutagenesis and V-79 mammalian cell mutagenesis assays, alkaline elution assays, or chromosomal aberrations assays, or in vivo in the bone marrow cells of male mice after administration of intravenous doses of up to 5 mg per kg of body weight (mg/kg) (about three times the maximum recommended daily human dose [MRHD] when compared on a body surface area basis).

**Pregnancy/Reproduction**
Fertility—Fertility and reproductive performance were not affected in studies with male and female rats given intravenous doses of up to 5 mg/kg per day (about five times the MRHD when compared on a body surface area basis).

Pregnancy—Adequate and well-controlled studies in humans have not been done.
Tirofiban crosses the placenta in pregnant rats and rabbits. Studies in rats and rabbits at intravenous doses of up to 5 mg/kg per day (about five and 13 times the MRHD, respectively, when compared on a body surface area basis) found no adverse effects on the fetus.
Risk-benefit should be considered before use of tirofiban during pregnancy.
FDA Pregnancy Category B.

**Breast-feeding**
It is not known whether tirofiban is distributed into breast milk. However, it is distributed in significant concentrations into the milk in lactating rats. Risk-benefit should be considered before breast-feeding during treatment with tirofiban.

**Pediatrics**
Safety and efficacy of tirofiban in children younger than 18 years of age have not been established.

**Geriatrics**
In clinical studies including elderly patients (42.8% were 65 years of age or older and 11.7% were 75 years of age and older), no apparent differences in efficacy were observed between elderly patients and younger adults.

An increased frequency of bleeding complications was observed in elderly patients in clinical trials, although the incremental risk of bleeding in patients treated with tirofiban in combination with heparin compared to the risk in patients treated with heparin alone was similar, regardless of age. The incidence of nonbleeding side effects was also increased in elderly patients.

Plasma clearance is approximately 19 to 26% lower in patients older than 65 years of age with coronary artery disease than it is in younger adults.

No dosage adjustment is recommended for the elderly population; however, elderly patients are more likely to have age-related renal function impairment, which may require adjustment of dosage in patients receiving tirofiban.

**Drug interactions and/or related problems**

The following drug interactions and/or related problems have been selected on the basis of their potential clinical significance (possible mechanism in parentheses where appropriate)—not necessarily inclusive (» = major clinical significance):

Note: Combinations containing any of the following medications, depending on the amount present, may also interact with this medication.

» Anticoagulants, coumarin- or indandione-derivative or
» Other medications that affect hemostasis
 (caution is recommended because of the increased risk of bleeding; tirofiban has been studied in settings that included the use of aspirin and heparin)
» Platelet aggregation inhibitors, other (especially inhibitors of platelet receptor GP IIb/IIIa)
 (concurrent use is not recommended)

**Medical considerations/Contraindications**

The medical considerations/contraindications included have been selected on the basis of their potential clinical significance (reasons given in parentheses where appropriate)—not necessarily inclusive (» = major clinical significance).

*Except under special circumstances, this medication should not be used when the following medical problems exist:*

» Aneurysm, history of or
» Aortic dissection, suggested by history, symptoms, or findings or
» Arteriovenous malformation, history of or
» Bleeding, internal, active or
» Bleeding diathesis within the last 30 days or
» Cerebrovascular accident (CVA) within the past 30 days or
» Hemorrhage, intracranial, history of or
» Hemorrhagic stroke, history of or
» Hypertension, severe, i.e., > 180 mm Hg systolic and/or > 110 mm Hg diastolic or
» Neoplasm, intracranial, history of or
» Pericarditis, acute or
» Surgery, major, recent (within 30 days) or
» Trauma, physical, severe (within 30 days)
 (increased risk of bleeding with tirofiban)
» Thrombocytopenia, tirofiban-induced, history of
 (risk of recurrence)

*Risk-benefit should be considered when the following medical problems exist:*

» Renal function impairment, severe or
 (plasma clearance of tirofiban is significantly decreased [50%] in patients with creatinine clearance < 30 mL per minute; it is recommended that dosage be reduced by half in these patients)
» Retinopathy, hemorrhagic
 (caution is recommended)
» Sensitivity to tirofiban
» Thrombocytopenia (< 150,000 per mm$^3$)
 (caution is recommended)

**Patient monitoring**

The following may be especially important in patient monitoring (other tests may be warranted in some patients, depending on condition; » = major clinical significance):

» Activated clotting time (ACT)
 (it is recommended that the ACT be checked before removal of the arterial sheath; the sheath should not be removed unless the ACT is less than 180 seconds)
» Activated partial thromboplastin time (aPTT)
 (should be monitored 6 hours after the start of the heparin infusion to monitor unfractionated heparin)
 (it is recommended that the aPTT be maintained at approximately two times the control value)
 (it is recommended that the aPTT be checked before removal of the arterial sheath; the sheath should not be removed unless the aPTT is less than 45 seconds)

» Hematocrit and
» Hemoglobin and
» Platelet count
 (recommended prior to initiation of tirofiban therapy, within 6 hours following the loading infusion, and at least daily during therapy, or more frequently if there is a significant decrease in counts; if the platelet count falls to < 90,000 per mm$^3$, additional platelet counts should be performed to exclude pseudothrombocytopenia)

## Side/Adverse Effects

The following side/adverse effects have been selected on the basis of their potential clinical significance (possible signs and symptoms in parentheses where appropriate)—not necessarily inclusive:

**Those indicating need for medical attention**
Incidence more frequent
 *Bleeding*
 Note: *Bleeding* is the most common complication of tirofiban therapy. Intracranial, gastrointestinal, genitourinary, and retroperitoneal bleeding are rare.
  Most *major bleeding* occurs at the arterial access site for cardiac catheterization.

Incidence less frequent
 *Coronary artery dissection; vasovagal reflex*

Incidence rare
 *Thrombocytopenia*

**Those indicating need for medical attention only if they continue or are bothersome**
Incidence less frequent
 *Bradycardia; dizziness; edema; fever; headache; leg pain; nausea; pelvic pain; sweating*

## Overdose

**Clinical effects of overdose**

The following effects have been selected on the basis of their potential clinical significance (possible signs and symptoms in parentheses where appropriate)—not necessarily inclusive:

Acute
 *Bleeding* (bleeding from gums; bleeding at the site of cardiac catheterization)
 Note: Inadvertent overdose has occurred in doses up to five times and two times the recommended dose for bolus administration and loading infusion, respectively. Inadvertent overdosage has occurred in doses up to 9.8 times the 0.15 mcg per kg of body weight per minute maintenance infusion rate. The most frequently reported effect was *bleeding*, which was usually minor.

**Treatment of overdose**

Following assessment of the patient's clinical condition, treatment consists of cessation or adjustment of the tirofiban infusion as appropriate.

Tirofiban can be removed by hemodialysis.

## General Dosing Information

Tirofiban intravenous solution should not be removed directly from the bag with a syringe.

Plastic containers should not be used in series connections, since such use can result in air embolism by drawing air from the first container if it is empty of solution.

Because of the risk of bleeding, arterial and venous punctures, intramuscular injections, and the use of urinary catheters, nasotracheal intubation, and nasogastric tubes should be minimized. Noncompressible sites, such as subclavian or jugular veins, should be avoided when obtaining intravenous access.

If bleeding occurs and cannot be controlled with pressure, it is recommended that the infusion of tirofiban and heparin be discontinued.

It is recommended that tirofiban intravenous infusion be continued through angiography and for 12 to 24 hours after angioplasty or atherectomy.

It is recommended that tirofiban and heparin therapy be discontinued, and appropriate monitoring and therapy initiated, if a confirmed platelet count decrease to less than 90,000 per mm$^3$ occurs and pseudothrombocytopenia has been ruled out.

**Care of femoral artery access site in patients undergoing percutaneous coronary intervention (PCI)**

Because tirofiban therapy is associated with increased bleeding rates, particularly at the site of arterial access for femoral sheath placement, care should be taken when attempting vascular access that only the anterior wall of the femoral artery is punctured. Prior to pulling the sheath, it is recommended that heparin be discontinued for 3 to 4 hours and an activated clotting time (ACT) of less than 180 seconds or an activated partial thromboplastin time (aPTT) of less than 45 seconds be documented. Care should also be taken to obtain proper hemostasis after removal of the sheaths using standard compressive techniques, followed by close observation. While the vascular sheath is in place, maintenance of patients on complete bed rest with the head of the bed elevated 30° and the affected limb restrained in a straight position is recommended. Sheath hemostasis should be achieved at least 4 hours before hospital discharge.

## Parenteral Dosage Forms

Note: Tirofiban hydrochloride injection contains tirofiban hydrochloride monohydrate. Strength and dosage are expressed in terms of tirofiban.

### TIROFIBAN HYDROCHLORIDE INJECTION

**Usual adult dose**

Note: For a dosing chart providing infusion rates in mL per hour by patient weight, see the *Aggrastat* package insert.

Acute coronary syndrome—
 Initial—
  Intravenous infusion, 0.4 micrograms per kg of body weight per minute for thirty minutes, immediately followed by—
 Maintenance—
  Intravenous infusion, 0.1 micrograms per kg of body weight per minute.

Note: In clinical studies, patients also received aspirin, unless it was contraindicated, and heparin.

It is recommended that the infusion rate be reduced by half in patients with severe renal function impairment (creatinine clearance less than 30 mL per minute).

**Usual pediatric dose**
Safety and efficacy have not been established in children younger than 18 years of age.

**Strength(s) usually available**
U.S.—
 50 mcg (0.05 mg) per mL (25 mg per 500-mL container) (Rx) [*Aggrastat* (premixed solution **for intravenous infusion**)].
 250 mcg (0.25 mg) per mL (12.5 mg per 50-mL vial) (Rx) [*Aggrastat* (concentrated solution **for dilution**)].

**Packaging and storage**
Store between 15 and 30°C (59 and 86°F), preferably at 25 °C (77 °F). Protect from light during storage. Protect from freezing.

**Preparation of dosage form**
- For tirofiban injection (250 mcg [0.25 mg] per mL, 50-mL vial):
  *This concentrated solution must be diluted prior to administration by intravenous infusion.*
  The solution is diluted for administration by first withdrawing and discarding 100 mL from a 500-mL bag of 0.9% sodium chloride injection or 5% dextrose injection, and then replacing this volume with 100 mL (2 vials) of tirofiban injection (total of 25 mg of tirofiban) and mixing well, to produce a solution containing 50 mcg (0.05 mg) of tirofiban per mL. Alternatively, a volume of 50 mL can be withdrawn from a 250-mL bag of 0.9% sodium chloride injection or 5% dextrose injection and replaced with 50 mL (1 vial) of concentrated tirofiban injection (total of 12.5 mg of tirofiban) and mixing well, to produce a solution containing 50 mcg (0.05 mg) of tirofiban per mL.

- For tirofiban injection premixed (50 mcg [0.05 mg] per mL, 500-mL container):
  This premixed solution may be administered undiluted by intravenous infusion.
  The plastic container is prepared by tearing off the dust cover and checking for leaks by squeezing the inner bag firmly. If any leaks are found, sterility cannot be guaranteed and the bag should be discarded. The plastic bag may appear somewhat opaque at first because of moisture absorption during sterilization, but should clear gradually. The container is then suspended by its eyelet support, the plastic protector is removed from the outlet port, and a conventional administration set is attached.

**Stability**
It is recommended that any unused solution be discarded 24 hours following the start of the infusion.

**Incompatibilities**
Tirofiban may be administered in the same intravenous line as heparin.
Tirofiban should not be administered in the same intravenous line as any other medications.

**Auxiliary labeling**
When dispensed, the 50-mL vial should carry a label indicating that it "MUST BE DILUTED BEFORE USE." When dispensed, the 500-mL container should carry a label indicating that it is "FOR CONTINUOUS INTRAVENOUS INFUSION."

**Caution**
*It is very important to distinguish between the 50-mL vial that must be diluted before administration and the 500-mL container that contains premixed infusion solution. The 50-mL vial must first be diluted to the same strength as the premixed solution.*

Developed: 08/28/98

---

# TIZANIDINE  Systemic†

VA CLASSIFICATION (Primary): MS900
Commonly used brand name(s): *Zanaflex*.
Note: For a listing of dosage forms and brand names by country availability, see *Dosage Forms* section(s).

†Not commercially available in Canada.

## Category
Antispastic.

## Indications

**Accepted**
Spasticity (treatment)—Tizanidine is indicated in the acute and intermittent management of increased muscle tone associated with spasticity related to multiple sclerosis and spinal cord injury. It is especially useful in relieving muscle spasms and clonus. Studies comparing the efficacy of tizanidine with that of other current treatment agents, such as baclofen and diazepam, found tizanidine to be as effective as the other agents in reducing spasticity. In addition, clinical studies have demonstrated that tizanidine reduces muscle tone without causing excessive muscle weakness.

**Acceptance not established**
Preliminary studies and case reports suggest that tizanidine may be used as an alternative treatment in patients with *chronic tension headaches and cluster headaches* who are resistant to other types of drug therapy. However, data are insufficient to establish safety and efficacy of tizanidine for these indications.

A preliminary study suggests tizanidine may be used as an alternative to clonidine as an *adjunct in anesthesia*. Results of a small study in healthy volunteers have shown that the effects of a single 12-mg dose of tizanidine were comparable to those of a 150-mcg dose of oral clonidine. However, data are currently insufficient to establish safety and efficacy for this indication.

## Pharmacology/Pharmacokinetics

**Physicochemical characteristics**
Chemical group—Imidazoline.
Molecular weight—290.18.

**Mechanism of action/Effect**
Tizanidine is an alpha-adrenergic agonist. It acts by increasing presynaptic inhibition of motor neurons at the alpha$_2$-adrenergic receptor sites, possibly by reducing the release of excitatory amino acids and inhibiting facilitory caeruleospinal pathways, resulting in a reduction in spasticity. Some studies suggest a possible postsynaptic action at the excitatory amino acid receptors. In addition, tizanidine may have some activity at the imidazoline receptors. A study in animals found that tizanidine acts mainly on the polysynaptic pathways, thereby reducing facilitation of spinal motor neurons. Tizanidine may also have minor effects on monosynaptic reflexes, which are associated with the facilitory effect of the caeruleospinal pathways. The exact mechanism of action of tizanidine is unknown.

### Other actions/effects
Tizanidine produces antihypotensive effects, possibly by binding to the imidazoline receptors. Pharmacologic studies done in animals found tizanidine to have one fiftieth to one tenth of the potency of clonidine, an alpha$_2$-adrenergic agonist, in lowering blood pressure. These antihypotensive effects are mild and transitory in relation to its activity as a muscle relaxant.

Tizanidine also has antinociceptive effects. However, these effects may be mediated through an alpha$_2$-adrenergic receptor mechanism rather than a narcotic or endorphin mechanism. The antinociceptive action has been confirmed at doses lower than those producing a muscle relaxant action.

In addition, various studies have shown that tizanidine has anticonvulsant, hypothermic, gastrointestinal, and sympatholytic effects.

### Absorption
Well-absorbed following oral administration. Due to extensive metabolism, bioavailability is low (approximately 40%). The presence of food has no effect on the extent of absorption. However, food affects the rate of absorption by decreasing the time to peak concentration and increasing the maximum plasma concentration, although these effects are not clinically significant.

### Distribution
Tizanidine is widely distributed. The apparent volume of distribution (Vol$_D$) following intravenous administration is approximately 2.4 L per kg of body weight (L/kg).

### Protein binding
Low (30%).

### Biotransformation
Hepatic; 95% metabolized to inactive metabolites.

### Half-life
Tizanidine—Approximately 2.5 hours.
Metabolites—Approximately 20 to 40 hours.

### Time to peak concentration
Approximately 1.5 hours.

Note: Following single doses of up to 8 mg, a linear relationship is observed among the dose, plasma concentration, and antispastic action.

### Elimination
Renal—Approximately 60%.
Fecal—Approximately 20%.

## Precautions to Consider

### Carcinogenicity
No evidence of carcinogenicity was found in rats and mice given tizanidine at doses of up to 16 mg per kg of body weight (mg/kg) (2 times the maximum recommended human dose [MRHD] on a mg per square meter of body surface area [mg/m$^2$] basis) for 78 weeks and doses of up to 9 mg/kg (2.5 times the MRHD on a mg/m$^2$ basis) for 104 weeks, respectively.

### Mutagenicity
Tizanidine demonstrated no mutagenic or clastogenic potential in *in vitro* studies, including the bacterial Ames test, the mammalian gene mutation test, and chromosomal aberration test in Chinese hamster cells. In addition, there was no evidence of mutagenic potential in *in vivo* studies in mice, including the bone marrow micronucleus test, dominant lethal mutagenicity test, and unscheduled DNA synthesis test; or in *in vivo* Chinese hamster studies, including the bone marrow micronucleus test and cytogenicity test.

### Pregnancy/Reproduction
Fertility—Studies in male and female rats given doses of 10 mg/kg (approximately 2.7 times the MRHD) and 3 mg/kg (approximately equal to the MRHD on a mg/m$^2$ basis), respectively, found no evidence of impairment of fertility. However, another study in male and female rats receiving 30 mg/kg (8 times the MRHD on a mg/m$^2$ basis) and 10 mg/kg (2.7 times the MRHD on a mg/m$^2$ basis), respectively, revealed reduced fertility. Abnormal maternal behavior, marked sedation, weight loss, and ataxia were also observed with doses used in the latter study.

Pregnancy—Adequate and well-controlled studies have not been done in humans.

Reproduction studies in rats and rabbits given doses of 3 mg/kg (equal to the MRHD) and 30 mg/kg (16 times the MRHD on a mg/m$^2$ basis), respectively, found no evidence of teratogenicity. However, a study in rats given doses equal to and up to eight times the MRHD on a mg/m$^2$ basis found an increase in gestation period. In addition, prenatal and postnatal pup loss increased and developmental retardation occurred. Another study in rabbits given doses of 1 mg/kg or greater (equal to or greater than 0.5 times the MRHD on a mg/m$^2$ basis) reported an increase in postimplantation loss.

FDA Pregnancy Category C.

Labor and delivery—The effect of tizanidine on labor and delivery is unknown.

### Breast-feeding
It is not known whether tizanidine is distributed into breast milk. Since tizanidine is lipid soluble, it may pass into the breast milk. However, problems in humans have not been documented.

### Pediatrics
Appropriate studies on the relationship of age to the effects of tizanidine have not been performed in the pediatric population. Safety and efficacy have not been established.

### Geriatrics
Tizanidine clearance is decreased fourfold in geriatric patients. In addition, geriatric patients are more likely to have age-related renal function impairment, which may require dosage adjustment.

### Dental
Prolonged use of tizanidine may decrease or inhibit salivary flow, thus contributing to the development of caries, periodontal disease, oral candidiasis, and discomfort.

### Drug interactions and/or related problems
The following drug interactions and/or related problems have been selected on the basis of their potential clinical significance (possible mechanism in parentheses where appropriate)—not necessarily inclusive (» = major clinical significance):

Note: Combinations containing any of the following medications, depending on the amount present, may also interact with this medication.

Acetaminophen
(in clinical trials, concurrent use of acetaminophen and tizanidine resulted in a delay in the time to peak effect of tizanidine by 16 minutes; the delay was not reported to be clinically significant)

Alcohol or
CNS depression–producing medications, other (see *Appendix II*)
(concurrent use with tizanidine may enhance the central nervous system [CNS] depressant effects)

» Hypotension-producing medications, other (see *Appendix II*)
(concurrent use may potentiate antihypertensive effects; caution is recommended; concurrent use with other alpha$_2$-adrenergic agonists is not recommended)

» Oral contraceptives
(concurrent use may reduce the clearance of tizanidine by approximately 50%; caution and dosage adjustments are recommended)

» Phenytoin
(in one study, a patient receiving 6 mg of phenytoin per day experienced an increase in the trough serum concentration of phenytoin from a baseline of approximately 75 micromoles per liter to 100 micromoles per liter, after one week of concurrent use with tizanidine; careful monitoring of serum hydantoin concentrations and dosage adjustments may be necessary)

### Laboratory value alterations
The following have been selected on the basis of their potential clinical significance (possible effect in parentheses where appropriate)—not necessarily inclusive (» = major clinical significance):

With physiology/laboratory test values
Alanine aminotransferase (ALT [SGPT]) and
Alkaline phosphatase and
Aspartate aminotransferase (AST [SGOT])
(in controlled clinical studies, the values have been increased up to three times the upper limit of normal)

### Medical considerations/Contraindications
The medical considerations/contraindications included have been selected on the basis of their potential clinical significance (reasons given in parentheses where appropriate)—not necessarily inclusive (» = major clinical significance).

*Risk-benefit should be considered when the following medical problems exist:*

» Hepatic function impairment or
» Renal function impairment
(studies have shown increased plasma concentrations of tizanidine in patients with hepatic or renal function impairment; a study evaluating six patients between 42 and 82 years of age receiving a single 4-mg dose of tizanidine reported an increase in mean maximum plasma concentration, mean elimination half-life, and mean area under the plasma concentration–time curve compared with those

patients without renal impairment; adjustment of tizanidine dosage may be necessary)

Sensitivity to tizanidine

**Patient monitoring**

The following may be especially important in patient monitoring (other tests may be warranted in some patients, depending on condition; » = major clinical significance):

Hepatic function determinations (recommended during the first 6 months of treatment and periodically thereafter)

## Side/Adverse Effects

Note: A study comparing tizanidine (single dose of 3 or 6 mg) with diazepam (10 mg) reported no evidence of psychological dependence associated with tizanidine.

The following side/adverse effects have been selected on the basis of their potential clinical significance (possible signs and symptoms in parentheses where appropriate)—not necessarily inclusive:

**Those indicating need for medical attention**
Incidence more frequent
*CNS effects, including nervousness; and paresthesias* (tingling, burning, or prickling sensations); *fever; hepatotoxicity* (loss of appetite; nausea and/or vomiting; yellow eyes or skin); *skin ulcers* (sores on the skin); *urinary tract infections* (pain or burning while urinating)

Incidence less frequent
*Arrhythmias* (irregular heartbeat); *blood dyscrasias, including anemia;* (unusual tiredness or weakness); *leukocytosis; or leukopenia* (chills, fever, or sore throat); *gastrointestinal hemorrhage* (black, tarry stools; bloody vomit); *hypothyroidism* (coldness; dry, puffy skin; unusual tiredness; weight gain); *mood or mental changes, including delusions; or visual hallucinations* (seeing things that are not there); *renal calculi* (kidney stones); *seizures; syncope* (fainting); *upper respiratory tract infections* (cough, fever, or sore throat); *visual disturbances, including amblyopia* (blurred vision); *eye pain; or visual field defects* (blurred vision)

**Those indicating need for medical attention only if they continue or are bothersome**
Incidence more frequent
*Anxiety; asthenia* (unusual tiredness and/or weakness)—dose-related; *back pain; constipation; depression; dizziness*—dose-related; *drowsiness*—dose-related; *dry mouth*—dose-related; *dyskinesia* (uncontrolled movements of the body); *dyspepsia* (heartburn); *hypotension* (dizziness or lightheadedness, especially when getting up from a lying or sitting position); *gastrointestinal effects* (diarrhea; stomach pain; vomiting); *increased muscle spasms or tone*—dose-related; *increased sweating; myasthenia* (muscle weakness); *pharyngitis* (pain or burning in throat); *rhinitis* (runny nose); *skin rash; somnolence* (sleepiness)—dose-related; *speech disorder* (difficulty in speaking)

Incidence less frequent
*Alopecia* (loss of hair); *arthritis* (joint or muscle pain or stiffness); *cellulitis* (swollen area that feels warm and tender); *dry skin; dysphagia* (difficulty swallowing); *edema* (swelling of feet or lower legs); *migraine headache; mood or mental changes, including agitation; euphoria* (unusual feeling of well-being); *or depersonalization; neck pain; tremor* (trembling or shaking); *weight loss*

## Overdose

For specific information on the agents used in the management of tizanidine overdose, see:
- *Furosemide* in *Diuretics, Loop (Systemic)* monograph; and/or
- *Mannitol (Systemic)* monograph.

For more information on the management of overdose or unintentional ingestion, **contact a Poison Control Center** (see *Poison Control Center Listing*).

**Clinical effects of overdose**
The following effects have been selected on the basis of their potential clinical significance (possible signs and symptoms in parentheses where appropriate)—not necessarily inclusive:

Acute and chronic
**Respiratory depression**

**Treatment of overdose**
To enhance elimination—Gastric lavage and forced diuresis with furosemide and mannitol.

Supportive care—May include maintaining an open airway and breathing, maintaining proper fluid and electrolyte balance, correcting hypotension, and controlling seizures. Patients in whom intentional overdose is confirmed or suspected should be referred for psychiatric consultation.

## Patient Consultation

As an aid to patient consultation, refer to *Advice for the Patient, Tizanidine (Systemic)*.

In providing consultation, consider emphasizing the following selected information (» = major clinical significance):

**Before using this medication**
» Conditions affecting use, especially:
Sensitivity to tizanidine
Breast-feeding—May be distributed into breast milk
Use in the elderly—Clearance may be reduced. Also, elderly people are more likely to have age-related renal function impairment, which may require dosage adjustment
Other medications, especially hypotension-producing medications, oral contraceptives, or phenytoin
Other medical problems, especially hepatic or renal function impairment

**Proper use of this medication**
Not taking more medication than the amount prescribed to minimize possibility of side effects
» Proper dosing
Missed dose: Taking if remembered within an hour; not taking if not remembered until later; not doubling doses
» Proper storage

**Precautions while using this medication**
Regular visits to physician to check progress during therapy
» Checking with physician before discontinuing medication; gradual dosage adjustment may be necessary
» Avoiding use of alcohol or other CNS depressants during therapy unless approved by physician
» Caution when driving or doing anything else requiring alertness because of possible drowsiness, dizziness, lightheadedness, impairment of physical or mental abilities, false sense of well-being, or visual disturbances
Possible dryness of mouth; using sugarless gum or candy, ice, or saliva substitute for relief; checking with physician or dentist if dry mouth continues for more than 2 weeks
» Caution when getting up suddenly from a lying or sitting position

**Side/adverse effects**
Signs of potential side effects, especially CNS effects, fever, hepatotoxicity, skin ulcer, urinary tract infections, arrhythmias, blood dyscrasias, gastrointestinal hemorrhage, hypothyroidism, mood or mental changes, renal calculi, seizures, syncope, upper respiratory tract infections, and visual disturbances

## Oral Dosage Forms

### TIZANIDINE TABLETS

**Usual adult dose**
Antispastic—
Oral, 8 mg every six to eight hours as needed.

Note: Due to the dose-related nature of the side effects and the various responses to doses among patients, the dose may be started at 4 mg and gradually titrated to optimum effect in 2- to 4-mg increments on an individual basis over a two- to four-week period.

**Usual adult prescribing limits**
36 mg per day.

**Usual pediatric dose**
Safety and efficacy have not been established.

**Usual geriatric dose**
See *Usual adult dose*.

Note: Dosage adjustment may be required.

**Strength(s) usually available**
U.S.—
4 mg (Rx) [*Zanaflex* (lactose; microcrystalline cellulose; silicone dioxide colloidal; stearic acid)].
Canada—
Not commercially available.

**Packaging and storage**
Store below 40 °C (104 °F), preferably between 15 and 30 °C (59 and 86 °F), unless otherwise specified by the manufacturer.

**Auxiliary labeling**
- May cause drowsiness.
- Avoid alcoholic beverages.

## Selected Bibliography

Lataste X, Emre M, Davis C, et al. Comparative profile of tizanidine in the management of spasticity. Neurology 1994; 44 Suppl 9: S53-S59.

Wagstaff AJ, Bryson HM. Tizanidine: a review of its pharmacology, clinical efficacy and tolerability in the management of spasticity associated with cerebral and spinal disorders. Drugs 1997; 53(3): 435-52.

Developed: 08/12/97

**TOBRAMYCIN**—See *Aminoglycosides (Systemic); Tobramycin (Ophthalmic)*

**TOBRAMYCIN**—The *Tobramycin (Ophthalmic)* monograph is not included in this published version of the USP DI database. Copies of the monograph are available on request from Micromedex, Inc. - Reprint Requests, 6200 S. Syracuse Way, Suite 300, Englewood, CO 80111; telephone (303) 486-6400; telefax (303) 486-6464; Email: USPDI@MDX.COM.

# TOCAINIDE Systemic

VA CLASSIFICATION (Primary): CV300
Commonly used brand name(s): *Tonocard*.
Note: For a listing of dosage forms and brand names by country availability, see *Dosage Forms* section(s).

## Category
Antiarrhythmic.

## Indications

**Accepted**

Arrhythmias, ventricular (treatment)—Tocainide is indicated for suppression of documented life-threatening ventricular arrhythmias, such as sustained ventricular tachycardia.

## Pharmacology/Pharmacokinetics

**Physicochemical characteristics**
Molecular weight—Tocainide: 192.26.
pKa—7.7.

**Mechanism of action/Effect**
Tocainide, like lidocaine, decreases sodium and potassium conductance, thereby decreasing the excitability of myocardial cells. It reduces the rate of rise and amplitude of the action potential and decreases automaticity (increases the threshold of excitability) in the Purkinje fibers. Tocainide shortens the action potential duration and, to a lesser extent, decreases the effective refractory period in the Purkinje fibers. Conduction velocity is usually not altered, although conduction may be slowed in patients with pre-existing conduction abnormalities. Tocainide does not significantly affect resting membrane potential or sinus node automaticity, left ventricular function, systolic arterial blood pressure, atrioventricular (AV) conduction velocity, or QRS or QT intervals. In the Vaughan Williams classification of antiarrhythmics, tocainide is considered to be a class IB agent.

**Absorption**
Bioavailability is close to 100%. Absorption is unaffected by food.

**Protein binding**
Low to moderate (10 to 50%).

**Biotransformation**
Hepatic; producing no active metabolites.

**Half-life**
Approximately 11 to 15 hours; may be prolonged up to 35 hours in patients with severe renal function impairment (creatinine clearance less than 30 mL per min per 1.73 square meters of body surface area.

**Time to peak plasma concentration**
30 minutes to 2 hours.

**Duration of action:**
8 hours.

**Elimination**
Renal (about 40% unchanged); alkalinization of urine significantly reduces percentage excreted unchanged.
In dialysis—Removable by hemodialysis.

## Precautions to Consider

**Cross-sensitivity and/or related problems**
Patients sensitive to other amide-type anesthetics may be sensitive to tocainide also. Cross-sensitivity with procainamide or quinidine has not been reported.

**Carcinogenicity**
Studies in mice at doses up to 300 mg per kg of body weight (mg/kg) per day (6 times the maximum human recommended dose) for up to 94 and 102 weeks in males and females, respectively, and in rats at doses up to 200 mg/kg per day for 24 months showed no evidence of carcinogenicity.

**Mutagenicity**
No evidence of mutagenicity was found in *in vivo* micronucleus tests in mice at oral doses of up to 187.5 mg/kg per day (about 7 times the usual human dose). The results of the *in vitro* Ames microbial mutagen test and mouse lymphoma forward mutation assay were also negative.

**Pregnancy/Reproduction**
Fertility—Studies in male and female rats given tocainide doses of 200 mg/kg per day (about 8 times the usual human dose) revealed no evidence of fertility impairment.

Pregnancy—Adequate and well-controlled studies in humans have not been done.

Studies in rabbits at doses of 25, 50, and 100 mg/kg per day (about 1 to 4 times the usual human dose) and in rats at doses of 200 and 300 mg/kg per day (about 8 and 12 times the usual human dose, respectively) produced an increased incidence of abortions, stillbirths, fetal resorptions, and decreased neonatal survival. There was no evidence of teratogenicity.

FDA Pregnancy Category C.

**Breast-feeding**
Studies have not been done to determine if tocainide is distributed into breast milk; however, concentrations in breast milk were documented in one woman at more than twice maternal blood concentrations.

**Pediatrics**
Appropriate studies on the relationship of age to the effects of tocainide have not been performed in the pediatric population. Safety and efficacy have not been established.

**Geriatrics**
Although appropriate studies on the relationship of age to the effects of tocainide have not been performed in geriatric patients, elderly patients are more likely to have age-related renal function impairment, which may require lower or less frequent doses in patients receiving tocainide. In addition, elderly patients may be more prone to dizziness and hypotension.

**Dental**
The leukopenic and thrombocytopenic effects of tocainide may result in an increased incidence of microbial infection, delayed healing, and gingival bleeding. If leukopenia or thrombocytopenia occurs, dental work should be deferred until blood counts have returned to normal and patients should be instructed in proper oral hygiene during treatment, including caution in use of regular toothbrushes, dental floss, and toothpicks.

**Drug interactions and/or related problems**
The following drug interactions and/or related problems have been selected on the basis of their potential clinical significance (possible mechanism in parentheses where appropriate)—not necessarily inclusive (» = major clinical significance):

Note: Combinations containing any of the following medications, depending on the amount present, may also interact with this medication.

Antiarrhythmics, other
(although some antiarrhythmic agents may be used in combination for therapeutic advantage, combined use may potentiate risk of adverse cardiac effects)

Beta-adrenergic blocking agents
(concurrent use with tocainide may result in an additive increase in pulmonary wedge pressure and reduction in cardiac index; caution is recommended, especially in patients with heart failure)

Bone marrow depressants (See *Appendix II* )
(although problems have not been reported, concurrent use with tocainide may increase the risk of leukopenia and thrombocytopenia)

**Medical considerations/Contraindications**
The medical considerations/contraindications included have been selected on the basis of their potential clinical significance (reasons given in parentheses where appropriate)—not necessarily inclusive (» = major clinical significance).

*Except under special circumstances, this medication should not be used when the following medical problem exists:*
» Atrioventricular (AV) block, pre-existing second or third degree without pacemaker
» Sensitivity to tocainide or to amide-type local anesthetics

*Risk-benefit should be considered when the following medical problems exist:*
Atrial flutter or fibrillation
(acceleration of ventricular rate occurs infrequently)
Congestive heart failure
(may be aggravated as a result of a small negative inotropic effect and slight increase in peripheral resistance caused by tocainide)
Hepatic function impairment
(reduced biotransformation; lower or less frequent doses may be required)
Renal function impairment
(reduced elimination; lower or less frequent doses may be required)

**Patient monitoring**
The following may be especially important in patient monitoring (other tests may be warranted in some patients, depending on condition; » = major clinical significance):
Blood counts, complete, including white blood cells with differential and platelets
(recommended at weekly intervals for the first 3 months of therapy and frequently thereafter to detect blood dyscrasias; also, recommended if patient develops any signs of infection)
Chest x-ray
(recommended if clinical signs or symptoms of adverse pulmonary effects occur)
Electrocardiogram (ECG)
(recommended prior to initiation of therapy and at periodic intervals during therapy to assess efficacy of tocainide)

## Side/Adverse Effects

Note: In the National Heart, Lung, and Blood Institute's Cardiac Arrhythmias Suppression Trial (CAST), treatment with encainide or flecainide in patients with asymptomatic, non–life-threatening ventricular arrhythmias who had a recent myocardial infarction was found to be associated with excessive mortality or nonfatal cardiac arrest rate (7.7%) as compared with placebo (3%). The implications of these results for other patient populations are uncertain; however, because of tocainide's proarrhythmogenic potential, tocainide should be reserved for patients with life-threatening ventricular arrhythmias.

The following side/adverse effects have been selected on the basis of their potential clinical significance (possible signs and symptoms in parentheses where appropriate)—not necessarily inclusive:

**Those indicating need for medical attention**
Incidence less frequent
*Trembling or shaking*
Note: *Trembling or shaking* may indicate that maximum dose is being reached.
Incidence rare
*Blood dyscrasias, including agranulocytosis* (fever or chills); *aplastic anemia; leukopenia* (fever or chills); *neutropenia; or thrombocytopenia* (unusual bleeding or bruising); *pneumonitis, pulmonary fibrosis, alveolitis, pulmonary edema, or pneumonia* (cough or shortness of breath); *skin reactions, severe, including erythema multiforme, exfoliative dermatitis, and Stevens-Johnson syndrome* (blisters on skin; peeling or scaling of skin; severe skin rash; sores in mouth; fever may also be associated with Stevens-Johnson syndrome); *ventricular arrhythmias* (irregular heartbeat)

Note: *Blood dyscrasias* usually occur within the first 12 weeks of therapy. Sequelae such as septicemia and septic shock, as well as fatalities, have been reported. Blood counts usually return to normal within 1 month of discontinuation of tocainide.
*Pulmonary* adverse effects usually occur after 3 to 18 weeks of therapy and are characterized by bilateral infiltrates on chest x-ray frequently associated with dyspnea and cough; fatalities have been reported.
Fatalities have been reported with *severe skin reactions*.

**Those indicating need for medical attention only if they continue or are bothersome**
Incidence more frequent
Anorexia (loss of appetite); *dizziness or lightheadedness; nausea*
Incidence less frequent
*Blurred vision; confusion; headache; nervousness; numbness or tingling of fingers and toes; skin rash; sweating; vomiting*

## Overdose
For more information on the management of overdose or unintentional ingestion, **contact a Poison Control Center** (see *Poison Control Center Listing*).

**Clinical effects of overdose**
The following effects have been selected on the basis of their potential clinical significance (possible signs and symptoms in parentheses where appropriate)—not necessarily inclusive:
*Cardiac arrest; cardiopulmonary depression; central nervous system effects; convulsions*
Note: *Central nervous system (CNS) effects* would be expected as the initial presentation of overdosage. Other adverse effects, such as gastrointestinal disturbances, may follow.

**Treatment of overdose**
Symptomatic and supportive, particularly airway patency and adequacy of ventilation.
Specific treatment—
For convulsions: If necessary, administering small increments of anticonvulsive agents, such as a benzodiazepine or an ultrashort- or short-acting barbiturate.

## Patient Consultation
As an aid to patient consultation, refer to *Advice for the Patient, Tocainide (Systemic)*.
In providing consultation, consider emphasizing the following selected information (» = major clinical significance):

**Before using this medication**
» Conditions affecting use, especially:
Sensitivity to tocainide or amide-type anesthetics
Pregnancy—Increased possibility of death in animal fetuses
Use in the elderly—Elderly may be more prone to dizziness and hypotension
Other medical problems, especially second or third degree atrioventricular (AV) block

**Proper use of this medication**
» Compliance with therapy; taking as directed even if feeling well
May be taken with food or milk to reduce stomach upset
» Importance of not missing doses and taking at evenly spaced intervals
» Proper dosing
Missed dose: Taking as soon as possible if remembered within 4 hours; not taking if remembered later; not doubling doses
» Proper storage

**Precautions while using this medication**
Regular visits to physician to check progress
Carrying medical identification card or bracelet
» Caution when driving or doing things requiring alertness because of possible dizziness
» Caution if any kind of surgery (including dental surgery) or emergency treatment is required

**Side/adverse effects**
Signs of potential side effects, especially trembling or shaking, agranulocytosis, aplastic anemia, leukopenia, neutropenia, thrombocytopenia, pulmonary problems, severe skin reactions, and ventricular arrhythmias

## General Dosing Information
Patients who experience adverse effects shortly after dosing with tocainide may require a shorter dosing interval (i.e., further division of the daily dose). Patients who experience worsening of arrhythmias shortly before

the next scheduled dose may require an increased dose and/or a shorter dosing interval.

The appearance of tremor may be used as an indication that the maximum dose is being reached.

It is recommended that tocainide therapy be withdrawn if bone marrow depression, pulmonary fibrosis, or a severe skin reaction occurs.

**Diet/Nutrition**
Tocainide may be taken with food or milk to reduce gastrointestinal irritation.

## Oral Dosage Forms

### TOCAINIDE HYDROCHLORIDE TABLETS USP

**Usual adult dose**
Antiarrhythmic—
 Initial: Oral, 400 mg every eight hours, the dose being adjusted as needed and tolerated.
 Maintenance: Oral, 1200 to 1800 mg per day in three divided doses.
Note: Some patients may tolerate twice daily dosing.
 Patients with renal or hepatic function impairment may be adequately treated with < 1200 mg a day. Dosage adjustments in these situations may be facilitated by the use of serum drug level determinations.
 Geriatric patients may be more sensitive to the effects of the usual adult dose.

**Usual pediatric dose**
Safety and efficacy have not been established.

**Strength(s) usually available**
U.S.—
 400 mg (Rx) [*Tonocard*].
 600 mg (Rx) [*Tonocard*].
Canada—
 400 mg (Rx) [*Tonocard*].
 600 mg (Rx) [*Tonocard*].

**Packaging and storage**
Store below 40 °C (104 °F), preferably between 15 and 30 °C (59 and 86 °F), unless otherwise specified by manufacturer. Store in a well-closed container.

Revised: 08/21/96

---

**TOLAZAMIDE**—See *Antidiabetic Agents, Sulfonylurea (Systemic)*

---

**TOLAZOLINE**—The *Tolazoline (Parenteral-Systemic)* monograph is not included in this published version of the USP DI database. Copies of the monograph are available on request from Micromedex, Inc. - Reprint Requests, 6200 S. Syracuse Way, Suite 300, Englewood, CO 80111; telephone (303) 486-6400; telefax (303) 486-6464; Email: USPDI@MDX.COM.

---

**TOLBUTAMIDE**—See *Antidiabetic Agents, Sulfonylurea (Systemic)*

---

# TOLCAPONE Systemic—INTRODUCTORY VERSION

VA CLASSIFICATION (Primary): CN500
Commonly used brand name(s): *Tasmar*.
Note: For a listing of dosage forms and brand names by country availability, see *Dosage Forms* section(s).

## Category
Antidyskinetic (COMT inhibitor).

## Indications
**Accepted**
Parkinson's disease (treatment adjunct)—Tolcapone is used as an adjunct to levodopa and carbidopa for the treatment of the symptoms of idiopathic Parkinson's disease.

## Pharmacology/Pharmacokinetics

**Physicochemical characteristics**
Molecular weight—273.25.

**Mechanism of action/Effect**
Tolcapone is a selective and reversible inhibitor of catechol-*O*-methyltransferase (COMT). COMT catalyzes the transfer of the methyl group of *S*-adenosyl-L-methionine to the phenolic group of substrates that contains a catechol structure. Physiological substrates of COMT include dopa, catecholamines (dopamine, norepinephrine, epinephrine) and their hydroxylated metabolites. The function of COMT is to eliminate biologically active catechols and some other hydroxylated metabolites. In the presence of a decarboxylase inhibitor, COMT becomes the major metabolizing enzyme (for levodopa) that catalyzes the metabolism to 3-methoxy-4-hydroxy-L-phenylalanine (3-OMD) in the brain and peripheral tissues. Although the precise mechanism of action of tolcapone is not known, it is believed to be related to its ability to inhibit COMT and alter the plasma pharmacokinetics of levodopa. Administration of tolcapone in conjunction with levodopa and an aromatic amino acid decarboxylase inhibitor, such as carbidopa, produces more sustained plasma levels of levodopa than administration of levodopa and an aromatic amino acid decarboxylase inhibitor alone. These sustained plasma levels of levodopa may result in more constant dopaminergic stimulation in the brain, leading to increased therapeutic effects on the symptoms of Parkinson's disease, as well as increased adverse effects; a decrease in the levodopa dosage may be required.

**Pharmacodynamics**
Studies in healthy volunteers have shown that tolcapone reversibly inhibits human erythrocyte catechol-*O*-methyltransferase (COMT) activity after oral administration, and that this inhibition is closely related to plasma tolcapone concentrations. Maximum inhibition of erythrocyte COMT activity averages > 80% following a single 200-mg dose of tolcapone. Following multiple doses of tolcapone (200 mg three times a day), erythrocyte COMT inhibition at trough tolcapone blood concentrations is 30 to 45%.

**Pharmacokinetics**
Tolcapone pharmacokinetics are linear over the dose range of 50 to 400 mg, independent of levodopa/carbidopa coadministration.

**Absorption**
Tolcapone is rapidly absorbed. Absolute bioavailability following oral administration is about 65%. Food given within 1 hour before or 2 hours after dosing of tolcapone decreases the relative bioavailability by 10 to 20%.

**Distribution**
Steady-state volume of distribution ($Vol_D$) is small, about 9 liters. Tolcapone is not widely distributed into tissues due to its high degree of plasma protein binding.

**Protein binding**
Very high (> 99.9%). *In vitro* studies have shown that tolcapone binds primarily to serum albumin.

**Biotransformation**
Tolcapone is almost completely metabolized. The primary metabolic pathway is glucuronidation to an inactive metabolite. Tolcapone is also methylated by COMT to 3-*O*-methyl-tolcapone. Hydroxylation of the methyl group on tolcapone results in a primary alcohol, which is subsequently oxidized to carboxylic acid. *In vitro* experiments have suggested that the oxidation may be catalyzed by cytochrome P450 3A4 and P450 2A6. Further reduction of the oxidized product to an amine and subsequent *N*-acetylation occur to a minor extent.

Polymorphic metabolism is not likely to occur, based on the metabolic pathways involved.

In patients with moderate cirrhotic liver disease (Child-Pugh Class B), clearance and $Vol_D$ of unbound tolcapone may be reduced by almost 50%, resulting in a twofold increase in the average concentration of unbound drug.

**Half-life**
Elimination—
2 to 3 hours. No significant accumulation occurs.

**Time to peak concentration**
Approximately 2 hours.

**Peak plasma concentration**
Peak plasma concentrations ($C_{max}$) were reported to be 3 micrograms per milliliter (mcg/mL) following tolcapone dosing of 100 mg three times a day, and 6 mcg/mL following tolcapone dosing of 200 mg three times a day.

**Elimination**
Renal. Following administration of an oral dose of radiolabeled tolcapone, 60% is excreted in urine. Only a very small amount (approximately 0.5% of a dose) is found unchanged in the urine.
Fecal. Following administration of an oral dose of radiolabeled tolcapone, 40% is excreted in feces.
In dialysis—
Because of the very high degree of protein binding of tolcapone, no significant removal by hemodialysis is expected.

**Effect of tolcapone on the pharmacokinetics of levodopa and its metabolites**
When administered together with levodopa/carbidopa, tolcapone increases the relative bioavailability (area under the plasma concentration–time curve [AUC]) of levodopa by approximately twofold. This increase in bioavailability is due to a decrease in levodopa clearance that prolongs the terminal elimination half-life of levodopa from approximately 2 hours to 3.5 hours. The average peak levodopa plasma concentration ($C_{max}$) and the time of its occurrence ($T_{max}$) generally are not affected. The onset of effect occurs after the first administration and is maintained during long-term treatment. The maximum effect occurs with 100 to 200 mg of tolcapone. When given with levodopa/carbidopa, tolcapone markedly decreases plasma levels of 3-methoxy-4-hydroxy-L-phenylalanine (3-OMD) in a dose-dependent manner.
Population pharmacokinetic analyses in patients with Parkinson's disease have shown the same effects of tolcapone on levodopa plasma concentrations as those that occur in healthy volunteers.

## Precautions to Consider

### Carcinogenicity
**Carcinogenicity/Tumorigenicity**
Carcinogenicity studies were conducted in rats that received tolcapone for 104 weeks at doses of 50, 250, and 450 milligrams per kilogram of body weight (mg/kg) per day; tolcapone exposures were 1, 6.3, and 13 times the human exposure in male rats, and 1.7, 11.8, and 26.4 times the human exposure in female rats, respectively. There was an increased incidence of uterine adenocarcinomas in female rats at 26.4 times the human exposure. Evidence of renal tubular injury and renal tubular tumor formation in rats also was reported. A low incidence of renal tubular cell adenomas occurred in middle- and high-dose male and high-dose female rats, with a statistically significant increase in high-dose males. No renal tumors were observed at exposures of 1 (males) or 1.7 (females) times the human exposure. Minimal to marked damage to the renal tubules, consisting of proximal tubule cell degeneration, single cell necrosis, hyperplasia, and karyocytomegaly, occurred at the doses associated with renal tumors. Renal tubule damage, characterized by proximal tubule cell degeneration and the presence of atypical nuclei, as well as one instance of adenocarcinoma in a high-dose male, were observed in a year-long study in rats receiving tolcapone doses of 150 and 450 mg/kg per day. These histopathologic changes suggest the possibility that renal tumor formation might be secondary to chronic cell damage and sustained repair, but this relationship has not been established, and the relevance of these findings to humans is not known.
Carcinogenicity studies in mice that received tolcapone in the diet at doses of 100, 300, and 800 mg/kg per day for 80 weeks (female) or 95 weeks (male) showed no evidence of carcinogenic effects.
The carcinogenic potential of tolcapone in combination with levodopa/carbidopa has not been studied.

### Mutagenicity
Tolcapone was clastogenic in the *in vitro* mouse lymphoma/thymidine kinase assay in the presence of metabolic activation. Tolcapone was not mutagenic in the Ames test, the *in vitro* V79/HPRT gene mutation assay, or the unscheduled DNA synthesis assay. It was not clastogenic in an *in vitro* chromosomal aberration assay in cultured human lymphocytes, or in an *in vivo* micronucleus assay in mice.

### Pregnancy/Reproduction
Fertility—Tolcapone did not affect fertility and general reproductive performance in rats receiving up to 300 mg/kg per day (5.7 times the human dose on a mg-per-square-meter of body surface area [mg/m$^2$] basis).

Pregnancy—Adequate and well-controlled studies in humans have not been done.
In rabbits receiving tolcapone doses ≥ 100 mg/kg per day (3.7 times the recommended daily clinical dose on a mg/m$^2$ basis), increased incidences of abortion occurred. Evidence of maternal toxicity (decreased weight gain and death) occurred at tolcapone doses of 300 mg/kg in rats (5.7 times the recommended daily clinical dose on a mg/m$^2$ basis) and 400 mg/kg in rabbits (15 times the recommended daily clinical dose on a mg/m$^2$ basis). Tolcapone was administered to female rats during the last part of gestation and throughout lactation at a dose that was decreased from 250 mg/kg (4.8 times the recommended clinical dose on a mg/m$^2$ basis) per day to 150 mg/kg (2.9 times the recommended clinical dose on a mg/m$^2$ basis) per day due to a high rate of maternal mortality; this resulted in decreased litter size, and impaired growth and learning performance in female pups.
Tolcapone is always given concomitantly with levodopa/carbidopa, which is known to cause visceral and skeletal malformations in rabbits. When pregnant rabbits were treated concomitantly with tolcapone (100 mg/kg per day) and levodopa/carbidopa (80/20 mg/kg per day) throughout organogenesis, an increased incidence of fetal malformations (primarily external and skeletal digit defects) occurred as compared to the incidence seen when levodopa/carbidopa was administered without tolcapone. Plasma exposures to tolcapone (based on area under the plasma concentration–time curve [AUC]) were 0.5 times the expected human exposure, and plasma exposures to levodopa were six times higher than those in humans under therapeutic conditions. In a combined embryo-fetal development study conducted in rats, fetal body weights were reduced by the combination of tolcapone (10, 30, and 50 mg/kg per day) and levodopa/carbidopa (120/30 mg/kg per day) and by levodopa/carbidopa administered alone. Tolcapone exposures were 0.5 times the expected human exposure or greater; levodopa exposures were 21 times the expected human exposure or greater. Tolcapone administered without levodopa/carbidopa at a dose of 50 mg/kg per day (plasma exposures of 1.4 times the expected human exposure) did not result in reduced fetal body weight.

FDA Pregnancy Category C.

### Breast-feeding
It is not known whether tolcapone is distributed into breast milk. In animal studies, tolcapone was shown to appear in maternal rat milk. Risk-benefit must be considered before administering tolcapone to a woman who is breast-feeding.

### Pediatrics
There is no identified potential use of tolcapone in pediatric patients.

### Geriatrics
The relative risk of hallucinations may be increased in patients older than 75 years of age.

### Pharmacogenetics
The pharmacokinetics of tolcapone are independent of sex, age, body weight, and race (Japanese, black, and Caucasian).

### Drug interactions and/or related problems
The following drug interactions and/or related problems have been selected on the basis of their potential clinical significance (possible mechanism in parentheses where appropriate)—not necessarily inclusive (» = major clinical significance):

Note: *In vitro* studies have shown that highly protein-bound tolcapone, at a concentration of 50 mcg per mL, did not displace other highly protein-bound agents (including warfarin, phenytoin, tolbutamide, and digitoxin) from their binding sites at therapeutic concentrations.

Tolcapone may influence the pharmacokinetics of agents metabolized by catechol-*O*-methyltransferase (COMT). However, no effects were seen on the COMT substrate carbidopa.

The potential of tolcapone to interact with the isoenzymes of cytochrome P450 (CYP) was assessed in *in vitro* experiments. No relevant interactions with substrates for CYP 2A6 (warfarin), CYP 1A2 (caffeine), CYP 3A4 (midazolam, terfenadine, cyclosporine), CYP 2C19 (*S*-mephenytoin), and CYP 2D6 (desipramine) were observed. Due to its affinity to cytochrome P450 2C9 *in vitro*, tolcapone potentially may interfere with agents whose clearance is dependent on this pathway, such as tolbutamide and warfarin. In an *in vivo* interaction study, however, tolcapone did not change the pharmacokinetics of tolbutamide; clinically relevant interactions involving cytochrome P450 2C9, therefore, appear unlikely.

Tolcapone did not alter the effects of ephedrine, an indirect sympathomimetic, on hemodynamic parameters or on plasma catecholamine levels, either at rest or during exercise.

Combinations containing any of the following medications, depending on the amount present, may also interact with this medication.

Desipramine
(when tolcapone was administered concomitantly with levodopa/carbidopa and desipramine, the frequency of adverse effects increased slightly; caution should be exercised when desipramine is administered to Parkinson's disease patients receiving this combination of medications)

Medications metabolized by catechol-*O*-methyltransferase [COMT], such as:
Apomorphine
Dobutamine
Isoproterenol
Methyldopa
(although the effect of tolcapone on these agents has not been evaluated, dose reductions of these medications may be needed when they are coadministered with tolcapone)

Monoamine oxidase inhibitors, nonselective, including phenelzine and tranylcypromine
(because monoamine oxidase [MAO] and catechol-*O*-methyltransferase [COMT] are the two major enzyme systems involved in the metabolism of catecholamines, it is theoretically possible that concurrent administration of tolcapone with these medications would result in inhibition of the majority of pathways needed for normal catecholamine metabolism; tolcapone may be taken concomitantly with a selective MAO-B inhibitor such as selegiline)

Warfarin
(clinical information is limited regarding concomitant use of warfarin and tolcapone; coagulation parameters should be monitored)

**Laboratory value alterations**
The following have been selected on the basis of their potential clinical significance (possible effect in parentheses where appropriate)—not necessarily inclusive (» = major clinical significance):
With physiology/laboratory test values
Alanine aminotransferase (ALT [SGPT]) or
Aspartate aminotransferase (AST [SGOT])
(values were increased to more than three times the upper limit of normal [ULN] in about 1% of patients treated with 100 mg of tolcapone three times a day, and in about 3% of patients treated with 200 mg of tolcapone three times a day, during Phase 3 controlled trials; female patients were more likely than male patients to have increased enzyme levels [5% as compared with 2%]; roughly one third of patients with elevated enzymes had diarrhea; increases of greater than eight times the ULN occurred in 0.3% of patients treated with 100 mg tolcapone three times a day and in 1.7% of patients treated with 200 mg tolcapone three times a day; elevations usually occurred within 6 weeks to 6 months of treatment initiation; in about one half of the cases with elevated hepatic enzymes, levels returned to baseline within 1 to 3 months while patients continued tolcapone treatment; when treatment was discontinued, enzyme levels generally declined within 2 to 3 weeks, but some cases took 1 to 2 months to return to normal)

**Medical considerations/Contraindications**
The medical considerations/contraindications included have been selected on the basis of their potential clinical significance (reasons given in parentheses where appropriate)—not necessarily inclusive (» = major clinical significance).

*Risk-benefit should be considered when the following medical problems exist:*
» Hallucinations
(condition may be exacerbated)
» Hepatic function impairment
(clearance may be impaired; dosage adjustments may be necessary)
» Hypotension or
» Orthostatic hypotension
(condition may be exacerbated)
» Renal function impairment, severe
(elimination may be impaired; caution should be exercised)
Sensitivity to tolcapone

**Patient monitoring**
The following may be especially important in patient monitoring (other tests may be warranted in some patients, depending on condition; » = major clinical significance):

Alanine aminotransferase (ALT [SGPT]) or
Aspartate aminotransferase (AST [SGOT])
(monthly monitoring of transaminases is recommended for the first 3 months of treatment; thereafter, liver function tests should be monitored every 6 weeks for the next 3 months; if elevations occur and treatment is continued, more frequent monitoring of complete liver function is recommended; tolcapone should be discontinued if ALT exceeds five times the upper limit of normal [ULN] or if jaundice develops)

## Side/Adverse Effects

Note: Patients with Parkinson's disease who are receiving dopaminergic therapy may experience orthostatic hypotension. Because tolcapone enhances levodopa bioavailability, it may increase the occurrence of orthostatic hypotension. In clinical trials, patients with orthostasis at baseline were more likely than patients without symptoms to experience orthostatic hypotension during the study. In addition, the effect was greater in tolcapone-treated patients than in placebo-treated patients. Baseline treatment with dopamine agonists or selegiline did not appear to increase the likelihood of orthostatic hypotension for patients treated with tolcapone. Syncope also was reported and generally occurred more frequently in patients who had a documented episode of hypotension.

Tolcapone may cause or exacerbate pre-existing dyskinesia. It may also potentiate the dopaminergic side effects of levodopa. Dyskinesia may be ameliorated by reducing the concomitant levodopa dose.

Four cases of a symptom complex characterized by elevated temperature, muscular rigidity, and altered consciousness, and resembling the neuroleptic malignant syndrome, have been reported in association with the abrupt withdrawal or lowering of the dose of tolcapone; similar symptoms have been reported in association with the rapid dose reduction or withdrawal of other dopaminergic medications. Three of these four patients also had elevated creatine kinase (CK). One patient died, and the other three patients recovered over periods ranging from 2 to 6 weeks.

Fibrotic complications, including retroperitoneal fibrosis, pulmonary infiltrates, pleural effusion, and pleural thickening, have been reported in some patients treated with ergot-derived dopaminergic agents. These complications may resolve upon discontinuation of the medication, but complete resolution does not always occur. Although these fibrotic effects are believed to be associated with the ergoline structure of these compounds, it is not known if non–ergot-derived medications that increase dopaminergic activity, such as tolcapone, may produce similar adverse effects. During clinical trials with tolcapone, three cases of pleural effusion, including one with pulmonary fibrosis, were reported. These patients also were taking concomitant dopamine agonists (pergolide or bromocriptine) and had a prior history of cardiac disease or pulmonary pathology (nonmalignant lung lesion).

The following side/adverse effects have been selected on the basis of their potential clinical significance (possible signs and symptoms in parentheses where appropriate)—not necessarily inclusive:

**Those indicating need for medical attention**
Incidence more frequent
***Abdominal pain; anorexia*** (loss of appetite); ***diarrhea; dizziness; dyskinesia*** (twitching, twisting, or other unusual body movements); ***dystonia*** (twisting or other unusual body movements); ***hallucinations*** (seeing, feeling, or hearing things that are not there); ***headache; insomnia*** (trouble in sleeping); ***nausea; orthostatic complaints*** (dizziness or lightheadedness when getting up from a lying or sitting position); ***somnolence*** (drowsiness); ***syncope*** (fainting); ***upper respiratory tract infection*** (cough; fever; nasal congestion; runny nose; sneezing; sore throat); ***vomiting***

Note: *Diarrhea* is usually of mild to moderate severity, but approximately 3 to 4% of patients in clinical trials had severe diarrhea. Typically, diarrhea presents 6 to 12 weeks after initiation of tolcapone therapy, but it may start as early as 2 weeks or as late as many months after tolcapone treatment is started. *Anorexia* may be associated with the diarrhea. No mechanism underlying these symptoms is known, and no consistent description of tolcapone-induced diarrhea has emerged from clinical trials of the medication. It is recommended that all cases of persistent diarrhea be evaluated with an appropriate medical work-up that includes checking for occult blood. A 55-year-old female patient who received tolcapone in doses of 200 mg three times a day for 53 days developed diarrhea followed 4 days later by yellowing of the skin and eyes; she died 7 days after the onset of diarrhea. No liver function tests were performed in this patient after the onset of symptoms.

*Hallucinations* may be more likely to develop in patients older than 75 years of age. In general, hallucinations present shortly after the initiation of tolcapone therapy, typically within the first 2 weeks. Hallucinations are commonly accompanied by confusion and, less commonly, by insomnia and excessive dreaming. Decreasing the concomitant dose of levodopa may help alleviate hallucinations.

*Dystonia* is more likely to develop in patients younger than 75 years of age. *Somnolence* is more likely to occur in female patients than in male patients.

Incidence less frequent
> *Chest pain; confusion; dyspnea* (troubled breathing); *fatigue* (unusual tiredness or weakness); *falling; hematuria* (blood in urine); *hyperkinesia* (hyperactivity); *influenza-like symptoms* (chills; fever; general feeling of discomfort or illness; headache; muscle pain); *loss of balance control*

Incidence rare
> *Agitation; arthritis* (joint pain, redness, or swelling); *burning of feet; chest discomfort; hyperactivity; hypotension* (low blood pressure); *irritability; mental deficiency* (difficulty in thinking or concentrating); *muscle cramps; neck pain; paresthesia* (burning, prickling, or tingling sensations); *sinus congestion* (headache; stuffy nose); *stiffness; urinary tract infection* (bloody or cloudy urine; difficult or painful urination; frequent urge to urinate)

**Those indicating need for medical attention only if they continue or are bothersome**
Incidence more frequent
> *Constipation; excessive dreaming; increased sweating; xerostomia* (dryness of mouth)

Incidence less frequent
> *Dyspepsia* (heartburn); *flatulence* (gas)

**Those not indicating need for medical attention**
Incidence more frequent
> *Discoloration of urine to bright yellow*

**Those indicating the need for medical attention if they occur together after medication is discontinued**
> *Confusion; fever; muscle rigidity*

## Overdose

For information on the management of overdose or unintentional ingestion, **contact a Poison Control Center** (see *Poison Control Center Listing*).

**Clinical effects of overdose**
The highest dose of tolcapone administered to humans was in a study in healthy elderly volunteers who received 800 mg of tolcapone three times a day (with or without concomitant levodopa/carbidopa administration) for 1 week. Nausea, vomiting, and dizziness were observed, particularly in combination with levodopa/carbidopa.

**Treatment of overdose**
To enhance elimination—Due to the very high degree of protein binding of tolcapone, hemodialysis is not likely to be beneficial.

Supportive care—Hospitalization is advised. General supportive care is indicated. Patients in whom intentional overdose is confirmed or suspected should be referred for psychiatric consultation.

## Patient Consultation

As an aid to patient consultation, refer to *Advice for the Patient, Tolcapone (Systemic)—Introductory Version*.
In providing consultation, consider emphasizing the following selected information (» = major clinical significance):

**Before using this medication**
» Conditions affecting use, especially:
  Sensitivity to tolcapone
  Pregnancy—Risk-benefit must be considered
  Breast-feeding—Risk-benefit must be considered
  Use in children—There is no identified potential use of tolcapone in the pediatric age group
  Use in the elderly—Hallucinations are more likely to occur in patients older than 75 years of age
  Other medical problems, especially hallucinations, hepatic function impairment, hypotension, orthostatic hypotension, or renal function impairment

**Proper use of this medication**
» Compliance with therapy; not taking more or less medicine than prescribed

» Proper dosing
  Missed dose: Taking as soon as possible; not taking if almost time for next dose; not doubling doses
» Proper storage

**Precautions while using this medication**
» Checking with physician before discontinuing medication; gradual dosage reduction may be needed
» Possible drowsiness, dizziness, lightheadedness, weakness, trouble in thinking or concentrating; caution when driving or doing jobs requiring alertness and coordination
» Caution when getting up suddenly from lying or sitting position
» Possible hallucinations, especially in older patients
» Medication causes urine to turn bright yellow

**Side/adverse effects**
Signs of potential side effects, especially abdominal pain, anorexia, diarrhea, dizziness, dyskinesia, dystonia, hallucinations, headache, insomnia, nausea, orthostatic complaints, somnolence, syncope, upper respiratory tract infection, vomiting, chest pain, confusion, dyspnea, fatigue, falling, hematuria, hyperkinesia, influenza-like symptoms, loss of balance control, agitation, arthritis, burning of feet, chest discomfort, hyperactivity, hypotension, irritability, mental deficiency, muscle cramps, neck pain, paresthesia, sinus congestion, stiffness, and urinary tract infection

## General Dosing Information

Tolcapone may be administered with either the immediate-release or the sustained-release formulation of levodopa/carbidopa.

In premarketing clinical trials, patients who were taking a daily dose of levodopa in excess of 600 mg, or who had moderate to severe dyskinesia before beginning treatment, were the most likely to require a decrease in their daily levodopa dose after tolcapone therapy was initiated. The average reduction of the daily levodopa dose needed was about 30%. Greater than 70% of patients with levodopa doses above 600 mg a day required such a reduction.

Rapid dose reduction or abrupt withdrawal of tolcapone may cause withdrawal-emergent hyperpyrexia and confusion.

**Diet/Nutrition**
Tolcapone may be taken with or without food.

## Oral Dosage Forms

### TOLCAPONE TABLETS

**Usual adult dose**
Parkinson's disease—
  Oral, initially 100 to 200 mg three times a day, always in conjunction with levodopa/carbidopa therapy. Although initial treatment with 200 mg of tolcapone three times a day generally is well tolerated, some clinicians may wish to initiate therapy with 100 mg of tolcapone three times a day because of the potential for increased dopaminergic side effects and the possible need to adjust the concomitant levodopa/carbidopa dose.

Note: In clinical trials, more than 70% of patients taking levodopa doses greater than 600 mg a day required decreases in the levodopa dose after tolcapone therapy was initiated. The average levodopa dose reduction needed in these patients was about 30%.

Patients with moderate to severe cirrhosis of the liver should not have treatment increased to 200 mg of tolcapone three times a day.

Tolcapone has not been evaluated in patients with a creatinine clearance less than 25 mL per minute (mL/min).

**Usual adult prescribing limits**
600 mg a day.

**Usual pediatric dose**
There is no identified potential use of tolcapone in the pediatric age group.

**Usual geriatric dose**
See *Usual adult dose*.

**Strength(s) usually available**
U.S.—
  100 mg (Rx) [*Tasmar* (film coated; dibasic calcium phosphate anhydrous; lactose monohydrate; magnesium stearate; microcrystalline cellulose; povidone K-30; sodium starch glycolate; talc)].
  200 mg (Rx) [*Tasmar* (film coated; dibasic calcium phosphate anhydrous; lactose monohydrate; magnesium stearate; microcrystalline cellulose; povidone K-30; sodium starch glycolate; talc)].

**Packaging and storage**
Store between 20 and 25 °C (68 and 77 °F) in a tight container, unless otherwise specified by manufacturer.

## Auxiliary labeling
- May cause drowsiness.
- May cause dizziness.

Developed: 05/15/98

**TOLMETIN**—See *Anti-inflammatory Drugs, Nonsteroidal (Systemic)*

**TOLNAFTATE**—The *Tolnaftate (Topical)* monograph is not included in this published version of the USP DI database. Copies of the monograph are available on request from Micromedex, Inc. - Reprint Requests, 6200 S. Syracuse Way, Suite 300, Englewood, CO 80111; telephone (303) 486-6400; telefax (303) 486-6464; Email: USPDI@MDX.COM.

# TOLTERODINE  Systemic—INTRODUCTORY VERSION

VA CLASSIFICATION (Primary): AU350
Commonly used brand name(s): *Detrol*.
Note: For a listing of dosage forms and brand names by country availability, see *Dosage Forms* section(s).

## Category
Antispasmodic (urinary bladder).

## Indications
### Accepted
Bladder hyperactivity (treatment)—Tolterodine is indicated for the treatment of overactive bladder with symptoms of urinary frequency, urgency, or urge incontinence.

## Pharmacology/Pharmacokinetics
**Physicochemical characteristics**
Molecular weight—325.5.
**Mechanism of action/Effect**
Both tolterodine and its active metabolite, 5-hydroxymethyl, exhibit similar antimuscarinic activity. In human studies, the effects of administration of a single, 5-mg dose were a decrease in detrusor pressure and an increase in residual urine, reflecting an incomplete emptying of the bladder.
**Absorption**
Rapid, at least 77% of a 5-mg radiolabeled oral dose was absorbed. It was found that food intake increased the bioavailability of tolterodine by an average of 53%, but did not affect the 5-hydroxymethyl metabolite concentrations in extensive metabolizers. There appeared to be no safety concerns related to this increased bioavailability and a dosage adjustment was not needed.
**Distribution**
$Vol_D$—113 ± 26.7 L following a 1.28 mg intravenous dose.
**Protein binding**
Very high (approximately 96.3%); to plasma proteins, primarily alpha acid glycoprotein. The 5-hydroxymethyl metabolite is approximately 64% protein bound.
**Biotransformation**
Tolterodine is transformed in the liver to 5-hydroxymethyl, its major pharmacologically active metabolite.
**Half-life**
Apparent—
 1.9 to 3.7 hours.
**Time to peak concentration**
1 to 2 hours.
**Elimination**
Following administration of a 5-mg oral, radioactive dose of tolterodine in healthy males, 77% was recovered in the urine and 17% was recovered in the feces. Less than 1% (< 2.5% in poor metabolizers) of the dose was recovered as intact tolterodine and 5 to 14% (< 1% in poor metabolizers) was recovered as the active 5-hydroxymethyl metabolite.

## Precautions to Consider
**Carcinogenicity**
Carcinogenicity studies with tolterodine in mice given 30 mg per kg of body weight (mg/kg) a day, female rats given 20 mg/kg a day, and male rats given 30 mg/kg a day (representing a 9- to 14-fold higher dose than the maximum tolerated dose in humans) found no increase in tumors.

**Mutagenicity**
Tolterodine was found nonmutagenic in the Ames test (using four strains of *Salmonella typhimurium* and two strains of *Escherichia coli*), a gene mutation assay in L5178Y mouse lymphoma cells, and chromosomal aberration tests in human lymphocytes. It was also negative in the bone marrow micronucleus test in the mouse.

**Pregnancy/Reproduction**
Fertility—In female mice treated with 20 mg/kg a day for 2 weeks before mating (a systemic exposure 15-fold higher in animals than in humans based on the area under the plasma concentration–time curve [AUC] of about 500 mcg • hour per L), no effects on fertility or on reproductive performance were observed. A dose of 30 mg/kg a day did not induce any adverse effects on fertility in male mice.
Pregnancy—Studies in humans have not been done. Tolterodine should be used during pregnancy only if the potential benefit for the mother justifies the potential risk for the fetus.
No anomalies or malformations were observed in mice given oral doses of 20 mg/kg a day (approximately 14 times the human exposure). Tolterodine was found to cause embryolethality, a reduced fetal weight, and an increased incidence of fetal abnormalities (cleft palate, digital abnormalities, intra-abdominal hemorrhage, and various skeletal abnormalities, primarily reduced ossification) in mice given doses of 30 to 40 mg/kg a day (approximately 20- to 25-fold higher than the human dose based on AUC). No embryotoxicity or teratogenicity was noted in rabbits treated with subcutaneous tolterodine doses of 0.8 mg/kg a day (threefold higher than the human dose based on AUC of 100 mcg • hour per L).
FDA Pregnancy Category C.

**Breast-feeding**
It is not known whether tolterodine is distributed into human breast milk; therefore its use should be discontinued during nursing. Tolterodine is distributed into the milk of mice. Offspring of female mice treated with 20 mg/kg a day of tolterodine during lactation had a slightly reduced body weight gain, but they regained the weight during the maturation phase.

**Pediatrics**
No information is available on the relationship of age to the effects of tolterodine in pediatric patients. Safety and efficacy have not been established.

**Geriatrics**
Appropriate studies performed to date have not demonstrated geriatrics-specific problems that would limit the usefulness of tolterodine in the elderly.

**Pharmacogenetics**
A subset of the population (approximately 7%) is devoid of cytochrome P450 2D6, the enzyme responsible for the formation of the 5-hydroxymethyl metabolite of tolterodine; the identified pathway of metabolism for these individuals is dealkylation via cytochrome P450 3A4 to *N*-dealkylated tolterodine. These individuals are referred to as poor metabolizers, while the remainder of the population is referred to as extensive metabolizers. Tolterodine is metabolized at a slower rate in poor metabolizers, resulting in significantly higher serum concentrations of tolterodine and negligible serum concentrations of the 5-hydroxymethyl metabolite. Because of differences in the protein binding characteristics of tolterodine and the 5-hydroxymethyl metabolite, the sum of unbound serum concentrations of tolterodine and the 5-hydroxymethyl metabolite is similar in extensive and poor metabolizers at steady state. Since tolterodine and the 5-hydroxymethyl metabolite have similar antimuscarinic effects, the net activity of tolterodine is expected to be similar in extensive and poor metabolizers.

**Drug interactions and/or related problems**
The following drug interactions and/or related problems have been selected on the basis of their potential clinical significance (possible mechanism

## Tolterodine (Systemic)—Introductory Version

in parentheses where appropriate)—not necessarily inclusive (» = major clinical significance):
  Clarithromycin or
  Erythromycin or
  Itraconazole or
  Ketoconazole or
  Miconazole
    (oral use of these medications may inhibit cytochrome P450 3A4, which could lead to increased tolterodine concentrations in certain subpopulations; if given concurrently, the dose for tolterodine should not be higher than 1 mg two times a day)
  Fluoxetine
    (fluoxetine, a selective serotonin reuptake inhibitor and cytochrome P450 2D6 inhibitor, significantly inhibits the metabolism of tolterodine in extensive metabolizers; however, no dosage adjustment is necessary)

### Medical considerations/Contraindications
The medical considerations/contraindications included have been selected on the basis of their potential clinical significance (reasons given in parentheses where appropriate)—not necessarily inclusive (» = major clinical significance).

*Except under special circumstances, this medication should not be used when the following medical problems exist:*
» Gastric retention or
» Glaucoma, narrow angle, uncontrolled or
» Urinary retention
    (tolterodine may aggravate these conditions)
» Hypersensitivity to tolterodine tartrate

*Risk-benefit should be considered when the following medical problems exist:*
  Gastrointestinal obstructive disease such as pyloric stenosis or
  Glaucoma, narrow-angle, controlled or
  Urinary bladder obstruction
    (tolterodine may aggravate these conditions)
» Hepatic function impairment, severe
    (patients with severe hepatic function impairment should not receive doses higher than 1 mg of tolterodine two times a day)

## Side/Adverse Effects
The following side/adverse effects have been selected on the basis of their potential clinical significance (possible signs and symptoms in parentheses where appropriate)—not necessarily inclusive:

### Those indicating need for medical attention
Incidence more frequent
  *Abnormal vision, including problems with accommodation* (difficulty adjusting to distances)—incidence 4.7%; *urinary tract infection* (difficult, burning, or painful urination; frequent urge to urinate; bloody or cloudy urine)—incidence 5.5%

### Those indicating need for medical attention only if they continue or are bothersome
Incidence more frequent
  *Chest pain*—incidence 3.4%; *dizziness*—incidence 8.6%; *dry mouth*—incidence 39.5%; *fatigue*—incidence 6.8%; *gastrointestinal symptoms, specifically abdominal pain*—incidence 7.6%; *constipation*—incidence 6.5%; *diarrhea*—incidence 4%; *dyspepsia* (upset stomach)—incidence 5.9%; *nausea*—incidence 4.2%; *headache*—incidence 11%; *influenza-like symptoms* (joint pain)—incidence 4.4%; *somnolence* (drowsiness)—incidence 3%; *xerophthalmia* (dry eyes)—incidence 3.8%
Incidence less frequent
  *Dysuria* (difficult urination)—incidence 2.5%; *hypertension* (dizziness)—incidence 1.5%

### Those not indicating need for medical attention
Incidence less frequent
  *Flatulence* (stomach gas)—incidence 1.3%

## Overdose
For more information on the management of overdose or unintentional ingestion, **contact a Poison Control Center** (see *Poison Control Center Listing*).

### Treatment of overdose
Tolterodine overdose has the potential to result in severe central anticholinergic effects and should be treated accordingly.
Monitoring—Monitoring of electrocardiogram (ECG) is recommended because QT interval changes were observed in animal studies, but not in humans at doses of up to 4 mg two times a day.
Supportive care—Patients in whom intentional overdose is confirmed or suspected should be referred for psychiatric consultation.

## Patient Consultation
As an aid to patient consultation, refer to *Advice for the Patient, Tolterodine (Systemic)—Introductory Version*.
In providing consultation, consider emphasizing the following selected information (» = major clinical significance):

### Before using this medication
» Conditions affecting use, especially:
    Pregnancy—Animal studies found increased embryo death, reduced fetal weight, and increased incidence of fetal abnormalities when tolterodine was given at high doses
    Breast-feeding—Tolterodine is distributed into the milk of animals, causing transient reduction in body weight gain of offspring
    Pharmacogenetics—7% of population devoid of cytochrome P450 2D6, the enzyme responsible for the formation of the 5-hydroxymethyl metabolite; overall effect is thought to be negligible
    Other medical problems, especially gastric retention; glaucoma, narrow angle (uncontrolled); hepatic function impairment (severe); hypersensitivity to tolterodine tartrate; or urinary retention

### Proper use of this medication
  Importance of not taking more medication than the amount prescribed
» Proper dosing
    Missed dose: Using as soon as possible; not using if almost time for next dose; not doubling doses
» Proper storage

### Precautions while using this medication
» Caution if vision problems occur
» Possible dizziness or drowsiness; caution when driving or doing things requiring alertness
  Possible dryness of mouth; using sugarless candy or gum, ice, or saliva substitute for relief; checking with physician or dentist if dry mouth continues for more than 2 weeks

### Side/adverse effects
  Signs of potential side effects, especially abnormal vision (including accommodation problems) or urinary tract infection

## Oral Dosage Forms

### TOLTERODINE TARTRATE TABLETS

**Usual adult and adolescent dose**
Urologic disorders, symptoms of—
  Oral, 2 mg two times a day; the dose may be lowered to 1 mg two times a day based on individual response and tolerance.
Note: For patients with significantly reduced hepatic function or those who are currently taking drugs that inhibit cytochrome P450 3A4, a dose no greater than of 1 mg two times a day is recommended.

**Usual pediatric dose**
Safety and efficacy have not been established.

**Strength(s) usually available**
U.S.—
  1 mg (Rx) [*Detrol*].
  2 mg (Rx) [*Detrol*].

**Packaging and storage**
Store below 40 °C (104 °F), preferably between 15 and 30 °C (59 and 86 °F), unless otherwise specified by manufacturer.

**Auxiliary labeling**
• May cause vision problems.
• May cause drowsiness.

Developed: 08/13/98

# TOPIRAMATE Systemic—INTRODUCTORY VERSION

VA CLASSIFICATION (Primary): CN400
Commonly used brand name(s): *Topamax*.
Note: For a listing of dosage forms and brand names by country availability, see *Dosage Forms* section(s).

## Category
Anticonvulsant.

## Indications

**Accepted**
Epilepsy (treatment adjunct)—Topiramate is indicated for use in the treatment of partial onset seizures.

## Pharmacology/Pharmacokinetics

**Physicochemical characteristics**
Chemical group—Sulfamate-substituted monosaccharide.
Molecular weight—339.36.

**Mechanism of action/Effect**
The precise mechanism of action is unknown. Electrophysiological and biochemical studies on cultured neurons demonstrated that topiramate blocks the action potentials elicited repetitively by a sustained depolarization of the neurons in a time-dependent manner; this effect suggests a state-dependent sodium channel blocking action. Also, topiramate increases the frequency at which gamma-aminobutyric acid (GABA) activates $GABA_A$ receptors, thereby enhancing GABA-induced influx of chloride ions into neurons. Thus, it appears that topiramate exerts its effects by potentiation of the activity of the inhibitory neurotransmitter, GABA. In addition, topiramate antagonizes the ability of kainate to activate the kainate/AMPA (alpha-amino-3-hydroxy-5-methylisoxazole-4-propionic acid; non-NMDA) subtype of excitatory amino acid (glutamate) receptor, but has no apparent effect on the activity of N-methyl-D-aspartate (NMDA) at the NMDA receptor subtype. These effects of topiramate are concentration-dependent within the range of 1 to 200 micromoles.

**Other actions/effects**
Topiramate also inhibits some isoenzymes of carbonic anhydrase (CA-II and CA-IV). This pharmacologic effect is generally weak and may not be a major contributing factor to the antiepileptic activity of topiramate.

**Absorption**
Rapid. The relative bioavailability of the tablet dosage form is about 80% as compared with that from a solution. Food does not affect the bioavailability of topiramate.

**Protein binding**
Low (13 to 17% over the concentration range of 1 to 250 mcg per mL).

**Biotransformation**
Topiramate is not extensively metabolized. Six metabolites (formed by hydroxylation, hydrolysis, and glucuronidation) have been identified in humans, with none constituting more than 5% of an administered dose.

**Half-life**
Elimination—
21 hours (mean) following single or multiple dosing.

**Time to peak concentration**
Approximately 2 hours following administration of a 400-mg oral dose.

**Time to steady state concentration**
In patients with normal renal function, steady state is reached in about 4 days.
Note: The pharmacokinetics of topiramate are linear, with dose-proportional increases in the plasma concentration over the range of 200 to 800 mg a day.

**Elimination**
Renal; approximately 70% of an administered dose is eliminated unchanged. Evidence from rat studies has shown that renal tubular reabsorption of topiramate occurs.
With impaired renal function—
Topiramate clearance was reduced by 42% in patients with moderate renal function impairment (creatinine clearance of 30 to 69 mL per minute per 1.73 square meters of body surface area), and by 54% in patients with severe renal impairment (creatinine clearance less than 30 mL per minute per 1.73 square meters of body surface area,) as compared with the clearance in subjects with normal renal function. Topiramate is presumed to undergo significant tubular reabsorption, but it is not certain if changes in clearance can be generalized to all cases of renal impairment. Some forms of renal disease may affect glomerular filtration rate and tubular reabsorption differently, resulting in a topiramate clearance rate not predicted by creatinine clearance. In general, one half of the usual dose is recommended in patients with moderate or severe renal impairment.
With impaired hepatic function—
The clearance of topiramate may be decreased in patients with impaired hepatic function; the mechanism of this effect is not well understood.
In hemodialysis—
120 mL per minute with blood flow through the dialyzer at 400 mL per minute (using a high efficiency, counterflow, single pass-dialysate hemodialysis procedure). This high clearance, as compared with 20 to 30 mL per minute total clearance of the oral dose in healthy adults, removes a clinically significant amount of topiramate from the patient over the hemodialysis treatment period; dosage adjustments may be necessary.

## Precautions to Consider

**Carcinogenicity**
An increase in urinary bladder tumors was observed in mice given topiramate (20, 75, and 300 mg per kg of body weight [mg/kg]) in the diet for 21 months. The statistically significant increased incidence of bladder tumors in male and female mice receiving 300 mg/kg was due primarily to the increased occurrence of a smooth muscle tumor considered histomorphologically unique to mice. Plasma exposures in mice receiving 300 mg/kg were approximately 0.5 to 1 time the steady-state exposures measured in patients receiving topiramate monotherapy at the recommended human dose of 400 mg, and 1.5 to 2 times the steady-state topiramate exposures in patients receiving 400 mg topiramate plus phenytoin. The relevance of this finding to human carcinogenic risk is uncertain. No evidence of carcinogenicity was seen in rats following oral administration of topiramate for 2 years at doses of up to 120 mg/kg (approximately three times the recommended human dose on a mg per square meter of body surface area [mg/m²] basis).

**Mutagenicity**
Topiramate did not demonstrate genotoxic potential when tested in a battery of *in vitro* and *in vivo* assays. Topiramate was not mutagenic in the Ames test or the *in vitro* mouse lymphoma assay; it did not increase unscheduled DNA synthesis in rat hepatocytes *in vitro*; and it did not increase chromosomal aberrations in human lymphocytes *in vitro* or in rat bone marrow *in vivo*.

**Pregnancy/Reproduction**
Fertility—No adverse effects on male or female fertility were observed in rats receiving up to 2.5 times the recommended human dose on a mg per square meter of body surface area (mg/m²) basis.

Pregnancy—Studies have not been done in humans.
Topiramate has demonstrated selective developmental toxicity, including teratogenicity, in animal studies.
Incidence of fetal malformations (primarily craniofacial defects) was increased in pregnant mice that received oral topiramate doses of 20, 100, or 500 mg/kg during the period of organogenesis. Fetal body weights and skeletal ossification were reduced at doses of 500 mg/kg; decreased maternal body weight gain also occurred at this dose. In studies in rats, the frequency of limb malformations (ectrodactyly, micromelia, and amelia) was increased among the offspring of dams treated with 400 mg of topiramate per kg or greater during the organogenesis period of pregnancy. Clinical signs of maternal toxicity were seen at doses of 400 mg/kg and above, and maternal body weight gain was reduced during treatment with doses of 100 mg/kg or greater. Embryotoxicity (reduced fetal body weights, increased incidence of structural variations) was observed at doses as low as 20 mg/kg.
In studies in rabbits receiving topiramate, embryo/fetal mortality was increased at doses of 35 mg/kg and greater, and teratogenic effects (primarily rib and vertebral malformations) were observed at doses of 120 mg/kg. Evidence of maternal toxicity (decreased body weight gain, clinical signs, and/or mortality) was seen at doses of 35 mg/kg and greater.
Offspring of female rats treated with topiramate during the latter part of gestation and throughout lactation exhibited decreased viability and delayed physical development at doses of 200 mg/kg, and reductions in pre- and/or postweaning body weight gain at doses of 2 mg/kg and greater. Maternal toxicity (decreased body weight gain, other clinical signs) was evident at doses of 100 mg/kg or greater.

In a rat embryo/fetal development study with a postnatal component, pups of dams receiving topiramate exhibited delayed physical development at doses of 400 mg/kg and persistent reductions in body weight gain at doses of 30 mg/kg and higher.

FDA Pregnancy Category C.

Labor and delivery—The effect of topiramate on labor and delivery in humans is unknown. In studies in rats in which dams were allowed to deliver pups naturally, no drug-related effects on gestation length or parturition were observed at doses of up to 200 mg/kg per day.

**Breast-feeding**
It is not known if topiramate is distributed into breast milk; however, it is distributed into the milk of lactating rats.

**Pediatrics**
Safety and efficacy of topiramate in pediatric patients have not been established.

Pharmacokinetic profiles obtained after 1 week at topiramate doses of 1, 3, and 9 mg per kg of body weight per day in patients aged 4 to 17 years receiving one or two other antiepileptic medications showed that clearance was independent of dose. Although the relationship between age and clearance among pediatric patients has not been systematically evaluated, it appears that the weight-adjusted clearance of topiramate is higher in pediatric patients than in adults.

**Geriatrics**
In clinical trials, 2% of patients were over 60 years of age. No age-related differences in the efficacy of topiramate were observed, and no pharmacokinetic differences related to age alone were found. However, elderly patients are more likely to have age-related renal function impairment, which may require topiramate dosage reductions.

**Pharmacogenetics**
The clearance of topiramate was not affected by race or gender.

**Drug interactions and/or related problems**
The following drug interactions and/or related problems have been selected on the basis of their potential clinical significance (possible mechanism in parentheses where appropriate)—not necessarily inclusive (» = major clinical significance):

Note: Combinations containing any of the following medications, depending on the amount present, may also interact with this medication.

Alcohol or
Central nervous system (CNS) depression–producing medications, other (see *Appendix II*)
(CNS depression may be enhanced)

» Carbamazepine
(mean carbamazepine area under the plasma concentration–time curve [AUC] was unchanged or changed by less than 10%, whereas the AUC of topiramate was decreased by 40% when these two medications were given concurrently during controlled clinical studies)

» Carbonic anhydrase inhibitors, such as:
Acetazolamide
Dichlorphenamide
(concurrent use with topiramate may increase the risk of renal stone formation)

» Contraceptives, estrogen-containing, oral
(efficacy of oral contraceptives may be compromised when used concurrently with topiramate; patients should be instructed to report any change in their bleeding patterns)

Digoxin
(in a single-dose study, serum digoxin area under the plasma concentration–time curve [AUC] was decreased by 12% with concomitant topiramate administration; clinical relevance has not been established)

» Phenytoin
(mean phenytoin area under the plasma concentration–time curve [AUC] was unchanged, changed by less than 10%, or increased by 25%, whereas the AUC of topiramate was decreased by 48% when these two medications were given concurrently during controlled clinical studies; increases in phenytoin plasma concentrations generally occurred in patients receiving phenytoin doses two times a day)

» Valproic acid
(mean valproic acid area under the plasma concentration–time curve [AUC] was decreased by 11%, whereas the AUC of topiramate was decreased by 14% when these two medications were given concurrently during controlled clinical studies)

**Medical considerations/Contraindications**
The medical considerations/contraindications included have been selected on the basis of their potential clinical significance (reasons given in parentheses where appropriate)—not necessarily inclusive (» = major clinical significance).

*Risk-benefit should be considered when the following medical problems exist:*

Hepatic function impairment or
» Renal function impairment
(clearance of topiramate and its metabolites may be decreased; dosage adjustments may be necessary)

Renal calculi, predisposition to
(increased risk of occurrence of renal calculi)

Sensitivity to topiramate

## Side/Adverse Effects

Note: Since topiramate is indicated for use as adjunctive therapy, the side/adverse effects reported in this section occurred in clinical trials in which patients were receiving additional antiepileptic medication.

The following side/adverse effects have been selected on the basis of their potential clinical significance (possible signs and symptoms in parentheses where appropriate)—not necessarily inclusive:

**Those indicating need for medical attention**
Incidence more frequent
*Asthenia* (unusual tiredness or weakness); *ataxia* (clumsiness or unsteadiness); *confusion; difficulty with concentration or attention; diplopia or other vision problems* (double vision or other vision problems); *dizziness; dysmenorrhea or other menstrual changes* (menstrual pain or other changes); *fatigue; memory problems; nervousness; nystagmus* (uncontrolled back-and-forth and/or rolling eye movements); *paresthesia* (burning, prickling, or tingling sensations); *psychomotor retardation* (generalized slowing of mental and physical activity); *somnolence* (drowsiness); *speech or language problems*—particularly word-finding difficulties

Note: *Fatigue* and *somnolence* are usually mild to moderate and appear early in therapy. The incidence of *fatigue* appears to increase at doses greater than 400 mg of topiramate a day. *Confusion, difficulty with concentration or attention, nervousness,* and *speech or language problems* appear to be dose-related.

Incidence less frequent
*Abdominal pain; anorexia* (loss of appetite); *chills; gingivitis* (red, irritated, or bleeding gums); *hypoesthesia* (lessening of sensations or perception); *leukopenia* (fever; chills; sore throat); *mood or mental changes, including aggression, agitation, apathy, irritability, and mental depression; pharyngitis* (sore throat); *weight loss*

Note: *Anorexia, mood or mental changes,* and *weight loss* appear to be dose-related.

Incidence rare
*Anemia* (pale skin; unusual tiredness or weakness); *conjunctivitis* (red or irritated eyes); *dyspnea* (troubled breathing); *edema* (swelling); *epistaxis* (nosebleeds); *eye pain; hematuria* (blood in urine); *impotence or decreased libido* (decrease in sexual performance or desire); *pruritus* (itching); *renal calculi* (flank pain; difficult or painful urination); *skin rash; tinnitus* (ringing or buzzing in ears; hearing loss); *urinary problems, including dysuria* (pain on urination); *urinary frequency* (frequent urination); *and incontinence* (loss of bladder control)

Note: *Renal calculi* occurred in about 1.5% of the patients exposed to topiramate during its development, an incidence which is about two to four times that expected in the general population. Incidence of stone formation was higher in males, as is usual for the general population. As a weak carbonic anhydrase inhibitor, topiramate may promote stone formation by reducing urinary citrate excretion and by increasing urinary pH. Concomitant use with other carbonic anhydrase inhibitors may increase the risk of stone formation and should be avoided. Hydration is recommended to reduce new stone formation; increased fluid intake increases urinary output, thus lowering the concentration of substances involved in stone formation.

**Those indicating need for medical attention only if they continue or are bothersome**
Incidence more frequent
*Breast pain in females; nausea; tremor*—appears to be dose-related

Incidence less frequent
*Back pain; chest pain; constipation; dyspepsia* (heartburn); *hot flushes; increased sweating; leg pain*

**Those not indicating need for medical attention**
Incidence less frequent
*Taste perversion* (change in sense of taste)

## Overdose

For more information on the management of overdose or unintentional ingestion, **contact a Poison Control Center** (see *Poison Control Center Listing*).

### Treatment of overdose

To decrease absorption—If ingestion is recent, the stomach should be emptied immediately by lavage or by induction of emesis. Since activated charcoal has not been shown to adsorb topiramate *in vitro*, its use in overdosage is not recommended.

To enhance elimination—Hemodialysis is an effective means of removing topiramate from the body.

Supportive care—Treatment should be appropriately supportive. Patients in whom intentional overdose is confirmed or suspected should be referred for psychiatric consultation.

## Patient Consultation

In providing consultation, consider emphasizing the following selected information (» = major clinical significance)

### Before using this medication
» Conditions affecting use, especially:
  - Sensitivity to topiramate
  - Pregnancy—In animal studies, topiramate has demonstrated selective developmental toxicity, including teratogenicity
  - Other medications, especially carbamazepine, carbonic anhydrase inhibitors, oral estrogen-containing contraceptives, phenytoin, or valproic acid
  - Other medical problems, especially renal function impairment

### Proper use of this medication
» Compliance with therapy; taking every day exactly as directed
Not breaking tablets, due to the bitter taste
» Proper dosing
Missed dose: Taking as soon as possible; not taking if almost time for next dose; not doubling doses
» Proper storage

### Precautions while using this medication
» Caution when driving, using machines, or doing other jobs requiring alertness
» Using alternative contraceptive method or additional means of birth control with oral estrogen-containing contraceptives
» Importance of adequate fluid intake during therapy to help prevent kidney stone formation

### Side/adverse effects
Signs of potential side effects, especially asthenia, ataxia, confusion, difficulty with concentration or attention, diplopia or other vision problems, dizziness, dysmenorrhea or other menstrual changes, fatigue, memory problems, nervousness, nystagmus, paresthesia, psychomotor retardation, somnolence, speech or language problems, abdominal pain, anorexia, chills, gingivitis, hypoesthesia, leukopenia, mood or mental changes, pharyngitis, weight loss, anemia, conjunctivitis, dyspnea, edema, epistaxis, eye pain, hematuria, impotence or decreased libido, pruritus, renal calculi, skin rash, tinnitus, and urinary problems

Taste perversion may be of concern to the patient, but usually does not require medical attention

## General Dosing Information

In the controlled trials, there was no correlation between trough plasma concentrations of topiramate and clinical efficacy; thus, monitoring of topiramate plasma concentrations to optimize therapy is not necessary.

Dosage adjustments may be required when topiramate is added to or withdrawn from antiepileptic dosing regimens. Similarly, when other agents are added to or withdrawn from a regimen that includes topiramate, dosage adjustments may be necessary (see *Drug Interactions* section).

Antiepileptic medications, including topiramate, should be withdrawn gradually to minimize the potential of increased seizure frequency.

Patients, particularly those with predisposing factors, should be instructed to maintain an adequate fluid intake in order to minimize the risk of renal stone formation.

Because of the bitter taste, tablets should not be broken.

### Diet/Nutrition
Topiramate may be taken without regard to meals.

## Oral Dosage Forms

### TOPIRAMATE TABLETS

#### Usual adult dose
Anticonvulsant—
Oral, 400 mg a day, administered in two divided doses. Dosage should be initiated at 50 mg a day for the first week, and increased at weekly intervals by 50 mg a day until an effective dose is reached.

Note: A daily dose of 200 mg has inconsistent effects and is less effective than 400 mg a day. Doses above 400 mg a day have not been shown to improve responses.

In patients with renal function impairment, one half of the usual adult dose is recommended. These patients will require a longer time to reach steady-state plasma concentrations at each dose. Similarly, patients with hepatic function impairment may have increased topiramate plasma concentrations, and dosage adjustments may be needed.

In patients undergoing hemodialysis, topiramate is cleared by hemodialysis at a rate four to six times greater than in a normal individual. Prolonged periods of dialysis may decrease topiramate concentrations below levels required to maintain seizure control. To avoid rapid decreases in topiramate plasma concentrations during hemodialysis, a supplemental topiramate dose may be required. The duration of dialysis, the clearance rate of the dialysis system employed, and the effective renal clearance of topiramate in the dialysis patient, should be considered when making dosage adjustments.

#### Usual pediatric dose
Safety and efficacy have not been established.

#### Usual geriatric dose
See *Usual adult dose*.

#### Strength(s) usually available
U.S.—
- 25 mg (Rx) [*Topamax* (coated; lactose monohydrate; pregelatinized starch; microcrystalline cellulose; sodium starch glycolate; magnesium stearate; purified water; carnauba wax; hydroxypropyl methylcellulose; titanium dioxide; polyethylene glycol; polysorbate 80)].
- 100 mg (Rx) [*Topamax* (coated; lactose monohydrate; pregelatinized starch; microcrystalline cellulose; sodium starch glycolate; magnesium stearate; purified water; carnauba wax; hydroxypropyl methylcellulose; titanium dioxide; polyethylene glycol; synthetic iron oxide; polysorbate 80)].
- 200 mg (Rx) [*Topamax* (coated; lactose monohydrate; pregelatinized starch; microcrystalline cellulose; sodium starch glycolate; magnesium stearate; purified water; carnauba wax; hydroxypropyl methylcellulose; titanium dioxide; polyethylene glycol; synthetic iron oxide; polysorbate 80)].

#### Packaging and storage
Store in tightly closed containers at 15 to 30 °C (59 to 86 °F). Protect from moisture.

#### Auxiliary labeling
- May cause drowsiness.
- Avoid alcoholic beverages.
- Do not break tablets.

Developed: 11/03/97

---

# TOPOTECAN  Systemic

VA CLASSIFICATION (Primary): AN900
Commonly used brand name(s): *Hycamtin*.
Note: For a listing of dosage forms and brand names by country availability, see *Dosage Forms* section(s).

## Category
Antineoplastic.

## Indications

Note: Bracketed information in the *Indications* section refers to uses that are not included in U.S. product labeling.

## Accepted

Carcinoma, ovarian (treatment)—Topotecan is indicated for the treatment of metastatic ovarian carcinoma after failure of first-line or subsequent chemotherapy.

[Carcinoma, lung, non–small cell (NSCLC) (treatment)][1] and
[Carcinoma, lung, small cell (SCLC) (treatment)][1]—Topotecan is indicated for the treatment of NSCLC (Evidence rating: IIIA) and SCLC (Evidence rating: IIIA). Topotecan is not recommended as first-line therapy, but may be considered for use at a later point in the management of patients with these diseases. In clinical trials, most responses in patients with SCLC were seen in those who had responded to, and relapsed more than 2 or 3 months after completion of, first-line therapy with other agents.

[Myelodysplastic syndrome (treatment)][1] and
[Chronic myelomonocytic leukemia (CMML) (treatment)][1]—Topotecan is indicated, alone or in combination with cytarabine, for the treatment of myelodysplastic syndrome (Evidence rating: IIID) and CMML (Evidence rating: IIID). Preliminary evidence indicates that topotecan may correct genetic abnormalities and prolong survival in patients with these diseases, for whom treatment options are limited.

---
[1]Not included in Canadian product labeling.

## Pharmacology/Pharmacokinetics

**Physicochemical characteristics**
Source—Semisynthetic analog of camptothecin, a plant alkaloid obtained from the *Camptotheca acuminata* tree.
Molecular weight—457.92.
pH—After reconstitution, topotecan injection has a pH of 2.5 to 3.5.
Solubility—Soluble in water.

**Mechanism of action/Effect**
Topotecan inhibits the action of topoisomerase I, an enzyme essential for cell growth and proliferation. Topoisomerase I produces single strand breaks in DNA, thereby relieving torsional strain and allowing DNA replication to proceed, then repairs the strand. Topotecan binds to the topoisomerase I–DNA complex and prevents religation of the DNA strand, resulting in double strand DNA breakage and cell death.

**Distribution**
Topotecan is evenly distributed between plasma and blood cells. Significant quantities of topotecan are distributed into cerebrospinal fluid.
Volume of distribution—130 liters; decreased by approximately 25% in patients with moderate renal function impairment (creatinine clearance 20 to 39 mL per minute [mL/min]).

**Protein binding**
Moderate (35%).

**Biotransformation**
Topotecan undergoes reversible, pH-dependent hydrolysis of the active lactone moiety, forming an open-ring hydroxyacid, which is inactive. Whereas only the lactone form is present at pH $\leq$ 4, the hydroxyacid form predominates at physiologic pH.
Relatively small quantities of topotecan are metabolized via hepatic microsomal enzymes to an *N*-demethylated derivative. Neither the lactone nor the hydroxyacid form of topotecan is metabolized to a significant extent.

**Half-life**
Terminal—
  Normal renal and hepatic function: Approximately 2 to 3 hours.
  Moderate renal function impairment (creatinine clearance 20 to 39 mL/min): Approximately 5 hours.
  Hepatic function impairment: May be increased slightly.

**Onset of action**
Tumor responses were observed at a median of 9 to 12 weeks (range, approximately 3 to 24 weeks) in clinical trials.

**Serum concentration**
Total exposure (as indicated by the area under the concentration-time curve [AUC]) is approximately proportional to the administered dose.

**Elimination**
Renal; approximately 30% of a dose. Some topotecan is also eliminated via the biliary route.
  Plasma clearance:
    Normal renal and hepatic function: Approximately 1030 mL/min; approximately 24% higher in males than in females because of differences in body size. Studies in female patients have not shown significant age-related differences in clearance.
    Renal function impairment:
      Mild (creatinine clearance 40 to 60 mL/min)—Decreased by approximately 33%.
      Moderate (creatinine clearance 20 to 39 mL/min)—Decreased by approximately 66%.
    Hepatic function impairment (serum bilirubin 1.7 to 15 mg per deciliter): Decreased by approximately 33%.

## Precautions to Consider

**Carcinogenicity**
Secondary malignancies are potential delayed effects of many antineoplastic agents, although it is not clear whether the effect is related to their mutagenic or immunosuppressive action. The effect of dose and duration of therapy is also unknown, although risk seems to increase with long-term use. There is some evidence linking therapy with topoisomerase I inhibitors such as topotecan to the development of acute leukemias associated with specific chromosomal translocations.
Long-term animal studies to evaluate the carcinogenic potential of topotecan have not been done. However, topotecan is genotoxic to mammalian cells and is a probable carcinogen.

**Mutagenicity**
*In vitro* studies have shown that topotecan, with or without metabolic activation, is mutagenic to L5178Y mouse lymphoma cells and clastogenic to cultured human lymphocytes. In an *in vivo* study, clastogenicity was also demonstrated in mouse bone marrow cells. However, topotecan did not cause mutations in bacterial cells.

**Pregnancy/Reproduction**
Fertility—Administration of 0.23 mg of topotecan per kg of body weight (mg/kg) per day to rats (equivalent to the recommended human dose on a mg per square meter of body surface area [mg/m$^2$] basis) from day 14 prior to conception through day 6 of gestation caused fetal resorptions and pre-implant losses.

Pregnancy—Studies in humans have not been done.
It is usually recommended that use of antineoplastics, especially combination chemotherapy, be avoided whenever possible, especially during the first trimester. Although information is limited because of the relatively few instances of antineoplastic therapy during pregnancy, the mutagenic, teratogenic, and carcinogenic potential of these medications must be considered.
Other potential hazards to the fetus include adverse reactions seen in adults.
In general, use of a contraceptive is recommended during therapy with cytotoxic medications.
Administration to rabbits of 0.1 mg/kg of topotecan per day (equivalent to the recommended human dose on a mg/m$^2$ basis) on days 6 through 20 of gestation resulted in maternal and fetal toxicity (diminished fetal body weight and embryolethality). Also, administration to rats of 0.23 mg/kg per day (equivalent to the recommended human dose on a mg/m$^2$ basis) from 14 days prior to conception through day 6 of gestation caused microphthalmia and mild maternal toxicity, and administration to rats of 0.1 mg/kg per day (approximately one half the recommended human dose on a mg/m$^2$ basis) from days 6 through 17 of gestation caused increases in post-implantation mortality and malformations of the eye (microphthalmia, anophthalmia, rosette formation of the retina, coloboma of the retina, ectopic orbit), brain (dilated lateral and third ventricles), skull, and vertebrae.

FDA Pregnancy Category D.

**Breast-feeding**
Although very little information is available regarding distribution of antineoplastic agents into breast milk, breast-feeding is not recommended while topotecan is being administered because of the risks to the infant (adverse effects, mutagenicity, carcinogenicity). It is not known whether topotecan is distributed into breast milk.

**Pediatrics**
Topotecan has been studied in a limited number of pediatric patients. One dose-finding study has shown that severe topotecan-induced myelotoxicity may occur at lower doses in children than in adults. Safety and efficacy have not been established.

**Geriatrics**
Clinical trials with topotecan have included patients 65 years of age and older. No geriatrics-specific problems have been documented to date. Pharmacokinetic studies have not been performed specifically in elderly individuals, but studies in female patients did not identify age as a significant factor in topotecan clearance. Dosage adjustment on the basis of advanced age is not necessary. However, elderly patients are more likely to have age-related renal function impairment, which may require dosage adjustment in patients receiving topotecan.

**Dental**
The bone marrow depressant effects of topotecan may result in an increased incidence of microbial infection, delayed healing, and gingival bleeding. Dental work, whenever possible, should be completed prior to initiation of therapy or deferred until blood counts have returned to nor-

mal. Patients should be instructed in proper oral hygiene during treatment, including caution in use of regular toothbrushes, dental floss, and toothpicks.

Topotecan may cause stomatitis, which is usually mild. In clinical trials, stomatitis occurred in 24% of the patients. The incidences of grade 3 and grade 4 stomatitis were 2% and < 1%, respectively.

**Drug interactions and/or related problems**
The following drug interactions and/or related problems have been selected on the basis of their potential clinical significance (possible mechanism in parentheses where appropriate)—not necessarily inclusive (» = major clinical significance):

Note: Combinations containing any of the following medications, depending on the amount present, may also interact with this medication.

Blood dyscrasia–causing medications (see *Appendix II*)
(leukopenic and/or thrombocytopenic effects of topotecan may be increased with concurrent or recent therapy if these medications cause the same effects; dosage adjustment of topotecan, if necessary, should be based on blood counts)

» Bone marrow depressants, other (see *Appendix II*) or
» Radiation therapy
(additive bone marrow depression may occur; dosage reduction may be required when two or more bone marrow depressants, including radiation, are used concurrently or consecutively)

(in a dose-finding study, concurrent use of topotecan and cisplatin caused unexpectedly severe myelosuppression and grade 3 or 4 nonhematologic effects, such as diarrhea, nausea, vomiting, and lethargy, without providing increased benefit over established regimens. A safe and effective regimen utilizing topotecan and cisplatin has not been established)

Filgrastim (rG-CSF)
(filgrastim may be used to decrease the incidence and shorten the duration of severe topotecan-induced neutropenia; however, filgrastim treatment must be started no sooner than 24 hours after the last dose of topotecan in a cycle because concurrent use of the two medications may actually prolong the duration of topotecan-induced neutropenia)

» Immunosuppressants, other, such as:
Azathioprine
Chlorambucil
Corticosteroids, glucocorticoid
Cyclophosphamide
Cyclosporine
Mercaptopurine
Muromonab CD-3
Tacrolimus
(concurrent use with topotecan may increase the risk of infection)

Probenecid
(in a study in mice, probenecid decreased renal clearance of topotecan by 50% and significantly increased systemic exposure to the medication, as demonstrated by an increase in the area under the topotecan concentration–time curve [AUC]; the possibility of a similar effect in humans leading to a higher risk of severe topotecan-induced myelotoxicity should be considered)

Vaccines, killed virus
(because normal defense mechanisms may be suppressed by topotecan therapy, the patient's antibody response to the vaccine may be decreased. The interval between discontinuation of medications that cause immunosuppression and restoration of the patient's ability to respond to the vaccine depends on the intensity and type of immunosuppression-causing medication used, the underlying disease, and other factors; estimates vary from 3 months to 1 year)

» Vaccines, live virus
(because normal defense mechanisms may be suppressed by topotecan therapy, concurrent use with a live virus vaccine may potentiate the replication of the vaccine virus, may increase the side/adverse effects of the vaccine virus, and/or may decrease the patient's antibody response to the vaccine; immunization of these patients should be undertaken only with extreme caution after careful review of the patient's hematologic status and only with the knowledge and consent of the physician managing the topotecan therapy. The interval between discontinuation of medications that cause immunosuppression and restoration of the patient's ability to respond to the vaccine depends on the intensity and type of immunosuppression-causing medication used, the underlying disease, and other factors; estimates vary from 3 months to 1 year. In addition, immunization with oral poliovirus vaccine should be postponed in persons in close contact with the patient, especially family members)

**Laboratory value alterations**
The following have been selected on the basis of their potential clinical significance (possible effect in parentheses where appropriate)—not necessarily inclusive (» = major clinical significance):

With physiology/laboratory test values
Alanine aminotransferase (ALT [SGPT]) and
Alkaline phosphatase and
Aspartate aminotransferase (AST [SGOT]) and
Bilirubin concentration, serum
(values may be increased; in clinical trials, transient grade 1 increases in aminotransferase values, grade 3 or 4 elevations of aminotransferase values, and grade 3 or 4 increases in bilirubin concentration occurred in 5%, < 1%, and < 3%, respectively, of the patients)

» Hematocrit/hemoglobin values and
» Leukocyte, especially neutrophil, count and
» Platelet count
(may be decreased; hematocrit or hemoglobin values, neutrophil count, and platelet count usually reach their nadirs at medians of 15, 11, and 15 days, respectively, after a treatment. The median durations of grade 3 or 4 anemia, neutropenia, and thrombocytopenia are generally 7, 7, and 5 days, respectively)

**Medical considerations/Contraindications**
The medical considerations/contraindications included have been selected on the basis of their potential clinical significance (reasons given in parentheses where appropriate)—not necessarily inclusive (» = major clinical significance).

*Except under special circumstances, this medication should not be used when the following medical problems exist:*

» Bone marrow depression, pre-existing or treatment-related
(topotecan therapy should not be initiated if baseline neutrophil and platelet counts are lower than 1500 cells per cubic millimeter [cells/mm$^3$] and 100,000 cells/mm$^3$, respectively. Also, if severe topotecan-induced anemia, neutropenia, or thrombocytopenia occurs during treatment, subsequent courses of therapy should be delayed until the hemoglobin concentration recovers to 9 grams per deciliter [with transfusion, if necessary], neutrophil counts recover to > 1000 cells/mm$^3$, and platelet counts recover to > 100,000 cells/mm$^3$)

» Renal function impairment, severe (creatinine clearance less than 20 mL per minute)
(topotecan elimination will be greatly decreased, resulting in increased and prolonged plasma concentrations and half-life and an increased risk of toxicity; use in patients with severe renal function impairment is not recommended, because a suitable dose for these patients has not been established)

*Risk-benefit should be considered when the following medical problems exist:*

» Chickenpox, existing or recent (including recent exposure) or
» Herpes zoster
(risk of severe, generalized disease)
» Hypersensitivity to topotecan
» Infection, pre-existing
(recovery may be impaired)
» Renal function impairment, moderate (creatinine clearance 20 to 39 mL per minute)
(topotecan elimination will be decreased by approximately 66%, resulting in increased and prolonged plasma concentrations and half-life and an increased risk of toxicity; a 50% reduction in dose is recommended for patients with moderate renal function impairment)

» Caution should also be used in patients who have had previous cytotoxic drug therapy or radiation therapy

**Patient monitoring**
The following may be especially important in patient monitoring (other tests may be warranted in some patients, depending on condition; » = major clinical significance):

» Hematocrit or hemoglobin and
» Leukocyte count, total and differential and
» Platelet count
(determinations recommended prior to initiation of therapy and at frequent intervals during therapy; topotecan therapy should not be initiated if baseline neutrophil and platelet counts are lower than 1500 cells/mm$^3$ and 100,000 cells/mm$^3$, respectively. Also, if severe topotecan-induced anemia, neutropenia, or thrombocytopenia occurs during treatment, subsequent courses of therapy should be delayed until the hemoglobin concentration recovers to 9 grams per deciliter [with transfusion, if necessary], neutrophil counts recover

to > 1000 cells/mm³, and platelet counts recover to > 100,000 cells/mm³. A reduction in dose or administration of a colony stimulating factor [e.g., filgrastim] is recommended for subsequent courses of therapy if severe neutropenia occurs)

## Side/Adverse Effects

The following side/adverse effects have been selected on the basis of their potential clinical significance (possible signs and symptoms in parentheses where appropriate)—not necessarily inclusive:

**Those indicating need for medical attention**
Incidence more frequent
*Anemia* (unusual tiredness or weakness); *dyspnea* (shortness of breath or troubled breathing); *fever*—not necessarily associated with neutropenia; *leukopenia or neutropenia, with or without infection (febrile neutropenia)* (fever or chills; cough or hoarseness; lower back or side pain; painful or difficult urination)—usually asymptomatic; *thrombocytopenia* (unusual bleeding or bruising; black, tarry stools; blood in urine or stools; pinpoint red spots on skin)—usually asymptomatic

Note: *Anemia* may be severe; red blood cell transfusions were required by 56% of patients in clinical trials. The red blood cell nadir occurred at a median of 15 days, and the median duration of grade 3 or 4 anemia was 7 days.

*Neutropenia*, the dose-limiting toxicity associated with topotecan therapy, is dose-related and not cumulative. In clinical trials, neutrophil counts of < 1500 cells per cubic millimeter (cells/mm³) and < 500 cells/mm³ occurred in 98% and 81%, respectively, of the patients, and febrile neutropenia (grade 4 neutropenia with fever and/or infection) occurred in 26%. The neutrophil nadir occurred at a median of 11 days. Severe neutropenia occurred primarily during the first course of therapy (filgrastim was not used until after the first cycle) and lasted for a median of 7 days.

In clinical trials, platelet count nadirs occurred at a median of 15 days, and *thrombocytopenia* lasted for a median of 5 days. Platelet transfusions were required by 13% of patients. There have been rare reports (postmarketing) of severe bleeding associated with topotecan-induced thrombocytopenia.

Incidence rare
*Allergic reactions, including anaphylactoid reactions* (changes in facial skin color; skin rash, hives, and/or itching; fast or irregular breathing; puffiness or swelling of the eyelids or around the eyes; shortness of breath, troubled breathing, tightness in chest, and/or wheezing); *angioedema* (large, hive-like swellings on face, eyelids, mouth, lips, and/or tongue); *and dermatitis, severe* (skin rash and/or itching, severe)

**Those indicating need for medical attention only if they continue or are bothersome**
Incidence more frequent
*Abdominal pain; anorexia* (loss of appetite); *constipation; diarrhea; fatigue; headache; nausea or vomiting; neurological effects, including asthenia* (muscle weakness); *or paresthesia* (burning or tingling in hands or feet); *stomatitis* (sores, ulcers, or white spots on lips or tongue or inside the mouth)

Incidence unknown
*Bruising or redness at place of injection*—if extravasation occurs

**Those not indicating need for medical attention**
Incidence more frequent
*Alopecia* (loss of hair)

## Overdose

For more information on the management of overdose or unintentional ingestion, **contact a Poison Control Center** (see *Poison Control Center Listing*).

**Clinical effects of overdose**
The following effects have been selected on the basis of their potential clinical significance (possible signs and symptoms in parentheses where appropriate)—not necessarily inclusive:

Acute and chronic
*Bone marrow suppression, including anemia* (unusual tiredness or weakness)*; leukopenia or neutropenia, including febrile neutropenia* (fever with or without chills; cough or hoarseness; lower back or side pain; painful or difficult urination)*; and/or thrombocytopenia* (black, tarry stools; blood in urine or stools; pinpoint red spots on skin; unusual bleeding or bruising)

**Treatment of overdose**
It is recommended that the patient be hospitalized for close monitoring of vital functions and treatment of observed effects. Severe bone marrow depression may require transfusion of required blood components. Febrile neutropenia should be treated empirically with broad-spectrum antibiotics, pending bacterial cultures and appropriate diagnostic tests.

## Patient Consultation

As an aid to patient consultation, refer to *Advice for the Patient, Topotecan (Systemic)*.
In providing consultation, consider emphasizing the following selected information (» = major clinical significance):

**Before using this medication**
» Conditions affecting use, especially:
Hypersensitivity to topotecan
Pregnancy—Use is not recommended because of embryotoxic, fetotoxic, and carcinogenic potential; advisability of using contraception; informing physician immediately if pregnancy is suspected
Breast-feeding—Not recommended because of potential serious adverse effects
Other medications, especially other bone marrow depressants and immunosuppressants, and radiation therapy
Other medical problems, especially chickenpox, herpes zoster, pre-existing infection, and renal function impairment

**Proper use of this medication**
Frequency of nausea and vomiting; importance of continuing treatment despite stomach upset
» Proper dosing

**Precautions while using this medication**
» Importance of close monitoring by the physician
» Avoiding immunizations unless approved by physician; other persons in patient's household should avoid immunizations with oral poliovirus vaccine; avoiding other persons who have taken oral poliovirus vaccine or wearing a protective mask that covers nose and mouth

*Caution if bone marrow depression occurs*
» Avoiding exposure to persons with infections, especially during periods of low blood counts; checking with physician immediately if fever with or without chills, cough or hoarseness, lower back or side pain, or painful or difficult urination occurs
» Checking with physician immediately if unusual bleeding or bruising; black, tarry stools; blood in urine or stools; or pinpoint red spots on skin occur
Caution in use of regular toothbrush, dental floss, or toothpick; physician, dentist, or nurse may suggest alternatives; checking with physician before having dental work done
Not touching eyes or inside of nose unless hands washed immediately before
Using caution to avoid accidental cuts when using sharp objects such as safety razor or fingernail or toenail cutters
Avoiding contact sports or other situations where bruising or injury could occur

**Side/adverse effects**
May cause adverse effects such as blood problems; importance of discussing possible effects with physician
Signs of potential side effects, especially anemia, dyspnea, fever, febrile neutropenia, thrombocytopenia, and allergic reactions
Some side effects may be asymptomatic, including anemia, leukopenia or neutropenia, and thrombocytopenia
Physician or nurse can help in dealing with side effects
Possibility of hair loss; regrowth should return after treatment has ended

## General Dosing Information

Topotecan should be administered only under the supervision of a physician experienced in cancer chemotherapy. Adequate facilities and medications for diagnosis and treatment of complications should be readily available.

Topotecan is to be administered only by intravenous infusion.

A reduction in subsequent doses is recommended for patients who develop severe neutropenia (neutrophil count < 500 cells per cubic millimeter) that persists for 7 days or more. Alternatively, a colony stimulating factor (e.g., filgrastim) may be administered during subsequent cycles, starting at least 24 hours after the last dose of topotecan (i.e, on day 6 of the cycle).

Patients who develop leukopenia should be observed carefully for signs and symptoms of infection. Antibiotic support may be required. In neutropenic patients who develop fever, broad-spectrum antibiotic coverage should be initiated empirically, pending bacterial cultures and appropriate diagnostic tests.

Special precautions are recommended for patients who develop thrombocytopenia as a result of topotecan therapy. These may include extreme care in performing invasive procedures; regular inspection of intravenous access sites, skin (including perirectal area), and mucous membrane surfaces for signs of bleeding or bruising; testing urine, emesis, stool, and secretions for occult blood; care in use of regular toothbrushes, dental floss, toothpicks, safety razors, and fingernail and toenail cutters; avoiding constipation; and using caution to prevent falls and other injuries. Such patients should avoid alcohol and aspirin intake because of the risk of gastrointestinal bleeding. Platelet transfusions may be required.

**Safety considerations for handling this medication**
There is limited but increasing evidence and concern that personnel involved in preparation and administration of parenteral antineoplastics may be at some risk because of the potential mutagenicity, teratogenicity, and/or carcinogenicity of these agents, although the actual risk is unknown. USP advisory panels recommend cautious handling both in preparation and disposal of antineoplastic agents. Precautions that have been suggested include:
- Use of a biological containment cabinet during reconstitution and dilution of parenteral medications and wearing of disposable surgical gloves and masks.
- Use of proper technique to prevent contamination of the medication, work area, and operator during transfer between containers (including proper training of personnel in this technique).
- Cautious and proper disposal of needles, syringes, vials, ampuls, and unused medication.

A number of medical centers have developed detailed guidelines for handling of antineoplastic agents.

If topotecan comes into contact with the skin, the skin should be washed immediately and thoroughly with soap and water. If the medication comes into contact with a mucous membrane, the area should be immediately and thoroughly flushed with water.

## Parenteral Dosage Forms

Note: Topotecan for injection contains topotecan hydrochloride. However, dosing and strengths are expressed in terms of topotecan base.

Bracketed information in the *Dosage Forms* section refers to uses that are not included in U.S. product labeling.

### TOPOTECAN FOR INJECTION

**Usual adult dose**
Carcinoma, ovarian
[Carcinoma, lung, non–small cell][1]—
    Intravenous infusion (over thirty minutes), 1.5 mg (base) per square meter of body surface area per day for five consecutive days, repeated every twenty-one days.
[Carcinoma, lung, small cell][1]—
    Intravenous infusion (over thirty minutes), 1.25 to 2 (usually 1.5) mg per square meter of body surface area per day for five consecutive days, repeated every twenty-one days.
[Myelodysplastic syndrome][1]
[Chronic myelomonocytic leukemia][1]—
    Intravenous infusion, 2 mg per square meter of body surface area per day as a twenty-four-hour continuous intravenous infusion for five consecutive days every three to four weeks until remission, then once a month.

Note: For patients with moderate renal function impairment (creatinine clearance 20 to 39 mL per minute), a reduction in dose to 0.75 mg (base) per square meter of body surface area is recommended. Adjustment of topotecan dosage is generally not required for patients with mild renal function impairment (creatinine clearance 40 to 60 mL per minute) or patients with hepatic function impairment (serum bilirubin concentration between 1.5 and 10 mg per deciliter).

If severe neutropenia occurs and persists for more than seven days, dosage for subsequent cycles should be reduced by 0.25 mg (base) per square meter of body surface area or therapy with a colony stimulating factor initiated no sooner than twenty-four hours after the last dose of topotecan.

Topotecan treatment should be continued for a minimum of four cycles. In clinical studies, the median time to response was nine to twelve weeks. Responses may be missed if therapy is discontinued prematurely.

**Usual pediatric dose**
Safety and efficacy have not been established.

**Usual geriatric dose**
See *Usual adult dose*.

**Size(s) usually available**
U.S.—
    4 mg (base) (Rx) [*Hycamtin* (mannitol 48 mg; tartaric acid 20 mg; hydrochloric acid and/or sodium hydroxide if needed to adjust pH)].
Canada—
    4 mg (base) (Rx) [*Hycamtin* (mannitol 48 mg; tartaric acid 20 mg; hydrochloric acid and/or sodium hydroxide if needed to adjust pH)].

**Packaging and storage**
Store between 20 and 25 °C (68 and 77 °F), protected from light, unless otherwise specified by manufacturer.

**Preparation of dosage form**
Topotecan for injection is reconstituted for intravenous use by adding 4 mL of sterile water for injection to the vial. The resulting yellow to yellow-green solution will contain 1 mg per mL. An appropriate volume of the injection should be further diluted with 5% dextrose injection or 0.9% sodium chloride injection. Final concentrations and volumes of 20 to 200 mcg per mL in 50 to 100 mL of diluent have been recommended.

**Stability**
Although topotecan for injection is stable after reconstitution, it contains no antimicrobial agent and preferably should be used immediately. However, the reconstituted injection may be stored in a refrigerator for up to 24 hours, if necessary. After further dilution for intravenous infusion, the product is stable for up to 24 hours when stored between 20 and 25 °C (68 and 77 °F).

[1]Not included in Canadian product labeling.

## Selected Bibliography

ten Bokkel Huinink W, Carmichael J, Armstrong D, Gordon A, Malfetano J. Efficacy and safety of topotecan in the treatment of advanced ovarian carcinoma. Semin Oncol 1997; 24(Suppl 5): S5-19-S5-25.

ten Bokkel Huinink W, Gore M, Carmichael J, et al. Topotecan versus paclitaxel for the treatment of recurrent epithelial ovarian cancer. J Clin Oncol 1997; 15: 2183-93.

Developed: 09/17/97
Revised: 07/02/98

# TOREMIFENE   Systemic—INTRODUCTORY VERSION

VA CLASSIFICATION (Primary): AN500
Commonly used brand name(s): *Fareston*.
Note: For a listing of dosage forms and brand names by country availability, see *Dosage Forms* section(s).

## Category
Antineoplastic.

## Indications

**Accepted**
Carcinoma, breast (treatment)—Toremifene is indicated for treatment of metastatic breast cancer in postmenopausal women with estrogen-receptor–positive or unknown tumors.

## Pharmacology/Pharmacokinetics

**Physicochemical characteristics**
Chemical group—Nonsteroidal triphenylethylene derivative.
Molecular weight—Toremifene citrate: 598.1.
pKa—8.
Solubility—Water solubility at 37 °C is 0.63 mg per mL (mg/mL) and solubility in hydrochloric acid at 37 °C is 0.38 mg/mL.

**Mechanism of action/Effect**
Toremifene binds to estrogen receptors. Its effects are mainly antiestrogenic (as indicated by a decrease in the estradiol-induced vaginal cornification index in some postmenopausal women), but it also has some estrogenic effects (as indicated by a decrease in serum gonadotropin [follicle-stimulating hormone (FSH) and luteinizing hormone (LH)] concentrations). The antitumor effect in breast cancer is thought to be related primarily to its antiestrogenic effects (i.e., competition with estrogen for binding sites in the cancer), thereby blocking the growth-stimulating effects of estrogen in the tumor.

**Absorption**
Well absorbed; not affected by food.

**Distribution**
Apparent volume of distribution is 580 liters.

**Protein binding**
Very high (more than 99.5%), mainly to albumin.

**Biotransformation**
Hepatic, extensive, mainly by cytochrome CYP3A4 to *N*-demethyltoremifene, which has antiestrogenic effects but weak *in vivo* antitumor activity.

**Half-life**
Distribution—
  Mean, about 4 hours.
Elimination—
  Toremifene: About 5 days.
  *N*-demethyltoremifene: 6 days.
  Deaminohydroxy toremifene: 4 days.
Note: Enterohepatic recirculation contributes to the slow elimination of toremifene.
Note: Mean total clearance of toremifene is approximately 5 liters per hour.

**Time to peak concentration**
Plasma—Within 3 hours.
Note: Time to steady-state concentrations is about 4 to 6 weeks. Serum concentrations of *N*-demethyltoremifene, the main metabolite, are two to four times higher than those of toremifene at steady state.
  Pharmacokinetics are linear after single oral doses of 10 to 680 mg; with multiple doses, dose proportionality occurs for doses of 10 to 400 mg.

**Elimination**
Fecal, as metabolites.
Renal, about 10% within 1 week.

## Precautions to Consider

**Carcinogenicity**
Studies in rats at doses of 0.12 to 12 mg per kg of body weight per day (mg/kg per day) (about .01 to 1.5 times the daily maximum recommended human dose [MRHD] on a mg per square meter of body surface area [mg/m²] basis) for up to 2 years did not find evidence of carcinogenicity. Studies in mice given doses of 1 to 30 mg/kg per day (about .07 to 2 times the daily MRHD on a mg/m² basis) for up to 2 years showed increased incidence of ovarian and testicular tumors, and an increased incidence of osteoma and osteosarcoma; the significance is uncertain because toremifene is predominantly estrogenic, rather than antiestrogenic, in mice.
Some patients treated with toremifene have developed endometrial cancer, but because of other factors present (short duration of treatment, prior antiestrogen therapy, premalignant conditions) a direct causal relationship has not been established.

**Mutagenicity**
Toremifene has not been found to be mutagenic in *in vitro* tests (Ames and *Escherichia coli* bacterial tests). It is clastogenic *in vitro* (chromosomal aberrations and micronuclei formation in human lymphoblastoid MCL-5 cells) and *in vivo* (chromosomal aberrations in rat hepatocytes). Use of ³²P post-labeling in liver DNA from rats given toremifene produced no detectable adduct formation compared with tamoxifen at similar doses. In addition, in a study in cultured human lymphocytes, adducting activity of toremifene (detected using ³²P post-labeling) was approximately one sixth that of tamoxifen at approximately equipotent concentrations. In a study in salmon sperm, adducting activity of toremifene (detected using ³²P post-labeling) was one sixth and one fourth that observed with tamoxifen at equivalent concentrations following activation by rat and human microsomal systems, respectively. However, toremifene exposure is fourfold that of tamoxifen based on human area under the plasma concentration–time curve (AUC) in serum at recommended clinical doses.

**Pregnancy/Reproduction**
Fertility—Studies in male and female rats at doses of 25 and 0.14 mg per kg of body weight per day (mg/kg per day) (about 3.5 times and .02 the daily MRHD on a mg/m² basis) or higher, respectively, found impairment of fertility and conception. At these doses, atrophy of seminal vesicles and prostate were seen in males and sperm counts, fertility indices, and conception rates were reduced. In females, fertility and reproductive indices were reduced markedly with increased pre- and postimplantation loss. Reproductive indices were also depressed in offspring of treated rats. Studies in dogs showed that doses of 3 mg/kg per day (about 1.5 times the daily MRHD on a mg/m² basis) or higher for 16 weeks produced ovarian atrophy. Studies in monkeys for 52 weeks at doses of 1 mg/kg per day (about one fourth of the daily MRHD on a mg/m² basis) or higher found cystic ovaries and reduction in endometrial stromal cellularity.

Pregnancy—Studies in humans have not been done.
Studies in rats at doses of 1 mg/kg per day (about one fourth of the daily MRHD on a mg/m² basis) or higher given during the period of organogenesis found toremifene to be embryotoxic and fetotoxic, as indicated by intrauterine mortality, increased resorption, reduced fetal weight, and fetal anomalies (including malformation of limbs, incomplete ossification, misshapen bones, ribs/spine anomalies, hydroureter, hydronephrosis, testicular displacement, and subcutaneous edema). Fetal anomalies may be the result of maternal toxicity. Toremifene crosses the placenta and accumulates in the rodent fetus.
In rodent models of fetal reproductive tract development, toremifene inhibits uterine development in female pups in a manner similar to that of diethylstilbestrol and tamoxifen, although the clinical relevance of these effects is unknown.
Studies in rabbits at doses of 1.25 mg/kg per day and 2.5 mg/kg per day (about one third and two thirds of the daily MRHD on a mg/m² basis) found embryotoxicity and fetotoxicity, respectively. Fetal anomalies included incomplete ossification and anencephaly.
Women who are or may become pregnant should be advised of the potential risks to the fetus or the risk for loss of the pregnancy.
FDA Pregnancy Category D.

**Breast-feeding**
It is not known whether toremifene is distributed into breast milk. However, it is distributed into the milk of lactating rats.

**Geriatrics**
The median ages in controlled clinical trials of toremifene ranged from 60 to 66 years; no age-related differences in efficacy or safety were noted.

**Drug interactions and/or related problems**
The following drug interactions and/or related problems have been selected on the basis of their potential clinical significance (possible mechanism in parentheses where appropriate)—not necessarily inclusive (» = major clinical significance):

Note: Combinations containing any of the following medications, depending on the amount present, may also interact with this medication.

» Anticoagulants, coumarin-derivative
    (concurrent use may result in an increased prothrombin time)
» Cytochrome P450 3A4 enzyme inducers, such as:
    Carbamazepine
    Phenobarbital
    Phenytoin
    (may increase the rate of metabolism of toremifene, leading to lower steady-state serum concentrations)
  Cytochrome P450 CYP3A4-6 inhibitors, such as:
    Erythromycin and similar macrolides
    Ketoconazole and similar antimycotics
    (theoretically may inhibit metabolism of toremifene; this interaction has not been studied)
  Medications that decrease renal excretion of calcium, such as
    Diuretics, thiazide
    (risk of hypercalcemia may be increased)

**Laboratory value alterations**
The following have been selected on the basis of their potential clinical significance (possible effect in parentheses where appropriate)—not necessarily inclusive (» = major clinical significance):

With physiology/laboratory test values
  Alkaline phosphatase values, serum, and
  Aspartate aminotransferase (AST [SGOT]) values, serum, and
  Bilirubin concentrations, serum
    (may be increased; dose-related)
  Calcium
    (serum concentrations may be increased infrequently, usually in patients with bone metastases)

**Medical considerations/Contraindications**
The medical considerations/contraindications included have been selected on the basis of their potential clinical significance (reasons given in parentheses where appropriate)—not necessarily inclusive (» = major clinical significance).

*Except under special circumstances, this medication should not be used when the following medical problem exists:*
» Thromboembolic disease, history of
    (use of toremifene is generally not recommended)

***Risk-benefit should be considered when the following medical problems exist:***

    Bone metastases
        (close monitoring for hypercalcemia is recommended during the first weeks of toremifene therapy)

» Endometrial hyperplasia, pre-existing
        (long-term use is not recommended)

    Leukopenia or
    Thrombocytopenia
        (since leukopenia and thrombocytopenia have been reported rarely during treatment with toremifene, monitoring of leukocyte and platelet counts is recommended)

    Sensitivity to toremifene

**Patient monitoring**

The following may be especially important in patient monitoring (other tests may be warranted in some patients, depending on condition; » = major clinical significance):

» Calcium concentrations, serum
        (recommended at periodic intervals during treatment)

    Complete blood count
        (recommended at periodic intervals during treatment)

    Hepatic function tests
        (recommended at periodic intervals during treatment)

## Side/Adverse Effects

Note: Side/adverse effects are mostly related to the antiestrogenic hormonal effects of toremifene and usually occur at the beginning of treatment.

    Some patients have developed endometrial cancer, but because of other factors present (short duration of treatment, prior antiestrogen therapy, premalignant conditions) a direct causal relationship with toremifene therapy has not been established.

    Leukopenia and thrombocytopenia have been reported but have not been attributed definitely to toremifene.

The following side/adverse effects have been selected on the basis of their potential clinical significance (possible signs and symptoms in parentheses where appropriate)—not necessarily inclusive:

**Those indicating need for medical attention**
Incidence more frequent
    *Hepatotoxicity*—usually asymptomatic
    Note: *Hepatotoxicity* usually consists of elevated hepatic enzyme and bilirubin levels. However, jaundice has been seen rarely.

Incidence less frequent
    *Endometrial hyperplasia* (change in vaginal discharge; pain or feeling of pressure in pelvis; vaginal bleeding); *hypercalcemia* (confusion; increased urination; loss of appetite; unusual tiredness); *ocular toxicity, including abnormal visual fields, cataracts, corneal keratopathy, glaucoma* (blurred vision; changes in vision)—may be asymptomatic initially
    Note: *Endometrial hyperplasia* of the uterus has also been seen in monkeys following doses of 1 mg per kg of body weight (mg/kg) (about one fourth of the daily maximum recommended human dose [MRHD] on a mg per square meter of body surface area [mg/m²] basis) or higher for 52 weeks, and in dogs following doses of 3 mg/kg (about 1.4 times the daily MRHD on a mg/m² basis) or higher for 16 weeks.
    *Hypercalcemia* may occur in some patients, usually those with bone metastases, during the first weeks of treatment.

Incidence rare
    *Cardiac failure* (swelling of feet or lower legs); *myocardial infarction* (chest pain); *pulmonary embolus* (shortness of breath); *thrombophlebitis or thrombosis* (pain or swelling in legs)

**Those indicating need for medical attention only if they continue or are bothersome**
Incidence more frequent
    *Hot flashes* (sudden sweating and feelings of warmth); *nausea*
    Note: *Nausea* is dose-related.

Incidence less frequent
    *Dizziness; dry eyes; tumor flare* (bone pain); *vomiting*
    Note: "Tumor flare," a transient increase in bone or tumor pain (characterized by diffuse musculoskeletal pain and erythema with increased size of tumor lesions) may occur during the first few weeks after initiation of therapy. It is often accompanied by hypercalcemia. This temporary "tumor flare" subsequently regresses and does not imply treatment failure or tumor progression.

## Overdose

For more information on the management of overdose or unintentional ingestion, **contact a Poison Control Center** (see *Poison Control Center Listing*).

**Clinical effects of overdose**
The following effects have been selected on the basis of their potential clinical significance (possible signs and symptoms in parentheses where appropriate)—not necessarily inclusive:

Acute and/or chronic
    *Dizziness; headache; nausea and/or vomiting*
    Note: The symptoms listed above have been reported with administration of a daily dose of 680 mg for 5 days; they appeared in two of five healthy subjects during the third day of treatment and disappeared within 2 days after withdrawal of the medication. In a study in postmenopausal breast cancer patients, a dose of 400 mg per square meter of body surface area per day caused similar symptoms, as well as reversible hallucinations and ataxia in one patient.
    Theoretical symptoms of toremifene overdose include antiestrogenic effects such as hot flashes, estrogenic effects such as vaginal bleeding, or nervous system disorders such as vertigo, dizziness, ataxia, or nausea.

**Treatment of overdose**
Treatment is symptomatic.
There is no specific antidote.

## Patient Consultation

As an aid to patient consultation, refer to *Advice for the Patient, Toremifene (Systemic)—Introductory Version*.

In providing consultation, consider emphasizing the following selected information (» = major clinical significance):

**Before using this medication**
» Conditions affecting use, especially:
    Sensitivity to toremifene
    Pregnancy—Risk of miscarriage, death of the fetus, and birth defects; telling physician immediately if pregnancy is suspected
    Other medications, especially anticoagulants (coumarin-derivative), carbamazepine, phenobarbital, or phenytoin
    Other medical problems, especially endometrial hyperplasia or history of thromboembolic disease

**Proper use of this medication**
» Proper dosing
» Proper storage

**Side/adverse effects**
    Possible increased risk of endometrial carcinoma
    Signs of potential side effects, especially endometrial hyperplasia, hypercalcemia, ocular toxicity, cardiac failure, myocardial infarction, pulmonary embolus, and thrombophlebitis or thrombosis
    Asymptomatic side effects including hepatotoxicity and ocular toxicity

## General Dosing Information

If hypercalcemia occurs, appropriate measures should be taken. If it is severe, toremifene should be discontinued.

## Oral Dosage Forms

**TOREMIFENE CITRATE TABLETS**

Note: The dosing and strengths available are expressed in terms of toremifene base (not the salt).

**Usual adult dose**
Breast carcinoma—
    Oral, 60 mg (base) once a day.

**Usual geriatric dose**
See *Usual adult dose*.

**Strength(s) usually available**
U.S.—
    60 mg (base) (Rx) [*Fareston* (lactose)].

**Packaging and storage**
Store at 25 °C (77 °F). Protect from light.

Developed: 03/23/98

# TORSEMIDE Systemic†

INN: Torasemide
BAN: Torasemide
VA CLASSIFICATION (Primary/Secondary): CV702/CV409
Commonly used brand name(s): *Demadex*.
Note: For a listing of dosage forms and brand names by country availability, see *Dosage Forms* section(s).

†Not commercially available in Canada.

## Category
Diuretic; antihypertensive.

## Indications

**Accepted**

Edema (treatment)—Torsemide is indicated in treatment of edema associated with congestive heart failure, renal disease, and hepatic disease (cirrhosis).

Hypertension (treatment)—Torsemide is indicated, alone or in combination with other antihypertensive agents, in the treatment of hypertension.

## Pharmacology/Pharmacokinetics

**Physicochemical characteristics**
Molecular weight—348.43.
pKa—7.1.

**Mechanism of action/Effect**

Diuretic—Torsemide is a loop diuretic. It inhibits reabsorption of sodium and chloride in the luminal membrane of the ascending limb of the loop of Henle by interfering with the chloride binding site of the $1Na+$, $1K+$, $2Cl-$ cotransport system. This increases the rate of delivery of tubular fluid and electrolytes to the distal sites of hydrogen and potassium ion secretion, while plasma volume contraction increases aldosterone production. The increased delivery and high aldosterone levels promote sodium reabsorption at the distal tubules, thus increasing the loss of potassium and hydrogen ions. Torsemide's effects in other portions of the nephron have not been demonstrated.

Antihypertensive—Diuretics lower blood pressure initially by reducing plasma and extracellular fluid volume; cardiac output also decreases. Eventually, cardiac output returns to normal with an accompanying decrease in peripheral resistance.

**Absorption**
Rapidly absorbed following oral administration; not affected by food. Bioavailability is approximately 80%.

**Distribution**
Volume of distribution ($Vol_D$)—0.14 to 0.19 L per kg.

**Protein binding**
Very high (97 to greater than 99%).

**Biotransformation**
Metabolized via the hepatic cytochrome P-450 system to 5 metabolites. The major metabolite, M5, is pharmacologically inactive. There are 2 minor metabolites, M1, possessing one-tenth the activity of torsemide, and M3, equal in activity to torsemide. Overall, torsemide appears to account for 80% of the total diuretic activity, while metabolites M1 and M3 account for 9% and 11%, respectively.

**Half-life**
Elimination—2.2 to 3.8 hours; not affected by moderate renal failure. However, metabolite M1 may accumulate in renal failure.

**Onset of action**
Diuretic:
  Oral: Within 1 hour.
  Intravenous: Within 10 minutes.

**Time to peak concentration**
Oral—1 to 2 hours.

**Time to peak effect**
Diuretic—
  Oral: 1 to 2 hours.
  Intravenous: Within 1 hour.

**Duration of action**
Diuretic—6 to 8 hours.

**Elimination**
Renal; 24% as parent compound.
In dialysis—Torsemide is not significantly removed by hemodialysis.

## Precautions to Consider

**Cross-sensitivity and/or related problems**
Patients sensitive to bumetanide, furosemide, or sulfonamides (including thiazide diuretics) may be sensitive to torsemide also.

**Carcinogenicity/Tumorigenicity**
Lifetime administration of torsemide to rats and mice at doses up to 9 and 32 mg per kg of body weight (mg/kg) per day, respectively, did not increase overall tumor incidence. These doses are equivalent to 27 and 96 times, respectively, a human dose of 20 mg on a body weight basis. However, renal tubular injury, interstitial inflammation, and a statistically significant increase in renal adenomas and carcinomas were observed in the high-dose female group of rats.

**Mutagenicity**
No mutagenic activity was seen in a variety of *in vitro* and *in vivo* tests.

**Pregnancy/Reproduction**

Fertility—No adverse effect on fertility was seen in male or female rats given doses up to 25 mg/kg per day (equivalent to 75 times a human dose of 20 mg on a body weight basis).

Pregnancy—Adequate and well-controlled studies have not been done in humans. Routine use of diuretics during normal pregnancy is not recommended because use may expose the mother and fetus to unnecessary hazard. However, diuretics may be continued during pregnancy if they were used to treat hypertension that existed prior to gestation. Diuretics do not prevent development of toxemia of pregnancy, and there is no satisfactory evidence that they are useful in the treatment of toxemia. Diuretics are indicated only in the treatment of edema due to pathologic causes or as a short course of treatment in patients with severe hypervolemia.

No fetotoxicity or teratogenicity was observed in rats and rabbits given doses up to 15 and 5 times, respectively, a human dose of 20 mg on a mg/kg basis. However, administration of doses 4 and 5 times larger in rats and rabbits, respectively, resulted in decreased average body weight, increased fetal resorption, and delayed fetal ossification.

FDA Pregnancy Category B.

**Breast-feeding**
It is not known whether torsemide is distributed into breast milk.

**Pediatrics**
No information is available on the relationship of age to the effects of torsemide in pediatric patients. Safety and efficacy have not been established.

**Geriatrics**
Studies that included patients over 65 years of age have not demonstrated geriatrics-specific problems that would limit the usefulness of torsemide in the elderly.

**Drug interactions and/or related problems**
The following drug interactions and/or related problems have been selected on the basis of their potential clinical significance (possible mechanism in parentheses where appropriate)—not necessarily inclusive (» = major clinical significance):

Note: Combinations containing any of the following medications, depending on the amount present, may also interact with this medication.

Alcohol or
Hypotension-producing medications, other (see *Appendix II* )
  (hypotensive and/or diuretic effects may be potentiated when these medications are used concurrently with torsemide; although some antihypertensive and/or diuretic combinations are frequently used for therapeutic advantage, dosage adjustments may be necessary during concurrent use)

» Amphotericin B, parenteral
  (concurrent and/or sequential administration with torsemide should be avoided since the potential for nephrotoxicity may be increased, especially in the presence of renal function impairment; in addition, concurrent use with torsemide may intensify electrolyte imbalance, particularly hypokalemia; frequent electrolyte determinations are recommended and potassium supplementation may be required)

Angiotensin-converting enzyme (ACE) inhibitors
  (sudden and severe hypotension may occur within the first 1 to 5 hours after the initial dose of an ACE inhibitor, particularly in patients who are sodium- and volume-depleted as a result of diuretic therapy. Withdrawal of the diuretic or increase of salt intake approximately 1 week before start of captopril therapy or 2 to 3 days before start of benazepril, enalapril, fosinopril, lisinopril, quinapril,

or ramipril therapy, or initiation of ACE inhibitor therapy at lower doses, will minimize the reaction; this reaction does not usually recur with subsequent doses, although caution in increasing doses is recommended; diuretics may be reinstituted as necessary)

(risk of renal failure may be increased in patients who are sodium- and volume-depleted as a result of diuretic therapy)

(ACE inhibitors may reduce the secondary aldosteronism and hypokalemia caused by diuretics)

Antiarrhythmic agents
(concurrent use with torsemide may lead to an increased risk of arrhythmias associated with hypokalemia)

» Anticoagulants, coumarin- or indandione-derivative, or
Heparin or
Streptokinase or
Urokinase
(anticoagulant effects may be decreased when these medications are used concurrently with torsemide, as a result of reduction of plasma volume leading to concentration of procoagulant factors in the blood; in addition, diuretic-induced improvement of hepatic congestion may lead to improved hepatic function, resulting in increased procoagulant factor synthesis; dosage adjustments may be necessary)

Antidiabetic agents, oral, or
Insulin
(torsemide may rarely raise blood glucose concentrations or interfere with the hypoglycemic effects of these agents; for non–insulin-dependent diabetics, dosage adjustment of hypoglycemic medications may be necessary)

Anti-inflammatory drugs, nonsteroidal (NSAIDs), especially indomethacin
(indomethacin, and possibly other NSAIDs, may reduce the natriuretic action of torsemide; NSAIDs may also reduce the antihypertensive effect or the increase in urine volume caused by torsemide, possibly by inhibiting renal prostaglandin synthesis and/or by causing sodium and fluid retention)

(in addition, concurrent use of NSAIDs with a diuretic may increase the risk of renal failure secondary to a decrease in renal blood flow caused by inhibition of renal prostaglandin synthesis)

Digitalis glycosides
(concurrent use with torsemide may enhance the possibility of digitalis toxicity associated with hypokalemia and hypomagnesemia)

» Hypokalemia-causing medications, other (see *Appendix II*)
(risk of severe hypokalemia due to other hypokalemia-causing medications may be increased; monitoring of serum potassium concentrations and cardiac function and potassium supplementation may be required)

» Lithium
(concurrent use with torsemide may promote lithium toxicity because of reduced renal clearance; concurrent use is not recommended unless patient can be closely monitored)

» Nephrotoxic medications, other, (see *Appendix II*) or
Ototoxic medications, other (see *Appendix II*)
(concurrent and/or sequential administration with torsemide is not recommended since the potential for ototoxicity and nephrotoxicity may be increased, especially in the presence of renal function impairment)

Neuromuscular blocking agents, nondepolarizing
(torsemide may induce hypokalemia, which may enhance the blockade of nondepolarizing neuromuscular blocking agents; serum potassium determinations may be necessary prior to administration of nondepolarizing neuromuscular blocking agents; careful postoperative monitoring of the patient may be necessary following concurrent or sequential use, especially if there is a possibility of incomplete reversal of neuromuscular blockade)

Probenecid
(concurrent use with torsemide may decrease the diuretic activity of torsemide because probenecid reduces secretion of torsemide into the proximal tubule)

» Salicylates, high-dose
(concurrent use with torsemide may increase the risk of salicylate toxicity because torsemide and salicylates compete for secretion by the renal tubules)

Sympathomimetics
(concurrent use may reduce the antihypertensive effects of torsemide; the patient should be carefully monitored to confirm that the desired effect is being obtained)

**Laboratory value alterations**
The following have been selected on the basis of their potential clinical significance (possible effect in parentheses where appropriate)—not necessarily inclusive (» = major clinical significance):

With physiology/laboratory test values
Blood urea nitrogen (BUN) and
Uric acid, serum
(concentrations may be increased)
Calcium and
Magnesium and
Potassium
(serum concentrations may be decreased)
Glucose
(blood glucose concentrations may be increased; hyperglycemia has been reported rarely)

**Medical considerations/Contraindications**
The medical considerations/contraindications included have been selected on the basis of their potential clinical significance (reasons given in parentheses where appropriate)—not necessarily inclusive (» = major clinical significance).

*Risk-benefit should be considered when the following medical problems exist:*

» Anuria
(may impair effectiveness of torsemide; possible reduced clearance may increase risk of ototoxicity)
Diabetes mellitus
(torsemide may increase serum glucose concentrations)
Gout, history of or
Hyperuricemia
(torsemide may increase serum uric acid concentrations)
Hearing function impairment
(condition may be exacerbated if ototoxic effects occur)
Hepatic function impairment with cirrhosis and ascites
(sudden alterations in fluid and electrolyte balance may precipitate hepatic coma; hospitalization during initiation of torsemide therapy is recommended)
Myocardial infarction, acute
(excessive diuresis should be avoided because of the danger of precipitating shock)
Sensitivity to torsemide, other loop diuretics, or sulfonylureas
Caution is recommended in patients who are at increased risk if hypokalemia occurs, including those taking concurrent digitalis and those with cardiovascular disease, because of the risk of arrhythmias.

**Patient monitoring**
The following may be especially important in patient monitoring (other tests may be warranted in some patients, depending on condition; » = major clinical significance):

Blood pressure measurements
(recommended at periodic intervals in patients being treated for hypertension; selected patients may be taught to monitor their blood pressure at home and report the results at regular physician visits)
Blood urea nitrogen (BUN) and
Glucose, serum and
Hepatic function and
Renal function and
Uric acid, serum
(determinations recommended at periodic intervals)
» Electrolytes, serum, especially potassium
(determinations recommended at periodic intervals)
Hearing examinations
(recommended at periodic intervals in patients receiving prolonged high-dose intravenous therapy)

*For use as a diuretic (in addition to the above)*
Weight measurements
(recommended prior to initiation of therapy and at periodic intervals during therapy to monitor fluid loss)

## Side/Adverse Effects

The following side/adverse effects have been selected on the basis of their potential clinical significance (possible signs and symptoms in parentheses where appropriate)—not necessarily inclusive:

## Those indicating need for medical attention
Incidence less frequent
> *Electrolyte imbalance such as hyponatremia, hypochloremic alkalosis, and hypokalemia* (dryness of mouth; fast or irregular heartbeat; increased thirst; mood or mental changes; muscle pain or cramps; nausea or vomiting; unusual tiredness or weakness)

Incidence rare
> *Allergic reaction* (skin rash); *gastrointestinal hemorrhage* (black, tarry stools); *hypotension, orthostatic* (dizziness when getting up from a sitting or lying position); *ototoxicity* (ringing or buzzing in the ears or any loss of hearing)
>
> Note: *Ototoxicity* may be more likely to occur with rapid intravenous administration or with use of very high doses.

## Those indicating need for medical attention only if they continue or are bothersome
Incidence more frequent
> *Constipation; dizziness; gastrointestinal disturbance* (stomach upset); *headache*

## Overdose
For more information on the management of overdose or unintentional ingestion, **contact a Poison Control Center** (see *Poison Control Center Listing*).

**Treatment of overdose**
Fluid and electrolyte replacement.
Symptomatic and supportive care.

## Patient Consultation
As an aid to patient consultation, refer to *Advice for the Patient, Torsemide (Systemic)*.
In providing consultation, consider emphasizing the following selected information (» = major clinical significance):

**Before using this medication**
» Conditions affecting use, especially:
  Sensitivity to loop diuretics or sulfonamides
  Pregnancy—Not recommended for routine use
  Other medications, especially amphotericin B, anticoagulants, hypokalemia-causing medications, lithium, other nephrotoxic medications, or high-dose salicylates
  Other medical problems, especially anuria

**Proper use of this medication**
Diuretic effects of the medication and timing of doses to minimize inconvenience of diuresis
Compliance with therapy; taking medication at the same time(s) each day to maintain the therapeutic effect
» Proper dosing
Missed dose: Taking as soon as possible; not taking if almost time for next dose; not doubling doses
» Proper storage

*For use as an antihypertensive*
Possible need for control of weight and diet, especially sodium intake
» Patient may not experience symptoms of hypertension; importance of taking medication even if feeling well
» Does not cure, but controls hypertension; possible need for lifelong therapy; serious consequences of untreated hypertension

**Precautions while using this medication**
Making regular visits to physician to check progress
» Possibility of hypokalemia; possible need for additional potassium in diet; not changing diet without first checking with physician
To prevent dehydration, notifying physician if severe nausea, vomiting, or diarrhea occurs and continues
Caution if any kind of surgery (including dental surgery) is required
» Caution when getting up suddenly from a lying or sitting position
» Caution in using alcohol, while standing for long periods or exercising, and during hot weather because of enhanced orthostatic hypotensive effects
Diabetics: May increase blood sugar levels

*For use as an antihypertensive*
» Not taking other medications, especially nonprescription sympathomimetics, unless discussed with physician

**Side/adverse effects**
Signs of potential side effects, especially electrolyte imbalance, allergic reaction, gastrointestinal hemorrhage, orthostatic hypotension, and ototoxicity

## General Dosing Information
Dosage must be adjusted to meet the individual requirements of each patient, on the basis of clinical response. The lowest effective dosage should be utilized to minimize potential fluid and electrolyte imbalance.

Concurrent administration of potassium supplements or potassium-sparing diuretics may be indicated in patients considered to be at higher risk for developing hypokalemia.

When torsemide is added to an antihypertensive regimen, the dose of other antihypertensive agents may have to be reduced to prevent an excessive drop in blood pressure.

**For parenteral dosage forms only**
Intravenous injections should be administered slowly, over a period of 2 minutes.

**Diet/Nutrition**
Torsemide may be taken at any time in relation to a meal.

**Bioequivalenence information**
Because of the high bioavailability of torsemide tablets, oral and intravenous doses of torsemide are equivalent.

## Oral Dosage Forms
### TORSEMIDE TABLETS
**Usual adult dose**
Diuretic—
  Congestive heart failure—
    Oral, 10 or 20 mg once a day, the dosage being increased as needed, up to 200 mg, for desired therapeutic effect.
  Hepatic cirrhosis—
    Oral, 5 or 10 mg once a day, administered with an aldosterone antagonist or a potassium-sparing diuretic.
  Renal failure, chronic—
    Oral, 20 mg once a day, the dosage being increased by doubling as needed until adequate diuretic response is achieved.
  Antihypertensive—
    Oral, 5 mg once a day for four to six weeks, the dosage being increased thereafter to 10 mg once a day if blood pressure response is not adequate.

**Usual adult prescribing limits**
Congestive heart failure—Single dose: 200 mg.
Hepatic cirrhosis—Single dose: 40 mg.
Renal failure, chronic—Single dose: 200 mg.

**Usual pediatric dose**
Safety and efficacy have not been established.

**Usual geriatric dose**
See *Usual adult dose*.

**Strength(s) usually available**
U.S.—
  5 mg (Rx) [*Demadex*].
  10 mg (Rx) [*Demadex*].
  20 mg (Rx) [*Demadex*].
  100 mg (Rx) [*Demadex*].
Canada—
  Not commercially available.

**Packaging and storage**
Store below 40 °C (104 °F), preferably between 15 and 30 °C (59 and 86 °F). Protect from freezing.

**Auxiliary labeling**
• Do not take other medicines without your doctor's advice.

## Parenteral Dosage Forms
### TORSEMIDE INJECTION
**Usual adult dose**
Diuretic—
  Congestive heart failure—
    Intravenous, 10 or 20 mg once a day, the dosage being increased as needed, up to 200 mg, for desired therapeutic effect.
  Hepatic cirrhosis—
    Intravenous, 5 or 10 mg once a day, administered with an aldosterone antagonist or a potassium-sparing diuretic.
  Renal failure, chronic—
    Intravenous, 20 mg once a day, the dosage being increased by doubling as needed until adequate diuretic response is achieved.

**Usual adult prescribing limits**
See *Torsemide Tablets*.

*USP DI*

**Usual pediatric dose**
Safety and efficacy have not been established.

**Usual geriatric dose**
See *Usual adult dose*.

**Strength(s) usually available**
U.S.—
  10 mg per mL (Rx) [*Demadex*].
Canada—
  Not commercially available.

**Packaging and storage**
Store below 40 °C (104 °F), preferably between 15 and 30 °C (59 and 86 °F). Protect from freezing.

**Stability**
Do not use if solution is discolored.

## Selected Bibliography
Friedel HA, Buckley MM. Torasemide. A review of its pharmacological properties and therapeutic potential. Drugs 1991; 41(1): 81-103.
The fifth report of the Joint National Committee on Detection, Evaluation, and Treatment of High Blood Pressure (JNC V). Arch Intern Med 1993; 153(2): 154-83.

Developed: 02/15/95
Interim revision: 08/01/95; 08/19/98

# TRAMADOL  Systemic†

VA CLASSIFICATION (Primary): CN103
Commonly used brand name(s): *Ultram*.
Note: For a listing of dosage forms and brand names by country availability, see *Dosage Forms* section(s).

†Not commercially available in Canada.

## Category
Analgesic.

## Indications

**Accepted**
Pain (treatment)—Tramadol is indicated for the management of moderate to moderately severe pain. It has been used to treat pain following orthopedic and gynecological procedures, including cesarean section.

**Acceptance not established**
Tramadol has been used for long-term treatment of *chronic pain* such as low back pain, neuropathic pain, orthopedic and joint conditions, and cancer pain. Tramadol may be a therapeutic option for patients who are intolerant to or inappropriate candidates for nonsteroidal anti-inflammatory drugs (NSAIDs); however, more studies evaluating safety and efficacy need to be established for long-term use.

Tramadol has been evaluated and has shown promise as an adjunct to NSAIDs for patients experiencing inadequate relief from *dental pain* with NSAIDs alone. Although tramadol would not be effective in patients needing only anti-inflammatory treatment, it would be effective in enhancing the suppression of pain. A small study found a single dose of tramadol given concomitantly with a single dose of ibuprofen enhanced suppression of dental pain caused by inflammation. However, additional studies need to be done to evaluate the use of tramadol and NSAIDs concomitantly as a therapeutic combination to enhance analgesic efficacy.

## Pharmacology/Pharmacokinetics

**Physicochemical characteristics**
Source—Synthetic.
Molecular weight—299.84.
pKa—9.41.

**Mechanism of action/Effect**
Tramadol is a centrally-acting analgesic that is not chemically related to opiates. The mechanism of action of tramadol is not completely understood, but it may bind to mu-opioid receptors and inhibit the reuptake of norepinephrine (NE) and serotonin (5-HT). The ability of tramadol to inhibit the neuronal uptake of monoamines in the same concentration range at which it binds to mu-opioid receptors differentiates it from typical opioids. Tramadol consists of (+) and (−) enantiomers that appear to interact synergistically to produce antinociception. The (+) enantiomer is five fold more potent in 5-HT uptake and has a greater affinity for mu receptor binding than for NE uptake. The (−) enantiomer is five to ten fold more potent in NE uptake inhibition and has less affinity for mu receptor binding than for 5-HT uptake. Electrophysiological studies show that tramadol, like morphine, depresses motor and sensory responses of the spinal nociceptive system by a spinal and a supraspinal action. Some opioid activity is derived from low affinity binding of the parent compound and higher affinity binding of the mono-*O*-desmethyltramadol (M1) metabolite to the opioid receptors. Although analgesic potency of M1 is about six times greater than that of tramadol in animal models, the relative potency in humans is unknown.

Note: It has been estimated that the analgesic potency of tramadol is one-tenth that of morphine.

**Other actions/effects**
Tramadol suppresses the cough reflex by binding to the mu-opioid receptor binding sites. Due to the high affinity binding of the M1 metabolite to the mu receptor, the metabolite has been found to have more cough suppressant activity than the parent compound.
Unlike morphine, tramadol has not been shown to cause histamine release.

**Absorption**
Oral—Rapid and almost complete. Mean absolute bioavailability of a 100-mg dose is approximately 75%. The rate or extent of absorption is not significantly affected by administration with food.

**Distribution**
The volume of distribution is 2.6 and 2.9 liters per kilogram of body weight (L/kg) in males and females, respectively, following a 100-mg intravenous dose. Tramadol crosses the blood-brain barrier in rats and possibly in humans.

**Protein binding**
Low (20%). Independent of concentration up to 10 micrograms per mL (mcg/mL); saturation of binding occurs only at concentrations outside of the clinically relevant range.

**Biotransformation**
Hepatic. Extensively metabolized via *N*- and *O*-demethylation and glucuronidation or sulfation. The production of the active metabolite mono-*O*-desmethyltramadol (M1) is dependent on the cyp2d6 isoenzyme of cytochrome *P*-450. The inactive metabolites are formed by *N*-demethylation.

**Half-life**
Terminal—
  Individuals with normal renal function:
    Tramadol—Approximately 6.3 hours (increased to 7 hours with multiple dosing [not clinically significant] and in individuals over 75 years of age [clinically significant]).
    M1 metabolite—Approximately 7.4 hours.

**Onset of action**
Dose-dependent; generally within 1 hour.

**Time to peak concentration**
Plasma—
  Following a single 100-mg dose:
    Tramadol—2 hours.
    M1 metabolite—3 hours.

**Time to steady state concentration**
Plasma—
  After administration of 100 mg four times a day:
    About 2 days.

**Peak serum concentration**
Plasma—
  Following a single 100-mg dose:
    Tramadol—308 nanograms per mL ±78 nanograms/mL.
    M1 metabolite—55 nanograms/mL ± 20 nanograms/mL.

**Time to peak effect**
Tramadol—2 hours.
M1 metabolite—3 hours.

**Elimination**
Renal—
  30% unchanged; 60% as metabolites. Clearance rate is slightly higher in females than in males.
In dialysis—
  7% of an administered dose is removed by hemodialysis.

## Precautions to Consider

### Tumorigenicity
Evidence of a statistically significant increase in two common murine tumors (pulmonary and hepatic) was observed in mice receiving oral doses up to 30 mg per kg of body weight (mg/kg) for approximately 2 years.

### Mutagenicity
No evidence of mutagenicity was found in the Ames test, CHO/HPRT mammalian cell assay, mouse lymphoma assay, or dominant lethal mutation test in mice. Weakly mutagenic results occurred in the presence of metabolic activation in the mouse lymphoma assay and micronucleus test in rats.

### Pregnancy/Reproduction
Fertility—No impairment of fertility was observed at oral dose levels up to 50 mg/kg in male rats and 75 mg/kg in female rats.

Pregnancy—Tramadol has been shown to cross the placenta. Well-controlled studies in humans have not been done.

Studies have shown tramadol to be embryotoxic and fetotoxic in mice, rats, and rabbits at maternally toxic doses (3 to 15 times the maximum human dose or higher); however, it was found not to be teratogenic at these levels. Studies done in progeny of mice, rats, and rabbits given tramadol by various routes (up to 140 mg/kg for mice, 80 mg/kg for rats, or 300 mg/kg for rabbits) found no drug-related teratogenic effects. Transient delays in the developmental and behavioral parameters during the delivery of pups from rat dams were observed. At maternally toxic levels, fetal toxicity and embryotoxicity primarily included decreased fetal weights, skeletal ossification, and increased supernumerary ribs. A study in rabbits reported embryo and fetal lethality caused by extreme maternal toxicity at doses of 300 mg/kg. In peri- and postnatal studies in rats, decreased weights were observed in the progeny of dams that received oral (gavage) doses of 50 mg/kg or greater. At doses of 80 mg/kg (6 to 10 times the maximum human dose), pup survival was decreased early in lactation. The progeny of dams receiving 8, 10, 20, 25, or 40 mg/kg showed no signs of toxicity. Evidence of severe maternal toxicity was observed at higher doses; however, maternal toxicity was found at all dose levels.

FDA Pregnancy Category C.

Labor and delivery—Tramadol is not recommended for use in pregnant women prior to or during labor unless the potential benefits outweigh the risks, because safe use in pregnancy has not been established.

### Breast-feeding
Following a single intravenous 100-mg dose of tramadol, the cumulative distribution in breast milk within 16 hours postdose was 100 micrograms (mcg) of tramadol (0.1% of the maternal dose) and 27 mcg of M1. Use of oral tramadol is not recommended for obstetrical preoperative medication or postdelivery analgesia in nursing mothers because of lack of studies on its safety in infants and newborns.

### Pediatrics
No information is available on the relationship of age to the effects of tramadol in patients under 16 years of age. Safety and efficacy have not been established.

### Geriatrics
Studies have shown that, in subjects over the age of 75 years, serum concentrations are slightly elevated and the elimination half-life is slightly prolonged. In addition, elderly patients are more likely to have age-related renal function impairment that may require dosage adjustment.

### Drug interactions and/or related problems
The following drug interactions and/or related problems have been selected on the basis of their potential clinical significance (possible mechanism in parentheses where appropriate)—not necessarily inclusive (» = major clinical significance):

» Alcohol or
» Anesthetic agents or
» Central nervous system (CNS) depression–producing medications, other (See *Appendix II*), such as:
  Antidepressants, tricyclics
  Opioid analgesics
  Phenothiazines
  Sedative hypnotics
  Tranquilizers
  (caution is recommended because concurrent use may potentiate the CNS depressant effects; tricyclic antidepressants, fluoxetine and sertraline may increase the risk of seizures; dosage reduction is recommended)

» Carbamazepine
  (causes a significant increase in tramadol metabolism, presumably through metabolic enzyme induction; dosage adjustment may be required [patients receiving chronic carbamazepine in doses up to 800 mg per day may require up to twice the recommended dose of tramadol])

» Monoamine oxidase (MAO) inhibitors, including furazolidone and procarbazine
  (tramadol inhibits the uptake of norepinephrine and serotonin; serotonin is believed to be the biogenic amine responsible for the toxic interactions; concurrent use may decrease seizure threshold; caution is recommended)

Quinidine
  (concurrent use may increase concentrations of tramadol and decrease concentration of the M1 metabolite by competitively inhibiting the cyp2d6 isoenzyme; inhibition of the formation of the M1 metabolite did not significantly alter the peak analgesic effect of a single 100-mg dose of tramadol in healthy volunteers)

Propafenone
  (concurrent use may increase concentrations of tramadol and decrease concentration of the M1 metabolite by inhibiting the cyp2d6 isoenzyme)

### Medical considerations/Contraindications
The medical considerations/contraindications included have been selected on the basis of their potential clinical significance (reasons given in parentheses where appropriate)—not necessarily inclusive (» = major clinical significance).

Note: Tramadol does not affect the bile duct sphincter, which indicates that it is less likely than opioids to cause urinary retention, constipation, or worsening of pancreatic or biliary disorders.

*Except under special circumstances, this medication should not be used when the following medical problems exist:*

» Acute intoxication with alcohol, hypnotics, centrally-acting analgesics, opioids, or psychotropic drugs
  (risk of respiratory depression)

» Drug abuse or dependence, current or history of, including alcoholism
  (patient predisposition to drug abuse)

*Risk-benefit should be considered when the following medical problems exist:*

Acute abdominal conditions
  (diagnosis may be obscured)

» Hepatic function impairment
  (metabolism of tramadol and M1 is reduced in patients with advanced cirrhosis of the liver; dosage reduction is recommended; delay in achievement of steady state may result from the prolonged half-life in this condition)

Increased intracranial pressure or
Head trauma
  (tramadol causes pupillary changes [miosis] that may obscure the existence, extent, or course of intracranial pathology; clinicians should consider the possibility of a drug effect when evaluating mental status)

» Renal function impairment
  (decreased rate and extent of excretion of tramadol and its active metabolite M1; dosage reduction is recommended in patients with creatinine clearance of less than 30 mL per minute [mL/min]; delay in achievement of steady-state may result from the prolonged half-life in this condition)

» Respiratory depression, risk of
  (tramadol may decrease respiratory drive and increase airway resistance in patients with this condition; although there is absence of significant respiratory depression following epidural and intravenous use, caution is still recommended with administration of oral tramadol in patients at risk for respiratory depression; may also occur with concurrent administration of anesthetic medication or alcohol)

» Seizures
  (tramadol may increase the risk of seizures in patients taking neuroleptics and other drugs that reduce the seizure threshold)

» Sensitivity to opioids or
» Sensitivity to tramadol
  (increased risk of anaphylactoid reactions)

Note: Caution is also recommended with the administration of tramadol in patients with a physical dependence on opioids. Withdrawal symptoms may occur in patients who have recently taken substantial amounts of opioids.

## Side/Adverse Effects

Note: Tramadol can produce drug dependence of the mu-opioid type and may potentially be abused. Tolerance development, drug seeking behavior and craving have been associated with the use of tramadol. The active metabolite of tramadol may be responsible for some delay in onset of activity and some extension of the duration of mu-opioid activity. Delayed mu-opioid activity is believed to reduce drug abuse liability. One case has been reported in which a patient developed tolerance to and dependence on oral tramadol (increase in daily dose by 500% over 6 years, from 50 to 300 mg per day). However, in a 3-week study no tolerance developed to oral tramadol. A few studies found no or very little development of tolerance with parenteral administration of tramadol.

The following side/adverse effects have been selected on the basis of their potential clinical significance (possible signs and symptoms in parentheses where appropriate)—not necessarily inclusive:

**Those indicating need for medical attention**
Incidence less frequent—1 to 5%
*Urinary frequency* (frequent urge to urinate); *urinary retention* (difficult urination); *visual disturbances* (blurred vision)

Incidence rare
*Abnormal gait* (change in walking and balance); *allergic reaction* (severe redness, swelling, and itching of the skin); *amnesia* (loss of memory); *cognitive dysfunction* (trouble performing routine tasks); *dyspnea* (shortness of breath); *hallucinations* (seeing, hearing, or feeling things that are not there); *orthostatic hypotension* (dizziness or lightheadedness when getting up from a lying or sitting position); *paresthesia* (numbness, tingling, pain, or weakness in hands or feet); *seizures*; *syncope* (fainting); *tachycardia* (fast heartbeat); *tremor* (trembling and shaking of hands or feet); *urticaria* (redness, swelling, and itching of the skin); *vesicles* (blisters under the skin)

**Those indicating need for medical attention only if they continue or are bothersome**
Incidence less frequent—1 to 5%
*Abdominal or stomach pain*; *anorexia* (loss of appetite); *anxiety*; *asthenia* (loss of strength or weakness); *confusion*; *constipation*; *coordination disturbance* (trouble in performing routine tasks); *diarrhea*; *dizziness or vertigo*; *drowsiness*; *dry mouth*; *dyspepsia* (heartburn); *euphoria* (unusual feeling of excitement); *flatulence* (excessive gas); *headache*; *malaise* (general feeling of bodily discomfort); *menopausal symptoms* (hot flashes); *nausea*; *nervousness*; *pruritis* (itching); *skin rash*; *sleep disorder* (trouble in sleeping); *sweating*; *vasodilation* (flushing or redness of the skin); *vomiting*

Note: Tramadol may produce opioid-like effects, including *constipation, dizziness, drowsiness, nausea, pruritus*, and *sweating*, but causes less respiratory depression than morphine.

**Those indicating possible withdrawal and the need for medical attention if they occur after medication is discontinued**
*Anxiety*; *body aches*; *diarrhea*; *fast heartbeat*; *fever, runny nose, or sneezing*; *gooseflesh*; *hypertension* (high blood pressure); *increased sweating*; *increased yawning*; *loss of appetite*; *nausea or vomiting*; *nervousness, restlessness, or irritability*; *shivering or trembling*; *stomach cramps*; *trouble in sleeping*; *unusually large pupils*; *weakness*

Note: The *signs and symptoms of withdrawal* listed above are characteristics of the abstinence syndrome produced by abrupt discontinuation of a mu-receptor agonist. Tramadol does have some activity involving the mu receptor; therefore, abrupt discontinuation may include some of these signs and symptoms. However, these effects may be milder compared with opiate agonists. Minimal withdrawal signs have been observed in naloxone-precipitation studies.

## Overdose

For specific information on the agents used in the management of tramadol overdose, see:
- *Diazepam* in *Benzodiazepines (Systemic)* monograph; and/or
- *Naloxone (Systemic)* monograph.

For more information on the management of overdose or unintentional ingestion, **contact a Poison Control Center** (see *Poison Control Center Listing*).

**Clinical effects of overdose**
The following effects have been selected on the basis of their potential clinical significance (possible signs and symptoms in parentheses where appropriate)—not necessarily inclusive:

Acute and chronic effects
*Cold, clammy skin*; *confusion*; *convulsions*; *dizziness, severe*; *drowsiness, severe*; *nervousness or restlessness, severe*; *pinpoint pupils of eyes*; *slow heartbeat*; *seizures*; *slow or troubled breathing*; *unconsciousness*; *weakness, severe*

Note: Studies have found the administration of intravenous tramadol may produce respiratory depression. However, morphine causes more clinically significant respiratory depression than tramadol. Clinical studies evaluating oral doses have not reported any clinically relevant respiratory depressant effects.

**Treatment of overdose**
Recommended treatment for tramadol overdose may consist of the following:

To decrease absorption—Gastric lavage may be performed.

Specific treatment—Administration of the opioid antagonist naloxone, which will reverse some, but not all, symptoms caused by overdosage with tramadol. Administer naloxone with caution because it may precipitate seizures. See the package insert or *Naloxone (Systemic)* for specific dosing guidelines for use of this product.

For treatment of convulsions caused by tramadol toxicity: Diazepam has been effective in treating convulsions. See the package insert or *Diazepam* in *Benzodiazepines (Systemic)* for specific dosing guidelines for use of this product.

Supportive care—Supportive measures such as establishing intravenous lines, hydration, correction of electrolyte imbalance, oxygenation, and support of ventilatory function are essential for maintaining the vital functions of the patient. Patients in whom intentional overdose is confirmed or suspected should be referred for psychiatric consultation.

Note: Hemodialysis is not recommended in overdose, since it removes less than 7% of the administered dose in a 4-hour dialysis period.

## Patient Consultation

As an aid to patient consultation, refer to *Advice for the Patient, Tramadol (Systemic)*.

In providing consultation, consider emphasizing the following selected information (» = major clinical significance):

**Before using this medication**
» Conditions affecting use, especially:
   Sensitivity to tramadol or opioids
   Pregnancy—Crosses the placenta; safe use in pregnancy has not been established
   Breast-feeding—Distributed into breast milk; use is not recommended
   Other medications, especially carbamazepine, CNS depressants or anesthetic agents, or MAO inhibitors
   Other medical problems, especially acute intoxication with alcohol, hypnotics, centrally-acting analgesics, opioids, or psychotropic drugs; hepatic function impairment; physical dependence on opioids; renal function impairment; risk of respiratory depression; or seizures

**Proper use of this medication**
» Not increasing dose if medication is less effective after a few weeks; checking with physician first
» Importance of not taking more medication than the amount prescribed because of danger of overdose
» Proper dosing
   Missed dose (if on scheduled dosing): Taking as soon as possible; not taking if almost time for next dose; not doubling doses
» Proper storage

**Precautions while using this medication**
» Avoiding use of alcoholic beverages or other CNS depressants during therapy unless prescribed or otherwise approved by physician
» Caution if dizziness, drowsiness, or lightheadedness occurs
» Caution when getting up from a lying or sitting position
   Lying down if nausea or vomiting, or dizziness or lightheadedness occurs
   Informing physician or dentist of use of medication if any kind of surgery (including dental surgery) or emergency treatment is required
» Suspected overdose: Getting emergency help at once

**Side/adverse effects**
Signs of potential side effects, especially urinary frequency, urinary retention, visual disturbances, abnormal gait, allergic reaction, amnesia, cognitive dysfunction, dyspnea, hallucinations, orthostatic hypotension, paresthesia, seizures, syncope, tachycardia, tremor, urticaria, and vesicles

## Oral Dosage Forms

### TRAMADOL HYDROCHLORIDE TABLETS

**Usual adult and adolescent dose**
Analgesic—Oral, 50 to 100 mg every six hours as needed.

# Tramadol (Systemic)

Note: A dose of 50 mg is usually more effective as the initial dose for moderate pain; a dose of 100 mg is usually more effective as the initial dose for more severe pain.

Patients with impaired renal function (creatinine clearance less than 30 mL/minute [mL/min]) should receive 50 to 100 mg every twelve hours.

An initial dose of 50 to 100 mg every twelve hours is usually adequate for patients with cirrhosis.

Patients on hemodialysis can receive their usual dose on the day of dialysis.

### Usual adult prescribing limits
Oral, 400 mg per day (200 mg per day in patients with creatinine clearance of less than 30 mL/min).

### Usual pediatric dose
Children up to 16 years of age—Safety and efficacy have not been established.

Children 16 years of age and over—See *Usual adult and adolescent dose*.

### Usual geriatric dose
See *Usual adult and adolescent dose*.

Note: In patients over 75 years of age the prescribing limit is 300 mg per day in divided doses.

### Strength(s) usually available
U.S.—
 50 mg (Rx) [*Ultram* (lactose)].
Canada—
 Not commercially available.

### Packaging and storage
Store between 15 and 30 °C (59 and 86 °F), in a tight container.

### Auxiliary labeling
- May cause drowsiness.
- Avoid alcoholic beverages.

Note: Tramadol is not a controlled substance in the U.S.

### Selected Bibliography
Levien TL, Baker DE. Reviews of tramadol and tretinoin. Hosp Pharm 1996; 31(1): 54-67.

Preston KL, Jasinski DR, Testa M. Abuse potential and pharmacological comparison of tramadol and morphine. Drug and Alcohol Depend 1991; 27: 7-17.

Sunshine A, Olson N, Zinghelboim I, et al. Analgesic oral efficacy of tramadol hydrochloride in postoperative pain. Clin Pharmacol Ther 1992; 51: 740-6.

Developed: 07/15/96

---

# TRANDOLAPRIL Systemic—INTRODUCTORY VERSION

VA CLASSIFICATION (Primary): CV800
Commonly used brand name(s): *Mavik*.
Note: For a listing of dosage forms and brand names by country availability, see *Dosage Forms* section(s).

## Category
Antihypertensive; vasodilator, congestive heart failure.

## Indications
### Accepted
Hypertension (treatment)—Trandolapril is indicated alone or in combination with other antihypertensive medication, such as hydrochlorothiazide, for the treatment of hypertension.

Left ventricular dysfunction, post–myocardial infarction (treatment) or
Congestive heart failure, post–myocardial infarction (treatment)—Trandolapril is indicated in stable patients who have evidence of left-ventricular systolic dysfunction (identified by wall motion abnormalities) or who are symptomatic from congestive heart failure within the first few days after sustaining acute myocardial infarction. Administration of trandolapril to Caucasian patients has been shown to decrease the risk of death (principally cardiovascular death) and to decrease the risk of heart failure–related hospitalization.

Note: In the Trandolapril Cardiac Evaluation (TRACE) trial, stable patients with echocardiographic evidence of left ventricular dysfunction 3 to 7 days after a myocardial infarction, who were tolerant of a 1-mg test dose of trandolapril, were randomized to receive a placebo or trandolapril, and followed for 24 months. Trandolapril-treated patients had a 16% reduction in the risk of all-cause mortality, primarily cardiovascular mortality. Treatment with trandolapril also was associated with a 20% reduction in the risk of progression of heart failure, defined by a time-to-first-event analysis of death attributed to heart failure, hospitalization for heart failure, or requirement for open-label angiotensin-converting enzyme (ACE) inhibitor treatment of heart failure. No significant effects on other end points, such as subsequent hospitalization, incidence of recurrent myocardial infarction, exercise tolerance, ventricular function, ventricular dimensions, or New York Heart Association (NYHA) class, occurred in trandolapril-treated patients. The patient population in this study was entirely Caucasian and had less usage of other postinfarction interventions that are typical in a U.S. population, such as thrombolysis (42%), beta-adrenergic blockade (16%), and percutaneous transluminal coronary angioplasty (PTCA) or coronary artery bypass graft (CABG) (6.7%), during the entire follow-up period.

## Pharmacology/Pharmacokinetics
### Physicochemical characteristics
Molecular weight—430.54.

### Mechanism of action/Effect
Antihypertensive—Trandolapril is a nonsulfhydryl angiotensin-converting enzyme (ACE) inhibitor. It is a prodrug for trandolaprilat, the active metabolite. Trandolaprilat is thought to lower blood pressure by inhibiting ACE activity. ACE catalyzes the conversion of angiotensin I to the potent vasoconstrictor, angiotensin II. Angiotensin II stimulates secretion of aldosterone and inhibits the release of renin through a negative feedback mechanism. When ACE activity is inhibited, angiotensin II formation is reduced and the interruption of the negative feedback mechanism results in increased plasma renin levels. The reduction of angiotensin II formation also decreases aldosterone secretion and vasoconstriction. The decrease in aldosterone secretion produces diuresis, natriuresis, and a slight increase in serum potassium concentrations.

### Other actions/effects
ACE is also known as kininase II, an enzyme that degrades bradykinin. Trandolapril may increase levels of bradykinin, producing a therapeutic vasodilating effect.

### Absorption
Bioavailability is approximately 10% for trandolapril. Trandolapril absorption is slowed by food, but this does not affect the area under the plasma concentration–time curve (AUC) or peak plasma concentration ($C_{max}$) of trandolaprilat or the $C_{max}$ of trandolapril.

### Distribution
Volume of distribution of trandolapril ($Vol_D$)—18 L.

### Protein binding
Trandolapril—High (80%), concentration-independent.
Trandolaprilat—Moderate to high (65 to 94%), concentration-dependent.

### Biotransformation
Trandolapril is converted, primarily in the liver, to trandolaprilat. Seven other metabolites, resulting primarily from glucuronidation or de-esterification, have been identified.

### Half-life
Elimination—
 Trandolapril: 6 hours.
 Trandolaprilat: 10 hours.

### Time to peak concentration
Trandolapril—1 hour.
Trandolaprilat—4 to 10 hours.

### Elimination
Renal—Approximately 33%.
Fecal—Approximately 66%.
In dialysis—
 Removable by hemodialysis.

## Precautions to Consider

### Cross-sensitivity and/or related problems
Patients hypersensitive to other angiotensin-converting enzyme (ACE) inhibitors may also be hypersensitive to trandolapril.

### Carcinogenicity
No evidence of carcinogenicity was found in long-term studies in mice at doses of up to 25 mg per kg of body weight (mg/kg) per day and in rats at doses of up to 8 mg/kg per day.

### Mutagenicity
Mutagenicity was not detected in the Ames test, the point mutation and chromosome aberration assays in Chinese hamster V79 cells, and the micronucleus test in mice.

### Pregnancy/Reproduction
Fertility—No impairment of fertility was found in rats administered doses of up to 100 mg/kg per day, which is 1250 times the maximum daily human dose based on weight.

Pregnancy—Fetal exposure to angiotensin-converting enzyme (ACE) inhibitors, including trandolapril, during the second and third trimesters can cause hypotension, reversible or irreversible renal failure, anuria, neonatal skull hypoplasia, and death in the fetus or neonate. Trandolapril should be discontinued as soon as possible when pregnancy is detected, unless no alternative therapy can be used. If trandolapril is continued, serial ultrasound examinations should be performed to assess the intra-amniotic environment. Perinatal diagnostic tests, such as contraction-stress testing (CST), a nonstress test (NST), or biophysical profiling (BPP) also may be appropriate during the applicable week of pregnancy.

Oligohydramnios, which may result from decreased fetal renal function, has been reported, and is associated with fetal limb contractures, craniofacial deformation, and hypoplastic lung development. If oligohydramnios is observed, trandolapril should be discontinued unless it is considered lifesaving for the mother. Oligohydramnios may not appear until after the fetus has sustained irreversible damage. Other adverse effects that have been reported are prematurity, intrauterine growth retardation, and patent ductus arteriosus, although it is not clear how these effects are related to drug exposure. When limited to the first trimester, exposure to ACE inhibitors does not appear to be associated with these adverse effects.

Infants exposed *in utero* to ACE inhibitors should be observed closely for hypotension, oliguria, and hyperkalemia. Oliguria should be treated with support of blood pressure and renal perfusion. Dialysis or exchange transfusion may be necessary to reverse hypotension and/or substitute for disordered renal function.

Teratogenic effects were not observed in rabbits given doses of 0.8 mg/kg per day, in rats given doses of 1000 mg/kg per day, or in monkeys given doses of 25 mg/kg per day. These doses represent 10, 1250, and 312 times the maximum projected human dose by weight, respectively.

FDA Pregnancy Category C (first trimester).

FDA Pregnancy Category D (second and third trimesters).

### Breast-feeding
It is not known whether trandolapril is distributed into breast milk. Trandolapril and/or its metabolites are distributed into the milk of lactating rats. It is not recommended that trandolapril be administered to women who are breast-feeding.

### Pediatrics
No information is available on the relationship of age to the effects of trandolapril in pediatric patients. Safety and efficacy have not been established.

### Geriatrics
Use of trandolapril in a limited number of patients 65 years of age and older (20.1% of patients in clinical studies) has not demonstrated geriatrics-specific problems that would limit the usefulness of trandolapril in the elderly. However, pharmacokinetic studies in patients over 65 years of age have shown higher plasma concentrations of trandolapril, but not of trandolaprilat, when compared with younger hypertensive patients.

### Pharmacogenetics
In controlled trials for which adequate data are available, black patients have been shown to have a higher incidence of ACE inhibitor–associated angioedema.

### Surgical
Excessive hypotension may occur in patients undergoing major surgery or during anesthesia and concurrently receiving trandolapril. If hypotension occurs, it can be corrected by volume expansion.

### Drug interactions and/or related problems
The following drug interactions and/or related problems have been selected on the basis of their potential clinical significance (possible mechanism in parentheses where appropriate)—not necessarily inclusive (» = major clinical significance):

Note: Combinations containing any of the following medications, depending on the amount present, may also interact with this medication.

» Diuretics
(concurrent use with trandolapril may produce additive hypotensive effects, especially when trandolapril therapy is initiated; withdrawal of diuretic therapy 2 to 3 days prior to beginning trandolapril therapy, cautiously increasing salt intake prior to initiation of trandolapril, or reducing the initial dose of trandolapril may minimize this effect)

» Diuretics, potassium-sparing or

» Potassium-containing salt substitutes or

» Potassium supplements
(concurrent use may increase the risk of hyperkalemia)

Lithium
(increases in serum lithium concentrations and symptoms of lithium toxicity have been reported during concurrent use; caution and frequent monitoring of serum lithium levels are recommended, especially if a diuretic is also used)

### Laboratory value alterations
The following have been selected on the basis of their potential clinical significance (possible effect in parentheses where appropriate)—not necessarily inclusive (» = major clinical significance):

With physiology/laboratory test values

Bilirubin and

Transaminases, serum
(concentrations may be increased)

Blood urea nitrogen (BUN) and

Creatinine, serum
(minor and transient increases in concentrations may occur, especially in patients concurrently receiving a calcium channel blocking agent and a diuretic, or in patients with compromised renal function)

Potassium, serum
(concentrations may be slightly increased as a result of reduced circulating aldosterone concentrations)

### Medical considerations/Contraindications
The medical considerations/contraindications included have been selected on the basis of their potential clinical significance (reasons given in parentheses where appropriate)—not necessarily inclusive (» = major clinical significance).

*Except under special circumstances, this medication should not be used when the following medical problems exist:*

» Angioedema, history of, related to previous ACE inhibitor therapy
(increased risk for development of trandolapril-related angioedema)

» Hypersensitivity to trandolapril

*Risk-benefit should be considered when the following medical problems exist:*

Aortic stenosis or

Cerebrovascular disease or

Ischemic heart disease
(reduction in blood pressure from ACE inhibitor therapy could aggravate these conditions)

Collagen-vascular disease, such as systemic lupus erythematosus (SLE) or scleroderma
(increased risk of developing agranulocytosis)

Congestive heart failure, with or without associated renal function impairment
(trandolapril therapy may cause excessive hypotension and may be associated with oliguria and/or progressive azotemia and, rarely, acute renal failure and/or death; these patients should be monitored closely during the first 2 weeks of treatment and when trandolapril or the diuretic dosage is increased)

Dehydration, sodium depletion, or volume depletion, due to excessive perspiration, vomiting, diarrhea, prolonged diuretic therapy, dialysis, or dietary salt restriction
(increased risk of symptomatic hypotension due to a reduction in salt or fluid volume)

Diabetes mellitus
(increased risk of hyperkalemia)

Dialysis with high-flux membranes or

Low-density lipoprotein apheresis with dextran sulfate absorption
(anaphylactoid reactions have been reported in patients undergoing these procedures who are concurrently taking an ACE inhibitor)

Hepatic function impairment
(increases in plasma concentrations of trandolapril and trandolaprilat have been observed; dosage adjustment of trandolapril may be necessary)

Hymenoptera venom
(life-threatening anaphylactoid reactions have been reported in two patients undergoing desensitizing treatment with hymenoptera venom while receiving ACE inhibitors)

» Renal artery stenosis, bilateral or in a solitary kidney or
» Renal function impairment
(increases in plasma concentration of trandolapril and trandolaprilat due to decreased elimination; increased risk of developing agranulocytosis; increased risk of hyperkalemia; increases in blood urea nitrogen [BUN] and serum creatinine may occur, especially in patients pretreated with a diuretic; renal function should be monitored during the first few weeks of trandolapril therapy; dosage adjustment and/or discontinuation of the diuretic may be necessary)

**Patient monitoring**

The following may be especially important in patient monitoring (other tests may be warranted in some patients, depending on condition; » = major clinical significance):

» Blood pressure measurements
(recommended to adjust the dose of trandolapril according to the patient's response)

Leucocyte count determinations
(recommended periodically in patients at risk for neutropenia, such as those with renal function impairment and/or collagen-vascular disease)

Potassium, serum concentrations
(recommended periodically in patients at risk for hyperkalemia, such as those with renal insufficiency, diabetes mellitus, or on concurrent potassium-sparing diuretic therapy, potassium supplements, and/or potassium-containing salt substitutes)

## Side/Adverse Effects

The following side/adverse effects have been selected on the basis of their potential clinical significance (possible signs and symptoms in parentheses where appropriate)—not necessarily inclusive:

**Those indicating need for medical attention**
Incidence less frequent
*Dizziness; hypotension* (lightheadedness or fainting)
Incidence rare
*Angioedema of the face, extremities, lips, tongue, glottis, and larynx* (sudden trouble in swallowing or breathing; swelling of face, mouth, hands, or feet; hoarseness); *bradycardia* (fainting, increased dizziness, and slow heart rate); *claudication, intermittent* (pain, tension, and weakness upon walking that subsides during periods of rest); *hepatotoxicity* (yellow eyes or skin; dark urine); *hyperkalemia* (confusion; irregular heartbeat; nervousness; numbness or tingling in hands, feet, or lips; shortness of breath or difficult breathing; weakness or heaviness of legs); *neutropenia or agranulocytosis* (fever; chills; sore throat); *syncope* (fainting)

Note: *Angioedema* involving the tongue, glottis, or larynx may cause airway obstruction, which could be fatal. Angioedema can occur at any time during treatment with ACE inhibitors and occurs at a higher rate in black patients than in nonblack patients. During clinical trials, 0.13% of trandolapril-treated patients experienced symptoms related to angioedema or facial edema. Two of four patients that experienced life-threatening symptoms improved without treatment or with medication (corticosteroids). In cases of angioedema, trandolapril therapy should be discontinued and appropriate treatment should be instituted until the swelling resolves.

*Hepatotoxicity* has been reported rarely in patients receiving ACE inhibitors. Although the syndrome is not understood, it has been associated with cholestatic jaundice, fulminant hepatic necrosis, and death. Patients who develop jaundice should discontinue therapy with trandolapril and receive appropriate medical follow-up.

*Hyperkalemia* occurred during clinical trials in approximately 0.4% of trandolapril-treated patients. Elevated serum potassium levels resolved, despite continued therapy, in most cases. None of these patients discontinued trandolapril therapy because of hyperkalemia.

**Those indicating need for medical attention only if they continue or are bothersome**
Incidence more frequent
*Cough, dry, persistent*
Incidence less frequent
*Asthenia* (weakness); *diarrhea; dyspepsia* (stomach discomfort, heartburn, belching); *fatigue; headache; myalgia* (muscle pain)

## Overdose

For more information on the management of overdose or unintentional ingestion, **contact a Poison Control Center** (see *Poison Control Center Listing*).

**Clinical effects of overdose**

The following effects have been selected on the basis of their potential clinical significance (possible signs and symptoms in parentheses where appropriate)—not necessarily inclusive:

*Hypotension* (dizziness, lightheadedness, or fainting)

**Treatment of overdose**

Treatment is symptomatic and supportive and may include infusion of normal saline solution to correct hypotension resulting from vasodilation and hypovolemia.

## Patient Consultation

As an aid to patient consultation, refer to *Advice for the Patient, Trandolapril (Systemic)—Introductory Version*.

In providing consultation, consider emphasizing the following selected information (» = major clinical significance):

**Before using this medication**
» Conditions affecting use, especially:
Hypersensitivity to trandolapril or other angiotensin-converting enzyme (ACE) inhibitors
Pregnancy—ACE inhibitor–associated fetal hypotension, renal failure, and death reported in humans
Breast-feeding—Trandolapril is distributed into the milk of lactating rats; administration to women who are breast-feeding is not recommended
Other medications, especially diuretics including potassium-sparing diuretics, potassium-containing medications or substances, potassium supplements, or potassium-containing salt substitutes
Other medical problems, especially history of angioedema related to ACE inhibitor therapy, renal artery stenosis, or renal function impairment

**Proper use of this medication**
Compliance with therapy; taking medication at same time each day to maintain the therapeutic effect
» Proper dosing
Missed dose
Taking as soon as possible; not taking if almost time for next dose; not doubling doses
» Proper storage

**Precautions while using this medication**
Regular visits to physician to check progress
» Not taking other medications, especially potassium supplements or salt substitutes that contain potassium, unless discussed with physician
Caution when driving or doing other things requiring alertness, because of possible dizziness, lightheadedness, and syncope, especially after initial dose of trandolapril and in patients concurrently taking diuretics
Reporting any signs of infection (fever, sore throat, chills) to physician because of risk of neutropenia
Checking with physician if severe nausea, vomiting, or diarrhea occurs and continues because of risk of dehydration, which may result in hypotension
Caution when exercising or during exposure to hot weather because of risk of dehydration, which may result in hypotension
Notifying physician immediately if pregnancy is suspected because of the possibility of fetal or neonatal injury and/or death
Reporting any signs of facial or extremity swelling and/or difficulty in swallowing or breathing because of risk of angioedema
Caution if any kind of surgery (including dental surgery) or emergency treatment is required

**Side/adverse effects**
Signs of potential side effects, especially, dizziness, hypotension, angioedema, bradycardia, intermittent claudication, hepatotoxicity, hyperkalemia, neutropenia or agranulocytosis, or syncope

## General Dosing Information

Dosage must be adjusted to meet the individual requirements of each patient, on the basis of clinical response.

### For treatment of adverse effects

For angioedema with swelling confined to the face and lips, treatment, other than withdrawal of the medication, usually is not necessary, although antihistamines may relieve the symptoms.

Treatment of angioedema involving the tongue, glottis, or larynx may include the following:
- Withdrawal of trandolapril and close observation of the patient to ensure full resolution of the symptoms.
- Administration of subcutaneous epinephrine.
- Administration of corticosteroids.
- Administration of antihistamines.

## Oral Dosage Forms

### TRANDOLAPRIL TABLETS

**Usual adult dose**
Antihypertensive—
  Oral, initially, in patients not receiving a diuretic: 1 mg once a day in nonblack patients and 2 mg once a day in black patients. Generally, dosage adjustments should be made at intervals of at least one week. Most patients require doses of 2 to 4 mg once a day. Patients inadequately treated with once-daily dosing of 4 mg may be treated with twice-daily dosing. If blood pressure is not controlled with trandolapril alone, a diuretic may be added.

  Note: It is recommended that previous diuretic therapy be withdrawn two to three days before trandolapril therapy is initiated to reduce the risk of hypotension. If blood pressure is not controlled with trandolapril alone, diuretic therapy should be resumed. If diuretic therapy cannot be discontinued, an initial trandolapril dose of 0.5 mg is recommended. The patient should remain under medical supervision for several hours until the blood pressure has stabilized.

  An initial dose of 0.5 mg once a day is recommended for patients with a creatinine clearance < 30 mL per min or with hepatic cirrhosis. Dosage may be cautiously titrated upward to achieve an optimal response.

Congestive heart failure, post–myocardial infarction or
Left ventricular dysfunction, post–myocardial infarction—
  Oral, initially, 1 mg once a day. Following the initial dose, all patients should be titrated, as tolerated, toward a target dose of 4 mg once a day or, if this dose is not tolerated, to the highest tolerated dose.

**Usual adult prescribing limits**
Doses above 8 mg have not been studied.

**Usual pediatric dose**
Safety and efficacy have not been established.

**Strength(s) usually available**
U.S.—
  1 mg (Rx) [*Mavik* (starch; croscarmellose sodium; hydroxypropyl methylcellulose; iron oxide; lactose; povidone; sodium stearyl fumarate)].
  2 mg (Rx) [*Mavik* (starch; croscarmellose sodium; hydroxypropyl methylcellulose; iron oxide; lactose; povidone; sodium stearyl fumarate)].
  4 mg (Rx) [*Mavik* (starch; croscarmellose sodium; hydroxypropyl methylcellulose; iron oxide; lactose; povidone; sodium stearyl fumarate)].

**Packaging and storage**
Store at controlled room temperature, 20 to 25 °C (68 to 77 °F).

**Auxiliary labeling**
- Do not take other medicines without your doctor's knowledge.

Developed: 06/01/98

---

# TRANDOLAPRIL AND VERAPAMIL   Systemic—INTRODUCTORY VERSION

VA CLASSIFICATION (Primary): CV401

Commonly used brand name(s): *Tarka*.

Note: For a listing of dosage forms and brand names by country availability, see *Dosage Forms* section(s).

## Category

Antihypertensive.

## Indications

**Accepted**

Hypertension (treatment)—The combination of trandolapril and verapamil is indicated for the treatment of hypertension. However, it is not indicated for initial treatment of hypertension.

## Pharmacology/Pharmacokinetics

**Physicochemical characteristics**
Molecular weight—Trandolapril: 430.54.
  Verapamil hydrochloride: 491.08.

**Mechanism of action/Effect**
Trandolapril is a nonsulfhydryl angiotensin-converting enzyme (ACE) inhibitor. It is a prodrug for trandolaprilat, the active metabolite. ACE catalyzes the conversion of angiotensin I to the vasoconstrictor, angiotensin II. Trandolaprilat is thought to lower blood pressure by inhibiting ACE activity. Angiotensin II stimulates secretion of aldosterone and inhibits the release of renin through a negative feedback mechanism. When ACE activity is inhibited, angiotensin II formation is reduced and the interruption of the negative feedback mechanism results in increased plasma renin concentrations. The reduction of angiotensin II formation also decreases aldosterone secretion and vasoconstriction. The decrease in aldosterone secretion produces a slight increase in serum potassium concentrations. Inhibition of ACE by trandolapril is not affected by verapamil.

Verapamil is a calcium channel blocking agent that inhibits the movement of calcium ions across cell membranes of arterial smooth muscle and cardiac muscle. The reduced influx of calcium ions results in a relaxation of arterial smooth muscle and a decrease in the contractility of cardiac muscle cells (a negative inotropic effect). Blood pressure is reduced with no change in heart rate. Verapamil reduces afterload, dilates the main coronary arteries and arterioles, and inhibits coronary artery spasm. The negative inotropic effect is offset by the decrease in afterload and a reflex increase in adrenergic tone. The inhibition of calcium ion movement also results in prolongation of the atrioventricular (AV) nodal effective refractory period and slowed AV conduction. However, verapamil may shorten the antegrade effective refractory period of accessory bypass tracts. The cardiac conduction effects of verapamil are not altered by trandolapril.

When trandolapril is given in combination with verapamil, the antihypertensive effects are additive.

**Other actions/effects**
ACE is also known as kininase II, an enzyme that degrades bradykinin. Therefore, trandolapril may increase concentrations of bradykinin, producing a therapeutic vasodilating effect.

**Absorption**
Trandolapril—Absolute bioavailability, approximately 10%.
Verapamil—Absolute bioavailability, range 20 to 35%. The area under the plasma concentration–time curve (AUC) for verapamil increases by approximately 65% when 4 mg of trandolapril is given in combination with 240 mg of extended-release verapamil.

Food decreases the bioavailability of verapamil, but does not alter the bioavailability of trandolapril.

**Protein binding**
Trandolapril—High (80%), concentration-independent.
Trandolaprilat—High (range, 65 to 94%), concentration-dependent.
Verapamil—High (90%).

**Biotransformation**
Trandolapril—Converted primarily in the liver (de-esterified) to its active metabolite, trandolaprilat. Trandolaprilat is approximately eight times more potent than trandolapril.
Verapamil—Extensively metabolized in the liver, producing 12 metabolites. The primary active metabolite of verapamil is norverapamil.

**Half-life**
Elimination—
  Effective: Trandolaprilat—Approximately 10 hours.
  Terminal: Verapamil—6 to 11 hours.
Note: In patients with hepatic function impairment, the elimination half-life of verapamil is prolonged up to 14 to 16 hours.

### Time to peak concentration
When 4 mg of trandolapril is given in combination with 240 mg of extended-release verapamil, the time to peak concentration ($C_{max}$) for verapamil increases by approximately 54%. Trandolapril's pharmacokinetics are not affected by concurrent administration of verapamil.

Trandolapril:
:   0.5 to 2 hours.

Trandolaprilat:
:   2 to 12 hours.

Verapamil:
:   4 to 15 hours; food delays the time to peak concentration by approximately 7 hours.

### Elimination
Trandolapril—
:   Renal: Approximately 33%.
:   Fecal: Approximately 66%.

Verapamil—
:   Renal: Approximately 70%.
:   Fecal: Approximately 16%.

In dialysis—
:   Verapamil: Not removable by hemodialysis.
:   Trandolapril or trandolaprilat: It is not known if removable by hemodialysis.

## Precautions to Consider

### Cross-sensitivity and/or related problems
Patients hypersensitive to other angiotensin-converting enzyme (ACE) inhibitors may also be hypersensitive to trandolapril.

### Carcinogenicity
No evidence of carcinogenicity was found in long-term studies with trandolapril in mice and rats given oral doses of 25 mg per kg (mg/kg) of body weight (85 mg per square meter of body surface area [mg/m$^2$]) per day and 8 mg/kg (60 mg/m$^2$) per day, respectively. Assuming a 50-kg individual, these doses represent 313 and 32 times for mice, and 100 and 23 times for rats, the maximum recommended human daily dose (MRHDD) of 4 mg based on body weight and body surface area, respectively.

No evidence of carcinogenicity was found in 2-year studies with verapamil in rats at dietary doses of 10, 35, and 120 mg/kg per day or approximately 1, 3.5, and 12 times the MRHDD (480 mg or 9.6 mg/kg per day), respectively.

### Tumorigenicity
Tumorigenic potential was not found in an 18-month study with verapamil in rats given a low (sixfold) multiple of the maximum recommended human dose, but not the maximum tolerated dose, of verapamil.

### Mutagenicity
Mutagenicity was not detected for trandolapril in the Ames test, the point mutation and chromosome aberration assays in Chinese hamster V79 cells, and the micronucleus test in mice.

Mutagenicity was not detected for verapamil in the Ames test, in five test strains at 3 mg per plate, with or without metabolic activation.

### Pregnancy/Reproduction
Fertility—No impairment of fertility was found in rats administered doses of trandolapril of up to 100 mg/kg (710 mg/m$^2$) per day, or 1250 and 260 times the MRHDD based on body weight and body surface area, respectively.

No impairment of fertility was found in female rats administered dietary doses of verapamil up to 55 mg/kg per day, which is 5.5 times the MRHDD. Effects of verapamil on male fertility have not been determined.

Pregnancy—Angiotensin-converting enzyme (ACE) inhibitors can cause fetal and neonatal morbidity and mortality when administered to pregnant women during the second and third trimesters. Trandolapril and verapamil combination should be discontinued as soon as possible when pregnancy is detected unless no alternative therapy can be used. In the latter instance, serial ultrasound examinations should be performed to assess the intra-amniotic environment. If oligohydramnios is observed, trandolapril and verapamil combination should be discontinued unless it is considered lifesaving for the mother. Perinatal diagnostics, such as contraction-stress testing (CST), a non-stress test (NST), or biophysical profiling (BPP) may also be appropriate during the applicable week of pregnancy. Oligohydramnios may not appear until after the fetus has sustained irreversible damage.

Fetal exposure to ACE inhibitors during the second and third trimesters can cause hypotension, reversible or irreversible renal failure, anuria, neonatal skull hypoplasia, and death in the fetus or neonate. Maternal oligohydramnios, which may result from decreased fetal renal function, has been reported and associated with fetal limb contractures, craniofacial deformation, and hypoplastic lung development. Other adverse effects that have been reported are prematurity, intrauterine growth retardation, and patent ductus arteriosus, although how these occurrences are related to ACE inhibitor exposure is not clear. These adverse effects do not appear to be associated with intrauterine ACE inhibitor exposure limited to the first trimester.

Infants exposed *in utero* to ACE inhibitors should be closely observed for hypotension, oliguria, and hyperkalemia. Oliguria should be treated with support of blood pressure and renal perfusion. Dialysis or exchange transfusion may be necessary to reverse hypotension and/or substitute for disordered renal function.

Teratogenic effects were not observed in rabbits given doses of 0.8 mg/kg per day, in rats given doses of 1000 mg/kg per day, or in monkeys given doses of 25 mg/kg per day of trandolapril. These doses represent 10, 1250, and 312 times the maximum projected human dose by weight (assuming a 50-kg woman), respectively.

FDA Pregnancy Category C (first trimester).
FDA Pregnancy Category D (second and third trimesters).

### Breast-feeding
Verapamil is distributed into human breast milk. Trandolapril and/or its metabolites are distributed into the milk of lactating rats.

It is recommended that trandolapril and verapamil combination not be administered to women who are breast-feeding.

### Pediatrics
No information is available on the relationship of age to the effects of the combination of trandolapril and verapamil in pediatric patients. Safety and efficacy in children younger than 18 years of age have not been established.

### Geriatrics
Use of trandolapril and verapamil combination in a limited number of patients 65 years of age and older (23% of patients in placebo-controlled studies) has not demonstrated geriatrics-specific problems that would limit the usefulness of this combination in the elderly. However, when compared with younger individuals, the bioavailability and area under the plasma concentration–time curve (AUC) of verapamil are increased by 87 and 80%, respectively, in the elderly. The bioavailability and AUC of trandolapril are increased by approximately 35% in the elderly. Verapamil clearance is reduced in the elderly, resulting in an increase in elimination half-life. The elderly may also experience greater sensitivity to the drug effects compared with younger individuals.

### Pharmacogenetics
Black patients, who may have predominantly low renin hypertension, have responded well to trandolapril therapy.

### Surgical
Patients taking an ACE inhibitor and undergoing major surgery or anesthesia with agents that produce hypotension may experience excessive hypotension. If hypotension in these patients is thought to be due to ACE inhibition, it can be corrected by volume expansion. Verapamil may prolong recovery from the neuromuscular blocking agent vecuronium.

### Drug interactions and/or related problems
The following drug interactions and/or related problems have been selected on the basis of their potential clinical significance (possible mechanism in parentheses where appropriate)—not necessarily inclusive (» = major clinical significance):

Note: Combinations containing any of the following medications, depending on the amount present, may also interact with this medication.

Anesthetics, inhalation
:   (concurrent use with verapamil has been shown to depress cardiovascular activity in animals by decreasing the inward movement of calcium ions; a dosage adjustment may be necessary)

» Beta-adrenergic blocking agents, systemic or ophthalmic
:   (heart rate, atrioventricular [AV] conduction, and cardiac contractility may be decreased with concurrent verapamil use; asymptomatic bradycardia with a wandering atrial pacemaker in a patient using both timolol eyedrops and oral verapamil has been reported; concurrent use with verapamil should be closely monitored)

Carbamazepine
:   (concurrent use with verapamil may increase carbamazepine serum concentrations; patient may experience carbamazepine side effects, such as diplopia, headache, ataxia, or dizziness)

Cimetidine
:   (concurrent use may decrease clearance of verapamil)

Cyclosporine
:   (concurrent use with verapamil may increase cyclosporine serum concentrations)

» Digitalis glycosides
(chronic verapamil therapy may increase serum digoxin concentrations by 50 to 75%; verapamil may reduce total body clearance and extrarenal clearance of digitoxin by 27% and 29%, respectively; the effect of this interaction is magnified in patients with hepatic cirrhosis; the patient should be monitored and the dose of digoxin or digitoxin may need to be reduced or temporarily discontinued)

» Disopyramide
(an interaction with verapamil is possible, although information on this interaction is not currently available; it is recommended that disopyramide not be given 48 hours before or 24 hours after trandolapril and verapamil combination administration)

» Diuretics
(concurrent use with ACE inhibitors may have additive hypotensive effects; the diuretic may need to be discontinued or salt intake cautiously increased prior to initiation of trandolapril and verapamil combination therapy; the initial combination dose may need to be reduced if it is not possible to discontinue the diuretic)

» Diuretics, potassium-sparing or
» Potassium-containing salt substitutes or
» Potassium supplements
(concurrent use with ACE inhibitor therapy may increase the risk of hyperkalemia; serum potassium concentrations should be monitored appropriately)

Flecainide
(concurrent use with verapamil may have additive effects on myocardial contractility, AV conduction, and repolarization [resulting in an additive negative inotropic effect and prolongation of AV conduction])

Lithium
(increased sensitivity to the neurotoxic effects of lithium has been reported when used concurrently with trandolapril and verapamil combination; concurrent ACE inhibitor use has resulted in increased serum lithium concentrations and symptoms of lithium toxicity; the risk of lithium toxicity may be increased if a diuretic is also used concurrently; frequent monitoring of serum lithium concentrations is recommended)

Neuromuscular blocking agents, especially vecuronium
(concurrent use with verapamil may have an additive neuromuscular blocking effect or prolong recovery from blockade; a dosage adjustment of either drug may be necessary)

Phenobarbital
(concurrent use may increase clearance of verapamil)

Quinidine
(concurrent use with verapamil has resulted in significant hypotension in a small number of patients with hypertrophic cardiomyopathy [HCM]; therefore, concurrent use is not recommended in these patients; increases in serum concentrations of quinidine have been reported with concurrent verapamil use; quinidine's effects on AV conduction are counteracted by concurrent verapamil use)

Rifampin
(concurrent use may reduce bioavailability of oral verapamil)

Theophylline
(concurrent use with verapamil may inhibit theophylline clearance and increase serum theophylline concentrations)

**Laboratory value alterations**
The following have been selected on the basis of their potential clinical significance (possible effect in parentheses where appropriate)—not necessarily inclusive (» = major clinical significance):

With physiology/laboratory test values
Liver function tests, including:
Alkaline phosphatase, serum and
Bilirubin, serum and
Lactate dehydrogenase (LDH), serum and
Transaminases, serum
(increases in values may be transient; however, significant increases may be the result of ACE inhibitor– or verapamil-associated hepatotoxicity)

Leukocyte count and
Lymphocyte count and
Neutrophil count and
Platelet count
(decreased counts may occur as a result of ACE inhibitor–associated bone marrow depression or agranulocytosis, especially in patients with a collagen-vascular disease or renal function impairment)

Potassium, serum
(concentrations may be slightly increased as a result of decreases in aldosterone secretion. In clinical trials, elevated serum potassium concentrations usually were isolated values and resolved despite continued therapy. None of the patients in clinical trials discontinued trandolapril and verapamil combined therapy because of hyperkalemia)

Sodium, serum
(concentrations may be slightly decreased)

Blood urea nitrogen (BUN) and
Creatinine, serum
(increases in concentrations may occur, especially in patients with renal insufficiency, diuretic pretreatment, and renal artery stenosis)

**Medical considerations/Contraindications**
The medical considerations/contraindications included have been selected on the basis of their potential clinical significance (reasons given in parentheses where appropriate)—not necessarily inclusive (» = major clinical significance).

*Except under extraordinary circumstances, this medication should not be used when the following medical problems exist:*

» Accessory bypass tract accompanied by atrial flutter or fibrillation
(patients receiving intravenous verapamil have developed a rapid ventricular response or ventricular fibrillation as a result of an increase in antegrade conduction over the accessory pathway, bypassing the AV node. Although this risk has not been established with oral verapamil, it should not be given to these patients)

» Angioedema, ACE inhibitor–associated, history of
(increased risk of development of trandolapril-related angioedema)

» Atrioventricular (AV) block, second- or third-degree, except in patients with a functioning artificial ventricular pacemaker
(risk of complete AV block with concurrent verapamil use)

» Cardiogenic shock or
» Hypotension (systolic pressure less than 90 mm Hg)
(concurrent verapamil use may aggravate these conditions)

» Hypersensitivity to trandolapril, any other ACE inhibitor, or verapamil

» Left ventricular dysfunction, severe (ejection fraction less than 30%, pulmonary wedge pressure above 20 mm Hg, or severe symptoms of cardiac failure) or

» Ventricular dysfunction with concurrent use of a beta-adrenergic blocking agent
(increased risk of further deterioration of ventricular function and of developing congestive heart failure or pulmonary edema with verapamil use)

» Sick sinus syndrome, except in patients with a functioning artificial ventricular pacemaker
(verapamil may interfere with sinus node impulse generation and precipitate sinus arrest or sinoatrial block)

*Risk-benefit should be considered when the following medical problems exist:*

Collagen vascular disease, such as systemic lupus erythematosus (SLE) or scleroderma
(increased risk of developing agranulocytosis and bone marrow depression with ACE inhibitor therapy)

» Congestive heart failure
(verapamil has a negative inotropic effect which may cause a worsening of symptoms, particularly in patients with an impaired inotropic state; patients with or without renal function impairment may experience excessive hypotension as a result of trandolapril therapy; excessive hypotension may be associated with oliguria, azotemia, acute renal failure, and/or death in patients who are particularly susceptible to changes in the renin-angiotensin-aldosterone system)

Dehydration (sodium or volume depletion due to excessive perspiration, vomiting, diarrhea, prolonged diuretic therapy, dialysis, or dietary salt restriction)
(increased risk of symptomatic hypotension with trandolapril)

Diabetes mellitus
(increased risk of hyperkalemia with ACE inhibitor therapy)

Dialysis with high-flux membranes or
Low-density lipoprotein apheresis with dextran sulfate absorption
(anaphylactoid reactions have been reported in patients undergoing these procedures and concurrently taking an ACE inhibitor)

Duchenne's muscular dystrophy
(verapamil may decrease neuromuscular transmission; verapamil component dosage may need to be decreased)

» Hepatic function impairment
(verapamil elimination half-life may be prolonged and clearance may be decreased due to decreased hepatic metabolism; PR interval may be prolonged or signs of overdosage may be seen with verapamil use; trandolapril and trandolaprilat serum concentrations may

be increased. In patients with mild to moderate alcoholic cirrhosis, plasma concentrations of trandolapril and trandolaprilat were ninefold and twofold greater, respectively, than in normal individuals; a dosage adjustment may be necessary)

Hymenoptera venom, treatment
(life-threatening anaphylactoid reactions have been reported in two patients undergoing desensitizing treatment with hymenoptera venom while receiving ACE inhibitors)

» Hypertrophic cardiomyopathy (HCM), especially in patients refractory to or intolerant of propranolol
(in clinical trials, 120 HCM patients receiving doses of up to 720 mg of verapamil per day experienced serious adverse effects, such as second-degree AV block, pulmonary edema with or without severe hypotension, severe hypotension, sinus arrest, and sinus bradycardia. See *Side/Adverse Effects* section)

» Renal function impairment
(clearance of verapamil metabolites may be reduced; PR interval may be prolonged or signs of overdosage may be seen with verapamil use; plasma concentrations of trandolapril and trandolaprilat may be increased due to reduced renal clearance; increased risk of developing hyperkalemia; increased risk of developing agranulocytosis and bone marrow depression; increases in blood urea nitrogen [BUN] and serum creatinine concentrations may occur, especially in patients on diuretic therapy; a dosage reduction or discontinuation of the diuretic and/or one or both components of trandolapril and verapamil combination may be necessary; renal function should be monitored during the initiation of therapy)

Ventricular dysfunction, mild
(increased risk of worsening ventricular function; this condition should be controlled with digitalis and/or diuretics before treatment with verapamil)

**Patient monitoring**
The following may be especially important in patient monitoring (other tests may be warranted in some patients, depending on condition; » = major clinical significance):

» Blood pressure measurements
(periodic monitoring is necessary for titration of dose according to the patient's response)

Electrocardiogram (ECG) determinations
(monitoring for abnormal PR interval prolongation associated with verapamil therapy may be necessary in patients with renal or hepatic function impairment)

Leukocyte count determinations
(periodic monitoring may be necessary in patients with a collagen-vascular disease or renal function impairment)

Potassium, serum concentrations
(monitoring may be necessary in patients at risk for hyperkalemia, such as those with renal insufficiency, diabetes mellitus, or those concurrently taking potassium-sparing diuretics, potassium supplements, and/or potassium-containing salt substitutes)

Renal function determinations
(monitoring may be necessary during the first few weeks of therapy in patients with renal function impairment)

## Side/Adverse Effects

Note: Asymptomatic atrioventricular (AV) block and transient bradycardia, sometimes accompanied by nodal escape rhythms, have occurred with verapamil therapy. This is a result of AV conduction slowing by verapamil. Patients without pre-existing conduction defects treated with verapamil can experience AV block. During the early titration period, prolongation of the PR interval can be correlated with verapamil plasma concentrations. Higher degrees of AV block have infrequently occurred (0.8%). Verapamil dosage should be reduced or the combination discontinued if marked first-degree AV block or progressive development to second- or third-degree AV block occurs.

In clinical trials, 120 hypertrophic cardiomyopathy (HCM) patients receiving doses of up to 720 mg of verapamil per day experienced serious adverse effects, such as second-degree AV block, pulmonary edema with or without severe hypotension, severe hypotension, sinus arrest, and sinus bradycardia. Most of these patients were refractory to or intolerant of propranolol. Three patients who had severe left ventricular outflow obstruction and a past history of left ventricular dysfunction experienced pulmonary edema and died. Eight other patients who had abnormally high (over 20 mm Hg) capillary wedge pressure and a severe left ventricular outflow obstruction experienced pulmonary edema and/or severe hypotension. Eleven percent of patients experienced sinus bradycardia, 4% experienced second-degree AV block, and 2% experienced sinus arrest. Most adverse effects were minimized by reducing the dosage of verapamil.

Verapamil has caused lenticular and/or suture line changes at doses of 30 mg/kg per day or greater and cataracts at doses of 62.5 mg/kg per day or greater in beagle dogs. These changes did not occur in long-term toxicology studies in rats and have not been reported to occur in humans.

The following side/adverse effects have been selected on the basis of their potential clinical significance (possible signs and symptoms in parentheses where appropriate)—not necessarily inclusive:

**Those indicating need for medical attention**
Incidence rare
*Angioedema* (sudden trouble in swallowing or breathing; swelling of face, mouth, hands, or feet; hoarseness); *bradycardia* (slow heartbeat); *bronchitis* (cough that produces mucus; shortness of breath; wheezing); *chest pain; dyspnea* (difficulty in breathing); *edema* (generalized swelling); *hepatotoxicity* (dark urine; fever; malaise; right upper quadrant pain; yellow eyes or skin); *hyperkalemia* (confusion; irregular heartbeat; nervousness; numbness or tingling in hands, feet, or lips; shortness of breath or difficulty in breathing; weakness or heaviness of legs)—hyperkalemia occurred during clinical trials in approximately 0.4% of trandolapril-treated patients and 0.8% of patients treated with trandolapril and verapamil combined; *hypotension* (lightheadedness or fainting)—hypotension and near-syncope occurred in 0.6% and 0.1% of patients, respectively, in clinical trials; *neutropenia or agranulocytosis* (chills; fever; sore throat)—occurs rarely in uncomplicated hypertension; occurs more frequently in patients with renal function impairment, especially if accompanied by a collagen-vascular disease

Note: *Angioedema* is associated with ACE inhibitor therapy and may involve the face, extremities, lips, tongue, glottis, or larynx. Angioedema associated with laryngeal edema, resulting in airway obstruction, could be fatal. During clinical trials, angioedema occurred in 0.15% of patients.

*Hepatotoxicity* has been reported in 3.2% of patients taking trandolapril and verapamil combination. Clinical symptoms of verapamil-associated hepatotoxicity include malaise, fever, and/or right upper quadrant pain. ACE inhibitor–associated hepatotoxicity occurs by a mechanism that is not understood, but is manifest as a syndrome of cholestatic jaundice, fulminant hepatic necrosis, and death. Trandolapril and verapamil combination therapy should be discontinued in patients who develop jaundice. Patients should receive appropriate medical follow-up.

**Those indicating need for medical attention only if they continue or are bothersome**
Incidence less frequent
*Constipation; cough, dry, persistent; dizziness; fatigue*

Note: *Cough* has been reported with ACE inhibitors and is thought to be due to increased concentrations of bradykinin as a result of kininase II inhibition. In clinical trials of combination therapy and trandolapril alone, the incidence of cough was 4.6% and 2%, respectively.

Incidence rare
*Diarrhea; extremity or joint pain; nausea; pruritus* (itching)

## Overdose

For specific information on the agents used in the management of trandolapril and verapamil combination overdose, see:
- *Atropine* in *Anticholinergics/Antispasmodics (Systemic)* monograph; and/or
- *Dobutamine, dopamine,* and/or *isoproterenol* in *Sympathomimetic Agents—Cardiovascular Use (Parenteral-Systemic)* monograph

For more information on the management of overdose or unintentional ingestion, **contact a Poison Control Center** (see *Poison Control Center Listing*).

**Clinical effects of overdose**
Acute and chronic

Note: No information is available on the clinical effects of overdose with trandolapril and verapamil combination. However, verapamil overdose has caused conduction system abnormalities, such as junctional rhythm with AV dissociation and high-degree AV block, including asystole. Effects secondary to hypoperfusion, such as convulsions, hyperglycemia, hyperkalemia, metabolic acidosis, and renal dysfunction, may also occur.

The following effects have been selected on the basis of their potential clinical significance (possible signs and symptoms in parentheses where appropriate)—not necessarily inclusive:

*Bradycardia* (slow heartbeat); *hypotension, severe* (dizziness or fainting)

### Treatment of overdose
Specific treatment—

Trandolapril overdose is clinically manifest as severe hypotension resulting from the hypotensive effects of vasodilation and hypovolemia. Trandolapril overdose is usually treated by infusion of normal saline solution.

Verapamil overdose has been effectively treated with beta-adrenergic stimulation or parenteral administration of calcium solutions to increase calcium ion flux across the slow channel.
- For bradycardia and conduction system abnormalities—Atropine, isoproterenol, and cardiac pacing.
- For cardiac failure—Inotropic agents, such as isoproterenol, dopamine, and dobutamine; and diuretics. Asystole should be managed by appropriate measures, including cardiopulmonary resuscitation.
- For hypotension—Intravenous fluids, calcium solutions (e.g. 10% calcium chloride injection), and vasopressors, such as dopamine and dobutamine.

Monitoring—

Patients with trandolapril and verapamil combination overdoses should be observed for at least 48 hours under continuous hospital care.

Overdoses with the extended-release formulation of verapamil have been associated with delayed pharmacodynamic effects. Verapamil slows gastrointestinal transit time and has been reported to form concretions within the stomach or intestines. Plain radiographs of the abdomen cannot detect concretions and no form of medical gastrointestinal emptying has proven efficacious in removing them. Endoscopy is a possible method for removing concretions when overdose symptoms are unusually prolonged.

Patients in whom intentional overdose is confirmed or suspected should be referred for psychiatric consultation.

## Patient Consultation
As an aid to patient consultation, refer to *Advice for the Patient, Trandolapril and Verapamil (Systemic)—Introductory Version*.

In providing consultation, consider emphasizing the following selected information (» = major clinical significance):

### Before using this medication
» Conditions affecting use, especially:

Hypersensitivity to trandolapril, other angiotensin-converting enzyme (ACE) inhibitors, or verapamil

Pregnancy—ACE inhibitor–associated fetal and neonatal hypotension, skull hypoplasia, renal failure, and death reported in humans

Breast-feeding—Verapamil is distributed into breast milk; use of the combination product is not recommended in nursing mothers

Use in the elderly—Bioavailability and AUC of trandolapril and verapamil are increased; increased elimination half-life of verapamil; elderly patients may experience greater sensitivity to drug effects

Other medications, especially beta-adrenergic blocking agents, digitalis glycosides, disopyramide, diuretics, potassium-containing salt substitutes, potassium-sparing diuretics, or potassium supplements

Other medical problems, especially accessory bypass tract accompanied by atrial flutter or fibrillation, cardiogenic shock, congestive heart failure, hepatic function impairment, history of ACE inhibitor–associated angioedema, hypertrophic cardiomyopathy (HCM), hypotension (systolic pressure less than 90 mm Hg), renal function impairment, second- or third-degree atrioventricular (AV) block (except in patients with a functioning artificial ventricular pacemaker), severe left ventricular dysfunction, sick sinus syndrome (except in patients with a functioning artificial ventricular pacemaker), and ventricular dysfunction with concurrent beta-adrenergic blocking agent use

Surgical—Anesthesia with hypotension-producing agents may cause excessive hypotension; prolonged recovery from neuromuscular blockade

### Proper use of this medication
» Compliance with therapy; taking medication at the same time each day to maintain the therapeutic effect

Swallowing tablets whole without crushing or chewing

Taking with food

» Proper dosing

Missed dose: Taking as soon as possible; not taking if almost time for next scheduled dose; not doubling doses

» Proper storage

### Precautions while using this medication
Regular visits to the physician to check progress

Notifying physician immediately if pregnancy is suspected

Not taking other medications, especially potassium supplements or salt substitutes that contain potassium, unless discussed with physician

Caution when driving or doing other things requiring alertness because of possible dizziness, lightheadedness, and syncope due to symptomatic hypotension

Reporting any signs of infection (fever, sore throat, chills) to physician because of risk of neutropenia

Reporting any signs of facial or extremity swelling and difficulty in swallowing or breathing because of risk of angioedema

To prevent dehydration and hypotension, checking with physician if severe nausea, vomiting, or diarrhea occurs and continues

Caution when exercising or during hot weather because of the risk of dehydration and hypotension due to reduced fluid volume

Caution if any kind of surgery (including dental surgery) or emergency treatment is required

### Side/adverse effects
Signs of potential side effects, especially angioedema, bradycardia, bronchitis, chest pain, dyspnea, edema, hepatotoxicity, hyperkalemia, hypotension, neutropenia or agranulocytosis

## General Dosing Information
Dosage must be adjusted to meet the individual requirements of each patient, on the basis of clinical response.

Combination trandolapril and verapamil therapy should only be used in patients who have failed to achieve the desired antihypertensive effect with one or the other as single therapy at its respective maximally recommended dose and shortest dosing interval, or when the dose of one or the other as single therapy cannot be increased further because of dose-limiting side effects. For dosage ranges for the individual agents when given as single therapy, see
- *Trandolapril (Systemic)* monograph; and/or
- *Verapamil* in *Calcium Channel Blocking Agents (Systemic)* monograph.

Black patients, who may have predominantly low renin hypertension, have responded well to trandolapril therapy.

Hepatic function impairment prolongs the elimination half-life of verapamil by up to 14 to 16 hours and decreases clearance by as much as 30%. Patients with hepatic function impairment should be administered approximately 30% of the normal dose. In clinical trials, patients with mild to moderate alcoholic cirrhosis had plasma concentrations of trandolapril and trandolaprilat ninefold and twofold greater, respectively, than in normal individuals. A dosage decrease should be considered in these patients.

In patients with a creatinine clearance below 30 mL per min (mL/min) and in hemodialysis patients, the plasma concentrations of trandolapril and trandolaprilat are approximately twofold greater and renal clearance is reduced by about 85% compared with normal individuals.

### Diet/Nutrition
Food decreases verapamil bioavailability; however, trandolapril and verapamil combination should be taken with food.

### For treatment of adverse effects
Recommended treatment consists of the following:
- For treatment of symptomatic hypotension; the patient should be placed in a supine position and, if necessary, normal saline may be administered intravenously. The individual component dose of trandolapril and/or verapamil or the concurrent diuretic may need to be reduced.
- For treatment of acute cardiovascular adverse effects, such as severe hypotension or AV block, emergency measures should be initiated; treatment involves intravenous administration of isoproterenol, norepinephrine, atropine, or 10% calcium gluconate solution. In patients with hypertrophic cardiomyopathy (HCM), treatment involves administration of alpha-adrenergic agonists, such as phenylephrine, metaraminol, or methoxamine to maintain blood pressure. Use of isoproterenol and norepinephrine should be avoided in these patients. Inotropic agents such as dopamine or dobutamine may be administered if needed.
- For treatment of ACE inhibitor–associated angioedema with swelling confined to the face and lips; treatment, other than withdrawal of the medication, is usually not necessary, although antihistamines may relieve the symptoms.

- Treatment of ACE inhibitor–associated angioedema involving the face, tongue, glottis, and/or larynx may include the following:
    — Withdrawal of trandolapril and verapamil combination and close observation of the patient to ensure full resolution of the symptoms.
    — Subcutaneous epinephrine.
    — Corticosteroids.
    — Antihistamines.

## Oral Dosage Forms

### TRANDOLAPRIL AND VERAPAMIL HYDROCHLORIDE EXTENDED-RELEASE TABLETS

**Usual adult dose**
Antihypertensive—
  Oral, 1 or 2 tablets a day, as determined by individual titration with the component agents.

**Usual adult prescribing limits**
4 mg trandolapril and 240 mg verapamil hydrochloride.

**Usual pediatric dose**
Safety and efficacy have not been established in patients below 18 years of age.

**Strength(s) usually available**
U.S.—
  1 mg trandolapril in immediate-release form and 240 mg verapamil hydrochloride in extended-release form (Rx) [*Tarka*].
  2 mg trandolapril in immediate-release form and 180 mg verapamil hydrochloride in extended-release form (Rx) [*Tarka*].
  2 mg trandolapril in immediate-release form and 240 mg verapamil hydrochloride in extended-release form (Rx) [*Tarka*].
  4 mg trandolapril in immediate-release form and 240 mg verapamil hydrochloride in extended-release form (Rx) [*Tarka*].

**Packaging and storage**
Store between 15 and 25 ºC (59 and 77 ºF), unless otherwise specified by the manufacturer. Store in a well closed container.

**Auxiliary labeling**
- Do not take other medicines without your doctor's advice.
- Take with food.

Developed: 10/21/97

# TRANEXAMIC ACID  Systemic

VA CLASSIFICATION (Primary/Secondary): BL116/IM900
Commonly used brand name(s): *Cyklokapron*.
Note:  For a listing of dosage forms and brand names by country availability, see *Dosage Forms* section(s).

## Category
Antifibrinolytic; antihemorrhagic.

## Indications
Note:  Bracketed information in the *Indications* section refers to uses that are not included in U.S. product labeling.

**Accepted**
Hemorrhage, following dental and [oral[1]] surgery, in patients with hemophilia (prophylaxis and treatment)
[Hemorrhage, oral, in patients with hemophilia (treatment)[1]]
[Hemorrhage, postsurgical (treatment)] or
[Hemorrhage, hyperfibrinolysis-induced (treatment)]—Tranexamic acid is indicated for the management of hemophilic patients (those having Factor VIII or Factor IX deficiency) who have [oral mucosal bleeding[1]], or are undergoing tooth extraction [or other oral surgical procedures[1]]. The medication prevents or decreases hemorrhaging in these patients and reduces the need for administration of clotting factors, particularly when desmopressin is also used.
[Tranexamic acid is indicated for the treatment of severe localized bleeding secondary to hyperfibrinolysis, including epistaxis, hyphema, or hypermenorrhea (menorrhagia) and hemorrhage following certain surgical procedures, such as conization of the cervix.]
[Antifibrinolytic agents are used to treat severe hemorrhaging caused by thrombolytic agents such as alteplase (tissue-type plasminogen activator, recombinant), anistreplase (anisoylated plasminogen-streptokinase activator complex), streptokinase, or urokinase.][1] However, controlled studies to demonstrate their efficacy have not been done in humans.
[Bleeding responsive to antifibrinolytic therapy also may occur following heart surgery (with or without cardiac bypass procedures) and portacaval shunt, prostatectomy, nephrectomy, or bladder surgery, and in association with hematologic disorders (such as aplastic anemia), abruptio placentae, hepatic cirrhosis, neoplastic disease, and polycystic or neoplastic diseases of the genitourinary system.][1]
[Angioedema, hereditary (treatment)]—Tranexamic acid is indicated for the treatment of hereditary angioedema. It is used to reduce the frequency and severity of acute attacks in patients with this disorder.
Note:  Antifibrinolytic agents are ineffective in bleeding caused by loss of vascular integrity; a definite clinical diagnosis or confirmation of hyperfibrinolysis (hyperplasminemia) via laboratory studies is required before tranexamic acid is used to treat hemorrhage. However, some conditions and laboratory findings suggestive of hyperfibrinolysis are also present in disseminated intravascular coagulation; differentiation between the two conditions is essential because antifibrinolytic agents may promote thrombus formation in patients with disseminated intravascular coagulation and must *not* be used unless heparin is administered concurrently. The following criteria may be useful in differential diagnosis:

| Test | Primary Hyperfibrinolysis Results | Disseminated Intravascular Coagulation Results |
|---|---|---|
| Platelet count* | Normal | Decreased |
| Protamine para-coagulation test | Negative | Positive |
| Euglobulin clot lysis time | Decreased | Normal |

*Following extracorporeal circulation (during cardiovascular surgery), decreased platelet count may not be useful for differentiating between primary hyperfibrinolysis and disseminated intravascular coagulation; the other criteria may be more useful in differential diagnosis in these patients.

[1]Not included in Canadian product labeling.

## Pharmacology/Pharmacokinetics

**Physicochemical characteristics**
Molecular weight—157.21.

**Mechanism of action/Effect**
Tranexamic acid competitively inhibits activation of plasminogen, thereby reducing conversion of plasminogen to plasmin (fibrinolysin), an enzyme that degrades fibrin clots, fibrinogen, and other plasma proteins, including the procoagulant factors V and VIII. Tranexamic acid also directly inhibits plasmin activity, but higher doses are required than are needed to reduce plasmin formation. *In vitro*, the antifibrinolytic potency of tranexamic acid is approximately 5 to 10 times that of aminocaproic acid.
In patients with hereditary angioedema, inhibition of the formation and activity of plasmin by tranexamic acid may prevent attacks of angioedema by decreasing plasmin-induced activation of the first complement protein (C1).

**Absorption**
Oral—30 to 50% of a dose is absorbed from the gastrointestinal tract. Bioavailability is not altered by food intake.

**Distribution**
In breast milk—Concentrations are approximately 1% of the maternal serum concentration.

**Protein binding**
Very low (<3%), primarily to plasminogen, at therapeutic plasma concentrations. Tranexamic acid does not bind to serum albumin.

**Biotransformation**
Less than 5% of a dose is metabolized.

**Half-life**
Elimination—Approximately 2 hours (following intravenous administration of a 1-gram dose).

**Time to peak concentration**
Oral—Approximately 3 hours.

**Peak plasma concentration**
Oral—8 mcg per mL (50.9 micromoles/L) following a dose of 1 gram; 15 mcg per mL (95.4 micromoles/L) following a dose of 2 grams.

**Therapeutic plasma concentration**
10 mcg per mL (63.6 micromoles/L). Therapeutic concentrations persist in serum for 7 to 8 hours, and in several other tissues for up to 17 hours, following administration of the last of 4 doses of 10 mg per kg of body weight (mg/kg) intravenously or 20 mg/kg orally.

**Elimination**
Renal, via glomerular filtration; > 95% of a dose is excreted as unchanged tranexamic acid.
Oral—39% of a dose (about 78% of the quantity absorbed) is excreted within 24 hours after administration of 10 to 15 mg/kg.
Intravenous—90% of a dose is excreted within 24 hours after administration of 10 mg/kg.

## Precautions to Consider

### Carcinogenicity/Tumorigenicity
An increased incidence of leukemia occurred in male mice receiving approximately 5 grams per kg of body weight per day of tranexamic acid (added to food in a concentration of 4.8%). Female mice were not included in that study. In another study, tranexamic acid produced adenomas, adenocarcinomas, and hyperplasia of the biliary tract when administered orally to one strain of rats in doses exceeding the maximum tolerated dose for a period of 22 months. Lower doses produced hyperplastic, but not neoplastic, changes. No hyperplastic or neoplastic changes were observed in subsequent long-term studies in which equivalent doses were administered to a different strain of rats.

### Mutagenicity
Studies using a variety of *in vivo* and *in vitro* test systems have not shown that tranexamic acid has mutagenic activity.

### Pregnancy/Reproduction
Fertility—Tranexamic acid has been detected in semen in antifibrinolytic concentrations but has no effect on the motility of spermatozoa. Reproductive studies in mice, rats, and rabbits have shown no evidence of impaired fertility.

Pregnancy—Tranexamic acid crosses the placenta. Following intravenous administration of 10 mg per kg of body weight (mg/kg) to pregnant women, 30 mcg of tranexamic acid per mL (190.8 micromoles/L) was measured in fetal serum. Adequate and well-controlled studies in humans have not been done. However, healthy infants have been born to women who received tranexamic acid during pregnancy for treatment of fibrinolytic bleeding or bleeding associated with abruptio placentae.

Studies in mice, rats, and rabbits have not shown that tranexamic acid causes adverse effects on the fetus.

FDA Pregnancy Category B.

### Breast-feeding
Tranexamic acid is distributed into breast milk; concentrations reach approximately 1% of the maternal plasma concentration.

### Pediatrics
Appropriate studies on the relationship of age to the effects of tranexamic acid have not been performed in the pediatric population. However, no pediatrics-specific problems have been documented to date.

### Geriatrics
Appropriate studies performed to date have not demonstrated geriatrics-specific problems that would limit the usefulness of tranexamic acid in the elderly.

### Drug interactions and/or related problems
The following drug interactions and/or related problems have been selected on the basis of their potential clinical significance (possible mechanism in parentheses where appropriate)—not necessarily inclusive (» = major clinical significance):

Anti-inhibitor coagulant complex or
Factor IX complex
(although tranexamic acid is often used in conjunction with clotting factor replacement for the perisurgical management of hemophilic patients, concurrent use may increase the risk of thrombotic complications; using tranexamic acid as an oral rinse for oral surgical procedures and tooth extractions may minimize this complication; some hematologists recommend that administration of tranexamic acid be delayed for 8 hours following injection of either of the clotting factor complexes)

Contraceptives, estrogen-containing, oral or
Estrogens
(concurrent use with tranexamic acid may increase the potential for thrombus formation)

Thrombolytic agents
(the actions of tranexamic acid and of thrombolytic agents [e.g., alteplase (tissue-type plasminogen activator, recombinant; tPA), anistreplase (anisoylated plasminogen-streptokinase activator complex; APSAC), streptokinase, or urokinase] are mutually antagonistic; although controlled studies to demonstrate its efficacy have not been done in humans, tranexamic acid may be useful in treating severe hemorrhage caused by a thrombolytic agent)

### Medical considerations/Contraindications
The medical considerations/contraindications included have been selected on the basis of their potential clinical significance (reasons given in parentheses where appropriate)—not necessarily inclusive (» = major clinical significance).

*Except under special circumstances, this medication should not be used when the following medical problem exists:*

» Intravascular clotting, active
(risk of serious, even fatal, thrombus formation)

*Risk-benefit should be considered when the following medical problems exist:*

» Defective color vision, acquired
(condition precludes assessment of color vision, which may be required to determine toxicity)

» Hematuria of upper urinary tract origin
(risk of intrarenal obstruction secondary to clot retention in the renal pelvis and ureters if hematuria is massive; also, if hematuria is associated with a disease of the renal parenchyma, intravascular precipitation of fibrin may occur and exacerbate the disease)

» Hemorrhage, subarachnoid
(increased risk of cerebral edema and cerebral infarction)

» Renal function impairment
(medication may accumulate; dosage adjustment based on the degree of impairment is recommended)

Sensitivity to tranexamic acid, history of

» Thrombosis, predisposition to or history of
(medication inhibits clot dissolution and may interfere with mechanisms for maintaining blood vessel patency; it is recommended that tranexamic acid be administered in conjunction with anticoagulant therapy, if at all)

### Patient monitoring
The following may be especially important in patient monitoring (other tests may be warranted in some patients, depending on condition; » = major clinical significance):

Ophthalmological examinations, including tests for visual acuity, color vision, eyeground, and visual fields
(recommended prior to and at regular intervals during therapy for patients receiving the medication for longer than several days because tranexamic acid has caused focal areas of retinal degeneration in animal studies and visual disturbances [although retinal lesions have not been reported] in humans)

## Side/Adverse Effects

Note: Patients receiving tranexamic acid should be monitored for signs of thromboembolic complications.

Focal areas of retinal degeneration have been reported in cats, dogs, and rats after oral or intravenous administration of tranexamic acid at doses of 250 to 1600 mg per kg of body weight (mg/kg) per day (6 to 40 times the recommended usual human dose) for 6 days to a year. The incidence and severity of the lesions are dose-dependent. Some lesions in animals receiving low doses have been reversible. Other studies in cats and rabbits have shown retinal changes to occur with doses as low as 126 mg/kg per day (about 3 times the recommended usual human dose) administered for several days to 2 weeks. However, no retinal changes occurred in patients receiving tranexamic acid for weeks to months in clinical trials.

The following side/adverse effects have been selected on the basis of their potential clinical significance (possible signs and symptoms in parentheses where appropriate)—not necessarily inclusive:

### Those indicating need for medical attention
Incidence less frequent or rare
*Blurred vision or other changes in vision; hypotension* (dizziness or lightheadedness; unusual tiredness or weakness)—may be associated with too-rapid intravenous administration; *thrombosis or thromboembolism* (pains in chest, groin, or legs [especially calves]; severe, sudden headache; sudden and unexplained shortness of breath, slurred speech, vision changes, and/or weakness or numbness in arm or leg; sudden

loss of coordination)—depending on site of thrombus formation or embolization

**Those indicating need for medical attention only if they continue or are bothersome**
Incidence more frequent
  *Diarrhea; nausea; vomiting*
Incidence unknown
  *Unusual menstrual discomfort*—caused by clotting of menstrual fluid

## Overdose

For more information on the management of overdose or unintentional ingestion, **contact a Poison Control Center** (see *Poison Control Center Listing*).

**Treatment of overdose**
Although there is no experience with overdose of tranexamic acid, discontinuing the medication is recommended.

For thromboembolic complications—Monitoring the patient carefully and administering appropriate therapy, depending on the location and size of the thrombus. Use of heparin or a thrombolytic agent may be considered in severe cases. However, these medications must be used with extreme caution, if at all, in patients receiving tranexamic acid to prevent or treat hemorrhaging, because of the risk of uncontrollable hemorrhage being induced in such patients.

If tranexamic acid had been administered orally, limiting absorption via induction of emesis, gastric lavage, and/or administration of activated charcoal may be helpful.

## Patient Consultation

As an aid to patient consultation, refer to *Advice for the Patient, Antifibrinolytic Agents (Systemic)*.
In providing consultation, consider emphasizing the following selected information (» = major clinical significance):

**Before using this medication**
» Conditions affecting use, especially:
    Sensitivity to tranexamic acid, history of
    Pregnancy—Tranexamic acid crosses the placenta, but has not been reported to cause problems when given to pregnant women
    Breast-feeding—Tranexamic acid is distributed into breast milk
    Other medical problems, especially defective color vision, hematuria of upper urinary tract origin, predisposition to or history of thrombosis, renal function impairment, and subarachnoid hemorrhage

**Proper use of this medication**
» Importance of not using more or less medication than the amount prescribed
» Proper dosing
    Missed dose: Taking as soon as possible, then returning to regular dosing schedule; not doubling doses
» Proper storage

**Precautions while using this medication**
Possible need for regular ophthalmologic examinations during long-term therapy

**Side/adverse effects**
Signs of potential side effects, especially blurred vision or other changes in vision, hypotension, and thrombosis or thromboembolism.

## General Dosing Information

A reduction in dosage may be required for patients with renal function impairment or if nausea, vomiting, or diarrhea occurs.

It is recommended that therapy be discontinued if thromboembolic complications occur or if changes in the results of ophthalmologic examinations are noted.

**For parenteral dosage forms only**
Tranexamic acid injection should be administered intravenously at a rate not to exceed 100 mg (1 mL) per minute, to avoid inducing hypotension.

## Oral Dosage Forms

Note: Bracketed uses in the *Dosage Forms* section refers to categories of use and/or indications that are not included in U.S. product labeling.

### TRANEXAMIC ACID TABLETS

**Usual adult and adolescent dose**
Prevention and treatment of [oral hemorrhage[1]], including hemorrhage following dental surgery, in hemophilic patients—
  Presurgical: Oral, 25 mg per kg of body weight every six to eight hours, beginning one day before the dental procedure. However, intravenous administration of the medication immediately prior to surgery may be preferred. When tranexamic acid is used, a single factor VIII infusion of 40 International Units per kg of body weight, or coagulation factor IX infusion of 60 International Units per kg of body weight prior to surgery is often enough for normal hemostasis.

  Note: Because of an increased risk of thrombotic complications when tranexamic acid and Factor IX or anti-inhibitor coagulant complex are administered concurrently, some hematologists recommend that tranexamic acid not be administered within eight hours of these clotting factor concentrates.

  Postsurgical: Oral, 25 mg per kg of body weight every six to eight hours for seven to ten days after surgery. In addition to systemic tranexamic acid, an oral rinse may be used topically (see *Tranexamic Acid Oral Solution*).

[Hemorrhage, postsurgical–conization of the cervix]—
  Oral, 1 to 1.5 grams every eight to twelve hours for twelve days after surgery.

[Hemorrhage, postsurgical–prostatectomy][1] or
[Bladder surgery][1]—
  Oral, 1 gram three to four times a day starting on the fourth day after surgery (the medication having been administered intravenously for the first three days postoperatively). Therapy should be continued until macroscopic hematuria is no longer present.

[Hemorrhage, hyperfibrinolysis-induced–epistaxis]—
  Oral, 1 to 1.5 grams three or four times a day for 10 days.

[Hemorrhage, hyperfibrinolysis-induced–hypermenorrhea]—
  Oral, 1 to 1.5 grams three or four times a day for three or four days, starting after copious bleeding has begun.

[Hemorrhage, hyperfibrinolysis-induced–hyphema]—
  Oral, 1 to 1.5 grams three or four times a day for seven days.

[Hemorrhage, hyperfibrinolysis-induced–other][1]—
  Oral, 20 to 25 mg two or three times a day. Therapy should be continued until there is evidence of cessation of bleeding or laboratory determinations of fibrinolysis indicate that treatment is no longer needed.

[Angioedema, hereditary]—
  Oral, 1 to 1.5 grams two or three times a day. Some patients can sense the onset of attacks and may be treated intermittently, with therapy being started at the first sign of an attack and continued for several days. Other patients should be treated on a continuing basis.

Note: Because of the risk of tranexamic acid accumulation, the following dosage regimens are recommended for patients with moderate to severe renal function impairment:

| Serum Creatinine (micromoles/L) | Dose |
| --- | --- |
| 120–250 (1.36–2.83 mg/dL) | 15 mg/kg two times a day |
| 250–500 (2.83–5.66 mg/dL) | 15 mg/kg a day |
| >500 (>5.66 mg/dL) | 15 mg/kg every 48 hours or 7.5 mg/kg every 24 hours |

**Usual pediatric dose**
Prevention and treatment of [oral hemorrhage[1]], including hemorrhage following dental surgery, in hemophilic patients—
  See *Usual adult and adolescent dose*.

**Strength(s) usually available**
U.S.—
  500 mg (Rx) [*Cyklokapron* (microcrystalline cellulose; talc; magnesium stearate; silicon dioxide; povidone)].
Canada—
  500 mg (Rx) [*Cyklokapron*].

**Packaging and storage**
Store between 15 and 30 °C (59 and 86 °F), in a well-closed container, unless otherwise specified by manufacturer.

### TRANEXAMIC ACID ORAL SOLUTION

**Usual adult and adolescent dose**
Prevention and treatment of [oral hemorrhage[1]], including hemorrhage following dental surgery, in hemophilic patients—
  Postsurgical: Topically, as an oral rinse, 10 mL of a 5% solution for two minutes four times a day for five to seven days after surgery, in addition to systemic tranexamic acid (see *Tranexamic Acid Tablets*).

**Usual pediatric dose**
Prevention and treatment of [oral hemorrhage[1]], including hemorrhage following dental surgery, in hemophilic patients—
  See *Usual adult and adolescent dose*.

**Strength(s) usually available**
U.S.—
    Dosage form not commercially available in the U.S. Compounding required for prescriptions.
Canada—
    Dosage form not commercially available in Canada. Compounding required for prescriptions.

**Preparation of dosage form**
A 5% oral rinse is prepared by diluting 5 mL of 10% tranexamic acid injection with 5 mL of sterile water.

## Parenteral Dosage Forms

Note: Bracketed uses in the *Dosage Forms* section refers to categories of use and/or indications that are not included in U.S. product labeling.

### TRANEXAMIC ACID INJECTION

**Usual adult and adolescent dose**
Prevention and treatment of [oral hemorrhage[1]], including hemorrhage following dental surgery, in hemophilic patients—
    Presurgical: Intravenous, 10 mg per kg of body weight, administered immediately prior to surgery. When tranexamic acid is used, a single factor VIII infusion of 40 International Units per kg of body weight, or coagulation factor IX infusion of 60 International Units per kg of body weight prior to surgery is often enough for normal hemostasis.
    Note: Because of an increased risk of thrombotic complications when tranexamic acid and Factor IX or anti-inhibitor coagulant complex are administered concurrently, some hematologists recommend that tranexamic acid not be administered within eight hours of these clotting factor concentrates.
    Postsurgical (for patients unable to take medication orally): Intravenous, 10 mg per kg of body weight every six to eight hours for seven to ten days.
[Hemorrhage, postsurgical]—
    Following prostatectomy or bladder surgery: Intravenous, 1 gram, administered during surgery initially, then every eight hours for three days. Therapy is then continued, using orally administered tranexamic acid, until macroscopic hematuria is no longer present.
    Note: Tranexamic acid injection may also be used as an irrigation following bladder surgery. One gram of tranexamic acid in one liter of 0.9% sodium chloride irrigation is instilled into the bladder at a rate of 1 mL per minute once a day for two to five days following surgery.
[Hemorrhage, hyperfibrinolysis-induced]—
    Intravenous, 15 mg per kg of body weight or 1 gram every six to eight hours. Therapy should be continued until there is evidence of cessation of bleeding or laboratory determinations of fibrinolysis indicate that treatment is no longer needed.
Note: For other specific indications listed under *Tranexamic Acid Tablets*, patients unable to take medication orally may receive intravenous administration of 10 mg per kg of body weight of tranexamic acid according to the dosing schedule recommended for that indication.
For relief of severe epistaxis, tranexamic acid injection has also been applied topically to the nasal mucosa, as a spray or by packing the nasal cavity with a gauze strip that has been soaked in the solution.
Because of the risk of tranexamic acid accumulation, the following dosage regimens are recommended for patients with moderate to severe renal function impairment:

| Serum Creatinine (micromoles/L) | Dose |
| --- | --- |
| 120–250 (1.36–2.83 mg/dL) | 10 mg/kg two times a day |
| 250–500 (2.83–5.66 mg/dL) | 10 mg/kg a day |
| >500 (>5.66 mg/dL) | 10 mg/kg every 48 hours or 5 mg/kg every 24 hours |

**Usual pediatric dose**
Prevention and treatment of [oral hemorrhage[1]], including hemorrhage following dental surgery, in hemophilic patients—
    See *Usual adult and adolescent dose*.

**Strength(s) usually available**
U.S.—
    100 mg per mL (in 10-mL ampuls) (Rx) [*Cyklokapron*].
Canada—
    100 mg per mL ( in 5- and 10-mL ampuls) (Rx) [*Cyklokapron*].

**Packaging and storage**
Store between 15 and 30 °C (59 and 86 °F), unless otherwise specified by manufacturer. Protect from freezing.

**Preparation of dosage form**
Tranexamic acid injection may be mixed with intravenous infusion solutions, including solutions containing electrolytes, carbohydrates, amino acids, or dextran.
Heparin may be added to the tranexamic acid injection, if necessary.

**Stability**
Intravenous infusion mixtures should be prepared the same day they are to be used.

**Incompatibilities**
Tranexamic acid should not be added to any solution containing penicillin or mixed with blood.

[1]Not included in Canadian product labeling.

Revised: 08/15/97

---

**TRANYLCYPROMINE**— See *Antidepressants, Monoamine Oxidase (MAO) Inhibitor (Systemic)*

---

# TRAZODONE Systemic

VA CLASSIFICATION (Primary/Secondary): CN609/CN103
Commonly used brand name(s): *Desyrel; Trazon; Trialodine*.
Note: For a listing of dosage forms and brand names by country availability, see *Dosage Forms* section(s).

## Category
Antidepressant; antineuralgic.

## Indications

Note: Bracketed information in the *Indications* section refers to uses that are not included in U.S. product labeling.

**Accepted**
Depression, mental (treatment)—Trazodone is indicated in the treatment of major depressive episodes with or without prominent anxiety.
[Pain, neurogenic (treatment)][1]—Trazodone has been used to treat painful diabetic neuropathy and other types of chronic pain.

[1]Not included in Canadian product labeling.

## Pharmacology/Pharmacokinetics

**Physicochemical characteristics**
Molecular weight—408.33.
Other characteristics—Trazodone is *not* chemically related to tricyclic, tetracyclic, or other known antidepressants.

**Mechanism of action/Effect**
Not completely established in humans. Animal studies indicate that trazodone selectively inhibits serotonin re-uptake in the brain, causes beta-receptor subsensitivity, and induces significant changes in serotonin-receptor binding with only a slight effect on alpha-adrenergic receptors. Also, trazodone potentiates the behavioral changes in animals induced by 5-hydroxytryptophan, a serotonin precursor.

**Absorption**
Well absorbed. When trazodone is taken with or shortly after ingestion of food, there may be an increase in the amount of drug absorbed, a decrease in maximum concentration, and a lengthening of time to reach peak concentration.

**Protein binding**
Very high (89 to 95%).

**Biotransformation**
Hepatic; extensive, by hydroxylation.

**Half-life**
Biphasic. More rapid, 3 to 6 hours; slower, 5 to 9 hours.

**Onset of therapeutic action**
In clinical trials, significant therapeutic results occurred after 2 weeks of therapy in 75% of the patients responsive to the medication, with some patients showing definite improvement after 1 week of therapy; 25% of the responding patients required 2 to 4 weeks of therapy before noticeable improvement occurred.

**Time to peak concentration**
Fasting, 1 hour; with food, 2 hours.

**Elimination**
Biliary—
   20%
Renal—
   75%, mostly as inactive metabolites.

# Precautions to Consider

**Carcinogenicity**
No evidence of carcinogenicity was observed in rats receiving up to 300 mg per kg of body weight (mg/kg) a day for 18 months.

**Pregnancy/Reproduction**
Pregnancy—Studies in humans have not been done.
Studies in animals have shown that trazodone causes congenital anomalies and increased fetal resorptions when given in doses up to 50 times those used in humans.
FDA Pregnancy Category C.

**Breast-feeding**
Problems in humans have not been documented; however, trazodone and its metabolites have been shown to be present in human milk and in the milk of lactating test animals.

**Pediatrics**
Appropriate studies on the relationship of age to the effects of trazodone have not been performed in the pediatric population.

**Geriatrics**
Elderly patients are more likely than younger adults to experience the sedative or hypotensive effects of trazodone; therefore, initial doses as low as half the recommended adult dose should be used in elderly patients, with adjustments made as needed and tolerated.

**Dental**
Peripheral anticholinergic effects, although they occur much less frequently with trazodone than with tricyclic antidepressants, may decrease or inhibit salivary flow, especially in middle-aged or elderly patients, thus contributing to the development of caries, periodontal disease, oral candidiasis, and discomfort.

**Drug interactions and/or related problems**
The following drug interactions and/or related problems have been selected on the basis of their potential clinical significance (possible mechanism in parentheses where appropriate)—not necessarily inclusive (» = major clinical significance):

Note: Combinations containing any of the following medications, depending on the amount present, may also interact with this medication.

» Alcohol or
» Central nervous system (CNS) depression–producing medications, other (See *Appendix II*)
   (concurrent use with trazodone may result in potentiation of CNS depressant effects)

Anticholinergics or other medications with anticholinergic activity (See *Appendix II*) or
Antidyskinetics or
Antihistamines
   (concurrent use with trazodone may intensify anticholinergic effects because of secondary anticholinergic activities of trazodone)
   (also, concurrent use of trazodone with antihistamines may potentiate the CNS depressant effects of either medication)

Antidepressants, tricyclic or
Haloperidol or
Loxapine or
Maprotiline or
Molindone or
Phenothiazines or
Pimozide or
Thioxanthenes
   (concurrent use may prolong and intensify the sedative and anticholinergic effects of either these medications or trazodone)

» Antihypertensives
   (concurrent use with trazodone may increase the likelihood of hypotension; dosage reduction of the antihypertensive medication may be necessary; also, antihypertensives with CNS depressant effects, such as clonidine, guanabenz, methyldopa, metyrosine, and rauwolfia alkaloids, may potentiate CNS depression when used concurrently with trazodone)

Digoxin
   (concurrent use with trazodone may increase serum concentration of digoxin and may result in digoxin toxicity)

Phenytoin and possibly other hydantoin anticonvulsants
   (increased plasma phenytoin concentrations have been reported when phenytoin was used concurrently with trazodone; caution and close monitoring are suggested)

**Laboratory value alterations**
The following have been selected on the basis of their potential clinical significance (possible effect in parentheses where appropriate)—not necessarily inclusive (» = major clinical significance):

With physiology/laboratory test values
Leukocyte counts and
Neutrophil counts
   (may occasionally be reduced, although not enough to be clinically significant)

**Medical considerations/Contraindications**
The medical considerations/contraindications included have been selected on the basis of their potential clinical significance (reasons given in parentheses where appropriate)—not necessarily inclusive (» = major clinical significance).

*Except under special circumstances, this medication should not be used when the following medical problem exists:*

» Myocardial infarction, during the acute recovery period

*Risk-benefit should be considered when the following medical problems exist:*

Alcoholism, active
   (possible excessive CNS depression)
» Cardiac disease, especially arrhythmias
   (ventricular arrhythmias, premature ventricular contractions, and ventricular tachycardia may be potentiated)
» Hepatic function impairment
   (possible serum trazodone accumulation resulting in potentiation of side effects)
» Renal function impairment
   (may result in prolonged trazodone effects)
Sensitivity to trazodone

**Patient monitoring**
The following may be especially important in patient monitoring (other tests may be warranted in some patients, depending on condition; » = major clinical significance):

Cardiac function
   (monitoring is recommended, especially for patients with pre-existing cardiac disease; reports indicate that trazodone may initiate arrhythmias, including isolated premature ventricular contractions [PVC], ventricular couplets, and short episodes of ventricular tachycardia, in such patients)

Careful supervision of depressed patients with suicidal tendencies
   (recommended especially during early weeks of treatment; hospitalization may be required as a protective measure)

Leukocyte and neutrophil counts
   (recommended particularly during extended treatment or if symptoms of systemic infection such as fever and sore throat develop; trazodone should be discontinued if patient's leukocyte or absolute neutrophil counts fall below normal)

# Side/Adverse Effects

The following side/adverse effects have been selected on the basis of their potential clinical significance (possible signs and symptoms in parentheses where appropriate)—not necessarily inclusive:

**Those indicating need for medical attention**
Incidence less frequent
   *CNS effects* (confusion; muscle tremors)
Incidence rare
   *Allergic reaction* (skin rash); *fast or slow heartbeat; hypotension* (fainting); *priapism* (prolonged, painful, inappropriate penile erection); *unusual excitement*

Note: When *abnormal erectile activity* occurs, the patient should be advised to discontinue medication immediately and consult with physician.

**Those indicating need for medical attention only if they continue or are bothersome**
Incidence more frequent
*Dizziness or lightheadedness; drowsiness; dryness of mouth, usually mild; headache; nausea and vomiting; unpleasant taste*

Incidence less frequent or rare
*Blurred vision; constipation; diarrhea; muscle aches or pains; unusual tiredness or weakness*

## Overdose

For specific information on the agents used in the management of trazodone overdose, see:
- *Charcoal, Activated (Oral-Local)* monograph.

For more information on the management of overdose or unintentional ingestion, **contact a Poison Control Center** (see *Poison Control Center Listing*).

**Clinical effects of overdose**
The following effects have been selected on the basis of their potential clinical significance (possible signs and symptoms in parentheses were appropriate)—not necessarily inclusive:

*Drowsiness; loss of muscle coordination; nausea and vomiting*

**Treatment of overdose**
There is no specific antidote for trazodone. Treatment may include:
To decrease absorption—
  Emptying stomach by gastric lavage.
  Administering activated charcoal slurry followed by a stimulant cathartic.
To enhance elimination—
  Forced diuresis may be helpful.
Supportive care—
  Maintaining respiratory and cardiac function.
  Providing symptomatic and supportive treatment in the event of hypotension or excessive sedation.
  Patients in whom intentional overdose is known or suspected should be referred for psychiatric consultation.

## Patient Consultation

As an aid to patient consultation, refer to *Advice for the Patient, Trazodone (Systemic)*.

In providing consultation, consider emphasizing the following selected information (» = major clinical significance):

**Before using this medication**
» Conditions affecting use, especially:
    Sensitivity to trazodone
    Pregnancy—Animal studies have shown congenital anomalies and increased fetal resorptions with large doses
    Breast-feeding—Excreted in breast milk
    Use in the elderly—Elderly are more prone to develop sedative and hypotensive effects
    Dental—Dry mouth may result in caries, periodontal disease, oral candidiasis, and discomfort
    Other medications, especially alcohol or other CNS depression–producing medications, or antihypertensives
    Other medical problems, especially myocardial infarction, arrhythmias or other cardiac disease, hepatic function impairment, or renal function impairment

**Proper use of this medication**
    Taking with or soon after a meal or light snack to minimize stomach upset and dizziness or lightheadedness
» Compliance with therapy
» May require up to 4 weeks to produce significant therapeutic results, although 75% of responding patients benefit within 2 weeks
» Proper dosing
    Missed dose: Taking as soon as possible; not taking if within 4 hours of next scheduled dose; not doubling doses
» Proper storage

**Precautions while using this medication**
    Regular visits to physician to check progress during therapy
» Checking with physician before discontinuing medication; gradual dosage reduction may be needed
» Caution if any kind of surgery, dental treatment, or emergency treatment is required
» Avoiding use of alcohol or other CNS depressants during therapy
» Possible drowsiness; caution when driving or doing other things requiring alertness

» Possible dizziness; caution when getting up suddenly from a lying or sitting position
    Possible dryness of mouth; using sugarless gum or candy, ice, or saliva substitute for relief; checking with physician or dentist if dry mouth continues for more than 2 weeks

**Side/adverse effects**
    Sedative and hypotensive side effects more likely to occur in the elderly
    Priapism may occur; discontinuing medication and checking with physician immediately
    Signs of potential side effects, especially CNS effects, fast or slow heartbeat, hypotension, priapism, unusual excitement, or allergic reaction

## General Dosing Information

Dosage of trazodone must be individualized for each patient by titration.

Potentially suicidal patients should not have access to large quantities of this medication since depressed patients, particularly those who may use alcohol excessively, may continue to exhibit suicidal tendencies until significant improvement occurs. Some clinicians recommend that the patient be supplied with the least amount of medication necessary for satisfactory patient management.

Daily dosage should be divided into at least two doses, because of trazodone's short elimination half-life. Trazodone should not be given as a single daily dose.

When side effects such as excessive drowsiness or dizziness might be bothersome or dangerous during waking hours, a larger portion (about two-thirds) of the total daily dose may be given at bedtime, with the balance being administered in the morning or during the day in divided doses.

To avoid a possible increase in side effects or aggravation of the patient's condition, any change or discontinuation of dosage should be accomplished gradually.

**Diet/Nutrition**
Each dose is best taken with or shortly after a meal or light snack. Food reduces the incidence and severity of side effects such as nausea or dizziness, by slowing trazodone's rate of absorption, decreasing the maximum concentration, and lengthening the time to maximum concentration.

**For treatment of priapism**
Treatment may include
- In patients with mild or no ischemia (as differentiated by intracorporeal blood gas and pressure monitoring)—Irrigation of the corpora with metaraminol or epinephrine.
- In patients with severe ischemia—Stagnant blood should be evacuated and a shunt procedure performed to allow metabolic replenishment of tissue.

## Oral Dosage Forms

### TRAZODONE HYDROCHLORIDE TABLETS USP

Note: The dosing and strengths of the dosage forms available are expressed in terms of trazodone hydrochloride.

**Usual adult and adolescent dose**
Antidepressant—
    Oral, initially 150 mg a day in divided doses, the dosage being increased by 50 mg per day at three- or four-day intervals, as needed and tolerated.

**Usual adult prescribing limits**
Outpatients—
    Up to 400 mg a day.
Inpatients—
    Up to 600 mg a day.

**Usual pediatric dose**
Antidepressant—
    Children up to 6 years of age: Dosage has not been established.
    Children 6 to 18 years of age: Oral, initially 1.5 to 2 mg per kg of body weight a day in divided doses, the dosage being increased gradually at three- or four-day intervals as needed and tolerated up to a maximum of 6 mg per kg of body weight a day.

**Usual geriatric dose**
Antidepressant—
    Oral, initially 75 mg a day in divided doses, the dosage being increased gradually at three- or four-day intervals, as needed and tolerated.

**Strength(s) usually available**
U.S.—
    50 mg (Rx) [*Desyrel* (scored); *Trazon; Trialodine* [GENERIC].
    100 mg (Rx) [*Desyrel* (scored); *Trazon; Trialodine* [GENERIC].

150 mg (Rx) [*Desyrel* (scored) [GENERIC].
300 mg (Rx) [*Desyrel* (scored) [GENERIC].
Canada—
  50 mg (Rx) [*Desyrel* (scored)].
  100 mg (Rx) [*Desyrel* (scored)].
  150 mg (Rx) [*Desyrel* (scored)].

**Packaging and storage**
Store below 40 °C (104 °F), preferably between 15 and 30 °C (59 and 86 °F), in a tight, light-resistant container, unless otherwise specified by manufacturer.

**Auxiliary labeling**
• May cause drowsiness.
• Avoid alcoholic beverages.
• Take with or immediately after food.

**Additional information**
The 150-mg tablet may be broken to yield doses of 50, 75, or 100 mg.
The 300-mg tablet may be broken to yield three 100-mg doses, two 150-mg doses, or one 200-mg dose.

Revised: 01/13/93
Interim revision: 01/19/95

# TRETINOIN   Systemic—INTRODUCTORY VERSION

VA CLASSIFICATION (Primary): AN900
Commonly used brand name(s): *Vesanoid*.
Note: For a listing of dosage forms and brand names by country availability, see *Dosage Forms* section(s).

## Category
Antineoplastic.

## Indications
**Accepted**
Leukemia, acute promyelocytic (treatment)—Tretinoin is indicated for induction of remission in patients with acute promyelocytic leukemia (APL) (French-American-British [FAB] subtype M3, including the M3 variant, of acute myelocytic leukemia. Responses to tretinoin have not been observed in patients who lack the genetic marker characteristic of APL, i.e., the t(15;17) translocation that produces the PML/RAR*alpha* gene; other treatment should be considered for patients in whom a diagnosis of APL cannot be confirmed by detection of t(15;17) translocation or PML/RAR*alpha* fusion. Tretinoin should be used only for patients who are refractory to, or who have relapsed from, anthracycline-based chemotherapy, or for whom anthracycline-based chemotherapy is contraindicated.
Note: After induction therapy with tretinoin has been completed, the patient should receive appropriate remission consolidation and/or maintenance therapy with other agent(s).

## Pharmacology/Pharmacokinetics
**Physicochemical characteristics**
Chemical group—Tretinoin (all-*trans* retinoic acid) is a retinoid chemically related to retinol (Vitamin A).
Molecular weight—300.44.

**Mechanism of action/Effect**
The precise mechanism of action has not been established. Tretinoin is not a cytolytic agent. It induces cytodifferentiation and decreases proliferation of acute promyelocytic leukemia cells. In patients who achieve complete remission, tretinoin therapy results in an initial maturation of the primitive promyelocytes derived from the leukemic clone, followed by a repopulation of the bone marrow and peripheral blood with normal, polyclonal hematopoietic cells.

**Absorption**
Tretinoin is well absorbed after oral administration. Whether coadministration with food affects tretinoin absorption has not been established. However, administration with food has been shown to enhance absorption of other retinoids.

**Protein binding**
Very high (> 95%), primarily to albumin.

**Biotransformation**
Hepatic, via oxidative metabolism by cytochrome *P*-450 (CYP) enzymes. Tretinoin probably induces its own metabolism; after 1 week of continuous therapy, the plasma concentration and the area under the tretinoin concentration–time curve (AUC) are substantially lower than on the first day of treatment.

**Half-life**
Elimination—0.5 to 2 hours.

**Time to peak plasma concentration:**
1 to 2 hours after an oral dose.

**Peak plasma concentration:**
Following a single oral dose of 45 mg per square meter of body surface area (mg/m$^2$)—347 ± 266 nanograms/mL.
Note: In a study in seven patients, plasma concentrations determined after 1 week of treatment with 45 mg/m$^2$ per day were approximately one-third of those measured on Day 1 of treatment.

**Time to peak effect**
Median time to complete remission in clinical trials was 40 to 50 days (range, 2 to 120 days).

**Elimination**
Renal and fecal; in studies using radiolabeled tretinoin, approximately 63% of the radioactivity was recovered in the urine within 72 hours and 31% in the feces within 6 days.

## Precautions to Consider
**Cross-sensitivity and/or related problems**
Patients sensitive to other retinoids may be sensitive to tretinoin also.

**Carcinogenicity/Tumorigenicity**
Long-term studies in animals have not been done. In short-term studies in mice receiving 30 mg per kg of body weight (mg/kg) per day (approximately twice the human dose on a mg per square meter of body surface area [mg/m$^2$] basis), tretinoin increased the rate of diethylnitrosamine-induced hepatic adenomas and carcinomas.

**Mutagenicity**
No evidence of mutagenicity was found in the Ames and Chinese hamster V79 cell HGPRT tests. Tretinoin produced a twofold increase in sister chromatid exchange in human diploid fibroblasts. However, no clastogenic or aneuploidogenic effect was demonstrated in other chromosome aberration assays, including an *in vitro* assay in human peripheral lymphocytes and an *in vivo* mouse micronucleus test.

**Pregnancy/Reproduction**
Fertility—Tretinoin caused increased fetal resorptions in all animal species studied (mice, rats, hamsters, rabbits, and pigtail monkeys), but caused no other adverse effects on fertility or on reproductive performance in rats given up to 5 mg/kg per day (approximately two-thirds the human dose on a mg/m$^2$ basis). Testicular degeneration and increased numbers of immature spermatozoa were observed in a 6-week study in dogs receiving 10 mg/kg per day (approximately 4 times the human dose on a mg/m$^2$ basis).
Pregnancy—Adequate and well-controlled studies with tretinoin have not been done in humans, but other retinoids have caused spontaneous abortions and major fetal abnormalities. Reported defects, some of which were fatal, include abnormalities of the central nervous system (CNS), musculoskeletal system, external ear, thymus, eye, and great vessels; facial dysmorphia; cleft palate; parathyroid hormone deficiency; and cases of below-average intelligence (intelligence quotient lower than 85) with or without apparent CNS abnormalities. **There is a high risk of a severely deformed infant being born to a woman receiving tretinoin during pregnancy.**
Administration of tretinoin to a female patient requires that the following criteria be met:
• Two reliable forms of contraception should be used simultaneously during, and for 1 month after discontinuation of, tretinoin therapy. Contraception should be used even after menopause, unless a hysterectomy has been performed.
• Pregnancy testing using a highly sensitive test should be performed within 1 week before treatment is started. If possible, treatment should be delayed until the test results are available. If treatment cannot be delayed, the patient should be placed on two forms of contraception.
• The patient must receive full information and warnings about the risk to the fetus if she becomes pregnant, the possibility of contraception

failure, and the need to use two forms of contraception simultaneously during and following treatment. Proof that the patient understands and acknowledges the need for using two methods of contraception simultaneously should be obtained.
- Pregnancy testing and contraception counseling should be repeated on a monthly basis during treatment.

If a patient becomes pregnant during tretinoin therapy, the physician and patient should discuss the advisability of continuing or terminating the pregnancy.

Tretinoin demonstrated teratogenic and embryotoxic effects and caused a decrease in the number of live fetuses in all animal species studied (mice, rats, hamsters, rabbits, and pigtail monkeys). Gross external, soft tissue, and skeletal abnormalities occurred with doses higher than 0.7 mg/kg per day in mice, 2 mg/kg per day in rats, and 7 mg/kg per day in hamsters, and with a dose of 10 mg/kg per day (the only dose studied) in pigtail monkeys. These doses are approximately equivalent to one-twentieth, one-fourth, one-half, and four times the human dose on a mg/m$^2$ basis, respectively.

FDA Pregnancy Category D.

### Breast-feeding
It is not known whether tretinoin is distributed into breast milk. However, because of the risk of serious adverse effects in nursing infants, it is recommended that breast-feeding be discontinued prior to initiation of tretinoin therapy.

### Pediatrics
Patients younger than 1 year of age: Safety and efficacy have not been established.

Patients 1 year of age and older: Clinical data in pediatric patients is limited. Fifteen patients 1 to 16 years of age received tretinoin in clinical trials. Complete remission was achieved in 10 patients (67%). However, particular caution is recommended when tretinoin is administered to children because the risk of retinoid-induced severe headache and pseudotumor cerebri is higher in this age group than in adults. Also, studies have shown that the maximal tolerated dose is lower in children than in adults (60 mg/m$^2$ per day versus 195 mg/m$^2$ per day, respectively). A reduction in dose may be considered if serious and/or intolerable toxicity occurs during treatment. However, the efficacy and safety of tretinoin in doses lower than 45 mg/m$^2$ per day have not been evaluated in pediatric patients.

### Drug interactions and/or related problems
The following drug interactions and/or related problems have been selected on the basis of their potential clinical significance (possible mechanism in parentheses where appropriate)—not necessarily inclusive (» = major clinical significance):

Note: Combinations containing any of the following medications, depending on the amount present, may also interact with this medication.

» Enzyme inducers, hepatic (see *Appendix II*)
(inducers of hepatic cytochrome *P*-450 [CYP] enzymes, such as glucocorticoids, pentobarbital, phenobarbital, and rifampin, may alter the pharmacokinetics of tretinoin; however, whether concurrent use of a hepatic CYP enzyme inducer alters the safety or efficacy of tretinoin has not been established)

» Enzyme inhibitors, hepatic (see *Appendix II*), especially
» Ketoconazole
(administration of 400 to 1000 mg of ketoconazole 1 hour prior to administration of tretinoin on the 29th day of tretinoin therapy resulted in a 72% increase in the mean area under the tretinoin concentration–time curve [AUC]; other medications that generally inhibit hepatic CYP enzymes, such as cimetidine, cyclosporine, diltiazem, erythromycin, and verapamil, may also alter the pharmacokinetics of tretinoin. However, whether concurrent use of a hepatic CYP enzyme inhibitor alters the safety or efficacy of tretinoin has not been established)

### Laboratory value alterations
The following have been selected on the basis of their potential clinical significance (possible effect in parentheses where appropriate)—not necessarily inclusive (» = major clinical significance):

With physiology/laboratory test values
» Cholesterol, serum, and
» Triglycerides, serum
(concentrations were increased in up to 60% of tretinoin-treated patients in clinical trials, but usually returned to pretreatment values after discontinuation of therapy; although the risks of temporary elevations of cholesterol and triglyceride concentrations have not been established, venous thrombosis and myocardial infarction have been reported in patients considered to be at low risk of developing these conditions)

Hepatic function tests
(elevated hepatic function test results occurred in 50 to 60% of tretinoin-treated patients in clinical trials, but values generally returned to normal during or following completion of therapy)
» Leukocyte count
(a rapidly evolving increase in leukocyte count may occur during treatment, especially in patients with pre-existing leukocytosis)

### Medical considerations/Contraindications
The medical considerations/contraindications included have been selected on the basis of their potential clinical significance (reasons given in parentheses where appropriate)—not necessarily inclusive (» = major clinical significance).

*Risk-benefit should be considered when the following medical problems exist:*

» Leukocytosis, pre-existing (leukocyte count > 5 x 10$^9$/L)
(high risk of further rapid increase in leukocyte count during therapy, which increases the risk of life-threatening complications, especially the retinoic acid–acute promyelocytic leukemia [RA-APL] syndrome; institution of concurrent full-dose chemotherapy, including an anthracycline if not contraindicated, on Day 1 or Day 2 of tretinoin treatment may decrease the risk of the RA-APL syndrome and should be considered for patients with pre-existing leukocytosis)

» Sensitivity to tretinoin or other retinoids
Sensitivity to parabens

### Patient monitoring
The following may be especially important in patient monitoring (other tests may be warranted in some patients, depending on condition; » = major clinical significance):

Cholesterol concentrations and
Triglyceride concentrations
(should be monitored frequently during therapy)

Hematopoietic profile, especially
» White blood cell (WBC) count
(should be monitored frequently during therapy; rapidly evolving leukocytosis occurs in approximately 40% of patients during tretinoin treatment, which increases the risk of life-threatening complications, especially the RA-APL syndrome. If the WBC count reaches ≥ 6 x 10$^9$/L by Day 5, ≥ 10 x 10$^9$/L by Day 10, or ≥ 15 x 10$^9$/L by Day 28 of tretinoin therapy, immediate institution of full-dose chemotherapy, including an anthracycline if not contraindicated, may decrease the risk of the RA-APL syndrome and should be considered)

» Hepatic function
(should be monitored frequently during therapy; although abnormalities detected in clinical trials usually resolved during or after treatment, approximately 3% of the patients developed hepatitis. Temporary withdrawal of tretinoin should be considered if hepatic function test values are elevated to more than five times the upper limit of normal)

## Side/Adverse Effects

Note: Almost all patients will experience tretinoin-related adverse effects during treatment, especially fatigue, fever, headache, and weakness. These effects are seldom permanent and generally do not require interruption of therapy.

In addition to the adverse effects listed below, adverse events that are common in patients with acute promyelocytic leukemia were reported in clinical trials, including hemorrhage (incidence 60%), infections (incidence 58%), gastrointestinal bleeding (incidence 34%), disseminated intravascular coagulation (incidence 26%), pneumonia (incidence 14%), cerebral hemorrhage (incidence 9%), hepatosplenomegaly (incidence 9%), and lymph disorders (incidence 6%).

The following side/adverse effects have been selected on the basis of their potential clinical significance (possible signs and symptoms in parentheses where appropriate)—not necessarily inclusive:

### Those indicating need for medical attention
Incidence more frequent (10% or higher)
*Abdominal distention* (swelling of abdomen); *cardiac arrhythmias* (irregular heartbeat); *earache or feeling of fullness in the ear; edema* (swelling of face, fingers, hands, feet, or lower legs); *fever; hypertension* (increase in blood pressure); *hypotension* (decrease in blood pressure); *mental depression; phlebitis* (pain and swelling in foot or leg); *renal insufficiency* (decreased urination; swelling of face, fingers, hands, feet, or lower legs); *retinoic acid–acute promyelocytic leukemia (RA-APL) syndrome* (bone pain; discomfort or pain in chest; fever;

shortness of breath, troubled breathing, tightness in chest, or wheezing; weight gain); *retinoid toxicity, including mucositis* (crusting, redness, pain, or sores in mouth or nose; cracked lips); *ocular disorders and visual disturbances* (any change in vision); *respiratory tract disorders* (coughing, sneezing, sore throat, stuffy or runny nose); *and skin rash*

Note: The *RA-APL syndrome* occurs in approximately 25% of tretinoin-treated patients and is characterized, in addition to the symptoms listed above, by radiographic pulmonary infiltrates and pleural and/or pericardial effusions. This syndrome has resulted in impaired myocardial contractility, episodic hypotension, progressive hypoxemia requiring respiratory assistance, and fatalities due to multiorgan failure. This complication usually occurs during the first month of treatment; a few cases have appeared following the first dose of tretinoin. Although the RA-APL syndrome may occur without concomitant leukocytosis, the risk may be increased if rapidly evolving leukocytosis occurs during treatment.

Incidence less frequent (3 to 9%)
*Bronchial asthma* (shortness of breath, troubled breathing, tightness in chest, or wheezing); *cardiac failure* (chest pain; shortness of breath or troubled breathing); *cellulitis* (swollen area that feels warm and tender); *coma* (loss of consciousness); *convulsions; dementia* (mood, mental, or personality changes); *difficult or painful urination; flank pain* (pain in lower back or side); *fluid imbalance; gastrointestinal tract ulcer* (cramping or pain in stomach, severe; heartburn, indigestion, or nausea, severe and continuing); *hallucinations; hearing loss*—may rarely be irreversible; *hepatitis or other hepatic disorder* (yellow eyes or skin); *laryngeal edema* (shortness of breath or troubled breathing); *myocardial infarction* (feeling of heaviness in chest; pain in back, chest, or left arm; shortness of breath or troubled breathing); *pseudotumor cerebri* (headache, severe; nausea and vomiting; papilledema; vision problems)—especially in children; *renal failure, acute* (decreased urination; swelling of face, hands, fingers, feet, or lower legs); *renal tubular necrosis; somnolence* (drowsiness, very severe and continuing); *stroke* (difficulty in speaking, slow speech, or inability to speak; inability to move arms, legs, or facial muscles)

**Those indicating need for medical attention only if they continue or are bothersome**
Incidence more frequent
*Anxiety; confusion; constipation; diarrhea; dizziness; flushing; general feeling of discomfort or illness; indigestion; insomnia* (trouble sleeping); *loss of appetite; muscle pain; paresthesia* (burning, crawling, or tingling feeling in the skin); *retinoid effects* (dryness of skin, mouth, or nose; hair loss; headache; itching of skin; nausea and vomiting); *shivering; weight loss*

Incidence less frequent
*Agitation* (anxiety and restlessness); *agnosia; clumsiness or unsteadiness when walking; forgetfulness; frequent urination; weakness in legs; trembling, sometimes with a flapping movement*

## Overdose

For information on the management of overdose or unintentional ingestion, **contact a Poison Control Center** (see *Poison Control Center listing*). There is no experience with acute overdose of tretinoin in humans. Overdose of other retinoids has caused symptoms such as abdominal pain, ataxia, cheilosis, dizziness, facial flushing, and transient headache. These symptoms resolved without apparent residual effects.

## Patient Consultation

As an aid to patient consultation, refer to *Advice for the Patient, Tretinoin (Systemic—Introductory Version)*.

In providing consultation, consider emphasizing the following selected information (» = major clinical significance):

**Before taking this medication**
» Conditions affecting use, especially:
   Sensitivity to tretinoin or other retinoids
   Pregnancy—High risk of fetal abnormalities if taken during pregnancy; need to use two effective methods of birth control simultaneously during and for 1 month following therapy
   Breast-feeding—Discontinuing breast-feeding prior to treatment because of the risk of adverse effects in nursing infants
   Use in children—Higher risk of severe headache and pseudotumor cerebri during treatment
   Other medications, especially hepatic enzyme inducers or inhibitors

**Proper use of this medication**
» Compliance with therapy; not taking more medication than the amount prescribed
» Proper dosing
   Missed dose: Taking as soon as possible; checking with physician if not remembered until almost time for next dose
» Proper storage

**Precautions while using this medication**
» Importance of regular visits to physician during therapy
» Continuing to take medication despite occurrence of expected side effects, such as fever, headache, tiredness, and weakness
» Notifying physician immediately if symptoms of retinoic acid–acute promyelocytic (RA-APL) syndrome or pseudotumor cerebri occur

**Side/adverse effects**
Notifying physician immediately if fever or symptoms of RA-APL syndrome, bronchial asthma, cardiac failure, convulsions, laryngeal edema, myocardial infarction, pseudotumor cerebri, or stroke occur
Signs of other potential side effects, especially abdominal distention, cardiac arrhythmias, earache or feeling of fullness in the ear, edema, hypertension, hypotension, mental depression, phlebitis, renal insufficiency, retinoid toxicity, cellulitis, dementia, difficult or painful urination, flank pain, gastrointestinal tract ulcer, hallucinations, hearing loss, hepatitis or other hepatic disorder, and somnolence

## General Dosing Information

Tretinoin is to be used only under the supervision of a physician experienced in the management of patients with acute leukemia. Use of this medication also requires the availability of laboratory and supportive services capable of monitoring drug tolerance and treating a patient compromised by drug toxicity, including respiratory impairment.

After remission has been achieved with tretinoin, the patient should receive a standard consolidation and/or maintenance chemotherapy regimen for acute promyelocytic leukemia, unless otherwise contraindicated.

**For treatment of adverse effects**
For the retinoic acid–acute promyelocytic leukemia syndrome: High-dose corticosteroid treatment may reduce morbidity and mortality. It is recommended that such therapy (e.g., 10 mg of dexamethasone intravenously every 12 hours for 3 days or until symptoms abate) be initiated at the first signs and symptoms suggestive of this complication. Discontinuation of tretinoin therapy is usually not necessary.

## Oral Dosage Forms

### TRETINOIN CAPSULES

**Usual adult and adolescent dose**
Leukemia, acute promyelocytic—
   Oral, 45 mg per square meter of body surface area per day, administered in two evenly divided doses. Treatment should be continued for thirty days after complete remission has been achieved or for a maximum of ninety days, whichever occurs first.

**Usual pediatric dose**
Leukemia, acute promyelocytic—
   See *Usual adult and adolescent dose*. A decrease in the dose may be considered for patients who experience serious or intolerable toxicity. However, the efficacy and safety of lower doses have not been established.

**Strength(s) usually available**
U.S.—
   10 mg (Rx) [*Vesanoid* (beeswax; butylated hydroxyanisole; edetate disodium; hydrogenated soybean oil flakes; hydrogenated vegetable oils and soybean oil; glycerin; yellow iron oxide; red iron oxide; titanium dioxide; methylparaben; propylparaben)].

**Packaging and storage**
Store between 15 and 30 °C (59 and 86 °F).

Developed: 07/03/96

# TRETINOIN Topical

VA CLASSIFICATION (Primary/Secondary):
  Oil-in-water cream—DE752/DE500
  Water-in-oil cream—DE900
  Gel—DE752/DE500
  Solution—DE752/DE500

Commonly used brand name(s): *Avita; Renova; Retin-A; Retin-A MICRO; Retisol-A; Stieva-A; Stieva-A Forte; Vitamin A Acid; Vitinoin.*

Some commonly used names are retinoic acid, all-*trans*-retinoic acid, and vitamin A acid.

Note: For a listing of dosage forms and brand names by country availability, see *Dosage Forms* section(s).

## Category

Antiacne agent (topical)—Cream (oil-in-water); Gel; Solution; Keratolytic (topical)—Cream (oil-in-water); Gel; Solution; Hypopigmenting agent (topical)—Cream (water-in-oil); Photoaging mitigative agent (topical)—Cream (water-in-oil).

## Indications

Note: Bracketed information in the *Indications* section refers to uses that are not included in U.S. product labeling.

**Accepted**

Acne vulgaris (treatment)—Tretinoin cream (oil-in-water formulation), gel, and topical solution are indicated in the topical treatment of acne vulgaris. Although use of tretinoin alone is effective in the topical treatment of mild acne vulgaris (Grades I to III), the therapeutic effect may be increased when tretinoin is used in combination with topical antibiotics or benzoyl peroxide when acne consists predominately of comedones, papules, and pustules. Tretinoin may be used with systemic antibiotics for treatment of all grades of acne, including severe (Grade IV) acne conglobata; however, tretinoin is not effective when used alone for severe acne conglobata. The water-in-oil formulation of the cream is not indicated for treatment of acne vulgaris.

Hyperpigmentation, mottled, facial, due to photoaging (treatment adjunct) or
Skin roughness, facial, due to photoaging (treatment adjunct) or
Wrinkling, fine facial, due to photoaging (treatment adjunct)—The water-in-oil formulation of tretinoin cream is indicated as palliative or adjunctive treatment to skin care and sun avoidance programs to lessen the roughness of facial skin, reduce hyperpigmentation, and decrease the number and severity of fine facial wrinkles caused by photoaging. Although studies to prevent photoaging were conducted with the water-in-oil formulation, there is no reason to expect other formulations to be inactive. Patients who have been compliant but unsuccessful when using skin care and sun avoidance programs alone may benefit by adding tretinoin to the regimen. Skin care and sun avoidance programs include use of sunscreens, protective clothing, and moisturizing lotions or creams. Tretinoin improves the histological process of photoaging but cannot completely repair sun-damaged skin or eliminate all wrinkles.

There are insufficient data to show tretinoin to be safe and effective for daily use longer than 48 weeks when used as a photoaging mitigative agent. Although the clinical significance is not known, some patients using the water-in-oil formulation of tretinoin cream 0.05% for longer than 48 weeks have experienced adverse effects, such as increased dermal elastosis and atypical changes in melanocytes and keratinocytes. Safety and efficacy have not been established for patients 50 years of age and older, for patients with a history of skin cancer, or for patients who have moderately to heavily pigmented skin.

[Keratosis follicularis (treatment)][1] or
[Verruca plana (treatment)][1]—Tretinoin as an oil-in-water cream, a gel, or a solution is used to treat disorders of keratinization, such as keratosis follicularis (Darier's disease, Darier-White disease), and verruca plana (flat warts).

**Acceptance not established**

The safety and efficacy of topical tretinoin for the treatment or prevention of *actinic keratoses* or *skin neoplasms* have not been established.

**Unaccepted**

Tretinoin is not indicated for and does not reduce coarse or deep wrinkling, skin yellowing, telangiectasia, skin laxity, melanocytic atypia, or dermal elastosis.

---

[1] Not included in Canadian product labeling.

## Pharmacology/Pharmacokinetics

**Physicochemical characteristics**

Molecular weight—300.44.
Chemical names—Retinoic acid or all-*trans*-retinoic acid.
Description—Aqueous gel formulation: Tretinoin is adsorbed on an acrylate copolymer, rendering the active ingredient water-soluble. May be referred to as a microsphere or microsponge system by the manufacturer.

**Mechanism of action/Effect**

The exact mechanism of tretinoin, a hormone and vitamin A analog, is not known. One possible explanation is altered gene expression causing changes in protein synthesis. Tretinoin diffuses across cell membranes and complexes with specific cytoplasmic receptors, which can then enter the cell's nucleus and bind to DNA. Depending on the tissue, either a transcription process begins—messenger RNA (mRNA) increases and results in subsequent protein synthesis—or transrepression occurs. Transrepression results when the hormone-receptor complex (i.e., cytoplasmic tretinoin receptor) cannot activate the gene transcription factors or the hormone-response element. When gene expression is suppressed, protein synthesis cannot occur. Transrepression is thought to contribute to the photoaging mitigative and hypopigmenting effects.

Antiacne agent or keratolytic agent—
  By stimulating the transcription process, tretinoin increases epidermal cell mitosis and epidermal cell turnover. The increased permeability of the skin causes water loss and weakens the horny cell layer, making it less cohesive and easier to peel. This action facilitates the removal of existing comedones and may inhibit the formation of new comedones. It has been proposed that increased turnover in the follicular epithelium prevents formation of keratinous plugs. Tretinoin has also been reported to suppress keratin synthesis.

Photoaging mitigative agent—
  Pretreatment of the skin with tretinoin inhibits a sun-induced effect of stimulating the gene transcription factor, AP-I. This transrepression effect stops the sun-induced production of the metalloproteinase enzymes, which responsively remove cells that potentially may be harmed by ultraviolet light from the skin's matrix. Tretinoin does not appreciably absorb ultraviolet light, cannot be regarded as a sunscreen, and will not protect the skin from redness. In addition, tretinoin is thought to increase the growth and differentiation of various epithelial cells, increase the glycosaminoglycan-like substance in the compacted stratum corneum, increase the number of anchoring fibrils, and improve epidermal dysplastic changes. Some studies showed no appreciable change in collagen or elastin tissue content in human skin; other studies did show an increase in collagen content.

  Whether tretinoin reverses, partially reverses, or only helps to mitigate the damage associated with ultraviolet light exposure is still considered controversial. This is partly because attentive skin care measures (sunscreens, protective clothing, moisturizers, mild soaps, and sun avoidance programs) used in the protocol of these studies also contributed to the overall efficacy against photoaging; even the placebo cream contributed positive effects. The long-term effects of suppressing the removal of potentially harmed DNA by the metalloproteinase enzymes within human skin are not known.

  In a placebo-controlled study in which the water-in-oil formulation of 0.05% tretinoin cream was applied for 24 weeks, patients averaged a 27.1% reduction in fine wrinkling, 37% decrease in mottled hyperpigmentation, and 29.3% decrease in roughness of skin. Total improvement of severity was considered mild and averaged only 1 to 2 units based on a scale of 0 to 9 units.

Hypopigmenting agent—
  Tretinoin inhibits melanogenesis. Lightening occurs because tretinoin reduces the melanin content in the epidermis, compacts the stratum corneum, and thickens the epidermis; it is not a result of a change of number or size of melanocytes. Tretinoin may improve but not clearly resolve hyperpigmented skin.

**Other actions/effects**

Tretinoin has shown some activity for increased wound healing, hair growth, and some antitumor effects that still need to be established. These actions may be due to increased rates of epidermal cell turnover, angiogenesis, protein synthesis, and increased cell differentiation.

**Absorption**

Systemic absorption—Up to 8% of the administered dose of the nonaqueous formulations may be absorbed systemically with repeated application for 10 days; only 1.41% of the administered dose was absorbed with the aqueous formulations. Absorption may be increased when

## 2872  Tretinoin (Topical)

medication is applied to large surface areas, or for long periods of time in chronic extensive dermatoses.

### Duration of action
Although gradual, most patients will show some improvement in skin condition within the first 6 to 7 weeks for the treatment of acne and within 24 weeks for the treatment of photoaging.

### Elimination
Renal—4.45% of applied dose.
Biliary—1.58% of applied dose.

## Precautions to Consider

### Cross-sensitivity and/or related problems
Patients sensitive to acitretin, etretinate, isotretinoin, or other vitamin A derivatives may be sensitive to tretinoin also, since it is a vitamin A derivative.

### Carcinogenicity/Tumorigenicity
A lifetime study in CD-1 mice receiving a topical tretinoin dose of 100 and 200 times the average recommended human dose resulted in a few skin tumors in female mice and liver tumors in male mice. These tumors occurred at a rate similar to that of the untreated mice. The clinical significance of this study as related to humans is not known.

In animal (hairless albino mice) studies, tretinoin has been shown to increase the rate of cutaneous tumor formation induced by ultraviolet radiation. However, the results have not been consistently reproduced in mouse skin *in vivo* or yeast cells *in vitro* and the significance of these studies as related to humans is unknown.

Dermal carcinogenicity studies for tretinoin aqueous gel, including the copolymer component, have not been done.

### Mutagenicity
The micronucleus assay in mice and the Ames assay are negative for tretinoin.

The Ames assay for the copolymer used in the tretinoin aqueous gel is negative. The copolymer's components, when individually evaluated, were not mutagenic in one study. Other studies show the copolymer to be potentially mutagenic and teratogenic if given long-term at doses several times greater than the recommended human dose. The copolymer is not considered a significant risk to humans when used topically at recommended doses, since the tretinoin aqueous gel contains less than 25 parts per million of the copolymer.

### Pregnancy/Reproduction
Pregnancy—Adequate and well-controlled studies in humans have not been done. Although not clearly associated, 30 cases of congenital malformations have been reported for topical tretinoin during 2 decades of clinical use. Five cases showed a rare defect of incomplete midline development of the forebrain, called holoprosencephaly. It is recommended that topical tretinoin not be used during pregnancy.

Rat, mouse, and rabbit studies have not shown tretinoin to be toxic or teratogenic when subchronic topical doses were used. Topical tretinoin has been shown to be fetotoxic in rabbits given 100 times the usual topical human dose. Teratogenicity studies in Wistar rabbits given 200 times the usual topical human dose showed evidence of a shortened or kinked tail. Doses 80 times the usual human topical dose resulted in domed head and hydrocephaly in the offspring of New Zealand white rabbits. Furthermore, topical tretinoin has caused delayed ossification in a number of bones in the offspring of rats and rabbits given 100 to 320 times the usual topical human dose, respectively. However, the delayed ossification is usually corrected after weaning.

FDA Pregnancy Category C.

### Breast-feeding
It is not known whether tretinoin is distributed into breast milk. Risk-benefit should be considered.

### Pediatrics
Appropriate studies on the relationship of age to the effects of tretinoin have not been performed in the pediatric population. However, no pediatrics-specific problems have been documented to date in children 12 years of age and older.

Safety and efficacy have not been established for children up to 12 years of age for all uses of tretinoin or for children 12 years of age and older for treatment of photoaging. Problems due to photoaging are unlikely to occur in children or adolescents.

### Geriatrics
Appropriate studies on the relationship of age to the effects of tretinoin have not been performed in the geriatric population. However, no geriatrics-specific problems have been documented to date. Significant acne vulgaris is not likely to occur in this age group. Safety and efficacy have not been established for tretinoin's use in treatment of photoaging for adults 50 years of age and older.

### Drug interactions and/or related problems
The following drug interactions and/or related problems have been selected on the basis of their potential clinical significance (possible mechanism in parentheses where appropriate)—not necessarily inclusive (» = major clinical significance):

Note: Combinations containing any of the following medications, depending on the amount present, may also interact with this medication.

Acne products, topical, or topical products containing a peeling agent, such as
   Antibiotics, topical, such as
»    Clindamycin, topical
»    Erythromycin, topical
   Benzoyl peroxide
   Resorcinol
   Salicylic acid
   Sulfur or
Alcohol-containing products, topical, such as
   After-shave lotions
   Astringents
   Cosmetics or soaps with a strong drying effect
   Shaving creams or lotions or
Hair products, skin-irritating, such as hair permanents or hair removal products or
Products containing lime or spices, topical or
Soaps or cleansers, abrasive
   (concurrent use with tretinoin may cause a cumulative irritant or drying effect, especially with the application of peeling, desquamating, or abrasive agents, resulting in excessive irritation of the skin. If irritation results, the strength or dose of tretinoin may need to be reduced or temporarily discontinued until the skin is less sensitive)

   (use of benzoyl peroxide or topical antibiotics with tretinoin on the same area of the skin at the same time is not recommended. A physical incompatibility between the medications or a change in pH may reduce tretinoin's efficacy if used simultaneously. When used together for clinical effect, it is recommended that these medications be used at different times of the day, such as morning and night, to minimize possible skin irritation. If irritation results, tretinoin's strength or dose may need to be reduced or temporarily discontinued until the skin is less sensitive)

Minoxidil, topical
   (tretinoin increases the rate and extent of systemic absorption of topical minoxidil and may enhance hair growth according to preliminary studies; however, increased skin irritation may occur. Use of these medications together is not recommended)

Photosensitizing medications, such as
   Fluoroquinolones
   Phenothiazines
   Sulfonamides
   Thiazide diuretics
   (concurrent use with these medications may increase risk of photosensitivity, partly due to tretinoin's ability to induce dryness, peeling, and scaling that is especially prominent during the first several months of use; if skin becomes sunburned or irritated, the strength or dose of tretinoin may need to be reduced or temporarily discontinued until the skin is less sensitive)

Retinoids, such as
»    Acitretin
»    Etretinate
   Isotretinoin
»    Tretinoin, oral
   (retinoids are not used together due to their cumulative mucocutaneous drying or irritative effects. Rarely, isotretinoin has been used together with topical tretinoin to treat acne; however, the strength or dose of one of the retinoids may need to be reduced or one or both retinoids temporarily discontinued if skin irritation results)

### Medical considerations/Contraindications
The medical considerations/contraindications included have been selected on the basis of their potential clinical significance (reasons given in parentheses where appropriate)—not necessarily inclusive (» = major clinical significance).

***Risk-benefit should be considered when the following medical problems exist:***

Dermatitis, seborrheic or
»    Eczema
   (tretinoin may cause severe irritation)
Sensitivity to tretinoin

» Sunburn
(irritation may be increased; tretinoin should be discontinued until the skin is less sensitive)

**Patient monitoring**

The following may be especially important in patient monitoring (other tests may be warranted in some patients, depending on condition; » = major clinical significance):

Monitoring for side/adverse effects and efficacy during prolonged therapy
(recommended for patients receiving tretinoin for prolonged periods, especially for treatment of photoaging, since long-term safety has not been established beyond 48 weeks)

## Side/Adverse Effects

The following side/adverse effects have been selected on the basis of their potential clinical significance (possible signs and symptoms in parentheses where appropriate)—not necessarily inclusive:

**Those indicating need for medical attention**
Incidence more frequent
*Burning or stinging sensation of skin, severe; erythema, severe* (redness of skin, severe); *hypopigmentation of treated skin* (lightening of treated skin)—may correspond with therapeutic use; *scaling of skin, severe* (severe peeling of skin); *unusually dry skin, severe*

Note: If the retinoid reaction (*erythema, stinging, or burning sensation of skin,* and *scaling of skin*) is severe, tretinoin should be discontinued for 1 to 3 days until the symptoms subside.

Not only does *hypopigmentation* occur in hyperpigmented skin but lightening of normal pigmented skin also may be statistically significant although clinically minimal. This may be a greater concern for patients with constitutionally dark complexions.

Incidence rare
*Hyperpigmentation of treated skin* (darkening of treated skin)

**Those indicating need for medical attention only if they continue or are bothersome**
Incidence more frequent
*Burning sensation, stinging, or tingling of skin, mild*—transient upon application; *erythema, mild* (redness of skin; unusually warm skin, mild); *scaling of skin, mild* (chapping and slight peeling of skin); *unusually dry skin, mild*

Note: A mild to moderate retinoid reaction (*erythema, mild burning sensation, stinging, or tingling of skin,* and *mild scaling*) occurs within the first few weeks in more than 70 to 90% of patients using therapeutic doses. This reaction peaks within 2 weeks for the 0.05% cream and at 2 months for the 0.1% cream; symptoms may occur less often and be less severe for weaker strengths. *Unusually dry skin* and *mild scaling of skin* are more persistent, peaking at 12 to 16 weeks for the 0.05% cream.

## Patient Consultation

As an aid to patient consultation, refer to *Advice for the Patient, Tretinoin (Topical)*.

In providing consultation, consider emphasizing the following selected information (» = major clinical significance):

**Before using this medication**
» Conditions affecting use, especially:
Sensitivity to etretinate, isotretinoin, tretinoin, or vitamin A derivatives
Pregnancy—Not recommended during pregnancy; although not clearly associated, rare cases of fetal problems have occurred with topical use of tretinoin
Breast-feeding—Consulting with physician before breast-feeding.
Other medications, especially acitretin, etretinate, and oral tretinoin
Other medical problems, especially eczema and sunburn

**Proper use of this medication**
» Importance of not using more medication than the amount prescribed
» Not applying medication to windburned or sunburned skin or on open wounds
» Avoiding contact with the eyes, mouth, and nose
Reading patient directions carefully before use
*Proper administration technique*
Before applying—Washing skin with mild or nonallergenic soap or cleanser and warm water; gently patting dry; avoid harsh scrubbing of face with washcloth or sponge
» Waiting 20 to 30 minutes for complete drying of skin; applying to wet skin can cause skin irritation

*For cream or gel dosage form*
Applying very sparingly to affected areas and rubbing in gently but well; a pea-sized amount is sufficient to cover the face
*For solution dosage form*
Using fingertips, gauze pad, or cotton swab and applying very sparingly to affected areas
Not oversaturating gauze pad or cotton swab to prevent medication from running into areas not intended for treatment
Washing hands afterwards to remove any lingering medication
» Proper dosing
Missed dose: Applying next dose at regularly scheduled time; not doubling doses
» Proper storage

**Precautions while using this medication**
Possibility that skin will become irritated or that acne may appear to worsen during the first 3 weeks of therapy; checking with health care professional at any time that skin irritation becomes severe or if acne does not improve within 8 to 12 weeks
Not washing the areas of the skin treated with tretinoin for at least 1 hour after application
» Avoiding use of any topical product on the same area within 1 hour before or after application of tretinoin to avoid physical incompatibilities or excessive skin irritation; applying tretinoin at bedtime helps to avoid this when other topical products are used during the day
» Either checking with health care professional before using or avoiding use of other topical acne or skin products containing a peeling agent (benzoyl peroxide, resorcinol, salicylic acid, or sulfur), irritating hair products (permanents or hair removal products), sun-sensitizing skin products (could contain limes or spices), alcohol-containing skin products, or drying or abrasive skin products (some cosmetics or soaps or skin cleansers); sometimes benzoyl peroxide is used with tretinoin for acne treatment but is applied at different times of the day to lessen skin irritation
» Minimizing exposure of treated areas to sunlight, wind, and cold temperatures to avoid sunburn, dryness, or irritation, especially during the first 6 months of treatment with tretinoin. Also, avoiding use of artificial sunlight or sunlamp
Using sunscreen preparations (minimum sun protection factor [SPF] of 15) or wearing protective clothing over treated areas when sunlight exposure cannot be avoided
» Checking with doctor at any time skin becomes too dry or irritated; choosing proper skin product to reduce skin dryness or irritation
*For patients using tretinoin to treat acne*
Using light water-based skin products, especially regular use of moisturizers, to help reduce skin irritation or dryness
*For patients using tretinoin to treat photoaging, hyperpigmentation, or fine wrinkling*
» Complying continually with sun avoidance measures
» Using oil-based skin products, especially regular use of moisturizers, to help reduce any skin irritation or dryness resulting from weather or tretinoin

**Side/adverse effects**
The side/adverse effects of tretinoin are reversible upon discontinuation of therapy; however, hyperpigmentation or hypopigmentation may persist for months
Signs of potential side effects, especially burning or stinging sensation of skin (severe); erythema (severe); hypopigmentation of treated skin—may correspond with therapeutic effect; scaling of skin (severe); unusually dry skin (mild or severe); hyperpigmentation of treated skin

## General Dosing Information

Since tretinoin potentially can cause severe irritation and peeling, therapy may be initiated or maintained on an alternate-day or, occasionally, every-third-day regimen, preferably with the less irritating and low-concentration cream or gel dosage form. If tolerated, the more potent liquid or higher-concentration cream or gel preparation may then be used. Alcohol-containing gels and solutions are considered more potent because of the dryness produced from the volatility of their vehicles, an effect appropriate for hot, wet climates and summer months.

If severe irritation occurs, tretinoin should not be applied until the skin is healed or less irritated. Tretinoin should not be applied to mucous membranes; contact near the eyes, lips, or nose should be avoided.

Patients should be counseled on the importance of protecting the skin from the sun, wind, cold temperatures, and excessive dryness by using sunscreens of at least SPF 15, moisturizers, and protective clothing. Artificial sunlight, such as sunlamps, should be avoided.

Any topical products, medications, or agents should not be applied simultaneously but should be delayed at least 1 hour after the application of tretinoin. Topical acne products, such as antibiotics or benzoyl peroxide, are used therapeutically with tretinoin to treat acne but can increase the risk of skin irritation.

The areas to be treated should be cleansed thoroughly before the medication is applied. Using the fingertips when washing the skin helps clean the skin and remove resulting scales and peeling of skin; harsh scrubbing of skin with sponges or cloths should be avoided. Tretinoin should be applied to dry skin (20 to 30 minutes should be allowed after washing) to reduce possible skin irritation that worsens or occurs more often if tretinoin is applied any earlier to nondry skin. Treated areas of skin should not be washed for at least 1 hour after applying tretinoin. When considering dosage adjustments, a pea-sized amount (0.4 inch or 1 centimeter) is enough to cover the entire face.

### For the treatment of acne
Within the first few weeks, acne can worsen because of exacerbation of deep, previously unseen lesions. Therapeutic results may be noticeable after 2 to 3 weeks of therapy, but more so after 6 weeks, with optimal results achieved after 3 months of therapy for most patients.

### For the treatment of photoaging, hyperpigmentation, or fine wrinkling
In a dose-response study of water-in-oil tretinoin cream, the 0.01% strength was marginally effective, the 0.001% strength showed no difference from the vehicle, and the 0.05% strength provided the best clinical response. Improvement persists for at least 2 months post-therapy, followed by partial and gradual regression.

### For the treatment of keratosis follicularis
Irritation caused by tretinoin may be minimized by use of adequate, yet threshold, concentrations of tretinoin or by concurrent use of topical steroids.

### For treatment of verruca plana
In the treatment of flat warts, therapy is initiated with a weak concentration of tretinoin. If there is no response, the concentration of the tretinoin preparation and/or frequency of application should be increased.

## Topical Dosage Forms
Note: Bracketed information in the *Dosage Forms* section refers to categories of use and/or indications that are not included in U.S. product labeling.

### TRETINOIN CREAM (Oil-in-water) USP
**Usual adult and adolescent dose**
Acne vulgaris—
  Initial: Topical, to the skin of affected areas, once a day at bedtime. After the first seven to ten days of use, dose may be increased to two times a day if excessive drying of skin has not occurred.
  Maintenance: Topical, to the skin of affected areas, once a day at bedtime or less often as needed.
[Keratosis follicularis][1] or
[Verruca plana][1]—
  Topical, to the skin of affected areas, one or two times a day.

**Strength(s) usually available**
U.S.—
  0.025% (Rx) [*Retin-A* (stearyl alcohol); *Avita* (stearyl alcohol)].
  0.05% (Rx) [*Retin-A* (stearyl alcohol)].
  0.1% (Rx) [*Retin-A* (stearyl alcohol)].
Canada—
  0.01% (Rx) [*Retin-A; Retisol-A; Stieva-A* (cetyl alcohol; edetate disodium; methylparaben; propylparaben; stearyl alcohol); *Vitamin A Acid*].
  0.025% (Rx) [*Retin-A; Retisol-A* (light mineral oil; Parsol MCX 7.5%; Parsol 1789 2%; sodium hydroxide; stearyl alcohol); *Stieva-A* (cetyl alcohol; edetate disodium; methylparaben; propylparaben; stearyl alcohol); *Vitamin A Acid; Vitinoin*].
  0.05% (Rx) [*Retin-A; Retisol-A* (light mineral oil; Parsol MCX 7.5%; Parsol 1789 2%; sodium hydroxide; stearyl alcohol); *Stieva-A* (cetyl alcohol; edetate disodium; methylparaben; propylparaben; stearyl alcohol); *Vitamin A Acid; Vitinoin*].
  0.1% (Rx) [*Retin-A; Retisol-A* (light mineral oil; Parsol MCX 7.5%; Parsol 1789 2%; sodium hydroxide; stearyl alcohol); *Stieva-A Forte* (cetyl alcohol; edetate disodium; methylparaben; propylparaben; stearyl alcohol; titanium dioxide); *Vitamin A Acid; Vitinoin*].
  Note: *Retisol-A* contains sunscreens with a sun protection factor (SPF) of 15.

**Packaging and storage**
Store between 15 and 27 °C (59 and 81 °F), unless otherwise specified by manufacturer. Store in a tight, light-resistant container. Protect from freezing.

**Incompatibilities**
Tretinoin and benzoyl peroxide should not be extemporaneously combined, since there is a physical incompatibility between the two medications.

**Auxiliary labeling**
• For external use only.
• Avoid prolonged or excessive exposure to direct and/or artificial sunlight while using this medication.

**Note**
Include patient instructions when dispensing.

### TRETINOIN CREAM (Water-in-oil) USP
**Usual adult and adolescent dose**
Hyperpigmentation, mottled, facial, due to photoaging (treatment adjunct) or
Skin roughness, facial, due to photoaging (treatment adjunct) or
Wrinkling, fine facial, due to photoaging (treatment adjunct)—
  Adults up to 50 years of age: Topical, to the skin of the face, a thin film once a day, usually at bedtime.
  Adults 50 years of age and older: Safety and efficacy have not been established.
Note: Dosing is individualized to minimize irritation while maintaining efficacy. Alternate-day dosing, a smaller volume, or a weaker strength can be used initially or when skin becomes too irritated. If irritation becomes severe, tretinoin should be discontinued until irritation substantially lessens or heals.
  Safety and efficacy have not been established for daily use for more than forty-eight weeks. Some clinicians recommend only two or three applications per week following use for eight to twelve months to maintain effects.

**Usual geriatric dose**
Hyperpigmentation, mottled, facial, due to photoaging (treatment adjunct) or
Skin roughness, facial, due to photoaging (treatment adjunct) or
Wrinkling, fine facial, due to photoaging (treatment adjunct)—
  Adults 50 years of age and older: Safety and efficacy have not been established.

**Strength(s) usually available**
U.S.—
  0.05% (Rx) [*Renova* (edetate disodium; light mineral oil; methylparaben; purified water; sorbital solution; stearyl alcohol)].
Canada—
  0.05% (Rx) [*Renova* (edetate disodium; light mineral oil; methylparaben; purified water; sorbital solution; stearyl alcohol)].

**Packaging and storage**
Store between 15 and 27 °C (59 and 81 °F), unless otherwise specified by manufacturer. Store in a tight, light-resistant container. Protect from freezing.

**Incompatibilities**
Tretinoin and benzoyl peroxide should not be extemporaneously combined, since there is a physical incompatibility between the two medications.
Insoluble in water, mineral oil, and glycerin.

**Auxiliary labeling**
• For external use only.
• Avoid prolonged or excessive exposure to direct and/or artificial sunlight while using this medication.

**Note**
Include patient instructions when dispensing.
For facial use only.

### TRETINOIN GEL USP
**Usual adult and adolescent dose**
Acne vulgaris or
[Keratosis follicularis][1] or
[Verruca plana][1]—
  See *Tretinoin Cream USP (Oil-in-water)*.

**Strength(s) usually available**
U.S.—
  0.01% (alcohol-based) (Rx) [*Retin-A* (butyl alcohol 90% w/w)].
  0.025% (alcohol-based) (Rx) [*Retin-A* (butyl alcohol 90% w/w); *Avita* (ethanol 83% w/w)].
  0.1% (aqueous-based) (Rx) [*Retin-A MICRO* (benzyl alcohol; butylated hydroxytoluene; carbomer 934P; cyclomethicone and dimethicone

copolyol; disodium EDTA; glycerin; PPG-20 methyl glucose ether distearate; propylene glycol; purified water; sorbic acid)].

Canada—
- 0.01% (alcohol-based) (Rx) [*Retin-A; Stieva-A* (alcohol); *Vitamin A Acid* (methylparaben; propylparaben)].
- 0.025% (alcohol-based) (Rx) [*Retin-A; Stieva-A* (alcohol); *Vitamin A Acid* (methylparaben; propylparaben); *Vitinoin*].
- 0.05% (alcohol-based) (Rx) [*Stieva-A* (alcohol); *Vitamin A Acid* (methylparaben; propylparaben)].

Note: *Vitinoin* gel contains moisturizers.

### Packaging and storage
Store between 15 and 25 °C (59 and 77 °F) unless otherwise specified by manufacturer. Store in a tight container. Protect from light.

### Incompatibilities
Tretinoin and benzoyl peroxide should not be extemporaneously combined, since there is a physical incompatibility between the two medications.

### Auxiliary labeling
- For external use only.
- Avoid prolonged or excessive exposure to direct and/or artificial sunlight while using this medication.

### Note
Include patient instructions when dispensing.
Protect from heat and flame.

## TRETINOIN TOPICAL SOLUTION USP

### Usual adult and adolescent dose
Acne vulgaris or
[Keratosis follicularis][1] or
[Verruca plana][1]—
See *Tretinoin Cream USP (Oil-in-water)*.

### Strength(s) usually available
U.S.—
- 0.05% (Rx) [*Retin-A* (alcohol 55% w/w)].

Canada—
- 0.025% (Rx) [*Stieva-A*].
- 0.05% (Rx) [*Stieva-A*].

### Packaging and storage
Store between 15 and 30 °C (59 and 86 °F), unless otherwise specified by manufacturer. Store in a tight, light-resistant container.

### Incompatibilities
Tretinoin and benzoyl peroxide should not be extemporaneously combined, since there is a physical incompatibility between the two medications.

### Auxiliary labeling
- For external use only.
- Keep container tightly closed.
- Avoid prolonged or excessive exposure to direct and/or artificial sunlight while using this medication.

### Note
Include patient instructions when dispensing.

[1]Not included in Canadian product labeling.

## Selected Bibliography
Fisher GJ, Datta SC, Talwar HS, et al. Molecular basis of sun-induced premature skin aging and retinoid antagonism. Nature 1996 Jan 25; 379: 335-9.

Olsen EA, Katz I, Levine N, et al. Tretinoin moisturizers cream: a new therapy for photodamaged skin. J Am Acad Dermatol 1992 Feb; 26(2Pt1): 283-4.

Muller SA, Belcher RW, Esterly NB. Keratinizing dermatoses. Arch Dermatol 1977 Aug; 113(8): 1052-4.

Revised: 08/21/97
Interim revision: 04/24/98

---

**TRIAMCINOLONE**—See *Corticosteroids—Glucocorticoid Effects (Systemic); Corticosteroids (Inhalation-Local); Corticosteroids (Nasal); Corticosteroids (Topical)*

---

**TRIAMTERENE**—See *Diuretics, Potassium-sparing (Systemic)*

---

**TRIAZOLAM**—See *Benzodiazepines (Systemic)*

---

**TRICHLORMETHIAZIDE**—See *Diuretics, Thiazide (Systemic)*

---

**TRICITRATES**—See *Citrates (Systemic)*

---

# TRIENTINE Systemic†

VA CLASSIFICATION (Primary): AD300
Commonly used brand name(s): *Syprine*.
Another commonly used name is trien.
Note: For a listing of dosage forms and brand names by country availability, see *Dosage Forms* section(s).

†Not commercially available in Canada.

## Category
Chelating agent.

## Indications

### Accepted
Wilson's disease (treatment)—Trientine is indicated in the treatment of symptomatic or asymptomatic patients when treatment with penicillamine has induced a serious side-effect. Trientine appears to be as therapeutically effective as penicillamine. However, except in patients who have not been previously treated with penicillamine, molar doses of trientine generally induce less cupriuresis than does penicillamine.

### Unaccepted
Trientine is *not* recommended for treatment of cystinuria since it lacks a sulfhydryl moiety and, unlike penicillamine or tiopronin, is incapable of binding with cystine to form a stable, soluble complex that is readily excreted.

Trientine was found to be ineffective in rheumatoid arthritis after administration for 12 weeks.

Trientine is *not* recommended for primary biliary cirrhosis.

## Pharmacology/Pharmacokinetics

### Physicochemical characteristics
Molecular weight—219.2.

### Mechanism of action/Effect
Trientine chelates excess copper in the body and facilitates its excretion. More recent evidence indicates that trientine may also decrease intestinal copper absorption. However, the exact mechanism of action of trientine is unknown.

### Other actions/effects
Trientine chelates and inhibits the absorption and metabolic action of iron and possibly other heavy metals. Trientine may produce a deficiency of copper in some storage pools, despite an overall bodily excess of copper in Wilson's disease.

### Elimination
Renal and possibly fecal.

## Precautions to Consider

### Carcinogenicity/Mutagenicity
Data on carcinogenicity and mutagenicity are not available.

### Pregnancy/Reproduction
Fertility—Data on impairment of fertility are not available.

Pregnancy—Problems in humans have not been documented. There have been reports of the delivery of normal infants to mothers treated with trientine during pregnancy, with no significant copper depletion in the infants. Pregnant women may be prone to develop iron deficiency anemia during trientine therapy, possibly due to the blocking of dietary iron absorption or to the low-copper diet recommended for Wilson's disease.

Trientine was found to be teratogenic in rats when administered in doses similar to the human dose. When trientine was included in the maternal diet, the frequency of resorptions and fetal abnormalities, including hemorrhage and edema, increased as fetal copper levels decreased.

FDA Pregnancy Category C.

### Breast-feeding
It is not known if trientine is distributed into breast milk. However, problems in nursing infants have not been documented.

### Pediatrics
Children have smaller body iron stores and need to get most of their iron from dietary sources. Since copper is essential for the absorption of iron and for the formation of red blood cells, children may be more prone than adults to develop sideroblastic anemia, which is characteristic of copper deficiency, during trientine therapy.

### Geriatrics
No information is available on the relationship of age to the effects of trientine in geriatric patients.

### Drug interactions and/or related problems
The following drug interactions and/or related problems have been selected on the basis of their potential clinical significance (possible mechanism in parentheses where appropriate)—not necessarily inclusive (» = major clinical significance):

Note: Combinations containing any of the following medications, depending on the amount present, may also interact with this medication.

» Copper supplements and
» Iron supplements, and possibly other minerals
   (concomitant administration with trientine may decrease trientine's effects; if iron supplementation becomes necessary, iron may be given in short courses, with at least a 2-hour interval between administration of iron and trientine)

### Medical considerations/Contraindications
The medical considerations/contraindications included have been selected on the basis of their potential clinical significance (reasons given in parentheses where appropriate)—not necessarily inclusive (» = major clinical significance).

*Risk-benefit should be considered when the following medical problem exists:*

» Iron deficiency
   (may be potentiated)

### Patient monitoring
The following may be especially important in patient monitoring (other tests may be warranted in some patients, depending on condition; » = major clinical significance):

Body temperature determination
   (recommended nightly during first month of treatment to detect fever caused by hypersensitivity reaction or systemic lupus erythematosus (SLE)–like syndrome; close observation is necessary to detect any other sign of hypersensitivity, such as skin rash)

Copper analyses, urinary, 24-hour
   (recommended prior to start of therapy and in first months of treatment, when initial measurement of 24-hour urinary copper exceeds 1 mg)

Free-copper concentrations, serum
   (recommended periodically as the most reliable index of patient compliance with therapy; value equals the difference between quantitatively determined total copper and ceruloplasmin copper; in compliant patients with proper treatment, serum free copper should be less than 10 mcg per dL; values consistently greater than 20 mcg per dL may be due to inadequate dosage or noncompliance)

Hemoglobin determinations and
Iron concentrations, serum and
Reticulocyte and siderocyte counts
   (hemoglobin determinations recommended monthly during first year of therapy and every 3 months thereafter; iron concentrations and reticulocyte and siderocyte counts suggested periodically during therapy to determine if anemia is present and to determine its cause)

## Side/Adverse Effects

Note: Hypersensitivity has not been reported in patients treated for Wilson's disease. However, asthma, bronchitis, and dermatitis have been reported in chemical workers after prolonged environmental exposure to trientine.

The following side/adverse effects have been selected on the basis of their potential clinical significance (possible signs and symptoms in parentheses where appropriate)—not necessarily inclusive:

### Those indicating need for medical attention
Incidence more frequent
   *Anemia* (unusually pale skin; unusual tiredness)
   Note: *Anemia* may be due to iron or copper deficiency, although diagnosis should not be based on symptoms alone since symptoms may relate to other disease states. Trientine-induced sideroblastic anemia may possibly be reversed with reduction of trientine dosage to 750 or 500 mg a day and addition of pyridoxine at a dosage of 100 mg a day.

Incidence rare
   *Hypersensitivity or systemic lupus erythematosus (SLE)–like syndrome* (fever; general feeling of discomfort, illness, or weakness; joint pain; skin rash, blisters, hives, or itching; swelling of the lymph glands)

## Patient Consultation

As an aid to patient consultation, refer to *Advice for the Patient, Trientine (Systemic)*.

In providing consultation, consider emphasizing the following selected information (» = major clinical significance):

### Before using this medication
» Conditions affecting use, especially:
     Pregnancy—Pregnant women more prone to develop iron deficiency anemia
     Use in children—Children more prone to develop sideroblastic anemia than adults
     Other medications, especially copper supplements, iron supplements, and possibly other minerals
     Other medical problems, especially iron deficiency

### Proper use of this medication
*Proper administration:*
   Taking with water
   Swallowing capsules whole
   Not opening, crushing, or chewing capsules
» Importance of taking on an empty stomach; taking at least one hour before or two hours after meals, and one hour apart from any other medication, food, or milk for maximum absorption and to prevent inactivation of trientine by metal binding in gastrointestinal tract
» Compliance with therapy; importance of continuing medication indefinitely; checking with physician before discontinuing medication since nontreatment of Wilson's disease may lead to fatal liver damage
» Possible need for low-copper diet; avoiding foods known to be high in copper, such as chocolate, mushrooms, liver, molasses, broccoli, cereals enriched with copper, shellfish, organ meats, and nuts
   Importance of taking only as directed by doctor; not taking more or less medication than the amount prescribed
» Proper dosing
   Missed dose: Doubling next dose; not making up more than one missed dose at a time
» Proper storage

### Precautions while using this medication
» Regular visits to physician to check progress during therapy
» Taking nightly temperature during first month of treatment; reporting to physician any symptoms of SLE–like syndrome, such as fever or skin eruption
» Avoiding concomitant administration of copper- or iron-containing medications or other vitamin-mineral or mineral supplements to prevent inactivation of trientine; taking iron supplements and trientine at least 2 hours apart
   Avoiding potential contact dermatitis from capsule contents; promptly washing site of exposure with water

### Side/adverse effects
Anemia is more likely to occur in children, menstruating women, and pregnant women

Signs of potential side effects, especially anemia, hypersensitivity, or systemic lupus erythematosus (SLE)–like syndrome

## General Dosing Information
To achieve and maintain a negative copper balance, optimal long-term maintenance dosage should be determined at 6- to 12-month intervals, depending on 24-hour urinary copper analysis.

The daily dose should be increased only when the clinical response is inadequate or the concentration of free copper in serum is persistently above 20 mcg per dL.

### Diet/Nutrition
Trientine should be taken on an empty stomach (at least 1 hour before meals or 2 hours after meals) and 1 hour apart from any other medication, food, or milk for maximum absorption and to prevent inactivation of trientine by metal binding in the gastrointestinal tract.

In conjunction with trientine therapy, a low-copper diet of less than 2 mg daily should be maintained. Patients should avoid foods known to be high in copper such as chocolate, nuts, shellfish, mushrooms, liver, molasses, broccoli, organ meats, and cereals enriched with copper. Distilled or demineralized water should be used if the patient's drinking water contains more than 1000 mcg (1 mg) of copper per liter.

## Oral Dosage Forms

### TRIENTINE HYDROCHLORIDE CAPSULES
**Usual adult and adolescent dose**
Chelating agent—
Oral, initially 750 mg to 1.25 grams a day, in two to four divided doses.

**Usual adult prescribing limits**
Up to 2 grams a day.

**Usual pediatric dose**
Chelating agent—
Oral, initially 500 to 750 mg a day, in two to four divided doses.

**Usual pediatric prescribing limits**
Children 12 years of age and under—1.5 grams a day.

**Strength(s) usually available**
U.S.—
250 mg (Rx) [*Syprine*].
Canada—
Not commercially available.

**Packaging and storage**
Store at 2 to 8 °C (36 to 46 °F). Store in a tight container, unless otherwise specified by manufacturer.

**Auxiliary labeling**
- Take on an empty stomach.
- Swallow capsule whole.

Revised: 09/17/92
Interim revision: 04/29/94

---

**TRIFLUOPERAZINE**—See *Phenothiazines (Systemic)*

---

**TRIFLUPROMAZINE**—See *Phenothiazines (Systemic)*

---

# TRIFLURIDINE   Ophthalmic

VA CLASSIFICATION (Primary): OP203
Commonly used brand name(s): *Viroptic*.
Another commonly used name is trifluorothymidine.
Note: For a listing of dosage forms and brand names by country availability, see *Dosage Forms* section(s).

## Category
Antiviral (ophthalmic).

## Indications
**Accepted**
Keratitis, herpes simplex virus (treatment) or
Keratoconjunctivitis, herpes simplex virus (treatment)—Trifluridine is indicated in the treatment of keratoconjunctivitis and recurrent epithelial keratitis caused by herpes simplex virus (HSV), types 1 and 2. Trifluridine may be useful in patients who do not respond to idoxuridine or vidarabine or when ocular toxicity or hypersensitivity to idoxuridine occurs.

**Unaccepted**
Trifluridine is not indicated in the prophylaxis of HSV keratoconjunctivitis or epithelial keratitis.

Trifluridine is not effective against bacterial, fungal, or chlamydial infections of the cornea or in nonviral trophic lesions.

## Pharmacology/Pharmacokinetics
**Physicochemical characteristics**
Molecular weight—296.20.

**Mechanism of action/Effect**
Trifluridine, also called trifluorothymidine, closely resembles thymidine. It inhibits thymidylic phosphorylase and specific DNA polymerases, which are necessary for the incorporation of thymidine into viral DNA. Trifluridine is incorporated in place of thymidine into viral DNA, resulting in faulty DNA and the inability to reproduce or to infect or destroy tissue. Trifluridine also is incorporated into mammalian DNA.

**Distribution**
Intraocular penetration occurs after topical administration of trifluridine. Decreased corneal integrity or stromal or uveal infections may increase trifluridine's penetration into the aqueous humor.

**Half-life**
Approximately 12 to 18 minutes.

## Precautions to Consider

**Carcinogenicity**
Lifetime carcinogenicity bioassays have been performed in rats and mice given daily subcutaneous doses of trifluridine. Rats given doses of 1.5, 7.5, or 15 mg per kg of body weight (mg/kg) per day had increased incidences of adenocarcinomas of the intestinal tract and mammary glands, hemangiosarcomas of the spleen and liver, carcinosarcomas of the prostate gland, and granulosa-thecal cell tumors of the ovary. Mice given doses of 10 mg/kg per day (but not those given 1 or 5 mg/kg per day) had significantly increased incidences of adenocarcinomas of the intestinal tract and uterus. These mice also had a significantly higher incidence of testicular atrophy than vehicle control mice.

**Mutagenicity**
Studies in various standard *in vitro* test systems have shown that trifluridine exerts mutagenic, DNA-damaging, and cell-transforming effects and that it is clastogenic in *Vicia faba* cells.

**Pregnancy/Reproduction**
Pregnancy—Adequate and well-controlled studies in humans have not been done.

Trifluridine has been shown to be teratogenic when injected directly into the yolk sac of developing chick embryos. Studies in rats and rabbits given trifluridine subcutaneously in doses of 2.5 mg/kg daily have shown that trifluridine causes delayed ossification. This dose also caused fetal death and resorption in rabbits. However, no effects were seen in rats and rabbits given doses of 1 mg/kg daily. Studies in rats and rabbits given trifluridine subcutaneously in doses of up to 5 mg/kg daily have not shown that trifluridine is teratogenic. Studies in rabbits, using 1% trifluridine applied to the eyes on days 6 to 18 of pregnancy, also have not shown that trifluridine is teratogenic.

FDA Pregnancy Category C.

**Breast-feeding**
Trifluridine is unlikely to be distributed into breast milk following ophthalmic administration, since the total daily dose is small (5 mg or less), and since trifluridine is diluted in body fluids and has an extremely short half-life (approximately 12 minutes).

## Trifluridine (Ophthalmic)

**Pediatrics**
Appropriate studies on the relationship of age to the effects of trifluridine have not been performed in the pediatric population. However, no pediatrics-specific problems have been documented to date.

**Geriatrics**
Appropriate studies on the relationship of age to the effects of trifluridine have not been performed in the geriatric population. However, no geriatrics-specific problems have been documented to date.

**Medical considerations/Contraindications**
The medical considerations/contraindications included have been selected on the basis of their potential clinical significance (reasons given in parentheses where appropriate)—not necessarily inclusive (» = major clinical significance).

*Risk-benefit should be considered when the following medical problem exists:*
  Sensitivity to trifluridine

**Patient monitoring**
The following may be especially important in patient monitoring (other tests may be warranted in some patients, depending on condition; » = major clinical significance):
  Ophthalmologic, including slit-lamp, examinations
    (may be required periodically during therapy)

### Side/Adverse Effects

The following side/adverse effects have been selected on the basis of their potential clinical significance (possible signs and symptoms in parentheses where appropriate)—not necessarily inclusive:

**Those indicating need for medical attention**
Incidence rare
  *Epithelial keratopathy; superficial punctate keratopathy* (blurred vision or other change in vision); *hyperemia* (redness of eye); *hypersensitivity* (itching, redness, swelling, or other sign of irritation not present before therapy); *increased intraocular pressure; keratitis sicca* (dryness of eye); *stromal edema* (irritation of eye)

**Those indicating need for medical attention only if they continue or are bothersome**
Incidence more frequent
  *Burning or stinging*

### Patient Consultation

As an aid to patient consultation, refer to *Advice for the Patient, Trifluridine (Ophthalmic)*.
In providing consultation, consider emphasizing the following selected information (» = major clinical significance):

**Before using this medication**
» Conditions affecting use, especially:
    Sensitivity to trifluridine

**Proper use of this medication**
  Proper administration technique for ophthalmic solution
» Not using more frequently or for longer than ordered by physician
» Compliance with full course of therapy
» Proper dosing
  Missed dose: Applying as soon as possible; not applying if almost time for next dose
» Proper storage

**Precautions while using this medication**
  Importance of keeping appointments with physician; checking with physician if symptoms become worse

**Side/adverse effects**
  Signs of potential side effects, especially epithelial keratopathy, superficial punctate keratopathy, hyperemia, hypersensitivity, increased intraocular pressure, keratitis sicca, or stromal edema

### General Dosing Information

Although some manufacturers recommend a dose of 2 drops of an ophthalmic solution at appropriate intervals, the conjunctival sac will usually hold only 1 drop.

Trifluridine may be administered concurrently with cycloplegics, mydriatics, antibiotics, sulfonamides, vasoconstrictors, miotics, adrenergics, and corticosteroids. Corticosteroids can accelerate the spread of viral infections and are usually contraindicated in superficial herpes simplex virus keratitis. However, steroids may be used concurrently with trifluridine in the treatment of herpes simplex stromal infections. Trifluridine should be continued for a few days after the steroid has been discontinued.

Treatment usually should not be continued for more than a total of 21 days or for more than 3 to 5 days after healing is complete. However, chronic or particularly difficult infections may require up to 3 to 6 weeks of treatment.

Herpetic keratitis may recur if trifluridine is discontinued before microscopic staining with fluorescein has cleared.

### Ophthalmic Dosage Forms

#### TRIFLURIDINE OPHTHALMIC SOLUTION

**Usual adult and adolescent dose**
Ophthalmic antiviral—
  Topical, to the conjunctiva, 1 drop every two hours while awake. Treatment should be continued until the cornea is completely re-epithelialized. Dose may then be reduced to 1 drop every four hours while awake (minimum of 5 drops daily) for an additional seven days.

**Usual adult prescribing limits**
Up to 9 drops daily.

**Usual pediatric dose**
See *Usual adult and adolescent dose*.

**Strength(s) usually available**
U.S.—
  1% (Rx) [*Viroptic* (thimerosal 0.001%)].
Canada—
  1% (Rx) [*Viroptic* (thimerosal 0.001%)].

**Packaging and storage**
Store between 2 and 8 °C (36 and 46 °F), unless otherwise specified by manufacturer.

**Auxiliary labeling**
• Refrigerate.
• For the eye.
• Continue medicine for full time of treatment.
• Do not use more often or longer than ordered.

**Note**
Dispense in original unopened container.

Revised: 07/01/93

---

**TRIHEXYPHENIDYL**—See *Antidyskinetics (Systemic)*

---

**TRIKATES**—See *Potassium Supplements (Systemic)*

---

**TRILOSTANE**—The *Trilostane (Systemic)* monograph is not included in this published version of the USP DI database. Copies of the monograph are available on request from Micromedex, Inc. - Reprint Requests, 6200 S. Syracuse Way, Suite 300, Englewood, CO 80111; telephone (303) 486-6400; telefax (303) 486-6464; Email: USPDI@MDX.COM.

---

**TRIMEPRAZINE**—See *Antihistamines, Phenothiazine-derivative (Systemic)*

# TRIMETHAPHAN  Systemic

VA CLASSIFICATION (Primary): CV409
Commonly used brand name(s): *Arfonad*.

Note:  For a listing of dosage forms and brand names by country availability, see *Dosage Forms* section(s).

## Category
Antihypertensive.

## Indications

**Accepted**

Hypotension, controlled (induction and maintenance)—Trimethaphan is indicated for production of controlled hypotension during surgery to reduce bleeding into the surgical field.

Hypertension (treatment)—Trimethaphan is indicated for rapid reduction of blood pressure in the treatment of hypertensive emergencies, especially in patients with acute dissecting aneurysm, and in the emergency treatment of pulmonary edema in patients with pulmonary hypertension associated with systemic hypertension.

## Pharmacology/Pharmacokinetics

**Physicochemical characteristics**
Molecular weight—596.80.

**Mechanism of action/Effect**
Ganglionic blocking agent; prevents stimulation of postsynaptic receptors by competing with acetylcholine for these receptor sites; additional effects may include direct peripheral vasodilation and release of histamine. Trimethaphan's hypotensive effect is due to reduction in sympathetic tone and vasodilation, and is primarily postural. Cardiac output may increase in patients with cardiac failure or decrease in patients with normal cardiac function.

**Biotransformation**
Exact metabolic fate unknown; however, possibly by pseudocholinesterase.

**Onset of action**
Immediate.

**Duration of action**
10 to 15 minutes.

**Elimination**
Renal, mostly unchanged.

## Precautions to Consider

**Carcinogenicity/Mutagenicity**
Adequate studies have not been done.

**Pregnancy/Reproduction**
Pregnancy—Trimethaphan crosses the placenta. Its ganglionic blocking effects may decrease gastrointestinal motility in the fetus, resulting in meconium ileus or neonatal paralytic ileus. Furthermore, trimethaphan-induced hypotension may have other serious adverse effects on the fetus. Risk-benefit must be carefully considered when this medication is required in life-threatening situations or in serious diseases for which other medications cannot be used.

FDA Pregnancy Category D.

**Breast-feeding**
It is not known whether trimethaphan is distributed into breast milk. Because of the potential for serious adverse effects in nursing infants, it is recommended that mothers who require trimethaphan refrain from nursing.

**Pediatrics**
Appropriate studies on the relationship of age to the effects of trimethaphan have not been performed in the pediatric population. However, caution may be required in pediatric patients.

**Geriatrics**
No information is available on the relationship of age to the effects of trimethaphan in geriatric patients. However, elderly patients may be more sensitive to the hypotensive effects of trimethaphan. Furthermore, these patients may have age-related renal function impairment, which may require caution in patients receiving trimethaphan.

**Drug interactions and/or related problems**
The following drug interactions and/or related problems have been selected on the basis of their potential clinical significance (possible mechanism in parentheses where appropriate)—not necessarily inclusive (» = major clinical significance):

Note:  Combinations containing any of the following medications, depending on the amount present, may also interact with this medication.

» Ambenonium or
» Neostigmine or
» Pyridostigmine
   (concurrent use may interfere with the antimyasthenic effect of ambenonium, neostigmine, or pyridostigmine, leading to weakness and sudden inability to swallow)

Anti-inflammatory drugs, nonsteroidal (NSAIDs), especially indomethacin
   (antihypertensive effects of trimethaphan may be reduced when it is used concurrently with these agents; indomethacin, and possibly other NSAIDs, may antagonize the antihypertensive effect by inhibiting renal prostaglandin synthesis and/or by causing sodium and fluid retention; the patient should be carefully monitored to confirm that the desired effect is being obtained)

Hypotension-producing medications, other (see *Appendix II* )
   (concurrent use with trimethaphan may result in enhanced hypotension; individual dosage adjustment is important; halothane may also reduce or prevent trimethaphan-induced tachycardia)
   (preanesthetic and anesthetic agents used in surgery, especially spinal anesthetics, may potentiate the hypotensive response to trimethaphan, with increased risk of severe hypotension, shock, and cardiovascular collapse during surgery)

Neuromuscular blocking agents
   (effects may be prolonged, especially by administration of large doses of trimethaphan, since trimethaphan appears to have a slight curare-like effect; careful postoperative monitoring of the patient may be necessary following concurrent or sequential use, especially if there is a possibility of incomplete reversal of neuromuscular blockade)

Sympathomimetics
   (trimethaphan may enhance the pressor response to sympathomimetic pressor amines, and the hypotensive effect of trimethaphan may be decreased or reversed by all sympathomimetics)

**Laboratory value alterations**
The following have been selected on the basis of their potential clinical significance (possible effect in parentheses where appropriate)—not necessarily inclusive (» = major clinical significance):

With physiology/laboratory test values
   Glucose, blood, concentrations
      (trimethaphan prevents surgically induced increase)
   Potassium, serum
      (concentrations may be slightly decreased)

**Medical considerations/Contraindications**
The medical considerations/contraindications included have been selected on the basis of their potential clinical significance (reasons given in parentheses where appropriate)—not necessarily inclusive (» = major clinical significance).

*Risk-benefit should be considered when the following medical problems exist:*

» Addison's disease

Allergies, history of
   (trimethaphan liberates histamine and has been reported to cause a histamine-like reaction along the vein where administered)

» Anemia, uncorrected or
» Asphyxia or
» Hypovolemia or
» Shock, frank or incipient
   (for use in producing controlled hypotension during anesthesia only; additional hypotension may result in hypoxia of vital organs)

Bladder neck obstruction or
Prostatic hypertrophy or
Urethral stricture
   (possible urinary retention caused by trimethaphan)

» Cardiovascular insufficiency, including coronary insufficiency or
» Cerebrovascular insufficiency or
» Myocardial infarction, recent
   (ischemia may be aggravated by hypotension)

» Degenerative disease of the central nervous system (CNS)

**2880 Trimethaphan (Systemic)**

» Diabetes mellitus
  Glaucoma
» Hepatic function impairment
    (the decrease in blood pressure secondary to trimethaphan administration may decrease hepatic perfusion and worsen this condition)
  Pyelonephritis, chronic
    (condition may be aggravated by urinary retention caused by trimethaphan)
» Renal function impairment
    (increased effects due to reduced excretion of trimethaphan)
» Respiratory insufficiency, uncorrected
    (aggravation of hypoxemia by trimethaphan)
  Sensitivity to trimethaphan
» Caution is required also in debilitated patients and those also receiving steroids.

**Patient monitoring**
The following may be especially important in patient monitoring (other tests may be warranted in some patients, depending on condition; » = major clinical significance):
» Blood pressure determinations
    (should be made frequently)
  Respiratory function determinations
    (recommended at periodic intervals, especially with large doses of trimethaphan, since respiratory arrest has been reported rarely with its use)

## Side/Adverse Effects
Note: Most side/adverse effects are due to parasympathetic blockade and respond to dosage reduction or withdrawal of trimethaphan.
  Overdosage may result in profound hypotension and respiratory arrest.

The following side/adverse effects have been selected on the basis of their potential clinical significance (possible signs and symptoms in parentheses where appropriate)—not necessarily inclusive:

**Incidence dose-related**
*Anorexia, nausea, and vomiting; constipation; cycloplegia and mydriasis; dryness of mouth; impotence; itching, urticaria; orthostatic hypotension; paralytic ileus; precipitation of angina; tachycardia; urinary retention, short-term*
  Note: Increased risk of *paralytic ileus* when the infusion is continued for longer than 48 hours.
    *Mydriasis* is common and does not necessarily indicate anoxia or depth of anesthesia.

## General Dosing Information
Trimethaphan Camsylate Injection USP must be diluted and administered by intravenous infusion.

To achieve optimal reduction in blood pressure, it is recommended that trimethaphan infusion be administered intravenously by means of an infusion pump, a micro-drip regulator, or a similar device to allow precise adjustment of the flow rate. Tilting the head of the bed up may enhance the hypotensive effect; the patient should be positioned to avoid cerebral anoxia.

**For use as an antihypertensive only**
It is recommended that patients receiving trimethaphan be in an intensive care unit and that blood pressure be monitored frequently.

It is recommended that oral antihypertensive therapy be instituted as soon as possible while the patient is receiving trimethaphan and that trimethaphan be withdrawn as soon as the blood pressure has stabilized. Patients receiving concomitant antihypertensive medication require lower doses of trimethaphan.

Pseudotolerance to the effects of trimethaphan occurs in some patients; tachyphylaxis may develop within 24 to 72 hours. Pseudotolerance with prolonged use may be prevented by use of a diuretic.

**For use to produce controlled hypotension during surgery only**
It is recommended that trimethaphan infusion be discontinued prior to wound closure to allow blood pressure to return to normal.

## Parenteral Dosage Forms

### TRIMETHAPHAN CAMSYLATE INJECTION USP

**Usual adult dose**
Controlled hypotension during surgery—
  Initial: Intravenous infusion, 3 to 4 mg per minute, adjusted according to response.
  Maintenance: Intravenous infusion, 300 mcg (0.3 mg) to 6 mg per minute.
Hypertensive emergency—
  Initial: Intravenous infusion, 500 mcg (0.5 mg) to 1 mg per minute, adjusted according to response.
  Maintenance: Intravenous infusion, 1 to 5 mg per minute.
Note: Geriatric patients may be more sensitive to the usual adult dose of trimethaphan.

**Usual pediatric dose**
Initial—Intravenous infusion, 50 mcg (0.05 mg) to 150 mcg (0.15 mg) per kg per minute, adjusted according to response.

**Strength(s) usually available**
U.S.—
  50 mg per mL (Rx) [*Arfonad*].
Canada—
  50 mg per mL (Rx) [*Arfonad*].

**Packaging and storage**
Store between 2 and 8 °C (36 and 46 °F). Protect from freezing (to avoid ampul breakage).

**Preparation of dosage form**
Trimethaphan Camsylate Injection USP is prepared for intravenous infusion by diluting the contents of a 500-mg ampul in 500 mL of 5% dextrose injection only to produce a solution containing 1 mg of trimethaphan camsylate per mL.

**Stability**
Intravenous solutions should be freshly prepared; unused portions should be discarded. After preparation, intravenous infusion solution is stable for 24 hours at room temperature.

**Auxiliary labeling**
• Dilute before using.

**Note**
Must be diluted before use.

Revised: 09/08/92
Interim revision: 08/19/98

---

# TRIMETHOBENZAMIDE Systemic†

INN: Trimethobenzamide
VA CLASSIFICATION (Primary): GA605
Commonly used brand name(s): *Arrestin; Benzacot; Bio-Gan; Stemetic; T-Gen; Tebamide; Tegamide; Ticon; Tigan; Tiject-20; Triban; Tribenzagan.*
Note: For a listing of dosage forms and brand names by country availability, see *Dosage Forms* section(s).

†Not commercially available in Canada.

## Category
Antiemetic.

## Indications
**Accepted**
Nausea and vomiting (prophylaxis and treatment)—Trimethobenzamide is indicated for the control of nausea and vomiting.

## Pharmacology/Pharmacokinetics
**Physicochemical characteristics**
Molecular weight—424.92.

**Mechanism of action/Effect**
Thought to inhibit the medullary chemoreceptor trigger zone.

**Biotransformation**
Hepatic.

**Elimination**
Renal; biliary.

## Precautions to Consider

**Cross-sensitivity and/or related problems**
The suppository dosage form contains 2% of benzocaine. Patients sensitive to benzocaine or similar local anesthetics should not use the suppository dosage form of trimethobenzamide.

**Pregnancy/Reproduction**
Pregnancy—Adequate and well-controlled studies in humans have not been done.
Reproduction studies in animals have not shown that trimethobenzamide causes teratogenic effects in the fetus; however, it has been shown to cause increased embryonic resorptions and stillbirths.

**Breast-feeding**
It is not known if trimethobenzamide is distributed into breast milk.

**Pediatrics**
Trimethobenzamide is not recommended for treatment of uncomplicated vomiting in children. Caution is required because of the suspicion that centrally acting antiemetics, when used in the presence of viral illnesses, may contribute to the development of Reye's syndrome.

**Geriatrics**
No information is available on the relationship of age to the effects of trimethobenzamide in geriatric patients.

**Drug interactions and/or related problems**
The following drug interactions and/or related problems have been selected on the basis of their potential clinical significance (possible mechanism in parentheses where appropriate)—not necessarily inclusive (» = major clinical significance):

Note: Combinations containing any of the following medications, depending on the amount present, may also interact with this medication.

Apomorphine
(prior administration of trimethobenzamide may decrease the emetic response to apomorphine; also, concurrent use may potentiate the central nervous system [CNS] effects of either apomorphine or trimethobenzamide)

» CNS depression–producing medications (See *Appendix II*)
(concurrent use may potentiate the effects of either these medications or trimethobenzamide; in addition, use of trimethobenzamide as well as other antiemetic agents in patients who have recently received other medications with CNS effects, such as phenothiazines, barbiturates, or the belladonna alkaloids, has resulted in opisthotonos, convulsions, coma, and extrapyramidal symptoms)

Ototoxic medications (See *Appendix II*)
(concurrent use with trimethobenzamide may mask the symptoms of ototoxicity, such as tinnitus, dizziness, and vertigo)

**Medical considerations/Contraindications**
The medical considerations/contraindications included have been selected on the basis of their potential clinical significance (reasons given in parentheses where appropriate)—not necessarily inclusive (» = major clinical significance).

*Risk-benefit should be considered when the following medical problems exist:*
Dehydration or
Electrolyte imbalance or
Encephalitis or
Fever, high or
Gastroenteritis
(CNS reactions such as opisthotonos, convulsions, coma, and extrapyramidal symptoms have been reported after administration of trimethobenzamide, especially in children and in elderly or debilitated patients, or in those who have recently received other medications with CNS effects)
Sensitivity to trimethobenzamide

Note: Antiemetic action of trimethobenzamide may impede diagnosis of such conditions as appendicitis and obscure signs of toxicity from overdosage of other medications.

## Side/Adverse Effects

The following side/adverse effects have been selected on the basis of their potential clinical significance (possible signs and symptoms in parentheses where appropriate)—not necessarily inclusive:

Those indicating need for medical attention
Incidence rare
*Allergic reactions* (skin rash); *blood dyscrasias* (sore throat or fever; unusual tiredness); *convulsions; hepatic function impairment* (yellow eyes or skin); *mental depression; opisthotonus* (body spasm with head and heels bent backward and body bowed forward); *Parkinson-like syndrome* (shakiness or tremors); *Reye's syndrome* (convulsions; severe or continuing vomiting)

**Those indicating need for medical attention only if they continue or are bothersome**
Incidence more frequent
*Drowsiness*
Incidence less frequent
*Blurred vision; diarrhea; dizziness; headache; muscle cramps*

## Patient Consultation

As an aid to patient consultation, refer to *Advice for the Patient, Trimethobenzamide (Systemic)*.

In providing consultation, consider emphasizing the following selected information (» = major clinical significance):

**Before using this medication**
» Conditions affecting use, especially:
Sensitivity to trimethobenzamide or to benzocaine (for suppository form)
Pregnancy—Animal studies have shown increased fetal resorptions and stillbirths
Use in children—Trimethobenzamide is not recommended for treatment of uncomplicated vomiting, due to the possible contribution of centrally acting antiemetics to the development of Reye's syndrome
Other medications, especially CNS depressants
Other medical problems, especially dehydration, electrolyte imbalance, encephalitis, high fever, or gastroenteritis

**Proper use of this medication**
Not giving to children unless prescribed; giving medication only as directed
Taking medication only as directed
Proper administration of this medication (for suppository dosage form only)
» Proper dosing
Missed dose: Taking as soon as possible; not taking if almost time for next dose; not doubling doses
» Proper storage

**Precautions while using this medication**
» Avoiding use of alcohol or other CNS depressants
» Possible dizziness, lightheadedness, or drowsiness; caution when driving or doing anything else requiring alertness
May mask ototoxic effects of large doses of salicylates

**Side/adverse effects**
Signs of potential side effects, especially allergic reactions, blood dyscrasias, convulsions, hepatic function impairment, mental depression, opisthotonus, Parkinson-like syndrome, and Reye's syndrome

## General Dosing Information

**For parenteral dosage form only**
Intravenous injection is not recommended.
Intramuscular administration should be made by deep injection into the upper outer quadrant of the gluteal area in order to minimize irritation at the site of injection.

## Oral Dosage Forms

### TRIMETHOBENZAMIDE HYDROCHLORIDE CAPSULES USP

**Usual adult and adolescent dose**
Antiemetic—
Oral, 250 mg three or four times a day as needed.

**Usual pediatric dose**
Antiemetic—
Oral, 15 mg per kg of body weight a day as needed, divided into three or four doses; or for
Children weighing 15 to 45 kg: Oral, 100 to 200 mg three or four times a day, as needed.

**Strength(s) usually available**
U.S.—
100 mg (Rx) [*Tigan*].
250 mg (Rx) [*Tigan*; GENERIC].

# 2882 Trimethobenzamide (Systemic)

Canada—
  Not commercially available.

**Packaging and storage**
Store below 40 °C (104 °F), preferably between 15 and 30 °C (59 and 86 °F), unless otherwise specified by manufacturer. Store in a well-closed container.

**Auxiliary labeling**
- May cause drowsiness.
- Avoid alcoholic beverages.

## Parenteral Dosage Forms

### TRIMETHOBENZAMIDE HYDROCHLORIDE INJECTION USP

**Usual adult and adolescent dose**
Antiemetic—
  Intramuscular, 200 mg three or four times a day as needed.

**Usual pediatric dose**
Use is not recommended.

**Strength(s) usually available**
U.S.—
  100 mg per mL (Rx) [*Arrestin; Benzacot; Stemetic; Tegamide; Ticon; Tigan* (parabens [methyl and propyl] 0.2%—in 2-mL ampuls; phenol 0.45%—in 20-mL vials; phenol 0.45%, disodium edetate 0.2 mg—in 2-mL syringes); *Tiject-20; Tribenzagan;* GENERIC].
Canada—
  Not commercially available.

**Packaging and storage**
Store between 15 and 30 °C (59 and 86 °F), unless otherwise specified by manufacturer. Protect from freezing.

## Rectal Dosage Forms

### TRIMETHOBENZAMIDE HYDROCHLORIDE SUPPOSITORIES

**Usual adult and adolescent dose**
Antiemetic—
  Rectal, 200 mg three or four times a day as needed.

**Usual pediatric dose**
Antiemetic—
  Rectal, 15 mg per kg of body weight a day as needed, divided into three or four doses; or for
  Children weighing less than 15 kg: Rectal, 100 mg three or four times a day as needed.
  Children weighing 15 to 45 kg: Rectal, 100 to 200 mg three or four times a day as needed.
Note: Premature and full-term neonates—Use is not recommended.

**Strength(s) usually available**
U.S.—
  100 mg (Rx) [*Bio-Gan; Tegamide; T-Gen; Tigan* (2% benzocaine); *Triban;* GENERIC].
  200 mg (Rx) [*Bio-Gan; Tebamide; Tegamide; T-Gen; Tigan* (2% benzocaine); *Triban;* GENERIC].
Canada—
  Not commercially available.

**Packaging and storage**
Store between 15 and 30 °C (59 and 86 °F), unless otherwise specified by manufacturer.

**Auxiliary labeling**
- May cause drowsiness.
- Avoid alcoholic beverages.

Revised: 05/12/93

---

# TRIMETHOPRIM  Systemic

VA CLASSIFICATION (Primary): AM900
Commonly used brand name(s): *Proloprim; Trimpex.*
Note: For a listing of dosage forms and brand names by country availability, see *Dosage Forms* section(s).

## Category
Antibacterial (systemic).

## Indications
Note: Bracketed information in the *Indications* section refers to uses that are not included in U.S. product labeling.

**Accepted**
Urinary tract infections, bacterial (treatment)—Trimethoprim is indicated in the treatment of initial, uncomplicated urinary tract infections caused by susceptible strains of *Escherichia coli, Proteus mirabilis, Klebsiella pneumoniae, Enterobacter* species, and coagulase-negative *Staphylococcus* species, including *S. saprophyticus.*

[Urinary tract infections, bacterial (prophylaxis)][1]—Trimethoprim is used in the prophylaxis of bacterial urinary tract infections.

[Pneumonia, *Pneumocystis carinii* (treatment)][1]—Trimethoprim is used in combination with dapsone in the treatment of mild to moderate pneumonia caused by *Pneumocystis carinii* (PCP).

Not all species or strains of a particular organism may be susceptible to trimethoprim.

**Unaccepted**
Trimethoprim is not effective against *Pseudomonas aeruginosa* or *Bacteroides fragilis.*

[1]Not included in Canadian product labeling.

## Pharmacology/Pharmacokinetics

**Physicochemical characteristics**
Molecular weight—290.32.

**Mechanism of action/Effect**
Bacteriostatic lipophilic weak base structurally related to pyrimethamine, binds to and reversibly inhibits the bacterial enzyme dihydrofolate reductase, selectively blocking conversion of dihydrofolic acid to its functional form, tetrahydrofolic acid. This depletes folate, an essential cofactor in the biosynthesis of nucleic acids, resulting in interference with bacterial nucleic acid and protein production. Bacterial dihydrofolate reductase is approximately 50,000 to 60,000 times more tightly bound by trimethoprim than by the corresponding mammalian enzyme.

Exerts its effect at a step in the folate biosynthesis immediately subsequent to the one in which sulfonamides exert their effect. When administered concurrently with sulfonamides, synergism occurs and is attributed to inhibition of tetrahydrofolate production at two sequential steps in its biosynthesis.

**Absorption**
Rapidly and almost completely (90 to 100%) absorbed from the gastrointestinal tract.

**Distribution**
Rapidly and widely distributed to various tissues and fluids, including kidneys, liver, spleen, bronchial secretions, saliva, and seminal fluid. Trimethoprim has also been demonstrated in bile; aqueous humor; bone marrow and spongy, but not compact, bone.
Cerebrospinal fluid (CSF) concentrations—30 to 50% of serum concentrations.
Prostatic tissue and fluid—2 to 3 times the serum concentration.
  Crosses the placenta and is excreted in breast milk.
Vol$_D$—
  Adults: 1.3 to 1.8 liters per kg.
Children:
  Newborns—Approximately 2.7 liters per kg.
  Age 1 to 10 years old—Approximately 1.0 liter per kg.

**Protein binding**
Moderate (approximately 45%).

**Biotransformation**
Hepatic; 10 to 20% metabolized to inactive metabolites by O-demethylation, ring N-oxidation, and alpha-hydroxylation; metabolites may be free or conjugated.

**Half-life**
Adults—
  Normal renal function: 8 to 10 hours.
  Anuric patients: 20 to 50 hours.

Children—
Newborns: Approximately 19 hours.
Age 1 to 10 years: 3 to 5.5 hours.

**Time to mean peak serum concentration**
1 to 4 hours.

**Mean peak serum concentration**
Approximately 1 mcg per mL, following a single 100-mg dose.

**Elimination**
Renal, 50 to 60% excreted within 24 hours, primarily by glomerular filtration and tubular secretion; of this amount, 80 to 90% excreted unchanged and remainder excreted as inactive metabolites. Excretion increased in acid urine and decreased in alkaline urine.
Small amounts excreted in the feces (approximately 4%) and bile.
In dialysis—Moderate amount of trimethoprim is removed from the blood by hemodialysis. Peritoneal dialysis is not effective in removing trimethoprim from the blood.

## Precautions to Consider

### Carcinogenicity
Long-term studies in animals to evaluate the carcinogenic potential of trimethoprim have not been done.

### Mutagenicity
Trimethoprim has not been shown to be mutagenic in the Ames assay. No chromosomal damage was seen in human leukocytes that were cultured *in vitro* with trimethoprim, using concentrations that exceeded serum concentrations following normal doses of trimethoprim.

### Pregnancy/Reproduction
Fertility—Trimethoprim has not been shown to cause adverse effects on fertility or reproductive performance in rats given oral doses as high as 70 mg per kg of body weight (mg/kg) daily in males and 14 mg/kg daily in females.
Pregnancy—Trimethoprim crosses the placenta. Adequate and well-controlled studies in humans have not been done. Trimethoprim may interfere with folic acid metabolism. However, a retrospective study of 186 pregnancies, in which mothers received trimethoprim plus sulfamethoxazole or placebo, has shown a lower incidence of congenital malformations (3.3% versus 4.5%) in the trimethoprim-treated group. There were no abnormalities in the 10 children whose mothers received trimethoprim during the first trimester. Also, another study found no congenital abnormalities in 35 children whose mothers received trimethoprim plus sulfamethoxazole at the time of conception or shortly thereafter.
Studies in rats given oral doses of 70 mg/kg daily during the third trimester and throughout parturition have not shown that trimethoprim causes adverse effects on gestation or pup growth and survival. However, studies in rats given doses of 40 times the human dose have shown that trimethoprim is teratogenic. Studies in rabbits given doses of 6 times the human dose have shown an increase in fetal loss (dead, resorbed, and malformed fetuses).
FDA Pregnancy Category C.

### Breast-feeding
Trimethoprim is excreted in breast milk in concentrations equal to or greater than those in the maternal serum and may interfere with folic acid metabolism in nursing infants. However, no significant problems in humans have been documented.

### Pediatrics
Safety has not been established in infants less than 2 months of age. Appropriate studies on the relationship of age to the effects of trimethoprim have not been performed in children up to 12 years of age. However, in studies performed in children over 12 years of age, no pediatrics-specific problems have been documented to date.

### Geriatrics
An increased incidence of thrombocytopenia with purpura has been reported in elderly patients who are receiving diuretics, primarily thiazides, concurrently with trimethoprim.

### Dental
The leukopenic and thrombocytopenic effects of trimethoprim may result in an increased incidence of certain microbial infections, delayed healing, and gingival bleeding. If leukopenia or thrombocytopenia occurs, dental work should be deferred until blood counts have returned to normal. Patients should be instructed in proper oral hygiene, including caution in use of regular toothbrushes, dental floss, and toothpicks.

### Drug interactions and/or related problems
The following drug interactions and/or related problems have been selected on the basis of their potential clinical significance (possible mechanism in parentheses where appropriate)—not necessarily inclusive (» = major clinical significance):

Note: Combinations containing any of the following medications, depending on the amount present, may also interact with this medication.

Bone marrow depressants (See *Appendix II*)
 (concurrent use of bone marrow depressants with trimethoprim may increase the leukopenic and/or thrombocytopenic effects; if concurrent use is required, close observation for myelotoxic effects should be considered)

Cyclosporine
 (concurrent use of cyclosporine with trimethoprim may increase the incidence of nephrotoxicity)

Dapsone
 (concurrent use with trimethoprim will usually increase the plasma concentrations of both dapsone and trimethoprim, possibly due to an inhibition in dapsone metabolism, and/or competition for renal secretion between the 2 medications; increased serum dapsone concentrations may increase the number and severity of side effects, especially methemoglobinemia)

» Folate antagonists, other (See *Appendix II*)
 (concurrent use with trimethoprim or use of trimethoprim between courses of other folic acid antagonists, such as methotrexate or pyrimethamine, is not recommended because of the possibility of an increased incidence of megaloblastic anemia)

Phenytoin
 (trimethoprim may inhibit the hepatic metabolism of phenytoin, increasing the half-life of phenytoin by up to 50% and decreasing its clearance by 30%)

Procainamide
 (concurrent use with trimethoprim may increase the plasma concentration of both procainamide and its metabolite NAPA by decreasing their renal clearance)

Rifampin
 (concurrent use may significantly increase the elimination and shorten the elimination half-life of trimethoprim)

Warfarin
 (trimethoprim may potentiate the anticoagulant activity of warfarin by inhibiting its metabolism)

### Laboratory value alterations
The following have been selected on the basis of their potential clinical significance (possible effect in parentheses where appropriate)—not necessarily inclusive (» = major clinical significance):

With diagnostic test results
 Creatinine determinations
  (trimethoprim may interfere with the Jaffé alkaline picrate assay for creatinine, resulting in creatinine values that are approximately 10% higher than actual values)
 Serum methotrexate assays
  (trimethoprim may interfere with serum methotrexate assays if measured by the competitive binding protein technique [CBPA] using a bacterial dihydrofolate reductase as the binding protein; no interference occurs if methotrexate is measured by radioimmunoassay [RIA])

With physiology/laboratory test values
 Alanine aminotransferase (ALT [SGPT]), serum and
 Aspartate aminotransferase (AST [SGOT]), serum and
 Bilirubin, serum and
 Blood urea nitrogen (BUN) and
 Creatinine, serum
  (concentrations may be increased)

### Medical considerations/Contraindications
The medical considerations/contraindications included have been selected on the basis of their potential clinical significance (reasons given in parentheses where appropriate)—not necessarily inclusive (» = major clinical significance).

*Risk-benefit should be considered when the following medical problems exist:*
 Hypersensitivity to trimethoprim
» Megaloblastic anemia due to folic acid deficiency
  (trimethoprim may worsen megaloblastic anemia caused by folic acid deficiency)
» Renal function impairment
  (trimethoprim is primarily renally excreted)

# Trimethoprim (Systemic)

### Patient monitoring
The following may be especially important in patient monitoring (other tests may be warranted in some patients, depending on condition; » = major clinical significance):

Complete blood counts (CBCs)
(may be required in patients on long-term treatment or those predisposed to folate deficiency if signs of blood dyscrasias occur during treatment; trimethoprim should be discontinued if there is a significant reduction in the count of any formed blood elements)

## Side/Adverse Effects

The following side/adverse effects have been selected on the basis of their potential clinical significance (possible signs and symptoms in parentheses where appropriate)—not necessarily inclusive:

### Those indicating need for medical attention
Incidence rare
*Aseptic meningitis* (headache; neck stiffness; malaise; nausea); **blood dyscrasias** (pale skin; sore throat and fever; unusual bleeding or bruising; unusual tiredness or weakness); *hypersensitivity* (skin rash or itching); *methemoglobinemia* (bluish fingernails, lips, or skin; difficult breathing; pale skin; sore throat and fever; unusual bleeding or bruising; unusual tiredness or weakness); *Stevens-Johnson syndrome* (aching joints and muscles; redness, blistering, peeling, or loosening of skin; unusual tiredness or weakness)

### Those indicating need for medical attention only if they continue or are bothersome
Incidence less frequent
*Gastrointestinal disturbances* (diarrhea; loss of appetite; nausea or vomiting; stomach cramps or pain); *headache*

## Overdose

For more information on the management of overdose or unintentional ingestion, **contact a Poison Control Center** (see *Poison Control Center Listing*).

### Treatment of overdose
Recommended treatment consists of the following:

To decrease absorption—Administering gastric lavage and general supportive measures.

Specific treatment—
Acidifying the urine to promote renal excretion of trimethoprim.
Using hemodialysis to remove a moderate amount of trimethoprim from the blood, although peritoneal dialysis is not effective.
Discontinuing trimethoprim and administering leucovorin, 3 to 6 mg intramuscularly per day for 5 to 7 days or as necessary, to restore normal hematopoiesis if signs of bone marrow depression occur.

Supportive care—Patients in whom intentional overdose is known or suspected should be referred for psychiatric consultation.

## Patient Consultation

As an aid to patient consultation, refer to *Advice for the Patient, Trimethoprim (Systemic)*.

In providing consultation, consider emphasizing the following selected information (» = major clinical significance):

### Before using this medication
» Conditions affecting use, especially:
Hypersensitivity to trimethoprim
Pregnancy—Trimethoprim crosses the placenta; may interfere with folic acid metabolism in the fetus
Breast-feeding—Trimethoprim is excreted in breast milk; may interfere with folic acid metabolism in the newborn
Other medications, especially folic acid antagonists
Other medical problems, especially megaloblastic anemia due to folic acid deficiency and renal function impairment

### Proper use of this medication
» Not giving this medication to infants or children unless directed by physician
Taking on an empty stomach or, if gastrointestinal irritation occurs, with food
» Compliance with full course of therapy
» Importance of not missing doses and taking at evenly spaced times
» Proper dosing
Missed dose: Taking as soon as possible; not taking if almost time for next dose; not doubling doses
» Proper storage

### Precautions while using this medication
Importance of regular visits to physician to check progress if on prolonged therapy
Checking with physician if no improvement within a few days
Importance of taking folic acid concurrently if anemia occurs
Using caution in use of regular toothbrushes, dental floss, and toothpicks; deferring dental work until blood counts have returned to normal; checking with physician or dentist concerning proper oral hygiene

### Side/adverse effects
Signs of potential side effects, especially blood dyscrasias, aseptic meningitis, hypersensitivity, Stevens-Johnson syndrome, and methemoglobinemia

## General Dosing Information

Trimethoprim may be taken on an empty stomach or, if gastrointestinal irritation occurs, it may be taken with food.

If trimethoprim causes folic acid deficiency, folates may be administered concurrently without interfering with the antibacterial activity of trimethoprim since bacteria are unable to utilize preformed folates. If signs of bone marrow depression occur, trimethoprim should be discontinued. Leucovorin (folinic acid) 3 to 6 mg may be given intramuscularly once a day for 3 days or as required to restore normal hematopoiesis. In chronic overdose of trimethoprim, leucovorin may be given in high doses and/or for an extended period of time.

## Oral Dosage Forms

Note: Bracketed uses in the *Dosage Forms* section refer to categories of use and/or indications that are not included in U.S. product labeling.

### TRIMETHOPRIM TABLETS USP

**Usual adult and adolescent dose**
Antibacterial—
Treatment of urinary tract infections: Oral, 100 mg every twelve hours for ten days; or 200 mg once a day for ten days.
[Pneumonia, *Pneumocystis carinii* (treatment)][1]: Oral, 20 mg per kg of body weight per day of trimethoprim in combination with 100 mg of dapsone once a day for 21 days.
[Prophylaxis of urinary tract infections][1]: Oral, 100 mg once a day.

Note: Adults with impaired renal function may require a reduction in dose as follows:

| Creatinine Clearance (mL/min)/(mL/sec) | Dose |
| --- | --- |
| >30/0.50 | See *Usual adult and adolescent dose* |
| 15–30/0.25–0.50 | 50% of usual dose |
| <15/<0.25 | Use is not recommended |

**Usual adult prescribing limits**
Doses greater than 600 mg are often used when treating *Pneumocystis carinii* pneumonia.

**Usual pediatric dose**
Antibacterial—
Infants and children up to 12 years of age: Dosage has not been established; however, a dose of 3 mg per kg of body weight two times a day has been effectively used in children.
Children 12 years of age and over: See *Usual adult and adolescent dose*.

Note: Safety has not been established in infants under 2 months of age. However, trimethoprim has been used extensively in combination with sulfamethoxazole in pediatric patients.

**Strength(s) usually available**
U.S.—
100 mg (Rx) [*Proloprim; Trimpex;* GENERIC].
200 mg (Rx) [*Proloprim;* GENERIC].
Canada—
100 mg (Rx) [*Proloprim* (scored)].
200 mg (Rx) [*Proloprim* (scored)].

**Packaging and storage**
Store below 40 °C (104 °F), preferably between 15 and 30 °C (59 and 86 °F), unless otherwise specified by manufacturer. Store in a tight, light-resistant container.

**Auxiliary labeling**
• Continue medicine for full time of treatment.

---

[1] Not included in Canadian product labeling.

Revised: 02/23/93

# TRIMETREXATE Systemic

VA CLASSIFICATION (Primary): AP109
Commonly used brand name(s): *Neutrexin*.

Note: For a listing of dosage forms and brand names by country availability, see *Dosage Forms* section(s).

## Category

Antiprotozoal (systemic).

## Indications

### Accepted

Pneumonia, *Pneumocystis carinii* (treatment)—Trimetrexate is indicated as an alternative treatment for moderate to severe *Pneumocystis carinii* pneumonia (PCP) in immunocompromised patients, including those with acquired immunodeficiency syndrome (AIDS), who are intolerant of, or are refractory to, sulfamethoxazole-trimethoprim therapy, or for whom sulfamethoxazole-trimethoprim therapy is contraindicated. Leucovorin must be given concurrently with trimetrexate to prevent potential serious side effects (bone marrow depression, oral and gastrointestinal mucosal ulceration) that could occur if trimetrexate were given alone.

### Acceptance not established

Trimetrexate has been used to treat colorectal, head and neck, non–small cell lung, and pancreatic carcinomas. However, data are limited and more comparative, randomized clinical studies are required to define the role of trimetrexate in these conditions.

## Pharmacology/Pharmacokinetics

### Physicochemical characteristics

Molecular weight—
  Trimetrexate: 369.43.
  Trimetrexate glucuronate: 563.57.
pKa—8.0.

### Mechanism of action/Effect

Trimetrexate is a nonclassical folate antagonist. It is a competitive inhibitor of dihydrofolate reductase (DHFR) from bacterial, protozoan, and mammalian sources. DHFR catalyzes the reduction of intracellular dihydrofolate to the active coenzyme tetrahydrofolate. Inhibition of DHFR results in the depletion of this coenzyme, leading directly to interference with thymidylate biosynthesis, as well as to inhibition of folate-dependent formyltransferases, and indirectly to inhibition of purine biosynthesis. The result is disruption of DNA, RNA, and protein synthesis, with consequent cell death. *In vitro*, trimetrexate binds to the DHFR of *Pneumocystis carinii* approximately 1500 times more potently than does trimethoprim.

Trimetrexate is chemically related to methotrexate but differs from it in several respects. Trimetrexate enters cells by a mechanism different from that of methotrexate. Trimetrexate penetrates the cell rapidly, in a manner that is independent of the folate carrier–mediated transport system required by methotrexate. The structure of trimetrexate does not resemble that of the substrates folic acid or dihydrofolic acid, and trimetrexate uptake is not affected by folic acid or calcium folinate. Also, trimetrexate does not interfere with folate polyglutamate formation or block folate entry by competitive inhibition of the reduced folate transport system. Further, unlike methotrexate, trimetrexate has sustained intracellular retention.

Note: Leucovorin (folinic acid) is transported into mammalian cells and can be assimilated into cellular folate pools following its metabolism. *In vitro* studies have shown that leucovorin provides a source of reduced folates necessary for normal cellular biosynthetic processes. Because *P. carinii* lacks the reduced folate carrier–mediated transport system, leucovorin is prevented from entering the organism. Therefore, at therapeutic doses of trimetrexate and leucovorin, the selective transport of trimetrexate, but not of leucovorin, into the *P. carinii* organism allows leucovorin to protect normal host cells from the cytotoxicity of trimetrexate without inhibiting trimetrexate's therapeutic effect.

### Distribution

Lipid-soluble; distributes readily into ascitic fluid. Penetrates poorly into the cerebrospinal fluid (CSF); the CSF concentration is < 5% of the simultaneous serum concentration.

The steady-state $Vol_D$ is variable and ranges from 9 to 33 liters per square meter of body surface area ($L/m^2$). One phase I study in cancer patients found the steady-state $Vol_D$ to be 0.62 L per kg of body weight.

### Protein binding

*In vitro* studies have found protein binding to vary from 80 to 98%, depending on the serum trimetrexate concentration.

### Biotransformation

Hepatic. Not fully characterized in humans; however, data suggest that the major metabolic pathway is oxidative *O*-demethylation, followed by conjugation to form either the glucuronide or sulfate metabolite. Preliminary findings in humans indicate the presence of a glucuronide conjugate with DHFR-inhibiting activity and a demethylated metabolite in urine.

### Half-life

Biphasic or triphasic elimination has been described; the terminal half-life ranges from 11 to 20 hours.

### Peak serum concentration

Approximately 10 to 12 micromoles per liter (3.7 to 4.4 mcg per mL) after intravenous administration of a dose of 30 mg per square meter of body surface area ($mg/m^2$).

### Elimination

Renal; active tubular secretion and tubular reabsorption are thought to be involved with renal clearance; however, only 10 to 20% of a dose is eliminated as unchanged trimetrexate within 48 hours. Urinary recovery of trimetrexate varies with the assay used, ranging from about 40% with a nonspecific DHFR inhibition assay, which suggests the presence of active metabolites, to about 10% with high pressure liquid chromatography (HPLC). Fecal excretion of the parent compound is < 6% of the dose over 48 hours.

## Precautions to Consider

### Cross-sensitivity and/or related problems

Patients sensitive to methotrexate also may be sensitive to trimetrexate.

### Carcinogenicity

Long-term studies in animals to evaluate the carcinogenic potential of trimetrexate have not been performed.

### Mutagenicity

Trimetrexate was not mutagenic when tested with the standard Ames *Salmonella* mutagenicity assay, with and without metabolic activation. It also did not induce mutations in Chinese hamster lung cells, or sister-chromatid exchange in Chinese hamster ovary cells. No clastogenic activity was found in a mouse micronucleus assay. However, trimetrexate did induce an increase in the incidence of chromosomal aberration in cultured Chinese hamster lung cells.

### Pregnancy/Reproduction

Fertility—No studies have been conducted to evaluate trimetrexate's effects on fertility. However, during standard toxicity studies conducted in mice and rats, degeneration of the testes and spermatocytes and arrest of spermatogenesis were observed.

Pregnancy—Trimetrexate can harm the fetus when administered to a pregnant woman. Women of childbearing potential should be counseled to avoid becoming pregnant during trimetrexate therapy.

Trimetrexate has been shown to be fetotoxic and teratogenic in rats and rabbits. Rats given 1.5 and 2.5 mg per kg of body weight (mg/kg) per day of intravenous trimetrexate on gestational days 6 through 15 showed substantial postimplantation losses and severe inhibition of maternal weight gain. In addition, administration to rats of 0.5 and 1 mg/kg per day on gestational days 6 through 15 caused teratogenicity and retarded fetal development. In rabbits, trimetrexate administered intravenously at doses of 2.5 and 5 mg/kg per day on gestational days 6 through 18 also caused significant maternal and fetal toxicity. Trimetrexate was teratogenic in rabbits given doses of 0.1 mg/kg per day in the absence of significant maternal toxicity. These effects were observed at doses 5 to 50% of the equivalent human therapeutic dose on a mg per square meter of body surface area ($mg/m^2$) basis. Teratogenic effects included skeletal, visceral, ocular, and cardiovascular abnormalities.

FDA Pregnancy Category D.

### Breast-feeding

It is not known if trimetrexate is distributed into breast milk. Breast-feeding is not recommended during trimetrexate therapy because of the potential for serious adverse effects in the nursing infant.

### Pediatrics

Appropriate studies on the relationship of age to the effects of trimetrexate have not been performed in children up to 18 years of age. However, 2 children, ages 9 months and 15 months, were both treated with 45 mg (base)/m² of trimetrexate for 21 days and 20 mg/m² of leucovorin every 6 hours for 24 days with no serious or unexpected adverse effects.

**Geriatrics**

No information is available on the relationship of age to the effects of trimetrexate in geriatric patients.

**Dental**

The bone marrow–depressant effects of trimetrexate may result in an increased incidence of microbial infection, delayed healing, and gingival bleeding. Dental work, whenever possible, should be completed prior to initiation of therapy or deferred until blood counts have returned to normal. Patients should be instructed in proper oral hygiene during treatment, including caution in use of regular toothbrushes, dental floss, and toothpicks.

Trimetrexate also commonly causes ulcerative stomatitis associated with considerable discomfort.

**Drug interactions and/or related problems**

The following drug interactions and/or related problems have been selected on the basis of their potential clinical significance (possible mechanism in parentheses where appropriate)—not necessarily inclusive (» = major clinical significance):

Note: Combinations containing any of the following medications, depending on the amount present, may also interact with this medication.

At this time, no clinically significant drug interactions and/or related problems have been documented in patients receiving trimetrexate. However, concurrent use with the medications listed below theoretically could produce life-threatening toxicity.

Blood dyscrasia–causing medications (see *Appendix II*)
(leukopenic and/or thrombocytopenic effects of trimetrexate may be increased with concurrent or recent therapy if these medications cause the same effects; dosage adjustment of trimetrexate, if necessary, should be based on blood counts)

» Bone marrow depressants, other (see *Appendix II*), or
Radiation therapy
(concurrent use may cause additive bone marrow depression; dosage reduction may be required when two or more bone marrow depressants, including radiation, are used concurrently or consecutively)

» Enzyme inhibitors, hepatic, cytochrome P450
(because trimetrexate is metabolized by the cytochrome P450 enzyme system, medications that affect this enzyme system may decrease, or compete with, the metabolism of trimetrexate, increasing the possibility of trimetrexate toxicity)

» Hepatotoxic medications (see *Appendix II*) such as
Zidovudine or
» Nephrotoxic medications (see *Appendix II*)
(trimetrexate is hepatically metabolized and renally excreted; hepatotoxic or nephrotoxic medications may decrease the clearance of trimetrexate, increasing the risk of trimetrexate toxicity)
(treatment with zidovudine should be discontinued during trimetrexate therapy)

Pyrimethamine or
Trimethoprim
(concurrent use potentially may increase the toxic effects of trimetrexate because of similar folic acid antagonist actions)

**Laboratory value alterations**

The following have been selected on the basis of their potential clinical significance (possible effect in parentheses where appropriate)—not necessarily inclusive (» = major clinical significance):

With physiology/laboratory test values
Alanine aminotransferase (ALT [SGPT]) and
Alkaline phosphatase and
Aspartate aminotransferase (AST [SGOT]) and
Bilirubin
(serum values may be transiently elevated)

Blood urea nitrogen and
Creatinine concentration, serum
(values rarely may be elevated)

» Hemoglobin or hematocrit and
» Leukocyte count, total and differential, and
» Platelet count
(values may be decreased)

**Medical considerations/Contraindications**

The medical considerations/contraindications included have been selected on the basis of their potential clinical significance (reasons given in parentheses where appropriate)—not necessarily inclusive (» = major clinical significance).

*Risk-benefit should be considered when the following medical problems exist:*

» Bone marrow depression
(increased risk of trimetrexate-induced bone marrow toxicity)
» Hepatic function impairment or
» Renal function impairment
(risk of trimetrexate toxicity is increased because clearance of trimetrexate may be impaired and accumulation may occur; even small doses may lead to severe myelosuppression and mucositis; larger doses and/or increased duration of leucovorin treatment may be necessary)
» Sensitivity to trimetrexate, methotrexate, or leucovorin

**Patient monitoring**

The following may be especially important in patient monitoring (other tests may be warranted in some patients, depending on condition; » = major clinical significance):

Alanine aminotransferase (ALT [SGPT]) and
Alkaline phosphatase and
Aspartate aminotransferase (AST [SGOT])
(serum transaminase and alkaline phosphatase values should be monitored approximately twice a week during therapy; trimetrexate therapy should be interrupted if transaminase or alkaline phosphatase values increase to 5 times the upper limit of normal)

Blood urea nitrogen (BUN) or
Creatinine concentration, serum
(blood urea nitrogen or serum creatinine concentrations should be monitored approximately twice a week during therapy; trimetrexate therapy should be interrupted if serum creatinine concentrations increase to ≥ 2.5 mg per dL and the elevation is considered to be secondary to trimetrexate)

» Hemoglobin or hematocrit and
» Leukocyte count, total and, if appropriate, differential, and
» Platelet counts
(determinations should be monitored approximately twice a week during therapy because trimetrexate causes neutropenia, thrombocytopenia, and anemia)

## Side/Adverse Effects

Note: Because many patients who participated in clinical trials had complications of advanced human immunodeficiency virus (HIV) disease, it was often difficult to differentiate between the manifestations of HIV infection and the adverse effects of trimetrexate.

One case of an anaphylactic reaction was observed in a cancer patient who received trimetrexate as a rapid injection.

The following side/adverse effects have been selected on the basis of their potential clinical significance (possible signs and symptoms in parentheses where appropriate)—not necessarily inclusive:

**Those indicating need for medical attention**

Incidence more frequent
*Neutropenia* (fever and sore throat)

Incidence less frequent
*Anemia* (unusual tiredness or weakness); *fever; mouth sores or ulcers; skin rash and itching; thrombocytopenia* (black, tarry stools; blood in urine or stools; pinpoint red spots on skin; unusual bleeding or bruising)

Note: Trimetrexate therapy should be interrupted in patients who experience severe mucosal toxicity that interferes with oral intake of leucovorin. Treatment should be discontinued if a fever develops (oral temperature ≥ 105 °F [40.5 °C]) that cannot be controlled by antipyretics.

**Those indicating need for medical attention only if they continue or are bothersome**

Incidence less frequent
*Confusion; nausea and vomiting; stomach pain*

## Overdose

**Treatment of overdose**

Specific treatment—There has been no extensive experience with patients receiving more than 90 mg per square meter of body surface area (mg/m²) per day of intravenous trimetrexate with concurrent administration of leucovorin. However, in the event of an overdose, the recommended treatment consists of discontinuing trimetrexate and administering leucovorin at a dose of 40 mg/m² every six hours for at least three days.

Supportive care—Patients in whom intentional overdose is confirmed or suspected should be referred for psychiatric consultation.

## Patient Consultation

As an aid to patient consultation, refer to *Advice for the Patient, Trimetrexate (Systemic)*. See also *Advice for the Patient, Leucovorin (Systemic)*.

In providing consultation, consider emphasizing the following selected information (» = major clinical significance):

### Before receiving this medication
» Conditions affecting use, especially:
- Sensitivity to trimetrexate, methotrexate, or leucovorin
- Pregnancy—Use is not recommended because of potential teratogenic and fetotoxic effects; using contraception during trimetrexate treatment; telling physician immediately if pregnancy is suspected
- Breast-feeding—Not recommended because of risk of serious side effects in nursing infants
- Dental—Risk of bleeding of gums and potential infection because of bone marrow–depressant effects
- Other medications, especially other bone marrow depressants, hepatic cytochrome P450 enzyme inhibitors, hepatotoxic medications, or nephrotoxic medications
- Other medical problems, especially bone marrow depression, hepatic function impairment, or renal function impairment

### Proper use of this medication
» *For leucovorin*
- Importance of taking or receiving leucovorin concurrently with trimetrexate, and for 3 days following the end of trimetrexate therapy
- Importance of not missing oral leucovorin doses and taking at evenly spaced times
- Compliance with full course of therapy
- Checking with physician if vomiting occurs shortly after oral dose of leucovorin is taken
» Proper dosing
- Missed dose of leucovorin: Taking oral leucovorin as soon as possible; not taking if almost time for next dose; not doubling doses
» Proper storage of leucovorin

### Precautions while receiving this medication
- Checking with physician if no improvement
» Importance of close monitoring by physician
*Caution if bone marrow depression occurs*
» Avoiding exposure to persons with bacterial infections, especially during periods of low blood counts; checking with physician immediately if fever or chills, cough or hoarseness, lower back or side pain, or painful or difficult urination occurs
» Checking with physician immediately if unusual bleeding or bruising; black, tarry stools; blood in urine or stools; or pinpoint red spots on skin occur
- Caution in use of regular toothbrush, dental floss, or toothpick; physician, dentist, or nurse may suggest alternatives; checking with physician before having dental work done
- Using caution to avoid accidental cuts with use of sharp objects such as safety razor or fingernail or toenail cutters

### Side/adverse effects
Signs of potential side effects, especially neutropenia, anemia, fever, mouth sores or ulcers, skin rash and itching, and thrombocytopenia

## General Dosing Information

**Leucovorin must be given concurrently with trimetrexate to avoid life-threatening toxicities.** Leucovorin therapy must also be continued for 72 hours after the last dose of trimetrexate.

Trimetrexate should be administered as an intravenous infusion, over 60 to 90 minutes. An anaphylactoid reaction was reported in a cancer patient receiving trimetrexate as a rapid injection.

Leucovorin may be administered prior to or following trimetrexate. To prevent formation of a precipitate, intravenous lines should be flushed with at least 10 mL of 5% dextrose injection between trimetrexate and leucovorin infusions. The oral dose of leucovorin (calculated on the basis of body surface area) should be rounded up to the next 25-mg increment to determine the actual dose.

Dosage must be adjusted to meet the individual requirements of each patient, based on clinical response and appearance or severity of toxicity.

Leucovorin tablets have an oral absorption that is saturable at doses above 25 mg. The bioavailability decreases as the dose increases: 97% for 25 mg, 75% for 50 mg, 37% for 100 mg. Because of the larger doses used with trimetrexate, saturable absorption may be a problem. Patients with AIDS may also have problems with malabsorption that could interfere with the absorption of leucovorin. If large doses (greater than 50 mg) are needed in patients with AIDS, intravenous leucovorin should be used.

### Safety considerations for handling this medication
In addition to being an antiprotozoal agent, trimetrexate is also an antineoplastic agent. There is limited but increasing evidence and concern that personnel involved in preparation and administration of parenteral antineoplastics may be at some risk because of the potential mutagenicity, teratogenicity, and/or carcinogenicity of these agents, although the actual risk is unknown. Medical experts recommend cautious handling in both preparation and disposal of antineoplastic agents. Precautions that have been suggested include:
- Use of a biological containment cabinet during reconstitution and dilution of parenteral medications and wearing of disposable surgical gloves and masks.
- Use of proper technique to prevent contamination of the medication, work area, and operator during transfer between containers (including proper training of personnel in this technique).
- Cautious and proper disposal of needles, syringes, vials, ampuls, and unused medication.

A number of medical centers have developed detailed guidelines for handling of antineoplastic agents.

## Parenteral Dosage Forms

Note: The dosing and strengths of the *dosage forms* available are expressed in terms of trimetrexate base (not the glucuronate salt).

### TRIMETREXATE GLUCURONATE FOR INJECTION
**Usual adult dose**
Antiprotozoal—
Intravenous infusion, 45 mg (base) per square meter of body surface area of trimetrexate once a day for twenty-one days. The dose should be administered by intravenous infusion over sixty to ninety minutes. During treatment with trimetrexate, leucovorin must be administered daily and for seventy-two hours after the last dose of trimetrexate (for a total period of twenty-four days). Leucovorin may be administered orally or by intravenous infusion, given over five to ten minutes, at a dose of 20 mg per square meter of body surface area every six hours.

Note: In the event of hematologic toxicity, the doses of trimetrexate and leucovorin should be modified as follows:

| Toxicity grade | Neutrophils (PMNs* and Bands) (per mm$^3$) | Platelets (per mm$^3$) | Trimetrexate dose (mg/m$^2$, once a day) | Leucovorin dose (mg/m$^2$, every 6 hours) |
|---|---|---|---|---|
| 1 | > 1000 | > 75,000 | 45 | 20 |
| 2 | 750-1000 | 50,000-75,000 | 45 | 40 |
| 3 | 500-749 | 25,000-49,999 | 22 | 40 |
| 4† | < 500 | < 25,000 | Day 1-9† Day 10-21† | 40 |

*Polymorphonuclear leukocytes.
†If grade 4 hematologic toxicity occurs prior to day 10, trimetrexate should be discontinued and leucovorin should be administered at a dose of 40 mg/m$^2$ every six hours for an additional seventy-two hours. If grade 4 hematologic toxicity occurs at day 10 or later, trimetrexate may be withheld for up to ninety-six hours to allow counts to recover. If counts recover to grade 3 within ninety-six hours, trimetrexate should be administered at a dose of 22 mg/m$^2$ and leucovorin maintained at 40 mg/m$^2$ every six hours. When counts recover to grade 2, trimetrexate may be increased to 45 mg/m$^2$, but the leucovorin dose should be maintained at 40 mg/m$^2$ for the duration of treatment. If counts do not improve to grade 3 within ninety-six hours, trimetrexate should be discontinued. Leucovorin at a dose of 40 mg/m$^2$ every six hours should be administered for seventy-two hours following the last dose of trimetrexate.

**Usual pediatric dose**
Safety and efficacy have not been established in children up to 18 years of age. However, two children, ages nine months and fifteen months, were treated with 45 mg (base) per square meter of body surface area (mg/m$^2$) of trimetrexate for twenty-one days and 20 mg/m$^2$ of leucovorin for twenty-four days with no serious or unexpected adverse effects.

**Strength(s) usually available**
U.S.—
25 mg per 5 mL (base) (Rx) [*Neutrexin*].
Canada—
25 mg per 5 mL (base) (Rx) [*Neutrexin*].

**Packaging and storage**
Store at room temperature between 15 and 30 °C (59 and 86 °F). Protect from light.

### Preparation of dosage form

Trimetrexate should be reconstituted with 2 mL of 5% dextrose injection or sterile water for injection, to yield a concentration of 12.5 mg per mL. Complete dissolution should occur within 30 seconds. The reconstituted product will appear as a pale greenish-yellow solution. The solution must be inspected visually for particulate matter prior to dilution; it should not be used if cloudiness or precipitation is observed. *The reconstituted solution should be filtered with a 0.22 micron filter prior to further dilution, even if the solution appears clear.*

The reconstituted solution should be further diluted with 5% dextrose injection, to yield a final concentration of 0.25 to 2 mg of trimetrexate per mL.

When reconstituting parenteral leucovorin, if bacteriostatic water for injection (which contains benzyl alcohol) is used, doses greater than 10 milligrams per square meter of body surface area are not recommended. If larger doses are required, leucovorin should be reconstituted with sterile water for injection and used immediately.

### Stability

After initial reconstitution, trimetrexate solution is stable under refrigeration or at room temperature for up to 24 hours. Do not freeze the reconstituted solution. The unused portions should be discarded after 24 hours.

A reconstituted solution that is further diluted with 5% dextrose is stable under refrigeration or at room temperature for up to 24 hours. Do not freeze. The unused portions should be discarded 24 hours after initial reconstitution.

### Incompatibilities

Trimetrexate should not be reconstituted or further diluted with solutions containing either the chloride ion (e.g., solutions containing sodium chloride) or leucovorin. Precipitation occurs instantly. Trimetrexate and leucovorin solutions must be administered separately. Intravenous lines should be flushed with at least 10 mL of 5% dextrose injection between trimetrexate and leucovorin infusions.

### Additional information

If trimetrexate comes in contact with the skin or mucosa, immediately wash thoroughly with soap and water. Procedures for proper disposal of cytotoxic drugs should be considered.

Revised: 05/26/98

---

**TRIMIPRAMINE**—See *Antidepressants, Tricyclic (Systemic)*

---

**TRIOXSALEN**—The *Trioxsalen (Systemic)* monograph is not included in this published version of the USP DI database. Copies of the monograph are available on request from Micromedex, Inc. - Reprint Requests, 6200 S. Syracuse Way, Suite 300, Englewood, CO 80111; telephone (303) 486-6400; telefax (303) 486-6464; Email: USPDI@MDX.COM.

---

**TRIPELENNAMINE**—See *Antihistamines (Systemic)*

---

**TRIPLE SULFA**—See *Sulfonamides (Vaginal)*

---

**TRIPROLIDINE**—See *Antihistamines (Systemic)*

---

# TROGLITAZONE  Systemic—INTRODUCTORY VERSION

VA CLASSIFICATION (Primary): HS505

Commonly used brand name(s): *Rezulin.*

Note:  For a listing of dosage forms and brand names by country availability, see *Dosage Forms* section(s).

## Category

Antidiabetic agent.

## Indications

### Accepted

Diabetes, type 2 (treatment)—Troglitazone is indicated as adjunctive therapy to diet and exercise in the management of patients with type 2 diabetes (previously referred to as non–insulin-dependent diabetes mellitus [NIDDM]). Troglitazone may be used as monotherapy or in combination with insulin or a sulfonylurea antidiabetic agent. In clinical trials, patients previously treated with a sulfonylurea or managed with diet alone were given troglitazone. There was no improvement in glycemic control in the former group. In the latter group, statistical significance versus placebo was seen only in those receiving the highest dose (600 mg per day) of troglitazone. Therefore, troglitazone may be added to, but not substituted for, sulfonylurea therapy in patients whose condition is inadequately controlled with a sulfonylurea alone, and should not be used as monotherapy in patients whose condition was previously well-controlled with a sulfonylurea.

## Pharmacology/Pharmacokinetics

### Physicochemical characteristics

Molecular weight—441.55 daltons.

Solubility—Soluble in *N,N*-dimethylformamide or acetone; sparingly soluble in ethyl acetate; slightly soluble in acetonitrile, anhydrous ethanol, or ether; practically insoluble in water.

### Mechanism of action/Effect

Troglitazone acts primarily by decreasing insulin resistance. It lowers blood glucose concentrations by improving target cell response to insulin. It decreases hepatic glucose output and increases insulin-dependent glucose utilization in skeletal muscle, possibly by binding to nuclear receptors that regulate the transcription of a number of insulin-responsive genes that are critical for the control of glucose and lipid metabolism. Unlike sulfonylureas, troglitazone is not an insulin secretagogue, and is dependent upon the presence of insulin for its activity.

In animal studies, troglitazone reduced the hyperglycemia, hyperinsulinemia, and hypertriglyceridemia characteristic of type 2 diabetes. Plasma lactate and ketone body formation were also decreased. In a rodent model of insulin resistance, no effect on pancreatic weight, islet cell number, or glucagon content was noted. However, an increase in the regranulation of the pancreatic beta cells was seen.

### Absorption

Rapid. The extent of absorption is increased by 30 to 85% in the presence of food.

### Distribution

The mean apparent volume of distribution following multiple-dose administration ranges from 10.5 to 26.5 L per kg of body weight. Radiolabeled troglitazone partitions into red blood cells with approximately 5% of whole blood radioactivity.

### Protein binding

Very high (> 99%); primarily to serum albumin.

### Biotransformation

A sulfate conjugate metabolite (Metabolite 1) and a quinone metabolite (Metabolite 3) have been detected in the plasma of healthy males. A glucuronide conjugate (Metabolite 2) has been detected in the urine and also in negligible amounts in the plasma. In healthy volunteers and in patients with type 2 diabetes, the steady-state concentration of Metabolite 1 is six to seven times that of troglitazone and Metabolite 3.

In *in vivo* drug interaction studies, troglitazone has been shown to induce cytochrome P450 CYP3A4 at clinically relevant doses.

### Half-life

Elimination—16 to 34 hours.

### Time to peak concentration

2 to 3 hours; the time to steady-state plasma concentration is 3 to 5 days.

### Peak plasma concentration

Mean concentrations were 0.9, 1.61, and 2.82 mcg per mL in healthy volunteers given 200, 400, and 600 mg per day, respectively; concentrations increased proportionally with increasing doses over the dose range.

**Elimination**
Fecal—85%.
Renal—3%, primarily as Metabolite 2. Unchanged troglitazone is not recovered in the urine.

## Precautions to Consider

### Carcinogenicity/Tumorigenicity
No evidence of carcinogenicity was found in male rats administered 100 or 400 mg per kg of body weight (mg/kg) per day or in female rats administered 25 or 50 mg/kg per day for 104 weeks. These doses represented area under the plasma concentration–time curve (AUC) values up to 24 times that of the 400-mg-per-day human dose. In a study in mice administered 50, 400, or 800 mg/kg for 104 weeks, the incidence of hemangiosarcoma was increased in females at the 400-mg/kg dose (corresponding to at least two times the 400-mg-per-day human dose based on AUC) and in both sexes at a dose of 800 mg/kg; the incidence of hepatocellular carcinoma was increased in females at the 800-mg/kg dose.

### Mutagenicity
No evidence of mutagenicity or clastogenicity was found in bacteria or in the bone marrow of mice, respectively. Increases in chromosomal aberrations were observed in an *in vitro* Chinese hamster lung cell assay; however, the significance of this finding is unknown. The results of a mouse lymphoma cell gene mutation assay were negative when conducted using an agar plate technique, but the significance of the findings was unknown when this assay was conducted using a microtiter technique. A liver unscheduled DNA synthesis assay in rats was negative.

### Pregnancy/Reproduction
Fertility—Troglitazone therapy may cause resumption of ovulation in premenopausal anovulatory patients with insulin resistance.
No evidence of impaired fertility or reproductive capability was found in male and female rats given 40, 200, or 1000 mg/kg per day (corresponding to three to nine times the human exposure based on AUC) before and during the mating and gestation periods.
Pregnancy—Studies have not been done in humans.
It is recommended that insulin alone be used during pregnancy for maintenance of blood glucose concentrations that are as close to normal as possible. Abnormal maternal blood glucose concentrations have been associated with a higher incidence of congenital anomalies and increased neonatal morbidity and mortality.
No evidence of teratogenicity was found in rats and rabbits given up to 2000 mg/kg and 1000 mg/kg (corresponding to nine and three times the 400-mg-per-day human dose based on AUC), respectively, during organogenesis. Decreased body weight was observed in the fetuses and offspring of rats given 2000 mg/kg during gestation and in the offspring of rats given 40, 200, or 1000 mg/kg during late gestation and lactation periods. The decreased body weight in the latter groups resulted in delayed postnatal development.
FDA Pregnancy Category B.

### Breast-feeding
It is not known whether troglitazone is distributed into human breast milk. However, it is distributed into the milk of lactating rats. Troglitazone is not recommended for use by nursing mothers.

### Pediatrics
Appropriate studies on the relationship of age to the effects of troglitazone have not been performed in the pediatric population. Safety and efficacy have not been established.

### Geriatrics
In clinical trials, 22% of patients were 65 years of age or older. These studies demonstrated no geriatrics-specific problems that would limit the usefulness of troglitazone in the elderly.

### Pharmacogenetics
The pharmacokinetics of troglitazone and its metabolites are similar among various ethnic groups.

### Drug interactions and/or related problems
The following drug interactions and/or related problems have been selected on the basis of their potential clinical significance (possible mechanism in parentheses where appropriate)—not necessarily inclusive (» = major clinical significance):

Note: Combinations containing any of the following medications, depending on the amount present, may also interact with this medication.

» Cholestyramine
(concurrent use may decrease the absorption of troglitazone by approximately 70% and is not recommended)

» Oral contraceptives, ethinyl estradiol– and norethindrone-containing or Other drugs metabolized by cytochrome P450 CYP3A4, such as:

  Astemizole
  Calcium channel blocking agents
  Cisapride
  Corticosteroids
  Cyclosporine
  HMG-CoA reductase inhibitors
  Tacrolimus
  Triazolam
  Trimetrexate or
» Terfenadine
(troglitazone may induce drug metabolism by cytochrome P450 isoenzyme CYP3A4; studies have not been performed with the other drugs metabolized by this enzyme; however, the possibility of altered safety and efficacy should be considered when troglitazone is used concurrently with these drugs; patients stable on one or more of these agents when troglitazone therapy is initiated should be closely monitored and their therapy adjusted as necessary)
(concurrent use may decrease the plasma concentrations of ethinyl estradiol and norethindrone by approximately 30%, resulting in a failure of contraception; a higher dose of oral contraceptive or an alternative method of contraception should be considered)
(concurrent use may decrease the plasma concentrations of terfenadine and its active metabolite by 50 to 70%)

### Laboratory value alterations
The following have been selected on the basis of their potential clinical significance (possible effect in parentheses where appropriate)—not necessarily inclusive (» = major clinical significance):

With physiology/laboratory test values
  Alanine aminotransferase (ALT [SGPT]) and
  Aspartate aminotransferase (AST [SGOT])
    (during controlled clinical trials, reversible elevations greater than three times the upper limit of normal were observed in 2.2% of troglitazone-treated patients versus 0.6% of patients receiving placebo; however, mean and median values at the final visit were decreased compared to baseline)
  Alkaline phosphatase and
  Gamma-glutamyltransferase (GGT)
    (values may be decreased)
  Bilirubin, serum
    (concentrations may initially be increased)
  Cholesterol, total and
  High-density lipoproteins (HDL) and
  Low-density lipoproteins (LDL)
    (concentrations may be increased; however, total cholesterol:HDL and LDL:HDL ratios will not change)
  Hematocrit and
  Hemoglobin concentration and
  Neutrophil count
    (values decreased slightly during the first 4 to 8 weeks of clinical trials but stabilized and remained unchanged for up to 2 years of continuing therapy; decreases have been attributed to dilutional effects of the increased plasma volume observed with troglitazone)
  Triglycerides
    (concentrations may be decreased; however, this decrease may be attenuated when the insulin dose is reduced in patients using combination therapy)

### Medical considerations/Contraindications
The medical considerations/contraindications included have been selected on the basis of their potential clinical significance (reasons given in parentheses where appropriate)—not necessarily inclusive (» = major clinical significance).

*Except under special circumstances, this medication should not be used when the following medical problems exist:*

» Diabetes, type 1 or
» Diabetic ketoacidosis
  (troglitazone lowers plasma glucose concentrations only in the presence of insulin)

» Hepatic function impairment
  (plasma concentrations of troglitazone and its metabolites may be increased; cases of severe idiosyncratic hepatocellular injury have been reported following both short- and long-term therapy with troglitazone; although injury has been rare and usually has been reversible, hepatic failure and death have been reported; troglitazone should be used with caution in patients with hepatic function impairment but should not be initiated in patients exhibiting clinical evidence of active liver disease or ALT values greater than 1.5 times the upper limit of normal; troglitazone should be discontinued if

transaminase values become greater than three times the upper limit of normal or if jaundice develops)
» Hypersensitivity to troglitazone

*Risk-benefit should be considered when the following medical problem exists:*
» Congestive heart failure
(troglitazone has been shown to increase plasma volume in healthy volunteers; use is not recommended in patients with New York Heart Association Class III or IV cardiac status unless the expected benefit is believed to outweigh the potential risk)

**Patient monitoring**
The following may be especially important in patient monitoring (other tests may be warranted in some patients, depending on condition; » = major clinical significance):
» Glucose concentrations, blood
(regular monitoring recommended to assess therapeutic efficacy)
» Glycosylated hemoglobin determinations
(recommended for monitoring long-term glycemic control)
» Liver function tests
(recommended if the patient develops symptoms, such as abdominal pain, anorexia, dark urine, fatigue, nausea, or vomiting, that are suggestive of hepatic dysfunction)
» Transaminase values
(recommended prior to the start of therapy, once a month for the first 8 months of therapy, every 2 months for the remainder of the first year of therapy, and periodically thereafter; troglitazone should not be initiated in patients exhibiting clinical evidence of active liver disease or ALT values greater than 1.5 times the upper limit of normal and should be discontinued if values become greater than three times the upper limit of normal or if the patient develops jaundice; if ALT values become greater than 1.5 to two times the upper limit of normal, the test should be repeated once a week until values return to normal)

## Side/Adverse Effects

Note: Troglitazone does not stimulate insulin secretion and, administered alone, is not expected to cause hypoglycemia. However, there is a potential for hypoglycemia when troglitazone is administered in conjunction with insulin or a sulfonylurea.

Cases of severe idiosyncratic hepatocellular injury have been reported following both short- and long-term therapy with troglitazone. Although injury has been rare and usually has been reversible, hepatic failure and death have been reported following use of troglitazone.

A 6 to 8% increase in plasma volume was observed in healthy volunteers given troglitazone versus those given placebo during clinical trials. This effect was not associated with an increase in the incidence of adverse effects potentially related to volume expansion, but patients with cardiac function impairment were not included in the trials. Use of troglitazone is not recommended in patients with New York Heart Association Class III or IV cardiac status unless the expected benefit is believed to outweigh the potential risk.

The following side/adverse effects have been selected on the basis of their potential clinical significance (possible signs and symptoms in parentheses where appropriate)—not necessarily inclusive:

**Those indicating need for medical attention**
Incidence more frequent
*Back pain*—incidence 6%; *infection*—incidence 18%; *pain*—incidence 10%
Incidence less frequent
*Peripheral edema* (swelling of feet or lower legs)—incidence 5%; *urinary tract infection* (painful or increased urination)—incidence 5%
Incidence rare
*Jaundice* (yellow eyes or skin)—reversible
Note: Troglitazone therapy should be discontinued if *jaundice* develops.

**Those indicating need for medical attention only if they continue or are bothersome**
Incidence more frequent
*Dizziness*—incidence 6%; *headache*—incidence 11%; *nausea*—incidence 6%; *unusual tiredness or weakness*—incidence 6%
Incidence less frequent
*Diarrhea*—incidence 5%; *pharyngitis* (sore throat)—incidence 5%; *rhinitis* (stuffy nose)—incidence 5%

## Patient Consultation
As an aid to patient consultation, refer to *Advice for the Patient, Troglitazone (Systemic)—Introductory Version.*
In providing consultation, consider emphasizing the following selected information (» = major clinical significance):

**Before using this medication**
» Conditions affecting use, especially:
Hypersensitivity to troglitazone
Pregnancy—Use of insulin alone is recommended during pregnancy for maintenance of blood glucose concentrations as close to normal as possible
Breast-feeding—Not recommended for use by nursing mothers
Other medications, especially cholestyramine, ethinyl estradiol- and norethindrone-containing oral contraceptives, or terfenadine
Other medical problems, especially congestive heart failure, diabetic ketoacidosis, hepatic function impairment, or type 1 diabetes

**Proper use of this medication**
» Importance of adherence to recommended regimens for diet, exercise, and glucose monitoring
» Taking medication with a meal
» Proper dosing
Missed dose: Taking with next meal if remembered the same day; if dose is missed on one day, not doubling dose the following day
» Proper storage

**Precautions while using this medication**
» Reporting symptoms, such as abdominal pain, anorexia, dark urine, fatigue, jaundice, nausea, or vomiting, that are suggestive of hepatic dysfunction to physician immediately
» Regular visits to physician to check progress and monitor liver function
» *Carefully following special instructions of health care team*
Discussing use of alcohol
Not taking other medications unless discussed with physician
Getting counseling for family members to help the patient with diabetes; also, special counseling for pregnancy planning and contraception
Making travel plans that include readiness for diabetic emergencies and eating meals at the usual times, even with changing time zones
» Preparing for and understanding what to do in case of diabetic emergency; carrying medical history and current medication list and wearing medical identification
» Recognizing what brings on symptoms of hypoglycemia, such as using other antidiabetic medication; delaying or missing a meal; exercising more than usual; drinking significant amounts of alcohol; or illness, including vomiting or diarrhea
» Recognizing symptoms of hypoglycemia: anxiety; behavior change similar to drunkenness; blurred vision; cold sweats; confusion; cool, pale skin; difficulty in concentrating; drowsiness; excessive hunger; fast heartbeat; headache; nausea; nervousness; nightmares; restless sleep; shakiness; slurred speech; or unusual tiredness or weakness
» Knowing what to do if symptoms of hypoglycemia occur, such as eating glucose tablets or gel, corn syrup, honey, or sugar cubes; drinking fruit juice, nondiet soft drink, or sugar dissolved in water; or injecting glucagon if symptoms are severe
» Recognizing what brings on symptoms of hyperglycemia, such as not taking enough or skipping a dose of antidiabetic medication, overeating or not following meal plan, having a fever or infection, or exercising less than usual
» Recognizing symptoms of hyperglycemia and ketoacidosis: blurred vision; drowsiness; dry mouth; flushed, dry skin; fruit-like breath odor; increased urination (frequency and volume); ketones in urine; loss of appetite; stomachache, nausea, or vomiting; tiredness; troubled breathing (rapid and deep); unconsciousness; and unusual thirst
» Knowing what to do if symptoms of hyperglycemia occur, such as checking blood glucose and contacting a member of the health care team

**Side/adverse effects**
Signs of potential side effects, especially back pain, infection, pain, peripheral edema, urinary tract infection, and jaundice

## General Dosing Information

**Diet/Nutrition**
Food increases the extent of absorption by 30 to 85%. Therefore, troglitazone should be taken with a meal to enhance its systemic bioavailability.

## Oral Dosage Forms

### TROGLITAZONE TABLETS

**Usual adult dose**
Antidiabetic agent—
As monotherapy:
    Oral, initially 400 or 600 mg once a day with a meal. After four weeks, if adequate response is not achieved with the 400-mg dose, it may be increased to 600 mg once a day with a meal; if adequate response is not achieved after four weeks at the 600-mg dose, troglitazone should be discontinued and alternative therapeutic options should be pursued.
In combination with insulin:
    Oral, initally 200 mg once a day with a meal. Dose may be increased after approximately two to four weeks to 400 mg once a day with a meal.
Note: The current insulin dose should be continued upon initiation of troglitazone therapy. However, the insulin dose should be decreased by 10 to 25% when the fasting plasma glucose concentration decreases to less than 120 mg per dL.
In combination with a sulfonylurea:
    Oral, 200 mg once a day with a meal. Dose may be increased after two to four weeks, if necessary.
Note: The current sulfonylurea dose should be continued upon initiation of troglitazone therapy. However, the sulfonylurea dose subsequently may be decreased.

**Usual adult prescribing limits**
600 mg once a day.

**Usual pediatric dose**
Safety and efficacy have not been established.

**Usual geriatric dose**
See *Usual adult dose.*

**Strength(s) usually available**
U.S.—
    200 mg (Rx) [*Rezulin* (croscarmellose sodium; hydroxypropyl methylcellulose; magnesium stearate; microcrystalline cellulose; polyethylene glycol 400; polysorbate 80; povidone; purified water; silicon dioxide; titanium dioxide; synthetic iron oxides)].
    300 mg (Rx) [*Rezulin* (croscarmellose sodium; hydroxypropyl methylcellulose; magnesium stearate; microcrystalline cellulose; polyethylene glycol 400; polysorbate 80; povidone; purified water; silicon dioxide; titanium dioxide; synthetic iron oxides)].
    400 mg (Rx) [*Rezulin* (croscarmellose sodium; hydroxypropyl methylcellulose; magnesium stearate; microcrystalline cellulose; polyethylene glycol 400; polysorbate 80; povidone; purified water; silicon dioxide; titanium dioxide; synthetic iron oxides)].

**Packaging and storage**
Store between 20 and 25 °C (68 and 77 °F). Protect from moisture and humidity.

**Auxiliary labeling**
• Take with a meal.

---

Developed: 04/18/97
Interim revision: 10/30/97; 11/17/97; 02/18/98; 08/12/98

---

**TROPICAMIDE**—The *Tropicamide (Ophthalmic)* monograph is not included in this published version of the USP DI database. Copies of the monograph are available on request from Micromedex, Inc. - Reprint Requests, 6200 S. Syracuse Way, Suite 300, Englewood, CO 80111; telephone (303) 486-6400; telefax (303) 486-6464; Email: USPDI@MDX.COM.

---

# TROVAFLOXACIN    Systemic—INTRODUCTORY VERSION

VA CLASSIFICATION (Primary): AM900
Note: This monograph contains dosage information for trovafloxacin and its prodrug alatrofloxacin.
Commonly used brand name(s): *Trovan.*
Note: For a listing of dosage forms and brand names by country availability, see *Dosage Forms* section(s).

## Category
Antibacterial (systemic).

## Indications

**General considerations**
Trovafloxacin and its prodrug alatrofloxacin are fluoronaphthyridones, which are related to the fluoroquinolone antibacterials. Trovafloxacin is active against a wide range of gram-positive and gram-negative microorganisms, both *in vitro* and in patients infected with them. The susceptible microorganisms include *Enterococcus faecalis, Escherichia coli, Gardnerella vaginalis, Haemophilus influenzae, Haemophilus parainfluenzae, Klebsiella pneumoniae, Moraxella catarrhalis, Neisseria gonorrhoeae, Proteus mirabilis, Pseudomonas aeruginosa,* methicillin-susceptible strains of *Staphylococcus aureus* and *Staphylococcus epidermidis, Streptococcus agalactiae,* penicillin-susceptible strains of *Streptococcus pneumoniae, Streptococcus pyogenes,* and viridans group streptococci; anaerobic microorganisms, including *Bacteroides fragilis* and *Peptostreptococcus* and *Prevotella* species; and other microorganisms such as *Chlamydia pneumoniae, Chlamydia trachomatis, Legionella pneumophila,* and *Mycoplasma pneumoniae.*

There is no evidence of microbial cross-resistance between trovafloxacin and aminoglycosides, cephalosporins, macrolides, penicillins, or tetracyclines. Cross-resistance has been observed between trovafloxacin and some other fluoroquinolones. However, some microorganisms that are resistant to other fluoroquinolones may be susceptible to trovafloxacin. *In vitro* bacterial resistance to trovafloxacin develops slowly via multiple-step mutation, in a manner similar to the development of resistance to other fluoroquinolones.

Results obtained from *in vitro* studies indicate that combinations of trovafloxacin with beta-lactam antibiotics or aminoglycosides may be synergistic when exposed to certain bacterial strains, but that such synergy is not commonly observed.

**Accepted**
Bronchitis, bacterial exacerbations (treatment)—Trovafloxacin is indicated in the treatment of bacterial exacerbations of chronic bronchitis due to *H. influenzae, H. parainfluenzae, M. catarrhalis, S. aureus,* or *S. pneumoniae.*

Cervicitis (treatment)—Trovafloxacin is indicated in the treatment of cervicitis due to *C. trachomatis.*

Gonorrhea, endocervical (treatment)
Gonorrhea, rectal, in females (treatment) or
Gonorrhea, urethral, uncomplicated (treatment)—Trovafloxacin is indicated in females for the treatment of endocervical and rectal gonorrhea, and in males for the treatment of uncomplicated urethral gonorrhea, due to *N. gonorrhoeae.*

Gynecologic infections (treatment)—Alatrofloxacin is indicated in the treatment of gynecologic and pelvic infections, including endomyometritis, parametritis, postpartum infections, and septic abortion, due to *B. fragilis, E. faecalis, E. coli, G. vaginalis, Peptostreptococcus* species, *Prevotella* species, *S. agalactiae,* or viridans group streptococci.

Intra-abdominal infections (treatment)—Alatrofloxacin is indicated in the treatment of complicated intra-abdominal infections, including postsurgical infections, due to *B. fragilis, E. coli, K. pneumoniae, Peptostreptococcus* species, *Prevotella* species, *P. aeruginosa,* or viridans group streptococci.

Pelvic inflammatory disease (treatment)—Trovafloxacin is indicated in the treatment of mild to moderate pelvic inflammatory disease due to *C. trachomatis* or *N. gonorrhoeae.*

Perioperative infections (prophylaxis)—Alatrofloxacin and trovafloxacin are indicated in the prevention of infection associated with elective abdominal or vaginal hysterectomy, or colorectal surgery.

Pneumonia, community-acquired (treatment)—Alatrofloxacin and trovafloxacin are indicated in the treatment of community-acquired pneumonia due to *C. pneumoniae, H. influenzae, K. pneumoniae, L. pneumophila, M. catarrhalis, M. pneumoniae, S. aureus,* or *S. pneumoniae.*

Pneumonia, nosocomial (treatment)—Alatrofloxacin is indicated in the treatment of nosocomial pneumonia due to *E. coli, H. influenzae, P. aeruginosa,* or *S. aureus.* Combination therapy with either an aminoglycoside or aztreonam may be clinically indicated when *P. aeruginosa* is a documented or presumptive pathogen.

**Prostatitis, bacterial, chronic (treatment)**—Trovafloxacin is indicated in the treatment of chronic bacterial prostatitis due to *E. faecalis*, *E. coli*, or *S. epidermidis*.

**Sinusitis, acute (treatment)**—Trovafloxacin is indicated in the treatment of acute sinusitis due to *H. influenzae*, *M. catarrhalis*, or *S. pneumoniae*.

**Skin and soft tissue infections (treatment)**—Trovafloxacin is indicated in the treatment of complicated skin and soft tissue infections, including diabetic foot infections, due to *E. faecalis*, *E. coli*, *P. mirabilis*, *P. aeruginosa*, *S. aureus*, or *S. agalactiae*. Trovafloxacin is also indicated in the treatment of uncomplicated skin and soft tissue infections due to *S. aureus*, *S. agalactiae*, or *S. pyogenes*.

**Urinary tract infections, bacterial (treatment)**—Trovafloxacin is indicated in the treatment of uncomplicated urinary tract infections, including cystitis, due to *E. coli*.

### Unaccepted
Trovafloxacin has not been studied in the treatment of osteomyelitis.

## Pharmacology/Pharmacokinetics

### Physicochemical characteristics
Chemical group—Fluoronaphthyridone, related to fluoroquinolone antibacterials. Alatrofloxacin is the L-alanyl-L-alanyl prodrug of trovafloxacin.
Molecular weight—Alatrofloxacin mesylate: 654.63.
Trovafloxacin mesylate: 512.47.

### Mechanism of action/Effect
The bactericidal action of trovafloxacin is due to its inhibition of the bacterial enzymes topoisomerase II (DNA gyrase) and topoisomerase IV, which are essential for duplication, transcription, and repair of bacterial DNA.

### Absorption
Oral trovafloxacin is well-absorbed from the gastrointestinal tract, and the rate of absorption is not altered by concomitant food intake. The absolute bioavailability is approximately 88%.

### Distribution
$Vol_D$—1.2 ± 0.2 to 1.3 ± 0.1 L per kg (L/kg) as trovafloxacin, following a 1-hour infusion of 200 mg of alatrofloxacin. 1.2 ± 0.1 to 1.4 ± 0.1 L/kg as trovafloxacin, following a 1-hour infusion of 300 mg of alatrofloxacin.

Trovafloxacin is widely distributed throughout the body; the highest concentrations are reached in bile, bronchial macrophages, lung epithelial lining fluid, and vaginal fluid. Rapid distribution into tissues results in significantly higher concentrations of trovafloxacin in most target tissues than in plasma or serum.

### Protein binding
High (approximately 76%); plasma protein binding is concentration-independent.

### Biotransformation
After intravenous administration, alatrofloxacin is rapidly converted to trovafloxacin.

Trovafloxacin is metabolized by conjugation; the role of the cytochrome P450 enzyme system in the oxidative metabolism of trovafloxacin is minimal. The major metabolites include the ester glucuronide, which appears in the urine (13% of the administered dose); and the *N*-acetyl metabolite, which appears in the feces and serum (9% and 2.5% of the administered dose, respectively). Other minor metabolites include diacid, hydroxycarboxylic acid, and sulfamate, which have been identified in both the feces and the urine in small amounts (< 4% of the administered dose).

### Serum half-life
Following intravenous administration, alatrofloxacin is rapidly converted to trovafloxacin. Plasma concentrations of alatrofloxacin are below quantifiable levels within 5 to 10 minutes of completion of a 1-hour infusion.

Alatrofloxacin injection (measured as trovafloxacin)—
Following a single 1-hour infusion of 200 mg: 9.4 hours.
Following multiple 1-hour infusions of 200 mg: 11.7 hours.
Following a single 1-hour infusion of 300 mg: 11.2 hours.
Following multiple 1-hour infusions of 300 mg: 12.7 hours.

Trovafloxacin tablets—
Following a single oral dose of 100 mg: 9.1 hours.
Following multiple oral doses of 100 mg: 10.5 hours.
Following a single oral dose of 200 mg: 9.6 hours.
Following multiple oral doses of 200 mg: 12.2 hours.

### Time to peak concentration
Alatrofloxacin injection (measured as trovafloxacin)—
Following a single 1-hour infusion of 200 mg: 1 hour.
Following multiple 1-hour infusions of 200 mg: 1 hour.
Following a single 1-hour infusion of 300 mg: 1.3 ± 0.4 hours.
Following multiple 1-hour infusions of 300 mg: 1.2 ± 0.2 hours.

Trovafloxacin tablets—
Following a single oral dose of 100 mg: 0.9 ± 0.4 hour.
Following multiple oral doses of 100 mg: 1 ± 0.5 hour.
Following a single oral dose of 200 mg: 1.8 ± 0.9 hours.
Following multiple oral doses of 200 mg: 1.2 ± 0.5 hours.

### Peak serum concentration
Serum concentrations of trovafloxacin are dose-proportional after oral administration of trovafloxacin in the dose range of 30 to 1000 mg, or after intravenous administration of alatrofloxacin in the dose range of 30 to 400 mg (trovafloxacin equivalents). Steady-state concentrations are achieved by the third daily oral or intravenous dose, with an accumulation factor of approximately 1.3 times the single dose concentrations.

Alatrofloxacin injection—
Following a single 1-hour infusion of 200 mg: 2.7 ± 0.4 mcg per mL (mcg/mL) of trovafloxacin.
Following multiple 1-hour infusions of 200 mg: 3.1 ± 0.6 mcg/mL of trovafloxacin.
Following a single 1-hour infusion of 300 mg: 3.6 ± 0.6 mcg/mL of trovafloxacin.
Following multiple 1-hour infusions of 300 mg: 4.4 ± 0.6 mcg/mL of trovafloxacin.

Trovafloxacin tablets—
Following a single oral dose of 100 mg: 1 ± 0.3 mcg/mL.
Following multiple oral doses of 100 mg: 1.1 ± 0.2 mcg/mL.
Following a single oral dose of 200 mg: 2.1 ± 0.5 mcg/mL.
Following multiple oral doses of 200 mg: 3.1 ± 1 mcg/mL.

### Elimination
Trovafloxacin is eliminated primarily by biliary excretion.
Fecal—Approximately 43% of an oral dose is recovered unchanged.
Renal—Approximately 6% of an oral dose is recovered unchanged. The mean cumulative urinary concentration is 12.1 ± 3.4 mcg/mL for healthy subjects receiving multiple doses of 200 mg.
In dialysis—Trovafloxacin is not efficiently removed by hemodialysis.

## Precautions to Consider

### Cross-sensitivity and/or related problems
Patients allergic to fluoroquinolones or other chemically related quinolone derivatives (e.g., cinoxacin, nalidixic acid) may be allergic to trovafloxacin or alatrofloxacin also.

### Carcinogenicity
Long-term studies in animals to determine the carcinogenic potential of alatrofloxacin or trovafloxacin have not been done.

### Mutagenicity
Alatrofloxacin—Alatrofloxacin was not mutagenic in a mouse micronucleus assay.
Trovafloxacin—Trovafloxacin was not mutagenic in the Ames *Salmonella* reversion assay or the CHO/HGPRT mammalian cell gene mutation assay, nor was it clastogenic in mitogen-stimulated human lymphocytes or mouse bone marrow cells. However, trovafloxacin was mutagenic in the *E. coli* bacterial mutagenicity assay.

### Pregnancy/Reproduction
Fertility—
*Alatrofloxacin*—
Intravenous doses of 50 mg per kg of body weight (mg/kg) per day did not affect the fertility of male or female rats. This dose is approximately 10 times the maximum recommended human dose (MRHD) on a mg/kg basis, or approximately two times the MRHD on a mg per square meter of body surface area (mg/m$^2$) basis.
*Trovafloxacin*—
Oral doses of 75 mg/kg per day did not affect the fertility of male or female rats. This dose is approximately 15 times the MRHD on a mg/kg basis, or approximately two times the MRHD on a mg/m$^2$ basis. However, oral doses of 200 mg/kg per day (40 times the MRHD on a mg/kg basis, or six times the MRHD on a mg/m$^2$ basis) were associated with increased preimplantation loss in rats.

Pregnancy—Adequate and well-controlled studies in humans have not been done. Trovafloxacin or alatrofloxacin should be used during pregnancy only if the potential benefit to the mother outweighs the potential risk to the fetus.
*Alatrofloxacin*—
An increase in skeletal variations was observed in rat fetuses following maternal intravenous doses of 20 mg/kg and greater per day (≥ four times the MRHD on a mg/kg basis, or ≥ 0.6 times

the MRHD on a mg/m² basis) given during the period of organogenesis. However, fetal skeletal variations or malformations were not observed following maternal intravenous doses of 6.5 mg/kg per day.

In rabbits, maternal intravenous doses of 20 mg/kg per day (approximately equal to the MRHD on a mg/m² basis) given during the period of organogenesis also were associated with an increased incidence of fetal skeletal malformations. However, fetal skeletal variations or malformations were not observed following maternal intravenous doses of 6.5 mg/kg per day.

*Trovafloxacin—*
An increase in skeletal variations was observed in rat fetuses following maternal oral doses of 75 mg/kg per day given during the period of organogenesis. Fetotoxicity, evidenced by increased perinatal mortality and decreased body weights of pups, was also observed for this level of dosing. However, fetal skeletal abnormalities were not observed in rats following maternal oral doses of 15 mg/kg per day. Oral doses greater than 5 mg/kg per day were associated with an increase in gestation time, and several rats given doses of 75 mg/kg per day experienced uterine dystocia.

In rabbits, maternal oral doses of 45 mg/kg per day (approximately nine times the MRHD on a mg/kg basis, or 2.7 times the MRHD on a mg/m² basis) were not associated with an increased incidence of fetal skeletal variations or malformations.

FDA Pregnancy Category C.

### Breast-feeding
Trovafloxacin is distributed into breast milk. The average measurable concentration was 0.8 mcg/mL (range, 0.3 to 2.1 mcg/mL) following a single intravenous dose of alatrofloxacin (equivalent to 300 mg trovafloxacin) and following multiple oral 200-mg doses of trovafloxacin. Breast-feeding is not recommended during treatment with trovafloxacin or alatrofloxacin because these medications have been reported to cause arthropathy in immature animals of several species.

### Pediatrics
Appropriate studies on the relationship of age to the effects of alatrofloxacin or trovafloxacin have not been performed in infants or children. Safety, efficacy, and pharmacokinetics of trovafloxacin or alatrofloxacin have not been established. Quinolones, including alatrofloxacin and trovafloxacin, cause arthropathy in immature animals of several species.

### Adolescents
Appropriate studies on the relationship of age to the effects of alatrofloxacin or trovafloxacin have not been performed in patients less than 18 years of age. Safety, efficacy, and pharmacokinetics have not been established. Quinolones, including alatrofloxacin and trovafloxacin, cause arthropathy in immature animals of several species.

### Geriatrics
Appropriate studies performed to date have not demonstrated geriatrics-specific problems that would limit the usefulness of alatrofloxacin or trovafloxacin in the elderly.

### Drug interactions and/or related problems
The following drug interactions and/or related problems have been selected on the basis of their potential clinical significance (possible mechanism in parentheses where appropriate)—not necessarily inclusive (» = major clinical significance):

Note: No significant pharmacokinetic interactions have been observed between oral trovafloxacin and cimetidine, cyclosporine, digoxin, theophylline, or warfarin. Minor pharmacokinetic interactions, most likely without clinical significance, were observed between oral trovafloxacin and caffeine, calcium carbonate, or omeprazole.

Combinations containing any of the following medications, depending on the amount present, may also interact with this medication.

» Antacids, aluminum- or magnesium-containing or
» Iron- or other metal–containing supplements or
» Sodium citrate and citric acid or
» Sucralfate
(the absorption of oral trovafloxacin is significantly reduced by concurrent administration of aluminum- or magnesium-containing antacids, iron- or other metal–containing supplements, sodium citrate and citric acid, or sucralfate; these oral agents should be taken at least 2 hours before or 2 hours after oral trovafloxacin is taken)

» Morphine
(concurrent administration of intravenous morphine significantly reduces the absorption of oral trovafloxacin; trovafloxacin has no effect on the pharmacokinetics of morphine or its metabolite morphine-6-beta-glucuronide; intravenous morphine should be administered at least 2 hours after oral trovafloxacin is taken in the fasted state, or at least 4 hours after oral trovafloxacin is taken with food)

### Laboratory value alterations
The following have been selected on the basis of their potential clinical significance (possible effect in parentheses where appropriate)—not necessarily inclusive (» = major clinical significance):

With physiology/laboratory test values
Liver function tests
(in a study on chronic bacterial prostatitis in which oral trovafloxacin was administered for 28 days, 9% of trovafloxacin-treated patients experienced elevations of serum transaminases [ALT (SGPT) and/or AST (SGOT)] ≥ three times the upper limit of normal; these abnormalities generally developed at the end of, or following completion of, the planned 28-day course of therapy, and were not associated with concurrent elevations of related measures of hepatic function; values generally returned to normal within 1 to 2 months after discontinuation of therapy)

### Medical considerations/Contraindications
The medical considerations/contraindications included have been selected on the basis of their potential clinical significance (reasons given in parentheses where appropriate)—not necessarily inclusive (» = major clinical significance).

Note: The safety and efficacy of alatrofloxacin or trovafloxacin given for more than 4 weeks have not been studied.

*Except under special circumstances, this medication should not be used when the following medical problem exists:*

» Hypersensitivity to alatrofloxacin, trovafloxacin, or other quinolone antimicrobial agents

*Risk-benefit should be considered when the following medical problems exist:*

Central nervous system (CNS) disorders, including:
» Cerebral arteriosclerosis, severe or
» Epilepsy or
» Other factors that predispose the patient to seizures
(convulsions, increased intracranial pressure, and toxic psychosis have been reported in patients receiving quinolones; quinolones may also cause CNS stimulation, which may lead to confusion, depression, hallucinations, insomnia, lightheadedness, nightmares, paranoia, restlessness, or tremors; alatrofloxacin and trovafloxacin should be used with caution in patients with known or suspected CNS disorders)

» Hepatic disease, chronic
(the area under the plasma concentration–time curve [AUC] for trovafloxacin was increased by approximately 45% in patients with mild cirrhosis [Child-Pugh class A] following daily administration of 100 mg for seven days; the AUC for trovafloxacin was increased by approximately 50% in patients with moderate cirrhosis [Child-Pugh class B] following daily administration of 200 mg for seven days; therefore, dosage adjustment is recommended in patients with mild or moderate cirrhosis; no data are available for patients with severe cirrhosis [Child-Pugh class C])

### Patient monitoring
The following may be especially important in patient monitoring (other tests may be warranted in some patients, depending on condition; » = major clinical significance):

Hepatic function tests
(alatrofloxacin or trovafloxacin may cause elevations of liver function tests during or soon after prolonged therapy [i.e., ≥ 21 days]; periodic assessment of hepatic function is recommended)

## Side/Adverse Effects
The following side/adverse effects have been selected on the basis of their potential clinical significance (possible signs and symptoms in parentheses where appropriate)—not necessarily inclusive:

### Those indicating need for medical attention
Incidence rare
**CNS stimulation, including acute psychosis** (confusion; hallucinations; restlessness; seizures; tremors); **hypersensitivity reaction** (difficulty in breathing or swallowing; rapid heartbeat; shortness of breath; skin itching, rash, or redness; swelling of face, throat, or tongue); **phlebitis** (pain at site of injection); **pseudomembranous colitis** (abdominal or stomach cramps and pain, severe; abdominal tenderness; diarrhea, watery and severe, which may also be bloody; fever); **tendinitis or tendon rupture** (pain in calves, radiating to heels; swelling of calves or lower legs)

Note: Trovafloxacin should be discontinued at the first appearance of skin rash or other sign of hypersensitivity reaction, or if the patient experiences pain, inflammation, or rupture of a tendon.

**Those indicating need for medical attention only if they continue or are bothersome**
Incidence more frequent
*Diarrhea, mild; dizziness or lightheadedness; headache; nausea or vomiting; vaginitis* (vaginal pain and discharge)
Incidence rare
*Photosensitivity reaction* (increased sensitivity of skin to sunlight)

**Those indicating possible pseudomembranous colitis and the need for medical attention if they occur after medication is discontinued**
*Abdominal or stomach cramps and pain, severe; abdominal tenderness; diarrhea, watery and severe, which may also be bloody; fever*

## Overdose
For more information on the management of overdose or unintentional ingestion, **contact a Poison Control Center** (see *Poison Control Center Listing*).

**Treatment of overdose**
To decrease absorption—The stomach may be emptied by emesis or by gastric lavage.
To enhance elimination—Trovafloxacin is not efficiently removed by hemodialysis.
Supportive care—Adequate hydration should be maintained. Patients in whom intentional overdose is confirmed or suspected should be referred for psychiatric consultation.

## Patient Consultation
As an aid to patient consultation, refer to *Advice for the Patient, Trovafloxacin (Systemic)—Introductory Version*.
In providing consultation, consider emphasizing the following selected information (» = major clinical significance):

**Before using this medication**
» Conditions affecting use, especially:
   Sensitivity to alatrofloxacin, trovafloxacin, or other quinolone antibiotics
   Pregnancy—Use is recommended only if the potential benefit to the mother outweighs the potential risk to the fetus
   Breast-feeding—Trovafloxacin is distributed into breast milk
   Use in children—Use is not recommended because fluoroquinolones have been shown to cause arthropathy in immature animals
   Use in adolescents—Use is not recommended in adolescents younger than 18 years of age because fluoroquinolones have been shown to cause arthropathy in immature animals
   Other medications, especially aluminum- or magnesium-containing antacids, iron- or other metal–containing supplements, morphine, sodium citrate and citric acid, or sucralfate
   Other medical problems, especially CNS disorders, including epilepsy, severe cerebral arteriosclerosis, and other factors that predispose the patient to seizures; or chronic hepatic disease

**Proper use of this medication**
» Not giving to infants, children, or adolescents
   Compliance with full course of therapy
» Proper dosing
   Missed dose: Taking as soon as possible if remembered the same day; if dose is missed on one day, not doubling dose the following day
» Proper storage

**Precautions while using this medication**
   Not taking antacids, citric acid buffered with sodium citrate, iron- or other metal–containing vitamins or supplements, or sucralfate within 2 hours before or 2 hours after taking oral trovafloxacin
   Possible photosensitivity reactions; importance of avoiding direct sunlight and using sunblock of SPF 15 or higher
   Caution if dizziness or lightheadedness occurs

**Side/adverse effects**
   Signs of potential side effects, especially CNS stimulation, including acute psychosis; hypersensitivity reaction; phlebitis; pseudomembranous colitis; or tendinitis or tendon rupture

## General Dosing Information
No dosage adjustment is necessary for patients with renal function impairment.
The safety and efficacy of alatrofloxacin or trovafloxacin given for more than 4 weeks have not been studied.

**For oral dosage forms only**
Oral trovafloxacin should be taken at least 2 hours before or 2 hours after aluminum- or magnesium-containing antacids, citric acid buffered with sodium citrate, iron- or other metal–containing supplements, or sucralfate is taken.
Intravenous morphine should be administered at least 2 hours after oral trovafloxacin is taken in the fasted state, or at least 4 hours after oral trovafloxacin is taken with food.

**For parenteral dosage forms only**
Alatrofloxacin injection should be administered only by intravenous infusion over a period of 60 minutes. Rapid or bolus intravenous infusion should be avoided.

**Diet/Nutrition**
Oral trovafloxacin may be taken with or without food.

**Bioequivalenence information**
Oral trovafloxacin and parenteral alatrofloxacin are bioequivalent, in terms of trovafloxacin base, on a mg-per-mg basis.

## Oral Dosage Forms
Note: The dosing and strengths of the dosage form available are expressed in terms of trovafloxacin base, not the mesylate salt.

### TROVAFLOXACIN MESYLATE TABLETS
**Usual adult dose**
Bronchitis, bacterial exacerbations or
Skin and soft tissue infections, uncomplicated—
   Oral, 100 mg (base) every twenty-four hours for seven to ten days.
Cervicitis—
   Oral, 200 mg (base) every twenty-four hours for five days.
Gonorrhea, endocervical or
Gonorrhea, rectal, in females or
Gonorrhea, urethral, uncomplicated—
   Oral, 100 mg (base) as a single dose.
Pelvic inflammatory disease, mild to moderate—
   Oral, 200 mg (base) every twenty-four hours for fourteen days.
Perioperative prophylaxis—
   Oral, 200 mg (base) one-half to four hours prior to the start of surgery.
Pneumonia, community-acquired—
   Oral, 200 mg (base) every twenty-four hours for seven to fourteen days.
Prostatitis, bacterial, chronic—
   Oral, 200 mg (base) every twenty-four hours for twenty-eight days.
Sinusitis, acute—
   Oral, 200 mg (base) every twenty-four hours for ten days.
Skin and soft tissue infections, complicated—
   Oral, 200 mg (base) every twenty-four hours for ten to fourteen days.
Urinary tract infections, uncomplicated, including cystitis—
   Oral, 100 mg (base) every twenty-four hours for three days.

Note: Adults with mild to moderate cirrhosis (Child-Pugh class A or B) may require a reduction in dose as follows:

| Indicated oral dose for patients with normal hepatic function | Recommended oral dose for patients with chronic hepatic disease |
|---|---|
| 100 mg | 100 mg |
| 200 mg | 100 mg |

There are no data available for patients with severe cirrhosis (Child-Pugh class C).

**Usual pediatric dose**
Children up to 18 years of age—Safety and efficacy have not been established.

**Usual geriatric dose**
See *Usual adult dose*.

**Strength(s) usually available**
U.S.—
   100 mg (base) (Rx) [*Trovan*].
   200 mg (base) (Rx) [*Trovan*].

**Packaging and storage**
Store between 15 and 30 °C (59 and 86 °F). Store in a tight container.

## Parenteral Dosage Form
Note: The dosing and strengths of the dosage form available are expressed in terms of trovafloxacin base.

### ALATROFLOXACIN MESYLATE INJECTION
Note: Alatrofloxacin is a prodrug of trovafloxacin.

**Usual adult dose**
Gynecologic infections or
Intra-abdominal infections—
  Intravenous infusion, 300 mg (base) every twenty-four hours, switching to 200 mg (oral dosage form) every twenty-four hours when clinically indicated, for a seven- to fourteen-day course of therapy.
Perioperative prophylaxis—
  Intravenous infusion, 200 mg (base) one-half to four hours prior to the start of surgery.
Pneumonia, community-acquired—
  Intravenous infusion, 200 mg (base) every twenty-four hours, switching to 200 mg (oral dosage form) every twenty-four hours when clinically indicated, for a seven- to fourteen-day course of therapy.
Pneumonia, nosocomial—
  Intravenous infusion, 300 mg (base) every twenty-four hours, switching to 200 mg (oral dosage form) when clinically indicated, for a ten- to fourteen-day course of therapy.
  Combination therapy with either an aminoglycoside or aztreonam may be clinically indicated when *Pseudomonas aeruginosa* is a documented or presumptive pathogen.
Note: Adults with mild to moderate cirrhosis (Child-Pugh class A or B) may require a reduction in dose as follows:

| Indicated intravenous dose for patients with normal hepatic function | Recommended intravenous dose for patients with chronic hepatic disease |
|---|---|
| 200 mg | 100 mg |
| 300 mg | 200 mg |

There are no data available for patients with severe cirrhosis (Child-Pugh class C).

**Usual pediatric dose**
Children up to 18 years of age—Safety and efficacy have not been established.

**Usual geriatric dose**
See *Usual adult dose*.

**Strength(s) usually available**
U.S.—
  200 mg (base) per 40 mL (Rx) [*Trovan* (requires dilution prior to administration)].
  300 mg (base) per 60 mL (Rx) [*Trovan* (requires dilution prior to administration)].

**Packaging and storage**
Store between 15 and 30 °C (59 and 86 °F). Protect from light. Do not freeze.

**Preparation of dosage form**
For intravenous infusion, the appropriate volume of concentrate should be withdrawn aseptically from the vial and diluted to a final concentration of 1 or 2 mg per mL with a suitable intravenous solution (see manufacturer's package insert) as follows:

| Dose (trovafloxacin base equivalent) | Infusion concentration | Volume of concentrate to withdraw | Volume of diluent to add |
|---|---|---|---|
| 100 mg | 2 mg/mL | 20 mL | 30 mL |
|  | 1 mg/mL | 20 mL | 80 mL |
| 200 mg | 2 mg/mL | 40 mL | 60 mL |
|  | 1 mg/mL | 40 mL | 160 mL |
| 300 mg | 2 mg/mL | 60 mL | 90 mL |
|  | 1 mg/mL | 60 mL | 240 mL |

The resulting solution should be infused over a period of 60 minutes by direct infusion or through a Y-type intravenous infusion set. If the same line is used for sequential infusion of several different medications, the line should be flushed before and after infusion of alatrofloxacin with an infusion solution compatible with all medications administered. If alatrofloxacin is to be administered concurrently with another medication, each medication should be given separately in accordance with the recommended dosage and route of administration for each medication.

**Stability**
After dilution to a concentration of 0.5 to 2 mg per mL with appropriate intravenous infusion fluids (see manufacturer's insert), solutions retain their potency for up to 7 days when refrigerated or up to 3 days at room temperature when stored in glass bottles or plastic (PVC type) intravenous containers.

**Incompatibilities**
Alatrofloxacin should not be administered concurrently through the same intravenous line as solutions containing multivalent cations, such as magnesium. Additives or other medications should not be added to alatrofloxacin in single use vials or infused concurrently through the same intravenous line.

Developed: 02/25/98

# TUBERCULIN, PURIFIED PROTEIN DERIVATIVE  Parenteral-Local

VA CLASSIFICATION (Primary): DX300
Commonly used brand name(s): *Aplisol; Aplitest; Tuberculin PPD TINE TEST; Tubersol*.
Note: For a listing of dosage forms and brand names by country availability, see *Dosage Forms* section(s).

## Category
Diagnostic aid (tuberculosis).

## Indications
**Accepted**
Tuberculosis (diagnosis)—Tuberculin, purified protein derivative (PPD) is indicated as a diagnostic aid in the detection of *Mycobacterium tuberculosis* infection. It is also indicated when BCG vaccination or isoniazid prophylaxis is being considered.

## Pharmacology/Pharmacokinetics
**Physicochemical characteristics**
Tuberculin PPD is a sterile isotonic solution of tuberculin. It is obtained from a human strain of *Mycobacterium tuberculosis* grown on a protein-free synthetic medium and buffered with potassium and sodium phosphates.

**Mechanism of action/Effect**
Intradermally injected tuberculin PPD causes a delayed (cellular) hypersensitivity reaction in individuals sensitized by mycobacterial infection. Following infection with mycobacteria, sensitization of T-cells occurs primarily in the regional lymph nodes. Natural infection with *M. tuberculosis* usually initiates a cell-mediated immune response against mycobacterial antigens. T-cells proliferate in response to the infection and give rise to T-cells specifically sensitized to mycobacterial antigens. After several weeks, these T-lymphocytes enter the bloodstream and circulate for a long period of time. Subsequent restimulation of these T-lymphocytes with intradermal injection of tuberculin PPD evokes a local reaction mediated by these cells.

**Onset of action**
5 to 6 hours after intradermal injection of tuberculin PPD. The reaction reaches its peak more than 24 (usually 48 to 72) hours after administration.

## Precautions to Consider

**Pregnancy/Reproduction**
Fertility—Studies on effects of tuberculin PPD on fertility have not been done.
Pregnancy—Studies have not been done in humans. It is not known whether tuberculin PPD can cause harm to the fetus when administered to a pregnant woman. However, during pregnancy known positive reactors may demonstrate a negative response to the PPD tine test.
Studies have not been done in animals.
FDA Pregnancy Category C.

**Breast-feeding**
It is not known whether tuberculin PPD is distributed into breast milk. However, problems in humans have not been documented.

**Pediatrics**
Appropriate studies on the relationship of age to the effects of tuberculin PPD have not been performed in the pediatric population. However, no pediatrics-specific problems have been documented to date.

**Geriatrics**
In geriatric patients, reactions may develop slowly and may not peak until after 72 hours.

### Drug interactions and/or related problems
The following drug interactions and/or related problems have been selected on the basis of their potential clinical significance (possible mechanism in parentheses where appropriate)—not necessarily inclusive (» = major clinical significance):

Note: Combinations containing any of the following medications, depending on the amount present, may also interact with this medication.

Bacillus Calmette-Guérin (BCG) vaccine
(individuals previously given BCG vaccine will usually show a positive reaction to tuberculin test administered within 6 to 12 weeks after BCG vaccination; a few years after BCG vaccination, reaction to tuberculin tests may be either positive or negative; a positive reaction to tuberculin PPD years after BCG vaccination suggests tuberculous infection)

Corticosteroids or
Immunosuppressive agents
(reactivity to the tuberculin test may be suppressed or enhanced in patients receiving these medications)

Vaccines, killed or live virus
(the reaction to tuberculin PPD may be suppressed if the test is given within 4 to 6 weeks following immunization with killed or live virus vaccines)

### Diagnostic interference
The following have been selected on the basis of their potential clinical significance (possible effect in parentheses where appropriate)—not necessarily inclusive (» = major clinical significance):

With results of this test
*Due to medical problems or conditions*

Acquired immunodeficiency syndrome (AIDS) or
Anergy or
Atopic dermatitis or sun-damaged skin or
Human immunodeficiency virus (HIV) infection or
Illness that affects the lymphoid system (Hodgkin's disease, lymphoma, chronic lymphocytic leukemia) or
Pregnancy or
Stress, severe
(may cause false-negative test results)

### Medical considerations/Contraindications
The medical considerations/contraindications included have been selected on the basis of their potential clinical significance (reasons given in parentheses where appropriate)—not necessarily inclusive (» = major clinical significance).

*Except under special circumstances, this medication should not be used when the following medical problem exists:*

» Known positive tuberculin reaction
(in highly sensitive persons the reaction at the test site can be severe, resulting in vesiculation, ulceration, or necrosis)

## Side/Adverse Effects
The following side/adverse effects have been selected on the basis of their potential clinical significance (possible signs and symptoms in parentheses where appropriate)—not necessarily inclusive:

### Those indicating need for medical attention
Incidence rare
*Allergic reactions* (skin rash or itching); *necrosis, ulceration, or vesiculation at the site of injection* (redness, blistering, peeling, or loosening of the skin)

### Those indicating need for medical attention only if they continue or are bothersome
Incidence less frequent
*Erythematous reaction* (redness at the site of injection); *granuloma* (sores at and around the site of injection); *pain; pruritus* (itching)

Note: Discomfort and transient bleeding may be observed at the PPD tine puncture site.

## Patient Consultation
As an aid to patient consultation, refer to *Advice for the Patient, Tuberculin, Purified Protein Derivative (PPD) Injection.*
In providing consultation, consider emphasizing the following selected information (» = major clinical significance):

### Before using this medication
» Conditions affecting use, especially:
Sensitivity to tuberculin PPD
Other medical problems, especially known positive tuberculin reaction

### Side/adverse effects
» Signs of potential side effects, especially allergic reactions and necrosis, ulceration, or vesiculation at the site of injection

## General Dosing Information
Anergy to tuberculin among asymptomatic HIV-positive persons is common, making interpretation of tuberculin tests difficult. Therefore, the Centers for Disease Control (CDC) has produced guidelines for assessing delayed-type hypersensitivity in these patients. Concurrent administration of at least 2 other skin test antigens is recommended. The CDC suggests choosing from among mumps skin test antigen, candida antigen, and tetanus toxoid. The test antigens are given concurrently with the tuberculin skin test and the response is measured 48 to 72 hours later. Any amount of induration is considered evidence of delayed-type hypersensitivity; failure to elicit a response is considered evidence of anergy. HIV-positive persons and others at risk of anergy are considered to have a significant reaction to a standard Mantoux test if the induration reaction measures 5 mm or more in diameter, regardless of the reaction to the other antigens. It is very important to perform anergy testing in a population at increased risk of tuberculosis.

Booster effect—The ability of persons who have TB infection to react to tuberculin may gradually wane. For example, if tested with tuberculin, adults who were infected during their childhood may have a negative reaction. However, the tuberculin could boost the hypersensitivity, and the size of the reaction could be larger on a subsequent test. This boosted reaction may be misinterpreted as a tuberculin test conversion from a newly acquired infection. Misinterpretation of a boosted reaction as a new infection could result in unnecessary investigations of laboratory and patient records in an attempt to identify the source of infection and in unnecessary prescription of preventive therapy for health care workers. Although this booster effect can occur among persons in any age group, the likelihood of the effect increases with the age of the person being tested.

Two-step testing—When tuberculin testing of an adult is to be repeated periodically, 2-step testing can be used to reduce the likelihood that a boosted reaction will be misinterpreted as a new infection. Two-step testing should be performed on all newly employed health care workers who have an initial negative tuberculin test at the time of employment and have not had a documented negative tuberculin test result during the 12 months preceding the initial test. A second test should be performed 1 to 3 weeks after the first test. If the second test result is positive, this is most likely a boosted reaction, and the patient should be classified as previously infected. If the second test result is negative, the patient is classified as uninfected, and a positive reaction to a subsequent test is likely to represent a new infection with *M. tuberculosis.*

It is recommended that children at high risk for tuberculosis be given tuberculin skin tests annually by the Mantoux method. Children considered at high risk include those from areas with a high prevalence of the disease; those from households with 1 or more cases of tuberculosis; black, Hispanic, Asian, native American, and native Alaskan children, and others who are socioeconomically deprived; children from Asia, Africa, the Middle East, Latin America, or the Caribbean and children of parents who have immigrated from these areas; and children with medical risk factors for tuberculosis.

It is recommended that individuals with signs and/or symptoms suggestive of current tuberculous disease be given tuberculin skin test routinely by the Mantoux method. These individuals include persons who are recent contacts of known cases of clinical tuberculosis or are suspected of having tuberculosis; persons with abnormal chest radiographs compatible with past tuberculosis; persons with medical conditions that increase the risk of tuberculosis; HIV-infected individuals; immigrants from Asia, Africa, Latin America, and Oceania; inner-city and skid row populations.

Tuberculin PPD is administered by intradermal injection (the Mantoux method) or by using a disposable multiple-puncture device. These 2 commonly used test methods are briefly described below.

*The Mantoux test method:* The test is performed by intradermally injecting exactly 0.1 mL of diluted tuberculin PPD. The result is read 48 to 72 hours later and only induration is considered in interpreting the test. Induration is a hard, raised area with clearly defined margins at, and around, the injection site. Erythema may develop at the injection site but has no diagnostic value. The test is performed as follows:

• The site of the test is usually the flexor surface of the forearm, about 4 inches below the elbow. Other skin sites may be used, but the flexor surface of the forearm is preferred. The site of the test should be free of lesions and away from the veins.

• The skin at the injection site is cleansed with 70% alcohol or another suitable antiseptic agent and allowed to dry.

- The test material is administered with a tuberculin syringe (0.5 or 1.0 mL) fitted with a short (one-half-inch) 26- or 27- gauge needle.
- The syringe and needle should be a sterile, disposable, single-use type or should have been sterilized by autoclaving, boiling, or the use of dry heat. A separate sterile unit should be used for each person tested.
- The diaphragm of the vial-stopper should be wiped with 70% alcohol.
- The needle is inserted through the stopper diaphragm of the inverted vial. Exactly 0.1 mL is added to the syringe, with care being taken to exclude air bubbles and to keep the lumen of the needle filled.
- The point of the needle is inserted into the most superficial layers of the skin with the needle bevel pointed upward. As the tuberculin solution is injected, a pale bleb 6 to 10 mm in size will rise over the point of the needle. This is quickly absorbed, and no dressing is required. In the event that the injection is delivered subcutaneously (in this case no bleb will form) or if a significant part of the dose leaks from the injection site, the test should be repeated immediately at another site at least 5 cm (2 inches) removed from the first site.
- The test site should be examined by trained personnel 48 to 72 hours after the injection. The examination should be performed in good light with the arm slightly flexed at the elbow. The reaction should be measured and recorded in millimeters. Any induration reaction that measures 5 mm or more in diameter is considered positive in persons who have had recent close contact with tuberculosis; persons who have chest radiographs consistent with tuberculosis (including stable lesions consistent with "inactive" tuberculosis); immunosuppressed persons (including HIV-infected persons and patients on immunosuppressive therapy); and persons with cancer (including leukemia or lymphoma), Hodgkin's disease, or end-stage renal disease. Induration of 10 mm or more is considered a positive reaction in foreign-born persons; substance abusers (alcoholics and intravenous drug users); residents and employees of correctional institutions and nursing homes; hospital employees; persons over age 70; low-income populations, including the homeless; and persons with medical conditions including diabetes mellitus, post gastrectomy, silicosis, prolonged corticosteroid therapy, and 10% or more below ideal body weight. Induration of 15 mm or more is considered a positive reaction in all other persons (general population with no known tuberculosis risk factors).

*The multiple-puncture (Tine) test method:* Each test unit provides for the intradermal administration of 1 test-dose of tuberculin PPD. The test is performed as follows:
- The preferred site of the test is the flexor surface of the forearm about 4 inches below the elbow. Other suitable skin sites, such as the dorsal surface of the forearm, may be used. Areas without adequate subcutaneous tissue, such as skin over a tendon, as well as hairy areas, should be avoided.
- The skin at the test site should be cleaned with 70% alcohol or another suitable antiseptic agent such as acetone, ether, or soap and water and allowed to dry thoroughly.
- To expose the 4 impregnated tines, remove the protective cap while holding the plastic handle.
- The patient's forearm should be grasped firmly to stretch the skin taut at the test site and to prevent any jerking motion of the arm that could cause scratching with the tines.
- The test unit should be applied firmly without twisting to the test area for approximately 1 second. Sufficient pressure should be exerted to ensure that all 4 tines have penetrated the skin.
- Used units should be disposed of carefully to avoid accidents. Do not reuse.
- The test site should be examined by trained personnel 48 to 72 hours after application of the test. The examination should be performed in good light with the arm slightly flexed at the elbow. The presence of vesiculation indicates a positive reaction to the test. The test reaction is negative if both induration and vesiculation are absent. Induration reactions less than 2 mm in diameter may be considered negative. However, unless vesiculation is present, individuals with any size induration reaction should be retested using a standard Mantoux test.

The dose of tuberculin PPD introduced into the skin with currently available multiple-puncture devices cannot be precisely controlled. Therefore, this test should not be used for the periodic surveillance of individuals likely to be exposed to clinical tuberculosis or for the evaluation of individuals who are suspected of having tuberculosis or are contacts of persons with clinical tuberculosis.

*The Heaf test method:* The test is performed using the Heaf multiple-puncture apparatus. The result is read 3 to 10 days later and only induration is considered in interpreting the test.
- The site of the test is usually the volar surface of the left forearm. The skin at the test site is cleansed with alcohol or another suitable antiseptic agent and allowed to dry. The undiluted tuberculin is transferred using a syringe needle or loop and smoothed over a circular area of about 1 cm in diameter.
- The needle points of the apparatus are placed on the forearm to give a puncture of 1 mm (for children under 2 years of age) or 2 mm (for older children and adults).
- With the apparatus held at a right angle to the skin, the end plate is placed firmly and evenly in the center of the film of tuberculin and the handle pressed to release the needles. No dressing need be applied. It is very important that the apparatus be properly sterilized after each application or that a disposable end plate be used.
- A positive result should be recorded only when there is palpable induration around at least 4 puncture points. The induration is best felt by passing the finger lightly over the punctures. If no resistance is felt, a negative result should be recorded.
- Four grades of positive response are recognized:
    Grade 1—At least 4 small indurated papules.
    Grade 2—An indurated ring formed by confluent papules.
    Grade 3—A solid induration 5 to 10 mm wide.
    Grade 4—Induration over 10 mm wide.

**For treatment of adverse effects**
Recommended treatment consists of the following:
- If strongly positive reactions, including vesiculation, ulceration, or necrosis, occur, cold packs or topical steroid preparations may be used for symptomatic relief of the associated pain, pruritus, and discomfort.

## Parenteral Dosage Forms

### TUBERCULIN (Purified Protein Derivative [PPD] Injection) USP

**Usual adult and adolescent dose**
Tuberculosis (diagnosis)—
    Intradermal, 5 U.S. units (tuberculin units [TU]).
Note: The 1-TU-per-test-dose preparation is used for individuals suspected of being highly sensitized, since larger initial doses may result in severe skin reactions. The preparation containing 250 TU per test dose should be used exclusively for the testing of individuals who fail to react to a previous injection of 5 TU; under no circumstances is it to be used for the initial injection.

**Usual pediatric dose**
See *Usual adult and adolescent dose*.

**Strength(s) usually available**
U.S.—
    1 U.S. unit (TU) per test dose (0.1 mL) (Rx) [*Tubersol*].
    5 U.S. units (TU) per test dose (0.1 mL) (Rx) [*Aplisol; Tubersol*].
    250 U.S. units (TU) per test dose (0.1 mL) (Rx) [*Tubersol*].
Canada—
    1 U.S. unit (TU) per test dose (0.1 mL) (Rx) [*Tubersol*].
    5 U.S. units (TU) per test dose (0.1 mL) (Rx) [*Tubersol*].
    250 U.S. units (TU) per test dose (0.1 mL) (Rx) [*Tubersol*].

**Packaging and storage**
Store between 2 and 8 °C (36 and 46 °F). Protect from light.

**Additional information**
Vials of tuberculin PPD that have been opened should be discarded after 1 month of use, since oxidation and degradation may have reduced the potency.

### TUBERCULIN (Purified Protein Derivative [PPD] Multiple-Puncture Device) USP

**Usual adult and adolescent dose**
Tuberculosis (diagnosis)—
    Intradermal, equivalent to or more potent than 5 U.S. units (tuberculin units [TU]).

**Usual pediatric dose**
See *Usual adult and adolescent dose*.

**Strength(s) usually available**
U.S.—
    Equivalent to or more potent than 5 U.S. units in individually capped test units (Rx) [*Aplitest; Tuberculin PPD TINE TEST*].
Canada—
    Not commercially available.

**Packaging and storage**
Store below 30 °C (86 °F). Do not refrigerate.

## Selected Bibliography
Menzies R, Vissandjee B, Rocher I, Germain YS. The booster effect in two-step tuberculin testing among young adults in Montreal. Ann Intern Med 1994; 120(3): 190-8.

Developed: 08/01/95

**TUBOCURARINE**—See *Neuromuscular Blocking Agents (Systemic)*

**TYPHOID VACCINE INACTIVATED**—The *Typhoid Vaccine Inactivated (Parenteral-Systemic)* monograph is not included in this published version of the USP DI database. Copies of the monograph are available on request from Micromedex, Inc. - Reprint Requests, 6200 S. Syracuse Way, Suite 300, Englewood, CO 80111; telephone (303) 486-6400; telefax (303) 486-6464; Email: USPDI@MDX.COM.

**TYPHOID VACCINE LIVE ORAL**—The *Typhoid Vaccine Live Oral (Systemic)* monograph is not included in this published version of the USP DI database. Copies of the monograph are available on request from Micromedex, Inc. - Reprint Requests, 6200 S. Syracuse Way, Suite 300, Englewood, CO 80111; telephone (303) 486-6400; telefax (303) 486-6464; Email: USPDI@MDX.COM.

**TYPHOID VI POLYSACCHARIDE VACCINE**—The *Typhoid Vi Polysaccharide Vaccine (Systemic)* monograph is not included in this published version of the USP DI database. Copies of the monograph are available on request from Micromedex, Inc. - Reprint Requests, 6200 S. Syracuse Way, Suite 300, Englewood, CO 80111; telephone (303) 486-6400; telefax (303) 486-6464; Email: USPDI@MDX.COM.

**TYROPANOATE**—See *Cholecystographic Agents, Oral (Systemic)*

**UNDECYLENIC ACID, COMPOUND**—The *Undecylenic Acid, Compound (Topical)* monograph is not included in this published version of the USP DI database. Copies of the monograph are available on request from Micromedex, Inc. - Reprint Requests, 6200 S. Syracuse Way, Suite 300, Englewood, CO 80111; telephone (303) 486-6400; telefax (303) 486-6464; Email: USPDI@MDX.COM.

**URACIL MUSTARD**—The *Uracil Mustard (Systemic)* monograph is not included in this published version of the USP DI database. Copies of the monograph are available on request from Micromedex, Inc. - Reprint Requests, 6200 S. Syracuse Way, Suite 300, Englewood, CO 80111; telephone (303) 486-6400; telefax (303) 486-6464; Email: USPDI@MDX.COM.

**UREA**—The *Urea (Parenteral-Local)* monograph is not included in this published version of the USP DI database. Copies of the monograph are available on request from Micromedex, Inc. - Reprint Requests, 6200 S. Syracuse Way, Suite 300, Englewood, CO 80111; telephone (303) 486-6400; telefax (303) 486-6464; Email: USPDI@MDX.COM.

# UREA  Systemic†

VA CLASSIFICATION (Primary/Secondary): CV709/OP115
Commonly used brand name(s): *Ureaphil*.
Note: For a listing of dosage forms and brand names by country availability, see *Dosage Forms* section(s).

†Not commercially available in Canada.

## Category
Diuretic; antiglaucoma agent (systemic).

## Indications

**Accepted**
Edema, cerebral (treatment)—Urea is indicated to treat cerebral edema and reduce brain mass and intracranial pressure.

Glaucoma, malignant (treatment) or
Glaucoma, secondary (treatment)—Urea is indicated to reduce elevated intraocular pressure (IOP) after other methods have failed or in preparation for intraocular surgery.

## Pharmacology/Pharmacokinetics

**Mechanism of action/Effect**
Cerebral edema—Elevates blood plasma osmolality, resulting in enhanced flow of water from tissues, including the brain and cerebrospinal fluid, into interstitial fluid and plasma. As a result, cerebral edema, elevated intracranial pressure, and cerebrospinal fluid volume and pressure may be reduced. This effect is evident early in the course of infusion as long as a gradient between plasma and intracellular urea exists. As urea diffuses into the cells and the gradient diminishes, the effect diminishes.
Glaucoma—Elevates blood plasma osmolality, resulting in enhanced flow of water from the eye into plasma and a consequent reduction in intraocular pressure.

**Distribution**
Urea is distributed into extracellular and intracellular fluids including lymph, bile, cerebral spinal fluid (CSF), and blood in approximately equal concentrations. Urea also crosses the placenta, penetrates the eyes, and appears in the milk of lactating women.

**Biotransformation**
Urea may be partially metabolized in the gastrointestinal tract by hydrolysis to ammonia and carbon dioxide, which may be resynthesized into urea.

**Half-life**
1.17 hours.

**Onset of action**
Reduction of intraocular and intracranial pressure—Within 10 minutes after infusion is started.

**Time to peak effect**
1 to 2 hours.

**Duration of action**
Diuresis—3 to 10 hours after infusion is stopped.
Reduction in cerebrospinal fluid pressure—3 to 10 hours after infusion is stopped.
Reduction in intraocular pressure—5 to 6 hours.

**Elimination**
Renal (reabsorption about 50%).

## Precautions to Consider

**Pregnancy/Reproduction**
Pregnancy—Studies have not been done in humans.
Studies have not been done in animals.
FDA Pregnancy Category C.

**Breast-feeding**
It is not known whether urea is distributed into breast milk. However, problems in humans have not been documented.

**Pediatrics**
Appropriate studies on the relationship of age to the effects of urea have not been performed in the pediatric population. However, pediatrics-specific problems that would limit the usefulness of urea in children are not expected.

**Geriatrics**
Urea should not be infused into veins of the lower extremities, especially in elderly patients, since phlebitis and thrombosis of superficial and deep veins may occur. In addition, elderly patients are more likely to have age-related renal function impairment, which may require caution in patients receiving urea.

**Drug interactions and/or related problems**
The following drug interactions and/or related problems have been selected on the basis of their potential clinical significance (possible mechanism in parentheses where appropriate)—not necessarily inclusive (» = major clinical significance):

Note: Combinations containing any of the following medications, depending on the amount present, may also interact with this medication.

Diuretics, other, including carbonic anhydrase inhibitors
  (diuretic and IOP–reducing effects may be potentiated when these medications are used concurrently with urea; dosage adjustments may be necessary)
Lithium
  (urea may increase renal excretion of lithium)

**Laboratory value alterations**
The following have been selected on the basis of their potential clinical significance (possible effect in parentheses where appropriate)—not necessarily inclusive (» = major clinical significance):

With physiology/laboratory test values
Blood urea nitrogen (BUN)
  (concentrations may be increased with excessive doses)
Potassium and
Sodium
  (serum concentrations may be decreased with prolonged administration)

**Medical considerations/Contraindications**
The medical considerations/contraindications included have been selected on the basis of their potential clinical significance (reasons given in parentheses where appropriate)—not necessarily inclusive (» = major clinical significance).

*Except under special circumstances, this medication should not be used when the following medical problems exist:*
» Dehydration, severe
  (this condition may increase risk of urea-induced electrolyte depletion)

» Hepatic function impairment, severe
(blood ammonia concentrations may be elevated)
» Intracranial bleeding, active, except during craniotomy
(reduction of brain edema by urea may increase bleeding)
» Renal function impairment, severe
(accumulation of urea solution may lead to circulatory overload)

*Risk-benefit should be considered when the following medical problems exist:*
Cardiovascular function impairment
(sudden expansion of extracellular fluid may lead to congestive heart failure)
Hepatic function impairment
(blood ammonia concentrations may be elevated)
» Hereditary fructose intolerance (aldolase deficiency)—for infusions prepared with invert sugar injection only
Hypovolemia
(may be masked and intensified)
Renal function impairment
(accumulation of urea may lead to overexpansion of extracellular fluid and circulatory overload)

**Patient monitoring**
The following may be especially important in patient monitoring (other tests may be warranted in some patients, depending on condition; » = major clinical significance):
Blood pressure measurements and
Electrolyte measurements, including sodium and potassium, and
Renal function determinations and
Urine output determinations
(recommended during intravenous infusion of urea, especially with repeated doses)
Blood urea nitrogen (BUN) determinations
(recommended before and frequently during intravenous administration; if a rapid increase occurs, the infusion should be slowed or stopped)

## Side/Adverse Effects

Note: Most side/adverse effects are related to the rate of administration.
Thrombosis may occur with administration into the superficial and deep veins of the lower extremities, especially in elderly patients.
Hemolysis may occur as a result of rapid administration; urea may also cause increased capillary bleeding, and rapid infusion has resulted in intraocular hemorrhage in patients with absolute glaucoma.
Side effects can be minimized by maintaining adequate hydration and keeping the patient horizontal.
Excessive diuresis can result from long-term urea therapy, which may lead to tissue dehydration, hypokalemia, and hyponatremia.

The following effects have been selected on the basis of their potential clinical significance (possible signs and symptoms in parentheses where appropriate)—not necessarily inclusive:

**Those indicating need for medical attention**
Incidence less frequent or rare
*Confusion, fast heartbeat, fever, or nervousness; electrolyte imbalance* (confusion; irregular heartbeat; muscle cramps or pain; numbness, tingling, pain, or weakness in hands or feet; seizures; trembling; unusual tiredness or weakness; weakness and heaviness of legs); *phlebitis or thrombosis, chemical, or extravasation* (redness, swelling, or pain at injection site)—for intravenous injection only; *subdural or subarachnoid hemorrhage, possible* (blurred vision; severe headache)
Note: *Confusion, fast heartbeat, fever, or nervousness* may be caused by too-rapid intravenous infusion.

**Those indicating need for medical attention only if they continue or are bothersome**
Incidence more frequent
*Dryness of mouth or increased thirst; headache; nausea or vomiting*
Incidence less frequent
*Dizziness or faintness; drowsiness*—with prolonged urea administration in patients with sickle cell crisis; *skin blemishes*
Note: In some cases, *headache, nausea or vomiting, blurred vision,* and *dizziness* may be symptoms of subdural or subarachnoid hemorrhage.

## Overdose

For more information on the management of overdose or unintentional ingestion, **contact a Poison Control Center** (see *Poison Control Center Listing*).

**Treatment of overdose**
In the event of overdose as reflected by elevated blood urea nitrogen (BUN) concentrations, recommended treatment consists of the following: discontinuation of medication; patient evaluation, and institution of corrective measures.

## General Dosing Information

**For intravenous injection only**
The dose used depends on the fluid and electrolyte and renal status of the patient.
An infusion rate of not greater than 4 mL per minute is recommended, since rapid infusion may cause hemolysis and cerebral vasomotor symptoms.
When urea is used preoperatively for reduction of intraocular or intracranial pressure, the dose should be started about 60 minutes prior to ocular surgery and at the time of scalp incision during intracranial surgery to achieve maximum reduction of pressure.
Urea should not be infused into veins of the lower extremities, especially in elderly patients, since phlebitis and thrombosis of superficial and deep veins may occur. Large veins should be used for infusion.
Caution should be used to prevent extravasation of urea infusion solution at the site of injection, which may result in irritation and tissue necrosis.
Use of an indwelling urethral catheter is recommended in comatose patients to ensure bladder emptying and adequacy of urine output.
The simultaneous use of hypothermia and urea infusion may increase the risk of venous thrombosis and hemoglobinuria.
If blood urea nitrogen (BUN) concentrations are elevated to 75 mg per 100 mL or more or if diuresis does not occur within 1 to 2 hours after administration of urea to patients with renal function impairment, dosage should be reduced or urea withheld until the patient is re-evaluated.

## Parenteral Dosage Forms

### UREA STERILE USP

**Usual adult and adolescent dose**
Diuretic or
Antiglaucoma agent—
Intravenous infusion, 500 mg to 1.5 grams per kg of body weight as a 30% solution in 5 or 10% Dextrose Injection USP or 10% invert sugar injection, administered at a rate of approximately 60 drops (4 or 6 mL, depending on manufacturer) per minute over a period of thirty minutes to two hours.

**Usual adult prescribing limits**
Up to 2 grams per kg of body weight per twenty-four-hour period.

**Usual pediatric dose**
Diuretic—
Children up to 2 years of age: Intravenous infusion, 100 mg to 1.5 grams per kg of body weight as a 30% solution in 5 or 10% dextrose injection or 10% invert sugar injection, administered at a rate of approximately 60 drops (4 or 6 mL, depending on manufacturer) per minute over a period of thirty minutes to two hours.
Children 2 years of age and over: See *Usual adult and adolescent dose*.

**Size(s) usually available**
U.S.—
40 grams (Rx) [*Ureaphil*].
Canada—
Not commercially available.

**Packaging and storage**
Prior to reconstitution, store below 40 °C (104 °F), preferably between 15 and 30 °C (59 and 86 °F), unless otherwise specified by manufacturer. Protect from freezing.

**Preparation of dosage form**
For preparation of product for injection, see manufacturer's package insert.
Use of 5% or 10% dextrose injection or invert sugar injection as a diluent reduces the risk of hemolysis that may occur with rapid administration of urea. However, invert sugar injection is contraindicated in patients with fructose intolerance due to aldolase deficiency.
One gram of urea is equivalent to approximately 16.7 mOsm (calculated on basis of urea being reconstituted with water for injection).
The number of mOsm of urea per liter of specified diluent is as follows:

| Urea (%) | Diluent | Total mOsm/liter (approx) |
|---|---|---|
| 30 | 5% Dextrose injection | 5250 |
| 30 | 10% Dextrose injection | 5500 |
| 30 | 10% Invert sugar injection | 5550 |

**Stability**
See manufacturer's package insert and/or label for stability of reconstituted solution.
Each dose of urea should be freshly prepared. Discard any unused portion.

**Incompatibilities**
When blood and urea are administered simultaneously, the urea infusion solution should not be administered through the same administration set through which the blood is being infused.

**Additional information**
Following reconstitution of urea powder for injection with 5 or 10% dextrose or 10% invert sugar injection, the solutions have a pH of 4.5 to 6.

Revised: 01/20/93

## URINE GLUCOSE AND KETONE TEST KITS FOR HOME USE
The *Urine Glucose and Ketone Test Kits for Home Use* monograph is not included in this published version of the USP DI database. Copies of the monograph are available on request from Micromedex, Inc. - Reprint Requests, 6200 S. Syracuse Way, Suite 300, Englewood, CO 80111; telephone (303) 486-6400; telefax (303) 486-6464; Email: USPDI@MDX.COM.

# UROFOLLITROPIN   Systemic

BAN: Urofollitrophin.
VA CLASSIFICATION (Primary): HS106
Note: Controlled substance in some states in the U.S.
U.S.—Schedule IV
Commonly used brand name(s): *Fertinex; Fertinorm HP; Metrodin.*
Other commonly used names are follicle-stimulating hormone (FSH) and urofollitrophin.
Note: For a listing of dosage forms and brand names by country availability, see *Dosage Forms* section(s).

## Category
Gonadotropin; infertility therapy adjunct.

## Indications
**Accepted**
Infertility, female (treatment)—Urofollitropin is indicated, in conjunction with human chorionic gonadotropin (hCG), for stimulation of ovulation and induction of pregnancy in patients with polycystic ovary syndrome who have an elevated luteinizing hormone/follicle-stimulating hormone (LH/FSH) ratio and who have failed to respond to adequate clomiphene citrate therapy. Urofollitropin is not useful in patients with primary ovarian failure.

Reproductive technologies, assisted[1]—Urofollitropin is indicated, in conjunction with hCG, to stimulate the development of multiple oocytes in ovulatory patients who are attempting to conceive by means of assisted reproductive technologies, such as gamete intrafallopian transfer (GIFT) or *in vitro* fertilization (IVF).

[1]Not included in Canadian product labeling.

## Pharmacology/Pharmacokinetics
**Physicochemical characteristics**
Source—Extracted from urine of postmenopausal women.

**Mechanism of action/Effect**
Urofollitropin contains follicle-stimulating hormone (FSH). The combination of FSH and luteinizing hormone (LH) stimulates follicular growth and maturation. Chorionic gonadotropin (hCG), whose actions are nearly identical to those of LH, is administered following urofollitropin treatment to mimic the naturally occurring surge of LH that triggers ovulation.

## Precautions to Consider
**Carcinogenicity**
Long-term studies have not been done in animals to evaluate the carcinogenic potential of urofollitropin.

**Pregnancy/Reproduction**
Fertility—Use of urofollitropin to stimulate ovulation is associated with a high incidence of multiple gestations and births. As a result, this may increase the risk of neonatal prematurity, as well as other complications associated with multiple gestations.

Pregnancy—Although problems in humans have not been documented, use of urofollitropin during pregnancy is unnecessary.

Ovarian hyperstimulation syndrome (OHS), which may be induced by urofollitropin therapy, is more common, more severe, and protracted in patients who conceive.

FDA Pregnancy Category X.

**Breast-feeding**
It is not known whether urofollitropin is distributed into breast milk. However, urofollitropin is not indicated during the course of breast-feeding.

**Medical considerations/Contraindications**
The medical considerations/contraindications included have been selected on the basis of their potential clinical significance (reasons given in parentheses where appropriate)—not necessarily inclusive (» = major clinical significance).

*Except under special circumstances, this medication should not be used when the following medical problems exist:*
» Abnormal vaginal bleeding, undiagnosed
(may indicate the presence of endometrial hyperplasia or carcinoma, which may be exacerbated by urofollitropin-induced increases in estrogen serum concentrations; other possible endocrinopathies should also be ruled out)
» Ovarian cyst or enlargement not associated with polycystic ovary syndrome
(risk of further enlargement)

*Risk-benefit should be considered when the following medical problem exists:*
Sensitivity to urofollitropin or other gonadotropins

**Patient monitoring**
The following may be especially important in patient monitoring (other tests may be warranted in some patients, depending on condition; » = major clinical significance):
» Estradiol
(measurement of serum concentrations is recommended as needed, continuing through the day of chorionic gonadotropin administration; recommended to determine optimal dose and to lessen the risk of ovarian hyperstimulation syndrome)
» Ultrasound examination
(recommended during urofollitropin therapy and prior to administration of chorionic gonadotropin to provide information on the number and size of mature follicles, to follow follicular development, and to lessen the risk of ovarian hyperstimulation syndrome and multiple gestation)
Daily basal body temperature
(can be used to determine if ovulation has occurred; pregnancy test is recommended if basal body temperature following a cycle of treatment is biphasic and not followed by menses)
Progesterone
(measurement of serum or urine concentrations can be used prior to urofollitropin therapy to confirm anovulation; serum concentrations can be used after urofollitropin therapy to detect luteinized ovarian follicles)

## Side/Adverse Effects
Note: Thromboembolism has not been reported in patients who have received urofollitropin, but has occurred with menotropins (LH/FSH) both in association with and separate from ovarian hyperstimulation syndrome. Complications resulting from thromboembolism have included venous thrombophlebitis, pulmonary embolism, pulmonary infarction, stroke, arterial occlusion necessitating limb amputation, and (rarely) death.

Serious respiratory complications have not been reported in patients who have received urofollitropin, but have occurred with menotropins (LH/FSH) therapy. These conditions included atelectasis and acute respiratory distress syndrome. Rarely, death has resulted.

The following side/adverse effects have been selected on the basis of their potential clinical significance (possible signs and symptoms in parentheses where appropriate)—not necessarily inclusive:

**Those indicating need for medical attention**
Incidence more frequent—about 10 to 20%
*Uncomplicated, mild to moderate ovarian enlargement or ovarian cysts* (mild bloating, abdominal or pelvic pain); *redness, pain, or swelling at injection site*

Note: *Ovarian enlargement* is usually mild to moderate and abates within 2 or 3 weeks. *Ovarian cysts* have also occurred, though less frequently.

Incidence less frequent or rare
*Severe ovarian hyperstimulation syndrome* (severe abdominal or stomach pain; feeling of indigestion; moderate to severe bloating; decreased amount of urine; continuing or severe nausea, vomiting, or diarrhea; severe pelvic pain; rapid weight gain; swelling of lower legs; shortness of breath); *fever and chills; skin rash or hives*

Note: In clinical trials, *ovarian hyperstimulation syndrome (OHS)* occurred in 6% of patients treated with urofollitropin for anovulation due to polycystic ovary syndrome and 0.25% of patients given urofollitropin for *in vitro* fertilization. OHS may often occur 7 to 10 days after ovulation or completion of therapy. OHS differs from uncomplicated ovarian enlargement and can progress rapidly to cause serious medical problems. With OHS, a marked increase in vascular permeability results in rapid accumulation of fluid in the peritoneal, pleural, and pericardial cavities (third spacing of fluids). Medical complications ultimately arising from this increased vascular permeability may include hypovolemia, hemoconcentration, electrolyte imbalance, ascites, hemoperitoneum, pleural effusions, hydrothorax, acute pulmonary distress, and thromboembolic events. OHS is more common, more severe, and protracted in patients who conceive.

**Those indicating need for medical attention only if they continue or are bothersome**
Incidence less frequent or rare
*Breast tenderness; diarrhea, mild; nausea; vomiting*

## Patient Consultation
As an aid to patient consultation, refer to *Advice for the Patient, Urofollitropin (Systemic)*.
In providing consultation, consider emphasizing the following selected information (» = major clinical significance):

**Before using this medication**
» Conditions affecting use, especially:
   Sensitivity to urofollitropin or other gonadotropins
   Other medical problems, especially abnormal vaginal bleeding or ovarian cyst or enlargement

**Proper use of this medication**
» Proper dosing

**Precautions while using this medication**
» Importance of close monitoring by physician
» Importance of following physician's instructions for recording of basal body temperature and timing of intercourse, when recommended by physician

**Side/adverse effects**
Signs of potential side effects, especially ovarian cysts, enlargement, or hyperstimulation syndrome

## General Dosing Information
Patients receiving urofollitropin should be under the supervision of a physician experienced in the treatment of gynecologic or endocrine disorders.

Dosage varies considerably and must be adjusted to meet the individual requirements of each patient, on the basis of clinical response.

Conception should be attempted within 48 hours of administration of hCG. It is recommended that the couple have intercourse or insemination be performed daily beginning the day after hCG is administered, until ovulation is thought to have occurred.

If ovulation does not occur after any cycle of therapy, the therapeutic regimen employed should be re-evaluated. After 3 to 6 cycles of non-ovulatory menses, the appropriateness of continuing the use of urofollitropin for ovulation induction should be reconsidered.

**For treatment of adverse effects**
Ovarian enlargement or ovarian cyst formation
• Discontinuing therapy until ovarian size has returned to baseline. Human chorionic gonadotropin should also be withheld for that cycle.
• Prohibiting intercourse until ovarian size has returned to baseline to prevent cyst rupture.
• Reducing dosage in next course of therapy.

Ovarian hyperstimulation syndrome (OHS)
Acute phase
• Discontinuing therapy.
• Prohibiting intercourse until ovarian size has returned to baseline to prevent cyst rupture.
• Most cases of OHS will spontaneously resolve when menses begins. In selected cases, hospitalization of the patient and bed rest may be necessary.
• Utilizing therapy to prevent hemoconcentration and minimize risk of thromboembolism and renal injury.
• Correcting (cautiously) electrolyte imbalance while maintaining acceptable intravascular volume; in the acute phase, intravascular volume deficit cannot be completely corrected without increasing third space fluid volume.
• Monitoring fluid intake and output, body weight, hematocrit, serum and urine electrolytes, urine specific gravity, blood urea nitrogen (BUN), creatinine, and abdominal girth daily or as often as required.
• Monitoring serum potassium concentrations for development of hyperkalemia.
• Limiting performance of pelvic examinations since they may result in rupture of ovarian cysts and hemoperitoneum.
• Administering intravenous fluids, electrolytes, and human serum albumin as needed to maintain adequate urine output and to avoid hemoconcentration.
• Administering analgesics as needed.
• Avoiding diuretic use since it reduces intravascular volume further.
• Removing ascitic, pleural, or pericardial fluid *only* if it is imperative for relief of symptoms such as respiratory distress or cardiac tamponade; to do so may increase risk of injury to the ovary.
• In patients who require surgery to control bleeding from ovarian cyst rupture, employing surgical measures that also maximally conserve ovarian tissue.

Intermediate phase
• Once patient is stabilized, minimizing third spacing of fluids by cautiously replacing potassium, sodium, and fluids as required, based on monitoring of serum electrolyte concentrations.
• Avoiding diuretic use.

Resolution phase
• The third space fluid shifts to intravascular compartment, resulting in decreased hematocrit value and increased urinary output.
• Peripheral and/or pulmonary edema may result if third space fluid volume mobilized exceeds renal output.
• Administering diuretics when required, to manage pulmonary edema.

## Parenteral Dosage Forms

### UROFOLLITROPIN FOR INJECTION

Note: According to the manufacturer, the purified product will replace this formulation of urofollitropin in 1997.

**Usual adult dose**
Infertility, female—
   Intramuscular, 75 Units once a day, usually for seven or more days, followed by 5000 to 10,000 Units of human chorionic gonadotropin (hCG) one day after the last dose of urofollitropin. If necessary, the dosage may then be increased to 150 Units once a day, usually for seven or more days.

Reproductive technologies, assisted[1]—
   Intramuscular, 150 Units once a day, beginning in the early follicular phase (cycle Day 2 or 3), until sufficient follicular development occurs, followed by 5000 to 10,000 Units of hCG one day after the last dose of urofollitropin.

Note: Dosage regimen may vary according to physician preference or patient response.

If the ovaries are abnormally enlarged or if serum estradiol concentrations are excessively elevated on the last day of urofollitropin therapy, human chorionic gonadotropin should not be given for that cycle.

## Size(s) usually available
U.S.—
- 75 Units (Rx) [*Metrodin*].
- 150 Units (Rx) [*Metrodin*].

Canada—
- 75 Units (Rx) [*Metrodin*].
- 150 Units (Rx) [*Metrodin*].

**Packaging and storage**
Store between 3 and 25 °C (37 and 77 °F), unless otherwise specified by manufacturer. Protect from light.

**Preparation of dosage form**
Using standard aseptic technique, reconstitute by adding 1 to 2 mL of Sodium Chloride Injection USP to the contents of 1 ampul of Urofollitropin for Injection.

**Stability**
Use immediately after reconstitution; discard any unused portion.

### UROFOLLITROPIN FOR INJECTION (Purified)

**Usual adult dose**
Infertility, female—
Subcutaneous, 75 Units once a day, usually for seven or more days, followed by 5000 to 10,000 Units of human chorionic gonadotropin (hCG) one day after the last dose of urofollitropin. If necessary, the dosage may then be increased to 150 Units once a day, usually for seven or more days.

Reproductive technologies, assisted[1]—
Subcutaneous, 150 Units once a day, beginning in the early follicular phase (cycle Day 2 or 3), until sufficient follicular development occurs, followed by 5000 to 10,000 Units of hCG one day after the last dose of urofollitropin.

Note: Dosage regimen may vary according to physician preference or patient response.

If the ovaries are abnormally enlarged or if serum estradiol concentrations are excessively elevated on the last day of urofollitropin therapy, human chorionic gonadotropin should not be given for that cycle.

Canadian labeling states that purified urofollitropin for injection can be given subcutaneously or intramuscularly; the subcutaneous route is less painful to the patient.

**Size(s) usually available**
U.S.—
- 75 Units (Rx) [*Fertinex*].
- 150 Units (Rx) [*Fertinex*].

Canada—
- 75 Units (Rx) [*Fertinorm HP*].
- 150 Units (Rx) [*Fertinorm HP*].

**Packaging and storage**
Store between 3 and 25 °C (37 and 77 °F), unless otherwise specified by manufacturer. Protect from light.

**Preparation of dosage form**
Using standard aseptic technique, reconstitute by adding 0.5 to 1 mL of Sodium Chloride Injection USP to the contents of 1 or more ampules. Do not exceed a strength of 225 Units urofollitropin per 0.5 mL.

**Stability**
Use immediately after reconstitution; discard any unused portion.

[1]Not included in Canadian product labeling.

Revised: 07/08/92
Interim revision: 06/30/94; 08/07/97

---

**UROKINASE**—See *Thrombolytic Agents (Systemic)*

---

# URSODIOL Systemic

INN: Ursodeoxycholic acid
BAN: Ursodeoxycholic acid
JAN: Ursodesoxycholic acid

VA CLASSIFICATION (Primary): GA900

Commonly used brand name(s): *Actigall*; *Ursofalk*.

Another commonly used name is UDCA.

Note: For a listing of dosage forms and brand names by country availability, see *Dosage Forms* section(s).

## Category
Anticholelithic.

## Indications
Note: Bracketed information in the *Indications* section refers to uses that are not included in U.S. product labeling.

**Accepted**
Gallstone disease (treatment)—Orally administered ursodiol is indicated for dissolution of cholesterol gallstones in selected patients with uncomplicated radiolucent gallstone disease. However, alternative therapies should be considered since gallstone dissolution with ursodiol may require many months of treatment, complete dissolution does not occur in all patients, and recurrence of stones occurs within 5 years in about 50% of patients who have had stones dissolved by use of bile acid therapy.

Ursodiol therapy is more likely to be effective if the stones are small (< 20 mm) and of the floatable type.

Body weight and dietary factors may influence gallstone formation and/or dissolution rate.

Gallstone formation (prophylaxis)[1]—Ursodiol is indicated for the prevention of gallstone formation in obese patients experiencing rapid weight loss.

[Atresia, biliary (treatment)][1]
[Cholangitis, sclerosing (treatment)][1]
[Cirrhosis, alcoholic (treatment)][1]
[Cirrhosis, biliary (treatment)][1]
[Hepatic disease, cholestatic (treatment)]
[Hepatic disease, cystic fibrosis–associated (treatment)][1] and
[Hepatitis, chronic (treatment)][1]—Ursodiol is used for the treatment of some chronic liver diseases, including primary biliary cirrhosis, primary sclerosing cholangitis, cystic fibrosis–associated liver disease, biliary atresia, chronic hepatitis, and alcoholic cirrhosis.

[Transplant rejection, liver (prophylaxis)][1]—Ursodiol is used as adjuvant therapy following orthotopic liver transplantation to prevent early graft rejection.

**Unaccepted**
Ursodiol is *not* indicated when there are calcified cholesterol stones, radiopaque stones (calcium-containing), or radiolucent bile pigment stones; when the gallbladder is not functioning; or when surgery for gallstones is clearly indicated.

[1]Not included in Canadian product labeling.

## Pharmacology/Pharmacokinetics

**Physicochemical characteristics**
Molecular weight—392.58.

**Mechanism of action/Effect**
Anticholelithic—Although the exact mechanism of ursodiol's anticholelithic action is not completely understood, it is known that when administered orally ursodiol is concentrated in bile and decreases biliary cholesterol saturation by suppressing hepatic synthesis and secretion of cholesterol, and by inhibiting its intestinal absorption. The reduced cholesterol saturation permits the gradual solubilization of cholesterol from gallstones, resulting in their eventual dissolution.

**Other actions/effects**
Ursodiol increases bile flow. In chronic cholestatic liver disease, ursodiol appears to reduce the detergent properties of the bile salts, thus reducing their cytotoxicity. Also, ursodiol may protect liver cells from the damaging activity of toxic bile acids (e.g., lithocholate, deoxycholate, and chenodeoxycholate), which increase in concentration in patients with chronic liver disease.

**Absorption**
Absorbed from the small bowel (about 90% of dose).

**Protein binding**
High.

**Biotransformation**

Hepatic (first-pass hepatic clearance). Exogenous ursodiol is metabolized in the liver to its taurine and glycine conjugates. The resulting conjugates are secreted into bile.

**Time to peak concentration**

1 to 3 hours.

**Elimination**

Primarily fecal; very small amounts are excreted into urine. Small amount of unabsorbed ursodiol passes into the colon where it undergoes bacterial degradation (7-dehydroxylation); the resulting lithocholic acid is partly absorbed from the colon but is sulfated in the liver and rapidly eliminated in the feces as the sulfolithocholyl glycine or sulfolithocholyl taurine conjugate.

## Precautions to Consider

**Cross-sensitivity and/or related problems**

Patients sensitive to other bile acid products may be sensitive to ursodiol also.

**Carcinogenicity/Tumorigenicity**

Studies in rats with intrarectal instillation of lithocholic acid and other metabolites of ursodiol and chenodiol did not show evidence of tumorigenicity, except when these substances were administered in conjunction with a carcinogenic agent. Epidemiologic studies suggest that bile acids might be involved in the pathogenesis of human colon cancer in patients who have undergone a cholecystectomy; however, conclusive evidence is lacking.

**Pregnancy/Reproduction**

Pregnancy—Adequate and well-controlled studies have not been done in humans.

Studies in rats at doses 20 to 100 times the human dose, and in rabbits at doses 5 times the human dose, have not shown that ursodiol causes adverse effects in the fetus.

FDA Pregnancy Category B.

**Breast-feeding**

It is not known whether ursodiol is distributed into breast milk. However, problems in humans have not been documented.

**Pediatrics**

Appropriate studies on the relationship of age to the effects of ursodiol when used as an anticholelithic have not been performed in the pediatric population. However, studies performed to date in children and infants with cholestatic liver disease and biliary atresia have not demonstrated pediatrics-specific problems that would limit the usefulness of ursodiol in children.

**Geriatrics**

Appropriate studies on the relationship of age to the effects of ursodiol have not been performed in the geriatric population. However, geriatrics-specific problems that would limit the usefulness of this medication in the elderly are not expected.

**Drug interactions and/or related problems**

The following drug interactions and/or related problems have been selected on the basis of their potential clinical significance (possible mechanism in parentheses where appropriate)—not necessarily inclusive (» = major clinical significance):

Note: Combinations containing any of the following medications, depending on the amount present, may also interact with this medication.

Antacids, aluminum-containing or
Cholestyramine or
Colestipol
(concurrent use may result in binding of ursodiol, thus decreasing its absorption)

Antihyperlipidemics, especially clofibrate or
Estrogens or
Neomycin or
Progestins
(concurrent use of these medications with ursodiol may decrease ursodiol's ability to dissolve cholesterol gallstones, since these medications tend to increase cholesterol saturation of bile)

**Laboratory value alterations**

The following have been selected on the basis of their potential clinical significance (possible effect in parentheses where appropriate)—not necessarily inclusive (» = major clinical significance):

With physiology/laboratory test values
Transaminase (mainly serum alanine aminotransferase [ALT (SGPT)])
(although this effect has not been clearly demonstrated, serum concentrations of liver enzymes may be increased due to the inability of some patients to form sulfate conjugates of lithocholic acid; however, these concentrations may be decreased in patients with primary biliary cirrhosis, with other cholestatic conditions, and with chronic active hepatitis)

**Medical considerations/Contraindications**

The medical considerations/contraindications included have been selected on the basis of their potential clinical significance (reasons given in parentheses where appropriate)—not necessarily inclusive (» = major clinical significance).

*Risk-benefit should be considered when the following medical problems exist:*

» Gallstone complications, such as:
  Biliary gastrointestinal fistula
  Biliary obstruction
  Cholangitis
  Cholecystitis
  Pancreatitis
    (medical treatment with ursodiol would be too lengthy; surgery may be indicated)

Hepatic function impairment, chronic
  (bile acid metabolism may be further impaired; however, in some studies ursodiol had a normalizing effect on previously abnormal liver test findings. Data suggest a possible therapeutic role for ursodiol in chronic cholestatic liver disease, in which cholestasis [impaired bile formation or flow] appears to play an important role)

Sensitivity to ursodiol or to other bile acids

**Patient monitoring**

The following may be especially important in patient monitoring (other tests may be warranted in some patients, depending on condition; » = major clinical significance):

Alanine aminotransferase (ALT [SGPT]) and
Alkaline phosphatase and
Aspartate aminotransferase (AST [SGOT]) and
Bilirubin and
Gamma-glutamyltransferase (GGT)
  (monitoring of serum values is recommended upon initiation of treatment, every 1 to 3 months for the first 3 months of treatment [depending on the indication for use], and then every 6 months during treatment; ursodiol must be discontinued if increased values persist)

Cholecystogram
  (recommended prior to treatment for gallstones to determine whether the gallbladder is functional, and whether gallstones are translucent or radiopaque)

Ultrasonograms
  (recommended prior to treatment to confirm the presence of gallstones, and at 6-month intervals during the first year of treatment to monitor stone dissolution; also recommended after gallstone dissolution to monitor for possible recurrence)

## Side/Adverse Effects

Note: Hepatotoxicity has not been associated with ursodiol therapy. However, in some individuals with a congenital or acquired reduction in ability to sulfate hepatotoxic lithocholic acid, the theoretical risk of lithocholate-induced liver damage may be increased.

The following side/adverse effects have been selected on the basis of their potential clinical significance (possible signs and symptoms in parentheses where appropriate)—not necessarily inclusive:

**Those indicating need for medical attention only if they continue or are bothersome**

Incidence more frequent
  *Back pain; diarrhea*—may be dose-related

Incidence less frequent or rare
  *Alopecia* (hair loss); *constipation; dizziness; dyspepsia* (heartburn); *nausea; psoriasis, exacerbation of pre-existing; vomiting*

## Overdose

No cases of ursodiol overdose have been reported.

For information on the management of overdose or unintentional ingestion, **contact a Poison Control Center** (see *Poison Control Center Listing*).

## Patient Consultation

As an aid to patient consultation, refer to *Advice for the Patient, Ursodiol (Systemic)*.

In providing consultation, consider emphasizing the following selected information (» = major clinical significance):

### Before using this medication
» Conditions affecting use, especially:
Sensitivity to ursodiol or to other bile acids
Other medical problems, especially gallstone complications

### Proper use of this medication
Taking with meals for optimal therapeutic effect
» Compliance with full course of therapy
» Proper dosing
Missed dose: Taking as soon as possible or doubling the next dose
» Proper storage

### Precautions while using this medication
» Regular visits to physician to check progress; laboratory tests may be required during therapy
Avoiding aluminum-containing antacids; may interfere with absorption of ursodiol
» Notifying physician immediately if symptoms of acute cholecystitis develop

## General Dosing Information
Ursodiol should be taken with meals or a snack since it dissolves more rapidly when bile and pancreatic juice are present in the intestinal chyme.

Gallstone dissolution may require 6 months to 2 years of continuous dosing depending on the size and composition of the stone(s). Response should be monitored by ultrasonograms performed at 6-month intervals during the first year of therapy. After complete dissolution, it is recommended that ursodiol be continued for at least 3 months to promote dissolution of particles that are too small to image.

Ursodiol therapy is unlikely to be effective if partial dissolution has not occurred after 6 to 12 months of treatment.

Gallbladder nonvisualization that develops during therapy is an indication that complete stone dissolution will not occur and therapy should be discontinued.

## Oral Dosage Forms
Note: Bracketed uses in the *Dosage Forms* section refer to categories of use and/or indications that are not included in U.S. product labeling.

### URSODIOL CAPSULES USP
#### Usual adult and adolescent dose
Gallstone disease (treatment)—
Oral, 8 to 10 mg per kg of body weight a day, divided into two or three doses, usually taken with meals.

Gallstone formation (prophylaxis)[1]—
Oral, 300 mg two times a day. Alternatively, some clinicians continue the dissolution dose of 8 to 10 mg per kg of body weight a day. Bedtime dosing has been reported to enhance dissolution.
[Hepatic disease, cholestatic (treatment)]—
Oral, 13 to 15 mg per kg of body weight a day, given in two divided doses (morning and bedtime) with food.

#### Usual pediatric dose
Anticholelithic—
Dosage has not been established.
Note: In children with cholestatic liver disease and extrahepatic biliary atresia, total daily doses have ranged from 10 to 18 mg per kg of body weight.

#### Usual geriatric dose
See *Usual adult and adolescent dose.*

#### Strength(s) usually available
U.S.—
300 mg (Rx) [*Actigall*].
Canada—
250 mg (Rx) [*Ursofalk*].

#### Packaging and storage
Store below 40 °C (104 °F), preferably between 15 and 30 °C (59 and 86 °F), in a tight container, unless otherwise specified by manufacturer.

#### Auxiliary labeling
• Continue medication for full time of treatment.
• Take with food.

[1]Not included in Canadian product labeling.

## Selected Bibliography
Rosenbaum CL, Cluxton RJ Jr. Ursodiol: a cholesterol gallstone solubilizing agent. Drug Intell Clin Pharm 1988 Dec; 22: 941-5.
Ward A, Brogden RN, Heel RC, et al. Ursodeoxycholic acid: a review of its pharmacological properties and therapeutic efficacy. Drugs 1984; 27: 95-131.

Revised: 08/12/97

# VALACYCLOVIR Systemic

INN: Valaciclovir
VA CLASSIFICATION (Primary): AM802
Commonly used brand name(s): *Valtrex*.

Note: For a listing of dosage forms and brand names by country availability, see *Dosage Forms* section(s).

## Category
Antiviral (systemic).

## Indications

**Accepted**

Herpes genitalis, initial episode (treatment)[1]—Valacyclovir is indicated in the treatment of initial episodes of genital herpes in immunocompetent adults.

Herpes genitalis, recurrent episodes (suppression)[1]—Valacyclovir is indicated in the suppression of recurrent episodes of genital herpes in immunocompetent adults.

Herpes genitalis, recurrent episodes (treatment)—Valacyclovir is indicated in the treatment of recurrent episodes of genital herpes in immunocompetent adults.

Herpes zoster (treatment)—Valacyclovir is indicated in the treatment of herpes zoster (shingles) infections caused by varicella-zoster virus (VZV) in immunocompetent adults. In patients older than 50 years of age, valacyclovir significantly reduced the duration of zoster-associated pain and the duration of postherpetic neuralgia lasting greater than 6 months when compared to acyclovir. Therapy is most effective when started within 48 hours of the onset of rash. There are no data on the safety and effectiveness of valacyclovir in children, immunocompromised patients, or patients with disseminated zoster.

[1]Not included in Canadian product labeling.

## Pharmacology/Pharmacokinetics

**Physicochemical characteristics**

Source—Valacyclovir is the hydrochloride salt of the L-valyl ester of acyclovir.
Molecular weight—Valacyclovir: 324.34.
Valacyclovir hydrochloride: 360.8.

**Mechanism of action/Effect**

Valacyclovir is a prodrug that is nearly completely converted to acyclovir and L-valine. Due to its more efficient phosphorylation by viral thymidine kinase, acyclovir's antiviral activity is greatest against herpes simplex virus type 1 (HSV-1), followed by herpes simplex virus type 2 (HSV-2), varicella-zoster virus (VZV), Epstein-Barr virus (EBV), and cytomegalovirus (CMV).

Acyclovir is phosphorylated by thymidine kinase to acyclovir monophosphate, which is then converted into acyclovir diphosphate and triphosphate by cellular enzymes. Acyclovir is selectively converted to the active triphosphate form by cells infected with herpes viruses. Acyclovir triphosphate inhibits herpes viral DNA replication by competitive inhibition of viral DNA polymerase, and by incorporation into and termination of the growing viral DNA chain.

**Absorption**

Valacyclovir is rapidly absorbed in the gastrointestinal tract; it is then converted to the active compound, acyclovir, by first-pass intestinal and hepatic metabolism. Administration of valacyclovir with food was not found to alter the bioavailability of acyclovir.

The bioavailability of acyclovir following administration of valacyclovir is approximately 54%, which is three to five times greater than its bioavailability following oral administration of acyclovir. After administration of 1 gram of valacyclovir given four times a day, the area under the plasma concentration–time curve (AUC) of acyclovir is approximately that obtained after intravenous administration of 5 mg per kg of body weight of acyclovir every 8 hours.

**Distribution**

Acyclovir is widely distributed to tissues and body fluids, including brain, kidneys, lungs, liver, aqueous humor, tears, intestines, muscle, spleen, breast milk, uterus, vaginal mucosa, vaginal secretions, semen, amniotic fluid, cerebrospinal fluid (CSF), and herpetic vesicular fluid. Highest concentrations are found in the kidneys, liver, and intestines. Acyclovir concentrations in the CSF are approximately 50% of plasma concentrations. In addition, acyclovir crosses the placenta.

**Protein binding**
Valacyclovir—Low (13 to 18%).
Acyclovir—Low (9 to 33%).

**Biotransformation**

Valacyclovir is rapidly and nearly completely (99%) converted to the active compound, acyclovir, and L-valine by first-pass intestinal and hepatic metabolism by enzymatic hydrolysis. Acyclovir is converted to inactive metabolites by alcohol and aldehyde dehydrogenase and, to a small extent, by aldehyde oxidase. The metabolism of valacyclovir and acyclovir is not associated with hepatic microsomal enzyme systems.

**Half-life**
Valacyclovir—
  Less than 30 minutes.
Acyclovir—
  After administration of valacyclovir:
    Normal renal function—2.5 to 3.3 hours.
    End-stage renal disease—Approximately 14 hours.
    Geriatric patients (65 to 83 years of age)—3.3 to 3.7 hours.

**Time to peak concentration**
1.6 to 2.1 hours.

**Peak plasma concentrations**
Valacyclovir—
  Plasma concentrations of unconverted valacyclovir are low, with peak concentrations of less than 0.5 mcg per mL (mcg/mL) after any dose. Plasma concentrations are nonquantifiable within 3 hours after administration.
Acyclovir—
  Peak plasma concentrations are not proportional to the dose.
  After a single dose of valacyclovir:
    500 mg: Approximately 3.3 mcg/mL.
    1 gram: 4.8 to 5.6 mcg/mL.
  After multiple doses of valacyclovir:
    500 mg: Approximately 3.7 mcg/mL.
    1 gram: 5 to 5.5 mcg/mL.

**Elimination**
Valacyclovir—
  Less than 1% of valacyclovir is recovered unchanged in the urine over 24 hours.
  In dialysis:
    It is not known if peritoneal dialysis removes valacyclovir from the blood.
Acyclovir—
  Renal; acyclovir accounts for 80 to 89% of the total urinary recovery. There was no accumulation of acyclovir after repeated administration of valacyclovir in patients with normal renal function.
  In dialysis:
    Hemodialysis—During a 4-hour hemodialysis session, approximately one third of acyclovir in the body is removed. The half-life of acyclovir is approximately 4 hours during hemodialysis.
    Peritoneal dialysis—Chronic ambulatory peritoneal dialysis (CAPD) and continuous arteriovenous hemofiltration/dialysis (CAVHD) do not substantially remove acyclovir, with pharmacokinetic parameters resembling those observed in patients with end-stage renal disease not receiving hemodialysis.

## Precautions to Consider

**Carcinogenicity/Tumorigenicity**

Valacyclovir was found to be noncarcinogenic in lifetime carcinogenicity bioassays at single daily doses of up to 120 mg per kg of body weight (mg/kg) per day for mice and 100 mg/kg per day for rats. There was no significant difference in the incidence of tumors between mice and rats treated with valacyclovir and control animals; also, valacyclovir did not shorten the latency of tumors. Plasma concentrations of acyclovir were equivalent to human levels in the mouse bioassay and 1.4 to 2.3 times human levels in the rat bioassay.

**Mutagenicity**

An *in vitro* cytogenetic study with human lymphocytes, a rat cytogenetic study after a single oral dose of 3000 mg/kg (eight to nine times human plasma concentrations), and Ames tests in the presence or absence of metabolic activation were all negative. Valacyclovir was also negative in the mouse lymphoma assay in the absence of metabolic activation. In the presence of metabolic activation (76 to 88% conversion to acyclovir), valacyclovir was weakly mutagenic. A mouse micronucleus assay was negative at 250 mg/kg, but weakly positive at 500 mg/kg (acyclovir concentrations of 26 and 51 times human plasma concentrations, respectively).

**Pregnancy/Reproduction**
Fertility—Valacyclovir did not impair fertility in rats given a dose of 200 mg/kg per day (six times human plasma concentrations).

Pregnancy—Acyclovir crosses the placenta. No adequate and well-controlled studies have been done with either valacyclovir or acyclovir in pregnant women. A prospective epidemiologic registry of acyclovir use during pregnancy from 1984 to December 1994 has documented 380 women with live births who were exposed to systemic acyclovir during the first trimester of pregnancy. The rate of birth defects in this group approximates that found in the general population. However, it is thought that the small size of the registry is insufficient to evaluate the risk for less common defects or to make definitive conclusions about the safety of acyclovir in developing fetuses.

FDA Pregnancy Category B.

**Breast-feeding**
It is not known whether valacyclovir is distributed into breast milk. Acyclovir has been found to pass into breast milk at concentrations ranging from 0.6 to 4.1 times the corresponding plasma concentration. At these concentrations, a nursing infant could potentially be exposed to a dose of acyclovir as high as 0.3 mg/kg per day. However, problems in humans have not been documented.

**Pediatrics**
No information is available on the relationship of age to the effects of valacyclovir in pediatric patients. Safety and efficacy have not been established.

**Geriatrics**
Studies performed to date have not demonstrated geriatrics-specific problems that would limit the usefulness of valacyclovir in the elderly. However, elderly patients are more likely to have an age-related decrease in renal function, which may require an adjustment of valacyclovir dosage or dosing interval.

**Drug interactions and/or related problems**
The following drug interactions and/or related problems have been selected on the basis of their potential clinical significance (possible mechanism in parentheses where appropriate)—not necessarily inclusive (» = major clinical significance):

Note: Combinations containing any of the following medications, depending on the amount present, may also interact with this medication.

Cimetidine and
Probenecid
   (cimetidine and probenecid have been found to decrease the rate, but not the extent, of conversion of valacyclovir to acyclovir; the renal clearance of acyclovir is reduced by approximately 24% and 33% by cimetidine and probenecid, respectively, resulting in an increase in the peak plasma concentration of acyclovir by approximately 8% and 22%, respectively; combined use of cimetidine and probenecid resulted in a reduced renal clearance of acyclovir by approximately 46% and an increase in the peak plasma concentration by approximately 30%)

**Medical considerations/Contraindications**
The medical considerations/contraindications included have been selected on the basis of their potential clinical significance (reasons given in parentheses where appropriate)—not necessarily inclusive (» = major clinical significance).

*Risk-benefit should be considered when the following medical problems exist:*

» Bone marrow transplantation or
» Human immunodeficiency virus (HIV) infection, advanced or
» Renal transplantation
   (thrombotic thrombocytopenic purpura/hemolytic uremic syndrome [TTP/HUS] has been reported in patients with these conditions who were taking high doses of valacyclovir for prolonged periods of time; in rare cases, death has occurred; therefore, valacyclovir is not indicated in immunocompromised patients; however, TTP/HUS has not been seen in immunocompetent patients treated with valacyclovir)

Hepatic function impairment
   (the rate, but not the extent, of conversion of valacyclovir to acyclovir is reduced in patients with moderate or severe liver disease [biopsy-proven cirrhosis]; however, the half-life of acyclovir is not affected and dosage modification is not recommended for patients with cirrhosis)

» Hypersensitivity to valacyclovir or acyclovir

» Renal function impairment
   (because valacyclovir is renally excreted, patients with renal function impairment may be at increased risk of toxicity; patients with a creatinine clearance of < 50 mL/min [< 0.83 mL/sec] require a reduction in dose)

## Side/Adverse Effects

Note: No serious side effects have been noted to date with the administration of valacyclovir in immunocompetent adults.

The following side/adverse effects have been selected on the basis of their potential clinical significance (possible signs and symptoms in parentheses where appropriate)—not necessarily inclusive:

**Those indicating need for medical attention**
Incidence less frequent
   *Dysmenorrhea* (painful menstruation, including abdominal cramps; diarrhea; nausea)

**Those indicating need for medical attention only if they continue or are bothersome**
Incidence more frequent
   *Headache; nausea*
Incidence less frequent
   *Arthralgia* (joint pain); *dizziness; fatigue* (unusual tiredness or weakness); *gastrointestinal disturbances* (constipation; diarrhea; loss of appetite; stomach pain; vomiting)

## Overdose

For more information on the management of overdose or unintentional ingestion, **contact a Poison Control Center** (see *Poison Control Center Listing*).

**Clinical effects of overdose**
To date, there have been no reports of overdosage with valacyclovir. However, precipitation of acyclovir in the renal tubules has occurred with rapid or high intravenous doses of acyclovir. No significant adverse effects have been seen with oral overdoses of acyclovir of up to 20 grams. If acute renal failure or anuria occurs, hemodialysis may be helpful until renal function is restored.

## Patient Consultation

As an aid to patient consultation, refer to Advice for the Patient, Valacyclovir (Systemic).

In providing consultation, consider emphasizing the following selected information (» = major clinical significance):

**Before using this medication**
» Conditions affecting use, especially:
   Hypersensitivity to valacyclovir or acyclovir
   Other medical problems, especially advanced human immunodeficiency virus infection, bone marrow transplantation, renal function impairment, or renal transplantation

**Proper use of this medication**
» Initiating use of valacyclovir at the earliest sign or symptom; within 48 hours of the onset of rash, pain, or burning when used to treat shingles or an initial episode of genital herpes, or within 24 hours of onset when used to treat recurrent genital herpes
   Valacyclovir may be taken with meals
» Compliance with full course of therapy; not using more often or for longer than prescribed
» Proper dosing
   Missed dose: Taking as soon as possible; not taking if almost time for next dose; not doubling doses
» Proper storage

**Precautions while using this medication**
Checking with physician if no improvement within a few days
Keeping affected areas as clean and dry as possible; wearing loose-fitting clothing to avoid irritating the lesions

**Side/adverse effects**
Signs of dysmenorrhea

## General Dosing Information

For treatment of initial or recurrent episodes of genital herpes, valacyclovir therapy should be initiated as soon as possible following the onset of signs and symptoms. In clinical studies, therapy for an initial episode was most effective when initiated within 48 hours of the onset of signs and symptoms; therapy for recurrent episodes was most effective when initiated within 24 hours.

Therapy should be initiated as soon as possible following the onset of signs and symptoms of varicella-zoster infection. In clinical studies, treatment was started within 72 hours of the onset of rash; however, valacyclovir was found to be more effective if started within 48 hours.

Valacyclovir may be taken with meals since absorption has not been shown to be significantly affected by food.

Adults with impaired renal function may require a change in dosing, as follows:

| Indication | Creatinine clearance (mL/min)/(mL/sec) ≥ 50/0.83 | 30–49/ 0.5–0.82 | 10–29/ 0.16–0.49 | < 10/0.16 |
|---|---|---|---|---|
| Genital herpes, treatment of initial episode | 1 gram every 12 hours | 1 gram every 12 hours | 1 gram every 24 hours | 500 mg every 24 hours |
| Genital herpes, treatment of recurrent episodes | 500 mg every 12 hours | 500 mg every 12 hours | 500 mg every 24 hours | 500 mg every 24 hours |
| Genital herpes, suppression | 500 mg every 24 hours* | 500 mg every 24 hours* | 500 mg every 48 hours* | 500 mg every 48 hours* |
|  | 1 gram every 24 hours | 1 gram every 24 hours | 500 mg every 24 hours | 500 mg every 24 hours |
| Herpes zoster treatment | 1 gram every 8 hours | 1 gram every 12 hours | 1 gram every 24 hours | 500 mg every 24 hours |
| Hemodialysis patients | Patients requiring hemodialysis should receive the recommended dose after hemodialysis. | | | |
| Peritoneal dialysis patients | Supplemental doses should not be required. | | | |

*Recommended for patients with a history of nine or fewer recurrent episodes of herpes genitalis per year.

## Oral Dosage Forms

Note: The dosing and strengths of the dosage forms available are expressed in terms of valacyclovir base (not the hydrochloride salt).

### VALACYCLOVIR HYDROCHLORIDE TABLETS

**Usual adult dose**
Herpes genitalis, treatment of initial episode[1]—
  Oral, 1 gram (base) two times a day for ten days.
Herpes genitalis, treatment of recurrent episodes—
  Oral, 500 mg (base) two times a day for five days.
Herpes genitalis, suppression of recurrent episodes[1]—
  Oral, 1 gram (base) once a day.
  Note: For patients with a history of nine or fewer recurrent episodes per year, 500 mg once a day may be given.
Herpes zoster, treatment—
  Oral, 1 gram (base) three times a day for seven days.

**Usual pediatric dose**
Safety and efficacy in patients younger than 18 years of age have not been established.

**Usual geriatric dose**
See *Usual adult dose*.

**Strength(s) usually available**
U.S.—
  500 mg (base) (Rx) [*Valtrex*].
  1 gram (base) (Rx) [*Valtrex*].
Canada—
  500 mg (base) (Rx) [*Valtrex*].

**Packaging and storage**
Store between 15 and 25 °C (59 and 77 °F), in a tight container. Protect from light.

**Auxiliary labeling**
• Continue medicine for full time of treatment.

[1]Not included in Canadian product labeling.

Developed: 05/28/96
Interim revision: 03/24/98

### VALPROATE SODIUM—See *Valproic Acid (Systemic)*

---

# VALPROIC ACID   Systemic

This monograph includes information on the following: 1) Divalproex; 2) Valproate Sodium†; 3) Valproic Acid.

INN: Divalproex Sodium—Valproate Semisodium
BAN: Divalproex Sodium—Semisodium Valproate
JAN: Valproate Sodium—Sodium Valproate
VA CLASSIFICATION (Primary/Secondary):
  Divalproex—CN400/CN105; CN900
  Valproate Sodium—CN400
  Valproic Acid—CN400

Commonly used brand name(s): *Alti-Valproic*[3]; *Depacon*[2]; *Depakene*[3]; *Depakote*[1]; *Depakote Sprinkle*[1]; *Deproic*[3]; *Dom-Valproic*[3]; *Epival*[1]; *Med Valproic*[3]; *Novo-Valproic*[3]; *Nu-Valproic*[3]; *PMS-Valproic Acid*[3]; *Penta-Valproic*[3]; *pms-Valproic Acid*[3]; *pms-Valproic Acid E.C.*[3].

Note: For a listing of dosage forms and brand names by country availability, see *Dosage Forms* section(s).

†Not commercially available in Canada.

## Category
Anticonvulsant; antimanic; migraine headache prophylactic.

## Indications
Note: Bracketed information in the *Indications* section refers to uses that are not included in U.S. product labeling.

**Accepted**
Epilepsy, absence seizure pattern (treatment)—Valproic acid, divalproex, and valproate sodium are indicated in the treatment of simple and complex absence (petit mal) seizures. Although these agents may be used alone or with other anticonvulsant medication, monotherapy with valproic acid, divalproex, or valproate sodium is preferred whenever possible because of unpredictable interactions with hepatic enzyme–inducing anticonvulsants and because of the increased risk of hepatotoxicity.

Epilepsy, mixed seizure pattern (treatment adjunct)—Valproic acid, divalproex, and valproate sodium are indicated as adjuncts in conditions of multiple seizures that include absence seizures.

[Epilepsy, myoclonic seizure pattern (treatment)]—Valproic acid, divalproex, and valproate sodium are used as primary agents for myoclonic seizures.

[Epilepsy, simple partial seizure pattern (treatment)] or
Epilepsy, complex partial seizure pattern (treatment)—Valproic acid, divalproex, and valproate sodium may be useful in patients with partial seizures that are refractory to other anticonvulsants.

[Epilepsy, tonic-clonic seizure pattern (treatment)]—Valproic acid, divalproex, and valproate sodium are used as primary agents in the treatment of tonic-clonic (grand mal) seizures.

Bipolar disorder, manic episodes (treatment)—Divalproex is indicated for the treatment of manic episodes associated with bipolar disorder.

[Bipolar disorder (prophylaxis and treatment)]—Valproic acid and divalproex may be useful in the prophylaxis and treatment of manic-depressive illness refractory to treatment with lithium or other agents.

Migraine headaches (prophylaxis)[1]—Divalproex is indicated in the prophylaxis of migraine headaches. There is no evidence that it may be useful in the treatment of acute migraine.

[1]Not included in Canadian product labeling.

## Pharmacology/Pharmacokinetics

Note: Divalproex sodium is a stable coordination compound composed of equal parts of valproic acid and sodium valproate. In the gastrointestinal tract, divalproex sodium dissociates into valproate and then produces the bioequivalent pharmacologic activity of valproic acid. Equivalent oral doses of divalproex sodium and valproic acid capsules deliver systemically equivalent quantities of valproate ion. Valproate sodium injection exists as the valproate ion in the blood and yields plasma levels equivalent to those of the oral valproic acid and divalproex products. In this monograph, the term valproate is used to designate the valproate ion in the body, whether administered as valproic acid, divalproex sodium, or valproate sodium.

**Physicochemical characteristics**
Molecular weight—
  Divalproex sodium: 310.41.
  Valproate sodium: 166.2.
  Valproic acid: 144.21.
pKa—
  Valproic acid: 4.8.
pH—
  Valproate sodium injection: 7.6.

**Mechanism of action/Effect**
The mechanism of action has not been established; however, it is thought to be related to a direct or secondary increase in concentrations of the inhibitory neurotransmitter, gamma-aminobutyric acid (GABA), possibly caused by its decreased metabolism or decreased reuptake in brain tissues. Another hypothesis is that valproate acts on postsynaptic receptor sites to mimic or enhance the inhibitory action of GABA. The effect on the neuronal membrane is not completely understood. Some studies suggest a possible direct effect on membrane activity related to changes in potassium conductance. Also, valproate has been shown in animal studies to block sustained neuronal bursting responses by reducing the amplitude of sodium-dependent action potentials in a voltage- and use-dependent manner.

**Other actions/effects**
Valproate is a weak inhibitor of some hepatic P450 isoenzymes, as well as epoxide hydrase and glucuronosyl transferase.

**Absorption**
Divalproex sodium—Enteric coating on the tablet delays absorption for about 1 to 4 hours after ingestion; concomitant administration with food may significantly slow the rate, but not the extent, of absorption.
Valproic acid—Rapid absorption from gastrointestinal tract; slight delay when taken with food.

**Distribution**
Valproate concentrations in the cerebrospinal fluid approximate unbound concentrations in plasma, which is about 10% of the total concentration. Valproate is distributed into breast milk in concentrations ranging from 1 to 10% of total maternal serum concentrations.

**Protein binding**
High (90 to 95%) at serum concentrations up to 50 micrograms (mcg) per mL; as the concentration increases from 50 to 100 mcg per mL, the percentage bound decreases to 80 to 85% and the free fraction becomes progressively larger, thus increasing the concentration gradient into the brain. Protein binding of valproate is reduced in the elderly, in patients with hypoalbuminemia, in patients with chronic hepatic diseases, and in patients with renal function impairment.

**Biotransformation**
Primarily hepatic. Some metabolites may have pharmacologic or toxic activity. Rate of metabolism is faster in children and in patients concurrently using hepatic enzyme–inducing medications, such as carbamazepine, phenobarbital, phenytoin, and primidone.

**Half-life**
Variable, from 6 to 16 hours; may be considerably longer in patients with hepatic function impairment, in the elderly, and in children up to 18 months of age; may be considerably shorter in patients receiving hepatic enzyme–inducing anticonvulsants.
Mean terminal half-life for valproate monotherapy following a 60-minute intravenous infusion of 1000 mg was 16 ± 3 hours.

**Time to peak serum concentration**
Capsules and syrup—1 to 4 hours.
Delayed-release capsules and tablets—3 to 4 hours.
Injection—At the end of a 1-hour intravenous infusion.

**Therapeutic plasma concentrations**
Variable. The therapeutic range in epilepsy is commonly considered to be 50 to 100 mcg per mL (347 to 693 micromoles per L) of total valproate, although some patients may require higher or lower plasma concentrations.
The relationship between plasma concentration and clinical response is not well documented. One contributing factor is the nonlinear, concentration-dependent protein binding of valproate, which affects the clearance of the medication. Monitoring of total serum valproate cannot provide a reliable index of the bioactive valproate species.

**Elimination**
Renal, mainly as glucuronide conjugate; small amounts excreted in feces and expired air.

## Precautions to Consider

**Carcinogenicity/Tumorigenicity**
Studies in rodents given valproic acid doses of 0, 80, and 170 mg per kg of body weight (mg/kg) a day for 2 years showed a variety of neoplasms and an increase in the incidence of subcutaneous fibrosarcomas in male rats receiving high doses, as well as a dose-related trend for benign pulmonary adenomas in male mice. The significance of these findings humans is not known.

**Mutagenicity**
Valproate was not mutagenic in an *in vitro* bacterial assay (Ames test), did not produce dominant lethal effects in mice, and did not increase chromosome aberration frequency in an *in vivo* cytogenetic study in rats. Increased frequency of sister chromatid exchange (SCE) has been reported in a study of epileptic children taking valproate, but this association was not observed in another study in adults. There is some evidence that increased SCE frequencies may be associated with epilepsy. The biological significance of an increase in SCE frequency is not known.

**Pregnancy/Reproduction**
Fertility—Long-term toxicity studies in rats given doses greater than 200 mg/kg a day and dogs given doses greater than 90 mg/kg a day have shown reduced spermatogenesis and testicular atrophy. Segment I fertility studies in rats given up to 350 mg/kg a day for 60 days have shown no effect on fertility. However, the effect of valproate on the development of the testes and on sperm production and fertility in humans is unknown.

Pregnancy—First trimester: Valproate crosses the placenta and has been reported to have caused teratogenic effects, including neural tube defects (anencephaly, meningomyelocele, and spina bifida) in the fetus when the mother received valproate during the first trimester of pregnancy. Risk-benefit must be carefully considered when these medications are required to treat epilepsy in pregnant patients for whom other medications are ineffective or cannot be used.

Studies in rodents have shown that skeletal abnormalities, primarily involving ribs and vertebrae, occurred in the offspring when the mother received doses exceeding 65 mg/kg per day during pregnancy.

FDA Pregnancy Category D.

**Breast-feeding**
Valproate is distributed into breast milk. Concentrations in breast milk have been reported to be 1 to 10% of the total maternal serum concentration.

**Pediatrics**
Children are at an increased risk of developing serious or fatal hepatotoxicity. Patients up to 2 years of age, especially those on polytherapy, those with congenital metabolic disorders, those with severe seizure disorders accompanied by mental retardation, and those with organic brain disease, appear to be at greatest risk. Experience in patients with epilepsy has shown that the risk of fatal hepatotoxicity decreases with advancing age.

**Geriatrics**
Geriatric patients tend to have increased free, unbound valproate concentrations and lowered intrinsic clearances, indicating a reduction of valproate metabolizing capacity and a fall in serum albumin. Therefore, these patients should receive a lower daily dosage, and the serum concentrations should be kept in the lower therapeutic range.

**Dental**
Valproate inhibits the secondary phase of platelet aggregation, which may be reflected in prolonged bleeding time and/or frank hemorrhaging.

In addition, the leukopenic and thrombocytopenic effects of valproate may result in an increased incidence of microbial infection, delayed healing, and gingival bleeding. If leukopenia or thrombocytopenia occurs, dental work, whenever possible, should be deferred until blood counts have returned to normal. Patients should be instructed in proper oral hygiene, including caution in use of regular toothbrushes, dental floss, and toothpicks.

**Surgical**
Because of the thrombocytopenic effects of valproate, as well as its inhibition of the secondary phase of platelet aggregation and production of abnormal coagulation parameters (e.g., low fibrinogen), monitoring of platelet counts and coagulation tests are recommended in patients prior to scheduled surgery.

**Drug interactions and/or related problems**
The following drug interactions and/or related problems have been selected on the basis of their potential clinical significance (possible mechanism

in parentheses where appropriate)—not necessarily inclusive (» = major clinical significance):

Note: In addition to the interactions listed below, additive or multiple effects leading to impaired blood clotting and/or increased risk of bleeding may occur if valproic acid, divalproex, or valproate sodium is used concurrently with any other medication having a significant potential for inhibiting platelet aggregation or for causing hypoprothrombinemia, thrombocytopenia, or gastrointestinal ulceration or hemorrhage.

Combinations containing any of the following medications, depending on the amount present, may also interact with this medication.

» Alcohol or
» Central nervous system (CNS) depression–producing medications, other (see *Appendix II*)
(concurrent use with valproic acid, divalproex, or valproate sodium may potentiate CNS depressant effects)

Anticoagulants, coumarin- or indandione-derivative or
» Heparin or
» Thrombolytic agents
(valproate-induced hypoprothrombinemia may increase the activity of coumarin- and indandione-derivative anticoagulants and may increase the risk of bleeding in patients receiving heparin or thrombolytic agents)
(inhibition of platelet aggregation and reduction of platelet numbers or thrombocytopenia may increase the risk of hemorrhage in patients receiving anticoagulant or thrombolytic therapy)

Antidepressants, tricyclic or
Bupropion or
Clozapine or
Haloperidol or
Loxapine or
Maprotiline or
Molindone or
Monoamine oxidase (MAO) inhibitors or
Phenothiazines or
Pimozide or
Thioxanthenes
(in addition to enhancing CNS depression when used concurrently with valproic acid, divalproex, or valproate sodium, these medications may lower the seizure threshold; dosage adjustments may be necessary to control seizures)

» Barbiturates or
» Primidone
(concurrent use with valproate causes higher serum concentrations of barbiturates or primidone, leading to increased CNS depression and neurological toxicity because of protein binding displacement of the barbiturate and reduced barbiturate metabolism; half-life of valproate is decreased; dosage adjustment of barbiturates or primidone may be necessary)

» Carbamazepine
(concurrent use may result in decreased serum concentrations and half-life of valproate due to increased metabolism induced by hepatic microsomal enzyme activity; valproate causes an increase in the active 10,11-epoxide metabolite of carbamazepine by inhibiting its breakdown; monitoring of serum concentrations as a guide to dosage is recommended, especially when either medication is added to or withdrawn from an existing regimen)

Clonazepam
(concurrent use with valproic acid, divalproex, or valproate sodium may produce absence status)

Diazepam
(valproate may displace diazepam from its plasma albumin binding sites and may inhibit its metabolism; coadministration was found to increase the free fraction of diazepam by 90% in healthy volunteers; plasma clearance of free diazepam was reduced by 25% and volume of distribution of free diazepam was reduced by 20% in the presence of valproate; the elimination half-life of diazepam remained unchanged)

Ethosuximide, and possibly other succinimide anticonvulsants
(concurrent use with valproic acid, divalproex, or valproate sodium has been reported to both increase and decrease ethosuximide concentrations; monitoring of serum concentrations as a guide to dosage is recommended)

» Felbamate
(coadministration of felbamate may increase valproate plasma concentrations by 35 to 50%; a decrease in valproic acid, divalproex, or valproate sodium dosage may be needed when felbamate therapy is initiated)

» Hepatotoxic medications, other (see *Appendix II*)
(concurrent use with valproic acid, divalproex, or valproate sodium may increase the risk of hepatotoxicity; patients on prolonged therapy or with a history of liver disease should be carefully monitored)

» Lamotrigine
(elimination half-life of lamotrigine was increased from 26 to 70 hours in a steady-state study in volunteers receiving both lamotrigine and valproate; when coadministered with valproate, the dose of lamotrigine should be reduced; concurrent use of lamotrigine with valproate may increase the risk of dangerous dermatologic reactions)

Levocarnitine
(requirements for carnitine may be increased in patients receiving valproic acid or divalproex)

» Mefloquine
(concurrent use with valproic acid, divalproex, or valproate sodium may result in low valproate serum concentrations and loss of seizure control; monitoring of valproate serum concentrations is recommended and dosage adjustments may be necessary during and after therapy with mefloquine)

» Phenytoin, and possibly other hydantoin anticonvulsants
(concurrent use with valproic acid, divalproex, or valproate sodium has resulted in breakthrough seizures or phenytoin toxicity because valproate may interfere with phenytoin protein binding, and phenytoin, through enzyme induction, will lower valproate levels; valproate increases unbound phenytoin concentrations and decreases intrinsic clearance by inhibiting metabolism of phenytoin; concurrent use requires close monitoring of the patient since variable serum phenytoin concentrations have resulted; total phenytoin serum concentrations may not reflect unbound phenytoin activity, and unbound phenytoin concentrations may be more reliable; dosage of phenytoin should be adjusted as required by clinical situation)

» Platelet aggregation inhibitors, other (see *Appendix II*)
(concurrent use with valproic acid, divalproex, or valproate sodium may increase the risk of hemorrhage because of additive or multiple actions that may decrease blood-clotting ability)
(the gastrointestinal ulcerative or hemorrhagic potential of aspirin, anti-inflammatory analgesics, or sulfinpyrazone may increase the risk of hemorrhage in patients receiving valproic acid, divalproex, or valproate sodium)
(in addition, aspirin may displace valproic acid, divalproex, or valproate sodium from protein binding sites, as well as altering valproate metabolism and excretion, resulting in increased levels of free [unbound] valproate, which may cause toxic effects)

Rifampin
(unpublished data obtained by the manufacturer suggest that increased clearance of single-dose oral valproate occurs following pretreatment with oral rifampin; dosage adjustments may be necessary if valproate and rifampin are used concurrently)

Sodium benzoate and sodium phenylacetate combination
(valproate-induced hyperammonemia may exacerbate urea cycle enzymopathy deficiency and antagonize the efficacy of sodium benzoate and sodium phenylacetate combination)

Zidovudine
(in six HIV-positive patients, the clearance of zidovudine was decreased by 38% following administration of valproate; the half-life of zidovudine was unaffected)

## Laboratory value alterations

The following have been selected on the basis of their potential clinical significance (possible effect in parentheses where appropriate)—not necessarily inclusive (» = major clinical significance):

With diagnostic test results
Metyrapone test
(increased metabolism of metyrapone by a hepatic enzyme inducer such as valproic acid, divalproex, or valproate sodium may decrease the response to metyrapone)

Thyroid function tests
(test results may be altered; decreased $T_4$, and free $T_3$ and $T_4$ concentrations have been reported; clinical significance is unknown)

Urine ketone tests
(use of valproic acid, divalproex, or valproate sodium may produce false-positive results because of a ketone metabolite excreted in urine)

With physiology/laboratory test values
Alanine aminotransferase (ALT [SGPT]) and
Aspartate aminotransferase (AST [SGOT]) and
Lactate dehydrogenase (LDH)
(minor elevations of serum concentrations occur frequently and appear to be dose-related; elevations may indicate asymptomatic hepatotoxicity)
Amino acid screening
(increases in glycine may occur)
Bilirubin
(serum concentrations may be increased; increase may indicate potentially serious hepatotoxicity)

**Medical considerations/Contraindications**
The medical considerations/contraindications included have been selected on the basis of their potential clinical significance (reasons given in parentheses where appropriate)—not necessarily inclusive (» = major clinical significance).

*Except under special circumstances, this medication should not be used when the following medical problems exist:*
» Hepatic disease or
» Hepatic function impairment, significant
(may be exacerbated)

*Risk-benefit should be considered when the following medical problems exist:*
Blood dyscrasias or
Brain disease, organic or
Hepatic disease, history of
(may be exacerbated)
Hypoalbuminemia
(alterations in protein binding may affect serum levels)
Renal function impairment
(metabolites may accumulate; valproate binding to serum albumin is decreased and volume of distribution is increased)
Sensitivity to valproic acid, divalproex, or valproate sodium

**Patient monitoring**
The following may be especially important in patient monitoring (other tests may be warranted in some patients, depending on condition; » = major clinical significance):
Ammonia concentrations, serum
(therapy should be discontinued if hyperammonemia occurs, with or without lethargy or coma)
Bleeding time determinations and
Blood cell counts, including platelets and
Renal function determinations
(recommended prior to therapy and periodically during therapy)
Hepatic function determinations
(should be performed prior to therapy and periodically thereafter, especially during the first 6 months of therapy; valproic acid, divalproex, or valproate sodium should be discontinued immediately if significant hepatic function impairment is apparent or suspected)
Valproate concentrations, serum
(since therapeutic concentrations vary widely, morning trough concentrations with values ranging from 50 to 100 mcg per mL [347 to 693 micromoles per L] may be useful when initiating therapy; doses may be raised gradually until patient achieves a predose serum concentration of at least 50 mcg per mL [347 micromoles per L], the dose then being increased as needed)
(total trough valproate plasma concentrations above 110 mcg/mL in females and 135 mcg/mL in males significantly increase the probability of thrombocytopenia; risk-benefit must be considered)
(since serum valproate concentrations do not always correspond with therapeutic effect, evaluation of dose adjustments must be based on total clinical assessment of the patient)

## Side/Adverse Effects
Note: Hepatic failure resulting in death has occurred in patients receiving valproic acid and divalproex. These incidents usually have occurred during the first 6 months of treatment. Patients at greatest risk are children receiving other anticonvulsants along with valproic acid, divalproex, or valproate sodium. Serious or fatal hepatotoxicity may be preceded by nonspecific symptoms such as loss of seizure control, malaise, weakness, lethargy, Reyes-like syndrome, anorexia, vomiting, jaundice, and edema. In some cases, hepatic function impairment has progressed despite discontinuation of medication.

The following side/adverse effects have been selected on the basis of their potential clinical significance (possible signs and symptoms in parentheses where appropriate)—not necessarily inclusive:

**Those indicating need for medical attention**
Incidence less frequent or rare
*Behavioral, mood, or mental changes; hepatotoxicity or hyperammonemia* (increase in frequency of seizures; loss of appetite; continuing nausea or vomiting; swelling of face; tiredness and weakness; yellow eyes or skin); *ophthalmological effects, specifically diplopia* (double vision); *nystagmus* (continuous, uncontrolled back-and-forth and/or rolling eye movements); *or spots before eyes; pancreatitis* (severe abdominal or stomach cramps; continuing nausea and vomiting); *platelet aggregation inhibition or thrombocytopenia* (unusual bleeding or bruising)

Note: Evidence of hemorrhage, bruising, or a disorder of coagulation or hemostasis is an indication for reduction of dosage or discontinuation of therapy.

**Those indicating need for medical attention only if they continue or are bothersome**
Incidence more frequent
*Abdominal or stomach cramps, mild*—may also indicate a risk of pancreatitis; less frequent with divalproex; *anorexia* (loss of appetite); *change in menstrual periods; diarrhea; hair loss; indigestion; nausea and vomiting; trembling of hands and arms; unusual weight loss or gain*

Incidence less frequent or rare
*Ataxia* (clumsiness or unsteadiness); *constipation; dizziness; drowsiness; headache; skin rash; unusual excitement, restlessness, or irritability*

## Overdose
For specific information on the agents used in the management of valproic acid overdose, see:
• *Naloxone (Systemic)* monograph.

For more information on the management of overdose or unintentional ingestion, **contact a Poison Control Center** (see *Poison Control Center Listing*).

**Treatment of overdose**
Treatment of overdose consists primarily of supportive and symptomatic measures.

To decrease absorption—The effectiveness of emesis or gastric lavage will depend upon the time elapsed since ingestion. The enteric-coated tablets will delay absorption about 1 to 4 hours.

To enhance elimination—Hemodialysis, or tandem hemodialysis and hemoperfusion, may result in significant reductions in valproate serum concentrations.

Specific treatment—Maintenance of adequate urinary output must be ensured. Naloxone has been administered to counteract severe CNS depression, but it also theoretically reverses the anticonvulsant effect and should be used with caution.

Supportive care—Patients in whom intentional overdose is confirmed or suspected should be referred for psychiatric consultation.

## Patient Consultation
As an aid to patient consultation, refer to *Advice for the Patient, Valproic Acid (Systemic).*
In providing consultation, consider emphasizing the following selected information (» = major clinical significance):

**Before using this medication**
» Conditions affecting use, especially:
Sensitivity to valproic acid, divalproex, or valproate sodium
Pregnancy—Pregnancy studies in animals have shown skeletal abnormalities involving ribs and vertebrae in offspring of mothers given large doses; in humans, crosses placenta in first trimester and may cause neural tube defects in fetus
Breast-feeding—Distributed into breast milk at concentrations up to 10% of the total maternal serum concentration
Use in children—Children are at an increased risk of serious hepatotoxicity
Use in the elderly—Elderly patients tend to have higher serum concentrations of free (unbound) valproic acid; lower daily dosages recommended
Dental—Prolonged bleeding time and/or hemorrhaging; leukopenia and thrombocytopenia may result in increased incidence of microbial infection, delayed healing, and gingival bleeding

Surgical—Prolonged bleeding time and/or hemorrhaging may occur; leukopenia and thrombocytopenia may cause surgical complications

Other medications, especially alcohol or other CNS depression–producing medications, heparin or thrombolytic agents, barbiturates, primidone, carbamazepine, felbamate, other hepatotoxic medications, lamotrigine, mefloquine, phenytoin, or other platelet aggregation inhibitors

Other medical problems, especially significant hepatic disease or hepatic function impairment

**Proper use of this medication**
*Proper administration*
For valproic acid capsules
Swallowing capsules whole with water only; not breaking, chewing, or crushing
For divalproex sodium delayed-release capsules
Swallowing capsules whole, or sprinkling the contents on a small amount of cool, soft food (such as applesauce or pudding) and swallowing, not chewing, immediately after preparation
For divalproex sodium delayed-release tablets
Swallowing tablets whole; not breaking, chewing, or crushing
For valproic acid syrup
Mixing with any liquid or adding to a small amount of food to enhance palatability
For all oral products
Taking with food if necessary to reduce gastrointestinal side effects
» Compliance with therapy; taking exactly as directed by physician
» Proper dosing
Missed dose: If dosing schedule is—
One dose a day: Taking as soon as possible; not taking if not remembered until next day; not doubling doses
Two or more doses a day: Taking if remembered within 6 hours; taking remaining doses for that day at equally spaced intervals; not doubling doses
» Proper storage

**Precautions while using this medication**
» Regular visits to physician to check progress of therapy
» Checking with physician before discontinuing medication; gradual dosage reduction may be necessary
» Possible prolonged bleeding or hemorrhage: caution if any kind of surgery, dental treatment, or emergency treatment is required
» Avoiding use of alcoholic beverages or other CNS depressants during therapy
Diabetic patients: When testing for urine ketones, possible false-positive test results
Caution if any laboratory tests required; possible interference with results of metyrapone or thyroid function tests
Possible need for carrying medical identification card or bracelet
» Possible drowsiness; caution when driving or doing other things requiring alertness

**Side/adverse effects**
Signs of potential side effects, especially behavioral, mood, or mental changes; hepatotoxicity; hyperammonemia; ophthalmological effects; pancreatitis; platelet aggregation inhibition; or thrombocytopenia

## General Dosing Information

Patients at primary risk for fatal liver failure with valproic acid, divalproex, or valproate sodium treatment include:
• Children up to 2 years of age, especially those on polytherapy, those with congenital metabolic disorders, those with severe epilepsy accompanied by mental retardation, and those with organic brain disease.
• All patients receiving concomitant anticonvulsants, especially those that enhance production of a toxic metabolite through induction of hepatic P450 isoenzymes (e.g., carbamazepine, felbamate, lamotrigine, phenobarbital, phenytoin, primidone)
• Patients with familial liver disease.

Recommendations for reducing the risk of serious hepatotoxicity with valproate include:
• Avoiding the administration of valproate with other anticonvulsants whenever possible, especially in children up to 3 years of age, unless monotherapy has failed or the benefits of polytherapy outweigh the risks.
• Avoiding valproate therapy in patients with pre-existing liver disease or a family history of childhood hepatic disease.
• Administering valproate in as low a dose as possible to achieve seizure control.
• Avoiding concurrent administration with other hepatotoxic medications, especially salicylates.
• Monitoring for prodromal symptoms (e.g., nausea or vomiting, headache, edema, jaundice, or seizure breakthrough, especially after a febrile illness).
• Avoiding administration to patients with congenital metabolic disorders, severe seizure disorders accompanied by mental retardation, or organic brain disease.

When valproic acid, divalproex, or valproate sodium is to be discontinued, dosage should be reduced gradually since abrupt withdrawal may precipitate seizures or status epilepticus.

The serum concentration of valproate does not always correspond with therapeutic effect; therefore, the evaluation of the patient's progress must be based on total clinical assessment.

When valproic acid, divalproex, or valproate sodium is used to replace or supplement other anticonvulsant therapy, the dosage should be increased gradually to achieve therapeutic serum concentrations, while that of the replaced medication is decreased gradually in order to maintain seizure control. The addition of valproic acid, divalproex, or valproate sodium may cause increases in the serum concentrations of hepatic enzyme–inducing anticonvulsants (e.g., carbamazepine, felbamate, lamotrigine, phenobarbital, phenytoin, primidone)

The possible prolongation of bleeding time, in addition to potentiation of depressant effect by CNS depressants, should be considered when surgery, dental treatment, or emergency treatment is required.

**Diet/Nutrition**
Valproic acid or divalproex may be taken with food to reduce gastrointestinal side effects.
The contents of divalproex sodium delayed-release capsules may be sprinkled on a small amount of cool, soft food (such as applesauce or pudding) and swallowed, not chewed, immediately after preparation.
Valproic acid syrup may be mixed with a small amount of food or liquid to enhance the palatability.
Requirements for carnitine may be increased in patients receiving valproic acid, divalproex, or valproate sodium.

---
### DIVALPROEX
---

## Oral Dosage Forms

**DIVALPROEX SODIUM DELAYED-RELEASE CAPSULES**

**Usual adult and adolescent dose**
Anticonvulsant—
Monotherapy: Oral, the equivalent of valproic acid—Initially, 5 to 15 mg per kg of body weight a day, the dosage being increased at one-week intervals by 5 to 10 mg per kg of body weight a day as needed and tolerated.
Polytherapy: Oral, the equivalent of valproic acid—Initially, 10 to 30 mg per kg of body weight a day, the dosage being increased at one-week intervals by 5 to 10 mg per kg of body weight a day as needed and tolerated.
Note: If the total daily dose exceeds 250 mg, it should be divided into two or more doses (usually given every 12 hours) to lessen the possibility of gastrointestinal irritation.
Geriatric patients may need lower doses.
Patients also taking a hepatic enzyme–inducing medication may need higher dosages depending on predose serum concentrations.

**Usual adult prescribing limits**
60 mg per kg of body weight a day.

**Usual pediatric dose**
Anticonvulsant: Children 1 to 12 years of age—
Monotherapy: Oral, the equivalent of valproic acid—Initially, 15 to 45 mg per kg of body weight a day, the dosage being increased at one-week intervals by 5 to 10 mg per kg of body weight a day as needed and tolerated.
Polytherapy: Oral, the equivalent of valproic acid—30 to 100 mg per kg of body weight a day.
Note: Dosage adjustments depend on clinical response and serum anticonvulsant concentrations.

**Usual geriatric dose**
Geriatric patients may need lower doses. See *Usual adult and adolescent dose.*

**Strength(s) usually available**
U.S.—
The equivalent of valproic acid:
125 mg (Rx) [*Depakote Sprinkle*].

Canada—
Not commercially available.

**Packaging and storage**
Store below 30 °C (86 °F), preferably between 15 and 30 °C (59 and 86 °F) in a tight, light-resistant container, unless otherwise specified by manufacturer.

**Auxiliary labeling**
- May cause drowsiness.
- Avoid alcoholic beverages.
- Do not chew contents of capsule.

### DIVALPROEX SODIUM DELAYED-RELEASE TABLETS

**Usual adult dose**
Anticonvulsant—
   Monotherapy: Oral, the equivalent of valproic acid—Initially, 5 to 15 mg per kg of body weight a day, the dosage being increased at one-week intervals by 5 to 10 mg per kg of body weight a day as needed and tolerated.
   Polytherapy: Oral, the equivalent of valproic acid—Initially, 10 to 30 mg per kg of body weight a day, the dosage being increased at one-week intervals by 5 to 10 mg per kg of body weight a day as needed and tolerated.
Antimanic—
   Oral, initially 750 mg a day in divided doses. The dose should be increased as rapidly as possible to achieve the lowest therapeutic dose that produces the desired clinical effect or a desired trough plasma concentration within the range of fifty to one hundred twenty-five micrograms/mL.
Migraine headache prophylactic—
   Oral, initially 250 mg two times a day. The dose may be increased as needed and tolerated; some patients may benefit from doses up to 1000 mg a day. However, daily doses above 1000 mg have not demonstrated increased efficacy in clinical trials.
Note: If the total daily dose exceeds 250 mg, it should be divided into two or more doses (usually given every 12 hours) to lessen the possibility of gastrointestinal irritation.
   Geriatric patients may need lower doses.
   Patients also taking a hepatic enzyme–inducing medication may need higher dosages depending on predose serum concentrations.

**Usual adult prescribing limits**
See *Divalproex Sodium Delayed-release Capsules*.

**Usual pediatric dose**
See *Divalproex Sodium Delayed-release Capsules*.

**Usual geriatric dose**
Geriatric patients may need lower doses. See *Usual adult dose*.

**Strength(s) usually available**
U.S.—
   The equivalent of valproic acid:
      125 mg (Rx) [*Depakote*].
      250 mg (Rx) [*Depakote*].
      500 mg (Rx) [*Depakote*].
Canada—
   The equivalent of valproic acid:
      125 mg (Rx) [*Epival* (enteric-coated)].
      250 mg (Rx) [*Epival* (enteric-coated)].
      500 mg (Rx) [*Epival* (enteric-coated)].

**Packaging and storage**
Store below 40 °C (104 °F), preferably between 15 and 30 °C (59 and 86 °F), in a tight, light-resistant container, unless otherwise specified by manufacturer.

**Auxiliary labeling**
- May cause drowsiness.
- Avoid alcoholic beverages.
- Swallow tablets whole. Do not break or chew.

---

## VALPROATE SODIUM

## Parenteral Dosage Forms

### VALPROATE SODIUM INJECTION

**Usual adult and adolescent dose**
Anticonvulsant—
   Initial exposure to valproate:
      Monotherapy—Intravenous infusion: Initially, 5 to 15 mg per kg of body weight a day, the dosage being increased at one-week intervals by 5 to 10 mg per kg of body weight a day as needed and tolerated.
      Polytherapy—Intravenous infusion: Initially, 10 to 30 mg per kg of body weight a day, the dosage being increased at one-week intervals by 5 to 10 mg per kg of body weight a day as needed and tolerated.
   Replacement for oral therapy:
      Intravenous infusion—The total daily dose should be equivalent to the total daily dose of the oral valproic acid or divalproex product and should be administered at the same frequency as the oral product. If the total daily dose exceeds 250 mg, it should be given in divided doses.
Note: Valproate sodium injection should be administered as a 60-minute intravenous infusion; the rate of infusion should not exceed 20 mg per minute. Plasma concentration monitoring and dosage adjustments may be necessary. Patients receiving doses approaching the maximum recommended daily dose of 60 mg per kg of body weight per day should be monitored closely, particularly those not receiving hepatic enzyme–inducing medications. Patients should be switched to oral valproate products as soon as clinically feasible.
   Geriatric patients may need lower doses.
   Patients also taking a hepatic enzyme–inducing medication may need higher dosages, depending on predose serum valproate concentrations.

**Usual adult prescribing limits**
60 mg per kg of body weight a day.

**Usual pediatric dose**
Anticonvulsant: Children 1 to 12 years of age—
   Monotherapy: Oral, initially, 15 to 45 mg per kg of body weight a day, the dosage being increased at one-week intervals by 5 to 10 mg per kg of body weight a day as needed and tolerated.
   Polytherapy: Oral, 30 to 100 mg per kg of body weight a day.
Note: Dosage adjustments depend on clinical response and serum anticonvulsant concentrations.

**Usual geriatric dose**
Geriatric patients may need lower doses. See *Usual adult and adolescent dose*.

**Strength(s) usually available**
U.S.—
   Equivalent to valproic acid:
      100 mg per mL (Rx) [*Depacon* (edetate disodium 0.4 mg per mL)].
Canada—
   Not commercially available.

**Packaging and storage**
Store between 15 and 30 °C (59 and 86 °F), unless otherwise specified by manufacturer.

**Preparation of dosage form**
Valproate sodium injection should be diluted with at least 50 mL of 5% Dextrose Injection USP, 0.9% Sodium Chloride Injection USP, or Lactated Ringers Injection USP. The product should be inspected visually for particulate matter and discoloration prior to administration.

**Stability**
Valproate sodium injection is stable in 5% Dextrose Injection USP, 0.9% Sodium Chloride Injection USP, or Lactated Ringers Injection USP for at least 24 hours when stored in glass or polyvinyl chloride (PVC) bags at controlled room temperature. Any valproate sodium remaining in the vial after preparing the intravenous infusion should be discarded.

---

## VALPROIC ACID

## Oral Dosage Forms

### VALPROIC ACID CAPSULES USP

**Usual adult and adolescent dose**
Anticonvulsant—
   Monotherapy: Oral, initially, 5 to 15 mg per kg of body weight a day, the dosage being increased at one-week intervals by 5 to 10 mg per kg of body weight a day as needed and tolerated.
   Polytherapy: Oral, initially, 10 to 30 mg per kg of body weight a day, the dosage being increased at one-week intervals by 5 to 10 mg per kg of body weight a day as needed and tolerated.
Note: If the total daily dose exceeds 250 mg, it should be divided into two or more doses (usually given every 12 hours) to lessen the possibility of gastrointestinal irritation.
   Geriatric patients may need lower doses.

## Valproic Acid (Systemic)

Patients also taking a hepatic enzyme–inducing medication may need higher dosages depending on predose serum concentrations.

**Usual adult prescribing limits**
60 mg per kg of body weight a day.

**Usual pediatric dose**
Anticonvulsant—Children 1 to 12 years of age—
  Monotherapy: Oral, initially, 15 to 45 mg per kg of body weight a day, the dosage being increased at one-week intervals by 5 to 10 mg per kg of body weight a day as needed and tolerated.
  Polytherapy: Oral, 30 to 100 mg per kg of body weight a day.
Note: Dosage adjustments depend on clinical response and serum anticonvulsant concentrations.

**Usual geriatric dose**
Geriatric patients may need lower doses. See *Usual adult and adolescent dose*.

**Strength(s) usually available**
U.S.—
  250 mg (Rx) [*Depakene* (parabens); GENERIC].
Canada—
  250 mg (Rx) [*Alti-Valproic; Depakene* (parabens); *Deproic* (parabens); *Dom-Valproic; Med Valproic; Novo-Valproic; Nu-Valproic; Penta-Valproic; pms-Valproic Acid*].
  500 mg (Rx) [*Alti-Valproic* (enteric-coated); *Depakene* (enteric-coated; parabens; tartrazine); *Deproic* (enteric-coated); *Dom-Valproic* (enteric-coated); *Novo-Valproic* (enteric-coated); *pms-Valproic Acid E.C.* (enteric-coated)].

**Packaging and storage**
Store between 15 and 30 °C (59 and 86 °F), in a tight container.

**Auxiliary labeling**
• May cause drowsiness.
• Avoid alcoholic beverages.
• Swallow capsules whole. Do not break or chew.

### VALPROIC ACID SYRUP USP

**Usual adult and adolescent dose**
See *Valproic Acid Capsules USP*.

**Usual adult prescribing limits**
See *Valproic Acid Capsules USP*.

**Usual pediatric dose**
See *Valproic Acid Capsules USP*.

**Usual geriatric dose**
See *Valproic Acid Capsules USP*.

**Strength(s) usually available**
U.S.—
  250 mg per 5 mL (Rx) [*Depakene* (parabens; sorbitol; sucrose); GENERIC].
Canada—
  250 mg per 5 mL (Rx) [*Alti-Valproic; Depakene* (parabens; sucrose); *PMS-Valproic Acid*].

**Packaging and storage**
Store below 40 °C (104 °F), preferably between 15 and 30 °C (59 and 86 °F), unless otherwise specified by manufacturer. Store in a tight container. Protect from freezing.

**Auxiliary labeling**
• May cause drowsiness.
• Avoid alcoholic beverages.

Revised: 08/15/97
Interim revision: 08/14/98

# VALSARTAN  Systemic—INTRODUCTORY VERSION

VA CLASSIFICATION (Primary/Secondary): CV805/CV409
Commonly used brand name(s): *Diovan*.
Note: For a listing of dosage forms and brand names by country availability, see *Dosage Forms* section(s).

## Category
Antihypertensive.

## Indications

**Accepted**
*Hypertension (treatment)*—Valsartan is indicated for the treatment of hypertension. It may be used alone or in combination with other antihypertensive medications.

## Pharmacology/Pharmacokinetics

**Physicochemical characteristics**
Molecular weight—435.5.

**Mechanism of action/Effect**
Valsartan is a nonpeptide angiotensin II antagonist that selectively blocks the binding of angiotensin II to the $AT_1$ receptors in tissues such as vascular smooth muscle and the adrenal gland. In the renin-angiotensin system, angiotensin I is converted by angiotensin-converting enzyme (ACE) to form angiotensin II. Angiotensin II stimulates the adrenal cortex to synthesize and secrete aldosterone, which decreases the excretion of sodium and increases the excretion of potassium. Angiotensin II also acts as a vasoconstrictor in vascular smooth muscle. Valsartan, by blocking the binding of angiotensin II to the $AT_1$ receptors, promotes vasodilation and decreases the effects of aldosterone. The negative feedback regulation of angiotensin II on renin secretion also is inhibited, resulting in a rise in plasma renin concentrations and a consequent rise in angiotensin II plasma concentrations; however, these effects do not counteract the blood pressure–lowering effect that occurs.

**Absorption**
Absolute bioavailability for the capsule formulation is approximately 25% (range, 10 to 35%).
Food decreases the area under the plasma concentration–time curve (AUC) and peak plasma concentration ($C_{max}$) by approximately 40 and 50%, respectively.

**Distribution**
$Vol_D$—Steady-state: 17 L.

**Protein binding**
Very high (95%), mainly to albumin.

**Biotransformation**
The enzymes responsible for the metabolism of valsartan have not been identified; however, valsartan is not believed to be metabolized by cytochrome P450 isozymes. The primary metabolite, valeryl 4-hydroxy valsartan, is inactive, with an affinity for the $AT_1$ receptor of about one-two hundredth that of valsartan itself. About 20% of a dose of valsartan is eliminated as metabolites.

**Half-life**
Elimination—
  Approximately 6 hours.

**Time to peak concentration**
2 to 4 hours.

**Elimination**
Renal—13%.
Fecal—83%.
In dialysis—
  It is not known if valsartan and/or its metabolites are removable by hemodialysis.

## Precautions to Consider

**Carcinogenicity**
No evidence of carcinogenicity was found in mice or rats given valsartan for up to 2 years in dietary doses of up to 160 and 200 mg per kg of body weight (mg/kg) per day, respectively. These doses represent 2.6 and 6 times the maximum recommended human dose (MRHD), respectively, on a mg per square meter of body surface area (mg/m$^2$) basis, assuming an oral dose of 320 mg per day and a 60-kg patient.

**Mutagenicity**
Mutagenicity was not detected at either the gene or chromosome level in bacterial mutagenicity tests with *Salmonella* (Ames test) and *E. coli*, a gene mutation test with Chinese hamster V79 cells, a cytogenetic test with Chinese hamster ovary cells, or a rat micronucleus test.

**Pregnancy/Reproduction**
*Fertility*—No impairment of reproductive performance was found in male or female rats given oral doses of up to 200 mg/kg per day. This dose represents six times the MRHD on a mg/m$^2$ basis, assuming an oral dose of 320 mg per day and a 60-kg patient.

*Pregnancy*—Medications that act directly on the renin-angiotensin system can cause fetal and neonatal morbidity and mortality when administered to pregnant women during the second and third trimesters. Valsartan should be discontinued as soon as possible when pregnancy is detected, unless no alternative therapy can be used. In the latter instance, serial ultrasound examinations should be performed to assess the intra-amniotic environment. If oligohydramnios is observed, valsartan should be discontinued unless it is considered lifesaving for the mother. Perinatal diagnostic tests, such as contraction-stress testing (CST), a nonstress test (NST), or biophysical profiling (BPP) also may be appropriate during the applicable week of pregnancy. Oligohydramnios may not appear until after the fetus has sustained irreversible damage.

Fetal exposure to drugs that act directly on the renin-angiotensin system during the second and third trimesters can cause hypotension, reversible or irreversible renal failure, anuria, neonatal skull hypoplasia, and death in the fetus or neonate. Maternal oligohydramnios, which may result from decreased fetal renal function, has been reported, and is associated with fetal limb contractures, craniofacial deformation, and hypoplastic lung development. Other adverse effects that have been reported are prematurity, intrauterine growth retardation, and patent ductus arteriosus, although it is not clear how these effects are related to drug exposure. When limited to the first trimester, exposure to this medication does not appear to be associated with these adverse effects.

Infants exposed *in utero* to angiotensin II receptor antagonists should be closely observed for hypotension, oliguria, and hyperkalemia. Oliguria should be treated with support of blood pressure and renal perfusion. Dialysis or exchange transfusion may be necessary to reverse hypotension and/or substitute for disordered renal function.

Teratogenic effects were not observed in pregnant mice or rats given oral doses of up to 600 mg/kg per day or to pregnant rabbits given oral doses of up to 10 mg/kg per day. Studies in rats given oral, maternally toxic (based on a reduction in body weight gain and food consumption) doses of 600 mg/kg per day of valsartan during organogenesis or late gestation and lactation periods resulted in significant decreases in fetal weight, pup birth weight, pup survival rate, and slight delays in developmental milestones. Studies in rabbits given maternally toxic (associated with mortality) doses of 5 and 10 mg/kg per day of valsartan resulted in fetotoxic effects, such as fetal resorptions, litter loss, abortions, and low body weight in pups. No adverse effects were observed in mice, rats, and rabbits given 600, 200, and 2 mg/kg per day, respectively, of valsartan. This represents 9, 6, and 0.1 times, respectively, the MRHD on a mg/m² basis, assuming an oral dose of 320 mg/day and a 60-kg patient.

FDA Pregnancy Category C (first trimester).
FDA Pregnancy Category D (second and third trimesters).

### Breast-feeding
It is not known whether valsartan is distributed into breast milk. However, valsartan is distributed into the milk of lactating rats. Because of the potential for adverse effects, it is recommended that valsartan not be administered to nursing mothers.

### Pediatrics
No information is available on the relationship of age to the effects of valsartan in pediatric patients. Safety and efficacy have not been established.

### Geriatrics
Use of valsartan in patients 65 years of age and older (36.2% of patients in clinical studies) has not demonstrated geriatrics-specific problems that would limit the usefulness of valsartan in the elderly. However, the area under the plasma concentration–time curve (AUC) and elimination half-life increased by 70 and 35%, respectively, when compared with those in younger patients. Elderly patients may also experience greater sensitivity to the effects of valsartan.

### Drug interactions and/or related problems
The following drug interactions and/or related problems have been selected on the basis of their potential clinical significance (possible mechanism in parentheses where appropriate)—not necessarily inclusive (» = major clinical significance):

Note: Combinations containing any of the following medications, depending on the amount present, may also interact with this medication.

» Diuretics
concurrent use with valsartan may have additive hypotensive effects

### Laboratory value alterations
The following have been selected on the basis of their potential clinical significance (possible effect in parentheses where appropriate)—not necessarily inclusive (» = major clinical significance):

With physiology/laboratory test values
Creatinine, serum
(minor increases in concentrations may occur)

Hematocrit and
Hemoglobin
(in clinical studies, decreases of greater than 20% occurred in 0.8 and 0.4% of hematocrit and hemoglobin values, respectively. Valsartan therapy was discontinued in one patient because of microcytic anemia)

Liver function tests
(in clinical studies, occasional elevations of greater than 150% have occurred in valsartan-treated patients; three patients discontinued valsartan because of elevated liver enzyme values)

Leukocyte counts
(in clinical studies, neutropenia occurred in 1.9% of patients who were taking valsartan)

Potassium, serum
(in clinical studies, increases in concentration of greater than 20% were observed in 4.4% of patients treated with valsartan; however, this did not require discontinuation of valsartan therapy)

### Medical considerations/Contraindications
The medical considerations/contraindications included have been selected on the basis of their potential clinical significance (reasons given in parentheses where appropriate)—not necessarily inclusive (» = major clinical significance).

*Except under special circumstances, this medication should not be used when the following medical problem exists:*
» Hypersensitivity to valsartan

*Risk-benefit should be considered when the following medical problems exist:*
» Congestive heart failure, severe
(therapy with angiotensin receptor antagonists in these patients, who may be especially susceptible to changes in the renin-angiotensin-aldosterone system, has been associated with oliguria, azotemia, acute renal failure, and/or death)

Dehydration (sodium or volume depletion, due to excessive perspiration, vomiting, diarrhea, prolonged diuretic therapy, dialysis, or dietary salt restriction)
(a reduction in salt or fluid volume may increase the risk of symptomatic hypotension)

Hepatic function impairment, mild to moderate, including biliary obstructive disorders or
Hepatic function impairment, severe
(in patients with mild to moderate chronic liver disease, decreased biliary elimination of valsartan may result in an increase in the AUC; the AUC in patients with mild to moderate chronic liver disease may be doubled, as compared with healthy volunteers; no information is available on the use of valsartan in patients with severe hepatic function impairment)

Renal artery stenosis, unilateral or bilateral or
Renal function impairment
(increases in serum creatinine or blood urea nitrogen [BUN] may occur; therapy with angiotensin receptor–antagonists in patients susceptible to changes in the renin-angiotensin-aldosterone system, such as patients with severe congestive heart failure, has been associated with oliguria, progressive azotemia, acute renal failure, and/or death)

### Patient monitoring
The following may be especially important in patient monitoring (other tests may be warranted in some patients, depending on condition; » = major clinical significance):

» Blood pressure measurements
periodic monitoring is necessary for titration of dose according to the patient's response

## Side/Adverse Effects
The following side/adverse effects have been selected on the basis of their potential clinical significance (possible signs and symptoms in parentheses where appropriate)—not necessarily inclusive:

### Those indicating need for medical attention
Incidence rare
*Hypotension* (dizziness, lightheadedness, or fainting)—usually seen in volume- or salt-depleted patients receiving high doses of a diuretic; *neutropenia* (chills; fever; sore throat)—incidence 1.9%

### Those indicating need for medical attention only if they continue or are bothersome
Incidence less frequent
*Abdominal pain; dizziness; fatigue; headache; viral infection*

**2916 Valsartan (Systemic)—Introductory Version**

Note: In clinical trials, the side effects that most often resulted in the discontinuation of valsartan were *headache* and *dizziness*.

## Overdose

For more information on the management of overdose or unintentional ingestion, **contact a Poison Control Center** (see *Poison Control Center Listing*).

### Clinical effects of overdose

The following effects have been selected on the basis of their potential clinical significance (possible signs and symptoms in parentheses where appropriate)—not necessarily inclusive:

Acute and/or chronic
  **Bradycardia** (slow heartbeat)—as a result of parasympathetic (vagal) stimulation; **hypotension** (dizziness, lightheadedness, or fainting); **tachycardia** (fast heartbeat)

### Treatment of overdose

Treatment should be symptomatic and supportive.

Supportive care—Patients in whom intentional overdose is confirmed or suspected should be referred for psychiatric consultation.

## Patient Consultation

As an aid to patient consultation, refer to *Advice for the Patient, Valsartan (Systemic)—Introductory Version*.

In providing consultation, consider emphasizing the following selected information (» = major clinical significance):

### Before using this medication

» Conditions affecting use, especially:
  Hypersensitivity to valsartan
  Pregnancy—Fetal and neonatal hypotension, skull hypoplasia, renal failure, and death have been reported in humans; valsartan should be discontinued as soon as possible when pregnancy is detected
  Breast-feeding—Valsartan is distributed into milk of lactating rats; not recommended in nursing mothers
  Use in the elderly—Area under the plasma concentration–time curve (AUC) and half-life may be increased; may experience greater sensitivity to the medication's effects
  Other medications, especially diuretics
  Other medical problems, especially severe congestive heart failure

### Proper use of this medication

» Compliance with therapy; taking medication at the same time each day to maintain the antihypertensive effect
» Proper dosing
  Missed dose: Taking as soon as possible; not taking if almost time for next scheduled dose; not doubling doses
» Proper storage

### Precautions while using this medication

Regular visits to physician to check progress
Notifying physician immediately if pregnancy is suspected
Not taking other medications without consulting the physician
Caution when driving or doing other things requiring alertness because of possible dizziness
To prevent dehydration and hypotension, checking with physician if severe nausea, vomiting, or diarrhea occurs and continues
Caution when exercising or during exposure to hot weather because of the risk of dehydration and hypotension due to reduced fluid volume

### Side/adverse effects

Signs of potential side effects, especially hypotension and neutropenia

## General Dosing Information

Dosage must be adjusted, on the basis of clinical response, to meet the individual requirements of each patient.

Studies using valsartan in patients with severe renal function impairment or in patients undergoing dialysis have not been done. Caution should be used when using valsartan in the treatment of these patients and in patients with hepatic function impairment.

The antihypertensive effect is considerable after 2 weeks of valsartan therapy. The maximum antihypertensive effect is usually attained after 4 weeks of therapy.

### Diet/Nutrition

Valsartan may be taken with or without food.

### For treatment of adverse effects

Recommended treatment consists of the following:
• Treatment of symptomatic hypotension involves placing the patient in a supine position and, if needed, administering normal saline intravenously.

## Oral Dosage Forms

### VALSARTAN CAPSULES

**Usual adult dose**
Antihypertensive—
  Oral, initially 80 mg once a day, when used as single therapy in patients who are not volume-depleted.

Note: For additional antihypertensive effect, the dosage may be increased to 160 or 320 mg, or a diuretic may be added. The added effect of a diuretic will be greater than that of dose increases above 80 mg.

**Usual adult prescribing limits**
320 mg per day.

**Usual pediatric dose**
Safety and efficacy have not been established.

**Strength(s) usually available**
U.S.—
  80 mg (Rx) [*Diovan*].
  160 mg (Rx) [*Diovan*].

**Packaging and storage**
Store below 30 °C (86 °F). Protect from moisture. Store in tight container.

**Auxiliary labeling**
• Do not take other medicines without your doctor's advice.

Developed: 10/31/97

---

# VANCOMYCIN   Oral-Local

VA CLASSIFICATION (Primary): AM900
Commonly used brand name(s): *Vancocin*.
Note: For a listing of dosage forms and brand names by country availability, see *Dosage Forms* section(s).

## Category

Antibacterial (oral-local).

## Indications

### Accepted

Colitis, antibiotic-associated (treatment)
Colitis, pseudomembranous (treatment) or
Diarrhea, antibiotic-associated (treatment)—Oral-local vancomycin is indicated in the treatment of antibiotic-associated diarrhea or colitis caused by *Clostridium difficile*. It is also indicated in the treatment of pseudomembranous colitis caused by *C. difficile*.

Oral metronidazole is considered the drug of choice by many clinicians because it has been found to be as effective as vancomycin in the treatment of patients with mild to moderate *C. difficile* colitis, and it is much more cost-effective. Also, the emergence of multidrug-resistant strains of enterococci, including vancomycin-resistant strains, is of concern.

Enterocolitis, staphylococcal (treatment)—Oral-local vancomycin is indicated in the treatment of staphylococcal enterocolitis.

Not all species or strains of a particular organism may be susceptible to vancomycin.

### Unaccepted

Oral vancomycin is not effective in the treatment of other intestinal infections or in systemic infections.

## Pharmacology/Pharmacokinetics

### Physicochemical characteristics

Molecular weight—Vancomycin hydrochloride: 1485.74.

### Mechanism of action/Effect

Oral vancomycin inhibits bacterial cell wall synthesis by binding tightly to the D-alanyl-D-alanine portion of cell wall precursors; this leads to destruction of the bacterial cell by lysis; vancomycin may also alter permeability of bacterial cytoplasmic membranes and may selectively inhibit ribonucleic acid (RNA) synthesis.

**Absorption**
Poorly absorbed from gastrointestinal tract.

**Peak serum concentration**
<1 mcg per mL; may be somewhat higher in patients with inflammatory disorders of the colonic mucosa or renal function impairment.

**Fecal concentration**
Approximately 350 mcg per gram following oral doses of 125 mg four times a day.
Approximately 3100 mcg per gram following oral doses of 2 grams daily.

**Elimination**
Primarily fecal.

## Precautions to Consider

**Carcinogenicity**
No long-term carcinogenicity studies have been performed in animals.

**Mutagenicity**
No mutagenic potential was found in standard laboratory tests.

**Pregnancy/Reproduction**
Fertility—No definitive fertility studies have been performed.

Pregnancy—Intravenous vancomycin crosses the placenta. In one small controlled study, infants of mothers treated with vancomycin in their second or third trimester of pregnancy had no sensorineural hearing loss or nephrotoxicity that was attributed to vancomycin.

Teratology studies revealed no evidence of harm to the fetuses of rats given the normal human dose and rabbits given 1.1 times the human dose on a mg per square meter of body surface area basis.

FDA Pregnancy Category B.

**Breast-feeding**
Orally administered vancomycin is poorly absorbed from the gastrointestinal tracts of the mother and infant, so the small amount of this medication that may be distributed into breast milk will result in only low blood levels in the nursing infant.

**Pediatrics**
Appropriate studies on the relationship of age to the effects of oral vancomycin have not been performed in the pediatric population. Safety and efficacy have not been established. However, no pediatrics-specific problems have been documented to date.

**Geriatrics**
Appropriate studies on the relationship of age to the effects of oral vancomycin have not been performed in the geriatric population. However, no geriatrics-specific problems have been documented to date.

**Drug interactions and/or related problems**
The following drug interactions and/or related problems have been selected on the basis of their potential clinical significance (possible mechanism in parentheses where appropriate)—not necessarily inclusive (» = major clinical significance):

Note: Combinations containing any of the following medications, depending on the amount present, may also interact with this medication.

» Cholestyramine or
» Colestipol
(cholestyramine and colestipol anion-exchange resins have been shown to bind oral vancomycin significantly when used concurrently, resulting in decreased stool concentrations and marked reduction in antibacterial activity; concurrent use is not recommended; patients should be advised to take oral vancomycin and these medications several hours apart)

Nephrotoxic medications, other (see *Appendix II*)
(concurrent use with oral vancomycin may, on rare occasions, increase the potential for nephrotoxicity; this is most likely to occur in patients also receiving aminoglycosides and in patients with severe colitis, which may increase vancomycin absorption; caution is recommended when these medications are used concurrently with oral vancomycin)

**Medical considerations/Contraindications**
The medical considerations/contraindications included have been selected on the basis of their potential clinical significance (reasons given in parentheses where appropriate)—not necessarily inclusive (» = major clinical significance):

*Risk-benefit should be considered when the following medical problems exist:*
Hypersensitivity to vancomycin
» Inflammatory intestinal disorders, other
(may result in increased absorption and toxicity)

Renal function impairment, severe
(serum concentrations may be significantly elevated in patients with severe colitis, possibly resulting in increased toxicity)

**Patient monitoring**
The following may be especially important in patient monitoring (other tests may be warranted in some patients, depending on condition; » = major clinical significance):

Renal function determinations
(may be required periodically during therapy in patients with renal function impairment)

For *Clostridium difficile* colitis
Colonoscopy and/or
Proctosigmoidoscopy
(proctosigmoidoscopy may be useful to document the presence of pseudomembranes and/or relapse in selected patients who have persistent symptoms of *C. difficile* colitis and do not respond to therapy; however, since proctosigmoidoscopy is not always reliable in the diagnosis of *C. difficile* colitis due to rectal sparing and the presence of colitis in the more distal portions of the colon, colonoscopy may also be required in patients with a negative proctosigmoidoscopy)

» Stool toxin assays
(enzyme immunoassay of stool samples for the presence of *C. difficile* toxins may be required prior to treatment of patients with antibiotic-associated diarrhea or colitis to document the presence of *C. difficile* toxins; however, *C. difficile* and its toxins may persist following treatment with oral vancomycin despite clinical improvement; follow-up cultures and toxin assays are not recommended if clinical improvement is complete)

## Side/Adverse Effects

Note: Since vancomycin is poorly absorbed from the gastrointestinal tract and serum concentrations are low, systemic side/adverse effects are unlikely to occur except perhaps during prolonged administration or administration of unusually large oral doses. For systemic side/adverse effects of vancomycin, see *Vancomycin (Systemic)*.

The following side/adverse effects have been selected on the basis of their potential clinical significance (possible signs and symptoms in parentheses where appropriate)—not necessarily inclusive:

**Those indicating need for medical attention**
Incidence rare
*Skin rash, including exfoliative dermatitis* (scaling of skin); *macular rash* (redness or discoloration of skin); *urticaria* (hives); *or vasculitis* (welting of skin)

**Those indicating need for medical attention only if they continue or are bothersome**
Incidence more frequent
*Bitter or unpleasant taste; mouth irritation*—with oral solution; *nausea or vomiting*

## Overdose

For more information on the management of overdose or unintentional ingestion, **contact a Poison Control Center** (see *Poison Control Center Listing*).

**Clinical effects of overdose**
Vancomycin overdose may cause acute renal failure and oliguria.

**Treatment of overdose**
To decrease absorption—Gastric emptying within the first 2 hours of overdose may decrease absorption; multiple doses of activated charcoal may also decrease absorption.

To enhance elimination—Poorly removed by dialysis; hemofiltration and hemoperfusion with polysulfone resin have been used to increase clearance.

Supportive care—Patients in whom intentional overdose is confirmed or suspected should be referred for psychiatric consultation.

## Patient Consultation

As an aid to patient consultation, refer to *Advice for the Patient, Vancomycin (Oral)*.

In providing consultation, consider emphasizing the following selected information (» = major clinical significance):

**Before using this medication**
» Conditions affecting use, especially:
Hypersensitivity to vancomycin
Other medications, especially cholestyramine and colestipol
Other medical problems, especially other inflammatory intestinal disorders

## Vancomycin (Oral-Local)

**Proper use of this medication**
*Proper administration technique*
For oral liquids—Using a calibrated liquid-measuring device; not using after expiration date
» Compliance with full course of therapy
» Proper dosing
Missed dose: Taking as soon as possible; not taking if almost time for next dose; not doubling doses
» Proper storage

**Precautions while using this medication**
Importance of physician checking progress during and after treatment
Checking with physician if no improvement within a few days
» Avoiding concurrent use of vancomycin and cholestyramine or colestipol; if concurrent use is necessary, taking vancomycin and these medications several hours apart
» Checking with physician or pharmacist before taking any other kind of diarrhea medication

**Side/adverse effects**
Signs of potential side effects, especially skin rash

# General Dosing Information

For *Clostridium difficile* colitis—
- Oral vancomycin is indicated in the treatment of *C. difficile* colitis, which may be caused by various antibiotics (e.g., cephalosporins, lincomycins, penicillins). *C. difficile* colitis may result in severe watery diarrhea, which may occur during therapy or up to several weeks after therapy is discontinued. If diarrhea occurs, administration of antiperistaltic antidiarrheals (e.g., atropine and diphenoxylate combination, loperamide, opiates) is not recommended since they may delay the removal of toxins from the colon, thereby prolonging and/or worsening the condition.
- Mild cases of *C. difficile* colitis may respond to discontinuation of the medication alone. Moderate to severe cases may require fluid, electrolyte, and protein replacement.
- In cases not responding to the above measures or in more severe cases, oral doses of vancomycin, metronidazole, or cholestyramine may be used. Oral vancomycin is usually effective at a dose of 125 mg every six hours for seven to ten days. The dose of metronidazole is 250 to 500 mg every eight hours and the dose of cholestyramine is 4 grams four times a day. Recurrences, which occur in approximately 25% of patients treated with vancomycin or metronidazole, may be treated with a second course of vancomycin, oral metronidazole, or oral bacitracin.
- Cholestyramine resin has been shown to bind *C. difficile* toxin *in vitro*. If cholestyramine resin is administered in conjunction with oral vancomycin, the medications should be administered several hours apart since the cholestyramine resin has been shown to bind oral vancomycin also.
- If a patient is too ill for oral therapy, vancomycin may be administered by enema, by passage of a long intestinal tube, or by direct instillation through a colonostomy or ileostomy. In addition, metronidazole may also be administered intravenously since 6 to 15% of metronidazole and its metabolites are excreted into the feces.

# Oral Dosage Forms

Note: The dosing and strengths of the dosage forms available are expressed in terms of vancomycin base, not the hydrochloride salt.

## VANCOMYCIN HYDROCHLORIDE CAPSULES USP

**Usual adult and adolescent dose**
*Clostridium difficile* colitis or diarrhea or
Staphylococcal enterocolitis—
Oral, 125 to 500 mg (base) every six hours for seven to ten days. May be repeated if necessary.
Note: Some studies suggest that this dose results in fecal concentrations of vancomycin that far exceed the minimum inhibitory concentration (MIC) for *C. difficile*. Also, studies have shown that 125 mg (base) every six hours is as effective as higher doses.

**Usual adult prescribing limits**
2 grams (base) per day.

**Usual pediatric dose**
*Clostridium difficile* colitis or diarrhea or
Staphylococcal enterocolitis—
Oral, 10 mg (base) per kg of body weight, up to 125 mg, every six hours for seven to ten days. May be repeated if necessary.
Note: Some medical experts recommend doses of up to 50 mg (base) per kg of body weight per day.

**Usual pediatric prescribing limits**
2 grams (base) per day.

**Strength(s) usually available**
U.S.—
  125 mg (base) (Rx) [*Vancocin*].
  250 mg (base) (Rx) [*Vancocin*].
Canada—
  125 mg (base) (Rx) [*Vancocin*].
  250 mg (base) (Rx) [*Vancocin*].

**Packaging and storage**
Store below 40 °C (104 °F), preferably between 15 and 30 °C (59 and 86 °F), unless otherwise specified by manufacturer. Store in a tight container.

**Auxiliary labeling**
- Continue medicine for full time of treatment.

## VANCOMYCIN HYDROCHLORIDE FOR ORAL SOLUTION USP

**Usual adult and adolescent dose**
See *Vancomycin Hydrochloride Capsules USP*.

**Usual adult prescribing limits**
See *Vancomycin Hydrochloride Capsules USP*.

**Usual pediatric dose**
See *Vancomycin Hydrochloride Capsules USP*.

**Usual pediatric prescribing limits**
See *Vancomycin Hydrochloride Capsules USP*.

**Strength(s) usually available**
U.S.—
  250 mg (base) per 5 mL (when reconstituted according to manufacturer's instructions) (Rx) [*Vancocin*].
  500 mg (base) per 6 mL (when reconstituted according to manufacturer's instructions) (Rx) [*Vancocin* (ethanol up to 40 mg per gram)].
Canada—
  Not commercially available.

**Packaging and storage**
Prior to reconstitution, store below 40 °C (104 °F), preferably between 15 and 30 °C (59 and 86 °F), unless otherwise specified by manufacturer. Store in a tight container.

**Preparation of dosage form**
Add 20 mL of distilled or deionized water to each 1-gram bottle to provide a concentration of 250 mg per 5 mL, or 115 mL of diluent to each 10-gram bottle to provide a concentration of 500 mg per 6 mL. Mix thoroughly to dissolve.
For intravenous dosage form used orally—To prepare initial dilution for oral use, the contents of each 500-mg vial may be diluted in distilled water. The resulting solution may be given to the patient to drink or it may be administered through a nasogastric tube to help prevent or minimize the bitter or unpleasant taste and nausea or vomiting.

**Stability**
After reconstitution, solutions retain their potency for 14 days if refrigerated.

**Auxiliary labeling**
- Refrigerate.
- Continue medicine for full time of treatment.
- Beyond-use date.

**Note**
When dispensing, include a calibrated liquid-measuring device.

Revised: 04/15/98

# VANCOMYCIN Systemic

VA CLASSIFICATION (Primary): AM900
Commonly used brand name(s): *Vancocin*.
Note: For a listing of dosage forms and brand names by country availability, see *Dosage Forms* section(s).

## Category
Antibacterial (systemic).

## Indications
Note: Bracketed information in the *Indications* section refers to uses that are not included in U.S. product labeling.

### General considerations
Vancomycin is a narrow-spectrum antibacterial agent that has excellent antimicrobial activity against gram-positive organisms, including *Clostridium difficile*, diphtheroids, most *Enterococcus* species, staphylococci, and streptococci. Vancomycin is used to treat enterococcal infections in patients with a history of hypersensitivity to beta-lactam antibiotics, and infections due to beta-lactam–resistant microorganisms, including methicillin-resistant *Staphylococcus aureus* (MRSA), methicillin-resistant *Staphylococcus epidermidis* (MRSE), and penicillin-resistant enterococci. The increase in prevalence of disease due to MRSA and MRSE and of antibiotic resistance in general has led to an increase in the use of vancomycin.

One of the consequences of increased vancomycin use has been the emergence of vancomycin-resistant microorganisms. From 1989 through 1993, the Centers for Disease Control and Prevention (CDC) reported an increase in the percentage of nosocomial enterococcal infections caused by vancomycin-resistant enterococci, from 0.3 to 7.9%. Since the determinants of vancomycin resistance in enterococci are located on a conjugative plasmid, vancomycin resistance may be transferred among enterococci and potentially to other gram-positive organisms. *Staphylococcus* species are among the most common causes of community- and hospital-acquired infection; thus, the potential emergence of vancomycin resistance in clinical isolates of *S. aureus* and *S. epidermidis* is a public health concern. Several strains of *S. aureus* with reduced susceptibility to vancomycin have been isolated from patients in Japan. In the U. S., two strains of *S. aureus* and several strains of *Staphylococcus hemolyticus* with intermediate levels of resistance to vancomycin have been reported. The CDC has responded by developing guidelines and recommendations for the detection and prevention of the spread of vancomycin-resistant organisms. The CDC concludes that reduction in the overuse and misuse of vancomycin, as well as of antimicrobials in general, will decrease the risk of emergence of staphylococci with reduced susceptibility to vancomycin.

### Accepted
Bone and joint infections (treatment)
Pneumonia (treatment)
Septicemia, bacterial (treatment) or
Skin and soft tissue infections (treatment)—Intravenous vancomycin is indicated in the treatment of bone and joint infections (including osteomyelitis), pneumonia, septicemia, and skin and soft tissue infections caused by susceptible strains of *Staphylococcus* species (including methicillin-resistant strains).

Endocarditis, bacterial (prophylaxis)—Intravenous vancomycin is indicated for prophylaxis of bacterial endocarditis in penicillin-allergic patients with prosthetic heart valves or congenital, rheumatic, or other acquired valvular heart disease who are undergoing dental procedures or surgical procedures of the upper respiratory tract. However, this use is no longer recommended by the American Heart Association or the American Dental Association. Medical experts agree that although vancomycin should not be used routinely in these patients, vancomycin should be available for use in selected patients (including penicillin-allergic patients) based on need for a life-saving medication when microorganisms are resistant to usual antibacterials.

[Vancomycin is used as a primary agent for the prophylaxis of bacterial endocarditis in penicillin-allergic patients with prosthetic heart valves or congenital or valvular heart disease who are undergoing gastrointestinal or genitourinary tract procedures; depending on the risk, gentamicin may be administered concurrently.][1]

Endocarditis, bacterial (treatment)—Intravenous vancomycin is indicated in the treatment of endocarditis caused by *Staphylococcus* species (including methicillin-resistant strains).

Vancomycin is also indicated as a primary agent, alone or concurrently with an aminoglycoside or rifampin, in endocarditis caused by *Corynebacterium* species (diphtheroids) (including penicillin- and cephalosporin-resistant strains) in penicillin-allergic patients, and as a secondary agent in endocarditis caused by *Streptococcus viridans* or *Streptococcus bovis*.

[Intravenous vancomycin is used as a primary agent, concurrently with gentamicin or streptomycin, in endocarditis caused by enterococci (*Enterococcus faecalis*) in penicillin-allergic patients.]

Intravenous vancomycin is indicated in the treatment of severe, potentially life-threatening staphylococcal infections in patients who cannot receive penicillins or cephalosporins or have failed to respond to them. Vancomycin is also indicated in the treatment of staphylococcal infections that are resistant to other antibacterials, including methicillin.

[Brain abscess (treatment)][1]
[Erysipelas (treatment)][1]
[Meningitis, staphylococcal (treatment)][1]
[Meningitis, streptococcal (treatment)][1] or
[Perioperative infections (prophylaxis)][1]—Intravenous vancomycin is used in the treatment of brain abscess, erysipelas, meningitis caused by staphylococci or streptococci, and in the prophylaxis of perioperative infections.

[Intravenous vancomycin, administered concurrently with an aminoglycoside (e.g., gentamicin) or rifampin, is also used in the treatment of serious infections caused by *Staphylococcus* species (including methicillin-resistant and multiresistant strains) in penicillin-allergic patients.][1]

Note: Not all species or strains of a particular organism may be susceptible to vancomycin.

### Unaccepted
Vancomycin is not effective against most gram-negative organisms, *Mycobacterium* species, *Bacteroides* species, *Rickettsia* species, *Chlamydia* species, or fungi.

The use of parenteral vancomycin is not recommended in the treatment of antibiotic-associated pseudomembranous colitis.

[1]Not included in Canadian product labeling.

## Pharmacology/Pharmacokinetics

### Physicochemical characteristics
Chemical group—Tricyclic glycopeptide.
Molecular weight—Vancomycin hydrochloride: 1485.74.

### Mechanism of action/Effect
Bactericidal for most organisms; bacteriostatic for enterococci; inhibits bacterial cell wall synthesis at a site different from that of penicillins and cephalosporins by binding tightly to the D-alanyl-D-alanine portion of cell wall precursors and interfering with bacterial growth; this leads to activation of bacterial autolysins that destroy the cell wall by lysis. Vancomycin also may alter the permeability of bacterial cytoplasmic membranes and may selectively inhibit ribonucleic acid (RNA) synthesis; vancomycin does not compete with penicillins for binding sites.

### Absorption
Intraperitoneal—Systemic absorption (up to 60%) may occur.

### Distribution
Widely distributed to most tissues and body fluids; adequate therapeutic concentrations in serum and in pleural, pericardial, peritoneal, ascitic, and synovial fluids; high concentrations in urine; inadequate concentrations in bile; does not readily cross normal blood-brain barrier into cerebrospinal fluid (CSF); however, penetrates into CSF when meninges are inflamed and may achieve therapeutic concentrations. Crosses the placenta.

Vol$_D$—Approximately 0.39 to 0.92 liter per kg.

### Protein binding
Moderate (approximately 37 to 55%) in healthy adults.
Low (approximately 20%) in adult patients with infections.

### Half-life
Normal renal function—
　Adults: Approximately 6 hours (range, 4 to 11 hours).
　Newborn infants: Approximately 6 to 10 hours.
　Older infants: Approximately 4 hours.
　Children: Approximately 2 to 3 hours.
Impaired renal function (oliguric or anuric)—
　Adults: 6 to 10 days.

**Peak serum concentration**
Approximately 49 mcg per mL immediately following a 500-mg intravenous dose infused over a 30-minute period; mean serum concentration is approximately 20 mcg per mL 1 to 2 hours after dosing.
Approximately 63 mcg per mL immediately following a 1-gram intravenous dose infused over a 60-minute period; mean serum concentration is approximately 23 to 30 mcg per mL 1 to 2 hours after dosing.

**Elimination**
Renal—Approximately 75 to 90% or more excreted by passive glomerular filtration unchanged in urine within 24 hours; slowly eliminated by unknown route and mechanism in anephric patients.
Biliary—Small to moderate amounts may be excreted in bile.
In dialysis—Not appreciably removed from the blood by hemodialysis or peritoneal dialysis.

## Precautions to Consider

**Carcinogenicity**
No long-term carcinogenicity studies have been performed in animals.

**Mutagenicity**
No mutagenic potential was found in standard laboratory tests.

**Pregnancy/Reproduction**
Fertility—No definitive fertility studies have been performed.
Pregnancy—Intravenous vancomycin crosses the placenta. In one small controlled study, infants of mothers treated with vancomycin in their second or third trimester of pregnancy had no sensorineural hearing loss or nephrotoxicity that was attributed to vancomycin therapy.
FDA Pregnancy Category C.

**Breast-feeding**
Parenteral vancomycin is distributed into breast milk. Although available data regarding the use of vancomycin while breast-feeding are limited, problems in humans have not been documented.

**Pediatrics**
Close monitoring of vancomycin serum concentrations is recommended in premature neonates and young infants.

**Geriatrics**
Elderly patients are more likely to have an age-related decrease in renal function, which may require dosage adjustments to avoid excessive vancomycin serum concentrations. Because of this, geriatric patients are at greater risk of vancomycin-induced ototoxicity (i.e., loss of hearing) and nephrotoxicity.

**Drug interactions and/or related problems**
The following drug interactions and/or related problems have been selected on the basis of their potential clinical significance (possible mechanism in parentheses where appropriate)—not necessarily inclusive (» = major clinical significance):
Note: Combinations containing any of the following medications, depending on the amount present, may also interact with this medication.

» Aminoglycosides or
» Amphotericin B, parenteral or
   Aspirin or other salicylates or
» Bacitracin, parenteral or
» Bumetanide, parenteral or
» Capreomycin or
   Carmustine or
» Cisplatin or
» Cyclosporine or
» Ethacrynic acid, parenteral or
» Furosemide, parenteral or
» Paromomycin or
» Polymyxins or
» Streptozocin
   (concurrent and/or sequential use of these medications with vancomycin may increase the potential for ototoxicity and/or nephrotoxicity; hearing loss may occur and may progress to deafness, even after discontinuation of the drug, and may be reversible, but usually is permanent; serial audiometric function determinations may be required with concurrent or sequential use of other ototoxic antibacterials)
   (however, vancomycin and aminoglycosides often must be administered concurrently in the prophylaxis of bacterial endocarditis, in the treatment of endocarditis caused by *Streptococcus* species and diphtheroids, in the treatment of resistant staphylococcal infections, or in penicillin-allergic patients; appropriate monitoring will help to reduce the possibility of an interaction between vancomycin and aminoglycosides; renal function determinations, monitoring of serum concentrations, dosage reductions and/or dosage interval adjustments, or alternate antibacterials may be required)

   Anesthetic agents or
» Vecuronium
   (some clinical studies report that patients experienced vancomycin-dependent hypotension or enhancement of neuromuscular depression with administration of anesthetic agents or vecuronium, respectively; however, other clinicians report no effects or significant differences between patients administered vancomycin before or after induction of anesthesia; it is recommended that vancomycin be administered by infusion over a period of at least 60 minutes, preferably prior to the induction of anesthesia, to minimize potential enhancement of the hypotensive or neuromuscular blockade effects of anesthetic agents or vecuronium)

   Antihistamines or
   Buclizine or
   Cyclizine or
   Meclizine or
   Phenothiazines or
   Thioxanthenes or
   Trimethobenzamide
   (concurrent use of these medications with vancomycin may mask the symptoms of ototoxicity, such as tinnitus, dizziness, or vertigo)

» Dexamethasone
   (studies in animals have demonstrated that concurrent administration of dexamethasone with vancomycin may impair the penetration of vancomycin into cerebrospinal fluid [CSF]; if dexamethasone is to be used as adjunctive therapy in bacterial meningitis, it is recommended that dexamethasone be administered either before or concurrently with the first dose of vancomycin)

**Laboratory value alterations**
The following have been selected on the basis of their potential clinical significance (possible effect in parentheses where appropriate)—not necessarily inclusive (» = major clinical significance):

With physiology/laboratory test values
   Blood urea nitrogen (BUN)
      (concentrations may be increased)

**Medical considerations/Contraindications**
The medical considerations/contraindications included have been selected on the basis of their potential clinical significance (reasons given in parentheses where appropriate)—not necessarily inclusive (» = major clinical significance).

*Risk-benefit should be considered when the following medical problems exist:*
   Hypersensitivity to vancomycin
» Loss of hearing, or deafness, history of
   (vancomycin may rarely cause hearing loss or deafness)
» Renal function impairment
   (because vancomycin is primarily excreted through the kidneys, patients with renal function impairment may need an adjustment in dosage)

**Patient monitoring**
The following may be especially important in patient monitoring (other tests may be warranted in some patients, depending on condition; » = major clinical significance):

» Audiograms and
» Renal function determinations
   (may be required prior to, periodically during, and following treatment in patients with pre-existing renal or eighth-cranial-nerve impairment, especially in patients older than 60 years of age, and with concurrent or sequential administration of other ototoxic antibacterials; twice-weekly or weekly audiometric testing to detect high-frequency hearing loss in patients old enough to be tested; daily renal function determinations may also be required in patients on high-dose or prolonged therapy, especially if renal function is changing or borderline)

» Urinalyses
   (may be required prior to treatment and periodically during treatment to detect albumin, casts, and cells in the urine, as well as decreased specific gravity)

» Vancomycin serum concentrations
   (may be required periodically in patients with renal function impairment, especially if renal function is changing or borderline, and in patients older than 60 years of age; peak concentrations should not be maintained in excess of approximately 40 mcg per mL, and trough concentrations should not exceed approximately 10 mcg per

mL; serum concentrations greater than 80 mcg per mL are considered to be in the toxic range)
White blood cell count
(should be monitored periodically to detect possible neutropenia)

## Side/Adverse Effects

Note: Side/adverse effects were relatively common with early formulations of vancomycin. Many of these side effects (e.g., chills, fever, hypotension, nephrotoxicity, skin rash, thrombophlebitis, pain at the injection site) were attributed to impurities. Because of subsequent purification, the incidence of these side effects has been substantially reduced.

The following side/adverse effects have been selected on the basis of their potential clinical significance (possible signs and symptoms in parentheses where appropriate)—not necessarily inclusive:

**Those indicating need for medical attention**
Incidence less frequent
*Nephrotoxicity* (change in frequency of urination or amount of urine; difficulty in breathing; drowsiness; increased thirst; loss of appetite; nausea or vomiting; weakness); *neutropenia* (chills; coughing; difficulty in breathing; fever; sore throat)—usually reversible; *"red man syndrome"* (chills or fever; fainting; fast heartbeat; hives; hypotension; itching of skin; nausea or vomiting; rash or redness of the face, base of neck, upper body, back, and arms)—may result from histamine release due to rapid infusion

Incidence rare
*Chemical peritonitis* (abdominal pain and cramps; abdominal tenderness)—in patients receiving high doses by intraperitoneal administration; *linear IgA bullous dermatosis* (large blisters on arms, legs, hands, feet, or upper body); *ototoxicity* (loss of hearing; ringing or buzzing or a feeling of fullness in the ears); *pseudomembranous colitis* (abdominal or stomach cramps and pain, severe; abdominal tenderness; diarrhea, watery and severe, which may also be bloody; fever); *thrombocytopenia* (abnormal bleeding or bruising)

**Those indicating possible ototoxicity, nephrotoxicity, or pseudomembranous colitis and the need for medical attention if they occur or progress after medication is discontinued**
*Abdominal or stomach cramps and pain, severe; abdominal tenderness; change in frequency of urination or amount of urine; diarrhea, watery and severe, which may also be bloody; difficulty in breathing; drowsiness; fever; increased thirst; loss of appetite; loss of hearing; nausea or vomiting; ringing or buzzing or a feeling of fullness in the ears; weakness*

## Overdose

For more information on the management of overdose or unintentional ingestion, **contact a Poison Control Center** (see *Poison Control Center Listing*).

**Clinical effects of overdose**
Vancomycin overdose may result in oliguria and acute renal function failure. Two cases of vancomycin overdose have been reported. An adult who received 1 gram of parenteral vancomycin every 4 hours, for a total of 56 grams over a 10-day period, developed acute renal failure. A 47-day-old premature infant inadvertently was given three 12-mg doses and six 240-mg doses of parenteral vancomycin. Both patients survived.

**Treatment of overdose**
To enhance elimination—Poorly removed by dialysis; hemofiltration and hemoperfusion with polysulfone resin have been used to reduce elevated serum concentrations of vancomycin.

Monitoring—Patients should be monitored for electrolytes, fluid, hearing function, hematologic status (especially platelet and white blood cell counts), renal function, and vestibular function.

Supportive care—Patients in whom intentional overdose is confirmed or suspected should be referred for psychiatric consultation.

## Patient Consultation

As an aid to patient consultation, refer to *Advice for the Patient, Vancomycin (Systemic)*.
In providing consultation, consider emphasizing the following selected information (» = major clinical significance):

**Before using this medication**
» Conditions affecting use, especially:
  Hypersensitivity to vancomycin
  Pregnancy—Vancomycin crosses the placenta
  Breast-feeding—Vancomycin is distributed into breast milk
  Use in the elderly—Elderly patients may be at greater risk of nephrotoxicity and ototoxicity
  Other medications, especially aminoglycosides, amphotericin B, anesthetic agents, bacitracin, bumetanide, capreomycin, cisplatin, cyclosporine, dexamethasone, ethacrynic acid, furosemide, paromomycin, polymyxins, streptozocin, or vecuronium
  Other medical problems, especially a history of hearing loss or deafness, or renal function impairment

**Proper use of this medication**
» If medication is being given at home, carefully following physician's instructions
» Importance of receiving medication for full course of therapy and on regular schedule
» Proper dosing
  Missed dose: Taking as soon as possible; not taking if almost time for next dose; not doubling doses

**Side/adverse effects**
Signs of potential side effects, especially nephrotoxicity, neutropenia, "red man syndrome," chemical peritonitis, linear IgA bullous dermatosis, ototoxicity, pseudomembranous colitis, and thrombocytopenia

## General Dosing Information

Since vancomycin is highly irritating to tissues and causes necrosis and severe pain on intramuscular administration or extravasation, parenteral vancomycin must be administered by intravenous [or intraperitoneal] infusion only. Avoid extravasation. Sterile vancomycin hydrochloride may also be administered orally for treatment of *Clostridium difficile* colitis, but oral vancomycin is not effective in systemic infections.

Parenteral vancomycin should be administered over a period of at least 60 minutes. To help reduce the incidence of administration rate–related side effects (e.g., cardiac arrest [rarely], hypotension, "red man syndrome"), this medication should not be administered rapidly or as a bolus injection. Vancomycin should be administered intermittently in at least 100 to 200 mL of 5% dextrose injection or 0.9% sodium chloride injection. Veins into which vancomycin is infused should be rotated to help prevent the development of thrombophlebitis, unless vancomycin is being administered via a central venous catheter.

Patients with impaired renal or auditory function may require (1) a reduction in the maintenance dose by administration of the usual dose at prolonged intervals, or (2) discontinuation of vancomycin. Since vancomycin is not metabolized and is excreted primarily in the urine, toxic concentrations may accumulate in patients with impaired renal function. Therapeutic concentrations of vancomycin may persist for 7 to 21 days after dosing, especially in anuric patients.

Serum concentrations should be monitored during therapy, especially during prolonged therapy or in patients with impaired renal function or a history of hearing loss or deafness. Peak concentrations should not be maintained in excess of approximately 40 mcg per mL, and trough concentrations should not exceed approximately 10 mcg per mL. Serum concentrations greater than 80 mcg per mL are considered to be in the toxic range.

Therapy should be continued for at least 4 weeks or longer in the treatment of staphylococcal endocarditis.

## Parenteral Dosage Forms

Note: Bracketed information in the *Dosage Forms* section refers to uses that are not included in U.S. product labeling.

Note: The dosing and strengths of the dosage forms available are expressed in terms of vancomycin base (not the hydrochloride salt).

### STERILE VANCOMYCIN HYDROCHLORIDE USP

**Usual adult and adolescent dose**
Antibacterial, treatment—
  Intravenous infusion, 7.5 mg (base) per kg of body weight or 500 mg every six hours; or 15 mg per kg of body weight or 1 gram every twelve hours.

Note: After an initial loading dose of 750 mg to 1 gram (base), but not less than 15 mg per kg of body weight, adults with impaired renal function may require a reduction in dose as indicated in the table below. However, the preferred method is to adjust dosage based on serum vancomycin concentrations.

## Vancomycin (Systemic)

| Creatinine clearance (mL/min)/(mL/sec) | Intravenous dose (base) |
|---|---|
| > 80/1.33 | See *Usual adult and adolescent dose* |
| 50–80/0.83–1.33 | 1 gram every 1 to 3 days |
| 10–50/0.17–0.83 | 1 gram every 3 to 7 days |
| < 10/0.17 | 1 gram every 7 to 14 days |

[Endocarditis, prophylaxis, in penicillin-allergic patients with prosthetic heart valves or congenital, rheumatic, or other acquired valvular heart disease who are undergoing gastrointestinal and genitourinary tract procedures][1]—
   Intravenous infusion, 1 gram (base) over a period of one to two hours, with or without gentamicin (administered intramuscularly or intravenously at a dose of 1.5 mg per kg of body weight up to 120 mg), depending on risk of bacterial endocarditis; the infusion/injection should be completed within one-half hour of the start of surgery.

### Usual adult prescribing limits
3 to 4 grams (base) a day have been used intravenously for short periods of time in very severe infections.

### Usual pediatric dose
Antibacterial, treatment—
   Neonates up to 1 week of age: Intravenous infusion, 15 mg (base) per kg of body weight initially, followed by 10 mg per kg of body weight every twelve hours.
   Infants 1 week to 1 month of age: Intravenous infusion, 15 mg (base) per kg of body weight initially, followed by 10 mg per kg of body weight every eight hours.
   Infants and children 1 month to 12 years of age: Intravenous infusion, 10 mg (base) per kg of body weight every six hours; or 20 mg per kg of body weight every twelve hours.
Note: Doses up to 60 mg (base) per kg of body weight per day have been used in some infections (e.g., staphylococcal infections of the central nervous system [CNS]).
[Endocarditis, prophylaxis, in penicillin-allergic patients with prosthetic heart valves or congenital, rheumatic, or other acquired valvular heart disease who are undergoing gastrointestinal and genitourinary tract procedures][1]—
   Intravenous infusion, 20 mg (base) per kg of body weight over a period of one to two hours, with or without gentamicin (administered intramuscularly or intravenously at a dose of 1.5 mg per kg of body weight), depending on degree of risk; the infusion/injection should be completed within one-half hour of the start of surgery.

### Strength(s) usually available
U.S.—
   500 mg (base) (may be available in ADD-Vantage® vials) (Rx) [*Vancocin*; GENERIC].
   1 gram (base) (may be available in ADD-Vantage® vials) (Rx) [*Vancocin*; GENERIC].
   5 grams (base) (Rx) [GENERIC].
Canada—
   500 mg (base) (may be available in ADD-Vantage® vials) (Rx) [*Vancocin*; GENERIC].
   1 gram (base) (may be available in ADD-Vantage® vials) (Rx) [*Vancocin*; GENERIC].
   5 grams (base) (Rx) [GENERIC].

### Packaging and storage
Prior to reconstitution, store below 40 °C (104 °F), preferably between 15 and 30 °C (59 and 86 °F), unless otherwise specified by manufacturer.

### Preparation of dosage form
For intravenous use—
   To prepare initial dilution for intravenous use, 10 or 20 mL of sterile water for injection should be added to each 500-mg or 1-gram vial, respectively. For intermittent intravenous infusion (preferred), the 10- or 20-mL solution should be further diluted in 100 or 200 mL, respectively, of 5% dextrose injection or 0.9% sodium chloride injection. The resulting solution should be administered over a 60-minute period or longer.
   For continuous intravenous infusion (used only when intermittent infusion is not feasible), 1 to 2 grams (20 to 40 mL) may be added to a sufficiently large volume of 5% dextrose injection or 0.9% sodium chloride injection to permit the total daily dose to be administered slowly by intravenous drip over a 24-hour period. Avoid extravasation.
   For reconstitution of ADD-Vantage® vials, see manufacturer's labeling for instructions.
For oral use—
   See *Vancomycin (Oral-Local)*.

### Stability
After reconstitution with 5% dextrose injection or 0.9% sodium chloride injection, solutions retain their potency for 14 days if refrigerated.

### Incompatibilities
The admixture of supplementary medication and vancomycin is not recommended. Vancomycin is incompatible with alkaline solutions and may be precipitated by heavy metals. It has also been found to be incompatible with aminophylline, amobarbital sodium, aztreonam, chloramphenicol sodium succinate, chlorothiazide sodium, dexamethasone sodium phosphate, heparin sodium, methicillin sodium, pentobarbital sodium, phenobarbital sodium, secobarbital sodium, and sodium bicarbonate.
Vancomycin should not be added to solutions containing albumin, cefepime, ceftazidime, foscarnet sodium, penicillin G, or piperacillin sodium–tazobactam sodium. If these solutions are administered concurrently, they should be administered at separate sites.

## VANCOMYCIN HYDROCHLORIDE FOR INJECTION USP

### Usual adult and adolescent dose
See *Sterile Vancomycin Hydrochloride USP*.

### Usual adult and adolescent prescribing limits
See *Sterile Vancomycin Hydrochloride USP*.

### Usual pediatric dose
See *Sterile Vancomycin Hydrochloride USP*.

### Strength(s) usually available
U.S.—
   10 grams (base) (Rx) [*Vancocin*; GENERIC].
Canada—
   10 grams (base) (Rx) [*Vancocin*].

### Packaging and storage
Prior to reconstitution, store below 40 °C (104 °F), preferably between 15 and 30 °C (59 and 86 °F), unless otherwise specified by manufacturer.

### Preparation of dosage form
For intravenous use—
   For reconstitution of pharmacy bulk vials, 95 mL of sterile water for injection should be added to each 10-gram vial to provide a solution of 100 mg per mL. Using aseptic technique, the closure should be penetrated only once after reconstitution using a suitable sterile dispensing set that allows measured dispensing of the contents. Use of a syringe and needle is not recommended as leakage may occur.
   Reconstituted solutions of 5 mL containing 500 mg of vancomycin should be diluted with at least 100 mL of suitable diluent (see manufacturer's labeling instructions), and reconstituted solutions of 10 mL containing 1 gram of vancomycin should be diluted with at least 200 mL of suitable diluent. The final dose should be administered by intermittent intravenous infusion over a period of at least 60 minutes.
For oral use—
   See *Vancomycin (Oral-Local)*.

### Stability
After reconstitution, the solution should be dispensed within 4 hours.

### Incompatibilities
The admixture of supplementary medication and vancomycin is not recommended. Vancomycin is incompatible with alkaline solutions and may be precipitated by heavy metals. It also has been found to be incompatible with aminophylline, amobarbital sodium, aztreonam, chloramphenicol sodium succinate, chlorothiazide sodium, dexamethasone sodium phosphate, heparin sodium, methicillin sodium, pentobarbital sodium, phenobarbital sodium, secobarbital sodium, and sodium bicarbonate.
Vancomycin should not be added to solutions containing albumin, cefepime, ceftazidime, foscarnet sodium, penicillin G, or piperacillin sodium–tazobactam sodium. If these solutions are administered concurrently, they should be administered at separate sites.

## VANCOMYCIN INJECTION USP

### Usual adult and adolescent dose
See *Sterile Vancomycin Hydrochloride USP*.

### Usual adult and adolescent prescribing limits
See *Sterile Vancomycin Hydrochloride USP*.

### Usual pediatric dose
See *Sterile Vancomycin Hydrochloride USP*.

### Strength(s) usually available
U.S.—
   500 mg per 100 mL (Rx) [*Vancocin*].
Canada—
   Not commercially available.

## Packaging and storage
Store between −20 and −10 °C (−4 and 14 °F), unless otherwise specified by manufacturer.

## Preparation of dosage form
Vancomycin Injection USP should be administered only by the intravenous route. For oral administration of parenteral vancomycin, see *Vancomycin (Oral-Local)*.

Frozen containers should be thawed at room temperature (25 °C [77 °F]) or under refrigeration (5 °C [41 °F]). Thawing should not be forced by immersion in water baths or by microwave irradiation.

Do not use plastic containers in series connections. Such use may result in an air embolism because of residual air being drawn from the primary container before administration of the fluid from the secondary container is complete.

## Stability
Once thawed, solutions remain stable for 72 hours at room temperature, or for 30 days when refrigerated. Thawed solutions should not be refrozen.

Do not use if solution is cloudy or contains a precipitate.

## Incompatibilities
The admixture of supplementary medication and vancomycin is not recommended. Vancomycin is incompatible with alkaline solutions and may be precipitated by heavy metals. It has also been found to be incompatible with aminophylline, amobarbital sodium, aztreonam, chloramphenicol sodium succinate, chlorothiazide sodium, dexamethasone sodium phosphate, heparin sodium, methicillin sodium, pentobarbital sodium, phenobarbital sodium, secobarbital sodium, and sodium bicarbonate.

Vancomycin should not be added to solutions containing albumin, cefepime, ceftazidime, foscarnet sodium, penicillin G, or piperacillin sodium–tazobactam sodium. If these solutions are administered concurrently, they should be administered at separate sites.

[1] Not included in Canadian product labeling.

## Selected Bibliography
Centers for Disease Control and Prevention. Recommendations for preventing the spread of vancomycin resistance. MMWR Morb Mortal Wkly Rep 1995; 44(RR–12): [20 screens]. Cited 11/18/97. Available from: URL: http://www.cdc.gov/epo/mmwr/ind95_rr.htm

Centers for Disease Control and Prevention. Interim guidelines for prevention and control of staphylococcal infection associated with reduced susceptibility to vancomycin. MMWR Morb Mortal Wkly Rep 1997; 46(27): [10 screens]. Cited 8/8/97. Available from: URL: http://www.cdc.gov/epo/mmwr/mmwr_wk.html

Revised: 06/17/98

# VARICELLA VIRUS VACCINE LIVE

## Systemic—INTRODUCTORY VERSION

VA CLASSIFICATION (Primary): IM100
Commonly used brand name(s): *Varivax*.
Note: For a listing of dosage forms and brand names by country availability, see *Dosage Forms* section(s).

## Category
Immunizing agent (active).

## Indications
**Accepted**
Varicella virus (prophylaxis)—Varicella virus vaccine live is indicated for immunization against varicella in individuals 12 months of age and older.

No information is available about the duration of protection for this vaccine. Studies are being conducted to evaluate the need for revaccination.

## Pharmacology/Pharmacokinetics
**Physicochemical characteristics**
Source—Varicella virus vaccine live is produced from the Oka/Merck strain of live, attenuated varicella virus. The initial virus was obtained from naturally occurring varicella, which was adapted and propagated in human diploid cell cultures (WI-38 and MRC-5). This live, attenuated vaccine is a lyophilized preparation.

**Mechanism of action/Effect**
A detectable humoral immune response was observed in most individuals between 1 and 55 years of age. A cell-mediated immune response also was induced by the vaccine.

**Protective effect**
Various clinical trials involving children were conducted using varicella virus vaccine live at doses between 1000 and 17,000 plaque-forming units (PFU). Results showed that children either were completely protected or only developed a mild form of chickenpox.

At doses of 1000 to 1625 PFU, approximately 3% of 4141 children developed mild cases of chickenpox. In a second study, ≤ 1% of 1164 children developed breakthrough cases of chickenpox after receiving a varicella vaccine dose of 2900 to 9000 PFU. These children were followed for 3 years after receiving the varicella vaccine.

Placebo-controlled trials have not been conducted using the current dose of varicella virus vaccine live (1350 PFU); however, a varicella vaccine containing 17,000 PFU was used in 956 children. This single dose protected 96 to 100% of children.

A placebo-controlled trial has not been conducted in adolescents or adults. A trial to determine efficacy was conducted by giving adolescents and adults two doses of varicella virus vaccine live either 4 or 8 weeks apart. This group was exposed to chickenpox in a household setting and was followed for up to 2 years. Results showed that 27% (17 of 64) reported a breakthrough case of chickenpox.

Seroconversion, defined as the detection of any varicella antibodies, was observed in 97% of 6889 susceptible children 1 to 12 years of age at approximately 4 to 6 weeks postvaccination. It is not known if administering the vaccine immediately after exposure to naturally occurring varicella will prevent illness.

In one study, adolescents and adults were given two doses of varicella virus vaccine live 4 to 8 weeks apart. A seroconversion rate of 75% was observed following the first dose, and 94% following the second dose. In a second study, a seroconversion rate of 94% was seen following the first dose and a rate of 99% was observed 6 weeks after the second dose.

**Duration of protective effect**
The duration of protection following immunization with varicella virus vaccine live is presently unknown. The need for a booster dose also is not known; however, studies are being conducted. In one study involving children, a seroconversion rate of 99.5% was present 4 years after vaccination. A similar study involving adolescents and adults showed antibody concentrations to be 97.2% 1 year following two doses of the vaccine given 4 to 8 weeks apart.

## Precautions to Consider
**Cross-sensitivity and/or related problems**
Since varicella virus vaccine live contains small amounts of gelatin and neomycin, patients allergic to gelatin and/or neomycin may be allergic to this vaccine.

**Carcinogenicity/Mutagenicity**
Studies have not been done to evaluate the carcinogenic and mutagenic potential of varicella virus vaccine live.

**Pregnancy/Reproduction**
Fertility—Varicella virus vaccine live has not been evaluated for its potential to impair fertility.

Pregnancy—Studies have not been done in humans. It is not known whether varicella virus vaccine live can cause fetal harm; however, naturally occurring varicella can sometimes cause harm to the developing fetus. It is recommended that pregnancy be avoided for 3 months following the vaccination.

Studies have not been done in animals.
FDA Pregnancy Category C.

**Breast-feeding**
It is not known whether varicella virus vaccine live is distributed into breast milk. Varicella virus vaccine live should be used with caution in nursing mothers.

**Pediatrics**
Appropriate studies on the relationship of age to the effects of varicella virus vaccine live have not been performed in children less than 12 months of age. Safety and efficacy have not been established.

**Geriatrics**
No information is available on the relationship of age to the effects of varicella virus vaccine live in geriatric patients.

## Drug interactions and/or related problems

The following drug interactions and/or related problems have been selected on the basis of their potential clinical significance (possible mechanism in parentheses where appropriate)—not necessarily inclusive (» = major clinical significance):

Note: Combinations containing any of the following medications, depending on the amount present, may also interact with this medication.

- » Blood or plasma transfusion or
- » Immune globulins

   (concurrent administration with varicella virus vaccine live may interfere with the patient's immune response to the virus because of the possibility of antibodies to varicella virus being present in these products; varicella virus vaccine live may be administered at least 5 months after blood or plasma transfusion, and 2 months following any immune globulin, including varicella zoster immune globulin [VZIG])

- » Immunosuppressive agents or
- » Radiation therapy

   (because normal defense mechanisms are suppressed by immunosuppressive agents or radiation therapy, concurrent use of the varicella virus vaccine live may potentiate the replication of the vaccine virus, may increase the side/adverse effects of the vaccine virus, and/or may decrease the patient's antibody response to varicella virus vaccine live; the interval between discontinuation of the medications that cause immunosuppression and restoration of the patient's ability to respond to varicella virus vaccine live depends on the intensity and type of immunosuppression-causing medication used, the underlying disease, and other factors; individuals who are taking immunosuppressive agents may develop a more extensive vaccine-associated rash or disseminated disease)

- » Live virus vaccines, other

   (although data are lacking on impairment of antibody responses to rubella, measles, mumps, oral polio, or varicella vaccine when these vaccines are administered on different days within 1 month of each other, there is a chance that the immune response may be impaired; therefore, when feasible, live virus vaccines not administered on the same day should be given at least 1 month apart)

- » Salicylates

   (use of salicylates should be avoided for 6 weeks following vaccination because Reye's Syndrome has occurred during natural varicella infection; however, there have been no reports of Reye's Syndrome in varicella virus vaccine live recipients)

## Medical considerations/Contraindications

The medical considerations/contraindications included have been selected on the basis of their potential clinical significance (reasons given in parentheses where appropriate)—not necessarily inclusive (» = major clinical significance).

*Except under special circumstances, this medication should not be used when the following medical problems exist:*

- » Blood dyscrasias or
- » Lymphomas or
- » Malignant neoplasm affecting the bone marrow or lymphatic system or
- » Febrile illness, active or
- » Febrile infection, respiratory

   (the presence of these conditions may create confusion in identifying possible side/adverse effects of the vaccine versus manifestations of the illness)

- » Immunodeficiency conditions, congenital or hereditary, history of
- » Immunodeficiency conditions, primary or acquired

   (because of reduced or suppressed defense mechanisms, the use of live virus vaccines may potentiate the replication of the vaccine virus, may increase the side/adverse effects of the vaccine virus, and/or may decrease the patient's antibody response to varicella)

   (when there is a family history of congenital or hereditary immune deficiency conditions, the patient should not be vaccinated until his or her immune competence is demonstrated)

   (safety and efficacy of the vaccine in patients with these conditions have not been established)

- » Leukemia

   (children and adolescents with acute lymphoblastic leukemia [ALL] in remission can receive the vaccine under an investigational protocol by contacting the Varivax Coordinating Center)

- » Tuberculosis, active, untreated

   (tuberculosis may be exacerbated by natural varicella infection, although there is no evidence that varicella virus vaccine live exacerbates tuberculosis)

*Risk-benefit should be considered when the following medical problem exists:*

   Sensitivity to varicella virus vaccine live, neomycin, or gelatin

## Side/Adverse Effects

Note: *Fever*, *pain at injection site*, and a *varicella-like rash* are the most common side effects and could occur within the first 42 days following vaccination. A fever of ≥ 39 °C (102 °F) occurred in approximately 15% of vaccinated children after receiving a single dose of varicella virus vaccine live. In general, side effects are minor.

The following side/adverse effects have been selected on the basis of their potential clinical significance (possible signs and symptoms in parentheses where appropriate)—not necessarily inclusive:

**Those indicating need for medical attention**
Incidence rare
   *Anaphylactic reaction* (difficulty in breathing or swallowing; hives; itching, especially soles of feet or palms of hands; swelling of eyes, face, or inside of nose); *febrile seizure*; *lymphadenopathy* (pain and swelling of lymph nodes); *myalgia* (pain in muscles); *varicella-like skin rash*—generalized or at injection site

**Those indicating need for medical attention only if they continue or are bothersome**
Incidence more frequent
   *Pain, redness, or soreness at injection site*
Incidence less frequent
   *Central nervous system effects* (headache; irritability; malaise; nervousness); *gastrointestinal effects* (abdominal pain; diarrhea; nausea; vomiting); *respiratory illness* (congestion; cough)

## Patient Consultation

In providing consultation, consider emphasizing the following selected information (» = major clinical significance):

**Before using this vaccine**
- » Conditions affecting use, especially:
   Sensitivity to varicella virus vaccine live or allergy to gelatin and/or neomycin
   Pregnancy—Natural varicella virus has been known to cause fetal harm; however, no studies have been conducted on the possible effects of this vaccine on fetal development; it is recommended that pregnancy be avoided for 3 months following immunization with the vaccine
   Breast-feeding—It is not known whether varicella virus vaccine live is distributed into breast milk; varicella virus vaccine live should be used with caution in nursing mothers
   Use in children—Use is not recommended for infants less than 12 months of age
   Other medications, especially blood or plasma transfusion, immune globulins including varicella zoster immune globulin, immunosuppressive agents, other live virus vaccines, radiation therapy, and salicylates
   Other medical problems, especially, blood dyscrasias, bone marrow neoplasm, congenital or hereditary immunodeficiency, febrile illness, febrile infection, leukemia, lymphatic system neoplasm, lymphomas, primary and acquired immunodeficiency conditions, or untreated tuberculosis

**Proper use of this vaccine**
- » Proper dosing

**Precautions while using this vaccine**
- » Not becoming pregnant for 3 months without first checking with physician because of possible birth defects

*Checking with a physician before receiving*
- » Blood or plasma transfusion; should be avoided for at least 5 months
- » Live virus vaccines, other; should be avoided for 1 month
- » Varicella zoster immune globulin; should be avoided for at least 2 months
- » Avoid salicylate products for 6 weeks following immunization with this vaccine

**Side/adverse effects**
   Signs of potential side effects, especially, anaphylactic reaction, febrile seizures, lymphadenopathy, myalgia, varicella-like skin rash

## General Dosing Information

The health care professional should inform the patient, parent, or guardian of the benefits and risks of varicella virus vaccine live and ask questions about reactions to a previous dose of varicella virus vaccine or a similar product. A previous immunization history should be obtained.

Patients, parents, or guardians should be instructed to report to their health care provider any adverse reactions.

Pregnancy should be avoided for 3 months following the vaccination.

The vaccine virus potentially can be transmitted from individuals receiving the vaccine to close contacts. Recipients should avoid contact with susceptible high risk individuals (newborns, pregnant women, and immunocompromised persons).

Varicella virus vaccine live can be given concurrently with the measles, mumps, and rubella virus vaccine live and the Haemophilus b conjugate vaccine (meningococcal protein conjugate), provided different syringes and injection sites are used. Oral poliovirus vaccine live (OPV) may also be given concurrently.

Varicella zoster immune globulin (VZIG) should not be given concurrently with varicella virus vaccine live.

When sterilizing syringes and skin before vaccination, care should be taken to avoid preservatives, antiseptics, detergents, and disinfectants, since the vaccine virus is easily inactivated by these substances.

To prevent inactivation of the vaccine, it is recommended that only the diluent provided by the manufacturer be used for vaccine reconstitution.

The reconstituted vaccine should be administered within 30 minutes after mixing to prevent loss of potency.

Varicella virus vaccine live is for subcutaneous administration. The preferred site of injection is the outer aspect (deltoid region) of the upper arm. The vaccine should not be injected intravenously.

The duration of protection from varicella virus vaccine live revaccination presently is not known.

## Parenteral Dosage Forms

### VARICELLA VIRUS VACCINE LIVE INJECTION

**Usual adult and adolescent dose**
Immunizing agent (active)—
    Subcutaneous 0.5 mL initially, followed by a second 0.5 mL dose four to eight weeks later. The preferred injection site is the outer aspect (deltoid region) of the upper arm.

**Usual pediatric dose**
Immunizing agent (active)—
    Infants up to 12 months of age: Use is not recommended. Safety and efficacy have not been established.
    Children 1 to 12 years of age: Subcutaneous, a single 0.5 mL dose. The preferred site of injection is the outer aspect (deltoid region) of the upper arm.

**Strength(s) usually available**
U.S.—
    Not less than 1350 plaque-forming units of Oka/Merck varicella virus per 0.5 mL (Rx) [*Varivax* (trace quantities of neomycin and gelatin)].

**Packaging and storage**
Store below −15 °C (+5 °F) until the time of reconstitution. The diluent should be stored below 40 °C (104 °F), preferably between 15 and 30 °C (59 and 86 °F).

**Preparation of dosage form**
To reconstitute, only the diluent provided by the manufacturer should be used because it is free of preservatives and other substances that might inactivate the vaccine.

0.7 mL of the diluent should be withdrawn into the syringe. All of the diluent should be injected into the vial of lyophilized vaccine and agitated to mix thoroughly. The entire contents should then be withdrawn into the syringe and the total volume of restored vaccine injected subcutaneously.

**Stability**
The vaccine should be administered immediately after reconstitution. The vaccine should be discarded if not used within 30 minutes after reconstitution. The reconstituted vaccine should not be frozen.

**Incompatibilities**
Preservatives or other substances may inactivate the vaccine; therefore, only the diluent supplied by the manufacturer should be used for reconstitution.

Also, a sterile syringe free of preservatives, antiseptics, and detergents should be used for each injection and/or reconstitution of the vaccine because these substances may inactivate the live virus vaccine.

**Auxiliary labeling**
• Keep frozen.
• Discard reconstituted vaccine if not used within 30 minutes.

**Note**
The date and time of reconstitution should be indicated on the vial if the vaccine is not used immediately.

Developed: 05/15/97

---

# VASCULAR HEADACHE SUPPRESSANTS, ERGOT DERIVATIVE–CONTAINING  Systemic

This monograph includes information on the following: 1) Dihydroergotamine; 2) Ergotamine; 3) Ergotamine and Caffeine; 4) Ergotamine, Caffeine, and Belladonna Alkaloids*; 5) Ergotamine, Caffeine, Belladonna Alkaloids, and Pentobarbital*; 6) Ergotamine, Caffeine, and Cyclizine*; 7) Ergotamine, Caffeine, and Dimenhydrinate*; 8) Ergotamine, Caffeine, and Diphenhydramine*.

VA CLASSIFICATION (Primary/Secondary):
    Dihydroergotamine—CN105/CV900
    Ergotamine—CN105
    Ergotamine and Caffeine—CN105
    Ergotamine, Caffeine, and Belladonna Alkaloids—CN105
    Ergotamine, Caffeine, Belladonna Alkaloids, and Pentobarbital—CN105
    Ergotamine, Caffeine, and Cyclizine—CN105
    Ergotamine, Caffeine, and Dimenhydrinate—CN105
    Ergotamine, Caffeine, and Diphenhydramine—CN105

Note: Controlled substance classification—, Canada—Ergotamine, Belladonna Alkaloids, Caffeine, and Pentobarbital—C.

Commonly used brand name(s): *Cafergot*[3]; *Cafergot-PB*[5]; *Cafertine*[3]; *Cafetrate*[3]; *D.H.E. 45*[1]; *Dihydroergotamine-Sandoz*[1]; *Ercaf*[3]; *Ergo-Caff*[3]; *Ergodryl*[8]; *Ergomar*[2]; *Ergostat*[2]; *Gotamine*[3]; *Gravergol*[7]; *Gynergen*[2]; *Medihaler Ergotamine*[2]; *Megral*[6]; *Migergot*[3]; *Wigraine*[3].

Note: For a listing of dosage forms and brand names by country availability, see *Dosage Forms* section(s).

*Not commercially available in U.S.

## Category

Vascular headache suppressant—Dihydroergotamine; Ergotamine; Ergotamine and Caffeine; Ergotamine, Caffeine, and Belladonna Alkaloids; Ergotamine, Caffeine, Belladonna Alkaloids, and Pentobarbital; Ergotamine, Caffeine, and Cyclizine; Ergotamine, Caffeine, and Dimenhydrinate; Ergotamine, Caffeine, and Diphenhydramine.

Thrombosis prophylaxis adjunct—Dihydroergotamine.

Antihypotensive—Dihydroergotamine.

Note: Some headache specialists question the validity of the term "vascular headache" because a correlation between dilatation of cerebral blood vessels and symptoms of migraine or cluster headaches has not been demonstrated conclusively. A clinical distinction between vascular, tension-type, and coexisting migraine and tension-type ("mixed") headaches may be difficult to ascertain in some patients.

## Indications

Note: Bracketed information in the *Indications* section refers to uses that are not included in U.S. product labeling.

### Accepted

Headache, vascular (treatment)—Ergot derivative–containing headache suppressants are indicated in the treatment of vascular headaches, such as migraine (with or without aura), cluster headache (histaminic cephalalgia, migrainous neuralgia, ciliary neuralgia, Horton's headache), and migraine variants.

For migraine: Ergot derivative–containing headache suppressants are used to relieve (abort) acute migraine headaches in patients who report that sufficient relief is not obtained with analgesics (e.g., acetaminophen, aspirin, other nonsteroidal anti-inflammatory drugs [NSAIDs]). When incapacitating migraines occur more frequently than twice a month, additional prophylactic treatment is recommended to reduce the severity and duration, as well as the number, of headaches. However, too frequent use of an ergotamine–containing headache suppressant may cause tolerance, leading to decreased efficacy, and physical dependence, leading to more frequent headaches (including withdrawal [rebound] headaches and chronic, intractable headaches) and medication abuse. Chronic use of ergot derivatives may also cause peripheral vasospasm, which may lead to arterial insufficiency, ischemia, and even gangrene. Therefore, these agents are not recommended for long-term migraine prophylaxis. Beta-adrenergic blocking agents, calcium channel blocking agents, tricyclic antidepressants, monoamine oxidase inhibitors, methysergide, pizotifen (pizotifen [not commercially available in the U.S.]), and sometimes cyproheptadine (especially in children) are used for prophylaxis.

Parenteral dihydroergotamine is used for rapid relief of severe, refractory migraine, including status migrainosus and chronic, intractable headaches resulting from overuse of ergotamine or analgesics. Some physicians consider it the treatment of choice in status migrainosus. Prophylactic treatment may also be needed to reduce recurrences.

For cluster headache: Ergot derivative–containing headache suppressants are indicated to abort headaches in patients who experience episodic or chronic cluster headaches. These headaches may occur daily, often more than once a day, for several months (a cluster period), followed by a headache-free interval. Cluster headaches often are unresponsive to simple analgesics. Prophylactic therapy is advisable during cluster periods, but many of the agents commonly used for migraine prophylaxis are ineffective in reducing the frequency or severity of cluster headaches (especially chronic cluster headaches), or lose efficacy after 1 or 2 cluster periods. [Ergotamine is therefore used prophylactically during cluster periods][1], alone or concurrently with a calcium channel blocking agent, usually verapamil, and/or lithium. Prophylactic administration of ergotamine during cluster periods is not likely to cause dependence of the type associated with its chronic use by migraine patients.

Ergot derivative–containing headache suppressants are generally not used in the treatment of chronic paroxysmal hemicrania, a cluster headache variant. Indomethacin is highly effective in relieving and preventing these headaches, and is considered the agent of choice for management of this condition.

Note: Other measures that may reduce the need for medication in headache patients include identification and avoidance of headache precipitants (for migraine or cluster headaches) and relaxation and/or biofeedback techniques (for migraine).

[Thrombosis, deep venous (prophylaxis adjunct)][1] and
[Thromboembolism, pulmonary (prophylaxis adjunct)][1]—Dihydroergotamine is used in combination with low-dose heparin for the prevention of postoperative deep-vein thrombosis and pulmonary embolism following elective orthopedic procedures, such as total hip replacement, or major abdominal, thoracic, or pelvic surgery. Prophylactic therapy with heparin is generally reserved for high-risk patients, such as patients with a history of thromboembolism or patients requiring prolonged immobilization following surgery, especially if they are 40 years of age or older. The combination of dihydroergotamine and heparin may be more effective than low-dose heparin alone in some cases, e.g., in hip replacement surgery. However, this combination of medications has been reported to cause serious complications, including severe peripheral ischemia, probably resulting from dihydroergotamine-induced vasospasm. Especially careful patient selection and careful monitoring throughout therapy are required to reduce the risk of such complications.

[Hypotension, orthostatic (prophylaxis and treatment)][1]—Dihydroergotamine is used to prevent or treat orthostatic hypotension that may occur in conjunction with spinal or epidural anesthesia. It is also used to treat orthostatic hypotension due to autonomic insufficiency or other causes.

### Unaccepted
Dihydroergotamine, ergotamine, and ergotamine-containing combinations are not recommended for long-term migraine prophylaxis.

Although ergotamine has oxytocic effects, it is not used clinically to produce these effects because other ergot alkaloids are more effective and less toxic.

---
[1] Not included in Canadian product labeling.

## Pharmacology/Pharmacokinetics

Note: Pharmacology/pharmacokinetics information for the adjuvants present in headache suppressant formulations (caffeine, belladonna alkaloids, cyclizine, dimenhydrinate, diphenhydramine, and pentobarbital) is limited to brief descriptions of the effects that may be pertinent to treatment of patients with vascular headaches. Gastric stasis that accompanies migraine headaches tends to inhibit absorption of orally administered medications and may therefore alter their pharmacokinetic profiles. For additional information on the actions of these agents, see—
Caffeine: *Caffeine (Systemic)*.
Belladonna alkaloids: *Anticholinergics/Antispasmodics (Systemic)*.
Cyclizine: *Cyclizine (Systemic)*.
Dimenhydrinate: *Antihistamines (Systemic)*.
Diphenhydramine: *Antihistamines (Systemic)*.
Pentobarbital: *Barbiturates (Systemic)*.

### Physicochemical characteristics
Source—
  Dihydroergotamine: Synthetic.
  Ergotamine: Semisynthetic alkaloid; derived from ergot, a product of the parasitic fungus *Claviceps purpurea*.
Molecular weight—
  Dihydroergotamine mesylate: 679.79.
  Ergotamine tartrate: 1313.43.
  Caffeine: 194.19.
  Cyclizine hydrochloride: 302.85.
  Dimenhydrinate: 469.97.
  Diphenhydramine hydrochloride: 291.82.
  Pentobarbital sodium: 248.26.

### Mechanism of action/Effect
Dihydroergotamine and Ergotamine—
  These ergot derivatives interact with several neurotransmitter receptors, including alpha-adrenergic, serotonergic (tryptaminergic), and dopaminergic receptors. Both agonistic (or partial agonistic) and antagonistic actions have been reported at different receptor types or subtypes. These medications directly stimulate vascular smooth muscle, causing constriction of both arteries and veins, and depress vasomotor centers in the brain. Dihydroergotamine's adrenergic blocking actions are somewhat more pronounced, and its vasoconstrictive actions (especially in arteries) are less pronounced, than those of ergotamine.
  Vascular headache suppressant:
    Ergot derivative–induced decreases in the firing of serotonergic (5-hydroxytryptaminergic, 5-HT) neurons may be responsible for headache suppression. Specifically, it is thought that agonist activity at the 5-HT$_{1D}$ receptor subtype provides relief of acute headache, whereas antagonist activity at the 5-HT$_2$ receptor subtype provides headache prophylaxis. It has been proposed that constriction of cerebral blood vessels by the ergot derivative (resulting from alpha-adrenergic stimulation as well as from activity at 5-HT receptors) reduces the pulsation in cerebral arteries that may be responsible for the pain of vascular headaches. However, studies have not consistently shown a significant correlation between dilatation of cerebral blood vessels and pain or other symptoms of migraine or cluster headaches, or between the vasoconstrictive effect of an ergot derivative and relief of these headaches.
  Dihydroergotamine and ergotamine may decrease hyperperfusion in the area of the basilar artery, but they do not reduce cerebral hemispheric blood flow.
  Thrombosis prophylaxis adjunct and Antihypotensive:
    Dihydroergotamine's constrictive effect on capacitance (venous) vasculature is significantly greater than its constrictive effect on resistance (arterial) vasculature. As a result, the velocity of venous blood flow in the legs is increased, venous return to the heart is enhanced, venous pooling (which may increase the risk of thrombus formation) is reduced, and arterial blood pressure is maintained or increased. It has also been proposed that dihydroergotamine may enhance the effects of heparin in preventing thrombosis.
Caffeine—
  Caffeine constricts the cerebral vasculature and decreases both cerebral blood flow and the oxygen tension of the brain. However, it is believed that the caffeine in many ergotamine-containing formulations acts primarily by increasing both the rate and extent of absorption of orally or rectally administered ergotamine, thereby hastening the onset of action and increasing the effect of ergotamine.
Belladonna alkaloids—
  Belladonna alkaloids are used in headache suppressant formulations for their antiemetic effects, because nausea and vomiting may occur in association with the migraine headache and/or as a result of ergotamine administration.

Cyclizine and Dimenhydrinate and Diphenhydramine—
  These antihistamines are used in headache suppressant formulations for their antiemetic and sedative effects.
Pentobarbital—
  This barbiturate is used in headache suppressant formulations for its sedative effects.

### Other actions/effects
Dihydroergotamine and Ergotamine—
  These medications may cause nausea and vomiting via direct stimulation of the chemoreceptor trigger zone.
  Like other ergot derivatives, dihydroergotamine and ergotamine stimulate uterine smooth muscle via an action on alpha-adrenergic receptors and/or 5-HT receptors. Ergotamine is much more potent than dihydroergotamine as a uterine stimulant.
  Peripheral vasoconstriction induced by dihydroergotamine and ergotamine may lead to decreased blood flow in various organs, increased peripheral vascular resistance, and increased blood pressure. However, with the doses usually used in the treatment of migraine or cluster headaches, increases in blood pressure are usually slight.
  Large doses of dihydroergotamine and ergotamine may cause constriction of the coronary vasculature and bradycardia. These effects may result from increased vagal activity as well as direct actions on the myocardium and the vasculature.
Caffeine—
  Caffeine has central nervous system (CNS) stimulant activity and may therefore inhibit sleep. Because sleep contributes to relief of migraine headaches, this action may be detrimental to the patient.
Belladonna alkaloids—
  Belladonna alkaloids have anticholinergic activity.
Cyclizine and Dimenhydrinate and Diphenhydramine—
  These medications have antihistaminic, anticholinergic, and CNS depressant activities.
Pentobarbital—
  Barbiturates have CNS depressant activity.

### Absorption
Dihydroergotamine—
  Intramuscular or subcutaneous: Rapid.
Ergotamine—
  Oral: Slow, incomplete, and subject to wide interpatient variability. Absorption is inhibited by the gastric stasis that accompanies migraine headaches. Concurrent administration of caffeine increases the rate and extent of absorption. Metoclopramide may also increase ergotamine absorption by accelerating gastrointestinal motility (and may also be useful as an antiemetic). Extensive first-pass metabolism of ergotamine also reduces bioavailability.
  Rectal: More rapid and extensive than after oral administration; increased by concurrent administration of caffeine.
  Sublingual: Very poor.

### Distribution
Ergotamine is distributed into breast milk.

### Protein binding
Dihydroergotamine—
  Very high (about 90%).
Ergotamine—
  Very high (93 to 98%).

### Biotransformation
Dihydroergotamine—
  Hepatic; extensive, with considerable first-pass metabolism. The principal metabolite, 8′-hydroxy-dihydroergotamine, is pharmacologically active.
Ergotamine—
  Hepatic; extensive, with considerable first-pass metabolism. At least some of the metabolites are pharmacologically active.

### Half-life
Note: Reported values vary widely, depending on the route of administration and study methodology. Values obtained after administration of radiolabeled dihydroergotamine or ergotamine represent metabolites as well as the parent compound, whereas values determined via specific radioimmunoassay (RIA) represent only the parent compound. At least 2 RIAs have been used to assess pharmacokinetics of dihydroergotamine, one of which is more sensitive (able to detect significantly smaller quantities of the compound) than the other.
Distribution—
  Dihydroergotamine:
    Intravenous—1 to 1.35 minutes in one study; 4 minutes in a second study. Different doses and RIAs were used in the 2 studies.
    Subcutaneous—Approximately 1 hour, measured via RIA.
  Ergotamine:
    2.7 hours, determined following oral administration of radiolabeled ergotamine.
Elimination—
  Dihydroergotamine:
    Intravenous—
      Alpha phase: Approximately 23 to 33 minutes in one study; 1.45 hours in a second study. Different doses and RIAs were used in the 2 studies.
      Beta phase: Approximately 15 hours, measured via the more sensitive RIA.
    Subcutaneous—About 7.25 hours, measured via RIA.
    Values ranging between 18 and 32 hours have been reported after administration of radiolabeled dihydroergotamine by various routes.
  Ergotamine: Determined after oral administration of radiolabeled ergotamine:
    Alpha phase: Approximately 2 hours.
    Beta phase: Approximately 21 hours.

### Onset of action
Acute headaches—
  Note: For relief of acute migraine or cluster headaches, the onset of action is highly dependent on the duration of the headache prior to initiation of therapy as well as on the route of administration. The most rapid onset of action is achieved when the medication is administered as soon as the first symptoms appear (during the prodrome, for migraine with aura).
  Dihydroergotamine:
    Intramuscular—15 to 30 minutes.
    Intravenous—Variable; usually less than 5 minutes.

### Time to peak concentration
Dihydroergotamine—
  Intramuscular: About 30 minutes.
  Intravenous: About 3 minutes.
  Subcutaneous: 15 to 45 minutes.
Ergotamine—
  Oral, administered without caffeine: About 2 hours.
  Oral, administered concurrently with caffeine: About 60 to 70 minutes.
  Rectal, administered concurrently with caffeine: About 1 hour.
Note: The pharmacokinetics of ergotamine after oral or rectal administration have been studied in healthy subjects and in migraine patients who were not experiencing an attack at the time of the study. During a migraine headache, peak concentrations after oral administration are likely to occur less rapidly than reported above, because the gastric stasis that accompanies migraine headaches inhibits absorption of medications.
  In a study investigating the association between pharmacokinetic variables and efficacy of ergotamine in migraine patients who were not experiencing an attack at the time of the study, plasma concentrations measured after a single oral or rectal dose of each patient's usual ergotamine-containing medication were subject to wide interindividual variability. Peak plasma concentrations of ergotamine occurred earlier, were higher, and were maintained for a longer time in patients who reported a good therapeutic response to their medications than in patients who reported a poor therapeutic response to the same medications. In most patients reporting a good therapeutic response, plasma concentrations of 200 picograms per mL or higher were measured within 1 hour after administration.

### Time to peak effect
Relief of acute headache—
  Dihydroergotamine: Parenteral—15 minutes to 2 hours.
  Ergotamine: Oral—Variable; usually within 1 to 2 hours, but up to 5 hours in some patients.

### Duration of action
Dihydroergotamine—Vasoconstrictive and antihypotensive effects—
  About 8 hours, following intravenous or subcutaneous administration.

### Elimination
Dihydroergotamine—
  Primarily via hepatic metabolism, followed by fecal (biliary) elimination of metabolites. Only 5 to 10% of a dose is excreted in the urine, with only trace amounts being excreted in the urine as unchanged dihydroergotamine.
Ergotamine—
  Primarily via hepatic metabolism, followed by fecal (biliary) elimination of metabolites. About 4% of an oral dose is excreted in the urine within 96 hours. Only trace amounts are eliminated in the

urine and feces as unmetabolized ergotamine. After sublingual administration, ergotamine is also eliminated, erratically, in saliva.

In dialysis—Ergotamine is dialyzable.

## Precautions to Consider

Note: Information in this section concerning the adjuvants present in ergotamine-containing headache suppressant formulations (caffeine, belladonna alkaloids, cyclizine, dimenhydrinate, diphenhydramine, and pentobarbital) is limited to brief summaries of the major precautions that may apply to their use in doses recommended for treatment of vascular headaches. For more complete information that may apply, especially if these agents are ingested frequently or in higher-than-recommended doses, see—

Caffeine: *Caffeine (Systemic)*.

Belladonna alkaloids: *Anticholinergics/Antispasmodics (Systemic)*.

Cyclizine: *Cyclizine (Systemic)*.

Dimenhydrinate: *Antihistamines (Systemic)*.

Diphenhydramine: *Antihistamines (Systemic)*.

Pentobarbital: *Barbiturates (Systemic)*.

### Mutagenicity
*Dimenhydrinate—*
Mutagenicity screening tests showed dimenhydrinate to be mutagenic in bacterial systems, but not mammalian systems. There are no human data showing that the medication is mutagenic.

### Pregnancy/Reproduction
Note: Information concerning use of adjuvants present in ergotamine-containing combinations by pregnant women is not included in this section because the potential adverse effects of ergotamine preclude the use of these combinations during pregnancy.

*Pregnancy—*
*Dihydroergotamine—*
Use during pregnancy is not recommended because dihydroergotamine stimulates the uterine musculature, although it has much less oxytocic activity than ergotamine. Also, constriction of the placental vasculature may cause fetotoxicity by reducing uterine blood flow.

*Ergotamine—*
Use during pregnancy is not recommended because of ergotamine's potent oxytocic activity. Ergotamine's uterine stimulating action and its vasoconstrictive activity, which may lead to reduced uterine blood flow, may both be harmful to the fetus. Although a definite causal relationship has not been established, use of ergotamine by pregnant women may have caused fetal growth retardation, intrauterine fetal deaths, miscarriages, and intestinal obstruction resulting in the death of a neonate.

In animal studies, ergotamine has caused retarded fetal growth and increases in the number of resorptions and intrauterine deaths.

FDA Pregnancy Category X.

### Breast-feeding
*Dihydroergotamine and Ergotamine—*
Ergot alkaloids are distributed into breast milk and have the potential to cause adverse effects (e.g., vomiting, diarrhea, weak pulse, unstable blood pressure, seizures) in the infant. These medications may also inhibit lactation.

*Caffeine—*
Caffeine is distributed into breast milk in small amounts. However, it is recommended that breast-feeding mothers limit their total daily intake of caffeine to 360 mg, because accumulation of caffeine in the infant, leading to hyperactivity, wakefulness, and other signs of caffeine stimulation, may occur when a breast-feeding mother ingests large quantities of caffeine.

*Belladonna alkaloids and Cyclizine and Dimenhydrinate and Diphenhydramine—*
Because of their anticholinergic activity, these medications have the potential to inhibit lactation. Dimenhydrinate is distributed into breast milk in small amounts. Cyclizine may also be distributed into breast milk.

*Pentobarbital—*
Barbiturates are distributed into breast milk in small amounts and may cause sedation or other signs of CNS depression in the infant.

### Pediatrics
*Dihydroergotamine—*
Although appropriate studies have not been done in the pediatric population, dihydroergotamine is being used to treat severe migraine headache in children as young as 6 years of age. No pediatrics-specific problems have been reported. However, it is recommended that an ergot derivative be used with caution and only in patients who are unresponsive to less toxic medications.

*Ergotamine—*
Ergotamine is being used in patients 6 years of age and older. No pediatrics-specific problems have been documented to date. However, it is recommended that an ergot derivative be used with caution and only in patients who are unresponsive to less toxic medications.

*Caffeine—*
Appropriate studies on the relationship of age to the effects of caffeine have not been performed in children up to 12 years of age. However, no pediatrics-specific problems have been documented to date.

*Belladonna alkaloids—*
Young children are especially susceptible to the toxic effects of anticholinergics. An increased response to anticholinergics has been reported in children with spastic paralysis or brain damage.

*Cyclizine and Dimenhydrinate and Diphenhydramine—*
A paradoxical reaction characterized by hyperexcitability may occur in children taking antihistamines.

*Pentobarbital—*
Some children react to barbiturates with paradoxical excitement.

### Geriatrics
*Dihydroergotamine and Ergotamine—*
Caution is recommended in the elderly, who are more likely to have occlusive peripheral vascular disease, and are therefore more likely to be adversely affected by peripheral vasoconstriction, than are younger adults. This increases the risk of hypothermia and other ischemic complications. The risk of cardiac ischemia is also increased in geriatric patients. Elderly patients are also more likely to have age-related renal function impairment, which requires caution in patients receiving these medications.

*Belladonna alkaloids—*
Geriatric patients may respond to usual doses of these medications with excitement, agitation, drowsiness, or confusion.

*Belladonna alkaloids and Cyclizine and Dimenhydrinate and Diphenhydramine—*
Caution is recommended when these medications are used in the elderly, who are especially sensitive to anticholinergic side effects. Also, the risk of precipitating undiagnosed glaucoma in the elderly must be considered. Dizziness, sedation, and hypotension are also more likely to occur in elderly patients receiving antihistamines such as cyclizine, dimenhydrinate, and diphenhydramine.

*Pentobarbital—*
Excitement, depression, and confusion may be more likely to occur in elderly patients, who are generally more susceptible than younger adults to the effects of barbiturates.

### Drug interactions and/or related problems
The following drug interactions and/or related problems have been selected on the basis of their potential clinical significance (possible mechanism in parentheses where appropriate)—not necessarily inclusive (» = major clinical significance):

Note: Combinations containing any of the following medications, depending on the amount present, may also interact with this medication.

Barbiturates such as pentobarbital induce hepatic chromosomal enzymes and may thereby increase the metabolism and decrease the efficacy of many medications that are metabolized by these enzymes. The most clinically significant interactions have been reported with adrenocorticoids, corticotropin, coumarin- or indandione-derivative anticoagulants, anticonvulsants (carbamazepine, divalproex sodium, valproic acid), and estrogen-containing oral contraceptives (see *Barbiturates [Systemic]* ). Although occasional use of a pentobarbital-containing headache suppressant may not cause significant interference with the effects of most of these agents, selection of a formulation that does not contain pentobarbital may be advisable in some cases.

*For dihydroergotamine and ergotamine*
Antibiotics, macrolide, especially
  Erythromycin
  Troleandomycin
  (these antibiotics may inhibit the metabolism of the ergot derivative and increase the risk of vasospasm)

Beta-adrenergic blocking agents
  (peripheral vasoconstriction and vasospastic reactions have occurred in a few patients receiving a beta-adrenergic blocking agent for migraine prophylaxis after administration of usual doses of dihydroergotamine or ergotamine; although most patients are able to tolerate the combination of medications without ill effects, closer monitoring of patients receiving both types of medication may be warranted)

» Ergot alkaloids, other or
» Vasoconstrictors, systemic, other, such as:
   Cocaine
   Epinephrine, parenteral
   Metaraminol
   Methoxamine
   Norepinephrine
   Phenylephrine, parenteral or
» Vasoconstrictor-containing local anesthetic solutions
   (concurrent use with dihydroergotamine or ergotamine may produce peripheral vascular ischemia and gangrene and is not recommended)
   (the pressor effect of sympathomimetic pressor amines may be potentiated, resulting in possible severe hypertension and rupture of cerebral blood vessels)
   Nitroglycerin
   (the vasoconstrictive effect of dihydroergotamine or ergotamine may oppose the vasodilating effect of nitroglycerin, thereby reducing nitroglycerin's efficacy as an antianginal agent)
   (nitroglycerin may also reduce hepatic metabolism of dihydroergotamine)
   Smoking, tobacco
   (administration of ergotamine to a patient who smokes heavily may increase the risk of peripheral vascular ischemia because nicotine also constricts blood vessels)

*For formulations containing caffeine*
   Caffeine from any other dietary or medicinal source or
   CNS stimulation–producing medications, other (See *Appendix II* )
   (excessive CNS stimulation, which may lead to nervousness, irritability, insomnia, or possibly convulsions or cardiac arrhythmias, may occur; close observation is recommended)
   Monoamine oxidase (MAO) inhibitors, including furazolidone, procarbazine and selegiline
   (the sympathomimetic side effects of caffeine may lead to cardiac arrhythmias or severe hypertension when large doses are used concurrently with MAO inhibitors; even small doses may cause tachycardia and a slight increase in blood pressure)

*For formulations containing belladonna alkaloids, cyclizine, dimenhydrinate, diphenhydramine, or pentobarbital*
   Anticholinergics or other medications with anticholinergic activity, other (See *Appendix II* ) or
   CNS depression–producing medications, other (See *Appendix II* ), including alcohol
   (the risk of additive anticholinergic effects must be considered when any medication having anticholinergic activity is used concurrently with belladonna alkaloids, cyclizine, dimenhydrinate, or diphenhydramine)
   (the risk of additive CNS depression must be considered when any medication having CNS depressant activity is used concurrently with cyclizine, dimenhydrinate, diphenhydramine, or pentobarbital)

**Laboratory value alterations**
The following have been selected on the basis of their potential clinical significance (possible effect in parentheses where appropriate)—not necessarily inclusive (» = major clinical significance):
With diagnostic test results
*For belladonna alkaloids*
» Gastric acid secretion test
   (belladonna alkaloids may antagonize the effects of pentagastrin and histamine in the evaluation of gastric acid secretory function; administration of belladonna alkaloids during the 24 hours preceding the test is not recommended)

*For caffeine*
   Myocardial perfusion studies, dipyridamole-assisted
   (caffeine may inhibit the effects of dipyridamole on myocardial blood flow, thereby interfering with test results; patients should be advised to avoid caffeine for at least 12 hours prior to the test)
   Urate, serum, determinations
   (false-positive elevations may occur when measured by the Bittner method)

*For cyclizine, dimenhydrinate, and diphenhydramine*
   Skin tests using allergen extracts
   (cyclizine, dimenhydrinate, and diphenhydramine may inhibit the cutaneous histamine response, thereby producing false-negative results; it is recommended that these medications not be administered for at least 72 hours before testing)

**Medical considerations/Contraindications**
The medical considerations/contraindications included have been selected on the basis of their potential clinical significance (reasons given in parentheses where appropriate)—not necessarily inclusive (» = major clinical significance).

*Except under special circumstances, this medication should not be used when the following medical problems exist:*
For dihydroergotamine and ergotamine
» Angioplasty, recent or contemplated or
» Vascular surgery, especially arterial, recent or contemplated
   (increased risk of ischemia)
» Hypertension, severe, uncontrolled
   (may be aggravated)

*Risk-benefit should be considered when the following medical problems exist:*
For dihydroergotamine and ergotamine
   Allergic reaction to dihydroergotamine or ergotamine, history of
» Coronary artery disease, especially:
» Angina pectoris, unstable or vasospastic, or other indication of coronary ischemia
   (vasospasm may aggravate existing angina pectoris, or cause angina pectoris or myocardial infarction)
   Diarrhea—for suppository dosage forms
   (impaired absorption of medications)
» Hepatic function impairment
   (impaired metabolism may result in ergot poisoning)
» Hypertension, not optimally controlled
   (may be aggravated)
   Hyperthyroidism
   (possible increased risk of ergotism)
   Malnutrition
   (risk of ergotism may be increased because malnutrition-associated metabolic disturbances may lead to increased concentrations of the ergot derivative and/or to hyperreactivity to the medication)
» Peripheral vascular disease, occlusive, or
» Pruritus, severe, especially when associated with hepatic disease, or
» Sepsis or other severe infection
   (increased risk of complications associated with vasospasm)
» Renal function impairment
   Caution is also recommended in geriatric patients, who may be especially susceptible to complications associated with vasospasm and to hypothermia.

*For dihydroergotamine only, when used concurrently with low-dose heparin for prophylaxis against perioperative thrombotic complications (in addition to the medical problems listed above)*
» Trauma
   (increased risk of vasospastic reactions, especially in an injured extremity of patients with multiple fractures)

*For formulations containing caffeine*
» Anxiety disorders, including
   Agoraphobia
   Panic attacks
   (increased risk of anxiety, nervousness, fear, nausea, palpitation, rapid heartbeat, restlessness, and trembling)
» Cardiac disease, severe
   (high doses of caffeine are not recommended because of an increased risk of tachycardia or extrasystoles, which may lead to heart failure)
» Insomnia
   (may be potentiated; this effect may be particularly detrimental to patients with a vascular headache, because sleep also helps relieve headache)
» Peptic ulcer
   (may be aggravated)
   Sensitivity to caffeine

*For formulations containing belladonna alkaloids, cyclizine, dimenhydrinate, or diphenhydramine*
   Any condition in which the anticholinergic effects of these medications may be detrimental, such as:
   Bladder neck obstruction
   Gastrointestinal tract obstructive disease
   Glaucoma, not optimally controlled, or predisposition to
   Prostatic hypertrophy
   Urinary retention
   Sensitivity to the agent considered for use

**Patient monitoring**
The following may be especially important in patient monitoring (other tests may be warranted in some patients, depending on condition; » = major clinical significance):

Blood pressure
(close monitoring is recommended when multiple doses of dihydroergotamine are administered for relief of chronic, intractable headache; antihypertensive therapy may be needed to assure that the patient is normotensive when each dose is given and/or to treat any rise in blood pressure that occurs after dihydroergotamine administration)

Electrocardiographic monitoring
(recommended, especially during the first few doses in patients older than 60 years of age, when multiple doses of dihydroergotamine are administered intravenously for relief of chronic, intractable headache)

Examination of extremities and
Palpation of peripheral pulses
(recommended periodically during therapy to detect vasospasm or ischemia in patients using frequent doses, especially when dihydroergotamine is administered daily as an adjunct to heparin prophylaxis against postoperative thrombotic complications or to treat orthostatic hypotension and when multiple doses of dihydroergotamine are administered intravenously for relief of chronic, intractable headache)

## Side/Adverse Effects

Note: Most side/adverse effects are dose-related and are usually relieved by a reduction in dose or withdrawal of the medication.

Although acute ergot poisoning is rare, patient sensitivity to the effects of ergotamine varies widely and symptoms of ergot toxicity (peripheral ischemia, paresthesia, headache, nausea and vomiting) may occur even with usual doses.

Nausea and vomiting may be caused by migraine headaches as well as by an ergot derivative.

The risk of side effects being induced by recommended doses of the adjuvants in ergotamine-containing combination formulations has not been determined. In general, it is expected that such effects, even in overdose situations, would be overshadowed by those of ergotamine. However, with acute overdose of formulations containing belladonna alkaloids, cyclizine, dimenhydrinate, or diphenhydramine, the possibility of severe symptoms associated with their anticholinergic activity should be considered. Also, with acute overdose of formulations containing pentobarbital, the possibility of severe CNS depression should be considered.

The following side/adverse effects have been selected on the basis of their potential clinical significance (possible signs and symptoms in parentheses where appropriate)—not necessarily inclusive:

**Those indicating need for medical attention**
Incidence more frequent
*Edema, localized* (swelling of face, fingers, feet, and/or lower legs)
Incidence less frequent or rare
*Cardiovascular effects, specifically angina pectoris, coronary vasospasm–induced* (chest pain); *fast or slow heartbeat; increase or decrease in blood pressure; rapid, weak pulse; ischemia, cerebral* (anxiety, confusion); *ischemia, peripheral vasospasm–induced* (itching of skin; numbness and tingling of fingers, toes, or face; pain in arms, legs, or lower back, especially pain in calves and/or heels upon exertion; pale, bluish-colored, or cold hands or feet; weak or absent pulses; weakness in legs); *and vasospasm, ocular* (changes in vision; miosis)
Note: *Myocardial infarction* and *cerebral infarction* have also been reported.

**Those indicating need for medical attention only if they continue or are bothersome**
Incidence more frequent
*CNS effects* (dizziness or drowsiness occurring without other signs and symptoms of overdose [especially with formulations containing cyclizine, dimenhydrinate, diphenhydramine, or pentobarbital]; rarely, nervousness, racing thoughts, and restlessness)—these dysphoric effects may be especially severe with repetitive administration of intravenous dihydroergotamine and metoclopramide for intractable headaches; *dryness of mouth*—especially likely with formulations containing belladonna alkaloids; *may also occur with formulations containing cyclizine, dimenhydrinate, or diphenhydramine; diarrhea, nausea, or vomiting*—occurring without other signs and symptoms of overdose; *peripheral vascular effects, mild and lasting 1 hour or less* (cold fingers or toes, itching of skin, numbness or tingling of fingers or toes, weakness in the legs occurring without other signs and symptoms of ischemia)

**Those indicating possible withdrawal and the need for medical attention if they occur after medication is discontinued**
*Headache*—severe withdrawal (rebound) headaches may occur in migraineurs who overuse ergotamine; they are generally most severe for the first 24 to 48 hours, and usually last about 72 hours, after the last dose of ergotamine, and may lead to increased use of ergotamine and/or analgesics, dependence, and chronic, intractable headaches

## Overdose

For specific information on the agents used in the management of vascular headache, suppressants, ergot derivative-containing overdose, see
- *Charcoal, Activated (Oral-Local)* monograph;
- *Diazepam* or *Lorazepam* in *Benzodiazepines (Systemic)* monograph;
- *Ipecac (Oral-Local)* monograph;
- *Neostigmine* in *Antimyasthenics (Systemic)* monograph;
- *Nitroglycerin* in *Nitrates (Systemic)* monograph;
- *Nitroprusside (Systemic)* monograph; and/or
- *Physostigmine (Systemic)* monograph.

For more information on the management of overdose or unintentional ingestion, **contact a Poison Control Center** (see *Poison Control Center Listing*).

**Clinical effects of overdose**
Note: *Cerebral ischemia* and/or *peripheral ischemia* may be signs of acute or chronic overdose. Continued chronic use of an ergot derivative after early signs and symptoms of peripheral ischemia appear may lead to *gangrene* (red or violet blisters on skin of hands or feet may be first signs) or to *thrombotic complications*.

In addition to vision changes associated with *ocular vasospasm* listed above, one case of reversible *bilateral papillitis with ring scotomata* has been reported in chronic overdose.

The following effects have been selected on the basis of their potential clinical significance (possible signs and symptoms in parentheses where appropriate)—not necessarily inclusive:

Acute
*CNS toxicity* (convulsions; severe confusion, dizziness, or drowsiness; weakness; one-sided paralysis; loss of consciousness); *diarrhea, vomiting, stomach pain or bloating; respiratory depression* (shortness of breath)

Note: After an acute overdose has been ingested, *CNS and gastrointestinal manifestations, hypotension,* and *tachycardia* may occur within a few hours, but signs and symptoms of *peripheral ischemia* may not appear until the next day.

*Hypotension* and sometimes *shock* may occur following initial *hypertension*.

Chronic
*Fibrosis, pleural or retroperitoneal* (shortness of breath; chest pain)—reported in isolated patients; *loss of appetite; nausea or vomiting, severe or continuing; headache; rectal ulceration* (abdominal pain, irregular bowel movements, rectal discomfort, difficulty in moving bowels)

Note: Increased frequency and/or severity of *migraine headaches* may indicate tolerance to ergotamine. Frequent use of ergotamine by migraineurs may also lead to the development of *chronic, intractable headaches* with both migrainous and nonmigrainous manifestations. These *chronic headaches* will not subside as long as ergotamine and/or analgesics continue to be taken. If specific treatment (e.g., intravenous dihydroergotamine) is not given after other headache-aborting medications are discontinued, the headaches usually become worse (being most severe on the third or fourth day) and may persist for 2 weeks or longer.

*Rectal ulceration* has been reported with chronic overuse of the rectal suppository dosage form of ergotamine and caffeine.

**Treatment of overdose**
To decrease absorption of orally administered ergotamine— Emesis may be induced with of syrup of ipecac. Alternatively, the stomach may be emptied via gastric lavage, provided that pharyngeal and laryngeal reflexes are present and the patient is conscious. If the patient is unconscious, gastric lavage should be performed only after intubation with a cuffed endotracheal tube has been performed. Activated charcoal, in water or a saline cathartic, such as sodium or magnesium sulfate in water, may then be introduced and left in the stomach.

To enhance elimination—There is no evidence that forced diuresis accelerates elimination of either dihydroergotamine or ergotamine. However, ergotamine is dialyzable.

Specific treatment—
For convulsions: Administering a benzodiazepine such as diazepam or lorazepam is recommended. The fact that intravenous benzodiazepines may cause circulatory depression when administered intravenously must be kept in mind. See the package inserts or *Diazepam* or *Lorazepam* in *Benzodiazepines (Systemic)* for specific dosing guidelines for use of these products.

For maintaining pulmonary ventilation: Mucus secretions may be removed via pharyngeal and tracheal suction. Oxygen may be administered if necessary, keeping in mind that further respiratory depression and hypercapnia may occur in the presence of hypoventilation hypoxia unless respiration is assisted. Very severe cases may require endotracheal intubation and tracheostomy, with or without assisted respiration.

For hypotension (in acute intoxication, may occur following initial hypertension): Mild to moderate hypotension may respond to positioning the patient in the Trendelenburg position and/or administering intravenous fluids. Volume expanders may be administered if necessary. Vasopressors may be considered if hypotension is very severe, keeping in mind the hazards of administering such substances in the presence of ergot derivative–induced peripheral vasoconstriction.

For peripheral vasospasm or ischemia: Warmth should be applied to ischemic extremities, taking care to avoid excessive heat. If necessary, a vasodilator may be administered, keeping in mind the risk of administering vasodilators in the presence of hypotension. Severe ischemia may require intravenous or intra-arterial nitroprusside; severe coronary ischemia or vasospasm may require intravenous nitroglycerin. Less severe cases may respond to oral vasodilators. Prazosin and captopril have been reported effective in a few patients. See the package inserts or *Nitroglycerin* in *Nitrates (Systemic)* or *Nitroprusside (Systemic)* for specific dosing guidelines for use of these products.

Careful nursing measures designed to prevent tissue damage should be instituted. Anticoagulant therapy may be warranted if ischemia is present, especially if the patient is unconscious; some emergency care physicians recommend low-dose heparin for ergot-induced vasospasm, even when arterial thrombosis has not been documented. Severe ischemia or gangrene unresponsive to treatment may require vascular surgery, catheter dilation, or even amputation.

Monitoring—Monitoring vital signs; monitoring cardiac rhythm (if vital signs are abnormal or the patient has a history of cardiovascular disease).

Supportive care—Supportive measures required to maintain pulmonary ventilation and correct hypotension; and measures to reduce additional absorption of orally ingested ergotamine, if an acute overdose had been ingested within the past 4 hours; and (in both acute and chronic intoxications) measures to ascertain the presence and/or extent of ischemia and to maintain adequate circulation. If no indication of vasospasm or ischemia is present 6 hours or longer following ingestion of an acute overdose, the patient should be informed about typical signs and symptoms, and instructed to seek medical attention immediately if they occur on a delayed basis.

For belladonna alkaloid–containing combinations—
Specific treatment—
Use of physostigmine or neostigmine methylsulfate to reverse severe anticholinergic symptoms. See package inserts or *Neostigmine* in *Antimyasthenics (Systemic)* or *Physostigmine (Systemic)* for specific dosing guidelines for use of these products.

Pentobarbital–containing formulations—
To enhance elimination—If renal function is normal, inducing forced diuresis, which may increase barbiturate elimination. Alkalinization of the urine increases renal excretion of some barbiturates.
Instituting hemodialysis or hemoperfusion in severe barbiturate poisoning or if the patient is anuric or in shock. However, hemodialysis or hemoperfusion is not recommended as a routine procedure.
Specific treatment—Administering chest physiotherapy. If pneumonia is suspected, appropriate cultures should be taken and antibiotics administered. Also, appropriate care should be taken to prevent hypostatic pneumonia, decubiti, aspiration, and other complications that may occur with altered states of consciousness.
Patients in whom intentional overdose is known or suspected should be referred for psychiatric consultation.

# Patient Consultation

As an aid to patient consultation, refer to *Advice for the Patient, Headache Medicines, Ergot Derivative-containing (Systemic)*.
In providing consultation, consider emphasizing the following selected information (» = major clinical significance):

### Before using this medication
» Conditions affecting use, especially:
  Sensitivity to any ingredient in the product considered for use
  Pregnancy—Use is not recommended because ergot derivatives have oxytocic activity, which may lead to miscarriage, and vasoconstrictive activity, which may result in fetotoxicity
  Breast-feeding—Ergot alkaloids are distributed into breast milk and may cause adverse effects in the infant; ergot alkaloids and medications having anticholinergic activity (belladonna alkaloids, cyclizine, dimenhydrinate, diphenhydramine) may also inhibit lactation; caffeine and pentobarbital are also distributed into breast milk and may cause CNS stimulation or CNS depression, respectively
  Use in children—Pediatrics-specific problems have not been reported in children 6 years of age or older, but dihydroergotamine and ergotamine are recommended only for patients unresponsive to less toxic medications; young children, especially those with spastic paralysis or brain damage, may be especially susceptible to the effects of belladonna alkaloids; also, risk of paradoxical hyperexcitability in children receiving cyclizine, dimenhydrinate, diphenhydramine, or pentobarbital
  Use in the elderly—Increased risk of hypothermia and other adverse effects associated with ergot derivative–induced peripheral and coronary vasoconstriction; increased susceptibility to effects of medications with anticholinergic activity and to barbiturates
  Other medications, especially other vasoconstrictors (including other ergot alkaloids and vasoconstrictors present in local anesthetic solutions)
  Other medical problems, especially angina pectoris or other coronary artery disease, hepatic function impairment, hypertension, severe infection, peripheral vascular disease, pruritus, renal function impairment, and recent or contemplated angioplasty or vascular surgery (for dihydroergotamine and ergotamine); anxiety disorders (e.g., agoraphobia, panic attacks), severe cardiac disease, insomnia, or peptic ulcer (for caffeine-containing formulations)

### Proper use of this medication
» Importance of not using more medication than the amount prescribed; risk of habituation with too frequent use and of peripheral vasoconstriction or other signs and symptoms of ergotism with acute or chronic overdosage
» Taking at first sign of headache (prodromal stage, for migraine with aura)
» Lying down in a quiet, dark room after taking initial dose
» Compliance with prophylactic therapy, if prescribed
  Proper administration techniques for—
    Dihydroergotamine injection
    Ergotamine inhalation: Reading patient directions; shaking container after removing cap; exhaling, placing mouthpiece in mouth aimed at back of throat, simultaneously inhaling and pressing vial down into the adapter; holding breath as long as possible after inhaling medication
    Ergotamine sublingual tablets: Allowing to dissolve under tongue; not chewing or swallowing whole; not eating, drinking, or smoking while tablet is dissolving
    Ergotamine-containing rectal suppositories
    If dividing suppository dosage form: Dividing lengthwise into pieces of equal size; easier to accomplish if suppositories have been refrigerated
» Proper dosing
» Proper storage

### Precautions while using this medication
» Checking with physician if usual dose fails to relieve headaches, or if frequency and/or severity of headaches increases; possibility that tolerance to or dependence on the medication has developed, leading to withdrawal (rebound) or chronic headaches
  Avoiding alcohol, which aggravates headache
  Avoiding smoking because nicotine constricts blood vessels
  Avoiding exposure to excessive cold, which may intensify peripheral vasoconstriction
  Notifying physician if infection develops; severe infection may cause increased sensitivity to medication
  For ergotamine inhalation—Possible hoarseness or throat irritation, which may be prevented by gargling and rinsing mouth after use; checking with physician if continuing or bothersome
  Possible interferences with laboratory tests; not taking caffeine for 12 hours prior to dipyridamole-assisted myocardial perfusion study, belladonna alkaloids for 24 hours prior to gastric acid secretion test, and cyclizine, dimenhydrinate, or diphenhydramine for 72 hours prior to skin tests using allergen extracts
» *For formulations containing cyclizine, dimenhydrinate, diphenhydramine, or pentobarbital*

Caution when driving or doing jobs requiring alertness because of possible dizziness, lightheadedness, or drowsiness, especially if taking other CNS depressants concurrently

*For formulations containing belladonna alkaloids, cyclizine, dimenhydrinate, or diphenhydramine*
- Possible dryness of mouth, nose, and throat; using sugarless candy or gum, ice, or saliva substitute for relief

**Side/adverse effects**
Signs and symptoms of potential side effects, especially edema, fast or slow heartbeat, cerebral or peripheral ischemia, gangrene, and coronary or ocular vasospasm

## General Dosing Information

Abortive therapy is most effective when initiated at the first symptoms of a migraine attack (during the prodrome, for migraine with aura). Delay in starting treatment increases the required dose and prolongs the onset of action of the ergot derivative.

After the first dose has been administered, it is recommended that the patient lie down and relax in a quiet, darkened room, because this contributes to relief of migraines.

To reduce the risk of adverse effects, the ergot derivative should be used in the lowest dose that provides adequate relief of headache. However, individual sensitivity to the effects of ergot derivatives varies, and signs and symptoms of toxicity may occur in some patients even with usual doses. Therapy should be withdrawn at the first sign of vasospasm.

Analgesics, antiemetics, antianxiety agents, and/or sedatives may be used concurrently with the ergot derivative, if needed, for relief of an acute migraine attack. Regimens used for relief of severe, refractory migraine utilize metoclopramide or prochlorperazine together with intravenous dihydroergotamine. However, medications having the potential to cause habituation (e.g., opioid analgesics, barbiturates, benzodiazepines) should be used with caution and as infrequently as possible.

Atropine, metoclopramide, or a phenothiazine antiemetic may be administered to prevent or relieve nausea and vomiting induced by an ergot derivative or by the migraine itself.

Tolerance to the effects of ergotamine may develop in migraineurs, leading to an increased dosage requirement, dependence, withdrawal (rebound) or chronic, intractable headaches, and abuse of the medication. The caffeine in many ergotamine-containing formulations may contribute to the development of dependence and withdrawal or chronic, intractable headaches, and the pentobarbital in some formulations may also be habit-forming. However, repetitive administration of intravenous dihydroergotamine over a 2- to 3-day period for treatment of chronic, intractable headaches associated with dependence on ergotamine or analgesics has not been reported to increase or prolong dependence.

To reduce the risk of dependence, it is recommended that ergotamine not be administered to migraine patients more frequently than every fifth day.

**For rectal dosage forms only**
Ergotamine-containing rectal suppositories are torpedo-shaped and are not scored. To assure proper dosage when a portion of a suppository is to be administered, the suppository should be cut lengthwise into pieces of equal size. This is easier to accomplish when the suppository has been refrigerated.

**For treatment of adverse effects**
Treatment of headaches associated with dependence on ergotamine may involve:
- Discontinuation of ergotamine and other headache medications, even acetaminophen or aspirin; in-patient treatment may be necessary during detoxification.
- Repetitive intravenous administration of dihydroergotamine (in conjunction with metoclopramide) is recommended by some headache specialists to relieve chronic, intractable headaches.
- Naproxen, alone or together with amitriptyline, may help relieve the headache pain. Overuse of acetaminophen or aspirin, especially in formulations containing caffeine in addition to the analgesic, may have contributed to the development of withdrawal headaches or chronic, intractable headaches; therefore, use of these agents is not recommended.
- Appropriate treatment for symptoms of withdrawal from other substances frequently used or abused by chronic headache patients may also be needed.
- Initiation or adjustment of appropriate prophylactic treatment is recommended to reduce the number and severity of future headaches.
- After a headache-prone patient has been detoxified from ergotamine and/or other abused substances, intramuscular or subcutaneous dihydroergotamine is recommended for treating future acute migraine headaches.

## DIHYDROERGOTAMINE

## Summary of Differences

Category/indications:
  May be agent of choice for treatment of status migrainosus or other severe, refractory headaches, including chronic headaches associated with dependence on ergotamine or analgesics.
  Also, indicated as a thrombosis prophylaxis adjunct, being used concurrently with low-dose heparin to prevent postoperative thrombotic complications.
  Also, indicated as an antihypotensive, to prevent or treat orthostatic hypotension.

Pharmacology/pharmacokinetics:
  Mechanism of action/effects—Adrenergic blocking actions are somewhat more pronounced, and vasoconstrictive actions less pronounced, than those of ergotamine.
  Other actions/effects—Much less potent as a uterine stimulant than ergotamine.
  Time to peak effect—Relieves acute headache in 15 minutes to 2 hours.
  Duration of action—Subcutaneous or intravenous: About 8 hours.

Precautions:
  Medical considerations/contraindications—When used concurrently with heparin to prevent postoperative thrombotic complications, caution also needed if trauma of an extremity is present because of the increased risk of vasospastic reactions.

Patient monitoring—
  Blood pressure monitoring needed when medication is administered repetitively for treatment of severe, intractable headache.
  Examination of extremities and palpation of peripheral pulses recommended when medication is administered daily for prophylaxis against postoperative thrombotic complications (concurrently with heparin) or for treatment of orthostatic hypotension.

## Additional Dosing Information

See also *General Dosing Information*.

Dihydroergotamine is administered via intramuscular, intravenous, or subcutaneous injection. Intra-arterial injection must be avoided.

When dihydroergotamine is used in conjunction with heparin for prophylaxis against postoperative thrombotic complications, all of the precautions pertinent to use of heparin must also be kept in mind.

## Parenteral Dosage Forms

Note: Bracketed uses in the *Dosage Forms* section refer to categories of use and/or indications that are not included in U.S. product labeling.

### DIHYDROERGOTAMINE MESYLATE INJECTION USP

**Usual adult dose**

Acute migraine or cluster headache (outpatient treatment)—
  Intramuscular (preferred) or subcutaneous, 1 mg at the start of the attack. May be repeated in one hour, if needed. The maximum recommended daily dose is 3 mg.
  Intravenous, 500 mcg (0.5 mg) at the start of the attack, administered in conjunction with an antiemetic. May be repeated in one hour, if necessary. The maximum recommended daily dose is 2 mg.

Chronic, intractable headache (inpatient treatment)—
  Intravenous, initially 500 mcg (0.5 mg), administered over one minute, three to five minutes after intravenous administration of an antiemetic (10 mg of metoclopramide is most commonly used). The dosage of dihydroergotamine and/or the antiemetic should be adjusted as needed to reduce the occurrence of side effects (especially to prevent nausea and vomiting) while providing adequate control of the headache; up to 1 mg of dihydroergotamine may be given for subsequent doses if needed and tolerated. This regimen may be repeated every eight hours until relief is obtained, although an antiemetic is usually no longer needed after six doses of dihydroergotamine have been administered. One specialist recommends an additional two or three doses of dihydroergotamine, administered at twelve-hour intervals after the headache is relieved, to reduce the likelihood of headache recurrence.

[Thrombosis prophylaxis adjunct][1]—
  To be administered concurrently with 5000 USP Units of subcutaneously administered heparin:
  Abdominal, thoracic, or pelvic surgery—Subcutaneous, 500 mcg (0.5 mg) two hours prior to surgery, then every twelve hours for five to seven days.
  Total hip replacement surgery—Subcutaneous, 500 mcg (0.5 mg) two hours prior to surgery, then every eight hours for seven to fourteen days.

[Prevention of orthostatic hypotension associated with spinal or epidural anesthesia][1]—
  Intravenous, 500 mcg (0.5 mg), administered a few minutes prior to the anesthetic.

[Treatment of orthostatic hypotension][1]—
  Intramuscular, 1 mg once a day.
  Subcutaneous, 6.5 to 13 mcg (0.0065 to 0.013 mg) per kg of body weight once a day, in the morning. Breakthrough episodes of hypotension may occur after meals when this dose is used, but can be prevented by oral administration of 250 mg of caffeine one-half hour before meals.

**Usual adult prescribing limits**
Vascular headache suppressant (migraine or cluster [acute])—6 mg per week.

**Usual pediatric dose**
Vascular headache suppressant (migraine [acute, severe])—
  Children 6 years of age and older:
    Intramuscular or subcutaneous, 500 mcg (0.5 mg) at the start of the attack. May be repeated in one hour if needed.
    Intravenous, 250 mcg (0.25 mg) at the start of the attack. May be repeated in one hour if needed.
Note:  Another regimen that has been advocated for treatment of children and adolescents with severe, acute migraine consists of:
    For children 6 to 9 years of age—Intravenous, 100 to 150 mcg (0.1 to 0.15 mg), with one or two additional doses being administered at twenty-minute intervals if needed.
    For children 9 to 12 years of age—Intravenous, 200 mcg (0.2 mg), with one or two additional doses being administered at twenty-minute intervals if needed.
    For adolescents 12 to 16 years of age—Intravenous, 250 to 500 mcg (0.25 to 0.5 mg), with one or two additional doses being administered at twenty-minute intervals if needed.
    Administration of an antiemetic (such as metoclopramide or a phenothiazine antiemetic) is recommended in conjunction with intravenous dihydroergotamine. Administering the antiemetic orally one hour prior to the first dose of dihydroergotamine, if feasible, may reduce the risk of severe side effects, including extrapyramidal reactions, that may be encountered after intravenous administration.

**Strength(s) usually available**
U.S.—
  1 mg per mL (Rx) [*D.H.E. 45* (alcohol; glycerin; methanesulfonic acid; and/or sodium hydroxide)].
Canada—
  1 mg per mL (Rx) [*Dihydroergotamine-Sandoz* (alcohol)].

**Packaging and storage**
Store below 40 °C (104 °F), preferably between 15 and 30 °C (59 and 86 °F), unless otherwise specified by manufacturer. Protect from light. Protect from freezing.

**Stability**
Do not use if solution is discolored.

---

[1]Not included in Canadian product labeling.

---

## ERGOTAMINE

### Summary of Differences
Pharmacology/pharmacokinetics:
  Mechanism of action/effects—Adrenergic blocking actions somewhat less pronounced, and vasoconstrictive actions more pronounced, than those of dihydroergotamine.
  Other actions/effects—Much more potent as a uterine stimulant than dihydroergotamine.
  Time to peak effect—Oral: Usually within 1 to 2 hours, but up to 5 hours in some patients.

### Inhalation Dosage Forms
#### ERGOTAMINE TARTRATE INHALATION AEROSOL USP

**Usual adult dose**
Vascular headache suppressant (migraine or cluster [acute])—
  Oral inhalation, 360 mcg (0.36 mg—1 metered spray) at the start of the attack, repeated at intervals of at least five minutes as needed for full relief, up to a total of 2.16 mg (6 metered sprays) per day.

**Usual adult prescribing limits**
To reduce the risk of dependence on ergotamine, it is recommended that the medication be used no more often than two times a week, preferably at least five days apart.

**Usual pediatric dose**
Dosage has not been established.

**Strength(s) usually available**
U.S.—
  Not commercially available.
Canada—
  360 mcg (0.36 mg) per metered spray (9 mg per mL) (Rx) [*Medihaler Ergotamine*].

**Packaging and storage**
Store below 40 °C (104 °F), preferably between 15 and 30 °C (59 and 86 °F), unless otherwise specified by manufacturer. Store in a light-resistant container.

**Auxiliary labeling**
• Shake well.

**Note**
Include patient instructions when dispensing.
Explain administration technique.

### Oral Dosage Forms
#### ERGOTAMINE TARTRATE TABLETS USP

**Usual adult dose**
Vascular headache suppressant (migraine or cluster [acute])—
  Oral, 1 or 2 tablets (1 or 2 mg of ergotamine) at the start of the attack, followed by an additional 1 or 2 tablets at intervals of at least thirty minutes, up to a total of 6 tablets (6 mg of ergotamine) per day. If an additional dose was needed, and the initial dose was well tolerated, a higher initial dose may be administered at the start of subsequent attacks. The maximum recommended initial dose is 3 tablets (3 mg of ergotamine).

**Usual adult prescribing limits**
To reduce the risk of dependence on ergotamine, it is recommended that the medication be used no more often than two times a week, preferably at least five days apart.

**Usual pediatric dose**
Dosage has not been established.

**Strength(s) usually available**
U.S.—
  Not commercially available.
Canada—
  1 mg (Rx) [*Gynergen*].

**Packaging and storage**
Store below 40 °C (104 °F), preferably between 15 and 30 °C (59 and 86 °F), unless otherwise specified by manufacturer. Store in a well-closed, light-resistant container.

#### ERGOTAMINE TARTRATE TABLETS (SUBLINGUAL) USP

**Usual adult dose**
Vascular headache suppressant (migraine or cluster [acute])—
  Sublingual, 2 mg at the start of the attack, repeated at intervals of at least thirty minutes, if necessary, up to a total of 6 mg per day.

**Usual adult prescribing limits**
To reduce the risk of dependence on ergotamine, it is recommended that the medication be used no more often than two times a week, preferably at least five days apart.

**Usual pediatric dose**
Product of suitable strength not available.

**Strength(s) usually available**
U.S.—
  2 mg (Rx) [*Ergostat* (lactose; saccharin)].
Canada—
  2 mg (Rx) [*Ergomar* (lactose)].

**Packaging and storage**
Store below 40 °C (104 °F), preferably between 15 and 30 °C (59 and 86 °F), unless otherwise specified by manufacturer. Store in a well-closed, light-resistant container.

## ERGOTAMINE AND CAFFEINE

### Summary of Differences
Pharmacology/pharmacokinetics:
   Mechanism of action/effects—
      Ergotamine: Adrenergic blocking actions somewhat less pronounced, and vasoconstrictive actions more pronounced, than those of dihydroergotamine.
      Caffeine: Probably contributes to efficacy of the combination by enhancing ergotamine absorption.
   Other actions/effects—
      Ergotamine: Much more potent as a uterine stimulant than dihydroergotamine.
      Caffeine: Has CNS stimulating effects; may inhibit sleep.
   Time to peak effect—Ergotamine: Oral—Usually within 1 to 2 hours, but up to 5 hours in some patients.
Precautions:
   Breast-feeding—Caffeine: Total daily intake by breast-feeding women should be limited, because accumulation and stimulant effects in the infant have been reported.
   Drug interactions and/or related problems—Caffeine: Potential excessive stimulation if used concurrently with other CNS stimulants; potential hypertension and arrhythmias if used concurrently with MAO inhibitors.
   Laboratory value alterations—Caffeine: May interfere with dipyridamole-assisted myocardial perfusion studies and serum urate determinations (Bittner method).
   Medical considerations/contraindications—Caffeine: Caution also recommended in patients with anxiety disorders, insomnia, peptic ulceration, and severe cardiac disease.

### Oral Dosage Forms
Note: Bracketed uses in the *Dosage Forms* section refer to categories of use and/or indications that are not included in U.S. product labeling.

#### ERGOTAMINE TARTRATE AND CAFFEINE TABLETS USP

**Usual adult dose**
Acute headache—
   Oral, 1 or 2 tablets (1 or 2 mg of ergotamine) at the start of the attack, followed by an additional 1 or 2 tablets (1 or 2 mg of ergotamine) at intervals of at least thirty minutes, up to a total of 6 tablets (6 mg of ergotamine) per day. If an additional dose was needed, and the initial dose was well tolerated, a higher initial dose may be administered at the start of subsequent attacks. The maximum recommended initial dose is 3 tablets (3 mg of ergotamine).
[Cluster headache prophylaxis][1]—
   Oral, 1 or 2 tablets (1 or 2 mg of ergotamine) one to three times a day, one or two hours prior to the time that attacks usually occur. Cluster headaches that occur only during the night may be prevented by a single dose, administered one or two hours before bedtime.

**Usual adult prescribing limits**
Acute migraine—
   To reduce the risk of dependence on ergotamine, it is recommended that the medication be used no more often than two times a week, preferably at least five days apart.

**Usual pediatric dose**
Vascular headache suppressant (migraine [acute, severe])—
   Children 6 to 12 years of age: Oral, 1 tablet (1 mg of ergotamine) initially; may be repeated one or two times, if necessary, up to a total of 3 tablets (3 mg of ergotamine) per day.

**Usual pediatric prescribing limits**
To reduce the risk of dependence on ergotamine, it is recommended that the medication be used no more often than two times a week, preferably at least five days apart.

**Strength(s) usually available**
U.S.—
   1 mg of ergotamine tartrate and 100 mg of caffeine (Rx) [*Cafergot; Ercaf; Ergo-Caff; Gotamine; Wigraine* (propylparaben ; sucrose; sugar); GENERIC].
   Note: In Canada, *Wigraine* tablets contain belladonna alkaloids in addition to ergotamine tartrate and caffeine.

Canada—
   1 mg of ergotamine tartrate and 100 mg of caffeine (Rx) [*Cafergot* (scored)].

**Packaging and storage**
Store below 40 °C (104 °F), preferably between 15 and 30 °C (59 and 86 °F), unless otherwise specified by manufacturer. Store in a well-closed, light-resistant container.

### Rectal Dosage Forms

#### ERGOTAMINE TARTRATE AND CAFFEINE SUPPOSITORIES USP

**Usual adult dose**
Vascular headache suppressant (migraine or cluster [acute])—
   Rectal, one-fourth to 1 suppository (500 mcg [0.5 mg] to 2 mg of ergotamine) initially, repeated at intervals of at least thirty minutes, if needed and tolerated, up to a total dose of 2 suppositories (4 mg of ergotamine) per day. Most patients respond well to an initial dose of one-half suppository (1 mg of ergotamine). However, if a repeat dose was necessary, and the first dose did not cause undue nausea, the initial dose for subsequent attacks may be increased. Up to 1½ suppositories (3 mg of ergotamine) may be administered as a single initial dose, if tolerated.
Note: One headache specialist recommends that the patient determine a dose that does not cause nausea (during a headache-free period) by inserting one-fourth of a suppository every 60 minutes, until nausea occurs or a maximum of 1 suppository has been used. The highest cumulative dose that does not cause nausea may then be used as the initial dose during an acute attack. For example, if nausea occurs after the third dose (a total of three-fourths of a suppository), the initial dose for that patient should be one-half suppository.

**Usual adult prescribing limits**
To reduce the risk of dependence on ergotamine, it is recommended that the medication be used no more often than two times a week, preferably at least five days apart.

**Usual pediatric dose**
Vascular headache suppressant (migraine [acute, severe])—
   Children 6 to 12 years of age: Rectal, one-fourth to one-half suppository (500 mcg [0.5 mg] to 1 mg of ergotamine) at the start of an attack. It is recommended that no more than one-half suppository be administered per day.

**Usual pediatric prescribing limits**
To reduce the risk of dependence on ergotamine, it is recommended that the medication be used no more often than two times a week, preferably at least five days apart.

**Strength(s) usually available**
U.S.—
   2 mg of ergotamine tartrate and 100 mg of caffeine (Rx) [*Cafergot; Cafertine; Cafetrate; Migergot; Wigraine;* GENERIC].
   Note: In Canada, *Wigraine* suppositories contain belladonna alkaloids in addition to ergotamine tartrate and caffeine.

Canada—
   2 mg of ergotamine tartrate and 100 mg of caffeine (Rx) [*Cafergot*].

**Packaging and storage**
Store at a temperature not above 25 °C (77 °F). Store in a tight container. Do not expose unwrapped suppositories to sunlight.

**Auxiliary labeling**
• For rectal use only.
• Store in a cool place.

[1]Not included in Canadian product labeling.

## ERGOTAMINE, CAFFEINE, AND BELLADONNA ALKALOIDS

### Summary of Differences
Pharmacology/pharmacokinetics:
   Mechanism of action/effects—
      Ergotamine: Adrenergic blocking actions somewhat less pronounced, and vasoconstrictive actions more pronounced, than those of dihydroergotamine.
      Caffeine: Probably contributes to efficacy of the combination by enhancing ergotamine absorption.
      Belladonna alkaloids: Provide an antiemetic effect.

Other actions/effects—
  Ergotamine: Much more potent as a uterine stimulant than dihydroergotamine.
  Caffeine: Has CNS stimulating effects; may inhibit sleep.
  Belladonna alkaloids: Have anticholinergic activity.
Time to peak effect—Ergotamine: Oral—Usually within 1 to 2 hours, but up to 5 hours in some patients.
Precautions:
  Breast-feeding—
    Caffeine: Total daily intake by breast-feeding women should be limited, because accumulation and stimulant effects in the infant have been reported.
    Belladonna alkaloids: May inhibit lactation.
  Pediatrics—Belladonna alkaloids: Young children, especially with spastic paralysis or brain damage, are especially susceptible to toxic effects of anticholinergics.
  Geriatrics—Belladonna alkaloids: Increased risk of excitement, agitation, drowsiness, or confusion; also, risk of precipitating undiagnosed glaucoma.
  Drug interactions and/or related problems—
    Caffeine: Potential excessive stimulation if used concurrently with other CNS stimulants; potential hypertension and arrhythmias if used concurrently with MAO inhibitors.
    Belladonna alkaloids: Potential additive anticholinergic effects if administered concurrently with other medications having similar activity.
  Laboratory value alterations—
    Caffeine: May interfere with dipyridamole-assisted myocardial perfusion studies and serum urate determinations (Bittner method).
    Belladonna alkaloids: Interfere with gastric acid secretion tests.
  Medical considerations/contraindications—
    Caffeine: Caution also recommended in patients with anxiety disorders, insomnia, peptic ulceration, and severe cardiac disease.
    Belladonna alkaloids: Caution also required in patients with conditions that may be adversely affected by anticholinergic effects.

## Oral Dosage Forms
### ERGOTAMINE TARTRATE, CAFFEINE, AND BELLADONNA ALKALOIDS TABLETS

**Usual adult dose**
Vascular headache suppressant (migraine or cluster [acute])—
  Oral, 1 or 2 tablets (1 or 2 mg of ergotamine) at the start of the attack, followed by an additional 1 or 2 tablets (1 or 2 mg of ergotamine) at intervals of at least thirty minutes, up to a total of 6 tablets (6 mg of ergotamine) per day. If an additional dose was needed, and the initial dose was well tolerated, a higher initial dose may be administered at the start of subsequent attacks. The maximum recommended initial dose is 3 tablets (3 mg of ergotamine).

**Usual adult prescribing limits**
To reduce the risk of dependence on ergotamine, it is recommended that the medication be used no more often than two times a week, preferably at least five days apart.

**Usual pediatric dose**
Vascular headache suppressant (migraine [acute, severe])—
  Children 6 to 12 years of age: Oral, 1 tablet (1 mg of ergotamine) initially; may be repeated one or two times, if necessary, up to a total of 3 tablets (3 mg of ergotamine) per day.

**Usual pediatric prescribing limits**
To reduce the risk of dependence on ergotamine, it is recommended that the medication be used no more often than two times a week, preferably at least five days apart.

**Strength(s) usually available**
U.S.—
  Not commercially available.
Canada—
  1 mg of ergotamine tartrate, 100 mg of caffeine, and 100 mcg (0.1 mg) of belladonna alkaloids (Rx) [*Wigraine* (scored)].
Note: In the U.S. *Wigraine* tablets contain only ergotamine tartrate and caffeine.

**Packaging and storage**
Store below 40 °C (104 °F), preferably between 15 and 30 °C (59 and 86 °F), unless otherwise specified by manufacturer.

## Rectal Dosage Forms
### ERGOTAMINE TARTRATE, CAFFEINE, AND BELLADONNA ALKALOIDS SUPPOSITORIES

**Usual adult dose**
Vascular headache suppressant (migraine or cluster [acute])—
  Rectal, one-half to 2 suppositories (500 mcg [0.5 mg] to 2 mg of ergotamine) initially, repeated at intervals of at least thirty minutes, if needed and tolerated, up to a total dose of 4 suppositories (4 mg of ergotamine) per day. Most patients respond well to an initial dose of one suppository (1 mg of ergotamine). However, if a repeat dose was necessary, and the first dose did not cause undue nausea, the initial dose for subsequent attacks may be increased. Up to 3 suppositories (3 mg of ergotamine) may be administered as a single initial dose, if tolerated.

Note: One headache specialist recommends that the patient determine a dose that does not cause nausea (during a headache-free period) by inserting one-half of a suppository every 60 minutes, until nausea occurs or a maximum of 2 suppositories has been used. The highest cumulative dose that does not cause nausea may then be used as the initial dose during an acute attack. For example, if nausea occurs after the third dose (a total of 1½ suppositories), the initial dose for that patient should be 1 suppository.

**Usual adult prescribing limits**
To reduce the risk of dependence on ergotamine, it is recommended that the medication be used no more often than two times a week, preferably at least five days apart.

**Usual pediatric dose**
Vascular headache suppressant (migraine [acute, severe])—
  Children 6 to 12 years of age: Rectal, one-half to one suppository (500 mcg [0.5 mg] to 1 mg of ergotamine) at the start of an attack. It is recommended that no more than one suppository be administered per day.

**Usual pediatric prescribing limits**
To reduce the risk of dependence on ergotamine, it is recommended that the medication be used no more often than two times a week, preferably at least five days apart.

**Strength(s) usually available**
U.S.—
  Not commercially available.
Canada—
  1 mg of ergotamine tartrate, 100 mg of caffeine, and 100 mcg (0.1 mg) of belladonna alkaloids. (Rx) [*Wigraine*].
Note: In the U.S., *Wigraine* suppositories contain only ergotamine tartrate and caffeine.

**Packaging and storage**
Store below 25 °C (77 °F), in a tight container, unless otherwise specified by manufacturer.

**Auxiliary labeling**
• For rectal use only.
• Store in a cool place.

---

### ERGOTAMINE, CAFFEINE, BELLADONNA ALKALOIDS, AND PENTOBARBITAL

## Summary of Differences
Pharmacology/pharmacokinetics:
  Mechanism of action/effects—
    Ergotamine: Adrenergic blocking actions somewhat less pronounced, and vasoconstrictive actions more pronounced, than those of dihydroergotamine.
    Caffeine: Probably contributes to efficacy of the combination by enhancing ergotamine absorption.
    Belladonna alkaloids: Provide an antiemetic effect.
    Pentobarbital: Provides a sedative effect.
  Other actions/effects—
    Ergotamine: Much more potent as a uterine stimulant than dihydroergotamine.
    Caffeine: Has CNS stimulating effects; may inhibit sleep.
    Belladonna alkaloids: Have anticholinergic activity.
    Pentobarbital: Has CNS depressant effects.
  Time to peak effect—Ergotamine: Oral—Usually within 1 to 2 hours, but up to 5 hours in some patients.

## Precautions:

Breast-feeding—
  Caffeine: Total daily intake by breast-feeding women should be limited, because accumulation and stimulant effects in the infant have been reported.
  Belladonna alkaloids: May inhibit lactation.
  Pentobarbital: May be distributed into breast milk.
Pediatrics—
  Belladonna alkaloids: Young children, especially with spastic paralysis or brain damage, are especially susceptible to toxic effects of anticholinergics.
  Pentobarbital: May cause paradoxical excitement.
Geriatrics—
  Belladonna alkaloids: Increased risk of excitement, agitation, drowsiness, or confusion; also, risk of precipitating undiagnosed glaucoma.
  Pentobarbital: Risk of excitement, depression, and/or confusion.
Drug interactions and/or related problems—
  Caffeine: Potential excessive stimulation if used concurrently with other CNS stimulants; potential hypertension and arrhythmias if used concurrently with MAO inhibitors.
  Belladonna alkaloids: Potential additive anticholinergic effects if administered concurrently with other medications having similar activity.
  Pentobarbital: Potential additive effects with other CNS depressants.
Laboratory value alterations—
  Caffeine: Interference with dipyridamole-assisted myocardial perfusion studies and serum urate determinations (Bittner method).
  Belladonna alkaloids: Interfere with gastric acid secretion tests.
Medical considerations/contraindications—
  Caffeine: Caution also recommended in patients with anxiety disorders, insomnia, peptic ulceration, and severe cardiac disease.
  Belladonna alkaloids: Caution also required in patients with conditions that may be adversely affected by anticholinergic effects.

## Oral Dosage Forms

### ERGOTAMINE TARTRATE, CAFFEINE, BELLADONNA ALKALOIDS, AND PENTOBARBITAL SODIUM TABLETS

#### Usual adult dose
Vascular headache suppressant (migraine or cluster [acute])—
  Oral, 1 or 2 tablets (1 or 2 mg of ergotamine) at the start of the attack, followed by an additional 1 or 2 tablets (1 or 2 mg of ergotamine) at intervals of at least thirty minutes, up to a total of 6 tablets (6 mg of ergotamine) per day. If an additional dose was needed, and the initial dose was well tolerated, a higher initial dose may be administered at the start of subsequent attacks. The maximum recommended initial dose is 3 tablets (3 mg of ergotamine).

Note: Geriatric and debilitated patients may react to usual doses of barbiturates with excitement, confusion, or mental depression. A reduction in dosage may be required in these patients.

#### Usual adult prescribing limits
To reduce the risk of dependence on ergotamine, it is recommended that the medication be used no more often than two times a week, preferably at least five days apart.

#### Usual pediatric dose
Vascular headache suppressant (migraine [acute, severe])—Children 6 to 12 years of age: Oral, 1 tablet (1 mg of ergotamine) initially; may be repeated one or two times, if necessary, up to a total of 3 tablets (3 mg of ergotamine) per day.

#### Usual pediatric prescribing limits
To reduce the risk of dependence on ergotamine, it is recommended that the medication be used no more often than two times a week, preferably at least five days apart.

#### Strength(s) usually available
U.S.—
  Not commercially available.
Canada—
  1 mg of ergotamine tartrate, 100 mg of caffeine, 125 mcg (0.125 mg) of belladonna alkaloids, and 30 mg of pentobarbital sodium (Rx) [*Cafergot-PB* (lactose; tartrazine)].

#### Packaging and storage
Store below 40 °C (104 °F), preferably between 15 and 30 °C (59 and 86 °F), in a well-closed container, unless otherwise specified by manufacturer. Protect from light.

#### Auxiliary labeling
- May cause drowsiness.
- Avoid alcoholic beverages.

## Rectal Dosage Forms

### ERGOTAMINE TARTRATE, CAFFEINE, BELLADONNA ALKALOIDS, AND PENTOBARBITAL SUPPOSITORIES

#### Usual adult dose
Vascular headache suppressant (migraine or cluster [acute])—
  Rectal, one-fourth to 1 suppository (500 mcg [0.5 mg] to 2 mg of ergotamine) initially, repeated at intervals of at least thirty minutes, if needed and tolerated, up to a total dose of 2 suppositories (4 mg of ergotamine) per day. Most patients respond well to an initial dose of one-half suppository (1 mg of ergotamine). However, if a repeat dose was necessary, and the first dose did not cause undue nausea, the initial dose for subsequent attacks may be increased. Up to 1½ suppositories (3 mg of ergotamine) may be administered as a single initial dose, if tolerated.

Note: One headache specialist recommends that the patient determine a dose that does not cause nausea (during a headache-free period) by inserting one-fourth of a suppository every 60 minutes, until nausea occurs or a maximum of 1 suppository has been used. The highest cumulative dose that does not cause nausea may then be used as the initial dose during an acute attack. For example, if nausea occurs after the third dose (a total of three-fourths of a suppository), the initial dose for that patient should be one-half suppository.

Geriatric and debilitated patients may react to usual doses of barbiturates with excitement, confusion, or mental depression. A reduction in dosage may be required in these patients.

#### Usual adult prescribing limits
To reduce the risk of dependence on ergotamine, it is recommended that the medication be used no more often than two times a week, preferably at least five days apart.

#### Usual pediatric dose
Vascular headache suppressant (migraine [acute, severe])—
  Children 6 to 12 years of age: Rectal, one-fourth to one-half suppository (500 mcg [0.5 mg] to 1 mg of ergotamine) at the start of an attack. It is recommended that no more than one-half suppository be administered per day.

#### Usual pediatric prescribing limits
To reduce the risk of dependence on ergotamine, it is recommended that the medication be used no more often than two times a week, preferably at least five days apart.

#### Strength(s) usually available
U.S.—
  Not commercially available.
Canada—
  2 mg of ergotamine tartrate, 100 mg of caffeine, 250 mcg (0.25 mg) of belladonna alkaloids, and 60 mg of pentobarbital (Rx) [*Cafergot-PB* (lactose)].

#### Packaging and storage
Store in a tight container at a temperature not exceeding 25 °C (77 °F), unless otherwise specified by manufacturer.

#### Auxiliary labeling
- For rectal use only.
- Store in a cool place.
- Avoid alcoholic beverages.
- May cause drowsiness.

---

## ERGOTAMINE, CAFFEINE, AND CYCLIZINE

## Summary of Differences

Pharmacology/pharmacokinetics:
  Mechanism of action/effects—
    Ergotamine: Adrenergic blocking actions somewhat less pronounced, and vasoconstrictive actions more pronounced, than those of dihydroergotamine.
    Caffeine: Probably contributes to efficacy of the combination by enhancing ergotamine absorption.
    Cyclizine: Provides antiemetic and sedative effects.
  Other actions/effects—
    Ergotamine: Much more potent as a uterine stimulant than dihydroergotamine.
    Caffeine: Has CNS stimulating effects; may inhibit sleep.
    Cyclizine: Has antihistaminic, anticholinergic, and CNS depressant activities.
  Time to peak effect—Ergotamine: Usually within 1 to 2 hours, but up to 5 hours in some patients.

Precautions:
  Breast-feeding—
    Caffeine: Total daily intake by breast-feeding women should be limited, because accumulation and stimulant effects in the infant have been reported.
    Cyclizine: May inhibit lactation and may be distributed into breast milk.
  Pediatrics—Cyclizine: May cause paradoxical excitement.
  Geriatrics—Cyclizine: Increased sensitivity to anticholinergic side effects; increased risk of dizziness, sedation, and hypotension.
  Drug interactions and/or related problems—
    Caffeine: Potential excessive stimulation if used concurrently with other CNS stimulants; potential hypertension and arrhythmias if used concurrently with MAO inhibitors.
    Cyclizine: Risk of additive anticholinergic and/or CNS effects if used concurrently with other medications having similar actions.
  Laboratory value alterations—
    Caffeine: May interfere with dipyridamole-assisted myocardial perfusion studies and serum urate determinations (Bittner method).
    Cyclizine: Interferes with skin tests using allergen extracts.
  Medical considerations/contraindications—
    Caffeine: Caution also recommended in patients with anxiety disorders, insomnia, peptic ulceration, and severe cardiac disease.
    Cyclizine: Caution also recommended in patients who may be adversely affected by anticholinergic effects.

## Oral Dosage Forms

### ERGOTAMINE TARTRATE, CAFFEINE, AND CYCLIZINE TABLETS

**Usual adult dose**
Vascular headache suppressant (migraine or cluster [acute])—
  Oral, one-half or 1 tablet (1 or 2 mg of ergotamine) at the start of the attack, followed by an additional one-half or 1 tablet (1 or 2 mg of ergotamine) at intervals of at least thirty minutes, up to a total of 3 tablets (6 mg of ergotamine) per day. If an additional dose was needed, and the initial dose was well tolerated, a higher initial dose may be administered at the start of subsequent attacks. The maximum recommended initial dose is 1½ tablets (3 mg of ergotamine).

**Usual adult prescribing limits**
To reduce the risk of dependence on ergotamine, it is recommended that the medication be used no more often than two times a week, preferably at least five days apart.

**Usual pediatric dose**
Vascular headache suppressant (migraine [acute, severe])—Children 6 to 12 years of age: Oral, one-half tablet (1 mg of ergotamine) initially; may be repeated one or two times, if necessary, up to a total of 1½ tablets (3 mg of ergotamine) per day.

**Usual pediatric prescribing limits**
To reduce the risk of dependence on ergotamine, it is recommended that the medication be used no more often than two times a week, preferably at least five days apart.

**Strength(s) usually available**
U.S.—
  Not commercially available.
Canada—
  2 mg of ergotamine tartrate, 100 mg of caffeine, and 50 mg of cyclizine hydrochloride (Rx) [*Megral* (scored)].

**Packaging and storage**
Store below 40 °C (104 °F), preferably between 15 and 30 °C (59 and 86 °F), in a well-closed container, unless otherwise specified by manufacturer.

**Auxiliary labeling**
• May cause drowsiness.
• Avoid alcoholic beverages.

---

### ERGOTAMINE, CAFFEINE, AND DIMENHYDRINATE

## Summary of Differences

Pharmacology/pharmacokinetics:
  Mechanism of action/effects—
    Ergotamine: Adrenergic blocking actions somewhat less pronounced, and vasoconstrictive actions more pronounced, than those of dihydroergotamine.
    Caffeine: Probably contributes to efficacy of the combination by enhancing ergotamine absorption.
    Dimenhydrinate: Provides antiemetic and sedative effects.

Other actions/effects—
  Ergotamine: Much more potent as a uterine stimulant than dihydroergotamine.
  Caffeine: Has CNS stimulating effects; may inhibit sleep.
  Dimenhydrinate: Has antihistaminic, anticholinergic, and CNS depressant activities.
Time to peak effect—Ergotamine: Usually 1 to 2 hours, but up to 5 hours in some patients.
Precautions:
  Breast-feeding—
    Caffeine: Total daily intake by breast-feeding women should be limited, because accumulation and stimulant effects in the infant have been reported.
    Dimenhydrinate: May inhibit lactation and is distributed into breast milk.
  Pediatrics—Dimenhydrinate: May cause paradoxical excitement.
  Geriatrics—Dimenhydrinate: Increased sensitivity to anticholinergic side effects; increased risk of dizziness, sedation, and hypotension.
  Drug interactions and/or related problems—
    Caffeine: Potential excessive stimulation if used concurrently with other CNS stimulants; potential hypertension and arrhythmias if used concurrently with MAO inhibitors.
    Dimenhydrinate: Risk of additive anticholinergic and/or CNS effects if used concurrently with other medications having similar actions.
  Laboratory value alterations—
    Caffeine: May interfere with dipyridamole-assisted myocardial perfusion studies and serum urate determinations (Bittner method).
    Dimenhydrinate: Interferes with skin tests using allergen extracts.
  Medical considerations/contraindications—
    Caffeine: Caution also recommended in patients with anxiety disorders, insomnia, peptic ulceration, and severe cardiac disease.
    Dimenhydrinate: Caution also recommended in patients who may be adversely affected by anticholinergic effects.

## Oral Dosage Forms

### ERGOTAMINE TARTRATE, CAFFEINE, AND DIMENHYDRINATE CAPSULES

**Usual adult dose**
Vascular headache suppressant (migraine or cluster [acute])—
  Oral, 1 or 2 capsules (1 or 2 mg of ergotamine) at the start of the attack, followed by an additional 1 or 2 capsules (1 or 2 mg of ergotamine) at intervals of at least thirty minutes, up to a total of 6 capsules (6 mg of ergotamine) per day. If an additional dose was needed, and the initial dose was well tolerated, a higher initial dose may be administered at the start of subsequent attacks. The maximum recommended initial dose is 3 capsules (3 mg of ergotamine).

**Usual adult prescribing limits**
To reduce the risk of dependence on ergotamine, it is recommended that the medication be used no more often than two times a week, preferably at least five days apart.

**Usual pediatric dose**
Vascular headache suppressant (migraine [acute, severe])—
  Children 6 to 12 years of age: Oral, 1 capsule (1 mg of ergotamine) initially; may be repeated one or two times, if necessary, up to a total of 3 capsules (3 mg of ergotamine) per day.

**Usual pediatric prescribing limits**
To reduce the risk of dependence on ergotamine, it is recommended that the medication be used no more often than two times a week, preferably at least five days apart.

**Strength(s) usually available**
U.S.—
  Not commercially available.
Canada—
  1 mg of ergotamine tartrate, 100 mg of caffeine, and 50 mg of dimenhydrinate (Rx) [*Gravergol*].

**Packaging and storage**
Store below 40 °C (104 °F), preferably between 15 and 30 °C (59 and 86 °F), in a well-closed container, unless otherwise specified by manufacturer.

**Auxiliary labeling**
• May cause drowsiness.
• Avoid alcoholic beverages.

## ERGOTAMINE, CAFFEINE, AND DIPHENHYDRAMINE

### Summary of Differences
Pharmacology/pharmacokinetics:
- Mechanism of action/effects—
  - Ergotamine: Adrenergic blocking actions somewhat less pronounced, and vasoconstrictive actions more pronounced, than those of dihydroergotamine.
  - Caffeine: Probably contributes to efficacy of the combination by enhancing ergotamine absorption.
  - Diphenhydramine: Provides antiemetic and sedative effects.
- Other actions/effects—
  - Ergotamine: Much more potent as a uterine stimulant than dihydroergotamine.
  - Caffeine: Has CNS stimulating effects; may inhibit sleep.
  - Diphenhydramine: Has antihistaminic, anticholinergic, and CNS depressant activities.
- Time to peak effect—Ergotamine: Usually within 1 to 2 hours, but up to 5 hours in some patients.

Precautions:
- Breast-feeding—
  - Caffeine: Total daily intake by breast-feeding women should be limited, because accumulation and stimulant effects in the infant have been reported.
  - Diphenhydramine: May inhibit lactation.
- Pediatrics—Diphenhydramine: May cause paradoxical excitement.
- Geriatrics—Diphenhydramine: Increased susceptibility to anticholinergic side effects; increased risk of dizziness, sedation, and hypotension.
- Drug interactions and/or related problems—
  - Caffeine: Potential excessive stimulation if used concurrently with other CNS stimulants; potential hypertension and arrhythmias if used concurrently with MAO inhibitors.
  - Diphenhydramine: Risk of additive anticholinergic and/or CNS effects if used concurrently with other medications having similar actions.
- Laboratory value alterations—
  - Caffeine: May interfere with dipyridamole-assisted myocardial perfusion studies and serum urate determinations (Bittner method).
  - Diphenhydramine: Interferes with skin tests using allergen extracts.
- Medical considerations/contraindications—
  - Caffeine: Caution also recommended in patients with anxiety disorders, insomnia, peptic ulceration, and severe cardiac disease.
  - Diphenhydramine: Caution also recommended in patients who may be adversely affected by anticholinergic effects.

### Oral Dosage Forms

#### ERGOTAMINE TARTRATE, CAFFEINE, AND DIPHENHYDRAMINE CAPSULES

**Usual adult dose**
Vascular headache suppressant (migraine or cluster [acute])—
  Oral, 1 or 2 capsules (1 or 2 mg of ergotamine) at the start of the attack, followed by an additional 1 or 2 capsules (1 or 2 mg of ergotamine) at intervals of at least thirty minutes, up to a total of 6 capsules (6 mg of ergotamine) per day. If an additional dose was needed, and the initial dose was well tolerated, a higher initial dose may be administered at the start of subsequent attacks. The maximum recommended initial dose is 3 capsules (3 mg of ergotamine).

**Usual adult prescribing limits**
To reduce the risk of dependence on ergotamine, it is recommended that the medication be used no more often than two times a week, preferably at least five days apart.

**Usual pediatric dose**
Vascular headache suppressant (migraine [acute, severe])—
  Children 6 to 12 years of age: Oral, 1 capsule (1 mg of ergotamine) initially; may be repeated one or two times, if necessary, up to a total of 3 capsules (3 mg of ergotamine) per day.

**Usual pediatric prescribing limits**
To reduce the risk of dependence on ergotamine, it is recommended that the medication be used no more often than two times a week, preferably at least five days apart.

**Strength(s) usually available**
U.S.—
  Not commercially available.
Canada—
  1 mg of ergotamine tartrate, 100 mg of caffeine, and 25 mg of diphenhydramine (Rx) [*Ergodryl*].

**Packaging and storage**
Store below 40 °C (104 °F), preferably between 15 and 30 °C (59 and 86 °F), in a well-closed container, unless otherwise specified by manufacturer.

**Auxiliary labeling**
- May cause drowsiness.
- Avoid alcoholic beverages.

### Selected Bibliography
Anthony M. The treatment of migraine and other headaches. Curr Opin Neurol Neurosurg 1991; 4: 245-52.
Diamond S. Migraine headache. Med Clin N Amer 1991; 75: 545-66.
Kudrow L. Diagnosis and treatment of cluster headache. Med Clin N Amer 1991; 75: 579-94.

Revised: 09/08/92

---

# VASOPRESSIN Systemic

VA CLASSIFICATION (Primary/Secondary): HS702/GA900; DX900
Commonly used brand name(s): *Pitressin; Pressyn*.
Note: For a listing of dosage forms and brand names by country availability, see *Dosage Forms* section(s).

## Category
Pituitary (posterior) hormone; antidiuretic (central diabetes insipidus); diagnostic aid (diabetes insipidus).

## Indications
Note: Bracketed information in the *Indications* section refers to uses that are not included in U.S. product labeling.

**Accepted**
Diabetes insipidus, central (treatment)—Vasopressin is indicated in the control or prevention of symptoms of central diabetes insipidus caused by insufficient antidiuretic hormone. It controls the polydipsia, polyuria, and dehydration associated with central diabetes insipidus.

Vasopressin injection may be used initially when diabetes insipidus is transient or due to surgery or head injury, or in unconscious patients receiving intravenous fluids. However, desmopressin is generally preferred for chronic therapy, since it lacks many of the effects on gastrointestinal and vascular smooth muscle vasopressin possesses.

[Diabetes insipidus (diagnosis)][1]—Vasopressin injection is used to differentially diagnose central and nephrogenic diabetes insipidus and psychogenic polydipsia.

**Unaccepted**
Vasopressin will not control polyuria associated with psychogenic polydipsia, renal disease, nephrogenic diabetes insipidus, hypokalemia, hypercalcemia, or the administration of demeclocycline or lithium.

Vasopressin injection was formerly used for the prevention and treatment of abdominal distention (in intestinal paresis, postoperatively, and complicating pneumonias or toxemias) and in abdominal roentgenography, urography, cholecystography, and kidney biopsy to disperse gas shadows. However, this use of vasopressin is no longer considered to be appropriate, because the risk of significant side effects does not outweigh the possible benefits of its use.

[1] Not included in Canadian product labeling.

## Pharmacology/Pharmacokinetics

**Physicochemical characteristics**
Source—Synthetic vasopressin (8-arginine vasopressin).
Molecular weight—1084.23.

### Mechanism of action/Effect
Antidiuretic (central diabetes insipidus) or

Diagnostic aid (diabetes insipidus)—Increases water reabsorption by increasing the cellular permeability of the collecting ducts, resulting in a decrease in urine volume with resultant increase in osmolality.

### Other actions/effects
At greater than physiologic doses, vasopressin has a pressor effect due to vasoconstriction and causes contraction of the smooth muscle of the gastrointestinal tract. It also increases secretion of corticotropin, growth hormone, and follicle-stimulating hormone (FSH).

### Biotransformation
Hepatic and renal.

### Half-life
Approximately 10 to 20 minutes.

### Duration of action
Approximately 2 to 8 hours.

### Elimination
Renal; approximately 5 to 15% excreted unchanged after intravenous administration.

## Precautions to Consider

### Pregnancy/Reproduction
Pregnancy—Problems in humans have not been documented; however, caution is recommended because of possible oxytocic effects, although these probably occur only with large doses. Vasopressin is inactivated by the placenta, possibly necessitating use of increased doses.

FDA Pregnancy Category C.

### Breast-feeding
Problems in humans have not been documented.

### Pediatrics
Caution is recommended in very young children because of the risk of water intoxication and hyponatremia.

### Geriatrics
Caution is recommended in the elderly because of the risk of water intoxication and hyponatremia.

### Drug interactions and/or related problems
The following drug interactions and/or related problems have been selected on the basis of their potential clinical significance (possible mechanism in parentheses where appropriate)—not necessarily inclusive (» = major clinical significance):

Note: Combinations containing any of the following medications, depending on the amount present, may also interact with this medication.

Carbamazepine or
Chlorpropamide or
Clofibrate
(may potentiate antidiuretic effect of vasopressin when used concurrently)

Demeclocycline or
Lithium or
Norepinephrine
(may decrease antidiuretic effect of vasopressin when used concurrently)

### Medical considerations/Contraindications
The medical considerations/contraindications included have been selected on the basis of their potential clinical significance (reasons given in parentheses where appropriate)—not necessarily inclusive (» = major clinical significance).

*Risk-benefit should be considered when the following medical problems exist:*

Allergy to vasopressin
Asthma or
Epilepsy or
Heart failure or
Migraine
(rapid addition of extracellular water may be hazardous)

» Coronary artery disease
(vasopressin may precipitate anginal pain; large doses may precipitate a myocardial infarction)

» Hypertensive cardiovascular disease
(vasopressin may increase blood pressure)

» Renal failure, chronic, with nitrogen retention

### Patient monitoring
The following may be especially important in patient monitoring (other tests may be warranted in some patients, depending on condition; » = major clinical significance):

Electrocardiograms (ECG) and
Fluid and electrolyte status determinations
(recommended at periodic intervals during therapy)

## Side/Adverse Effects
Note: Intra-arterial administration has been reported to cause local gangrene, coronary thrombosis, mesenteric infarction, venous thrombosis, infarction and necrosis of the small bowel, and peripheral emboli.

Large doses may cause increases in blood pressure, cardiac arrhythmias, and myocardial infarction.

The following side/adverse effects have been selected on the basis of their potential clinical significance (possible signs and symptoms in parentheses where appropriate)—not necessarily inclusive:

### Those indicating need for medical attention
Incidence rare
*Allergic reaction* (fever; redness of skin; skin rash, hives, or itching; swelling of face, feet, hands, or mouth; wheezing or troubled breathing); *angina or myocardial infarction* (chest pain); *water intoxication* (coma; confusion; drowsiness; continuing headache; problems with urination; seizures; weight gain)

### Those indicating need for medical attention only if they continue or are bothersome
Incidence less frequent—dose related
*Abdominal or stomach cramps; belching; diarrhea; dizziness or lightheadedness; increased sweating; increased urge for bowel movement; nausea or vomiting; pale skin; passage of gas; "pounding" in head; trembling; white-colored area around mouth*

## Overdose
For specific information on the agents used in the management of vasopressin overdose, see:
- *Furosemide* in *Diuretics, Loop (Systemic)* monograph;
- *Mannitol (Systemic)* monograph; and/or
- *Urea (Parenteral-Local)* monograph.

For more information on the management of overdose or unintentional ingestion, **contact a Poison Control Center** (see *Poison Control Center Listing*).

### Treatment of overdose
Specific treatment—Severe water intoxication may require osmotic diuresis with mannitol, hypertonic dextrose, or urea, alone or with furosemide.

Supportive care—Water intoxication may be treated with water restriction and temporary withdrawal of vasopressin until polyuria occurs. Patients in whom intentional overdose is confirmed or suspected should be referred for psychiatric consultation.

## Patient Consultation
As an aid to patient consultation, refer to *Advice for the Patient, Vasopressin (Systemic)*.

In providing consultation, consider emphasizing the following selected information (» = major clinical significance):

### Before using this medication
» Conditions affecting use, especially:
Allergy to vasopressin
Use in children—Very young children may be at greater risk of water intoxication and hyponatremia
Use in the elderly—May be at greater risk of water intoxication and hyponatremia
Other medical problems, especially coronary artery disease, hypertensive cardiovascular disease, or chronic renal failure

### Proper use of this medication
» Importance of not using more medication than the amount prescribed
Missed dose: Using as soon as possible; not using at all if almost time for next dose; not doubling doses
» Proper dosing
» Proper storage

### Side/adverse effects
Signs of potential side effects, especially allergic reaction, angina, myocardial infarction, and water intoxication

## General Dosing Information

Aqueous Vasopressin Injection USP may be administered intramuscularly, subcutaneously, intravenously, or intra-arterially. It may also be administered intranasally for treatment of diabetes insipidus, although this route is now mainly of historical interest.

To achieve optimal control of effect, aqueous Vasopressin Injection USP may be administered intravenously or intra-arterially by means of an infusion pump, a micro-drip regulator, or a similar device to allow precise adjustment of the flow rate.

Caution is recommended to avoid extravasation because of the risk of necrosis and gangrene.

Vasopressin injection is recommended at the onset of the illness in diabetes insipidus, to decrease the risk of water intoxication until the severity of the disease is established, or when close monitoring and a short duration of action are desired (e.g., after skull fracture or surgery).

## Parenteral Dosage Forms

Note: Bracketed uses in the *Dosage Forms* section refer to categories of use and/or indications that are not included in U.S. product labeling.

### VASOPRESSIN INJECTION USP

**Usual adult dose**
Antidiuretic (central diabetes insipidus)—
  Intramuscular or subcutaneous, 5 to 10 Units two or three times a day as needed.

[Diagnostic aid (diabetes insipidus [central])][1]—
  Subcutaneous, 5 Units.

**Usual pediatric dose**
Antidiuretic (central diabetes insipidus)—
  Intramuscular or subcutaneous, 2.5 to 10 Units three or four times a day.

**Strength(s) usually available**
U.S.—
  20 USP Posterior Pituitary Units per mL (Rx) [*Pitressin*; GENERIC].
Canada—
  20 USP Posterior Pituitary Units per mL (Rx) [*Pitressin*; *Pressyn*].

**Packaging and storage**
Store below 40 °C (104 °F), preferably between 15 and 30 °C (59 and 86 °F), unless otherwise specified by manufacturer. Protect from freezing.

[1]Not included in Canadian product labeling.

Revised: 8/26/93
Interim revision: 06/30/94

---

**VECURONIUM**—See *Neuromuscular Blocking Agents (Systemic)*

---

# VENLAFAXINE  Systemic

VA CLASSIFICATION (Primary): CN609
Commonly used brand name(s): *Effexor; Effexor XR*.
Note: For a listing of dosage forms and brand names by country availability, see *Dosage Forms* section(s).

## Category
Antidepressant.

## Indications

**Accepted**
Depressive disorder, major (treatment)—Venlafaxine is indicated for the treatment of major depressive disorder. Treatment of acute depressive episodes typically requires 6 to 12 months of antidepressant therapy. Patients with recurrent or chronic depression may require long-term treatment.

## Pharmacology/Pharmacokinetics

Note: A large degree of interpatient variability has been observed in the pharmacokinetic parameters of venlafaxine in patients with hepatic or renal function impairment.

**Physicochemical characteristics**
Chemically unrelated to tricyclic, tetracyclic, or other currently available antidepressants.
Chemical group—Phenethylamine.
Molecular weight—Venlafaxine hydrochloride: 313.87.
Venlafaxine: 277.
*O*-desmethylvenlafaxine (ODV): 263.
pKa—9.4.

**Mechanism of action/Effect**
The antidepressant action of venlafaxine is believed to be associated with its ability to potentiate neurotransmitter activity in the central nervous system (CNS). Venlafaxine and its active metabolite, *O*-desmethylvenlafaxine (ODV), are potent inhibitors of neuronal serotonin (5-hydroxytryptamine; 5-HT) reuptake, slightly less potent inhibitors of neuronal norepinephrine reuptake, and weak inhibitors of neuronal dopamine reuptake. Venlafaxine inhibits serotonin reuptake less potently than do the selective serotonin reuptake inhibitors. Studies in rats indicate that venlafaxine induces reduced sensitivity of the adenylate-cyclase coupled beta-adrenergic system after single doses. Many other currently available antidepressants induce this change in beta-receptor sensitivity only after repeated dosing. However, not all antidepressants produce beta-adrenergic subsensitivity, and the clinical significance of this effect remains to be determined.

Neither venlafaxine nor ODV has demonstrated specific affinity for adrenergic alpha$_1$ receptors, muscarinic receptors, or histaminergic H$_1$ receptors. Venlafaxine has demonstrated no specific affinity for adrenergic alpha$_2$ or beta receptors, dopaminergic D$_2$ receptors, serotonergic 5HT$_1$ or 5HT$_2$ receptors, benzodiazepine receptors, opiate receptors, phencyclidine (PCP) receptors, or N-methyl-D-aspartic acid (NMDA) receptors *in vitro*. Neither venlafaxine nor ODV inhibits monoamine oxidase.

**Other actions/effects**
Venlafaxine induces hypertension at a rate of incidence that increases with dosage from 3% at dosages below 100 mg/day to 13% at dosages above 300 mg/day.

**Absorption**
Venlafaxine is rapidly and well absorbed. At least 92% of a single dose is absorbed, based on mass balance studies. The bioavailability of venlafaxine is the same with a tablet or with an oral solution and is about 45%. Food delays absorption, but does not impair extent of absorption of venlafaxine.

Venlafaxine release from the extended-release dosage form is membrane-controlled and is not pH-dependent. Although absorption from the extended-release dosage form occurs at a slower rate and results in a lower maximum plasma concentration of venlafaxine, the extent of absorption is the same as with the prompt-release tablet.

**Distribution**
Venlafaxine Vol$_D$—7.5 ± 3.7 L per kg of body weight (L/kg).
ODV Vol$_D$—5.7 ± 1.8 L/kg.

**Protein binding**
Low to moderate.
Venlafaxine—25 to 30%.
ODV—18 to 42%.

**Biotransformation**
Venlafaxine is extensively metabolized in the liver and undergoes significant first-pass metabolism. The primary metabolite is *O*-desmethylvenlafaxine (ODV), which is approximately equivalent in pharmacologic activity and potency to venlafaxine. ODV is formed by *O*-demethylation via the cytochrome P450 2D6 (CYP2D6) isoenzyme. Biotransformation of venlafaxine to ODV is saturable to a modest degree. *In vitro* studies indicate that the CYP3A4 isoenzyme is involved in the metabolism of venlafaxine to a minor, less active metabolite than ODV, *N*-desmethylvenlafaxine.

In nine patients with cirrhosis, hepatic clearance of venlafaxine was decreased by about 50%, and that of ODV was decreased by about 30%. Clearance of venlafaxine in three patients with more severe cirrhosis was decreased by about 90%.

**Half-life**
Elimination—
  Venlafaxine: 5 ± 2 hours.
  ODV: 11 ± 2 hours.
  In nine patients with cirrhosis, elimination half-lives were increased by about 30% for venlafaxine, and by about 60% for ODV.

In patients with renal function impairment, elimination half-lives were increased by about 50% for venlafaxine, and by about 40% for ODV. In dialysis patients, venlafaxine elimination half-life was increased by up to 1.5 times that of patients with normal renal function.

**Onset of action**
Although some symptoms of major depression may improve within about 2 weeks, significant overall improvement may take several weeks.

**Time to peak concentration**
Prompt-release dosage form:
 Venlafaxine: Approximately 2 hours.
 ODV: 3 to 4 hours.
Extended-release dosage form:
 Venlafaxine: Approximately 5.5 hours.
 ODV: Approximately 9 hours.

**Peak plasma concentration**
Mean peak plasma concentrations ($C_{max}$) following administration of 25, 75, or 150 mg of the prompt-release dosage form of venlafaxine to 18 healthy males every 8 hours for three days were 53, 167, and 393 nanograms/mL (0.19, 0.603, and 1.42 micromoles/L), respectively, for venlafaxine, and 148, 397, and 686 nanograms/mL (0.563, 1.51, and 2.61 micromoles/L), respectively, for ODV. $C_{max}$ is generally lower following administration of the extended-release dosage form. Both venlafaxine and ODV exhibit linear pharmacokinetics over the dose range of 75 to 450 mg of venlafaxine per day.

Steady-state concentrations of venlafaxine and ODV are attained within 3 days with regular oral dosing.

**Elimination**
Renal—
 Approximately 87% of a dose is recovered in the urine within 48 hours, with unchanged venlafaxine comprising about 5%, unconjugated ODV comprising about 29%, conjugated ODV comprising about 26%, and other minor inactive metabolites comprising about 27% of the amount excreted.
 In patients with renal function impairment, the clearance of venlafaxine was decreased by about 24%, but the clearance of ODV was unchanged. In patients with end-stage renal disease, total clearance of venlafaxine and ODV was decreased by about 55%.
 In dialysis: In one study of six patients on maintenance hemodialysis, a 4-hour dialysis treatment removed only about 5% of a single 50-mg dose of venlafaxine.
Fecal—
 Approximately 2% of a dose of venlafaxine is recovered in feces after 35 days.

## Precautions to Consider

**Carcinogenicity/Tumorigenicity**
Studies in rats and mice that received venlafaxine for 24 and 18 months, respectively, have shown no evidence of an increased risk of tumor development.

**Mutagenicity**
Venlafaxine and its major metabolite, O-desmethylvenlafaxine (ODV), were not mutagenic in a battery of *in vivo* and *in vitro* tests. However, there was a clastogenic response in the *in vivo* chromosomal aberration assay in rat bone marrow in male rats receiving 200 times, on a mg per kg of body weight (mg/kg) basis, or 50 times, on a mg per square meter of body surface area (mg/m²) basis, the maximum recommended human dose (MRHD) of venlafaxine. The no-effect dose was 67 times (mg/kg) or 17 times (mg/m²) the MRHD.

**Pregnancy/Reproduction**
Fertility—No effects on male or female fertility were reported in rats administered oral doses of up to eight times the MRHD of venlafaxine on a mg/kg basis, or up to two times the MRHD on a mg/m² basis.
Pregnancy—Adequate and well-controlled studies in humans have not been done.
No teratogenic effects were observed in rats or rabbits given up to 11 or 12 times, respectively, the MRHD of venlafaxine on a mg/kg basis (2.5 or 4 times, respectively, the MRHD on a mg/m² basis). However, when dosing in rats began during pregnancy and continued until weaning, a decrease in pup weight, an increase in stillborn pups, and an increase in pup deaths during the first 5 days of lactation occurred. The cause of these deaths is not known.
FDA Pregnancy Category C.
Labor and delivery—The effect of venlafaxine on labor and delivery in humans is unknown.

**Breast-feeding**
It is not known whether venlafaxine is distributed into breast milk. However, problems in humans have not been documented.

**Pediatrics**
No information is available on the relationship of age to the effects of venlafaxine in pediatric patients. Safety and efficacy in children up to 18 years of age have not been established.

**Geriatrics**
No geriatrics-specific problems have been documented in studies done to date that have included geriatric patients.

**Pharmacogenetics**
Subjects with low cytochrome P450 2D6 (CYP2D6) activity, known as poor metabolizers, showed decreased ODV and increased venlafaxine concentrations as compared with concentrations in subjects with normal CYP2D6 activity, known as extensive metabolizers. However, since the sums of the concentrations of ODV and venlafaxine in the two groups were similar, this difference in metabolism is not likely to be of clinical significance.

**Drug interactions and/or related problems**
The following drug interactions and/or related problems have been selected on the basis of their potential clinical significance (possible mechanism in parentheses where appropriate)—not necessarily inclusive (» = major clinical significance):

Note: Possible interactions with medications that inhibit cytochrome P450 2D6 (CYP2D6) metabolism potentially may result in increased plasma concentrations of venlafaxine and decreased plasma concentrations of O-desmethylvenlafaxine (ODV). However, the sum of the venlafaxine and ODV concentrations is not expected to change significantly, and dosage adjustments are not recommended.

CYP3A4 is involved to a lesser extent in the metabolism of venlafaxine and the effects of concomitant use of venlafaxine and a potent inhibitor of both CYP2D6 and CYP3A4 on venlafaxine pharmacokinetics are unknown.

*In vivo* and *in vitro* studies indicate that venlafaxine weakly inhibits CYP2D6 but does not inhibit CYP1A2, CYP2C9, CYP2C19, or CYP3A4.

Combinations containing any of the following medications, depending on the amount present, may also interact with this medication.

Alcohol or
CNS depression–producing medications (see *Appendix II*)
 (although venlafaxine has not been shown to increase impairment of mental and motor skills, concomitant use with alcohol in depressed patients is not recommended)
 (similarly, CNS depressants should be administered with caution, since the potential for interactions in clinical practice is not known)

Cimetidine
 (in 18 healthy subjects, cimetidine inhibited the first-pass metabolism of venlafaxine, resulting in a decrease in clearance of about 43% and an increase in maximum plasma concentrations of about 60%; however, there was no apparent effect on the pharmacokinetics of ODV, which was present in the circulation in much greater quantities; thus, the overall pharmacologic activity of venlafaxine plus ODV was only slightly increased; dosage adjustments are not needed for most patients)
 (this interaction potentially could be more pronounced in the elderly, in patients with pre-existing hypertension, or in patients with hepatic or renal function impairment; caution should be exercised when venlafaxine and cimetidine are used concurrently in these patients)

Haloperidol
 (the area under the plasma concentration–time curve [AUC] of haloperidol was increased by 70%, the maximum plasma concentration [$C_{max}$] was increased by 88%, the oral-dose clearance [Cl/F] was decreased by 42%, and the half-life was unchanged when a single 2-mg dose of haloperidol was administered to 24 healthy subjects who were at steady-state on a venlafaxine dosage of 150 mg per day administered as 75 mg every 12 hours)

» Moclobemide
 (because of the potentially fatal consequences of combining nonselective, irreversible monoamine oxidase inhibitors with venlafaxine, and the increased risk of developing the serotonin syndrome with combined use of venlafaxine and the reversible monoamine oxidase-A inhibitor moclobemide, concurrent use is not recommended and a wash-out period of 3 to 7 days is advised between the use of one medication and the other)

## Venlafaxine (Systemic)

» Monoamine oxidase (MAO) inhibitors, including furazolidone, procarbazine, and selegiline
(concurrent use of MAO inhibitors with venlafaxine may result in confusion, agitation, restlessness, and gastrointestinal symptoms, or possibly hyperpyretic episodes, severe convulsions, hypertensive crises, or the serotonin syndrome; concurrent use of an MAO inhibitor with venlafaxine is **contraindicated**; at least 14 days should elapse between discontinuation of an MAO inhibitor and initiation of venlafaxine; at least 7 days should elapse between discontinuation of venlafaxine and initiation of an MAO inhibitor)

» Serotonergics or other medications or substances with serotonergic activity (see *Appendix II*)
(increased risk of development of the serotonin syndrome, a rare but potentially fatal hyperserotonergic state which may occur in patients receiving serotonergic medications, usually in combination; symptoms typically occur shortly [hours to days] after the addition of a serotonergic agent to a regimen that includes serotonin-enhancing drugs; symptoms include agitation, diaphoresis, diarrhea, fever, hyperreflexia, incoordination, mental status changes [confusion, hypomania], myoclonus, shivering, or tremor; effects including cardiac arryhthmias, coma, disseminated intravascular coagulation, hyper- or hypo-tension, renal failure, respiratory failure, seizures, and severe hyperthermia have been reported also)

### Laboratory value alterations
The following have been selected on the basis of their potential clinical significance (possible effect in parentheses where appropriate)—not necessarily inclusive (» = major clinical significance):

With physiology/laboratory test values
Blood pressure
(dose-related sustained hypertension, defined as supine diastolic blood pressure measurements on three consecutive visits that are ≥ 90 mm Hg and that are increased over baseline by ≥ 10 mm Hg, has been reported)

Cholesterol, serum
(mean increases in serum cholesterol concentrations of 3 mg/dL from baseline have been reported; the clinical significance of this finding is not known)

Electrocardiogram (ECG)
(mean change in corrected QT interval [QT$_c$] in 357 patients receiving the extended-release dosage form of venlafaxine was an increase of 4.7 milliseconds [msec] as opposed to a 1.9 msec decrease in 285 placebo-treated patients)

Pulse
(heart rate increases of three to nine beats per minute have been reported, with a mean increase of four beats per minute)

### Medical considerations/Contraindications
The medical considerations/contraindications included have been selected on the basis of their potential clinical significance (reasons given in parentheses where appropriate)—not necessarily inclusive (» = major clinical significance).

*Risk-benefit should be considered when the following medical problems exist:*

» Blood pressure problems or
» Cardiac disease
(sustained hypertension or orthostatic hypotension induced by venlafaxine may exacerbate these conditions)

» Hepatic function impairment
(metabolism of venlafaxine may be altered; large interindividual variation in venlafaxine clearance is seen in these patients; patients with moderate to severe impairment may require dosage reductions of 50% or more)

» Mania, history of
(activation of hypomania or mania has been reported in depressed patients treated with venlafaxine)

Neurological impairment, including mental retardation
(risk of seizures may be increased)

» Renal function impairment
(excretion of venlafaxine may be altered; large interindividual variation in venlafaxine clearance is seen in these patients; patients with mild to moderate impairment may require dosage reductions of 25 to 50%; patients undergoing hemodialysis should receive a dosage reduction of 50% and the dose should be administered after the dialysis session is completed)

Seizures, history of
(as with other antidepressants, venlafaxine should be introduced with caution; if seizures develop, venlafaxine should be discontinued)

Sensitivity to venlafaxine
Weight loss
(loss of ≥ 5% of baseline body weight occurred in 6% of patients receiving venlafaxine in clinical trials and in 1% of patients receiving placebo; significant weight loss, if it occurs, may be undesirable in some patients)

### Patient monitoring
The following may be especially important in patient monitoring (other tests may be warranted in some patients, depending on condition; » = major clinical significance):

Blood pressure measurements
(recommended at regular intervals because of sustained increases in blood pressure associated with venlafaxine treatment; dosage reduction or discontinuation of venlafaxine treatment should be considered in patients who develop sustained increases in blood pressure)

Careful supervision of depressed patients with suicidal tendencies
(recommended especially during early treatment phase before peak effectiveness of venlafaxine is achieved; prescribing the smallest number of tablets necessary for good patient management is recommended to decrease the risk of overdose)

## Side/Adverse Effects
Note: Venlafaxine is generally well-tolerated, with evidence of dose-dependency for some of the most common adverse effects. In addition, there is evidence of adaptation with continuing therapy to some effects such as nausea, vomiting, somnolence, and dizziness.

The following side/adverse effects have been selected on the basis of their potential clinical significance (possible signs and symptoms in parentheses where appropriate)—not necessarily inclusive:

### Those indicating need for medical attention
Incidence more frequent
*Headache; hypertension* (high blood pressure)—usually asymptomatic; *sexual dysfunction, including anorgasmia; decreased libido; delayed ejaculation; or impotence* (decrease in sexual desire or ability); *vision disturbances, including abnormal accommodation; and blurred vision*

Note: *Sexual dysfunction* may be dose-related and does not show evidence of adaptation with continuing venlafaxine therapy.
Venlafaxine-induced sustained *hypertension*, defined as supine diastolic blood pressure measurements on three consecutive visits that are ≥ 90 mm Hg and that are increased over baseline by ≥ 10 mm Hg, is reported to be dose-dependent.

Probability of Sustained Hypertension*

| Venlafaxine Dose (mg/day) | Incidence (%) |
|---|---|
| < 100 | 3 |
| 101 to 200 | 5 |
| 201 to 300 | 7 |
| > 300 | 13 |
| Placebo | 2 |

*Estimated by the manufacturer from pooled data of premarketing studies of the prompt-release dosage form.

Incidence less frequent
*Cardiovascular effects, other, including chest pain; palpitation* (feeling of fast or irregular heartbeat); *and tachycardia* (fast heartbeat); *CNS effects* (mood or mental changes); *including abnormal thinking; agitation; confusion; depersonalization; and emotional lability; tinnitus* (ringing or buzzing in ears)

Incidence rare
*Dyspnea* (trouble in breathing); *edema* (swelling); *itching or skin rash; mania or hypomania* (talking, feeling, and acting with excitement and activity one cannot control); *menstrual changes; orthostatic hypotension* (lightheadedness or fainting)—especially when getting up suddenly from a sitting or lying position; *seizures* (convulsions); *trismus* (lockjaw); *urinary effects, including impaired urination; urinary frequency; urinary incontinence; or urinary retention* (problems in urinating or in holding urine)

### Those indicating need for medical attention only if they continue or are bothersome
Incidence more frequent
*Abnormal dreams; anorexia* (loss of appetite); *anxiety or nervousness; asthenia* (unusual tiredness or weakness); *chills; constipation; diarrhea; dizziness; dryness of mouth; dyspepsia* (heartburn); *increased sweating; insomnia* (trouble in sleeping); *nausea; paresthesia* (tingling, burning, or prickly sensations); *rhinitis* (stuffy or runny nose); *somnolence* (drowsiness); *stomach pain or gas; tremor* (trembling or shaking); *vomiting; weight loss*

Note: *Anorexia, chills, dizziness, nausea, somnolence, sweating, tremor, vomiting,* and *weight loss* may be dose-related. Loss of ≥ 5% of baseline body weight occurred in 6% of patients in clinical trials of venlafaxine.

Incidence less frequent
  *Hypertonia* (muscle tension); *taste perversion* (change in sense of taste); *yawning*

**Those indicating the need for medical attention if they occur after medication is discontinued**
  *Asthenia* (unusual tiredness or weakness); *changes in dreaming; dizziness; dryness of mouth; headache; increased sweating; insomnia* (trouble in sleeping); *nausea; nervousness*

## Overdose

For specific information on the agents used in the management of venlafaxine overdose, see *Charcoal, Activated (Oral-Local)* monograph.

For more information on the management of overdose or unintentional ingestion, **contact a Poison Control Center** (see *Poison Control Center Listing*).

**Clinical effects of overdose**
The following effects have been selected on the basis of their potential clinical significance (possible signs and symptoms in parentheses where appropriate)—not necessarily inclusive:

  *Agitation; electrocardiogram (ECG) changes, specifically $QT_c$ prolongation; lethargy* (extreme tiredness or weakness); *paresthesia* (tingling, burning, or prickling sensations); *seizures; sinus tachycardia* (fast heartbeat); *somnolence* (drowsiness); *tremor* (trembling or shaking)

  Note: Only a small number of overdose cases were reported during premarketing studies of venlafaxine. In most of these cases, no symptoms were reported. However, there have been postmarketing reports of fatalities occurring with venlafaxine overdose, predominantly when alcohol or other drugs were co-ingested.

  Overdosage with venlafaxine may result in development of the serotonin syndrome, a potentially fatal hyperserotonergic state. Symptoms include agitation, diaphoresis, diarrhea, fever, hyperreflexia, incoordination, mental status changes (confusion, hypomania), myoclonus, shivering, and tremor. The non-specific serotonergic receptor antagonists cyproheptadine and methysergide have been reported to be of some use in shortening the duration of the serotonin syndrome.

**Treatment of overdose**
There is no specific antidote for venlafaxine. Treatment is essentially symptomatic and supportive.
  To decrease absorption—
    Considering use of activated charcoal or gastric lavage.
  Monitoring—
    Monitoring cardiac function and vital signs.
  Supportive care—
    Ensuring adequate airway patency, oxygenation, and ventilation. Patients in whom intentional overdose is known or suspected should be referred for psychiatric consultation.
  Note: Due to the large volume of distribution of venlafaxine, forced diuresis, dialysis, hemoperfusion, or exchange transfusion is not likely to be of benefit. In six patients undergoing hemodialysis, less than 5% of an administered dose of venlafaxine was recovered in dialysis fluid as venlafaxine and *O*-desmethylvenlafaxine (ODV).

## Patient Consultation

As an aid to patient consultation, refer to *Advice for the Patient, Venlafaxine (Systemic)*.

In providing consultation, consider emphasizing the following selected information (» = major clinical significance):

**Before using this medication**
» Conditions affecting use, especially:
    Sensitivity to venlafaxine
    Contraindicated medications—MAO inhibitors
    Other medications, especially serotonergics and other medications or substances with serotonergic activity
    Other medical problems, especially blood pressure problems, cardiac disease, or hepatic or renal function impairment

**Proper use of this medication**
» Compliance with therapy; not taking more or less medicine than prescribed
» Four weeks or more of therapy may be required before antidepressant effects are achieved
  Taking with food to lessen gastrointestinal effects

» For extended-release dosage form: Swallowing capsule whole with fluid; not dividing, crushing, chewing, or placing in liquid
» Proper dosing
  Missed dose:
    For prompt-release dosage form—Taking as soon as possible unless it is within 2 hours of next dose; continuing on regular schedule with next dose; not doubling doses
    For extended-release dosage form—Taking as soon as possible if remembered the same day; continuing on regular schedule with next dose; not doubling doses
» Proper storage

**Precautions while using this medication**
  Regular visits to physician to check progress of therapy
» Notifying physician immediately if any signs or symptoms of allergic reaction, such as skin rash or hives, occur
  Checking with physician before discontinuing medication
  Avoiding use of alcoholic beverages; not taking other CNS depressants unless prescribed by physician
» Caution when driving or doing other jobs requiring alertness, judgment, or clear vision until effects of medication are known
» Possible dizziness or lightheadedness; caution when getting up from a lying or sitting position

**Side/adverse effects**
  Possibility of discontinuation symptoms
  Signs of potential side effects, especially headache; hypertension; sexual dysfunction; vision disturbances; cardiovascular effects, other; CNS effects; tinnitus; dyspnea; edema; itching or skin rash; mania or hypomania; menstrual changes; orthostatic hypotension; seizures; urinary effects

## General Dosing Information

Abrupt discontinuation of venlafaxine may result in symptoms of withdrawal, including asthenia, changes in dreaming, dizziness, dryness of mouth, headache, increased sweating, insomnia, nausea, and nervousness. It is recommended that patients taking venlafaxine for longer than 1 week be tapered off the drug; venlafaxine should be discontinued gradually over 2 weeks or longer in patients receiving therapy for 6 weeks or longer. In clinical trials, the extended-release dosage form was tapered in decrements of 75 mg per day at 1-week intervals.

Potentially suicidal patients should not have access to large quantities of this medication since depressed patients, particularly those who may use alcohol excessively, may continue to exhibit suicidal tendencies until significant improvement occurs. Some clinicians recommend that the patient be supplied with the smallest quantity of medication necessary for satisfactory patient management.

Activation of hypomania or mania has been reported in depressed patients treated with venlafaxine.

Patients receiving the prompt-release dosage form of venlafaxine may change to the extended-release dosage form at the most nearly equivalent mg per day dosage available.

**Diet/Nutrition**
Venlafaxine should be taken with food to lessen gastrointestinal side effects.

## Oral Dosage Forms

Note: The available dosage forms contain venlafaxine hydrochloride, but dosage and strength are expressed in terms of the base.

### VENLAFAXINE EXTENDED-RELEASE CAPSULES

**Usual adult dose**
Antidepressant—
  Oral, initially 75 mg (base) a day in a single dose, taken with food, in the morning or evening. Some patients may require an initial dosage of 37.5 mg (base) a day for four to seven days in order to adjust to the medication. The dosage may be increased, as needed and tolerated, in increments of 75 mg a day at intervals of at least four days.

Note: Patients with moderate hepatic function impairment should receive an initial dosage reduction of 50%. Patients with renal function impairment should receive an initial dosage reduction of 25 to 50%. The total daily dose for patients undergoing hemodialysis should be reduced by 50% and the dose should be administered after completion of the dialysis session.

**Usual adult prescribing limits**
225 mg per day. The maximum recommended dosage of 225 mg per day reflects experience in moderately depressed outpatients. However, severely depressed inpatients in a study using the prompt-release dosage form responded to dosages up to 375 mg per day. There is little expe-

## Venlafaxine (Systemic)

rience with the extended-release dosage form at dosages above 225 mg per day, and whether severely depressed patients will respond to higher dosages has not been established.

**Usual pediatric dose**
Safety and efficacy have not been established.

**Usual geriatric dose**
See *Usual adult dose*.

Note: Although no special dosage adjustments based on age are recommended generally, some clinicians recommend a reduced initial dosage and more gradual dosage increases in elderly patients.

**Strength(s) usually available**
U.S.—
- 37.5 mg (base) (Rx) [*Effexor XR* (cellulose; ethylcellulose; gelatin; hydroxypropyl methylcellulose; iron oxide; titanium dioxide)].
- 75 mg (base) (Rx) [*Effexor XR* (cellulose; ethylcellulose; gelatin; hydroxypropyl methylcellulose; iron oxide; titanium dioxide)].
- 150 mg (base) (Rx) [*Effexor XR* (cellulose; ethylcellulose; gelatin; hydroxypropyl methylcellulose; iron oxide; titanium dioxide)].

Canada—
- 37.5 mg (base) (Rx) [*Effexor XR*].
- 75 mg (base) (Rx) [*Effexor XR*].
- 150 mg (base) (Rx) [*Effexor XR*].

**Packaging and storage**
Store between 20 and 25 °C (68 and 77 °F) in a well-closed container unless otherwise specified by manufacturer.

**Auxiliary labeling**
- Avoid alcoholic beverages.
- May cause drowsiness.
- Swallow capsules whole. Do not break or chew.
- Take with food.

Note: Release of venlafaxine from extended-release capsule is membrane-controlled and is not dependent upon pH.

### VENLAFAXINE TABLETS

**Usual adult dose**

Antidepressant—
Oral, initially 75 mg a day, administered in two or three divided doses and taken with food. The dosage may be increased, as needed and tolerated, in increments up to 75 mg a day at intervals of no less than four days, up to 225 mg a day. Although dosages over 225 mg a day have not been shown to be useful in moderately depressed outpatients, more severely depressed patients may respond to dosages of up to 375 mg a day, administered in three divided doses.

Note: Some clinicians recommend an initial dosage of 50 mg a day administered in two divided doses in the treatment of mild depression in order to minimize nausea.

In patients with moderate to severe hepatic function impairment—Dosage reductions of 50% or more are recommended.

In patients with renal function impairment—Mild to moderate: Dosage reductions of 25% are recommended. Moderate to severe ($CL_{cr}$ < 30 mL/min): Dosage should be reduced by 50%. The dose may be administered once a day because of the prolonged half-life. In dialysis patients: Total daily dose should be reduced by 50%, and administration withheld until dialysis treatment is completed.

**Usual adult prescribing limits**
375 mg a day.

**Usual pediatric dose**
Safety and efficacy in children up to 18 years of age have not been established.

**Usual geriatric dose**
See *Usual adult dose*.

Note: Although no special dosage adjustments based on age are recommended generally, some clinicians recommend a reduced initial dosage and more gradual dosage increases in elderly patients.

**Strength(s) usually available**
U.S.—
- 25 mg (base) (Rx) [*Effexor* (scored; cellulose; iron oxides; lactose; magnesium stearate; sodium starch glycolate)].
- 37.5 mg (base) (Rx) [*Effexor* (scored; cellulose; iron oxides; lactose; magnesium stearate; sodium starch glycolate)].
- 50 mg (base) (Rx) [*Effexor* (scored; cellulose; iron oxides; lactose; magnesium stearate; sodium starch glycolate)].
- 75 mg (base) (Rx) [*Effexor* (scored; cellulose; iron oxides; lactose; magnesium stearate; sodium starch glycolate)].
- 100 mg (base) (Rx) [*Effexor* (scored; cellulose; iron oxides; lactose; magnesium stearate; sodium starch glycolate)].

Canada—
- 37.5 mg (base) (Rx) [*Effexor* (scored; cosmetic brown iron oxide; ferric oxide NF yellow; lactose NF hydrous; magnesium stearate NF; microcrystalline cellulose NF; sodium starch glycolate NF)].
- 75 mg (base) (Rx) [*Effexor* (scored; cosmetic brown iron oxide; ferric oxide NF yellow; lactose NF hydrous; magnesium stearate NF; microcrystalline cellulose NF; sodium starch glycolate NF)].

**Packaging and storage**
Store in a dry place between 20 and 25 °C (68 and 77 °F) in a well-closed container unless otherwise specified by manufacturer.

**Auxiliary labeling**
- Avoid alcoholic beverages.
- May cause drowsiness.
- Take with food.

### Selected Bibliography

Ellingrod VL, Perry PJ. Venlafaxine: a heterocyclic antidepressant. Am J Hosp Pharm 1994 Dec 15; 51: 3033-46.

Holliday SM, Benfield P. Venlafaxine. A review of its pharmacology and therapeutic potential in depression. Drugs 1995; 49(2): 280-94.

Developed: 05/24/95
Revised: 05/21/98
Interim revision: 08/07/98

---

**VERAPAMIL**—See *Calcium Channel Blocking Agents (Systemic)*

---

# VIDARABINE Ophthalmic

VA CLASSIFICATION (Primary): OP203

Commonly used brand name(s): *Vira-A*.

Other commonly used names are arabinoside and ara-A.

Note: For a listing of dosage forms and brand names by country availability, see *Dosage Forms* section(s).

## Category
Antiviral (ophthalmic).

## Indications

**Accepted**
Keratitis, herpes simplex virus (treatment) or
Keratoconjunctivitis, herpes simplex virus (treatment)—Ophthalmic vidarabine is indicated in the treatment of acute keratoconjunctivitis and recurrent epithelial keratitis caused by herpes simplex virus (HSV), types 1 and 2.

Vidarabine also may be indicated in patients with superficial herpetic keratitis who do not respond to idoxuridine or who develop ocular toxicity or hypersensitivity to idoxuridine.

**Unaccepted**
Vidarabine is not indicated for the treatment of infections caused by RNA viruses or adenoviruses, in other infections (bacterial, fungal, chlamydial), or in nonviral trophic ulcers.

## Pharmacology/Pharmacokinetics

**Physicochemical characteristics**
Molecular weight—285.26.

**Mechanism of action/Effect**
Vidarabine is phosphorylated intracellularly to arabinosyl adenosine monophosphate (ara-AMP) or the triphosphate (ara-ATP). These cause preferential inhibition of viral DNA polymerase, inhibition of virus-induced ribonucleotide reductase, or inhibition of other virus-specific enzymes involved in DNA synthesis that are more sensitive to inhibition than the corresponding host cell enzymes. This inhibition prevents length-

ening of the DNA chain. Vidarabine may also be incorporated into both mammalian and viral DNA.

**Absorption**
Systemic absorption is unlikely following ocular administration even when nasolacrimal secretions are swallowed, since vidarabine is rapidly deaminated in the gastrointestinal tract.

**Distribution**
Because of low solubility, trace amounts of vidarabine and its metabolite, ara-hx, can be detected in the aqueous humor only if there is a corneal epithelial defect. When the cornea is intact, trace amounts of the metabolite only are found in the aqueous humor.

**Biotransformation**
Vidarabine is rapidly deaminated by adenosine deaminase to arabinosyl hypoxanthine (ara-hx). Ara-hx is the primary metabolite, which also has antiviral activity, although much less than vidarabine. Vidarabine and arabinosyl hypoxanthine may act synergistically to inhibit DNA viral replication.

## Precautions to Consider

**Carcinogenicity/Tumorigenicity**
Chronic studies in mice given vidarabine intramuscularly have shown that vidarabine causes a statistically significant increase in hepatic tumors in female mice and renal neoplasia in male mice.
Chronic studies in rats given vidarabine intramuscularly have shown that intestinal, testicular, and thyroid neoplasia occurred more frequently in rats given vidarabine than in control animals. Male rats given doses of 50 mg per kg of body weight (mg/kg) per day and female rats given doses of 30 mg/kg per day showed statistically significant increases in the incidence of thyroid adenomas.

**Mutagenicity**
In vitro studies have shown that vidarabine may be incorporated into mammalian DNA and may induce mutations in mammalian cells (mouse L5178Y cell line). The in vivo dominant lethal assay in mice, although not as conclusive, has shown some evidence that vidarabine may cause mutagenic effects in male germ cells.
In vitro studies also have shown that vidarabine causes chromosome breaks and gaps when added to human leukocytes.

**Pregnancy/Reproduction**
Pregnancy—Adequate and well-controlled studies in humans have not been done. The possibility of embryonic or fetal damage in pregnant women is remote, since the ophthalmic dose of vidarabine is small, vidarabine is relatively insoluble, and ocular penetration of vidarabine is very low.
Studies in rats and rabbits have shown that vidarabine given parenterally is teratogenic. Fetal abnormalities have been reported in rabbits that had 10% vidarabine ointment applied to 10% of the body surface during organogenesis. There were no fetal abnormalities reported when the ointment was applied to only 2 to 3% of the body surface, a dose that greatly exceeds the total recommended human ophthalmic dose.
FDA Pregnancy Category C.

**Breast-feeding**
It is not known whether vidarabine, applied ophthalmically, is absorbed systemically and distributed into breast milk. However, it is unlikely, since the ophthalmic dose of vidarabine is small, vidarabine is relatively insoluble, ocular penetration of vidarabine is very low, and vidarabine is rapidly deaminated in the gastrointestinal tract even when nasolacrimal secretions are swallowed.

**Pediatrics**
Appropriate studies on the relationship of age to the effects of vidarabine have not been performed in the pediatric population. However, no pediatrics-specific problems have been documented to date.

**Geriatrics**
Appropriate studies on the relationship of age to the effects of vidarabine have not been performed in the geriatric population. However, no geriatrics-specific problems have been documented to date.

**Medical considerations/Contraindications**
The medical considerations/contraindications included have been selected on the basis of their potential clinical significance (reasons given in parentheses where appropriate)—not necessarily inclusive (» = major clinical significance):

*Risk-benefit should be considered when the following medical problem exists:*
   Sensitivity to vidarabine

**Patient monitoring**
The following may be especially important in patient monitoring (other tests may be warranted in some patients, depending on condition; » = major clinical significance):

   Ophthalmologic, including slit-lamp, examinations
      (may be required periodically during therapy)

## Side/Adverse Effects

The following side/adverse effects have been selected on the basis of their potential clinical significance (possible signs and symptoms in parentheses where appropriate)—not necessarily inclusive:

**Those indicating need for medical attention**
Incidence not reported
   *Hypersensitivity* (itching, redness, swelling, pain, burning, or other signs of irritation not present before therapy); *increased sensitivity of eyes to light*

**Those indicating need for medical attention only if they continue or are bothersome**
Incidence not reported
   *Feeling of something in the eye; lacrimal punctal stenosis or occlusion* (excess flow of tears)

## Patient Consultation

As an aid to patient consultation, refer to *Advice for the Patient, Vidarabine (Ophthalmic)*.
In providing consultation, consider emphasizing the following selected information (» = major clinical significance):

**Before using this medication**
» Conditions affecting use, especially:
   Sensitivity to vidarabine

**Proper use of this medication**
   Proper administration technique for ophthalmic ointment
» Not using more frequently or for longer than ordered by physician
» Compliance with full course of therapy
» Proper dosing
   Missed dose: Applying as soon as possible; not applying if almost time for next dose
» Proper storage

**Precautions while using this medication**
   Blurred vision after application of ophthalmic ointments
   Importance of keeping appointments with physician; checking with physician if symptoms become worse
   Possible photophobic reactions; wearing sunglasses and avoiding prolonged exposure to bright light

**Side/adverse effects**
   Signs of potential side effects, especially hypersensitivity or increased sensitivity of eyes to light

## General Dosing Information

Vidarabine may be administered concurrently with antibiotics (gentamicin, erythromycin, and chloramphenicol) and corticosteroids (prednisolone and dexamethasone). Corticosteroids can accelerate the spread of viral infections and usually are contraindicated alone in superficial herpes simplex virus keratitis. However, corticosteroids may be used concurrently with vidarabine in the treatment of herpes simplex infections. Vidarabine should be continued for a few days after the corticosteroid has been discontinued.

Treatment should usually not be continued for more than a total of 21 days or for more than 3 to 5 days after healing is complete. However, chronic or particularly difficult infections may require a longer treatment period. Too frequent administration may result in small, punctate defects in the cornea.

## Ophthalmic Dosage Forms

### VIDARABINE OPHTHALMIC OINTMENT USP

**Usual adult and adolescent dose**
Ophthalmic antiviral—
   Topical, to the conjunctiva, a thin strip (approximately 1.25 cm) of ointment every three hours (five times a day). Treatment should be continued until the cornea is completely re-epithelialized. Dose then may be reduced to 1.25 cm of ointment two times a day for an additional seven days.

**Usual pediatric dose**
See *Usual adult and adolescent dose*.

## Vidarabine (Ophthalmic)

**Strength(s) usually available**
U.S.—
 3% (monohydrate) (each gram of ophthalmic ointment contains 30 mg of vidarabine monohydrate, equivalent to 28.11 mg of anhydrous vidarabine) (Rx) [*Vira-A*].

Canada—
 3% (monohydrate) (each gram of ophthalmic ointment contains 30 mg of vidarabine monohydrate, equivalent to 28.11 mg of anhydrous vidarabine) (Rx) [*Vira-A*].

**Packaging and storage**
Store below 40 °C (104 °F), preferably between 15 and 30 °C (59 and 86 °F), unless otherwise specified by manufacturer. Protect from freezing.

**Auxiliary labeling**
- For the eye.
- Continue medicine for full time of treatment.
- Do not use more often or longer than ordered.

Revised: 07/01/93

---

# VINBLASTINE Systemic

VA CLASSIFICATION (Primary): AN900
Commonly used brand name(s): *Velban; Velbe*.

Note: For a listing of dosage forms and brand names by country availability, see *Dosage Forms* section(s).

## Category
Antineoplastic.

## Indications

Note: Bracketed information in the *Indications* section refers to uses that are not included in U.S. product labeling.

**Accepted**
Carcinoma, breast (treatment)
Tumors, trophoblastic, gestational (treatment)
Carcinoma, testicular (treatment)
[Carcinoma, bladder (treatment)][1]
[Carcinoma, lung, non–small cell (treatment)][1] or
[Carcinoma, renal (treatment)][1]—Vinblastine is indicated for treatment of breast carcinoma unresponsive to appropriate endocrine surgery and hormonal therapy, choriocarcinoma resistant to other chemotherapeutic agents, and advanced testicular germ cell carcinomas (embryonal carcinoma, teratocarcinoma, and choriocarcinoma). Vinblastine also is indicated for treatment of bladder carcinoma, non–small cell lung carcinoma, and renal carcinoma.

Lymphomas, Hodgkin's (treatment) or
Lymphomas, non-Hodgkin's (treatment)—Vinblastine is indicated for treatment of generalized Hodgkin's disease (Stages III and IV, Ann Arbor modification of Rye staging system) and for treatment of lymphocytic lymphoma (nodular and diffuse, poorly and well differentiated) and histiocytic lymphoma.

Sarcoma, Kaposi's (treatment)—Vinblastine is indicated for treatment of Kaposi's sarcoma, including [acquired immunodeficiency syndrome (AIDS)-associated Kaposi's sarcoma][1] by intravenous or intralesional injection.

Letterer-Siwe disease (treatment)—Vinblastine is indicated for treatment of Letterer-Siwe disease (histiocytosis X; Langerhans' cell histiocytoses).

Mycosis fungoides (treatment)—Vinblastine is indicated for treatment of advanced stages of mycosis fungoides.

[Carcinoma, prostatic (treatment)][1]—Vinblastine is indicated as reasonable medical therapy for treatment of prostatic carcinoma (Evidence rating: IIID).

[Melanoma, malignant (treatment)][1]—Vinblastine is indicated for treatment of metastatic malignant melanoma.

[Tumors, germ cell, ovarian (treatment)][1]—Vinblastine is indicated for treatment of germ cell ovarian tumors.

[1]Not included in Canadian product labeling.

## Pharmacology/Pharmacokinetics

**Physicochemical characteristics**
Source—Vinblastine is a vinca alkaloid.
Molecular weight—909.07.

**Mechanism of action/Effect**
Vinblastine blocks mitosis by arresting cells in metaphase, and may also interfere with amino acid metabolism; it is cell cycle–specific for the M phase of cell division.

**Distribution**
Does not cross the blood-brain barrier in significant amounts.

**Biotransformation**
Hepatic; metabolism of vinca alkaloids has been shown to be mediated by hepatic cytochrome P450 3A isoenzymes.

**Half-life**
Following rapid intravenous administration—
 Initial phase: 3.7 minutes.
 Middle phase: 1.6 hours.
 Terminal phase: 24.8 hours.

**Elimination**
Primary route—Biliary/fecal.
Secondary route—Renal.

## Precautions to Consider

**Carcinogenicity/Mutagenicity**
Secondary malignancies are potential delayed effects of many antineoplastic agents, although it is not clear whether the effect is related to their mutagenic or immunosuppressive action. The effects of dose and duration of therapy are also unknown, although risk seems to increase with long-term use.

In studies in rats and mice, administration of the maximum tolerated dose of vinblastine and half of the maximum tolerated dose for 6 months did not show a clear relationship between vinblastine and tumor development. The test demonstrated that other agents were clearly carcinogenic; however, vinblastine was one of the drugs in the group of drugs that caused slightly increased or the same tumor incidence as controls.

**Pregnancy/Reproduction**
Fertility—Gonadal suppression, resulting in amenorrhea or azoospermia, has occurred in patients taking vinblastine. In general, these effects appear to be related to dose and length of therapy and may be irreversible. Prediction of the degree of testicular or ovarian function impairment is complicated by the common use of combinations of several antineoplastics, which makes it difficult to assess the effects of individual agents. Vinblastine also has been reported to cause aspermia.

Pregnancy—In general, use of a contraceptive is recommended during cytotoxic drug therapy.

First trimester: It is usually recommended that use of antineoplastics, especially combination chemotherapy, be avoided whenever possible, especially during the first trimester. Although information is limited because of the relatively few instances of antineoplastic administration during pregnancy, the mutagenic, teratogenic, and carcinogenic potential of these medications must be considered.

Administration of vinblastine to animals early in pregnancy results in fetal resorption with surviving fetuses showing gross deformities.

Other hazards to the fetus include adverse reactions seen in adults.

FDA Pregnancy Category D.

**Breast-feeding**
Although very little information is available regarding distribution of antineoplastic agents into breast milk, breast-feeding is not recommended while vinblastine is being administered because of the risks to the infant (adverse effects, mutagenicity, carcinogenicity). It is not known whether vinblastine is distributed into breast milk.

**Pediatrics**
Studies performed to date have not demonstrated pediatrics-specific problems that would limit the usefulness of this medication in children.

**Geriatrics**
Although appropriate studies with vinblastine have not been performed in the geriatric population, the leukopenic response may be increased in elderly patients suffering from malnutrition or skin ulcers.

**Dental**
The bone marrow depressant effects of vinblastine may result in an increased incidence of microbial infection, delayed healing, and gingival bleeding. Dental work, whenever possible, should be completed prior

to initiation of therapy or deferred until blood counts have returned to normal. Patients should be instructed in proper oral hygiene during treatment, including caution in use of regular toothbrushes, dental floss, and toothpicks.

Vinblastine may also cause stomatitis associated with considerable discomfort.

### Drug interactions and/or related problems

The following drug interactions and/or related problems have been selected on the basis of their potential clinical significance (possible mechanism in parentheses where appropriate)—not necessarily inclusive (» = major clinical significance):

Note: Combinations containing any of the following medications, depending on the amount present, may also interact with this medication.

Allopurinol or
Colchicine or
» Probenecid or
» Sulfinpyrazone
(vinblastine may raise the concentration of blood uric acid; dosage adjustment of antigout agents may be necessary to control hyperuricemia and gout; allopurinol may be preferred to prevent or reverse vinblastine-induced hyperuricemia because of risk of uric acid nephropathy with uricosuric antigout agents)

Blood dyscrasia–causing medications (see *Appendix II*)
(leukopenic and/or thrombocytopenic effects of vinblastine may be increased with concurrent or recent therapy if these medications cause the same effects; dosage adjustment of vinblastine, if necessary, should be based on blood counts)

» Bone marrow depressants, other (see *Appendix II*) or
Radiation therapy
(additive bone marrow depression may occur; dosage reduction may be required when two or more bone marrow depressants, including radiation, are used concurrently or consecutively)

Vaccines, killed virus
(because normal defense mechanisms may be suppressed by vinblastine therapy, the patient's antibody response to the vaccine may be decreased. The interval between discontinuation of medications that cause immunosuppression and restoration of the patient's ability to respond to the vaccine depends on the intensity and type of immunosuppression-causing medication used, the underlying disease, and other factors; estimates vary from 3 months to 1 year)

» Vaccines, live virus
(because normal defense mechanisms may be suppressed by vinblastine therapy, concurrent use with a live virus vaccine may potentiate the replication of the vaccine virus, may increase the side/adverse effects of the vaccine virus, and/or may decrease the patient's antibody response to the vaccine; immunization of these patients should be undertaken only with extreme caution after careful review of the patient's hematologic status and only with the knowledge and consent of the physician managing the vinblastine therapy. The interval between discontinuation of medications that cause immunosuppression and restoration of the patient's ability to respond to the vaccine depends on the intensity and type of immunosuppression-causing medication used, the underlying disease, and other factors; estimates vary from 3 months to 1 year. Immunization with oral poliovirus vaccine should also be postponed in persons in close contact with the patient, especially family members)

### Laboratory value alterations

The following have been selected on the basis of their potential clinical significance (possible effect in parentheses where appropriate)—not necessarily inclusive (» = major clinical significance):

With physiology/laboratory test values
Uric acid concentrations in blood and urine
(may be increased)

### Medical considerations/Contraindications

The medical considerations/contraindications included have been selected on the basis of their potential clinical significance (reasons given in parentheses where appropriate)—not necessarily inclusive (» = major clinical significance).

***Risk-benefit should be considered when the following medical problems exist:***

» Bone marrow depression
» Chickenpox, existing or recent (including recent exposure) or
» Herpes zoster
(risk of severe generalized disease)

Gout, history of or
Urate renal stones, history of
(risk of hyperuricemia)

» Hepatic function impairment
(a 50% dosage reduction is recommended for patients with a direct serum bilirubin concentration greater than 3 mg per 100 mL)

» Infection
Sensitivity to vinblastine

» Tumor cell infiltration of bone marrow
(in patients with malignant-cell infiltration of bone marrow, leukocyte and platelet counts have been reported to fall precipitously following administration of moderate doses of vinblastine; further administration of vinblastine in such patients is not recommended)

» Caution should be used also in patients who have had previous cytotoxic drug therapy or radiation therapy.

### Patient monitoring

The following may be especially important in patient monitoring (other tests may be warranted in some patients, depending on condition; » = major clinical significance):

Alanine aminotransferase (ALT [SGPT]), serum and
Aspartate aminotransferase (AST [SGOT]), serum and
Bilirubin, serum and
Lactate dehydrogenase (LDH)
(determinations recommended prior to initiation of therapy and at periodic intervals during therapy; frequency varies according to clinical state, agent, dose, and other agents being used concurrently; toxicity may be enhanced in the presence of hepatic insufficiency)

» Hematocrit or hemoglobin and
» Platelet count and
» Total and, if appropriate, differential leukocyte count
(determinations recommended prior to initiation of therapy and at periodic intervals during therapy; frequency varies according to clinical state, agent, dose, and other agents being used concurrently)

Uric acid concentrations, serum
(determinations recommended prior to initiation of therapy and at periodic intervals during therapy; frequency varies according to clinical state, agent, dose, and other agents being used concurrently)

## Side/Adverse Effects

Note: Many "side effects" of antineoplastic therapy are unavoidable and represent the medication's pharmacologic action. Some of these (for example, leukopenia and thrombocytopenia) are actually used as parameters to aid in individual dosage titration.
Incidence of side effects is generally dose-related.

The following side/adverse effects have been selected on the basis of their potential clinical significance (possible signs and symptoms in parentheses where appropriate)—not necessarily inclusive:

### Those indicating need for medical attention

Incidence more frequent
*Leukopenia* (fever or chills; cough or hoarseness; lower back or side pain; painful or difficult urination)—usually asymptomatic

Note: With *leukopenia*, the nadir of the leukocyte count occurs 5 to 10 days after the last day of administration, and recovery is usually complete within another 7 to 14 days.

Incidence less frequent
*Cellulitis* (pain or redness at site of injection)—caused by extravasation; *hyperuricemia or uric acid nephropathy* (joint pain; lower back or side pain; swelling of feet or lower legs); *stomatitis* (sores in mouth and on lips); *thrombocytopenia, transient* (unusual bleeding or bruising; black, tarry stools; blood in urine or stools; pinpoint red spots on skin)—usually asymptomatic

Note: *Hyperuricemia or uric acid nephropathy* occurs most commonly during initial treatment of patients with lymphoma as a result of rapid cell breakdown that leads to elevated serum uric acid concentrations.

Incidence rare
*Rectal bleeding, hemorrhagic colitis, or bleeding from a previously existing peptic ulcer* (black, tarry stools); *neurotoxicity* (difficulty in walking; dizziness; double vision; drooping eyelids; headache; jaw pain; mental depression; numbness or tingling in fingers and toes; pain in fingers and toes; pain in testicles; weakness)

### Those indicating need for medical attention only if they continue or are bothersome

Incidence less frequent
*Nausea and vomiting; pain in bone or tumor-containing tissues*

# Vinblastine (Systemic)

**Those not indicating need for medical attention**
Incidence more frequent
*Loss of hair*
Note: *Hair growth* should return after treatment has ended and possibly during therapy.

## Patient Consultation

As an aid to patient consultation, refer to *Advice for the Patient, Vinblastine (Systemic)*.

In providing consultation, consider emphasizing the following selected information (» = major clinical significance):

**Before using this medication**
Conditions affecting use, especially:
Sensitivity to vinblastine
Pregnancy—Advisability of using contraception; telling physician immediately if pregnancy is suspected
Breast-feeding—Not recommended because of risk of serious side effects
Other medications, especially other bone marrow depressants, probenecid, or sulfinpyrazone
Other medical problems, especially chickenpox or recent exposure, hepatic function impairment, herpes zoster, other infections, previous cytotoxic medication or radiation therapy, or tumor cell infiltration of bone marrow

**Proper use of this medication**
Caution in taking combination therapy; taking each medication at the right time
Importance of ample fluid intake and subsequent increase in urine output to aid in excretion of uric acid
Frequency of nausea and vomiting; importance of continuing medication despite stomach upset
» Proper dosing

**Precautions while using this medication**
» Importance of close monitoring by physician
» Avoiding immunizations unless approved by physician; other persons in patient's household should avoid immunizations with oral poliovirus vaccine; avoiding other persons who have taken oral poliovirus vaccine within the past several months or wearing a protective mask that covers nose and mouth

*Caution if bone marrow depression occurs*
» Avoiding exposure to persons with infections, especially during periods of low blood counts; checking with physician immediately if fever or chills, cough or hoarseness, lower back or side pain, or painful or difficult urination occurs
» Checking with physician immediately if unusual bleeding or bruising; black, tarry stools; blood in urine or stools; or pinpoint red spots on skin occur
Caution in use of regular toothbrush, dental floss, or toothpick; physician, dentist, or nurse may suggest alternatives; checking with physician before having dental work done
Not touching eyes or inside of nose unless hands washed immediately before
Using caution to avoid accidental cuts with use of sharp objects such as safety razor or fingernail or toenail cutters
Avoiding contact sports or other situations where bruising or injury could occur
» Possibility of local tissue injury and scarring if infiltration of intravenous solution occurs; telling physician or nurse right away about redness, swelling, or pain at site of injection

**Side/adverse effects**
May cause adverse effects such as blood problems, loss of hair, and cancer; importance of discussing possible effects with physician
Signs of potential side effects, especially leukopenia, cellulitis caused by extravasation, hyperuricemia, uric acid nephropathy, stomatitis, transient thrombocytopenia, rectal bleeding, hemorrhagic colitis, bleeding from existing peptic ulcer, and neurotoxicity
Physician or nurse can help in dealing with side effects
Possibility of hair loss; growth should return after treatment has ended and possibly during therapy

## General Dosing Information

Vinblastine may be administered by intravenous push or injected into the tubing of a running intravenous infusion, over a 1-minute period. *Do not administer vinblastine intrathecally because death of the patient will occur.*

Patients receiving vinblastine should be under supervision of a physician experienced in cancer chemotherapy.

Dosage must be adjusted to meet the individual requirements of each patient, on the basis of clinical response and degree of bone marrow depression.

Development of uric acid nephropathy in patients with lymphoma may be prevented by adequate oral hydration and, in some cases, administration of allopurinol. Alkalinization of urine may be necessary if serum uric acid concentrations are elevated.

It is recommended that vinblastine be administered no more frequently than every 7 days, to allow the full effect of each dose on the leukocyte count to be seen.

Dilution in larger volumes (100 to 250 mL) or administration over longer periods (30 to 60 minutes and longer) is recommended only with great caution because of irritation to the vein and increased risk of extravasation.

To minimize the risk of extravasation, rinsing of the syringe and needle with venous blood before withdrawal of the needle is recommended.

If extravasation of vinblastine occurs during intravenous administration, the injection should be stopped immediately and the remaining dose injected into another vein.

Injection of vinblastine into an extremity in which circulation is compromised by conditions such as compressing or invading neoplasm, phlebitis, or viscosity is not recommended because of the increased risk of thrombosis.

If marked leukopenia (particularly granulocytopenia) or thrombocytopenia occurs, it is recommended that vinblastine therapy be withdrawn until leukocyte counts return to satisfactory levels (at least 4000 per cubic millimeter).

Special precautions are recommended in patients who develop thrombocytopenia as a result of administration of vinblastine. These may include extreme care in performing invasive procedures; regular inspection of intravenous sites, skin (including perirectal area), and mucous membrane surfaces for signs of bleeding or bruising; limiting frequency of venipuncture and avoiding intramuscular injections; testing urine, emesis, stool, and secretions for occult blood; care in use of regular toothbrushes, dental floss, toothpicks, safety razors, and fingernail and toenail cutters; avoiding constipation; and using caution to prevent falls and other injuries. Such patients should avoid alcohol and aspirin intake because of the risk of gastrointestinal bleeding. Platelet transfusions may be required.

Patients who develop leukopenia should be observed carefully for signs of infection. Antibiotic support may be required. In neutropenic patients who develop fever, broad-spectrum antibiotic coverage should be initiated empirically, pending bacterial cultures and appropriate diagnostic tests.

**Safety considerations for handling this medication**

There is limited but increasing evidence and concern that personnel involved in preparation and administration of parenteral antineoplastics may be at some risk because of the potential mutagenicity, teratogenicity, and/or carcinogenicity of these agents, although the actual risk is unknown. USP advisory panels recommend cautious handling both in preparation and disposal of antineoplastic agents. Precautions that have been suggested include:
• Use of a biological containment cabinet during reconstitution and dilution of parenteral medications and wearing of disposable surgical gloves and masks.
• Use of proper technique to prevent contamination of the medication, work area, and operator during transfer between containers (including proper training of personnel in this technique).
• Cautious and proper disposal of needles, syringes, vials, ampuls, and unused medication.

A number of medical centers have developed detailed guidelines for handling of antineoplastic agents.

**Combination chemotherapy**

Vinblastine may be used in combination with other agents in various regimens. As a result, incidence and/or severity of side effects may be altered and different dosages (usually reduced) may be used. For example, vinblastine is part of the following chemotherapeutic combinations (some commonly used acronyms are in parentheses):
—doxorubicin, bleomycin, vinblastine, and dacarbazine (ABVD).
—carmustine, cyclophosphamide, vinblastine, procarbazine, and prednisone (BCVPP).

For specific dosages and schedules, consult the literature. For information regarding each agent, consult the individual monograph.

## Parenteral Dosage Forms

Note: Bracketed uses in the *Dosage Forms* section refer to categories of use and/or indications that are not included in U.S. product labeling.

## VINBLASTINE SULFATE INJECTION
### Usual adult dose
Carcinoma, breast or
Tumors, trophoblastic, gestational or
Carcinoma, testicular or
[Carcinoma, renal][1] or
Lymphomas, Hodgkin's or
Lymphomas, non-Hodgkin's or
Sarcoma, Kaposi's or
Letterer-Siwe disease or
Mycosis fungoides or
[Tumors, germ cell, ovarian][1]—
- Initial: Intravenous, 100 mcg (0.1 mg) per kg of body weight or 3.7 mg per square meter of body surface area a week, with successive weekly doses increased by increments of 50 mcg (0.05 mg) per kg of body weight or 1.8 to 1.9 mg per square meter of body surface area until the leukocyte count falls to 3000 per cubic millimeter, or a decrease in tumor size occurs, or a maximum dose of 500 mcg (0.5 mg) per kg of body weight or 18.5 mg per square meter of body surface area is reached (usual range 150 to 200 mcg [0.15 to 0.2 mg] per kg of body weight or 5.5 to 7.4 mg per square meter of body surface area).
- Maintenance: Intravenous, dosage one increment smaller than the final initial dosage every seven days, or 10 mg one or two times a month.

Note: Each subsequent dose should not be given until the leukocyte count after the preceding dose returns to 4000 per cubic millimeter, even if seven days have passed.

A reduction in dosage of 50% is recommended in patients with a direct serum bilirubin concentration above 3 mg per 100 mL.

A variety of dosage schedules and regimens of vinblastine, alone or in combination with other antitumor agents, are used. The prescriber may consult the medical literature in choosing a specific dosage.

[Carcinoma, bladder][1] or
[Carcinoma, lung, non–small cell][1] or
[Carcinoma, prostatic][1] or
[Melanoma, malignant][1]—
- Consult medical literature or manufacturer's literature for appropriate dosage.

### Usual pediatric and adolescent dose
Carcinoma, breast or
Tumors, trophoblastic, gestational or
Carcinoma, testicular or
[Carcinoma, renal][1] or
Lymphomas, Hodgkin's or
Lymphomas, non-Hodgkin's or
Sarcoma, Kaposi's or
Letterer-Siwe disease or
Mycosis fungoides or
[Tumors, germ cell, ovarian][1]—
- Initial: Intravenous, 2.5 mg per square meter of body surface area a week, with successive weekly doses increased by increments of 1.25 mg per square meter of body surface area until the leukocyte count falls to 3000 per cubic millimeter, or a decrease in tumor size occurs, or a maximum dose of 7.5 mg per square meter of body surface area is reached.
- Maintenance: Intravenous, dosage one increment smaller than the final initial dosage every seven days.

Note: Each subsequent dose should not be given until the leukocyte count after the preceding dose returns to 4000 per cubic millimeter, even if seven days have passed.

A reduction in dosage of 50% is recommended in patients with a direct serum bilirubin concentration above 3 mg per 100 mL.

A variety of dosage schedules and regimens of vinblastine, alone or in combination with other antitumor agents, are used. The prescriber may consult the medical literature in choosing a specific dosage.

[Carcinoma, bladder][1] or
[Carcinoma, lung, non–small cell][1] or
[Carcinoma, prostatic][1] or
[Melanoma, malignant][1]—
- Consult medical literature or manufacturer's literature for appropriate dosage.

### Strength(s) usually available
U.S.—
- 1 mg per mL (Rx) [GENERIC].

Canada—
- Not commercially available.

### Packaging and storage
Store between 2 and 8 °C (36 and 46 °F).

### Stability
After withdrawal of the first dose, the remainder of the vial may be stored for 30 days between 2 and 8 °C (36 and 46 °F) without significant loss of potency.

### Caution
When dispensed, the container or the syringe holding the individual dose prepared for administration to the patient must be enclosed in an overwrap bearing the statement: "DO NOT REMOVE COVERING UNTIL THE MOMENT OF INJECTION. FATAL IF GIVEN INTRATHECALLY. FOR INTRAVENOUS USE ONLY." USP does not specifically define the term "overwrap," but it is believed a ziplock bag or similar wrap utilized in hospitals may suffice to meet this requirement.

### Note
If accidental contamination of the eye with vinblastine occurs, the eye should be immediately and thoroughly flushed with water to prevent severe irritation and possible corneal ulceration.

## STERILE VINBLASTINE SULFATE USP
### Usual adult dose
Carcinoma, breast or
Tumors, trophoblastic, gestational or
Carcinoma, testicular or
[Carcinoma, renal][1] or
Lymphomas, Hodgkin's or
Lymphomas, non-Hodgkin's or
Sarcoma, Kaposi's or
Letterer-Siwe disease or
Mycosis fungoides or
[Tumors, germ cell, ovarian][1]—
- Initial: Intravenous, 100 mcg (0.1 mg) per kg of body weight or 3.7 mg per square meter of body surface area a week, with successive weekly doses increased by increments of 50 mcg (0.05 mg) per kg of body weight or 1.8 to 1.9 mg per square meter of body surface area until the leukocyte count falls to 3000 per cubic millimeter, or a decrease in tumor size occurs, or a maximum dose of 500 mcg (0.5 mg) per kg of body weight or 18.5 mg per square meter of body surface area is reached (usual range 150 to 200 mcg [0.15 to 0.2 mg] per kg of body weight or 5.5 to 7.4 mg per square meter of body surface area).
- Maintenance: Intravenous, dosage one increment smaller than the final initial dosage every seven days, or 10 mg one or two times a month.

Note: Each subsequent dose should not be given until the leukocyte count after the preceding dose returns to 4000 per cubic millimeter, even if seven days have passed.

A reduction in dosage of 50% is recommended in patients with a direct serum bilirubin concentration above 3 mg per 100 mL.

A variety of dosage schedules and regimens of vinblastine, alone or in combination with other antitumor agents, are used. The prescriber may consult the medical literature in choosing a specific dosage.

[Carcinoma, bladder][1] or
[Carcinoma, lung, non–small cell][1] or
[Carcinoma, prostatic][1] or
[Melanoma, malignant][1]—
- Consult medical literature or manufacturer's literature for appropriate dosage.

### Usual pediatric and adolescent dose
Carcinoma, breast or
Tumors, trophoblastic, gestational or
Carcinoma, testicular or
[Carcinoma, renal][1] or
Lymphomas, Hodgkin's or
Lymphomas, non-Hodgkin's or
Sarcoma, Kaposi's or
Letterer-Siwe disease or
Mycosis fungoides or
[Tumors, germ cell, ovarian][1]—
- Initial: Intravenous, 2.5 mg per square meter of body surface area a week, with successive weekly doses increased by increments of 1.25 mg per square meter of body surface area until the leukocyte count falls to 3000 per cubic millimeter, or a decrease in tumor size occurs, or a maximum dose of 7.5 mg per square meter of body surface area is reached.
- Maintenance: Intravenous, dosage one increment smaller than the final initial dosage every seven days.

Note: Each subsequent dose should not be given until the leukocyte count after the preceding dose returns to 4000 per cubic millimeter, even if seven days have passed.

A reduction in dosage of 50% is recommended in patients with a direct serum bilirubin concentration above 3 mg per 100 mL.

A variety of dosage schedules and regimens of vinblastine, alone or in combination with other antitumor agents, are used. The prescriber may consult the medical literature in choosing a specific dosage.

[Carcinoma, bladder][1] or
[Carcinoma, lung, non–small cell][1] or
[Carcinoma, prostatic][1] or
[Melanoma, malignant][1]—
  Consult medical literature or manufacturer's literature for appropriate dosage.

### Size(s) usually available
U.S.—
  10 mg (Rx) [*Velban;* GENERIC].
Canada—
  10 mg (Rx) [*Velbe*].

### Packaging and storage
Store between 2 and 8 °C (36 and 46 °F).

### Preparation of dosage form
Sterile Vinblastine Sulfate USP is reconstituted for intravenous use by adding 10 mL of 0.9% sodium chloride injection preserved with benzyl alcohol to the vial to produce a solution containing 1 mg of vinblastine sulfate per mL. It is not necessary to use preservative-containing 0.9% sodium chloride injection if unused solution is discarded immediately.

### Stability
Solutions of vinblastine that are reconstituted with sodium chloride injection containing a preservative may be stored for 28 days between 2 and 8 °C (36 and 46 °F). Preservative-free solutions should be discarded immediately.

### Caution
When dispensed, the container or the syringe holding the individual dose prepared for administration to the patient must be enclosed in an overwrap bearing the statement: "DO NOT REMOVE COVERING UNTIL THE MOMENT OF INJECTION. FATAL IF GIVEN INTRATHECALLY. FOR INTRAVENOUS USE ONLY." USP does not specifically define the term "overwrap," but it is believed a ziplock bag or similar wrap utilized in hospitals may suffice to meet this requirement.

Use of diluents containing benzyl alcohol is not recommended for preparation of medications for use in neonates. A fatal toxic syndrome consisting of metabolic acidosis, central nervous system (CNS) depression, respiratory problems, renal failure, hypotension, and possibly seizures and intracranial hemorrhages has been associated with this use.

### Note
If accidental contamination of the eye with vinblastine occurs, the eye should be immediately and thoroughly flushed with water to prevent severe irritation and possible corneal ulceration.

---

[1]Not included in Canadian product labeling.

Revised: 07/02/98

# VINCRISTINE  Systemic

VA CLASSIFICATION (Primary): AN900
Commonly used brand name(s): *Oncovin; Vincasar PFS*.
Note: For a listing of dosage forms and brand names by country availability, see *Dosage Forms* section(s).

## Category
Antineoplastic.

## Indications
Note: Bracketed information in the *Indications* section refers to uses that are not included in U.S. product labeling.

### Accepted
Leukemia, acute lymphocytic (treatment)
[Leukemia, chronic lymphocytic (treatment)][1] or
[Leukemia, chronic myelocytic (treatment)][1]—Vincristine is indicated for treatment of acute lymphocytic, chronic lymphocytic, and chronic myelocytic (blastic phase) leukemias.

Neuroblastoma (treatment)
Wilms' tumor (treatment)
[Carcinoma, breast (treatment)]
[Carcinoma, lung, small cell (treatment)]
[Carcinoma, ovarian, epithelial (treatment)][1]
[Carcinoma, cervical (treatment)] or
[Carcinoma, colorectal (treatment)]—Vincristine is indicated for treatment of neuroblastoma, Wilms' tumor, breast carcinoma, small cell lung carcinoma, epithelial carcinoma of the ovaries, cancer of the uterine cervix, and colorectal carcinoma.

Lymphomas, Hodgkin's (treatment) or
Lymphomas, non-Hodgkin's (treatment)—Vincristine is indicated for treatment of Hodgkin's and non-Hodgkin's lymphomas.

Kaposi's sarcoma, acquired immunodeficiency syndrome (AIDS)–associated (treatment)
Rhabdomyosarcoma (treatment)
[Ewing's sarcoma (treatment)] or
[Osteosarcoma (treatment)]—Vincristine is indicated for treatment of AIDS-associated Kaposi's sarcoma, rhabdomyosarcoma, Ewing's sarcoma, and osteogenic sarcoma.

[Hepatoblastoma (treatment)][1]
[Retinoblastoma (treatment)][1]
[Tumors, trophoblastic, gestational (treatment)][1] or
[Tumors, brain, primary (treatment)][1]—
Vincristine is used for the treatment of hepatoblastoma, retinoblastoma, gestational trophoblastic tumors, and primary brain tumors.

[Melanoma, malignant (treatment)]—Vincristine is indicated for treatment of malignant melanoma.

[Multiple myeloma (treatment)][1] or
[Waldenström's macroglobulinemia (treatment)][1]—Vincristine is used for treatment of multiple myeloma and Waldenström's macroglobulinemia.

[Tumors, germ cell, ovarian (treatment)][1]—Vincristine is used for treatment of germ cell ovarian tumors.

[Mycosis fungoides (treatment)][1]—Vincristine is used for treatment of mycosis fungoides.

[Thrombocytopenic purpura, idiopathic (treatment)]—Vincristine is used to treat true idiopathic thrombocytopenic purpura (ITP) resistant to the usual treatment of splenectomy and short-term treatment with adrenocorticoids.

  [However, although it may raise the platelet count in patients with chronic ITP, vincristine is recommended for use only in severe hematological disorders.][1]

---

[1]Not included in Canadian product labeling.

## Pharmacology/Pharmacokinetics

### Physicochemical characteristics
Source—Vincristine is a vinca alkaloid.
Molecular weight—Vincristine sulfate: 923.04.

### Mechanism of action/Effect
Vincristine blocks mitosis by arresting cells in metaphase, and may also interfere with amino acid metabolism; it is cell cycle–specific for the M phase of cell division.

### Distribution
Within 15 to 30 minutes after injection, > 90% distributed from blood into tissue; does not cross the blood-brain barrier in significant amounts.

### Protein binding
High (75%); extensive tissue binding.

### Biotransformation
Hepatic; metabolism of vinca alkaloids has been shown to be mediated by hepatic cytochrome P450 3A isoenzymes.

### Half-life
Following rapid intravenous administration—
  Initial phase: 5 minutes.
  Middle phase: 2.3 hours.
  Terminal phase: 85 hours.

### Elimination
Primary route—Biliary/fecal (about 80%).
Secondary route—Renal (about 10 to 20%).

## Precautions to Consider

### Carcinogenicity/Mutagenicity
Secondary malignancies are potential delayed effects of many antineoplastic agents, although it is not clear whether the effect is related to their mutagenic or immunosuppressive action. The effects of dose and duration of therapy are also unknown, although risk seems to increase with long-term use. Some patients who received chemotherapy with vincristine in combination with other medications known to be carcinogenic have developed second malignancies.

In a limited study in rats and mice, intraperitoneal administration of vincristine showed no evidence of carcinogenicity.

### Pregnancy/Reproduction
Fertility—Gonadal suppression, resulting in amenorrhea or azoospermia, may occur in patients taking combination antineoplastic therapy that includes vincristine. In general, these effects appear to be related to dose and length of therapy and may be irreversible. Prediction of the degree of testicular or ovarian function impairment is complicated by the common use of combinations of several antineoplastics, which makes it difficult to assess the effects of individual agents.

Pregnancy—Adequate and well-controlled studies in humans have not been done. However, studies in animals have shown that vincristine causes fetal resorption, fetal malformations, and embryo death, even at doses that are not toxic to the pregnant animal.

First trimester: It is usually recommended that use of antineoplastics, especially combination chemotherapy, be avoided whenever possible, especially during the first trimester. Although information is limited because of the relatively few instances of antineoplastic administration during pregnancy, the mutagenic, teratogenic, and carcinogenic potential of these medications must be considered.

Other hazards to the fetus include adverse reactions seen in adults.

In general, use of a contraceptive is recommended during cytotoxic drug therapy.

FDA Pregnancy Category D.

### Breast-feeding
Although very little information is available regarding distribution of antineoplastic agents into breast milk, breast-feeding is not recommended while vincristine is being administered because of the risks to the infant (adverse effects, mutagenicity, carcinogenicity). It is not known whether vincristine is distributed into breast milk.

### Pediatrics
Studies performed to date have not demonstrated pediatrics-specific problems that would limit the usefulness of vincristine in children.

### Geriatrics
Although appropriate studies with vincristine have not been performed in the geriatric population, elderly patients appear to be more susceptible to the neurotoxic effects.

### Dental
Vincristine may cause stomatitis, which is associated with considerable discomfort.

### Drug interactions and/or related problems
The following drug interactions and/or related problems have been selected on the basis of their potential clinical significance (possible mechanism in parentheses where appropriate)—not necessarily inclusive (» = major clinical significance):

Note: Combinations containing any of the following medications, depending on the amount present, may also interact with this medication.

Allopurinol or
Colchicine or
» Probenecid or
» Sulfinpyrazone
(vincristine may raise the concentration of blood uric acid; dosage adjustment of antigout agents may be necessary to control hyperuricemia and gout; allopurinol may be preferred to prevent or reverse vincristine-induced hyperuricemia because of risk of uric acid nephropathy with uricosuric antigout agents)

» Asparaginase
(concurrent use may result in additive neurotoxicity; if vincristine and asparaginase are to be used concurrently, toxicity appears to be less pronounced when asparaginase is administered after vincristine rather than before or with it)

Bleomycin
(sequential administration of vincristine prior to bleomycin arrests cells in mitosis so that they are more susceptible to bleomycin; frequently used to therapeutic advantage)

Blood dyscrasia–causing medications (see *Appendix II*)
(leukopenic and/or thrombocytopenic effects of vincristine may be increased with concurrent or recent therapy if these medications cause the same effects; dosage adjustment of vincristine, if necessary, should be based on blood counts)

Bone marrow depressants, other (see *Appendix II*) or
Radiation therapy
(concurrent use may increase the bone marrow depressant effects of these medications and radiation therapy, although myelosuppressive effects of vincristine are mild)

» Doxorubicin
(concurrent use with vincristine and prednisone may produce increased myelosuppression; it is recommended that the combination be avoided)

Neurotoxic medications, other (see *Appendix II*) or
Spinal cord irradiation
(concurrent use with vincristine may produce additive neurotoxicity)

Vaccines, killed virus
(because normal defense mechanisms may be suppressed by vincristine therapy, the patient's antibody response to the vaccine may be decreased. The interval between discontinuation of medications that cause immunosuppression and restoration of the patient's ability to respond to the vaccine depends on the intensity and type of immunosuppression-causing medication used, the underlying disease, and other factors; estimates vary from 3 months to 1 year)

» Vaccines, live virus
(because normal defense mechanisms may be suppressed by vincristine therapy, concurrent use with a live virus vaccine may potentiate the replication of the vaccine virus, may increase the side/adverse effects of the vaccine virus, and/or may decrease the patient's antibody response to the vaccine; immunization of these patients should be undertaken only with extreme caution after careful review of the patient's hematologic status and only with the knowledge and consent of the physician managing the vincristine therapy. The interval between discontinuation of medications that cause immunosuppression and restoration of the patient's ability to respond to the vaccine depends on the intensity and type of immunosuppression-causing medication used, the underlying disease, and other factors; estimates vary from 3 months to 1 year. Patients with leukemia in remission should not receive live virus vaccine until at least 3 months after their last chemotherapy. Immunization with oral poliovirus vaccine should also be postponed in persons in close contact with the patient, especially family members)

### Laboratory value alterations
The following have been selected on the basis of their potential clinical significance (possible effect in parentheses where appropriate)—not necessarily inclusive (» = major clinical significance):

With physiology/laboratory test values
Uric acid concentrations in blood and urine
(may be increased)

### Medical considerations/Contraindications
The medical considerations/contraindications included have been selected on the basis of their potential clinical significance (reasons given in parentheses where appropriate)—not necessarily inclusive (» = major clinical significance).

*Risk-benefit should be considered when the following medical problems exist:*

» Chickenpox, existing or recent, including recent exposure or
» Herpes zoster
(risk of severe generalized disease)

Gout, history of or
Urate renal stones, history of
(risk of hyperuricemia)

» Hepatic function impairment
(a 50% dosage reduction is recommended for patients with a direct bilirubin concentration in serum greater than 3 mg per 100 mL)

» Infection
» Leukopenia
» Neuromuscular disease
Sensitivity to vincristine
» Caution should be used also in patients who have had previous cytotoxic drug therapy or radiation therapy, and in those with existing neuromuscular problems who appear to be more susceptible to the neurotoxic effects of vincristine.

**Patient monitoring**
The following may be especially important in patient monitoring (other tests may be warranted in some patients, depending on condition; » = major clinical significance):
» Hematocrit or hemoglobin and
» Platelet count and
» Total and, if appropriate, differential leukocyte count
(determinations recommended prior to initiation of therapy and at periodic intervals during therapy; frequency varies according to clinical state, agent, dose, and other agents being used concurrently)
   Alanine aminotransferase (ALT [SGPT]) and
   Aspartate aminotransferase (AST [SGOT]) and
   Bilirubin, serum and
   Lactate dehydrogenase (LDH)
   (determinations recommended prior to initiation of therapy and at periodic intervals during therapy; frequency varies according to clinical state, agent, dose, and other agents being used concurrently)
   Uric acid, serum
   (determinations recommended prior to initiation of therapy and at periodic intervals during therapy; frequency varies according to clinical state, agent, dose, and other agents being used concurrently)

## Side/Adverse Effects

Note: Many "side effects" of antineoplastic therapy are unavoidable and represent the medication's pharmacologic action. Some of these (for example, leukopenia and thrombocytopenia) are actually used as parameters to aid in individual dosage titration.
Incidence of side effects is generally dose-related.

The following side/adverse effects have been selected on the basis of their potential clinical significance (possible signs and symptoms in parentheses where appropriate)—not necessarily inclusive:

**Those indicating need for medical attention**
Incidence more frequent
*Constipation, severe; decrease or increase in or painful or difficult urination; hyperuricemia or uric acid nephropathy* (joint pain; lower back or side pain); *neurotoxicity, progressive* (blurred or double vision; difficulty in walking; drooping eyelids; headache; jaw pain; numbness or tingling in fingers and toes; pain in fingers and toes; pain in testicles; weakness)

Note: *Hyperuricemia or uric acid nephropathy* occurs most commonly during initial treatment of patients with leukemia or lymphoma as a result of rapid cell breakdown that leads to elevated serum uric acid concentrations.
*Neurotoxicity* may become more severe with continued treatment; although most symptoms usually disappear by about 6 weeks following discontinuation of treatment with vincristine, some neuromuscular symptoms may persist for prolonged periods.

Incidence less frequent
*Cellulitis* (pain or redness at site of injection)—caused by extravasation
Incidence rare
*Leukopenia* (fever or chills; cough or hoarseness; lower back or side pain; painful or difficult urination)—usually asymptomatic; *thrombocytopenia* (unusual bleeding or bruising; black, tarry stools; blood in urine or stools; pinpoint red spots on skin)—usually asymptomatic; *stomatitis* (sores in mouth and lips); *syndrome of inappropriate antidiuretic hormone (SIADH)*

Note: Although *thrombocytopenia* is possible, platelet count changes little and may actually increase in some patients.

**Those indicating need for medical attention only if they continue or are bothersome**
Incidence less frequent
*Bloating; diarrhea; loss of weight; nausea and vomiting; skin rash*
**Those not indicating need for medical attention**
Incidence more frequent
*Loss of hair*
Note: *Hair growth* should return after treatment has ended and possibly during therapy.

## Overdose

For more information on the management of overdose or unintentional ingestion, **contact a Poison Control Center** (see *Poison Control Center Listing*).

**Treatment of overdose**
Treatment of overdose is symptomatic and supportive; it may include:
   Administration of anticonvulsants.
   Enemas to prevent ileus.
   Cardiovascular function and blood count monitoring.

## Patient Consultation

As an aid to patient consultation, refer to *Advice for the Patient, Vincristine (Systemic)*.
In providing consultation, consider emphasizing the following selected information (» = major clinical significance):
**Before using this medication**
   Conditions affecting use, especially:
      Sensitivity to vincristine
      Pregnancy—Advisability of using contraception; telling physician immediately if pregnancy is suspected
      Breast-feeding—Not recommended because of risk of serious side effects
      Use in the elderly—Elderly patients may be more susceptible to the neurotoxic effects
      Other medications, especially asparaginase, doxorubicin, previous cytotoxic medication or radiation therapy, probenecid, or sulfinpyrazone
      Other medical problems, especially chickenpox or recent exposure, hepatic function impairment, herpes zoster, other infection, leukopenia, or neuromuscular disease
**Proper use of this medication**
   Caution in taking combination therapy; taking each medication at the right time
   Importance of ample fluid intake and subsequent increase in urine output to aid in excretion of uric acid
   Possible nausea and vomiting; importance of continuing medication despite stomach upset
   Checking with physician about using laxative if constipation and stomach pain occur
» Proper dosing
**Precautions while using this medication**
» Importance of close monitoring by physician
» Avoiding immunizations unless approved by physician; other persons in patient's household should avoid immunizations with oral poliovirus vaccine; avoiding other persons who have taken oral poliovirus vaccine or wearing a protective mask that covers nose and mouth
» Possibility of local tissue injury and scarring if infiltration of intravenous solution occurs; telling physician or nurse right away about redness, swelling, or pain at site of injection
**Side/adverse effects**
   Signs of potential side effects, especially severe constipation, decrease or increase in or painful or difficult urination, hyperuricemia, uric acid nephropathy, neurotoxicity, cellulitis caused by extravasation, leukopenia, thrombocytopenia, stomatitis, and SIADH
   Physician or nurse can help in dealing with side effects
   Possibility of hair loss; growth should return after treatment has ended and possibly during therapy

## General Dosing Information

Vincristine may be administered by intravenous push or injected into the tubing of a running intravenous infusion, over a 1-minute period. *Do not administer vincristine intrathecally, because death of the patient will occur.*

Patients receiving vincristine should be under supervision of a physician experienced in cancer chemotherapy.

A variety of dosage schedules and regimens of vincristine, alone or in combination with other antitumor agents, are used. The prescriber may consult the medical literature as well as the manufacturer's literature in choosing a specific dosage.

Dosage must be adjusted to meet the individual requirements of each patient, on the basis of clinical response and appearance or severity of toxicity.

The needle should be carefully positioned in the vein to avoid extravasation and tissue damage.

If extravasation of vincristine occurs during intravenous administration, the injection should be stopped immediately and the remaining dose injected into another vein. Local discomfort and cellulitis may be minimized by local injection of hyaluronidase and application of moderate heat.

Development of uric acid nephropathy in patients with leukemia or lymphoma may be prevented by adequate oral hydration and, in some cases, administration of allopurinol. Alkalinization of urine may be necessary if serum uric acid concentrations are elevated.

Caution is required in encouraging large fluid intake because of the risk of inappropriate secretion of antidiuretic hormone (ADH), which is treated with fluid deprivation.

If signs of hyponatremia or inappropriate ADH secretion occur, vincristine therapy should be temporarily discontinued and the patient treated with fluid restriction and, if necessary, a diuretic affecting the loop of Henle and distal tubule.

If depression of reflexes, paresthesia, hypotension, and/or motor weakness develops, a reduction in dosage or withdrawal of vincristine is recommended.

Prophylactic administration of a laxative or enema is recommended to prevent upper colon impaction.

### Safety considerations for handling this medication

There is limited but increasing evidence and concern that personnel involved in preparation and administration of parenteral antineoplastics may be at some risk because of the potential mutagenicity, teratogenicity, and/or carcinogenicity of these agents, although the actual risk is unknown. USP advisory panels recommend cautious handling both in preparation and disposal of antineoplastic agents. Precautions that have been suggested include:
- Use of a biologic containment cabinet during reconstitution and dilution of parenteral medications and wearing of disposable surgical gloves and masks.
- Use of proper technique to prevent contamination of the medication, work area, and operator during transfer between containers (including proper training of personnel in this technique).
- Cautious and proper disposal of needles, syringes, vials, ampuls, and unused medication.

A number of medical centers have developed detailed guidelines for handling of antineoplastic agents.

### Combination chemotherapy

Vincristine may be used in combination with other agents in various regimens. As a result, incidence and/or severity of side effects may be altered and different dosages (usually reduced) may be used. For example, vincristine is part of the following chemotherapeutic combinations (some commonly used acronyms are in parentheses):
- cyclophosphamide, doxorubicin, vincristine, and prednisone (CHOP).
- cyclophosphamide, methotrexate, fluorouracil, vincristine, and prednisone (CMFVP).
- cyclophosphamide, vincristine, and prednisone (COP or CVP).
- cyclophosphamide, vincristine, procarbazine, and prednisone (COPP).
- cyclophosphamide, vincristine, doxorubicin, and dacarbazine (CyVADIC).
- mechlorethamine, vincristine, procarbazine, and prednisone (MOPP).
- vincristine, dactinomycin, and cyclophosphamide (VAC).

For specific dosages and schedules, consult the literature. For information regarding each agent, consult the individual monographs.

## Parenteral Dosage Forms

Note: Bracketed uses in the *Dosage Forms* section refer to categories of use and/or indications that are not included in U.S. product labeling.

### VINCRISTINE SULFATE INJECTION USP

**Usual adult dose**
Leukemia, acute lymphocytic or
Neuroblastoma or
Wilms' tumor or
[Carcinoma, breast] or
[Carcinoma, lung, small cell] or
[Carcinoma, ovarian, epithelial] or
[Carcinoma, cervical] or
[Carcinoma, colorectal] or
Lymphomas, Hodgkin's or
Lymphomas, non-Hodgkin's or
Rhabdomyosarcoma or
[Ewing's sarcoma] or
[Osteosarcoma] or
[Melanoma, malignant] or
[Tumors, germ cell, ovarian][1] or
[Mycosis fungoides][1] or
[Thrombocytopenic purpura, idiopathic]—
  Intravenous, 10 to 30 mcg (0.01 to 0.03 mg) per kg of body weight or 400 mcg (0.4 mg) to 1.4 mg per square meter of body surface area a week as a single dose.

Note: A 50% reduction in dose is recommended in patients with direct bilirubin concentrations in serum above 3 mg per 100 mL.

**Usual pediatric dose**
Leukemia, acute lymphocytic or
Neuroblastoma or
Wilms' tumor or
[Carcinoma, breast] or
[Carcinoma, lung, small cell] or
[Carcinoma, ovarian, epithelial] or
[Carcinoma, cervical] or
[Carcinoma, colorectal] or
Lymphomas, Hodgkin's or
Lymphomas, non-Hodgkin's or
Rhabdomyosarcoma or
[Ewing's sarcoma] or
[Osteosarcoma] or
[Melanoma, malignant] or
[Tumors, germ cell, ovarian][1] or
[Mycosis fungoides][1] or
[Thrombocytopenic purpura, idiopathic]—
  Intravenous, 1.5 to 2 mg per square meter of body surface area a week as a single dose.

Note: For children weighing 10 kg or less, the initial dose is 50 mcg (0.05 mg) per kg of body weight intravenously once a week.

A 50% reduction in dose is recommended in patients with direct bilirubin concentrations in serum above 3 mg per 100 mL.

**Strength(s) usually available**
U.S.—
  1 mg per mL (Rx) [*Oncovin* (mannitol; methylparaben; propylparaben); *Vincasar PFS;* GENERIC].
Canada—
  1 mg per mL (Rx) [*Oncovin* (mannitol; methylparaben; propylparaben)].

**Packaging and storage**
Store between 2 and 8 °C (36 and 46 °F), in a light-resistant, glass container.

**Caution**
When dispensed, the container or the syringe holding the individual dose prepared for administration to the patient must be enclosed in an overwrap bearing the statement: "DO NOT REMOVE COVERING UNTIL THE MOMENT OF INJECTION. FATAL IF GIVEN INTRATHECALLY. FOR INTRAVENOUS USE ONLY." USP does not specifically define the term "overwrap," but it is believed a ziplock bag or similar wrap utilized in hospitals may suffice to meet this requirement.

**Note**
If accidental contamination of the eye with vincristine occurs, the eye should be immediately and thoroughly flushed with water to prevent severe irritation and possible corneal ulceration.

---

[1]Not included in Canadian product labeling.

Revised: 09/26/97
Interim revision: 07/08/98

---

# VINORELBINE  Systemic

VA CLASSIFICATION (Primary): AN900
Commonly used brand name(s): *Navelbine*.
Note: For a listing of dosage forms and brand names by country availability, see *Dosage Forms* section(s).

## Category
Antineoplastic.

## Indications
Note: Bracketed information in the *Indications* section refers to uses that are not included in U.S. product labeling.

## Accepted

Carcinoma, lung (treatment)—Vinorelbine is indicated, as a single agent or in combination with cisplatin, for first-line treatment of ambulatory patients with unresectable, advanced non–small cell lung carcinoma (NSCLC). Vinorelbine is indicated as a single agent in Stage IV NSCLC and in combination with cisplatin in Stage III or IV NSCLC.

[Carcinoma, breast (treatment)]—Vinorelbine is indicated for the treatment of patients with metastatic breast cancer who did not respond to standard first-line chemotherapy for metastatic disease. Vinorelbine is also indicated for the treatment of patients with metastatic breast cancer who have relapsed within 6 months of anthracycline-based adjuvant therapy.

## Pharmacology/Pharmacokinetics

Note: Vinorelbine pharmacokinetics were analyzed in preclinical animal studies and in patients enrolled in disparate clinical trials. Concentrations of vinorelbine and its metabolites in biological fluids have been determined by measuring total radioactivity, by radioimmunoassay, and by high-performance liquid chromatography (HPLC). Most of the early studies involved the total-radioactivity assay, which measures both unchanged vinorelbine and all metabolites that retain the labeled moiety. The total-radioactivity assay is highly sensitive but lacks the specificity needed in pharmacokinetic studies. Radioimmunoassay was primarily used in animal studies and in some early clinical studies. Although radioimmunoassay is more specific than measuring total radioactivity, there is cross-sensitivity with metabolites of the vindoline ring structure. Three HPLC methods were developed for analyzing vinorelbine. HPLC has complete specificity for the parent drug and allows for measurement of its metabolites. Therefore, clinical studies in which HPLC is used are thought to provide the most valid pharmacokinetic estimates for vinorelbine.

**Physicochemical characteristics**
Source—Vinorelbine is a semisynthetic vinca alkaloid, derived from vinblastine. Vinorelbine differs in structure from other vinca alkaloids in that it contains an eight-member catharanthine ring structure, whereas vincristine and vinblastine contain a nine-member catharanthine ring structure.
Molecular weight—1079.13.

**Mechanism of action/Effect**
Vinca alkaloids appear to exert their antitumor activity by binding to tubulin with high affinity. Two types of tubulin, alpha and beta, exist as dimers that polymerize to form microtubules, of which many cellular structures, including the mitotic spindle, are constituted. The cellular functions of microtubules include neurotransmission and mitosis. Vinca alkaloids are cell cycle–specific agents that arrest mitosis by interfering with microtubule assembly and inducing depolarization of microtubules. Like other vinca alkaloids, vinorelbine may also interfere with amino acid, cyclic adenosine monophosphate (cAMP), and glutathione metabolism; with calmodulin-dependent calcium-transport–adenosinetriphosphatase activity; with cellular respiration; and with nucleic acid and lipid biosynthesis.

All vinca alkaloids are thought to have slightly different mechanisms of action due in part to differences in their interaction with microtubule-associated proteins, which are believed to modify the interaction of vinca alkaloids with tubulin. At least two sites of vinca alkaloid fixation on tubulin have been reported: one site with high affinity, which is responsible for depolymerization activity, and one site with low affinity, which induces unwinding of microtubules and spiral formation. Researchers found that vinorelbine was as active as vincristine and vinblastine in inducing the assembly of tubulin *in vitro* but was uniquely inefficient in causing spiral formation. This observation led to the hypothesis that vinorelbine may have a mechanism of action differing slightly from that of other vinca alkaloids and may be potentially less toxic.

Vinorelbine appears to have selective activity against mitotic microtubules. Researchers compared the effect of vinorelbine, vinblastine, and vincristine on mitotic and axonal microtubules in postimplantation mouse embryos at the earliest stage of neuronal development. Mitotic microtubule activity appeared to be correlated with antitumor activity, while axonal microtubule activity was thought to be correlated with neurotoxicity. At low concentrations (2 micromolar), vincristine, vinblastine, and vinorelbine inhibited spindle assembly by arresting cell division at metaphase. At higher concentrations (25 micromolar), only vinorelbine arrested mitosis at prophase. Depolymerization of axonal microtubules was concentration-dependent and occurred at markedly higher concentrations of vinorelbine (40 micromolar) than of vincristine (5 micromolar) or vinblastine (30 micromolar); presumably this accounts for the decreased neurotoxicity of vinorelbine. Further research is needed to describe clearly the interaction of vinorelbine with tubulin and to determine the clinical relevance of this activity.

**Distribution**
Preclinical tissue distribution studies in mice, rats, and monkeys showed that radiolabeled vinorelbine was widely distributed in the body after intravenous administration. High amounts of radioactivity were localized in the spleen, liver, kidneys, lungs, and thymus; moderate amounts in the heart and muscles; and minimal amounts in fat, the brain, and bone marrow.

In human hepatocytes, the degree of cellular accumulation of the vinca alkaloids increases with increasing lipophilicity of the compound. Since vinorelbine is one of the most lipid-soluble vinca alkaloids, there is rapid uptake and extensive distribution in cells. Measurements in human lung tissue show that vinorelbine has up to a 300-fold greater concentration in lung than in serum.

**Protein binding**
Vinorelbine is highly bound to platelets and lymphocytes, and is also bound to alpha$_1$-acid glycoprotein, albumin, and lipoproteins. In one study in 24 cancer patients, serum binding of vinorelbine ranged from 79.6 to 91.2%. The fraction of unbound vinorelbine averaged 0.135 (range 0.088 to 0.204). Because of high binding to platelets, the fraction bound in blood was 98.3%. Concurrent administration of other anticancer agents is unlikely to cause displacement of vinorelbine from its binding sites in serum. In control serum, vinorelbine binding (85.2%) was not significantly different from binding in the presence of 5-fluorouracil (87.4%), doxorubicin (85%), or cisplatin (85.6%).

**Biotransformation**
Hepatic. Metabolism of vinorelbine was initially suggested by *in vitro* studies that used human hepatic subcellular fractions and identified two metabolites. Radiochromatography of urine and fecal samples found at least three unidentified vinorelbine metabolites after intravenous and oral administration of the agent to cancer patients. An HPLC method was developed for the measurement of two likely vinorelbine metabolites, vinorelbine N-oxide and deacetylvinorelbine. Although vinorelbine N-oxide appears to be inactive, evidence indicates that deacetylvinorelbine possesses pharmacologic activity similar to that of vinorelbine. However, this finding may have minimal clinical significance, since a pharmacokinetics study in 20 patients who received intravenous vinorelbine revealed no vinorelbine N-oxide in serum or urine and no deacetylvinorelbine in serum. A small amount of deacetylvinorelbine, however, was found in urine.

**Half-life**
There is a prolonged terminal phase due to relatively slow efflux of vinorelbine from peripheral compartments, which results in a long terminal phase half-life, with average value ranging from 27.7 to 43.6 hours.

**Elimination**
Preclinical animal studies indicated that vinorelbine and its metabolites are excreted in the bile. Significant amounts of vinorelbine and metabolites were found in the feces of all species studied and in the bile of cannulated rats after intravenous administration of vinorelbine. Researchers used an HPLC method to study the biliary excretion of vinorelbine in micropigs following administration of doses comparable to those used in humans and found that 25.8% of the vinorelbine dose was excreted unchanged in the bile. Low amounts of deacetylvinorelbine ($< 5\%$) were found, and treatment of urine with beta-glucuronidase did not indicate glucuronidation of vinorelbine. Most likely, biliary excretion also occurs in humans, since, as mentioned above, a large percentage of radiolabeled vinorelbine administered intravenously is eliminated in the feces.

## Precautions to Consider

**Carcinogenicity/Tumorigenicity**
Carcinogenicity studies with vinorelbine have not been done.

**Mutagenicity**
*In vivo* studies found that vinorelbine affected chromosome number and possibly structure (polyploidy in bone marrow cells from Chinese hamsters and a positive micronucleus test in mice). Results of the Ames mutagenicity test were negative and results were inconclusive in the mouse lymphoma TK Locus assay.

**Pregnancy/Reproduction**
Fertility—Studies in rats given either 9 mg per square meter of body surface area (mg/m$^2$) (approximately one third the human dose) once a week or 4.2 mg/m$^2$ (approximately one seventh the human dose) every other day, prior to and during mating, found no significant effect on fertility. However, studies in male rats given 2.1 and 7.2 mg/m$^2$ (approximately one fifteenth and one fourth the human dose, respectively) biweekly for 13 or 26 weeks found decreased spermatogenesis and prostate/seminal vesicle secretion.

Pregnancy—Studies have not been done in humans.

Vinorelbine has been shown to be embryotoxic and/or fetotoxic in animals; nonmaternotoxic doses of vinorelbine caused a reduction in fetal weight and a delay in ossification. However, vinorelbine has not been shown to be teratogenic. Women of childbearing potential should be informed about the potential hazard to the fetus if they become pregnant during vinorelbine therapy. They should also be advised to avoid becoming pregnant during vinorelbine therapy.

FDA Pregnancy Category D.

**Breast-feeding**
It is not known whether vinorelbine is distributed into breast milk. However, because of vinorelbine's potential for serious adverse reactions in nursing infants, it is recommended that nursing be discontinued in women receiving vinorelbine therapy.

**Pediatrics**
Appropriate studies on the relationship of age to the effects of vinorelbine have not been performed in the pediatric population. Safety and efficacy in children have not been established.

**Geriatrics**
Approximately one third of the patients enrolled in the North American clinical trials of vinorelbine were over the age of 65 years. Although this subset of patients did experience a slight increase in grade 3 and 4 leukopenia and granulocytopenia compared with patients under 65 years of age, the overall safety profile and antitumor efficacy were not significantly different for the older people. Furthermore, examination of pharmacokinetic parameters from the clinical trials did not suggest any differences in drug metabolism in older patients. As a result, no specific dosage adjustments are recommended for geriatric patients. The safety profile of vinorelbine suggests that vinorelbine may be particularly well suited to elderly patients, as this patient population is typically intolerant of severe side effects.

**Dental**
The leukopenic and thrombocytopenic effects of vinorelbine may result in an increased incidence of certain microbial infections of the mouth, delayed healing, and gingivial bleeding. If leukopenia or thrombocytopenia occurs, dental work should be deferred until blood counts have returned to normal. Patients should be instructed in proper oral hygiene, including caution in use of regular toothbrushes, dental floss, and toothpicks.

**Drug interactions and/or related problems**
The following drug interactions and/or related problems have been selected on the basis of their potential clinical significance (possible mechanism in parentheses where appropriate)—not necessarily inclusive (» = major clinical significance):

Note: Combinations containing any of the following medications, depending on the amount present, may also interact with this medication.

Blood dyscrasia–causing medications (see *Appendix II*)
(leukopenic effects of vinorelbine may be increased with concurrent or recent therapy if these medications cause the same effects; dosage adjustment of vinorelbine, if necessary, should be based on blood count)

» Bone marrow depressants, other (see *Appendix II*) or
Radiation therapy
(concurrent use may increase the bone marrow depressant effect of these medications and radiation therapy)

Cisplatin
(although the pharmacokinetics of vinorelbine are not influenced by the concurrent administration of cisplatin, the incidence of toxicities, specifically granulocytopenia, with the combination of vinorelbine and cisplatin is significantly higher than with single-agent vinorelbine)

» Mitomycin
(acute pulmonary reactions have been reported with vinorelbine used in conjunction with mitomycin; vinorelbine should be administered with caution in combination with mitomycin)

Vaccines, killed virus
(because normal defense mechanisms may be suppressed by vinorelbine therapy, the patient's antibody response to the vaccine may be decreased. The interval between discontinuation of medications that cause immunosuppression and restoration of the patient's ability to respond to the vaccine depends on the intensity and type of immunosuppression-causing medication used, the underlying disease, and other factors; estimates vary from 3 months to 1 year)

» Vaccines, live virus
(because normal defense mechanisms may be suppressed by vinorelbine therapy, concurrent use with a live virus vaccine may potentiate the replication of the vaccine virus, may increase the side/adverse effects of the vaccine virus, and/or may decrease the patient's antibody response to the vaccine; immunization of these patients should be undertaken only with extreme caution after careful review of the patient's hematologic status and only with the knowledge and consent of the physician managing the vinorelbine therapy. The interval between discontinuation of medications that cause immunosuppression and restoration of the patient's ability to respond to the vaccine depends on the intensity and type of immunosuppression-causing medication used, the underlying disease, and other factors; estimates vary from 3 months to 1 year. Patients with leukemia in remission should not receive live virus vaccine until at least 3 months after their last chemotherapy. Immunization with oral poliovirus vaccine should also be postponed in persons in close contact with the patient, especially family members)

**Laboratory value alterations**
The following have been selected on the basis of their potential clinical significance (possible effect in parentheses where appropriate)—not necessarily inclusive (» = major clinical significance):

With physiology/laboratory test values
Alanine aminotransferase (ALT [SGPT]) and
Alkaline phosphatase and
Aspartate aminotransferase (AST [SGOT])
(values may be increased)

Bilirubin, serum
(concentrations may be increased)

Note: Transient increases in alanine aminotransferase and aspartate aminotransferase values were reported in approximately 50% of patients, but patients with elevated liver enzymes values were typically asymptomatic and did not require discontinuation of therapy. A somewhat greater effect was observed on total bilirubin concentrations, with 6% of patients developing concentrations of grade 3 or 4 severity. Although vinorelbine treatment may have contributed to these increases in bilirubin concentrations, these abnormalities also may be related to disease progression in the liver.

**Medical considerations/Contraindications**
The medical considerations/contraindications included have been selected on the basis of their potential clinical significance (reasons given in parentheses where appropriate)—not necessarily inclusive (» = major clinical significance).

*Risk-benefit should be considered when the following medical problems exist:*

» Chickenpox, existing or recent (including recent exposure) or
» Herpes zoster
(risk of severe generalized disease)

» Granulocytopenia or
» Thrombocytopenia
(administration of vinorelbine is not recommended if pretreatment granulocyte counts are less than 1000 cells per cubic millimeter; as with other vinca alkaloids, vinorelbine should not be used in patients who have drug-induced severe granulocytopenia or severe thrombocytopenia)

» Sensitivity to vinorelbine

» Tumor cell infiltration of the bone marrow

» Caution should be used also in patients with inadequate bone marrow reserves due to previous cytotoxic drug or radiation therapy.

**Patient monitoring**
The following may be especially important in patient monitoring (other tests may be warranted in some patients, depending on condition; » = major clinical significance):

Alanine aminotransferase (ALT [SGPT]) values, and
Alkaline phosphatase values, serum and
Aspartate aminotransferase (AST [SGOT]) values, and
Bilirubin concentrations, serum
(recommended prior to initiation of therapy and at periodic intervals during therapy)

» Leukocyte count, total and differential
(determinations and review recommended on the day of treatment prior to administering each dose of vinorelbine)

## Side/Adverse Effects

Note: Extensive clinical experience has been obtained with the antineoplastic agent vinorelbine in Europe and elsewhere. This experience has been supplemented by more clinical trials of patients with advanced non–small cell lung cancer or breast cancer conducted in North America. Data from these trials indicate that vinorelbine is safe and well tolerated in the outpatient population. Granulocytopenia is the dose-limiting toxicity. Although the incidence of this condition is high among vinorelbine-treated patients, it is uncommonly associated with severe complications. Elevations in alkaline phosphatase values are seen in the majority of patients, but this effect may be due in part to liver and bone metastases. Nonhematologic toxicities are mostly mild or moderate. Injection site reactions have been noted in some patients, but improved administration techniques may help reduce the incidence of the effect. Gastrointestinal and respiratory effects are seldom severe and usually respond to treatment. Drug-associated neurotoxicity occurs less often than with other commonly used vinca alkaloid compounds. Overall, vinorelbine is associated with few severe toxicities which, for the most part, are easily managed.

The following side/adverse effects have been selected on the basis of their potential clinical significance (possible signs and symptoms in parentheses where appropriate)—not necessarily inclusive:

**Those indicating need for medical attention**
Incidence more frequent
*Anemia* (unusual tiredness or weakness); *asthenia* (loss of strength and energy); *granulocytopenia or leukopenia* (sore throat and fever); *injection site reactions* (redness, increased warmth, pain, or discoloration of vein at place of injection)

Note: *Asthenia* is one of the most common adverse effects of vinorelbine, occurring in one third of patients. The fatigue is generally mild or moderate but increases with repeated administration.

*Injection site reactions* are common with vinorelbine treatment, although, in one study, only approximately 2% of patients experienced severe reactions. Like other vinca alkaloids, vinorelbine is a vesicant that can cause extravasation injuries as well as local effects at the injection site. The occurrence and severity of venous irritation appear to be reduced when vinorelbine is administered as a 6- to 10-minute infusion with a free-flowing intravenous fluid to ensure proper flushing of veins. Phlebitis occurs in approximately 6% of patients; however, the frequency of phlebitis was notably greater in clinical trials in which vinorelbine was administered over 1 hour.

The most notable toxicity associated with vinorelbine treatment is hematologic. *Granulocytopenia* is the dose-limiting toxicity, with grade 3 or 4 granulocytopenia occurring in 64% of treated patients. White blood cell counts are also severely affected; grade 3 or 4 *leukopenia* was reported in 50% of vinorelbine-treated patients. A lesser effect was observed in red blood cells, as indicated by hemoglobin concentrations; only 9% of patients reached grade 3 or 4 toxicity. Although *anemia* was fairly common among vinorelbine-treated patients, it was rarely severe, and transfusions were required rarely. Platelets are relatively unaffected.

Incidence less frequent
***Chest pain; neuropathy, peripheral, mild to moderate, including paresthesia and hypesthesia*** (numbness or tingling in fingers and toes); ***pulmonary reactions*** (shortness of breath); ***stomatitis*** (sores in mouth and on lips)

Note: *Chest pain* has been reported in 5% of patients receiving vinorelbine therapy. The majority of patients reporting chest pain have either a history of cardiovascular disease or a tumor within the chest. One report describes a fatal myocardial infarction in a patient with a previous infarction who received two courses of vinorelbine. It is unclear what role vinorelbine played in the patient's myocardial infarction. Cardiovascular toxicity has been rarely reported with vincristine and vinblastine. The pathogenesis of cardiovascular toxicity is postulated to involve transitory coronary artery spasm.

Shortness of breath has been noted in 5% of patients; 2% of these patients described severe shortness of breath. As with other vinca alkaloids, vinorelbine can produce both acute and subacute *pulmonary reactions*. The acute reaction resembles an allergic reaction and responds to bronchodilators. Subacute pulmonary reactions generally occur within 1 hour after drug administration and are characterized by cough, dyspnea, hypoxemia, and interstitial infiltration. Subacute pulmonary reactions typically respond to corticosteroid therapy.

The neurotoxic effects of vinorelbine, such as *peripheral neuropathy*, seem to be reversible on discontinuation of vinorelbine. The addition of cisplatin does not appear to increase the neurotoxic effects of vinorelbine. However, prior treatment with paclitaxel may result in cumulative neurotoxicity.

Incidence rare
*Hemorrhagic cystitis* (inflammation and bleeding of the urinary bladder)—reported in less than 1% of patients; *skin rash*—reported in 4% of patients; *thrombocytopenia* (unusual bleeding or bruising; black, tarry stools; blood in urine or stools; pinpoint red spots on skin)

Note: Grade 3 and 4 *thrombocytopenia* has been reported in less than 1% of patients; however, in one study no grade 3 or 4 thrombocytopenia was observed in vinorelbine recipients.

**Those indicating need for medical attention only if they continue or are bothersome**
Incidence more frequent
*Anorexia* (loss of appetite); *constipation; nausea and vomiting*

Note: Prophylactic antiemetic therapy has not been used routinely in clinical trials of vinorelbine. Nausea and vomiting occur in approximately 40% and 20% of patients, respectively. Vinorelbine-associated *nausea and vomiting* are typically mild to moderate and appear to respond to conventional antiemetic therapy; serotonin-receptor antagonists are not generally required.

Incidence less frequent
*Diarrhea; jaw pain; joint or muscle pain*

**Those not indicating need for medical attention**
Incidence more frequent
*Alopecia* (loss of hair)

Note: Vinorelbine has caused *alopecia* in about 10% of patients, manifested as a gradual thinning of hair. Few patients suffer total hair loss. Alopecia appears to occur with cumulative toxicity of vinorelbine.

## Overdose

### Clinical effects of vinorelbine overdose
The following effects have been selected on the basis of their potential clinical significance (possible signs and symptoms in parentheses where appropriate)—not necessarily inclusive:

Acute and chronic effects
*Bone marrow suppression* (sore throat or fever; unusual bleeding or bruising; unusual tiredness or weakness); *neurotoxicity, peripheral* (numbness or tingling in fingers and toes)

### Treatment of overdose
There are no known antidotes for the treatment of vinorelbine overdosage. Therefore, treatment of overdose is supportive and may include appropriate blood transfusions and antibiotics.

## Patient Consultation
As an aid to patient consultation, refer to *Advice for the Patient, Vinorelbine (Systemic)*.

In providing consultation, consider emphasizing the following selected information (» = major clinical significance):

### Before using this medication
» Conditions affecting use, especially:
  Sensitivity to vinorelbine
  Pregnancy—Advisability of using contraception; telling physician immediately if pregnancy is suspected
  Breast-feeding—Not recommended because of the risk of serious side effects
  Other medications, especially bone marrow depressants, mitomycin, or previous cytotoxic or radiation therapy
  Other medical problems, especially chickenpox; granulocytopenia; herpes zoster; thrombocytopenia; or tumor cell infiltration of the bone marrow

### Proper use of this medication
Caution in taking combination therapy; taking each medication at the right time
Importance of ample fluid intake and subsequent increase in urine output to aid in excretion of uric acid
Possible nausea and vomiting; importance of continuing medication despite stomach upset
» Proper dosing

### Precautions while using this medication
» Importance of close monitoring by physician
» Possibility of local tissue injury if infiltration of intravenous solution occurs; telling physician or nurse right away about redness, swelling, or pain at site of injection
» Avoiding immunizations unless approved by physician; other persons in patient's household should avoid immunizations with oral poliovirus vaccine; avoiding other persons who have taken oral poliovirus vaccine or wearing a protective mask that covers nose and mouth

*Caution if bone marrow depression occurs*
» Avoiding exposure to persons with infections, especially during periods of low blood counts; checking with physician immediately if fever or chills, cough or hoarseness, lower back or side pain, or painful or difficult urination occurs
» Checking with physician immediately if unusual bleeding or bruising; black, tarry stools; blood in urine or stools; or pinpoint red spots on skin occur
- Caution in use of regular toothbrush, dental floss, or toothpick; physician, dentist, or nurse may suggest alternatives; checking with physician before having dental work done
- Not touching eyes or inside of nose unless hands washed immediately before
- Using caution to avoid accidental cuts with use of sharp objects such as safety razor or fingernail or toenail cutters
- Avoiding contact sports or other situations where bruising or injury could occur

### Side/adverse effects
Signs of potential side effects, especially anemia, asthenia, granulocytopenia or leukopenia, injection site reaction, chest pain, peripheral neuropathy, pulmonary reactions, stomatitis, hemorrhagic cystitis, skin rash, and thrombocytopenia

## General Dosing Information

Patients receiving vinorelbine should be under the supervision of a physician experienced in cancer chemotherapy. Patients and/or family members should be instructed to report any side/adverse effects immediately.

Clinical trials have demonstrated that vinorelbine is an effective chemotherapeutic agent in the treatment of patients with advanced non–small cell lung cancer (NSCLC). Vinorelbine has also been shown to increase survival without compromising quality of life (QOL) in several randomized, controlled trials. A summary of preliminary QOL findings for two vinorelbine (randomized and single-arm) trials in patients with NSCLC shows that symptoms status was as good or better for patients receiving vinorelbine as for those receiving 5-fluorouracil/leucovorin in the randomized study.

Although vinorelbine is effective as monotherapy, a higher overall response rate and median duration of survival are seen when it is combined with cisplatin. Data from some clinical studies indicate that vinorelbine plus cisplatin is superior to vindesine plus cisplatin and to vinorelbine alone.

Patients with renal insufficiency do not require dosage adjustments. However, in patients with hepatic insufficiency, the dosage of vinorelbine should be adjusted on the basis of degree of hyperbilirubinemia.

Vinorelbine should be administered intravenously. Intrathecal administration of other vinca alkaloids has resulted in death.

It is very important that the intravenous needle or catheter be positioned properly before any vinorelbine is injected. Leakage into surrounding tissue during intravenous administration of vinorelbine may cause considerable irritation, local tissue necrosis and/or thrombophlebitis. If extravasation occurs, the injection should be discontinued immediately, and any remaining portion of the dose should then be introduced into another vein. Local injection of hyaluronidase and the application of moderate heat to the area of leakage has been reported to help disperse the agent and minimize discomfort associated with the extravasation of other vinca alkaloids.

Although venous irritation is a problem associated with peripherally administered vinorelbine, it does not necessitate central line placement. Incidence of this problem can be reduced with a shorter duration of administration. Vinorelbine should be diluted in either a syringe or intravenous bag and administered by intravenous injection, over a period of 6 to 10 minutes. However, if a central line is to be considered for patients receiving vinorelbine, the following can be used as a guide:
• If the patient has poor venous access, early placement of a central line should be considered.
• If the patient has reasonable venous access, treatment should be started with peripheral administration (especially until therapeutic response is determined). Placement of a central line should be considered only if difficulty in venous access is encountered.

After vinorelbine has been infused, flushing of the vein should be continued with at least 100 mL of normal saline or 5% dextrose in water to prevent injection site reactions. Inadequate flushing may increase the risk of phlebitis; therefore, the catheter should not be removed without flushing the vein.

Vinorelbine has shown reduced neurotoxicity, at both the cellular and clinical levels, compared with other vinca alkaloids. However, physicians should make clinical judgment before initiating vinorelbine treatment in patients with pre-existing neurologic disorders. Patients who previously have received neurologic chemotherapy are at high risk for developing neurologic complications. It is recommended that vinorelbine be discontinued if moderate or severe neurotoxicity occurs during treatment.

Granulocytopenia is the major dose-limiting adverse effect with vinorelbine therapy; however, it is reversible and not cumulative over time. Patients who develop leukopenia (particularly granulocytopenia) should be observed carefully for signs of infection. Prophylactic hematologic growth factors have not been used routinely with vinorelbine; however, if medically necessary, growth factors may be administered at recommended doses no earlier than 24 hours after the administration of cytotoxic chemotherapy.

### Safety considerations for handling this medication

Note: As with other toxic compounds, caution should be exercised in handling and preparing the solution of vinorelbine. The use of gloves is recommended since skin reactions are reported with accidental exposure. If the solution of vinorelbine contacts the skin or mucosa, the skin or mucosa should be washed immediately with soap and water. Severe irritation of the eye has been reported with accidental contamination of the eye with another vinca alkaloid. If this happens with vinorelbine, the affected eye should be washed with water immediately and thoroughly.

There is limited but increasing evidence and concern that personnel involved in preparation and administration of parenteral antineoplastics may be at some risk because of the potential mutagenicity, teratogenicity, and/or carcinogenicity of these agents, although the actual risk is unknown. USP advisory panels recommend cautious handling both in preparation and disposal of antineoplastic agents. Precautions that have been suggested include:
• Use of a biologic containment cabinet during reconstitution and dilution of parenteral medications and wearing of disposable surgical gloves and masks.
• Use of proper technique to prevent contamination of the medication, work area, and operator during transfer between containers (including proper training of personnel in this technique).
• Cautious and proper disposal of needles, syringes, vials, ampuls, and unused medication.

A number of medical centers have developed detailed guidelines for handling of antineoplastic agents.

### For treatment of adverse effects
If shortness of breath or bronchospasm occurs during concurrent treatment with vinorelbine and mitomycin, treatment with supplemental oxygen, bronchodilators, and/or corticosteroids may be required.

## Parenteral Dosage Forms

Note: Bracketed use in the *Dosage Forms* section refers to category of use and/or indication that is not included in U.S. product labeling.

### VINORELBINE TARTRATE INJECTION

Note: The dosing and strength of the dosage form available are expressed in terms of vinorelbine base (not the tartrate salt).

#### Usual adult dose
Carcinoma, lung, non–small cell or
[Carcinoma, breast]—
Intravenous (over six to ten minutes), 30 mg (base) per square meter of body surface area once a week, as a single agent. The same dose is used in combination therapy with cisplatin, which is given in a dose of 120 mg (base) per square meter of body surface area on Days 1 and 29, followed by one dose every six weeks.
Dosage adjustment is recommended according to hematologic toxicity or hepatic function impairment, as outlined below, whichever results in a lower dose. (If both hematologic and hepatic toxicity occur, the lower of the doses determined from the following is recommended.)
Dosage adjustment for hematologic toxicity is—
Granulocytes 1500 cells per cubic millimeter (cells/mm$^3$) or more on days of treatment:
Give 30 mg (base) per square meter of body surface area.
Granulocytes 1000 to 1499 cells/mm$^3$ on days of treatment:
Give 15 mg (base) per square meter of body surface area.
Granulocytes less than 1000 cells/mm$^3$ on days of treatment:
Do not administer vinorelbine. Repeat granulocyte count in one week. If three consecutive weekly doses have to be held because of low granulocyte counts, it is recommended that vinorelbine be discontinued.

Note: In patients who have experienced fever and/or sepsis while granulocytopenic during vinorelbine therapy, or have had two consecutive doses held because of granulocytopenia, subsequent doses should be 22.5 mg (base) per square meter of body surface area (for granulocytes greater than or equal to 1500 cells/mm$^3$) or 11.25 mg (base) per square meter of body surface area (for granulocytes 1000 to 1499 cells/mm³).

Dosage adjustment for hepatic insufficiency is—
Total bilirubin 2 mg per deciliter (mg/dL) or less:
Give 30 mg (base) per square meter of body surface area.
Total bilirubin 2.1 to 3 mg/dL:
Give 15 mg (base) per square meter of body surface area.
Total bilirubin 3 mg/dL or more:
Give 7.5 mg (base) per square meter of body surface area.

**Usual pediatric dose**
Safety and efficacy have not been established.

**Strength(s) usually available**
U.S.—
10 mg (base) per mL (1- and 5-mL vials) (Rx) [*Navelbine*].
Canada—
10 mg (base) per mL (1- and 5-mL vials) (Rx) [*Navelbine*].

**Packaging and storage**
Store between 2 and 8 °C (36 and 46 °F), in the carton. Protect from light. Protect from freezing.

**Preparation of dosage form**
For intravenous administration via syringe, the calculated dose of vinorelbine tartrate injection is diluted to a concentration of 1.5 to 3 mg per mL (mg/mL) with either 5% dextrose injection or 0.9% sodium choride injection. For administration via an intravenous bag, the calculated dose of vinorelbine tartrate injection is diluted to a concentration of 0.5 to 2 mg/mL with 5% dextrose injection, 0.9% sodium chloride injection, 0.45% sodium chloride injection, 5% dextrose in 0.45% sodium chloride injection, Ringer's injection, or lactated Ringer's injection.

**Stability**
Unopened vials of vinorelbine tartrate injection are stable for up to 72 hours at 25 °C (77 °F). Diluted injection is stable for up to 24 hours at 5 to 30 °C (41 to 86 °F) under normal room light when stored in polypropylene syringes or polyvinyl chloride bags.

**Incompatibilities**
Vinorelbine tartrate is not compatible with acyclovir sodium, aminophylline, amphotericin B, ampicillin sodium, cefoperazone sodium, ceforanide, cefotetan sodium, ceftriaxone sodium, fluorouracil, furosemide, ganciclovir sodium, methylprednisolone sodium succinate, mitomycin, piperacillin sodium, sodium bicarbonate, thiotepa, and sulfamethoxazole and trimethoprim when administered with these medications via Y-site injection. Therefore, vinorelbine should not be administered simultaneously with these medications via a Y-site injection.

**Note**
If accidental contamination of the eye with vinorelbine occurs, the eye should be immediately and thoroughly washed with water to prevent severe irritation.

Developed: 08/29/97
Interim revision: 07/01/98

# VITAMIN A  Systemic

VA CLASSIFICATION (Primary): VT050
Commonly used brand name(s): *Aquasol A*.
Another commonly used name is retinol.
Note: For a listing of dosage forms and brand names by country availability, see *Dosage Forms* section(s).

## Category
Nutritional supplement (vitamin).
Note: Vitamin A is a fat-soluble vitamin.

## Indications

### Accepted
Vitamin A deficiency (prophylaxis and treatment)—Vitamin A is indicated only for prevention or treatment of vitamin A deficiency states. Vitamin A deficiency may occur as a result of inadequate nutrition or intestinal malabsorption but does not occur in healthy individuals receiving an adequate balanced diet. For prophylaxis of vitamin A deficiency, dietary improvement, rather than supplementation, is advisable. For treatment of vitamin A deficiency, supplementation is preferred.

Deficiency of vitamin A may lead to keratomalacia, xerophthalmia, and nyctalopia (night blindness).

Recommended intakes may be increased and/or supplementation may be necessary in infants receiving unfortified formula or in individuals with the following conditions (based on documented vitamin A deficiency):
Diarrhea
Gastrectomy
Hyperthyroidism
Infections, chronic
Intestinal diseases—celiac, diarrhea, topical sprue, regional enteritis
Malabsorption syndromes associated with pancreatic insufficiency—pancreatic disease, cystic fibrosis
Measles
Protein deficiency, severe
Stress, prolonged
Xerophthalmia

Vitamin A absorption will be impaired in any condition in which fat malabsorption (steatorrhea) occurs.

Some studies have shown that vitamin A supplementation in the presence of vitamin A deficiency may reduce morbidity and mortality from certain diseases in children, including diarrhea and measles. Vitamin A deficiency is more likely to be a problem where malnutrition is prevalent.

Some unusual diets (e.g., reducing diets that drastically restrict food selection, especially the fat-containing foods) may not supply minimum daily recommended intakes of vitamin A. Supplementation is necessary in patients receiving total parenteral nutrition (TPN) or undergoing rapid weight loss or in those with malnutrition, because of inadequate dietary intake.

Recommended intakes for most vitamins and minerals are increased during pregnancy. Many physicians recommend that pregnant women receive multivitamin and mineral supplements, especially those pregnant women who do not consume an adequate diet and those in high-risk categories (i.e., women carrying more than one fetus, heavy cigarette smokers, and alcohol and drug abusers). Taking excessive amounts of a multivitamin and mineral supplement may be harmful to the mother and/or fetus and should be avoided.

Recommended intakes for all vitamins and most minerals are increased during breast-feeding.

Recommended intakes may be increased by the following medications: Cholestyramine, colestipol, mineral oil, and neomycin.

### Acceptance not established
There are insufficient data to show that vitamin A may reduce the occurrence of certain types of *cancer*.

### Unaccepted
Vitamin A is not useful for treatment of dry or wrinkled skin, eye problems, or prevention or treatment of infections not related to vitamin A deficiency. Large doses of vitamin A have been used for treatment of acne but, because of potential toxicity, this use is not recommended; topical retinoic acid (tretinoin) or isotretinoin, related compounds, are probably more useful. Vitamin A has not been proven effective for treatment of renal calculi, hyperthyroidism, anemia, degenerative conditions of the nervous system, sunburn, lung diseases, deafness, osteoarthritis, inflammatory bowel disease, or psoriasis.

## Pharmacology/Pharmacokinetics

### Mechanism of action/Effect
Vitamin A is essential for normal function of the retina. In the form of retinal, it combines with opsin (red pigment in the retina) to form rhodopsin (visual purple), which is necessary for visual adaptation to darkness. Other forms (retinol, retinoic acid) are necessary for growth of bone, testicular and ovarian function, and embryonic development, and for regulation of growth and differentiation of epithelial tissues. Retinol and retinoic acid may act as cofactors in biochemical reactions.

### Absorption
Vitamin A is readily absorbed from healthy gastrointestinal tract (duodenum and jejunum). Absorption of retinol requires presence of bile salts, pancreatic lipase, protein, and dietary fat. Excess, unabsorbed vitamin is excreted in feces. Water-miscible preparations are absorbed more readily than oil solutions.

### Protein binding
Less than 5% of circulating vitamin A is bound to lipoproteins in blood (normal), but may be up to 65% when hepatic stores are saturated be-

cause of excessive intake. The amount of vitamin A bound to lipoproteins may be increased in hyperlipoproteinemia. When released from liver, vitamin A is bound to retinol-binding protein (RBP). Most vitamin A circulates in the form of retinol bound to RBP.

**Storage**
Hepatic (approximately 2 years' adult requirements), with small amounts stored in kidney and lung tissues. Zinc is required for mobilization of vitamin A reserves in the liver.

**Biotransformation**
Hepatic.

**Elimination**
Fecal/renal.

## Precautions to Consider

**Pregnancy/Reproduction**
Pregnancy—Problems in humans have not been documented with intake of normal daily recommended amounts. Vitamin A crosses the placenta to only a limited extent. Fetal abnormalities (including urinary tract malformations), growth retardation, and early epiphyseal closure have been reported in children whose mothers took excessive amounts during pregnancy. Daily amounts from supplements exceeding 1800 RE (6000 Units) are not recommended because of potential fetotoxicity.

Maternal overdosage in animals has been reported to result in central nervous system (CNS) malformations, as well as malformations of the spinal column, rib cage, heart, eye, palate, and genitourinary tract of the fetus.

FDA Pregnancy Category X (parenteral vitamin A).

**Breast-feeding**
Vitamin A is distributed into breast milk; however, problems in humans have not been documented with intake of normal daily recommended amounts.

**Pediatrics**
Problems in pediatrics have not been documented with intake of normal daily recommended amounts. However, caution is recommended in young children, who are more likely to develop toxicity from higher-than-recommended doses and/or prolonged use of vitamin A.

**Geriatrics**
Problems in geriatrics have not been documented with intake of normal daily recommended amounts. However, long-term vitamin A use in the elderly may increase the risk of vitamin A overload due to delayed retinyl ester clearance.

**Dental**
High doses and/or prolonged use of vitamin A may cause bleeding from the gums; dry or sore mouth; or drying, cracking, or peeling of the lips.

**Drug interactions and/or related problems**
The following drug/dietary supplement interactions and/or related problems have been selected on the basis of their potential clinical significance (possible mechanism in parentheses where appropriate)—not necessarily inclusive (» = major clinical significance):

Note: Combinations containing any of the following medications or dietary supplements, depending on the amount present, may also interact with vitamin A supplements.

Calcium supplements
(excessive intake [more than 7500 RE or 25,000 Units per day] of vitamin A may stimulate bone loss and counteract the effects of calcium supplementation and may cause hypercalcemia)

Cholestyramine or
Colestipol or
Mineral oil or
Neomycin, oral
(concurrent use may interfere with absorption of vitamin A; recommended intakes for vitamin A may be increased or a water-miscible form of vitamin A may be needed in patients receiving these medications)

Contraceptives, oral
(concurrent use may increase plasma vitamin A concentrations)

» Etretinate or
» Isotretinoin
(concurrent use with vitamin A may result in additive toxic effects)

Tetracycline
(concurrent use with vitamin A 50,000 Units a day and higher has been reported to cause benign intracranial hypertension)

Vitamin E
(concurrent use of vitamin E may facilitate absorption, hepatic storage, and utilization of vitamin A, and reduce toxicity; excessive doses may deplete vitamin A stores)

**Laboratory value alterations**
The following have been selected on the basis of their potential clinical significance (possible effect in parentheses where appropriate)—not necessarily inclusive (» = major clinical significance):

With physiology/laboratory test values
Blood urea nitrogen (BUN) and
Calcium, serum and
Cholesterol and triglyceride, serum
(concentrations may be increased in chronic toxicity)

Erythrocyte counts and
Leukocyte counts
(may be decreased by high doses)

**Medical considerations/Contraindications**
The medical considerations/contraindications included have been selected on the basis of their potential clinical significance (reasons given in parentheses where appropriate)—not necessarily inclusive (» = major clinical significance).

*Except under special circumstances, vitamin A supplements should not be used when the following medical problem exists:*
» Hypervitaminosis A

*Risk-benefit should be considered when the following medical problems exist:*

Alcoholism, chronic or
Cirrhosis or
Hepatic disease or
Viral hepatitis
(use of vitamin A in these conditions may potentiate hepatotoxicity; however, this may not apply in cases of chronic cholestatic liver disease with accompanying vitamin A malabsorption)

» Renal failure, chronic
(serum vitamin A concentrations are increased)

Sensitivity to vitamin A

**Patient monitoring**
The following may be especially important in patient monitoring (other tests may be warranted in some patients, depending on condition; » = major clinical significance):

Carotene determinations, plasma and
» Vitamin A determinations, plasma
(recommended to confirm deficiency; plasma vitamin A concentrations are not necessarily indicative of vitamin A nutritional status because of significant hepatic storage, although low concentrations correlate with deficiency)

Dark adaptation tests

## Overdose

For more information on the management of overdose or unintentional ingestion **contact a Poison Control Center** (see *Poison Control Center Listing*).

**Clinical effects of overdose**
The following effects have been selected on the basis of their potential clinical significance (possible signs and symptoms in parentheses where appropriate)—not necessarily inclusive:

Note: Ingestion of excessive doses of vitamin A acutely (greater than 450,000 RE [1,500,000 Units] in adults and 22,500 RE [75,000 Units] to 105,100 RE [350,000 Units] in children, depending on age) or over prolonged periods (greater than 7500 RE [25,000 Units] a day for eight months in adults and 5400 RE [18,000 Units] to 15,000 RE [50,000 Units] a day for several months in children, depending on age) can result in severe toxicity and even death. Daily doses higher than 1800 RE (6000 Units) in pregnant women are not recommended because of potential fetotoxicity.

Acute effects
*Bleeding from gums or sore mouth; bulging soft spot on head*—in babies; *confusion or unusual excitement; diarrhea; dizziness or drowsiness; double vision; severe headache; severe irritability; peeling of skin, especially on lips and palms; severe vomiting*

Note: Toxicity usually occurs about 6 hours after ingestion of acute overdoses of vitamin A. Acute overdose also results in hydrocephalus in infants and increased intracranial pressure (pseudotumor cerebri) in older children and adults. Acute toxicity is reversible on withdrawal of vitamin A.

**Chronic effects**
*Bone or joint pain; drying or cracking of skin or lips; dry mouth; fever; general feeling of discomfort or illness or weakness; headache; increased sensitivity of skin to sunlight; increase in frequency of urination, especially at night, or in amount of urine; irritability; loss of appetite; loss of hair; seizures; stomach pain; unusual tiredness; vomiting; yellow-orange patches on soles of feet, palms of hands, or skin around nose and lips*

Note: Chronic overdose may also result in any of the following: hepatotoxicity, papilledema, intracranial hypertension, hypomenorrhea, portal hypertension, hemolysis and anemia, radiographic bone changes, and, in children, premature closure of epiphyses. Chronic toxicity is slowly reversible on withdrawal of vitamin A, but may persist for several weeks.

**Treatment of overdose**
Hypervitaminosis A is treated by withdrawing vitamin A and instituting symptomatic and supportive treatment. Some signs and symptoms disappear within 1 week, while others may persist for several weeks to months.

For female patients of childbearing potential, it is recommended that a pregnancy test be performed and a blood sample collected for the determination of vitamin A concentrations at the time of overdose and at one complete menstrual cycle after the overdose. Effective contraception should be used for at least one complete menstrual cycle after the overdose and continued if necessary until vitamin A concentrations are no longer measurable in the blood. Patients with a positive pregnancy test should be counseled on the risk of fetotoxicity.

# Patient Consultation

As an aid to patient consultation, refer to *Advice for the Patient, Vitamin A (Systemic)*.
In providing consultation, consider emphasizing the following selected information (» = major clinical significance):

**Description of use**
Description should include function in the body, signs of deficiency, and unproven uses

**Importance of diet**
Importance of proper nutrition; supplement may be needed because of inadequate dietary intake
Food sources of vitamin A; difference between retinols and beta-carotene; effects of processing
Not using vitamins as substitute for balanced diet
Recommended daily intake for vitamin A

**Before using this dietary supplement**
» Conditions affecting use, especially:
 Sensitivity to vitamin A
 Pregnancy—Fetal abnormalities, growth retardation, early epiphyseal closure reported in children of mothers taking excessive amounts during pregnancy; daily doses above 1800 retinol equivalents (RE) (6000 Units) not recommended
 Use in children—Children may be more sensitive to effects of high doses and/or prolonged use
 Use in the elderly—Use of high doses may cause vitamin A overload
 Dental—High doses and/or prolonged use of vitamin A may cause bleeding from the gums; dry or sore mouth; or drying, cracking, or peeling of the lips
 Other medications, especially etretinate and isotretinoin
 Other medical problems, especially hypervitaminosis A or chronic renal failure

**Proper use of this dietary supplement**
» Proper dosing
 Missed dose: No cause for concern because of length of time necessary for depletion; remembering to take as directed
  Proper administration of oral solution dosage form: Taking by mouth even though it comes in dropper bottle; may be dropped directly into the mouth or mixed with cereal, fruit juice, or other food
» Proper storage

**Precautions while using this dietary supplement**
Risk of toxicity with chronic overdose; upper limits for chronic and acute vitamin A toxicity; upper limits for use in pregnancy

# General Dosing Information

**For oral dosage forms only**
When oral absorption or storage of vitamin A is impaired, higher doses or parenteral administration may be required.

Water-miscible preparations may be useful for prevention of vitamin A deficiency in individuals with fat malabsorption, although if bile acid depletion is present, high doses may still be necessary.

**For parenteral dosage forms only**
Parenteral administration is indicated when oral administration is not acceptable (for example, in nausea, vomiting, preoperative and postoperative conditions) or possible, or when ocular damage is severe.

The administration of intravenous vitamin A is restricted to special intravenous preparations.

**Diet/Nutrition**
Recommended dietary intakes for vitamin A are defined differently worldwide.
For U.S.—
 The Recommended Dietary Allowances (RDAs) for vitamins and minerals are determined by the Food and Nutrition Board of the National Research Council and are intended to provide adequate nutrition in most healthy persons under usual environmental stresses. In addition, a different designation may be used by the FDA for food labeling purposes, as with Daily Value (DV). DVs replace the previous labeling terminology United States Recommended Daily Allowances (USRDAs).
For Canada—
 Recommended Nutrient Intakes (RNIs) for vitamins, minerals, and protein are determined by Health and Welfare Canada and provide recommended amounts of a specific nutrient while minimizing the risk of chronic diseases.
The expression of vitamin A activity has changed from Units to retinol equivalents (RE) or micrograms (mcg) of retinol, with 1 RE equal to 1 mcg of retinol. One RE of vitamin A is equal to 3.33 Units of retinol and 10 Units of vitamin A activity as beta-carotene. This conversion was made because the term Units did not take into account the poor absorption and bioavailability of carotenoids. Most commercially available vitamin A products continue to be labeled in Units.
Daily recommended dietary intakes for vitamin A are generally defined according to age or condition and form of vitamin A as follows

*For the U.S.*

| Age or Condition | Form of Vitamin A |||
|---|---|---|---|
| | RE or mcg of Retinol | Amount in Units as Retinol | Amount in Units as a Combination of Retinol and Beta-carotene* |
| Infants and children | | | |
| Birth to 3 years | 375–400 | 1250–1330 | 1875–2000 |
| 4 to 6 years | 500 | 1665 | 2500 |
| 7 to 10 years | 700 | 2330 | 3500 |
| Adolescent and adult males | 1000 | 3330 | 5000 |
| Adolescent and adult females | 800 | 2665 | 4000 |
| Pregnant females | 800 | 2665 | 4000 |
| Breast-feeding females | 1200–1300 | 4000–4330 | 6000–6500 |

*Based on 1980 Recommended Dietary Allowances (RDAs) for vitamin A in the diet that is a combination of retinol and beta-carotene.

*For Canada*

| Age or Condition | Form of Vitamin A |||
|---|---|---|---|
| | RE or mcg of Retinol | Amount in Units as Retinol | Amount in Units as a Combination of Retinol and Beta-carotene* |
| Infants and children | | | |
| Birth to 3 years | 400 | 1330 | 2000 |
| 4 to 6 years | 500 | 1665 | 2500 |
| 7 to 10 years | 700–800 | 2330–2665 | 3500 |
| Adolescent and adult males | 1000 | 3330 | 5000 |
| Adolescent and adult females | 800 | 2665 | 4000 |
| Pregnant females | 900 | 2665–3000 | 4000–4500 |
| Breast-feeding females | 1200 | 4000 | 6000 |

*Based on 1980 U.S. Recommended Dietary Allowances (RDAs) for vitamin A in the diet that is a combination of retinol and beta-carotene.

The above recommended dietary intakes are usually provided by nutritionally adequate diets.

Best dietary sources of vitamin A activity include yellow-orange fruits and vegetables; dark green, leafy vegetables; vitamin A-fortified milk; liver; and margarine. Approximately 20% of beta-carotene, which is found in green and yellow vegetables, is converted to retinol after absorption from the gastrointestinal tract. Ordinary cooking does not destroy vitamin A activity in vegetables, but frozen foods lose 5 to 10% during storage for 12 months at −23 °C.

## Oral Dosage Forms

### VITAMIN A CAPSULES USP

**Usual adult and adolescent dose**
Deficiency (prophylaxis)—
    Oral, amount based on normal daily recommended intakes:
*For the U.S.*

| Age or Condition | Form of Vitamin A |||
|---|---|---|---|
| | RE or mcg of Retinol | Amount in Units as Retinol | Amount in Units as a Combination of Retinol and Beta-carotene* |
| Adolescent and adult males | 1000 | 3330 | 5000 |
| Adolescent and adult females | 800 | 2665 | 4000 |
| Pregnant females | 800 | 2665 | 4000 |
| Breast-feeding females | 1200–1300 | 4000–4330 | 6000–6500 |

*Based on 1980 Recommended Dietary Allowances (RDAs) for vitamin A in the diet that is a combination of retinol and beta-carotene.

*For Canada*

| Age or Condition | Form of Vitamin A |||
|---|---|---|---|
| | RE or mcg of Retinol | Amount in Units as Retinol | Amount in Units as a Combination of Retinol and Beta-carotene* |
| Adolescent and adult males | 1000 | 3330 | 5000 |
| Adolescent and adult females | 800 | 2665 | 4000 |
| Pregnant females | 900 | 2665–3000 | 4000–4500 |
| Breast-feeding females | 1200 | 4000 | 6000 |

*Based on 1980 U.S. Recommended Dietary Allowances (RDAs) for vitamin A in the diet that is a combination of retinol and beta-carotene.

Deficiency (treatment)—
    Treatment dose is individualized by prescriber based on severity of deficiency. The following dosage has been established:
Xerophthalmia—
    Oral, 7500 to 15,000 RE (25,000 to 50,000 Units) a day.
Note:   Acute toxicity has been reported at a single dose of 450,000 RE (1,500,000 Units). Chronic toxicity has been reported at doses of 7500 RE (25,000 Units) a day for eight months. However, individuals with compromised liver function may develop toxicity at lower doses.

**Usual pediatric dose**
Deficiency (prophylaxis)—
    Oral, amount based on intake of normal daily recommended intakes:
*For the U.S.*

| Age or Condition | Form of Vitamin A |||
|---|---|---|---|
| | RE or mcg of Retinol | Amount in Units as Retinol | Amount in Units as a Combination of Retinol and Beta-carotene* |
| Infants and children | | | |
| Birth to 3 years | 375–400 | 1250–1330 | 1875–2000 |
| 4 to 6 years | 500 | 1665 | 2500 |
| 7 to 10 years | 700 | 2330 | 3500 |

*Based on 1980 Recommended Dietary Allowances (RDAs) for vitamin A in the diet that is a combination of retinol and beta-carotene.

*For Canada*

| Age or Condition | Form of Vitamin A |||
|---|---|---|---|
| | RE or mcg of Retinol | Amount in Units as Retinol | Amount in Units as a Combination of Retinol and Beta-carotene* |
| Infants and children | | | |
| Birth to 3 years | 400 | 1330 | 2000 |
| 4 to 6 years | 500 | 1665 | 2500 |
| 7 to 10 years | 700–800 | 2330–2665 | 3500 |

*Based on 1980 U.S. Recommended Dietary Allowances (RDAs) for vitamin A in the diet that is a combination of retinol and beta-carotene.

Deficiency (treatment)—
    Treatment dose is individualized by prescriber based on severity of deficiency. The following dosages have been established:
Measles:
    Children 6 months to 1 year of age: Oral, 30,000 RE (100,000 Units) as a single dose when measles are diagnosed.
    Children 1 year of age and older: Oral, 60,000 RE (200,000 Units) as a single dose when measles are diagnosed.
Xerophthalmia:
    Children 6 months to 1 year of age: Oral, 30,000 RE (100,000 Units) as a single dose, repeated the next day, and again at 4 weeks.
    Children 1 year of age and older: Oral, 60,000 RE (200,000 Units) as a single dose, repeated the next day, and again at 4 weeks.
Note:   The vitamin A doses recommended for measles and xerophthalmia are based on World Health Organization (WHO) guidelines and are used when vitamin A deficiency may be a problem, such as in malnutrition or selected disease states.
    Acute toxicity has been reported at a single dose of 22,500 to 105,100 RE (75,000 to 350,000 Units), depending on age. Chronic toxicity has been reported at doses of 5400 to 15,000 RE (18,000 to 50,000 Units) a day for several months. However, individuals with compromised liver function may develop toxicity at lower doses.

**Strength(s) usually available**
U.S.—
    10,000 Units (3000 RE) (Rx/OTC) [GENERIC].
    25,000 Units (7500 RE) [*Aquasol A (Rx);* GENERIC].
    50,000 Units (15,000 RE) (Rx) [*Aquasol A;* GENERIC].
Canada—
    10,000 Units (3000 RE) (Rx/OTC) [GENERIC].
    25,000 Units (7500 RE) (Rx) [*Aquasol A;* GENERIC].
    50,000 Units (15,000 RE) (Rx) [*Aquasol A;* GENERIC].
Note:   A water-miscible product is available.
    Some strengths of these vitamin A preparations may exceed the dosage range recommended by USP DI Advisory Panels based on the amount necessary to meet normal nutritional needs.

**Packaging and storage**
Store below 40 °C (104 °F), preferably between 15 and 30 °C (59 and 86 °F), unless otherwise specified by manufacturer. Store in a tight, light-resistant container. Protect from light.

### VITAMIN A ORAL SOLUTION

**Usual adult and adolescent dose**
See *Vitamin A Capsules USP*.

**Usual pediatric dose**
See *Vitamin A Capsules USP*.

**Strength(s) usually available**
U.S.—
    5000 Units (1500 RE) per 0.1 mL (Rx) [*Aquasol A*].
Canada—
    Not commercially available.
Note:   Product is water-miscible.
    The strength of this vitamin A preparation may exceed the dosage range recommended by USP DI Advisory Panels based on the amount necessary to meet normal nutritional needs.

**Packaging and storage**
Store below 40 °C (104 °F), preferably between 15 and 30 °C (59 and 86 °F), unless otherwise specified by manufacturer. Store in a tight container. Protect from light. Protect from freezing.

## VITAMIN A TABLETS

**Usual adult and adolescent dose**
See *Vitamin A Capsules USP*.

**Usual pediatric dose**
See *Vitamin A Capsules USP*.

**Strength(s) usually available**
U.S.—
　10,000 Units (3000 RE) (Rx/OTC) [GENERIC].
　25,000 Units (7500 RE) (Rx/OTC) [GENERIC].
　50,000 Units (15,000 RE) (Rx) [GENERIC].
Canada—
　Not commercially available.

Note: Some strengths of these vitamin A preparations may exceed the dosage range recommended by USP DI Advisory Panels based on the amount necessary to meet normal nutritional needs.

**Packaging and storage**
Store below 40 °C (104 °F), preferably between 15 and 30 °C (59 and 86 °F), unless otherwise specified by manufacturer. Store in a tight container. Protect from light.

## Parenteral Dosage Forms

### VITAMIN A INJECTION

**Usual adult and adolescent dose**
Deficiency (prophylaxis or treatment)—
　Intravenous infusion, as part of total parenteral nutrition solutions, the specific amount determined by individual patient need.
　Intramuscular, 15,000 to 30,000 RE (50,000 to 100,000 Units) a day for three days, followed by 15,000 RE (50,000 Units) a day for two weeks.

**Usual pediatric dose**
Deficiency (prophylaxis or treatment)—
　Children up to 1 year of age:
　　Intramuscular, 1500 to 3000 RE (5000 to 10,000 Units) a day for ten days.
　　In severe deficiency—Intramuscular, 2250 to 4500 RE (7500 to 15,000 Units) a day for ten days.
　Children 1 to 8 years of age:
　　Intramuscular, 1500 to 4500 RE (5000 to 15,000 Units) a day for ten days.
　　In severe deficiency—Intramuscular, 5250 to 10,500 RE (17,500 to 35,000 Units) a day for ten days.
　Children 8 years of age and over:
　　See *Usual adult and adolescent dose*.

**Strength(s) usually available**
U.S.—
　50,000 Units (15,000 RE) per mL (Rx) [*Aquasol A*].
Canada—
　Not commercially available.

Note: Product is water-miscible.

**Packaging and storage**
Store below 40 °C (104 °F), preferably between 15 and 30 °C (59 and 86 °F), unless otherwise specified by manufacturer. Protect from light. Protect from freezing.

**Stability**
Vitamin A has been found to adsorb to PVC containers and tubing. Exposure to light causes degradation of vitamin A; therefore, total parenteral solutions that contain vitamin A should be protected from light. Total parenteral nutrition solutions containing vitamin A should be used within 24 hours of admixture.

Revised: 07/29/94
Interim revision: 05/26/95

---

# VITAMIN B$_{12}$　Systemic

This monograph includes information on the following: 1) Cyanocobalamin; 2) Hydroxocobalamin†.

VA CLASSIFICATION (Primary/Secondary): VT101/DX900

Commonly used brand name(s): *Alphamin*[2]; *Anacobin*[1]; *Bedoz*[1]; *Cobex*[1]; *Cobolin-M*[1]; *Crystamine*[1]; *Crysti-12*[1]; *Cyanoject*[1]; *Cyomin*[1]; *Hydro-Cobex*[2]; *Hydro-Crysti-12*[2]; *Hydrobexan*[2]; *Hydroxy-Cobal*[2]; *LA-12*[2]; *Neuroforte-R*[1]; *Primabalt*[1]; *Rubesol-1000*[1]; *Rubramin PC*[1]; *Shovite*[1]; *Vibal*[1]; *Vibal LA*[2]; *Vitabee 12*[1].

Note: For a listing of dosage forms and brand names by country availability, see *Dosage Forms* section(s).

†Not commercially available in Canada.

## Category

Nutritional supplement (vitamin); antianemic; diagnostic aid (vitamin B$_{12}$ deficiency)

Note: Vitamin B$_{12}$ (also known as the cobalamins) is a water-soluble vitamin.

## Indications

Note: Bracketed information in the *Indications* section refers to uses that are not included in U.S. product labeling.

Note: Indications for cyanocobalamin and hydroxocobalamin are the same, although hydroxocobalamin may be preferred for treatment of vitamin B$_{12}$ deficiency since optic neuropathies may degenerate with administration of cyanocobalamin. However, some patients develop antibodies to the hydroxocobalamin-transcobalamin II complex.

**Accepted**
Anemia, pernicious (treatment)—Vitamin B$_{12}$ is indicated for treatment of pernicious anemia (due to lack of or inhibition of intrinsic factor).
Vitamin B$_{12}$ deficiency (prophylaxis and treatment)—Vitamin B$_{12}$ is indicated for prevention and treatment of vitamin B$_{12}$ deficiency.

Deficiency of vitamin B$_{12}$ may lead to macrocytic, megaloblastic anemia and possible irreversible neurologic damage.

Vitamin B$_{12}$ deficiency may occur as a result of inadequate nutrition or intestinal malabsorption but does not occur in healthy individuals receiving an adequate balanced diet. However, simple vitamin B$_{12}$ deficiency may occur in strict vegetarians (vegan-vegetarians) and their breast-fed infants since vitamin B$_{12}$ is found in animal protein and not in vegetables. For prophylaxis of vitamin B$_{12}$ deficiency, dietary improvement, rather than supplementation, is advisable. For treatment of vitamin B$_{12}$ deficiency, supplementation is preferred.

Recommended intakes may be increased and/or supplementation may be necessary in the following conditions (based on documented vitamin B$_{12}$ deficiency):
Alcoholism
Anemia, hemolytic
Fever, chronic
Fish tapeworm infestation
Gastrectomy
Gastritis, atropic with achlorhydria
Genetic disorders—homocystinuria and/or methylmalonic aciduria
Hepatic-biliary tract disease—hepatic function impairment, alcoholism with cirrhosis
Hyperthyroidism
Intestinal diseases—celiac, tropical sprue, regional enteritis, bacterial overgrowth of small intestine, persistent diarrhea, ileal resection
Infection, prolonged
Malabsorption syndromes associated with pancreatic insufficiency
Malignancy of pancreas or bowel
Renal disease
Stress, prolonged

Some unusual diets (e.g., vegan-vegetarian, macrobiotic, or reducing diets that drastically restrict food selection) may not supply minimum daily requirements of vitamin B$_{12}$. Supplementation is necessary in patients receiving total parenteral nutrition (TPN) or undergoing rapid weight loss or in those with malnutrition, because of inadequate dietary intake.

Recommended intakes for all vitamins and most minerals are increased during pregnancy. Many physicians recommend that pregnant women receive multivitamin and mineral supplements, especially those pregnant women who do not consume an adequate diet and those in high-risk categories (i.e., women carrying more than one fetus, heavy cigarette smokers, and alcohol and drug abusers). Taking excessive amounts of a multivitamin and mineral supplement may be harmful to the mother and/or fetus and should be avoided.

Pregnant women who are strict vegetarians (vegan-vegetarians) may need vitamin $B_{12}$ supplementation.

Recommended intakes for all vitamins and most minerals are increased during breast-feeding.

Recommended intakes may be increased by the following medications: Aminosalicylates, colchicine, and epoetin.

Vitamin $B_{12}$ should not be administered as a dietary supplement before pernicious anemia or folic acid deficiency has been ruled out.

[Vitamin $B_{12}$ deficiency (diagnosis)]—Cyanocobalamin or hydroxocobalamin may be used as the flushing dose in the Schilling test for vitamin $B_{12}$ malabsorption.

### Unaccepted
Cyanocobalamin has not been proven effective for treatment of acute viral hepatitis; aging; allergies; amblyopia; delayed growth, poor appetite, or malnutrition; dermatologic disorders; fatigue; mental disorders; multiple sclerosis; sterility; thyrotoxicosis; and trigeminal neuralgia and other neuropathies.

## Pharmacology/Pharmacokinetics

### Physicochemical characteristics
Molecular weight—
  Cyanocobalamin: 1355.39.
  Hydroxocobalamin: 1346.38.

### Mechanism of action/Effect
Vitamin $B_{12}$ acts as a coenzyme for various metabolic functions, including fat and carbohydrate metabolism and protein synthesis. It is necessary for growth, cell replication, hematopoiesis, and nucleoprotein and myelin synthesis, largely due to its effects on metabolism of methionine, folic acid, and malonic acid.

### Absorption
The B vitamins are readily absorbed from the gastrointestinal tract, except in malabsorption syndromes. Vitamin $B_{12}$ is absorbed in the lower half of the ileum.

Dietary vitamin $B_{12}$ is released from the proteins to which it is bound by gastric acid and pancreatic proteases, before being bound to the intrinsic factor (IF).

A vitamin $B_{12}$–IF complex is formed and passes down the intestine where it binds with receptor sites on the ileal mucosa so that vitamin $B_{12}$ can be absorbed into the systemic circulation. Calcium and a pH greater than 5.4 are required for attachment to the receptor sites.

The enterohepatic circulation conserves vitamin $B_{12}$ by reabsorbing vitamin $B_{12}$ from bile.

### Protein binding
Very high (to specific plasma proteins called transcobalamins); binding of hydroxocobalamin is slightly higher than cyanocobalamin.

### Storage
Hepatic (90%); some renal.

### Biotransformation
Hepatic.

### Half-life
Approximately 6 days (400 days in the liver).

### Time to peak plasma concentration
After oral administration—8 to 12 hours.
After intramuscular administration—60 minutes.

### Elimination
Biliary. Excess beyond daily needs is excreted, largely unchanged, in urine.

## Precautions to Consider

### Cross-sensitivity and/or related problems
Individuals sensitive to other cobalamins (found naturally in foods) may be sensitive to vitamin $B_{12}$ also.

### Carcinogenicity
Studies have not been done in either animals or humans.

### Pregnancy/Reproduction
Pregnancy—Studies have not been done in humans. Problems in humans have not been documented with intake of normal daily recommended amounts.

Studies have not been done in animals.
FDA Pregnancy Category C (parenteral).

### Breast-feeding
Vitamin $B_{12}$ is distributed into breast milk; however, problems in humans have not been documented with intake of normal daily recommended amounts.

### Pediatrics
Problems in pediatrics have not been documented with intake of normal daily recommended amounts.

Cyanocobalamin injection that contains benzyl alcohol as a preservative should not be used in newborn and immature infants. The use of benzyl alcohol in neonates has been associated with a fatal toxic syndrome consisting of metabolic acidosis and central nervous system (CNS), respiratory, circulatory, and renal function impairment.

### Geriatrics
Problems in geriatrics have not been documented with intake of normal daily recommended amounts.

### Drug interactions and/or related problems
The following drug interactions and/or related problems have been selected on the basis of their potential clinical significance (possible mechanism in parentheses where appropriate)—not necessarily inclusive (» = major clinical significance):

Note: Combinations containing any of the following, depending on the amount present, may also interact with vitamin $B_{12}$ supplements.

Alcohol, excessive intake for longer than 2 weeks or
Aminosalicylates or
Colchicine, especially in combination with aminoglycosides
  (may act to reduce absorption of vitamin $B_{12}$ from the gastrointestinal tract; requirements for vitamin $B_{12}$ may be increased in patients receiving these medications)
Antibiotics
  (may interfere with the microbiologic method of assay for serum and erythrocyte vitamin $B_{12}$ concentrations and cause falsely low results)
Folic acid
  (large and continuous doses may reduce vitamin $B_{12}$ concentrations in blood)

### Medical considerations/Contraindications
The medical considerations/contraindications included have been selected on the basis of their potential clinical significance (reasons given in parentheses where appropriate)—not necessarily inclusive (» = major clinical significance).

*Except under special circumstances, this medication should not be used when the following medical problem exists:*

For cyanocobalamin
» Leber's disease
  (optic nerve atrophy has occurred rapidly after administration; cyanocobalamin concentrations are already elevated)

*Risk-benefit should be considered when the following medical problem exists:*

Sensitivity to cyanocobalamin or hydroxocobalamin

### Patient monitoring
The following may be especially important in patient monitoring (other tests may be warranted in some patients, depending on condition; » = major clinical significance):

Folic acid concentrations, plasma and
Hematocrit and
Reticulocyte count, plasma and
Vitamin $B_{12}$ concentrations, plasma
  (determinations recommended prior to treatment and between the 5th and 7th days of therapy)
Potassium concentrations, serum
  (determinations recommended during first 48 hours of treatment of megaloblastic anemia to detect possible serious hypokalemia, which could result in sudden death)

## Side/Adverse Effects

Note: Water-soluble vitamins seldom cause toxicity in persons with normal renal function.

  Treatment with vitamin $B_{12}$ may unmask the signs of polycythemia vera.

The following side/adverse effects have been selected on the basis of their potential clinical significance (possible signs and symptoms in parentheses where appropriate)—not necessarily inclusive:

## Those indicating need for medical attention
Incidence rare
   *Anaphylactic reaction* (skin rash; itching; wheezing)—after parenteral administration

## Those indicating need for medical attention only if they continue or are bothersome
Incidence less frequent
   *Diarrhea; itching of skin*

# Patient Consultation
As an aid to patient consultation, refer to *Advice for the Patient, Vitamin B₁₂ (Systemic)*.
In providing consultation, consider emphasizing the following selected information (» = major clinical significance):

### Description of use
   Description should include function in the body, signs of deficiency, and unproven uses

### Importance of diet
   Importance of proper nutrition; supplement may be needed because of inadequate dietary intake
   Food sources of vitamin $B_{12}$; effects of processing
   Not using vitamins as substitute for balanced diet
   Recommended daily intake for vitamin $B_{12}$

### Before using this dietary supplement
» Conditions affecting use, especially:
      Sensitivity to cobalamins
      Other medical problems, especially Leber's disease

### Proper use of this dietary supplement
» Proper dosing
» Need for lifelong therapy for pernicious anemia or following gastrectomy or ileal resection
   Missed dose: No cause for concern because of length of time necessary for depletion; remembering to take as directed
» Proper storage

### Side/adverse effects
   Signs of potential side effects, especially anaphylactic reaction

# General Dosing Information
Because of the infrequency of single B vitamin deficiencies, combinations are commonly administered. Many commercial combinations of B vitamins are available.

Vitamin $B_{12}$ is also synthesized by bacteria in the gastrointestinal tract but is not absorbed and is excreted in the feces.

A diagnosis of vitamin $B_{12}$ deficiency should be confirmed by laboratory investigations before institution of vitamin $B_{12}$ therapy; vitamin $B_{12}$ administration may mask folic acid deficiency.

### For oral dosage forms only
The oral route is useful only for treating nutritional vitamin $B_{12}$ deficiency (when gastrointestinal absorption is normal or in vegan-vegetarians); it is not useful in small bowel disease, malabsorption syndromes, or following gastric or ileal resection. Oral preparations containing intrinsic factor have little reliable continuous efficacy in pernicious anemia.

### For parenteral dosage forms only
Cyanocobalamin or hydroxocobalamin injection should not be administered intravenously, although small amounts of cyanocobalamin are sometimes included in total parenteral nutrition (TPN) solutions.

### Diet/Nutrition
Recommended dietary intakes for vitamin $B_{12}$ are defined differently worldwide.

For U.S.—
   The Recommended Dietary Allowances (RDAs) for vitamins and minerals are determined by the Food and Nutrition Board of the National Research Council and are intended to provide adequate nutrition in most healthy persons under usual environmental stresses. In addition, a different designation may be used by the FDA for food and dietary supplement labeling purposes, as with Daily Value (DV). DVs replace the previous labeling terminology United States Recommended Daily Allowances (USRDAs).

For Canada—
   Recommended Nutrient Intakes (RNIs) for vitamins, minerals, and protein are determined by Health and Welfare Canada and provide recommended amounts of a specific nutrient while minimizing the risk of chronic diseases.

Daily recommended intakes for vitamin $B_{12}$ are generally defined as follows:

| Persons | U.S. (mcg) | Canada (mcg) |
|---|---|---|
| Infants and children | | |
|   Birth to 3 years of age | 0.3–0.7 | 0.3–0.4 |
|   4 to 6 years of age | 1 | 0.5 |
|   7 to 10 years of age | 1.4 | 0.8–1 |
| Adolescent and adult males | 2 | 1–2 |
| Adolescent and adult females | 2 | 1–2 |
| Pregnant females | 2.2 | 2–3 |
| Breast-feeding females | 2.6 | 1.5–2.5 |

These are usually provided by adequate diets.

Best dietary sources of vitamin $B_{12}$ are fish, seafood, egg yolk, milk, and fermented cheeses. Vitamin $B_{12}$ is not found in vegetables; however, bacteria found on vegetables may be a source of vitamin $B_{12}$ for vegan-vegetarians. There is little loss of vitamin $B_{12}$ from foods with ordinary cooking; however, severe heating may cause degeneration.

---

## CYANOCOBALAMIN

# Summary of Differences
Indications for cyanocobalamin and hydroxocobalamin are the same, although hydroxocobalamin may be preferred for treatment of vitamin $B_{12}$ deficiency since optic neuropathies may degenerate with administration of cyanocobalamin. However, some patients develop antibodies to the hydroxocobalamin-transcobalamin II complex.

# Oral Dosage Forms
## CYANOCOBALAMIN TABLETS
### Usual adult and adolescent dose
Deficiency (prophylaxis)—
   Oral, amount based on normal daily recommended intakes:

| Persons | U.S. (mcg) | Canada (mcg) |
|---|---|---|
| Adolescent and adult males | 2 | 1–2 |
| Adolescent and adult females | 2 | 1–2 |
| Pregnant females | 2.2 | 2–3 |
| Breast-feeding females | 2.6 | 1.5–2.5 |

Deficiency (treatment)—
   Treatment dose is individualized by prescriber based on severity of deficiency.

### Usual pediatric dose
Deficiency (prophylaxis)—
   Oral, amount based on normal daily recommended intakes:

| Persons | U.S. (mcg) | Canada (mcg) |
|---|---|---|
| Infants and children | | |
|   Birth to 3 years of age | 0.3–0.7 | 0.3–0.4 |
|   4 to 6 years of age | 1 | 0.5 |
|   7 to 10 years of age | 1.4 | 0.8–1 |

Deficiency (treatment)—
   Treatment dose is individualized by prescriber based on severity of deficiency.

### Strength(s) usually available
U.S.—
   25 mcg (0.025 mg) (OTC) [GENERIC].
   50 mcg (0.05 mg) (OTC) [GENERIC].
   100 mcg (0.1 mg) (OTC) [GENERIC].
   200 mcg (0.2 mg) (OTC) [GENERIC].
   250 mcg (0.25 mg) (OTC) [GENERIC].
   500 mcg (0.5 mg) (OTC) [GENERIC].
   1000 mcg (1 mg) (OTC) [GENERIC].
   1500 mcg (1.5 mg) (OTC) [GENERIC].
Canada—
   10 mcg (0.01 mg) (OTC) [GENERIC].
   25 mcg (0.025 mg) (OTC) [GENERIC].
   100 mcg (0.1 mg) (OTC) [GENERIC].
   250 mcg (0.25 mg) (OTC) [GENERIC].

Note: Some strengths of these cyanocobalamin preparations may exceed the dosage range recommended by USP DI Advisory Panels based on the amount necessary to meet normal nutritional needs.

**Packaging and storage**
Store below 40 °C (104 °F), preferably between 15 and 30 °C (59 and 86 °F), in a tight container, unless otherwise specified by manufacturer. Protect from light.

## CYANOCOBALAMIN EXTENDED-RELEASE TABLETS
**Usual adult and adolescent dose**
See *Cyanocobalamin Tablets*.

**Usual pediatric dose**
Dosage form not suitable for use in children.

**Strength(s) usually available**
U.S.—
  100 mcg (0.1 mg) (OTC) [GENERIC].
  200 mcg (0.2 mg) (OTC) [GENERIC].
  500 mcg (0.5 mg) (OTC) [GENERIC].
  1000 mcg (1 mg) (OTC) [GENERIC].
Canada—
  Not commercially available.

Note: Some strengths of these cyanocobalamin preparations may exceed the dosage range recommended by USP DI Advisory Panels based on the amount necessary to meet normal nutritional needs.

**Packaging and storage**
Store below 40 °C (104 °F), preferably between 15 and 30 °C (59 and 86 °F), in a tight container, unless otherwise specified by manufacturer. Protect from light.

# Parenteral Dosage Forms
Note: Bracketed uses in the *Dosage Forms* section refer to categories of use and/or indications that are not included in U.S. product labeling.

## CYANOCOBALAMIN INJECTION USP
**Usual and adolescent adult dose**
Deficiency (prophylaxis)—
  Intravenous infusion, as part of total parenteral nutrition solutions, the specific amount determined by individual patient need.
Deficiency (treatment)—
  Initial: Intramuscular or deep subcutaneous, 100 mcg (0.1 mg) per day for six or seven days, followed by 100 mcg (0.1 mg) every other day for seven doses if clinical improvement and a reticulocyte response occur, then 100 mcg (0.1 mg) every three or four days for another two to three weeks.
  Maintenance: Intramuscular, 100 to 200 mcg (0.1 to 0.2 mg) once a month (in pernicious anemia and following total gastrectomy and extensive ileal resection, parenteral maintenance supplementation is continued for life).
[Diagnostic aid (vitamin B$_{12}$ deficiency)]—
  Intramuscular, 1 mcg (0.001 mg) per day for ten days plus low dietary folic acid and vitamin B$_{12}$. The flushing dose for the Schilling test is 1000 mcg (1 mg) intramuscularly.

**Usual pediatric dose**
Deficiency (prophylaxis)—
  Intravenous infusion, as part of total parenteral nutrition solutions, the specific amount determined by individual patient need.
Deficiency (treatment)—
  Initial: Intramuscular or deep subcutaneous, 30 to 50 mcg (0.03 to 0.05 mg) per day for two or more weeks (total dose of 1 to 5 mg).
  Maintenance: Intramuscular or deep subcutaneous, 100 mcg (0.1 mg) once a month as necessary (for life in the case of pernicious anemia and following total gastrectomy and extensive ileal resection).

Note: Cyanocobalamin injection that contains benzyl alcohol as a preservative should not be used in newborn and immature infants. The use of benzyl alcohol in neonates has been associated with a fatal toxic syndrome consisting of metabolic acidosis and CNS, respiratory, circulatory, and renal function impairment.

**Strength(s) usually available**
U.S.—
  30 mcg (0.03 mg) per mL (Rx) [GENERIC].
  100 mcg (0.1 mg) per mL (Rx) [*Rubramin PC* (benzyl alcohol); GENERIC].
  1000 mcg (1 mg) per mL (Rx) [*Cobex; Cobolin-M; Crystamine; Crysti-12; Cyanoject* (benzyl alcohol); *Cyomin* (benzyl alcohol); *Neuroforte-R; Primabalt; Rubesol-1000* (benzyl alcohol); *Rubramin PC* (benzyl alcohol); *Shovite; Vibal; Vitabee 12;* GENERIC].
Canada—
  100 mcg (0.1 mg) per mL (Rx) [GENERIC].
  1000 mcg (1 mg) per mL (Rx) [*Anacobin; Bedoz;* GENERIC].

**Packaging and storage**
Store below 40 °C (104 °F), preferably between 15 and 30 °C (59 and 86 °F), unless otherwise specified by manufacturer. Store in a light-resistant container. Protect from freezing.

**Incompatibilities**
Cyanocobalamin injection is physically incompatible with warfarin sodium for injection.

---

## *HYDROXOCOBALAMIN*

## Summary of Differences
Indications for cyanocobalamin and hydroxocobalamin are the same, although hydroxocobalamin may be preferred for treatment of vitamin B$_{12}$ deficiency since optic neuropathies may degenerate with administration of cyanocobalamin. However, some patients develop antibodies to the hydroxocobalamin-transcobalamin II complex.

# Parenteral Dosage Forms
Note: Bracketed uses in the *Dosage Forms* section refer to categories of use and/or indications that are not included in U.S. product labeling.

## HYDROXOCOBALAMIN INJECTION USP
**Usual adult and adolescent dose**
Deficiency (prophylaxis)—
  Intravenous infusion, as part of total parenteral nutrition solutions, the specific amount determined by individual patient need.
Deficiency (treatment)—
  Initial: Intramuscular or deep subcutaneous, 30 to 50 mcg (0.03 to 0.05 mg) per day (100 mcg [0.1 mg] if megaloblastic anemia is severe) for five to ten days.
  Maintenance: Intramuscular, 100 to 200 mcg (0.1 to 0.2 mg) once a month (in pernicious anemia and following total gastrectomy and extensive ileal resection, parenteral maintenance supplementation is continued for life).
[Diagnostic aid (vitamin B$_{12}$ deficiency)]—
  Intramuscular, 1 mcg (0.001 mg) per day for ten days plus low dietary folic acid and vitamin B$_{12}$. The flushing dose for the Schilling test is 1000 mcg (1 mg) intramuscularly.

**Usual pediatric dose**
Deficiency (prophylaxis)—
  Intravenous infusion, as part of total parenteral nutrition solutions, the specific amount determined by individual patient need.
Deficiency (treatment)—
  Initial: Intramuscular or deep subcutaneous, 30 to 50 mcg (0.03 to 0.05 mg) per day for two or more weeks (total dose of 1 to 5 mg).
  Maintenance: Intramuscular or deep subcutaneous, 100 mcg (0.1 mg) once a month as necessary (for life in the case of pernicious anemia and following total gastrectomy and extensive ileal resection).

**Strength(s) usually available**
U.S.—
  100 mcg (0.1 mg) per mL (Rx) [*Alphamin;* GENERIC].
  1000 mcg (1 mg) per mL (Rx) [*Alphamin; Hydrobexan; Hydro-Cobex; Hydro-Crysti-12; Hydroxy-Cobal; LA-12; Vibal LA;* GENERIC].
Canada—
  Not commercially available.

**Packaging and storage**
Store below 40 °C (104 °F), preferably between 15 and 30 °C (59 and 86 °F), unless otherwise specified by manufacturer. Protect from light. Protect from freezing.

---

Revised: 01/29/92
Interim revision: 04/15/92; 06/02/92; 06/19/95

# VITAMIN D AND ANALOGS   Systemic

This monograph includes information on the following: 1) Alfacalcidol*; 2) Calcifediol†; 3) Calcitriol; 4) Dihydrotachysterol; 5) Ergocalciferol.

VA CLASSIFICATION (Primary):
  Alfacalcidol—VT509
  Calcifediol—VT501
  Calcitriol—VT502
  Dihydrotachysterol—VT503
  Ergocalciferol—VT504

Commonly used brand name(s): *Calciferol*[5]; *Calciferol Drops*[5]; *Calcijex*[3]; *Calderol*[2]; *DHT*[4]; *DHT Intensol*[4]; *Drisdol*[5]; *Drisdol Drops*[5]; *Hytakerol*[4]; *One-Alpha*[1]; *Ostoforte*[5]; *Radiostol Forte*[5]; *Rocaltrol*[3].

Note: For a listing of dosage forms and brand names by country availability, see *Dosage Forms* section(s).

*Not commercially available in U.S.
†Not commercially available in Canada.

## Category

Note: Vitamin D is a fat-soluble vitamin.

Antihypocalcemic—Alfacalcidol; Calcifediol; Calcitriol; Dihydrotachysterol; Ergocalciferol.
Nutritional supplement (vitamin)—Calcifediol; Calcitriol; Ergocalciferol.
Antihypoparathyroid—Calcitriol; Dihydrotachysterol; Ergocalciferol.

## Indications

Note: Bracketed information in the *Indications* section refers to uses that are not included in U.S. product labeling.

**Accepted**

Hypocalcemia, chronic (treatment)
Hypophosphatemia (treatment)
Osteodystrophy (treatment) or
Rickets (prophylaxis and treatment)—Therapeutic doses of specific vitamin D analogs are used in the treatment of chronic hypocalcemia, hypophosphatemia, rickets, and osteodystrophy associated with various medical conditions including chronic renal failure, familial hypophosphatemia, and hypoparathyroidism (postsurgical or idiopathic, or pseudohypoparathyroidism). Some analogs have been found to reduce elevated parathyroid hormone concentrations in patients with renal osteodystrophy associated with hyperparathyroidism.

Theoretically, any of the vitamin D analogs may be used for the above conditions. However, because of their pharmacologic properties, some may be more useful in certain situations than others. Alfacalcidol, calcitriol, and dihydrotachysterol are usually preferred in patients with renal failure since these patients have impaired ability to synthesize calcitriol from cholecalciferol and ergocalciferol; therefore, the response is more predictable. In addition, their shorter half-lives may make toxicity easier to manage (hypercalcemia reverses more quickly). Ergocalciferol may not be the preferred agent in the treatment of familial hypophosphatemia or hypoparathyroidism because the large doses needed are associated with a risk of overdose and hypercalcemia; dihydrotachysterol and calcitriol may be preferred.

Tetany (prophylaxis and treatment)—Dihydrotachysterol is indicated [and ergocalciferol and calcitriol are used] for treatment of chronic and latent forms of postoperative tetany and idiopathic tetany.

Vitamin D deficiency (prophylaxis and treatment)—Ergocalciferol is indicated for prevention and treatment of vitamin D deficiency states. Vitamin D deficiency may occur as a result of inadequate nutrition, intestinal malabsorption, or lack of exposure to sunlight, but does not occur in healthy individuals receiving an adequate balanced diet and exposure to sunlight. Vitamin D therapy, alone, as treatment for osteoporosis is not generally recommended; however, vitamin D supplements in doses of 400 to 800 Units may be used as part of the prevention and treatment of osteoporosis in patients with an inadequate vitamin D and/or calcium intake. For prophylaxis of vitamin D deficiency, dietary improvement, rather than supplementation, is advisable. For treatment of vitamin D deficiency, supplementation is preferred.

Deficiency of vitamin D may lead to rickets and osteomalacia.

Recommended intakes may be increased and/or supplementation may be necessary in the following persons or conditions (based on documented vitamin D deficiency):
Alcoholism
Dark-skinned individuals
Hepatic-biliary tract disease—hepatic function impairment, cirrhosis, obstructive jaundice
Infants, breast-fed, with inadequate exposure to sunlight
Intestinal diseases—celiac, tropical sprue, regional enteritis, persistent diarrhea
Lack of exposure to sunlight combined with reduced vitamin D intake
Renal function impairment
In general, vitamin D absorption will be impaired in any condition in which fat malabsorption (steatorrhea) occurs.

Some unusual diets (e.g., strict vegetarian diets with no milk intake such as vegan-vegetarian or macrobiotic, or reducing diets that drastically restrict food selection) may not supply minimum daily requirements of vitamin D. Supplementation may be necessary in patients receiving total parenteral nutrition (TPN) or undergoing rapid weight loss or in those with malnutrition, because of inadequate dietary intake.

Recommended intakes for all vitamins and most minerals are increased during pregnancy. Many physicians recommend that pregnant women receive multivitamin and mineral supplements, especially those pregnant women who do not consume an adequate diet and those in high-risk categories (i.e., women carrying more than one fetus, heavy cigarette smokers, and alcohol and drug abusers). Taking excessive amounts of a multivitamin and mineral supplement may be harmful to the mother and/or fetus and should be avoided.

Pregnant women who are strict vegetarians (vegan-vegetarians) and/or have minimal exposure to sunlight may need vitamin D supplementation.

Congenital rickets have been reported in newborns whose mothers had low serum levels of vitamin D.

Recommended intakes for all vitamins and most minerals are increased during breast-feeding.

Recommended intakes may be increased by the following medications: Barbiturates, cholestyramine, colestipol, hydantoin anticonvulsants, mineral oil, and primidone.

**Acceptance not established**

There are insufficient data to show that vitamin D supplementation is beneficial in the treatment of *psoriasis*.

**Unaccepted**

Ergocalciferol has not been proven effective for treatment of lupus vulgaris or rheumatoid arthritis, or prevention of nearsightedness or nervousness.

**Table 1. Indications**

Note: Bracketed information in the *Category/Indications* section refers to uses that are not included in U.S. product labeling.

| | I | II | III | IV | V |
|---|---|---|---|---|---|
| Legend: I=Alfacalcidol; II=Calcifediol; III=Calcitriol; IV=Dihydrotachysterol; V=Ergocalciferol | | | | | |
| Vitamin D deficiency (prophylaxis and treatment) | | [✔] | | | ✔ |
| Vitamin D–dependent rickets (prophylaxis and treatment) | | | [✔] | | |
| Familial hypophosphatemia (vitamin D–resistant rickets) (treatment) | | [✔] | [✔] | [✔] | ✔ |
| Hypocalcemia associated with hypoparathyroidism (treatment) | ✔ | [✔] | ✔ | ✔ | ✔ |
| Chronic renal failure (treatment adjunct) | ✔ | | ✔ | [✔] | |
| Chronic, and latent forms of postoperative tetany and idiopathic tetany (treatment) | | | | ✔ | [✔] |

## Pharmacology/Pharmacokinetics

**Physicochemical characteristics**
Molecular weight—
  Alfacalcidol: 400.64.
  Calcifediol: 418.66.

Calcitriol: 416.64.
Dihydrotachysterol: 398.67.
Ergocalciferol: 396.65.

### Mechanism of action/Effect
Vitamin D is essential for promoting absorption and utilization of calcium and phosphate and for normal calcification of bone. Along with parathyroid hormone and calcitonin, it regulates serum calcium concentrations by increasing serum calcium and phosphate concentrations as needed. Vitamin D stimulates calcium and phosphate absorption from the small intestine and mobilizes calcium from bone.

Exposure of the skin to ultraviolet rays in sunlight results in formation of cholecalciferol (vitamin $D_3$). Ergocalciferol (calciferol, vitamin $D_2$) is found in commercial vitamin preparations and is used as a food additive; cholecalciferol is found in vitamin D–fortified milk. Cholecalciferol and ergocalciferol are transferred to the liver where they are converted to calcifediol (25-hydroxycholecalciferol), which is then transferred to the kidneys and converted to calcitriol (1,25-dihydroxycholecalciferol, thought to be the most active form) and 24,25-dihydroxycholecalciferol (physiologic role not determined). Dihydrotachysterol is a synthetic reduction product of ergocalciferol; it has only weak antirachitic activity; it is metabolically activated by 25-hydroxylation in the liver. Alfacalcidol is rapidly converted to 1,25-dihydroxycholecalciferol in the liver.

Calcitriol appears to act by binding to a specific receptor in the cytoplasm of the intestinal mucosa and subsequently being incorporated into the nucleus, probably leading to formation of the calcium-binding protein that results in increased absorption of calcium from the intestine. Also, calcitriol may regulate the transfer of calcium ion from bone and stimulate reabsorption of calcium in the distal renal tubule, thereby effecting calcium homeostasis in the extracellular fluid.

### Absorption
Readily absorbed from small intestine (proximal or distal); cholecalciferol may be absorbed more rapidly and completely than ergocalciferol. Ergocalciferol requires presence of bile salts.

There is evidence that some metabolites of vitamin D are reabsorbed from bile; however, the benefit to overall vitamin D status is thought to be negligible.

### Protein binding
Bound to specific alpha globulins for transport.

### Storage
Stored mainly in liver and other fat depots.

### Biotransformation
Metabolic activation of cholecalciferol and ergocalciferol occurs in 2 steps, the first in the liver and the second in the kidneys. Metabolic activation of calcifediol occurs in the kidneys; dihydrotachysterol and alfacalcidol are activated in the liver. Calcitriol does not require metabolic activation. Degradation also occurs partly in the kidneys.

### Plasma half-life
Calcifediol—Approximately 16 days (10 to 22 days).
Calcitriol—3 to 6 hours.
Ergocalciferol—19 to 48 hours (however, stored in fat deposits in body for prolonged periods).

### Onset of action
Hypercalcemic—
Calcitriol: Oral—2 to 6 hours.
Dihydrotachysterol: Several hours (maximal after 1 to 2 weeks).
Ergocalciferol: 12 to 24 hours; therapeutic effect may take 10 to 14 days.

### Time to peak serum concentration
Alfacalcidol—Approximately 12 hours after a single dose.
Calcifediol—Approximately 4 hours.
Calcitriol—Oral: Approximately 3 to 6 hours.

### Duration of action
Following oral administration—
Alfacalcidol: Up to 48 hours.
Calcifediol: 15 to 20 days (increased 2 to 3 times in renal failure).
Calcitriol: 3 to 5 days.
Dihydrotachysterol: Up to 9 weeks.
Ergocalciferol: Up to 6 months; repeated doses have a cumulative action.

### Elimination
Biliary/renal.

## Precautions to Consider

### Mutagenicity
Studies with calcitriol have found no evidence of mutagenicity.

### Pregnancy/Reproduction
Pregnancy—Problems in humans have not been documented with intake of normal daily recommended amounts. There are insufficient data on acute and chronic vitamin D toxicity in pregnant women. Maternal hypercalcemia during pregnancy in humans may be associated with increased sensitivity to effects of vitamin D, suppression of parathyroid function, or a syndrome of peculiar (elfin) facies, mental retardation, and congenital aortic stenosis in infants.

Overdosage of vitamin D has been associated with fetal abnormalities in animals. Animal studies have shown calcitriol to be teratogenic when given in doses 4 and 15 times the dose recommended for human use. Excessive doses of dihydrotachysterol are also teratogenic in animals. Animal studies have also shown calcifediol to be teratogenic when given in doses of 6 to 12 times the human dose.

FDA Pregnancy Category C.

### Breast-feeding
Only small amounts of vitamin D metabolites appear in human milk. Infants who are totally breast-fed and have little exposure to the sun may require vitamin D supplementation.

### Pediatrics
Some studies have shown that infants who are exclusively breast-fed, especially from dark-skinned mothers, and/or have little exposure to sunlight may be at risk for vitamin D deficiency.

Because of varying sensitivity, some infants may be sensitive to even small doses.

Also, growth may be arrested in children, especially after prolonged administration of 1800 Units of ergocalciferol a day.

### Geriatrics
Studies have shown that the elderly may have an increased need for vitamin D due to a possible decrease in the capacity of the skin to produce previtamin $D_3$ ora decrease in exposure to the sun or impaired renal function or impaired vitamin D absorption.

### Drug interactions and/or related problems
The following drug interactions and/or related problems have been selected on the basis of their potential clinical significance (possible mechanism in parentheses where appropriate)—not necessarily inclusive (» = major clinical significance):

Note: Combinations containing any of the following, depending on the amount present, may also interact with vitamin D.

Antacids, aluminum-containing
(long-term use of aluminum-containing antacids as phosphate binders in hyperphosphatemia in conjunction with vitamin D has been found to increase blood levels for aluminum and may lead to aluminum bone toxicity, especially in patients with chronic renal failure)

» Antacids, magnesium-containing
(concurrent use with vitamin D may result in hypermagnesemia, especially in patients with chronic renal failure)

Anticonvulsants, hydantoin or
Barbiturates or
Primidone
(may reduce effect of vitamin D by accelerating metabolism by hepatic microsomal enzyme induction; patients on long-term anticonvulsant therapy may require vitamin D supplementation to prevent osteomalacia)

Calcitonin or
Etidronate or
Gallium nitrate or
Pamidronate or
Plicamycin
(concurrent use with vitamin D may antagonize these medications in the treatment of hypercalcemia)

» Calcium-containing preparations, in high doses or
» Diuretics, thiazide
(concurrent use with vitamin D may increase the risk of hypercalcemia; however, it may be therapeutically advantageous in elderly and high-risk groups when it is necessary to prescribe vitamin D or its derivatives together with calcium; careful monitoring of serum calcium concentrations is essential during long-term therapy)

Cholestyramine or
Colestipol or
Mineral oil
(concurrent use may impair intestinal absorption of vitamin D since these medications have been reported to reduce intestinal absorption of fat-soluble vitamins; requirements for vitamin D may be increased in patients receiving these medications)

Corticosteroids
(vitamin D supplementation may be recommended by some clinicians for prolonged corticosteroids use, because corticosteroids may interfere with vitamin D action)

Digitalis glycosides
(caution is recommended in patients being treated with these medications since the hypercalcemia that may be caused by vitamin D may potentiate the effects of digitalis glycosides, resulting in cardiac arrhythmias)

Phosphorus-containing preparations, in high doses
(concurrent use with vitamin D may increase the potential for hyperphosphatemia, because of vitamin D enhancement of phosphate absorption)

» Vitamin D and analogs, other
(concurrent use of one analog with another, especially calcifediol, is not recommended because of additive effects and increased potential for toxicity)

## Laboratory value alterations

The following have been selected on the basis of their potential clinical significance (possible effect in parentheses where appropriate)—not necessarily inclusive (» = major clinical significance):

With physiology/laboratory test values
Alkaline phosphatase
(serum concentrations may be decreased prior to development of hypercalcemia in patients receiving excessive doses)

Calcium concentrations, serum and
Cholesterol concentrations, serum and
Phosphate concentrations, serum
(may be increased with high doses)

Calcium concentrations, urinary and
Phosphate concentrations, urinary
(may be increased with therapeutic doses, even when serum concentrations are still low)

Magnesium
(serum concentrations may be increased)

## Medical considerations/Contraindications

The medical considerations/contraindications included have been selected on the basis of their potential clinical significance (reasons given in parentheses where appropriate)—not necessarily inclusive (» = major clinical significance).

*Except under special circumstances, this medication should not be used when the following medical problems exist:*

» Hypercalcemia
» Hypervitaminosis D
» Renal osteodystrophy with hyperphosphatemia
(risk of metastatic calcification; however, vitamin D therapy can begin once serum phosphate levels have stabilized)

*Risk-benefit should be considered when the following medical problems exist:*

» Arteriosclerosis or
» Cardiac function impairment
(conditions may be exacerbated due to possibility of hypercalcemia and elevated serum cholesterol concentrations)

» Hyperphosphatemia
(risk of metastatic calcification; dietary phosphate restriction or administration of intestinal phosphate binders is recommended to produce normal serum phosphorus concentrations)

» Hypersensitivity to effects of vitamin D
(may be involved in causing idiopathic hypercalcemia in infants)

» Renal function impairment
(toxicity may occur in patients receiving vitamin D for nonrenal problems, although toxicity is also possible during treatment of renal osteodystrophy because of increased requirements and decreased renal function)

Sarcoidosis, and possibly other granulomatous diseases
(increased sensitivity to effects of vitamin D)

## Patient monitoring

The following may be especially important in patient monitoring (other tests may be warranted in some patients, depending on condition; » = major clinical significance):

Blood urea nitrogen (BUN) and
Creatinine, serum
(determinations recommended at periodic intervals in patients receiving therapeutic doses)

Alkaline phosphatase concentrations, serum and
Phosphorus concentrations, serum and
Calcium concentrations, urinary, 24-hour and
Calcium/creatinine, urinary ratio
(determinations recommended every 1 to 3 months during therapy, as long as the patient remains stable)

» Calcium concentrations, serum or
Ionized calcium concentration, serum
(determinations recommended at least once weekly in early period of treatment to aid in dosage adjustment because of narrow therapeutic range, then at periodic intervals during therapy in patients receiving therapeutic doses; serum calcium concentrations should be maintained at 8.8 to 10.3 mg per 100 mL, depending on lab variability; serum ionized calcium concentrations are preferable to determine free and bound calcium, but may not be readily available from a reliable lab)

X-rays of bones
(recommended by some clinicians every 3 to 6 months until patient is stable, then yearly to determine when treatment of familial hypophosphatemia or hypoparathyroidism is sufficient)

# Side/Adverse Effects

Note: Ingestion of excessive doses of vitamin D over prolonged periods (20,000 to 60,000 Units a day or more for several weeks or months in adults and 2,000 to 4,000 Units a day for several months in children) can result in severe toxicity. Acute excessive doses of vitamin D can also result in severe toxicity, but there are insufficient data to determine at what dose.

Chronic vitamin D–induced hypercalcemia may result in generalized vascular calcification, nephrocalcinosis, and other soft tissue calcification that may lead to hypertension and renal failure. These effects are more likely to occur when the hypercalcemia is accompanied by hyperphosphatemia.

Growth may be arrested in children, especially after prolonged administration of 1800 Units of ergocalciferol per day.

Death may occur as a result of renal or cardiovascular failure caused by vitamin D toxicity.

Dosage necessary to cause toxicity varies with individual sensitivity, but in individuals without malabsorption problems, 10,000 Units a day for more than several weeks or months is the maximum dose.

Toxicity may occur with therapeutic doses of calcitriol.

The following side/adverse effects have been selected on the basis of their potential clinical significance (possible signs and symptoms in parentheses where appropriate)—not necessarily inclusive:

## Those indicating need for medical attention

Early symptoms of vitamin D toxicity associated with hypercalcemia
*Constipation*—usually more frequent in children and adolescents; *diarrhea; dryness of mouth; headache, continuing; increased thirst; increase in frequency of urination, especially at night, or in amount of urine; loss of appetite; metallic taste; nausea or vomiting*—usually more frequent in children and adolescents; *unusual tiredness or weakness*

Late symptoms of vitamin D toxicity associated with hypercalcemia
*Bone pain; cloudy urine; high blood pressure; increased sensitivity of eyes to light or irritation of eyes; irregular heartbeat; itching of skin; lethargy* (drowsiness); *muscle pain; nausea or vomiting and pancreatitis* (stomach pain, severe); *psychosis, overt* (mood or mental changes)—rare; *weight loss*

# Patient Consultation

As an aid to patient consultation, refer to *Advice for the Patient, Vitamin D and Related Compounds (Systemic)*.

In providing consultation, consider emphasizing the following selected information (» = major clinical significance):

## Description of use
*For ergocalciferol*
Description should include function in the body, signs of deficiency, and unproven uses

## Importance of diet
*For ergocalciferol*
Importance of proper nutrition; supplement may be needed because of inadequate dietary intake

Food sources of vitamin D; importance of sunlight exposure; effects of processing

Recommended daily intake for vitamin D

» Importance of not exceeding recommended daily intake if self-medicating with vitamin supplements

### Before using this dietary supplement
» Conditions affecting use, especially:
Sensitivity to vitamin D or any vitamin D analog
Pregnancy—No problems documented with normal intake; overdose associated with increased sensitivity to vitamin D, suppression of parathyroid function, or syndrome of peculiar facies, mental retardation, and congenital aortic stenosis in infants
Breast-feeding—Possible vitamin D deficiency in totally breast-fed infants
Use in children—Possible vitamin D deficiency in breast-fed infants especially of dark-skinned mothers; varying sensitivity in infants may make some children sensitive to small doses; children may show slowed growth when receiving high doses of vitamin D for long periods
Other medications, especially calcium-containing preparations, magnesium-containing antacids, thiazide diuretics, or other vitamin D analogs
Other medical problems, especially hypercalcemia, hypervitaminosis D, renal or cardiac impairment, arteriosclerosis, or hyperphosphatemia

### Proper use of this dietary supplement
» Proper storage
*For the oral solution dosage form*
*Proper administration*
Taking by mouth even though dietary supplement comes in a dropper bottle
May be dropped directly into the mouth or mixed with cereal, fruit juice, or other food
*For use as an antihypocalcemic*
» Importance of not taking more medication than the amount prescribed
Carefully following instructions for special diet or calcium supplementation, if prescribed
Making sure physician knows if calcium supplement or any calcium-containing preparation is already being taken
» Proper dosing
Missed dose: If dosing schedule is—
Every other day: Taking as soon as possible if remembered same day; if remembered later, not taking until next day, then skipping a day; not doubling doses
Once a day: Taking as soon as possible; taking next day if not remembered until then; not doubling doses
Several times a day: Taking as soon as possible; not taking if almost time for next dose; not doubling doses
*For use as a dietary supplement*
» Importance of not taking more dietary supplement than the amount recommended; risk of toxicity with chronic overdose
Missed dose: No cause for concern because of length of time necessary for depletion; remembering to take as directed

### Precautions while using this dietary supplement
Avoiding concurrent use of nonprescription medications or dietary supplements containing calcium, phosphorus, or vitamin D, unless otherwise directed by health care professional
» Avoiding concurrent use of magnesium-containing antacids
*For use as a dietary supplement*
Risk of toxicity with overdose; upper limits for vitamin D toxicity
*For use as an antihypocalcemic*
» Regular visits to physician to check progress during therapy

### Side/adverse effects
Signs of potential side effects, especially signs of vitamin D toxicity

## General Dosing Information

### For use as an antihypocalcemic
Before vitamin D therapy is begun, elevated serum phosphate concentrations must be controlled.

Clinical response to vitamin D depends on adequate dietary calcium.

Because of individual variation in sensitivity to its effects, dosage of vitamin D must be adjusted on the basis of clinical response. Some infants are hyperreactive to even small doses. Careful titration is necessary to avoid overdosage, which induces hypercalcemia and can cause hypercalciuria and hyperphosphatemia.

Dosage of vitamin D from dietary and other sources should be evaluated in determining the therapeutic dosage.

The serum calcium times phosphorus (Ca × P, in mg/dL) product should not exceed 60.

To control elevated serum phosphate concentrations in patients undergoing dialysis, a phosphate binding agent should be used. The dosage of the binding agent may need to be increased during vitamin D therapy since phosphate absorption is enhanced.

### For use as a dietary supplement
Because of the infrequency of vitamin D deficiency alone, combinations of several vitamins are commonly administered. Many commercial vitamin complexes are available.

### Diet/Nutrition
Recommended dietary intakes for vitamin D are defined differently worldwide:
For U.S.—
The Recommended Dietary Allowances (RDAs) for vitamins and minerals are determined by the Food and Nutrition Board of the National Research Council and are intended to provide adequate nutrition in most healthy persons under usual environmental stresses. In addition, a different designation may be used by the FDA for food and dietary supplement labeling purposes, as with Daily Value (DV). DVs replace the previous labeling terminology United States Recommended Daily Allowances (USRDAs).
For Canada—
Recommended Nutrient Intakes (RNIs) for vitamins, minerals, and protein are determined by Health and Welfare Canada and provide recommended amounts of a specific nutrient while minimizing the risk of chronic diseases.
The expression of vitamin D activity has changed from Units to micrograms (mcg), with 1 Unit of vitamin D equal to the activity of 0.025 mcg of cholecalciferol (vitamin $D_3$). This change was made to reflect a broader activity for vitamin $D_3$ compared to vitamin $D_2$.
Normal daily recommended intakes in mcg and Units are generally defined as follows:

|  | U.S. |  | Canada |  |
| --- | --- | --- | --- | --- |
| Persons | (mcg) | Units | (mcg) | Units |
| Infants and children |  |  |  |  |
| Birth to 3 years of age | 7.5–10 | 300–400 | 5–10 | 200–400 |
| 4 to 6 years of age | 10 | 400 | 5 | 200 |
| 7 to 10 years of age | 10 | 400 | 2.5–5 | 100–200 |
| Adolescents and adults | 5–10 | 200–400 | 2.5–5 | 100–200 |
| Pregnant and breast-feeding females | 10 | 400 | 5–7.5 | 200–300 |

These are usually provided by adequate diets and adequate exposure to sunlight (1.5 to 2 hours of exposure per week is sufficient for most people).

Best dietary sources of vitamin D (as cholecalciferol) include some fish and fish liver oils and vitamin D–fortified milk. The vitamin D content of foods is not affected by cooking.

### For parenteral dosage forms only
Parenteral administration may be indicated in patients with malabsorption problems.

### For treatment of adverse effects
Recommended treatment includes the following:
• Hypervitaminosis D is treated by withdrawal of the vitamin, low-calcium diet, and generous fluid intake.
• If hypercalcemia persists, prednisone may be started. Severe hypercalcemia may be treated with calcitonin, etidronate, pamidronate, or gallium nitrate.
• Hypercalcemic crisis requires vigorous hydration with intravenous saline to increase calcium excretion, with or without a loop diuretic.
• Cardiac arrhythmias may be treated with small doses of potassium with continuous cardiac monitoring.
• Therapy may be reinstituted at a lower dose when serum calcium concentrations return to normal. Serum or urinary calcium levels should be obtained twice weekly after dosage changes.

## *ALFACALCIDOL*

## Oral Dosage Forms

### ALFACALCIDOL CAPSULES

**Usual adult and adolescent dose**
Initial—Oral, 1 mcg per day, the dosage being increased in increments of 0.5 mcg every two to four weeks as necessary, up to 2 mcg a day. In rare cases, a maximum dose of 3 mcg per day may be needed.
Maintenance—Oral, 0.25 to 1 mcg per day.

**Strength(s) usually available**
U.S.—
Not commercially available.

Canada—
    0.25 mcg (Rx) [*One-Alpha*].
    1 mcg (Rx) [*One-Alpha*].

**Packaging and storage**
Store below 40 °C (104 °F), preferably between 15 and 30 °C (59 and 86 °F), unless otherwise specified by manufacturer. Store in a tight, light-resistant container.

### ALFACALCIDOL ORAL SOLUTION

**Usual adult and adolescent dose**
Initial—Oral, 1 mcg per day, the dosage being increased in increments of 0.5 mcg every two to four weeks as necessary, up to 2 mcg a day. In rare cases, a maximum dose of 3 mcg per day may be needed.
Maintenance—Oral, 0.25 to 1 mcg per day.

**Usual pediatric dose**
Oral, 0.25 mcg per day.

**Strength(s) usually available**
U.S.—
    Not commercially available.
Canada—
    0.2 mcg per mL (Rx) [*One-Alpha*].

**Packaging and storage**
Store below 40 °C (104 °F), preferably between 15 and 30 °C (59 and 86 °F), unless otherwise specified by manufacturer. Store in a tight, light-resistant container.

---
## CALCIFEDIOL
---

## Oral Dosage Forms

### CALCIFEDIOL CAPSULES USP

**Usual adult and adolescent dose**
Oral, initially 300 to 350 mcg (0.3 to 0.35 mg) per week administered on a once-a-day or alternate-day schedule, the dosage being increased, if necessary, at four-week intervals.
Note: Most patients respond to doses of 50 to 100 mcg (0.05 to 0.1 mg) per day or 100 to 200 mcg (0.1 to 0.2 mg) on alternate days; as low as 20 mcg (0.02 mg) every other day may be sufficient in patients with normal serum calcium concentrations.

**Usual pediatric dose**
Children up to 2 years of age—Oral, 20 to 50 mcg (0.02 to 0.05 mg) per day.
Children 2 to 10 years of age—Oral, 50 mcg (0.05 mg) per day.
Note: For use of calcifediol in hypoparathyroidism, a dose of 3 to 6 mcg per kilogram of body weight a day in children less than 10 years of age may be necessary.
Children 10 years of age and over—See *Usual adult and adolescent dose*.

**Strength(s) usually available**
U.S.—
    20 mcg (0.02 mg) (Rx) [*Calderol*].
    50 mcg (0.05 mg) (Rx) [*Calderol*].
Canada—
    Not commercially available.

**Packaging and storage**
Store below 40 °C (104 °F), preferably between 15 and 30 °C (59 and 86 °F), unless otherwise specified by manufacturer. Store in a tight, light-resistant container.

---
## CALCITRIOL
---

## Oral Dosage Forms

Note: Bracketed uses in the *Dosage Forms* section refer to categories of use and/or indications that are not included in U.S. product labeling.

### CALCITRIOL CAPSULES

**Usual adult and adolescent dose**
Initial—Oral, 0.25 mcg per day, the dosage being increased in increments of 0.25 mcg every two to four weeks as necessary, up to the following usual doses:
[Familial hypophosphatemia]—
    Oral, 2 mcg per day.
Hypocalcemia in chronic dialysis—
    Oral, 0.5 to 3 mcg or more per day.
Hypoparathyroidism—
    Oral, 0.25 to 2.7 mcg per day.
Renal osteodystrophy—
    Oral, 0.25 mcg every other day to 3 mcg or more per day.
Note: Some clinicians believe that in order for calcitriol to be most effective, it should be given in divided doses, at least two or three times a day.

**Usual pediatric dose**
Oral, 0.25 mcg per day, the dosage being increased in increments of 0.25 mcg every two to four weeks as necessary up to the following usual doses:
[Vitamin D–dependent rickets]—
    Oral, 1 mcg per day.
Hypocalcemia in chronic dialysis—
    Oral, 0.25 to 2 mcg per day.
Hypoparathyroidism—
    Oral, 0.04 to 0.08 mcg per kg of body weight per day.
Renal osteodystrophy—
    Oral, 0.014 to 0.041 mcg per kg of body weight per day.
Note: Pediatric patients with liver disease may need initial doses of up to 0.1 to 0.2 mcg per kilogram of body weight per day.

**Strength(s) usually available**
U.S.—
    0.25 mcg (Rx) [*Rocaltrol*].
    0.5 mcg (Rx) [*Rocaltrol*].
Canada—
    0.25 mcg (Rx) [*Rocaltrol*].
    0.5 mcg (Rx) [*Rocaltrol*].

**Packaging and storage**
Store below 40 °C (104 °F), preferably between 15 and 30 °C (59 and 86 °F), in a tight container, unless otherwise specified by manufacturer. Protect from light.

### CALCITRIOL ORAL SOLUTION

**Usual adult and adolescent dose**
See *Calcitriol Capsules*.

**Usual pediatric dose**
See *Calcitriol Capsules*.

**Strength(s) usually available**
U.S.—
    Not commercially available.
Canada—
    1 mcg per mL (Rx) [*Rocaltrol*].

**Packaging and storage**
Store below 40 °C (104 °F), preferably between 15 and 30 °C (59 and 86 °F), unless otherwise specified by manufacturer. Protect from light.

## Parenteral Dosage Forms

### CALCITRIOL INJECTION

**Usual adult and adolescent dose**
Antihypocalcemic—
    Initial: Intravenous (rapid), 0.5 mcg (or 0.01 mcg per kg of body weight) three times a week, the dosage being increased in increments of 0.25 to 0.5 mcg every two to four weeks as necessary.
    Maintenance: Intravenous (rapid), 0.5 to 3.0 mcg (or 0.01 to 0.05 mcg per kg of body weight) three times a week.

**Usual pediatric dose**
Dosage has not been established.

**Strength(s) usually available**
U.S.—
    1 mcg per mL (Rx) [*Calcijex*].
    2 mcg per mL (Rx) [*Calcijex*].
Canada—
    1 mcg per mL (Rx) [*Calcijex*].
    2 mcg per mL (Rx) [*Calcijex*].

**Packaging and storage**
Store below 40 °C (104 °F), preferably between 15 and 30 °C (59 and 86 °F), unless otherwise specified by manufacturer. Protect from light.

---
## DIHYDROTACHYSTEROL
---

## Oral Dosage Forms

Note: Bracketed uses in the *Dosage Forms* section refer to categories of use and/or indications that are not included in U.S. product labeling.

## DIHYDROTACHYSTEROL CAPSULES USP

### Usual adult and adolescent dose
Oral, 125 mcg (0.125 mg) to 2 mg per day.
[Familial hypophosphatemia]—
  Initial: Oral, 500 mcg (0.5 mg) to 2 mg per day.
  Maintenance: Oral, 200 mcg (0.2 mg) to 1.5 mg per day.
Hypocalcemic tetany—
  Initial: Acute—Oral, 750 mcg (0.75 mg) to 2.5 mg per day for three days.
  Less acute—Oral, 250 to 500 mcg (0.25 to 0.5 mg) per day for three days.
  Maintenance: Oral, 250 mcg (0.25 mg) per week to 1 mg per day, as necessary.
Hypoparathyroidism—
  Initial: Oral, 750 mcg (0.75 mg) to 2.5 mg per day for several days.
  Maintenance: Oral, 200 mcg (0.2 mg) to 1 mg per day.
[Renal osteodystrophy]—
  Initial: Oral, 100 to 250 mcg (0.1 to 0.25 mg) per day.
  Maintenance: Oral, 200 mcg (0.2 mg) to 1 mg per day.

### Usual pediatric dose
[Familial hypophosphatemia]—
  See *Usual adult and adolescent dose*.
Hypoparathyroidism—
  Initial: Oral, 1 to 5 mg per day for four days, then continued or decreased to one-fourth the dose.
  Maintenance: Oral, 500 mcg (0.5 mg) to 1.5 mg per day.

### Strength(s) usually available
U.S.—
  125 mcg (0.125 mg) (Rx) [*Hytakerol*].
Canada—
  125 mcg (0.125 mg) (Rx) [*Hytakerol*].

### Packaging and storage
Store below 40 °C (104 °F), preferably between 15 and 30 °C (59 and 86 °F), unless otherwise specified by manufacturer. Store in a well-closed, light-resistant container.

## DIHYDROTACHYSTEROL ORAL SOLUTION USP

### Usual adult and adolescent dose
Oral, 125 mcg (0.125 mg) to 2 mg per day.
[Familial hypophosphatemia]—
  Initial: Oral, 500 mcg (0.5 mg) to 2 mg per day.
  Maintenance: Oral, 200 mcg (0.2 mg) to 1.5 mg per day.
Hypocalcemic tetany—
  Initial: Acute—Oral, 750 mcg (0.75 mg) to 2.5 mg per day for three days.
  Less acute—Oral, 250 to 500 mcg (0.25 to 0.5 mg) per day for three days.
  Maintenance: Oral, 250 mcg (0.25 mg) per week to 1 mg per day, as necessary.
Hypoparathyroidism—
  Initial: Oral, 750 mcg (0.75 mg) to 2.5 mg per day for several days.
  Maintenance: Oral, 200 mcg (0.2 mg) to 1 mg per day.
[Renal osteodystrophy]—
  Initial: Oral, 100 to 250 mcg (0.1 to 0.25 mg) per day.
  Maintenance: Oral, 200 mcg (0.2 mg) to 1 mg per day.

### Usual pediatric dose
[Familial hypophosphatemia]—
  See *Usual adult and adolescent dose*.
Hypoparathyroidism—
  Initial: Oral, 1 to 5 mg per day for four days, then continued or decreased to one-fourth the dose.
  Maintenance: Oral, 500 mcg (0.5 mg) to 1.5 mg per day.

### Strength(s) usually available
U.S.—
  200 mcg (0.2 mg) per mL (Rx) [*DHT Intensol* (alcohol 20%)].
Canada—
  Not commercially available.

### Packaging and storage
Store below 40 °C (104 °F), preferably between 15 and 30 °C (59 and 86 °F), unless otherwise specified by manufacturer. Store in a tight, light-resistant glass container. Protect from freezing.

## DIHYDROTACHYSTEROL TABLETS USP

### Usual adult and adolescent dose
Oral, 125 mcg (0.125 mg) to 2 mg per day.
[Familial hypophosphatemia]—
  Initial: Oral, 500 mcg (0.5 mg) to 2 mg per day.
  Maintenance: Oral, 200 mcg (0.2 mg) to 1.5 mg per day.
Hypocalcemic tetany—
  Initial: Acute—Oral, 750 mcg (0.75 mg) to 2.5 mg per day for three days.
  Less acute—Oral, 250 to 500 mcg (0.25 to 0.5 mg) per day for three days.
  Maintenance: Oral, 250 mcg (0.25 mg) per week to 1 mg per day, as necessary.
Hypoparathyroidism—
  Initial: Oral, 750 mcg (0.75 mg) to 2.5 mg per day for several days.
  Maintenance: Oral, 200 mcg (0.2 mg) to 1 mg per day.
[Renal osteodystrophy]—
  Initial: Oral, 100 to 250 mcg (0.1 to 0.25 mg) per day.
  Maintenance: Oral, 200 mcg (0.2 mg) to 1 mg per day.

### Usual pediatric dose
[Familial hypophosphatemia]—
  See *Usual adult and adolescent dose*.
Hypoparathyroidism—
  Initial: Oral, 1 to 5 mg per day for four days, then continued or decreased to one-fourth the dose.
  Maintenance: Oral, 500 mcg (0.5 mg) to 1.5 mg per day.

### Strength(s) usually available
U.S.—
  125 mcg (0.125 mg) (Rx) [*DHT*].
  200 mcg (0.2 mg) (Rx) [*DHT*].
  400 mcg (0.4 mg) (Rx) [*DHT*].
Canada—
  Not commercially available.

### Packaging and storage
Store below 40 °C (104 °F), preferably between 15 and 30 °C (59 and 86 °F), unless otherwise specified by manufacturer. Store in a well-closed, light-resistant container.

---

# ERGOCALCIFEROL

## Oral Dosage Forms

Note: Bracketed uses in the *Dosage Forms* section refer to categories of use and/or indications that are not included in U.S. product labeling.

## ERGOCALCIFEROL CAPSULES USP

### Usual adult and adolescent dose
Deficiency (prophylaxis)—
  Oral, amount based on normal daily recommended intakes:

| Persons | U.S. (mcg) | U.S. Units | Canada (mcg) | Canada Units |
|---|---|---|---|---|
| Adolescents and adults | 5–10 | 200–400 | 2.5–5 | 100–200 |
| Pregnant and breast-feeding females | 10 | 400 | 5–7.5 | 200–300 |

Deficiency (treatment)—
  Treatment dose is individualized by prescriber based on severity of deficiency.
Vitamin D–resistant rickets—
  Oral, 12,000 to 150,000 Units per day.
Vitamin D–dependent rickets—
  Oral, 10,000 to 60,000 Units per day (up to 150,000 Units per day).
Osteomalacia due to prolonged use of anticonvulsants—
  Oral, 1000 to 4000 Units per day.
Familial hypophosphatemia—
  Oral, 50,000 to 100,000 Units per day.
Hypoparathyroidism—
  Oral, 50,000 to 150,000 Units per day.
[Renal function impairment]—
  Oral, 40,000 to 100,000 Units per day.
[Renal osteodystrophy]—
  Initial: Oral, 20,000 Units per day.
  Maintenance: Oral, 10,000 to 300,000 Units per day.

### Usual pediatric dose
Deficiency (prophylaxis)—
  Oral, amount based on normal daily recommended intakes:

| Persons | U.S. (mcg) | U.S. Units | Canada (mcg) | Canada Units |
|---|---|---|---|---|
| Infants and children | | | | |
| Birth to 3 years of age | 7.5–10 | 300–400 | 5–10 | 200–400 |
| 4 to 6 years of age | 10 | 400 | 5 | 200 |
| 7 to 10 years of age | 10 | 400 | 2.5–5 | 100–200 |

## Vitamin D and Analogs (Systemic)

Deficiency (treatment)—
  Treatment dose in individualized by prescriber based on severity of deficiency.
Vitamin D–dependent rickets—
  Oral, 3000 to 10,000 Units per day (up to 50,000 Units per day).
Osteomalacia due to prolonged use of anticonvulsants—
  Oral, 1000 Units per day.
Hypoparathyroidism—
  Oral, 50,000 to 200,000 Units per day.
[Renal osteodystrophy]—
  Oral, 4000 to 40,000 Units per day.

### Strength(s) usually available
U.S.—
  50 Units (OTC) [GENERIC].
  400 Units (0.01 mg) (OTC) [GENERIC].
  25,000 Units (0.625 mg) (Rx) [GENERIC].
  50,000 Units (1.25 mg) (Rx) [*Drisdol* (tartrazine); GENERIC].
Canada—
  50,000 Units (1.25 mg) (Rx) [*Ostoforte*].
Note: Lower strengths are also available as over-the-counter dietary supplements.

### Packaging and storage
Store below 40 °C (104 °F), preferably between 15 and 30 °C (59 and 86 °F), unless otherwise specified by manufacturer. Store in a tight, light-resistant container.

### ERGOCALCIFEROL ORAL SOLUTION USP

**Usual adult and adolescent dose**
Deficiency (prophylaxis or treatment)—
  See *Ergocalciferol Capsules USP*.
Vitamin D–resistant rickets—
  Oral, 12,000 to 500,000 Units per day.
Vitamin D–dependent rickets—
  Oral, 10,000 to 60,000 Units per day (up to 500,000 Units per day).
Osteomalacia due to prolonged use of anticonvulsants—
  Oral, 1000 to 4000 Units per day.
Familial hypophosphatemia—
  Oral, 50,000 to 100,000 Units per day.
Hypoparathyroidism—
  Oral, 50,000 to 150,000 Units per day.
[Renal function impairment]—
  Oral, 40,000 to 100,000 Units per day.
[Renal osteodystrophy]—
  Initial: Oral, 20,000 Units per day.
  Maintenance: Oral, 10,000 to 300,000 Units per day.

**Usual pediatric dose**
See *Ergocalciferol Capsules USP*.

**Strength(s) usually available**
U.S.—
  8000 Units (0.2 mg) per mL (OTC) [*Calciferol Drops; Drisdol Drops*].
Canada—
  8000 Units (0.2 mg) per mL (OTC) [*Drisdol*].
  300,000 Units (7.5 mg) per mL (Rx) [*Radiostol Forte* (alcohol)].

**Packaging and storage**
Store below 40 °C (104 °F), preferably between 15 and 30 °C (59 and 86 °F), unless otherwise specified by manufacturer. Store in a tight, light-resistant container. Protect from freezing.

### ERGOCALCIFEROL TABLETS USP

**Usual adult and adolescent dose**
See *Ergocalciferol Oral Solution USP*.

**Usual pediatric dose**
See *Ergocalciferol Capsules USP*.

**Strength(s) usually available**
U.S.—
  400 Units (0.01 mg) (OTC) [GENERIC].
  50,000 Units (1.25 mg) [*Calciferol (Rx)*; GENERIC].
Canada—
  1,000 Units (0.025 mg) (OTC) [GENERIC].
  50,000 Units (1.25 mg) (Rx) [*Calciferol*].

**Packaging and storage**
Store below 40 °C (104 °F), preferably between 15 and 30 °C (59 and 86 °F), unless otherwise specified by manufacturer. Store in a tight, light-resistant container.

## Parenteral Dosage Forms

### ERGOCALCIFEROL INJECTION

**Usual adult and adolescent dose**
Deficiency (prophylaxis or treatment)—
  Intravenous infusion, as part of total parenteral nutrition solutions, the specific amount determined by individual patient need.
Malabsorption—
  Intramuscular, 10,000 Units per day.

**Usual pediatric dose**
See *Usual adult and adolescent dose*.

**Strength(s) usually available**
U.S.—
  500,000 Units (12.5 mg) per mL (Rx) [*Calciferol*].
Canada—
  500,000 Units (12.5 mg) per mL (Rx) [*Calciferol*].

**Packaging and storage**
Store below 40 °C (104 °F), preferably between 15 and 30 °C (59 and 86 °F), unless otherwise specified by manufacturer. Protect from light. Protect from freezing.

Revised: 08/03/92
Interim revision: 08/18/92; 08/07/95

---

# VITAMIN E   Systemic

VA CLASSIFICATION (Primary): VT600

Commonly used brand name(s): *Amino-Opti-E; Aquasol E; E-1000 I.U. Softgels; E-200 I.U. Softgels; E-400 I.U. in a Water Soluble Base; E-Complex-600; E-Vitamin Succinate; Liqui-E; Pheryl E; Vita-Plus E; Webber Vitamin E*.

Another commonly used name is alpha tocopherol.

Note: For a listing of dosage forms and brand names by country availability, see *Dosage Forms* section(s).

## Category
Nutritional supplement (vitamin).
Note: Vitamin E is a fat-soluble vitamin.

## Indications

**Accepted**
Vitamin E deficiency (prophylaxis and treatment)— Vitamin E (also known as alpha tocopherol) is indicated for prevention and treatment of vitamin E deficiency. For prophylaxis of vitamin E deficiency, dietary improvement, rather than supplementation, is advisable. For treatment of vitamin E deficiency, supplementation is preferred. Although dietary vitamin E deficiency usually does not occur, even with inadequate nutrition, it may occur rarely in newborn, premature, or low-birthweight babies fed unfortified formulas or when transfer from the mother to the fetus is insufficient, and in severe fat malabsorption.

Deficiency of vitamin E may lead to peripheral neuropathy, decreased proprioception, ophthalmoplegia, and necrotizing myopathy.

Recommended intakes may be increased and/or supplementation may be necessary in the following persons or conditions (based on documented vitamin E deficiency):
Abetalipoproteinemia
Acanthocytosis
Gastrectomy
Hepatic-biliary tract disease—chronic cholestasis, hepatic cirrhosis, biliary atresia, obstructive jaundice
Infants receiving formula not sufficiently fortified with vitamin E
Intestinal diseases—celiac, tropical sprue, regional enteritis
Malabsorption syndromes associated with pancreatic insufficiency—cystic fibrosis

In general, vitamin E absorption will be impaired in any condition in which fat malabsorption (steatorrhea) occurs.

Vitamin E supplementation may be necessary in patients receiving total parenteral nutrition (TPN).

Recommended intakes for all vitamins and most minerals are increased during pregnancy. Many physicians recommend that pregnant women receive multivitamin and mineral supplements, especially those pregnant women who do not consume an adequate diet and those in high-risk categories (i.e., women carrying more than one fetus, heavy cigarette smokers, and alcohol and drug abusers). Taking excessive amounts of a multivitamin and mineral supplement may be harmful to the mother and/or fetus and should be avoided.

Recommended intakes for all vitamins and most minerals are increased during breast-feeding.

Recommended intakes may be increased by the following medications: Cholestyramine, colestipol, mineral oil, and iron supplements.

Recommended intakes for vitamin E are directly related to amounts of polyunsaturated fatty acids (PUFA) in the diet. A high intake of PUFA may increase vitamin E requirements.

Recommended intakes may be decreased in diets containing selenium, sulfur-containing amino acids, or antioxidants.

Routine administration of vitamin E to low-birthweight premature infants is being recommended by some clinicians for prevention of hemolytic anemia due to vitamin E deficiency and to reduce the severity of retrolental fibroplasia (which may cause blindness) and bronchopulmonary dysplasia due to oxygen toxicity. However, benefits of routine prophylactic use have not been conclusively proven, and there are significant potential risks, such as necrotizing enterocolitis, associated with its use. Further study is necessary.

**Acceptance not established**
There are insufficient data to show that vitamin E may prevent the occurrence of certain types of *cancer*.

**Unaccepted**
Although a large number of unsubstantiated claims for vitamin E have been made, it has not been proven effective for treatment of beta-thalassemia, cancer, fibrocystic disease of the breast, inflammatory skin disorders, loss of hair, habitual abortion, heart disease, intermittent claudication, menopausal syndrome, infertility, peptic ulcer, sickle cell disease, burns, porphyria, neuromuscular disorders, thrombophlebitis, impotence, bee stings, liver spots on the hands, bursitis, diaper rash, lung toxicity from air pollution, or for prevention of arteriosclerosis, or deterioration from aging. Vitamin E has also not been shown to increase physical endurance or sexual ability.

## Pharmacology/Pharmacokinetics

**Mechanism of action/Effect**
Vitamin E is considered an essential nutritional element, although its exact function is unknown. As an antioxidant, in conjunction with dietary selenium, vitamin E protects polyunsaturated fatty acids in membranes and other cellular structures from attack by free radicals and protects red blood cells against hemolysis. Protection against oxygen radical damage appears to be important for the development and maintenance of nerve and muscle function. Vitamin E may also act as a cofactor in some enzyme systems.

**Absorption**
50 to 80% absorbed from gastrointestinal tract (duodenum); requires presence of bile salts, dietary fat, and normal pancreatic function for efficient absorption.

**Protein binding**
Bound to betalipoproteins in blood.

**Storage**
All body tissues, especially fatty tissues.

**Biotransformation**
Hepatic.

**Elimination**
Biliary/renal.

## Precautions to Consider

**Pregnancy/Reproduction**
Pregnancy—Problems in humans have not been documented with intake of normal daily recommended amounts. Placental transfer is incomplete; neonates receive 20 to 30% of maternal concentrations. Low-birthweight infants may be deficient in vitamin E because of low stores at birth.

**Breast-feeding**
Vitamin E is distributed into breast milk; however, problems in humans have not been documented with intake of normal daily recommended amounts.

**Pediatrics**
Problems in pediatrics have not been documented with intake of normal daily recommended amounts. Plasma vitamin E concentrations in newborn infants are about one-third those of adults and are even lower in premature or low-birthweight infants. The Committee on Nutrition of the American Academy of Pediatrics recommends that the full-term infant receive 0.3 U of vitamin E per 100 kilocalories and at least 1 U of vitamin E per gram of linoleic acid; it also recommends that formula fed to premature infants provide 0.7 U of vitamin E per 100 kilocalories and at least 1 U of vitamin E per gram of linoleic acid. In addition, it has been suggested that premature infants receive 5 to 25 U of supplemental vitamin E per day because of concerns about the adequacy of its intestinal absorption.

**Geriatrics**
Problems in geriatrics have not been documented with intake of normal daily recommended amounts.

**Drug interactions and/or related problems**
The following drug interactions and/or related problems have been selected on the basis of their potential clinical significance (possible mechanism in parentheses where appropriate)—not necessarily inclusive (» = major clinical significance):

Note: Combinations containing any of the following, depending on the amount present, may also interact with vitamin E supplements.

Anticoagulants, coumarin- or indandione-derivative
 (concurrent use with doses of vitamin E greater than 400 U a day should be avoided to prevent a possible hypoprothrombinemic response)

Cholestyramine or
Colestipol or
Mineral oil
 (may interfere with absorption of vitamin E; recommended intakes for vitamin E may be increased in patients receiving these medications)

Iron supplements
 (large doses of iron may catalyze the oxidation of and possibly increase daily requirements for vitamin E; observation of individuals receiving both is recommended)

Vitamin A
 (vitamin E may facilitate absorption, hepatic storage, and utilization, and reduce toxicity of vitamin A; excessive doses of vitamin E may deplete vitamin A stores)

**Medical considerations/Contraindications**
The medical considerations/contraindications included have been selected on the basis of their potential clinical significance (reasons given in parentheses where appropriate)—not necessarily inclusive (» = major clinical significance).

*Risk-benefit should be considered when the following medical problems exist:*

Hypoprothrombinemia due to vitamin K deficiency
 (may be aggravated by doses of vitamin E greater than 400 U a day)

Sensitivity to vitamin E

## Side/Adverse Effects

The following side/adverse effects have been selected on the basis of their potential clinical significance (possible signs and symptoms in parentheses where appropriate)—not necessarily inclusive:

**Those indicating need for medical attention only if they continue or are bothersome**

With large doses (between 400 and 800 Units per day for prolonged periods)
 *Blurred vision; diarrhea; dizziness; headache; nausea or stomach cramps; unusual tiredness or weakness*

Note: Although data have not been established, very high doses of vitamin E (greater than 800 Units per day for prolonged periods) have been reported to increase bleeding tendencies in vitamin K–deficient patients, alter metabolism of thyroid hormones, impair sexual function, and may increase the risk of thrombophlebitis or thromboembolism in susceptible patients.

## Patient Consultation

As an aid to patient consultation, refer to *Advice for the Patient, Vitamin E (Systemic).*

In providing consultation, consider emphasizing the following selected information (» = major clinical significance):

**Description of use**
 Description should include function in the body, signs of deficiency, and unproven uses

## Importance of diet
Importance of proper nutrition; supplement may be needed because of inadequate intake
Food sources of vitamin E; effects of processing
Not using vitamins as substitute for balanced diet
Recommended daily intake for vitamin E

## Before using this dietary supplement
» Conditions affecting use, especially:
Sensitivity to vitamin E
Use in children—Premature infants may need additional supplementation

## Proper use of this dietary supplement
» Proper dosing
Proper administration of oral solution dosage form: Taking by mouth even though dietary supplement comes in a dropper bottle; may be dropped directly into the mouth or mixed with cereal, fruit juice, or other food
Missed dose: No cause for concern because of length of time necessary for depletion; remembering to take as directed
» Proper storage

# General Dosing Information

In spite of the infrequency of vitamin E deficiency, combinations of vitamins may contain vitamin E. Many commercial vitamin complexes are available.

Vitamin E is available in various forms, including d- or dl-alpha tocopheryl acetate, d- or dl-alpha tocopherol, and d- or dl-alpha tocopheryl acid succinate. The synthetic form of vitamin E is dl-alpha tocopherol, while the natural form of vitamin E is d-alpha tocopherol.

## For oral dosage forms only
Water-miscible preparations may be useful for prevention of vitamin E deficiency in individuals with fat malabsorption; if bile acid depletion is present, high doses of vitamin E may still be necessary.

## Diet/Nutrition
Recommended dietary intakes for vitamin E are defined differently worldwide.
For U.S.—
The Recommended Dietary Allowances (RDAs) for vitamins and minerals are determined by the Food and Nutrition Board of the National Research Council and are intended to provide adequate nutrition in most healthy persons under usual environmental stresses. In addition, a different designation may be used by the FDA for food and dietary supplement labeling purposes, as with Daily Value (DV). DVs replace the previous labeling terminology United States Recommended Daily Allowances (USRDAs).
For Canada—
Recommended Nutrient Intakes (RNIs) for vitamins, minerals, and protein are determined by Health and Welfare Canada and provide recommended amounts of a specific nutrient while minimizing the risk of chronic diseases.

The expression of vitamin E activity has changed from Units to alpha tocopherol equivalents (alpha-TE), with 1 alpha-TE equal to the activity of 1 mg of d-alpha tocopherol, 1.4 mg dl-alpha tocopherol, 1.7 mg dl-alpha tocopheryl acid succinate, 1.1 mg d-alpha tocopheryl acetate, 1.5 mg dl-alpha tocopheryl acetate, or 1.2 mg d-alpha tocopheryl acid succinate. One Unit of vitamin E is equal to 1 mg of dl-alpha tocopherol acetate, 0.7 mg of d-alpha tocopherol, 0.9 mg dl-alpha tocopherol, 1.1 mg dl-alpha tocopheryl acid succinate, 0.7 mg d-alpha tocopheryl, or 0.8 mg d-alpha tocopheryl acid succinate. This change was made to reflect the total activity of all forms of vitamin E. Most commercially available vitamin E products continue to be labeled in Units.

Daily recommended intakes for vitamin E are generally defined as follows:

| Persons | U.S. mg alpha-TE | U.S. Units | Canada mg alpha-TE | Canada Units |
|---|---|---|---|---|
| Infants and children | | | | |
| Birth to 3 years of age | 3–6 | 5–10 | 3–4 | 5–6.7 |
| 4 to 6 years of age | 7 | 11.7 | 5 | 8.3 |
| 7 to 10 years of age | 7 | 11.7 | 6–8 | 10–13 |
| Adolescent and adult males | 10 | 16.7 | 6–10 | 10–16.7 |
| Adolescent and adult females | 8 | 13 | 5–7 | 8.3–11.7 |
| Pregnant females | 10 | 16.7 | 8–9 | 13–15 |
| Breast-feeding females | 11–12 | 18–20 | 9–10 | 15–16.7 |

These are usually provided by adequate diets.

The best dietary sources of vitamin E include vegetable oils (corn, cottonseed, soybean, safflower), wheat germ, whole-grain cereals, and green leafy vegetables. Foods may lose significant amounts of vitamin E activity during cooking and storage.

## Oral Dosage Forms

Note: Dosages and strengths are expressed in terms of USP Units of vitamin E activity.

### VITAMIN E CAPSULES USP
**Usual adult and adolescent dose**
Deficiency (prophylaxis)—
Oral, amount based on normal daily recommended intakes:

| Persons | U.S. mg alpha-TE | U.S. Units | Canada mg alpha-TE | Canada Units |
|---|---|---|---|---|
| Adolescent and adult males | 10 | 16.7 | 6–10 | 10–16.7 |
| Adolescent and adult females | 8 | 13 | 5–7 | 8.3–11.7 |
| Pregnant females | 10 | 16.7 | 8–9 | 13–15 |
| Breast-feeding females | 11–12 | 18–20 | 9–10 | 15–16.7 |

Deficiency (treatment)—
Treatment dose is individualized by prescriber based on severity of deficiency.

**Usual pediatric dose**
Dosage form not appropriate for use in children.

**Strength(s) usually available**
U.S.—
100 Units (OTC) [*Aquasol E* (d-alpha tocopheryl acetate); GENERIC].
200 Units (OTC) [*Amino-Opti-E* (d-alpha tocopheryl acid succinate); *E-200 I.U. Softgels* (d-alpha tocopheryl acetate); *E-Vitamin Succinate* (d-alpha tocopheryl acid succinate); GENERIC].
400 Units (OTC) [*Aquasol E* (d-alpha tocopheryl acetate); *E-Vitamin Succinate* (d-alpha tocopheryl acid succinate); *E-400 I.U. in a Water Soluble Base; Vita-Plus E* (d-alpha tocopheryl acetate); GENERIC].
500 Units (OTC) [GENERIC].
600 Units (OTC) [*E-Complex-600*; GENERIC].
1000 Units (OTC) [*E-1000 I.U. Softgels*; GENERIC].
Canada—
100 Units (OTC) [*Aquasol E* (d-alpha tocopheryl acetate); GENERIC].
200 Units (OTC) [GENERIC].
400 Units (OTC) [GENERIC].
800 Units (OTC) [GENERIC].
1000 Units (OTC) [GENERIC].

Note: A water-miscible dosage form is available.
Some strengths of these vitamin E preparations may exceed the dosage range recommended by USP DI Advisory Panels based on the amount necessary to meet normal nutritional needs.

**Packaging and storage**
Store below 40 °C (104 °F), preferably between 15 and 30 °C (59 and 86 °F), unless otherwise specified by manufacturer. Store in a tight container. Protect from light.

### VITAMIN E ORAL SOLUTION
**Usual adult and adolescent dose**
See *Vitamin E Capsules USP*.

**Usual pediatric dose**
Deficiency (prophylaxis)—
Premature infants receiving formulas high in polyunsaturated fatty acids (PUFA)—Oral, 15 to 25 Units per day, or 7 Units per Liter of formula.
Infants with chronic cholestasis—Oral, 15 to 25 Units of a water-miscible preparation per kg of body weight per day.
Normal birthweight infants—Oral, 5 Units per Liter of formula.
Other children—Oral, amount based on normal daily recommended intakes:

| Persons | U.S. mg alpha-TE | U.S. Units | Canada mg alpha-TE | Canada Units |
|---|---|---|---|---|
| Infants and children | | | | |
| Birth to 3 years of age | 3–6 | 5–10 | 3–4 | 5–6.7 |
| 4 to 6 years of age | 7 | 11.7 | 5 | 8.3 |
| 7 to 10 years of age | 7 | 11.7 | 6–8 | 10–13 |

Deficiency (treatment)—
  Treatment dose is individualized by prescriber based on severity of deficiency.

**Strength(s) usually available**
U.S.—
  26.6 Units per mL (OTC) [*Liqui-E* (*d*-alpha tocopheryl polyethylene glycol 1000 succinate)].
  50 Units per mL (OTC) [*Aquasol E* (*dl*-alpha tocopheryl acetate)].
Canada—
  50 Units per mL (OTC) [*Aquasol E* (*dl*-alpha tocopheryl acetate)].
  77 Units per mL (OTC) [*Webber Vitamin E* (*d*-alpha tocopheryl polyethylene glycol 1000 succinate)].
Note: *d*-Alpha tocopheryl polyethylene glycol 1000 succinate is a water-miscible form of vitamin E.
  Some strengths of these vitamin E preparations may exceed the dosage range recommended by USP DI Advisory Panels based on the amount necessary to meet normal nutritional needs.

**Packaging and storage**
Store below 40 °C (104 °F), preferably between 15 and 30 °C (59 and 86 °F), unless otherwise specified by manufacturer. Store in a tight container. Protect from light. Protect from freezing.

## VITAMIN E TABLETS

**Usual adult and adolescent dose**
See *Vitamin E Capsules USP*.

**Usual pediatric dose**
See *Vitamin E Oral Solution*.

**Strength(s) usually available**
U.S.—
  100 Units (OTC) [GENERIC].
  200 Units (OTC) [GENERIC].
  400 Units (OTC) [*Pheryl E* (*d*-alpha tocopheryl acid succinate); GENERIC].
  500 Units (OTC) [GENERIC].
  800 Units (OTC) [GENERIC].
Canada—
  Not commercially available.
Note: Some strengths of these vitamin E preparations may exceed the dosage range recommended by USP DI Advisory Panels based on the amount necessary to meet normal nutritional needs.

**Packaging and storage**
Store below 40 °C (104 °F), preferably between 15 and 30 °C (59 and 86 °F), unless otherwise specified by manufacturer. Store in a tight container. Protect from light.

## VITAMIN E CHEWABLE TABLETS

**Usual adult and adolescent dose**
See *Vitamin E Capsules USP*.

**Usual pediatric dose**
See *Vitamin E Oral Solution*.

**Strength(s) usually available**
U.S.—
  400 Units (OTC) [GENERIC].
Canada—
  Not commercially available.
Note: The strength of this vitamin E preparation may exceed the dosage range recommended by USP DI Advisory Panels based on the amount necessary to meet normal nutritional needs.

**Packaging and storage**
Store below 40 °C (104 °F), preferably between 15 and 30 °C (59 and 86 °F), unless otherwise specified by manufacturer. Store in a tight container. Protect from light.

Revised: 06/22/93
Interim revision: 07/20/94; 05/26/95

---

# VITAMIN K  Systemic

This monograph includes information on the following: 1) Menadiol†; 2) Phytonadione.
INN: Phytonadione—Phytomenadione
VA CLASSIFICATION (Primary):
  Menadiol—VT701
  Phytonadione—VT702
Commonly used brand name(s): *AquaMEPHYTON*[2]; *Konakion*[2]; *Mephyton*[2]; *Synkayvite*[1].

Other commonly used names are: Phytomenadione [Phytonadione] Vitamin $K_1$ [Phytonadione] Vitamin $K_4$ [Menadiol]

Note: For a listing of dosage forms and brand names by country availability, see *Dosage Forms* section(s).

†Not commercially available in Canada.

## Category

Nutritional supplement (vitamin), prothrombogenic—Menadiol Sodium Diphosphate; Phytonadione.
Antidote (to drug-induced hypoprothrombinemia)—Menadiol Sodium Diphosphate; Phytonadione.
Antihemorrhagic—Phytonadione
Note: Vitamin K is a fat-soluble vitamin. Phytonadione (vitamin $K_1$) is a synthetic lipid-soluble form of vitamin K. Menadiol sodium diphosphate (vitamin $K_4$) is a water-soluble derivative converted in the body to menadione (vitamin $K_3$).

## Indications

**Accepted**
Hypoprothrombinemia (prophylaxis and treatment)—Vitamin K is indicated for treatment and prevention of various coagulation disorders involving impaired formation of factors II, VII, IX, and X resulting from vitamin K deficiency or impairment of vitamin K activity, including hypoprothrombinemia due to oral anticoagulants, salicylates, and some antibiotics. Vitamin K does not return abnormal platelet function to normal. Vitamin K does not counteract the anticoagulant activity of heparin. Vitamin K may not be effective in hepatic function impairment since prothrombin synthesis occurs in the liver.

Deficiency may occur in the following persons or conditions: Patients receiving total parenteral nutrition (TPN); in malabsorption syndromes associated with pancreatic insufficiency (including cystic fibrosis), hepatic-biliary tract disease (obstructive jaundice, internal biliary fistula), diseases of the small intestine (celiac disease, tropical sprue, regional enteritis, ulcerative colitis, persistent diarrhea or dysentery, short bowel syndrome after extensive bowel resection); prolonged T-tube drainage; abetalipoproteinemia; infants receiving milk substitute formulas and those who are breast-fed.

Deficiency may occur when vitamin K activity is impaired by salicylates, sulfonamides, quinine, quinidine, dactinomycin or broad-spectrum antibiotic therapy, or when absorption is decreased by concurrent administration of cholestyramine, colestipol, mineral oil, or sucralfate.

Hemorrhagic disease of the newborn (prophylaxis)—The American Academy of Pediatrics recommends routine phytonadione administration at birth to prevent hemorrhagic disease of the newborn, since vitamin K from the mother may be inadequate because of poor passage through the placenta and because intestinal bacteria responsible for natural synthesis of vitamin K are not present for 5 to 8 days following birth. In addition, the risk of hemorrhagic disease of the newborn is increased in infants of mothers who received anticonvulsants (e.g., phenobarbital, phenytoin) during pregnancy. Phytonadione is preferred over menadiol because the risk of causing hyperbilirubinemia and hemolytic anemia is less, especially in premature infants.

**Unaccepted**
Menadiol sodium diphosphate may be used as a liver function test, although it has generally been replaced by newer methods.

## Pharmacology/Pharmacokinetics

**Physicochemical characteristics**
Molecular weight—
  Menadiol sodium diphosphate: 530.18.
  Phytonadione: 450.70.

**Mechanism of action/Effect**
Naturally-occurring vitamin K is normally synthesized by intestinal flora. Vitamin K promotes hepatic formation of active prothrombin (factor II), proconvertin (factor VII), plasma thromboplastin component or Christmas factor (factor IX), and Stuart factor (factor X), which are essential for normal blood clotting.

## Absorption
Readily absorbed from healthy gastrointestinal tract (duodenum); phytonadione requires presence of bile salts.

## Biotransformation
Hepatic (rapid).

## Onset of action
Menadiol sodium diphosphate—
  Parenteral: 8 to 24 hours.
Phytonadione—
  Oral: 6 to 12 hours.
  Parenteral: 1 to 2 hours, with hemorrhage usually controlled in 3 to 6 hours; normal prothrombin concentrations are often obtained in 12 to 14 hours.

## Elimination
Renal/biliary. Bacterial synthesis of vitamin K in the intestine may result in high fecal concentrations.

# Precautions to Consider

### Pregnancy/Reproduction
Pregnancy—Studies have not been done in either animals or humans. In general, administration before delivery to prevent hemorrhagic disease of the newborn is not recommended because of possible neonatal toxicity.

### Breast-feeding
Problems in humans have not been documented. Vitamin K is especially needed in breast-fed infants since there is no vitamin K in breast milk.

### Pediatrics
Caution is recommended with use of menadiol sodium diphosphate in children because of the risk of hepatotoxicity and hemolytic anemia; administration to newborns (especially premature infants) is not recommended.

### Geriatrics
No information is available on the relationship of age to the effects of vitamin K in geriatric patients.

### Drug interactions and/or related problems
The following drug interactions and/or related problems have been selected on the basis of their potential clinical significance (possible mechanism in parentheses where appropriate)—not necessarily inclusive (» = major clinical significance):

Note: Combinations containing any of the following medications, depending on the amount present, may also interact with this medication.

Antacids
  (large amounts of aluminum hydroxide may precipitate bile acids in the upper small intestine, thereby decreasing absorption of fat-soluble vitamins)
Antibiotics, broad-spectrum, or
Quinidine or
Quinine or
Salicylates, high doses, or
Sulfonamides, antibacterial
  (requirements for vitamin K may be increased in patients receiving these medications)
» Anticoagulants, coumarin- or indandione-derivative
  (concurrent use with vitamin K may decrease the effects of these anticoagulants as a result of increased hepatic synthesis of procoagulant factors; dosage adjustments may be necessary, especially when vitamin K has been used to counteract excessive effects of anticoagulants)
Cholestyramine or
Colestipol or
Mineral oil or
Sucralfate
  (concurrent use may decrease absorption of vitamin K; requirements for vitamin K may be increased in patients receiving these medications)
Dactinomycin
  (concurrent use may decrease the effects of vitamin K; evidence is inconclusive, observation of patients is recommended and a higher dose of vitamin K may be required)
» Hemolytics, other (See *Appendix II*)
  (concurrent use with vitamin K, especially menadiol, may increase the potential for toxic side effects)

### Medical considerations/Contraindications
The medical considerations/contraindications included have been selected on the basis of their potential clinical significance (reasons given in parentheses where appropriate)—not necessarily inclusive (» = major clinical significance).

*Risk-benefit should be considered when the following medical problems exist:*
Glucose-6-phosphate dehydrogenase (G6PD) deficiency
  (menadiol sodium diphosphate may induce erythrocyte hemolysis)
» Hepatic function impairment
  (large doses may increase impairment of function)
Sensitivity to the vitamin K analog considered for use, history of

### Patient monitoring
The following may be especially important in patient monitoring (other tests may be warranted in some patients, depending on condition; » = major clinical significance):
Prothrombin time (PT) determinations
  (recommended to determine responsiveness to and need for additional vitamin K therapy)

## Side/Adverse Effects
Note: A rare hypersensitivity-like reaction, which has occasionally resulted in death, has been reported after intravenous administration of phytonadione, especially when rapid.
  In newborns, especially premature infants, menadiol sodium diphosphate has been associated with hemolytic anemia, hyperbilirubinemia, and kernicterus because of immature hepatic function in these infants. There is less risk with phytonadione, unless high doses are given.

The following side/adverse effects have been selected on the basis of their potential clinical significance (possible signs and symptoms in parentheses where appropriate)—not necessarily inclusive:

**Those indicating need for medical attention only if they continue or are bothersome**
Incidence less frequent
  *Flushing of face; redness, pain, or swelling at place of injection; unusual taste*

## Patient Consultation
As an aid to patient consultation, refer to *Advice for the Patient, Vitamin K (Systemic)*.
In providing consultation, consider emphasizing the following selected information (» = major clinical significance):

### Description of use
Description should include function in the body, food sources, and signs of deficiency

### Before using this medication
» Conditions affecting use, especially:
  Sensitivity to the vitamin K analog considered for use, history of
  Use in children—Menadiol may cause hepatotoxicity and hemolytic anemia and is not recommended for newborns, especially premature neonates; the risk of hemolytic anemia is lower with phytonadione
  Other medications, especially coumarin- or indandione-derivative anticoagulants and hemolytics
  Other medical problems, especially hepatic function impairment

### Proper use of this medication
» Importance of not taking more medication than the amount prescribed
» Regular prothrombin time tests and regular visits to physician to check progress
» Proper dosing
  Missed dose: Taking as soon as remembered; not taking if almost time for next dose; not doubling doses; telling physician about any missed doses
» Proper storage

### Precautions while using this medication
» Need for patient to inform all physicians and dentists that this medication is being used
» Not taking any other medications unless discussed with physician since they may alter the effect

### Side/adverse effects
Signs of potential side effects, especially hemolytic anemia

## General Dosing Information
There are no Recommended Dietary Allowances (RDA) for vitamin K since a normal diet and intestinal bacterial synthesis supply more than enough. The minimum daily requirement is estimated to be 0.03 mcg per kg of body weight for adults and 1 to 5 mcg per kg of body weight for infants.

Best dietary sources of vitamin K include green leafy vegetables, meats, and dairy products. There is little loss of vitamin K from foods with ordinary cooking.

Dosage of vitamin K should be based on laboratory tests of clotting function. Intake of vitamin K from dietary and other sources should also be evaluated in determining the therapeutic dosage.

When used to counteract anticoagulant-induced hypoprothrombinemia, use of the smallest effective dose is recommended since excessive dosage may result in temporary refractoriness to subsequent anticoagulant therapy.

Administration of fresh whole blood or plasma may also be required when bleeding is severe, because of the delay in onset of vitamin K activity.

**For parenteral dosage forms only**
The parenteral route of administration is preferred whenever possible, especially when oral administration is not possible because of malabsorption problems.

Because of the risk of severe hypersensitivity-like reactions, intravenous administration is not recommended.

## MENADIOL

## Oral Dosage Forms
### MENADIOL SODIUM DIPHOSPHATE TABLETS USP

**Usual adult and adolescent dose**
Hypoprothrombinemia secondary to obstructive jaundice and biliary fistulas—
 Oral, 5 mg per day.
Hypoprothrombinemia secondary to the administration of antibacterials or salicylates—
 Oral, 5 to 10 mg per day.

**Usual pediatric dose**
Vitamin (prothrombogenic); or
Antidote (to drug-induced hypoprothrombinemia)—
 Oral, 5 to 10 mg per day.

**Strength(s) usually available**
U.S.—
 5 mg (Rx) [*Synkayvite*].
Canada—
 Not commercially available.

**Packaging and storage**
Store below 40 °C (104 °F), preferably between 15 and 30 °C (59 and 86 °F), unless otherwise specified by manufacturer. Store in a well-closed, light-resistant container.

## Parenteral Dosage Forms
### MENADIOL SODIUM DIPHOSPHATE INJECTION USP

**Usual adult and adolescent dose**
Nutritional supplement (vitamin), prothrombogenic; or
Antidote (to drug-induced hypoprothrombinemia)—
 Intramuscular or subcutaneous, 5 to 15 mg one or two times a day.

**Usual pediatric dose**
Vitamin (prothrombogenic); or
Antidote (to drug-induced hypoprothrombinemia)—
 Intramuscular or subcutaneous, 5 to 10 mg one or two times a day.

**Strength(s) usually available**
U.S.—
 5 mg per mL (Rx) [*Synkayvite*].
 10 mg per mL (Rx) [*Synkayvite*].
 37.5 mg per mL (75 mg per 2-mL ampul) (Rx) [*Synkayvite*].
Canada—
 Not commercially available.

**Packaging and storage**
Store below 40 °C (104 °F), preferably between 15 and 30 °C (59 and 86 °F), unless otherwise specified by manufacturer. Store in a light-resistant container. Protect from freezing.

**Incompatibilities**
Incompatible with protein hydrolysate.

## PHYTONADIONE

## Oral Dosage Forms
### PHYTONADIONE TABLETS USP

**Usual adult and adolescent dose**
Hypoprothrombinemia, anticoagulant-induced—
 Oral, 2.5 to 10 mg (up to 25 mg); may be repeated after twelve to forty-eight hours if necessary.

**Usual pediatric dose**
Nutritional supplement (vitamin), prothrombogenic; or
Antidote (to drug-induced hypoprothrombinemia)—
 Children: Oral, 5 to 10 mg.

**Strength(s) usually available**
U.S.—
 5 mg (Rx) [*Mephyton*].
Canada—
 Not commercially available.

**Packaging and storage**
Store below 40 °C (104 °F), preferably between 15 and 30 °C (59 and 86 °F), unless otherwise specified by manufacturer. Store in a well-closed, light-resistant container.

## Parenteral Dosage Forms
### PHYTONADIONE INJECTION USP

Note: Some preparations are for intramuscular use only.

**Usual adult and adolescent dose**
Hypoprothrombinemia, anticoagulant-induced (except heparin type)—
 Intramuscular or subcutaneous, 2.5 to 10 mg (up to 25 mg); may be repeated after six to eight hours if necessary.
Hypoprothrombinemia due to malabsorption syndrome or other medications—
 Intramuscular or subcutaneous, 2 to 25 mg; may be repeated if necessary.
Prevention of hypoprothrombinemia during prolonged total parenteral nutrition—
 Intramuscular, 5 to 10 mg once a week.

**Usual pediatric dose**
Infants receiving milk substitutes or who are breast-fed—
 Intramuscular or subcutaneous, 1 mg per month if vitamin K content of diet is less than 0.1 mg per L.
Prevention of hypoprothrombinemia during prolonged total parenteral nutrition—
 Intramuscular, 2 to 5 mg once a week.
Treatment of hypoprothrombinemia—
 Infants—Intramuscular or subcutaneous, 1 to 2 mg.
 Children—Intramuscular or subcutaneous, 5 to 10 mg.
Prevention of hemorrhagic disease of the newborn—
 Intramuscular or subcutaneous, 0.5 to 1 mg immediately after delivery; may be repeated after six to eight hours if necessary (e.g., if mothers received anticonvulsants during pregnancy).

Note: Higher doses may be needed for infants whose mothers received anticoagulants or anticonvulsants during pregnancy.

**Strength(s) usually available**
U.S.—
 2 mg per mL (1 mg per 0.5-mL ampul) (Rx) [*AquaMEPHYTON* (benzyl alcohol); *Konakion*].
 10 mg per mL (Rx) [*AquaMEPHYTON* (benzyl alcohol); *Konakion*].
Canada—
 2 mg per mL (1 mg per 0.5-mL ampul) (Rx) [GENERIC].
 10 mg per mL (Rx) [GENERIC].

**Packaging and storage**
Store below 40 °C (104 °F), preferably between 15 and 30 °C (59 and 86 °F), unless otherwise specified by manufacturer. Protect from light. Protect from freezing.

**Preparation of dosage form**
Phytonadione injection may be diluted with sodium chloride injection, 5% dextrose injection, or 5% dextrose and sodium chloride injection.

**Stability**
Solutions should be prepared immediately prior to use and any unused portion discarded.

**Incompatibilities**
Phytonadione injection is physically incompatible with phenytoin injection.

# VITAMINS, MULTIPLE, AND FLUORIDE  Systemic

This monograph includes information on the following: 1) Multiple Vitamins and Fluoride; 2) Vitamins A, D, and C and Fluoride.

VA CLASSIFICATION (Primary): VT802

Commonly used brand name(s): *Adeflor*[1]; *Cari-Tab*[2]; *Mulvidren-F*[1]; *Poly-Vi-Flor*[1]; *Tri-Vi-Flor*[2]; *ViDaylin/F*[1].

Note: For a listing of dosage forms and brand names by country availability, see *Dosage Forms* section(s).

## Category
Vitamin replenisher–dental caries prophylactic.

## Indications

### Accepted
Vitamin deficiency (prophylaxis and treatment) or

Dental caries (prophylaxis)—This combination has been used as a dietary supplement for prevention of dental caries in children in those areas where the level of naturally occurring fluoride in the drinking water is inadequate, and for prophylaxis and treatment of deficiencies of essential fat- and water-soluble vitamins. In optimally fluoridated communities, fluoride supplementation may be necessary in infants that are totally breast-fed or receive ready-to-use formulas or in children consuming nonfluoridated bottled water rather than tap water. Fluoride supplementation may also be indicated in those situations where home water filtration systems remove fluoride. This usually occurs with reverse osmosis or distillation units, but not with carbon charcoal filters.

Evidence that oral systemic fluoride supplements reduce dental caries in adults is lacking.

## Pharmacology/Pharmacokinetics
Note: See also information in individual vitamin monographs.

### Mechanism of action/Effect
Sodium fluoride—Fluoride ion becomes incorporated into and stabilizes apatite crystal of bone and teeth. Deposition in the enamel surface of teeth appears to increase resistance to acid and to development of caries. Fluorides may also promote remineralization of decalcified enamel and may interfere with growth and development of dental plaque bacteria.

Vitamins, multiple—Essential to meet nutritional requirements for normal growth and development and maintenance of good health.

### Absorption
Fluorides in solution or in the form of rapidly soluble salts are readily and almost completely absorbed from the gastrointestinal tract.

### Storage
Fluoride—In bone and developing teeth.

### Elimination
Fluoride—Renal.

## Precautions to Consider
Note: Also see information in individual vitamin monographs.

### Carcinogenicity
Fluoride in the concentrations shown to be effective against tooth decay has not been shown to cause cancer in individuals who receive fluoride over prolonged periods. A recent study directed by the National Toxicology program has determined no carcinogenic activity in female rats and male or female mice receiving 25, 100, or 175 parts per million (ppm) sodium fluoride in drinking water over a period of 2 years. In this same study, male rats receiving the same doses of sodium fluoride, also over 2 years, showed a marginal increase in bone neoplasms in the 2 higher dose groups that may have been chemically related.

### Pregnancy/Reproduction
Fluoride crosses the placenta to a limited extent; however, problems in humans have not been documented. There is conflicting evidence as the whether administration of fluoride supplements to women during pregnancy will help prevent caries in the child.

### Breast-feeding
Trace amounts of fluoride are excreted in breast milk, although the concentration is not high enough to provide benefits to the infant. Problems in humans have not been documented.

### Pediatrics
No pediatrics-specific information is available. However, chronic overdose of fluoride may cause fluorosis of the teeth and osseous changes.

### Geriatrics
Appropriate studies with fluoride have not been performed in the geriatric population. However, no geriatrics-specific problems have been documented to date.

### Dental
Excessive doses of sodium fluoride may result in fluorosis of teeth if taken during tooth formation years.

### Drug interactions and/or related problems
The following drug interactions and/or related problems have been selected on the basis of their potential clinical significance (possible mechanism in parentheses where appropriate)—not necessarily inclusive (» = major clinical significance):

Note: Combinations containing any of the following medications, depending on the amount present, may also interact with this medication.

Aluminum hydroxide
(may decrease absorption and increase fecal excretion of fluoride; large amounts of aluminum hydroxide may precipitate bile acids in the upper small intestine, thereby decreasing absorption of fat-soluble vitamins, especially vitamin A)

» Anticoagulants, coumarin- or indandione-derivative
(concurrent use with vitamin K may decrease the effects of oral anticoagulants as a result of increased hepatic synthesis of procoagulant factors; concurrent use with large doses of vitamin A or E may lead to a possible hypoprothrombinemic response; dosage adjustments may be necessary)

Anticonvulsants, hydantoin
(concurrent use with folic acid may decrease the effects of hydantoins by antagonism of their central nervous system [CNS] effects; concurrent use with vitamin D may accelerate metabolism by hepatic microsomal enzyme induction, and prolonged use may increase vitamin D requirements)

Calcitonin
(concurrent use with vitamin D may antagonize the effect of calcitonin in the treatment of hypercalcemia)

Calcium ions
(may complex with and inhibit absorption of fluoride; concurrent use of high doses of calcium-containing preparations with vitamin D may increase the risk of hypercalcemia)

Chloramphenicol
(concurrent use may antagonize hematopoietic response to vitamin $B_{12}$; monitoring of hematologic status or use of an alternate antibiotic is recommended)

Diuretics, thiazide
(concurrent use with vitamin D may increase the risk of hypercalcemia)

» Iron supplements
(vitamin E may impair the hematologic response in patients with iron deficiency anemia; large doses of iron may increase daily requirements of vitamin E; observation of patients receiving both is recommended)

» Vitamin D and analogs
(concurrent use of one with another, especially calcifediol, is not

recommended because of additive effects and increased potential for toxicity)

**Laboratory value alterations**

The following have been selected on the basis of their potential clinical significance (possible effect in parentheses where appropriate)—not necessarily inclusive (» = major clinical significance):

With diagnostic test results
*For sodium fluoride*
Serum acid phosphatase concentrations
(may be falsely decreased)
Serum aspartate aminotransferase (AST [SGOT]) concentrations
(may be falsely increased)

**Medical considerations/Contraindications**

The medical considerations/contraindications included have been selected on the basis of their potential clinical significance (reasons given in parentheses where appropriate)—not necessarily inclusive (» = major clinical significance).

*Risk-benefit should be considered when the following medical problems exist:*
High dental fluorosis, or prevalence in other members of the immediate community
Sensitivity to fluorides

**Patient monitoring**

The following may be especially important in patient monitoring (other tests may be warranted in some patients, depending on condition; » = major clinical significance):

Dental examination
(recommended once or twice a year in most patients, and more frequently in those highly prone to developing caries)

## Side/Adverse Effects

Note: See also information contained in monographs on the individual vitamins.

The following side/adverse effects have been selected on the basis of their potential clinical significance (possible signs and symptoms in parentheses where appropriate)—not necessarily inclusive:

**Those indicating need for medical attention**

Incidence rare
*Allergic reaction* (skin rash); **mucous membrane ulceration** (sores in the mouth and on the lips)

## Overdose

For specific information on the agents used in the management of multiple vitamins and fluoride overdose, see:
• *Calcium Supplements (Systemic)* monograph.

For more information on the management of overdose or unintentional ingestion, **contact a Poison Control Center** (see *Poison Control Center Listing*).

**Clinical effects of overdose**

Note: Gastrointestinal distress may occur with ingestion of 4 to 20 mg of sodium fluoride. The lethal dose is not known but has been estimated as 5 to 10 grams in untreated adults and 500 mg in children, depending on the weight of the child.

Severe acute fluoride overdose can cause hypocalcemia and tetany and bone pain, especially in the feet and ankles, of uncertain cause; electrolyte disturbances and cardiac arrhythmias have been reported, progressing to cardiac failure or respiratory arrest in some cases.

The following effects have been selected on the basis of their potential clinical significance (possible signs and symptoms in parentheses where appropriate)—not necessarily inclusive:

Chronic effects (fluorosis and osteosclerosis)
***Pain and aching of bones or stiffness or white, brown, or black discoloration of teeth***

Acute effects
***Black, tarry stools; bloody vomit; diarrhea; drowsiness; faintness; increased watering of mouth; nausea or vomiting; shallow breathing; stomach cramps or pain; tremors; unusual excitement; watery eyes; weakness***

**Treatment of overdose**

Specific treatment—
Administration of intravenous dextrose. Isotonic sodium chloride gastric lavage with lime water to precipitate fluoride. Intravenous calcium gluconate if hypocalcemia occurs.

Supportive care—
Maintenance of high urine output. Patients in whom intentional overdose is confirmed or suspected should be referred for psychiatric consultation.

## Patient Consultation

As an aid to patient consultation, refer to *Advice for the Patient, Vitamins and Fluoride (Systemic)*.

In providing consultation, consider emphasizing the following selected information (» = major clinical significance):

**Before using this dietary supplement**
» Conditions affecting use, especially:
Sensitivity to fluorides
Pregnancy—Fluoride crosses the placenta to a limited extent
Breast-feeding—Trace amount of fluoride excreted in breast milk
Use in children—Chronic overdose may cause dental fluorosis and osseous changes
Dental—Excessive doses taken during tooth formation years may result in tooth fluorosis

**Proper use of this dietary supplement**
» Importance of not using more dietary supplement than the amount prescribed
Taking multiple vitamins and fluoride products 1 hour before or 2 hours after taking foods that contain calcium
Missed dose: Taking as soon as possible; not taking if almost time for next dose; not doubling doses
» Proper storage

*For patients taking the chewable tablet dosage form*
Chewing or crushing tablets before swallowing
Advisability of taking at bedtime after brushing teeth; not eating or drinking for at least 15 minutes after taking

*For patients taking the oral solution dosage form*
Proper use of the dropper bottle
» Avoiding use of glass with fluoride-containing solutions
May be dropped directly into the mouth or mixed with cereal, fruit juice, or other food

**Precautions while using this dietary supplement**
Checking with physician or dentist as soon as possible after move to another area to see if continued treatment at the same dosage is necessary, since fluoride levels of community drinking water vary; also checking if changing infant feeding habits, drinking water, or filtration
» Informing physician or dentist if teeth show signs of mottling

**Side/adverse effects**
Signs of potential side effects, especially allergic reaction or oral mucous membrane ulceration

## General Dosing Information

Optimum benefit of both fluorides and vitamins must be established on an individual basis taking into consideration both the fluoride content of the water supply and the nutritional status of the patient when determining the dose.

The amount of fluoride from all sources should be taken into account when determining the therapeutic dose. For example, infant formulas made with fluoridated water provide a significant amount. Also, some schools in communities without water fluoridation have added up to 4.5 times the optimal fluoride level of 1.0 ppm fluoride to the school's water supply to ensure that children receive adequate fluoride.

Use of this preparation is not recommended in infants less than 3 years of age who consume drinking water containing 0.3 parts per million (ppm) of fluoride or more.

A fluoride level of approximately 1 ppm (0.7 to 1.2 ppm) in water is generally considered optimal for development of decay-resistant teeth without causing fluorosis, the actual value depending on the annual mean maximum daily temperature of the geographic area.

2.2 mg of sodium fluoride is equivalent to 1 mg of fluoride ion.

Use of fixed-dosage combination products of fluoride and vitamins is generally not recommended because of the difficulty in adjustment of dosage.

Since therapy with oral systemic fluoride supplements is most effective on unerupted teeth, it is recommended that children receive oral fluoride supplementation until the age of 13 to 16 (when the second molars have erupted) to provide maximum benefit to both deciduous and permanent teeth. Subsequent periodic topical application of fluoride for life may be advisable to prolong the cariostatic benefits, since beneficial effects, particularly in caries-prone individuals, appear to be lost a year or two after topical use is discontinued.

Effects of dietary and topical fluorides may be additive in children, and combination use may be of benefit in those highly susceptible to caries.

The recommended dose should not be exceeded, since prolonged overdosage may cause dental fluorosis and osseous changes.

Mottling of tooth enamel (dental fluorosis) occurs only with excessive ingestion of fluoride (e.g., continual use of drinking water containing greater than 2 ppm of fluoride) during the period of tooth development in children.

Stiffness (skeletal fluorosis) occurs with chronic ingestion of water containing 4 to 14 ppm of fluoride.

Generalized effects (renal damage, albuminuria, goiter) occur only after chronic ingestion of large amounts of fluoride over 10 to 20 years.

It is recommended that fluoride preparations (especially the chewable tablets) taken on a once-a-day basis be taken at bedtime after the teeth have been thoroughly brushed, in order to provide some topical benefit from the fluoride as well.

### Diet/Nutrition

Nausea (although rare with the doses taken for dental caries) may be reduced by taking sodium fluoride with or just after meals, provided that the foods do not contain calcium, since calcium may interfere with fluoride absorption.

The oral solution may be administered undiluted or mixed with cereal, fluids, or other food. However, absorption of sodium fluoride may be reduced when the medication is taken with calcium-rich foods or beverages.

---

### MULTIPLE VITAMINS AND SODIUM OR POTASSIUM FLUORIDE

---

## Oral Dosage Forms

### MULTIPLE VITAMINS AND SODIUM OR POTASSIUM FLUORIDE ORAL SOLUTION

**Usual pediatric dose**
Oral, 0.6 or 1 mL once a day.
Dosage of fluoride recommended by the American Dental Association for communities where the recommended optimal level of fluoride in drinking water is 1 ppm—
Children up to 2 years of age: Oral, 1 ppm of fluoride in water used for drinking and for preparing food or formula; as follows:

| Water Fluoride (ppm) | Age (yrs) | Dose of Fluoride Ion (mg per day) |
|---|---|---|
| <0.3 | Birth to 2 | 0.25 |
|  | 2 to 3 | 0.5 |
|  | 3 to 13 | 1.0 |
| 0.3–0.7 | Birth to 2 | 0 |
|  | 2 to 3 | 0.25 |
|  | 3 to 13 | 0.5 |
| >0.7 | Birth to 2 | 0 |
|  | 2 to 3 | 0 |
|  | 3 to 13 | 0 |

**Strength(s) usually available**
U.S.—
  0.25 mg per mL (Rx) [*Poly-Vi-Flor; ViDaylin/F*].
  0.5 mg per mL (Rx) [*Adeflor; Poly-Vi-Flor*].
Canada—
  0.5 mg per 0.6 mL (Rx) [*Poly-Vi-Flor*].

**Packaging and storage**
Store below 40 °C (104 °F), preferably between 15 and 30 °C (59 and 86 °F), in tight plastic containers, unless otherwise specified by manufacturer. Protect from freezing.

**Stability**
A slight darkening in color of the solution does not indicate reduced potency.

**Auxiliary labeling**
• Keep out of reach of children.

**Note**
To reduce the risk associated with accidental ingestion and overdosage, it is recommended that no more than 264 mg of sodium fluoride be dispensed at one time. The American Dental Association Council on Dental Therapeutics considers a limit of 300 mg acceptable when sodium fluoride is dispensed in prepackaged containers.

### MULTIPLE VITAMINS AND SODIUM OR POTASSIUM FLUORIDE CHEWABLE TABLETS

**Usual pediatric dose**
Children up to 3 years of age—Use is not recommended.
Children 3 years of age and over—Oral, 1 tablet a day.

**Strength(s) usually available**
U.S.—
  0.5 mg (Rx) [*Adeflor; Poly-Vi-Flor*].
  1 mg (Rx) [*Adeflor; Mulvidren-F; Poly-Vi-Flor; Vi-Daylin/F*].
Canada—
  1 mg (Rx) [*Adeflor; Poly-Vi-Flor*].

**Packaging and storage**
Store below 40 °C (104 °F), preferably between 15 and 30 °C (59 and 86 °F), in a tight container, unless otherwise specified by manufacturer. Protect from light.

**Auxiliary labeling**
• Keep out of reach of children.

**Note**
To reduce the risk associated with accidental ingestion and overdosage, it is recommended that no more than 264 mg of sodium fluoride be dispensed at one time. The American Dental Association Council on Dental Therapeutics considers a limit of 300 mg acceptable when sodium fluoride is dispensed in prepackaged containers.

---

### VITAMINS A, D, AND C AND SODIUM OR POTASSIUM FLUORIDE

---

## Oral Dosage Forms

### VITAMINS A, D, AND C AND SODIUM OR POTASSIUM FLUORIDE ORAL SOLUTION

**Usual pediatric dose**
Oral, 0.6 or 1 mL once a day.
Dosage of fluoride recommended by the American Dental Association for communities where the recommended optimal level of fluoride in drinking water is 1 ppm—
Children up to 2 years of age: Oral, 1 ppm of fluoride in water used for drinking and for preparing food or formula; as follows:

| Water Fluoride (ppm) | Age (yrs) | Dose of Fluoride Ion (mg per day) |
|---|---|---|
| <0.3 | Birth to 2 | 0.25 |
|  | 2 to 3 | 0.5 |
|  | 3 to 13 | 1.0 |
| 0.3–0.7 | Birth to 2 | 0 |
|  | 2 to 3 | 0.25 |
|  | 3 to 13 | 0.5 |
| >0.7 | Birth to 2 | 0 |
|  | 2 to 3 | 0 |
|  | 3 to 13 | 0 |

Note: May be dropped directly into the mouth or mixed with cereal, fruit juice, or other food.

**Strength(s) usually available**
U.S.—
  0.25 mg per mL (Rx) [*Tri-Vi-Flor*].
  0.5 mg per mL (Rx) [*Tri-Vi-Flor*].
Canada—
  0.5 mg per 0.6 mL (Rx) [*Tri-Vi-Flor*].

**Packaging and storage**
Store below 40 °C (104 °F), preferably between 15 and 30 °C (59 and 86 °F), in a tight plastic container, unless otherwise specified by manufacturer. Protect from light. Protect from freezing.

**Stability**
A slight darkening of the solution does not indicate reduced potency.

**Auxiliary labeling**
• Keep out of reach of children.

**Note**
To reduce the risk associated with accidental ingestion and overdosage, it is recommended that no more than 264 mg of sodium fluoride be dispensed at one time. The American Dental Association Council on Dental Therapeutics considers a limit of 300 mg acceptable when sodium fluoride is dispensed in prepackaged containers.

## VITAMINS A, D, AND C AND SODIUM OR POTASSIUM FLUORIDE CHEWABLE TABLETS

**Usual pediatric dose**
Children up to 3 years of age—Use is not recommended.
Children 3 years of age and over—Oral, 1 tablet a day.

**Strength(s) usually available**
U.S.—
  0.5 mg (Rx) [*Cari-Tab; Tri-Vi-Flor*].
Canada—
  1 mg (Rx) [*Tri-Vi-Flor*].

**Packaging and storage**
Store below 40 °C (104 °F), preferably between 15 and 30 °C (59 and 86 °F), in a tight container, unless otherwise specified by manufacturer. Protect from light.

**Auxiliary labeling**
• Keep out of reach of children.

**Note**
To reduce the risk associated with accidental ingestion and overdosage, it is recommended that no more than 264 mg of sodium fluoride be dispensed at one time. The American Dental Association Council on Dental Therapeutics considers a limit of 300 mg acceptable when sodium fluoride is dispensed in prepackaged containers.

Revised: september 1990
Interim revision: 08/21/92

# WARFARIN—See *Anticoagulants (Systemic)*

# XENON Xe 127  Systemic*

VA CLASSIFICATION (Primary): DX201
Commonly used brand name(s): *Xenon Xe 127 Gas*.
Note:  For a listing of dosage forms and brand names by country availability, see *Dosage Forms* section(s).

*Not commercially available in U.S.

## Category
Diagnostic aid, radioactive (pulmonary disease).

## Indications
**Accepted**
Pulmonary function studies and
Lung imaging, radionuclide—Xenon Xe 127 for inhalation (in ventilation studies) is indicated in the evaluation and assessment of suspected pulmonary emboli. Lung ventilation imaging is almost always performed in conjunction with lung perfusion imaging in order to better differentiate pulmonary embolism from obstructive-type lung diseases.

Pulmonary ventilation imaging is also beneficial in the evaluation of lung diseases that affect ventilation, such as asthma, pulmonary emphysema, bronchiectasis, and carcinoma of the lung.

## Physical Properties
**Nuclear data**

| Radionu-clide* (half-life) | Decay constant | Mode of decay | Principal photons (keV) | Mean number of photons/ disintegration |
|---|---|---|---|---|
| Xe 127 (36.41 days) | 0.000793 h$^{-1}$ | Electron capture (to Iodine I 127) | Gamma (172.1) | 0.247 |
|  |  |  | Gamma (202.8) | 0.681 |
|  |  |  | Gamma (375) | 0.174 |

*Xenon Xe 127 is produced by the proton bombardment of cesium Cs 133; xenon Xe 127 gas contains less than 10% xenon Xe 129m (half-life, 8.89 days) and less than 10% xenon Xe 133m (half-life, 11.84 days).

## Pharmacology/Pharmacokinetics
**Mechanism of action/Effect**
Xenon Xe 127 is a physiologically inert gas that is relatively insoluble. It diffuses easily, passing through cell membranes and exchanging freely between blood and tissue. It is distributed in the lungs in a manner similar to that of air, thus representing the regions of the lung that are aerated. The gamma photons of xenon Xe 127 can then be employed to obtain an image of lung ventilation. Xenon Xe 127's presence in various stages of breathing is thus determined. Scintigraphs taken during the washout period, as the patient breathes room air, will show any obstruction in the airways as regions of radioactive gas trapping or retention. (In the presence of an abnormal or near normal Tc 99m albumin aggregated perfusion study, a normal ventilation study favors a diagnosis of pulmonary emboli. However, the presence of xenon Xe 127 gas trapping, during washout imaging, in areas of abnormal perfusion, favors a diagnosis of chronic-type obstructive pulmonary disease.)

**Distribution**
When inhaled, xenon Xe 127 passes through the airways into the alveoli. Because of its insolubility, very little passes into the pulmonary venous circulation via capillaries. Most of it returns to the lungs and is exhaled after passing through the peripheral circulation. Inhaled xenon Xe 127 gas will mix with the air in the lungs and come to an equilibrium distribution if the patient is in a closed ventilation system.

## Radiation dosimetry

| | Estimated absorbed radiation dose* With single inhalation (30 sec breath-hold) | |
|---|---|---|
| Organ | mGy/MBq | rad/mCi |
| Lungs | 0.00034 | 0.0013 |
| Pancreas | 0.00014 | 0.00052 |
| Red marrow | 0.00014 | 0.00052 |
| Adrenals | 0.00013 | 0.00048 |
| Bone surfaces | 0.00012 | 0.00044 |
| Stomach wall | 0.00012 | 0.00044 |
| Small intestine | 0.00012 | 0.00044 |
| Large intestine wall (upper) | 0.00012 | 0.00044 |
| Liver | 0.00012 | 0.00044 |
| Spleen | 0.00012 | 0.00044 |
| Uterus | 0.00012 | 0.00044 |
| Bladder wall | 0.00011 | 0.00041 |
| Breast | 0.00011 | 0.00041 |
| Large intestine wall (lower) | 0.00011 | 0.00041 |
| Kidneys | 0.00011 | 0.00041 |
| Ovaries | 0.00011 | 0.00041 |
| Thyroid | 0.000089 | 0.00033 |
| Testes | 0.000083 | 0.00031 |
| Other tissue | 0.000099 | 0.00037 |

Effective dose: 0.00014 mSv/MBq (0.00052 rem/mCi)*

| | Estimated absorbed radiation dose* With inhalation (rebreathing from closed spirometer) | | | |
|---|---|---|---|---|
| Organ | For 5 minutes | | For 10 minutes | |
| | mGy/MBq | rad/mCi | mGy/MBq | rad/mCi |
| Red marrow | 0.00090 | 0.0033 | 0.0015 | 0.0056 |
| Pancreas | 0.00088 | 0.0033 | 0.0014 | 0.0052 |
| Uterus | 0.00087 | 0.0032 | 0.0014 | 0.0052 |
| Small intestine | 0.00085 | 0.0031 | 0.0014 | 0.0052 |
| Lungs | 0.00082 | 0.0030 | 0.0011 | 0.0041 |
| Bone surfaces | 0.00081 | 0.0030 | 0.0013 | 0.0048 |
| Stomach wall | 0.00081 | 0.0030 | 0.0013 | 0.0048 |
| Adrenals | 0.00080 | 0.0030 | 0.0013 | 0.0048 |
| Large intestine wall (upper) | 0.00080 | 0.0030 | 0.0013 | 0.0048 |
| Ovaries | 0.00080 | 0.0030 | 0.0013 | 0.0048 |
| Spleen | 0.00078 | 0.0029 | 0.0013 | 0.0048 |
| Bladder wall | 0.00077 | 0.0029 | 0.0013 | 0.0048 |
| Large intestine wall (lower) | 0.00077 | 0.0029 | 0.0013 | 0.0048 |
| Kidneys | 0.00075 | 0.0028 | 0.0012 | 0.0044 |
| Liver | 0.00075 | 0.0028 | 0.0012 | 0.0044 |
| Breast | 0.00065 | 0.0024 | 0.0010 | 0.0037 |
| Thyroid | 0.00060 | 0.0022 | 0.00098 | 0.0036 |
| Testes | 0.00058 | 0.0021 | 0.00096 | 0.0036 |
| Other tissue | 0.00065 | 0.0024 | 0.0011 | 0.0041 |

| | Effective dose* | | | |
|---|---|---|---|---|
| Radionuclide | Rebreathing for 5 minutes | | Rebreathing for 10 minutes | |
| | mSv/MBq | rem/mCi | mSv/MBq | rem/mCi |
| Xe 127 | 0.00077 | 0.0028 | 0.0012 | 0.0044 |

*In adults. Data based on the International Commission on Radiological Protection (ICRP) Publication 53—Radiation dose to patients from radiopharmaceuticals.

**Elimination**
Pulmonary.

## Precautions to Consider

### Carcinogenicity/Mutagenicity
Long-term animal studies to evaluate carcinogenic or mutagenic potential of xenon Xe 127 have not been performed.

### Pregnancy/Reproduction
Pregnancy—Studies have not been done with xenon Xe 127 in humans. The possibility of pregnancy should be assessed in women of child-bearing potential. Clinical situations exist where the benefit to the patient and fetus, based on information derived from radiopharmaceutical use, outweighs the risks from fetal exposure to radiation. In these situations, the physician should use discretion and reduce the radiopharmaceutical dose to the lowest possible amount.

Studies have not been done in animals.

FDA Pregnancy Category C.

### Breast-feeding
It is not known whether xenon Xe 127 is distributed into breast milk. However, risk to the infant from radiation exposure is considered negligible. Because of xenon Xe 127's poorly soluble nature, the amount that enters the venous circulation is not significant. Also, the small amount of xenon Xe 127 gas that passes into the venous circulation returns rapidly to the lungs to be exhaled.

### Pediatrics
There have been no specific studies evaluating the safety and efficacy of xenon Xe 127 in pediatric patients. When this radiopharmaceutical is used in children, the diagnostic benefit should be judged to outweigh the potential risk of radiation.

### Geriatrics
Appropriate studies on the relationship of age to the effects of xenon Xe 127 have not been performed in the geriatric population. However, no geriatrics-specific problems have been documented to date.

### Drug interactions and/or related problems
See *Diagnostic interference*.

### Diagnostic interference
The following have been selected on the basis of their potential clinical significance (possible effect in parentheses where appropriate)—not necessarily inclusive (» = major clinical significance):

With results of *this* test
*Due to other medications*
  Anesthetics, inhalation or
  Diazepam
    (distribution of xenon Xe 127 in the lung may be affected, with more activity shifting to the top of the lung and less to the bottom, due to a change in the gradient of ventilation, from nondependent to dependent lung, caused by these medications)
  Alcohol, chronic use or
  Clofibrate or
  Parenteral nutrition, total (TPN)
    (these medications may alter hepatic function [e.g., fatty liver disease as a result of TPN therapy]; because xenon is lipid soluble, appearance of radioactivity in liver during washout phase of ventilation study is theoretically possible; hepatic retention of xenon Xe 127 may be incorrectly attributed to other disorders associated with fatty liver infiltration [e.g., diabetes mellitus] that may also promote accumulation of xenon Xe 127 in the liver)

*Due to medical problems or conditions*
  Diabetes mellitus or
  Hyperlipidemia or
  Obesity
    (fatty liver infiltration associated with these disorders may promote accumulation of lipid-soluble xenon in the liver)

### Medical considerations/Contraindications
See *Diagnostic interference*.

## Side/Adverse Effects

There are no known side/adverse effects associated with the use of xenon Xe 127 as a diagnostic aid.

## Patient Consultation

As an aid to patient consultation, refer to *Advice for the Patient, Radiopharmaceuticals (Diagnostic)*.

In providing consultation, consider emphasizing the following selected information (» = major clinical significance):

### Description of use
Action in the body: Localization in airways of the lung
Visualization of radioactivity in lungs
Small amounts of radioactivity used in diagnosis; radiation received is low and considered safe

### Before having this test
» Conditions affecting use, especially:
    Pregnancy—Risk to fetus from radiation exposure as opposed to benefit derived from use should be considered
    Breast-feeding—Not known if distributed into breast milk; however, risk to infant from radiation exposure is considered negligible
    Use in children—Risk of radiation exposure as opposed to benefit derived from use should be considered

### Preparation for this test
Special preparatory instructions may be given; patient should inquire in advance

### Precautions after having this test
No special precautions

## General Dosing Information

Radiopharmaceuticals are to be administered only by or under the supervision of physicians who have had extensive training in the safe use and handling of radioactive materials and who are authorized by the appropriate Federal or State agency, if required, or, outside the U.S., the appropriate authority.

Xenon Xe 127 should not be allowed to stand in tubing or respirator containers since it adheres to some plastics and rubber, causing a reduction in the administered activity.

Xenon Xe 127 is administered by inhalation, as a mixture with air, from a shielded, closed respirator system or spirometer.

Adequate trapping or exhausting of exhaled xenon Xe 127 in accordance with state requirements is essential to reduce contamination of air by airborne Xe 127.

Ventilation imaging is performed as the patient inhales the radioactive xenon. Successive images are obtained while the patient holds his or her breath (single-breath-hold image) and during various phases of breathing (rebreathing and washout from lungs).

### Safety considerations for handling this radiopharmaceutical
Improper handling of this radiopharmaceutical may cause radioactive contamination. Guidelines for handling radioactive material have been prepared by scientific, professional, state, federal, and international bodies and are available to the specially qualified and authorized users who have access to radiopharmaceuticals.

## Inhalation Dosage Forms

### XENON Xe 127

#### Usual adult and adolescent administered activity
Inhalation, 185 to 370 megabecquerels (5 to 10 millicuries).

Note: When the ventilation study with xenon Xe 127 is combined with a lung perfusion study using technetium Tc 99m albumin aggregated, xenon Xe 127 may be administered immediately following Tc 99m perfusion imaging.

#### Usual pediatric administered activity
Dosage must be individualized by physician. The minimum recommended total dosage is 74 megabecquerels (2 millicuries).

#### Usual geriatric administered activity
See *Usual adult and adolescent administered activity*.

#### Size(s) usually available
U.S.—
  Not commercially available.
Canada—
  185 megabecquerels (5 millicuries) per 2-mL-size vial (Rx) [*Xenon Xe 127 Gas*].

#### Packaging and storage
Store between 15 and 30 °C (59 and 86 °F).

#### Stability
Xenon Xe 127 gas should not be administered after 120 days from the date of calibration stated on the label.

Adheres to some plastics and rubber; to avoid a reduction in the administered activity, do not allow to stand in tubing or respirator container.

#### Note
Caution—Radioactive material.

# XENON Xe 133 Systemic

VA CLASSIFICATION (Primary): DX201

Commonly used brand name(s): *MPI Xenon Xe 133 Gas; MPI Xenon Xe 133 Gas Ampul; Xenon Xe 133-V.S.S.*.

Note: For a listing of dosage forms and brand names by country availability, see *Dosage Forms* section(s).

## Category
Diagnostic aid, radioactive (pulmonary disease; cerebrovascular disease).

## Indications

**Accepted**

Pulmonary function studies and

Lung imaging, radionuclide—Xenon Xe 133 for inhalation (in ventilation studies) is indicated to assess and evaluate pulmonary function and to provide images of the lungs in both cardiac and pulmonary diseases, such as asthma, pulmonary emphysema, bronchiectasis, carcinoma of the lung, and pulmonary embolism. Lung ventilation imaging is almost always performed in conjunction with lung perfusion imaging in order to better differentiate pulmonary embolism from obstructive-type lung diseases.

Blood flow studies, cerebral—Xenon Xe 133 for inhalation is indicated to assess and evaluate regional cerebral blood flow, mainly in patients with cerebrovascular disease.

## Physical Properties

**Nuclear data**

| Radionuclide (half-life)* | Decay constant | Mode of decay | Principal photons (keV) | Mean number of photons/ disintegration |
|---|---|---|---|---|
| Xe 133 (5.24 days) | 0.00551 h$^{-1}$ | Beta emission | Gamma (81.0) | 0.37 |

*Xenon Xe 133 is produced by the fission of uranium U 235. At time of calibration, it contains no more than 0.3% xenon Xe 133m, 1.5% xenon Xe 131m, 0.06% krypton Kr 85, and 0.01% iodine I 131.

## Pharmacology/Pharmacokinetics

**Mechanism of action/Effect**

Xenon Xe 133 diffuses easily, passing through cell membranes and exchanging freely between blood and tissue. It is distributed in the lungs in a manner similar to that of air, thus representing the regions of the lung that are aerated. The gamma photons of xenon Xe 133 can then be employed to obtain counts per minute per lung or region of the lung, or to display their distribution as a scan. Scintigraphs taken during the washout period, as the patient breathes room air, will show any obstruction in the airways as regions of radioactive gas trapping or retention. (In the presence of an abnormal or near normal Tc 99m albumin aggregated perfusion study, a normal ventilation study favors a diagnosis of pulmonary emboli. However, the presence of xenon Xe 133 gas trapping, during washout imaging, in areas of abnormal perfusion, favors a diagnosis of chronic-type obstructive pulmonary disease.)

**Distribution**

When inhaled, xenon Xe 133 passes through the airways into the alveoli. Because of its insolubility, very little passes into the pulmonary venous circulation via capillaries. Most of it returns to the lungs and is exhaled after passing through the peripheral circulation. Inhaled xenon Xe 133 gas will mix with the air in the lungs and come to an equilibrium distribution if the patient is in a closed ventilation system.

## Radiation dosimetry

Estimated absorbed radiation dose*
With single inhalation
(30 sec breath-hold)

| Organ | mGy/MBq | rad/mCi |
|---|---|---|
| Lungs | 0.00077 | 0.0029 |
| Bone surfaces | 0.00012 | 0.00044 |
| Breast | 0.00012 | 0.00044 |
| Red marrow | 0.00012 | 0.00044 |
| Small intestine | 0.00011 | 0.00041 |
| Large intestine wall (upper) | 0.00011 | 0.00041 |
| Large intestine wall (lower) | 0.00011 | 0.00041 |
| Liver | 0.00011 | 0.00041 |
| Pancreas | 0.00011 | 0.00041 |
| Spleen | 0.00011 | 0.00041 |
| Uterus | 0.00011 | 0.00041 |
| Adrenals | 0.00010 | 0.00037 |
| Bladder wall | 0.00010 | 0.00037 |
| Stomach wall | 0.00010 | 0.00037 |
| Kidneys | 0.00010 | 0.00037 |
| Ovaries | 0.00010 | 0.00037 |
| Testes | 0.000099 | 0.00037 |
| Thyroid | 0.000099 | 0.00037 |
| Other tissue | 0.00010 | 0.00037 |

Effective dose: 0.00019 mSv/MBq (0.00070 rem/mCi)*

| Organ | Estimated absorbed radiation dose* With inhalation (rebreathing from closed spirometer) ||||
|---|---|---|---|---|
| | For 5 minutes || For 10 minutes ||
| | mGy/MBq | rad/mCi | mGy/MBq | rad/mCi |
| Lungs | 0.0011 | 0.0041 | 0.0012 | 0.0044 |
| Red marrow | 0.00084 | 0.0031 | 0.0014 | 0.0052 |
| Breast | 0.00083 | 0.0031 | 0.0014 | 0.0052 |
| Bone surfaces | 0.00080 | 0.0030 | 0.0013 | 0.0048 |
| Small intestine | 0.00074 | 0.0027 | 0.0012 | 0.0044 |
| Large intestine wall (upper) | 0.00074 | 0.0027 | 0.0012 | 0.0044 |
| Large intestine wall (lower) | 0.00074 | 0.0027 | 0.0012 | 0.0044 |
| Pancreas | 0.00074 | 0.0027 | 0.0012 | 0.0044 |
| Uterus | 0.00074 | 0.0027 | 0.0012 | 0.0044 |
| Bladder wall | 0.00073 | 0.0027 | 0.0012 | 0.0044 |
| Liver | 0.00073 | 0.0027 | 0.0012 | 0.0044 |
| Ovaries | 0.00073 | 0.0027 | 0.0012 | 0.0044 |
| Spleen | 0.00073 | 0.0027 | 0.0012 | 0.0044 |
| Stomach wall | 0.00072 | 0.0027 | 0.0012 | 0.0044 |
| Kidneys | 0.00072 | 0.0027 | 0.0012 | 0.0044 |
| Adrenals | 0.00071 | 0.0026 | 0.0012 | 0.0044 |
| Testes | 0.00069 | 0.0026 | 0.0011 | 0.0041 |
| Thyroid | 0.00069 | 0.0026 | 0.0011 | 0.0041 |
| Other tissue | 0.00070 | 0.0026 | 0.0012 | 0.0044 |

| Radionuclide | Effective dose* |||| 
|---|---|---|---|---|
| | Rebreathing for 5 minutes || Rebreathing for 10 minutes ||
| | mSv/MBq | rem/mCi | mSv/MBq | rem/mCi |
| Xe 133 | 0.00080 | 0.0030 | 0.0013 | 0.0048 |

*In adults. Data based on the International Commission on Radiological Protection (ICRP) Publication 53—Radiation dose to patients from radiopharmaceuticals.

**Elimination**
Pulmonary.

## Precautions to Consider

**Carcinogenicity/Mutagenicity**
Long-term animal studies to evaluate carcinogenic or mutagenic potential of xenon Xe 133 have not been performed.

**Pregnancy/Reproduction**
Pregnancy—Studies have not been done with xenon Xe 133 in humans. The possibility of pregnancy should be assessed in women of child-bearing potential. Clinical situations exist where the benefit to the patient and fetus, based on information derived from radiopharmaceutical use, outweighs the risks from fetal exposure to radiation. In these situations, the physician should use discretion and reduce the radiopharmaceutical dose to the lowest possible amount.
Studies have not been done in animals.
FDA Pregnancy Category C.

**Breast-feeding**
It is not known whether xenon Xe 133 is distributed into breast milk. However, risk to the infant from radiation exposure is considered negligible. Because of xenon Xe 133's poorly soluble nature, the amount that enters the venous circulation is not significant. Also, the small amount of xenon Xe 133 gas that passes into the venous circulation returns rapidly to the lungs to be exhaled.

**Pediatrics**
There have been no specific studies evaluating the safety and efficacy of xenon Xe 133 in pediatric patients. However, no pediatrics-specific problems have been documented to date. When this radiopharmaceutical is used in children, the diagnostic benefit should be judged to outweigh the potential risk of radiation.

**Geriatrics**
Appropriate studies on the relationship of age to the effects of xenon Xe 133 have not been performed in the geriatric population. However, no geriatrics-specific problems have been documented to date.

**Drug interactions and/or related problems**
See *Diagnostic interference*.

**Diagnostic interference**
The following have been selected on the basis of their potential clinical significance (possible effect in parentheses where appropriate)—not necessarily inclusive (» = major clinical significance):

With results of *this* test
*Due to other medications*
Anesthetics, inhalation or
Diazepam
(distribution of xenon Xe 133 in the lung may be affected, with more activity shifting to the top of the lung and less to the bottom, due to a change in the gradient of ventilation, from nondependent to dependent lung, caused by these medications)
Alcohol, chronic use or
Clofibrate or
Parenteral nutrition, total (TPN)
(these medications may alter hepatic function [e.g., fatty liver disease as a result of TPN therapy]; because xenon is lipid soluble, appearance of radioactivity in liver during washout phase of ventilation study is theoretically possible; hepatic retention of xenon Xe 133 may be incorrectly attributed to other disorders associated with fatty liver infiltration [e.g., diabetes mellitus] that may also promote accumulation of xenon Xe 133 in the liver)

*Due to medical problems or conditions*
Diabetes mellitus or
Hyperlipidemia or
Obesity
(fatty liver infiltration associated with these disorders may promote accumulation of lipid-soluble xenon in the liver)

**Medical considerations/Contraindications**
See *Diagnostic interference*.

## Side/Adverse Effects

There are no known side/adverse effects associated with the use of xenon Xe 133 as a diagnostic aid.

## Patient Consultation

As an aid to patient consultation, refer to *Advice for the Patient, Radiopharmaceuticals (Diagnostic)*.
In providing consultation, consider emphasizing the following selected information (» = major clinical significance):

**Description of use**
Action in the body: Localization in airways of the lung
Visualization of radioactivity in lungs and brain
Small amounts of radioactivity used in diagnosis; radiation received is low and considered safe

**Before having this test**
» Conditions affecting use, especially:
Pregnancy—Risk to fetus from radiation exposure as opposed to benefit derived from use should be considered
Breast-feeding—Not known if distributed into breast milk; however, risk to infant from radiation exposure is considered negligible
Use in children—Risk of radiation exposure as opposed to benefit derived from use should be considered

**Preparation for this test**
Special preparatory instructions may be given; patient should inquire in advance

**Precautions after having this test**
No special precautions when used for diagnosis

## General Dosing Information

Radiopharmaceuticals are to be administered only by or under the supervision of physicians who have had extensive training in the safe use and handling of radioactive materials and who are authorized by the Nuclear Regulatory Commission (NRC) or the appropriate Agreement State agency, if required, or, outside the U.S., the appropriate authority.

Xenon Xe 133 should not be allowed to stand in tubing or respirator containers since it adheres to some plastics and rubber, causing a reduction in the administered activity.

Adequate trapping or exhausting of exhaled xenon Xe 133 is essential to reduce contamination of air by airborne Xe 133.

Ventilation imaging is performed as the patient inhales the radioactive xenon. Successive images are obtained while the patient holds his or her breath (single-breath-hold image) and during various phases of breathing (rebreathing and washout from lungs).

**Safety considerations for handling this radiopharmaceutical**
Improper handling of this radiopharmaceutical may cause radioactive contamination. Guidelines for handling radioactive material have been prepared by scientific, professional, state, federal, and international bodies and are available to the specially qualified and authorized users who have access to radiopharmaceuticals.

## Inhalation Dosage Forms

### XENON Xe 133 USP

**Usual adult and adolescent administered activity**
Pulmonary function studies and imaging—
Inhalation, 74 megabecquerels to 1.1 gigabecquerels (2 to 30 millicuries) per 3 liters of air.
Blood flow studies, cerebral—
Inhalation, 370 megabecquerels to 1.1 gigabecquerels (10 to 30 millicuries) per 3 liters of air.

**Usual pediatric administered activity**
Dosage must be individualized by physician. The minimum recommended total dosage is 74 megabecquerels (2 millicuries).

**Usual geriatric administered activity**
See *Usual adult and adolescent administered activity*.

**Size(s) usually available**
U.S.—
370 megabecquerels (10 millicuries) per 2-mL-size vial (Rx) [*MPI Xenon Xe 133 Gas*].
370 megabecquerels (10 millicuries) ±20% per ampul capsule (Rx) [*Xenon Xe 133-V.S.S.*].

370 megabecquerels (10 millicuries) per 3-mL size vial (Rx) [GENERIC].
740 megabecquerels (20 millicuries) per 2-mL size vial (Rx) [*MPI Xenon Xe 133 Gas*].
740 megabecquerels (20 millicuries) per 3-mL size vial (Rx) [GENERIC].
1.11 gigabecquerels (30 millicuries) per 3-mL size vial (Rx) [GENERIC].
1.48 gigabecquerels (40 millicuries) per 3-mL size vial (Rx) [GENERIC].
1.85 gigabecquerels (50 millicuries) per 3-mL size vial (Rx) [GENERIC].
9.25 gigabecquerels (0.25 Curie) per mL per 4-mL size ampul (Rx) [*MPI Xenon Xe 133 Gas Ampul*].
12.33 gigabecquerels (0.333 Curie) per mL per 3-mL size ampul (Rx) [*MPI Xenon Xe 133 Gas Ampul*].

Canada—
370 megabecquerels (10 millicuries) per 2-mL size vial (Rx) [GENERIC].
740 megabecquerels (20 millicuries) per 2-mL size vial (Rx) [GENERIC].

**Packaging and storage**
Store between 15 and 30 °C (59 and 86 °F).

**Stability**
Adheres to some plastics and rubber; to avoid a reduction in the administered activity, do not allow to stand in tubing or respirator container.
Xenon Xe 133 gas should not be administered 14 days from the date of calibration stated on the label.

**Note**
Caution—Radioactive material.

## Selected Bibliography
Alderson PO, Line BR. Scintigraphic evaluation of regional pulmonary ventilation. Semin Nucl Med 1980; 10(3): 218-42.
Hayes M, Taplin GV. Lung imaging with radioaerosols for the assessment of airway disease. Semin Nucl Med 1980; 10(3): 243-51.

Revised: 02/23/94
Interim revision: 08/02/94

---

**XYLOMETAZOLINE**—The *Xylometazoline (Nasal)* monograph is not included in this published version of the USP DI database. Copies of the monograph are available on request from Micromedex, Inc. - Reprint Requests, 6200 S. Syracuse Way, Suite 300, Englewood, CO 80111; telephone (303) 486-6400; telefax (303) 486-6464; Email: USPDI@MDX.COM.

---

**YELLOW FEVER VACCINE**—The *Yellow Fever Vaccine (Systemic)* monograph is not included in this published version of the USP DI database. Copies of the monograph are available on request from Micromedex, Inc. - Reprint Requests, 6200 S. Syracuse Way, Suite 300, Englewood, CO 80111; telephone (303) 486-6400; telefax (303) 486-6464; Email: USPDI@MDX.COM.

---

**YOHIMBINE**—The *Yohimbine (Systemic)* monograph is not included in this published version of the USP DI database. Copies of the monograph are available on request from Micromedex, Inc. - Reprint Requests, 6200 S. Syracuse Way, Suite 300, Englewood, CO 80111; telephone (303) 486-6400; telefax (303) 486-6464; Email: USPDI@MDX.COM.

# ZAFIRLUKAST Systemic†

VA CLASSIFICATION (Primary): RE108
Commonly used brand name(s): *Accolate*.
Note: For a listing of dosage forms and brand names by country availability, see *Dosage Forms* section(s).

†Not commercially available in Canada.

## Category
Antiasthmatic (leukotriene receptor antagonist).

## Indications

**Accepted**

*Asthma, chronic (prophylaxis and treatment)*—Zafirlukast is indicated in patients with chronic asthma to improve daytime asthma symptoms, forced expiratory volume in 1 second ($FEV_1$), and morning peak expiratory flow rates, and to decrease nighttime awakenings, mornings with asthma symptoms, and use of a rescue $beta_2$ agonist. When used daily with an as-needed, inhaled $beta_2$ agonist in patients with mild-to-moderate asthma, zafirlukast significantly reduces asthma symptoms and use of an as-needed, inhaled $beta_2$ agonist as compared with use of an as-needed, inhaled $beta_2$ agonist alone.

Only patients with mild-to-moderate asthma have been treated with zafirlukast in clinical trials; therefore, its use in the management of patients with more severe asthma and in those receiving antiasthma therapy other than as-needed, inhaled $beta_2$ agonists remains to be studied, as does use of zafirlukast as an oral or inhaled corticosteroid-sparing agent.

**Unaccepted**

Zafirlukast is not indicated for the treatment of bronchospasm in acute asthma attacks, including status asthmaticus; however, use of zafirlukast can be continued during an acute exacerbation.

## Pharmacology/Pharmacokinetics

**Physicochemical characteristics**
Molecular weight—575.69.

**Mechanism of action/Effect**
Zafirlukast is a selective and competitive receptor antagonist of the cysteinyl leukotrienes $D_4$ and $E_4$. The cysteinyl leukotrienes, originally described as slow-reacting substances of anaphylaxis, produce airway edema, smooth muscle constriction, and altered cellular activity associated with the inflammatory process, all of which are associated with the pathophysiology of asthma. In humans, pretreatment with single oral doses of zafirlukast inhibited bronchoconstriction caused by sulfur dioxide and cold air and reduced the early- and late-phase reaction in patients with asthma caused by inhalation of various antigens, such as grass, cat dander, and ragweed. Zafirlukast reduced the increase in bronchial hyperresponsiveness to inhaled histamine that followed inhaled allergen challenge.

**Absorption**
Rapid.
Bioavailability is reduced following administration with a high-fat or high-protein meal.

**Protein binding**
High (more than 99% bound to plasma proteins, predominantly albumin).

**Biotransformation**
Hepatic; extensively metabolized by the cytochrome P450 2C9 enzyme pathway to metabolites that are 90 times less potent antagonists of leukotriene $D_4$ receptors than zafirlukast *in vitro*.

**Half-life**
*Elimination*—The mean terminal elimination half-life is approximately 10 hours.

**Onset of action**
In clinical trials, improvement in asthma symptoms was seen within 1 week of starting treatment with zafirlukast.

**Time to peak plasma concentration**
3 hours after dosing.

**Elimination**
*Fecal*—Approximately 90%.
*Renal*—Approximately 10%.

## Precautions to Consider

**Carcinogenicity/Tumorigenicity**
A 2-year study in mice given zafirlukast orally in doses of 10, 100, and 300 mg per kg of body weight (mg/kg) per day showed a greater incidence of hepatocellular adenomas in males and whole-body histocytic sarcomas in females given the highest dose, as compared with controls. Plasma concentrations of zafirlukast following the 100- and 300-mg-per-kg-per-day doses were approximately 70 and 220 times, respectively, the plasma concentrations found at the maximum recommended human daily oral dose.

A 2-year study in rats given zafirlukast orally in doses of 40, 400, and 2000 mg/kg per day found a greater incidence of urinary bladder transitional cell papillomas at doses of 2000 mg/kg per day, as compared with controls. Plasma concentrations of zafirlukast following the 400- and 2000-mg-per-kg-per-day doses were approximately 170 and 200 times, respectively, the plasma concentrations found at the maximum recommended human daily oral dose.

**Mutagenicity**
Zafirlukast was not mutagenic in reverse or forward point mutation assays or in human and rat assays for chromosomal abnormalities.

**Pregnancy/Reproduction**
*Fertility*—Reproduction studies in rats given oral zafirlukast in doses approximately 400 times the maximum recommended human daily oral dose on a mcg per square meter of body surface area ($mcg/m^2$) basis showed no effect on fertility.

*Pregnancy*—Adequate and well-controlled studies have not been done in humans.

No teratogenicity was observed in mice, rats, or monkeys given oral zafirlukast in doses up to approximately 160, 400, and 800 times the maximum recommended human daily oral dose on a mg per square meter of body surface area ($mg/m^2$) basis.

In rats given oral doses of 2000 mg/kg per day, maternal toxicity and deaths were seen, as well as an increased incidence of early fetal resorptions. In monkeys, the same dose resulted in maternal toxicity and an increased incidence of spontaneous abortions.

FDA Pregnancy Category B.

**Breast-feeding**
Zafirlukast is distributed into human breast milk. Steady-state concentrations of zafirlukast in breast milk and plasma were 50 and 255 nanograms per mL, respectively, after administration of 40 mg two times a day. Because of the potential for tumorigenicity and adverse effects in the neonate shown in animal studies, use of zafirlukast during breast-feeding is not recommended.

**Pediatrics**
Appropriate studies on the relationship of age to the effects of zafirlukast have not been performed in the pediatric population. Safety and efficacy in children up to 12 years of age have not been established.

**Geriatrics**
In patients 65 years of age and older, the clearance of zafirlukast is reduced, resulting in peak plasma concentration and area under the plasma concentration–time curve (AUC) values that are approximately two to three times greater than those of younger patients. However, the recommended dose of 20 mg two times a day did not result in increased adverse effects or withdrawal from the study in elderly patients during clinical trials when compared with patients younger than 65 years of age.

In clinical trials, a greater incidence of mild or moderate infections, predominantly affecting the respiratory tract, occurred in patients older than 55 years of age treated with zafirlukast, as compared with other age groups and placebo-treated patients. The number of infections was proportional to the amount, in milligrams, of zafirlukast administered and was associated with concurrent use of inhaled corticosteroids. The clinical significance of this finding is unknown.

**Drug interactions and/or related problems**
The following drug interactions and/or related problems have been selected on the basis of their potential clinical significance (possible mechanism in parentheses where appropriate)—not necessarily inclusive (» = major clinical significance):

Note: In *in vitro* studies using human liver microsomes, zafirlukast has been shown to inhibit the cytochrome P450 3A4 and 2C9 isoenzymes at concentrations close to those achieved following recommended dosing.

In a 3-week study in females taking oral contraceptives, 40 mg of zafirlukast two times a day had no significant effect on ethinyl estradiol plasma concentrations or contraceptive efficacy.

Aspirin
(concurrent administration of 40 mg a day of zafirlukast with aspirin at a dosage of 650 mg four times a day increased mean plasma concentrations of zafirlukast by approximately 45%)

» Astemizole or
» Cisapride or
» Cyclosporine or
Dihydropyridine calcium channel blocking agents, such as:
» Felodipine or
» Isradipine or
» Nicardipine or
» Nifedipine or
» Nimodipine
(although studies have not been done with zafirlukast and medications known to be metabolized by the cytochrome P450 3A4 isoenzyme, such as astemizole, cisapride, cyclosporine, and the dihydropyridine calcium channel blocking agents, concurrent use of these medications with zafirlukast should be monitored carefully, since zafirlukast is known to inhibit cytochrome P450 3A4 *in vitro*)

» Carbamazepine or
» Phenytoin or
» Tolbutamide
(although studies have not been done with zafirlukast and medications known to be metabolized by the cytochrome P450 2C9 isoenzyme, such as carbamazepine, phenytoin, and tolbutamide, patients in whom these medications are coadministered with zafirlukast should be appropriately monitored clinically, since zafirlukast is known to inhibit cytochrome P450 2C9 *in vitro*)

Erythromycin
(administration of a single 40-mg dose of zafirlukast during steady-state erythromycin therapy resulted in a 40% decrease in the mean plasma concentration of zafirlukast, due to decreased zafirlukast bioavailability)

Terfenadine
(concurrent administration of zafirlukast with terfenadine resulted in a 66% and 54% decrease in the mean peak plasma concentration and area under the plasma concentration–time curve, respectively, of zafirlukast; no effect was observed on terfenadine plasma concentrations or electrocardiogram results)

Theophylline
(concurrent administration of 80 mg a day of zafirlukast with a single 6-mg-per-kg dose of theophylline decreased the mean plasma concentration of zafirlukast by approximately 30%; no effect on theophylline plasma concentration was observed)

» Warfarin
(the concurrent use of a single 25-mg warfarin dose with multiple doses of zafirlukast resulted in an increase of approximately 35% in the mean prothrombin time, due to an inhibition of the cytochrome P450 2C9 isoenzyme; prothrombin times should be monitored closely and warfarin dose adjusted accordingly)

## Side/Adverse Effects

Note: In clinical trials, a greater incidence of mild or moderate infections, predominantly affecting the respiratory tract, occurred in patients older than 55 years of age treated with zafirlukast, as compared with other age groups and placebo-treated patients. The number of infections was proportional to the amount, in milligrams, of zafirlukast administered and was associated with concurrent use of inhaled corticosteroids. The clinical significance of this finding is unknown.

Rarely, elevation of one or more hepatic transaminases has occurred in patients receiving zafirlukast at doses four times higher than the recommended dose during controlled clinical trials. Most patients were asymptomatic. Hepatic enzyme values returned to normal after a variable period of time following discontinuation of zafirlukast. Rare cases of symptomatic hepatitis and hyperbilirubinemia have been reported in patients who received the recommended dosage of zafirlukast. In these patients, the hepatic transaminase elevations returned to normal or near-normal after discontinuation of the medication.

At least six cases of Churg-Strauss syndrome have been reported in adult asthma patients *whose corticosteroid asthma medications were being gradually reduced or discontinued* and who were also taking zafirlukast. Churg-Strauss syndrome is a systemic eosinophilic vasculitis, which may present as generalized, flu-like symptoms (fever, muscle aches or pains, and weight loss), eosinophilia, vasculitic rash, worsening pulmonary symptoms, cardiac complications, or neuropathy. If left untreated, Churg-Strauss syndrome can result in damage to major organs and death. Although a causal relationship between the use of zafirlukast and the development of Churg-Strauss syndrome has not been established, adult asthma patients should be monitored carefully when corticosteroids are being reduced or discontinued.

The following side/adverse effects have been selected on the basis of their potential clinical significance (possible signs and symptoms in parentheses where appropriate)—not necessarily inclusive:

**Those indicating need for medical attention only if they continue or are bothersome**
Incidence less frequent
*Headache; nausea*

## Patient Consultation

As an aid to patient consultation, refer to *Advice for the Patient*, *Zafirlukast (Systemic)*.

In providing consultation, consider emphasizing the following selected information (» = major clinical significance):

**Before using this medication**
» Conditions affecting use, especially:
Breast-feeding—Distributed into breast milk; use not recommended
Use in the elderly—Mild to moderate respiratory infections may be more likely to develop in patients older than 55 years of age; whether this is related to taking zafirlukast or to other factors, such as use of inhaled corticosteroids, is not clear
Other medications, especially astemizole, carbamazepine, cisapride, cyclosporine, felodipine, isradipine, nicardipine, nifedipine, nimodipine, phenytoin, tolbutamide, and warfarin

**Proper use of this medication**
» Importance of not using this medication to treat acute asthma symptoms
» Taking medication on an empty stomach, 1 hour before or 2 hours after meals
» Proper dosing
Missed dose: Taking as soon as possible; if almost time for next dose, skipping missed dose; not doubling doses
» Proper storage

**Precautions while using this medication**
» Compliance with therapy by using every day in regularly spaced doses, even during symptom-free periods
» Checking with health care professional before stopping or reducing therapy with any other asthma medications

**Side/adverse effects**
Signs of potential side effects, especially headache or nausea

## General Dosing Information

**Diet/Nutrition**
In two separate studies, administration of zafirlukast with a high-fat and a high-protein meal resulted in a reduction of the mean bioavailability by approximately 40%; therefore, the medication should be taken on an empty stomach at least 1 hour before or 2 hours after meals.

## Oral Dosage Forms

### ZAFIRLUKAST TABLETS

**Usual adult and adolescent dose**
Antiasthmatic—
Oral, 20 mg two times a day, one hour before or two hours after a meal.

**Usual adult and adolescent prescribing limits**
20 mg two times a day.

**Usual pediatric dose**
Children up to 12 years of age—Safety and efficacy have not been established.

**Usual geriatric dose**
See *Usual adult and adolescent dose*.

**Strength(s) usually available**
U.S.—
20 mg (Rx) [*Accolate* (film-coated)].
Canada—
Not commercially available.

**Packaging and storage**
Store between 20 and 25 °C (68 and 77 °F). Protect from light and moisture.

**Auxiliary labeling**
- Take on empty stomach.

**Selected Bibliography**
Holgate ST, Bradding P, Sampson AP. Leukotriene antagonists and synthesis inhibitors: new directions in asthma therapy. J Allergy Clin Immunol 1996; 98: 1-13.

Developed: 07/18/97
Interim revision: 8/21/97

# ZALCITABINE   Systemic

VA CLASSIFICATION (Primary): AM809
Commonly used brand name(s): *HIVID*.
Another commonly used name is ddC.
Note: For a listing of dosage forms and brand names by country availability, see *Dosage Forms* section(s).

## Category
Antiviral (systemic).

## Indications
**Accepted**
Human immunodeficiency virus (HIV) infection (treatment)—Zalcitabine is indicated, in combination with zidovudine, for the treatment of HIV infection in patients with limited prior exposure (< 3 months) to zidovudine. Zalcitabine is also indicated, in combination with antiretroviral protease inhibitors, for the treatment of HIV infection.

Human immunodeficiency virus (HIV) infection, advanced (treatment)—Zalcitabine is indicated as a monotherapy for the treatment of advanced HIV infection in patients who are intolerant of, or who have disease progression while receiving, alternative antiretroviral therapy.

The duration of clinical benefit from antiretroviral therapy may be limited. Alterations in antiretroviral therapy should be considered if disease progression occurs during treatment with zalcitabine.

## Pharmacology/Pharmacokinetics
**Physicochemical characteristics**
Molecular weight—211.22.

**Mechanism of action/Effect**
Zalcitabine is phosphorylated by cellular enzymes to its active moiety, 2,3-dideoxycytidine-5-triphosphate (ddCTP). It then competes with the natural substrates for formation of viral DNA by reverse transcriptase, thereby inhibiting viral replication. It also acts as a terminator of chain elongation. *In vitro*, zalcitabine is approximately 10 times more potent than zidovudine against HIV.

**Absorption**
Bioavailability in adults is greater than 80%; one small study done in children found a mean bioavailability of approximately 54%.
Administration with food resulted in a decrease in peak plasma concentration ($C_{max}$) of 39%, a decrease in the mean area under the plasma concentration–time curve (AUC) of 14%, and a twofold increase in time to peak plasma concentration ($T_{max}$).

**Distribution**
Crosses the blood-brain barrier and distributes into the cerebrospinal fluid (CSF); the mean CSF plasma concentration ratio is 20 (range, 7 to 37).
$Vol_D$—
  Adults: Approximately 0.54 L per kg (L/kg).
  Children: Approximately 9.3 L per square meter of body surface (L/m²).

**Plasma protein binding**
Low (< 4%)

**Biotransformation**
Phosphorylated intracellularly to ddCTP, the active substrate for HIV reverse transcriptase. Zalcitabine does not appear to undergo significant metabolism by the liver. The primary metabolite that has been identified is dideoxyuridine (ddU).

**Half-life**
Normal renal function—
  Adults: 1 to 3 hours.
  Children (ages 6 months to 13 years): Approximately 0.8 hour.
Renal function impairment in adults (creatinine clearance < 55 mL/min [0.92 mL/sec])—
  Up to 8.5 hours.
Intracellular half-life of ddCTP is 2.6 to 10 hours.

**Time to peak concentration**
1 to 2 hours.

**Peak serum concentration**
7.6 nanograms/mL after a single oral dose of 0.5 mg.
25.2 nanograms/mL after a single oral dose of 1.5 mg.

**Elimination**
Renal; approximately 70% of zalcitabine is excreted in the urine as the parent drug. Less than 10% (as ddCTP and ddU) is found in the feces.
In dialysis—It is not known whether zalcitabine is removed by hemodialysis or peritoneal dialysis.

## Precautions to Consider
**Carcinogenicity**
Carcinogenicity studies in animals have not yet been completed.

**Tumorigenicity**
High doses of zalcitabine administered for 3 months to $B_6C_3F_1$ mice (resulting in plasma concentrations of over 1000 times those seen in patients taking the recommended doses of zalcitabine) induced an increased incidence of thymic lymphoma.

**Mutagenicity**
No evidence of mutagenicity was found in the Ames test, in the mouse lymphoma cell test, or in the Chinese hamster lung cell test. An unscheduled DNA synthesis assay showed no increases in DNA repair when the assay was performed in rat hepatocytes. However, an *in vitro* mammalian cell transformation assay was positive at doses of 500 mg per mL and higher. Dose-related increases in chromosomal aberration were seen when human peripheral blood lymphocytes were exposed to zalcitabine, with and without metabolic activation, at concentrations of 1.5 mcg per mL and higher. Oral doses of zalcitabine at 2500 and 4500 mg per kg of body weight (mg/kg) were clastogenic in the mouse micronucleus assay.

**Pregnancy/Reproduction**
Fertility—No adverse effects on the rate of conception or general reproductive performance were observed in rats at concentrations of zalcitabine up to 2142 times those achieved with the maximum recommended human dose (MRHD). The fertility of F1 males was significantly reduced at a calculated dose of 2142 (but not 485) times the MRHD (based on area under the plasma concentration–time curve [AUC] measurements) in a teratology study in which rat mothers were dosed on gestation days 7 to 15. No adverse effects were observed on the fertility of parents or F1 generation in the study of fertility and general reproductive performance or in the perinatal and postnatal reproduction study.

Pregnancy—It is not known whether zalcitabine crosses the placenta. Adequate and well-controlled studies have not been done in pregnant women. Unlike zidovudine, it is not known whether zalcitabine reduces perinatal transmission of HIV infection. Zalcitabine should be used in pregnancy only if the potential benefit to the mother outweighs the potential risk to the fetus. Fertile women should not receive zalcitabine unless they are using effective contraception during therapy.

Zalcitabine was teratogenic in mice at calculated exposure levels 1365 and 2730 times the MRHD. It was teratogenic in rats at a calculated exposure level 2142 times the MRHD, but not 485 times the MRHD. Increased embryolethality was seen in pregnant mice at doses 2730 times the MRHD and in rats at doses above 485 times the MRHD. Average fetal body weight was significantly decreased in mice at doses 1365 times the MRHD and in rats at 2142 times the MRHD.

FDA Pregnancy Category C.

**Breast-feeding**
It is not known whether zalcitabine is distributed into breast milk.
There have been case reports of HIV being transmitted from an infected mother to her nursing infant through breast milk. Therefore, breast-feeding is not recommended in HIV-infected mothers, to avoid potential postnatal transmission of HIV to the nursing infant.

## Pediatrics
Safety and efficacy of zalcitabine in combination with zidovudine or as monotherapy have not been fully established in HIV-infected children up to 12 years of age. However, zalcitabine has been both given as a monotherapy and alternated with zidovudine in children 6 months to 12 years of age. Preliminary data show that zalcitabine appears to be well tolerated, and there was clinical improvement and improvement in immunologic and virologic indicators of disease activity. The side effects profile appears to be similar in children and adults.

## Geriatrics
No information is available on the relationship of age to the effects of zalcitabine in geriatric patients. However, elderly patients are more likely to have an age-related decrease in renal function, which may require a reduction in dose.

## Drug interactions and/or related problems
The following drug interactions and/or related problems have been selected on the basis of their potential clinical significance (possible mechanism in parentheses where appropriate)—not necessarily inclusive (» = major clinical significance):

Note: Combinations containing any of the following medications, depending on the amount present, may also interact with this medication.

» Alcohol or
» Asparaginase or
» Azathioprine or
» Estrogens or
» Furosemide or
» Methyldopa or
» Pentamidine, intravenous or
» Sulfonamides or
» Sulindac or
» Tetracyclines or
» Thiazide diuretics or
» Valproic acid or
  Other drugs associated with pancreatitis
    (medications associated with the development of pancreatitis should be avoided during zalcitabine therapy or, if concurrent use is necessary, used with caution since zalcitabine may cause pancreatitis, which, on rare occasion, has been fatal)
    (treatment with zalcitabine should be interrupted if intravenous pentamidine is required)

» Aminoglycosides, parenteral or
» Amphotericin B or
» Foscarnet
    (these medications may increase the toxicity of zalcitabine by interfering with its renal clearance)

» Antacids, aluminum- and/or magnesium-containing
    (concurrent administration of antacids and zalcitabine resulted in a 25% reduction in zalcitabine absorption; it is recommended that antacids and zalcitabine not be administered together)

» Chloramphenicol or
» Cisplatin or
» Dapsone or
» Didanosine or
» Disulfiram or
» Ethambutol or
» Ethionamide or
» Gold or
» Hydralazine or
» Isoniazid or
» Lithium or
» Metronidazole or
» Nitrous oxide or
» Phenytoin or
» Ribavirin or
» Stavudine or
» Vincristine or
  Other drugs associated with peripheral neuropathy
    (since zalcitabine has been shown to cause peripheral neuropathy, other medications associated with the development of neuropathy should be avoided during zalcitabine therapy or, if concurrent use is necessary, used with caution)

» Cimetidine or
» Probenecid
    (use of these medications with zalcitabine has been shown to decrease the clearance of zalcitabine; this is thought to be due to decreased renal clearance; patients should be monitored for signs of toxicity and the dose of zalcitabine may need to be reduced)

» Nitrofurantoin
    (concurrent use of nitrofurantoin with zalcitabine may increase the risk of pancreatitis and peripheral neuropathy; if concurrent use is necessary, patients should be monitored for signs of toxicity and the dose of zalcitabine may need to be reduced)

## Laboratory value alterations
The following have been selected on the basis of their potential clinical significance (possible effect in parentheses where appropriate)—not necessarily inclusive (» = major clinical significance):

With physiology/laboratory test values
  Alanine aminotransferase (ALT [SGPT]) and
  Alkaline phosphatase and
  Aspartate aminotransferase (AST [SGOT])
    (serum values may be increased; values greater than five times the upper normal limit occurred more frequently in patients with abnormal baseline values)

» Amylase and
  Lipase and
  Triglycerides
    (serum values may be increased)

## Medical considerations/Contraindications
The medical considerations/contraindications included have been selected on the basis of their potential clinical significance (reasons given in parentheses where appropriate)—not necessarily inclusive (» = major clinical significance).

*Risk-benefit should be considered when the following medical problems exist:*

» Alcoholism, active or
» Hypertriglyceridemia, or history of or
» Pancreatitis, or history of
    (zalcitabine has caused pancreatitis, which, on rare occasion, has been fatal; patients who have pancreatitis or a history of pancreatitis, or are at risk for pancreatitis, either should not take zalcitabine or should take it with extreme caution)

» Alcoholism, history of or
» Hepatic function impairment
    (rare occurrences of lactic acidosis, in the absence of hypoxemia, and severe hepatomegaly with steatosis have been reported with the use of nucleoside analogues, including zalcitabine, and are potentially fatal; in addition, rare cases of hepatic failure and death considered possibly related to underlying hepatitis B and zalcitabine monotherapy have been reported)

» Peripheral neuropathy
    (zalcitabine may cause peripheral neuropathy; patients with mild peripheral neuropathy should consider alternative agents; patients with moderate to severe peripheral neuropathy should not take zalcitabine)

  Renal function impairment
    (patients with renal function impairment may be at increased risk of toxicity due to decreased clearance of zalcitabine through the kidneys; patients with a creatinine clearance of < 55 mL/min [0.92 mL/sec] may require a reduction in dose)

## Patient monitoring
The following may be especially important in patient monitoring (other tests may be warranted in some patients, depending on condition; » = major clinical significance):

» Alanine aminotransferase (ALT [SGPT]) and
» Alkaline phosphatase and
» Aspartate aminotransferase (AST [SGOT])
    (serum values may be increased to greater than five times the upper normal limit; the incidence of laboratory abnormalities is higher in patients with preexisting abnormal baseline values or a history of alcohol abuse)

» Amylase, serum and
» Lipase, serum and
  Triglycerides, serum
    (zalcitabine administration has been associated with pancreatitis; patients should be monitored for laboratory changes consistent with pancreatitis, such as elevated amylase, lipase, and triglyceride concentrations; zalcitabine should be discontinued if amylase concentration is elevated by 1.5 to 2 times normal limits and/or the patient has symptoms consistent with pancreatitis)

» Blood urea nitrogen (BUN) and
» Creatinine, serum
    (blood urea nitrogen and serum creatinine concentrations should be monitored in patients with renal function impairment; an adjustment in dosage or dosage interval may be required)

## Side/Adverse Effects

Note: In general, patients with decreased CD4 cell counts appear to have an increased incidence of adverse events related to zalcitabine.

Some side effects of zalcitabine (ddC), such as peripheral neuropathy, may also be seen with severe HIV disease; therefore, differentiation between the side effects of ddC and the complications of HIV disease may be difficult. Also, toxicities associated with zidovudine monotherapy are likely to occur when zidovudine is administered concurrently with zalcitabine; these side effects should also be monitored.

Dose-related peripheral neuropathy occurred in 17 to 31% of adult patients treated with zalcitabine monotherapy. Sensorimotor neuropathy starts with numbness and a burning sensation in the distal extremities, followed by sharp shooting pain or severe continuous burning pain if the drug is not discontinued. Peripheral neuropathy is usually dose-related and slowly reversible; however, it is potentially irreversible if zalcitabine is not stopped promptly, and may initially progress despite discontinuation of the drug. Patients with a very low CD4 count (< 50 cells/mm$^3$) are at the greatest risk of developing peripheral neuropathy. Zalcitabine should be discontinued as soon as there is mild progressive discomfort from numbness, tingling, burning, or pain of the extremities.

Fatal pancreatitis has been observed when zalcitabine was given alone and in combination with zidovudine. Pancreatitis is relatively uncommon with zalcitabine monotherapy, occurring in < 1% of patients; asymptomatic elevations in serum amylase also occurred in < 1% of patients. Of the patients treated in the expanded access trial (n=633) who had a prior history of pancreatitis or an elevated serum amylase, 1.6% developed pancreatitis and 1.6% developed an asymptomatic increase in serum amylase.

Severe hepatotoxicity has occurred rarely. Lactic acidosis, in the absence of hypoxemia, and severe hepatomegaly with steatosis have been reported with the use of nucleoside analogues, including zidovudine and zalcitabine, and are potentially fatal. In addition, rare cases of hepatic failure and death considered possibly related to underlying hepatitis B and zalcitabine monotherapy have been reported.

The following side/adverse effects have been selected on the basis of their potential clinical significance (possible signs and symptoms in parentheses where appropriate)—not necessarily inclusive:

**Those indicating need for medical attention**
Incidence more frequent
 *Peripheral neuropathy* (tingling, burning, numbness, or pain in the hands, arms, feet, or legs)
Incidence less frequent
 *Arthralgia* (joint pain); *hypersensitivity* (fever; skin rash); *myalgia* (muscle pain); *ulceration of the mouth and throat*
Incidence rare
 *Hepatotoxicity* (yellow eyes or skin); *leukopenia or neutropenia* (fever and sore throat); *pancreatitis* (abdominal pain, severe; nausea; vomiting)

**Those indicating need for medical attention only if they continue or are bothersome**
Incidence less frequent
 *Gastrointestinal disturbances* (abdominal pain, mild; diarrhea; nausea); *headache*

## Overdose

For more information on the management of overdose or unintentional ingestion, **contact a Poison Control Center** (see *Poison Control Center Listing*).

**Clinical effects of overdose**
Doses of up to 1.5 mg per kg of body weight have inadvertently been given to pediatric patients. The children received prompt gastric lavage and treatment with activated charcoal and had no sequelae. Mixed overdoses of zalcitabine with other medications have caused drowsiness and vomiting, increased gamma-glutamyltransferase values, or increased creatine kinase (CK) serum values. There is no known antidote for zalcitabine overdosage.

Chronic
 *Peripheral neuropathy* (tingling, burning, numbness, or pain in the hands, arms, feet, or legs)

**Treatment of overdose**
Supportive care—Patients in whom intentional overdose is confirmed or suspected should be referred for psychiatric consultation.

## Patient Consultation

As an aid to patient consultation, refer to *Advice for the Patient, Zalcitabine (Systemic)*.
In providing consultation, consider emphasizing the following selected information (» = major clinical significance):

**Before using this medication**
» Conditions affecting use, especially:
 Pregnancy—Zalcitabine should be used during pregnancy only if the benefit to the mother outweighs the potential risk to the fetus; fertile women should not receive zalcitabine unless they are using effective contraception during therapy
 Breast-feeding—Not recommended, because of the potential for postnatal transmission of HIV to the nursing infant
 Use in children—Preliminary data suggest zalcitabine is well tolerated and produces clinical improvement in some children; the side effect profile is similar to that for adults
 Other medications, especially parenteral aminoglycosides, amphotericin B, antacids, cimetidine, foscarnet, nitrofurantoin, other drugs associated with pancreatitis, other drugs associated with peripheral neuropathy, and probenecid
 Other medical problems, especially active alcoholism or a history of alcoholism, hepatic function impairment, hypertriglyceridemia or a history of hypertriglyceridemia, pancreatitis or a history of pancreatitis, or peripheral neuropathy

**Proper use of this medication**
» Importance of not taking more medication than prescribed; importance of not discontinuing medication without checking with physician
» Compliance with full course of therapy
» Importance of not missing doses and of taking at evenly spaced times
 Not sharing medication with others
» Proper dosing
 Missed dose: Taking as soon as possible; not taking if almost time for next dose; not doubling doses
» Proper storage

**Precautions while using this medication**
» Regular visits to physician for blood tests
» Importance of not taking other medications concurrently without checking with physician
» Taking steps to avoid spreading HIV infection

**Side/adverse effects**
Signs of potential side effects, especially peripheral neuropathy, arthralgia, hypersensitivity, myalgia, ulceration of the mouth and throat, hepatotoxicity, leukopenia or neutropenia, and pancreatitis

## General Dosing Information

No adjustment in dose needs to be made for patients who weigh 30 kg or more; this is based on pharmacokinetic weight-ranging data.

If patients receiving zalcitabine and zidovudine combination therapy develop what are thought to be medication-related side effects, the dose of the medication associated with that particular toxicity profile should be modified. When the toxicity is more likely to be caused by zalcitabine, the dose of that drug should be reduced or the drug should be discontinued; the same is true for zidovudine. For severe toxicity in which the causative drug cannot be identified, or side effects continue despite dose reduction or discontinuation of one medication, the dose of the other medication should also be reduced or the medication discontinued.

Patients with mild, new onset, or progressive symptoms of peripheral neuropathy should discontinue taking zalcitabine, especially if the symptoms last for more than 3 days and are bilateral. Zalcitabine may be reintroduced at 50% of the regular dose (0.375 mg every 8 hours) only if the peripheral neuropathy improves to very mild symptoms.

## Oral Dosage Forms

### ZALCITABINE TABLETS USP
**Usual adult and adolescent dose**
Human immunodeficiency virus (HIV) infection—
 Oral, 0.75 mg in combination with 200 mg zidovudine, every eight hours.

# Zalcitabine (Systemic)

Human immunodeficiency virus (HIV) infection, advanced—
Oral, 0.75 mg every eight hours.

Note: Adults with acute or chronic renal impairment may require a reduction in dose of zalcitabine as follows:

| Creatinine clearance (mL/min)/(mL/sec) | Dose (mg) | Dosing interval (hr) |
|---|---|---|
| > 40/0.67 | 0.75 | 8 |
| 10–40/0.17–0.67 | 0.75 | 12 |
| 0–10/0–0.17 | 0.75 | 24 |

### Usual pediatric dose
Safety and effectiveness of zalcitabine given alone or in combination with zidovudine have not been established in children up to 13 years of age. The doses being studied in ongoing clinical trials are 0.005 and 0.01 mg per kg of body weight every eight hours.

### Strength(s) usually available
U.S.—
0.375 mg (Rx) [*HIVID* (lactose)].
0.75 mg (Rx) [*HIVID* (lactose)].
Canada—
0.375 mg (Rx) [*HIVID* (lactose)].
0.75 mg (Rx) [*HIVID* (lactose)].

### Packaging and storage
Store between 15 and 30 °C (59 and 86 °F), in a tight, light-resistant container.

### Auxiliary labeling
- Continue medicine for full time of treatment.

Revised: 02/01/95
Interim revision: 04/17/98

# ZIDOVUDINE  Systemic

VA CLASSIFICATION (Primary): AM800
Commonly used brand name(s): *Apo-Zidovudine*; *Novo-AZT*; *Retrovir*.
Another commonly used name is AZT.

Note: For a listing of dosage forms and brand names by country availability, see *Dosage Forms* section(s).

## Category
Antiviral (systemic).

## Indications
Note: Bracketed information in the *Indications* section refers to uses that are not included in U.S. product labeling.

### Accepted
Human immunodeficiency virus (HIV) infection, asymptomatic (treatment) or
Immunodeficiency syndrome, acquired, (AIDS) (treatment)—Zidovudine is indicated as a primary agent in the treatment of human immunodeficiency virus (HIV) disease in adult patients with a CD4 lymphocyte count of 500 per mm$^3$ or less who are asymptomatic, who have early symptoms of HIV disease, or who have advanced symptoms of HIV disease (AIDS). Also, zalcitabine (ddC) is indicated in combination with zidovudine in adult patients with advanced HIV disease (CD4 lymphocyte count of 300 per mm$^3$ or less). [Didanosine (ddI) is also used in combination with zidovudine.][1] Zidovudine (alone) is indicated in children over 3 months of age who have HIV-related symptoms or who are asymptomatic with abnormal laboratory values indicating significant HIV-related immunosuppression.

Maternal-fetal human immunodeficiency virus (HIV) transmission (prophylaxis)—Zidovudine is indicated for the prevention of maternal-fetal HIV transmission as part of a regimen that includes oral zidovudine beginning between 14 and 34 weeks gestation, continuous intravenous infusion of zidovudine during labor, and administration of zidovudine syrup to the neonate for the first six weeks of life. However, transmission to infants may still occur in some cases despite the use of this regimen.

[Human immunodeficiency virus (HIV) infection, occupational exposure (prophylaxis)][1]—Zidovudine has been used prophylactically in health care workers at risk of acquiring HIV infection after occupational exposure to the virus. Risk of transmission from a single needlestick is approximately 0.3%. Efficacy, and optimal dose and duration of prophylactic treatment are unknown at this time; however, HIV infection has occurred in persons who received zidovudine prophylaxis after a needlestick or other parenteral exposure.

*In vitro* resistance of HIV isolates to zidovudine has been reported in AIDS patients receiving zidovudine treatment for 6 months or longer. Deterioration of clinical status has been observed in some patients with resistant virus; evidence of a direct association of viral resistance with lack of drug effect continues to mount. Patients can simultaneously carry several viral strains with different susceptibilities to zidovudine. Reduced *in vitro* sensitivity of HIV to zidovudine develops at a slower rate and to a lesser degree in patients with early stages of infection than in those with advanced disease. A low level of cross-resistance between zidovudine, didanosine, and zalcitabine has been observed. However, data suggest that HIV develops resistance to zidovudine more readily than to either didanosine or zalcitabine.

Zidovudine is not a cure for HIV infection. Patients treated with zidovudine may continue to develop complications of AIDS, including opportunistic infections. The treatment or prevention of these infections may require the concurrent administration of other anti-infectives.

### Unaccepted
Zidovudine is not effective in the treatment of infections caused by gram-positive organisms, gram-negative organisms, cytomegalovirus, vaccinia, herpes simplex, varicella zoster, anaerobes, mycobacteria, or fungi.

Zidovudine has not been shown to reduce the risk of transmission of HIV to others through sexual contact or blood contamination.

[1] Not included in Canadian product labeling.

## Pharmacology/Pharmacokinetics

### Physicochemical characteristics
Molecular weight—267.24.

### Mechanism of action/Effect
Virustatic; zidovudine, a structural analog of thymidine, is phosphorylated intracellularly by cellular thymidine kinase to zidovudine monophosphate. The monophosphate is converted to the diphosphate by cellular thymidylate kinase and is further converted to the triphosphate by other cellular enzymes. Zidovudine triphosphate competes with the natural substrate, thymidine triphosphate, for incorporation into growing chains of viral RNA-dependent DNA polymerase (reverse transcriptase), thereby inhibiting viral DNA replication. Once incorporated, zidovudine triphosphate also prematurely terminates the growing DNA chain since the 3'-azido group prevents further 5' to 3' phosphodiester linkages. Zidovudine has a 100- to 300-fold greater affinity for inhibiting HIV reverse transcriptase than it does for inhibiting human DNA polymerase.

### Other actions/effects
Zidovudine has been found to have activity against hepatitis B virus and Epstein-Barr virus *in vitro*; however, one small study found that zidovudine did not markedly inhibit hepatitis B virus replication when used alone in patients with AIDS. Low concentrations of zidovudine have also been shown to inhibit many strains of Enterobacteriaceae *in vitro*, including strains of *Shigella*, *Salmonella*, *Klebsiella*, *Enterobacter*, and *Citrobacter* species, and *Escherichia coli*. However, bacterial resistance to zidovudine develops rapidly. No activity was seen against *Pseudomonas aeruginosa in vitro*. At very high concentrations (1.9 mcg/mL [7 micromoles per L]), zidovudine has also been shown to inhibit *Giardia lamblia*, although no activity has been observed against other protozoal pathogens.

### Absorption
Rapid and nearly complete absorption from the gastrointestinal tract following oral administration; however, because of first-pass metabolism, systemic bioavailability of zidovudine capsules and solution is approximately 65% (range, 52 to 75%). Bioavailability in neonates up to 14 days old is approximately 89%, and in neonates over 14 days of age, it decreases to approximately 61%. Administration with a high-fat meal may decrease the rate and extent of absorption.

### Distribution
Crosses the blood-brain barrier; distribution to cerebrospinal fluid (CSF) averages approximately 24% of the plasma concentration in children.
Crosses the placenta. One case report and a study in 3 pregnant women found that the zidovudine concentrations in the infant cord blood were

slightly higher than simultaneous maternal serum concentrations, and that the amniotic fluid concentrations were several times higher than the simultaneous umbilical cord concentrations. The concentration of zidovudine in the central nervous system tissue of a gestational 13-week fetus (0.01 micromole per liter) was below effective antiviral concentrations.

Also shown to concentrate in the semen of HIV-infected patients, with concentrations ranging from 1.3 to 20.4 times those found in the serum; zidovudine does not appear to affect the recovery of HIV from the semen, and, therefore, may not prevent sexual transmission of HIV.

Vol$_D$—Adults and children: 1.4 to 1.7 liters per kg (42 to 52 liters per m$^2$).

**Protein binding**
Low (30 to 38%).

**Biotransformation**
Hepatic; metabolized by glucuronide conjugation to major, inactive metabolite, 3'-azido-3'-deoxy-5'-O-beta-D-glucopyranuronosylthymidine (GAZT).

In children under 1 year of age—The glucuronide conjugation pathway is underdeveloped at birth; however, a study done in infants older than 30 days of age found that the clearance and half-life of zidovudine were comparable to those in adults.

**Half-life**
Intracellular zidovudine-triphosphate—
   Approximately 3.3 hours.
Zidovudine (serum)—
   Adults (oral and intravenous):
      Normal renal function—Approximately 1 hour (range, 0.8 to 1.2 hours).
      Renal function impairment (creatinine clearance <30 mL per min)—1.4 to 2.9 hours.
      Cirrhosis—Variable, depending on the degree of liver function impairment; however, one study found the half-life to be approximately 2.4 hours.
   Children age 2 weeks to 13 years (oral and intravenous):
      Approximately 1 to 1.8 hours.
   Children up to 14 days of age:
      Approximately 3 hours.
   Neonates (mother receiving zidovudine):
      Approximately 13 hours.
GAZT (serum)—
   Adults (oral and intravenous) Normal renal function:
      Approximately 1 hour.
   Renal function impairment:
      Approximately 8 hours.
   Anuria:
      29 to 94 hours.
   Cirrhosis:
      Variable, depending on the degree of liver function impairment; however, one study found the half-life to be approximately 2.4 hours.

**Time to peak concentration**
Serum—0.5 to 1.5 hours.
CSF—1 hour after end of 1 hour infusion.

**Peak serum concentration**
(linear kinetics)—
   Intravenous infusion: 1 mg per kg of body weight (mg/kg) (over 1 hour)—1.5 to 2.5 micromoles per L (0.40 to 0.68 mcg/mL).
   Oral (capsules and solution): 2 mg/kg—1.5 to 2 micromoles per L (0.41 to 0.54 mcg/mL).
   Continuous intravenous infusion in children (age 14 months to 12 years): Steady state concentrations—0.5 mg/kg/hr (360 mg/m$^2$/day): 1.9 micromoles per L (0.51 mcg/mL).

**Elimination**
Adults—
   Zidovudine: Renal; approximately 14 to 18% excreted by glomerular filtration and active tubular secretion in urine.
   GAZT: Renal; approximately 60 to 74% recovered in urine.
   Total of zidovudine and GAZT: Approximately 63 to 95% recovered in urine.
   In dialysis: Current available data vary; it appears that hemodialysis and peritoneal dialysis have a negligible effect on the removal of zidovudine. Hemodialysis does enhance the elimination of GAZT; however, dialysis clearance of GAZT is minimal compared to the clearance of GAZT in patients with normal renal function.
Children (age 14 months to 12 years)—
   Zidovudine: Renal; approximately 30% excreted by the kidneys.
   GAZT: Renal; approximately 45% recovered in the urine.

## Precautions to Consider

### Carcinogenicity
Long-term carcinogenicity studies found five malignant and two benign vaginal squamous cell tumors in 60 female mice given zidovudine in doses of 120 mg per kg of body weight (mg/kg) per day, later reduced to 40 mg/kg per day. Two out of 60 rats were found to have vaginal squamous cell carcinoma after receiving doses of 600 mg/kg per day, later reduced to 450, then 300 mg/kg per day. The tumors occurred at the end of the life span of the animals. No treatment-related tumors were seen in the 60 male mice or 60 male rats. Zidovudine was positive for carcinogenicity at concentrations of 0.5 mcg/mL and higher in *in vitro* mammalian-cell transformation assays.

### Mutagenicity
Zidovudine has not been shown to be mutagenic, with or without metabolic activation, in the Ames *Salmonella* mutagenicity assay.

In the absence of metabolic activation, zidovudine was shown to be weakly mutagenic only at the highest concentrations tested (4000 and 5000 mcg/mL) in the mutagenicity assay in L5178Y/TK +/− mouse lymphoma cells. In the presence of metabolic activation, zidovudine was shown to be weakly mutagenic at concentrations of 1000 mcg/mL and higher.

Zidovudine has been shown to induce dose-related structural chromosomal abnormalities at concentrations of 3 mcg/mL and higher in *in vitro* cytogenetic studies in cultured human lymphocytes. No mutagenic effects were noted at the 2 lowest concentrations tested (0.3 and 1 mcg/mL).

In *in vivo* cytogenetic studies in rats given single intravenous doses of 37.5 to 300 mg/kg, zidovudine has not been shown to cause treatment-related structural or numerical chromosomal alterations, in spite of plasma concentrations as high as 453 mcg/mL 5 minutes after dosing.

In 2 *in vivo* micronucleus studies in male mice designed to measure chromosome breakage or mitotic spindle apparatus damage, oral doses of zidovudine of 100 to 1000 mg/kg per day administered once daily for approximately 4 weeks induced dose-related increases in micronucleated erythrocytes. Similar results were also seen after 4 or 7 days of dosing at 500 mg/kg per day in rats and mice.

### Pregnancy/Reproduction
Fertility—The effects of zidovudine on fertility have not been studied in humans.

Studies in rats given oral zidovudine at dosages up to 450 mg/kg per day showed no effect on male or female fertility.

Pregnancy—Zidovudine crosses the placenta. Adequate and well-controlled studies in humans have not been completed. However, the rate of HIV transmission from pregnant women to their infants has been shown to be decreased in women treated with zidovudine compared to women treated with placebo. One survey of 43 women who took zidovudine (300 to 1200 mg per day) during various stages of pregnancy found that zidovudine was well tolerated by the mothers and was not associated with teratogenic abnormalities, premature birth, or fetal distress. Three small studies done in women given zidovudine during their last trimester of pregnancy found that peak plasma concentrations and the elimination half-life were similar to values reported in nonpregnant adults, although volume of distribution and plasma clearance were significantly increased during pregnancy in 2 of the studies. Therapeutic plasma concentrations have been measured in the newborn infant. Therapeutic levels have also been measured in the amniotic fluid of a gestational 13-week fetus; however, the concentration of zidovudine in this fetus' CNS tissue (0.01 micromole per liter) was below effective antiviral concentrations.

Studies in rats and rabbits given oral doses of up to 500 mg/kg per day have not shown zidovudine to be teratogenic. There was an increased incidence of fetal resorption in rats given 150 or 450 mg/kg per day of zidovudine, rabbits given 500 mg/kg per day, and mice given 0.25 mg/mL in drinking water, producing serum concentrations of 0.12 mcg/mL.

FDA Pregnancy Category C.

### Breast-feeding
It is not known whether zidovudine is distributed into human breast milk. There have been case reports of HIV being transmitted from an infected mother to her nursing infant through breast milk. Therefore, breast-feeding is not recommended in HIV-infected mothers where safe infant formula is available and affordable.

### Pediatrics
Zidovudine is approved for use in children 3 months of age and older. Results of uncontrolled studies showed that children with symptomatic HIV disease and a CD4 lymphocyte count of 500 per mm$^3$ or less had a positive response to zidovudine, including improvement in neuropsychological function, immunological function, p24 antigen concentrations, and weight gain. No studies have been published addressing the

efficacy of zidovudine in asymptomatic children with a CD4 lymphocyte count of 500 per mm³ or less. It is also not known whether doses lower than 180 mg per square meter of body surface every 6 hours would maintain adequate CNS concentrations of zidovudine to provide improvement of HIV-related CNS disease in children. The pharmacokinetics of zidovudine in children 14 days of age and older have been found to be similar to those in adults. The half-life in newborns was found to be 10 times that of the mother (13 vs 1.3 hours, respectively). The side effects seen in children, including the hematologic effects, were also similar to those seen in adults.

### Geriatrics
Studies have not been performed to determine the safety and effectiveness of zidovudine in the geriatric population. However, 1 case reports that a 90-year-old patient responded well to zidovudine therapy. Preliminary data indicate that the elimination rate of zidovudine may be decreased in the elderly.

### Dental
The bone marrow–depressant effects of zidovudine may result in an increased incidence of certain microbial infections and delayed healing.

### Drug interactions and/or related problems
The following drug interactions and/or related problems have been selected on the basis of their potential clinical significance (possible mechanism in parentheses where appropriate)—not necessarily inclusive (» = major clinical significance):

Note: Combinations containing any of the following medications, depending on the amount present, may also interact with this medication.

Blood dyscrasia–causing medications (See *Appendix II*) or
» Bone marrow depressants, other (See *Appendix II*) or
Radiation therapy
(concurrent use of these medications and/or radiation therapy with zidovudine may cause an additive or synergistic myelosuppression; dosage reductions may be required)

» Clarithromycin
(initial results of a dose escalation study in HIV-infected patients showed that concurrent use of zidovudine and clarithromycin resulted in a lower peak serum concentration [$C_{max}$], lower area under the plasma-concentration-time curve [AUC], and delayed time to peak concentration [$T_{max}$] of zidovudine)

» Ganciclovir
(concurrent use with zidovudine has caused severe hematologic toxicity even when the zidovudine dose was reduced to 300 mg per day; this effect is thought to be the result of synergistic myelosuppressive toxicity rather than a pharmacokinetic interaction; concurrent administration should be used with extreme caution)

Hepatic glucuronidation–metabolized medications, other
(other medications metabolized by hepatic glucuronidation, such as acetaminophen, aspirin, benzodiazepines, cimetidine, indomethacin, morphine, and sulfonamides, may, in theory, compete with zidovudine for metabolism and decrease the clearance of zidovudine or the other medication; this could potentially increase the risk of toxicity of either zidovudine or the other medication)

» Probenecid
(concurrent use inhibits hepatic glucuronidation and secretion of zidovudine through the renal tubules, resulting in increased serum concentrations and a prolonged elimination half-life; this may increase the risk of toxicity, or possibly permit a reduction in daily zidovudine dosage; however, in 1 small trial, a very high incidence of rash was observed in patients receiving probenecid concurrently with zidovudine)

Ribavirin
(*in vitro* studies have shown that, when combined, ribavirin and zidovudine are reproducibly antagonistic and should not be used concurrently; ribavirin inhibits the phosphorylation of zidovudine to its active triphosphate form)

Stavudine (d4T)
(*in vitro* studies detected an antagonistic antiviral effect between stavudine and zidovudine at a molar ratio of 20 to 1, respectively; concurrent use is not recommended until *in vivo* studies demonstrate that these medications are not antagonistic in their anti-HIV activity)

### Laboratory value alterations
The following have been selected on the basis of their potential clinical significance (possible effect in parentheses where appropriate)—not necessarily inclusive (» = major clinical significance):

With physiology/laboratory test values
Mean corpuscular volume (MCV)
(usually will be increased)

### Medical considerations/Contraindications
The medical considerations/contraindications included have been selected on the basis of their potential clinical significance (reasons given in parentheses where appropriate)—not necessarily inclusive (» = major clinical significance).

*Risk-benefit should be considered when the following medical problems exist:*

» Bone marrow depression
(zidovudine may cause bone marrow depression, worsening any pre-existing granulocytopenia and anemia)

Folic acid deficiency or
Vitamin $B_{12}$ deficiency
(patients with folic acid or vitamin $B_{12}$ deficiency may be more prone to anemia since zidovudine can cause impaired erythrocyte maturation, resulting in a macrocytic anemia)

» Hepatic function impairment
(because zidovudine is metabolized in the liver to an inactive metabolite, GAZT, hepatic function impairment may lead to accumulation of zidovudine and increased toxicity)

Hypersensitivity to zidovudine

### Patient monitoring
The following may be especially important in patient monitoring (other tests may be warranted in some patients, depending on condition; » = major clinical significance):

» Complete blood counts (CBCs)
(in patients with HIV disease who are asymptomatic or have early symptoms, CBCs are recommended monthly during the first 3 months, then every 3 months thereafter, unless indicated for other reasons. CBCs are recommended at least every 2 weeks during the first 8 weeks of therapy to detect serious anemia or granulocytopenia in patients with advanced HIV disease taking zidovudine; the frequency of CBCs may be decreased to every 4 weeks after the first 2 months if zidovudine is well tolerated. Decreases in hemoglobin concentrations may occur as early as 2 to 4 weeks after the beginning of therapy, and peak falls in hemoglobin usually occur during the first 4 to 6 weeks. Granulocytopenia usually occurs after 6 to 8 weeks; when significant anemia [hemoglobin of < 7.5 grams/dL] and/or significant granulocytopenia [granulocyte count of < 750/mm³] occurs, dosage adjustments, discontinuation of the drug, blood transfusions, or, in selected patients, treatment with epoetin [recombinant human erythropoietin] or GM-CSF [granulocyte-macrophage colony-stimulating factor] may be necessary. Zidovudine should not be restarted until some evidence of bone marrow recovery is evident; if bone marrow recovery occurs following dosage adjustments, gradual increases in dose may be appropriate, depending on blood counts and patient tolerance; patients should be informed of the importance of having blood counts followed closely during therapy)

Liver function tests
(liver function tests, including serum ALT [SGPT], alkaline phosphatase, and AST [SGOT] values, and serum bilirubin concentration, should be monitored periodically since elevations, usually reversible, have been reported on rare occasions with zidovudine therapy; however, in 2 large placebo-controlled studies, the difference in incidence of aminotransferase elevation between the treatment and the placebo groups was not statistically significant; elevations in liver function tests in some cases may be related to reactivation of hepatitis virus or due to HIV infection itself)

## Side/Adverse Effects

Note: Because of the complexity of this disease state, it is often difficult to differentiate between the manifestations of HIV infection and the adverse effects of zidovudine. In addition, very little placebo-controlled data are available to assess this difference, with most of the information coming from uncontrolled studies and case reports. The long-term effects of zidovudine are still not known; however, hematologic side effects are more likely to occur with higher doses, and in patients with more advanced disease.

The most frequent side/adverse effects of zidovudine are granulocytopenia and anemia. These have been shown to be inversely related to the CD4 lymphocyte count, hemoglobin concentration, and granulocyte count at the time of therapy initiation, and directly related to dosage and duration of therapy. Significant anemia most commonly occurs after 4 to 6 weeks of therapy.

The following side/adverse effects have been selected on the basis of their potential clinical significance (possible signs and symptoms in parentheses where appropriate)—not necessarily inclusive:

### Those indicating need for medical attention
Incidence more frequent
> *Anemia* (pale skin; unusual tiredness or weakness); *leukopenia or neutropenia* (fever, chills, or sore throat)

Incidence less frequent
> *Changes in platelet count*—often increased with therapy, however, may be decreased infrequently

Incidence rare
> *Hepatotoxicity* (abdominal discomfort; nausea; decreased appetite; general feeling of discomfort); *myopathy* (muscular atrophy, tenderness, and weakness); *neurotoxicity* (confusion; mood or mental changes; seizures)

### Those indicating need for medical attention only if they continue or are bothersome
Incidence more frequent
> *Headache, severe; insomnia* (trouble in sleeping); *myalgia* (muscle soreness); *nausea*

Incidence less frequent
> *Hyperpigmentation of nails* (bluish-brownish bands)

### Those indicating need for medical attention if they occur after medication is discontinued
> *Bone marrow depression* (fever, chills, or sore throat; pale skin; unusual tiredness or weakness)

## Overdose

For more information on the management of overdose or unintentional ingestion, **contact a Poison Control Center** (see *Poison Control Center Listing*).

**Clinical effects of overdose**
The following effects have been selected on the basis of their potential clinical significance (possible signs and symptoms in parentheses where appropriate)—not necessarily inclusive:

Symptoms of overdose
> *Bone marrow toxicity, specifically anemia, leukopenia, thrombocytopenia* (pale skin; unusual tiredness or weakness; fever, chills, or sore throat; increase in bleeding or bruising); *gastrointestinal disturbances* (severe nausea and vomiting); *neurotoxicity, specifically ataxia, fatigue, lethargy, nystagmus, seizures* (lack of coordination; involuntary, rapid, rhythmic movement of the eyes; convulsions)

Note: At this time, the information available on acute zidovudine overdose is limited to several case reports. These patients took between 6 and 50 grams of zidovudine. Severe *nausea and vomiting* are the most common symptoms after an overdose. Other reported symptoms include *ataxia, nystagmus, lethargy, fatigue,* and, in one patient, a single *tonic-clonic seizure*. One patient who took a chronic overdose of zidovudine, 500 mg five times a day for 16 days, had an increase in liver transaminases, which resolved when the dose was reduced. There is also one case report of a patient who ingested 6 grams in a suicide attempt who experienced *hematologic toxicity*; the lowest blood cell count occurred 8 days after the ingestion and returned to previous levels by day 20.

**Treatment of overdose**
Specific treatment—Zidovudine is not removed from the blood by peritoneal dialysis or hemodialysis in sufficient amounts to warrant the use of dialysis in an overdose situation.

Monitoring—Close observation of the patient for evidence of neurotoxicity and bone marrow suppression.

Supportive care—Supportive therapy. Patients in whom intentional overdose is known or suspected should be referred for psychiatric consultation.

## Patient Consultation

As an aid to patient consultation, refer to *Advice for the Patient, Zidovudine (Systemic)*.

In providing consultation, consider emphasizing the following selected information (» = major clinical significance):

### Before using this medication
» Conditions affecting use, especially:
  Hypersensitivity to zidovudine
  Pregnancy—Zidovudine crosses the placenta and reaches concentrations in the fetus similar to those observed in adults; zidovudine has been shown to decrease perinatal transmission of HIV
  Breast-feeding—It is not known whether zidovudine is distributed into breast milk; however, breast-feeding is not recommended in HIV-infected mothers where safe infant formula is available and affordable
  Dental—The bone marrow–depressant effects of zidovudine may result in an increased incidence of certain microbial infections and delayed healing
  Other medications, especially other bone marrow depressants, clarithromycin, ganciclovir, or probenecid
  Other medical problems, especially bone marrow depression or hepatic function impairment

### Proper use of this medication
Supplying patient information about zidovudine
» Importance of not taking more medication than prescribed; importance of not discontinuing medication without checking with physician
» Compliance with full course of therapy
» Importance of not missing doses and taking at evenly spaced times
» Proper dosing
  Missed dose: Taking as soon as possible; not taking if almost time for next dose; not doubling doses
» Proper storage

### Precautions while using this medication
» Regular visits to physician for blood tests
» Importance of not taking other medications concurrently without checking with physician
  Using caution in use of regular toothbrushes, dental floss, and toothpicks; checking with physician or dentist concerning proper oral hygiene
» Avoiding sexual intercourse or using a condom to help prevent transmission of the AIDS virus to others; not sharing needles with anyone

### Side/adverse effects
Signs of potential side effects, especially anemia, leukopenia or neutropenia, changes in platelet count, hepatotoxicity, myopathy, and neurotoxicity

## General Dosing Information

The optimal dosage and dosing schedule for zidovudine have not been established at this time. Also, the long-term effects of early zidovudine intervention on delaying clinical progression, prolonging survival, and the potential side effects, as well as the clinical implications of drug resistance, are unknown at this time.

Patients should be advised of the importance of taking zidovudine exactly as prescribed. Patients should not exceed the prescribed dose.

Zidovudine infusion should be administered at a constant rate over one hour. It should not be administered intramuscularly or by rapid infusion or direct injection.

Patients with significant anemia (hemoglobin < 7.5 grams/dL) and/or significant granulocytopenia (granulocyte count of < 750/mm$^3$) may require a dose reduction until bone marrow recovery is seen or dose interruption with reinstitution of therapy at a lower dose (300 mg per day has been used) after bone marrow recovery has occurred.

Granulocytopenia and anemia have been shown to be inversely related to the CD4 lymphocyte count, hemoglobin concentration, and granulocyte count at time of therapy initiation, and directly related to dosage and duration of therapy. Significant anemia most commonly occurs after 4 to 6 weeks of therapy.

Patients with anemia usually improve when zidovudine is discontinued or the dose is reduced. However, even with lower doses, patients may require blood transfusions or, in selected patients, treatment with epoetin (recombinant human erythropoietin). Patients with granulocytopenia may require interruption of therapy or treatment with GM-CSF (granulocyte-macrophage colony-stimulating factor).

## Oral Dosage Forms

### ZIDOVUDINE CAPSULES

**Usual adult and adolescent dose**
Antiviral—
  Monotherapy:
    Symptomatic HIV infection—Oral, 100 mg every four hours (600 mg per day).
    Asymptomatic HIV infection—Oral, 100 mg every four hours while awake (500 mg per day).
  Note: Zidovudine has also been given in doses of 200 mg every eight hours.
  Combination therapy with zalcitabine:
    Oral, 200 mg of zidovudine and 0.75 mg of zalcitabine given together every eight hours.

Maternal-fetal HIV transmission (prophylaxis)—
  Oral, 100 mg five times a day beginning after fourteen weeks of gestation and continuing until the start of labor. At that time, intravenous zidovudine should be administered (see *Zidovudine Injection*).

**Usual pediatric dose**
Antiviral—
Symptomatic HIV infection or
Asymptomatic HIV infection:
  Infants up to 3 months of age—Dosage has not been established.
  Children 3 months to 12 years of age—Oral, 90 to 180 mg per square meter of body surface every six hours.
  Children 13 years of age and older— See *Usual adult and adolescent dose*.
Note: Dosage should not exceed 200 mg every six hours.
  Pediatric patients with granulocytopenia may require a dose reduction to 120 mg per square meter of body surface every six hours.

**Strength(s) usually available**
U.S.—
  100 mg (Rx) [*Retrovir*].
Canada—
  100 mg (Rx) [*Apo-Zidovudine; Novo-AZT; Retrovir*].

**Packaging and storage**
Store between 15 and 25 °C (59 and 77 °F), in a tight container. Protect from light and moisture.

**Auxiliary labeling**
• Continue medicine for full time of treatment.

### ZIDOVUDINE SYRUP

**Usual adult and adolescent dose**
See *Zidovudine Capsules*.

**Usual pediatric dose**
Antiviral—
Symptomatic HIV infection; or
Asymptomatic HIV infection: See *Zidovudine Capsules*.
Maternal-fetal HIV transmission (prophylaxis), infant dosing: Oral, 2 mg per kg of body weight every six hours starting within twelve hours after birth and continuing through six weeks of age. If the infant cannot receive zidovudine syrup, intravenous zidovudine may be administered (see *Zidovudine Injection*).

**Strength(s) usually available**
U.S.—
  50 mg per 5 mL (Rx) [*Retrovir*].
Canada—
  50 mg per 5 mL (Rx) [*Retrovir*].

**Packaging and storage**
Store between 15 and 25 °C (59 and 77 °F), in a tight container. Protect from light.

**Auxiliary labeling**
• Continue medicine for full time of treatment.

## Parenteral Dosage Forms

### ZIDOVUDINE INJECTION

**Usual adult and adolescent dose**
Antiviral—
  Symptomatic HIV infection: Intravenous infusion, 1 mg per kg of body weight, infused over one hour, every four hours around the clock until oral therapy can be administered.
  Maternal-fetal HIV transmission (prophylaxis), maternal dose at the start of labor and delivery: Intravenous, 2 mg per kg of total body weight over one hour, followed by a continuous infusion of 1 mg per kg of total body weight per hour until clamping of the umbilical cord.

**Usual pediatric dose**
Antiviral—
Symptomatic HIV infection:
  Intravenous infusion, 120 mg per square meter of body surface, infused over one hour, every six hours.
Note: Dosage should not exceed 160 mg for any individual dose.
  Pediatric patients with granulocytopenia may require a dose reduction to 90 mg per square meter of body surface every six hours.
Maternal-fetal HIV transmission (prophylaxis), if the infant is unable to receive zidovudine syrup (See *Zidovudine Syrup*):
  Intravenous, 1.5 mg per kg of body weight over thirty minutes every six hours.

**Strength(s) usually available**
U.S.—
  200 mg in 20 mL (Rx) [*Retrovir*].
Canada—
  200 mg in 20 mL (Rx) [*Retrovir*].

**Packaging and storage**
Store between 15 and 25 °C (59 and 77 °F). Protect from light.

**Preparation of dosage form**
Zidovudine injection must be diluted prior to administration to a concentration of no greater than 4 mg per mL in 5% dextrose injection, 0.9% sodium chloride injection, 5% dextrose and 0.9% sodium chloride injection, lactated Ringer's injection, or 5% dextrose and lactated Ringer's injection.

**Stability**
After dilution, solutions are physically and chemically stable for 24 hours at room temperature (25 °C [77 °F]) and 48 hours if refrigerated (2 to 8 °C [36 to 46 °F]).
It is recommended that diluted solutions be administered within 8 hours if stored at 25 °C (77 °F) or 24 hours if refrigerated (2 to 8 °C [36 to 46 °F]) to minimize potential microbial contamination.
Do not use if the solution is discolored.

**Incompatibilities**
Zidovudine injection should not be admixed with biological or colloidal solutions (e.g., blood products, protein-containing solutions).

## Selected Bibliography

Wilde MI, Langtry HD. Zidovudine. An update of its pharmacodynamic and pharmacokinetic properties, and therapeutic efficacy. Drugs 1993; 46(3): 515-78.
Matthews SJ, Cersosimo RJ, Spivack ML. Zidovudine and other reverse transcriptase inhibitors in the management of human immunodeficiency virus-related disease. Pharmacotherapy 1991; 11(6): 419-49.
Morse GD, Lechner JL, Santora JA, Rozed SL. Zidovudine update: 1990. DICP Ann Pharmacother 1990; 24: 754-60.

Revised: 06/22/94
Interim revision: 01/11/95

# ZILEUTON  Systemic†

VA CLASSIFICATION (Primary): RE108
Commonly used brand name(s): *Zyflo*.
Note: For a listing of dosage forms and brand names by country availability, see *Dosage Forms* section(s).

†Not commercially available in Canada.

## Category
Antiasthmatic (leukotriene inhibitor).

## Indications

**Accepted**
Asthma, chronic (prophylaxis and treatment)—Zileuton is indicated in patients with chronic asthma to improve asthma symptoms, improve pulmonary function (forced expiratory volume in 1 second [$FEV_1$], morning and evening peak expiratory flow rates), and to decrease the use of an inhaled beta$_2$-agonist. In clinical trials, zileuton was used to treat patients with mild to moderate persistent asthma.

**Unaccepted**
Zileuton is not indicated for the treatment of bronchospasm in acute asthma attacks, including status asthmaticus; however, zileuton does not need to be discontinued during an acute exacerbation.

## Pharmacology/Pharmacokinetics

**Physicochemical characteristics**
Molecular weight—236.29.

**Mechanism of action/Effect**
Zileuton is a selective inhibitor of 5-lipoxygenase, which is the enzyme that catalyzes the formation of leukotrienes from arachidonic acid. Specifically, it inhibits the formation of leukotrienes $LTC_4$, $LTD_4$, and $LTE_4$, which are the active constituents of slow-reacting substances of anaphylaxis, and $LTB_4$, a substance that attracts neutrophils and eosinophils. Leukotrienes produce numerous biological effects, including augmentation of neutrophil and eosinophil migration, neutrophil and monocyte aggregation, leukocyte adhesion, increased capillary permeability, and smooth muscle contraction. These effects contribute to inflammation, edema, mucus secretion, and bronchoconstriction in the airways of asthmatic patients.

**Absorption**
Rapidly and almost completely absorbed.

**Protein binding**
High (93%). Bound primarily to albumin.

**Biotransformation**
Hepatic. *In vitro* studies using human liver microsomes have shown that zileuton and its *N*-dehydroxylated metabolite are oxidatively metabolized by the cytochrome P450 isoenzymes 1A2, 2C9, and 3A4.

**Half-life**
Mean terminal half-life is 2.5 hours.

**Onset of action**
Significant improvement from baseline in $FEV_1$ occurred 2 hours after initial administration in clinical trials.

**Time to peak plasma concentration**
1.7 hours.

## Precautions to Consider

**Carcinogenicity/Tumorigenicity**
A 2-year study in female mice given zileuton in doses of approximately four times the systemic exposure achieved at the maximum recommended human daily oral dose showed an increased incidence of liver, kidney, and vascular tumors. The same study in male mice given zileuton in doses of approximately seven times the systemic exposure achieved at the maximum recommended human daily oral dose showed a trend toward an increase in the incidence of liver tumors. Zileuton was not tumorigenic in mice given zileuton in doses of approximately two times the systemic exposure achieved at the maximum recommended human daily oral dose.

In rats, an increased incidence of kidney tumors was shown in females and males given zileuton in doses of approximately 14 and 6 times, respectively, the systemic exposure achieved at the maximum recommended human daily oral dose. Zileuton was not tumorigenic in male and female rats given doses of approximately four and six times, respectively, the systemic exposure achieved at the maximum recommended human daily oral dose.

**Mutagenicity**
Zileuton was not mutagenic in multiple *in vivo* and *in vitro* assays; however, the livers and kidneys of female mice treated with zileuton showed a dose-related increase in DNA adduct formation. Although some evidence of DNA damage was shown in the hepatocytes of *Aroclor 1254*–treated rats in an unscheduled DNA synthesis assay, the results of a similar study in monkeys were negative.

**Pregnancy/Reproduction**
Fertility—Zileuton produced no effects on fertility in male and female rats given oral doses of up to approximately 8 and 18 times, respectively, the systemic exposure achieved at the maximum recommended human daily oral dose. However, a reduction in rat fetal implantations was seen with oral doses of approximately nine times the systemic exposure achieved at the maximum recommended human daily oral dose. In addition, reduced rat pup survival and growth were noted following maternal oral doses of approximately 18 times the systemic exposure achieved at the maximum recommended human daily oral dose.

Pregnancy—Adequate and well-controlled studies have not been done in humans.

Zileuton and its metabolites cross the placenta in rats. When zileuton was administered orally to pregnant rats in doses of approximately 18 times the systemic exposure achieved at the maximum recommended human daily oral dose, the fetuses showed reduced body weight and increased skeletal variations.

Administration of zileuton to pregnant rabbits in doses equivalent to the maximum recommended human daily oral dose produced cleft palate in 2.5% of the fetuses.

FDA Pregnancy Category C.

**Breast-feeding**
It is not known whether zileuton is distributed into the breast milk of humans; however, the drug and its metabolites are distributed into the milk of lactating rats. Because of the potential for tumorigenicity shown in animal studies, use of zileuton during breast-feeding is not recommended.

**Pediatrics**
Appropriate studies on the relationship of age to the effects of zileuton have not been performed in the pediatric population. Safety and efficacy in children up to 12 years of age have not been established.

**Geriatrics**
In clinical studies, the pharmacokinetics of zileuton in healthy adults 65 years of age and older were similar to those of adults 18 to 40 years of age.

**Drug interactions and/or related problems**
The following drug interactions and/or related problems have been selected on the basis of their potential clinical significance (possible mechanism in parentheses where appropriate)—not necessarily inclusive (» = major clinical significance):

Note: Drug interaction studies have been conducted with zileuton and prednisone and with zileuton and ethinyl estradiol, an oral contraceptive; no significant interactions were shown.

Combinations containing any of the following medications, depending on the amount present, may also interact with this medication.

» Astemizole or
» Cisapride or
» Cyclosporine or
Dihydropyridine calcium channel blocking agents, such as:
» Felodipine or
» Isradipine or
» Nicardipine or
» Nifedipine or
» Nimodipine
(these medications are metabolized by the cytochrome P450 isoenzyme 3A4; although studies have not been done with zileuton and these medications, concurrent use should be monitored carefully, since zileuton is known to inhibit CYP3A4 *in vitro*)

» Beta-adrenergic blocking agents (systemic and ophthalmic)
(concurrent administration of zileuton and propranolol doubles the area under the plasma concentration–time curve and increases the pharmacologic effects of propranolol; although studies have not been done with other beta-adrenergic blocking agents, patients using beta-adrenergic blocking agents and zileuton should be monitored carefully)

» Terfenadine
(concurrent administration of recommended doses of terfenadine and zileuton for 7 days increased the mean area under the plasma concentration–time curve and peak serum concentration of terfenadine by approximately 35%; although no cardiac effects were noted, concurrent administration of these medications is not recommended)

» Theophylline
(concurrent administration of zileuton and theophylline approximately doubles the serum theophylline concentration; theophylline dosage should be reduced approximately by half and serum theophylline concentrations monitored closely in patients using these medications concurrently)

» Warfarin
(concurrent administration of zileuton and warfarin results in a clinically significant increase in the prothrombin time; prothrombin times should be monitored closely and warfarin dose adjusted accordingly in patients using these medications concurrently)

**Laboratory value alterations**
The following have been selected on the basis of their potential clinical significance (possible effect in parentheses where appropriate)—not necessarily inclusive (» = major clinical significance):

With physiology/laboratory test values
Transaminases, hepatic
(elevations of one or more liver function tests may occur during therapy with zileuton; the values may continue to rise, remain unchanged, or return to normal during continued therapy)

(if clinical signs or symptoms of hepatic function impairment or ALT values ≥ five times the upper limit of normal develop, therapy with zileuton should be stopped and ALT monitored until values return to normal)

(in clinical trials involving more than 5000 patients treated with zileuton, there was a 3.2% incidence of serum ALT values at least three times the upper limit of normal. One patient developed symptomatic hepatitis with jaundice that resolved following discontinuation of zileuton. Three patients with transaminase elevations developed hyperbilirubinemia that was less than three times the upper limit of normal. In subset analyses, females older than 65 years of age and patients with pre-existing transaminase elevations appeared to be at increased risk for ALT elevations)

**Medical considerations/Contraindications**
The medical considerations/contraindications included have been selected on the basis of their potential clinical significance (reasons given in parentheses where appropriate)—not necessarily inclusive (» = major clinical significance).

*Except under special circumstances, this medication should not be used when the following medical problems exist:*
» Hepatic disease, active
» Hepatic function impairment
(zileuton is not recommended in patients with active hepatic disease or transaminase elevations three times the upper limit of normal or greater)

*Risk-benefit should be considered when the following medical problems exist:*
» Alcoholism, active
(caution is recommended in patients taking zileuton who consume substantial quantities of alcohol because of possible hepatic function impairment)
Hypersensitivity to zileuton

**Patient monitoring**
The following may be especially important in patient monitoring (other tests may be warranted in some patients, depending on condition; » = major clinical significance):
» Alanine aminotransferase, serum (ALT [SGPT])
**(serum ALT determinations are recommended before treatment starts, once a month for the first 3 months, every 2 to 3 months for the remainder of the first year, and periodically thereafter during zileuton therapy)**
(if clinical signs or symptoms of hepatic function impairment or ALT values ≥ five times the upper limit of normal develop, therapy with zileuton should be stopped and ALT monitored until values return to normal)

## Side/Adverse Effects

Note: In clinical trials involving more than 5000 patients treated with zileuton, there was a 3.2% incidence of serum ALT values at least three times the upper limit of normal. One patient developed symptomatic hepatitis with jaundice that resolved following discontinuation of zileuton. Three patients with transaminase elevations developed hyperbilirubinemia that was less than three times the upper limit of normal. In subset analyses, females older than 65 years of age and patients with pre-existing transaminase elevations appeared to be at increased risk for ALT elevations.

The following side/adverse effects have been selected on the basis of their potential clinical significance (possible signs and symptoms in parentheses where appropriate)—not necessarily inclusive:

**Those indicating need for medical attention**
Incidence rare
*Hepatic function impairment* (flu-like symptoms; itching; nausea; right upper abdominal pain; unusual tiredness or weakness; yellow eyes or skin)

**Those indicating need for medical attention only if they continue or are bothersome**
Incidence more frequent
*Dyspepsia* (upset stomach); *nausea*
Incidence less frequent
*Abdominal pain; asthenia* (weakness)

## Patient Consultation

In providing consultation, consider emphasizing the following selected information (» = major clinical significance):

**Before using this medication**
» Conditions affecting use, especially:
Hypersensitivity to zileuton
Pregnancy—Risk-benefit should be considered because of the potential for fetal abnormalities shown in animal studies
Breast-feeding—Use is not recommended
Other medications, especially astemizole, beta-adrenergic blocking agents, cisapride, cyclosporine, felodipine, isradipine, nicardipine, nifedipine, nimodipine, terfenadine, theophylline, or warfarin
Other medical problems, especially active alcoholism, hepatic function impairment, or hepatic disease

**Proper use of this medication**
» Importance of not using this medication to treat acute asthma symptoms
» Proper dosing
Missed dose: Taking as soon as possible; if almost time for next dose, skipping missed dose; not doubling doses
» Proper storage

**Precautions while using this medication**
» Compliance with therapy by using every day in regularly spaced doses, even during symptom-free periods
» Importance of regular visits to physician to check progress and to test liver enzymes
» Checking with health care professional if more inhalations than usual of an inhaled, short-acting bronchodilator are needed to relieve an acute attack or if more than the maximum number of inhalations of the bronchodilator prescribed for a 24-hour period are needed
» Checking with health care professional before stopping or reducing therapy with any other asthma medications

**Side/adverse effects**
Signs of potential side effects, especially hepatic function impairment

## Oral Dosage Forms

### Zileuton Tablets

**Usual adult and adolescent dose**
Antiasthmatic—
Oral, 600 mg four times a day.

**Usual adult and adolescent prescribing limits**
2400 mg a day.

**Usual pediatric dose**
Children up to 12 years of age—Safety and efficacy have not been established.

**Usual geriatric dose**
Antiasthmatic—
See *Usual adult and adolescent dose*.

**Strength(s) usually available**
U.S.—
600 mg (Rx) [*Zyflo*].
Canada—
Not commercially available.

**Packaging and storage**
Store at controlled room temperature, between 20 and 25 °C (68 and 77 °F). Protect from light.

## Selected Bibliography

Sorkness CA. The use of 5-lipoxygenase inhibitors and leukotriene receptor antagonists in the treatment of chronic asthma. Pharmacotherapy 1997; 17(1 Pt 2): 50S-54S.

Developed: 12/29/97

---

**ZINC CHLORIDE**—See *Zinc Supplements (Systemic)*

---

**ZINC GLUCONATE**—See *Zinc Supplements (Systemic)*

---

**ZINC SULFATE**—See *Zinc Supplements (Systemic)*

# ZINC SUPPLEMENTS  Systemic

This monograph includes information on the following: 1) Zinc Chloride†; 2) Zinc Gluconate; 3) Zinc Sulfate.

VA CLASSIFICATION (Primary/Secondary): TN405/AD300

Commonly used brand name(s): *Orazinc*[2]; *PMS Egozinc*[3]; *Verazinc*[3]; *Zinc 15*[3]; *Zinc-220*[3]; *Zinca-Pak*[3]; *Zincate*[3].

Note: For a listing of dosage forms and brand names by country availability, see *Dosage Forms* section(s).

†Not commercially available in Canada.

## Category

Nutritional supplement (mineral); copper absorption inhibitor.

## Indications

Note: Bracketed information in the *Indications* section refers to uses that are not included in U.S. product labeling.

**Accepted**

Zinc deficiency (prophylaxis and treatment)—Zinc supplements are indicated in the prevention and treatment of zinc deficiency, which may result from inadequate nutrition or intestinal malabsorption and other conditions that interfere with zinc utilization or increase zinc losses from the body, but does not occur in healthy individuals receiving an adequate balanced diet. For prophylaxis of zinc deficiency, dietary improvement, rather than supplementation, is advisable. For treatment of zinc deficiency, supplementation is preferred.

Deficiency of zinc may lead to growth retardation, hypogonadism in males, anorexia (possibly due to changes in taste and smell), depressed mental function, dermatitis, impaired wound-healing, suppressed immune function, diarrhea, and abnormal vitamin A metabolism with impaired night vision.

Recommended intakes may be increased and/or supplementation may be necessary in the following conditions (based on documented zinc deficiency):
 Alcoholism
 Burns
 Cirrhosis of the liver
 Diabetes mellitus
 Eating disorders—anorexia nervosa, bulimia
 Gastrectomy
 Genetic disorders—acrodermatitis enteropathica, Down's syndrome, sickle cell anemia, thalassemia
 Hemodialysis
 Infants—premature
 Infections, chronic, due to decreased immune responses
 Intestinal diseases—celiac, Crohn's, diarrhea, sprue, ulcerative colitis
 Intestinal parasitism
 Malabsorption syndromes associated with pancreatic insufficiency—pancreatic disease, cystic fibrosis
 Renal diseases—nephrotic syndrome, renal failure, uremia
 Short bowel syndrome
 Skin disorders—exfoliative dermatoses, psoriasis
 Stress, prolonged
 Trauma, prolonged

Some unusual diets (e.g., reducing diets that drastically restrict food selection) may not supply minimum daily requirements of zinc. Supplementation may be necessary in patients receiving total parenteral nutrition (TPN) or undergoing rapid weight loss or in those with malnutrition, because of inadequate dietary intake.

Recommended intakes for all vitamins and most minerals are increased during pregnancy. Many physicians recommend that pregnant women receive multivitamin and mineral supplements, especially those pregnant women who do not consume an adequate diet and those in high-risk categories (i.e., women carrying more than one fetus, heavy cigarette smokers, and alcohol and drug abusers). However, taking excessive amounts of multivitamin and mineral supplements may be harmful to the mother and/or fetus and should be avoided.

There is some evidence that low serum zinc levels may lead to complications of pregnancy or congenital malformations.

Recommended intakes for all vitamins and most minerals are increased during breast-feeding.

Recommended intakes may be increased by the following: Folic acid, penicillamine, iron supplements, or thiazide diuretics.

[Wilson's disease (treatment adjunct)][1]—Zinc supplements have been used along with a reduced copper diet in the treatment of Wilson's disease in patients who are unable to tolerate penicillamine.

**Unaccepted**

A potential role for zinc in retarding the progression of age-related macular degeneration has not been proven. Zinc salts have not been found to be beneficial in the treatment of acute intermittent porphyria.

[1]Not included in Canadian product labeling.

## Pharmacology/Pharmacokinetics

**Physicochemical characteristics**

Molecular weight—
 Elemental zinc: 65.37.
 Zinc chloride: 136.3.
 Zinc gluconate: 455.68.
 Zinc sulfate: 287.5.

**Mechanism of action/Effect**

Nutritional supplement—Zinc is necessary for the proper functioning of over 200 metalloenzymes, including carbonic anhydrase, carboxypeptidase A, alcohol dehydrogenase, alkaline phosphatase, and RNA polymerase. It is also required to maintain structure in nucleic acids, proteins, and cell membranes. Physiological functions that are zinc dependent include cell growth and division, sexual maturation and reproduction, dark adaptation and night vision, wound-healing, host immunity, taste acuity, and possibly olfactory acuity.

Copper absorption inhibitor—Large doses of zinc inhibit the absorption of copper.

**Absorption**

Approximately 20 to 30% of dietary zinc is absorbed, primarily from the duodenum and ileum. The amount absorbed is dependent on the bioavailability from food. Zinc is the most bioavailable from red meat and oysters. Phytates may impair absorption by chelation and formation of insoluble complexes at an alkaline pH.

After absorption, zinc is bound in the intestine to the protein metallothionein.

Endogenous zinc can be reabsorbed in the ileum and colon, creating an enteropancreatic circulation of zinc.

**Protein binding**

Zinc is 60% bound to albumin; 30 to 40% bound to alpha-2 macroglobulin or transferrin; and 1% bound to amino acids, primarily histidine and cysteine.

**Storage**

Zinc is stored primarily in red and white blood cells, but also in the muscle, bone, skin, kidney, liver, pancreas, retina, and prostate.

**Time to peak concentration**

Approximately 2 hours.

**Elimination**

Primarily fecal (approximately 90%); to a lesser extent in the urine and in perspiration.

## Precautions to Consider

**Pregnancy/Reproduction**

Pregnancy—Problems in humans have not been documented with intake of normal daily recommended amounts. However, adequate and well controlled studies in humans have not been done.

Studies have not been done in animals.

FDA Pregnancy Category C (parenteral zinc).

**Breast-feeding**

Problems in humans have not been documented with intake of normal daily recommended amounts.

**Pediatrics**

Problems in pediatrics have not been documented with intake of normal daily recommended amounts.

Zinc injection that contains benzyl alcohol as a preservative should not be used in newborn and immature infants. The use of benzyl alcohol in neonates has been associated with a fatal toxic syndrome consisting of metabolic acidosis and CNS, respiratory, circulatory, and renal function impairment.

**Geriatrics**

Problems in geriatrics have not been documented with intake of normal daily recommended amounts. The elderly may be at risk of zinc deficiency due to poor food selection, decreased intestinal absorption of zinc, or medications which may decrease absorption or increase urinary loss of zinc.

**Drug interactions and/or related problems**
The following drug interactions and/or related problems have been selected on the basis of their potential clinical significance (possible mechanism in parentheses where appropriate)—not necessarily inclusive (» = major clinical significance):

Note: Combinations containing any of the following, depending on the amount present, may also interact with zinc supplements.

» Copper supplements
(large doses of zinc may inhibit copper absorption in the intestine; zinc supplements should be taken at least 2 hours after the administration of copper supplements)

Diuretics, thiazide
(thiazide diuretics have been found to increase urinary zinc excretion)

Fiber, found in bran, whole-grain breads and cereals or
Phosphorus-containing foods, such as milk or poultry or
Phytates, found in bran and whole-grain breads and cereals
(concurrent use of large amounts of fiber, phosphorus, or phytates with zinc supplements may reduce zinc absorption by formation of nonabsorbable complexes; foods containing fiber, phosphorus, or phytates should be taken at least 2 hours after zinc supplements)

Folic acid
(some studies have found that folate can decrease the absorption of zinc, but not in the presence of excessive zinc; other studies have found no inhibition)

Iron supplements, oral
(large doses of iron supplements can inhibit the intestinal absorption of zinc; this, at one time, was a problem in individuals taking commercial multivitamin-mineral preparations or infant formulas that had a high iron to zinc ratio; however, most firms in the U.S. have reformulated their products; zinc supplements should be taken at least 2 hours after iron supplements)

Penicillamine, and possibly other heavy metal chelators
(concurrent use may decrease the absorption of zinc; a period of 2 hours should elapse between administration of penicillamine and zinc)

Phosphorus-containing preparations
(concurrent use of phosphorus-containing preparations with zinc supplements may reduce zinc absorption by formation of nonabsorbable complexes; phosphorus-containing preparations should be taken 2 hours after zinc supplements)

» Tetracycline, oral
(zinc salts may decrease the absorption of tetracycline by forming insoluble chelates; zinc supplements should be given 2 hours after the administration of tetracycline)

Zinc-containing medications, other
(concurrent use with zinc supplements may increase serum zinc concentration)

**Laboratory value alterations**
The following have been selected on the basis of their potential clinical significance (possible effect in parentheses where appropriate)—not necessarily inclusive (» = major clinical significance):

With physiology/laboratory test values
Copper
(serum concentrations may be reduced with long-term, high-dose therapy with zinc)

**Medical considerations/Contraindications**
The medical considerations/contraindications included have been selected on the basis of their potential clinical significance (reasons given in parentheses where appropriate)—not necessarily inclusive (» = major clinical significance):

*Risk-benefit should be considered when the following medical problem exists:*

» Copper deficiency
(zinc supplementation may induce copper deficiency or further decrease serum copper concentrations)

**Patient monitoring**
The following may be especially important in patient monitoring (other tests may be warranted in some patients, depending on condition; » = major clinical significance):

Alkaline phosphatase
(monthly monitoring in patients with zinc deficiency is recommended; serum concentrations have been found to increase with zinc therapy)

Copper
(serum copper concentrations may be decreased with prolonged zinc therapy; monthly monitoring of copper may be required with long-term use)

High-density lipoprotein (HDL)
(serum concentrations may be decreased; monthly monitoring is recommended for patients receiving high doses of zinc for long periods of time)

Zinc, plasma or serum or urinary
(monthly monitoring is recommended; however, concentrations may not accurately reflect zinc status since plasma, serum, or urinary zinc concentrations are subject to many variables; zinc concentrations may be subject to a renal regulatory mechanism to conserve zinc; these factors should be considered when monitoring zinc status)

## Side/Adverse Effects

The following side/adverse effects have been selected on the basis of their potential clinical significance (possible signs and symptoms in parentheses where appropriate)—not necessarily inclusive:

**Those indicating need for medical attention**
Incidence rare—with large doses
*Gastrointestinal abnormalities, specifically dyspepsia* (indigestion); *epigastric pain* (heartburn); *or nausea; hematologic abnormalities, secondary to zinc-induced copper deficiency, specifically leukopenia* (fever, chills, or sore throat); *neutropenia* (continuing ulcers or sores in mouth or throat); *sideroblastic anemia* (unusual tiredness or weakness)

## Overdose

For specific information on the agents used in the management of zinc overdose, see:
• *Edetate Calcium Disodium (Systemic)* monograph.

For more information on the management of overdose or unintentional ingestion, **contact a Poison Control Center** (See *Poison Control Center Listing*).

**Clinical effects of overdose**
The following effects have been selected on the basis of their potential clinical significance (possible signs and symptoms in parentheses where appropriate)—not necessarily inclusive:
*Hypotension* (dizziness or fainting); *jaundice* (yellow eyes or skin); *pulmonary edema* (chest pain or shortness of breath); *vomiting*

**Treatment of overdose**
Dilute with milk or water.
Specific treatment—
Intramuscular or intravenous edetate calcium disodium at a dose of 50 to 75 mg per kg (mg/kg) of body weight per day, in 3 to 6 divided doses, for up to 5 days.

## Patient Consultation

As an aid to patient consultation, refer to *Advice for the Patient, Zinc Supplements (Systemic)*.
In providing consultation, consider emphasizing the following selected information (» = major clinical significance):

**Description of use**
Description should include function in the body, signs of deficiency, conditions that may cause zinc deficiency, and unproven uses

**Importance of diet**
Importance of proper nutrition; supplement may be needed because of inadequate dietary intake
Food sources of zinc; effects of processing
Recommended daily intake for zinc

**Before using this dietary supplement**
» Conditions affecting use, especially:
Pregnancy—Low serum zinc levels may be associated with pregnancy complications or congenital malformations
Use in the elderly—May be at risk for zinc deficiency
Other medications or dietary supplements, especially oral copper supplements and oral tetracycline
Other medical problems, especially copper deficiency

**Proper use of this dietary supplement**
» Proper dosing
Taking at least 1 hour before or 2 hours after meals, unless gastrointestinal irritation develops
Missed dose: No cause for concern because of length of time necessary for depletion; remembering to take as directed

» Proper storage

**Precautions while using this dietary supplement**
Taking zinc supplements 2 hours before eating fiber-containing foods, such as bran or whole-grain breads and cereals or phosphorus-containing foods such as milk, or poultry
Not taking zinc supplements within 2 hours of iron, copper, or phosphorus supplements

**Side/adverse effects**
Signs of potential side effects, especially gastrointestinal or hematologic abnormalities

## General Dosing Information

Because of the infrequency of zinc deficiency alone, combinations of several vitamins and/or minerals are commonly administered. Many commercial vitamin-mineral complexes are available.

**For parenteral dosage forms only**
In most cases, parenteral administration is indicated only when oral administration is not acceptable (for example, in nausea, vomiting, preoperative and postoperative conditions) or possible (for example, in malabsorption syndromes or following gastric resection).

**Diet/Nutrition**
Zinc supplements should be taken at least 1 hour before or 2 hours after meals, since many foods may impair the absorption of zinc. If gastric irritation occurs, then zinc supplements may be taken with meals; however, the zinc will be less bioavailable.
Recommended dietary intakes for zinc are defined differently worldwide.
For U.S—
The Recommended Dietary Allowances (RDAs) for vitamins and minerals are determined by the Food and Nutrition Board of the National Research Council and are intended to provide adequate nutrition in most healthy persons under usual environmental stresses. In addition, a different designation may be used by the FDA for food and dietary supplement labeling purposes, as with Daily Value (DV). DVs replace the previous labeling terminology United States Recommended Daily Allowances (USRDAs).
For Canada—
Recommended Nutrient Intakes (RNIs) for vitamins, minerals, and protein are determined by Health and Welfare Canada and provide recommended amounts of a specific nutrient while minimizing the risk of chronic diseases.
Daily recommended intakes for elemental zinc are generally defined as follows:

| Persons | U.S. (mg) | Canada (mg) |
|---|---|---|
| Infants and children | | |
| Birth to 3 years of age | 5–10 | 2–4 |
| 4 to 6 years of age | 10 | 5 |
| 7 to 10 years of age | 10 | 7–9 |
| Adolescent and adult males | 15 | 9–12 |
| Adolescent and adult females | 12 | 9 |
| Pregnant females | 15 | 15 |
| Breast-feeding females | 16–19 | 15 |

The best sources of zinc include lean red meats, seafoods (especially herring and oysters), peas, and beans. Zinc is found in whole-grains; however, large amounts of whole-grain foods have been found to reduce zinc absorption. Zinc has been reported to leach from galvanized cookware or storage containers in the presence of acidic foods, causing toxicity. Foods stored in unlacquered tin containers may cause a decrease in zinc available for absorption.

---

### ZINC CHLORIDE

## Parenteral Dosage Forms

Note: Injectable zinc products must be diluted prior to intravenous administration.

### ZINC CHLORIDE INJECTION USP

**Usual adult and adolescent dose**
Deficiency (prophylaxis or treatment)—
Intravenous infusion, 2.5 to 4 mg of elemental zinc a day, added to total parenteral nutrition (TPN).
Note: Some clinicians recommend doses as high as 12 mg per day to allow for excessive zinc losses that may occur with conditions such as diarrhea.

**Usual pediatric dose**
Deficiency (prophylaxis or treatment)—
Intravenous infusion: For full term infants and children up to 5 years of age—100 mcg of elemental zinc per kg of body weight a day, added to TPN.
For premature infants (up to 3 kg of body weight)—300 mcg of elemental zinc per kg of body weight a day, added to TPN.
Note: Zinc injection that contains benzyl alcohol as a preservative should not be used in newborn and immature infants. The use of benzyl alcohol in neonates has been associated with a fatal toxic syndrome consisting of metabolic acidosis and CNS, respiratory, circulatory, and renal function impairment.

**Strength(s) usually available**
U.S.—
1 mg of elemental zinc (2.09 mg zinc chloride) per mL (Rx) [GENERIC].
Canada—
Not commercially available.

**Packaging and storage**
Store below 40 °C (104 °F), preferably between 15 and 30 °C (59 and 86 °F), unless otherwise specified by manufacturer. Protect from freezing.

**Preparation of dosage form**
Zinc chloride is physically compatible with amino acid solutions, dextrose solutions, and injectable vitamin preparations.

---

### ZINC GLUCONATE

## Oral Dosage Forms

Note: Bracketed uses in the *Dosage Forms* section refer to categories of use and/or indications that are not included in U.S. product labeling.

### ZINC GLUCONATE LOZENGES

**Usual adult and adolescent dose**
Deficiency (prophylaxis)—
Oral, amount based on normal daily recommended intakes of elemental zinc:

| Persons | U.S. (mg) | Canada (mg) |
|---|---|---|
| Adolescent and adult males | 15 | 9–12 |
| Adolescent and adult females | 12 | 9 |
| Pregnant females | 15 | 15 |
| Breast-feeding females | 16–19 | 15 |

Deficiency (treatment)—
Treatment dose is individualized by prescriber based on severity of deficiency.
[Copper absorption inhibitor][1]—
Oral, 50 mg of elemental zinc three times a day.

**Usual pediatric dose**
Deficiency (prophylaxis)—
Oral, amount based on normal daily recommended intakes of elemental zinc:

| Persons | U.S. (mg) | Canada (mg) |
|---|---|---|
| Infants and children | | |
| Birth to 3 years of age | 5–10 | 2–4 |
| 4 to 6 years of age | 10 | 5 |
| 7 to 10 years of age | 10 | 7–9 |

Deficiency (treatment)—
Treatment dose is individualized by prescriber based on severity of deficiency.
[Copper absorption inhibitor][1]—
Oral, 22.5 to 34 mg of elemental zinc three times a day.

**Strength(s) usually available**
U.S.—
1.4 mg elemental zinc (10 mg zinc gluconate) (OTC) [*Orazinc*].
Canada—
Not commercially available.

Note: The strength of this zinc preparation may exceed the dosage range recommended by USP DI Advisory Panels based on the amount necessary to meet normal nutritional needs.

**Packaging and storage**
Store below 40 °C (104 °F), preferably between 15 and 30 °C (59 and 86 °F), unless otherwise specified by manufacturer. Store in a tight container.

## ZINC GLUCONATE TABLETS

**Usual adult and adolescent dose**
See *Zinc Gluconate Lozenges*.

**Usual pediatric dose**
See *Zinc Gluconate Lozenges*.

**Strength(s) usually available**
U.S.—
    1.4 mg of elemental zinc (10 mg zinc gluconate) (OTC) [GENERIC].
    2 mg of elemental zinc (15 mg zinc gluconate) (OTC) [GENERIC].
    4 mg of elemental zinc (30 mg zinc gluconate) (OTC) [GENERIC].
    7 mg of elemental zinc (50 mg zinc gluconate) (OTC) [GENERIC].
    8 mg of elemental zinc (60 mg zinc gluconate) (OTC) [GENERIC].
    11 mg of elemental zinc (78 mg zinc gluconate) (OTC) [GENERIC].
    13 mg of elemental zinc (100 mg zinc gluconate) (OTC) [GENERIC].
    31 mg of elemental zinc (235 mg zinc gluconate) (OTC) [GENERIC].
    52 mg of elemental zinc (390 mg zinc gluconate) (OTC) [GENERIC].
Canada—
    10 mg of elemental zinc (70 mg zinc gluconate) (OTC) [GENERIC].
    50 mg of elemental zinc (350 mg zinc gluconate) (OTC) [GENERIC].

Note: The strength of these zinc preparations may exceed the dosage range recommended by USP DI Advisory Panels based on the amount necessary to meet normal nutritional needs.

**Packaging and storage**
Store below 40 °C (104 °F), preferably between 15 and 30 °C (59 and 86 °F), unless otherwise specified by manufacturer. Store in a tight container.

[1]Not included in Canadian product labeling.

---

## ZINC SULFATE

# Oral Dosage Forms

Note: Bracketed uses in the *Dosage Forms* section refer to categories of use and/or indications that are not included in U.S. product labeling.

## ZINC SULFATE CAPSULES

**Usual adult and adolescent dose**
Deficiency (prophylaxis)—
    Oral, amount based on normal daily recommended intakes of elemental zinc:

| Persons | U.S. (mg) | Canada (mg) |
|---|---|---|
| Adolescent and adult males | 15 | 9–12 |
| Adolescent and adult females | 12 | 9 |
| Pregnant females | 15 | 15 |
| Breast-feeding females | 16–19 | 15 |

Deficiency (treatment)—
    Treatment dose is individualized by prescriber based on severity of deficiency.
[Copper absorption inhibitor][1]—
    Oral, 50 mg elemental zinc three times a day.

**Usual pediatric dose**
Deficiency (prophylaxis)—
    Oral, amount based on normal daily recommended intakes of elemental zinc:

| Persons | U.S. (mg) | Canada (mg) |
|---|---|---|
| Infants and children | | |
|   Birth to 3 years of age | 5–10 | 2–4 |
|   4 to 6 years of age | 10 | 5 |
|   7 to 10 years of age | 10 | 7–9 |

Deficiency (treatment)—
    Treatment dose is individualized by prescriber based on severity of deficiency.
[Copper absorption inhibitor][1]—
    Oral, 22.5 to 34 mg elemental zinc three times a day.

**Strength(s) usually available**
U.S.—
    25 mg elemental zinc (110 mg zinc sulfate) (OTC) [*Orazinc;* GENERIC].
    50 mg elemental zinc (220 mg zinc sulfate) [*Orazinc (OTC)* (OTC); *Verazinc (OTC)* (OTC); *Zinc-220 (OTC)* (OTC); *Zincate (Rx)* (Rx); GENERIC (Rx/OTC)].
Canada—
    Not commercially available.

Note: The strength of these zinc preparations may exceed the dosage range recommended by USP DI Advisory Panels based on the amount necessary to meet normal nutritional needs.

**Packaging and storage**
Store below 40 °C (104 °F), preferably between 15 and 30 °C (59 and 86 °F), unless otherwise specified by manufacturer. Store in a tight container.

## ZINC SULFATE TABLETS

**Usual adult and adolescent dose**
See *Zinc Sulfate Capsules*.

**Usual pediatric dose**
See *Zinc Sulfate Capsules*.

**Strength(s) usually available**
U.S.—
    15 mg elemental zinc (66 mg zinc sulfate) (OTC) [*Zinc 15*].
    25 mg elemental zinc (110 mg zinc sulfate) (OTC) [*Orazinc;* GENERIC].
    45 mg elemental zinc (200 mg zinc sulfate) (Rx/OTC) [].
    50 mg elemental zinc (220 mg zinc sulfate) (Rx) [GENERIC].
Canada—
    50 mg elemental zinc (220 mg zinc sulfate) (OTC) [*PMS Egozinc*].

Note: The strength of these zinc preparations may exceed the dosage range recommended by USP DI Advisory Panels based on the amount necessary to meet normal nutritional needs.

**Packaging and storage**
Store below 40 °C (104 °F), preferably between 15 and 30 °C (59 and 86 °F), unless otherwise specified by manufacturer. Store in a tight container.

## ZINC SULFATE EXTENDED-RELEASE TABLETS

**Usual adult and adolescent dose**
See *Zinc Sulfate Capsules*.

**Usual pediatric dose**
See *Zinc Sulfate Capsules*.

**Strength(s) usually available**
U.S.—
    50 mg elemental zinc (220 mg zinc sulfate) (OTC) [GENERIC].
Canada—
    Not commercially available.

Note: The strength of this zinc preparation may exceed the dosage range recommended by USP DI Advisory Panels based on the amount necessary to meet normal nutritional needs.

**Packaging and storage**
Store below 40 °C (104 °F), preferably between 15 and 30 °C (59 and 86 °F), unless otherwise specified by manufacturer. Store in a tight container.

# Parenteral Dosage Forms

## ZINC SULFATE INJECTION USP

Note: **Injectable zinc products must be diluted prior to intravenous administration.**

**Usual adult and adolescent dose**
Deficiency (prophylaxis or treatment)—
    Intravenous infusion, 2.5 to 4 mg of elemental zinc a day, added to total parenteral nutrition (TPN).

Note: Some clinicians recommend doses as high as 12 mg per day to allow for excessive zinc losses that may occur with conditions such as diarrhea.

**Usual pediatric dose**
Deficiency (prophylaxis or treatment)—
    Intravenous infusion: For full term infants and children up to 5 years of age: 100 mcg of elemental zinc per kg of body weight a day, added to TPN.
    For premature infants (up to 3 kg of body weight): 300 mcg of elemental zinc per kg of body weight a day added to TPN.

Note: Zinc injection that contains benzyl alcohol as a preservative should not be used in newborn and immature infants. The use of benzyl alcohol in neonates has been associated with a fatal toxic syndrome consisting of metabolic acidosis and CNS, respiratory, circulatory, and renal function impairment.

**Strength(s) usually available**
U.S.—
    1 mg of elemental zinc (4.39 mg zinc sulfate) per mL (Rx) [*Zinca-Pak* (0.9% benzyl alcohol); GENERIC].
    5 mg of elemental zinc (21.95 mg zinc sulfate) per mL (Rx) [*Zinca-Pak;* GENERIC].

# ZOLMITRIPTAN Systemic—INTRODUCTORY VERSION

VA CLASSIFICATION (Primary): CN105

Note: For a listing of dosage forms and brand names by country availability, see *Dosage Forms* section(s).

## Category
Antimigraine agent.

## Indications

**General considerations**
Zolmitriptan should only be prescribed for patients who have an established clear diagnosis of migraine.

**Accepted**
Headache, migraine (treatment)—Zolmitriptan is indicated to relieve (abort) acute migraine headaches (with or without aura).

**Unaccepted**
Zolmitriptan is not recommended for treatment of basilar artery migraine or hemiplegic migraine. Efficacy and safety of zolmitriptan in these conditions have not been established.

Zolmitriptan is not recommended for treatment of cluster headaches. Efficacy and safety of zolmitriptan in this condition have not been established.

## Pharmacology/Pharmacokinetics

**Physicochemical characteristics**
Source—Synthetic. Zolmitriptan is structurally related to serotonin (5-hydroxytryptamine, 5-HT).
Molecular weight—287.36.

**Mechanism of action/Effect**
Zolmitriptan's mechanism of action has not been established. It is thought that agonist activity at the $5-HT_{1D}$ and $5-HT_{1B}$ receptor subtypes provides relief of headaches. Zolmitriptan is a highly selective agonist at these receptor subtypes; it has no significant activity at $5-HT_2$, $5-HT_3$, or $5-HT_4$ receptor subtypes or at adrenergic, dopaminergic, histamine, or muscarinic receptors. However, zolmitriptan has moderate activity at the $5-HT_{1A}$ receptor subtype. It has been proposed that constriction of cerebral blood vessels resulting from $5-HT_{1D/1B}$ receptor stimulation reduces the pulsation that may be responsible for the pain of vascular headaches. It has also been proposed that zolmitriptan may relieve migraines by decreasing the release of neuropeptides.

**Absorption**
Oral—Rapid; bioavailability is moderate (40%). The rate and extent of absorption are not affected by administration with food.

**Protein binding**
Low (25%).

**Biotransformation**
Hepatic; three metabolites have been identified: indole acetic acid, *N*-oxide, and *N*-desmethyl metabolites. However, *N*-desmethyl is the only active metabolite.

**Half-life**
Elimination—
 Zolmitriptan: Approximately 3 hours.
 *N*-desmethyl metabolite: Approximately 3 hours.

**Time to peak concentration**
Within 2 hours.

**Elimination**
Renal—65% (8% of the dose as unchanged zolmitriptan; 31% as the indole acetic acid metabolite; 7% as the *N*-oxide metabolite; 4% as the *N*-desmethyl metabolite.
Fecal—30%.

## Precautions to Consider

**Carcinogenicity/Tumorigenicity**
In 85- and 92-week carcinogenicity studies in male and female mice, respectively, given zolmitriptan by oral gavage at doses of 400 mg per kg of body weight (mg/kg) (quantities sufficient to achieve peak concentrations of up to 800 times the maximum recommended human dose [MRHD]), no evidence of tumorigenicity was found. However, in a 104- to 105-week study in rats, the high-dose male and female rats were sacrificed, due to excess mortality, after receiving zolmitriptan 400 mg/kg per day for 101 weeks and 86 weeks, respectively. Although there was no evidence of tumorigenicity in male rats receiving 400 mg/kg per day of zolmitriptan (quantities sufficient to achieve peak concentrations approximately 3000 times the MRHD), an increased incidence of thyroid follicular cell hyperplasia and thyroid follicular cell adenomas occurred in male rats.

**Mutagenicity**
Zolmitriptan demonstrated mutagenic effects in two of five strains of *Salmonella typhimurium* tested in an Ames test in the presence of metabolic activation. However, no mutagenic activity was found in an *in vitro* mammalian gene cell mutation assay. There was evidence of clastogenic activity in an *in vitro* human lymphocyte assay, with and without metabolic activation, but no evidence of clastogenic activity was observed in the *in vivo* mouse micronucleus assay. Also, there was no genotoxicity observed in an unscheduled DNA synthesis study.

**Pregnancy/Reproduction**
Fertility—Reproduction studies in male and female rats given zolmitriptan doses of up to 400 mg per kg of body weight (mg/kg) per day (approximately 3000 times the maximum recommended human dose [MRHD]) found no effect on fertility.

Pregnancy—Adequate and well-controlled trials have not been done in pregnant women.

Reproductive toxicity studies in pregnant rats and rabbits found evidence of embryolethality and fetal abnormalities. During the organogenesis period, studies in pregnant rats receiving doses of 100, 400, and 1200 mg/kg per day (approximately 280, 1100, and 5000 times the MRHD, respectively) resulted in a dose-related increase in embryolethality. The higher dose was found to be maternotoxic, which resulted in decreased maternal body weight gain during gestation. In a study in rabbits, embryolethality was increased at maternally toxic doses of 10 and 30 mg/kg per day (equivalent to 11 and 42 times the MRHD, respectively). In addition, at doses of 30 mg/kg per day there was evidence of an increase in fetal malformations, such as fused sternebrae, rib anomalies, major blood vessel variations, and an irregular ossification pattern of ribs. Also, hydronephrosis was observed in the offspring of female rats receiving zolmitriptan 400 mg/kg per day (approximately 1100 times the MRHD).

FDA Pregnancy Category C.

**Breast-feeding**
It is not known whether zolmitriptan is distributed into breast milk.
Zolmitriptan was found to be distributed into the milk of lactating rats. The concentration of zolmitriptan in the rat milk was equivalent to maternal plasma concentrations at 1 hour and four times higher than maternal plasma concentrations at 4 hours.

**Pediatrics**
Appropriate studies on the relationship of age to the effects of zolmitriptan have not been performed in children up to 12 years of age.

**Adolescents**
Appropriate studies performed to date have not demonstrated pediatrics-specific problems that would limit the usefulness of zolmitriptan in adolescents.

**Geriatrics**
No information is available on the relationship of age to the effects of zolmitriptan in geriatric patients.

### Drug interactions and/or related problems
The following drug interactions and/or related problems have been selected on the basis of their potential clinical significance (possible mechanism in parentheses where appropriate)—not necessarily inclusive (» = major clinical significance):

Note: Combinations containing any of the following medications, depending on the amount present, may also interact with this medication.

Cimetidine
(concurrent use of cimetidine and zolmitriptan may cause an increase in half-life and area under the plasma concentration–time curve of zolmitriptan)

Dihydroergotamine or
Ergotamine or
Methysergide or
Other 5-hydroxytryptamine agonists such as:
Sumatriptan
(a delay of 24 hours between administration of dihydroergotamine, ergotamine, methysergide, or other 5-hydroxytryptamine agonists and zolmitriptan is recommended because of the possibility of additive and/or prolonged vasoconstriction)

Selective serotonin reuptake inhibitors, such as:
Fluoxetine
Fluvoxamine
Paroxetine
Sertraline
(concurrent use may result in weakness, hyperreflexia, and incoordination; monitoring is recommended)

» Monoamine oxidase-A (MAO-A) inhibitors, including furazolidone, procarbazine, and selegiline
(concurrent use may increase systemic exposure of zolmitriptan; zolmitriptan should not be taken during or within 14 days following administration of an MAO-A inhibitor)

### Laboratory value alterations
The following have been selected on the basis of their potential clinical significance (possible effect in parentheses where appropriate)—not necessarily inclusive (» = major clinical significance):

With physiology/laboratory test values
Blood pressure
(may be increased; in healthy volunteers blood pressure elevations [increase in systolic and diastolic by 1 mm Hg and 5 mm Hg, respectively] occurred in patients receiving a 5-mg dose; however, a small study evaluating patients with moderate to severe liver disease receiving a 10-mg dose, resulted in elevations in systolic and/or diastolic pressure [20 mm Hg to 80 mm Hg]; monitoring is recommended in patients with hepatic impairment and hepatic disease)

### Medical considerations/Contraindications
The medical considerations/contraindications included have been selected on the basis of their potential clinical significance (reasons given in parentheses where appropriate)—not necessarily inclusive (» = major clinical significance).

*Except under special circumstances, this medication should not be used when the following medical problems exist:*

» Cardiac arrythmias or
» Wolff-Parkinson-White syndrome
(may exacerbate condition)

» Coronary artery disease, especially:
Angina pectoris
Myocardial infarction, history of
Myocardial ischemia, silent, documented
Prinzmetal's angina or

» Other conditions in which coronary vasoconstriction would be detrimental
(zolmitriptan may cause coronary vasospasms)

» Hypertension, uncontrolled
(may be exacerbated)

*Risk-benefit should be considered when the following medical problems exist:*

» Cerebrovascular accident, history of
(zolmitriptan may cause cerebral hemorrhage, subarachnoid hemorrhage, or stroke; caution should be used when administering in patients at risk for cerebrovascular events)

» Coronary artery disease, predisposition to
(zolmitriptan may cause serious coronary adverse effects; patients in whom coronary artery disease is a possibility on the basis of age or the presence of other risk factors, such as diabetes, hypercholesterolemia, obesity, a strong family history of coronary artery disease, or tobacco smoking, should be evaluated for the presence of cardiovascular disease before zolmitriptan is prescribed; even after a satisfactory evaluation, the advisability of administering the patient's first dose under medical supervision should be considered)

» Hepatic disease or
» Hepatic function impairment, severe or
Renal function impairment, severe
(studies have shown a decreased clearance in zolmitriptan in patients with severe renal or hepatic impairment; caution is recommended; a dosage adjustment is recommended in patients with hepatic impairment and hepatic disease)

» Hypertension, controlled
(may precipitate an increase in systolic and diastolic blood pressure)

» Hypersensitivity to zolmitriptan

### Patient monitoring
The following may be especially important in patient monitoring (other tests may be warranted in some patients, depending on condition; » = major clinical significance):

Blood pressure determinations
(monitoring is recommended for patients with hepatic impairment)

Electrocardiogram (ECG)
(monitoring is recommended for long-term intermittent users of zolmitriptan)

## Side/Adverse Effects
The following side/adverse effects have been selected on the basis of their potential clinical significance (possible signs and symptoms in parentheses where appropriate)—not necessarily inclusive:

### Those indicating need for medical attention
Incidence more frequent
*Chest pain, severe; heaviness, tightness, or pressure in chest and/or neck; paresthesias* (sensation of burning, warmth, heat, numbness, tightness, or tingling)

Note: Although *chest pain and heaviness, tightness, or pressure in the chest and/or neck* are suggestive of angina pectoris, monitoring of the electrocardiogram (ECG) during such symptoms in clinical studies failed to detect evidence of myocardial ischemia or arrythmias. Zolmitriptan-induced coronary artery vasospasm resulting in symptomatic myocardial ischemia and myocardial infarction have not been documented in patients taking zolmitriptan.

Incidence less frequent
*Arrythmias* (irregular heartbeat); *gastroenteritis* (severe abdominal pain; diarrhea; loss of appetite; nausea; weakness)

Incidence rare
*Leukopenia* (fever or chills; cough or hoarseness; lower back or side pain; painful or difficult urination)

### Those indicating need for medical attention only if they continue or are bothersome
Incidence more frequent
*Asthenia* (unusual tiredness or muscle weakness); *dizziness; nausea; somnolence* (sleepiness)

Incidence less frequent
*Central nervous system effects, including agitation; anxiety; and depression; discomfort in jaw, mouth, or throat; dry mouth; dyspepsia* (heartburn); *dysphagia* (difficulty swallowing); *ecchymosis* (large, nonelevated blue or purplish patches in the skin); *edema* (swelling of face, fingers, feet and/or lower legs); *hypertension* (increased blood pressure); *myalgia* (muscle aches); *palpitations* (pounding heartbeat); *polyuria* (sudden, large increase in frequency and quantity of urine); *pruritus* (itching of the skin); *skin rash; sweating; syncope* (fainting)

## Overdose
For more information on the management of overdose or unintentional ingestion, **contact a Poison Control Center** (see *Poison Control Center Listing*).

### Treatment of overdose
Monitoring—Patients should be monitored for at least 15 hours after an overdose of zolmitriptan.

Supportive care—Maintaining an open airway and breathing, maintaining proper fluid and electrolyte balance, and/or correcting hypertension. Patients in whom intentional overdose is confirmed or suspected should be referred for psychiatric consultation.

## Patient Consultation

As an aid to patient consultation, refer to *Advice for the Patient, Zolmitriptan (Systemic)—Introductory Version*.

In providing consultation, consider emphasizing the following selected information (» = major clinical significance):

### Before using this medication
» Conditions affecting use, especially:
    Sensitivity to zolmitriptan
    Other medications, especially monamine oxidase inhibitors
    Other medical problems, especially cardiac arrythmias, cerebrovascular accident (history of), coronary artery disease, predisposition to coronary artery disease, or other conditions that may be adversely affected by coronary artery constriction, hepatic disease, hepatic function impairment (severe), hypertension, Wolf-Parkinson-White syndrome

### Proper use of this medication
» Not administering if atypical headache symptoms are present; checking with physician instead
    Administering after onset of headache pain
    Additional benefit may be obtained if the patient lies down in a quiet, dark room after administering medication
» Not using additional doses if first dose does not provide substantial relief; additional zolmitriptan is not likely to be effective in these circumstances; taking alternate medication as previously advised by physician, then checking with physician as soon as possible
    Taking additional doses, if needed, for return of migraine after initial relief was obtained, provided that prescribed limits (quantity used and frequency of administration) are not exceeded
    Compliance with prophylactic therapy, if prescribed
» Proper dosing
» Proper storage

### Precautions while using this medication
Avoiding alcohol, which aggravates headache
» Caution when driving or doing anything else requiring alertness because of possible drowsiness, dizziness, lightheadedness, impairment of physical or mental abilities

### Side/adverse effects
Signs of potential side effects, especially chest pain, severe; heaviness, tightness, or pressure in chest and/or neck; paresthesias; arrhythmias; gastroenteritis; leukopenia

## Oral Dosage Forms

### ZOLMITRIPTAN TABLETS

**Usual adult**
Antimigraine agent—
    Oral, initially 2.5 mg or lower (tablet may be broken in half). If necessary, additional doses may be taken at intervals of at least two hours.
    A single dose of less than 2.5 mg is recommended for patients with hepatic disease or impairment.

**Usual adult limits**
10 mg in twenty-four hours.

**Usual pediatric dose**
Safety and efficacy have not been established in children up to 12 years of age.

**Usual geriatric dose**
See *Usual adult dose*.

**Strength(s) usually available**
U.S.—
    2.5 mg (Rx) [*Zomig* (anhydrous lactose; microcrystalline cellulose; sodium starch glycolate; magnesium stearate; hydroxypropyl methylcellulose; titanium dioxide; polyethylene glycol 400; yellow iron oxide; red iron oxide; polyethylene glycol 8000)].
    5 mg (Rx) [*Zomig* (anhydrous lactose; microcrystalline cellulose; sodium starch glycolate; magnesium stearate; hydroxypropyl methylcellulose; titanium dioxide; polyethylene glycol 400; yellow iron oxide; red iron oxide; polyethylene glycol 8000)].

**Packaging and storage**
Store at room temperature, preferably between 20 and 25 °C (68 and 77 °F).

Developed: 04/09/98

---

# ZOLPIDEM Systemic†

VA CLASSIFICATION (Primary): CN309
Note: Controlled substance in the U.S.—Schedule IV.
Commonly used brand name(s): *Ambien*.
Note: For a listing of dosage forms and brand names by country availability, see *Dosage Forms* section(s).

†Not commercially available in Canada.

## Category
Sedative-hypnotic.

## Indications

**Accepted**
Insomnia (treatment)—Zolpidem is indicated for short-term treatment of insomnia. Failure of insomnia to remit after 7 to 10 days of treatment may indicate the presence of a primary psychiatric or medical illness. Worsening of insomnia or the emergence of new abnormalities of thinking or behavior may be the consequence of an unrecognized psychiatric or physical disorder.

## Pharmacology/Pharmacokinetics

**Physicochemical characteristics**
Chemical group—Imidazopyridinesedative hypnotic structurally unrelated to benzodiazepines, barbiturates, or other available sedative-hypnotics.
Molecular weight—764.9.
pKa—6.16.

**Mechanism of action/Effect**
Zolpidem is a potent agonist with high intrinsic activity at the omega ($\omega$) 1 subtype (also called the benzodiazepine 1 [$BZ_1$] subtype) of the gamma-aminobutyric acid type A ($GABA_A$) receptor-chloride ionophore complex. The omega 1 $GABA_A$ receptor is thought to be located primarily in the cerebellum, sensory-motor cortex, substantia nigra, inferior colliculus, olfactory bulb, ventral thalamic complex, pons, and globus pallidus in the central nervous system (CNS). The receptor complex resides on neuronal membranes and functions in the gating of the chloride channel. Activation of the $GABA_A$ receptor results in the opening of the chloride channel, allowing the flow of chloride ions through the neuronal membrane and into the neuron. This results in hyperpolarization, which inhibits firing of that neuron.
In contrast to the benzodiazepines, which bind non-selectively to the omega 1, omega 2, and omega 3 $GABA_A$ receptors, zolpidem possesses relative selectivity for the omega 1 $GABA_A$ receptor. This preference for the omega 1 $GABA_A$ receptor may account for zolpidem's relative lack of anticonvulsant, myorelaxant, and anxiolytic effects at therapeutic doses, and for the general preservation of sleep architecture seen with zolpidem use.

**Absorption**
Rapid and complete, although first-pass metabolism results in 70% bioavailability. Food may decrease the rate and extent of absorption.

**Distribution**
The volume of distribution ($Vol_D$) of zolpidem in healthy volunteers was 0.54 L per kg (L/kg) following an 8 mg intravenous dose. Zolpidem is distributed into breast milk; amounts ranging from 0.004 to 0.019% of a 20-mg oral dose were present in milk samples taken 3 hours following administration.

**Protein binding**
Very high (92%).

**Biotransformation**
Hepatic, resulting in 3 major and several minor metabolites, all of which are inactive.

**Half-life**
Elimination—
    2.6 hours (range, 1.4 to 4.5 hours). The elimination half-life of zolpidem is prolonged in the elderly and in patients with impaired hepatic or renal function.

**Onset of action**
Rapid.

### Time to peak concentration
30 minutes to 2 hours; may be longer if zolpidem is taken with food

### Peak serum concentration
Mean peak plasma concentration ($C_{max}$) following oral administration of 5 mg of zolpidem to healthy volunteers was 59 nanograms per mL (nanograms/mL) (0.077 micromoles per L [micromoles/L]), with a range of 29 to 113 nanograms/mL (0.038 to 0.148 micromoles/L); $C_{max}$ following administration of 10 mg of zolpidem was 121 nanograms/mL (0.158 micromoles/L) with a range of 58 to 272 nanograms/mL (0.076 to 0.356 micromoles/L).

### Elimination
Renal—
   48 to 67% of a single dose is eliminated in the urine. Unchanged zolpidem is present in trace amounts in urine and feces.
Fecal—
   29 to 42% of a single dose is eliminated in the feces. Unchanged zolpidem is present in trace amounts in urine and feces.
In dialysis—
   Not hemodialyzable.

## Precautions to Consider

### Carcinogenicity/Tumorigenicity
No evidence of carcinogenic potential was observed in mice administered zolpidem in doses of 4, 18, and 80 mg per kg of body weight (mg/kg) per day (26 to 520 times the recommended human dose of 10 mg per day on a mg/kg basis) for 2 years. In rats administered zolpidem in doses of 4, 18, and 80 mg/kg per day (43 to 876 times the recommended human dose on a mg/kg basis) for 2 years, the incidences of lipoma and liposarcoma were comparable to those seen in historical controls.

### Mutagenicity
Zolpidem showed no evidence of mutagenicity based on unscheduled DNA synthesis in rat hepatocytes *in vitro*, the Ames test, or the micronucleus test in mice. Zolpidem showed no evidence of genotoxicity in mouse lymphoma cells *in vitro*; and caused no chromosomal aberrations in cultured human lymphocytes.

### Pregnancy/Reproduction
Fertility—In rats given daily oral doses of 4 to 100 mg/kg of zolpidem base (5 to 130 times the recommended human dose in mg per square meter of body surface area [mg/m$^2$]), neither male nor female fertility was affected. However, female rats receiving 100 mg/kg of zolpidem base per day displayed irregular estrus cycles and prolonged precoital intervals. The significance to humans is not known.

Pregnancy—Zolpidem has not been studied in pregnant women.
No frank teratogenicity was seen in rat and rabbit studies. Rats administered 20 and 100 mg/kg of zolpidem base (25 to 125 times the recommended human dose in mg/m$^2$) showed maternal lethargy and ataxia as well as a dose-related trend toward incomplete ossification of fetal skull bones, which was believed to be secondary to delayed maturation. Rabbits administered 16 mg/kg of zolpidem base (28 times the recommended human dose in mg/m$^2$) showed an increase in postimplantation fetal loss and underossification of fetal sternebrae. These effects were believed to be secondary to decreased maternal weight gain.

FDA Pregnancy Category B.
Postpartum—Studies of children whose mothers received zolpidem during pregnancy have not been conducted. However, flaccidity and withdrawal symptoms have been reported in neonates born to mothers receiving other sedative-hypnotics during pregnancy.

### Breast-feeding
One study in 5 nursing mothers showed <0.02% of a single oral dose of zolpidem was distributed into breast milk. The effect of zolpidem on the infant is not known.
In rats, zolpidem doses greater than 4 mg/kg (6 times the recommended human dose in mg/m$^2$) inhibited milk secretion.

### Pediatrics
Appropriate studies on the relationship of age to the effects of zolpidem have not been performed in children up to 18 years of age. Safety and efficacy have not been established.

### Geriatrics
Studies have shown zolpidem to have an increased half-life, peak plasma concentration, and area under the plasma concentration time curve in geriatric patients. Elderly patients may be more likely to experience confusion or falls while taking zolpidem. A reduced starting dosage and careful monitoring are recommended. In addition, geriatric patients are more likely to have age-related renal function impairment, which may require dosage reductions.

### Drug interactions and/or related problems
The following drug interactions and/or related problems have been selected on the basis of their potential clinical significance (possible mechanism in parentheses where appropriate)—not necessarily inclusive (» = major clinical significance):

Note: Combinations containing any of the following medications, depending on the amount present, may also interact with this medication.

» Alcohol or
» CNS depression–producing medications, other (See *Appendix II*)
   (concurrent use may increase the CNS depressant effects of either these medications or zolpidem; caution is recommended, and dosage of one or both agents should be reduced)

Chlorpromazine
   (concurrent use may prolong elimination half-life of chlorpromazine)

Imipramine
   (concurrent use may increase drowsiness and incidence of anterograde amnesia, and decrease peak concentrations of imipramine)

### Medical considerations/Contraindications
The medical considerations/contraindications included have been selected on the basis of their potential clinical significance (reasons given in parentheses where appropriate)—not necessarily inclusive (» = major clinical significance):

*Risk-benefit should be considered when the following medical problems exist:*

» Alcohol intoxication, acute, with depressed vital signs
   (additive CNS depression may occur)

Alcohol or drug abuse or dependence, history of
   (predisposition to habituation and dependence may exist)

Hepatic function impairment
   (zolpidem elimination may be prolonged due to biphasic elimination with prolonged terminal half-life)

Mental depression
   (condition may be exacerbated)

Pulmonary disease, severe chronic obstructive
   (ventilatory failure may be exacerbated)

Renal function impairment
   (zolpidem elimination may be prolonged)

» Sensitivity to zolpidem
» Sleep apnea, established or suspected
   (condition may be exacerbated)

## Side/Adverse Effects
The following side/adverse effects have been selected on the basis of their potential clinical significance (possible signs and symptoms in parentheses where appropriate)—not necessarily inclusive:

### Those indicating need for medical attention
Incidence less frequent
   *Ataxia* (clumsiness or unsteadiness); *confusion*—higher incidence in the elderly; *mental depression*

Incidence rare
   *Allergic reaction or rash; anaphylaxis* (fast heartbeat; swelling of face; wheezing or difficulty in breathing); *falling*—higher incidence in the elderly; *hypotension* (dizziness, lightheadedness, or fainting); *paradoxical reactions, including agitation* (unusual excitement or nervousness); *or irritability; hallucinations* (seeing, hearing, or feeling things that are not there); *or insomnia* (trouble in sleeping)

### Those indicating need for medical attention only if they continue or are bothersome
Incidence less frequent
   *Abnormal dreams, including nightmares; anterograde amnesia* (memory problems); *daytime drowsiness; dizziness; lightheadedness; or vertigo; drugged feelings; dryness of mouth; gastrointestinal effects, including abdominal or gastric pain; diarrhea; nausea; or vomiting; headache; malaise* (general feeling of discomfort or illness); *vision abnormalities, including diplopia* (double vision)

### Those indicating possible withdrawal and/or the need for medical attention if they occur after medication is discontinued, usually within 48 hours
*Abdominal or stomach cramps or discomfort; agitation, nervousness, or feelings of panic; flushing; lightheadedness; muscle cramps; nausea; psychotic exacerbation* (worsening of mental or emotional problems); *seizures; sweating; tremors; uncontrolled crying; unusual tiredness or weakness; or vomiting*

## Overdose

For specific information on the agents used in the management of zolpidem overdose, see:
- *Charcoal, Activated (Oral-Local)* monograph; and/or
- *Flumazenil (Systemic)* monograph.

For more information on the management of overdose or unintentional ingestion, **contact a Poison Control Center** (see *Poison Control Center Listing*).

### Clinical effects of overdose

The following effects have been selected on the basis of their potential clinical significance (possible signs and symptoms in parentheses where appropriate)—not necessarily inclusive:

*Ataxia, severe* (clumsiness or unsteadiness); *cardiovascular compromise* (slow heartbeat); *diplopia* (double vision); *or disturbed vision; dizziness, severe; drowsiness, severe; nausea, severe; respiratory problems* (troubled breathing); *unconsciousness; vomiting, severe*

### Treatment of overdose

Treatment is essentially symptomatic and supportive, possibly including:
 To decrease absorption—
  Inducing emesis or performing gastric lavage as appropriate.
 To enhance elimination—
  Administering activated charcoal to increase clearance and decrease absorption of zolpidem.
  Zolpidem is not dialyzable.
 Specific treatment—
  Withholding sedating drugs even if excitation occurs.
  Flumazenil may be useful in reversing zolpidem's sedative and respiratory depressant effects.
 Monitoring—
  Monitoring respiratory, cardiac, and CNS status.
 Supportive care—
  Providing general supportive therapy as indicated. Patients in whom intentional overdose is known or suspected should be referred for psychiatric consultation.

## Patient Consultation

As an aid to patient consultation, refer to *Advice for the Patient, Zolpidem (Systemic)*.

In providing consultation, consider emphasizing the following selected information (» = major clinical significance):

### Before using this medication
» Conditions affecting use, especially:
  Sensitivity to zolpidem
  Breast-feeding—Small amounts of zolpidem are distributed into breast milk; effect on infant is not known
  Use in the elderly—Elderly patients are usually more sensitive to CNS effects of zolpidem
  Other medications, especially other CNS depression–producing medications
  Other medical problems, especially acute alcohol intoxication or sleep apnea

### Proper use of this medication
» Not taking more medication than the amount prescribed, because of habit-forming potential
» Not increasing dose if medication becomes less effective over time; checking with physician
  Being prepared to go to sleep immediately after taking medicine
» Proper dosing
  Missed dose—Skipping missed dose; not doubling doses
» Proper storage

### Precautions while using this medication
» Avoiding use of alcohol or other CNS depressants during therapy
» Caution if clumsiness or unsteadiness, drowsiness, dizziness, or visual disturbances occur, especially in the elderly
  Checking with physician before discontinuing medication after more than 1 to 2 weeks of use; gradual dosage reduction may be necessary to avoid withdrawal symptoms

### Side/adverse effects
 Signs of potential side effects, especially ataxia, confusion, mental depression, allergic reaction or rash, anaphylaxis, falling, hypotension, or paradoxical reactions

## General Dosing Information

Geriatric or debilitated patients, or patients with hepatic or renal function impairment should receive decreased initial dosage since elimination of zolpidem may be prolonged, resulting in increased CNS and gastrointestinal side effects.

Optimal dosage of zolpidem varies with patient response. Individual dosage adjustments should be made. The minimal effective dose should be used for the shortest period, with the need for continuing therapy with zolpidem reviewed regularly.

Because of zolpidem's rapid onset of action, the patient should be ready for sleep when the dose is taken.

To minimize the occurrence of anterograde amnesia and hang-over effects, zolpidem should be taken only when the patient's schedule will allow for a full night's sleep (7 to 8 hours).

For the most rapid effect, zolpidem should be taken on an empty stomach.

Following prolonged administration, zolpidem should be withdrawn gradually to lessen the possibility of precipitating withdrawal symptoms.

Potentially suicidal patients, particularly those who use alcohol excessively, should not have access to large quantities of zolpidem.

## Oral Dosage Forms

### ZOLPIDEM TARTRATE TABLETS

**Usual adult dose**
Hypnotic—
 Oral, 10 mg at bedtime.
Note: Debilitated patients or patients with hepatic or renal function impairment—Oral, initially 5 mg at bedtime, the dosage being adjusted as needed and tolerated.

**Usual adult prescribing limits**
Up to 20 mg a day.

**Usual pediatric dose**
Children up to 18 years of age—
 Safety and efficacy have not been established.

**Usual geriatric dose**
Hypnotic—
 Oral, initially 5 mg at bedtime, the dosage being adjusted as needed and tolerated.

**Usual geriatric prescribing limits**
Up to 10 mg a day.

**Strength(s) usually available**
U.S.—
 5 mg (Rx) [*Ambien* (hydroxypropyl methylcellulose; lactose; magnesium stearate; microcrystalline cellulose; polyethylene glycol; sodium starch glycolate; titanium dioxide; FD&C Red No. 40; iron oxide colorant; and polysorbate 80)].
 10 mg (Rx) [*Ambien* (hydroxypropyl methylcellulose; lactose; magnesium stearate; microcrystalline cellulose; polyethylene glycol; sodium starch glycolate; titanium dioxide)].
Canada—
 Not commercially available.

**Packaging and storage**
Store below 40 °C (104 °F), preferably between 15 and 30 °C (59 and 86 °F), unless otherwise specified by manufacturer. Store in a well-closed container.

**Auxiliary labeling**
- Avoid alcoholic beverages.
- May cause daytime drowsiness.

**Note**
Controlled substance in the U.S.

## Selected Bibliography

Langtry HD, Benfield P. Zolpidem: A review of its pharmacodynamic and pharmacokinetic properties and therapeutic potential. Drugs 1990; 40(2): 291-313.

Hoehns JD, Perry PJ. Zolpidem: A nonbenzodiazepine hypnotic for treatment of insomnia [published erratum appears in Clin Pharm 1993 Dec; 12: 881]. Clin Pharm 1993 Nov; 12: 814-28.

Developed: 06/29/94

USP DI             **Additional Products and Indications**     3009

# Appendix I

## ADDITIONAL PRODUCTS AND INDICATIONS

The following information is based on the product's package insert. It has not gone through the USP DI review process. It is essential to refer to the product literature for additional information until a full monograph is developed. The term "new" as used in this chart means that the product in question is not currently included in the main text of USP DI; it does not necessarily imply that the product has just recently been marketed.

| GENERIC NAME (*Brand name*, manufacturer [country]) VA Classification (Primary/Secondary) | DOSAGE FORMS AND STRENGTHS | CATEGORIES— INDICATIONS | USUAL ADULT DOSE | USUAL PEDIATRIC DOSE | COMMENTS |
|---|---|---|---|---|---|
| Acenocoumarol* (*Sintrom*, Geigy [Canada]) BL114 | Tablets: 1 and 4 mg | Anticoagulant—Deep venous thrombosis†‡; Pulmonary embolism†‡; Thromboembolism associated with chronic atrial fibrillation or myocardial infarction†; Transient cerebral ischemic attacks‡ | Oral, 8 to 12 mg on the first day; 4 to 8 mg on the second day; then 1 to 10 mg a day as determined by prothrombin-time tests | | For general information that may apply to all coumarin-derivative anticoagulants, see *Anticoagulants (Systemic)* Also known as acenocoumarin and nicoumalone |
| Acetaminophen, Aspirin, and Caffeine (*Excedrin Migraine*, Bristol-Myers [U.S.]) CN105 | Tablets USP: 250 mg, 250 mg, and 65 mg§ | Antimigraine agent—Headache, migraine‡ | Oral, 2 tablets every 6 hours as needed | Safety and efficacy have not been established | New OTC brand name product; same formulation as *Extra Strength Excedrin* |
| Albendazole (*Albenza*, SmithKline Beecham [U.S.]) AP200 | Tablets: 200 mg | Anthelmintic (systemic)—Hydatid disease‡; Neurocysticercosis‡ | Oral: Hydatid disease—Patients up to 60 kg of body weight: 7.5 mg per kg of body weight twice a day for 28 days followed by a 14-day albendazole-free interval, for a total of 3 cycles Patients 60 kg of body weight or more: 400 mg twice a day for 28 days followed by a 14-day albendazole-free interval, for a total of 3 cycles Neurocysticercosis—Patients up to 60 kg of body weight: 7.5 mg per kg of body weight twice a day for 8 to 30 days Patients 60 kg of body weight or more: 400 mg twice a day for 8 to 30 days | Oral: Hydatid disease—Patients up to 60 kg of body weight: 7.5 mg per kg of body weight twice a day for 28 days followed by a 14-day albendazole-free interval, for a total of 3 cycles Neurocysticercosis—Patients up to 60 kg of body weight: 7.5 mg per kg of body weight twice a day for 8 to 30 days | Approved for the U.S. |
| Albuterol Sulfate (*Volmax*, Muro [U.S.]) RE103 | Extended-release Tablets: 4 and 8 mg (base) | Bronchodilator—Bronchospasm‡ in patients with reversible obstructive airway disease | | Children 6 to 12 years of age—4 mg (base) every 12 hours | New pediatric dosing |
| Aminosalicylic Acid (*Paser*, Jacobus Pharmaceutical [U.S.]) AM500 | Granules: 4 grams per packet | Antibacterial (antimycobacterial)—Multi-drug-resistant tuberculosis in combination with other antimycobacterials | Oral, 4 grams (one packet) 3 times a day | To be determined by the physician | For general information that may apply to this product see *Aminosalicylate Sodium (Systemic)* |

*Not commercially available in the United States.
†Prophylactic.
‡Therapeutic.
§Respectively.
#Diagnostic.

## Additional Products and Indications (continued)

| GENERIC NAME (Brand name, manufacturer [country]) VA Classification (Primary/Secondary) | DOSAGE FORMS AND STRENGTHS | CATEGORIES—INDICATIONS | USUAL ADULT DOSE | USUAL PEDIATRIC DOSE | COMMENTS |
|---|---|---|---|---|---|
| Amoxicillin<br><br>(*Amoxil*, SmithKline Beecham [U.S.])<br><br><br><br><br><br>(*Trimox*, Apothecon [U.S.]; *Wymox*, Wyeth-Ayerst [U.S.])<br><br>(*Polymox*, Bristol [U.S.])<br><br>(*Mylan* [U.S.])<br><br><br><br>(Warner Chilcott [U.S.])<br>AM112 | Capsules USP: 250 and 500 mg<br>Oral Suspension USP: 25 and 50 mg per mL<br>Tablets USP (chewable): 125 and 250 mg<br>Capsules USP: 250 and 500 mg<br>Oral Suspension USP: 25 and 50 mg per mL<br>Oral Suspension USP: 25 and 50 mg per mL<br>Capsules USP: 250 and 500 mg<br>Oral Suspension USP: 25 and 50 mg per mL<br>Tablets USP (chewable): 250 mg | Antiulcer agent—<br><br>Ulcer, duodenal, associated with *Helicobacter pylori* infection‡: for concurrent use with clarithromycin and lansoprazole<br>Ulcer, duodenal, associated with *Helicobacter pylori* infection in patients either allergic or intolerant to clarithromycin, or in whom resistance to clarithromycin is known or suspected‡: for concurrent use with lansoprazole | Oral, 1000 mg in combination with clarithromycin 500 mg and lansoprazole 30 mg, taken every 12 hours for 14 days<br><br>Oral, 1000 mg in combination with lansoprazole 30 mg, taken every 8 hours for 14 days | Safety and efficacy have not been established | Additional FDA-approved indications |
| Amoxicillin and Clavulanate (*Augmentin*, SmithKline Beecham [U.S.])<br>AM112 | Oral suspension: 200 mg of amoxicillin and 28.6 mg of clavulanic acid per 5 mL; and 400 mg of amoxicillin and 57.1 mg of clavulanic acid per 5 mL<br>Tablets (Chewable): 200 mg of amoxicillin and 28.6 mg of clavulanic acid; and 400 mg of amoxicillin and 57.1 mg of clavulanic acid<br>Tablets: 875 mg of amoxicillin and 125 mg of clavulanic acid | Antibacterial (systemic)—Bronchitis‡; Otitis media, acute‡; Pneumonia, bacterial‡; Sinusitis‡; Skin and soft tissue infections‡; Urinary tract infections, bacterial‡ | Oral, 500 mg of amoxicillin and 125 mg of clavulanic acid to 875 mg of amoxicillin and 125 mg of clavulanic acid every 12 hours; or 250 mg of amoxicillin and 125 mg of clavulanic acid to 500 mg of amoxicillin and 125 mg of clavulanic acid every 8 hours | Neonates and infants less than 12 weeks of age: 15 mg per kg of body weight twice a day, based on the amoxicillin content<br>Children 12 weeks of age and older: 12.5 to 22.5 mg per kg of body weight twice a day, based on amoxicillin content; or 6.7 to 13.3 mg per kg of body weight 3 times a day, based on amoxicillin content<br>Children weighing 40 kg or more: See *Usual adult dose* | Additional twice-a-day dosing option approved by FDA<br>Additional strengths of oral suspension, chewable tablets, and tablets, as listed |
| Amsacrine* (*Amsa P-D*, PD [Canada])<br>AN900 | Injection: 50 mg per mL | Antineoplastic—Leukemia, acute lymphocytic‡ | Induction—IV infusion (over 60 to 90 minutes), 75, 100, or 125 mg per square meter of body surface per day for 5 days, the course being repeated every 3 to 4 weeks<br>Maintenance—IV infusion, one-half the dose used for induction, each course being repeated every 4 to 8 weeks | Not intended for pediatric use | Canadian drug product |
| Anagrelide (*Agrylin*, Roberts Pharmaceutical [Canada])<br>BL400 | Capsules: 0.5 mg | Platelet reducing agent—Thrombocythemia, essential‡ | | | Approved for use in Canada |

## Additional Products and Indications (continued)

| GENERIC NAME (Brand name, manufacturer [country]) VA Classification (Primary/Secondary) | DOSAGE FORMS AND STRENGTHS | CATEGORIES—INDICATIONS | USUAL ADULT DOSE | USUAL PEDIATRIC DOSE | COMMENTS |
|---|---|---|---|---|---|
| Anileridine* (Leritine, Frosst [Canada]) CN101/CN205 | Tablets USP: 25 mg (base) Injection USP: 25 mg (base) per mL | Analgesic—Moderate to severe pain‡; Obstetrical pain‡ Anesthesia adjunct | Oral, 25 to 50 mg (base) every 6 hours as needed Parenteral— Analgesic: IM or SC, 25 to 50 mg (base) every 4 to 6 hours as needed, adjusted according to severity of pain but not exceeding 200 mg per day Preoperative—IM or SC, 50 to 75 mg (base) In obstetrics—IM or SC, 50 mg (base); may be repeated at 3- to 4-hour intervals up to a maximum of 200 mg Anesthesia adjunct: IV infusion, 5 to 10 mg (base) administered at a rate of 600 mcg per minute | Dosage has not been established | An opioid agonist analgesic; Canadian Controlled Substance Classification: N For general information that may apply to all opioid agonist analgesics, see Opioid (Narcotic) Analgesics (Systemic) |
| Antihemophilic Factor (Recombinant) (Helixate, Bayer [Canada]) BL116 | for Injection: 250, 500, and 1000 IU per single-dose bottle | | | | Now available in Canada |
| Aztreonam (Azactam, Squibb [U.S.]) AM119 | Injection: 1 gram per 50 mL and 2 grams per 50 mL for Injection: 500 mg, 1 gram, and 2 grams | Antibacterial (systemic)‡ | | IV— Mild-to-moderate infections: 30 mg per kg of body weight every 8 hours Moderate-to-severe infections: 30 mg per kg of body weight every 6 or 8 hours | Pediatric dosing |
| BCG Live (Montreal Strain) (PACIS, IAF Biovac [Canada]) AN900 | 120 mg (semi-dry weight) or 2–10×10⁶ colony-forming units (CFU) per vial | | | | Additional brand name product For additional information, see Bacillus Calmette-Guérin (BCG) Live (Mucosal-Local) |
| Beclomethasone Dipropionate Monohydrate (Vancenase AQ, Schering [U.S.]) NT201 | Nasal Solution: 84 mcg (0.084 mg) per metered spray | Anti-inflammatory (steroidal); corticosteroid (nasal)—Rhinitis, seasonal allergic‡; Rhinitis, vasomotor‡; Polyps, nasal, postsurgical recurrence of† | Nasal, 1 or 2 metered sprays in each nostril once a day (total daily dose, 168 to 336 mcg) | Children up to 6 years of age: Safety and efficacy have not been established Children 6 years of age and older: See Usual adult dose | Additional strength Name change—Formerly Vancenase AQ Double Strength |
| Benzoyl Peroxide (Triaz, Medicis Dermatologics [U.S.]) DE752/DE500 | Gel: 6% and 10% Cleansing Lotion: 10% | | | | Additional brand name product; Rx; 6% is an additional strength |
| Benzydamine Hydrochloride* (Tantum, Riker/3M [Canada]) OR900 | Oral Topical Solution: 0.15% | Analgesic (oral-local)—Sore throat pain‡; Mucositis, oropharyngeal, radiation therapy–induced‡ | Sore throat—Topical, as a gargle, 15 mL every 1.5 to 3 hours. To be expelled after gargling Mucositis, oropharyngeal—Topical, to the mucosa, 15 mL 3 or 4 times a day, to be kept in contact with the mucosa for 30 seconds, then expelled, starting 1 day prior to radiation therapy | Children up to 6 years of age—Dosage has not been established Children 6 years of age and over—See Usual adult dose | Canadian drug product |

*Not commercially available in the United States.
†Prophylactic.
‡Therapeutic.
§Respectively.
#Diagnostic.

## Additional Products and Indications (continued)

| GENERIC NAME (Brand name, manufacturer [country]) VA Classification (Primary/Secondary) | DOSAGE FORMS AND STRENGTHS | CATEGORIES— INDICATIONS | USUAL ADULT DOSE | USUAL PEDIATRIC DOSE | COMMENTS |
|---|---|---|---|---|---|
| Betamethasone Dipropionate (Occlucort, Genderm [Canada]) DE200 | Lotion: 0.05% (base) | | | | Canadian brand name product; film-forming lotion |
| Betamethasone Disodium Phosphate (Betnesol*, Glaxo [Canada]) OR900 | Dental Pellets: 100 mcg (base)* | Corticosteroid (topical); Anti-inflammatory (steroidal)—Aphthous ulcers‡ | Topical, to the oral mucous membranes, 1 pellet 4 times a day, to be dissolved close to the ulcer | Dosage has not been established | Dosage form available in Canada. For general information that may apply to all topical corticosteroids, see Corticosteroids (Topical) |
| Betaxolol Hydrochloride (Betoptic S, Alcon [Canada]) OP110 | Ophthalmic Suspension: 0.25% | | | | Available in Canada |
| Budesonide (Entocort, Astra Pharma [Canada]) HS051 | Extended-release Capsules: 3 mg | Anti-inflammatory (steroidal)—Crohn's disease, mild to moderate‡: Affecting the ileum and/or the ascending colon | Initial: Oral, 9 mg once a day before the morning meal for up to 8 weeks. Maintenance: Oral, 6 mg once a day before the morning meal | Safety and efficacy have not been established | Additional dosage form |
| Budesonide (Rhinocort Nasal Inhaler, Astra [U.S.]) | Nasal Aerosol; 32 mcg per metered spray | Anti-inflammatory (steroidal), nasal; Corticosteroid (nasal)—Rhinitis, seasonal allergic‡; Rhinitis, perennial allergic‡; Rhinitis, perennial nonallergic‡; Rhinitis, vasomotor‡; Polyps, nasal‡; Polyps, nasal, postsurgical recurrence of† | Initially, 64 mcg (2 metered sprays) in each nostril 2 times a day; or 128 mcg (4 metered sprays) in each nostril once a day in the morning (total daily dose, 256 mcg), the dosage then being decreased to the lowest effective dose according to patient response | Infants and children up to 6 years of age—Safety and efficacy have not been established. Children 6 years of age and older—See Usual adult dose | Additional dosage form; additional brand name product; additional strength. Medication is indicated for perennial nonallergic rhinitis in adults only, since adequate numbers of children have not been studied |
| (Rhinocort Aqua, Astra [Canada]) | Nasal Solution: 100 mcg per metered spray | | Rhinitis: Initially, 200 mcg (2 metered sprays) in each nostril once a day in the morning; or 100 mcg (1 metered spray) in each nostril 2 times a day (total daily dose, 400 mcg), the dosage then being decreased to the lowest effective dose according to patient response. Polyps: 100 mcg (1 metered spray) in each nostril 2 times a day (total daily dose, 400 mcg) | | Change in indications and dosage |
| (Rhinocort Turbuhaler, Astra [Canada]) NT201 | Nasal Powder: 100 mcg per metered inhalation | | Rhinitis: Initially, 200 mcg (2 metered inhalations) in each nostril once a day in the morning (total daily dose, 400 mcg), the dosage then being decreased to the lowest effective dose according to patient response. Polyps: 100 mcg (1 metered inhalation) in each nostril 2 times a day (total daily dose, 400 mcg) | | Change in indications and dosage |

## Additional Products and Indications (continued)

| GENERIC NAME (Brand name, manufacturer [country]) VA Classification (Primary/Secondary) | DOSAGE FORMS AND STRENGTHS | CATEGORIES— INDICATIONS | USUAL ADULT DOSE | USUAL PEDIATRIC DOSE | COMMENTS |
|---|---|---|---|---|---|
| Bufexamac* (Norfemac, Nordic [Canada]; Parfenac, Lederle [Canada]) DE200 | Cream: 50 mg per gram Ointment: 50 mg per gram | Anti-inflammatory (nonsteroidal)—Dermatoses‡; Vulvitis‡; Pruritus vulvae‡; Hemorrhoids‡; Pruritus, anorectal‡; Fissures, anorectal‡; Thrombophlebitis, superficial‡; Radiodermatitis‡ | Topical, to the affected area, 2 or 3 times a day | See Usual adult dose | Canadian drug product |
| Calfactant (Infasurf, Forest Pharmaceuticals [U.S.]) RE700 | 35 mg of phospholipids per mL | Pulmonary surfactant—Respiratory distress syndrome, neonatal†‡ |  | Children up to 72 hours of age—Intratracheal, 3 mL per kg of body weight, administered in two aliquots of 1.5 mL per kg of body weight each, given as soon as possible after birth, preferably within 30 minutes For treatment of respiratory distress syndrome, repeat doses of 3 mL per kg of body weight may be administered at 12-hour intervals up to a total of 3 doses if the patient is still intubated | New drug After each aliquot of medication is instilled, the patient should be positioned with either the right or the left side dependent. The administration is made while ventilation is continued over 20 to 30 breaths for each aliquot, with small bursts timed only during the inspiratory cycles After administration of the first aliquot, respiratory status and repositioning should be evaluated before the second aliquot is instilled |
| Carbachol (Miostat, Alcon [U.S.]) | Intraocular Solution USP: 0.01% | Antiglaucoma agent (ophthalmic)—Hypertension, ocular, postsurgical‡ | Intraocular irrigation, no more than 0.5 mL of a 0.01% solution instilled into the anterior chamber. May be instilled before or after securing sutures | See Usual adult dose | Additional FDA-approved indication: In addition to miosis during surgery, carbachol intraocular solution reduces the intensity of intraocular pressure elevation in the first 24 hours after cataract surgery |
| (Carbastat, CIBA Vision [U.S. and Canada]) OP118/OP900 |  |  |  |  | Additional brand name product |
| Carbidopa and Levodopa (Nu-Levocarb, Nu-pharm Inc. [Canada]) CN500 | Tablets USP: 25 mg and 100 mg; 10 mg and 100 mg; 25 mg and 250 mg§ | Antidyskinetic— Parkinsonism‡ |  |  | Additional brand name product |
| Carboxymethylcellulose | Ophthalmic Solution: | Tears (artificial)— Keratoconjunctivitis sicca‡ |  |  | U.S. drug product; OTC |
| (Celluvisc, Allergan [U.S.]) | 1% |  |  |  |  |
| (Refresh Plus, Allergan [U.S.]) OP500 | 0.5% |  |  |  | Brand name change— formerly Cellufresh |

*Not commercially available in the United States.
†Prophylactic.
‡Therapeutic.
§Respectively.
#Diagnostic.

## Additional Products and Indications (continued)

| GENERIC NAME (Brand name, manufacturer [country]) VA Classification (Primary/Secondary) | DOSAGE FORMS AND STRENGTHS | CATEGORIES— INDICATIONS | USUAL ADULT DOSE | USUAL PEDIATRIC DOSE | COMMENTS |
|---|---|---|---|---|---|
| Cefdinir (Omnicef, Parke-Davis [U.S.]) AM103 | Capsules: 300 mg for Oral Suspension: After reconstitution, 125 mg per 5 mL | Antibacterial (systemic)—Bronchitis, exacerbations of‡; Otitis media‡; Pharyngitis‡; Pneumonia, community-acquired‡; Sinusitis, acute maxillary‡; Skin and soft tissue infections, uncomplicated‡; Tonsillitis‡ | Bronchitis, exacerbations of, or sinusitis—Oral, 300 mg every 12 hours, or 600 mg every 24 hours, for 10 days Community-acquired pneumonia or skin and soft tissue infections—Oral, 300 mg every 12 hours for 10 days Pharyngitis or tonsillitis—Oral, 300 mg every 12 hours for 5 to 10 days, or 600 mg every 24 hours for 10 days | Otitis media or sinusitis—Oral, 7 mg per kg of body weight every 12 hours, or 14 mg per kg of body weight every 24 hours, for 10 days Pharyngitis or tonsillitis—Oral, 7 mg per kg of body weight every 12 hours for 5 to 10 days, or 14 mg per kg of body weight every 24 hours for 10 days Skin and soft tissue infections—Oral, 7 mg per kg of body weight every 12 hours for 10 days | New drug |
| Cervical Cap, Cavity-rim (Prentif, Cervical Cap Ltd. [U.S.]) GU400 | | Contraceptive—Pregnancy† | Contraceptive—Vaginal, 1 cervical cap inserted so as to cover the cervix prior to intercourse, being filled one-third full with contraceptive cream or jelly prior to insertion | | Cervical cap should be left in place a minimum of 8 hours after last act of intercourse. May be left in place for 48 hours after initial insertion Additional contraceptive cream or jelly is not necessary prior to repeat acts of intercourse. However, proper cervical cap placement should be confirmed before and after each act of intercourse |
| Chloramphenicol (Diochloram, Dioptic [Canada]) OP201 | Ophthalmic Ointment USP: 1% Ophthalmic Solution USP: 0.5% | | | | Additional brand name product |
| Chlorhexidine Gluconate (PerioChip, Astra [U.S.]) OR900 | Implants (periodontal): 2.5 mg | Antibacterial (dental)—Periodontal disease‡ | Implantation, 2.5 mg (1 implant) inserted into a periodontal pocket that has a probing depth of ≥ 5 mm. Up to 20 mg (8 implants) may be inserted in a single visit. Treatment may be repeated every 3 months to pockets still having a depth of ≥ 5 mm | Safety and efficacy have not been established | New dosage form New FDA-approved indication |
| Choline Salicylate and Cetyl-dimethyl-benzyl-ammonium Chloride* (Teejel, Purdue Frederick [Canada]) OR900 | Gel: 87 mg and 100 mcg per gram§ | Analgesic (oral-local)—Pain, teething‡; Pain, dental prosthetic‡; Pain, gingival or oral mucosal‡ | Topical, to the affected mucosa, 1 cm of gel applied gently with a finger every 3 to 4 hours as needed | See Usual adult dose | Contains 39% alcohol Should not be used in patients intolerant of other salicylates |
| Citalopram Hydrobromide (Celexa, Forest Laboratories [U.S.]) CN603 | Tablets: 20 and 40 mg (base) | Antidepressant—Depressive disorder, major‡ | Oral, initially 20 mg as a single dose in the morning or evening. Dose may be increased by 20 mg a day at intervals of at least one week, if needed; generally increased to 40 mg a day; may be increased to 60 mg a day in nonresponding patients | Safety and efficacy have not been established | New drug Dosing is once a day at all dosages |
| Citric Acid and D-Gluconic Acid (Renacidin Powder for Irrigation, United Guardian [U.S.]) GU900 | for Topical Solution | Antiurolithic—Calcifications on indwelling urethral catheters†‡ | Instillation into the indwelling urethral catheter, 1 or 2 ounces of a 10% solution 1 to 3 times a day as needed | Dosage has not been established | Contraindicated for treatment or prophylaxis of renal or biliary calculi. Contraindicated for use in ureteral catheters or in ureterostomy, pyelostomy, or nephrostomy tubes |

## Additional Products and Indications (continued)

| GENERIC NAME (Brand name, manufacturer [country]) VA Classification (Primary/Secondary) | DOSAGE FORMS AND STRENGTHS | CATEGORIES— INDICATIONS | USUAL ADULT DOSE | USUAL PEDIATRIC DOSE | COMMENTS |
|---|---|---|---|---|---|
| Citric Acid, Glucono-delta-lactone, and Magnesium Carbonate (Renacidin Irrigation, United Guardian [U.S.]) GU900 | Solution | Antiurolithic (apatite calculi; struvite calculi)—Renal calculi, apatite‡; Renal calculi, struvite‡ | | | Ready-to-use solution for local irrigation for dissolution of renal calculi |
| Clioquinol and Flumethasone Pivalate* (Locorten Vioform, CIBA [Canada]) DE250 | Cream: 3% and 0.02%§ Ointment: 3% and 0.02%§ | Antibacterial-antifungal-corticosteroid (topical)—Dermatitis, atopic‡; Dermatitis, contact‡; Folliculitis‡; Intertrigo‡; Pruritus, anogenital‡; Skin infections, bacterial, minor‡ | Topical, to the skin, 3 or 4 times a day | See Usual adult dose | Canadian combination product  For general information that may apply to this combination, see Clioquinol and Hydrocortisone (Topical) |
| Clioquinol and Flumethasone Pivalate* (Locorten Vioform, CIBA [Canada]) OT250 | Otic Solution: 1% and 0.02%§ | Antibacterial-antifungal-corticosteroid (otic)—Furunculosis of the ear canal‡; Mastoidectomy cavity infections‡; Otitis externa‡; Otitis media, acute (treatment adjunct); Otitis media, chronic suppurative‡; Otomycosis‡ | Topical, to the ear canal, 2 or 3 drops every 12 hours or more frequently | Dosage has not been established | Canadian combination product  For general information that may apply to all otic corticosteroids, see Corticosteroids (Otic) |
| Clobetasol Propionate (Cormax, Oclassen [U.S.]) (Taro [U.S.]) DE200 | Ointment USP: 0.05% | | | | Additional brand name product  Available generically |
| Clobetasol Propionate (Temovate E, Glaxo Wellcome [U.S.]) DE200 | Cream USP: 0.05% | | | | New brand name product |
| Condom, female, polyurethane (Reality, Female Health Company [U.S.]) XA900 | | Contraceptive— Pregnancy† | | | U.S. product; OTC; caution should be taken not to use after the expiration date  The closed ring of the device is instilled against the pubic bone of the vagina by using the index finger; the open ring plus about one inch of the device stays outside of the vagina; caution should be taken not to twist the device  The product is removed by squeezing and twisting the outer ring to keep sperm inside the condom and pulling gently; should not be flushed down toilet  A new condom must be used with each act of sexual intercourse; lubricant may be added; a male condom should not be used with the female condom because the female condom may not stay in place or work as well  Estimated one year pregnancy rate is 21 to 26% |

*Not commercially available in the United States.
†Prophylactic.
‡Therapeutic.
§Respectively.
#Diagnostic.

## Additional Products and Indications (continued)

| GENERIC NAME (Brand name, manufacturer [country]) VA Classification (Primary/Secondary) | DOSAGE FORMS AND STRENGTHS | CATEGORIES— INDICATIONS | USUAL ADULT DOSE | USUAL PEDIATRIC DOSE | COMMENTS |
|---|---|---|---|---|---|
| Condom, male, polyurethane (*Avanti*, London International U.S. Holdings [U.S.]; *Avanti Super Thin*, London International U.S. Holdings [U.S.]) XA900 | | Contraceptive— Pregnancy† | | | Product is made of polyurethane; OTC; caution should be taken not to use after the expiration date |
| | | | | | Oil or water-based lubricants may be used; caution should be taken not to twist the condom; directions to apply or remove these condoms are the same as for latex condoms. For general information that may apply to all condoms, see *Condoms* |
| Cromolyn Sodium (*Nasalcrom*, McNeil [U.S.]) NT900 | Nasal Solution: 4% (40 mg of Cromolyn Sodium per mL; 5.2 mg per metered spray) | | | | Schedule change from Rx to OTC |
| Cyproterone Acetate* (*Androcur*, Berlex [Canada]) AN500 | Injection: 100 mg per mL Tablets: 50 mg | Antineoplastic—Carcinoma, prostatic‡ | IM, 300 mg per week, the dosage being reduced after orchiectomy to 300 mg every 2 weeks | Not intended for pediatric use | Canadian drug product |
| | | | Oral, 200 to 300 mg per day in 2 or 3 divided doses taken after meals, the dosage being reduced after orchiectomy to 100 to 200 mg per day | | |
| Desmopressin (*DDAVP*, Rhône-Poulenc Rorer [U.S.]) HS702 | Tablets: 0.1 and 0.2 mg | Antidiuretic (central diabetes insipidus)—Diabetes insipidus, central‡ | Oral, initially 0.05 mg two times a day, increased to 0.1 to 1.2 mg in divided doses two or three times a day, as needed | See *Usual adult dose* | Additional dosage form |
| | | | The dosage must be determined for each individual patient and adjusted according to the diurnal pattern of response estimated by adequate duration of sleep and adequate, not excessive, water turnover | | |
| | | | Patients previously on intranasal desmopressin therapy should begin oral therapy 12 hours after the last intranasal dose | | |
| Desoximetasone (Taro [U.S.]) DE200 | Ointment USP: 0.25% | | | | Available generically |
| Dexamethasone Sodium Phosphate (*Dexacort Turbinaire*, Adams [U.S.]) NT201 | Nasal Aerosol: 100 mcg phosphate per metered spray | | | | Brand name change— formerly *Decadron Turbinaire*; change in manufacturer/distributor |

## Additional Products and Indications *(continued)*

| GENERIC NAME (Brand name, manufacturer [country]) VA Classification (Primary/Secondary) | DOSAGE FORMS AND STRENGTHS | CATEGORIES— INDICATIONS | USUAL ADULT DOSE | USUAL PEDIATRIC DOSE | COMMENTS |
|---|---|---|---|---|---|
| Dextromethorphan Hydrobromide and Guaifenesin (*Touro DM,* Dartmouth Pharmaceuticals [U.S.]) RE302 | Extended-release Tablets: 30 mg and 575 mg§ | Antitussive-expectorant—Cough‡ | Oral, 1 or 2 tablets every 12 hours, not to exceed 4 tablets in 24 hours | Children up to 2 years of age: Use is not recommended. Children 2 to 6 years of age: Oral, ½ tablet every 12 hours, not to exceed 1 tablet in 24 hours. Children 6 to 12 years of age: Oral, 1 tablet every 12 hours, not to exceed 2 tablets in 24 hours | New brand name product. Tablets should not be crushed or chewed prior to swallowing. For additional information that may apply to this combination, see *Cough/Cold Combinations (Systemic)* |
| Diethylamine Salicylate* (*Algesal,* Solvay Kingswood [Canada]) DE650 | Cream: 10% | Analgesic (topical)—Muscular strains, sprains‡; Pain, arthritic, mild‡ | Topical, massaged into the affected area for 5 to 10 minutes several times a day as required | See *Usual adult dose* | Caution required in patients intolerant of other salicylates |
| Diflorasone Diacetate (*Psorcon,* Dermik [U.S.]) DE200 | Cream USP: 0.05% | | | | Additional brand name product |
| Diltiazem Hydrochloride (*Tiazac,* Forest [U.S.]) CV200/CV250 | Extended-release Capsules: 120, 180, 240, 300, and 360 mg | Antihypertensive—Hypertension‡ Antianginal—Angina pectoris, chronic stable‡ | Hypertension—Oral, initially 120 to 240 mg once daily, as tolerated. Dose may be increased to 540 mg once daily, if needed. The full antihypertensive effect is usually seen after 2 weeks. Angina pectoris, chronic stable—Oral, initially 120 to 180 mg once daily, as tolerated. Dose may be increased to 540 mg once daily, if needed. Titration should be carried out over 7 to 14 days | Safety and efficacy have not been established | New brand name product and strength |
| Dimethyl Sulfoxide (*Kemsol,* Horner [Canada]) DE900 | Solution: 70% | Antifibrotic (topical)—Morphea‡; Scleroderma‡ | Topical, to the skin, 2 mL of a 70% solution, 3 times a day. Apply medication with a swab held by forceps to clean, dry skin free of any other medication or chemical. Doses exceeding 30 mL per day are not recommended | | This information refers to uses that appear only in Canadian product labeling |
| Dipivefrin Hydrochloride (*AKPro,* Akorn [U.S.]; *DPE,* Alcon Canada [Canada]) OP114 | Ophthalmic Solution USP: 0.1% | | | | Additional brand name products |

*Not commercially available in the United States.
†Prophylactic.
‡Therapeutic.
§Respectively.
#Diagnostic.

## Additional Products and Indications (continued)

| GENERIC NAME (Brand name, manufacturer [country]) VA Classification (Primary/Secondary) | DOSAGE FORMS AND STRENGTHS | CATEGORIES— INDICATIONS | USUAL ADULT DOSE | USUAL PEDIATRIC DOSE | COMMENTS |
|---|---|---|---|---|---|
| Dipyridamole and Aspirin* (Asasantine, Boehringer Ingelheim [Canada]) BL117 | Capsules: 75 mg and 330 mg§ | Platelet aggregation inhibitor—Myocardial reinfarction†; Saphenous vein coronary artery bypass graft occlusion† | Myocardial reinfarction prophylaxis—Oral, 1 capsule 3 times a day Saphenous vein graft occlusion prophylaxis— Oral, 1 capsule 7 hours postoperatively, then 3 times a day for 12 months (Prior to initiation of Asasantine, single ingredient dipyridamole is given as follows: Oral, 100 mg 4 times a day for 2 days preoperatively, and 100 mg on the morning of surgery; then, via a nasogastric tube, 100 mg 1 hour postoperatively) | Dosage has not been established | For general information that may apply to this combination, see Dipyridamole (Systemic) and Salicylates (Systemic) |
| Docusate Sodium (Colace, Roberts [U.S.]) RS300 | Enema: 250 mg per 5 mL | Laxative— Constipation‡ | Rectally, 5 mL as needed for relief of occasional constipation | Children 3 years of age and older: See Usual Adult Dose | Additional OTC product in the U.S. |
| Domperidone* (Motilium, Janssen [Canada]) AU300 | Tablets: 10 mg | Dopaminergic blocking agent; Gastrointestinal emptying (delayed) adjunct; Peristaltic stimulant; Antiemetic—Gastrointestinal motility disorders‡; Nausea and vomiting, antiparkinson agent– induced‡ | Gastrointestinal motility disorders—Oral, 10 mg 3 to 4 times a day, 15 to 30 minutes before meals and at bedtime Nausea and vomiting, antiparkinson agent– induced—Oral, 20 mg 3 to 4 times a day | Dosage has not been established | Canadian drug product |
| Dorzolamide Hydrochloride and Timolol Maleate (Cosopt, Merck [U.S.]) OP160 | Ophthalmic Solution: 20 mg and 6 mg§ per mL | Antiglaucoma agent (ophthalmic)—Glaucoma, open-angle‡; Hypertension, ocular‡ | Topical, to the conjunctiva, 1 drop in the affected eye(s) 2 times daily | Safety and efficacy have not been established | New combination product |
| Epirubicin Hydrochloride* (Pharmorubicin PFS, Adria [Canada]) (Pharmorubicin RDF, Adria [Canada]) AN200 | Injection: 2 mg per mL for Injection: 10, 20, 50, and 150 mg | Antineoplastic—Carcinoma, breast‡; Carcinoma, lung‡; Lymphomas, Hodgkin's‡; Lymphomas, non-Hodgkin's‡; Carcinoma, gastric‡; Carcinoma, ovarian‡ | ** | Dosage has not been established | Canadian drug product |
| Erythromycin (E/Gel, Fulton [U.S.]; Emgel, Glaxo [U.S.]) (Theramycin Z, Medicis [U.S.]; Erythro-Statin, High-Tech Pharmacal [U.S.]) (Erythra-Derm, Paddock [U.S.]) (Stiefel [U.S.]) DE752/DE101 | Topical Gel: 2% Topical Solution USP: 2% Topical Solution: 2% (erythromycin base) Topical Gel: 2% | | | | Additional brand name products Additional brand name products Additional brand name product Available generically |

## Additional Products and Indications (continued)

| GENERIC NAME (Brand name, manufacturer [country]) VA Classification (Primary/Secondary) | DOSAGE FORMS AND STRENGTHS | CATEGORIES— INDICATIONS | USUAL ADULT DOSE | USUAL PEDIATRIC DOSE | COMMENTS |
|---|---|---|---|---|---|
| Etodolac | | | | Safety and efficacy have not been established | |
| (Lodine, Wyeth-Ayerst [U.S.]) | Capsules: 200 and 300 mg Tablets: 400 and 500 mg | Capsules and Tablets: Analgesic—Pain‡ Antirheumatic— Rheumatoid arthritis‡; Osteoarthritis‡ | Capsules and Tablets: Analgesic—Oral, 200 to 400 mg every 6 to 8 hours Antirheumatic—Oral, 300 mg 2 to 3 times a day or 400 to 500 mg twice a day | | Management of the treatment of the signs and symptoms of rheumatoid arthritis is an additional FDA-approved indication 500 mg tablet is additional strength |
| (Lodine XL, Wyeth-Ayerst [U.S.]) MS102/CN104; MS400; CN105 | Extended-release Tablets: 400 and 600 mg | Extended-release Tablets: Antirheumatic— Rheumatoid arthritis‡; Osteoarthritis‡ | Extended-release Tablets: Antirheumatic—Oral, 400 to 1000 mg a day | | Extended-release tablet is an additional dosage form |
| Ferumoxsil (Gastromark, Advanced Magnetics [U.S.]) DX900 | Injection: 175 mcg iron, 1.4 mg parabens, per mL | Diagnostic aid, superparamagnetic (gastrointestinal disorders)—Bowel imaging, magnetic resonance# | Oral, 105 mg of iron (600 mL), administered at a rate of 300 mL over 15 minutes | Safety and efficacy have not been established | U.S. drug product |

\*Not commercially available in the United States.
† Prophylactic.
‡ Therapeutic.
§ Respectively.
# Diagnostic.
\*\* Breast carcinoma:
    Single agent—IV, 75 to 90 mg per square meter of body surface area every 21 days; or 12.5 to 25 mg per square meter of body surface area every 7 days
    Combination therapy—IV, 50 to 60 mg per square meter of body surface area on Days 1 and 8 every 4 weeks, in combination with cyclophosphamide and fluorouracil
Small cell lung carcinoma:
    Single agent —IV, 90 to 120 mg per square meter of body surface area every 21 days
    Combination therapy—IV, 50 to 90 mg per square meter of body surface area, in combination with cisplatin; ifosfamide; cyclophosphamide and vincristine; cyclophosphamide and etoposide; or cisplatin and etoposide
Non-small cell lung carcinoma:
    Single agent—IV, 120 to 150 mg per square meter of body surface area every 3 to 4 weeks
    Combination therapy—IV, 90 to 120 mg per square meter of body surface area on Day 1 every 3 to 4 weeks, in combination with etoposide, cisplatin, mitomycin, vindesine, and vinblastine
Hodgkin's lymphoma:
    Combination therapy—IV, 35 mg per square meter of body surface area every 2 weeks, or 70 mg per square meter of body surface area every 3 to 4 weeks, in combination with bleomycin, vinblastine, and dacarbazine
Non-Hodgkin's lymphoma:
    Single agent—IV, 75 to 90 mg per square meter of body surface area every 21 days
    Combination therapy—IV, 60 to 75 mg per square meter of body surface area, in combination with cyclophosphamide, vincristine, and prednisone, with or without bleomycin
Gastric carcinoma:
    Single agent —IV, 75 to 100 mg per square meter of body surface area
    Combination therapy—IV, 80 mg per square meter of body surface area, in combination with fluorouracil
Ovarian carcinoma:
    Single agent—IV, 50 to 90 mg per square meter of body surface area every 3 to 4 weeks
    Combination therapy—IV, 50 to 90 mg per square meter of body surface area every 3 to 4 weeks, in combination with cisplatin and cyclophosphamide

## Additional Products and Indications (continued)

| GENERIC NAME (Brand name, manufacturer [country]) VA Classification (Primary/Secondary) | DOSAGE FORMS AND STRENGTHS | CATEGORIES— INDICATIONS | USUAL ADULT DOSE | USUAL PEDIATRIC DOSE | COMMENTS |
|---|---|---|---|---|---|
| Fibrin Sealant (Tisseel VH Kit, Baxter [U.S.]) BL116/XX000 | for Solution: 0.5 mL, 1 mL, 2 mL, and 5 mL kits containing 1 vial each of Sealer Protein Concentrate (Human), Vapor Heated, freeze-dried, sterile; Fibrinolysis Inhibitor Solution (Bovine), sterile, 3000 KIU of aprotinin per mL; Thrombin (Human), Vapor Heated, freeze-dried, sterile, 500 IU per mL; and Calcium Chloride Solution, sterile, 40 micromoles per mL | Antihemorrhagic adjunct (local); Sealant (local)—Hemorrhage, surgical-associated, involving cardiopulmonary bypass (treatment adjunct)‡; Hemorrhage, during surgical repair of spleen (treatment adjunct)‡; Sealant, colostomy closure (treatment adjunct)‡ | Locally, to the involved area, as follows: 0.5 mL for up to 4 cm$^2$ area 1 mL for up to 8 cm$^2$ area 2 mL for up to 16 cm$^2$ area 5 mL for up to 40 cm$^2$ area | Safety and efficacy have not been established | New drug |
| Flunisolide (Nasarel, Roche [U.S.]) NT201 | Nasal Solution USP: 0.025% (25 mcg) per metered spray | | | | Additional brand name product |
| Fluocinonide (Lemmon [U.S.]) DE200 | Ointment: 0.05% | | | | Available generically |
| Fluocinonide, Procinonide, and Ciprocinonide* (Trisyn, Medican [Canada]) DE200 | Cream: 0.015% (total corticosteroids) | Corticosteroid (topical); Anti-inflammatory (steroidal)— Corticosteroid-responsive dermatoses‡ | Topical, to the skin, as a 0.015% cream 1 to 3 times a day | | For general information that may apply to all topical corticosteroids, see Corticosteroids (Topical) |
| Flurbiprofen Sodium (Bausch & Lomb [U.S.]) OP302/OP900 | Ophthalmic Solution USP: 0.03% | | | | Available generically |
| Fluspirilene* (Imap, McNeil [Canada]) (Imap Forte, McNeil [Canada]) CN709 | Injection: 2 mg per mL Injection: 10 mg per mL | Antipsychotic—Psychotic disorders‡ | IM, initially 2 to 3 mg once a week, the dose being increased by 1 to 2 mg per week, as needed and tolerated | | A long-acting diphenylbutylpiperidine neuroleptic, with side effects similar to other neuroleptics; extrapyramidal symptoms tend to occur or peak during the first 2 days after injection |
| Fluticasone Propionate (Flonase, Glaxo [Canada]) NT201 | Nasal Suspension: 50 mcg per metered spray | | | | Additional dosage form For general information that may apply to all nasal corticosteroids, see Corticosteroids (Nasal) |
| Foscarnet (Foscavir, Astra [U.S.]) AM802 | Injection: 6000 mg per 250 mL and 12,000 mg per 500 mL | Antiviral (systemic)—Herpes simplex infections, mucocutaneous acyclovir-resistant‡ | IV, 40 mg per kg of body weight, administered over at least 1 hour, every 8 or 12 hours for 2 to 3 weeks or until healed | | Additional FDA-approved indication |
| Framycetin Sulfate* (Soframycin, Roussel [Canada]) OP201 | Ophthalmic Ointment: 0.5% Ophthalmic Solution: 0.5% | Antibacterial (ophthalmic)—Abrasions, corneal‡; Blepharitis, bacterial‡; Burns, corneal‡; Conjunctivitis, bacterial‡; Hordeolum‡; Ocular infections‡; Ocular infections following foreign body removal†; Ulcer, corneal‡ | Ophthalmic ointment— Topical, to the conjunctiva, a thin strip of ointment every 8 to 12 hours; or at bedtime, concurrently with the ophthalmic solution Ophthalmic solution— Topical, to the conjunctiva, 1 or 2 drops every 1 to 2 hours, for 2 or 3 days, then decreased to 1 or 2 drops every 6 to 8 hours | See Usual adult dose | Canadian drug product Belongs to the group of Streptomyces-derived antibiotics (including neomycin, paromomycin, kanamycin) |

## Additional Products and Indications (continued)

| GENERIC NAME (Brand name, manufacturer [country]) VA Classification (Primary/Secondary) | DOSAGE FORMS AND STRENGTHS | CATEGORIES—INDICATIONS | USUAL ADULT DOSE | USUAL PEDIATRIC DOSE | COMMENTS |
|---|---|---|---|---|---|
| Framycetin Sulfate* (Sofra-Tulle, Roussel [Canada]) DE101 | Impregnated Gauze: 1% | Antibacterial (topical)—Burn wound infections‡; Skin infections, bacterial, minor‡ | Topical, to the skin, once a day or more frequently. May be applied less frequently in non-exudative lesions | See Usual adult dose | Canadian drug product Belongs to the group of Streptomyces-derived antibiotics (including neomycin, paromomycin, kanamycin) |
| Framycetin Sulfate and Gramicidin* (Soframycin, Roussel [Canada]) DE101 | Ointment: 1.5% and 0.005%§ | Antibacterial (topical)—Burn wound infections‡; Folliculitis‡; Paronychia‡; Skin infections, bacterial, minor‡ | Topical, to the skin, 2 to 4 times a day | See Usual adult dose | Canadian combination product |
| Framycetin Sulfate, Gramicidin, and Dexamethasone* (Sofracort Eye-Ear, Roussel [Canada]) OP350 | Ophthalmic Ointment: 5 mg, 50 mcg, and 500 mcg per gram§ Ophthalmic Solution: 5 mg, 50 mcg, and 500 mcg per mL§ | Antibacterial-adrenocorticoid (ophthalmic)—Ocular infections‡ | Ophthalmic ointment—Topical, to the conjunctiva, a thin strip of ointment every 8 to 12 hours; or at bedtime, concurrently with the ophthalmic solution Ophthalmic solution—Topical, to the conjunctiva, 1 or 2 drops every 1 to 2 hours for 2 or 3 days, then decreased to 1 or 2 drops every 6 to 8 hours | Dosage has not been established | Canadian combination product |
| Framycetin Sulfate, Gramicidin, and Dexamethasone* (Sofracort Eye-Ear, Roussel [Canada]) OT250 | Otic Ointment: 5 mg, 50 mcg, and 500 mcg per gram§ Otic Solution: 5 mg, 50 mcg, and 500 mcg per mL§ | Antibacterial-corticosteroid (otic)—Otitis externa, acute‡; Otitis externa, chronic‡; Inflammatory and seborrheic conditions of the external ear, other‡ | Otic ointment—Topical, to the ear, every 8 to 12 hours Otic solution—Topical, to the ear canal, 2 or 3 drops every 6 to 8 hours | Dosage has not been established | Canadian combination product |
| Fusidic Acid* (Fucidin, Leo [Canada]) AM900 | for Injection: 482 mg (base) Oral Suspension: 246 mg per 5 mL Tablets: 240 mg (base) | Antibacterial (systemic)—Bone infections‡; Burn wound infections‡; Endocarditis, bacterial‡; Pneumonia, staphylococcal‡; Septicemia, bacterial‡; Skin and soft-tissue infections‡ | for Injection—IV infusion, 482 mg (base) every 8 hours Oral suspension—Oral, 738 mg every 8 hours Tablets—Oral, 480 mg (base) every 8 hours | for Injection— Infants and children up to 12 years of age: IV infusion, 5.53 mg (base) per kg of body weight every 8 hours, administered over a 6-hour period Oral suspension— Infants and children up to 1 year of age: Oral, 16.4 mg per kg of body weight every 8 hours Children 1 to 5 years of age: Oral, 246 mg every 8 hours Children 6 to 12 years of age: Oral, 492 mg every 8 hours | Canadian drug product Because of incomplete absorption (approximately 70%), the dose of the oral suspension dosage form is correspondingly higher |
| Fusidic Acid* (Fucidin, Leo [Canada]) DE101 | Cream: 2% (as fusidic acid) Impregnated Gauze: 2% (as sodium fusidate) Ointment: 2% (as sodium fusidate) | Antibacterial (topical)—Burn wound infections‡; Erythrasma‡; Skin infections, bacterial, minor‡ | Cream and ointment—Topical, to the skin, 3 or 4 times a day Impregnated gauze—Topical, to the skin, once a day or more frequently. May be applied less frequently in non-exudative lesions | See Usual adult dose | Canadian drug product |

*Not commercially available in the United States.
†Prophylactic.
‡Therapeutic.
§Respectively.
#Diagnostic.

## Additional Products and Indications (continued)

| GENERIC NAME (Brand name, manufacturer [country]) VA Classification (Primary/Secondary) | DOSAGE FORMS AND STRENGTHS | CATEGORIES—INDICATIONS | USUAL ADULT DOSE | USUAL PEDIATRIC DOSE | COMMENTS |
|---|---|---|---|---|---|
| Ganciclovir (Cytovene, Roche [U.S.]) | Capsules: 250 mg | Antiviral (systemic)—Cytomegalovirus (CMV) disease in individuals with advanced HIV infection and transplant patients at risk for developing CMV disease† | Oral, 1000 mg 3 times a day | Safety and efficacy have not been established | Additional FDA-approved indication for the oral dosage form |
| (Cytovene, Roche [Canada]) AM809 | | Antiviral (systemic)—Cytomegalovirus (CMV) retinitis, maintenance treatment in imunocompromised patients where retinitis is stable following at least 3 weeks of therapy with intravenous ganciclovir‡ | | | Additional dosage form in Canada |
| Glyburide (Novopharm [U.S. and Canada]) HS502 | Tablets: 1.25, 2.5, and 5 mg | | | | Available generically |
| Haemophilus b Conjugate Vaccine (Omnihib, SmithKline [U.S.]) IM100 | Injection: 10 mcg of purified haemophilus b capsular polysaccharide and 20 mcg of tetanus protein, per 0.5 mL dose | | | | Additional brand name product |
| Halofantrine Hydrochloride (Halfan, SmithKline Beecham [U.S.]) AP101 | Tablets: 250 mg | Antimalarial—Mild to moderate malaria caused by *Plasmodium falciparum* or *plasmodium vivax*‡ | Oral— Non-immune patients: 500 mg every 6 hours for 3 doses; repeat in 7 days Semi-immune patients: 500 mg every 6 hours for 3 doses Tablets should be taken on an empty stomach at least 1 hour before or 2 hours after food | Safety and efficacy have not been established | Now available in the U.S. and Canada |
| Hemin (Panhematin, Abbott [U.S.]) BL900 | for Injection: Approximately 7 mg hematin equivalents per mL when reconstituted | Porphyrin synthesis inhibitor—Porphyria, acute intermittent‡; Coproporphyria, hereditary‡; Porphyria variegata‡ | IV, 1 to 4 mg per kg of body weight a day for 3 to 14 days. In severe cases may be administered at intervals of not less than 12 hours, but total dosage per 24 hours should not exceed 6 mg per kg of body weight | Dosage has not been established | To be administered only by physicians experienced in the management of porphyrias, in hospitals where the recommended clinical and laboratory monitoring techniques are available. To be considered only for patients who do not respond satisfactorily to an appropriate period of alternate therapy, i.e., 400 grams of glucose per day for 1 or 2 days. Filtering the reconstituted solution through a sterile 0.45-micron (or smaller) filter is recommended |
| Hydrocodone Bitartrate and Acetaminophen (Lortab 10/500, UCB Pharma [U.S.]) CN101/RE301 | Tablets USP: 10 mg and 500 mg§ | Analgesic—Moderate to moderately severe pain‡ | Oral, 1 tablet every 4 to 6 hours as needed for pain Total daily dose should not exceed 6 tablets | Safety and efficacy have not been established | Additional strength |

## Additional Products and Indications *(continued)*

| GENERIC NAME (Brand name, manufacturer [country]) VA Classification (Primary/Secondary) | DOSAGE FORMS AND STRENGTHS | CATEGORIES— INDICATIONS | USUAL ADULT DOSE | USUAL PEDIATRIC DOSE | COMMENTS |
|---|---|---|---|---|---|
| Hydrocortisone (*Anusol-HC 2.5%*, PD [U.S.]) | Cream USP: 2.5% | Corticosteroid (topical); Anti-inflammatory, steroidal (topical)—Skin disorders‡ | Topical, to the affected area(s), 2 to 4 times a day | | Additional brand name product |
| (*Prevex HC*, Trans-CanaDerm [Canada]) DE200 | Cream USP: 1% | | | | Canadian brand name product |
| Hydrocortisone Acetate (*Gynecort 10*, Combe [U.S.]; *Lanacort 10*, Combe [U.S.]) DE200 | Cream USP: 1% | Corticosteroid (topical); Anti-inflammatory, steroidal (topical)—Skin disorders‡ | Topical, to the skin or affected areas, as a 1% cream, 1 to 4 times a day | Children up to 2 years of age—Dosage has not been established Children 2 years of age and older—See *Usual adult dose* | Additional brand name products; OTC |
| Hydrocortisone Buteprate (*Pandel*, Savage [U.S.]) DE200 | Cream: 0.1% | Corticosteroid (topical); Anti-inflammatory, steroidal (topical)—Dermatoses, corticosteroid-responsive‡ | Topical, to the affected area as a thin film once or twice a day | Safety and efficacy have not been established | U.S. drug product |
| Hydrocortisone Butyrate (*Locoid*, Yamanouchi Europe B.V. [U.S.]) DE200 | Topical Solution: 0.1% | Corticosteroid (topical); Anti-inflammatory, steroidal (topical)—Dermatitis, seborrheic‡ | Topical, to the affected area as a thin film 2 or 3 times a day | | Additional dosage form |
| Hydrocortisone and Acetic Acid (*Acetasol HC*, Barre [U.S.]; *Otomycet-HC*, Marin [U.S.]; *Vasotate HC*, Major [U.S.]) (Bausch & Lomb [U.S.]) OT250 | Otic Solution USP: 1% and 2%§ | | | | Additional brand name products Available generically |
| Hydrocortisone and Urea (*Sential*, Pharmacia [Canada]) DE200 | Cream: 0.5% and 4%§ | | | | Canadian brand name product For general information that may apply to this medication, see *Corticosteroids (Topical)* |
| Hydroxypropyl Methylcellulose (*Ocucoat*, Storz [U.S.]) OP900 | Injection: 20 mg per mL | Surgical aid (ophthalmic)—Anterior segment, surgical procedures of, including cataract extraction and intraocular lens (IOL) implantation | Intracavitary, a sufficient quantity injected into the anterior chamber at any time during intraocular surgery to maintain patency of, or to replace fluids lost from, the anterior chamber during the surgical procedure | See *Usual adult dose* | Additional FDA-approved indication; additional dosage form Brand name change—formerly *Occucoat*; Rx For general information that may apply, see *Hydroxypropyl Methylcellulose (Ophthalmic)* |

*Not commercially available in the United States.
†Prophylactic.
‡Therapeutic.
§Respectively.
#Diagnostic.

## Additional Products and Indications (continued)

| GENERIC NAME (Brand name, manufacturer [country]) VA Classification (Primary/Secondary) | DOSAGE FORMS AND STRENGTHS | CATEGORIES— INDICATIONS | USUAL ADULT DOSE | USUAL PEDIATRIC DOSE | COMMENTS |
|---|---|---|---|---|---|
| Hydroxyurea (*Droxia*, Bristol-Myers Squibb [U.S.]) XX000 | Capsules: 200, 300, and 400 mg | Sickle cell disease therapy agent— Sickle cell disease‡ | Oral, initially, 15 mg per kg of body weight per day, as a single dose. If blood counts are in acceptable range, dose may be increased by 5 mg per kg of body weight per day every 12 weeks until a maximum tolerated dose (i.e. the highest dose that does not produce toxic blood counts over 24 consecutive weeks) or 35 mg per kg of body weight per day is reached. If toxic blood counts occur, dosing should be discontinued until hematological recovery. Treatment may be resumed after dose is reduced by 2.5 mg per kg of body weight per day from the dose associated with the toxicity. Dose may be increased or decreased in increments of 2.5 mg per kg of body weight per day every 12 weeks, until patient does not experience hematological toxicity for 24 weeks | Safety and efficacy have not been established | Additional brand name product<br>Additional FDA-approved indication and dose<br>Used for reduction in frequency of painful crises and need for blood transfusions in adult patients with generally at least 3 moderate to severe painful crises within last 12 months<br>Dosing should be based on actual or ideal body weight, whichever is less<br>Blood counts should be monitored every two weeks; acceptable range of blood counts: neutrophils ≥2500 cells per cubic millimeter; platelets ≥95,000 cells per cubic millimeter; hemoglobin >5.3 grams per dL; and reticulocytes ≥95,000 cells per cubic millimeter, if the hemoglobin concentration is <9 grams per dL<br>Toxic range of blood counts: neutrophils <2000 cells per cubic millimeter; platelets <80,000 cells per cubic millimeter; hemoglobin <4.5 grams per dL; and reticulocytes <80,000 cells per cubic millimeter, if the hemoglobin concentration is <9 grams per dL<br>Dose should not be increased if blood counts are between the acceptable and toxic range |
| Immune Globulin Intravenous (Human) (*Gamimune N*, Bayer [U.S. and Canada]) | Injection: 5 and 10% | Immunizing agent (passive); Antibacterial (systemic)— Immunodepression, bone marrow transplantation (BMT)† | For adults 20 years of age and older—IV, 500 mg (10 mL for 5% solution, 5 mL for 10% solution) per kg of body weight each day on Days 7 through 2 before transplantation (or beginning at the time conditioning therapy for transplantation is begun), then 500 mg (10 mL for 5% solution, 5 mL for 10% solution) per kg of body weight each week through Day 90 after transplantation | Use is not recommended | Additional FDA-approved indication |
| | | Immunizing agent (passive); Antibacterial (systemic)— Human immunodeficiency virus (HIV) disease, pediatric, infections in† | | IV, 400 mg (8 mL for 5% solution, 4 mL for 10% solution) per kg of body weight as a single infusion every 28 days | Additional FDA-approved indication |

## Additional Products and Indications (continued)

| GENERIC NAME (Brand name, manufacturer [country]) VA Classification (Primary/Secondary) | DOSAGE FORMS AND STRENGTHS | CATEGORIES—INDICATIONS | USUAL ADULT DOSE | USUAL PEDIATRIC DOSE | COMMENTS |
|---|---|---|---|---|---|
| Immune Globulin Intravenous (Human) (*Gammagard SD*, Baxter [U.S.]; *SD Polygam*, Baxter [U.S.]) | for Injection: 0.5, 2.5, 5, and 10 grams, with a suitable amount of diluent | | | | Additional brand name products; *SD Polygam* is distributed by the American Red Cross<br><br>The products replace *Gammagard* and *Polygam*, respectively, which were withdrawn from the market worldwide because of possible association with hepatitis C virus<br><br>For these new products, an organic solvent detergent virally-inactivated purification process is used to inactivate lipid-enveloped viruses such as hepatitis C virus |
| (*Iveegam*, Immuno [U.S.]) | for Injection: 0.5, 1, 2.5, and 5 grams, along with a suitable amount of diluent | Anti-Kawasaki disease agent (systemic)—Kawasaki disease‡ | | IV, 400 mg per kg of body weight a day for 4 days; alternatively, a single dose of 2 grams per kg of body weight may be administered over a ten-hour period. Treatment should be initiated within 10 days of onset of the disease. The treatment regimen should include 100 mg of aspirin per kg of body weight a day through the fourteenth day of illness, then 3 to 5 mg of aspirin per kg of body weight a day thereafter for 5 weeks | Additional FDA-approved indication |
| (*Venoglobulin-S*, Alpha [U.S.]) IM500/AM900; BL900; CV900 | Injection: 5 and 10% | Immunizing agent (passive); Platelet count stimulator (systemic)—Immunodeficiency, primary‡; Thrombocytopenic purpura, idiopathic (ITP)‡ | For ITP:<br>Induction—IV, a maximum cumulative dose of 2 grams (40 mL for 5% solution, 20 mL for 10% solution) per kg of body weight, administered over a maximum of 5 days<br>Maintenance—IV, 1 gram (20 mL for 5% solution, 10 mL for 10% solution) per kg of body weight as a single infusion, repeated intermittently as needed | See *Usual adult dose* | Additional brand name product; additional dosage for ITP |
| Insulin Lispro (*Humalog*, Eli Lilly [Canada]) HS501 | Injection: 100 USP Insulin Human Units per mL | Antidiabetic agent—Diabetes mellitus‡ | SC, dosage must be determined by the physician based on individual patient requirements<br>When used as a mealtime insulin, insulin lispro should be administered within 15 minutes before the meal | | Canadian drug product |

*Not commercially available in the United States.
†Prophylactic.
‡Therapeutic.
§Respectively.
#Diagnostic.

## Additional Products and Indications (continued)

| GENERIC NAME (Brand name, manufacturer [country]) VA Classification (Primary/Secondary) | DOSAGE FORMS AND STRENGTHS | CATEGORIES— INDICATIONS | USUAL ADULT DOSE | USUAL PEDIATRIC DOSE | COMMENTS |
|---|---|---|---|---|---|
| Interferon, Beta-1a (Rebif, Serono Canada Inc. [Canada]) CN900/IM700 | for Injection: 11 mcg (3 million International Units [IU]) and 44 mcg (12 million IU) Injection: 22 mcg (6 million IU) and 44 mcg (12 million IU) per 0.5 mL | Multiple sclerosis therapy agent—Multiple sclerosis‡ Biological response modifier—Condyloma acuminatum‡ | Multiple sclerosis: Subcutaneous, 22 mcg (6 million IU) 3 times a week Condyloma acuminatum: Intra- or peri-lesional, 3.67 mcg (1 million IU) per lesion 3 times a week for 3 weeks | Children up to 16 years of age—Safety and efficacy have not been established | Available in Canada |
| Interferon Beta-1b (Betaseron, Berlex [Canada]) IM900 | for Injection: 0.3 mg (9.6 million units) | Immunomodulator— Multiple sclerosis‡ | SC, 0.25 mg (8 million units) every other day | Safety and efficacy have not been established | Canadian drug product |
| Ipratropium Bromide (Atrovent, Boehringer Ingelheim [U.S.]) NT900 | Nasal Solution: | Anticholinergic (nasal)— | Nasal, | Children up to 12 years of age: Safety and efficacy have not been established | Additional dosage form; additional strengths; additional FDA-approved indications |
| | 0.03% per metered spray | Rhinorrhea (associated with perennial allergic rhinitis and perennial non-allergic rhinitis)‡ | 42 mcg (2 metered sprays) into each nostril 2 or 3 times a day | Children 12 years of age and older: See Usual adult dose | Does not relieve nasal congestion, sneezing, or postnasal drip associated with perennial allergic rhinitis and perennial non-allergic rhinitis |
| | 0.06% per metered spray | Rhinorrhea (associated with the common cold)‡ | 84 mcg (2 metered sprays) into each nostril 3 or 4 times a day | Children 12 years of age and older: See Usual adult dose | Does not relieve nasal congestion or sneezing associated with the common cold Safety and efficacy beyond 4 days in patients with the common cold have not been established |
| Isotretinoin (Isotrex, Stiefel [Canada]) DE752 | Gel: 0.05% | Antiacne agent (topical)—Acne vulgaris‡ | Topical, to the skin, 2 times a day, morning and at bedtime | Dosage has not been established | Canadian brand name product; additional dosage form |
| Ivermectin (Stromectol, Merck [U.S.]) AP200 | Tablets: 6 mg | Anthelmintic—Strongyloidiasis (nondisseminated intestinal threadworm)‡; Onchocerciasis (river blindness)‡ | Oral— Strongyloidiasis: A single dose based on body weight, 200 mcg per kg of body weight Onchocerciasis: A single dose based on body weight, 150 mcg per kg of body weight | Safety and efficacy have not been established in pediatric patients weighing less than 15 kg | U.S. drug product |
| Ketoconazole (Nizoral, Janssen [U.S.]) DE102 | Shampoo: 2% | Antifungal—Tinea versicolor (pityriasis)‡ | Topical, to damp skin of the affected area and to surrounding area, as a single application. Lather and leave in place for 5 minutes, then rinse off with water | Safety and efficacy have not been established | New FDA-approved indication |
| Ketorolac Tromethamine (Acular, Allergan [U.S.]) OP302/OP900 | Ophthalmic Solution: 0.5% | Anti-inflammatory, nonsteroidal (ophthalmic)—Inflammation, ocular (following cataract surgery)‡ | Topical, to the conjunctiva, 1 drop in the affected eye 4 times a day, beginning 24 hours after cataract surgery and continuing through the first 2 weeks of the postoperative period | Children 12 years of age and older: See Usual Adult Dose Children under 12 years of age: Safety and efficacy have not been established | Additional FDA-approved indication |
| Ketotifen Fumarate* (Zaditen, Sandoz [Canada]) RE109 | Syrup: 1 mg (base) per 5 mL Tablets: 1 mg (base) | Asthma prophylactic; Antiallergic (systemic)—Asthma, atopic, in children† | | Children up to 3 years of age—Dosage has not been established Children 3 years of age and older—Oral, 1 mg 2 times a day with morning and evening meals | Canadian drug product |
| Latanoprost (Xalatan, Pharmacia & Upjohn [Canada]) OP116 | Ophthalmic Solution: 0.005% | | | | Available in Canada |

# Additional Products and Indications *(continued)*

| GENERIC NAME (*Brand name*, manufacturer [country]) VA Classification (Primary/Secondary) | DOSAGE FORMS AND STRENGTHS | CATEGORIES— INDICATIONS | USUAL ADULT DOSE | USUAL PEDIATRIC DOSE | COMMENTS |
|---|---|---|---|---|---|
| Levobunolol Hydrochloride (Bausch & Lomb [U.S.]) (*AKBeta*, Akorn [U.S.]) OP110 | Ophthalmic Solution USP: 0.25 and 0.5% | | | | Available generically Additional brand name product |
| Levocabastine (*Livostin*, Janssen [Canada]) NT900 | Nasal Suspension: 0.05% | Antihistaminic (H₁-receptor) (nasal)—Rhinitis, allergic‡ | Adolescents and adults 12 to 65 years of age—Intranasal, 2 sprays into each nostril 2 times a day<br>Adults over 65 years of age—Safety and efficacy have not been established | Children up to 12 years of age—Safety and efficacy have not been established | Canadian drug product |
| Levocabastine Hydrochloride (*Livostin*, CIBA Vision [U.S. and Canada]) OP801 | Ophthalmic Suspension: 0.05% (0.5 mg/mL [base]) | Antihistaminic (H₁-receptor) (ophthalmic); Antiallergic (ophthalmic)—Conjunctivitis, seasonal allergic‡ | In the U.S.—Topical, to the conjunctiva, 1 drop 4 times a day | | FDA-approved labeling no longer restricts use to 2 weeks<br>Change in manufacturer/distributor |
| Levodopa and Benserazide* (*Prolopa*, Roche [Canada]) CN500 | Capsules: 50 mg and 12.5 mg§; 100 mg and 25 mg§; 200 mg and 50 mg§ | Antidyskinetic—Parkinsonism‡ | For patients not being converted from levodopa therapy—Oral, 100 mg of levodopa and 25 mg of benserazide 1 or 2 times a day initially, the dosage per day being increased gradually by 1 capsule every third or fourth day, as needed and tolerated<br>For patients being converted from levodopa therapy (levodopa must be discontinued for at least 12 hours prior to conversion to levodopa and benserazide therapy)—Dosage should provide approximately 15% of the previous levodopa daily dosage | Dosage has not been established | The 50/12.5 and 200/50 mg capsules are intended only for maintenance therapy once the optimal dosage has been determined |
| Levonorgestrel and Ethinyl Estradiol (*Levlite*, Berlex [U.S.]) HS200/HS900 | Tablets: Monophasic formulation—100 mcg of levonorgestrel and 20 mcg of ethinyl estradiol<br>Note: Available in 21- or 28-day cycles. The 28-day cycle includes 7 days of placebo tablets | Contraceptive, systemic—Pregnancy, prevention of† | | | Additional brand name product |

*Not commercially available in the United States.
†Prophylactic.
‡Therapeutic.
§Respectively.
#Diagnostic.

## Additional Products and Indications *(continued)*

| GENERIC NAME (*Brand name*, manufacturer [country]) VA Classification (Primary/Secondary) | DOSAGE FORMS AND STRENGTHS | CATEGORIES— INDICATIONS | USUAL ADULT DOSE | USUAL PEDIATRIC DOSE | COMMENTS |
|---|---|---|---|---|---|
| Liothyronine Sodium (*Triostat*, SmithKline Beecham [U.S.]) HS851 | Injection: 10 mcg per mL (base) | Thyroid hormone— Myxedema coma/ precoma‡ | IV, initially 25 to 50 mcg. Initial and subsequent doses should be titrated to patient status and response. Lower initial dosing (10 to 20 mcg) is recommended for patients with known or suspected cardiovascular disease. Dosing interval is generally between 4 and 12 hours | | Additional dosage form |
| Lodoxamide Tromethamine (*Alomide*, Alcon Canada [Canada]) OP900 | Ophthalmic Solution: 0.1% | | | | Available in Canada |
| Loperamide and Simethicone (*Imodium Advanced*, McNeil Consumer [U.S.]) GA400/GA900 | Chewable Tablets: 2 mg and 125 mg§ | Antidiarrheal/ Antiflatulent— Diarrhea‡; Gas, gastrointestinal‡ | Oral, 2 tablets after first loose stool; if needed, 1 tablet after next loose stool. Not to exceed 4 tablets a day. Tablets should be chewed, then taken with water | Children 6 to 8 years of age (48 to 59 pounds)—Oral, 1 tablet after first loose stool; if needed, ½ tablet after next loose stool. Not to exceed 2 tablets a day. Children 9 to 11 years of age (60 to 95 pounds)—Oral, 1 tablet after first loose stool; if needed, ½ tablet after next loose stool. Not to exceed 3 tablets a day. Children 12 years of age and older—See *Usual adult dose*. Tablets should be chewed, then taken with water | New OTC drug combination |
| Methylprednisolone Sodium Succinate (*Solu-Medrol*, Upjohn [Canada]) HS051/IM600 | for Injection USP: 40, 125, and 500 mg and 1 gram (base) | Corticosteroid (systemic); Anti-inflammatory (steroidal); Immunosuppressant— Spinal cord injury‡ | Spinal cord injury (acute) —IV, 30 mg (base) per kg of body weight administered over 15 minutes, followed in 45 minutes by a continuous infusion of 5.4 mg per kg per hour, for 23 hours | | HPB-approved indication in Canada; treatment should begin within 8 hours of injury |
| Metronidazole (*MetroCream*, Galderma [U.S.]) DE752 | Cream: 0.75% | Antirosacea agent (topical)—Rosacea‡ | Topical, to the affected area(s), 2 times daily | Safety and efficacy have not been established | New dosage form |
| Metronidazole and Nystatin* (*Flagystatin*, Rhone-Poulenc [Canada]) GU309 | Vaginal Cream: 500 mg and 100,000 Units§ per applicatorful. Vaginal Suppositories: 500 mg and 100,000 Units§. Vaginal Tablets: 500 mg and 100,000 Units§ | Antiprotozoal-antifungal (vaginal)—Candidiasis, vulvovaginal‡; Trichomoniasis‡ | Intravaginal, 1 applicatorful of cream, 1 vaginal suppository, or 1 vaginal tablet once a day for 10 days | Dosage has not been established | Canadian combination product |
| Moclobemide* (*Manerex*, Hoffmann-La Roche, [Canada]) CN609 | Tablets: 100 and 150 mg (scored) | Antidepressant— Depression‡ | Oral, initially 300 mg a day given in 2 or 3 divided doses, the dose being increased, as needed and tolerated, to a maximum of 600 mg a day | Children up to 18 years of age—Safety and efficacy have not been established | Canadian drug product |

## Additional Products and Indications (continued)

| GENERIC NAME (Brand name, manufacturer [country]) VA Classification (Primary/Secondary) | DOSAGE FORMS AND STRENGTHS | CATEGORIES—INDICATIONS | USUAL ADULT DOSE | USUAL PEDIATRIC DOSE | COMMENTS |
|---|---|---|---|---|---|
| Morphine Sulfate (Kadian, Purepac Pharmaceutical [U.S. and Canada]) CN101 | Extended-release Capsules: 20, 50, and 100 mg | | | | Available in the U.S. For general information that may apply to all opioid analgesics, see Opioid (Narcotic) Analgesics (Systemic) |
| Mupirocin Calcium (Bactroban, SmithKline Beecham [U.S.]) DE101 | Cream: 2% (mupirocin free acid) | Antibacterial (topical)—Skin lesions, traumatic, secondarily infected‡ | Topical, to the affected area, 3 times daily for 10 days | Children up to 3 months of age: Dosage has not been established  Children 3 months of age and older: See Usual adult dose | New dosage form Patients not showing a clinical response within 3 to 5 days should be re-evaluated |
| Naltrexone Hydrochloride (Barr [U.S.]) CN102/AD100 | Tablets: 50 mg | | | | Now available generically |
| Naproxen (Naprelan, Wyeth-Ayerst [U.S.]) MS102/CN104; MS400 | Extended-release Tablets: 375 and 500 mg | Analgesic—Pain‡ Antigout—Acute gout‡ Anti-inflammatory—Bursitis‡; Tendinitis‡ Antidysmenorrheal—Dysmenorrhea‡ Antirheumatic—Rheumatoid arthritis‡; Osteoarthritis‡; Ankylosing spondylitis‡ | Analgesic and Antirheumatic—Oral, two 375-mg tablets once daily, or two 500-mg tablets once daily  Anti-inflammatory and Antidysmenorrheal—Oral, two 500-mg tablets once daily. For patients that require greater analgesic benefit, three 500-mg tablets once daily for a limited period. Thereafter, the daily dose should not exceed two 500-mg tablets  Antigout—Oral, initially two to three 500-mg tablets once daily, followed by two 500-mg tablets once daily, until attack has subsided | Safety and efficacy have not been established | Additional dosage form |
| Nefazodone (Serzone, Bristol-Myers Squibb [Canada]) CN609 | Tablets: 100 and 150 mg (scored); 200 mg | Antidepressant—Depression, mental‡ | Oral, initially 100 mg twice a day, the dose being increased as needed and tolerated, to 300 to 600 mg a day | Safety and efficacy have not been established | Available in Canada |
| Neomycin and Polymyxin B Sulfates and Gramicidin (Triple Antibiotic, Steris [U.S.]) OP201 | Ophthalmic Solution USP: 1.75 mg of neomycin (base), 10,000 Units of polymyxin B (base), and 25 mcg of gramicidin, per mL | | | | Additional brand name product |
| Nicardipine Hydrochloride (Cardene SR, Roche [U.S.]) CV200/CV409 | Extended-release Capsules: 30, 45, and 60 mg | Antihypertensive—Hypertension‡ | Oral, initially 30 mg twice a day, the dosage being adjusted as needed and tolerated | Safety and efficacy have not been established | Additional dosage form |
| Nicotinamide* (Papulex, GenDerm [Canada]) DE752 | Gel: 4% | Antiacne agent (topical)—Acne vulgaris‡ | Topical, to the skin, 2 times a day | Dosage has not been established | Canadian drug product |

*Not commercially available in the United States.
†Prophylactic.
‡Therapeutic.
§Respectively.
#Diagnostic.

## Additional Products and Indications (continued)

| GENERIC NAME (Brand name, manufacturer [country]) VA Classification (Primary/Secondary) | DOSAGE FORMS AND STRENGTHS | CATEGORIES— INDICATIONS | USUAL ADULT DOSE | USUAL PEDIATRIC DOSE | COMMENTS |
|---|---|---|---|---|---|
| Nicotine<br><br>(NicoDerm CQ, SmithKline Beecham [U.S.])<br><br>(SANO Corporation [U.S.])<br><br>(Habitrol, Novartis [Canada])<br><br>(Nicotrol, McNeil [U.S.])<br>AD900 | Transdermal Systems: 7, 14, and 21 mg<br><br><br><br><br><br><br><br>Transdermal System: 15 mg | Smoking cessation adjunct—Nicotine dependence‡ | <br><br><br><br><br><br><br><br><br><br>Topical, to intact skin, 1 patch applied for 16 hours per day for 6 weeks | <br><br><br><br><br><br><br><br><br><br>Safety and efficacy have not been established | Available OTC; brand name change<br><br>Now available generically<br><br>Now available OTC<br><br>Available OTC; additional dosing regimen |
| Nystatin (Nystop, Paddock Laboratories [U.S.])<br>DE102 | Topical Powder USP: 100,000 USP nystatin units per gram | | | | Additional brand name product |
| Ofloxacin (Ocuflox, Allergan [U.S. and Canada])<br>OP201 | Ophthalmic Solution: 0.3% (3 mg/mL) | Antibacterial (ophthalmic)—Corneal ulcers, bacterial‡ | Topical, to the conjunctiva. On days 1 and 2, 1 drop in the affected eye every 30 minutes while awake and 1 drop 4 to 6 hours after retiring. On days 3 through 7, 8, or 9, 1 drop every hour while awake. On days 7, 8, or 9 through treatment completion, 1 drop 4 times a day | Infants and children up to 1 year of age: Safety and efficacy have not been established<br><br>Children 1 year of age and older—See Usual adult dose | Additional FDA-approved indication for treatment of corneal ulcers, bacterial<br><br>Drug available in Canada |
| Oxaprozin (Daypro, Searle [Canada])<br>MS102 | Tablets: 600 mg | | | | Available in Canada |
| Oxiconazole Nitrate (Oxistat, Glaxo Wellcome [U.S.])<br>DE102 | Cream: 1% | Antifungal—Tinea (pityriasis) versicolor due to Malassezia furfur‡ | Topical, apply to the affected area once daily for 2 weeks | Tinea versicolor—Topical, apply to affected area once daily for 2 weeks. Cream also may be used for tinea corporis and tinea cruris<br><br>Tinea pedis—Topical, apply to affected area once daily for 1 month | New FDA-approved indication for tinea versicolor and pediatric dosage information |
| Oxycodone Hydrochloride (OxyContin SR, Purdue Pharma L.P. [U.S.])<br>CN101 | Extended-release Tablets: 10, 20, 40, and 80 mg | Analgesic—Moderate to severe pain‡ | Oral, administer dose every 12 hours<br><br>Dosage must be individualized by the physician according to the severity of pain and patient response<br><br>The 80-mg dose should be used in opioid tolerant patients only | Safety and efficacy have not been established | Additional dosage form<br><br>For general information that may apply to all opioid analgesics, see Opioid (Narcotic) Analgesics (Systemic) |
| Oxymetazoline Hydrochloride (Nasal Decongestant Spray, Taro [U.S.])<br>NT100 | Nasal Solution USP: 0.05% (nasal spray) | | | | Additional brand name product; OTC |
| Oxymetazoline Hydrochloride (12 Hour Nostrilla Nasal Decongestant, Novartis [U.S.])<br>NT100 | Nasal Solution USP: 0.05% (nasal spray) | | | | OTC<br><br>Formerly Nostrilla Long-Acting Nasal Decongestant |

## Additional Products and Indications (continued)

| GENERIC NAME (Brand name, manufacturer [country]) VA Classification (Primary/Secondary) | DOSAGE FORMS AND STRENGTHS | CATEGORIES—INDICATIONS | USUAL ADULT DOSE | USUAL PEDIATRIC DOSE | COMMENTS |
|---|---|---|---|---|---|
| Pantoprazole (Pantoloc, Solvay [Canada]) GA900/GA309 | Enteric-coated Tablets: 40 mg | Gastric acid pump inhibitor; Antiulcer agent—Ulcer, duodenal‡; Ulcer, gastric‡; Reflux, gastroesophageal‡ | Oral— Ulcer, duodenal: 40 mg once a day in the morning. Healing usually occurs within 2 weeks. If the ulcer has not healed after initial course of therapy, an additional 2-week course of pantoprazole may be given Ulcer, gastric or reflux esophagitis: 40 mg once a day in the morning. Healing usually occurs within 4 weeks. If the patient is not healed after the initial course of therapy, an additional 4-week course of pantoprazole may be given Pantoprazole is not indicated for use as maintenance therapy | Safety and efficacy have not been established | New drug |
| Paricalcitol (Zemplar, Abbott [U.S.]) VT509 | Injection: 5 mcg per mL | Antihyperparathyroid agent—Hyperparathyroidism, secondary†‡ | Intravenous, 0.04 to 0.1 mcg per kg of body weight (approximately 2.8 to 7 mcg) as a bolus dose, given no more frequently than every other day at any time during dialysis If a satisfactory response is not observed, the dose may be increased by 2 to 4 mcg at 2- to 4-week intervals | Safety and efficacy have not been established | New drug |
| Pentastarch (Pentaspan, Du Pont Critical Care [U.S.]) BL900 | Injection: 10%, in 0.9% sodium chloride injection | Leukapheresis adjunct (red cell sedimenting agent)—Improve harvesting and increase yield of leukocytes by centrifugal means | 250 to 700 mL, injected aseptically into the input line of the centrifugation apparatus at a ratio of 1:8 to 1:13 to venous whole blood | Dosage has not been established | Citrate anticoagulant should be added to and thoroughly mixed with the pentastarch, to ensure effective anticoagulation of blood as it flows through the leukapheresis machine |

*Not commercially available in the United States.
†Prophylactic.
‡Therapeutic.
§Respectively.
#Diagnostic.

## Additional Products and Indications (continued)

| GENERIC NAME (Brand name, manufacturer [country]) VA Classification (Primary/Secondary) | DOSAGE FORMS AND STRENGTHS | CATEGORIES— INDICATIONS | USUAL ADULT DOSE | USUAL PEDIATRIC DOSE | COMMENTS |
|---|---|---|---|---|---|
| Permethrin (Acticin, Alpharma [U.S.]) (Elimite, Herbert [U.S.]; Nix Dermal Cream, BW [Canada]) AP300 | Cream; 5% | Scabicide— Scabies‡ | Topical, to the skin from the head to the soles of the feet. Remove, by washing, 8 to 14 hours later | Children up to 2 months of age: Safety and efficacy have not been established. Children 2 months of age and older: See Usual adult dose. One application is generally curative. Usually 30 grams is sufficient for the average adult. Infants 2 months of age and over should be treated also on the scalp, temple, and forehead | Additional FDA-approved indication; additional dosage form in U.S. and Canada. Note—Permethrin 0.5% is used also as a repellent in the form of a contact spray for clothing (not skin) to prevent the bites of ixodid ticks. The bites of ixodid ticks infected with Borrelia burgdorferi cause Lyme disease |
| Phenylephrine Hydrochloride (Dionephrine, Dioptic [Canada]) (Minims Phenylephrine, Smith & Nephew [Canada]) (Neofrin, Ocusoft [U.S.]) OP600/OP802; DX900 | Ophthalmic Solution USP: 2.5% 2.5% 2.5 and 10% | | | | Additional brand name product Additional strength Additional brand name product |
| Pilocarpine Hydrochloride (Salagen, MGI Pharma, Inc. [U.S.], Pharmacia & Upjohn [Canada]) AU300 | Tablets: 5 mg | Cholinergic—Xerostomia, radiation induced‡; Xerostomia in Sjogren's syndrome‡; Xerophthalmia in Sjogren's syndrome‡ | Oral, 1 tablet 4 times a day | Safety and efficacy have not been established | Available in Canada; government-approved indications in Canada |
| Piperacillin and Tazobactam (Zosyn, Wyeth-Ayerst [U.S.]) AM114 | for Injection: 2.25, 3.375, and 4.5 grams | Antibacterial (systemic)—Pneumonia, nosocomial, moderate to severe‡ | IV, 3.375 grams every 4 hours in combination with an aminoglycoside | Dosage has not been established | Additional FDA-approved indication |
| Pizotyline Malate* (Sandomigran, Sandoz [Canada]) (Sandomigran DS, Sandoz [Canada]) CN105 | Tablets: 500 mcg Tablets: 1 mg | Vascular headache prophylactic— Migraine† | Oral, 500 mcg at bedtime, initially; increased gradually to 500 mcg 3 times a day. Maintenance dosage may range from 1 to 6 mg (average 1.5 mg) a day | Dosage has not been established | Dosage should be decreased gradually over a 2-week period prior to discontinuation, to prevent rebound headache |
| Polyacrylamide (Orcolon, Optical Radiation [U.S.]; Dispersa [Canada]) OP900 | Injection: 0.75 mL (4.5% polyacrylamide) | Surgical aid (ophthalmic)—Anterior segment, surgical procedures of, including cataract extraction and intraocular lens (IOL) implantation | Intracavitary, a sufficient quantity injected into the anterior chamber at any time during intraocular surgery to maintain patency of, or to replace fluids lost from, the anterior chamber during the surgical procedure | See Usual adult dose | U.S. and Canadian drug product |
| Polymyxin B Sulfate (Aerosporin, Wellcome [U.S.]) OP201 | for Ophthalmic Solution: 0.1 to 0.25%, depending on amount of diluent used | Antibacterial (ophthalmic)—Ocular infections caused by Pseudomonas aeruginosa‡ | Topical, to the conjunctiva, 1 to 3 drops in each eye every hour, increasing the intervals as response indicates | See Usual adult dose | U.S. drug product |

## Additional Products and Indications (continued)

| GENERIC NAME (Brand name, manufacturer [country]) VA Classification (Primary/Secondary) | DOSAGE FORMS AND STRENGTHS | CATEGORIES— INDICATIONS | USUAL ADULT DOSE | USUAL PEDIATRIC DOSE | COMMENTS |
|---|---|---|---|---|---|
| Pramipexole Dihydrochloride (*Mirapex*, Boehringer-Ingelheim Ltd [Canada]) CN500 | Tablets: 0.25, 1, and 1.5 mg | | | | Available in Canada For general information that may apply, see *Pramipexole (Systemic)—Introductory Version* |
| Prednicarbate (*Dermatop*, Hoechst-Roussel [U.S.]) DE200 | Emollient Cream: 0.1% | Anti-inflammatory, steroidal, topical; Antipruritic, topical—Dermatoses, corticosteroid-responsive‡ | Topical, to the affected skin areas, 2 times a day | Safety and efficacy have not been established | U.S. drug product |
| Pseudoephedrine Hydrochloride and Guaifenesin (*Humibid Guaifenesin Plus*, Menley & James Laboratories [U.S.]) RE516 | Tablets: 60 mg and 400 mg§ | Decongestant-expectorant—Cough‡; Congestion, nasal‡ | Oral, 1 tablet every 4 to 6 hours, not to exceed 4 tablets in 24 hours | Children up to 6 years of age: Use as directed by physician Children 6 to 12 years of age: Oral, ½ tablet every 4 to 6 hours, not to exceed 2 tablets in 24 hours | New OTC brand name product For additional information that may apply to this combination, see *Cough/Cold Combinations (Systemic)* |
| Quetiapine (*Seroquel*, Zeneca Pharma [Canada]) CN709 | Tablets: 25, 100, and 200 mg | | | | Available in Canada |
| Ranitidine Bismuth Citrate (*Pylorid*, Glaxo Wellcome [Canada]) GA303 | Tablets: 400 mg | Antiulcer agent—Active duodenal ulcer associated with *Helicobacter pylori* infection‡, in combination with clarithromycin | Oral, 400 mg twice a day for 4 weeks, taken in combination with clarithromycin (500 mg three times a day or 250 mg four times a day) for the first 2 weeks | Safety and efficacy have not been established | New drug in Canada |
| Ribavirin/Interferon Alfa-2b (*Rebetron*, Schering [U.S.]) AM800 | Capsules: 200 mg/ Injection: 3 million IU of interferon alfa-2b per 0.2 mL and 3 million IU of interferon alfa-2b per 0.5 mL | Antiviral (systemic)—Hepatitis C, chronic‡: In patients with compensated liver disease who have relapsed following alpha interferon therapy | Hepatitis C— For patients ≤ 75 kg of body weight: Oral, 400 mg of ribavirin in the morning and 600 mg of ribavirin in the evening, and subcutaneous, 3 million IU of interferon alfa-2b 3 times per week, for a total of 24 weeks of treatment For patients > 75 kg of body weight: Oral, 600 mg of ribavirin 2 times a day, and subcutaneous, 3 million IU of interferon alfa-2b 3 times per week, for a total of 24 weeks of treatment | Children up to 18 years of age: Safety and efficacy have not been established | New FDA-approved combination therapy product |
| Sacrosidase (*Sucraid*, Orphan Medical [U.S.]) HS551 | Oral Solution: 8500 International Units (IU) per mL | Enzyme replenisher—Sucrase deficiency, a part of congenital sucrase-isomaltase deficiency (CSID)‡ | Oral, 17,000 IU (2 mL) taken with each meal or snack. The dose should be diluted with 2 to 4 ounces of water or milk | Children up to 15 kg of body weight—Oral, 8500 IU (1 mL) taken with each meal or snack. The dose should be diluted with 2 to 4 ounces of water, milk, or infant formula Children over 15 kg of body weight—See *Usual adult dose* | New drug The beverage used for dilution of the medication should be served cold or at room temperature, because heating may decrease the potency; the dose should not be reconstituted or consumed with fruit juices because the acidity may reduce the enzyme activity It is recommended that approximately one-half of the dosage be taken at the beginning of each meal or snack, and the remainder taken at the end of each meal or snack |

\*Not commercially available in the United States.
†Prophylactic.
‡Therapeutic.
§Respectively.
#Diagnostic.

## Additional Products and Indications (continued)

| GENERIC NAME (*Brand name*, manufacturer [country]) VA Classification (Primary/Secondary) | DOSAGE FORMS AND STRENGTHS | CATEGORIES— INDICATIONS | USUAL ADULT DOSE | USUAL PEDIATRIC DOSE | COMMENTS |
|---|---|---|---|---|---|
| Salmeterol Xinafoate (*Serevent*, Glaxo Wellcome [U.S.]) RE102 | Inhalation Aerosol: 21 mcg (base) per metered spray | Bronchodilator— Bronchospasm, chronic bronchitis-associated†; Bronchospasm, chronic obstructive pulmonary disease (COPD)-associated†; Bronchospasm, pulmonary emphysema-associated† | Oral inhalation, 42 mcg (base) (2 inhalations) 2 times a day, morning and evening, approximately 12 hours apart | Children up to 12 years of age—Safety and efficacy have not been established | New FDA-approved indication For general information that may apply to all inhalation-local adrenergic bronchodilators, see *Bronchodilators, Adrenergic (Inhalation-Local)* |
| Sodium Fluoride and Triclosan (*Total*, Colgate [U.S.]) OR300/OR100; DE101 | Dental Paste (Toothpaste): 0.24% and 0.3%§ | Dental caries prophylactic; Antibacterial, dental— Dental caries†; Gingivitis†; Plaque, dental† | As a toothpaste, brush teeth thoroughly, preferably after each meal or at least twice a day, or as directed | Children up to 6 years of age—Do not use unless directed by a dentist or doctor Children 6 years of age and older—Dental caries: See *Usual adult dose* | New OTC drug combination Should not be swallowed |
| Somatropin, Recombinant (*Genotropin*, Pharmacia & Upjohn [U.S.]) | for Injection: 1.5 mg (approximately 4.5 IU per cartridge), 5.8 mg (approximately 17.4 IU per cartridge), and 13.8 mg (approximately 41.4 IU per cartridge) | Growth hormone— Growth hormone deficiency, in adults | SC (in thigh, buttocks, or abdomen), initially not more than 0.04 mg per kg of body weight per week. Dose may be increased at 4- to 8-week intervals, according to individual patient requirements, up to a maximum of 0.08 mg per kg of body weight per week Weekly doses should be divided into 6 or 7 injections, given on a daily basis Intravenous administration is not recommended | | New FDA-approved indication For general information that may apply, see *Growth Hormone (Systemic)* |
| (*Humatrope*, Eli Lilly [U.S.]) | for Injection: 5 mg per vial | Growth hormone— Somatropin deficiency syndrome in adults‡ | SC, initially 0.006 mg (0.018 International Unit [IU]) per kg of body weight per day; dose may be increased based on individual patient requirements to a maximum of 0.0125 mg (0.0375 IU) per kg of body weight per day | | Additional FDA-approved indication |
| (*Nutropin*, Genentech [U.S.]) | for Injection: 5 mg (approximately 15 International Units [IU]) and 10 mg (approximately 30 IU) per vial | Growth hormone— Short stature associated with Turner's syndrome‡ | | SC, up to 0.375 mg (approximately 1.125 IU) per kg of body weight per week in 3 to 7 equally divided doses | Additional FDA-approved indication |
| (*Nutropin AQ*, Genentech [U.S.]) | Injection: 5 mg (approximately 15 International Units [IU]) per mL | Growth hormone— Growth failure‡: Associated with growth hormone deficiency; Growth failure‡: Associated with chronic renal failure | | Growth failure (growth hormone deficiency): SC, 0.3 mg (0.9 IU) per kg of body weight once a day; dose and dosage should be individualized according to the patient's needs Growth failure (chronic renal failure): SC, 0.35 mg (1.05 IU) per kg of body weight once a week with duration of therapy individualized according to the patient's needs | Additional dosage form Hemodialysis patients should receive somatropin at night just before going to sleep or at least 3 to 4 hours after hemodialysis; chronic cycling peritoneal dialysis patients should receive somatropin in the morning after having completed dialysis; chronic ambulatory peritoneal dialysis patients should receive somatropin in the evening at the time of the overnight exchange |

## Additional Products and Indications (continued)

| GENERIC NAME (Brand name, manufacturer [country]) VA Classification (Primary/Secondary) | DOSAGE FORMS AND STRENGTHS | CATEGORIES—INDICATIONS | USUAL ADULT DOSE | USUAL PEDIATRIC DOSE | COMMENTS |
|---|---|---|---|---|---|
| Somatropin, Recombinant (Genotropin, Pharmacia & Upjohn [U.S.]) (continued) (Serostim, Serono [U.S.]) HS701 | for Injection: 5 mg (approximately 15 International Units [IU]) and 6 mg (approximately 18 IU) per vial | Growth hormone—Cachexia, AIDS-associated‡ | Patients weighing more than 55 kg—SC, 6 mg at bedtime. Patients weighing 45 to 55 kg—SC, 5 mg at bedtime. Patients weighing 35 to 45 kg—SC, 4 mg at bedtime. Patients weighing less than 35 kg—SC, 0.1 mg per kg of body weight at bedtime | Safety and efficacy have not been established | Additional FDA-approved indication |
| Somatropin, Recombinant (Saizen, Serono [U.S.]) HS701 | for Injection: 5 mg (approximately 15 International Units [IU]) per vial | Growth hormone—Growth failure‡ |  | Intramuscular or subcutaneous, 0.06 mg (0.18 IU) per kg of body weight 3 times a week. Treatment should be discontinued once the epiphyses are fused | New brand name product |
| Sufentanil Citrate (Sufenta, Janssen [U.S. and Canada]) CN101/CN206 | Injection USP: 50 mcg (base) per mL | Anesthesia adjunct (opioid analgesic)—Anesthesia, local, adjunct, for labor and delivery | Anesthesia, local, adjunct: Labor and delivery—Epidural, 10 to 15 mcg (base), mixed with and given together with 10 mL of 0.125% bupivacaine with or without epinephrine. May be repeated at intervals of not less than 1 hour, up to a total of 3 doses |  | Additional indication in U.S. and Canada |
|  |  | Analgesic—Pain, acute, postoperative‡ | Analgesic: Acute pain—Epidural, 30 to 60 mcg (base) in 10 mL of 0.9% sodium chloride injection. Additional 25-mcg doses may be administered at intervals of not less than 1 hour if there is evidence of lightening of analgesia, but recommended initial dose usually provides 4 to 6 hours of pain relief |  | Additional indication in Canada |
| Teniposide (Vumon, Bristol [Canada]) AN900 | Injection: 10 mg per mL (50-mg ampul) | Antineoplastic—Neuroblastoma‡; Lymphomas, non-Hodgkin's‡; Leukemia, acute lymphocytic‡ | Neuroblastoma—IV infusion (over at least 30 minutes), 130 to 180 mg per square meter of body surface (mg/m²) per day once a week (single agent) or 100 mg/m² per day every 21 days (in combination). Lymphomas, non-Hodgkin's—IV infusion (over at least 30 minutes), 30 mg/m² per day for 10 days, or 30 mg/m² per day every 5 days, or 50 to 100 mg/m² once a week (single agent); or 60 to 70 mg/m² per day once a week (in combination). Leukemia, acute lymphocytic—IV infusion (over at least 30 minutes), 165 mg/m² per day 2 times a week (in combination) |  | Canadian drug product |

*Not commercially available in the United States.
†Prophylactic.
‡Therapeutic.
§Respectively.
#Diagnostic.

# Additional Products and Indications (continued)

| GENERIC NAME (Brand name, manufacturer [country]) VA Classification (Primary/Secondary) | DOSAGE FORMS AND STRENGTHS | CATEGORIES— INDICATIONS | USUAL ADULT DOSE | USUAL PEDIATRIC DOSE | COMMENTS |
|---|---|---|---|---|---|
| Terbinafine (Lamisil, Novartis [U.S.]) AM700 | Tablets: 250 mg | Antifungal (systemic)—Onychomycosis‡ | Oral, 250 mg once a day for 6 to 12 weeks | Safety and efficacy have not been established | Available in U.S. |
| Terbinafine Hydrochloride (Lamisil, Novartis [U.S.]) DE102 | Solution: 1% (pump spray) | Antifungal (topical)—Tinea corporis‡; Tinea cruris‡; Tinea pedis‡; Tinea versicolor‡ | Tinea corporis or tinea cruris—Topical, to the affected area(s), once a day for 1 week. Tinea pedis or tinea versicolor—Topical, to the affected area(s), 2 times a day for 1 week | Safety and efficacy have not been established | New dosage form. If successful outcome is not achieved during the post-treatment period, the diagnosis should be reviewed |
| Timolol Hemihydrate (Betimol, CIBA Vision [U.S.]) OP110 | Ophthalmic Solution: 0.25 and 0.5% | Antiglaucoma agent (ophthalmic)—Glaucoma, open-angle‡; Hypertension, ocular‡ | Topical, to the conjunctiva, 1 drop in the affected eye(s) 2 times a day | Safety and efficacy have not been established | Additional dosage form; additional brand name product |
| Timolol Maleate | | Antiglaucoma agent (ophthalmic)—Glaucoma, open-angle‡; Hypertension, ocular‡ | | | Additional brand name products |
| (Timoptic-XE, Merck [U.S. and Canada]) | Ophthalmic Gel-forming Solution: 0.25 and 0.5% | | Topical, to the conjunctiva, 1 drop in each eye once a day | Safety and efficacy have not been established | Additional dosage form |
| (Beta-Tim, Ciba Vision [Canada]; Med Timolol, Medican [Canada]; Novo-Timol, Novopharm [Canada]; Nu-Timolol, Nu-Pharm [Canada]; Timodal, Pharmascience [Canada]) | Ophthalmic Solution USP: 0.25 and 0.5% | | | | |
| (Akorn; Alcon; Fougera [U.S.]) OP110 | | | | | Available generically |
| Tioconazole (Trosyd Dermal Cream, Pfizer [Canada]) DE102 | Cream: 1% | Antifungal (topical)—Candidiasis, cutaneous‡; Tinea corporis‡; Tinea cruris‡; Tinea pedis‡; Tinea versicolor‡ | Topical, to the skin and surrounding areas, 2 times a day, morning and evening | See Usual adult dose | Canadian drug product |
| Tirofiban Hydrochloride (Aggrastat, Merck & Co. [U.S.]) BL700 | Injection: 50 mcg per mL (25 mg per 500 mL) in a premixed 500 mL container; 250 mcg per mL (12.5 mg per 50 mL) in 50 mL vials | Platelet aggregation inhibitor—Unstable angina or non-Q-wave myocardial infarction‡, in patients to be managed medically and those undergoing PTCA or atherectomy | IV infusion (continuous), at an initial rate of 0.4 mcg per kg of body weight per minute for 30 minutes and then continued at 0.1 mcg per kg of body weight per minute for 48 to 108 hours; in patients undergoing PTCA or atherectomy, the infusion should be continued through angiography and for 12 to 24 hours after PTCA or atherectomy | Safety and efficacy have not been established | New drug. Tirofiban is administered in combination with aspirin (unless contraindicated) and heparin. Patients with severe renal insufficiency (CrCl < 30 mL per minute) should receive half the usual rate of infusion. The 50-mL vial containing 250 mcg per mL must first be diluted to 50 mcg per mL, the same strength as the premixed solution, prior to use |
| Tobramycin (AKTob, Akorn [U.S.]) OP201 | Ophthalmic Solution USP: 0.3% | | | | Additional brand name product |
| Tolbutamide Sodium (Orinase Diagnostic, Upjohn [U.S.]) DX900 | Sterile Powder USP: 1 gram (base) | Diagnostic aid (pancreatic islet cell function)—Adenoma, pancreatic islet cell (insulinoma)# | IV, 1 gram (20 mL of a 50-mg-per-mL solution), injected at a constant rate over 2 to 3 minutes | | Multiple blood samples are drawn to determine fasting blood glucose and serum insulin concentrations and to monitor changes in these concentrations after the administration of tolbutamide sodium. Sterile diluent provided (sterile water for injection) |

## Additional Products and Indications *(continued)*

| GENERIC NAME (*Brand name*, manufacturer [country]) VA Classification (Primary/Secondary) | DOSAGE FORMS AND STRENGTHS | CATEGORIES— INDICATIONS | USUAL ADULT DOSE | USUAL PEDIATRIC DOSE | COMMENTS |
|---|---|---|---|---|---|
| Triamcinolone Acetonide (Taro [U.S.]) OR900 | Dental Paste USP: 0.1% | | | | Available generically |
| Triamcinolone Acetonide (*Nasacort*, Rhone-Poulenc Rorer [U.S.]) | Nasal Aerosol: 55 mcg per metered spray | Anti-inflammatory (steroidal), nasal; Corticosteroid (nasal)—Rhinitis, perennial allergic‡; Rhinitis, seasonal allergic‡ | | Children up to 6 years of age: Safety and efficacy have not been established. Children 6 through 11 years of age: Nasal, 110 mcg (2 metered sprays) in each nostril once a day (total daily dose, 220 mcg). Once the maximal effect has been achieved, the minimum effective dose should be administered. Children 12 years of age and older: See *Usual adult dose* | Additional FDA-approved pediatric dose |
| (*Nasacort AQ*, Rhone-Poulenc Rorer [U.S.]) NT201 | Nasal Solution: 55 mcg per metered spray | | 110 mcg (2 metered sprays) in each nostril once a day (total daily dose, 220 mcg). When symptoms have been controlled, patients may be maintained on 55 mcg (1 metered spray) in each nostril once a day (total daily dose, 110 mcg) | Children up to 12 years of age: Safety and efficacy have not been established. Children 12 years of age and older: See *Usual adult dose* | Additional dosage form and brand name product |
| Verapamil Hydrochloride (*Chronovera*, Searle [Canada]) CV200; CV250 | Extended-release Tablets: 180 and 240 mg | Antihypertensive— Hypertension‡ Antianginal—Angina pectoris, chronic stable‡ | Hypertension—Oral, initially 180 mg once daily at bedtime. Dose may be gradually titrated up to 480 mg, as tolerated, once daily at bedtime. Angina pectoris, chronic stable—Oral, initially 180 mg once daily at bedtime. Dose may be gradually titrated up to 360 mg, as tolerated, once daily at bedtime; however, some patients may require a dose of 480 mg once daily | Safety and efficacy have not been established | New brand name product and strength. Verapamil should be administered cautiously to patients with hepatic or renal function impairment and should not be used in patients with severe hepatic function impairment |
| Vindesine Sulfate* (*Eldisine*, Lilly [Canada]) AN900 | for Injection: 5 mg | Antineoplastic— Leukemia, acute lymphocytic‡ | IV (rapid), 3 mg per square meter of body surface (mg/m$^2$), the dosage being repeated every 7 to 10 days for 8 cycles | IV (rapid), 4 mg/m$^2$ repeated every 7 to 10 days for 8 cycles, or 2 mg/m$^2$ per day for 2 days followed by 5 to 7 days without the drug, the dosage being repeated for 8 cycles | Canadian drug product |

*Not commercially available in the United States.
†Prophylactic.
‡Therapeutic.
§Respectively.
#Diagnostic.

## Additional Products and Indications (continued)

| GENERIC NAME (*Brand name*, manufacturer [country]) VA Classification (Primary/Secondary) | DOSAGE FORMS AND STRENGTHS | CATEGORIES— INDICATIONS | USUAL ADULT DOSE | USUAL PEDIATRIC DOSE | COMMENTS |
|---|---|---|---|---|---|
| Warfarin Sodium (*Coumadin*, DuPont [U.S.]) BL114 | Tablets USP: 1, 2, 2.5, 3, 4, 5, 6, 7.5, and 10 mg | Anticoagulant— Thromboembolism, associated with cardiac valve replacement††‡ | Oral, initially 2 to 5 mg per day, then 2 to 10 mg per day, with dosage adjustments based on the results of International Normalized Ratio (INR) and/or prothrombin time (PT) determinations. The INR should be maintained at 2.5 to 3.5 times the control value in patients with mechanical heart valves, and at 2 to 3 times the control value for 12 weeks after valve insertion in patients with bioprosthetic heart valves | Dosage has not been established | Additional FDA-approved indications; 3 and 6 mg are additional strengths |
| | | Risk reduction, after myocardial infarction†, of death, recurrent myocardial infarction, and thromboembolic events such as stroke or systemic embolization | Oral, therapy should be initiated early (2 to 4 weeks post-infarction), initially 2 to 5 mg per day, then 2 to 10 mg per day, with dosage adjustments based on the results of International Normalized Ratio (INR) and/or prothrombin time (PT) determinations. The INR should be maintained at 2.5 to 3.5 times the control value. Patients at an increased risk of bleeding complications or on aspirin therapy should be maintained at the lower end of this INR range. Long-term therapy is recommended | | |
| | for Injection USP: 2 mg per mL when reconstituted | | IV, as an alternate route of administration for patients who cannot receive oral medications. Dosages would be the same as those that would be used orally. The medication should be administered slowly over 1 to 2 minutes into a peripheral vein. IM administration is not recommended | | Additional dosage form |
| Warfarin Sodium (Barr [U.S.]) BL114 | Tablets USP: 1, 2, 2.5, 4, 5, 7.5, and 10 mg | Anticoagulant | | | Now available generically |
| Xylometazoline Hydrochloride (*Inspire*, Quintex [U.S.]) NT100 | Nasal Solution: 0.1% | Decongestant (topical)—Congestion, nasal‡ | Nasal, 2 or 3 sprays into each nostril every 8 to 10 hours as needed | Children 12 years of age and older: See *Usual Adult Dose* Children under 12 years of age: Use is not recommended | Additional brand name product |
| Zidovudine (*Retrovir*, Glaxo Wellcome [U.S.]) AM800 | Tablets: 300 mg | Antiviral—Human immunodeficiency virus (HIV) infection, asymptomatic‡; Immunodeficiency syndrome, acquired (AIDS)‡ | | | Additional dosage form |

## Additional Products and Indications *(continued)*

| GENERIC NAME (*Brand name*, manufacturer [country]) VA Classification (Primary/Secondary) | DOSAGE FORMS AND STRENGTHS | CATEGORIES— INDICATIONS | USUAL ADULT DOSE | USUAL PEDIATRIC DOSE | COMMENTS |
|---|---|---|---|---|---|
| Zinc Acetate (*Galzin*, Gate [U.S.]) AD300 | Capsules: 25 and 50 mg (elemental zinc) | Copper absorption inhibitor—Wilson's disease (treatment adjunct) | Oral, 50 mg elemental zinc 3 times a day on an empty stomach Note: Pregnant women should be started on 25 mg elemental zinc 3 times a day; the dose can be raised to 50 mg 3 times a day if needed | Children 10 years of age or older—Oral, 25 mg elemental zinc 3 times a day on an empty stomach Children under 10 years of age—Safety and efficacy have not been established | New drug |
| Zopiclone* (*Imovane*, Rhône-Poulenc Pharma [Canada]) CN309 | Tablets: 7.5 mg (scored) | Sedative-hypnotic— Insomnia‡ | Oral, 7.5 mg at bedtime. Dose may be lowered to 3.75 mg at bedtime Geriatric patient and patients with hepatic insufficiency—Oral, 3.75 mg at bedtime | Safety and efficacy have not been established | Canadian drug product |

*Not commercially available in the United States.
† Prophylactic.
‡ Therapeutic.
§ Respectively.
# Diagnostic.
** Breast carcinoma:
    Single agent—IV, 75 to 90 mg per square meter of body surface area every 21 days; or 12.5 to 25 mg per square meter of body surface area every 7 days
    Combination therapy—IV, 50 to 60 mg per square meter of body surface area on Days 1 and 8 every 4 weeks, in combination with cyclophosphamide and fluorouracil
Small cell lung carcinoma:
    Single agent—IV, 90 to 120 mg per square meter of body surface area every 21 days
    Combination therapy—IV, 50 to 90 mg per square meter of body surface area, in combination with cisplatin; ifosfamide; cyclophosphamide and vincristine; cyclophosphamide and etoposide; or cisplatin and etoposide
Non-small cell lung carcinoma:
    Single agent—IV, 120 to 150 mg per square meter of body surface area every 3 to 4 weeks
    Combination therapy—IV, 90 to 120 mg per square meter of body surface area on Day 1 every 3 to 4 weeks, in combination with etoposide, cisplatin, mitomycin, vindesine, and vinblastine
Hodgkin's lymphoma:
    Combination therapy—IV, 35 mg per square meter of body surface area every 2 weeks, or 70 mg per square meter of body surface area every 3 to 4 weeks, in combination with bleomycin, vinblastine, and dacarbazine
Non-Hodgkin's lymphoma:
    Single agent—IV, 75 to 90 mg per square meter of body surface area every 21 days
    Combination therapy—IV, 60 to 75 mg per square meter of body surface area, in combination with cyclophosphamide, vincristine, and prednisone, with or without bleomycin
Gastric carcinoma:
    Single agent—IV, 75 to 100 mg per square meter of body surface area
    Combination therapy—IV, 80 mg per square meter of body surface area, in combination with fluorouracil
Ovarian carcinoma:
    Single agent—IV, 50 to 90 mg per square meter of body surface area every 3 to 4 weeks
    Combination therapy—IV, 50 to 90 mg per square meter of body surface area every 3 to 4 weeks, in combination with cisplatin and cyclophosphamide

# Appendix II

## SELECTED LIST OF DRUG-INDUCED EFFECTS

The following list of selected drug-induced side effects has been compiled for use in conjunction with the drug interactions section of *USP DI* monographs. This listing gives examples of certain substances that may contribute to additive effects of the medication being referred to where such an effect has been identified as posing a potentially clinically significant problem with the concurrent use of two or more medications. The listing of drugs is not meant to be inclusive.

**Anticholinergics**
  Anisotropine
  Atropine
  Belladonna
  Clidinium
  Dicyclomine
  Glycopyrrolate
  Homatropine
  Hyoscyamine
  Ipratropium
  Mepenzolate
  Methantheline
  Methscopolamine
  Pirenzepine
  Propantheline
  Scopolamine

  Other medications with anticholinergic activity
   Antidepressants, monoamine oxidase (MAO) inhibitor
   Antidepressants, tricyclic
   Antihistamines, H₁-receptor, except astemizole, cetirizine, loratidine, and terfenadine
   Benztropine
   Biperiden
   Buclizine
   Carbamazepine
   Clozapine
   Cyclizine
   Cyclobenzaprine
   Digoxin
   Disopyramide
   Dronabinol
   Ethopropazine
   Loxapine
   Maprotiline
   Meclizine
   Molindone
   Olanzapine
   Orphenadrine
   Oxybutynin
   Phenothiazines
   Pimozide
   Procainamide
   Procyclidine
   Quinidine
   Thioxanthenes
   Trihexyphenidyl

**Blood dyscrasia–causing medications—** Defined as those drugs causing unpredictable myelotoxicity that usually occurs in a minority of patients and is not dose-dependent
  Aminopyrine
  Amodiaquine
  Amphotericin B lipid complex
  Angiotensin-converting enzyme (ACE) inhibitors
  Anticonvulsants, dione
  Anticonvulsants, hydantoin

**Blood dyscrasia–causing medications—** Defined as those drugs causing unpredictable myelotoxicity that usually occurs in a minority of patients and is not dose-dependent *(continued)*
  Anticonvulsants, succinimide
  Antidepressants, tricyclic
  Antidiabetic agents, sulfonylurea
  Anti-inflammatory drugs, nonsteroidal (NSAIDS), especially phenylbutazone
  Antithyroid agents
  Carbamazepine
  Chloramphenicol
  Clozapine
  Dapsone
  Divalproex
  Felbamate
  Flecainide
  Foscarnet
  Gold compounds
  Levamisole
  Loxapine
  Maprotiline
  Mirtazapine
  Penicillamine
  Pentamidine
  Phenacemide
  Phenothiazines
  Pimozide
  Primaquine
  Primidone
  Procainamide
  Propafenone
  Pyrimethamine (with high doses)
  Rifampin
  Rituximab
  Sulfasalazine
  Sulfamethoxazole and trimethoprim
  Sulfonamides, systemic
  Thioxanthenes
  Ticlopidine
  Tiopronin
  Tocainide
  Trimethobenzamide
  Trimethoprim
  Valproic acid

**Bone marrow depressants—**Defined as those drugs producing a predictable dose-related myelotoxicity
  Aldesleukin
  Altretamine
  Amphotericin B, systemic
  Amphotericin B cholestryl complex
  Amphotericin B lipid complex
  Amphotericin B liposomal complex
  Anastrozole
  Azathioprine
  Busulfan
  Carboplatin
  Carmustine, systemic
  Chlorambucil
  Chloramphenicol

**Bone marrow depressants—**Defined as those drugs producing a predictable dose-related myelotoxicity *(continued)*
  Chromic phosphate P 32
  Cisplatin
  Cladribine
  Clozapine
  Colchicine
  Cyclophosphamide
  Cytarabine
  Dacarbazine
  Dactinomycin
  Daunorubicin
  Daunorubicin, liposomal
  Didanosine
  Docetaxel
  Doxorubicin
  Doxorubicin, liposomal
  Eflornithine
  Etoposide
  Floxuridine
  Flucytosine
  Fludarabine
  Fluorouracil, systemic
  Ganciclovir
  Gemcitabine
  Hydroxyurea
  Idarubicin
  Ifosfamide
  Interferon, gamma
  Interferons, alpha
  Irinotecan
  Lomustine
  Mechlorethamine, systemic
  Melphalan
  Mercaptopurine
  Methotrexate
  Mitomycin
  Mitoxantrone
  Paclitaxel
  Pegasparagase
  Pentostatin
  Plicamycin
  Procarbazine
  Sodium iodide I 131
  Sodium phosphate P 32
  Strontium 89 chloride
  Streptozocin
  Teniposide
  Thioguanine
  Thiotepa
  Topotecan
  Trimetrexate
  Uracil mustard
  Vidarabine, systemic (with high doses)
  Vinblastine
  Vincristine
  Vinorelbine
  Zidovudine
  Zidovudine and lamivudine

## CNS depression–producing medications
Alcohol
Aminoglutethimide
Anesthetics, general
Anesthetics, parenteral-local
Anticonvulsants
Antidepressants, monoamine oxidase (MAO) inhibitor
Antidepressants, tricyclic
Antidyskinetics (except amantadine)
Antihistamines, H₁-receptor, except astemizole, cetirizine, fexofenadine, loratadine, and terfenadine
Apomorphine
Azelastine
Baclofen
Barbiturates
Benzodiazepines
Beta-adrenergic blocking agents
Brimonidine
Buclizine
Carbamazepine
Chlophedianol
Chloral hydrate
Chlorzoxazone
Clonidine
Clozapine
Cyclizine
Difenoxin and atropine
Diphenoxylate and atropine
Disulfiram
Donepezil
Dronabinol
Droperidol
Ethchlorvynol
Ethinamate
Etomidate
Guanabenz
Guanfacine
Haloperidol
Hydroxyzine
Interferons, alpha
Loxapine
Magnesium sulfate, parenteral
Maprotiline
Meclizine
Meprobamate
Methyldopa
Methyprylon
Metoclopramide
Metyrosine
Mirtazapine
Mitotane
Molindone
Nabilone
Nefazodone
Olanzapine
Opioid (narcotic) analgesics
Paraldehyde
Paregoric
Pargyline
Phenothiazines
Pimozide
Procarbazine
Promethazine
Propiomazine
Propofol
Quetiapine
Rauwolfia alkaloids
Risperidone
Scopolamine
Skeletal muscle relaxants (centrally acting)
Thioxanthenes
Trazodone
Trimeprazine

## CNS depression–producing medications (continued)
Trimethobenzamide
Zolpidem

## CNS stimulation–producing medications
Amantadine
Amphetamines
Anesthetics, local
Appetite suppressants (except fenfluramine)
Bronchodilators, theophylline
Bupropion
Caffeine
Chlophedianol
Cocaine
Doxapram
Dronabinol
Dyphylline
Fluoroquinolones
Meropenem
Methylphenidate
Nabilone
Pemoline
Selegiline
Sympathomimetics

## Enzyme inducers, hepatic, cytochrome P450
Alcohol (with chronic use)
Barbiturates, especially phenobarbital
Carbamazepine
Glutethimide
Griseofulvin
Nevirapine
Phenylbutazone (mixed inducing and inhibiting effect)
Phenytoin (and possibly other hydantoins)
Primidone
Rifampin
Troglitazone

## Enzyme inhibitors, hepatic, various
Note: The following agents may affect single or multiple enzymes.
Alcohol (with acute, high-dose use)
Allopurinol
Antidepressants, monoamine oxidase (MAO) inhibitor
Antifungals, azole
Chloramphenicol
Cimetidine
Clarithromycin
Contraceptives, estrogen-containing, oral
Diltiazem
Disulfiram
Divalproex
Erythromycins
Fluoroquinolones
Fluoxetine
Fluvoxamine
Indinavir
Isoniazid
Letrozole
Metoprolol
Mibefradil
Nefazodone
Nelfinavir
Omeprazole
Paroxetine
Phenylbutazone (mixed inducing and inhibiting effect)
Propranolol
Quinidine
Ritonavir

## Enzyme inhibitors, hepatic, various (continued)
Note: The following agents may affect single or multiple enzymes.
Saquinavir
Sertraline
Valproic acid
Venlafaxine
Verapamil

## Extrapyramidal reaction–causing medications
Amoxapine
Droperidol
Haloperidol
Loxapine
Metoclopramide
Metyrosine
Molindone
Olanzapine
Phenothiazines
Pimozide
Rauwolfia alkaloids
Risperidone
Tacrine
Thioxanthenes

## Folate antagonists
Anticonvulsants, dione
Anticonvulsants, hydantoin
Anticonvulsants, succinimide
Divalproex
Methotrexate
Phenobarbital (with long-term use)
Pyrimethamine
Sulfonamides
Triamterene
Trimethoprim
Trimetrexate
Valproic acid

## Hemolytics
Acetohydroxamic acid
Antidiabetic agents, sulfonylurea
Doxapram
Furazolidone
Mefenamic acid
Menadiol
Methyldopa
Nitrofurans
Primaquine
Procainamide
Quinidine
Quinine
Sulfonamides, systemic
Sulfones

## Hepatotoxic medications
Acetaminophen (with long-term, high-dose use or acute overdose)
Acitretin
Alcohol
Aldesleukin
Amiodarone
Anabolic steroids
Androgens
Angiotensin-converting enzyme (ACE) inhibitors
Anticonvulsants, dione
Anti-inflammatory drugs, nonsteroidal (NSAIDS)
Asparaginase
Carbamazepine
Carmustine
Cytarabine
Dantrolene

### Hepatotoxic medications (continued)
Dapsone
Daunorubicin
Disulfiram
Divalproex
Erythromycins
Estrogens
Ethionamide
Etretinate
Fat emulsions, intravenous (with prolonged use)
Felbamate
Fluconazole
Flutamide
Gold compounds
Halothane
HMG-CoA reductase inhibitors
Iron (overdose)
Isoniazid
Itraconazole
Ketoconazole, oral
Labetalol
Mercaptopurine
Methimazole
Methotrexate
Methyldopa
Naltrexone (with long-term, high-dose use)
Nevirapine
Niacin (with high doses, sustained release, and antihyperlipidemic use)
Nilutamide
Nitrofurans
Pemoline
Phenothiazines
Phenytoin
Plicamycin
Propylthiouracil
Rifampin
Sulfamethoxazole and trimethoprim
Sulfonamides, systemic
Tacrine
Tizanidine
Toremifene
Tretinoin
Troleandomycin
Valproic acid
Vitamin A (with chronic overdose)
Zidovudine
Zidovudine and lamivudine

### Hyperkalemia-causing medications
Angiotensin-converting enzyme (ACE) inhibitors
Anti-inflammatory drugs, nonsteroidal (NSAIDS), especially indomethacin
Cyclosporine
Digitalis glycosides (with acute overdose)
Diuretics, potassium-sparing
Heparin
Penicillins, potassium-containing (with high doses)
Pentamidine
Phosphates, potassium-containing
Potassium citrate-containing medications
Potassium iodide
Potassium supplements
Succinylcholine chloride
Tacrolimus

### Hypokalemia-causing medications
Alcohol
Amphotericin B, systemic
Amphotericin B cholestryl complex
Amphotericin B lipid complex
Amphotericin B liposomal complex
Bronchodilators, adrenergic, beta-2 selective
Capreomycin
Carbenicillin, parenteral
Carbonic anhydrase inhibitors
Corticosteroids, systemic
Diuretics, loop
Diuretics, thiazide
Edetate disodium (with prolonged use)
Foscarnet
Indapamide
Insulin
Insulin lispro
Laxatives (with acute overdose or chronic misuse)
Mannitol
Mezlocillin
Piperacillin
Piperacillin and tazobactam
Salicylates
Sodium bicarbonate
Sodium polystyrene sulfonate
Ticarcillin
Ticarcillin and clavulanate
Urea, systemic

### Hypotension-producing medications
Alcohol
Aldesleukin
Alprostadil
Amantadine
Amifostine
Anesthetics, general
Angiotensin-converting enzyme (ACE) inhibitors
Antidepressants, monoamine oxidase (MAO) inhibitor
Antidepressants, tricyclic
Antihypertensives
Benzodiazepines used as preanesthetics
Beta-adrenergic blocking agents
Bretylium
Brimonidine
Bromocriptine
Cabergoline
Calcium channel blocking agents
Calcium supplements, parenteral
Carbidopa and levodopa
Clozapine
Contrast agents, radiopaque, water-soluble organic iodides (with intravascular use)
Contrast agents, paramagnetic
Contrast agents, superparamagnetic
Deferoxamine (when given IV at doses >15 mg/kg/hr)
Diuretics
Droperidol
Edetate calcium disodium
Edetate disodium
Gadopentetate
Haloperidol
Hydralazine
Levodopa
Lidocaine, systemic
Loxapine
Magnesium sulfate, parenteral
Mirtazapine
Molindone
Nabilone (with high doses)
Nefazodone
Nitrates
Nitrites
Olanzapine
Opioid (narcotic) analgesics (including alfentanil, fentanyl, and sufentanil)
Paclitaxel
Pentamidine
Phenothiazines
Pimozide
Pramipexole
Procainamide
Propofol
Protamine (with too rapid administration)
Quetiapine
Quinidine
Ranitidine bismuth citrate
Risperidone
Rituximab
Ropinirole
Thioxanthenes
Thrombolytic agents
Tizanidine
Tocainide
Tolcapone

### Hypothermia-producing medications
Alcohol, ethyl
Alpha-adrenergic blocking agents (dihydroergotamine, ergotamine, labetalol, phenoxybenzamine, phentolamine, prazosin, tolazoline)
Anesthetics, general
Barbiturates (with high doses or acute overdose)
Beta-adrenergic blocking agents
Clonidine
Insulin
Minoxidil, systemic
Opioid analgesics (with overdose)
Polyethylene glycol and electrolytes (with large amounts of refrigerated solution)
Vasodilators

### Methemoglobinemia-causing medications
Acetaminophen
Acetanilid
Aminosalicylic acid
Articaine
Benzocaine
Castellani solution
Cetrimide
Chloroquine
Coal tar
Dapsone
Flutamide
Lidocaine
Mafenide
Methylene blue (with high doses)
Nitrates
Nitrites
Nitrofurantoin
Nitroglycerin
Nitroprusside
Pamaquine
Phenacetin
Phenobarbital
Prilocaine
Primaquine
Quinine
Silver nitrate
Sulfonamides
Thiopental
Triclocarban

### Nephrotoxic medications
Acetaminophen (in acute high doses)
Acyclovir, parenteral
Aldesleukin
Aminoglycosides, parenteral and topical irrigation (only on denuded surfaces or mucous membranes)
Amphotericin B, parenteral
Amphotericin B cholestryl complex
Amphotericin B lipid complex
Amphotericin B liposomal complex
Analgesic combinations containing acetaminophen and aspirin or other salicylates (with chronic high-dose use)
Anticonvulsants, dione
Anti-inflammatory drugs, nonsteroidal (NSAIDS)
Bacitracin, parenteral
Capreomycin
Carmustine
Cholecystographic agents, oral
Cidofovir
Ciprofloxacin
Cisplatin
Contrast agents, radiopaque, water-soluble organic iodides (with intravascular administration)
Cyclosporine
Deferoxamine (with long-term use)
Demeclocycline (in nephrogenic diabetes insipidus)
Edetate calcium disodium (with high doses)
Edetate disodium (with high doses)
Foscarnet
Gallium nitrate
Gold compounds
Ifosfamide
Lithium
Methotrexate (with high-dose therapy)
Methoxyflurane
Neomycin, oral
Pamidronate
Penicillamine
Pentamidine
Phenacetin
Plicamycin
Polymyxins, parenteral
Rifampin
Streptozocin
Sulfamethoxazole and trimethoprim
Sulfonamides, systemic
Tacrolimus
Tetracyclines, other (except doxycycline and minocycline)
Tiopronin
Tretinoin
Vancomycin, parenteral

### Neurotoxic medications
Altretamine
Aminoglycosides, parenteral and topical irrigation (only on denuded surfaces or mucous membranes)
Anticonvulsants, hydantoin
Asparaginase
Capreomycin

### Neurotoxic medications (continued)
Carbamazepine
Carboplatin
Chloramphenicol, systemic
Chloroquine
Cilastatin
Ciprofloxacin
Cisplatin
Cycloserine
Cyclosporine
Cytarabine
Didanosine
Disulfiram
Docetaxel
Ethambutol
Ethionamide
Fludarabine
Hydroxychloroquine
Imipenem
Interferon, gamma
Interferons, alpha
Isoniazid
Lincomycins
Lindane, topical
Lithium
Methotrexate, intrathecal
Metronidazole
Mexiletine
Nitrofurantoin
Oxamniquine
Pemoline
Penicillins, parenteral
Polymyxins, parenteral
Pyridoxine (with long-term, high-dose use)
Quinacrine
Quinidine
Quinine
Stavudine
Tacrolimus
Tetracyclines
Vincristine
Zalcitabine

### Ototoxic medications
Aminoglycosides, parenteral and topical irrigation (only on denuded surfaces or mucous membranes)
Anti-inflammatory drugs, nonsteroidal (NSAIDS)
Bumetanide, parenteral
Capreomycin
Carboplatin
Chloroquine
Cisplatin
Deferoxamine (with long-term, high-dose use)
Erythromycins (with high doses and renal function impairment)
Ethacrynic acid
Furosemide
Hydroxychloroquine
Quinidine
Quinine
Salicylates (especially with long-term, high-dose use or overdose)
Vancomycin, parenteral (with high doses and renal function impairment)

### Platelet aggregation inhibitors or Other medications with platelet aggregation–inhibiting activity
Abciximab
Alprostadil, systemic
Anagrelide
Anti-inflammatory drugs, nonsteroidal (NSAIDS)
Aspirin
Clopidogrel
Contrast agents, radiopaque, water-soluble organic iodides (with intravascular administration)
Dextran
Dipyridamole
Divalproex
Epoprostenol
Eptifibatide
Mezlocillin
Pentoxifylline
Piperacillin
Plicamycin
Sulfinpyrazone
Ticarcillin
Ticlopidine
Tirofiban
Valproic acid

### Serotonergics
Citalopram
Clomipramine
Fluoxetine
Fluvoxamine
Lysergic acid diethylamide (LSD)
Methylenedioxymethamphetamine (MDMA ["ecstasy"])
Moclobemide
Monoamine oxidase inhibitors, irreversible (furazolidone, phenelzine, procarbazine, selegiline, tranylcypromine)
Nefazodone
Paroxetine
Sertraline
Sibutramine
Tryptophan
Venlafaxine
Other medications or substances with serotonergic activity
Ademetionine
Amitriptyline
Bromocriptine
Buspirone
Dextromethorphan
Imipramine
Levodopa
Lithium
Marijuana
Meperidine
Naratriptan
Pentazocine
Sumatriptan
Tramadol
Trazodone
Zomitriptan

# Appendix III

## THERAPEUTIC GUIDELINES

### Hyperlipidemia

In the second report of the National Cholesterol Education Program Expert Panel on Detection, Evaluation, and Treatment of High Blood Cholesterol in Adults (Adult Treatment Panel II), the following guidelines for the treatment of high blood cholesterol are recommended:

Nonpharmacologic management, especially reduction in dietary intake of saturated fat and cholesterol, weight reduction, increase in physical activity, and cessation of smoking, is recommended initially for all patients and as an adjunct to all pharmacologic therapy.

If an adequate response is not achieved after 6 months of dietary therapy, then medication therapy is recommended to be added to dietary therapy. The combination of nonpharmacologic and medication therapy should be started earlier in patients with severe elevations in low density lipoprotein (LDL) cholesterol or in patients with established coronary heart disease or other clinical atherosclerotic disease.

The major classes of medications available for pharmacologic therapy are: bile acid sequestrants (cholestyramine, colestipol), nicotinic acid, HMG-CoA reductase inhibitors (fluvastatin, lovastatin, pravastatin, simvastatin), fibric acid derivatives (clofibrate, gemfibrozil), and probucol. Bile acid sequestrants are especially useful for treatment of isolated elevations of LDL cholesterol. Nicotinic acid is useful in patients in whom LDL cholesterol concentrations are moderately elevated combined with an increase in triglycerides and low high density lipoprotein (HDL) cholesterol concentrations. The HMG-CoA reductase inhibitors are particularly useful in achieving substantial LDL cholesterol reduction in patients with severe forms of hypercholesterolemia or in patients with established coronary heart disease and lesser degrees of LDL cholesterol elevation. The fibric acid derivatives are primarily effective in lowering triglyceride concentrations and, to a lesser extent, increasing HDL cholesterol concentrations. Therapy with probucol is generally reserved for patients who do not tolerate or respond to other cholesterol-lowering medications.

If patient response to initial medication therapy is not adequate, the patient may be switched to another class of medications or to a combination of two medications. Most antihyperlipidemic agents may be used in combination. The combination of a bile acid sequestrant with either nicotinic acid or an HMG-CoA reductase inhibitor may be particularly effective. However, the use of an HMG-CoA reductase inhibitor plus a fibric acid derivative or nicotinic acid may increase the risk of myopathy.

Consultation with a lipid specialist may be necessary in cases of unusually severe, complex, or refractory lipid disorders.

In postmenopausal women who qualify for consideration of medication therapy to lower LDL cholesterol, estrogen replacement therapy may be considered. Estrogen may decrease LDL and increase HDL concentrations. An individualized approach to selection of patients for estrogen replacement therapy is recommended, taking into consideration risk of coronary heart disease and potential risks of prolonged estrogen therapy.

**Reference:** National Cholesterol Education Program. Second Report of the Expert Panel on Detection, Evaluation, and Treatment of High Blood Cholesterol in Adults (Adult Treatment Panel II). Circulation 1994; 89(3): 1329-445.

### Hypertension

**Initial treatment**—In the fifth report of the Joint National Committee on the Detection, Evaluation, and Treatment of High Blood Pressure (JNC V), a varied selection of antihypertensive agents is recommended for the initial treatment of essential hypertension. A choice is presented from 6 classes of agents: diuretics, beta-adrenergic blocking agents, angiotensin-converting enzyme (ACE) inhibitors, calcium channel blocking agents, alpha-1 adrenergic blocking agents, and the alpha-beta receptor blocking agent. The medications in each of these classes are effective in reducing and controlling arterial pressure. However, the diuretics and beta-adrenergic blocking agents are preferred since a reduction in cardiovascular morbidity and mortality have been demonstrated with these classes of agents in controlled clinical trials. The ACE inhibitors, calcium channel blocking agents, alpha-1 adrenergic blocking agents, and the alpha-beta adrenergic blocking agent have not been tested to demonstrate a reduction in morbidity and mortality. Factors such as the cost of medication, side effects, drug interactions, concomitant diseases, additional risk factors, and other prescribed medications should be considered in choosing an initial antihypertensive agent. In addition, special population groups and situations such as ethnic, demographic, and other clinical situations should be considered in that choice. The direct acting smooth muscle vasodilators, the alpha-2 agonists, and the peripherally acting adrenergic blocking agents are considered supplemental antihypertensive agents but may be used for initial monotherapy in selected patients.

If an adequate response (achieved goal blood pressure or progress towards goal) is not achieved after 1 to 3 months of initial monotherapy the dose of the initial agent may be increased, an agent from another class may be substituted, or a second agent from another class may be added. If addition of a second agent produces adequate blood pressure control, withdrawal of the first agent may be considered. If an adequate response is still not achieved, a second or third agent and/or diuretic, if not already prescribed, may be added. If blood pressure has been effectively controlled for 1 year and at least 4 clinician visits, a deliberate, slow, and progressive reduction in antihypertensive medication therapy may be attempted.

Life-style modifications, including weight reduction, increased physical activity, smoking cessation, and moderation of dietary sodium and alcohol intake, are important therapeutic modalities in the treatment of hypertension. Life-style modifications alone may adequately control hypertension in some cases. However, even when not adequate in themselves, they may reduce the number and doses of antihypertensive medications required to manage hypertension. Furthermore, life-style modifications may be particularly helpful in hypertensive patients with additional cardiovascular risk factors.

**Reference:** The fifth report of the Joint National Committee on Detection, Evaluation, and Treatment of High Blood Pressure (JNC V). Arch Intern Med 1993; 153(2): 154-83.

# Appendix IV

## VA MEDICATION CLASSIFICATION SYSTEM

### INTRODUCTION

The Veterans Administration Medication Classification system was developed to provide a systematic and management approach to the classification of medications, including investigational and over-the-counter drugs, prosthetic items, and expendable supplies for hospital patients. The system was designed to:

1. Support the inpatient and outpatient pharmacy activities;
2. Facilitate the identification of drug-drug, drug-allergy, drug-lab, and drug-food interactions;
3. Uphold the requirements for inventory accountability;
4. Substantiate and improve all patient medication-related activity;
5. Provide an improved database to assist the physician;
6. Provide a coordinated method of database communication for VA management;
7. Facilitate the monitoring of investigational drugs; and
8. Facilitate the control of prosthetic and supply items.

Each 5-character alpha-numeric code specifies a broad classification and a specific type of product. The first two characters are letters and form the mnemonic for the major classification (e.g., AM for antimicrobials). Characters 3 through 5 are numbers and form the basis for subclassification. For example, the classification system for the penicillins is as follows:

AM000 ANTIMICROBIALS
    AM100 Beta-Lactam Antimicrobials
        AM111 Penicillin G-related Penicillins
        AM112 Penicillins, Amino Derivatives
        AM113 Penicillinase-resistant Penicillins
        AM114 Extended Spectrum Penicillins

Descriptive comments are included in the following listing only when the classification system itself is not considered to be self-explanatory. The VA Drug Classification system classifies drug products, not generic ingredients. Drug products with local effects are classified by route of administration (e.g., dermatological, ophthalmic, otic, nasal and throat, rectal-local). If a product is not classified by route of administration, in most instances it is classified under a specific chemical or pharmacological classification (e.g., beta-blockers, cephalosporins). If a product is not classified by route of administration or chemical or pharmacological subclassification, it may be classified under a therapeutic category (e.g., antilipemic agents, antiparkinson agents).

Most combination products are found in the "other" subclassification under each major classification unless a specific subcategory for combination products has been added or a descriptive comment indicates inclusion elsewhere. In addition, products which are not adequately described by a minor category or subcategory within the major classification are classified as "other" (e.g., metronidazole, vancomycin).

The "notes" included in the following master classification list define assignment of codes for *primary* classifications only. These notes may or may not be applicable to any *secondary* classifications.

AD000 ANTIDOTES, DETERRENTS, AND POISON CONTROL
    Note: Includes nicotine polacrilex and other deterrents (AD900).

        Excludes anticoagulant antagonists (BL200, VT700); antifolate antagonists (VT102); antivenins (IM300); dialysis solutions (IR200); emetics (GA600); opioid antagonists (CN102).

    AD100 Alcohol Deterrents
    AD200 Cyanide Antidotes
    AD300 Heavy Metal Antagonists
    AD400 Exchange Resins
    AD500 Antivenins
    AD600 Smoking Deterrents
    AD700 Benzodiazepine Antagonists
    AD800 Opioid Antagonists
    AD900 Antidotes/Deterrents, Other

AH000 ANTIHISTAMINES
    Note: Excludes H$_2$-antagonists (GA301); combination cold products (RE500).
    AH101 Antihistamines, Phenothiazine
    AH102 Antihistamines, Non-Sedating
    AH109 Antihistamines, Other

AM000 ANTIMICROBIALS
    Note: Combination products containing two or more active ingredients from the same product are classified in that product (e.g., triple sulfas in AM650). Products containing two or more active ingredients from different products are classified under "anti-infectives, other" (e.g., tetracycline and amphotericin B in AM900). Products containing probenecid or clavulanic acid are classified under the product of the antimicrobial agent. Beta-lactam antibiotics not classified under penicillins or cephalosporins are classified under AM130.

    Excludes topical anti-infectives (DE100); topical anti-infective/anti-inflammatory combinations (DE250); ophthalmic anti-infectives (OP200); ophthalmic anti-infective/anti-inflammatory combinations (OP350); otic anti-infectives (OT100); otic anti-infective/anti-inflammatory combinations (OT250); vaginal anti-infectives (GU300).

    AM100 Beta-Lactam Antimicrobials
        AM111 Penicillin G-related Penicillins
        AM112 Penicillins, Amino Derivatives
        AM113 Penicillinase-resistant Penicillins
        AM114 Extended Spectrum Penicillins
        AM115 Cephalosporins, 1st Generation
        AM116 Cephalosporins, 2nd Generation
        AM117 Cephalosporins, 3rd Generation
        AM118 Cephalosporins, 4th Generation
        AM119 Beta-lactam Antimicrobials, Other
    AM200 Macrolides
    AM250 Tetracyclines
    AM300 Aminoglycosides
    AM350 Lincomycins
    AM400 Quinolones
        AM401 Quinolones
        AM402 Quinolones, Extended Spectrum
    AM500 Antituberculars
    AM550 Methenamine Salts
    AM600 Nitrofurans
    AM650 Sulfonamide/Related
    AM700 Antifungals
    AM800 Antivirals
        AM801 Antivirals, Antihepatitis Agents
        AM802 Antivirals, Antiherpetic Agents
        AM803 Antivirals, Protease Inhibitors
        AM804 Antivirals, Reverse Transcriptase Inhibitors
        AM809 Antivirals, Other
    AM900 Anti-infectives, Other

AN000 ANTINEOPLASTICS
    Note: Includes antineoplastic hormones (AN500) which are only used as antineoplastics (e.g., tamoxifen).
    Excludes other hormones (HS000).
    AN100 Alkylating Agents
    AN200 Antineoplastic Antibiotics
    AN300 Antimetabolites
    AN400 Antineoplastic Adjuvants
    AN500 Antineoplastic Hormones
    AN600 Antineoplastic Radiopharmaceuticals
    AN700 Protective Agents
    AN900 Antineoplastics, Other

AP000 ANTIPARASITICS
    Note: Includes topical pediculicides (AP300).
    AP100 Antiprotozoals
        AP101 Antimalarials
        AP109 Antiprotozoals, Other
    AP200 Anthelmintics
    AP300 Pediculicides
    AP900 Antiparasitics, Other

AS000 ANTISEPTICS/DISINFECTANTS
    Note: Includes products used only for the disinfection of inanimate objects and surfaces (e.g., benzalkonium chloride).
    Excludes products used for the cleansing or disinfection of animate objects (e.g., hexachlorophene [DE400]) and products used for the cleansing or disinfection of both animate and inanimate objects (e.g., povidone iodine [DE101]).

## AU000 AUTONOMIC MEDICATIONS

Note: Includes single ingredient anticholinergic products used as antiparkinson agents (e.g., benztropine, trihexyphenidyl) and single ingredient anticholinergic products used as antispasmodics in the gastrointestinal tract (e.g., glycopyrrolate).

Excludes those products classified under selected cardiovascular (beta-blockers [CV100], alpha-blockers [CV150], antihypertensives [CV400, CV490]), respiratory (sympathomimetic bronchodilators [RE103], anticholinergic bronchodilators [RE105]), or ophthalmic (beta-blockers [OP101, OP107]) products; gastrointestinal tract antispasmodic combinations (GA802); and urinary tract antispasmodics (GU200).

- AU100 Sympathomimetics (Adrenergics)
- AU150 Antiadrenergics
- AU300 Parasympathomimetics (Cholinergics)
- AU350 Anticholinergics
- AU900 Autonomic Agents, Other

## BL000 BLOOD PRODUCTS/MODIFIERS/VOLUME EXPANDERS

- BL100 Blood Coagulation Modifiers
  - BL110 Heparin
  - BL111 Low Molecular Weight Heparin
  - BL112 Heparinoid Fragments
  - BL113 Hiruidin Anticoagulants
  - BL114 Anticoagulants, Oral
  - BL115 Thrombolytics
  - BL116 Antihemorrhagics
  - BL117 Platelet Aggregation Inhibitors
  - BL118 Heparin Antagonists
  - BL119 Blood Coagulation Modifiers, Other
- BL400 Blood Formation
- BL500 Blood Derivatives
- BL800 Volume Expanders
- BL900 Blood Products, Other

## CN000 CENTRAL NERVOUS SYSTEM MEDICATIONS

Note: Includes all single-entity and combination analgesic products containing an opioid agonist or partial agonist (CN101); nonopioid single-entity and combination analgesic products containing acetaminophen and/or salicylates (CN103); single-entity monocyclic, bicyclic, or tetracyclic antidepressants (CN609); and single-entity products containing a phenothiazine or thioxanthene (CN701).

Excludes antitussive products containing an agonist or partial agonist opioid (RE301); antidiarrheal products containing tincture of opium or paregoric (GA400); single-entity anticholinergic products and dopamine agonists (AU350); pargyline (CV490); procarbazine (AN900); "anesthetics, local topical" (DE700).

- CN100 Analgesics
  - CN101 Opioid Analgesics
  - CN102 Opioid Antagonists
  - CN103 Non-opioid Analgesics
  - CN104 Nonsteroidal Anti-inflammatories
  - CN105 Antimigraine Agents
- CN200 Anesthetics
  - CN201 Gaseous Anesthetics
  - CN202 Barbituric Acid Derivatives, Anesthetic
  - CN203 General Anesthetics, Other
  - CN204 Local Anesthetics
  - CN205 Peripheral Nerve Blocking Agents
  - CN206 Anesthetic Adjuncts
- CN300 Sedatives/Hypnotics/Anxiolytics
  - CN301 Barbituric Acid Derivatives, Sedatives/Anxiolytics
  - CN302 Benzodiazepine Derivatives, Sedatives/Anxiolytics
  - CN303 Benzodiazepine Antagonists
  - CN304 Anxiolytics
  - CN309 Sedatives/Hypnotics, Other
- CN400 Anticonvulsants
- CN500 Antiparkinson Agents
- CN550 Antivertigo Agents
- CN600 Antidepressants
  - CN601 Tricyclic Antidepressants
  - CN602 Monoamine Oxidase Inhibitors
  - CN603 Selective Serotonin Reuptake Inhibitors
  - CN609 Antidepressants, Other
- CN700 Antipsychotics
  - CN701 Phenothiazine Antipsychotics
  - CN709 Antipsychotics, Other
- CN750 Lithium Salts
- CN800 CNS Stimulants
  - CN801 Amphetamines
  - CN802 Amphetamine-like Stimulants
  - CN809 CNS Stimulants, Other
- CN850 Antipyretics
- CN900 CNS Medications, Other

## CV000 CARDIOVASCULAR MEDICATIONS

Note: The beta-blockers/related product (CV100) includes all single-entity beta-blockers and alpha-beta-blockers. Combinations containing a beta-blocker are included with the combination antihypertensives (CV400). The alpha-blockers/related product (CV150) includes both peripheral and central single-entity products. All antihypertensive combinations, with the exception of potassium-sparing diuretics in combination with other diuretics (CV704), are included in the CV400 product.

- CV050 Cardiac Inotropic Agents
  - CV051 Digitalis Glycosides
  - CV052 Cardiac Inotropic Agents, Phosphodiasterase Inhibitors
  - CV053 Cardiac Inotropic Agents, Adrenergics
  - CV059 Cardiac Inotropic Agents, Other
- CV100 Beta-blockers/Related
- CV150 Alpha-blockers/Related
- CV200 Calcium Channel Blockers
- CV250 Antianginals
- CV300 Antiarrhythmics
  - CV351 Antilipemic Agents, HMG CoA Reductase Inhibitors
  - CV359 Antilipemic Agents, Other
- CV400 Antihypertensives, Combinations
  - CV402 Antihypetensives, Direct Acting Vasodilators
  - CV408 Antihypertensives, Combinations
  - CV409 Antihypertensives, Other
- CV490 Antihypertensives, Other
- CV500 Peripheral Vasodilators
- CV600 Sclerosing Agents
- CV700 Diuretics
  - CV701 Thiazides/Related
  - CV702 Loop Diuretics
  - CV703 Carbonic Anhydrase Inhibitors
  - CV704 Potassium-sparing/Combinations
  - CV709 Diuretics, Other
- CV800 ACE Inhibitors
  - CV805 Angiotensin II Inhibitors
- CV900 Cardiovascular Agents, Other

## DE000 DERMATOLOGICAL AGENTS

Note: The topical anti-inflammatory product (DE200) includes all single-entity anti-inflammatory agents and all combinations containing an adrenocorticoid except those which also contain an anti-infective agent (DE250) or an antipsoriatic agent (DE802). The topical antipsoriatic product (DE802) includes products containing adrenocorticoids in combination with coal tar or salicylic acid and products containing coal tar. The "anti-infective, topical, other" product (DE109) includes products containing combinations of agents from any one or more products of "anti-infectives, topical" (DE101, DE102, DE103). Topical pediculicides are included under AP300.

- DE100 Anti-infective, Topical
  - DE101 Antibacterial, Topical
  - DE102 Antifungal, Topical
  - DE103 Antiviral, Topical
  - DE109 Anti-infective, Topical, Other
- DE200 Anti-inflammatories, Topical
- DE250 Anti-infective/Anti-inflammatory Combinations, Topical
- DE300 Sun Protectants/Screens
- DE350 Emollients
- DE400 Soaps/Shampoos
- DE450 Deodorants/Antiperspirants
- DE500 Keratolytics/Caustics
- DE600 Antineoplastics, Topical
- DE650 Analgesics, Topical
- DE700 Local Anesthetics, Topical
- DE750 Antiacne Agents
  - DE751 Antiacne Agents, Systemic
  - DE752 Antiacne Agents, Topical
- DE800 Antipsoriatics
  - DE801 Antipsoriatics, Systemic
  - DE802 Antipsoriatics, Topical
- DE890 Dermatologicals, Systemic, Other
- DE900 Dermatologicals, Topical, Other

## DX000 DIAGNOSTIC AGENTS

Note: DX401 includes control solutions. DX409 includes combination blook test strips. DX509 includes combination urine test strips.

- DX100 Radiological/Contrast Media
  - DX101 Non-ionic Contrast Media
  - DX102 Ionic Contrast Media
- DX200 Radiopharmaceuticals, Diagnostic
  - DX201 Imaging Agents (in vivo), Radiopharmaceutical
  - DX202 Non-imaging Agents, Radiopharmaceutical
- DX300 Diagnostic Antigens
- DX400 Blood Test Strips/Reagents
  - DX401 Blood Glucose Test Strips/Reagents
  - DX409 Blood Test Strips/Reagents, Other
- DX500 Urine Test Strips/Reagents
  - DX501 Urine Glucose Test Strips/Reagents
  - DX509 Urine Test Strips/Reagents, Other
- DX900 Diagnostics, Other

## GA000 GASTRIC MEDICATIONS

Note: The "laxatives, other" product (GA209) includes combination products. The digestant product (GA500) includes any single-entity or combination product containing a digestive enzyme. Antacid and simethicone combinations are included in product "antacids, other" (GA199). GA303 includes combination products.

- GA100 Antacids
  - GA101 Aluminum-containing Antacids
  - GA102 Aluminum/Calcium/Magnesium-containing Antacids
  - GA103 Aluminum/Magnesium-containing Antacids
  - GA104 Aluminum/Magnesium/Sodium Bicarbonate-containing Antacids
  - GA105 Calcium-containing Antacids
  - GA106 Calcium/Magnesium-containing Antacids
  - GA107 Magaldrate-containing Antacids
  - GA108 Magnesium-containing Antacids
  - GA109 Magnesium/Sodium Bicarbonate-containing Antacids
  - GA110 Sodium Bicarbonate-containing Antacids
  - GA199 Antacids, Other
- GA200 Laxatives/Antidiarrheal Agents
  - GA201 Bulk-forming Laxatives
  - GA202 Hyperosmotic Laxatives
  - GA203 Lubricant Laxatives
  - GA204 Stimulant Laxatives
  - GA205 Stool Softeners
  - GA208 Antidiarrheal Agents
  - GA209 Laxatives/Antidiarrheal Agents, Other
- GA300 Antiulcer Agents
  - GA301 Histamine Antagonists
  - GA302 Protectants, Ulcer
  - GA303 Anti-*H. pylori* Antiulcer Agents
  - GA304 Antiulcer Agents, Proton Pumping Inhibitors
  - GA309 Antiulcer Agents, Other
- GA400 Inflammatory Bowel Disease Agents

GA500 Digestants
GA600 Emetics
　GA605 Antiemetics
GA700 Appetite Stimulants
GA750 Appetite Suppressants
　GA751 Centrally-acting Appetite Suppressants
　GA752 Bulking Agent Appetite Suppressants
　GA759 Appetite Suppressants, Other
GA800 Antimuscarinics/Antispasmodics
　GA801 Antimuscarinics/Antispasmodics
　GA802 Antimuscarinic/Antispasmodic Combinations
GA900 Gastric Medications, Other

GU000 GENITOURINARY MEDICATIONS
　Note: The oxytocic product (GU600) includes 20% sodium chloride, 40 to 60% urea solutions, ergonovine, and methylergonovine but does not include oxytocin (HS702) or prostaglandins (HS875). The "antispasmodics, urinary" product (GU201) includes single-entity products. The "antispasmodics, urinary, other" product (GU209) includes any combination containing an anticholinergic ingredient that is intended for genitourinary use.

GU100 Analgesics, Urinary
GU200 Antispasmodics, Urinary
　GU201 Antispasmodics, Urinary
　GU202 Antispasmodic, Urinary, Other
GU300 Anti-infectives, Vaginal
　GU301 Antimicrobials, Vaginal
　GU302 Antifungals, Vaginal
　GU309 Anti-Infectives, Vaginal, Other
GU400 Contraceptives, Non-Hormonal
GU500 Estrogens, Vaginal
GU600 Oxytocics
GU650 Labor Suppressants
GU700 Benign Prostatic Hypertrophy Agents
GU900 Genitourinary Agents, Other

HS000 HORMONES/SYNTHETICS/MODIFIERS
HS050 Adrenal Corticosteroids
　HS051 Glucocorticoids
　HS052 Mineralocorticoids
HS100 Sex Hormones/Modifiers
　HS101 Androgens/Anabolics
　HS102 Estrogens
　HS103 Progestins
　HS104 Contraceptives, Hormonal
　HS105 Estrogen/Progestin Replacement Combinations
　HS106 Gonadotropins
　HS109 Sex Hormones, Modifiers, Other
HS200 Prostaglandins
HS300 Calcium Regulating Agents
　HS301 Biphosphonates, Osteoporosis Agent
　HS302 Biphosphanates, Hypercalcemia Agent
　HS303 Biphosphanates, Pagets Disease
　HS304 Calcium Regulating Hormones
　HS305 Calcium Regulating Antineoplastics
　HS309 Calcium Regulating Agents, Other
HS450 Enzyme Replacements/Modifiers
　HS451 Enzyme Replacement Agents
　HS452 Enzyme Modifiers/Inhibitors
　HS459 Enzyme Replacements/Modifiers, Other
HS500 Blood Glucose Regulation Agents
　HS501 Insulin
　HS502 Oral Antidiabetic Agents, Sulfonylureas
　HS503 Oral Antidiabetic Agents, Biguanides
　HS504 Oral Antidiabetic Agents, Alpha Glucosidase Inhibitors
　HS505 Oral Antidiabetic Agents, Insulin Sensitizing
　HS508 Antihypoglycemics
　HS509 Blood Glucose Regulation Agents, Other
HS600 Parathyroid
HS700 Pituitary
　HS701 Anterior Pituitary
　HS702 Posterior Pituitary
HS850 Thyroid Modifiers
　HS851 Thyroid Supplements
　HS852 Antithyroid Agents
HS900 Hormones/Synthetics/Modifiers, Other

IM000 IMMUNOLOGICAL AGENTS
IM100 Vaccines
IM200 Toxoids
IM300 Antitoxins
IM400 Immune Serums
IM500 Immunoglobulins
IM600 Immune Suppressants
IM700 Immune Stimulants
IM900 Immunological Agents, Other

IN000 INVESTIGATIONAL AGENTS
　Note: Drugs/devices used for investigational purposes are included in this classification.

IP000 INTRAPLEURAL MEDICATIONS
　Note: Includes all medications introduced into the intrapleural space.
IP100 Intrapleural Sclerosing Agents
IP900 Intrapleural Agents, Other

IR000 IRRIGATION/DIALYSIS SOLUTIONS
　Note: Excludes 50% dimethyl sulfoxide (GU900).
IR100 Irrigation Solutions
IR200 Peritoneal Dialysis Solutions
IR300 Hemodialysis Solutions
IR900 Irrigation/Dialysis Solutions, Other

MS000 MUSCULOSKELETAL MEDICATIONS
　Note: The antigout product (MS400) includes colchicine, uricosuric agents, and xanthine-oxidase inhibitors. The skeletal muscle relaxant product includes all combinations, except those containing an opioid ingredient (CN101).
MS100 Antirheumatics
　MS101 Salicylates, Antirheumatic
　MS102 Nonsalicylate NSAIs, Antirheumatic
　MS103 Cytotoxics, Antirheumatic
　MS109 Antirheumatics, Other
MS200 Skeletal Muscle Relaxants
MS300 Neuromuscular Blockers
MS400 Antigout Agents
MS900 Musculoskeletal Agents, Other

NT000 NASAL AND THROAT AGENTS, TOPICAL
NT100 Decongestants, Nasal
NT200 Anti-inflammatories, Nasal
　NT201 Anti-inflammatories, Steroid-containing, Nasal, Topical
　NT209 Anti-inflammatories, Nasal, Topical, Other
NT300 Anesthetics, Mucosal
NT400 Antihistamines, Nasal
NT900 Nasal and Throat, Topical, Other

OP000 OPHTHALMIC AGENTS
　Note: The "anti-infectives, other" product (OP209) includes products containing combinations from any one or more products (OP201, OP202, OP203) of anti-infectives, topical. The "ophthalmic, other" product (OP900) includes all combination ophthalmics except those classified under antiglaucoma combinations (OP105), anti-infective/anti-inflammatory combinations (OP350), or "anti-infectives, other" (OP209).

OP100 Intraocular Pressure Modifiers
　OP110 Antiglaucoma Beta-blockers, Topical
　OP111 Antiglaucoma Beta-blockers, Systemic
　OP112 Antiglaucoma Carbonic Anhydrase Inhibitors, Topical
　OP113 Antiglaucoma Carbonic Anhydrase Inhibitors, Systemic
　OP114 Antiglaucoma Adrenergics
　OP115 Antiglaucoma Osmotic Agents, Systemic
　OP116 Antiglaucoma Prostaglandins, Topical
　OP117 Antiglaucoma Combinations, Topical
　OP118 Miotics, Topical
　OP119 Intraocular Pressure Modifiers, Other
OP200 Anti-infective, Topical Ophthalmic
　OP201 Antibacterials, Topical Ophthalmic
　OP202 Antifungal, Topical Ophthalmic
　OP203 Antivirals, Topical Ophthalmic
　OP209 Anti-infective, Topical Ophthalmic, Other
OP300 Anti-inflammatory, Topical Ophthalmic
　OP301 Anti-inflammatory, Steroidal, Topical Ophthalmic
　OP302 Anti-inflammatory, Non-Steroidal, Topical Ophthalmic
OP350 Anti-infective/Anti-inflammatory Combinations, Topical Ophthalmic
OP400 Contact Lens Solutions
OP500 Eye Washes/Lubricants
OP600 Mydriatics/Cycloplegics, Topical Ophthalmic
OP700 Anesthetics, Topical Ophthalmic
OP800 Antihistamine/Decongestants, Topical Ophthalmic
　OP801 Antihistamine, Topical Ophthalmic
　OP802 Decongestant, Topical Ophthalmic
　OP809 Antihistamine/Decongestant Combinations, Topical Ophthalmic
OP900 Ophthalmics, Other

OR000 DENTAL AND ORAL AGENTS, TOPICAL
　Note: The cariostatic product (OR100) includes topical fluoride products only. Sodium fluoride tablets are included under TN407 Dental and oral anesthetics, topical OR600 includes combinations.
OR100 Cariostatics
OR200 Dental Protectants
OR300 Dentifrices
OR400 Denture Adhesives
OR500 Mouthwashes
OR600 Dental/Oral Anesthetics, Topical
OR900 Dental and Oral Agents, Topical, Other

OT000 OTIC AGENTS
　Note: The "anti-infectives, other" product (OT109) includes products containing combinations from any one or more products (OT101, OT102) of "anti-infectives, otic." The "otic, other" product (OT900) includes all combination otic products except those classified under anti-infective/anti-inflammatory combinations (OT250), otic analgesics (OT400), or "anti-infectives, otic, other" (OT109).
OT100 Anti-infective, Topical Otic
　OT101 Antibacterials, Topical Otic
　OT102 Antifungals, Topical Otic
　OT109 Anti-infective, Topical Otic, Other
OT200 Anti-inflammatories, Topical Otic
OT250 Anti-infective/Anti-inflammatory Combinations, Topical Otic
OT300 Ceruminolytics
OT400 Analgesics, Topical Otic
OT900 Otic Agents, Other

PH000 PHARMACEUTICAL AIDS/REAGENTS
　Note: Includes agents used in the preparation or reconstitution of pharmaceutical products. All diluents with separate NDC codes are included.

RE000 RESPIRATORY TRACT MEDICATIONS
　Note: The xanthine bronchodilator product (RE104) includes single-entity dyphylline-containing products. Antiasthma combination products containing two or more active ingredients from different products are included in the "antiasthma, other" product (RE109). Both single-entity and combinations of antitussives and expectorants will be included in products RE301 or RE302. Any of these products with at least one

opioid is included in product RE301. The "cold remedies, other" product (RE599) contains all cold/cough preparations which are not included in product RE200, RE301, RE302, or RE500 through RE516.
- RE100 Antiasthma/Bronchodilators
  - RE101 Anti-inflammatories, Inhalation
  - RE102 Bronchodilators, Sympathomimetic, Inhalation
  - RE103 Bronchodilators, Sympathomimetic, Oral/Parenteral
  - RE104 Bronchodilators, Xanthine-derivative
  - RE105 Bronchodilators, Anticholinergic
  - RE106 Mast Cell Stabilizers, Inhalation
  - RE108 Antiasthma, Antileukotrienes
  - RE109 Antiasthma, Other
- RE200 Decongestants, Systemic
- RE300 Antitussives/Expectorants
  - RE301 Antitussives/Expectorants, Opioid-containing
  - RE302 Antitussives/Expectorants, Non-opioid-containing
- RE400 Mucolytics
- RE500 Cold Remedies, Combinations
  - RE501 Antihistamine/Decongestant
  - RE502 Antihistamine/Decongestant/Antitussive
  - RE503 Antihistamine/Decongestant/Expectorant
  - RE504 Antihistamine/Decongestant/Antitussive/Expectorant
  - RE505 Antihistamine/Decongestant/Antitussive/Expectorant/Analgesic
  - RE506 Antihistamine/Decongestant/Antitussive/Analgesic
  - RE507 Antihistamine/Antitussive
  - RE508 Antihistamine/Antitussive/Expectorant
  - RE509 Antihistamine/Antitussive/Analgesic
  - RE510 Antitussive/Antimuscarinic
  - RE511 Antitussive/Bronchodilator
  - RE512 Decongestant/Antitussive
  - RE513 Decongestant/Antitussive/Expectorant
  - RE514 Decongestant/Antitussive/Expectorant/Analgesic
  - RE515 Decongestant/Antitussive/Analgesic
  - RE516 Decongestant/Expectorant
  - RE599 Cold Remedies, Other
- RE600 Non-anesthetic Gases
- RE700 Respiratory Surfactants
- RE900 Respiratory Agents, Other

RS000 RECTAL, LOCAL
Note: Includes only those products administered rectally with local activity. Products administered rectally for their systemic effect are classified under the appropriate pharmacological or therapeutic category (e.g., acetaminophen suppositories [CN103]).
- RS100 Anti-inflammatories, Rectal
- RS200 Hemorrhoidal Preparations, Rectal
- RS201 Hemorrhoidal Preparations without Steroid
- RS202 Hemorrhoidal Preparations with Steroid
- RS300 Laxatives, Rectal
- RS900 Rectal, Local, Other

TN000 THERAPEUTIC NUTRIENTS/MINERALS/ELECTROLYTES
Note: products TN501 and TN502 include kits and products containing dextrose.
- TN100 IV Solutions
  - TN101 IV Solutions without Electrolytes
  - TN102 IV Solutions with Electrolytes
- TN200 Enteral Nutrition
- TN300 Lipid Supplements
- TN400 Electrolytes/Minerals
  - TN401 Iron
  - TN402 Calcium
  - TN403 Potassium
  - TN404 Sodium
  - TN405 Zinc
  - TN406 Magnesium
  - TN407 Fluoride
  - TN408 Phosphorus
  - TN409 Bicarbonates
  - TN410 Citrates
  - TN490 Electrolytes/Minerals, Combinations
  - TN499 Electrolytes/Minerals, Other
- TN500 Amino Acids/Proteins
  - TN501 Amino Acids/Proteins, Parenteral, without added electrolytes
  - TN502 Amino Acids/Proteins, Parenteral, with added electrolytes
  - TN503 Amino Acids/Proteins, Oral
  - TN509 Amino Acids/Proteins, Other
- TN900 Therapeutic Nutrients/Minerals/Electrolytes, Other

VT000 VITAMINS
Note: The "vitamin B, other" product (VT109) includes combinations containing only vitamin B complex. Combinations containing only vitamin D are included in product (VT509) and product (VT709) includes combinations of vitamin K only. The "vitamins, other" product (VT809) includes any product in which a vitamin is found in combination with an ingredient which is neither a vitamin nor a mineral.
- VT050 Vitamin A
- VT100 Vitamin B
  - VT101 Cyanocobalamin
  - VT102 Folic Acid/Leucovorin
  - VT103 Nicotinic Acid
  - VT104 Pyridoxine
  - VT105 Thiamine
  - VT106 Riboflavin
  - VT107 Pantothenic Acid
  - VT109 Vitamin B, Other
- VT400 Vitamin C
- VT500 Vitamin D
  - VT501 Calcifediol
  - VT502 Calcitriol
  - VT503 Dihydrotachysterol
  - VT504 Ergocalciferol
  - VT509 Vitamin D, Other
- VT600 Vitamin E
- VT700 Vitamin K
  - VT701 Menadiol
  - VT702 Phytonadione
  - VT709 Vitamin K, Other
- VT800 Vitamins, Combinations
  - VT801 Multivitamins
  - VT802 Multivitamins with Minerals
  - VT809 Vitamin Combinations, Other
- VT900 Vitamins, Other

XA000 PROSTHETICS/SUPPLIES/DEVICES
- XA100 Bandages/Dressings
  - XA101 Pads, Gauze, Sterile
  - XA102 Pads, Gauze, Non-Sterile
  - XA103 Pads, Gauze with Adhesive
  - XA104 Pads, Gauze with Medication Added
  - XA105 Gauze, Fine Mesh
  - XA106 Bandage, Film
  - XA107 Bandage, Elastic
  - XA108 Bandage, Stretch
  - XA109 Foam with Adhesive
  - XA110 Packing, Gauze, Plain
  - XA111 Packing, Gauze, Medicated
  - XA199 Bandages/Dressing, Other
- XA200 Tape
  - XA201 Tape, Paper
  - XA202 Tape, Cloth
  - XA203 Tape, Plastic
  - XA204 Tape, Foam
  - XA205 Straps, Montgomery
  - XA206 Tape, Trach
  - XA299 Tape, Other
- XA300 Pads/Diapers
  - XA301 Pads, Bed
  - XA302 Pads, Combination
  - XA303 Pants, Rubber
  - XA304 Liner, Rubber Pants
  - XA305 Diapers
  - XA306 Pads, Mattress
  - XA399 Pads/Diapers, Other
- XA400 Colostomy/Ileostomy Collection Devices
  - XA401 Bag, Drainable with Adhesive, Colostomy/Ileostomy
  - XA402 Bag, Drainable without Adhesive, Colostomy/Ileostomy
  - XA403 Bags, Closed, with Adhesive, Colostomy/Ileostomy
  - XA404 Bags, Closed without Adhesive, Colostomy/Ileostomy
  - XA405 Bags, Disposable with Adhesive, Colostomy/Ileostomy
  - XA406 Bags, Disposable without Adhesive, Colostomy/Ileostomy
  - XA407 Sets, Appliances
  - XA499 Colostomy/Ileostomy Collection Devices, Other
- XA500 Urostomy/Urinary Collection Devices
Note: Includes urinary catheters and irrigation syringes. Excludes suction catheters.
  - XA501 Bag, Bedside Urinary COllection Device
  - XA502 Bottles/Other Bedside Urinary Collection Devices
  - XA503 Sets, Appliance, Urostomy
  - XA504 Bag, Drainable with Adhesive, Urostomy
  - XA505 Bag, Drainable without Adhesive, Urostomy
  - XA506 Bag, Closed with Adhesive, Urostomy
  - XA507 Bag, Closed without Adhesive, Urostomy
  - XA508 Bag, Urinary Collection Device
  - XA509 Catheter, Foley
  - XA510 Catheter, Coude-tip
  - XA511 Catheter, Balloon
  - XA512 Catheter, Red Rubber
  - XA513 Catheter, External Urinary
  - XA514 Plug, Catheter
  - XA515 Kit, Catheter Care
  - XA516 Set, Irrigation
  - XA599 Urostomy/Urinary Collection Devices, Other
- XA600 Ostomy Supplies, Other
  - XA601 Rings, Ostomy
  - XA602 Discs, Ostomy
  - XA603 Adhesive, Ostomy
  - XA604 Protectants, Skin, Ostomy
  - XA605 Belts, Ostomy
  - XA606 Odor Control Products, Ostomy
  - XA607 Irrigators/Sets, Ostomy
  - XA608 Caps, Ostomy
  - XA699 Ostomy Supplies, Other
- XA700 Bags/Tubes/Supplies for Oral Nutrition, Other
  - XA701 Bags, Feeding
  - XA702 Pumps, Feeding
  - XA703 Tubes, Feeding
  - XA799 Bags/Tubes/Supplies for Oral Nutrition, Other
- XA800 Intravenous Sets
  - XA801 Sets, Volumetric, Intravenous
  - XA802 Sets, Maxi Drip, Intravenous
  - XA803 Sets, Mini Drip, Intravenous
  - XA804 Sets, Filter, Intravenous
  - XA805 Sets, Butterfly, Intravenous
  - XA809 Intravenous Sets, Other
- XA850 Syringes/Needles
Note: Includes only syringes for injectable use.
  - XA851 Syringes, Slip Tip, Injection
  - XA852 Syringes, Luer Lock, Injection
  - XA853 Syringes with Needle, Injection
  - XA854 Syringe, Insulin, Injection
  - XA855 Caps, Syringe
  - XA856 Needles, Injection
  - XA859 Syringes/Needles, Other
- XA900 Supplies, Other

XX000 MISCELLANEOUS AGENTS
Note: Includes all products not elsewhere classified.

# VA Medication Classification System

The following list identifies all drugs in the USP DI database by their primary and secondary VA code assignments. This list groups all drugs by their VA code; an asterisk identifies primary assignments.

## DRUG LISTING BY VA CODE
(* = primary)

|  |  |
|---|---|
| AD100 | *Disulfiram (Systemic) |
| | Naltrexone (Systemic) |
| AD200 | Amyl Nitrite (Systemic) |
| | *Sodium Nitrite (Systemic) |
| | *Sodium Thiosulfate (Systemic) |
| AD300 | *Deferoxamine (Systemic) |
| | *Dimercaprol (Systemic) |
| | *Edetate Calcium Disodium (Systemic) |
| | *Edetate Disodium (Systemic) |
| | Penicillamine (Systemic) |
| | *Prussian Blue (Oral-Local) |
| | *Succimer (Systemic) |
| | *Trientine (Systemic) |
| | *Zinc Acetate (Systemic) |
| | Zinc Chloride (Systemic) |
| | Zinc Gluconate (Systemic) |
| | Zinc Sulfate (Systemic) |
| AD400 | Cholestyramine (Oral-Local) |
| | *Sodium Polystyrene Sulfonate (Local) |
| AD500 | *Antivenin (Chironex Fleckeri) (Systemic) |
| | *Antivenin (Crotalidae) Polyvalent (Systemic) |
| | *Antivenin (Enhydrina Schistosa) (Systemic) |
| | *Antivenin (Latrodectus Mactans) (Systemic) |
| | *Antivenin (Micrurus Fulvius) (Systemic) |
| | *Antivenin (Notechis Scutatus) (Systemic) |
| | *Antivenin (Pseudonaja Textilis) (Systemic) |
| AD600 | Bupropion (Systemic) |
| | *Nicotine (Inhalation-Systemic) |
| | *Nicotine (Nasal) |
| AD700 | *Flumazenil (Systemic) |
| AD800 | *Nalmefene (Systemic) |
| | *Naloxone (Systemic) |
| | *Naltrexone (Systemic) |
| AD900 | Acetylcysteine, Oral (Systemic) |
| | *Acetylcysteine, Parenteral (Systemic) |
| | Ascorbic Acid (Systemic) |
| | Atropine (Systemic) |
| | *Charcoal, Activated (Oral-Local) |
| | *Charcoal, Activated, and Sorbitol (Oral-Local) |
| | *Digoxin Immune Fab (Ovine) (Systemic) |
| | Edrophonium (Systemic) |
| | Edrophonium and Atropine (Systemic) |
| | *Fomepizole (Systemic) |
| | Glucagon (Systemic) |
| | Glycopyrrolate, Parenteral (Systemic) |
| | Hyoscyamine, Parenteral (Systemic) |
| | Iodine, Strong (Systemic) |
| | Leucovorin (Systemic) |
| | *Mesna (Systemic) |
| | Methadone (Systemic) |
| | *Methylene Blue (Systemic) |
| | *Nicotine (Systemic) |
| | Potassium Iodide (Systemic) |
| | *Pralidoxime (Systemic) |
| | Prazosin (Systemic) |
| | Racemethionine (Systemic) |
| | Sodium Ascorbate (Systemic) |
| | *Sodium Benzoate and Sodium Phenylacetate (Systemic) |
| | *Sodium Phenylbutyrate (Systemic) |
| | Sodium Thiosulfate (Systemic) |
| AH101 | *Methdilazine (Systemic) |
| | *Promethazine (Systemic) |
| | *Trimeprazine (Systemic) |
| AH102 | *Astemizole (Systemic) |
| | *Fexofenadine (Systemic) |
| | *Loratadine (Systemic) |
| | *Terfenadine (Systemic) |
| AH109 | *Acrivastine (Systemic) |
| | *Azatadine (Systemic) |
| | *Bromodiphenhydramine (Systemic) |
| | *Brompheniramine (Systemic) |
| | *Carbinoxamine (Systemic) |
| | *Cetirizine (Systemic) |
| | *Chlorpheniramine (Systemic) |
| | *Clemastine (Systemic) |
| | *Cyproheptadine (Systemic) |
| | *Dexchlorpheniramine (Systemic) |
| | *Dimenhydrinate (Systemic) |
| | *Diphenhydramine, Oral (Systemic) |
| | *Diphenylpyraline (Systemic) |
| | *Doxylamine (Systemic) |
| | *Hydroxyzine (Systemic) |
| | *Phenindamine (Systemic) |
| | *Pyrilamine (Systemic) |
| | *Tripelennamine (Systemic) |
| | *Triprolidine (Systemic) |
| AH900 | Olopatadine (Ophthalmic) |
| AM103 | *Cefdinir (Systemic) |
| AM111 | *Penicillin G (Systemic) |
| | *Penicillin V (Systemic) |
| AM112 | *Amoxicillin (Systemic) |
| | *Amoxicillin and Clavulanate (Systemic) |
| | *Ampicillin (Systemic) |
| | *Ampicillin and Sulbactam (Systemic) |
| | *Bacampicillin (Systemic) |
| | *Pivampicillin (Systemic) |
| | *Pivmecillinam (Systemic) |
| AM113 | *Cloxacillin (Systemic) |
| | *Dicloxacillin (Systemic) |
| | *Flucloxacillin (Systemic) |
| | *Methicillin (Systemic) |
| | *Nafcillin (Systemic) |
| | *Oxacillin (Systemic) |
| AM114 | *Carbenicillin (Systemic) |
| | *Mezlocillin (Systemic) |
| | *Piperacillin (Systemic) |
| | *Piperacillin and Tazobactam (Systemic) |
| | *Ticarcillin (Systemic) |
| | *Ticarcillin and Clavulanate (Systemic) |
| AM115 | *Cefadroxil (Systemic) |
| | *Cefazolin (Systemic) |
| | *Cephalexin (Systemic) |
| | *Cephalothin (Systemic) |
| | *Cephapirin (Systemic) |
| | *Cephradine (Systemic) |
| AM116 | *Cefaclor (Systemic) |
| | *Cefamandole (Systemic) |
| | *Cefonicid (Systemic) |
| | *Cefotetan (Systemic) |
| | *Cefoxitin (Systemic) |
| | *Cefprozil (Systemic) |
| | *Cefuroxime (Systemic) |
| AM117 | *Cefixime (Systemic) |
| | *Cefoperazone (Systemic) |
| | *Cefotaxime (Systemic) |
| | *Cefpodoxime (Systemic) |
| | *Ceftazidime (Systemic) |
| | Ceftibuten (Systemic) |
| | *Ceftizoxime (Systemic) |
| | *Ceftriaxone (Systemic) |
| AM118 | *Cefepime (Systemic) |
| AM119 | Aztreonam (Systemic) |
| | *Imipenem and Cilastatin (Systemic) |
| | *Loracarbef (Systemic) |
| | *Meropenem (Systemic) |
| AM130 | *Aztreonam (Systemic) |
| AM200 | *Azithromycin (Systemic) |
| | *Clarithromycin (Systemic) |
| | *Dirithromycin (Systemic) |
| | *Erythromycin Base (Systemic) |
| | *Erythromycin Estolate (Systemic) |
| | *Erythromycin Ethylsuccinate (Systemic) |
| | *Erythromycin Gluceptate (Systemic) |
| | *Erythromycin Lactobionate (Systemic) |
| | *Erythromycin Stearate (Systemic) |
| | *Spiramycin (Systemic) |
| AM250 | *Demeclocycline (Systemic) |
| | *Doxycycline (Systemic) |
| | *Minocycline (Systemic) |
| | *Oxytetracycline (Systemic) |
| | *Tetracycline (Systemic) |
| AM300 | *Amikacin (Systemic) |
| | *Gentamicin (Systemic) |
| | *Kanamycin (Oral-Local) |
| | *Kanamycin (Systemic) |
| | *Neomycin (Oral-Local) |
| | *Neomycin (Systemic) |
| | *Netilmicin (Systemic) |
| | *Streptomycin (Systemic) |
| | *Tobramycin (Systemic) |
| AM350 | *Clindamycin (Systemic) |
| | *Lincomycin (Systemic) |
| AM401 | *Cinoxacin (Systemic) |
| AM402 | *Ciprofloxacin (Systemic) |
| | *Enoxacin (Systemic) |
| | *Grepafloxacin (Systemic) |
| | *Levofloxacin (Systemic) |
| | *Lomefloxacin (Systemic) |
| | *Norfloxacin (Systemic) |
| | *Ofloxacin (Systemic) |
| | *Sparfloxacin (Systemic) |
| AM500 | *Aminosalicylate Sodium (Systemic) |
| | *Aminosalicylic Acid (Systemic) |
| | *Capreomycin (Systemic) |
| | *Cycloserine (Systemic) |
| | *Ethambutol (Systemic) |
| | *Ethionamide (Systemic) |
| | *Isoniazid (Systemic) |
| | *Isoniazid and Thiacetazone (Systemic) |
| | *Pyrazinamide (Systemic) |
| | *Rifampin (Systemic) |
| | *Rifampin and Isoniazid (Systemic) |
| | *Rifampin, Isoniazid, and Pyrazinamide (Systemic) |
| | *Rifapentine (Systemic) |
| | Streptomycin (Systemic) |
| AM550 | *Methenamine (Systemic) |
| AM600 | *Furazolidone (Oral-Local) |
| | *Nitrofurantoin (Systemic) |
| AM650 | *Sulfadiazine (Systemic) |
| | *Sulfadiazine and Trimethoprim (Systemic) |
| | *Sulfamethizole (Systemic) |
| | *Sulfamethoxazole (Systemic) |
| | *Sulfamethoxazole and Phenazopyridine (Systemic) |
| | *Sulfamethoxazole and Trimethoprim (Systemic) |
| | *Sulfisoxazole (Systemic) |
| | *Sulfisoxazole and Phenazopyridine (Systemic) |
| AM700 | *Amphotericin B (Systemic) |
| | *Amphotericin B Cholesteryl Complex (Systemic) |
| | *Amphotericin B Lipid Complex (Systemic) |
| | *Amphotericin B Liposomal Complex (Systemic) |
| | *Clotrimazole (Oral-Local) |
| | Dapsone (Systemic) |
| | *Fluconazole (Systemic) |
| | *Flucytosine (Systemic) |
| | *Griseofulvin (Systemic) |
| | *Itraconazole (Systemic) |
| | *Ketoconazole (Systemic) |
| | Nystatin (Oral-Local) |
| | Potassium Iodide (Systemic) |
| | *Terbinafine (Systemic) |
| AM800 | *Nevirapine (Systemic) |
| | *Zidovudine (Systemic) |
| AM802 | *Acyclovir (Systemic) |
| | *Cidofovir (Systemic) |
| | *Famciclovir (Systemic) |
| | *Foscarnet (Systemic) |
| | *Valacyclovir (Systemic) |
| AM803 | *Indinavir (Systemic) |
| | *Nelfinavir (Systemic) |
| | *Ritonavir (Systemic) |
| | *Saquinavir (Systemic) |
| AM804 | *Delavirdine (Systemic) |
| | *Didanosine (Systemic) |
| | *Lamivudine (Systemic) |
| AM809 | *Amantadine (Systemic) |
| | *Ganciclovir (Systemic) |
| | *Lamivudine and Zidovudine (Systemic) |
| | *Ribavirin (Systemic) |
| | *Rimantadine (Systemic) |
| | *Stavudine (Systemic) |
| | *Zalcitabine (Systemic) |
| AM900 | *Alatrofloxacin (Systemic) |
| | *Chloramphenicol (Systemic) |
| | *Clarithromycin (Systemic) |
| | *Clofazimine (Systemic) |
| | *Dapsone (Systemic) |
| | *Erythromycin and Sulfisoxazole (Systemic) |
| | *Fosfomycin (Systemic) |
| | *Fusidic Acid (Systemic) |
| | Immune Globulin Intravenous (Human) (Systemic) |
| | *Metronidazole (Systemic) |
| | *Nalidixic Acid (Systemic) |
| | *Rifabutin (Systemic) |
| | Rifampin (Systemic) |
| | *Spectinomycin (Systemic) |
| | *Trimethoprim (Systemic) |
| | *Trovafloxacin (Systemic) |
| | Vancomycin (Oral-Local) |
| | *Vancomycin (Systemic) |
| AN100 | *Busulfan (Systemic) |

# VA Medication Classification System

|  |  |  |  |  |  |
|---|---|---|---|---|---|
| | *Carmustine (Implantation-Local) | | *Mesna (Systemic) | | *Dopamine (Parenteral-Systemic) |
| | *Carmustine (Systemic) | | Methoxsalen (Systemic) | | *Ephedrine, Parenteral (Systemic) |
| | *Chlorambucil (Systemic) | | Methyltestosterone (Systemic) | | *Epinephrine, Parenteral (Systemic) |
| | *Cyclophosphamide (Systemic) | | *Mitotane (Systemic) | | *Isoproterenol (Systemic) |
| | *Ifosfamide (Systemic) | | *Mitoxantrone (Systemic) | | *Mephentermine (Parenteral-Systemic) |
| | *Lomustine (Systemic) | | Nandrolone (Systemic) | | *Metaraminol (Parenteral-Systemic) |
| | *Mechlorethamine (Systemic) | | *Nilutamide (Systemic) | | *Methoxamine (Parenteral-Systemic) |
| | *Melphalan (Systemic) | | *Paclitaxel (Systemic) | | *Norepinephrine (Parenteral-Systemic) |
| | *Uracil Mustard (Systemic) | | *Pegaspargase (Systemic) | | *Phenylephrine (Parenteral-Systemic) |
| AN200 | *Bleomycin (Systemic) | | *Pentostatin (Systemic) | | *Phenylpropanolamine (Systemic) |
| | *Dactinomycin (Systemic) | | *Porfimer (Systemic) | | *Ritodrine (Systemic) |
| | *Daunorubicin (Systemic) | | *Procarbazine (Systemic) | | *Terbutaline, Parenteral (Systemic) |
| | *Daunorubicin, Liposomal (Systemic) | | *Rituximab (Systemic) | AU150 | *Phentolamine (Intracavernosal) |
| | *Doxorubicin (Systemic) | | *Teniposide (Systemic) | AU200 | *Phentolamine (Systemic) |
| | *Doxorubicin, Liposomal (Systemic) | | *Testosterone (Systemic) | AU300 | *Ambenonium (Systemic) |
| | *Epirubicin (Systemic) | | Testosterone Cypionate (Systemic) | | *Bethanechol (Systemic) |
| | *Idarubicin (Systemic) | | Testosterone Enanthate (Systemic) | | *Domperidone (Systemic) |
| | *Mitomycin (Systemic) | | Testosterone Propionate (Systemic) | | *Edrophonium (Systemic) |
| | *Plicamycin (Systemic) | | *Thiotepa (Systemic) | | *Edrophonium and Atropine (Systemic) |
| | *Streptozocin (Systemic) | | Thyrotropin (Systemic) | | *Metoclopramide (Systemic) |
| AN300 | *Capecitabine (Systemic) | | *Topotecan (Systemic) | | *Neostigmine (Systemic) |
| | *Cladribine (Systemic) | | *Tretinoin (Systemic) | | *Physostigmine (Systemic) |
| | *Cytarabine (Systemic) | | *Vinblastine (Systemic) | | *Pilocarpine (Systemic) |
| | *Floxuridine (Systemic) | | *Vincristine (Systemic) | | *Pyridostigmine (Systemic) |
| | *Fludarabine (Systemic) | | *Vindesine (Systemic) | AU350 | Amantadine (Systemic) |
| | *Fluorouracil (Systemic) | | *Vinorelbine (Systemic) | | *Anisotropine (Systemic) |
| | Gemcitabine (Systemic) | AP100 | *Benznidazole (Systemic) | | *Atropine (Systemic) |
| | *Hydroxyurea (Systemic) | | *Diloxanide (Systemic) | | *Belladonna (Systemic) |
| | *Mercaptopurine (Systemic) | | *Meglumine Antimoniate (Systemic) | | *Benztropine (Systemic) |
| | *Methotrexate—For Cancer (Systemic) | | *Melarsoprol (Systemic) | | *Biperiden (Systemic) |
| | *Thioguanine (Systemic) | | *Nifurtimox (Systemic) | | Chlorpromazine (Systemic) |
| AN400 | Leucovorin (Systemic) | | *Suramin (Systemic) | | *Clidinium (Systemic) |
| | Levamisole (Systemic) | AP101 | *Chloroquine (Systemic) | | *Dicyclomine (Systemic) |
| AN500 | Aminoglutethimide (Systemic) | | Clindamycin (Systemic) | | Diphenhydramine, Oral (Systemic) |
| | *Anastrazole (Systemic) | | Dapsone (Systemic) | | *Ethopropazine (Systemic) |
| | *Anastrozole (Systemic) | | *Halofantrine (Systemic) | | *Glycopyrrolate (Systemic) |
| | *Buserelin (Systemic) | | *Hydroxychloroquine (Systemic) | | *Homatropine (Systemic) |
| | *Cyproterone (Systemic) | | *Mefloquine (Systemic) | | *Hyoscyamine (Systemic) |
| | Diethylstilbestrol (Systemic) | | *Primaquine (Systemic) | | *Mepenzolate (Systemic) |
| | Estradiol (Systemic) | | *Proguanil (Systemic) | | *Methantheline (Systemic) |
| | Estrogens, Conjugated (Systemic) | | *Pyrimethamine (Systemic) | | *Methscopolamine (Systemic) |
| | Estrogens, Esterified (Systemic) | | Quinidine (Systemic) | | *Orphenadrine Hydrochloride (Systemic) |
| | Estrone (Systemic) | | *Quinine (Systemic) | | *Pirenzepine (Systemic) |
| | Ethinyl Estradiol (Systemic) | | *Sulfadoxine and Pyrimethamine (Systemic) | | *Procyclidine (Systemic) |
| | Goserelin (Systemic) | AP109 | Amphotericin B (Systemic) | | *Propantheline (Systemic) |
| | Letrozole (Systemic) | | Amphotericin B Liposomal Complex (Systemic) | | *Scopolamine, Oral (Systemic) |
| | Leuprolide (Systemic) | | *Atovaquone (Systemic) | | *Scopolamine, Parenteral (Systemic) |
| | Levothyroxine (Systemic) | | Dapsone (Systemic) | | *Scopolamine, Rectal (Systemic) |
| | Liothyronine (Systemic) | | Demeclocycline (Systemic) | | Thioridazine (Systemic) |
| | Liotrix (Systemic) | | Doxycycline (Systemic) | | *Tolterodine (Systemic) |
| | Medroxyprogesterone (Systemic) | | *Eflornithine (Systemic) | | *Trihexyphenidyl (Systemic) |
| | Megestrol (Systemic) | | Furazolidone (Oral-Local) | AU900 | *Bromocriptine (Systemic) |
| | *Tamoxifen (Systemic) | | *Iodoquinol (Oral-Local) | | *Cabergoline (Systemic) |
| | *Testolactone (Systemic) | | Metronidazole (Systemic) | | Ergotamine, Belladonna Alkaloids, and Phenobarbital (Systemic) |
| | Thyroglobulin (Systemic) | | Minocycline (Systemic) | BL100 | *Anisindione (Systemic) |
| | Thyroid (Systemic) | | Oxytetracycline (Systemic) | | *Dicumarol (Systemic) |
| | Toremifene (Systemic) | | *Pentamidine (Inhalation) | | *Warfarin (Systemic) |
| | Trilostane (Systemic) | | *Pentamidine (Systemic) | BL110 | *Heparin (Systemic) |
| AN600 | *Chromic Phosphate P 32 (Parenteral-Local) | | Pyrimethamine (Systemic) | BL111 | *Ardeparin (Systemic) |
| | *Iobenguane I 131 Sulfate (Systemic—Therapeutic) | | *Quinacrine (Systemic) | | *Dalteparin (Systemic) |
| | *Sodium Iodide I 131 (Systemic—Therapeutic) | | Tetracycline (Systemic) | | *Enoxaparin (Systemic) |
| | *Sodium Phosphate P 32 (Systemic) | | *Trimetrexate (Systemic) | BL112 | *Danaparoid (Systemic) |
| | *Strontium Chloride Sr 89 (Systemic) | AP200 | *Albendazole (Systemic) | BL113 | *Lepirudin (Systemic) |
| AN700 | *Amifostine (Systemic) | | *Diethylcarbamazine (Systemic) | BL114 | *Acenocoumarol (Systemic) |
| | *Dexrazoxane (Systemic) | | *Ivermectin (Systemic) | | *Warfarin (Systemic) |
| AN900 | *Aldesleukin (Systemic) | | *Mebendazole (Systemic) | BL115 | *Alteplase, Recombinant (Systemic) |
| | *Altretamine (Systemic) | | Metronidazole (Systemic) | | *Anistreplase (Systemic) |
| | *Amsacrine (Systemic) | | *Niclosamide (Oral-Local) | | *Reteplase, Recombinant (Systemic) |
| | Asparaginase (Systemic) | | *Oxamniquine (Systemic) | | *Streptokinase (Systemic) |
| | *Bacillus Calmette-Guérin (BCG) Live (Mucosal-Local) | | Piperazine (Systemic) | | *Urokinase (Systemic) |
| | *BCG Live (Montreal Strain) (Mucosal-Local) | | *Praziquantel (Systemic) | BL116 | *Aminocaproic Acid (Systemic) |
| | | | *Pyrantel (Oral-Local) | | *Antihemophilic Factor (Systemic) |
| | *Bicalutamide (Systemic) | | *Pyrvinium (Oral-Local) | | *Anti-inhibitor Coagulant Complex (Systemic) |
| | *Carboplatin (Systemic) | | *Thiabendazole (Systemic) | | *Aprotinin (Systemic) |
| | *Cisplatin (Systemic) | | *Thiabendazole (Topical) | | Desmopressin (Systemic) |
| | *Dacarbazine (Systemic) | AP300 | *Benzyl Benzoate (Topical) | | *Factor IX (Systemic) |
| | *Docetaxel (Systemic) | | *Lindane (Topical) | | Fibrin Sealant (Local) |
| | *Estramustine (Systemic) | | *Malathion (Topical) | | *Tranexamic Acid (Systemic) |
| | *Etoposide (Systemic) | | *Permethrin (Topical) | BL117 | *Abciximab (Systemic) |
| | Fluoxymesterone (Systemic) | | *Pyrethrins and Piperonyl Butoxide (Topical) | | *Clopidogrel (Systemic) |
| | *Flutamide (Systemic) | AP900 | Benzyl Benzoate (Topical) | | *Dipyridamole (Systemic) |
| | Interferon Alfa-2a, Recombinant (Systemic) | | *Crotamiton (Topical) | | *Dipyridamole and Aspirin (Systemic) |
| | Interferon Alfa-2b, Recombinant (Systemic) | | Lindane (Topical) | | *Eptifibatide (Systemic) |
| | | | Permethrin (Topical) | | *Protamine (Systemic) |
| | Interferon Alfa-n1 (Ins) (Systemic) | | Spiramycin (Systemic) | | *Ticlopidine (Systemic) |
| | Interferon Alfa-n3 (Systemic) | | Sulfurated Lime Topical Solution (Topical) | | *Tirofiban (Systemic) |
| | *Irinotecan (Systemic) | | Sulfur Ointment (Topical) | BL119 | *Antithrombin III (Systemic) |
| | Ketoconazole (Systemic) | AU100 | *Arbutamine (Systemic) | BL160 | Aspirin, Sodium Bicarbonate, and Citric Acid (Systemic) |
| | | | *Dobutamine (Parenteral-Systemic) | BL170 | Aspirin, Buffered (Systemic) |

## VA Medication Classification System

|       | |       | |       | |
|---|---|---|---|---|---|
| | Aspirin and Caffeine, Buffered (Systemic) | | *Acetaminophen, Sodium Bicarbonate, and Citric Acid (Systemic) | | Flunarizine (Systemic) |
| | Aspirin Delayed-release Tablets USP (Systemic) | | Amitriptyline (Systemic) | | Ibuprofen (Systemic) |
| | Aspirin Tablets USP (Systemic) | | *Aspirin (Systemic) | | Indomethacin (Systemic) |
| | Aspirin Tablets USP (Chewable) (Systemic) | | *Aspirin, Buffered (Systemic) | | Indomethacin—For Patent Ductus Arteriosus, Oral (Systemic) |
| BL400 | *Anagrelide (Systemic) | | *Aspirin and Caffeine, Buffered (Systemic) | | Isometheptene, Dichloralphenazone, and Acetaminophen (Systemic) |
| | *Epoetin (Systemic) | | *Aspirin, Sodium Bicarbonate, and Citric Acid (Systemic) | | Ketoprofen (Systemic) |
| | *Filgrastim (Systemic) | | Baclofen (Systemic) | | Meclofenamate (Systemic) |
| | Fluoxymesterone (Systemic) | | *Butalbital and Acetaminophen (Systemic) | | Mefenamic Acid (Systemic) |
| | Leucovorin (Systemic) | | *Butalbital and Aspirin (Systemic) | | *Methysergide (Systemic) |
| | Lithium (Systemic) | | Carbamazepine (Systemic) | | Metoprolol (Systemic) |
| | Nandrolone (Systemic) | | *Choline Salicylate (Systemic) | | Nadolol (Systemic) |
| | *Oprelvekin (Systemic) | | *Choline and Magnesium Salicylates (Systemic) | | Naproxen (Systemic) |
| | Oxymetholone (Systemic) | | Clomipramine (Systemic) | | Naratriptan (Systemic) |
| | *Sargramostim (Systemic) | | *Clonidine (Parenteral-Local) | | *Pizotyline (Systemic) |
| | Stanozolol (Systemic) | | Desipramine (Systemic) | | Propranolol (Systemic) |
| | Testosterone Cypionate (Systemic) | | Doxepin (Systemic) | | Sumatriptan (Systemic) |
| | Testosterone Enanthate (Systemic) | | Fluphenazine (Systemic) | | Timolol (Systemic) |
| BL800 | *Albumin Human (Systemic) | | Imipramine (Systemic) | | Verapamil (Systemic) |
| BL900 | *Hemin (Systemic) | | *Isometheptene, Dichloralphenazone, and Acetaminophen (Systemic) | | Zolmitriptan (Systemic) |
| | *Imiglucerase (Systemic) | | *Ketorolac (Systemic) | CN201 | *Desflurane (Inhalation-Systemic) |
| | Immune Globulin Intravenous (Human) (Systemic) | | *Magnesium Salicylate (Systemic) | | *Enflurane (Systemic) |
| | *Pentastarch | | Maprotiline (Systemic) | | *Halothane (Systemic) |
| CN101 | *Acetaminophen and Codeine (Systemic) | | *Meprobamate and Aspirin (Systemic) | | *Isoflurane (Systemic) |
| | *Alfentanil (Systemic) | | Methotrimeprazine (Systemic) | | *Methoxyflurane (Systemic) |
| | *Anileridine (Systemic) | | Nortriptyline (Systemic) | | Nitrous Oxide (Systemic) |
| | *Aspirin and Codeine (Systemic) | | Salsalate (Systemic) | | *Sevoflurane (Inhalation-Systemic) |
| | *Aspirin and Codeine, Buffered (Systemic) | | Sodium Salicylate (Systemic) | CN202 | *Methohexital (Systemic) |
| | *Aspirin and Dihydrocodeine (Systemic) | | *Tramadol (Systemic) | | *Thiopental (Systemic) |
| | *Buprenorphine (Systemic) | | Trazodone (Systemic) | CN203 | *Etomidate (Systemic) |
| | *Butalbital, Acetaminophen, Caffeine, and Codeine (Systemic) | | Trimipramine (Systemic) | | *Ketamine (Systemic) |
| | *Butalbital, Aspirin, Caffeine, and Codeine (Systemic) | CN104 | Aspirin, Buffered (Systemic) | | *Propofol (Systemic) |
| | *Butorphanol (Nasal-Systemic) | | Aspirin and Caffeine, Buffered (Systemic) | CN204 | *Articaine (Parenteral-Local) |
| | *Butorphanol (Systemic) | | Aspirin and Caffeine Capsules (Systemic) | | *Articaine and Epinephrine (Parenteral-Local) |
| | *Codeine (Systemic) | | Aspirin and Caffeine Tablets (Systemic) | | *Bupivacaine (Parenteral-Local) |
| | *Dezocine (Systemic) | | Aspirin Delayed-release Tablets USP (Systemic) | | *Chloroprocaine (Parenteral-Local) |
| | *Dihydrocodeine and Acetaminophen (Systemic) | | Aspirin Extended-release Tablets USP (Systemic) | | *Diphenhydramine, Parenteral (Systemic) |
| | *Fentanyl (Systemic) | | Aspirin Suppositories USP (Systemic) | | *Etidocaine (Parenteral-Local) |
| | *Fentanyl (Transdermal-Systemic) | | Aspirin Tablets USP (Systemic) | | *Lidocaine (Parenteral-Local) |
| | *Hydrocodone (Systemic) | | Aspirin Tablets USP (Chewable) (Systemic) | | *Mepivacaine (Parenteral-Local) |
| | *Hydrocodone and Acetaminophen (Systemic) | | *Bromfenac (Systemic) | CN205 | *Prilocaine (Parenteral-Local) |
| | *Hydrocodone and Aspirin (Systemic) | | Choline Salicylate (Systemic) | | *Procaine (Parenteral-Local) |
| | *Hydromorphone (Systemic) | | Choline and Magnesium Salicylates (Systemic) | | *Ropivacaine (Parenteral-Local) |
| | *Levomethadyl (Systemic) | | Diclofenac (Systemic) | | *Tetracaine (Parenteral-Local) |
| | *Levorphanol (Systemic) | | Diflunisal (Systemic) | CN205 | Alfentanil (Systemic) |
| | *Meperidine (Systemic) | | Etodolac (Systemic) | | Anileridine (Systemic) |
| | *Methadone (Systemic) | | Fenoprofen (Systemic) | | Epinephrine, Parenteral (Systemic) |
| | *Morphine (Systemic) | | *Floctafenine (Systemic) | | Fentanyl (Systemic) |
| | *Nalbuphine (Systemic) | | Ibuprofen (Systemic) | CN206 | Buprenorphine (Systemic) |
| | Opium, Oral (Systemic) | | Ketoprofen (Systemic) | | Butorphanol (Systemic) |
| | *Opium, Parenteral (Systemic) | | Magnesium Salicylate (Systemic) | | *Droperidol (Systemic) |
| | *Oxycodone (Systemic) | | Meclofenamate (Systemic) | | Etomidate (Systemic) |
| | *Oxycodone and Acetaminophen (Systemic) | | *Mefenamic Acid (Systemic) | | Hydromorphone, Parenteral (Systemic) |
| | *Oxycodone and Aspirin (Systemic) | | Naproxen (Systemic) | | Ketamine (Systemic) |
| | *Oxymorphone (Systemic) | | Salsalate (Systemic) | | Levorphanol, Parenteral (Systemic) |
| | Paregoric (Systemic) | | Sodium Salicylate (Systemic) | | Meperidine, Parenteral (Systemic) |
| | *Pentazocine (Systemic) | CN105 | *Acetaminophen, Aspirin, and Caffeine (Systemic) | | Midazolam (Systemic) |
| | *Pentazocine and Acetaminophen (Systemic) | | Atenolol (Systemic) | | Morphine, Parenteral (Systemic) |
| | *Pentazocine and Aspirin (Systemic) | | Clonidine, Oral (Systemic) | | Nalbuphine (Systemic) |
| | *Phenobarbital, Aspirin, and Codeine (Systemic) | | Diclofenac (Systemic) | | Oxymorphone, Parenteral (Systemic) |
| | *Propoxyphene (Systemic) | | Diflunisal (Systemic) | | Pentazocine, Parenteral (Systemic) |
| | *Propoxyphene and Acetaminophen (Systemic) | | *Dihydroergotamine (Nasal–Systemic) | | Propofol (Systemic) |
| | *Propoxyphene and Aspirin (Systemic) | | *Dihydroergotamine (Systemic) | | *Remifentanil (Systemic) |
| | Remifentanil (Systemic) | | Divalproex (Systemic) | | Scopolamine, Parenteral (Systemic) |
| | Sufentanil (Systemic) | | *Ergotamine (Systemic) | | Sufentanil (Systemic) |
| CN102 | *Naltrexone (Systemic) | | *Ergotamine, Belladonna Alkaloids, and Phenobarbital (Systemic) | CN301 | *Amobarbital, Oral (Systemic) |
| CN103 | *Acetaminophen (Systemic) | | *Ergotamine and Caffeine (Systemic) | | *Amobarbital, Parenteral (Systemic) |
| | *Acetaminophen and Aspirin (Systemic) | | *Ergotamine, Caffeine, and Belladonna Alkaloids (Systemic) | | *Aprobarbital, Oral (Systemic) |
| | *Acetaminophen, Aspirin, and Caffeine (Systemic) | | *Ergotamine, Caffeine, Belladonna Alkaloids, and Pentobarbital (Systemic) | | *Butabarbital, Oral (Systemic) |
| | *Acetaminophen, Aspirin, and Caffeine, Buffered (Systemic) | | *Ergotamine, Caffeine, and Cyclizine (Systemic) | | *Pentobarbital, Oral (Systemic) |
| | *Acetaminophen, Aspirin, and Salicylamide, Buffered (Systemic) | | *Ergotamine, Caffeine, and Dimenhydrinate (Systemic) | | *Pentobarbital, Parenteral (Systemic) |
| | *Acetaminophen, Aspirin, Salicylamide, and Caffeine (Systemic) | | *Ergotamine, Caffeine, and Diphenhydramine (Systemic) | | *Phenobarbital, Oral (Systemic) |
| | *Acetaminophen and Salicylamide (Systemic) | | Etodolac (Systemic) | | *Phenobarbital, Parenteral (Systemic) |
| | *Acetaminophen, Salicylamide, and Caffeine (Systemic) | | Fenoprofen (Systemic) | | *Secobarbital, Oral (Systemic) |
| | | | Floctafenine (Systemic) | | *Secobarbital, Parenteral (Systemic) |
| | | | | CN302 | *Alprazolam Oral (Systemic) |
| | | | | | *Bromazepam, Oral (Systemic) |
| | | | | | *Chlordiazepoxide, Oral (Systemic) |
| | | | | | *Chlordiazepoxide, Parenteral (Systemic) |
| | | | | | *Clonazepam, Oral (Systemic) |
| | | | | | *Clorazepate, Oral (Systemic) |
| | | | | | *Diazepam, Oral (Systemic) |
| | | | | | *Diazepam, Parenteral (Systemic) |
| | | | | | *Estazolam, Oral (Systemic) |
| | | | | | *Flurazepam, Oral (Systemic) |
| | | | | | *Halazepam, Oral (Systemic) |
| | | | | | *Ketazolam, Oral (Systemic) |
| | | | | | *Lorazepam, Oral (Systemic) |
| | | | | | *Lorazepam, Parenteral (Systemic) |
| | | | | | *Midazolam (Systemic) |
| | | | | | *Nitrazepam, Oral (Systemic) |

## 3052 VA Medication Classification System

|  |  |
|---|---|
| | *Oxazepam, Oral (Systemic) |
| | *Prazepam, Oral (Systemic) |
| | *Quazepam, Oral (Systemic) |
| | *Temazepam, Oral (Systemic) |
| | *Triazolam, Oral (Systemic) |
| | Flumazenil (Systemic) |
| CN304 | *Buspirone (Systemic) |
| | *Meprobamate (Systemic) |
| CN309 | *Chloral Hydrate (Systemic) |
| | Diphenhydramine, Oral (Systemic) |
| | Doxylamine (Systemic) |
| | *Ethchlorvynol (Systemic) |
| | *Ethinamate (Systemic) |
| | *Glutethimide (Systemic) |
| | Hydroxyzine (Systemic) |
| | Methotrimeprazine (Systemic) |
| | *Methyprylon (Systemic) |
| | Promethazine (Systemic) |
| | *Propiomazine (Systemic) |
| | Propofol (Systemic) |
| | *Zolpidem (Systemic) |
| | *Zopiclone (Systemic) |
| CN400 | Acetazolamide (Systemic) |
| | Amobarbital, Parenteral (Systemic) |
| | *Carbamazepine (Systemic) |
| | *Clobazam (Systemic) |
| | Clonazepam, Oral (Systemic) |
| | Clorazepate, Oral (Systemic) |
| | *Corticotropin, Repository, Injection USP (Systemic) |
| | Diazepam, Oral (Systemic) |
| | Diazepam, Parenteral (Systemic) |
| | Diazepam, Rectal (Systemic) |
| | *Divalproex (Systemic) |
| | *Ethosuximide (Systemic) |
| | *Ethotoin (Systemic) |
| | *Felbamate (Systemic) |
| | *Fosphenytoin (Systemic) |
| | *Gabapentin (Systemic) |
| | *Lamotrigine (Systemic) |
| | Lorazepam, Parenteral (Systemic) |
| | Magnesium Sulfate (Systemic) |
| | *Mephenytoin (Systemic) |
| | *Mephobarbital, Oral (Systemic) |
| | *Metharbital, Oral (Systemic) |
| | *Methsuximide (Systemic) |
| | Nitrazepam, Oral (Systemic) |
| | *Paraldehyde (Systemic) |
| | *Paramethadione (Systemic) |
| | Pentobarbital, Parenteral (Systemic) |
| | *Phenacemide (Systemic) |
| | Phenobarbital, Oral (Systemic) |
| | Phenobarbital, Parenteral (Systemic) |
| | *Phenytoin (Systemic) |
| | *Primidone (Systemic) |
| | Secobarbital, Parenteral (Systemic) |
| | *Tiagabine (Systemic) |
| | *Trimethadione (Systemic) |
| | Topiramate (Systemic) |
| | *Valproate Sodium (Systemic) |
| | *Valproic Acid (Systemic) |
| CN500 | *Carbidopa and Levodopa (Systemic) |
| | *Levodopa (Systemic) |
| | *Levodopa and Benserazide (Systemic) |
| | *Pergolide (Systemic) |
| | *Pramipexole (Systemic) |
| | *Ropinirole (Systemic) |
| | *Selegiline (Systemic) |
| | *Tolcapone (Systemic) |
| CN550 | Dimenhydrinate (Systemic) |
| | Diphenhydramine, Oral (Systemic) |
| | *Diphenidol (Systemic) |
| | *Meclizine (Systemic) |
| | Scopolamine, Oral (Systemic) |
| | Scopolamine, Parenteral (Systemic) |
| | *Scopolamine, Transdermal (Systemic) |
| CN601 | *Amitriptyline (Systemic) |
| | *Amoxapine (Systemic) |
| | *Clomipramine (Systemic) |
| | *Desipramine (Systemic) |
| | *Doxepin (Systemic) |
| | *Imipramine (Systemic) |
| | *Nortriptyline (Systemic) |
| | *Protriptyline (Systemic) |
| | *Trimipramine (Systemic) |
| CN602 | *Phenelzine (Systemic) |
| | *Tranylcypromine (Systemic) |
| CN603 | *Citalopram (Systemic) |
| | *Fluoxetine (Systemic) |
| | Fluvoxamine (Systemic) |
| | *Paroxetine (Systemic) |
| | *Sertraline (Systemic) |
| CN609 | *Bupropion (Systemic) |

|  |  |
|---|---|
| | *Maprotiline (Systemic) |
| | *Mirtazapine (Systemic) |
| | *Moclobemide (Systemic) |
| | *Nefazodone (Systemic) |
| | *Trazodone (Systemic) |
| | Venlafaxine (Systemic) |
| CN701 | *Acetophenazine (Systemic) |
| | *Chlorpromazine (Systemic) |
| | *Fluphenazine (Systemic) |
| | *Mesoridazine (Systemic) |
| | *Methotrimeprazine (Systemic) |
| | *Pericyazine (Systemic) |
| | *Perphenazine (Systemic) |
| | *Pipotiazine (Systemic) |
| | *Prochlorperazine (Systemic) |
| | *Promazine (Systemic) |
| | *Thiopropazate (Systemic) |
| | *Thioproperazine (Systemic) |
| | *Thioridazine (Systemic) |
| | *Trifluoperazine (Systemic) |
| | *Triflupromazine (Systemic) |
| CN709 | *Chlorprothixene (Systemic) |
| | *Clozapine (Systemic) |
| | Droperidol (Systemic) |
| | *Flupenthixol (Systemic) |
| | *Fluspirilene (Systemic) |
| | *Haloperidol (Systemic) |
| | *Loxapine (Systemic) |
| | *Molindone (Systemic) |
| | *Olanzapine (Systemic) |
| | *Quetiapine (Systemic) |
| | Pimozide (Systemic) |
| | *Risperidone (Systemic) |
| | *Thiothixene (Systemic) |
| CN750 | *Lithium (Systemic) |
| CN801 | *Amphetamine (Systemic) |
| | *Amphetamine and Dextroamphetamine (Systemic) |
| | *Dextroamphetamine (Systemic) |
| | *Methamphetamine (Systemic) |
| CN802 | *Methylphenidate (Systemic) |
| CN809 | *Caffeine (Systemic) |
| | *Caffeine, Citrated (Systemic) |
| | *Caffeine and Sodium Benzoate (Systemic) |
| | Ephedrine, Oral (Systemic) |
| | *Pemoline (Systemic) |
| CN850 | Acetaminophen (Systemic) |
| | Acetaminophen and Aspirin (Systemic) |
| | Acetaminophen, Aspirin, and Caffeine (Systemic) |
| | Acetaminophen, Aspirin, and Caffeine, Buffered (Systemic) |
| | Acetaminophen, Aspirin, and Salicylamide, Buffered (Systemic) |
| | Acetaminophen, Aspirin, Salicylamide, and Caffeine (Systemic) |
| | Acetaminophen and Salicylamide (Systemic) |
| | Acetaminophen, Salicylamide, and Caffeine (Systemic) |
| | Aspirin, Buffered (Systemic) |
| | Aspirin and Caffeine, Buffered (Systemic) |
| | Aspirin and Caffeine Capsules (Systemic) |
| | Aspirin and Caffeine Tablets (Systemic) |
| | Aspirin Delayed-release Tablets USP (Systemic) |
| | Aspirin Extended-release Tablets USP (Systemic) |
| | Aspirin Suppositories USP (Systemic) |
| | Aspirin Tablets USP (Systemic) |
| | Aspirin Tablets USP (Chewable) (Systemic) |
| | Choline Salicylate (Systemic) |
| | Choline and Magnesium Salicylates (Systemic) |
| | Ibuprofen (Systemic) |
| | Indomethacin (Systemic) |
| | Indomethacin—For Patent Ductus Arteriosus, Oral (Systemic) |
| | Magnesium Salicylate (Systemic) |
| | Naproxen (Systemic) |
| | Salsalate (Systemic) |
| | Sodium Salicylate (Systemic) |
| | Tiludronate (Systemic) |
| CN900 | Acebutolol (Systemic) |
| | Amantadine (Systemic) |
| | Amitriptyline (Systemic) |
| | Atenolol (Systemic) |
| | Carbamazepine (Systemic) |

|  |  |
|---|---|
| | *Chlordiazepoxide and Amitriptyline (Systemic) |
| | Clomipramine (Systemic) |
| | Clonidine, Oral (Systemic) |
| | Desipramine (Systemic) |
| | Divalproex (Systemic) |
| | *Donepezil (Systemic) |
| | Doxepin (Systemic) |
| | *Ergoloid Mesylates (Systemic) |
| | Fluoxetine (Systemic) |
| | *Fluvoxamine (Systemic) |
| | Glatiramer Acetate (Systemic) |
| | Haloperidol (Systemic) |
| | *Hydrocodone and Ibuprofen (Systemic) |
| | Imipramine (Systemic) |
| | *Interferon Beta-1a (Systemic) |
| | *Interferon Beta-1b (Systemic) |
| | Lithium (Systemic) |
| | Loxapine (Systemic) |
| | Metoprolol (Systemic) |
| | Nadolol (Systemic) |
| | Nortriptyline (Systemic) |
| | Oxprenolol (Systemic) |
| | Paroxetine (Systemic) |
| | *Perphenazine and Amitriptyline (Systemic) |
| | Phenelzine (Systemic) |
| | *Pimozide (Systemic) |
| | Pindolol (Systemic) |
| | Propranolol (Systemic) |
| | Protriptyline (Systemic) |
| | *Riluzole (Systemic) |
| | Sertraline (Systemic) |
| | Sotalol (Systemic) |
| | *Tacrine (Systemic) |
| | Timolol (Systemic) |
| | Tranylcypromine (Systemic) |
| CV050 | *Digitoxin (Systemic) |
| | Digoxin (Systemic) |
| CV052 | *Milrinone (Systemic) |
| CV053 | Arbutamine (Systemic) |
| CV100 | *Acebutolol (Systemic) |
| | *Atenolol (Systemic) |
| | *Betaxolol (Systemic) |
| | *Bisoprolol (Systemic) |
| | *Carteolol (Systemic) |
| | *Carvedilol (Systemic) |
| | *Esmolol (Systemic) |
| | *Labetalol (Systemic) |
| | *Metoprolol (Systemic) |
| | *Nadolol (Systemic) |
| | *Oxprenolol (Systemic) |
| | *Penbutolol (Systemic) |
| | *Pindolol (Systemic) |
| | *Propranolol (Systemic) |
| | *Sotalol (Systemic) |
| | *Timolol (Systemic) |
| CV150 | *Doxazosin (Systemic) |
| | Phentolamine (Systemic) |
| | Phenoxybenzamine (Systemic) |
| | *Prazosin (Systemic) |
| | *Terazosin (Systemic) |
| CV200 | Amlodipine (Systemic) |
| | *Bepridil (Systemic) |
| | *Diltiazem (Systemic) |
| | Felodipine (Systemic) |
| | *Flunarizine (Systemic) |
| | *Isradipine (Systemic) |
| | Mibefradil (Systemic) |
| | *Nicardipine (Systemic) |
| | *Nifedipine (Systemic) |
| | *Nimodipine (Systemic) |
| | *Verapamil (Systemic) |
| CV250 | Acebutolol (Systemic) |
| | Amlodipine (Systemic) |
| | *Amyl Nitrite (Systemic) |
| | Atenolol (Systemic) |
| | Bepridil (Systemic) |
| | Diltiazem (Systemic) |
| | *Erythrityl Tetranitrate (Systemic) |
| | *Isosorbide Dinitrate (Systemic) |
| | *Isosorbide Mononitrate (Systemic) |
| | Labetalol (Systemic) |
| | Metoprolol (Systemic) |
| | Mibefradil (Systemic) |
| | Nadolol (Systemic) |
| | Nicardipine (Systemic) |
| | Nifedipine (Systemic) |
| | *Nitroglycerin (Systemic) |
| | Oxprenolol (Systemic) |
| | *Pentaerythritol Tetranitrate (Systemic) |
| | Pindolol (Systemic) |
| | Propranolol (Systemic) |

USP DI

## VA Medication Classification System

Sotalol (Systemic)
Timolol (Systemic)
Verapamil (Systemic)
CV300 Acebutolol (Systemic)
*Adenosine (Systemic)
*Amiodarone (Systemic)
Atenolol (Systemic)
Atropine, Parenteral (Systemic)
*Bretylium (Systemic)
Digitoxin (Systemic)
Digoxin (Systemic)
Diltiazem (Systemic)
*Disopyramide (Systemic)
*Encainide (Systemic)
Esmolol (Systemic)
*Flecainide (Systemic)
Glycopyrrolate, Parenteral (Systemic)
Hyoscyamine, Parenteral (Systemic)
*Ibutilide (Systemic)
Isoproterenol (Parenteral-Systemic)
*Lidocaine (Systemic)
Magnesium Sulfate (Systemic)
Metoprolol (Systemic)
*Mexiletine (Systemic)
*Moricizine (Systemic)
Nadolol (Systemic)
Oxprenolol (Systemic)
Phenylephrine (Parenteral-Systemic)
Phenytoin (Systemic)
*Procainamide (Systemic)
*Propafenone (Systemic)
Propranolol (Systemic)
*Quinidine (Systemic)
Scopolamine, Parenteral (Systemic)
Sotalol (Systemic)
Timolol (Systemic)
*Tocainide (Systemic)
Verapamil (Systemic)
CV351 *Atorvastatin (Systemic)
*Cerivastatin (Systemic)
CV352 Cholestyramine (Oral-Local)
CV400 *Deserpidine and Hydrochlorothiazide (Systemic)
*Deserpidine and Methyclothiazide (Systemic)
*Guanethidine and Hydrochlorothiazide (Systemic)
CV401 *Amlodipine and Benazepril (Systemic)
*Atenolol and Chlorthalidone (Systemic)
*Bisoprolol and Hydrochlorothiazide (Systemic)
*Captopril and Hydrochlorothiazide (Systemic)
*Clonidine and Chlorthalidone (Systemic)
*Enalapril and Diltiazem (Systemic)
*Enalapril and Felodipine (Systemic)
*Enalapril and Hydrochlorothiazide (Systemic)
*Hydralazine and Hydrochlorothiazide (Systemic)
*Lisinopril and Hydrochlorothiazide (Systemic)
*Losartan and Hydrochlorothiazide (Systemic)
*Methyldopa and Chlorothiazide (Systemic)
*Methyldopa and Hydrochlorothiazide (Systemic)
Metoprolol and Hydrochlorothiazide (Systemic)
*Moexipril and Hydrochlorothiazide (Systemic)
Nadolol and Bendroflumethiazide (Systemic)
Pindolol and Hydrochlorothiazide (Systemic)
*Prazosin and Polythiazide (Systemic)
Propranolol and Hydrochlorothiazide (Systemic)
*Rauwolfia Serpentina and Bendroflumethiazide (Systemic)
*Reserpine and Chlorothiazide (Systemic)
*Reserpine and Chlorthalidone (Systemic)
*Reserpine, Hydralazine, and Hydrochlorothiazide (Systemic)
*Reserpine and Hydrochlorothiazide (Systemic)
*Reserpine and Hydroflumethiazide (Systemic)
*Reserpine and Methyclothiazide (Systemic)
*Reserpine and Polythiazide (Systemic)

*Reserpine and Trichlormethiazide (Systemic)
Timolol and Hydrochlorothiazide (Systemic)
Trandolapril and Verapamil (Systemic)
*Valsartan and Hydrochlorothiazide (Systemic)
CV402 *Fenoldopam (Systemic)
*Nitroprusside (Systemic)
CV409 Acebutolol (Systemic)
Amlodipine (Systemic)
Atenolol (Systemic)
Benazepril (Systemic)
Bendroflumethiazide (Systemic)
Betaxolol (Systemic)
Bisoprolol (Systemic)
Bumetanide (Systemic)
Captopril (Systemic)
Carteolol (Systemic)
Carvedilol (Systemic)
Chlorothiazide (Systemic)
Chlorthalidone (Systemic)
*Clonidine, Oral (Systemic)
*Clonidine, Transdermal (Systemic)
*Deserpidine (Systemic)
*Diazoxide (Parenteral-Systemic)
Diltiazem (Systemic)
Doxazosin (Systemic)
Enalapril (Systemic)
Ethacrynic Acid (Systemic)
Felodipine (Systemic)
Fosinopril (Systemic)
Furosemide (Systemic)
*Guanabenz (Systemic)
*Guanadrel (Systemic)
*Guanethidine (Systemic)
*Guanfacine (Systemic)
Hydrochlorothiazide (Systemic)
Hydroflumethiazide (Systemic)
Irbesartan (Systemic)
Isradipine (Systemic)
Labetalol (Systemic)
Lisinopril (Systemic)
Losartan (Systemic)
Methyclothiazide (Systemic)
*Methyldopa (Systemic)
Metolazone (Systemic)
Metoprolol (Systemic)
Mibefradil (Systemic)
Minoxidil (Systemic)
Moexipril (Systemic)
Nadolol (Systemic)
Nicardipine (Systemic)
Nifedipine (Systemic)
Oxprenolol (Systemic)
Penbutolol (Systemic)
Phenoxybenzamine (Systemic)
Pindolol (Systemic)
Polythiazide (Systemic)
Propranolol (Systemic)
Quinapril (Systemic)
Quinethazone (Systemic)
Prazosin (Systemic)
Ramipril (Systemic)
*Rauwolfia Serpentina (Systemic)
*Reserpine (Systemic)
Sotalol (Systemic)
Timolol (Systemic)
Terazosin (Systemic)
Torsemide (Systemic)
Trichlormethiazide (Systemic)
Valsartan (Systemic)
Verapamil (Systemic)
CV490 Amiloride (Systemic)
Amiloride and Hydrochlorothiazide (Systemic)
*Hydralazine (Systemic)
Indapamide (Systemic)
*Mecamylamine (Systemic)
*Metyrosine (Systemic)
Nitroglycerin (Systemic)
Spironolactone (Systemic)
Spironolactone and Hydrochlorothiazide (Systemic)
Triamterene (Systemic)
Triamterene and Hydrochlorothiazide (Systemic)
CV500 Alprostadil (Local)
*Cyclandelate (Systemic)
Fenoldopam (Systemic)
*Isoxsuprine (Systemic)
*Nicotinyl Alcohol (Systemic)
Nitroprusside (Systemic)

*Nylidrin (Systemic)
*Papaverine (Intracavernosal)
*Papaverine (Systemic)
*Tolazoline (Parenteral-Systemic)
CV601 *Atorvastatin (Systemic)
*Cerivastatin (Systemic)
*Fluvastatin (Systemic)
*Lovastatin (Systemic)
*Pravastatin (Systemic)
*Simvastatin (Systemic)
CV602 *Cholestyramine (Oral-Local)
*Colestipol (Oral-Local)
CV603 *Clofibrate (Systemic)
*Fenofibrate (Systemic)
*Gemfibrozil (Systemic)
CV609 *Dextrothyroxine (Systemic)
Niacin (Systemic)
Niacinamide (Systemic)
*Probucol (Systemic)
Psyllium Hydrophilic Mucilloid (Local)
CV701 *Bendroflumethiazide (Systemic)
*Chlorothiazide (Systemic)
*Chlorthalidone (Systemic)
*Hydrochlorothiazide (Systemic)
*Hydroflumethiazide (Systemic)
*Indapamide (Systemic)
*Methyclothiazide (Systemic)
*Metolazone (Systemic)
*Polythiazide (Systemic)
*Quinethazone (Systemic)
*Trichlormethiazide (Systemic)
CV702 *Bumetanide (Systemic)
*Ethacrynic Acid (Systemic)
*Furosemide (Systemic)
*Torsemide (Systemic)
CV703 *Acetazolamide (Systemic)
*Dichlorphenamide (Systemic)
*Methazolamide (Systemic)
CV704 *Amiloride (Systemic)
*Amiloride and Hydrochlorothiazide (Systemic)
*Spironolactone (Systemic)
*Spironolactone and Hydrochlorothiazide (Systemic)
*Triamterene (Systemic)
*Triamterene and Hydrochlorothiazide (Systemic)
CV709 *Glycerin (Systemic)
*Mannitol (Systemic)
*Urea (Systemic)
CV800 *Benazepril (Systemic)
*Captopril (Systemic)
*Enalapril (Systemic)
*Fosinopril (Systemic)
*Lisinopril (Systemic)
*Moexipril (Systemic)
*Quinapril (Systemic)
*Ramipril (Systemic)
*Trandolapril (Systemic)
CV805 *Irbesartan (Systemic)
*Losartan (Systemic)
*Valsartan (Systemic)
CV900 Abciximab (Systemic)
Acebutolol (Systemic)
*Amrinone (Systemic)
Atenolol (Systemic)
Benazepril (Systemic)
Bendroflumethiazide (Systemic)
Calcium Chloride, Parenteral (Systemic)
Calcium Gluconate, Parenteral (Systemic)
Captopril (Systemic)
Captopril and Hydrochlorothiazide (Systemic)
Chlorothiazide (Systemic)
Chlorpropamide (Systemic)
Chlorthalidone (Systemic)
Desmopressin (Systemic)
Dihydroergotamine (Systemic)
Digitoxin (Systemic)
Digoxin (Systemic)
Dobutamine (Parenteral-Systemic)
Dopamine (Parenteral-Systemic)
Enalapril (Systemic)
Enalapril and Hydrochlorothiazide (Systemic)
Ephedrine (Parenteral-Systemic)
Epinephrine (Parenteral-Systemic)
Erythrityl Tetranitrate (Systemic)
*Ethanolamine Oleate (Parenteral-Local)
Fludrocortisone (Systemic)
Fosinopril (Systemic)
Hydralazine (Systemic)

# VA Medication Classification System

Hydrochlorothiazide (Systemic)
Hydroflumethiazide (Systemic)
Immune Globulin Intravenous (Human) (Systemic)
Indomethacin (Systemic)
Indomethacin—For Patent Ductus Arteriosus, Oral (Systemic)
*Indomethacin—For Patent Ductus Arteriosus, Parenteral (Systemic)
Isosorbide Dinitrate (Systemic)
Lisinopril (Systemic)
Lisinopril and Hydrochlorothiazide (Systemic)
Lypressin (Systemic)
Mephentermine (Parenteral-Systemic)
Metaraminol (Parenteral-Systemic)
Methoxamine (Parenteral-Systemic)
Methyclothiazide (Systemic)
Metolazone (Systemic)
Metoprolol (Systemic)
*Midodrine (Systemic)
Moexipril (Systemic)
Nadolol (Systemic)
Nitroglycerin (Systemic)
Nitroprusside (Systemic)
Norepinephrine (Parenteral-Systemic)
Octreotide (Systemic)
Oxprenolol (Systemic)
Pentaerythritol Tetranitrate (Systemic)
*Pentoxifylline (Systemic)
*Perfluorochemical Emulsion (Systemic)
Phentolamine (Systemic)
Phenylephrine (Parenteral-Systemic)
Polythiazide (Systemic)
Prazosin (Systemic)
Propranolol (Systemic)
Quinapril (Systemic)
Quinethazone (Systemic)
Ramipril (Systemic)
Sotalol (Systemic)
Timolol (Systemic)
Trichlormethiazide (Systemic)
Verapamil (Systemic)

DE100 *Iodine (Topical)
DE101 *Ammoniated Mercury (Systemic)
Chlorhexidine (Mucosal-Local)
*Chlortetracycline (Topical)
Clindamycin (Topical)
*Clioquinol (Topical)
Erythromycin (Topical)
*Framycetin (Topical)
*Framycetin and Gramicidin (Topical)
*Fusidic Acid (Topical)
*Gentamicin (Topical)
*Mafenide (Topical)
*Mupirocin (Topical)
*Neomycin (Topical)
*Neomycin and Polymyxin B (Topical)
*Neomycin, Polymyxin B, and Bacitracin (Topical)
*Silver Sulfadiazine (Topical)
Sodium Fluoride and Triclosan (Systemic)
Tetracycline (Topical)
Tetracycline Periodontal Fibers (Mucosal-Local)

DE102 *Amphotericin B (Topical)
*Butenafine (Topical)
*Carbol-Fuchsin (Topical)
*Ciclopirox (Topical)
Clioquinol (Topical)
*Clotrimazole (Topical)
*Econazole (Topical)
*Gentian Violet (Topical)
*Haloprogin (Topical)
*Ketoconazole (Topical)
Mafenide (Topical)
*Miconazole (Topical)
*Naftifine (Topical)
*Nystatin (Topical)
*Oxiconazole (Topical)
Silver Sulfadiazine (Topical)
*Sulconazole (Topical)
*Terbinafine (Topical)
*Tioconazole (Topical)
*Tolnaftate (Topical)
*Undecylenic Acid, Compound (Topical)

DE103 *Acyclovir (Topical)
*Penciclovir (Topical)

DE200 *Alclometasone (Topical)
Amcinonide (Topical)
*Beclomethasone (Topical)
*Betamethasone (Topical)
*Bufexamac (Topical)
*Clobetasol (Topical)
*Clobetasone (Topical)
*Clocortolone (Topical)
*Desonide (Topical)
*Desoximetasone (Topical)
*Dexamethasone (Topical)
*Diflorasone (Topical)
*Diflucortolone (Topical)
*Flumethasone (Topical)
*Fluocinolone (Topical)
*Fluocinonide (Topical)
*Fluocinonide, Procinonide, and Ciprocinonide (Topical)
*Flurandrenolide (Topical)
*Fluticasone (Topical)
*Halcinonide (Topical)
*Halobetasol (Topical)
*Hydrocortisone (Topical)
*Hydrocortisone Acetate (Topical)
*Hydrocortisone and Urea (Topical)
*Mometasone (Topical)
*Prednicarbate (Topical)
*Triamcinolone (Topical)

DE250 *Clioquinol and Flumethasone (Topical)
*Clioquinol and Hydrocortisone (Topical)
*Clotrimazole and Betamethasone (Topical)
*Nystatin and Triamcinolone (Topical)

DE300 *Aminobenzoic Acid, Padimate O, and Oxybenzone (Topical)
*Aminobenzoic Acid and Titanium Dioxide (Topical)
*Avobenzone, Octocrylene, Octyl Salicylate, and Oxybenzone (Topical)
*Avobenzone and Octyl Methoxycinnamate (Topical)
*Avobenzone, Octyl Methoxycinnamate, Octyl Salicylate, and Oxybenzone (Topical)
*Avobenzone, Octyl Methoxycinnamate, and Oxybenzone (Topical)
*Dioxybenzone, Oxybenzone, and Padimate O (Topical)
*Homosalate (Topical)
*Homosalate, Menthyl Anthranilate, and Octyl Methoxycinnamate (Topical)
*Homosalate, Menthyl Anthranilate, Octyl Methoxycinnamate, Octyl Salicylate, and Oxybenzone (Topical)
*Homosalate, Octocrylene, Octyl Methoxycinnamate, and Oxybenzone (Topical)
*Homosalate, Octyl Methoxycinnamate, Octyl Salicylate, and Oxybenzone (Topical)
*Homosalate, Octyl Methoxycinnamate, and Oxybenzone (Topical)
*Homosalate and Oxybenzone (Topical)
*Lisadimate, Oxybenzone, and Padimate O (Topical)
*Lisadimate and Padimate O (Topical)
*Menthyl Anthranilate (Topical)
*Menthyl Anthranilate, Octocrylene, and Octyl Methoxycinnamate (Topical)
*Menthyl Anthranilate, Octocrylene, Octyl Methoxycinnamate, and Oxybenzone (Topical)
*Menthyl Anthranilate and Octyl Methoxycinnamate (Topical)
*Menthyl Anthranilate, Octyl Methoxycinnamate, and Octyl Salicylate (Topical)
*Menthyl Anthranilate, Octyl Methoxycinnamate, Octyl Salicylate, and Oxybenzone (Topical)
*Menthyl Anthranilate, Octyl Methoxycinnamate, and Oxybenzone (Topical)
*Menthyl Anthranilate and Padimate O (Topical)
*Menthyl Anthranilate and Titanium Dioxide (Topical)
*Octocrylene and Octyl Methoxycinnamate (Topical)
*Octocrylene, Octyl Methoxycinnamate, Octyl Salicylate, and Oxybenzone (Topical)
*Octocrylene, Octyl Methoxycinnamate, Octyl Salicylate, Oxybenzone, and Titanium Dioxide (Topical)
*Octocrylene, Octyl Methoxycinnamate, and Oxybenzone (Topical)
*Octocrylene, Octyl Methoxycinnamate, Oxybenzone, and Titanium Dioxide (Topical)
*Octocrylene, Octyl Methoxycinnamate, and Titanium Dioxide (Topical)
*Octyl Methoxycinnamate (Topical)
*Octyl Methoxycinnamate and Octyl Salicylate (Topical)
*Octyl Methoxycinnamate, Octyl Salicylate, and Oxybenzone (Topical)
*Octyl Methoxycinnamate, Octyl Salicylate, Oxybenzone, and Padimate O (Topical)
*Octyl Methoxycinnamate, Octyl Salicylate, Oxybenzone, Padimate O, and Titanium Dioxide (Topical)
*Octyl Methoxycinnamate, Octyl Salicylate, Oxybenzone, Phenylbenzimidazole, and Titanium Dioxide (Topical)
*Octyl Methoxycinnamate, Octyl Salicylate, Oxybenzone, and Titanium Dioxide (Topical)
*Octyl Methoxycinnamate, Octyl Salicylate, Phenylbenzimidazole, and Titanium Dioxide (Topical)
*Octyl Methoxycinnamate, Octyl Salicylate, and Titanium Dioxide (Topical)
*Octyl Methoxycinnamate and Oxybenzone (Topical)
*Octyl Methoxycinnamate, Oxybenzone, and Padimate O (Topical)
*Octyl Methoxycinnamate, Oxybenzone, Padimate O, and Titanium Dioxide (Topical)
*Octyl Methoxycinnamate, Oxybenzone, and Titanium Dioxide (Topical)
*Octyl Methoxycinnamate and Padimate O (Topical)
*Octyl Methoxycinnamate and Phenylbenzimidazole (Topical)
*Octyl Salicylate (Topical)
*Octyl Salicylate and Padimate O (Topical)
*Oxybenzone and Padimate O (Topical)
*Oxybenzone and Roxadimate (Topical)
*Padimate O (Topical)
*Phenylbenzimidazole (Topical)
*Phenylbenzimidazole and Sulisobenzone (Topical)
*Titanium Dioxide (Topical)
*Titanium Dioxide and Zinc Oxide (Topical)
*Trolamine Salicylate (Topical)

DE400 *Chloroxine (Topical)
*Pyrithione (Topical)
*Selenium Sulfide (Topical)

DE500 Alcohol and Sulfur (Topical)
Benzoyl Peroxide (Topical)
Coal Tar (Topical)
*Podofilox (Topical)
*Podophyllum (Topical)
Resorcinol (Topical)
Resorcinol and Sulfur (Topical)
*Salicylic Acid Cream (Topical)
*Salicylic Acid Gel (Topical)
*Salicylic Acid Lotion (Topical)
*Salicylic Acid Ointment (Topical)
*Salicylic Acid Pads (Topical)
*Salicylic Acid Plaster (Topical)
*Salicylic Acid Shampoo (Topical)
*Salicylic Acid Soap (Topical)
*Salicylic Acid and Sulfur (Topical)
*Salicylic Acid, Sulfur, and Coal Tar (Topical)
*Salicylic Acid Topical Solution (Topical)
*Sulfurated Lime (Topical)
*Sulfur Bar Soap (Topical)
*Sulfur Cream (Topical)
*Sulfur Lotion (Topical)
*Sulfur Ointment (Topical)
Tretinoin Cream USP (Oil-in-water) (Topical)
Tretinoin Gel USP (Topical)
Tretinoin Topical Solution USP (Topical)

DE600 Bleomycin (Systemic)
Carmustine (Systemic)
*Fluorouracil (Topical)
*Masoprocol (Topical)
Mechlorethamine (Systemic)
*Mechlorethamine (Topical)
Mitomycin (Systemic)

DE650 *Diethylamine (Topical)

DE700 *Benzocaine Cream USP (Topical)

# VA Medication Classification System

*Benzocaine and Menthol (Topical)
Benzocaine Ointment (Mucosal-Local)
Benzocaine Ointment USP (Topical)
*Benzocaine Topical Aerosol (Mucosal-Local)
*Benzocaine Topical Aerosol USP (Topical)
*Benzocaine Topical Spray Solution (Topical)
*Butamben (Topical)
*Dibucaine Cream USP (Topical)
Dibucaine Ointment (Mucosal-Local)
Dibucaine Ointment USP (Topical)
*Lidocaine Hydrochloride Film-forming Gel (Topical)
Lidocaine Hydrochloride Jelly USP (Topical)
*Lidocaine Hydrochloride Ointment (Topical)
*Lidocaine Hydrochloride Topical Aerosol (Topical)
Lidocaine Ointment (Mucosal-Local)
*Lidocaine 2.5% Ointment USP (Topical)
Lidocaine 5% Ointment USP (Topical)
*Lidocaine and Prilocaine (Topical)
*Lidocaine Topical Spray Solution (Topical)
Pramoxine Cream (Mucosal-Local)
Pramoxine Cream (Topical)
*Pramoxine Lotion (Topical)
Pramoxine Hydrochloride Cream USP (Topical)
*Pramoxine Hydrochloride Lotion USP (Topical)
*Pramoxine and Menthol (Topical)
*Pramoxine and Menthol Gel (Topical)
*Pramoxine and Menthol Lotion (Topical)
Tetracaine (Topical)
Tetracaine Cream (Mucosal-Local)
Tetracaine Cream (Topical)
Tetracaine and Menthol (Topical)
Tetracaine and Menthol Ointment (Mucosal-Local)
Tetracaine and Menthol Ointment (Topical)

DE751 Erythromycin Base (Systemic)
Erythromycin Estolate (Systemic)
Erythromycin Ethylsuccinate (Systemic)
Erythromycin Stearate (Systemic)
*Isotretinoin (Systemic)
Minocycline (Systemic)
Tetracycline (Systemic)

DE752 *Adapalene (Topical)
*Alcohol and Acetone (Topical)
*Alcohol and Sulfur (Topical)
*Azelaic Acid (Topical)
*Benzoyl Peroxide (Topical)
*Clindamycin (Topical)
*Erythromycin (Topical)
*Erythromycin and Benzoyl Peroxide (Topical)
*Isotretinoin (Topical)
*Meclocycline (Topical)
*Metronidazole (Topical)
*Nicotinamide (Topical)
*Resorcinol (Topical)
*Resorcinol and Sulfur (Topical)
Salicylic Acid Gel (Topical)
Salicylic Acid Lotion (Topical)
Salicylic Acid Ointment (Topical)
Salicylic Acid Pads (Topical)
Salicylic Acid Soap (Topical)
Salicylic Acid and Sulfur Bar Soap (Topical)
Salicylic Acid and Sulfur Cleansing Cream (Topical)
Salicylic Acid and Sulfur Cleansing Lotion (Topical)
Salicylic Acid and Sulfur Cleansing Suspension (Topical)
Salicylic Acid and Sulfur Cream (Topical)
Salicylic Acid and Sulfur Lotion (Topical)
Salicylic Acid and Sulfur Topical Suspension (Topical)
Salicylic Acid Topical Solution (Topical)
Sulfurated Lime (Topical)
Sulfur Bar Soap (Topical)
Sulfur Cream (Topical)
Sulfur Lotion (Topical)
Sulfur Ointment (Topical)
Tazarotene (Systemic)
*Tetracycline (Topical)

*Tretinoin Cream USP (Oil-in-water)
*Tretinoin Gel USP (Topical)
Tretinoin Topical Solution USP (Topical)

DE801 *Acitretin (Systemic)
Cyclophosphamide (Systemic)
Cyclosporine (Systemic)
*Etretinate (Systemic)
*Methotrexate—For Noncancerous Conditions (Systemic)
*Methoxsalen (Systemic)
Trioxsalen (Systemic)

DE802 *Anthralin (Topical)
*Calcipotriene (Topical)
*Coal Tar (Topical)
Methoxsalen (Topical)
Salicylic Acid Gel (Topical)
Salicylic Acid Ointment (Topical)
Salicylic Acid, Sulfur, and Coal Tar (Topical)
*Tazarotene (Systemic)

DE890 *Aminobenzoate Potassium (Systemic)
Beta-carotene (Systemic)
Cholestyramine (Oral-Local)
Cimetidine (Systemic)
Colestipol (Oral-Local)
Doxepin (Systemic)
Ephedrine, Oral (Systemic)
Ephedrine, Parenteral (Systemic)
Etretinate (Systemic)
Finasteride (Systemic)
Isotretinoin (Systemic)
Methoxsalen (Systemic)
*Sulfapyridine (Systemic)
*Trioxsalen (Systemic)

DE900 Anthralin (Topical)
Azelaic Acid (Topical)
*Becaplermin (Topical)
*Bentoquatam (Topical)
*Calamine (Topical)
*Capsaicin (Topical)
Coal Tar (Topical)
*Diethyltoluamide (Topical)
*Dimethyl Sulfoxide (Topical)
*Doxepin (Topical)
Epinephrine, Parenteral (Systemic)
*Methoxsalen (Topical)
*Minoxidil (Topical)
Salicylic Acid Lotion (Topical)
Salicylic Acid Ointment (Topical)
Salicylic Acid Shampoo (Topical)
Salicylic Acid, Sulfur, and Coal Tar (Topical)
Salicylic Acid and Sulfur Cream (Topical)
Salicylic Acid and Sulfur Cream Shampoo (Topical)
Salicylic Acid and Sulfur Lotion Shampoo (Topical)
Salicylic Acid and Sulfur Suspension Shampoo (Topical)
Sulfur Ointment (Topical)

DX101 *Barium Sulfate (Local)
*Iodixanol (Systemic)
*Iohexol (Local)
*Iohexol (Systemic)
*Iopamidol (Systemic)
*Iopromide (Systemic)
*Ioversol (Systemic)
*Ioxilan (Systemic)
*Metrizamide (Systemic)

DX102 *Diatrizoate and Iodipamide (Local)
*Diatrizoate Meglumine (Local)
*Diatrizoate Meglumine (Systemic)
*Diatrizoate Meglumine and Diatrizoate Sodium (Systemic)
*Diatrizoate Sodium (Local)
*Diatrizoate Sodium (Systemic)
*Iocetamic Acid (Systemic)
*Iodipamide (Systemic)
*Iopanoic Acid (Systemic)
*Iothalamate (Local)
*Iothalamate (Systemic)
*Ioxaglate (Local)
*Ioxaglate (Systemic)
*Ipodate (Systemic)
*Tyropanoate (Systemic)

DX201 *Ammonia N 13 (Systemic)
*Cyanocobalamin Co 57 (Systemic)
*Ferrous Citrate Fe 59 (Systemic)
*Fludeoxyglucose F 18 (Systemic)
*Gallium Citrate Ga 67 (Systemic)
*Indium In 111 Capromab Pendetide (Systemic)

*Indium In 111 Oxyquinoline (Systemic)
*Indium In 111 Pentetate (Systemic)
*Indium In 111 Pentetreotide (Systemic)
*Indium In 111 Satumomab Pendetide (Systemic)
*Iobenguane I 123 (Systemic—Diagnostic)
*Iobenguane I 131 (Systemic—Diagnostic)
*Iodohippurate Sodium I 123 (Systemic)
*Iodohippurate Sodium I 131 (Systemic)
*Iofetamine I 123 (Systemic)
*Krypton Kr 81m (Systemic)
*Rubidium Rb 82 (Systemic)
*Sodium Chromate Cr 51 (Systemic)
*Sodium Fluoride F 18 (Systemic)
*Sodium Iodide I 123 (Systemic)
*Sodium Iodide I 131 (Systemic—Diagnostic)
Sodium Pertechnetate Tc 99m (Mucosal-Local)
*Sodium Pertechnetate Tc 99m (Ophthalmic)
*Sodium Pertechnetate Tc 99m (Systemic)
*Technetium Tc 99m Albumin (Systemic)
*Technetium Tc 99m Albumin Aggregated (Systemic)
*Technetium Tc 99m Albumin Colloid (Systemic)
*Technetium Tc 99m Arcitumomab (Systemic)
*Technetium Tc 99m Bicisate (Systemic)
*Technetium Tc 99m Disofenin (Systemic)
*Technetium Tc 99m Exametazime (Systemic)
*Technetium Tc 99m Gluceptate (Systemic)
*Technetium Tc 99m Lidofenin (Systemic)
*Technetium Tc 99m Mebrofenin (Systemic)
*Technetium Tc 99m Medronate (Systemic)
*Technetium Tc 99m Mertiatide (Systemic)
*Technetium Tc 99m Nofetumomab Merpentan (Systemic)
*Technetium Tc 99m Oxidronate (Systemic)
*Technetium Tc 99m Pentetate (Systemic)
*Technetium Tc 99m Pyrophosphate (Systemic)
*Technetium Tc 99m (Pyro- and Trimeta-) Phosphates (Systemic)
*Technetium Tc 99m Sestamibi (Systemic)
*Technetium Tc 99m Succimer (Systemic)
*Technetium Tc 99m Sulfur Colloid (Systemic)
*Technetium Tc 99m Teboroxime (Systemic)
*Technetium Tc 99m Tetrofosmin (Systemic)
*Thallous Chloride Tl 201 (Systemic)
*Xenon Xe 127 (Systemic)
*Xenon Xe 133 (Systemic)

DX202 *Iodinated I 125 Albumin (Systemic)
*Iodinated I 131 Albumin (Systemic)

DX300 *Tuberculin, Purified Protein Derivative (Parenteral-Local)

DX501 Urine Glucose and Ketone (Combined) Test Kits for Home Use

DX900 Acetylcysteine (Local)
Adenosine (Systemic)
Alprostadil (Local)
Amyl Nitrite (Systemic)
*Apomorphine (Systemic)
Ascorbic Acid (Systemic)
*Bentiromide (Systemic)
Cholecystokinin (Systemic)
Chorionic Gonadotropin (Systemic)
Clomiphene (Systemic)
Clonidine, Oral (Systemic)
*Corticorelin Ovine (Systemic-Diagnostic)
Corticotropin for Injection (Systemic)
*Cosyntropin (Systemic)
Cyanocobalamin (Systemic)
Demecarium (Ophthalmic)
Dexamethasone (Systemic)
Dinoprost (Parenteral-Local)

# VA Medication Classification System

Dipyridamole (Systemic)
Echothiophate (Ophthalmic)
Edetate Calcium Disodium (Systemic)
Edrophonium (Systemic)
Ergonovine (Systemic)
Fecal Occult Blood Test Kits for Clinic Use
Fecal Occult Blood Test Kits for Home Use
*Ferumoxides (Systemic)
Fludrocortisone (Systemic)
*Gadodiamide (Systemic)
*Gadopentetate (Systemic)
*Gadoteridol (Systemic)
Glucagon (Systemic)
Gonadorelin (Systemic)
*Histamine (Systemic)
Hydroxocobalamin (Systemic)
Insulin (Systemic)
Insulin Human (Systemic)
Insulin Human, Buffered (Systemic)
Insulin, Isophane (Systemic)
Insulin, Isophane, Human (Systemic)
Insulin, Isophane, Human, and Insulin Human (Systemic)
Insulin Zinc (Systemic)
Insulin Zinc, Extended (Systemic)
Insulin Zinc, Extended, Human (Systemic)
Insulin Zinc, Human (Systemic)
Insulin Zinc, Prompt (Systemic)
*Inulin (Systemic)
Isoflurophate (Ophthalmic)
Levothyroxine (Systemic)
Liothyronine (Systemic)
*Methacholine (Inhalation-Local)
Methylene Blue (Systemic)
*Metyrapone (Systemic)
Oxytocin (Systemic)
*Pentagastrin (Systemic)
Perflubron (Oral-Local)
*Phenolsulfonphthalein (Systemic)
Phenylephrine (Ophthalmic)
*Protirelin (Systemic)
Simethicone (Oral-Local)
Sincalide (Systemic)
*Teriparatide (Systemic)
*Thyrotropin (Systemic)
*Tolbutamide (Systemic)
Tropicamide (Ophthalmic)
Tubocurarine (Systemic)
Vasopressin (Systemic)

GA101 *Alumina, Calcium Carbonate, and Sodium Bicarbonate (Oral-Local)
*Alumina and Sodium Bicarbonate (Oral-Local)
*Aluminum Carbonate, Basic (Oral-Local)
*Aluminum Hydroxide (Oral-Local)
GA103 *Alumina and Magnesia (Oral-Local)
*Alumina, Magnesia, and Magnesium Carbonate (Oral-Local)
*Alumina, Magnesium Alginate, and Magnesium Carbonate (Oral-Local)
*Alumina and Magnesium Carbonate (Oral-Local)
*Alumina and Magnesium Trisilicate (Oral-Local)
GA104 *Alumina, Magnesium Carbonate, and Sodium Bicarbonate (Oral-Local)
*Alumina, Magnesium Trisilicate, and Sodium Bicarbonate (Oral-Local)
GA105 *Calcium Carbonate (Oral-Local)
Calcium Carbonate, Oral (Systemic)
GA106 *Calcium Carbonate and Magnesia (Oral-Local)
*Calcium and Magnesium Carbonates (Oral-Local)
GA107 *Magaldrate (Oral-Local)
GA108 *Magnesium Hydroxide (Local)
*Magnesium Hydroxide (Oral-Local)
Magnesium Oxide (Local)
*Magnesium Oxide (Oral-Local)
GA109 *Magnesium Carbonate and Sodium Bicarbonate (Oral-Local)
GA110 Alumina, Calcium Carbonate, and Sodium Bicarbonate (Oral-Local)
Alumina and Sodium Bicarbonate (Oral-Local)
*Sodium Bicarbonate (Systemic)
GA199 *Alumina, Calcium Carbonate, and Sodium Bicarbonate (Oral-Local)
*Alumina, Magnesia, Calcium Carbonate, and Simethicone (Oral-Local)

*Alumina, Magnesia, Magnesium Carbonate, and Simethicone (Oral-Local)
*Alumina, Magnesia, and Simethicone (Oral-Local)
*Alumina and Sodium Bicarbonate (Oral-Local)
*Alumina, Magnesium Carbonate, and Simethicone (Oral-Local)
*Alumina and Simethicone (Oral-Local)
*Aluminum Carbonate, Basic and Simethicone (Oral-Local)
*Calcium Carbonate, Magnesia, and Simethicone (Oral-Local)
*Calcium Carbonate and Simethicone (Oral-Local)
*Magaldrate and Simethicone (Oral-Local)
GA201 *Malt Soup Extract (Local)
*Malt Soup Extract and Psyllium (Local)
*Methylcellulose (Local)
*Polycarbophil (Local)
*Psyllium (Local)
*Psyllium Hydrophilic Mucilloid (Local)
*Psyllium Hydrophilic Mucilloid and Carboxymethylcellulose (Local)
GA202 *Lactulose (Local)
*Magnesium Citrate (Local)
*Magnesium Hydroxide (Local)
Magnesium Hydroxide (Oral-Local)
*Magnesium Oxide (Local)
Magnesium Oxide (Oral-Local)
*Magnesium Sulfate (Local)
*Sodium Phosphate, Oral (Local)
GA203 *Mineral Oil, Oral (Local)
GA204 *Bisacodyl, Oral (Local)
*Casanthranol, Oral (Local)
*Cascara Sagrada (Local)
*Cascara Sagrada and Aloe (Local)
*Cascara Sagrada and Phenolphthalein (Local)
*Castor Oil (Local)
*Dehydrocholic Acid (Local)
*Phenolphthalein (Local)
*Phenolphthalein and Senna (Local)
*Senna, Oral (Local)
*Sennosides (Local)
GA205 *Docusate, Oral (Local)
*Poloxamer 188 (Local)
GA208 Aluminum Hydroxide (Oral-Local)
*Attapulgite (Local)
*Bismuth Subsalicylate (Oral-Local)
Cholestyramine (Oral-Local)
Colestipol (Oral-Local)
*Difenoxin and Atropine (Systemic)
*Diphenoxylate and Atropine (Systemic)
Glycopyrrolate (Systemic)
*Kaolin and Pectin (Oral-Local)
*Kaolin, Pectin, and Belladonna Alkaloids (Systemic)
*Kaolin, Pectin, and Paregoric (Systemic)
*Loperamide (Oral-Local)
Polycarbophil (Local)
GA209 *Bisacodyl and Docusate, Oral (Local)
*Casanthranol and Docusate (Local)
*Danthron and Docusate (Local)
*Dehydrocholic Acid and Docusate (Local)
*Dehydrocholic Acid, Docusate, and Phenolphthalein (Local)
*Magnesium Hydroxide and Cascara Sagrada (Local)
*Magnesium Hydroxide and Mineral Oil (Local)
*Mineral Oil and Glycerin (Local)
*Mineral Oil, Glycerin, and Phenolphthalein (Local)
*Mineral Oil and Phenolphthalein (Local)
*Phenolphthalein and Docusate (Local)
*Polyethylene Glycol and Electrolytes (Local)
*Psyllium Hydrophilic Mucilloid and Senna (Local)
*Psyllium Hydrophilic Mucilloid and Sennosides (Local)
*Psyllium and Senna (Local)
*Sennosides and Docusate (Local)
GA250 Aluminum Hydroxide (Oral-Local)
Glycopyrrolate (Systemic)
*Octreotide (Systemic)
Psyllium Hydrophilic Mucilloid (Local)
GA301 *Cimetidine (Systemic)
*Famotidine (Systemic)
*Nizatidine (Systemic)

*Ranitidine (Systemic)
GA302 *Sucralfate (Oral-Local)
GA303 *Bismuth Subsalicylate, Metronidazole, and Tetracycline—For *H. pylori* (Systemic)
*Ranitidine Bismuth Citrate (Systemic)
GA304 *Lansoprazole (Systemic)
*Omeprazole (Systemic)
GA309 Amitriptyline (Systemic)
Doxepin (Systemic)
Lansoprazole (Systemic)
Pantoprazole (Systemic)
Trimipramine (Systemic)
GA400 Azathioprine (Systemic)
Cholestyramine (Oral-Local)
Codeine (Systemic)
*Loperamide and Simethicone (Oral-Local)
*Mesalamine (Oral-Local)
Morphine, Oral (Systemic)
Morphine, Parenteral (Systemic)
*Olsalazine (Oral-Local)
*Opium, Oral (Systemic)
*Paregoric (Systemic)
*Sulfasalazine (Systemic)
GA500 Pancrelipase (Systemic)
GA600 *Ipecac (Oral-Local)
GA605 *Buclizine (Systemic)
*Cyclizine (Systemic)
Dexamethasone (Systemic)
Diphenidol (Systemic)
*Dolasetron (Systemic)
Droperidol (Systemic)
*Fructose, Dextrose, and Phosphoric Acid (Oral-Local)
*Granisetron (Systemic)
Haloperidol (Systemic)
Hydrocortisone (Systemic)
Lorazepam, Parenteral (Systemic)
*Meclizine (Systemic)
Metoclopramide (Systemic)
*Nabilone (Systemic)
*Ondansetron (Systemic)
Prednisone (Systemic)
Scopolamine, Oral (Systemic)
Scopolamine, Parenteral (Systemic)
*Thiethylperazine (Systemic)
trimethobenzamide
GA650 Scopolamine (Systemic)
GA700 Chlorpromazine (Systemic)
*Dronabinol (Systemic)
Perphenazine (Systemic)
Prochlorperazine (Systemic)
Promethazine (Systemic)
Triflupromazine (Systemic)
GA751 *Benzphetamine (Systemic)
*Diethylpropion (Systemic)
*Fenfluramine (Systemic)
*Mazindol (Systemic)
*Phendimetrazine (Systemic)
*Phentermine (Systemic)
Phenylpropanolamine (Systemic)
*Sibutramine (Systemic)
GA801 Anisotropine (Systemic)
Atropine (Systemic)
Belladonna (Systemic)
Clidinium (Systemic)
Dicyclomine (Systemic)
Glucagon (Systemic)
Glycopyrrolate (Systemic)
Homatropine (Systemic)
Hyoscyamine (Systemic)
Mepenzolate (Systemic)
Methantheline (Systemic)
Methscopolamine (Systemic)
Pirenzepine (Systemic)
Scopolamine, Oral (Systemic)
Scopolamine, Parenteral (Systemic)
GA802 *Atropine, Hyoscyamine, Scopolaine, and Phenobarbital (Systemic)
*Atropine and Phenobarbital (Systemic)
*Belladonna and Butabarbital (Systemic)
*Belladonna and Phenobarbital (Systemic)
*Chlordiazepoxide and Clidinium (Systemic)
*Hyoscyamine and Phenobarbital (Systemic)
GA900 *Chenodiol (Systemic)
*Cisapride (Systemic)
Dehydrocholic Acid (Local)
Diazoxide (Oral-Systemic)
Dronabinol (Systemic)

Insulin (Systemic)
Insulin Human (Systemic)
Insulin Human, Buffered (Systemic)
Insulin, Isophane (Systemic)
Insulin, Isophane, Human (Systemic)
Insulin, Isophane, Human, and Insulin Human (Systemic)
Insulin Zinc (Systemic)
Insulin Zinc, Extended (Systemic)
Insulin Zinc, Extended, Human (Systemic)
Insulin Zinc, Human (Systemic)
Insulin Zinc, Prompt (Systemic)
Kanamycin (Oral-Local)
Lactulose (Local)
Loperamide and Simethicone (Oral-Local)
Mercaptopurine (Systemic)
Metronidazole (Systemic)
*Monoctanoin (Local)
Neomycin (Oral-Local)
*Pantoprazole (Systemic)
Phenobarbital (Systemic)
*Simethicone (Oral-Local)
*Ursodiol (Systemic)
Vasopressin (Systemic)

GU100 *Phenazopyridine (Systemic)
GU200 *Atropine, Hyoscyamine, Methenaine, Methylene Blue, Phenyl Salicylte, and Benzoic Acid (Systemic)
GU201 Atropine, Oral (Systemic)
Atropine, Parenteral (Systemic)
*Flavoxate (Systemic)
Hyoscyamine, Oral (Systemic)
Hyoscyamine, Parenteral (Systemic)
Methantheline (Systemic)
*Oxybutynin (Systemic)
Scopolamine, Oral (Systemic)
GU301 *Metronidazole (Vaginal)
*Sulfanilamide (Vaginal)
*Triple Sulfa (Vaginal)
GU302 *Butoconazole (Vaginal)
*Clotrimazole (Vaginal)
*Econazole (Vaginal)
*Gentian Violet (Vaginal)
*Miconazole (Vaginal)
*Nystatin (Vaginal)
*Terconazole (Vaginal)
*Tioconazole (Vaginal)
GU309 *Clindamycin (Vaginal)
*Metronidazole and Nystatin (Vaginal)
GU400 *Benzalkonium Chloride (Vaginal)
*Cervical Cap, Cavity-rim (Vaginal)
*Copper-T 200 Intrauterine Device
*Copper-T 200Ag Intrauterine Device
*Copper-T 380A Intrauterine Device
*Copper-T 380S Intrauterine Device
*Lamb Cecum Condoms and Nonoxynol 9
*Latex Condoms and Nonoxynol 9
*Nonoxynol 9 (Vaginal)
*Octoxynol 9 (Vaginal)
*Progesterone Intrauterine Device (IUD)
GU500 *Conjugated Estrogens (Vaginal)
*Dienestrol (Vaginal)
*Estradiol (Vaginal)
*Estrogens, Conjugated (Vaginal)
*Estrone (Vaginal)
*Estropipate (Vaginal)
GU600 Carboprost (Systemic)
Dinoprost (Parenteral-Local)
Dinoprostone (Cervical/Vaginal)
Ergonovine (Systemic)
*Methylergonovine (Systemic)
Oxytocin (Systemic)
*Sodium Chloride (Parenteral-Local)
*Urea (Parenteral-Local)
GU700 *Finasteride (Systemic)
*Tamsulosin (Systemic)
GU900 Acetazolamide (Systemic)
*Acetohydroxamic Acid (Systemic)
Allopurinol (Systemic)
Alprostadil (Local)
Aluminum Carbonate, Basic (Oral-Local)
Aluminum Hydroxide (Oral-Local)
Amitriptyline (Systemic)
Bendroflumethiazide (Systemic)
Benzocaine, Butamben, and Tetracaine Gel (Mucosal-Local)
Benzocaine Gel (Mucosal-Local)
*Cellulose Sodium Phosphate (Systemic)
Chlorothiazide (Systemic)
Chlorthalidone (Systemic)

Cholestyramine (Oral-Local)
*Citric Acid and D-Gluconic Acid (Local)
*Citric Acid, Glucono-delta-lactone, and Magnesium Carbonate (Local)
Diethylstilbestrol and Methyltestosterone (Systemic)
*Dimethyl Sulfoxide (Mucosal-Local)
Dinoprostone (Cervical/Vaginal)
Doxazosin (Systemic)
Dyclonine Topical Solution (Mucosal-Local)
Ergonovine (Systemic)
Estrogens, Conjugated, and Methyltestosterone (Systemic)
Estrogens, Esterified, and Methyltestosterone (Systemic)
Fluoxymesterone and Ethinyl Estradiol (Systemic)
Hydrochlorothiazide (Systemic)
Hydroflumethiazide (Systemic)
Imipramine (Systemic)
Isoxsuprine (Systemic)
Lidocaine Hydrochloride Jelly (Mucosal-Local)
Lidocaine Hydrochloride Jelly USP (Topical)
Magnesium Hydroxide (Oral-Local)
Magnesium Sulfate (Systemic)
Methyclothiazide (Systemic)
Metolazone (Systemic)
Papaverine (Intracavernosal)
Penicillamine (Systemic)
*Pentosan (Systemic)
Phenoxybenzamine (Systemic)
Phentolamine (Intracavernosal)
Polythiazide (Systemic)
Potassium Citrate (Systemic)
Potassium Citrate and Citric Acid (Systemic)
Potassium Citrate and Sodium Citrate (Systemic)
Potassium Phosphates (Systemic)
Potassium and Sodium Phosphates (Systemic)
Prazosin (Systemic)
Quinethazone (Systemic)
*Racemethionine (Systemic)
Ritodrine (Systemic)
*Sildenafil (Systemic)
Sodium Citrate and Citric Acid (Systemic)
Terazosin (Systemic)
Terbutaline (Systemic)
Testosterone and Estradiol (Systemic)
*Tiopronin (Systemic)
Trichlormethiazide (Systemic)
Tricitrates (Systemic)
*Yohimbine (Systemic)

HS051 *Betamethasone (Systemic)
*Budesonide (Oral)
*Cortisone (Systemic)
*Budesonide (Systemic)
*Dexamethasone (Systemic)
*Hydrocortisone (Systemic)
*Methylprednisolone (Systemic)
*Prednisolone (Systemic)
*Prednisone (Systemic)
*Triamcinolone (Systemic)
HS052 *Fludrocortisone (Systemic)
HS101 *Fluoxymesterone (Systemic)
*Methyltestosterone (Systemic)
*Nandrolone (Systemic)
*Oxandrolone (Systemic)
*Oxymetholone (Systemic)
*Stanozolol (Systemic)
*Testosterone (Systemic)
*Testosterone Cypionate (Systemic)
*Testosterone Enanthate (Systemic)
*Testosterone Propionate (Systemic)
*Testosterone Undecanoate (Systemic)
HS102 *Diethylstilbestrol (Systemic)
*Estradiol (Systemic)
Estradiol (Vaginal)
*Estrogens, Conjugated (Systemic)
Estrogens, Conjugated (Vaginal)
*Estrogens, Esterified (Systemic)
*Estrone (Systemic)
Estrone (Vaginal)
*Estropipate (Systemic)
Estropipate (Vaginal)
*Ethinyl Estradiol (Systemic)
HS103 *Hydroxyprogesterone (Systemic)
*Levonorgestrel (Systemic)

*Medrogestone (Systemic)
*Medroxyprogesterone (Systemic)
*Megestrol (Systemic)
*Norethindrone (Systemic)
*Norgestrel (Systemic)
*Progesterone (Systemic)
HS104 *Desogestrel and Ethinyl Estradiol (Systemic)
Diethylstilbestrol (Systemic)
Estrogens, Conjugated (Systemic)
Ethinyl Estradiol (Systemic)
*Ethynodiol Diacetate and Ethinyl Estradiol (Systemic)
Levonorgestrel (Systemic)
*Levonorgestrel and Ethinyl Estradiol (Systemic)
Medroxyprogesterone (Systemic)
Norethindrone (Systemic)
*Norethindrone Acetate and Ethinyl Estradiol (Systemic)
*Norethindrone and Ethinyl Estradiol (Systemic)
*Norethindrone and Mestranol (Systemic)
*Norgestimate and Ethinyl Estradiol (Systemic)
Norgestrel (Systemic)
*Norgestrel and Ethinyl Estradiol (Systemic)
HS105 *Conjugated Estrogens and Medroxyprogesterone Acetate (Systemic)
*Conjugated Estrogens Tablets USP, and Conjugated Estrogens and Medroxyprogesterone Tablets (Systemic)
Dienestrol (Vaginal)
HS106 *Chorionic Gonadotropin (Systemic)
*Clomiphene (Systemic)
*Follitropin Alfa (Systemic)
*Follitropin Beta (Systemic)
*Menotropins (Systemic)
*Urofollitropin (Systemic)
HS109 *Danazol (Systemic)
Desogestrel and Ethinyl Estradiol (Systemic)
Ethynodiol Diacetate and Ethinyl Estradiol (Systemic)
*Histrelin (Systemic)
Levonorgestrel and Ethinyl Estradiol (Systemic)
Norethindrone Acetate and Ethinyl Estradiol (Systemic)
Norethindrone and Ethinyl Estradiol (Systemic)
Norethindrone and Mestranol (Systemic)
Norgestimate and Ethinyl Estradiol (Systemic)
Norgestrel and Ethinyl Estradiol (Systemic)
HS200 *Alprostadil (Local)
*Alprostadil (Systemic)
*Carboprost (Systemic)
*Dinoprost (Parenteral-Local)
*Dinoprostone (Cervical/Vaginal)
*Levonorgestrel and Ethinyl Estradiol (Systemic)
*Misoprostol (Systemic)
HS301 *Alendronate (Systemic)
HS302 Etidronate (Systemic)
*Pamidronate (Systemic)
HS303 Alendronate (Systemic)
*Etidronate (Systemic)
Pamidronate (Systemic)
*Risedronate (Systemic)
*Tiludronate (Systemic)
HS304 *Calcitonin-Human (Systemic)
*Calcitonin-Salmon (Systemic)
HS305 Plicamycin
HS309 *Gallium Nitrate (Systemic)
HS451 *Alglucerase (Systemic)
*Imiglucerase (Systemic)
*Pancrelipase (Systemic)
HS452 *Betaine (Systemic)
HS501 *Insulin (Systemic)
*Insulin Human (Systemic)
*Insulin Human, Buffered (Systemic)
*Insulin, Isophane (Systemic)
*Insulin, Isophane, Human (Systemic)
*Insulin, Isophane, Human, and Insulin Human (Systemic)
*Insulin Lispro (Systemic)
*Insulin Zinc (Systemic)
*Insulin Zinc, Extended (Systemic)
*Insulin Zinc, Extended, Human (Systemic)

# VA Medication Classification System

|  |  |
|---|---|
| | *Insulin Zinc, Human (Systemic) |
| | *Insulin Zinc, Prompt (Systemic) |
| HS502 | *Acetohexamide (Systemic) |
| | *Chlorpropamide (Systemic) |
| | *Gliclazide (Systemic) |
| | *Glimepiride (Systemic) |
| | *Glipizide (Systemic) |
| | *Glyburide (Systemic) |
| | *Miglitol (Oral-Local) |
| | *Tolazamide (Systemic) |
| | *Tolbutamide, Oral (Systemic) |
| | *Troglitazone (Systemic) |
| HS503 | *Metformin (Systemic) |
| HS504 | *Acarbose (Systemic) |
| HS505 | *Troglitazone (Systemic) |
| HS508 | *Diazoxide (Oral-Systemic) |
| | *Glucagon (Systemic) |
| HS509 | *Repaglinide (Systemic) |
| HS521 | *Acetohexamide (Systemic) |
| | *Chlorpropamide (Systemic) |
| | *Gliclazide (Systemic) |
| | *Glipizide (Systemic) |
| | *Glyburide (Systemic) |
| | *Tolazamide (Systemic) |
| | *Tolbutamide (Systemic) |
| HS551 | *Sacrosidase (Systemic) |
| HS600 | Teriparatide (Systemic) |
| HS701 | Cosyntropin (Systemic) |
| | *Somatrem (Systemic) |
| | *Somatropin, Recombinant (Systemic) |
| HS702 | *Desmopressin (Systemic) |
| | *Lypressin (Systemic) |
| | *Vasopressin (Systemic) |
| HS850 | Thyrotropin (Systemic) |
| HS851 | *Levothyroxine (Systemic) |
| | *Liothyronine (Systemic) |
| | *Liotrix (Systemic) |
| | *Thyroglobulin (Systemic) |
| | *Thyroid (Systemic) |
| HS852 | *Iodine, Strong (Systemic) |
| | Iopodate (Systemic) |
| | *Methimazole (Systemic) |
| | *Potassium Iodide (Systemic) |
| | *Propylthiouracil (Systemic) |
| | Sodium Iodide (Systemic) |
| HS900 | *Aminoglutethimide (Systemic) |
| | Bromocriptine (Systemic) |
| | Cabergoline (Systemic) |
| | *Calcitonin (Nasal-Systemic) |
| | *Calcitonin-Salmon (Nasal-Systemic) |
| | Carbamazepine (Systemic) |
| | *Cholecystokinin (Systemic) |
| | Chorionic Gonadotropin (Systemic) |
| | Clomiphene (Systemic) |
| | *Gonadorelin (Systemic) |
| | *Goserelin (Systemic) |
| | Ketoconazole (Systemic) |
| | *Leuprolide (Systemic) |
| | Levonorgestrel and Ethinyl Estradiol (Systemic) |
| | Metyrapone (Systemic) |
| | Mitotane (Systemic) |
| | *Nafarelin (Systemic) |
| | Octreotide (Systemic) |
| | Oxytocin (Systemic) |
| | *Raloxifene (Systemic) |
| | *Sermorelin (Systemic) |
| | *Sincalide (Systemic) |
| | Sodium Iodide (Systemic) |
| | Spironolactone (Systemic) |
| | *Trilostane (Systemic) |
| HS950 | *Diethylstilbestrol and Methyltestosterone (Systemic) |
| | *Estrogens, Conjugated, and Methyltestosterone (Systemic) |
| | *Estrogens, Esterified, and Methyltestosterone (Systemic) |
| | *Fluoxymesterone and Ethinyl Estradiol (Systemic) |
| | *Testosterone and Estradiol (Systemic) |
| IM100 | *Bacillus Calmette-Guéerin (BCG) Live (Systemic) |
| | *Cholera Vaccine (Systemic) |
| | *Haemophilus b Conjugate Vaccine (HbOC—Diphtheria CRM$_{197}$ Protein Conjugate) (Systemic) |
| | *Haemophilus b Conjugate Vaccine (PRP-D—Diphtheria Toxoid Conjugate) (Systemic) |
| | *Haemophilus b Conjugate Vaccine (PRP-OMP—Meningococcal Protein Conjugate) (Systemic) |
| | *Haemophilus b Conjugate Vaccine (PRP-T—Tetanus Protein Conjugate) (Systemic) |
| | *Haemophilus b Conjugate Vaccine (Systemic) |
| | *Haemophilus b Polysaccharide Vaccine (Systemic) |
| | *Hepatitis A Vaccine, Inactivated (Systemic) |
| | *Hepatitis A Vaccine Inactivated (Systemic) |
| | *Hepatitis B Vaccine Recombinant (Systemic) |
| | *Influenza Virus Vaccine (Systemic) |
| | *Japanese Encephalitis Virus Vaccine (Systemic) |
| | *Measles, Mumps, and Rubella Virus Vaccine Live (Systemic) |
| | *Measles and Rubella Virus Vaccine Live (Systemic) |
| | *Measles Virus Vaccine Live (Systemic) |
| | *Meningococcal Polysaccharide Vaccine (Systemic) |
| | *Mumps Virus Vaccine Live (Systemic) |
| | *Plague Vaccine (Systemic) |
| | *Pneumococcal Vaccine Polyvalent (Systemic) |
| | *Poliovirus Vaccine Inactivated (Systemic) |
| | *Poliovirus Vaccine Inactivated Enhanced Potency (Systemic) |
| | *Poliovirus Vaccine Live Oral (Systemic) |
| | *Rabies Vaccine Adsorbed (Systemic) |
| | *Rabies Vaccine, Human Diploid Cell (Systemic) |
| | *Rubella and Mumps Virus Vaccine Live (Systemic) |
| | *Rubella Virus Vaccine Live (Systemic) |
| | *Typhoid Vaccine Inactivated (Parenteral-Systemic) |
| | *Typhoid Vaccine Live Oral (Systemic) |
| | *Typhoid Vi Polysaccharide Vaccine (Systemic) |
| | *Varicella Virus Vaccine (Systemic) |
| | *Varicella Virus Vaccine Live (Oka/Merck) (Systemic) |
| | *Varicella Virus Vaccine Live (Systemic) |
| | *Yellow Fever Vaccine (Systemic) |
| IM200 | *Diphtheria and Tetanus Toxoids for Pediatric Use (DT) (Systemic) |
| | *Tetanus and Diphtheria Toxoids for Adult Use (Td) (Systemic) |
| | *Tetanus Toxoid (Systemic) |
| IM300 | *Diphtheria Antitoxin (Systemic) |
| IM500 | *Immune Globulin Intravenous (Human) (Systemic) |
| | *Palivizumab (Systemic) |
| | *Rabies Immune Globulin (Systemic) |
| | *Rh$_o$(D) Immune Globulin (Human) (Systemic) |
| | *Rh$_o$(D) Immune Globulin (Systemic) |
| | *Respiratory Syncytial Virus IG IV (Systemic) |
| | *Tetanus Immune Globulin (Systemic) |
| IM600 | *Azathioprine (Systemic) |
| | *Basiliximab (Systemic) |
| | Betamethasone (Systemic) |
| | Chlorambucil (Systemic) |
| | Cortisone (Systemic) |
| | Cyclophosphamide (Systemic) |
| | *Cyclosporine (Systemic) |
| | *Daclizumab (Systemic) |
| | Dexamethasone (Systemic) |
| | Hydrocortisone (Systemic) |
| | Mercaptopurine (Systemic) |
| | Methylprednisolone (Systemic) |
| | *Muromonab-CD3 (Systemic) |
| | *Mycophenolate (Systemic) |
| | Prednisolone (Systemic) |
| | Prednisone (Systemic) |
| | Tacrolimus (Systemic) |
| | Triamcinolone (Systemic) |
| IM700 | *Imiquimod (Topical) |
| | *Interferon Alfa-2a, Recombinant (Systemic) |
| | *Interferon Alfa-2b, Recombinant (Systemic) |
| | *Interferon Alfa-n1 (Ins) (Systemic) |
| | *Interferon Alfa-n3 (Systemic) |
| | *Interferon, Alfacon-1 (Systemic) |
| | Interferon Beta-1a (Systemic) |
| | *Interferon, Gamma (Systemic) |
| | *Levamisole (Systemic) |
| IM900 | *Cromolyn (Systemic/Oral-Local) |
| | Danazol (Systemic) |
| | *Diphtheria and Tetanus Toxoids and Pertussis Vaccine Adsorbed (Systemic) |
| | *Diphtheria and Tetanus Toxoids and Pertussis Vaccine Adsorbed and Haemophilus b Conjugate Vaccine (Systemic) |
| | *Glatiramer Acetate (Systemic) |
| | *Interferon Beta-1a (Systemic) |
| | *Interferon Beta-1b (Systemic) |
| | Oxymetholone (Systemic) |
| | *Pegademase (Systemic) |
| | Stanozolol (Systemic) |
| | *Thalidomide (Systemic) |
| | Tranexamic Acid (Systemic) |
| MS101 | Aspirin, Buffered (Systemic) |
| | Aspirin and Caffeine, Buffered (Systemic) |
| | Aspirin and Caffeine Capsules (Systemic) |
| | Aspirin and Caffeine Tablets (Systemic) |
| | Aspirin Delayed-release Tablets USP (Systemic) |
| | Aspirin Extended-release Tablets USP (Systemic) |
| | Aspirin Suppositories USP (Systemic) |
| | Aspirin Tablets USP (Systemic) |
| | Aspirin Tablets USP (Chewable) (Systemic) |
| | Choline Salicylate (Systemic) |
| | Choline and Magnesium Salicylates (Systemic) |
| | Magnesium Salicylate (Systemic) |
| | *Salsalate (Systemic) |
| | Sodium Salicylate (Systemic) |
| MS102 | *Diclofenac (Systemic) |
| | *Diflunisal (Systemic) |
| | *Etodolac (Systemic) |
| | *Fenoprofen (Systemic) |
| | *Flurbiprofen (Systemic) |
| | *Ibuprofen (Systemic) |
| | *Indomethacin (Systemic) |
| | *Indomethacin—For Patent Ductus Arteriosus, Oral (Systemic) |
| | *Ketoprofen (Systemic) |
| | *Meclofenamate (Systemic) |
| | *Nabumetone (Systemic) |
| | *Naproxen (Systemic) |
| | *Oxaprozin (Systemic) |
| | *Phenylbutazone (Systemic) |
| | *Piroxicam (Systemic) |
| | *Sulindac (Systemic) |
| | *Tenoxicam (Systemic) |
| | *Tiaprofenic Acid (Systemic) |
| | Thalidomide (Systemic) |
| | *Tolmetin (Systemic) |
| MS105 | Cyclophosphamide (Systemic) |
| | Mercaptopurine (Systemic) |
| | Methotrexate—For Noncancerous Conditions (Systemic) |
| MS109 | *Auranofin (Systemic) |
| | *Aurothioglucose (Systemic) |
| | Azathioprine (Systemic) |
| | Chloroquine (Systemic) |
| | Cyclosporine (Systemic) |
| | *Diclofenac and Misoprostol (Systemic) |
| | *Gold Sodium Thiomalate (Systemic) |
| | Hydroxychloroquine (Systemic) |
| | Minocycline (Systemic) |
| | *Penicillamine (Systemic) |
| | Sulfasalazine (Systemic) |
| MS200 | *Baclofen (Intrathecal-Systemic) |
| | *Baclofen (Systemic) |
| | *Carisoprodol (Systemic) |
| | *Chlorphenesin (Systemic) |
| | *Chlorzoxazone (Systemic) |
| | *Chlorzoxazone and Acetaminophen (Systemic) |
| | *Cyclobenzaprine (Systemic) |
| | *Dantrolene (Systemic) |
| | Diazepam (Systemic) |
| | Lorazepam (Systemic) |
| | *Metaxalone (Systemic) |
| | *Methocarbamol (Systemic) |
| | *Orphenadrine, Aspirin, and Caffeine (Systemic) |
| | *Orphenadrine Citrate (Systemic) |
| | Phenytoin (Systemic) |
| MS300 | *Atracurium (Systemic) |
| | *Cisatracurium (Systemic) |
| | *Doxacurium (Systemic) |

## VA Medication Classification System

|  |  |
|---|---|
| | *Gallamine (Systemic) |
| | *Metocurine (Systemic) |
| | *Mivacurium (Systemic) |
| | *Pancuronium (Systemic) |
| | *Pipecuronium (Systemic) |
| | *Rocuronium (Systemic) |
| | *Succinylcholine (Systemic) |
| | *Tubocurarine (Systemic) |
| | *Vecuronium (Systemic) |
| MS400 | *Allopurinol (Systemic) |
| | *Colchicine (Systemic) |
| | Diclofenac (Systemic) |
| | Diflunisal (Systemic) |
| | Etodolac (Systemic) |
| | Fenoprofen (Systemic) |
| | Floctafenine (Systemic) |
| | Ibuprofen (Systemic) |
| | Indomethacin (Systemic) |
| | Indomethacin—For Patent Ductus Arteriosus, Oral (Systemic) |
| | Ketoprofen (Systemic) |
| | Naproxen (Systemic) |
| | Phenylbutazone (Systemic) |
| | Piroxicam (Systemic) |
| | *Probenecid (Systemic) |
| | *Probenecid and Colchicine (Systemic) |
| | *Sulfinpyrazone (Systemic) |
| | Sulindac (Systemic) |
| MS900 | Acetazolamide (Systemic) |
| | Chondrocytes, Autologous Cultured (Implantation-Local) |
| | *Chymopapain (Parenteral-Local) |
| | Conjugated Estrogens and Medroxyprogesterone Acetate (Systemic) |
| | Diethylstilbestrol (Systemic) |
| | Estradiol (Systemic) |
| | Estrogens, Conjugated (Systemic) |
| | Estrogens, Esterified (Systemic) |
| | Estropipate (Systemic) |
| | Ethinyl Estradiol (Systemic) |
| | *Hyaluronate Sodium (Systemic) |
| | *Hyaluronate Sodium Derivative (Systemic) |
| | Quinine (Systemic) |
| | *Tizanidine (Systemic) |
| NT100 | *Oxymetazoline (Nasal) |
| | *Phenylephrine (Nasal) |
| | *Xylometazoline (Nasal) |
| NT201 | *Beclomethasone (Nasal) |
| | *Budesonide (Nasal) |
| | *Dexamethasone (Nasal) |
| | *Flunisolide (Nasal) |
| | *Fluticasone (Nasal) |
| | *Mometasone (Nasal) |
| | *Triamcinolone (Nasal) |
| NT300 | *Benzocaine, Butamben, and Tetracaine Gel (Mucosal-Local) |
| | *Benzocaine, Butamben, and Tetracaine Ointment (Mucosal-Local) |
| | *Benzocaine, Butamben, and Tetracaine Topical Aerosol (Mucosal-Local) |
| | *Benzocaine, Butamben, and Tetracaine Topical Solution (Mucosal-Local) |
| | *Benzocaine Gel (Mucosal-Local) |
| | Benzocaine Topical Aerosol (Mucosal-Local) |
| | Benzocaine Topical Aerosol USP (Topical) |
| | *Benzocaine Topical Solution (Mucosal-Local) |
| | *Cocaine (Mucosal-Local) |
| | *Dyclonine Topical Solution (Mucosal-Local) |
| | *Lidocaine Hydrochloride Jelly (Mucosal-Local) |
| | *Lidocaine Hydrochloride Jelly USP (Topical) |
| | *Lidocaine Hydrochloride Topical Solution (Mucosal-Local) |
| | *Lidocaine Hydrochloride Topical Spray Solution (Mucosal-Local) |
| | *Lidocaine Ointment (Mucosal-Local) |
| | *Lidocaine 5% Ointment USP (Topical) |
| | *Lidocaine Topical Aerosol (Mucosal-Local) |
| | *Tetracaine Hydrochloride Topical Solution (Mucosal-Local) |
| NT400 | *Azelastine (Nasal) |
| NT900 | *Cromolyn (Nasal) |
| | *Ipratropium (Nasal) |
| | *Levocabastine (Nasal) |
| | *Mupirocin (Nasal) |
| OP101 | *Betaxolol (Ophthalmic) |

|  |  |
|---|---|
| | *Carteolol (Ophthalmic) |
| | *Levobunolol (Ophthalmic) |
| | *Metipranolol (Ophthalmic) |
| | *Timolol (Ophthalmic) |
| OP102 | *Carbachol (Ophthalmic) |
| OP110 | *Betaxolol (Ophthalmic) |
| | *Carteolol (Ophthalmic) |
| | *Levobunolol (Ophthalmic) |
| | *Metipranolol (Ophthalmic) |
| | *Timolol (Ophthalmic) |
| OP112 | *Brinzolamide (Ophthalmic) |
| | *Dorzolamide (Ophthalmic) |
| OP113 | Acetazolamide (Systemic) |
| | Dichlorphenamide (Systemic) |
| | Methazolamide (Systemic) |
| OP114 | *Apraclonidine (Ophthalmic) |
| | *Brimonidine (Ophthalmic) |
| | *Dipivefrin (Ophthalmic) |
| | *Epinephrine (Ophthalmic) |
| | *Epinephryl Borate (Ophthalmic) |
| OP115 | Glycerin (Systemic) |
| | Urea (Systemic) |
| OP116 | *Latanoprost (Ophthalmic) |
| OP118 | *Carbachol (Ophthalmic) |
| | *Demecarium (Ophthalmic) |
| | *Echothiophate (Ophthalmic) |
| | *Isoflurophate (Ophthalmic) |
| | *Physostigmine (Ophthalmic) |
| | *Pilocarpine (Ophthalmic) |
| OP140 | Mannitol (Ophthalmic) |
| OP160 | Dorzolamide Hydrochloride and Timolol Maleate (Ophthalmic) |
| OP180 | Demecarium (Ophthalmic) |
| | Echothiophate (Ophthalmic) |
| | Isoflurophate (Ophthalmic) |
| OP201 | *Chloramphenicol (Ophthalmic) |
| | *Chlortetracycline (Ophthalmic) |
| | *Ciprofloxacin (Ophthalmic) |
| | *Erythromycin (Ophthalmic) |
| | *Framycetin (Ophthalmic) |
| | *Gentamicin (Ophthalmic) |
| | *Neomycin (Ophthalmic) |
| | *Neomycin, Polymyxin B, and Bacitracin (Ophthalmic) |
| | *Neomycin, Polymyxin B, and Gramicidin (Ophthalmic) |
| | *Norfloxacin (Ophthalmic) |
| | *Ofloxacin (Ophthalmic) |
| | *Polymyxin B (Ophthalmic) |
| | *Sulfacetamide (Ophthalmic) |
| | *Sulfisoxazole (Ophthalmic) |
| | *Tetracycline (Ophthalmic) |
| | *Tobramycin (Ophthalmic) |
| OP202 | *Natamycin (Ophthalmic) |
| OP203 | *Idoxuridine (Ophthalmic) |
| | *Trifluridine (Ophthalmic) |
| | *Vidarabine (Ophthalmic) |
| OP301 | *Betamethasone (Ophthalmic) |
| | *Dexamethasone (Ophthalmic) |
| | *Fluorometholone (Ophthalmic) |
| | *Hydrocortisone (Ophthalmic) |
| | *Loteprednol (Ophthalmic) |
| | *Medrysone (Ophthalmic) |
| | *Prednisolone (Ophthalmic) |
| | *Rimexolone (Ophthalmic) |
| OP302 | *Diclofenac (Ophthalmic) |
| | *Flurbiprofen (Ophthalmic) |
| | *Indomethacin (Ophthalmic) |
| | *Ketorolac (Ophthalmic) |
| OP350 | *Framycetin, Gramicidin, and Dexamethasone (Ophthalmic) |
| | *Neomycin, Polymyxin B, and Hydrocortisone (Ophthalmic) |
| OP500 | *Carboxymethylcellulose (Ophthalmic) |
| | *Hydroxypropyl Cellulose (Ophthalmic) |
| | *Hydroxypropyl Methylcellulose (Ophthalmic) |
| OP600 | *Atropine (Ophthalmic) |
| | *Cyclopentolate (Ophthalmic) |
| | *Homatropine (Ophthalmic) |
| | *Phenylephrine (Ophthalmic) |
| | *Scopolamine (Ophthalmic) |
| | *Tropicamide (Ophthalmic) |
| OP700 | *Proparacaine (Ophthalmic) |
| | *Tetracaine (Ophthalmic) |
| OP801 | *Emedastine (Ophthalmic) |
| | *Levocabastine (Ophthalmic) |
| | *Olopatadine (Ophthalmic) |
| OP802 | *Naphazoline (Ophthalmic) |
| | *Oxymetazoline (Ophthalmic) |
| | *Phenylephrine (Ophthalmic) |
| OP900 | *Botulinum Toxin Type A (Parenteral-Local) |

|  |  |
|---|---|
| | Carbachol (Ophthalmic) |
| | *Cromolyn (Ophthalmic) |
| | *Dapiprazole (Ophthalmic) |
| | Demecarium (Ophthalmic) |
| | Diclofenac (Ophthalmic) |
| | Echothiophate (Ophthalmic) |
| | *Edetate Disodium (Ophthalmic) |
| | Epinephrine (Ophthalmic) |
| | Epinephrine, Parenteral (Systemic) |
| | Flurbiprofen (Ophthalmic) |
| | *Ganciclovir (Implantation-Ophthalmic) |
| | Hydroxypropyl Methylcellulose (Ophthalmic) |
| | *Indomethacin (Ophthalmic) |
| | Isoflurophate (Ophthalmic) |
| | Ketorolac (Ophthalmic) |
| | *Lodoxamide (Ophthalmic) |
| | *Polyacrylamide (Ophthalmic) |
| | *Silicone Oil 5000 Centistokes (Parenteral-Local) |
| | *Suprofen (Ophthalmic) |
| OR100 | Sodium Fluoride and Triclosan (Systemic) |
| OR300 | *Sodium Fluoride and Triclosan (Systemic) |
| OR500 | *Chlorhexidine (Mucosal-Local) |
| OR600 | Benzocaine, Butamben, and Tetracaine Gel (Mucosal-Local) |
| | Benzocaine, Butamben, and Tetracaine Ointment (Mucosal-Local) |
| | Benzocaine, Butamben, and Tetracaine Topical Aerosol (Mucosal-Local) |
| | Benzocaine, Butamben, and Tetracaine Topical Solution (Mucosal-Local) |
| | *Benzocaine Dental Paste (Mucosal-Local) |
| | Benzocaine Gel (Mucosal-Local) |
| | *Benzocaine Lozenges (Mucosal-Local) |
| | *Benzocaine and Menthol Lozenges (Mucosal-Local) |
| | Benzocaine Ointment (Mucosal-Local) |
| | *Benzocaine and Phenol Gel (Mucosal-Local) |
| | *Benzocaine and Phenol Topical Solution (Mucosal-Local) |
| | Benzocaine Topical Aerosol (Mucosal-Local) |
| | Benzocaine Topical Aerosol USP (Topical) |
| | Benzocaine Topical Solution (Mucosal-Local) |
| | Cocaine (Mucosal-Local) |
| | *Dyclonine Lozenges (Mucosal-Local) |
| | Dyclonine Topical Solution (Mucosal-Local) |
| | Lidocaine Hydrochloride Oral Topical Solution (Mucosal-Local) |
| | Lidocaine Hydrochloride Topical Solution (Mucosal-Local) |
| | Lidocaine Ointment (Mucosal-Local) |
| | Lidocaine 5% Ointment USP (Topical) |
| | *Lidocaine Oral Topical Solution (Mucosal-Local) |
| | Lidocaine Topical Aerosol (Mucosal-Local) |
| | *Tetracaine Topical Aerosol (Mucosal-Local) |
| OR900 | *Amlexanox (Mucosal-Local) |
| | *Benzydamine (Oral-Local) |
| | *Betamethasone (Dental) |
| | Chlorhexidine (Systemic) |
| | *Choline Salicylate and Cetyl-dimethyl-benzyl-ammonium Chloride (Mucosal-Local) |
| | *Hydrocortisone (Dental) |
| | *Tetracycline Periodontal Fibers (Mucosal-Local) |
| | *Triamcinolone (Dental) |
| OT101 | *Chloramphenicol (Otic) |
| | *Gentamicin (Otic) |
| | *Ofloxacin (Otic) |
| OT200 | *Betamethasone (Otic) |
| | *Dexamethasone (Otic) |
| | *Hydrocortisone (Otic) |
| OT250 | *Clioquinol and Flumethasone (Otic) |
| | *Colistin, Neomycin, and Hydrocortisone (Otic) |
| | *Desonide and Acetic Acid (Otic) |
| | *Framycetin, Gramicidin, and Dexamethasone (Otic) |
| | *Hydrocortisone and Acetic Acid (Otic) |
| | *Neomycin, Polymyxin B, and Hydrocortisone (Otic) |

# VA Medication Classification System

| | |
|---|---|
| OT300 | Antipyrine and Benzocaine (Otic) |
| OT400 | *Antipyrine and Benzocaine (Otic) |
| RE101 | *Beclomethasone (Inhalation-Local) |
| | *Budesonide (Inhalation-Local) |
| | *Cromolyn (Inhalation-Local) |
| | *Dexamethasone (Inhalation-Local) |
| | *Flunisolide (Inhalation-Local) |
| | *Fluticasone (Inhalation-Local) |
| | *Nedocromil (Inhalation-Local) |
| | *Triamcinolone (Inhalation-Local) |
| RE102 | *Albuterol (Inhalation-Local) |
| | *Bitolterol (Inhalation-Local) |
| | *Epinephrine (Inhalation-Local) |
| | *Fenoterol (Inhalation-Local) |
| | *Isoetharine (Inhalation-Local) |
| | *Isoproterenol (Inhalation-Local) |
| | *Metaproterenol (Inhalation-Local) |
| | *Pirbuterol (Inhalation-Local) |
| | *Procaterol (Inhalation-Local) |
| | *Salmeterol (Inhalation-Local) |
| | *Terbutaline (Inhalation-Local) |
| RE103 | *Albuterol, Oral (Systemic) |
| | *Ephedrine, Oral (Systemic) |
| | *Fenoterol, Oral (Systemic) |
| | Isoproterenol, Oral (Systemic) |
| | *Metaproterenol, Oral (Systemic) |
| | *Terbutaline, Oral (Systemic) |
| RE104 | *Aminophylline (Systemic) |
| | *Dyphylline (Systemic) |
| | *Oxtriphylline (Systemic) |
| | *Theophylline (Systemic) |
| | *Theophylline in Dextrose (Systemic) |
| RE105 | *Ipratropium (Inhalation-Local) |
| RE106 | Cromolyn (Inhalation-Local) |
| RE108 | *Montelukast (Systemic) |
| | Zafirlukast (Systemic) |
| | Zileuton (Systemic) |
| RE109 | Aminophylline, Oral (Systemic) |
| | Beclomethasone (Inhalation-Local) |
| | Budesonide (Inhalation-Local) |
| | Dexamethasone (Inhalation-Local) |
| | Flunisolide (Inhalation-Local) |
| | Fluticasone (Inhalation-Local) |
| | *Ipratropium and Albuterol (Inhalation-Local) |
| | *Ketotifen (Systemic) |
| | Nedocromil (Inhalation-Local) |
| | Oxtriphylline (Systemic) |
| | *Oxtriphylline and Guaifenesin (Systemic) |
| | *Theophylline, Ephedrine, Guaifenesin, and Phenobarbital (Systemic) |
| | *Theophylline, Ephedrine, and Hydroxyzine (Systemic) |
| | *Theophylline, Ephedrine, and Phenobarbital (Systemic) |
| | *Theophylline and Guaifenesin (Systemic) |
| | Theophylline, Oral (Systemic) |
| | Triamcinolone (Inhalation-Local) |
| RE200 | Ephedrine, Oral (Systemic) |
| | Phenylpropanolamine (Systemic) |
| | *Pseudoephedrine (Systemic) |
| RE301 | *Bromodiphenhydramine and Codeine (Systemic) |
| | *Bromodiphenhydramine, Diphenhydramine, Codeine, Ammonium Chloride, and Potassium Guaiacolsulfonate (Systemic) |
| | *Brompheniramine, Phenylephrine, Phenylpropanolamine, and Codeine (Systemic) |
| | *Brompheniramine, Phenylephrine, Phenylpropanolamine, Codeine, and Guaifenesin (Systemic) |
| | *Brompheniramine, Phenylephrine, Phenylpropanolamine, and Dextromethorphan (Systemic) |
| | *Brompheniramine, Phenylephrine, Phenylpropanolamine, Hydrocodone, and Guaifenesin (Systemic) |
| | *Brompheniramine, Phenylpropanolamine, and Codeine (Systemic) |
| | *Chlorpheniramine and Hydrocodone (Systemic) |
| | *Chlorpheniramine, Pheniramine, Pyrilamine, Phenylephrine, Hydrocodone, Salicylamide, Caffeine, and Ascorbic Acid (Systemic) |
| | *Chlorpheniramine, Phenylephrine, Codeine, and Ammonium Chloride (Systemic) |
| | *Chlorpheniramine, Phenylephrine, Codeine, and Potassium Iodide (Systemic) |
| | *Chlorpheniramine, Phenylephrine, and Hydrocodone (Systemic) |
| | *Chlorpheniramine, Phenylephrine, Hydrocodone, Acetaminophen, and Caffeine (Systemic) |
| | *Chlorpheniramine, Phenylephrine, Phenylpropanolamine, and Codeine (Systemic) |
| | *Chlorpheniramine, Phenylephrine, Phenylpropanolamine, and Dihydrocodeine (Systemic) |
| | *Chlorpheniramine, Phenyltoloxamine, Ephedrine, Codeine, and Guaiacol Carbonate (Systemic) |
| | *Chlorpheniramine, Pseudoephedrine, and Codeine (Systemic) |
| | *Chlorpheniramine, Pseudoephedrine, and Hydrocodone (Systemic) |
| | *Codeine, Ammonium Chloride, and Guaifenesin (Systemic) |
| | *Codeine and Calcium Iodide (Systemic) |
| | *Codeine and Guaifenesin (Systemic) |
| | *Codeine and Iodinated Glycerol (Systemic) |
| | Codeine, Oral (Systemic) |
| | *Diphenhydramine, Codeine, and Ammonium Chloride (Systemic) |
| | Hydrocodone (Systemic) |
| | Hydrocodone and Acetaminophen (Systemic) |
| | *Hydrocodone and Guaifenesin (Systemic) |
| | *Hydrocodone and Homatropine (Systemic) |
| | *Hydrocodone and Potassium Guaiacolsulfonate (Systemic) |
| | *Hydromorphone and Guaifenesin (Systemic) |
| | Hydromorphone, Oral (Systemic) |
| | Hydromorphone, Parenteral (Systemic) |
| | Methadone (Systemic) |
| | Morphine (Systemic) |
| | *Pheniramine, Codeine, and Guaifenesin (Systemic) |
| | *Pheniramine, Phenylephrine, Codeine, Sodium Citrate, Sodium Salicylate, and Caffeine (Systemic) |
| | *Pheniramine, Phenylephrine, Phenylpropanolamine, Hydrocodone, and Guaifenesin (Systemic) |
| | *Pheniramine, Pyrilamine, Hydrocodone, Potassium Citrate, and Ascorbic Acid (Systemic) |
| | *Pheniramine, Pyrilamine, Phenylephrine, Phenylpropanolamine, and Hydrocodone (Systemic) |
| | *Pheniramine, Pyrilamine, Phenylpropanolamine, and Codeine (Systemic) |
| | *Pheniramine, Pyrilamine, Phenylpropanolamine, and Hydrocodone (Systemic) |
| | *Pheniramine, Pyrilamine, Phenylpropanolamine, Hydrocodone, and Guaifenesin (Systemic) |
| | *Phenylephrine, Hydrocodone, and Guaifenesin (Systemic) |
| | *Phenylpropanolamine, Codeine, and Guaifenesin (Systemic) |
| | *Phenylpropanolamine and Hydrocodone (Systemic) |
| | *Phenyltoloxamine and Hydrocodone (Systemic) |
| | *Promethazine and Codeine (Systemic) |
| | *Promethazine, Codeine, and Potassium Guaiacolsulfonate (Systemic) |
| | *Promethazine, Phenylephrine, and Codeine (Systemic) |
| | *Promethazine, Phenylephrine, Codeine, and Potassium Guaiacolsulfonate (Systemic) |
| | *Pseudoephedrine and Codeine (Systemic) |
| | *Pseudoephedrine, Codeine, and Guaifenesin (Systemic) |
| | *Pseudoephedrine and Hydrocodone (Systemic) |
| | *Pseudoephedrine, Hydrocodone, and Guaifenesin (Systemic) |
| | *Pseudoephedrine, Hydrocodone, and Potassium Guaiacolsulfonate (Systemic) |
| | *Pyrilamine and Codeine (Systemic) |
| | *Pyrilamine, Phenylephrine, and Codeine (Systemic) |
| | *Pyrilamine, Phenylephrine, and Hydrocodone (Systemic) |
| | *Pyrilamine, Phenylephrine, Hydrocodone, and Ammonium Chloride (Systemic) |
| | *Triprolidine, Pseudoephedrine, and Codeine (Systemic) |
| | *Triprolidine, Pseudoephedrine, Codeine, and Guaifenesin (Systemic) |
| RE302 | *Benzonatate (Systemic) |
| | *Chlophedianol (Systemic) |
| | *Dextromethorphan (Systemic) |
| | *Dextromethorphan and Acetaminophen (Systemic) |
| | *Dextromethorphan and Guaifenesin (Systemic) |
| | *Dextromethorphan and Iodinated Glycerol (Systemic) |
| | Diphenhydramine, Oral (Systemic) |
| | *Guaifenesin (Systemic) |
| RE400 | *Acetylcysteine (Local) |
| | *Acetylcysteine, Oral (Systemic) |
| | *Iodinated Glycerol (Systemic) |
| RE501 | *Acrivastine and Pseudoephedrine (Systemic) |
| | *Azatadine and Pseudoephedrine (Systemic) |
| | *Brompheniramine and Phenylephrine (Systemic) |
| | *Brompheniramine, Phenylephrine, and Phenylpropanolamine (Systemic) |
| | *Brompheniramine and Phenylpropanolamine (Systemic) |
| | *Brompheniramine and Pseudoephedrine (Systemic) |
| | *Carbinoxamine and Pseudoephedrine (Systemic) |
| | *Chlorpheniramine, Phenindamine, and Phenylpropanolamine (Systemic) |
| | *Chlorpheniramine and Phenylephrine (Systemic) |
| | *Chlorpheniramine, Phenylephrine, and Phenylpropanolamine (Systemic) |
| | *Chlorpheniramine and Phenylpropanolamine (Systemic) |
| | *Chlorpheniramine, Phenyltoloxamine, and Phenylephrine (Systemic) |
| | *Chlorpheniramine, Phenyltoloxamine, Phenylephrine, and Phenylpropanolamine (Systemic) |
| | *Chlorpheniramine and Pseudoephedrine (Systemic) |
| | *Chlorpheniramine, Pyrilamine, and Phenylephrine (Systemic) |
| | *Chlorpheniramine, Pyrilamine, Phenylephrine, and Phenylpropanolamine (Systemic) |
| | *Clemastine and Phenylpropanolamine (Systemic) |
| | *Dexbrompheniramine and Pseudoephedrine (Systemic) |
| | *Diphenhydramine and Pseudoephedrine (Systemic) |
| | *Fexofenadine and Pseudoephedrine (Systemic) |
| | *Loratadine and Pseudoephedrine (Systemic) |
| | *Pheniramine and Phenylephrine (Systemic) |
| | *Pheniramine, Phenyltoloxamine, Pyrilamine, and Phenylpropanolamine (Systemic) |
| | *Pheniramine, Pyrilamine, and Phenylpropanolamine (Systemic) |
| | *Promethazine and Phenylephrine (Systemic) |
| | *Terfenadine and Pseudoephedrine (Systemic) |
| | *Triprolidine and Pseudoephedrine (Systemic) |
| RE502 | *Brompheniramine, Phenylpropanolmine, and Dextromethorphan (Systemic) |
| | *Brompheniramine, Pseudoephedrine, and Dextromethorphan (Systemic) |
| | *Carbinoxamine, Pseudoephedrine, and Dextromethorphan (Systemic) |
| | *Chlorpheniramine, Ephedrine, Phenylephrine, and Carbetapentane (Systemic) |
| | *Chlorpheniramine, Phenylephrine, and Dextromethorphan (Systemic) |

*USP DI*                  VA Medication Classification System    3061

|  |  |
|---|---|
|  | *Chlorpheniramine, Phenylpropanolamine, and Caramiphen (Systemic) |
|  | *Chlorpheniramine, Phenylpropanolamine, and Dextromethorphan (Systemic) |
|  | *Chlorpheniramine, Pseudoephedrine, and Dextromethorphan (Systemic) |
|  | *Diphenhydramine, Dextromethorphan, and Ammonium Chloride (Systemic) |
|  | *Diphenhydramine, Phenylephrine, and Dextromethorphan (Systemic) |
|  | *Doxylamine, Etafedrine, and Hydrocodone (Systemic) |
|  | *Pheniramine, Phenylephrine, and Dextromethorphan (Systemic) |
|  | *Pheniramine, Pyrilamine, Phenylpropanolamine, and Dextromethorphan (Systemic) |
|  | *Promethazine, Psuedoephedrine, and Dextromethorphan (Systemic) |
|  | *Pyrilamine, Phenylephrine, and Dextromethorphan (Systemic) |
|  | *Triprolidine, Pseudoephedrine, and Dextromethorphan (Systemic) |
| RE503 | *Brompheniramine, Phenylephrine, Phenylpropanolamine, and Guaifenesin (Systemic) |
|  | *Chlorpheniramine, Ephedrine, and Guaifenesin (Systemic) |
|  | *Chlorpheniramine, Phenylephrine, and Guaifenesin (Systemic) |
|  | *Chlorpheniramine, Phenylpropanolamine, and Guaifenesin (Systemic) |
|  | *Chlorpheniramine, Phenylpropanolamine, Guaifenesin, Sodium Citrate, and Citric Acid (Systemic) |
|  | *Chlorpheniramine, Pseudoephedrine, and Guaifenesin (Systemic) |
|  | *Dexchlorpheniramine, Pseudoephedrine, and Guaifenesin (Systemic) |
|  | *Promethazine, Phenylephrine, and Potassium Guaiacolsulfonate (Systemic) |
| RE504 | *Chlorpheniramine, Ephedrine, Phenylephrine, Dextromethorphan, Ammonium Chloride, and Ipecac (Systemic) |
|  | *Chlorpheniramine, Phenylephrine, Dextromethorphan, and Guaifenesin (Systemic) |
|  | *Chlorpheniramine, Phenylephrine, Dextromethorphan, Guaifenesin, and Ammonium Chloride (Systemic) |
|  | *Chlorpheniramine, Phenylephrine, Phenylpropanolamine, Carbetapentane, and Potassium Guaiacolsulfonate (Systemic) |
|  | *Chlorpheniramine, Phenylephrine, Phenylpropanolamine, Dextromethorphan, Potassium Guaiacolsulfonate, and Ipecac (Systemic) |
|  | *Chlorpheniramine, Pseudoephedrine, Dextromethorphan, and Guaifenesin(Systemic) |
|  | *Pheniramine, Pyrilamine, Phenylpropanolamine, Dextromethorphan, and Ammonium Chloride (Systemic) |
|  | *Pyrilamine, Phenylpropanolamine, Dextromethorphan, Guaifenesin, Potassium Citrate, and Citric Acid (Systemic) |
| RE506 | *Chlorpheniramine, Phenindamine, Phenylephrine, Dextromethorphan, Acetaminophen, Salicylamide, Cafeine, and Ascorbic Acid (Systemic) |
|  | *Chlorpheniramine, Phenylephrine, Dextromethorphan, Acetaminophen, and Salicylamide (Systemic) |
|  | *Chlorpheniramine, Phenylpropanolamine, Dextromethorphan, and Acetaminophen (Systemic) |
|  | *Chlorpheniramine, Phenylpropanolamine, Dextromethorphan, and Aspirin (Systemic) |
|  | *Chlorpheniramine, Pseudoephedrine, Codeine, and Acetaminophen(Systemic) |
|  | *Chlorpheniramine, Pseudoephedrine, Dextromethorphan, and Acetaminophen (Systemic) |
|  | *Doxylamine, Phenylpropanolamine, Dextromethorphan, and Aspirin (Systemic) |
|  | *Doxylamine, Pseudoephedrine, Dextromethorphan, and Acetaminophen (Systemic) |
|  | *Pyrilamine, Pseudoephedrine, Dextromethorphan, and Acetaminophen (Systemic) |
| RE507 | *Chlorpheniramine and Codeine (Systemic) |
|  | *Chlorpheniramine and Dextromethorphan (Systemic) |
|  | *Promethazine and Dextromethorphan (Systemic) |
| RE509 | *Doxylamine, Codeine, and Acetaminphen (Systemic) |
| RE512 | *Phenylephrine and Codeine (Systemic) |
|  | *Phenylephrine and Hydrocodone (Systemic) |
|  | *Phenylpropanolamine and Caramiphen (Systemic) |
|  | *Phenylpropanolamine and Dextromethorphan (Systemic) |
|  | *Pseudoephedrine and Dextromethorphan (Systemic) |
| RE513 | *Ephedrine, Carbetapentane, and Guaifenesin (Systemic) |
|  | *Phenylephrine, Dextromethorphan, and Guaifenesin (Systemic) |
|  | *Phenylephrine, Phenylpropanolamine, Carbetapentane, and Potassium Guaiacolsulfonate (Systemic) |
|  | *Phenylpropanolamine, Dextromethorphan, and Guaifenesin (Systemic) |
|  | *Pseudoephedrine, Dextromethorphan, and Guaifenesin (Systemic) |
| RE514 | *Phenylpropanolamine, Dextromethorhan, Guaifenesin, and Acetaminophen (Systemic) |
|  | *Pseudoephedrine, Dextromethorphan, Guaifenesin, and Acetaminophen (Systemic) |
| RE515 | *Phenylpropanolamine, Dextromethorhan, and Acetaminophen (Systemic) |
|  | *Phenylpropanolamine, Hydrocodone, Dextromethorphan, and Acetaminophen (Systemic) |
|  | *Pseudoephedrine, Dextromethorphan, and Acetaminophen (Systemic) |
| RE516 | *Ephedrine and Guaifenesin (Systemic) |
|  | *Ephedrine and Potassium Iodide (Systemic) |
|  | *Phenylephrine and Guaifenesin (Systemic) |
|  | *Phenylephrine, Phenylpropanolamine, and Guaifenesin (Systemic) |
|  | *Phenylpropanolamine and Guaifenesin (Systemic) |
|  | *Pseudoephedrine and Guaifenesin (Systemic) |
| RE599 | *Brompheniramine, Phenylpropanolmine, and Acetaminophen (Systemic) |
|  | *Brompheniramine, Pseudoephedrine, and Acetaminophen (Systemic) |
|  | *Chlorpheniramine, Phenylephrine, and Acetaminophen (Systemic) |
|  | *Chlorpheniramine, Phenylephrine, and Methscopolamine (Systemic) |
|  | *Chlorpheniramine, Phenylephrine, Phenylpropanolamine, Atropine, Hyoscyamine, and Scopolamine (Systemic) |
|  | *Chlorpheniramine, Phenylpropanolamine, and Acetaminophen (Systemic) |
|  | *Chlorpheniramine, Phenylpropanolamine, Acetaminophen, and Caffeine (Systemic) |
|  | *Chlorpheniramine, Phenylpropanolamine, and Aspirin (Systemic) |
|  | *Chlorpheniramine, Phenylpropanolamine, Guaifenesin, and Acetaminophen (Systemic) |
|  | *Chlorpheniramine, Phenylpropanolamine, and Methscopolamine (Systemic) |
|  | *Chlorpheniramine, Phenyltoxamine, Phenylpropanolamine, and Acetaminophen (Systemic) |
|  | *Chlorpheniramine, Pseudoephedrine, and Acetaminophen (Systemic) |
|  | *Chlorpheniramine, Pseudoephedrine, and Methscopolamine (Systemic) |
|  | *Chlorpheniramine, Pyrilamine, Phenylephrine, and Acetaminophen (Systemic) |
|  | *Chlorpheniramine, Pyrilamine, Phenylephrine, Phenylpropanolamine, and Acetaminophen (Systemic) |
|  | *Pyrilamine, Pseudoephedrine, Dextromethorphan, and Acetaminophen (Systemic) |
|  | *Dexbrompheniramine, Pseudoephedrine, and Acetaminophen (Systemic) |
|  | *Diphenhydramine, Phenylpropanolamine, and Aspirin (Systemic) |
|  | *Diphenhydramine, Pseudoephedrine, and Acetaminophen (Systemic) |
|  | *Diphenylpyraline, Phenylpropanolamine, Acetaminophen, and Caffeine (Systemic) |
|  | *Pheniramine, Phenylephrine, and Acetaminophen |
|  | *Pheniramine, Phenylephrine, Sodium Salicylate, and Caffeine (Systemic) |
|  | *Pheniramine, Pyrilamine, Phenylpropanolamine, Acetaminophen, and Caffeine (Systemic) |
|  | *Phenylephrine and Acetaminophen (Systemic) |
|  | *Phenylephrine, Guaifenesin, Acetaminophen, Salicylamide, and Caffeine (Systemic) |
|  | *Phenylephrine, Phenylpropanolamine, and Acetaminophen (Systemic) |
|  | *Phenylpropanolamine and Acetaminophen (Systemic) |
|  | *Phenylpropanolamine, Acetaminophen, and Aspirin (Systemic) |
|  | *Phenylpropanolamine, Acetaminophen, and Caffeine (Systemic) |
|  | *Phenylpropanolamine, Acetaminophen, Salicylamide, and Caffeine (Systemic) |
|  | *Phenylpropanolamine and Aspirin (Systemic) |
|  | *Phenyltoloxamine, Phenylpropanolamine, and Acetaminophen (Systemic) |
|  | *Promethazine and Potassium Guaiacolsulfonate (Systemic) |
|  | *Pseudoephedrine and Acetaminophen (Systemic) |
|  | *Pseudoephedrine and Aspirin (Systemic) |
|  | *Pseudoephedrine and Ibuprofen (Systemic) |
|  | *Pyrilamine, Phenylephrine, Aspirin, and Caffeine (Systemic) |
|  | *Pyrilamine, Phenylpropanolamine, Acetaminophen, and Caffeine (Systemic) |
|  | *Triprolidine, Pseudoephedrine, and Acetaminophen (Systemic) |
| RE700 | *Beractant (Intratracheal-Local) |
|  | *Calfactant (Intratracheal-Local) |
|  | *Colfosceril, Cetyl Alcohol, and Tyloxapol (Intratracheal-Local) |
| RE900 | *Albuterol, Parenteral (Systemic) |
|  | *Alpha,-proteinase Inhibitor, Human (Systemic) |
|  | Aminophylline Oral Solution USP (Systemic) |
|  | Aminophylline, Parenteral (Systemic) |
|  | *Ammonia Spirit, Aromatic (Inhalation-Systemic) |
|  | Caffeine (Systemic) |
|  | Caffeine, Citrated (Systemic) |
|  | *Dornase Alfa (Inhalation-Local) |
|  | *Doxapram (Systemic) |
|  | Ephedrine, Parenteral (Systemic) |
|  | Epinephrine (Inhalation-Local) |
|  | Epinephrine, Parenteral (Systemic) |
|  | *Ethylnorepinephrine, Parenteral (Systemic) |
|  | Isoproterenol, Parenteral (Systemic) |
|  | Terbutaline, Parenteral (Systemic) |
|  | Tetracaine (Topical) |
|  | Tetracaine and Menthol (Topical) |
|  | Theophylline Elixir (Systemic) |
|  | Theophylline Oral Solution (Systemic) |
|  | Theophylline, Parenteral (Systemic) |
|  | Theophylline Syrup (Systemic) |
|  | Theophylline in Dextrose (Systemic) |
| RS100 | *Betamethasone (Rectal) |
|  | *Budesonide (Rectal) |
|  | *Hydrocortisone (Rectal) |
|  | *Mesalamine (Rectal-Local) |
|  | *Tixocortol (Rectal) |
| RS201 | *Benzocaine Ointment (Mucosal-Local) |
|  | *Benzocaine Ointment USP (Topical) |
|  | *Dibucaine Ointment (Mucosal-Local) |
|  | *Dibucaine Ointment USP (Topical) |
|  | *Pramoxine Aerosol Foam (Mucosal-Local) |
|  | *Pramoxine Cream (Mucosal-Local) |

## VA Medication Classification System

|        |                                                             |
|--------|-------------------------------------------------------------|
|        | *Pramoxine Hydrochloride Cream USP (Topical)                |
|        | *Pramoxine Ointment (Mucosal-Local)                         |
|        | *Tetracaine (Topical)                                       |
|        | *Tetracaine Cream (Mucosal-Local)                           |
|        | *Tetracaine and Menthol (Topical)                           |
|        | *Tetracaine and Menthol Ointment (Mucosal-Local)            |
| RS300  | *Bisacodyl, Rectal (Local)                                  |
|        | *Docusate, Rectal (Local)                                   |
|        | *Glycerin (Local)                                           |
|        | *Mineral Oil, Rectal (Local)                                |
|        | *Potassium Bitartrate and Sodium Bicarbonate (Local)        |
|        | *Senna, Rectal (Local)                                      |
|        | *Sodium Phosphate, Rectal (Local)                           |
| RS900  | Benzocaine, Butamben, and Tetracaine Gel (Mucosal-Local)    |
|        | Benzocaine Gel (Mucosal-Local)                              |
|        | Benzocaine Ointment (Mucosal-Local)                         |
|        | Benzocaine Ointment USP (Topical)                           |
|        | Dibucaine Ointment (Mucosal-Local)                          |
|        | Dibucaine Ointment USP (Topical)                            |
|        | Dyclonine Topical Solution (Mucosal-Local)                  |
|        | Pramoxine Aerosol Foam (Mucosal-Local)                      |
|        | Pramoxine Cream (Mucosal-Local)                             |
|        | Pramoxine Hydrochloride Cream USP (Topical)                 |
|        | Tetracaine Cream (Mucosal-Local)                            |
|        | Tetracaine and Menthol Ointment (Mucosal-Local)             |
| TN200  | *Enteral Nutrition Formula, Blenderized (Systemic)          |
|        | *Enteral Nutrition Formula, Disease-specific (Systemic)     |
|        | *Enteral Nutrition Formula, Fiber-containing (Systemic)     |
|        | *Enteral Nutrition Formula, Milk-based (Systemic)           |
|        | *Enteral Nutrition Formula, Modular (Systemic)              |
|        | *Enteral Nutrition Formula, Monomeric (Elemental) (Systemic)|
|        | *Enteral Nutrition Formula, Polymeric (Systemic)            |
|        | *Infant Formulas, Hypoallergenic (Systemic)                 |
|        | *Infant Formulas, Milk-based (Systemic)                     |
|        | *Infant Formulas, Soy-based (Systemic)                      |
| TN300  | *Fat Emulsions (Systemic)                                   |
| TN401  | *Ferrous Fumarate (Systemic)                                |
|        | *Ferrous Gluconate (Systemic)                               |
|        | *Ferrous Sulfate (Systemic)                                 |
|        | *Iron Dextran (Systemic)                                    |
|        | *Iron-Polysaccharide (Systemic)                             |
|        | *Iron Sorbitol (Systemic)                                   |
| TN402  | Calcium Acetate (Systemic)                                  |
|        | *Calcium Acetate, Parenteral (Systemic)                     |
|        | Calcium Carbonate (Oral-Local)                              |
|        | *Calcium Carbonate, Oral (Systemic)                         |
|        | *Calcium Chloride, Parenteral (Systemic)                    |
|        | *Calcium Citrate, Oral (Systemic)                           |
|        | *Calcium Glubionate, Oral (Systemic)                        |

|        |                                                             |
|--------|-------------------------------------------------------------|
|        | *Calcium Gluceptate, Parenteral (Systemic)                  |
|        | *Calcium Gluceptate and Calcium Gluconate, Oral (Systemic)  |
|        | *Calcium Gluconate, Oral (Systemic)                         |
|        | *Calcium Gluconate, Parenteral (Systemic)                   |
|        | *Calcium Glycerophosphate and Calcium Lactate, Parenteral (Systemic) |
|        | *Calcium Lactate, Oral (Systemic)                           |
|        | *Calcium Lactate-Gluconate and Calcium Carbonate, Oral (Systemic) |
|        | *Calcium Phosphate, Dibasic (Systemic)                      |
|        | *Calcium Phosphate, Tribasic (Systemic)                     |
| TN403  | *Potassium Acetate (Systemic)                               |
|        | *Potassium Bicarbonate (Systemic)                           |
|        | *Potassium Bicarbonate and Potassium Chloride (Systemic)    |
|        | *Potassium Bicarbonate and Potassium Citrate (Systemic)     |
|        | *Potassium Chloride (Systemic)                              |
|        | *Potassium Gluconate (Systemic)                             |
|        | *Potassium Gluconate and Potassium Chloride (Systemic)      |
|        | *Potassium Gluconate and Potassium Citrate (Systemic)       |
|        | *Trikates (Systemic)                                        |
| TN405  | *Zinc Chloride (Systemic)                                   |
|        | *Zinc Gluconate (Systemic)                                  |
|        | *Zinc Sulfate (Systemic)                                    |
| TN406  | *Magnesium Chloride (Systemic)                              |
|        | *Magnesium Citrate (Systemic)                               |
|        | *Magnesium Gluceptate (Systemic)                            |
|        | *Magnesium Gluconate (Systemic)                             |
|        | *Magnesium Hydroxide (Systemic)                             |
|        | *Magnesium Lactate (Systemic)                               |
|        | *Magnesium Oxide (Systemic)                                 |
|        | *Magnesium Pidolate (Systemic)                              |
|        | *Magnesium Sulfate (Systemic)                               |
| TN407  | *Sodium Fluoride (Systemic)                                 |
| TN408  | *Potassium Phosphates (Systemic)                            |
|        | *Potassium and Sodium Phosphates (Systemic)                 |
|        | *Sodium Phosphates (Systemic)                               |
| TN409  | Sodium Bicarbonate (Systemic)                               |
| TN410  | *Potassium Citrate (Systemic)                               |
|        | *Potassium Citrate and Citric Acid (Systemic)               |
|        | *Potassium Citrate and Sodium Citrate (Systemic)            |
|        | *Sodium Citrate and Citric Acid (Systemic)                  |
|        | *Tricitrates (Systemic)                                     |
| TN490  | *Chromic Chloride (Systemic)                                |
|        | *Chromium (Systemic)                                        |
|        | *Dextrose and Electrolytes (Systemic)                       |
|        | *Oral Rehydration Salts (Systemic)                          |
|        | *Rice Syrup Solids and Electrolytes (Systemic)              |
| TN499  | *Ammonium Molybdate (Systemic)                              |
|        | *Copper Gluconate (Systemic)                                |
|        | *Cupric Sulfate (Systemic)                                  |
|        | Iodine, Strong (Systemic)                                   |
|        | *Manganese Chloride (Systemic)                              |
|        | *Manganese Sulfate (Systemic)                               |

|        |                                                             |
|--------|-------------------------------------------------------------|
|        | Potassium Iodide (Systemic)                                 |
|        | *Selenious Acid (Systemic)                                  |
|        | *Selenium (Systemic)                                        |
|        | *Sodium Iodide (Systemic)                                   |
| TN900  | Amiloride (Systemic)                                        |
|        | Amiloride and Hydrochlorothiazide (Systemic)                |
|        | Bumetanide (Systemic)                                       |
|        | Chloroquine (Systemic)                                      |
|        | Ethacrynic Acid (Systemic)                                  |
|        | Furosemide (Systemic)                                       |
|        | Hydroxychloroquine (Systemic)                               |
|        | *Levocarnitine (Systemic)                                   |
|        | Potassium Citrate and Citric Acid (Systemic)                |
|        | Sodium Citrate and Citric Acid (Systemic)                   |
|        | Spironolactone (Systemic)                                   |
|        | Spironolactone and Hydrochlorothiazide (Systemic)           |
|        | Triamterene (Systemic)                                      |
|        | Triamterene and Hydrochlorothiazide (Systemic)              |
|        | Tricitrates (Systemic)                                      |
| VT050  | *Beta-carotene (Systemic)                                   |
|        | *Vitamin A (Systemic)                                       |
| VT101  | *Cyanocobalamin (Systemic)                                  |
|        | *Hydroxocobalamin (Systemic)                                |
| VT102  | *Folic Acid (Systemic)                                      |
|        | *Leucovorin (Systemic)                                      |
| VT103  | *Niacin (Systemic)                                          |
|        | *Niacinamide (Systemic)                                     |
| VT104  | *Pyridoxine (Systemic)                                      |
| VT105  | *Thiamine (Systemic)                                        |
| VT106  | *Riboflavin (Systemic)                                      |
| VT107  | *Calcium Pantothenate (Systemic)                            |
|        | *Pantothenic Acid (Systemic)                                |
| VT109  | *Biotin (Systemic)                                          |
| VT400  | *Ascorbic Acid (Systemic)                                   |
|        | *Sodium Ascorbate (Systemic)                                |
| VT501  | *Calcifediol (Systemic)                                     |
| VT502  | *Calcitriol (Systemic)                                      |
| VT503  | *Dihydrotachysterol (Systemic)                              |
| VT504  | *Ergocalciferol (Systemic)                                  |
| VT509  | *Alfacalcidol (Systemic)                                    |
|        | *Paricalcitriol (Systemic)                                  |
| VT600  | *Vitamin E (Systemic)                                       |
| VT701  | *Menadiol (Systemic)                                        |
| VT702  | *Phytonadione (Systemic)                                    |
| VT802  | *Vitamins A, D, and C and Fluoride (Systemic)               |
|        | *Vitamins, Multiple, and Fluoride (Systemic)                |
| XA900  | *Condom, Female, Polyurethane                               |
|        | *Condom, Male, Polyurethane                                 |
|        | *Lamb Cecum Condoms                                         |
|        | *Latex Condoms                                              |
| XX000  | *Cysteamine (Systemic)                                      |
|        | Fibrin Sealant (Local)                                      |
|        | Hydroxyurea (Systemic)                                      |
|        | Immune Globulin Intravenous (Human) (Systemic)              |
|        | *Talc, Sterile (Intrapleural-Local)                         |

# Appendix V

## POISON CONTROL CENTER LISTING

The following is a list of emergency telephone numbers of poison control centers, as of May 1998. Center names in **bold print** are Certified Regional Poison Centers. Source: American Association of Poison Control Centers, Inc.

### ALABAMA
**Alabama Poison Center, Tuscaloosa**
Area: Alabama state
2503 Phoenix Dr.
Tuscaloosa, AL 35405
(205) 345-0600; (800) 462-0800 (AL only)

**Regional Poison Control Center**
Area: Alabama state
The Children's Hospital of Alabama
1600 Seventh Ave. South
Birmingham, AL 35233
(205) 933-4050; (205) 939-9201; (800) 292-6678 (AL only)

### ALASKA
Anchorage Poison Control Center
Area: Alaska state
3200 Providence Dr., P.O. Box 196604
Anchorage, AK 99519-6604
(907) 261-3193; (800) 478-3193

### ARIZONA
**Arizona Poison and Drug Information Center**
Area: Arizona state, except Phoenix
Arizona Health Sciences Center, Room 1156
1501 N. Campbell Ave.
Tucson, AZ 85724
(520) 626-6016; (800) 322-0101 (AZ only)

**Samaritan Regional Poison Center**
Area: Maricopa County (Phoenix)
Good Samaritan Regional Medical Center
1111 E. McDowell Rd., Ancillary 1
Phoenix, AZ 85006
(602) 253-3334; (800) 362-0101 (AZ only)

### ARKANSAS
Arkansas Poison and Drug Information Center
Area: Arkansas state
University of Arkansas for Medical Sciences
4301 West Markham- Slot 522
Little Rock, AR 72205
(800) 376-4766

Southern Poison Center, Inc.
Area: Eastern Arkansas
847 Monroe Ave., Suite 230
Memphis, TN 38163
(901) 528-6048; (800) 288-9999 (TN only)

### CALIFORNIA
**California Poison Control System—Fresno Division**
Area: Central California
Valley Children's Hospital
3151 N. Millbrook, IN31
Fresno, CA 93703
(800) 876-4766 (CA only)

**California Poison Control System—Sacramento Division**
Area: Northeastern California
UCDMC—HSF Room 1024
2315 Stockton Blvd.
Sacramento, CA 95817
(800) 876-4766 (CA only)

**California Poison Control System—San Diego Division**
Area: San Diego County and Imperial County
UCSD Medical Center
200 West Arbor Dr.
San Diego, CA 92103-8925
(800) 876-4766 (CA only)

**California Poison Control System—San Francisco Division**
Area: San Francisco Bay area
San Francisco General Hospital
1001 Potrero Ave., Building 80, Room 230
San Francisco, CA 94110
(800) 876-4766 (CA only)

### COLORADO
**Rocky Mountain Poison and Drug Center**
Area: Colorado state
8802 E. Ninth Ave.
Denver, CO 80220-6800
(303) 739-1123 (Denver metro area); (800) 332-3073 (Outside metro-CO only)

### CONNECTICUT
**Connecticut Poison Control Center**
Area: Connecticut state
University of Connecticut Health Center
263 Farmington Ave.
Farmington, CT 06030-5365
(800) 343-2722 (CT only)

### DELAWARE
**The Poison Control Center**
Area: Delaware state
3600 Market St., Suite 220
Philadelphia, PA 19104
(215) 386-2100; (800) 722-7112

### DISTRICT OF COLUMBIA
**National Capital Poison Center**
Area: Washington, DC and surrounding metro area
3201 New Mexico Ave., NW, Suite #310
Washington, DC 20016
(202) 625-3333

### FLORIDA
**Florida Poison Information Center—Jacksonville**
Area: Northern and eastern coastal areas of Florida
655 West Eighth St.
Jacksonville, FL 32209
(904) 549-4480; (800) 282-3171 (FL only)

**Florida Poison Information Center—Miami**
Area: Miami and surrounding metro counties
University of Miami, Department of Pediatrics
P.O. Box 016960 (R-131)
Miami, FL 33101
(305) 585-5253; (800) 282-3171 (FL only)

**Florida Poison Information Center—Tampa**
Area: Tampa and surrounding metro counties
Tampa General Hospital
P.O. Box 1289
Tampa, FL 33601
(813) 253-4444; (800) 282-3171 (FL only)

### GEORGIA
**Georgia Poison Center**
Area: Georgia state
Hughes Spalding Children's Hospital
Grady Health System
80 Butler St. SE, P.O. Box 26066
Atlanta, GA 30335-3801
(404) 616-9000; (800) 282-5846 (GA only)

### HAWAII
Hawaii Poison Center
1319 Punahou St.
Honolulu, HI 96813
(808) 941-4411

### IDAHO
**Rocky Mountain Poison and Drug Center**
Area: Idaho state
8802 E. Ninth Ave.
Denver, CO 80220-6800
(303) 739-1123; (800) 860-0620 (ID only)

### ILLINOIS
Illinois Poison Control Center
Area: Illinois state
222 S. Riverside Plaza, Suite 1900
Chicago, IL 60606
(800) 942-5969 (IL only)

### INDIANA
**Indiana Poison Center**
Area: Indiana state
Methodist Hospital of Indiana
I-65 at 21st St.
Indianapolis, IN 46206-1367
(317) 929-2323; (800) 382-9097 (IN only)

### IOWA
St. Luke's Poison Center
Area: Iowa state
St. Luke's Regional Medical Center
2720 Stone Park Blvd.
Sioux City, IA 51104
(712) 277-2222; (800) 352-2222

Poison Control Center
The University of Iowa Hospitals and Clinics
Department of Pharmaceutical Care
200 Hawkins Dr.
Iowa City, IA 52242
(800) 272-6477 (IA only)

### KANSAS
Mid-America Poison Control Center
Area: Kansas state
University of Kansas Medical Center
3901 Rainbow Blvd., Room B-400
Kansas City, KS 66160-7231
(913) 588-6633; (800) 332-6633 (KS only)

## KENTUCKY

**Kentucky Regional Poison Center**
Medical Towers South, Suite 572
234 East Gray St.
Louisville, KY 40202
(502) 589-8222

## LOUISIANA

**Louisiana Drug and Poison Information Center**
Area: Louisiana state
Northeast Louisiana University School of Pharmacy
Sugar Hall
Monroe, LA 71209-6430
(800) 256-9822 (LA only)

## MAINE

**Maine Poison Control Center**
Area: Maine state
Maine Medical Center, Department of Emergency Medicine
22 Bramhall St.
Portland, ME 04102
(207) 871-2950; (800) 442-6305 (ME only)

## MARYLAND

**Maryland Poison Center**
Area: Maryland state
20 N. Pine St.
Baltimore, MD 21201
(410) 706-7701; (800) 492-2414 (MD only)

**National Capital Poison Center**
Area: Washington, DC and surrounding metro area
3201 New Mexico Ave., NW, Suite #310
Washington, DC 20016
(202) 625-3333

## MASSACHUSETTS

**Massachusetts Poison Control System**
Area: Massachusetts state
Children's Hospital
300 Longwood Ave.
Boston, MA 02115
(617) 232-2120; (800) 682-9211 (MA only)

## MICHIGAN

**Spectrum Health Regional Poison Center**
Area: Eastern Michigan and peninsula
1840 Wealthy, SE
Grand Rapids, MI 49506-2968
(800) 764-7661 (MI only)

**Children's Hospital of Michigan Poison Control Center**
Area: Southeastern and thumb area of Michigan
4160 John R. Harper Office Building, Suite 616
Detroit, MI 48201
(313) 745-5711; (800) 764-7661 (MI only)

## MINNESOTA

**Hennepin Regional Poison Center**
Area: Minneapolis and surrounding counties
Hennepin County Medical Center
701 Park Ave.
Minneapolis, MN 55415
(612) 347-3141; (800) 764-7661 (MN only)

**International Poison Control Center**
(Does not take calls from the public)
1295 Bandana Blvd., Suite 335
Minneapolis, MN 55425
(888) 779-7921

**Minnesota Regional Poison Center**
Area: Eastern metro area of Twin Cities, greater Minnesota
8100 34th Ave. S., P.O. Box 1309
Minneapolis, MN 55440-1309
(612) 221-2113; (800) 222-1222 (MN only); (800) 764-7661 (MN only)

**North Dakota Poison Information Center**
Area: Northwestern Minnesota
MeritCare Medical Center
720 Fourth St. North
Fargo, ND 58122
(701) 234-5575; (800) 732-2200 (MN only)

## MISSISSIPPI

**Mississippi Regional Poison Control Center**
Area: Mississippi state
University of Mississippi Medical Center
2500 North State St.
Jackson, MS 39216
(601) 354-7660

**Southern Poison Center, Inc.**
Area: Northern Mississippi
847 Monroe Ave., Suite 230
Memphis, TN 38163
(901) 528-6048

## MISSOURI

**Cardinal Glennon Children's Hospital Regional Poison Center**
Area: Missouri state
1465 S. Grand Blvd.
St. Louis, MO 63104
(314) 772-5200; (800) 366-8888 (MO only)

**Children's Mercy Hospital Poison Control Center**
Area: Western Missouri
2401 Gillham Rd.
Kansas City, MO 64108
(816) 234-3430

## MONTANA

**Rocky Mountain Poison and Drug Center**
Area: Montana state
8802 E. Ninth Ave.
Denver, CO 80220-6800
(800) 525-5042 (MT only)

## NEBRASKA

**The Poison Center**
Area: Nebraska state
8301 Dodge St.
Omaha, NE 68114
(402) 354-5555; (800) 955-9119 (NE and WY only)

## NEVADA

**Rocky Mountain Poison and Drug Center**
Area: Nevada state
8802 E. Ninth Ave.
Denver, CO 80220-6800
(800) 446-6179 (NV only)

## NEW HAMPSHIRE

**New Hampshire Poison Information Center**
Area: New Hampshire state
Dartmouth-Hitchcock Medical Center
One Medical Center Drive
Lebanon, NH 03756
(603) 650-8000; (800) 562-8236 (NH only)

## NEW JERSEY

**New Jersey Poison Information and Education System**
Area: New Jersey state
201 Lyons Ave.
Newark, NJ 07112
(800) 764-7661 (NJ only)

## NEW MEXICO

**New Mexico Poison and Drug Information Center**
Area: New Mexico state
University of New Mexico
Health Science Center Library, Room 125
Albuquerque, NM 87131-1076
(505) 272-2222; (800) 432-6866 (NM only)

## NEW YORK

**Central New York Poison Control Center**
Area: Central New York
750 East Adams St.
Syracuse, NY 13210
(815) 476-4766; (800) 252-5655 (NY only)

**Finger Lakes Poison and Drug Information Center**
Area: Finger Lakes region of New York
University of Rochester Medical Center
601 Elmwood Ave., Box 321
Rochester, NY 14642
(716) 275-3232; (800) 333-0542 (NY only)

**Hudson Valley Regional Poison Center**
Area: Eastern New York from New York City to Canada
Phelps Memorial Hospital Center
701 North Broadway
Sleepy Hollow, NY 10591
(914) 366-3030; (800) 336-6997 (NY only)

**Long Island Regional Poison Control Center**
Area: Long Island
Winthrop University Hospital
259 First St.
Mineola, NY 11501
(516) 542-2323

**New York City Poison Control Center**
Area: New York City
New York City Department of Health
455 First Ave., Room 123
New York, NY 10016
(212) POISONS; (212) 340-4494

**Western New York Regional Poison Control Center**
Area: Western New York
219 Bryant St.
Buffalo, NY 14222-2099
(716) 878-7654; (800) 888-7655 (NY western regions only)

## NORTH CAROLINA

**Carolinas Poison Center**
Area: North Carolina state
Carolinas Medical Center
5000 Airport Center Pkwy., Suite B
P.O. Box 32861
Charlotte, NC 28232-2861
(704) 355-4000; (800) 848-6946 (NC only)

**Poison Center for North Carolina**
Area: Western North Carolina
St. Joseph's Hospital
428 Biltmore Ave., Box 60
Asheville, NC 28801
(828) 255-4490; (800) 542-4225 (NC only)

## NORTH DAKOTA
**North Dakota Poison Information Center**
Area: North Dakota state
MeritCare Medical Center
720 Fourth St. North
Fargo, ND 58122
(701) 234-5575; (800) 732-2200 (ND only)

## OHIO
**Central Ohio Poison Center**
Area: Central Ohio
700 Children's Dr.
Columbus, OH 43205-2696
(614) 228-1323; (800) 682-7625 (OH only)

**Cincinnati Drug and Poison Information Center Regional Poison Control System**
Area: Southwestern Ohio
2368 Victory Pkwy., Suite 300
Cincinnati, OH 45206
(513) 558-5111; (800) 872-5111 (OH only)

**Greater Cleveland Poison Control Center**
Area: Cleveland and surrounding metro area
11100 Euclid Ave.
Cleveland, OH 44106-6010
(216) 231-4455; (888) 234-4455 (OH only)

**Medical College of Ohio Poison and Drug Information Center**
Area: Toledo and surrounding metro areas
3000 Arlington Ave.
Toledo, OH 43614
(419) 381-3897; (800) 589-3897 (419 and 513 area codes only)

## OKLAHOMA
**Oklahoma Poison Control Center**
Area: Oklahoma state
Children's Hospital of Oklahoma
940 NE 13th St., Room 3512
Oklahoma City, OK 73104
(405) 271-5454; (800) 764-7661 (OK only)

## OREGON
**Oregon Poison Center**
Area: Oregon state
Oregon Health Sciences University
3181 SW Sam Jackson Park Rd.
Portland, OR 97201
(503) 494-8968; (800) 452-7165 (OR only)

## PENNSYLVANIA
**Central Pennsylvania Poison Center**
Area: Central Pennsylvania
Pennsylvania State University Hospital
Milton S. Hershey Medical Center
Hershey, PA 17033
(717) 531-6111; (800) 521-6110 (PA only)

**Pittsburgh Poison Center**
Area: Western Pennsylvania
3705 Fifth Ave.
Pittsburgh, PA 15213
(412) 681-6669

**The Poison Control Center**
Area: Southeastern Pennsylvania and Lehigh Valley
3600 Market St., Suite 220
Philadelphia, PA 19104
(215) 386-2100; (800) 722-7112

## PUERTO RICO
San Jorge Children's Hospital Poison Center
258 San Jorge St.
Santurce, PR 00912
(787) 726-5660; (787) 726-5674

## RHODE ISLAND
**Lifespan Poison Center**
Area: Rhode Island state
Rhode Island Hospital
593 Eddy St.
Providence, RI 02903
(401) 444-5727

## SOUTH CAROLINA
**Palmetto Poison Center**
Area: South Carolina state
University of South Carolina College of Pharmacy
Columbia, SC 29208
(803) 777-1117; (800) 922-1117 (SC only)

## SOUTH DAKOTA
**St. Luke's Poison Center**
Area: Southeastern South Dakota
St. Luke's Regional Medical Center
2720 Stone Park Blvd.
Sioux City, IA 51104
(712) 277-2222; (800) 352-2222

## TENNESSEE
**Middle Tennessee Poison Center**
Area: Middle Tennessee state
The Center for Clinical Toxicology
501 Oxford House, 1161 21st Ave. South
Nashville, TN 37232-4632
(615) 936-2034; (800) 288-9999 (TN only)

**Southern Poison Center, Inc.**
Area: Western and eastern Tennessee
847 Monroe Ave., Suite 230
Memphis, TN 38163
(901) 528-6048; (800) 288-9999 (TN only)

## TEXAS
**Central Texas Poison Center**
Area: Central Texas
Scott and White Memorial Hospital
2401 South 31st St.
Temple, TX 76508
(254) 724-7401; (800) 764-7661 (TX only)

**North Texas Poison Center**
Area: Northern Texas
Parkland Health and Hospital System
5201 Harry Hines Blvd., P.O. Box 35926
Dallas, TX 75235
(800) 764-7661 (TX only)

**South Texas Poison Center**
Area: Southern Texas
University of Texas Health Science Center
Forensic Science Building
7703 Floyd Curl Dr., Room 146
San Antonio, TX 78284-7849
(800) 764-7661 (TX only)

**Southeast Texas Poison Center**
Area: Southeastern Texas
The University of Texas Medical Branch
301 University Blvd.
Galveston, TX 77555-1175
(409) 765-1420; (800) 764-7661 (TX only)

**Texas Panhandle Poison Center**
Area: Amarillo and surrounding area
1501 S. Coulter, P.O. Box 1110
Amarillo, TX 79175
(800) 764-7661 (TX only)

**West Texas Regional Poison Center**
Area: Western Texas
4815 Alameda Ave.
El Paso, TX 79905
(800) 764-7661 (TX only)

## UTAH
**Utah Poison Control Center**
Area: Utah state
410 Chipeta Way, Suite 230
Salt Lake City, UT 84108
(801) 581-2151; (800) 456-7707 (UT only)

## VERMONT
**Vermont Poison Center**
Area: Vermont state
Fletcher Allen Health Care
111 Colchester Ave.
Burlington, VT 05401
(802) 656-5656

## VIRGINIA
**Blue Ridge Poison Center**
Area: Central western Virginia
University of Virginia Health System, Box 437
Charlottesville, VA 22908
(804) 924-5543; (800) 451-1428 (VA only)

**National Capital Poison Center**
Area: Washington, DC and surrounding metro area
3201 New Mexico Ave., NW, Suite #310
Washington, DC 20016
(202) 625-3333

**Virginia Poison Center**
Area: Eastern and central Virginia
Virginia Commonwealth University
P.O. Box 980522
Richmond, VA 23298-0522
(804) 828-9123; (800) 552-6337 (VA only)

## WASHINGTON
**Washington Poison Center**
Area: Washington state
155 NE 100th St., Suite #400
Seattle, WA 98125-8012
(206) 526-2121; (800) 732-6985 (WA only)

## WEST VIRGINIA
**West Virginia Poison Center**
Area: West Virginia state
3110 MacCorkle Ave., SE
Charleston, WV 25304
(304) 348-4211; (800) 642-3625 (WV only)

## WISCONSIN
Children's Hospital of Wisconsin Poison Center
Area: Eastern Wisconsin
P.O. Box 1997
Milwaukee, WI 53201
(414) 266-2222; (800) 815-8855 (WI only)

**University of Wisconsin Hospital Regional Poison Center**
Area: Western Wisconsin
600 Highland Ave., Room F6/133 CSC
Madison, WI 53792
(800) 815-8855 (WI only)

## WYOMING
**The Poison Center**
Area: Wyoming state
8301 Dodge St.
Omaha, NE 68114
(402) 354-5555; (800) 955-9119 (NE and WY only)

# Appendix VI

## COMBINATION CROSS-REFERENCE LISTING

The following alphabetic listing identifies the therapeutically active ingredients found in combination products included in the 1999 edition of *USP DI*, along with a cross-reference to the title of the monograph where the specific combination product can be found.

**Acetaminophen-containing Combinations**
Acetaminophen and Aspirin (Systemic)—*See* Acetaminophen and Salicylates (Systemic)
Acetaminophen, Aspirin, and Caffeine (Systemic)—*See* Acetaminophen and Salicylates (Systemic)
Acetaminophen, Aspirin, and Caffeine, Buffered (Systemic)—*See* Acetaminophen and Salicylates (Systemic)
Acetaminophen, Aspirin, and Salicylamide, Buffered (Systemic)—*See* Acetaminophen and Salicylates (Systemic)
Acetaminophen, Aspirin, Salicylamide, and Caffeine (Systemic)—*See* Acetaminophen and Salicylates (Systemic)
Acetaminophen and Caffeine (Systemic)—*See* Acetaminophen (Systemic)
Acetaminophen and Codeine (Systemic)—*See* Opioid (Narcotic) Analgesics and Acetaminophen (Systemic)
Acetaminophen, Codeine, and Caffeine (Systemic)—*See* Opioid (Narcotic) Analgesics and Acetaminophen (Systemic)
Acetaminophen and Salicylamide (Systemic)—*See* Acetaminophen and Salicylates (Systemic)
Acetaminophen, Salicylamide, and Caffeine (Systemic)—*See* Acetaminophen and Salicylates (Systemic)
Acetaminophen, Sodium Bicarbonate, and Citric Acid (Systemic)
Brompheniramine, Phenylpropanolamine, and Acetaminophen (Systemic)—*See* Antihistamines, Decongestants, and Analgesics (Systemic)
Brompheniramine, Pseudoephedrine, and Acetaminophen (Systemic)—*See* Antihistamines, Decongestants, and Analgesics (Systemic)
Butalbital and Acetaminophen (Systemic)—*See* Barbiturates and Analgesics (Systemic)
Butalbital, Acetaminophen, and Caffeine (Systemic)—*See* Barbiturates and Analgesics (Systemic)
Butalbital, Acetaminophen, Caffeine, and Codeine (Systemic)—*See* Barbiturates and Analgesics (Systemic)
Chlorpheniramine, Phenindamine, Phenylephrine, Dextromethorphan, Acetaminophen, Salicylamide, Caffeine, and Ascorbic Acid (Systemic)—*See* Cough/Cold Combinations (Systemic)
Chlorpheniramine, Phenylephrine, and Acetaminophen (Systemic)—*See* Antihistamines, Decongestants, and Analgesics (Systemic)
Chlorpheniramine, Phenylephrine, Acetaminophen, and Salicylamide (Systemic)—*See* Antihistamines, Decongestants, and Analgesics (Systemic)
Chlorpheniramine, Phenylephrine, Acetaminophen, Salicylamide, and Caffeine (Systemic)—*See* Antihistamines, Decongestants, and Analgesics (Systemic)
Chlorpheniramine, Phenylephrine, Dextromethorphan, Acetaminophen, and Salicylamide (Systemic)—*See* Cough/Cold Combinations (Systemic)
Chlorpheniramine, Phenylephrine, Hydrocodone, Acetaminophen, and Caffeine (Systemic)—*See* Cough/Cold Combinations (Systemic)

**Acetaminophen-containing Combinations** (continued)
Chlorpheniramine, Phenylpropanolamine, and Acetaminophen (Systemic)—*See* Antihistamines, Decongestants, and Analgesics (Systemic)
Chlorpheniramine, Phenylpropanolamine, Acetaminophen, and Caffeine (Systemic)—*See* Antihistamines, Decongestants, and Analgesics (Systemic)
Chlorpheniramine, Phenylpropanolamine, Dextromethorphan, and Acetaminophen (Systemic)—*See* Cough/Cold Combinations (Systemic)
Chlorpheniramine, Phenylpropanolamine, Dextromethorphan, Acetaminophen, and Caffeine (Systemic)—*See* Cough/Cold Combinations (Systemic)
Chlorpheniramine, Phenylpropanolamine, Guaifenesin, and Acetaminophen (Systemic)—*See* Cough/Cold Combinations (Systemic)
Chlorpheniramine, Phenyltoloxamine, Phenylpropanolamine, and Acetaminophen (Systemic)—*See* Antihistamines, Decongestants, and Analgesics (Systemic)
Chlorpheniramine, Pseudoephedrine, and Acetaminophen (Systemic)—*See* Antihistamines, Decongestants, and Analgesics (Systemic)
Chlorpheniramine, Pseudoephedrine, Codeine, and Acetaminophen (Systemic)—*See* Cough/Cold Combinations (Systemic)
Chlorpheniramine, Pseudoephedrine, Dextromethorphan, and Acetaminophen (Systemic)—*See* Cough/Cold Combinations (Systemic)
Chlorpheniramine, Pyrilamine, Phenylephrine, and Acetaminophen (Systemic)—*See* Antihistamines, Decongestants, and Analgesics (Systemic)
Chlorpheniramine, Pyrilamine, Phenylephrine, Phenylpropanolamine, and Acetaminophen (Systemic)—*See* Antihistamines, Decongestants, and Analgesics (Systemic)
Chlorzoxazone and Acetaminophen (Systemic)
Dexbrompheniramine, Pseudoephedrine, and Acetaminophen (Systemic)—*See* Antihistamines, Decongestants, and Analgesics (Systemic)
Dextromethorphan and Acetaminophen (Systemic)—*See* Cough/Cold Combinations (Systemic)
Dihydrocodeine, Acetaminophen, and Caffeine (Systemic)—*See* Opioid (Narcotic) Analgesics and Acetaminophen (Systemic)
Diphenhydramine, Pseudoephedrine, and Acetaminophen (Systemic)—*See* Antihistamines, Decongestants, and Analgesics (Systemic)
Diphenylpyraline, Phenylpropanolamine, Acetaminophen, and Caffeine (Systemic)—*See* Antihistamines, Decongestants, and Analgesics (Systemic)
Doxylamine, Codeine, and Acetaminophen (Systemic)—*See* Cough/Cold Combinations (Systemic)
Doxylamine, Pseudoephedrine, Dextromethorphan, and Acetaminophen (Sys-

**Acetaminophen-containing Combinations** (continued)
temic)—*See* Cough/Cold Combinations (Systemic)
Hydrocodone and Acetaminophen (Systemic)—*See* Opioid (Narcotic) Analgesics and Acetaminophen (Systemic)
Isometheptene, Dichloralphenazone, and Acetaminophen (Systemic)
Oxycodone and Acetaminophen (Systemic)—*See* Opioid (Narcotic) Analgesics and Acetaminophen (Systemic)
Pentazocine and Acetaminophen (Systemic)—*See* Opioid (Narcotic) Analgesics and Acetaminophen (Systemic)
Pheniramine, Phenylephrine, and Acetaminophen (Systemic)—*See* Antihistamines, Decongestants, and Analgesics (Systemic)
Pheniramine, Pyralimine, Phenylpropanolamine, Acetaminophen, and Caffeine (Systemic)—*See* Antihistamines, Decongestants, and Analgesics (Systemic)
Phenylephrine and Acetaminophen (Systemic)—*See* Decongestants and Analgesics (Systemic)
Phenylephrine, Guaifenesin, Acetaminophen, Salicylamide, and Caffeine (Systemic)—*See* Cough/Cold Combinations (Systemic)
Phenylephrine, Phenylpropanolamine, and Acetaminophen (Systemic)—*See* Decongestants and Analgesics (Systemic)
Phenylpropanolamine and Acetaminophen (Systemic)—*See* Decongestants and Analgesics (Systemic)
Phenylpropanolamine, Acetaminophen, and Aspirin (Systemic)—*See* Decongestants and Analgesics (Systemic)
Phenylpropanolamine, Acetaminophen, and Caffeine (Systemic)—*See* Decongestants and Analgesics (Systemic)
Phenylpropanolamine, Acetaminophen, Salicylamide, and Caffeine (Systemic)—*See* Decongestants and Analgesics (Systemic)
Phenylpropanolamine, Dextromethorphan, and Acetaminophen (Systemic)—*See* Cough/Cold Combinations (Systemic)
Phenylpropanolamine, Dextromethorphan, Guaifenesin, and Acetaminophen (Systemic)—*See* Cough/Cold Combinations (Systemic)
Phenylpropanolamine, Hydrocodone, Dextromethorphan, and Acetaminophen (Systemic)—*See* Cough/Cold Combinations (Systemic)
Phenyltoloxamine, Phenylpropanolamine, and Acetaminophen (Systemic)—*See* Antihistamines, Decongestants, and Analgesics (Systemic)
Propoxyphene and Acetaminophen (Systemic)—*See* Opioid (Narcotic) Analgesics and Acetaminophen (Systemic)
Pseudoephedrine and Acetaminophen (Systemic)—*See* Decongestants and Analgesics (Systemic)
Pseudoephedrine, Dextromethorphan, and Acetaminophen (Systemic)—*See* Cough/Cold Combinations (Systemic)
Pseudoephedrine, Dextromethorphan, Guaifenesin, and Acetaminophen (Systemic)—*See* Cough/Cold Combinations (Systemic)

**Acetaminophen-containing Combinations** *(continued)*
Pyrilamine, Phenylpropanolamine, Acetaminophen, and Caffeine (Systemic)—*See* Antihistamines, Decongestants, and Analgesics (Systemic)
Pyrilamine, Pseudoephedrine, Dextromethorphan, and Acetaminophen (Systemic)—*See* Cough/Cold Combinations (Systemic)
Triprolidine, Pseudoephedrine, and Acetaminophen (Systemic)—*See* Antihistamines, Decongestants, and Analgesics (Systemic)

**Acetic Acid–containing Combinations**
Desonide and Acetic Acid (Otic)—*See* Corticosteroids and Acetic Acid (Otic)
Hydrocortisone and Acetic Acid (Otic)—*See* Corticosteroids and Acetic Acid (Otic)

**Acetone-containing Combinations**
Alcohol and Acetone (Topical)

**Acrivastine-containing Combinations**
Acrivastine and Pseudoephedrine (Systemic)—*See* Antihistamines and Decongestants (Systemic)

**Alumina-containing Combinations**
Acetaminophen, Aspirin, and Salicylamide, Buffered (Systemic)—*See* Acetaminophen and Salicylates (Systemic)
Alumina and Magnesia (Oral-Local)—*See* Antacids (Oral-Local)
Alumina, Magnesia, and Calcium Carbonate (Oral-Local)—*See* Antacids (Oral-Local)
Alumina, Magnesia, Calcium Carbonate, and Simethicone (Oral-Local)—*See* Antacids (Oral-Local)
Alumina, Magnesia, and Simethicone (Oral-Local)—*See* Antacids (Oral-Local)
Alumina and Magnesium Carbonate (Oral-Local)—*See* Antacids (Oral-Local)
Alumina and Magnesium Trisilicate (Oral-Local)—*See* Antacids (Oral-Local)
Alumina, Magnesium Trisilicate, and Sodium Bicarbonate (Oral-Local)—*See* Antacids (Oral-Local)
Aspirin, Buffered (Systemic)—*See* Salicylates (Systemic)
Aspirin and Codeine, Buffered (Systemic)—*See* Opioid (Narcotic) Analgesics and Aspirin (Systemic)
Simethicone, Alumina, Magnesium Carbonate, and Magnesia (Oral-Local)—*See* Antacids (Oral-Local)

**Amiloride-containing Combinations**
Amiloride and Hydrochlorothiazide (Systemic)—*See* Diuretics, Potassium-sparing, and Hydrochlorothiazide (Systemic)

**Aminobenzoic Acid-containing Combinations**
Aminobenzoic Acid, Padimate O, and Oxybenzone (Topical)—*See* Sunscreen Agents (Topical)
Aminobenzoic Acid and Titanium Dioxide (Topical)—*See* Sunscreen Agents (Topical)

**Amitriptyline-containing Combinations**
Chlordiazepoxide and Amitriptyline (Systemic)
Perphenazine and Amitriptyline (Systemic)

**Ammonium Chloride—containing Combinations**
Bromodiphenhydramine, Diphenhydramine, Codeine, Ammonium Chloride, and Potassium Guaiacolsulfonate (Systemic)—*See* Cough/Cold Combinations (Systemic)
Chlorpheniramine, Ephedrine, Phenylephrine, Dextromethorphan, Ammonium Chloride, and Ipecac (Systemic)—*See* Cough/Cold Combinations (Systemic)
Chlorpheniramine, Phenylephrine, Codeine, and Ammonium Chloride (Systemic)—*See* Cough/Cold Combinations (Systemic)
Chlorpheniramine, Phenylephrine, Dextromethorphan, Guaifenesin, and Ammonium Chloride (Systemic)—*See* Cough/Cold Combinations (Systemic)

**Ammonium Chloride—containing Combinations** *(continued)*
Codeine, Ammonium Chloride, and Guaifenesin (Systemic)—*See* Cough/Cold Combinations (Systemic)
Diphenhydramine, Codeine, and Ammonium Chloride (Systemic)—*See* Cough/Cold Combinations (Systemic)
Diphenhydramine, Dextromethorphan, and Ammonium Chloride (Systemic)—*See* Cough/Cold Combinations (Systemic)
Pheniramine, Pyrilamine, Phenylpropanolamine, Dextromethorphan, and Ammonium Chloride (Systemic)—*See* Cough/Cold Combinations (Systemic)
Pyrilamine, Phenylephrine, Hydrocodone, and Ammonium Chloride (Systemic)—*See* Cough/Cold Combinations (Systemic)

**Amobarbital-containing Combinations**
Secobarbital and Amobarbital (Systemic)—*See* Barbiturates (Systemic)

**Amoxicillin-containing Combinations**
Amoxicillin and Clavulanate (Systemic)—*See* Penicillins and Beta-lactamase Inhibitors (Systemic)

**Ampicillin-containing Combinations**
Ampicillin and Sulbactam (Systemic)—*See* Penicillins and Beta-lactamase Inhibitors (Systemic)

**Antipyrine-containing Combinations**
Antipyrine and Benzocaine (Otic)

**Articaine-containing Combinations**
Articaine and Epinephrine (Systemic)

**Ascorbic Acid–containing Combinations**
Chlorpheniramine, Phenindamine, Phenylephrine, Dextromethorphan, Acetaminophen, Salicylamide, Caffeine, and Ascorbic Acid (Systemic)—*See* Cough/Cold Combinations (Systemic)
Chlorpheniramine, Pheniramine, Pyrilamine, Phenylephrine, Hydrocodone, Salicylamide, Caffeine, and Ascorbic Acid (Systemic)—*See* Cough/Cold Combinations (Systemic)
Pheniramine, Pyrilamine, Hydrocodone, Potassium Citrate, and Ascorbic Acid (Systemic)—*See* Cough/Cold Combinations (Systemic)

**Aspirin-containing Combinations**
Acetaminophen and Aspirin (Systemic)—*See* Acetaminophen and Salicylates (Systemic)
Acetaminophen, Aspirin, and Caffeine (Systemic)—*See* Acetaminophen and Salicylates (Systemic)
Acetaminophen, Aspirin, and Caffeine, Buffered (Systemic)—*See* Acetaminophen and Salicylates (Systemic)
Acetaminophen, Aspirin, and Salicylamide, Buffered (Systemic)—*See* Acetaminophen and Salicylates (Systemic)
Acetaminophen, Aspirin, Salicylamide, and Caffeine (Systemic)—*See* Acetaminophen and Salicylates (Systemic)
Aspirin, Buffered (Systemic)—*See* Salicylates (Systemic)
Aspirin and Caffeine (Systemic)—*See* Salicylates (Systemic)
Aspirin and Caffeine, Buffered (Systemic)—*See* Salicylates (Systemic)
Aspirin, Caffeine, and Dihydrocodeine (Systemic)—*See* Opioid (Narcotic) Analgesics and Aspirin (Systemic)
Aspirin and Codeine (Systemic)—*See* Opioid (Narcotic) Analgesics and Aspirin (Systemic)
Aspirin and Codeine, Buffered (Systemic)—*See* Opioid (Narcotic) Analgesics and Aspirin (Systemic)
Aspirin, Codeine, and Caffeine (Systemic)—*See* Opioid (Narcotic) Analgesics and Aspirin (Systemic)
Aspirin, Sodium Bicarbonate, and Citric Acid (Systemic)

**Aspirin-containing Combinations** *(continued)*
Brompheniramine, Phenylpropanolamine, and Aspirin (Systemic)
Butalbital and Aspirin (Systemic)—*See* Barbiturates and Analgesics (Systemic)
Butalbital, Aspirin, and Caffeine (Systemic)—*See* Barbiturates and Analgesics (Systemic)
Butalbital, Aspirin, Caffeine, and Codeine (Systemic)—*See* Barbiturates and Analgesics (Systemic)
Chlorpheniramine, Phenylpropanolamine, and Aspirin (Systemic)—*See* Antihistamines, Decongestants, and Analgesics (Systemic)
Chlorpheniramine, Phenylpropanolamine, Aspirin, and Caffeine (Systemic)—*See* Antihistamines, Decongestants, and Analgesics (Systemic)
Chlorpheniramine, Phenylpropanolamine, Dextromethorphan, and Aspirin (Systemic)—*See* Cough/Cold Combinations (Systemic)
Diphenhydramine, Phenylpropanolamine, and Aspirin (Systemic)—*See* Antihistamines, Decongestants, and Analgesics (Systemic)
Dipyridamole and Aspirin (Systemic)
Doxylamine, Phenylpropanolamine, Dextromethorphan, and Aspirin (Systemic)—*See* Cough/Cold Combinations (Systemic)
Hydrocodone and Aspirin (Systemic)—*See* Opioid (Narcotic) Analgesics and Aspirin (Systemic)
Meprobamate and Aspirin (Systemic)
Orphenadrine, Aspirin, and Caffeine (Systemic)—*See* Orphenadrine and Aspirin (Systemic)
Oxycodone and Aspirin (Systemic)—*See* Opioid (Narcotic) Analgesics and Aspirin (Systemic)
Pentazocine and Aspirin (Systemic)—*See* Opioid (Narcotic) Analgesics and Aspirin (Systemic)
Phenobarbital, ASA, and Codeine (Systemic)—*See* Barbiturates and Analgesics (Systemic)
Phenylpropanolamine, Acetaminophen, and Aspirin (Systemic)—*See* Decongestants and Analgesics (Systemic)
Phenylpropanolamine, Acetaminophen, and Caffeine (Systemic)—*See* Decongestants and Analgesics (Systemic)
Phenylpropanolamine and Aspirin (Systemic)—*See* Decongestants and Analgesics (Systemic)
Propoxyphene and Aspirin (Systemic)—*See* Opioid (Narcotic) Analgesics and Aspirin (Systemic)
Propoxyphene, Aspirin, and Caffeine (Systemic)—*See* Opioid (Narcotic) Analgesics and Aspirin (Systemic)
Pseudoephedrine and Aspirin (Systemic)—*See* Decongestants and Analgesics (Systemic)
Pyrilamine, Phenylephrine, Aspirin, and Caffeine (Systemic)—*See* Antihistamines, Decongestants, and Analgesics (Systemic)

**Atenolol-containing Combinations**
Atenolol and Chlorthalidone (Systemic)—*See* Beta-adrenergic Blocking Agents and Thiazide Diuretics (Systemic)

**Atropine-containing Combinations**
Atropine, Hyoscyamine, Methenamine, Methylene Blue, Phenyl Salicylate, and Benzoic Acid (Systemic)
Atropine, Hyoscyamine, Scopolamine, and Phenobarbital (Systemic)—*See* Belladonna Alkaloids and Barbiturates (Systemic)
Atropine and Phenobarbital (Systemic)—*See* Belladonna Alkaloids and Barbiturates (Systemic)
Chlorpheniramine, Phenylephrine, Phenylpropanolamine, Atropine, Hyoscyamine, and Scopolamine (Systemic)—*See* Antihista-

# 3068 Combination Cross-reference Listing

**Atropine-containing Combinations**
*(continued)*
  mines, Decongestants, and Anticholinergics (Systemic)
  Difenoxin and Atropine (Systemic)
  Diphenoxylate and Atropine (Systemic)
  Kaolin, Pectin, Hyoscyamine, Atropine, and Scopolamine (Systemic)—*See* Kaolin, Pectin, and Belladonna Alkaloids (Systemic)
  Magnesium Sulfate Tablets (Oral-Local)—*See* Laxatives (Local)

**Avobenzone-containing Combinations**
  Avobenzone, Octocrylene, Octyl Salicylate, and Oxybenzone (Topical)—*See* Sunscreen Agents (Topical)
  Avobenzone and Octyl Methoxycinnamate (Topical)—*See* Sunscreen Agents (Topical)
  Avobenzone, Octyl Methoxycinnamate, Octyl Salicylate, and Oxybenzone (Topical)—*See* Sunscreen Agents (Topical)
  Avobenzone, Octyl Methoxycinnamate, and Oxybenzone (Topical)—*See* Sunscreen Agents (Topical)

**Azatadine-containing Combinations**
  Azatadine and Pseudoephedrine (Systemic)—*See* Antihistamines and Decongestants (Systemic)

**Bacitracin-containing Combinations**
  Neomycin, Polymyxin B, and Bacitracin (Ophthalmic)
  Neomycin, Polymyxin B, and Bacitracin (Topical)

**Belladonna Alkaloid–containing Combinations**
  Atropine, Hyoscyamine, Methenamine, Methylene Blue, Phenyl Salicylate, and Benzoic Acid (Systemic)
  Atropine, Hyoscyamine, Scopolamine, and Phenobarbital (Systemic)—*See* Belladonna Alkaloids and Barbiturates (Systemic)
  Atropine and Phenobarbital (Systemic)—*See* Belladonna Alkaloids and Barbiturates (Systemic)
  Belladonna and Butabarbital (Systemic)—*See* Belladonna Alkaloids and Barbiturates (Systemic)
  Belladonna and Phenobarbital (Systemic)—*See* Belladonna Alkaloids and Barbiturates (Systemic)
  Chlorpheniramine, Phenylephrine, Phenylpropanolamine, Atropine, Hyoscyamine, and Scopolamine (Systemic)—*See* Antihistamines, Decongestants, and Anticholinergics (Systemic)
  Chlorpheniramine, Phenylpropanolamine, and Methscopolamine (Systemic)—*See* Antihistamines, Decongestants, and Anticholinergics (Systemic)
  Difenoxin and Atropine (Systemic)
  Diphenoxylate and Atropine (Systemic)
  Ergotamine, Belladonna Alkaloids, and Phenobarbital (Systemic)
  Ergotamine, Caffeine, and Belladonna Alkaloids (Systemic)—*See* Vascular Headache Suppressants, Ergot Derivative–containing (Systemic)
  Ergotamine, Caffeine, Belladonna Alkaloids, and Pentobarbital (Systemic)—*See* Vascular Headache Suppressants, Ergot Derivative–containing (Systemic)
  Hydrocodone and Homatropine (Systemic)—*See* Cough/Cold Combinations (Systemic)
  Hyoscyamine and Phenobarbital (Systemic)—*See* Belladonna Alkaloids and Barbiturates (Systemic)
  Kaolin, Pectin, Hyoscyamine, Atropine, and Scopolamine (Systemic)—*See* Kaolin, Pectin, and Belladonna Alkaloids (Systemic)
  Magnesium Sulfate Tablets (Oral-Local)—*See* Laxatives (Local)

**Belladonna–containing Combinations**
  Chlorpheniramine, Phenylephrine, and Methscopolamine (Systemic)—*See* Antihistamines, Decongestants, and Anticholinergics (Systemic)
  Chlorpheniramine, Pseudoephedrine, and Methscopolamine (Systemic)—*See* Antihistamines, Decongestants, and Anticholinergics (Systemic)

**Bendroflumethiazide-containing Combinations**
  Nadolol and Bendroflumethiazide (Systemic)—*See* Beta-adrenergic Blocking Agents and Thiazide Diuretics (Systemic)
  Rauwolfia Serpentina and Bendroflumethiazide (Systemic)—*See* Rauwolfia Alkaloids and Thiazide Diuretics (Systemic)

**Benserazide-containing Combinations**
  Levodopa and Benserazide (Systemic)

**Benzocaine-containing Combinations**
  Antipyrine and Benzocaine (Otic)
  Benzocaine, Butamben, and Tetracaine (Mucosal-Local)—*See* Anesthetics (Mucosal-Local)

**Benzoyl Peroxide–containing Combinations**
  Erythromycin and Benzoyl Peroxide (Topical)

**Betamethasone-containing Combinations**
  Clotrimazole and Betamethasone (Topical)

**Bisacodyl-containing Combinations**
  Bisacodyl and Docusate (Oral-Local)—*See* Laxatives (Local)

**Bisoprolol-containing Combinations**
  Bisoprolol and Hydrochlorothiazide (Systemic)—*See* Beta-adrenergic Blocking Agents and Thiazide Diuretics (Systemic)

**Bromodiphenhydramine-containing Combinations**
  Bromodiphenhydramine and Codeine (Systemic)—*See* Cough/Cold Combinations (Systemic)
  Bromodiphenhydramine, Diphenhydramine, Codeine, Ammonium Chloride, and Potassium Guaiacolsulfonate (Systemic)—*See* Cough/Cold Combinations (Systemic)

**Brompheniramine-containing Combinations**
  Brompheniramine and Phenylephrine (Systemic)—*See* Antihistamines and Decongestants (Systemic)
  Brompheniramine, Phenylephrine, and Phenylpropanolamine (Systemic)—*See* Antihistamines and Decongestants (Systemic)
  Brompheniramine, Phenylephrine, Phenylpropanolamine, and Codeine (Systemic)—*See* Cough/Cold Combinations (Systemic)
  Brompheniramine, Phenylephrine, Phenylpropanolamine, Codeine, and Guaifenesin (Systemic)—*See* Cough/Cold Combinations (Systemic)
  Brompheniramine, Phenylephrine, Phenylpropanolamine, and Dextromethorphan (Systemic)—*See* Cough/Cold Combinations (Systemic)
  Brompheniramine, Phenylephrine, Phenylpropanolamine, Dextromethorphan, Potassium Guaiacolsulfonate, and Ipecac (Systemic)—*See* Cough/Cold Combinations (Systemic)
  Brompheniramine, Phenylephrine, Phenylpropanolamine, and Guaifenesin (Systemic)—*See* Cough/Cold Combinations (Systemic)
  Brompheniramine, Phenylephrine, Phenylpropanolamine, Hydrocodone, and Guaifenesin (Systemic)—*See* Cough/Cold Combinations (Systemic)
  Brompheniramine and Phenylpropanolamine (Systemic)—*See* Antihistamines and Decongestants (Systemic)
  Brompheniramine, Phenylpropanolamine, and Acetaminophen (Systemic)—*See* Antihistamines, Decongestants, and Analgesics (Systemic)

**Brompheniramine-containing Combinations**
*(continued)*
  Brompheniramine, Phenylpropanolamine, and Aspirin (Systemic)
  Brompheniramine, Phenylpropanolamine, and Codeine (Systemic)—*See* Cough/Cold Combinations (Systemic)
  Brompheniramine, Phenylpropanolamine, and Dextromethorphan (Systemic)—*See* Cough/Cold Combinations (Systemic)
  Brompheniramine and Pseudoephedrine (Systemic)—*See* Antihistamines and Decongestants (Systemic)
  Brompheniramine, Pseudoephedrine, and Acetaminophen (Systemic)—*See* Antihistamines, Decongestants, and Analgesics (Systemic)
  Brompheniramine, Pseudoephedrine, and Dextromethorphan (Systemic)—*See* Cough/Cold Combinations (Systemic)

**Bupivacaine-containing Combinations**
  Bupivacaine and Epinephrine (Parenteral-Local)—*See* Anesthetics (Parenteral-Local)

**Butabarbital-containing Combinations**
  Belladonna and Butabarbital (Systemic)—*See* Belladonna Alkaloids and Barbiturates (Systemic)

**Butalbital-containing Combinations**
  Butalbital and Acetaminophen (Systemic)—*See* Barbiturates and Analgesics (Systemic)
  Butalbital, Acetaminophen, and Caffeine (Systemic)—*See* Barbiturates and Analgesics (Systemic)
  Butalbital, Acetaminophen, Caffeine, and Codeine (Systemic)—*See* Barbiturates and Analgesics (Systemic)
  Butalbital and Aspirin (Systemic)—*See* Barbiturates and Analgesics (Systemic)
  Butalbital, Aspirin, and Caffeine (Systemic)—*See* Barbiturates and Analgesics (Systemic)
  Butalbital, Aspirin, Caffeine, and Codeine (Systemic)—*See* Barbiturates and Analgesics (Systemic)

**Butamben-containing Combinations**
  Benzocaine, Butamben, and Tetracaine (Mucosal-Local)—*See* Anesthetics (Mucosal-Local)

**Caffeine-containing Combinations**
  Acetaminophen, Aspirin, and Caffeine (Systemic)—*See* Acetaminophen and Salicylates (Systemic)
  Acetaminophen, Aspirin, and Caffeine, Buffered (Systemic)—*See* Acetaminophen and Salicylates (Systemic)
  Acetaminophen, Aspirin, Salicylamide, and Caffeine (Systemic)—*See* Acetaminophen and Salicylates (Systemic)
  Acetaminophen and Caffeine (Systemic)—*See* Acetaminophen (Systemic)
  Acetaminophen, Codeine, and Caffeine (Systemic)—*See* Opioid (Narcotic) Analgesics and Acetaminophen (Systemic)
  Acetaminophen, Salicylamide, and Caffeine (Systemic)—*See* Acetaminophen and Salicylates (Systemic)
  Aspirin and Caffeine (Systemic)—*See* Salicylates (Systemic)
  Aspirin and Caffeine, Buffered (Systemic)—*See* Salicylates (Systemic)
  Aspirin, Caffeine, and Dihydrocodeine (Systemic)—*See* Opioid (Narcotic) Analgesics and Aspirin (Systemic)
  Aspirin and Codeine, Buffered (Systemic)—*See* Opioid (Narcotic) Analgesics and Aspirin (Systemic)
  Aspirin, Codeine, and Caffeine (Systemic)—*See* Opioid (Narcotic) Analgesics and Aspirin (Systemic)
  Butalbital, Acetaminophen, and Caffeine (Systemic)—*See* Barbiturates and Analgesics (Systemic)

USP DI

**Caffeine-containing Combinations**
(continued)
Butalbital, Acetaminophen, Caffeine, and Codeine (Systemic)—See Barbiturates and Analgesics (Systemic)
Butalbital, Aspirin, and Caffeine (Systemic)—See Barbiturates and Analgesics (Systemic)
Butalbital, Aspirin, Caffeine, and Codeine (Systemic)—See Barbiturates and Analgesics (Systemic)
Caffeine and Sodium Benzoate (Systemic)—See Caffeine (Systemic)
Chlorpheniramine, Phenindamine, Phenylephrine, Dextromethorphan, Acetaminophen, Salicylamide, Caffeine, and Ascorbic Acid (Systemic)—See Cough/Cold Combinations (Systemic)
Chlorpheniramine, Pheniramine, Pyrilamine, Phenylephrine, Hydrocodone, Salicylamide, Caffeine, and Ascorbic Acid (Systemic)—See Cough/Cold Combinations (Systemic)
Chlorpheniramine, Phenylephrine, Acetaminophen, Salicylamide, and Caffeine (Systemic)—See Antihistamines, Decongestants, and Analgesics (Systemic)
Chlorpheniramine, Phenylephrine, Hydrocodone, Acetaminophen, and Caffeine (Systemic)—See Cough/Cold Combinations (Systemic)
Chlorpheniramine, Phenylpropanolamine, Acetaminophen, and Caffeine (Systemic)—See Antihistamines, Decongestants, and Analgesics (Systemic)
Chlorpheniramine, Phenylpropanolamine, Aspirin, and Caffeine (Systemic)—See Antihistamines, Decongestants, and Analgesics (Systemic)
Chlorpheniramine, Phenylpropanolamine, Dextromethorphan, Acetaminophen, and Caffeine (Systemic)—See Cough/Cold Combinations (Systemic)
Dihydrocodeine, Acetaminophen, and Caffeine (Systemic)—See Opioid (Narcotic) Analgesics and Acetaminophen (Systemic)
Diphenylpyraline, Phenylpropanolamine, Acetaminophen, and Caffeine (Systemic)—See Antihistamines, Decongestants, and Analgesics (Systemic)
Ergotamine and Caffeine (Systemic)—See Vascular Headache Suppressants, Ergot Derivative–containing (Systemic)
Ergotamine, Caffeine, and Belladonna Alkaloids (Systemic)—See Vascular Headache Suppressants, Ergot Derivative–containing (Systemic)
Ergotamine, Caffeine, Belladonna Alkaloids, and Pentobarbital (Systemic)—See Vascular Headache Suppressants, Ergot Derivative–containing (Systemic)
Ergotamine, Caffeine, and Cyclizine (Systemic)
Ergotamine, Caffeine, and Cyclizine (Systemic)—See Vascular Headache Suppressants, Ergot Derivative–containing (Systemic)
Ergotamine, Caffeine, and Dimenhydrinate (Systemic)
Ergotamine, Caffeine, and Dimenhydrinate (Systemic)—See Vascular Headache Suppressants, Ergot Derivative–containing (Systemic)
Ergotamine, Caffeine, and Diphenhydramine (Systemic)
Ergotamine, Caffeine, and Diphenhydramine (Systemic)—See Vascular Headache Suppressants, Ergot Derivative–containing (Systemic)
Orphenadrine, Aspirin, and Caffeine (Systemic)—See Orphenadrine and Aspirin (Systemic)
Pheniramine, Phenylephrine, Codeine, Sodium Citrate, Sodium Salicylate, and Caf-

**Caffeine-containing Combinations**
(continued)
feine (Systemic)—See Cough/Cold Combinations (Systemic)
Pheniramine, Phenylephrine, Sodium Salicylate, and Caffeine (Systemic)—See Antihistamines, Decongestants, and Analgesics (Systemic)
Pheniramine, Pyrilamine, Phenylpropanolamine, Acetaminophen, and Caffeine (Systemic)—See Antihistamines, Decongestants, and Analgesics (Systemic)
Phenylephrine, Guaifenesin, Acetaminophen, Salicylamide, and Caffeine (Systemic)—See Cough/Cold Combinations (Systemic)
Phenylpropanolamine, Acetaminophen, and Caffeine (Systemic)—See Decongestants and Analgesics (Systemic)
Phenylpropanolamine, Acetaminophen, Salicylamide, and Caffeine (Systemic)—See Decongestants and Analgesics (Systemic)
Propoxyphene, Aspirin, and Caffeine (Systemic)—See Opioid (Narcotic) Analgesics and Aspirin (Systemic)
Pyrilamine, Phenylephrine, Aspirin, and Caffeine (Systemic)—See Antihistamines, Decongestants, and Analgesics (Systemic)
Pyrilamine, Phenylpropanolamine, Acetaminophen, and Caffeine (Systemic)—See Antihistamines, Decongestants, and Analgesics (Systemic)

**Calcium Carbonate–containing Combinations**
Alumina, Magnesia, and Calcium Carbonate (Oral-Local)—See Antacids (Oral-Local)
Alumina, Magnesia, Calcium Carbonate, and Simethicone (Oral-Local)—See Antacids (Oral-Local)
Calcium Carbonate and Magnesia (Oral-Local)—See Antacids (Oral-Local)
Calcium Carbonate, Magnesia, and Simethicone (Oral-Local)—See Antacids (Oral-Local)
Calcium and Magnesium Carbonates (Oral-Local)—See Antacids (Oral-Local)
Calcium and Magnesium Carbonates and Magnesium Oxide (Oral-Local)—See Antacids (Oral-Local)
Calcium Carbonate and Simethicone (Oral-Local)—See Antacids (Oral-Local)

**Captopril-containing Combinations**
Captopril and Hydrochlorothiazide (Systemic)—See Angiotensin-converting Enzyme (ACE) Inhibitors and Hydrochlorothiazide (Systemic)

**Caramiphen-containing Combinations**
Chlorpheniramine, Phenylpropanolamine, and Caramiphen (Systemic)—See Cough/Cold Combinations (Systemic)
Phenylpropanolamine and Caramiphen (Systemic)—See Cough/Cold Combinations (Systemic)

**Carbetapentane-containing Combinations**
Chlorpheniramine, Ephedrine, Phenylephrine, and Carbetapentane (Systemic)—See Cough/Cold Combinations (Systemic)
Chlorpheniramine, Phenindamine, Phenylpropanolamine, Carbetapentane, and Potassium Guaiacolsulfonate (Systemic)—See Cough/Cold Combinations (Systemic)
Ephedrine, Carbetapentane, and Guaifenesin (Systemic)—See Cough/Cold Combinations (Systemic)
Phenylephrine, Phenylpropanolamine, Carbetapentane, and Potassium Guaiacolsulfonate (Systemic)—See Cough/Cold Combinations (Systemic)

**Carbidopa-containing Combinations**
Carbidopa and Levodopa (Systemic)

**Carbinoxamine-containing Combinations**
Carbinoxamine and Pseudoephedrine (Systemic)—See Antihistamines and Decongestants (Systemic)
Carbinoxamine, Pseudoephedrine, and Dextromethorphan (Systemic)—See Cough/Cold Combinations (Systemic)

**Carboxymethylcellulose-containing Combinations**
Psyllium Hydrophilic Mucilloid and Carboxymethylcellulose (Oral-Local)—See Laxatives (Local)

**Casanthranol-containing Combinations**
Casanthranol and Docusate (Oral-Local)—See Laxatives (Local)

**Cascara Sagrada–containing Combinations**
Cascara Sagrada and Aloe (Oral-Local)—See Laxatives (Local)
Cascara Sagrada and Phenolphthalein (Oral-Local)—See Laxatives (Local)
Magnesium Hydroxide and Cascara Sagrada (Oral-Local)—See Laxatives (Local)

**Charcoal-containing Combinations**
Activated Charcoal and Sorbitol (Oral-Local)—See Charcoal, Activated (Oral-Local)

**Chlordiazepoxide-containing Combinations**
Chlordiazepoxide and Amitriptyline (Systemic)
Chlordiazepoxide and Clidinium (Systemic)

**Chlorothiazide-containing Combinations**
Methyldopa and Chlorothiazide (Systemic)—See Methyldopa and Thiazide Diuretics (Systemic)
Reserpine and Chlorothiazide (Systemic)—See Rauwolfia Alkaloids and Thiazide Diuretics (Systemic)

**Chlorpheniramine-containing Combinations**
Chlorpheniramine and Codeine (Systemic)—See Cough/Cold Combinations (Systemic)
Chlorpheniramine and Dextromethorphan (Systemic)—See Cough/Cold Combinations (Systemic)
Chlorpheniramine, Ephedrine, and Guaifenesin (Systemic)—See Cough/Cold Combinations (Systemic)
Chlorpheniramine, Ephedrine, Phenylephrine, and Carbetapentane (Systemic)—See Cough/Cold Combinations (Systemic)
Chlorpheniramine, Ephedrine, Phenylephrine, Dextromethorphan, Ammonium Chloride, and Ipecac (Systemic)—See Cough/Cold Combinations (Systemic)
Chlorpheniramine and Hydrocodone (Systemic)—See Cough/Cold Combinations (Systemic)
Chlorpheniramine, Phenindamine, Phenylephrine, Dextromethorphan, Acetaminophen, Salicylamide, Caffeine, and Ascorbic Acid (Systemic)—See Cough/Cold Combinations (Systemic)
Chlorpheniramine, Phenindamine, and Phenylpropanolamine (Systemic)—See Antihistamines and Decongestants (Systemic)
Chlorpheniramine, Pheniramine, Pyrilamine, Phenylephrine, Hydrocodone, Salicylamide, Caffeine, and Ascorbic Acid (Systemic)—See Cough/Cold Combinations (Systemic)
Chlorpheniramine and Phenylephrine (Systemic)—See Antihistamines and Decongestants (Systemic)
Chlorpheniramine, Phenylephrine, and Acetaminophen (Systemic)—See Antihistamines, Decongestants, and Analgesics (Systemic)
Chlorpheniramine, Phenylephrine, Codeine, and Ammonium Chloride (Systemic)—See Cough/Cold Combinations (Systemic)
Chlorpheniramine, Phenylephrine, Codeine, and Potassium Iodide (Systemic)—See Cough/Cold Combinations (Systemic)
Chlorpheniramine, Phenylephrine, and Dextromethorphan (Systemic)—See Cough/Cold Combinations (Systemic)

**Chlorpheniramine-containing Combinations**
(continued)
Chlorpheniramine, Phenylephrine, Dextromethorphan, Acetaminophen, and Salicylamide (Systemic)—*See* Cough/Cold Combinations (Systemic)
Chlorpheniramine, Phenylephrine, Dextromethorphan, and Guaifenesin (Systemic)—*See* Cough/Cold Combinations (Systemic)
Chlorpheniramine, Phenylephrine, Dextromethorphan, Guaifenesin, and Ammonium Chloride (Systemic)—*See* Cough/Cold Combinations (Systemic)
Chlorpheniramine, Phenylephrine, and Guaifenesin (Systemic)—*See* Cough/Cold Combinations (Systemic)
Chlorpheniramine, Phenylephrine, and Hydrocodone (Systemic)—*See* Cough/Cold Combinations (Systemic)
Chlorpheniramine, Phenylephrine, Hydrocodone, Acetaminophen, and Caffeine (Systemic)—*See* Cough/Cold Combinations (Systemic)
Chlorpheniramine, Phenylephrine, and Methscopolamine (Systemic)—*See* Antihistamines, Decongestants, and Anticholinergics (Systemic)
Chlorpheniramine, Phenylephrine, and Phenylpropanolamine (Systemic)—*See* Antihistamines and Decongestants (Systemic)
Chlorpheniramine, Phenylephrine, Phenylpropanolamine, Atropine, Hyoscyamine, and Scopolamine (Systemic)—*See* Antihistamines, Decongestants, and Anticholinergics (Systemic)
Chlorpheniramine, Phenylephrine, Phenylpropanolamine, Carbetapentane, and Potassium Guaiacolsulfonate (Systemic)—*See* Cough/Cold Combinations (Systemic)
Chlorpheniramine, Phenylephrine, Phenylpropanolamine, and Codeine (Systemic)—*See* Cough/Cold Combinations (Systemic)
Chlorpheniramine, Phenylephrine, Phenylpropanolamine, and Dextromethorphan (Systemic)—*See* Cough/Cold Combinations (Systemic)
Chlorpheniramine, Phenylephrine, Phenylpropanolamine, Dextromethorphan, Potassium Guaiacolsulfonate, and Ipecac (Systemic)—*See* Cough/Cold Combinations (Systemic)
Chlorpheniramine, Phenylephrine, Phenylpropanolamine, and Dihydrocodeine (Systemic)—*See* Cough/Cold Combinations (Systemic)
Chlorpheniramine and Phenylpropanolamine (Systemic)—*See* Antihistamines and Decongestants (Systemic)
Chlorpheniramine, Phenylpropanolamine, and Acetaminophen (Systemic)—*See* Antihistamines, Decongestants, and Analgesics (Systemic)
Chlorpheniramine, Phenylpropanolamine, Acetaminophen, and Caffeine (Systemic)—*See* Antihistamines, Decongestants, and Analgesics (Systemic)
Chlorpheniramine, Phenylpropanolamine, and Aspirin (Systemic)—*See* Antihistamines, Decongestants, and Analgesics (Systemic)
Chlorpheniramine, Phenylpropanolamine, and Caramiphen (Systemic)—*See* Cough/Cold Combinations (Systemic)
Chlorpheniramine, Phenylpropanolamine, and Dextromethorphan (Systemic)—*See* Cough/Cold Combinations (Systemic)
Chlorpheniramine, Phenylpropanolamine, Dextromethorphan, and Acetaminophen (Systemic)—*See* Cough/Cold Combinations (Systemic)
Chlorpheniramine, Phenylpropanolamine, Dextromethorphan, Acetaminophen, and

**Chlorpheniramine-containing Combinations**
(continued)
Caffeine (Systemic)—*See* Cough/Cold Combinations (Systemic)
Chlorpheniramine, Phenylpropanolamine, Dextromethorphan, and Aspirin (Systemic)—*See* Cough/Cold Combinations (Systemic)
Chlorpheniramine, Phenylpropanolamine, and Guaifenesin (Systemic)—*See* Cough/Cold Combinations (Systemic)
Chlorpheniramine, Phenylpropanolamine, Guaifenesin, and Acetaminophen (Systemic)—*See* Cough/Cold Combinations (Systemic)
Chlorpheniramine, Phenylpropanolamine, Guaifenesin, Sodium Citrate, and Citric Acid (Systemic)—*See* Cough/Cold Combinations (Systemic)
Chlorpheniramine, Phenylpropanolamine, and Methscopolamine (Systemic)—*See* Antihistamines, Decongestants, and Anticholinergics (Systemic)
Chlorpheniramine, Phenyltoloxamine, Ephedrine, Codeine, and Guaiacol Carbonate (Systemic)—*See* Cough/Cold Combinations (Systemic)
Chlorpheniramine, Phenyltoloxamine, and Phenylephrine (Systemic)—*See* Antihistamines and Decongestants (Systemic)
Chlorpheniramine, Phenyltoloxamine, Phenylephrine, and Phenylpropanolamine (Systemic)—*See* Antihistamines and Decongestants (Systemic)
Chlorpheniramine, Phenyltoloxamine, Phenylpropanolamine, and Acetaminophen (Systemic)—*See* Antihistamines, Decongestants, and Analgesics (Systemic)
Chlorpheniramine and Pseudoephedrine (Systemic)—*See* Antihistamines and Decongestants (Systemic)
Chlorpheniramine, Pseudoephedrine, and Acetaminophen (Systemic)—*See* Antihistamines, Decongestants, and Analgesics (Systemic)
Chlorpheniramine, Pseudoephedrine, and Codeine (Systemic)—*See* Cough/Cold Combinations (Systemic)
Chlorpheniramine, Pseudoephedrine, Codeine, and Acetaminophen (Systemic)—*See* Cough/Cold Combinations (Systemic)
Chlorpheniramine, Pseudoephedrine, and Dextromethorphan (Systemic)—*See* Cough/Cold Combinations (Systemic)
Chlorpheniramine, Pseudoephedrine, Dextromethorphan, and Acetaminophen (Systemic)—*See* Cough/Cold Combinations (Systemic)
Chlorpheniramine, Pseudoephedrine, Dextromethorphan, and Guaifenesin (Systemic)—*See* Cough/Cold Combinations (Systemic)
Chlorpheniramine, Pseudoephedrine, and Guaifenesin (Systemic)—*See* Cough/Cold Combinations (Systemic)
Chlorpheniramine, Pseudoephedrine, and Hydrocodone (Systemic)—*See* Cough/Cold Combinations (Systemic)
Chlorpheniramine, Pseudoephedrine, and Methscopolamine (Systemic)—*See* Antihistamines, Decongestants, and Anticholinergics (Systemic)
Chlorpheniramine, Pyrilamine, and Phenylephrine (Systemic)—*See* Antihistamines and Decongestants (Systemic)
Chlorpheniramine, Pyrilamine, Phenylephrine, and Acetaminophen (Systemic)—*See* Antihistamines, Decongestants, and Analgesics (Systemic)
Chlorpheniramine, Pyrilamine, Phenylephrine, and Phenylpropanolamine (Systemic)—*See* Antihistamines and Decongestants (Systemic)

**Chlorpheniramine-containing Combinations**
(continued)
Chlorpheniramine, Pyrilamine, Phenylephrine, Phenylpropanolamine, and Acetaminophen (Systemic)—*See* Antihistamines, Decongestants, and Analgesics (Systemic)

**Chlorthalidone-containing Combinations**
Atenolol and Chlorthalidone (Systemic)—*See* Beta-adrenergic Blocking Agents and Thiazide Diuretics (Systemic)
Clonidine and Chlorthalidone (Systemic)
Reserpine and Chlorthalidone (Systemic)—*See* Rauwolfia Alkaloids and Thiazide Diuretics (Systemic)

**Chlorzoxazone-containing Combinations**
Chlorzoxazone and Acetaminophen (Systemic)

**Choline Salicylate–containing Combinations**
Choline and Magnesium Salicylates (Systemic)—*See* Salicylates (Systemic)
Choline Salicylate and Cetyl-dimethylbenzylammonium Chloride (Oral-Local)

**Cilastatin-containing Combinations**
Imipenem and Cilastatin (Systemic)

**Citric Acid–containing Combinations**
Acetaminophen, Sodium Bicarbonate, and Citric Acid (Systemic)
Aspirin, Sodium Bicarbonate, and Citric Acid (Systemic)
Chlorpheniramine, Phenylpropanolamine, Guaifenesin, Sodium Citrate, and Citric Acid (Systemic)—*See* Cough/Cold Combinations (Systemic)
Citric Acid, Glucono-deltalactone, and Magnesium Carbonate (Systemic)
Potassium Citrate and Citric Acid (Systemic)—*See* Citrates (Systemic)
Pyrilamine, Phenylpropanolamine, Dextromethorphan, Guaifenesin, Potassium Citrate, and Citric Acid (Systemic)—*See* Cough/Cold Combinations (Systemic)
Sodium Citrate and Citric Acid (Systemic)—*See* Citrates (Systemic)
Tricitrates (Systemic)—*See* Citrates (Systemic)

**Clavulanate-containing Combinations**
Amoxicillin and Clavulanate (Systemic)—*See* Penicillins and Beta-lactamase Inhibitors (Systemic)
Ticarcillin and Clavulanate (Systemic)—*See* Penicillins and Beta-lactamase Inhibitors (Systemic)

**Clemastine-containing Combinations**
Clemastine and Phenylpropanolamine (Systemic)—*See* Antihistamines and Decongestants (Systemic)

**Clidinium-containing Combinations**
Chlordiazepoxide and Clidinium (Systemic)

**Clioquinol-containing Combinations**
Clioquinol and Flumethasone (Otic)
Clioquinol and Flumethasone (Topical)
Clioquinol and Hydrocortisone (Topical)

**Clonidine-containing Combinations**
Clonidine and Chlorthalidone (Systemic)

**Clotrimazole-containing Combinations**
Clotrimazole and Betamethasone (Topical)

**Coal Tar–containing Combinations**
Salicylic Acid, Sulfur, and Coal Tar (Topical)

**Codeine-containing Combinations**
Acetaminophen and Codeine (Systemic)—*See* Opioid (Narcotic) Analgesics and Acetaminophen (Systemic)
Acetaminophen, Codeine, and Caffeine (Systemic)—*See* Opioid (Narcotic) Analgesics and Acetaminophen (Systemic)
Aspirin and Codeine (Systemic)—*See* Opioid (Narcotic) Analgesics and Aspirin (Systemic)
Aspirin and Codeine, Buffered (Systemic)—*See* Opioid (Narcotic) Analgesics and Aspirin (Systemic)
Aspirin, Codeine, and Caffeine (Systemic)—*See* Opioid (Narcotic) Analgesics and Aspirin (Systemic)

**Codeine-containing Combinations**
(continued)
Bromodiphenhydramine and Codeine (Systemic)—See Cough/Cold Combinations (Systemic)
Bromodiphenhydramine, Diphenhydramine, Codeine, Ammonium Chloride, and Potassium Guaiacolsulfonate (Systemic)—See Cough/Cold Combinations (Systemic)
Brompheniramine, Phenylephrine, Phenylpropanolamine, and Codeine (Systemic)—See Cough/Cold Combinations (Systemic)
Brompheniramine, Phenylephrine, Phenylpropanolamine, Codeine, and Guaifenesin (Systemic)—See Cough/Cold Combinations (Systemic)
Brompheniramine, Phenylpropanolamine, and Codeine (Systemic)—See Cough/Cold Combinations (Systemic)
Butalbital, Acetaminophen, Caffeine, and Codeine (Systemic)—See Barbiturates and Analgesics (Systemic)
Butalbital, Aspirin, Caffeine, and Codeine (Systemic)—See Barbiturates and Analgesics (Systemic)
Chlorpheniramine and Codeine (Systemic)—See Cough/Cold Combinations (Systemic)
Chlorpheniramine, Phenylephrine, Codeine, and Ammonium Chloride (Systemic)—See Cough/Cold Combinations (Systemic)
Chlorpheniramine, Phenylephrine, Codeine, and Potassium Iodide (Systemic)—See Cough/Cold Combinations (Systemic)
Chlorpheniramine, Phenylephrine, Phenylpropanolamine, and Codeine (Systemic)—See Cough/Cold Combinations (Systemic)
Chlorpheniramine, Phenylephrine, Phenylpropanolamine, and Dihydrocodeine (Systemic)—See Cough/Cold Combinations (Systemic)
Chlorpheniramine, Phenyltoloxamine, Ephedrine, Codeine, and Guaiacol Carbonate (Systemic)—See Cough/Cold Combinations (Systemic)
Chlorpheniramine, Pseudoephedrine, and Codeine (Systemic)—See Cough/Cold Combinations (Systemic)
Chlorpheniramine, Pseudoephedrine, Codeine, and Acetaminophen (Systemic)—See Cough/Cold Combinations (Systemic)
Codeine, Ammonium Chloride, and Guaifenesin (Systemic)—See Cough/Cold Combinations (Systemic)
Codeine and Calcium Iodide (Systemic)—See Cough/Cold Combinations (Systemic)
Codeine and Guaifenesin (Systemic)—See Cough/Cold Combinations (Systemic)
Codeine and Iodinated Glycerol (Systemic)—See Cough/Cold Combinations (Systemic)
Diphenhydramine, Codeine, and Ammonium Chloride (Systemic)—See Cough/Cold Combinations (Systemic)
Doxylamine, Codeine, and Acetaminophen (Systemic)—See Cough/Cold Combinations (Systemic)
Pheniramine, Codeine, and Guaifenesin (Systemic)—See Cough/Cold Combinations (Systemic)
Pheniramine, Phenylephrine, Codeine, Sodium Citrate, Sodium Salicylate, and Caffeine (Systemic)—See Cough/Cold Combinations (Systemic)
Pheniramine, Pyrilamine, Phenylpropanolamine, and Codeine (Systemic)—See Cough/Cold Combinations (Systemic)
Phenobarbital, ASA, and Codeine (Systemic)—See Barbiturates and Analgesics (Systemic)
Phenylephrine and Codeine (Systemic)—See Cough/Cold Combinations (Systemic)

**Codeine-containing Combinations**
(continued)
Phenylpropanolamine, Codeine, and Guaifenesin (Systemic)—See Cough/Cold Combinations (Systemic)
Promethazine and Codeine (Systemic)—See Cough/Cold Combinations (Systemic)
Promethazine, Codeine, and Potassium Guaiacolsulfonate (Systemic)—See Cough/Cold Combinations (Systemic)
Promethazine, Phenylephrine, and Codeine (Systemic)—See Cough/Cold Combinations (Systemic)
Promethazine, Phenylephrine, Codeine, and Potassium Guaiacolsulfonate (Systemic)—See Cough/Cold Combinations (Systemic)
Pseudoephedrine and Codeine (Systemic)—See Cough/Cold Combinations (Systemic)
Pseudoephedrine, Codeine, and Guaifenesin (Systemic)—See Cough/Cold Combinations (Systemic)
Pyrilamine and Codeine (Systemic)—See Cough/Cold Combinations (Systemic)
Pyrilamine, Phenylephrine, and Codeine (Systemic)—See Cough/Cold Combinations (Systemic)
Triprolidine, Pseudoephedrine, and Codeine (Systemic)—See Cough/Cold Combinations (Systemic)
Triprolidine, Pseudoephedrine, Codeine, and Guaifenesin (Systemic)—See Cough/Cold Combinations (Systemic)
**Colchicine-containing Combinations**
Probenecid and Colchicine (Systemic)
**Colistin-containing Combinations**
Colistin, Neomycin, and Hydrocortisone (Otic)
**Conjugated Estrogen–containing Combinations**
Conjugated Estrogens and Medroxyprogesterone Tablets (Systemic)—See Conjugated Estrogens and Medroxyprogesterone for Ovarian Hormone Therapy (OHT) (Systemic)
Conjugated Estrogens and Methyltestosterone (Systemic)—See Androgens and Estrogens (Systemic)
Conjugated Estrogens Tablets USP, and Conjugated Estrogens and Medroxyprogesterone Tablets (Systemic)—See Conjugated Estrogens and Medroxyprogesterone for Ovarian Hormone Therapy (OHT) (Systemic)
**Cyclizine-containing Combinations**
Ergotamine, Caffeine, and Cyclizine (Systemic)
Ergotamine, Caffeine, and Cyclizine (Systemic)—See Vascular Headache Suppressants, Ergot Derivative–containing (Systemic)
**Danthron-containing Combinations**
Danthron and Docusate (Oral-Local)—See Laxatives (Local)
**Dehydrocholic Acid–containing Combinations**
Dehydrocholic Acid and Docusate (Oral-Local)—See Laxatives (Local)
Dehydrocholic Acid, Docusate, and Phenolphthalein (Oral-Local)—See Laxatives (Local)
**Deserpidine-containing Combinations**
Deserpidine and Hydrochlorothiazide (Systemic)—See Rauwolfia Alkaloids and Thiazide Diuretics (Systemic)
Deserpidine and Methyclothiazide (Systemic)—See Rauwolfia Alkaloids and Thiazide Diuretics (Systemic)
**Desonide-containing Combinations**
Desonide and Acetic Acid (Otic)—See Corticosteroids and Acetic Acid (Otic)

**Dexamethasone-containing Combinations**
Framycetin, Gramicidin, and Dexamethasone (Ophthalmic)
Framycetin, Gramicidin, and Dexamethasone (Otic)
**Dexbrompheniramine-containing Combinations**
Dexbrompheniramine and Pseudoephedrine (Systemic)—See Antihistamines and Decongestants (Systemic)
Dexbrompheniramine, Pseudoephedrine, and Acetaminophen (Systemic)—See Antihistamines, Decongestants, and Analgesics (Systemic)
**Dexchlorpheniramine-containing Combinations**
Dexchlorpheniramine, Pseudoephedrine, and Guaifenesin (Systemic)—See Cough/Cold Combinations (Systemic)
**Dextromethorphan-containing Combinations**
Brompheniramine, Phenylephrine, Phenylpropanolamine, and Dextromethorphan (Systemic)—See Cough/Cold Combinations (Systemic)
Brompheniramine, Phenylephrine, Phenylpropanolamine, Dextromethorphan, Potassium Guaiacolsulfonate, and Ipecac (Systemic)—See Cough/Cold Combinations (Systemic)
Brompheniramine, Phenylpropanolamine, and Dextromethorphan (Systemic)—See Cough/Cold Combinations (Systemic)
Brompheniramine, Pseudoephedrine, and Dextromethorphan (Systemic)—See Cough/Cold Combinations (Systemic)
Carbinoxamine, Pseudoephedrine, and Dextromethorphan (Systemic)—See Cough/Cold Combinations (Systemic)
Chlorpheniramine and Dextromethorphan (Systemic)—See Cough/Cold Combinations (Systemic)
Chlorpheniramine, Ephedrine, Phenylephrine, Dextromethorphan, Ammonium Chloride, and Ipecac (Systemic)—See Cough/Cold Combinations (Systemic)
Chlorpheniramine, Phenindamine, Phenylephrine, Dextromethorphan, Acetaminophen, Salicylamide, Caffeine, and Ascorbic Acid (Systemic)—See Cough/Cold Combinations (Systemic)
Chlorpheniramine, Phenylephrine, and Dextromethorphan (Systemic)—See Cough/Cold Combinations (Systemic)
Chlorpheniramine, Phenylephrine, Dextromethorphan, Acetaminophen, and Salicylamide (Systemic)—See Cough/Cold Combinations (Systemic)
Chlorpheniramine, Phenylephrine, Dextromethorphan, and Guaifenesin (Systemic)—See Cough/Cold Combinations (Systemic)
Chlorpheniramine, Phenylephrine, Dextromethorphan, Guaifenesin, and Ammonium Chloride (Systemic)—See Cough/Cold Combinations (Systemic)
Chlorpheniramine, Phenylephrine, Phenylpropanolamine, and Dextromethorphan (Systemic)—See Cough/Cold Combinations (Systemic)
Chlorpheniramine, Phenylephrine, Phenylpropanolamine, Dextromethorphan, Potassium Guaiacolsulfonate, and Ipecac (Systemic)—See Cough/Cold Combinations (Systemic)
Chlorpheniramine, Phenylpropanolamine, and Dextromethorphan (Systemic)—See Cough/Cold Combinations (Systemic)
Chlorpheniramine, Phenylpropanolamine, Dextromethorphan, and Acetaminophen (Systemic)—See Cough/Cold Combinations (Systemic)
Chlorpheniramine, Phenylpropanolamine, Dextromethorphan, Acetaminophen, and

## Dextromethorphan-containing Combinations (continued)

Caffeine (Systemic)—*See* Cough/Cold Combinations (Systemic)
Chlorpheniramine, Phenylpropanolamine, Dextromethorphan, and Aspirin (Systemic)—*See* Cough/Cold Combinations (Systemic)
Chlorpheniramine, Pseudoephedrine, and Dextromethorphan (Systemic)—*See* Cough/Cold Combinations (Systemic)
Chlorpheniramine, Pseudoephedrine, Dextromethorphan, and Acetaminophen (Systemic)—*See* Cough/Cold Combinations (Systemic)
Chlorpheniramine, Pseudoephedrine, Dextromethorphan, and Guaifenesin (Systemic)—*See* Cough/Cold Combinations (Systemic)
Dextromethorphan and Acetaminophen (Systemic)—*See* Cough/Cold Combinations (Systemic)
Dextromethorphan and Guaifenesin (Systemic)—*See* Cough/Cold Combinations (Systemic)
Dextromethorphan and Iodinated Glycerol (Systemic)—*See* Cough/Cold Combinations (Systemic)
Diphenhydramine, Dextromethorphan, and Ammonium Chloride (Systemic)—*See* Cough/Cold Combinations (Systemic)
Diphenhydramine, Phenylephrine, and Dextromethorphan (Systemic)—*See* Cough/Cold Combinations (Systemic)
Diphenylpyraline, Phenylephrine, and Dextromethorphan (Systemic)—*See* Cough/Cold Combinations (Systemic)
Doxylamine, Phenylpropanolamine, Dextromethorphan, and Aspirin (Systemic)—*See* Cough/Cold Combinations (Systemic)
Doxylamine, Pseudoephedrine, Dextromethorphan, and Acetaminophen (Systemic)—*See* Cough/Cold Combinations (Systemic)
Pheniramine, Phenylephrine, and Dextromethorphan (Systemic)—*See* Cough/Cold Combinations (Systemic)
Pheniramine, Pyrilamine, Phenylpropanolamine, and Dextromethorphan (Systemic)—*See* Cough/Cold Combinations (Systemic)
Pheniramine, Pyrilamine, Phenylpropanolamine, Dextromethorphan, and Ammonium Chloride (Systemic)—*See* Cough/Cold Combinations (Systemic)
Phenylephrine, Dextromethorphan, and Guaifenesin (Systemic)—*See* Cough/Cold Combinations (Systemic)
Phenylpropanolamine and Dextromethorphan (Systemic)—*See* Cough/Cold Combinations (Systemic)
Phenylpropanolamine, Dextromethorphan, and Acetaminophen (Systemic)—*See* Cough/Cold Combinations (Systemic)
Phenylpropanolamine, Dextromethorphan, and Guaifenesin (Systemic)—*See* Cough/Cold Combinations (Systemic)
Phenylpropanolamine, Dextromethorphan, Guaifenesin, and Acetaminophen (Systemic)—*See* Cough/Cold Combinations (Systemic)
Phenylpropanolamine, Hydrocodone, Dextromethorphan, and Acetaminophen (Systemic)—*See* Cough/Cold Combinations (Systemic)
Promethazine and Dextromethorphan (Systemic)—*See* Cough/Cold Combinations (Systemic)
Promethazine, Pseudoephedrine, and Dextromethorphan (Systemic)—*See* Cough/Cold Combinations (Systemic)
Pseudoephedrine and Dextromethorphan (Systemic)—*See* Cough/Cold Combinations (Systemic)

## Dextromethorphan-containing Combinations (continued)

Pseudoephedrine, Dextromethorphan, and Acetaminophen (Systemic)—*See* Cough/Cold Combinations (Systemic)
Pseudoephedrine, Dextromethorphan, and Guaifenesin (Systemic)—*See* Cough/Cold Combinations (Systemic)
Pseudoephedrine, Dextromethorphan, Guaifenesin, and Acetaminophen (Systemic)—*See* Cough/Cold Combinations (Systemic)
Pyrilamine, Phenylephrine, and Dextromethorphan (Systemic)—*See* Cough/Cold Combinations (Systemic)
Pyrilamine, Phenylpropanolamine, Dextromethorphan, Guaifenesin, Potassium Citrate, and Citric Acid (Systemic)—*See* Cough/Cold Combinations (Systemic)
Pyrilamine, Pseudoephedrine, Dextromethorphan, and Acetaminophen (Systemic)—*See* Cough/Cold Combinations (Systemic)
Triprolidine, Pseudoephedrine, and Dextromethorphan (Systemic)—*See* Cough/Cold Combinations (Systemic)

## Diatrizoate-containing Combinations
Diatrizoate and Iodipamide (Local)

## Dichloralphenazone-containing Combinations
Isometheptene, Dichloralphenazone, and Acetaminophen (Systemic)

## Diethylstilbestrol-containing Combinations
Diethylstilbestrol and Methyltestosterone (Systemic)—*See* Androgens and Estrogens (Systemic)

## Difenoxin-containing Combinations
Difenoxin and Atropine (Systemic)

## Dihydrocodeine-containing Combinations
Aspirin, Caffeine, and Dihydrocodeine (Systemic)—*See* Opioid (Narcotic) Analgesics and Aspirin (Systemic)
Chlorpheniramine, Phenylephrine, Phenylpropanolamine, and Dihydrocodeine (Systemic)—*See* Cough/Cold Combinations (Systemic)
Dihydrocodeine, Acetaminophen, and Caffeine (Systemic)—*See* Opioid (Narcotic) Analgesics and Acetaminophen (Systemic)

## Dimenhydrinate-containing Combinations
Ergotamine, Caffeine, and Dimenhydrinate (Systemic)
Ergotamine, Caffeine, and Dimenhydrinate (Systemic)—*See* Vascular Headache Suppressants, Ergot Derivative–containing (Systemic)

## Dioxybenzone-containing Combinations
Dioxybenzone, Oxybenzone, and Padimate O (Topical)—*See* Sunscreen Agents (Topical)

## Diphenhydramine-containing Combinations
Bromodiphenhydramine, Diphenhydramine, Codeine, Ammonium Chloride, and Potassium Guaiacolsulfonate (Systemic)—*See* Cough/Cold Combinations (Systemic)
Diphenhydramine, Codeine, and Ammonium Chloride (Systemic)—*See* Cough/Cold Combinations (Systemic)
Diphenhydramine, Dextromethorphan, and Ammonium Chloride (Systemic)—*See* Cough/Cold Combinations (Systemic)
Diphenhydramine, Phenylephrine, and Dextromethorphan (Systemic)—*See* Cough/Cold Combinations (Systemic)
Diphenhydramine, Phenylpropanolamine, and Aspirin (Systemic)—*See* Antihistamines, Decongestants, and Analgesics (Systemic)
Diphenhydramine and Pseudoephedrine (Systemic)—*See* Antihistamines and Decongestants (Systemic)
Diphenhydramine, Pseudoephedrine, and Acetaminophen (Systemic)—*See* Antihistamines, Decongestants, and Analgesics (Systemic)
Ergotamine, Caffeine, and Diphenhydramine (Systemic)
Ergotamine, Caffeine, and Diphenhydramine (Systemic)—*See* Vascular Headache Suppressants, Ergot Derivative–containing (Systemic)

## Diphenoxylate-containing Combinations
*See* Diphenoxylate and Atropine (Systemic), 2230, XR

## Diphenylpyraline-containing Combinations
Diphenylpyraline, Phenylephrine, and Dextromethorphan (Systemic)—*See* Cough/Cold Combinations (Systemic)
Diphenylpyraline, Phenylpropanolamine, Acetaminophen, and Caffeine (Systemic)—*See* Antihistamines, Decongestants, and Analgesics (Systemic)

## Docusate-containing Combinations
Bisacodyl and Docusate (Oral-Local)—*See* Laxatives (Local)
Casanthranol and Docusate (Oral-Local)—*See* Laxatives (Local)
Danthron and Docusate (Oral-Local)—*See* Laxatives (Local)
Dehydrocholic Acid and Docusate (Oral-Local)—*See* Laxatives (Local)
Dehydrocholic Acid, Docusate, and Phenolphthalein (Oral-Local)—*See* Laxatives (Local)
Phenolphthalein and Docusate (Oral-Local)—*See* Laxatives (Local)
Sennosides and Docusate (Oral-Local)—*See* Laxatives (Local)

## Doxylamine-containing Combinations
Doxylamine, Codeine, and Acetaminophen (Systemic)—*See* Cough/Cold Combinations (Systemic)
Doxylamine, Etafedrine, and Codeine (Systemic)—*See* Cough/Cold Combinations (Systemic)
Doxylamine, Phenylpropanolamine, Dextromethorphan, and Aspirin (Systemic)—*See* Cough/Cold Combinations (Systemic)
Doxylamine, Pseudoephedrine, Dextromethorphan, and Acetaminophen (Systemic)—*See* Cough/Cold Combinations (Systemic)

## Enalapril-containing Combinations
Enalapril and Hydrochlorothiazide (Systemic)—*See* Angiotensin-converting Enzyme (ACE) Inhibitors and Hydrochlorothiazide (Systemic)

## Ephedrine-containing Combinations
Chlorpheniramine, Ephedrine, and Guaifenesin (Systemic)—*See* Cough/Cold Combinations (Systemic)
Chlorpheniramine, Ephedrine, Phenylephrine, and Carbetapentane (Systemic)—*See* Cough/Cold Combinations (Systemic)
Chlorpheniramine, Ephedrine, Phenylephrine, Dextromethorphan, Ammonium Chloride, and Ipecac (Systemic)—*See* Cough/Cold Combinations (Systemic)
Chlorpheniramine, Phenyltoloxamine, Ephedrine, Codeine, and Guaiacol Carbonate (Systemic)—*See* Cough/Cold Combinations (Systemic)
Ephedrine, Carbetapentane, and Guaifenesin (Systemic)—*See* Cough/Cold Combinations (Systemic)
Ephedrine and Guaifenesin (Systemic)—*See* Cough/Cold Combinations (Systemic)
Ephedrine and Potassium Iodide (Systemic)—*See* Cough/Cold Combinations (Systemic)
Theophylline, Ephedrine, Guaifenesin, and Phenobarbital (Systemic)
Theophylline, Ephedrine, and Hydroxyzine (Systemic)
Theophylline, Ephedrine, and Phenobarbital (Systemic)

## Epinephrine-containing Combinations
Articaine and Epinephrine (Systemic)
Bupivacaine and Epinephrine (Parenteral-Local)—*See* Anesthetics (Parenteral-Local)
Etidocaine and Epinephrine (Parenteral-Local)—*See* Anesthetics (Parenteral-Local)
Lidocaine and Epinephrine (Parenteral-Local)—*See* Anesthetics (Parenteral-Local)
Prilocaine and Epinephrine (Parenteral-Local)—*See* Anesthetics (Parenteral-Local)

**Ergotamine-containing Combinations**
　Ergotamine, Belladonna Alkaloids, and Phenobarbital (Systemic)
　Ergotamine and Caffeine (Systemic)—*See* Vascular Headache Suppressants, Ergot Derivative–containing (Systemic)
　Ergotamine, Caffeine, and Belladonna Alkaloids (Systemic)—*See* Vascular Headache Suppressants, Ergot Derivative–containing (Systemic)
　Ergotamine, Caffeine, Belladonna Alkaloids, and Pentobarbital (Systemic)—*See* Vascular Headache Suppressants, Ergot Derivative–containing (Systemic)
　Ergotamine, Caffeine, and Cyclizine (Systemic)
　Ergotamine, Caffeine, and Cyclizine (Systemic)—*See* Vascular Headache Suppressants, Ergot Derivative–containing (Systemic)
　Ergotamine, Caffeine, and Dimenhydrinate (Systemic)
　Ergotamine, Caffeine, and Dimenhydrinate (Systemic)—*See* Vascular Headache Suppressants, Ergot Derivative–containing (Systemic)
　Ergotamine, Caffeine, and Diphenhydramine (Systemic)
　Ergotamine, Caffeine, and Diphenhydramine (Systemic)—*See* Vascular Headache Suppressants, Ergot Derivative–containing (Systemic)

**Erythromycin-containing Combinations**
　Erythromycin and Benzoyl Peroxide (Topical)
　Erythromycin and Sulfisoxazole (Systemic)

**Esterified Estrogen–containing Combinations**
　Esterified Estrogens and Methyltestosterone (Systemic)—*See* Androgens and Estrogens (Systemic)

**Estradiol-containing Combinations**
　Testosterone and Estradiol (Systemic)—*See* Androgens and Estrogens (Systemic)

**Etafedrine-containing Combinations**
　Doxylamine, Etafedrine, and Hydrocodone (Systemic)—*See* Cough/Cold Combinations (Systemic)

**Ethinyl Estradiol–containing Combinations**
　Desogestrel and Ethinyl Estradiol (Systemic)—*See* Estrogens and Progestins (Systemic)
　Ethynodiol Diacetate and Ethinyl Estradiol (Systemic)—*See* Estrogens and Progestins (Systemic)
　Fluoxymesterone and Ethinyl Estradiol (Systemic)—*See* Androgens and Estrogens (Systemic)
　Levonorgestrel and Ethinyl Estradiol (Systemic)—*See* Estrogens and Progestins (Systemic)
　Norethindrone Acetate and Ethinyl Estradiol (Systemic)—*See* Estrogens and Progestins (Systemic)
　Norethindrone and Ethinyl Estradiol (Systemic)—*See* Estrogens and Progestins (Systemic)
　Norgestimate and Ethinyl Estradiol (Systemic)—*See* Estrogens and Progestins (Systemic)
　Norgestrel and Ethinyl Estradiol (Systemic)—*See* Estrogens and Progestins (Systemic)

**Etidocaine-containing Combinations**
　Etidocaine and Epinephrine (Parenteral-Local)—*See* Anesthetics (Parenteral-Local)

**Flumethasone-containing Combinations**
　Clioquinol and Flumethasone (Otic)
　Clioquinol and Flumethasone (Topical)

**Fluocinonide-containing Combinations**
　Fluocinonide, Procinonide, and Ciprocinonide (Topical)

**Fluoxymesterone-containing Combinations**
　Fluoxymesterone and Ethinyl Estradiol (Systemic)—*See* Androgens and Estrogens (Systemic)

**Framycetin-containing Combinations**
　Framycetin and Gramicidin (Topical)
　Framycetin, Gramicidin, and Dexamethasone (Ophthalmic)
　Framycetin, Gramicidin, and Dexamethasone (Otic)

**Glycerin-containing Combinations**
　Mineral Oil and Glycerin (Oral-Local)—*See* Laxatives (Local)
　Mineral Oil, Glycerin, and Phenolphthalein (Oral-Local)—*See* Laxatives (Local)

**Gramicidin-containing Combinations**
　Framycetin and Gramicidin (Topical)
　Framycetin, Gramicidin, and Dexamethasone (Ophthalmic)
　Framycetin, Gramicidin, and Dexamethasone (Otic)
　Neomycin, Polymyxin B, and Gramicidin (Ophthalmic)

**Guaifenesin-containing Combinations**
　Brompheniramine, Phenylephrine, Phenylpropanolamine, Codeine, and Guaifenesin (Systemic)—*See* Cough/Cold Combinations (Systemic)
　Brompheniramine, Phenylephrine, Phenylpropanolamine, and Guaifenesin (Systemic)—*See* Cough/Cold Combinations (Systemic)
　Brompheniramine, Phenylephrine, Phenylpropanolamine, Hydrocodone, and Guaifenesin (Systemic)—*See* Cough/Cold Combinations (Systemic)
　Chlorpheniramine, Ephedrine, and Guaifenesin (Systemic)—*See* Cough/Cold Combinations (Systemic)
　Chlorpheniramine, Phenylephrine, Dextromethorphan, and Guaifenesin (Systemic)—*See* Cough/Cold Combinations (Systemic)
　Chlorpheniramine, Phenylephrine, Dextromethorphan, Guaifenesin, and Ammonium Chloride (Systemic)—*See* Cough/Cold Combinations (Systemic)
　Chlorpheniramine, Phenylephrine, and Guaifenesin (Systemic)—*See* Cough/Cold Combinations (Systemic)
　Chlorpheniramine, Phenylpropanolamine, and Guaifenesin (Systemic)—*See* Cough/Cold Combinations (Systemic)
　Chlorpheniramine, Phenylpropanolamine, Guaifenesin, and Acetaminophen (Systemic)—*See* Cough/Cold Combinations (Systemic)
　Chlorpheniramine, Phenylpropanolamine, Guaifenesin, Sodium Citrate, and Citric Acid (Systemic)—*See* Cough/Cold Combinations (Systemic)
　Chlorpheniramine, Pseudoephedrine, Dextromethorphan, and Guaifenesin (Systemic)—*See* Cough/Cold Combinations (Systemic)
　Chlorpheniramine, Pseudoephedrine, and Guaifenesin (Systemic)—*See* Cough/Cold Combinations (Systemic)
　Codeine, Ammonium Chloride, and Guaifenesin (Systemic)—*See* Cough/Cold Combinations (Systemic)
　Codeine and Guaifenesin (Systemic)—*See* Cough/Cold Combinations (Systemic)
　Dexchlorpheniramine, Pseudoephedrine, and Guaifenesin (Systemic)—*See* Cough/Cold Combinations (Systemic)
　Dextromethorphan and Guaifenesin (Systemic)—*See* Cough/Cold Combinations (Systemic)
　Ephedrine, Carbetapentane, and Guaifenesin (Systemic)—*See* Cough/Cold Combinations (Systemic)
　Ephedrine and Guaifenesin (Systemic)—*See* Cough/Cold Combinations (Systemic)

**Guaifenesin-containing Combinations**
*(continued)*
　Hydrocodone and Guaifenesin (Systemic)—*See* Cough/Cold Combinations (Systemic)
　Hydromorphone and Guaifenesin (Systemic)—*See* Cough/Cold Combinations (Systemic)
　Oxtriphylline and Guaifenesin (Systemic)
　Pheniramine, Codeine, and Guaifenesin (Systemic)—*See* Cough/Cold Combinations (Systemic)
　Pheniramine, Phenylephrine, Phenylpropanolamine, Hydrocodone, and Guaifenesin (Systemic)—*See* Cough/Cold Combinations (Systemic)
　Pheniramine, Pyrilamine, Phenylpropanolamine, Hydrocodone, and Guaifenesin (Systemic)—*See* Cough/Cold Combinations (Systemic)
　Phenylephrine, Dextromethorphan, and Guaifenesin (Systemic)—*See* Cough/Cold Combinations (Systemic)
　Phenylephrine and Guaifenesin (Systemic)—*See* Cough/Cold Combinations (Systemic)
　Phenylephrine, Guaifenesin, Acetaminophen, Salicylamide, and Caffeine (Systemic)—*See* Cough/Cold Combinations (Systemic)
　Phenylephrine, Hydrocodone, and Guaifenesin (Systemic)—*See* Cough/Cold Combinations (Systemic)
　Phenylephrine, Phenylpropanolamine, and Guaifenesin (Systemic)—*See* Cough/Cold Combinations (Systemic)
　Phenylpropanolamine, Codeine, and Guaifenesin (Systemic)—*See* Cough/Cold Combinations (Systemic)
　Phenylpropanolamine, Dextromethorphan, and Guaifenesin (Systemic)—*See* Cough/Cold Combinations (Systemic)
　Phenylpropanolamine, Dextromethorphan, Guaifenesin, and Acetaminophen (Systemic)—*See* Cough/Cold Combinations (Systemic)
　Phenylpropanolamine and Guaifenesin (Systemic)—*See* Cough/Cold Combinations (Systemic)
　Pseudoephedrine, Codeine, and Guaifenesin (Systemic)—*See* Cough/Cold Combinations (Systemic)
　Pseudoephedrine, Dextromethorphan, and Guaifenesin (Systemic)—*See* Cough/Cold Combinations (Systemic)
　Pseudoephedrine, Dextromethorphan, Guaifenesin, and Acetaminophen (Systemic)—*See* Cough/Cold Combinations (Systemic)
　Pseudoephedrine and Guaifenesin (Systemic)—*See* Cough/Cold Combinations (Systemic)
　Pseudoephedrine, Hydrocodone, and Guaifenesin (Systemic)—*See* Cough/Cold Combinations (Systemic)
　Pyrilamine, Phenylpropanolamine, Dextromethorphan, Guaifenesin, Potassium Citrate, and Citric Acid (Systemic)—*See* Cough/Cold Combinations (Systemic)
　Theophylline, Ephedrine, Guaifenesin, and Phenobarbital (Systemic)
　Theophylline and Guaifenesin (Systemic)
　Triprolidine, Pseudoephedrine, Codeine, and Guaifenesin (Systemic)—*See* Cough/Cold Combinations (Systemic)

**Guanethidine-containing Combinations**
　Guanethidine and Hydrochlorothiazide (Systemic)

**Homatropine-containing Combinations**
　Hydrocodone and Homatropine (Systemic)—*See* Cough/Cold Combinations (Systemic)

## Homosalate-containing Combinations
Homosalate, Menthyl Anthranilate, and Octyl Methoxycinnamate (Topical)—*See* Sunscreen Agents (Topical)
Homosalate, Menthyl Anthranilate, Octyl Methoxycinnamate, Octyl Salicylate, and Oxybenzone (Topical)—*See* Sunscreen Agents (Topical)
Homosalate, Octocrylene, Octyl Methoxycinnamate, and Oxybenzone (Topical)—*See* Sunscreen Agents (Topical)
Homosalate, Octyl Methoxycinnamate, Octyl Salicylate, and Oxybenzone (Topical)—*See* Sunscreen Agents (Topical)
Homosalate, Octyl Methoxycinnamate, and Oxybenzone (Topical)—*See* Sunscreen Agents (Topical)
Homosalate and Oxybenzone (Topical)—*See* Sunscreen Agents (Topical)

## Hydralazine-containing Combinations
Hydralazine and Hydrochlorothiazide (Systemic)
Reserpine, Hydralazine, and Hydrochlorothiazide (Systemic)

## Hydrochlorothiazide-containing Combinations
Amiloride and Hydrochlorothiazide (Systemic)—*See* Diuretics, Potassium-sparing, and Hydrochlorothiazide (Systemic)
Bisoprolol and Hydrochlorothiazide (Systemic)—*See* Beta-adrenergic Blocking Agents and Thiazide Diuretics (Systemic)
Captopril and Hydrochlorothiazide (Systemic)—*See* Angiotensin-converting Enzyme (ACE) Inhibitors and Hydrochlorothiazide (Systemic)
Deserpidine and Hydrochlorothiazide (Systemic)—*See* Rauwolfia Alkaloids and Thiazide Diuretics (Systemic)
Enalapril and Hydrochlorothiazide (Systemic)—*See* Angiotensin-converting Enzyme (ACE) Inhibitors and Hydrochlorothiazide (Systemic)
Guanethidine and Hydrochlorothiazide (Systemic)
Hydralazine and Hydrochlorothiazide (Systemic)
Lisinopril and Hydrochlorothiazide (Systemic)—*See* Angiotensin-converting Enzyme (ACE) Inhibitors and Hydrochlorothiazide (Systemic)
Methyldopa and Hydrochlorothiazide (Systemic)—*See* Methyldopa and Thiazide Diuretics (Systemic)
Metoprolol and Hydrochlorothiazide (Systemic)—*See* Beta-adrenergic Blocking Agents and Thiazide Diuretics (Systemic)
Pindolol and Hydrochlorothiazide (Systemic)—*See* Beta-adrenergic Blocking Agents and Thiazide Diuretics (Systemic)
Propranolol and Hydrochlorothiazide (Systemic)—*See* Beta-adrenergic Blocking Agents and Thiazide Diuretics (Systemic)
Reserpine, Hydralazine, and Hydrochlorothiazide (Systemic)
Reserpine and Hydrochlorothiazide (Systemic)—*See* Rauwolfia Alkaloids and Thiazide Diuretics (Systemic)
Spironolactone and Hydrochlorothiazide (Systemic)—*See* Diuretics, Potassium-sparing, and Hydrochlorothiazide (Systemic)
Timolol and Hydrochlorothiazide (Systemic)—*See* Beta-adrenergic Blocking Agents and Thiazide Diuretics (Systemic)
Triamterene and Hydrochlorothiazide (Systemic)—*See* Diuretics, Potassium-sparing, and Hydrochlorothiazide (Systemic)

## Hydrocodone-containing Combinations
Brompheniramine, Phenylephrine, Phenylpropanolamine, Hydrocodone, and Guaifenesin (Systemic)—*See* Cough/Cold Combinations (Systemic)
Chlorpheniramine and Hydrocodone (Systemic)—*See* Cough/Cold Combinations (Systemic)
Chlorpheniramine, Pheniramine, Pyrilamine, Phenylephrine, Hydrocodone, Salicylamide, Caffeine, and Ascorbic Acid (Systemic)—*See* Cough/Cold Combinations (Systemic)
Chlorpheniramine, Phenylephrine, and Hydrocodone (Systemic)—*See* Cough/Cold Combinations (Systemic)
Chlorpheniramine, Phenylephrine, Hydrocodone, Acetaminophen, and Caffeine (Systemic)—*See* Cough/Cold Combinations (Systemic)
Chlorpheniramine, Pseudoephedrine, and Hydrocodone (Systemic)—*See* Cough/Cold Combinations (Systemic)
Doxylamine, Etafedrine, and Hydrocodone (Systemic)—*See* Cough/Cold Combinations (Systemic)
Hydrocodone and Acetaminophen (Systemic)—*See* Opioid (Narcotic) Analgesics and Acetaminophen (Systemic)
Hydrocodone and Aspirin (Systemic)—*See* Opioid (Narcotic) Analgesics and Aspirin (Systemic)
Hydrocodone and Guaifenesin (Systemic)—*See* Cough/Cold Combinations (Systemic)
Hydrocodone and Homatropine (Systemic)—*See* Cough/Cold Combinations (Systemic)
Hydrocodone and Potassium Guaiacolsulfonate (Systemic)—*See* Cough/Cold Combinations (Systemic)
Pheniramine, Phenylephrine, Phenylpropanolamine, Hydrocodone, and Guaifenesin (Systemic)—*See* Cough/Cold Combinations (Systemic)
Pheniramine, Pyrilamine, Hydrocodone, Potassium Citrate, and Ascorbic Acid (Systemic)—*See* Cough/Cold Combinations (Systemic)
Pheniramine, Pyrilamine, Phenylephrine, Phenylpropanolamine, and Hydrocodone (Systemic)—*See* Cough/Cold Combinations (Systemic)
Pheniramine, Pyrilamine, Phenylpropanolamine, and Hydrocodone (Systemic)—*See* Cough/Cold Combinations (Systemic)
Pheniramine, Pyrilamine, Phenylpropanolamine, Hydrocodone, and Guaifenesin (Systemic)—*See* Cough/Cold Combinations (Systemic)
Phenylephrine and Hydrocodone (Systemic)—*See* Cough/Cold Combinations (Systemic)
Phenylephrine, Hydrocodone, and Guaifenesin (Systemic)—*See* Cough/Cold Combinations (Systemic)
Phenylpropanolamine and Hydrocodone (Systemic)—*See* Cough/Cold Combinations (Systemic)
Phenylpropanolamine, Hydrocodone, Dextromethorphan, and Acetaminophen (Systemic)—*See* Cough/Cold Combinations (Systemic)
Phenyltoloxamine and Hydrocodone (Systemic)—*See* Cough/Cold Combinations (Systemic)
Pseudoephedrine and Hydrocodone (Systemic)—*See* Cough/Cold Combinations (Systemic)
Pseudoephedrine, Hydrocodone, and Guaifenesin (Systemic)—*See* Cough/Cold Combinations (Systemic)
Pseudoephedrine, Hydrocodone, and Potassium Guaiacolsulfonate (Systemic)—*See* Cough/Cold Combinations (Systemic)
Pyrilamine, Phenylephrine, and Hydrocodone (Systemic)—*See* Cough/Cold Combinations (Systemic)
Pyrilamine, Phenylephrine, Hydrocodone, and Ammonium Chloride (Systemic)—*See* Cough/Cold Combinations (Systemic)

## Hydrocortisone-containing Combinations
Clioquinol and Hydrocortisone (Topical)
Colistin, Neomycin, and Hydrocortisone (Otic)
Hydrocortisone and Acetic Acid (Otic)—*See* Corticosteroids and Acetic Acid (Otic)
Hydrocortisone and Urea (Topical)
Neomycin, Polymyxin B, and Hydrocortisone (Ophthalmic)
Neomycin, Polymyxin B, and Hydrocortisone (Otic)

## Hydroflumethiazide-containing Combinations
Reserpine and Hydroflumethiazide (Systemic)—*See* Rauwolfia Alkaloids and Thiazide Diuretics (Systemic)

## Hydromorphone-containing Combinations
Hydromorphone and Guaifenesin (Systemic)—*See* Cough/Cold Combinations (Systemic)

## Hydroxyzine-containing Combinations
Theophylline, Ephedrine, and Hydroxyzine (Systemic)

## Hyoscyamine-containing Combinations
Atropine, Hyoscyamine, Methenamine, Methylene Blue, Phenyl Salicylate, and Benzoic Acid (Systemic)
Atropine, Hyoscyamine, Scopolamine, and Phenobarbital (Systemic)—*See* Belladonna Alkaloids and Barbiturates (Systemic)
Chlorpheniramine, Phenylephrine, Phenylpropanolamine, Atropine, Hyoscyamine, and Scopolamine (Systemic)—*See* Antihistamines, Decongestants, and Anticholinergics (Systemic)
Hyoscyamine and Phenobarbital (Systemic)—*See* Belladonna Alkaloids and Barbiturates (Systemic)
Kaolin, Pectin, Hyoscyamine, Atropine, and Scopolamine (Systemic)—*See* Kaolin, Pectin, and Belladonna Alkaloids (Systemic)

## Ibuprofen-containing Combinations
Pseudoephedrine and Ibuprofen (Systemic)—*See* Decongestants and Analgesics (Systemic)

## Imipenem-containing Combinations
Imipenem and Cilastatin (Systemic)

## Iodine-containing Combinations
Chlorpheniramine, Phenylephrine, Codeine, and Potassium Iodide (Systemic)—*See* Cough/Cold Combinations (Systemic)
Codeine and Calcium Iodide (Systemic)—*See* Cough/Cold Combinations (Systemic)
Codeine and Iodinated Glycerol (Systemic)—*See* Cough/Cold Combinations (Systemic)
Dextromethorphan and Iodinated Glycerol (Systemic)—*See* Cough/Cold Combinations (Systemic)
Ephedrine and Potassium Iodide (Systemic)—*See* Cough/Cold Combinations (Systemic)

## Iodipamide-containing Combinations
Diatrizoate and Iodipamide (Local)

## Ipecac-containing Combinations
Brompheniramine, Phenylephrine, Phenylpropanolamine, Dextromethorphan, Potassium Guaiacolsulfonate, and Ipecac (Systemic)—*See* Cough/Cold Combinations (Systemic)
Chlorpheniramine, Ephedrine, Phenylephrine, Dextromethorphan, Ammonium Chloride, and Ipecac (Systemic)—*See* Cough/Cold Combinations (Systemic)
Chlorpheniramine, Phenylephrine, Phenylpropanolamine, Dextromethorphan, Potassium Guaiacolsulfonate, and Ipecac (Systemic)—*See* Cough/Cold Combinations (Systemic)

### Isometheptene-containing Combinations
Isometheptene, Dichloralphenazone, and Acetaminophen (Systemic)

### Isoniazid-containing Combinations
Isoniazid and Thiacetazone (Systemic)
Rifampin and Isoniazid (Systemic)
Rifampin, Isoniazid, and Pyrazinamide (Systemic)

### Isoproterenol-containing Combinations
Isoproterenol and Phenylephrine (Systemic)

### Kaolin-containing Combinations
Kaolin and Pectin (Oral-Local)
Kaolin, Pectin, Hyoscyamine, Atropine, and Scopolamine (Systemic)—*See* Kaolin, Pectin, and Belladonna Alkaloids (Systemic)
Kaolin, Pectin, and Paregoric (Systemic)

### Levodopa-containing Combinations
Carbidopa and Levodopa (Systemic)
Levodopa and Benserazide (Systemic)

### Levonordefrin-containing Combinations
Mepivacaine and Levonordefrin (Parenteral-Local)—*See* Anesthetics (Parenteral-Local)
Propoxycaine, Procaine, and Levonordefrin (Parenteral-Local)—*See* Anesthetics (Parenteral-Local)

### Lidocaine-containing Combinations
Lidocaine and Epinephrine (Parenteral-Local)—*See* Anesthetics (Parenteral-Local)
Lidocaine and Prilocaine (Topical)

### Lisadimate-containing Combinations
Lisadimate, Oxybenzone, and Padimate O (Topical)—*See* Sunscreen Agents (Topical)
Lisadimate and Padimate O (Topical)—*See* Sunscreen Agents (Topical)

### Lisinopril-containing Combinations
Lisinopril and Hydrochlorothiazide (Systemic)—*See* Angiotensin-converting Enzyme (ACE) Inhibitors and Hydrochlorothiazide (Systemic)

### Loratadine-containing Combinations
Loratadine and Pseudoephedrine (Systemic)—*See* Antihistamines and Decongestants (Systemic)

### Magaldrate-containing Combinations
Magaldrate and Simethicone (Oral-Local)—*See* Antacids (Oral-Local)

### Magnesia-containing Combinations
Alumina and Magnesia (Oral-Local)—*See* Antacids (Oral-Local)
Alumina, Magnesia, and Calcium Carbonate (Oral-Local)—*See* Antacids (Oral-Local)
Alumina, Magnesia, Calcium Carbonate, and Simethicone (Oral-Local)—*See* Antacids (Oral-Local)
Alumina, Magnesia, and Simethicone (Oral-Local)—*See* Antacids (Oral-Local)
Aspirin, Buffered (Systemic)—*See* Salicylates (Systemic)
Aspirin and Codeine, Buffered (Systemic)—*See* Opioid (Narcotic) Analgesics and Aspirin (Systemic)
Calcium Carbonate and Magnesia (Oral-Local)—*See* Antacids (Oral-Local)
Calcium Carbonate, Magnesia, and Simethicone (Oral-Local)—*See* Antacids (Oral-Local)
Magnesium Hydroxide and Cascara Sagrada (Oral-Local)—*See* Laxatives (Local)
Magnesium Hydroxide and Mineral Oil (Oral-Local)—*See* Laxatives (Local)
Simethicone, Alumina, Magnesium Carbonate, and Magnesia (Oral-Local)—*See* Antacids (Oral-Local)

### Magnesium Carbonate–containing Combinations
Alumina and Magnesium Carbonate (Oral-Local)—*See* Antacids (Oral-Local)
Calcium and Magnesium Carbonates (Oral-Local)—*See* Antacids (Oral-Local)
Calcium and Magnesium Carbonates and Magnesium Oxide (Oral-Local)—*See* Antacids (Oral-Local)
Citric Acid, Glucono-deltalactone, and Magnesium Carbonate (Systemic)

### Magnesium Carbonate–containing Combinations *(continued)*
Magnesium Carbonate and Sodium Bicarbonate (Oral-Local)—*See* Antacids (Oral-Local)
Simethicone, Alumina, Magnesium Carbonate, and Magnesia (Oral-Local)—*See* Antacids (Oral-Local)

### Magnesium Oxide–containing Combinations
Aspirin, Buffered (Systemic)—*See* Salicylates (Systemic)
Calcium and Magnesium Carbonates and Magnesium Oxide (Oral-Local)—*See* Antacids (Oral-Local)

### Magnesium Salicylate–containing Combinations
Choline and Magnesium Salicylates (Systemic)—*See* Salicylates (Systemic)

### Magnesium Trisilicate–containing Combinations
Alumina and Magnesium Trisilicate (Oral-Local)—*See* Antacids (Oral-Local)
Alumina, Magnesium Trisilicate, and Sodium Bicarbonate (Oral-Local)—*See* Antacids (Oral-Local)

### Malt Soup Extract–containing Combinations
Malt Soup Extract and Psyllium (Oral-Local)—*See* Laxatives (Local)

### Medroxyprogesterone–containing Combinations
Conjugated Estrogens and Medroxyprogesterone Tablets (Systemic)—*See* Conjugated Estrogens and Medroxyprogesterone for Ovarian Hormone Therapy (OHT) (Systemic)
Conjugated Estrogens Tablets USP, and Conjugated Estrogens and Medroxyprogesterone Tablets (Systemic)—*See* Conjugated Estrogens and Medroxyprogesterone for Ovarian Hormone Therapy (OHT) (Systemic)

### Menthyl Anthranilate-containing Combinations
Homosalate, Menthyl Anthranilate, and Octyl Methoxycinnamate (Topical)—*See* Sunscreen Agents (Topical)
Homosalate, Menthyl Anthranilate, Octyl Methoxycinnamate, and Octyl Salicylate (Topical)—*See* Sunscreen Agents (Topical)
Homosalate, Menthyl Anthranilate, Octyl Methoxycinnamate, Octyl Salicylate, and Oxybenzone (Topical)—*See* Sunscreen Agents (Topical)
Homosalate, Menthyl Anthranilate, Octyl Methoxycinnamate, and Oxybenzone (Topical)—*See* Sunscreen Agents (Topical)
Menthyl Anthranilate, Octocrylene, and Octyl Methoxycinnamate (Topical)—*See* Sunscreen Agents (Topical)
Menthyl Anthranilate, Octocrylene, Octyl Methoxycinnamate, and Oxybenzone (Topical)—*See* Sunscreen Agents (Topical)
Menthyl Anthranilate and Octyl Methoxycinnamate (Topical)—*See* Sunscreen Agents (Topical)
Menthyl Anthranilate, Octyl Methoxycinnamate, and Octyl Salicylate (Topical)—*See* Sunscreen Agents (Topical)
Menthyl Anthranilate, Octyl Methoxycinnamate, Octyl Salicylate, and Oxybenzone (Topical)—*See* Sunscreen Agents (Topical)
Menthyl Anthranilate, Octyl Methoxycinnamate, and Oxybenzone (Topical)—*See* Sunscreen Agents (Topical)
Menthyl Anthranilate and Padimate O (Topical)—*See* Sunscreen Agents (Topical)
Menthyl Anthranilate and Titanium Dioxide (Topical)—*See* Sunscreen Agents (Topical)

### Mepivacaine-containing Combinations
Mepivacaine and Levonordefrin (Parenteral-Local)—*See* Anesthetics (Parenteral-Local)

### Meprobamate-containing Combinations
Meprobamate and Aspirin (Systemic)

### Mestranol–containing Combinations
Norethindrone and Mestranol (Systemic)—*See* Estrogens and Progestins (Systemic)

### Methenamine-containing Combinations
Atropine, Hyoscyamine, Methenamine, Methylene Blue, Phenyl Salicylate, and Benzoic Acid (Systemic)

### Methscopolamine-containing Combinations
Chlorpheniramine, Phenylephrine, and Methscopolamine (Systemic)—*See* Antihistamines, Decongestants, and Anticholinergics (Systemic)
Chlorpheniramine, Phenylpropanolamine, and Methscopolamine (Systemic)—*See* Antihistamines, Decongestants, and Anticholinergics (Systemic)
Chlorpheniramine, Pseudoephedrine, and Methscopolamine (Systemic)—*See* Antihistamines, Decongestants, and Anticholinergics (Systemic)

### Methyclothiazide-containing Combinations
Deserpidine and Methyclothiazide (Systemic)—*See* Rauwolfia Alkaloids and Thiazide Diuretics (Systemic)
Reserpine and Methyclothiazide (Systemic)—*See* Rauwolfia Alkaloids and Thiazide Diuretics (Systemic)

### Methyldopa-containing Combinations
Methyldopa and Chlorothiazide (Systemic)—*See* Methyldopa and Thiazide Diuretics (Systemic)
Methyldopa and Hydrochlorothiazide (Systemic)—*See* Methyldopa and Thiazide Diuretics (Systemic)

### Methyltestosterone-containing Combinations
Conjugated Estrogens and Methyltestosterone (Systemic)—*See* Androgens and Estrogens (Systemic)
Diethylstilbestrol and Methyltestosterone (Systemic)—*See* Androgens and Estrogens (Systemic)
Esterified Estrogens and Methyltestosterone (Systemic)—*See* Androgens and Estrogens (Systemic)

### Metoprolol-containing Combinations
Metoprolol and Hydrochlorothiazide (Systemic)—*See* Beta-adrenergic Blocking Agents and Thiazide Diuretics (Systemic)

### Metronidazole-containing Combinations
Metronidazole and Nystatin (Vaginal)

### Mineral Oil–containing Combinations
Magnesium Hydroxide and Mineral Oil (Oral-Local)—*See* Laxatives (Local)
Mineral Oil and Cascara Sagrada (Oral-Local)—*See* Laxatives (Local)
Mineral Oil and Glycerin (Oral-Local)—*See* Laxatives (Local)
Mineral Oil, Glycerin, and Phenolphthalein (Oral-Local)—*See* Laxatives (Local)
Mineral Oil and Phenolphthalein (Oral-Local)—*See* Laxatives (Local)

### Nadolol-containing Combinations
Nadolol and Bendroflumethiazide (Systemic)—*See* Beta-adrenergic Blocking Agents and Thiazide Diuretics (Systemic)

### Naloxone-containing Combinations
Pentazocine and Naloxone (Systemic)—*See* Opioid (Narcotic) Analgesics (Systemic)

### Neomycin-containing Combinations
Colistin, Neomycin, and Hydrocortisone (Otic)
Neomycin and Polymyxin B (Topical)
Neomycin, Polymyxin B, and Bacitracin (Ophthalmic)
Neomycin, Polymyxin B, and Bacitracin (Topical)
Neomycin, Polymyxin B, and Gramicidin (Ophthalmic)
Neomycin, Polymyxin B, and Hydrocortisone (Ophthalmic)
Neomycin, Polymyxin B, and Hydrocortisone (Otic)

## Norepinephrine-containing Combinations
Propoxycaine, Procaine, and Norepinephrine (Parenteral-Local)—*See* Anesthetics (Parenteral-Local)

## Nystatin-containing Combinations
Metronidazole and Nystatin (Vaginal)
Nystatin and Triamcinolone (Topical)

## Octocrylene-containing Combinations
Avobenzone, Octocrylene, Octyl Salicylate, and Oxybenzone (Topical)—*See* Sunscreen Agents (Topical)
Homosalate, Octocrylene, Octyl Methoxycinnamate, and Oxybenzone (Topical)—*See* Sunscreen Agents (Topical)
Menthyl Anthranilate, Octocrylene, and Octyl Methoxycinnamate (Topical)—*See* Sunscreen Agents (Topical)
Menthyl Anthranilate, Octocrylene, Octyl Methoxycinnamate, and Oxybenzone (Topical)—*See* Sunscreen Agents (Topical)
Octocrylene and Octyl Methoxycinnamate (Topical)—*See* Sunscreen Agents (Topical)
Octocrylene, Octyl Methoxycinnamate, Octyl Salicylate, and Oxybenzone (Topical)—*See* Sunscreen Agents (Topical)
Octocrylene, Octyl Methoxycinnamate, Octyl Salicylate, Oxybenzone, and Titanium Dioxide (Topical)—*See* Sunscreen Agents (Topical)
Octocrylene, Octyl Methoxycinnamate, and Oxybenzone (Topical)—*See* Sunscreen Agents (Topical)
Octocrylene, Octyl Methoxycinnamate, Oxybenzone, and Titanium Dioxide (Topical)—*See* Sunscreen Agents (Topical)
Octocrylene, Octyl Methoxycinnamate, and Titanium Dioxide (Topical)—*See* Sunscreen Agents (Topical)

## Octyl Methoxycinnamate-containing Combinations
Avobenzone and Octyl Methoxycinnamate (Topical)—*See* Sunscreen Agents (Topical)
Avobenzone, Octyl Methoxycinnamate, Octyl Salicylate, and Oxybenzone (Topical)—*See* Sunscreen Agents (Topical)
Avobenzone, Octyl Methoxycinnamate, and Oxybenzone (Topical)—*See* Sunscreen Agents (Topical)
Homosalate, Menthyl Anthranilate, and Octyl Methoxycinnamate (Topical)—*See* Sunscreen Agents (Topical)
Homosalate, Menthyl Anthranilate, Octyl Methoxycinnamate, Octyl Salicylate, and Oxybenzone (Topical)—*See* Sunscreen Agents (Topical)
Homosalate, Octocrylene, Octyl Methoxycinnamate, and Oxybenzone (Topical)—*See* Sunscreen Agents (Topical)
Homosalate, Octyl Methoxycinnamate, Octyl Salicylate, and Oxybenzone (Topical)—*See* Sunscreen Agents (Topical)
Homosalate, Octyl Methoxycinnamate, and Oxybenzone (Topical)—*See* Sunscreen Agents (Topical)
Menthyl Anthranilate, Octocrylene, and Octyl Methoxycinnamate (Topical)—*See* Sunscreen Agents (Topical)
Menthyl Anthranilate, Octocrylene, Octyl Methoxycinnamate, and Oxybenzone (Topical)—*See* Sunscreen Agents (Topical)
Menthyl Anthranilate and Octyl Methoxycinnamate (Topical)—*See* Sunscreen Agents (Topical)
Menthyl Anthranilate, Octyl Methoxycinnamate, and Octyl Salicylate (Topical)—*See* Sunscreen Agents (Topical)
Menthyl Anthranilate, Octyl Methoxycinnamate, Octyl Salicylate, and Oxybenzone (Topical)—*See* Sunscreen Agents (Topical)
Menthyl Anthranilate, Octyl Methoxycinnamate, and Oxybenzone (Topical)—*See* Sunscreen Agents (Topical)
Octocrylene and Octyl Methoxycinnamate (Topical)—*See* Sunscreen Agents (Topical)

## Octyl Methoxycinnamate-containing Combinations *(continued)*
Octocrylene, Octyl Methoxycinnamate, Octyl Salicylate, and Oxybenzone (Topical)—*See* Sunscreen Agents (Topical)
Octocrylene, Octyl Methoxycinnamate, Octyl Salicylate, Oxybenzone, and Titanium Dioxide (Topical)—*See* Sunscreen Agents (Topical)
Octocrylene, Octyl Methoxycinnamate, and Oxybenzone (Topical)—*See* Sunscreen Agents (Topical)
Octocrylene, Octyl Methoxycinnamate, Oxybenzone, and Titanium Dioxide (Topical)—*See* Sunscreen Agents (Topical)
Octocrylene, Octyl Methoxycinnamate, and Titanium Dioxide (Topical)—*See* Sunscreen Agents (Topical)
Octyl Methoxycinnamate and Octyl Salicylate (Topical)—*See* Sunscreen Agents (Topical)
Octyl Methoxycinnamate, Octyl Salicylate, and Oxybenzone (Topical)—*See* Sunscreen Agents (Topical)
Octyl Methoxycinnamate, Octyl Salicylate, Oxybenzone, and Padimate O (Topical)—*See* Sunscreen Agents (Topical)
Octyl Methoxycinnamate, Octyl Salicylate, Oxybenzone, Padimate O, and Titanium Dioxide (Topical)—*See* Sunscreen Agents (Topical)
Octyl Methoxycinnamate, Octyl Salicylate, Oxybenzone, Phenylbenzimidazole, and Titanium Dioxide (Topical)—*See* Sunscreen Agents (Topical)
Octyl Methoxycinnamate, Octyl Salicylate, Oxybenzone, and Titanium Dioxide (Topical)—*See* Sunscreen Agents (Topical)
Octyl Methoxycinnamate, Octyl Salicylate, Phenylbenzimidazole, and Titanium Dioxide (Topical)—*See* Sunscreen Agents (Topical)
Octyl Methoxycinnamate, Octyl Salicylate, and Titanium Dioxide (Topical)—*See* Sunscreen Agents (Topical)
Octyl Methoxycinnamate and Oxybenzone (Topical)—*See* Sunscreen Agents (Topical)
Octyl Methoxycinnamate, Oxybenzone, and Padimate O (Topical)—*See* Sunscreen Agents (Topical)
Octyl Methoxycinnamate, Oxybenzone, Padimate O, and Titanium Dioxide (Topical)—*See* Sunscreen Agents (Topical)
Octyl Methoxycinnamate, Oxybenzone, and Titanium Dioxide (Topical)—*See* Sunscreen Agents (Topical)
Octyl Methoxycinnamate and Padimate O (Topical)—*See* Sunscreen Agents (Topical)
Octyl Methoxycinnamate and Phenylbenzimidazole (Topical)—*See* Sunscreen Agents (Topical)

## Octyl Salicylate-containing Combinations
Avobenzone, Octocrylene, Octyl Salicylate, and Oxybenzone (Topical)—*See* Sunscreen Agents (Topical)
Avobenzone, Octyl Methoxycinnamate, Octyl Salicylate, and Oxybenzone (Topical)—*See* Sunscreen Agents (Topical)
Homosalate, Menthyl Anthranilate, Octyl Methoxycinnamate, Octyl Salicylate, and Oxybenzone (Topical)—*See* Sunscreen Agents (Topical)
Homosalate, Octyl Methoxycinnamate, Octyl Salicylate, and Oxybenzone (Topical)—*See* Sunscreen Agents (Topical)
Menthyl Anthranilate, Octyl Methoxycinnamate, and Octyl Salicylate (Topical)—*See* Sunscreen Agents (Topical)
Menthyl Anthranilate, Octyl Methoxycinnamate, Octyl Salicylate, and Oxybenzone (Topical)—*See* Sunscreen Agents (Topical)
Octocrylene, Octyl Methoxycinnamate, Octyl Salicylate, and Oxybenzone (Topical)—*See* Sunscreen Agents (Topical)
Octocrylene, Octyl Methoxycinnamate, Octyl Salicylate, Oxybenzone, and Titanium Diox-

## Octyl Salicylate-containing Combinations *(continued)*
ide (Topical)—*See* Sunscreen Agents (Topical)
Octyl Methoxycinnamate and Octyl Salicylate (Topical)—*See* Sunscreen Agents (Topical)
Octyl Methoxycinnamate, Octyl Salicylate, and Oxybenzone (Topical)—*See* Sunscreen Agents (Topical)
Octyl Methoxycinnamate, Octyl Salicylate, Oxybenzone, and Padimate O (Topical)—*See* Sunscreen Agents (Topical)
Octyl Methoxycinnamate, Octyl Salicylate, Oxybenzone, Padimate O, and Titanium Dioxide (Topical)—*See* Sunscreen Agents (Topical)
Octyl Methoxycinnamate, Octyl Salicylate, Oxybenzone, Phenylbenzimidazole, and Titanium Dioxide (Topical)—*See* Sunscreen Agents (Topical)
Octyl Methoxycinnamate, Octyl Salicylate, Oxybenzone, and Titanium Dioxide (Topical)—*See* Sunscreen Agents (Topical)
Octyl Methoxycinnamate, Octyl Salicylate, Phenylbenzimidazole, and Titanium Dioxide (Topical)—*See* Sunscreen Agents (Topical)
Octyl Methoxycinnamate, Octyl Salicylate, and Titanium Dioxide (Topical)—*See* Sunscreen Agents (Topical)
Octyl Salicylate and Padimate O (Topical)—*See* Sunscreen Agents (Topical)

## Orphenadrine-containing Combinations
Orphenadrine, Aspirin, and Caffeine (Systemic)—*See* Orphenadrine and Aspirin (Systemic)

## Oxtriphylline-containing Combinations
Oxtriphylline and Guaifenesin (Systemic)

## Oxybenzone-containing Combinations
Aminobenzoic Acid, Padimate O, and Oxybenzone (Topical)—*See* Sunscreen Agents (Topical)
Avobenzone, Octocrylene, Octyl Salicylate, and Oxybenzone Sunscreen Agents (Topical)
Avobenzone, Octyl Methoxycinnamate, Octyl Salicylate, and Oxybenzone (Topical)—*See* Sunscreen Agents (Topical)
Avobenzone, Octyl Methoxycinnamate, and Oxybenzone Sunscreen Agents (Topical)
Dioxybenzone, Oxybenzone, and Padimate O (Topical)—*See* Sunscreen Agents (Topical)
Homosalate, Menthyl Anthranilate, Octyl Methoxycinnamate, Octyl Salicylate, and Oxybenzone (Topical)—*See* Sunscreen Agents (Topical)
Homosalate, Octocrylene, Octyl Methoxycinnamate, and Oxybenzone (Topical)—*See* Sunscreen Agents (Topical)
Homosalate, Octyl Methoxycinnamate, Octyl Salicylate, and Oxybenzone (Topical)—*See* Sunscreen Agents (Topical)
Homosalate, Octyl Methoxycinnamate, and Oxybenzone (Topical)—*See* Sunscreen Agents (Topical)
Homosalate and Oxybenzone (Topical)—*See* Sunscreen Agents (Topical)
Lisadimate, Oxybenzone, and Padimate O (Topical)—*See* Sunscreen Agents (Topical)
Menthyl Anthranilate, Octocrylene, Octyl Methoxycinnamate, and Oxybenzone (Topical)—*See* Sunscreen Agents (Topical)
Menthyl Anthranilate, Octyl Methoxycinnamate, Octyl Salicylate, and Oxybenzone (Topical)—*See* Sunscreen Agents (Topical)
Menthyl Anthranilate, Octyl Methoxycinnamate, and Oxybenzone (Topical)—*See* Sunscreen Agents (Topical)
Octocrylene, Octyl Methoxycinnamate, Octyl Salicylate, and Oxybenzone (Topical)—*See* Sunscreen Agents (Topical)
Octocrylene, Octyl Methoxycinnamate, Octyl Salicylate, Oxybenzone, and Titanium Dioxide (Topical)—*See* Sunscreen Agents (Topical)

## Oxybenzone-containing Combinations
(continued)
Octocrylene, Octyl Methoxycinnamate, and Oxybenzone (Topical)—See Sunscreen Agents (Topical)
Octocrylene, Octyl Methoxycinnamate, Oxybenzone, and Titanium Dioxide (Topical)—See Sunscreen Agents (Topical)
Octyl Methoxycinnamate, Octyl Salicylate, and Oxybenzone (Topical)—See Sunscreen Agents (Topical)
Octyl Methoxycinnamate, Octyl Salicylate, Oxybenzone, and Padimate O (Topical)—See Sunscreen Agents (Topical)
Octyl Methoxycinnamate, Octyl Salicylate, Oxybenzone, Padimate O, and Titanium Dioxide (Topical)—See Sunscreen Agents (Topical)
Octyl Methoxycinnamate, Octyl Salicylate, Oxybenzone, Phenylbenzimidazole, and Titanium Dioxide (Topical)—See Sunscreen Agents (Topical)
Octyl Methoxycinnamate, Octyl Salicylate, Oxybenzone, and Titanium Dioxide (Topical)—See Sunscreen Agents (Topical)
Octyl Methoxycinnamate and Oxybenzone (Topical)—See Sunscreen Agents (Topical)
Octyl Methoxycinnamate, Oxybenzone, and Padimate O (Topical)—See Sunscreen Agents (Topical)
Octyl Methoxycinnamate, Oxybenzone, Padimate O, and Titanium Dioxide (Topical)—See Sunscreen Agents (Topical)
Octyl Methoxycinnamate, Oxybenzone, and Titanium Dioxide (Topical)—See Sunscreen Agents (Topical)
Oxybenzone and Padimate O (Topical)—See Sunscreen Agents (Topical)
Oxybenzone and Roxadimate (Topical)—See Sunscreen Agents (Topical)

## Oxycodone-containing Combinations
Oxycodone and Acetaminophen (Systemic)—See Opioid (Narcotic) Analgesics and Acetaminophen (Systemic)
Oxycodone and Aspirin (Systemic)—See Opioid (Narcotic) Analgesics and Aspirin (Systemic)

## Padimate O-containing Combinations
Aminobenzoic Acid, Padimate O, and Oxybenzone (Topical)—See Sunscreen Agents (Topical)
Dioxybenzone, Oxybenzone, and Padimate O (Topical)—See Sunscreen Agents (Topical)
Lisadimate, Oxybenzone, and Padimate O (Topical)—See Sunscreen Agents (Topical)
Lisadimate and Padimate O (Topical)—See Sunscreen Agents (Topical)
Menthyl Anthranilate and Padimate O (Topical)—See Sunscreen Agents (Topical)
Octyl Methoxycinnamate, Octyl Salicylate, Oxybenzone, and Padimate O (Topical)—See Sunscreen Agents (Topical)
Octyl Methoxycinnamate, Octyl Salicylate, Oxybenzone, Padimate O, and Titanium Dioxide (Topical)—See Sunscreen Agents (Topical)
Octyl Methoxycinnamate, Oxybenzone, and Padimate O (Topical)—See Sunscreen Agents (Topical)
Octyl Methoxycinnamate, Oxybenzone, Padimate O, and Titanium Dioxide (Topical)—See Sunscreen Agents (Topical)
Octyl Methoxycinnamate and Padimate O (Topical)—See Sunscreen Agents (Topical)
Octyl Salicylate and Padimate O (Topical)—See Sunscreen Agents (Topical)
Oxybenzone and Padimate O (Topical)—See Sunscreen Agents (Topical)

## Paregoric-containing Combinations
Kaolin, Pectin, and Paregoric (Systemic)

## Pectin-containing Combinations
Kaolin and Pectin (Oral-Local)
Kaolin, Pectin, Hyoscyamine, Atropine, and Scopolamine (Systemic)—See Kaolin, Pectin, and Belladonna Alkaloids (Systemic)
Kaolin, Pectin, and Paregoric (Systemic)

## Pentazocine-containing Combinations
Pentazocine and Acetaminophen (Systemic)—See Opioid (Narcotic) Analgesics and Acetaminophen (Systemic)
Pentazocine and Aspirin (Systemic)—See Opioid (Narcotic) Analgesics and Aspirin (Systemic)
Pentazocine and Naloxone (Systemic)—See Opioid (Narcotic) Analgesics (Systemic)

## Pentobarbital-containing Combinations
Ergotamine, Caffeine, Belladonna Alkaloids, and Pentobarbital (Systemic)—See Vascular Headache Suppressants, Ergot Derivative–containing (Systemic)

## Perphenazine-containing Combinations
Perphenazine and Amitriptyline (Systemic)

## Phenazopyridine-containing Combinations
Sulfamethoxazole and Phenazopyridine (Systemic)—See Sulfonamides and Phenazopyridine (Systemic)
Sulfisoxazole and Phenazopyridine (Systemic)—See Sulfonamides and Phenazopyridine (Systemic)

## Phenindamine-containing Combinations
Chlorpheniramine, Phenindamine, Phenylephrine, Dextromethorphan, Acetaminophen, Salicylamide, Caffeine, and Ascorbic Acid (Systemic)—See Cough/Cold Combinations (Systemic)
Chlorpheniramine, Phenindamine, and Phenylpropanolamine (Systemic)—See Antihistamines and Decongestants (Systemic)

## Pheniramine-containing Combinations
Chlorpheniramine, Pheniramine, Pyrilamine, Phenylephrine, Hydrocodone, Salicylamide, Caffeine, and Ascorbic Acid (Systemic)—See Cough/Cold Combinations (Systemic)
Pheniramine, Codeine, and Guaifenesin (Systemic)—See Cough/Cold Combinations (Systemic)
Pheniramine and Phenylephrine (Systemic)—See Antihistamines and Decongestants (Systemic)
Pheniramine, Phenylephrine, and Acetaminophen (Systemic)—See Antihistamines, Decongestants, and Analgesics (Systemic)
Pheniramine, Phenylephrine, Codeine, Sodium Citrate, Sodium Salicylate, and Caffeine (Systemic)—See Cough/Cold Combinations (Systemic)
Pheniramine, Phenylephrine, and Dextromethorphan (Systemic)—See Cough/Cold Combinations (Systemic)
Pheniramine, Phenylephrine, Phenylpropanolamine, Hydrocodone, and Guaifenesin (Systemic)—See Cough/Cold Combinations (Systemic)
Pheniramine, Phenylephrine, Sodium Salicylate, and Caffeine (Systemic)—See Antihistamines, Decongestants, and Analgesics (Systemic)
Pheniramine, Phenyltoloxamine, Pyrilamine, and Phenylpropanolamine (Systemic)—See Antihistamines and Decongestants (Systemic)
Pheniramine, Pyrilamine, Hydrocodone, Potassium Citrate, and Ascorbic Acid (Systemic)—See Cough/Cold Combinations (Systemic)
Pheniramine, Pyrilamine, Phenylephrine, Phenylpropanolamine, and Hydrocodone (Systemic)—See Cough/Cold Combinations (Systemic)
Pheniramine, Pyrilamine, and Phenylpropanolamine (Systemic)—See Antihistamines and Decongestants (Systemic)

## Pheniramine-containing Combinations
(continued)
Pheniramine, Pyrilamine, Phenylpropanolamine, Acetaminophen, and Caffeine (Systemic)—See Antihistamines, Decongestants, and Analgesics (Systemic)
Pheniramine, Pyrilamine, Phenylpropanolamine, and Codeine (Systemic)—See Cough/Cold Combinations (Systemic)
Pheniramine, Pyrilamine, Phenylpropanolamine, and Dextromethorphan (Systemic)—See Cough/Cold Combinations (Systemic)
Pheniramine, Pyrilamine, Phenylpropanolamine, Dextromethorphan, and Ammonium Chloride (Systemic)—See Cough/Cold Combinations (Systemic)
Pheniramine, Pyrilamine, Phenylpropanolamine, and Hydrocodone (Systemic)—See Cough/Cold Combinations (Systemic)
Pheniramine, Pyrilamine, Phenylpropanolamine, Hydrocodone, and Guaifenesin (Systemic)—See Cough/Cold Combinations (Systemic)

## Phenobarbital-containing Combinations
Atropine, Hyoscyamine, Scopolamine, and Phenobarbital (Systemic)—See Belladonna Alkaloids and Barbiturates (Systemic)
Atropine and Phenobarbital (Systemic)—See Belladonna Alkaloids and Barbiturates (Systemic)
Belladonna and Phenobarbital (Systemic)—See Belladonna Alkaloids and Barbiturates (Systemic)
Ergotamine, Belladonna Alkaloids, and Phenobarbital (Systemic)
Hyoscyamine and Phenobarbital (Systemic)—See Belladonna Alkaloids and Barbiturates (Systemic)
Phenobarbital, ASA, and Codeine (Systemic)—See Barbiturates and Analgesics (Systemic)
Theophylline, Ephedrine, Guaifenesin, and Phenobarbital (Systemic)
Theophylline, Ephedrine, and Phenobarbital (Systemic)

## Phenolphthalein-containing Combinations
Cascara Sagrada and Phenolphthalein (Oral-Local)—See Laxatives (Local)
Dehydrocholic Acid, Docusate, and Phenolphthalein (Oral-Local)—See Laxatives (Local)
Docusate and Phenolphthalein (Oral-Local)—See Laxatives (Local)
Mineral Oil, Glycerin, and Phenolphthalein (Oral-Local)—See Laxatives (Local)
Mineral Oil and Phenolphthalein (Oral-Local)—See Laxatives (Local)
Phenolphthalein and Senna (Oral-Local)—See Laxatives (Local)

## Phenylbenzimidazole-containing Combinations
Octyl Methoxycinnamate, Octyl Salicylate, Oxybenzone, Phenylbenzimidazole, and Titanium Dioxide (Topical)—See Sunscreen Agents (Topical)
Octyl Methoxycinnamate, Octyl Salicylate, Phenylbenzimidazole, and Titanium Dioxide (Topical)—See Sunscreen Agents (Topical)
Octyl Methoxycinnamate and Phenylbenzimidazole (Topical)—See Sunscreen Agents (Topical)
Phenylbenzimidazole and Sulisobenzone (Topical)—See Sunscreen Agents (Topical)

## Phenylephrine-containing Combinations
Brompheniramine and Phenylephrine (Systemic)—See Antihistamines and Decongestants (Systemic)
Brompheniramine, Phenylephrine, and Phenylpropanolamine (Systemic)—See Antihistamines and Decongestants (Systemic)

**Phenylephrine-containing Combinations**
*(continued)*

Brompheniramine, Phenylephrine, Phenylpropanolamine, and Codeine (Systemic)—*See* Cough/Cold Combinations (Systemic)

Brompheniramine, Phenylephrine, Phenylpropanolamine, Codeine, and Guaifenesin (Systemic)—*See* Cough/Cold Combinations (Systemic)

Brompheniramine, Phenylephrine, Phenylpropanolamine, and Dextromethorphan (Systemic)—*See* Cough/Cold Combinations (Systemic)

Brompheniramine, Phenylephrine, Phenylpropanolamine, Dextromethorphan, Potassium Guaiacolsulfonate, and Ipecac (Systemic)—*See* Cough/Cold Combinations (Systemic)

Brompheniramine, Phenylephrine, Phenylpropanolamine, and Guaifenesin (Systemic)—*See* Cough/Cold Combinations (Systemic)

Brompheniramine, Phenylephrine, Phenylpropanolamine, Hydrocodone, and Guaifenesin (Systemic)—*See* Cough/Cold Combinations (Systemic)

Chlorpheniramine, Ephedrine, Phenylephrine, and Carbetapentane (Systemic)—*See* Cough/Cold Combinations (Systemic)

Chlorpheniramine, Ephedrine, Phenylephrine, Dextromethorphan, Ammonium Chloride, and Ipecac (Systemic)—*See* Cough/Cold Combinations (Systemic)

Chlorpheniramine, Phenindamine, Phenylephrine, Dextromethorphan, Acetaminophen, Salicylamide, Caffeine, and Ascorbic Acid (Systemic)—*See* Cough/Cold Combinations (Systemic)

Chlorpheniramine, Pheniramine, Pyrilamine, Phenylephrine, Hydrocodone, Salicylamide, Caffeine, and Ascorbic Acid (Systemic)—*See* Cough/Cold Combinations (Systemic)

Chlorpheniramine and Phenylephrine (Systemic)—*See* Antihistamines and Decongestants (Systemic)

Chlorpheniramine, Phenylephrine, and Acetaminophen (Systemic)—*See* Antihistamines, Decongestants, and Analgesics (Systemic)

Chlorpheniramine, Phenylephrine, Acetaminophen, and Salicylamide (Systemic)—*See* Antihistamines, Decongestants, and Analgesics (Systemic)

Chlorpheniramine, Phenylephrine, Acetaminophen, Salicylamide, and Caffeine (Systemic)—*See* Antihistamines, Decongestants, and Analgesics (Systemic)

Chlorpheniramine, Phenylephrine, Codeine, and Ammonium Chloride (Systemic)—*See* Cough/Cold Combinations (Systemic)

Chlorpheniramine, Phenylephrine, Codeine, and Potassium Iodide (Systemic)—*See* Cough/Cold Combinations (Systemic)

Chlorpheniramine, Phenylephrine, and Dextromethorphan (Systemic)—*See* Cough/Cold Combinations (Systemic)

Chlorpheniramine, Phenylephrine, Dextromethorphan, Acetaminophen, and Salicylamide (Systemic)—*See* Cough/Cold Combinations (Systemic)

Chlorpheniramine, Phenylephrine, Dextromethorphan, and Guaifenesin (Systemic)—*See* Cough/Cold Combinations (Systemic)

Chlorpheniramine, Phenylephrine, Dextromethorphan, Guaifenesin, and Ammonium Chloride (Systemic)—*See* Cough/Cold Combinations (Systemic)

Chlorpheniramine, Phenylephrine, and Guaifenesin (Systemic)—*See* Cough/Cold Combinations (Systemic)

Chlorpheniramine, Phenylephrine, and Hydrocodone (Systemic)—*See* Cough/Cold Combinations (Systemic)

**Phenylephrine-containing Combinations**
*(continued)*

Chlorpheniramine, Phenylephrine, Hydrocodone, Acetaminophen, and Caffeine (Systemic)—*See* Cough/Cold Combinations (Systemic)

Chlorpheniramine, Phenylephrine, and Methscopolamine (Systemic)—*See* Antihistamines, Decongestants, and Anticholinergics (Systemic)

Chlorpheniramine, Phenylephrine, and Phenylpropanolamine (Systemic)—*See* Antihistamines and Decongestants (Systemic)

Chlorpheniramine, Phenylephrine, Phenylpropanolamine, Atropine, Hyoscyamine, and Scopolamine (Systemic)—*See* Antihistamines, Decongestants, and Anticholinergics (Systemic)

Chlorpheniramine, Phenylephrine, Phenylpropanolamine, Carbetapentane, and Potassium Guaiacolsulfonate (Systemic)—*See* Cough/Cold Combinations (Systemic)

Chlorpheniramine, Phenylephrine, Phenylpropanolamine, and Codeine (Systemic)—*See* Cough/Cold Combinations (Systemic)

Chlorpheniramine, Phenylephrine, Phenylpropanolamine, and Dextromethorphan (Systemic)—*See* Cough/Cold Combinations (Systemic)

Chlorpheniramine, Phenylephrine, Phenylpropanolamine, Dextromethorphan, Potassium Guaiacolsulfonate, and Ipecac (Systemic)—*See* Cough/Cold Combinations (Systemic)

Chlorpheniramine, Phenylephrine, Phenylpropanolamine, and Dihydrocodeine (Systemic)—*See* Cough/Cold Combinations (Systemic)

Chlorpheniramine, Phenyltoloxamine, and Phenylephrine (Systemic)—*See* Antihistamines and Decongestants (Systemic)

Chlorpheniramine, Phenyltoloxamine, Phenylephrine, and Phenylpropanolamine (Systemic)—*See* Antihistamines and Decongestants (Systemic)

Chlorpheniramine, Pyrilamine, and Phenylephrine (Systemic)—*See* Antihistamines and Decongestants (Systemic)

Chlorpheniramine, Pyrilamine, Phenylephrine, and Acetaminophen (Systemic)—*See* Antihistamines, Decongestants, and Analgesics (Systemic)

Chlorpheniramine, Pyrilamine, Phenylephrine, and Phenylpropanolamine (Systemic)—*See* Antihistamines and Decongestants (Systemic)

Chlorpheniramine, Pyrilamine, Phenylephrine, Phenylpropanolamine, and Acetaminophen (Systemic)—*See* Antihistamines, Decongestants, and Analgesics (Systemic)

Diphenhydramine, Phenylephrine, and Dextromethorphan (Systemic)—*See* Cough/Cold Combinations (Systemic)

Diphenylpyraline, Phenylephrine, and Dextromethorphan (Systemic)—*See* Cough/Cold Combinations (Systemic)

Isoproterenol and Phenylephrine (Systemic)

Pheniramine and Phenylephrine (Systemic)—*See* Antihistamines and Decongestants (Systemic)

Pheniramine, Phenylephrine, and Acetaminophen (Systemic)—*See* Antihistamines, Decongestants, and Analgesics (Systemic)

Pheniramine, Phenylephrine, Codeine, Sodium Citrate, Sodium Salicylate, and Caffeine (Systemic)—*See* Cough/Cold Combinations (Systemic)

Pheniramine, Phenylephrine, and Dextromethorphan (Systemic)—*See* Cough/Cold Combinations (Systemic)

Pheniramine, Phenylephrine, Phenylpropanolamine, Hydrocodone, and Guaifenesin

**Phenylephrine-containing Combinations**
*(continued)*

(Systemic)—*See* Cough/Cold Combinations (Systemic)

Pheniramine, Phenylephrine, Sodium Salicylate, and Caffeine (Systemic)—*See* Antihistamines, Decongestants, and Analgesics (Systemic)

Pheniramine, Pyrilamine, Phenylephrine, Phenylpropanolamine, and Hydrocodone (Systemic)—*See* Cough/Cold Combinations (Systemic)

Phenylephrine and Acetaminophen (Systemic)—*See* Decongestants and Analgesics (Systemic)

Phenylephrine and Codeine (Systemic)—*See* Cough/Cold Combinations (Systemic)

Phenylephrine, Dextromethorphan, and Guaifenesin (Systemic)—*See* Cough/Cold Combinations (Systemic)

Phenylephrine and Guaifenesin (Systemic)—*See* Cough/Cold Combinations (Systemic)

Phenylephrine, Guaifenesin, Acetaminophen, Salicylamide, and Caffeine (Systemic)—*See* Cough/Cold Combinations (Systemic)

Phenylephrine and Hydrocodone (Systemic)—*See* Cough/Cold Combinations (Systemic)

Phenylephrine, Hydrocodone, and Guaifenesin (Systemic)—*See* Cough/Cold Combinations (Systemic)

Phenylephrine, Phenylpropanolamine, and Acetaminophen (Systemic)—*See* Decongestants and Analgesics (Systemic)

Phenylephrine, Phenylpropanolamine, Carbetapentane, and Potassium Guaiacolsulfonate (Systemic)—*See* Cough/Cold Combinations (Systemic)

Phenylephrine, Phenylpropanolamine, and Guaifenesin (Systemic)—*See* Cough/Cold Combinations (Systemic)

Promethazine and Phenylephrine (Systemic)—*See* Antihistamines and Decongestants (Systemic)

Promethazine, Phenylephrine, and Codeine (Systemic)—*See* Cough/Cold Combinations (Systemic)

Promethazine, Phenylephrine, Codeine, and Potassium Guaiacolsulfonate (Systemic)—*See* Cough/Cold Combinations (Systemic)

Promethazine, Phenylephrine, and Potassium Guaiacolsulfonate (Systemic)—*See* Cough/Cold Combinations (Systemic)

Pyrilamine, Phenylephrine, Aspirin, and Caffeine (Systemic)—*See* Antihistamines, Decongestants, and Analgesics (Systemic)

Pyrilamine, Phenylephrine, and Codeine (Systemic)—*See* Cough/Cold Combinations (Systemic)

Pyrilamine, Phenylephrine, and Dextromethorphan (Systemic)—*See* Cough/Cold Combinations (Systemic)

Pyrilamine, Phenylephrine, and Hydrocodone (Systemic)—*See* Cough/Cold Combinations (Systemic)

Pyrilamine, Phenylephrine, Hydrocodone, and Ammonium Chloride (Systemic)—*See* Cough/Cold Combinations (Systemic)

**Phenylpropanolamine-containing Combinations**

Brompheniramine, Phenylephrine, and Phenylpropanolamine (Systemic)—*See* Antihistamines and Decongestants (Systemic)

Brompheniramine, Phenylephrine, Phenylpropanolamine, and Codeine (Systemic)—*See* Cough/Cold Combinations (Systemic)

Brompheniramine, Phenylephrine, Phenylpropanolamine, Codeine, and Guaifenesin (Systemic)—*See* Cough/Cold Combinations (Systemic)

**Phenylpropanolamine-containing Combinations** (continued)
 Brompheniramine, Phenylephrine, Phenylpropanolamine, and Dextromethorphan (Systemic)—See Cough/Cold Combinations (Systemic)
 Brompheniramine, Phenylephrine, Phenylpropanolamine, Dextromethorphan, Potassium Guaiacolsulfonate, and Ipecac (Systemic)—See Cough/Cold Combinations (Systemic)
 Brompheniramine, Phenylephrine, Phenylpropanolamine, and Guaifenesin (Systemic)—See Cough/Cold Combinations (Systemic)
 Brompheniramine, Phenylephrine, Phenylpropanolamine, Hydrocodone, and Guaifenesin (Systemic)—See Cough/Cold Combinations (Systemic)
 Brompheniramine and Phenylpropanolamine (Systemic)—See Antihistamines and Decongestants (Systemic)
 Brompheniramine, Phenylpropanolamine, and Acetaminophen (Systemic)—See Antihistamines, Decongestants, and Analgesics (Systemic)
 Brompheniramine, Phenylpropanolamine, and Aspirin (Systemic)
 Brompheniramine, Phenylpropanolamine, and Codeine (Systemic)—See Cough/Cold Combinations (Systemic)
 Brompheniramine, Phenylpropanolamine, and Dextromethorphan (Systemic)—See Cough/Cold Combinations (Systemic)
 Chlorpheniramine, Phenindamine, and Phenylpropanolamine (Systemic)—See Antihistamines and Decongestants (Systemic)
 Chlorpheniramine, Phenylephrine, and Phenylpropanolamine (Systemic)—See Antihistamines and Decongestants (Systemic)
 Chlorpheniramine, Phenylephrine, Phenylpropanolamine, Atropine, Hyoscyamine, and Scopolamine (Systemic)—See Antihistamines, Decongestants, and Anticholinergics (Systemic)
 Chlorpheniramine, Phenylephrine, Phenylpropanolamine, Carbetapentane, and Potassium Guaiacolsulfonate (Systemic)—See Cough/Cold Combinations (Systemic)
 Chlorpheniramine, Phenylephrine, Phenylpropanolamine, and Codeine (Systemic)—See Cough/Cold Combinations (Systemic)
 Chlorpheniramine, Phenylephrine, Phenylpropanolamine, and Dextromethorphan (Systemic)—See Cough/Cold Combinations (Systemic)
 Chlorpheniramine, Phenylephrine, Phenylpropanolamine, Dextromethorphan, Potassium Guaiacolsulfonate, and Ipecac (Systemic)—See Cough/Cold Combinations (Systemic)
 Chlorpheniramine, Phenylephrine, Phenylpropanolamine, and Dihydrocodeine (Systemic)—See Cough/Cold Combinations (Systemic)
 Chlorpheniramine and Phenylpropanolamine (Systemic)—See Antihistamines and Decongestants (Systemic)
 Chlorpheniramine, Phenylpropanolamine, and Acetaminophen (Systemic)—See Antihistamines, Decongestants, and Analgesics (Systemic)
 Chlorpheniramine, Phenylpropanolamine, Acetaminophen, and Caffeine (Systemic)—See Antihistamines, Decongestants, and Analgesics (Systemic)
 Chlorpheniramine, Phenylpropanolamine, and Aspirin (Systemic)—See Antihistamines, Decongestants, and Analgesics (Systemic)
 Chlorpheniramine, Phenylpropanolamine, Aspirin, and Caffeine (Systemic)—See Antihistamines, Decongestants, and Analgesics (Systemic)
 Chlorpheniramine, Phenylpropanolamine, and Caramiphen (Systemic)—See Cough/Cold Combinations (Systemic)
 Chlorpheniramine, Phenylpropanolamine, and Dextromethorphan (Systemic)—See Cough/Cold Combinations (Systemic)
 Chlorpheniramine, Phenylpropanolamine, Dextromethorphan, and Acetaminophen (Systemic)—See Cough/Cold Combinations (Systemic)
 Chlorpheniramine, Phenylpropanolamine, Dextromethorphan, Acetaminophen, and Caffeine (Systemic)—See Cough/Cold Combinations (Systemic)
 Chlorpheniramine, Phenylpropanolamine, Dextromethorphan, and Aspirin (Systemic)—See Cough/Cold Combinations (Systemic)
 Chlorpheniramine, Phenylpropanolamine, and Guaifenesin (Systemic)—See Cough/Cold Combinations (Systemic)
 Chlorpheniramine, Phenylpropanolamine, Guaifenesin, and Acetaminophen (Systemic)—See Cough/Cold Combinations (Systemic)
 Chlorpheniramine, Phenylpropanolamine, Guaifenesin, Sodium Citrate, and Citric Acid (Systemic)—See Cough/Cold Combinations (Systemic)
 Chlorpheniramine, Phenylpropanolamine, and Methscopolamine (Systemic)—See Antihistamines, Decongestants, and Anticholinergics (Systemic)
 Chlorpheniramine, Phenyltoloxamine, Phenylephrine, and Phenylpropanolamine (Systemic)—See Antihistamines and Decongestants (Systemic)
 Chlorpheniramine, Phenyltoloxamine, Phenylpropanolamine, and Acetaminophen (Systemic)—See Antihistamines, Decongestants, and Analgesics (Systemic)
 Chlorpheniramine, Pseudoephedrine, and Methscopolamine (Systemic)—See Antihistamines, Decongestants, and Anticholinergics (Systemic)
 Chlorpheniramine, Pyrilamine, Phenylephrine, and Phenylpropanolamine (Systemic)—See Antihistamines and Decongestants (Systemic)
 Chlorpheniramine, Pyrilamine, Phenylephrine, Phenylpropanolamine, and Acetaminophen (Systemic)—See Antihistamines, Decongestants, and Analgesics (Systemic)
 Clemastine and Phenylpropanolamine (Systemic)—See Antihistamines and Decongestants (Systemic)
 Diphenhydramine, Phenylpropanolamine, and Aspirin (Systemic)—See Antihistamines, Decongestants, and Analgesics (Systemic)
 Diphenylpyraline, Phenylpropanolamine, Acetaminophen, and Caffeine (Systemic)—See Antihistamines, Decongestants, and Analgesics (Systemic)
 Doxylamine, Phenylpropanolamine, Dextromethorphan, and Aspirin (Systemic)—See Cough/Cold Combinations (Systemic)
 Pheniramine, Phenylephrine, Phenylpropanolamine, Hydrocodone, and Guaifenesin (Systemic)—See Cough/Cold Combinations (Systemic)
 Pheniramine, Phenyltoloxamine, Pyrilamine, and Phenylpropanolamine (Systemic)—See Antihistamines and Decongestants (Systemic)
 Pheniramine, Pyrilamine, Phenylephrine, Phenylpropanolamine, and Hydrocodone (Systemic)—See Cough/Cold Combinations (Systemic)
 Pheniramine, Pyrilamine, and Phenylpropanolamine (Systemic)—See Antihistamines and Decongestants (Systemic)
 Pheniramine, Pyrilamine, Phenylpropanolamine, Acetaminophen, and Caffeine (Systemic)—See Antihistamines, Decongestants, and Analgesics (Systemic)
 Pheniramine, Pyrilamine, Phenylpropanolamine, and Codeine (Systemic)—See Cough/Cold Combinations (Systemic)
 Pheniramine, Pyrilamine, Phenylpropanolamine, and Dextromethorphan (Systemic)—See Cough/Cold Combinations (Systemic)
 Pheniramine, Pyrilamine, Phenylpropanolamine, Dextromethorphan, and Ammonium Chloride (Systemic)—See Cough/Cold Combinations (Systemic)
 Pheniramine, Pyrilamine, Phenylpropanolamine, and Hydrocodone (Systemic)—See Cough/Cold Combinations (Systemic)
 Pheniramine, Pyrilamine, Phenylpropanolamine, Hydrocodone, and Guaifenesin (Systemic)—See Cough/Cold Combinations (Systemic)
 Phenylephrine, Phenylpropanolamine, and Acetaminophen (Systemic)—See Decongestants and Analgesics (Systemic)
 Phenylephrine, Phenylpropanolamine, Carbetapentane, and Potassium Guaiacolsulfonate (Systemic)—See Cough/Cold Combinations (Systemic)
 Phenylephrine, Phenylpropanolamine, and Guaifenesin (Systemic)—See Cough/Cold Combinations (Systemic)
 Phenylpropanolamine and Acetaminophen (Systemic)—See Decongestants and Analgesics (Systemic)
 Phenylpropanolamine, Acetaminophen, and Aspirin (Systemic)—See Decongestants and Analgesics (Systemic)
 Phenylpropanolamine, Acetaminophen, and Caffeine (Systemic)—See Decongestants and Analgesics (Systemic)
 Phenylpropanolamine, Acetaminophen, Salicylamide, and Caffeine (Systemic)—See Decongestants and Analgesics (Systemic)
 Phenylpropanolamine and Aspirin (Systemic)—See Decongestants and Analgesics (Systemic)
 Phenylpropanolamine and Caramiphen (Systemic)—See Cough/Cold Combinations (Systemic)
 Phenylpropanolamine, Codeine, and Guaifenesin (Systemic)—See Cough/Cold Combinations (Systemic)
 Phenylpropanolamine and Dextromethorphan (Systemic)—See Cough/Cold Combinations (Systemic)
 Phenylpropanolamine, Dextromethorphan, and Acetaminophen (Systemic)—See Cough/Cold Combinations (Systemic)
 Phenylpropanolamine, Dextromethorphan, and Guaifenesin (Systemic)—See Cough/Cold Combinations (Systemic)
 Phenylpropanolamine, Dextromethorphan, Guaifenesin, and Acetaminophen (Systemic)—See Cough/Cold Combinations (Systemic)
 Phenylpropanolamine and Guaifenesin (Systemic)—See Cough/Cold Combinations (Systemic)
 Phenylpropanolamine and Hydrocodone (Systemic)—See Cough/Cold Combinations (Systemic)
 Phenylpropanolamine, Hydrocodone, Dextromethorphan, and Acetaminophen (Systemic)—See Cough/Cold Combinations (Systemic)
 Phenyltoloxamine, Phenylpropanolamine, and Acetaminophen (Systemic)—See Antihista-

**Phenylpropanolamine-containing Combinations** *(continued)*
mines, Decongestants, and Analgesics (Systemic)
Pyrilamine, Phenylpropanolamine, Acetaminophen, and Caffeine (Systemic)—*See* Antihistamines, Decongestants, and Analgesics (Systemic)
Pyrilamine, Phenylpropanolamine, Dextromethorphan, Guaifenesin, Potassium Citrate, and Citric Acid (Systemic)—*See* Cough/Cold Combinations (Systemic)

**Phenyl Salicylate–containing Combinations**
Atropine, Hyoscyamine, Methenamine, Methylene Blue, Phenyl Salicylate, and Benzoic Acid (Systemic)

**Phenyltoloxamine-containing Combinations**
Chlorpheniramine, Phenyltoloxamine, Ephedrine, Codeine, and Guaiacol Carbonate (Systemic)—*See* Cough/Cold Combinations (Systemic)
Chlorpheniramine, Phenyltoloxamine, and Phenylephrine (Systemic)—*See* Antihistamines and Decongestants (Systemic)
Chlorpheniramine, Phenyltoloxamine, Phenylephrine, and Phenylpropanolamine (Systemic)—*See* Antihistamines and Decongestants (Systemic)
Chlorpheniramine, Phenyltoloxamine, Phenylpropanolamine, and Acetaminophen (Systemic)—*See* Antihistamines, Decongestants, and Analgesics (Systemic)
Pheniramine, Phenyltoloxamine, Pyrilamine, and Phenylpropanolamine (Systemic)—*See* Antihistamines and Decongestants (Systemic)
Phenyltoloxamine and Hydrocodone (Systemic)—*See* Cough/Cold Combinations (Systemic)
Phenyltoloxamine, Phenylpropanolamine, and Acetaminophen (Systemic)—*See* Antihistamines, Decongestants, and Analgesics (Systemic)

**Pindolol-containing Combinations**
Pindolol and Hydrochlorothiazide (Systemic)—*See* Beta-adrenergic Blocking Agents and Thiazide Diuretics (Systemic)

**Piperacillin-containing Combinations**
Piperacillin and Tazobactam (Systemic)—*See* Penicillins and Beta-lactamase Inhibitors (Systemic)

**Polymyxin B–containing Combinations**
Neomycin and Polymyxin B (Topical)
Neomycin, Polymyxin B, and Bacitracin (Ophthalmic)
Neomycin, Polymyxin B, and Bacitracin (Topical)
Neomycin, Polymyxin B, and Gramicidin (Ophthalmic)
Neomycin, Polymyxin B, and Hydrocortisone (Ophthalmic)
Neomycin, Polymyxin B, and Hydrocortisone (Otic)

**Polythiazide-containing Combinations**
Prazosin and Polythiazide (Systemic)
Reserpine and Polythiazide (Systemic)—*See* Rauwolfia Alkaloids and Thiazide Diuretics (Systemic)

**Potassium Guaiacolsulfonate–containing Combinations**
Bromodiphenhydramine, Diphenhydramine, Codeine, Ammonium Chloride, and Potassium Guaiacolsulfonate (Systemic)—*See* Cough/Cold Combinations (Systemic)
Brompheniramine, Phenylephrine, Phenylpropanolamine, Dextromethorphan, Potassium Guaiacolsulfonate, and Ipecac (Systemic)—*See* Cough/Cold Combinations (Systemic)
Chlorpheniramine, Phenylephrine, Phenylpropanolamine, Carbetapentane, and Potassium Guaiacolsulfonate (Systemic)—*See* Cough/Cold Combinations (Systemic)

**Potassium Guaiacolsulfonate–containing Combinations** *(continued)*
Chlorpheniramine, Phenylephrine, Phenylpropanolamine, Dextromethorphan, Potassium Guaiacolsulfonate, and Ipecac (Systemic)—*See* Cough/Cold Combinations (Systemic)
Hydrocodone and Potassium Guaiacolsulfonate (Systemic)—*See* Cough/Cold Combinations (Systemic)
Phenylephrine, Phenylpropanolamine, Carbetapentane, and Potassium Guaiacolsulfonate (Systemic)—*See* Cough/Cold Combinations (Systemic)
Promethazine, Codeine, and Potassium Guaiacolsulfonate (Systemic)—*See* Cough/Cold Combinations (Systemic)
Promethazine, Phenylephrine, Codeine, and Potassium Guaiacolsulfonate (Systemic)—*See* Cough/Cold Combinations (Systemic)
Promethazine, Phenylephrine, and Potassium Guaiacolsulfonate (Systemic)—*See* Cough/Cold Combinations (Systemic)
Promethazine and Potassium Guaiacolsulfonate (Systemic)—*See* Cough/Cold Combinations (Systemic)
Pseudoephedrine, Hydrocodone, and Potassium Guaiacolsulfonate (Systemic)—*See* Cough/Cold Combinations (Systemic)

**Prazosin-containing Combinations**
Prazosin and Polythiazide (Systemic)

**Prilocaine-containing Combinations**
Lidocaine and Prilocaine (Topical)
Prilocaine and Epinephrine (Parenteral-Local)—*See* Anesthetics (Parenteral-Local)

**Probenecid-containing Combinations**
Probenecid and Colchicine (Systemic)

**Procaine-containing Combinations**
Propoxycaine, Procaine, and Levonordefrin (Parenteral-Local)—*See* Anesthetics (Parenteral-Local)
Propoxycaine, Procaine, and Norepinephrine (Parenteral-Local)—*See* Anesthetics (Parenteral-Local)

**Promethazine-containing Combinations**
Promethazine and Codeine (Systemic)—*See* Cough/Cold Combinations (Systemic)
Promethazine, Codeine, and Potassium Guaiacolsulfonate (Systemic)—*See* Cough/Cold Combinations (Systemic)
Promethazine and Dextromethorphan (Systemic)—*See* Cough/Cold Combinations (Systemic)
Promethazine and Phenylephrine (Systemic)—*See* Antihistamines and Decongestants (Systemic)
Promethazine, Phenylephrine, and Codeine (Systemic)—*See* Cough/Cold Combinations (Systemic)
Promethazine, Phenylephrine, Codeine, and Potassium Guaiacolsulfonate (Systemic)—*See* Cough/Cold Combinations (Systemic)
Promethazine, Phenylephrine, and Potassium Guaiacolsulfonate (Systemic)—*See* Cough/Cold Combinations (Systemic)
Promethazine and Potassium Guaiacolsulfonate (Systemic)—*See* Cough/Cold Combinations (Systemic)
Promethazine, Pseudoephedrine, and Dextromethorphan (Systemic)—*See* Cough/Cold Combinations (Systemic)

**Propoxycaine-containing Combinations**
Propoxycaine, Procaine, and Levonordefrin (Parenteral-Local)—*See* Anesthetics (Parenteral-Local)
Propoxycaine, Procaine, and Norepinephrine (Parenteral-Local)—*See* Anesthetics (Parenteral-Local)

**Propoxyphene-containing Combinations**
Propoxyphene and Acetaminophen (Systemic)—*See* Opioid (Narcotic) Analgesics and Acetaminophen (Systemic)
Propoxyphene and Aspirin (Systemic)—*See* Opioid (Narcotic) Analgesics and Aspirin (Systemic)
Propoxyphene, Aspirin, and Caffeine (Systemic)—*See* Opioid (Narcotic) Analgesics and Aspirin (Systemic)

**Propranolol-containing Combinations**
Propranolol and Hydrochlorothiazide (Systemic)—*See* Beta-adrenergic Blocking Agents and Thiazide Diuretics (Systemic)

**Pseudoephedrine-containing Combinations**
Acrivastine and Pseudoephedrine (Systemic)—*See* Antihistamines and Decongestants (Systemic)
Azatadine and Pseudoephedrine (Systemic)—*See* Antihistamines and Decongestants (Systemic)
Brompheniramine and Pseudoephedrine (Systemic)—*See* Antihistamines and Decongestants (Systemic)
Brompheniramine, Pseudoephedrine, and Acetaminophen (Systemic)—*See* Antihistamines, Decongestants, and Analgesics (Systemic)
Brompheniramine, Pseudoephedrine, and Dextromethorphan (Systemic)—*See* Cough/Cold Combinations (Systemic)
Carbinoxamine and Pseudoephedrine (Systemic)—*See* Antihistamines and Decongestants (Systemic)
Carbinoxamine, Pseudoephedrine, and Dextromethorphan (Systemic)—*See* Cough/Cold Combinations (Systemic)
Chlorpheniramine and Pseudoephedrine (Systemic)—*See* Antihistamines and Decongestants (Systemic)
Chlorpheniramine, Pseudoephedrine, and Acetaminophen (Systemic)—*See* Antihistamines, Decongestants, and Analgesics (Systemic)
Chlorpheniramine, Pseudoephedrine, and Codeine (Systemic)—*See* Cough/Cold Combinations (Systemic)
Chlorpheniramine, Pseudoephedrine, Codeine, and Acetaminophen (Systemic)—*See* Cough/Cold Combinations (Systemic)
Chlorpheniramine, Pseudoephedrine, and Dextromethorphan (Systemic)—*See* Cough/Cold Combinations (Systemic)
Chlorpheniramine, Pseudoephedrine, Dextromethorphan, and Acetaminophen (Systemic)—*See* Cough/Cold Combinations (Systemic)
Chlorpheniramine, Pseudoephedrine, Dextromethorphan, and Guaifenesin (Systemic)—*See* Cough/Cold Combinations (Systemic)
Chlorpheniramine, Pseudoephedrine, and Guaifenesin (Systemic)—*See* Cough/Cold Combinations (Systemic)
Chlorpheniramine, Pseudoephedrine, and Hydrocodone (Systemic)—*See* Cough/Cold Combinations (Systemic)
Chlorpheniramine, Pseudoephedrine, and Methscopolamine (Systemic)—*See* Antihistamines, Decongestants, and Anticholinergics (Systemic)
Dexbrompheniramine and Pseudoephedrine (Systemic)—*See* Antihistamines and Decongestants (Systemic)
Dexbrompheniramine, Pseudoephedrine, and Acetaminophen (Systemic)—*See* Antihistamines, Decongestants, and Analgesics (Systemic)
Dexchlorpheniramine, Pseudoephedrine, and Guaifenesin (Systemic)—*See* Cough/Cold Combinations (Systemic)

*USP DI*                                                                                                    **Combination Cross-reference Listing**

**Pseudoephedrine-containing Combinations**
*(continued)*
Diphenhydramine and Pseudoephedrine (Systemic)—*See* Antihistamines and Decongestants (Systemic)
Diphenhydramine, Pseudoephedrine, and Acetaminophen (Systemic)—*See* Antihistamines, Decongestants, and Analgesics (Systemic)
Doxylamine, Pseudoephedrine, Dextromethorphan, and Acetaminophen (Systemic)—*See* Cough/Cold Combinations (Systemic)
Loratadine and Pseudoephedrine (Systemic)—*See* Antihistamines and Decongestants (Systemic)
Promethazine, Pseudoephedrine, and Dextromethorphan (Systemic)—*See* Cough/Cold Combinations (Systemic)
Pseudoephedrine and Acetaminophen (Systemic)—*See* Decongestants and Analgesics (Systemic)
Pseudoephedrine and Aspirin (Systemic)—*See* Decongestants and Analgesics (Systemic)
Pseudoephedrine and Codeine (Systemic)—*See* Cough/Cold Combinations (Systemic)
Pseudoephedrine, Codeine, and Guaifenesin (Systemic)—*See* Cough/Cold Combinations (Systemic)
Pseudoephedrine and Dextromethorphan (Systemic)—*See* Cough/Cold Combinations (Systemic)
Pseudoephedrine, Dextromethorphan, and Acetaminophen (Systemic)—*See* Cough/Cold Combinations (Systemic)
Pseudoephedrine, Dextromethorphan, and Guaifenesin (Systemic)—*See* Cough/Cold Combinations (Systemic)
Pseudoephedrine, Dextromethorphan, Guaifenesin, and Acetaminophen (Systemic)—*See* Cough/Cold Combinations (Systemic)
Pseudoephedrine and Guaifenesin (Systemic)—*See* Cough/Cold Combinations (Systemic)
Pseudoephedrine and Hydrocodone (Systemic)—*See* Cough/Cold Combinations (Systemic)
Pseudoephedrine, Hydrocodone, and Guaifenesin (Systemic)—*See* Cough/Cold Combinations (Systemic)
Pseudoephedrine, Hydrocodone, and Potassium Guaiacolsulfonate (Systemic)—*See* Cough/Cold Combinations (Systemic)
Pseudoephedrine and Ibuprofen (Systemic)—*See* Decongestants and Analgesics (Systemic)
Pyrilamine, Pseudoephedrine, Dextromethorphan, and Acetaminophen (Systemic)—*See* Cough/Cold Combinations (Systemic)
Terfenadine and Pseudoephedrine (Systemic)—*See* Antihistamines and Decongestants (Systemic)
Triprolidine and Pseudoephedrine (Systemic)—*See* Antihistamines and Decongestants (Systemic)
Triprolidine, Pseudoephedrine, and Acetaminophen (Systemic)—*See* Antihistamines, Decongestants, and Analgesics (Systemic)
Triprolidine, Pseudoephedrine, and Codeine (Systemic)—*See* Cough/Cold Combinations (Systemic)
Triprolidine, Pseudoephedrine, Codeine, and Guaifenesin (Systemic)—*See* Cough/Cold Combinations (Systemic)
Triprolidine, Pseudoephedrine, and Dextromethorphan (Systemic)—*See* Cough/Cold Combinations (Systemic)

**Psyllium-containing Combinations**
Malt Soup Extract and Psyllium (Oral-Local)—*See* Laxatives (Local)

**Psyllium-containing Combinations**
*(continued)*
Psyllium Hydrophilic Mucilloid and Carboxymethylcellulose (Oral-Local)—*See* Laxatives (Local)
Psyllium Hydrophilic Mucilloid and Senna (Oral-Local)—*See* Laxatives (Local)
Psyllium Hydrophilic Mucilloid and Sennosides (Oral-Local)—*See* Laxatives (Local)
Psyllium and Senna (Oral-Local)—*See* Laxatives (Local)

**Pyrazinamide-containing Combinations**
Rifampin, Isoniazid, and Pyrazinamide (Systemic)

**Pyrilamine-containing Combinations**
Chlorpheniramine, Pheniramine, Pyrilamine, Phenylephrine, Hydrocodone, Salicylamide, Caffeine, and Ascorbic Acid (Systemic)—*See* Cough/Cold Combinations (Systemic)
Chlorpheniramine, Pyrilamine, and Phenylephrine (Systemic)—*See* Antihistamines and Decongestants (Systemic)
Chlorpheniramine, Pyrilamine, Phenylephrine, and Acetaminophen (Systemic)—*See* Antihistamines, Decongestants, and Analgesics (Systemic)
Chlorpheniramine, Pyrilamine, Phenylephrine, and Phenylpropanolamine (Systemic)—*See* Antihistamines and Decongestants (Systemic)
Chlorpheniramine, Pyrilamine, Phenylephrine, Phenylpropanolamine, and Acetaminophen (Systemic)—*See* Antihistamines, Decongestants, and Analgesics (Systemic)
Pheniramine, Phenyltoloxamine, Pyrilamine, and Phenylpropanolamine (Systemic)—*See* Antihistamines and Decongestants (Systemic)
Pheniramine, Pyrilamine, Hydrocodone, Potassium Citrate, and Ascorbic Acid (Systemic)—*See* Cough/Cold Combinations (Systemic)
Pheniramine, Pyrilamine, Phenylephrine, Phenylpropanolamine, and Hydrocodone (Systemic)—*See* Cough/Cold Combinations (Systemic)
Pheniramine, Pyrilamine, and Phenylpropanolamine (Systemic)—*See* Antihistamines and Decongestants (Systemic)
Pheniramine, Pyrilamine, Phenylpropanolamine, and Codeine (Systemic)—*See* Cough/Cold Combinations (Systemic)
Pheniramine, Pyrilamine, Phenylpropanolamine, and Dextromethorphan (Systemic)—*See* Cough/Cold Combinations (Systemic)
Pheniramine, Pyrilamine, Phenylpropanolamine, Dextromethorphan, and Ammonium Chloride (Systemic)—*See* Cough/Cold Combinations (Systemic)
Pheniramine, Pyrilamine, Phenylpropanolamine, and Hydrocodone (Systemic)—*See* Cough/Cold Combinations (Systemic)
Pheniramine, Pyrilamine, Phenylpropanolamine, Hydrocodone, and Guaifenesin (Systemic)—*See* Cough/Cold Combinations (Systemic)
Pyrilamine and Codeine (Systemic)—*See* Cough/Cold Combinations (Systemic)
Pyrilamine, Phenylephrine, Aspirin, and Caffeine (Systemic)—*See* Antihistamines, Decongestants, and Analgesics (Systemic)
Pyrilamine, Phenylephrine, and Codeine (Systemic)—*See* Cough/Cold Combinations (Systemic)
Pyrilamine, Phenylephrine, and Dextromethorphan (Systemic)—*See* Cough/Cold Combinations (Systemic)
Pyrilamine, Phenylephrine, and Hydrocodone (Systemic)—*See* Cough/Cold Combinations (Systemic)

**Pyrilamine-containing Combinations**
*(continued)*
Pyrilamine, Phenylephrine, Hydrocodone, and Ammonium Chloride (Systemic)—*See* Cough/Cold Combinations (Systemic)
Pyrilamine, Phenylpropanolamine, Acetaminophen, and Caffeine (Systemic)—*See* Antihistamines, Decongestants, and Analgesics (Systemic)
Pyrilamine, Phenylpropanolamine, Dextromethorphan, Guaifenesin, Potassium Citrate, and Citric Acid (Systemic)—*See* Cough/Cold Combinations (Systemic)
Pyrilamine, Pseudoephedrine, Dextromethorphan, and Acetaminophen (Systemic)—*See* Cough/Cold Combinations (Systemic)

**Pyrimethamine-containing Combinations**
Sulfadoxine and Pyrimethamine (Systemic)

**Rauwolfia Serpentina–containing Combinations**
Rauwolfia Serpentina and Bendroflumethiazide (Systemic)—*See* Rauwolfia Alkaloids and Thiazide Diuretics (Systemic)

**Reserpine-containing Combinations**
Reserpine and Chlorothiazide (Systemic)—*See* Rauwolfia Alkaloids and Thiazide Diuretics (Systemic)
Reserpine and Chlorthalidone (Systemic)—*See* Rauwolfia Alkaloids and Thiazide Diuretics (Systemic)
Reserpine, Hydralazine, and Hydrochlorothiazide (Systemic)
Reserpine and Hydrochlorothiazide (Systemic)—*See* Rauwolfia Alkaloids and Thiazide Diuretics (Systemic)
Reserpine and Hydroflumethiazide (Systemic)—*See* Rauwolfia Alkaloids and Thiazide Diuretics (Systemic)
Reserpine and Methyclothiazide (Systemic)—*See* Rauwolfia Alkaloids and Thiazide Diuretics (Systemic)
Reserpine and Polythiazide (Systemic)—*See* Rauwolfia Alkaloids and Thiazide Diuretics (Systemic)
Reserpine and Trichlormethiazide (Systemic)—*See* Rauwolfia Alkaloids and Thiazide Diuretics (Systemic)

**Resorcinol-containing Combinations**
Resorcinol and Sulfur (Topical)

**Rifampin-containing Combinations**
Rifampin and Isoniazid (Systemic)
Rifampin, Isoniazid, and Pyrazinamide (Systemic)

**Roxadimate-containing Combinations**
Oxybenzone and Roxadimate (Topical)—*See* Sunscreen Agents (Topical)

**Salicylamide-containing Combinations**
Acetaminophen, Aspirin, and Salicylamide, Buffered (Systemic)—*See* Acetaminophen and Salicylates (Systemic)
Acetaminophen, Aspirin, Salicylamide, and Caffeine (Systemic)—*See* Acetaminophen and Salicylates (Systemic)
Acetaminophen and Salicylamide (Systemic)—*See* Acetaminophen and Salicylates (Systemic)
Acetaminophen, Salicylamide, and Caffeine (Systemic)—*See* Acetaminophen and Salicylates (Systemic)
Chlorpheniramine, Phenindamine, Phenylephrine, Dextromethorphan, Acetaminophen, Salicylamide, Caffeine, and Ascorbic Acid (Systemic)—*See* Cough/Cold Combinations (Systemic)
Chlorpheniramine, Pheniramine, Pyrilamine, Phenylephrine, Hydrocodone, Salicylamide, Caffeine, and Ascorbic Acid (Systemic)—*See* Cough/Cold Combinations (Systemic)
Chlorpheniramine, Phenylephrine, Acetaminophen, and Salicylamide (Systemic)—*See* Antihistamines, Decongestants, and Analgesics (Systemic)

**Salicylamide-containing Combinations**
*(continued)*
Chlorpheniramine, Phenylephrine, Acetaminophen, Salicylamide, and Caffeine (Systemic)—*See* Antihistamines, Decongestants, and Analgesics (Systemic)
Chlorpheniramine, Phenylephrine, Dextromethorphan, Acetaminophen, and Salicylamide (Systemic)—*See* Cough/Cold Combinations (Systemic)
Phenylephrine, Guaifenesin, Acetaminophen, Salicylamide, and Caffeine (Systemic)—*See* Cough/Cold Combinations (Systemic)
Phenylpropanolamine, Acetaminophen, Salicylamide, and Caffeine (Systemic)—*See* Decongestants and Analgesics (Systemic)

**Salicylic Acid–containing Combinations**
Salicylic Acid and Sulfur (Topical)
Salicylic Acid, Sulfur, and Coal Tar (Topical)

**Scopolamine-containing Combinations**
Atropine, Hyoscyamine, Scopolamine, and Phenobarbital (Systemic)—*See* Belladonna Alkaloids and Barbiturates (Systemic)
Chlorpheniramine, Phenylephrine, Phenylpropanolamine, Atropine, Hyoscyamine, and Scopolamine (Systemic)—*See* Antihistamines, Decongestants, and Anticholinergics (Systemic)
Kaolin, Pectin, Hyoscyamine, Atropine, and Scopolamine (Systemic)—*See* Kaolin, Pectin, and Belladonna Alkaloids (Systemic)

**Secobarbital-containing Combinations**
Secobarbital and Amobarbital (Systemic)—*See* Barbiturates (Systemic)

**Senna-containing Combinations**
Phenolphthalein and Senna (Oral-Local)—*See* Laxatives (Local)
Psyllium Hydrophilic Mucilloid and Senna (Oral-Local)—*See* Laxatives (Local)
Psyllium and Senna (Oral-Local)—*See* Laxatives (Local)

**Sennosides-containing Combinations**
Psyllium Hydrophilic Mucilloid and Sennosides (Oral-Local)—*See* Laxatives (Local)
Sennosides and Docusate (Oral-Local)—*See* Laxatives (Local)

**Simethicone-containing Combinations**
Alumina, Magnesia, Calcium Carbonate,, and Simethicone (Oral-Local)—*See* Antacids (Oral-Local)
Alumina, Magnesia, and Simethicone (Oral-Local)—*See* Antacids (Oral-Local)
Calcium Carbonate, Magnesia, and Simethicone (Oral-Local)—*See* Antacids (Oral-Local)
Calcium Carbonate and Simethicone (Oral-Local)—*See* Antacids (Oral-Local)
Magaldrate and Simethicone (Oral-Local)—*See* Antacids (Oral-Local)
Simethicone, Alumina, Magnesium Carbonate, and Magnesia (Oral-Local)—*See* Antacids (Oral-Local)

**Sodium Bicarbonate–containing Combinations**
Acetaminophen, Sodium Bicarbonate, and Citric Acid (Systemic)
Alumina, Magnesium Carbonate, and Sodium Bicarbonate (Oral-Local)—*See* Antacids (Oral-Local)
Alumina, Magnesium Trisilicate, and Sodium Bicarbonate (Oral-Local)—*See* Antacids (Oral-Local)
Aspirin, Sodium Bicarbonate, and Citric Acid (Systemic)
Magnesium Carbonate and Sodium Bicarbonate (Oral-Local)—*See* Antacids (Oral-Local)
Potassium Bitartrate and Sodium Bicarbonate (Rectal-Local)—*See* Laxatives (Local)

**Sodium Salicylate–containing Combinations**
Pheniramine, Phenylephrine, Codeine, Sodium Citrate, Sodium Salicylate, and Caffeine (Systemic)—*See* Cough/Cold Combinations (Systemic)
Pheniramine, Phenylephrine, Sodium Salicylate, and Caffeine (Systemic)—*See* Antihistamines, Decongestants, and Analgesics (Systemic)

**Sorbitol-containing Combinations**
Activated Charcoal and Sorbitol (Oral-Local)—*See* Charcoal, Activated (Oral-Local)

**Spironolactone-containing Combinations**
Spironolactone and Hydrochlorothiazide (Systemic)—*See* Diuretics, Potassium-sparing, and Hydrochlorothiazide (Systemic)

**Sulbactam-containing Combinations**
Ampicillin and Sulbactam (Systemic)—*See* Penicillins and Beta-lactamase Inhibitors (Systemic)

**Sulfabenzamide-containing Combinations**
Triple Sulfa (Vaginal)—*See* Sulfonamides (Vaginal)

**Sulfacetamide-containing Combinations**
Triple Sulfa (Vaginal)—*See* Sulfonamides (Vaginal)

**Sulfadiazine-containing Combinations**
Sulfadiazine and Trimethoprim (Systemic)

**Sulfadoxine-containing Combinations**
Sulfadoxine and Pyrimethamine (Systemic)

**Sulfamethoxazole-containing Combinations**
Sulfamethoxazole and Phenazopyridine (Systemic)—*See* Sulfonamides and Phenazopyridine (Systemic)
Sulfamethoxazole and Trimethoprim (Systemic)

**Sulfanilamide-containing Combinations**
Sulfanilamide, Aminacrine, and Allantoin (Vaginal)—*See* Sulfonamides (Vaginal)

**Sulfathiazole-containing Combinations**
Triple Sulfa (Vaginal)—*See* Sulfonamides (Vaginal)

**Sulfisoxazole-containing Combinations**
Erythromycin and Sulfisoxazole (Systemic)
Sulfisoxazole and Phenazopyridine (Systemic)—*See* Sulfonamides and Phenazopyridine (Systemic)

**Sulfur-containing Combinations**
Alcohol and Sulfur (Topical)
Resorcinol and Sulfur (Topical)
Salicylic Acid and Sulfur (Topical)
Salicylic Acid, Sulfur, and Coal Tar (Topical)

**Sulisobenzone-containing Combinations**
Phenylbenzimidazole and Sulisobenzone (Topical)—*See* Sunscreen Agents (Topical)

**Tazobactam-containing Combinations**
Piperacillin and Tazobactam (Systemic)—*See* Penicillins and Beta-lactamase Inhibitors (Systemic)

**Testosterone-containing Combinations**
Testosterone and Estradiol (Systemic)—*See* Androgens and Estrogens (Systemic)

**Tetracaine-containing Combinations**
Benzocaine, Butamben, and Tetracaine (Mucosal-Local)—*See* Anesthetics (Mucosal-Local)

**Theophylline-containing Combinations**
Theophylline, Ephedrine, Guaifenesin, and Phenobarbital (Systemic)
Theophylline, Ephedrine, and Hydroxyzine (Systemic)
Theophylline, Ephedrine, and Phenobarbital (Systemic)
Theophylline and Guaifenesin (Systemic)

**Thiacetazone-containing Combinations**
Isoniazid and Thiacetazone (Systemic)

**Ticarcillin-containing Combinations**
Ticarcillin and Clavulanate (Systemic)—*See* Penicillins and Beta-lactamase Inhibitors (Systemic)

**Timolol-containing Combinations**
Timolol and Hydrochlorothiazide (Systemic)—*See* Beta-adrenergic Blocking Agents and Thiazide Diuretics (Systemic)

**Titanium Dioxide-containing Combinations**
Aminobenzoic Acid and Titanium Dioxide (Topical)—*See* Sunscreen Agents (Topical)
Menthyl Anthranilate and Titanium Dioxide (Topical)—*See* Sunscreen Agents (Topical)
Octocrylene, Octyl Methoxycinnamate, Octyl Salicylate, Oxybenzone, and Titanium Dioxide (Topical)—*See* Sunscreen Agents (Topical)
Octocrylene, Octyl Methoxycinnamate, Oxybenzone, and Titanium Dioxide (Topical)—*See* Sunscreen Agents (Topical)
Octocrylene, Octyl Methoxycinnamate, and Titanium Dioxide (Topical)—*See* Sunscreen Agents (Topical)
Octyl Methoxycinnamate, Octyl Salicylate, Oxybenzone, Padimate O, and Titanium Dioxide (Topical)—*See* Sunscreen Agents (Topical)
Octyl Methoxycinnamate, Octyl Salicylate, Oxybenzone, Phenylbenzimidazole, and Titanium Dioxide (Topical)—*See* Sunscreen Agents (Topical)
Octyl Methoxycinnamate, Octyl Salicylate, Oxybenzone, and Titanium Dioxide (Topical)—*See* Sunscreen Agents (Topical)
Octyl Methoxycinnamate, Octyl Salicylate, Phenylbenzimidazole, and Titanium Dioxide (Topical)—*See* Sunscreen Agents (Topical)
Octyl Methoxycinnamate, Octyl Salicylate, and Titanium Dioxide (Topical)—*See* Sunscreen Agents (Topical)
Octyl Methoxycinnamate, Oxybenzone, Padimate O, and Titanium Dioxide (Topical)—*See* Sunscreen Agents (Topical)
Octyl Methoxycinnamate, Oxybenzone, and Titanium Dioxide (Topical)—*See* Sunscreen Agents (Topical)
Titanium Dioxide and Zinc Oxide (Topical)—*See* Sunscreen Agents (Topical)

**Triamcinolone-containing Combinations**
Nystatin and Triamcinolone (Topical)

**Triamterene-containing Combinations**
Triamterene and Hydrochlorothiazide (Systemic)—*See* Diuretics, Potassium-sparing, and Hydrochlorothiazide (Systemic)

**Trichlormethiazide-containing Combinations**
Reserpine and Trichlormethiazide (Systemic)—*See* Rauwolfia Alkaloids and Thiazide Diuretics (Systemic)

**Trimethoprim-containing Combinations**
Sulfadiazine and Trimethoprim (Systemic)
Sulfamethoxazole and Trimethoprim (Systemic)

**Triprolidine-containing Combinations**
Triprolidine and Pseudoephedrine (Systemic)—*See* Antihistamines and Decongestants (Systemic)
Triprolidine, Pseudoephedrine, and Acetaminophen (Systemic)—*See* Antihistamines, Decongestants, and Analgesics (Systemic)
Triprolidine, Pseudoephedrine, and Codeine (Systemic)—*See* Cough/Cold Combinations (Systemic)
Triprolidine, Pseudoephedrine, Codeine, and Guaifenesin (Systemic)—*See* Cough/Cold Combinations (Systemic)
Triprolidine, Pseudoephedrine, and Dextromethorphan (Systemic)—*See* Cough/Cold Combinations (Systemic)

**Urea-containing Combinations**
Hydrocortisone and Urea (Topical)

**Zinc Oxide-containing Combinations**
Titanium Dioxide and Zinc Oxide (Topical)—*See* Sunscreen Agents (Topical)

USP DI                                                                                                                    The Medicine Chart    3083

# Appendix VII

## THE MEDICINE CHART

*The Medicine Chart* presents photographs of the most frequently prescribed medicines in the United States. In general, commonly used brand name products and a representative sampling of generic products have been included. The pictorial listing is not intended to be inclusive and does not represent all products on the market. Only selected solid oral dosage forms (capsules and tablets) have been included. The inclusion of a product does not mean the authors have any particular knowledge that the product included has properties different from other products, nor should it be interpreted as an endorsement. Similarly, the fact that a particular product has not been included does not indicate that the product has been judged to be unsatisfactory or unacceptable.

The drug products in *The Medicine Chart* are listed alphabetically by generic name of active ingredient(s). To quickly locate a particular medicine, check the product listing index that follows. This listing provides brand and generic names and directs the user to the appropriate page and chart location. In addition, any identifying code found on the surface of a capsule or tablet that might be useful in making a correct identification is included in the parentheses that follow the product's index entry. Only the identifying alphanumeric codes have been indexed; if a product also bears the brand name or manufacturer's name, this information has not been indexed. Please note that these codes may change as manufacturers reformulate or redesign their products. In addition, some companies may not manufacture all of their own products. In some of these cases, the imprinting on the tablet or capsule may be that of the actual manufacturer and not of the company marketing the product.

Brand names are in *italics*. An asterisk next to the generic name of the active ingredient(s) indicates that the solid oral dosage forms containing the ingredient(s) are available only from a single source with no generic equivalents currently available in the U.S. Where multiple source products are shown, it must be kept in mind that other products may also be available.

The size and color of the products shown are intended to match the actual product as closely as possible; however, there may be some differences due to variations caused by the photographic process. Also, manufacturers may occasionally change the color, imprinting, or shape of their products, and for a period of time both the "old" and the newly changed dosage forms may be on the market. Such changes may not occur uniformly thoughout the different dosages of the product. These types of changes will be incorporated in subsequent versions of the chart as they are brought to our attention.

> Use of this chart is limited to serving as an initial guide in identifying drug products. The identity of a product should be verified further before any action is taken.

**Acarbose**..............MC-1, A1-2
**Accolate** Tablets—
  20 mg (ZENECA/
    ACCOLATE 20).......MC-32, D1
**Accupril** Tablets—
  5 mg (PD 527/5).......MC-27, A5
  10 mg (PD 530/10)....MC-27, A5
  20 mg (PD 532/20)....MC-27, A5
**Accutane** Capsules—
  10 mg (ACCUTANE 10
    ROCHE)............MC-16, B5
  20 mg (ACCUTANE 20
    ROCHE)............MC-16, B5
  40 mg (ACCUTANE 40
    ROCHE)............MC-16, B5
**Acebutolol**...........MC-1, A3-5
  Mylan Capsules—
    200 mg (MYLAN
      1200).............MC-1, A3
    400 mg (MYLAN
      1400).............MC-1, A3
  Watson Capsules—
    200 mg (WATSON 437/
      200 mg)...........MC-1, A4
    400 mg (WATSON 438/
      400 mg)...........MC-1, A4
**Acetaminophen and
  Codeine**..............MC-1, A6-B2
  Purepac Tablets—
    300/30 mg (Logo
      001/3).............MC-1, B1
    300/60 mg (Logo
      003/4).............MC-1, B1
**Acetohexamide**.........MC-1, B3
  Barr Tablets—
    250 mg (barr 442).....MC-1, B3
    500 mg (barr 443).....MC-1, B3
**Achromycin V** Capsules—
  250 mg (Lederle 250 mg/
    Lederle A3).........MC-29, C6
  500 mg (Lederle 500 mg/
    Lederle A5).........MC-29, C6
**Acitretin**.............MC-1, B4
**Actigall** Capsules—
  300 mg (ACTIGALL/
    300 mg).............MC-32, A4

**Acyclovir**.............MC-1, B5-C1
**Apothecon** Capsules—
  200 mg (AP 4168).......MC-1, B5
**Apothecon** Tablets—
  400 mg (AP 4165).......MC-1, B6
  800 mg (AP 4166).......MC-1, B6
**Adalat** Capsules—
  10 mg (ADALAT 10)...MC-22, A3
  20 mg (ADALAT 20)...MC-22, A3
**Adalat CC Extended-release**
  Tablets—
    30 mg (ADALAT CC/
      30)...............MC-22, A4
    60 mg (ADALAT CC
      /60)..............MC-22, A4
    90 mg (ADALAT CC
      /90)..............MC-22, A5
**Albuterol**.............MC-1, C2-5
  Mylan Tablets—
    2 mg (M 255).........MC-1, C3
    4 mg (M 572).........MC-1, C3
  Novopharm Tablets—
    2 mg (N 480/2).......MC-1, C4
    4 mg (N 499/4).......MC-1, C4
**Aldactazide** Tablets—
  25/25 mg (SEARLE 1011/
    ALDACTAZIDE 25)....MC-28, C3
  50/50 mg (SEARLE 1021/
    ALDACTAZIDE 50)....MC-28, C3
**Aldactone** Tablets—
  25 mg (SEARLE 1001/
    ALDACTONE 25).....MC-28, C1
  50 mg (SEARLE 1041/
    ALDACTONE 50).....MC-28, C1
  100 mg (SEARLE 1031/
    ALDACTONE 100)....MC-28, C1
**Aldomet** Tablets—
  125 mg (MSD 135/
    ALDOMET)...........MC-19, B5
  250 mg (MSD 140/
    ALDOMET)...........MC-19, B5
  500 mg (MSD 516/
    ALDOMET)...........MC-19, B5

**Aldoril** Tablets—
  250/15 mg (MSD 423/
    ALDORIL)...........MC-19, B6
  250/25 mg (MSD 456/
    ALDORIL)...........MC-19, B6
  500/30 mg (MSD 694/
    ALDORIL)...........MC-19, B7
  500/50 mg (MSD 935/
    ALDORIL)...........MC-19, B7
**Alendronate**..............MC-1, C6
**Alkeran** Tablets—
  2 mg (ALKERAN
    A2A)................MC-18, C6
**Allegra** Capsules—
  60 mg (60 mg/1102)...MC-12, D5
**Allegra-D Extended-release**
  Capsules—
    60/120 mg (allegra-D)..MC-12, D6
**Allopurinol**...........MC-1, C7-D2
  Mutual Tablets—
    100 mg (Logo 71).....MC-1, D1
    300 mg (Logo 80).....MC-1, D1
  Mylan Tablets—
    100 mg (M 31)........MC-1, D2
    300 mg (M 71)........MC-1, D2
**Alprazolam**............MC-1, D3-5
  Lederle Tablets—
    0.25 mg (Logo/A 51)...MC-1, D3
    0.5 mg (Logo/A 52)....MC-1, D3
    1 mg (Logo/A 53)......MC-1, D3
    2 mg (Logo/A 54)......MC-1, D3
  Purepac Tablets—
    0.25 mg (Logo/027)....MC-1, D5
    0.5 mg (Logo/029).....MC-1, D5
    1 mg (Logo/031).......MC-1, D5
    2 mg (Logo 039).......MC-1, D5
**Altace** Capsules—
  1.25 mg (HOECHST/ALTACE
    1.25 mg).............MC-27, B4
  2.5 mg (HOECHST/ALTACE
    2.5 mg)..............MC-27, B4
  5 mg (HOECHST/ALTACE
    5 mg)................MC-27, B4
  10 mg (HOECHST/ALTACE
    10 mg)...............MC-27, B4

**Alupent** Tablets—
  10 mg (BI 74)..........MC-18, D6
  20 mg (BI 72).........MC-18, D6
**Amantadine**...........MC-1, D6-7
  Rosemont Capsules—
    100 mg (C-122)........MC-1, D7
**Amaryl** Tablets—
  1 mg (Logo/AMARYL)..MC-13, D4
  2 mg (Logo/AMARYL)..MC-13, D4
  4 mg (Logo/AMARYL)..MC-13, D4
**Ambien** Tablets
  5 mg (AMB 5/5401)....MC-32, D7
  10 mg (AMB 10/5421)..MC-32, D7
**Amerge** Tablets—
  1 mg (GX CE3).........MC-21, D2
  2.5 mg (GX CE5).......MC-21, D2
**Amicar** Tablets—
  500 mg (Logo (LL)/
    A 10)................MC-2, A4
**Amiloride**................MC-2, A1
**Amiloride and
  Hydrochlorothiazide**...MC-2, A2-3
  Barr Tablets—
    5/50 mg (barr/555
      483)................MC-2, A2
**Aminocaproic Acid**......MC-2, A4
**Amiodarone**............MC-2, A5-6
**Amitriptyline**..........MC-2, A7-B3
  Rugby Tablets—
    10 mg (RUGBY/3071)..MC-2, A7
    25 mg (RUGBY/3072)..MC-2, A7
    50 mg (RUGBY/3073)..MC-2, A7
    75 mg (RUGBY/3074)..MC-2, B1
    100 mg (RUGBY/3075)..MC-2, B1
    150 mg (RUGBY/M39)..MC-2, B1
**Amlodipine**.................MC-2, B4
**Amlodipine and
  Benazepril**..............MC-2, B5
**Amoxapine**.............MC-2, B6-7
  Schein Tablets
    50 mg (DAN 50/5714)..MC-2, B7
    100 mg (DAN 100/
      5715)..............MC-2, B7
**Amoxicillin**............MC-2, C1-6
  Novopharm Capsules—
    250 mg (N 724/250)...MC-2, C3
    500 mg (N 176/500)...MC-2, C3

**Amoxicillin and Clavulanate** .......... MC-2, C7-D3
**Amoxil** Capsules—
　250 mg (AMOXIL 250) ... MC-2, C4
　500 mg (AMOXIL 500) ... MC-2, C4
**Amoxil** Chewable Tablets—
　125 mg (AMOXIL/125) .. MC-2, C5
　250 mg (AMOXIL/250) .. MC-2, C5
**Ampicillin** ............ MC-2, D4-7
　Warner Chilcott Capsules—
　　500 mg (WC 404) ... MC-2, D5
　Warner Chilcott Chewable Tablets—
　　250 mg (B L/222) ...... MC-2, D6
**Anafranil** Capsules—
　25 mg (ANAFRANIL 25 mg) .............. MC-7, C7
　50 mg (ANAFRANIL 50 mg) .............. MC-7, C7
　75 mg (ANAFRANIL 75 mg) .............. MC-7, C7
**Anaprox** Tablets—
　275 mg (ANAPROX/ROCHE) ........... MC-21, C7
　550 mg (ANAPROX DS/ROCHE) ........... MC-21, C7
**Anastrozole** ............... MC-3, A1
**Ansaid** Tablets—
　50 mg (ANSAID 50 mg) .............. MC-13, B7
　100 mg (ANSAID 100 mg) ............. MC-13, B7
**Antivert** Tablets—
　25 mg (ANTIVERT/211) ................ MC-18, B6
　50 mg (ANTIVERT/214) ................ MC-18, B6
**Apresazide** Capsules—
　25/25 mg (CIBA 139/APRESAZIDE 25/25) ........ MC-14, C1
　50/50 mg (CIBA 149/APRESAZIDE 50/50) ........ MC-14, C1
　100/50 mg (CIBA 159/APRESAZIDE 100/50) ....... MC-14, C1
**Apresoline** Tablets—
　10 mg (CIBA/37) ....... MC-14, B7
　25 mg (CIBA/39) ....... MC-14, B7
　50 mg (CIBA/73) ....... MC-14, B7
　100 mg (CIBA/101) ..... MC-14, B7
**Aricept** Tablets—
　10 mg (E 246/10) ...... MC-10, B7
**Arimidex** Tablets—
　1 mg (Logo/Adx 1) ...... MC-3, A1
**Arthrotec** Tablets—
　50 mg/200 mcg (SEARLE 1411/A50) ............. MC-9, A7
　75 mg/200 mcg (SEARLE 1421/75) ............... MC-9, A2
**Asacol** Delayed-release Tablets—
　400 mg (ASACOL NE) MC-18, D3
**Asendin** Tablets—
　50 mg (LL 50/A 15) ...... MC-2, B6
**Aspirin, Caffeine, and Dihydrocodeine** .......... MC-3, A2
**Astemizole** ............... MC-3, A3
**Atacand** Tablets—
　4 mg (ACF/004) ....... MC-5, A3
　8 mg (ACG/008) ....... MC-5, A3
　16 mg (ACH/016) ...... MC-5, A4
　32 mg (ACL/032) ...... MC-5, A4
**Atenolol** ................ MC-3, A4-6
　Lederle Tablets—
　　25 mg (Logo/A7) ...... MC-3, A4
　　50 mg (Logo/A 49) .... MC-3, A4
　　100 mg (Logo/A 71) ... MC-3, A4
　Mutual Tablets—
　　25 mg (Logo 9) ....... MC-3, A5
　　50 mg (Logo 146) ..... MC-3, A5
　　100 mg (Logo 147) .... MC-3, A5
**Atenolol and Chlorthalidone** ........ MC-3, A7-B2
　Mutual Tablets—
　　50/25 mg (Logo 153) .. MC-3, A7
　　100/25 mg (Logo 152) . MC-3, A7
　Mylan Tablets—
　　50/25 mg (M 63) ...... MC-3, B1
　　100/25 mg (M 64) ..... MC-3, B1

**Ativan** Tablets—
　0.5 mg (WYETH 81/Logo) ............... MC-18, A4
　1 mg (WYETH 64/Logo) ............... MC-18, A4
　2 mg (WYETH 65/Logo 2) ............. MC-18, A4
**Atorvastatin** .............. MC-3, B3
**Atropine, Hyoscyamine, Scopolamine, and Phenobarbital** ........ MC-3, B4-6
**Augmentin** Chewable Tablets—
　200/28.5 mg (AUGMENTIN 200) ................. MC-2, D2
　400/57.0 mg (AUGMENTIN 400) ................. MC-2, D2
　125/31.25 mg (BMP 189) ................... MC-2, D3
　250/62.5 mg (BMP 190) ................... MC-2, D3
**Augmentin** Tablets—
　875/125 mg (AUGMENTIN 875) ................. MC-2, C7
　250/125 mg (AUGMENTIN/250/125) ............. MC-2, C7
　500/125 mg (AUGMENTIN/500/125) ............. MC-2, D1
**Axid** Capsules—
　150 mg (Lilly 3144/AXID 150 mg) ............. MC-22, C4
　300 mg (Lilly 3145/AXID 300 mg) ............. MC-22, C4
**Azatadine** ................ MC-3, B7
**Azatadine and Pseudoephedrine** .... MC-3, C1
**Azathioprine** ............. MC-3, C2-3
　Roxane Tablets—
　　50 mg (54 043) ....... MC-3, C3
**Azithromycin** ............. MC-3, C4
**Azulfidine** Tablets—
　500 mg (Logo/101) ..... MC-28, D3
**Azulfidine EN-Tabs** Enteric-coated Tablets—
　500 mg (Logo/102) ..... MC-28, D4
**Baclofen** ................ MC-3, C5-6
　Rugby Tablets—
　　10 mg (RUGBY/4959) .. MC-3, C6
　　20 mg (RUGBY/4960) .. MC-3, C6
**Bactrim** Tablets—
　400/80 mg (ROCHE/BACTRIM) ............ MC-28, D1
　800/160 mg (ROCHE/BACTRIM-DS) ......... MC-28, D1
**Benazepril** ............... MC-3, C7
**Benazepril and Hydrochlorothiazide** .. MC-3, D1-2
**Bendroflumethiazide** ...... MC-3, D3
**Bentyl** Capsules—
　10 mg (BENTYL 10) .... MC-9, B1
**Bentyl** Tablets—
　20 mg (BENTYL 20) .... MC-9, B2
**Benzphetamine** ........... MC-3, B7
**Benztropine** ............. MC-3, D5-7
　Goldline Tablets—
　　1 mg (par 165) ....... MC-3, D5
　　2 mg (INV 210) ....... MC-3, D5
　Mutual Tablets—
　　1 mg (Logo 44) ....... MC-3, D7
　　2 mg (Logo 142) ...... MC-3, D7
**Bepridil** ................. MC-4, A1
**Betapace** Tablets—
　80 mg (BETAPACE/80 mg) ............. MC-28, B4
　120 mg (BETAPACE/120 mg) ............ MC-28, B4
　160 mg (BETAPACE/160 mg) ............ MC-28, B5
　240 mg (BETAPACE/240 mg) ............ MC-28, B5
**Betaxolol** ................ MC-4, A2
**Biaxin** Tablets—
　250 mg (Logo KT) ..... MC-7, C1
　500 mg (Logo KL) ..... MC-7, C1

**Bicalutamide** ............ MC-4, A3
**Bismuth Subsalicylate/Metronidazole/Tetracycline** .... MC-4, A4-5
**Bisoprolol** ............... MC-4, A7
**Bisoprolol and Hydrochlorothiazide** ...... MC-4, B1
**Blocadren** Tablets—
　5 mg (MSD 59/BLOCADREN) ......... MC-30, C2
　10 mg (MSD 136/BLOCADREN) ......... MC-30, C2
　20 mg (MSD 437/BLOCADREN) ......... MC-30, C2
**Brethine** Tablets—
　2.5 mg (Geigy 72) ..... MC-29, C2
　5 mg (Geigy 105) ..... MC-29, C2
**Bromocriptine** .......... MC-4, B2-4
　Rosemont Tablets—
　　2.5 mg (BCT 2) ....... MC-4, B4
**Bumetanide** ............ MC-4, B5-6
　Mylan Tablets—
　　0.5 mg (MYLAN/245) .. MC-4, B5
　　1 mg (MYLAN/370) .... MC-4, B5
　　2 mg (MYLAN/417) .... MC-4, B5
**Bumex** Tablets—
　0.5 mg (ROCHE/BUMEX 0.5) .......... MC-4, B6
　1 mg (ROCHE/BUMEX 1) ............. MC-4, B6
　2 mg (ROCHE/BUMEX 2) ............. MC-4, B6
**Bupropion** .............. MC-4, B7-C2
**BuSpar** Tablets—
　5 mg (MJ5/BUSPAR) ... MC-4, C3
　10 mg (MJ10/BUSPAR) . MC-4, C3
**Buspirone** ................ MC-4, C3
**Busulfan** ................. MC-4, C4
**Butalbital, Acetaminophen, and Caffeine** ........ MC-4, C5-D1
　Qualitest Capsules—
　　50/325/40 mg (59743/004) ................ MC-4, C6
　Qualitest Tablets—
　　50/325/40 mg (HD 567) ................. MC-4, C7
　Teva USA Tablets—
　　50/325/50 mg (West-Ward 787) ............ MC-4, D1
**Butalbital, Acetaminophen, Caffeine, and Codeine** ..... MC-4, D2
**Butalbital, Aspirin, and Caffeine** ............. MC-4, D3-5
　Qualitest Tablets—
　　50/325/40 mg (West-Ward 785) ............ MC-4, D5
**Butalbital, Aspirin, Caffeine, and Codeine** .......... MC-4, D6-7
　Watson Capsules—
　　50/325/40/30 mg (WATSON 425) ............. MC-4, D7
**Calan** Tablets—
　40 mg (CALAN/40) ..... MC-32, B6
　80 mg (CALAN/80) ..... MC-32, B6
　120 mg (CALAN 120) ... MC-32, B6
**Calan SR** Extended-release Tablets—
　120 mg (CALAN/SR 120) ............... MC-32, B7
　180 mg (CALAN/SR 180) ............... MC-32, B7
　240 mg (CALAN/SR 240) ............... MC-32, B7
**Calcitriol** ................ MC-5, A1
**Calcium Acetate** .......... MC-5, A2
**Candesartan** ............ MC-5, A3-4
**Capecitabine** ............. MC-5, A5
**Capoten** Tablets—
　12.5 mg (CAPOTEN/12.5) ................. MC-5, A7
　25 mg (CAPOTEN 25) .. MC-5, A7
　50 mg (CAPOTEN 50) .. MC-5, A7
　100 mg (CAPOTEN 100) ................. MC-5, A7
**Capozide** Tablets—
　25/15 mg (CAPOZIDE 25/25) ............... MC-5, B2
　25/25 mg (CAPOZIDE 25/15) ............... MC-5, B2

**Capozide** Tablets (continued)
　50/15 mg (CAPOZIDE 50/15) ............... MC-5, B3
　50/25 mg (CAPOZIDE 50/25) ............... MC-5, B3
**Captopril** ............... MC-5, A6-B1
　Apothecon Tablets—
　　12.5 mg (AP/7045) .... MC-5, A6
　　25 mg (AP 7046) ...... MC-5, A6
　　50 mg (AP 7047) ...... MC-5, A6
　　100 mg (AP 7048) ..... MC-5, A6
　West-ward Tablets—
　　12.5 mg (W7) ......... MC-5, B1
　　25 mg (WW 172) ....... MC-5, B1
　　50 mg (WW 173) ....... MC-5, B1
　　100 mg (WW 174) ...... MC-5, B1
**Captopril and Hydrochlorothiazide** ... MC-5, B2-4
　Endo Tablets—
　　25/15 mg (Endo 733) ... MC-5, B4
　　25/25 mg (Endo 741) ... MC-5, B4
　　50/15 mg (Endo 739) ... MC-5, B4
　　50/25 mg (Endo 731) ... MC-5, B4
**Carafate** Tablets—
　1 gram (CARAFATE/1712) ............... MC-28, C5
**Carbamazepine** ......... MC-5, B5-C2
　Purepac Tablets—
　　200 mg (Logo/143) .... MC-5, C1
　Warner Chilcott Chewable Tablets—
　　100 mg (WC 242) ..... MC-5, C2
**Carbidopa and Levodopa** ............ MC-5, C3-5
　Purepac Tablets—
　　10/100 mg (93 292) .... MC-5, C5
　　25/100 mg (Logo/539) .. MC-5, C5
　　25/250 mg (Logo/540) .. MC-5, C5
**Carbinoxamine and Pseudoephedrine** ..... MC-5, C6
**Cardene** Capsules—
　20 mg (CARDENE 20 mg/ROCHE) ............ MC-21, D7
　30 mg (CARDENE 30 mg/ROCHE) ............ MC-21, D7
**Cardene SR** Extended-release Capsules—
　30 mg (CARDENE SR 30 mg/ROCHE) ............ MC-22, A1
　45 mg (CARDENE SR 45 mg/ROCHE) ............ MC-22, A1
　60 mg (CARDENE SR 60 mg/ROCHE) ............ MC-22, A2
**Cardizem** Tablets—
　30 mg (MARION/1771) ... MC-9, D3
　60 mg (MARION/1772) ... MC-9, D3
　90 mg (CARDIZEM/90 mg) ................ MC-9, D4
　120 mg (CARDIZEM/120 mg) ............... MC-9, D4
**Cardizem CD** Capsules—
　120 mg (Logo/cardizem CD 120 mg) ......... MC-9, C7
　180 mg (Logo/cardizem CD 180 mg) ......... MC-9, C7
　240 mg (Logo/cardizem CD 240 mg) ......... MC-9, D1
　300 mg (Logo/cardizem CD 300 mg) ......... MC-9, D1
**Cardizem SR** Extended-release Capsules
　60 mg (Logo/cardizem SR 60 mg) .......... MC-9, D2
　90 mg (Logo/cardizem SR 90 mg) .......... MC-9, D2
　120 mg (Logo/cardizem SR 120 mg) ......... MC-9, D2
**Cardura** Tablets—
　1 mg (CARDURA/1 mg) ............... MC-10, C1
　2 mg (CARDURA/2 mg) ............... MC-10, C1
　4 mg (CARDURA/4 mg) ............... MC-10, C1
　8 mg (CARDURA/8 mg) ............... MC-10, C1
**Carisoprodol** ........... MC-5, C7-D1
　Mutual Tablets—
　　350 mg (Logo 58) ..... MC-5, C7

**Carisoprodol and Aspirin** .............. MC-5, D2-3
  Qualitest Tablets—
    200/325 mg (par 246) MC-5, D2
**Carisoprodol, Aspirin, and Codeine**............ MC-5, D4
**Carteolol** .................... MC-5, D5
**Cartrol** Tablets—
  2.5 mg (Logo 1A)....... MC-5, D5
  5 mg (Logo 1C)......... MC-5, D5
**Carvedilol** ................. MC-5, D6-7
**Casodex** Tablets—
  50 mg (Logo/Cdx 50) .... MC-4, A3
**Catapres** Tablets—
  0.1 mg (BI 6) ........... MC-7, D4
  0.2 mg (BI 7) ........... MC-7, D4
  0.3 mg (BI 11) .......... MC-7, D4
**Ceclor** Capsules—
  250 mg (Lilly 3061/
    CECLOR 250 mg) ...... MC-6, A1
  500 mg (Lilly 3062/
    CECLOR 500 mg) ...... MC-6, A1
**Cedax** Capsules—
  400 mg (Cedax/
    400 mg)................MC-6, B2
**Cefaclor** ..................MC-6, A1-2
  Mylan Capsules—
    250 mg (MYLAN 7250/
      MYLAN 7250) ........ MC-6, A2
    500 mg (MYLAN 7500/
      MYLAN 7500)........MC-6, A2
**Cefadroxil** ..............MC-6, A3-5
  Apothecon Capsules—
    500 mg (500 mg/
      BRISTOL 7271)........MC-6, A3
**Cefixime**...................MC-6, A6
**Cefpodoxime**...............MC-6, A7
**Cefprozil** ...................MC-6, B1
**Ceftibuten** ..................MC-6, B2
**Ceftin** Tablets—
  125 mg (Glaxo/395) ...MC-6, B3
  250 mg (Glaxo/387) ...MC-6, B3
  500 mg (Glaxo/394) ...MC-6, B4
**Cefuroxime Axetil** .......MC-6, B3-4
**Cefzil** Tablets—
  250 mg (7720 BMS
    250).................MC-6, B1
  500 mg (7721 BMS
    500).................MC-6, B1
**CellCept** Capsules—
  250 mg (CellCept 250/
    Roche) ............. MC-21, A7
**CellCept** Tablets—
  500 mg (CellCept 500/
    Roche) .............. MC-21, B1
**Cephalexin** ............. MC-6, B5-C1
  Apothecon Capsules—
    250 mg (SQUIBB
      181 ................MC-6, B5
    500 mg (SQUIBB
      239).................MC-6, B5
  Barr Capsules—
    250 mg (barr/514).......MC-6, B6
    500 mg (barr/515)......MC-6, B6
  Biocraft Capsules—
    250 mg (biocraft 115/
      biocraft 115) ..........MC-6, B7
    500 mg (biocraft 117/
      biocraft 117)..........MC-6, B7
  Novopharm Capsules—
    250 mg (N 084/250)... MC-6, C1
    500 mg (N 114/500)... MC-6, C1
**Cephradine**............ MC-6, C2-3
  Biocraft Capsules—
    250 mg (biocraft 112/
      biocraft 112) ..........MC-6, C3
    500 mg (biocraft 113/
      biocraft 113) ..........MC-6, C3
**Cetirizine** .................. MC-6, C4
**Chlor-Trimeton** Tablets—
  8 mg (Logo 374)........MC-6, D3
  12 mg (Logo 009) ......MC-6, D3
**Chlorambucil** ...............MC-6, C5
**Chlordiazepoxide** ........MC-6, C6
  Barr Capsules—
    5 mg (barr/158) .........MC-6, C6
    10 mg (barr/033).......MC-6, C6
    25 mg (barr/159)........MC-6, C6

**Chlordiazepoxide and Amitriptyline** ............. MC-6, C7
  Mylan Tablets—
    5/12.5 mg (MYLAN/
      211).................MC-6, C7
    10/25 mg (MYLAN/
      277)................. MC-6, C7
**Chlordiazepoxide and Clidinium** ............ MC-6, D1-2
**Chlorpheniramine**........ MC-6, D3
**Chlorpheniramine, Phenylpropanolamine, Phenylephrine, and Phenyltoloxamine**....... MC-6, D4
  Geneva Extended-release Tablets—
    5/15/10/40 mg (GG
      118)................. MC-6, D4
**Chlorpheniramine, Phenyltoloxamine, Phenylephrine, and Phenylpropanolamine** .. MC-6, D5
**Chlorpheniramine, Pyrilamine, and Phenylephrine** ..... MC-6, D6
**Chlorpromazine** .........MC-6, D7, MC-7, A1
**Chlorpropamide**............MC-7, A2
  Mylan Tablets—
    100mg (MYLAN 197/
      100)..................MC-7, A2
    250 mg (MYLAN 210/
      250)..................MC-7, A2
**Chlorthalidone** ..........MC-7, A3-5
  Barr Tablets—
    25 mg (Barr/267).......MC-7, A3
    50 mg (Barr/268).......MC-7, A3
**Chlorzoxazone** ........ MC-7, A6-B1
  Barr Tablets—
    500 mg (barr/555
      585).................MC-7, A6
  Mutual Tablets—
    500 mg (Logo 74) ......MC-7, A7
**Cimetidine** ...............MC-7, B2-4
  Mylan Tablets—
    200 mg (M/53)........MC-7, B2
    300 mg (M/317).......MC-7, B2
    400 mg (M/372).......MC-7, B2
    800 mg (M 541)........MC-7, B2
**Cipro** Tablets—
  100 mg (CIPRO/100)....MC-7, B5
  250 mg (CIPRO/250)....MC-7, B5
  500 mg (CIPRO/500).....MC-7, B6
  750 mg (CIPRO/750)....MC-7, B6
**Ciprofloxacin**............MC-7, B5-6
**Cisapride**..................MC-7, B7
**Clarithromycin** ..........MC-7, C1
**Claritin** Tablets—
  10 mg (CLARITIN 10/
    458)................ MC-17, D7
**Claritin-D** Tablets—
  5/120 mg (CLARITIN
    D) ................ MC-18, A1
**Cleocin** Capsules—
  75 mg (CLEOCIN 75 mg/
    CLEOCIN 75 mg)...... MC-7, C3
  150 mg (CLEOCIN 150 mg/
    CLEOCIN 150 mg)..... MC-7, C3
  300 mg (CLEOCIN 300 mg/
    CLEOCIN 300 mg)..... MC-7, C4
**Clindamycin** ........... MC-7, C2-4
  Biocraft Capsules—
    150 mg (biocraft 149).. MC-7, C2
**Clindex** Capsules—
  5/2.5 mg (RUGBY
    3490) ............... MC-6, D2
**Clinoril** Tablets—
  150 mg (MSD 941/
    CLINORIL) ............ MC-29, A1
  200 mg (MSD 942/
    CLINORIL) ........... MC-29, A1
**Clomid** Tablets—
  50 mg (CLOMID 50).... MC-7, C5
**Clomiphene** .............MC-7, C5
**Clomipramine** ........ MC-7, C6-7
  Invamed Capsules—
    25 mg (INV 321/
      INV 321)........... MC-7, C6
    75 mg (INV 323/
      INV 323).............. MC-7, C6

**Clonazepam**............. MC-7, D1-3
  Teva USA Tablets—
    0.5 mg (93 832) ....... MC-7, D3
    2 mg (93 834)......... MC-7, D3
**Clonidine**.............. MC-7, D4-7
  Lederle Tablets—
    0.1 mg (Logo/C 42).... MC-7, D5
    0.2 mg (Logo/C 43).... MC-7, D5
    0.3 mg (Logo/C 44).... MC-7, D5
  Mylan Tablets
    0.1 mg (MYLAN 152)... MC-7, D6
    0.2 mg (MYLAN 186).. MC-7, D6
    0.3 mg (MYLAN 199)... MC-7, D6
  Purepac Tablets—
    0.1 mg (Logo/127) .... MC-7, D7
    0.2 mg (Logo/128) .... MC-7, D7
    0.3 mg (Logo/129) .... MC-7, D7
**Clonidine and Chlorthalidone** .........MC-8, A1-2
**Clorazepate** ...............MC-8, A3-5
  Mylan Tablets—
    3.75 mg (M 30).........MC-8, A5
    7.5 mg (M 40)..........MC-8, A5
    15 mg (M 70)...........MC-8, A5
    0.2/15 mg (M 27)......MC-8, A1
    0.1/15 mg (M 1).......MC-8, A1
**Clorpres** Tablets—
  0.3/15 mg (M 72) .......MC-8, A1
**Clotrimazole**..............MC-8, A6
**Clozapine** .................MC-8, A7
**Clozaril** Tablets—
  25 mg (CLOZARIL/25) .. MC-8, A7
  100 mg (CLOZARIL/
    100)..................MC-8, A7
**Cogentin** Tablets—
  0.5 mg (MSD 21/
    COGENTIN) .......... MC-3, D6
  1 mg (MSD 635/
    COGENTIN)........... MC-3, D6
  2 mg (COGENTIN/60)... MC-3, D6
**Cognex** Capsules—
  10 mg (COGNEX 10) ..MC-29, A5
  20 mg (COGNEX 20) ..MC-29, A5
  30 mg (COGNEX 30) ..MC-29, A6
  40 mg (COGNEX 40) ..MC-29, A6
**Colestid** Tablets—
  1000 mg (1 gm) (U) ....MC-8, B1
**Colestipol** ...................MC-8, B1
**Combipres** Tablets—
  0.1/15 mg (BI 8) ........MC-8, A2
  0.2/15 mg (BI 9) ........MC-8, A2
  0.3/15 mg (BI 10) ......MC-8, A2
**Combivir** Tablets—
  150/300 mg (GX FC3).. MC-16, D3
**Compazine** Extended-release Capsules—
  10 mg (SKB logo 10 mg/
    3344 10 mg)......... MC-26, B1
  15 mg (SKB logo 15 mg/
    3346 15 mg)......... MC-26, B1
**Compazine** Tablets—
  5 mg (SKF C66) ....... MC-26, B2
  10 mg (SKF C67)...... MC-26, B2
**Cordarone** Tablets—
  200 mg (WYETH 4188/
    200)...................MC-2, A6
**Coreg** Tablets—
  3.125 mg (SB/39) ....... MC-5, D6
  6.25 mg (SB 4140/SB
    4140).................MC-5, D6
  12.5 mg (SB 4141/SB
    4141)................ MC-5, D7
  25 mg (SB 4142/SB
    4142).................MC-5, D7
**Corgard** Tablets—
  20 mg (CORGARD 20/
    BL 232) ............. MC-21, B5
  40 mg (CORGARD 40/
    BL 207) ............. MC-21, B5
  80 mg (CORGARD 80/
    BL 241) ............. MC-21, B5
  120 mg (CORGARD 120 MG/
    BL 208) ............ MC-21, B6
  160 mg (CORGARD 160 MG/
    BL 246) ............ MC-21, B6
**Cortef** Tablets—
  5 mg (CORTEF 5) ..... MC-15, A1
  10 mg (CORTEF 10) .. MC-15, A1
  20 mg (CORTEF 20) .. MC-15, A1

**Corzide** Tablets—
  40/5 mg (CORZIDE 40-5/
    PPP 283) ........... MC-21, B7
  80/5 mg (CORZIDE 80-5/
    PPP 284) ........... MC-21, B7
**Cotazym** Capsules—
  8/30/30 units (Organon
    (Logo)/381) .......... MC-24, B6
**Coumadin** Tablets—
  1 mg (DuPont/
    COUMADIN 1) ....... MC-32, C4
  2 mg (DuPont/
    COUMADIN 2) ....... MC-32, C4
  2.5 mg (DuPont/
    COUMADIN 2) ...... MC-32, C4
  5 mg (DuPont/
    COUMADIN 5) ....... MC-32, C5
  7.5 mg (DuPont/
    COUMADIN 7) ....... MC-32, C5
  10 mg (DuPont/
    COUMADIN 10) ..... MC-32, C5
**Covera-HS** Extended-release Tablets—
  180 mg (COVERA-HS
    2011) ............... MC-32, C1
  240 mg (COVERA-HS
    2021) ............... MC-32, C1
**Cozaar** Tablets—
  25 mg (MRK/951) ...... MC-18, A5
  50 mg (MRK952/
    COZAAR) ............ MC-18, A5
**Creon** Capsules—
  5/16.6/18.75 (000) Units
    (SOLVAY/1205) ...... MC-24, B5
  10/32.2/37.5 (000) Units
    (SOLVAY/1210) ...... MC-24, B5
  20/66.4/75 (000) Units
    (SOLVAY/1220) ...... MC-24, B5
**Crixivan** Capsules—
  200 mg (CRIXIVAN
    200 mg) ............. MC-15, D5
  400 mg (CRIXIVAN
    400 mg) ............. MC-15, D5
**Cyclobenzaprine** .........MC-8, B2-5
  Endo Tablets—
    10 mg (WPPh/156) ....MC-8, B2
  Invamed Tablets—
    10 mg (INV 252) .......MC-8, B3
  Mylan Tablets—
    10 mg (Logo/751) ......MC-8, B5
**Cyclophosphamide** .........MC-8, B6
**Cyclosporine**...........MC-8, B7-C1
**Cylert** Chewable Tablets—
  37.5 mg (Logo/TK) .... MC-24, C5
**Cylert** Tablets—
  18.75 mg (Logo/TH) ... MC-24, C4
  37.5 mg (Logo/TI) .... MC-24, C4
  75 mg (Logo/TJ) ..... MC-24, C4
**Cytotec** Tablets—
  0.1 mg (SEARLE/
    1451)................ MC-20, D3
  0.2 mg (Logo/SEARLE
    1461)................ MC-20, D3
**Cytovene** Capsules—
  250 mg (CYTOVENE
    250 mg) ............. MC-13, C7
**Cytoxan** Tablets—
  50 mg (MJ (Logo) 503/
    50)...................MC-8, B6
**Dalmane** Capsules—
  15 mg (DALMANE 15
    ROCHE) ............. MC-13, B5
  30 mg (DALMANE 30
    ROCHE) ............. MC-13, B5
**Danazol** ................... MC-8, C2
**Danocrine** Capsules—
  50 mg (Logo D 03/DANO-
    CRINE 50 mg)......... MC-8, C2
  100 mg (Logo D 04/DANO-
    CRINE 100 mg) ........MC-8, C2
  200 mg (Logo D 05/DANO-
    CRINE 200 mg) ....... MC-8, C2
**Dantrium** Capsules—
  25 mg (DANTRIUM 25 mg/
    0149 0030)............ MC-8, C3
  50 mg (DANTRIUM 50 mg/
    0149 0031)............ MC-8, C3
  100 mg (DANTRIUM 100 mg/
    0149 0033)............ MC-8, C3

**Dantrolene** .......... MC-8, C3
**Daraprim** Tablets—
 25 mg (DARAPRIM
  A3A) .......... MC-27, A3
**Darvocet-N** Tablets—
 50/325 mg (Lilly DARVOCET-N
  50) .......... MC-26, C1
 100/650 mg (Lilly/DARVOCET-N
  100) .......... MC-26, C1
**Daypro** Tablets—
 600 mg (DAYPRO/
  1381) .......... MC-23, C7
**DDAVP** Tablets—
 0.2 mg (Logo/DDAVP
  0.2) .......... MC-8, D1
 0.1 mg (Logo/DDAVP
  0.1) .......... MC-8, D1
**Decadron** Tablets—
 0.5 mg (MSD 41/
  DECADRON) .......... MC-8, D4
 0.75 mg (MSD 63/
  DECADRON) .......... MC-8, D4
 1.5 mg (MSD 95/
  DECADRON) .......... MC-8, D4
 4 mg (MSD 97/
  DECADRON) .......... MC-8, D4
**Declomycin** Tablets—
 150 mg (LL/D 11) .......... MC-8, C4
 300 mg (LL/D12) .......... MC-8, C4
**Deltasone** Tablets—
 2.5 mg (DELTASONE
  2.5) .......... MC-25, D6
 5 mg (DELTASONE
  5) .......... MC-25, D6
 10 mg (DELTASONE
  10) .......... MC-25, D6
 20 mg (DELTASONE
  20) .......... MC-25, D7
 50 mg (DELTASONE
  50) .......... MC-25, D7
**Demadex** Tablets—
 5 mg (ROCHE/5) .......... MC-31, A5
 10 mg (ROCHE DEMADEX/
  10) .......... MC-31, A5
 20 mg (ROCHE DEMADEX/
  20) .......... MC-31, A6
 100 mg (ROCHE DEMADEX/
  100) .......... MC-31, A6
**Demeclocycline** .......... MC-8, C4
**Demerol** Tablets—
 50 mg (Logo/D35) .......... MC-18, D1
 100 mg (Logo/D37) .......... MC-18, D1
**Demulen 1/35-21 and -28**
 Tablets—
 1/0.035 mg (SEARLE/
  151) .......... MC-12, A6
 Inert (SEARLE/P) .......... MC-12, A6
**Demulen 1/50-21 and -28**
 Tablets—
 1/0.05 mg (SEARLE/
  71) .......... MC-12, A7
 Inert (SEARLE/P) .......... MC-12, A7
**Depakene** Delayed-release
 Capsules—
 250 mg (DEPAKENE) .. MC-32, A6
**Depakote** Delayed-release Tablets—
 125 mg (Logo NT) .......... MC-10, B5
 250 mg (Logo NR) .......... MC-10, B5
 500 mg (Logo NS) .......... MC-10, B6
**Depakote Sprinkle** Delayed-release
 Capsules—
 125 mg (DEPAKOTE SPRINKLE
  125 mg/THIS END
  UP) .......... MC-10, B4
**Desipramine** .......... MC-8, C5-7
 Geneva Tablets—
 100 mg (GG 167) .......... MC-8, C5
 150 mg (GG 168) .......... MC-8, C5
**Desmopressin** .......... MC-8, D1
**Desogen** Tablets—
 0.15/0.03 mg (ORGANON*/
  TR 5) .......... MC-8, D2
 Inert (ORGANON*/
  KH 2) .......... MC-8, D2

**Desogestrel and Ethinyl
 Estradiol** .......... MC-8, D2-3
**Desyrel** Tablets—
 50 mg (DESYREL
  MJ775) .......... MC-31, B5
 100 mg (DESYREL
  MJ776) .......... MC-31, B5
**Desyrel Dividose** Tablets—
 150 mg (L800/778) .......... MC-31, B6
**Dexamethasone** .......... MC-8, D4-5
 Roxane Tablets—
 0.5 mg (54 299) .......... MC-8, D5
 0.75 mg (54 960) .......... MC-8, D5
 1 mg (54 489) .......... MC-8, D5
 1.5 mg (54 943) .......... MC-8, D5
 2 mg (54 662) .......... MC-8, D5
 4 mg (54 892) .......... MC-8, D5
**DiaBeta** Tablets—
 1.25 mg (HOECHST/
  Dia) .......... MC-14, A2
 2.5 mg (HOECHST/
  Dia) .......... MC-14, A2
 5 mg (HOECHST/Dia) .. MC-14, A2
**Diazepam** .... MC-8, D6, MC-9, A1
 Barr Tablets—
 5 mg (barr/555 363) .. MC-8, D6
 10 mg (barr/555 164) .. MC-8, D6
 Purepac Tablets—
 2 mg (Logo/051) .......... MC-8, D7
 5 mg (Logo/052) .......... MC-8, D7
 10 mg (Logo/053) .......... MC-8, D7
**Diclofenac and
 Misoprostol** .......... MC-9, A2
**Diclofenac Sodium** .... MC-9, A3-6
 Geneva Enteric-coated Tablets—
 50 mg (GG 738) .......... MC-9, A4
 75 mg (GG 739) .......... MC-9, A3
 Purepac Delayed-release Tablets—
 50 mg (Logo/550) .......... MC-9, A6
 75 mg (Logo/551) .......... MC-9, A6
**Diclofenac Sodium
 and Misoprostol** .......... MC-9, A7
**Dicyclomine** .......... MC-9, B1-4
 Rugby Capsules—
 10 mg (RUGBY
  3367) .......... MC-9, B3
 Rugby Tablets—
 20 mg (RUGBY/3377) .. MC-9, B4
**Didanosine** .......... MC-9, B5
**Didrex** Tablets—
 50 mg (DIDREX 50) .... MC-3, D4
**Didronel** Tablets—
 200 mg (P & G/402) .... MC-12, B1
 400 mg (N E/406) .... MC-12, B1
**Diethylpropion** .......... MC-9, B6-7
**Diflucan** Tablets—
 50 mg (ROERIG/DIFLUCAN
  50) .......... MC-13, A3
 100 mg (ROERIG/DIFLUCAN
  100) .......... MC-13, A3
 150 mg (ROERIG/DIFLUCAN
  150) .......... MC-13, A4
 200 mg (ROERIG/DIFLUCAN
  200) .......... MC-13, A4
**Diflunisal** .......... MC-9, C1-2
 Roxane Tablets—
 250 mg (54 010) .......... MC-9, C2
 500 mg (54 093) .......... MC-9, C2
**Digoxin** .......... MC-9, C3-4
**Dilantin Infatabs**
 Chewable Tablets—
 50 mg (P-D 007) .......... MC-25, B5
**Dilantin Kapseals** Extended-
 release Capsules—
 30 mg (P-D 365) .......... MC-25, B4
 100 mg (P-D 362) .......... MC-25, B4
**Dilatrate-SR** Extended-release
 Capsules—
 40 mg (SCHWARZ/
  0920) .......... MC-16, A4
**Dilaudid** Tablets—
 2 mg (Logo/2) .......... MC-15, A3
 4 mg (Logo/4) .......... MC-15, A3
 8 mg (Logo/8) .......... MC-15, A3
**Diltiazem** .......... MC-9, C5-D7
 Mylan Extended-release Capsules—
 60 mg (MYLAN 6060) ... MC-9, D5
 90 mg (MYLAN 6090) ... MC-9, D5
 120 mg (MYLAN
  6120) .......... MC-9, D5

Mylan Tablets—
 30 mg (M 23) .......... MC-9, D6
 60 mg (M 45) .......... MC-9, D6
 90 mg (M 135) .......... MC-9, D7
 120 mg (M 525) .......... MC-9, D7
**Dipentum** Capsules—
 250 mg (DIPENTUM
  250mg) .......... MC-23, C3
**Diphenhist** Tablets—
 25 mg (RUGBY/3597) .. MC-10, A2
**Diphenhydramine** ..... MC-10, A1-2
 Rugby Capsules—
 25 mg (RUGBY
  3758) .......... MC-10, A1
 50 mg (RUGBY
  3762) .......... MC-10, A1
**Diphenoxylate and
 Atropine** .......... MC-10, A3-4
 Mylan Tablets—
 2.5/0.025 mg (M 15) .. MC-10, A3
**Dipyridamole** .......... MC-10, A5-6
 Barr Tablets—
 25 mg (Logo/252) .......... MC-10, A5
 50 mg (Logo/285) .......... MC-10, A5
 75 mg (BARR/286) .... MC-10, A5
**Dirithromycin** .......... MC-10, A7
**Disopyramide** .......... MC-10, B1-3
 Geneva Capsules—
 100 mg (GG 56) .......... MC-10, B1
 150 mg (GG 57) .......... MC-10, B1
**Divalproex** .......... MC-10, B4-6
**Dolobid** Tablets—
 250 mg (MSD 675/
  DOLOBID) .......... MC-9, C1
 500 mg (MSD 697/
  DOLOBID) .......... MC-9, C1
**Donepezil** .......... MC-10, B7
**Donnatal** Capsules—
 0.0194/0.1037/0.0065/
 16.2 mg (AHR 4207) ... MC-3, B4
**Donnatal** Extended-release
 Tablets—
 0.0582/0.3111/0.0195/
 48.6 mg (AHR DONNATAL
  EXTENTAB) .......... MC-3, B6
**Donnatal** Tablets—
 0.0194/0.1037/0.0065/16.2 mg
  (R 4250) .......... MC-3, B5
**Doxazosin** .......... MC-10, C1
**Doxepin** .......... MC-10, C2-D2
 Mylan Capsules—
 10 mg (MYLAN
  1049) .......... MC-10, C2
 25 mg (MYLAN
  3125) .......... MC-10, C2
 50 mg (MYLAN
  4250) .......... MC-10, C2
 75 mg (MYLAN
  5375) .......... MC-10, C3
 100 mg (MYLAN
  6410) .......... MC-10, C3
 Par Capsules—
 10 mg (par 217) .......... MC-10, C4
 25 mg (par 218) .......... MC-10, C4
 50 mg (par 219) .......... MC-10, C4
 75 mg (par 220) .......... MC-10, C5
 100 mg (par 221) .......... MC-10, C5
 150 mg (par 222) .......... MC-10, C5
 Rugby Capsules—
 10 mg (RUGBY
  4563) .......... MC-10, D1
 25 mg (RUGBY
  4564) .......... MC-10, D1
 50 mg (RUGBY
  4565) .......... MC-10, D1
 75 mg (RUGBY
  3737) .......... MC-10, D2
 100 mg (RUGBY
  4566) .......... MC-10, D2
 150 mg (RUGBY
  3738) .......... MC-10, D2
**Doxycycline** .......... MC-10, D3-5
 Purepac Delayed-release
 Capsules—
 100 mg (Logo 2598) .. MC-10, D3
 Rugby Capsules—
 50 mg (RUGBY/0280) .. MC-10, D4
 100 mg (RUGBY/
  0230) .......... MC-10, D4

West-ward Capsules—
 50 mg (West-ward/
  3141) .......... MC-10, D5
 100 mg (West-ward/
  3142) .......... MC-10, D5
**Drisdol** Capsules—
 1.25 mg (W (Logo)/
  D92) .......... MC-11, A5
**Duricef** Capsules—
 500 mg (MJ 784) .......... MC-6, A4
**Duricef** Tablets—
 1 gram (MJ 785) .......... MC-6, A5
**Dyazide** Capsules—
 37.5/25 mg (DYAZIDE
  Logo) .......... MC-31, D1
**Dynabac** Tablets—
 250 mg (DYNABAC
  UC5364) .......... MC-10, A7
**DynaCirc** Capsules—
 2.5 mg (Logo 2.5/DynaCirc
  Logo) .......... MC-16, B6
 5 mg (Logo 5/DynaCirc
  Logo) .......... MC-16, B6
**Dyphylline** .......... MC-10, D6
**Dyphylline and
 Guaifenesin** .......... MC-10, D7
**Dyrenium** Capsules—
 50 mg (DYRENIUM 50
  SKF) .......... MC-31, C4
 100 mg (DYRENIUM 100
  SKF) .......... MC-31, C4
**E-C Naprosyn** Delayed-release
 Tablets—
 375 mg (EC-NAPROSYN/
  375) .......... MC-21, C4
 500 mg (EC-NAPROSYN/
  500) .......... MC-21, C4
**E-Mycin** Delayed-release Tablets—
 250 mg (E-MYCIN
  250 mg) .......... MC-11, C1
 333 mg (E-MYCIN
  333 mg) .......... MC-11, C1
**E.E.S.** Tablets—
 400 mg (Logo EE) .... MC-11, C7
**Effexor** Tablets—
 25 mg (Logo 25/701) .. MC-32, B1
 37.5 mg (Logo 37.5/
  781) .......... MC-32, B1
 50 mg (Logo 50/703) .. MC-32, B1
 75 mg (Logo 75/704) .. MC-32, B2
 100 mg (Logo 100/
  705) .......... MC-32, B2
**Elavil** Tablets—
 10 mg (MSD 23/
  ELAVIL) .......... MC-2, B2
 25 mg (MSD 45/
  ELAVIL) .......... MC-2, B2
 50 mg (MSD 102/
  ELAVIL) .......... MC-2, B2
 75 mg (MSD 430/
  ELAVIL) .......... MC-2, B3
 100 mg (MSD 435/
  ELAVIL) .......... MC-2, B3
 150 mg (MSD 673/
  ELAVIL) .......... MC-2, B3
**Eldepryl** Capsules—
 5 mg (Logo Somerset/
  Eldepryl 5 mg) .......... MC-28, A6
**Elmiron** Capsules—
 100 mg (BNP 7600/
  BNP 7600) .......... MC-24, D7
**Enalapril** .......... MC-11, A1
**Enalapril and
 Felodipine** .......... MC-11, A2
**Enalapril and
 Hydrochlorothiazide** .. MC-11, A3
**Enduron** Tablets—
 2.5 mg (Logo
  ENDURON) .......... MC-19, B2
 5 mg (Logo
  ENDURON) .......... MC-19, B2
**Enoxacin** .......... MC-11, A4
**Entex** Capsules—
 5/45/200 mg (ENTEX/
  0149 0412) .......... MC-25, B1
**Entex LA** Extended-release
 Tablets—
 75/400mg (entex LA/
  0149 0436) .......... MC-25, B2

**Entex PSE** Tablets—
120/600 mg (entex
PSE) .................. MC-27, A1
*Epivir* Tablets—
150 mg (GX CJ7/150) .. MC-16, D2
*Ercaf* Tablets—
1/100 mg (Logo/400) ... MC-11, B2
*Ergocalciferol* ........... MC-11, B2
*Ergoloid Mesylates* ... MC-11, A6-B1
Mutual Tablets—
1 mg (Logo 20) ....... MC-11, A6
**Ergotamine and
Caffeine** ........... MC-11, B2
*Ery-Tab* Delayed-release
Tablets—
250 mg (Logo EC) ..... MC-11, B6
333 mg (Logo EH) ..... MC-11, B6
500 mg (Logo ED) ..... MC-11, B6
*Eryc* Delayed-release Capsules—
250 mg (Eryc/P-D
696) ................... MC-11, C3
*EryPed* Chewable Tablets—
200 mg (Logo/CHEW
EZ) .................. MC-11, D1
*Erythrocin* Tablets—
250 mg (Logo/ES) ..... MC-11, D2
500 mg (Logo/ET) ..... MC-11, D2
**Erythromycin** ......... MC-11, B3-C3
Abbott Delayed-release Capsules—
250 mg (Logo ER) ..... MC-11, B3
Abbott Tablets—
250 mg (Logo EB) .... MC-11, B4
500 mg (Logo EA) .... MC-11, B4
Barr Delayed-release Capsules—
250 mg (barr/584) ..... MC-11, B7
Purepac Delayed-release
Capsules—
250 mg (Logo 553) ... MC-11, C2
**Erythromycin
Estolate** .............. MC-11, C4-6
Barr Capsules—
250 mg (barr 230/
barr 230) ............. MC-11, C4
**Erythromycin
Ethylsuccinate** ....... MC-11, C7-D1
**Erythromycin
Stearate** ............. MC-11, D2
*Esidrix* Tablets—
25 mg (CIBA/22) ....... MC-14, C5
50 mg (CIBA/46) ....... MC-14, C5
100 mg (CIBA/192) .... MC-14, C5
*Eskalith* Capsules—
300 mg (ESKALITH
SKB Logo) ........... MC-17, C6
*Eskalith CR* Extended-release
Tablets—
450 mg (SKF J10) ..... MC-17, C7
*Estazolam* ............... MC-11, D3
*Estrace* Tablets—
0.5 mg (Logo 021) ...... MC-11, D4
1 mg (Logo 755) ....... MC-11, D4
2 mg (Logo 756) ....... MC-11, D4
*Estradiol* ............ MC-11, D4-5
Watson Tablets—
0.5 mg (WATSON
528) ................. MC-11, D5
1 mg (WATSON
487) ................. MC-11, D5
2 mg (WATSON
488) ................. MC-11, D5
*Estratab* Tablets—
0.3 mg (SOLVAY
1014) ................. MC-12, A2
0.625 mg (SOLVAY
1022) ................. MC-12, A2
2.5 mg (SOLVAY
1025) ................. MC-12, A2
*Estratest* Tablets—
1.25/0.625 mg
(SOLVAY 1023) ....... MC-19, D4
2.5/1.25 mg (SOLVAY
1026) ................. MC-19, D4

**Estrogens,
Conjugated** ......... MC-11, D6-7
**Estrogens,
Esterified** .......... MC-12, A1-2
*Estropipate* ........... MC-12, A3-5
Watson Tablets—
0.75 mg (WATSON
414) .................. MC-12, A5
1.5 mg (WATSON
415) .................. MC-12, A5
3 mg (WATSON 416) .. MC-12, A5
*Estrostep Fe* Tablets—
1/0.035 mg ........... MC-23, A4
1/0.03 mg ............. MC-23, A4
75 mg .................. MC-23, A4
1/0.02 mg ............. MC-23, A4
*Ethmozine* Tablets—
200 mg (ETHMOZINE
200) .................. MC-21, A1
250 mg (ETHMOZINE
250) .................. MC-21, A1
300 mg (ETHMOZINE
300) .................. MC-21, A2
**Ethynodiol Diacetate and
Ethinyl Estradiol** .... MC-12, A6-7
*Etidronate* ............. MC-12, B1
*Etodolac* .............. MC-12, B2-5
*Etretinate* .............. MC-12, B6
*Famciclovir* .......... MC-12, B7-C1
*Famotidine* ............. MC-12, C2
*Famvir* Tablets—
125 mg (FAMVIR/
125) .................. MC-12, B7
250 mg (FAMVIR/
250) .................. MC-12, B7
500 mg (FAMVIR/
500) .................. MC-12, C1
*Fansidar* Tablets—
500/25 mg (FANSIDAR
ROCHE) .............. MC-28, C6
*Felbamate* .............. MC-12, C3
*Felbatol* Tablets—
400 mg (WALLACE/
0430) ................. MC-12, C3
600 mg (WALLACE/
0431) ................. MC-12, C3
*Feldene* Capsules—
10 mg (PFIZER 322/
FELDENE) ........... MC-25, C2
20 mg (PFIZER 323/
FELDENE) ........... MC-25, C2
*Felodipine* ............ MC-12, C4-5
*Fenofibrate* ............ MC-12, C6
*Fenoprofen* .......... MC-12, C7-D3
Geneva Capsules—
300 mg
GG 559) .............. MC-12, D1
Geneva Tablets—
600 mg (GG 254) .... MC-12, D2
Purepac Tablets—
600 mg (Logo 317) ... MC-12, D3
*Ferrous Sulfate* ........ MC-12, D4
Paddock Tablets—
324 mg (B-3) .......... MC-12, D4
*Fexofenadine* .......... MC-12, D5
**Fexofenadine and
Pseudoephedrine** .... MC-12, D6
*Finasteride* .. MC-12, D7-MC-13, A1
*Fioricet* Tablets—
50/325/40 mg (Logo/
78-84) ................ MC-4, C5
*Fioricet with Codeine* Capsules—
50/325/40/30 mg (Logo/
Fioricet Codeine) ....... MC-4, D2
*Fiorinal* Capsules—
50/325/40 mg (FIORINAL
78-103) ............... MC-4, D3
*Fiorinal* Tablets—
50/325/40 mg (FIORINAL/
78-104) ............... MC-4, D3
*Fiorinal with Codeine* Capsules—
50/325/40/30 mg (Logo F-C/
SANDOZ 78-107) ..... MC-4, D6

*Flagyl* Tablets—
250 mg (SEARLE 1831/
FLAGYL 250) ......... MC-20, B6
500 mg (FLAGYL/
500) .................. MC-20, B6
*Flagyl ER* Extended-release
Tablets—
750 mg (FLAGYL ER/SEARLE
1961) ................. MC-20, B7
*Flagyl 375* Capsules—
375 mg (FLAGYL/
375 mg) .............. MC-20, B5
*Flecainide* .............. MC-13, A2
*Flexeril* Tablets—
10 mg (MSD 931/
FLEXERIL) ........... MC-8, B4
*Floxin* Tablets—
200 mg (FLOXIN
200 mg) .............. MC-23, B7
300 mg (FLOXIN
300 mg) .............. MC-23, B7
400 mg (FLOXIN
400 mg) .............. MC-23, B7
*Fluconazole* .......... MC-13, A3-4
*Flumadine* Tablets—
100 mg (FLUMADINE
100/FOREST) ........ MC-27, D3
*Fluoxetine* ............. MC-13, A5
*Fluoxymesterone* ...... MC-13, A6-7
Rosemont Tablets—
10 mg (832/86) ........ MC-13, A7
*Fluphenazine* .......... MC-13, B1-3
Mylan Tablets—
1 mg (MYLAN/4) ...... MC-13, B2
2.5 mg (MYLAN/9) .... MC-13, B2
5 mg (MYLAN/74) .... MC-13, B3
10 mg (MYLAN/97) ... MC-13, B3
*Flurazepam* ........... MC-13, B4-5
Purepac Capsules—
15 mg (Logo-021) ..... MC-13, B4
30 mg (Logo-022) ..... MC-13, B4
*Flurbiprofen* .......... MC-13, B6-7
Mylan Tablets—
50 mg (M 76) ......... MC-13, B6
100 mg (M 93) ........ MC-13, B6
*Fluvastatin* ............ MC-13, C1
*Fluvoxamine* .......... MC-13, C2
*Fortovase* Capsules—
200 mg (ROCHE
0246) ................. MC-28, A3
*Fosamax* Tablets—
5 mg (Logo MRK) ..... MC-1, C6
10 mg (Logo MRK
936) .................. MC-1, C6
40 mg (MRK 212) ..... MC-1, C6
*Fosinopril* ............. MC-13, C3
*Furosemide* ........... MC-13, C4-5
Schein Tablets—
20 mg (M2) ........... MC-13, C5
40 mg (DAN/5575) ... MC-13, C5
80 mg (WATSON
302) .................. MC-13, C5
*Gabapentin* ............ MC-13, C6
*Gabitril* Tablets—
4 mg (Logo/FK) ....... MC-30, B6
12 mg (Logo/FL) ...... MC-30, B6
16 mg (Logo/FM) ..... MC-30, B7
20 mg (Logo/FN) ..... MC-30, B7
*Ganciclovir* ............ MC-13, C7
*Gantanol* Tablets—
500 mg (ROCHE
GANTANOL) ......... MC-28, C7
*Gemfibrozil* ........... MC-13, D1-3
Invamed Tablets—
600 mg (INV 320) .... MC-13, D1
Rugby Tablets—
600 mg (RUGBY/
3854) ................. MC-13, D3
*Genora 0.5/35-28* Tablets—
0.5/0.035 mg (SGP/0.5/
35) .................... MC-22, D3
Inert (S G P) .......... MC-22, D3
*Genora 1/35-28* Tablets—
1/0.035 mg (SFP/1/
35) .................... MC-22, D4
Inert (S G P) .......... MC-22, D4
*Genora 1/50-28* Tablets—
1/0.05 mg (SGP/1/50).. MC-22, D6
Inert (SGP) ........... MC-22, D6

*Glimepiride* ............ MC-13, D4
*Glipizide* .............. MC-13, D5-7
Mylan Tablets—
5 mg (MYLAN G1) ... MC-13, D5
10 mg (MYLAN G2) .. MC-13, D5
*Glucophage* Tablets—
500 mg (BMS 6060/
500) .................. MC-19, A1
850 mg (BMS 6070/
850) .................. MC-19, A1
*Glucotrol* Tablets—
5 mg (PFIZER 411) .... MC-13, D6
10 mg (PFIZER 412) ... MC-13, D6
*Glucotrol XL* Extended-release
Tablets—
5 mg (GLUCOTROL XL
5) ..................... MC-13, D7
10 mg (GLUCOTROL XL
10) .................... MC-13, D7
*Glyburide* ............. MC-14, A1-3
Geneva Tablets—
2.5 mg (GG 239) ...... MC-14, A1
5 mg (GG 240) ....... MC-14, A1
*Granisetron* ............ MC-14, A4
*Grepafloxacin* .......... MC-14, A5
*Grifulvin V* Tablets—
250 mg (Ortho 211) ... MC-14, A7
500 mg (Ortho 214) ... MC-14, B1
*Griseofulvin* ........ MC-14, A6-B1
ESI Tablets—
500 mg (59911
5808) ................. MC-14, A6
*Guaifen PSE* Tablets—
120/600 mg (V/6211) ... MC-27, A2
*Guanabenz* ............. MC-14, B2
*Guanfacine* ........... MC-14, B3-4
Watson Tablets—
1 mg (WATSON
444) .................. MC-14, B4
2 mg (WATSON
453) .................. MC-14, B4
*Halcion* Tablets—
0.125 mg (HALCION
0.125) ................. MC-31, D2
0.25 mg (HALCION
0.25) .................. MC-31, D2
*Haloperidol* ............ MC-14, B5
Mylan Tablets—
0.5 mg (MYLAN
351) .................. MC-14, B5
1 mg (MYLAN 257) ... MC-14, B5
2 mg (MYLAN 214) ... MC-14, B5
5 mg (MYLAN 327) ... MC-14, B5
*Halotestin* Tablets—
2 mg (HALOTESTIN
2) ..................... MC-13, A6
5 mg (HALOTESTIN
5) ..................... MC-13, A6
10 mg (HALOTESTIN
10) .................... MC-13, A6
*Helidac Therapy* Capsules—
500 mg (PG 12) ....... MC-4, A4
*Helidac Therapy* Chewable
Tablets—
262.4 mg (PG 11) ..... MC-4, A6
*Helidac Therapy* Tablets—
250 mg (PG 10) ....... MC-4, A5
*Hismanal* Tablets—
10 mg (JANSSEN/Ast
10) .................... MC-3, A3
*Hivid* Tablets—
0.75 mg (ROCHE/HIVID
0.750) ................. MC-32, D2
0.375 mg (ROCHE/HIVID
0.375) ................. MC-32, D2
*Hycodan* Tablets—
5/1.5 mg (Du Pont/
HYCODAN) .......... MC-14, D5
*Hydergine* Tablets—
1 mg (Logo/HYDERGINE
1) ..................... MC-11, B1
*Hydergine LC* Capsules—
1 mg (Logo/HYDERGINE LC
1 mg) ................. MC-11, A7
*Hydralazine* ........... MC-14, B6-7
Lederle Tablets—
25 mg (Logo/H11) .... MC-14, B6
50 mg (Logo/H12) .... MC-14, B6

Hydralazine and
  Hydrochlorothiazide... MC-14, C1
Hydrea Capsules—
  500 mg (HYDREA
    830)................. MC-15, A6
Hydrochlorothiazide.. MC-14, C2-5
  Geneva Tablets—
    25 mg (GG 28)...... MC-14, C3
    50 mg (GG 27)...... MC-14, C3
Hydrocodone and
  Acetaminophen..... MC-14, C6-D4
  Endo Tablets—
    5/500 mg (KPI 1).... MC-14, C7
    7.5/650 mg (KPI 4).. MC-14, C7
    7.5/750 mg (KPI 2).. MC-14, C7
Hydrocodone and
  Homatropine......... MC-14, D5
Hydrocodone and
  Ibuprofen............ MC-14, D6
Hydrocortisone....... MC-14, D7-
                      MC-15, A1
Hydrocortone Tablets—
  10 mg (HYDROCORTONE/
    MSD 619)......... MC-14, D7
HydroDIURIL Tablets—
  25 mg (MSD 42/
    HYDRODIURIL)... MC-14, C4
  50 mg (MSD 105/
    HYDRODIURIL)... MC-14, C4
Hydromorphone...... MC-15, A2-3
  Endo Tablets—
    2 mg (752/2)........ MC-15, A2
    4 mg (757/4)........ MC-15, A2
Hydroxychloroquine. MC-15, A4-5
  Invamed Tablets—
    200 mg (INV 250).... MC-15, A4
Hydroxyurea.......... MC-15, A6-7
  Roxane Capsules—
    500 mg (54 072).... MC-15, A7
Hydroxyzine........... MC-15, B1-2
  Barr Capsules—
    25 mg (barr 323/25).. MC-15, B1
    100 mg (barr 324/
      100)............... MC-15, B1
  Qualitest Tablets—
    10 mg (SL/07)...... MC-15, B2
    25 mg (SL/08 (80))... MC-15, B2
Hygroton Tablets—
  25 mg (Logo/H 22r)...MC-7, A5
  50 mg (Logo/H 20r)...MC-7, A5
  100 mg (Logo/21)......MC-7, A5
Hyoscyamine
  Sulfate................ MC-15, B3-4
Hytrin Capsules—
  1 mg (Logo/DF)........ MC-29, B6
  2 mg (Logo/HY)....... MC-29, B6
  5 mg (Logo/HK)........ MC-29, B7
  10 mg (Logo/HN)...... MC-29, B7
Hyzaar Tablets—
  50/12.5 mg (MRK 717/
    HYZAAR)........... MC-18, A6
Ibuprofen................ MC-15, B5-C5
  Mylan Tablets—
    400 mg (MYLAN
      1401)............. MC-15, B5
    600 mg (MYLAN
      1601)............. MC-15, B5
    800 mg (MYLAN
      1801)............. MC-15, B6
  Rugby Tablets—
    400 mg (RUGBY/
      4604)............. MC-15, C2
    600 mg (RUGBY/
      4605)............. MC-15, C2
    800 mg (RUGBY/
      4606)............. MC-15, C3
  Schein Tablets—
    200 mg (DAN/5585).. MC-15, C4
    400 mg (DAN/5584).. MC-15, C4
    600 mg (DAN/5586).. MC-15, C4
    800 mg (DAN/5644).. MC-15, C5
Ilosone Capsules—
  250 mg (DISTA H09/
    ILOSONE 250 mg).... MC-11, C5
Ilosone Tablets—
  500 mg (DISTA U26)... MC-11, C6
Imipramine............MC-15, C6-D2
  Geneva Tablets—
    10 mg (GG/41)...... MC-15, C6
    25 mg (GG/47)...... MC-15, C6

Imitrex Tablets—
  25 mg (Logo/25)...... MC-29, A4
  50 mg (Imitrex/50)..... MC-29, A4
Imodium Capsules—
  2 mg (JANSSEN/
    IMODIUM)........... MC-17, D5
Imuran Tablets—
  50 mg (IMURAN 50).... MC-3, C2
Indapamide........... MC-15, D3-4
Invamed Tablets—
  1.25 mg (INV 246).... MC-15, D3
Inderal Tablets—
  10 mg (Logo/INDERAL
    10)................. MC-26, C7
  20 mg (Logo/INDERAL
    20)................. MC-26, C7
  40 mg (Logo/INDERAL
    40)................. MC-26, C7
  60 mg (Logo/INDERAL
    60)................. MC-26, C7
  80 mg (Logo/INDERAL
    80)................. MC-26, C7
Inderal LA Extended-release
  Capsules—
  60 mg (INDERAL LA
    60)................. MC-26, C5
  80 mg (INDERAL LA
    80)................. MC-26, C5
  120 mg (INDERAL LA
    120)................ MC-26, C6
  160 mg (INDERAL LA
    160)................ MC-26, C6
Inderide Tablets—
  40/25 mg (Logo/INDERIDE
    40/25).............. MC-26, D5
  80/25 mg (Logo/INDERIDE
    80/25).............. MC-26, D5
Inderide LA Extended-release
  Capsules—
  80/50 mg (INDERIDE LA
    80/50).............. MC-26, D4
  120/50 mg (INDERIDE LA
    120/50)............. MC-26, D4
  160/50 mg (INDERIDE LA
    160/50)............. MC-26, D4
Indinavir................ MC-15, D5
Indocin Capsules—
  25 mg (MSD 25/
    INDOCIN).......... MC-15, D7
  50 mg (MSD 50/
    INDOCIN).......... MC-15, D7
Indocin SR Extended-release
  Capsules—
  75 mg (MSD 693/
    INDOCIN SR)....... MC-16, A1
Indomethacin........ MC-15, D6-
                    MC-16, A1
  Geneva Capsules—
    25 mg (GG 517)..... MC-15, D6
    50 mg (GG 518)..... MC-15, D6
Invirase Capsules—
  200 mg (ROCHE
    0245).............. MC-28, A4
ISMO Tablets—
  20 mg (Logo/ISMO 20)..MC-16, B4
Isoniazid.............. MC-16, A2-3
  Barr Tablets—
    100 mg (Barr 066/
      100)............. MC-16, A2
    300 mg (Barr 071/
      300)............. MC-16, A2
  Paddock Tablets—
    300 mg (Logo 4350).. MC-16, A3
Isoptin SR Extended-release
  Tablets—
  120 mg (KNOLL/120
    SR)................ MC-32, B3
  180 mg (ISOPTIN SR/
    180 MG)........... MC-32, B3
  240 mg (Logo/
    ISOPTIN SR)....... MC-32, B3
Isordil Extended-release Tablets—
  40 mg (WYETH
    4125).............. MC-16, A6
Isordil Sublingual Tablets—
  2.5 mg (W/2.5)....... MC-16, A7
  5 mg (W/5).......... MC-16, A7
  10 mg (WYETH/10)... MC-16, A7

Isordil Tablets—
  5 mg (WYETH 4152).. MC-16, A5
  10 mg (WYETH
    4153).............. MC-16, A5
  20 mg (WYETH
    4154).............. MC-16, A5
  30 mg (WYETH
    4159).............. MC-16, A5
  40 mg (WYETH
    4192).............. MC-16, A5
Isosorbide
  Dinitrate............ MC-16, A4-B2
Isosorbide
  Mononitrate........ MC-16, B3-4
Isotretinoin........... MC-16, B5
Isradipine............. MC-16, B6
Itraconazole.......... MC-16, B7
K-Dur Extended-release Tablets—
  750 mg (K-DUR 10)... MC-25, C5
  1500 mg (K-DUR
    20)................. MC-25, C5
K-Tab Extended-release Tablets—
  750 mg (K-TAB)..... MC-25, C3
Kerlone Tablets—
  10 mg (KERLONE 10)...MC-4, A2
  20 mg (Logo/KERLONE
    20)................. MC-4, A2
Ketoconazole......... MC-16, C1
Ketoprofen........... MC-16, C2-5
Ketorolac............. MC-16, C6
Klonopin Tablets—
  0.5 mg (KLONOPIN 1/2
    ROCHE)........... MC-7, D2
  1 mg (KLONOPIN 1/
    ROCHE)........... MC-7, D2
  2 mg (KLONOPIN 2/
    ROCHE)........... MC-7, D2
Klor-Con Extended-release
  Tablets—
  600 mg (KLOR-CON
    8)................. MC-25, D1
  750 mg (KLOR-CON
    10)................ MC-25, D1
Klotrix Extended-release Tablets—
  750 mg (Logo KLOTRIX 10
    mEq 710)......... MC-25, C4
Kytril Tablets—
  1 mg (K1).......... MC-14, A4
Labetalol............. MC-16, C7-D1
Lamictal Tablets—
  25 mg (LAMICTAL
    25)................ MC-16, D4
  100 mg (LAMICTAL
    100)............... MC-16, D4
  150 mg (LAMICTAL
    150)............... MC-16, D5
  200 mg (LAMICTAL
    200)............... MC-16, D5
Lamisil Tablets—
  250 mg (LAMISIL/
    250)............... MC-29, C1
Lamivudine.......... MC-16, D2
Lamivudine/
  Zidovudine........ MC-16, D3
Lamotrigine......... MC-16, D4-5
Lanoxicaps Capsules—
  0.05 mg (A2C)...... MC-9, C3
  0.1 mg (B2C)....... MC-9, C3
  0.2 mg (C2C)....... MC-9, C3
Lanoxin Tablets—
  0.125 mg (LANOXIN
    Y3B).............. MC-9, C4
  0.25 mg (LANOXIN
    X3A).............. MC-9, C4
Lansoprazole........ MC-16, D6
Lariam Tablets—
  250 mg (LARIAM
    ROCHE 250)..... MC-18, C3
Lasix Tablets—
  20 mg (HOECHST/
    LASIX)........... MC-13, C4
  40 mg (HOECHST/
    LASIX 40)....... MC-13, C4
  80 mg (HOESCHST/
    LASIX 80)....... MC-13, C4
Ledercillin VK Tablets—
  250 mg (Logo/L10)... MC-24, D1
  500 mg (Logo/L9).... MC-24, D1

Lescol Capsules—
  20 mg (Logo 20/
    LESCOL Logo)...... MC-13, C1
  40 mg (Logo 40/
    LESCOL Logo)...... MC-13, C1
Leucovorin.. MC-16, D7-MC-17, A1
  Barr Tablets—
    5 mg (Logo/484).... MC-16, D7
    25 mg (Logo/485).... MC-16, D7
Immunex Tablets—
  5 mg (LL 5/C 33).... MC-17, A1
  15 mg (LL 15/C 35)... MC-17, A1
Leukeran Tablets—
  2 mg (635)........... MC-6, C5
Levaquin Tablets—
  250 mg (McNEIL 1520/
    250)................ MC-17, A2
Levatol Tablets—
  20 mg (Logo 22)..... MC-24, C6
  0.375 mg (SP 538)... MC-15, B4
Levbid Extended-release Tablets—
Levlen 21 and 28 Tablets—
  0.15/0.03 mg (B/21).... MC-17, A3
  Inert (B/28)........ MC-17, A3
Levofloxacin........ MC-17, A2
Levonorgestrel and
  Ethinyl Estradiol... MC-17, A3-6
Levothyroxine....... MC-17, A7-B4
  Rugby Tablets—
    0.1 mg (RUGBY/
      3952)............. MC-17, B4
    0.15 mg (RUGBY/
      3953)............. MC-17, B4
    0.2 mg (RUGBY/
      4381)............. MC-17, B4
    0.3 mg (RUGBY/
      3958)............. MC-17, B4
Levoxyl Tablets—
  0.025 mg (LEVOXYL/
    Logo 25).......... MC-17, A7
  0.05 mg (LEVOXYL/
    Logo 50).......... MC-17, A7
  0.075 mg (LEVOXYL/
    Logo 75).......... MC-17, A7
  0.088 mg (LEVOXYL/
    Logo 88).......... MC-17, A7
  0.1 mg (LEVOXYL/
    Logo 100)......... MC-17, B1
  0.112 mg (LEVOXYL/
    Logo 112)......... MC-17, B1
  0.125 mg (LEVOXYL/
    Logo 125)......... MC-17, B1
  0.137 mg (LEVOXYL/
    Logo 137)......... MC-17, B1
Lexxel Extended-release Tablets—
  5/5 mg (LEXXEL 1
    5-5)............... MC-11, A2
Librax Capsules—
  5/2.5 mg (ROCHE
    LIBRAX).......... MC-6, D1
Lioresal Tablets—
  10 mg (Geigy 23).... MC-3, C5
  20 mg (Geigy/33).... MC-3, C5
Lipitor Tablets—
  10 mg (PD155/10).... MC-3, B3
  20 mg (PD156)...... MC-3, B3
  40 mg (PD 157/40)... MC-3, B3
Lisinopril............MC-17, B5-C1
Lisinopril and Hydro-
  chlorothiazide....... MC-17, C2-3
Lithium................MC-17, C4-D3
  Roxane Capsules—
    150 mg (54 213).... MC-17, C4
    300 mg (54 463).... MC-17, C4
    600 mg (54 702).... MC-17, C4
  Roxane Tablets—
    300 mg (54 452).... MC-17, C5
Lithobid Extended-release Tablets—
  300 mg (SOLVAY
    4492).............. MC-17, D3
Lithonate Capsules—
  300 mg (SOLVAY
    7512).............. MC-17, D1
Lithotab Tablets—
  300 mg (SOLVAY
    7516).............. MC-17, D2
Lo-Ovral-21 and -28 Tablets—
  0.3/0.03 mg (WYETH/
    78)................ MC-23, B1
  Inert (WYETH/486)... MC-23, B1

**Lodine** Capsules—
200 mg (LODINE 200)............ MC-12, B4
300 mg (LODINE 300)............ MC-12, B4
**Lodine** Tablets—
400 mg (LODINE 400)............ MC-12, B5
500 mg (LODINE 500)............ MC-12, B5
**Loestrin 21 1.0/20** Tablets—
1/0.02 mg (P-D 915)... MC-22, D7
**Loestrin 21 1.5/30** Tablets—
1.5/0.03mg (P-D 916).. MC-23, A1
**Loestrin Fe 1.0/20** Tablets—
75 mg (P-D 622)...... MC-23, A2
1/0.02 mg (P-D 915)... MC-23, A2
**Loestrin Fe 1.5/30** Tablets—
75 mg (P-D 622)...... MC-23, A3
1.5/0.03 mg (P-D 916)............. MC-23, A3
**Lomefloxacin** ........... MC-17, D4
**Lomotil** Tablets—
2.5/0.025 mg (Searle/ 61)............... MC-10, A4
**Loniten** Tablets—
2.5 mg (U121/2)........ MC-20, C7
10 mg (LONITEN 10) .. MC-20, C7
**Loperamide** ............. MC-17, D5
**Lopid** Tablets—
600 mg (Lopid)........ MC-13, D2
**Lopressor** Tablets—
50 mg (GEIGY/51 51)............... MC-20, A7
100 mg (GEIGY/71 71)............... MC-20, A7
**Lopressor HCT** Tablets—
100/25 mg (GEIGY/53 53)............... MC-20, B3
100/50 mg (GEIGY/73 73)............... MC-20, B3
**Lorabid** Capsules—
200 mg (Lilly 3170/ LORABID 200 mg).... MC-17, D6
400 mg (Lilly 3171/ LORABID 400 mg).... MC-17, D6
**Loracarbef** ............. MC-17, D6
**Loratadine** ............. MC-17, D7
**Loratadine and Pseudoephedrine**...... MC-18, A1
**Lorazepam** ........... MC-18, A2-4
Mylan Tablets—
0.5 mg (M/321) ...... MC-18, A2
1 mg (MYLAN 457).. MC-18, A2
2 mg (MYLAN 777)... MC-18, A2
Purepac Tablets—
0.5 mg (Logo/57) .... MC-18, A3
1 mg (Logo/59) ..... MC-18, A3
2 mg (Logo/063) .... MC-18, A3
**Lortab** Tablets—
2.5/500 mg (ucb/901).. MC-14, D4
5/500 mg (ucb/902).. MC-14, D4
7.5/500 mg (ucb/903).. MC-14, D4
10/500 mg (ucb/910) ..... MC-14, D4
**Losartan** ............. MC-18, A5
**Losartan and Hydrochlorothiazide** ... MC-18, A6
**Lotensin** Tablets—
5 mg (LOTENSIN/5) .... MC-3, C7
10 mg (LOTENSIN/10) .. MC-3, C7
20 mg (LOTENSIN/20) .. MC-3, C7
40 mg (LOTENSIN/40) .. MC-3, C7
**Lotensin HCT** Tablets—
5/6.25 mg (LOTENSIN HCT/57)............ MC-3, D1
10/12.5 mg (LOTENSIN HCT/72)............ MC-3, D1
20/12.5 mg (LOTENSIN HCT/74)............ MC-3, D2
20/25 mg (LOTENSIN HCT/75)............ MC-3, D2
**Lotrel** Capsules—
2.5/10 mg (LOTREL 2255).............. MC-2, B5
5/10 mg (LOTREL 2260).............. MC-2, B5
5/20 mg (LOTREL 2265).............. MC-2, B5

**Lovastatin**............... MC-18, A7
**Loxapine** ............ MC-18, B1-3
Watson Capsules—
5 mg (WATSON 369/ 5 mg)............ MC-18, B2
10 mg (WATSON 370/ 10 mg)........... MC-18, B2
25 mg (WATSON 371/ 25 mg)........... MC-18, B3
50 mg (WATSON 372/ 50 mg)........... MC-18, B3
**Loxitane** Capsules—
25 mg (Lederle L3/ 25 mg)............ MC-18, B1
**Lozol** Tablets—
1.25 mg (R/7)....... MC-15, D4
2.5 mg (R/8)........ MC-15, D4
**Ludiomil** Tablets—
25 mg (CIBA/110)...... MC-18, B4
50 mg (CIBA/26)...... MC-18, B4
75 mg (CIBA/135)..... MC-18, B4
**Lufyllin** Tablets—
200 mg (WALLACE 521)............... MC-10, D6
**Luvox** Tablets—
25 mg (SOLVAY 4202)............ MC-13, C2
50 mg (SOLVAY 4205)............ MC-13, C2
100 mg (SOLVAY 4210)............ MC-13, C2
**Macrobid** Capsules—
100 mg (Norwich Eaton/ Macrobid)......... MC-22, B6
**Macrodantin** Capsules—
25 mg (MACRODANTIN 25 mg/ 0149 0007)........... MC-22, B7
50 mg (MACRODANTIN 50 mg/ 0149 0008)........... MC-22, B7
100 mg (MACRODANTIN 100 mg/ 0149 0009)........... MC-22, B7
**Maprotiline** ........... MC-18, B4
**Mavik** Tablets—
1 mg (KNOLL 1)....... MC-31, B1
2 mg (KNOLL 2)....... MC-31, B1
4 mg (KNOLL 4)....... MC-31, B1
**Maxaquin** Tablets—
400 mg (MAXAQUIN 400).............. MC-17, D4
**Maxzide** Tablets—
37.5/25 mg (MAXZIDE/ B M9)............ MC-31, C6
75/50 mg (MAXZIDE/B M8)............. MC-31, C6
**Meclizine** ............ MC-18, B5-6
Geneva Tablets—
12.5 mg (GG 141).... MC-18, B5
25 mg (GG 261)..... MC-18, B5
**Meclofenamate**......... MC-18, B7-C1
Mylan Capsules—
50 mg (MYLAN 2150)............ MC-18, B7
100 mg (MYLAN 3000)............ MC-18, B7
Schein Capsules—
50 mg (DAN 5636).. MC-18, C1
100 mg (DAN 5637).. MC-18, C1
**Medrol** Tablets—
2 mg (MEDROL 2) ..... MC-19, D2
4 mg (MEDROL 4) ..... MC-19, D2
8 mg (MEDROL 8) ..... MC-19, D2
16 mg (MEDROL 16).... MC-19, D3
24 mg (MEDROL 24)... MC-19, D3
32 mg (MEDROL 32)... MC-19, D3
**Medroxyprogesterone** .... MC-18, C2
**Mefloquine** ............. MC-18, C3
**Megace** Tablets—
20 mg (MJ 595) ..... MC-18, C5
40 mg (MEGACE/40) .. MC-18, C5
**Megestrol** ............ MC-18, C4-5
Barr Tablets—
40 mg (barr/555 607)............. MC-18, C4
**Mellaril** Tablets—
10 mg (Logo/78-2) ..... MC-30, A6
15 mg (Logo/78-8) ..... MC-30, A6
25 mg (Logo/MELLARIL 25)............... MC-30, A6
50 mg (Logo/MELLARIL 50)............... MC-30, A6

**Mellaril** Tablets (continued)
100 mg (Logo/MELLARIL 100)............... MC-30, A7
150 mg (Logo/MELLARIL 150)............... MC-30, A7
200 mg (Logo/MELLARIL 200)............... MC-30, A7
**Melphalan** ............ MC-18, C6
0.625 mg (BMP 126).... MC-12, A1
**Menest** Tablets—
**Meperidine** ............MC-18, C7-D1
Barr Tablets—
50 mg (Logo/381) ..... MC-18, C7
100 mg (barr/382) ..... MC-18, C7
**Mercaptopurine** ......... MC-18, D2
**Meridia** Capsules—
5 mg (MERIDIA/5) ..... MC-28, B1
10 mg (MERIDIA/10)... MC-28, B1
15 mg (MERIDIA/15)... MC-28, B1
**Mesalamine** ........... MC-18, D3-4
**Mesoridazine**........... MC-18, D5
**Metaproterenol** ...... MC-18, D6-7
Goldline Tablets—
10 mg (BL/132) ..... MC-18, D7
**Metformin** ............. MC-19, A1
0.2 mg (SANDOZ/78 54)................ MC-19, C3
**Methergine** Tablets—
**Methocarbamol** ...... MC-19, A2-3
Geneva Tablets—
500 mg (GG 190) ..... MC-19, A2
750 mg (GG 101) ..... MC-19, A2
**Methocarbamol and Aspirin** .............. MC-19, A4-5
Zenith Tablets—
400/325 mg (Z 2813) MC-19, A5
**Methotrexate** ........MC-19, A6-B1
Barr Tablets—
2.5 mg (Logo 572).... MC-19, A6
Roxane Tablets—
2.5 mg (54 323) ..... MC-19, A7
**Methyclothiazide**....... MC-19, B2-3
Geneva Tablets—
2.5 mg (GG 244) ..... MC-19, B3
5 mg (GG 242) ..... MC-19, B3
**Methyldopa**............ MC-19, B4-5
Goldline Tablets—
250 mg (Z 2931) ..... MC-19, B4
500 mg (Z 2932) ..... MC-19, B4
**Methyldopa and Hydro- chlorothiazide**........MC-19, B6-C2
Qualitest Tablets—
250/15 mg (par 186)... MC-19, C1
250/25 mg (INV 206) MC-19, C1
Schein Tablets—
250/15 mg (DAN 15/ 5607)............. MC-19, C2
**Methylergonovine Maleate** ............. MC-19, C3
**Methylphenidate** ...... MC-19, C4-7
Apothecon Extended-release Tablets—
20 mg (MD/562) ..... MC-19, C5
Apothecon Tablets—
5 mg (MD/530) ..... MC-19, C4
10 mg (MD/531) ..... MC-19, C4
20 mg (MD/532) ..... MC-19, C4
**Methylprednisolone**... MC-19, D1-3
Invamed Tablets—
4 mg (INV 351)...... MC-19, D1
**Methyltestosterone and Esterified Estrogens** .... MC-19, D4
**Metoclopramide**........ MC-19, D5-7
Purepac Tablets—
10 mg (Logo/269)..... MC-19, D5
Rugby Tablets—
10 mg (RUGBY/ 4042)............. MC-19, D7
**Metoprolol Succinate** ........... MC-20, A1-3
**Metoprolol Tartrate**............MC-20, A4-B2
Geneva Tablets—
50 mg (GG 414)..... MC-20, A4
100 mg (GG 415)..... MC-20, A4
Mutual Tablets—
50 mg (Logo 184)..... MC-20, A5
100 mg (Logo 185)... MC-20, A5

Mylan Tablets—
50 mg (M 32)......... MC-20, A6
100 mg (M 47) ....... MC-20, A6
Novopharm Tablets—
100 mg (N 734/100).. MC-20, B1
Purepac Tablets—
100 mg (Logo/555).... MC-20, B2
**Metoprolol and Hydrochlorothiazide**.... MC-20, B3
**Metronidazole**......... MC-20, B4-7
Rugby Tablets—
250 mg (RUGBY/ 4018)............. MC-20, B4
500 mg (RUGBY/ 4019)............. MC-20, B4
**Mevacor** Tablets—
10 mg (MSD 730/ MEVACOR)......... MC-18, A7
20 mg (MSD 731/ MEVACOR)......... MC-18, A7
40 mg (MSD 732/ MEVACOR)......... MC-18, A7
**Mexiletine** ............. MC-20, C1-3
Novopharm Capsules—
250 mg (N 741/250).. MC-20, C1
**Mexitil** Capsules—
150 mg (BI 66) ..... MC-20, C2
200 mg (BI 67) ..... MC-20, C3
250 mg (BI 68) ..... MC-20, C3
**Micro-K** Extended-release Capsules—
600 mg (MICRO-K/AHR 5720)............. MC-25, C6
750 mg (MICRO-K 10/AHR 5730)............. MC-25, C6
**Micronase** Tablets—
1.25 mg (MICRONASE 1.25)............. MC-14, A3
2.5 mg (MICRONASE 2.5) ............. MC-14, A3
5 mg (MICRONASE 5) ............... MC-14, A3
**Midamor** Tablets—
5 mg (MSD 92/ MIDAMOR).........MC-2, A1
**Minizide** Capsules—
1/0.5 mg (PFIZER 430/ MINIZIDE).............. MC-25, D5
**Minocin** Tablets—
50 mg (Lederle M45/ Lederle 50 mg) ....... MC-20, C4
100 mg (Lederle M46/ Lederle 100 mg) ...... MC-20, C4
**Minocycline** ........... MC-20, C4-6
Lederle Tablets—
50 mg (Logo/M 45) .. MC-20, C5
100 mg (Logo/M 46).. MC-20, C5
Warner Chilcott Capsules—
50 mg (WC 615/ WC 615)........... MC-20, C6
100 mg (WC 616/ WC 616)........... MC-20, C6
**Minoxidil** .............MC-20, C7-D1
Schein Tablets—
2.5 mg (DAN 5642)... MC-20, D1
10 mg (DAN 5643) ... MC-20, D1
**Mirtazapine** ........... MC-20, D2
**Misoprostol** ........... MC-20, D3
**Moduretic** Tablets—
5/50 mg (MSD 917/ Logo)..............MC-2, A3
**Moexipril** .............. MC-20, D4
**Moexipril and Hydrochlorothiazide**.... MC-20, D5
**Mono-gesic** Tablets—
750 mg (SP 2164/ 750 mg)............ MC-28, A1
**Monoket** Tablets—
10 mg (Schwarz 610/ 10).............. MC-16, B3
20 mg (Schwarz 620/ 20).............. MC-16, B3
**Monopril** Tablets—
10 mg (BMS/MONOPRIL 10)............. MC-13, C3
20 mg (BMS/MONOPRIL 20)............. MC-13, C3

| | |
|---|---|
| Montelukast | MC-20, D6-7 |
| Moricizine | MC-21, A1-2 |
| Morphine | MC-21, A3-6 |
| *Motrin* Tablets— | |
| 300 mg (MOTRIN 300 mg) | MC-15, B7 |
| 400 mg (MOTRIN 400 mg) | MC-15, B7 |
| 600 mg (MOTRIN 600 mg) | MC-15, C1 |
| 800 mg (MOTRIN 800 mg) | MC-15, C1 |
| *MS Contin* Extended-release Tablets— | |
| 15 mg (PF/M 15) | MC-21, A5 |
| 30 mg (PF/M 30) | MC-21, A5 |
| 60 mg (PF/M 60) | MC-21, A5 |
| 100 mg (PF/100) | MC-21, A6 |
| 200 mg (PF/M 200) | MC-21, A6 |
| *MSIR* Capsules— | |
| 15 mg (PF MSIR 15/THIS END UP) | MC-21, A3 |
| 30 mg (PF MSIR 30/THIS END UP) | MC-21, A3 |
| *MSIR* Tablets— | |
| 15 mg (PF/MI 15) | MC-21, A4 |
| 30 mg (PF/MI 30) | MC-21, A4 |
| *Mycelex Troche* Lozenges— | |
| 10 mg (MYCELEX 10) | MC-8, A6 |
| *Mycobutin* Capsules— | |
| 150 mg (Adria MYCOBUTIN) | MC-27, C4 |
| Mycophenolate | MC-21, A7-B1 |
| *Myleran* Tablets— | |
| 2 mg (MYLERAN K2A) | MC-4, C4 |
| Nabumetone | MC-21, B2 |
| Nadolol | MC-21, B3-6 |
| Apothecon Tablets— | |
| 20 mg (AP 2461) | MC-21, B3 |
| 40 mg (AP 2462) | MC-21, B3 |
| 80 mg (AP 2463) | MC-21, B3 |
| 120 mg (AP 2464) | MC-21, B4 |
| 160 mg (AP 2465) | MC-21, B4 |
| Nadolol and Bendroflumethiazide | MC-21, B7 |
| *Nalfon* Capsules— | |
| 200 mg (DISTA H76/NALFON 200) | MC-12, C7 |
| 300 mg (DISTA H77/NALFON) | MC-12, C7 |
| Nalidixic Acid | MC-21, C1 |
| *Naprelan* Extended-release Tablets— | |
| 375 mg (W/901) | MC-21, D1 |
| 500 mg (W/902) | MC-21, D1 |
| *Naprosyn* Tablets— | |
| 250 mg (SYNTEX/NAPROSYN 250) | MC-21, C3 |
| 375 mg (NAPROSYN/375) | MC-21, C3 |
| 500 mg (NAPROSYN/500) | MC-21, C3 |
| Naproxen | MC-21, C2-5 |
| Mylan Tablets— | |
| 250 mg (MYLAN/377) | MC-21, C2 |
| 375 mg (MYLAN/555) | MC-21, C2 |
| 500 mg (MYLAN/451) | MC-21, C2 |
| Teva USA Tablets— | |
| 250 mg (93/147) | MC-21, C5 |
| 375 mg (93/148) | MC-21, C5 |
| Naproxen Sodium | MC-21, C6-D1 |
| Mylan Tablets— | |
| 275 mg (M/537) | MC-21, C6 |
| 550 mg (MYLAN/733) | MC-21, C6 |
| Naratriptan | MC-21, D2 |
| *Naturetin* Tablets— | |
| 5 mg (PPP 606/NATURETIN 5) | MC-3, D3 |
| 10 mg (PPP 618/NATURETIN 10) | MC-3, D3 |
| *Navane* Capsules— | |
| 1 mg (ROERIG 571/NAVANE) | MC-30, B2 |
| 2 mg (ROERIG 572/NAVANE) | MC-30, B2 |
| 5 mg (ROERIG 573/NAVANE) | MC-30, B2 |

| | |
|---|---|
| *Navane* Capsules *(continued)* | |
| 10 mg (ROERIG 574/NAVANE) | MC-30, B3 |
| 20 mg (ROERIG 577/NAVANE) | MC-30, B3 |
| Nefazodone | MC-21, D3-4 |
| *NegGram* Tablets— | |
| 1 gram (Logo/N 23) | MC-21, C1 |
| 250 mg (Logo/N 21) | MC-21, C1 |
| 500 mg (Logo/N 22) | MC-21, C1 |
| *Neoral* Capsules— | |
| 25 mg (NEORAL 25 mg) | MC-8, B7 |
| 100 mg (NEORAL 100 mg) | MC-8, B7 |
| *Neurontin* Capsules— | |
| 100 mg (Logo/Neurontin 100 mg) | MC-13, C6 |
| 300 mg (Logo/Neurontin 300 mg) | MC-13, C6 |
| 400 mg (Logo/Neurontin 400 mg) | MC-13, C6 |
| Niacin | MC-21, D5-6 |
| Apothecon Tablets— | |
| 50 mg (SQUIBB 611) | MC-21, D5 |
| 100 mg (SQUIBB 612) | MC-21, D5 |
| 500 mg (SQUIBB 537) | MC-21, D5 |
| Nicardipine | MC-21, D7-MC-22, A2 |
| Nifedipine | MC-22, A3-B1 |
| Purepac Capsules— | |
| 10 mg (Logo 497) | MC-22, B1 |
| 20 mg (Logo 530) | MC-22, B1 |
| *Nilandron* Tablets— | |
| 50 mg (Logo/168) | MC-22, B2 |
| Nilutamide | MC-22, B2 |
| Nimodipine | MC-22, B3 |
| *Nimotop* Capsules— | |
| 30 mg (NIMOTOP) | MC-22, B3 |
| Nisoldipine | MC-22, B4-5 |
| Nitrofurantoin | MC-22, B6-C1 |
| Schein Capsules— | |
| 25 mg (DAN 25 mg/NITROFURANTOIN MACROCRYSTALS) | MC-22, C1 |
| 50 mg (DAN 50 mg/NITROFURANTOIN MACROCRYSTALS) | MC-22, C1 |
| 100 mg (DAN 100 mg/NITROFURANTOIN MACROCRYSTALS) | MC-22, C1 |
| Nitroglycerin | MC-22, C2-3 |
| Goldline Extended-release Capsules— | |
| 6.5 mg (TCL/1222) | MC-22, C2 |
| 9 mg (TCL/1223) | MC-22, C2 |
| *Nitrostat Sublingual* Tablets— | |
| 0.3 mg | MC-22, C3 |
| 0.4 mg | MC-22, C3 |
| 0.6 mg | MC-22, C3 |
| Nizatidine | MC-22, C4 |
| *Nizoral* Tablets— | |
| 200 mg (JANSSEN/NIZORAL) | MC-16, C1 |
| *Nolvadex* Tablets— | |
| 10 mg (NOLVADEX 600) | MC-29, B2 |
| 20 mg (Logo/NOLVADEX 604) | MC-29, B2 |
| *Nordette-21 and -28* Tablets— | |
| 0.15/0.03 mg (WYETH/75) | MC-17, A5 |
| Inert (WYETH/486) | MC-17, A5 |

| | |
|---|---|
| Norethindrone and Ethinyl Estradiol | MC-22, C5-D4 |
| Norethindrone and Mestranol | MC-22, D5-6 |
| Norethindrone Acetate and Ethinyl Estradiol | MC-22, D7-MC-23, A1 |
| Norethindrone Acetate, Ethinyl Estradiol and Ferrous Fumarate | MC-23, A2-4 |
| Norfloxacin | MC-23, A5 |
| Norgestimate and Ethinyl Estradiol | MC-23, A6-7 |
| Norgestrel and Ethinyl Estradiol | MC-23, B1-2 |
| *Normodyne* Tablets— | |
| 100 mg (SCHERING 244/NORMODYNE 100) | MC-16, D1 |
| 200 mg (SCHERING 752/NORMODYNE 200) | MC-16, D1 |
| 300 mg (SCHERING 438/NORMODYNE 300) | MC-16, D1 |
| *Noroxin* Tablets— | |
| 400 mg (MSD 705/NOROXIN) | MC-23, A5 |
| *Norpace* Capsules— | |
| 100 mg (SEARLE 2752/NORPACE 100 mg) | MC-10, B2 |
| 150 mg (SEARLE 2762/NORPACE 150 mg) | MC-10, B2 |
| *Norpace CR* Extended-release Capsules— | |
| 100 mg (SEARLE 2732/NORPACE CR 100 mg) | MC-10, B3 |
| 150 mg (SEARLE 2742/NORPACE CR 150 mg) | MC-10, B3 |
| *Norpramin* Tablets— | |
| 10 mg (68-7) | MC-8, C6 |
| 25 mg (NORPRAMIN 25) | MC-8, C6 |
| 50 mg (NORPRAMIN 50) | MC-8, C6 |
| 75 mg (NORPRAMIN 75) | MC-8, C7 |
| 100 mg (NORPRAMIN 100) | MC-8, C7 |
| 150 mg (NORPRAMIN 150) | MC-8, C7 |
| Nortriptyline | MC-23, B3-6 |
| Mylan Capsules— | |
| 10 mg (MYLAN 1410) | MC-23, B3 |
| 25 mg (MYLAN 2325) | MC-23, B3 |
| 50 mg (MYLAN 3250) | MC-23, B4 |
| 75 mg (MYLAN 4175) | MC-23, B4 |
| *Norvasc* Tablets— | |
| 2.5 mg (NORVASC/2.5) | MC-2, B4 |
| 5 mg (NORVASC 5) | MC-2, B4 |
| 10 mg (NORVASC 10) | MC-2, B4 |
| *Norvir* Capsules— | |
| 100 mg (Logo 100 mg PI) | MC-27, D6 |
| Ofloxacin | MC-23, B7 |
| Olanzapine | MC-23, C1-2 |
| Olsalazine | MC-23, C3 |
| Omeprazole | MC-23, C4 |
| *Omnipen* Capsules— | |
| 250 mg (Wyeth/53) | MC-2, D7 |
| 500 mg (Wyeth/309) | MC-2, D7 |
| Ondansetron | MC-23, C5 |
| *Optimine* Tablets— | |
| 1 mg (SCHERING Logo/282) | MC-3, B7 |
| *Oretic* Tablets— | |
| 25 mg (Logo) | MC-14, C2 |
| 50 mg (Logo) | MC-14, C2 |
| *Orinase* Tablets— | |
| 500 mg (ORINASE 500) | MC-30, D3 |
| *Ortho-Cyclen* Tablets— | |
| 0.250/0.035 mg (Ortho 250) | MC-23, A6 |
| Inert (Ortho) | MC-23, A6 |

| | |
|---|---|
| *Ortho Tri-Cyclen* Tablets— | |
| 0.180/0.035 mg (Ortho 180) | MC-23, A7 |
| 0.215/0.035 mg (Ortho 215) | MC-23, A7 |
| 0.25/0.035 mg (Ortho 250) | MC-23, A7 |
| Inert (Ortho) | MC-23, A7 |
| *Ortho-Cept* Tablets— | |
| 0.15/ 0.03 mg (ORTHO/D 150) | MC-8, D3 |
| Inert (ORTHO P) | MC-8, D3 |
| *Ortho-Est* Tablets— | |
| 0.625 mg (equivalent to 0.75 mg estropipate) (Ortho 1801) | MC-12, A4 |
| 1.25 mg (equivalent to 1.5 mg estropipate) (Ortho 1800) | MC-12, A3 |
| *Ortho-Novum 1/35-21 and -28* Tablets— | |
| 1/0.035 mg (Ortho 135) | MC-22, C7 |
| Inert (Ortho) | MC-22, C7 |
| *Ortho-Novum 1/50-21 and -28* Tablets— | |
| 1/0.05 mg (Ortho 150) | MC-22, D5 |
| Inert (Ortho) | MC-22, D5 |
| *Ortho-Novum 7/7/7-21 and -28* Tablets— | |
| 0.5/0.035 mg (Ortho 535) | MC-22, D1 |
| 0.75/0.035 mg (Ortho 75) | MC-22, D1 |
| 1/0.035 mg (Ortho 135) | MC-22, D2 |
| Inert (Ortho) | MC-22, D2 |
| *Orudis* Capsules— | |
| 25 mg (WYETH 4186/ORUDIS 25) | MC-16, C2 |
| 50 mg (WYETH 4181/ORUDIS 50) | MC-16, C2 |
| 75 mg (WYETH 4187/ORUDIS 75) | MC-16, C3 |
| *Oruvail* Extended-release Capsules— | |
| 100 mg (ORUVAIL 100) | MC-16, C4 |
| 150 mg (ORUVAIL 150) | MC-16, C4 |
| 200 mg (ORUVAIL 200) | MC-16, C5 |
| *Ovcon 35-21 and -28* Tablets— | |
| 0.4/0.035 mg (MJ/583) | MC-22, C5 |
| Inert (MJ/850) | MC-22, C5 |
| *Ovcon 50-21 and -28* Tablets— | |
| 1/0.05 mg (MJ/584) | MC-22, C6 |
| Inert (MJ/850) | MC-22, C6 |
| *Ovral-21 and -28* Tablets— | |
| 0.5/0.05 mg (WYETH/56) | MC-23, B2 |
| 0.5/0.05 mg (WYETH/56) | MC-23, B2 |
| Oxacillin | MC-23, C6 |
| Oxaprozin | MC-23, C7 |
| Oxazepam | MC-23, D1-3 |
| Purepac Capsules— | |
| 10 mg (Logo-067) | MC-23, D1 |
| 15 mg (Logo-069) | MC-23, D1 |
| 30 mg (Logo-073) | MC-23, D1 |
| Oxybutynin | MC-23, D4-5 |
| Qualitest Tablets— | |
| 5 mg (SL 456) | MC-23, D4 |
| Rosemont Tablets— | |
| 5 mg (832/38) | MC-23, D5 |
| Oxycodone | MC-23, D6-MC-24, A4 |
| Oxycodone and Acetaminophen | MC-24, A5-B1 |
| Oxycodone and Aspirin | MC-24, B2-4 |
| *OxyContin* Extended-release Tablets— | |
| 10 mg (OC/10) | MC-24, A2 |
| 20 mg (OC/20) | MC-24, A2 |
| 40 mg (OC/40) | MC-24, A3 |
| 80 mg (OC/80) | MC-24, A3 |
| *OxyIR* Capsules— | |
| 5 mg (O-IR/PF 5 mg) | MC-23, D7 |

**Pacerone** Tablets—
200 mg (P200/U-S
0147)..................MC-2, A5
**Pamelor** Capsules—
10 mg (Logo SANDOZ/
Logo PAMELOR)......MC-23, B5
25 mg (Logo SANDOZ/
PAMELOR)...........MC-23, B5
50 mg (Logo SANDOZ/
PAMELOR)...........MC-23, B6
75 mg (Logo SANDOZ/
PAMELOR)...........MC-23, B6
**Pancrease** Delayed-release
Capsules—
4/12/12 (McNEIL Pancrease
MT 4)................MC-24, B7
4/20/25 (McNEIL/
Pancrease)...........MC-24, B7
10/30/30 (McNEIL/Pancrease
MT 10)...............MC-24, B7
16/48/48 (McNEIL/Pancrease
MT 16)...............MC-24, C1
25/75/75 (McNEIL/Pancrease
MT 25)...............MC-24, C1
**Pancreatin**..............MC-24, B5
**Pancrelipase**.........MC-24, B6-C1
**Panfil-G** Capsules—
200/100 mg (PAL/
0305).................MC-10, D7
**Panmycin** Capsules—
250 mg (PANMYCIN
250 mg)..............MC-29, C7
**Parafon Forte DSC** Tablets—
500 mg (McNEIL/PARAFON
FORTE DSC)...........MC-7, B1
**Parlodel** Capsules—
5 mg (Logo/PARLODEL
5 mg)..................MC-4, B2
**Parlodel** Tablets—
2.5 mg (PARLODEL 2)..MC-4, B3
**Parnate** Tablets—
10 mg (PARNATE
SKF)..................MC-31, B4
**Paroxetine**...........MC-24, C2-3
**Paxil** Tablets—
10 mg (PAXIL/10).....MC-24, C2
20 mg (PAXIL/20).....MC-24, C2
30 mg (PAXIL/30).....MC-24, C3
40 mg (PAXIL/40).....MC-24, C3
**PCE** Tablets—
333 mg (Logo PCE)...MC-11, B5
500 mg (Logo EK)....MC-11, B5
**Pemoline**..............MC-24, C4-5
**Pen-Vee K** Tablets—
250 mg (WYETH/
59)....................MC-24, D4
500 mg (WYETH/
390)...................MC-24, D4
**Penbutolol**.............MC-24, C6
**Penetrex** Tablets—
200 mg (Logo/5100)...MC-11, A4
400 mg (Logo/5140)...MC-11, A4
**Penicillin V**............MC-24, C7-D4
Warner Chilcott Tablets—
250 mg (WC648).....MC-24, D3
500 mg (WC673).....MC-24, D3
**Pentasa** Extended-release
Capsules—
250 mg (Logo 2010/PENTASA
250 mg Logo)........MC-18, D4
**Pentazocine and
Acetaminophen**.......MC-24, D5
**Pentazocine and
Naloxone**.............MC-24, D6
**Pentosan**...............MC-24, D7
**Pentoxifylline**..........MC-25, A1
**Pepcid** Tablets—
20 mg (PEPCID/MSD
963)....................MC-12, C2
40 mg (PEPCID/MSD
964)....................MC-12, C2
**Percocet** Tablets—
5/325 mg (DuPont/
PERCOCET)..........MC-24, A5
**Percodan** Tablets—
4.88/325 mg
(Percodan)...........MC-24, B2

**Percodan-Demi** Tablets—
2.44/325 mg (PERCODAN
DEMI).................MC-24, B3
**Percolone** Tablets—
5 mg (EPI/1132).......MC-23, D6
**Pergolide**................MC-25, A2
0.05 mg (A615).........MC-25, A2
0.25 mg (Logo (A)
625)....................MC-25, A2
**Permax** Tablets—
1 mg (A630)............MC-25, A2
**Perphenazine and
Amitriptyline**..........MC-25, A3-4
Mylan Tablets—
2/10 mg (MYLAN/
330)..................MC-25, A3
2/25 mg (MYLAN/
442)..................MC-25, A3
4/25 mg (MYLAN/
574)..................MC-25, A3
4/10 mg (MYLAN/
727)..................MC-25, A4
4/50 mg (MYLAN/73)..MC-25, A4
**Persantine** Tablets—
25 mg (BI/17)..........MC-10, A6
50 mg (BI/18)..........MC-10, A6
75 mg (BI/19)..........MC-10, A6
**Phenaphen with Codeine**
Capsules—
325/15 mg (AHR 6242/
AHR 6242)...........MC-1, B2
325/30 mg (AHR 6257/
AHR 6257)...........MC-1, B2
**Phendimetrazine**.........MC-25, A5
**Phenergan** Tablets—
12.5 mg (WYETH/19)..MC-26, B4
25 mg (WYETH 27)...MC-26, B4
50 mg (WYETH/227)...MC-26, B4
**Phenobarbital**..........MC-25, A6-7
Lilly Tablets—
15 mg (Lilly J31).......MC-25, A6
Warner Chilcott Tablets—
15 mg (WC 699)......MC-25, A7
30 mg (WC 700)......MC-25, A7
60 mg (WC 607)......MC-25, A7
100 mg (WC 698)....MC-25, A7
**Phenylephrine,
Phenylpropanolamine and
Guaifenesin**............MC-25, B1
**Phenylpropanolamine and
Guaifenesin**...........MC-25, B2-3
Sidmak Extended-release Tablets—
75/400 mg (SL 385)..MC-25, B3
**Phenytoin**...............MC-25, B4-5
**PhosLo** Tablets—
667 mg (BRA 200)......MC-5, A2
**Pindolol**..................MC-25, B6-7
Mutual Tablets—
5 mg (Logo 178).......MC-25, B6
10 mg (Logo 183).....MC-25, B6
**Piroxicam**................MC-25, C1-2
Mylan Capsules—
10 mg (MYLAN
1010)................MC-25, C1
20 mg (MYLAN
2020)................MC-25, C1
**Plaquenil** Tablets—
200 mg (PLA-
QUENIL).............MC-15, A5
**Plendil** Extended-release Tablets—
2.5 mg (PLENDIL/
450)..................MC-12, C4
5 mg (PLENDIL/451)...MC-12, C4
10 mg (PLENDIL/
452)..................MC-12, C5
**Potassium
Chloride**..............MC-25, C3-D1
**Pravachol** Tablets—
10 mg (Logo/PRAVACHOL
10)...................MC-25, D2
20 mg (PRAVACHOL 20/
Logo)..................MC-25, D2
40 mg (Logo/PRAVACHOL
40)...................MC-25, D2
**Pravastatin**..............MC-25, D2
**Prazosin**..................MC-25, D3-4
Mylan Capsules—
1 mg (MYLAN 1101)...MC-25, D3
2 mg (MYLAN 2302)...MC-25, D3
5 mg (MYLAN 3205)...MC-25, D3

Purepac Capsules—
1 mg (Logo-500).......MC-25, D4
2 mg (Logo-501).......MC-25, D4
5 mg (Logo-502).......MC-25, D4
**Prazosin and
Polythiazide**...........MC-25, D5
**Precose** Tablets—
50 mg (PRECOSE
50)....................MC-1, A1
100 mg (PRECOSE
100)...................MC-1, A2
**Prednisone**..........MC-25, D6-MC-26, A1
Rugby Tablets—
5 mg (Logo 189).......MC-26, A1
10 mg (RUGBY/
4325).................MC-26, A1
20 mg (RUGBY/
4326).................MC-26, A1
50 mg (Logo 527).....MC-26, A1
**Prelu-2** Extended-release
Capsules—
105 mg (BI/64)........MC-25, A5
**Premarin** Tablets—
0.3 mg (PREMARIN
0.3)....................MC-11, D6
0.625 mg (PREMARIN
0.625).................MC-11, D6
0.9 mg (PREMARIN
0.9)....................MC-11, D6
1.25 mg (PREMARIN
1.25)...................MC-11, D7
2.5 mg (PREMARIN
2.5)....................MC-11, D7
**Prevacid** Delayed-release
Capsules—
15 mg (Logo/PREVACID
15)....................MC-16, D6
30 mg (Logo/PREVACID
30)....................MC-16, D6
**Prilosec** Delayed-release
Capsules—
10 mg (PRILOSEC 10/
606)..................MC-23, C4
20 mg (PRILOSEC 20/
742)..................MC-23, C4
40 mg (PRILOSEC 40/
743)..................MC-23, C4
**Principen** Capsules—
250 mg (BRISTOL
7992)..................MC-2, D4
500 mg (BRISTOL
7993)..................MC-2, D4
**Prinivil** Tablets—
2.5 mg (MSD/15).....MC-17, B5
5 mg (MSD 19/
PRINIVIL).............MC-17, B5
10 mg (MSD 106/
PRINIVIL).............MC-17, B5
20 mg (MSD 207/
PRINIVIL).............MC-17, B6
40 mg (MSD 237/
PRINIVIL).............MC-17, B6
**Prinzide** Tablets—
10/12.5 mg (MSD 145/
PRINZIDE)............MC-17, C2
20/12.5 mg (MSD 140/
PRINZIDE)............MC-17, C2
20/25 mg (MSD 142/
PRINZIDE)............MC-17, C2
**Pro-Banthine** Tablets—
7.5 mg (SEARLE/
611)..................MC-26, B6
15 mg (SEARLE/
601)..................MC-26, B6
**Procainamide**.........MC-26, A2-6
Copley Extended-release Tablets—
500 mg (COPLEY/
188)..................MC-26, A5
750 mg (COPLEY/
114)..................MC-26, A5
Qualitest Extended-release
Tablets—
750 mg (COPLEY/
114)..................MC-26, A6
**Procardia** Capsules—
10 mg (PROCARDIA
PFIZER 260).........MC-22, A6
20 mg (PROCARDIA 20
PFIZER 261).........MC-22, A6

**Procardia XL** Extended-release
Tablets—
30 mg (PROCARDIA XL
30)....................MC-22, A7
60 mg (PROCARDIA XL/
60)....................MC-22, A7
90 mg (PROCARDIA XL
90)....................MC-22, A7
**Prochlorperazine**.....MC-26, A7-B2
Invamed Tablets—
5 mg (INV 275/5).....MC-26, A7
10 mg (INV 276/10)..MC-26, A7
**Prograf** Capsules—
1 mg (1 mg/Logo
617)..................MC-29, A7
5 mg (5 mg/Logo
657)..................MC-29, A7
**Prolixin** Tablets—
1 mg (PPP 863)......MC-13, B1
2.5 mg (PPP 864)....MC-13, B1
5 mg (PPP 865)......MC-13, B1
10 mg (PPP 956)....MC-13, B1
**Promethazine**........MC-26, B3-4
ESI Tablets—
12.5 mg (59911/
5871).................MC-26, B3
25 mg (59911 5872)..MC-26, B3
**Pronestyl** Capsules—
250 mg (PPP 758)...MC-26, A2
375 mg (PPP 756)...MC-26, A2
500 mg (PPP 757)...MC-26, A2
**Pronestyl** Tablets—
250 mg (PPP 431)...MC-26, A3
375 mg (PPP 434)...MC-26, A3
500 mg (SQUIBB
438)..................MC-26, A3
**Pronestyl-SR** Extended-release
Tablets—
500 mg (PPP 775)...MC-26, A4
**Propafenone**............MC-26, B5
**Propantheline**.........MC-26, B6-7
Roxane Tablets—
15 mg (54 303).......MC-26, B7
**Propecia** Tablets—
1 mg (PROPECIA/MRK
71)....................MC-12, D7
**Propoxyphene Napsylate and
Acetaminophen**......MC-26, C1-2
Mylan Tablets—
100/650 mg (1155)...MC-26, C2
**Propranolol**.............MC-26, C3-7
Lederle Tablets—
20 mg (Logo/P 45)...MC-26, C3
40 mg (Logo/P 46)...MC-26, C3
80 mg (Logo/P 47)...MC-26, C3
Rugby Tablets—
10 mg (RUGBY/4309)..MC-26, C4
20 mg (RUGBY/4313)..MC-26, C4
40 mg (RUGBY/4314)..MC-26, C4
60 mg (RUGBY/4315)..MC-26, C4
80 mg (RUGBY/4316)..MC-26, C4
**Propranolol and Hydro-
chlorothiazide**........MC-26, D1-5
Barr Tablets—
40/25 mg (barr/555
427)..................MC-26, D1
80/25 mg (barr/555
428)..................MC-26, D1
Purepac Tablets—
40/25 mg (Logo/358)..MC-26, D2
80/25 mg (Logo/360)..MC-26, D2
Rugby Tablets—
40/25 mg (RUGBY/
4402).................MC-26, D3
80/25 mg (RUGBY/
4403).................MC-26, D3
**Propulsid** Tablets—
10 mg (JANSSEN/
P10)...................MC-7, B7
20 mg (JANSSEN/
P20)...................MC-7, B7
**Proscar** Tablets—
5 mg (MSD 72/
PROSCAR)...........MC-13, A1
**ProSom** Tablets—
1 mg (Logo UC).....MC-11, D3
2 mg (Logo UD)....MC-11, D3

*Prostaphlin* Capsules—
  250 mg (BRISTOL
  7977).................. MC-23, C6
  500 mg (BRISTOL
  7982).................. MC-23, C6
*Protriptyline*........... MC-26, D6-7
  Sidmak Tablets—
  5 mg (SL 523)........ MC-26, D7
  10 mg (SL 524)...... MC-26, D7
*Proventil* Extended-release
  Tablets—
  4 mg (Logo 431)........ MC-1, C5
*Provera* Tablets—
  2.5 mg (PROVERA
  2.5).................. MC-18, C2
  5 mg (PROVERA 5)... MC-18, C2
  10 mg (PROVERA
  10).................. MC-18, C2
*Prozac* Capsules—
  20 mg (DISTA 3105/PROZAC
  20 mg)... MC-13, A5
  10 mg (DISTA 3104/PROZAC
  10 mg)... MC-13, A5
*Pseudoephedrine and
  Guaifenesin*.......... MC-27, A1-2
*Purinethol* Tablets—
  50 mg (PURINETHOL
  04A)................ MC-18, D2
*Pyrimethamine*.......... MC-27, A3
*Quetiapine*............. MC-27, A4
*Quibron* Capsules—
  150/90 mg (BRISTOL
  516).................. MC-30, A2
  300/180 mg (BRISTOL
  515).................. MC-30, A2
*Quibron-T Dividose* Tablets—
  300 mg (BL 512)..... MC-29, D5
*Quibron-T/SR Dividose* Extended-
  release Tablets—
  300 mg (BL 519).... MC-29, D6
*Quinaglute Dura-Tabs* Extended-
  release Tablets—
  324 mg (Logo/Clock-
  face)................ MC-27, A6
*Quinapril*.............. MC-27, A5
*Quinidex* Extended-release
  Tablets—
  300 mg (AHR
  QUINIDEX)........... MC-27, B2
*Quinidine
  Gluconate*........... MC-27, A6-B1
  Mutual Extended-release Tablets—
  324 mg (Logo 66).... MC-27, A7
  Schein Extended-release Tablets—
  324 mg (DAN/5538).. MC-27, B1
*Quinidine Sulfate*..... MC-27, B2-3
  Roxane Tablets—
  300 mg (54 053/300). MC-27, B3
*Ramipril*................ MC-27, B4
*Ranitidine*............. MC-27, B5-C1
  Apothecon Tablets—
  150 mg (APO/025)... MC-27, B5
  300 mg (APO 26)... MC-27, B5
*Ranitidine Bismuth
  Citrate*............. MC-27, C2
*Raxar* Tablets—
  200 mg (GX CK3)..... MC-14, A5
*Reglan* Tablets—
  5 mg (AHR/REGLAN
  5).................... MC-19, D6
  10 mg (AHR 10/
  REGLAN)............. MC-19, D6
*Relafen* Tablets—
  500 mg (RELAFEN/
  500)................ MC-21, B2
  750 mg (RELAFEN/
  750)................ MC-21, B2
*Remeron* Tablets—
  15 mg (Organon/TZ 3
  TZ 3)................ MC-20, D2
*Reserpine, Hydralazine and
  Hydrochlorothiazide*... MC-27, C3
*Restoril* Capsules—
  7.5 mg (RESTORIL 7.5mg/
  FOR SLEEP)......... MC-29, B4
  15 mg (RESTORIL 15 mg/
  FOR SLEEP)......... MC-29, B4
  30 mg (RESTORIL 30 mg/
  FOR SLEEP)......... MC-29, B4

*Retrovir* Capsules—
  100 mg (Logo Wellcome/
  Y9C 100)............ MC-32, D3
*Retrovir* Tablets—
  300 mg (GX CW3/
  300)................ MC-32, D4
*Rezulin* Tablets—
  200 mg (PD 352/
  200)................ MC-32, A2
  300 mg (PD 357/
  300)................ MC-32, A2
  400 mg (PD 353/
  400)................ MC-32, A2
*Rheumatrex* Tablets—
  2.5 mg (Logo/M 1).... MC-19, B1
*Rifabutin*.............. MC-27, C4
*Rifadin* Capsules—
  150 mg (RIFADIN
  150)................ MC-27, C5
  300 mg (RIFADIN
  300)................ MC-27, C5
*Rifamate* Capsules—
  300/150 mg (RIFA-
  MATE)............... MC-27, C7
*Rifampin*............... MC-27, C5-6
*Rifampin and
  Isoniazid*........... MC-27, C7
*Rifampin, Isoniazid,
  and Pyrazinamide*... MC-27, D1
*Rifater* Tablets—
  120/50/300 mg
  (RIFATER).......... MC-27, D1
*Rilutek* Tablets—
  50 mg (RPR 202)..... MC-27, D2
*Riluzole*............... MC-27, D2
*Rimactane* Capsules—
  300 mg (CIBA 154/
  CIBA 154).......... MC-27, C6
*Rimantadine*.......... MC-27, D3
*Risperdal* Tablets—
  1 mg (JANSSEN/R 1).. MC-27, D4
  2 mg (JANSSEN/R 2).. MC-27, D4
  3 mg (JANSSEN/R 3).. MC-27, D5
  4 mg (JANSSEN/R 4).. MC-27, D5
*Risperidone*........... MC-27, D4-5
*Ritalin* Tablets—
  5 mg (CIBA/7)........ MC-19, C6
  10 mg (CIBA/3)....... MC-19, C6
  20 mg (CIBA/34)..... MC-19, C6
*Ritalin-SR* Extended-release
  Tablets—
  20 mg (CIBA 16)..... MC-19, C7
*Ritonavir*............. MC-27, D6
*Robaxin* Tablets—
  500 mg (AHR
  ROBAXIN).......... MC-19, A3
  750 mg (AHR/ROBAXIN
  750)............... MC-19, A3
*Robaxisal* Tablets—
  400/325 mg (AHR
  ROBAXISAL)........ MC-19, A4
*Rocaltrol* Capsules—
  0.25 mg (ROCALTROL
  0.25 ROCHE)........ MC-5, A1
  0.5 mcg (ROCALTROL 0.5
  ROCHE).............. MC-5, A1
*Rondec-TR* Tablets—
  8/120 mg (R/6240)..... MC-5, C6
*Roxicet* Tablets—
  5/325 mg (54 543)... MC-24, B1
  5/500 mg (54 730)... MC-24, B1
*Roxicodone* Tablets—
  5 mg (54 582)........ MC-24, A4
*Roxiprin* Tablets—
  4.88/325 mg (54
  902)................ MC-24, B4
*Rynatan* Tablets—
  8/25/25 mg (WALLACE
  713)................ MC-6, D6
*Rythmol* Tablets—
  150 mg (Logo 150)... MC-26, B5
  225 mg (Logo/225)... MC-26, B5
  300 mg (Logo 300)... MC-26, B5
*Salsalate*............. MC-27, D7-MC-28, A2
  Mutual Tablets—
  500 mg (Logo 174)... MC-27, D7
  750 mg (Logo 177)... MC-27, D7
  Sidmak Tablets—
  500 mg (SL 390)..... MC-28, A2

*Sandimmune SGC* Capsules—
  25 mg (Logo 78 240)... MC-8, C1
  50 mg (Logo 78 242)... MC-8, C1
  100 mg (Logo 78
  241)................ MC-8, C1
*Saquinavir*............ MC-28, A3
*Saquinavir Mesylate*... MC-28, A4
*Sectral* Capsules—
  200 mg (WYETH 4177/
  SECTRAL 200)...... MC-1, A5
  400 mg (WYETH 4179/
  SECTRAL 400)...... MC-1, A5
*Selegiline*............. MC-28, A5-6
  Novopharm Tablets—
  5 mg (N 179/5)...... MC-28, A5
*Ser-Ap-Es* Tablets—
  0.1/25/15 mg (CIBA/
  71)................. MC-27, C3
*Serax* Capsules—
  10 mg (WYETH-51 Logo/
  SERAX 10)......... MC-23, D2
  15 mg (WYETH-6 Logo/
  SERAX 15)......... MC-23, D2
  30 mg (WYETH-52 Logo/
  SERAX 30)......... MC-23, D2
*Serax* Tablets—
  15 mg (WYETH 317/
  15)................. MC-23, D3
*Serentil* Tablets—
  10 mg (BI/10)........ MC-18, D5
  25 mg (BI/25)........ MC-18, D5
  50 mg (BI/50)........ MC-18, D5
*Seroquel* Tablets—
  25 mg (SEROQUEL
  25)................. MC-27, A4
  100 mg (SEROQUEL
  100)................ MC-27, A4
  200 mg (SEROQUEL
  200)................ MC-27, A4
*Sertraline*............ MC-28, A7
*Serzone* Tablets—
  100 mg (BMS 100/32).. MC-21, D3
  150 mg (BMS 150/39).. MC-21, D3
  200 mg (BMS 200/33).. MC-21, D4
  250 mg (BMS 250/41).. MC-21, D4
*Sibutramine*........... MC-28, B1
*Sildenafil*............ MC-28, B2
*Simvastatin*........... MC-28, B3
*Sinemet* Tablets—
  10/100 mg (SINEMET/
  647)................ MC-5, C3
  25/100 mg (SINEMET/
  650)................ MC-5, C3
  25/250 mg (SINEMET/
  654)................ MC-5, C3
*Sinemet CR* Extended-release
  Tablets—
  25/100 mg (SINEMET CR/
  601)................ MC-5, C4
  50/200 mg (SINEMET CR/
  521)................ MC-5, C4
*Sinequan* Capsules—
  10 mg (SINEQUAN/ROERIG
  534)................ MC-10, C6
  25 mg (SINEQUAN/ROERIG
  535)................ MC-10, C6
  50 mg (SINEQUAN/ROERIG
  536)................ MC-10, C6
  75 mg (SINEQUAN/ROERIG
  539)................ MC-10, C7
  100 mg (SINEQUAN/ROERIG
  538)................ MC-10, C7
  150 mg (SINEQUAN/ROERIG
  537)................ MC-10, C7
*Singulair Chewable* Tablets—
  5 mg (SINGULAIR/MRK
  275)................ MC-20, D7
*Singulair* Tablets—
  10 mg (SINGULAIR/MRK
  117)................ MC-20, D6
*Slo-bid* Extended-release
  Capsules—
  50 mg (RORER/Slo-bid
  50)................. MC-29, D2
  75 mg (Logo/Slo-bid
  75 mg).............. MC-29, D2
  100 mg (Logo/Slo-bid
  100 mg)............. MC-29, D2
  125 mg (Logo/Slo-bid
  125 mg)............. MC-29, D3

*Slo-bid* Extended-release
  Capsules *(continued)*
  200 mg (Logo/Slo-bid
  200 mg)............. MC-29, D3
  300 mg (Logo/Slo-bid
  300 mg)............. MC-29, D3
*Slo-Niacin* Extended-release
  Tablets—
  250 mg (250)........ MC-21, D6
  500 mg (500)........ MC-21, D6
  750 mg (750)........ MC-21, D6
*Slo-Phyllin* Tablets—
  100 mg (Logo 351).... MC-29, D4
  200 mg (Logo 352)... MC-29, D4
*Slow-K* Extended-release Tablets—
  600 mg (Slow-K)..... MC-25, C7
*Soma* Tablets—
  350 mg (37 WALLACE 2001/
  SOMA)............... MC-5, D1
*Soma Compound* Tablets—
  200/325 mg (WALLACE 2103/
  SOMA C)............ MC-5, D3
*Soma Compound with Codeine*
  Tablets—
  200/325/16 mg (WALLACE 2403/
  SOMA CC).......... MC-5, D4
*Sorbitrate* Chewable Tablets—
  5 mg (S/810)........ MC-16, B2
*Sorbitrate* Tablets—
  5 mg (S/770)........ MC-16, B1
  10 mg (S/780)....... MC-16, B1
  20 mg (S/820)....... MC-16, B1
  30 mg (S/773)....... MC-16, B1
  40 mg (S/774)....... MC-16, B1
*Soriatane* Capsules—
  10 mg (SORIATANE 10
  ROCHE)............. MC-1, B4
  25 mg (SORIATANE 25
  ROCHE)............. MC-1, B4
*Sotalol*............... MC-28, B4-5
*Sparfloxacin*.......... MC-28, B6
*Spironolactone*........ MC-28, B7-C1
  Mylan Tablets—
  25 mg (MYLAN 146/
  25)................ MC-28, B7
*Spironolactone and Hydro-
  chlorothiazide*...... MC-28, C2-3
  Geneva Tablets—
  25/25 mg (GG 95).... MC-28, C2
*Sporanox* Capsules—
  100 mg (JANSSEN SPORANOX
  100)................ MC-16, B7
*Stavudine*............ MC-28, C4
*Stelazine* Tablets—
  2 mg (SKF 504)...... MC-31, D5
*Sucralfate*........... MC-28, C5
*Sular* Extended-release Tablets—
  10 mg (ZENECA 10/
  891)................ MC-22, B4
  20 mg (Zeneca 20/
  892)................ MC-22, B4
  30 mg (ZENECA 30/
  893)................ MC-22, B5
  40 mg (ZENECA 40/
  894)................ MC-22, B5
*Sulfadoxine &
  Pyrimethamine*...... MC-28, C6
*Sulfamethoxazole*...... MC-28, C7
*Sulfamethoxazole and
  Trimethoprim*........ MC-28, D1-2
  Schein Tablets—
  400/80 mg (DAN/
  5546)............... MC-28, D2
  800/160 mg (DAN/
  5547)............... MC-28, D2
*Sulfasalazine*......... MC-28, D3-5
  Rugby Tablets—
  500 mg (RUGBY/
  4617)............... MC-28, D5
*Sulfinpyrazone*........ MC-28, D6-7
  Barr Capsules—
  200 mg (barr/272)... MC-28, D6
  Barr Tablets—
  100 mg (barr/555
  271)............... MC-28, D7
*Sulindac*............. MC-29, A1-3
  Mutual Tablets—
  150 mg (Logo 112)... MC-29, A2
  200 mg (Logo 116)... MC-29, A2

Schein Tablets—
150 mg (DAN/5661) .. MC-29, A3
200 mg (DAN/5660) .. MC-29, A3
**Sumatriptan** ............. MC-29, A4
**Sumycin** Capsules—
250 mg (SQUIBB
655) .................. MC-29, C3
500 mg (SQUIBB
763) .................. MC-29, C3
**Sumycin** Tablets—
250 mg (SQUIBB
663) .................. MC-29, C4
500 mg (SQUIBB
603) .................. MC-29, C4
**Suprax** Tablets—
200 mg (Logo 200/
SUPRAX) ............. MC-6, A6
400 mg (Logo 400/
SUPRAX) ............. MC-6, A6
**Surmontil** Capsules—
25 mg (WYETH/4132) ...MC-32, A1
50 mg (WYETH/4133) ..MC-32, A1
100 mg (WYETH/4158) ..MC-32, A1
**Symmetrel** Tablets—
100 mg (SYM-
METREL) ............. MC-1, D6
**Synalgos-DC** Capsules—
356.4/30/16 mg (WYETH/
4191) ................. MC-3, A2
**Synthroid** Tablets—
0.088 mg (FLINT/88) .. MC-17, B2
0.025 mg (FLINT/25) .. MC-17, B2
0.05 mg (FLINT/50) ... MC-17, B2
0.075 mg (FLINT/75) .. MC-17, B2
0.1 mg (FLINT/100) ... MC-17, B2
0.112 mg (FLINT/112) ..MC-17, B2
0.125 mg (FLINT/125) ..MC-17, B3
0.15 mg (FLINT/150) .. MC-17, B3
0.175 mg (FLINT/175) ..MC-17, B3
0.2 mg (FLINT/200) ... MC-17, B3
0.3 mg (FLINT/300) ... MC-17, B3
**Tacrine** ............. MC-29, A5-6
**Tacrolimus** ........... MC-29, A7
**Tagamet** Tablets—
200 mg (TAGAMET 200
SKF) ................. MC-7, B3
300 mg (TAGAMET 300
SB) .................. MC-7, B3
400 mg (TAGAMET 400
SB) .................. MC-7, B4
800 mg (TAGAMET 800
SB) .................. MC-7, B4
**Talacen** Tablets—
25/650 mg (Winthrop/
T37) ................. MC-24, D5
**Talwin-Nx** Tablets—
50/0.5 mg (Logo/T 51).. MC-24, D6
**Tambocor** Tablets—
50 mg (3M/TR 50) ..... MC-13, A2
100 mg (3M/TR 100) .. MC-13, A2
**Tamoxifen** ........... MC-29, B1-2
Barr Tablets—
10 mg (barr/446) ...... MC-29, B1
**Tarka** Extended-release Tablets—
1/240 mg (Logo 241/
TARKA) .............. MC-31, B2
2/180 mg (Logo 182/
TARKA) .............. MC-31, B3
2/240 mg (Logo 242/
TARKA) .............. MC-31, B2
4/240 mg (Logo 244/
TARKA) .............. MC-31, B3
**Tasmar** Tablets—
100 mg (ROCHE/TASMAR
100) .................. MC-30, D4
200 mg (ROCHE/TASMAR
200) .................. MC-30, D4
**Tegison** Capsules—
10 mg (TEGISON 10 ROCHE/
TEGISON 10
ROCHE) ............. MC-12, B6
**Tegretol** Chewable Tablets—
100 mg (TEGRETOL/52
52) .................. MC-5, B6
**Tegretol** Tablets—
200 mg (TEGRETOL/27
27) .................. MC-5, B5

**Tegretol-XR** Extended-release
Tablets—
200 mg (T (Logo)/
200 mg) .............. MC-5, B7
**Temazepam** ......... MC-29, B3-5
Mylan Capsules—
15 mg (MYLAN
4010) ............... MC-29, B3
30 mg (MYLAN
5050) ............... MC-29, B3
Purepac Capsules—
15 mg (Logo-076) ..... MC-29, B5
30 mg (Logo-077) ..... MC-29, B5
**Tenex** Tablets—
1 mg (AHR 1/TENEX) ..MC-14, B3
2 mg (AHR 2/TENEX) ..MC-14, B3
**Tenoretic** Tablets—
50/25 mg (TENORETIC/
115) .................. MC-3, B2
100/25 mg (TENORETIC/
117) .................. MC-3, B2
**Tenormin** Tablets—
25 mg (Logo/107) ..... MC-3, A6
50 mg (TENORMIN/
105) .................. MC-3, A6
100 mg (TENORMIN/
101) .................. MC-3, A6
**Tenuate** Tablets—
25 mg (TENUATE 25) ..MC-9, B6
**Tenuate Dospan** Extended-release
Tablets—
75 mg (TENUATE 75) ...MC-9, B7
**Terazosin** ............ MC-29, B6-7
**Terbinafine** ............ MC-29, C1
**Terbutaline** ............ MC-29, C2
**Tetracycline** .......... MC-29, C3-7
Barr Capsules—
250 mg (barr/011) ..... MC-29, C5
500 mg (barr/010) ..... MC-29, C5
**Thalitone** Tablets—
25 mg (BI/76) .......... MC-7, A4
**Theo-24** Extended-release
Capsules—
100 mg (ucb 2832/Theo-24
100) .................. MC-29, D7
200 mg (ucb 2842/Theo-24
200) .................. MC-29, D7
300 mg (ucb 2852/Theo-24
300) .................. MC-30, A1
400 mg (ucb 2902/Theo-24
400) .................. MC-30, A1
**Theophylline**. MC-29, D1-MC-30, A1
**Theophylline and
Guaifenesin** ........... MC-30, A2
**Thioridazine** .......... MC-30, A3-7
Creighton Tablets—
10 mg (Logo/264) ..... MC-30, A3
25 mg (Logo/266) ..... MC-30, A3
100 mg (CP/268) ...... MC-30, A3
Geneva Tablets—
150 mg (GG 35) ...... MC-30, A4
200 mg (GG 36) ...... MC-30, A4
Mylan Tablets—
10 mg (M 54/10) ..... MC-30, A5
25 mg (M 58/25) ..... MC-30, A5
50 mg (M 59/50) ..... MC-30, A5
100 mg (M 61/100) ... MC-30, A5
**Thiothixene** ........... MC-30, B1-5
Geneva Capsules—
1 mg (GG 589) ...... MC-30, B1
2 mg (GG 596) ...... MC-30, B1
5 mg (GG 597) ...... MC-30, B1
10 mg (GG 598) ..... MC-30, B1
Schein Capsules—
1 mg (DAN 5593) .... MC-30, B4
2 mg (DAN 5592) .... MC-30, B4
5 mg (DAN 5595) .... MC-30, B5
10 mg (DAN 5594) .. MC-30, B5
**Thorazine** Extended-release
Capsules—
75 mg (SKF T64) ...... MC-6, D7
150 mg (SKF T66) ..... MC-6, D7
**Thorazine** Tablets—
10 mg (SKF T73) ...... MC-7, A1
25 mg (SKF T74) ...... MC-7, A1
50 mg (SKF T76) ...... MC-7, A1

**Tiagabine** ............ MC-30, B6-7
**Tiazac** Extended-release Capsules—
120 mg (Tiazac 120).... MC-9, C5
180 mg (Tiazac 180)... MC-9, C5
240 mg (Tiazac 240)... MC-9, C5
300 mg (Tiazac 300)... MC-9, C6
360 mg (Tiazac 360)... MC-9, C6
**Ticlid** Tablets—
250 mg (Ticlid/250) ..... MC-30, C1
**Ticlopidine** ............. MC-30, C1
**Timolol** ............... MC-30, C2-3
Mylan Tablets—
5 mg (M 55) .......... MC-30, C3
10 mg (M 221) ....... MC-30, C3
20 mg (M 715) ....... MC-30, C3
**Tizanidine** ............. MC-30, C4
**Tocainide** .............. MC-30, C5
**Tofranil** Tablets—
10 mg (GEIGY/32) .... MC-15, D2
25 mg (GEIGY/140) .. MC-15, D2
50 mg (GEIGY/136) .. MC-15, D2
**Tofranil-PM** Capsules—
75 mg (GEIGY/20) .... MC-15, C7
100 mg (GEIGY/40) ... MC-15, C7
125 mg (GEIGY/45) ... MC-15, D1
150 mg (GEIGY/22) ... MC-15, D1
**Tolazamide** ......... MC-30, C6-D1
Zenith Tablets—
100 mg (Z 2978) ...... MC-30, D1
250 mg (Z 2979) ...... MC-30, D1
**Tolbutamide** ........ MC-30, D2-3
Mylan Tablets—
500 mg (M 13) ....... MC-30, D2
**Tolcapone** ............. MC-30, D4
**Tolectin** Tablets—
200 mg (McNEIL/TOLECTIN
200) ................. MC-31, A1
600 mg (McNEIL 600
TOLECTIN) .......... MC-31, A1
**Tolectin DS** Capsules—
400 mg (McNEIL/TOLECTIN
DS) .................. MC-30, D7
**Tolinase** Tablets—
100 mg (TOLINASE
100) .................. MC-30, C6
250 mg (TOLINASE
250) .................. MC-30, C6
500 mg (TOLINASE
500) .................. MC-30, C7
**Tolmetin**... MC-30, D5-MC-31, A3
Mutual Capsules—
400 mg (MUTUAL
179) .................. MC-30, D5
Mutual Tablets—
200 mg (Logo 50) .... MC-30, D6
Purepac Capsules—
400 mg (Logo-520) ... MC-31, A2
Purepac Tablets—
600 mg (Logo/480) ... MC-31, A3
**Tonocard** Tablets—
400 mg (TONOCARD/
707) .................. MC-30, C5
600 mg (TONOCARD/
709) .................. MC-30, C5
**Toprol XL** Extended-release
Tablets—
100 mg (A MS) ....... MC-20, A3
200 mg (A MY) ....... MC-20, A3
**Toprol-XL** Extended-release
Tablets—
50 mg (A MO) ........ MC-20, A1
**Toradol** Tablets—
10 mg (TORADOL/
SYNTEX) ............. MC-16, C6
**Torsemide** ............. MC-31, A4-6
**Tramadol** ............... MC-31, A7
**Trandate** Tablets—
100 mg (TRANDATE
100) .................. MC-16, C7
200 mg (TRANDATE
200) .................. MC-16, C7
300 mg (TRANDATE
300) .................. MC-16, C7
**Trandolapril** ............ MC-31, B1
**Trandolapril and
Verapamil** ........... MC-31, B2-3
**Tranxene SD** Tablets—
11.25 mg (Logo TX) ....MC-8, A3
22.5 mg (Logo TY) ..... MC-8, A3

**Tranxene T-Tab** Tablets—
3.75 mg (Logo/TL) .......MC-8, A4
7.5 mg (Logo/TM) ...... MC-8, A4
15 mg (Logo/TN) ....... MC-8, A4
**Tranylcypromine** ........ MC-31, B4
**Trazodone**. ........... MC-31, B5-C2
Barr Tablets—
50 mg (barr/555
489) .................. MC-31, B7
100 mg (barr/555
490) .................. MC-31, B7
Mutual Tablets—
50 mg (Logo 118) .... MC-31, C1
100 mg (Logo 114) ... MC-31, C1
150 mg (MP 168/25-25
50-50) ............... MC-31, C1
Purepac Tablets—
50 mg (Logo/439) .... MC-31, C2
100 mg (Logo/441) ... MC-31, C2
**Trental** Extended-release Tablets—
400 mg (HOECHST/
TRENTAL) ........... MC-25, A1
**Tretinoin** ............... MC-31, C3
**Tri-Levlen 21 and 28** Tablets—
0.05/0.03 mg (B/95).... MC-17, A4
0.075/0.04 mg (B/96).. MC-17, A4
0.125/0.03 mg (B/97).. MC-17, A4
Inert (B/11) ............ MC-17, A4
**Tri-phen-mine** Extended-release
Tablets—
5/15/10/40 mg (832
PPPC) ................ MC-6, D5
**Triamterene** ............. MC-31, C4
**Triamterene and Hydro-
chlorothiazide**...... MC-31, C5-D1
Barr Tablets—
75/50 mg (barr/555
444) .................. MC-31, C5
Geneva Tablets—
75/50 mg (GG 172)... MC-31, C7
**Triazolam** ............. MC-31, D2-3
Qualitest Tablets—
0.25 mg (Logo/TR
250) .................. MC-31, D3
**Tricor** Capsules—
67 mg (Logo FR) ...... MC-12, C6
**Trifluoperazine** ......... MC-31, D4-5
Geneva Tablets—
1 mg (GG 51/1) ...... MC-31, D4
2 mg (GG 53/2) ...... MC-31, D4
5 mg (GG 55/5) ...... MC-31, D4
10 mg (GG 58/10) ... MC-31, D4
**Trimethoprim**........ MC-31, D6-7
Schein Tablets—
100 mg (DAN/5571) .. MC-31, D7
**Trimipramine** .......... MC-32, A1
**Trimox** Capsules—
250 mg (BRISTOL
7278) ................. MC-2, C1
500 mg (BRISTOL
7279) ................. MC-2, C1
**Trimox** Chewable Tablets—
125 mg (BMS 37)..... MC-2, C2
250 mg (BMS 38)..... MC-2, C2
**Trimpex** Tablets—
100 mg (ROCHE/TRIMPEX
100) .................. MC-31, D6
**Trinalin** Extended-release Tablets—
1/120 mg (TRINALIN
703) .................. MC-3, C1
**Triphasil-21 and -28** Tablets—
0.05/0.03 mg (Logo/
641) .................. MC-17, A6
0.075/0.04 mg (Logo/
642) .................. MC-17, A6
0.125/0.03 mg (Logo/
643) .................. MC-17, A6
Inert (Logo/650) ...... MC-17, A6
**Tritec** Tablets—
400 mg (Logo/
TRITEC) .............. MC-27, C2
**Troglitazone** ........... MC-32, A2
**Trovafloxacin** ........... MC-32, A3
**Trovan** Tablets—
100 mg (PFIZER/378) ..MC-32, A3
200 mg (PFIZER/379) ..MC-32, A3

**Tylenol with Codeine** Tablets—
  300/7.5 mg (McNEIL/TYLENOL
    CODEINE 1)............MC-1, A6
  300/15 mg (McNEIL/TYLENOL
    CODEINE 2)............MC-1, A6
  300/30 mg (McNEIL/TYLENOL
    CODEINE 3)............MC-1, A7
  300/60 mg (McNEIL/TYLENOL
    CODEINE 4)............MC-1, A7
**Tylox** Capsules—
  5/500 mg (TYLOX
    McNEIL)................MC-24, A7
**Ultram** Tablets—
  50 mg (McNEIL/
    659)...................MC-31, A7
**Uniphyl** Extended-release Tablets—
  400 mg (PF/U 400)....MC-29, D1
  600 mg (PF/U 600)....MC-29, D1
**Uniretic** Tablets—
  7.5/12.5 mg (S P/
    712)...................MC-20, D5
  15/25 mg (S P/725)....MC-20, D5
**Univasc** Tablets—
  7.5 mg (SP 7.5/707)..MC-20, D4
  15 mg (SP 15/715)....MC-20, D4
**Ursodiol**................MC-32, A4
**V-Cillin K** Tablets—
  250 mg (V-CILLIN K 250
    Lilly)................MC-24, D2
  500 mg (V-CILLIN K 500
    Lilly)................MC-24, D2
**Valacyclovir**............MC-32, A5
**Valium** Tablets—
  2 mg (ROCHE/2
    Valium)...............MC-9, A1
  5 mg (ROCHE/5
    Valium)...............MC-9, A1
  10 mg (ROCHE/10
    Valium)...............MC-9, A1
**Valproic Acid**...MC-32, A6-7
  Goldline Capsules—
    250 mg (0665 4120)..MC-32, A7
**Valtrex** Tablets—
  1 gram (VALTREX
    1 gram)...............MC-32, A5
  500 mg (VALTREX
    500 mg)...............MC-32, A5
**Vantin** Tablets—
  100 mg (U 3617).........MC-6, A7
  200 mg (U 3618).........MC-6, A7
**Vascor** Tablets—
  200 mg (VASCOR
    200)..................MC-4, A1
  300 mg (VASCOR
    300)..................MC-4, A1
  400 mg (VASCOR
    400)..................MC-4, A1
**Vaseretic** Tablets—
  5/12.5 mg (MSD/173)..MC-11, A3
  10/25 mg (MSD 720/
    VASERETIC)..........MC-11, A3
**Vasotec** Tablets—
  2.5 mg (MSD 14/
    VASOTEC)............MC-11, A1
  5 mg (MSD 712/
    VASOTEC)............MC-11, A1
  10 mg (MSD 713/
    VASOTEC)............MC-11, A1
  20 mg (MSD 714/
    VASOTEC)............MC-11, A1

**Veetids** Tablets—
  250 mg (BL V1).........MC-24, C7
  500 mg (BL V2).........MC-24, C7
**Velosef** Capsules—
  250 mg (SQUIBB 113)...MC-6, C2
  500 mg (SQUIBB 114)...MC-6, C2
**Venlafaxine**..........MC-32, B1-2
**Ventolin** Tablets—
  2 mg (Glaxo/
    VENTOLIN 2).........MC-1, C2
  4 mg (Glaxo/
    VENTOLIN 4).........MC-1, C2
**Verapamil**............MC-32, B3-C3
  Purepac Tablets—
    80 mg (Logo/473).....MC-32, B4
    120 mg (Logo/475)....MC-32, B4
  Rugby Tablets—
    80 mg (RUGBY/4812)..MC-32, B5
    120 mg (RUGBY/
      4932)..............MC-32, B5
**Verelan** Extended-release
  Capsules—
    120 mg (Lederle V8/VERELAN
      120 mg)............MC-32, C2
    180 mg (Lederle V7/VERELAN
      180 mg)............MC-32, C2
    240 mg (Lederle V9/VERELAN
      240 mg)............MC-32, C3
    360 mg (Lederle V6/VERELAN
      360 mg)............MC-32, C3
**Vesanoid** Capsules—
  10 mg (VESANOID 10
    ROCHE)...............MC-31, C3
**Viagra** Tablets—
  25 mg (PFIZER/VGR
    25)..................MC-28, B2
  50 mg (PFIZER/VGR
    50)..................MC-28, B2
  100 mg (PFIZER/VGR
    100).................MC-28, B2
**Vicodin** Tablets—
  5/500 mg (VICODIN)...MC-14, D1
**Vicodin ES** Tablets—
  7.5/750 mg (VICODIN
    ES)..................MC-14, D2
**Vicodin HP** Tablets—
  10/660 mg (VICODIN
    HP)..................MC-14, D3
**Vicoprofen** Tablets—
  7.5/200 mg (Logo
    VP)..................MC-14, D6
**Videx** Tablets—
  100 mg (VIDEX/100)....MC-9, B5
  150 mg (VIDEX/150)....MC-9, B5
**Visken** Tablets—
  5 mg (VISKEN 5).......MC-25, B7
  10 mg (VISKEN 10/
    V)...................MC-25, B7
**Vivactil** Tablets—
  5 mg (MSD 26/
    VIVACTIL)............MC-26, D6
**Voltaren** Enteric-coated Tablets—
  25 mg (VOLTAREN
    25)..................MC-9, A5
  50 mg (VOLARTEN
    50)..................MC-9, A5
  75 mg (VOLTAREN
    75)..................MC-9, A5

**Warfarin Sodium**......MC-32, C4-7
  Invamed Tablets—
    1 mg (INV 309/1).....MC-32, C6
    2 mg (INV 310/2).....MC-32, C6
    2.5 mg (INV 311/2.5).MC-32, C6
    4 mg (INV 312/4).....MC-32, C
    65 mg (INV 313/5)....MC-32, C7
    7.5 mg (INV 314/7.5).MC-32, C7
    10 mg (INV 315/10)...MC-32, C7
**Wellbutrin** Tablets—
  75 mg (WELLBUTRIN
    75)..................MC-4, B7
  100 mg (WELLBUTRIN
    100).................MC-4, B7
**Wellbutrin SR** Extended-release
  Tablets—
  100 mg (WELLBUTRIN
    SR 100)..............MC-4, C2
  150 mg (WELLBUTRIN
    SR 150)..............MC-4, C2
**Wymox** Capsules—
  250 mg (WYETH 559)...MC-2, C6
  500 mg (WYETH 560)...MC-2, C6
**Wytensin** Tablets—
  4 mg (WYETH 73/W4)..MC-14, B2
  8 mg (WYETH 74/W8)..MC-14, B2
**Xanax** Tablets—
  0.25 mg (XANAX 0.25)..MC-1, D4
  0.5 mg (XANAX 0.5)....MC-1, D4
  1 mg (XANAX 1.0)......MC-1, D4
  2 mg (XANAX/2)........MC-1, D4
**Xeloda** Tablets—
  150 mg (XELODA/150)..MC-5, A5
  500 mg (XELODA/500)..MC-5, A5
**Zafirlukast**...............MC-32, D1
**Zagam** Tablets—
  200 mg (RPR 201).....MC-28, B6
**Zalcitabine**..............MC-32, D2
**Zanaflex** Tablets—
  4 mg (Logo/594).......MC-30, C4
**Zantac** Tablets—
  150 mg (Glaxo/ZANTAC
    150).................MC-27, B7
  300 mg (Glaxo/ZANTAC
    300).................MC-27, B7
**Zantac EFFERdose** Effervescent
  Tablets—
  150 mg (ZANTAC 150/
    427).................MC-27, C1
**Zantac Geldose** Capsules—
  150 mg (Glaxo/ZANTAC
    150).................MC-27, B6
  300 mg (Glaxo/ZANTAC
    300).................MC-27, B6
**Zebeta** Tablets—
  5 mg (Logo/B1)........MC-4, A7
  10 mg (Logo/B3).......MC-4, A7
**Zerit** Capsules—
  30 mg (BMS 1966/
    30)..................MC-28, C4
  40 mg (BMS 1967/
    40)..................MC-28, C4
**Zestoretic** Tablets—
  10/12.5 mg (STUART 141/
    ZESTORETIC).........MC-17, C3
  20/25 mg (ZESTORETIC
    145).................MC-17, C3
  20/12.5 mg (ZESTORETIC
    142).................MC-17, C3

**Zestril** Tablets—
  2.5 mg (Zestril 2/
    135).................MC-17, B7
  5 mg (ZESTRIL/130)...MC-17, B7
  10 mg (ZESTRIL 10/
    131).................MC-17, B7
  20 mg (ZESTRIL 20/
    132).................MC-17, C1
  40 mg (ZESTRIL 40/
    134).................MC-17, C1
**Ziac** Tablets—
  2.5/6.25 mg (Logo/
    B12).................MC-4, B1
  5/6.25 mg (Logo/B13)..MC-4, B1
  10/6.25 mg (Logo/B14).MC-4, B1
**Zidovudine**...........MC-32, D3-4
**Zileuton**..............MC-32, D5
**Zithromax** Tablets—
  250 mg (PFIZER/306)..MC-3, C4
**Zocor** Tablets—
  5 mg (MSD 726/
    ZOCOR)...............MC-28, B3
  10 mg (MSD 735/
    ZOCOR)...............MC-28, B3
  20 mg (MSD 740/
    ZOCAR)...............MC-28, B3
  40 mg (MSD 749/
    ZOCOR)...............MC-28, B3
**Zofran** Tablets—
  4 mg (Zofran/4).......MC-23, C5
  8 mg (Zofran/8).......MC-23, C5
**Zolmitriptan**..........MC-32, D6
**Zoloft** Tablets—
  25 mg (ZOLOFT/
    25 MG)...............MC-28, A7
  50 mg (ZOLOFT/
    50 MG)...............MC-28, A7
  100 mg (ZOLOFT/
    100 MG)..............MC-28, A7
**Zolpidem**..............MC-32, D7
**Zomig** Tablets—
  2.5 mg (ZOMIG 2.5)...MC-32, D6
  5 mg (ZOMIG 5).......MC-32, D6
**Zovirax** Capsules—
  200 mg (Logo Wellcome/
    ZOVIRAX 200).........MC-1, B7
**Zovirax** Tablets—
  400 mg (Logo/
    ZOVIRAX).............MC-1, C1
  800 mg (ZOVIRAX
    800).................MC-1, C1
**Zyban** Extended-release Tablets—
  150 mg (ZYBAN 150)....MC-4, C1
**Zydone** Capsules—
  5/500 mg (DUPONT
    ZYDONE)..............MC-14, C6
**Zyflo** Tablets—
  600 mg (Logo ZL)......MC-32, D5
**Zyloprim** Tablets—
  100 mg (ZYLOPRIM
    100).................MC-1, C7
  300 mg (ZYLOPRIM
    300).................MC-1, C7
**Zyprexa** Tablets—
  2.5 mg (LILLY 4112)..MC-23, C1
  5 mg (LILLY 4115)....MC-23, C1
  7.5 mg (LILLY 4116)..MC-23, C2
  10 mg (LILLY 4117)...MC-23, C2
**Zyrtec** Tablets—
  5 mg (PFIZER/550)....MC-6, C4
  10 mg (PFIZER/551)...MC-6, C4

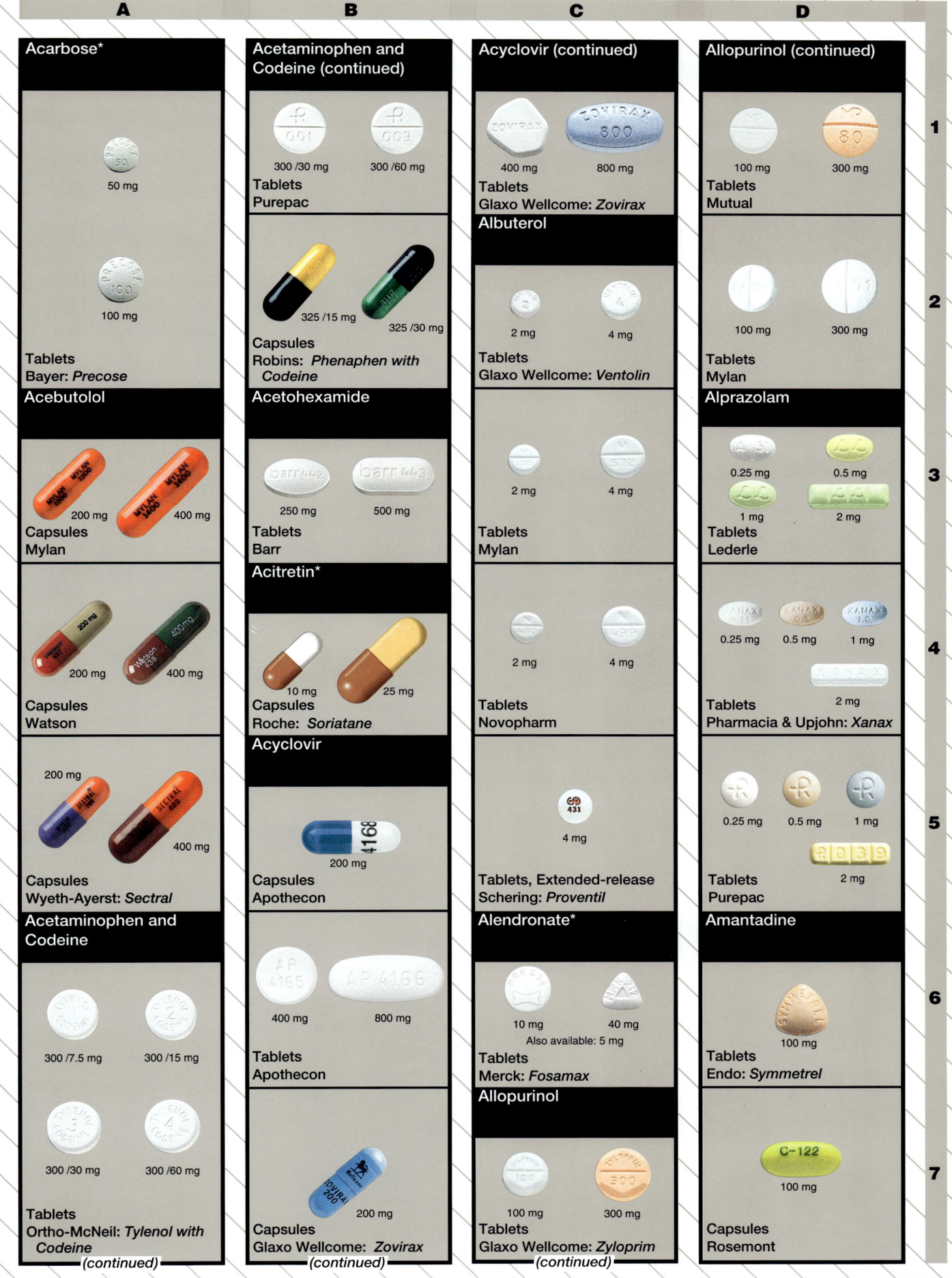

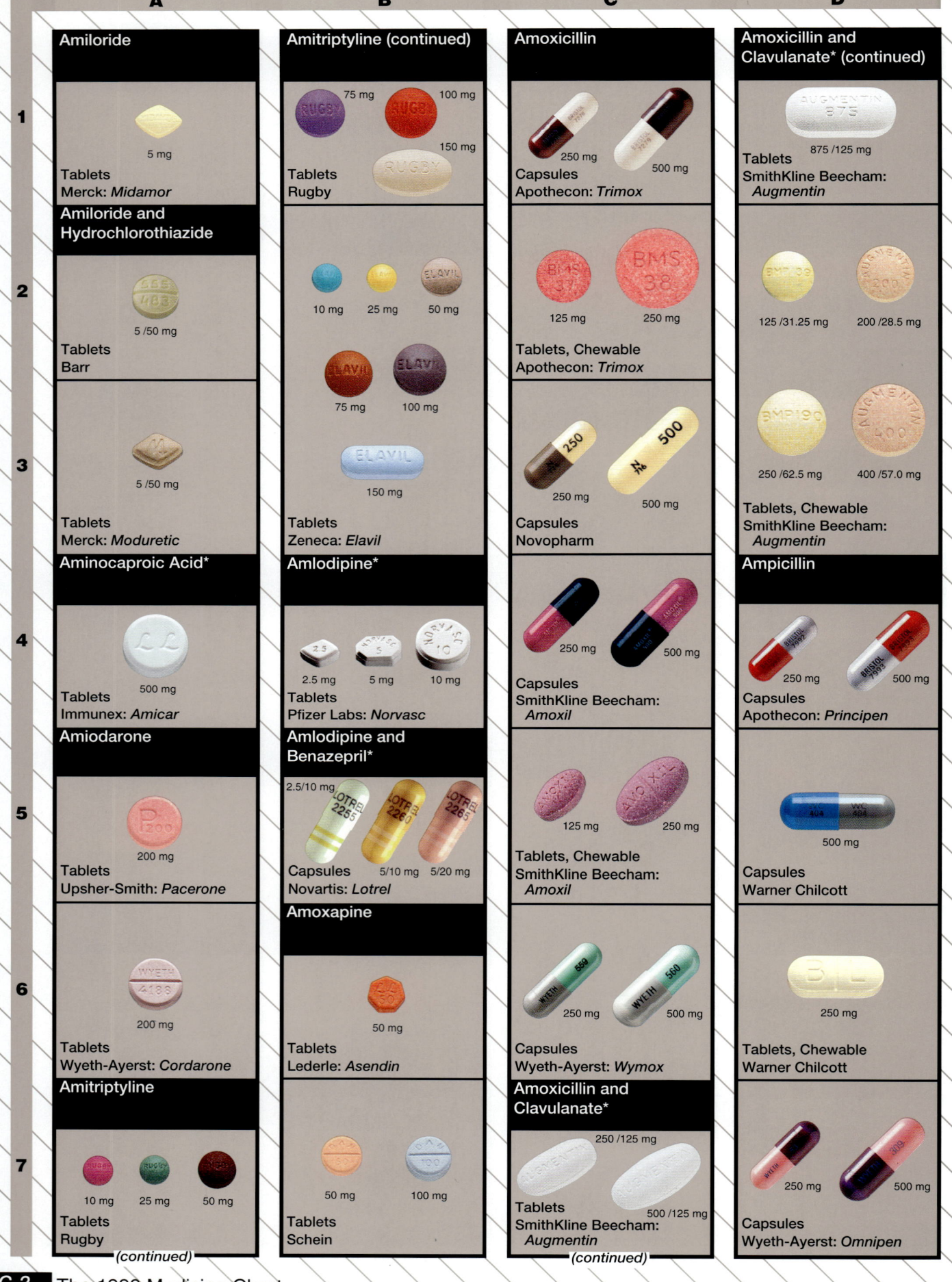

The 1999 Medicine Chart
© 1998 Micromedex, Inc.

*Single source product for solid oral dosage forms in the U.S.

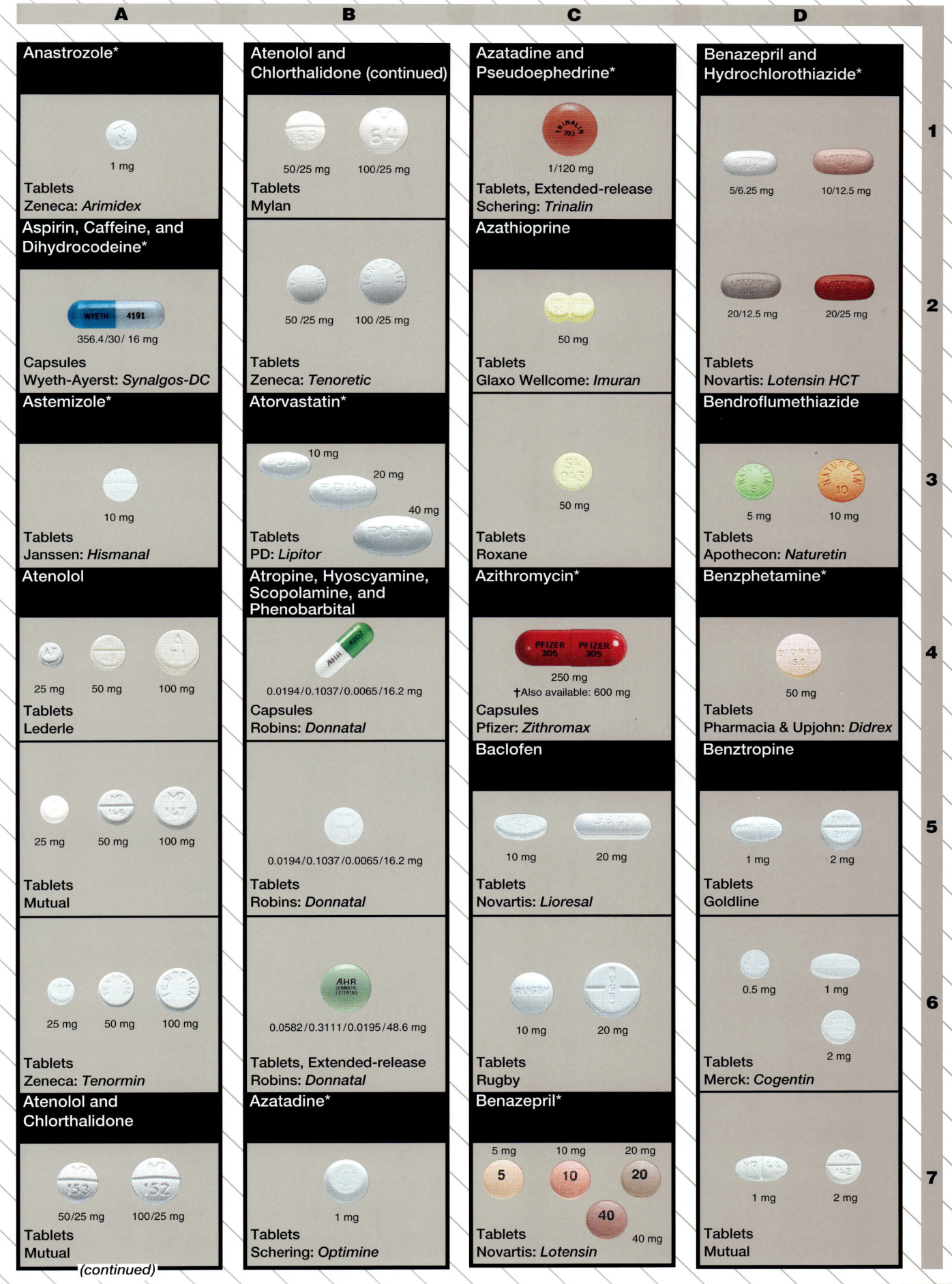

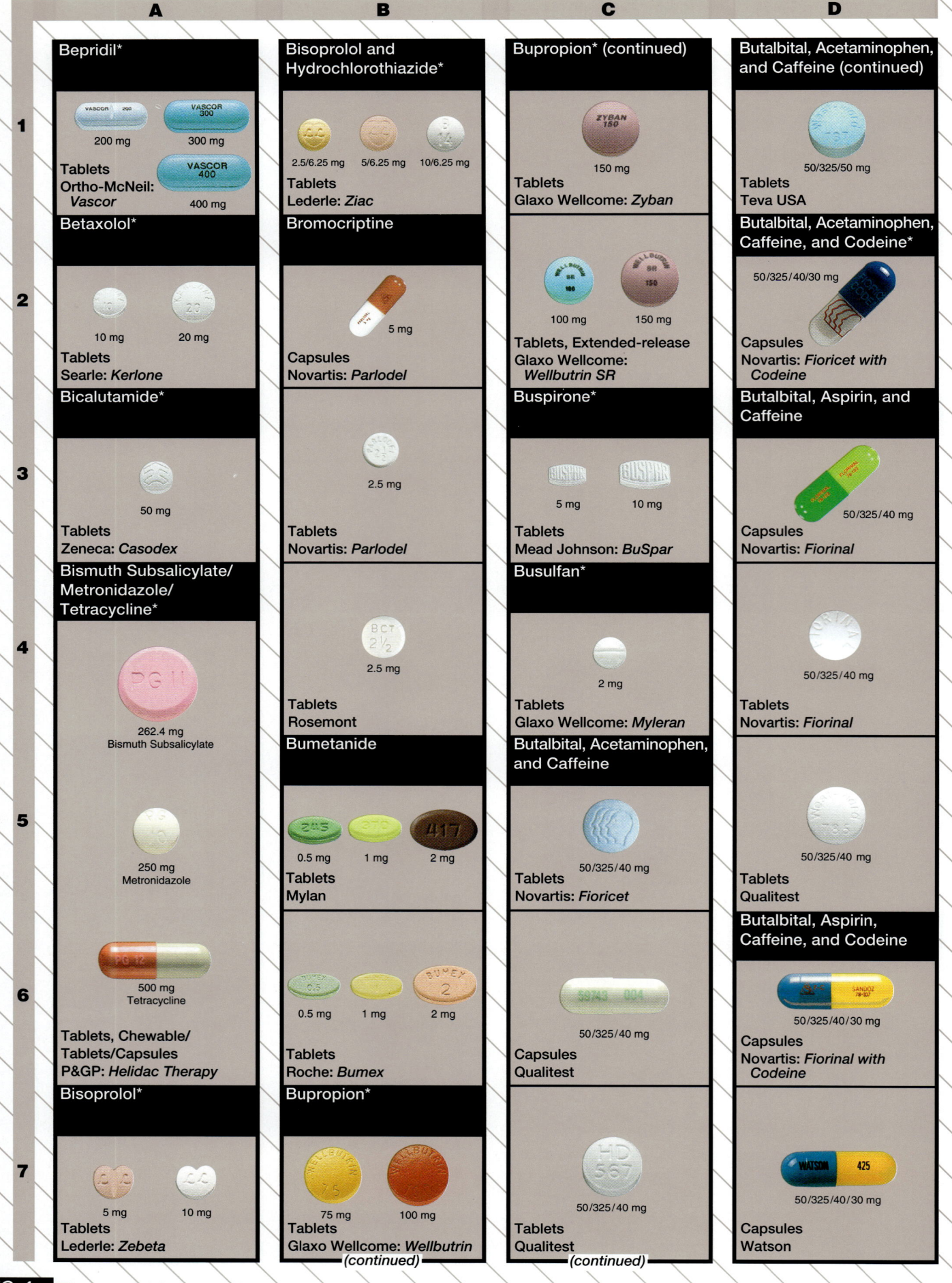

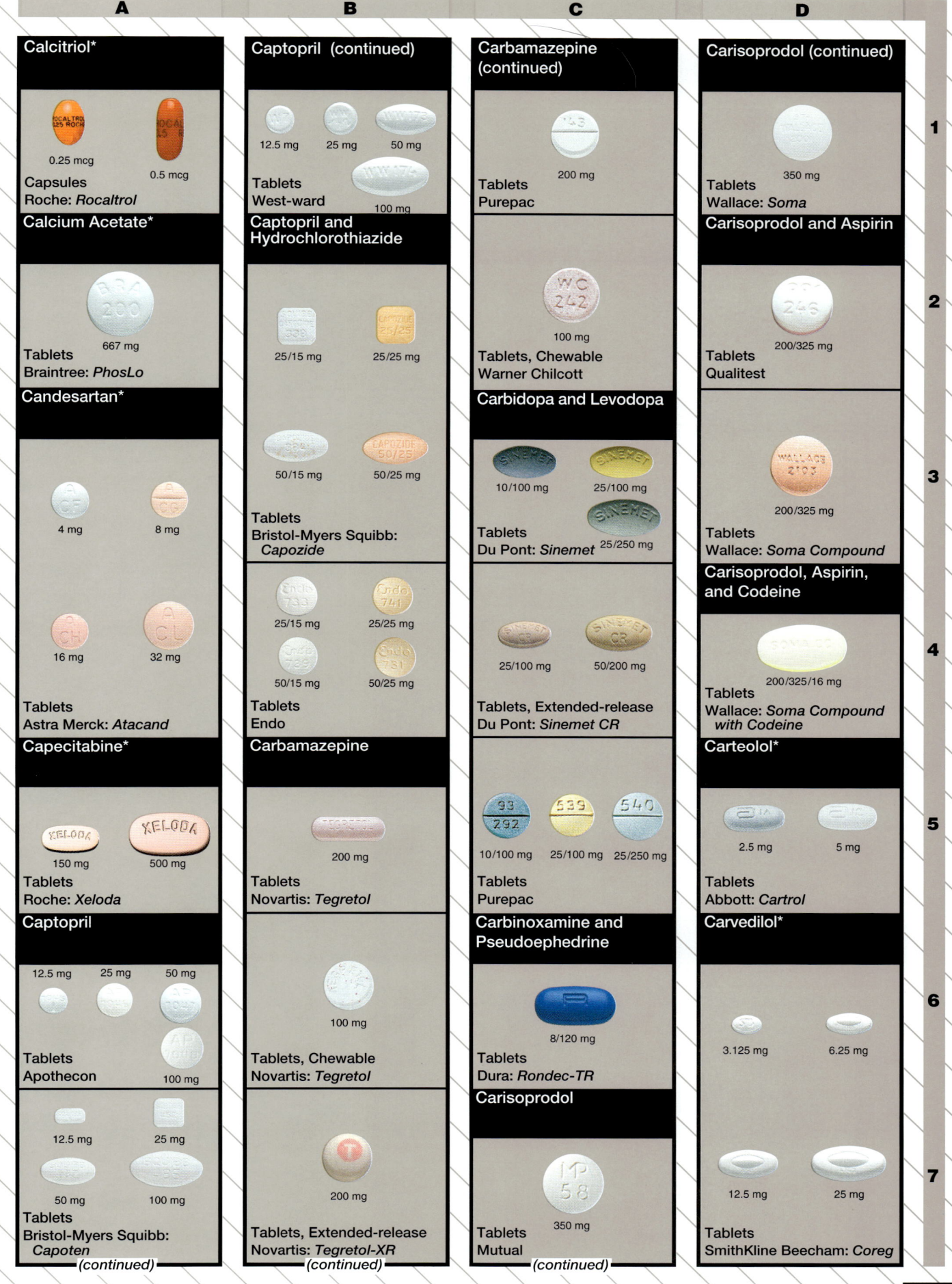

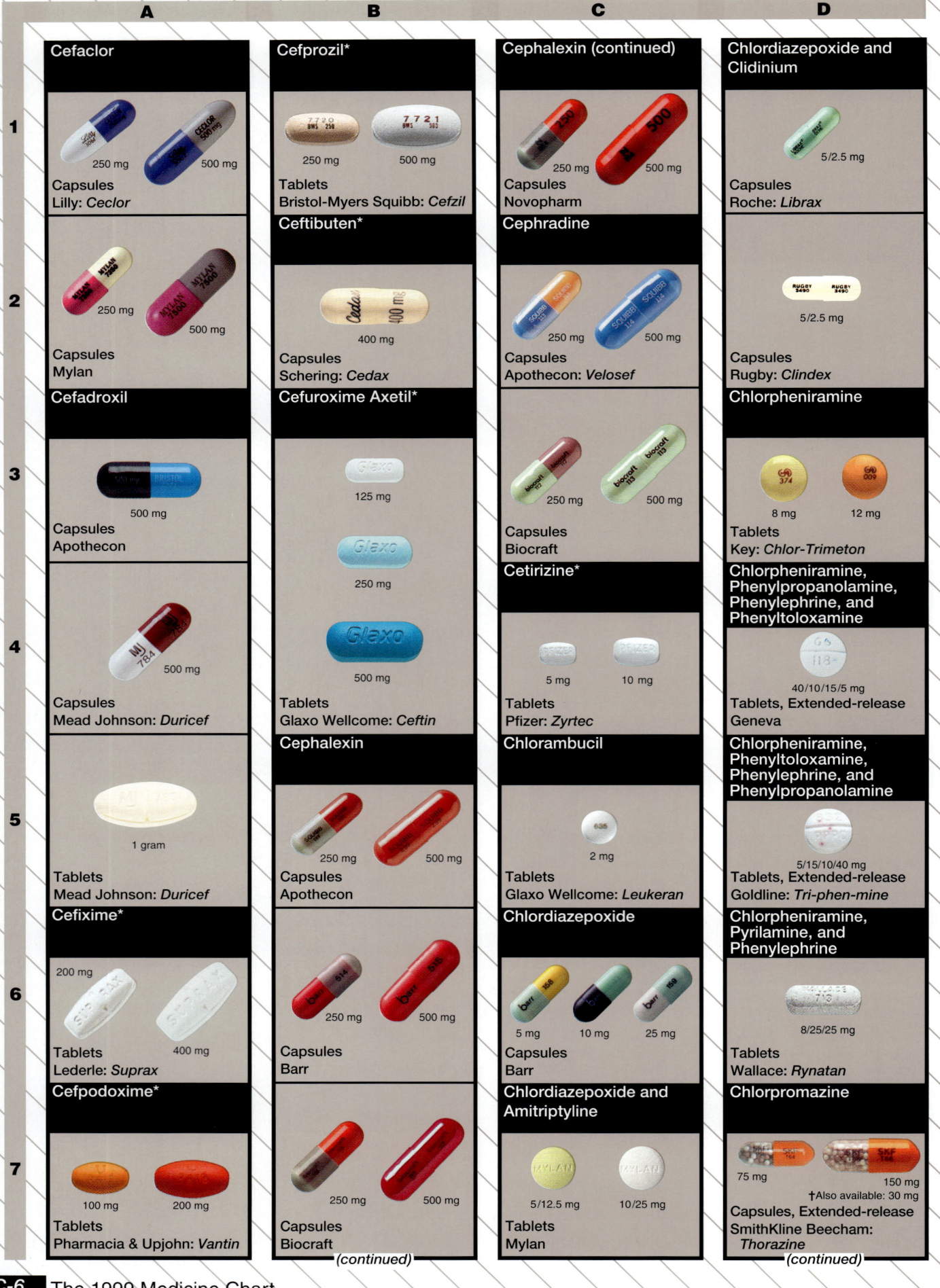

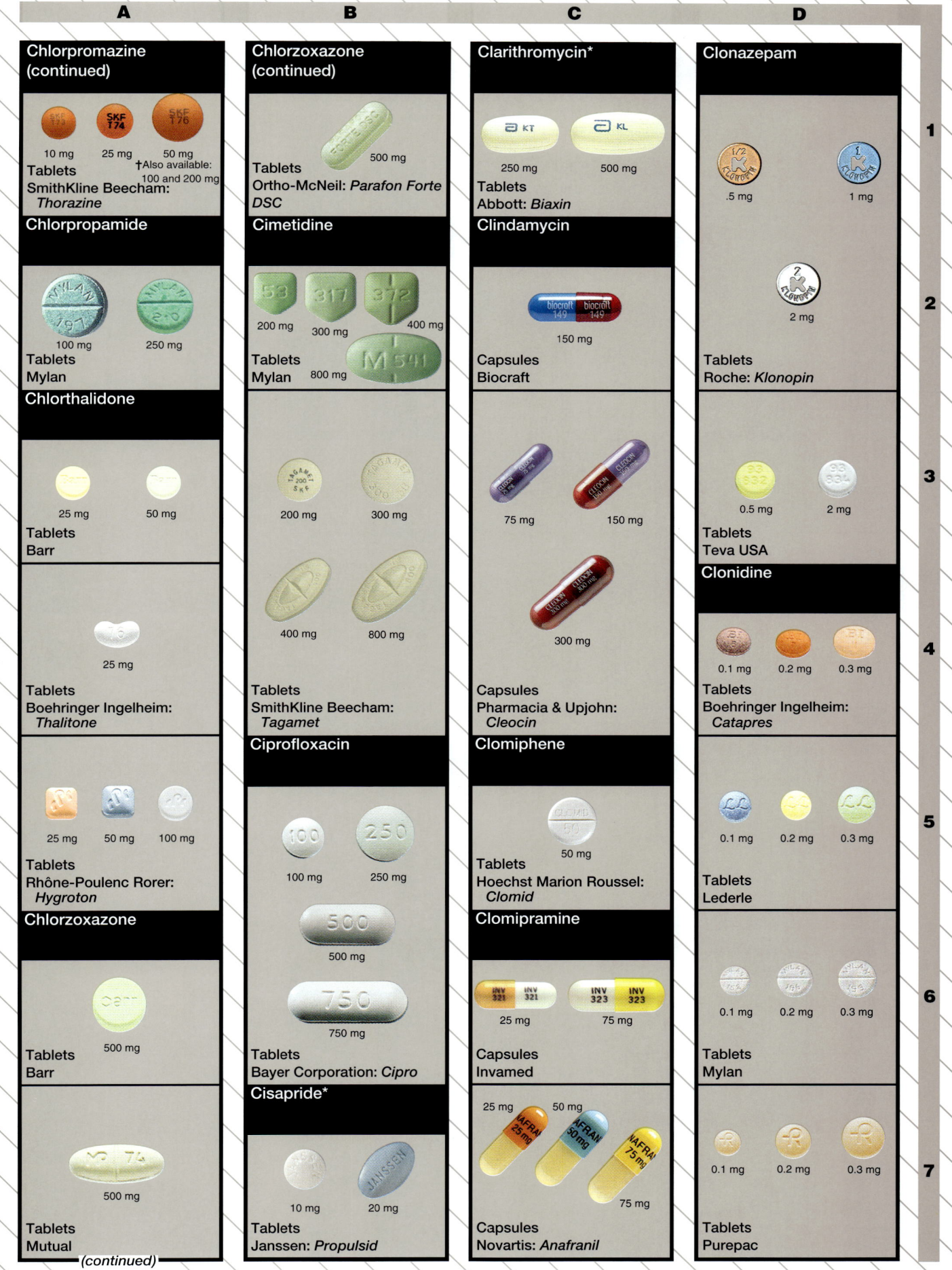

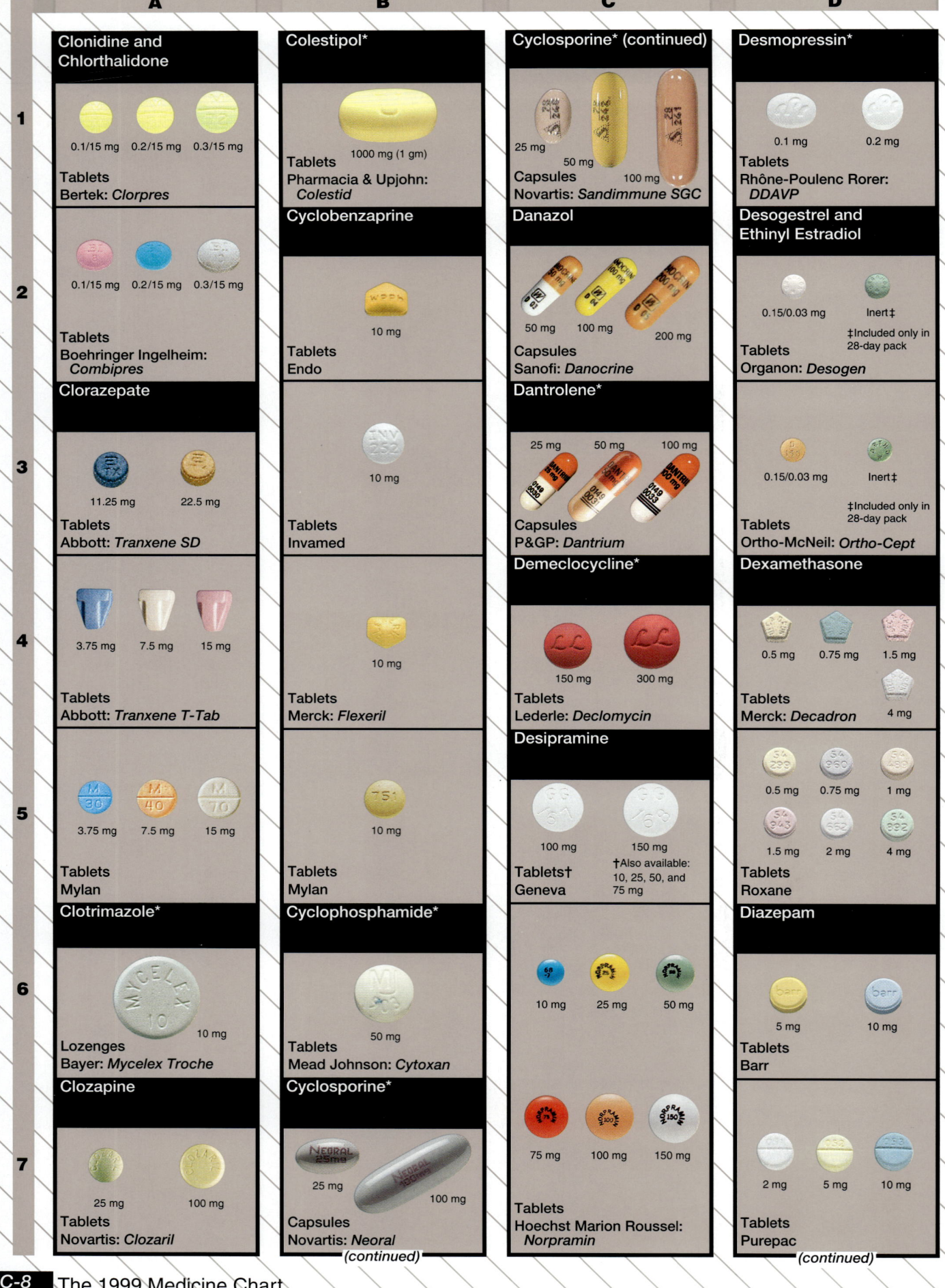

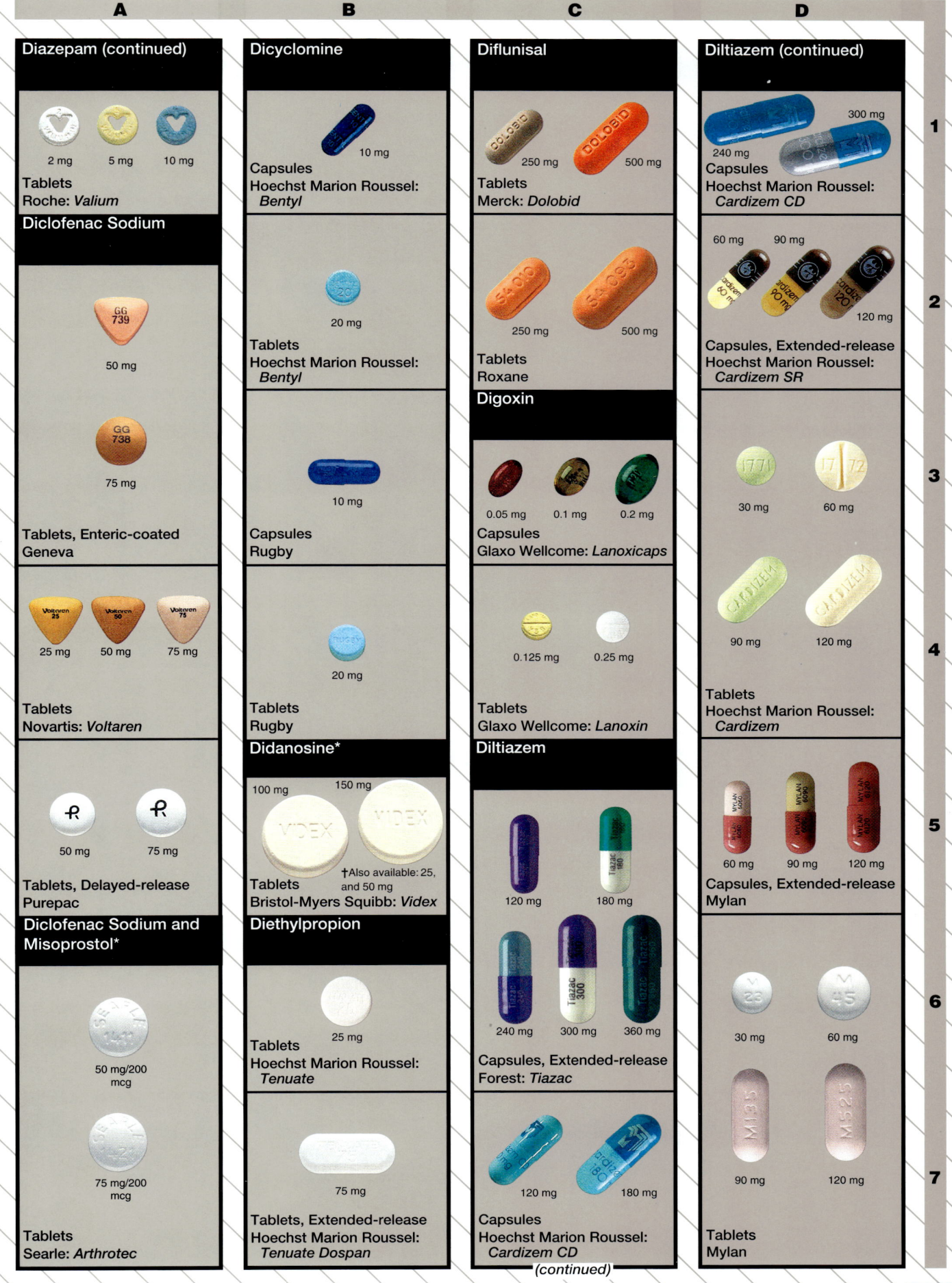

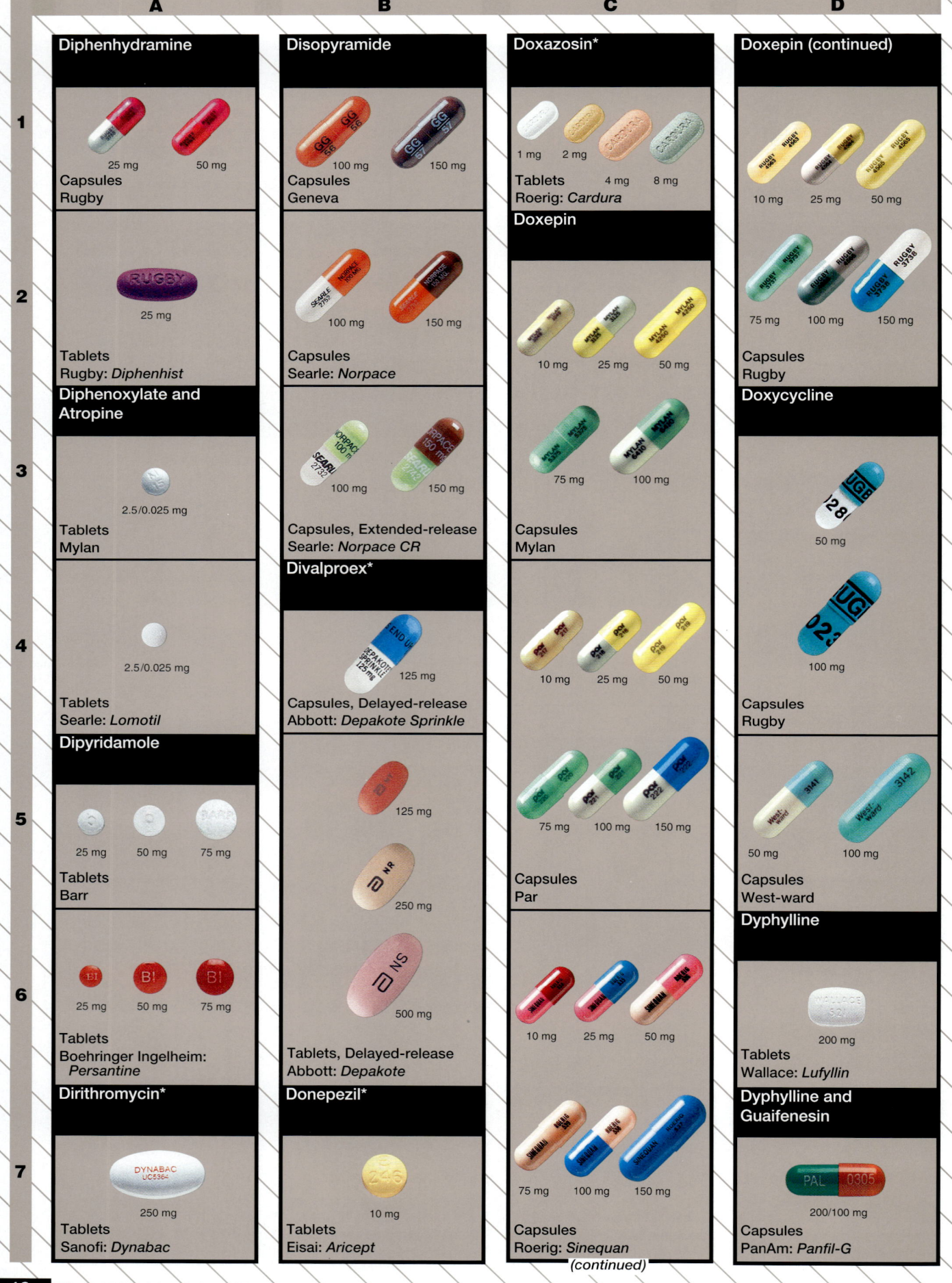

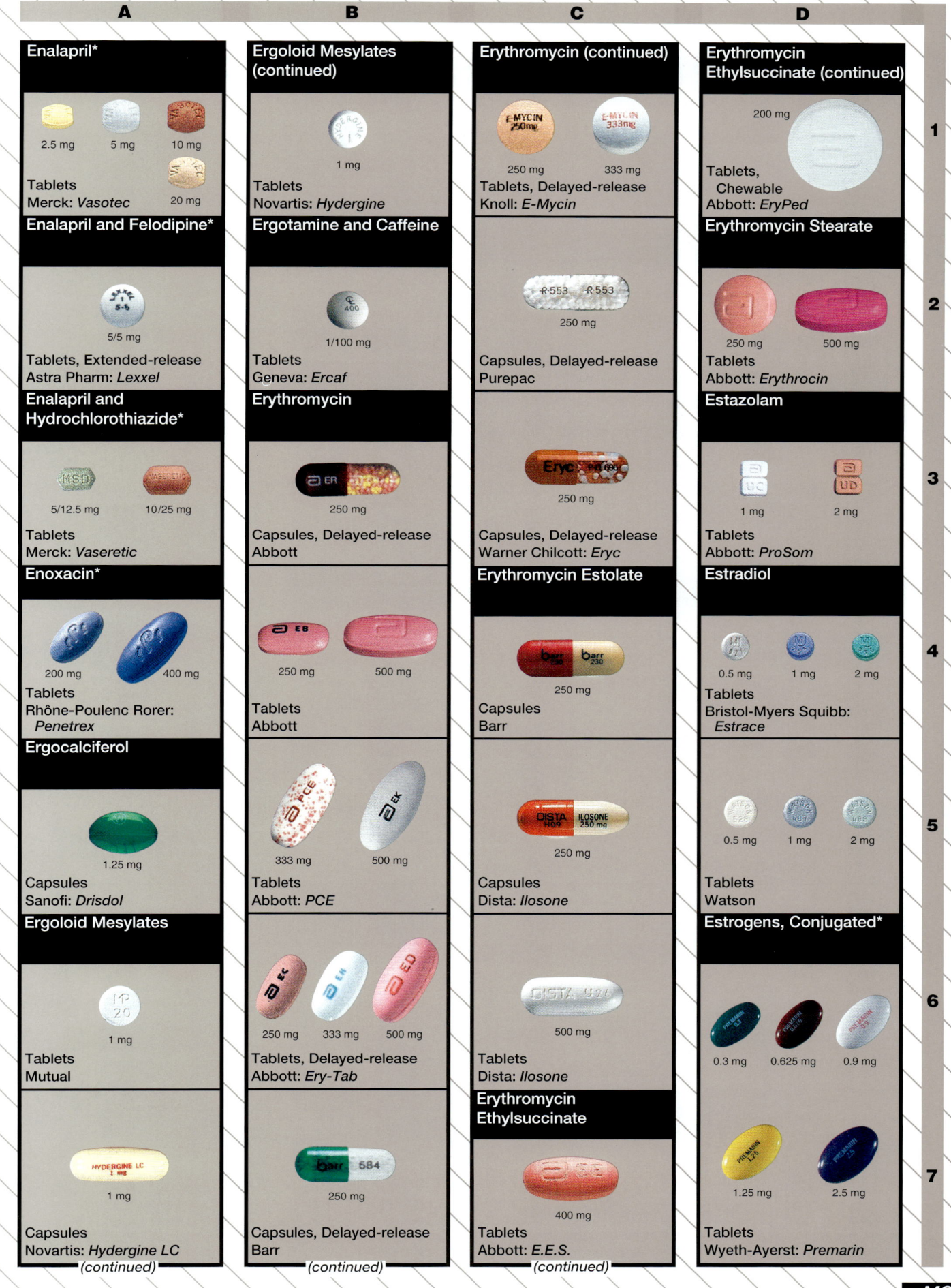

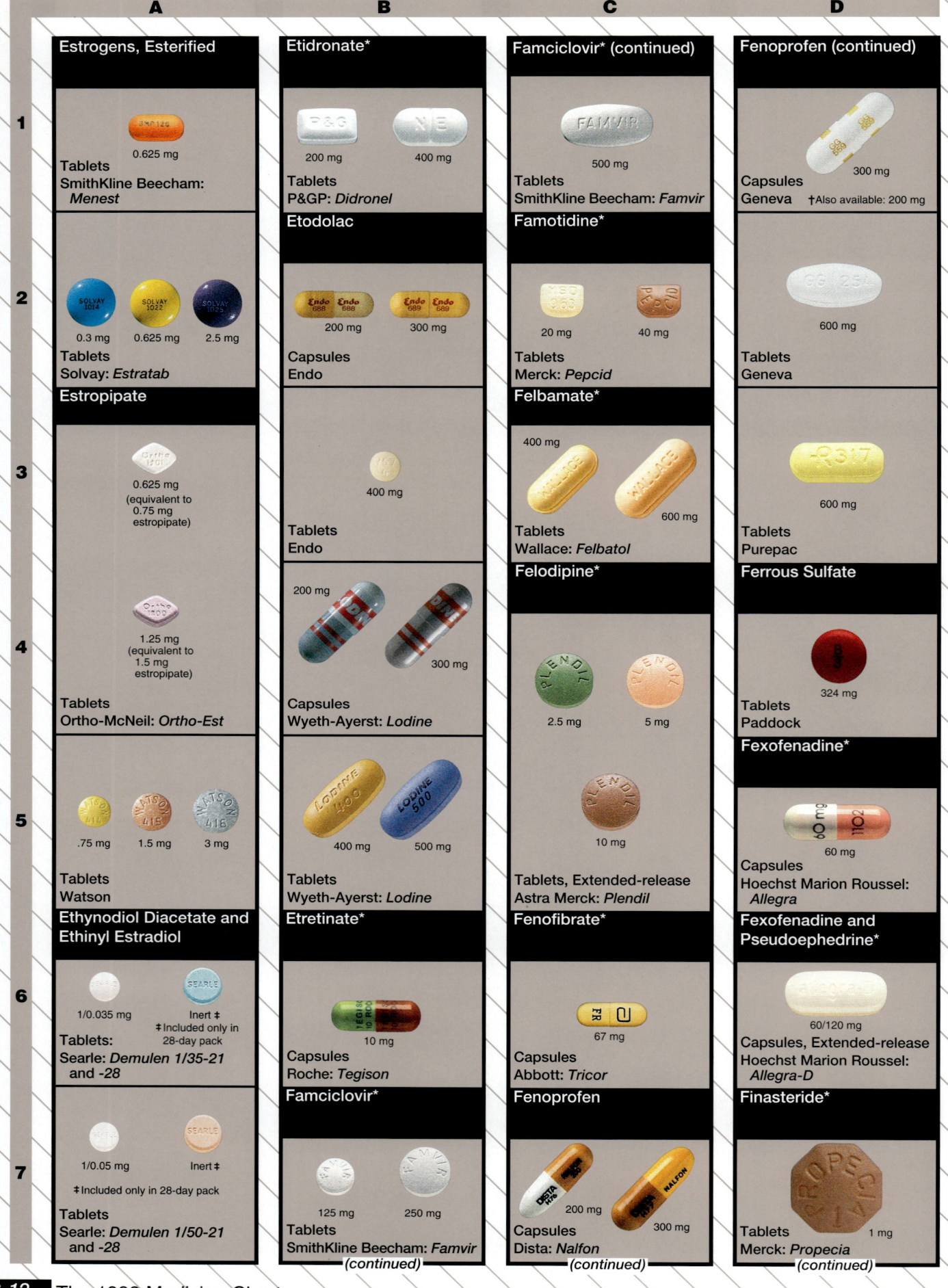

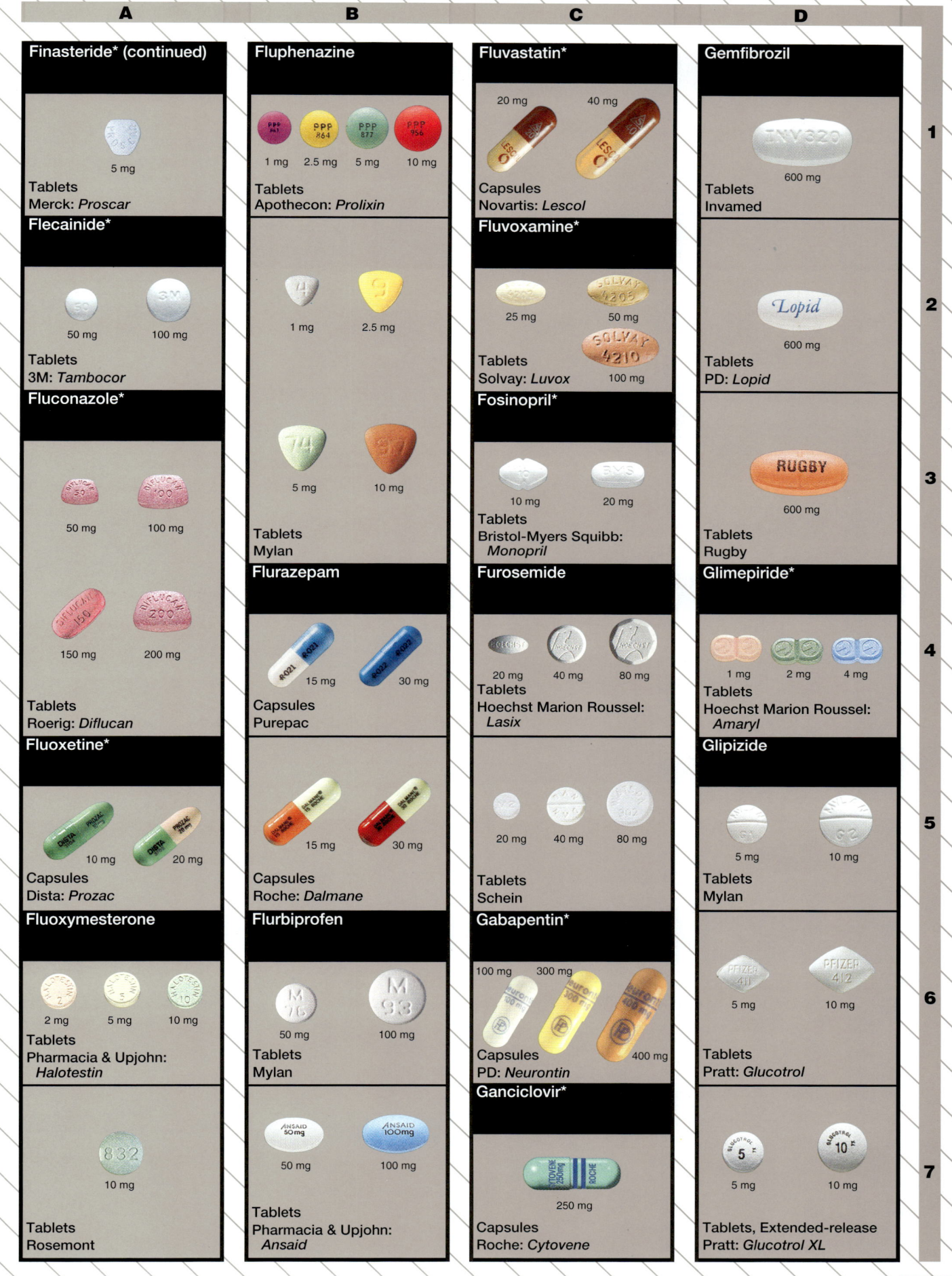

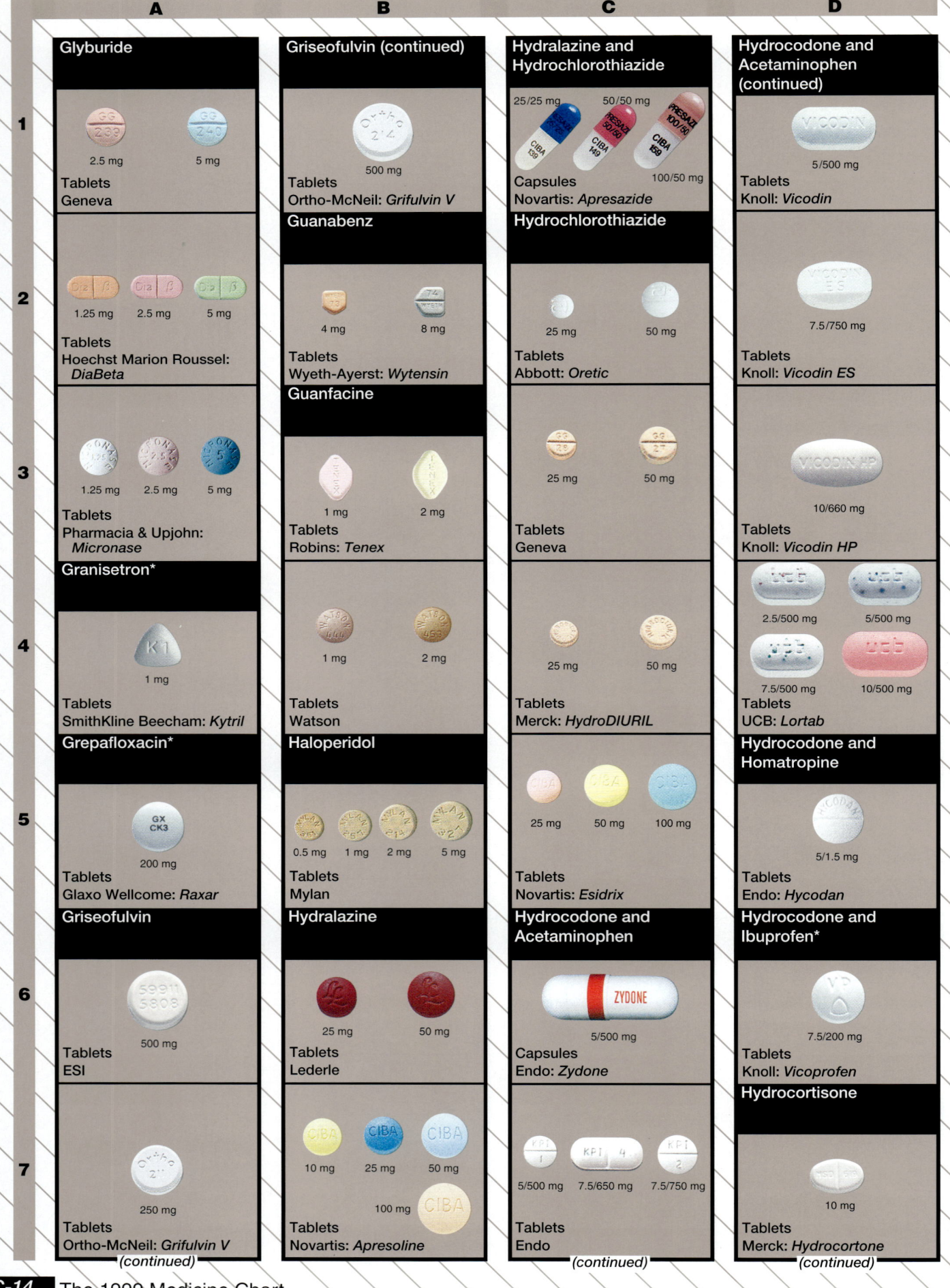

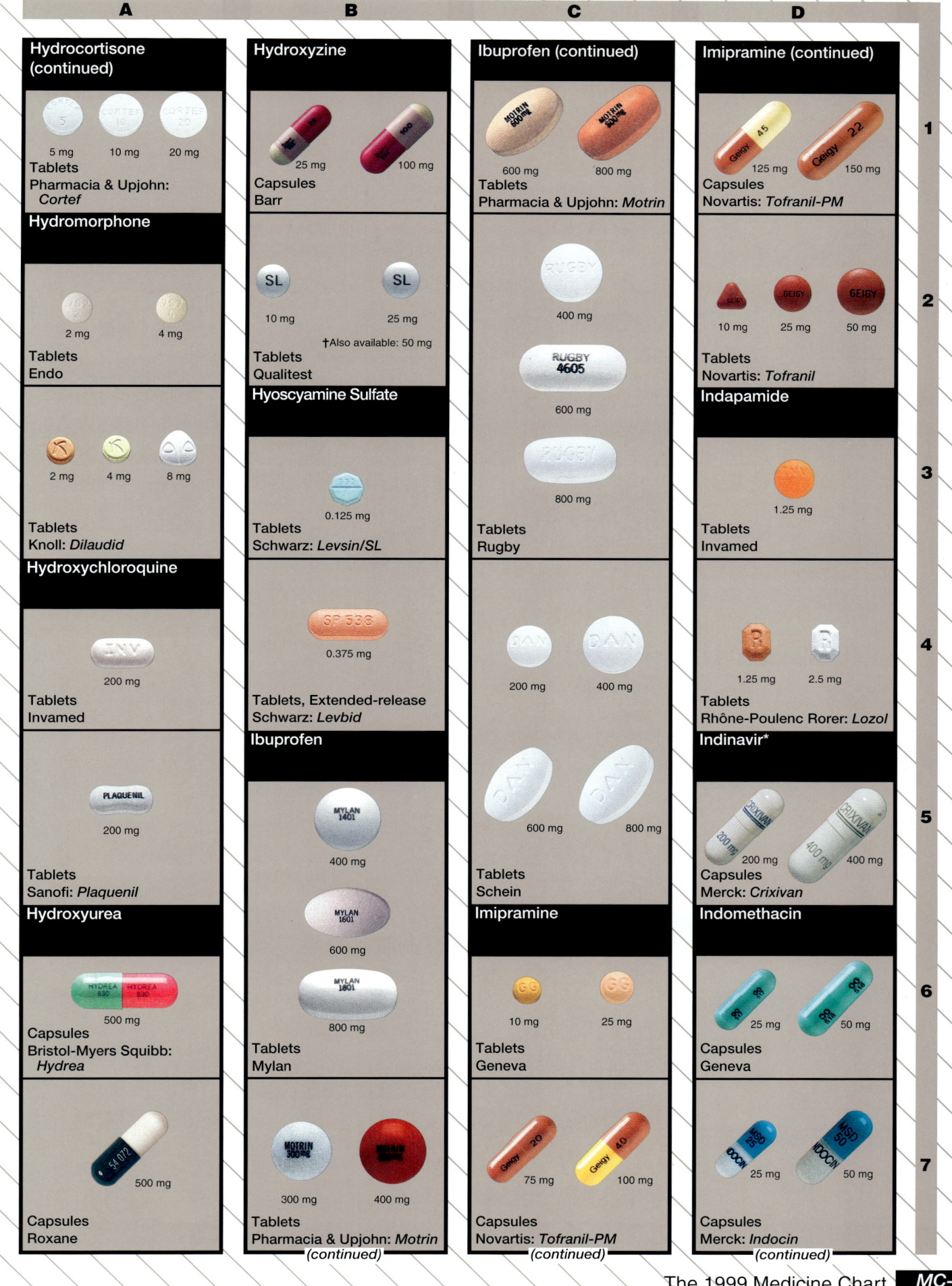

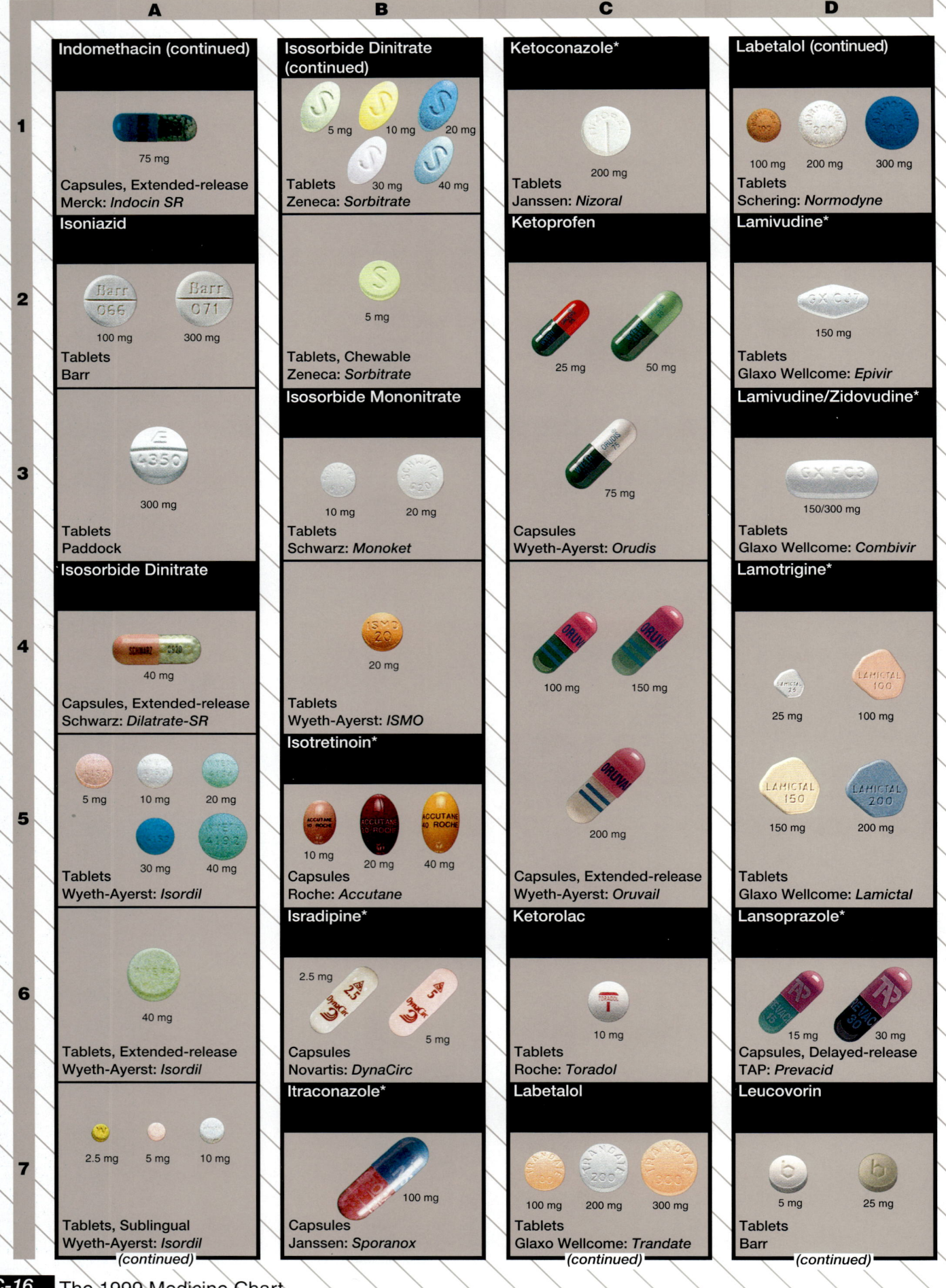

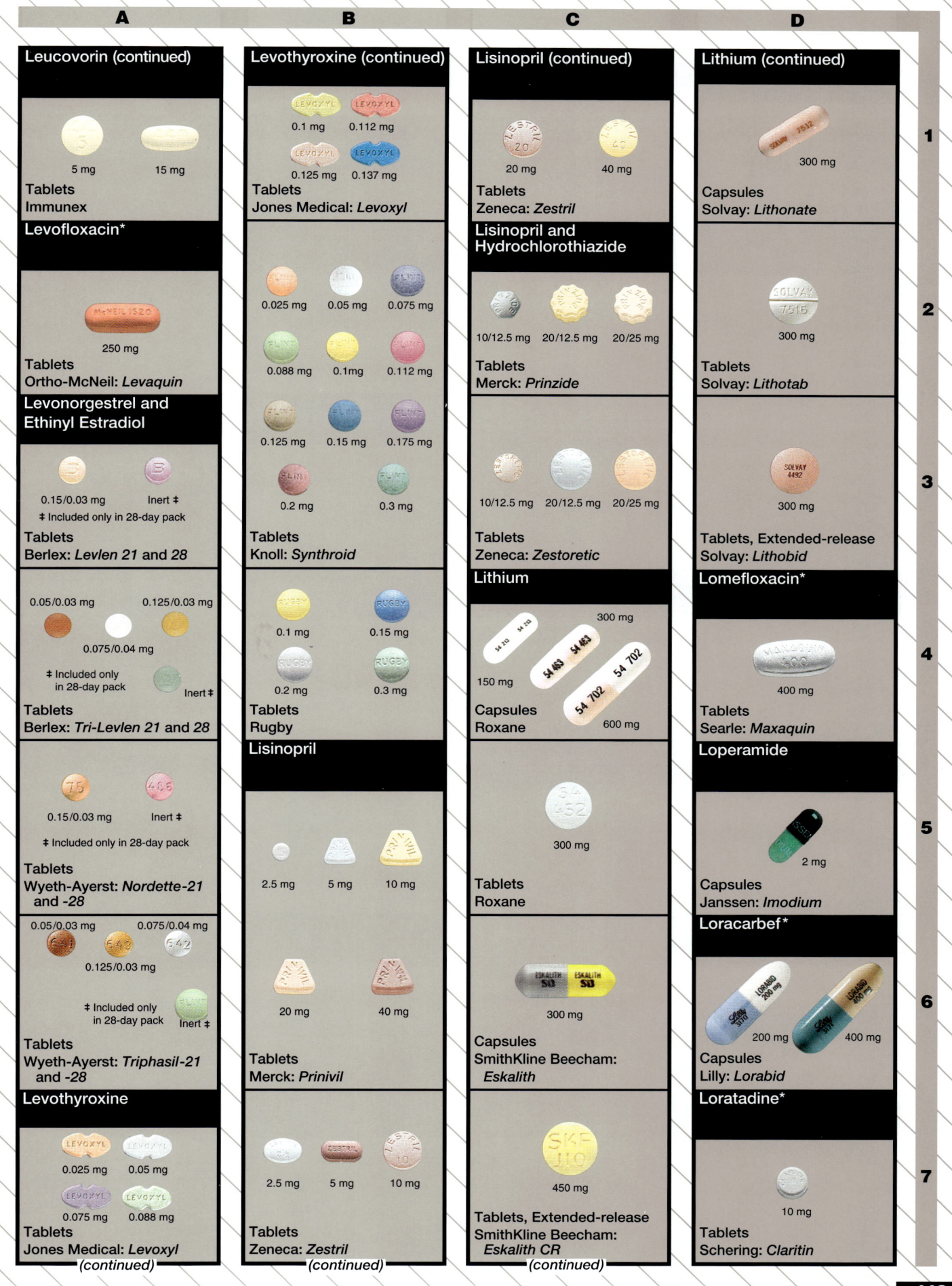

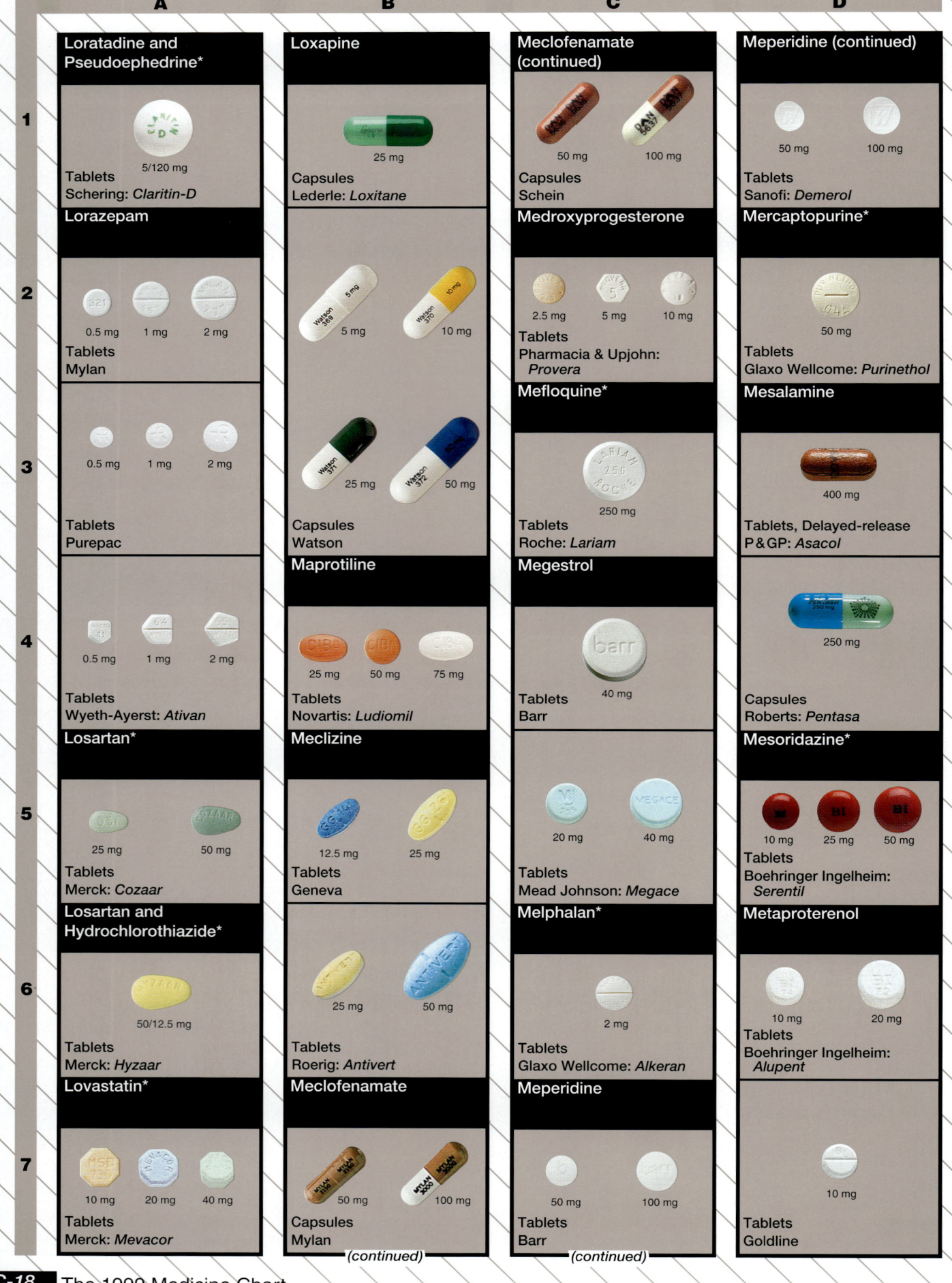

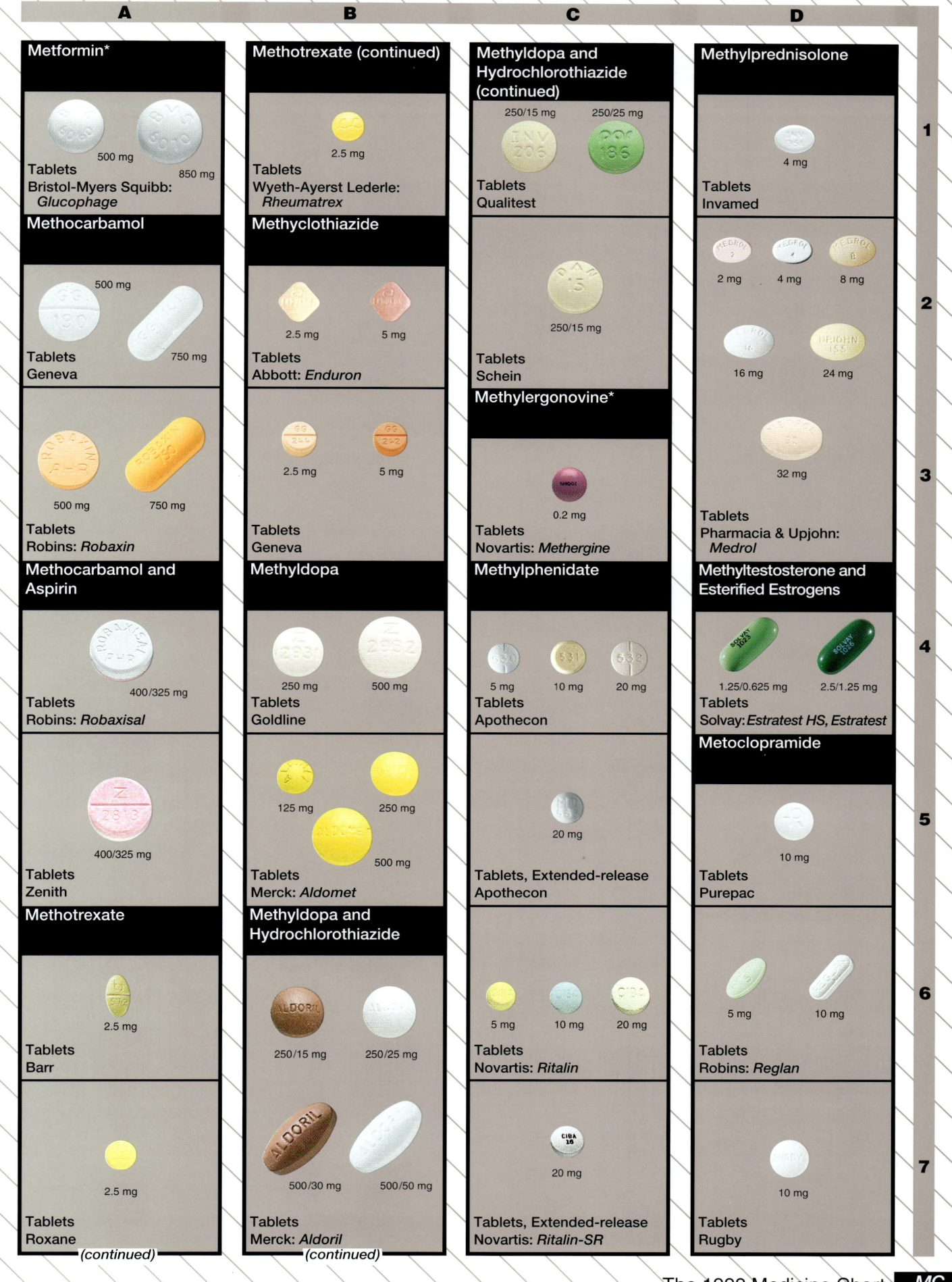

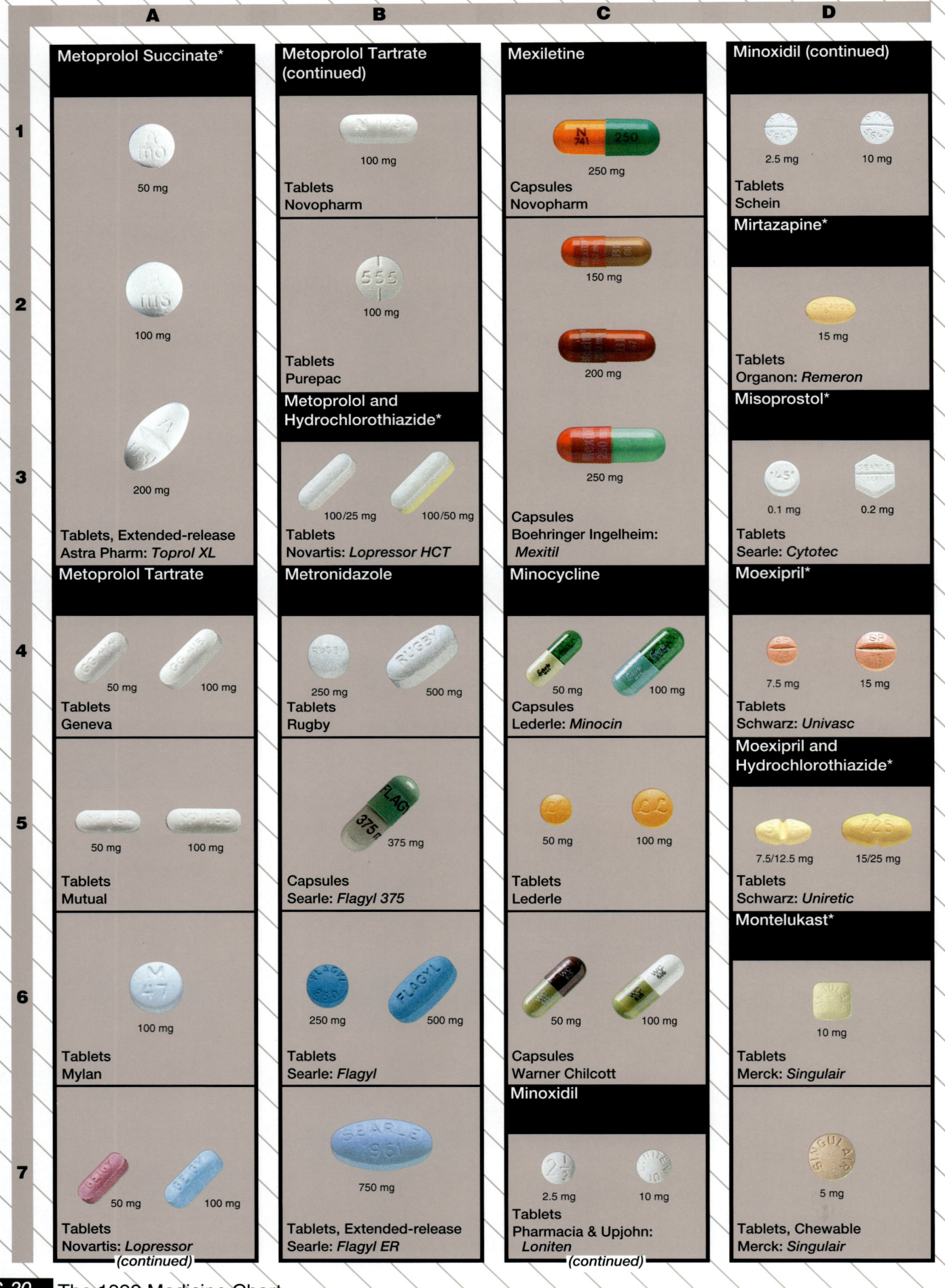

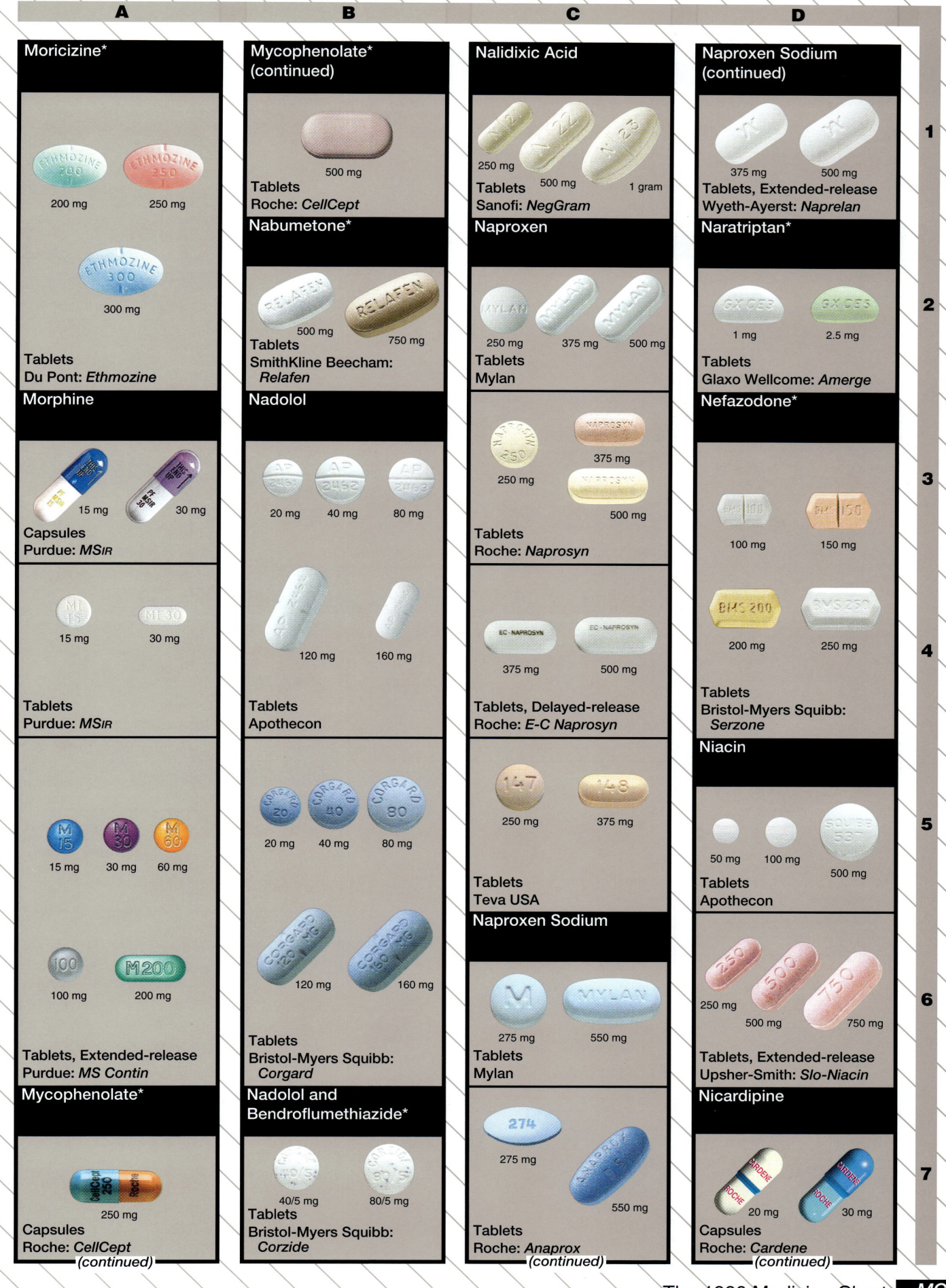

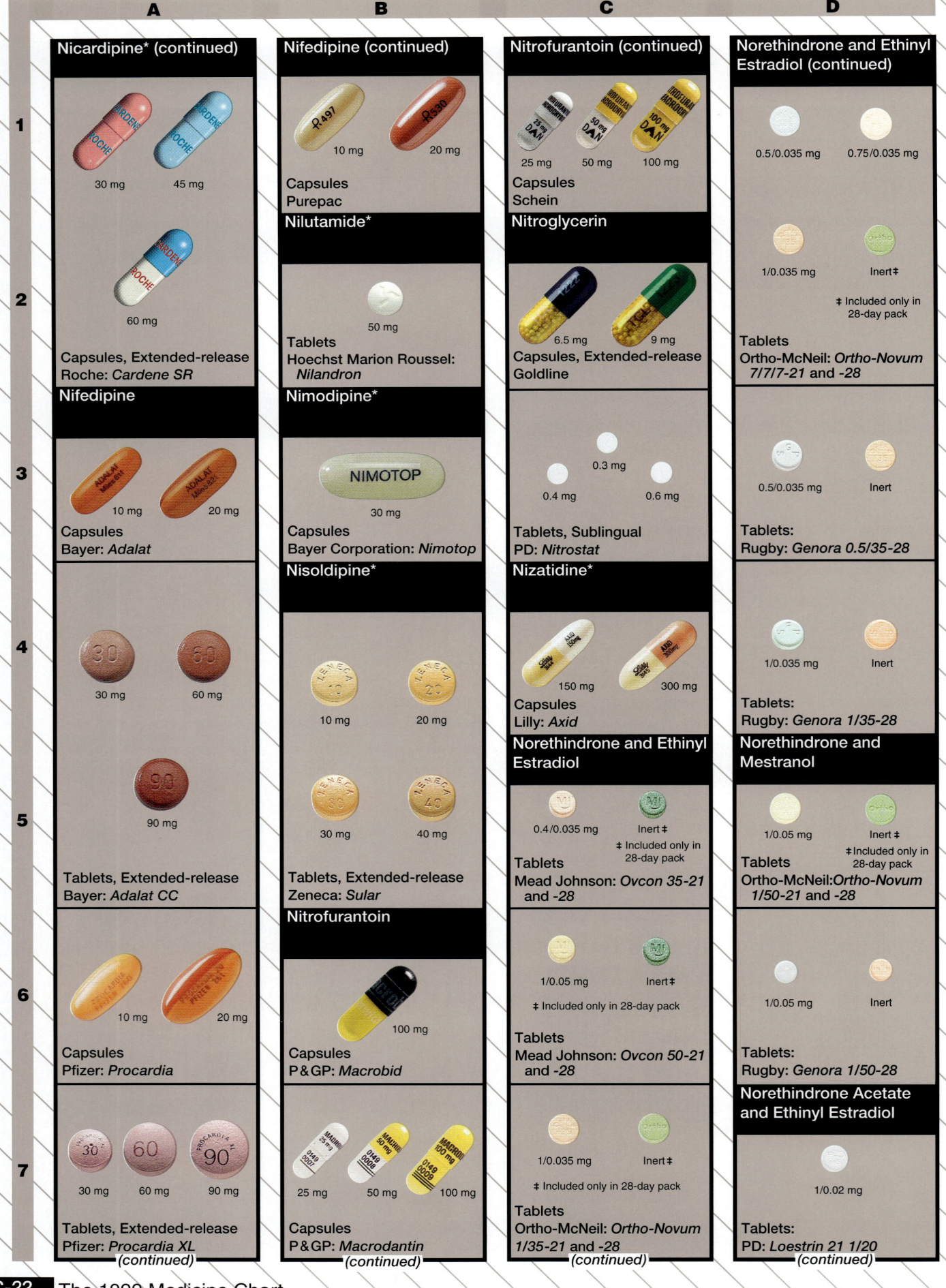

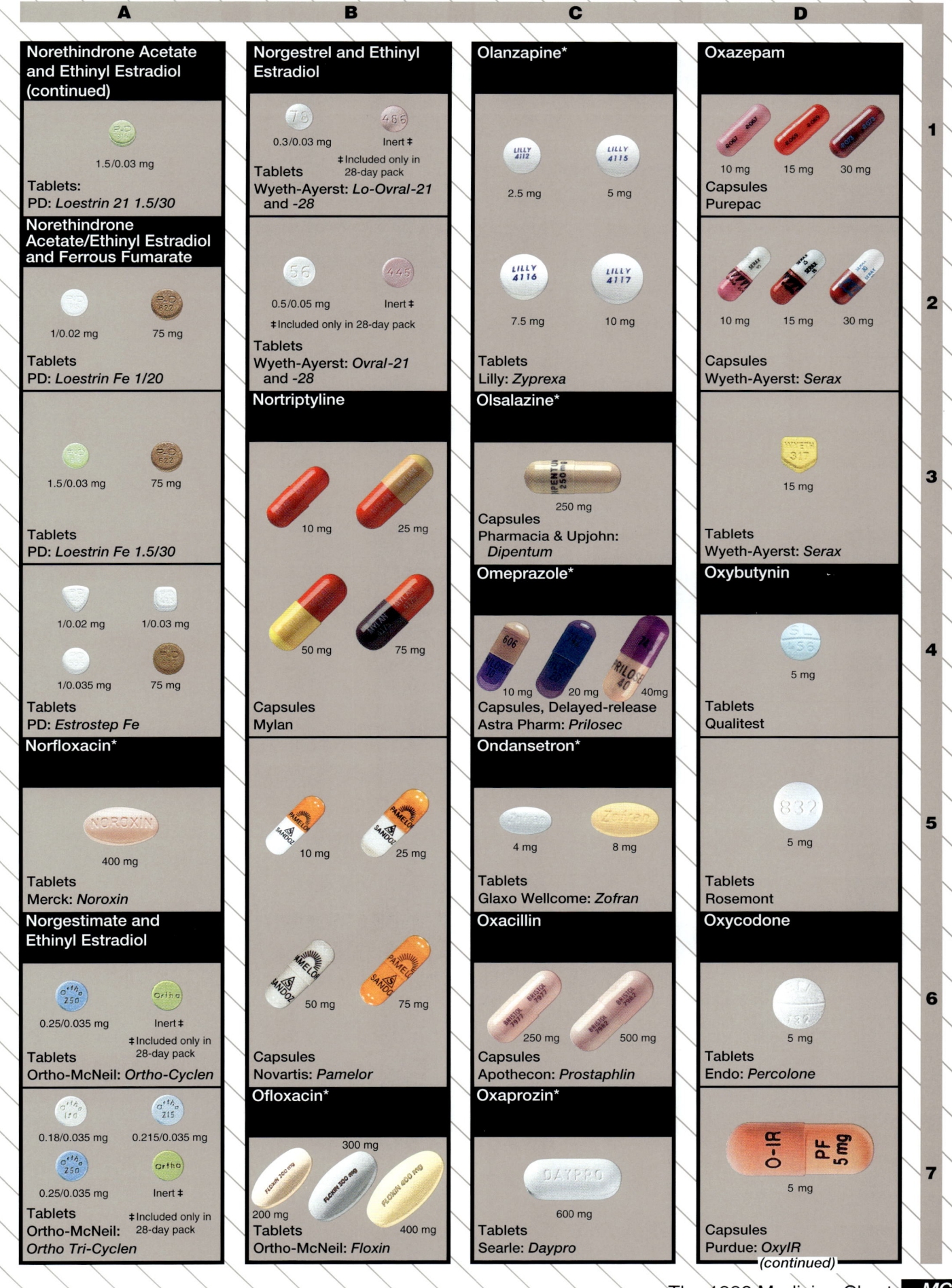

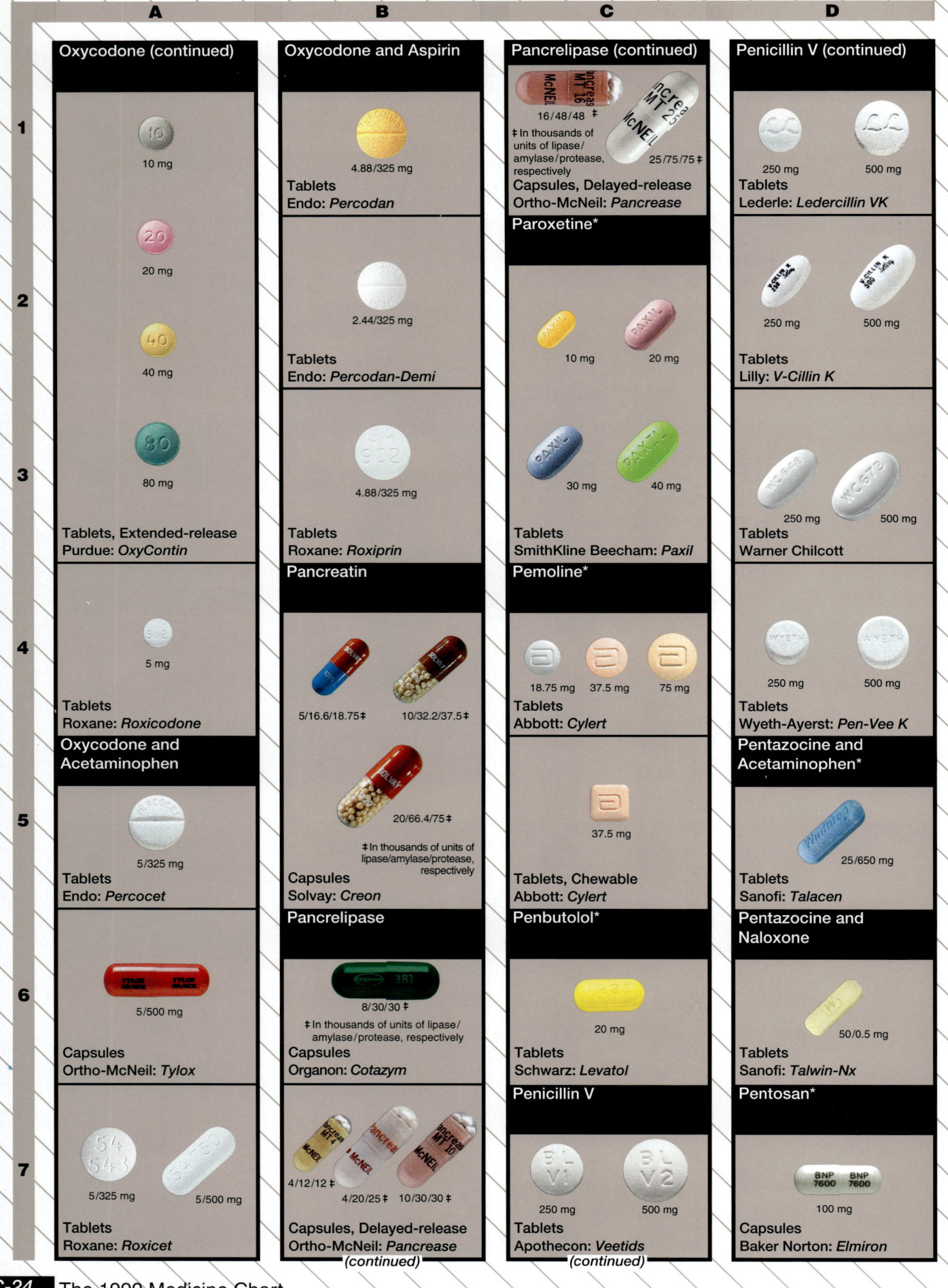

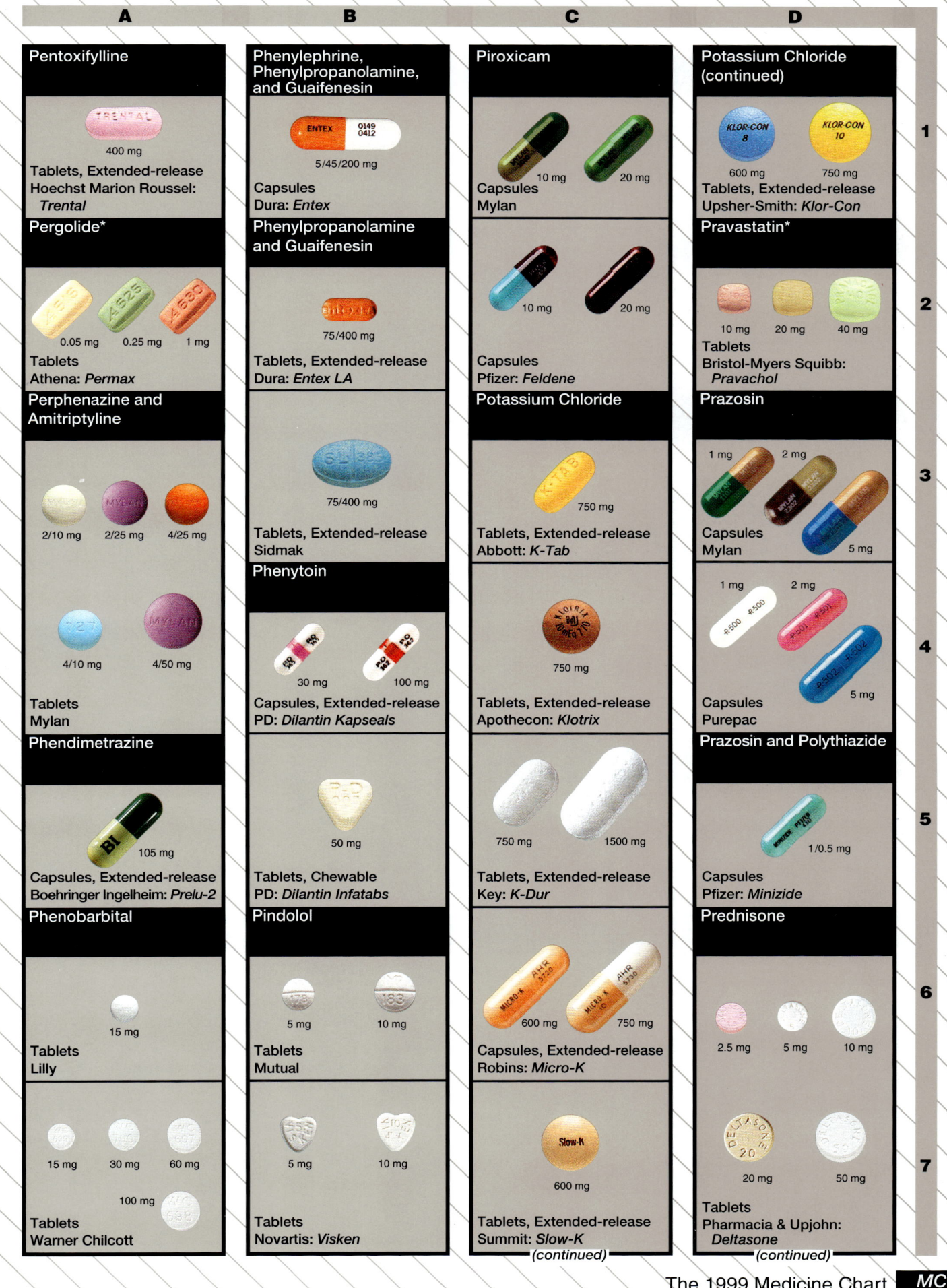

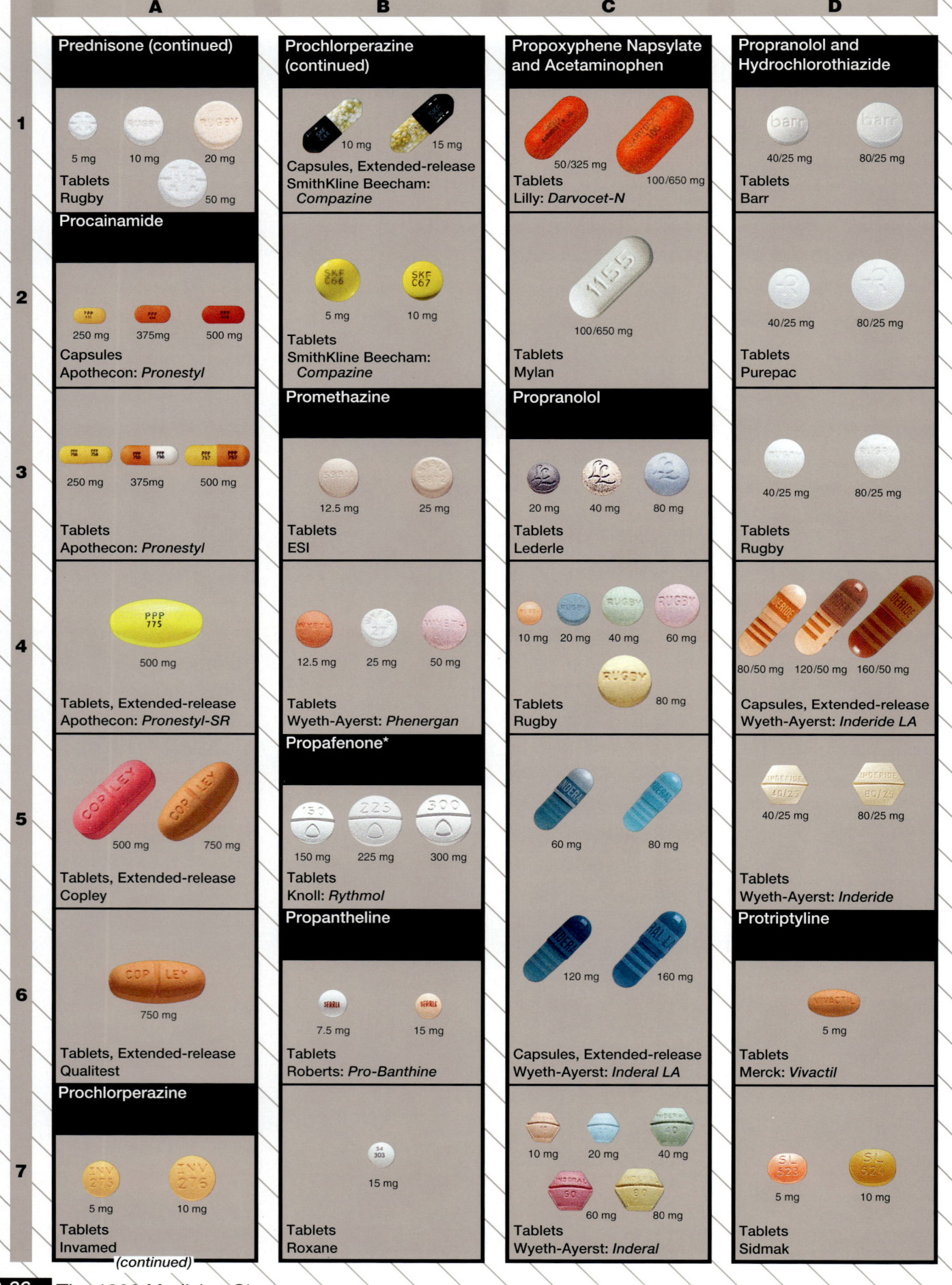

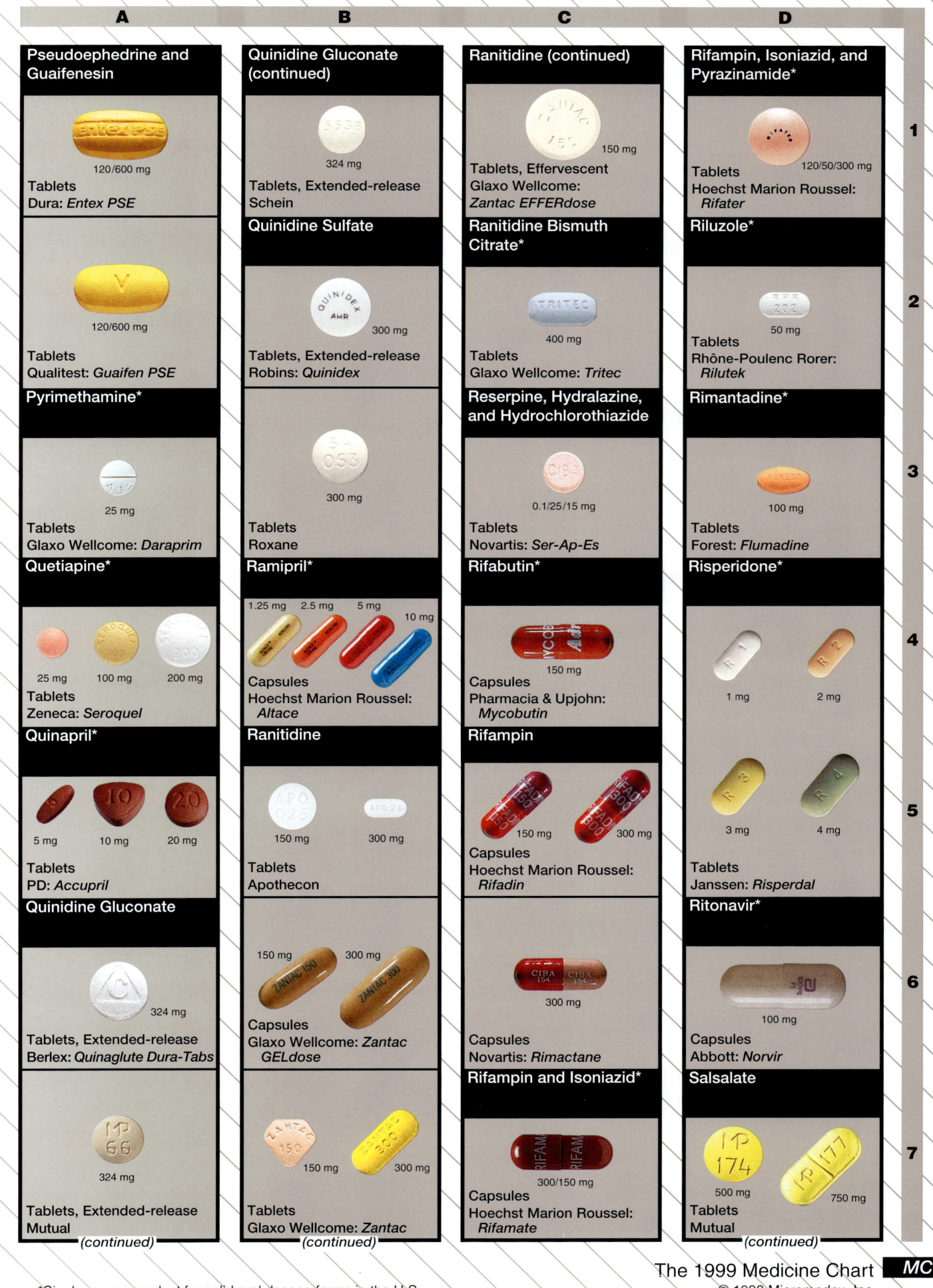

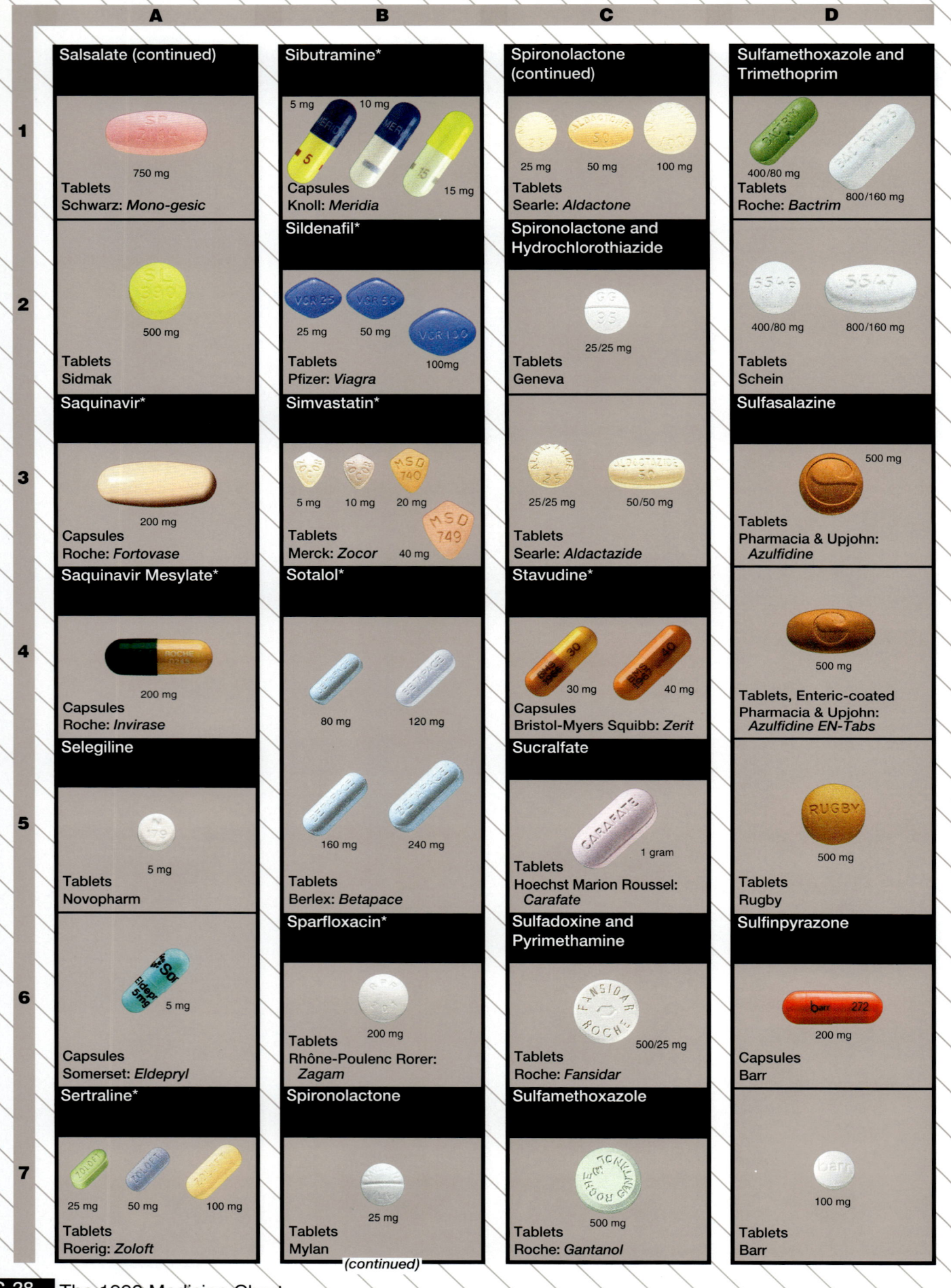

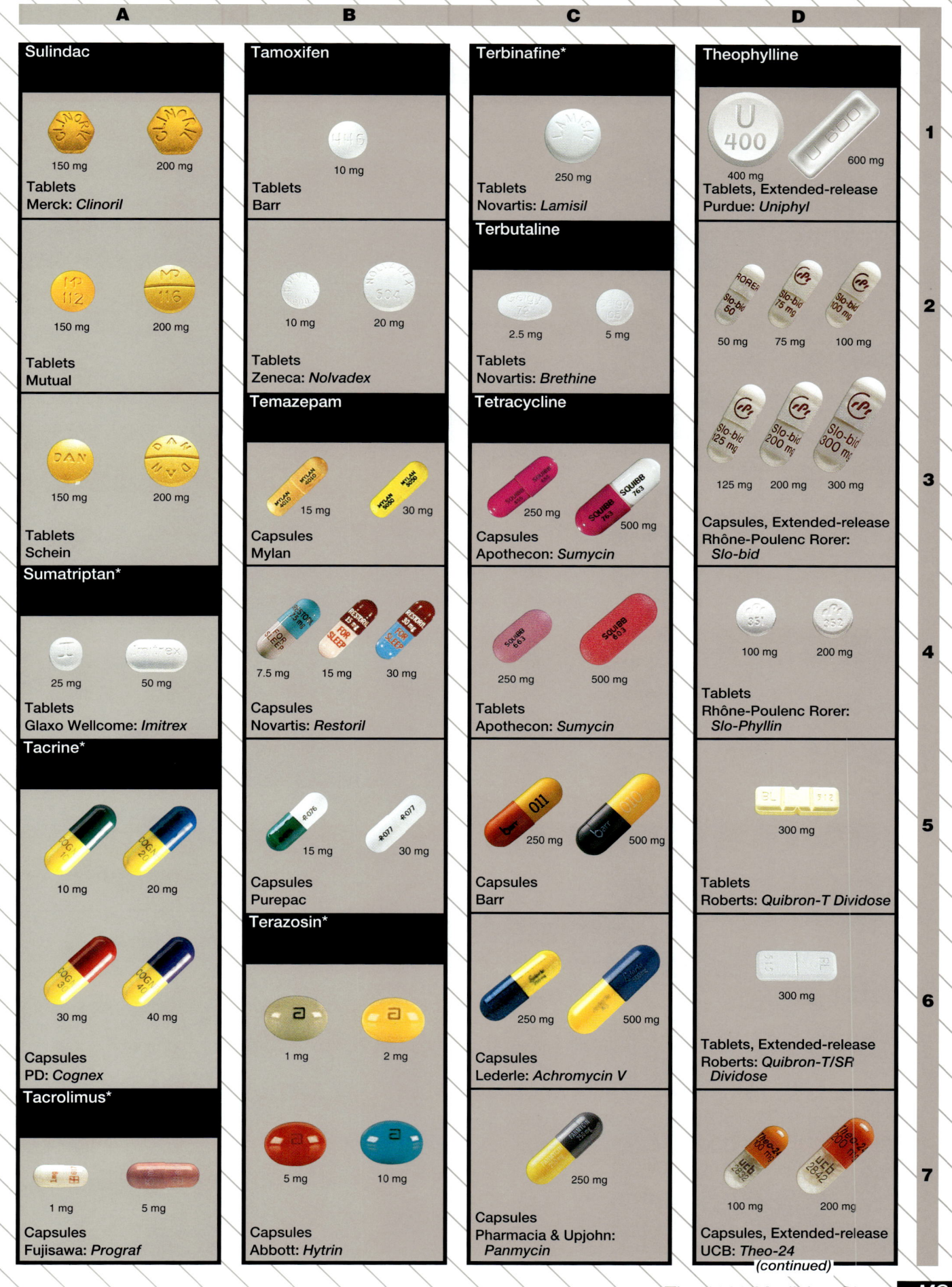

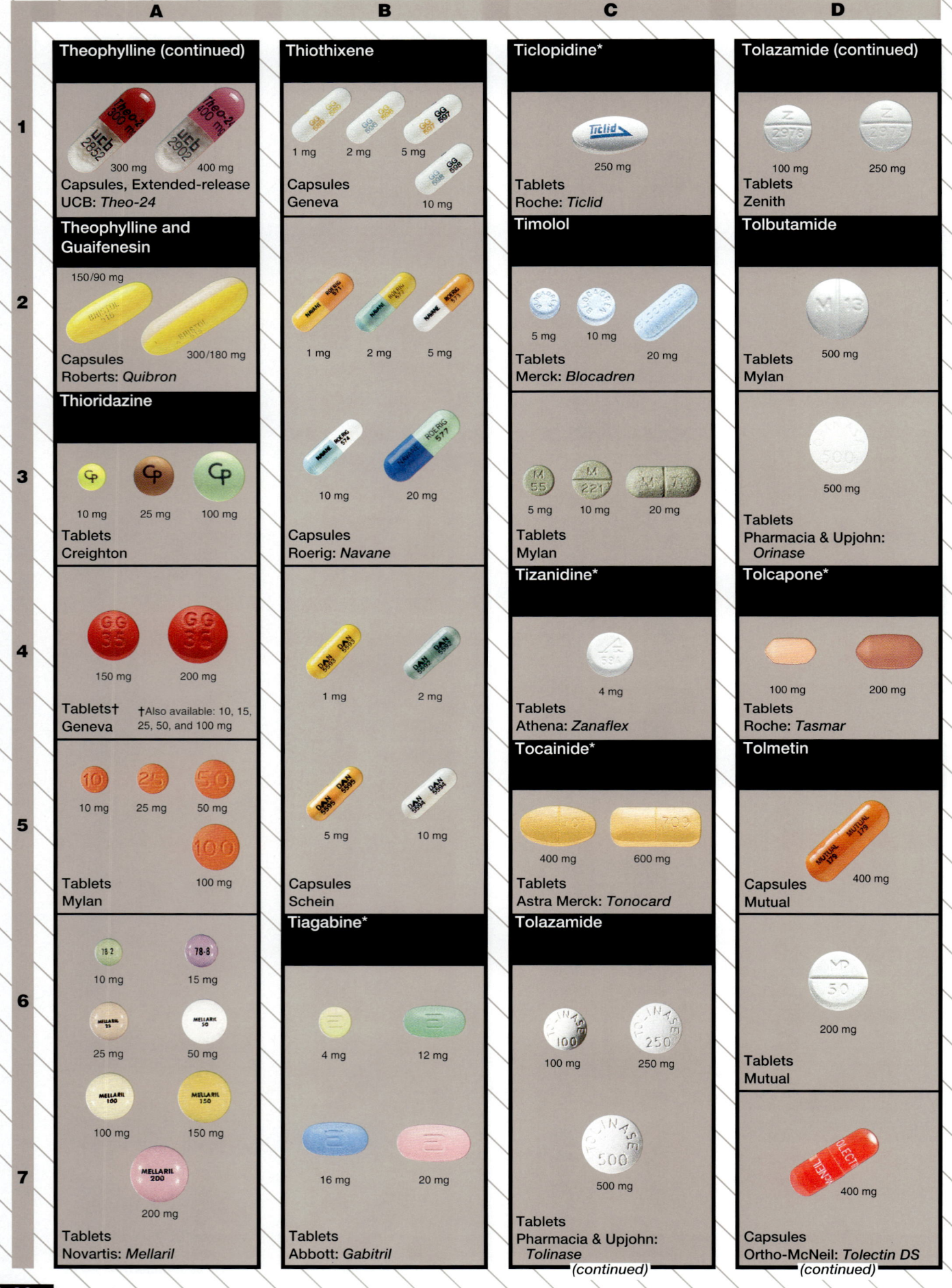

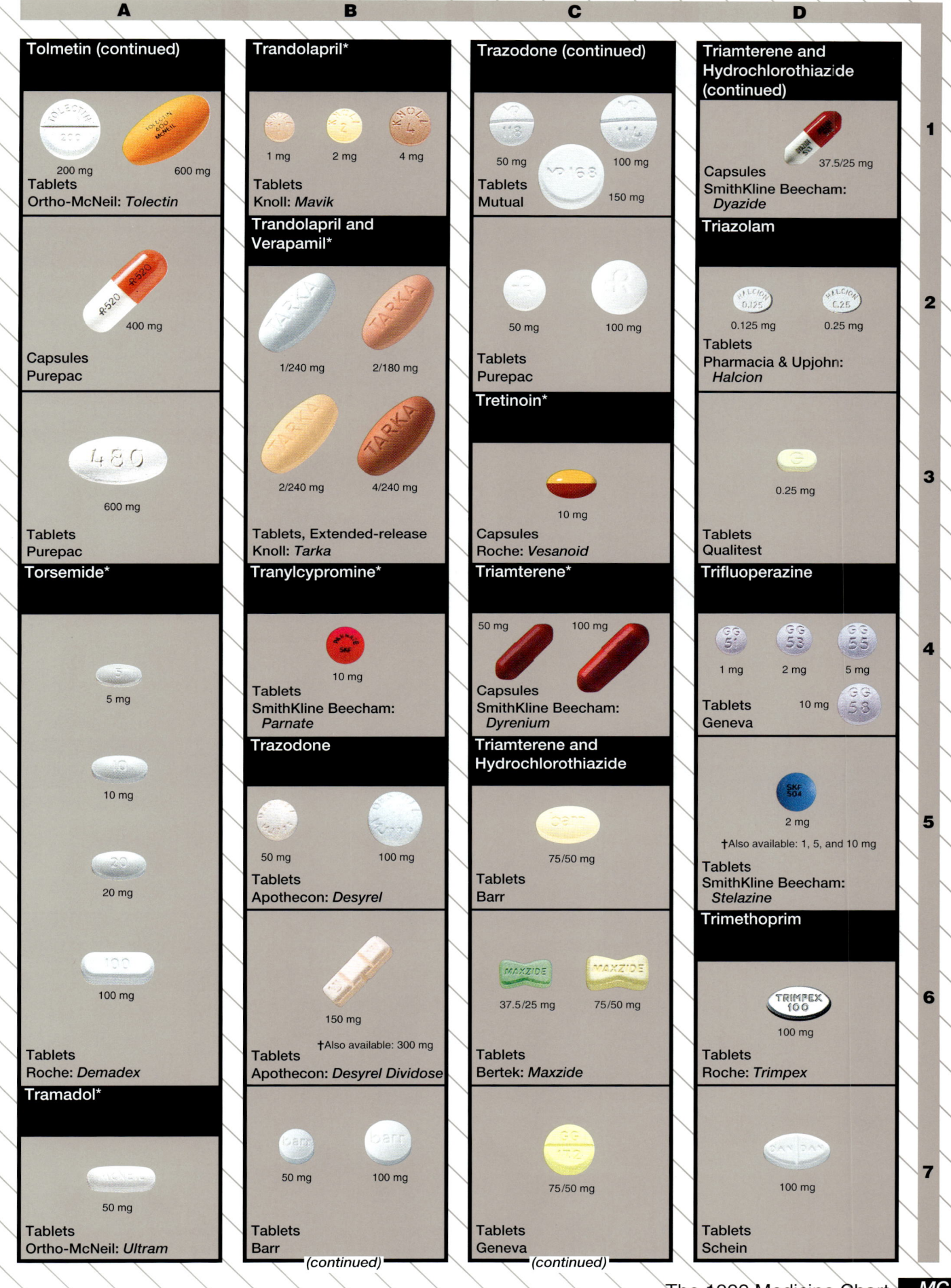

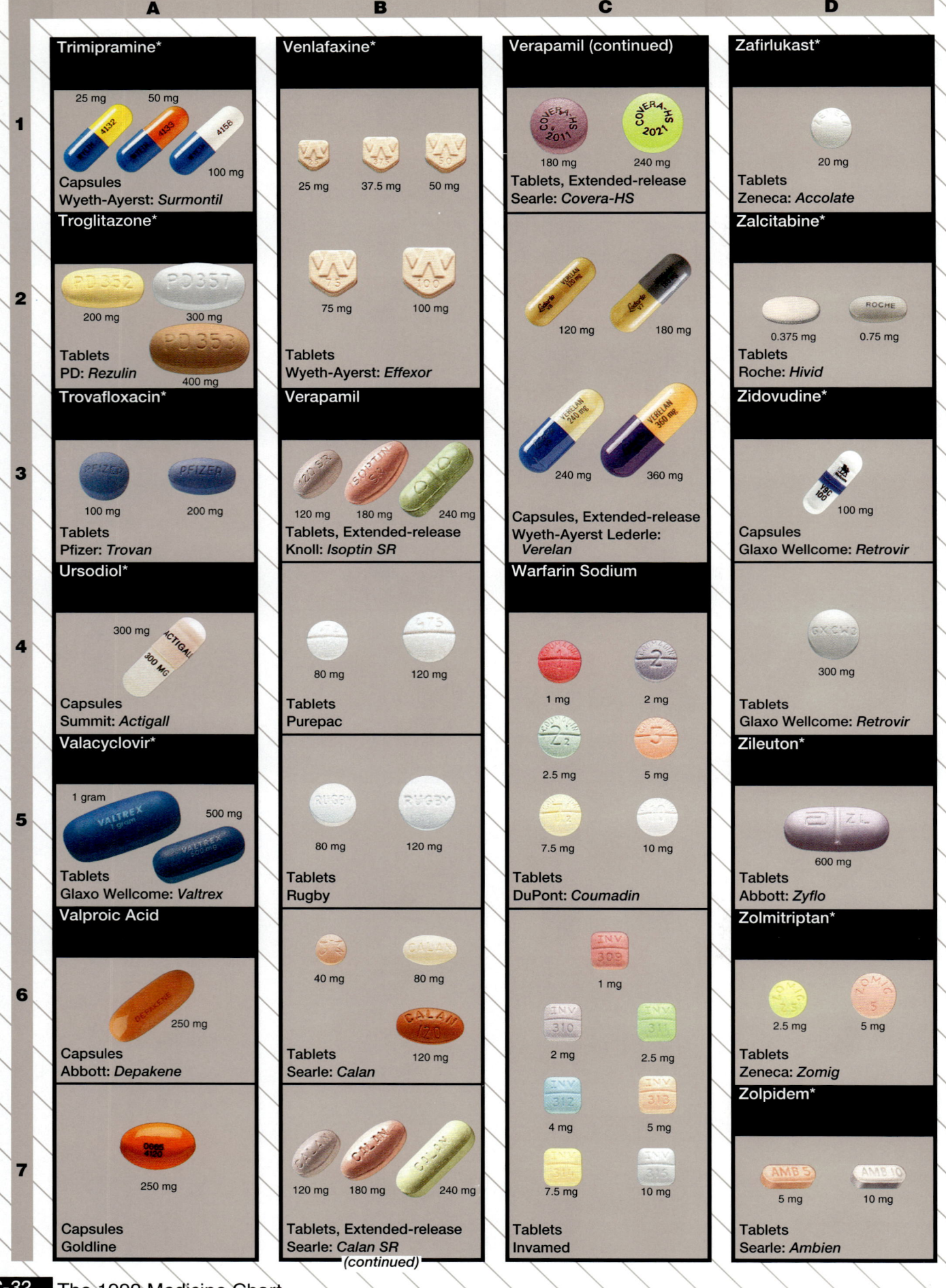
The 1999 Medicine Chart

# Appendix VIII

## ORPHAN DRUG AND BIOLOGICAL LISTING

The Orphan Drug Act (Public Law 97-414), which amends the Federal Food, Drug, and Cosmetic Act, was enacted into law in January 1983. The law provides incentives to drug manufacturers to develop and market drugs for the diagnosis, treatment, or prevention of rare diseases or conditions (orphan drugs). Section 526 of the Orphan Drug Act establishes a process by which a drug manufacturer or sponsor may obtain designation of its drug as an orphan drug.

Public Law 98-551 amended the Orphan Drug Act in 1984 to define a rare disease or condition as (a) one which affects less than 200,000 persons in the United States or (b) one which affects more than 200,000 persons in the United States and for which there is no reasonable expectation that the cost of developing the drug and making it available in the United States will be recovered from the sales of that drug in the United States.

This appendix to *USP DI* reproduces the list of orphan drug and biological designations as issued by the United States Food and Drug Administration (FDA). This listing includes the names of the substances, designated uses, and the names and addresses of sponsors. The information included is inclusive for all orphan/drug biological designations made since the inception of the program through August 31, 1995.

The designated uses identified in this listing have been reproduced as originally identified by FDA. If sponsors are limiting investigational use to a more restricted group of patients than for which the original designation was issued, this fact is not known by USP and therefore is not included in this listing. Other information included in the original FDA designation has been updated where appropriate. For example, in some cases, the sponsor, the sponsor's address, and/or the brand name specified by the sponsor have changed.

Some of the orphan drug products in this cumulative listing have since been approved by the FDA and are currently being marketed. Others remain under investigation or are no longer being actively studied. The current status of each orphan drug/biological, where known, is included in this listing.

It should be noted that the names used in this listing for products that have not been approved for marketing may not be the established or proper names approved by FDA for these products if they are eventually approved or licensed for marketing. Since these products are investigational, some may not have been reviewed by FDA for purposes of assigning the most appropriate name.

## CUMULATIVE LIST OF ORPHAN PRODUCT DESIGNATIONS AND APPROVALS
[Through October 31, 1998]

| NAME<br>*Generic/Chemical*<br>*TN is Trade Name* | INDICATION DESIGNATED | SPONSOR AND ADDRESS<br>*DD is Date Designated*<br>*MA is Marketing Approval* |
|---|---|---|
| 15AU81 | TREATMENT OF PRIMARY PULMONARY HYPERTENSION | LUNG RX, INC.<br>2 DAVIS DRIVE<br>P.O. BOX 13169<br>RESEARCH TRIANGLE PARK NC 27709 |
| 1,5-(BUTYLIMINO-1,5 DIDEOXY, D-GLUCITOL | TREATMENT OF FABRY'S DISEASE | OXFORD GLYCOSCIENCES<br>10, THE QUADRANT<br>ABINGTON SCIENCE PARK, ABINGTON<br>OXFORDSHIRE OX14 3YS<br>UNITED KINGDOM |
| 1,5-(BUTYLIMINO)-1,5 DIDEOXY, D-GLUCITOL | TREATMENT OF GAUCHER DISEASE | OXFORD GLYCOSCIENCES<br>10, THE QUADRANT<br>ABINGTON SCIENCE PARK, ABINGTON<br>OXFORDSHIRE OX14 3YS<br>UNITED KINGDOM |
| 2-0-DESULFATED HEPARIN<br>TN is AEROPIN | TREATMENT OF CYSTIC FIBROSIS | KENNEDY & HOIDAL, MDs.<br>CAROLINAS MEDICAL CENTER<br>CHARLOTTE NC 28232-2861<br>DD 09/17/93 |
| 2-CHLORODEOXYADENOSINE | TREATMENT OF ACUTE MYELOID LEUKEMIA | R.W. JOHNSON RESEARCH INSTITUTE<br>ROUTE 202 SOUTH, P.O. BOX 670<br>RARITAN NJ 08869-0670<br>DD 07/20/90 |
| 2'-DEOXYCYTIDINE | FOR USE AS A HOST-PROTECTIVE AGENT IN THE TREATMENT OF ACUTE MYELOGENOUS LEUKEMIA | GRANT, STEVEN M.D.<br>MASSEY CANCER CENTER, VCU<br>P.O. BOX 980230<br>RICHMOND VA 23298 |
| 24,25 DIHYDROXYCHOLE-CALCIFEROL | TREATMENT OF UREMIC OSTEODYSTROPHY | LEMMON COMPANY<br>650 CATHILL ROAD<br>SELLERSVILLE PA 18960<br>DD 02/27/87 |
| 3,4-DIAMINOPYRIDINE | TREATMENT OF LAMBERT-EATON MYASTHENIC SYNDROME | JACOBUS PHARMACEUTICAL COMPANY<br>P.O. BOX 5290<br>PRINCETON NJ 08540<br>DD 12/18/90 |

# CUMULATIVE LIST OF ORPHAN PRODUCT DESIGNATIONS AND APPROVALS
[Through October 31, 1998] *(continued)*

| NAME<br>*Generic/Chemical*<br>*TN is Trade Name* | INDICATION DESIGNATED | SPONSOR AND ADDRESS<br>*DD is Date Designated*<br>*MA is Marketing Approval* |
|---|---|---|
| 4-AMINOSALICYLIC ACID<br>TN is PAMISYL (P-D), REZIPAS (SQUIBB) | TREATMENT OF MILD TO MODERATE ULCERATIVE COLITIS IN PATIENTS INTOLERANT TO SULFASALAZINE | BEEKEN, WARREN, M.D.<br>UNIVERSITY OF VERMONT<br>BURLINGTON VT 05405-0068<br>DD 12/13/89 |
| 4-METHYLPYRAZOLE | TREATMENT OF METHANOL OR ETHYLENE GLYCOL POISONING | ORPHAN MEDICAL<br>13911 RIDGEDALE DRIVE<br>MINNETONKA MN 55305<br>DD 12/22/88 |
| 5, 6-DIHYDRO-5-AZACYTIDINE | TREATMENT OF MALIGNANT MESOTHELIOMA | ILEX ONCOLOGY INC.<br>14785 OMICRON DRIVE<br>SAN ANTONIO TX 78245-3217<br>DD 05/11/92 |
| 5-AZA-2'-DEOXYCYTIDINE | TREATMENT OF ACUTE LEUKEMIA | PHARMACHEMIE U.S.A., INCORP.<br>P.O. BOX 145<br>ORADELL NJ 07049<br>DD 08/03/87 |
| 5a8, MONOCLONAL ANTIBODY TO CD4 | FOR USE IN POST-EXPOSURE PROPHYLAXIS FOR OCCUPATIONAL EXPOSURE TO HUMAN IMMUNODEFICIENCY VIRUS | BIOGEN, INC.<br>14 CAMBRIDGE CENTER<br>CAMBRIDGE MA 02142<br>DD 12/20/93 |
| 8 CYCLOPENTYL 1,3-DIPROPYL-XANTHINE | TREATMENT OF CYSTIC FIBROSIS | SCICLONE PHARMACEUTICALS, INC.<br>901 MARINER'S ISLAND BOULEVARD<br>SUITE 315<br>SAN MATEO CA 94404 |
| 8-METHOXSALEN<br>TN is UVADEX | FOR USE IN CONJUNCTION WITH THE UVAR PHOTOPHERESIS TO TREAT DIFFUSE SYSTEMIC SCLEROSIS | THERAKOS, INCORPORATED<br>201 BRANDYWINE PARKWAY<br>WEST CHESTER PA 19380<br>DD 06/22/93 |
| 8-METHOXSALEN<br>TN is UVADEX | FOR THE PREVENTION OF ACUTE REJECTION OF CARDIAC ALLOGRAFTS | THERAKOS, INCORPORATED<br>201 BRANDYWINE PARKWAY<br>WEST CHESTER PA 19380<br>DD 05/12/94 |
| 9-CIS-RETINOIC ACID | PREVENTION OF RETINAL DETACHMENT DUE TO PROLIFERATIVE VITREORETINOPATHY | ALLERGAN<br>2525 DUPONT DRIVE<br>P.O. BOX 19534<br>IRVINE CA 92623 |
| 9-CIS RETINOIC ACID | TREATMENT OF ACUTE PROMYELOCYTIC LEUKEMIA | LIGAND PHARMACEUTICALS, INC.<br>9393 TOWNE CENTRE DRIVE<br>SUITE 100<br>SAN DIEGO CA 92121<br>DD 04/10/92 |
| 9-CIS-RETINOIC ACID | FOR THE TOPICAL TREATMENT OF CUTANEOUS LESIONS IN PATIENTS WITH AIDS-RELATED KAPOSI'S SARCOMA | LIGAND PHARMACEUTICALS INC.<br>10275 SCIENCE CENTER DRIVE<br>SAN DIEGO CA 92121 |
| 9-NITRO-20-(S)-CAMPTOTHECIN (9-NC) | TREATMENT OF PANCREATIC CANCER | STEHLIN FOUNDATION FOR CANCER RESEARCH<br>1315 CALHOUN, SUITE 1818<br>HOUSTON TX 77002 |
| 9-[3-PYRIDYLMETHYL]-9-DEAZAGUANINE | TREATMENT OF CUTANEOUS T-CELL LYMPHOMA | BIOCRYST PHARMACEUTICALS, INCORPORATED<br>2190 PARKWAY LAKE DRIVE<br>BIRMINGHAM AL 35244<br>DD 10/05/93 |
| ACETYLCYSTEINE<br>TN is MUCOMYST/MUCOMYST 10 IV | INTRAVENOUS TREATMENT OF PATIENTS PRESENTING WITH MODERATE TO SEVERE ACETAMINOPHEN OVERDOSE | APOTHECON<br>P.O. BOX 4500<br>PRINCETON NJ 08543-4500<br>DD 08/13/87 |
| ACONIAZIDE | TREATMENT OF TUBERCULOSIS | LINCOLN DIAGNOSTICS<br>P.O. BOX 1128<br>DECATUR IL 62525<br>DD 06/20/88 |
| ADENO-AS'TED VIRAL-BASED VECTOR CYSTIC FIBROSIS GENE THERAPY | TREATMENT OF CYSTIC FIBROSIS | TARGETED GENETICS CORPORATION<br>1100 OLIVE WAY, SUITE 100<br>SEATTLE WA 98101<br>DD 02/15/95 |
| AI-RSA | TREATMENT OF AUTOIMMUNE UVEITIS | AUTOIMMUNE, INC.<br>128 SPRING STREET<br>BOSTON MA 02115<br>DD 10/08/92 |

# CUMULATIVE LIST OF ORPHAN PRODUCT DESIGNATIONS AND APPROVALS
[Through October 31, 1998] *(continued)*

| NAME<br>*Generic/Chemical*<br>*TN is Trade Name* | INDICATION DESIGNATED | SPONSOR AND ADDRESS<br>*DD is Date Designated*<br>*MA is Marketing Approval* |
|---|---|---|
| ALBENDAZOLE | TREATMENT OF HYDATID CYST DISEASE (CYSTIC ECHINOCOCCOSIS DUE TO E. GRANULOSUS LARVAE OR ALVEOLAR ECHINOCOCCOSIS DUE TO E. MULTILOCULARIS LARVAE) | SMITHKLINE BEECHAM PHARMACEUTICALS<br>ONE FRANKLIN PLAZA<br>P.O. BOX 7929<br>PHILADELPHIA PA 19101 |
| ALBENDAZOLE | TREATMENT OF NEUROCYSTICERCOSIS DUE TO TAENIA SOLIUM AS: 1) CHEMOTHERAPY OF PARENCHYMAL, SUBARACHNOIDAL AND RACEMOSE (CYSTS IN SPINAL FLUID) NEUROCYSTICERCOSIS IN SYMPTOMATIC CASES AND 2) PROPHYLAXIS OF EPILEPSY AND OTHER SEQUELAE IN ASYMPTOMATIC NEUROCYSTICERCOSIS | SMITHKLINE BEECHAM PHARMACEUTICALS<br>ONE FRANKLIN PLAZA<br>P.O. BOX 7929<br>PHILADELPHIA PA 19101 |
| ALDESLEUKIN<br>TN is PROLEUKIN | TREATMENT OF METASTATIC RENAL CELL CARCINOMA | CHIRON CORPORATION<br>4560 HORTON STREET<br>EMERYVILLE CA 94608-2916<br>DD 09/14/88 MA 05/05/92 |
| ALDESLEUKIN<br>TN is PROLEUKIN | TREATMENT OF PRIMARY IMMUNODEFICIENCY DISEASE ASSOCIATED WITH T-CELL DEFECTS | CHIRON CORPORATION<br>4560 HORTON STREET<br>EMERYVILLE CA 94608<br>DD 03/22/89 |
| ALDESLEUKIN<br>TN is PROLEUKIN | TREATMENT OF ACUTE MYELOGENOUS LEUKEMIA | CHIRON CORPORATION<br>4560 HORTON STREET<br>EMERYVILLE CA 94608 |
| ALGLUCERASE INJECTION<br>TN is CEREDASE | REPLACEMENT THERAPY IN PATIENTS WITH GAUCHER'S DISEASE TYPE I | GENZYME COPORATION<br>ONE KENDALL SQUARE<br>CAMBRIDGE MA 02139<br>DD 03/11/85 MA 04/05/91 |
| ALGLUCERASE INJECTION<br>TN is CEREDASE | REPLACEMENT THERAPY IN PATIENTS WITH TYPE II AND TYPE III GAUCHER'S DISEASE | GENZYME CORPORATION<br>ONE KENDALL SQUARE<br>CAMBRIDGE MA 02139-1562<br>DD 07/21/95 |
| ALLOGENEIC PERIPHERAL BLOOD MONONUCLEAR CELLS SENSITIZED AGAINST PATIENT ALLOANTIGENS BY MIXED LYMPHOCYTE CULTURE<br>TN is CYTOIMPLANT | TREATMENT OF PANCREATIC CANCER | APPLIED IMMUNOTHERAPEUTICS, LLC<br>14132 E. FIRESTONE BOULEVARD<br>SANTA FE SPRINGS CA 90670 |
| ALLOPURINOL SODIUM<br>TN is ZYLOPRIM FOR INJECTION | MANAGEMENT OF PATIENTS WITH LEUKEMIA, LYMPHOMA, AND SOLID TUMOR MALIGNANCIES WHO ARE RECEIVING CANCER THERAPY WHICH CAUSES ELEVATIONS OF SERUM AND URINARY URIC ACID LEVELS AND WHO CANNOT TOLERATE ORAL THERAPY | BURROUGHS WELLCOME COMPANY<br>3030 CORNWALLIS ROAD<br>RESEARCH TRIANGLE PK NC 27709<br>DD 10/16/92 |
| ALPHA-1-ANTITRYPSIN (RECOMBINANT DNA ORIGIN) | SUPPLEMENTATION THERAPY FOR ALPHA-1-ANTITRYPSIN DEFICIENCY IN THE ZZ PHENOTYPE POPULATION | CHIRON CORPORATION<br>4560 HORTON STREET<br>EMERYVILLE CA 94608-2916<br>DD 01/01/84 |
| ALPHA-1-PROTEINASE INHIBITOR<br>TN is PROLASTIN | REPLACEMENT THERAPY IN THE ALPHA-1-PROTEINASE INHIBITOR CONGENITAL DEFICIENCY STATE | MILES, INC.<br>4TH & PARKER STREETS<br>BERKELEY CA 94710<br>DD 12/07/84 MA 12/02/87 |
| ALPHA-GALACTOSIDASE A<br>TN is FABRase | TREATMENT OF FABRY'S DISEASE | DESNICK, ROBERT J., M.D.<br>MOUNT SINAI SCHOOL OF MEDICINE<br>NEW YORK NY 10029-6574<br>DD 07/20/90 |
| ALPHA-GALACTOSIDASE A<br>TN is CC-GALACTOSIDASE | TREATMENT OF ALPHA-GALACTOSIDASE A DEFICIENCY (FABRY'S DISEASE) | CALHOUN, DAVID H., PH.D.<br>CONVENT AVE. & 138TH STREET<br>NEW YORK NY 10031-9127<br>DD 06/17/91 |
| ALPHA-GALACTOSIDASE A | LONG-TERM ENZYME REPLACEMENT THERAPY FOR THE TREATMENT OF FABRY DISEASE | TRANSKARYOTIC THERAPIES INC.<br>195 ALBANY STREET<br>CAMBRIDGE MA 02139 |
| ALPHA-MELANOCYTE STIMULATING HORMONE | PREVENTION AND TREATMENT OF INTRINSIC ACUTE RENAL FAILURE DUE TO ISCHEMIA | STAR, ROBERT A., M.D.<br>UNIVERSITY OF TEXAS-SOUTHWESTERN MEDICAL SCHOOL<br>5323 HARRY HINES BLVD.<br>DALLAS TX 75235 |
| ALPROSTADIL<br>TN is VASOPROST | TREATMENT OF SEVERE PERIPHERAL ARTERIAL OCCLUSIVE DISEASE (CRITICAL LIMB ISCHEMIA) IN PATIENTS WHERE OTHER PROCEDURES, GRAFTS OR ANGIOPLASTY, ARE NOT INDICATED | SCHWARZ PHARMA<br>5600 WEST COUNTY LINE ROAD<br>MEQUON WI 53092<br>DD 10/20/93 |
| ALTRETAMINE<br>TN is HEXALEN | TREATMENT OF ADVANCED ADENOCARCINOMA OF THE OVARY | U.S. BIOSCIENCE, INC.<br>100 FRONT STREET<br>WEST CONSHOHOCKEN PA 19428<br>DD 02/09/84 MA 12/26/90 |

# CUMULATIVE LIST OF ORPHAN PRODUCT DESIGNATIONS AND APPROVALS
[Through October 31, 1998] *(continued)*

| NAME<br>*Generic/Chemical*<br>*TN is Trade Name* | INDICATION DESIGNATED | SPONSOR AND ADDRESS<br>*DD is Date Designated*<br>*MA is Marketing Approval* |
|---|---|---|
| AMIFOSTINE<br>TN is ETHYOL | FOR USE AS A CHEMOPROTECTIVE AGENT FOR CISPLATIN IN THE TREATMENT OF ADVANCED OVARIAN CARCINOMA | U.S. BIOSCIENCE, INC.<br>100 FRONT STREET<br>WEST CONSHOHOCKEN PA 19428<br>DD 05/30/90 |
| AMIFOSTINE<br>TN is ETHYOL | FOR USE AS A CHEMOPROTECTIVE AGENT FOR CYCLOPHOSPHAMIDE IN THE TREATMENT OF ADVANCED OVARIAN CARCINOMA | U.S. BIOSCIENCE, INC.<br>100 FRONT STREET<br>WEST CONSHOHOCKEN PA 19428<br>DD 05/30/90 |
| AMIFOSTINE<br>TN is ETHYOL | FOR USE AS A CHEMOPROTECTIVE AGENT FOR CISPLATIN IN THE TREATMENT OF METASTATIC MELANOMA | U.S. BIOSCIENCE, INC.<br>100 FRONT STREET<br>WEST CONSHOHOCKEN PA 19428<br>DD 05/30/90 |
| AMIFOSTINE<br>TN is ETHYOL | REDUCTION OF THE INCIDENCE AND SEVERITY OF RADIATION-INDUCED XEROSTOMIA | U.S. BIOSCIENCE, INC.<br>100 FRONT STREET<br>WEST CONSHOHOCKEN PA 19428 |
| AMILORIDE HCL SOLUTION FOR INHALATION | TREATMENT OF CYSTIC FIBROSIS | GLAXO, INC.<br>5 MOORE DRIVE<br>RESEARCH TRIANGLE PK NC 27709<br>DD 07/18/90 |
| AMINOCAPROIC ACID | FOR THE TOPICAL TREATMENT OF TRAUMATIC HYPHEMA OF THE EYE | ORPHAN MEDICAL<br>13911 RIDGEDALE DRIVE<br>MINNETONKA MN 55305<br>DD 01/06/95 |
| AMINOSALICYLATE SODIUM | TREATMENT OF CROHN'S DISEASE | SYNCOM PHARMACEUTICALS, INC.<br>66 HANOVER ROAD<br>FLORHAM PARK NJ 07932-1522<br>DD 04/06/93 |
| AMINOSALICYLIC ACID<br>TN is PASER GRANULES | TREATMENT OF TUBERCULOSIS INFECTIONS | JACOBUS PHARMACEUTICAL COMPANY<br>37 CLEVELAND LANE<br>PRINCETON NJ 08540<br>DD 02/19/92 MA 06/30/94 |
| AMINOSIDINE<br>TN is GABBROMICINA | TREATMENT OF TUBERCULOSIS | KANYOK, THOMAS P., PHARM.D<br>UNIVERSITY OF ILLINOIS AT CHICAGO<br>CHICAGO IL 60612<br>DD 05/14/93 |
| AMINOSIDINE<br>TN is GABBROMICINA | TREATMENT OF MYCOBACTERIUM AVIUM COMPLEX | KANYOK, THOMAS P., PHARM.D.<br>UNIVERSITY OF ILLINOIS AT CHICAGO<br>CHICAGO IL 60612<br>DD 11/15/93 |
| AMINOSIDINE<br>TN is PAROMOMYCIN | TREATMENT OF VISCERAL LEISHMANIASIS (KALA-AZAR) | KANYOK, THOMAS P., PHARM.D.<br>UNIV. OF ILLINOIS AT CHICAGO<br>CHICAGO IL 60612<br>DD 09/09/94 |
| AMIODARONE<br>TN is AMIO-AQUEOUS | TREATMENT OF INCESSANT VENTRICULAR TACHYCARDIA | ACADEMIC PHARMACEUTICALS, INC.<br>25720 SAUNDERS ROAD NORTH<br>LAKE FOREST IL 60045<br>DD 08/17/93 |
| AMIODARONE HCL<br>TN is CORDARONE | FOR THE ACUTE TREATMENT AND PROPHYLAXIS OF LIFE-THREATENING VENTRICULAR TACHYCARDIA OR VENTRICULAR FIBRILLATION | WYETH-AYERST LABORATORIES<br>P.O. BOX 8299<br>PHILADELPHIA PA 19101-1245<br>DD 03/16/94 MA 08/03/95 |
| AMMONIUM TETRATHIO-MOLYBDATE | TREATMENT OF WILSON'S DISEASE | BREWER, GEORGE J., M.D.<br>UNIVERSITY OF MICHIGAN MEDICAL SCHOOL<br>ANN ARBOR MI 48109-0618<br>DD 01/31/94 |
| AMPHOTERICIN B LIPID COMPLEX<br>TN is ABELCET | TREATMENT OF INVASIVE CANDIDIASIS | THE LIPOSOME COMPANY, INC.<br>ONE RESEARCH WAY<br>PRINCETON NJ 08540 |
| AMPHOTERICIN B LIPID COMPLEX<br>TN is ABELCET | TREATMENT OF INVASIVE COCCIDIOIDOMYCOSIS | THE LIPOSOME COMPANY, INC.<br>ONE RESEARCH WAY<br>PRINCETON NJ 08540 |
| AMPHOTERICIN B LIPID COMPLEX<br>TN is ABLC | TREATMENT OF CRYPTOCOCCAL MENINGITIS | THE LIPOSOME COMPANY<br>ONE RESEARCH WAY<br>PRINCETON NJ 08540-6619<br>DD 12/05/91 |
| AMPHOTERICIN B LIPID COMPLEX<br>TN is ABELCET | TREATMENT OF INVASIVE PROTOTHECOSIS | THE LIPOSOME COMPANY, INC.<br>ONE RESEARCH WAY<br>PRINCETON NJ 08540 |
| AMPHOTERICIN B LIPID COMPLEX<br>TN is ABELCET | TREATMENT OF INVASIVE SPOROTRICHOSIS | THE LIPOSOME COMPANY, INC.<br>ONE RESEARCH WAY<br>PRINCETON NJ 08540 |

# CUMULATIVE LIST OF ORPHAN PRODUCT DESIGNATIONS AND APPROVALS
[Through October 31, 1998] *(continued)*

| NAME<br>*Generic/Chemical*<br>*TN is Trade Name* | INDICATION DESIGNATED | SPONSOR AND ADDRESS<br>*DD is Date Designated*<br>*MA is Marketing Approval* |
|---|---|---|
| AMPHOTERICIN B LIPID COMPLEX<br>TN is ABELCET | TREATMENT OF INVASIVE ZYGOMYCOSIS | THE LIPOSOME COMPANY, INC.<br>ONE RESEARCH WAY<br>PRINCETON NJ 08540 |
| ANAGRELIDE | TREATMENT OF THROMBOCYTOSIS IN CHRONIC MYCLOGENOUS LEUKEMIA | ROBERTS PHARMACEUTICAL CORP.<br>6 INDUSTRIAL WAY WEST<br>EATONTOWN NJ 07724<br>DD 07/14/86 |
| ANAGRELIDE | TREATMENT OF ESSENTIAL THROMBOCYTHEMIA (ET) | ROBERTS PHARMACEUTICAL CORP.<br>6 INDUSTRIAL WAY WEST<br>EATONTOWN NJ 07724<br>DD 01/27/88 |
| ANAGRELIDE | TREATMENT OF THROMBOCYTOSIS IN CHRONIC MYELOGENOUS LEUKEMIA | ROBERTS PHARMACEUTICAL CORP.<br>6 INDUSTRIAL WAY WEST<br>EATONTOWN NJ 07724<br>DD 07/14/86 |
| ANANAIN, COMOSAIN<br>TN is VIANAIN | FOR THE ENZYMATIC DEBRIDEMENT OF SEVERE BURNS | GENZYME CORPORATION<br>ONE KENDALL SQUARE<br>CAMBRIDGE MA 02139<br>DD 01/21/92 |
| ANARITIDE ACETATE<br>TN is AURICULIN | IMPROVEMENT OF EARLY RENAL ALLOGRAFT FUNCTION FOLLOWING RENAL TRANSPLANTATION | SCIOS NOVA, INC.<br>2450 BAYSHORE PARKWAY<br>MOUNTAIN VIEW CA 94043<br>DD 04/10/92 |
| ANARITIDE ACETATE<br>TN is AURICULIN | TREATMENT OF PATIENTS WITH ACUTE RENAL FAILURE | SCIOS NOVA, INC.<br>2450 BAYSHORE PARKWAY<br>MOUNTAIN VIEW CA 94043<br>DD 08/27/92 |
| ANCROD | TO ESTABLISH AND MAINTAIN ANTICOAGULATION IN HEPARIN-INTOLERANT PATIENTS UNDERGOING CARDIOPULMONARY BYPASS | KNOLL PHARMACEUTICALS<br>30 NORTH JEFFERSON ROAD<br>WHIPPANY NJ 07981 |
| ANCROD<br>TN is ARVIN | FOR USE AS AN ANTITHROMBOTIC IN PATIENTS WITH HEPARIN INDUCED THROMBOCYTOPENIA OR THROMBOSIS WHO REQUIRE IMMEDIATE AND CONTINUED ANTICOAGULATION | KNOLL PHARMACEUTICALS<br>30 NORTH JEFFERSON ROAD<br>WHIPPANY NJ 07981<br>DD 10/20/89 |
| ANTI-CD45 MONOCLONAL ANTIBODIES | PREVENTION OF ACUTE GRAFT REJECTION OF HUMAN ORGAN TRANSPLANTS | BAXTER HEALTHCARE CORPORATION<br>1620 WAUKEGAN ROAD<br>MCGAW PARK IL 60085<br>DD 09/10/90 |
| ANTI-THYMOCYTE SERUM<br>TN is NASHVILLE RABBIT ANTI-THYMOCYTE SERUM | TREATMENT OF ALLOGRAFT REJECTION, INCLUDING SOLID ORGAN (KIDNEY, LIVER, HEART, LUNG, AND PANCREAS) AND BONE MARROW TRANSPLANTATION | APPLIED MEDICAL RESEARCH<br>1600 HAYES STREET<br>NASHVILLE TN 37203<br>DD 06/02/93 |
| ANTIEPILEPSIRINE | TREATMENT OF DRUG RESISTANT GENERALIZED TONIC-CLONIC (GTC) EPILEPSY IN CHILDREN AND ADULTS | CHILDREN'S HOSPITAL<br>700 CHILDREN'S DRIVE<br>COLUMBUS OH 43205<br>DD 03/23/89 |
| ANTIHEMOPHILIC FACTOR (RECOMBINANT)<br>TN is KOGENATE | PROPHYLAXIS AND TREATMENT OF BLEEDING IN INDIVIDUALS WITH HEMOPHILIA A OR FOR PROPHYLAXIS WHEN SURGERY IS REQUIRED IN INDIVIDUALS WITH HEMOPHILIA A | MILES, INC.<br>4TH & PARKER STREETS<br>BERKELEY CA 94710<br>DD 09/25/89 MA 02/25/93 |
| ANTIHEMOPHILIC FACTOR (HUMAN)<br>TN is ALPHANATE | TREATMENT OF VON WILLEBRAND'S DISEASE | ALPHA THERAPEUTIC CORPORATION<br>5555 VALLEY BOULEVARD<br>LOS ANGELES CA 90032 |
| ANTIHEMOPHILIC FACTOR, HUMAN<br>TN is HUMATE P | TREATMENT OF PATIENTS WITH VON WILLEBRAND'S DISEASE | BEHRINGWERKE AKTIENGESELLSCHAFT (AG)<br>500 ARCOLA ROAD, P.O. BOX 1200<br>COLLEGEVILLE PA 19426-0107<br>DD 10/16/92 |
| ANTITHROMBIN III (HUMAN)<br>TN is THROMBATE III | REPLACEMENT THERAPY IN CONGENITAL DEFICIENCY OF AT-III FOR PREVENTION AND TREATMENT OF THROMBOSIS AND PULMONARY EMBOLI | MILES, INC.<br>4TH & PARKER STREETS<br>BERKELEY CA 94710<br>DD 11/26/84 MA 12/30/91 |
| ANTITHROMBIN III CONCENTRATE IV<br>TN is KYBERNIN | PROPHYLAXIS AND TREATMENT OF THROMBOEMBOLIC EPISODES IN PATIENTS WITH GENETIC AT-III DEFICIENCY | BEHRINGWERKE (ARMOUR-U.S. AGENT)<br>500 ARCOLA ROAD, PO BOX 1200<br>COLLEGEVILLE PA 19426-0107<br>DD 07/02/85 |
| ANTITHROMBIN III HUMAN<br>TN is ATnativ | FOR THE TREATMENT OF PATIENTS WITH HEREDITARY ANTITHROMBIN III DEFICIENCY IN CONNECTION WITH SURGICAL OR OBSTETRICAL PROCEDURES OR WHEN THEY SUFFER FROM THROMBOEMBOLISM | KABIVITRUM, INC.<br>P.O. BOX 430<br>DANVILLE CA 94526<br>DD 02/08/85 MA 12/13/89 |

# CUMULATIVE LIST OF ORPHAN PRODUCT DESIGNATIONS AND APPROVALS
[Through October 31, 1998] *(continued)*

| NAME<br>*Generic/Chemical*<br>*TN is Trade Name* | INDICATION DESIGNATED | SPONSOR AND ADDRESS<br>*DD is Date Designated*<br>*MA is Marketing Approval* |
|---|---|---|
| ANTITHROMBIN III HUMAN<br>TN is ANTITHROMBIN III HUMAN | PREVENTING OR ARRESTING EPISODES OF THROMBOSIS IN PATIENTS WITH CONGENITAL AT-III DEFICIENCY AND/OR TO PREVENT THE OCCURRENCE OF THROMBOSIS IN PATIENTS WITH AT-III DEFICIENCY WHO HAVE UNDERGONE TRAUMA OR WHO ARE ABOUT TO UNDERGO SURGERY OR PARTURITION | AMERICAN NATIONAL RED CROSS<br>9312 OLD GEORGETOWN ROAD<br>BETHESDA MD 20814<br>DD 01/02/86 |
| ANTIVENIN, POLYVALENT CROTALID (OVINE) FAB<br>TN is CROTAB | TREATMENT OF ENVENOMATIONS INFLICTED BY NORTH AMERICAN CROTALID SNAKES | THERAPEUTIC ANTIBODIES INC.<br>1500 21ST AVENUE SOUTH<br>SUITE 310<br>NASHVILLE TN 37212<br>DD 01/12/94 |
| ANTIVENOM (CROTALIDAE) PURIFIED (AVIAN) | TREATMENT OF ENVENOMATION BY POISONOUS SNAKES BELONGING TO THE CROTALIDAE FAMILY | OPHIDIAN PHARMACEUTICALS, INC.<br>5445 EAST CHERYL PARKWAY<br>MADISON WI 53711<br>DD 02/12/91 |
| APL 400-020 | TREATMENT OF CUTANEOUS T CELL LYMPHOMA | APOLLON, INC.<br>ONE GREAT VALLEY PARKWAY<br>MALVERN PA 19355<br>DD 03/08/95 |
| APOMORPHINE<br>TN is ZYDIS | FOR USE AS RESCUE TREATMENT FOR EARLY MORNING MOTOR DYSFUNCTION IN LATE-STAGE PARKINSON'S DISEASE | SCHERER DDS<br>FRANKLAND ROAD<br>SWINDON<br>WILTSHIRE UK SN5 8RU |
| APOMORPHINE HCL | TREATMENT OF THE ON-OFF FLUCTUATIONS ASSOCIATED WITH LATE-STAGE PARKINSON'S DISEASE | FORUM PRODUCTS, INC.<br>33 FLYING POINT ROAD<br>SOUTHAMPTON NY 11968<br>DD 04/22/93 |
| APOMORPHINE HCL | TREATMENT OF ON-OFF FLUCTUATIONS ASSOCIATED WITH LATE-STAGE PARKINSON'S DISEASE | PENTECH PHARMACEUTICALS, INC.<br>417 HARVESTER COURT<br>WHEELING IL 60090<br>DD 07/17/95 |
| APROTININ<br>TN is TRASYLOL | FOR PROPHYLACTIC USE TO REDUCE PERIOPERATIVE BLOOD LOSS AND THE HOMOLOGOUS BLOOD TRANSFUSION REQUIREMENT IN PATIENTS UNDERGOING CARDIOPULMONARY BYPASS SURGERY IN THE COURSE OF REPEAT CORONARY ARTERY BYPASS GRAFT SURGERY, AND IN SELECTED CASES OF PRIMARY CORONARY ARTERY BYPASS GRAFT SURGERY WHERE THE RISK OF BLEEDING IS ESPECIALLY HIGH (IMPAIRED HEMOSTASIS) OR WHERE TRANSFUSION IS UNAVAILABLE OR UNACCEPTABLE | MILES, INC.<br>400 MORGAN LANE<br>WEST HAVEN CT 06516<br>DD 11/17/93 MA 12/29/93 |
| ARCITUMOMAB | DIAGNOSIS AND LOCALIZATION OF PRIMARY, RESIDUAL, RECURRENT AND METASTATIC MEDULLARY THYROID CARCINOMA | IMMUNOMEDICS, INC.<br>300 AMERICAN ROAD<br>MORRIS PLAINS NJ 07950 |
| ARGININE BUTYRATE | TREATMENT OF BETA-HEMOGLOBINOPATHIES AND BETA-THALASSEMIA | PERRINE, SUSAN P., M.D.<br>BOSTON UNIVERSITY<br>BOSTON MA 02118<br>DD 04/07/92 |
| ARGININE BUTYRATE | TREATMENT OF SICKLE CELL DISEASE AND BETA THALASSEMIA | VERTEX PHARMACEUTICALS INC.<br>40 ALLSTON STREET<br>CAMBRIDGE MA 02139-4211<br>DD 05/25/94 |
| ARSENIC TRIOXIDE | TREATMENT OF ACUTE PROMYELOCYTIC LEUKEMIA | POLARX, INC.<br>787 SEVENTH AVE., 48TH FLOOR<br>NEW YORK NY 10019 |
| ATOVAQUONE<br>TN is MEPRON | TREATMENT OF AIDS ASSOCIATED PNEUMOCYSTIS CARINII PNEUMONIA (PCP) | BURROUGHS WELLCOME COMPANY<br>3030 CORNWALLIS ROAD<br>RESEARCH TRIANGLE PK NC 27709<br>DD 09/10/90 MA 11/25/92 |
| ATOVAQUONE<br>TN is MEPRON | PREVENTION OF PNEUMOCYSTIS CARINII PNEUMONIA (PCP) IN HIGH-RISK, HIV-INFECTED PATIENTS DEFINED BY A HISTORY OF ONE OR MORE EPISODES OF PCP AND/OR A PERIPHERAL CD4+ (T4 HELPER/INDUCER) LYMPHOCYTE COUNT LESS THAN OR EQUAL TO 200/MM3 | BURROUGHS WELLCOME COMPANY<br>3030 CORNWALLIS ROAD<br>RESEARCH TRIANGLE PK NC 27709<br>DD 08/14/91 |
| ATOVAQUONE<br>TN is MEPRON | TREATMENT AND SUPPRESSION OF TOXOPLASMA GONDII ENCEPHALITIS | BURROUGHS WELLCOME COMPANY<br>3030 CORNWALLIS ROAD<br>RESEARCH TRIANGLE PK NC 27709<br>DD 03/16/93 |
| ATOVAQUONE<br>TN is MEPRON | PRIMARY PROPHYLAXIS OF HIV-INFECTED PERSONS AT HIGH RISK FOR DEVELOPING TOXOPLASMA GONDII ENCEPHALITIS | BURROUGHS WELLCOME COMPANY<br>3030 CORNWALLIS ROAD<br>RESEARCH TRIANGLE PK NC 27709<br>DD 03/16/93 |
| AUTOLYMPHOCYTE THERAPY | TREATMENT OF RENAL CELL CARCINOMA | CELLCOR INCORPORATED<br>200 WELLS AVENUE<br>NEWTON MA 02159<br>DD 07/12/94 |

# CUMULATIVE LIST OF ORPHAN PRODUCT DESIGNATIONS AND APPROVALS
[Through October 31, 1998] *(continued)*

| NAME<br>*Generic/Chemical*<br>*TN is Trade Name* | INDICATION DESIGNATED | SPONSOR AND ADDRESS<br>*DD is Date Designated*<br>*MA is Marketing Approval* |
|---|---|---|
| B2036-PEG<br>TN is TROVERT | TREATMENT OF ACROMEGALY | SENSUS CORPORATION<br>98 SAN JACINTO BOULEVARD,<br>SUITE 430<br>AUSTIN TX 78701 |
| BACITRACIN<br>TN is ALTRACIN | ANTIBIOTIC-ASSOCIATED PSEUDOMEMBRANOUS ENTEROCOLITIS CAUSED BY TOXINS A AND B ELABORATED BY CLOSTRIDIUM DIFFICILE | A.L. LABORATORIES, INC.<br>ONE EXECUTIVE DR.<br>P.O. BOX 1399<br>FORT LEE NJ 07024<br>DD 03/13/84 |
| BACLOFEN<br>TN is LIORESAL INTRATHECAL | TREATMENT OF INTRACTABLE SPASTICITY CAUSED BY SPINAL CORD INJURY, MULTIPLE SCLEROSIS, AND OTHER SPINAL DISEASES (INCLUDING SPINAL ISCHEMIA, SPINAL TUMOR, TRANSVERSE MYELITIS, CERVICAL SPONDYLOSIS, AND DEGENERATIVE MYELOPATHY) | MEDTRONIC, INC.<br>7000 CENTRAL AVE N.E.<br>MINNEAPOLIS MN 55432<br>DD 11/10/87 MA 06/25/92 |
| BACLOFEN | TREATMENT OF INTRACTABLE SPASTICITY DUE TO MULTIPLE SCLEROSIS OR SPINAL CORD INJURY | INFUSAID, INC.<br>1400 PROVIDENCE HIGHWAY<br>NORWOOD MA 02062<br>DD 12/16/91 |
| BACLOFEN<br>TN is LIORESAL INTRATHECAL | TREATMENT OF SPASTICITY ASSOCIATED WITH CEREBRAL PALSY | MEDTRONIC, INCORPORATED<br>800 53RD AVENUE N.E.<br>MINNEAPOLIS MN 55432<br>DD 09/26/94 |
| BECLOMETHASONE DIPROPIONATE | FOR ORAL ADMINISTRATION IN THE TREATMENT OF INTESTINAL GRAFT-VERSUS-HOST DISEASE | GEORGE B. MCDONALD, M.D.<br>FRED HUTCHINSON CANCER RESEARCH CENTER<br>1100 FAIRVIEW AVENUE NORTH<br>(SC-113)<br>P.O. BOX 19024<br>SEATTLE WA 98109 |
| BENZOATE AND PHENYLACETATE<br>TN is UCEPHAN | ADJUNCTIVE THERAPY IN THE PREVENTION AND TREATMENT OF HYPERAMMONEMIA IN PATIENTS WITH UREA CYCLE ENZYMOPATHY (UCE) DUE TO CARBAMYLPHOSPHATE SYNTHETASE, ORNITHINE, TRANSCARBAMYLASE, OR ARGINOSUCCINATE SYNTHETASE DEFICIENCY | KENDALL McGAW LABORATORIES<br>2525 McGAW AVENUE<br>P.O. BOX 19791<br>IRVINE CA 92713-9791<br>DD 01/21/86 MA 12/23/87 |
| BENZYDAMINE HYDROCHLORIDE<br>TN is TANTUM | PROPHYLACTIC TREATMENT OF ORAL MUCOSITIS RESULTING FROM RADIATION THERAPY FOR HEAD AND NECK CANCER | ANGELINI PHARMACEUTICALS, INC.<br>70 GRAND AVENUE<br>RIVER EDGE NJ 07661 |
| BENZYLPENICILLIN, BENZYLPENICILLOIC, BENZYLPENILLOIC ACID<br>TN is PRE-PEN/MDM | ASSESSING THE RISK OF ADMINISTERING PENICILLIN WHEN IT IS THE PREFERRED DRUG OF CHOICE IN ADULT PATIENTS WHO HAVE PREVIOUSLY RECEIVED PENICILLIN AND HAVE A HISTORY OF CLINICAL SENSITIVITY | KREMERS-URBAN COMPANY<br>P.O. BOX 2038<br>MILWAUKEE WI 53201<br>DD 09/29/87 |
| BERACTANT<br>TN is SURVANTA INTRATRACHEAL SUSPENSION | TREATMENT OF NEONATAL RESPIRATORY DISTRESS SYNDROME (RDS) | ROSS LABORATORIES<br>625 CLEVELAND AVENUE<br>COLUMBUS OH 43215<br>DD 02/05/86 MA 07/01/91 |
| BERACTANT<br>TN is SURVANTA INTRATRACHEAL SUSPENSION | PREVENTION OF NEONATAL RESPIRATORY DISTRESS SYNDROME (RDS) | ROSS LABORATORIES<br>625 CLEVELAND AVENUE<br>COLUMBUS OH 43215<br>DD 02/05/86 MA 07/01/91 |
| BERACTANT<br>TN is SURVANTA INTRATRACHEAL SUSPENSION | TREATMENT OF FULL-TERM NEWBORN INFANTS WITH RESPIRATORY FAILURE CAUSED BY MECONIUM ASPIRATION SYNDROME, PERSISTENT PULMONARY HYPERTENSION OF THE NEWBORN, OR PNEUMONIA AND SEPSIS | ROSS LABORATORIES<br>625 CLEVELAND AVENUE<br>COLUMBUS OH 43215<br>DD 12/20/93 |
| BETA ALETHINE<br>TN is BETATHINE | TREATMENT OF METASTATIC MELANOMA | DOVETAIL TECHNOLOGIES, INC.<br>10615 MANTZ ROAD<br>SILVER SPRING MD 20903 |
| BETA ALETHINE<br>TN is BETATHINE | TREATMENT OF MULTIPLE MYELOMA | DOVETAIL TECHNOLOGIES, INC.<br>10615 MANTZ ROAD<br>SILVER SPRING MD 20903 |
| BETAINE | TREATMENT OF HOMOCYSTINURIA | ORPHAN MEDICAL<br>13911 RIDGEDALE DRIVE<br>MINNETONKA MN 55305<br>DD 05/16/94 |
| BINDARIT | TREATMENT OF LUPUS NEPHRITIS | ANGELINI PHARMACEUTICALS, INC.<br>70 GRAND AVENUE<br>RIVER EDGE NJ 07661 |
| BIODEL IMPLANT/CARMUSTINE (BCNU)<br>TN is GLIADEL | FOR THE LOCALIZED PLACEMENT IN THE BRAIN FOR THE TREATMENT OF RECURRENT MALIGNANT GLIOMA | GUILFORD PHARMACEUTICALS, INC.<br>6611 TRIBUTARY STREET<br>BALTIMORE MD 21224<br>DD 12/13/89 |
| BISPECIFIC ANTIBODY<br>520C9x22 | IN VIVO SEROTHERAPY OF PATIENTS WITH OVARIAN CANCER | MEDAREX<br>1545 ROUTE 22 EAST<br>ANNANDALE NJ 08801-0992<br>DD 10/05/93 |

# CUMULATIVE LIST OF ORPHAN PRODUCT DESIGNATIONS AND APPROVALS
[Through October 31, 1998] *(continued)*

| NAME<br>*Generic/Chemical*<br>*TN is Trade Name* | INDICATION DESIGNATED | SPONSOR AND ADDRESS<br>*DD is Date Designated*<br>*MA is Marketing Approval* |
|---|---|---|
| BLEOMYCIN SULFATE<br>TN is BLENOXANE | TREATMENT OF MALIGNANT PLEURAL EFFUSION | BRISTOL-MYERS SQUIBB<br>P.O. BOX 4000<br>PRINCETON NJ 08543-4000<br>DD 09/17/93 |
| BOTULINUM TOXIN TYPE A<br>TN is BOTOX | TREATMENT OF BLEPHAROSPASM ASSOCIATED WITH DYSTONIA IN ADULTS (PATIENTS 12 YEARS OF AGE AND ABOVE) | ALLERGAN, INC.<br>2525 DUPONT DRIVE<br>P.O. BOX 19534<br>IRVINE CA 92713-9534<br>DD 03/22/84 MA 12/29/89 |
| BOTULINUM TOXIN TYPE A<br>TN is BOTOX | TREATMENT OF STRABISMUS ASSOCIATED WITH DYSTONIA IN ADULTS (PATIENTS 12 YEARS OF AGE AND ABOVE) | ALLERGAN, INC.<br>2525 DUPONT DRIVE<br>P.O. BOX 19534<br>IRVINE CA 92713-9534<br>DD 03/22/84 MA 12/29/89 |
| BOTULINUM TOXIN TYPE A<br>TN is BOTOX | TREATMENT OF CERVICAL DYSTONIA | ALLERGAN, INC.<br>2525 DUPONT DRIVE<br>P.O. BOX 19534<br>IRVINE CA 92713-9534<br>DD 08/20/86 |
| BOTULINUM TOXIN TYPE A<br>TN is DYSPORT | TREATMENT OF ESSENTIAL BLEPHAROSPASM | PORTON INTERNATIONAL, INC.<br>816 CONNECTICUT AVENUE NW<br>WASHINGTON DC 20006<br>DD 03/23/89 |
| BOTULINUM TOXIN TYPE A<br>TN is BOTOX | TREATMENT OF DYNAMIC MUSCLE CONTRACTURE IN PEDIATRIC CEREBRAL PALSY PATIENTS | ALLERGAN, INC.<br>2525 DUPONT DR.<br>P.O. BOX 19534<br>IRVINE CA 92713-9534<br>DD 12/06/91 |
| BOTULINUM TOXIN TYPE A | TREATMENT OF SYNKINETIC CLOSURE OF THE EYELID ASSOCIATED WITH VII CRANIAL NERVE ABERRANT REGENERATION | ASSOCIATED SYNAPSE BIOLOGICS<br>68 HARRISON AVENUE<br>BOSTON MA 02111<br>DD 09/15/92 |
| BOTULINUM TOXIN TYPE B | TREATMENT OF CERVICAL DYSTONIA | ATHENA NEUROSCIENCES, INC.<br>800F GATEWAY BOULEVARD<br>SOUTH SAN FRANCISCO CA 94080<br>DD 01/16/92 |
| BOTULINUM TOXIN TYPE F | TREATMENT OF ESSENTIAL BLEPHAROSPASM | PORTON INTERNATIONAL, INC.<br>816 CONNECTICUT AVENUE N.W.<br>WASHINGTON DC 20006<br>DD 12/05/91 |
| BOTULINUM TOXIN TYPE F | TREATMENT OF SPASMODIC TORTICOLLIS (CERVICAL DYSTONIA) | PORTON INTERNATIONAL, INC.<br>816 CONNECTICUT AVENUE N.W.<br>WASHINGTON DC 20006<br>DD 10/24/91 |
| BOTULISM IMMUNE GLOBULIN | TREATMENT OF INFANT BOTULISM | CALIFORNIA DEPT HEALTH SERVICE<br>2151 BERKELEY WAY<br>BERKELEY CA 94704<br>DD 01/31/89 |
| BOVINE COLOSTRUM | TREATMENT OF AIDS-RELATED DIARRHEA | HASTINGS, DONALD, DVM<br>1030 NORTH PARKVIEW DRIVE<br>BISMARCK ND 58501<br>DD 11/19/90 |
| BOVINE IMMUNOGLOBULIN CONCENTRATE, CRYPTOSPORIDIUM PARVUM<br>TN is SPORIDIN-G | TREATMENT AND SYMPTOMATIC RELIEF OF CRYPTOSPORIDIUM PARVUM INFECTION OF THE GASTROINTESTINAL TRACT IN IMMUNOCOMPROMISED PATIENTS | GALAGEN, INCORPORATED<br>4001 LEXINGTON AVENUE NORTH<br>ARDEN HILLS MN 55126-2998<br>DD 03/01/94 |
| BOVINE WHEY PROTEIN CONCENTRATE<br>TN is IMMUNO-C | TREATMENT OF CRYPTOSPORIDIOSIS CAUSED BY THE PRESENCE OF CRYPTOSPORIDIUM PARVUM IN THE GASTROINTESTINAL TRACT OF PATIENTS WHO ARE IMMUNODEFICIENT/IMMUNOCOMPROMISED OR IMMUNOCOMPETENT | BIOMUNE SYSTEMS, INCORPORATED<br>540 ARAPEEN DRIVE<br>SUITE 202<br>SALT LAKE CITY UT 84108<br>DD 09/30/93 |
| BRANCHED CHAIN AMINO ACIDS | TREATMENT OF AMYOTROPHIC LATERAL SCLEROSIS | MOUNT SINAI MEDICAL CENTER<br>ONE GUSTAVE L. LEVY PLACE<br>NEW YORK NY 10029-6574<br>DD 12/23/88 |
| BROMHEXINE | TREATMENT OF MILD TO MODERATE KERATOCONJUNCTIVITIS SICCA IN PATIENTS WITH SJOGREN'S SYNDROME | BOEHRINGER INGELHEIM<br>900 RIDGEBURY ROAD, BOX 368<br>RIDGEFIELD CT 06877<br>DD 05/15/89 |
| BROMODEOXYURIDINE | RADIATION SENSITIZER IN THE TREATMENT OF PRIMARY BRAIN TUMORS | NEOPHARM, INC.<br>225 EAST DEERPATH, SUITE 250<br>LAKE FOREST IL 60045 |

# CUMULATIVE LIST OF ORPHAN PRODUCT DESIGNATIONS AND APPROVALS
[Through October 31, 1998] *(continued)*

| NAME<br>*Generic/Chemical*<br>*TN is Trade Name* | INDICATION DESIGNATED | SPONSOR AND ADDRESS<br>*DD is Date Designated*<br>*MA is Marketing Approval* |
|---|---|---|
| BUPRENORPHINE HYDROCHLORIDE | TREATMENT OF OPIATE ADDICTION IN OPIATE USERS | RECKITT & COLMAN PHARMACEUTICALS, INC.<br>1901 HUGUENOT ROAD<br>RICHMOND VA 23235<br>DD 06/15/94 |
| BUPRENORPHINE IN COMBINATION WITH NALOXONE | TREATMENT OF OPIATE ADDICTION IN OPIATE USERS | RECKITT & COLMAN PHARMACEUTICALS INC.<br>1901 HUGUENOT ROAD<br>RICHMOND VA 23235<br>DD 10/27/94 |
| BUSULFAN | FOR USE AS PREPARATIVE THERAPY FOR MALIGNANCIES TREATED WITH BONE MARROW TRANSPLANTATION | SPARTA PHARMACEUTICALS, INC.<br>P.O. BOX 13288<br>RESEARCH TRIANGLE PK NC 27709<br>DD 04/21/94 |
| BUSULFAN | AS PREPARATIVE THERAPY IN THE TREATMENT OF MALIGNANCIES WITH BONE MARROW TRANSPLANTATION | ORPHAN MEDICAL<br>13911 RIDGEDALE DRIVE<br>MINNETONKA MN 55305<br>DD 07/28/94 |
| BUSULFAN | TREATMENT OF PRIMARY BRAIN MALIGNANCIES | SPARTA PHARMACEUTICALS, INC.<br>111 ROCK ROAD<br>HORSHAM PA 19044 |
| BUTYRYLCHOLINESTERASE | FOR THE REDUCTION AND CLEARANCE OF TOXIC BLOOD LEVELS OF COCAINE ENCOUNTERED DURING A DRUG OVERDOSE | PHARMAVENE, INC.<br>35 WEST WATKINS MILL ROAD<br>GAITHERSBURG MD 20878<br>DD 03/25/92 |
| BUTYRYLCHOLINESTERASE | TREATMENT OF POST-SURGICAL APNEA | PHARMAVENE, INC.<br>35 WEST WATKINS MILL ROAD<br>GAITHERSBURG MD 20878<br>DD 09/30/92 |
| C1-ESTERASE INHIBITOR (HUMAN) | TREATMENT AND PREVENTION OF ANGIOEDEMA CAUSED BY C1-ESTERASE INHIBITOR DEFICIENCY | ALPHA THERAPEUTIC CORPORATION<br>5555 VALLEY BOULEVARD<br>LOS ANGELES CA 90032 |
| C1-ESTERASE-INHIBITOR, HUMAN, PASTEURIZED | PREVENTION AND/OR TREATMENT OF ACUTE ATTACKS OF HEREDITARY ANGIOEDEMA | BEHRINGWERKE AKTIENGESELLSCHAFT (AG)<br>500 ARCOLA ROAD<br>P.O. BOX 1200<br>COLLEGEVILLE PA 19426-0107<br>DD 10/16/92 |
| C1-INHIBITOR<br>TN is C1-INHIBITOR (HUMAN) VAPOR HEATED, IMMUNO | PREVENTION OF ACUTE ATTACKS OF ANGIOEDEMA, INCLUDING SHORT-TERM PROPHYLAXIS FOR PATIENTS REQUIRING DENTAL OR OTHER SURGICAL PROCEDURES | IMMUNO CLINICAL RESEARCH CORP.<br>750 LEXINGTON AVENUE, 19TH FLOOR<br>NEW YORK NY 10022<br>DD 08/30/90 |
| C1-INHIBITOR<br>TN is C1-INHIBITOR (HUMAN) VAPOR HEATED, IMMUNO | TREATMENT OF ACUTE ATTACKS OF ANGIOEDEMA | OSTERREICHISCHES INSTITUTE FUR HAEMODER.<br>750 LEXINGTON AVENUE, 19TH FLOOR<br>NEW YORK NY 10022<br>DD 08/30/90 |
| CAFFEINE<br>TN is NEOCAF | TREATMENT OF APNEA OF PREMATURITY | O.P.R. DEVELOPMENT, L.P.<br>BECKLOFF ASSOCIATES<br>OVERLAND PARK KS 66210<br>DD 09/20/88 |
| CALCITONIN-HUMAN FOR INJECTION<br>TN is CIBACALCIN | TREATMENT OF SYMPTOMATIC PAGET'S DISEASE (OSTEITIS DEFORMANS) | CIBA-GEIGY CORPORATION<br>556 MORRIS AVE<br>SUMMIT NJ 07901<br>DD 01/20/87 MA 10/31/86 |
| CALCIUM ACETATE<br>TN is PHOS-LO | TREATMENT OF HYPERPHOSPHATEMIA IN END STAGE RENAL FAILURE | BRAINTREE LABORATORIES<br>60 COLUMBIAN STREET<br>P.O. BOX 361<br>BRAINTREE MA 02184<br>DD 12/22/88 MA 12/10/90 |
| CALCIUM ACETATE | TREATMENT OF HYPERPHOSPHATEMIA IN END STAGE RENAL DISEASE (ESRD) | PHARMEDIC COMPANY<br>28101 BALLARD ROAD<br>SUITE F<br>LAKE FOREST IL 60045<br>DD 06/27/89 |
| CALCIUM CARBONATE<br>TN is R & D CALCIUM CARBONATE/600 | TREATMENT OF HYPERPHOSPHATEMIA IN PATIENTS WITH END STAGE RENAL DISEASE | R & D LABORATORIES, INC.<br>4204 GLENCOE AVENUE<br>MARINA DEL REY CA 90292<br>DD 06/06/90 |
| CALCIUM GLUCONATE<br>TN is CALGONATE | FOR USE AS A WASH FOR HYDROFLUORIC ACID SPILLS ON HUMAN SKIN | CALGONATE CORP.<br>190 COMMERCE DRIVE<br>WARWICK RI 02886 |

# CUMULATIVE LIST OF ORPHAN PRODUCT DESIGNATIONS AND APPROVALS
[Through October 31, 1998] *(continued)*

| NAME<br>*Generic/Chemical*<br>*TN is Trade Name* | INDICATION DESIGNATED | SPONSOR AND ADDRESS<br>*DD is Date Designated*<br>*MA is Marketing Approval* |
|---|---|---|
| CALCIUM GLUCONATE GEL<br>TN is H-F GEL | FOR USE IN THE EMERGENCY TOPICAL TREATMENT OF HYDROGEN FLUORIDE (HYDROFLUORIC ACID) BURNS | LTR PHARMACEUTICALS, INC.<br>145 SAKONNET BLVD.<br>NARRAGANSETT RI 02882<br>DD 05/21/91 |
| CALCIUM GLUCONATE GEL 2.5% | EMERGENCY TOPICAL TREATMENT OF HYDROGEN FLUORIDE (HYDROFLUORIC ACID) BURNS | PADDOCK LABORATORIES, INC.<br>3940 QUEBEC AVENUE NORTH<br>MINNEAPOLIS MN 55427<br>DD 09/10/90 |
| CAMPATH-1H | TREATMENT OF CHRONIC LYMPHOCYTIC LEUKEMIA | L&I PARTNERS, LP<br>11550 IH 10 WEST, SUITE 300<br>SAN ANTONIO TX 78230 |
| CARBAMYLGLUTAMIC ACID | TREATMENT OF N-ACETYLGLUTAMATE SYNTHETASE DEFICIENCY | ORPHAN EUROPE<br>IMMEUBLE "LEGUILLAUMET"<br>60 AVENUE DU PRESIDENT WILSON<br>92046 PARIS FRANCE |
| CARBOVIR | TREATMENT OF PERSONS WITH AIDS AND IN PATIENTS WITH SYMPTOMATIC HIV INFECTION AND A CD4 COUNT LESS THAN 200/MM3 | GLAXO, INC.<br>5 MOORE DRIVE, P.O. BOX 13358<br>RESEARCH TRIANGLE PK NC 27709<br>DD 12/13/89 |
| CASCARA SAGRADA FLUID EXTRACT | TREATMENT OF ORAL DRUG OVERDOSAGE TO SPEED LOWER BOWEL EVACUATION | INTRAMED CORPORATION<br>102 TREMONT WAY<br>AUGUSTA GA 30907<br>DD 03/21/89 |
| CCD 1042 | TREATMENT OF INFANTILE SPASMS | COCENSYS, INC.<br>213 TECHNOLOGY DRIVE<br>IRVINE CA 92718<br>DD 05/25/94 |
| CD5-T LYMPHOCYTE IMMUNOTOXIN<br>TN is XOMAZYME-H65 | TREATMENT OF GRAFT VERSUS HOST DISEASE (GVHD) AND/OR REJECTION IN PATIENTS WHO HAVE RECEIVED BONE MARROW TRANSPLANTS | XOMA CORPORATION<br>2910 SEVENTH STREET<br>BERKELEY CA 94710<br>DD 08/27/87 |
| CERAMIDE TRIHEXOSIDASE/ALPHA-GALACTOSIDASE A | TREATMENT OF FABRY'S DISEASE | GENZYME CORPORATION<br>ONE KENDALL SQUARE<br>CAMBRIDGE MA 02139-1562<br>DD 01/19/88 |
| CHENODIOL<br>TN is CHENIX | FOR PATIENTS WITH RADIOLUCENT STONES IN WELL OPACIFYING GALLBLADDERS, IN WHOM ELECTIVE SURGERY WOULD BE UNDERTAKEN EXCEPT FOR THE PRESENCE OF INCREASED SURGICAL RISK DUE TO SYSTEMIC DISEASE OR AGE | SOLVAY<br>901 SAWYER ROAD<br>MARIETTA GA 30062-2224<br>DD 09/21/84 MA 07/28/83 |
| CHIMERIC A2 (HUMAN-MURINE) IgG MONOCLONAL ANTI-TNF ANTIBODY (cA2) | TREATMENT OF CROHN'S DISEASE | CENTOCOR, INC.<br>200 GREAT VALLEY PARKWAY<br>MALVERN PA 19355 |
| CHIMERIC (MURINE VARIABLE, HUMAN CONSTANT) MAB TO CD20 | TREATMENT OF NON-HODGKIN'S B-CELL LYMPHOMA | IDEC PHARMACEUTICALS CORPORATION<br>11011 TORREYANA ROAD<br>SAN DIEGO CA 92121<br>DD 06/13/94 |
| CHIMERIC M-T412 (HUMAN-MURINE) IgG MONOCLONAL ANTI-CD4 | TREATMENT OF MULTIPLE SCLEROSIS | CENTOCOR, INC.<br>244 GREAT VALLEY PARKWAY<br>MALVERN PA 19355<br>DD 06/05/91 |
| CHLORHEXIDINE GLUCONATE MOUTHRINSE<br>TN is PERIDEX | FOR USE IN THE AMELIORATION OF ORAL MUCOSITIS ASSOCIATED WITH CYTOREDUCTIVE THERAPY USED IN CONDITIONING PATIENTS FOR BONE MARROW TRANSPLANTATION THERAPY | PROCTER & GAMBLE COMPANY<br>11370 REED HARTMAN HIGHWAY<br>CINCINNATI OH 45241-2422<br>DD 08/18/86 |
| CHOLINE CHLORIDE | TREATMENT OF CHOLINE DEFICIENCY, SPECIFICALLY THE CHOLINE DEFICIENCY, HEPATIC STEATOSIS, AND CHOLESTASIS, ASSOCIATED WITH LONG-TERM PARENTERAL NUTRITION | ORPHAN MEDICAL<br>13911 RIDGEDALE DRIVE<br>MINNETONKA MN 55305<br>DD 02/10/94 |
| CHONDROITINASE | TREATMENT OF PATIENTS UNDERGOING VITRECTOMY | STORZ OPHTHALMICS<br>AMERICAN CYANAMID COMPANY<br>PEARL RIVER NY 10965<br>DD 02/09/95 |
| CILIARY NEUROTROPHIC FACTOR | TREATMENT OF AMYOTROPHIC LATERAL SCLEROSIS | REGENERON PHARMACEUTICALS, INC<br>777 OLD SAW MILL RIVER ROAD<br>TARRYTOWN NY 10591-6707<br>DD 01/30/92 |
| CILIARY NEUROTROPHIC FACTOR, RECOMBINANT HUMAN | TREATMENT OF SPINAL MUSCULAR ATROPHIES | SYNTEX-SYNERGEN NEUROSCIENCE<br>3200 WALNUT STREET<br>BOULDER CO 80301<br>DD 04/02/92 |

# CUMULATIVE LIST OF ORPHAN PRODUCT DESIGNATIONS AND APPROVALS
[Through October 31, 1998] *(continued)*

| NAME<br>*Generic/Chemical*<br>*TN is Trade Name* | INDICATION DESIGNATED | SPONSOR AND ADDRESS<br>*DD is Date Designated*<br>*MA is Marketing Approval* |
|---|---|---|
| CILIARY NEUROTROPHIC FACTOR, RECOMBINANT HUMAN | TREATMENT OF MOTOR NEURON DISEASE (INCLUDING AMYOTROPHIC LATERAL SCLEROSIS, PROGRESSIVE MUSCULAR ATROPHY, PROGRESSIVE BULBAR PALSY, AND PRIMARY LATERAL SCLEROSIS) | SYNTEX-SYNERGEN NEUROSCIENCE<br>3200 WALNUT STREET<br>BOULDER CO 80301<br>DD 05/08/92 |
| CITRIC ACID, GLUCONO-DELTA-LACTONE AND MAGNESIUM CARBONATE<br>TN is RENACIDIN IRRIGATION | TREATMENT OF RENAL AND BLADDER CALCULI OF THE APATITE OR STRUVITE VARIETY | UNITED-GUARDIAN, INC.<br>P.O. BOX 2500<br>SMITHTOWN NY 11787<br>DD 08/28/89 MA 10/02/90 |
| CLADRIBINE<br>TN is LEUSTATIN INJECTION | TREATMENT OF HAIRY CELL LEUKEMIA | R.W. JOHNSON RESEARCH INSTITUTE<br>ROUTE 202<br>P.O. BOX 300<br>RARITAN NJ 08869-0602<br>DD 11/15/90 MA 02/26/93 |
| CLADRIBINE<br>TN is LEUSTATIN INJECTION | TREATMENT OF CHRONIC LYMPHOCYTIC LEUKEMIA | R.W. JOHNSON RESEARCH INSTITUTE<br>ROUTE 202, P.O. BOX 300<br>RARITAN NJ 08869-0602<br>DD 12/31/90 |
| CLADRIBINE<br>TN is LEUSTATIN INJECTION | TREATMENT OF NON-HODGKIN'S LYMPHOMA | R.W. JOHNSON RESEARCH INSTITUTE<br>ROUTE 202 SOUTH, P.O. BOX 300<br>RARITAN NJ 08869-0602<br>DD 04/19/93 |
| CLADRIBINE<br>TN is LEUSTATIN | TREATMENT OF THE CHRONIC PROGRESSIVE FORM OF MULTIPLE SCLEROSIS | R.W. JOHNSON RESEARCH INSTITUTE<br>700 ROUTE 200 SOUTH<br>P.O. BOX 670<br>RARITAN NJ 08869-0670<br>DD 04/19/94 |
| CLINDAMYCIN<br>TN is CLEOCIN | TREATMENT OF PNEUMOCYSTIS CARINII PNEUMONIA ASSOCIATED WITH AIDS PATIENTS | UPJOHN COMPANY<br>7000 PORTAGE ROAD<br>KALAMAZOO MI 49001<br>DD 10/28/88 |
| CLINDAMYCIN<br>TN is CLEOCIN | PREVENTION OF PNEUMOCYSTIS CARINII PNEUMONIA IN AIDS PATIENTS | UPJOHN COMPANY<br>7000 PORTAGE ROAD<br>KALAMAZOO MI 49001<br>DD 10/28/88 |
| CLOFAZIMINE<br>TN is LAMPRENE | TREATMENT OF LEPROMATOUS LEPROSY, INCLUDING DAPSONE-RESISTANT LEPROMATOUS LEPROSY AND LEPROMATOUS LEPROSY COMPLICATED BY ERYTHEMA NODOSUM LEPROSUM | CIBA-GEIGY CORPORATION<br>556 MORRIS AVE<br>SUMMIT NJ 07901<br>DD 06/11/84 MA 12/15/86 |
| CLONAZEPAM<br>TN is KLONOPIN | TREATMENT OF HYPEREKPLEXIA (STARTLE DISEASE) | HOFFMAN-LA ROCHE, INCORPORATED<br>340 KINGSLAND STREET<br>NUTLEY NJ 07110-1199<br>DD 08/04/94 |
| CLONIDINE | FOR CONTINUOUS EPIDURAL ADMINISTRATION AS ADJUNCTIVE THERAPY WITH INTRASPINAL OPIATES FOR THE TREATMENT OF PAIN IN CANCER PATIENTS TOLERANT TO, OR UNRESPONSIVE TO, INTRASPINAL OPIATES | FUJISAWA PHARMACEUTICAL CO.<br>3 PARKWAY NORTH<br>DEERFIELD IL 60015-2548<br>DD 01/24/89 |
| CLOSTRIDIAL COLLAGENASE | TREATMENT OF ADVANCED (INVOLUTIONAL OR RESIDUAL STAGE) DUPUYTREN'S DISEASE | HURST, L. M.D. & BADALAMENTE, M. PH.D.<br>STATE UNIVERSITY OF NEW YORK AT STONY BROOK<br>SCHOOL OF MEDICINE, HEALTH SCIENCES CENTER<br>T18-020<br>STONY BROOK NY 11794 |
| CLOTRIMIDAZOLE | TREATMENT OF SICKLE CELL DISEASE | BRUGNARA, CARLO, M.D.<br>THE CHILDREN'S HOSPITAL<br>BOSTON MA 02115<br>DD 04/24/95 |
| COAGULATION FACTOR IX<br>TN is MONONINE | REPLACEMENT TREATMENT AND PROPHYLAXIS OF THE HEMORRHAGIC COMPLICATIONS OF HEMOPHILIA B | ARMOUR PHARMACEUTICAL COMPANY<br>500 ARCOLA ROAD, P.O. BOX 1200<br>COLLEGEVILLE PA 19426-0107<br>DD 06/27/89 MA 08/20/92 |
| COAGULATION FACTOR IX (HUMAN)<br>TN is ALPHANINE | FOR USE AS REPLACEMENT THERAPY IN PATIENTS WITH HEMOPHILIA B FOR THE PREVENTION AND CONTROL OF BLEEDING EPISODES, AND DURING SURGERY TO CORRECT DEFECTIVE HEMOSTASIS | ALPHA THERAPEUTIC CORPORATION<br>555 VALLEY BLVD<br>LOS ANGELES CA 90032<br>DD 07/05/90 MA 12/31/90 |
| COAGULATION FACTOR IX (RECOMBINANT) | TREATMENT OF HEMOPHILIA B | GENETICS INSTITUTE, INCORPORATED<br>87 CAMBRIDGE PARK DRIVE<br>CAMBRIDGE MA 02140<br>DD 10/03/94 |

## CUMULATIVE LIST OF ORPHAN PRODUCT DESIGNATIONS AND APPROVALS
[Through October 31, 1998] *(continued)*

| NAME<br>*Generic/Chemical*<br>*TN is Trade Name* | INDICATION DESIGNATED | SPONSOR AND ADDRESS<br>*DD is Date Designated*<br>*MA is Marketing Approval* |
|---|---|---|
| COLCHICINE | ARRESTING THE PROGRESSION OF NEUROLOGIC DISABILITY CAUSED BY CHRONIC PROGRESSIVE MULTIPLE SCLEROSIS | PHARMACONTROL CORPORATION<br>661 PALISADE AVE.<br>P.O. BOX 931<br>ENGLEWOOD CLIFFS NJ 07632<br>DD 12/09/85 |
| COLFOSCERIL PALMITATE, CETYL ALCOHOL, TYLOXAPOL<br>TN is EXOSURF NEONATAL FOR INTRATRACHEAL SUSPENSION | PREVENTION OF HYALINE MEMBRANE DISEASE (HMD), ALSO KNOWN AS RESPIRATORY DISTRESS SYNDROME (RDS), IN INFANTS BORN AT 32 WEEKS GESTATION OR LESS | BURROUGHS WELLCOME COMPANY<br>3030 CORNWALLIS ROAD<br>RESEARCH TRIANGLE PK NC 27709<br>DD 10/20/89 MA 08/02/90 |
| COLFOSCERIL PALMITATE, CETYL ALCOHOL, TYLOXAPOL<br>TN is EXOSURF NEONATAL FOR INTRATRACHEAL SUSPENSION | TREATMENT OF ESTABLISHED HYALINE MEMBRANE DISEASE (HMD) AT ALL GESTATIONAL AGES | BURROUGHS WELLCOME COMPANY<br>3030 CORNWALLIS ROAD<br>RESEARCH TRIANGLE PK NC 27709<br>DD 10/20/89 MA 08/02/90 |
| COLFOSCERIL PALMITATE, CETYL ALCOHOL, TYLOXAPOL<br>TN is EXOSURF | TREATMENT OF ADULT RESPIRATORY DISTRESS SYNDROME | BURROUGHS WELLCOME COMPANY<br>3030 CORNWALLIS ROAD<br>RESEARCH TRIANGLE PK NC 27709<br>DD 01/11/93 |
| COLLAGENASE (LYOPHILIZED) FOR INJECTION<br>TN is PLAQUASC | TREATMENT OF PEYRONIC'S DISEASE | ADVANCE BIOFACTURES CORPORATION<br>35 WILBUR STREET<br>LYNBROOK NY 11563 |
| COPOLYMER-1<br>TN is COPAXONE | TREATMENT OF MULTIPLE SCLEROSIS | TEVA PHARMACEUTICALS USA<br>1510 DELP DRIVE<br>KULPSVILLE PA 19443<br>DD 11/12/87 |
| CORTICORELIN OVINE TRIFLUTATE<br>TN is ACTHREL | FOR USE IN DIFFERENTIATING PITUITARY AND ECTOPIC PRODUCTION OF ACTH IN PATIENTS WITH ACTH-DEPENDENT CUSHINGS SYNDROME | FERRING LABORATORIES, INC.<br>400 RELLA BOULEVARD, SUITE 201<br>SUFFERN NY 10901<br>DD 11/24/89 |
| CORTICOTROPIN-RELEASING FACTOR, HUMAN<br>TN is XERECEPT | TREATMENT OF PERITUMORAL BRAIN EDEMA | NEUROBIOLOGICAL TECHNOLOGIES, INC.<br>1387 MARINA WAY SOUTH<br>RICHMOND CA 94804 |
| COUMARIN<br>TN is ONCOSTATE | TREATMENT OF RENAL CELL CARCINOMA | SCHAPER AND BRUMMER GmbH & CO., KG<br>1425 BROAD STREET<br>CLIFTON NJ 07013<br>DD 12/22/94 |
| CROMOLYN SODIUM<br>TN is GASTROCROM | TREATMENT OF MASTOCYTOSIS | FISONS CORPORATION<br>755 JEFFERSON RD.<br>P.O. BOX 1710<br>ROCHESTER NY 14603<br>DD 03/08/84 MA 12/22/89 |
| CROMOLYN SODIUM 4% OPHTHALMIC SOLUTION<br>TN is OPTICROM 4% OPHTHALMIC SOLUTION | TREATMENT OF VERNAL KERATOCONJUNCTIVITIS (VKC) | FISONS CORPORATION<br>755 JEFFERSON RD.<br>P.O. BOX 1710<br>ROCHESTER NY 14603<br>DD 07/24/85 MA 10/03/84 |
| CRYPTOSPORIDIUM HYPERIMMUNE BOVINE COLOSTRUM IgG CONCENTRATE | TREATMENT OF DIARRHEA IN AIDS PATIENTS CAUSED BY INFECTION WITH CRYPTOSPORIDIUM PARVUM | IMMUCELL CORPORATION<br>56 EVERGREEN DRIVE<br>PORTLAND ME 04103-1066<br>DD 12/30/91 |
| CY-1503<br>TN is CYLEXIN | TREATMENT OF NEONATES AND INFANTS UNDERGOING CARDIOPULMONARY BYPASS DURING SURGICAL REPAIR OF CONGENITAL HEART LESIONS | CYTEL CORPORATION<br>3525 JOHN HOPKINS COURT<br>SAN DIEGO CA 92121 |
| CY-1503 | TREATMENT OF POST-ISCHEMIC PULMONARY REPERFUSION EDEMA FOLLOWING SURGICAL TREATMENT FOR CHRONIC THROMBOEMBOLIC PULMONARY HYPERTENSION | CYTEL CORPORATION<br>3525 JOHN HOPKINS COURT<br>SAN DIEGO CA 92121<br>DD 12/22/93 |
| CY-1899 | TREATMENT OF CHRONIC ACTIVE HEPATITIS B INFECTION IN HLA-A2 POSITIVE PATIENTS | CYTEL CORPORATION<br>3525 JOHN HOPKINS COURT<br>SAN DIEGO CA 92121<br>DD 03/16/94 |
| CYCLOSPORINE 2% OPHTHALMIC OINTMENT | TREATMENT OF PATIENTS AT HIGH RISK OF GRAFT REJECTION FOLLOWING PENETRATING KERATOPLASTY | ALLERGAN, INC.<br>2525 DUPONT DRIVE<br>P.O. BOX 19534<br>IRVINE CA 92713-9534<br>DD 08/01/91 |
| CYCLOSPORINE 2% OPHTHALMIC OINTMENT | FOR USE IN CORNEAL MELTING SYNDROMES OF KNOWN OR PRESUMED IMMUNOLOGIC ETIOPATHOGENESIS, INCLUDING MOOREN'S ULCER | ALLERGAN, INC.<br>2525 DUPONT DRIVE<br>P.O. BOX 19534<br>IRVINE CA 92713-9534<br>DD 08/01/91 |

# CUMULATIVE LIST OF ORPHAN PRODUCT DESIGNATIONS AND APPROVALS
[Through October 31, 1998] *(continued)*

| NAME<br>*Generic/Chemical*<br>*TN is Trade Name* | INDICATION DESIGNATED | SPONSOR AND ADDRESS<br>*DD is Date Designated*<br>*MA is Marketing Approval* |
|---|---|---|
| CYCLOSPORINE OPHTHALMIC<br>TN is OPTIMMUNE | TREATMENT OF SEVERE KERATOCONJUNCTIVITIS SICCA ASSOCIATED WITH SJOGREN'S SYNDROME | UNIVERSITY OF GEORGIA<br>COLLEGE OF VETERINARY MEDICINE<br>ATHENS GA 30602-7390<br>DD 11/09/88 |
| CYSTEAMINE | TREATMENT OF NEPHROPATHIC CYSTINOSIS | THOENE, JESS, M.D.<br>UNIVERSITY OF MICHIGAN<br>ANN ARBOR MI 48109-0408<br>DD 05/01/86 |
| CYSTEAMINE<br>TN is CYSTAGON | TREATMENT OF NEPHROPATHIC CYSTINOSIS | MYLAN LABORATORIES, INC<br>781 CHESTNUT RIDGE ROAD<br>P.O. BOX 4310<br>MORGANTOWN WV 26504-4310<br>DD 01/25/91 MA 08/15/94 |
| CYSTEAMINE HYDROCHLORIDE | TREATMENT OF CORNEAL CYSTINE CRYSTAL ACCUMULATION IN CYSTINOSIS PATIENTS | SIGMA-TAU PHARMACEUTICALS, INC.<br>800 SOUTH FREDERICK AVENUE<br>GAITHERSBURG MD 20877 |
| CYSTIC FIBROSIS GENE THERAPY | TREATMENT OF CYSTIC FIBROSIS | GENZYME CORPORATION<br>ONE KENDALL SQUARE<br>CAMBRIDGE MA 02139-1562<br>DD 06/30/92 |
| CYSTIC FIBROSIS TR GENE THERAPY (RECOMBINANT ADENOVIRUS)<br>TN is ADgvCFTR.10 | TREATMENT OF CYSTIC FIBROSIS | GENVAC, INCORPORATED<br>12111 PARKLAWN DRIVE<br>ROCKVILLE MD 20852<br>DD 03/09/95 |
| CYSTIC FIBROSIS TRANSMEMBRANE CONDUCTANCE REGULATOR | FOR CYSTIC FIBROSIS TRANSMEMBRANE CONDUCTANCE REGULATOR PROTEIN REPLACEMENT THERAPY IN CYSTIC FIBROSIS PATIENTS | GENZYME CORPORATION<br>ONE KENDALL SQUARE<br>CAMBRIDGE MA 02139<br>DD 01/14/92 |
| CYSTIC FIBROSIS TRANSMEMBRANE CONDUCTANCE REGULATOR GENE | TREATMENT OF CYSTIC FIBROSIS | GENETIC THERAPY, INC.<br>938 CLOPPER ROAD<br>GAITHERSBURG MD 20878<br>DD 01/08/93 |
| CYTOMEGALOVIRUS IMMUNE GLOBULIN (HUMAN) | PREVENTION OR ATTENUATION OF PRIMARY CYTOMEGALOVIRUS DISEASE IN IMMUNOSUPPRESSED RECIPIENTS OF ORGAN TRANSPLANTS | MASS PUB HEALTH BIO LABS<br>305 SOUTH STREET<br>BOSTON MA 02130<br>DD 08/03/87 MA 04/17/90 |
| CYTOMEGALOVIRUS IMMUNE GLOBULIN INTRAVENOUS (HUMAN) | FOR USE IN CONJUNCTION WITH GANCICLOVIR SODIUM FOR THE TREATMENT OF CYTOMEGALOVIRUS PNEUMONIA IN BONE MARROW TRANSPLANT PATIENTS | MILES, INC.<br>4TH & PARKER STREETS<br>BERKELEY CA 94710<br>DD 01/28/91 |
| DAB389IL-2 | TREATMENT OF CUTANEOUS T-CELL LYMPHOMA | SERAGEN, INC.<br>97 SOUTH STREET<br>HOPKINTON MA 01748 |
| DAPSONE | PROPHYLAXIS OF TOXOPLASMOSIS IN SEVERELY IMMUNOCOMPROMISED PATIENTS WITH CD4 COUNTS BELOW 100 | JACOBUS PHARMACEUTICAL COMPANY<br>37 CLEVELAND LANE<br>P.O. BOX 5290<br>PRINCETON NJ 08540<br>DD 11/07/94 |
| DAPSONE USP<br>TN is DAPSONE | PROPHYLAXIS FOR PNEUMOCYSTIS CARINII PNEUMONIA | JACOBUS PHARMACEUTICAL COMPANY<br>P.O. BOX 5290<br>PRINCETON NJ 08540<br>DD 12/24/91 |
| DAPSONE USP<br>TN is DAPSONE | FOR THE COMBINATION TREATMENT OF PNEUMOCYSTIS CARINII PNEUMONIA IN CONJUNCTION WITH TRIMETHOPRIM | JACOBUS PHARMACEUTICAL COMPANY<br>P.O. BOX 5290<br>PRINCETON NJ 08540<br>DD 01/08/92 |
| DEFIBROTIDE | TREATMENT OF THROMBOTIC THROMBOCYTOPENIC PURPURA | CRINOS INTERNATIONAL<br>VIA BELVEDERE 1<br>VILLA GUARDIA ITALY 22079<br>DD 07/05/85 |
| DEHYDREX | TREATMENT OF RECURRENT CORNEAL EROSION UNRESPONSIVE TO CONVENTIONAL THERAPY | HOLLES LABORATORIES, INC.<br>30 FOREST NOTCH<br>COHASSET MA 02025<br>DD 03/05/90 |
| DEHYDROEPIANDROSTERONE | TREATMENT OF SYSTEMIC LUPUS ERYTHEMATOSUS (SLE) AND THE REDUCTION IN THE USE OF STEROIDS IN STEROID-DEPENDENT SLE PATIENTS | GENELABS TECHNOLOGIES, INC.<br>505 PENOBSCOT DRIVE<br>REDWOOD CITY CA 94063<br>DD 07/13/94 |
| DEHYDROEPIANDROSTERONE SULFATE SODIUM | TO ACCELERATE THE RE-EPITHELIALIZATION OF DONOR SITES IN THOSE HOSPITALIZED BURN PATIENTS WHO MUST UNDERGO AUTOLOGOUS SKIN GRAFTING | PARADIGM, INC.<br>2401 FOOTHILL DRIVE<br>SALT LAKE CITY UT 84109 |

## CUMULATIVE LIST OF ORPHAN PRODUCT DESIGNATIONS AND APPROVALS
[Through October 31, 1998] *(continued)*

| NAME<br>*Generic/Chemical*<br>*TN is Trade Name* | INDICATION DESIGNATED | SPONSOR AND ADDRESS<br>*DD is Date Designated*<br>*MA is Marketing Approval* |
| --- | --- | --- |
| DEHYDROEPIANDROSTERONE SULFATE SODIUM | TREATMENT OF SERIOUS BURNS REQUIRING HOSPITALIZATION | PARADIGM, INC.<br>2401 FOOTHILL DRIVE<br>SALT LAKE CITY UT 84109 |
| DEPOFOAM ENCAPSULATED CYTARABINE | TREATMENT OF NEOPLASTIC MENINGITIS | DEPOTECH CORPORATION<br>10450 SCIENCE CENTER DRIVE<br>SAN DIEGO CA 92121<br>DD 06/02/93 |
| DESLORELIN<br>TN is SOMAGARD | TREATMENT OF CENTRAL PRECOCIOUS PUBERTY | ROBERTS PHARMACEUTICAL CORP.<br>6 INDUSTRIAL WAY WEST<br>EATONTOWN NJ 07724<br>DD 11/05/87 |
| DESMOPRESSIN ACETATE | TREATMENT OF MILD HEMOPHILIA A AND VON WILLEBRAND'S DISEASE | RHONE-POULENC RORER PHARM.<br>500 ARCOLA ROAD<br>COLLEGEVILLE PA 19426<br>DD 01/22/91 MA 03/07/94 |
| DEXRAZOXANE<br>TN is ZINECARD | FOR THE PREVENTION OF CARDIOMYOPATHY ASSOCIATED WITH DOXORUBICIN ADMINISTRATION | PHARMACIA, INC.<br>P.O. BOX 16529<br>COLUMBUS OH 43216-6529<br>DD 12/17/91 MA 05/26/95 |
| DEXTRAN AND DEFEROXAMINE<br>TN is BIO-RESCUE | TREATMENT OF ACUTE IRON POISONING | BIOMEDICAL FRONTIERS, INC.<br>1095 10TH AVENUE S.E.<br>MINNEAPOLIS MN 55414<br>DD 03/08/91 |
| DEXTRAN SULFATE (INHALED, AEROSOLIZED)<br>TN is UENDEX | AS AN ADJUNCT TO THE TREATMENT OF CYSTIC FIBROSIS | KENNEDY & HOIDAL, MDs.<br>UNIVERSITY OF UTAH MEDICAL CENTER<br>SALT LAKE CITY UT 84132-1001<br>DD 10/05/90 |
| DEXTRAN SULFATE SODIUM | TREATMENT OF ACQUIRED IMMUNODEFICIENCY SYNDROME (AIDS) | UENO FINE CHEMICALS<br>2-31 KORAIBASHI, HIGASHI-KU<br>OSAKA 541 JAPAN<br>DD 11/19/87 |
| DIANEAL PD-2 PERITONEAL DIALYSIS SOLN WITH 1.1% AMINO ACIDS<br>TN is NUTRINEAL PD-2 PERITONEAL DIALYSIS SOLN WITH 1.1% AMINO ACID | FOR USE AS A NUTRITIONAL SUPPLEMENT FOR THE TREATMENT OF MALNOURISHMENT IN PATIENTS UNDERGOING CONTINUOUS AMBULATORY PERITONEAL DIALYSIS | BAXTER HEALTHCARE CORP.<br>1620 WAUKEGAN ROAD<br>MCGAW PARK IL 60085-6730<br>DD 06/11/92 |
| DIAZEPAM VISCOUS SOLUTION FOR RECTAL ADMINISTRATION | TREATMENT OF ACUTE REPETITIVE SEIZURES | ATHENA NEUROSCIENCES, INC.<br>800F GATEWAY BOULEVARD<br>SOUTH SAN FRANCISCO CA 94080<br>DD 02/25/92 |
| DIBROMODULCITOL | TREATMENT OF RECURRENT INVASIVE OR METASTATIC SQUAMOUS CARCINOMA OF THE CERVIX | BIOPHARMACEUTICS, INC.<br>990 STATION ROAD<br>BELLPORT NY 11713<br>DD 01/23/89 |
| DIETHYLDITHIOCARBAMATE<br>TN is IMUTHIOL | TREATMENT OF ACQUIRED IMMUNODEFICIENCY SYNDROME (AIDS) | CONNAUGHT LABORATORIES<br>ROUTE 611, P.O. BOX 187<br>SWIFTWATER PA 18370-0187<br>DD 04/03/86 |
| DIGOXIN IMMUNE FAB (OVINE)<br>TN is DIGIDOTE | TREATMENT OF LIFE-THREATENING ACUTE CARDIAC GLYCOSIDE INTOXICATION MANIFESTED BY CONDUCTION DISORDERS, ECTOPIC VENTRICULAR ACTIVITY AND (IN SOME CASES) HYPERKALEMIA | BOEHRINGER MANNHEIM CORP.<br>1301 PICCARD DRIVE<br>ROCKVILLE MD 20850<br>DD 03/11/85 |
| DIGOXIN IMMUNE FAB (OVINE)<br>TN is DIGIBIND | TREATMENT OF POTENTIALLY LIFE THREATENING DIGITALIS INTOXICATION IN PATIENTS WHO ARE REFRACTORY TO MANAGEMENT BY CONVENTIONAL THERAPY | BURROUGHS WELLCOME COMPANY<br>3030 CORNWALLIS ROAD<br>RESEARCH TRIANGLE PK NC 27709<br>DD 11/01/84 MA 03/21/86 |
| DIHYDROTESTOSTERONE<br>TN is ANDROGEL-DHT | TREATMENT OF WEIGHT LOSS IN AIDS PATIENTS WITH HIV-ASSOCIATED WASTING | UNIMED PHARMACEUTICALS, INC.<br>2150 EAST LAKE COOK ROAD<br>SUITE 210<br>BUFFALO GROVE IL 60089 |
| DIMETHYL SULFOXIDE | TOPICAL TREATMENT FOR THE PREVENTION OF SOFT TISSUE INJURY FOLLOWING EXTRAVASATION OF CYTOTOXIC DRUGS | CANCER TECHNOLOGIES, INC.<br>7301 EAST 22ND STREET,<br>SUITE 10E<br>TUCSON AZ 85710 |
| DIMETHYL SULFOXIDE | TREATMENT OF INCREASED INTRACRANIAL PRESSURE IN PATIENTS WITH SEVERE, CLOSED-HEAD INJURY, ALSO KNOWN AS TRAUMATIC BRAIN COMA, FOR WHOM NO OTHER EFFECTIVE TREATMENT IS AVAILABLE | PHARMA 21<br>4850 S.W. SCHOLLS FERRY ROAD<br>SUITE 301<br>PORTLAND OR 97225-1686<br>DD 11/22/94 |
| DIMETHYLSULFOXIDE | TREATMENT OF PALMAR-PLANTAR ERYTHRODYSETHESIA SYNDROME | CANCER TECHNOLOGIES, INC.<br>7301 EAST 22ND STREET, SUITE 10E<br>TUCSON AZ 85710 |

# CUMULATIVE LIST OF ORPHAN PRODUCT DESIGNATIONS AND APPROVALS
[Through October 31, 1998] *(continued)*

| NAME<br>*Generic/Chemical*<br>TN is Trade Name | INDICATION DESIGNATED | SPONSOR AND ADDRESS<br>DD is Date Designated<br>MA is Marketing Approval |
|---|---|---|
| DIPALMITOYLPHOSPHATIDYLCHOLINE/PHOSPHATIDYLGLYCEROL<br>TN is ALEC | PREVENTION AND TREATMENT OF NEONATAL RESPIRATORY DISTRESS SYNDROME (RDS) | FORUM PRODUCTS, INC.<br>33 FLYING POINT ROAD<br>SOUTHAMPTON NY 11968<br>DD 07/28/88 |
| DISACCHARIDE TRIPEPTIDE GLYCEROL DIPALMITOYL<br>TN is IMMTHER | TREATMENT OF PULMONARY AND HEPATIC METASTASES IN PATIENTS WITH COLORECTAL ADENOCARCINOMA | IMMUNO THERAPEUTICS, INC.<br>3505 RIVERVIEW CIRCLE<br>MOORHEAD MN 56560-5560<br>DD 03/01/90 |
| DISODIUM CLODRONATE | TREATMENT OF HYPERCALCEMIA OF MALIGNANCY | DISCOVERY EXPERIMENTAL & DEVELOPMENT, INC<br>29949 S.R. 54 WEST<br>WESLEY CHAPEL FL 33543<br>DD 06/16/93 |
| DISODIUM CLODRONATE TETRAHYDRATE<br>TN is BONEFOS | TREATMENT OF INCREASED BONE RESORPTION DUE TO MALIGNANCY | LEIRAS, INCORPORATED<br>1805 CENTENNIAL PARK DRIVE<br>SUITE 450<br>RESTON VA 22091<br>DD 03/05/90 |
| DISODIUM SILIBININ DIHEMISUCCINATE<br>TN is LEGALON | TREATMENT OF HEPATIC INTOXICATION BY AMANITA PHALLOIDES (MUSHROOM POISONING) | PHARMAQUEST CORPORATION<br>4470 REDWOOD HIGHWAY<br>SAN RAFAEL CA 94903<br>DD 07/10/86 |
| DMP 777 | THERAPEUTIC MANAGEMENT OF PATIENTS WITH LUNG DISEASE ATTRIBUTABLE TO CYSTIC FIBROSIS | DUPONT MERCK PHARMACEUTICAL COMPANY<br>DUPONT MERCK PLAZA, MAPLE RUN 2110<br>WILMINGTON DE 19805 |
| DORNASE ALFA<br>TN is PULMOZYME | TO REDUCE MUCOUS VISCOSITY AND ENABLE THE CLEARANCE OF AIRWAY SECRETIONS IN PATIENTS WITH CYSTIC FIBROSIS | GENENTECH, INC.<br>460 POINT SAN BRUNO BOULEVARD<br>SOUTH SAN FRANCISCO CA 94080<br>DD 01/16/91 MA 12/30/93 |
| DRONABINOL<br>TN is MARINOL | FOR THE STIMULATION OF APPETITE AND PREVENTION OF WEIGHT LOSS IN PATIENTS WITH A CONFIRMED DIAGNOSIS OF ACQUIRED IMMUNODEFICIENCY SYNDROME (AIDS) | UNIMED, INC.<br>2150 EAST LAKE COOK ROAD<br>BUFFALO GROVE IL 60089<br>DD 01/15/91 MA 12/22/92 |
| DYNAMINE | TREATMENT OF LAMBERT EATON MYASTHENIC SYNDROME | MAYO FOUNDATION<br>200 S.W. 1ST AVENUE<br>ROCHESTER MN 55905<br>DD 02/05/90 |
| DYNAMINE | TREATMENT OF HEREDITARY MOTOR AND SENSORY NEUROPATHY TYPE I (CHARCOT-MARIE-TOOTH DISEASE) | MAYO FOUNDATION<br>200 FIRST STREET SOUTHWEST<br>ROCHESTER MN 55905<br>DD 10/16/91 |
| EFLORNITHINE HCL<br>TN is ORNIDYL | TREATMENT OF TRYPANOSOMA BRUCEI GAMBIENSE INFECTION (SLEEPING SICKNESS) | MARION MERRELL DOW, INC.<br>P.O. BOX 9707, MARION PARK DRIVE<br>KANSAS CITY MO 64134-0707<br>DD 04/23/86 MA 11/28/90 |
| ELCATONIN | INTRATHECAL TREATMENT OF INTRACTABLE PAIN | INNAPHARMA, INC.<br>75 MONTEBELLO ROAD<br>SUFFERN NY 10901 |
| ELLIOTT'S B SOLUTION | TREATMENT OF ACUTE LYMPHOCYTIC LEUKEMIAS AND ACUTE LYMPHOBLASTIC LYMPHOMAS | ORPHAN MEDICAL<br>13911 RIDGEDALE DRIVE<br>MINNETONKA MN 55305<br>DD 08/24/94 |
| ENADOLINE HYDROCHLORIDE | TREATMENT OF SEVERE HEAD INJURY | WARNER-LAMBERT COMPANY<br>PARKE-DAVIS PHARMACEUTICAL RESEARCH DIVISION<br>2800 PLYMOUTH ROAD<br>ANN ARBOR MI 48105 |
| ENCAPSULATED PORCINE ISLET PREPARATION<br>TN is BETARX | TREATMENT OF TYPE I DIABETIC PATIENTS WHO ARE ALREADY ON IMMUNOSUPPRESSION | VIVORX<br>3212 NEBRASKA AVENUE<br>SANTA MONICA CA 90404<br>DD 07/05/95 |
| EPIDERMAL GROWTH FACTOR (HUMAN) | ACCELERATION OF CORNEAL EPITHELIAL REGENERATION AND THE HEALING OF STROMAL TISSUE IN THE CONDITION OF NON-HEALING CORNEAL DEFECTS | CHIRON VISION<br>500 IOLAB DRIVE<br>CLAREMONT CA 91711<br>DD 10/05/87 |
| EPOETIN ALFA<br>TN is EPOGEN | TREATMENT OF ANEMIA ASSOCIATED WITH END STAGE RENAL DISEASE (ESRD) | AMGEN, INC.<br>1840 DEHAVILLAND DRIVE<br>THOUSAND OAKS CA 91320-1789<br>DD 04/10/86 MA 06/01/89 |

# CUMULATIVE LIST OF ORPHAN PRODUCT DESIGNATIONS AND APPROVALS
[Through October 31, 1998] *(continued)*

| NAME<br>*Generic/Chemical*<br>*TN is Trade Name* | INDICATION DESIGNATED | SPONSOR AND ADDRESS<br>*DD is Date Designated*<br>*MA is Marketing Approval* |
|---|---|---|
| EPOETIN ALFA<br>TN is EPOGEN | TREATMENT OF ANEMIA ASSOCIATED WITH HIV INFECTION OR HIV TREATMENT | AMGEN, INC.<br>1840 DEHAVILLAND DRIVE<br>THOUSAND OAKS CA 91320-1789<br>DD 07/01/91 MA 12/31/90 |
| EPOETIN ALFA | TREATMENT OF MYELODYSPLASTIC SYNDROME | R.W. JOHNSON RESEARCH INSTITUTE<br>ROUTE 202, P.O. BOX 300<br>RARITAN NJ 08869-0602<br>DD 12/20/93 |
| EPOETIN ALFA<br>TN is PROCRIT | TREATMENT OF ANEMIA ASSOCIATED WITH END STAGE RENAL DISEASE | R.W. JOHNSON RESEARCH INSTITUTE<br>ROUTE 202, P.O. BOX 300<br>RARITAN NJ 08869-0602<br>DD 08/27/87 |
| EPOETIN ALFA<br>TN is PROCRIT | TREATMENT OF ANEMIA OF PREMATURITY IN PRETERM INFANTS | R.W. JOHNSON RESEARCH INSTITUTE<br>ROUTE 202, P.O. BOX 300<br>RARITAN NJ 08869-0602<br>DD 07/21/88 |
| EPOETIN ALFA<br>TN is PROCRIT | TREATMENT OF HIV ASSOCIATED ANEMIA RELATED TO HIV INFECTION OR HIV TREATMENT | R.W. JOHNSON RESEARCH INSTITUTE<br>ROUTE 202, P.O. BOX 300<br>RARITAN NJ 08869-0602<br>DD 03/07/89 |
| EPOETIN BETA<br>TN is MAROGEN | TREATMENT OF ANEMIA ASSOCIATED WITH END STAGE RENAL DISEASE (ESRD) | CHUGAI-USA, INC.<br>3780 HAWTHORN COURT<br>WAUKEGAN IL 60087<br>DD 10/22/87 |
| EPOPROSTENOL<br>TN is FLOLAN | TREATMENT OF PRIMARY PULMONARY HYPERTENSION (PPH) | BURROUGHS WELLCOME COMPANY<br>3030 CORNWALLIS ROAD<br>RESEARCH TRIANGLE PK NC 27709<br>DD 09/25/85 |
| EPOPROSTENOL<br>TN is FLOLAN | REPLACEMENT OF HEPARIN IN PATIENTS REQUIRING HEMODIALYSIS AND WHO ARE AT INCREASED RISK OF HEMORRHAGE | BURROUGHS WELLCOME COMPANY<br>3030 CORNWALLIS ROAD<br>RESEARCH TRIANGLE PK NC 27709<br>DD 03/29/84 |
| ERWINIA L-ASPARAGINASE<br>TN is ERWINASE | TREATMENT OF ACUTE LYMPHOCYTIC LEUKEMIA | PORTON INTERNATIONAL, INC.<br>816 CONNECTICUT AVENUE NW<br>WASHINGTON DC 20006<br>DD 07/30/86 |
| ERYTHROPOIETIN (RECOMBINANT HUMAN) | TREATMENT OF ANEMIA ASSOCIATED WITH END STAGE RENAL DISEASE | MCDONNELL DOUGLAS CORP<br>P.O. BOX 516<br>ST. LOUIS MO 63166<br>DD 08/19/87 |
| ETHANOLAMINE OLEATE<br>TN is ETHAMOLIN | TREATMENT OF PATIENTS WITH ESOPHAGEAL VARICES THAT HAVE RECENTLY BLED, TO PREVENT REBLEEDING | BLOCK DRUG COMPANY, INC.<br>257 CORNELISON AVENUE<br>JERSEY CITY NJ 07302<br>DD 03/22/84 MA 12/12/88 |
| ETHINYL ESTRADIOL, USP | TREATMENT OF TURNER'S SYNDROME | BIO-TECHNOLOGY GENERAL CORP.<br>70 WOOD AVENUE, SOUTH<br>ISELIN NJ 08830<br>DD 06/22/88 |
| ETIDRONATE DISODIUM<br>TN is DIDRONEL | TREATMENT OF HYPERCALCEMIA OF A MALIGNANCY INADEQUATELY MANAGED BY DIETARY MODIFICATION AND/OR ORAL HYDRATION | MGI PHARMA, INC.<br>9900 BREN ROAD EAST, SUITE 300E<br>MINNEAPOLIS MN 55343-9667<br>DD 03/21/86 MA 04/21/87 |
| ETIOCHOLANEDIONE | TREATMENT OF APLASTIC ANEMIA | SUPERGEN, INC.<br>3158 DES PLAINES AVENUE<br>SUITE 10<br>DES PLAINES IL 60018 |
| ETIOCHOLANEDIONE | TREATMENT OF PRADER-WILLI SYNDROME | SUPERGEN, INC.<br>3158 DES PLAINES AVENUE<br>SUITE 10<br>DES PLAINES IL 60018 |
| EXEMESTANE | HORMONAL THERAPY OF METASTATIC CARCINOMA OF THE BREAST | PHARMACIA, INC.<br>P.O. BOX 16529<br>COLUMBUS OH 43216-6529<br>DD 09/19/91 |
| FACTOR VIIa (RECOMBINANT, DNA ORIGIN) | TREATMENT OF PATIENTS WITH HEMOPHILIA A AND B WITH AND WITHOUT ANTIBODIES AGAINST FACTORS VIII/IX, AND PATIENTS WITH VON WILLEBRAND'S DISEASE | NOVO NORDISK PHARMACEUTICALS<br>100 OVERLOOK CENTER, SUITE 200<br>PRINCETON NJ 08540-7810<br>DD 06/06/88 |
| FACTOR XIII (PLACENTA-DERIVED)<br>TN is FIBROGAMMIN P | TREATMENT OF CONGENITAL FACTOR XIII DEFICIENCY | BEHRINGWERKE (ARMOUR, U.S. AGENT)<br>500 ARCOLA ROAD<br>P.O. BOX 1200<br>COLLEGEVILLE PA 19426-0107<br>DD 01/16/85 |

# CUMULATIVE LIST OF ORPHAN PRODUCT DESIGNATIONS AND APPROVALS
[Through October 31, 1998] *(continued)*

| NAME<br>*Generic/Chemical*<br>*TN is Trade Name* | INDICATION DESIGNATED | SPONSOR AND ADDRESS<br>*DD is Date Designated*<br>*MA is Marketing Approval* |
|---|---|---|
| FAMPRIDINE<br>TN is NEURELAN | RELIEF OF SYMPTOMS OF MULTIPLE SCLEROSIS | ELAN PHARMACEUTICAL RESEARCH<br>1300 GOULD DRIVE<br>GAINESVILLE GA 30501<br>DD 06/02/87 |
| FAMPRIDINE | TREATMENT OF CHRONIC, INCOMPLETE SPINAL CORD INJURY | ACORDA THERAPEUTICS, INC.<br>145 WEST 58TH STREET,<br>SUITE 8J<br>NEW YORK NY 10019 |
| FELBAMATE<br>TN is FELBATOL | TREATMENT OF LENNOX-GASTAUT SYNDROME | WALLACE LABORATORIES<br>301B COLLEGE ROAD EAST<br>PRINCETON NJ 08540<br>DD 01/24/89 MA 07/29/93 |
| FGN-1 | FOR THE SUPPRESSION AND CONTROL OF COLONIC ADENOMATOUS POLYPS IN THE INHERITED DISEASE ADENOMATOUS POLYPOSIS COLI | CELL PATHWAYS, INC.<br>1300 SOUTH POTOMAC<br>SUITE 110<br>AURORA CO 80012-4256<br>DD 02/14/94 |
| FIAU | ADJUNCTIVE TREATMENT OF CHRONIC ACTIVE HEPATITIS B | OCLASSEN PHARMACEUTICALS, INC.<br>ELI LILLY AND COMPANY<br>INDIANAPOLIS IN 46285<br>DD 07/24/92 |
| FIBRINOGEN (HUMAN) | FOR THE CONTROL OF BLEEDING AND PROPHYLACTIC TREATMENT OF PATIENTS DEFICIENT IN FIBRINOGEN | ALPHA THERAPEUTIC CORPORATION<br>5555 VALLEY BOULEVARD<br>LOS ANGELES CA 90032<br>DD 08/21/95 |
| FIBRONECTIN (HUMAN PLASMA DERIVED) | TREATMENT OF NON-HEALING CORNEAL ULCERS OR EPITHELIAL DEFECTS WHICH HAVE BEEN UNRESPONSIVE TO CONVENTIONAL THERAPY AND THE UNDERLYING CAUSE HAS BEEN ELIMINATED | NEW YORK BLOOD CENTER<br>310 E. 67TH STREET<br>NEW YORK NY 10021<br>DD 09/05/88 |
| FILGRASTIM<br>TN is NEUPOGEN | TREATMENT OF MYELODYSPLASTIC SYNDROME | AMGEN, INC.<br>1840 DEHAVILLAND DRIVE<br>THOUSAND OAKS CA 91320-1789<br>DD 08/30/90 |
| FILGRASTIM<br>TN is NEUPOGEN | REDUCTION IN THE DURATION OF NEUTROPENIA, FEVER, ANTIBIOTIC USE, AND HOSPITALIZATION, FOLLOWING INDUCTION AND CONSOLIDATION TREATMENT FOR ACUTE MYELOID LEUKEMIA | AMGEN, INC.<br>1840 DEHAVILAND DRIVE<br>THOUSAND OAKS CA 91320 |
| FILGRASTIM<br>TN is NEUPOGEN | TREATMENT OF PATIENTS WITH SEVERE CHRONIC NEUTROPENIA (ABSOLUTE NEUTROPHIL COUNT LESS THAN 500/MM3) | AMGEN, INC.<br>1840 DEHAVILLAND DRIVE<br>THOUSAND OAKS CA 91320-1789<br>DD 11/07/90 MA 12/19/94 |
| FILGRASTIM<br>TN is NEUPOGEN | TREATMENT OF NEUTROPENIA ASSOCIATED WITH BONE MARROW TRANSPLANTS | AMGEN, INC.<br>1840 DEHAVILLAND DRIVE<br>THOUSAND OAKS CA 91320-1789<br>DD 10/01/90 MA 06/15/94 |
| FILGRASTIM<br>TN is NEUPOGEN | TREATMENT OF PATIENTS WITH ACQUIRED IMMUNODEFICIENCY SYNDROME (AIDS) WHO, IN ADDITION, ARE AFFLICTED WITH CYTOMEGALOVIRUS RETINITIS (CMV RETINITIS) AND ARE BEING TREATED WITH GANCICLOVIR | AMGEN, INC.<br>1840 DEHAVILLAND DRIVE<br>THOUSAND OAKS CA 91320-1789<br>DD 09/03/91 |
| FILGRASTIM<br>TN is NEUPOGEN | FOR USE IN THE MOBILIZATION OF PERIPHERAL BLOOD PROGENITOR CELLS FOR COLLECTION IN PATIENTS WHO WILL RECEIVE MYELOABLATIVE OR MYELOSUPPRESSIVE CHEMOTHERAPY | AMGEN, INCORPORATED<br>1840 DEHAVILLAND DRIVE<br>THOUSAND OAKS CA 91320-1789<br>DD 07/17/95 |
| FLUDARABINE PHOSPHATE<br>TN is FLUDARA | TREATMENT OF CHRONIC LYMPHOCYTIC LEUKEMIA (CLL), INCLUDING REFRACTORY CLL | BERLEX LABORATORIES, INC.<br>15049 SAN PABLO AVENUE<br>P.O. BOX 4099<br>RICHMOND CA 94804-0099<br>DD 04/18/89 MA 04/18/91 |
| FLUDARABINE PHOSPHATE<br>TN is FLUDARA | TREATMENT AND MANAGEMENT OF PATIENTS WITH NON-HODGKINS LYMPHOMA | BERLEX LABORATORIES, INC.<br>15049 SAN PABLO AVENUE<br>P.O. BOX 4099<br>RICHMOND CA 94804-0099<br>DD 04/18/89 |
| FLUMECINOL<br>TN is ZIXORYN | TREATMENT OF HYPERBILIRUBINEMIA IN NEWBORN INFANTS UNRESPONSIVE TO PHOTOTHERAPY | FARMACON, INC.<br>90 GROVE STREET, SUITE 109<br>RIDGEFIELD CT 06877-4118<br>DD 01/15/85 |
| FLUNARIZINE<br>TN is SIBELIUM | TREATMENT OF ALTERNATING HEMIPLEGIA | JANSSEN RESEARCH FOUNDATION<br>1125 TRENTON-HARBOURTON ROAD<br>P.O. BOX 200<br>TITUSVILLE NJ 08560-0200<br>DD 01/06/86 |

# CUMULATIVE LIST OF ORPHAN PRODUCT DESIGNATIONS AND APPROVALS
[Through October 31, 1998] *(continued)*

| NAME<br>*Generic/Chemical*<br>*TN is Trade Name* | INDICATION DESIGNATED | SPONSOR AND ADDRESS<br>*DD is Date Designated*<br>*MA is Marketing Approval* |
|---|---|---|
| FLUOROURACIL<br>TN is ADRUCIL | FOR USE IN COMBINATION WITH LEUCOVORIN FOR THERAPY OF METASTATIC ADENOCARCINOMA OF THE COLON AND RECTUM | LEDERLE LABORATORIES DIVISION<br>AMERICAN CYANAMID COMPANY<br>PEARL RIVER NY 10965<br>DD 02/06/89 |
| FLUOROURACIL | FOR USE IN COMBINATION WITH INTERFERON ALPHA-2A, RECOMBINANT, FOR THE TREATMENT OF ESOPHAGEAL CARCINOMA | HOFFMANN-LA ROCHE, INC.<br>340 KINGSLAND STREET<br>NUTLEY NJ 07110-1199<br>DD 10/27/89 |
| FLUOROURACIL | FOR USE IN COMBINATION WITH INTERFERON ALPHA-2A, RECOMBINANT, FOR THE TREATMENT OF ADVANCED COLORECTAL CARCINOMA | HOFFMANN-LA ROCHE, INC.<br>340 KINGSLAND STREET<br>NUTLEY NJ 07110-1199<br>DD 04/18/90 |
| FOSPHENYTOIN | ACUTE TREATMENT OF PATIENTS WITH STATUS EPILEPTICUS OF THE GRAND MAL TYPE | WARNER-LAMBERT COMPANY<br>2800 PLYMOUTH ROAD<br>ANN ARBOR MI 48105-1047<br>DD 06/04/91 |
| FRUCTOSE-1,6-DIPHOSPHATE | TREATMENT OF PAINFUL VASO-OCCLUSIVE EPISODES ASSOCIATED WITH SICKLE CELL DISEASE | CYPROS PHARMACEUTICAL CORPORATION<br>2714 LOKER AVENUE WEST<br>CARLSBAD CA 92008 |
| GABAPENTIN<br>TN is NEURONTIN | TREATMENT OF AMYOTROPHIC LATERAL SCLEROSIS | WARNER-LAMBERT COMPANY<br>PARKE-DAVIS PHARMACEUTICAL RESEARCH DIV.<br>ANN ARBOR MI 48105-2430<br>DD 07/05/95 |
| GALLIUM NITRATE INJECTION<br>TN is GANITE | TREATMENT OF HYPERCALCEMIA OF MALIGNANCY | SOLOPAK PHARMACEUTICAL CO.<br>1845 TONNE ROAD<br>ELK GROVE VILLAGE IL 60007<br>DD 12/05/88 MA 01/17/91 |
| GAMMA-HYDROXYBUTYRATE | TREATMENT OF NARCOLEPSY | ORPHAN MEDICAL<br>13911 RIDGEDALE DRIVE<br>MINNETONKA MN 55305<br>DD 11/07/94 |
| GAMMALINOLENIC ACID | TREATMENT OF JUVENILE RHEUMATOID ARTHRITIS | ZURIER, ROBERT B., M.D.<br>55 LAKE AVE.<br>UNIV. OF MASS. MED. CTR.<br>WORCESTER MA 01655<br>DD 07/27/94 |
| GENTAMICIN IMPREGNATED PMMA BEADS ON SURGICAL WIRE<br>TN is SEPTOPAL | TREATMENT OF CHRONIC OSTEOMYELITIS OF POST-TRAUMATIC, POSTOPERATIVE, OR HEMATOGENOUS ORIGIN | EM INDUSTRIES, INC.<br>5 SKYLINE DRIVE<br>HAWTHORNE NY 10532<br>DD 01/31/91 |
| GENTAMICIN LIPOSOME INJECTION<br>TN is MAITEC | TREATMENT OF DISSEMINATED MYCOBACTERIUM AVIUM-INTRACELLULARE INFECTION | THE LIPOSOME COMPANY, INC.<br>ONE RESEARCH WAY<br>PRINCETON NJ 08540<br>DD 07/10/90 |
| GLUTAMINE | FOR USE WITH HUMAN GROWTH HORMONE IN THE TREATMENT OF SHORT BOWEL SYNDROME (NUTRIENT MALABSORPTION FROM THE GASTROINTESTINAL TRACT RESULTING FROM AN INADEQUATE ABSORPTIVE SURFACE) | RESEARCH TRIANGLE PHARMACEUTICALS<br>4364 SOUTH ALSTON AVENUE<br>DURHAM NC 27713<br>DD 03/06/95 |
| GLYCERYL TRIOLEATE AND GLYCERYL TRIERUCATE<br>TN is LORENZO'S OIL | TREATMENT OF ADRENOLEUKODYSTROPHY | MOSER, HUGO W., M.D.<br>JOHNS HOPKINS UNIVERSITY<br>BALTIMORE MD 21205<br>DD 02/14/95 |
| GONADORELIN ACETATE<br>TN is LUTREPULSE | INDUCTION OF OVULATION IN WOMEN WITH HYPOTHALAMIC AMENORRHEA DUE TO A DEFICIENCY OR ABSENCE IN THE QUANTITY OR PULSE PATTERN OF ENDOGENOUS GNRH SECRETION | FERRING LABORATORIES, INC.<br>400 RELLA BOULEVARD, SUITE 201<br>SUFFERN NY 10901-4249<br>DD 04/22/87 MA 10/10/89 |
| GOSSYPOL | TREATMENT OF CANCER OF THE ADRENAL CORTEX | REIDENBERG, MARCUS M., M.D.<br>525 EAST 68TH STREET, BOX 70<br>NEW YORK NY 10021<br>DD 10/22/90 |
| GP 100 ADENOVIRAL GENE THERAPY | TREATMENT OF METASTATIC MELANOMA | GENZYME<br>P.O. BOX 9322<br>ONE MOUNTAIN ROAD<br>FRAMINGHAM MA 01701 |
| GROUP B STREPTOCOCCUS IMMUNE GLOBULIN | TREATMENT OF NEONATES FOR DISSEMINATED GROUP B STREPTOCOCCAL INFECTION | UNIVAX BIOLOGICS, INC.<br>12280 WILKINS AVENUE<br>ROCKVILLE MD 20852<br>DD 05/08/90 |

# CUMULATIVE LIST OF ORPHAN PRODUCT DESIGNATIONS AND APPROVALS
[Through October 31, 1998] *(continued)*

| NAME<br>*Generic/Chemical*<br>*TN is Trade Name* | INDICATION DESIGNATED | SPONSOR AND ADDRESS<br>*DD is Date Designated*<br>*MA is Marketing Approval* |
|---|---|---|
| GROWTH HORMONE RELEASING FACTOR | FOR THE LONG-TERM TREATMENT OF CHILDREN WHO HAVE GROWTH FAILURE DUE TO A LACK OF ADEQUATE ENDOGENOUS GROWTH HORMONE SECRETION | ICN PHARMACEUTICALS<br>3300 HYLAND AVENUE<br>COSTA MESA CA 92626<br>DD 08/07/89 |
| GUANETHIDINE MONOSULFATE<br>TN is ISMELIN | TREATMENT OF MODERATE TO SEVERE REFLEX SYMPATHETIC DYSTROPHY AND CAUSALGIA | CIBA-GEIGY CORPORATION<br>556 MORRIS AVENUE<br>SUMMIT NJ 07901<br>DD 01/06/86 |
| GUSPERIMUS<br>TN is SPANIDIN | TREATMENT OF ACUTE RENAL GRAFT REJECTION EPISODES | BRISTOL-MYERS SQUIBB COMPANY<br>5 RESEARCH PARKWAY<br>P.O. BOX 5100<br>WALLINGFORD CT 06492 |
| HALOFANTRINE<br>TN is HALFAN | TREATMENT OF MILD TO MODERATE ACUTE MALARIA CAUSED BY SUSCEPTIBLE STRAINS OF P. FALCIPARUM AND P. VIVAX | SMITHKLINE BEECHAM<br>P.O. BOX 1510<br>KING OF PRUSSIA PA 19406<br>DD 11/04/91 MA 07/24/92 |
| HEME ARGINATE<br>TN is NORMOSANG | TREATMENT OF SYMPTOMATIC STAGE OF ACUTE PORPHYRIA | LEIRAS, INCORPORATED<br>1850 CENTENNIAL PARK DRIVE<br>SUITE 450<br>RESTON VA 22091<br>DD 03/10/88 |
| HEME ARGINATE<br>TN is NORMOSANG | TREATMENT OF MYELODYSPLASTIC SYNDROMES | LEIRAS, INCORPORATED<br>1850 CENTENNIAL PARK DRIVE<br>SUITE 450<br>RESTON VA 22091<br>DD 03/01/94 |
| HEMIN<br>TN is PANHEMATIN | AMELIORIATION OF RECURRENT ATTACKS OF ACUTE INTERMITTENT PORPHYRIA (AIP) TEMPORARILY RELATED TO THE MENSTRUAL CYCLE IN SUSCEPTIBLE WOMEN AND SIMILAR SYMPTOMS WHICH OCCUR IN OTHER PATIENTS WITH AIP, PORPHYRIA VARIEGATA AND HEREDITA COPROPORPHYRIA | ABBOTT LABORATORIES<br>DIAGNOSTICS DIVISION<br>ABBOTT PARK IL 60064<br>DD 03/16/84 MA 07/20/83 |
| HEMIN AND ZINC MESOPORPHYRIN<br>TN is HEMEX | TREATMENT OF ACUTE PORPHYRIC SYNDROMES | BONKOVSKY, HERBERT L., M.D.<br>UNIV. OF MASS. MED. CTR.<br>WORCESTER MA 01655<br>DD 12/20/93 |
| HEPATITIS B IMMUNE GLOBULIN, INTRAVENOUS<br>TN is H-BIGIV | PROPHYLAXIS AGAINST HEPATITIS B VIRUS REINFECTION IN LIVER TRANSPLANT PATIENTS | NORTH AMERICAN BIOLOGICS, INC.<br>16500 N.W. 15TH AVENUE<br>MIAMI FL 33169<br>DD 03/08/95 |
| HERPES SIMPLEX VIRUS GENE | TREATMENT OF PRIMARY AND METASTATIC BRAIN TUMORS | GENETIC THERAPY, INC.<br>938 CLOPPER ROAD<br>GAITHERSBURG MD 20878<br>DD 10/16/92 |
| HISTRELIN | TREATMENT OF ACUTE INTERMITTENT PORPHYRIA, HEREDITARY COPROPORPHYRIA, AND VARIEGATE PORPHYRIA | ANDERSON, KARL E., M.D.<br>U. OF TEXAS MEDICAL BRANCH<br>GALVESTON TX 77550<br>DD 05/03/91 |
| HISTRELIN ACETATE<br>TN is SUPPRELIN INJECTION | TREATMENT OF CENTRAL PRECOCIOUS PUBERTY | ROBERTS PHARMACEUTICAL CORP.<br>6 INDUSTRIAL WAY WEST<br>EATONTOWN NJ 07724<br>DD 08/10/88 MA 12/24/91 |
| HIV NEUTRALIZING ANTIBODIES<br>TN is IMMUPATH | TREATMENT OF ACQUIRED IMMUNODEFICIENCY SYNDROME (AIDS) | HEMACARE CORPORATION<br>4954 VAN NUYS BOULEVARD<br>SHERMAN OAKS CA 91403<br>DD 03/24/92 |
| HUMAN ACID ALPHA-GLUCOSIDASE | TREATMENT OF GLYCOGEN STORAGE DISEASE TYPE II | PHARMING B.V.<br>NIELS BOHRWEG 11-13<br>2333 CA LEIDEN<br>THE NETHERLANDS |
| HUMAN GROWTH HORMONE | FOR USE WITH GLUTAMINE IN THE TREATMENT OF SHORT BOWEL SYNDROME (NUTRIENT MALABSORPTION FROM THE GASTROINTESTINAL TRACT RESULTING FROM AN INADEQUATE ABSORPTIVE SURFACE) | RESEARCH TRIANGLE PHARMACEUTICALS<br>4364 SOUTH ALSTON AVENUE<br>DURHAM NC 27713<br>DD 03/06/95 |
| HUMAN IMMUNODEFICIENCY VIRUS IMMUNE GLOBULIN | TREATMENT OF AIDS | NORTH AMERICAN BIOLOGICALS, INC.<br>16500 N.W. 15TH AVENUE<br>MIAMI FL 33169<br>DD 11/21/89 |
| HUMAN IMMUNODEFICIENCY VIRUS IMMUNE GLOBULIN | TREATMENT OF HIV-INFECTED PREGNANT WOMEN AND INFANTS OF HIV-INFECTED MOTHERS | NORTH AMERICAN BIOLOGICALS, INC.<br>16500 N.W. 15TH AVENUE<br>MIAMI FL 33169<br>DD 03/25/92 |

# CUMULATIVE LIST OF ORPHAN PRODUCT DESIGNATIONS AND APPROVALS
[Through October 31, 1998] *(continued)*

| NAME<br>*Generic/Chemical*<br>*TN is Trade Name* | INDICATION DESIGNATED | SPONSOR AND ADDRESS<br>*DD is Date Designated*<br>*MA is Marketing Approval* |
|---|---|---|
| HUMAN IMMUNODEFICIENCY VIRUS IMMUNE GLOBULIN<br>TN is HIVIG | TREATMENT OF HIV-INFECTED PEDIATRIC PATIENTS | NORTH AMERICAN BIOLOGICALS, INC.<br>16500 N.W. 15TH AVENUE<br>MIAMI FL 33169<br>DD 01/04/95 |
| HUMAN RETINAL PIGMENTED EPITHELIAL CELLS ON COLLAGEN MICROCARRIERS<br>TN is SPHERAMINE | TREATMENT OF HOEHN AND YAHR STAGE 3 AND 4 PARKINSON'S DISEASE | THERACELL, INC.<br>50 DIVISION STREET, SUITE 503<br>SOMERVILLE NJ 08876 |
| HUMAN T-LYMPHOTROPIC VIRUS TYPE III gp160 ANTIGENS<br>TN is VAXSYN HIV-1 | TREATMENT OF ACQUIRED IMMUNODEFICIENCY SYNDROME (AIDS) | MICROGENESYS, INC.<br>1000 RESEARCH PARKWAY<br>MERIDEN CT 06450<br>DD 11/20/89 |
| HUMAN THYROID STIMULATING HORMONE (TSH)<br>TN is THYROGEN | AS AN ADJUNCT IN THE DIAGNOSIS OF THYROID CANCER | GENZYME CORPORATION<br>ONE KENDALL SQUARE<br>CAMBRIDGE MA 02139<br>DD 02/24/92 |
| HUMANIZED ANTI-TAC<br>TN is ZENAPAX | PREVENTION OF ACUTE RENAL ALLOGRAFT REJECTION | HOFFMANN-LA ROCHE, INC.<br>340 KINGSLAND STREET<br>NUTLEY NJ 07110<br>DD 03/05/93 |
| HUMANIZED ANTI-TAC<br>TN is ZENAPAX | PREVENTION OF ACUTE GRAFT-VS-HOST DISEASE FOLLOWING BONE MARROW TRANSPLANTATION | HOFFMANN-LA ROCHE, INC.<br>340 KINGSLAND STREET<br>NUTLEY NJ 07110<br>DD 03/05/93 |
| HYDROXYCOBALAMIN/SODIUM THIOSULFATE | TREATMENT OF SEVERE ACUTE CYANIDE POISONING | HALL, ALAN H., M.D.<br>6200 SOUTH SYRACUSE WAY<br>SUITE 300<br>ENGLEWOOD CO 80111-4740<br>DD 10/04/85 |
| HYDROXYUREA<br>TN is HYDREA | TREATMENT OF PATIENTS WITH SICKLE CELL ANEMIA AS SHOWN BY THE PRESENCE OF HEMOGLOBIN S | BRISTOL-MYERS SQUIBB<br>2400 WEST LLOYD EXPRESSWAY<br>EVANSVILLE IN 47721-0001<br>DD 10/01/90 |
| I-131 RADIOLABELED B1 MONOCLONAL ANTIBODY | TREATMENT OF NON-HODGKIN'S B-CELL LYMPHOMA | COULTER CORPORATION<br>11800 S.W. 147 AVENUE<br>P.O. BOX 169015<br>MIAMI FL 33116-9015<br>DD 05/16/94 |
| IBUPROFEN I.V. SOLUTION<br>TN is SALPROFEN | PREVENTION OF PATENT DUCTUS ARTERIOSUS | FARMACON, INC.<br>90 GROVE STREET, SUITE 109<br>RIDGEFIELD CT 06877 |
| IBUPROFEN I.V. SOLUTION | TREATMENT OF PATENT DUCTUS ARTERIOSUS | FARMACON, INC.<br>90 GROVE STREET<br>RIDGEFIELD CT 06877 |
| ICODEXTRIN 7.5% WITH ELECTROLYTES PERITONEAL DIALYSIS SOLUTION<br>TN is EXTRANEAL (WITH 7.5% ICODEXTRIN) PERITONEAL DIALYSIS SOLUTION) | TREATMENT OF THOSE PATIENTS HAVING END-STAGE RENAL DISEASE AND REQUIRING PERITONEAL DIALYSIS TREATMENT | BAXTER HEALTHCARE CORPORATION<br>RENAL DIVISION<br>1620 WAUKEGAN ROAD<br>WAUKEGAN IL 60085 |
| IDARUBICIN<br>TN is IDAMYCIN | TREATMENT OF MYELODYSPLASTIC SYNDROMES | ADRIA LABORATORIES, INC.<br>P.O. BOX 16529<br>COLUMBUS OH 43216-6529<br>DD 12/01/92 |
| IDARUBICIN<br>TN is IDAMYCIN | TREATMENT OF CHRONIC MYELOGENOUS LEUKEMIA | ADRIA LABORATORIES, INC.<br>P.O. BOX 16529<br>COLUMBUS OH 42316-6529<br>DD 12/02/92 |
| IDARUBICIN HCL FOR INJECTION<br>TN is IDAMYCIN | TREATMENT OF ACUTE MYELOGENOUS LEUKEMIA (AML), ALSO REFERRED TO AS ACUTE NONLYMPHOCYTIC LEUKEMIA (ANLL) | ADRIA LABORATORIES, INC.<br>P.O. BOX 16529<br>COLUMBUS OH 43216-6529<br>DD 07/25/88 MA 09/27/90 |
| IDARUBICIN HCL FOR INJECTION<br>TN is IDAMYCIN | TREATMENT OF ACUTE LYMPHOBLASTIC LEUKEMIA IN PEDIATRIC PATIENTS | ADRIA LABORATORIES, INC.<br>P.O. BOX 16529<br>COLUMBUS OH 43216-6529<br>DD 02/12/91 |
| IDOXURIDINE | TREATMENT OF NONPARENCHYMATOUS SARCOMAS | NEOPHARM, INC.<br>225 EAST DEERPATH, SUITE 250<br>LAKE FOREST IL 60045 |

# CUMULATIVE LIST OF ORPHAN PRODUCT DESIGNATIONS AND APPROVALS
[Through October 31, 1998] *(continued)*

| NAME<br>*Generic/Chemical*<br>*TN is Trade Name* | INDICATION DESIGNATED | SPONSOR AND ADDRESS<br>*DD is Date Designated*<br>*MA is Marketing Approval* |
|---|---|---|
| IFOSFAMIDE<br>TN is IFEX | IN COMBINATION WITH CERTAIN OTHER APPROVED ANTINEOPLASTIC AGENTS, FOR THIRD LINE CHEMOTHERAPY IN THE TREATMENT OF GERM CELL TESTICULAR CANCER | BRISTOL-MYERS SQUIBB<br>P.O. BOX 4000<br>PRINCETON NJ 08543-4000<br>DD 01/20/87 MA 12/30/88 |
| IFOSFAMIDE<br>TN is IFEX | TREATMENT OF BONE SARCOMAS | BRISTOL-MYERS SQUIBB<br>P.O. BOX 4000<br>PRINCETON NJ 08543-4000<br>DD 08/07/85 |
| IFOSFAMIDE<br>TN is IFEX | TREATMENT OF SOFT TISSUE SARCOMAS | BRISTOL-MYERS SQUIBB<br>P.O. BOX 4000<br>PRINCETON NJ 08543-4000<br>DD 08/07/85 |
| IMCIROMAB PENTETATE<br>TN is MYOSCINT | DETECTING EARLY NECROSIS AS AN INDICATION OF REJECTION OF ORTHOTOPIC CARDIAC TRANSPLANTS | CENTOCOR, INC.<br>244 GREAT VALLEY PARKWAY<br>MALVERN PA 19355-1307<br>DD 01/25/89 |
| IMIGLUCERASE<br>TN is CEREZYME | FOR REPLACEMENT THERAPY IN PATIENTS WITH TYPES I, II, AND III GAUCHER'S DISEASE | GENZYME CORPORATION<br>ONE KENDALL SQUARE<br>CAMBRIDGE MA 02139<br>DD 11/05/91 MA 05/23/94 |
| IMMUNE GLOBULIN INTRAVENOUS (HUMAN)<br>TN is IVEEGAM, IMMUNO | TREATMENT OF JUVENILE RHEUMATOID ARTHRITIS | IMMUNO CLINICAL RESEARCH CORP.<br>155 EAST 56TH STREET<br>NEW YORK NY 10022<br>DD 12/16/92 |
| IMMUNE GLOBULIN INTRAVENOUS (HUMAN)<br>TN is IVEEGAM, IMMUNO | TREATMENT OF POLYMYOSITIS/DERMATOMYOSITIS | IMMUNO CLINICAL RESEARCH CORP.<br>155 EAST 56TH STREET<br>NEW YORK NY 10022<br>DD 10/13/92 |
| IMMUNE GLOBULIN INTRAVENOUS (HUMAN)<br>TN is IMMUNE GLOBULIN INTRAVENOUS (HUMAN) IMMUNO, IVEEGAM | TREATMENT OF PATIENTS WITH ACUTE MYOCARDITIS | IMMUNO CLINICAL RESEARCH CORP.<br>750 LEXINGTON AVENUE<br>NEW YORK NY 10022<br>DD 11/22/93 |
| IMMUNE GLOBULIN INTRAVENOUS HUMAN<br>TN is GAMIMUNE N | INFECTION PROPHYLAXIS IN PEDIATRIC PATIENTS AFFECTED WITH THE HUMAN IMMUNODEFICIENCY VIRUS | MILES, INC.<br>4TH & PARKER STREETS<br>BERKELEY CA 94710<br>DD 02/18/93 MA 12/27/93 |
| IMPORTED FIRE ANT VENOM, ALLERGENIC EXTRACT | FOR SKIN TESTING OF VICTIMS OF FIRE ANT STINGS TO CONFIRM FIRE ANT SENSITIVITY AND IF POSITIVE, FOR USE AS IMMUNOTHERAPY FOR THE PREVENTION OF IgE-MEDIATED ANAPHYLACTIC REACTIONS | ALK LABORATORIES, INC.<br>RESEARCH CENTER<br>27 VILLAGE LANE<br>WALLINGFORD CT 06492<br>DD 05/12/92 |
| IN-111 MURINE MAB(2B8-MX-DTPA) & Y-90 MURINE MAB(2B8-MX-DTPA)<br>TN is MELIMMUNE | TREATMENT OF B-CELL NON-HODGKIN'S LYMPHOMA | IDEC PHARMACEUTICALS CORPORATION<br>11011 TORREYANA ROAD<br>SAN DIEGO CA 92121<br>DD 09/06/94 |
| INDIUM IN 111 MURINE MONOCLONAL ANTIBODY FAB TO MYOSIN<br>TN is MYOSCINT | TO AID IN THE DIAGNOSIS OF MYOCARDITIS | CENTOCOR, INC.<br>244 GREAT VALLEY PARKWAY<br>MALVERN PA 19355<br>DD 08/07/89 |
| INDIUM IN-111 ALTUMOMAB PENTETATE<br>TN is HYBRI-CEAker | DETECTION OF SUSPECTED AND PREVIOUSLY UNIDENTIFIED TUMOR FOCI OF RECURRENT COLORECTAL CARCINOMA | HYBRITECH, INC.<br>11095 TORREYANNA ROAD<br>SAN DIEGO CA 92196-9006<br>DD 02/06/90 |
| INOSINE PRANOBEX<br>TN is ISOPRINOSINE | TREATMENT OF SUBACUTE SCLEROSING PANENCEPHALITIS (SSPE) | NEWPORT PHARMACEUTICALS<br>897 WEST SIXTEENTH STREET<br>NEWPORT BEACH CA 92663<br>DD 09/20/88 |
| INSULIN-LIKE GROWTH FACTOR-1<br>TN is MYOTROPHIN | TREATMENT OF AMYOTROPHIC LATERAL SCLEROSIS (ALS) | CEPHALON, INC.<br>145 BRANDYWINE PARKWAY<br>WEST CHESTER PA 19380-4245<br>DD 08/05/91 |
| INTERFERON ALFA-2A (RECOMBINANT)<br>TN is ROFERON-A | TREATMENT OF AIDS RELATED KAPOSI'S SARCOMA | HOFFMANN-LA ROCHE, INC.<br>340 KINGSLAND STREET<br>NUTLEY NJ 07110<br>DD 12/14/87 MA 11/21/88 |
| INTERFERON ALFA-2A (RECOMBINANT)<br>TN is ROFERON-A | TREATMENT OF RENAL CELL CARCINOMA | HOFFMANN-LA ROCHE, INC.<br>340 KINGSLAND STREET<br>NUTLEY NJ 07110-1199<br>DD 04/18/88 |

# CUMULATIVE LIST OF ORPHAN PRODUCT DESIGNATIONS AND APPROVALS
[Through October 31, 1998] *(continued)*

| NAME<br>*Generic/Chemical*<br>*TN is Trade Name* | INDICATION DESIGNATED | SPONSOR AND ADDRESS<br>*DD is Date Designated*<br>*MA is Marketing Approval* |
|---|---|---|
| INTERFERON ALFA-2A (RECOMBINANT)<br>TN is ROFERON A | TREATMENT OF CHRONIC MYELOGENOUS LEUKEMIA | HOFFMANN-LA ROCHE, INC.<br>340 KINGSLAND STREET<br>NUTLEY NJ 07110-1199<br>DD 06/06/89 |
| INTERFERON ALFA-2A (RECOMBINANT)<br>TN is ROFERON-A | FOR USE IN COMBINATION WITH FLUOROURACIL FOR THE TREATMENT OF ESOPHAGEAL CARCINOMA | HOFFMANN-LA ROCHE, INC.<br>340 KINGSLAND STREET<br>NUTLEY NJ 07110-1199<br>DD 10/27/89 |
| INTERFERON ALFA-2A (RECOMBINANT)<br>TN is ROFERON-A | FOR THE CONCOMITANT ADMINISTRATION WITH FLUOROURACIL FOR THE TREATMENT OF ADVANCED COLORECTAL CANCER | HOFFMANN-LA ROCHE, INC.<br>340 KINGSLAND STREET<br>NUTLEY NJ 07110-1199<br>DD 05/14/90 |
| INTERFERON ALFA-2A (RECOMBINANT)<br>TN is ROFERON-A | FOR THE CONCOMITANT ADMINISTRATION WITH TECELEUKIN FOR THE TREATMENT OF METASTATIC RENAL CELL CARCINOMA | HOFFMANN-LA ROCHE, INC.<br>340 KINGSLAND STREET<br>NUTLEY NJ 07119-1199<br>DD 05/02/90 |
| INTERFERON ALFA-2A (RECOMBINANT)<br>TN is ROFERON-A | FOR THE TREATMENT OF METASTATIC MALIGNANT MELANOMA IN COMBINATION WITH TECELEUKIN | HOFFMANN-LA ROCHE, INC.<br>340 KINGSLAND STREET<br>NUTLEY NJ 07110-1199<br>DD 05/11/90 |
| INTERFERON ALFA-2B (RECOMBINANT)<br>TN is INTRON A | TREATMENT OF AIDS-RELATED KAPOSI'S SARCOMA | SCHERING CORPORATION<br>2000 GALLOPING HILL ROAD<br>KENILWORTH NJ 07033<br>DD 06/24/87 MA 11/21/88 |
| INTERFERON ALFA-NL<br>TN is WELLFERON | TREATMENT OF HUMAN PAPILLOMAVIRUS (HPV) IN PATIENTS WITH SEVERE RESISTANT/RECURRENT RESPIRATORY (LARYNGEAL) PAPILLOMATOSIS | BURROUGHS WELLCOME COMPANY<br>3030 CORNWALLIS ROAD<br>RESEARCH TRIANGLE PK NC 27709<br>DD 10/16/87 |
| INTERFERON BETA (RECOMBINANT HUMAN) | TREATMENT OF ACUTE NON-A, NON-B HEPATITIS | BIOGEN, INC.<br>14 CAMBRIDGE CENTER<br>CAMBRIDGE MA 02142<br>DD 07/24/92 |
| INTERFERON BETA (RECOMBINANT HUMAN) | TREATMENT OF PRIMARY BRAIN TUMORS | BIOGEN, INC.<br>14 CAMBRIDGE CENTER<br>CAMBRIDGE MA 02142<br>DD 01/13/93 |
| INTERFERON BETA (RECOMBINANT)<br>TN is r-IFN-beta | SYSTEMIC TREATMENT OF CUTANEOUS T-CELL LYMPHOMA | BIOGEN, INC.<br>14 CAMBRIDGE CENTER<br>CAMBRIDGE MA 02142<br>DD 04/18/91 |
| INTERFERON BETA (RECOMBINANT)<br>TN is r-IFN-beta | SYSTEMIC TREATMENT OF CUTANEOUS MALIGNANT MELANOMA | BIOGEN, INC.<br>14 CAMBRIDGE CENTER<br>CAMBRIDGE MA 02142<br>DD 04/03/91 |
| INTERFERON BETA (RECOMBINANT)<br>TN is r-IFN-beta | FOR THE INTRALESIONAL AND/OR SYSTEMIC TREATMENT OF AIDS-RELATED KAPOSI'S SARCOMA | BIOGEN, INC.<br>14 CAMBRIDGE CENTER<br>CAMBRIDGE MA 02142<br>DD 05/09/91 |
| INTERFERON BETA (RECOMBINANT)<br>TN is r-IFN-beta | SYSTEMIC TREATMENT OF METASTATIC RENAL CELL CARCINOMA | BIOGEN, INC.<br>14 CAMBRIDGE CENTER<br>CAMBRIDGE MA 02142<br>DD 02/12/91 |
| INTERFERON BETA (RECOMBINANT)<br>TN is R-FRONE | TREATMENT OF SYMPTOMATIC PATIENTS WITH ACQUIRED IMMUNODEFICIENCY SYNDROME INCLUDING ALL PATIENTS WITH CD4 T-CELL COUNTS LESS THAN 200 CELLS PER MM3 | SERONO LABORATORIES, INC.<br>100 LONGWATER CIRCLE<br>NORWELL MA 02061<br>DD 12/02/92 |
| INTERFERON BETA-1A<br>TN is AVONEX | TREATMENT OF MULTIPLE SCLEROSIS | BIOGEN, INC.<br>14 CAMBRIDGE CENTER<br>CAMBRIDGE MA 02142<br>DD 12/16/91 |
| INTERFERON BETA-1B<br>TN is BETASERON | TREATMENT OF MULTIPLE SCLEROSIS | CHIRON CORP. & BERLEX LABORATORIES<br>4560 HORTON STREET<br>EMERYVILLE CA 94608<br>DD 11/17/88 MA 07/23/93 |
| INTERFERON BETA-1A<br>TN is REBIF | TREATMENT OF PATIENTS WITH SECONDARY PROGRESSIVE MULTIPLE SCLEROSIS | SERONO LABORATORIES, INC.<br>100 LONGWATER CIRCLE<br>NORWELL MA 02061 |
| INTERFERON GAMMA 1-B<br>TN is ACTIMMUNE | TREATMENT OF CHRONIC GRANULOMATOUS DISEASE | GENENTECH, INC.<br>460 POINT SAN BRUNO BOULEVARD<br>SOUTH SAN FRANCISCO CA 94080<br>DD 09/30/88 MA 12/20/90 |

# CUMULATIVE LIST OF ORPHAN PRODUCT DESIGNATIONS AND APPROVALS
[Through October 31, 1998] *(continued)*

| NAME<br>*Generic/Chemical*<br>*TN is Trade Name* | INDICATION DESIGNATED | SPONSOR AND ADDRESS<br>*DD is Date Designated*<br>*MA is Marketing Approval* |
|---|---|---|
| INTERFERON GAMMA-1B<br>TN is ACTIMMUNE | TREATMENT OF RENAL CELL CARCINOMA | GENENTECH, INC.<br>460 POINT SAN BRUNO BOULEVARD<br>SOUTH SAN FRANCISCO CA 94080 |
| INTERFERON GAMMA-1B<br>TN is ACTIMMUNE | TREATMENT OF SEVERE CONGENITAL OSTEOPETROSIS | GENENTECH, INC.<br>460 POINT SAN BRUNO BOULEVARD<br>SOUTH SAN FRANCISCO CA 94080 |
| INTERLEUKIN-1 RECEPTOR ANTAGONIST, HUMAN RECOMBINANT<br>TN is ANTRIL | TREATMENT OF JUVENILE RHEUMATOID ARTHRITIS | SYNERGEN, INC.<br>1885 33RD STREET<br>BOULDER CO 80301<br>DD 09/23/91 |
| INTERLEUKIN-1 RECEPTOR ANTAGONIST, HUMAN RECOMBINANT<br>TN is ANTRIL | PREVENTION AND TREATMENT OF GRAFT VERSUS HOST DISEASE IN TRANSPLANT RECIPIENTS | SYNERGEN, INC.<br>1885 33RD STREET<br>BOULDER CO 80301<br>DD 10/16/92 |
| INTERLEUKIN-2<br>TN is TECELEUKIN | TREATMENT OF METASTATIC RENAL CELL CARCINOMA | HOFFMANN-LA ROCHE, INC.<br>340 KINGSLAND STREET<br>NUTLEY NJ 07110-1199<br>DD 02/05/90 |
| INTERLEUKIN-2<br>TN is TECELEUKIN | TREATMENT OF METASTATIC MALIGNANT MELANOMA | HOFFMANN-LA ROCHE, INC.<br>340 KINGSLAND STREET<br>NUTLEY NJ 07110-1199<br>DD 02/06/90 |
| INTERLEUKIN-2<br>TN is TECELEUKIN | IN COMBINATION WITH INTERFERON ALFA-2A FOR THE TREATMENT OF METASTATIC RENAL CELL CARCINOMA | HOFFMANN-LA ROCHE, INC.<br>340 KINGSLAND STREET<br>NUTLEY NJ 07110-1199<br>DD 05/03/90 |
| INTERLEUKIN-2<br>TN is TECELEUKIN | IN COMBINATION WITH INTERFERON ALFA-2A FOR THE TREATMENT OF METASTATIC MALIGNANT MELANOMA | HOFFMANN-LA ROCHE, INC.<br>340 KINGSLAND STREET<br>NUTLEY NJ 07110-1199<br>DD 05/11/90 |
| INTERLEUKIN-3 HUMAN, RECOMBINANT | FOR SEQUENTIAL ADMINISTRATION WITH SARGRAMOSTIM TO ACCELERATE NEUTROPHIL AND PLATELET RECOVERY IN PATIENTS UNDERGOING AUTOLOGOUS BONE MARROW TRANSPLANTATION FOR THE TREATMENT OF HODGKIN'S DISEASE OR NON-HODGKIN'S LYMPHOMA | SANDOZ PHARMACEUTICALS CORP.<br>59 ROUTE 10<br>EAST HANOVER NJ 07936-1080<br>DD 09/30/93 |
| INTRAVITREAL GANCICLOVIR FREE ACID IMPLANT<br>TN is VITRASERT IMPLANT | TREATMENT OF CYTOMEGALOVIRUS RETINITIS | CHIRON VISION<br>500 IOLAB DRIVE<br>CLAREMONT CA 91711<br>DD 06/07/95 |
| IOBENGUANE SULFATE I 131 | DIAGNOSTIC ADJUNCT IN PATIENTS WITH PHEOCHROMOCYTOMA | CIS-US, INC.<br>10 DE ANGELO DRIVE<br>BEDFORD MA 01730<br>DD 11/14/84 MA 03/25/94 |
| IODINE 131 6B-IODOMETHYL-19-NORCHOLESTEROL | ADRENAL CORTICAL IMAGING | BEIERWALTES, WILLIAM, M.D.<br>1405 E. ANN STREET<br>ANN ARBOR MI 48109<br>DD 08/01/84 |
| IODINE I 123 MURINE MONOCLONAL ANTIBODY TO ALPHA-FETOPROTEIN | DETECTION OF HEPATOCELLULAR CARCINOMA AND HEPATOBLASTOMA | IMMUNOMEDICS, INC.<br>300 AMERICAN ROAD<br>MORRIS PLAINS NJ 07950<br>DD 09/30/88 |
| IODINE I 123 MURINE MONOCLONAL ANTIBODY TO ALPHA-FETOPROTEIN | DETECTION OF ALPHA-FETOPROTEIN PRODUCING GERM CELL TUMORS | IMMUNOMEDICS, INC.<br>300 AMERICAN ROAD<br>MORRIS PLAINS NJ 07950<br>DD 09/30/88 |
| IODINE I 123 MURINE MONOCLONAL ANTIBODY TO HCG | DETECTION OF HCG PRODUCING TUMORS SUCH AS GERM CELL AND TROPHOBLASTIC CELL TUMORS | IMMUNOMEDICS, INC.<br>300 AMERICAN ROAD<br>MORRIS PLAINS NJ 07950<br>DD 11/07/88 |
| IODINE I 131 MURINE MONOCLONAL ANTIBODY IgG2a TO B CELL<br>TN is IMMURAIT, LL-2-I-131 | TREATMENT OF B-CELL LEUKEMIA AND B-CELL LYMPHOMA | IMMUNOMEDICS, INC.<br>300 AMERICAN ROAD<br>MORRIS PLAINS NJ 07950<br>DD 09/18/89 |
| IODINE I 131 MURINE MONOCLONAL ANTIBODY TO ALPHA-FETOPROTEIN | TREATMENT OF HEPATOCELLULAR CARCINOMA AND HEPATOBLASTOMA | IMMUNOMEDICS, INC.<br>300 AMERICAN ROAD<br>MORRIS PLAINS NJ 07950<br>DD 09/30/88 |
| IODINE I 131 MURINE MONOCLONAL ANTIBODY TO ALPHA-FETOPROTEIN | TREATMENT OF ALPHA-FETOPROTEIN PRODUCING GERM CELL TUMORS | IMMUNOMEDICS, INC.<br>300 AMERICAN ROAD<br>MORRIS PLAINS NJ 07950<br>DD 09/30/88 |

## CUMULATIVE LIST OF ORPHAN PRODUCT DESIGNATIONS AND APPROVALS
[Through October 31, 1998] *(continued)*

| NAME<br>*Generic/Chemical*<br>*TN is Trade Name* | INDICATION DESIGNATED | SPONSOR AND ADDRESS<br>*DD is Date Designated*<br>*MA is Marketing Approval* |
|---|---|---|
| IODINE I 131 MURINE MONO-CLONAL ANTIBODY TO HCG | TREATMENT OF HCG PRODUCING TUMORS SUCH AS GERM CELL AND TROPHOBLASTIC CELL TUMORS | IMMUNOMEDICS, INC.<br>300 AMERICAN ROAD<br>MORRIS PLAINS NJ 07950<br>DD 11/07/88 |
| ISOBUTYRAMIDE<br>TN is ISOBUTYRAMIDE ORAL SOLUTION | TREATMENT OF BETA-HEMOGLOBINOPATHIES AND BETA-THALASSEMIA SYNDROMES | PERRINE, SUSAN P., M.D.<br>BOSTON UNIVERSITY<br>BOSTON MA 02118<br>DD 12/18/92 |
| ISOBUTYRAMIDE | TREATMENT OF SICKLE CELL DISEASE AND BETA THALASSEMIA | VERTEX PHARMACEUTICALS INC.<br>40 ALLSTON STREET<br>CAMBRIDGE MA 02139-4211<br>DD 05/25/94 |
| KL4-SURFACTANT | TREATMENT OF ACUTE RESPIRATORY DISTRESS SYNDROME IN ADULTS | R.W. JOHNSON RESEARCH INSTITUTE<br>ROUTE 202, P.O. BOX 300<br>RARITAN NJ 08869-0602<br>DD 07/17/95 |
| KL4-SURFACTANT | TREATMENT OF MECONIUM ASPIRATION SYNDROME IN NEWBORN INFANTS | COCHRANE, CHARLES M.D.<br>THE SCRIPPS RESEARCH INSTITUTE<br>10666 TORREY PINES ROAD<br>LA JOLLA CA 92037 |
| KL4-SURFACTANT | TREATMENT OF RESPIRATORY DISTRESS SYNDROME IN PREMATURE INFANTS | COCHRANE, CHARLES G., M.D.<br>THE SCRIPPS RESEARCH INSTITUTE<br>10666 NORTH TORREY PINES ROAD,<br>IMM 12<br>LA JOLLA CA 92037 |
| L-2 OXOTHIAZOLIDINE-4-CARBOXYLIC ACID<br>TN is PROCYSTEINE | TREATMENT OF ADULT RESPIRATORY DISTRESS SYNDROME | TRANSCEND THERAPEUTICS, INC.<br>640 MEMORIAL DRIVE<br>3RD FLOOR WEST<br>CAMBRIDGE MA 02139<br>DD 06/14/94 |
| L-2-OXOTHIAZOLIDINE-4-CARBOXYLIC ACID<br>TN is PROCYSTEINE | TREATMENT OF AMYOTROPHIC LATERAL SCLEROSIS | TRANSCEND THERAPEUTICS, INC.<br>640 MEMORIAL DRIVE,<br>3rd FLOOR WEST<br>CAMBRIDGE MA 02139 |
| L-5 HYDROXYTRYPTOPHAN | TREATMENT OF POSTANOXIC INTENTION MYOCLONUS | CIRCA PHARMACEUTICALS, INC.<br>33 RALPH AVENUE<br>P.O. BOX 30<br>COPIAQUE NY 11726<br>DD 11/01/84 |
| L-BACLOFEN | TREATMENT OF TRIGEMINAL NEURALGIA | FROMM, GERHARD, M.D.<br>UNIVERSITY OF PITTSBURGH<br>PITTSBURGH PA 15261<br>DD 07/13/90 |
| L-BACLOFEN | TREATMENT OF TRIGEMINAL NEURALGIA | PHARMASCIENCE, INC.<br>8400 DARNLEY ROAD<br>MONTREAL QUEBEC<br>CANADA H4T 1M4 |
| L-BACLOFEN<br>TN is NEURALGON | TREATMENT OF INTRACTABLE SPASTICITY ASSOCIATED WITH SPINAL CORD INJURY OR MULTIPLE SCLEROSIS | WTD, INCORPORATED<br>8819 NORTH PIONEER ROAD<br>PEORIA IL 61615<br>DD 12/17/91 |
| L-BACLOFEN<br>TN is NEURALGON | TREATMENT OF INTRACTABLE SPASTICITY IN CHILDREN WITH CEREBRAL PALSY | WTD, INCORPORATED<br>8819 NORTH PIONEER ROAD<br>PEORIA IL 61615<br>DD 01/30/92 |
| L-CYCLOSERINE | TREATMENT OF GAUCHER'S DISEASE | LEV, MEIR, M.D.<br>CITY UNIVERSITY OF NY MEDICAL SCHOOL<br>NEW YORK NY 10031<br>DD 08/01/89 |
| L-CYSTEINE | FOR THE PREVENTION AND LESSENING OF PHOTOSENSITIVITY IN ERYTHROPOIETIC PROTOPORPHYRIA | TYSON AND ASSOCIATES<br>12832 SOUTH CHADRON AVENUE<br>HAWTHORNE CA 90250<br>DD 05/16/94 |
| L-LEUCOVORIN<br>TN is ISOVORIN | FOR USE IN CONJUNCTION WITH HIGH-DOSE METHOTREXATE IN THE TREATMENT OF OSTEOSARCOMA | LEDERLE LABORATORIES DIVISION<br>AMERICAN CYANAMID CORPORATION<br>PEARL RIVER NY 10965<br>DD 08/01/91 |
| L-LEUCOVORIN<br>TN is ISOVORIN | FOR USE IN COMBINATION CHEMOTHERAPY WITH THE APPROVED AGENT 5-FLUOROURACIL IN THE PALLIATIVE TREATMENT OF METASTATIC ADENOCARCINOMA OF THE COLON AND RECTUM | LEDERLE LABORATORIES DIVISION<br>AMERICAN CYANAMID COMPANY<br>PEARL RIVER NY 10965<br>DD 12/18/90 |

# CUMULATIVE LIST OF ORPHAN PRODUCT DESIGNATIONS AND APPROVALS
[Through October 31, 1998] *(continued)*

| NAME<br>*Generic/Chemical*<br>*TN is Trade Name* | INDICATION DESIGNATED | SPONSOR AND ADDRESS<br>*DD is Date Designated*<br>*MA is Marketing Approval* |
|---|---|---|
| L-THREONINE<br>TN is THREOSTAT | TREATMENT OF AMYOTROPHIC LATERAL SCLEROSIS | TYSON AND ASSOCIATES<br>12832 CHADRON AVENUE<br>HAWTHORNE CA 90250<br>DD 02/06/89 |
| L-THREONINE | TREATMENT OF SPASTICITY ASSOCIATED WITH FAMILIAL SPASTIC PARAPARESIS | INTERNEURON PHARMACEUTICALS<br>99 HAYDEN AVENUE, SUITE 340<br>LEXINGTON MA 02173<br>DD 07/24/92 |
| LACTOBIN<br>TN is LACTOBIN | TREATMENT OF AIDS-ASSOCIATED DIARRHEA UNRESPONSIVE TO INITIAL ANTIDIARRHEAL THERAPY | ROXANE LABORATORIES, INC.<br>1809 WILSON ROAD<br>P.O. BOX 16532<br>COLUMBUS OH 43216-6532<br>DD 09/12/90 |
| LAMOTRIGINE<br>TN is LAMICTAL | TREATMENT OF LENNOX-GASTAUT SYNDROME | BURROUGHS-WELLCOME COMPANY<br>3030 CORNWALLIS ROAD<br>P.O. BOX 12700<br>RESEARCH TRIANGLE PK NC 27709<br>DD 08/23/95 |
| LEFLUNOMIDE | PREVENTION OF ACUTE AND CHRONIC REJECTION IN PATIENTS WHO HAVE RECEIVED SOLID ORGAN TRANSPLANTS | JAMES W. WILLIAMS, M.D.<br>655 SUPERIOR<br>OAK PARK IL 60302 |
| LEPIRUDIN<br>TN is REFLUDAN | TREATMENT OF HEPARIN-ASSOCIATED THROMBOCYTOPENIA TYPE II | BEHRINGWERKE AG<br>P.O. BOX 1140<br>D-35001 MARBURG<br>GERMANY |
| LEUCOVORIN<br>TN is LEUCOVORIN CALCIUM | FOR USE IN COMBINATION WITH 5-FLUOROURACIL FOR THE TREATMENT OF METASTATIC COLORECTAL CANCER | IMMUNEX CORPORATION<br>51 UNIVERSITY STREET<br>SEATTLE WA 98101<br>DD 12/08/86 MA 12/12/91 |
| LEUCOVORIN<br>TN is LEUCOVORIN CALCIUM | FOR RESCUE USE AFTER HIGH DOSE METHOTREXATE THERAPY IN THE TREATMENT OF OSTEOSARCOMA | IMMUNEX CORPORATION<br>51 UNIVERSITY STREET<br>SEATTLE WA 98101<br>DD 08/17/88 MA 08/31/88 |
| LEUCOVORIN CALCIUM<br>TN is WELLCOVORIN | FOR USE IN COMBINATION WITH 5-FLUOROURACIL FOR THE TREATMENT OF METASTATIC COLORECTAL CANCER | BURROUGHS WELLCOME COMPANY<br>3030 CORNWALLIS ROAD<br>RESEARCH TRIANGLE PK NC 27709<br>DD 06/23/88 |
| LEUPEPTIN | AS AN ADJUNCT TO MICROSURGICAL PERIPHERAL NERVE REPAIR | RESEARCH TRIANGLE PHARMACEUTICALS<br>4364 SOUTH ALSTON AVENUE<br>DURHAM NC 27713<br>DD 09/18/90 |
| LEUPROLIDE ACETATE<br>TN is LUPRON INJECTION | TREATMENT OF CENTRAL PRECOCIOUS PUBERTY | TAP PHARMACEUTICALS, INC.<br>2355 WAUKEGAN ROAD<br>DEERFIELD IL 60015<br>DD 07/25/88 MA 04/16/93 |
| LEVOCARNITINE<br>TN is CARNITOR | TREATMENT OF ZIDOVUDINE-INDUCED MITOCHONDRIAL MYOPATHY | SIGMA-TAU PHARMACEUTICALS, INC.<br>800 S. FREDERICK AVENUE<br>SUITE 300<br>GAITHERSBURG MD 20877 |
| LEVOCARNITINE<br>TN is VITA CARN | TREATMENT OF GENETIC CARNITINE DEFICIENCY | SIGMA-TAU PHARMACEUTICALS, INC.<br>200 ORCHARD RIDGE DRIVE<br>SUITE 300<br>GAITHERSBURG MD 20878-1978<br>DD 02/28/84 MA 04/10/86 |
| LEVOCARNITINE<br>TN is CARNITOR | TREATMENT OF PRIMARY AND SECONDARY CARNITINE DEFICIENCY OF GENETIC ORIGIN | SIGMA-TAU PHARMACEUTICALS, INC.<br>200 ORCHARD RIDGE DRIVE<br>SUITE 300<br>GAITHERSBURG MD 20878-1978<br>DD 07/26/84 MA 12/16/92 |
| LEVOCARNITINE<br>TN is CARNITOR | TREATMENT OF MANIFESTATIONS OF CARNITINE DEFICIENCY IN PATIENTS WITH END STAGE RENAL DISEASE (ESRD) WHO REQUIRE DIALYSIS | SIGMA-TAU PHARMACEUTICALS, INC.<br>200 ORCHARD RIDGE DRIVE<br>SUITE 300<br>GAITHERSBURG MD 20878-1978<br>DD 09/06/88 |
| LEVOCARNITINE<br>TN is VITACARN | FOR THE PREVENTION OF SECONDARY CARNITINE DEFICIENCY IN VALPROIC ACID TOXICITY | SIGMA-TAU PHARMACEUTICALS, INC.<br>200 ORCHARD RIDGE DRIVE<br>SUITE 300<br>GAITHERSBURG MD 20878-1978<br>DD 11/15/89 |

# CUMULATIVE LIST OF ORPHAN PRODUCT DESIGNATIONS AND APPROVALS
[Through October 31, 1998] *(continued)*

| NAME<br>*Generic/Chemical*<br>*TN is Trade Name* | INDICATION DESIGNATED | SPONSOR AND ADDRESS<br>*DD is Date Designated*<br>*MA is Marketing Approval* |
|---|---|---|
| LEVOCARNITINE<br>TN is VITACARN | FOR THE TREATMENT OF SECONDARY CARNITINE DEFICIENCY IN VALPROIC ACID TOXICITY | SIGMA-TAU PHARMACEUTICALS, INC.<br>200 ORCHARD RIDGE DRIVE<br>SUITE 300<br>GAITHERSBURG MD 20878-1978<br>DD 11/15/89 |
| LEVOCARNITINE<br>TN is CARNITOR | TREATMENT OF PEDIATRIC CARDIOMYOPATHY | SIGMA-TAU PHARMACEUTICALS, INC.<br>200 ORCHARD RIDGE DRIVE<br>SUITE 300<br>GAITHERSBURG MD 20878<br>DD 11/22/93 |
| LEVOMETHADYL ACETATE HYDROCHLORIDE<br>TN is ORLAAM | TREATMENT OF HEROIN ADDICTS SUITABLE FOR MAINTENANCE ON OPIATE AGONISTS | BIODEVELOPMENT CORPORATION<br>8180 GREENSBORO DRIVE<br>SUITE 1000<br>MCLEAN VA 22102<br>DD 01/24/84 MA 07/09/93 |
| LIDOCAINE PATCH 5%<br>TN is LIDODERM PATCH | TREATMENT OF POST-HERPETIC NEURALGIA RESULTING FROM HERPES ZOSTER INFECTION | HIND HEALTH CARE, INC.<br>165 GIBRALTAR COURT<br>SUNNYVALE CA 94089 |
| LIOTHYRONINE SODIUM INJECTION<br>TN is TRIOSTAT | TREATMENT OF MYXEDEMA COMA/PRECOMA | SMITHKLINE BEECHAM<br>P.O. BOX 1510<br>KING OF PRUSSIA PA 19406<br>DD 07/30/90 MA 12/31/91 |
| LIPID/DNA HUMAN CYSTIC FIBROSIS GENE | TREATMENT OF CYSTIC FIBROSIS | GENZYME CORPORATION<br>ONE KENDALL SQUARE<br>CAMBRIDGE MA 02139 |
| LIPOSOMAL AMPHOTERICIN B<br>TN is AMBISOME | TREATMENT OF CRYPTOCOCCAL MENINGITIS | FUJISAWA USA, INC.<br>3 PARKWAY NORTH CENTER<br>DEERFIELD IL 60015 |
| LIPOSOMAL AMPHOTERICIN B<br>TN is AMBISOME | TREATMENT OF HISTOPLASMOSIS | FUJISAWA USA, INC.<br>3 PARKWAY NORTH CENTER<br>DEERFIELD IL 60015 |
| LIPOSOMAL AMPHOTERICIN B<br>TN is AMBISOME | TREATMENT OF VISCERAL LEISHMANIASIS | FUJISAWA USA, INC.<br>3 PARKWAY NORTH CENTER<br>DEERFIELD IL 60015 |
| LIPOSOMAL CYCLOSPORIN A<br>TN is CYCLOSPIRE | FOR AEROSOLIZED ADMINISTRATION IN THE PREVENTION AND TREATMENT OF LUNG ALLOGRAFT REJECTION AND PULMONARY REJECTION EVENTS ASSOCIATED WITH BONE MARROW TRANSPLANTATION | VERNON KNIGHT, M.D.<br>BAYLOR COLLEGE OF MEDICINE<br>DEPT. OF MOLECULAR PHYSIOLOGY<br>ONE BAYLOR PLAZA<br>HOUSTON TX 77030 |
| LIPOSOMAL DAUNORUBICIN<br>TN is DAUNOXOME | TREATMENT OF PATIENTS WITH ADVANCED HIV-ASSOCIATED KAPOSI'S SARCOMA | VESTAR, INC.<br>650 CLIFFSIDE DRIVE<br>SAN DIMAS CA 91773<br>DD 05/14/93 |
| LIPOSOMAL N-ACETYLGLUCOSMINYL-N-ACETYLMURAMYL-L-ALA-D-ISOGLN-L-ALA-GLYCEROLID-PALMITOYL<br>TN is IMMTHER | TREATMENT OF OSTEOSARCOMA | ENDOREX CORPORATION<br>900 NORTH SHORE DRIVE<br>LAKE BLUFF IL 60044 |
| LIPOSOMAL N-ACETYLGLUCOSMINYL-N-ACETYLMURAMYL-L-ALA-D-ISO-GLN-L-ALA-GLYCEROLID-PALMITOYL<br>TN is IMMTHER | TREATMENT OF EWING'S SARCOMA | ENDOREX CORPORATION<br>900 NORTH SHORE DRIVE<br>LAKE BLUFF, IL 60044 |
| LIPOSOMAL PROSTAGLANDIN E1 INJECTION | TREATMENT OF ACUTE RESPIRATORY DISTRESS SYNDROME | THE LIPOSOME COMPANY, INC.<br>ONE RESEARCH WAY<br>PRINCETON NJ 08540 |
| LIPOSOME ENCAPSULATED RECOMBINANT INTERLEUKIN-2 | TREATMENT OF BRAIN AND CNS TUMORS | ONCOTHERAPEUTICS, INC.<br>1002 EASTPARK BOULEVARD<br>CRANBURY NJ 08512<br>DD 11/25/91 |
| LIPOSOME ENCAPSULATED RECOMBINANT INTERLEUKIN-2 | TREATMENT OF CANCERS OF THE KIDNEY AND RENAL PELVIS | ONCOTHERAPEUTICS, INC.<br>1002 EASTPARK BOULEVARD<br>CRANBURY NJ 08512<br>DD 06/20/94 |
| LODOXAMIDE TROMETHAMINE<br>TN is ALOMIDE OPHTHALMIC SOLUTION | TREATMENT OF VERNAL KERATOCONJUNCTIVITIS | ALCON LABORATORIES, INC.<br>6201 SOUTH FREEWAY<br>FORT WORTH TX 76134<br>DD 10/16/91 |
| MAFENIDE ACETATE SOLUTION<br>TN is SULFAMYLON SOLUTION | FOR THE CONTROL OF BACTERIAL COLONIZATION UNDER MOIST DRESSINGS OVER MESHED AUTOGRAFTS ON EXCISED BURN WOUNDS | DOW B. HICKAM, INC.<br>10410 CORPORATE DRIVE<br>SUGAR LAND TX 77478<br>DD 07/18/90 |

# CUMULATIVE LIST OF ORPHAN PRODUCT DESIGNATIONS AND APPROVALS
[Through October 31, 1998] *(continued)*

| NAME<br>*Generic/Chemical*<br>*TN is Trade Name* | INDICATION DESIGNATED | SPONSOR AND ADDRESS<br>*DD is Date Designated*<br>*MA is Marketing Approval* |
|---|---|---|
| MART-1 ADENOVIRAL GENE THERAPY FOR MALIGNANT MELANOMA | TREATMENT OF METASTATIC MELONOMA | GENZYME CORPORATION<br>ONE KENDALL SQUARE<br>CAMBRIDGE MA 02139 |
| MATRIX METALLOPROTEINASE INHIBITOR<br>TN is GALARDIN | TREATMENT OF CORNEAL ULCERS | GLYCOMED, INC<br>860 ATLANTIC AVENUE<br>ALAMEDA CA 94501<br>DD 12/05/91 |
| MAZINDOL<br>TN is SANOREX | TREATMENT OF DUCHENNE MUSCULAR DYSTROPHY (DMD) | COLLIPP, PLATON J., M.D.<br>176 MEMORIAL DRIVE<br>JESUP GA 31545<br>DD 12/08/86 |
| MECASERMIN | TREATMENT OF GROWTH HORMONE INSUFFICENCY SYNDROME | GENENTECH, INC.<br>460 POINT SAN BRUNO BOULEVARD<br>SOUTH SAN FRANCISCO CA 94080 |
| MEFLOQUINE HCL<br>TN is MEPHAQUIN | TREATMENT OF CHLOROQUINE-RESISTANT FALCIPARUM MALARIA | MEPHA AG<br>4143 DORNACH, POSTFASH 137<br>AESCH BASEL SWITZERLAND<br>DD 07/22/87 |
| MEFLOQUINE HCL<br>TN is LARIAM | TREATMENT OF ACUTE MALARIA DUE TO PLASMODIUM FALCIPARUM AND PLASMODIUM VIVAX | HOFFMANN-LA ROCHE, INC.<br>340 KINGSLAND STREET<br>NUTLEY NJ 07110<br>DD 04/13/88 MA 05/02/89 |
| MEFLOQUINE HCL<br>TN is LARIAM | PROPHYLAXIS OF PLASMODIUM FALCIPARUM MALARIA WHICH IS RESISTANT TO OTHER AVAILABLE DRUGS | HOFFMANN-LA ROCHE, INC.<br>340 KINGSLAND STREET<br>NUTLEY NJ 07110<br>DD 04/13/88 MA 05/02/89 |
| MEFLOQUINE HCL<br>TN is MEPHAQUIN | PREVENTION OF CHLOROQUINE-RESISTANT FALCIPARUM MALARIA | MEPHA AG<br>4143 DORNACH, POSTFASH 137<br>AESCH BASEL SWITZED<br>DD 07/22/87 |
| MEGESTROL ACETATE<br>TN is MEGACE | TREATMENT OF PATIENTS WITH ANOREXIA, CACHEXIA, OR SIGNIFICANT WEIGHT LOSS (=/10% OF BASELINE BODY WEIGHT) AND CONFIRMED DIAGNOSIS OF ACQUIRED IMMUNODEFICIENCY SYNDROME (AIDS) | BRISTOL-MYERS SQUIBB<br>2400 WEST LLOYD EXPRESSWAY<br>EVANSVILLE IN 47721-0001<br>DD 04/13/88 |
| MELANOMA CELL VACCINE | TREATMENT OF INVASIVE MELANOMA | MORTON, DONALD L., M.D.<br>JOHN WAYNE CANCER INSTITUTE<br>SANTA MONICA CA 90404<br>DD 10/13/94 |
| MELANOMA VACCINE<br>TN is MELACINE | TREATMENT OF STAGE III - IV MELANOMA | RIBI IMMUNOCHEM RESEARCH, INC.<br>533 OLD CORVALLIS ROAD<br>HAMILTON MT 59840<br>DD 12/20/89 |
| MELATONIN | TREATMENT OF CIRCADIAN RHYTHM SLEEP DISORDERS IN BLIND PEOPLE WITH NO LIGHT PERCEPTION | SACK, ROBERT, M.D.<br>3181 S.W. SAM JACKSON PARK ROAD<br>PORTLAND OR 97201-3098<br>DD 11/15/93 |
| MELPHALAN<br>TN is ALKERAN FOR INJECTION | TREATMENT OF PATIENTS WITH MULTIPLE MYELOMA FOR WHOM ORAL THERAPY IS INAPPROPRIATE | BURROUGHS WELLCOME COMPANY<br>3030 CORNWALLIS ROAD<br>RESEARCH TRIANGLE PK NC 27709<br>DD 02/24/92 MA 11/18/92 |
| MELPHALAN<br>TN is ALKERAN FOR INJECTION | FOR USE IN HYPERTHERMIC REGIONAL LIMB PERFUSION TO TREAT METASTATIC MELANOMA OF THE EXTREMITY | BURROUGHS WELLCOME COMPANY<br>3030 CORNWALLIS ROAD<br>RESEARCH TRIANGLE PK NC 27709<br>DD 03/03/92 |
| MESNA<br>TN is MESNEX | FOR USE AS A PROPHYLACTIC AGENT IN REDUCING THE INCIDENCE OF IFOSFAMIDE-INDUCED HEMORRHAGIC CYSTITIS | DEGUSSA CORPORATION<br>65 CHALLENGER ROAD<br>RIDGEFIELD NJ 07660<br>DD 11/14/85 MA 12/30/88 |
| MESNA | INHIBITION OF THE UROTOXIC EFFECTS INDUCED BY OXAZAPHOSPHORINE COMPOUNDS SUCH AS CYCLOPHOSPHAMIDE | ASTA MEDICAL<br>401 HACKENSACK AVENUE<br>HACKENSACK NJ 07601<br>DD 12/16/87 |
| METHIONINE/L-METHIONINE | TREATMENT OF AIDS MYELOPATHY | DI ROCCO, ALESSANDRO, M.D.<br>THE MOUNT SINAI MEDICAL CENTER<br>ONE GUSTAVE L. LEVY PLACE,<br>BOX 1139<br>NEW YORK NY 10029 |
| METHOTREXATE<br>TN is RHEUMATREX | TREATMENT OF JUVENILE RHEUMATOID ARTHRITIS | LEDERLE LABORATORIES DIVISION<br>AMERICAN CYANAMID COMPANY<br>PEARL RIVER NY 10965-1299<br>DD 08/23/93 |

# CUMULATIVE LIST OF ORPHAN PRODUCT DESIGNATIONS AND APPROVALS
[Through October 31, 1998] *(continued)*

| NAME<br>*Generic/Chemical*<br>*TN is Trade Name* | INDICATION DESIGNATED | SPONSOR AND ADDRESS<br>*DD is Date Designated*<br>*MA is Marketing Approval* |
|---|---|---|
| METHOTREXATE SODIUM<br>TN is METHOTREXATE | TREATMENT OF OSTEOGENIC SARCOMA | LEDERLE LABORATORIES DIVISION<br>AMERICAN CYANAMID COMPANY<br>PEARL RIVER NY 10965<br>DD 10/21/85 MA 04/07/88 |
| METHOTREXATE USP WITH LAUROCAPRAM<br>TN is METHOTREXATE/AZONE | TOPICAL TREATMENT OF MYCOSIS FUNGOIDES | DISCOVERY THERAPEUTICS, INC.<br>911 EAST LEIGH STREET<br>RICHMOND VA 23219<br>DD 10/15/90 |
| METHYLNALTREXONE | TREATMENT OF CHRONIC OPIOID-INDUCED CONSTIPATION UNRESPONSIVE TO CONVENTIONAL THERAPY | THE UNIVERSITY OF CHICAGO<br>5841 SOUTH MARYLAND AVENUE<br>MC 4028<br>CHICAGO IL 60637 |
| METRONIDAZOLE<br>TN is METROGEL | TREATMENT OF PERIORAL DERMATITIS | GALDERMA LABORATORIES, INC.<br>P.O. BOX 331329<br>FORT WORTH TX 76163<br>DD 10/24/91 |
| METRONIDAZOLE (TOPICAL)<br>TN is METROGEL | TREATMENT OF ACNE ROSACEA | GALDERMA LABORATORIES, INC.<br>P.O. BOX 331329<br>FORT WORTH TX 76163<br>DD 10/22/87 MA 11/22/88 |
| METRONIDAZOLE (TOPICAL)<br>TN is FLAGYL | TREATMENT OF GRADE III AND IV, ANAEROBICALLY INFECTED, DECUBITUS ULCERS | G.D. SEARLE & COMPANY<br>4901 SEARLE PARKWAY<br>SKOKIE IL 60077<br>DD 11/24/87 |
| MICROBUBBLE CONTRAST AGENT<br>TN is FILMIX NEUROSONO-GRAPHIC CONTRAST AGENT | INTRAOPERATIVE AID IN THE IDENTIFICATION AND LOCALIZATION OF INTRACRANIAL TUMORS | CAV-CON, INC.<br>55 KNOLLWOOD ROAD<br>FARMINGTON CT 06032<br>DD 11/16/90 |
| MIDODRINE HCL<br>TN is AMATINE | TREATMENT OF IDIOPATHIC ORTHOSTATIC HYPOTENSION | ROBERTS PHARMACEUTICAL CORP.<br>6 INDUSTRIAL WAY WEST<br>EATONTOWN NJ 07724<br>DD 06/21/85 |
| MITOGUAZONE | TREATMENT OF DIFFUSE NON-HODGKIN'S LYMPHOMA, INCLUDING AIDS-RELATED DIFFUSE NON-HODGKIN'S LYMPHOMA | ILEX ONCOLOGY, INC.<br>14960 OMICRON DRIVE<br>SAN ANTONIO TX 78245-3217<br>DD 03/18/94 |
| MITOLACTOL | AS ADJUVANT THERAPY IN THE TREATMENT OF PRIMARY BRAIN TUMORS | BIOPHARMACEUTICS, INC.<br>990 STATION ROAD<br>BELLPORT NY 11713<br>DD 07/12/95 |
| MITOMYCIN-C | TREATMENT OF REFRACTORY GLAUCOMA AS AN ADJUNCT TO AB EXTERNO GLAUCOMA SURGERY | IOP INCORPORATED<br>3100 AIRWAY AVENUE<br>COSTA MESA CA 92626<br>DD 08/20/93 |
| MITOXANTRONE<br>TN is NOVANTRONE | TREATMENT OF HORMONE REFRACTORY PROSTATE CANCER | IMMUNEX CORPORATION<br>51 UNIVERSITY STREET<br>SEATTLE WA 98101 |
| MITOXANTRONE HCL<br>TN is NOVANTRONE | TREATMENT OF ACUTE MYELOGENOUS LEUKEMIA (AML), ALSO REFERRED TO AS ACUTE NONLYMPHOCYTIC LEUKEMIA (ANLL) | LEDERLE LABORATORIES DIVISION<br>AMERICAN CYANAMID COMPANY<br>PEARL RIVER NY 10965<br>DD 07/13/87 MA 12/23/87 |
| MODAFINIL | TREATMENT OF EXCESSIVE DAYTIME SLEEPINESS IN NARCOLEPSY | CEPHALON, INC.<br>145 BRANDYWINE PARKWAY<br>WEST CHESTER PA 19380-4245<br>DD 03/15/93 |
| MONOCLONAL AB (MURINE) ANTI-IDIOTYPE MELANOMA ASS'TED ANTIGEN<br>TN is MELIMMUNE | TREATMENT OF INVASIVE CUTANEOUS MELANOMA | IDEC PHARMACEUTICALS CORPORATION<br>11011 TORREYANA ROAD<br>SAN DIEGO CA 92121<br>DD 09/19/94 |
| MONOCLONAL ANTIBODY-B43.13<br>TN is OVAREX MAB-B43.13 | TREATMENT OF EPITHELIAL OVARIAN CANCER | ALTAREX, INC.<br>1134 DENTISTRY-PHARMACY BUILDING<br>UNIVERSITY OF ALBERTA<br>EDMONTON ALBERTA CANADA |
| MONOCLONAL ANTIBODIES PM-81 AND AML-2-23 | FOR THE EXOGENOUS DEPLETION OF CD14 AND CD15 POSITIVE ACUTE MYELOID LEUKEMIC BONE MARROW CELLS FROM PATIENTS UNDERGOING BONE MARROW TRANSPLANTATION | MEDAREX, INC.<br>1545 ROUTE 22 EAST<br>P.O. BOX 992<br>ANNANDALE NJ 08801-0992<br>DD 03/12/90 |
| MONOCLONAL ANTIBODY 17-1A<br>TN is PANOREX | TREATMENT OF PANCREATIC CANCER | CENTOCOR, INC.<br>244 GREAT VALLEY PARKWAY<br>MALVERN PA 19355<br>DD 04/04/88 |

# CUMULATIVE LIST OF ORPHAN PRODUCT DESIGNATIONS AND APPROVALS
[Through October 31, 1998] *(continued)*

| NAME<br>*Generic/Chemical*<br>*TN is Trade Name* | INDICATION DESIGNATED | SPONSOR AND ADDRESS<br>*DD is Date Designated*<br>*MA is Marketing Approval* |
|---|---|---|
| MONOCLONAL ANTIBODY FOR IMMUNIZATION AGAINST LUPUS NEPHRITIS | TREATMENT OF LUPUS NEPHRITIS | MEDCLONE, INC.<br>2435 MILITARY AVENUE<br>LOS ANGELES CA 90064<br>DD 01/07/93 |
| MONOCLONAL ANTIBODY PM-81 | ADJUNCTIVE TREATMENT OF ACUTE MYELOGENOUS LEUKEMIA | MEDAREX, INC.<br>1545 ROUTE 22 EAST<br>P.O. BOX 992<br>ANNANDALE NJ 08801-0992<br>DD 06/27/91 |
| MONOCLONAL ANTIBODY TO CYTOMEGALOVIRUS (HUMAN) | PROPHYLAXIS OF CYTOMEGALOVIRUS DISEASE IN PATIENTS UNDERGOING SOLID ORGAN TRANSPLANTATION | PROTEIN DESIGN LABS, INC.<br>2375 GARCIA AVENUE<br>MOUNTAIN VIEW CA 94043<br>DD 09/13/91 |
| MONOCLONAL ANTIBODY TO CYTOMEGALOVIRUS (HUMAN) | TREATMENT OF CYTOMEGALOVIRUS RETINITIS IN PATIENTS WITH ACQUIRED IMMUNODEFICIENCY SYNDROME | PROTEIN DESIGN LABS, INC.<br>2375 GARCIA AVENUE<br>MOUNTAIN VIEW CA 94043<br>DD 11/15/91 |
| MONOCLONAL ANTIBODY TO HEPATITIS B VIRUS (HUMAN) | PROPHYLAXIS OF HEPATITIS B REINFECTION IN PATIENTS UNDERGOING LIVER TRANSPLANTATION SECONDARY TO END-STAGE CHRONIC HEPATITIS B INFECTION | PROTEIN DESIGN LABS, INC.<br>2375 GARCIA AVENUE<br>MOUNTAIN VIEW CA 94043<br>DD 06/17/91 |
| MONOLAURIN<br>TN is GLYLORIN | TREATMENT OF CONGENITAL PRIMARY ICHTHYOSIS | CELLEGY PHARMACEUTICALS, INC.<br>371 BEL MARIN KEYS, SUITE 210<br>NOVATO CA 94949<br>DD 04/29/93 |
| MONOOCTANOIN<br>TN is MOCTANIN | DISSOLUTION OF CHOLESTEROL GALLSTONES RETAINED IN THE COMMON BILE DUCT | ETHITEK PHARMACEUTICALS, INC.<br>7855 GROSS POINT ROAD, UNIT L<br>SKOKIE IL 60077<br>DD 05/30/84 MA 10/31/85 |
| MORPHINE SULFATE CONCENTRATE (PRESERVATIVE FREE)<br>TN is INFUMORPH | FOR USE IN MICROINFUSION DEVICES FOR INTRASPINAL ADMINISTRATION IN THE TREATMENT OF INTRACTABLE CHRONIC PAIN | ELKINS-SINN, INC.<br>2 ESTERBROOK LANE<br>CHERRY HILL NJ 08003-4099<br>DD 07/12/90 MA 07/19/91 |
| MUCOID EXOPOLYSACCHARIDE PSEUDOMONAS HYPERIMMUNE GLOBULIN<br>TN is MEPIG | TREATMENT OF PULMONARY INFECTIONS DUE TO PSEUDOMONAS AERUGINOSA IN PATIENTS WITH CYSTIC FIBROSIS | UNIVAX BIOLOGICS, INC.<br>12280 WILKINS AVENUE<br>ROCKVILLE MD 20852<br>DD 01/09/91 |
| MUCOID EXOPOLYSACCHARIDE PSEUDOMONAS HYPERIMMUNE GLOBULIN<br>TN is MEPIG | PREVENTION OF PULMONARY INFECTIONS DUE TO PSEUDOMONAS AERUGINOSA IN PATIENTS WITH CYSTIC FIBROSIS | UNIVAX BIOLOGICS, INC.<br>12280 WILKINS AVENUE<br>ROCKVILLE MD 20852<br>DD 11/07/90 |
| MULTI-VITAMIN INFUSION (NEONATAL FORMULA) | FOR ESTABLISHMENT AND MAINTENANCE OF TOTAL PARENTERAL NUTRITION IN VERY LOW BIRTH WEIGHT INFANTS | ASTRA PHARMACEUTICAL PRODUCTS, INC.<br>50 OTIS STREET<br>WESTBOROUGH MA 01581-4500<br>DD 12/12/89 |
| MYCOBACTERIUM AVIUM SENSITIN RS-10 | FOR USE IN THE DIAGNOSIS OF INVASIVE MYCOBACTERIUM AVIUM DISEASE IN IMMUNOCOMPETENT INDIVIDUALS | STATENS SERUMINSTITUT<br>5 ARTILLERIVEJ<br>DK-2300 COPENHAGEN S<br>DENMARK |
| MYELIN | TREATMENT OF MULTIPLE SCLEROSIS | AUTOIMMUNE, INC.<br>128 SPRING STREET<br>LEXINGTON MA 02173<br>DD 06/27/91 |
| N-ACETYL-PROCAINAMIDE | PREVENTION OF LIFE-THREATENING VENTRICULAR ARRHYTHMIAS IN PATIENTS WITH DOCUMENTED PROCAINAMIDE-INDUCED LUPUS | NAPA OF THE BAHAMAS<br>3560 PENNSYLVANIA AVENUE, SUITE 7<br>DUBUQUE IA 52002 |
| N-TRIFLUOROACETYLADRIAMYCIN-14-VALERATE | TREATMENT OF CARCINOMA IN SITU OF THE URINARY BLADDER | ANTHRA PHARMACEUTICALS, INC.<br>19 CARSON ROAD<br>PRINCETON NJ 08540<br>DD 05/23/94 |
| NAFARELIN ACETATE<br>TN is SYNAREL NASAL SOLUTION | TREATMENT OF CENTRAL PRECOCIOUS PUBERTY | SYNTEX (USA), INC.<br>3401 HILLVIEW AVENUE<br>PALO ALTO CA 94303<br>DD 07/20/88 MA 02/26/92 |
| NALTREXONE HCL<br>TN is TREXAN | BLOCKADE OF THE PHARMACOLOGICAL EFFECTS OF EXOGENOUSLY ADMINISTERED OPIOIDS AS AN ADJUNCT TO THE MAINTENANCE OF THE OPIOID-FREE STATE IN DETOXIFIED FORMERLY OPIOID-DEPENDENT INDIVIDUALS | DU PONT PHARMACEUTICALS<br>E.I. du PONT de NEMOURS & CO.<br>WILMINGTON DE 19880-0026<br>DD 03/11/85 MA 11/30/84 |
| NEBACUMAB<br>TN is CENTOXIN | TREATMENT OF PATIENTS WITH GRAM-NEGATIVE BACTEREMIA WHICH HAS PROGRESSED TO ENDOTOXIN SHOCK | CENTOCOR, INC.<br>200 GREAT VALLEY PARKWAY<br>MALVERN PA 19355-1307<br>DD 10/01/86 |

# CUMULATIVE LIST OF ORPHAN PRODUCT DESIGNATIONS AND APPROVALS
[Through October 31, 1998] *(continued)*

| NAME<br>*Generic/Chemical*<br>*TN is Trade Name* | INDICATION DESIGNATED | SPONSOR AND ADDRESS<br>*DD is Date Designated*<br>*MA is Marketing Approval* |
|---|---|---|
| NEUROTROPHIN-1 | TREATMENT OF MOTOR NEURON DISEASE/AMYOTROPHIC LATERAL SCLEROSIS | ERICSSON, ARTHUR DALE, M.D.<br>6560 FANNIN, SCURLOCK TOWER<br>SUITE 720<br>HOUSTON TX 77303<br>DD 09/13/94 |
| NG-29<br>TN is SOMATREL | DIAGNOSTIC MEASURE OF THE CAPACITY OF THE PITUITARY GLAND TO RELEASE GROWTH HORMONE | FERRING LABORATORIES, INC.<br>400 RELLA BOULEVARD, SUITE 201<br>SUFFERN NY 10901<br>DD 08/08/89 |
| NIFEDIPINE | TREATMENT OF INTERSTITIAL CYSTITIS | FLEISCHMANN, JONATHAN, M.D.<br>3395 SCRANTON ROAD<br>CLEVELAND OH 44109<br>DD 06/13/91 |
| NITAZOXANIDE | TREATMENT OF CRYPTOSPORIDIOSIS IN HIV-POSITIVE AND AIDS PATIENTS | UNIMED PHARMACEUTICALS, INC.<br>2150 EAST LAKE COOK ROAD, SUITE 210<br>BUFFALO GROVE IL 60089 |
| NITAZOXANIDE | TREATMENT OF IMMUNOCOMPROMISED PATIENTS WITH CRYPTO-SPORIDIOSIS | UNIMED PHARMACEUTICALS, INC.<br>2150 EAST LAKE COOK ROAD, SUITE 210<br>BUFFALO GROVE IL 60089 |
| NITRIC OXIDE | TREATMENT OF PERSISTENT PULMONARY HYPERTENSION IN THE NEWBORN | OHMEDA PHARMACEUTICAL PRODUCTS DIVISION<br>110 ALLEN ROAD, P.O. BOX 804<br>LIBERTY CORNER NJ 07938-0804<br>DD 06/22/93 |
| NITRIC OXIDE | TREATMENT OF ACUTE RESPIRATORY DISTRESS SYNDROME IN ADULTS | OHMEDA PHARMACEUTICAL PRODUCTS DIVISION<br>110 ALLEN ROAD<br>LIBERTY CORNER NJ 07938-0804<br>DD 07/10/95 |
| NTBC | TREATMENT OF TYROSINEMIA TYPE 1 | SWEDISH ORPHAN AB<br>ORPHAN PHARMACEUTICAL, USA, INC.<br>NASHVILLE TN 37217<br>DD 05/16/95 |
| OFLOXACIN<br>TN is OCUFLOX OPHTHALMIC SOLUTION | TREATMENT OF BACTERIAL CORNEAL ULCERS | ALLERGAN, INC.<br>2525 DUPONT DRIVE<br>IRVINE CA 92715<br>DD 04/18/91 |
| OM 401<br>TN is DREPANOL | PROPHYLACTIC TREATMENT OF SICKLE CELL DISEASE | OMEX INTERNATIONAL, INC.<br>6001 SAVOY, SUITE 110<br>HOUSTON TX 77036<br>DD 10/24/91 |
| OMEGA-3 (n-3) POLYUNSATURATED FATTY ACID WITH ALL DOUBLE BONDS IN THE CIS CONFIGURATION | PREVENTION OF ORGAN GRAFT REJECTION | RESEARCH TRIANGLE PHARMACEUTICALS<br>4364 SOUTH ALSTON AVENUE<br>DURHAM NC 27713 |
| ONCORAD OV103 | TREATMENT OF OVARIAN CANCER | CYTOGEN CORPORATION<br>600 COLLEGE ROAD EAST<br>PRINCETON NJ 08540-5308<br>DD 04/24/90 |
| ORGOTEIN FOR INJECTION | TREATMENT OF FAMILIAL AMYOTROPHIC LATERAL SCLEROSIS ASSOCIATED WITH A MUTATION OF THE GENE (ON CHROMOSOME 21q) FOR COPPER, ZINC SUPEROXIDE DISMUTASE | OXIS INTERNATIONAL, INC.<br>6040 N. CUTTER CIRCLE<br>SUITE 317<br>PORTLAND OR 97217<br>DD 12/22/94 |
| OXALIPLATIN | TREATMENT OF OVARIAN CANCER | AXION PHARMACEUTICALS<br>395 OYSTER POINT BOULEVARD<br>SUITE 405<br>SOUTH SAN FRANCISCO CA 94080<br>DD 10/06/92 |
| OXANDROLONE<br>TN is OXANDRIN | TREATMENT OF PATIENTS WITH DUCHENNE'S MUSCULAR DYSTROPHY AND BECKER'S MUSCULAR DYSTROPHY | BIO-TECHNOLOGY GENERAL CORPORATION<br>70 WOOD AVENUE SOUTH<br>ISELIN NJ 08830 |
| OXANDROLONE<br>TN is OXANDRIN | TREATMENT OF SHORT STATURE ASSOCIATED WITH TURNER'S SYNDROME | BIO-TECHNOLOGY GENERAL CORP.<br>70 WOOD AVENUE, SOUTH<br>ISELIN NJ 08830<br>DD 07/05/90 |
| OXANDROLONE | TREATMENT OF CONSTITUTIONAL DELAY OF GROWTH AND PUBERTY | BIO-TECHNOLOGY GENERAL CORP.<br>70 WOOD AVENUE, SOUTH<br>ISELIN NJ 08830<br>DD 10/05/90 |

# CUMULATIVE LIST OF ORPHAN PRODUCT DESIGNATIONS AND APPROVALS
[Through October 31, 1998] *(continued)*

| NAME<br>*Generic/Chemical*<br>*TN is Trade Name* | INDICATION DESIGNATED | SPONSOR AND ADDRESS<br>*DD is Date Designated*<br>*MA is Marketing Approval* |
|---|---|---|
| OXANDROLONE<br>TN is OXANDRIN | ADJUNCTIVE THERAPY FOR AIDS PATIENTS SUFFERING FROM HIV-WASTING SYNDROME | BIO-TECHNOLOGY GENERAL CORP.<br>70 WOOD AVENUE, SOUTH<br>ISELIN NJ 08830<br>DD 09/06/91 |
| OXANDROLONE<br>TN is HEPANDRIN | TREATMENT OF MODERATE/SEVERE ACUTE ALCOHOLIC HEPATITIS IN THE PRESENCE OF MODERATE PROTEIN CALORIE MALNUTRITION | BIO-TECHNOLOGY GENERAL CORP.<br>700 WOOD AVENUE SOUTH<br>ISELIN NJ 08830<br>DD 03/18/94 |
| OXYMORPHONE HCL<br>TN is NUMORPHAN H.P | RELIEF OF SEVERE INTRACTABLE PAIN IN NARCOTIC-TOLERANT PATIENTS | DU PONT MERCK PHARMACEUTICALS<br>P.O. BOX 80027<br>WILMINGTON DE 19880-0027<br>DD 03/19/85 |
| PACLITAXEL<br>TN is PAXENE | TREATMENT OF AIDS-RELATED KAPOSI'S SARCOMA | BAKER NORTON PHARMACEUTICALS, INC.<br>4400 BISCAYNE BOULEVARD<br>MIAMI FL 33137 |
| PACLITAXEL<br>TN is TAXOL | TREATMENT OF AIDS-RELATED KAPOSI'S SARCOMA | BRISTOL-MYERS SQUIBB PHARMACEUTICAL RESEARCH INSTITUTE<br>5 RESEARCH PARKWAY<br>P.O. BOX 5100<br>WALLINGFORD CT 06492 |
| PATUL-END | TREATMENT OF PATULOUS EUSTACHIAN TUBE | THE EAR FOUNDATION<br>24209 CASTILLO STREET<br>SUITE 100<br>SANTA BARBARA CA 93105 |
| PEG-GLUCOCEREBROSIDASE | FOR USE AS CHRONIC ENZYME REPLACEMENT THERAPY IN PATIENTS WITH GAUCHER'S DISEASE WHO ARE DEFICIENT IN GLUCOCEREBROSIDASE | ENZON, INC.<br>40 KINGSBRIDGE ROAD<br>PISCATAWAY NJ 08854-3998<br>DD 12/09/92 |
| PEG-INTERLEUKIN-2 | TREATMENT OF PRIMARY IMMUNODEFICIENCIES ASSOCIATED WITH T-CELL DEFECTS | CHIRON CORPORATION<br>4560 HORTON STREET<br>EMERYVILLE CA 94608<br>DD 02/01/90 |
| PEGADEMASE BOVINE<br>TN is ADAGEN | ENZYME REPLACEMENT THERAPY FOR ADA DEFICIENCY IN PATIENTS WITH SEVERE COMBINED IMMUNODEFICIENCY (SCID) | ENZON, INC.<br>40 KINGSBRIDGE ROAD<br>PISCATAWAY NJ 08854-3998<br>DD 05/29/94 MA 03/21/90 |
| PEGASPARGASE<br>TN is ONCASPAR | TREATMENT OF ACUTE LYMPHOCYTIC LEUKEMIA (ALL) | ENZON, INC.<br>40 KINGSBRIDGE ROAD<br>PISCATAWAY NJ 08854-3998<br>DD 10/20/89 |
| PEGASYS | TREATMENT OF RENAL CELL CARCINOMA | HOFFMAN-LA ROCHE INC.<br>340 KINGSLAND STREET<br>NUTLEY NJ 07110 |
| PEGYLATED RECOMBINANT HUMAN MEGAKARYOCYTE GROWTH AND DEVELOPMENT FACTOR<br>TN is MEGAGEN | FOR REDUCING THE PERIOD OF THROMBOCYTOPENIA IN PATIENTS UNDERGOING HEMATOPOIETIC STEM CELL TRANSPLANTATION | AMGEN, INC.<br>1840 DEHAVILLAND DRIVE<br>THOUSAND OAKS CA 91320 |
| PENTAMIDINE ISETHIONATE<br>TN is PENTAM 300 | TREATMENT OF PNEUMOCYSTIS CARINII PNEUMONIA | FUJISAWA PHARMACEUTICAL CO.<br>3 PARKWAY NORTH<br>DEERFIELD IL 60015-2548<br>DD 02/28/84 MA 10/16/84 |
| PENTAMIDINE ISETHIONATE | TREATMENT OF PNEUMOCYSTIS CARINII PNEUMONIA | RHONE-POULENC RORER PHARM.<br>500 ARCOLA ROAD<br>COLLEGEVILLE PA 19426<br>DD 10/29/84 |
| PENTAMIDINE ISETHIONATE<br>TN is NEBUPENT | PREVENTION OF PNEUMOCYSTIS CARINII PNEUMONIA IN PATIENTS AT HIGH RISK OF DEVELOPING THIS DISEASE | FUJISAWA PHARMACEUTICAL CO.<br>3 PARKWAY NORTH<br>DEERFIELD IL 60015-2548<br>DD 01/12/88 MA 06/15/89 |
| PENTAMIDINE ISETHIONATE (INHALATION)<br>TN is PNEUMOPENT | PREVENTION OF PNEUMOCYSTIS CARINII PNEUMONIA IN PATIENTS AT HIGH RISK OF DEVELOPING THIS DISEASE | FISONS CORPORATION<br>755 JEFFERSON RD., P.O. BOX 1710<br>ROCHESTER NY 14603<br>DD 10/05/87 |
| PENTASTARCH<br>TN is PENTASPAN | ADJUNCT IN LEUKAPHERESIS TO IMPROVE THE HARVESTING AND INCREASE THE YIELD OF LEUKOCYTES BY CENTRIFUGAL MEANS | DU PONT PHARMACEUTICALS<br>E.I. du PONT de NEMOURS & CO.<br>WILMINGTON DE 19898<br>DD 08/28/85 MA 05/19/87 |
| PENTOSAN POLYSULPHATE<br>TN is ELMIRON | TREATMENT OF INTERSTITIAL CYSTITIS | BAKER NORTON PHARMACEUTICALS<br>8800 NORTHWEST 36TH STREET<br>MIAMI FL 33178<br>DD 08/07/85 |

## CUMULATIVE LIST OF ORPHAN PRODUCT DESIGNATIONS AND APPROVALS
[Through October 31, 1998] *(continued)*

| NAME<br>*Generic/Chemical*<br>*TN is Trade Name* | INDICATION DESIGNATED | SPONSOR AND ADDRESS<br>*DD is Date Designated*<br>*MA is Marketing Approval* |
|---|---|---|
| PENTOSTATIN | TREATMENT OF PATIENTS WITH CHRONIC LYMPHOCYTIC LEUKEMIA | WARNER-LAMBERT COMPANY<br>2800 PLYMOUTH ROAD<br>ANN ARBOR MI 48106-1047<br>DD 01/29/91 |
| PENTOSTATIN | TREATMENT OF CUTANEOUS T-CELL LYMPHOMA | SUPERGEN, INC.<br>TWO ANABEL LANE, SUITE 220<br>SAN RAMON CA 94583 |
| PENTOSTATIN FOR INJECTION<br>TN is NIPENT | TREATMENT OF HAIRY CELL LEUKEMIA | WARNER-LAMBERT COMPANY<br>2800 PLYMOUTH RD.,<br>P.O. BOX 1047<br>ANN ARBOR MI 48106<br>DD 09/10/87 MA 10/11/91 |
| PERGOLIDE<br>TN is PERMAX | TREATMENT OF TOURETTE'S SYNDROME | SALLE, FLOYD R., M.D., PH.D.<br>MEDICAL UNIVERSITY OF SOUTH CAROLINA<br>171 ASHLEY AVENUE, ROOM PH246<br>CHARLESTON SC 29425 |
| PHENYLACETATE | FOR USE AS AN ADJUNCT TO SURGERY, RADIATION THERAPY, AND CHEMOTHERAPY FOR THE TREATMENT OF PATIENTS WITH PRIMARY OR RECURRENT MALIGNANT GLIOMA | TARGON CORPORATION<br>307 COLLEGE ROAD EAST<br>PRINCETON NJ 08540 |
| PHENYLALANINE AMMONIA-LYASE<br>TN is PHENYLASE | TREATMENT OF HYPERPHENYLALANINEMIA | IBEX TECHNOLOGIES, INC.<br>5485 PARE<br>MONTREAL QUEBEC<br>DD 03/08/95 |
| PHOSPHOCYSTEAMINE | TREATMENT OF CYSTINOSIS | MEDEA RESEARCH LABORATORIES<br>200 WILSON STREET, BLDG D-6<br>PORT JEFFERSON NY 11776<br>DD 09/12/88 |
| PHYSOSTIGMINE SALICYLATE<br>TN is ANTILIRIUM | FRIEDREICH'S AND OTHER INHERITED ATAXIAS | FOREST PHARMACEUTICALS, INC.<br>150 EAST 58TH STREET<br>NEW YORK NY 10155<br>DD 01/16/85 |
| PILOCARPINE<br>TN is SALAGEN | TREATMENT OF XEROSTOMIA INDUCED BY RADIATION THERAPY FOR HEAD AND NECK CANCER | MGI PHARMA, INC.<br>SUITE 300 E, 9900 BREN ROAD EAST<br>MINNEAPOLIS MN 55343-9667<br>DD 09/24/90 |
| PILOCARPINE HCL<br>TN is SALAGEN | TREATMENT OF XEROSTOMIA AND KERATOCONJUNCTIVITIS SICCA IN SJOGREN'S SYNDROME PATIENTS | MGI PHARMA, INC.<br>9900 BREN ROAD EAST, SUITE 900E<br>MINNEAPOLIS MN 55343-9667<br>DD 02/28/92 |
| PIRACETAM<br>TN is NOOTROPIL | TREATMENT OF MYOCLONUS | UCB PHARMACEUTICALS, INC.<br>1950 LAKE PARK DRIVE<br>SMYRNA GA 30080<br>DD 10/02/87 |
| POLOXAMER 188 | TREATMENT OF VASOSPASM IN SUBARACHNOID HEMORRHAGE PATIENTS FOLLOWING SURGICAL REPAIR OF A RUPTURED CEREBRAL ANEURYSM | CYTRX CORPORATION<br>154 TECHNOLOGY PARKWAY<br>NORCROSS GA 30092 |
| POLOXAMER 188<br>TN is RHEOTHRX COPOLYMER | TREATMENT OF SICKLE CELL CRISIS | BURROUGHS WELLCOME COMPANY<br>3030 CORNWALLIS ROAD<br>RESEARCH TRIANGLE PK NC 27709<br>DD 06/27/89 |
| POLOXAMER 188<br>TN is RHEOTHRX COPOLYMER | TREATMENT OF SEVERE BURNS REQUIRING HOSPITALIZATION | BURROUGHS WELLCOME COMPANY<br>3030 CORNWALLIS ROAD<br>RESEARCH TRIANGLE PK NC 27709<br>DD 02/22/90 |
| POLOXAMER 331<br>TN is PROTOX | INITIAL THERAPY OF TOXOPLASMOSIS IN PATIENTS WITH ACQUIRED IMMUNODEFICIENCY SYNDROME (AIDS) | CYTRX CORPORATION<br>150 TECHNOLOGY PARKWAY<br>NORCROSS GA 30092<br>DD 03/21/91 |
| POLY-ICLC | TREATMENT OF PRIMARY BRAIN TUMORS | SALAZAR, ANDRES M., M.D., AND LEVY, HILTON B., PH.D.<br>3202 CLEVELAND AVENUE, N.W.<br>WASHINGTON DC 20008 |
| POLY I: POLY C12U<br>TN is AMPLIGEN | TREATMENT OF ACQUIRED IMMUNODEFICIENCY SYNDROME (AIDS) | HEM PHARMACEUTICALS CORP.<br>1617 JFK BOULEVARD, SUITE 600<br>PHILADELPHIA PA 19103<br>DD 07/19/88 |
| POLY I: POLY C12U<br>TN is AMPLIGEN | TREATMENT OF RENAL CELL CARCINOMA | HEM PHARMACEUTICALS CORP.<br>1617 JFK BOULEVARD, SUITE 600<br>PHILADELPHIA PA 19103<br>DD 05/20/91 |

# CUMULATIVE LIST OF ORPHAN PRODUCT DESIGNATIONS AND APPROVALS
[Through October 31, 1998] *(continued)*

| NAME<br>*Generic/Chemical*<br>*TN is Trade Name* | INDICATION DESIGNATED | SPONSOR AND ADDRESS<br>*DD is Date Designated*<br>*MA is Marketing Approval* |
|---|---|---|
| POLY I: POLY C12U<br>TN is AMPLIGEN | TREATMENT OF CHRONIC FATIGUE SYNDROME | HEM PHARMACEUTICALS CORP.<br>ONE PENN CENTER, SUITE 660<br>PHILADELPHIA PA 19103<br>DD 12/09/93 |
| POLY I; POLY C12U<br>TN is AMPLIGEN | TREATMENT OF INVASIVE METASTATIC MELANOMA (STAGE IIB, III, IV) | HEM PHARMACEUTICALS CORP.<br>ONE PENN CENTER<br>SUITE 660<br>PHILADELPHIA PA 19103<br>DD 12/09/93 |
| POLYMERIC OXYGEN | TREATMENT OF SICKLE CELL ANEMIA | CAPMED USA<br>P.O. BOX 14<br>BRYN MAWR PA 19010<br>DD 03/25/92 |
| PORCINE FETAL NEURAL DOPAMINERGIC CELLS AND/OR PRECURSORS ASEPTICALLY PREPARED AND COATED WITH ANTI-MHC-1 AB FOR INTRACEREBRAL IMPLANTATION<br>TN is NEUROCELL-PD | TREATMENT OF HOEHN AND YAHR STAGE 4 AND 5 PARKINSON'S DISEASE | DIACRIN, INC.<br>BUILDING 39, 13TH STREET<br>CHARLESTOWN MA 02129 |
| PORCINE FETAL NEURAL DOPAMINERGIC CELLS AND/OR PRECURSORS ASEPTICALLY PREPARED FOR INTRACEREBRAL IMPLANTATION<br>TN is NEUROCELL-PD | TREATMENT OF HOEHN AND YAHR STAGE 4 AND 5 PARKINSON'S DISEASE | DIACRIN, INC.<br>BUILDING 96, 13TH STREET<br>CHARLESTOWN NAVY YARD<br>CHARLESTOWN MA 02129 |
| PORCINE FETAL NEURAL GABAERGIC CELLS AND/OR PRECURSORS ASEPTICALLY PREPARED AND COATED WITH ANTI-MHC-1 AB FOR INTRACEREBRAL IMPLANTATION<br>TN is NEUROCELL-HD | TREATMENT OF HUNTINGTON'S DISEASE | DIACRIN, INC.<br>BUILDING 96, 13TH STREET<br>CHARLESTOWN MA 02129 |
| PORCINE FETAL NEURAL GABAERGIC CELLS AND/OR PRECURSORS ASEPTICALLY PREPARED FOR INTRACEREBRAL IMPLANTATION FOR HUNTINGTON'S DISEASE<br>TN is NEUROCELL-HD | TREATMENT OF HUNTINGTON'S DISEASE | DIACRIN, INC.<br>BUILDING 96, 13TH STREET<br>CHARLESTOWN NAVY YARD<br>CHARLESTOWN MA 02129 |
| PORCINE SERTOLI CELLS<br>TN is N-GRAFT | TREATMENT OF HOEHN AND YAHR STAGES FOUR AND FIVE PARKINSON'S DISEASE | THERACELL, INC.<br>50 DIVISION STREET<br>SUITE 503<br>SOMERVILLE NJ 08876 |
| PORFIMER SODIUM<br>TN is PHOTOFRIN | FOR THE PHOTODYNAMIC THERAPY OF PATIENTS WITH PRIMARY OR RECURRENT OBSTRUCTING (EITHER PARTIALLY OR COMPLETELY) ESOPHAGEAL CARCINOMA | QLT PHOTOTHERAPEUTICS, INC.<br>401 NORTH MIDDLETOWN ROAD<br>PEARL RIVER NY 10965<br>DD 06/06/89 |
| PORFIMER SODIUM<br>TN is PHOTOFRIN | FOR THE PHOTODYNAMIC THERAPY OF PATIENTS WITH TRANSITIONAL CELL CARCINOMA IN SITU OF URINARY BLADDER | QLT PHOTOTHERAPEUTICS, INC.<br>401 NORTH MIDDLETOWN ROAD<br>PEARL RIVER NY 10965<br>DD 11/15/89 |
| PORFIROMYCIN<br>TN is PROMYCIN | TREATMENT OF CERVICAL CANCER | VION PHARMACEUTICALS, INC.<br>FOUR SCIENCE PARK<br>NEW HAVEN CT 06511 |
| PORFIROMYCIN | TREATMENT OF HEAD AND NECK CANCER | ONCORX, INC.<br>4 SCIENCE PARK<br>NEW HAVEN CT 06511 |
| POTASSIUM CITRATE<br>TN is UROCIT-K | PREVENTION OF URIC ACID NEPHROLITHIASIS | UNIV. OF TEXAS HEALTH SCIENCES<br>5323 HARRY HINES BLVD<br>DALLAS TX 75235<br>DD 11/01/84 MA 08/30/85 |
| POTASSIUM CITRATE<br>TN is UROCIT-K | PREVENTION OF CALCIUM RENAL STONES IN PATIENTS WITH HYPOCITRATURIA | UNIV. OF TEXAS HEALTH SCIENCES<br>5323 HARRY HINES BLVD<br>DALLAS TX 75235<br>DD 09/16/85 MA 08/30/85 |
| POTASSIUM CITRATE<br>TN is UROCIT K | AVOIDANCE OF THE COMPLICATION OF CALCIUM STONE FORMATION IN PATIENTS WITH URIC LITHIASIS | UNIV. OF TEXAS HEALTH SCIENCES<br>5323 HARRY HINES BLVD.<br>DALLAS TX 75235<br>DD 05/29/84 MA 08/30/85 |
| PREDNIMUSTINE<br>TN is STERECYT | TREATMENT OF MALIGNANT NON-HODGKIN'S LYMPHOMAS | PHARMACIA, INC.<br>P.O. BOX 16529<br>COLUMBUS OH 43216-6529<br>DD 06/17/85 |

# CUMULATIVE LIST OF ORPHAN PRODUCT DESIGNATIONS AND APPROVALS
[Through October 31, 1998] *(continued)*

| NAME<br>*Generic/Chemical*<br>*TN is Trade Name* | INDICATION DESIGNATED | SPONSOR AND ADDRESS<br>*DD is Date Designated*<br>*MA is Marketing Approval* |
|---|---|---|
| PRIMAQUINE PHOSPHATE | FOR USE IN COMBINATION WITH CLINDAMYCIN HYDROCHLORIDE IN THE TREATMENT OF PNEUMOCYSTIS CARINII PNEUMONIA ASSOCIATED WITH ACQUIRED IMMUNODEFICIENCY SYNDROME | SANOFI WINTHROP INC.<br>90 PARK AVENUE<br>NEW YORK NY 10016-1389<br>DD 07/23/93 |
| PROGESTERONE | ESTABLISHMENT AND MAINTENANCE OF PREGNANCY IN WOMEN UNDERGOING IN VITRO FERTILIZATION OR EMBRYO TRANSFER PROCEDURES | WATSON LABORATORIES, INC.<br>311 BONNIE CIRCLE<br>CORONA CA 91720<br>DD 12/22/94 |
| PROPAMIDINE ISETHIONATE 0.1% OPHTHALMIC SOLUTION<br>TN is BROLENE | TREATMENT OF ACANTHAMOEBA KERATITIS | BAUSCH & LOMB PHARMACEUTICALS<br>1400 NORTH GOODMAN STREET<br>ROCHESTER NY 14692<br>DD 03/10/88 |
| PROSTAGLANDIN EL ENOL ESTER (AS-013) | TREATMENT OF FONTAINE STAGE IV CHRONIC CRITICAL LIMB ISCHEMIA | ALPHA THERAPEUTIC CORP.<br>5555 VALLEY BLVD.<br>LOS ANGELES CA 90032 |
| PROSTAGLANDIN E1 IN LIPID EMULSION | TREATMENT OF ISCHEMIC ULCERATION OF THE LOWER LIMBS DUE TO PERIPHERAL ARTERIAL DISEASE | ALPHA THERAPEUTIC CORPORATION<br>5555 VALLEY BOULEVARD<br>LOS ANGELES CA 90032 |
| PROTEIN C CONCENTRATE<br>TN is PROTEIN C CONCENTRATE (HUMAN) VAPOR HEATED, IMMUNO | FOR REPLACEMENT THERAPY IN PATIENTS WITH CONGENITAL OR ACQUIRED PROTEIN C DEFICIENCY FOR THE PREVENTION AND TREATMENT OF WARFARIN-INDUCED SKIN NECROSIS DURING ORAL ANTICOAGULATION | IMMUNO CLINICAL RESEARCH CORP.<br>750 LEXINGTON AVENUE, 19TH FLOOR<br>NEW YORK NY 10022<br>DD 06/19/92 |
| PROTEIN C CONCENTRATE<br>TN is PROTEIN C CONCENTRATE (HUMAN) VAPOR HEATED, IMMUNO | FOR USE IN THE PREVENTION AND TREATMENT OF PURPURA FULMINANS IN MENINGOCOCCEMIA | IMMUNO CLINICAL RESEARCH CORP.<br>750 LEXINGTON AVENUE, 19TH FLOOR<br>NEW YORK NY 10022<br>DD 04/22/93 |
| PROTEIN C CONCENTRATE<br>TN is PROTEIN C CONCENTRATE (HUMAN) VAPOR HEATED, IMMUNO | FOR REPLACEMENT THERAPY IN CONGENITAL PROTEIN C DEFICIENCY FOR THE PREVENTION AND TREATMENT OF THROMBOSIS, PULMONARY EMBOLI, AND PURPURA FULMINANS | IMMUNO CLINICAL RESEARCH CORP.<br>750 LEXINGTON AVENUE, 19TH FLOOR<br>NEW YORK NY 10022<br>DD 06/23/92 |
| PROTIRELIN | PREVENTION OF INFANT RESPIRATORY DISTRESS SYNDROME ASSOCIATED WITH PREMATURITY | UCB PHARMACEUTICALS, INC.<br>1950 LAKE PARK DRIVE<br>ATLANTA GA 30080<br>DD 08/24/93 |
| PULMONARY SURFACTANT REPLACEMENT | PREVENTION AND TREATMENT OF INFANT RESPIRATORY DISTRESS SYNDROME (RDS) | SCIOS NOVA, INC.<br>2450 BAYSHORE PARKWAY<br>MOUNTAIN VIEW CA 94043<br>DD 12/05/88 |
| PULMONARY SURFACTANT REPLACEMENT, PORCINE<br>TN is CUROSURF | FOR THE TREATMENT AND PREVENTION OF RESPIRATORY DISTRESS SYNDROME IN PREMATURE INFANTS | DEY LABORATORIES<br>2751 NAPA VALLEY CORPORATE DRIVE<br>NAPA CA 94550<br>DD 08/02/93 |
| PURIFIED EXTRACT OF PSEUDOMONAS AERUGINOSA<br>TN is IMMUDYN | TREATMENT OF IMMUNE THROMBOCYTOPENIA PURPURA WHERE IT IS REQUIRED TO INCREASE PLATELET COUNTS | DYNAGEN, INC.<br>99 ERIE STREET<br>CAMBRIDGE MA 02139 |
| PURIFIED TYPE II COLLAGEN<br>TN is COLLORAL | TREATMENT OF JUVENILE RHEUMATOID ARTHRITIS | AUTOIMMUNE, INCORPORATED<br>128 SPRING STREET<br>LEXINGTON MA 02173<br>DD 02/09/95 |
| RADIOLABELED MONOCLONAL ANTIBODY TO CD22 ANTIGEN ON B-CELLS<br>TN is LYMPHOCIDE | TREATMENT OF NON-HODGKIN'S LYMPHOMA | IMMUNOMEDICS, INC.<br>300 AMERICAN ROAD<br>MORRIS PLAINS NJ 07950 |
| RECOMBINANT BACTERICIDAL/PERMEABILITY-INCREASING PROTEIN<br>TN is NEUPREX | TREATMENT OF SEVERE MENINGOCOCCAL DISEASE | XOMA CORPORATION<br>2910 SEVENTH STREET<br>BERKELEY CA 94710 |
| RECOMBINANT HUMAN ACID ALPHA-GLUCOSIDASE | TREATMENT OF GLYCOGEN STORAGE DISEASE TYPE II | CHEN, Y. T., M.D., PHD.<br>DEPARTMENT OF PEDIATRICS<br>DUKE UNIVERSITY MEDICAL CENTER<br>DURHAM NC 27710 |
| RECOMBINANT HUMAN ALPHA-L-IDURONIDASE | TREATMENT OF PATIENTS WITH MUCOPOLYSACCHARIDOSIS-I | BIOMARIN PHARMACEUTICALS, INC.<br>11 PIMENTAL COURT<br>NOVATA CA 94949 |
| RECOMBINANT HUMAN CD4 IMMUNOGLOBULIN G | TREATMENT OF ACQUIRED IMMUNODEFICIENCY SYNDROME (AIDS) RESULTING FROM INFECTION WITH THE HUMAN IMMUNODEFICIENCY VIRUS (HIV-1) | GENENTECH, INC.<br>460 POINT SAN BRUNO BOULEVARD<br>SO. SAN FRANCISCO CA 94080<br>DD 08/30/90 |
| RECOMBINANT HUMAN CLARA CELL 10KDA PROTEIN | PREVENTION OF NEONATAL BRONCHOPULMONARY DYSPLASIA IN PREMATURE NEONATES WITH RESPIRATORY DISTRESS SYNDROME | CLARAGEN, INC.<br>335 PAINT BRANCH DRIVE<br>COLLEGE PARK MD 20742 |

# CUMULATIVE LIST OF ORPHAN PRODUCT DESIGNATIONS AND APPROVALS
[Through October 31, 1998] *(continued)*

| NAME<br>*Generic/Chemical*<br>*TN is Trade Name* | INDICATION DESIGNATED | SPONSOR AND ADDRESS<br>*DD is Date Designated*<br>*MA is Marketing Approval* |
|---|---|---|
| RECOMBINANT HUMAN GELSOLIN | TREATMENT OF THE RESPIRATORY SYMTOMS OF CYSTIC FIBROSIS | BIOGEN, INC.<br>14 CAMBRIDGE CENTER<br>CAMBRIDGE MA 02124<br>DD 01/12/94 |
| RECOMBINANT HUMAN GELSOLIN | TREATMENT OF ACUTE AND CHRONIC RESPIRATORY SYMPTOMS OF BRONCHIECTASIS | BIOGEN, INCORPORATED<br>14 CAMBRIDGE CENTER<br>CAMBRIDGE MA 02142<br>DD 03/06/95 |
| RECOMBINANT HUMAN INSULIN-LIKE GROWTH FACTOR I<br>TN is IGEF | TREATMENT OF GROWTH HORMONE RECEPTOR DEFICIENCY | PHARMACIA, INC.<br>P.O. BOX 16529<br>COLUMBUS OH 43216-6529<br>DD 06/07/95 |
| RECOMBINANT HUMAN INSULIN-LIKE GROWTH FACTOR I<br>TN is IGEF | TREATMENT OF ANTIBODY-MEDIATED GROWTH HORMONE RESISTANCE IN PATIENTS WITH ISOLATED GROWTH HORMONE DEFICIENCY IA | PHARMACIA, INC.<br>P.O. BOX 16529<br>COLUMBUS OH 43216-6529<br>DD 06/07/95 |
| RECOMBINANT HUMAN INSULIN-LIKE GROWTH FACTOR-I | TREATMENT OF POST-POLIOMYELITIS SYNDROME | CEPHALON, INC.<br>145 BRANDYWINE PARKWAY<br>WEST CHESTER PA 19380 |
| RECOMBINANT HUMAN INTERLEUKIN-11<br>TN is NEUMEGA RHIL-11 GROWTH FACTOR | PREVENTION OF SEVERE CHEMOTHERAPY-INDUCED THROMBOCYTOPENIA | GENETICS INSTITUTE, INC.<br>87 CAMBRIDGE PARK DRIVE<br>CAMBRIDGE MA 02140 |
| RECOMBINANT HUMAN INTERLEUKIN-12 | TREATMENT OF RENAL CELL CARCINOMA | GENETICS INSTITUTE<br>87 CAMBRIDGE PARK DRIVE<br>CAMBRIDGE MA 02140 |
| RECOMBINANT HUMAN LUTEINIZING HORMONE | FOR USE IN ASSOCATION WITH RECOMBINANT HUMAN FOLLICLE STIMULATING HORMONE FOR THE TREATMENT OF WOMEN WITH CHRONIC ANOVULATION DUE TO HYPOGONADOTROPIC HYPOGONADISM | SERONO LABORATORIES, INCORPORATED<br>100 LONGWATER CIRCLE<br>NORWELL MA 02061<br>DD 10/07/94 |
| RECOMBINANT HUMAN RELAXIN | TREATMENT OF PROGRESSIVE SYSTEMIC SCLEROSIS | CONNECTIVE TECHNOLOGIES, INC.<br>3400 WEST BAYSHORE ROAD<br>PALO ALTO CA 94303 |
| RECOMBINANT HUMAN THROMBOPOIETIN | FOR USE IN ACCELERATING PLATELET RECOVERY IN PATIENTS UNDERGOING HEMATOPOIETIC STEM CELL TRANSPLANTATION | GENENTECH, INC.<br>ONE DNA WAY<br>SAN FRANCISCO CA 94080 |
| RECOMBINANT HUMANIZED MONOCLONAL ANTIBODY 5C8 | TREATMENT OF IMMUNE THROMBOCYTOPENIC PURPURA | BIOGEN, INC.<br>14 CAMBRIDGE CENTER<br>CAMBRIDGE MA 02142 |
| RECOMBINANT HUMANIZED MONOCLONAL ANTIBODY 5C8 | TREATMENT OF SYSTEMIC LUPUS ERYTHEMATOSUS | BIOGEN, INC.<br>14 CAMBRIDGE CENTER<br>CAMBRIDGE MA 02142 |
| RECOMBINANT METHIONYL BRAIN-DERIVED NEUROTROPHIC FACTOR | TREATMENT OF AMYOTROPHIC LATERAL SCLEROSIS | AMGEN, INCORPORATED<br>1840 DEHAVILLAND DRIVE<br>THOUSAND OAKS CA 91320-1789<br>DD 11/28/94 |
| RECOMBINANT METHIONYL HUMAN STEM CELL FACTOR | FOR USE IN COMBINATION WITH FILGRASTIM TO DECREASE THE NUMBER OF PHERESES REQUIRED TO COLLECT PERIPHERAL BLOOD PROGENITOR CELLS CAPABLE OF PROVIDING RAPID MULTI-LINEAGE HEMATOPOIETIC RECONSTITUTION FOLLOWING MYELOSUPPRESSIVE OR MYELOABLATIVE THERAPY | AMGEN, INCORPORATED<br>1840 DEHAVILLAND DRIVE<br>THOUSAND OAKS CA 91320-1789<br>DD 07/05/95 |
| RECOMBINANT METHIONYL HUMAN STEM CELL FACTOR | TREATMENT OF PRIMARY BONE MARROW FAILURE | AMGEN, INC.<br>1840 DEHAVILLAND DRIVE<br>THOUSAND OAKS CA 91320 |
| RECOMBINANT RETROVIRAL VECTOR—GLUCOCEREBROSIDASE | FOR USE AS ENZYME REPLACEMENT THERAPY FOR PATIENTS WITH TYPES I, II, OR III GAUCHER DISEASE | GENETIC THERAPY, INC.<br>938 CLOPPER ROAD<br>GAITHERSBURG MD 20878<br>DD 11/15/93 |
| RECOMBINANT SECRETORY LEUCOCYTE PROTEASE INHIBITOR | TREATMENT OF CONGENITAL ALPHA-1 ANTITRYPSIN DEFICIENCY | AMGEN BOULDER INC.<br>3200 WALNUT STREET<br>BOULDER CO 80301<br>DD 03/29/91 |
| RECOMBINANT SECRETORY LEUCOCYTE PROTEASE INHIBITOR | TREATMENT OF CYSTIC FIBROSIS | AMGEN BOULDER INC.<br>3200 WALNUT STREET<br>BOULDER CO 80301<br>DD 03/29/91 |
| RECOMBINANT SOLUBLE HUMAN CD 4 (rCD4) | TREATMENT OF AIDS IN PATIENTS INFECTED WITH HIV VIRUS | GENENTECH, INC.<br>460 POINT SAN BRUNO BOULEVARD<br>SOUTH SAN FRANCISCO CA 94080<br>DD 03/23/89 |

## CUMULATIVE LIST OF ORPHAN PRODUCT DESIGNATIONS AND APPROVALS
[Through October 31, 1998] (continued)

| NAME<br>Generic/Chemical<br>TN is Trade Name | INDICATION DESIGNATED | SPONSOR AND ADDRESS<br>DD is Date Designated<br>MA is Marketing Approval |
|---|---|---|
| RECOMBINANT SOLUBLE HUMAN CD4<br>TN is RECEPTIN | TREATMENT OF ACQUIRED IMMUNODEFICIENCY SYNDROME (AIDS) | BIOGEN, INC.<br>14 CAMBRIDGE CENTER<br>CAMBRIDGE MA 02142<br>DD 11/20/89 |
| RECOMBINANT VACCINIA (HUMAN PAPILLOMAVIRUS)<br>TN is TA-HPV | TREATMENT OF CERVICAL CANCER | CANTAB PHARMACEUTICALS RESEARCH, LTD.<br>184 CAMBRIDGE SCIENCE PARK<br>CAMBRIDGE CB4 4GN UK<br>DD 08/24/94 |
| REDUCED L-GLUTATHIONE<br>TN is CACHEXON | TREATMENT OF AIDS-ASSOCIATED CACHEXIA | TELLURIDE PHARMACEUTICAL CORPORATION<br>146 FLANDERS DRIVE<br>HILLSBOROUGH NJ 08876-4656<br>DD 02/14/94 |
| REFAXIMIN<br>TN is NORMIX | TREATMENT OF HEPATIC ENCEPHALOPATHY | SALIX PHARMACEUTICALS, INC.<br>3600 W. BAYSHORE ROAD<br>PALO ALTO CA 94303 |
| RESPIRATORY SYNCYTIAL VIRUS IMMUNE GLOBULIN (HUMAN)<br>TN is RESPIGAN | PROPHYLAXIS OF RESPIRATORY SYNCYTIAL VIRUS (RSV) LOWER RESPIRATORY TRACT INFECTIONS IN INFANTS AND YOUNG CHILDREN AT HIGH RISK OF RSV DISEASE | MEDIMMUNE, INC.<br>35 WEST WATKINS MILL ROAD<br>GAITHERSBURG MD 20878<br>DD 09/27/90 |
| RESPIRATORY SYNCYTIAL VIRUS IMMUNE GLOBULIN (HUMAN)<br>TN is HYPERMUNE RSV | TREATMENT OF RESPIRATORY SYNCYTIAL VIRUS (RSV) LOWER RESPIRATORY TRACT INFECTIONS IN HOSPITALIZED INFANTS AND YOUNG CHILDREN | MEDIMMUNE, INC.<br>35 WEST WATKINS MILL ROAD<br>GAITHERSBURG MD 20878<br>DD 09/27/90 |
| RETINOIN | TREATMENT OF SQUAMOUS METAPLASIA OF THE OCULAR SURFACE EPITHELIA (CONJUNCTIVA AND/OR CORNEA) WITH MUCOUS DEFICIENCY AND KERATINIZATION | HANNAN OPHTHALMIC MARKETING SERVICES, INC.<br>163 MEETINGHOUSE ROAD<br>DUXBURY MA 02332<br>DD 04/15/85 |
| RETROVIRAL VECTOR, R-GC AND GC GENE 1750 | TREATMENT OF GAUCHER DISEASE | GENZYME CORPORATION<br>ONE KENDALL SQUARE<br>CAMBRIDGE MA 02139 |
| RGG0853, E1A LIPID COMPLEX | TREATMENT OF ADVANCED OVARIAN CANCER THAT OVEREXPRESSES THE HER-2/NEU ONCOGENE | RGENE THERAPEUTICS, INC.<br>2170 BLACKTHORNE PLACE, SUITE 230<br>THE WOODLANDS TX 77380 |
| RGG0853, E1A LIPID COMPLEX | TREATMENT OF OVARIAN CANCER | TARGETED GENETICS CORPORATION<br>1100 OLIVE WAY, SUITE 100<br>SEATTLE WA 98101 |
| RHO(D) IMMUNE GLOBULIN (HUMAN)<br>TN is WINRho SD | TREATMENT OF IMMUNE THROMBOCYTOPENIC PURPURA | RH PHARMACEUTICALS, INC.<br>104 CHANCELLOR MATHESON ROAD<br>WINNIPEG MANITOBA<br>DD 11/09/93 MA 03/24/95 |
| RIBAVIRIN<br>TN is VIRAZOLE | TREATMENT OF HEMORRHAGIC FEVER WITH RENAL SYNDROME | ICN PHARMACEUTICALS, INC.<br>3300 HYLAND AVENUE<br>COSTA MESA CA 92626<br>DD 04/12/91 |
| RICIN (BLOCKED) CONJUGATED MURINE MCA (ANTI-B4) | TREATMENT OF B-CELL LEUKEMIA AND B-CELL LYMPHOMA | IMMUNOGEN, INC.<br>148 SIDNEY STREET<br>CAMBRIDGE MA 02139<br>DD 11/17/88 |
| RICIN (BLOCKED) CONJUGATED MURINE MCA (ANTI-B4) | FOR THE EX-VIVO PURGING OF LEUKEMIC CELLS FROM THE BONE MARROW OF NON-T CELL ACUTE LYMPHOCYTIC LEUKEMIA PATIENTS WHO ARE IN COMPLETE REMISSION | IMMUNOGEN, INC.<br>148 SIDNEY STREET<br>CAMBRIDGE MA 02139<br>DD 01/24/91 |
| RICIN (BLOCKED) CONJUGATED MURINE MCA (ANTI-MY9) | TREATMENT OF MYELOID LEUKEMIA, INCLUDING AML, AND BLAST CRISIS OF CML | IMMUNOGEN, INC.<br>148 SIDNEY STREET<br>CAMBRIDGE MA 02139<br>DD 08/03/89 |
| RICIN (BLOCKED) CONJUGATED MURINE MCA (ANTI-MY9) | FOR USE IN THE EX-VIVO TREATMENT OF AUTOLOGOUS BONE MARROW AND SUBSEQUENT REINFUSION IN PATIENTS WITH ACUTE MYELOGENOUS LEUKEMIA (AML) | IMMUNOGEN, INC.<br>148 SIDNEY STREET<br>CAMBRIDGE MA 02139<br>DD 02/01/90 |
| RICIN (BLOCKED) CONJUGATED MURINE MCA (N901) | TREATMENT OF SMALL CELL LUNG CANCER | IMMUNOGEN, INC.<br>148 SIDNEY STREET<br>CAMBRIDGE MA 02139<br>DD 01/25/91 |
| RICIN (BLOCKED) CONJUGATED MURINE MOAB (CD6) | TREATMENT OF CUTANEOUS T-CELL LYMPHOMAS, ACUTE T-CELL LEUKEMIA-LYMPHOMA, AND RELATED MATURE T-CELL MALIGNANCIES | IMMUNOGEN, INC.<br>148 SIDNEY STREET<br>CAMBRIDGE MA 02139-4239<br>DD 09/06/94 |

# CUMULATIVE LIST OF ORPHAN PRODUCT DESIGNATIONS AND APPROVALS
[Through October 31, 1998] *(continued)*

| NAME<br>*Generic/Chemical*<br>*TN is Trade Name* | INDICATION DESIGNATED | SPONSOR AND ADDRESS<br>*DD is Date Designated*<br>*MA is Marketing Approval* |
|---|---|---|
| RIFABUTIN | TREATMENT OF DISSEMINATED MYCOBACTERIUM AVIUM COMPLEX (MAC) DISEASE | ADRIA LABORATORIES, INC.<br>P.O. BOX 16529<br>COLUMBUS OH 43216-6529<br>DD 12/18/89 |
| RIFABUTIN<br>TN is MYCOBUTIN | PREVENTION OF DISSEMINATED MYCOBACTERIUM AVIUM COMPLEX (MAC) DISEASE IN PATIENTS WITH ADVANCED HIV INFECTION | ADRIA LABORATORIES, INC.<br>P.O. BOX 16529<br>COLUMBUS OH 43216-6529<br>DD 12/18/89 MA 12/23/92 |
| RIFAMPIN<br>TN is RIFADIN I.V | ANTITUBERCULOSIS TREATMENT WHERE USE OF THE ORAL FORM OF THE DRUG IS NOT FEASIBLE | MARION MERRELL DOW, INC.<br>P.O. BOX 9707, MARION PARK DRIVE<br>KANSAS CITY MO 64134-0707<br>DD 12/09/85 MA 05/25/89 |
| RIFAMPIN, ISONIAZID, PYRA-ZINAMIDE<br>TN is RIFATER | SHORT COURSE TREATMENT OF TUBERCULOSIS | MARION MERRELL DOW, INC.<br>P.O. BOX 9627<br>KANSAS CITY MO 64134-0627<br>DD 09/12/85 |
| RIFAPENTINE | PROPHYLACTIC TREATMENT OF MYCOBACTERIUM AVIUM COMPLEX IN PATIENTS WITH ACQUIRED IMMUNODEFICIENCY SYNDROME AND A CD4+ COUNT LESS THAN OR EQUAL TO 75/MM3 | MARION MERRELL DOW INC.<br>P.O. BOX 9627 (PARK A)<br>KANSAS CITY MO 64137 |
| RIFAPENTINE | TREATMENT OF PULMONARY TUBERCULOSIS | MARION MERRELL DOW INC.<br>P.O. BOX 9627 (PARK A)<br>KANSAS CITY MO 64137<br>DD 06/09/95 |
| RIFAPENTINE | TREATMENT OF MYCOBACTERIUM AVIUM COMPLEX IN PATIENTS WITH ACQUIRED IMMUNODEFICIENCY SYNDROME | MARION MERRELL DOW INC.<br>P.O. BOX 9627 (PARK A)<br>KANSAS CITY MO 64137<br>DD 06/09/95 |
| RII RETINAMIDE | TREATMENT OF MYELODYSPLASTIC SYNDROMES | SPARTA PHARMACEUTICALS, INCORPORATED<br>P.O. BOX 13288<br>RESEARCH TRIANGLE PK NC 27709<br>DD 05/06/93 |
| RILUZOLE | TREATMENT OF AMYOTROPHIC LATERAL SCLEROSIS | RHONE-POULENC RORER PHARM.<br>500 ARCOLA ROAD,<br>P.O. BOX 1200<br>COLLEGEVILLE PA 19426-0107<br>DD 03/16/93 |
| RILUZOLE<br>TN is RILUTEK | TREATMENT OF HUNTINGTON'S DISEASE | RHONE-POULENC RORER PHARMACEUTICALS, INC.<br>500 ARCOLA ROAD<br>COLLEGEVILLE PA 19426 |
| ROQUINIMEX<br>TN is LINOMIDE | TO PROLONG TIME TO RELAPSE IN LEUKEMIA PATIENTS WHO HAVE UNDERGONE AUTOLOGOUS BONE MARROW TRANSPLANTATION | PHARMACIA, INC.<br>P.O. BOX 16529<br>COLUMBUS OH 43216-6529<br>DD 07/01/93 |
| R-VIII SQ<br>TN is REFACTO | FOR LONG-TERM AND/OR HOSPITAL TREATMENT OF HEMOPHILIA A OR FOR TREATMENT OF PATIENTS WITH HEMOPHILIA A IN CONNECTION WITH SURGICAL PROCEDURES | PHARMACIA, INC.<br>P.O. BOX 16529<br>COLUMBUS OH 43216 |
| S-ADENOSYLMETHIONINE | TREATMENT OF AIDS MYELOPATHY | DI ROCCO, ALESSANDRO, M.D.<br>BETH ISRAEL MEDICAL CENTER<br>DEPT. OF NEUROLOGY<br>PHILIPS BUILDING, SUITE 2Q<br>10 UNION SQUARE<br>NEW YORK NY 10003 |
| SARGRAMOSTIM<br>TN is LEUKINE | TREATMENT OF NEUTROPENIA ASSOCIATED WITH BONE MARROW TRANSPLANT, FOR THE TREATMENT OF GRAFT FAILURE AND DELAY OF ENGRAFTMENT, AND FOR THE PROMOTION OF EARLY ENGRAFTMENT | IMMUNEX CORPORATION<br>51 UNIVERSITY STREET<br>SEATTLE WA 98101<br>DD 05/03/90 MA 03/05/91 |
| SARGRAMOSTIM<br>TN is LEUKINE | TO REDUCE NEUTROPENIA AND LEUKOPENIA AND DECREASE THE INCIDENCE OF DEATH DUE TO INFECTION IN PATIENTS WITH ACUTE MYELOGENOUS LEUKEMIA | IMMUNEX CORPORATION<br>51 UNIVERSITY STREET<br>SEATTLE WA 98101<br>DD 03/06/95 |
| SATUMOMAB PENDETIDE<br>TN is ONCOSCINT CR/OV | DETECTION OF OVARIAN CARCINOMA | CYTOGEN CORPORATION<br>600 COLLEGE ROAD EAST<br>PRINCETON NJ 08540-5308<br>DD 09/25/89 MA 12/29/92 |
| SECALCIFEROL<br>TN is OSTEO-D | TREATMENT OF FAMILIAL HYPOPHOSPHATEMIC RICKETS | LEMMON COMPANY<br>650 CATHILL ROAD<br>SELLERSVILLE PA 18960<br>DD 07/26/93 |

# CUMULATIVE LIST OF ORPHAN PRODUCT DESIGNATIONS AND APPROVALS
[Through October 31, 1998] *(continued)*

| NAME<br>*Generic/Chemical*<br>*TN is Trade Name* | INDICATION DESIGNATED | SPONSOR AND ADDRESS<br>*DD is Date Designated*<br>*MA is Marketing Approval* |
|---|---|---|
| SECRETORY LEUKOCYTE PROTEASE INHIBITOR | TREATMENT OF BRONCHOPULMONARY DYSPLASIA | SYNERGEN, INC.<br>1885 33RD STREET<br>BOULDER CO 80301-2546<br>DD 06/30/92 |
| SELEGILINE HCL<br>TN is ELDEPRYL | ADJUVANT TO LEVODOPA AND CARBIDOPA TREATMENT OF IDIOPATHIC PARKINSON'S DISEASE (PARALYSIS AGITANS), POSTENCEPHALITIC PARKINSONISM, AND SYMPTOMATIC PARKINSONISM | SOMERSET PHARMACEUTICALS, INC.<br>777 SOUTH HARBOR ISLAND BOULEVARD<br>TAMPA FL 33602<br>DD 11/07/84 MA 06/05/89 |
| SERMORELIN ACETATE<br>TN is GEREF | TREATMENT OF IDIOPATHIC OR ORGANIC GROWTH HORMONE DEFICIENCY (GHD) IN CHILDREN WITH GROWTH FAILURE | SERONO LABORATORIES, INC.<br>100 LONGWATER CIRCLE<br>NORWELL MA 02061<br>DD 09/14/88 |
| SERMORELIN ACETATE<br>TN is GEREF | ADJUNCT TO GONADOTROPIN THERAPY IN THE INDUCTION OF OVULATION IN WOMEN WITH ANOVULATORY OR OLIGO-OVULATORY INFERTILITY WHO FAIL TO OVULATE IN RESPONSE TO ADEQUATE TREATMENT WITH CLOMIPHENE CITRATE ALONE AND GONADOTROPIN THERAPY ALONE | SERONO LABORATORIES, INC.<br>100 LONGWATER CIRCLE<br>NORWELL MA 02061<br>DD 02/13/90 |
| SERMORELIN ACETATE<br>TN is GEREF | TREATMENT OF AIDS-ASSOCIATED CATABOLISM/WEIGHT LOSS | SERONO LABORATORIES, INC.<br>100 LONGWATER CIRCLE<br>NORWELL MA 02061<br>DD 12/05/91 |
| SERRATIA MARCESCENS EXTRACT (POLYRIBOSOMES)<br>TN is IMUVERT | TREATMENT OF PRIMARY BRAIN MALIGNANCIES | CELL TECHNOLOGY, INC.<br>1668 VALTEC LANE<br>BOULDER CO 80306<br>DD 09/07/88 |
| SHORT CHAIN FATTY ACID ENEMA<br>TN is COLOMED | TREATMENT OF CHRONIC RADIATION PROCTITIS | ORPHAN MEDICAL, INC.<br>13911 RIDGEDALE DRIVE, SUITE 475<br>MINNETONKA MN 55305 |
| SHORT CHAIN FATTY ACID SOLUTION | TREATMENT OF THE ACTIVE PHASE OF ULCERATIVE COLITIS WITH INVOLVEMENT RESTRICTED TO THE LEFT SIDE OF THE COLON | ORPHAN MEDICAL<br>13911 RIDGEDALE DRIVE<br>MINNETONKA MN 55305<br>DD 05/29/90 |
| SODIUM BENZOATE/SODIUM PHENYLACETATE | TREATMENT OF UREA CYCLE DISORDERS: CARBAMYLPHOSPHATE SYNTHETASE DEFICIENCY, ORNITHINE TRANSCARBAMYLASE DEFICIENCY, AND ARGININOSUCCINIC ACID SYNTHETASE DEFICIENCY | BRUSILOW, SAUL W., M.D.<br>JOHNS HOPKINS MEDICAL INSTITUTIONS<br>BALTIMORE MD 21205<br>DD 11/22/93 |
| SODIUM DICHLOROACETATE | TREATMENT OF CONGENITAL LACTIC ACIDOSIS | STACPOOLE, PETER, M.D.<br>U. OF FLORIDA<br>P.O. BOX 100226<br>GAINESVILLE FL 32610-0226<br>DD 06/11/90 |
| SODIUM DICHLOROACETATE | TREATMENT OF HOMOZYGOUS FAMILIAL HYPERCHOLESTEROLEMIA | STACPOOLE, PETER, M.D.<br>U. OF FLORIDA<br>P.O. BOX 100226<br>GAINESVILLE FL 32610-0226<br>DD 06/11/90 |
| SODIUM DICHLOROACETATE | TREATMENT OF LACTIC ACIDOSIS IN PATIENTS WITH SEVERE MALARIA | STACPOOLE, PETER W., PH.D., M.D.<br>UNIVERSITY OF FLORIDA<br>GAINESVILLE FL 32610-0277<br>DD 11/10/94 |
| SODIUM MONOMERCAPTOUNDECAHYDRO-CLOSO-DODECABORATE<br>TN is BOROCELL | FOR USE IN BORON NEUTRON CAPTURE THERAPY (BNCT) IN THE TREATMENT OF GLIOBLASTOMA MULTIFORME | NEUTRON TECH. CORP.& NEUTRON R&D PARTNER<br>877 MAIN STREET<br>BOISE ID 83702<br>DD 04/15/92 |
| SODIUM PHENYLBUTYRATE | TREATMENT FOR SICKLING DISORDERS, WHICH INCLUDE S-S HEMOGLOBINOPATHY, S-C HEMOGLOBINOPATHY, AND S-THALASSEMIA HEMOGLOBINOPATHY | BRUSILOW, SAUL W., M.D.<br>JOHNS HOPKINS MEDICAL INSTITUTIONS<br>BALTIMORE MD 21205<br>DD 07/02/92 |
| SODIUM PHENYLBUTYRATE | TREATMENT OF UREA CYCLE DISORDERS: CARBAMYLPHOSPHATE SYNTHETASE DEFICIENCY, ORNITHINE TRANSCARBAMYLASE DEFICIENCY, AND ARGINIOSUCCINIC ACID SYNTHETASE DEFICIENCY | BRUSILOW, SAUL W., M.D.<br>JOHNS HOPKINS MEDICAL INSTITUTIONS<br>BALTIMORE MD 21205<br>DD 11/22/93 |
| SODIUM PHENYLBUTYRATE | FOR USE AS AN ADJUNCT TO SURGERY, RADIATION THERAPY, AND CHEMOTHERAPY FOR THE TREATMENT OF PATIENTS WITH PRIMARY OR RECURRENT MALIGNANT GLIOMA | TARGON CORPORATION<br>307 COLLEGE ROAD EAST<br>PRINCETON NJ 08540 |
| SODIUM TETRADECYL SULFATE<br>TN is SOTRADECOL | TREATMENT OF BLEEDING ESOPHAGEAL VARICES | ELKINS-SINN, INC.<br>2 ESTERBROOK LANE<br>CHERRY HILL NJ 08003-4099<br>DD 06/10/86 |

# CUMULATIVE LIST OF ORPHAN PRODUCT DESIGNATIONS AND APPROVALS
[Through October 31, 1998] *(continued)*

| NAME<br>*Generic/Chemical*<br>*TN is Trade Name* | INDICATION DESIGNATED | SPONSOR AND ADDRESS<br>*DD is Date Designated*<br>*MA is Marketing Approval* |
|---|---|---|
| SODIUM/GAMMA HYDROXY-BUTYRATE | TREATMENT OF NARCOLEPSY AND THE AUXILIARY SYMPTOMS OF CATAPLEXY, SLEEP PARALYSIS, HYPNAGOGIC HALLUCINATIONS AND AUTOMATIC BEHAVIOR | BIOCRAFT LABORATORIES, INC.<br>18-01 RIVER ROAD<br>FAIR LAWN NJ 07410<br>DD 12/22/87 |
| SOLUBLE RECOMBINANT HUMAN COMPLEMENT RECEPTOR TYPE 1 | PREVENTION OR REDUCTION OF ADULT RESPIRATORY DISTRESS SYNDROME | T CELL SCIENCES, INC.<br>38 SIDNEY STREET<br>CAMBRIDGE MA 02139-4135<br>DD 11/21/94 |
| SOMATOSTATIN<br>TN is ZECNIL | ADJUNCT TO THE NON-OPERATIVE MANAGEMENT OF SECRETING CUTANEOUS FISTULAS OF THE STOMACH, DUODENUM, SMALL INTESTINE (JEJUNUM AND ILEUM), OR PANCREAS | FERRING LABORATORIES, INC.<br>400 RELLA BOULEVARD, SUITE 201<br>SUFFERN NY 10901<br>DD 06/20/88 |
| SOMATOSTATIN | TREATMENT OF BLEEDING ESOPHAGEAL VARICES | UCB PHARMA, INC.<br>1950 LAKE PARK DRIVE<br>ATLANTA GA 30080<br>DD 12/22/94 |
| SOMATROPIN<br>TN is SAIZEN | TREATMENT OF IDIOPATHIC OR ORGANIC GROWTH HORMONE DEFICIENCY IN CHILDREN WITH GROWTH FAILURE | SERONO LABORATORIES, INC.<br>100 LONGWATER CIRCLE<br>NORWELL MA 02061<br>DD 03/06/87 |
| SOMATROPIN<br>TN is NUTROPIN | FOR USE IN THE LONG-TERM TREATMENT OF CHILDREN WHO HAVE GROWTH FAILURE DUE TO A LACK OF ADEQUATE ENDOGENOUS GROWTH HORMONE SECRETION | GENENTECH, INC.<br>460 POINT SAN BRUNO BOULEVARD<br>SOUTH SAN FRANCISCO CA 94080<br>DD 03/06/87 MA 03/09/94 |
| SOMATROPIN<br>TN is NORDITROPIN | TREATMENT OF GROWTH FAILURE IN CHILDREN DUE TO INADEQUATE GROWTH HORMONE SECRETION | NOVO NORDISK PHARMACEUTICALS<br>100 OVERLOOK CENTER, SUITE 200<br>PRINCETON NJ 08540-7810<br>DD 07/10/87 |
| SOMATROPIN<br>TN is SAIZEN | FOR THE ENHANCEMENT OF NITROGEN RETENTION IN HOSPITALIZED PATIENTS SUFFERING FROM SEVERE BURNS | SERONO LABORATORIES, INC.<br>100 LONGWATER CIRCLE<br>NORWELL MA 02061<br>DD 05/03/89 |
| SOMATROPIN<br>TN is HUMATROPE | TREATMENT OF SHORT STATURE ASSOCIATED WITH TURNER'S SYNDROME | ELI LILLY AND COMPANY<br>LILLY CORPORATE CENTER<br>INDIANAPOLIS IN 46285<br>DD 05/08/90 |
| SOMATROPIN<br>TN is BIOTROPIN | TREATMENT OF CACHEXIA ASSOCIATED WITH AIDS | BIO-TECHNOLOGY GENERAL CORP.<br>70 WOOD AVENUE, SOUTH<br>ISELIN NJ 08830<br>DD 02/12/93 |
| SOMATROPIN<br>TN is GENOTROPIN/GENOTONORM | TREATMENT OF ADULTS WITH GROWTH HORMONE DEFICIENCY | PHARMACIA, INC.<br>P.O. BOX 16529<br>COLUMBUS OH 43216-6529<br>DD 09/06/94 |
| SOMATROPIN FOR INJECTION<br>TN is NUTROPIN | FOR USE AS REPLACEMENT THERAPY FOR GROWTH HORMONE DEFICIENCY IN ADULTS AFTER EPIPHYSEAL CLOSURE | GENENTECH, INC.<br>460 POINT SAN BRUNO BOULEVARD<br>SOUTH SAN FRANCISCO CA 94080 |
| SOMATROPIN FOR INJECTION<br>TN is HUMATROPE | LONG-TERM TREATMENT OF CHILDREN WHO HAVE GROWTH FAILURE DUE TO INADEQUATE SECRETION OF NORMAL ENDOGENOUS GROWTH HORMONE | ELI LILLY AND COMPANY<br>LILLY CORPORATE CENTER<br>INDIANAPOLIS IN 46285<br>DD 06/12/86 MA 03/08/87 |
| SOMATROPIN FOR INJECTION<br>TN is NUTROPIN | TREATMENT OF GROWTH RETARDATION ASSOCIATED WITH CHRONIC RENAL FAILURE | GENENTECH, INC.<br>460 POINT SAN BRUNO BOULEVARD<br>SOUTH SAN FRANCISCO CA 94080<br>DD 08/04/89 MA 11/17/93 |
| SOMATROPIN FOR INJECTION<br>TN is NUTROPIN | TREATMENT OF SHORT STATURE ASSOCIATED WITH TURNER'S SYNDROME | GENENTECH, INC.<br>460 POINT SAN BRUNO BOULEVARD<br>SOUTH SAN FRANCISCO CA 94080<br>DD 03/23/89 |
| SOMATREM FOR INJECTION<br>TN is PROTROPIN | FOR LONG-TERM TREATMENT OF CHILDREN WHO HAVE GROWTH FAILURE DUE TO A LACK OF ADEQUATE ENDOGENOUS GROWTH HORMONE SECRETION | GENENTECH, INC.<br>460 POINT SAN BRUNO BOULEVARD<br>SOUTH SAN FRANCISCO CA 94080<br>DD 12/09/85 MA 10/17/85 |
| SOMATREM FOR INJECTION<br>TN is PROTROPIN | TREATMENT OF SHORT STATURE ASSOCIATED WITH TURNER'S SYNDROME | GENENTECH, INC.<br>460 POINT SAN BRUNO BOULEVARD<br>SOUTH SAN FRANCISCO CA 94080<br>DD 12/09/85 |
| SOMATROPIN FOR INJECTION<br>TN is SAIZEN | TREATMENT OF AIDS-ASSOCIATED CATABOLISM/WEIGHT LOSS | SERONO LABORATORIES, INC.<br>100 LONGWATER CIRCLE<br>NORWELL MA 02061<br>DD 11/15/91 |

## CUMULATIVE LIST OF ORPHAN PRODUCT DESIGNATIONS AND APPROVALS
[Through October 31, 1998] (continued)

| NAME<br>Generic/Chemical<br>TN is Trade Name | INDICATION DESIGNATED | SPONSOR AND ADDRESS<br>DD is Date Designated<br>MA is Marketing Approval |
|---|---|---|
| SOMATROPIN FOR INJECTION<br>TN is SCROSTIM | TREATMENT OF CHILDREN WITH AIDS-ASSOCIATED FAILURE-TO-THRIVE INCLUDING AIDS-ASSOCIATED WASTING | SERONO LABORATORIES, INC.<br>100 LONGWATER CIRCLE<br>NORWELL MA 02061 |
| SORIVUDINE<br>TN is BRAVADIR | TREATMENT OF HERPES ZOSTER (SHINGLES) IN IMMUNOCOMPROMISED PATIENTS | BRISTOL-MEYERS SQUIBB<br>5 RESEARCH PARKWAY<br>P.O. BOX 5100<br>WALLINGFORD CT 06492 |
| SOTALOL HCL<br>TN is BETAPACE | TREATMENT OF LIFE-THREATENING VENTRICULAR TACHYARRHYTHMIAS | BERLEX LABORATORIES<br>300 FAIRFIELD ROAD<br>WAYNE NJ 07470-4100<br>DD 09/23/88 MA 10/30/92 |
| SOTALOL HCL<br>TN is BETAPACE | PREVENTION OF LIFE THREATENING VENTRICULAR TACHYARRHYTHMIAS | BERLEX LABORATORIES<br>300 FAIRFIELD ROAD<br>WAYNE NJ 07470-4100<br>DD 09/23/88 |
| STERILE AEROSOL TALC | TREATMENT OF MALIGNANT PLEURAL EFFUSION | BRYAN CORPORATION<br>4 PLYMPTON STREET<br>WOBURN MA 01801 |
| ST1-RTA IMMUNOTOXIN (SR-44163) | PREVENTION OF ACUTE GRAFT VERSUS HOST DISEASE (GVHD) IN ALLOGENIC BONE MARROW TRANSPLANTATION | SANOFI PHARMACEUTICALS, INC.<br>1250 S. COLLEGEVILLE ROAD<br>COLLEGEVILLE PA 19426-0900<br>DD 08/12/87 |
| ST1-RTA IMMUNOTOXIN (SR 44163) | TREATMENT OF PATIENTS WITH B-CHRONIC LYMPHOCYTIC LEUKEMIA (CLL) | SANOFI PHARMACEUTICALS, INC.<br>1250 S. COLLEGEVILLE ROAD<br>COLLEGEVILLE PA 19426-0900<br>DD 08/12/87 |
| SU-101 | TREATMENT OF MALIGNANT GLIOMA | SUGEN, INC.<br>515 GALVESTON DRIVE<br>REDWOOD CITY CA 94063-4720<br>DD 05/25/95 |
| SU101 | TREATMENT OF OVARIAN CANCER | SUGEN, INC.<br>515 GALVESTON DRIVE<br>REDWOOD CITY CA 94063 |
| SUCCIMER<br>TN is CHEMET CAPSULES | TREATMENT OF LEAD POISONING IN CHILDREN | MCNEIL CONSUMER PRODUCTS CO.<br>CAMP HILL ROAD<br>FORT WASHINGTON PA 19034<br>DD 05/09/84 MA 01/30/91 |
| SUCCIMER<br>TN is CHEMET | PREVENTION OF CYSTINE KIDNEY STONE FORMATION IN PATIENTS WITH HOMOZYGOUS CYSTINURIA WHO ARE PRONE TO STONE DEVELOPMENT | MCNEIL CONSUMER PRODUCTS CO.<br>CAMP HILL ROAD<br>FORT WASHINGTON PA 19034<br>DD 11/05/90 |
| SUCCIMER<br>TN is CHEMET | TREATMENT OF MERCURY INTOXICATION | MCNEIL CONSUMER PRODUCTS CO.<br>CAMP HILL ROAD<br>FORT WASHINGTON PA 19034<br>DD 03/22/91 |
| SUCRALFATE | TREATMENT OF ORAL MUCOSITIS AND STOMATITIS FOLLOWING RADIATION THERAPY FOR HEAD AND NECK CANCER | FUISZ TECHNOLOGIES, LTD.<br>3810 CONCORDE PARKWAY<br>SUITE 100<br>CHANTILLY VA 22021<br>DD 07/15/93 |
| SUCRALFATE SUSPENSION | TREATMENT OF ORAL COMPLICATIONS OF CHEMOTHERAPY IN BONE MARROW TRANSPLANT PATIENTS | DARBY PHARMACEUTICALS, INC.<br>100 BANKS AVENUE<br>ROCKVILLE CENTRE NY 11570<br>DD 03/12/90 |
| SUCRALFATE SUSPENSION | TREATMENT OF ORAL ULCERATIONS AND DYSPHAGIA IN PATIENTS WITH EPIDERMOLYSIS BULLOSA | DARBY PHARMACEUTICALS, INC.<br>100 BANKS AVENUE<br>ROCKVILLE CENTRE NY 11570<br>DD 03/04/91 |
| SUCRASE (YEAST-DERIVED)<br>TN is SACARASA | TREATMENT OF CONGENITAL SUCRASE-ISOMALTASE DEFICIENCY | ORPHAN MEDICAL<br>13911 RIDGEDALE DRIVE<br>MINNETONKA MN 55305<br>DD 12/10/93 |
| SULFADIAZINE | FOR USE IN COMBINATION WITH PYRIMETHAMINE FOR THE TREATMENT OF TOXOPLASMA GONDII ENCEPHALITIS IN PATIENTS WITH AND WITHOUT ACQUIRED IMMUNODEFICIENCY SYNDROME | EON LABS MANUFACTURING, INC.<br>227-15 NORTH CONDUIT AVENUE<br>LAURELTON NY 11413<br>DD 03/14/94 MA 07/29/94 |
| SULFAPYRIDINE | TREATMENT OF DERMATITIS HERPETIFORMIS | JACOBUS PHARMACEUTICAL COMPANY<br>P.O. BOX 5290<br>PRINCETON NJ 08540<br>DD 09/10/90 |

# CUMULATIVE LIST OF ORPHAN PRODUCT DESIGNATIONS AND APPROVALS
[Through October 31, 1998] *(continued)*

| NAME<br>*Generic/Chemical*<br>*TN is Trade Name* | INDICATION DESIGNATED | SPONSOR AND ADDRESS<br>*DD is Date Designated*<br>*MA is Marketing Approval* |
|---|---|---|
| SUPEROXIDE DISMUTASE (HUMAN) | PROTECTION OF DONOR ORGAN TISSUE FROM DAMAGE OR INJURY MEDIATED BY OXYGEN-DERIVED FREE RADICALS THAT ARE GENERATED DURING THE NECESSARY PERIODS OF ISCHEMIA (HYPOXIA, ANOXIA), AND ESPECIALLY REPERFUSION, ASSOCIATED WITH THE OPERATIVE PROCEDURE | PHARMACIA-CHIRON PARTNERSHIP<br>4560 HORTON STREET<br>EMERYVILLE CA 94608<br>DD 03/06/85 |
| SUPEROXIDE DISMUTASE (RECOMBINANT HUMAN) | PREVENTION OF REPERFUSION INJURY TO DONOR ORGAN TISSUE | BIO-TECHNOLOGY GENERAL CORP.<br>70 WOOD AVENUE, SOUTH<br>ISELIN NJ 08830<br>DD 05/17/88 |
| SUPEROXIDE DISMUTASE (RECOMBINANT HUMAN) | FOR THE PREVENTION OF BRONCHOPULMONARY DYSPLASIA IN PREMATURE NEONATES WEIGHING LESS THAN 1500 GRAMS | BIO-TECHNOLOGY GENERAL CORP.<br>70 WOOD AVENUE, SOUTH<br>ISELIN NJ 08830<br>DD 04/18/91 |
| SURAMIN | TREATMENT OF METASTATIC HORMONE-REFRACTORY PROSTATE CANCER | WARNER-LAMBERT COMPANY<br>PARKE-DAVIS PHARMACEUTICAL RESEARCH DIVISION<br>2800 PLYMOUTH ROAD<br>ANN ARBOR MI 48105 |
| SURFACE ACTIVE EXTRACT OF SALINE LAVAGE OF BOVINE LUNGS<br>TN is INFASURF | TREATMENT AND PREVENTION OF RESPIRATORY FAILURE DUE TO PULMONARY SURFACTANT DEFICIENCY IN PRETERM INFANTS | ONY, INC.<br>1576 SWEET HOME ROAD<br>AMHERST NY 14228<br>DD 06/07/85 |
| SYNSORB PK | TREATMENT OF VEROCYTOTOXOGENIC E. COLI INFECTIONS | SYNSORB BIOTECH INC.<br>FOURTH FLOOR<br>140 4TH AVENUE SW<br>CALGARY ALBERTA<br>DD 07/17/95 |
| TACROLIMUS<br>TN is PROGRAF | PROPHYLAXIS OF GRAFT-VERSUS-HOST DISEASE | FUJISAWA USA, INC.<br>THREE PARKWAY NORTH CENTER<br>DEERFIELD IL 60015 |
| TAK-603 | TREATMENT OF CROHN'S DISEASE | TAP HOLDINGS INC.<br>2355 WAUKEGAN ROAD<br>DEERFIELD IL 60015 |
| T4 ENDONUCLEASE V, LIPOSOME ENCAPSULATED | TO PREVENT CUTANEOUS NEOPLASMS AND OTHER SKIN ABNORMALITIES IN XERODERMA PIGMENTOSUM | APPLIED GENETICS, INC.<br>205 BUFFALO AVENUE<br>FREEPORT NY 11520<br>DD 06/27/89 |
| TECHNETIUM TC 99M ANTI-MELANOMA MURINE MONOCLONAL ANTIBODY<br>TN is ONCOTRAC MELANOMA IMAGING KIT | FOR USE IN DETECTING, BY IMAGING, METASTASES OF MALIGNANT MELANOMA | NEORX CORPORATION<br>410 WEST HARRISON<br>SEATTLE WA 98119<br>DD 06/02/87 |
| TECHNETIUM Tc-99m MURINE MONOCLONAL ANTIBODY (IgG2a) TO BCE<br>TN is IMMURAID-LL-2[99mTc] | DIAGNOSTIC IMAGING IN THE EVALUATION OF THE EXTENT OF DISEASE IN PATIENTS WITH HISTOLOGICALLY CONFIRMED DIAGNOSIS OF NON-HODGKIN'S B-CELL LYMPHOMA, ACUTE B-CELL LYMPHOBLASTIC LEUKEMIA (IN CHILDREN AND ADULTS), AND CHRONIC B-CELL LYMPHOCYTIC LEUKEMIA | IMMUNOMEDICS, INC.<br>300 AMERICAN ROAD<br>MORRIS PLAINS NJ 07950<br>DD 04/07/92 |
| TECHNETIUM Tc-99m MURINE MONOCLONAL ANTIBODY TO HUMAN AFP<br>TN is IMMURAID, AFP-Tc99m | DETECTION OF HEPATOCELLULAR CARCINOMA AND HEPATOBLASTOMA | IMMUNOMEDICS, INC.<br>300 AMERICAN ROAD<br>MORRIS PLAINS NJ 07950<br>DD 08/01/89 |
| TECHNETIUM Tc-99m MURINE MONOCLONAL ANTIBODY TO HUMAN AFP<br>TN is IMMURAID, AFP-Tc99m | DETECTION OF ALPHA-FETOPROTEIN PRODUCING GERM CELL TUMORS | IMMUNOMEDICS, INC.<br>300 AMERICAN ROAD<br>MORRIS PLAINS NJ 07950<br>DD 08/01/89 |
| TECHNETIUM Tc-99m MURINE MONOCLONAL ANTIBODY TO hCG<br>TN is IMMURAID, hCG-Tc-99m | DETECTION OF HCG PRODUCING TUMORS SUCH AS GERM CELL AND TROPHOBLASTIC CELL TUMORS | IMMUNOMEDICS, INC.<br>300 AMERICAN ROAD<br>MORRIS PLAINS NJ 07950<br>DD 08/07/89 |
| TENIPOSIDE<br>TN is VUMON FOR INJECTION | TREATMENT OF REFRACTORY CHILDHOOD ACUTE LYMPHOCYTIC LEUKEMIA (ALL) | BRISTOL-MYERS SQUIBB<br>5 RESEARCH PARKWAY<br>P.O. BOX 5100<br>WALLINGFORD CT 06492-7660<br>DD 11/01/84 MA 07/14/92 |
| TERIPARATIDE<br>TN is PARATHAR | DIAGNOSTIC AGENT TO ASSIST IN ESTABLISHING THE DIAGNOSIS IN PATIENTS PRESENTING WITH CLINICAL AND LABORATORY EVIDENCE OF HYPOCALCEMIA DUE TO EITHER HYPOPARATHYROIDISM OR PSEUDOHYPOPARATHYROIDISM | RHONE-POULENC RORER PHARM.<br>500 ARCOLA ROAD<br>COLLEGEVILLE PA 19426<br>DD 01/09/87 MA 12/23/87 |
| TERLIPRESSIN<br>TN is GLYPRESSIN | TREATMENT OF BLEEDING ESOPHAGEAL VARICES | FERRING LABORATORIES, INC.<br>400 RELLA BOULEVARD, SUITE 201<br>SUFFERN NY 10901<br>DD 03/06/86 |

## CUMULATIVE LIST OF ORPHAN PRODUCT DESIGNATIONS AND APPROVALS
[Through October 31, 1998] (continued)

| NAME<br>Generic/Chemical<br>TN is Trade Name | INDICATION DESIGNATED | SPONSOR AND ADDRESS<br>DD is Date Designated<br>MA is Marketing Approval |
|---|---|---|
| TESTOSTERONE<br>TN is ANDROGEL | TREATMENT OF WEIGHT LOSS IN AIDS PATIENTS WITH HIV-ASSOCIATED WASTING | UNIMED PHARMACEUTICALS, INC.<br>2150 EAST LAKE COOK ROAD<br>SUITE 210<br>BUFFALO GROVE IL 60089 |
| TESTOSTERONE<br>TN is THERADERM TESTOSTERONE TRANSDERMAL SYSTEM | FOR USE AS PHYSIOLOGIC TESTOSTERONE REPLACEMENT IN ANDROGEN DEFICIENT HIV+ PATIENTS WITH AN ASSOCIATED WEIGHT LOSS | THERATECH, INC.<br>417 WAKARA WAY<br>SALT LAKE CITY UT 84108 |
| TESTOSTERONE PROPIONATE OINTMENT 2% | TREATMENT OF VULVAR DYSTROPHIES | STAR PHARMACEUTICALS, INC.<br>1990 N.W. 44TH STREET<br>POMPANO BEACH FL 33064<br>DD 07/31/91 |
| TESTOSTERONE SUBLINGUAL | TREATMENT OF CONSTITUTIONAL DELAY OF GROWTH AND PUBERTY IN BOYS | BIO-TECHNOLOGY GENERAL CORP.<br>70 WOOD AVENUE, SOUTH<br>ISELIN NJ 08830<br>DD 01/16/91 |
| TETRABENAZINE | TREATMENT OF MODERATE-TO-SEVERE TARDIVE DYSKINESIA | LIFEHEALTH LIMITED<br>RICHMOND HOUSE, OLD BREWERY COURT<br>SANDYFORD ROAD<br>NEWCASTLE-UPON-TYNE NE2 1XG<br>UNITED KINGDOM |
| THALIDOMIDE | TREATMENT OF GRAFT VERSUS HOST DISEASE (GVHD) IN PATIENTS RECEIVING BONE MARROW TRANSPLANTATION (BMT) | PEDIATRIC PHARMACEUTICALS, INC.<br>718 BRADFORD AVENUE<br>WESTFIELD NJ 07090<br>DD 09/19/88 |
| THALIDOMIDE | PREVENTION OF GRAFT VERSUS HOST DISEASE (GVHD) IN PATIENTS RECEIVING BONE MARROW TRANSPLANTATION | PEDIATRIC PHARMACEUTICALS, INC.<br>718 BRADFORD AVENUE<br>WESTFIELD NJ 07090<br>DD 09/19/88 |
| THALIDOMIDE | TREATMENT AND MAINTENANCE OF REACTIONAL LEPROMATOUS LEPROSY | PEDIATRIC PHARMACEUTICALS, INC.<br>718 BRADFORD AVENUE<br>WESTFIELD NJ 07090<br>DD 11/15/88 |
| THALIDOMIDE | TREATMENT OF GRAFT VERSUS HOST DISEASE | ANDRULIS PHARMACEUTICALS CORPORATION<br>11800 BALTIMORE AVENUE<br>BELTSVILLE MD 20705<br>DD 03/05/90 |
| THALIDOMIDE | PREVENTION OF GRAFT VERSUS HOST DISEASE | ANDRULIS PHARMACEUTICALS CORPORATION<br>11800 BALTIMORE AVENUE<br>BELTSVILLE MD 20705<br>DD 03/05/90 |
| THALIDOMIDE | TREATMENT OF THE CLINICAL MANIFESTATIONS OF MYCOBACTERIAL INFECTION CAUSED BY MYCOBACTERIUM TUBERCULOSIS AND NON-TUBERCULOUS MYCOBACTERIA | CELGENE CORPORATION<br>7 POWDER HORN DRIVE<br>WARREN NJ 07059<br>DD 01/12/93 |
| THALIDOMIDE | TREATMENT OF SEVERE RECURRENT APHTHOUS STOMATITIS IN SEVERELY, TERMINALLY IMMUNOCOMPROMISED PATIENTS | CELGENE CORPORATION<br>P.O. BOX 4914<br>WARREN NJ 07059<br>DD 05/01/95 |
| THALIDOMIDE | TREATMENT AND PREVENTION OF RECURRENT APHTHOUS ULCERS IN SEVERELY, TERMINALLY IMMUNOCOMPROMISED PATIENTS | ANDRULIS RESEARCH CORPORATION<br>11800 BALTIMORE AVENUE<br>SUITE 113<br>BELTSVILLE MD 20705<br>DD 05/15/95 |
| THALIDOMIDE | TREATMENT OF PRIMARY BRAIN MALIGNANCIES | ENTREMED, INC.<br>9610 MEDICAL CENTER DRIVE, SUITE 200<br>ROCKVILLE MD 20850 |
| THALIDOMIDE<br>TN is SYNOVIR | TREATMENT OF ERYTHEMA NODOSUM LEPROSUM | CELGENE CORPORATION<br>7 POWDER HORN DRIVE<br>P.O. BOX 4914<br>WARREN NJ 07059<br>DD 07/26/95 |
| THALIDOMIDE<br>TN is SYNOVIR | TREATMENT OF HIV-ASSOCIATED WASTING SYNDROME | CELGENE CORPORATION<br>P.O. BOX 4914<br>7 POWDER HORN DRIVE<br>WARREN NJ 07059 |
| THALIDOMIDE | TREATMENT OF KAPOSI'S SARCOMA | ENTREMED, INC.<br>9610 MEDICAL CENTER DR., SUITE 200<br>ROCKVILLE MD 20850 |

# CUMULATIVE LIST OF ORPHAN PRODUCT DESIGNATIONS AND APPROVALS
[Through October 31, 1998] *(continued)*

| NAME<br>*Generic/Chemical*<br>*TN is Trade Name* | INDICATION DESIGNATED | SPONSOR AND ADDRESS<br>*DD is Date Designated*<br>*MA is Marketing Approval* |
|---|---|---|
| THYMALFASIN<br>TN is ZADAXIN | TREATMENT OF DIGEORGE ANOMALY WITH IMMUNE DEFECTS | SCICLONE PHARMACEUTICALS, INC.<br>901 MARINER'S ISLAND BLVD.<br>SAN MATEO CA 94404 |
| THYMOSIN ALPHA-1 | TREATMENT OF CHRONIC ACTIVE HEPATITIS B | ALPHA 1 BIOMEDICALS, INC.<br>6903 ROCKLEDGE DRIVE, SUITE 1200<br>BETHESDA MD 20817-1818<br>DD 05/03/91 |
| TIAPRIDE | TREATMENT OF TOURETTE'S SYNDROME | SYNTHELABO RESEARCH, INC.<br>400 PLAZA DRIVE<br>SECAUCUS NJ 07094 |
| TIOPRONIN<br>TN is THIOLA | PREVENTION OF CYSTINE NEPHROLITHIASIS IN PATIENTS WITH HOMOZYGOUS CYSTINURIA | PAK, CHARLES Y.C., M.D.<br>5323 HARRY HINES BOULEVARD<br>DALLAS TX 75235<br>DD 01/17/86 MA 08/11/88 |
| TIRATRICOL<br>TN is TRIACANA | FOR USE IN COMBINATION WITH LEVO-THYROXINE TO SUPPRESS THYROID STIMULATING HORMONE (TSH) IN PATIENTS WITH WELL-DIFFERENTIATED THYROID CANCER WHO ARE INTOLERANT TO ADEQUATE DOSES OF LEVO-THYROXINE ALONE | MARCOFINA LABORATORIES<br>48 BIS RUE DES BELLES FEUILLES<br>75116 PARIS FRANCE<br>DD 08/13/91 |
| TIZANIDINE HCL<br>TN is ZANAFLEX | TREATMENT OF SPASTICITY ASSOCIATED WITH MULTIPLE SCLEROSIS AND SPINAL CORD INJURY | ATHENA NEUROSCIENCES, INC.<br>800F GATEWAY BOULEVARD<br>SOUTH SAN FRANCISCO CA 94080<br>DD 01/31/94 |
| TOBRAMYCIN FOR INHALATION | TREATMENT OF BRONCHOPULMONARY INFECTIONS OF PSEUDOMONAS AERUGINOSA IN CYSTIC FIBROSIS PATIENTS | PATHOGENESIS CORPORATION<br>201 ELLIOTT AVENUE WEST<br>SUITE 150<br>SEATTLE WA 98119<br>DD 10/13/94 |
| TOPIRAMATE<br>TN is TOPIMAX | TREATMENT OF LENNOX-GASTAUT SYNDROME | R.W. JOHNSON RESEARCH INSTITUTE<br>WELSH AND MCKEAN ROADS<br>SPRING HOUSE PA 19477-0776<br>DD 11/25/92 |
| TOREMIFENE | HORMONAL THERAPY OF METASTATIC CARCINOMA OF THE BREAST | ORION CORPORATION<br>400 OYSTER POINT BLVD.<br>SUITE 325<br>SOUTH SAN FRANCISCO CA 94080-1919<br>DD 09/19/91 |
| TOREMIFENE | TREATMENT OF DESMOID TUMORS | ORION CORPORATION<br>400 OYSTER POINT BLVD.<br>SUITE 325<br>SOUTH SAN FRANCISCO CA 94080-1919<br>DD 08/17/93 |
| TRANEXAMIC ACID<br>TN is CYKLOKAPRON | TREATMENT OF PATIENTS WITH CONGENITAL COAGULOPATHIES WHO ARE UNDERGOING SURGICAL PROCEDURES, E.G. DENTAL EXTRACTIONS | PHARMACIA, INC.<br>P.O. BOX 16529<br>COLUMBUS OH 43216-6529<br>DD 10/29/85 MA 12/30/86 |
| TRANSFORMING GROWTH FACTOR-BETA 2 | TREATMENT OF FULL THICKNESS MACULAR HOLES | CELTRIX PHARMACEUTICALS, INC.<br>3055 PATRICK HENRY DRIVE<br>SANTA CLARA CA 95054<br>DD 12/18/92 |
| TRANSGENIC HUMAN ALPHA 1 ANTITRYPSIN | TREATMENT OF CYSTIC FIBROSIS | PPL THERAPEUTICS (SCOTLAND) LIMITED<br>ROSLIN, EDINBURGH<br>EH25 9PP SCOTLAND UK |
| TREOSULFAN<br>TN is OVASTAT | TREATMENT OF OVARIAN CANCER | MEDAC GmbH<br>C/O PRINCETON REG. ASSOC.<br>65 SOUTH MAIN STREET<br>PENNINGTON NJ 08534<br>DD 05/16/94 |
| TRETINOIN<br>TN is VESANOID | TREATMENT OF ACUTE PROMYELOCYTIC LEUKEMIA | HOFFMAN-LA ROCHE, INC.<br>340 KINGSLAND STREET<br>NUTLEY NJ 07110<br>DD 10/24/90 |
| TRETINOIN<br>TN is TRETINOIN LF, IV | TREATMENT OF ACUTE AND CHRONIC LEUKEMIA | ARGUS PHARMACEUTICALS, INC.<br>3400 RESEARCH FOREST DRIVE<br>THE WOODLANDS TX 77381<br>DD 01/14/93 |
| TRIENTINE HCL<br>TN is CUPRID | TREATMENT OF PATIENTS WITH WILSON'S DISEASE WHO ARE INTOLERANT, OR INADEQUATELY RESPONSIVE TO PENICILLAMINE | MERCK SHARP & DOHME RESEARCH DIVISION OF MERCK AND COMPANY<br>WEST POINT PA 19486<br>DD 12/24/84 MA 11/08/85 |

## CUMULATIVE LIST OF ORPHAN PRODUCT DESIGNATIONS AND APPROVALS
[Through October 31, 1998] *(continued)*

| NAME<br>*Generic/Chemical*<br>*TN is Trade Name* | INDICATION DESIGNATED | SPONSOR AND ADDRESS<br>*DD is Date Designated*<br>*MA is Marketing Approval* |
|---|---|---|
| TRIMETREXATE GLUCURONATE<br>TN is NEUTREXIN | TREATMENT OF PNEUMOCYSTIS CARINII PNEUMONIA IN AIDS PATIENTS | U.S. BIOSCIENCE, INC.<br>100 FRONT STREET<br>WEST CONSHOHOCKEN PA 19428<br>DD 05/15/86 MA 12/17/93 |
| TRIMETREXATE GLUCURONATE | TREATMENT OF METASTATIC CARCINOMA OF THE HEAD AND NECK (I.E., BUCCAL CAVITY, PHARYNX, AND LARYNX) | U.S. BIOSCIENCE, INC.<br>100 FRONT STREET<br>WEST CONSHOHOCKEN PA 19428<br>DD 07/25/85 |
| TRIMETREXATE GLUCURONATE | TREATMENT OF METASTATIC COLORECTAL ADENOCARCINOMA | U.S. BIOSCIENCE, INC.<br>100 FRONT STREET<br>WEST CONSHOHOCKEN PA 19428<br>DD 07/25/85 |
| TRIMETREXATE GLUCURONATE | TREATMENT OF PANCREATIC ADENOCARCINOMA | U.S. BIOSCIENCE, INC.<br>100 FRONT STREET<br>WEST CONSHOHOCKEN PA 19428<br>DD 07/25/85 |
| TRIMETREXATE GLUCURONATE | TREATMENT OF PATIENTS WITH ADVANCED NON-SMALL CELL CARCINOMA OF THE LUNG | U.S. BIOSCIENCE, INC.<br>100 FRONT STREET<br>WEST CONSHOHOCKEN PA 19428<br>DD 01/13/88 |
| TRISACCHARIDES A AND B<br>TN is BIOSYNJECT | TREATMENT OF MODERATE TO SEVERE CLINICAL FORMS OF HEMOLYTIC DISEASE OF THE NEWBORN ARISING FROM PLACENTAL TRANSFER OF ANTIBODIES AGAINST BLOOD GROUP SUBSTANCES A AND B | CHEMBIOMED, LTD.<br>P.O. BOX 8050<br>EDMONTON ALBERTA<br>CANADA T6H4NP<br>DD 04/12/87 |
| TRISACCHARIDES A AND B<br>TN is BIOSYNJECT | FOR USE IN ABO-INCOMPATIBLE SOLID ORGAN TRANSPLANTATION, INCLUDING KIDNEY, HEART, LIVER AND PANCREAS | CHEMBIOMED, LTD.<br>P.O. BOX 8050<br>EDMONTON ALBERTA<br>CANADA T6H4N9<br>DD 04/20/87 |
| TRISACCHARIDES A AND B<br>TN is BIOSYNJECT | PREVENTION OF ABO MEDICAL HEMOLYTIC REACTIONS ARISING FROM ABO-INCOMPATIBLE BONE MARROW TRANSPLANTATION | CHEMBIOMED, LTD.<br>P.O. BOX 8050<br>EDMONTON ALBERTA<br>CANADA T6H4N9<br>DD 04/15/88 |
| TRISODIUM CITRATE CONCENTRATION<br>TN is HEMOCITRATE | FOR USE IN LEUKAPHERESIS PROCEDURES | HEMOTEC MEDICAL PRODUCTS, INC.<br>BOX 19255<br>JOHNSTON RI 02919<br>DD 06/15/95 |
| TROLEANDOMYCIN | TREATMENT OF SEVERE STEROID-REQUIRING ASTHMA | SZEFLER, STANLEY M., M.D.<br>1400 JACKSON STREET<br>DENVER CO 80206<br>DD 09/21/89 |
| TUMOR NECROSIS FACTOR-BINDING PROTEIN 1 | TREATMENT OF SYMPTOMATIC PATIENTS WITH ACQUIRED IMMUNODEFICIENCY SYNDROME INCLUDING ALL PATIENTS WITH CD4 COUNTS LESS THAN 200 CELLS PER MM3 | SERONO LABORATORIES, INC.<br>100 LONGWATER CIRCLE<br>NORWELL MA 02061<br>DD 01/06/93 |
| TUMOR NECROSIS FACTOR-BINDING PROTEIN II | TREATMENT OF SYMPTOMATIC PATIENTS WITH THE ACQUIRED IMMUNODEFICIENCY SYNDROME INCLUDING ALL PATIENTS WITH CD4 T-CELL COUNTS LESS THAN 200 CELLS PER MM3 | SERONO LABORATORIES, INC.<br>100 LONGWATER CIRCLE<br>NORWELL MA 02061<br>DD 01/06/93 |
| TYLOXAPOL | TREATMENT OF CYSTIC FIBROSIS | KENNEDY & HOIDAL, MDs<br>50 NORTH MEDICAL DRIVE<br>U OF UTAH<br>SALT LAKE CITY UT 84132<br>DD 03/08/95 |
| URIDINE 5'-TRIPHOSPHATE | TREATMENT OF CYSTIC FIBROSIS | INSPIRE PHARMACEUTICALS, INC.<br>P.O. BOX 14285<br>RESEARCH TRIANGLE PARK, NC 27709 |
| URIDINE 5'-TRIPHOSPHATE | TO FACILITATE THE REMOVAL OF LUNG SECRETIONS IN THE TREATMENT OF PATIENTS WITH PRIMARY CILIARY DYSKINESIA | INSPIRE PHARMACEUTICALS, INC.<br>4222 EMPEROR BOULEVARD,<br>SUITE 470<br>DURHAM NC 27703 |
| UROFOLLITROPIN<br>TN is FERTINEX | FOR THE INITIATION AND RE-INITIATION OF SPERMATOGENESIS IN ADULT MALES WITH REPRODUCTIVE FAILURE DUE TO HYPOTHALAMIC OR PITUITARY DYSFUNCTION, HYPOGONADOTROPIC HYPOGONADISM | SERONO LABORATORIES, INC.<br>100 LONGWATER CIRCLE<br>NORWELL MA 02061 |
| UROFOLLITROPIN<br>TN is METRODIN | INDUCTION OF OVULATION IN PATIENTS WITH POLYCYSTIC OVARIAN DISEASE WHO HAVE AN ELEVATED LH/FSH RATIO AND WHO HAVE FAILED TO RESPOND TO ADEQUATE CLOMIPHENE CITRATE THERAPY | SERONO LABORATORIES, INC.<br>100 LONGWATER CIRCLE<br>NORWELL MA 02061<br>DD 11/25/87 MA 09/18/86 |

# CUMULATIVE LIST OF ORPHAN PRODUCT DESIGNATIONS AND APPROVALS
[Through October 31, 1998] *(continued)*

| NAME<br>*Generic/Chemical*<br>*TN is Trade Name* | INDICATION DESIGNATED | SPONSOR AND ADDRESS<br>*DD is Date Designated*<br>*MA is Marketing Approval* |
|---|---|---|
| UROGASTRONE | ACCELERATION OF CORNEAL EPITHELIAL REGENERATION AND HEALING OF STROMAL INCISIONS FROM CORNEAL TRANSPLANT SURGERY | CHIRON OPHTHALMICS<br>500 IOLAB DRIVE<br>CLAREMONT CA 91711<br>DD 11/01/84 |
| URSODEOXYCHOLIC ACID<br>TN is URSOFALK | TREATMENT OF PATIENTS WITH PRIMARY BILIARY CIRRHOSIS | AXCAN PHARMA, INC.<br>25 MARGARET STREET<br>PLATTSBURGH NY 12901-1206<br>DD 06/20/91 |
| URSODIOL<br>TN is ACTIGALL | MANAGEMENT OF THE CLINICAL SIGNS AND SYMPTOMS ASSOCIATED WITH PRIMARY BILIARY CIRRHOSIS | CIBA-GEIGY CORPORATION<br>556 MORRIS AVENUE<br>SUMMIT NJ 07901<br>DD 02/19/91 |
| VALINE, ISOLEUCINE AND LEUCINE<br>TN is VIL | TREATMENT OF HYPERPHENYLALAMINEMIA | LEAS RESEARCH PRODUCTS<br>4 BROOKVIEW LANE<br>TROY NY 12180 |
| VASOACTIVE INTESTINAL POLYPEPTIDE | TREATMENT OF ACUTE ESOPHAGEAL FOOD IMPACTION | RESEARCH TRIANGLE PHARMACEUTICALS<br>200 WESTPARK CORPORATE CENTER<br>DURHAM NC 27713<br>DD 06/23/93 |
| ZALCITABINE | TREATMENT OF ACQUIRED IMMUNODEFICIENCY SYNDROME (AIDS) | NATIONAL CANCER INSTITUTE, DCT<br>NIH, EXEC. PLAZA N., ROOM 7-18<br>BETHESDA MD 20892<br>DD 12/09/86 |
| ZALCITABINE<br>TN is HIVID | TREATMENT OF ACQUIRED IMMUNODEFICIENCY SYNDROME (AIDS) | HOFFMANN-LA ROCHE, INC.<br>340 KINGSLAND STREET<br>NUTLEY NJ 07110-1199<br>DD 06/28/88 MA 06/19/92 |
| ZIDOVUDINE<br>TN is RETROVIR | TREATMENT OF ACQUIRED IMMUNODEFICIENCY SYNDROME (AIDS) | BURROUGHS WELLCOME COMPANY<br>3030 CORNWALLIS ROAD<br>RESEARCH TRIANGLE PK NC 27709<br>DD 07/17/85 MA 03/19/87 |
| ZIDOVUDINE<br>TN is RETROVIR | TREATMENT OF AIDS RELATED COMPLEX (ARC) | BURROUGHS WELLCOME COMPANY<br>3030 CORNWALLIS ROAD<br>RESEARCH TRIANGLE PK NC 27709<br>DD 05/12/87 MA 03/19/87 |
| ZINC ACETATE | TREATMENT OF WILSON'S DISEASE | LEMMON COMPANY<br>650 CATHILL ROAD<br>SELLERSVILLE PA 18960<br>DD 11/06/85 |

# Appendix IX

## THE USP PRACTITIONERS' REPORTING NETWORK℠ (USP PRN®):
## An FDA MedWatch Partner

Health care professionals are encouraged to report problems that they observe with the use of medications or medical devices. Without such input, manufacturers, government, the compendia, and colleagues may not be aware of problems that are experienced. This exchange of meaningful information is an integral part of improving the safety, efficacy, and quality of medical products. The individual practitioner is in the best position to recognize that a problem may exist and to report it.

The **USP Practitioners' Reporting Network℠ (USP PRN®)** is a singular, nationwide network designed to serve all reporting needs of health care professionals. USP PRN comprises three separate programs: the Drug Product Problem Reporting Program, the Medication Errors Reporting Program, and the Veterinary Practitioners' Reporting Program. The USP PRN publishes the *USP Quality Review*, a timely, educational newsletter based on case reports received through the programs and for your convenience has current practitioner reporting news available on the Internet at *www.usp.org/prn*.

**The USP Drug Product Problem Reporting (DPPR) Program:**
This program has been in existence for more than 27 years thanks to the active involvement of health care practitioners across the nation. The program has evolved into an effective tool for regulatory bodies, the pharmaceutical industry, and the USP to monitor the quality of drug products in the marketplace.

All reports received at USP become part of the DPPR database. The database allows for tracking, analysis, and comparison of product problems occurring nationwide. These reports have identified problems such as the presence of foreign matter, suspected contamination, color variation, broken tablets, packaging and labeling that is inadequate or incomplete, adverse drug reactions, questionable potency, and suspected bioinequivalence based on observed therapeutic response. Unlike any other drug quality reporting program, the DPPR can directly impact the development and revision of USP standards and information.

**The USP Medication Errors Reporting (MER) Program:**
This nationwide program makes it possible for health professionals who encounter actual or potential medication errors to report confidentially to USP. By sharing these experiences, pharmacists, nurses, physicians, and other health care professionals can contribute to improved patient safety and to the development of valuable educational services for the prevention of future errors. The program encompasses a wide variety of problems such as misinterpretations, miscalculations, misadministrations, difficulty interpreting handwritten orders, or misunderstanding verbal orders. The MER Program is presented in cooperation with the Institute for Safe Medication Practices.

USP has just introduced **MedMARx™**, an Internet-accessible database software program designed to anonymously collect, track, and "benchmark" medication error data for hospitals nationwide. MedMARx is based on and consistent with the current USP medication error database. To receive additional information on the MedMARx Program see the MedMARx homepage at www.usp.org/medmarx or call USP at 1-800-487-7776.

In an effort to keep the health care population informed and educated regarding the effects of medication errors on the public and on the health care practitioners, USP has developed an education resource, *Understanding and Preventing Medication Errors*. Every day a disturbing number of medication errors occur throughout the health care system. In response to this serious problem, USP offers an in-depth program of interactive lecture and study material on this topic especially tailored to the health care professional. For additional information on this resource or to place an order call 800-227-8772.

**The Veterinary Practitioners' Reporting (VPR) Program:**
The Veterinary Practitioners' Reporting Program, presented in co-operation with the American Veterinary Medical Association (AVMA), is designed to detect product quality problems, medication mishaps, and adverse reactions associated with drugs, biologics, pesticides, and other products used in the practice of veterinary medicine. The program accepts reports regarding any type of problem observed in any species of animal. USP shares reported information with the manufacturer/labeler, the appropriate federal regulatory agency (USDA-Center for Veterinary Biologics, FDA-Center for Veterinary Medicine, EPA), and the AVMA. The information is also entered into USP's national database of veterinary reports where it is available for analysis.

The USP PRN reporting forms are available on diskette free of charge. These forms are designed to run using Microsoft Word for Windows Version 6.0 or Novell WordPerfect Windows Version 6.0/6.1. Call toll free (800-487-7776) to receive your free diskette.

To report or receive information, call 800-487-7776 (800-4 USP PRN). The USP PRN reporting forms are now available **on-line** at:

| | |
|---|---|
| www.usp.org/prn/dppr.htm | Drug Product Problem Reporting Program |
| www.usp.org/prn/mer.htm | Medication Errors Reporting Program |
| www.usp.org/prn/vprp.htm | Veterinary Practitioners' Reporting Program |
| www.usp.org/medmarx | MedMARx™ |

In 1993, USP became an active partner in MedWatch, the FDA's medical product reporting program. As a partner, USP supports the FDA's efforts to protect the public health by helping to identify serious adverse events.

USP PRN... call us when you need us.

# USP PRACTITIONERS' REPORTING NETWORK℠
*An FDA MEDWATCH partner*

**DRUG PRODUCT PROBLEM REPORTING PROGRAM**

1. PRODUCT NAME (include generic name)

2. DOSAGE FORM (tablet, capsule, injectable, etc.)

3. SIZE/TYPE OF CONTAINER

4. STRENGTH

5. NDC NUMBER

6. LOT NUMBER(S)

7. EXPIRATION DATE(S)

8. NAME AND ADDRESS OF THE MANUFACTURER

9. NAME AND ADDRESS OF LABELER (if different from manufacturer)

10. PROBLEMS NOTED OR SUSPECTED (if more space is needed, please attach separate page)

11. YOUR NAME AND TITLE (please type or print)

12. YOUR PRACTICE LOCATION (include establishment name, address, and ZIP code)

Days and times available _____

13. PHONE NUMBER AT PRACTICE LOCATION (include area code)

14. A copy of your report is routinely sent to the manufacturer/labeler and to the FDA. USP may release my identity to: (check boxes that apply)
   - ❏ The manufacturer and/or labeler as listed above.
   - ❏ The Food and Drug Administration.
   - ❏ Other persons requesting a copy of this report.
   - ❏ None of the above.

15. If requested, will the actual product involved be available for examination by the manufacturer or FDA? ❏ Yes ❏ No (Do not send samples to USP)

15a. This event has been reported to:
   - ❏ Manufacturer ❏ FDA
   - ❏ Other _____

15b. Date problem occurred or observed: _____

16. SIGNATURE OF REPORTER (as listed in question 11)

17. DATE

Return to the attention of:
Diane D. Cousins, R.Ph.
USP PRN
12601 Twinbrook Parkway
Rockville, MD 20852-1790

Call Toll Free: **800-4-USP PRN** (800-487-7776)
or FAX 301-816-8532
USP home page: http://www.usp.org/prn
Electronic reporting forms are available. Please call for additional information and/or your *free* diskette.

File Access Number:

Date Received by USP:

USP DI 1999

# USP MEDICATION ERRORS REPORTING PROGRAM

Presented in cooperation with the Institute for Safe Medication Practices
The USP Practitioners' Reporting Network℠ is an FDA MEDWATCH partner

**MEDICATION ERRORS REPORTING PROGRAM**

☐ ACTUAL ERROR  ☐ POTENTIAL ERROR

Please describe the error. Include sequence of events, personnel involved, and work environment (e.g., code situation, change of shift, short staffing, no 24-hr. pharmacy, floor stock). If more space is needed, please attach separate page.

Was the medication administered to or used by the patient? ☐ No ☐ Yes   Date and time of event: _____

What type of staff or health care practitioner made the initial error? _____

Describe outcome (e.g., death, type of injury, adverse reaction). _____

If the medication did not reach the patient, describe the intervention. _____

Who discovered the error? _____

When and how was error discovered? _____

Where did the error occur (e.g., hospital, outpatient or retail pharmacy, nursing home, patient's home)? _____

Was another practitioner involved in the error ? ☐ No ☐ Yes  If yes, what type of practitioner? _____

Was patient counseling provided? ☐ No ☐ Yes  If yes, before or after error was discovered? _____

If a product was involved, please complete the following:

|  | Product #1 | Product #2 |
|---|---|---|
| Brand name of product involved | | |
| Generic name | | |
| Manufacturer | | |
| Labeler (if different from mfr.) | | |
| Dosage form | | |
| Strength/concentration | | |
| Type and size of container | | |
| NDC number | | |

If available, please provide relevant patient information (age, gender, diagnosis, etc.). Patient identification not required.

Reports are most useful when relevant materials such as product label, copy of prescription/order, etc. can be reviewed.
Can these materials be provided? ☐ No ☐ Yes  If yes, please specify. _____

Suggest any recommendations you have to prevent recurrence of this error or describe policies or procedures you have instituted to prevent future similar errors.

A copy of this report is routinely sent to the Institute for Safe Medication Practices (ISMP), to the manufacturer/labeler, and to the Food and Drug Administration (FDA). **USP may release my identity to: (check boxes that apply)**
☐ ISMP ☐ The manufacturer and/or labeler as listed above ☐ FDA ☐ Other persons requesting a copy of this report ☐ Anonymous to all

Your name and title

Your facility name, address, and ZIP

Telephone number (include area code)

Signature                                                                 Date

Return to the attention of:
Diane D. Cousins, R.Ph.
USP PRN
12601 Twinbrook Parkway
Rockville, MD 20852-1790

Call Toll Free: **800-23-ERROR** (800-233-7767)
or FAX 301-816-8532
USP home page: http://www.usp.org/prn
Electronic reporting forms are available. Please call for additional information and/or your free diskette.

Date Received by USP:

File Access Number:

USP DI 1999

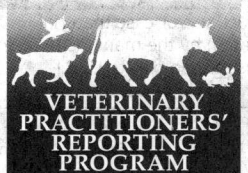

# USP PRACTITIONERS' REPORTING NETWORK℠

The Veterinary Practitioners' Reporting Program is presented in cooperation with
the American Veterinary Medical Association (AVMA)

page 1

**VETERINARY PRACTITIONERS' REPORTING PROGRAM**

1. Describe the reaction, problem, or medication error. See page 2 for guidelines. Attach separate sheet if necessary.

2. Please complete the following for **all** suspected products relevant to the problem:

| | Product 1 | Product 2 | Product 3 |
|---|---|---|---|
| Brand name | | | |
| Generic name | | | |
| Manufacturer | | | |
| Labeler (if different) | | | |
| Dosage form | | | |
| Strength/concentration | | | |
| Lot/serial no. & Exp. date | | | |

Please provide one of the following for each product (see product label):
Biologics: US Vet. Lic. No.
Drugs: (A)NADA or NDC
Pesticides: EPA Reg. No.

**Complete numbers 3–14 in the boxed area to report an adverse event. Skip to page 2 for other problems.**

3. Date of product administration:
4. Date of onset of adverse event:
5. Animal/Case ID:
6. Reason for product usage:
7. Administered by: ❑ Veterinarian ❑ Technician ❑ Owner ❑ Other _____
8. Product administration
   Dose & interval: _____ Length of treatment: _____
   Route: _____
   For animals managed in a group (herd, flock, litter, etc.), number of animals treated: _____

   Concurrent procedures and clinical problems/products administered, including pesticides, chemicals, feed additives, etc.:

9. Species:
10. Breed:
11. Age:
12. Sex:
13. Weight: _____ kg. _____ lbs.

14. Reaction/Problem information
    a. Number of affected animals described in this report: _____
    b. Overall state of health at time of product administration:
       ❑ Good ❑ Fair ❑ Poor ❑ Critical
    c. Time between the initial administration of the suspected product and the onset of reaction: _____
    d. Time between last administration of suspected product and onset of reaction (if different from 14c): _____
    e. When the reaction appeared, administration of suspected product:
       ❑ had already been completed
       ❑ was discontinued due to reaction
       ❑ was discontinued and replaced with another product
       ❑ was discontinued and reintroduced later
       ❑ was continued at altered dose

    f. The reaction continued: ❑ until death
       ❑ other: _____
       stopped: ❑ with specific treatment
       ❑ with nonspecific treatment
       ❑ with no treatment
       recurred: ❑ (comment in item 1)
    g. Was the reaction treated?
       ❑ No ❑ Yes (describe treatment in item 1)
    h. Outcome:
       ❑ Recovered from reaction ❑ Other (comment in item 1)
       ❑ Died from reaction ❑ Euthanized due to this adverse event
       ❑ Euthanized/culled for other reasons (comment in item 1)
    i. Veterinarian's level of suspicion that product(s) caused the reaction:
       ❑ High ❑ Medium ❑ Low
    j. Has the animal received this product in the past?
       ❑ No ❑ Yes If yes, describe reaction, if any, in item 1.

Return to the attention of:
Diane D. Cousins, R.Ph.
USP PRN
12601 Twinbrook Parkway
Rockville, MD 20852-1790

Call Toll Free: **800-4-USP PRN** (800-487-7776)
or FAX: 301-816-8532
USP PRN home page: http://www.usp.org/prn/vprp.htm
Electronic reporting forms are available. Please call for additional information and/or your free diskette.

File Access Number:

Date Processed by USP:

*Please complete other side*

USP DI 1999

| 15. Reporter's name, title, and address: | 16. If requested, will the actual product and/or case material involved be available for examination by the manufacturer or regulatory agency? (Do not send samples to USP.) ❏ No ❏ Yes |
|---|---|
| Telephone number: _____ | 17. This event has already been reported to: ❏ Manufacturer ❏ FDA ❏ USDA ❏ EPA ❏ Other: _____ |

18. A copy of your report is routinely sent to the manufacturer/labeler, to the appropriate regulatory agency (FDA, USDA, or EPA), and AVMA. USP may release my identity to: (check boxes that apply)

❏ The manufacturer and/or labeler as listed in item 2   ❏ Regulatory agency   ❏ AVMA   ❏ Other persons requesting a copy of this report   ❏ None of these

Signature of reporter:                                                   Date:

## Animal Safety and Quality Products Through the USP Practitioners' Reporting Network℠ (USP PRN®)

To further enhance the USP Practitioners' Reporting Network, the United States Pharmacopeia has added the Veterinary Practitioners' Reporting Program. Through the combined efforts of the American Veterinary Medical Association and the USP, this program is aimed at detecting product quality problems, medication mishaps, and adverse reactions to drugs, biologics, chemicals, pesticides, and other products used in the practice of veterinary medicine. This program covers products used in companion and other household pets, food-producing and farm animals, zoo animals, and exotic pets. The USP shares reports with the product manufacturer/labeler and the appropriate regulatory agency to provide a safer environment for the various animal populations in the U.S. Reports may be submitted anonymously, and USP will act as your intermediary.

## Where Vital INPUT Enhances Valuable OUTPUT

A call to USP PRN puts you in touch with a USP health care professional, who will take your report and respond to your concerns. Your phoned, faxed, or written report rapidly and effectively communicates a potential health hazard or product defect to the appropriate regulating agency, the product manufacturer, and the AVMA for review and any necessary follow-up. Your report can result in product improvement or correction and, if necessary, product recall. Unlike any other reporting program, the USP Veterinary Practitioners' Reporting Program can directly impact the development and revision of *USP-NF* standards for quality, strength, purity, packaging, labeling, and identity, and information monographs in the *USP DI®*.

## USP: A Partner in MEDWATCH

The USP PRN is a partner in MEDWATCH, the FDA's medical products reporting program. As a partner, USP PRN contributes to the FDA's efforts to protect the public health by helping to identify serious adverse events for the agency. This means that all reports on FDA-regulated products are shared with the FDA on a daily basis or immediately if necessary.

## Contribute to a Nationwide Database

The report you submit becomes part of a database that serves to provide insight into product problems that can affect the quality of veterinary care. This database captures all fields of reported information to allow for tracking, analysis, and comparison of product problems occurring nationwide. The product information received through the program is available under the USP Document Disclosure Policy.*

*Fees may be required for disclosure of any information pursuant to the USP Document Disclosure Policy.

## Guidelines: Products and Problems That Can Be Reported

**All products used in your practice, such as:**

Drugs                Vaccines              Syringes
Chemicals            Surgical gloves       Anesthesia products
Pet dips             Vitamins              Salves/ointments
Feed additives       Serums/antivenins

**Product problems:**

Ineffectiveness/lack of efficacy    Contamination
Product failure/malfunction         Color/odor changes
Suspected counterfeit drugs         Foreign material
Product mix-ups                     Therapeutic failures
Inaccurate/confusing labeling       Particulate matter/precipitate
Adverse reactions (including human reactions to animal products)

**Therapy errors:**

Misadministration, similar products and names, miscalculations, wrong product administered, etc.

**Potential medication errors — before an adverse event occurs:**

Incomplete/confusing label information, confusing/similar product names, similar labels, similar/confusing containers, inappropriate product design.

**Valuable information:**

Practitioners are asked to provide specific information on species, age, breed, sex, histopathology, clinical pathology or necropsy results, etc., which add value to reported incidents.

---

### Just a Phone Call Away (800-487-7776)

The USP PRN® is designed to collect experiences and observations from health care providers through three separate reporting programs:

- The USP Veterinary Practitioners' Reporting Program
- The USP Drug Product Problem Reporting Program
- The USP Medication Errors Reporting Program

The American Veterinary Medical Association and the Institute for Safe Medication Practices cooperate in presenting programs of the USP PRN.

Your Input Could Make the Difference!

**USP PRN...CALL US WHEN YOU NEED US.**

## MedWatch, the FDA Medical Products Reporting Program

For health care providers wishing to report serious adverse events or product problems directly to the FDA, a MedWatch form is provided.

Report experiences with:
- medications (drugs or biologics)
- medical devices (including *in vitro* diagnostics)
- special nutritional products (dietary supplements, medical foods, infant formulas)
- other products regulated by FDA

Report SERIOUS adverse events. An event is serious when the patient outcome is:
- death
- life-threatening (real risk of dying)
- hospitalization (initial or prolonged)
- disability (significant, persistent or permanent)
- congenital anomaly
- required intervention to prevent permanent impairment or damage

How to report:
- fill in the sections that apply to your report
- use section C for all products except medical devices
- attach additional blank pages if needed
- use a separate form for each patient
- report either to FDA or the manufacturer (or both)

Important numbers:
- 1-800-FDA-0178 to FAX report
- 1-800-FDA-1088 for more information or to report quality problems
- 1-800-822-7967 for a VAERS form for vaccines

If your report involves a serious adverse event with a device and it occurred in a facility outside a doctor's office, that facility may be legally required to report to FDA and/or the manufacturer. Please notify the person in that facility who would handle such reporting.

To report a medical device problem, you may submit an FDA MedWatch form.

*Confidentiality:* The patient's identity is held in strict confidence by FDA and protected to the fullest extent of the law. The reporter's identity may be shared with the manufacturer unless requested otherwise. However, FDA will not disclose the reporter's identity in reponse to a request from the public pursuant to the Freedom of Information Act.

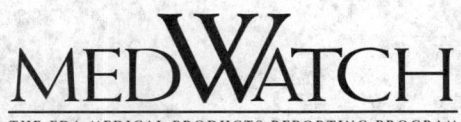

**For VOLUNTARY reporting by health professionals of adverse events and product problems**

Form Approved: OMB No. 0910-0291 Expires: 4/30/96
See OMB statement on reverse

FDA Use Only
Triage unit sequence #

Page ___ of ___

### A. Patient information
1. Patient identifier  In confidence
2. Age at time of event: ___ or Date of birth: ___
3. Sex: ☐ female ☐ male
4. Weight: ___ lbs or ___ kgs

### B. Adverse event or product problem
1. ☐ Adverse event and/or ☐ Product problem (e.g., defects/malfunctions)
2. Outcomes attributed to adverse event (check all that apply)
   ☐ death ___ (mo/day/yr)
   ☐ life-threatening
   ☐ hospitalization – initial or prolonged
   ☐ disability
   ☐ congenital anomaly
   ☐ required intervention to prevent permanent impairment/damage
   ☐ other ___
3. Date of event (mo/day/yr)
4. Date of this report (mo/day/yr)
5. Describe event or problem

6. Relevant tests/laboratory data, including dates

7. Other relevant history, including preexisting medical conditions (e.g., allergies, race, pregnancy, smoking and alcohol use, hepatic/renal dysfunction, etc.)

PLEASE TYPE OR USE BLACK INK

### C. Suspect medication(s)
1. Name (give labeled strength & mfr/labeler, if known)
   #1
   #2
2. Dose, frequency & route used
   #1
   #2
3. Therapy dates (if unknown, give duration) from/to (or best estimate)
   #1
   #2
4. Diagnosis for use (indication)
   #1
   #2
5. Event abated after use stopped or dose reduced
   #1 ☐ yes ☐ no ☐ doesn't apply
   #2 ☐ yes ☐ no ☐ doesn't apply
6. Lot # (if known)
   #1
   #2
7. Exp. date (if known)
   #1
   #2
8. Event reappeared after reintroduction
   #1 ☐ yes ☐ no ☐ doesn't apply
   #2 ☐ yes ☐ no ☐ doesn't apply
9. NDC # (for product problems only)
10. Concomitant medical products and therapy dates (exclude treatment of event)

### D. Suspect medical device
1. Brand name
2. Type of device
3. Manufacturer name & address
4. Operator of device
   ☐ health professional
   ☐ lay user/patient
   ☐ other: ___
5. Expiration date (mo/day/yr)
6. model # ___
   catalog # ___
   serial # ___
   lot # ___
   other # ___
7. If implanted, give date (mo/day/yr)
8. If explanted, give date (mo/day/yr)
9. Device available for evaluation? (Do not send to FDA)
   ☐ yes ☐ no ☐ returned to manufacturer on ___ (mo/day/yr)
10. Concomitant medical products and therapy dates (exclude treatment of event)

### E. Reporter (see confidentiality section on back)
1. Name & address
   phone #
2. Health professional? ☐ yes ☐ no
3. Occupation
4. Also reported to
   ☐ manufacturer
   ☐ user facility
   ☐ distributor
5. If you do NOT want your identity disclosed to the manufacturer, place an "X" in this box. ☐

**FDA**  Mail to: MEDWATCH  5600 Fishers Lane  Rockville, MD 20852-9787  or FAX to: 1-800-FDA-0178

FDA Form 3500 (1/96)  Submission of a report does not constitute an admission that medical personnel or the product caused or contributed to the event.

# Indications Index

The indications listed have been extracted from the monographs included in *USP DI*. Since the USP DI data base does not yet include monographs on every therapeutic agent available, users should not assume that all medications which are appropriate for a given indication are listed or that those not listed are inappropriate. In addition, since any indication listed may encompass varying degrees of severity and since different medications may not be appropriate for differing degrees of severity or because of other patient-related factors, it can not be assumed that the agents listed for any specific indication are interchangeable. *This indications index can not be used by itself to determine the appropriateness of therapy;* rather, it should be used as a tool in searching out more information about the therapies available.

Drugs are listed alphabetically. Brackets are used to identify a medication available in the U.S. whose FDA-approved labeling does not include the stated indication but which is included in the *USP DI* monograph. Symbols denote the following:

* \* — Products not available in the U.S.
* [1] — Indications not included in Canadian product labeling.
* † — Products not available in Canada.
* ‡ — FDA orphan use designations.
* # — Drugs for which monographs are not included in this published version of the USP DI database. Copies of the monographs are available on request from Micromedex, Inc.—Reprint Requests, 6200 S. Syracuse Way, Suite 300, Englewood, CO 80111; telephone (303) 486-6400; telefax (303) 486-6464; Email: USPDI@MDS.COM.

## A

**Abdominal imaging, computed tomographic, adjunct**
[Glucagon (Systemic)][1], 1563
Iohexol (Systemic)[1], #
**Abdominal imaging, digital angiographic, adjunct**
[Glucagon (Systemic)][1], 1563
**Abdominal imaging, magnetic resonance, adjunct**
[Glucagon (Systemic)][1], 1563
**Abortion**
Carboprost (Systemic), 782
**Abortion, elective**
Dinoprost (Parenteral-Local)*, #
Dinoprostone Vaginal Suppositories (Cervical/Vaginal), 1228
Sodium Chloride (Parenteral-Local), #
[Urea (Parenteral-Local)], #
**Abortion, incomplete (treatment)**
[Carboprost (Systemic)][1], 782
Dinoprost (Parenteral-Local)*[1], #
[Ergonovine (Systemic)][1], 1360
[Methylergonovine (Systemic)]†, 1984
Oxytocin, Parenteral (Systemic), 2211
**Abortion, missed (treatment)**
Dinoprostone Vaginal Suppositories (Cervical/Vaginal), 1228
**Abortion, therapeutic**
Dinoprost (Parenteral-Local)*[1], #
Dinoprostone Vaginal Suppositories (Cervical/Vaginal), 1228
Oxytocin, Parenteral (Systemic), 2211
**Abrasions, corneal (treatment)**
Framycetin (Ophthalmic)*, 3020
**Achlorhydria**—*See* Anacidity; Gastric histamine test
**Acidosis, lactic (treatment)**
Sodium Dichloroacetate (Systemic), 3164‡
[Thiamine (Systemic)], 2787
**Acidosis, metabolic (treatment)**
Sodium Bicarbonate, Oral (Systemic), 2586
**Acidosis, in renal tubular disorders (diagnosis)**
[Fludrocortisone (Systemic)][1], 1481
**Acidosis, in renal tubular disorders (treatment)**
[Fludrocortisone (Systemic)][1], 1481
Potassium Citrate and Citric Acid (Systemic), 881
Sodium Citrate and Citric Acid (Systemic), 881
Tricitrates (Systemic), 881
**Acne, adult**—*See* Rosacea
**Acne rosacea**—*See* Rosacea
**Acne vulgaris (treatment)**
Adapalene (Topical), 30
Alcohol and Acetone (Topical)†, #
Alcohol and Sulfur (Topical), #
Azelaic Acid (Topical)†, 495
Benzoyl Peroxide (Topical), 579
Clindamycin (Topical), 896
Demeclocycline (Systemic), 2765
Doxycycline (Systemic), 2765
Erythromycin (Topical), 1365
Erythromycin and Benzoyl Peroxide (Topical)†, 1367
[Erythromycin, Oral (Systemic)], 1368
Isotretinoin (Systemic), 1796
Isotretinoin (Topical), 3026
Meclocycline (Topical)†, 2774
Minocycline, Oral (Systemic), 2765
Nicotinamide (Topical)*, 3029
Norgestrel and Ethinyl Estradiol, Triphasic (Systemic)[1], 1397

**Acne vulgaris (treatment)** *(continued)*
Oxytetracycline (Systemic)†, 2765
Resorcinol (Topical), #
Resorcinol and Sulfur (Topical), #
Salicylic Acid Gel USP (Topical), #
Salicylic Acid Lotion (Topical), #
Salicylic Acid Ointment (Topical), #
Salicylic Acid Pads (Topical), #
Salicylic Acid Soap (Topical), #
Salicylic Acid Topical Solution (Topical), #
Salicylic Acid and Sulfur Bar Soap (Topical), #
Salicylic Acid and Sulfur Cleansing Cream (Topical), #
Salicylic Acid and Sulfur Cleansing Lotion (Topical), #
Salicylic Acid and Sulfur Cleansing Suspension (Topical), #
Salicylic Acid and Sulfur Lotion (Topical), #
Salicylic Acid and Sulfur Topical Suspension (Topical), #
Sulfurated Lime (Topical), #
Sulfur (Topical), #
Tazarotene (Topical), 2692
Tetracycline Hydrochloride for Topical Solution (Topical), 2774
Tetracycline, Oral (Systemic), 2765
Tretinoin (Topical), 2871
**Acromegaly (treatment)**
B2036-PEG (Systemic), 3133‡
Bromocriptine (Systemic), 636
Octreotide (Systemic)[1], 2152
**ACTH**—*See* Adrenocorticotropic hormone
**Actinic cheilitis (treatment)**
[Fluorouracil (Topical)][1], 1500
**Actinic keratoses, multiple (treatment)**
Fluorouracil (Topical), 1500
Masoprocol (Topical)†, 1912
**Actinomycosis (treatment)**
[Clindamycin (Systemic)][1], 893
Demeclocycline (Systemic), 2765
Doxycycline (Systemic), 2765
[Erythromycin (Systemic)][1], 1368
Minocycline (Systemic), 2765
Oxytetracycline (Systemic)†, 2765
Penicillin G, Parenteral (Systemic), 2240
[Penicillin V (Systemic)][1], 2240
Tetracycline (Systemic), 2765
**Actinomycotic mycetoma (treatment)**
[Dapsone (Systemic)], 1170
**Acute nonlymphocytic leukemia**—*See* Leukemia, acute nonlymphocytic
**Addison's disease**—*See* Adrenocortical insufficiency, chronic primary
**Adenoma, multiple endocrine (treatment)**
Cimetidine (Systemic), 1633
Famotidine (Systemic), 1633
[Nizatidine (Systemic)][1], 1633
Omeprazole (Systemic), 2163
Ranitidine (Systemic), 1633
**Adenoma, multiple endocrine (treatment adjunct)**
Alumina, Calcium Carbonate, and Sodium Bicarbonate (Oral-Local)*, 188
Alumina and Magnesia (Oral-Local), 188
Alumina, Magnesia, Calcium Carbonate, and Simethicone (Oral-Local)*, 188
Alumina, Magnesia, and Magnesium Carbonate (Oral-Local)*, 188
Alumina, Magnesia, Magnesium Carbonate, and Simethicone (Oral-Local)*, 188

**Adenoma, multiple endocrine (treatment adjunct)** *(continued)*
Alumina, Magnesia, and Simethicone (Oral-Local), 188
Alumina, Magnesium Alginate, and Magnesium Carbonate (Oral-Local)*, 188
Alumina and Magnesium Carbonate (Oral-Local)†, 188
Alumina, Magnesium Carbonate, and Simethicone (Oral-Local)†, 188
Alumina, Magnesium Carbonate, and Sodium Bicarbonate (Oral-Local)†, 188
Alumina and Magnesium Trisilicate (Oral-Local)†, 188
Alumina, Magnesium Trisilicate, and Sodium Bicarbonate (Oral-Local)†, 188
Alumina and Simethicone (Oral-Local)†, 188
Alumina and Sodium Bicarbonate (Oral-Local)*, 188
Aluminum Carbonate, Basic (Oral-Local)†, 188
Aluminum Carbonate, Basic and Simethicone (Oral-Local)†, 188
Aluminum Hydroxide (Oral-Local), 188
Calcium Carbonate (Oral-Local)†, 188
Calcium Carbonate and Magnesia (Oral-Local)†, 188
Calcium Carbonate, Magnesia, and Simethicone (Oral-Local)†, 188
Calcium and Magnesium Carbonates (Oral-Local)†, 188
Calcium Carbonate and Simethicone (Oral-Local)†, 188
Magaldrate (Oral-Local), 188
Magaldrate and Simethicone (Oral-Local), 188
Magnesium Carbonate and Sodium Bicarbonate (Oral-Local)*, 188
Magnesium Hydroxide (Oral-Local), 188
Magnesium Oxide (Oral-Local)†, 188
**Adenoma, pancreatic islet cell (diagnostic)**
Tolbutamide (Systemic), 3036
**Adenosine deaminase deficiency (treatment)**
Pegademase (Systemic)†, #
Pegademase Bovine (Systemic), 3157‡
**ADHD**—*See* Attention-deficit hyperactivity disorder
**Adrenal hyperplasia, congenital**—*See* Adrenogenital syndrome
**Adrenocortical imaging**
Iodine I 131 6B-Iodomethyl-19-Norcholesterol (Systemic), 3149dd
**Adrenocortical insufficiency (diagnosis)**
Corticotropin for Injection USP (Systemic), 1021
Cosyntropin (Systemic), 1023
**Adrenocortical insufficiency, acute (treatment)**
Betamethasone, Parenteral (Systemic), 998
Cortisone, Parenteral (Systemic), 998
Dexamethasone, Parenteral (Systemic), 998
Hydrocortisone, Parenteral (Systemic), 998
Methylprednisolone, Parenteral (Systemic), 998
Prednisolone, Parenteral (Systemic), 998
Triamcinolone, Parenteral (Systemic), 998
**Adrenocortical insufficiency, chronic primary (treatment)**
Betamethasone, Oral (Systemic), 998
Betamethasone, Parenteral (Systemic), 998
Cortisone (Systemic), 998
Dexamethasone, Oral (Systemic), 998
Dexamethasone, Parenteral (Systemic), 998
Fludrocortisone (Systemic), 1481
Hydrocortisone, Oral (Systemic), 998

## Adrenocortical insufficiency, chronic primary (treatment) (continued)
Hydrocortisone, Parenteral (Systemic), 998
Methylprednisolone, Oral (Systemic), 998
Methylprednisolone, Parenteral (Systemic), 998
Prednisolone, Oral (Systemic), 998
Prednisolone, Parenteral (Systemic), 998
Prednisone (Systemic), 998
Triamcinolone, Oral (Systemic), 998
Triamcinolone, Parenteral (Systemic), 998

## Adrenocortical insufficiency, chronic secondary (treatment)
Fludrocortisone (Systemic), 1481

## Adrenocortical insufficiency, secondary (diagnosis)
Metyrapone (Systemic), #

## Adrenocortical insufficiency, secondary (treatment)
Betamethasone, Oral (Systemic), 998
Betamethasone, Parenteral (Systemic), 998
Cortisone (Systemic), 998
Dexamethasone, Oral (Systemic), 998
Dexamethasone, Parenteral (Systemic), 998
Hydrocortisone, Oral (Systemic), 998
Hydrocortisone, Parenteral (Systemic), 998
Methylprednisolone, Oral (Systemic), 998
Methylprednisolone, Parenteral (Systemic), 998
Prednisolone, Oral (Systemic), 998
Prednisolone, Parenteral (Systemic), 998
Prednisone (Systemic), 998
Triamcinolone, Oral (Systemic), 998
Triamcinolone, Parenteral (Systemic), 998

## Adrenocorticotropic hormone (ACTH) production, origin of (diagnosis)
Corticorelin Ovine (Systemic-Diagnostic), 954

## Adrenogenital syndrome (treatment)
Betamethasone, Oral (Systemic), 998
Betamethasone, Parenteral (Systemic), 998
Cortisone (Systemic), 998
Dexamethasone, Oral (Systemic), 998
Dexamethasone, Parenteral (Systemic), 998
Fludrocortisone (Systemic), 1481
Hydrocortisone, Oral (Systemic), 998
Hydrocortisone, Parenteral (Systemic), 998
Methylprednisolone, Oral (Systemic), 998
Methylprednisolone, Parenteral (Systemic), 998
Prednisolone, Oral (Systemic), 998
Prednisolone, Parenteral (Systemic), 998
Prednisone (Systemic), 998
Triamcinolone, Oral (Systemic), 998
Triamcinolone, Parenteral (Systemic), 998

## Adrenoleukodystrophy (treatment)
Glyceryl Trioleate and Glyceryl Trierucate (Systemic), 3144‡

**African sleeping sickness**—See Trypanosomiasis, African

**AIDS**—See Immunodeficiency syndrome, acquired (AIDS)

**AIDS-associated Kaposi's sarcoma**—See Kaposi's sarcoma, AIDS-associated

## Akathisia, neuroleptic-induced (treatment)
[Betaxolol (Systemic)]†, 593
[Metoprolol (Systemic)]1, 593
[Nadolol (Systemic)]1, 593
[Propranolol (Systemic)]1, 593

## Alcoholism (treatment)
Disulfiram (Systemic), 1256

## Alcohol withdrawal (treatment)
[Carbamazepine (Systemic)]1, 757
Chlordiazepoxide (Systemic), 556
Clorazepate (Systemic), 556
Diazepam (Systemic), 556
Hydroxyzine, Parenteral (Systemic), 325
[Lorazepam (Systemic)]1, 556
Oxazepam (Systemic), 556

## Allergic disorders, nasal (treatment)
Beclomethasone (Nasal), 961
Budesonide (Nasal)*, 961
Cromolyn Nasal Solution USP (Nasal), 1118
Dexamethasone (Nasal)†, 961
Flunisolide (Nasal), 961
Triamcinolone (Nasal), 961

## Allergic disorders, ophthalmic (treatment)
Betamethasone (Ophthalmic)*, 966
Cromolyn (Ophthalmic), 1120
Dexamethasone (Ophthalmic), 966
Fluorometholone (Ophthalmic), 966
Hydrocortisone (Ophthalmic)*, 966
Prednisolone (Ophthalmic), 966

## Allergic disorders, ophthalmic, severe (treatment)
Betamethasone, Oral (Systemic), 998
Betamethasone, Parenteral (Systemic), 998
Cortisone (Systemic), 998
Dexamethasone, Oral (Systemic), 998
Dexamethasone, Parenteral (Systemic), 998
Hydrocortisone, Oral (Systemic), 998

## Allergic disorders, ophthalmic, severe (treatment) (continued)
Hydrocortisone, Parenteral (Systemic), 998
Methylprednisolone, Oral (Systemic), 998
Methylprednisolone, Parenteral (Systemic), 998
Prednisolone, Oral (Systemic), 998
Prednisolone, Parenteral (Systemic), 998
Prednisone (Systemic), 998
Triamcinolone, Oral (Systemic), 998
Triamcinolone, Parenteral (Systemic), 998

## Allergic reactions, drug-induced (treatment)
Betamethasone, Oral (Systemic), 998
Betamethasone, Parenteral (Systemic), 998
Cortisone (Systemic), 998
Dexamethasone, Oral (Systemic), 998
Dexamethasone, Parenteral (Systemic), 998
Epinephrine Injection USP (Systemic), 651
Hydrocortisone, Oral (Systemic), 998
Hydrocortisone, Parenteral (Systemic), 998
Methylprednisolone, Oral (Systemic), 998
Methylprednisolone, Parenteral (Systemic), 998
Prednisolone, Oral (Systemic), 998
Prednisolone, Parenteral (Systemic), 998
Prednisone (Systemic), 998
Triamcinolone, Oral (Systemic), 998
Triamcinolone, Parenteral (Systemic), 998

## Allergy, human seminal plasma (treatment)
[Condoms, Lamb Cecum]1, 1474
[Condoms, Lamb Cecum, and Nonoxynol 9]1, 1474
[Condoms, Latex]1, 1474
[Condoms, Latex, and Nonoxynol 9]1, 1474

## Allergy, penicillin (diagnosis)
Benzylpenicillin, Benzylpenicilloic Acid, and Benzylpenilloic Acid (Systemic), 3133‡

## Alopecia androgenetica (treatment)
Finasteride (Systemic), 1465
Minoxidil (Topical), 2021

## Alopecia areata (treatment)
Amcinonide (Topical), 978
Beclomethasone Dipropionate (Topical), 978
Betamethasone Benzoate (Topical), 978
Betamethasone Dipropionate (Topical), 978
Betamethasone, Parenteral-Local (Systemic), 998
Betamethasone Valerate (Topical), 978
Clobetasol Propionate (Topical), 978
Clobetasone Butyrate (Topical), 978
Desoximetasone (Topical), 978
Dexamethasone, Parenteral-Local (Systemic), 998
Diflorasone Diacetate (Topical), 978
Diflucortolone Valerate (Topical), 978
Fluocinolone Acetonide (Topical), 978
Fluocinonide (Topical), 978
Flurandrenolide (except 0.0125% cream and ointment) (Topical), 978
Fluticasone Propionate (Topical), 978
Halcinonide (Topical), 978
Halobetasol Propionate (Topical), 978
Hydrocortisone Butyrate (Topical), 978
Hydrocortisone, Parenteral-Local (Systemic), 998
Hydrocortisone Valerate (Topical), 978
[Methoxsalen (Systemic)]1, 1973
[Methoxsalen (Topical)]1, 1977
Methylprednisolone, Parenteral-Local (Systemic), 998
Mometasone Furoate (Topical), 978
Prednisolone, Parenteral-Local (Systemic), 998
Triamcinolone Acetonide (Topical), 978
Triamcinolone, Parenteral-Local (Systemic), 998

## Alpha-1-antitrypsin deficiency (treatment)
Alpha-1-antitrypsin (Recombinant DNA Origin) (Systemic), 3129‡
Recombinant Secretory Leucocyte Protease Inhibitor (Systemic), 3161‡

**Alpha-galactosidase A deficiency**—See Fabry's disease

## Alpha-1-proteinase inhibitor deficiency (treatment)
Alpha-1-proteinase Inhibitor (Systemic), 3129‡

**ALS**—See Amyotrophic lateral sclerosis

## Altitude sickness (prophylaxis)
Acetazolamide, Oral (Systemic)1, 773

## Altitude sickness (treatment)
Acetazolamide, Oral (Systemic)1, 773

## Amebiasis, extraintestinal (treatment)
Chloroquine (Systemic), 849
[Iodoquinol (Oral-Local)]1, #
Metronidazole (Systemic), 1996
[Tetracycline (Systemic)], 2765

## Amebiasis, intestinal (treatment)
Diloxanide (Systemic)*†, #
Iodoquinol (Oral-Local), #
Metronidazole, Oral (Systemic), 1996

**Amebiasis, invasive**—See Amebiasis, extraintestinal

## Amenorrhea (treatment)
[Desogestrel and Ethinyl Estradiol (Systemic)]1, 1397
[Ethynodiol Diacetate and Ethinyl Estradiol (Systemic)]1, 1397
Gonadorelin (Systemic)1, 3144‡
[Levonorgestrel and Ethinyl Estradiol (Systemic)]1, 1397
[Norethindrone Acetate and Ethinyl Estradiol (Systemic)]1, 1397
[Norethindrone and Ethinyl Estradiol (Systemic)]1, 1397
[Norethindrone and Mestranol (Systemic)]], 1397
[Norgestimate and Ethinyl Estradiol (Systemic)]1, 1397
[Norgestrel and Ethinyl Estradiol (Systemic)]1, 1397

## Amenorrhea, primary hypothalamic (treatment)
Gonadorelin (Systemic), 1571

## Amenorrhea, secondary (treatment)
Bromocriptine (Systemic), 636
Hydroxyprogesterone (Systemic)†, 2400
Medrogestone (Systemic)*, 2400
Medroxyprogesterone, Oral (Systemic), 2400
Norethindrone Acetate Tablets USP (Systemic), 2400
Progesterone (Systemic), 2400

**American hookworm**—See Hookworm infection

## Amnesia, in cardioversion
Diazepam, Parenteral (Systemic), 556

## Amnesia, in endoscopic procedures
Diazepam, Parenteral (Systemic), 556
[Lorazepam, Parenteral (Systemic)]1, 556

## Amniography
[Diatrizoate Meglumine, Parenteral (Systemic)]1, #

## Amyloidosis (treatment)
[Colchicine (Systemic)]1, 928

## Amyloidosis, primary, of lung (treatment adjunct)
Acetylcysteine (Inhalation-Local), #

## Amyotrophic lateral sclerosis (treatment)
Branched Chain Amino Acids (Systemic), 3134‡
Ciliary Neurotrophic Factor (Systemic), 3136‡, 3137‡
Ciliary Neurotrophic Factor, Recombinant Human (Systemic), 3136‡
Gabapentin (Systemic), 3144‡
Insulin-like Growth Factor-1 (Systemic), 3147‡
L-2-Oxothiazolidine-4-Carboxylic Acid (Systemic), 3150‡
L-Threonine (Systemic), 3150‡, 3151‡
Neurotrophin-1 (Systemic), 3156‡
Orgotein (Systemic), 3156‡
Recombinant Methionyl Brain-derived Neurotrophic Factor (Systemic), 3161‡
Riluzole (Systemic), 2500†, 3163‡

## Anacidity (diagnosis)
See also Gastric histamine test
Histamine (Systemic)*, #
Pentagastrin (Systemic), #

## Analgesia adjunct, during labor
Propiomazine (Systemic)†, #

## Analgesia adjunct, during surgery
Hydroxyzine, Parenteral (Systemic), 325
Promethazine, Parenteral (Systemic), 377

## Anaphylactic reactions (treatment)
Epinephrine Injection USP (Systemic), 651

## Anaphylactic or anaphylactoid reactions (treatment adjunct)
Acrivastine (Systemic)*†, 325
Astemizole (Systemic), 325
Azatadine (Systemic), 325
Betamethasone, Oral (Systemic), 998
Betamethasone, Parenteral (Systemic), 998
Bromodiphenhydramine (Systemic)*†, 325
Brompheniramine (Systemic), 325
Carbinoxamine (Systemic)*†, 325
Cetirizine (Systemic), 325
Chlorpheniramine (Systemic), 325
Clemastine (Systemic), 325
Cortisone (Systemic), 998
Cyproheptadine (Systemic), 325
Dexamethasone, Oral (Systemic), 998
Dexamethasone, Parenteral (Systemic), 998
Dexchlorpheniramine (Systemic), 325
Dimenhydrinate (Systemic), 325
Diphenhydramine (Systemic), 325
Diphenylpyraline (Systemic)*†, 325
Doxylamine (Systemic)†, 325
Hydrocortisone, Oral (Systemic), 998
Hydrocortisone, Parenteral (Systemic), 998
Hydroxyzine (Systemic), 325
Loratadine (Systemic), 325
Methdilazine (Systemic)†, 377
Methylprednisolone, Oral (Systemic), 998
Methylprednisolone, Parenteral (Systemic), 998
Phenindamine (Systemic)†, 325

**Anaphylactic or anaphylactoid reactions (treatment adjunct)** (continued)
Prednisolone, Oral (Systemic), 998
Prednisolone, Parenteral (Systemic), 998
Prednisone (Systemic), 998
Promethazine (Systemic), 377
Pyrilamine (Systemic)*†, 325
Triamcinolone, Oral (Systemic), 998
Triamcinolone, Parenteral (Systemic), 998
Trimeprazine (Systemic), 377
Tripelennamine (Systemic), 325
Triprolidine (Systemic)*†, 325
**Anaphylactic shock (treatment adjunct)**
Epinephrine (Parenteral-Systemic), 2669
**Androgen deficiency, due to primary or secondary hypogonadism (treatment)**
Fluoxymesterone (Systemic), 118
Methyltestosterone (Systemic), 118
Testosterone (Systemic), 118
**Anemia (diagnosis)**
See also Bone marrow imaging, radionuclide; Red blood cell survival time determinations
Cyanocobalamin Co 57 (Systemic), 1123
Ferrous Citrate Fe 59 (Systemic)*, 1460
**Anemia (treatment)**
[Fluoxymesterone (Systemic)][1], 118
Nandrolone Decanoate (Systemic)[1], 110
[Nandrolone Phenpropionate (Systemic)], 110
Oxymetholone (Systemic)*, 110
[Stanozolol (Systemic)]†, 110
[Testosterone Cypionate (Systemic)][1], 118
[Testosterone Enanthate (Systemic)][1], 118
**Anemia, aplastic (treatment)**
Etiocholanedione (Systemic), 3142‡
**Anemia, associated with chemotherapy in cancer patients (treatment)**
Epoetin Alfa (Systemic), 1352
**Anemia, associated with end-stage renal disease (treatment)**
Epoetin Alfa (Systemic), 3142‡
Epoetin Beta (Systemic), 3142‡
Erythropoietin, Recombinant Human (Systemic), 3142‡
**Anemia, associated with frequent blood donation (prophylaxis)**
[Epoetin Alfa (Systemic)], 1352
**Anemia, associated with malignancy (treatment)**
[Epoetin Alfa (Systemic)], 1352
**Anemia, associated with renal failure (treatment)**
Epoetin Alfa (Systemic), 1352
**Anemia, erythroid**—See Anemia, hypoplastic, congenital
**Anemia, hemolytic, acquired (treatment)**
Betamethasone, Oral (Systemic), 998
Betamethasone, Parenteral (Systemic), 998
Cortisone (Systemic), 998
Dexamethasone, Oral (Systemic), 998
Dexamethasone, Parenteral (Systemic), 998
Hydrocortisone, Oral (Systemic), 998
Hydrocortisone, Parenteral (Systemic), 998
Methylprednisolone, Oral (Systemic), 998
Methylprednisolone, Parenteral (Systemic), 998
Prednisolone, Oral (Systemic), 998
Prednisolone, Parenteral (Systemic), 998
Prednisone (Systemic), 998
Triamcinolone, Oral (Systemic), 998
Triamcinolone, Parenteral (Systemic), 998
**Anemia, hemolytic, autoimmune**—See Anemia, hemolytic, acquired
**Anemia, HIV-associated (treatment)**
Epoetin Alfa (Systemic), 3142‡
**Anemia, HIV treatment–associated (treatment)**
Epoetin Alfa (Systemic), 3142‡
**Anemia, hypoplastic, congenital (treatment)**
Betamethasone, Oral (Systemic), 998
Betamethasone, Parenteral (Systemic), 998
Cortisone (Systemic), 998
Dexamethasone, Oral (Systemic), 998
Dexamethasone, Parenteral (Systemic), 998
Hydrocortisone, Oral (Systemic), 998
Hydrocortisone, Parenteral (Systemic), 998
Methylprednisolone, Oral (Systemic), 998
Methylprednisolone, Parenteral (Systemic), 998
Prednisolone, Oral (Systemic), 998
Prednisolone, Parenteral (Systemic), 998
Prednisone (Systemic), 998
Triamcinolone, Oral (Systemic), 998
Triamcinolone, Parenteral (Systemic), 998
**Anemia, megaloblastic (treatment)**
Leucovorin (Systemic), 1837
**Anemia, pernicious (treatment)**
Cyanocobalamin (Systemic), 2962
Hydroxocobalamin (Systemic)†, 2962
**Anemia of prematurity (treatment)**
Epoetin Alfa (Systemic), 3142‡

**Anemia, red blood cell (treatment)**
Betamethasone, Oral (Systemic), 998
Betamethasone, Parenteral (Systemic), 998
Cortisone (Systemic), 998
Dexamethasone, Oral (Systemic), 998
Dexamethasone, Parenteral (Systemic), 998
Hydrocortisone, Oral (Systemic), 998
Hydrocortisone, Parenteral (Systemic), 998
Methylprednisolone, Oral (Systemic), 998
Methylprednisolone, Parenteral (Systemic), 998
Prednisolone, Oral (Systemic), 998
Prednisolone, Parenteral (Systemic), 998
Prednisone (Systemic), 998
Triamcinolone, Oral (Systemic), 998
Triamcinolone, Parenteral (Systemic), 998
**Anemia, severe, associated with zidovudine therapy in HIV-infected patients (treatment)**
Epoetin Alfa (Systemic), 1352
**Anemia, sickle cell**—See Sickle cell disease
**Anesthesia adjunct**
Anileridine (Systemic)*, 3011
Chlordiazepoxide, Parenteral (Systemic), 556
Diazepam, Parenteral (Systemic), 556
Lorazepam, Parenteral (Systemic), 556
Remifentanil (Systemic), 2464
**Anesthesia, basal**
Methohexital Sodium for Rectal Solution (Systemic)*†, 161
Thiamylal Sodium for Rectal Solution (Systemic)*†, 161
Thiopental Sodium for Rectal Solution (Systemic)*†, 161
Thiopental Sodium Rectal Suspension (Systemic), 161
**Anesthesia, general**
Desflurane (Inhalation-Systemic)†, #
Enflurane (Systemic), 168
Etomidate (Systemic)†, 1422
Halothane (Systemic), 168
Isoflurane (Systemic), 168
Ketamine (Systemic), 1805
Methohexital (Systemic), 161
Methoxyflurane (Systemic), 168
Nitrous Oxide (Systemic), 168
Propofol (Systemic), 2416
Sevoflurane (Inhalation-Systemic), #
Thiamylal (Systemic), 161
Thiopental (Systemic), 161
**Anesthesia, general, adjunct**
Alfentanil (Systemic), 1452
Amobarbital (Systemic), 518
[Buprenorphine (Systemic)], 683
Butabarbital (Systemic), 518
Butorphanol (Systemic)†, 2168
Chloral Hydrate (Systemic), 834
Droperidol (Systemic), 1319
Etomidate (Systemic)†, 1422
Fentanyl (Systemic), 1452
[Hydromorphone, Parenteral (Systemic)], 2168
Hydroxyzine, Parenteral (Systemic), 325
Ketamine (Systemic), 1805
Levorphanol (Systemic), 2168
Meperidine, Parenteral (Systemic), 2168
[Methotrimeprazine, Parenteral (Systemic)], 2289
Midazolam (Systemic), 2007
Morphine, Parenteral (Systemic), 2168
Nalbuphine (Systemic), 2168
Oxymorphone, Parenteral (Systemic), 2168
Pentazocine, Parenteral (Systemic), 2168
Pentobarbital (Systemic), 518
Phenobarbital, Parenteral (Systemic), 518
Promethazine (Systemic), 377
Propiomazine (Systemic)†, #
Propofol (Systemic), 2416
Scopolamine, Parenteral (Systemic)1, 226
Secobarbital (Systemic), 518
Sufentanil (Systemic), 1452
**Anesthesia, local**
Benzocaine (Mucosal-Local), 128
Benzocaine, Butamben, and Tetracaine (Mucosal-Local), 128
Cocaine (Mucosal-Local)[1], 923
Dyclonine (Mucosal-Local), 128
Lidocaine (Mucosal-Local), 128
Lidocaine and Prilocaine (Topical), #
Proparacaine (Ophthalmic), #
Tetracaine (Mucosal-Local), 128
Tetracaine (Ophthalmic), #
**Anesthesia, local, adjunct**
Amobarbital (Systemic), 518
[Buprenorphine (Systemic)], 683
Butabarbital (Systemic), 518
Butorphanol (Systemic)†, 2168
Chloral Hydrate (Systemic), 834
Droperidol (Systemic), 1319
Epinephrine Injection USP (Systemic), 651

**Anesthesia, local, adjunct** (continued)
Fentanyl (Systemic), 1452
[Hydromorphone, Parenteral (Systemic)], 2168
Hydroxyzine, Parenteral (Systemic), 325
[Ketamine (Systemic)][1], 1805
Levorphanol, Parenteral (Systemic), 2168
Meperidine, Parenteral (Systemic), 2168
[Midazolam (Systemic)][1], 2007
Morphine, Parenteral (Systemic), 2168
Nalbuphine (Systemic), 2168
Oxymorphone, Parenteral (Systemic), 2168
Pentazocine, Parenteral (Systemic), 2168
Pentobarbital (Systemic), 518
Phenobarbital, Parenteral (Systemic), 518
Promethazine, Parenteral (Systemic), 377
Propiomazine (Systemic)†, #
Secobarbital (Systemic), 518
[Sufentanil (Systemic)][1], 1452, 3035
**Anesthesia, surgical**
Ropivacaine (Parenteral-Local), #
**Anesthesia, surgical, cesarean section**
Ropivacaine (Parenteral-Local), #
**Aneurysm, ventricular (diagnosis)**—See Cardiac blood pool imaging, radionuclide
**Angina pectoris (diagnosis)**
See also Cardiac imaging, radionuclide
[Ergonovine (Systemic)][1], 1360
**Angina pectoris, acute (prophylaxis)**
Erythrityl Tetranitrate, Sublingual (Systemic), 2129
Isosorbide Dinitrate Chewable Tablets USP (Systemic), 2129
Isosorbide Dinitrate, Sublingual (Systemic), 2129
Nitroglycerin, Buccal (Systemic), 2129
Nitroglycerin, Lingual (Systemic)[1], 2129
Nitroglycerin, Sublingual (Systemic), 2129
**Angina pectoris, acute (treatment)**
Amyl Nitrite (Systemic), #
Isosorbide Dinitrate Chewable Tablets USP (Systemic), 2129
Isosorbide Dinitrate, Sublingual (Systemic)[1], 2129
Nitroglycerin, Buccal (Systemic)[1], 2129
Nitroglycerin, Lingual (Systemic), 2129
Nitroglycerin, Sublingual (Systemic), 2129
**Angina pectoris, chronic (treatment)**
[Acebutolol (Systemic)], 593
Amlodipine (Systemic)†, 86
Atenolol (Systemic), 593
Bepridil (Systemic)†, 720
[Carteolol (Systemic)]†, 593
Diltiazem (Systemic), 720
Erythrityl Tetranitrate (Systemic), 2129
Felodipine (Systemic), 720
Isosorbide Dinitrate (Systemic), 2129
Isosorbide Mononitrate (Systemic)†, 2129
[Isradipine (Systemic)]†, 720
[Labetalol (Systemic)][1], 593
Metoprolol (Systemic), 593
Nadolol (Systemic), 593
Nicardipine (Systemic), 720
Nifedipine (Systemic), 720
Nitroglycerin, Buccal (Systemic), 2129
Nitroglycerin, Oral (Systemic), 2129
Nitroglycerin, Parenteral (Systemic), 2129
Nitroglycerin, Topical (Systemic), 2129
Oxprenolol (Systemic)*[1], 593
[Penbutolol (Systemic)]†, 593
[Pindolol (Systemic)], 593
Propranolol (Systemic), 593
[Sotalol (Systemic)], 593
[Timolol (Systemic)], 593
Verapamil (Systemic), 720
**Angina pectoris, chronic stable (treatment)**
Diltiazem (Systemic), 3017
Mibefradil (Systemic), 4#
Verapamil (Systemic), 3037
**Angina, unstable (treatment)**
Tirofiban (Systemic), 3036
**Angina, vasospastic (treatment)**
Amlodipine (Systemic)†, 86
**Angiocardiography**
Diatrizoate Meglumine and Diatrizoate Sodium, Parenteral (Systemic), #
Diatrizoate Meglumine, Parenteral (Systemic), #
Iodixanol (Systemic), #
Iohexol (Systemic), #
Iopamidol (Systemic), #
Iothalamate Meglumine and Iothalamate Sodium (Systemic)†, #
Iothalamate Sodium (Systemic), #
Ioversol (Systemic), #
Ioxaglate (Systemic), #
Metrizamide (Systemic)†, #
**Angiocardiography, radionuclide**—See Cardiac blood pool imaging, radionuclide

## Angioedema (treatment)
Acrivastine (Systemic)*†, 325
Astemizole (Systemic), 325
Azatadine (Systemic), 325
Bromodiphenhydramine (Systemic)*†, 325
Brompheniramine (Systemic), 325
Carbinoxamine (Systemic)*†, 325
Cetirizine (Systemic), 325
Chlorpheniramine (Systemic), 325
Clemastine (Systemic), 325
Cyproheptadine (Systemic), 325
Dexchlorpheniramine (Systemic), 325
Dimenhydrinate (Systemic), 325
Diphenhydramine (Systemic), 325
Diphenylpyraline (Systemic)*†, 325
Doxylamine (Systemic)†, 325
Epinephrine Injection USP (Systemic), 651
Hydroxyzine (Systemic), 325
Loratadine (Systemic), 325
Methdilazine (Systemic)†, 377
Phenindamine (Systemic)†, 325
Promethazine (Systemic), 377
Pyrilamine (Systemic)*†, 325
Trimeprazine (Systemic), 377
Tripelennamine (Systemic), 325
Triprolidine (Systemic)*†, 325

## Angioedema (treatment adjunct)
Betamethasone, Oral (Systemic), 998
Betamethasone, Parenteral (Systemic), 998
Cortisone (Systemic), 998
Dexamethasone, Oral (Systemic), 998
Dexamethasone, Parenteral (Systemic), 998
Hydrocortisone, Oral (Systemic), 998
Hydrocortisone, Parenteral (Systemic), 998
Methylprednisolone, Oral (Systemic), 998
Methylprednisolone, Parenteral (Systemic), 998
Prednisolone, Oral (Systemic), 998
Prednisolone, Parenteral (Systemic), 998
Prednisone (Systemic), 998
Triamcinolone, Oral (Systemic), 998
Triamcinolone, Parenteral (Systemic), 998

## Angioedema, C1-esterase inhibitor deficiency–induced (prophylaxis)
C1-Esterase Inhibitor (Human) (Systemic), 3135‡

## Angioedema, C1-esterase inhibitor deficiency–induced (treatment)
C1-Esterase Inhibitor (Human) (Systemic), 3135‡

## Angioedema, hereditary (prophylaxis)
C1-Esterase-Inhibitor, Human, Pasteurized (Systemic), 3135‡
C1-Inhibitor (Systemic), 3135‡
Danazol (Systemic)[1], 1163
Oxymetholone (Systemic)*[1], 110
Stanozolol (Systemic)†, 110

## Angioedema, hereditary (treatment)
C1-Esterase-Inhibitor, Human, Pasteurized (Systemic), 3135‡
C1-Inhibitor (Systemic), 3135‡
Oxymetholone (Systemic)*[1], 110
[Stanozolol (Systemic)]†, 110
[Tranexamic Acid (Systemic)], 2862

## Angiography
Diatrizoate Meglumine and Diatrizoate Sodium, Parenteral (Systemic), #
Diatrizoate Meglumine, Parenteral (Systemic), #
Diatrizoate Sodium, Parenteral (Systemic), #
Iodixanol (Systemic), #
Iohexol (Systemic), #
Iopamidol (Systemic), #
Iopromide (Systemic), #
Iothalamate Meglumine (Systemic), #
Iothalamate Meglumine and Iothalamate Sodium (Systemic)†, #
Ioversol (Systemic), #
Ioxaglate (Systemic), #
Ioxilan (Systemic), #

## Angiography adjunct
Dinoprost (Parenteral-Local)*[1], #

## Angiography, cerebral, radionuclide
Sodium Pertechnetate Tc 99m (Systemic), 2612

## Angiography, radionuclide—See Blood pool imaging, radionuclide

## Ankylosing spondylitis (treatment)
Betamethasone, Oral (Systemic), 998
Betamethasone, Parenteral (Systemic), 998
Cortisone (Systemic), 998
Dexamethasone, Oral (Systemic), 998
Dexamethasone, Parenteral (Systemic), 998
Diclofenac (Systemic)[1], 388
[Diflunisal (Systemic)][1], 388
[Fenoprofen (Systemic)][1], 388
[Flurbiprofen (Systemic)][1], 388
Hydrocortisone, Oral (Systemic), 998
Hydrocortisone, Parenteral (Systemic), 998
[Ibuprofen (Systemic)][1], 388
Indomethacin (Systemic), 388

## Ankylosing spondylitis (treatment) (continued)
[Ketoprofen (Systemic)], 388
Methylprednisolone, Oral (Systemic), 998
Methylprednisolone, Parenteral (Systemic), 998
Naproxen (Systemic), 388, 3029
Phenylbutazone (Systemic), 388
[Piroxicam (Systemic)], 388
Prednisolone, Oral (Systemic), 998
Prednisolone, Parenteral (Systemic), 998
Prednisone (Systemic), 998
[Sulfasalazine (Systemic)][1], 2643
Sulindac (Systemic), 388
Tenoxicam (Systemic)*, 388
[Tolmetin (Systemic)], 388
Triamcinolone, Oral (Systemic), 998
Triamcinolone, Parenteral (Systemic), 998

## Anorexia (treatment)
Megestrol (Systemic), 2400

## Anorexia, AIDS-associated (treatment)
See also Weight loss, AIDS-associated (prophylaxis)
See also Weight loss, AIDS-associated (treatment)
Dronabinol (Systemic), 1316
Megestrol (Systemic), 3153‡

## Anovulation, chronic (treatment)
Human Luteinizing Hormone, Recombinant, 3161‡

## Anterior segment disease, inflammatory (treatment)
Betamethasone (Ophthalmic)*, 966
Dexamethasone (Ophthalmic), 966
Fluorometholone (Ophthalmic), 966
Hydrocortisone (Ophthalmic)*, 966
Prednisolone (Ophthalmic), 966

## Anterior segment, surgical procedures of
Hydroxypropyl Methylcellulose (Ophthalmic), 3023
Polyacrylamide (Ophthalmic), 3032

## Anthrax (treatment)
Demeclocycline (Systemic), 2765
Doxycycline (Systemic), 2765
[Erythromycin (Systemic)], 1368
Minocycline (Systemic), 2765
Oxytetracycline (Systemic)†, 2765
Penicillin G, Parenteral (Systemic), 2240
Penicillin G Procaine (Systemic), 2240
[Penicillin V (Systemic)][1], 2240
Tetracycline (Systemic), 2765

## Antibiotic therapy, adjunct
Probenecid (Systemic), 2380

## Antithrombin III deficiency (treatment)
Antithrombin III (Human) (Systemic), 3131‡
[Stanozolol (Systemic)]†, 110

## ANUG—See Gingivitis, necrotizing ulcerative, acute

## Anxiety (treatment)
Alprazolam (Systemic), 556
Bromazepam (Systemic)*, 556
Buspirone (Systemic), 693
Chlordiazepoxide (Systemic), 556
Clorazepate (Systemic), 556
Diazepam (Systemic), 556
Halazepam (Systemic)†, 556
Hydroxyzine (Systemic), 325
[Ketazolam (Systemic)][1]*, 556
Lorazepam (Systemic), 556
Meprobamate (Systemic), #
Oxazepam (Systemic), 556
[Prazepam (Systemic)][1]†, 556

## Anxiety (treatment adjunct)
[Acebutolol (Systemic)][1], 593
[Metoprolol (Systemic)][1], 593
Oxprenolol (Systemic)*[1], 593
[Propranolol (Systemic)][1], 593
[Sotalol (Systemic)][1], 593
[Timolol (Systemic)][1], 593

## Anxiety, associated with mental depression (treatment)
Chlordiazepoxide and Amitriptyline (Systemic)†, 845
[Loxapine (Systemic)][1], 1889
Maprotiline (Systemic), 1909
Perphenazine and Amitriptyline (Systemic), 2286

## Anxiety, associated with mental depression (treatment adjunct)
Alprazolam (Systemic)[1], 556
Lorazepam, Oral (Systemic)[1], 556
Oxazepam (Systemic)[1], 556

## Anxiety, in cardioversion (treatment)
Diazepam, Parenteral (Systemic), 556

## Anxiety, in endoscopic procedures (treatment adjunct)
Diazepam, Parenteral (Systemic), 556
[Lorazepam, Parenteral (Systemic)][1], 556

## Aortography
Diatrizoate Meglumine and Diatrizoate Sodium, Parenteral (Systemic), #
Diatrizoate Meglumine, Parenteral (Systemic), #
Diatrizoate Sodium, Parenteral (Systemic), #

## Aortography (continued)
Iodixanol (Systemic), #
Iohexol (Systemic), #
Iopamidol (Systemic)[1], #
Iopromide (Systemic), #
Iothalamate Meglumine and Iothalamate Sodium (Systemic)†, #
Iothalamate Sodium (Systemic), #
Ioversol (Systemic), #
Ioxaglate (Systemic), #
Ioxilan (Systemic), #

## Aphthous ulceration—See Stomatitis, aphthous

## Apnea, infant, postoperative (prophylaxis)
[Caffeine (Systemic)], 706
[Caffeine, Citrated (Systemic)], 706

## Apnea, neonatal (treatment adjunct)
[Aminophylline Injection USP (Systemic)][1], 668
[Aminophylline Oral Solution USP (Systemic)][1], 668
[Caffeine (Systemic)], 706, 3135‡
[Caffeine, Citrated (Systemic)], 706
[Theophylline Elixir (Systemic)][1], 668
[Theophylline Oral Solution (Systemic)][1], 668
[Theophylline Syrup (Systemic)][1], 668

## Apnea, post-surgical (treatment)
Butyrylcholinesterase (Systemic), 3135‡

## Appetite, lack of (treatment)
[Cyproheptadine (Systemic)], 325

## ARDS—See Respiratory distress syndrome, adult

## Arrhythmias, in anesthesia (treatment)
Atropine, Parenteral (Systemic), 226
Glycopyrrolate, Parenteral (Systemic), 226
Lidocaine (Systemic), 1860

## Arrhythmias, atrial (treatment)
Ibutilide (Systemic), 1670

## Arrhythmias, cardiac (prophylaxis)
See also specific arrhythmias, e.g., Atrial contractions, premature; Atrioventricular (AV) junctional rhythm, paroxysmal; Fibrillation; Flutter, atrial; Tachyarrhythmias; Tachycardia; Ventricular contractions, premature
[Acebutolol (Systemic)][1], 593
[Atenolol (Systemic)][1], 593
Bretylium (Systemic), 630
Digitoxin (Systemic), 1213
Digoxin (Systemic), 1213
Diltiazem, Parenteral (Systemic), 720
[Metoprolol (Systemic)][1], 593
[Nadolol (Systemic)][1], 593
Oxprenolol (Systemic)*[1], 593
Propranolol (Systemic), 593
Sotalol (Systemic)[1], 593
[Timolol (Systemic)][1], 593
Verapamil (Systemic), 720

## Arrhythmias, cardiac (treatment)
See also specific arrhythmias, e.g., Atrial contractions, premature; Atrioventricular (AV) junctional rhythm, paroxysmal; Bradycardia, sinus; Extrasystoles, ventricular; Fibrillation; Flutter, atrial; Tachyarrhythmias; Tachycardia; Ventricular contractions, premature
[Acebutolol (Systemic)][1], 593
Adenosine (Systemic)†, 32
[Atenolol (Systemic)][1], 593
Atropine, Parenteral (Systemic), 226
Bretylium (Systemic), 630
Digitoxin (Systemic), 1213
Digoxin (Systemic), 1213
Diltiazem, Parenteral (Systemic), 720
Disopyramide (Systemic), 1252
Encainide (Systemic)*†, 1344
Esmolol (Systemic)†, 1377
Flecainide (Systemic), 1469
Lidocaine (Systemic), 1860
[Metoprolol (Systemic)][1], 593
Mexiletine (Systemic), 2005
Moricizine (Systemic)†, 2060
[Nadolol (Systemic)][1], 593
Oxprenolol (Systemic)*[1], 593
Procainamide (Systemic), 2387
Propafenone (Systemic), 2413
Propranolol (Systemic), 593
Quinidine (Systemic), 2440
Sotalol (Systemic)[1], 593
[Timolol (Systemic)][1], 593
Tocainide (Systemic), 2831
Verapamil (Systemic), 720

## Arrhythmias, cardiac, in anesthesia (treatment)
Procainamide, Parenteral (Systemic), 2387

## Arrhythmias, cardiac, in surgery (treatment)
Procainamide, Parenteral (Systemic), 2387

## Arrhythmias, digitalis-induced (treatment)
See also Tachyarrhythmias, digitalis-induced
Lidocaine (Systemic), 1860
[Phenytoin (Systemic)][1], 253

**Arrhythmias, succinylcholine-induced (prophylaxis)**
Atropine, Parenteral (Systemic), 226
**Arrhythmias, supraventricular (prophylaxis)**
See also Atrial contractions, premature; Fibrillation, atrial; Flutter, atrial; Tachycardia, atrial, paroxysmal; Tachycardia, supraventricular
[Acebutolol (Systemic)][1], 593
[Amiodarone (Systemic)][1], 79
[Atenolol (Systemic)][1], 593
Flecainide (Systemic), 1469
[Metoprolol (Systemic)][1], 593
[Nadolol (Systemic)][1], 593
Oxprenolol (Systemic)*[1], 593
Propranolol (Systemic), 593
Quinidine (Systemic), 2440
Sotalol (Systemic)[1], 593
[Timolol (Systemic)][1], 593
**Arrhythmias, supraventricular (treatment)**
See also Atrial contractions, premature; Fibrillation, atrial; Fibrillation, atrial, paroxysmal; Flutter, atrial; Tachycardia, atrial, paroxysmal; Tachycardia, supraventricular
[Acebutolol (Systemic)][1], 593
Adenosine (Systemic)†, 32
[Amiodarone (Systemic)][1], 79
[Atenolol (Systemic)][1], 593
Esmolol (Systemic)†, 1377
[Metoprolol (Systemic)][1], 593
[Nadolol (Systemic)][1], 593
Oxprenolol (Systemic)*[1], 593
[Procainamide (Systemic)], 2387
[Propafenone (Systemic)][1], 2413
Propranolol (Systemic), 593
Quinidine (Systemic), 2440
Sotalol (Systemic)[1], 593
[Timolol (Systemic)][1], 593
**Arrhythmias, in surgery (treatment)**
Atropine, Parenteral (Systemic), 226
Glycopyrrolate, Parenteral (Systemic), 226
Lidocaine (Systemic), 1860
**Arrhythmias, surgical procedure–induced (prophylaxis)**
Atropine, Parenteral (Systemic), 226
**Arrhythmias, ventricular (prophylaxis)**
See also Fibrillation, ventricular; Tachycardia, ventricular; Ventricular contractions, premature
Amiodarone (Systemic), 79
Bretylium (Systemic), 630
Flecainide (Systemic), 1469
Quinidine (Systemic), 2440
**Arrhythmias, ventricular (treatment)**
See also Extrasystoles, ventricular; Fibrillation, ventricular; Tachycardia, ventricular; Ventricular contractions, premature
Amiodarone (Systemic), 79
Bretylium (Systemic), 630
Disopyramide (Systemic), 1252
Encainide (Systemic)*†, 1344
Flecainide (Systemic), 1469
Lidocaine (Systemic), 1860
Mexiletine (Systemic), 2005
Moricizine (Systemic)†, 2060
N-Acetyl-Procainamide (Systemic), 3155‡
Procainamide (Systemic), 2387
Propafenone (Systemic), 2413
Quinidine (Systemic), 2440
Tocainide (Systemic), 2831
**Arterial blood flow, hepatic, regional, assessment**
Ammonia N 13 (Systemic)*†, 91
**Arteriography**
Diatrizoate Meglumine and Diatrizoate Sodium, Parenteral (Systemic), #
Diatrizoate Meglumine, Parenteral (Systemic), #
Diatrizoate Sodium, Parenteral (Systemic), #
Iodixanol (Systemic), #
Iohexol (Systemic), #
Iopamidol (Systemic), #
Iopromide (Systemic), #
Iothalamate Meglumine (Systemic), #
Iothalamate Meglumine and Iothalamate Sodium (Systemic)†, #
Ioversol (Systemic), #
Ioxaglate (Systemic), #
Ioxilan (Systemic), #
Metrizamide (Systemic)†, #
**Arteritis, giant-cell (treatment)**
[Betamethasone, Oral (Systemic)]1, 998
[Betamethasone, Parenteral (Systemic)][1], 998
[Cortisone (Systemic)][1], 998
[Dexamethasone, Oral (Systemic)][1], 998
[Dexamethasone, Parenteral (Systemic)][1], 998
[Hydrocortisone, Oral (Systemic)][1], 998
[Hydrocortisone, Parenteral (Systemic)][1], 998
[Methylprednisolone, Oral (Systemic)][1], 998
[Methylprednisolone, Parenteral (Systemic)][1], 998

**Arteritis, giant-cell (treatment)** (continued)
[Prednisolone, Oral (Systemic)][1], 998
[Prednisolone, Parenteral (Systemic)][1], 998
[Prednisone (Systemic)][1], 998
[Triamcinolone, Oral (Systemic)][1], 998
[Triamcinolone, Parenteral (Systemic)][1], 998
**Arteritis, temporal**—See Arteritis, giant-cell
**Arthritis, gonococcal (treatment)**
[Demeclocycline (Systemic)], 2765
[Doxycycline (Systemic)], 2765
[Minocycline (Systemic)], 2765
[Oxytetracycline (Systemic)]†, 2765
Penicillin G, Parenteral (Systemic), 2240
[Tetracycline (Systemic)], 2765
**Arthritis, gouty, acute**—See Gouty arthritis, acute
**Arthritis, gouty, chronic**—See Gouty arthritis, chronic
**Arthritis, juvenile**—See also Arthritis, rheumatoid
**Arthritis, juvenile (treatment)**
Aspirin (Systemic), 2538
Aspirin, Buffered (Systemic), 2538
[Auranofin (Systemic)][1], 1566
Aurothioglucose (Systemic), 1566
[Chloroquine, Oral (Systemic)][1], 849
Choline Salicylate (Systemic)†, 2538
Choline and Magnesium Salicylates (Systemic), 2538
Gammalinolenic Acid (Systemic), 3144‡
Gold Sodium Thiomalate (Systemic), 1566
[Hydroxychloroquine (Systemic)][1], 1663
Ibuprofen (Systemic), 388
Immune Globulin Intravenous (Human) (Systemic), 3147‡
Indomethacin (Systemic)[1], 388
Interleukin-1 Receptor Antagonist, Human Recombinant (Systemic), 3149‡
Magnesium Salicylate (Systemic), 2538
Methotrexate—for Noncancerous Conditions (Systemic), 3152‡
Naproxen (Systemic), 388
Purified Type II Collagen (Systemic), 3160‡
Salsalate (Systemic), 2538
Sodium Salicylate (Systemic), 2538
Tolmetin (Systemic), 388
**Arthritis, psoriatic (treatment)**
[Auranofin (Systemic)][1], 1566
[Aurothioglucose (Systemic)][1], 1566
Betamethasone, Oral (Systemic), 998
Betamethasone, Parenteral (Systemic), 998
Betamethasone, Parenteral-Local (Systemic), 998
Cortisone (Systemic), 998
Dexamethasone (Systemic), 998
[Diflunisal (Systemic)][1], 388
Fenoprofen (Systemic), 388
[Gold Sodium Thiomalate (Systemic)][1], 1566
Hydrocortisone, Oral (Systemic), 998
Hydrocortisone, Parenteral (Systemic), 998
Hydrocortisone, Parenteral-Local (Systemic), 998
[Ibuprofen (Systemic)][1], 388
[Indomethacin (Systemic)][1], 388
[Ketoprofen (Systemic)][1], 388
[Meclofenamate (Systemic)]†, 388
[Mercaptopurine (Systemic)][1], 1946
[Methotrexate—For Noncancerous Conditions (Systemic)][1], 1969
Methylprednisolone, Oral (Systemic), 998
Methylprednisolone, Parenteral (Systemic), 998
Methylprednisolone, Parenteral-Local (Systemic), 998
[Phenylbutazone (Systemic)][1], 388
Prednisolone (Systemic), 998
Prednisone (Systemic), 998
[Tolmetin (Systemic)][1], 388
Triamcinolone (Systemic), 998
**Arthritis, rheumatoid (treatment)**
See also Osteoarthritis
Aspirin (Systemic), 2538
Aspirin, Buffered (Systemic), 2538
Auranofin (Systemic), 1566
Aurothioglucose (Systemic), 1566
Azathioprine (Systemic), 491
Betamethasone, Oral (Systemic), 998
Betamethasone, Parenteral (Systemic), 998
Betamethasone, Parenteral-Local (Systemic), 998
Capsaicin (Topical), 753
[Chloroquine, Oral (Systemic)]1, 849
Choline Salicylate (Systemic)†, 2538
Choline and Magnesium Salicylates (Systemic), 2538
Cortisone (Systemic), 998
[Cyclophosphamide (Systemic)][1], 1128
Cyclosporine (Systemic), 1136
Dexamethasone (Systemic), 998
Diclofenac (Systemic), 388
Diclofenac and Misoprostol (Systemic), 1202
Diflunisal (Systemic), 388

**Arthritis, rheumatoid (treatment)** (continued)
Etodolac (Systemic), 3019
Fenoprofen (Systemic), 388
Flurbiprofen (Systemic), 388
Gold Sodium Thiomalate (Systemic), 1566
Hydrocortisone, Oral (Systemic), 998
Hydrocortisone, Parenteral (Systemic), 998
Hydrocortisone, Parenteral-Local (Systemic), 998
Hydroxychloroquine (Systemic), 1663
Ibuprofen (Systemic), 388
Indomethacin (Systemic), 388
Ketoprofen (Systemic), 388
Magnesium Salicylate (Systemic), 2538
Meclofenamate (Systemic)†, 388
Methotrexate, Oral—For Noncancerous Conditions (Systemic), 1969
[Methotrexate, Parenteral—For Noncancerous Conditions (Systemic)][1], 1969
Methylprednisolone, Oral (Systemic), 998
Methylprednisolone, Parenteral (Systemic), 998
Methylprednisolone, Parenteral-Local (Systemic), 998
Nabumetone (Systemic), 388
Naproxen (Systemic), 388, 3029
Oxaprozin (Systemic)*, 388
Penicillamine (Systemic), 2237
Phenylbutazone (Systemic)[1], 388
Piroxicam (Systemic), 388
Prednisolone (Systemic), 998
Prednisone (Systemic), 998
Salsalate (Systemic), 2538
Sodium Salicylate (Systemic), 2538
[Sulfasalazine (Systemic)], 2643
Sulindac (Systemic), 388
Tenoxicam (Systemic)*, 388
Tiaprofenic Acid (Systemic)*, 388
Tolmetin (Systemic), 388
Triamcinolone (Systemic), 998
**Arthritis, rheumatoid (treatment adjunct)**
[Cimetidine (Systemic)][1], 1633
[Ranitidine (Systemic)][1], 1633
[Sucralfate (Oral-Local)][1], 2635
**Arthritis, sarcoid (treatment)**
See also Sarcoidosis
[Colchicine (Systemic)][1], 928
**Arthrography**
Diatrizoate Meglumine, Parenteral (Systemic), #
Iohexol (Systemic), #
[Iopamidol (Systemic)][1], #
Iothalamate Meglumine (Systemic), #
[Ioversol (Systemic)][1], #
Ioxaglate (Systemic), #
**Ascariasis (treatment)**
Albendazole (Systemic)*†, #
Mebendazole (Systemic), 1926
Piperazine (Systemic), #
Pyrantel (Oral-Local), #
**Ascites (treatment adjunct)**
Albumin Human (Systemic)[1], 34
**Aspergillosis (treatment)**
Amphotericin B (Systemic), 98
Amphotericin B Cholesteryl Complex (Systemic), 101
Amphotericin B Liposomal Complex (Systemic), 105
Itraconazole (Systemic), 302
**Assisted reproductive technologies, female (treatment)**
Progesterone Gel (Systemic), 2400
[Progesterone Suppositories (Systemic)][1], 2400
**Asthma (diagnosis)**
Methacholine (Inhalation-Local)†, 4#
**Asthma (prophylaxis)**
Cromolyn (Inhalation-Local), 1116
Oxtriphylline and Guaifenesin (Systemic), #
Theophylline and Guaifenesin (Systemic)†, #
**Asthma (treatment)**
Oxtriphylline and Guaifenesin (Systemic), #
Theophylline and Guaifenesin (Systemic)†, #
**Asthma (treatment adjunct)**
[Ipratropium (Inhalation-Local)], 1761
**Asthma, atropic, in children (prophylaxis)**
Ketotifen (Systemic)*, 3026
**Asthma, bronchial (prophylaxis)**
Aminophylline (Systemic), 668
Nedocromil (Inhalation-Local), 2090
Oxtriphylline (Systemic), 668
Theophylline (Systemic), 668
**Asthma, bronchial (treatment)**
Albuterol (Systemic), 651
Aminophylline (Systemic), 668
Betamethasone, Oral (Systemic), 998
Betamethasone, Parenteral (Systemic), 998
Cortisone (Systemic), 998
Dexamethasone, Oral (Systemic), 998
Dexamethasone, Parenteral (Systemic), 998

**Asthma, bronchial (treatment)** *(continued)*
  Ephedrine (Systemic), 651
  Epinephrine (Systemic), 651
  Ethylnorepinephrine (Systemic)†, 651
  Fenoterol (Systemic)*, 651
  Hydrocortisone, Oral (Systemic), 998
  Hydrocortisone, Parenteral (Systemic), 998
  Isoproterenol (Systemic), 651
  Metaproterenol (Systemic), 651
  Methylprednisolone, Oral (Systemic), 998
  Methylprednisolone, Parenteral (Systemic), 998
  Oxtriphylline (Systemic), 668
  Prednisolone, Oral (Systemic), 998
  Prednisolone, Parenteral (Systemic), 998
  Prednisone (Systemic), 998
  Terbutaline (Systemic), 651
  Theophylline (Systemic), 668
  Triamcinolone, Oral (Systemic), 998
  Triamcinolone, Parenteral (Systemic), 998
**Asthma, bronchial (treatment adjunct)**
  [Astemizole (Systemic)][1], 325
  [Cetirizine (Systemic)][1], 325
  [Loratadine (Systemic)][1], 325
**Asthma, bronchial, chronic (prophylaxis)**
  Montelukast (Systemic), 2057
**Asthma, bronchial, chronic (treatment)**
  Beclomethasone (Inhalation-Local), 955
  Budesonide (Inhalation-Local)*, 955
  Flunisolide (Inhalation-Local), 955
  Montelukast (Systemic), 2057
  Triamcinolone (Inhalation-Local), 955
**Asthma, chronic (prophylaxis)**
  Zafirlukast (Systemic), 2987
  Zileuton (Systemic)†, 2996
**Asthma, chronic (treatment)**
  Fluticasone (Inhalation-Local), 1508
  Zafirlukast (Systemic), 2987
  Zileuton (Systemic)†, 2996
**Asthma, severe (treatment)**
  Troleandomycin (Systemic), 3170‡
**Astrocytoma**—*See* Tumors, brain, primary
**Ataxias, Friedreich's**—*See* Ataxias, hereditary
**Ataxias, hereditary (treatment)**
  [Physostigmine (Systemic)][1], 2322, 3158‡
**Atelectasis due to mucous obstruction (treatment adjunct)**
  Acetylcysteine (Inhalation-Local), #
**Atherosclerotic disease (prophylaxis)**
  [Diethylstilbestrol (Systemic)][1], 1383
  [Estradiol (Systemic)][1], 1383
  [Estradiol Cypionate (Systemic)][1], 1383
  [Estradiol Valerate (Systemic)][1], 1383
  [Estrogens, Conjugated (Systemic)][1], 1383
  [Estrogens, Esterified (Systemic)][1], 1383
  [Estrone (Systemic)][1]†, 1383
  [Estropipate (Systemic)][1], 1383
  [Ethinyl Estradiol (Systemic)][1], 1383
**Athetosis, congenital (treatment)**
  [Ethopropazine (Systemic)][1], 297
**Athlete's foot**—*See* Skin and nail infections, fungal, minor; Tinea pedis
**Atony, postoperative, gastric (treatment)**
  [Bethanechol (Systemic)][1], 614
**Atresia, biliary (treatment)**
  [Ursodiol (Systemic)][1], 2903
**Atrial contractions, premature (prophylaxis)**
  Quinidine (Systemic), 2440
**Atrial contractions, premature (treatment)**
  Quinidine (Systemic), 2440
**Atrioventricular (AV) junctional rhythm, paroxysmal (prophylaxis)**
  Quinidine (Systemic), 2440
**Atrioventricular (AV) junctional rhythm, paroxysmal (treatment)**
  Quinidine (Systemic), 2440
**Atrophic dystrophy of the vulva, menopausal**—
  *See* Vulvar squamous hyperplasia
**Attention-deficit hyperactivity disorder (treatment)**
  Amphetamine (Systemic)†, 94
  Amphetamine and Dextroamphetamine (Systemic)†, 94
  [Desipramine (Systemic)][1], 271
  Dextroamphetamine (Systemic), 94
  [Imipramine (Systemic)][1], 271
  Methamphetamine (Systemic)†, 94
  Methylphenidate (Systemic), 1987
  Pemoline (Systemic), 2233
  [Protriptyline (Systemic)][1], 271
**Autism, infantile (treatment)**
  [Haloperidol (Systemic)][1], 1611
**Autologous skin grafts (treatment)**
  Dehydroepiandrosterone Sulfate Sodium (Topical), 3139‡

## B

**Babesiosis (treatment)**
  [Clindamycin (Systemic)][1], 893
  [Quinine (Systemic)][1], 2444
**Bacteremia**—*See* Septicemia, bacterial
**Balantidiasis (treatment)**
  [Iodoquinol (Oral-Local)][1], #
  [Metronidazole (Systemic)][1], 1996
**Baldness, male pattern**—*See* Alopecia androgenetica
**Bartter's syndrome (treatment)**
  [Indomethacin (Systemic)][1], 388
**Bay sore**—*See* Leishmaniasis, cutaneous
**Behcet's syndrome (treatment)**
  [Thalidomide (Systemic)][1]†, 2776
**Becker's muscular dystrophy (treatment)**
  Oxandrolone (Systemic), 3156‡
**Beef tapeworm**—*See* Taeniasis
**Behavior-metabolism relationship studies**
  [Fludeoxyglucose F 18 (Systemic)][1]*†, 1478
**Behavior problems, severe (treatment)**
  Haloperidol (Systemic), 1611
**Behet's syndrome (treatment)**
  [Colchicine (Systemic)][1], 928
**Bejel (treatment)**
  [Demeclocycline (Systemic)], 2765
  [Doxycycline (Systemic)], 2765
  [Minocycline (Systemic)], 2765
  [Oxytetracycline (Systemic)]†, 2765
  Penicillin G Benzathine (Systemic), 2240
  Penicillin G Procaine (Systemic), 2240
  [Tetracycline (Systemic)], 2765
**Benign prostatic hyperplasia (treatment)**
  Doxazosin (Systemic)[1], 1303
  Finasteride (Systemic), 1465
  [Phenoxybenzamine (Systemic)], 2312
  [Prazosin (Systemic)][1], 2370
  Tamsulosin (Systemic), 2690
  Terazosin (Systemic), 2750
**Benign prostatic hypertrophy**—*See* Benign prostatic hyperplasia
**Beriberi**—*See* Thiamine deficiency
**Berylliosis (treatment)**
  Betamethasone, Oral (Systemic), 998
  Betamethasone, Parenteral (Systemic), 998
  Cortisone (Systemic), 998
  Dexamethasone, Oral (Systemic), 998
  Dexamethasone, Parenteral (Systemic), 998
  Hydrocortisone, Oral (Systemic), 998
  Hydrocortisone, Parenteral (Systemic), 998
  Methylprednisolone, Oral (Systemic), 998
  Methylprednisolone, Parenteral (Systemic), 998
  Prednisolone, Oral (Systemic), 998
  Prednisolone, Parenteral (Systemic), 998
  Prednisone (Systemic), 998
  Triamcinolone, Oral (Systemic), 998
  Triamcinolone, Parenteral (Systemic), 998
**Beta-hemoglobinopathies (treatment)**
  Arginine Butyrate (Systemic), 3132‡
  Isobutyramide (Systemic), 3150‡
**Beta-thalassemia (treatment)**
  Arginine Butyrate (Systemic), 3132‡
  Isobutyramide (Systemic), 3150‡
**Bier block**—*See* Intravenous regional anesthesia
**Bilharziasis**—*See* Schistosomiasis
**Biliary tract disorders (diagnosis)**—*See* Cholangiography, direct; Cholangiography, oral; Cholangiography, percutaneous transhepatic; Hepatobiliary imaging, radionuclide
**Biliary tract disorders (treatment)**
  Dehydrocholic Acid (Local)†, #
**Biliary tract infections (treatment)**
  Amikacin (Systemic), 69
  Cefazolin (Systemic)[1], 69, 794
  [Demeclocycline (Systemic)], 2765
  [Doxycycline (Systemic)], 2765
  Gentamicin (Systemic), 69
  Kanamycin (Systemic)†, 69
  [Minocycline (Systemic)], 2765
  Netilmicin (Systemic), 69
  [Oxytetracycline (Systemic)]†, 2765
  Streptomycin (Systemic), 69
  [Sulfamethoxazole and Trimethoprim (Systemic)], 2661
  [Tetracycline (Systemic)], 2765
  Tobramycin (Systemic), 69
**Biotin deficiency (prophylaxis)**
  Biotin (Systemic), #
**Biotin deficiency (treatment)**
  Biotin (Systemic), #
**Bipolar disorder (prophylaxis)**
  [Carbamazepine (Systemic)][1], 757
  [Divalproex (Systemic)], 2908
  [Valproic Acid (Systemic)], 2908

**Bipolar disorder (treatment)**
  [Carbamazepine (Systemic)][1], 757
  [Divalproex (Systemic)], 2908
  Lithium (Systemic), 1869
  [Valproic Acid (Systemic)], 2908
**Bipolar disorder, depressed type (treatment)**
  *See also* Depression, mental
  Maprotiline (Systemic), 1909
  [Tranylcypromine (Systemic)], 266
**Bipolar disorder, manic episodes (treatment)**
  Divalproex (Systemic), 2908
**Bites, insect (treatment)**
  Benzocaine (Topical), 155
  Benzocaine and Menthol (Topical), 155
  Butamben (Topical), 155
  Dibucaine (Topical), 155
  Epinephrine Injection USP (Systemic), 651
  Lidocaine (Topical), 155
  Pramoxine (Topical), 155
  Pramoxine and Menthol (Topical), 155
  Tetracaine (Topical), 155
  Tetracaine and Menthol (Topical), 155
**Black sickness**—*See* Leishmaniasis, visceral
**Bladder calculi, apatite (treatment)**
  Citric Acid, Glucono-delta-lactone, and Magnesium Carbonate (Local), 3137‡
**Bladder calculi, struvite (treatment)**
  Citric Acid, Glucono-delta-lactone, and Magnesium Carbonate (Local), 3137‡
**Bladder hyperactivity (treatment)**
  Tolterodine (Systemic), 2837
**Bladder urine, residual, determinations**
  Phenolsulfonphthalein (Systemic), #
**Blastomycosis (treatment)**
  Amphotericin B (Systemic), 98
  Itraconazole (Systemic), 302
  Ketoconazole (Systemic)[1], 302
**Bleeding, gastrointestinal (diagnosis)**
  Fecal Occult Blood Test Kits, #
  Sodium Chromate Cr 51 (Systemic), 2590
  [Sodium Pertechnetate Tc 99m (Systemic)][1], 2612
  Technetium Tc 99m Pyrophosphate (Systemic)†, 2729
  Technetium Tc 99m (Pyro- and trimeta-) Phosphates (Systemic), 2733
  [Technetium Tc 99m Sulfur Colloid (Systemic)][1], 2740
**Bleeding, gastrointestinal (diagnosis adjunct)**
  [Glucagon (Systemic)][1], 1563
**Bleeding, upper gastrointestinal (treatment)**
  Cimetidine (Systemic), 1633
  [Famotidine (Systemic)][1], 1633
  [Ranitidine (Systemic)], 1633
**Bleeding, uterine, dysfunctional (treatment)**
  [Desogestrel and Ethinyl Estradiol (Systemic)][1], 1397
  [Ethynodiol Diacetate and Ethinyl Estradiol (Systemic)][1], 1397
  Hydroxyprogesterone (Systemic)†, 2400
  [Levonorgestrel and Ethinyl Estradiol (Systemic)][1], 1397
  Medrogestone (Systemic)*, 2400
  Medroxyprogesterone, Oral (Systemic), 2400
  [Norethindrone Acetate and Ethinyl Estradiol (Systemic)][1], 1397
  Norethindrone Acetate Tablets USP (Systemic), 2400
  [Norethindrone and Ethinyl Estradiol (Systemic)][1], 1397
  [Norethindrone and Mestranol (Systemic)], 1397
  [Norgestimate and Ethinyl Estradiol (Systemic)][1], 1397
  [Norgestrel and Ethinyl Estradiol (Systemic)][1], 1397
  Progesterone (Systemic), 2400
**Bleeding, uterine, hormonal imbalance–induced (treatment)**
  Estrogens, Conjugated, Parenteral (Systemic), 1383
  Estrone (Systemic)†, 1383
**Blepharitis, bacterial (treatment)**
  [Chloramphenicol (Ophthalmic)], #
  [Chlortetracycline (Ophthalmic)], 2763
  [Erythromycin (Ophthalmic)][1], 1364
  Framycetin (Ophthalmic)*, 3020
  Gentamicin (Ophthalmic), 1555
  Neomycin (Ophthalmic)*†, #
  [Neomycin, Polymyxin B, and Bacitracin (Ophthalmic)], #
  [Neomycin, Polymyxin B, and Gramicidin (Ophthalmic)], #
  [Sulfacetamide (Ophthalmic)], 2651
  [Sulfisoxazole (Ophthalmic)], 2651
  [Tetracycline (Ophthalmic)], 2763
  [Tobramycin (Ophthalmic)], #

**Blepharitis, fungal (treatment)**
   Natamycin (Ophthalmic)†, #
**Blepharoconjunctivitis (treatment)**
   [Chloramphenicol (Ophthalmic)], #
   [Chlortetracycline (Ophthalmic)], 2763
   [Erythromycin (Ophthalmic)][1], 1364
   Gentamicin (Ophthalmic), 1555
   Neomycin (Ophthalmic)*†, #
   [Neomycin, Polymyxin B, and Bacitracin (Ophthalmic)], #
   [Neomycin, Polymyxin B, and Gramicidin (Ophthalmic)], #
   [Sulfacetamide (Ophthalmic)], 2651
   [Sulfisoxazole (Ophthalmic)], 2651
   [Tetracycline (Ophthalmic)], 2763
   [Tobramycin (Ophthalmic)]†, #
**Blepharospasm (treatment)**
   Botulinum Toxin Type A (Parenteral-Local), 627, 3134‡
   Botulinum Toxin Type F (Parenteral-Local), 3134‡
**Blood clotting, in arterial surgery (prophylaxis)**
   Heparin (Systemic), 1617
**Blood clotting, during extracorporeal circulation (prophylaxis)**
   Heparin (Systemic), 1617
**Blood clotting in heparin-intolerant patients (prophylaxis)**
   Ancrod (Systemic), 3131‡
**Blood flow studies, cerebral**
   Xenon Xe 133 (Systemic), 2984
**Blood and plasma volumes determinations**
   Iodinated I 125 Albumin (Systemic), 2453
   Iodinated I 131 Albumin (Systemic), 2453
**Blood pool imaging, radionuclide**
   See also Bleeding, gastrointestinal (diagnosis); Cardiac blood pool imaging, radionuclide
   Sodium Pertechnetate Tc 99m (Systemic), 2612
**Blood transfusions, allogenic, in anemic surgery patients, reduction of**
   Epoetin Alfa (Systemic), 1352
**Body imaging, computed tomographic**
   Barium Sulfate Oral Suspension (Local), #
   Barium Sulfate Rectal Suspension (Local), #
   Barium Sulfate for Suspension USP (Oral) (Local), #
   Barium Sulfate for Suspension USP (Rectal) (Local), #
   Diatrizoate Meglumine and Diatrizoate Sodium, Parenteral (Systemic), #
   Diatrizoate Meglumine, Parenteral (Systemic), #
   Iodixanol (Systemic), #
   Iohexol (Systemic), #
   Iopamidol (Systemic)[1], #
   Iopromide (Systemic), #
   Iothalamate Meglumine (Systemic), #
   Iothalamate Sodium (Systemic), #
   Ioversol (Systemic), #
   Ioxaglate (Systemic), #
   Ioxilan (Systemic), #
**Body imaging, computed tomographic, adjunct**
   Diatrizoate Meglumine and Diatrizoate Sodium, Oral (Systemic), #
**Body imaging, magnetic resonance**
   Gadopentetate (Systemic)†, #
**Bone infections (treatment)**
   See also Bone and joint infections
   Fusidic Acid (Systemic)*, 3021
   Gentamicin Impregnated PMMA Beads on Surgical Wire, 3144‡
**Bone and joint infections (treatment)**
   Amikacin (Systemic), 69
   [Ampicillin and Sulbactam (Systemic)]†, 2263
   [Aztreonam (Systemic)]†, 502
   Carbenicillin, Parenteral (Systemic), 2240
   [Cefaclor (Systemic)][1], 794
   [Cefadroxil (Systemic)][1], 794
   Cefamandole (Systemic), 794
   Cefazolin (Systemic), 794
   [Cefixime (Systemic)][1], 794
   Cefonicid (Systemic)[1]†, 794
   [Cefoperazone (Systemic)][1], 794
   Cefotaxime (Systemic)[1], 794
   Cefotetan (Systemic), 794
   Cefoxitin (Systemic), 794
   [Cefpodoxime (Systemic)][1]†, 794
   [Cefprozil (Systemic)][1]†, 794
   Ceftazidime (Systemic), 794
   Ceftizoxime (Systemic), 794
   Ceftriaxone (Systemic), 794
   Cefuroxime (Systemic), 794
   Cephalexin (Systemic), 794
   [Cephalothin (Systemic)][1], 794
   Cephapirin (Systemic)[1]†, 794
   [Cephradine (Systemic)][1], 794
   Ciprofloxacin (Systemic), 1487
   Clindamycin, Parenteral (Systemic), 893

**Bone and joint infections (treatment)** (continued)
   Cloxacillin, Parenteral (Systemic), 2240
   Gentamicin (Systemic), 69
   Imipenem and Cilastatin (Systemic), 1681
   Kanamycin (Systemic)†, 69
   [Methicillin (Systemic)]†, 2240
   Metronidazole (Systemic), 1996
   [Nafcillin, Parenteral (Systemic)][1], 2240
   Netilmicin (Systemic), 69
   [Oxacillin, Parenteral (Systemic)]†, 2240
   [Penicillin G, Parenteral (Systemic)][1], 2240
   Piperacillin (Systemic), 2240
   Streptomycin (Systemic), 69
   [Sulfamethoxazole and Trimethoprim (Systemic)], 2661
   Ticarcillin and Clavulanate (Systemic), 2263
   Tobramycin (Systemic), 69
   Vancomycin (Systemic), 2919
**Bone lesions, metastatic (diagnosis)**—See Skeletal imaging, radionuclide
**Bone lesions, metastatic (treatment)**
   Sodium Phosphate P 32 (Systemic), 2616
   Strontium Chloride Sr 89 (Systemic), 2632
**Bone marrow failure, primary (treatment)**
   Recombinant Methionyl Human Stem Cell Factor (Systemic), 3161‡
**Bone marrow imaging, radionuclide**
   Technetium Tc 99m Albumin Colloid (Systemic)†, 2699
   Technetium Tc 99m Sulfur Colloid (Systemic), 2740
**Bone marrow toxicity, antineoplastic agent–induced (prophylaxis)**
   [Amifostine (Systemic)][1], 61
**Bone marrow transplant adjunct**
   [Chlorhexidine (Mucosal-Local)]†, 3136‡
   Interleukin-3 Human, Recombinant (Systemic), 3149‡
**Bone marrow transplant adjunct, in leukemia**
   Monoclonal Antibodies PM-81 and AML-2-23 (Systemic), 3155‡
   Roquinimex (Systemic), 3163‡
**Bone marrow transplant preparation**
   Busulfan (Systemic), 3135‡
**Botulism, infant (treatment)**
   Botulism Immune Globulin (Systemic), 3135‡
**Bowel disease, inflammatory (diagnosis)**
   Technetium Tc 99m Exametazime (Systemic)[1], 2708
**Bowel disease, inflammatory (prophylaxis)**
   Mesalamine (Oral-Local), 1952
   [Mesalamine (Rectal-Local)], 1954
   Olsalazine (Oral-Local), 2161
   Sulfasalazine (Systemic), 2643
**Bowel disease, inflammatory (treatment)**
   Aminosalicylate Sodium (Systemic), 3130‡
   4-Aminosalicylic Acid (Systemic), 3128‡
   [Azathioprine (Systemic)]1, 491
   Betamethasone, Oral (Systemic), 998
   Betamethasone, Parenteral (Systemic), 998
   Cortisone (Systemic), 998
   Dexamethasone, Oral (Systemic), 998
   Fatty Acids, Short Chain (Systemic), 3164‡
   Hydrocortisone, Oral (Systemic), 998
   Hydrocortisone, Parenteral (Systemic), 998
   [Mercaptopurine (Systemic)][1], 1946
   Mesalamine (Oral-Local), 1952
   Mesalamine (Rectal-Local), 1954
   Methylprednisolone, Oral (Systemic), 998
   Methylprednisolone, Parenteral (Systemic), 998
   [Metronidazole (Systemic)][1], 1996
   [Olsalazine (Oral-Local)], 2161
   Prednisolone, Oral (Systemic), 998
   Prednisolone, Parenteral (Systemic), 998
   Prednisone (Systemic), 998
   Sulfasalazine (Systemic), 2643
   TAK-603 (Systemic), 3167‡
   Triamcinolone, Oral (Systemic), 998
   Triamcinolone, Parenteral (Systemic), 998
**Bowel evacuation, preoperative**
   Bisacodyl (Local), #
   Bisacodyl and Docusate (Local)*, #
   Casanthranol (Local)†, #
   Casanthranol and Docusate (Local), #
   Cascara Sagrada (Local)†, #
   Cascara Sagrada and Aloe (Local)†, #
   Cascara Sagrada and Phenolphthalein (Local)†, #
   Castor Oil (Local), #
   Danthron and Docusate (Local)*, #
   Dehydrocholic Acid (Local)†, #
   Dehydrocholic Acid and Docusate (Local)†, #
   Dehydrocholic Acid, Docusate, and Phenolphthalein (Local), #
   Docusate, Rectal (Local), #
   Glycerin (Local), #
   Magnesium Citrate (Local), #

**Bowel evacuation, preoperative** (continued)
   Magnesium Hydroxide (Local), #
   Magnesium Hydroxide and Cascara Sagrada (Local)†, #
   Magnesium Oxide (Local)†, #
   Magnesium Sulfate (Local)†, #
   Mineral Oil, Glycerin, and Phenolphthalein (Local)*, #
   Mineral Oil and Phenolphthalein (Local)†, #
   Phenolphthalein (Local), #
   Phenolphthalein and Docusate (Local), #
   Phenolphthalein and Senna (Local)*, #
   Polyethylene Glycol and Electrolytes (Local), 2349
   Potassium Bitartrate and Sodium Bicarbonate (Local)†, #
   Psyllium Hydrophilic Mucilloid and Senna (Local)*, #
   Psyllium Hydrophilic Mucilloid and Sennosides (Local)†, #
   Psyllium and Senna (Local)†, #
   Senna (Local), #
   Sennosides (Local), #
   Sennosides and Docusate (Local), #
   Sodium Phosphate (Local)†, #
**Bowel evacuation, pre- and postpartum**
   Potassium Bitartrate and Sodium Bicarbonate (Local)†, #
**Bowel evacuation, pre-radiography**
   Bisacodyl (Local), #
   Bisacodyl and Docusate (Local)*, #
   Casanthranol (Local)†, #
   Casanthranol and Docusate (Local), #
   Cascara Sagrada (Local)†, #
   Cascara Sagrada and Aloe (Local)†, #
   Cascara Sagrada and Phenolphthalein (Local)†, #
   Castor Oil (Local), #
   Danthron and Docusate (Local)*, #
   Dehydrocholic Acid (Local)†, #
   Dehydrocholic Acid and Docusate (Local)†, #
   Dehydrocholic Acid, Docusate, and Phenolphthalein (Local)†, #
   Docusate, Rectal (Local), #
   Glycerin (Local), #
   Magnesium Citrate (Local), #
   Magnesium Hydroxide (Local), #
   Magnesium Hydroxide and Cascara Sagrada (Local)†, #
   Magnesium Oxide (Local)†, #
   Magnesium Sulfate (Local)†, #
   Mineral Oil, Glycerin, and Phenolphthalein (Local)*, #
   Mineral Oil and Phenolphthalein (Local)†, #
   Phenolphthalein (Local), #
   Phenolphthalein and Docusate (Local), #
   Phenolphthalein and Senna (Local)*, #
   Polyethylene Glycol and Electrolytes (Local), 2349
   Potassium Bitartrate and Sodium Bicarbonate (Local)†, #
   Psyllium Hydrophilic Mucilloid and Senna (Local)*, #
   Psyllium Hydrophilic Mucilloid and Sennosides (Local)†, #
   Psyllium and Senna (Local)†, #
   Senna (Local), #
   Sennosides (Local), #
   Sennosides and Docusate (Local), #
   Sodium Phosphate (Local)†, #
**Bowel imaging, magnetic resonance (diagnosis)**
   Ferumoxsil (Systemic), 3019
**Bowel preparation, preoperative**
   Erythromycin Base (Systemic), 1368
   Kanamycin (Oral-Local)†, #
   Neomycin (Oral-Local), #
**Bowel syndrome, irritable (treatment)**
   Atropine (Systemic), 226
   Belladonna (Systemic)†, 226
   Chlordiazepoxide and Clidinium (Systemic), 846
   [Clidinium (Systemic)]†, 226
   Dicyclomine (Systemic), 226
   [Glycopyrrolate (Systemic)], 226
   Hyoscyamine (Systemic), 226
   [Propantheline (Systemic)], 226
   Scopolamine (Systemic), 226
**Bowel syndrome, irritable (treatment adjunct)**
   Atropine, Hyoscyamine, Scopolamine, and Phenobarbital (Systemic), 551
   Atropine and Phenobarbital (Systemic)†, 551
   Belladonna and Butabarbital (Systemic), 551
   Belladonna and Phenobarbital (Systemic)†, 551
   Hyoscyamine and Phenobarbital (Systemic)†, 551
   [Malt Soup Extract (Local)]†, #
   [Malt Soup Extract and Psyllium (Local)]†, #
   [Methylcellulose (Local)]†, #
   Polycarbophil (Local), #
   [Psyllium (Local)], #
   [Psyllium Hydrophilic Mucilloid (Local)], #

**Bowel syndrome, irritable (treatment adjunct)** *(continued)*
　[Psyllium Hydrophilic Mucilloid and Carboxymethylcellulose (Local)]†, #
**Bowen's disease (treatment)**
　[Fluorouracil (Topical)]1, 1500
**BPH**—See Benign prostatic hyperplasia
**Bradycardia (treatment)**
　Isoproterenol (Parenteral-Systemic), 2669
**Bradycardia, sinus (treatment)**
　Atropine, Parenteral (Systemic), 226
**Brain abscess (treatment)**
　Chloramphenicol (Systemic), 841
　Metronidazole (Systemic), 1996
　[Vancomycin (Systemic)]1, 2919
**Brain damage, minimal**—See Attention-deficit hyperactivity disorder
**Brain death (diagnosis)**
　[Technetium Tc 99m Exametazime (Systemic)]1, 2708
**Brain edema, peritumoral (treatment)**
　Corticotropin-releasing Factor, Human (Systemic), 3138‡
**Brain imaging, computed tomographic**
　Diatrizoate Meglumine and Diatrizoate Sodium, Parenteral (Systemic), #
　Diatrizoate Meglumine, Parenteral (Systemic), #
　Diatrizoate Sodium, Parenteral (Systemic), #
　Iodixanol (Systemic), #
　Iohexol (Systemic), #
　Iopamidol (Systemic)1, #
　Iopromide (Systemic), #
　Iothalamate Meglumine (Systemic), #
　Iothalamate Meglumine and Iothalamate Sodium (Systemic)†, #
　Iothalamate Sodium (Systemic), #
　Ioversol (Systemic), #
　Ioxaglate (Systemic), #
　Ioxilan (Systemic), #
**Brain imaging, magnetic resonance**
　Gadodiamide (Systemic), #
　Gadopentetate (Systemic)†, #
　Gadoteridol (Systemic)†, #
**Brain imaging, positron emission tomographic**
　Ammonia N 13 (Systemic)*†, 91
　[Fludeoxyglucose F 18 (Systemic)]1*†, 1478
　[Methionine C 11]1*†, 4233
**Brain imaging, radionuclide**
　Iofetamine I 123 (Systemic), 1757
　Sodium Pertechnetate Tc 99m (Systemic), 2612
　Technetium Tc 99m Bicisate (Systemic), 2703
　Technetium Tc 99m Exametazime (Systemic), 2708
　Technetium Tc 99m Gluceptate (Systemic), 2711
　Technetium Tc 99m Pentetate (Systemic), 2727
**Brain malignancies, primary (treatment)**
　Busulfan (Systemic), 3134‡
　Thalidomide (Systemic), 3168‡
**Brain perfusion studies**
　Technetium Tc 99m Gluceptate (Systemic), 2711
**Branched-chain aminoacidopathy**—See Maple syrup urine disease
**Breast disease, fibrocystic (treatment)**
　Danazol (Systemic), 1163
**Breast imaging, magnetic resonance**—See Body imaging, magnetic resonance
**Broad tapeworm**—See Diphyllobothriasis
**Bronchial airway hyperreactivity (diagnosis)**
　Methacholine (Inhalation-Local)†, #
**Bronchial studies**
　Acetylcysteine (Inhalation-Local), #
**Bronchiectasis (treatment)**
　Albuterol (Systemic), 651
　Ephedrine (Systemic), 651
　Epinephrine (Systemic), 651
　Ethylnorepinephrine (Systemic)†, 651
　Fenoterol (Systemic)*, 651
　Gelsolin, Recombinant Human (Systemic), 3161‡
　Isoproterenol (Systemic), 651
　Metaproterenol (Systemic), 651
　Terbutaline (Systemic), 651
**Bronchiectasis (treatment adjunct)**
　Acetylcysteine (Inhalation-Local), #
**Bronchitis (treatment), 794**
　Albuterol (Systemic), 651
　[Amoxicillin and Clavulanate (Systemic)]1, 2263
　Amoxicillin and Clavulanate (Systemic), 3010
　Aztreonam (Systemic)†, 502
　Cefaclor (Systemic), 794
　Cefixime (Systemic), 794
　Cefprozil (Systemic)1†, 794
　Cefuroxime Axetil (Systemic), 794
　Demeclocycline (Systemic), 2765
　Doxycycline (Systemic), 2765
　Ephedrine (Systemic), 651
　Epinephrine (Systemic), 651

**Bronchitis (treatment)** *(continued)*
　Ethylnorepinephrine (Systemic)†, 651
　Fenoterol (Systemic)*, 651
　Ipratropium (Inhalation-Local), 1761
　Isoproterenol (Systemic), 651
　Metaproterenol (Systemic), 651
　Minocycline (Systemic), 2765
　Oxytetracycline (Systemic)†, 2765
　Sulfamethoxazole and Trimethoprim, Oral (Systemic), 2661
　Terbutaline (Systemic), 651
　Tetracycline (Systemic), 2765
**Bronchitis (treatment adjunct)**
　Acetylcysteine (Inhalation-Local), #
**Bronchitis, asthmatic (treatment)**
　[Betamethasone, Oral (Systemic)]1, 998
　[Betamethasone, Parenteral (Systemic)]1, 998
　[Cortisone (Systemic)]1, 998
　[Dexamethasone, Oral (Systemic)]1, 998
　[Dexamethasone, Parenteral (Systemic)]1, 998
　[Hydrocortisone, Oral (Systemic)]1, 998
　[Hydrocortisone, Parenteral (Systemic)]1, 998
　[Methylprednisolone, Oral (Systemic)]1, 998
　[Methylprednisolone, Parenteral (Systemic)]1, 998
　[Prednisolone, Oral (Systemic)]1, 998
　[Prednisolone, Parenteral (Systemic)]1, 998
　[Prednisone (Systemic)]1, 998
　[Triamcinolone, Oral (Systemic)]1, 998
　[Triamcinolone, Parenteral (Systemic)]1, 998
**Bronchitis, asthmatic (treatment adjunct)**
　Acetylcysteine (Inhalation-Local), #
**Bronchitis, bacterial exacerbations (treatment)**
　Amoxicillin (Systemic), 2240
　Ampicillin (Systemic), 2240
　Azithromycin (Systemic), 499
　Bacampicillin (Systemic), 2240
　Cefaclor (Systemic)1, 794
　Cefdinir (Systemic), 3014
　[Cefepime (Systemic)]1, 794
　Cefixime (Systemic)1, 794
　Cefpodoxime (Systemic)1, 794
　Cefprozil (Systemic)1, 794
　Ceftibuten (Systemic)1, 794
　Cefuroxime Axetil (Systemic)1, 794
　Ciprofloxacin (Systemic), 1487
　Clarithromycin (Systemic), 889
　Cloxacillin, Oral (Systemic), 2240
　Dicloxacillin (Systemic)†, 2240
　Dirithromycin (Systemic)†, 1250
　Erythromycin (Systemic), 1368
　Grepafloxacin (Systemic), 1580
　Levofloxacin (Systemic), 1852
　Lomefloxacin (Systemic), 1487
　Loracarbef (Systemic)†, 1880
　Ofloxacin (Systemic), 1487
　Penicillin V (Systemic), 2240
　Pivampicillin (Systemic)*, 2240
　Sparfloxacin (Systemic), 2620
**Bronchitis, chronic (treatment)**
　Aminophylline (Systemic), 668
　Oxtriphylline (Systemic), 668
　Oxtriphylline and Guaifenesin (Systemic), #
　Theophylline (Systemic), 668
　Theophylline and Guaifenesin (Systemic)†, #
　Trovafloxacin (Systemic), 2891
**Bronchopulmonary dysplasia, in neonates with respiratory distress syndrome (prophylaxis)**
　Human Clara Cell 10KDA Protein, Recombinant (Systemic), 3160‡
**Bronchospasm (prophylaxis)**
　Cromolyn (Inhalation-Local), 1116
　[Nedocromil (Inhalation-Local)], 2090
**Bronchospasm (treatment)**
　Albuterol (Systemic), 651
　Ephedrine (Systemic), 651
　Epinephrine (Systemic), 651
　Ethylnorepinephrine (Systemic)†, 651
　Fenoterol (Systemic)*, 651
　Isoproterenol (Systemic), 651
　Metaproterenol (Systemic), 651
　Terbutaline (Systemic), 651
**Bronchospasm, asthma-associated (prophylaxis)**
　Salmeterol (Inhalation-Local), 640
**Bronchospasm, asthma-associated (treatment)**
　Albuterol (Inhalation-Local), 640
　Bitolterol (Inhalation-Local)†, 640
　Fenoterol (Inhalation-Local)*, 640
　Metaproterenol (Inhalation-Local), 640
　Pirbuterol (Inhalation-Local), 640
　Terbutaline (Inhalation-Local), 640
**Bronchospasm, chronic, bronchitis-associated (prophylaxis)**
　Bitolterol (Inhalation-Local)†, 640
　Fenoterol (Inhalation-Local)*, 640
　Procaterol (Inhalation-Local)*, 640
　Salmeterol (Inhalation-Local), 3034

**Bronchospasm, chronic, bronchitis-associated (prophylaxis)** *(continued)*
　Terbutaline (Inhalation-Local), 640
**Bronchospasm, chronic, bronchitis-associated (treatment)**
　Albuterol (Inhalation-Local), 640
　Bitolterol (Inhalation-Local)†, 640
　Fenoterol (Inhalation-Local)*, 640
　Metaproterenol (Inhalation-Local), 640
　Pirbuterol (Inhalation-Local), 640
　Procaterol (Inhalation-Local)*, 640
　Terbutaline (Inhalation-Local), 640
**Bronchospasm, chronic obstructive pulmonary disease–associated (prophylaxis)**
　Albuterol (Inhalation-Local), 640
　Fenoterol (Inhalation-Local)*, 640
　Metaproterenol (Inhalation-Local), 640
　Salmeterol (Inhalation-Local), 3034
　Terbutaline (Inhalation-Local), 640
**Bronchospasm, chronic obstructive pulmonary disease–associated (treatment)**
　Albuterol (Inhalation-Local), 640
　Bitolterol (Inhalation-Local)†, 640
　Fenoterol (Inhalation-Local)*, 640
　Procaterol (Inhalation-Local)*, 640
　Terbutaline (Inhalation-Local), 640
**Bronchospasm, during anesthesia (treatment)**
　[Epinephrine, Parenteral (Systemic)], 651
　Isoproterenol, Parenteral (Systemic), 651
　[Terbutaline, Parenteral (Systemic)], 651
**Bronchospasm, exercise-induced (prophylaxis)**
　Albuterol (Inhalation-Local), 640
　[Bitolterol (Inhalation-Local)]†, 640
　[Pirbuterol (Inhalation-Local)], 640
　Procaterol (Inhalation-Local)*, 640
　Salmeterol (Inhalation-Local)1, 640
　[Terbutaline (Inhalation-Local)]1, 640
**Bronchospasm, pulmonary emphysema–associated (prophylaxis)**
　Albuterol (Inhalation-Local), 640
　Bitolterol (Inhalation-Local)†, 640
　Fenoterol (Inhalation-Local)*, 640
　Metaproterenol (Inhalation-Local), 640
　Pirbuterol (Inhalation-Local), 640
　Salmeterol (Inhalation-Local), 3034
**Bronchospasm, pulmonary emphysema–associated (treatment)**
　Bitolterol (Inhalation-Local)†, 640
　Fenoterol (Inhalation-Local)*, 640
　Metaproterenol (Inhalation-Local), 640
　Pirbuterol (Inhalation-Local), 640
　Procaterol (Inhalation-Local)*, 640
**Bronchospasm, reversible obstructive airway disease–associated (treatment)**
　Albuterol (Systemic), 3009
**Brucellosis (treatment)**
　Demeclocycline (Systemic), 2765
　Doxycycline (Systemic), 2765
　Minocycline (Systemic), 2765
　Oxytetracycline (Systemic)†, 2765
　Streptomycin (Systemic), 69
　Tetracycline (Systemic), 2765
**Bulbar palsy, progressive (treatment)**
　Ciliary Neurotrophic Factor, Recombinant Human (Systemic), 3137‡
**Bulimia nervosa (treatment)**
　[Amitriptyline (Systemic)]1, 271
　[Clomipramine (Systemic)]1, 271
　[Desipramine (Systemic)]1, 271
　Fluoxetine (Systemic), 1503
　[Imipramine (Systemic)]1, 271
**Burkitt's lymphoma**—See Lymphomas, non-Hodgkin's
**Burns, corneal (treatment)**
　Framycetin (Ophthalmic)*, 3020
**Burns, excised, bacterial colonization with grafts (treatment)**
　Mafenide (Topical), 3152‡
**Burns, hydrogen fluoride (treatment)**
　Calcium Gluconate (Topical), 3136‡
**Burns, minor (treatment)**
　Benzocaine (Topical), 155
　Benzocaine and Menthol (Topical), 155
　Butamben (Topical), 155
　Dibucaine (Topical), 155
　Lidocaine (Topical), 155
　Pramoxine (Topical), 155
　Pramoxine and Menthol (Topical), 155
　Tetracaine (Topical), 155
　Tetracaine and Menthol (Topical), 155
**Burns, severe (treatment)**
　Ananain, Comosain (Topical), 3131‡
　Dehydroepiandrosterone Sulfate Sodium (Topical), 3139‡, 3140‡
　Poloxamer 188 (Systemic), 3158‡
　Somatropin (Systemic), 3165‡

**Burns, severe (treatment adjunct)**
  Albumin Human (Systemic), 34
**Burn wound infections (prophylaxis)**
  *See also* Skin and soft tissue infections
  Mafenide (Topical)†, #
  Silver Sulfadiazine (Topical), #
**Burn wound infections (treatment)**
  *See also* Skin and soft tissue infections
  Framycetin (Topical), 3021
  Framycetin and Gramicidin (Topical)*, 3021
  Fusidic Acid (Systemic)*, 3021
  Mafenide (Topical)†, #
  Silver Sulfadiazine (Topical), #
**Bursitis (treatment)**
  *See also* Inflammation, nonrheumatic
  Betamethasone, Oral (Systemic), 998
  Betamethasone, Parenteral (Systemic), 998
  Betamethasone, Parenteral-Local (Systemic), 998
  Cortisone (Systemic), 998
  Dexamethasone, Oral (Systemic), 998
  Dexamethasone, Parenteral (Systemic), 998
  Dexamethasone, Parenteral-Local (Systemic), 998
  Hydrocortisone, Oral (Systemic), 998
  Hydrocortisone, Parenteral (Systemic), 998
  Hydrocortisone, Parenteral-Local (Systemic), 998
  Methylprednisolone, Oral (Systemic), 998
  Methylprednisolone, Parenteral (Systemic), 998
  Methylprednisolone, Parenteral-Local (Systemic), 998
  Naproxen (Systemic), 3029
  Prednisolone (Systemic), 998
  Prednisone (Systemic), 998
  Triamcinolone (Systemic), 998

# C

**Cachexia (treatment)**
  Megestrol (Systemic), 2400
**Cachexia, AIDS-associated (treatment)**
  L-Glutathione, Reduced (Systemic), 3162‡
  Megestrol (Systemic), 3153‡
  Somatropin (Systemic), 3165‡
  Somatropin, Recombinant (Systemic), 3035
**Calcifications, on indwelling urethral catheters (prophylaxis)**
  Citric Acid and D-Gluconic Acid (Local), 3014
**Calcifications, on indwelling urethral catheters (treatment)**
  Citric Acid and D-Gluconic Acid (Local), 3014
**Calcium deficiency (prophylaxis)**
  Calcium Carbonate (Systemic), 736
  Calcium Citrate (Systemic)†, 736
  Calcium Glubionate (Systemic), 736
  Calcium Gluceptate and Calcium Gluconate (Systemic)*, 736
  Calcium Gluconate, Oral (Systemic), 736
  Calcium Lactate (Systemic), 736
  Calcium Lactate-Gluconate and Calcium Carbonate (Systemic)*, 736
  Calcium Phosphate, Dibasic (Systemic)†, 736
  Calcium Phosphate, Tribasic (Systemic)†, 736
**Calcium deposits, corneal (treatment)**
  [Edetate Disodium (Ophthalmic)*†][1], 550
**Calcium hydroxide burns, in eye (treatment)**
  [Edetate Disodium (Ophthalmic)*†][1], 550
**Calcium pyrophosphate deposition disease, acute (prophylaxis)**
  [Colchicine (Systemic)][1], 928
**Calcium pyrophosphate deposition disease, acute (treatment)**
  [Betamethasone, Oral (Systemic)][1], 998
  [Betamethasone, Parenteral (Systemic)][1], 998
  [Betamethasone, Parenteral-Local (Systemic)][1], 998
  [Colchicine (Systemic)][1], 928
  [Cortisone (Systemic)][1], 998
  [Dexamethasone (Systemic)][1], 998
  [Diclofenac (Systemic)][1], 388
  [Diflunisal (Systemic)][1], 388
  [Etodolac (Systemic)]†, 388
  [Fenoprofen (Systemic)][1], 388
  Floctafenine (Systemic)*[1], 388
  [Hydrocortisone, Oral (Systemic)][1], 998
  [Hydrocortisone, Parenteral (Systemic)][1], 998
  [Hydrocortisone, Parenteral-Local (Systemic)][1], 998
  [Ibuprofen (Systemic)][1], 388
  [Indomethacin (Systemic)][1], 388
  [Ketoprofen (Systemic)][1], 388
  [Meclofenamate (Systemic)]†, 388
  [Mefenamic Acid (Systemic)][1], 388
  [Methylprednisolone, Oral (Systemic)][1], 998
  [Methylprednisolone, Parenteral (Systemic)][1], 998
  [Methylprednisolone, Parenteral-Local (Systemic)][1], 998
  [Naproxen (Systemic)][1], 388

**Calcium pyrophosphate deposition disease, acute (treatment)** *(continued)*
  [Phenylbutazone (Systemic)][1], 388
  [Piroxicam (Systemic)][1], 388
  [Prednisolone (Systemic)][1], 998
  [Prednisone (Systemic)][1], 998
  [Sulindac (Systemic)][1], 388
  [Triamcinolone (Systemic)][1], 998
**Calluses (treatment)**
  Resorcinol (Topical), 1#
**Candidiasis (prophylaxis)**
  Fluconazole (Systemic), 302
**Candidiasis (treatment)**
  Amphotericin B Lipid Complex (Systemic), 3130‡
  Amphotericin B Liposomal Complex (Systemic), 105
**Candidiasis, cutaneous (treatment)**
  Ciclopirox (Topical), 863
  Clotrimazole (Topical), 916
  [Clotrimazole and Betamethasone (Topical)][1], 918
  Econazole (Topical), 1323
  Ketoconazole (Topical)[1], 1807
  Miconazole (Topical), #
  Nystatin (Topical), 2148
  Nystatin and Triamcinolone (Topical)†, 2150
  [Sulconazole (Topical)]†, #
  Tioconazole (Topical), 3036
**Candidiasis, disseminated (treatment)**
  Amphotericin B (Systemic), 98
  Fluconazole (Systemic), 302
  [Flucytosine (Systemic)][1], #
  Ketoconazole (Systemic), 302
**Candidiasis, esophageal (treatment)**
  Fluconazole (Systemic), 302
  Itraconazole (Systemic), 302
  Ketoconazole (Systemic), 302
**Candidiasis, mucocutaneous, chronic (treatment)**
  [Fluconazole (Systemic)][1], 302
  [Itraconazole (Systemic)][1], 302
  Ketoconazole (Systemic), 302
  Nystatin (Topical), 2148
**Candidiasis, oropharyngeal (prophylaxis)**
  Clotrimazole (Oral-Local)†, 915
  [Nystatin Lozenges (Pastilles) (Oral-Local)]†, 2146
  [Nystatin Oral Suspension (Oral-Local)], 2146
  [Nystatin for Oral Suspension (Oral-Local)], 2146
**Candidiasis, oropharyngeal (treatment)**
  Clotrimazole (Oral-Local)†, 915
  Fluconazole (Systemic), 302
  Itraconazole (Systemic), 302
  Ketoconazole (Systemic), 302
  Nystatin Lozenges (Pastilles) (Oral-Local)†, 2146
  Nystatin Oral Suspension (Oral-Local), 2146
  Nystatin for Oral Suspension (Oral-Local), 2146
  [Nystatin Tablets (Vaginal)], 2149
**Candidiasis, vulvovaginal (treatment)**
  Butoconazole (Vaginal)†, 310
  Clotrimazole (Vaginal), 310
  Econazole (Vaginal)*, 310
  Fluconazole (Systemic), 302
  Gentian Violet (Vaginal), #
  [Itraconazole (Systemic)][1], 302
  [Ketoconazole (Systemic)][1], 302
  Metronidazole and Nystatin (Vaginal), 3028
  Miconazole (Vaginal), 310
  Nystatin (Vaginal), 2149
  Terconazole (Vaginal), 310
  Tioconazole (Vaginal), 310
**Canker sores (treatment)**
  Benzocaine Gel (Dental) (Mucosal-Local), 128
  Benzocaine and Phenol Gel (Mucosal-Local), 128
  Benzocaine and Phenol Topical Solution (Mucosal-Local), 128
  Benzocaine Topical Solution USP (Dental) (Mucosal-Local), 128
  Lidocaine 2.5% Oral Topical Solution USP (Mucosal-Local), 128
**Cannula, arteriovenous, clearance**
  Streptokinase (Systemic), 2799
  [Urokinase (Systemic)][1], 2799
**Capillariasis (treatment)**
  Albendazole (Systemic)*†, #
  [Mebendazole (Systemic)][1], 1926
  [Thiabendazole (Systemic)]†, 2784
**Capsulitis**—*See* Inflammation, nonrheumatic
**Carcinoid syndrome (treatment)**
  *See also* Tumors, gastrointestinal; Tumors, neuroendocrine
  Iobenguane I 131 Sulfate (Systemic)—Therapeutic)*†, 1749
**Carcinoid tumors**—*See* Tumors, gastrointestinal
**Carcinoid tumors (treatment)**
  *See also* Tumors, gastrointestinal; Tumors, neuroendocrine

**Carcinoma, adrenal cortex (treatment)**
  Gossypol (Systemic), 3144‡
  [Trilostane (Systemic)]†, #
**Carcinoma, adrenocortical (treatment)**
  [Cisplatin (Systemic)][1], 876
  [Etoposide (Systemic)][1], 1424
  Mitotane (Systemic), 2031
**Carcinoma, anal (treatment)**
  [Fluorouracil (Systemic)], 1497
  [Mitomycin (Systemic)][1], 2028
**Carcinoma, biliary (treatment)**
  [Mitomycin (Systemic)][1], 2028
**Carcinoma, bladder (prophylaxis)**
  Bacillus Calmette-Guérin (BCG) Live (Mucosal-Local), 507
  [Thiotepa (Systemic)][1], 2790
**Carcinoma, bladder (treatment)**
  Bacillus Calmette-Guérin (BCG) Live (Mucosal-Local), 507
  Cisplatin (Systemic), 876
  [Cyclophosphamide (Systemic)][1], 1128
  Doxorubicin (Systemic), 1308
  [Fluorouracil (Systemic)], 1497
  [Gemcitabine (Systemic)][1], 1548
  [Interferon Alfa-2a, Recombinant (Systemic)][1], 1740
  [Interferon Alfa-2b, Recombinant (Systemic)][1], 1740
  Interferon Alfa-n1 (Ins) (Systemic)*[1], 1740
  [Interferon Alfa-n3 (Systemic)]†, 1740
  [Methotrexate—For Cancer (Systemic)], 1962
  [Mitomycin (Systemic)], 2028
  N-Trifluoroacetyladriamycin-14-Valerate (Systemic), 3155‡
  [Paclitaxel (Systemic)][1], 2215
  Porfimer Sodium (Systemic), 3159‡
  Thiotepa (Systemic)[1], 2790
  [Vinblastine (Systemic)][1], 2946
**Carcinoma, breast (diagnosis)**
  [Fludeoxyglucose F 18 (Systemic)][1]*†, 1478
**Carcinoma, breast (treatment)**
  [Aminoglutethimide (Systemic)], 67
  Anastrozole (Systemic), 116
  [Betamethasone, Oral (Systemic)][1], 998
  [Betamethasone, Parenteral (Systemic)][1], 998
  Capecitabine (Systemic), 748
  [Cisplatin (Systemic)][1], 876
  [Cortisone (Systemic)][1], 998
  Cyclophosphamide (Systemic), 1128
  [Dexamethasone, Oral (Systemic)][1], 998
  [Dexamethasone, Parenteral (Systemic)][1], 998
  Docetaxel (Systemic), 1282
  Doxorubicin (Systemic), 1308
  Epirubicin (Systemic)*, 3018
  Estradiol, Oral (Systemic), 1383
  Estrogens, Conjugated, Oral (Systemic), 1383
  Estrogens, Esterified (Systemic)[1], 1383
  Ethinyl Estradiol (Systemic), 1383
  Exemestane (Systemic), 3142‡
  Fluorouracil (Systemic), 1497
  Fluoxymesterone (Systemic), 118
  Goserelin (Systemic)[1], 1575
  [Hydrocortisone, Oral (Systemic)][1], 998
  [Hydrocortisone, Parenteral (Systemic)][1], 998
  [Ifosfamide (Systemic)][1], 1677
  Letrozole (Systemic), 1836
  [Leuprolide (Systemic)][1], 1840
  [Lomustine (Systemic)][1], 1874
  [Medroxyprogesterone (Systemic)], 2400
  Megestrol (Systemic), 2400
  [Melphalan (Systemic)][1], 1938
  Methotrexate—For Cancer (Systemic), 1962
  [Methylprednisolone, Oral (Systemic)][1], 998
  [Methylprednisolone, Parenteral (Systemic)][1], 998
  Methyltestosterone (Systemic), 118
  [Mitomycin (Systemic)][1], 2028
  [Mitoxantrone (Systemic)], 2033
  [Nandrolone Decanoate (Systemic)][1], 110
  Nandrolone Phenpropionate (Systemic), 110
  Paclitaxel (Systemic), 2215, 3159‡
  [Prednisolone, Oral (Systemic)][1], 998
  [Prednisolone, Parenteral (Systemic)][1], 998
  [Prednisone (Systemic)][1], 998
  Tamoxifen (Systemic), 2688
  Testosterone (Systemic), 118
  Thiotepa (Systemic), 2790
  Toremifene (Systemic), 2845, 3169‡
  [Triamcinolone, Oral (Systemic)][1], 998
  [Triamcinolone, Parenteral (Systemic)][1], 998
  Vinblastine (Systemic), 2946
  [Vincristine (Systemic)], 2950
  [Vinorelbine (Systemic)], 2953

**Carcinoma, cervical (treatment)**
Bleomycin (Systemic), 624
[Cisplatin (Systemic)][1], 876
[Cyclophosphamide (Systemic)][1], 1128
Dibromodulcitol (Systemic), 3140‡
[Doxorubicin (Systemic)], 1308
[Fluorouracil (Systemic)][1], 1497
[Hydroxyurea (Systemic)][1], 1666
[Ifosfamide (Systemic)], 1677
[Methotrexate—For Cancer (Systemic)][1], 1962
[Mitomycin (Systemic)][1], 2028
[Paclitaxel (Systemic)][1], 2215
Porfiromycin (Systemic), 3159‡
Vaccinia, Recombinant (Human Papillomavirus) (Systemic), 3162‡
[Vincristine (Systemic)], 2950

**Carcinoma, colorectal (diagnosis)**
[Fludeoxyglucose F 18 (Systemic)][1]*†, 1478
Indium In 111 Altumomab Pentetate (Systemic), 3147‡

**Carcinoma, colorectal (diagnosis adjunct)**
Fecal Occult Blood Test Kits, #
Technetium Tc 99m Arcitumomab (Systemic), 2701

**Carcinoma, colorectal (treatment)**
[Carmustine (Systemic)], 786
Disaccharide Tripeptide Glycerol Dipalmitoyl (Systemic), 3141‡
Floxuridine (Systemic)†, 1472
Fluorouracil (Systemic), 1497, 3144‡
Interferon Alfa-2a, Recombinant (Systemic), 3148‡
Irinotecan (Systemic), 1769
[Lomustine (Systemic)][1], 1874
[Methotrexate—For Cancer (Systemic)][1], 1962
[Mitomycin (Systemic)], 2028
Trimetrexate (Systemic), 3170‡
[Vincristine (Systemic)], 2950

**Carcinoma, colorectal (treatment adjunct)**
Leucovorin (Systemic), 1837, 3152‡
Leucovorin Calcium (Systemic), 3150‡
Levamisole (Systemic), 1844
L-Leucovorin (Systemic), 3150‡

**Carcinoma, endometrial (treatment)**
[Cisplatin (Systemic)][1], 876
[Cyclophosphamide (Systemic)][1], 1128
[Doxorubicin (Systemic)][1], 1308
[Fluorouracil (Systemic)][1], 1497
[Medroxyprogesterone, Oral (Systemic)], 2400
Medroxyprogesterone, Parenteral (Systemic), 2400
Megestrol (Systemic), 2400
[Paclitaxel (Systemic)][1], 2215

**Carcinoma, esophageal (treatment)**
Bleomycin (Systemic), 624
[Cisplatin (Systemic)][1], 876
[Fluorouracil (Systemic)][1], 1497
Fluorouracil (Systemic), 3144‡
Interferon Alfa-2a (Recombinant) (Systemic), 3148‡
[Methotrexate—For Cancer (Systemic)][1], 1962
[Mitomycin (Systemic)][1], 2028
[Paclitaxel (Systemic)][1], 2215
Porfimer (Systemic), 2351, 3159‡

**Carcinoma, gastric (treatment)**
[Carmustine (Systemic)], 786
[Cisplatin (Systemic)][1], 876
Doxorubicin (Systemic), 1308
Epirubicin (Systemic)*, 3018
[Etoposide (Systemic)][1], 1424
Fluorouracil (Systemic), 1497
[Methotrexate—For Cancer (Systemic)], 1962
Mitomycin (Systemic), 2028

**Carcinoma, head and neck (treatment)**
Bleomycin (Systemic), 624
[Carboplatin (Systemic)][1], 779
[Cisplatin (Systemic)][1], 876
[Doxorubicin (Systemic)][1], 1308
[Fluorouracil (Systemic)], 1497
[Ifosfamide (Systemic)][1], 1677
Methotrexate—For Cancer (Systemic), 1962
[Mitomycin (Systemic)][1], 2028
[Paclitaxel (Systemic)][1], 2215
Porfiromycin (Systemic), 3159‡
Trimetrexate (Systemic), 3170‡

**Carcinoma, hepatic (diagnosis)**
[Fludeoxyglucose F 18 (Systemic)][1]*†, 1478
Iodine I 123 Murine Monoclonal Antibody to Alpha-fetoprotein (Systemic), 3149‡
Technetium Tc 99m Murine Monoclonal Antibody to Human Alpha-fetoprotein (Systemic), 3167‡

**Carcinoma, hepatic (treatment)**
[Floxuridine (Systemic)][1]†, 1472
Iodine I 131 Murine Monoclonal Antibody to Alpha-fetoprotein (Systemic), 3149‡

**Carcinoma, hepatocellular (diagnosis)**
Ammonia N 13 (Systemic)*†, 91

**Carcinoma, hepatocellular, primary (treatment)**
[Cisplatin (Systemic)][1], 876
[Doxorubicin (Systemic)][1], 1308
[Fluorouracil (Systemic)][1], 1497

**Carcinoma, islet cell (treatment)**
[Dacarbazine (Systemic)][1], 1148
Streptozocin (Systemic), 2629

**Carcinoma, laryngeal (treatment)**
Bleomycin (Systemic), 624

**Carcinoma, lung (diagnosis)**
[Fludeoxyglucose F 18 (Systemic)][1]*†, 1478

**Carcinoma, lung (treatment)**
Epirubicin (Systemic)*, 3018
Ricin (Blocked) Conjugated Murine Monoclonal Antibody (N901) (Systemic), 3162‡
Trimetrexate (Systemic), 3170‡
[Vinblastine (Systemic)][1], 2946
Vinorelbine (Systemic), 2953

**Carcinoma, lung, metastatic (diagnosis adjunct)**
Technetium Tc 99m Nofetumomab Merpentan (Systemic)†, 2701, 2722

**Carcinoma, lung, non–small cell (treatment)**
[Carboplatin (Systemic)][1], 779
[Cisplatin (Systemic)][1], 876
[Cyclophosphamide (Systemic)], 1128
[Docetaxel (Systemic)], 1282
[Doxorubicin (Systemic)], 1308
[Etoposide (Systemic)], 1424
Gemcitabine (Systemic), 1548
[Ifosfamide (Systemic)][1], 1677
Lomustine (Systemic), 1874
Methotrexate—For Cancer (Systemic)[1], 1962
[Mitomycin (Systemic)][1], 2028
[Paclitaxel (Systemic)][1], 2215
Porfimer (Systemic), 2351
[Topotecan (Systemic)][1], 2841
[Vinblastine (Systemic)][1], 2946

**Carcinoma, lung, primary (diagnosis adjunct)**
Technetium Tc 99m Nofetumomab Merpentan (Systemic), 2701
Technetium Tc 99m Nofetumomab Merpentan (Systemic)†, 2722

**Carcinoma, lung, small cell (treatment)**
[Carboplatin (Systemic)][1], 779
[Cisplatin (Systemic)][1], 876
[Cyclophosphamide (Systemic)], 1128
[Docetaxel (Systemic)][1], 1282
Doxorubicin (Systemic), 1308
Etoposide (Systemic), 1424
[Ifosfamide (Systemic)][1], 1677
Methotrexate—For Cancer (Systemic)[1], 1962
[Paclitaxel (Systemic)][1], 2215
[Topotecan (Systemic)][1], 2841
[Vincristine (Systemic)], 2950

**Carcinoma, musculoskeletal (diagnosis)**
[Fludeoxyglucose F 18 (Systemic)][1]*†, 1478

**Carcinoma, ovarian (diagnosis)**
[Fludeoxyglucose F 18 (Systemic)][1]*†, 1478
Satumomab Pendetide (Systemic), 3163‡

**Carcinoma, ovarian (treatment)**
Altretamine (Systemic), 55, 3129‡
Amifostine (Systemic), 3130‡
Bispecific Antibody 520C9x22 (Systemic), 3133‡
Chromic Phosphate P 32 (Parenteral-Local)†, #
Cisplatin (Systemic), 876
[Dactinomycin (Systemic)][1], 1153
[Docetaxel (Systemic)][1], 1282
[Doxorubicin, Liposomal (Systemic)][1], 1312
Epirubicin (Systemic)*, 3018
Monoclonal Antibody-B43.13 (Systemic), 3154‡
OncoRad OV103 (Systemic), 3156‡
Oxaliplatin (Systemic), 3156‡
RGG0853, E1A Lipid Complex (Systemic), 3162‡
SU101 (Systemic), 3166‡
Topotecan (Systemic), 2841
Treosulfan (Systemic), 3169‡

**Carcinoma, ovarian, epithelial (treatment)**
Carboplatin (Systemic), 779
[Chlorambucil (Systemic)][1], 837
Cyclophosphamide (Systemic), 1128
Doxorubicin (Systemic), 1308
[Floxuridine (Systemic)]†, 1472
[Fluorouracil (Systemic)][1], 1497
Hydroxyurea (Systemic), 1666
[Ifosfamide (Systemic)][1], 1677
[Interferon Alfa-2a, Recombinant (Systemic)][1], 1740
[Interferon Alfa-2b, Recombinant (Systemic)][1], 1740
[Interferon Alfa-n1 (Ins) (Systemic)][1]*, 1740
[Interferon Alfa-n3 (Systemic)][1]†, 1740
Melphalan (Systemic), 1938
[Methotrexate—For Cancer (Systemic)][1], 1962
Paclitaxel (Systemic), 2215
Thiotepa (Systemic), 2790
[Vincristine (Systemic)][1], 2950

**Carcinoma, pancreatic (diagnosis)**
[Fludeoxyglucose F 18 (Systemic)][1]*†, 1478

**Carcinoma, pancreatic (treatment)**
Allogeneic Peripheral Blood Mononuclear Cells Sensitized Against Patient Alloantigens By Mixed Lymphocyte Culture (Systemic), 3129‡
[Cisplatin (Systemic)][1], 876
[Doxorubicin (Systemic)][1], 1308
Fluorouracil (Systemic), 1497
Gemcitabine (Systemic), 1548
[Methotrexate—For Cancer (Systemic)][1], 1962
Mitomycin (Systemic), 2028
Monoclonal Antibody 17-1A (Systemic), 3154‡
9-Nitro-20-(S)-Camptothecin (9-NC) (Systemic), 3128‡
Streptozocin (Systemic), 2629
Trimetrexate (Systemic), 3170‡

**Carcinoma, paralaryngeal (treatment)**
[Bleomycin (Systemic)], 624

**Carcinoma, penile (treatment)**
Bleomycin (Systemic), 624
[Methotrexate—For Cancer (Systemic)][1], 1962

**Carcinoma, prostatic (treatment)**
[Aminoglutethimide (Systemic)][1], 67
[Betamethasone, Oral (Systemic)][1], 998
[Betamethasone, Parenteral (Systemic)][1], 998
Bicalutamide (Systemic), 220
Buserelin (Systemic)*, 691
Chromic Phosphate P 32 (Parenteral-Local)†, #
[Cisplatin (Systemic)][1], 876
[Cortisone (Systemic)][1], 998
[Cyclophosphamide (Systemic)][1], 1128
Cyproterone (Systemic)*, 3016
[Dexamethasone, Oral (Systemic)][1], 998
[Dexamethasone, Parenteral (Systemic)][1], 998
Diethylstilbestrol (Systemic), 1383
[Doxorubicin (Systemic)][1], 1308
Estradiol, Oral (Systemic)[1], 1383
Estradiol Valerate (Systemic), 1383
Estramustine (Systemic), 1380
Estrogens, Conjugated, Oral (Systemic), 1383
Estrogens, Esterified (Systemic)[1], 1383
Estrone (Systemic)†, 1383
Ethinyl Estradiol (Systemic), 1383
[Fluorouracil (Systemic)], 1497
Flutamide (Systemic), 220
Goserelin (Systemic), 1575
[Hydrocortisone, Oral (Systemic)][1], 998
[Hydrocortisone, Parenteral (Systemic)][1], 998
[Ketoconazole (Systemic)][1], 302
Leuprolide (Systemic), 1840
[Megestrol (Systemic)], 2400
[Methylprednisolone, Oral (Systemic)][1], 998
[Methylprednisolone, Parenteral (Systemic)][1], 998
Mitoxantrone (Systemic), 3154‡
Nilutamide (Systemic), 220
[Prednisolone, Oral (Systemic)][1], 998
[Prednisolone, Parenteral (Systemic)][1], 998
[Prednisone (Systemic)][1], 998
Suramin (Systemic), 3167‡
[Triamcinolone, Oral (Systemic)][1], 998
[Triamcinolone, Parenteral (Systemic)][1], 998
[Vinblastine (Systemic)][1], 2946

**Carcinoma, prostatic, advanced hormone-refractory (treatment)**
Mitoxantrone (Systemic)[1], 2033

**Carcinoma, prostatic, intra-pelvic metastases (diagnosis)**
Indium In 111 Capromab Pendetide (Systemic), #

**Carcinoma, prostatic, occult, recurrence (diagnosis)**
Indium In 111 Capromab Pendetide (Systemic), #

**Carcinoma, renal (treatment)**
Aldesleukin (Systemic)†, 36, 3129‡
Autolymphocyte Therapy (Systemic), 3132‡
Coumarin (Systemic), 3138‡
[Floxuridine (Systemic)]†, 1472
[Interferon Alfa-2a, Recombinant (Systemic)], 1740, 3148‡
[Interferon Alfa-2b, Recombinant (Systemic)][1], 1740
Interferon Alfa-n1 (Ins) (Systemic)*[1], 1740
[Interferon Alfa-n3 (Systemic)]†, 1740
Interferon Beta (Recombinant) (Systemic), 3148‡
Interferon Gamma-1b (Systemic), 3149‡
Interleukin-2 (Systemic), 3149‡
Interleukin-2, Recombinant, Liposome Encapsulated (Systemic), 3149‡
Medroxyprogesterone, Parenteral (Systemic), 2400
Poly I: Poly C12U (Systemic), 3158‡
[Vinblastine (Systemic)][1], 2946

**Carcinoma, renal cell (treatment)**
Human Interleukin-12, Recombinant (Systemic), 3161‡
Pegasys (Systemic), 3157‡

**Carcinoma, skin (treatment)**
[Bleomycin (Systemic)], 624
[Fluorouracil (Systemic)], 1497
Fluorouracil (Topical), 1500
Interferon Alfa-2b, Recombinant (Systemic), 3148‡
[Interferon Alfa-2b, Recombinant (Systemic)], 1740
**Carcinoma, testicular (treatment)**
Bleomycin (Systemic), 624
[Carboplatin (Systemic)][1], 779
Cisplatin (Systemic), 876
[Cyclophosphamide (Systemic)][1], 1128
Dactinomycin (Systemic), 1153
Etoposide Injection (Systemic), 1424
Plicamycin (Systemic)†, 2334
Vinblastine (Systemic), 2946
**Carcinoma, thyroid (diagnosis)**
Arcitumomab (Systemic), 3132‡
[Fludeoxyglucose F 18 (Systemic)][1]*†, 1478
[Iobenguane I 123 (Systemic)—Diagnostic]†, 1747
[Iobenguane I 131 (Systemic)—Diagnostic]†, 1747
Thyrotropin (Systemic), #
**Carcinoma, thyroid (diagnosis adjunct)**
Human Thyroid-Stimulating Hormone (Systemic), 3146‡
**Carcinoma, thyroid (prophylaxis)**
Levothyroxine (Systemic)[1], 2809
Liothyronine (Systemic)[1], 2809
Liotrix (Systemic)†, 2809
Thyroglobulin (Systemic)*†, 2809
Thyroid (Systemic)[1], 2809
**Carcinoma, thyroid (treatment)**
[Bleomycin (Systemic)][1], 624
[Cisplatin (Systemic)][1], 876
Doxorubicin (Systemic), 1308
Levothyroxine (Systemic)[1], 2809
Liothyronine (Systemic)[1], 2809
Liotrix (Systemic)†, 2809
Sodium Iodide I 131 (Systemic—Therapeutic), 2606
Thyroglobulin (Systemic)*†, 2809
Thyroid (Systemic)[1], 2809
**Carcinoma, thyroid (treatment adjunct)**
[Thyrotropin (Systemic)], #
Tiratricol (Systemic), 3169‡
**Carcinomatous meningitis (treatment)**
[Methotrexate—For Cancer (Systemic)][1], 1962
**Carcinoma, uterine**—See Carcinoma, endometrial
**Carcinoma, vulvar (treatment)**
Bleomycin (Systemic), 624
**Cardiac arrest (treatment)**
Epinephrine (Parenteral-Systemic), 2669
**Cardiac arrest (treatment adjunct)**
Calcium Chloride (Systemic), 736
[Calcium Gluconate, Parenteral (Systemic)], 736
**Cardiac blood pool imaging, positron emission tomographic**
Ammonia N 13 (Systemic)*†, 91
**Cardiac blood pool imaging, radionuclide**
[Sodium Pertechnetate Tc 99m (Systemic)][1], 2612
Technetium Tc 99m Albumin (Systemic), 2695
Technetium Tc 99m Pyrophosphate (Systemic)†, 2729
Technetium Tc 99m (Pyro- and trimeta-) Phosphates (Systemic), 2733
**Cardiac bypass surgery assessment**
Ammonia N 13 (Systemic)*†, 91
[Fludeoxyglucose F 18 (Systemic)][1]*†, 1478
**Cardiac function studies**
See also Cardiac blood pool imaging, radionuclide
[Amyl Nitrite (Systemic)][1], #
**Cardiac graft rejection**—See Transplant rejection, cardiac allograft
**Cardiac imaging**—See Angiocardiography; Cardiac imaging, radionuclide
**Cardiac imaging, magnetic resonance**
[Gadopentetate (Systemic)]†, #
**Cardiac imaging, positron emission tomographic**
Ammonia N 13 (Systemic)*†, 91
[Fludeoxyglucose F 18 (Systemic)][1]*†, 1478
Rubidium Rb 82 (Systemic)†, 2536
**Cardiac imaging, radionuclide**
See also Cardiac blood pool imaging, radionuclide
Imciromab Pentetate (Systemic), 3147‡
Indium In 111 Murine Monoclonal Antibody Fab to Myosin (Systemic), 3147‡
Technetium Tc 99m Pyrophosphate (Systemic)†, 2729
Technetium Tc 99m (Pyro- and trimeta-) Phosphates (Systemic), 2733
Technetium Tc 99m Sestamibi (Systemic), 2736
Technetium Tc 99m Teboroxime (Systemic)†, 2743
Technetium Tc 99m Tetrofosmin (Systemic)†, 2745
Thallous Chloride Tl 201 (Systemic), 2781

**Cardiac output, low (treatment)**
Dobutamine (Parenteral-Systemic), 2669
Dopamine (Parenteral-Systemic), 2669
Norepinephrine (Parenteral-Systemic), 2669
**Cardiac ventricular function assessment**
Technetium Tc 99m Sestamibi (Systemic)1, 2736
**Cardiac wall-motion abnormalities assessment**
Ammonia N 13 (Systemic)*†, 91
[Fludeoxyglucose F 18 (Systemic)][1]*†, 1478
[Technetium Tc 99m Sestamibi (Systemic)][1], 2736
**Cardiomyopathy (prophylaxis)**
Dexrazoxane (Systemic), 1190
**Cardiomyopathy, doxorubicin-induced (prophylaxis)**
Dexrazoxane (Systemic), 3140‡
**Cardiomyopathy, hypertrophic (treatment)**
[Acebutolol (Systemic)][1], 593
[Atenolol (Systemic)][1], 593
[Metoprolol (Systemic)][1], 593
[Nadolol (Systemic)][1], 593
[Oxprenolol (Systemic)]*[1], 593
[Pindolol (Systemic)][1], 593
Propranolol (Systemic), 593
[Sotalol (Systemic)][1], 593
[Timolol (Systemic)][1], 593
**Cardiomyopathy, hypertrophic (treatment adjunct)**
[Verapamil (Systemic)], 720
**Cardiomyopathy, pediatric (treatment)**
Levocarnitine (Systemic), 3152‡
**Cardiopulmonary bypass (treatment adjunct)**
Albumin Human (Systemic), 34
**Carditis, nonrheumatic, acute (treatment)**
[Betamethasone, Oral (Systemic)][1], 998
[Betamethasone, Parenteral (Systemic)][1], 998
[Cortisone (Systemic)][1], 998
[Dexamethasone, Oral (Systemic)][1], 998
[Dexamethasone, Parenteral (Systemic)][1], 998
[Hydrocortisone, Oral (Systemic)][1], 998
[Hydrocortisone, Parenteral (Systemic)][1], 998
[Methylprednisolone, Oral (Systemic)][1], 998
[Methylprednisolone, Parenteral (Systemic)][1], 998
[Prednisolone, Oral (Systemic)][1], 998
[Prednisolone, Parenteral (Systemic)][1], 998
[Prednisone (Systemic)][1], 998
[Triamcinolone, Oral (Systemic)][1], 998
[Triamcinolone, Parenteral (Systemic)][1], 998
**Carditis, rheumatic, acute (treatment)**
Betamethasone, Oral (Systemic), 998
Betamethasone, Parenteral (Systemic), 998
Cortisone (Systemic), 998
Dexamethasone, Oral (Systemic), 998
Dexamethasone, Parenteral (Systemic), 998
Hydrocortisone, Oral (Systemic), 998
Hydrocortisone, Parenteral (Systemic), 998
Methylprednisolone, Oral (Systemic), 998
Methylprednisolone, Parenteral (Systemic), 998
Prednisolone, Oral (Systemic), 998
Prednisone (Systemic), 998
Triamcinolone, Oral (Systemic), 998
**Carnitine deficiency (treatment)**
Levocarnitine (Systemic), 1847
**Carnitine deficiency, associated with end-stage renal disease (prophylaxis)**
Levocarnitine (Systemic), 3151‡
**Carnitine deficiency, associated with end-stage renal disease (treatment)**
Levocarnitine (Systemic), 3151‡
**Carnitine deficiency, genetic (treatment)**
Levocarnitine (Systemic), 3151‡, 3152‡
**Carnitine deficiency, secondary to valproic acid toxicity (prophylaxis)**
Levocarnitine (Systemic), 3151‡
[Levocarnitine Oral Solution USP (Systemic)][1], 1847
**Carnitine deficiency, secondary to valproic acid toxicity (treatment)**
Levocarnitine (Systemic), 3151‡
[Levocarnitine Oral Solution USP (Systemic)][1], 1847
**Cartilaginous defects, femoral (treatment)**
Chondrocytes, Autologous Cultured (Implantation-Local), 856
**Catabolic or tissue-depleting processes (treatment)**
[Nandrolone Decanoate (Systemic)], 110
Oxandrolone (Systemic)†, 110
[Stanozolol (Systemic)]†, 110
**Cataplexy (treatment)**
Sodium/Gamma Hydroxybutyrate (Systemic), 3165‡
**Cat and dog hookworm**—See Hookworm infection; Larva migrans, cutaneous
**Catheter, intravenous, clearance**
[Streptokinase (Systemic)][1], 2799
Urokinase (Systemic), 2799

**Causalgia (treatment)**
Guanethidine Monosulfate (Systemic), 3145‡
**Celiac disease, severe (treatment)**
[Betamethasone, Oral (Systemic)][1], 998
[Betamethasone, Parenteral (Systemic)][1], 998
[Cortisone (Systemic)][1], 998
[Dexamethasone, Oral (Systemic)][1], 998
[Dexamethasone, Parenteral (Systemic)][1], 998
[Hydrocortisone, Oral (Systemic)][1], 998
[Hydrocortisone, Parenteral (Systemic)][1], 998
[Methylprednisolone, Oral (Systemic)][1], 998
[Methylprednisolone, Parenteral (Systemic)][1], 998
[Prednisolone, Oral (Systemic)][1], 998
[Prednisolone, Parenteral (Systemic)][1], 998
[Prednisone (Systemic)][1], 998
[Triamcinolone, Oral (Systemic)][1], 998
[Triamcinolone, Parenteral (Systemic)][1], 998
**Central nervous system (CNS) infections (treatment)**
Amikacin (Systemic), 69
Gentamicin (Systemic), 69
Kanamycin (Systemic)†, 69
Metronidazole (Systemic), 1996
Netilmicin (Systemic), 69
Streptomycin (Systemic), 69
Tobramycin (Systemic), 69
**Central neural blocks**
Bupivacaine and Dextrose (Parenteral-Local), 139
Bupivacaine and Epinephrine (Parenteral-Local), 139
Bupivicaine (Parenteral-Local), 139
Chloroprocaine (Parenteral-Local), 139
Etidocaine (Parenteral-Local), 139
Etidocaine and Epinephrine (Parenteral-Local), 139
Lidocaine (Parenteral-Local), 139
Lidocaine and Dextrose (Parenteral-Local), 139
Lidocaine and Epinephrine (Parenteral-Local), 139
Mepivacaine (Parenteral-Local), 139
Procaine (Parenteral-Local)[1], 139
Tetracaine (Parenteral-Local), 139
Tetracaine and Dextrose (Parenteral-Local), 139
**Cerebral dysfunction, minimal**—See Attention-deficit hyperactivity disorder
**Cerebral dysfunction, minor**—See Attention-deficit hyperactivity disorder
**Cerebral infarction (diagnosis)**—See Brain imaging, computed tomographic
**Cerebral infections (diagnosis)**—See Brain imaging, computed tomographic
**Cerebral perfusion, regional, abnormalities of (diagnosis)**—See Brain imaging, radionuclide
**Cerebrospinal fluid flow disorders (diagnosis)**—See Cisternography; Cisternography, computed tomographic; Cisternography, radionuclide
**Cerebrovascular disease (diagnosis)**—See Angiography; Angiography, cerebral, radionuclide; Brain imaging, radionuclide
**Cerebrovascular insufficiency (treatment)**
Isoxsuprine (Systemic), #
**Cervical neoplasia (prophylaxis)**
[Condoms, Lamb Cecum][1], 1474
[Condoms, Lamb Cecum, and Nonoxynol 9][1], 1474
[Condoms, Latex][1], 1474
[Condoms, Latex, and Nonoxynol 9][1], 1474
**Cervical neoplasia (treatment)**
[Condoms, Lamb Cecum][1], 1474
[Condoms, Lamb Cecum, and Nonoxynol 9][1], 1474
[Condoms, Latex][1], 1474
[Condoms, Latex, and Nonoxynol 9][1], 1474
**Cervical ripening**
[Carboprost (Systemic)][1], 782
Dinoprostone Cervical Gel (Cervical/Vaginal)*, 1228
Dinoprostone Vaginal System (Cervical/Vaginal)*, 1228
**Cervicitis (treatment)**
Trovafloxacin (Systemic), 2891
**Cervicitis, gonococcal (treatment)**
Azithromycin (Systemic), 499
**Cervicitis, nongonococcal (treatment)**
Azithromycin (Systemic), 499
Grepafloxacin (Systemic), 1580
**CGD**—See Chronic granulomatous disease
**Chagas' disease**—See Trypanosomiasis, American

## Indications Index

**Chancroid (treatment)**
[Amoxicillin and Clavulanate (Systemic)]¹, 2263
Azithromycin (Systemic), 499
[Ciprofloxacin (Systemic)]¹, 1487
[Enoxacin (Systemic)]¹, 1487
[Erythromycin (Systemic)]¹, 1368
Sulfadiazine (Systemic), 2653
Sulfamethoxazole (Systemic), 2653
[Sulfamethoxazole and Trimethoprim (Systemic)]¹, 2661
Sulfisoxazole (Systemic), 2653
**Chemotherapy, intra-arterial, infusion adjunct**
[Technetium Tc 99m Albumin Aggregated (Systemic)]¹, 2697
**Chickenpox**—See Varicella
**Chiclero ulcer**—See Leishmaniasis, cutaneous
**Chilblains**—See Frostbite
**Chinese liver fluke**—See Clonorchiasis
**Chlamydial infections (treatment)**
[Amoxicillin (Systemic)]¹, 2240
[Ampicillin (Systemic)]¹, 2240
[Erythromycin (Ophthalmic)]¹, 1364
Sulfacetamide (Ophthalmic), 2651
[Sulfamethoxazole and Trimethoprim (Systemic)]¹, 2661
Sulfisoxazole (Ophthalmic), 2651
[Tetracycline (Ophthalmic)], 2763
[Tetracycline (Systemic)], 2765
**Chlamydial infections, endocervical (treatment)**
Erythromycin (Systemic), 1368
Ofloxacin (Systemic), 1487
Sulfadiazine (Systemic)¹, 2653
Sulfamethoxazole (Systemic), 2653
Sulfisoxazole (Systemic), 2653
**Chlamydial infections, urethral (treatment)**
Erythromycin (Systemic), 1368
Ofloxacin (Systemic), 1487
Sulfadiazine (Systemic)¹, 2653
Sulfamethoxazole (Systemic), 2653
Sulfisoxazole (Systemic), 2653
**Cholangiography adjunct**
Cholecystokinin (Systemic)*, #
**Cholangiography, direct**
Diatrizoate Meglumine and Diatrizoate Sodium, Parenteral (Systemic)¹, #
Diatrizoate Meglumine, Parenteral (Systemic), #
Diatrizoate Sodium, Parenteral (Systemic), #
Iothalamate Meglumine (Systemic), #
**Cholangiography, intravenous**
Iodipamide (Systemic), #
**Cholangiography, percutaneous transhepatic**
Diatrizoate Meglumine and Diatrizoate Sodium, Parenteral (Systemic)¹, #
Diatrizoate Meglumine, Parenteral (Systemic)¹, #
Diatrizoate Sodium, Parenteral (Systemic)¹, #
Iothalamate Meglumine (Systemic), #
**Cholangiography, radionuclide**—See Hepatobiliary imaging, radionuclide
**Cholangiopancreatography, endoscopic retrograde**
Iohexol (Systemic)¹, #
[Iopamidol (Systemic)]¹, #
Iothalamate Meglumine (Systemic), #
[Ioversol (Systemic)]¹, #
**Cholangitis, sclerosing (treatment)**
[Ursodiol (Systemic)]¹, 2903
**Cholecystitis, acute (diagnosis)**—See Hepatobiliary imaging, radionuclide
**Cholecystography, intravenous**
Iodipamide (Systemic), #
**Cholecystography, oral**
Iocetamic Acid (Systemic)†, #
Iopanoic Acid (Systemic), #
Ipodate (Systemic)†, #
Tyropanoate (Systemic)†, #
**Cholecystography, oral, adjunct**
Cholecystokinin (Systemic)*, #
**Cholera (treatment)**
Furazolidone (Oral-Local)†, 1533
**Choline deficiency (treatment)**
Choline Chloride (Systemic), 3136‡
**Chondrocalcinosis articularis**—See Calcium pyrophosphate deposition disease, acute
**Chorea, Huntington's (treatment)**
[Haloperidol (Systemic)]¹, 1611
**Choreoathetosis, paroxysmal (treatment)**
[Phenytoin (Systemic)]¹, 253
**Chorioadenoma destruens**—See Tumors, trophoblastic, gestational
**Choriocarcinoma**—See Tumors, trophoblastic, gestational
**Chorioretinitis (treatment)**
Betamethasone, Oral (Systemic), 998
Betamethasone, Parenteral (Systemic), 998

**Chorioretinitis (treatment)** *(continued)*
Cortisone (Systemic), 998
Dexamethasone, Oral (Systemic), 998
Dexamethasone, Parenteral (Systemic), 998
Hydrocortisone, Oral (Systemic), 998
Hydrocortisone, Parenteral (Systemic), 998
Methylprednisolone, Oral (Systemic), 998
Methylprednisolone, Parenteral (Systemic), 998
Prednisolone, Oral (Systemic), 998
Prednisolone, Parenteral (Systemic), 998
Prednisone (Systemic), 998
Triamcinolone, Oral (Systemic), 998
Triamcinolone, Parenteral (Systemic), 998
**Choroiditis, posterior, diffuse (treatment)**
Betamethasone, Oral (Systemic), 998
Betamethasone, Parenteral (Systemic), 998
Cortisone (Systemic), 998
Dexamethasone, Oral (Systemic), 998
Dexamethasone, Parenteral (Systemic), 998
Hydrocortisone, Oral (Systemic), 998
Hydrocortisone, Parenteral (Systemic), 998
Methylprednisolone, Oral (Systemic), 998
Methylprednisolone, Parenteral (Systemic), 998
Prednisolone, Oral (Systemic), 998
Prednisolone, Parenteral (Systemic), 998
Prednisone (Systemic), 998
Triamcinolone, Oral (Systemic), 998
Triamcinolone, Parenteral (Systemic), 998
**Christmas disease**—See Hemophilia B, hemorrhagic complications of
**Chromium deficiency (prophylaxis)**
Chromic Chloride (Systemic)†, 861
Chromium (Systemic), 861
**Chromium deficiency (treatment)**
Chromic Chloride (Systemic)†, 861
Chromium (Systemic), 861
**Chromomycosis (treatment)**
[Flucytosine (Systemic)]1, #
[Itraconazole (Systemic)], 302
Ketoconazole (Systemic), 302
**Chronic fatigue syndrome (treatment)**
Poly I: Poly C12U (Systemic), 3159‡
**Chronic granulomatous disease (treatment)**
Interferon, Gamma (Systemic)†, 1737
Interferon Gamma-1b (Systemic), 3148‡
**Cicatricial pemphigoid (treatment)**
[Dapsone (Systemic)]¹, 1170
**Cirrhosis, alcoholic (treatment)**
[Ursodiol (Systemic)]¹, 2903
**Cirrhosis, biliary (treatment)**
[Azathioprine (Systemic)]¹, 491
[Colchicine (Systemic)]¹, 928
Ursodeoxycholic Acid (Systemic), 3171‡
[Ursodiol (Systemic)]¹, 2903, 3171‡
**Cisplatin toxicity (prophylaxis)**
Amifostine (Systemic), 3130‡
**Cisternography**
Metrizamide (Systemic)†, #
**Cisternography, computed tomographic**
Iopamidol (Systemic)¹, #
Metrizamide (Systemic)†, #
**Cisternography, radionuclide**
Indium In 111 Pentetate (Systemic)†, 1698
[Technetium Tc 99m Pentetate (Systemic)]¹, 2727
**Clonorchiasis (treatment)**
Praziquantel (Systemic)†, 2368
**Clostridium tetani infection (prophylaxis)**
[Tetanus Antitoxin (Systemic)]¹*†, #
Tetanus Immune Globulin (Systemic)*, 2758
**Clostridium tetani infection (treatment)**
[Tetanus Antitoxin (Systemic)]¹*†, 6141
**CMV disease**—See Cytomegalovirus disease, primary
**CMV gastrointestinal disease**—See Cytomegalovirus disease, primary
**CMV pneumonia**—See Cytomegalovirus disease, primary; Cytomegalovirus pneumonia, in bone marrow transplant patients
**Coagulation, disseminated intravascular (treatment)**
Heparin (Systemic), 1617
**Coagulation, disseminated intravascular (treatment adjunct)**
[Antihemophilic Factor, Cryoprecipitated (Systemic)]¹, 319
**Cocaine withdrawal (treatment)**
[Desipramine (Systemic)]¹, 271
[Imipramine (Systemic)]¹, 271
**Coccidioidomycosis (treatment)**
Amphotericin B (Systemic), 98
Amphotericin B Lipid Complex (Systemic), 3130‡
[Fluconazole (Systemic)]¹, 302
[Itraconazole (Systemic)]¹, 302
Ketoconazole (Systemic), 302

**Cold sores (treatment)**
Benzocaine Gel (Dental) (Mucosal-Local), 128
Benzocaine and Phenol Gel (Mucosal-Local), 128
Benzocaine and Phenol Topical Solution (Mucosal-Local), 128
Benzocaine Topical Solution USP (Dental) (Mucosal-Local), 128
Lidocaine 2.5% Oral Topical Solution USP (Mucosal-Local), 128
**Cold symptoms (treatment)**
*See also* Congestion, nasal; Cough; Cough and nasal congestion
Bromodiphenhydramine and Codeine (Systemic)†, 1024
Bromodiphenhydramine, Diphenhydramine, Codeine, Ammonium Chloride, and Potassium Guaiacolsulfonate (Systemic)*, 1024
Brompheniramine, Phenylephrine, Phenylpropanolamine, and Codeine (Systemic)*, 1024
Brompheniramine, Phenylephrine, Phenylpropanolamine, Codeine, and Guaifenesin (Systemic)*, 1024
Brompheniramine, Phenylephrine, Phenylpropanolamine, and Dextromethorphan (Systemic)*, 1024
Brompheniramine, Phenylephrine, Phenylpropanolamine, and Guaifenesin (Systemic)*, 1024
Brompheniramine, Phenylephrine, Phenylpropanolamine, Hydrocodone, and Guaifenesin (Systemic)*, 1024
Brompheniramine, Phenylpropanolamine, and Acetaminophen (Systemic)†, 366
Brompheniramine, Phenylpropanolamine, and Codeine (Systemic)†, 1024
Brompheniramine, Phenylpropanolamine, and Dextromethorphan (Systemic)†, 1024
Brompheniramine, Pseudoephedrine, and Acetaminophen (Systemic)†, 366
Brompheniramine, Pseudoephedrine, and Dextromethorphan (Systemic)†, 1024
Carbinoxamine, Pseudoephedrine, and Dextromethorphan (Systemic)†, 1024
Chlorpheniramine and Codeine (Systemic)*, 1024
Chlorpheniramine and Dextromethorphan (Systemic)†, 1024
Chlorpheniramine, Ephedrine, and Guaifenesin (Systemic)†, 1024
Chlorpheniramine, Ephedrine, Phenylephrine, and Carbetapentane (Systemic)†, 1024
Chlorpheniramine, Ephedrine, Phenylephrine, Dextromethorphan, Ammonium Chloride, and Ipecac (Systemic)†, 1024
Chlorpheniramine and Hydrocodone (Systemic)†, 1024
Chlorpheniramine, Phenindamine, Phenylephrine, Dextromethorphan, Acetaminophen, Salicylamide, Caffeine, and Ascorbic Acid (Systemic)†, 1024
Chlorpheniramine, Pheniramine, Pyrilamine, Phenylephrine, Hydrocodone, Salicylamide, Caffeine, and Ascorbic Acid (Systemic)†, 1024
Chlorpheniramine, Phenylephrine, and Acetaminophen (Systemic), 366
Chlorpheniramine, Phenylephrine, Codeine, and Potassium Iodide (Systemic)†, 1024
Chlorpheniramine, Phenylephrine, and Dextromethorphan (Systemic)†, 1024
Chlorpheniramine, Phenylephrine, Dextromethorphan, Acetaminophen, and Salicylamide (Systemic)†, 1024
Chlorpheniramine, Phenylephrine, Dextromethorphan, and Guaifenesin (Systemic)†, 1024
Chlorpheniramine, Phenylephrine, Dextromethorphan, Guaifenesin, and Ammonium Chloride (Systemic)†, 1024
Chlorpheniramine, Phenylephrine, and Guaifenesin (Systemic)†, 1024
Chlorpheniramine, Phenylephrine, and Hydrocodone (Systemic)†, 1024
Chlorpheniramine, Phenylephrine, Hydrocodone, Acetaminophen, and Caffeine (Systemic)†, 1024
Chlorpheniramine, Phenylephrine, and Methscopolamine (Systemic)†, 373
Chlorpheniramine, Phenylephrine, Phenylpropanolamine, Atropine, Hyoscyamine, and Scopolamine (Systemic)†, 373
Chlorpheniramine, Phenylephrine, Phenylpropanolamine, Carbetapentane, and Potassium Guaiacolsulfonate (Systemic)†, 1024
Chlorpheniramine, Phenylephrine, Phenylpropanolamine, and Codeine (Systemic)†, 1024
Chlorpheniramine, Phenylephrine, Phenylpropanolamine, Dextromethorphan, Potassium Guaiacolsulfonate, and Ipecac (Systemic)†, 1024
Chlorpheniramine, Phenylephrine, Phenylpropanolamine, and Dihydrocodeine (Systemic)†, 1024

**Cold symptoms (treatment)** *(continued)*
   Chlorpheniramine, Phenylpropanolamine, and Acetaminophen (Systemic), 366
   Chlorpheniramine, Phenylpropanolamine, and Aspirin (Systemic), 366
   Chlorpheniramine, Phenylpropanolamine, and Caramiphen (Systemic)*, 1024
   Chlorpheniramine, Phenylpropanolamine, and Dextromethorphan (Systemic), 1024
   Chlorpheniramine, Phenylpropanolamine, Dextromethorphan, and Acetaminophen (Systemic)†, 1024
   Chlorpheniramine, Phenylpropanolamine, Dextromethorphan, and Aspirin (Systemic)†, 1024
   Chlorpheniramine, Phenylpropanolamine, and Guaifenesin (Systemic)*, 1024
   Chlorpheniramine, Phenylpropanolamine, Guaifenesin, and Acetaminophen (Systemic)†, 1024
   Chlorpheniramine, Phenylpropanolamine, Guaifenesin, Sodium Citrate, and Citric Acid (Systemic)†, 1024
   Chlorpheniramine, Phenyltoloxamine, Ephedrine, Codeine, and Guaiacol Carbonate (Systemic)*, 1024
   Chlorpheniramine, Phenyltoloxamine, Phenylpropanolamine, and Acetaminophen (Systemic)†, 366
   Chlorpheniramine, Pseudoephedrine, and Codeine (Systemic)†, 1024
   Chlorpheniramine, Pseudoephedrine, Codeine, and Acetaminophen (Systemic)*, 1024
   Chlorpheniramine, Pseudoephedrine, and Dextromethorphan (Systemic), 1024
   Chlorpheniramine, Pseudoephedrine, Dextromethorphan, and Acetaminophen (Systemic), 1024
   Chlorpheniramine, Pseudoephedrine, Dextromethorphan, and Guaifenesin (Systemic)*, 1024
   Chlorpheniramine, Pseudoephedrine, and Guaifenesin (Systemic)*, 1024
   Chlorpheniramine, Pseudoephedrine, and Hydrocodone (Systemic)†, 1024
   Chlorpheniramine, Pyrilamine, Phenylephrine, and Acetaminophen (Systemic)†, 366
   Codeine, Ammonium Chloride, and Guaifenesin (Systemic)*, 1024
   Codeine and Calcium Iodide (Systemic)†, 1024
   Codeine and Guaifenesin (Systemic)†, 1024
   Dexbrompheniramine, Pseudoephedrine, and Acetaminophen (Systemic)†, 366
   Dexchlorpheniramine, Pseudoephedrine, and Guaifenesin (Systemic)†, 1024
   Dextromethorphan and Acetaminophen (Systemic), 1024
   Dextromethorphan and Iodinated Glycerol (Systemic)†, 1024
   Diphenhydramine, Dextromethorphan, and Ammonium Chloride (Systemic)*, 1024
   Diphenhydramine, Phenylpropanolamine, and Aspirin (Systemic)†, 366
   Diphenhydramine, Pseudoephedrine, and Acetaminophen (Systemic), 366
   Diphenylpyraline, Phenylephrine, and Dextromethorphan (Systemic)*, 1024
   Diphenylpyraline, Phenylpropanolamine, Acetaminophen, and Caffeine (Systemic), 366
   Doxylamine, Codeine, and Acetaminophen (Systemic)*, 1024
   Doxylamine, Etafedrine, and Hydrocodone (Systemic)*, 1024
   Doxylamine, Phenylpropanolamine, Dextromethorphan, and Aspirin (Systemic)†, 1024
   Doxylamine, Pseudoephedrine, Dextromethorphan, and Acetaminophen (Systemic), 1024
   Ephedrine, Carbetapentane, and Guaifenesin (Systemic)*, 1024
   Ephedrine and Potassium Iodide (Systemic)†, 1024
   Hydrocodone and Guaifenesin (Systemic)†, 1024
   Hydrocodone and Homatropine (Systemic), 1024
   Hydrocodone and Potassium Guaiacolsulfonate (Systemic)†, 1024
   Hydromorphone and Guaifenesin (Systemic)†, 1024
   Pheniramine, Codeine, and Guaifenesin (Systemic)*, 1024
   Pheniramine, Phenylephrine, and Acetaminophen (Systemic), 366
   Pheniramine, Phenylephrine, Codeine, Sodium Citrate, Sodium Salicylate, and Caffeine (Systemic)†, 1024
   Pheniramine, Phenylephrine, and Dextromethorphan (Systemic)*, 1024
   Pheniramine, Phenylephrine, Phenylpropanolamine, Hydrocodone, and Guaifenesin (Systemic)†, 1024
   Pheniramine, Phenylephrine, Sodium Salicylate, and Caffeine (Systemic)†, 366

**Cold symptoms (treatment)** *(continued)*
   Pheniramine, Pyrilamine, Hydrocodone, Potassium Citrate, and Ascorbic Acid (Systemic)†, 1024
   Pheniramine, Pyrilamine, Phenylephrine, Phenylpropanolamine, and Hydrocodone (Systemic)†, 1024
   Pheniramine, Pyrilamine, Phenylpropanolamine, Acetaminophen, and Caffeine (Systemic), 366
   Pheniramine, Pyrilamine, Phenylpropanolamine, and Codeine (Systemic)*, 1024
   Pheniramine, Pyrilamine, Phenylpropanolamine, and Dextromethorphan (Systemic)*, 1024
   Pheniramine, Pyrilamine, Phenylpropanolamine, Dextromethorphan, and Ammonium Chloride (Systemic)†, 1024
   Pheniramine, Pyrilamine, Phenylpropanolamine, and Hydrocodone (Systemic)*, 1024
   Pheniramine, Pyrilamine, Phenylpropanolamine, Hydrocodone, and Guaifenesin (Systemic), 1024
   Phenylephrine and Codeine (Systemic)*, 1024
   Phenylephrine, Dextromethorphan, and Guaifenesin (Systemic)†, 1024
   Phenylephrine and Guaifenesin (Systemic)†, 1024
   Phenylephrine, Guaifenesin, Acetaminophen, Salicylamide, and Caffeine (Systemic)†, 1024
   Phenylephrine and Hydrocodone (Systemic)†, 1024
   Phenylephrine, Hydrocodone, and Guaifenesin (Systemic), 1024
   Phenylephrine, Phenylpropanolamine, Carbetapentane, and Potassium Guaiacolsulfonate (Systemic)†, 1024
   Phenylephrine, Phenylpropanolamine, and Guaifenesin (Systemic)†, 1024
   Phenylpropanolamine and Caramiphen (Systemic)†, 1024
   Phenylpropanolamine, Codeine, and Guaifenesin (Systemic)†, 1024
   Phenylpropanolamine and Dextromethorphan (Systemic)†, 1024
   Phenylpropanolamine, Dextromethorphan, and Acetaminophen (Systemic)†, 1024
   Phenylpropanolamine, Dextromethorphan, and Guaifenesin (Systemic), 1024
   Phenylpropanolamine, Dextromethorphan, Guaifenesin, and Acetaminophen (Systemic)†, 1024
   Phenylpropanolamine and Guaifenesin (Systemic), 1024
   Phenylpropanolamine and Hydrocodone (Systemic)†, 1024
   Phenylpropanolamine, Hydrocodone, Dextromethorphan, and Acetaminophen (Systemic), 1024
   Phenyltoloxamine and Hydrocodone (Systemic)*, 1024
   Phenyltoloxamine, Phenylpropanolamine, and Acetaminophen (Systemic), 366
   Promethazine and Codeine (Systemic)†, 1024
   Promethazine, Codeine, and Potassium Guaiacolsulfonate (Systemic)*, 1024
   Promethazine and Dextromethorphan (Systemic)†, 1024
   Promethazine, Phenylephrine, and Codeine (Systemic)†, 1024
   Promethazine, Phenylephrine, Codeine, and Potassium Guaiacolsulfonate (Systemic)*, 1024
   Promethazine, Phenylephrine, and Potassium Guaiacolsulfonate (Systemic)*, 1024
   Promethazine and Potassium Guaiacolsulfonate (Systemic)*, 1024
   Promethazine, Pseudoephedrine, and Dextromethorphan (Systemic)*, 1024
   Pseudoephedrine and Codeine (Systemic), 1024
   Pseudoephedrine, Codeine, and Guaifenesin (Systemic), 1024
   Pseudoephedrine and Dextromethorphan (Systemic), 1024
   Pseudoephedrine, Dextromethorphan, and Acetaminophen (Systemic), 1024
   Pseudoephedrine, Dextromethorphan, and Guaifenesin (Systemic), 1024
   Pseudoephedrine, Dextromethorphan, Guaifenesin, and Acetaminophen (Systemic), 1024
   Pseudoephedrine and Guaifenesin (Systemic), 1024
   Pseudoephedrine and Hydrocodone (Systemic)†, 1024
   Pseudoephedrine, Hydrocodone, and Guaifenesin (Systemic)†, 1024
   Pseudoephedrine, Hydrocodone, and Potassium Guaiacolsulfonate (Systemic)†, 1024
   Pyrilamine and Codeine (Systemic)†, 1024
   Pyrilamine, Phenylephrine, Aspirin, and Caffeine (Systemic), 366
   Pyrilamine, Phenylephrine, and Codeine (Systemic)†, 1024
   Pyrilamine, Phenylephrine, and Dextromethorphan (Systemic)†, 1024

**Cold symptoms (treatment)** *(continued)*
   Pyrilamine, Phenylephrine, and Hydrocodone (Systemic)†, 1024
   Pyrilamine, Phenylephrine, Hydrocodone, and Ammonium Chloride (Systemic)*, 1024
   Pyrilamine, Phenylpropanolamine, Acetaminophen, and Caffeine (Systemic)†, 366
   Pyrilamine, Phenylpropanolamine, Dextromethorphan, Guaifenesin, Potassium Citrate, and Citric Acid (Systemic)†, 1024
   Pyrilamine, Pseudoephedrine, Dextromethorphan, and Acetaminophen (Systemic)†, 1024
   Triprolidine, Pseudoephedrine, and Acetaminophen (Systemic), 366
   Triprolidine, Pseudoephedrine, and Codeine (Systemic), 1024
   Triprolidine, Pseudoephedrine, Codeine, and Guaifenesin (Systemic)*, 1024
   Triprolidine, Pseudoephedrine, and Dextromethorphan (Systemic)*, 1024
**Cold urticaria (treatment)**
   Cyproheptadine (Systemic), 325
**Colic, renal**—*See* Urologic disorders, symptoms
**Colic, ureteral**—*See* Urologic disorders, symptoms
**Colitis, antibiotic-associated (treatment)**
   Vancomycin (Oral-Local), 2916
**Colitis, antibiotic-associated pseudomembranous (treatment)**
   Bacitracin (Systemic), 3133‡
   [Metronidazole (Systemic)]1, 1996
**Colitis, mucous**—*See* Bowel syndrome, irritable
**Colitis, pseudomembranous (treatment)**
   Vancomycin (Oral-Local), 2916
**Colitis, regional**—*See* Bowel disease, inflammatory
**Colitis, ulcerative (treatment)**
   *See also* Bowel disease
   Betamethasone (Rectal)*, 973
   Budesonide (Rectal)*, 973
   Hydrocortisone (Rectal), 973
   Methylprednisolone, Rectal (Systemic), 998
   Tixocortol (Rectal)*, 973
**Colon, irritable**—*See* Bowel syndrome, irritable
**Colon, spastic**—*See* Bowel syndrome, irritable
**Common hookworm**—*See* Hookworm infection
**Common roundworm**—*See* Ascariasis
**Condyloma acuminata (treatment)**
   Interferon Alfa-2b, Recombinant (Systemic)[1], 1740
   Interferon Alfa-n1 (Ins) (Systemic)*, 1740
   Interferon Alfa-n3 (Systemic)†, 1740
   Podophyllum (Topical)†, 2341
**Condyloma acuminatum (treatment)**
   Imiquimod (Topical), 1685
   Interferon Beta-1a (Systemic), 3026
   Podofilox (Topical), 2339
   Podophyllum (Topical)†, 2341
**Congestion, conjunctival, during surgery (treatment)**
   [Epinephrine (Ophthalmic)][1], 1350
   Epinephrine Injection USP (Systemic), 651
**Congestion, eustachian tube (treatment)**
   Phenylephrine (Nasal), #
   Pseudoephedrine (Systemic), 2422
**Congestion, nasal (treatment)**
   Acrivastine and Pseudoephedrine (Systemic)†, 343
   Azatadine and Pseudoephedrine (Systemic), 343
   Brompheniramine and Phenylephrine (Systemic)†, 343
   Brompheniramine, Phenylephrine, and Phenylpropanolamine (Systemic), 343
   Brompheniramine and Phenylpropanolamine (Systemic), 343
   Brompheniramine, Phenylpropanolamine, and Acetaminophen (Systemic)†, 366
   Brompheniramine and Pseudoephedrine (Systemic)†, 343
   Brompheniramine, Pseudoephedrine, and Acetaminophen (Systemic)†, 366
   Carbinoxamine and Pseudoephedrine (Systemic)†, 343
   Chlorpheniramine, Phenindamine, and Phenylpropanolamine (Systemic)†, 343
   Chlorpheniramine and Phenylephrine (Systemic)†, 343
   Chlorpheniramine, Phenylephrine, and Acetaminophen (Systemic), 366
   Chlorpheniramine, Phenylephrine, and Methscopolamine (Systemic)†, 373
   Chlorpheniramine, Phenylephrine, and Phenylpropanolamine (Systemic)†, 343
   Chlorpheniramine and Phenylpropanolamine (Systemic), 343
   Chlorpheniramine, Phenylpropanolamine, and Acetaminophen (Systemic), 366
   Chlorpheniramine, Phenylpropanolamine, Acetaminophen, and Caffeine (Systemic)†, 366

**Congestion, nasal (treatment)** *(continued)*
  Chlorpheniramine, Phenylpropanolamine, and Aspirin (Systemic), 366
  Chlorpheniramine, Phenylpropanolamine, and Methscopolamine (Systemic)†, 373
  Chlorpheniramine, Phenyltoxamine, and Phenylephrine(Systemic)†, 343
  Chlorpheniramine, Phenyltoxamine, Phenylephrine, and Phenylpropanolamine (Systemic)†, 343
  Chlorpheniramine, Phenyltoxamine, Phenylpropanolamine, and Acetaminophen (Systemic)†, 366
  Chlorpheniramine and Pseudoephedrine (Systemic), 343
  Chlorpheniramine, Pseudoephedrine, and Acetaminophen (Systemic), 366
  Chlorpheniramine, Pseudoephedrine, and Methscopolamine (Systemic)†, 373
  Chlorpheniramine, Pyrilamine, and Phenylephrine (Systemic)†, 343
  Chlorpheniramine, Pyrilamine, Phenylephrine, and Acetaminophen (Systemic)†, 366
  Chlorpheniramine, Pyrilamine, Phenylephrine, andPhenylpropanolamine (Systemic)†, 343
  Chlorpheniramine, Pyrilamine, Phenylephrine, Phenylpropanolamine, and Acetaminophen (Systemic)†, 366
  Clemastine and Phenylpropanolamine (Systemic)†, 343
  Dexbrompheniramine and Pseudoephedrine (Systemic), 343
  Dexbrompheniramine, Pseudoephedrine, and Acetaminophen (Systemic)†, 366
  Diphenhydramine, Phenylpropanolamine, and Aspirin (Systemic)†, 366
  Diphenhydramine and Pseudoephedrine (Systemic), 343
  Diphenhydramine, Pseudoephedrine, and Acetaminophen (Systemic), 366
  Diphenylpyraline, Phenylpropanolamine, Acetaminophen, and Caffeine (Systemic), 366
  Ephedrine, Oral (Systemic), 651
  Loratadine and Pseudoephedrine (Systemic), 343
  Oxymetazoline (Nasal), #
  Pheniramine and Phenylephrine (Systemic), 343
  Pheniramine, Phenylephrine, and Acetaminophen (Systemic), 366
  Pheniramine, Phenylephrine, Sodium Salicylate, and Caffeine (Systemic)†, 366
  Pheniramine, Phenyltoxamine, Pyrilamine, and Phenylpropanolamine (Systemic)†, 343
  Pheniramine, Pyrilamine, and Phenylpropanolamine (Systemic), 343
  Pheniramine, Pyrilamine, Phenylpropanolamine, Acetaminophen, and Caffeine (Systemic), 366
  Phenylephrine (Nasal), #
  Phenylephrine, Phenylpropanolamine, and Acetaminophen (Systemic), 1180
  Phenylpropanolamine (Systemic)†, 2314
  Phenylpropanolamine and Acetaminophen (Systemic), 1180
  Phenylpropanolamine, Acetaminophen, and Aspirin (Systemic)†, 1180
  Phenyltoxamine, Phenylpropanolamine, and Acetaminophen (Systemic), 366
  Promethazine and Phenylephrine (Systemic)†, 343
  Pseudoephedrine (Systemic), 2422
  Pseudoephedrine and Guaifenesin (Systemic), 3033
  Pseudoephedrine and Ibuprofen (Systemic), 1180
  Pyrilamine, Phenylephrine, Aspirin, and Caffeine (Systemic), 366
  Pyrilamine, Phenylephrine, Acetaminophen, and Caffeine (Systemic)†, 366
  Triprolidine and Pseudoephedrine (Systemic), 343
  Triprolidine, Pseudoephedrine, and Acetaminophen (Systemic), 366
  Xylometazoline (Nasal), #, 3038
**Congestion, sinus (treatment)**
  Brompheniramine, Phenylpropanolamine, and Acetaminophen (Systemic)†, 366
  Brompheniramine, Pseudoephedrine, and Acetaminophen (Systemic)†, 366
  Chlorpheniramine, Phenylephrine, and Acetaminophen (Systemic), 366
  Chlorpheniramine, Phenylpropanolamine, and Acetaminophen (Systemic), 366
  Chlorpheniramine, Phenylpropanolamine, Acetaminophen, and Caffeine (Systemic)†, 366
  Chlorpheniramine, Phenylpropanolamine, and Aspirin (Systemic), 366
  Chlorpheniramine, Phenyltoxamine, Phenylpropanolamine, and Acetaminophen (Systemic)†, 366
  Chlorpheniramine, Pseudoephedrine, and Acetaminophen (Systemic), 366
  Chlorpheniramine, Pyrilamine, Phenylephrine, and Acetaminophen (Systemic)†, 366

**Congestion, sinus (treatment)** *(continued)*
  Chlorpheniramine, Pyrilamine, Phenylephrine, Phenylpropanolamine, and Acetaminophen (Systemic)†, 366
  Dexbrompheniramine, Pseudoephedrine, and Acetaminophen (Systemic)†, 366
  Diphenhydramine, Phenylpropanolamine, and Aspirin (Systemic)†, 366
  Diphenylpyraline, Phenylpropanolamine, Acetaminophen, and Caffeine (Systemic), 366
  Ephedrine, Oral (Systemic), 651
  [Oxymetazoline (Nasal)], #
  Pheniramine, Phenylephrine, and Acetaminophen (Systemic), 366
  Pheniramine, Phenylephrine, Sodium Salicylate, and Caffeine (Systemic)†, 366
  Pheniramine, Pyrilamine, Phenylpropanolamine, Acetaminophen, and Caffeine (Systemic), 366
  [Phenylephrine (Nasal)], #
  Phenylephrine, Phenylpropanolamine, and Acetaminophen (Systemic), 1180
  Phenylpropanolamine and Acetaminophen (Systemic), 1180
  Phenylpropanolamine, Acetaminophen, and Aspirin (Systemic)†, 1180
  Phenylpropanolamine, Acetaminophen, and Caffeine (Systemic), 1180
  Phenylpropanolamine, Acetaminophen, Salicylamide, and Caffeine (Systemic)†, 1180
  Phenylpropanolamine and Aspirin (Systemic), 1180
  Phenyltoxamine, Phenylpropanolamine, and Acetaminophen (Systemic), 366
  Pseudoephedrine (Systemic), 2422
  Pseudoephedrine and Acetaminophen (Systemic), 1180
  Pseudoephedrine and Aspirin (Systemic)†, 1180
  Pseudoephedrine and Ibuprofen (Systemic), 1180
  Pyrilamine, Phenylephrine, Aspirin, and Caffeine (Systemic), 366
  Pyrilamine, Phenylephrine, Acetaminophen, and Caffeine (Systemic)†, 366
  Triprolidine, Pseudoephedrine, and Acetaminophen (Systemic), 366
  [Xylometazoline (Nasal)], #
**Congestive heart failure (treatment)**
  *See also* related indications, e.g., Edema
  Amrinone (Systemic), 108
  [Benazepril (Systemic)]†, 177
  Captopril (Systemic), 177
  [Captopril and Hydrochlorothiazide (Systemic)]†, 187
  Carvedilol (Systemic), 790
  Digitoxin (Systemic), 1213
  Digoxin (Systemic), 1213
  Dobutamine (Parenteral-Systemic), 2669
  Dopamine (Parenteral-Systemic), 2669
  Enalapril (Systemic), 177
  [Enalapril and Hydrochlorothiazide (Systemic)]†, 187
  [Erythrityl Tetranitrate (Systemic)][1], 2129
  [Hydralazine (Systemic)][1], 1655
  [Isosorbide Dinitrate Capsules (Systemic)][1], 2129
  [Isosorbide Dinitrate Chewable Tablets USP (Systemic)], 2129
  [Isosorbide Dinitrate, Sublingual (Systemic)][1], 2129
  [Isosorbide Dinitrate Tablets USP (Systemic)][1], 2129
  Lisinopril (Systemic), 177
  [Lisinopril and Hydrochlorothiazide (Systemic)]†, 187
  Milrinone (Systemic), 2016
  [Nitroglycerin, Lingual (Systemic)][1], 2129
  Nitroglycerin, Parenteral (Systemic), 2129
  [Nitroglycerin, Sublingual (Systemic)][1], 2129
  [Nitroglycerin, Topical (Systemic)][1], 2129
  Nitroprusside (Systemic)[1], 2142
  Norepinephrine (Parenteral-Systemic), 2669
  [Pentaerythritol Tetranitrate Tablets USP (Systemic)][1], 2129
  [Phentolamine (Systemic)][1], #
  [Prazosin (Systemic)][1], 2370
  [Quinapril (Systemic)]†, 177
  [Ramipril (Systemic)]†, 177
**Congestive heart failure, post–myocardial infarction (treatment)**
  Trandolapril (Systemic), 2854
**Conjunctivitis, allergic (prophylaxis)**
  *See also* Allergic disorders, ophthalmic
  Acrivastine (Systemic)*†, 325
  Astemizole (Systemic), 325
  Azatadine (Systemic), 325
  Bromodiphenhydramine (Systemic)*†, 325
  Brompheniramine (Systemic), 325
  Carbinoxamine (Systemic)*†, 325
  Cetirizine (Systemic), 325
  Chlorpheniramine (Systemic), 325

**Conjunctivitis, allergic (prophylaxis)** *(continued)*
  Clemastine (Systemic), 325
  Cyproheptadine (Systemic), 325
  Dexchlorpheniramine (Systemic), 325
  Dimenhydrinate (Systemic), 325
  Diphenhydramine (Systemic), 325
  Diphenylpyraline (Systemic)*†, 325
  Doxylamine (Systemic)†, 325
  Hydroxyzine (Systemic), 325
  Loratadine (Systemic), 325
  Phenindamine (Systemic)†, 325
  Pyrilamine (Systemic)*†, 325
  Tripelennamine (Systemic), 325
  Triprolidine (Systemic)*†, 325
**Conjunctivitis, allergic (treatment)**
  *See also* Allergic disorders, ophthalmic
  Acrivastine (Systemic)*†, 325
  Astemizole (Systemic), 325
  Azatadine (Systemic), 325
  Betamethasone (Ophthalmic)*, 966
  Betamethasone, Oral (Systemic), 998
  Betamethasone, Parenteral (Systemic), 998
  Bromodiphenhydramine (Systemic)*†, 325
  Brompheniramine (Systemic), 325
  Carbinoxamine (Systemic)*†, 325
  Cetirizine (Systemic), 325
  Chlorpheniramine (Systemic), 325
  Clemastine (Systemic), 325
  Cortisone (Systemic), 998
  Cyproheptadine (Systemic), 325
  Dexamethasone (Ophthalmic), 966
  Dexamethasone, Oral (Systemic), 998
  Dexamethasone, Parenteral (Systemic), 998
  Dexchlorpheniramine (Systemic), 325
  Dimenhydrinate (Systemic), 325
  Diphenhydramine (Systemic), 325
  Diphenylpyraline (Systemic)*†, 325
  Doxylamine (Systemic)†, 325
  Emedastine (Ophthalmic), 1333
  Fluorometholone (Ophthalmic), 966
  Hydrocortisone (Ophthalmic)*, 966
  Hydrocortisone, Oral (Systemic), 998
  Hydrocortisone, Parenteral (Systemic), 998
  Hydroxyzine (Systemic), 325
  Ketorolac (Ophthalmic)1, 1809
  Loratadine (Systemic), 325
  Medrysone (Ophthalmic), 966
  Methdilazine (Systemic)†, 377
  Methylprednisolone, Oral (Systemic), 998
  Methylprednisolone, Parenteral (Systemic), 998
  Olopatadine (Ophthalmic), 2160
  Phenindamine (Systemic)†, 325
  Prednisolone (Ophthalmic), 966
  Prednisolone, Oral (Systemic), 998
  Prednisolone, Parenteral (Systemic), 998
  Prednisone (Systemic), 998
  Promethazine (Systemic), 377
  Pyrilamine (Systemic)*†, 325
  Triamcinolone, Oral (Systemic), 998
  Triamcinolone, Parenteral (Systemic), 998
  Trimeprazine (Systemic), 377
  Tripelennamine (Systemic), 325
  Triprolidine (Systemic)*†, 325
**Conjunctivitis, bacterial (treatment)**
  [Chloramphenicol (Ophthalmic)], #
  [Chlortetracycline (Ophthalmic)], 2763
  Ciprofloxacin (Ophthalmic), 868
  [Erythromycin (Ophthalmic)][1], 1364
  Framycetin (Ophthalmic)*, 3020
  Gentamicin (Ophthalmic), 1555
  Neomycin (Ophthalmic)*†, #
  [Neomycin, Polymyxin B, and Bacitracin (Ophthalmic)], #
  [Neomycin, Polymyxin B, and Gramicidin (Ophthalmic)], #
  Norfloxacin (Ophthalmic), #
  Ofloxacin (Ophthalmic)†, #
  Sulfacetamide (Ophthalmic), 2651
  Sulfisoxazole (Ophthalmic), 2651
  [Tetracycline (Ophthalmic)], 2763
  [Tobramycin (Ophthalmic)], #
**Conjunctivitis, chlamydial (treatment)**
  Erythromycin (Systemic), 1368
**Conjunctivitis, fungal (treatment)**
  Natamycin (Ophthalmic)†, #
**Conjunctivitis, inclusion (treatment)**
  Demeclocycline (Systemic), 2765
  Doxycycline (Systemic), 2765
  Minocycline (Systemic), 2765
  Oxytetracycline (Systemic)†, 2765
  Sulfadiazine (Systemic), 2653
  Sulfamethoxazole (Systemic), 2653
  Sulfisoxazole (Systemic), 2653
  Tetracycline (Systemic), 2765
**Conjunctivitis, neonatal (prophylaxis)**
  Erythromycin (Ophthalmic), 1364

**Conjunctivitis, seasonal allergic (treatment)**
See also Allergic disorders, ophthalmic
[Cromolyn (Ophthalmic)], 1120
Levocabastine (Ophthalmic), 3#, 3027
Loteprednol (Ophthalmic), 1887
**Conjunctivitis, vernal (treatment)**
Cromolyn (Ophthalmic)[1], 1120
Lodoxamide (Ophthalmic)†, #
**Connective tissue disease, mixed (treatment)**
[Betamethasone, Oral (Systemic)][1], 998
[Betamethasone, Parenteral (Systemic)][1], 998
[Cortisone (Systemic)][1], 998
[Dexamethasone, Oral (Systemic)][1], 998
[Dexamethasone, Parenteral (Systemic)][1], 998
[Hydrocortisone, Oral (Systemic)][1], 998
[Hydrocortisone, Parenteral (Systemic)][1], 998
[Methylprednisolone, Oral (Systemic)][1], 998
[Methylprednisolone, Parenteral (Systemic)][1], 998
[Prednisolone, Oral (Systemic)][1], 998
[Prednisolone, Parenteral (Systemic)][1], 998
[Prednisone (Systemic)][1], 998
[Triamcinolone, Oral (Systemic)][1], 998
[Triamcinolone, Parenteral (Systemic)][1], 998
**Constipation (prophylaxis)**
Docusate, Oral (Local), #
Magnesium Hydroxide and Mineral Oil (Local)†, #
Malt Soup Extract (Local)†, #
Malt Soup Extract and Psyllium (Local)†, #
Methylcellulose (Local)†, #
Mineral Oil and Glycerin (Local)*, #
Mineral Oil, Oral (Local), #
Poloxamer 188 (Local)†, #
Polycarbophil (Local), #
Psyllium (Local), #
Psyllium Hydrophilic Mucilloid (Local), #
Psyllium Hydrophilic Mucilloid and Carboxymethylcellulose (Local)†, #
**Constipation (treatment)**
Bisacodyl (Local), #
Bisacodyl and Docusate (Local)*, #
Casanthranol (Local)†, #
Casanthranol and Docusate (Local), #
Cascara Sagrada (Local)†, #
Cascara Sagrada and Aloe (Local)†, #
Cascara Sagrada and Phenolphthalein (Local)†, #
Castor Oil (Local), #
Danthron and Docusate (Local)*, #
Dehydrocholic Acid (Local)†, #
Dehydrocholic Acid and Docusate (Local)†, #
Dehydrocholic Acid, Docusate, and Phenolphthalein (Local)†, #
Docusate (Local), #, 3018
Glycerin (Local), #
Lactulose (Local), #
Magnesium Citrate (Local), #
Magnesium Hydroxide (Local), #
Magnesium Hydroxide and Cascara Sagrada (Local)†, #
Magnesium Hydroxide and Mineral Oil (Local)†, #
Magnesium Oxide (Local)†, #
Magnesium Sulfate (Local), #
Malt Soup Extract (Local)†, #
Malt Soup Extract and Psyllium (Local)†, #
Methylcellulose (Local)†, #
Mineral Oil (Local), #
Mineral Oil and Glycerin (Local)*, #
Mineral Oil, Glycerin, and Phenolphthalein (Local)*, #
Mineral Oil and Phenolphthalein (Local)†, #
Phenolphthalein (Local), #
Phenolphthalein and Docusate (Local), #
Phenolphthalein and Senna (Local)*, #
Poloxamer 188 (Local)†, #
Polycarbophil (Local), #
Potassium Bitartrate and Sodium Bicarbonate (Local)†, #
Psyllium (Local), #
Psyllium Hydrophilic Mucilloid (Local), #
Psyllium Hydrophilic Mucilloid and Carboxymethylcellulose (Local)†, #
Psyllium Hydrophilic Mucilloid and Senna (Local)*, #
Psyllium Hydrophilic Mucilloid and Sennosides (Local)†, #
Psyllium and Senna (Local)†, #
Senna (Local), #
Sennosides (Local), #
Sennosides and Docusate (Local), #
Sodium Phosphate (Local)†, #
**Constipation, opioid-induced (treatment)**
Methylnaltrexone (Systemic), 3154‡
**Contraception, emergency postcoital**
[Levonorgestrel and Ethinyl Estradiol (Systemic)], 1397
[Norgestrel and Ethinyl Estradiol (Systemic)], 1397

**Convulsions (treatment)**
See also Epilepsy
Amobarbital, Parenteral (Systemic), 518
[Atracurium (Systemic)]1, 2098
[Gallamine (Systemic)], 2098
Metocurine (Systemic), 2098
[Pancuronium (Systemic)][1], 2098
Paraldehyde (Systemic), #
Pentobarbital, Parenteral (Systemic), 518
Phenobarbital, Parenteral (Systemic), 518
Secobarbital, Parenteral (Systemic), 518
[Succinylcholine (Systemic)], 2098
[Thiamylal, Parenteral (Systemic)][1], 161
Thiopental, Parenteral (Systemic), 161
Tubocurarine (Systemic), 2098
[Vecuronium (Systemic)][1], 2098
**Convulsions (treatment adjunct)**
[Clonazepam (Systemic)][1], 556
Diazepam (Systemic)[1], 556
**COPD**—See Chronic obstructive pulmonary disease
**Copper deficiency (prophylaxis)**
Copper Gluconate (Systemic)†, 952
Cupric Sulfate (Systemic)†, 952
**Copper deficiency (treatment)**
Copper Gluconate (Systemic)†, 952
Cupric Sulfate (Systemic)†, 952
**Coproporphyria, hereditary (treatment)**
Hemin (Systemic), 3022, 3144‡, 3145
Histrelin (Systemic), 3145‡
**Corneal cysteine accumulation in cystinosis patients (treatment)**
Cysteamine Hydrochloride (Systemic), 3139‡
**Corneal epithelial defects (treatment)**
Epidermal Growth Factor (Human) (Ophthalmic), 3141‡
Fibronectin (Human Plasma Derived), 3143‡
**Corneal epithelial regeneration**
Epidermal Growth Factor (Human) (Ophthalmic), 3141‡
Urogastrone (Ophthalmic), 3171‡
**Corneal erosions, recurrent (treatment)**
Dehydrex (Ophthalmic), 3139‡
Hydroxypropyl Cellulose (Ophthalmic)[1], #
[Hydroxypropyl Methylcellulose (Ophthalmic)][1], #
**Corneal graft rejection (prophylaxis)**
Cyclosporine (Ophthalmic), 3138‡
**Corneal injuries (treatment)**
Betamethasone (Ophthalmic)*, 966
Dexamethasone (Ophthalmic), 966
Fluorometholone (Ophthalmic), 966
Hydrocortisone (Ophthalmic)*, 966
Prednisolone (Ophthalmic), 966
**Corneal sensitivity, decreased (treatment)**
Hydroxypropyl Cellulose (Ophthalmic), #
[Hydroxypropyl Methylcellulose (Ophthalmic)][1], #
**Corneal ulcers (treatment)**
Cyclosporine (Ophthalmic), 3138‡
Matrix Metalloproteinase Inhibitor (Ophthalmic), 3153
**Corneal ulcers, bacterial (treatment)**
Ciprofloxacin (Ophthalmic), 868
Ofloxacin (Ophthalmic), 3156
**Corneal ulcers, nonhealing (treatment)**
Fibronectin (Human Plasma Derived), 3143‡
**Corns (treatment)**
Resorcinol (Topical), 1#
**Coronary artery disease (diagnosis)**
See also Cardiac imaging, radionuclide; Cardiac imaging, positron emission tomographic
Ammonia N 13 (Systemic)*†, 91
Arbutamine (Systemic), 464
[Rubidium Rb 82 (Systemic)]†, 2536
Thallous Chloride Tl 201 (Systemic), 2781
**Coronary artery disease, atherosclerotic**—See Angina pectoris; Heart disease, ischemic
**Corpus luteum insufficiency (treatment)**
[Chorionic Gonadotropin (Systemic)][1], 858
[Clomiphene (Systemic)][1], 903
[Progesterone (Systemic)][1], 2400
**Cough (treatment)**
See also Cough and nasal congestion
Benzonatate (Systemic), #
Bromodiphenhydramine and Codeine (Systemic)†, 1024
Bromodiphenhydramine, Diphenhydramine, Codeine, Ammonium Chloride, and Potassium Guaiacolsulfonate (Systemic)*, 1024
Brompheniramine, Phenylephrine, Phenylpropanolamine, and Codeine (Systemic)*, 1024
Brompheniramine, Phenylephrine, Phenylpropanolamine, Codeine, and Guaifenesin (Systemic)*, 1024
Brompheniramine, Phenylephrine, Phenylpropanolamine, and Dextromethorphan (Systemic)*, 1024

**Cough (treatment)** (continued)
Brompheniramine, Phenylephrine, Phenylpropanolamine, Dextromethorphan, Potassium Guaiacolsulfonate, and Ipecac (Systemic), 1024
Brompheniramine, Phenylephrine, Phenylpropanolamine, and Guaifenesin (Systemic)*, 1024
Brompheniramine, Phenylephrine, Phenylpropanolamine, Hydrocodone, and Guaifenesin (Systemic)*, 1024
Brompheniramine, Phenylpropanolamine, and Codeine (Systemic)†, 1024
Brompheniramine, Phenylpropanolamine, and Dextromethorphan (Systemic)†, 1024
Brompheniramine, Pseudoephedrine, and Dextromethorphan (Systemic)†, 1024
Carbinoxamine, Pseudoephedrine, and Dextromethorphan (Systemic)†, 1024
Chlophedianol (Systemic)*, #
Chlorpheniramine and Codeine (Systemic)*, 1024
Chlorpheniramine and Dextromethorphan (Systemic)†, 1024
Chlorpheniramine, Ephedrine, and Guaifenesin (Systemic)†, 1024
Chlorpheniramine, Ephedrine, Phenylephrine, and Carbetapentane (Systemic)†, 1024
Chlorpheniramine, Ephedrine, Phenylephrine, Dextromethorphan, Ammonium Chloride, and Ipecac (Systemic)†, 1024
Chlorpheniramine and Hydrocodone (Systemic)†, 1024
Chlorpheniramine, Phenindamine, Phenylephrine, Dextromethorphan, Acetaminophen, Salicylamide, Caffeine, and Ascorbic Acid (Systemic)†, 1024
Chlorpheniramine, Pheniramine, Pyrilamine, Phenylephrine, Hydrocodone, Salicylamide, Caffeine, and Ascorbic Acid (Systemic)†, 1024
Chlorpheniramine, Phenylephrine, Codeine, and Ammonium Chloride (Systemic)†, 1024
Chlorpheniramine, Phenylephrine, Codeine, and Potassium Iodide (Systemic)†, 1024
Chlorpheniramine, Phenylephrine, and Dextromethorphan (Systemic)†, 1024
Chlorpheniramine, Phenylephrine, Dextromethorphan, Acetaminophen, and Salicylamide (Systemic)†, 1024
Chlorpheniramine, Phenylephrine, Dextromethorphan, and Guaifenesin (Systemic)†, 1024
Chlorpheniramine, Phenylephrine, Dextromethorphan, Guaifenesin, and Ammonium Chloride (Systemic)†, 1024
Chlorpheniramine, Phenylephrine, and Guaifenesin (Systemic)†, 1024
Chlorpheniramine, Phenylephrine, and Hydrocodone (Systemic)†, 1024
Chlorpheniramine, Phenylephrine, Hydrocodone, Acetaminophen, and Caffeine (Systemic)†, 1024
Chlorpheniramine, Phenylephrine, Phenylpropanolamine, Carbetapentane, and Potassium Guaiacolsulfonate (Systemic)†, 1024
Chlorpheniramine, Phenylephrine, Phenylpropanolamine, and Codeine (Systemic)†, 1024
Chlorpheniramine, Phenylephrine, Phenylpropanolamine, and Dextromethorphan (Systemic)†, 1024
Chlorpheniramine, Phenylephrine, Phenylpropanolamine, Dextromethorphan, Potassium Guaiacolsulfonate, and Ipecac (Systemic)†, 1024
Chlorpheniramine, Phenylephrine, Phenylpropanolamine, and Dihydrocodeine (Systemic)†, 1024
Chlorpheniramine, Phenylpropanolamine, and Caramiphen (Systemic)*, 1024
Chlorpheniramine, Phenylpropanolamine, and Dextromethorphan (Systemic), 1024
Chlorpheniramine, Phenylpropanolamine, Dextromethorphan, and Acetaminophen (Systemic)†, 1024
Chlorpheniramine, Phenylpropanolamine, Dextromethorphan, Acetaminophen, and Caffeine (Systemic), 1024
Chlorpheniramine, Phenylpropanolamine, Dextromethorphan, and Aspirin (Systemic)†, 1024
Chlorpheniramine, Phenylpropanolamine, and Guaifenesin (Systemic)*, 1024
Chlorpheniramine, Phenylpropanolamine, Guaifenesin, and Acetaminophen (Systemic)†, 1024
Chlorpheniramine, Phenylpropanolamine, Guaifenesin, Sodium Citrate, and Citric Acid (Systemic)†, 1024
Chlorpheniramine, Phenyltoloxamine, Ephedrine, Codeine, and Guaiacol Carbonate (Systemic)*, 1024
Chlorpheniramine, Pseudoephedrine, and Codeine (Systemic)†, 1024
Chlorpheniramine, Pseudoephedrine, Codeine, and Acetaminophen (Systemic)*, 1024

**Cough (treatment)** *(continued)*
Chlorpheniramine, Pseudoephedrine, and Dextromethorphan (Systemic), 1024
Chlorpheniramine, Pseudoephedrine, Dextromethorphan, and Acetaminophen (Systemic), 1024
Chlorpheniramine, Pseudoephedrine, Dextromethorphan, and Guaifenesin (Systemic)*, 1024
Chlorpheniramine, Pseudoephedrine, and Guaifenesin (Systemic)*, 1024
Chlorpheniramine, Pseudoephedrine, and Hydrocodone (Systemic)†, 1024
Codeine, Ammonium Chloride, and Guaifenesin (Systemic)*, 1024
Codeine and Calcium Iodide (Systemic)†, 1024
Codeine and Guaifenesin (Systemic)†, 1024
Codeine and Iodinated Glycerol (Systemic)†, 1024
Codeine, Oral (Systemic), 2168
Dexchlorpheniramine, Pseudoephedrine, and Guaifenesin (Systemic)†, 1024
Dextromethorphan (Systemic), 1191
Dextromethorphan and Acetaminophen (Systemic), 1024
Dextromethorphan and Guaifenesin (Systemic), 1024, 3017
Dextromethorphan and Iodinated Glycerol (Systemic)†, 1024
Diphenhydramine, Codeine, and Ammonium Chloride (Systemic)*, 1024
Diphenhydramine, Dextromethorphan, and Ammonium Chloride (Systemic)*, 1024
Diphenhydramine Hydrochloride Syrup (Systemic), 325
Diphenhydramine, Phenylephrine, and Dextromethorphan (Systemic), 1024
Diphenylpyraline, Phenylephrine, and Dextromethorphan (Systemic)*, 1024
Doxylamine, Codeine, and Acetaminophen (Systemic)*, 1024
Doxylamine, Etafedrine, and Hydrocodone (Systemic)*, 1024
Doxylamine, Phenylpropanolamine, Dextromethorphan, and Aspirin (Systemic)†, 1024
Doxylamine, Pseudoephedrine, Dextromethorphan, and Acetaminophen (Systemic), 1024
Ephedrine, Carbetapentane, and Guaifenesin (Systemic)*, 1024
Ephedrine and Guaifenesin (Systemic)†, 1024
Ephedrine and Potassium Iodide (Systemic)†, 1024
Guaifenesin (Systemic), 1588
Hydrocodone (Systemic)*, 2168
Hydrocodone and Guaifenesin (Systemic)†, 1024
Hydrocodone and Homatropine (Systemic), 1024
Hydrocodone and Potassium Guaiacolsulfonate (Systemic)†, 1024
Hydromorphone (Systemic), 2168
Hydromorphone and Guaifenesin (Systemic)†, 1024
[Methadone (Systemic)], 2168
[Morphine (Systemic)], 2168
Pheniramine, Codeine, and Guaifenesin (Systemic)*, 1024
Pheniramine, Phenylephrine, Codeine, Sodium Citrate, Sodium Salicylate, and Caffeine (Systemic)†, 1024
Pheniramine, Phenylephrine, and Dextromethorphan (Systemic)*, 1024
Pheniramine, Phenylephrine, Phenylpropanolamine, Hydrocodone, and Guaifenesin (Systemic), 1024
Pheniramine, Pyrilamine, Hydrocodone, Potassium Citrate, and Ascorbic Acid (Systemic)†, 1024
Pheniramine, Pyrilamine, Phenylephrine, Phenylpropanolamine, and Hydrocodone (Systemic)†, 1024
Pheniramine, Pyrilamine, Phenylpropanolamine, and Codeine (Systemic)*, 1024
Pheniramine, Pyrilamine, Phenylpropanolamine, and Dextromethorphan (Systemic)*, 1024
Pheniramine, Pyrilamine, Phenylpropanolamine, Dextromethorphan, and Ammonium Chloride (Systemic)†, 1024
Pheniramine, Pyrilamine, Phenylpropanolamine, and Hydrocodone (Systemic)*, 1024
Pheniramine, Pyrilamine, Phenylpropanolamine, Hydrocodone, and Guaifenesin (Systemic), 1024
Phenylephrine and Codeine (Systemic)*, 1024
Phenylephrine, Dextromethorphan, and Guaifenesin (Systemic)†, 1024
Phenylephrine and Guaifenesin (Systemic)†, 1024
Phenylephrine, Guaifenesin, Acetaminophen, Salicylamide, and Caffeine (Systemic)†, 1024
Phenylephrine and Hydrocodone (Systemic), 1024
Phenylephrine, Hydrocodone, and Guaifenesin (Systemic), 1024

**Cough (treatment)** *(continued)*
Phenylephrine, Phenylpropanolamine, Carbetapentane, and Potassium Guaiacolsulfonate (Systemic)†, 1024
Phenylephrine, Phenylpropanolamine, and Guaifenesin (Systemic)†, 1024
Phenylpropanolamine and Caramiphen (Systemic)†, 1024
Phenylpropanolamine, Codeine, and Guaifenesin (Systemic)†, 1024
Phenylpropanolamine and Dextromethorphan (Systemic)†, 1024
Phenylpropanolamine, Dextromethorphan, and Acetaminophen (Systemic), 1024
Phenylpropanolamine, Dextromethorphan, and Guaifenesin (Systemic)†, 1024
Phenylpropanolamine, Dextromethorphan, Guaifenesin, and Acetaminophen (Systemic)†, 1024
Phenylpropanolamine and Guaifenesin (Systemic), 1024
Phenylpropanolamine and Hydrocodone (Systemic)†, 1024
Phenylpropanolamine, Hydrocodone, Dextromethorphan, and Acetaminophen (Systemic), 1024
Phenyltoloxamine and Hydrocodone (Systemic)*, 1024
Promethazine and Codeine (Systemic)†, 1024
Promethazine, Codeine, and Potassium Guaiacolsulfonate (Systemic)*, 1024
Promethazine and Dextromethorphan (Systemic)†, 1024
Promethazine, Phenylephrine, and Codeine (Systemic)†, 1024
Promethazine, Phenylephrine, Codeine, and Potassium Guaiacolsulfonate (Systemic)*, 1024
Promethazine, Phenylephrine, and Potassium Guaiacolsulfonate (Systemic)*, 1024
Promethazine and Potassium Guaiacolsulfonate (Systemic)*, 1024
Promethazine, Pseudoephedrine, and Dextromethorphan (Systemic)*, 1024
Pseudoephedrine and Codeine (Systemic), 1024
Pseudoephedrine, Codeine, and Guaifenesin (Systemic), 1024
Pseudoephedrine and Dextromethorphan (Systemic), 1024
Pseudoephedrine, Dextromethorphan, and Acetaminophen (Systemic), 1024
Pseudoephedrine, Dextromethorphan, and Guaifenesin (Systemic), 1024
Pseudoephedrine, Dextromethorphan, Guaifenesin, and Acetaminophen (Systemic), 1024
Pseudoephedrine and Guaifenesin (Systemic), 1024, 3033
Pseudoephedrine and Hydrocodone (Systemic)†, 1024
Pseudoephedrine, Hydrocodone, and Guaifenesin (Systemic)†, 1024
Pseudoephedrine, Hydrocodone, and Potassium Guaiacolsulfonate (Systemic)†, 1024
Pyrilamine and Codeine (Systemic)†, 1024
Pyrilamine, Phenylephrine, and Codeine (Systemic)†, 1024
Pyrilamine, Phenylephrine, and Dextromethorphan (Systemic)†, 1024
Pyrilamine, Phenylephrine, and Hydrocodone (Systemic)†, 1024
Pyrilamine, Phenylephrine, Hydrocodone, and Ammonium Chloride (Systemic)*, 1024
Pyrilamine, Phenylpropanolamine, Dextromethorphan, Guaifenesin, Potassium Citrate, and Citric Acid (Systemic)†, 1024
Pyrilamine, Pseudoephedrine, Dextromethorphan, and Acetaminophen (Systemic)†, 1024
Triprolidine, Pseudoephedrine, and Codeine (Systemic), 1024
Triprolidine, Pseudoephedrine, Codeine, and Guaifenesin (Systemic)*, 1024
Triprolidine, Pseudoephedrine, and Dextromethorphan (Systemic)*, 1024

**Cough and nasal congestion (treatment)**
Bromodiphenhydramine and Codeine (Systemic)†, 1024
Bromodiphenhydramine, Diphenhydramine, Codeine, Ammonium Chloride, and Potassium Guaiacolsulfonate (Systemic)*, 1024
Brompheniramine, Phenylephrine, Phenylpropanolamine, and Codeine (Systemic)*, 1024
Brompheniramine, Phenylephrine, Phenylpropanolamine, Codeine, and Guaifenesin (Systemic)*, 1024
Brompheniramine, Phenylephrine, Phenylpropanolamine, and Dextromethorphan (Systemic)*, 1024
Brompheniramine, Phenylephrine, Phenylpropanolamine, Dextromethorphan, Potassium Guaiacolsulfonate, and Ipecac (Systemic), 1024

**Cough and nasal congestion (treatment)** *(continued)*
Brompheniramine, Phenylephrine, Phenylpropanolamine, and Guaifenesin (Systemic)*, 1024
Brompheniramine, Phenylephrine, Phenylpropanolamine, Hydrocodone, and Guaifenesin (Systemic)*, 1024
Brompheniramine, Phenylpropanolamine, and Codeine (Systemic)†, 1024
Brompheniramine, Phenylpropanolamine, and Dextromethorphan (Systemic)*, 1024
Brompheniramine, Pseudoephedrine, and Dextromethorphan (Systemic)†, 1024
Carbinoxamine, Pseudoephedrine, and Dextromethorphan (Systemic)†, 1024
Chlorpheniramine and Codeine (Systemic)*, 1024
Chlorpheniramine and Dextromethorphan (Systemic)†, 1024
Chlorpheniramine, Ephedrine, and Guaifenesin (Systemic)†, 1024
Chlorpheniramine, Ephedrine, Phenylephrine, and Carbetapentane (Systemic)†, 1024
Chlorpheniramine, Ephedrine, Phenylephrine, Dextromethorphan, Ammonium Chloride, and Ipecac (Systemic)†, 1024
Chlorpheniramine and Hydrocodone (Systemic)†, 1024
Chlorpheniramine, Phenindamine, Phenylephrine, Dextromethorphan, Acetaminophen, Salicylamide, Caffeine, and Ascorbic Acid (Systemic)†, 1024
Chlorpheniramine, Pheniramine, Pyrilamine, Phenylephrine, Hydrocodone, Salicylamide, Caffeine, and Ascorbic Acid (Systemic)†, 1024
Chlorpheniramine, Phenylephrine, Codeine, and Ammonium Chloride (Systemic)*, 1024
Chlorpheniramine, Phenylephrine, Codeine, and Potassium Iodide (Systemic)†, 1024
Chlorpheniramine, Phenylephrine, and Dextromethorphan (Systemic)†, 1024
Chlorpheniramine, Phenylephrine, Dextromethorphan, Acetaminophen, and Salicylamide (Systemic)†, 1024
Chlorpheniramine, Phenylephrine, Dextromethorphan, and Guaifenesin (Systemic)†, 1024
Chlorpheniramine, Phenylephrine, Dextromethorphan, Guaifenesin, and Ammonium Chloride (Systemic)†, 1024
Chlorpheniramine, Phenylephrine, and Guaifenesin (Systemic)†, 1024
Chlorpheniramine, Phenylephrine, and Hydrocodone (Systemic)†, 1024
Chlorpheniramine, Phenylephrine, Hydrocodone, Acetaminophen, and Caffeine (Systemic)†, 1024
Chlorpheniramine, Phenylephrine, Phenylpropanolamine, Carbetapentane, and Potassium Guaiacolsulfonate (Systemic)†, 1024
Chlorpheniramine, Phenylephrine, Phenylpropanolamine, and Codeine (Systemic)†, 1024
Chlorpheniramine, Phenylephrine, Phenylpropanolamine, and Dextromethorphan (Systemic), 1024
Chlorpheniramine, Phenylephrine, Phenylpropanolamine, Dextromethorphan, Potassium Guaiacolsulfonate, and Ipecac (Systemic)†, 1024
Chlorpheniramine, Phenylephrine, Phenylpropanolamine, and Dihydrocodeine (Systemic)†, 1024
Chlorpheniramine, Phenylpropanolamine, and Caramiphen (Systemic)*, 1024
Chlorpheniramine, Phenylpropanolamine, and Dextromethorphan (Systemic), 1024
Chlorpheniramine, Phenylpropanolamine, Dextromethorphan, and Acetaminophen (Systemic)†, 1024
Chlorpheniramine, Phenylpropanolamine, Dextromethorphan, Acetaminophen, and Caffeine (Systemic), 1024
Chlorpheniramine, Phenylpropanolamine, Dextromethorphan, and Aspirin (Systemic)†, 1024
Chlorpheniramine, Phenylpropanolamine, and Guaifenesin (Systemic)*, 1024
Chlorpheniramine, Phenylpropanolamine, Guaifenesin, and Acetaminophen (Systemic)†, 1024
Chlorpheniramine, Phenylpropanolamine, Guaifenesin, Sodium Citrate, and Citric Acid (Systemic)†, 1024
Chlorpheniramine, Phenyltoloxamine, Ephedrine, Codeine, and Guaiacol Carbonate (Systemic)*, 1024
Chlorpheniramine, Pseudoephedrine, and Codeine (Systemic)†, 1024
Chlorpheniramine, Pseudoephedrine, Codeine, and Acetaminophen (Systemic)*, 1024
Chlorpheniramine, Pseudoephedrine, and Dextromethorphan (Systemic), 1024
Chlorpheniramine, Pseudoephedrine, Dextromethorphan, and Acetaminophen (Systemic), 1024

**Cough and nasal congestion (treatment)** *(continued)*
- Chlorpheniramine, Pseudoephedrine, Dextromethorphan, and Guaifenesin (Systemic)*, 1024
- Chlorpheniramine, Pseudoephedrine, and Guaifenesin (Systemic)*, 1024
- Chlorpheniramine, Pseudoephedrine, and Hydrocodone (Systemic)†, 1024
- Codeine, Ammonium Chloride, and Guaifenesin (Systemic)*, 1024
- Codeine and Calcium Iodide (Systemic)†, 1024
- Codeine and Guaifenesin (Systemic)†, 1024
- Codeine and Iodinated Glycerol (Systemic)†, 1024
- Dexchlorpheniramine, Pseudoephedrine, and Guaifenesin (Systemic)†, 1024
- Dextromethorphan and Acetaminophen (Systemic), 1024
- Dextromethorphan and Guaifenesin (Systemic), 1024
- Dextromethorphan and Iodinated Glycerol (Systemic)†, 1024
- Diphenhydramine, Codeine, and Ammonium Chloride (Systemic)*, 1024
- Diphenhydramine, Dextromethorphan, and Ammonium Chloride (Systemic)*, 1024
- Diphenhydramine, Phenylephrine, and Dextromethorphan (Systemic), 1024
- Diphenylpyraline, Phenylephrine, and Dextromethorphan (Systemic)*, 1024
- Doxylamine, Codeine, and Acetaminophen (Systemic)*, 1024
- Doxylamine, Etafedrine, and Hydrocodone (Systemic)*, 1024
- Doxylamine, Phenylpropanolamine, Dextromethorphan, and Aspirin (Systemic)†, 1024
- Doxylamine, Pseudoephedrine, Dextromethorphan, and Acetaminophen (Systemic), 1024
- Ephedrine, Carbetapentane, and Guaifenesin (Systemic)*, 1024
- Ephedrine and Guaifenesin (Systemic)†, 1024
- Ephedrine and Potassium Iodide (Systemic)†, 1024
- Hydrocodone and Guaifenesin (Systemic)†, 1024
- Hydrocodone and Homatropine (Systemic), 1024
- Hydrocodone and Potassium Guaiacolsulfonate (Systemic)†, 1024
- Hydromorphone and Guaifenesin (Systemic)†, 1024
- Pheniramine, Codeine, and Guaifenesin (Systemic)*, 1024
- Pheniramine, Phenylephrine, Codeine, Sodium Citrate, Sodium Salicylate, and Caffeine (Systemic)†, 1024
- Pheniramine, Phenylephrine, and Dextromethorphan (Systemic)*, 1024
- Pheniramine, Phenylephrine, Phenylpropanolamine, Hydrocodone, and Guaifenesin (Systemic)†, 1024
- Pheniramine, Pyrilamine, Hydrocodone, Potassium Citrate, and Ascorbic Acid (Systemic)†, 1024
- Pheniramine, Pyrilamine, Phenylephrine, Phenylpropanolamine, and Hydrocodone (Systemic)†, 1024
- Pheniramine, Pyrilamine, Phenylpropanolamine, and Codeine (Systemic)*, 1024
- Pheniramine, Pyrilamine, Phenylpropanolamine, and Dextromethorphan (Systemic)*, 1024
- Pheniramine, Pyrilamine, Phenylpropanolamine, Dextromethorphan, and Ammonium Chloride (Systemic)†, 1024
- Pheniramine, Pyrilamine, Phenylpropanolamine, and Hydrocodone (Systemic)*, 1024
- Pheniramine, Pyrilamine, Phenylpropanolamine, Hydrocodone, and Guaifenesin (Systemic), 1024
- Phenylephrine and Codeine (Systemic)*, 1024
- Phenylephrine, Dextromethorphan, and Guaifenesin (Systemic)†, 1024
- Phenylephrine and Guaifenesin (Systemic)†, 1024
- Phenylephrine, Guaifenesin, Acetaminophen, Salicylamide, and Caffeine (Systemic)†, 1024
- Phenylephrine and Hydrocodone (Systemic), 1024
- Phenylephrine, Hydrocodone, and Guaifenesin (Systemic), 1024
- Phenylephrine, Phenylpropanolamine, Carbetapentane, and Potassium Guaiacolsulfonate (Systemic)†, 1024
- Phenylephrine, Phenylpropanolamine, and Guaifenesin (Systemic)†, 1024
- Phenylpropanolamine and Caramiphen (Systemic)†, 1024
- Phenylpropanolamine, Codeine, and Guaifenesin (Systemic)†, 1024
- Phenylpropanolamine and Dextromethorphan (Systemic)†, 1024
- Phenylpropanolamine, Dextromethorphan, and Acetaminophen (Systemic)†, 1024

**Cough and nasal congestion (treatment)** *(continued)*
- Phenylpropanolamine, Dextromethorphan, and Guaifenesin (Systemic)†, 1024
- Phenylpropanolamine, Dextromethorphan, Guaifenesin, and Acetaminophen (Systemic)†, 1024
- Phenylpropanolamine and Guaifenesin (Systemic), 1024
- Phenylpropanolamine and Hydrocodone (Systemic)†, 1024
- Phenylpropanolamine, Hydrocodone, Dextromethorphan, and Acetaminophen (Systemic), 1024
- Phenyltoloxamine and Hydrocodone (Systemic)*, 1024
- Promethazine and Codeine (Systemic)†, 1024
- Promethazine, Codeine, and Potassium Guaiacolsulfonate (Systemic)*, 1024
- Promethazine and Dextromethorphan (Systemic)†, 1024
- Promethazine, Phenylephrine, and Codeine (Systemic)†, 1024
- Promethazine, Phenylephrine, Codeine, and Potassium Guaiacolsulfonate (Systemic)*, 1024
- Promethazine, Phenylephrine, and Potassium Guaiacolsulfonate (Systemic)*, 1024
- Promethazine and Potassium Guaiacolsulfonate (Systemic)*, 1024
- Promethazine, Pseudoephedrine, and Dextromethorphan (Systemic)*, 1024
- Pseudoephedrine and Codeine (Systemic), 1024
- Pseudoephedrine, Codeine, and Guaifenesin (Systemic), 1024
- Pseudoephedrine and Dextromethorphan (Systemic), 1024
- Pseudoephedrine, Dextromethorphan, and Acetaminophen (Systemic), 1024
- Pseudoephedrine, Dextromethorphan, and Guaifenesin (Systemic), 1024
- Pseudoephedrine, Dextromethorphan, Guaifenesin, and Acetaminophen (Systemic), 1024
- Pseudoephedrine and Guaifenesin (Systemic), 1024
- Pseudoephedrine and Hydrocodone (Systemic)†, 1024
- Pseudoephedrine, Hydrocodone, and Guaifenesin (Systemic)†, 1024
- Pseudoephedrine, Hydrocodone, and Potassium Guaiacolsulfonate (Systemic)†, 1024
- Pyrilamine and Codeine (Systemic)†, 1024
- Pyrilamine, Phenylephrine, and Codeine (Systemic)†, 1024
- Pyrilamine, Phenylephrine, and Dextromethorphan (Systemic)†, 1024
- Pyrilamine, Phenylephrine, and Hydrocodone (Systemic)†, 1024
- Pyrilamine, Phenylephrine, Hydrocodone, and Ammonium Chloride (Systemic)*, 1024
- Pyrilamine, Phenylpropanolamine, Dextromethorphan, Guaifenesin, Potassium Citrate, and Citric Acid (Systemic)†, 1024
- Pyrilamine, Pseudoephedrine, Dextromethorphan, and Acetaminophen (Systemic)†, 1024
- Triprolidine, Pseudoephedrine, and Codeine (Systemic), 1024
- Triprolidine, Pseudoephedrine, Codeine, and Guaifenesin (Systemic)*, 1024

**Coughing measles**—*See* Measles
**Creeping eruption**—*See* Larva migrans, cutaneous
**Crohn's disease (treatment)**
*See also* Bowel disease, inflammatory; Enteritis, regional
- Budesonide (Systemic), 3012‡
- Tak-603 (Systemic), 30121‡

**Crohn's disease (treatment adjunct)**
- [Hydrocortisone, Enema (Rectal)], 973

**Croup (treatment)**
- [Epinephrine (Inhalation-Local)]1, 640
- Racepinephrine (Inhalation-Local), 640

**Cryptitis (treatment)**
- Hydrocortisone (Rectal), 973

**Cryptococcosis (treatment)**
- Amphotericin B (Systemic), 98
- Amphotericin B Liposomal Complex (Systemic), 105
- [Fluconazole (Systemic)]1, 302
- [Flucytosine (Systemic)]1, #
- [Itraconazole (Systemic)]1, 302

**Cryptorchidism (diagnosis)**
- [Chorionic Gonadotropin (Systemic)]1, 858

**Cryptorchidism (treatment)**
- Chorionic Gonadotropin (Systemic), 858

**Cryptosporidiosis (treatment)**
- Nitazoxanide (Systemic), 3156

**Cryptosporidiosis, associated with immunodeficiency (treatment)**
- Bovine Immunoglobulin, *Cryptosporidium parvum* (Systemic), 3134‡
- Bovine Whey Protein Concentrate (Systemic), 3134‡
- Nitazoxanide (Systemic), 3156‡

**CT of the abdomen**—*See* Abdominal imaging, computed tomographic, adjunct
**CT of the body**—*See* Body imaging, computed tomographic
**CT of the brain**—*See* Brain imaging, computed tomographic

**Cushing's syndrome (diagnosis)**
- Corticorelin Ovine Triflutate (Systemic), 3138‡
- Dexamethasone, Oral (Systemic), 998
- Dexamethasone, Parenteral (Systemic), 998
- [Metyrapone (Systemic)]1, #

**Cushing's syndrome (treatment)**
- Aminoglutethimide (Systemic), 67
- [Ketoconazole (Systemic)]1, 302
- [Metyrapone (Systemic)]1, #
- [Mitotane (Systemic)]1, 2031
- Trilostane (Systemic)†, #

**Cyclitis (treatment)**
- Betamethasone (Ophthalmic)*, 966
- Dexamethasone (Ophthalmic), 966
- Fluorometholone (Ophthalmic), 966
- Hydrocortisone (Ophthalmic)*, 966
- Prednisolone (Ophthalmic), 966

**Cyclophosphamide toxicity (prophylaxis)**
- Amifostine (Systemic), 3130‡

**Cyclospora infections (treatment)**
- [Sulfamethoxazole and Trimethoprim (Systemic)]1, 2661

**Cysticercosis (treatment)**
- [Praziquantel (Systemic)]†, 2368

**Cystic fibrosis (treatment)**
- Adeno-associated Viral-based Vector Cystic Fibrosis Gene Therapy (Systemic), 3128‡
- Amiloride Hydrochloride (Inhalation), 3130‡
- 8-Cyclopentyl 1,3-Dipropylxanthine (Systemic), 3128‡
- Cystic Fibrosis Gene, Lipid/DNA, Human (Systemic), 3152‡
- Cystic Fibrosis Gene Therapy (Systemic), 3139‡
- Cystic Fibrosis Transmembrane Conductance Regulator (Systemic), 3139‡
- Cystic Fibrosis TR Gene Therapy (Recombinant Adenovirus) (Systemic), 3139‡
- 2-0-Desulfated Heparin (Systemic), 3127‡
- Human Alpha 1 Antitrypsin, Transgenic (Systemic)‡, 3169‡
- Recombinant Secretory Leucocyte Protease Inhibitor (Systemic), 3161‡
- Transgenic Human Alpha 1 Antitrypsin, 3169‡
- Tyloxapol (Systemic), 3170‡
- Uridine 5'-Triphosphate (Systemic), 3170‡

**Cystic fibrosis (treatment adjunct)**
- Dextran Sulfate (Inhalation), 3140‡
- Dornase Alfa (Inhalation-Local), 1292

**Cystic fibrosis, pulmonary complications of (prophylaxis)**
- Mucoid Exopolysaccharide Pseudomonas Hyperimmune Globulin (Systemic), 3155‡

**Cystic fibrosis, pulmonary complications of (treatment)**
- DMP 777 (Systemic), 3141‡
- Dornase Alfa (Inhalation-Local), 3141‡
- Gelsolin, Recombinant Human (Systemic), 3161‡
- Mucoid Exopolysaccharide Pseudomonas Hyperimmune Globulin (Systemic), 3155‡
- Tobramycin (Systemic), 3169‡

**Cystic fibrosis, pulmonary complications of (treatment adjunct)**
- Acetylcysteine (Inhalation-Local), #

**Cystinosis (treatment)**
- Phosphocysteamine (Systemic), 3158‡

**Cystinosis, nephropathic (prophylaxis)**
- Cysteamine (Systemic), #

**Cystinosis, nephropathic (treatment)**
- Cysteamine (Systemic), 3139‡

**Cystinuria (treatment)**
- Penicillamine (Systemic), 2237
- Tiopronin (Systemic)†, 2824

**Cystitis (treatment)**—*See also* Irritative voiding, symptoms of; Urologic disorders, symptoms of
- Aztreonam (Systemic)†, 502

**Cystitis, hemorrhagic**
*See* Hemorrhagic cystitis

**Cystitis, interstitial (treatment)**
- Dimethyl Sulfoxide (Mucosal-Local), 1227
- Nifedipine (Systemic), 3156‡
- Pentosan (Systemic), 2277
- Pentosan Polysulphate (Systemic), 3157‡

**3196  Indications Index**  USP DI

**Cystography, radionuclide**—See Urinary bladder imaging, radionuclide
**Cystography, retrograde**
  Iothalamate (Local), #
**Cystography, voiding, indirect, radionuclide**
  [Technetium Tc 99m Mertiatide (Systemic)], 2720
**Cystourethrography, retrograde**
  Diatrizoate Meglumine (Local), #
  Iohexol (Local)[1], #
  Iothalamate (Local), #
**Cytomegalovirus disease (prophylaxis)**
  Ganciclovir (Systemic), 3022
**Cytomegalovirus disease, primary (prophylaxis)**
  Cytomegalovirus Immune Globulin (Human) (Systemic), 3139‡
  Ganciclovir, Parenteral (Systemic)[1], 1544
**Cytomegalovirus disease, primary (treatment)**
  Cytomegalovirus Immune Globulin (Human) (Systemic), 3139‡
  [Foscarnet (Systemic)]†, 1528
  [Ganciclovir, Parenteral (Systemic)][1], 1544
**Cytomegalovirus infection, human, in immunosuppressed patients (prophylaxis)**
  Monoclonal Antibody to Cytomegalovirus (Human) (Systemic), 3155‡
**Cytomegalovirus pneumonia, in bone marrow transplant patients (treatment)**
  Cytomegalovirus Immune Globulin Intravenous (Human) (Systemic), 3139‡
**Cytomegalovirus retinitis (treatment)**
  Cidofovir (Systemic), 865
  Filgrastim (Systemic), 3143‡
  Foscarnet (Systemic)†, 1528
  Ganciclovir (Implantation-Ophthalmic), 2948
  Ganciclovir (Systemic), 1544, 3022
  Intravitreal Ganciclovir Free Acid Implant (Ophthalmic), 3149‡
  Monoclonal Antibody to Cytomegalovirus (Human) (Systemic), 3155‡

# D

**Dacryocystitis (treatment)**
  Gentamicin (Ophthalmic), 1555
  [Tobramycin (Ophthalmic)], #
**Dacryoscintigraphy**
  Sodium Pertechnetate Tc 99m (Ophthalmic), 2611
**Dandruff (treatment)**
  Chloroxine (Topical)†, #
  Coal Tar (Topical), #
  Ketoconazole (Topical), 1807
  Pyrithione (Topical), #
  Salicylic Acid Lotion (Topical), #
  Salicylic Acid Shampoo (Topical), #
  Salicylic Acid, Sulfur, and Coal Tar (Topical), #
  Salicylic Acid and Sulfur Cream Shampoo (Topical), #
  Salicylic Acid and Sulfur Lotion Shampoo (Topical), #
  Salicylic Acid and Sulfur Suspension Shampoo (Topical), #
  Selenium Sulfide (Topical), #
**Darier's disease**—See Keratosis follicularis
**Darier-White disease**—See Keratosis follicularis
**Degeneration, hepatolenticular (treatment)**
  See also Wilson's disease
  [Ethopropazine (Systemic)][1], 297
**Dementia, Alzheimer-type (diagnosis)**
  [Fludeoxyglucose F 18 (Systemic)][1]†, 1478
  [Iofetamine I 123 (Systemic)][1], 1757
  [Technetium Tc 99m Exametazime (Systemic)][1], 2708
**Dementia, Alzheimer-type (treatment)**
  Donepezil (Systemic), 1290
  Tacrine (Systemic)†, 2680
**Dementia, early (treatment adjunct)**
  Ergoloid Mesylates (Systemic), 1358
**Dental caries (prophylaxis)**
  Sodium Fluoride (Systemic), 2592
  Sodium Fluoride and Triclosan (Dental), 3034
  Vitamins A, D, and C and Potassium Fluoride (Systemic), 2978
  Vitamins A, D, and C and Sodium Fluoride (Systemic), 2978
  Vitamins, Multiple, and Potassium Fluoride (Systemic), 2978
  Vitamins, Multiple, and Sodium Fluoride (Systemic), 2978
**Dental infiltration or nerve block**
  [Articaine and Epinephrine (Parenteral-Local)], 139
  Bupivacaine and Epinephrine (Parenteral-Local), 139
  Chloroprocaine (Parenteral-Local), 139
  Chloroprocaine and Epinephrine (Parenteral-Local), 139
  Etidocaine and Epinephrine (Parenteral-Local), 139

**Dental infiltration or nerve block** (continued)
  Lidocaine (Parenteral-Local), 139
  Lidocaine and Epinephrine (Parenteral-Local), 139
  Mepivacaine (Parenteral-Local), 139
  Mepivacaine and Levonordefrin (Parenteral-Local), 139
  Prilocaine (Parenteral-Local), 139
  Prilocaine and Epinephrine (Parenteral-Local), 139
**Dependence, on opioid drugs**—See Opioid (narcotic) abstinence syndrome; Opioid (narcotic) dependence, neonatal; Opioid (narcotic) drug use, illicit
**Depression, atypical**—See Depression, mental
**Depression, mental**—See Depressive disorder, major
**Depression, mental (diagnosis)**
  [Fludeoxyglucose F 18 (Systemic)][1]*†, 1478
**Depression, mental (treatment)**
  Amitriptyline (Systemic), 271
  Amoxapine (Systemic), 271
  [Clomipramine (Systemic)], 271
  Desipramine (Systemic), 271
  Doxepin (Systemic), 271
  Ephedrine, Oral (Systemic), 651
  [Fluvoxamine (Systemic)], 1513
  Imipramine (Systemic), 271
  [Lithium (Systemic)][1], 1869
  Moclobemide (Systemic), 3028
  Nefazodone (Systemic), 3029
  Nortriptyline (Systemic), 271
  Phenelzine (Systemic), 266
  Protriptyline (Systemic), 271
  Tranylcypromine (Systemic), 266
  Trazodone (Systemic), 2865
  Trimipramine (Systemic), 271
**Depression, mental, endogenous (diagnosis)**
  [Dexamethasone, Oral (Systemic)][1], 998
**Depression, mental, secondary to medical illness (treatment)**
  [Methylphenidate (Systemic)][1], 1987
**Depression, nonendogenous**—See Depression, mental
**Depressive disorder, major**—See Depression, mental
**Depressive disorder, major (treatment)**
  Bupropion (Systemic)†, 687
  Citalopram (Systemic), 3014
  Fluoxetine (Systemic), 1503
  Maprotiline (Systemic), 1909
  Mirtazapine (Systemic), 2023
  Nefazodone (Systemic), 2092
  Paroxetine (Systemic), 2225
  Sertraline (Systemic), 2566
  Venlafaxine (Systemic), 2940
**Depressive neurosis**—See Depression, mental
**Dermatitis, allergic contact (prophylaxis)**
  Bentoquatam (Topical), 555
**Dermatitis, atopic (treatment)**
  Betamethasone, Oral (Systemic), 998
  Betamethasone, Parenteral (Systemic), 998
  Clioquinol and Flumethasone (Topical)*, 3015
  Clioquinol and Hydrocortisone (Topical), #
  Coal Tar (Topical), #
  Cortisone (Systemic), 998
  Dexamethasone, Oral (Systemic), 998
  Dexamethasone, Parenteral (Systemic), 998
  Hydrocortisone, Oral (Systemic), 998
  Hydrocortisone, Parenteral (Systemic), 998
  [Methoxsalen (Systemic)], 1973
  Methylprednisolone, Oral (Systemic), 998
  Methylprednisolone, Parenteral (Systemic), 998
  Prednisolone, Oral (Systemic), 998
  Prednisolone, Parenteral (Systemic), 998
  Prednisone (Systemic), 998
  Triamcinolone, Oral (Systemic), 998
  Triamcinolone, Parenteral (Systemic), 998
**Dermatitis, atopic, mild to moderate (treatment)**
  Alclometasone Dipropionate (Topical), 978
  Beclomethasone Dipropionate (Topical), 978
  Betamethasone Benzoate (Topical), 978
  Betamethasone Valerate (Topical), 978
  Clobetasone Butyrate (Topical), 978
  Clocortolone Pivalate (Topical), 978
  Desonide (Topical), 978
  Desoximetasone (0.05% cream only) (Topical), 978
  Dexamethasone (Topical), 978
  Dexamethasone Sodium Phosphate (Topical), 978
  Diflucortolone Valerate (Topical), 978
  Flumethasone Pivalate (Topical), 978
  Fluocinolone Acetonide (except 0.2% cream) (Topical), 978
  Flurandrenolide (Topical), 978
  Fluticasone Propionate (Topical), 978
  Hydrocortisone (Topical), 978
  Hydrocortisone Acetate (Topical), 978

**Dermatitis, atopic, mild to moderate (treatment)** (continued)
  Hydrocortisone Butyrate (Topical), 978
  Hydrocortisone Valerate (Topical), 978
  Methylprednisolone Acetate (Topical), 978
  Mometasone Furoate (Topical), 978
  Triamcinolone Acetonide (except 0.5% cream and ointment) (Topical), 978
**Dermatitis, atopic, moderate to severe (treatment)**
  Amcinonide (Topical), 978
  Beclomethasone Dipropionate (Topical), 978
  Betamethasone Benzoate (Topical), 978
  Betamethasone Dipropionate (Topical), 978
  Betamethasone Valerate (Topical), 978
  Clobetasol Propionate (Topical), 978
  Clobetasone Butyrate (Topical), 978
  Desoximetasone (Topical), 978
  Diflorasone Diacetate (Topical), 978
  Diflucortolone Valerate (Topical), 978
  Fluocinolone Acetonide (Topical), 978
  Fluocinonide (Topical), 978
  Flurandrenolide (except 0.0125% cream and ointment) (Topical), 978
  Fluticasone Propionate (Topical), 978
  Halcinonide (Topical), 978
  Halobetasol Propionate (Topical), 978
  Hydrocortisone Butyrate (Topical), 978
  Hydrocortisone Valerate (Topical), 978
  Mometasone Furoate (Topical), 978
  Triamcinolone Acetonide (Topical), 978
**Dermatitis, contact (treatment)**
  Alclometasone Dipropionate (Topical), 978
  Beclomethasone Dipropionate (Topical), 978
  Benzocaine (Topical), 155
  Benzocaine and Menthol (Topical), 155
  Betamethasone Benzoate (Topical), 978
  Betamethasone, Oral (Systemic), 998
  Betamethasone, Parenteral (Systemic), 998
  Betamethasone Valerate (Topical), 978
  Butamben (Topical), 155
  Calamine (Topical), #
  Clioquinol and Flumethasone (Topical)*, 3015
  Clioquinol and Hydrocortisone (Topical), #
  Clobetasone Butyrate (Topical), 978
  Clocortolone Pivalate (Topical), 978
  Cortisone (Systemic), 998
  Desonide (Topical), 978
  Desoximetasone (0.05% cream only) (Topical), 978
  Dexamethasone (Topical), 978
  Dexamethasone, Oral (Systemic), 998
  Dexamethasone, Parenteral (Systemic), 998
  Dexamethasone Sodium Phosphate (Topical), 978
  Dibucaine (Topical), 155
  Diflucortolone Valerate (Topical), 978
  Flumethasone Pivalate (Topical), 978
  Fluocinolone Acetonide (except 0.2% cream) (Topical), 978
  Flurandrenolide (Topical), 978
  Fluticasone Propionate (Topical), 978
  Hydrocortisone (Topical), 978
  Hydrocortisone Acetate (Topical), 978
  Hydrocortisone Butyrate (Topical), 978
  Hydrocortisone, Oral (Systemic), 998
  Hydrocortisone, Parenteral (Systemic), 998
  Hydrocortisone Valerate (Topical), 978
  Lidocaine (Topical), 155
  Methylprednisolone Acetate (Topical), 978
  Methylprednisolone, Oral (Systemic), 998
  Methylprednisolone, Parenteral (Systemic), 998
  Mometasone Furoate (Topical), 978
  Pramoxine (Topical), 155
  Pramoxine and Menthol (Topical), 155
  Prednisolone, Oral (Systemic), 998
  Prednisolone, Parenteral (Systemic), 998
  Prednisone (Systemic), 998
  Racemethionine (Systemic)†, #
  Tetracaine (Topical), 155
  Tetracaine and Menthol (Topical), 155
  Triamcinolone Acetonide (except 0.5% cream and ointment) (Topical), 978
  Triamcinolone, Oral (Systemic), 998
  Triamcinolone, Parenteral (Systemic), 998
**Dermatitis, exfoliative (treatment)**
  Amcinonide (Topical), 978
  Beclomethasone Dipropionate (Topical), 978
  Betamethasone Benzoate (Topical), 978
  Betamethasone Dipropionate (Topical), 978
  Betamethasone, Oral (Systemic), 998
  Betamethasone, Parenteral (Systemic), 998
  Betamethasone Valerate (Topical), 978
  Clobetasol Propionate (Topical), 978
  Clobetasone Butyrate (Topical), 978
  Cortisone (Systemic), 998
  Desoximetasone (Topical), 978
  Dexamethasone, Oral (Systemic), 998

**Dermatitis, exfoliative (treatment)** *(continued)*
   Dexamethasone, Parenteral (Systemic), 998
   Diflorasone Diacetate (Topical), 978
   Diflucortolone Valerate (Topical), 978
   Fluocinolone Acetonide (Topical), 978
   Fluocinonide (Topical), 978
   Flurandrenolide (except 0.0125% cream and ointment) (Topical), 978
   Fluticasone Propionate (Topical), 978
   Halcinonide (Topical), 978
   Halobetasol Propionate (Topical), 978
   Hydrocortisone Butyrate (Topical), 978
   Hydrocortisone, Oral (Systemic), 998
   Hydrocortisone, Parenteral (Systemic), 998
   Hydrocortisone Valerate (Topical), 978
   Methylprednisolone, Oral (Systemic), 998
   Methylprednisolone, Parenteral (Systemic), 998
   Mometasone Furoate (Topical), 978
   Prednisolone, Oral (Systemic), 998
   Prednisolone, Parenteral (Systemic), 998
   Prednisone (Systemic), 998
   Triamcinolone Acetonide (Topical), 978
   Triamcinolone, Oral (Systemic), 998
   Triamcinolone, Parenteral (Systemic), 998
**Dermatitis herpetiformis (treatment)**
   Dapsone (Systemic), 1170
   Sulfapyridine (Systemic), 2640, 3166‡
**Dermatitis herpetiformis, bullous (treatment)**
   Betamethasone, Oral (Systemic), 998
   Betamethasone, Parenteral (Systemic), 998
   Cortisone (Systemic), 998
   Dexamethasone, Oral (Systemic), 998
   Dexamethasone, Parenteral (Systemic), 998
   Hydrocortisone, Oral (Systemic), 998
   Hydrocortisone, Parenteral (Systemic), 998
   Methylprednisolone, Oral (Systemic), 998
   Methylprednisolone, Parenteral (Systemic), 998
   Prednisolone, Oral (Systemic), 998
   Prednisolone, Parenteral (Systemic), 998
   Prednisone (Systemic), 998
   Triamcinolone, Oral (Systemic), 998
   Triamcinolone, Parenteral (Systemic), 998
**Dermatitis, mild to moderate (treatment)**
   Alclometasone Dipropionate (Topical), 978
   Beclomethasone Dipropionate (Topical), 978
   Betamethasone Benzoate (Topical), 978
   Betamethasone Valerate (Topical), 978
   Clobetasone Butyrate (Topical), 978
   Clocortolone Pivalate (Topical), 978
   Desonide (Topical), 978
   Desoximetasone (0.05% cream only) (Topical), 978
   Dexamethasone (Topical), 978
   Dexamethasone Sodium Phosphate (Topical), 978
   Diflucortolone Valerate (Topical), 978
   Flumethasone Pivalate (Topical), 978
   Fluocinolone Acetonide (except 0.2% cream) (Topical), 978
   Flurandrenolide (Topical), 978
   Fluticasone Propionate (Topical), 978
   Hydrocortisone (Topical), 978
   Hydrocortisone Acetate (Topical), 978
   Hydrocortisone Butyrate (Topical), 978
   Hydrocortisone Valerate (Topical), 978
   Methylprednisolone Acetate (Topical), 978
   Mometasone Furoate (Topical), 978
   Triamcinolone Acetonide (except 0.5% cream and ointment) (Topical), 978
**Dermatitis, moderate to severe (treatment)**
   Amcinonide (Topical), 978
   Beclomethasone Dipropionate (Topical), 978
   Betamethasone Benzoate (Topical), 978
   Betamethasone Dipropionate (Topical), 978
   Betamethasone Valerate (Topical), 978
   Clobetasol Propionate (Topical), 978
   Clobetasone Butyrate (Topical), 978
   Desoximetasone (Topical), 978
   Diflorasone Diacetate (Topical), 978
   Diflucortolone Valerate (Topical), 978
   Fluocinolone Acetonide (Topical), 978
   Fluocinonide (Topical), 978
   Flurandrenolide (except 0.0125% cream and ointment) (Topical), 978
   Fluticasone Propionate (Topical), 978
   Halcinonide (Topical), 978
   Halobetasol Propionate (Topical), 978
   Hydrocortisone Butyrate (Topical), 978
   Hydrocortisone Valerate (Topical), 978
   Mometasone Furoate (Topical), 978
   Triamcinolone Acetonide (Topical), 978
**Dermatitis, nummular, mild (treatment)**
   Alclometasone Dipropionate (Topical), 978
   Beclomethasone Dipropionate (Topical), 978
   Betamethasone Benzoate (Topical), 978
   Betamethasone Valerate (Topical), 978
   Clobetasone Butyrate (Topical), 978

**Dermatitis, nummular, mild (treatment)** *(continued)*
   Clocortolone Pivalate (Topical), 978
   Desonide (Topical), 978
   Desoximetasone (0.05% cream only) (Topical), 978
   Dexamethasone (Topical), 978
   Dexamethasone Sodium Phosphate (Topical), 978
   Diflucortolone Valerate (Topical), 978
   Flumethasone Pivalate (Topical), 978
   Fluocinolone Acetonide (except 0.2% cream) (Topical), 978
   Flurandrenolide (Topical), 978
   Fluticasone Propionate (Topical), 978
   Hydrocortisone (Topical), 978
   Hydrocortisone Acetate (Topical), 978
   Hydrocortisone Butyrate (Topical), 978
   Hydrocortisone Valerate (Topical), 978
   Methylprednisolone Acetate (Topical), 978
   Mometasone Furoate (Topical), 978
   Triamcinolone Acetonide (except 0.5% cream and ointment) (Topical), 978
**Dermatitis, nummular, moderate to severe (treatment)**
   Amcinonide (Topical), 978
   Beclomethasone Dipropionate (Topical), 978
   Betamethasone Benzoate (Topical), 978
   Betamethasone Dipropionate (Topical), 978
   Betamethasone Valerate (Topical), 978
   Clobetasol Propionate (Topical), 978
   Clobetasone Butyrate (Topical), 978
   Desoximetasone (Topical), 978
   Diflorasone Diacetate (Topical), 978
   Diflucortolone Valerate (Topical), 978
   Fluocinolone Acetonide (Topical), 978
   Fluocinonide (Topical), 978
   Flurandrenolide (except 0.0125% cream and ointment) (Topical), 978
   Fluticasone Propionate (Topical), 978
   Halcinonide (Topical), 978
   Halobetasol Propionate (Topical), 978
   Hydrocortisone Butyrate (Topical), 978
   Hydrocortisone Valerate (Topical), 978
   Mometasone Furoate (Topical), 978
   Triamcinolone Acetonide (Topical), 978
**Dermatitis, perioral (treatment)**
   Metronidazole (Topical), 3154‡
**Dermatitis, seborrheic (treatment)**
   Alclometasone Dipropionate (Topical), 978
   Beclomethasone Dipropionate (Topical), 978
   Betamethasone Benzoate (Topical), 978
   Betamethasone Valerate (Topical), 978
   Clobetasone Butyrate (Topical), 978
   Clocortolone Pivalate (Topical), 978
   Coal Tar (Topical), #
   Desonide (Topical), 978
   Desoximetasone (0.05% cream only) (Topical), 978
   Dexamethasone (Topical), 978
   Dexamethasone Sodium Phosphate (Topical), 978
   Diflucortolone Valerate (Topical), 978
   Flumethasone Pivalate (Topical), 978
   Fluocinolone Acetonide (except 0.2% cream) (Topical), 978
   Flurandrenolide (Topical), 978
   Fluticasone Propionate (Topical), 978
   Hydrocortisone (Topical), 978
   Hydrocortisone Acetate (Topical), 978
   Hydrocortisone Butyrate (Topical), 978, 3023
   Hydrocortisone Valerate (Topical), 978
   Ketoconazole (Topical), 1807
   Methylprednisolone Acetate (Topical), 978
   Mometasone Furoate (Topical), 978
   Pyrithione (Topical), #
   Resorcinol (Topical), 1#
   Salicylic Acid Ointment (Topical), #
   Sulfurated Lime Topical Solution (Topical)†, #
   Sulfur Ointment USP (Topical)†, #
   Triamcinolone Acetonide (except 0.5% cream and ointment) (Topical), 978
**Dermatitis, seborrheic, of scalp (treatment)**
   Chloroxine (Topical)†, #
   Salicylic Acid Lotion (Topical), #
   Salicylic Acid Shampoo (Topical), #
   Salicylic Acid, Sulfur, and Coal Tar (Topical), #
   Salicylic Acid and Sulfur Lotion Shampoo (Topical), #
   Salicylic Acid and Sulfur Suspension Shampoo (Topical), #
   Selenium Sulfide (Topical), #
**Dermatitis, seborrheic, severe (treatment)**
   Betamethasone, Oral (Systemic), 998
   Betamethasone, Parenteral (Systemic), 998
   Cortisone (Systemic), 998
   Dexamethasone, Oral (Systemic), 998
   Dexamethasone, Parenteral (Systemic), 998
   Hydrocortisone, Oral (Systemic), 998

**Dermatitis, seborrheic, severe (treatment)** *(continued)*
   Hydrocortisone, Parenteral (Systemic), 998
   Methylprednisolone, Oral (Systemic), 998
   Methylprednisolone, Parenteral (Systemic), 998
   Prednisolone, Oral (Systemic), 998
   Prednisolone, Parenteral (Systemic), 998
   Prednisone (Systemic), 998
   Triamcinolone, Oral (Systemic), 998
   Triamcinolone, Parenteral (Systemic), 998
**Dermatographism (treatment)**
   Acrivastine (Systemic)*†, 325
   Astemizole (Systemic), 325
   Azatadine (Systemic), 325
   Bromodiphenhydramine (Systemic)*†, 325
   Brompheniramine (Systemic), 325
   Carbinoxamine (Systemic)*†, 325
   Cetirizine (Systemic), 325
   Chlorpheniramine (Systemic), 325
   Clemastine (Systemic), 325
   Cyproheptadine (Systemic), 325
   Dexchlorpheniramine (Systemic), 325
   Dimenhydrinate (Systemic), 325
   Diphenhydramine (Systemic), 325
   Diphenylpyraline (Systemic)*†, 325
   Doxylamine (Systemic)†, 325
   Hydroxyzine (Systemic), 325
   Loratadine (Systemic), 325
   Methdilazine (Systemic)†, 377
   Phenindamine (Systemic)†, 325
   Promethazine (Systemic), 377
   Pyrilamine (Systemic)*†, 325
   Trimeprazine (Systemic), 377
   Tripelennamine (Systemic), 325
   Triprolidine (Systemic)*†, 325
**Dermatomyositis, fibrosis and/or nonsuppurative inflammation in (treatment)**
   Aminobenzoate Potassium (Systemic), #
**Dermatomyositis, systemic (treatment)**
   [Azathioprine (Systemic)][1], 491
   Betamethasone, Oral (Systemic), 998
   Betamethasone, Parenteral (Systemic), 998
   Cortisone (Systemic), 998
   [Cyclophosphamide (Systemic)][1], 1128
   Dexamethasone, Oral (Systemic), 998
   Dexamethasone, Parenteral (Systemic), 998
   Hydrocortisone, Oral (Systemic), 998
   Hydrocortisone, Parenteral (Systemic), 998
   Immune Globulin Intravenous (Human) (Systemic), 3147‡
   [Methotrexate—For Noncancerous Conditions (Systemic)][1], 1969
   Methylprednisolone, Oral (Systemic), 998
   Methylprednisolone, Parenteral (Systemic), 998
   Prednisolone, Oral (Systemic), 998
   Prednisolone, Parenteral (Systemic), 998
   Prednisone (Systemic), 998
   Triamcinolone, Oral (Systemic), 998
   Triamcinolone, Parenteral (Systemic), 998
**Dermatoses (treatment)**
   Bufexamac (Topical), 3013
**Dermatoses, corticosteroid-responsive (treatment)**
   Fluocinolone, Procinonide, and Ciprocinonide (Topical)*, 3020
   Hydrocortisone Buteprate (Topical), 3023
   Prednicarbate (Topical), 3033
**Dermatoses, ichthyosiform (treatment)**
   [Etretinate (Systemic)], #
**Dermatoses, inflammatory (treatment)**
   [Methoxsalen (Systemic)][1], 1973
   [Methoxsalen (Topical)][1], 1977
**Dermatoses, inflammatory, mild to moderate (treatment)**
   Alclometasone Dipropionate (Topical), 978
   Beclomethasone Dipropionate (Topical), 978
   Betamethasone Benzoate (Topical), 978
   Betamethasone Valerate (Topical), 978
   Clobetasone Butyrate (Topical), 978
   Clocortolone Pivalate (Topical), 978
   Desonide (Topical), 978
   Desoximetasone (0.05% cream only) (Topical), 978
   Dexamethasone (Topical), 978
   Dexamethasone Sodium Phosphate (Topical), 978
   Diflucortolone Valerate (Topical), 978
   Flumethasone Pivalate (Topical), 978
   Fluocinolone Acetonide (except 0.2% cream) (Topical), 978
   Flurandrenolide (Topical), 978
   Fluticasone Propionate (Topical), 978
   Hydrocortisone (Topical), 978
   Hydrocortisone Acetate (Topical), 978
   Hydrocortisone Valerate (Topical), 978
   Methylprednisolone Acetate (Topical), 978

## Indications Index

**Dermatoses, inflammatory, mild to moderate (treatment)** *(continued)*
Mometasone Furoate (Topical), 978
Triamcinolone Acetonide (except 0.5% cream and ointment) (Topical), 978

**Dermatoses, inflammatory, moderate to severe (treatment)**
Amcinonide (Topical), 978
Beclomethasone Dipropionate (Topical), 978
Betamethasone Benzoate (Topical), 978
Betamethasone Dipropionate (Topical), 978
Betamethasone Valerate (Topical), 978
Clobetasol Propionate (Topical), 978
Clobetasone Butyrate (Topical), 978
Desoximetasone (Topical), 978
Diflorasone Diacetate (Topical), 978
Diflucortolone Valerate (Topical), 978
Fluocinolone Acetonide (Topical), 978
Fluocinonide (Topical), 978
Flurandrenolide (except 0.0125% cream and ointment) (Topical), 978
Fluticasone Propionate (Topical), 978
Halcinonide (Topical), 978
Halobetasol Propionate (Topical), 978
Hydrocortisone Butyrate (Topical), 978
Hydrocortisone Valerate (Topical), 978
Mometasone Furoate (Topical), 978
Triamcinolone Acetonide (Topical), 978

**Dermatoses, inflammatory, severe (treatment)**
Betamethasone, Oral (Systemic), 998
Betamethasone, Parenteral (Systemic), 998
Betamethasone, Parenteral-Local (Systemic), 998
Cortisone (Systemic), 998
Dexamethasone (Systemic), 998
Hydrocortisone, Oral (Systemic), 998
Hydrocortisone, Parenteral (Systemic), 998
Hydrocortisone, Parenteral-Local (Systemic), 998
Methylprednisolone, Oral (Systemic), 998
Methylprednisolone, Parenteral (Systemic), 998
Methylprednisolone, Parenteral-Local (Systemic), 998
Prednisolone (Systemic), 998
Prednisone (Systemic), 998
Triamcinolone (Systemic), 998

**Dermatosis, subcorneal pustular (treatment)**
[Dapsone (Systemic)][1], 1170
[Sulfapyridine (Systemic)][1], 2640

**Diabetes insipidus (diagnosis)**
[Vasopressin (Systemic)][1], 2938

**Diabetes insipidus, central (treatment)**
[Bendroflumethiazide (Systemic)][1], 1273
[Carbamazepine (Systemic)][1], 757
[Chlorothiazide (Systemic)]†, 1273
[Chlorpropamide (Systemic)][1], 283
[Chlorthalidone (Systemic)][1], 1273
Desmopressin (Systemic), 1187, 3016
[Hydrochlorothiazide (Systemic)][1], 1273
[Hydroflumethiazide (Systemic)]†, 1273
Lypressin (Systemic), 1893
[Methyclothiazide (Systemic)][1], 1273
[Metolazone (Systemic)][1], 1273
[Polythiazide (Systemic)]†, 1273
[Quinethazone (Systemic)]†, 1273
[Trichlormethiazide (Systemic)]†, 1273
Vasopressin (Systemic), 2938

**Diabetes insipidus, nephrogenic (treatment)**
[Bendroflumethiazide (Systemic)][1], 1273
[Chlorothiazide (Systemic)]†, 1273
[Chlorthalidone (Systemic)][1], 1273
[Hydrochlorothiazide (Systemic)][1], 1273
[Hydroflumethiazide (Systemic)]†, 1273
[Methyclothiazide (Systemic)][1], 1273
[Metolazone (Systemic)][1], 1273
[Polythiazide (Systemic)]†, 1273
[Quinethazone (Systemic)]†, 1273
[Trichlormethiazide (Systemic)]†, 1273

**Diabetes mellitus (treatment)**
Encapsulated Porcine Islet Preparation (Systemic), 3141‡
Insulin Lispro (Systemic), 3025

**Diabetes mellitus (treatment adjunct)**
Insulin Lispro (Systemic), 1727

**Diabetes mellitus, gestational (treatment)**
Insulin (Systemic), 1713
Insulin Human (Systemic), 1713
Insulin Human, Buffered (Systemic), 1713
Insulin, Isophane (Systemic), 1713
Insulin, Isophane, Human (Systemic), 1713
Insulin, Isophane, Human, and Insulin Human (Systemic), 1713
Insulin Zinc (Systemic), 1713
Insulin Zinc, Extended (Systemic), 1713
Insulin Zinc, Extended, Human (Systemic), 1713

**Diabetes mellitus, gestational (treatment)** *(continued)*
Insulin Zinc, Human (Systemic), 1713
Insulin Zinc, Prompt (Systemic)*, 1713

**Diabetes mellitus, insulin-dependent (treatment)**
Insulin (Systemic), 1713
Insulin Human (Systemic), 1713
Insulin Human, Buffered (Systemic), 1713
Insulin, Isophane (Systemic), 1713
Insulin, Isophane, Human (Systemic), 1713
Insulin, Isophane, Human, and Insulin Human (Systemic), 1713
Insulin Zinc (Systemic), 1713
Insulin Zinc, Extended (Systemic)*, 1713
Insulin Zinc, Extended, Human (Systemic), 1713
Insulin Zinc, Human (Systemic), 1713
Insulin Zinc, Prompt (Systemic)*, 1713

**Diabetes mellitus, non–insulin-dependent (treatment)**
See also Diabetes, type 2
Acetohexamide (Systemic), 283
Chlorpropamide (Systemic), 283
Gliclazide (Systemic)*, 283
Glipizide (Systemic)†, 283
Glyburide (Systemic), 283
Insulin (Systemic), 1713
Insulin Human (Systemic), 1713
Insulin Human, Buffered (Systemic), 1713
Insulin, Isophane (Systemic), 1713
Insulin, Isophane, Human (Systemic), 1713
Insulin, Isophane, Human, and Insulin Human (Systemic), 1713
Insulin Zinc (Systemic), 1713
Insulin Zinc, Extended (Systemic)*, 1713
Insulin Zinc, Extended, Human (Systemic), 1713
Insulin Zinc, Human (Systemic), 1713
Insulin Zinc, Prompt (Systemic)*, 1713
Metformin (Systemic), 1957
Miglitol (Oral-Local), 4441
Tolazamide (Systemic)†, 283
Tolbutamide (Systemic), 283

**Diabetes, type 2 (treatment)**
See also Diabetes mellitus, non–insulin dependent
Acarbose (Systemic), 3
Glimepiride (Systemic), 1560
Repaglinide (Systemic), 2467
Troglitazone (Systemic), 2888

**Diagnostic procedure–induced symptoms, urinary (treatment)**
Atropine, Hyoscyamine, Methenamine, Methylene Blue, Phenyl Salicylate, and Benzoic Acid (Systemic)†, 488

**Diarrhea (treatment)**
Attapulgite (Oral-Local), #
Bismuth Subsalicylate (Oral-Local), 616
Charcoal, Activated (Oral-Local), 831
[Codeine (Systemic)][1], 2168
Dextrose and Electrolytes (Systemic), 769
Kaolin and Pectin (Oral-Local), 1802
Loperamide (Oral-Local), 1877
Loperamide and Simethicone (Systemic), 3028
[Morphine (Systemic)], 2168
Opium Tincture USP (Systemic), 2168
Oral Rehydration Salts (Systemic)*, 769
Polycarbophil (Local), #
[Psyllium Hydrophilic Mucilloid (Local)], #
Rice Syrup Solids and Electrolytes (Systemic)†, 769

**Diarrhea (treatment adjunct)**
Difenoxin and Atropine (Systemic)†, 1210
Diphenoxylate and Atropine (Systemic), 1233
Sodium Bicarbonate, Parenteral (Systemic), 2586

**Diarrhea, AIDS-associated (treatment)**
Bovine Colostrum (Systemic), 3134‡
Cryptosporidium Hyperimmune Bovine Colostrum IgG Concentrate (Systemic), 3138‡
Lactobin (Systemic), 3151‡
[Octreotide (Systemic)][1], 2152

**Diarrhea, antibiotic-associated (treatment)**
Vancomycin (Oral-Local), 2916

**Diarrhea, bacterial (treatment)**
Furazolidone (Oral-Local)†, 1533

**Diarrhea, due to bile acids (treatment)**
[Cholestyramine (Oral-Local)], 853
[Colestipol (Oral-Local)][1], 934

**DiGeorge anomaly with immune defects (treatment)**
Thymalfasin (Systemic), 3169‡

**Diphtheria (prophylaxis)**
Diphtheria Antitoxin (Systemic), 2236
Erythromycin (Systemic), 1368
[Penicillin G Benzathine (Systemic)][1], 2240
Penicillin G, Parenteral (Systemic), 2240
Penicillin G Procaine (Systemic), 2240
Penicillin V (Systemic), 2240

**Diphtheria (treatment)**
Diphtheria Antitoxin (Systemic), 2236
Erythromycin (Systemic), 1368

**Diphtheria and tetanus (prophylaxis)**
Diphtheria and Tetanus Toxoids (Systemic), 1236
Tetanus and Diphtheria Toxoids (Systemic), 1236

**Diphtheria, tetanus, and pertussis (prophylaxis)**
Diphtheria and Tetanus Toxoids and Pertussis Vaccine Adsorbed (Systemic), 1240

**Diphtheria, tetanus, pertussis, and *Haemophilus influenzae* type b diseases (prophylaxis)**
Diphtheria and Tetanus Toxoids and Pertussis Vaccine Adsorbed and Haemophilus b Conjugate Vaccine (Systemic), 1244

**Diphyllobothriasis (treatment)**
Niclosamide (Oral-Local)†, #
[Praziquantel (Systemic)]†, 2368

**Dipylidiasis (treatment)**
[Niclosamide (Oral-Local)]†, #
[Praziquantel (Systemic)]†, 2368

**Disk, herniated lumbar intervertebral (treatment)**
Chymopapain (Parenteral-Local), 9710

**Diskography**
Diatrizoate Meglumine, Parenteral (Systemic), #

**Dog and cat hookworm**—See Hookworm infection; Larva migrans, cutaneous

**Dog and cat roundworm**—See Larva migrans, visceral

**Dog and cat tapeworm**—See Dipylidiasis

**Dracunculiasis (treatment)**
[Metronidazole (Systemic)][1], 1996
[Thiabendazole (Systemic)]†, 2784

**Drowsiness (treatment)**
Caffeine (Systemic), 706
Caffeine, Citrated (Systemic), 706

**DUB**—See Bleeding, uterine, dysfunctional

**Duchenne's muscular dystrophy (treatment)**
Mazindol (Systemic), 3153‡
Oxandrolone (Systemic), 3156‡

**Ductus arteriosus, patent (maintenance)**
Alprostadil (Systemic), 52

**Ductus arteriosus, patent (prophylaxis)**
Ibuprofen (Systemic), 3146‡

**Ductus arteriosus, patent (treatment)**
Ibuprofen (Systemic), 3146‡
[Indomethacin Capsules USP—For Patent Ductus Arteriosus (Systemic)][1], 1704
Sterile Indomethacin Sodium—For Patent Ductus Arteriosus (Systemic), 1704

**Duhring's disease**—See Dermatitis herpetiformis

**Dupuytren's disease (treatment)**
Clostridial Collagenase (Systemic), 3137‡

**Dwarf tapeworm**—See Hymenolepiasis

**Dyskinesia, ciliary (prophylaxis)**
Uridine 5'-Triphosphate (Systemic), 3170‡

**Dysmenorrhea (treatment)**
See also Pain
[Clonidine, Oral (Systemic)][1], 908
[Desogestrel and Ethynyl Estradiol (Systemic)][1], 1397
Diclofenac (Systemic), 388
[Diflunisal (Systemic)][1], 388
[Ethynodiol Diacetate and Ethinyl Estradiol (Systemic)][1], 1397
[Etodolac (Systemic)]†, 388
Fenoprofen (Systemic)[1], 388
Floctafenine (Systemic)*[1], 388
[Flurbiprofen (Systemic)], 388
Ibuprofen (Systemic), 388
[Indomethacin (Systemic)][1], 388
[Isoxsuprine (Systemic)][1], #
Ketoprofen (Systemic), 388
[Levonorgestrel and Ethinyl Estradiol (Systemic)][1], 1397
Meclofenamate (Systemic)†, 388
Mefenamic Acid (Systemic), 388
Naproxen (Systemic), 388, 3029
[Norethindrone Acetate and Ethinyl Estradiol (Systemic)][1], 1397
[Norethindrone and Ethinyl Estradiol (Systemic)][1], 1397
[Norethindrone and Mestranol (Systemic)], 1397
[Norgestimate and Ethinyl Estradiol (Systemic)][1], 1397
[Norgestrel and Ethinyl Estradiol (Systemic)][1], 1397
[Piroxicam (Systemic)], 388

**Dysplasia, bronchopulmonary (treatment)**
Secretory Leukocyte Protease Inhibitor (Systemic), 3164‡

**Dysplasia, bronchopulmonary, neonatal (prophylaxis)**
Superoxide Dismutase (Recombinant Human) (Intratracheal-Local), 3167‡

**Dysthymia**—See Depression, mental

**Dysthymia (treatment)**
Maprotiline (Systemic), 1909
**Dystonia, cervical (treatment)**
Botulinum Toxin Type A (Parenteral-Local), 3134‡
Botulinum Toxin Type B (Parenteral-Local), 3134‡
Botulinum Toxin Type F (Parenteral-Local), 3134‡
**Dystrophy, reflex sympathetic, moderate to severe (treatment)**
Guanethidine Monosulfate (Systemic), 3145‡

# E

***E. coli* infections, verocytotoxogenic (treatment)**
Synsorb PK (Systemic), 3167‡
**Ear canal infections, external (prophylaxis)**
[Hydrocortisone and Acetic Acid (Otic)], 996
**Ear canal infections, external (treatment)**
Chloramphenicol (Otic), #
Colistin, Neomycin, and Hydrocortisone (Otic), 939
Desonide and Acetic Acid (Otic), 996
Hydrocortisone and Acetic Acid (Otic), 996
Neomycin, Polymyxin B, and Hydrocortisone (Otic), #
**Ear, external, inflammatory and seborrheic conditions of (treatment)**
Framycetin, Gramicidin, and Dexamethasone (Otic)*, 3021
**Ear, inner, circulatory disturbances of (treatment)**
Diphenidol (Systemic), 1232
Nicotinyl Alcohol (Systemic)*, #
**Ear, nose, and throat infections**—See Otitis media, acute; Pharyngitis, bacterial; Sinusitis
**Echinococcosis**—See Hydatid disease
**Ectopic calcification**—See Ossification, heterotopic
**Eczema (treatment)**
Clioquinol and Hydrocortisone (Topical), #
Coal Tar (Topical), #
[Methoxsalen (Systemic)][1], 1973
[Methoxsalen (Topical)][1], 1977
Resorcinol (Topical), 1#
**Eczema, infected (treatment)**
[Mupirocin (Topical)], 4253
**Eczema, severe (treatment)**
[Betamethasone, Oral (Systemic)], 998
[Cortisone, Oral (Systemic)], 998
[Dexamethasone, Oral (Systemic)], 998
[Hydrocortisone, Oral (Systemic)], 998
[Methylprednisolone, Oral (Systemic)][1], 998
[Prednisolone, Oral (Systemic)], 998
[Prednisone (Systemic)], 998
[Triamcinolone, Oral (Systemic)], 998
**Edema (treatment)**
Amiloride (Systemic), 1266
Amiloride and Hydrochlorothiazide (Systemic), 1272
Bendroflumethiazide (Systemic), 1273
Bumetanide (Systemic)†, 1259
Chlorothiazide (Systemic)†, 1273
Chlorthalidone (Systemic), 1273
Ethacrynic Acid (Systemic), 1259
Furosemide (Systemic), 1259
Hydrochlorothiazide (Systemic), 1273
Hydroflumethiazide (Systemic)†, 1273
Indapamide (Systemic), 1691
Methyclothiazide (Systemic), 1273
Metolazone Tablets, Extended (Systemic), 1273
Polythiazide (Systemic)†, 1273
Quinethazone (Systemic)†, 1273
Spironolactone (Systemic), 1266
Spironolactone and Hydrochlorothiazide (Systemic), 1272
Torsemide (Systemic)†, 2848
Triamterene (Systemic), 1266
Triamterene and Hydrochlorothiazide (Systemic), 1272
Trichlormethiazide (Systemic)†, 1273
**Edema, cerebral (prophylaxis)**
[Dexamethasone, Oral (Systemic)][1], 998
[Dexamethasone Sodium Phosphate Injection USP (Systemic)][1], 998
[Prednisone (Systemic)][1], 998
**Edema, cerebral (treatment)**
See also Hypertension, cerebral
Dexamethasone, Oral (Systemic), 998
Dexamethasone, Parenteral (Systemic), 998
[Glycerin (Systemic)], #
Mannitol (Systemic), 1906
[Prednisone (Systemic)][1], 998
Urea (Systemic)†, 2899
**Edema, cerebral, associated with primary or metastatic brain tumor, craniotomy, or head injury (prophylaxis)**
[Dexamethasone, Oral (Systemic)][1], 998
[Dexamethasone, Parenteral (Systemic)][1], 998
[Prednisone (Systemic)][1], 998

**Edema, cerebral, associated with primary or metastatic brain tumor, craniotomy, or head injury (treatment)**
Dexamethasone, Oral (Systemic), 998
Dexamethasone, Parenteral (Systemic), 998
[Prednisone (Systemic)][1], 998
**Edema, cystoid macular, following cataract surgery (prophylaxis)**
[Diclofenac (Ophthalmic)], 383
Indomethacin (Ophthalmic)*, 383
**Edema, cystoid macular, following cataract surgery (treatment)**
[Diclofenac (Ophthalmic)], 383
Indomethacin (Ophthalmic)*, 383
**Edema, pulmonary, acute (treatment adjunct)**
See also Edema
Morphine (Systemic), 2168
**Edema, pulmonary, following surgery for pulmonary hypertension (treatment)**
CY-1503 (Systemic), 3138‡
**Edema, pulmonary, noncardiogenic (treatment)**
[Betamethasone, Oral (Systemic)][1], 998
[Betamethasone, Parenteral (Systemic)][1], 998
[Cortisone (Systemic)][1], 998
[Dexamethasone, Oral (Systemic)][1], 998
[Dexamethasone, Parenteral (Systemic)][1], 998
[Hydrocortisone, Oral (Systemic)][1], 998
[Hydrocortisone, Parenteral (Systemic)][1], 998
[Methylprednisolone, Oral (Systemic)][1], 998
[Methylprednisolone, Parenteral (Systemic)][1], 998
[Prednisolone, Oral (Systemic)][1], 998
[Prednisolone, Parenteral (Systemic)][1], 998
[Prednisone (Systemic)][1], 998
[Triamcinolone, Oral (Systemic)][1], 998
[Triamcinolone, Parenteral (Systemic)][1], 998
**Edema, pulmonary, protamine sensitivity-induced**—See Edema, pulmonary, noncardiogenic
**Ehrlichiosis (treatment)**
Chloramphenicol (Systemic), 841
**Ekbom's syndrome**—See Pain, neurogenic
**Electroconvulsive therapy (treatment adjunct)**
[Caffeine (Systemic)], 706
**Electrolyte depletion (prophylaxis)**
Dextrose and Electrolytes (Systemic), 769
Oral Rehydration Salts (Systemic)*, 769
Rice Syrup Solids and Electrolytes (Systemic)†, 769
**Electrolyte depletion (treatment)**
Calcium Acetate (Systemic)†, 736
Calcium Chloride (Systemic), 736
Calcium Gluceptate (Systemic)†, 736
Calcium Gluconate, Parenteral (Systemic), 736
Dextrose and Electrolytes (Systemic), 769
Magnesium Chloride, Parenteral (Systemic)†, 1897
Magnesium Sulfate, Parenteral (Systemic), 1897
Oral Rehydration Salts (Systemic)*, 769
Rice Syrup Solids and Electrolytes (Systemic)†, 769
**Embolism, pulmonary (diagnosis)**
See also Lung imaging, radionuclide
[Krypton Kr 81m (Systemic)], 1816
**Embolism, thrombosis-induced**—See Thromboembolism
**Emphysema, panacinar, due to alpha₁-antitrypsin deficiency (treatment)**
Alpha₁-Proteinase Inhibitor, Human (Systemic), #
**Emphysema, pulmonary (treatment)**
Albuterol (Systemic), 651
Aminophylline (Systemic), 668
Ephedrine (Systemic), 651
Epinephrine (Systemic), 651
Ethylnorepinephrine (Systemic)†, 651
Fenoterol (Systemic)*, 651
Ipratropium (Inhalation-Local), 1761
Isoproterenol (Systemic), 651
Metaproterenol (Systemic), 651
Oxtriphylline (Systemic), 668
Oxtriphylline and Guaifenesin (Systemic), #
Terbutaline (Systemic), 651
Theophylline (Systemic), 668
Theophylline and Guaifenesin (Systemic)†, #
**Emphysema, pulmonary (treatment adjunct)**
Acetylcysteine (Inhalation-Local), #
**Encephalomyelopathy, subacute necrotizing (treatment)**
[Thiamine (Systemic)], 2787
**Endocarditis, bacterial (prophylaxis)**
[Amoxicillin (Systemic)][1], 2240
[Ampicillin (Systemic)][1], 2240
[Cefadroxil (Systemic)][1], 794
[Cefazolin (Systemic)][1], 794
[Cephalexin (Systemic)][1], 794
Erythromycin (Systemic), 1368
Penicillin G, Parenteral (Systemic), 2240
Penicillin V (Systemic), 2240
Vancomycin (Systemic), 2919

**Endocarditis, bacterial (treatment)**
Ampicillin, Parenteral (Systemic), 2240
Carbenicillin, Parenteral (Systemic), 2240
Cefazolin (Systemic), 794
[Cephalothin (Systemic)], 794
Cephapirin (Systemic)¹†, 794
[Cephradine (Systemic)][1], 794
Cloxacillin, Parenteral (Systemic), 2240
Fusidic Acid (Systemic)*, 3021
Imipenem and Cilastatin (Systemic), 1681
[Methicillin (Systemic)][1], 2240
Metronidazole (Systemic), 1996
[Nafcillin, Parenteral (Systemic)][1], 2240
[Oxacillin, Parenteral (Systemic)]¹†, 2240
[Penicillin G, Parenteral (Systemic)][1], 2240
Penicillin G Procaine (Systemic), 2240
[Sulfamethoxazole and Trimethoprim (Systemic)][1], 2661
Vancomycin (Systemic), 2919
**Endocarditis, fungal (treatment)**
Amphotericin B (Systemic), 98
Flucytosine (Systemic), #
**Endocervical infections**—See Genitourinary tract infections
**Endometrial thinning**
[Goserelin (Systemic)], 1575
**Endometriosis (prophylaxis)**
[Desogestrel and Ethinyl Estradiol (Systemic)][1], 1397
[Ethynodiol Diacetate and Ethinyl Estradiol (Systemic)][1], 1397
[Levonorgestrel and Ethinyl Estradiol (Systemic)][1], 1397
[Norethindrone Acetate and Ethinyl Estradiol (Systemic)][1], 1397
[Norethindrone and Ethinyl Estradiol (Systemic)][1], 1397
[Norethindrone and Mestranol (Systemic)], 1397
[Norgestimate and Ethinyl Estradiol (Systemic)][1], 1397
[Norgestrel and Ethinyl Estradiol (Systemic)][1], 1397
**Endometriosis (treatment)**
Danazol (Systemic), 1163
[Desogestrel and Ethinyl Estradiol (Systemic)][1], 1397
[Ethynodiol Diacetate and Ethinyl Estradiol (Systemic)][1], 1397
Goserelin (Systemic), 1575
Leuprolide (Systemic), 1840
[Levonorgestrel and Ethinyl Estradiol (Systemic)][1], 1397
[Medroxyprogesterone (Oral) (Systemic)][1], 2400
[Medroxyprogesterone (Parenteral) (Systemic)], 2400
Nafarelin (Systemic), 2076
[Norethindrone Acetate and Ethinyl Estradiol (Systemic)][1], 1397
Norethindrone Acetate Tablets USP (Systemic), 2400
[Norethindrone and Ethinyl Estradiol (Systemic)][1], 1397
[Norethindrone and Mestranol (Systemic)][1], 1397
[Norgestimate and Ethinyl Estradiol (Systemic)][1], 1397
[Norgestrel and Ethinyl Estradiol (Systemic)][1], 1397
**Endophthalmitis, candidal (treatment)**
Amphotericin B (Systemic), 98
**ENL**—See Erythema nodosum leprosum
**Enteritis, *Campylobacter* (treatment)**
[Erythromycin (Systemic)][1], 1368
**Enteritis, regional (treatment)**
See also Bowel disease, inflammatory
Aminosalicylate Sodium (Systemic), 3130‡
Betamethasone, Oral (Systemic), 998
Betamethasone, Parenteral (Systemic), 998
Chimeric A2 (Human-Murine) IgG Monoclonal Anti-TNF Antibody (cA2) (Systemic), 3136‡
Cortisone, (Systemic), 998
Dexamethasone, Oral (Systemic), 998
Dexamethasone, Parenteral (Systemic), 998
Hydrocortisone, Oral (Systemic), 998
Hydrocortisone, Parenteral (Systemic), 998
Methylprednisolone, Oral (Systemic), 998
Methylprednisolone, Parenteral (Systemic), 998
Prednisolone, Oral (Systemic), 998
Prednisolone, Parenteral (Systemic), 998
Prednisone (Systemic), 998
Triamcinolone, Oral (Systemic), 998
Triamcinolone, Parenteral (Systemic), 998
**Enterobiasis (treatment)**
Albendazole (Systemic)*†, #
Mebendazole (Systemic), 1926
Piperazine (Systemic), #
Pyrantel (Oral-Local), #

**Enterobiasis (treatment)** *(continued)*
  Pyrvinium (Oral-Local)*, #
**Enterocolitis,** *Shigella* **species (treatment)**
  [Demeclocycline (Systemic)], 2765
  [Doxycycline (Systemic)], 2765
  [Minocycline (Systemic)], 2765
  [Oxytetracycline (Systemic)]†, 2765
  Sulfamethoxazole and Trimethoprim (Systemic), 2661
  [Tetracycline (Systemic)], 2765
**Enterocolitis, staphylococcal (treatment)**
  Vancomycin (Oral-Local), 2916
**Enuresis (treatment adjunct)**
  [Amitriptyline (Systemic)], 271
  Imipramine Hydrochloride (Systemic), 271
**Enuresis, primary nocturnal (treatment)**
  Desmopressin, Nasal (Systemic), 1187
**Envenomation, black widow spider (treatment)**
  Antivenin (Latrodectus Mactans) (Systemic), #
**Envenomation, box jellyfish (treatment)**
  Antivenin (Chironex Fleckeri) (Systemic)*†, #
**Envenomation, brown snake (treatment)**
  Antivenin (Pseudonaja Textilis) (Systemic)*†, #
**Envenomation,** *Crotalidae* **venom (treatment)**
  Antivenin, Polyvalent Crotalid (Ovine) Fab (Systemic), 3132‡
  Antivenom (*Crotalidae*) Purified (Avian) (Systemic), 3132‡
**Envenomation, North American coral snake (treatment)**
  Antivenin (*Micrurus Fulvius*) (Systemic)†, #
**Envenomation, pit viper (treatment)**
  Antivenin (*Crotalidae*) Polyvalent (Systemic), #
**Envenomation, sea snake (treatment)**
  Antivenin (*Enhydrina Schistosa*) (Systemic)*†, #
**Envenomation, sea wasp (treatment)**
  See Envenomation, box jellyfish (Systemic)*†, #
**Envenomation, tiger snake (treatment)**
  [Antivenin (*Notechis Scutatus*) (Systemic)]1, #
**Eosinophilia, tropical pulmonary**—See Tropical eosinophilia
**Eosinophilic lung**—See Tropical eosinophilia
**Ependymoma**—See Tumors, brain, primary
**Epicondylitis (treatment)**
  Betamethasone, Oral (Systemic), 998
  Betamethasone, Parenteral (Systemic), 998
  Betamethasone, Parenteral-Local (Systemic), 998
  Cortisone (Systemic), 998
  Dexamethasone (Systemic), 998
  Hydrocortisone, Oral (Systemic), 998
  Hydrocortisone, Parenteral (Systemic), 998
  Hydrocortisone, Parenteral-Local (Systemic), 998
  Methylprednisolone, Oral (Systemic), 998
  Methylprednisolone, Parenteral (Systemic), 998
  Methylprednisolone, Parenteral-Local (Systemic), 998
  Prednisolone (Systemic), 998
  Prednisone (Systemic), 998
  Triamcinolone (Systemic), 998
**Epididymo-orchitis**—See Genitourinary tract infections
**Epilepsy**
  See also Status epilepticus
**Epilepsy (diagnosis)**
  [Technetium Tc 99m Exametazime (Systemic)]1, 2708
**Epilepsy (treatment adjunct)**
  Tiagabine (Systemic), 2815
  Topiramate (Systemic), 2839
**Epilepsy, absence seizure pattern (treatment)**
  Acetazolamide (Systemic), 773
  Clonazepam (Systemic), 556
  Divalproex (Systemic), 2908
  Ethosuximide (Systemic), #
  Methsuximide (Systemic), #
  Paramethadione (Systemic)*†, #
  Trimethadione (Systemic)*†, #
  Valproate Sodium (Systemic)†, 2908
  Valproic Acid (Systemic), 2908
**Epilepsy, akinetic seizure pattern (treatment)**
  Clonazepam (Systemic), 556
**Epilepsy, complex partial seizure pattern (treatment)**
  Carbamazepine (Systemic), 757
  [Clonazepam (Systemic)]1, 556
  Divalproex (Systemic), 2908
  Ethotoin (Systemic)†, 253
  Felbamate (Systemic)†, 1436
  Mephenytoin (Systemic), 253
  [Methsuximide (Systemic)]1, #
  [Phenacemide (Systemic)]1*†, #
  Phenytoin (Systemic), 253
  Primidone (Systemic), 2376
  Valproate Sodium (Systemic)†, 2908
  [Valproic Acid (Systemic)], 2908

**Epilepsy, complex partial seizure pattern (treatment adjunct)**
  Clorazepate (Systemic)1, 556
  Gabapentin (Systemic), 1536
**Epilepsy, cortical focal seizure pattern**—See Epilepsy, simple partial seizure pattern
**Epilepsy, grand mal**—See Epilepsy, tonic-clonic seizure pattern
**Epilepsy, Jacksonian**—See Epilepsy, simple partial seizure pattern
**Epilepsy, Lennox-Gastaut syndrome (treatment)**
  Clonazepam (Systemic), 556
  Felbamate (Systemic), 3143‡
  Lamotrigine (Systemic), 3151‡
  Topiramate (Systemic), 3169‡
**Epilepsy, Lennox-Gastaut syndrome (treatment adjunct)**
  Felbamate (Systemic)†, 1436
**Epilepsy, mixed seizure pattern (treatment)**
  Acetazolamide (Systemic), 773
  Carbamazepine (Systemic), 757
**Epilepsy, mixed seizure pattern (treatment adjunct)**
  Divalproex (Systemic), 2908
  Valproate Sodium (Systemic)†, 2908
  Valproic Acid (Systemic), 2908
**Epilepsy, myoclonic seizure pattern (treatment)**
  Acetazolamide (Systemic), 773
  Clonazepam (Systemic), 556
  [Divalproex (Systemic)], 2908
  Nitrazepam (Systemic)*, 556
  Valproate Sodium (Systemic)†, 2908
  [Valproic Acid (Systemic)], 2908
**Epilepsy, myoclonic seizure pattern (treatment adjunct)**
  [Diazepam, Oral (Systemic)]1, 556
**Epilepsy, nocturnal myoclonic (treatment)**
  Primidone (Systemic), 2376
**Epilepsy, petit mal**—See Epilepsy, absence seizure pattern
**Epilepsy, psychomotor**—See Epilepsy, complex partial seizure pattern
**Epilepsy, simple partial seizure pattern (treatment)**
  Acetazolamide (Systemic), 773
  Carbamazepine (Systemic), 757
  [Clonazepam (Systemic)]1, 556
  [Divalproex (Systemic)], 2908
  Ethotoin (Systemic)†, 253
  Felbamate (Systemic)†, 1436
  Fosphenytoin (Systemic)†, 253
  Mephenytoin (Systemic), 253
  Mephobarbital (Systemic), 518
  Metharbital (Systemic)*†, 518
  Phenobarbital (Systemic), 518
  Primidone (Systemic), 2376
  Valproate Sodium (Systemic)†, 2908
  [Valproic Acid (Systemic)], 2908
**Epilepsy, simple partial seizure pattern (treatment adjunct)**
  Clorazepate (Systemic)1, 556
  Gabapentin (Systemic), 1536
  Lamotrigine (Systemic), 1824
**Epilepsy, temporal lobe**—See Epilepsy, complex partial seizure pattern
**Epilepsy, tonic-clonic seizure pattern (treatment)**
  Acetazolamide (Systemic), 773
  Carbamazepine (Systemic), 757
  [Clonazepam (Systemic)]1, 556
  [Divalproex (Systemic)], 2908
  Ethotoin (Systemic)†, 253
  Fosphenytoin (Systemic)†, 253
  Mephenytoin (Systemic), 253
  Mephobarbital (Systemic), 518
  Metharbital (Systemic)*†, 518
  Phenobarbital (Systemic), 518
  Phenytoin (Systemic), 253
  Primidone (Systemic), 2376
  [Valproic Acid (Systemic)], 2908
**Epilepsy, tonic-clonic seizure pattern, drug-resistant (treatment)**
  Antiepilepsirine (Systemic), 3131‡
**Episcleritis (treatment)**
  Betamethasone (Ophthalmic)*, 966
  Dexamethasone (Ophthalmic), 966
  Fluorometholone (Ophthalmic), 966
  Hydrocortisone (Ophthalmic)*, 966
  Medrysone (Ophthalmic), 966
  Prednisolone (Ophthalmic), 966
**Episodic dyscontrol (treatment)**
  [Phenytoin (Systemic)]1, 253
**Epistaxis secondary to hyperfibrinolysis**—See Hemorrhage, hyperfibrinolysis-induced
**Epitheliomatosis, multiple superficial (treatment)**
  Podophyllum (Topical)†, 2341

**Erectile dysfunction (diagnosis)**
  Alprostadil (Local), 48
**Erectile dysfunction (treatment)**
  Alprostadil (Local), 48
  Sildenafil (Systemic), 2574
**Erysipelas (treatment)**
  [Clindamycin (Systemic)]1, 893
  Penicillin G, Parenteral (Systemic), 2240
  Penicillin G Procaine (Systemic), 2240
  Penicillin V (Systemic), 2240
  [Vancomycin (Systemic)]1, 2919
**Erysipeloid (treatment)**
  [Penicillin G Benzathine (Systemic)]1, 2240
  [Penicillin G, Parenteral (Systemic)]1, 2240
  [Penicillin G Procaine (Systemic)]1, 2240
  [Penicillin V (Systemic)]1, 2240
**Erythema multiforme, severe (treatment)**
  Betamethasone, Oral (Systemic), 998
  Betamethasone, Parenteral (Systemic), 998
  Cortisone (Systemic), 998
  Dexamethasone, Oral (Systemic), 998
  Dexamethasone, Parenteral (Systemic), 998
  Hydrocortisone, Oral (Systemic), 998
  Hydrocortisone, Parenteral (Systemic), 998
  Methylprednisolone, Oral (Systemic), 998
  Methylprednisolone, Parenteral (Systemic), 998
  Prednisolone, Oral (Systemic), 998
  Prednisolone, Parenteral (Systemic), 998
  Prednisone (Systemic), 998
  Triamcinolone, Oral (Systemic), 998
  Triamcinolone, Parenteral (Systemic), 998
**Erythema nodosum (treatment)**
  [Potassium Iodide (Systemic)]1, 2354
**Erythema nodosum leprosum (treatment)**
  Thalidomide (Systemic)*†, 2776, 3168‡
**Erythema nodosum leprosum, recurrent (suppression)**
  Thalidomide (Systemic)1†, 2776
**Erythrasma (treatment)**
  Erythromycin (Systemic), 1368
  Fusidic Acid (Topical)*, 3021
**Erythroblastopenia**—See Anemia, red blood cell
**Erythroderma, congenital ichthyosiform (treatment)**
  [Etretinate (Systemic)], #
  [Isotretinoin (Systemic)]1, 1796
**Erythroderma, ichthyosiform (treatment)**
  [Acitretin (Systemic)]1, 18
**Erythroleukemia (treatment)**
  Daunorubicin (Systemic)1, 1173
**Erythroplasia of Queyrat (treatment)**
  [Fluorouracil (Topical)]1, 1500
**Esophageal imaging, radionuclide**
  Technetium Tc 99m Sulfur Colloid (Systemic)1, 2740
**Esophageal obstruction, foreign body (treatment)**
  [Glucagon (Systemic)]1, 1563
  Vasoactive Intestinal Polypeptide (Systemic), 3171‡
**Esophageal transit studies**—See Esophageal imaging, radionuclide
**Esophageal varices, bleeding (treatment)**
  Ethanolamine Oleate (Parenteral-Local), #, 3142‡
  Sodium Tetradecyl Sulfate, 3164‡
  Somatostatin (Systemic), 3165‡
  Terlipressin, 3167‡
**Esophagitis, reflux**—See Reflux, gastroesophageal
**Esotropia, accommodative (diagnosis)**
  Demecarium (Ophthalmic), 315
  Echothiophate (Ophthalmic), 315
  Isoflurophate (Ophthalmic), 315
**Esotropia, accommodative (treatment)**
  Demecarium (Ophthalmic), 315
  Echothiophate (Ophthalmic), 315
  Isoflurophate (Ophthalmic), 315
**Espundia**—See Leishmaniasis, mucosal
**Essential tremor (treatment)**
  [Primidone (Systemic)]1, 2376
**Estrogen production, endogenous (diagnosis)**
  Hydroxyprogesterone (Systemic)†, 2400
  [Medroxyprogesterone, Oral (Systemic)], 2400
  [Progesterone, Parenteral (Systemic)], 2400
**Eustachian tube, patulous (treatment)**
  Patul-end (Systemic), 3157‡
**Ewing's sarcoma (treatment)**
  [Cyclophosphamide (Systemic)]1, 1128
  Dactinomycin (Systemic), 1153
  [Daunorubicin (Systemic)], 1173
  [Doxorubicin (Systemic)]1, 1308
  [Etoposide (Systemic)]1, 1424
  [Ifosfamide (Systemic)]1, 1677
  N-Acetylglucosminyl-N-Acetylmuramyl-L-Ala-D-IsoGln-L-Ala-Glycerolid-Palmitoyl, Liposomal (Systemic), 3152‡
  [Vincristine (Systemic)], 2950

**Extrahepatic malignant disease (diagnosis)**
Indium In 111 Satumomab Pendetide (Systemic)†, 1702
**Extrapyramidal reactions, drug-induced (treatment)**
Amantadine (Systemic), 58
Benztropine (Systemic), 297
Biperiden (Systemic), 297
Diphenhydramine (Systemic)[1], 325
Ethopropazine (Systemic), 297
Procyclidine (Systemic), 297
Trihexyphenidyl (Systemic), 297
**Extrasystoles, ventricular (treatment)**
Procainamide, Parenteral (Systemic), 2387
**Eyelid closure, synkinetic (treatment)**
Botulinum Toxin Type A (Systemic), 3134‡

## F

**Fabry's disease (treatment)**
1,5-(Butylimino-1,5 Dideoxy, D-Glucitol (Systemic), 3127‡
Alpha-Galactosidase A (Systemic), 3129‡
Ceramide Trihexosidase and Alpha-Galactosidase A (Systemic), 3136‡
**Facial spasm (treatment)**
[Botulinum Toxin Type A (Parenteral-Local)], 627
**Factor XIII deficiency (treatment)**
Antihemophilic Factor, Cryoprecipitated (Systemic), 319
Factor XIII (Systemic), 3142‡
**Familial tremor**—See Essential tremor
**Fatigue (treatment)**
Caffeine (Systemic), 706
Caffeine, Citrated (Systemic), 706
**Fatigue, multiple sclerosis–associated (treatment)**
[Amantadine (Systemic)][1], 58
**Fatty acid deficiency (prophylaxis)**
Fat Emulsions (Systemic), #
**Fatty acid deficiency (treatment)**
Fat Emulsions (Systemic), #
**Felty's syndrome (treatment)**
[Auranofin (Systemic)][1], 1566
[Aurothioglucose (Systemic)][1], 1566
[Gold Sodium Thiomalate (Systemic)][1], 1566
[Penicillamine (Systemic)][1], 2237
**Fetal distress (diagnosis)**
[Oxytocin, Parenteral (Systemic)][1], 2211
**Fever (treatment)**
Acetaminophen (Systemic), 6
Acetaminophen and Aspirin (Systemic)†, 11
Acetaminophen, Aspirin, and Caffeine (Systemic)†, 11
Acetaminophen, Aspirin, and Caffeine, Buffered (Systemic)†, 11
Acetaminophen, Aspirin, and Salicylamide, Buffered (Systemic)†, 11
Acetaminophen, Aspirin, Salicylamide, and Caffeine (Systemic)†, 11
Acetaminophen and Caffeine (Systemic), 6
Acetaminophen and Salicylamide (Systemic)†, 11
Acetaminophen, Salicylamide, and Caffeine (Systemic)†, 11
Aspirin (Systemic), 2538
Aspirin, Buffered (Systemic), 2538
Choline Salicylate (Systemic)†, 2538
Choline and Magnesium Salicylates (Systemic), 2538
Ibuprofen (Systemic), 388
Magnesium Salicylate (Systemic), 2538
Naproxen (Systemic)[1], 388
Salsalate (Systemic), 2538
Sodium Salicylate (Systemic), 2538
**Fever blisters (treatment)**
Benzocaine Gel (Dental) (Mucosal-Local), 128
Benzocaine and Phenol Gel (Mucosal-Local), 128
Benzocaine and Phenol Topical Solution (Mucosal-Local), 128
Benzocaine Topical Solution USP (Dental) (Mucosal-Local), 128
Lidocaine 2.5% Oral Topical Solution USP (Mucosal-Local), 128
**Fever, due to malignancy (treatment)**
[Indomethacin (Systemic)][1], 388
**Fever, due to malignancy (treatment adjunct)**
[Betamethasone, Oral (Systemic)][1], 998
[Betamethasone, Parenteral (Systemic)][1], 998
[Cortisone (Systemic)][1], 998
[Dexamethasone, Oral (Systemic)][1], 998
[Dexamethasone, Parenteral (Systemic)][1], 998
[Hydrocortisone, Oral (Systemic)][1], 998
[Hydrocortisone, Parenteral (Systemic)][1], 998
[Methylprednisolone, Oral (Systemic)][1], 998
[Methylprednisolone, Parenteral (Systemic)][1], 998
[Prednisolone, Oral (Systemic)][1], 998
[Prednisolone, Parenteral (Systemic)][1], 998

**Fever, due to malignancy (treatment adjunct)** (continued)
[Prednisone (Systemic)][1], 998
[Triamcinolone, Oral (Systemic)][1], 998
[Triamcinolone, Parenteral (Systemic)][1], 998
**Fever, hemorrhagic, nephrotic syndrome–associated (treatment)**
Ribavirin (Systemic), 3162‡
**Fever, unknown origin, source of (diagnosis)**
[Gallium Citrate Ga 67 (Systemic)], 1538
**Fibrillation, atrial (prophylaxis)**
Digitoxin (Systemic), 1213
Digoxin (Systemic), 1213
Diltiazem, Parenteral (Systemic), 720
Quinidine (Systemic), 2440
Verapamil (Systemic), 720
**Fibrillation, atrial (treatment)**
See also Arrhythmias, supraventricular
Digitoxin (Systemic), 1213
Digoxin (Systemic), 1213
Diltiazem, Parenteral (Systemic), 720
Esmolol (Systemic)†, 1377
[Procainamide (Systemic)], 2387
Quinidine (Systemic), 2440
Verapamil (Systemic), 720
**Fibrillation, atrial, paroxysmal (prophylaxis)**
Diltiazem, Parenteral (Systemic), 720
Flecainide (Systemic)[1], 1469
Quinidine (Systemic), 2440
Verapamil (Systemic), 720
**Fibrillation, atrial, paroxysmal (treatment)**
Diltiazem, Parenteral (Systemic), 720
Quinidine (Systemic), 2440
Verapamil (Systemic), 720
**Fibrillation, ventricular (prophylaxis)**
Amiodarone Hydrochloride (Systemic), 3130‡
Bretylium (Systemic), 630
**Fibrillation, ventricular (treatment)**
Amiodarone Hydrochloride (Systemic), 3130‡
Bretylium (Systemic), 630
**Fibrinogen deficiency, hemorrhagic complications of (prophylaxis)**
Fibrinogen (Human) (Systemic), 3143‡
**Fibrinogen deficiency, hemorrhagic complications of (treatment)**
Fibrinogen (Human) (Systemic), 3143‡
**Fibrinogen excess (treatment)**
[Stanozolol (Systemic)]†, 110
**Fibromyalgia syndrome**
[Cyclobenzaprine (Systemic)][1], 1126
**Filariasis, Bancroft's (treatment)**
Diethylcarbamazine (Systemic), #
Ivermectin (Systemic)*†, #
**Fire ant sensitivity (diagnosis)**
Imported Fire Ant Venom, Allergenic Extract (Systemic), 3147‡
**Fire ant sensitivity (treatment)**
Imported Fire Ant Venom, Allergenic Extract (Systemic), 3147‡
**Fish tapeworm**—See Diphyllobothriasis
**Fissures, anorectal (treatment)**
Bufexamac (Topical)*, 3013
**Fistulas, secreting cutaneous, nonoperative (treatment adjunct)**
Somatostatin (Systemic), 3165‡
**Flutter, atrial (prophylaxis)**
Digitoxin (Systemic), 1213
Digoxin (Systemic), 1213
Diltiazem, Parenteral (Systemic), 720
Quinidine (Systemic), 2440
Verapamil (Systemic), 720
**Flutter, atrial (treatment)**
See also Arrhythmias, supraventricular
Digitoxin (Systemic), 1213
Digoxin (Systemic), 1213
Diltiazem, Parenteral (Systemic), 720
Esmolol (Systemic)†, 1377
Quinidine (Systemic), 2440
Verapamil (Systemic), 720
**Folate deficiency (diagnosis)**
[Folic Acid (Systemic)][1], 1517
**Folic acid deficiency (prophylaxis)**
Folic Acid (Systemic), 1517
**Folic acid deficiency (treatment)**
Folic Acid (Systemic), 1517
**Folliculitis (treatment)**
Clioquinol and Flumethasone (Topical)*, 3015
Clioquinol and Hydrocortisone (Topical), #
Framycetin and Gramicidin (Topical)*, 3021
[Isotretinoin (Systemic)][1], 1796
Gentamicin (Topical), 1557
[Mupirocin (Topical)][1], 4253
**Fontaine state IV chronic critical limb ischemia**
Prostaglandin E1 Enol Ester (AS-013) (Systemic), 3160‡

**Frostbite (treatment)**
Nicotinyl Alcohol (Systemic)*, #
Nylidrin (Systemic)*, #
**Fungal infection, presumed, in febrile neutropenia (treatment)**
Amphotericin B Liposomal Complex (Systemic), 105
**Fungal infections, invasive (treatment)**
Amphotericin B Lipid Complex (Systemic), 103
**Furunculosis (treatment)**
Gentamicin (Topical), 1557
**Furunculosis of the ear canal (treatment)**
Clioquinol and Flumethasone (Otic)*, 3015

## G

**Gag reflex suppression**
Benzocaine, Butamben, and Tetracaine Hydrochloride Topical Aerosol USP (Mucosal-Local), 128
Benzocaine Gel (Mucosal-Local), 128
Benzocaine Topical Aerosol USP (Mucosal-Local), 128
Benzocaine Topical Solution USP (Mucosal-Local), 128
Dyclonine Hydrochloride 0.5% Topical Solution USP (Mucosal-Local), 128
Lidocaine Hydrochloride Oral Topical Solution USP (Mucosal-Local), 128
Lidocaine Hydrochloride Topical Spray Solution (Mucosal-Local), 128
[Lidocaine Topical Aerosol (Mucosal-Local)], 128
Tetracaine Hydrochloride Topical Solution USP (Mucosal-Local), 128
Tetracaine Topical Aerosol (Mucosal-Local), 128
**Galactorrhea, due to hyperprolactinemia (treatment)**
Bromocriptine (Systemic), 636
**Gallbladder disorders (diagnosis)**
See also Cholangiography, preoperative; Cholecystography, intravenous; cholecystography, oral
Sincalide (Systemic) #
**Gallstone disease (treatment)**
Chenodiol (Systemic)*†, #, 3136‡
Monoctanoin (Local)†, #
Monooctanoin (Local), 3155‡
Ursodiol (Systemic), 2903
**Gallstone formation (prophylaxis)**
[Ursodiol (Systemic)][1], 2903
Ursodiol (Systemic)[1], 2903
**Gas gangrene infections (treatment)**
[Penicillin G, Parenteral (Systemic)][1], 2240
**Gas, gastrointestinal (treatment)**
Charcoal, Activated (Oral-Local), 831
Loperamide and Simethicone (Systemic), 3028
Simethicone (Oral-Local), #
**Gastric distress (treatment)**
Bismuth Subsalicylate (Oral-Local), 616
**Gastric emptying, slow (treatment)**
[Metoclopramide (Systemic)], 1992
**Gastric emptying studies**
[Technetium Tc 99m Sulfur Colloid (Systemic)][1], 2740
**Gastric histamine test**
Histamine (Systemic)*, #
**Gastric mucosa imaging, radionuclide**
[Sodium Pertechnetate Tc 99m (Systemic)][1], 2612
**Gastric stasis, in preterm infants (treatment)**
[Metoclopramide (Systemic)], 1992
**Gastritis, Helicobacter pylori–associated (treatment adjunct)**
[Amoxicillin (Systemic)][1], 2240
[Bismuth Subsalicylate (Oral-Local)][1], 616
[Metronidazole (Systemic)][1], 1996
**Gastroenteritis, bacterial (treatment)**
Ciprofloxacin (Systemic), 1487
[Norfloxacin (Systemic)][1], 1487
**Gastroesophageal reflux disease (prophylaxis)**
Lansoprazole (Systemic), 1828
Omeprazole (Systemic), 2163
**Gastroesophageal reflux disease (treatment)**
Lansoprazole (Systemic), 1828
Omeprazole (Systemic), 2163
**Gastrointestinal imaging, magnetic resonance**
Perflubron (Oral-Local)†, #
**Gastrointestinal motility disorders (treatment)**
Domperidone (Systemic)*, 3018
**Gastroparesis (treatment)**
See also Gastric emptying, slow; Gastric stasis, in preterm infants
[Cisapride (Systemic)], 869
[Erythromycin (Systemic)][1], 1368
Metoclopramide (Systemic)[1], 1992
**Gastroscopy adjunct**
[Simethicone (Oral-Local)][1], #

### Gaucher's disease (treatment)
1,5-(Butylimino-1,5 Dideoxy, D-Glucitol (Systemic), 3127‡
Alglucerase (Systemic), #, 3129‡
Imiglucerase (Systemic)†, 1680, 3147‡
L-Cycloserine (Systemic), 3150‡
PEG-Glucocerebrosidase (Systemic), 3157‡
Retroviral Vector—Glucocerebrosidase, Recombinant (Systemic), 3161‡
Retroviral Vector, R-GC and GC (Systemic), 3162‡

### Gender change, female-to-male
[Testosterone (Systemic)][1], 118

### Genitourinary disorders, spastic—See Urologic disorders, symptoms

### Genitourinary tract infections (treatment)
See also Gynecologic infections; Pelvic infections, female
Cefazolin (Systemic), 794
Cefoperazone (Systemic)[1], 794
Cefotaxime (Systemic), 794
Cephalexin (Systemic), 794
[Cephalothin (Systemic)], 794
Cephradine (Systemic)[1], 794
Demeclocycline (Systemic), 2765
Doxycycline (Systemic), 2765
Minocycline (Systemic), 2765
Oxytetracycline (Systemic)†, 2765
Tetracycline (Systemic), 2765

### GERD—See Gastroesophageal reflux disease (GERD)

### Giardiasis (treatment)
Furazolidone (Oral-Local)†, 1533
[Metronidazole, Oral (Systemic)][1], 1996
Quinacrine (Systemic), #

### Gilles de la Tourette's syndrome (treatment)
[Clonidine, Oral (Systemic)][1], 908
Haloperidol (Systemic), 1611
Pergolide (Systemic)‡, 3158‡
Pimozide (Systemic)[1], 2326

### Gingival disorders (treatment)
[Corticosteroids (Topical)], 978
Hydrocortisone Acetate Dental Paste (Topical), 978
Triamcinolone Acetonide Dental Paste (Topical), 978

### Gingivitis (prophylaxis)
Sodium Fluoride and Triclosan (Dental), 3034

### Gingivitis (treatment)
Chlorhexidine (Mucosal-Local)†, 847

### Gingivitis, desquamative (treatment)
[Betamethasone, Oral (Systemic)][1], 998
[Cortisone, Oral (Systemic)][1], 998
[Dexamethasone, Oral (Systemic)][1], 998
[Hydrocortisone, Oral (Systemic)][1], 998
[Hydrocortisone Acetate Dental Paste (Topical)], 978
[Methylprednisolone, Oral (Systemic)][1], 998
[Prednisolone, Oral (Systemic)][1], 998
[Prednisone (Systemic)][1], 998
[Triamcinolone Acetonide Dental Paste (Topical)], 978
[Triamcinolone, Oral (Systemic)][1], 998

### Gingivitis, necrotizing ulcerative, acute (treatment)
See also Gingivostomatitis, necrotizing ulcerative
[Chlorhexidine (Mucosal-Local)]†, 847
Penicillin G (Systemic), 2240
Penicillin G Procaine (Systemic), 2240
Penicillin V (Systemic), 2240

### Gingivostomatitis, necrotizing ulcerative (treatment)
Demeclocycline (Systemic), 2765
Doxycycline (Systemic), 2765
Minocycline (Systemic), 2765
Oxytetracycline (Systemic)†, 2765
Tetracycline (Systemic), 2765

### Glaucoma, angle-closure (treatment)
Acetazolamide (Systemic), 773
[Carbachol Ophthalmic Solution USP (Ophthalmic)][1], 755
Dichlorphenamide (Systemic)†, 773
Glycerin (Systemic), #
Methazolamide (Systemic), 773
Pilocarpine (Ophthalmic), #

### Glaucoma, angle-closure (treatment adjunct)
[Betaxolol (Ophthalmic)][1], 585
[Carteolol (Ophthalmic)]†, 585
[Levobunolol (Ophthalmic)][1], 585
[Metipranolol (Ophthalmic)]†, 585
[Timolol (Ophthalmic)], 585

### Glaucoma, angle-closure, after iridectomy (treatment)
Demecarium (Ophthalmic), 315
Echothiophate (Ophthalmic), 315
Isoflurophate (Ophthalmic), 315

### Glaucoma, angle-closure, before iridectomy (treatment)
Glycerin (Systemic), #

### Glaucoma, angle-closure, during or after iridectomy (treatment)
[Betaxolol (Ophthalmic)][1], 585
[Carbachol Ophthalmic Solution USP (Ophthalmic)][1], 755
[Carteolol (Ophthalmic)]†, 585
Glycerin (Systemic), #
[Levobunolol (Ophthalmic)][1], 585
[Metipranolol (Ophthalmic)]†, 585
[Physostigmine (Ophthalmic)]†, #
Pilocarpine (Ophthalmic), #
[Timolol (Ophthalmic)][1], 585

### Glaucoma, in aphakic eyes (treatment)
[Betaxolol (Ophthalmic)][1], 585
[Carteolol (Ophthalmic)]†, 585
[Levobunolol (Ophthalmic)][1], 585
[Metipranolol (Ophthalmic)]†, 585
Timolol (Ophthalmic), 585

### Glaucoma, chronic simple—See Glaucoma, open-angle
### Glaucoma, ciliary block—See Glaucoma, malignant
### Glaucoma, closed-angle—See Glaucoma, angle-closure

### Glaucoma, malignant (treatment)
[Acetazolamide (Systemic)], 773
Atropine (Ophthalmic), 485
[Betaxolol (Ophthalmic)][1], 585
[Carteolol (Ophthalmic)]†, 585
Glycerin (Systemic), #
[Levobunolol (Ophthalmic)][1], 585
[Metipranolol (Ophthalmic)]†, 585
[Timolol (Ophthalmic)][1], 585
Urea (Systemic)†, 2899

### Glaucoma, narrow-angle—See Glaucoma, angle-closure
### Glaucoma, narrow-angle, after iridectomy—See Glaucoma, angle-closure, after iridectomy
### Glaucoma, narrow-angle, during or after iridectomy—See Glaucoma, angle-closure, during or after iridectomy

### Glaucoma, open-angle (treatment)
(Systemic), 773
Acetazolamide (Systemic), 773
Apraclonidine (Ophthalmic), 459
Betaxolol (Ophthalmic), 585
Brimonidine (Ophthalmic), 632
Brinzolamide (Ophthalmic), 634
Carbachol Ophthalmic Solution USP (Ophthalmic), 755
Carteolol (Ophthalmic)†, 585
Demecarium (Ophthalmic), 315
Dichlorphenamide (Systemic)†, 773
Dipivefrin (Ophthalmic), 1249
Dorzolamide (Ophthalmic), 1294
Dorzolamide and Timolol (Ophthalmic), 3018
Echothiophate (Ophthalmic), 315
Epinephrine (Ophthalmic), 1350
Glycerin (Systemic), #
Isoflurophate (Ophthalmic), 315
Latanoprost (Ophthalmic), 1831
Levobunolol (Ophthalmic), 585
Methazolamide (Systemic), 773
Metipranolol (Ophthalmic)†, 585
Physostigmine (Ophthalmic)†, #
Pilocarpine (Ophthalmic), #
Timolol (Ophthalmic), 585, 3036
[Timolol (Ophthalmic)][1], 593

### Glaucoma, refractory (treatment)
Mitomycin-C (Ophthalmic), 3154‡

### Glaucoma, secondary (treatment)
Acetazolamide (Systemic), 773
[Betaxolol (Ophthalmic)][1], 585
[Carbachol Ophthalmic Solution USP (Ophthalmic)][1], 755
[Carteolol (Ophthalmic)]†, 585
Dichlorphenamide (Systemic)†, 773
[Dipivefrin (Ophthalmic)][1], 1249
Echothiophate (Ophthalmic), 315
[Epinephrine (Ophthalmic)][1], 1350
Glycerin (Systemic), #
[Levobunolol (Ophthalmic)][1], 585
Methazolamide (Systemic), 773
[Metipranolol (Ophthalmic)]†, 585
[Physostigmine (Ophthalmic)]†, #
Pilocarpine (Ophthalmic), #
Timolol (Ophthalmic), 585
Urea (Systemic)†, 2899

### Glioblastoma—See Tumors, brain, primary
### Glioma, brainstem—See Tumors, brain, primary

### Glioma, malignant (treatment adjunct)
Phenylacetate (Systemic)‡, 3158
Sodium Phenylbutyrate (Systemic)‡, 3164‡

### Glomerular filtration rate determination
Technetium Tc 99m Pentetate (Systemic), 2727

### Glomerulonephritis (treatment)
[Azathioprine (Systemic)][1], 491

### Glycogen storage disease, type II (treatment)
Human Acid Alpha-Glucosidase, 3145‡
Human Acid Alpha-Glucosidase, Recombinant (Systemic), 3160‡

### Glycosuria (diagnosis)
Copper Reduction Urine Glucose Test, #
Glucose Oxidase Urine Glucose Test, #
Urine Glucose and Ketone (Combined) Test, #

### Gnathostomiasis (treatment)
[Mebendazole (Systemic)][1], 1926

### Goiter (prophylaxis)
Levothyroxine (Systemic)[1], 2809
Liothyronine (Systemic)[1], 2809
Liotrix (Systemic)†, 2809
Thyroglobulin (Systemic)*†, 2809
Thyroid (Systemic)[1], 2809

### Goiter (treatment)
Levothyroxine (Systemic), 2809
Liothyronine (Systemic), 2809
Liotrix (Systemic)†, 2809
Thyroglobulin (Systemic)*†, 2809
Thyroid (Systemic), 2809

### Gonadal dysgenesis—See Turner's syndrome

### Gonadal function studies
See also Hypogonadism, female (diagnosis); Hypogonadism, male (diagnosis); Ovarian function studies
[Clomiphene (Systemic)], 903

### Gonorrhea (treatment)
[Doxycycline (Systemic)], 2765
[Tetracycline (Systemic)], 2765

### Gonorrhea, disseminated (treatment)
Cefuroxime (Systemic)[1], 794
[Spectinomycin (Systemic)][1], 2622

### Gonorrhea, endocervical (treatment)
[Ampicillin and Sulbactam (Systemic)]†, 2263
Ciprofloxacin (Systemic), 1487
Enoxacin (Systemic), 1487
Erythromycin (Systemic), 1368
Norfloxacin (Systemic), 1487
Ofloxacin (Systemic), 1487
Spectinomycin (Systemic), 2622
[Sulfamethoxazole and Trimethoprim (Systemic)], 2661
Trovafloxacin (Systemic), 2891

### Gonorrhea, endocervical, uncomplicated (treatment)
Amoxicillin (Systemic), 2240
Grepafloxacin (Systemic), 1580
[Penicillin G, Parenteral (Systemic)][1], 2240

### Gonorrhea, rectal (treatment)
Spectinomycin (Systemic), 2622

### Gonorrhea, rectal, in females
Trovafloxacin (Systemic), 2891

### Gonorrhea, rectal, uncomplicated (treatment)
Grepafloxacin (Systemic), 1580
Spectinomycin (Systemic), 2622

### Gonorrhea, uncomplicated (treatment)
Cefixime (Systemic), 794
Cefotaxime (Systemic), 794
Cefpodoxime (Systemic)[1], 794
Ceftizoxime (Systemic)[1], 794
Ceftriaxone (Systemic), 794
Cefuroxime (Systemic), 794
Cefuroxime Axetil (Systemic), 794

### Gonorrhea, urethral (treatment)
[Ampicillin and Sulbactam (Systemic)]†, 2263
Ciprofloxacin (Systemic), 1487
Enoxacin (Systemic), 1487
Erythromycin (Systemic), 1368
Norfloxacin (Systemic), 1487
Ofloxacin (Systemic), 1487
Spectinomycin (Systemic), 2622

### Gonorrhea, urethral, uncomplicated (treatment)
Amoxicillin (Systemic), 2240
Grepafloxacin (Systemic), 1580
[Penicillin G, Parenteral (Systemic)][1], 2240
Spectinomycin (Systemic), 2622
Trovafloxacin (Systemic), 2891

### Gout, acute—See Gouty arthritis, acute

### Gout, acute (treatment)
Naproxen (Systemic), 3029

### Gout, chronic—See Gouty arthritis, chronic

### Gouty arthritis, acute (prophylaxis)
Colchicine (Systemic), 928

### Gouty arthritis, acute (treatment)
Betamethasone, Oral (Systemic), 998
Betamethasone, Parenteral (Systemic), 998
Betamethasone, Parenteral-Local (Systemic), 998
Colchicine (Systemic), 928
Cortisone (Systemic), 998
Dexamethasone (Systemic), 998

**Gouty arthritis, acute (treatment)** (continued)
[Diclofenac (Systemic)]1, 388
[Diflunisal (Systemic)]¹, 388
[Etodolac (Systemic)]†, 388
[Fenoprofen (Systemic)]¹, 388
Floctafenine (Systemic)*¹, 388
Hydrocortisone, Oral (Systemic), 998
Hydrocortisone, Parenteral (Systemic), 998
Hydrocortisone, Parenteral-Local (Systemic), 998
[Ibuprofen (Systemic)]¹, 388
Indomethacin (Systemic), 388
[Ketoprofen (Systemic)]¹, 388
[Meclofenamate (Systemic)]†, 388
[Mefenamic Acid (Systemic)]¹, 388
Methylprednisolone, Oral (Systemic), 998
Methylprednisolone, Parenteral (Systemic), 998
Methylprednisolone, Parenteral-Local (Systemic), 998
Naproxen (Systemic)¹, 388
Phenylbutazone (Systemic), 388
[Piroxicam (Systemic)]¹, 388
Prednisolone (Systemic), 998
Prednisone (Systemic), 998
Sulindac (Systemic), 388
Triamcinolone (Systemic), 998
**Gouty arthritis, chronic (treatment)**
Allopurinol (Systemic), 44
Colchicine (Systemic), 928
Probenecid (Systemic), 2380
Probenecid and Colchicine (Systemic), 2384
Sulfinpyrazone (Systemic), 2646
**Graft rejection, burn wounds (treatment)**
Mafenide (Topical), 3152‡
**Graft rejection, corneal (prophylaxis)**
Cyclosporine (Ophthalmic), 3138‡
**Graft rejection, organ (prophylaxis)**
See also Transplant rejection, kidney; organ
Anti-CD45 Monoclonal Antibodies (Systemic), 3131‡
Omega-3 (n-3) Polyunsaturated Fatty Acid with All Double Bonds in the cis Configuration (Systemic), 3156‡
**Graft versus host disease (prophylaxis)**
[Cyclosporine (Systemic)], 1136
Interleukin-1 Receptor Antagonist, Human Recombinant (Systemic), 3149‡
[Tacrolimus (Systemic)]¹, 2683, 3167‡
Thalidomide (Systemic), 3168‡
**Graft versus host disease (treatment)**
[Cyclosporine (Systemic)], 1136
Interleukin-1 Receptor Antagonist, Human Recombinant (Systemic), 3149‡
[Tacrolimus (Systemic)]¹, 2683
Thalidomide (Systemic), 3168‡
**Graft versus host disease, in bone marrow transplantation (prophylaxis)**
Humanized Anti-TAC (Systemic), 3146‡
ST1-RTA Immunotoxin (SR-44163) (Systemic), 3166‡
Thalidomide (Systemic), 3168‡
**Graft versus host disease, in bone marrow transplantation (treatment)**
CD5-T Lymphocyte Immunotoxin (Systemic), 3136‡
Thalidomide (Systemic), 3168‡
**Graft versus host disease, intestinal (treatment)**
Beclomethasone Dipropionate (Systemic)‡, 3133
**Granuloma annulare (treatment)**
Amcinonide (Topical), 978
Beclomethasone Dipropionate (Topical), 978
Betamethasone Benzoate (Topical), 978
Betamethasone Dipropionate (Topical), 978
Betamethasone, Parenteral-Local (Systemic), 998
Betamethasone Valerate (Topical), 978
Clobetasol Propionate (Topical), 978
Clobetasone Butyrate (Topical), 978
[Dapsone (Systemic)]1, 1170
Desoximetasone (Topical), 978
Dexamethasone, Parenteral-Local (Systemic), 998
Diflorasone Diacetate (Topical), 978
Diflucortolone Valerate (Topical), 978
Fluocinolone Acetonide (Topical), 978
Fluocinonide (Topical), 978
Flurandrenolide (except 0.0125% cream and ointment) (Topical), 978
Fluticasone Propionate (Topical), 978
Halcinonide (Topical), 978
Halobetasol Propionate (Topical), 978
Hydrocortisone Butyrate (Topical), 978
Hydrocortisone, Parenteral-Local (Systemic), 998
Hydrocortisone Valerate (Topical), 978
Methylprednisolone, Parenteral-Local (Systemic), 998
Mometasone Furoate (Topical), 978
Prednisolone, Parenteral-Local (Systemic), 998
Triamcinolone Acetonide (Topical), 978

**Granuloma annulare (treatment)** (continued)
Triamcinolone, Parenteral-Local (Systemic), 998
**Granuloma inguinale (treatment)**
Demeclocycline (Systemic), 2765
Doxycycline (Systemic), 2765
Minocycline (Systemic), 2765
Oxytetracycline (Systemic)†, 2765
Streptomycin (Systemic), 69
[Sulfamethoxazole and Trimethoprim (Systemic)]¹, 2661
Tetracycline (Systemic), 2765
**Growth, constitutional delay in (treatment)**
[Fluoxymesterone (Systemic)]¹, 118
[Methyltestosterone (Systemic)]¹, 118
[Testosterone (Systemic)]¹, 118
**Growth failure (treatment)**
Growth Hormone Releasing Factor (Systemic), 3145‡
[Oxandrolone (Systemic)]†, 3156‡
Sermorelin (Systemic), 3164‡
Somatrem (Systemic), 1586, 3165‡
Somatropin (Systemic), 3165‡
Somatropin, Recombinant (Systemic), 1586, 3034, 3035
Testosterone Sublingual (Systemic), 3168‡
**Growth failure (treatment adjunct)**
See also Turner's syndrome
[Nandrolone (Systemic)], 110
[Oxandrolone (Systemic)]†, 110
[Oxymetholone (Systemic)*], 110
[Stanozolol (Systemic)]†, 110
**Growth failure, renal failure–associated (treatment)**
Somatropin, Recombinant (Systemic), 3034
**Growth hormone deficiency (diagnosis)**
[Insulin (Systemic)]¹, 1713
[Insulin Human (Systemic)]¹, 1713
NG-29 (Systemic), 3156‡
**Growth hormone deficiency (treatment)**
Mecasermin (Systemic), 3153‡
Sermorelin (Systemic), 2565, 3164‡
Somatrem (Systemic), 3165‡
Somatropin (Systemic), 3165‡
**Growth hormone deficiency, in adults (treatment)**
Somatropin, Recombinant (Systemic), 3034
**Growth hormone receptor deficiency (treatment)**
Recombinant Human Insulin-like Growth Factor I (Systemic), 3161‡
**Growth hormone resistance (treatment)**
Recombinant Human Insulin-like Growth Factor I (Systemic), 3161‡
**Growth retardation, renal failure–associated (treatment)**
Somatropin (Systemic), 3165‡
**Guillain-Barré syndrome, pain of**—See Pain, neurogenic
**Guinea worm infection**—See Dracunculiasis
**Gynecologic infections (treatment)**
See also Genitourinary tract infections; Pelvic infections, female
Alatrofloxacin (Systemic), 2891
Aztreonam (Systemic)†, 502
Trovafloxacin (Systemic), 2891
**Gynecomastia (treatment)**
[Danazol (Systemic)]¹, 1163

# H

**Haemophilus influenzae type b infection (prophylaxis)**
Haemophilus b Conjugate Vaccine (HbOC—Diphtheria CRM$_{197}$ Protein Conjugate) (Systemic), 1601
Haemophilus b Conjugate Vaccine (PRP-D—Diphtheria Toxoid Conjugate) (Systemic), 1601
Haemophilus b Conjugate Vaccine (PRP-OMP—Meningococcal Protein Conjugate) (Systemic), 1601
Haemophilus b Conjugate Vaccine (PRP-T—Tetanus Protein Conjugate) (Systemic), 1601
Haemophilus b Polysaccharide Vaccine (Systemic)*†, 1606
[Rifampin (Systemic)]¹, 2485
**Hallucinations, hypnagogic (treatment)**
Sodium/Gamma Hydroxybutyrate (Systemic), 3165‡
**Hansen's disease**—See Leprosy
**Hard measles**—See Measles
**Headache (prophylaxis)**
[Amitriptyline (Systemic)]¹, 271
[Amoxapine (Systemic)]¹, 271
[Clomipramine (Systemic)]¹, 271
[Desipramine (Systemic)]¹, 271
[Doxepin (Systemic)]¹, 271
[Imipramine (Systemic)]¹, 271
[Nortriptyline (Systemic)]¹, 271

**Headache (prophylaxis)** (continued)
[Protriptyline (Systemic)]¹, 271
[Trimipramine (Systemic)]¹, 271
**Headache, cluster**—See also Headache, vascular
See Headache, vascular, 1363, 1869, 1990
**Headache, cluster (treatment)**
Sumatriptan (Systemic), 2664
**Headache, migraine (prophylaxis)**
Divalproex (Systemic), 2908
Pizotyline (Systemic)*, 3032
**Headache, migraine (treatment)**
See also Headache, vascular
Acetaminophen, Aspirin, and Caffeine (Systemic), 3009
[Butalbital and Acetaminophen (Systemic)]†, 532
[Butalbital, Acetaminophen, and Caffeine (Systemic)]†, 532
[Butalbital, Acetaminophen, Caffeine, and Codeine (Systemic)]†, 532
[Butalbital and Aspirin (Systemic)]†, 532
[Butalbital, Aspirin, and Caffeine (Systemic)]¹, 532
[Butalbital, Aspirin, Caffeine, and Codeine (Systemic)]¹, 532
Dihydroergotamine (Nasal-Systemic), 1221
Isometheptene, Dichloralphenazone, and Acetaminophen (Systemic), 1786
Naratriptan (Systemic), 2087
Phenobarbital, ASA, and Codeine (Systemic)*¹, 532
Sumatriptan (Systemic), 2664
Zolmitriptan (Systemic), 3003
**Headache, mixed syndrome (treatment)**
See also Headache, migraine; Headache, tension-type
Isometheptene, Dichloralphenazone, and Acetaminophen (Systemic), 1786
**Headache, muscle contraction**—See Headache, tension-type
**Headache, sinus (treatment)**
Phenylephrine and Acetaminophen (Systemic), 1180
Phenylephrine, Phenylpropanolamine, and Acetaminophen (Systemic), 1180
Phenylpropanolamine, Acetaminophen, and Aspirin (Systemic)†, 1180
Phenylpropanolamine, Acetaminophen, and Caffeine (Systemic), 1180
Phenylpropanolamine, Acetaminophen, Salicylamide, and Caffeine (Systemic)†, 1180
Phenylpropanolamine and Aspirin (Systemic), 1180
Pseudoephedrine and Acetaminophen (Systemic), 1180
Pseudoephedrine and Aspirin (Systemic)†, 1180
**Headache, tension (prophylaxis)**
[Phenelzine (Systemic)]¹, 266
[Tranylcypromine (Systemic)]¹, 266
**Headache, tension (treatment)**
See also Pain; Pain, with anxiety and tension
[Chlordiazepoxide (Systemic)], 556
[Diazepam (Systemic)]¹, 556
[Lorazepam (Systemic)]¹, 556
Meprobamate and Aspirin (Systemic), #
**Headache, tension-type (treatment)**
See also Pain; Pain, with anxiety and tension
Butalbital and Acetaminophen (Systemic)†, 532
Butalbital, Acetaminophen, and Caffeine (Systemic)†, 532
Butalbital, Acetaminophen, Caffeine, and Codeine (Systemic)†, 532
Butalbital and Aspirin (Systemic)†, 532
Butalbital, Aspirin, and Caffeine (Systemic), 532
Butalbital, Aspirin, Caffeine, and Codeine (Systemic), 532
Isometheptene, Dichloralphenazone, and Acetaminophen (Systemic), 1786
Phenobarbital, ASA, and Codeine (Systemic)*, 532
**Headache, vascular (prophylaxis)**
[Atenolol (Systemic)]¹, 593
[Clonidine, Oral (Systemic)]¹, 908
Ergotamine, Belladonna Alkaloids, and Phenobarbital (Systemic), 1363
[Fenoprofen (Systemic)]¹, 388
Flunarizine (Systemic)*, 720
[Ibuprofen (Systemic)]¹, 388
[Indomethacin (Systemic)]¹, 388
[Lithium (Systemic)]¹, 1869
[Mefenamic Acid (Systemic)]¹, 388
Methysergide (Systemic), 1990
[Metoprolol (Systemic)]¹, 593
[Nadolol (Systemic)]¹, 593
Naproxen (Systemic)¹, 388
[Phenelzine (Systemic)]¹, 266
Propranolol (Systemic), 593
Timolol (Systemic), 593
[Tranylcypromine (Systemic)]¹, 266
[Verapamil (Systemic)], 720

**Headache, vascular (treatment)**
See also Headache, migraine
[Cyproheptadine (Systemic)], 325
[Diclofenac (Systemic)]1, 388
[Diflunisal (Systemic)]1, 388
Dihydroergotamine (Systemic), 2925
Ergotamine (Systemic), 2925
Ergotamine and Caffeine (Systemic), 2925
Ergotamine, Caffeine, and Belladonna Alkaloids (Systemic)*, 2925
Ergotamine, Caffeine, Belladonna Alkaloids, and Pentobarbital (Systemic)*, 2925
Ergotamine, Caffeine, and Cyclizine (Systemic)*, 2925
Ergotamine, Caffeine, and Dimenhydrinate (Systemic)*, 2925
Ergotamine, Caffeine, and Diphenhydramine (Systemic)*, 2925
[Etodolac (Systemic)]†, 388
[Fenoprofen (Systemic)]1, 388
Floctafenine (Systemic)*1, 388
[Ibuprofen (Systemic)]1, 388
[Indomethacin (Systemic)]1, 388
[Ketoprofen (Systemic)]1, 388
[Meclofenamate (Systemic)]†, 388
[Mefenamic Acid (Systemic)]1, 388
[Naproxen (Systemic)]1, 388
**Headache, vascular (treatment adjunct)**
[Metoclopramide (Systemic)]1, 1992
**Head injury, severe (treatment)**
Enadoline Hydrochloride (Systemic), 3141‡
**Heartburn, acid indigestion, and sour stomach, hyperacidity–associated (prophylaxis)**
Cimetidine (Systemic), 1633
Famotidine (Systemic), 1633
Nizatidine (Systemic), 1633
Ranitidine (Systemic), 1633
**Heartburn, acid indigestion, and sour stomach, hyperacidity–associated (treatment)**
Cimetidine (Systemic), 1633
Famotidine (Systemic), 1633
Ranitidine (Systemic), 1633
**Heart lesions, congenital, in neonates and infants, surgical repair of, cardiopulmonary bypass during (treatment)**
CY-1503 (Systemic), 3138‡
**Helminth infections, multiple (treatment)**
Pyrantel (Oral-Local), #
**Hemangioma, airway-obstructing, in infants (treatment)**
[Betamethasone, Oral (Systemic)]1, 998
[Betamethasone, Parenteral (Systemic)]1, 998
[Cortisone (Systemic)]1, 998
[Dexamethasone, Oral (Systemic)]1, 998
[Dexamethasone, Parenteral (Systemic)]1, 998
[Hydrocortisone, Oral (Systemic)]1, 998
[Hydrocortisone, Parenteral (Systemic)]1, 998
[Methylprednisolone, Oral (Systemic)]1, 998
[Methylprednisolone, Parenteral (Systemic)]1, 998
[Prednisolone, Oral (Systemic)]1, 998
[Prednisolone, Parenteral (Systemic)]1, 998
[Prednisone (Systemic)]1, 998
[Triamcinolone, Oral (Systemic)]1, 998
[Triamcinolone, Parenteral (Systemic)]1, 998
**Hemifacial spasm (treatment)**
[Botulinum Toxin Type A (Parenteral-Local)], 627
**Hemiplegia, alternating (treatment)**
Flunarizine (Systemic), 3143‡
**Hemodialysis**
Albumin Human (Systemic), 34
**Hemolysis (prophylaxis)**
Mannitol (Systemic), 1906
**Hemolysis (treatment)**
[Betamethasone, Oral (Systemic)]1, 998
[Betamethasone, Parenteral (Systemic)]1, 998
[Cortisone, (Systemic)]1, 998
[Dexamethasone, Oral (Systemic)]1, 998
[Dexamethasone, Parenteral (Systemic)]1, 998
[Hydrocortisone, Oral (Systemic)]1, 998
[Hydrocortisone, Parenteral (Systemic)]1, 998
[Methylprednisolone, Oral (Systemic)]1, 998
[Methylprednisolone, Parenteral (Systemic)]1, 998
[Prednisolone, Oral (Systemic)]1, 998
[Prednisolone, Parenteral (Systemic)]1, 998
[Prednisone (Systemic)]1, 998
[Triamcinolone, Oral (Systemic)]1, 998
[Triamcinolone, Parenteral (Systemic)]1, 998
**Hemolytic disease, in neonates (treatment)**
Trisaccharides A and B (Systemic), 3170‡
**Hemophilia A (treatment)**
Desmopressin, Parenteral (Systemic), 1187
R-VIII SQ (Systemic), 3163‡

**Hemophilia A, hemorrhagic complications of (prophylaxis)**
Antihemophilic Factor (Recombinant) (Systemic), 3131‡
Antihemophilic Factor (Systemic), 319
Factor IX (Systemic), 1430
**Hemophilia A, hemorrhagic complications of (treatment)**
Antihemophilic Factor (Recombinant) (Systemic), 3131‡
Antihemophilic Factor (Systemic), 319
Desmopressin (Inhalation/Systemic), 3140‡
Factor VIIa (Recombinant, DNA Origin) (Systemic), 3142‡
Factor IX (Systemic), 1430
**Hemophilia B, hemorrhagic complications of (prophylaxis)**
Coagulation Factor IX (Human) (Systemic), 3137‡
Coagulation Factor IX (Systemic), 3137‡
Coagulation Factor IX, Recombinant (Systemic), 3137‡
Factor IX (Systemic), 1430
**Hemophilia B, hemorrhagic complications of (treatment)**
Coagulation Factor IX (Human) (Systemic), 3137‡
Coagulation Factor IX (Systemic), 3137‡
Coagulation Factor IX, Recombinant (Systemic), 3137‡
Factor VIIa (Recombinant, DNA Origin) (Systemic), 3142‡
Factor IX (Systemic), 1430
**Hemophilia, classical**—See Hemophilia A, hemorrhagic complications of
**Hemophilus**—See Haemophilus influenzae type b infection
**Hemorrhage, anticoagulant-induced (treatment)**
Factor IX (Systemic), 1430
**Hemorrhage, coronary artery bypass graft surgery–associated (prophylaxis)**
Aprotinin (Systemic)1, 461, 3132‡
**Hemorrhage, during extracorporeal circulation (prophylaxis)**
Epoprostenol (Systemic), 3142‡
**Hemorrhage, fibrinolytic agent–induced**—See Hemorrhage, hyperfibrinolysis-induced
**Hemorrhage, following dental surgery, in hemophiliacs (prophylaxis)**
[Aminocaproic Acid (Systemic)], 64
Tranexamic Acid (Systemic), 2862
**Hemorrhage, following dental surgery, in hemophiliacs (treatment)**
[Aminocaproic Acid (Systemic)], 64
Tranexamic Acid (Systemic), 2862, 3169‡
**Hemorrhage, gingival (treatment adjunct)**
[Epinephrine Injection USP (Systemic) used topically]1, 651
**Hemorrhage, hyperfibrinolysis-induced (treatment)**
Aminocaproic Acid (Systemic), 64
[Tranexamic Acid (Systemic)], 2862
**Hemorrhage, oral, in hemophiliacs (treatment)**
[Aminocaproic Acid (Systemic)], 64
[Tranexamic Acid (Systemic)]1, 2862
**Hemorrhage, postabortion (prophylaxis)**
Ergonovine (Systemic), 1360
Methylergonovine (Systemic)†, 1984
**Hemorrhage, postabortion (treatment)**
[Dinoprostone Vaginal Suppositories (Cervical/Vaginal)], 1228
Ergonovine (Systemic), 1360
Methylergonovine (Systemic)†, 1984
Oxytocin, Parenteral (Systemic), 2211
**Hemorrhage, postpartum (prophylaxis)**
Ergonovine (Systemic), 1360
Methylergonovine (Systemic)†, 1984
**Hemorrhage, postpartum (treatment)**
Carboprost (Systemic)1, 782
[Dinoprostone Vaginal Suppositories (Cervical/Vaginal)], 1228
Ergonovine (Systemic), 1360
Methylergonovine (Systemic)†, 1984
Oxytocin, Parenteral (Systemic), 2211
**Hemorrhage, postsurgical (prophylaxis)**
Aminocaproic Acid (Systemic), 64
**Hemorrhage, postsurgical (treatment)**
Aminocaproic Acid (Systemic), 64
[Tranexamic Acid (Systemic)], 2862, 3169‡
**Hemorrhage, pulpal (treatment)**
[Epinephrine Injection USP (Systemic) used topically]1, 651
**Hemorrhage, subarachnoid, recurrence (prophylaxis)**
[Aminocaproic Acid (Systemic)], 64
**Hemorrhage, superficial (treatment)**
Epinephrine Injection USP (Systemic) used topically, 651

**Hemorrhage, superficial, in ocular surgery (treatment)**
Epinephrine Injection USP (Systemic), 651
**Hemorrhage, surgical-associated (treatment adjunct)**
Fibrin Sealant (Local), 3020
**Hemorrhage, thrombolytic agent–induced**—See Hemorrhage, hyperfibrinolysis-induced
**Hemorrhagic complications of factor VII deficiency (prophylaxis)**
Factor IX (Systemic), 1430
**Hemorrhagic complications of factor VII deficiency (treatment)**
Factor IX (Systemic), 1430
**Hemorrhagic complications in hemophilic patients with factor VIII or factor IX inhibitors (prophylaxis)**
Anti-inhibitor Coagulant Complex (Systemic), 435
**Hemorrhagic complications in hemophilic patients with factor VIII or factor IX inhibitors (treatment)**
Anti-inhibitor Coagulant Complex (Systemic), 435
**Hemorrhagic complications in non-hemophilic patients with acquired inhibitors (prophylaxis)**
Anti-inhibitor Coagulant Complex (Systemic), 435
**Hemorrhagic complications in non-hemophilic patients with acquired inhibitors (treatment)**
Anti-inhibitor Coagulant Complex (Systemic), 435
**Hemorrhagic complications in patients with factor VIII inhibitors (prophylaxis)**
Antihemophilic Factor, Porcine (Systemic), 319
**Hemorrhagic complications in patients with factor VIII inhibitors (treatment)**
Antihemophilic Factor, Porcine (Systemic), 319
**Hemorrhagic cystitis, ifosfamide-induced (prophylaxis)**
Mesna (Systemic), 3153‡
**Hemorrhagic cystitis, oxazaphosphorine-induced (prophylaxis)**
Mesna (Systemic), 3153‡
**Hemorrhagic cystitis, oxazaphosphorine–induced (prophylaxis)**
Mesna (Systemic), 1956
**Hemorrhagic disease of the newborn (prophylaxis)**
Phytonadione, Parenteral (Systemic), 2975
**Hemorrhoids (treatment)**
Benzocaine Ointment USP (Rectal) (Mucosal-Local), 128
Bufexamac (Topical)*, 3013
Dibucaine (Mucosal-Local), 128
Hydrocortisone (Rectal), 973
Pramoxine (Mucosal-Local), 128
Tetracaine, Rectal (Mucosal-Local), 128
**Hepatic coma (treatment)**
Kanamycin (Oral-Local)†, #
**Hepatic disease, cholestatic (treatment)**
[Ursodiol (Systemic)], 2903
**Hepatic disease, cholestatic, chronic (treatment)**
[Ursodiol (Systemic)]1, 2903
**Hepatic disease, cystic fibrosis–associated (treatment)**
[Ursodiol (Systemic)]1, 2903
**Hepatic encephalopathy (treatment)**
Refaximin (Systemic), 3162‡
**Hepatic encephalopathy (treatment adjunct)**
Neomycin (Oral-Local), #
**Hepatitis (diagnosis)**—See Hepatobiliary imaging, radionuclide; Liver imaging, radionuclide
**Hepatitis A (prophylaxis)**
Hepatitis A Vaccine Inactivated (Systemic), 1625
**Hepatitis, alcoholic (treatment)**
Oxandrolone (Systemic), 3157‡
**Hepatitis, alcoholic, with encephalopathy (treatment)**
[Methylprednisolone, Oral (Systemic)]1, 998
[Methylprednisolone, Parenteral (Systemic)]1, 998
[Prednisolone, Oral (Systemic)]1, 998
[Prednisolone, Parenteral (Systemic)]1, 998
[Prednisone (Systemic)]1, 998
**Hepatitis B (prophylaxis)**
Hepatitis B Immune Globulin (Systemic), 3145‡
Monoclonal Antibody to Hepatitis B Virus (Human) (Systemic), 3155‡
**Hepatitis B (treatment adjunct)**
Thymosin Alpha-1 (Systemic), 3169‡
**Hepatitis B, chronic (treatment)**
Interferon Alfa-2b, Recombinant (Systemic)1, 1740
**Hepatitis B, chronic (treatment adjunct)**
Fiau (Systemic), 3143‡
**Hepatitis B, chronic, active, in HLA-A2 positive patients (treatment)**
CY-1899 (Systemic), 3138‡
**Hepatitis B virus (prophylaxis)**
Hepatitis B Vaccine Recombinant (Systemic), 1628

**Hepatitis C, chronic (treatment)**
Ribavirin/Interferon Alfa-2b (Systemic), 3033
**Hepatitis, chronic (treatment)**
[Ursodiol (Systemic)][1], 2903
**Hepatitis, chronic, active (treatment)**
[Azathioprine (Systemic)][1], 491
[Interferon Alfa-2a, Recombinant (Systemic)][1], 1740
Interferon Alfa-2b, Recombinant (Systemic), 1740
Interferon Alfacon-1 (Systemic), 1730
Interferon Alfa-n1 (Ins) (Systemic)*[1], 1740
[Interferon Alfa-n3 (Systemic)]†, 1740
[Methylprednisolone, Oral (Systemic)][1], 998
[Methylprednisolone, Parenteral (Systemic)][1], 998
[Prednisolone, Oral (Systemic)][1], 998
[Prednisolone, Parenteral (Systemic)][1], 998
[Prednisone (Systemic)][1], 998
**Hepatitis D virus (prophylaxis)**
Hepatitis B Vaccine Recombinant (Systemic), 1628
**Hepatitis, nonalcoholic, in women (treatment)**
[Methylprednisolone, Oral (Systemic)][1], 998
[Methylprednisolone, Parenteral (Systemic)][1], 998
[Prednisolone, Oral (Systemic)][1], 998
[Prednisolone, Parenteral (Systemic)][1], 998
[Prednisone (Systemic)][1], 998
**Hepatitis, non-A, non-B (treatment)**
Interferon Beta (Recombinant Human) (Systemic), 3148‡
**Hepatobiliary imaging, radionuclide**
Technetium Tc 99m Disofenin (Systemic)†, 2705
Technetium Tc 99m Lidofenin (Systemic), 2713
Technetium Tc 99m Mebrofenin (Systemic), 2716
**Hepatoblastoma (treatment)**
[Cisplatin (Systemic)][1], 876
[Doxorubicin (Systemic)][1], 1308
[Etoposide (Systemic)][1], 1424
[Fluorouracil (Systemic)][1], 1497
[Vincristine (Systemic)][1], 2950
**Herniography**
Iohexol (Systemic)[1], #
[Iopamidol (Systemic)][1], #
[Ioversol (Systemic)][1], #
**Herpes genitalis (suppression)**
[Famciclovir (Systemic)][1], 1434
**Herpes genitalis (treatment)**
Famciclovir (Systemic), 1434
**Herpes genitalis, initial episode (treatment)**
Acyclovir (Systemic), 24
Valacyclovir (Systemic)[1], 2906
**Herpes genitalis, recurrent episodes (suppression)**
Valacyclovir (Systemic)[1], 2906
**Herpes genitalis, recurrent episodes (treatment)**
Acyclovir, Oral (Systemic), 24
Valacyclovir (Systemic), 2906
**Herpes labialis (treatment)**
Penciclovir (Topical), 2236
**Herpes simplex (prophylaxis)**
[Acyclovir (Systemic)][1], 24
**Herpes simplex (treatment)**
[Acyclovir, Oral (Systemic)], 24
Acyclovir, Parenteral (Systemic), 24
[Foscarnet (Systemic)]†, 1528, 3020
**Herpes simplex encephalitis (treatment)**
Acyclovir, Parenteral (Systemic)[1], 24
**Herpes simplex virus, disseminated neonatal infection (treatment)**
[Acyclovir, Parenteral (Systemic)][1], 24
**Herpes zoster (prophylaxis)**
[Acyclovir (Systemic)][1], 24
**Herpes zoster (treatment)**
Acyclovir (Systemic), 24
Famciclovir (Systemic), 1434
Sorivudine (Systemic), 3166‡
Valacyclovir (Systemic)[1], 2906
**Herpes zoster (treatment adjunct)**
[Acyclovir (Topical)], 28
**Herpes zoster, ocular (treatment)**
Betamethasone, Oral (Systemic), 998
Betamethasone, Parenteral (Systemic), 998
Cortisone (Systemic), 998
Dexamethasone, Oral (Systemic), 998
Dexamethasone, Parenteral (Systemic), 998
Hydrocortisone, Oral (Systemic), 998
Hydrocortisone, Parenteral (Systemic), 998
Methylprednisolone, Oral (Systemic), 998
Methylprednisolone, Parenteral (Systemic), 998
Prednisolone, Oral (Systemic), 998
Prednisolone, Parenteral (Systemic), 998
Prednisone (Systemic), 998
Triamcinolone, Oral (Systemic), 998
Triamcinolone, Parenteral (Systemic), 998
**Herpes zoster ophthalmicus (treatment)**
[Acyclovir (Systemic)][1], 24

**Hiccups, intractable (treatment)**
Chlorpromazine (Systemic), 2289
[Metoclopramide (Systemic)][1], 1992
**Hidradenitis suppurativa (treatment)**
[Isotretinoin (Systemic)][1], 1796
**Hirsutism (treatment)**
[Ketoconazole (Systemic)][1], 302
**Hirsutism, female (treatment)**
[Desogestrel and Ethinyl Estradiol (Systemic)][1], 1397
[Ethynodiol Diacetate and Ethinyl Estradiol (Systemic)][1], 1397
[Levonorgestrel and Ethinyl Estradiol (Systemic)][1], 1397
[Norethindrone Acetate and Ethinyl Estradiol (Systemic)][1], 1397
[Norethindrone and Ethinyl Estradiol (Systemic)][1], 1397
[Norethindrone and Mestranol (Systemic)][1], 1397
[Norgestimate and Ethinyl Estradiol (Systemic)][1], 1397
[Norgestrel and Ethinyl Estradiol (Systemic)][1], 1397
[Spironolactone (Systemic)][1], 1266
**Hirsutism, female (treatment adjunct)**
[Desogestrel and Ethinyl Estradiol (Systemic)][1], 1397
[Ethynodiol Diacetate and Ethinyl Estradiol (Systemic)][1], 1397
[Levonorgestrel and Ethinyl Estradiol (Systemic)][1], 1397
[Norethindrone Acetate and Ethinyl Estradiol (Systemic)][1], 1397
[Norethindrone and Ethinyl Estradiol (Systemic)][1], 1397
[Norethindrone and Mestranol (Systemic)][1], 1397
[Norgestimate and Ethinyl Estradiol (Systemic)][1], 1397
[Norgestrel and Ethinyl Estradiol (Systemic)][1], 1397
**Histiocytosis, Langerhan's cell**—See Letterer-Siwe disease
**Histiocytosis X**—See Letterer-Siwe disease
**Histoplasmosis (suppression)**
[Itraconazole (Systemic)][1], 302
**Histoplasmosis (treatment)**
Amphotericin B (Systemic), 98
Amphotericin B, Liposomal (Systemic), 3152‡
Itraconazole (Systemic), 302
Ketoconazole (Systemic), 302
**HIV infection**—See Human immunodeficiency virus (HIV) infection
**Hodgkin's disease**—See Lymphomas, Hodgkin's
**Homocystinuria (treatment)**
Betaine (Systemic), 3133‡
Betaine (Systemic)†, #
**Hookworm infection (treatment)**
See also Larva migrans, cutaneous
Albendazole (Systemic)*†, #
Mebendazole (Systemic), 1926
[Pyrantel (Oral-Local)], #
**Hordeolum (treatment)**
Framycetin (Ophthalmic)*, 3020
**HTLV-III**—See Human immunodeficiency virus (HIV) infection
**Human immunodeficiency virus (HIV)–associated wasting syndrome (treatment)**
See also Cachexia, AIDS-associated (treatment)
Somatropin (Systemic), 3166‡
[Thalidomide (Systemic)][1]†, 2776
Thalidomide (Systemic), 3168‡
**Human immunodeficiency virus (HIV) infection (treatment)**
See also Immunodeficiency syndrome, acquired (AIDS) (treatment)
Delavirdine (Systemic), 1184
Human Immunodeficiency Virus Immune Globulin (Systemic), 3145‡, 3146‡
Indinavir (Systemic), 1693
Lamivudine and Zidovudine (Systemic), 1822
Nelfinavir (Systemic), 2095
Nevirapine (Systemic), 2113
Ritonavir (Systemic), 2516
Saquinavir (Systemic), 2564
Stavudine (Systemic), 2627
Zalcitabine (Systemic), 2989
**Human immunodeficiency virus (HIV) infection, advanced (treatment)**
Didanosine (Systemic), 1206
Zalcitabine (Systemic), 2989
**Human immunodeficiency virus (HIV) infection, asymptomatic (treatment)**
Zidovudine (Systemic), 2992, 3038

**Human immunodeficiency virus (HIV) infection, occupational exposure (prophylaxis)**
5a8, Monoclonal Antibody to CD4 (Systemic), 3128‡
[Zidovudine (Systemic)]1, 2992
**Human immunodeficiency virus (HIV) infection, pediatric (prophylaxis)**
Immune Globulin Intravenous (Human) (Systemic), 3024
**Human immunodeficiency virus (HIV), maternal-fetal transmission (prophylaxis)**
Zidovudine (Systemic), 2992
**Huntington's disease (treatment)**
Porcine Fetal Neural GABAergic Cells (Systemic), 3159‡
Riluzole (Systemic), 3163‡
**Huntington's disease, choreiform movement of (treatment)**
[Chlorpromazine (Systemic)][1], 2289
[Thioridazine (Systemic)][1], 2289
**Hyaline membrane disease**—See Respiratory distress syndrome, neonatal
**Hydatid disease (treatment)**
Albendazole (Systemic)*†, #, 3009, 3129‡
**Hydatid disease, alveolar (treatment)**
[Mebendazole (Systemic)][1], 1926
**Hydatid disease, unilocular (treatment)**
[Mebendazole (Systemic)][1], 1926
**Hydatidiform mole**—See Tumors, trophoblastic, gestational
**Hydatidiform mole, benign (treatment)**
[Carboprost (Systemic)][1], 782
Dinoprostone Vaginal Suppositories (Cervical/Vaginal), 1228
**Hymenolepiasis (treatment)**
Niclosamide (Oral-Local)†, #
[Praziquantel (Systemic)][1], 2368
**Hyperacidity (treatment)**
Alumina, Calcium Carbonate, and Sodium Bicarbonate (Oral-Local)*, 188
Alumina and Magnesia (Oral-Local), 188
Alumina, Magnesia, Calcium Carbonate, and Simethicone (Oral-Local)*, 188
Alumina, Magnesia, and Magnesium Carbonate (Oral-Local)*, 188
Alumina, Magnesia, Magnesium Carbonate, and Simethicone (Oral-Local)*, 188
Alumina, Magnesia, and Simethicone (Oral-Local), 188
Alumina, Magnesium Alginate, and Magnesium Carbonate (Oral-Local)*, 188
Alumina and Magnesium Carbonate (Oral-Local)†, 188
Alumina, Magnesium Carbonate, and Simethicone (Oral-Local)†, 188
Alumina, Magnesium Carbonate, and Sodium Bicarbonate (Oral-Local)†, 188
Alumina and Magnesium Trisilicate (Oral-Local)†, 188
Alumina, Magnesium Trisilicate, and Sodium Bicarbonate (Oral-Local)†, 188
Alumina and Simethicone (Oral-Local)†, 188
Alumina and Sodium Bicarbonate (Oral-Local)*, 188
Aluminum Carbonate, Basic (Oral-Local)†, 188
Aluminum Carbonate, Basic, and Simethicone (Oral-Local)†, 188
Aluminum Hydroxide (Oral-Local), 188
Calcium Carbonate (Oral-Local)†, 188
Calcium Carbonate and Magnesia (Oral-Local)†, 188
Calcium Carbonate, Magnesia, and Simethicone (Oral-Local)†, 188
Calcium and Magnesium Carbonates (Oral-Local)†, 188
Calcium Carbonate and Simethicone (Oral-Local)†, 188
Magaldrate (Oral-Local), 188
Magaldrate and Simethicone (Oral-Local), 188
Magnesium Carbonate and Sodium Bicarbonate (Oral-Local)*, 188
Magnesium Hydroxide (Local), #
Magnesium Hydroxide (Oral-Local), 188
Magnesium Oxide (Local)†, #
Magnesium Oxide (Oral-Local)†, 188
Sodium Bicarbonate, Oral (Systemic), 2586
**Hyperalaninemia (treatment)**
[Thiamine (Systemic)], 2787
**Hyperaldosteronism, primary (diagnosis)**
Spironolactone (Systemic), 1266
**Hyperaldosteronism, primary (treatment)**
Spironolactone (Systemic), 1266
**Hyperammonemia (prophylaxis)**
Lactulose (Local), #
Sodium Benzoate and Sodium Phenylacetate (Systemic)†, #, 3132‡

**Hyperammonemia (treatment)**
Lactulose (Local), #
Sodium Benzoate and Sodium Phenylacetate (Systemic)†, #, 3132‡

**Hyperandrogenism, ovarian (treatment)**
[Desogestrel and Ethinyl Estradiol (Systemic)][1], 1397
[Ethynodiol Diacetate and Ethinyl Estradiol (Systemic)][1], 1397
[Levonorgestrel and Ethinyl Estradiol (Systemic)][1], 1397
[Norethindrone Acetate and Ethinyl Estradiol (Systemic)][1], 1397
[Norethindrone and Ethinyl Estradiol (Systemic)][1], 1397
[Norethindrone and Mestranol (Systemic)][1], 1397
[Norgestimate and Ethinyl Estradiol (Systemic)][1], 1397
[Norgestrel and Ethinyl Estradiol (Systemic)][1], 1397

**Hyperandrogenism, ovarian (treatment adjunct)**
[Desogestrel and Ethinyl Estradiol (Systemic)][1], 1397
[Ethynodiol Diacetate and Ethinyl Estradiol (Systemic)][1], 1397
[Levonorgestrel and Ethinyl Estradiol (Systemic)][1], 1397
[Norethindrone Acetate and Ethinyl Estradiol (Systemic)][1], 1397
[Norethindrone and Ethinyl Estradiol (Systemic)][1], 1397
[Norethindrone and Mestranol (Systemic)][1], 1397
[Norgestimate and Ethinyl Estradiol (Systemic)][1], 1397
[Norgestrel and Ethinyl Estradiol (Systemic)][1], 1397

**Hyperbilirubinemia (prophylaxis)**
[Phenobarbital (Systemic)][1], 518

**Hyperbilirubinemia (treatment)**
Albumin Human (Systemic), 34
Flumecinol (Systemic), 3143‡
[Phenobarbital (Systemic)][1], 518

**Hypercalcemia (treatment)**
[Bumetanide (Systemic)]†, 1259
Edetate Disodium (Systemic)†, 1327
[Ethacrynic Acid (Systemic)][1], 1259
[Furosemide (Systemic)][1], 1259

**Hypercalcemia (treatment adjunct)**
[Calcitonin-Human (Systemic)]†, 716
Calcitonin-Salmon (Systemic), 716

**Hypercalcemia, associated with neoplasms (treatment)**
Betamethasone, Oral (Systemic), 998
Betamethasone, Parenteral (Systemic), 998
Cortisone (Systemic), 998
Dexamethasone, Oral (Systemic), 998
Dexamethasone, Parenteral (Systemic), 998
Disodium Clodronate (Systemic), 3141‡
Disodium Clodronate Tetrahydrate (Systemic), 3141‡
Etidronate (Systemic), 3142‡
Gallium Nitrate (Systemic), 3144‡
Gallium Nitrate (Systemic)†, 1540
Hydrocortisone, Oral (Systemic), 998
Hydrocortisone, Parenteral (Systemic), 998
Methylprednisolone, Oral (Systemic), 998
Methylprednisolone, Parenteral (Systemic), 998
Pamidronate (Systemic), 2220
Plicamycin (Systemic)†, 2334
Prednisolone, Oral (Systemic), 998
Prednisolone, Parenteral (Systemic), 998
Prednisone (Systemic), 998
Triamcinolone, Oral (Systemic), 998
Triamcinolone, Parenteral (Systemic), 998

**Hypercalcemia, associated with neoplasms (treatment adjunct)**
Etidronate (Systemic), 1419

**Hypercalcemia, sarcoid-associated (treatment)**
[Betamethasone, Oral (Systemic)][1], 998
[Betamethasone, Parenteral (Systemic)][1], 998
[Chloroquine, Oral (Systemic)][1], 849
[Cortisone (Systemic)][1], 998
[Dexamethasone, Oral (Systemic)][1], 998
[Dexamethasone, Parenteral (Systemic)][1], 998
[Hydrocortisone, Oral (Systemic)][1], 998
[Hydrocortisone, Parenteral (Systemic)][1], 998
[Hydroxychloroquine (Systemic)][1], 1663
[Methylprednisolone, Oral (Systemic)][1], 998
[Methylprednisolone, Parenteral (Systemic)][1], 998
[Prednisolone, Oral (Systemic)][1], 998
[Prednisolone, Parenteral (Systemic)][1], 998
[Prednisone (Systemic)][1], 998
[Triamcinolone, Oral (Systemic)][1], 998
[Triamcinolone, Parenteral (Systemic)][1], 998

**Hypercalciuria, associated with neoplasms (treatment)**
Plicamycin (Systemic)†, 2334

**Hyperekplexia (treatment)**
Clonazepam (Systemic), 3137‡

**Hypereosinophilic syndrome**—See Loeffler syndrome

**Hyperkalemia (treatment)**
Calcium Chloride (Systemic), 736
Calcium Gluconate, Parenteral (Systemic), 736
Sodium Polystyrene Sulfonate (Local), 2618

**Hyperkeratotic skin disorders (treatment)**
Salicylic Acid Cream (Topical), #
Salicylic Acid Gel USP (Topical), #
Salicylic Acid Ointment (Topical), #
Salicylic Acid Plaster USP (Topical), #
Salicylic Acid Topical Solution (Topical), #

**Hyperkinetic child syndrome**—See Attention-deficit hyperactivity disorder

**Hyperlipidemia (treatment)**
Atorvastatin (Systemic), 479
Cerivastatin (Systemic), 827
Cholestyramine (Oral-Local), 853
Clofibrate (Systemic), 900
Colestipol (Oral-Local), 934
Fenofibrate (Systemic), 1439
[Fluvastatin (Systemic)]†, 1647
Gemfibrozil (Systemic), 1552
Lovastatin (Systemic), 1647
Niacin (Systemic), 2116
Pravastatin (Systemic), 1647
Probucol (Systemic), 2385
[Psyllium Hydrophilic Mucilloid (Local)], #
Simvastatin (Systemic), 1647
Sodium Dichloroacetate (Systemic), 3164‡

**Hypermagnesemia (treatment adjunct)**
Calcium Chloride (Systemic), 736
[Calcium Gluceptate (Systemic)]†, 736
Calcium Gluconate, Parenteral (Systemic), 736

**Hypermenorrhea (treatment)**
[Desogestrel and Ethinyl Estradiol (Systemic)][1], 1397
[Diclofenac (Systemic)][1], 388
[Ethynodiol Diacetate and Ethinyl Estradiol (Systemic)][1], 1397
[Etodolac (Systemic)]†, 388
[Floctafenine (Systemic)][*1], 388
[Flurbiprofen (Systemic)][1], 388
[Ibuprofen (Systemic)][1], 388
[Indomethacin (Systemic)][1], 388
[Ketoprofen (Systemic)][1], 388
[Levonorgestrel and Ethinyl Estradiol (Systemic)][1], 1397
[Meclofenamate (Systemic)]†, 388
[Mefenamic Acid (Systemic)][1], 388
[Naproxen (Systemic)][1], 388
[Norethindrone Acetate and Ethinyl Estradiol (Systemic)][1], 1397
[Norethindrone and Ethinyl Estradiol (Systemic)][1], 1397
[Norethindrone and Mestranol (Systemic)][1], 1397
[Norgestimate and Ethinyl Estradiol (Systemic)][1], 1397
[Norgestrel and Ethinyl Estradiol (Systemic)][1], 1397
[Piroxicam (Systemic)][1], 388

**Hypermenorrhea secondary to hyperfibrinolysis**—See Hemorrhage, hyperfibrinolysis-induced

**Hyperoxaluria (treatment)**
[Cholestyramine (Oral-Local)][1], 853

**Hyperparathyroidism, secondary (treatment)**
Paricalcitol (Systemic), 3031

**Hyperphenylalaninemia (treatment)**
Phenlalanine Ammonia-Lyase (Systemic), 3158‡
Valine, Isoleucine, and Leucine (Systemic), 3171‡

**Hyperphosphatemia (treatment)**
[Aluminum Carbonate, Basic (Oral-Local)]†, 188
[Aluminum Hydroxide (Oral-Local)][1], 188
Calcium Acetate (Systemic), 719, 3135‡
[Calcium Carbonate (Systemic)], 736, 3135‡
[Calcium Citrate (Systemic)]†, 736

**Hyperpigmentation, mottled, facial, due to photoaging (treatment adjunct)**
Tretinoin (Topical), 2871

**Hyperplasia, adrenal medulla (diagnosis)**
[Iobenguane I 123 (Systemic—Diagnostic)]†, 1747
[Iobenguane I 131 (Systemic—Diagnostic)]†, 1747

**Hyperplasia, endometrial (treatment)**
[Medroxyprogesterone, Oral (Systemic)][1], 2400
[Megestrol (Systemic)][1], 2400

**Hyperplasia, endometrial, estrogen-induced (prophylaxis)**
[Medrogesterone, Oral (Systemic)], 2400
[Medroxyprogesterone (Oral) (Systemic)][1], 1747
[Norethindrone (Systemic)][1], 1747, 2400

**Hyperprolactinemic disorders (treatment)**
Cabergoline (Systemic), 704

**Hypersecretory conditions, gastric (diagnosis)**
See also Gastric histamine test
Histamine (Systemic)*, #
Pentagastrin (Systemic), #

**Hypersecretory conditions, gastric (treatment)**
See also Ulcer, peptic
Cimetidine (Systemic), 1633
Famotidine (Systemic), 1633
Lansoprazole (Systemic), 1828
[Nizatidine (Systemic)][1], 1633
Omeprazole (Systemic), 2163
Ranitidine (Systemic), 1633

**Hypersecretory conditions, gastric (treatment adjunct)**
Alumina, Calcium Carbonate, and Sodium Bicarbonate (Oral-Local)*, 188
Alumina and Magnesia (Oral-Local), 188
Alumina, Magnesia, Calcium Carbonate, and Simethicone (Oral-Local)*, 188
Alumina, Magnesia, and Magnesium Carbonate (Oral-Local)*, 188
Alumina, Magnesia, Magnesium Carbonate, and Simethicone (Oral-Local)*, 188
Alumina, Magnesia, and Simethicone (Oral-Local), 188
Alumina, Magnesium Alginate, and Magnesium Carbonate (Oral-Local)*, 188
Alumina and Magnesium Carbonate (Oral-Local)†, 188
Alumina, Magnesium Carbonate, and Simethicone (Oral-Local)†, 188
Alumina, Magnesium Carbonate, and Sodium Bicarbonate (Oral-Local)†, 188
Alumina and Magnesium Trisilicate (Oral-Local)†, 188
Alumina, Magnesium Trisilicate, and Sodium Bicarbonate (Oral-Local)†, 188
Alumina and Simethicone (Oral-Local)†, 188
Alumina and Sodium Bicarbonate (Oral-Local)*, 188
Aluminum Carbonate, Basic (Oral-Local)†, 188
Aluminum Carbonate, Basic, and Simethicone (Oral-Local)†, 188
Aluminum Hydroxide (Oral-Local), 188
Calcium Carbonate (Oral-Local)†, 188
Calcium Carbonate and Magnesia (Oral-Local)†, 188
Calcium Carbonate, Magnesia, and Simethicone (Oral-Local)†, 188
Calcium and Magnesium Carbonates (Oral-Local)†, 188
Calcium Carbonate and Simethicone (Oral-Local)†, 188
Magaldrate (Oral-Local), 188
Magaldrate and Simethicone (Oral-Local), 188
Magnesium Carbonate and Sodium Bicarbonate (Oral-Local)*, 188
Magnesium Hydroxide (Oral-Local), 188
Magnesium Oxide (Oral-Local)†, 188

**Hypersecretory conditions, gastric, in anesthesia (prophylaxis)**
Glycopyrrolate, Parenteral (Systemic), 226

**Hypertension (treatment)**
Acebutolol (Systemic), 593
Amiloride and Hydrochlorothiazide (Systemic)1, 1272
Amlodipine (Systemic)†, 86
Amlodipine and Benazepril (Systemic), 88
Atenolol (Systemic), 593
Atenolol and Chlorthalidone (Systemic), 609
Benazepril (Systemic)†, 177
Bendroflumethiazide (Systemic), 1273
Betaxolol (Systemic)†, 593
Bisoprolol (Systemic)†, 593
Bisoprolol and Hydrochlorothiazide (Systemic)†, 609
[Bumetanide (Systemic)]†, 1259
Captopril (Systemic), 177
Captopril and Hydrochlorothiazide (Systemic)†, 187
Carteolol (Systemic)†, 593
Carvedilol (Systemic), 790
Chlorothiazide (Systemic)†, 1273
Chlorthalidone (Systemic), 1273
Clonidine (Systemic), 908
Clonidine and Chlorthalidone (Systemic), 912
Deserpidine (Systemic)†, 2460
Deserpidine and Hydrochlorothiazide (Systemic)†, #
Deserpidine and Methyclothiazide (Systemic), #
Diazoxide (Parenteral-Systemic), 1200
Diltiazem (Systemic), 720, 3017
Doxazosin (Systemic), 1303
Enalapril (Systemic), 177

**Hypertension (treatment)** *(continued)*
  Enalapril and Diltiazem (Systemic), 1334
  Enalapril and Felodipine (Systemic), 1339
  Enalapril and Hydrochlorothiazide (Systemic)†, 187
  [Ethacrynic Acid (Systemic)][1], 1259
  Felodipine (Systemic), 720
  Fenoldopam (Systemic), 1443
  Fosinopril (Systemic)†, 177
  Furosemide (Systemic), 1259
  Guanabenz (Systemic)†, 1590
  Guanadrel (Systemic)†, 1592
  Guanethidine (Systemic), 1595
  Guanethidine and Hydrochlorothiazide (Systemic), 3971
  Guanfacine (Systemic)†, 1598
  Hydralazine (Systemic), 1655
  Hydralazine and Hydrochlorothiazide (Systemic)†, 1658
  Hydrochlorothiazide (Systemic), 1273
  Hydroflumethiazide (Systemic)†, 1273
  Indapamide (Systemic), 1691
  Irbesartan (Systemic), 1767
  Isradipine (Systemic)†, 720
  Labetalol (Systemic), 593
  Lisinopril (Systemic), 177
  Lisinopril and Hydrochlorothiazide (Systemic)†, 187
  Losartan (Systemic)†, 1882
  Losartan and Hydrochlorothiazide (Systemic), 1884
  Mecamylamine (Systemic)†, #
  Methyclothiazide (Systemic), 1273
  Methyldopa (Systemic), 1979
  Methyldopa and Chlorothiazide (Systemic), 1983
  Methyldopa and Hydrochlorothiazide (Systemic), 1983
  Metolazone (Systemic), 1273
  Metoprolol (Systemic), 593
  Metoprolol and Hydrochlorothiazide (Systemic)†, 609
  Mibefradil (Systemic), #
  Minoxidil (Systemic), 2018
  Moexipril (Systemic)†, 2042
  Moexipril and Hydrochlorothiazide (Systemic), 2045
  Nadolol (Systemic), 593
  Nadolol and Bendroflumethiazide (Systemic), 609
  Nicardipine (Systemic), 720, 3029
  Nifedipine (Systemic), 720
  Nitroglycerin, Parenteral (Systemic), 2129
  Nitroprusside (Systemic), 2142
  Oxprenolol (Systemic)*, 593
  Penbutolol (Systemic)†, 593
  Pindolol (Systemic), 593
  Pindolol and Hydrochlorothiazide (Systemic)*, 609
  Polythiazide (Systemic)†, 1273
  Prazosin (Systemic), 2370
  Prazosin and Polythiazide (Systemic)†, 2374
  Propranolol (Systemic), 593
  Propranolol and Hydrochlorothiazide (Systemic), 609
  Quinapril (Systemic)†, 177
  Quinethazone (Systemic)†, 1273
  Ramipril (Systemic)†, 177
  Rauwolfia Serpentina (Systemic)†, 2460
  Rauwolfia Serpentina and Bendroflumethiazide (Systemic)†, #
  Reserpine (Systemic), 2460
  Reserpine and Chlorothiazide (Systemic)†, #
  Reserpine and Chlorthalidone (Systemic)†, #
  Reserpine, Hydralazine, and Hydrochlorothiazide (Systemic), #
  Reserpine and Hydrochlorothiazide (Systemic), #
  Reserpine and Hydroflumethiazide (Systemic)†, #
  Reserpine and Methyclothiazide (Systemic)†, #
  Reserpine and Polythiazide (Systemic)†, #
  Reserpine and Trichlormethiazide (Systemic)†, #
  [Sotalol (Systemic)], 593
  Spironolactone and Hydrochlorothiazide (Systemic), 1272
  Terazosin (Systemic), 2750
  Timolol (Systemic), 593
  Timolol and Hydrochlorothiazide (Systemic), 609
  Torsemide (Systemic)†, 2848
  Trandolapril (Systemic), 2854
  Trandolapril and Verapamil (Systemic), 2857
  Triamterene and Hydrochlorothiazide (Systemic), 1272
  Trichlormethiazide (Systemic)†, 1273
  Trimethaphan (Systemic), 2879
  Valsartan (Systemic), 2914
  Verapamil (Systemic), 720, 3037
**Hypertension (treatment adjunct)**
  Amiloride (Systemic), 1266
  Spironolactone (Systemic), 1266
  [Triamterene (Systemic)][1], 1266

**Hypertension, cerebral (treatment)**
  *See also* Edema, cerebral
  Dimethyl Sulfoxide (Systemic), 3140‡
  [Pentobarbital, Parenteral (Systemic)][1], 518
  Thiopental, Parenteral (Systemic)[1], 161
  Urea (Systemic)†, 2899
**Hypertension, intraoperative (treatment)**
  Esmolol (Systemic)†, 1377
**Hypertension, ocular (prophylaxis)**
  Apraclonidine (Ophthalmic), 459
**Hypertension, ocular (treatment)**
  Apraclonidine (Ophthalmic), 459
  Betaxolol (Ophthalmic), 585
  Brimonidine (Ophthalmic), 632
  Brinzolamide (Ophthalmic), 634
  Carteolol (Ophthalmic)†, 585
  Dorzolamide (Ophthalmic), 1294
  Dorzolamide and Timolol (Ophthalmic), 3018
  Latanoprost (Ophthalmic), 1831
  Levobunolol (Ophthalmic), 585
  Metipranolol (Ophthalmic)†, 585
  Timolol (Ophthalmic), 585, 3036
  Urea (Systemic)†, 2899
**Hypertension, ocular, during surgery (treatment)**
  Epinephrine Injection USP (Systemic), 651
**Hypertension, ocular, postsurgical (treatment)**
  Carbachol (Ophthalmic), 3013
**Hypertension, paroxysmal, in surgery for pheochromocytoma (prophylaxis)**
  Phentolamine (Systemic), #
**Hypertension, paroxysmal, in surgery for pheochromocytoma (treatment)**
  [Nitroprusside (Systemic)][1], 2142
  Phentolamine (Systemic), #
**Hypertension, postoperative (treatment)**
  Esmolol (Systemic)†, 1377
**Hypertension, pulmonary, neonatal (treatment)**
  Nitric Oxide (Systemic), 3156‡
**Hypertension, pulmonary, persistent (treatment)**
  Tolazoline (Parenteral-Systemic)†, #
**Hypertension, pulmonary, primary (treatment)**
  15AU81 (Systemic), 3127‡
  Epoprostenol (Systemic)[1], 3142‡
**Hyperthermia, malignant (prophylaxis)**
  Dantrolene (Systemic), 1165
**Hyperthermia, malignant (treatment adjunct)**
  Dantrolene, Parenteral (Systemic), 1165
**Hyperthyroidism (diagnosis)**
  *See also* Thyroid function studies; Thyroid uptake tests; Thyroid imaging, radionuclide
  Sodium Iodide I 131 (Systemic—Diagnostic), 2603
**Hyperthyroidism (treatment)**
  Methimazole (Systemic), 446
  Potassium Iodide (Systemic)[1], 2354
  Propylthiouracil (Systemic), 446
  Sodium Iodide I 131 (Systemic—Therapeutic), 2606
**Hyperthyroidism (treatment adjunct)**
  [Iodine, Strong (Systemic)][1], 1751
**Hyperthyroidism, in Graves' disease (treatment)**
  [Iopanoic Acid (Systemic)], #
  [Ipodate (Systemic)]†, #
  [Tyropanoate (Systemic)]†, #
**Hypertrophic subaortic stenosis**—*See* Cardiomyopathy, hypertrophic
**Hyperuricemia (prophylaxis)**
  Allopurinol (Systemic), 44, 3129‡
**Hyperuricemia (treatment)**
  Allopurinol (Systemic), 44
  Allopurinol Sodium (Systemic), 3129‡
  Probenecid (Systemic), 2380
  Sulfinpyrazone (Systemic), 2646
**Hyphema secondary to hyperfibrinolysis**—*See* Hemorrhage, hyperfibrinolysis-induced
**Hyphema, traumatic (treatment)**
  Aminocaproic Acid (Ophthalmic), 3130‡
**Hypocalcemia, acute (treatment)**
  Calcium Acetate (Systemic)†, 736
  Calcium Chloride (Systemic), 736
  Calcium Gluceptate (Systemic)†, 736
  Calcium Gluconate, Parenteral (Systemic), 736
  Calcium Glycerophosphate and Calcium Lactate (Systemic)†, 736
**Hypocalcemia, associated with hypoparathyroidism (treatment)**
  Alfacalcidol (Systemic)*, 2966
  [Calcifediol (Systemic)]†, 2966
  Calcitriol (Systemic), 2966
  Dihydrotachysterol (Systemic), 2966
  Ergocalciferol (Systemic), 2966
**Hypocalcemia, chronic (treatment)**
  *See also* Calcium deficiency; Hypoparathyroidism; Osteodystrophy; Osteoporosis; Pseudohypoparathyroidism; Tetany, hypocalcemic
  Alfacalcidol (Systemic)*, 2966
  Calcifediol (Systemic)†, 2966

**Hypocalcemia, chronic (treatment)** *(continued)*
  Calcitriol (Systemic), 2966
  Calcium Carbonate (Systemic), 736
  Calcium Citrate (Systemic)†, 736
  Calcium Glubionate (Systemic), 736
  Calcium Gluceptate and Calcium Gluconate (Systemic)*, 736
  Calcium Gluconate, Oral (Systemic), 736
  Calcium Lactate (Systemic), 736
  Calcium Lactate-Gluconate and Calcium Carbonate (Systemic)*, 736
  Calcium Phosphate, Dibasic (Systemic)†, 736
  Calcium Phosphate, Tribasic (Systemic)†, 736
  Dihydrotachysterol (Systemic), 2966
  Ergocalciferol (Systemic), 2966
**Hypocitraturia (prophylaxis)**
  Potassium Citrate (Systemic), 881, 3159‡
  Potassium Citrate and Citric Acid (Systemic), 881
**Hypocitraturia (treatment)**
  Potassium Citrate (Systemic), 881
  Potassium Citrate and Citric Acid (Systemic), 881
**Hypofibrinogenemia (treatment)**
  Antihemophilic Factor, Cryoprecipitated (Systemic), 319
**Hypoglycemia (treatment)**
  Diazoxide (Oral-Systemic), 1197
  Glucagon (Systemic), 1563
**Hypogonadism (diagnosis)**
  Gonadorelin (Systemic), 1571
**Hypogonadism, female (treatment)**
  Estradiol Cypionate (Systemic), 1383
  Estradiol Cypionate (Systemic)[1], 1383
  Estradiol, Oral (Systemic)[1], 1383
  Estradiol, Transdermal (Systemic)[1], 1383
  Estradiol, Transdermal System (Matrix-type) (Systemic)[1], 1383
  Estradiol, Transdermal System (Reservoir-type) (Systemic), 1383
  Estradiol Valerate (Systemic)[1], 1383
  Estrogens, Conjugated, Oral (Systemic), 1383
  Estrogens, Esterified (Systemic), 1383
  Estrone (Systemic)†, 1383
  Estropipate (Systemic)[1], 1383
  Ethinyl Estradiol (Systemic)[1], 1383
**Hypogonadism, male**—*See* Cryptorchidism; Infertility, male; Puberty, delayed, male
**Hypogonadism, male (diagnosis)**
  [Chorionic Gonadotropin (Systemic)][1], 858
**Hypogonadism, male, due to hyperprolactinemia (treatment)**
  Bromocriptine (Systemic), 636
**Hypokalemia (prophylaxis)**
  [Amiloride (Systemic)][1], 1266
  Potassium Acetate (Systemic), 2357
  Potassium Bicarbonate (Systemic), 2357
  Potassium Bicarbonate and Potassium Chloride (Systemic), 2357
  Potassium Bicarbonate and Potassium Citrate (Systemic)†, 2357
  Potassium Chloride (Systemic), 2357
  Potassium Gluconate (Systemic), 2357
  Potassium Gluconate and Potassium Chloride (Systemic)†, 2357
  Potassium Gluconate and Potassium Citrate (Systemic)†, 2357
  Spironolactone (Systemic), 1266
  [Triamterene (Systemic)][1], 1266
  Trikates (Systemic)†, 2357
**Hypokalemia (treatment)**
  [Amiloride (Systemic)][1], 1266
  Amiloride and Hydrochlorothiazide (Systemic)[1], 1272
  Potassium Acetate (Systemic), 2357
  Potassium Bicarbonate (Systemic), 2357
  Potassium Bicarbonate and Potassium Chloride (Systemic), 2357
  Potassium Bicarbonate and Potassium Citrate (Systemic)†, 2357
  Potassium Chloride (Systemic), 2357
  Potassium Gluconate (Systemic), 2357
  Potassium Gluconate and Potassium Chloride (Systemic)†, 2357
  Potassium Gluconate and Potassium Citrate (Systemic)†, 2357
  Spironolactone (Systemic), 1266
  Spironolactone and Hydrochlorothiazide (Systemic)[1], 1272
  [Triamterene (Systemic)][1], 1266
  Triamterene and Hydrochlorothiazide (Systemic)[1], 1272
  Trikates (Systemic)†, 2357
**Hypomagnesemia (prophylaxis)**
  Magnesium Chloride (Systemic)†, 1897
  Magnesium Citrate (Systemic), 1897
  Magnesium Gluceptate (Systemic)*, 1897
  Magnesium Gluconate (Systemic), 1897

## Hypomagnesemia (prophylaxis) (continued)
Magnesium Hydroxide (Systemic), 1897
Magnesium Lactate (Systemic)†, 1897
Magnesium Oxide (Systemic), 1897
Magnesium Pidolate (Systemic)*, 1897
Magnesium Sulfate (Systemic), 1895, 1897

## Hypomagnesemia (treatment)
Magnesium Chloride (Systemic)†, 1897
Magnesium Citrate (Systemic), 1897
Magnesium Gluceptate (Systemic)*, 1897
Magnesium Gluconate (Systemic), 1897
Magnesium Hydroxide (Systemic), 1897
Magnesium Lactate (Systemic)†, 1897
Magnesium Oxide (Systemic), 1897
Magnesium Pidolate (Systemic)*, 1897
Magnesium Sulfate (Systemic), 1895, 1897

## Hypoparathyroidism (treatment)
[Calcifediol (Systemic)]†, 2966
Calcitriol (Systemic), 2966
Dihydrotachysterol (Systemic), 2966
Ergocalciferol (Systemic), 2966

## Hypoparathyroidism, idiopathic (diagnosis)
Teriparatide (Systemic)†, #, 3167‡

## Hypophosphatemia (prophylaxis)
Potassium Phosphates (Systemic), 2317
Potassium and Sodium Phosphates (Systemic), 2317
Sodium Phosphates (Systemic)†, 2317

## Hypophosphatemia (treatment)
Alfacalcidol (Systemic)*, 2966
Calcifediol (Systemic)†, 2966
Calcitriol (Systemic), 2966
Dihydrotachysterol (Systemic), 2966
Ergocalciferol (Systemic), 2966
Potassium Phosphates (Systemic), 2317
Potassium and Sodium Phosphates (Systemic), 2317
Sodium Phosphates (Systemic)†, 2317

## Hypophosphatemia, familial (treatment)
[Calcifediol (Systemic)]†, 2966
[Calcitriol (Systemic)], 2966
[Dihydrotachysterol (Systemic)], 2966
Ergocalciferol (Systemic), 2966
Secalciferol (Systemic), 3163‡

## Hypoproteinemia (treatment)
Albumin Human (Systemic), 34

## Hypoprothrombinemia (prophylaxis)
Menadiol (Systemic)†, 2975
Phytonadione (Systemic), 2975

## Hypoprothrombinemia (treatment)
Menadiol (Systemic)†, 2975
Phytonadione (Systemic), 2975

## Hypotension (treatment)
Midodrine (Systemic), 2014
[Octreotide (Systemic)][1], 2152

## Hypotension, acute (prophylaxis)
Metaraminol (Parenteral-Systemic)†, 2669
Methoxamine (Parenteral-Systemic), 2669

## Hypotension, acute (treatment)
See also Shock
Dobutamine (Parenteral-Systemic), 2669
Dopamine (Parenteral-Systemic), 2669
Ephedrine (Parenteral-Systemic), 2669
Epinephrine (Parenteral-Systemic), 2669
Mephentermine (Parenteral-Systemic)†, 2669
Metaraminol (Parenteral-Systemic)†, 2669
Methoxamine (Parenteral-Systemic), 2669
Norepinephrine (Parenteral-Systemic), 2669
Phenylephrine (Parenteral-Systemic), 2669

## Hypotension, controlled
Nitroglycerin, Parenteral (Systemic), 2129
Nitroprusside (Systemic), 2142

## Hypotension, controlled (induction)
[Labetalol, Parenteral (Systemic)][1], 593
Trimethaphan (Systemic), 2879

## Hypotension, controlled (maintenance)
[Labetalol, Parenteral (Systemic)][1], 593
Trimethaphan (Systemic), 2879

## Hypotension, idiopathic orthostatic (treatment)
[Fludrocortisone (Systemic)][1], 1481
Midodrine (Systemic), 3154‡

## Hypotension, orthostatic (prophylaxis)
[Dihydroergotamine (Systemic)][1], 2925

## Hypotension, orthostatic (treatment)
[Dihydroergotamine (Systemic)][1], 2925

## Hypothalamic-pituitary-gonadal axis function studies
[Clomiphene (Systemic)][1], 903

## Hypothyroidism (diagnosis)
Levothyroxine (Systemic), 2809
Liothyronine (Systemic), 2809
Thyrotropin (Systemic), #

## Hypothyroidism (treatment)
Levothyroxine (Systemic), 2809
Liothyronine (Systemic), 2809

## Hypovolemia (treatment)
Albumin Human (Systemic), 34

## Hypoxia, cerebral (treatment)
[Thiopental, Parenteral (Systemic)][1], 161

## Hysterosalpingography
Diatrizoate Meglumine (Local), #
Diatrizoate Meglumine and Iodipamide Meglumine (Local), #
Diatrizoate Sodium (Mucosal-Local), #
Iohexol (Local)[1], #
Ioxaglate (Local), #

## Hysterosalpingography, adjunct
[Glucagon (Systemic)][1], 1563

# I

## Ichthyosis, lamellar (treatment)
[Acitretin (Systemic)]†, 18
[Etretinate (Systemic)], #

## Ichthyosis, lamellar, and other ichthyoses (treatment)
[Isotretinoin (Systemic)][1], 1796

## Ichthyosis, primary, congenital (treatment)
Monolaurin (Systemic), 3155‡

## Ileus, gastrointestinal, postoperative (prophylaxis)
Neostigmine, Parenteral (Systemic), 437

## Ileus, gastrointestinal, postoperative (treatment)
Neostigmine, Parenteral (Systemic), 437
[Sincalide (Systemic)], #

## Immunodeficiency, combined, severe (treatment adjunct)
Pegademase Bovine (Systemic), 3157‡

## Immunodeficiency, primary (treatment)
Aldesleukin (Systemic), 3129‡
Immune Globulin Intravenous (Human) (Systemic), 1686, 3025
PEG-Interleukin-2 (Systemic), 3157‡

## Immunodeficiency syndrome, acquired (AIDS) (treatment)
Carbovir (Systemic), 3136‡
CD 4, Human Recombinant Soluble (rCD4) (Systemic), 3161‡, 3162‡
CD4 Immunoglobulin G (Recombinant Human) (Systemic), 3160‡
Dextran Sulfate Sodium (Systemic), 3140‡
Didanosine (Systemic), 1206
Diethyldithiocarbamate (Systemic), 3140‡
Human Immunodeficiency Virus Immune Globulin (Systemic), 3145‡
Human Immunodeficiency Virus (HIV) Neutralizing Antibodies (Systemic), 3145‡
Human T-Lymphotropic Virus Type III gp160 Antigens (Systemic), 3146‡
[Immune Globulin Intravenous (Human) (Systemic)][1], 1686
Indinavir (Systemic), 1693
Interferon Beta, Recombinant (Systemic), 3148‡
Nevirapine (Systemic), 2113
Poly I: Poly C12U (Systemic), 3158‡
Ritonavir (Systemic), 2516
Saquinavir (Systemic), 2454
Tumor Necrosis Factor Binding Protein I (Systemic), 3170‡
Tumor Necrosis Factor Binding Protein II (Systemic), 3170‡
Zalcitabine (Systemic), 3171‡
Zidovudine (Systemic), 2992, 3038, 3171‡

## Immunodeficiency syndrome, acquired (AIDS), related disorders—See Anorexia, AIDS-associated; Cachexia, AIDS-associated; Kaposi's sarcoma; Pneumonia, Pneumocystis carinii; Stomatitis, aphthous, immunodeficiency-associated; Toxoplasmosis, AIDS-associated; Weight loss, AIDS-associated

## Immunodeficiency syndrome, acquired (AIDS), related disorders (diagnosis)
Gallium Citrate Ga 67 (Systemic), 1538

## Immunodeficiency syndrome, acquired (AIDS), related disorders (prophylaxis)
See Weight loss, AIDS-associated, 3141‡

## Immunodeficiency syndrome, acquired (AIDS), related infections (prophylaxis)
See also Mycobacterium avium complex (MAC) disease, in AIDS patients; Pneumonia, Pneumocystis carinii; Stomatitis, aphthous, immunodeficiency-associated
Immune Globulin Intravenous (Human) (Systemic), 3147‡

## Immunodeficiency syndrome—related complex, acquired (ARC) (treatment)
[Immune Globulin Intravenous (Human) (Systemic)][1], 1686
Zidovudine (Systemic), 3171‡

## Immunodepression, bone marrow transplantation (prophylaxis)
Immune Globulin Intravenous (Human) (Systemic), 3024

## Immunodepression, iatrogenically induced or disease-associated (treatment)
[Immune Globulin Intravenous (Human) (Systemic)][1], 1686

## Immunodepression, iatrogenically induced or disease-associated (treatment adjunct)
[Immune Globulin Intravenous (Human) (Systemic)][1], 1686

## Impetigo (treatment)
Cefadroxil (Systemic)[1], 794
Cefuroxime Axetil (Systemic)[1], 794
[Cephalexin (Systemic)][1], 794
Mupirocin (Topical), 4253

## Impotence (diagnosis)
[Papaverine (Intracavernosal)][1], #
[Phentolamine (Intracavernosal)][1], #

## Impotence (treatment)
See also Erectile dysfunction
[Papaverine (Intracavernosal)][1], #
[Yohimbine (Systemic)][1], #

## Impotence (treatment adjunct)
[Phentolamine (Intracavernosal)][1], #

## Infection, insect-bite–transmitted (prophylaxis)
Diethyltoluamide (Topical), #

## Infertility, female (treatment)
See also Amenorrhea; Corpus luteum insufficiency; Endometriosis; Hypogonadism, female
Chorionic Gonadotropin (Systemic), 858
Clomiphene (Systemic), 903
Follitropin Alfa (Systemic), 1520
Follitropin Beta (Systemic), 1523
[Gonadorelin (Systemic)][1], 3144‡
Menotropins (Systemic), 1943
Progesterone (Systemic), 3160‡
Urofollitropin (Systemic), 2901, 3170‡

## Infertility, female (treatment adjunct)
Ovulation Prediction Test Kits for Home Use, #
Sermorelin (Systemic), 3164‡

## Infertility, female, due to primary hypothalamic hypogonadism (treatment)
Gonadorelin (Systemic), 1571

## Infertility, due to hyperprolactinemia (treatment)
Bromocriptine (Systemic), 636

## Infertility, male (treatment)
Chorionic Gonadotropin (Systemic), 858
[Clomiphene (Systemic)][1], 903
[Gonadorelin (Systemic)][1], 1571
Menotropins (Systemic), 1943
Urofollitropin (Systemic), 3170‡

## Infertility, male (treatment adjunct)
Ovulation Prediction Test Kits for Home Use, #

## Infestation, arthropod (prophylaxis)
Diethyltoluamide (Topical), #

## Infestation, insect (prophylaxis)
Diethyltoluamide (Topical), #

## Inflammation, anorectal (treatment)
Benzocaine Ointment USP (Rectal) (Mucosal-Local), 128
Dibucaine (Mucosal-Local), 128
Pramoxine (Mucosal-Local), 128
Tetracaine, Rectal (Mucosal-Local), 128

## Inflammation, nonrheumatic—See Bursitis; Epicondylitis; Tenosynovitis, specific, nonacute

## Inflammation, nonrheumatic (treatment)
Aspirin (Systemic), 2538
Aspirin, Buffered (Systemic), 2538
Choline Salicylate (Systemic)†, 2538
Choline and Magnesium Salicylates (Systemic), 2538
[Diclofenac (Systemic)][1], 388
[Diflunisal (Systemic)][1], 388
[Etodolac (Systemic)]†, 388
[Fenoprofen (Systemic)][1], 388
Floctafenine (Systemic)*[1], 388
[Flurbiprofen (Systemic)], 388
[Ibuprofen (Systemic)][1], 388
Indomethacin (Systemic)[1], 388
[Ketoprofen (Systemic)][1], 388
Magnesium Salicylate (Systemic), 2538
[Meclofenamate (Systemic)]†, 388
[Mefenamic Acid (Systemic)][1], 388
[Nabumetone (Systemic)][1], 388
Naproxen (Systemic), 388
[Oxaprozin (Systemic)]†, 388
[Phenylbutazone (Systemic)][1], 388
[Piroxicam (Systemic)][1], 388
Salsalate (Systemic), 2538
Sodium Salicylate (Systemic), 2538
Sulindac (Systemic), 388
Tenoxicam (Systemic)*, 388
Tiaprofenic Acid (Systemic)*[1], 388
[Tolmetin (Systemic)][1], 388

**Inflammation, ocular (prophylaxis)**
 [Ketorolac (Ophthalmic)], 1809
**Inflammation, ocular (treatment)**
 Diclofenac (Ophthalmic), 383
 [Flurbiprofen (Ophthalmic)], 383
 Indomethacin (Ophthalmic)*[1], 383
 [Ketorolac (Ophthalmic)], 1809
**Inflammation, ocular, following cataract surgery (treatment)**
 Ketorolac (Ophthalmic), 3026
**Inflammation, postoperative (treatment)**
 Loteprednol (Ophthalmic), 1887
 Rimexolone (Ophthalmic), 2504
**Inflammatory conditions, noninfectious, nasal (treatment)**
 Beclomethasone (Nasal), 961
 Budesonide (Nasal)*, 961
 Dexamethasone (Nasal)†, 961
 Flunisolide (Nasal), 961
 Triamcinolone (Nasal), 961
**Inflammatory disease, pelvic (prophylaxis)**
 [Condoms, Lamb Cecum][1], 1474
 [Condoms, Lamb Cecum, and Nonoxynol 9][1], 1474
 [Condoms, Latex][1], 1474
 [Condoms, Latex, and Nonoxynol 9][1], 1474
**Inflammatory lesions (diagnosis)**
 Gallium Citrate Ga 67 (Systemic), 1538
 Indium In 111 Oxyquinoline (Systemic)†, 1695
 Technetium Tc 99m Exametazime (Systemic)[1], 2708
**Influenza (prophylaxis)**
 Influenza Virus Vaccine (Systemic), 1707
**Influenza A (prophylaxis)**
 Amantadine (Systemic), 58
 Rimantadine (Systemic)†, 2502
**Influenza A (treatment)**
 Amantadine (Systemic), 58
 [Ribavirin (Systemic)][1], 2478
 Rimantadine (Systemic)†, 2502
**Influenza B (treatment)**
 [Ribavirin (Systemic)][1], 2478
**Injuries, athletic**—See Inflammation, nonrheumatic
**Insomnia (treatment)**
 [Alprazolam (Systemic)][1], 556
 Bromazepam (Systemic)*[1], 556
 [Diazepam (Systemic)][1], 556
 Diphenhydramine (Systemic), 325
 Doxylamine (Systemic), 325
 Estazolam (Systemic)†, 556
 Flurazepam (Systemic), 556
 [Halazepam (Systemic)]†, 556
 Ketazolam (Systemic)*[1], 556
 Lorazepam (Systemic)[1], 556
 [Nitrazepam (Systemic)][1]*, 556
 [Prazepam (Systemic)]†, 556
 Quazepam (Systemic)†, 556
 Temazepam (Systemic), 556
 Triazolam (Systemic), 556
 Zolpidem (Systemic)†, 3005
 Zopiclone (Systemic)*, 3039
**Intertrigo (treatment)**
 Alclometasone Dipropionate (Topical), 978
 Beclomethasone Dipropionate (Topical), 978
 Betamethasone Benzoate (Topical), 978
 Betamethasone Valerate (Topical), 978
 Clioquinol and Flumethasone (Topical)*, 3015
 Clioquinol and Hydrocortisone (Topical), #
 Clobetasone Butyrate (Topical), 978
 Clocortolone Pivalate (Topical), 978
 Desonide (Topical), 978
 Desoximetasone (0.05% cream only) (Topical), 978
 Dexamethasone (Topical), 978
 Dexamethasone Sodium Phosphate (Topical), 978
 Diflucortolone Valerate (Topical), 978
 Flumethasone Pivalate (Topical), 978
 Fluocinolone Acetonide (except 0.2% cream) (Topical), 978
 Flurandrenolide (Topical), 978
 Fluticasone Propionate (Topical), 978
 Hydrocortisone (Topical), 978
 Hydrocortisone Acetate (Topical), 978
 Hydrocortisone Butyrate (Topical), 978
 Hydrocortisone Valerate (Topical), 978
 Methylprednisolone Acetate (Topical), 978
 Mometasone Furoate (Topical), 978
 Triamcinolone Acetonide (except 0.5% cream and ointment) (Topical), 978
**Intestinal fluke**—See Metagonimiasis
**Intestinal roundworm, multiple (treatment)**
 Mebendazole (Systemic), 1926

**Intra-abdominal infections (treatment)**
 Alatrofloxacin, 2891
 Amikacin (Systemic), 69
 Amphotericin B (Systemic), 98
 Ampicillin and Sulbactam (Systemic)†, 2263
 Aztreonam (Systemic)†, 502
 Carbenicillin, Parenteral (Systemic), 2240
 Cefamandole (Systemic), 794
 Cefepime (Systemic), 794
 Cefoperazone (Systemic)[1], 794
 Cefotaxime (Systemic), 794
 Cefotetan (Systemic), 794
 Cefoxitin (Systemic), 794
 Ceftazidime (Systemic), 794
 Ceftizoxime (Systemic), 794
 Ceftriaxone (Systemic), 794
 Cephalothin (Systemic), 794
 Clindamycin (Systemic), 893
 [Demeclocycline (Systemic)], 2765
 [Doxycycline (Systemic)], 2765
 Gentamicin (Systemic), 69
 Imipenem and Cilastatin (Systemic), 1681
 Kanamycin (Systemic)†, 69
 Meropenem (Systemic), 1949
 Metronidazole (Systemic), 1996
 Mezlocillin (Systemic)†, 2240
 [Minocycline (Systemic)], 2765
 Netilmicin (Systemic), 69
 [Oxytetracycline (Systemic)]†, 2765
 [Penicillin G, Parenteral (Systemic)][1], 2240
 Piperacillin (Systemic), 2240
 Piperacillin and Tazobactam (Systemic), 2263
 Streptomycin (Systemic), 69
 [Tetracycline (Systemic)], 2765
 Ticarcillin (Systemic), 2240
 Ticarcillin and Clavulanate (Systemic), 2263
 Tobramycin (Systemic), 69
 Trovafloxacin (Systemic), 2891
**Intra-abdominal infections (treatment adjunct)**
 Albumin Human (Systemic), 34
**Intracranial abnormalities (diagnosis)**—See Angiography; Angiography, cerebral, radionuclide; Brain imaging, radionuclide
**Intracranial pressure**—See Hypertension, cerebral
**Intracranial pressure, elevated (treatment)**
 Mannitol (Systemic), 1906
**Intraocular pressure, elevated**—See Hypertension, ocular
**Intravenous regional anesthesia**
 [Chloroprocaine (Parenteral-Local)][1], 139
 Lidocaine (Parenteral-Local)[1], 139
 [Mepivacaine (Parenteral-Local)][1], 139
**Intubation, intestinal**
 Metoclopramide, Parenteral (Systemic), 1992
**In vitro fertilization**—See Reproductive technologies, assisted
**Iodine deficiency (prophylaxis)**
 Sodium Iodide (Systemic)†, 2597
**Iodine deficiency (treatment)**
 [Iodine, Strong (Systemic)], 1751
 [Potassium Iodide (Systemic)]†, 2354
 Sodium Iodide (Systemic)†, 2597
**Iridocyclitis (treatment)**
 Betamethasone (Ophthalmic)*, 966
 Betamethasone, Oral (Systemic), 998
 Betamethasone, Parenteral (Systemic), 998
 Cortisone (Systemic), 998
 Dexamethasone (Ophthalmic), 966
 Dexamethasone, Oral (Systemic), 998
 Dexamethasone, Parenteral (Systemic), 998
 Fluorometholone (Ophthalmic), 966
 Hydrocortisone (Ophthalmic)*, 966
 Hydrocortisone, Oral (Systemic), 998
 Hydrocortisone, Parenteral (Systemic), 998
 [Medrysone (Ophthalmic)][1], 966
 Methylprednisolone, Oral (Systemic), 998
 Methylprednisolone, Parenteral (Systemic), 998
 Prednisolone (Ophthalmic), 966
 Prednisolone, Oral (Systemic), 998
 Prednisolone, Parenteral (Systemic), 998
 Prednisone (Systemic), 998
 [Scopolamine (Ophthalmic)]†, 2557
 Triamcinolone, Oral (Systemic), 998
 Triamcinolone, Parenteral (Systemic), 998
**Iridocyclitis, postoperative (treatment)**
 Scopolamine (Ophthalmic)†, 2557
**Iridocyclitis, preoperative (treatment)**
 Scopolamine (Ophthalmic)†, 2557
**Iron absorption studies**
 Ferrous Citrate Fe 59 (Systemic)*, 1460
**Iron deficiency anemia (prophylaxis)**
 Ferrous Fumarate (Systemic), 1774
 Ferrous Gluconate (Systemic), 1774
 Ferrous Sulfate (Systemic), 1774
 Iron Dextran (Systemic), 1774
 Iron-Polysaccharide (Systemic)†, 1774

**Iron deficiency anemia (prophylaxis)** (continued)
 Iron Sorbitol (Systemic)*, 1774
**Iron deficiency anemia (treatment)**
 Ferrous Fumarate (Systemic), 1774
 Ferrous Gluconate (Systemic), 1774
 Ferrous Sulfate (Systemic), 1774
 Iron Dextran (Systemic), 1774
 Iron-Polysaccharide (Systemic)†, 1774
 Iron Sorbitol (Systemic)*, 1774
**Iron metabolism studies**
 Ferrous Citrate Fe 59 (Systemic)*, 1460
**Irritative voiding, symptoms of (treatment)**
 Atropine, Hyoscyamine, Methenamine, Methylene Blue, Phenyl Salicylate, and Benzoic Acid (Systemic)†, 488
 Flavoxate (Systemic), 1468
 Oxybutynin (Systemic), 2209
**Isaac's syndrome**—See Neuromyotonia
**Ischemia, cerebral (treatment)**
 [Dexamethasone, Oral (Systemic)][1], 998
 [Dexamethasone, Parenteral (Systemic)][1], 998
 [Pentobarbital, Parenteral (Systemic)][1], 518
 [Thiopental, Parenteral (Systemic)][1], 161
**Ischemia, myocardial (diagnosis)**
 See also Cardiac imaging, radionuclide; Cardiac imaging, positron emission tomographic
 Ammonia N 13 (Systemic)*†, 91
 [Fludeoxyglucose F 18 (Systemic)][1]*†, 1478
 [Rubidium Rb 82 (Systemic)]†, 2536
 Technetium Tc 99m Sestamibi (Systemic)[1], 2736
**Ischemia, myocardial (prophylaxis)**
 Perfluorochemical Emulsion (Systemic), #
**Ischemia, myocardial (treatment)**
 Perfluorochemical Emulsion (Systemic), #
**Ischemic attacks, transient, in females (treatment)**
 [Dipyridamole (Systemic)][1], #
 [Warfarin (Systemic)], 243
**Ischemic attacks, transient, in males (prophylaxis)**
 Aspirin, Buffered (Systemic), 2538
 Aspirin Delayed-release Tablets USP (Systemic), 2538
 Aspirin, Sodium Bicarbonate, and Citric Acid (Systemic)[1], 477
 Aspirin Tablets USP (Systemic), 2538
 Aspirin Tablets USP (Chewable) (Systemic), 2538
**Ischemic attacks, transient, in males (treatment)**
 [Dipyridamole (Systemic)][1], #
 [Warfarin (Systemic)], 243
**Isosporiasis (prophylaxis)**
 [Pyrimethamine (Systemic)][1], 2433
 [Sulfadoxine and Pyrimethamine (Systemic)][1], 2637
 [Sulfamethoxazole and Trimethoprim (Systemic)][1], 2661
**Isosporiasis (treatment)**
 [Pyrimethamine (Systemic)][1], 2433
 [Sulfamethoxazole and Trimethoprim (Systemic)][1], 2661

# J–L

**Japanese encephalitis (prophylaxis)**
 Japanese Encephalitis Virus Vaccine (Systemic), #
**Jock itch**—See Tinea cruris
**Joint infections**—See Bone and joint infections
**Kala-azar**—See Leishmaniasis, visceral
**Kaposi's sarcoma (treatment)**
 Thalidomide (Systemic)‡, 1837, 3168
 Vinblastine (Systemic), 2946
**Kaposi's sarcoma, AIDS-associated (treatment)**
 Bleomycin (Systemic), 624
 [Cisplatin (Systemic)][1], 876
 9-Cis-Retinoic Acid (Topical)‡, 3128
 [Dactinomycin (Systemic)][1], 1153
 Daunorubicin, Liposomal (Systemic), 1992, 3152‡
 [Doxorubicin (Systemic)][1], 1308
 Doxorubicin, Liposomal (Systemic), 1312
 [Etoposide (Systemic)][1], 1424
 Interferon Alfa-2a, Recombinant (Systemic), 1740, 3147‡
 Interferon Alfa-2b, Recombinant (Systemic), 1740, 3148‡
 Interferon Alfa-n1 (Ins) (Systemic)*[1], 1740
 [Interferon Alfa-n3 (Systemic)]†, 1740
 Interferon Beta (Recombinant) (Systemic), 3148‡
 Paclitaxel (Systemic)[1], 2215, 3157‡
 Vinblastine (Systemic), 2946
 Vincristine (Systemic), 2950
**Kasabach-Merritt syndrome (treatment adjunct)**
 [Antihemophilic Factor, Cryoprecipitated (Systemic)][1], 319

## Indications Index

**Kawasaki disease (treatment)**
[Aspirin (Systemic)][1], 2538
[Aspirin, Buffered (Systemic)][1], 2538
Immune Globulin Intravenous (Human) (Systemic), 3025

**Kawasaki disease (treatment adjunct)**
[Immune Globulin Intravenous (Human) (Systemic)][1], 1686

**Kawasaki syndrome**—See Kawasaki disease

**Keloids (treatment)**
Betamethasone, Parenteral-Local (Systemic), 998
Dexamethasone, Parenteral-Local (Systemic), 998
Hydrocortisone, Parenteral-Local (Systemic), 998
Methylprednisolone, Parenteral-Local (Systemic), 998
Prednisolone, Parenteral-Local (Systemic), 998
Triamcinolone, Parenteral-Local (Systemic), 998

**Keloids, reduction of associated itching (treatment)**
Amcinonide (Topical), 978
Beclomethasone Dipropionate (Topical), 978
Betamethasone Benzoate (Topical), 978
Betamethasone Dipropionate (Topical), 978
Betamethasone Valerate (Topical), 978
Clobetasol Propionate (Topical), 978
Clobetasone Butyrate (Topical), 978
Desoximetasone (Topical), 978
Diflorasone Diacetate (Topical), 978
Diflucortolone Valerate (Topical), 978
Fluocinolone Acetonide (Topical), 978
Fluocinonide (Topical), 978
Flurandrenolide (except 0.0125% cream and ointment) (Topical), 978
Fluticasone Propionate (Topical), 978
Halcinonide (Topical), 978
Halobetasol Propionate (Topical), 978
Hydrocortisone Butyrate (Topical), 978
Hydrocortisone Valerate (Topical), 978
Mometasone Furoate (Topical), 978
Triamcinolone Acetonide (Topical), 978

**Keratitis, *Acanthamoeba* (treatment)**
Propamidine (Ophthalmic), 3160‡

**Keratitis, bacterial (treatment)**
[Chloramphenicol (Ophthalmic)], #
[Chlortetracycline (Ophthalmic)], 2763
[Erythromycin (Ophthalmic)][1], 1364
Gentamicin (Ophthalmic), 1555
Neomycin (Ophthalmic)*†, #
[Neomycin, Polymyxin B, and Bacitracin (Ophthalmic)], #
[Neomycin, Polymyxin B, and Gramicidin (Ophthalmic)], #
[Sulfacetamide (Ophthalmic)], 2651
[Sulfisoxazole (Ophthalmic)], 2651
[Tetracycline (Ophthalmic)], 2763
[Tobramycin (Ophthalmic)], #

**Keratitis, exposure (treatment)**
[Chloramphenicol (Ophthalmic)], #
Hydroxypropyl Cellulose (Ophthalmic), #
Hydroxypropyl Methylcellulose (Ophthalmic), #
[Tobramycin (Ophthalmic)], #

**Keratitis, fungal (treatment)**
Natamycin (Ophthalmic)†, #

**Keratitis, herpes simplex virus (treatment)**
Idoxuridine (Ophthalmic), 1675
Trifluridine (Ophthalmic), 2877
Vidarabine (Ophthalmic), 2944

**Keratitis, herpes zoster (treatment)**
Dexamethasone (Ophthalmic), 966
Fluorometholone (Ophthalmic), 966
Hydrocortisone (Ophthalmic)*, 966
[Medrysone (Ophthalmic)][1], 966
Prednisolone (Ophthalmic), 966

**Keratitis, neuroparalytic (treatment)**
[Chloramphenicol (Ophthalmic)], #
[Hydroxypropyl Cellulose (Ophthalmic)][1], #
Hydroxypropyl Methylcellulose (Ophthalmic), #
[Tobramycin (Ophthalmic)], #

**Keratitis, not associated with herpes simplex or fungal infection (treatment)**
Betamethasone, Oral (Systemic), 998
Betamethasone, Parenteral (Systemic), 998
Cortisone (Systemic), 998
Dexamethasone (Ophthalmic), 966
Dexamethasone, Oral (Systemic), 998
Dexamethasone, Parenteral (Systemic), 998
Fluorometholone (Ophthalmic), 966
Hydrocortisone (Ophthalmic)*, 966
Hydrocortisone, Oral (Systemic), 998
Hydrocortisone, Parenteral (Systemic), 998
[Medrysone (Ophthalmic)][1], 966
Methylprednisolone, Oral (Systemic), 998
Methylprednisolone, Parenteral (Systemic), 998
Prednisolone (Ophthalmic), 966
Prednisolone, Oral (Systemic), 998
Prednisolone, Parenteral (Systemic), 998

**Keratitis, not associated with herpes simplex or fungal infection (treatment)** *(continued)*
Prednisone (Systemic), 998
Triamcinolone, Oral (Systemic), 998
Triamcinolone, Parenteral (Systemic), 998

**Keratitis, punctate, superficial (treatment)**
Betamethasone (Ophthalmic)*, 966
Dexamethasone (Ophthalmic), 966
Fluorometholone (Ophthalmic), 966
Hydrocortisone (Ophthalmic)*, 966
[Medrysone (Ophthalmic)][1], 966
Prednisolone (Ophthalmic), 966

**Keratitis, vaccinia virus (treatment)**
[Idoxuridine (Ophthalmic)][1], 1675

**Keratitis, vernal (treatment)**
Betamethasone (Ophthalmic)*, 966
Cromolyn (Ophthalmic)[1], 1120
Dexamethasone (Ophthalmic), 966
Fluorometholone (Ophthalmic), 966
Hydrocortisone (Ophthalmic)*, 966
Lodoxamide (Ophthalmic)†, #
[Medrysone (Ophthalmic)][1], 966
Prednisolone (Ophthalmic), 966

**Keratoconjunctivitis (treatment)**
[Tobramycin (Ophthalmic)], #

**Keratoconjunctivitis, allergic (treatment)**
Betamethasone (Ophthalmic)*, 966
Dexamethasone (Ophthalmic), 966
Fluorometholone (Ophthalmic), 966
Hydrocortisone (Ophthalmic)*, 966
[Medrysone (Ophthalmic)][1], 966
Prednisolone (Ophthalmic), 966

**Keratoconjunctivitis, bacterial (treatment)**
[Chloramphenicol (Ophthalmic)], #
[Chlortetracycline (Ophthalmic)], 2763
[Erythromycin (Ophthalmic)][1], 1364
Gentamicin (Ophthalmic), 1555
Neomycin (Ophthalmic)*†, #
[Neomycin, Polymyxin B, and Bacitracin (Ophthalmic)], #
[Neomycin, Polymyxin B, and Gramicidin (Ophthalmic)], #
[Sulfacetamide (Ophthalmic)], 2651
[Sulfisoxazole (Ophthalmic)], 2651
[Tetracycline (Ophthalmic)], 2763

**Keratoconjunctivitis, herpes simplex virus (treatment)**
[Idoxuridine (Ophthalmic)][1], 1675
Trifluridine (Ophthalmic), 2877
Vidarabine (Ophthalmic), 2944

**Keratoconjunctivitis sicca (treatment)**
Bromhexine (Ophthalmic), 3134‡
Carboxymethylcellulose (Ophthalmic), 3013
Cromolyn (Ophthalmic), 3139‡
Hydroxypropyl Cellulose (Ophthalmic), #
Hydroxypropyl Methylcellulose (Ophthalmic), #
Pilocarpine (Systemic), 3158‡

**Keratoconjunctivitis, vernal (treatment)**
Betamethasone (Ophthalmic)*, 966
Cromolyn (Ophthalmic), 1120, 3138‡
Dexamethasone (Ophthalmic), 966
Fluorometholone (Ophthalmic), 966
Hydrocortisone (Ophthalmic)*, 966
Lodoxamide (Ophthalmic)†, #, 3152‡
Medrysone (Ophthalmic), 966
Prednisolone (Ophthalmic), 966

**Keratoses, pre-epitheliomatosis (treatment)**
Podophyllum (Topical)†, 2341

**Keratoses, solar**—See Actinic keratoses, multiple

**Keratosis follicularis (treatment)**
[Acitretin (Systemic)][1], 18
[Etretinate (Systemic)], #
[Isotretinoin (Systemic)][1], 1796
[Tretinoin (Topical)][1], 2871

**Keratosis palmaris et plantaris (treatment)**
[Etretinate (Systemic)], #
[Isotretinoin (Systemic)][1], 1796

**Ketonuria (diagnosis)**
Nitroprusside Urine Ketone Test, #
Urine Glucose and Ketone (Combined) Test, #

**Kidney stones**—See Renal calculi

**Kraurosis vulvae**—See Vulvar atrophy

**Labor, augmentation of**
Oxytocin, Parenteral (Systemic), 2211

**Labor, induction of**
[Carboprost (Systemic)][1], 782
Dinoprost (Parenteral-Local)*[1], #
[Dinoprostone Vaginal Gel (Cervical/Vaginal)], 1228
Oxytocin, Parenteral (Systemic), 2211

**Labor, premature (prophylaxis)**
[Isoxsuprine (Systemic)], #
Ritodrine (Systemic), 2513
[Terbutaline, Oral (Systemic)][1], 651
[Terbutaline, Parenteral (Systemic)][1], 651

**Labor, premature (treatment)**
[Isoxsuprine (Systemic)], #
[Magnesium Sulfate (Systemic)][1], 1895
Ritodrine (Systemic), 2513
[Terbutaline, Oral (Systemic)][1], 651
[Terbutaline, Parenteral (Systemic)][1], 651

**Lactation, after second- or third-trimester pregnancy loss (prophylaxis)**
[Bromocriptine (Systemic)][1], 636

**Lactation deficiency (treatment)**
Oxytocin, Nasal (Systemic), 2211

**Lambert-Eaton myasthenic syndrome (treatment)**
3,4-Diaminopyridine (Systemic), 3127‡
Dynamine (Systemic), 3141‡

**Larva migrans, cutaneous (treatment)**
Thiabendazole (Systemic)†, 2784
Thiabendazole (Topical)*, 2786

**Larva migrans, visceral (treatment)**
Thiabendazole (Systemic)†, 2784

**Laryngeal edema, acute noninfectious (treatment)**
Epinephrine Injection USP (Systemic), 651

**Laryngeal edema, acute noninfectious (treatment adjunct)**
Betamethasone, Oral (Systemic), 998
Betamethasone, Parenteral (Systemic), 998
Cortisone (Systemic), 998
Dexamethasone, Parenteral (Systemic), 998
Hydrocortisone, Oral (Systemic), 998
Hydrocortisone, Parenteral (Systemic), 998
Methylprednisolone, Oral (Systemic), 998
Methylprednisolone, Parenteral (Systemic), 998
Prednisolone, Oral (Systemic), 998
Prednisolone, Parenteral (Systemic), 998
Prednisone (Systemic), 998
Triamcinolone, Oral (Systemic), 998
Triamcinolone, Parenteral (Systemic), 998

**Lassa fever (prophylaxis)**
[Ribavirin (Systemic)][1], 2478

**Lassa fever (treatment)**
[Ribavirin (Systemic)][1], 2478

**LAV**—See Human immunodeficiency virus (HIV) infection

**Laxative dependency (treatment)**
Glycerin Suppositories (Local), #

**Lead mobilization determination**
[Edetate Calcium Disodium (Systemic)][1], 1324

**Left ventricular dysfunction, post–myocardial infarction (treatment)**
Trandolapril (Systemic), 2854

**Leg cramps (prophylaxis)**
[Quinine (Systemic)], 2444

**Leg cramps (treatment)**
Nylidrin (Systemic)*, #
[Quinine (Systemic)], 2444

**Legionnaires' disease (treatment)**
[Clarithromycin (Systemic)][1], 889
Dirithromycin (Systemic)†, 1250
Erythromycin (Systemic), 1368

**Leigh's disease**—See Encephalomyelopathy, subacute necrotizing

**Leiomyomata, uterine (treatment)**
Leuprolide (Systemic)[1], 1840

**Leishmaniasis, American mucocutaneous (treatment)**
Amphotericin B (Systemic), 98

**Leishmaniasis, cutaneous (treatment)**
[Itraconazole (Systemic)][1], 302
[Ketoconazole (Systemic)][1], 302
Meglumine Antimoniate (Systemic)*†, #
[Pentamidine (Systemic)][1], 2274

**Leishmaniasis, diffuse cutaneous (treatment)**
Meglumine Antimoniate (Systemic)*†, #

**Leishmaniasis, mucosal (treatment)**
Meglumine Antimoniate (Systemic)*†, #

**Leishmaniasis, visceral (treatment)**
Aminosidine (Systemic), 3130‡
Amphotericin B, Liposomal (Systemic), 3152‡
Amphotericin B Liposomal Complex (Systemic), 105
Meglumine Antimoniate (Systemic)*†, #
[Pentamidine (Systemic)][1], 2274

**Lennox-Gastaut syndrome**—See Epilepsy, Lennox-Gastaut syndrome

**Lens opacities, axial (treatment)**
Homatropine (Ophthalmic), 1651

**Leprosy (treatment)**
Clofazimine (Systemic)†, #, 3137‡
Dapsone (Systemic), 1170
[Ethionamide (Systemic)]†, 1417
[Rifampin (Systemic)][1], 2485
Thalidomide (Systemic), 3168‡

**Leptospirosis (treatment)**
[Ampicillin, Parenteral (Systemic)][1], 2240
[Penicillin G, Parenteral (Systemic)][1], 2240

**Lesions, oral, associated with corticosteroid-responsive disorders (treatment)**
[Betamethasone, Oral (Systemic)][1], 998
[Cortisone, Oral (Systemic)][1], 998
[Dexamethasone, Oral (Systemic)][1], 998
[Hydrocortisone, Oral (Systemic)][1], 998
[Methylprednisolone, Oral (Systemic)][1], 998
[Prednisolone, Oral (Systemic)][1], 998
[Prednisone (Systemic)][1], 998
[Triamcinolone, Oral (Systemic)][1], 998

**Lesions, oral, inflammatory (treatment)**
Hydrocortisone Acetate Dental Paste (Topical), 978
Triamcinolone Acetonide Dental Paste (Topical), 978

**Lesions, oral, ulcerative (treatment)**
Hydrocortisone Acetate Dental Paste (Topical), 978
Triamcinolone Acetonide Dental Paste (Topical), 978

**Letterer-Siwe disease (treatment)**
Vinblastine (Systemic), 2946

**Leukemia (diagnosis)**—See Bone marrow imaging, radionuclide

**Leukemia, acute (treatment)**
5-AZA-2′-deoxycytidine (Systemic), 3128‡
Tretinoin (Systemic), 3169‡

**Leukemia, acute erythroid (treatment)**
Mitoxantrone (Systemic), 2033

**Leukemia, acute lymphoblastic (treatment)**
Pegaspargase (Systemic)†, 2230

**Leukemia, acute lymphocytic (diagnosis)**
Technetium Tc 99m Murine Monoclonal Antibody (IgG2a) to BCE (Systemic), 3167‡

**Leukemia, acute lymphocytic (treatment)**
Amsacrine (Systemic)*, 3010
Asparaginase (Systemic), 474
Betamethasone, Oral (Systemic), 998
Betamethasone, Parenteral (Systemic), 998
Cortisone (Systemic), 998
Cyclophosphamide (Systemic), 1128
Cytarabine (Systemic), 1143
Daunorubicin (Systemic), 1173
Dexamethasone, Oral (Systemic), 998
Dexamethasone, Parenteral (Systemic), 998
Doxorubicin (Systemic), 1308
Elliott's B Solution (Systemic), 3141‡
Erwinia l-Asparaginase (Systemic), 3142‡
[Etoposide (Systemic)][1], 1424
Hydrocortisone, Oral (Systemic), 998
Hydrocortisone, Parenteral (Systemic), 998
[Idarubicin (Systemic)][1], 1671, 3146‡
[Ifosfamide (Systemic)][1], 1677
Mercaptopurine (Systemic), 1946
Methotrexate—For Cancer (Systemic), 1962
Methylprednisolone, Oral (Systemic), 998
Methylprednisolone, Parenteral (Systemic), 998
[Mitoxantrone (Systemic)], 2033
Pegaspargase (Systemic), 3157‡
Prednisolone, Oral (Systemic), 998
Prednisolone, Parenteral (Systemic), 998
Prednisone (Systemic), 998
Ricin (Blocked) Conjugated Murine MOAB (CD6) (Systemic), 3162‡
Ricin (Blocked) Conjugated Murine Monoclonal Antibody (Anti-B4) (Systemic), 3162‡
Teniposide (Systemic), 2747, 3035, 3167‡
Triamcinolone, Oral (Systemic), 998
Triamcinolone, Parenteral (Systemic), 998
Vincristine (Systemic), 2950
Vindesine (Systemic)*, 3037

**Leukemia, acute monocytic (treatment)**
Cyclophosphamide (Systemic), 1128
Daunorubicin (Systemic)[1], 1173
Mitoxantrone (Systemic), 2033

**Leukemia, acute myelocytic (treatment)**
See also Leukemia, acute nonlymphocytic
2-Chlorodeoxyadenosine (Systemic), 3127‡
Cyclophosphamide (Systemic), 1128
Daunorubicin (Systemic), 1173
Idarubicin (Systemic), 3146‡
Mitoxantrone (Systemic), 2033, 3154‡
Monoclonal Antibodies PM-81 and AML-2-23 (Systemic), 3155‡
Ricin (Blocked) Conjugated Murine Monoclonal Antibody (Anti-My9) (Systemic), 3162‡

**Leukemia, acute myelocytic (treatment adjunct)**
Monoclonal Antibody PM-81 (Systemic), 3154‡
Ricin (Blocked) Conjugated Murine Monoclonal Antibody (Anti-My9) (Systemic), 3162‡

**Leukemia, acute myelocytic, leukopenia of (treatment)**
Sargramostim (Systemic)†, 3163‡

**Leukemia, acute myelogenous (treatment)**
Aldesleukin (Systemic), 3129‡
2′-Deoxycytidine (Systemic), 3127‡

**Leukemia, acute myeloid (treatment)**
Filgrastim (Systemic), 3143‡

**Leukemia, acute nonlymphocytic (treatment)**
[Busulfan (Systemic)][1], 695
Cyclophosphamide (Systemic), 1128
Cytarabine, 1143
Daunorubicin (Systemic), 1173
Doxorubicin (Systemic), 1308
[Etoposide (Systemic)][1], 1424
Idarubicin (Systemic), 1671
Mercaptopurine (Systemic), 1946
[Methotrexate—For Cancer (Systemic)][1], 1962
Mitoxantrone (Systemic), 2033
Thioguanine (Systemic), #

**Leukemia, acute promyelocytic (treatment)**
Arsenic Trioxide (Systemic)‡, 3132
9-Cis Retinoic Acid (Systemic), 3128‡
Mitoxantrone (Systemic), 2033
Tretinoin (Systemic), 2868, 3169‡

**Leukemia, B-cell (treatment)**
Iodine I 131 Murine Monoclonal Antibody IgG$_{2a}$ to B Cell (Systemic), 3149‡
Ricin (Blocked) Conjugated Murine Monoclonal Antibody (Anti-B4) (Systemic), 3162‡

**Leukemia, chronic (treatment)**
Tretinoin (Systemic), 3169‡

**Leukemia, chronic lymphocytic (diagnosis)**
Technetium Tc 99m Murine Monoclonal Antibody (IgG2a) to BCE (Systemic), 3167‡

**Leukemia, chronic lymphocytic (treatment)**
Betamethasone, Oral (Systemic), 998
Betamethasone, Parenteral (Systemic), 998
CAMPATH-1H (Systemic), 3136‡
Chlorambucil (Systemic), 837
[Cladribine (Systemic)][1], 886, 3136‡
Cortisone (Systemic), 998
Cyclophosphamide (Systemic), 1128
Dexamethasone, Oral (Systemic), 998
Dexamethasone, Parenteral (Systemic), 998
[Doxorubicin (Systemic)][1], 1308
Fludarabine (Systemic), 1475, 3143‡
Hydrocortisone, Oral (Systemic), 998
Hydrocortisone, Parenteral (Systemic), 998
Methylprednisolone, Oral (Systemic), 998
Methylprednisolone, Parenteral (Systemic), 998
Pentostatin (Systemic), 3158‡
Prednisolone, Oral (Systemic), 998
Prednisolone, Parenteral (Systemic), 998
Prednisone (Systemic), 998
Sodium Phosphate P 32 (Systemic), 2616
ST1-RTA Immunotoxin (SR 44163) (Systemic), 3166‡
Triamcinolone, Oral (Systemic), 998
Triamcinolone, Parenteral (Systemic), 998
[Vincristine (Systemic)][1], 2950

**Leukemia, chronic lymphocytic (treatment adjunct)**
Immune Globulin Intravenous (Human) (Systemic)[1], 1686

**Leukemia, chronic myelocytic (treatment)**
Busulfan (Systemic), 695
Cyclophosphamide (Systemic), 1128
Cytarabine (Systemic), 1143
[Daunorubicin (Systemic)], 1173
Hydroxyurea (Systemic), 1666
Idarubicin (Systemic), 3146‡
[Interferon Alfa-2a, Recombinant (Systemic)], 1740, 3148‡
[Interferon Alfa-2b, Recombinant (Systemic)][1], 1740
Interferon Alfa-n1 (Ins) (Systemic)*[1], 1740
[Interferon Alfa-n3 (Systemic)]†, 1740
[Mercaptopurine (Systemic)], 1946
[Mitomycin (Systemic)][1], 2028
Ricin (Blocked) Conjugated Murine Monoclonal Antibody (Anti-My9) (Systemic), 3162‡
Sodium Phosphate P 32 (Systemic), 2616
[Vincristine (Systemic)][1], 2950

**Leukemia, chronic myelomonocytic (treatment)**
[Topotecan (Systemic)][1], 2841

**Leukemia, hairy cell (treatment)**
[Chlorambucil (Systemic)][1], 837
Cladribine (Systemic), 886, 3137‡
Interferon Alfa-2a, Recombinant (Systemic), 1740
Interferon Alfa-2b, Recombinant (Systemic), 1740
Interferon Alfa-n1 (Ins) (Systemic)*, 1740
[Interferon Alfa-n3 (Systemic)]†, 1740
Pentostatin (Systemic), 2279, 3158‡

**Leukemia, meningeal (prophylaxis)**
Cytarabine (Systemic), 1143
Methotrexate—For Cancer (Systemic), 1962

**Leukemia, meningeal (treatment)**
Cytarabine (Systemic), 1143
Methotrexate—For Cancer (Systemic), 1962

**Leukocytes, labeling of**
Indium In 111 Oxyquinoline (Systemic)†, 1695
Technetium Tc 99m Exametazime (Systemic), 2708

**Leukopenia, acute myelogenous leukemia–associated (treatment)**
Sargramostim (Systemic)†, 3163‡

**Leukoplakia, mucosal (treatment)**
[Fluorouracil (Topical)][1], 1500

**LeVeen peritoneovenous shunt patency assessment**
Technetium Tc 99m Albumin Aggregated (Systemic)[1], 2697
Technetium Tc 99m Sulfur Colloid (Systemic)[1], 2740

**Lice, body**—See Pediculosis corporis
**Lice, crab**—See Pediculosis pubis
**Lice, head**—See Pediculosis capitis
**Lice, pubic**—See Pediculosis pubis

**Lichen planus (treatment)**
Amcinonide (Topical), 978
Beclomethasone Dipropionate (Topical), 978
Betamethasone Benzoate (Topical), 978
Betamethasone Dipropionate (Topical), 978
Betamethasone, Parenteral-Local (Systemic), 998
Betamethasone Valerate (Topical), 978
Clobetasol Propionate (Topical), 978
Clobetasone Butyrate (Topical), 978
Desoximetasone (Topical), 978
Dexamethasone, Parenteral-Local (Systemic), 998
Diflorasone Diacetate (Topical), 978
Diflucortolone Valerate (Topical), 978
Fluocinolone Acetonide (Topical), 978
Fluocinonide (Topical), 978
Flurandrenolide (except 0.0125% cream and ointment) (Topical), 978
Fluticasone Propionate (Topical), 978
Halcinonide (Topical), 978
Halobetasol Propionate (Topical), 978
Hydrocortisone Butyrate (Topical), 978
Hydrocortisone, Parenteral-Local (Systemic), 998
Hydrocortisone Valerate (Topical), 978
[Methoxsalen (Systemic)][1], 1973
[Methoxsalen (Topical)][1], 1977
Methylprednisolone, Parenteral-Local (Systemic), 998
Mometasone Furoate (Topical), 978
Prednisolone, Parenteral-Local (Systemic), 998
Triamcinolone Acetonide (Topical), 978
Triamcinolone, Parenteral-Local (Systemic), 998

**Lichen planus, facial and intertriginous areas (treatment)**
Alclometasone Dipropionate (Topical), 978
Beclomethasone Dipropionate (Topical), 978
Betamethasone Benzoate (Topical), 978
Betamethasone Valerate (Topical), 978
Clobetasone Butyrate (Topical), 978
Clocortolone Pivalate (Topical), 978
Desonide (Topical), 978
Desoximetasone (0.05% cream only) (Topical), 978
Dexamethasone (Topical), 978
Dexamethasone Sodium Phosphate (Topical), 978
Diflucortolone Valerate (Topical), 978
Flumethasone Pivalate (Topical), 978
Fluocinolone Acetonide (except 0.2% cream) (Topical), 978
Flurandrenolide (Topical), 978
Fluticasone Propionate (Topical), 978
Hydrocortisone (Topical), 978
Hydrocortisone Acetate (Topical), 978
Hydrocortisone Butyrate (Topical), 978
Hydrocortisone Valerate (Topical), 978
Methylprednisolone Acetate (Topical), 978
Mometasone Furoate (Topical), 978
Triamcinolone Acetonide (except 0.5% cream and ointment) (Topical), 978

**Lichen planus, oral (treatment)**
[Desoximetasone Gel (Topical)], 978
[Etretinate (Systemic)][1], #
[Fluocinonide Gel (Topical)], 978
[Hydrocortisone Acetate Dental Paste (Topical)], 978
[Triamcinolone Acetonide Dental Paste (Topical)], 978

**Lichen sclerosus (treatment adjunct)**
[Testosterone, Topical (Systemic)][1], 118

**Lichen simplex chronicus (treatment)**
Amcinonide (Topical), 978
Beclomethasone Dipropionate (Topical), 978
Betamethasone Benzoate (Topical), 978
Betamethasone Dipropionate (Topical), 978
Betamethasone, Parenteral-Local (Systemic), 998
Betamethasone Valerate (Topical), 978
Clobetasol Propionate (Topical), 978
Clobetasone Butyrate (Topical), 978

## Indications Index

**Lichen simplex chronicus (treatment)** *(continued)*
　Desoximetasone (Topical), 978
　Dexamethasone, Parenteral-Local (Systemic), 998
　Diflorasone Diacetate (Topical), 978
　Diflucortolone Valerate (Topical), 978
　Fluocinolone Acetonide (Topical), 978
　Fluocinonide (Topical), 978
　Flurandrenolide (except 0.0125% cream and ointment) (Topical), 978
　Fluticasone Propionate (Topical), 978
　Halcinonide (Topical), 978
　Halobetasol Propionate (Topical), 978
　Hydrocortisone Butyrate (Topical), 978
　Hydrocortisone, Parenteral-Local (Systemic), 998
　Hydrocortisone Valerate (Topical), 978
　Methylprednisolone, Parenteral-Local (Systemic), 998
　Mometasone Furoate (Topical), 978
　Prednisolone, Parenteral-Local (Systemic), 998
　Triamcinolone Acetonide (Topical), 978
　Triamcinolone, Parenteral-Local (Systemic), 998

**Lichen simplex chronicus, localized (treatment)**
　Betamethasone (Otic)*, 971
　[Dexamethasone (Otic)], 971
　Hydrocortisone (Otic)*, 971

**Lichen striatus (treatment)**
　Amcinonide (Topical), 978
　Beclomethasone Dipropionate (Topical), 978
　Betamethasone Benzoate (Topical), 978
　Betamethasone Dipropionate (Topical), 978
　Betamethasone Valerate (Topical), 978
　Clobetasol Propionate (Topical), 978
　Clobetasone Butyrate (Topical), 978
　Desoximetasone (Topical), 978
　Diflorasone Diacetate (Topical), 978
　Diflucortolone Valerate (Topical), 978
　Fluocinolone Acetonide (Topical), 978
　Fluocinonide (Topical), 978
　Flurandrenolide (except 0.0125% cream and ointment) (Topical), 978
　Fluticasone Propionate (Topical), 978
　Halcinonide (Topical), 978
　Halobetasol Propionate (Topical), 978
　Hydrocortisone Butyrate (Topical), 978
　Hydrocortisone Valerate (Topical), 978
　Mometasone Furoate (Topical), 978
　Triamcinolone Acetonide (Topical), 978

**Listeriosis (treatment)**
　[Ampicillin, Parenteral (Systemic)][1], 2240
　Erythromycin (Systemic), 1368
　Penicillin G, Parenteral (Systemic), 2240

**Liver abscess, amebic (treatment)**
　Chloroquine (Systemic), 849
　Metronidazole (Systemic), 1996

**Liver failure, acute (treatment adjunct)**
　Albumin Human (Systemic), 34

**Liver fluke**—*See* Opisthorchiasis

**Liver imaging, magnetic resonance**
　*See also* Body imaging, magnetic resonance
　Ferumoxides (Systemic)†, #

**Liver imaging, positron emission tomographic**
　Ammonia N 13 (Systemic)*†, 91

**Liver imaging, radionuclide**
　Technetium Tc 99m Albumin Colloid (Systemic)†, 2699
　Technetium Tc 99m Sulfur Colloid (Systemic), 2740

**Local infiltration**
　Bupivacaine (Parenteral-Local), 139
　Bupivacaine and Epinephrine (Parenteral-Local), 139
　Chloroprocaine (Parenteral-Local), 139
　Etidocaine (Parenteral-Local), 139
　Etidocaine and Epinephrine (Parenteral-Local), 139
　Lidocaine (Parenteral-Local), 139
　Lidocaine and Epinephrine (Parenteral-Local), 139
　Mepivacaine (Parenteral-Local), 139
　Procaine Parenteral (Systemic), 139

**Loeffler syndrome (treatment)**
　Betamethasone, Oral (Systemic), 998
　Betamethasone, Parenteral (Systemic), 998
　Cortisone (Systemic), 998
　Dexamethasone, Oral (Systemic), 998
　Dexamethasone, Parenteral (Systemic), 998
　Hydrocortisone, Oral (Systemic), 998
　Hydrocortisone, Parenteral (Systemic), 998
　Methylprednisolone, Oral (Systemic), 998
　Methylprednisolone, Parenteral (Systemic), 998
　Prednisolone, Oral (Systemic), 998
　Prednisolone, Parenteral (Systemic), 998
　Prednisone (Systemic), 998
　Triamcinolone, Oral (Systemic), 998
　Triamcinolone, Parenteral (Systemic), 998

**Loiasis (treatment)**
　Diethylcarbamazine (Systemic), #

**Lou Gehrig's disease**—*See* Amyotrophic lateral sclerosis

**Low birth weight (treatment)**
　Multi-Vitamin Infusion (Neonatal Formula) (Systemic), 3155‡

**Lower respiratory infections**—*See* Pneumonia, bacterial

**Lung abscess (treatment adjunct)**
　[Acetylcysteine (Inhalation-Local)], #

**Lung imaging, radionuclide**
　Technetium Tc 99m Albumin Aggregated (Systemic), 2697
　[Technetium Tc 99m Pentetate (Systemic)][1], 2727
　Xenon Xe 127 (Systemic), 2982
　Xenon Xe 133 (Systemic), 2984

**Lung perfusion studies**
　*See also* Lung imaging, radionuclide
　Xenon Xe 133 (Systemic), 2984

**Lupus erythematosus, discoid (treatment)**
　Amcinonide (Topical), 978
　Beclomethasone Dipropionate (Topical), 978
　Betamethasone Benzoate (Topical), 978
　Betamethasone Dipropionate (Topical), 978
　Betamethasone, Parenteral-Local (Systemic), 998
　Betamethasone Valerate (Topical), 978
　[Chloroquine, Oral (Systemic)][1], 849
　Clobetasol Propionate (Topical), 978
　Clobetasone Butyrate (Topical), 978
　Desoximetasone (Topical), 978
　Dexamethasone, Parenteral-Local (Systemic), 998
　Diflorasone Diacetate (Topical), 978
　Diflucortolone Valerate (Topical), 978
　Fluocinolone Acetonide (Topical), 978
　Fluocinonide (Topical), 978
　Flurandrenolide (except 0.0125% cream and ointment) (Topical), 978
　Fluticasone Propionate (Topical), 978
　Halcinonide (Topical), 978
　Halobetasol Propionate (Topical), 978
　Hydrocortisone, Parenteral-Local (Systemic), 998
　Hydrocortisone Valerate (Topical), 978
　Hydroxychloroquine (Systemic), 1663
　Methylprednisolone, Parenteral-Local (Systemic), 998
　Mometasone Furoate (Topical), 978
　Prednisolone, Parenteral-Local (Systemic), 998
　[Quinacrine (Systemic)][1], #
　Triamcinolone Acetonide (Topical), 978
　Triamcinolone, Parenteral-Local (Systemic), 998

**Lupus erythematosus, discoid, facial and intertriginous areas (treatment)**
　Alclometasone Dipropionate (Topical), 978
　Beclomethasone Dipropionate (Topical), 978
　Betamethasone Benzoate (Topical), 978
　Betamethasone Valerate (Topical), 978
　Clobetasone Butyrate (Topical), 978
　Clocortolone Pivalate (Topical), 978
　Desonide (Topical), 978
　Desoximetasone (0.05% cream only) (Topical), 978
　Dexamethasone (Topical), 978
　Dexamethasone Sodium Phosphate (Topical), 978
　Diflucortolone Valerate (Topical), 978
　Flumethasone Pivalate (Topical), 978
　Fluocinolone Acetonide (except 0.2% cream) (Topical), 978
　Flurandrenolide (Topical), 978
　Fluticasone Propionate (Topical), 978
　Hydrocortisone (Topical), 978
　Hydrocortisone Acetate (Topical), 978
　Hydrocortisone Butyrate (Topical), 978
　Hydrocortisone Valerate (Topical), 978
　Methylprednisolone Acetate (Topical), 978
　Mometasone Furoate (Topical), 978
　Triamcinolone Acetonide (except 0.5% cream and ointment) (Topical), 978

**Lupus erythematosus, subacute cutaneous (treatment)**
　Amcinonide (Topical), 978
　Beclomethasone Dipropionate (Topical), 978
　Betamethasone Benzoate (Topical), 978
　Betamethasone Dipropionate (Topical), 978
　Betamethasone Valerate (Topical), 978
　Clobetasol Propionate (Topical), 978
　Clobetasone Butyrate (Topical), 978
　Desoximetasone (Topical), 978
　Diflorasone Diacetate (Topical), 978
　Diflucortolone Valerate (Topical), 978
　Fluocinolone Acetonide (Topical), 978
　Fluocinonide (Topical), 978
　Flurandrenolide (except 0.0125% cream and ointment) (Topical), 978
　Fluticasone Propionate (Topical), 978
　Halcinonide (Topical), 978
　Halobetasol Propionate (Topical), 978

**Lupus erythematosus, subacute cutaneous (treatment)** *(continued)*
　Hydrocortisone Butyrate (Topical), 978
　Hydrocortisone Valerate (Topical), 978
　Mometasone Furoate (Topical), 978
　Triamcinolone Acetonide (Topical), 978

**Lupus erythematosus, systemic (treatment)**
　[Azathioprine (Systemic)][1], 491
　Betamethasone, Oral (Systemic), 998
　Betamethasone, Parenteral (Systemic), 998
　[Chloroquine, Oral (Systemic)][1], 849
　Cortisone (Systemic), 998
　[Cyclophosphamide (Systemic)][1], 1128
　[Dapsone (Systemic)][1], 1170
　Dehydroepiandrosterone (Systemic), 3139‡
　Dexamethasone, Oral (Systemic), 998
　Dexamethasone, Parenteral (Systemic), 998
　Humanized Monoclonal Antibody 5C8, Recombinant (Systemic), 3161‡
　Hydrocortisone, Oral (Systemic), 998
　Hydrocortisone, Parenteral (Systemic), 998
　Hydroxychloroquine (Systemic), 1663
　Methylprednisolone, Oral (Systemic), 998
　Methylprednisolone, Parenteral (Systemic), 998
　Prednisolone, Oral (Systemic), 998
　Prednisolone, Parenteral (Systemic), 998
　Prednisone (Systemic), 998
　Triamcinolone, Oral (Systemic), 998
　Triamcinolone, Parenteral (Systemic), 998

**Lupus nephritis (treatment)**
　Bindarit (Systemic), 3133‡
　Monoclonal Antibody for Immunization against Lupus Nephritis (Systemic), 3155‡

**Lyme disease (treatment)**
　[Amoxicillin (Systemic)][1], 2240
　[Cefotaxime (Systemic)][1], 794
　[Ceftriaxone (Systemic)][1], 794
　Cefuroxime Axetil (Systemic)[1], 794
　[Doxycycline (Systemic)], 2765
　[Erythromycin (Systemic)][1], 1368
　[Penicillin G, Parenteral (Systemic)][1], 2240
　[Penicillin V (Systemic)][1], 2240
　[Tetracycline (Systemic)][1], 2765

**Lymphogranuloma venereum (treatment)**
　Demeclocycline (Systemic), 2765
　Doxycycline (Systemic), 2765
　[Erythromycin (Systemic)][1], 1368
　Minocycline (Systemic), 2765
　Oxytetracycline (Systemic)†, 2765
　[Sulfadiazine (Systemic)][1], 2653
　Sulfamethoxazole (Systemic), 2653
　[Sulfamethoxazole and Trimethoprim (Systemic)][1], 2661
　Sulfisoxazole (Systemic), 2653
　Tetracycline (Systemic), 2765

**Lymphoma (diagnosis)**
　[Fludeoxyglucose F 18 (Systemic)][1]*†, 1478

**Lymphoma, B-cell**—*See* Lymphomas, non-Hodgkin's

**Lymphoma, Burkitt's**—*See* Lymphomas, non-Hodgkin's

**Lymphoma, follicular**—*See* Lymphomas, non-Hodgkin's

**Lymphoma, giant follicular**—*See* Lymphomas, non-Hodgkin's

**Lymphoma, histiocytic**—*See* Lymphomas, non-Hodgkin's

**Lymphoma, lymphocytic**—*See* Lymphomas, non-Hodgkin's

**Lymphoma, mixed-cell type**—*See* Lymphomas, non-Hodgkin's

**Lymphoma, nodular or diffuse**—*See* Lymphomas, non-Hodgkin's

**Lymphomas, acute lymphocytic (treatment adjunct)**
　Ricin (Blocked) Conjugated Murine Monoclonal Antibody (Anti-B4) (Systemic), 3162‡

**Lymphomas, acute T-cell (treatment)**
　Ricin (Blocked) Conjugated Murine MOAB (CD6), 3162‡

**Lymphomas, cutaneous T-cell (treatment)**
　APL 400-020 (Systemic), 3132‡
　[Chlorambucil (Systemic)][1], 837
　DAB389IL-2 (Systemic), 3139‡
　[Etoposide (Systemic)][1], 1424
　Interferon Beta (Recombinant) (Systemic), 3148‡
　9-[3-Pyridylmethyl]-9-Deazaguanine (Systemic), 3128‡
　Pentostatin (Systemic)‡, 3159
　Ricin (Blocked) Conjugated Murine MOAB (CD6) (Systemic), 3162‡

**Lymphomas, Hodgkin's (treatment)**
　Betamethasone, Oral (Systemic), 998
　Betamethasone, Parenteral (Systemic), 998
　Bleomycin (Systemic), 624
　Carmustine (Systemic), 786

**Lymphomas, Hodgkin's (treatment)** *(continued)*
  Chlorambucil (Systemic), 837
  [Cisplatin (Systemic)]1, 876
  Cortisone (Systemic), 998
  Cyclophosphamide (Systemic), 1128
  Dacarbazine (Systemic)1, 1148
  Dexamethasone, Oral (Systemic), 998
  Dexamethasone, Parenteral (Systemic), 998
  Doxorubicin (Systemic), 1308
  Epirubicin (Systemic)*, 3018
  [Etoposide (Systemic)]1, 1424
  Hydrocortisone, Oral (Systemic), 998
  Hydrocortisone, Parenteral (Systemic), 998
  [Ifosfamide (Systemic)]1, 1677
  Interleukin-3 Human, Recombinant (Systemic), 3149‡
  Lomustine (Systemic), 1874
  Mechlorethamine (Systemic), 1929
  [Melphalan (Systemic)]1, 1938
  [Methotrexate—For Cancer (Systemic)]1, 1962
  Methylprednisolone, Oral (Systemic), 998
  Methylprednisolone, Parenteral (Systemic), 998
  Prednisolone, Oral (Systemic), 998
  Prednisolone, Parenteral (Systemic), 998
  Prednisone (Systemic), 998
  Procarbazine (Systemic), 2391
  Thiotepa (Systemic), 2790
  Triamcinolone, Oral (Systemic), 998
  Triamcinolone, Parenteral (Systemic), 998
  Vinblastine (Systemic), 2946
  Vincristine (Systemic), 2950
**Lymphomas, non-Hodgkin's (diagnosis)**
  Technetium Tc 99m Murine Monoclonal Antibody (IgG2a) to BCE (Systemic), 3167‡
**Lymphomas, non-Hodgkin's (treatment)**
  [Asparaginase (Systemic)], 474
  Betamethasone, Oral (Systemic), 998
  Betamethasone, Parenteral (Systemic), 998
  Bleomycin (Systemic), 624
  Carmustine (Systemic), 786
  Chimeric (Murine Variable, Human Constant) MAB to CD20 (Systemic), 3136‡
  Chlorambucil (Systemic), 837
  [Cisplatin (Systemic)]1, 876
  [Cladribine (Systemic)]1, 886, 3137‡
  Cortisone (Systemic), 998
  Cyclophosphamide (Systemic), 1128
  [Cytarabine (Systemic)], 1143
  [Daunorubicin (Systemic)], 1173
  Dexamethasone, Oral (Systemic), 998
  Dexamethasone, Parenteral (Systemic), 998
  Doxorubicin (Systemic), 1308
  Epirubicin (Systemic)*, 3018
  [Etoposide (Systemic)], 1424
  [Fludarabine (Systemic)]1, 1475
  Fludarabine (Systemic), 3143‡
  Hydrocortisone, Oral (Systemic), 998
  Hydrocortisone, Parenteral (Systemic), 998
  [Ifosfamide (Systemic)]1, 1677
  In-111 Murine MAB(2B8-MXDTPA) and Y-90 Murine MAB(2B8-MXDTPA) (Systemic), 3147‡
  [Interferon Alfa-2a, Recombinant (Systemic)]1, 1740
  [Interferon Alfa-2b, Recombinant (Systemic)]1, 1740
  Interferon Alfa-n1 (Ins) (Systemic)*1, 1740
  [Interferon Alfa-n3 (Systemic)]†, 1740
  Interleukin-3 Human, Recombinant (Systemic), 3149‡
  Iodine I 131 Murine Monoclonal Antibody IgG2a to B Cell (Systemic), 3150‡
  I-131 Radiolabeled B1 Monoclonal Antibody (Systemic), 3146‡
  Mechlorethamine (Systemic), 1929
  [Mercaptopurine (Systemic)]1, 1946
  Methotrexate—For Cancer (Systemic), 1962
  Methylprednisolone, Oral (Systemic), 998
  Methylprednisolone, Parenteral (Systemic), 998
  Mitoguazone (Systemic), 3154‡
  [Mitoxantrone (Systemic)], 2033
  Prednimustine (Systemic), 3158‡
  Prednisolone, Oral (Systemic), 998
  Prednisolone, Parenteral (Systemic), 998
  Prednisone (Systemic), 998
  [Procarbazine (Systemic)]1, 2391
  Radiolabeled Monoclonal Antibody to CD 22 (Systemic), 3162‡
  Ricin (Blocked) Conjugated Murine Monoclonal Antibody (Anti-B4) (Systemic), 3160‡
  Rituximab (Systemic), INN-2519
  Teniposide (Systemic), 3035
  Triamcinolone, Oral (Systemic), 998
  Triamcinolone, Parenteral (Systemic), 998
  Vinblastine (Systemic), 2946
  Vincristine (Systemic), 2950
**Lymphosarcoma**—*See* Lymphomas, non-Hodgkin's

**Lymphosarcoma, lymphoblastic**—*See* Lymphomas, non-Hodgkin's
**Lymphosarcoma, lymphocytic**—*See* Lymphomas, non-Hodgkin's

## M

**Macerations (treatment adjunct)**
  Carbol-Fuchsin (Topical), #
**Macular hole disease (treatment)**
  Transforming Growth Factor-Beta 2 (Systemic), 3169‡
**Malaria (prophylaxis)**
  Chloroquine (Systemic), 849
  [Dapsone (Systemic)]1, 1170
  Doxycycline (Systemic), 2765
  Hydroxychloroquine (Systemic), 1663
  Mefloquine (Systemic)†, 1935, 3153‡
  Proguanil (Systemic)*, #
  Sulfadoxine and Pyrimethamine (Systemic), 2637
**Malaria (treatment)**
  Chloroquine (Systemic), 849
  [Clindamycin (Systemic)]1, 893
  [Doxycycline (Systemic)], 2765
  Halofantrine (Systemic), 3022
  Halofantrine (Systemic)*†, 1608, 3145‡
  Hydroxychloroquine (Systemic), 1663
  Mefloquine (Systemic)†, 1935, 3153‡
  Primaquine (Systemic), 2375
  Pyrimethamine (Systemic), 2433
  Quinidine, Parenteral (Systemic)1, 2440
  Quinine (Systemic), 2444
  Sulfadiazine (Systemic), 2653
  Sulfadoxine and Pyrimethamine (Systemic), 2637
  Sulfamethoxazole (Systemic), 2653
  Sulfisoxazole (Systemic), 2653
  [Tetracycline (Systemic)], 2765
**Malignant effusions, pericardial (treatment)**
  [Bleomycin (Systemic)]1, 624
  Mechlorethamine (Systemic), 1929
  Thiotepa (Systemic), 2790
**Malignant effusions, peritoneal (treatment)**
  [Bleomycin (Systemic)]1, 624
  Chromic Phosphate P 32 (Parenteral-Local)†, #
  Mechlorethamine (Systemic), 1929
**Malignant effusions, pleural (treatment)**
  Bleomycin (Systemic), 624
  Chromic Phosphate P 32 (Parenteral-Local)†, #
  [Doxycycline (Systemic)], 2765
  [Fluorouracil (Systemic)]1, 1497
  Mechlorethamine (Systemic), 1929
  Thiotepa (Systemic), 2790
**Manganese deficiency (prophylaxis)**
  Manganese Chloride (Systemic)†, 1905
  Manganese Sulfate (Systemic)†, 1905
**Manganese deficiency (treatment)**
  Manganese Chloride (Systemic)†, 1905
  Manganese Sulfate (Systemic)†, 1905
**Maple syrup urine disease (treatment)**
  [Thiamine (Systemic)], 2787
**Mastocytosis, systemic (treatment)**
  Cimetidine (Systemic), 1633
  Cromolyn (Systemic/Oral-Local)1, 1121, 3138‡
  Famotidine (Systemic), 1633
  [Nizatidine (Systemic)]1, 1633
  Omeprazole (Systemic), 2163
  Ranitidine (Systemic), 1633
**Mastocytosis, systemic (treatment adjunct)**
  Alumina, Calcium Carbonate, and Sodium Bicarbonate (Oral-Local)*, 188
  Alumina and Magnesia (Oral-Local), 188
  Alumina, Magnesia, Calcium Carbonate, and Simethicone (Oral-Local)†, 188
  Alumina, Magnesia, and Magnesium Carbonate (Oral-Local)*, 188
  Alumina, Magnesia, Magnesium Carbonate, and Simethicone (Oral-Local)*, 188
  Alumina, Magnesia, and Simethicone (Oral-Local), 188
  Alumina, Magnesium Alginate, and Magnesium Carbonate (Oral-Local)*, 188
  Alumina and Magnesium Carbonate (Oral-Local)†, 188
  Alumina, Magnesium Carbonate, and Simethicone (Oral-Local)†, 188
  Alumina, Magnesium Carbonate, and Sodium Bicarbonate (Oral-Local)†, 188
  Alumina and Magnesium Trisilicate (Oral-Local)†, 188
  Alumina, Magnesium Trisilicate, and Sodium Bicarbonate (Oral-Local)†, 188
  Alumina and Simethicone (Oral-Local)†, 188
  Alumina and Sodium Bicarbonate (Oral-Local)*, 188
  Aluminum Carbonate, Basic (Oral-Local)†, 188

**Mastocytosis, systemic (treatment adjunct)** *(continued)*
  Aluminum Carbonate, Basic, and Simethicone (Oral-Local)†, 188
  Aluminum Hydroxide (Oral-Local), 188
  Calcium Carbonate (Oral-Local)†, 188
  Calcium Carbonate and Magnesia (Oral-Local)†, 188
  Calcium Carbonate, Magnesia, and Simethicone (Oral-Local)†, 188
  Calcium and Magnesium Carbonates (Oral-Local)†, 188
  Calcium Carbonate and Simethicone (Oral-Local)†, 188
  Magaldrate (Oral-Local), 188
  Magaldrate and Simethicone (Oral-Local), 188
  Magnesium Carbonate and Sodium Bicarbonate (Oral-Local)*, 188
  Magnesium Hydroxide (Oral-Local), 188
  Magnesium Oxide (Oral-Local)†, 188
**Mastoidectomy cavity infections (treatment)**
  [Chloramphenicol (Otic)], #
  Clioquinol and Flumethasone (Otic)*, 3015
  Colistin, Neomycin, and Hydrocortisone (Otic)1, 939
  Gentamicin (Otic)*, 1556
  Neomycin, Polymyxin B, and Hydrocortisone (Otic), #
**Measles (prophylaxis)**
  Measles Virus Vaccine Live (Systemic), 1922
  **Measles, German**—*See* Measles, mumps, and rubella; Measles and rubella; Rubella
**Measles, mumps, and rubella (prophylaxis)**
  Measles, Mumps, and Rubella Virus Vaccine Live (Systemic), 1914
**Measles and rubella (prophylaxis)**
  Measles and Rubella Virus Vaccine Live (Systemic), 1918
**Meconium aspiration syndrome (treatment)**
  KL4-Surfactant (Intratracheal-Local), 3150‡
**Meconium ileus (treatment)**
  [Diatrizoate Meglumine and Diatrizoate Sodium, Rectal (Systemic)]1, #
  [Diatrizoate Sodium, Rectal (Systemic)]1, #
**Mediterranean fever, familial (prophylaxis)**
  [Colchicine (Systemic)], 928
**Mediterranean fever, familial (treatment)**
  [Colchicine (Systemic)], 928
**Medulloblastoma**—*See* Tumors, brain, primary
**Megacolon, congenital (treatment)**
  [Bethanechol (Systemic)]1, 614
**Meibomianitis (treatment)**
  [Chlortetracycline (Ophthalmic)], 2763
  [Erythromycin (Ophthalmic)]1, 1364
  Gentamicin (Ophthalmic), 1555
  [Tetracycline (Ophthalmic)], 2763
  [Tobramycin (Ophthalmic)], #
**Melanoma, of the extremity (treatment)**
  Melphalan (Systemic), 3153‡
**Melanoma, malignant (diagnosis)**
  [Fludeoxyglucose F 18 (Systemic)]1*†, 1478
  Technetium Tc 99m Anti-melanoma Murine Monoclonal Antibody (Systemic), 3167‡
**Melanoma, malignant (treatment)**
  [Carboplatin (Systemic)]1, 779
  [Carmustine (Systemic)], 786
  [Cisplatin (Systemic)]1, 876
  Dacarbazine (Systemic), 1148
  [Interferon Alfa-2a, Recombinant (Systemic)]1, 1740, 3148‡
  [Interferon Alfa-2b, Recombinant (Systemic)]1, 1740
  Interferon Alfa-n1 (Ins) (Systemic)*1, 1740
  [Interferon Alfa-n3 (Systemic)]†, 1740
  Interleukin-2 (Systemic), 3149‡
  [Lomustine (Systemic)], 1874
  Melanoma Cell Vaccine (Systemic), 3153‡
  Melanoma Vaccine (Systemic), 3153‡
  [Melphalan (Systemic)], 1938
  Poly I: Poly C12U (Systemic), 3159‡
  [Tamoxifen (Systemic)]1, 2688
  [Vinblastine (Systemic)]1, 2946
  [Vincristine (Systemic)], 2950
**Melanoma, malignant, cutaneous (treatment)**
  Interferon Beta (Recombinant) (Systemic), 3148‡
  Monoclonal AB (Murine) Anti-Idiotype Melanoma Associated Antigen (Systemic), 3154‡
**Melanoma, metastatic (treatment)**
  Amifostine (Systemic), 3130‡
  Beta Alethine (Systemic), 3133‡
  gp 100 Adenoviral Gene Therapy (Systemic), 3144‡
  MART-1 Adenoviral Gene Therapy for Malignant Melanoma (Systemic), 3153‡
**Melasma (treatment)**
  [Azelaic Acid (Topical)]†, 495

**Ménière's disease**—See Ear, inner, circulatory disturbances of; Vertigo
**Meningitis (prophylaxis)**
  Sulfadiazine (Systemic)[1], 2653
  Sulfamethoxazole (Systemic)[1], 2653
  Sulfisoxazole (Systemic)[1], 2653
**Meningitis (treatment)**
  See also Central nervous system (CNS) infections
  Cefotaxime (Systemic), 794
  Ceftazidime (Systemic), 794
  Ceftizoxime (Systemic)[1], 794
  Ceftriaxone (Systemic), 794
  Cefuroxime (Systemic), 794
  [Sulfamethoxazole and Trimethoprim (Systemic)], 2661
**Meningitis, bacterial (treatment)**
  Ampicillin, Parenteral (Systemic), 2240
  Carbenicillin, Parenteral (Systemic), 2240
  Meropenem (Systemic), 1949
  [Nafcillin, Parenteral (Systemic)][1], 2240
  [Oxacillin, Parenteral (Systemic)]†, 2240
  Penicillin G, Parenteral (Systemic), 2240
  [Piperacillin (Systemic)][1], 2240
  [Ticarcillin (Systemic)][1], 2240
**Meningitis, cryptococcal (suppression)**
  Amphotericin B (Systemic), 98
  Fluconazole (Systemic), 302
  [Itraconazole (Systemic)][1], 302
**Meningitis, cryptococcal (treatment)**
  Amphotericin B (Systemic), 98
  Amphotericin B, Liposomal (Systemic), 3152‡
  Amphotericin B Lipid Complex (Systemic), 3130‡
  Fluconazole (Systemic), 302
**Meningitis, fungal (treatment)**
  Amphotericin B (Systemic), 98
  Flucytosine (Systemic), #
**Meningitis, Haemophilus influenzae (treatment)**
  Chloramphenicol (Systemic), 841
**Meningitis, meningococcal (prophylaxis)**
  Meningococcal Polysaccharide Vaccine (Systemic), 1941
**Meningitis, Neisseria meningitidis (treatment)**
  Chloramphenicol (Systemic), 841
**Meningitis, neoplastic (treatment)**
  Depofoam Encapsulated Cytarabine (Systemic), 3140‡
**Meningitis, staphylococcal (treatment)**
  [Vancomycin (Systemic)], 2919
**Meningitis, streptococcal (treatment)**
  [Vancomycin (Systemic)], 2919
**Meningitis, Streptococcus pneumoniae (treatment)**
  Chloramphenicol (Systemic), 841
**Meningitis, tuberculous (treatment)**
  [Rifampin (Systemic)][1], 2485
**Meningitis, tuberculous (treatment adjunct)**
  Betamethasone, Oral (Systemic), 998
  Betamethasone, Parenteral (Systemic), 998
  Cortisone (Systemic), 998
  Dexamethasone, Oral (Systemic), 998
  Dexamethasone, Parenteral (Systemic), 998
  Hydrocortisone, Oral (Systemic), 998
  Hydrocortisone, Parenteral (Systemic), 998
  Methylprednisolone, Oral (Systemic), 998
  Methylprednisolone, Parenteral (Systemic), 998
  Prednisolone, Oral (Systemic), 998
  Prednisolone, Parenteral (Systemic), 998
  Prednisone (Systemic), 998
  Triamcinolone, Oral (Systemic), 998
  Triamcinolone, Parenteral (Systemic), 998
**Meningococcal carriers (treatment)**
  Minocycline, Oral (Systemic), 2765
**Meningococcal disease, severe (treatment)**
  Bactericidal/Permeability-increasing Protein, Recombinant (Systemic), 3160‡
**Meningococcal infections (prophylaxis)**
  Rifampin (Systemic), 2485
**Meningococcemia (treatment)**
  Protein C Concentrate (Systemic), 3160‡
**Meningoencephalitis, primary amebic (treatment)**
  [Amphotericin B (Systemic)][1], 98
**Menopausal symptoms (treatment)**
  Ergotamine, Belladonna Alkaloids, and Phenobarbital (Systemic), 1363
**Menopause, vasomotor symptoms of (treatment)**
  [Clonidine, Oral (Systemic)], 908
  Conjugated Estrogens and Medroxyprogesterone Tablets (Systemic)†, 946
  Conjugated Estrogens Tablets USP, and Conjugated Estrogens and Medroxyprogesterone Tablets (Systemic)†, 946
  Estradiol Cypionate (Systemic), 1383
  Estradiol, Oral (Systemic), 1383
  Estradiol, Parenteral (Systemic), 1383
  Estradiol, Transdermal Systems (Systemic), 1383
  Estradiol Valerate (Systemic), 1383

**Menopause, vasomotor symptoms of (treatment)** (continued)
  Estrogens, Conjugated, Oral (Systemic), 1383
  Estrogens, Esterified (Systemic), 1383
  Estrone (Systemic)†, 1383
  Estropipate (Systemic), 1383
  Ethinyl Estradiol (Systemic)1, 1383
**Menorrhagia (treatment)**
  [Danazol (Systemic)][1], 1163
**Menses, induction of (treatment)**
  Hydroxyprogesterone (Systemic)†, 2400
  Medrogestone (Systemic)*, 2400
  Medroxyprogesterone, Oral (Systemic), 2400
  Norethindrone Acetate Tablets USP (Systemic), 2400
  Progesterone (Systemic), 2400
**Mesothelioma, malignant (treatment)**
  5,6-Dihydro-5-Azacytidine (Systemic), 3128‡
**Metabolic acidosis (treatment**
  Sodium Bicarbonate, Oral (Systemic), 2586
**Metagonimiasis (treatment)**
  [Praziquantel (Systemic)]†, 2368
**Metaplasia, squamous, of ocular epithelia (treatment)**
  Retinoin (Ophthalmic), 3162‡
**Metastases, osteolytic (treatment adjunct)**
  Pamidronate (Systemic)[1], 2220
**Methemoglobinemia, acquired (treatment)**
  Methylene Blue (Systemic), 1391
**Methemoglobinemia, idiopathic (treatment)**
  Methylene Blue (Systemic), 1391
**Methotrexate toxicity**—See Toxicity, methotrexate
**Microphallus (treatment)**
  [Testosterone Enanthate, Parenteral (Systemic)][1], 118
  [Testosterone, Topical (Systemic)][1], 118
**Middle ear infections**—See Otitis media
**Migraine**—See Headache, migraine; Headache, vascular
**Miosis, during ophthalmic surgery (prophylaxis)**
  [Diclofenac (Ophthalmic)], 383
  Flurbiprofen (Ophthalmic), 383
  Indomethacin (Ophthalmic)*, 383
  Suprofen (Ophthalmic)†, 383
**Miosis induction, during surgery**
  Carbachol Intraocular Solution USP (Ophthalmic), 755
**Miosis induction, following ophthalmoscopy**
  Pilocarpine Hydrochloride Ophthalmic Solution USP (Ophthalmic), #
  Pilocarpine Nitrate (Ophthalmic), #
**Miosis induction, postoperative**
  Pilocarpine Hydrochloride Ophthalmic Solution USP (Ophthalmic), #
  Pilocarpine Nitrate (Ophthalmic), #
**Mitochondrial myopathy, zidovudine-induced (treatment)**
  Levocarnitine (Systemic), 3151‡
**Mitral valve prolapse syndrome (treatment)**
  [Acebutolol (Systemic)][1], 593
  [Atenolol (Systemic)][1], 593
  [Metoprolol (Systemic)][1], 593
  [Nadolol (Systemic)][1], 593
  Oxprenolol (Systemic)*[1], 593
  [Pindolol (Systemic)][1], 593
  [Propranolol (Systemic)][1], 593
  [Sotalol (Systemic)][1], 593
  [Timolol (Systemic)][1], 593
**Molybdenum deficiency (prophylaxis)**
  Ammonium Molybdate (Systemic)†, 2053
**Molybdenum deficiency (treatment)**
  Ammonium Molybdate (Systemic)†, 2053
**Moniliasis, cutaneous**—See Candidiasis, cutaneous
**Mooren's ulcer**—See Corneal ulcers
**Morbilli**—See Measles
**Morphea (treatment)**
  Dimethyl Sulfoxide (Topical), 3017
**Morphea, fibrosis and/or nonsuppurative inflammation in (treatment)**
  Aminobenzoate Potassium (Systemic), #
**Motion sickness (prophylaxis)**
  Buclizine (Systemic)†, #
  Cyclizine (Systemic), #
  Dimenhydrinate (Systemic), 325
  Diphenhydramine (Systemic), 325
  Meclizine (Systemic), 1933
  Promethazine (Systemic), 377
  Scopolamine, Transdermal (Systemic), 226
**Motion sickness (treatment)**
  Cyclizine (Systemic), #
  Dimenhydrinate (Systemic), 325
  Diphenhydramine (Systemic), 325
  Meclizine (Systemic), 1933
  Promethazine (Systemic), 377
**Mouth infections (prophylaxis)**
  [Chlorhexidine (Mucosal-Local)]†, 847

**Mouth infections (treatment)**
  [Chlorhexidine (Mucosal-Local)]†, 847
**MRI**—See Magnetic resonance imaging
**Mucocutaneous lymph node syndrome**—See Kawasaki disease
**Mucopolysaccharidosis-I (treatment)**
  Human Alpha-L-Iduronidase, Recombinant (Systemic), 3160‡
**Mucormycosis (treatment)**
  Amphotericin B (Systemic), 98
**Mucositis, oropharyngeal, radiation therapy–induced (treatment)**
  Benzydamine (Oral-Local)*, 3011
**Multiple myeloma (treatment)**
  [Betamethasone, Oral (Systemic)][1], 998
  [Betamethasone, Parenteral (Systemic)][1], 998
  Carmustine (Systemic), 786
  [Cortisone (Systemic)][1], 998
  Cyclophosphamide (Systemic), 1128
  [Dexamethasone, Oral (Systemic)][1], 998
  [Dexamethasone, Parenteral (Systemic)][1], 998
  Doxorubicin (Systemic), 1308
  [Etoposide (Systemic)][1], 1424
  [Hydrocortisone, Oral (Systemic)][1], 998
  [Hydrocortisone, Parenteral (Systemic)][1], 998
  [Interferon Alfa-2a, Recombinant (Systemic)][1], 1740
  [Interferon Alfa-2b, Recombinant (Systemic)][1], 1740
  Interferon Alfa-n1 (Ins) (Systemic)*[1], 1740
  [Interferon Alfa-n3 (Systemic)]†, 1740
  [Lomustine (Systemic)][1], 1874
  Melphalan (Systemic), 1938, 3153‡
  [Methylprednisolone, Oral (Systemic)][1], 998
  [Methylprednisolone, Parenteral (Systemic)][1], 998
  [Prednisolone, Oral (Systemic)][1], 998
  [Prednisolone, Parenteral (Systemic)][1], 998
  [Prednisone (Systemic)][1], 998
  [Procarbazine (Systemic)][1], 2391
  [Triamcinolone, Oral (Systemic)][1], 998
  [Triamcinolone, Parenteral (Systemic)][1], 998
  [Vincristine (Systemic)][1], 2950
**Multiple sclerosis (treatment)**
  Betamethasone, Oral (Systemic)[1], 998
  Betamethasone, Parenteral (Systemic)[1], 998
  Chimeric M-T412 (Human-Murine) IgG Monoclonal Anti-CD4 (Systemic), 3136‡
  Cladribine (Systemic), 3137‡
  Colchicine (Systemic), 3138‡
  Copolymer-1 (Systemic), 3138‡
  Cortisone (Systemic)[1], 998
  [Cyclophosphamide (Systemic)][1], 1128
  Dexamethasone, Oral (Systemic)[1], 998
  Dexamethasone, Parenteral (Systemic)[1], 998
  Fampridine (Systemic), 3143‡
  Glatiramer Acetate (Systemic), 1558
  Hydrocortisone, Oral (Systemic)[1], 998
  Hydrocortisone, Parenteral (Systemic)[1], 998
  Interferon Beta-1a (Systemic), 1732, 3026, 3148‡
  Interferon Beta-1b (Systemic), 1735, 3026, 3148‡
  Methylprednisolone, Oral (Systemic)[1], 998
  Methylprednisolone, Parenteral (Systemic)[1], 998
  Myelin (Systemic), 3155‡
  Prednisolone, Oral (Systemic)[1], 998
  Prednisolone, Parenteral (Systemic)[1], 998
  Prednisone (Systemic)[1], 998
  Triamcinolone, Oral (Systemic)[1], 998
  Triamcinolone, Parenteral (Systemic)[1], 998
**Multiple sclerosis, pain of**—See Pain, neurogenic
**Mumps (prophylaxis)**
  See also Measles, mumps, and rubella
  Mumps Virus Vaccine Live (Systemic), 2062
**Muscle fiber activity syndrome, continuous**—See Neuromyotonia
**Muscle (skeletal) relaxation, for intensive care**
  Cisatracurium (Systemic), 872
**Muscle (skeletal) relaxation, for surgery**
  Atracurium (Systemic), 2098
  Cisatracurium (Systemic), 872
  Doxacurium (Systemic)†, 1296
  Gallamine (Systemic), 2098
  Metocurine (Systemic), 2098
  Mivacurium (Systemic)†, 2036
  Pancuronium (Systemic), 2098
  Pipecuronium (Systemic)†, 2330
  Rocuronium (Systemic), 2522
  Succinylcholine (Systemic), 2098
  Tubocurarine (Systemic), 2098
  Vecuronium (Systemic), 2098
**Muscular atrophy, progressive (treatment)**
  Ciliary Neurotrophic Factor, Recombinant Human (Systemic), 3136‡
**Muscular atrophy, spinal (treatment)**
  Ciliary Neurotrophic Factor, Recombinant Human (Systemic), 3136‡
**Muscular spasm**—See Spasm, skeletal muscle

## Indications Index

**Muscular sprains, strains (treatment)**
  Diethylamine Salicylate (Topical)*, 3017
**Mushroom poisoning**—See Toxicity, *Amanita phalloides*
**Myasthenia gravis (diagnosis)**
  Edrophonium (Systemic), 1329
  [Neostigmine, Parenteral (Systemic)][1], 437
  Tubocurarine (Systemic), 2098
**Myasthenia gravis (treatment)**
  Ambenonium (Systemic)†, 437
  [Azathioprine (Systemic)][1], 491
  [Betamethasone, Oral (Systemic)][1], 998
  [Cortisone, Oral (Systemic)][1], 998
  [Dexamethasone, Oral (Systemic)][1], 998
  [Hydrocortisone, Oral (Systemic)][1], 998
  [Methylprednisolone, Oral (Systemic)][1], 998
  Neostigmine (Systemic), 437
  [Prednisolone, Oral (Systemic)][1], 998
  [Prednisone (Systemic)][1], 998
  Pyridostigmine (Systemic), 437
  [Triamcinolone, Oral (Systemic)][1], 998
**Mycobacterial infections, atypical (treatment)**
  Clofazimine (Systemic)†, 
  [Cycloserine (Systemic)]†, 1134
  [Doxycycline (Systemic)], 2765
  [Ethambutol (Systemic)], 1412
  [Ethionamide (Systemic)]†, 1417
  [Minocycline (Systemic)], 2765
  [Rifampin (Systemic)][1], 2485
**Mycobacterial infections, nontuberculous (treatment)**
  Thalidomide (Systemic), 3168‡
**Mycobacterium avium complex (MAC) disease (diagnosis)**
  *Mycobacterium avium* Sensitin RS-10 (Systemic), 3155‡
**Mycobacterium avium complex (MAC) disease (prophylaxis)**
  Rifabutin (Systemic), 2483
**Mycobacterium avium complex (MAC) disease (treatment)**
  Aminosidine (Systemic), 3130‡
**Mycobacterium avium complex (MAC) disease, in AIDS patients (prophylaxis)**
  Rifabutin (Systemic), 3163‡
  Rifapentine (Systemic), 3163‡
**Mycobacterium avium complex disease, disseminated (prophylaxis)**
  Azithromycin (Systemic)[1], 499
**Mycobacterium avium complex (MAC) disease, disseminated (prophylaxis)**
  Clarithromycin (Systemic)[1], 889
  Rifabutin (Systemic), 3163‡
**Mycobacterium avium complex (MAC) disease, disseminated (treatment)**
  Clarithromycin (Systemic), 889
  Gentamicin Liposomes (Systemic), 3144‡
  Rifabutin (Systemic), 3163‡
**Mycosis fungoides (treatment)**
  Betamethasone, Oral (Systemic), 998
  Betamethasone, Parenteral (Systemic), 998
  [Bleomycin (Systemic)][1], 624
  [Carmustine (Systemic)][1], 786
  Cortisone (Systemic), 998
  Cyclophosphamide (Systemic), 1128
  Dexamethasone, Oral (Systemic), 998
  Dexamethasone, Parenteral (Systemic), 998
  Hydrocortisone, Oral (Systemic), 998
  Hydrocortisone, Parenteral (Systemic), 998
  [Interferon Alfa-2a, Recombinant (Systemic)][1], 1740
  [Interferon Alfa-2b, Recombinant (Systemic)][1], 1740
  Interferon Alfa-n1 (Ins) (Systemic)*[1], 1740
  [Interferon Alfa-n3 (Systemic)]†, 1740
  Mechlorethamine (Systemic), 1929
  Mechlorethamine (Topical)*†, #
  Methotrexate—For Cancer (Systemic), 1962
  Methotrexate with Laurocapram (Topical), 3154‡
  [Methoxsalen (Topical)][1], 1977
  Methoxsalen Capsules USP (XXI) (Hard Gelatin) (Systemic)[1], 1973
  [Methoxsalen Capsules USP (XXII) (Soft Gelatin) (Systemic)][1], 1973
  Methylprednisolone, Oral (Systemic), 998
  Methylprednisolone, Parenteral (Systemic), 998
  Prednisolone, Oral (Systemic), 998
  Prednisolone, Parenteral (Systemic), 998
  Prednisone (Systemic), 998
  Triamcinolone, Oral (Systemic), 998
  Triamcinolone, Parenteral (Systemic), 998
  Vinblastine (Systemic), 2946
  [Vincristine (Systemic)][1], 2950

**Mydriasis, in diagnostic procedures**
  Cyclopentolate (Ophthalmic), #
  Phenylephrine (Ophthalmic), #
  Scopolamine (Ophthalmic)†, 2557
  Tropicamide (Ophthalmic), #
**Mydriasis, during surgery**
  Epinephrine Injection USP (Systemic), 651
**Mydriasis, postoperative**
  [Atropine (Ophthalmic)], 485
  Homatropine (Ophthalmic), 1651
  Scopolamine (Ophthalmic)†, 2557
  Tropicamide (Ophthalmic), #
**Mydriasis, preoperative**
  [Atropine (Ophthalmic)], 485
  Homatropine (Ophthalmic), 1651
  Phenylephrine (Ophthalmic), #
  Tropicamide (Ophthalmic), #
**Mydriasis, reversal of**
  Dapiprazole (Ophthalmic), 1168
**Myelodysplastic syndrome (treatment)**
  [Cytarabine (Systemic)][1], 1143
  Epoetin Alfa (Systemic), 3142‡
  [Filgrastim (Systemic)][1], 941
  Filgrastim (Systemic), 3143‡
  Heme Arginate (Systemic), 3145‡
  Idarubicin (Systemic), 3146‡
  RII Retinamide (Systemic), 3163‡
  Sargramostim (Systemic)†, 941
**Myelofibrosis (diagnosis)**—See Bone marrow imaging, radionuclide
**Myelography, cervical**
  Iohexol (Systemic), #
  Iopamidol (Systemic)[1], #
  Metrizamide (Systemic)†, #
**Myelography, lumbar**
  Iohexol (Systemic), #
  Iopamidol (Systemic)[1], #
  Metrizamide (Systemic)†, #
**Myelography, thoracic**
  Iohexol (Systemic), #
  Iopamidol (Systemic)[1], #
  Metrizamide (Systemic)†, #
**Myelography, total columnar**
  Iohexol (Systemic), #
  Iopamidol (Systemic)[1], #
  Metrizamide (Systemic)†, #
**Myeloid engraftment following bone marrow transplantation, failure or delay of (treatment)**
  [Filgrastim (Systemic)][1], 941
  Sargramostim (Systemic)†, 941
**Myeloid engraftment following bone marrow transplantation, promotion of (treatment adjunct)**
  Filgrastim (Systemic), 941
  Sargramostim (Systemic)†, 941
**Myeloid engraftment following hematopoietic stem cell transplantation, failure or delay of (treatment)**
  Sargramostim (Systemic)†, 941
**Myeloid engraftment following hematopoietic stem cell transplantation, promotion of (treatment adjunct)**
  [Filgrastim (Systemic)], 941
  Sargramostim (Systemic)†, 941
**Myeloma, multiple**—See Multiple myeloma
**Myeloma, multiple (treatment)**
  Beta Alethine (Systemic), 3133‡
**Myelopathy, AIDS-associated (treatment)**
  Methionine/L-Methionine, 3153‡
  S-Adenosylmethionine (Systemic), 3163‡
**Myocardial infarction (diagnosis)**
  See also Cardiac imaging, radionuclide; Cardiac imaging, positron emission tomographic
  Ammonia N 13 (Systemic)*†, 91
  Rubidium Rb 82 (Systemic)†, 2536
  Technetium Tc 99m Sestamibi (Systemic), 2736
  Technetium Tc 99m Teboroxime (Systemic)†, 2743
  Technetium Tc 99m Tetrofosmin (Systemic)†, 2745
  Thallous Chloride Tl 201 (Systemic), 2781
**Myocardial infarction (prophylaxis)**
  [Acebutolol (Systemic)][1], 593
  Aspirin, Buffered (Systemic), 2538
  Aspirin Delayed-release Tablets USP (Systemic), 2538
  Aspirin, Sodium Bicarbonate, and Citric Acid (Systemic)[1], 477
  Aspirin Tablets USP (Systemic), 2538
  Aspirin Tablets USP (Chewable) (Systemic), 2538
  Atenolol (Systemic)[1], 593
  Clodpidogrel (Systemic), 913
  Metoprolol (Systemic), 593
  [Nadolol (Systemic)][1], 593
  Oxprenolol (Systemic)*[1], 593
  Propranolol (Systemic), 593

**Myocardial infarction (prophylaxis)** *(continued)*
  [Sotalol (Systemic)][1], 593
  Timolol (Systemic), 593
**Myocardial infarction (treatment)**
  [Acebutolol (Systemic)][1], 593
  Atenolol (Systemic)[1], 593
  Metoprolol (Systemic), 593
  [Nadolol (Systemic)][1], 593
  Oxprenolol (Systemic)*[1], 593
  Propranolol (Systemic), 593
  [Sotalol (Systemic)][1], 593
  Timolol (Systemic), 593
**Myocardial infarction (treatment adjunct)**
  [Erythrityl Tetranitrate (Systemic)][1], 2129
  [Isosorbide Dinitrate Capsules (Systemic)][1], 2129
  [Isosorbide Dinitrate Chewable Tablets USP (Systemic)], 2129
  [Isosorbide Dinitrate, Sublingual (Systemic)][1], 2129
  [Isosorbide Dinitrate Tablets USP (Systemic)][1], 2129
  [Nitroglycerin, Lingual (Systemic)][1], 2129
  Nitroglycerin, Parenteral (Systemic), 2129
  [Nitroglycerin, Sublingual (Systemic)][1], 2129
  [Nitroglycerin, Topical (Systemic)][1], 2129
  [Nitroprusside (Systemic)][1], 2142
  [Pentaerythritol Tetranitrate Tablets USP (Systemic)][1], 2129
**Myocardial infarction, non-Q wave (treatment)**
  Tirofiban (Systemic), 3036
**Myocardial perfusion imaging, positron emission tomographic**
  Ammonia N 13 (Systemic)*†, 91
  Rubidium Rb 82 (Systemic)†, 2536
**Myocardial perfusion imaging, radionuclide**
  Technetium Tc 99m Sestamibi (Systemic), 2736
  Technetium Tc 99m Teboroxime (Systemic)†, 2743
  Technetium Tc 99m Tetrofosmin (Systemic)†, 2745
  Thallous Chloride Tl 201 (Systemic), 2781
**Myocardial perfusion imaging, radionuclide, adjunct**
  [Adenosine (Systemic)]†, 32
  Dipyridamole (Systemic), #
**Myocardial reinfarction (prophylaxis)**
  [Anisindione (Systemic)]†, 243
  Aspirin, Buffered (Systemic), 2538
  Aspirin Delayed-release Tablets USP (Systemic), 2538
  Aspirin, Sodium Bicarbonate, and Citric Acid (Systemic)[1], 477
  Aspirin Tablets USP (Systemic), 2538
  Aspirin Tablets USP (Chewable) (Systemic), 2538
  [Dicumarol (Systemic)]†, 243
  Dipyridamole and Aspirin (Systemic)*, 3018
  [Warfarin (Systemic)], 243
  Warfarin (Systemic), 3038
**Myocardial reinfarction (prophylaxis adjunct)**
  [Dipyridamole (Systemic)], #
**Myocarditis (diagnosis)**—See Cardiac imaging, radionuclide
  Indium In 111 Murine Monoclonal Antibody Fab to Myosin, 3147‡
**Myocarditis, acute (treatment)**
  Immune Globulin Intravenous (Human) (Systemic), 3147‡
**Myoclonus (treatment)**
  Piracetam (Systemic), 3158‡
**Myoclonus, postanoxic intention (treatment)**
  L-5 Hydroxytryptophan (Systemic), 3150‡
**Myodysplastic syndrome (treatment)**
  [Topotecan (Systemic)][1], 2841
**Myopathy, inflammatory (treatment)**
  [Azathioprine (Systemic)][1], 491
**Myositis ossificans**—See Ossification, heterotopic
**Myotonia congenita (treatment)**
  [Phenytoin (Systemic)][1], 253
**Myotonic muscular dystrophy (treatment)**
  [Phenytoin (Systemic)][1], 253
**Myxedema coma/precoma (treatment)**
  Liothyronine (Systemic), 3028, 3152‡
**Myxedema, pretibial (treatment)**
  Amcinonide (Topical), 978
  Beclomethasone Dipropionate (Topical), 978
  Betamethasone Benzoate (Topical), 978
  Betamethasone Dipropionate (Topical), 978
  Betamethasone Valerate (Topical), 978
  Clobetasol Propionate (Topical), 978
  Clobetasone Butyrate (Topical), 978
  Desoximetasone (Topical), 978
  Diflorasone Diacetate (Topical), 978
  Diflucortolone Valerate (Topical), 978
  Fluocinolone Acetonide (Topical), 978
  Fluocinonide (Topical), 978
  Flurandrenolide (except 0.0125% cream and ointment) (Topical), 978

**Myxedema, pretibial (treatment)** *(continued)*
    Fluticasone Propionate (Topical), 978
    Halcinonide (Topical), 978
    Halobetasol Propionate (Topical), 978
    Hydrocortisone Butyrate (Topical), 978
    Hydrocortisone Valerate (Topical), 978
    Mometasone Furoate (Topical), 978
    Triamcinolone Acetonide (Topical), 978

# N

**N-acetylglutamate synthetase deficiency (treatment)**
    Carbamylglutamic Acid (Systemic), 3136‡
**Narcoanalysis**
    Amobarbital, Parenteral (Systemic), 518
    Thiopental, Parenteral (Systemic)[1], 161
**Narcolepsy (treatment)**
    Amphetamine (Systemic)†, 94
    Amphetamine and Dextroamphetamine (Systemic)†, 94
    Dextroamphetamine (Systemic), 94
    Ephedrine, Oral (Systemic), 651
    Gamma-Hydroxybutyrate (Systemic), 3144‡
    Methylphenidate (Systemic), 1987
    Modafinil (Systemic), 3154‡
    Sodium/Gamma Hydroxybutyrate (Systemic), 3165‡
**Narcolepsy/cataplexy syndrome (treatment)**
    [Clomipramine (Systemic)][1], 271
    [Desipramine (Systemic)][1], 271
    [Imipramine (Systemic)][1], 271
    [Protriptyline (Systemic)][1], 271
**Narcolepsy/cataplexy syndrome (treatment adjunct)**
    [Clopramine (Systemic)][1], 271
    [Desipramine (Systemic)][1], 271
    [Imipramine (Systemic)][1], 271
**Narcosis, basal**
    Thiopental Sodium for Rectal Solution (Systemic)*†, 161
    Thiopental Sodium Rectal Suspension (Systemic), 161
**Nasolacrimal imaging, radionuclide**—See Dacryoscintigraphy
**Nausea and vomiting (prophylaxis)**
    Droperidol (Systemic), 1319
    Hydroxyzine, Parenteral (Systemic), 325
    Promethazine (Systemic), 377
    Thiethylperazine (Systemic), #
    Trimethobenzamide (Systemic)†, 2880
**Nausea and vomiting (treatment)**
    Chlorpromazine (Systemic), 2289
    Diphenidol (Systemic), 1232
    Hydroxyzine, Parenteral (Systemic), 325
    Perphenazine (Systemic), 2289
    Prochlorperazine (Systemic), 2289
    Promethazine (Systemic), 377
    Thiethylperazine (Systemic), #
    Triflupromazine (Systemic)†, 2289
    Trimethobenzamide (Systemic)†, 2880
**Nausea and vomiting, antiparkinson agent–induced (treatment)**
    Domperidone (Systemic)*, 3018
**Nausea and vomiting, cancer chemotherapy–induced (prophylaxis)**
    [Dexamethasone, Oral (Systemic)][1], 998
    [Dexamethasone, Parenteral (Systemic)][1], 998
    Diphenidol (Systemic), 1232
    Dolasetron (Systemic), 1287
    Dronabinol (Systemic), 1316
    Granisetron (Systemic), 1578
    [Haloperidol (Systemic)][1], 1611
    [Hydrocortisone, Oral (Systemic)][1], 998
    [Hydrocortisone, Parenteral (Systemic)][1], 998
    [Lorazepam, Parenteral (Systemic)][1], 556
    Metoclopramide, Parenteral (Systemic), 1992
    Nabilone (Systemic)*, 2074
    Ondansetron (Systemic), 2165
    [Prednisone (Systemic)][1], 998
**Nausea and vomiting, cancer chemotherapy–induced (treatment)**
    Diphenidol (Systemic), 1232
    [Haloperidol (Systemic)][1], 1611
**Nausea and vomiting, cancer radiotherapy–induced (prophylaxis)**
    [Granisetron (Systemic)][1], 1578
**Nausea and vomiting, postoperative (prophylaxis)**
    Cyclizine (Systemic), #
    Dolasetron (Systemic), 1287
    Metoclopramide (Systemic), 1992
    Ondansetron (Systemic), 2165
**Nausea and vomiting, postoperative (treatment)**
    Cyclizine (Systemic), #
    Dolasetron (Systemic), 1287
    Ondansetron (Systemic), 2165

**Nausea and vomiting, postoperative, drug-related (treatment)**
    [Metoclopramide (Systemic)], 1992
**Nausea and vomiting, radiotherapy-induced (prophylaxis)**
    [Meclizine (Systemic)], 1933
    Ondansetron (Systemic), 2165
**Nausea and vomiting, radiotherapy-induced (treatment)**
    [Meclizine (Systemic)], 1933
**Necrobiosis lipoidica diabeticorum (treatment)**
    Amcinonide (Topical), 978
    Beclomethasone Dipropionate (Topical), 978
    Betamethasone Benzoate (Topical), 978
    Betamethasone Dipropionate (Topical), 978
    Betamethasone, Parenteral-Local (Systemic), 998
    Betamethasone Valerate (Topical), 978
    Clobetasol Propionate (Topical), 978
    Clobetasone Butyrate (Topical), 978
    Desoximetasone (Topical), 978
    Dexamethasone, Parenteral-Local (Systemic), 998
    Diflorasone Diacetate (Topical), 978
    Diflucortolone Valerate (Topical), 978
    Fluocinolone Acetonide (Topical), 978
    Fluocinonide (Topical), 978
    Flurandrenolide (except 0.0125% cream and ointment) (Topical), 978
    Fluticasone Propionate (Topical), 978
    Halcinonide (Topical), 978
    Halobetasol Propionate (Topical), 978
    Hydrocortisone Butyrate (Topical), 978
    Hydrocortisone, Parenteral-Local (Systemic), 998
    Hydrocortisone Valerate (Topical), 978
    Methylprednisolone, Parenteral-Local (Systemic), 998
    Mometasone Furoate (Topical), 978
    Prednisolone, Parenteral-Local (Systemic), 998
    Triamcinolone Acetonide (Topical), 978
    Triamcinolone, Parenteral-Local (Systemic), 998
**Necrosis, dermal (prophylaxis)**
    Phentolamine (Systemic), #
**Necrosis, hepatic, subacute (treatment)**
    [Methylprednisolone, Oral (Systemic)][1], 998
    [Methylprednisolone, Parenteral (Systemic)][1], 998
    [Prednisolone, Oral (Systemic)][1], 998
    [Prednisolone, Parenteral (Systemic)][1], 998
    [Prednisone (Systemic)][1], 998
**Necrosis, indicating cardiac transplant rejection (diagnosis)**
    Imciromab Pentetate (Systemic), 3147‡
**Necrosis, skin, warfarin-induced (prophylaxis)**
    Protein C Concentrate (Systemic), 3160‡
**Necrosis, skin, warfarin-induced (treatment)**
    Protein C Concentrate (Systemic), 3160‡
**Neonates, high-risk, preterm, low-birthweight, infections in (prophylaxis)**
    [Immune Globulin Intravenous (Human) (Systemic)][1], 1686
**Neonates, high-risk, preterm, low-birthweight, infections in (treatment adjunct)**
    [Immune Globulin Intravenous (Human) (Systemic)][1], 1686
**Neoplastic disease (diagnosis)**
    Gallium Citrate Ga 67 (Systemic), 1538
**Nephropathy, diabetic (treatment)**
    [Captopril (Systemic)][1], 177
**Nephropathy, uric acid (prophylaxis)**
    Allopurinol (Systemic), 44
**Nephropathy, uric acid (treatment)**
    Allopurinol (Systemic), 44
**Nephrosis, acute (treatment adjunct)**
    Albumin Human (Systemic), 34
**Nephrotic syndrome (treatment)**
    [Azathioprine (Systemic)][1], 491
    Betamethasone, Oral (Systemic), 998
    Betamethasone, Parenteral (Systemic), 998
    [Chlorambucil (Systemic)][1], 837
    Cortisone (Systemic), 998
    Cyclophosphamide (Systemic)[1], 1128
    [Cyclosporine (Systemic)], 1136
    Dexamethasone, Oral (Systemic), 998
    Dexamethasone, Parenteral (Systemic), 998
    Hydrocortisone, Oral (Systemic), 998
    Hydrocortisone, Parenteral (Systemic), 998
    Methylprednisolone, Oral (Systemic), 998
    Methylprednisolone, Parenteral (Systemic), 998
    Prednisolone, Oral (Systemic), 998
    Prednisolone, Parenteral (Systemic), 998
    Prednisone (Systemic), 998
    Triamcinolone, Oral (Systemic), 998
    Triamcinolone, Parenteral (Systemic), 998
**Nephrotic syndrome, acute (treatment adjunct)**
    Albumin Human (Systemic), 34
**Nephrotic syndrome, hemorrhagic fever of (treatment)**
    Ribavirin (Systemic), 3162‡

**Nephrotomography**
    Diatrizoate Meglumine and Diatrizoate Sodium, Parenteral (Systemic), #
    Diatrizoate Meglumine, Parenteral (Systemic), #
**Nephrotoxicity, cisplatin-induced (prophylaxis)**
    Amifostine (Systemic), 61
    Sodium Thiosulfate (Systemic)[1], #
**Nerve repair, microsurgical peripheral, adjunct**
    Leupeptin, 3151‡
**Neuralgia (treatment)**
    Capsaicin (Topical), 753
**Neuralgia, glossopharyngeal**—See Pain, neurogenic
**Neuralgia, post-herpetic (treatment)**
    See also Pain, neurogenic
    Lidocaine (Systemic), 3152‡
**Neuralgia, post-traumatic**—See Pain, neurogenic
**Neuralgia, trigeminal (treatment)**
    See also Pain, neurogenic
    [Baclofen (Systemic)][1], 515
    Carbamazepine (Systemic), 757
    L-Baclofen (Systemic), 3150‡
    [Phenytoin (Systemic)][1], 253
**Neuritis, idiopathic, acute**—See Pain, neurogenic
**Neuritis, optic (treatment)**
    Betamethasone, Oral (Systemic), 998
    Betamethasone, Parenteral (Systemic), 998
    Cortisone (Systemic), 998
    Dexamethasone, Oral (Systemic)‡
    Dexamethasone, Parenteral (Systemic), 998
    Hydrocortisone, Oral (Systemic), 998
    Hydrocortisone, Parenteral (Systemic), 998
    Methylprednisolone, Oral (Systemic), 998
    Methylprednisolone, Parenteral (Systemic), 998
    Prednisolone, Oral (Systemic), 998
    Prednisolone, Parenteral (Systemic), 998
    Prednisone (Systemic), 998
    Triamcinolone, Oral (Systemic), 998
    Triamcinolone, Parenteral (Systemic), 998
**Neuroblastoma (treatment)**
    [Cisplatin (Systemic)][1], 876
    Cyclophosphamide (Systemic), 1128
    [Daunorubicin (Systemic)][1], 1173
    Doxorubicin (Systemic), 1308
    [Etoposide (Systemic)][1], 1424
    [Ifosfamide (Systemic)][1], 1677
    Iobenguane I 131 Sulfate (Systemic—Therapeutic)*†, 1749
    Teniposide (Systemic), 3035
    Vincristine (Systemic), 2950
**Neurocysticercosis (treatment)**
    Albendazole (Systemic), 3009, 3129‡
    Albendazole (Systemic)*†, #
    [Praziquantel (Systemic)]†, 2368
**Neuroleptic malignant syndrome (treatment)**
    [Bromocriptine (Systemic)][1], 636
    [Dantrolene (Systemic)][1], 1165
**Neuromuscular blockade, nondepolarizing (treatment)**
    Edrophonium (Systemic), 1329
    Edrophonium and Atropine (Systemic)†, 1331
    Neostigmine, Parenteral (Systemic), 437
    Pyridostigmine, Parenteral (Systemic), 437
**Neuromyotonia (treatment)**
    [Phenytoin (Systemic)][1], 253
**Neuropathy, peripheral, diabetic**—See Pain, neurogenic
**Neuropathy, post-traumatic**—See Pain, neurogenic
**Neuropathy type I, motor and sensory, hereditary (treatment)**
    Dynamine (Systemic), 3141‡
**Neurotoxicity, cisplatin-induced (prophylaxis)**
    [Amifostine (Systemic)][1], 61
**Neutropenia (treatment)**
    [Lithium (Systemic)][1], 1869
**Neutropenia, acute myelogenous leukemia–related (treatment)**
    Filgrastim (Systemic), 3143‡
**Neutropenia, AIDS-associated (treatment)**
    [Filgrastim (Systemic)][1], 941
    [Sargramostim (Systemic)]†, 941
**Neutropenia, bone marrow transplant–related (treatment)**
    Filgrastim (Systemic), 3143‡
    Sargramostim (Systemic)†, 3163‡
**Neutropenia, chemotherapy-related (treatment)**
    Filgrastim (Systemic), 941
    [Sargramostim (Systemic)]†, 941
    Sargramostim (Systemic)†, 3163‡
**Neutropenia, chronic, severe (treatment)**
    Filgrastim (Systemic), 941, 3143‡
    [Sargramostim (Systemic)][1], 941
**Neutropenia, drug-induced (treatment)**
    [Filgrastim (Systemic)][1], 941
    [Sargramostim (Systemic)]†, 941

**Neutropenia, febrile, (treatment)**
Cefepime (Systemic), 794
[Ceftazidime (Systemic)][1], 794
**Neutrophil and platelet deficiency, following bone marrow transplantation (treatment)**
Interleukin-3 Human, Recombinant (Systemic), 3149‡
**New World hookworm**—See Hookworm infection
**NIA**—See Akathisia, neuroleptic-induced
**Niacin deficiency (prophylaxis)**
Niacin (Systemic), 2116
Niacinamide (Systemic), 2116
**Niacin deficiency (treatment)**
Niacin (Systemic), 2116
Niacinamide (Systemic), 2116
**Nicotine dependence (treatment)**
Bupropion (Systemic), 687
Nicotine (Systemic), 3030
**Nicotine dependence (treatment adjunct)**
[Clonidine, Oral (Systemic)][1], 908
Nicotine (Inhalation-Systemic), 2120
Nicotine (Nasal), 2122
Nicotine (Systemic), 2125
**NIDDM**—See Diabetes mellitus, non–insulin-dependent
Diabetes mellitus, non–insulin-dependent, 1957
**Nitrogen retention, enhancement of, in severe burn patients**
Somatropin (Systemic), 3165‡
**Nocardiosis (treatment)**
[Minocycline (Systemic)], 2765
Sulfadiazine (Systemic), 2653
Sulfamethoxazole (Systemic), 2653
[Sulfamethoxazole and Trimethoprim (Systemic)][1], 2661
Sulfisoxazole (Systemic), 2653
**Nutritional deficiency (prophylaxis)**
Enteral Nutrition Formulas (Systemic), #
Infant Formulas, Hypoallergenic (Systemic), #
Infant Formulas, Milk-based (Systemic), #
Infant Formulas, Soy-based (Systemic), #
**Nutritional deficiency (treatment)**
Dianeal PD-2 Peritoneal Dialysis Solution with Amino Acids (Systemic), 3140‡
Enteral Nutrition Formulas (Systemic), #
Infant Formulas, Hypoallergenic (Systemic), #
Infant Formulas, Milk-based (Systemic), #
Infant Formulas, Soy-based (Systemic), #
Multi-Vitamin Infusion (Neonatal Formula) (Systemic), 3155‡

# O

**Obesity, exogenous (treatment)**
Benzphetamine (Systemic)†, 452
Diethylpropion (Systemic), 452
Mazindol (Systemic), 452
Phendimetrazine (Systemic)†, 452
Phentermine (Systemic), 452
Phenylpropanolamine (Systemic)†, 2314
Sibutramine (Systemic), 2571
**Obsessive-compulsive disorder (treatment)**
Clomipramine (Systemic), 271
Fluoxetine (Systemic), 1503
Fluvoxamine (Systemic), 1513
Paroxetine (Systemic), 2225
Sertraline (Systemic), 2566
**Ocular conditions, inflammatory (treatment)**
Loteprednol (Ophthalmic), 1887
**Ocular infections (treatment)**
Chloramphenicol (Ophthalmic), #
Chlortetracycline (Ophthalmic), 2763
Erythromycin (Ophthalmic), 1364
Framycetin (Ophthalmic)*, 3020
Framycetin, Gramicidin, and Dexamethasone (Ophthalmic)*, 3021
Neomycin (Ophthalmic)*†, #
Neomycin, Polymyxin B, and Bacitracin (Ophthalmic), #
Neomycin, Polymyxin B, and Gramicidin (Ophthalmic), #
Neomycin, Polymyxin B, and Hydrocortisone (Ophthalmic), #
Sulfacetamide (Ophthalmic), 2651
Sulfisoxazole (Ophthalmic), 2651
Tetracycline (Ophthalmic), 2763
Tobramycin (Ophthalmic), #
**Ocular infections, following foreign body removal (prophylaxis)**
Framycetin (Ophthalmic)*, 3020
**Ocular infections, Pseudomonas aeruginosa–associated (treatment)**
Polymyxin B (Ophthalmic), 3032

**Ocular infections, superficial (treatment adjunct)**
Betamethasone (Ophthalmic)*, 966
Dexamethasone (Ophthalmic), 966
Fluorometholone (Ophthalmic), 966
Hydrocortisone (Ophthalmic)*, 966
[Medrysone (Ophthalmic)][1], 966
Prednisolone (Ophthalmic), 966
**Ocular lubrication**
[Hydroxypropyl Cellulose (Ophthalmic)][1], #
Hydroxypropyl Methylcellulose (Ophthalmic)[1], #
**Ocular redness (treatment)**
Naphazoline (Ophthalmic), #
Oxymetazoline (Ophthalmic), #
Phenylephrine (Ophthalmic), #
**Ocular sensitivity to epinephrine (treatment)**
Betamethasone (Ophthalmic)*, 966
Dexamethasone (Ophthalmic), 966
Fluorometholone (Ophthalmic), 966
Hydrocortisone (Ophthalmic)*, 966
Medrysone (Ophthalmic), 966
Prednisolone (Ophthalmic), 966
**Oily skin (treatment)**
Alcohol and Acetone (Topical)†, #
Alcohol and Sulfur (Topical), #
Salicylic Acid and Sulfur Bar Soap (Topical), #
Salicylic Acid and Sulfur Cleansing Cream (Topical), #
Salicylic Acid and Sulfur Cleansing Lotion (Topical), #
Salicylic Acid and Sulfur Cleansing Suspension (Topical), #
Salicylic Acid and Sulfur Lotion (Topical), #
Salicylic Acid and Sulfur Topical Suspension (Topical), #
**Old World hookworm**—See Hookworm infection
**Onchocerciasis (treatment)**
Diethylcarbamazine (Systemic), #
Ivermectin (Systemic), 3026
Ivermectin (Systemic)*†, #
Suramin (Systemic)*†, #
**Onychomycosis (treatment)**
See also Tinea unguium
[Ciclopirox (Topical)], 863
[Fluconazole (Systemic)], 302
Itraconazole (Systemic)[1], 302
[Ketoconazole (Systemic)], 302
Terbinafine (Systemic), 3036
Terbinafine (Systemic)*, 2752
**Ophthalmia neonatorum (prophylaxis)**
[Chlortetracycline (Ophthalmic)], 2763
Erythromycin (Ophthalmic), 1364
Tetracycline (Ophthalmic), 2763
**Ophthalmia, sympathetic (treatment)**
Betamethasone (Ophthalmic)*, 966
Betamethasone, Oral (Systemic), 998
Betamethasone, Parenteral (Systemic), 998
Cortisone (Systemic), 998
Dexamethasone (Ophthalmic), 966
Dexamethasone, Oral (Systemic), 998
Dexamethasone, Parenteral (Systemic), 998
Fluorometholone (Ophthalmic), 966
Hydrocortisone (Ophthalmic)*, 966
Hydrocortisone, Oral (Systemic), 998
Hydrocortisone, Parenteral (Systemic), 998
[Medrysone (Ophthalmic)][1], 966
Methylprednisolone, Oral (Systemic), 998
Methylprednisolone, Parenteral (Systemic), 998
Prednisolone (Ophthalmic), 966
Prednisolone, Oral (Systemic), 998
Prednisolone, Parenteral (Systemic), 998
Prednisone (Systemic), 998
Triamcinolone, Oral (Systemic), 998
Triamcinolone, Parenteral (Systemic), 998
**Opioid (narcotic) abstinence syndrome (prophylaxis)**
Methadone (Systemic), 2168
**Opioid (narcotic) abstinence syndrome (treatment)**
[Clonidine, Oral (Systemic)][1], 908
Methadone (Systemic), 2168
**Opioid (narcotic) dependence, neonatal (treatment)**
[Opium Tincture USP (Systemic)], 2168
**Opioid depression, postoperative (treatment)**
Nalmefene (Systemic), 2080
**Opioid (narcotic) drug use, illicit (diagnosis)**
[Naloxone (Systemic)][1], 2082
**Opioid (narcotic) drug use, illicit (treatment)**
Buprenorphine (Systemic), 3135‡
Buprenorphine and Naloxone (Systemic), 3135‡
Levomethadyl Acetate Hydrochloride (Systemic), 3152‡
Methadone, Oral (Systemic), 2168

**Opioid (narcotic) drug use, illicit (treatment adjunct)**
Levomethadyl (Systemic)†, 1855
Naltrexone (Systemic), 2084, 3155‡
**Opioid (narcotic) overdose (treatment)**
Nalmefene (Systemic), 2080
**Opisthorchiasis (treatment)**
Praziquantel (Systemic)†, 2368
**Oral complications of epidermolysis bullosa (treatment)**
Sucralfate (Oral-Local), 3166‡
**Oral mucositis, due to bone marrow transplant therapy (treatment)**
[Chlorhexidine (Mucosal-Local)]†, 3136‡
Sucralfate (Oral-Local), 3166‡
**Oral mucositis, due to head and neck cancer chemotherapy (treatment)**
Sucralfate (Oral-Local), 3166‡
**Oral mucositis, due to head and neck cancer radiation therapy (prophylaxis)**
Benzydamine (Systemic), 3133‡
**Oriental liver fluke**—See Clonorchiasis
**Oriental lung fluke**—See Paragonimiasis
**Oriental sore**—See Leishmaniasis, cutaneous
**Ossification, heterotopic (prophylaxis)**
Etidronate, Oral (Systemic), 1419
**Ossification, heterotopic (treatment)**
Etidronate, Oral (Systemic), 1419
**Osteitis deformans**—See Paget's disease of bone
**Osteoarthritis (treatment)**
See also Pain, arthritic, mild
Aspirin (Systemic), 2538
Aspirin, Buffered (Systemic), 2538
Capsaicin (Topical), 753
Choline Salicylate (Systemic)†, 2538
Choline and Magnesium Salicylates (Systemic), 2538
Diclofenac (Systemic), 388
Diclofenac and Misoprostol (Systemic), 1202
Diflunisal (Systemic), 388
Etodolac (Systemic), 3019
Etodolac (Systemic)†, 388
Fenoprofen (Systemic), 388
Flurbiprofen (Systemic), 388
Ibuprofen (Systemic), 388
Indomethacin (Systemic), 388
Ketoprofen (Systemic), 388
Magnesium Salicylate (Systemic), 2538
Meclofenamate (Systemic)†, 388
Nabumetone (Systemic), 388
Naproxen (Systemic), 388, 3029
Oxaprozin (Systemic)†, 388
Phenylbutazone (Systemic)[1], 388
Piroxicam (Systemic), 388
Salsalate (Systemic), 2538
Sodium Salicylate (Systemic), 2538
Sulindac (Systemic), 388
Tenoxicam (Systemic)*, 388
Tiaprofenic Acid (Systemic)*, 388
Tolmetin (Systemic), 388
**Osteoarthritis, post-traumatic (treatment)**
See also Osteoarthritis
Betamethasone, Oral (Systemic), 998
Betamethasone, Parenteral (Systemic), 998
Betamethasone, Parenteral-Local (Systemic), 998
Cortisone (Systemic), 998
Dexamethasone (Systemic), 998
Hydrocortisone, Oral (Systemic), 998
Hydrocortisone, Parenteral (Systemic), 998
Hydrocortisone, Parenteral-Local (Systemic), 998
Methylprednisolone, Oral (Systemic), 998
Methylprednisolone, Parenteral (Systemic), 998
Methylprednisolone, Parenteral-Local (Systemic), 998
Prednisolone (Systemic), 998
Prednisone (Systemic), 998
Triamcinolone (Systemic), 998
**Osteodystrophy (treatment)**
Alfacalcidol (Systemic)*, 2966
Calcifediol (Systemic)†, 2966
Calcitriol (Systemic), 2966
Dihydrotachysterol (Systemic), 2966
24,25 Dihydroxycholecalciferol (Systemic), 3127‡
Ergocalciferol (Systemic), 2966
**Osteomyelitis**—See Bone and joint infections
**Osteopetrosis, severe congenital (treatment)**
Interferon Gamma-1b (Systemic), 3149‡
**Osteoporosis, postmenopausal (prophylaxis)**
Alendronate (Systemic), 42
Conjugated Estrogens and Medroxyprogesterone Tablets (Systemic)†, 946
Conjugated Estrogens Tablets USP, and Conjugated Estrogens and Medroxyprogesterone Tablets (Systemic)†, 946
Estradiol, Oral (Systemic)1, 1383
Estradiol, Transdermal Systems (Systemic), 1383

**Osteoporosis, postmenopausal (prophylaxis)** *(continued)*
   Estrogens, Conjugated, Oral (Systemic), 1383
   [Estrogens, Esterified (Systemic)]1, 1383
   Estropipate (Systemic)1, 1383
   Raloxifene (Systemic), 2455
**Osteoporosis, postmenopausal (treatment adjunct)**
   Alendronate (Systemic), 42
   [Calcitonin-Human (Systemic)]†, 716
   Calcitonin-Salmon (Nasal-Systemic), 714
   Calcitonin-Salmon (Systemic)1, 716
**Osteoporosis, premenopausal, estrogen deficiency–induced (prophylaxis)**
   [Estradiol, Oral (Systemic)]1, 1383
   [Estradiol, Transdermal Systems (Systemic)]1, 1383
   [Estrogens, Conjugated, Oral (Systemic)]1, 1383
   [Estrogens, Esterified (Systemic)]1, 1383
   [Estropipate (Systemic)]1, 1383
**Osteoporosis, secondary (treatment adjunct)**
   [Calcitonin-Human (Systemic)]†, 716
   [Calcitonin-Salmon (Systemic)]1, 716
**Osteosarcoma (treatment)**
   [Bleomycin (Systemic)]1, 624
   [Cisplatin (Systemic)]1, 876
   [Cyclophosphamide (Systemic)]1, 1128
   [Dactinomycin (Systemic)]1, 1153
   Doxorubicin (Systemic), 1308
   [Ifosfamide (Systemic)]1, 1677
   Ifosfamide (Systemic), 3147‡
   Leucovorin (Systemic), 3151‡
   Methotrexate—For Cancer (Systemic), 1962
   Methotrexate—for Cancer (Systemic)1, 3154‡
   N-Acetylglucosminyl-N-Acetylmuramyl-L-Ala-D-Isogln-L-Ala-Glycerolid-Palmitoyl, Liposomal (Systemic), 3152‡
   [Vincristine (Systemic)], 2950
**Osteosarcoma (treatment adjunct)**
   Leucovorin (Systemic), 3150‡
   L-Leucovorin (Systemic), 3150‡
**Otitis externa (treatment)**
   Clioquinol and Flumethasone (Otic)*, 3015
   Ofloxacin (Otic), 2154
**Otitis externa, acute (treatment)**
   Framycetin, Gramicidin, and Dexamethasone (Otic)*, 3021
**Otitis externa, allergic (treatment)**
   Betamethasone (Otic)*, 971
   Dexamethasone (Otic), 971
   Hydrocortisone (Otic)*, 971
**Otitis externa, chronic (treatment)**
   Framycetin, Gramidicin, and Dexamethasone (Otic), 3021
**Otitis externa, eczematoid, chronic (prophylaxis)**
   [Hydrocortisone and Acetic Acid (Otic)], 996
**Otitis externa, eczematoid, chronic (treatment)**
   Betamethasone (Otic)*, 971
   [Dexamethasone (Otic)], 971
   Hydrocortisone (Otic)*, 971
   [Hydrocortisone and Acetic Acid (Otic)], 996
**Otitis, external (treatment)**
   Gentamicin (Otic)*, 1556
**Otitis externa, seborrheic (prophylaxis)**
   [Hydrocortisone and Acetic Acid (Otic)], 996
**Otitis externa, seborrheic (treatment)**
   Betamethasone (Otic)*, 971
   [Dexamethasone (Otic)], 971
   Hydrocortisone (Otic)*, 971
   [Hydrocortisone and Acetic Acid (Otic)], 996
**Otitis, infective (treatment adjunct)**
   Betamethasone (Otic)*, 971
   Dexamethasone (Otic), 971
   Hydrocortisone (Otic)*, 971
**Otitis media (treatment)**
   Cefaclor (Systemic), 794
   [Cefadroxil (Systemic)]1, 794
   [Cefazolin (Systemic)]1, 794
   Cefdinir (Systemic), 3014
   Cefixime (Systemic), 794
   Cefpodoxime (Systemic)sd1, 794
   Cefprozil (Systemic)†, 794
   Ceftibuten (Systemic) 1, 1880
   Ceftriaxone (Systemic) 1, 2653
   Cefuroxime Axetil (Systemic), 794
   Cephalexin (Systemic), 794
   [Cephalothin (Systemic)]1, 794
   [Cephapirin (Systemic)]†1, 794
   Cephradine (Systemic) 1, 794
   Clarithromycin (Systemic), 889
   Loracarbef (Systemic)†, 1880
   Sulfadiazine (Systemic)1, 2653
   Sulfamethoxazole (Systemic)1, 2653
   Sulfisoxazole (Systemic)1, 2653

**Otitis media, acute (treatment)**
   Amoxicillin (Systemic), 2240
   Amoxicillin and Clavulanate (Systemic), 2263, 3010
   Ampicillin (Systemic), 2240
   Bacampicillin (Systemic), 2240
   Demeclocycline (Systemic), 2765
   Doxycycline (Systemic), 2765
   Erythromycin (Systemic), 1368
   Erythromycin and Sulfisoxazole (Systemic), 1376
   Minocycline (Systemic), 2765
   Ofloxacin (Otic), 2154
   Oxytetracycline (Systemic)†, 2765
   Penicillin G, Oral (Systemic), 2240
   Penicillin G Procaine (Systemic), 2240
   Penicillin V (Systemic), 2240
   Pivampicillin (Systemic)*, 2240
   Sulfamethoxazole and Trimethoprim, Oral (Systemic), 2661
   Tetracycline (Systemic), 2765
**Otitis media, acute (treatment adjunct)**
   Clioquinol and Flumethasone (Otic)*, 3015
**Otitis media, chronic suppurative (treatment)**
   [Chloramphenicol (Otic)], #
   [Clindamycin (Systemic)], 893
   Clioquinol and Flumethasone (Otic)*, 3015
   [Colistin, Neomycin, and Hydrocortisone (Otic)]1, 939
   Gentamicin (Otic)*, 1556
   [Neomycin, Polymyxin B, and Hydrocortisone (Otic)]1, #
   Ofloxacin (Otic), 2154
**Otitis media, subacute purulent (treatment)**
   Gentamicin (Otic)*, 1556
**Otomycosis (treatment)**
   Clioquinol and Flumethasone (Otic)*, 3015
**Ovarian failure, primary (treatment)**
   Estradiol, Oral (Systemic), 1383
   Estradiol, Transdermal (Systemic), 1383
   Estradiol, Transdermal System (Matrix-type) (Systemic)1, 1383
   Estradiol, Transdermal System (Reservoir-type) (Systemic), 1383
   Estradiol Valerate (Systemic), 1383
   Estrogens, Conjugated, Oral (Systemic), 1383
   Estrogens, Esterified (Systemic), 1383
   Estrone (Systemic)†, 1383
   Estropipate (Systemic), 1383
   Ethinyl Estradiol (Systemic), 1383
   Ethinyl Estradiol (Systemic)1, 1383
**Ovarian function studies**
   [Clomiphene (Systemic)]1, 903
**Ovariectomy (treatment)**
   Estradiol, Oral (Systemic)1, 1383
   Estradiol, Transdermal (Systemic), 1383
   Estradiol Valerate (Systemic), 1383
   Estrogens, Conjugated, Oral (Systemic), 1383
   Estrogens, Esterified (Systemic), 1383
   Estrone (Systemic)†, 1383
   Estropipate (Systemic)1, 1383
   Ethinyl Estradiol (Systemic)1, 1383
**Oxyuriasis**—*See* Enterobiasis

# P

**Paget's disease of bone (diagnosis)**—*See* Skeletal imaging, radionuclide
**Paget's disease of bone (treatment)**
   Alendronate (Systemic), 42
   Calcitonin-Human (Systemic)†, 716, 3135‡
   Calcitonin-Salmon (Systemic), 716
   Etidronate, Oral (Systemic), 1419
   Pamidronate (Systemic), 2220
   [Plicamycin (Systemic)]†, 2334
   Risedronate (Systemic), 2506
   Tiludronate (Systemic), 2822
**Paget's disease of bone, rheumatologic complications associated with (treatment)**
   [Indomethacin (Systemic)]1, 388
**Pain (treatment)**
   Acetaminophen (Systemic), 6
   Acetaminophen and Aspirin (Systemic)†, 11
   Acetaminophen, Aspirin, and Caffeine (Systemic)†, 11
   Acetaminophen, Aspirin, and Caffeine, Buffered (Systemic)†, 11
   Acetaminophen, Aspirin, and Salicylamide, Buffered (Systemic)†, 11
   Acetaminophen, Aspirin, Salicylamide, and Caffeine (Systemic)†, 11
   Acetaminophen and Caffeine (Systemic), 6
   Acetaminophen and Codeine (Systemic), 2198
   Acetaminophen and Salicylamide (Systemic)†, 11
   Acetaminophen, Salicylamide, and Caffeine (Systemic)†, 11

**Pain (treatment)** *(continued)*
   Anileridine (Systemic)*, 3011
   Aspirin (Systemic), 2538
   Aspirin, Buffered (Systemic), 2538
   Aspirin and Codeine (Systemic), 2202
   Aspirin and Codeine, Buffered (Systemic)*, 2202
   Aspirin and Dihydrocodeine (Systemic)†, 2202
   Bromfenac (Systemic), #
   Buprenorphine (Systemic), 683
   [Butalbital and Acetaminophen (Systemic)]†, 532
   [Butalbital, Acetaminophen, and Caffeine (Systemic)]†, 532
   [Butalbital, Acetaminophen, Caffeine, and Codeine (Systemic)]†, 532
   [Butalbital and Aspirin (Systemic)]†, 532
   [Butalbital, Aspirin, and Caffeine (Systemic)], 532
   [Butalbital, Aspirin, Caffeine, and Codeine (Systemic)], 532
   Butorphanol (Nasal-Systemic), 700
   Butorphanol (Systemic)†, 2168
   Choline Salicylate (Systemic)†, 2538
   Choline and Magnesium Salicylates (Systemic), 2538
   Codeine (Systemic), 2168
   Dezocine (Systemic)†, 1193
   Diclofenac (Systemic), 388
   Diflunisal (Systemic), 388
   Dihydrocodeine and Acetaminophen (Systemic)†, 2198
   Elcatonin (Systemic), 3141‡
   Etodolac (Systemic), 3019
   Etodolac (Systemic)†, 388
   Fenoprofen (Systemic)1, 388
   Floctafenine (Systemic)*, 388
   Hyaluronate Sodium (Systemic), #97
   Hyaluronate Sodium Derivative, 1654
   Hydrocodone (Systemic)*, 2168
   Hydrocodone and Acetaminophen (Systemic), 3022
   Hydrocodone and Acetaminophen (Systemic)†, 2198
   Hydrocodone and Aspirin (Systemic)†, 2202
   Hydrocodone and Ibuprofen (Systemic), 1659
   Hydromorphone (Systemic), 2168
   Ibuprofen (Systemic), 388
   Ketoprofen (Systemic), 388
   Ketorolac (Systemic), 1810
   Levorphanol (Systemic), 2168
   Magnesium Salicylate (Systemic), 2538
   Meclofenamate (Systemic)†, 388
   Mefenamic Acid (Systemic), 388
   Meperidine (Systemic), 2168
   Methadone (Systemic), 2168
   Methotrimeprazine (Systemic), 2289
   Morphine (Systemic), 2168, 3155‡
   Nalbuphine (Systemic), 2168
   Naproxen (Systemic), 388, 3029
   Opium, Parenteral (Systemic), 2168
   Oxycodone (Systemic), 2168, 3030
   Oxycodone and Acetaminophen (Systemic), 2198
   Oxycodone and Aspirin (Systemic), 2202
   Oxymorphone (Systemic), 2168, 3157‡
   Pentazocine (Systemic), 2168
   Pentazocine and Acetaminophen (Systemic)†, 2198
   Pentazocine and Aspirin (Systemic)†, 2202
   Phenobarbital, ASA, and Codeine (Systemic)*, 532
   Propoxyphene (Systemic), 2168
   Propoxyphene and Acetaminophen (Systemic)†, 2198
   Propoxyphene and Aspirin (Systemic), 2202
   Salsalate (Systemic), 2538
   Sodium Salicylate (Systemic), 2538
   Tramadol (Systemic), 2851
**Pain, acute, postoperative (treatment)**
   Sufentanil (Systemic), 3035
**Pain, anogenital, external (treatment)**
   Benzocaine Ointment USP (Rectal) (Mucosal-Local), 128
   Dibucaine (Mucosal-Local), 128
   Pramoxine Hydrochloride Aerosol Foam (Mucosal-Local), 128
   Pramoxine Hydrochloride Cream USP (Mucosal-Local), 128
   Tetracaine, Rectal (Mucosal-Local), 128
**Pain, anogenital lesion–associated (treatment)**
   Dyclonine Hydrochloride 0.5% Topical Solution USP (Mucosal-Local), 128
**Pain, anorectal (treatment)**
   Benzocaine Ointment USP (Rectal) (Mucosal-Local), 128
   Dibucaine (Mucosal-Local), 128
   Pramoxine (Mucosal-Local), 128
   Tetracaine, Rectal (Mucosal-Local), 128

**Pain, with anxiety and tension (treatment)**
Meprobamate and Aspirin (Systemic), #
**Pain, arthritic, mild (treatment)**
See also Osteoarthritis
Acetaminophen (Systemic), 6
Acetaminophen and Aspirin (Systemic)†, 11
Acetaminophen, Aspirin, and Caffeine (Systemic)†, 11
Acetaminophen, Aspirin, and Caffeine, Buffered (Systemic)†, 11
Acetaminophen, Aspirin, and Salicylamide, Buffered (Systemic)†, 11
Acetaminophen, Aspirin, Salicylamide, and Caffeine (Systemic)†, 11
Acetaminophen and Caffeine (Systemic), 6
Acetaminophen and Salicylamide (Systemic)†, 11
Acetaminophen, Salicylamide, and Caffeine (Systemic)†, 11
Diethylamine Salicylate (Topical)*, 3017
**Pain, cancer (treatment adjunct)**
Clonidine (Parenteral-Local), 905
Clonidine (Systemic), 3137‡
**Pain, chronic (treatment)**
Fentanyl (Transdermal-Systemic), 1446
**Pain, dental prosthetic (treatment)**
Benzocaine Dental Paste (Mucosal-Local), 128
Benzocaine Gel (Dental) (Mucosal-Local), 128
Benzocaine Ointment USP (Dental) (Mucosal-Local), 128
Benzocaine and Phenol Gel (Mucosal-Local), 128
Benzocaine and Phenol Topical Solution (Mucosal-Local), 128
Benzocaine Topical Solution USP (Dental) (Mucosal-Local), 128
Choline and Cetyl-dimethyl-benzyl-ammonium (Mucosal-Local)*, 3013
Lidocaine Ointment USP (Mucosal-Local), 128
**Pain, esophageal (treatment)**
Dyclonine Hydrochloride Topical Solution USP (Mucosal-Local), 128
[Lidocaine Hydrochloride Oral Topical Solution USP (Mucosal-Local)], 128
**Pain, exercise-induced, in Duchenne muscular dystrophy (treatment)**
[Dantrolene, Oral (Systemic)][1], 1165
**Pain, exercise-induced, in muscle phosphorylase deficiency (treatment)**
[Dantrolene, Oral (Systemic)][1], 1165
**Pain, gingival or oral mucosal (treatment)**
Benzocaine Dental Paste (Mucosal-Local), 128
Benzocaine Gel (Mucosal-Local), 128
Benzocaine Lozenges (Mucosal-Local), 128
Benzocaine and Phenol Gel (Mucosal-Local), 128
Benzocaine and Phenol Topical Solution (Mucosal-Local), 128
Benzocaine Topical Solution USP (Dental) (Mucosal-Local), 128
Choline and Cetyl-dimethyl-benzyl-ammonium (Mucosal-Local)*, 3013
Dyclonine Hydrochloride Lozenges (Mucosal-Local), 128
Dyclonine Hydrochloride 0.5% Topical Solution USP (Mucosal-Local), 128
Lidocaine Hydrochloride Oral Topical Solution USP (Mucosal-Local), 128
Lidocaine Oral Topical Solution USP (Mucosal-Local), 128
**Pain, neurogenic (treatment)**
[Amitriptyline (Systemic)][1], 271
[Carbamazepine (Systemic)][1], 757
[Clomipramine (Systemic)][1], 271
[Desipramine (Systemic)][1], 271
[Doxepin (Systemic)][1], 271
[Imipramine (Systemic)][1], 271
[Maprotiline (Systemic)][1], 1909
[Nortriptyline (Systemic)][1], 271
[Trazodone (Systemic)][1], 2865
[Trimipramine (Systemic)][1], 271
**Pain, neurogenic (treatment adjunct)**
[Fluphenazine (Systemic)][1], 2289
**Pain, neurogenic, other (treatment)**
[Capsaicin (Topical)][1], 753
**Pain, obstetrical (treatment)**
Anileridine (Systemic)*, 3011
Ropivacaine (Parenteral-Local), 1926
**Pain, pharyngeal (treatment)**
Benzocaine Lozenges (Mucosal-Local), 128
Benzocaine and Menthol Lozenges (Mucosal-Local), 128
Dyclonine Hydrochloride Lozenges (Mucosal-Local), 128
Lidocaine Hydrochloride Oral Topical Solution USP (Mucosal-Local), 128
**Pain, postoperative (treatment)**
Fentanyl (Systemic), 1452
Ropivacaine (Parenteral-Local), 1926

**Pain, postoperative (treatment adjunct)**
Promethazine (Systemic), 377
**Pain, sore throat (treatment)**
Benzydamine (Oral-Local)*, 3011
**Pain, teething (treatment)**
Benzocaine 7.5% Gel (Dental) (Mucosal-Local), 128
Benzocaine 10% Gel (Dental) (Mucosal-Local), 128
Choline and Cetyl-dimethyl-benzyl-ammonium (Mucosal-Local)*, 3013
**Pain and upset stomach (treatment)**
Aspirin, Sodium Bicarbonate, and Citric Acid (Systemic), 477
**Pain, vaginal (treatment)**
Benzocaine Topical Aerosol USP (Mucosal-Local), 128
Benzocaine Topical Solution USP (Mucosal-Local), 128
Dyclonine Hydrochloride Topical Solution USP (Mucosal-Local), 128
**Palmar-plantar brain erythrodysethesia syndrome (treatment)**
Corticotropin-releasing Factor, Human (Systemic), 3138‡
Dimethylsulfoxide (Systemic), 3140‡
**Pancreas disorders (diagnosis)**
Sincalide (Systemic), #
**Pancreatic insufficiency (diagnosis)**
Bentiromide (Systemic)†, #
[Pancrelipase (Systemic)][1], 2222
**Pancreatic insufficiency (diagnosis adjunct)**
Cholecystokinin (Systemic)*, #
**Pancreatic insufficiency (treatment)**
Pancrelipase (Systemic), 2222
**Pancreatic insufficiency (treatment adjunct)**
[Cimetidine (Systemic)][1], 1633
**Pancreatitis (treatment adjunct)**
Albumin Human (Systemic), 34
**Pancreatography, endoscopic retrograde**
Iohexol (Systemic)[1], #
[Iopamidol (Systemic)][1], #
[Ioversol (Systemic)][1], #
**Panencephalitis, subacute sclerosing (treatment)**
Inosine Pranobex (Systemic), 3147‡
**Panic disorder (treatment)**
Alprazolam (Systemic), 556
[Chlordiazepoxide, Parenteral (Systemic)], 556
[Clomipramine (Systemic)][1], 271
[Clonazepam (Systemic)][1], 556
[Desipramine (Systemic)][1], 271
Diazepam (Systemic)[1], 556
[Doxepin (Systemic)][1], 271
[Imipramine (Systemic)][1], 271
[Lorazepam (Systemic)][1], 556
[Nortriptyline (Systemic)][1], 271
Paroxetine (Systemic), 2225
[Phenelzine (Systemic)][1], 266
Sertraline (Systemic), 2566
[Tranylcypromine (Systemic)][1], 266
**Pantothenic acid deficiency (prophylaxis)**
Calcium Pantothenate (Systemic)†, #
Pantothenic Acid (Systemic)†, #
**Pantothenic acid deficiency (treatment)**
Calcium Pantothenate (Systemic)†, #
Pantothenic Acid (Systemic)†, #
**Papilloma, of the larynx, juvenile (treatment)**
Podophyllum (Topical)†, 2341
**Papillomatosis, laryngeal (treatment)**
[Interferon Alfa-2b, Recombinant (Systemic)][1], 1740
Interferon Alfa-n1 (Ins) (Systemic)*, 1740, 3148‡
[Interferon Alfa-n3 (Systemic)]†, 1740
**Paracoccidioidomycosis (treatment)**
[Amphotericin B (Systemic)][1], 98
[Itraconazole (Systemic)], 302
Ketoconazole (Systemic), 302
[Sulfadiazine (Systemic)][1], 2653
[Sulfamethoxazole and Trimethoprim (Systemic)][1], 2661
**Paragonimiasis (treatment)**
[Praziquantel (Systemic)]†, 2368
**Paralysis agitans**—See Parkinsonism
**Paralysis, familial periodic (treatment)**
[Acetazolamide (Systemic)][1], 773
**Paraosteoarthropathy**—See Ossification, heterotopic
**Parasites, intestinal (treatment adjunct)**
Magnesium Citrate (Local), #
Magnesium Hydroxide (Local), #
Magnesium Oxide (Local)†, #
Magnesium Sulfate (Local)†, #
Sodium Phosphate (Local), #
**Parathyroid imaging, radionuclide**
[Technetium Tc 99m Sestamibi (Systemic)][1], 2736
Thallous Chloride Tl 201 (Systemic)[1], 2781

**Paratyphoid fever (treatment)**
Chloramphenicol (Systemic), 841
[Sulfamethoxazole and Trimethoprim (Systemic)], 2661
**Parenchymal disorders, renal (diagnosis)**—See Renal imaging, radionuclide
**Parkinsonism (diagnosis)**
Apomorphine (Systemic)*, #
**Parkinsonism (treatment)**
Amantadine (Systemic), 58
Benztropine (Systemic), 297
Biperiden (Systemic), 297
Bromocriptine (Systemic), 636
Carbidopa and Levodopa (Systemic), 765, 3013
Diphenhydramine (Systemic)[1], 325
Ethopropazine (Systemic), 297
Levodopa (Systemic), 1848
Levodopa and Benserazide (Systemic)*, 3027
Procyclidine (Systemic), 297
Trihexyphenidyl (Systemic), 297
**Parkinsonism (treatment adjunct)**
Apomorphine Hydrochloride (Systemic), 3132‡
Orphenadrine Hydrochloride (Systemic)*, 2577
Pergolide (Systemic), 2284
Selegiline (Systemic)*, 2560, 3164‡
**Parkinsonism, associated with cerebral arteriosclerosis**—See Parkinsonism
**Parkinsonism, idiopathic**—See Parkinsonism
**Parkinsonism, postencephalitic**—See Parkinsonism
**Parkinsonism, symptomatic**—See Parkinsonism
**Parkinson's disease (treatment)**
Human Retinal Pigmented Epithelial Cells on Collagen Microcarriers (Systemic), 3146‡
Porcine Fetal Neural Dopaminergic Cells (Systemic), 3159‡
Porcine Sertoli Cells (Systemic), 3159‡
**Parkinson's disease (treatment adjunct)**
Tolcapone (Systemic), 2833
**Parkinson's disease, idiopathic (treatment)**
Pramipexole (Systemic), 2718
Ropinirole (Systemic), 2525
**Parkinson's disease, late-stage, early morning dysfunction in (treatment)**
Apomorphine (Systemic), 3132‡
**Parkinson's disease, late-stage, early morning motor dysfunction in (treatment)**
Apomorphine (Systemic), 3132‡
**Paronychia (treatment)**
[Clotrimazole (Topical)][1], 916
[Econazole (Topical)][1], 1323
Framycetin and Gramicidin (Topical)*, 3021
Gentamicin (Topical), 1557
[Itraconazole (Systemic)][1], 302
[Ketoconazole (Systemic)][1], 302
[Ketoconazole (Topical)][1], 1807
[Miconazole (Topical)], #
**Pasteurella multocida infections (treatment)**
[Ampicillin, Parenteral (Systemic)][1], 2240
Penicillin G, Parenteral (Systemic), 2240
[Penicillin V (Systemic)][1], 2240
**PCP**—See Pneumonia, Pneumocystis carinii
**Pediculosis capitis (treatment)**
Benzyl Benzoate (Topical)*†, #
[Lindane Cream USP (Topical)], 1866
[Lindane Lotion USP (Topical)], 1866
Lindane Shampoo USP (Topical), 1866
Malathion (Topical)†, #
Permethrin (Topical), #
Pyrethrins and Piperonyl Butoxide (Topical), #
**Pediculosis corporis (treatment)**
Pyrethrins and Piperonyl Butoxide (Topical), #
**Pediculosis pubis (treatment)**
Benzyl Benzoate (Topical)*†, #
[Lindane Cream USP (Topical)], 1866
[Lindane Lotion USP (Topical)], 1866
Lindane Shampoo USP (Topical), 1866
Pyrethrins and Piperonyl Butoxide (Topical), #
**Pelvic imaging, magnetic resonance, adjunct**
[Glucagon (Systemic)][1], 1563
**Pelvic infections, female (treatment)**
See also Genitourinary tract infections; Gynecologic infections
Ampicillin and Sulbactam (Systemic)†, 2263
[Carbenicillin, Parenteral (Systemic)]1†, 2240
Cefoperazone (Systemic) [1], 794
Cefotaxime (Systemic), 794
Cefotetan (Systemic), 794
Cefoxitin (Systemic), 794
Cefpodoxime (Systemic) [1], 794
Ceftazidime (Systemic) [1], 794
Ceftizoxime (Systemic) [1], 794
Ceftriaxone (Systemic) [1], 794
Clindamycin (Systemic), 893
Imipenem and Cilastatin (Systemic), 1681
Metronidazole (Systemic), 1996

**Pelvic infections, female (treatment)** *(continued)*
  Mezlocillin (Systemic)†, 2240
  Piperacillin (Systemic), 2240
  Piperacillin and Tazobactam (Systemic), 2263
  Ticarcillin (Systemic), 2240
  Ticarcillin and Clavulanate (Systemic), 2263
**Pelvic inflammatory disease (prophylaxis)**
  Benzalkonium Chloride (Vaginal)*[1], #
  [Nonoxynol 9 (Vaginal)][1], #
  [Octoxynol 9 (Vaginal)][1], #
**Pelvic inflammatory disease (treatment)**
  Azithromycin (Systemic)[1], 499
  Trovafloxacin (Systemic), 2891
**Pemphigoid (treatment)**
  Amcinonide (Topical), 978
  [Azathioprine (Systemic)][1], 491
  Beclomethasone Dipropionate (Topical), 978
  Betamethasone Benzoate (Topical), 978
  Betamethasone Dipropionate (Topical), 978
  [Betamethasone, Oral (Systemic)][1], 998
  [Betamethasone, Parenteral (Systemic)][1], 998
  Betamethasone Valerate (Topical), 978
  Clobetasol Propionate (Topical), 978
  Clobetasone Butyrate (Topical), 978
  [Cortisone (Systemic)][1], 998
  [Dapsone (Systemic)][1], 1170
  Desoximetasone (Topical), 978
  [Dexamethasone, Oral (Systemic)][1], 998
  [Dexamethasone, Parenteral (Systemic)][1], 998
  Diflorasone Diacetate (Topical), 978
  Diflucortolone Valerate (Topical), 978
  Fluocinolone Acetonide (Topical), 978
  Fluocinonide (Topical), 978
  Flurandrenolide (except 0.0125% cream and ointment) (Topical), 978
  Fluticasone Propionate (Topical), 978
  Halcinonide (Topical), 978
  Halobetasol Propionate (Topical), 978
  Hydrocortisone Butyrate (Topical), 978
  [Hydrocortisone, Oral (Systemic)][1], 998
  [Hydrocortisone, Parenteral (Systemic)][1], 998
  Hydrocortisone Valerate (Topical), 978
  [Methylprednisolone, Oral (Systemic)][1], 998
  [Methylprednisolone, Parenteral (Systemic)][1], 998
  Mometasone Furoate (Topical), 978
  [Prednisolone, Oral (Systemic)][1], 998
  [Prednisone (Systemic)][1], 998
  [Sulfapyridine (Systemic)][1], 2640
  Triamcinolone Acetonide (Topical), 978
  [Triamcinolone, Oral (Systemic)][1], 998
  [Triamcinolone, Parenteral (Systemic)][1], 998
**Pemphigus (treatment)**
  Amcinonide (Topical), 978
  [Azathioprine (Systemic)]1, 491
  Beclomethasone Dipropionate (Topical), 978
  Betamethasone Benzoate (Topical), 978
  Betamethasone Dipropionate (Topical), 978
  Betamethasone, Oral (Systemic), 998
  Betamethasone, Parenteral (Systemic), 998
  Betamethasone Valerate (Topical), 978
  Clobetasol Propionate (Topical), 978
  Clobetasone Butyrate (Topical), 978
  Cortisone (Systemic), 998
  Desoximetasone (Topical), 978
  Dexamethasone, Oral (Systemic), 998
  Dexamethasone, Parenteral (Systemic), 998
  Diflorasone Diacetate (Topical), 978
  Diflucortolone Valerate (Topical), 978
  Fluocinolone Acetonide (Topical), 978
  Fluocinonide (Topical), 978
  Flurandrenolide (except 0.0125% cream and ointment) (Topical), 978
  Fluticasone Propionate (Topical), 978
  Halcinonide (Topical), 978
  Halobetasol Propionate (Topical), 978
  Hydrocortisone Butyrate (Topical), 978
  Hydrocortisone, Oral (Systemic), 998
  Hydrocortisone, Parenteral (Systemic), 998
  Hydrocortisone Valerate (Topical), 978
  Methylprednisolone, Oral (Systemic), 998
  Methylprednisolone, Parenteral (Systemic), 998
  Mometasone Furoate (Topical), 978
  Prednisolone, Oral (Systemic), 998
  Prednisolone, Parenteral (Systemic), 998
  Prednisone (Systemic), 998
  Triamcinolone Acetonide (Topical), 978
  Triamcinolone, Oral (Systemic), 998
  Triamcinolone, Parenteral (Systemic), 998
**Pemphigus, fibrosis and/or nonsuppurative inflammation in (treatment)**
  Aminobenzoate Potassium (Systemic)[1], #
**Penile vasculature imaging (diagnostic adjunct)**
  Alprostadil (Local), 48
**Percutaneous transluminal coronary angioplasty assessment**
  [Fludeoxyglucose F 18 (Systemic)][1]*†, 1478

**Periarticular ossification**—*See* Ossification, heterotopic
**Pericardial effusion studies**—*See* Cardiac blood pool imaging, radionuclide
**Pericarditis (treatment)**
  [Betamethasone, Oral (Systemic)][1], 998
  [Betamethasone, Parenteral (Systemic)][1], 998
  [Cortisone (Systemic)][1], 998
  [Dexamethasone, Oral (Systemic)][1], 998
  [Dexamethasone, Parenteral (Systemic)][1], 998
  [Hydrocortisone, Oral (Systemic)][1], 998
  [Hydrocortisone, Parenteral (Systemic)][1], 998
  [Methylprednisolone, Oral (Systemic)][1], 998
  [Methylprednisolone, Parenteral (Systemic)][1], 998
  [Prednisolone, Oral (Systemic)][1], 998
  [Prednisolone, Parenteral (Systemic)][1], 998
  [Prednisone (Systemic)][1], 998
  [Triamcinolone, Oral (Systemic)][1], 998
  [Triamcinolone, Parenteral (Systemic)][1], 998
**Pericarditis, bacterial (treatment)**
  [Nafcillin, Parenteral][1], 2240
  Penicillin G, Parenteral (Systemic), 2240
  Penicillin G Procaine (Systemic), 2240
**Pericarditis, inflammation, pain, and fever associated with (treatment)**
  [Indomethacin (Systemic)][1], 388
**Pericarditis, recurrent (treatment)**
  [Colchicine (Systemic)][1], 928
**Periodontal disease (treatment)**
  Chlorhexidine (Mucosal-Local), 3014
**Periodontal infections (treatment)**
  [Metronidazole (Systemic)][1], 1996
**Periodontitis (treatment adjunct)**
  Tetracycline Periodontal Fibers (Mucosal-Local)†, #
**Perioperative infections (prophylaxis)**
  Alatrofloxacin (Systemic), 2891
  Cefamandole (Systemic) [1], 794
  Cefazolin (Systemic), 794
  Cefonicid (Systemic)†[1], 794
  Cefotaxime (Systemic), 794
  Cefotetan (Systemic), 794
  Cefoxitin (Systemic), 794
  Ceftriaxone (Systemic), 794
  Cefuroxime (Systemic), 794
  Cephalothin (Systemic), 794
  Cephapirin (Systemic)†[1], 794
  [Ticarcillin and Clavulanate (Systemic)], 2263
  Trovafloxacin (Systemic), 2891
  [Vancomycin (Systemic)][1], 2919
**Perioperative infections, colorectal (prophylaxis)**
  Metronidazole, Parenteral (Systemic), 1996
**Peripheral arterial occlusive disease (treatment)**
  Alprostadil (Systemic), 3129‡
**Peripheral nerve block**
  Bupivacaine (Parenteral-Local), 139
  Bupivacaine and Epinephrine (Parenteral-Local), 139
  Chloroprocaine (Parenteral-Local), 139
  Etidocaine (Parenteral-Local), 139
  Etidocaine and Epinephrine (Parenteral-Local), 139
  Lidocaine (Parenteral-Local), 139
  Lidocaine and Epinephrine (Parenteral-Local), 139
  Mepivacaine (Parenteral-Local), 139
  Procaine (Parenteral-Local), 139
**Peripheral progenitor cell yield, enhancement of**
  Sargramostim (Systemic)†, 941
**Peripheral progenitor cell yield, enhancement of (treatment adjunct)**
  Filgrastim (Systemic), 941
**Peripheral progenitor cell yield enhancement adjunct**
  Filgrastim (Systemic), 3143‡
**Peripheral progenitor cell yield, enhancement of, adjunct**
  Recombinant Methionyl Human Stem Cell Factor (Systemic), 3161‡
**Peritonitis**—*See* Intra-abdominal infections
**Pertussis (treatment)**
  Erythromycin (Systemic), 1368
**Petriellidiosis**—*See* Pseudoallescheriasis
**Peyronic's disease (treatment)**
  Collagenase (lyophilized) (Systemic), 3138‡
**Peyronie's disease, fibrosis and/or nonsuppurative inflammation in (treatment)**
  Aminobenzoate Potassium (Systemic), #
**Phantom limb pain**—*See* Pain, neurogenic
**Pharyngitis (treatment)**
  Azithromycin (Systemic), 499
  Cefdinir (Systemic), 3014
  Clarithromycin (Systemic), 889
**Pharyngitis, bacterial (treatment)**
  Amoxicillin (Systemic), 2240
  Ampicillin (Systemic), 2240
  Bacampicillin (Systemic), 2240
  Cefaclor (Systemic), 794

**Pharyngitis, bacterial (treatment)** *(continued)*
  Cefadroxil (Systemic), 794
  Cefixime (Systemic), 794
  Cefpodoxime (Systemic)†[1], 794
  Cefprozil (Systemic)†[1], 794
  Ceftibuten (Systemic) [1], 794
  Cefuroxime Axetil (Systemic), 794
  Cephalexin (Systemic), 794
  Cephradine (Systemic) [1], 794
  Cloxacillin, Oral (Systemic), 2240
  Demeclocycline (Systemic), 2765
  Dicloxacillin (Systemic)†, 2240
  Doxycycline (Systemic), 2765
  Flucloxacillin (Systemic)*, 2240
  Minocycline (Systemic), 2765
  Oxytetracycline (Systemic)†, 2765
  Penicillin G Benzathine (Systemic), 2240
  Penicillin G, Oral (Systemic), 2240
  Penicillin V (Systemic), 2240
  Pivampicillin (Systemic)*, 2240
  Tetracycline (Systemic), 2765
**Pharyngitis, streptococcal (treatment)**
  Dirithromycin (Systemic)†, 1250
  Erythromycin (Systemic), 1368
  Loracarbef (Systemic)†, 1880
**Pheochromocytoma (diagnosis)**
  *See also* Tumors, adrenal medulla
  [Clonidine, Oral (Systemic)][1], 908
  I 131 Iobenguane (Systemic—Diagnostic), 1747
  Iobenguane Sulfate I 131 (Systemic), R-22‡
**Pheochromocytoma (diagnostic adjunct)**
  Iobenguane Sulfate I 131 (Diagnostic), 3149‡
**Pheochromocytoma (treatment)**
  *See also* Hypertension, paroxysmal, in surgery for pheochromocytoma
  Iobenguane I 131 Sulfate (Systemic—Therapeutic)*†, 1749
  Metyrosine (Systemic)†, #
  Phenoxybenzamine (Systemic), 2312
  [Prazosin (Systemic)][1], 2370
**Pheochromocytoma (treatment adjunct)**
  [Acebutolol (Systemic)][1], 593
  [Atenolol (Systemic)][1], 593
  [Labetalol (Systemic)][1], 593
  [Metoprolol (Systemic)][1], 593
  [Nadolol (Systemic)][1], 593
  [Oxprenolol (Systemic)*[1], 593
  Propranolol (Systemic), 593
  [Sotalol (Systemic)][1], 593
  [Timolol (Systemic)][1], 593
**Phlebography**—*See* Venography
**Photosensitivity reactions in erythropoietic protoporphyria (prophylaxis)**
  [Beta-carotene (Systemic)][1], 612
  L-Cysteine (Systemic), 3150‡
**Photosensitivity reactions in erythropoietic protoporphyria (treatment)**
  [Beta-carotene (Systemic)][1], 612
  L-Cysteine (Systemic), 3150‡
**Phycomycosis**—*See* Mucormycosis
**Pinta (treatment)**
  [Demeclocycline (Systemic)], 2765
  [Doxycycline (Systemic)], 2765
  [Minocycline (Systemic)], 2765
  [Oxytetracycline (Systemic)]†, 2765
  Penicillin G Benzathine (Systemic), 2240
  Penicillin G Procaine (Systemic), 2240
  [Tetracycline (Systemic)], 2765
**Pinworm**—*See* Enterobiasis
**Pituitary function studies**
  Protirelin (Systemic), #
***Pityriasis rosea* (treatment)**
  Amcinonide (Topical), 978
  Beclomethasone Dipropionate (Topical), 978
  Betamethasone Benzoate (Topical), 978
  Betamethasone Dipropionate (Topical), 978
  Betamethasone Valerate (Topical), 978
  Clobetasol Propionate (Topical), 978
  Clobetasone Butyrate (Topical), 978
  Desoximetasone (Topical), 978
  Diflorasone Diacetate (Topical), 978
  Diflucortolone Valerate (Topical), 978
  Fluocinolone Acetonide (Topical), 978
  Fluocinonide (Topical), 978
  Flurandrenolide (except 0.0125% cream and ointment) (Topical), 978
  Fluticasone Propionate (Topical), 978
  Halcinonide (Topical), 978
  Halobetasol Propionate (Topical), 978
  Hydrocortisone Butyrate (Topical), 978
  Hydrocortisone Valerate (Topical), 978
  Mometasone Furoate (Topical), 978
  Triamcinolone Acetonide (Topical), 978
***Pityriasis rubra pilaris* (treatment)**
  [Etretinate (Systemic)], #
  [Isotretinoin (Systemic)]1, 1796

USP DI
Indications Index 3221

**Pityriasis versicolor (treatment)**
See also Tinea versicolor
Haloprogin (Topical), #
Ketoconazole (Systemic), 302
Ketoconazole (Topical), 1807
**Placenta localization**
Sodium Pertechnetate Tc 99m (Systemic), 2612
**Plague (prophylaxis)**
Plague Vaccine (Systemic), #
**Plague (treatment)**
[Demeclocycline (Systemic)], 2765
[Doxycycline (Systemic)], 2765
[Minocycline (Systemic)], 2765
[Oxytetracycline (Systemic)]†, 2765
Streptomycin (Systemic), 69
[Tetracycline (Systemic)], 2765
**Plaque, dental (prophylaxis)**
[Chlorhexidine (Mucosal-Local)]†, 847
Sodium Fluoride and Triclosan (Dental), 3034
**Platelet aggregation (prophylaxis)**
Aspirin, Buffered (Systemic), 2538
Aspirin Delayed-release Tablets USP (Systemic), 2538
Aspirin, Sodium Bicarbonate, and Citric Acid (Systemic)[1], 477
Aspirin Tablets USP (Systemic), 2538
Aspirin Tablets USP (Chewable) (Systemic), 2538
Dipyridamole (Systemic), #
**Platelet recovery, accelerating, in hematopoietic stem cell transplantation**
Human Thrombopoietin, Recombinant (Systemic), 3161‡
**Platelets, labeling of**
[Indium In 111 Oxyquinoline (Systemic)]†, 1695
[Sodium Chromate Cr 51 (Systemic)], 2590
**Platelet survival studies**
See also Platelets, labeling of
[Sodium Chromate Cr 51 (Systemic)], 2590
**Pleural effusion, malignant (treatment)**
Bleomycin Sulfate (Systemic), 3134‡
Talc, Sterile, Aerosol (Systemic), 3166‡
**Pleural effusions, malignant, recurrence (prophylaxis)**
Talc (Intrapleural-Local), 6319
**Pneumococcal disease (prophylaxis)**
Pneumococcal Vaccine Polyvalent (Systemic), 2337
**Pneumonia (treatment)**
Vancomycin (Systemic), 2919
**Pneumonia (treatment adjunct)**
Acetylcysteine (Inhalation-Local), #
**Pneumonia, anaerobic (treatment)**
Clindamycin (Systemic), 893
**Pneumonia, bacterial (treatment)**
Amoxicillin (Systemic), 2240
Amoxicillin and Clavulanate (Systemic), 2263, 3010
Ampicillin (Systemic), 2240
Bacampicillin (Systemic), 2240
Carbenicillin, Parenteral (Systemic), 2240
Cefaclor (Systemic), 794
[Cefadroxil (Systemic)], 794
Cefamandole (Systemic), 794
Cefazolin (Systemic), 794
[Cefepime (Systemic)], 794
Cefotaxime (Systemic), 794
Cefoxitin (Systemic), 794
Cefpodoxime (Systemic)†[1], 794
[Cefprozil (Systemic)]†[1], 794
Ceftazidime (Systemic), 794
Ceftriaxone (Systemic) [1], 794
Cefuroxime (Systemic), 794
[Cefuroxime Axetil (Systemic)], 794, 2240
[Cephalothin (Systemic)], 794
Cephradine (Systemic) [1], 794
Clarithromycin (Systemic), 889
Cloxacillin (Systemic), 2240
Dicloxacillin (Systemic)†, 2240
Grepafloxacin (Systemic), 1580
Mezlocillin (Systemic)†, 2240
Penicillin G, Parenteral (Systemic), 2240
Penicillin G Procaine (Systemic), 2240
Piperacillin (Systemic), 2240
Piperacillin and Tazobactam (Systemic), 2263
Ticarcillin (Systemic), 2240
Ticarcillin and Clavulanate (Systemic), 2263
**Pneumonia, bacterial, gram-negative (treatment)**
Amikacin (Systemic), 69
Aztreonam (Systemic)†, 502
Ciprofloxacin (Systemic), 1487
Gentamicin (Systemic), 69
Imipenem and Cilastatin (Systemic), 1681
Kanamycin (Systemic)†, 69
Netilmicin (Systemic), 69
Ofloxacin (Systemic), 1487
Streptomycin (Systemic), 69

**Pneumonia, bacterial, gram-negative (treatment)** (continued)
Tobramycin (Systemic), 69
**Pneumonia, Bacteroides species (treatment)**
Metronidazole (Systemic), 1996
**Pneumonia, chlamydial (treatment)**
Erythromycin (Systemic), 1368
**Pneumonia, community-acquired (treatment)**
Alatrofloxacin (Systemic), 2891
Azithromycin (Systemic), 499
Cefdinir (Systemic), 3014
Levofloxacin (Systemic), 1852
Sparfloxacin (Systemic), 2620
Trovafloxacin (Systemic), 2891
**Pneumonia, fungal (treatment)**
[Fluconazole (Systemic)][1], 302
Flucytosine (Systemic), #
[Itraconazole (Systemic)][1], 302
[Ketoconazole (Systemic)][1], 302
**Pneumonia, Haemophilus influenzae (treatment)**
Demeclocycline (Systemic), 2765
Doxycycline (Systemic), 2765
Imipenem and Cilastatin (Systemic), 1681
Loracarbef (Systemic)†, 1880
Minocycline (Systemic), 2765
Oxytetracycline (Systemic)†, 2765
Tetracycline (Systemic), 2765
**Pneumonia, Klebsiella species (treatment)**
Demeclocycline (Systemic), 2765
Doxycycline (Systemic), 2765
Minocycline (Systemic), 2765
Oxytetracycline (Systemic)†, 2765
Tetracycline (Systemic), 2765
**Pneumonia, mycoplasmal (treatment)**
[Demeclocycline (Systemic)], 2765
Dirithromycin (Systemic)†, 1250
[Doxycycline (Systemic)], 2765
Erythromycin (Systemic), 1368
[Minocycline (Systemic)], 2765
[Oxytetracycline (Systemic)]†, 2765
[Tetracycline (Systemic)], 2765
**Pneumonia, nosocomial (treatment)**
Alatrofloxacin (Systemic), 2891
Piperacillin and Tazobactam (Systemic), 3032
Trovafloxacin (Systemic), 2891
**Pneumonia, pneumococcal (treatment)**
Clindamycin (Systemic), 893
Erythromycin (Systemic), 1368
**Pneumonia, Pneumocystis carinii (prophylaxis)**
Atovaquone (Systemic), 3132‡
Clindamycin (Systemic), 3137‡
[Dapsone (Systemic)][1], 1170, 3139‡
Pentamidine (Inhalation), 2272, 3157‡
Sulfamethoxazole and Trimethoprim (Systemic)[1], 2661
**Pneumonia, Pneumocystis carinii (treatment)**
Atovaquone (Systemic), 483, 3132‡
[Clindamycin (Systemic)][1], 893
[Dapsone (Systemic)][1], 1170, 3139‡
[Pentamidine (Inhalation)][1], 2272
Pentamidine (Systemic), 2274, 3157‡
[Primaquine (Systemic)][1], 2375
[Pyrimethamine (Systemic)][1], 2433
Sulfamethoxazole and Trimethoprim (Systemic), 2661
[Trimethoprim (Systemic)][1], 2882
Trimetrexate (Systemic), 2885, 3170‡
**Pneumonia, Pneumocystis carinii (treatment adjunct)**
Primaquine (Systemic), 3160‡
**Pneumonia, Pneumocystis carinii, AIDS-associated (treatment)**
[Clindamycin (Systemic)][1], 3137‡
**Pneumonia, Pneumocystis carinii, AIDS-associated (treatment adjunct)**
[Betamethasone, Oral (Systemic)][1], 998
[Betamethasone, Parenteral (Systemic)][1], 998
[Cortisone (Systemic)][1], 998
[Dexamethasone, Oral (Systemic)][1], 998
[Dexamethasone, Parenteral (Systemic)][1], 998
[Hydrocortisone, Oral (Systemic)][1], 998
[Hydrocortisone, Parenteral (Systemic)][1], 998
[Methylprednisolone, Oral (Systemic)][1], 998
[Methylprednisolone, Parenteral (Systemic)][1], 998
[Prednisolone, Oral (Systemic)][1], 998
[Prednisolone, Parenteral (Systemic)][1], 998
[Prednisone (Systemic)][1], 998
[Triamcinolone, Oral (Systemic)][1], 998
[Triamcinolone, Parenteral (Systemic)][1], 998
**Pneumonia, staphylococcal (treatment)**
Clindamycin (Systemic), 893
Fusidic Acid (Systemic)*, 3021
Imipenem and Cilastatin (Systemic), 1681

**Pneumonia, streptococcal (treatment)**
Ciprofloxacin (Systemic), 1487
Clindamycin (Systemic), 893
Imipenem and Cilastatin (Systemic), 1681
Ofloxacin (Systemic), 1487
**Pneumonia, Streptococcus pneumoniae (treatment)**
Dirithromycin (Systemic)†, 1250
Loracarbef (Systemic)†, 1880
**Pneumonitis, aspiration (prophylaxis)**
[Cimetidine (Systemic)], 1633
[Famotidine (Systemic)], 1633
Glycopyrrolate, Parenteral (Systemic), 226
[Metoclopramide (Systemic)][1], 1992
[Ranitidine (Systemic)], 1633
Sodium Citrate and Citric Acid (Systemic), 881
Tricitrates (Systemic), 881
**Pneumonitis, aspiration (treatment)**
Betamethasone, Oral (Systemic), 998
Betamethasone, Parenteral (Systemic), 998
Cortisone (Systemic), 998
Dexamethasone, Oral (Systemic), 998
Dexamethasone, Parenteral (Systemic), 998
Hydrocortisone, Oral (Systemic), 998
Hydrocortisone, Parenteral (Systemic), 998
Methylprednisolone, Oral (Systemic), 998
Methylprednisolone, Parenteral (Systemic), 998
Prednisolone, Oral (Systemic), 998
Prednisolone, Parenteral (Systemic), 998
Prednisone (Systemic), 998
Triamcinolone, Oral (Systemic), 998
Triamcinolone, Parenteral (Systemic), 998
**Pneumonitis, eosinophilic**—See Loeffler syndrome
**Pneumothorax (prophylaxis)**
[Quinacrine (Systemic)][1], #
**Poisoning**—See Toxicity, nonspecific
**Poison ivy**—See Dermatitis, contact
**Poison oak**—See Dermatitis, contact
**Poison sumac**—See Dermatitis, contact
**Poliomyelitis (prophylaxis)**
Poliovirus Vaccine (Systemic), 2343
**Polyarteritis nodosa (treatment)**
[Betamethasone, Oral (Systemic)][1], 998
[Betamethasone, Parenteral (Systemic)][1], 998
[Cortisone (Systemic)][1], 998
[Dexamethasone, Oral (Systemic)][1], 998
[Dexamethasone, Parenteral (Systemic)][1], 998
[Hydrocortisone, Oral (Systemic)][1], 998
[Hydrocortisone, Parenteral (Systemic)][1], 998
[Methylprednisolone, Oral (Systemic)][1], 998
[Methylprednisolone, Parenteral (Systemic)][1], 998
[Prednisolone, Oral (Systemic)][1], 998
[Prednisolone, Parenteral (Systemic)][1], 998
[Prednisone (Systemic)][1], 998
[Triamcinolone, Oral (Systemic)][1], 998
[Triamcinolone, Parenteral (Systemic)][1], 998
**Polychondritis, relapsing (treatment)**
[Betamethasone, Oral (Systemic)][1], 998
[Betamethasone, Parenteral (Systemic)][1], 998
[Cortisone (Systemic)][1], 998
[Dapsone (Systemic)][1], 1170
[Dexamethasone, Oral (Systemic)][1], 998
[Dexamethasone, Parenteral (Systemic)][1], 998
[Hydrocortisone, Oral (Systemic)][1], 998
[Hydrocortisone, Parenteral (Systemic)][1], 998
[Methylprednisolone, Oral (Systemic)][1], 998
[Methylprednisolone, Parenteral (Systemic)][1], 998
[Prednisolone, Oral (Systemic)][1], 998
[Prednisolone, Parenteral (Systemic)][1], 998
[Prednisone (Systemic)][1], 998
[Triamcinolone, Oral (Systemic)][1], 998
[Triamcinolone, Parenteral (Systemic)][1], 998
**Polycystic ovary syndrome (treatment)**
[Desogestrel and Ethinyl Estradiol (Systemic)][1], 1397
[Ethynodiol Diacetate and Ethinyl Estradiol (Systemic)][1], 1397
[Levonorgestrel and Ethinyl Estradiol (Systemic)][1], 1397
[Medroxyprogesterone (Systemic)][1], 2400
[Norethindrone Acetate and Ethinyl Estradiol (Systemic)][1], 1397
[Norethindrone and Ethinyl Estradiol (Systemic)][1], 1397
[Norethindrone and Mestranol (Systemic)][1], 1397
[Norgestimate and Ethinyl Estradiol (Systemic)][1], 1397
[Norgestrel and Ethinyl Estradiol (Systemic)][1], 1397
[Spironolactone (Systemic)][1], 1266
Urofollitropin (Systemic), 2901, 3170‡
**Polycythemia rubra vera (treatment)**
Sodium Phosphate P 32 (Systemic), 2616
**Polycythemia vera (diagnosis)**—See Bone marrow imaging, radionuclide; Red blood cell volume or mass determinations

## Polycythemia vera (treatment)
[Hydroxyurea (Systemic)]1, 1666
[Interferon Alfa-2a, Recombinant (Systemic)]1, 1740
[Interferon Alfa-2b, Recombinant (Systemic)]1, 1740

## Polymorphous light eruption (prophylaxis)
[Beta-carotene (Systemic)]1, 612

## Polymorphous light eruption (treatment)
Alclometasone Dipropionate (Topical), 978
Beclomethasone Dipropionate (Topical), 978
[Beta-carotene (Systemic)]1, 612
Betamethasone Benzoate (Topical), 978
Betamethasone Valerate (Topical), 978
[Chloroquine, Oral (Systemic)]1, 849
Clobetasone Butyrate (Topical), 978
Clocortolone Pivalate (Topical), 978
Desonide (Topical), 978
Desoximetasone (0.05% cream only) (Topical), 978
Dexamethasone (Topical), 978
Dexamethasone Sodium Phosphate (Topical), 978
Diflucortolone Valerate (Topical), 978
Flumethasone Pivalate (Topical), 978
Fluocinolone Acetonide (except 0.2% cream) (Topical), 978
Flurandrenolide (Topical), 978
Fluticasone Propionate (Topical), 978
Hydrocortisone (Topical), 978
Hydrocortisone Acetate (Topical), 978
Hydrocortisone Butyrate (Topical), 978
Hydrocortisone Valerate (Topical), 978
[Hydroxychloroquine (Systemic)]1, 1663
Methylprednisolone Acetate (Topical), 978
Mometasone Furoate (Topical), 978
Triamcinolone Acetonide (except 0.5% cream and ointment) (Topical), 978

## Polymyalgia rheumatica (treatment)
[Betamethasone, Oral (Systemic)]1, 998
[Betamethasone, Parenteral (Systemic)]1, 998
[Cortisone (Systemic)]1, 998
[Dexamethasone, Oral (Systemic)]1, 998
[Dexamethasone, Parenteral (Systemic)]1, 998
[Hydrocortisone, Oral (Systemic)]1, 998
[Hydrocortisone, Parenteral (Systemic)]1, 998
[Methylprednisolone, Oral (Systemic)]1, 998
[Methylprednisolone, Parenteral (Systemic)]1, 998
[Prednisolone, Oral (Systemic)]1, 998
[Prednisolone, Parenteral (Systemic)]1, 998
[Prednisone (Systemic)]1, 998
[Triamcinolone, Oral (Systemic)]1, 998
[Triamcinolone, Parenteral (Systemic)]1, 998

## Polymyositis—See Dermatomyositis, systemic

## Polyneuropathies, chronic inflammatory demyelinating (treatment)
[Immune Globulin Intravenous (Human) (Systemic)]1, 1686

## Polyposis coli, adenomatous (treatment)
FGN-1 (Systemic), 3143‡

## Polyps, nasal (treatment)
Beclomethasone (Nasal), 961
Betamethasone, Oral (Systemic)1, 998
Betamethasone, Parenteral (Systemic)1, 998
Budesonide (Nasal), 3012
Budesonide (Nasal)*, 961
Cortisone (Systemic)1, 998
Dexamethasone (Nasal)†, 961
Dexamethasone, Oral (Systemic)1, 998
Dexamethasone, Parenteral (Systemic)1, 998
Flunisolide (Nasal), 961
Hydrocortisone, Oral (Systemic)1, 998
Hydrocortisone, Parenteral (Systemic)1, 998
Methylprednisolone, Oral (Systemic)1, 998
Methylprednisolone, Parenteral (Systemic)1, 998
Prednisolone, Oral (Systemic)1, 998
Prednisolone, Parenteral (Systemic)1, 998
Prednisone (Systemic)1, 998
Triamcinolone (Nasal), 961
Triamcinolone, Oral (Systemic)1, 998
Triamcinolone, Parenteral (Systemic)1, 998

## Polyps, nasal, postsurgical recurrence of (prophylaxis)
Beclomethasone (Nasal), 961, 3011
Budesonide (Nasal), 3012
Budesonide Nasal Solution (Nasal)*, 961
[Dexamethasone (Nasal)]†, 961
[Flunisolide (Nasal)], 961
[Triamcinolone (Nasal)], 961

## Polyps, nasal, severe (treatment)
[Betamethasone, Parenteral-Local (Systemic)]1, 998
[Dexamethasone, Parenteral-Local (Systemic)]1, 998
[Methylprednisolone, Parenteral-Local (Systemic)]1, 998
[Prednisolone, Parenteral-Local (Systemic)]1, 998

## Polyps, nasal, severe (treatment) (continued)
[Triamcinolone, Parenteral-Local (Systemic)]1, 998

## Polyradiculopathy (treatment)
[Ganciclovir, Parenteral (Systemic)]1, 1544

## Polyserositis, recurrent, familial—See Mediterranean fever, familial

## Pork tapeworm—See Taeniasis
## Pork worm—See Trichinosis

## Porphyria, acute, intermittent (treatment)
Chlorpromazine (Systemic), 2289
Hemin (Systemic), 3022, 3145‡
Histrelin (Systemic), 3145‡

## Porphyria, acute, symptomatic stage (treatment)
Heme Arginate (Systemic), 3145‡

## Porphyria cutanea tarda (treatment)
[Chloroquine, Oral (Systemic)]1, 849
[Hydroxychloroquine (Systemic)]1, 1663

## Porphyria variegata (treatment)
Hemin (Systemic), 3022, 3145‡
Histrelin (Systemic), 3145‡

## Porphyric syndromes, acute (treatment)
Hemin and Zinc Mesoporphyrin (Systemic), 3145‡

## Post-poliomyelitis syndrome (treatment)
Recombinant Human Insulin-like Growth Factor-I (Systemic), 3161‡

## Prader-Willi syndrome (treatment)
Etiocholanedione (Systemic), 3142‡

## Pregnancy (diagnosis)
Immunoassay Pregnancy Test Kits, #

## Pregnancy (prophylaxis)
Benzalkonium Chloride (Vaginal)*, #
Cervical Cap, Cavity-rim, 3014
Condom, Female, Polyurethane, 3015
Condom, Male, Polyurethane, 3016
Condoms, Lamb Cecum, 1474
Condoms, Lamb Cecum, and Nonoxynol 9, 1474
Condoms, Latex, 1474
Condoms, Latex, and Nonoxynol 9, 1474
Copper-T 200 Intrauterine Device*, #
Copper-T 200Ag Intrauterine Device*, #
Copper-T 380A Intrauterine Device†, #
Copper-T 380S Intrauterine Device*, #
Desogestrel and Ethinyl Estradiol (Systemic), 1397
Ethynodiol Diacetate and Ethinyl Estradiol (Systemic), 1397
Levonorgestrel (Systemic), 2400
Levonorgestrel and Ethinyl Estradiol (Systemic), 1397, 3027
Medroxyprogesterone, Parenteral (Systemic), 2400
Nonoxynol 9 (Vaginal), #
Norethindrone Acetate and Ethinyl Estradiol (Systemic), 1397
Norethindrone and Ethinyl Estradiol (Systemic), 1397
Norethindrone and Mestranol (Systemic), 1397
Norethindrone Tablets USP (Systemic), 2400
Norgestimate and Ethinyl Estradiol (Systemic), 1397
Norgestrel (Systemic)†, 2400
Norgestrel and Ethinyl Estradiol (Systemic), 1397
Octoxynol 9 (Vaginal), #
Progesterone Intrauterine Device (IUD)†, 2396

## Premenstrual dysphoric disorder (treatment)
[Fluoxetine (Systemic)]1, 1503

## Priapism (treatment)
[Epinephrine Injection USP (Systemic)]1, 651

## Primary lateral sclerosis (treatment)
Ciliary Neurotrophic Factor, Recombinant Human (Systemic), 3137‡

## Proctitis (treatment)—See Bowel disease, inflammatory

## Proctitis, factitial (treatment)
Hydrocortisone (Rectal), 973

## Proctitis, radiation, chronic (treatment)
Short Chain Fatty Acid Enema (Systemic), 3164‡

## Proctosigmoiditis—See Bowel disease, inflammatory

## Prolactinomas, pituitary (treatment)
Bromocriptine (Systemic), 636
Cabergoline (Systemic), 704

## Prostatic hyperplasia, benign—See Benign prostatic hyperplasia
## Prostatic hypertrophy, benign—See Benign prostatic hyperplasia

## Prostatitis (treatment)
Carbenicillin, Oral (Systemic), 2240

## Prostatitis (treatment adjunct)—See Irritative voiding, symptoms of

## Prostatitis, bacterial (treatment)
[Ciprofloxacin (Systemic)]1, 1487
Norfloxacin (Systemic)1, 1487
Ofloxacin (Systemic), 1487
Trovafloxacin (Systemic), 2891

## Protein C deficiency (prophylaxis)
Protein C Concentrate (Systemic), 3158‡

## Protein C deficiency (treatment)
Protein C Concentrate (Systemic), 3160‡

## Prototheocosis, invasive (treatment)
Amphotericin B Lipid Complex (Systemic), 3130‡

## PRP—See Pityriasis rubra pilaris

## Pruritus, aquagenic (treatment)
[Capsaicin (Topical)], 753

## Pruritus, hemodialysis-induced (treatment)
[Capsaicin (Topical)], 753

## Pruritus (treatment)
Acrivastine (Systemic)*†, 325
Astemizole (Systemic), 325
Azatadine (Systemic), 325
Bromodiphenhydramine (Systemic)*†, 325
Brompheniramine (Systemic), 325
Carbinoxamine (Systemic)*†, 325
Cetirizine (Systemic), 325
Chlorpheniramine (Systemic), 325
Clemastine (Systemic), 325
Cyproheptadine (Systemic), 325
Dexchlorpheniramine (Systemic), 325
Dimenhydrinate (Systemic), 325
Diphenhydramine (Systemic), 325
Diphenylpyraline (Systemic)*†, 325
[Doxepin (Systemic)]1, 271
Doxylamine (Systemic)†, 325
Hydroxyzine (Systemic), 325
Loratadine (Systemic), 325
Methdilazine (Systemic)†, 377
Phenindamine (Systemic)†, 325
Promethazine (Systemic), 377
Pyrilamine (Systemic)*†, 325
Trimeprazine (Systemic), 377
Tripelennamine (Systemic), 325
Triprolidine (Systemic)*†, 325

## Pruritus ani—See Pruritus, anogenital

## Pruritus, anogenital (treatment)
Alclometasone Dipropionate (Topical), 978
Beclomethasone Dipropionate (Topical), 978
Benzocaine Ointment USP (Rectal) (Mucosal-Local), 128
Betamethasone Benzoate (Topical), 978
Betamethasone Valerate (Topical), 978
Clioquinol and Flumethasone (Topical)*, 3015
Clioquinol and Hydrocortisone (Topical), #
Clobetasone Butyrate (Topical), 978
Clocortolone Pivalate (Topical), 978
Desonide (Topical), 978
Desoximetasone (0.05% cream only) (Topical), 978
Dexamethasone (Topical), 978
Dexamethasone Sodium Phosphate (Topical), 978
Dibucaine (Mucosal-Local), 128
Diflucortolone Valerate (Topical), 978
Flumethasone Pivalate (Topical), 978
Fluocinolone Acetonide (except 0.2% cream) (Topical), 978
Flurandrenolide (Topical), 978
Fluticasone Propionate (Topical), 978
Hydrocortisone (Rectal), 973
Hydrocortisone (Topical), 978
Hydrocortisone Acetate (Topical), 978
Hydrocortisone Butyrate (Topical), 978
Hydrocortisone Rectal Ointment (Topical)*, 978
Hydrocortisone Suppositories (Topical), 978
Hydrocortisone Valerate (Topical), 978
Methylprednisolone Acetate (Topical), 978
Mometasone Furoate (Topical), 978
Pramoxine Hydrochloride Aerosol Foam (Mucosal-Local), 128
Pramoxine Hydrochloride Cream USP (Mucosal-Local), 128
Tetracaine, Rectal (Mucosal-Local), 128
Triamcinolone Acetonide (except 0.5% cream and ointment) (Topical), 978

## Pruritus, anorectal (treatment)
Bufexamac (Topical)*, 3013

## Pruritus, associated with eczema (treatment)
Doxepin (Topical), 1305

## Pruritus, associated with partial biliary obstruction (treatment)
Cholestyramine (Oral-Local), 853
[Colestipol (Oral-Local)]1, 934

## Pruritus, associated with pityriasis rosea (treatment)
Acrivastine (Systemic)*†, 325
[Astemizole (Systemic)]1, 325
[Azatadine (Systemic)]1, 325
Bromodiphenhydramine (Systemic)*†, 325
[Brompheniramine (Systemic)]1, 325
Carbinoxamine (Systemic)*†, 325
Cetirizine (Systemic)1, 325
[Chlorpheniramine (Systemic)]1, 325
[Clemastine (Systemic)]1, 325
[Cyproheptadine (Systemic)]1, 325
[Dexchlorpheniramine (Systemic)]1, 325

**Pruritus, associated with** *pityriasis rosea* **(treatment)** *(continued)*
  [Dimenhydrinate (Systemic)][1], 325
  [Diphenhydramine (Systemic)][1], 325
  Diphenylpyraline (Systemic)*†, 325
  [Doxylamine (Systemic)]†, 325
  [Hydroxyzine (Systemic)][1], 325
  [Loratadine (Systemic)][1], 325
  Methdilazine (Systemic)†, 377
  [Phenindamine (Systemic)]†, 325
  [Pyrilamine (Systemic)]†, 325
  [Tripelennamine (Systemic)][1], 325
  [Triprolidine (Systemic)]*†, 325
**Pruritus senilis (treatment)**
  Alclometasone Dipropionate (Topical), 978
  Beclomethasone Dipropionate (Topical), 978
  Betamethasone Benzoate (Topical), 978
  Betamethasone Valerate (Topical), 978
  Clobetasone Butyrate (Topical), 978
  Clocortolone Pivalate (Topical), 978
  Desonide (Topical), 978
  Desoximetasone (0.05% cream only) (Topical), 978
  Dexamethasone (Topical), 978
  Dexamethasone Sodium Phosphate (Topical), 978
  Diflucortolone Valerate (Topical), 978
  Flumethasone Pivalate (Topical), 978
  Fluocinolone Acetonide (except 0.2% cream) (Topical), 978
  Flurandrenolide (Topical), 978
  Fluticasone Propionate (Topical), 978
  Hydrocortisone (Topical), 978
  Hydrocortisone Acetate (Topical), 978
  Hydrocortisone Butyrate (Topical), 978
  Hydrocortisone Valerate (Topical), 978
  Methylprednisolone Acetate (Topical), 978
  Mometasone Furoate (Topical), 978
  Triamcinolone Acetonide (except 0.5% cream and ointment) (Topical), 978
**Pruritus vulvae (treatment)**
  *See also* Vulvar atrophy
  Bufexamac (Topical)*, 3013
**Pseudogout**—*See* Calcium pyrophosphate deposition disease, acute
**Pseudohypoparathyroidism (diagnosis)**
  Teriparatide (Systemic)†, #, 3167‡
**Pseudohypoparathyroidism (treatment)**
  Alfacalcidol (Systemic)*, 2966
  [Calcifediol (Systemic)]†, 2966
  Calcitriol (Systemic), 2966
  Dihydrotachysterol (Systemic), 2966
  Ergocalciferol (Systemic), 2966
**Pseudotumor cerebri (treatment)**
  [Dexamethasone, Oral (Systemic)][1], 998
  [Dexamethasone, Parenteral (Systemic)][1], 998
**Psittacosis (treatment)**
  Demeclocycline (Systemic), 2765
  Doxycycline (Systemic), 2765
  Minocycline (Systemic), 2765
  Oxytetracycline (Systemic)†, 2765
  Tetracycline (Systemic), 2765
**Psoriasis (treatment)**
  Amcinonide (Topical), 978
  Anthralin (Topical), 218
  Beclomethasone Dipropionate (Topical), 978
  Betamethasone Benzoate (Topical), 978
  Betamethasone Dipropionate (Topical), 978
  Betamethasone Valerate (Topical), 978
  Calcipotriene (Topical), 711
  Clobetasol Propionate (Topical), 978
  Clobetasone Butyrate (Topical), 978
  Coal Tar (Topical), #
  Desoximetasone (Topical), 978
  Diflorasone Diacetate (Topical), 978
  Diflucortolone Valerate (Topical), 978
  Etretinate (Systemic), #
  Fluocinolone Acetonide (Topical), 978
  Fluocinonide (Topical), 978
  Flurandrenolide (except 0.0125% cream and ointment) (Topical), 978
  Fluticasone Propionate (Topical), 978
  Halcinonide (Topical), 978
  Halobetasol Propionate (Topical), 978
  Hydrocortisone Butyrate (Topical), 978
  Hydrocortisone Valerate (Topical), 978
  Methotrexate—For Noncancerous Conditions (Systemic), 1969
  [Methoxsalen (Topical)], 1977
  Methoxsalen (Systemic), 1973
  Mometasone Furoate (Topical), 978
  Resorcinol (Topical), 1#
  Salicylic Acid Gel USP (Topical), #
  Salicylic Acid Ointment (Topical), #
  Tazarotene (Topical), 2692
  Triamcinolone Acetonide (Topical), 978
  [Trioxsalen (Systemic)], #

**Psoriasis, facial and intertriginous areas (treatment)**
  Alclometasone Dipropionate (Topical), 978
  Beclomethasone Dipropionate (Topical), 978
  Betamethasone Benzoate (Topical), 978
  Betamethasone Valerate (Topical), 978
  Clobetasone Butyrate (Topical), 978
  Clocortolone Pivalate (Topical), 978
  Desonide (Topical), 978
  Desoximetasone (0.05% cream only) (Topical), 978
  Dexamethasone (Topical), 978
  Dexamethasone Sodium Phosphate (Topical), 978
  Diflucortolone Valerate (Topical), 978
  Flumethasone Pivalate (Topical), 978
  Fluocinolone Acetonide (except 0.2% cream) (Topical), 978
  Flurandrenolide (Topical), 978
  Fluticasone Propionate (Topical), 978
  Hydrocortisone (Topical), 978
  Hydrocortisone Acetate (Topical), 978
  Hydrocortisone Butyrate (Topical), 978
  Hydrocortisone Valerate (Topical), 978
  Methylprednisolone Acetate (Topical), 978
  Mometasone Furoate (Topical), 978
  Triamcinolone Acetonide (except 0.5% cream and ointment) (Topical), 978
**Psoriasis, of scalp (treatment)**
  Calcipotriene (Topical), 711
  Salicylic Acid, Sulfur, and Coal Tar (Topical), #
**Psoriasis, severe (treatment)**
  Acitretin (Systemic), 18
  Betamethasone, Oral (Systemic), 998
  Betamethasone, Parenteral (Systemic), 998
  Betamethasone, Parenteral-Local (Systemic), 998
  Cortisone (Systemic), 998
  Cyclosporine (Systemic), 1136
  Dexamethasone (Systemic), 998
  Hydrocortisone, Oral (Systemic), 998
  Hydrocortisone, Parenteral (Systemic), 998
  Hydrocortisone, Parenteral-Local (Systemic), 998
  Methylprednisolone, Oral (Systemic), 998
  Methylprednisolone, Parenteral (Systemic), 998
  Methylprednisolone, Parenteral-Local (Systemic), 998
  Prednisolone (Systemic), 998
  Prednisone (Systemic), 998
  Triamcinolone (Systemic), 998
**Psychotic disorders (treatment)**
  Acetophenazine (Systemic)†, 2289
  [Carbamazepine (Systemic)][1], 757
  Chlorpromazine (Systemic), 2289
  Chlorprothixene (Systemic)†, 2793
  [Droperidol (Systemic)][1], 1319
  Flupenthixol (Systemic)*, 2793
  Fluphenazine (Systemic), 2289
  Fluspirilene (Systemic)*, 3020
  Haloperidol (Systemic), 1611
  Loxapine (Systemic), 1889
  Mesoridazine (Systemic), 2289
  [Methotrimeprazine (Systemic)], 2289
  Molindone (Systemic)†, 2050
  Olanzapine (Systemic), 2156
  Pericyazine (Systemic)*, 2289
  Perphenazine (Systemic), 2289
  [Pimozide (Systemic)], 2326
  Pipotiazine (Systemic)*, 2289
  Prochlorperazine (Systemic), 2289
  Promazine (Systemic), 2289
  Quetiapine (Systemic), 2437
  Risperidone (Systemic), 2508
  Thiopropazate (Systemic)*, 2289
  Thioproperazine (Systemic)*, 2289
  Thioridazine (Systemic), 2289
  Thiothixene (Systemic), 2793
  Trifluoperazine (Systemic), 2289
  Triflupromazine (Systemic)†, 2289
**Puberty, central precocious (treatment)**
  Histrelin (Systemic), 1644
  Nafarelin (Systemic), 2076
**Puberty, delayed (treatment)**
  [Gonadorelin (Systemic)][1], 1571
  Oxandrolone (Systemic), 3156‡
**Puberty, delayed, male (treatment)**
  Fluoxymesterone (Systemic), 118
  Methyltestosterone (Systemic), 118
  Testosterone (Systemic), 118
  Testosterone Sublingual (Systemic), 3168‡
**Puberty, precocious (treatment)**
  [Danazol (Systemic)][1], 1163
  Deslorelin (Systemic), 3140‡
  Histrelin (Systemic), 3145‡
  Leuprolide (Systemic), 1840
  Leuprolide Acetate (Systemic), 3151‡
  [Medroxyprogesterone, Parenteral (Systemic)][1], 2400

**Puberty, precocious (treatment)** *(continued)*
  Nafarelin (Systemic), 3155‡
**Pulmonary disease (diagnosis)**—*See* Lung imaging, radionuclide
**Pulmonary disease, chronic obstructive (treatment)**
  Aminophylline (Systemic), 668
  [Betamethasone, Oral (Systemic)], 998
  [Betamethasone, Parenteral (Systemic)], 998
  [Cortisone (Systemic)], 998
  [Dexamethasone, Oral (Systemic)], 998
  [Dexamethasone, Parenteral (Systemic)], 998
  [Hydrocortisone, Oral (Systemic)], 998
  [Hydrocortisone, Parenteral (Systemic)], 998
  Ipratropium (Inhalation-Local), 1761
  Ipratropium and Albuterol (Inhalation-Local), 1765
  [Methylprednisolone, Oral (Systemic)], 998
  [Methylprednisolone, Parenteral (Systemic)], 998
  Oxtriphylline (Systemic), 668
  Oxtriphylline and Guaifenesin (Systemic), #
  [Prednisolone, Oral (Systemic)], 998
  [Prednisolone, Parenteral (Systemic)], 998
  [Prednisone (Systemic)], 998
  Theophylline (Systemic), 668
  [Triamcinolone, Oral (Systemic)], 998
  [Triamcinolone, Parenteral (Systemic)], 998
**Pulmonary disease, chronic obstructive, other (treatment)**
  Theophylline and Guaifenesin (Systemic)†, #
**Pulmonary disease, obstructive (treatment)**
  Albuterol (Systemic), 651
  Ephedrine (Systemic), 651
  Epinephrine (Systemic), 651
  Ethylnorepinephrine (Systemic)†, 651
  Fenoterol (Systemic)*, 651
  Isoproterenol, Oral (Systemic), 651
  Metaproterenol (Systemic), 651
  Terbutaline (Systemic), 651
**Pulmonary emboli (prophylaxis)**
  Acenocoumarol (Systemic)*, 3009
**Pulmonary emboli (treatment)**
  Acenocoumarol (Systemic)*, 3009
**Pulmonary emboli, due to Protein C deficiency (prophylaxis)**
  Protein C Concentrate (Systemic), 3160‡
**Pulmonary emboli, due to Protein C deficiency (treatment)**
  Protein C Concentrate (Systemic), 3160‡
**Pulmonary function studies**
  Krypton Kr 81m (Systemic), 1816
  Xenon Xe 127 (Systemic), 2982
  Xenon Xe 133 (Systemic), 2984
**Pulmonary function studies, fetal**
  [Oxytocin, Parenteral (Systemic)][1], 2211
**Pulmonary imaging, radionuclide**—*See* Lung imaging, radionuclide
**Pulmonary infections, in cystic fibrosis (treatment)**
  [Cefaclor (Systemic)], 794
  [Cefamandole (Systemic)], 794
  Ceftazidime (Systemic)[1], 794
**Pulmonary infections,** *Pseudomonas aeruginosa* **(prophylaxis)**
  Mucoid Exopolysaccharide Pseudomonas Hyperimmune Globulin (Systemic), 3155‡
**Pulmonary infections,** *Pseudomonas aeruginosa* **(treatment)**
  Mucoid Exopolysaccharide Pseudomonas Hyperimmune Globulin (Systemic), 3155‡
**Purpura fulminans, associated with Protein C deficiency (prophylaxis)**
  Protein C Concentrate (Systemic), 3160‡
**Purpura fulminans, associated with Protein C deficiency (treatment)**
  Protein C Concentrate (Systemic), 3160‡
**Purpura fulminans, in meningococcemia (prophylaxis)**
  Protein C Concentrate (Systemic), 3160‡
**Purpura fulminans, in meningococcemia (treatment)**
  Protein C Concentrate (Systemic), 3160‡
**Pustular infections (treatment)**
  Sulfurated Lime Topical Solution (Topical)†, #
**Pustulosis, palmoplantar (treatment)**
  [Etretinate (Systemic)], #
**Pyelography, retrograde**
  Diatrizoate Meglumine (Local), #
  Diatrizoate Sodium (Local), #
  Iothalamate (Local), #
**Pyelonephritis (treatment)**
  Levofloxacin (Systemic), 1852
**Pyoderma gangrenosum (treatment)**
  [Dapsone (Systemic)][1], 1170
  [Sulfapyridine (Systemic)][1], 2640
**Pyridoxine deficiency (prophylaxis)**
  Pyridoxine (Systemic), 2430

## Q–R

**Pyridoxine deficiency (treatment)**
Pyridoxine (Systemic), 2430
**Pyrimethamine toxicity**—See Toxicity, pyrimethamine
**Pyruvate carboxylase deficiency (treatment)**
[Thiamine (Systemic)], 2787

**Q fever (treatment)**
Chloramphenicol (Systemic), 841
Demeclocycline (Systemic), 2765
Doxycycline (Systemic), 2765
Minocycline (Systemic), 2765
Oxytetracycline (Systemic)†, 2765
Tetracycline (Systemic), 2765
**Rabies (prophylaxis)**
Rabies Immune Globulin (Systemic), 2448
Rabies Vaccine Adsorbed (Systemic)†, 2449
Rabies Vaccine, Human Diploid Cell (Systemic), 2449
**Radiation protectant, thyroid gland**
[Iodine, Strong (Systemic)][1], 1751
Potassium Iodide (Systemic), 2354
**Radiodermatitis (treatment)**
Bufexamac (Topical)*, 3013
[Fluorouracil (Topical)][1], 1500
**Radiography, bowel, adjunct**
[Simethicone (Oral-Local)][1], #
**Radiography, gastrointestinal**
Barium Sulfate (Local), #
Diatrizoate Meglumine and Diatrizoate Sodium, Oral or Rectal (Systemic), #
Diatrizoate Sodium, Oral or Rectal (Systemic), #
Iohexol (Systemic)[1], #
**Radiography, gastrointestinal, adjunct**
Glucagon (Systemic), 1563
Metoclopramide, Parenteral (Systemic), 1992
**Rat-bite fever (treatment)**
Penicillin G, Parenteral (Systemic), 2240
Penicillin G Procaine (Systemic), 2240
[Penicillin V (Systemic)][1], 2240
**Rat tapeworm**—See Hymenolepiasis
**Raynaud's phenomenon (treatment)**
[Felodipine (Systemic)], 720
[Isradipine (Systemic)]†, 720
[Nicardipine (Systemic)], 720
[Nifedipine (Systemic)][1], 720
Nylidrin (Systemic)*, #
[Prazosin (Systemic)][1], 2370
[Reserpine (Systemic)][1], 2460
**RDS**—See Respiratory distress syndrome
**Rectal infections, uncomplicated (treatment)**
Doxycycline (Systemic), 2765
Minocycline (Systemic), 2765
Oxytetracycline (Systemic)†, 2765
Tetracycline (Systemic), 2765
**Red blood cell resuspension**
Albumin Human (Systemic), 34
**Red blood cell sequestration studies**
Sodium Chromate Cr 51 (Systemic), 2590
**Red blood cells, labeling of**
See also Cardiac blood pool imaging, radionuclide; Bleeding, gastrointestinal
Sodium Chromate Cr 51 (Systemic), 2590
[Sodium Pertechnetate Tc 99m (Systemic)][1], 2612
Technetium Tc 99m Pyrophosphate (Systemic)†, 2729
Technetium Tc 99m (Pyro- and trimeta-) Phosphates (Systemic), 2733
**Red blood cells, labeling of, adjunct**
Ascorbic Acid, Parenteral (Systemic), 469
**Red blood cell survival time determinations**
Sodium Chromate Cr 51 (Systemic), 2590
**Red blood cell volume or mass determinations**
Sodium Chromate Cr 51 (Systemic), 2590
**Red measles**—See Measles
**Reflux, gastroesophageal (diagnosis)**—See Esophageal imaging, radionuclide
**Reflux, gastroesophageal (prophylaxis)**
Cisapride (Systemic), 869
**Reflux, gastroesophageal (treatment)**
Alumina, Calcium Carbonate, and Sodium Bicarbonate (Oral-Local)*, 188
Alumina and Magnesia (Oral-Local), 188
Alumina, Magnesia, Calcium Carbonate, and Simethicone (Oral-Local)†, 188
Alumina, Magnesia, and Magnesium Carbonate (Oral-Local)*, 188
Alumina, Magnesia, Magnesium Carbonate, and Simethicone (Oral-Local)*, 188
Alumina, Magnesia, and Simethicone (Oral-Local), 188
Alumina, Magnesia Alginate, and Magnesium Carbonate (Oral-Local)*, 188

**Reflux, gastroesophageal (treatment)** (continued)
Alumina and Magnesium Carbonate (Oral-Local)†, 188
Alumina, Magnesium Carbonate, and Simethicone (Oral-Local)†, 188
Alumina, Magnesium Carbonate, and Sodium Bicarbonate (Oral-Local)†, 188
Alumina and Magnesium Trisilicate (Oral-Local)†, 188
Alumina, Magnesium Trisilicate, and Sodium Bicarbonate (Oral-Local)†, 188
Alumina and Simethicone (Oral-Local)†, 188
Alumina and Sodium Bicarbonate (Oral-Local)*, 188
Aluminum Carbonate, Basic (Oral-Local)†, 188
Aluminum Carbonate, Basic and Simethicone (Oral-Local)†, 188
Aluminum Hydroxide (Oral-Local), 188
[Bethanechol, Oral (Systemic)], 614
Calcium Carbonate (Oral-Local)†, 188
Calcium Carbonate and Magnesia (Oral-Local)†, 188
Calcium Carbonate, Magnesia, and Simethicone (Oral-Local)†, 188
Calcium and Magnesium Carbonates (Oral-Local)†, 188
Calcium Carbonate and Simethicone (Oral-Local)†, 188
Cimetidine (Systemic), 1633
Cisapride (Systemic), 869
Famotidine (Systemic), 1633
Magaldrate (Oral-Local), 188
Magaldrate and Simethicone (Oral-Local), 188
Magnesium Carbonate and Sodium Bicarbonate (Oral-Local)*, 188
Magnesium Hydroxide (Oral-Local), 188
Magnesium Oxide (Oral-Local)†, 188
Metoclopramide, Oral (Systemic)[1], 1992
Nizatidine (Systemic)[1], 1633
Pantoprazole (Systemic), 3031
Ranitidine (Systemic), 1633
[Sucralfate (Oral-Local)], 2635
**Reflux, vesico-ureteral (diagnosis)**—See Urinary bladder imaging, radionuclide
**Refraction, cycloplegic**
Atropine (Ophthalmic), 485
Cyclopentolate (Ophthalmic), #
Homatropine (Ophthalmic), 1651
Scopolamine (Ophthalmic)†, 2557
Tropicamide (Ophthalmic), #
**Reiter's disease (treatment)**
[Betamethasone, Oral (Systemic)][1], 998
[Betamethasone, Parenteral (Systemic)][1], 998
[Cortisone (Systemic)][1], 998
[Dexamethasone, Oral (Systemic)][1], 998
[Dexamethasone, Parenteral (Systemic)][1], 998
[Hydrocortisone, Oral (Systemic)][1], 998
[Hydrocortisone, Parenteral (Systemic)][1], 998
[Indomethacin (Systemic)][1], 388
[Methylprednisolone, Oral (Systemic)][1], 998
[Methylprednisolone, Parenteral (Systemic)][1], 998
[Prednisolone, Oral (Systemic)][1], 998
[Prednisolone, Parenteral (Systemic)][1], 998
[Prednisone (Systemic)][1], 998
[Triamcinolone, Oral (Systemic)][1], 998
[Triamcinolone, Parenteral (Systemic)][1], 998
**Relapsing fever (treatment)**
Demeclocycline (Systemic), 2765
Doxycycline (Systemic), 2765
[Erythromycin (Systemic)][1], 1368
Minocycline (Systemic), 2765
Oxytetracycline (Systemic)†, 2765
[Penicillin V (Systemic)][1], 2240
Tetracycline (Systemic), 2765
**Renal abnormalities (diagnosis)**—See Renal function studies; Renal imaging, radionuclide; Renal perfusion studies; Urography, excretory
**Renal calculi, apatite (treatment)**
Citric Acid, Glucono-delta-lactone, and Magnesium Carbonate (Local), 3015, 3137‡
**Renal calculi, calcium (prophylaxis)**
[Bendroflumethiazide (Systemic)][1], 1273
Cellulose Sodium Phosphate (Systemic)†, #
[Chlorothiazide (Systemic)]†, 1273
[Chlorthalidone (Systemic)][1], 1273
[Hydrochlorothiazide (Systemic)][1], 1273
[Hydroflumethiazide (Systemic)][1], 1273
[Methyclothiazide (Systemic)][1], 1273
[Metolazone (Systemic)][1], 1273
Monobasic Potassium Phosphate Tablets for Oral Solution (Systemic)†, 2317
[Polythiazide (Systemic)]†, 1273
Potassium Citrate (Systemic), 881, 3159‡
Potassium Citrate and Citric Acid (Systemic), 881
Potassium and Sodium Phosphates (Systemic), 2317

**Renal calculi, calcium (prophylaxis)** (continued)
[Quinethazone (Systemic)]†, 1273
[Trichlormethiazide (Systemic)]†, 1273
**Renal calculi, calcium (treatment)**
Potassium Citrate (Systemic), 881
Potassium Citrate and Citric Acid (Systemic), 881
**Renal calculi, calcium oxalate, recurrence (prophylaxis)**
Allopurinol (Systemic), 44
**Renal calculi, cystine (prophylaxis)**
[Acetazolamide, Oral (Systemic)][1], 773
Potassium Citrate (Systemic), 881
Potassium Citrate and Citric Acid (Systemic), 881
Potassium Citrate and Sodium Citrate (Systemic), 881
Sodium Citrate and Citric Acid (Systemic), 881
Succimer (Systemic), 3166‡
Tiopronin (Systemic)†, 2824, 3169‡
Tricitrates (Systemic), 881
**Renal calculi, cystine (treatment)**
Potassium Citrate (Systemic), 881
Potassium Citrate and Citric Acid (Systemic), 881
Potassium Citrate and Sodium Citrate (Systemic), 881
Sodium Citrate and Citric Acid (Systemic), 881
Tricitrates (Systemic), 881
**Renal calculi, cystine, recurrence (prophylaxis)**
Penicillamine (Systemic), 2237
**Renal calculi, struvite (prophylaxis)**
Acetohydroxamic Acid (Systemic)†, #
**Renal calculi, struvite (treatment)**
Citric Acid, Glucono-delta-lactone, and Magnesium Carbonate (Local), 3015, 3137‡
**Renal calculi, uric acid (prophylaxis)**
[Acetazolamide, Oral (Systemic)][1], 773
Allopurinol (Systemic), 44
Potassium Citrate (Systemic), 881, 3159‡
Potassium Citrate and Citric Acid (Systemic), 881
Potassium Citrate and Sodium Citrate (Systemic), 881
Sodium Bicarbonate, Oral (Systemic), 2586
Sodium Citrate and Citric Acid (Systemic), 881
Tricitrates (Systemic), 881
**Renal calculi, uric acid (treatment)**
Potassium Citrate (Systemic), 881
Potassium Citrate and Citric Acid (Systemic), 881
Potassium Citrate and Sodium Citrate (Systemic), 881
Sodium Citrate and Citric Acid (Systemic), 881
Tricitrates (Systemic), 881
**Renal disease, end-stage, requiring peritoneal dialysis treatment (treatment)**
Icodextrin 7.5% with Electrolytes Peritoneal Dialysis Solution (Systemic), 3146‡
**Renal failure, acute (treatment)**
Anaritide Acetate (Systemic), 3131‡
**Renal failure, acute, oliguric phase (prophylaxis)**
Mannitol (Systemic), 1906
**Renal failure, acute, oliguric phase (treatment)**
Mannitol (Systemic), 1906
**Renal failure, chronic (treatment adjunct)**
Alfacalcidol (Systemic)*, 2966
Calcitriol (Systemic), 2966
[Dihydrotachysterol (Systemic)], 2966
**Renal failure, growth retardation associated with (treatment)**
Somatropin (Systemic), 3165‡
**Renal failure, intrinsic acute, due to ischemia (prophylaxis)**
Alpha-Melanocyte Stimulating Hormone (Systemic), 3129‡
**Renal failure, intrinsic acute, due to ischemia (treatment)**
Alpha-Melanocyte Stimulating Hormone (Systemic), 3129‡
**Renal function studies**
See also Renal imaging, radionuclide
Inulin (Systemic)†, #
Phenolsulfonphthalein (Systemic), #
Technetium Tc 99m Mertiatide (Systemic), 2720
**Renal imaging, radionuclide**
Iodohippurate Sodium I 123 (Systemic)*, 1753
Iodohippurate Sodium I 131 (Systemic), 1755
Technetium Tc 99m Gluceptate (Systemic), 2711
Technetium Tc 99m Mertiatide (Systemic), 2720
Technetium Tc 99m Pentetate (Systemic), 2727
Technetium Tc 99m Succimer (Systemic)†, 2738
**Renal imaging, radionuclide, adjunct**
[Furosemide (Systemic)][1], 1259
**Renal perfusion studies**
Technetium Tc 99m Gluceptate (Systemic), 2711
Technetium Tc 99m Pentetate (Systemic), 2727
**Renography**
Iodohippurate Sodium I 123 (Systemic)*, 1753
Iodohippurate Sodium I 131 (Systemic), 1755

**Renography, adjunct**
[Furosemide (Systemic)][1], 1259
**Reproductive technologies, assisted**
See also Infertility, female (treatment)
Chorionic Gonadotropin (Systemic), 858
Follitropin Alfa (Systemic), 1520
Follitropin Beta (Systemic), 1523
Menotropins (Systemic)[1], 1943
Urofollitropin (Systemic)[1], 2901
**Respiratory depression, opioid (narcotic)-induced (treatment)**
Naloxone (Systemic), 2082
**Respiratory depression, opioid (narcotic)-induced, post-anesthesia (treatment)**
Naloxone (Systemic), 2082
**Respiratory depression, post-anesthesia (treatment)**
Doxapram (Systemic), 1301
**Respiratory distress syndrome (treatment)**
KL4-Surfactant (Intratracheal-Local), 3150‡
Prostaglandin E1 Injection, Liposomal (Systemic), 3152‡
**Respiratory distress syndrome, acute (treatment)**
N-Acetylglucosminyl-N-Acetylmuramyl-L-Ala-D-Isogln-L-Ala-Glycerolid-Palmitoyl, Liposomal (Systemic), 3152‡
**Respiratory distress syndrome, adult (prophylaxis)**
Soluble Recombinant Human Complement Receptor Type 1 (Systemic), 3165‡
**Respiratory distress syndrome, adult (treatment)**
Colfosceril, Cetyl Alcohol, and Tyloxapol (Intratracheal-Local), 3138‡
[Dexamethasone, Parenteral (Systemic)][1], 998
KL4-Surfactant (Intratracheal-Local), 3150‡
L-2 Oxothiazolidine-4-Carboxylic Acid (Intratracheal-Local), 3150‡
Nitric Oxide (Systemic), 3156‡
Soluble Recombinant Human Complement Receptor Type 1 (Systemic), 3165‡
**Respiratory distress syndrome, adult (treatment adjunct)**
Albumin Human (Systemic), 34
**Respiratory distress syndrome, neonatal (prophylaxis)**
Beractant (Intratracheal-Local), 583, 3133‡
[Betamethasone, Parenteral (Systemic)][1], 998
Calfactant (Intratracheal-Local), 3013
Colfosceril, Cetyl Alcohol, and Tyloxapol (Intratracheal-Local), 937, 3138‡
[Dexamethasone, Parenteral (Systemic)][1], 998
Dipalmitoylphosphatidylcholine and Phosphatidylglycerol (Intratracheal-Local), 3141‡
[Hydrocortisone, Parenteral (Systemic)][1], 998
Protirelin (Systemic), 3158‡
Pulmonary Surfactant Replacement (Intratracheal-Local), 3160‡
Pulmonary Surfactant Replacement, Porcine (Intratracheal-Local), 3160‡
Surface Active Extract of Saline Lavage of Bovine Lungs (Intratracheal-Local), 3167‡
**Respiratory distress syndrome, neonatal (treatment)**
Beractant (Intratracheal-Local), 583, 3133‡
Calfactant (Intratracheal-Local), 3013
Colfosceril, Cetyl Alcohol, and Tyloxapol (Intratracheal-Local), 937, 3138‡
Dipalmitoylphosphatidylcholine and Phosphatidylglycerol (Intratracheal-Local), 3141‡
KL4-Surfactant (Intratracheal-Local), 3150‡
Pulmonary Surfactant Replacement (Intratracheal-Local), 3160‡
Pulmonary Surfactant Replacement, Porcine (Intratracheal-Local), 3160‡
Surface Active Extract of Saline Lavage of Bovine Lungs (Intratracheal-Local), 3167‡
**Respiratory insufficiency, acute (treatment)**
Doxapram (Systemic), 1301
**Respiratory syncytial virus infection (prophylaxis)**
Palivizumab (Systemic), 2219
Respiratory Syncytial Virus Immune Globulin Intravenous (Systemic), 2471
**Respiratory syncytial virus (RSV) infections, lower respiratory tract (prophylaxis)**
Respiratory Syncytial Virus Immune Globulin (Human) (Systemic), 3162‡
**Respiratory syncytial virus (RSV) infections, lower respiratory tract (treatment)**
Respiratory Syncytial Virus Immune Globulin (Human) (Systemic), 3162‡
Ribavirin (Systemic), 2478
**Respiratory tract infections**—See Otitis media, acute; Otitis media, chronic suppurative; Pharyngitis, bacterial; Pneumonia; Sinusitis

**Respiratory tract secretions, excessive, in anesthesia (prophylaxis)**
Atropine (Systemic), 226
Glycopyrrolate, Parenteral (Systemic), 226
Scopolamine, Parenteral (Systemic)[1], 226
**Restless leg syndrome**—See Pain, neurogenic
**Retinal detachment (treatment)**
Silicone Oil 5000 Centistokes (Parenteral-Local), #
**Retinal detachment, proliferative vitreretinopathy–related (prophylaxis)**
9-Cis-Retinoic Acid (Systemic), 3128‡
**Retinoblastoma (treatment)**
Cyclophosphamide (Systemic), 1128
[Vincristine (Systemic)][1], 2950
**Retrobulbar block**
Bupivacaine (Parenteral-Local), 139
Etidocaine (Parenteral-Local), 139
Lidocaine (Parenteral-Local), 139
[Procaine (Parenteral-Local)][1], 139
**Rhabdomyosarcoma**
See also Sarcoma, soft tissue
Dactinomycin (Systemic), 1153
Vincristine (Systemic), 2950
**Rheumatic fever (prophylaxis)**
Erythromycin (Systemic), 1368
Penicillin G Benzathine (Systemic), 2240
Penicillin V (Systemic), 2240
Sulfadiazine (Systemic)[1], 2653
[Sulfamethoxazole (Systemic)], 2653
[Sulfisoxazole (Systemic)], 2653
**Rheumatic fever (treatment)**
Aspirin (Systemic), 2538
Aspirin, Buffered (Systemic), 2538
[Betamethasone, Oral (Systemic)], 998
[Betamethasone, Parenteral (Systemic)], 998
Choline Salicylate (Systemic)†, 2538
Choline and Magnesium Salicylates (Systemic), 2538
[Cortisone (Systemic)], 998
[Dexamethasone, Oral (Systemic)], 998
[Dexamethasone, Parenteral (Systemic)], 998
[Hydrocortisone, Oral (Systemic)], 998
[Hydrocortisone, Parenteral (Systemic)], 998
Magnesium Salicylate (Systemic), 2538
[Methylprednisolone, Oral (Systemic)], 998
[Methylprednisolone, Parenteral (Systemic)], 998
[Prednisolone, Oral (Systemic)], 998
[Prednisolone, Parenteral (Systemic)], 998
[Prednisone (Systemic)], 998
Salsalate (Systemic), 2538
Sodium Salicylate (Systemic), 2538
[Triamcinolone, Oral (Systemic)], 998
[Triamcinolone, Parenteral (Systemic)], 998
**Rh hemolytic disease of the newborn (prophylaxis)**
Rh₀(D) Immune Globulin (Systemic), 2476
**Rhinitis, allergic (prophylaxis)**
Cromolyn (Nasal), 1118
**Rhinitis, allergic (treatment)**
Cromolyn Sodium Nasal Solution USP (Nasal), 1118
Levocabastine (Nasal), 3027
**Rhinitis, allergic, severe (treatment)**
Betamethasone, Oral (Systemic), 998
Betamethasone, Parenteral (Systemic), 998
[Betamethasone, Parenteral-Local (Systemic)][1], 998
Cortisone (Systemic), 998
Dexamethasone, Oral (Systemic), 998
Dexamethasone, Parenteral (Systemic), 998
[Dexamethasone, Parenteral-Local (Systemic)][1], 998
Hydrocortisone, Oral (Systemic), 998
Hydrocortisone, Parenteral (Systemic), 998
[Hydrocortisone, Parenteral-Local (Systemic)][1], 998
Methylprednisolone, Oral (Systemic), 998
Methylprednisolone, Parenteral (Systemic), 998
[Methylprednisolone, Parenteral-Local (Systemic)][1], 998
Prednisolone, Oral (Systemic), 998
Prednisolone, Parenteral (Systemic), 998
[Prednisolone, Parenteral-Local (Systemic)][1], 998
Prednisone (Systemic), 998
Triamcinolone, Oral (Systemic), 998
Triamcinolone, Parenteral (Systemic), 998
[Triamcinolone, Parenteral-Local (Systemic)][1], 998
**Rhinitis, perennial (treatment)**
Beclomethasone (Nasal), 961
Budesonide (Nasal)*, 961
Dexamethasone (Nasal)†, 961
Flunisolide (Nasal), 961
Triamcinolone (Nasal), 961

**Rhinitis, perennial allergic (prophylaxis)**
Acrivastine (Systemic)*†, 325
Astemizole (Systemic), 325
Azatadine (Systemic), 325
Bromodiphenhydramine (Systemic)*†, 325
Brompheniramine (Systemic), 325
Carbinoxamine (Systemic)*†, 325
Cetirizine (Systemic), 325
Chlorpheniramine (Systemic), 325
Clemastine (Systemic), 325
Cyproheptadine (Systemic), 325
Dexchlorpheniramine (Systemic), 325
Dimenhydrinate (Systemic), 325
Diphenhydramine (Systemic), 325
Diphenylpyraline (Systemic)*†, 325
Doxylamine (Systemic)†, 325
Hydroxyzine (Systemic), 325
Loratadine (Systemic), 325
Phenindamine (Systemic)†, 325
Pyrilamine (Systemic)*†, 325
Tripelennamine (Systemic), 325
Triprolidine (Systemic)*†, 325
**Rhinitis, perennial allergic (treatment)**
Acrivastine (Systemic)*†, 325
Astemizole (Systemic), 325
Azatadine (Systemic), 325
Bromodiphenhydramine (Systemic)*†, 325
Brompheniramine (Systemic), 325
Budesonide (Nasal), 3012
Carbinoxamine (Systemic)*†, 325
Cetirizine (Systemic), 325
Chlorpheniramine (Systemic), 325
Chlorpheniramine, Phenylephrine, and Methscopolamine (Systemic)†, 373
Chlorpheniramine, Phenylephrine, Phenylpropanolamine, Atropine, Hyoscyamine, and Scopolamine (Systemic)†, 373
Chlorpheniramine, Phenylpropanolamine, and Methscopolamine (Systemic)†, 373
Chlorpheniramine, Pseudoephedrine, and Methscopolamine (Systemic)†, 373
Clemastine (Systemic), 325
Cyproheptadine (Systemic), 325
Dexchlorpheniramine (Systemic), 325
Dimenhydrinate (Systemic), 325
Diphenhydramine (Systemic), 325
Diphenylpyraline (Systemic)*†, 325
Doxylamine (Systemic)†, 325
Fluticasone (Nasal), 1511
Hydroxyzine (Systemic), 325
Loratadine (Systemic), 325
Methdilazine (Systemic)†, 377
Mometasone (Nasal), 2055
Phenindamine (Systemic)†, 325
Promethazine (Systemic), 377
Pyrilamine (Systemic)*†, 325
Triamcinolone (Nasal), 3037
Trimeprazine (Systemic), 377
Tripelennamine (Systemic), 325
Triprolidine (Systemic)*†, 325
**Rhinitis, perennial nonallergic (treatment)**
Budesonide (Nasal), 3012
**Rhinitis, seasonal (prophylaxis)**
[Beclomethasone (Nasal)], 961
Budesonide (Nasal)*, 961
[Dexamethasone (Nasal)]†, 961
[Flunisolide (Nasal)], 961
[Triamcinolone (Nasal)], 961
**Rhinitis, seasonal (treatment)**
Beclomethasone (Nasal), 961
Budesonide (Nasal)*, 961
Flunisolide (Nasal), 961
Triamcinolone (Nasal), 961
**Rhinitis, seasonal allergic (prophylaxis)**
Acrivastine (Systemic)*†, 325
Astemizole (Systemic), 325
Azatadine (Systemic), 325
Bromodiphenhydramine (Systemic)*†, 325
Brompheniramine (Systemic), 325
Carbinoxamine (Systemic)*†, 325
Cetirizine (Systemic), 325
Chlorpheniramine (Systemic), 325
Clemastine (Systemic), 325
Cyproheptadine (Systemic), 325
Dexchlorpheniramine (Systemic), 325
Dimenhydrinate (Systemic), 325
Diphenhydramine (Systemic), 325
Diphenylpyraline (Systemic)*†, 325
Doxylamine (Systemic)†, 325
Hydroxyzine (Systemic), 325
Loratadine (Systemic), 325
Mometasone (Nasal), 2055
Phenindamine (Systemic)†, 325
Pyrilamine (Systemic)*†, 325
Tripelennamine (Systemic), 325
Triprolidine (Systemic)*†, 325

**Rhinitis, seasonal allergic (treatment)**
  Acrivastine (Systemic)*†, 325
  Astemizole (Systemic), 325
  Azatadine (Systemic), 325
  Azelastine (Nasal), 497
  Beclomethasone (Nasal), 3011
  Bromodiphenhydramine (Systemic)*†, 325
  Brompheniramine (Systemic), 325
  Budesonide (Nasal), 3012
  Carbinoxamine (Systemic)*†, 325
  Cetirizine (Systemic), 325
  Chlorpheniramine (Systemic), 325
  Chlorpheniramine, Phenylephrine, Phenylpropanolamine, Atropine, Hyoscyamine, and Scopolamine (Systemic)†, 373
  Chlorpheniramine, Phenylpropanolamine, and Methscopolamine (Systemic)†, 373
  Clemastine (Systemic), 325
  Cyproheptadine (Systemic), 325
  Dexchlorpheniramine (Systemic), 325
  Dimenhydrinate (Systemic), 325
  Diphenhydramine (Systemic), 325
  Diphenylpyraline (Systemic)*†, 325
  Doxylamine (Systemic)†, 325
  Fexofenadine (Systemic), 1461
  Fexofenadine and Pseudoephedrine (Systemic), 1463
  Fluticasone (Nasal), 1511
  Hydroxyzine (Systemic), 325
  Loratadine (Systemic), 325
  Methdilazine (Systemic)†, 377
  Mometasone (Nasal), 2055
  Phenindamine (Systemic)†, 325
  Promethazine (Systemic), 377
  Pyrilamine (Systemic)*†, 325
  Triamcinolone (Nasal), 3037
  Trimeprazine (Systemic), 377
  Tripelennamine (Systemic), 325
  Triprolidine (Systemic)*†, 325

**Rhinitis, vasomotor (prophylaxis)**
  Acrivastine (Systemic)*†, 325
  Astemizole (Systemic), 325
  Azatadine (Systemic), 325
  Bromodiphenhydramine (Systemic)*†, 325
  Brompheniramine (Systemic), 325
  Carbinoxamine (Systemic)*†, 325
  Cetirizine (Systemic), 325
  Chlorpheniramine (Systemic), 325
  Clemastine (Systemic), 325
  Cyproheptadine (Systemic), 325
  Dexchlorpheniramine (Systemic), 325
  Dimenhydrinate (Systemic), 325
  Diphenhydramine (Systemic), 325
  Diphenylpyraline (Systemic)*†, 325
  Doxylamine (Systemic)†, 325
  Hydroxyzine (Systemic), 325
  Loratadine (Systemic), 325
  Phenindamine (Systemic)†, 325
  Pyrilamine (Systemic)*†, 325
  Tripelennamine (Systemic), 325
  Triprolidine (Systemic)*†, 325

**Rhinitis, vasomotor (treatment)**
  Acrivastine (Systemic)*†, 325
  Astemizole (Systemic), 325
  Azatadine (Systemic), 325
  Beclomethasone (Nasal), 3011
  Bromodiphenhydramine (Systemic)*†, 325
  Brompheniramine (Systemic), 325
  Budesonide (Nasal), 3012
  Budesonide (Systemic)*, 961
  Carbinoxamine (Systemic)*†, 325
  Cetirizine (Systemic), 325
  Chlorpheniramine (Systemic), 325
  Chlorpheniramine, Phenylephrine, and Methscopolamine (Systemic)†, 373
  Chlorpheniramine, Phenylephrine, Phenylpropanolamine, Atropine, Hyoscyamine, and Scopolamine (Systemic)†, 373
  Chlorpheniramine, Phenylpropanolamine, and Methscopolamine (Systemic)†, 373
  Chlorpheniramine, Pseudoephedrine, and Methscopolamine (Systemic)†, 373
  Clemastine (Systemic), 325
  Cyproheptadine (Systemic), 325
  Dexchlorpheniramine (Systemic), 325
  Dimenhydrinate (Systemic), 325
  Diphenhydramine (Systemic), 325
  Diphenylpyraline (Systemic)*†, 325
  Doxylamine (Systemic)†, 325
  Hydroxyzine (Systemic), 325
  Loratadine (Systemic), 325
  Methdilazine (Systemic)†, 377
  Phenindamine (Systemic)†, 325
  Promethazine (Systemic), 377
  Pyrilamine (Systemic)*†, 325
  Trimeprazine (Systemic), 377

**Rhinitis, vasomotor (treatment)** *(continued)*
  Tripelennamine (Systemic), 325
  Triprolidine (Systemic)*†, 325

**Rhinorrhea (treatment)**
  Acrivastine (Systemic)*†, 325
  Acrivastine and Pseudoephedrine (Systemic)†, 343
  Astemizole (Systemic), 325
  Azatadine (Systemic), 325
  Azatadine and Pseudoephedrine (Systemic), 343
  Bromodiphenhydramine (Systemic)*†, 325
  Brompheniramine (Systemic), 325
  Brompheniramine and Phenylephrine (Systemic)†, 343
  Brompheniramine, Phenylephrine, and Phenylpropanolamine (Systemic), 343
  Brompheniramine and Phenylpropanolamine (Systemic), 343
  Brompheniramine and Pseudoephedrine (Systemic)†, 343
  Carbinoxamine (Systemic)*†, 325
  Carbinoxamine and Pseudoephedrine (Systemic)†, 343
  Cetirizine (Systemic), 325
  Chlorpheniramine (Systemic), 325
  Chlorpheniramine, Phenindamine, and Phenylpropanolamine (Systemic)†, 343
  Chlorpheniramine and Phenylephrine (Systemic)†, 343
  Chlorpheniramine, Phenylephrine, and Phenylpropanolamine (Systemic)†, 343
  Chlorpheniramine and Phenylpropanolamine (Systemic), 343
  Chlorpheniramine and Pseudoephedrine (Systemic), 343
  Chlorpheniramine, Pyrilamine, and Phenylephrine (Systemic)†, 343
  Chlorpheniramine, Pyrilamine, Phenylephrine, and Phenylpropanolamine (Systemic)†, 343
  Clemastine (Systemic), 325
  Clemastine and Phenylpropanolamine (Systemic)†, 343
  Cyproheptadine (Systemic), 325
  Dexbrompheniramine and Pseudoephedrine (Systemic), 343
  Dexchlorpheniramine (Systemic), 325
  Dimenhydrinate (Systemic), 325
  Diphenhydramine (Systemic), 325
  Diphenhydramine and Pseudoephedrine (Systemic), 343
  Diphenylpyraline (Systemic)*†, 325
  Doxylamine (Systemic)†, 325
  Hydroxyzine (Systemic), 325
  Ipratropium (Nasal)*, 1764
  Loratadine and Pseudoephedrine (Systemic), 343
  Methdilazine (Systemic)†, 377
  Phenindamine (Systemic)†, 325
  Pheniramine and Phenylephrine (Systemic), 343
  Pheniramine, Phenyltoloxamine, Pyrilamine, and Phenylpropanolamine (Systemic)†, 343
  Pheniramine, Pyrilamine, and Phenylpropanolamine (Systemic), 343
  Promethazine (Systemic), 377
  Promethazine and Phenylephrine (Systemic)†, 343
  Pyrilamine (Systemic)*†, 325
  Trimeprazine (Systemic), 377
  Tripelennamine (Systemic), 325
  Triprolidine (Systemic)*†, 325
  Triprolidine and Pseudoephedrine (Systemic), 343

**Rhinorrhea, common cold–associated (treatment)**
  Ipratropium (Inhalation-Local), 3026

**Rhinorrhea, perennial allergic rhinitis–associated (treatment)**
  Ipratropium (Inhalation-Local), 3026

**Rhinorrhea, perennial nonallergic rhinitis–associated (treatment)**
  Ipratropium (Inhalation-Local), 3026

**Riboflavin deficiency (prophylaxis)**
  Riboflavin (Systemic), 2481

**Riboflavin deficiency (treatment)**
  Riboflavin (Systemic), 2481

**Rickets, vitamin D–dependent (prophylaxis)**
  [Calcitriol (Systemic)], 2966

**Rickets, vitamin D–dependent (treatment)**
  [Calcitriol (Systemic)], 2966

**Rickets, vitamin D–resistant**—See Hypophosphatemia, familial

**Rickettsial infections (treatment)**
  Chloramphenicol (Systemic), 841

**Rickettsial pox (treatment)**
  Demeclocycline (Systemic), 2765
  Doxycycline (Systemic), 2765
  Minocycline (Systemic), 2765
  Oxytetracycline (Systemic)†, 2765
  Tetracycline (Systemic), 2765

**Ringworm of the beard**—See Tinea barbae
**Ringworm of the body**—See Tinea corporis
**Ringworm of the foot**—See Skin and nail infections, fungal, minor; Tinea pedis
**Ringworm of the groin**—See Tinea cruris
**Ringworm of the hand**—See Tinea manuum
**Ringworm of the nails**—See Onychomycosis; Skin and nail infections, fungal, minor
**Ringworm of the scalp**—See Tinea capitis
**River blindness**—See Onchocerciasis

**Rocky Mountain spotted fever (treatment)**
  Chloramphenicol (Systemic), 841
  Demeclocycline (Systemic), 2765
  Doxycycline (Systemic), 2765
  Minocycline (Systemic), 2765
  Oxytetracycline (Systemic)†, 2765
  Tetracycline (Systemic), 2765

**Rosacea (treatment)**
  Metronidazole (Topical), 2000, 3028, 3154‡
  [Sulfur (Topical)], #

**Rosacea, ocular (treatment)**
  Betamethasone (Ophthalmic)*, 966
  Dexamethasone (Ophthalmic), 966
  Fluorometholone (Ophthalmic), 966
  Hydrocortisone (Ophthalmic)*, 966
  [Medrysone (Ophthalmic)][1], 966
  Prednisolone (Ophthalmic), 966
  [Tetracycline (Ophthalmic)], 2763
  [Tetracycline (Systemic)], 2765

**Rosacea, severe (treatment)**
  [Isotretinoin (Systemic)][1], 1796

**Rubella (prophylaxis)**—See Measles, mumps, and rubella; Measles and rubella; Rubella Virus Vaccine Live (Systemic)

**Rubella and mumps (prophylaxis)**
  Rubella and Mumps Virus Vaccine Live (Systemic)†, 2528

**Rubeola**—See Measles; Measles, mumps, and rubella; Measles and rubella

## S

**Salivary gland imaging, radionuclide**
  Sodium Pertechnetate Tc 99m (Systemic), 2612

**Salivation, excessive, in anesthesia (prophylaxis)**
  Atropine (Systemic), 226
  Glycopyrrolate, Parenteral (Systemic), 226
  Scopolamine, Parenteral (Systemic)[1], 226

**Salivation, excessive, in dental procedures (prophylaxis)**
  [Atropine, Oral (Systemic)]†, 226
  [Glycopyrrolate, Oral (Systemic)][1], 226
  [Methantheline (Systemic)]†, 226
  [Propantheline (Systemic)][1], 226

**Salivation, excessive, medical condition–related (prophylaxis)**
  [Scopolamine, Transdermal (Systemic)][1], 226

**Salivation, excessive, post-surgical (prophylaxis)**
  [Scopolamine, Transdermal (Systemic)][1], 226

*Salmonella typhi* **(prophylaxis)**
  Typhoid Vaccine Inactivated (Parenteral-Systemic), #
  Typhoid Vi Polysaccharide Vaccine (Systemic)†, #

*Salmonella typhi* **infection (prophylaxis)**
  Typhoid Vaccine Live Oral (Systemic), #

**Saphenous vein coronary artery bypass graft occlusion (prophylaxis)**
  Dipyridamole and Aspirin (Systemic)*, 3018

**Sarcoid, localized cutaneous (treatment)**
  [Bethamethasone, Parenteral-Local (Systemic)][1], 998
  [Dexamethasone, Parenteral-Local (Systemic)][1], 998
  [Hydrocortisone, Parenteral-Local (Systemic)][1], 998
  [Methylprednisolone, Parenteral-Local (Systemic)][1], 998
  [Prednisolone, Parenteral-Local (Systemic)][1], 998
  [Triamcinolone, Parenteral-Local (Systemic)][1], 998

**Sarcoidosis (treatment)**
  Amcinonide (Topical), 978
  Beclomethasone Dipropionate (Topical), 978
  Betamethasone Benzoate (Topical), 978
  Betamethasone Dipropionate (Topical), 978
  Betamethasone Valerate (Topical), 978
  Clobetasol Propionate (Topical), 978
  Clobetasone Butyrate (Topical), 978
  Desoximetasone (Topical), 978
  Diflorasone Diacetate (Topical), 978
  Diflucortolone Valerate (Topical), 978
  Fluocinolone Acetonide (Topical), 978
  Fluocinonide (Topical), 978
  Flurandrenolide (except 0.0125% cream and ointment) (Topical), 978
  Fluticasone Propionate (Topical), 978
  Halcinonide (Topical), 978
  Halobetasol Propionate (Topical), 978
  Hydrocortisone Butyrate (Topical), 978

## Sarcoidosis (treatment) (continued)
Hydrocortisone Valerate (Topical), 978
Mometasone Furoate (Topical), 978
Triamcinolone Acetonide (Topical), 978
## Sarcoidosis, symptomatic (treatment)
See also Hypercalcemia, sarcoid-associated
Betamethasone, Oral (Systemic), 998
Betamethasone, Parenteral (Systemic), 998
Cortisone (Systemic), 998
Dexamethasone, Oral (Systemic), 998
Dexamethasone, Parenteral (Systemic), 998
Hydrocortisone, Oral (Systemic), 998
Hydrocortisone, Parenteral (Systemic), 998
Methylprednisolone, Oral (Systemic), 998
Methylprednisolone, Parenteral (Systemic), 998
Prednisolone, Oral (Systemic), 998
Prednisolone, Parenteral (Systemic), 998
Prednisone (Systemic), 998
Triamcinolone, Oral (Systemic), 998
Triamcinolone, Parenteral (Systemic), 998
## Sarcoma botryoides (treatment)
Dactinomycin (Systemic), 1153
## Sarcoma, Ewing's—See Ewing's sarcoma
## Sarcoma, Kaposi's, AIDS-associated—See Kaposi's sarcoma, AIDS-associated
## Sarcoma, nonparenchymatous (treatment)
Idoxuridine (Systemic), 3146‡
## Sarcoma, osteogenic—See Osteosarcoma
## Sarcoma, reticulum cell—See Lymphomas, non-Hodgkin's
## Sarcoma, soft tissue (treatment)
[Cyclophosphamide (Systemic)][1], 1128
[Dacarbazine (Systemic)][1], 1148
Dactinomycin (Systemic), 1153
Doxorubicin (Systemic), 1308
[Etoposide (Systemic)][1], 1424
[Ifosfamide (Systemic)][1], 1677, 3147‡
[Methotrexate—For Cancer (Systemic)][1], 1962
Vinblastine (Systemic), 2946
Vincristine (Systemic), 2950
## Scabies (treatment)
Benzyl Benzoate (Topical)*†, #
Crotamiton (Topical), #
Lindane Cream USP (Topical), 1866
Lindane Lotion USP (Topical), 1866
Permethrin (Topical), 3032
Sulfurated Lime Topical Solution (Topical)†, #
Sulfur Ointment USP (Topical)†, #
## Scarlet fever
Penicillin G Procaine (Systemic), 2240
Penicillin V (Systemic), 2240
## Scarlet fever (treatment)
[Penicillin G, Parenteral (Systemic)][1], 2240
## Schilling test—See Anemia; Vitamin B$_{12}$ deficiency
## Schistosomiasis (treatment)
Oxamniquine (Systemic)†, #
Praziquantel (Systemic)†, 2368
## Schizophrenia (treatment)
See also Psychotic disorders
Clozapine (Systemic), 919
## SCID—See Immunodeficiency, combined, severe
## Scleroderma (treatment)
Dimethyl Sulfoxide (Topical), 3017
## Scleroderma, fibrosis and/or nonsuppurative inflammation in (treatment)
Aminobenzoate Potassium (Systemic), #
## Scleroderma, hypertension in (treatment)
[Benazepril (Systemic)]†, 177
[Captopril (Systemic)][1], 177
[Enalapril (Systemic)][1], 177
[Fosinopril (Systemic)]†, 177
[Lisinopril (Systemic)][1], 177
[Quinapril (Systemic)]†, 177
[Ramipril (Systemic)]†, 177
## Scleroderma, linear, fibrosis and/or nonsuppurative inflammation in (treatment)
Aminobenzoate Potassium (Systemic), #
## Scleroderma, renal crisis in (treatment)
[Benazepril (Systemic)]†, 177
[Captopril (Systemic)][1], 177
[Enalapril (Systemic)][1], 177
[Fosinopril (Systemic)]†, 177
[Lisinopril (Systemic)][1], 177
[Quinapril (Systemic)]†, 177
[Ramipril (Systemic)]†, 177
## Sclerosis, systemic, diffuse (treatment adjunct)
8-Methoxsalen (Systemic), 3128‡
## Sclerosis, systemic, progressive (treatment)
Recombinant Human Relaxin (Systemic), 3161‡
## Scurvy—See Vitamin C deficiency
## Sealant, colostomy closure (treatment adjunct)
Fibrin Sealant (Local), 3020
## Sedation
Diphenhydramine (Systemic), 325
Hydroxyzine (Systemic), 325
Methotrimeprazine (Systemic), 2289

## Sedation (continued)
Promethazine (Systemic), 377
[Propofol (Systemic)][1], 2416
[Trimeprazine (Systemic)][1], 377
## Sedation and amnesia
Midazolam (Systemic), 2007
## Sedation, benzodiazepine-induced, reversal of
Flumazenil (Systemic), 1483
## Sedation, conscious
[Diazepam, Parenteral (Systemic)][1], 556
Droperidol (Systemic), 1319
Midazolam (Systemic), 2007
## Sedation for procedures in pediatric patients
[Chloral Hydrate (Systemic)], 834
## Seizures (diagnosis)
[Fludeoxyglucose F 18 (Systemic)][1]*†, 1478
[Iofetamine I 123 (Systemic)][1], 1757
## Seizures (prophylaxis)
See also Epilepsy
Phenobarbital (Systemic)[1], 518
## Seizures (treatment)
See also Epilepsy
Diazepam Injection USP (Systemic), 556
Diazepam, Rectal (Systemic), 3140‡
[Diazepam for Rectal Solution (Systemic)], 556
Phenobarbital (Systemic)[1], 518
## Seizures, myoclonic, infantile (treatment)
[Corticotropin, Repository, Injection USP (Systemic)][1], 1021
## Seizures, in neurosurgery (prophylaxis)
Phenytoin (Systemic), 253
## Seizures, in neurosurgery (treatment)
Phenytoin (Systemic), 253
## Seizures, in toxemia of pregnancy (prophylaxis)
Magnesium Sulfate (Systemic), 1895
## Seizures, in toxemia of pregnancy (treatment)
Magnesium Sulfate (Systemic), 1895
## Selenium deficiency (prophylaxis)
Selenious Acid (Systemic)†, 2563
Selenium (Systemic), 2563
## Selenium deficiency (treatment)
Selenious Acid (Systemic)†, 2563
Selenium (Systemic), 2563
## Seminoma (treatment)
[Carboplatin (Systemic)][1], 779
## Sensitization of Rh$_o$(D)–negative females to Rh$_o$(D)–positive blood (prophylaxis)
Rh$_o$(D) Immune Globulin (Systemic), 2476
## Sepsis, gram-negative, progressed to shock (treatment)
Nebacumab (Systemic), 3155‡
## Septicemia, bacterial (treatment)
Amikacin (Systemic), 69
Ampicillin, Parenteral (Systemic), 2240
Aztreonam (Systemic)†, 502
Carbenicillin, Parenteral (Systemic), 2240
Cefamandole (Systemic), 794
Cefazolin (Systemic), 794
Cefepime (Systemic), 794
Cefonicid (Systemic)†[1], 794
Cefoperazone (Systemic)[1], 794
Cefotaxime (Systemic), 794
[Cefotetan (Systemic)][1], 794
Cefoxitin (Systemic), 794
Ceftazidime (Systemic), 794
Ceftizoxime (Systemic), 794
Ceftriaxone (Systemic), 794
Cefuroxime (Systemic)[1], 794
[Cephalothin (Systemic)], 794
Cephapirin (Systemic)†[1], 794
[Cephradine (Systemic)][1], 794
Clindamycin (Systemic), 893
Cloxacillin, Parenteral (Systemic), 2240
[Demeclocycline (Systemic)], 2765
[Doxycycline (Systemic)], 2765
Fusidic Acid (Systemic)*, 3021
Gentamicin (Systemic), 69
Imipenem and Cilastatin (Systemic), 1681
Kanamycin (Systemic)†, 69
Methicillin (Systemic), 2240
Metronidazole (Systemic), 1996
Mezlocillin (Systemic)†, 2240
[Minocycline (Systemic)], 2765
Nafcillin, Parenteral (Systemic), 2240
Netilmicin (Systemic), 69
Oxacillin, Parenteral (Systemic)†, 2240
[Oxytetracycline (Systemic)]†, 2765
Penicillin G, Parenteral (Systemic), 2240
Penicillin G Procaine (Systemic), 2240
Piperacillin (Systemic), 2240
[Piperacillin and Tazobactam (Systemic)][1], 2263
Streptomycin (Systemic), 69
[Sulfamethoxazole and Trimethoprim (Systemic)], 2661
[Tetracycline (Systemic)], 2765
Ticarcillin (Systemic), 2240

## Septicemia, bacterial (treatment) (continued)
Ticarcillin and Clavulanate (Systemic), 2263
Tobramycin (Systemic), 69
Vancomycin (Systemic), 2919
## Septicemia, fungal (treatment)
Amphotericin B (Systemic), 98
[Fluconazole (Systemic)][1], 302
Flucytosine (Systemic), #
[Itraconazole (Systemic)][1], 302
[Ketoconazole (Systemic)][1], 302
## Serum sickness (treatment)
Betamethasone, Oral (Systemic), 998
Betamethasone, Parenteral (Systemic), 998
Cortisone (Systemic), 998
Dexamethasone, Oral (Systemic), 998
Dexamethasone, Parenteral (Systemic), 998
Hydrocortisone, Oral (Systemic), 998
Hydrocortisone, Parenteral (Systemic), 998
Methylprednisolone, Oral (Systemic), 998
Methylprednisolone, Parenteral (Systemic), 998
Prednisolone, Oral (Systemic), 998
Prednisolone, Parenteral (Systemic), 998
Prednisone (Systemic), 998
Triamcinolone, Oral (Systemic), 998
Triamcinolone, Parenteral (Systemic), 998
## Sexual anomalies, congenital (diagnosis)
[Diatrizoate Meglumine and Iodipamide Meglumine (Local)][1], #
## Sexually transmitted diseases (STDs) (prophylaxis)
Benzalkonium Chloride (Vaginal)*[1], #
[Condoms, Lamb Cecum], 1474
[Condoms, Lamb Cecum, and Nonoxynol 9], 1474
Condoms, Latex, 1474
Condoms, Latex, and Nonoxynol 9, 1474
[Nonoxynol 9 (Vaginal)][1], #
[Octoxynol 9 (Vaginal)][1], #
## Shaking palsy—See Parkinsonism
## Shingles—See Herpes zoster
## Shock (treatment)
Dobutamine (Parenteral-Systemic), 2669
Dopamine (Parenteral-Systemic), 2669
Ephedrine (Parenteral-Systemic), 2669
Epinephrine (Parenteral-Systemic), 2669
Mephentermine (Parenteral-Systemic)†, 2669
Metaraminol (Parenteral-Systemic)†, 2669
Methoxamine (Parenteral-Systemic), 2669
Norepinephrine (Parenteral-Systemic), 2669
Phenylephrine (Parenteral-Systemic), 2669
## Shock, adrenocortical insufficiency–induced (treatment)
Betamethasone, Oral (Systemic), 998
Betamethasone, Parenteral (Systemic), 998
Cortisone (Systemic), 998
Dexamethasone, Oral (Systemic), 998
Dexamethasone, Parenteral (Systemic), 998
Hydrocortisone, Oral (Systemic), 998
Hydrocortisone, Parenteral (Systemic), 998
Methylprednisolone, Oral (Systemic), 998
Methylprednisolone, Parenteral (Systemic), 998
Prednisolone, Oral (Systemic), 998
Prednisolone, Parenteral (Systemic), 998
Prednisone (Systemic), 998
Triamcinolone, Oral (Systemic), 998
Triamcinolone, Parenteral (Systemic), 998
## Shock, septic (treatment adjunct)
[Betamethasone, Parenteral (Systemic)], 998
[Dexamethasone, Parenteral (Systemic)], 998
[Hydrocortisone, Parenteral (Systemic)], 998
Naloxone (Systemic)[1], 2082
[Prednisolone, Parenteral (Systemic)], 998
[Triamcinolone, Parenteral (Systemic)], 998
## Short bowel syndrome (treatment adjunct)
Glutamine (Systemic), 3144‡
Growth Hormone, Human (Systemic), 3146‡
## Short stature, Turner's syndrome–associated (treatment)
Somatropin, Recombinant (Systemic), 3034
## Sickle cell disease (treatment)
Arginine Butyrate (Systemic), 3132‡
Clotrimidazole (Systemic), 3137‡
Fructose-1,6-Diphosphate (Systemic), 3144‡
Hydroxyurea (Systemic), 3024, 3146‡
Isobutyramide (Systemic), 3150
OM 401 (Systemic), 3156‡
Polymeric Oxygen (Systemic), 3159‡
Sodium Phenylbutyrate (Systemic), 3164‡
## Sickle cell disease crisis (treatment)
Poloxamer 188 (Systemic), 3158‡
## Sinusitis (treatment)
Amoxicillin (Systemic), 2240
Amoxicillin and Clavulanate (Systemic), 2263, 3010
Ampicillin (Systemic), 2240
Bacampicillin (Systemic), 2240
[Cefixime (Systemic)], 794

**Sinusitis (treatment)** *(continued)*
  Cefprozil (Systemic), 794
  Cefuroxime Axetil (Systemic), 794
  [Clindamycin (Systemic)]1, 893
  Cloxacillin (Systemic), 2240
  Demeclocycline (Systemic), 2765
  Doxycycline (Systemic), 2765
  Erythromycin (Systemic), 1368
  [Erythromycin and Sulfisoxazole (Systemic)]1, 1376
  Flucloxacillin (Systemic)*, 2240
  Levofloxacin (Systemic), 1852
  Loracarbef (Systemic)†, 1880
  Methicillin (Systemic)†, 2240
  Minocycline (Systemic), 2765
  Nafcillin (Systemic), 2240
  Oxacillin (Systemic)†, 2240
  Oxytetracycline (Systemic)†, 2765
  Penicillin V (Systemic), 2240
  [Sulfamethoxazole and Trimethoprim (Systemic)]1, 2661
  Tetracycline (Systemic), 2765
**Sinusitis, acute (treatment)**
  Trovafloxacin (Systemic), 2891
**Sinusitis, acute maxillary (treatment)**
  Cefdinir (Systemic), 3014
  Clarithromycin (Systemic), 889
**Sinusitis, amoxicillin-resistant (treatment)**
  [Cefaclor (Systemic)]1, 794
**Skeletal imaging, positron emission tomographic**
  [Sodium Fluoride F 18 (Systemic)]1, 2595
**Skeletal imaging, radionuclide**
  Technetium Tc 99m Medronate (Systemic), 2718
  Technetium Tc 99m Oxidronate (Systemic)†, 2724
  Technetium Tc 99m Pyrophosphate (Systemic)†, 2729
  Technetium Tc 99m (Pyro- and trimeta-) Phosphates (Systemic), 2733
**Skin conditions related to acne (treatment)**
  Resorcinol and Sulfur (Topical), #
**Skin disorders (treatment)**
  Hydrocortisone (Topical), 3023
  Hydrocortisone Acetate (Topical), 3023
**Skin disorders, inflammatory (treatment)**
  Clioquinol (Topical), #
  Resorcinol (Topical), 1#
**Skin, increased tolerance to sunlight**
  [Methoxsalen (Topical)]1, 1977
  Trioxsalen (Systemic), #
**Skin infections, bacterial, minor (prophylaxis)**
  [Chlortetracycline (Topical)], 2774
  [Clioquinol (Topical)], #
  [Erythromycin Ointment USP (Topical)]†, 1365
  [Gentamicin (Topical)]1, 1557
  Iodine (Topical)†, #
  [Mupirocin (Topical)], 4253
  Neomycin (Topical), #
  Neomycin and Polymyxin B (Topical)†, #
  Neomycin, Polymyxin B, and Bacitracin (Topical), #
  [Tetracycline Hydrochloride Ointment (Topical)], 2774
**Skin infections, bacterial, minor (treatment)**
  Chlortetracycline (Topical), 2774
  [Clindamycin (Topical)]1, 896
  [Clioquinol (Topical)], #
  Clioquinol and Flumethasone (Topical)*, 3015
  Clioquinol and Hydrocortisone (Topical), #
  [Erythromycin Ointment USP (Topical)]†, 1365
  Framycetin (Topical)*, 3021
  Framycetin and Gramicidin (Topical)*, 3021
  Fusidic Acid (Topical)*, 3021
  Gentamicin (Topical), 1557
  Iodine (Topical)†, #
  [Neomycin (Topical)], #
  [Neomycin, Polymyxin B, and Bacitracin (Topical)], #
  [Silver Sulfadiazine (Topical)], #
  Tetracycline Hydrochloride Ointment (Topical), 2774
**Skin, intolerance to sunlight**
  [Methoxsalen (Systemic)]1, 1973
**Skin irritation, minor**—*See* Dermatitis, contact
**Skin lesions, infected (treatment)**
  Mupirocin (Topical), 3029
**Skin lesions, traumatic, secondarily infected (treatment)**
  Mupirocin (Topical), 3029
**Skin and nail infections, fungal, minor (treatment)**
  *See also* Onychomycosis; Tinea pedis
  Carbol-Fuchsin (Topical), #
  Clioquinol (Topical), #
**Skin pigmentation, enhancement of**
  Trioxsalen (Systemic), #
**Skin roughness, facial, due to photoaging (treatment adjunct)**
  Tretinoin (Topical), 2871

**Skin and soft tissue infections (treatment)**
  Amikacin (Systemic), 69
  Amoxicillin and Clavulanate (Systemic), 2263, 3010
  Ampicillin and Sulbactam (Systemic)†, 2263
  Azithromycin (Systemic), 499
  Aztreonam (Systemic)†, 502
  Carbenicillin, Parenteral (Systemic), 2240
  Cefaclor (Systemic), 794
  Cefadroxil (Systemic), 794
  Cefamandole (Systemic), 794
  Cefazolin (Systemic), 794
  [Cefepime (Systemic)]1, 889
  Cefipime (Systemic), 794
  [Cefixime (Systemic)]†, 794
  Cefonicid (Systemic)†1, 794
  Cefoperazone (Systemic)1, 794
  Cefotaxime (Systemic), 794
  Cefotetan (Systemic), 794
  Cefoxitin (Systemic), 794
  Cefpodoxime (Systemic)†1, 794
  Cefprozil (Systemic)†, 794
  Ceftazidime (Systemic), 794
  Ceftizoxime (Systemic), 794
  Ceftriaxone (Systemic), 794
  Cefuroxime (Systemic), 794
  Cefuroxime Axetil (Systemic), 794, 893
  Cephalexin (Systemic), 794
  [Cephalothin (Systemic)], 794
  Cephapirin (Systemic)†1, 794
  Cephradine (Systemic)1, 794
  Ciprofloxacin (Systemic), 1487
  Cloxacillin (Systemic), 2240
  Demeclocycline (Systemic), 2765
  Dicloxacillin (Systemic)†, 2240
  Dirithromycin (Systemic)†, 1250
  Doxycycline (Systemic), 2765
  Erythromycin (Systemic), 1368
  Flucloxacillin (Systemic)*, 2240
  Fusidic Acid (Systemic)*, 3021
  Gentamicin (Systemic), 69
  Imipenem and Cilastatin (Systemic), 1681
  Kanamycin (Systemic)†, 69
  Levofloxacin (Systemic), 1852
  Loracarbef (Systemic)†, 1880
  Methicillin (Systemic)†, 2240
  Metronidazole (Systemic), 1996
  Mezlocillin (Systemic)†, 2240
  Minocycline (Systemic), 2765
  Nafcillin (Systemic), 2240
  Netilmicin (Systemic), 69
  Ofloxacin (Systemic), 1487
  Oxacillin (Systemic), 2240
  Oxytetracycline (Systemic)†, 2765
  Penicillin G, Parenteral (Systemic), 2240
  Penicillin G Procaine (Systemic), 2240
  Penicillin V (Systemic), 2240
  Piperacillin (Systemic), 2240
  Piperacillin and Tazobactam (Systemic), 2263
  Pivampicillin (Systemic)*, 2240
  Streptomycin (Systemic), 69
  [Sulfamethoxazole and Trimethoprim (Systemic)], 2661
  Tetracycline (Systemic), 2765
  Ticarcillin (Systemic), 2240
  Ticarcillin and Clavulanate (Systemic), 2263
  Tobramycin (Systemic), 69
  Trovafloxacin (Systemic), 2891
  Vancomycin (Systemic), 2919
**Skin and soft tissue infections, uncomplicated (treatment)**
  Cefdinir (Systemic), 3014
**SLA syndrome**—*See* Adrenogenital syndrome, congenital
**Sleep disorders, circadian rhythm (treatment)**
  Melatonin (Systemic), 3153‡
**Sleep paralysis (treatment)**
  Sodium/Gamma Hydroxybutyrate (Systemic), 3165‡
**Small intestine studies**
  Cholecystokinin (Systemic)*, #
**Snakebite**
  *See* Envenomation, *Crotadilae* venom (treatment), 3132‡
**SNE**—*See* Encephalomyelopathy, subacute necrotizing
**Sneddon-Wilkinson disease**—*See* Dermatosis, subcorneal pustular
**Sneezing (treatment)**
  Acrivastine (Systemic)*†, 325
  Acrivastine and Pseudoephedrine (Systemic)†, 343
  Azatadine (Systemic), 325
  Azatadine and Pseudoephedrine (Systemic), 343
  Bromodiphenhydramine (Systemic)*†, 325
  Brompheniramine (Systemic), 325

**Sneezing (treatment)** *(continued)*
  Brompheniramine and Phenylephrine (Systemic)†, 343
  Brompheniramine and Phenylpropanolamine (Systemic), 343
  Brompheniramine and Pseudoephedrine (Systemic)†, 343
  Carbinoxamine (Systemic)*†, 325
  Carbinoxamine and Pseudoephedrine (Systemic)†, 343
  Cetirizine (Systemic), 325
  Chlorpheniramine (Systemic), 325
  Chlorpheniramine, Phenindamine, and Phenylpropanolamine (Systemic)†, 343
  Chlorpheniramine and Phenylephrine (Systemic)†, 343
  Chlorpheniramine, Phenylephrine, and Phenylpropanolamine (Systemic)†, 343
  Chlorpheniramine and Phenylpropanolamine (Systemic), 343
  Chlorpheniramine, Phenyltoloxamine, and Phenylephrine (Systemic)†, 343
  Chlorpheniramine, Phenyltoloxamine, Phenylephrine, and Phenylpropanolamine (Systemic)†, 343
  Chlorpheniramine and Pseudoephedrine (Systemic), 343
  Chlorpheniramine, Pyrilamine, and Phenylephrine (Systemic)†, 343
  Chlorpheniramine, Pyrilamine, Phenylephrine, and Phenylpropanolamine (Systemic)†, 343
  Clemastine and Phenylpropanolamine (Systemic)†, 343
  Cyproheptadine (Systemic), 325
  Dexbrompheniramine and Pseudoephedrine (Systemic), 343
  Dexchlorpheniramine (Systemic), 325
  Dimenhydrinate (Systemic), 325
  Diphenhydramine (Systemic), 325
  Diphenhydramine and Pseudoephedrine (Systemic), 343
  Diphenylpyraline (Systemic)*†, 325
  Doxylamine (Systemic)†, 325
  Hydroxyzine (Systemic), 325
  Loratadine and Pseudoephedrine (Systemic), 343
  Methdilazine (Systemic)†, 377
  Phenindamine (Systemic), 325
  Pheniramine and Phenylephrine (Systemic), 343
  Pheniramine, Phenyltoloxamine, Pyrilamine, and Phenylpropanolamine (Systemic)†, 343
  Pheniramine, Pyrilamine, and Phenylpropanolamine (Systemic), 343
  Promethazine (Systemic), 377
  Promethazine and Phenylephrine (Systemic)†, 343
  Pyrilamine (Systemic)*†, 325
  Trimeprazine (Systemic), 377
  Tripelennamine (Systemic), 325
  Triprolidine (Systemic)*†, 325
  Triprolidine and Pseudoephedrine (Systemic), 343
**Soft tissue injury, following extravasation of cytotoxic drugs (treatment)**
  Dimethyl Sulfoxide (Mucosal-Local), 3140‡
**Somatropin deficiency syndrome, adult (treatment)**
  Somatropin, Recombinant (Systemic), 3034
**Spasm, flexor (treatment)**
  [Dantrolene, Oral (Systemic)]1, 1165
**Spasm, hemifacial**—*See* Pain, neurogenic
**Spasm, infantile (treatment)**
  CCD 1042 (Systemic), 3136‡
**Spasmodic dysphonia (treatment)**
  [Botulinum Toxin Type A (Parenteral-Local)], 627
**Spasmodic torticollis (treatment)**
  [Botulinum Toxin Type A (Parenteral-Local)], 627
**Spasm, skeletal muscle (treatment)**
  Carisoprodol (Systemic), 2577
  Chlorphenesin (Systemic)†, 2577
  Chlorzoxazone (Systemic)†, 2577
  Cyclobenzaprine (Systemic), 1126
  Metaxalone (Systemic)†, 2577
  Methocarbamol (Systemic), 2577
  Orphenadrine (Systemic), 2577
**Spasm, skeletal muscle (treatment adjunct)**
  Diazepam (Systemic), 556
  [Lorazepam (Systemic)]1, 556
**Spasm, skeletal muscle, accompanied by pain (treatment)**
  Chlorzoxazone and Acetaminophen (Systemic)*, 853
  Orphenadrine, Aspirin, and Caffeine (Systemic), 2208
**Spasticity (treatment)**
  Baclofen (Systemic), 515, 3133‡
  Botulinum Toxin Type A (Parenteral-Local), 3134‡
  Dantrolene, Oral (Systemic), 1165
  L-Baclofen (Systemic), 3150‡
  L-Threonine (Systemic), 3151‡

**Spasticity (treatment)** *(continued)*
Tizanidine (Systemic)†, 2828
Tizanidine Hydrochloride (Systemic), 3169‡
**Spasticity, severe (treatment)**
Baclofen (Intrathecal-Systemic), 513
**Spasticity of spinal cord origin (treatment)**
Baclofen (Systemic), 3133‡
Baclofen, Intrathecal (Systemic), 3133‡
**Spherocytosis, hereditary (diagnosis)**—*See* Red blood cell survival time determinations
**Spills, hydrofluoric acid (treatment)**
Calcium Gluconate (Topical), 3135‡
**Spinal cord injury (treatment)**
Methylprednisolone (Systemic), 3028
[Methylprednisolone, Oral (Systemic)][1], 998
[Methylprednisolone, Parenteral (Systemic)][1], 998
**Spinal cord injury, chronic, incomplete (treatment)**
Fampridine (Systemic), 3143‡
**Spinal lesions imaging, magnetic resonance**
Gadodiamide (Systemic), #
Gadopentetate (Systemic)†, #
Gadoteridol (Systemic)†, #
**Spleen imaging, radionuclide**
Technetium Tc 99m Albumin Colloid (Systemic)†, 2699
Technetium Tc 99m Sulfur Colloid (Systemic), 2740
**Splenic infarct (diagnosis)**—*See* Spleen imaging, radionuclide
**Splenic lesions (diagnosis)**—*See* Spleen imaging, radionuclide
**Splenic rupture (diagnosis)**—*See* Spleen imaging, radionuclide
**Splenoportography**
Diatrizoate Meglumine and Diatrizoate Sodium, Parenteral (Systemic), #
Diatrizoate Meglumine, Parenteral (Systemic), #
Diatrizoate Sodium, Parenteral (Systemic)[1], #
[Iothalamate Meglumine (Systemic)][1], #
[Iothalamate Meglumine and Iothalamate Sodium (Systemic)]†, #
[Iothalamate Sodium (Systemic)][1], #
**Sporotrichosis (treatment)**
Amphotericin B Lipid Complex (Systemic), 3130‡
**Sporotrichosis, cutaneous lymphatic (treatment)**
[Potassium Iodide (Systemic)][1], 2354
**Sporotrichosis, disseminated (treatment)**
Amphotericin B (Systemic), 98
[Itraconazole (Systemic)], 302
[Ketoconazole (Systemic)], 302
***Staphylococcus aureus* methicillin-resistent (treatment)**
Mupirocin (Nasal), 2066
**Staphylococcus infection (treatment)**
[Rifampin (Systemic)][1], 2485
**Startle disease**—*See* Hyperekplexia
**Status asthmaticus (treatment)**
Albuterol, Parenteral (Systemic)*, 651
[Betamethasone, Parenteral (Systemic)], 998
[Cortisone, Parenteral (Systemic)], 998
[Dexamethasone, Parenteral (Systemic), 998
[Hydrocortisone, Parenteral (Systemic)], 998
[Methylprednisolone, Parenteral (Systemic)], 998
[Prednisolone, Parenteral (Systemic)], 998
[Triamcinolone, Parenteral (Systemic)], 998
**Status epilepticus (treatment)**
Amobarbital, Parenteral (Systemic), 518
Diazepam Injection USP (Systemic), 556
[Diazepam for Rectal Solution (Systemic)], 556
Fosphenytoin (Systemic), 3144‡
Fosphenytoin, Parenteral (Systemic)†, 253
[Lorazepam, Parenteral (Systemic)], 556
Paraldehyde, Parenteral (Systemic), #
Pentobarbital, Parenteral (Systemic), 518
Phenobarbital, Parenteral (Systemic), 518
Phenytoin, Parenteral (Systemic), 253
Secobarbital, Parenteral (Systemic), 518
**Steatorrhea (treatment)**
Pancrelipase (Systemic), 2222
**Sterilizing agent, female**
[Quinacrine (Systemic)][1], #
**Stevens-Johnson syndrome**—*See* Erythema multiforme, severe
**Stiff man syndrome**—*See* Neuromyotonia
**Stings, insect (treatment)**
*See also* Bites, insect
Epinephrine Injection USP (Systemic), 651
**Stomatitis, aphthous (treatment)**
Amlexanox (Mucosal-Local), 85
Betamethasone Dipropionate (Diprolene ointment only) (Topical), 978
[Chlorhexidine (Mucosal-Local)]†, 847
Clobetasol Propionate (0.05% ointment only) (Topical), 978
Desoximetasone (0.05% gel only) (Topical), 978

**Stomatitis, aphthous (treatment)** *(continued)*
Diflorasone Diacetate (Psorcon ointment only) (Topical), 978
Fluocinonide (0.05% gel only) (Topical), 978
Halobetasol Propionate (0.05% ointment only) (Topical), 978
Hydrocortisone Acetate Dental Paste (Topical), 978
[Thalidomide (Systemic)][1]†, 2776
Triamcinolone Acetonide Dental Paste (Topical), 978
**Stomatitis, aphthous, immunodeficiency-associated (prophylaxis)**
Thalidomide (Systemic), 3168‡
**Stomatitis, aphthous, immunodeficiency-associated (treatment)**
[Thalidomide (Systemic)][1]†, 2776
Thalidomide (Systemic), 3168‡
**Stomatitis, aphthous, recurrent (treatment)**
[Betamethasone, Oral (Systemic)][1], 998
[Cortisone, Oral (Systemic)][1], 998
[Dexamethasone, Oral (Systemic)][1], 998
Hydrocortison Acetate Dental Paste (Topical), 978
[Hydrocortisone, Oral (Systemic)][1], 998
[Methylprednisolone, Oral (Systemic)][1], 998
[Prednisolone, Oral (Systemic)][1], 998
[Prednisone (Systemic)][1], 998
Triamcinolone Acetonide Dental Paste (Topical), 978
[Triamcinolone, Oral (Systemic)][1], 998
**Stomatitis, associated with head and neck cancer chemotherapy (treatment)**
Sucralfate (Oral-Local), 3166‡
**Stomatitis, denture (treatment)**
[Chlorhexidine (Mucosal-Local)]†, 847
**Strabismus (treatment)**
Botulinum Toxin Type A (Parenteral-Local), 627
**Strabismus, associated with dystonia (treatment)**
Botulinum Toxin Type A (Parenteral-Local), 3134‡
**Streptococcal infection, Group B, disseminated, in neonates (treatment)**
Group B Streptococcus Immune Globulin (Systemic), 3144‡
**Stress echocardiography adjunct**
[Adenosine (Systemic)]†, 32
[Dipyridamole (Systemic)][1], #
**Stress electrocardiography adjunct**
[Technetium Tc 99m Sestamibi (Systemic)][1], 2736
**Stress-related mucosal damage (prophylaxis)**
Alumina, Calcium Carbonate, and Sodium Bicarbonate (Oral-Local)*, 188
Alumina and Magnesia (Oral-Local), 188
Alumina, Magnesia, Calcium Carbonate, and Simethicone (Oral-Local)†, 188
Alumina, Magnesia, and Magnesium Carbonate (Oral-Local)*, 188
Alumina, Magnesia, Magnesium Carbonate, and Simethicone (Oral-Local)*, 188
Alumina, Magnesia, and Simethicone (Oral-Local), 188
Alumina, Magnesium Alginate, and Magnesium Carbonate (Oral-Local)*, 188
Alumina and Magnesium Carbonate (Oral-Local)†, 188
Alumina, Magnesium Carbonate, and Simethicone (Oral-Local)†, 188
Alumina, Magnesium Carbonate, and Sodium Bicarbonate (Oral-Local)†, 188
Alumina and Magnesium Trisilicate (Oral-Local)†, 188
Alumina, Magnesium Trisilicate, and Sodium Bicarbonate (Oral-Local)†, 188
Alumina and Simethicone (Oral-Local)†, 188
Alumina and Sodium Bicarbonate (Oral-Local), 188
Aluminum Carbonate, Basic (Oral-Local)†, 188
Aluminum Carbonate, Basic and Simethicone (Oral-Local)†, 188
Aluminum Hydroxide (Oral-Local), 188
Calcium Carbonate (Oral-Local)†, 188
Calcium Carbonate and Magnesia (Oral-Local)†, 188
Calcium Carbonate, Magnesia, and Simethicone (Oral-Local)†, 188
Calcium and Magnesium Carbonates (Oral-Local)†, 188
Calcium Carbonate and Simethicone (Oral-Local)†, 188
Cimetidine, Parenteral (Systemic), 1633
Magaldrate (Oral-Local), 188
Magaldrate and Simethicone (Oral-Local), 188
Magnesium Carbonate and Sodium Bicarbonate (Oral-Local)*, 188
Magnesium Hydroxide (Oral-Local), 188
Magnesium Oxide (Oral-Local)†, 188
[Ranitidine, Parenteral (Systemic)], 1633
[Sucralfate (Oral-Local)], 2635

**Stress-related mucosal damage (treatment)**
Alumina, Calcium Carbonate, and Sodium Bicarbonate (Oral-Local)*, 188
Alumina and Magnesia (Oral-Local), 188
Alumina, Magnesia, Calcium Carbonate, and Simethicone (Oral-Local)†, 188
Alumina, Magnesia, and Magnesium Carbonate (Oral-Local)*, 188
Alumina, Magnesia, Magnesium Carbonate, and Simethicone (Oral-Local)*, 188
Alumina, Magnesia, and Simethicone (Oral-Local), 188
Alumina, Magnesium Alginate, and Magnesium Carbonate (Oral-Local)*, 188
Alumina and Magnesium Carbonate (Oral-Local)†, 188
Alumina, Magnesium Carbonate, and Sodium Bicarbonate (Oral-Local)†, 188
Alumina, Magnesium Carbonate, and Simethicone (Oral-Local)†, 188
Alumina and Magnesium Trisilicate (Oral-Local)†, 188
Alumina, Magnesium Trisilicate, and Sodium Bicarbonate (Oral-Local)†, 188
Alumina and Simethicone (Oral-Local)†, 188
Alumina and Sodium Bicarbonate (Oral-Local)*, 188
Aluminum Carbonate, Basic (Oral-Local)†, 188
Aluminum Carbonate, Basic and Simethicone (Oral-Local)†, 188
Aluminum Hydroxide (Oral-Local), 188
Calcium Carbonate (Oral-Local)†, 188
Calcium Carbonate and Magnesia (Oral-Local)†, 188
Calcium Carbonate, Magnesia, and Simethicone (Oral-Local)†, 188
Calcium and Magnesium Carbonates (Oral-Local)†, 188
Calcium Carbonate and Simethicone (Oral-Local)†, 188
Magaldrate (Oral-Local), 188
Magaldrate and Simethicone (Oral-Local), 188
Magnesium Carbonate and Sodium Bicarbonate (Oral-Local)*, 188
Magnesium Hydroxide (Oral-Local), 188
Magnesium Oxide (Oral-Local)†, 188
[Ranitidine, Parenteral (Systemic)], 1633
[Sucralfate (Oral-Local)], 2635
**Stroke (diagnosis)**
[Fludeoxyglucose F 18 (Systemic)][1]*†, 1478
**Stroke, acute ischemic (treatment)**
Alteplase, Recombinant (Systemic), 2799
**Stroke, thromboembolic, initial or recurrent (prophylaxis)**
Ticlopidine (Systemic), 2818
**Stroke, thromboembolic (prophylaxis)**
Clodpidogrel (Systemic), 913
**Stromal incisions (treatment)**
Epidermal Growth Factor (Human) (Ophthalmic), 3141‡
Urogastrone (Ophthalmic), 3171‡
**Strongyloidiasis (treatment)**
Albendazole (Systemic)*†, #
Ivermectin (Systemic), 3026
Ivermectin (Systemic)*†, #
Thiabendazole (Systemic)†, 2784
**Subarachnoid hemorrhage–associated neurologic deficits (treatment)**
Flunarizine (Systemic)*, 720
[Nicardipine (Systemic)], 720
Nimodipine (Systemic), 720
**Sucrase deficiency (treatment)**
Sacrosidase (Systemic), 3033
**Sucrase-isomaltase deficiency, congenital (treatment)**
Sucrase (Yeast-derived) (Systemic), 3166‡
**Sunburn (prophylaxis)**
Aminobenzoic Acid, Padimate O, and Oxybenzone (Topical), #
Aminobenzoic Acid and Titanium Dioxide (Topical), #
Avobenzone, Octocrylene, Octyl Salicylate, and Oxybenzone (Topical), #
Avobenzone and Octyl Methoxycinnamate (Topical), #
Avobenzone, Octyl Methoxycinnamate, Octyl Salicylate, and Oxybenzone (Topical), #
Avobenzone, Octyl Methoxycinnamate, and Oxybenzone (Topical), #
Dioxybenzone, Oxybenzone, and Padimate O (Topical), #
Homosalate (Topical), #
Homosalate, Menthyl Anthranilate, and Octyl Methoxycinnamate (Topical), #

**Sunburn (prophylaxis)** *(continued)*
   Homosalate, Menthyl Anthranilate, Octyl Methoxycinnamate, Octyl Salicylate, and Oxybenzone (Topical), #
   Homosalate, Octocrylene, Octyl Methoxycinnamate, and Oxybenzone (Topical), #
   Homosalate, Octyl Methoxycinnamate, Octyl Salicylate, and Oxybenzone (Topical), #
   Homosalate, Octyl Methoxycinnamate, and Oxybenzone (Topical), #
   Homosalate and Oxybenzone (Topical), #
   Lisadimate, Oxybenzone, and Padimate O (Topical), #
   Lisadimate and Padimate O (Topical), #
   Menthyl Anthranilate (Topical), #
   Menthyl Anthranilate, Octocrylene, and Octyl Methoxycinnamate (Topical), #
   Menthyl Anthranilate, Octocrylene, Octyl Methoxycinnamate, and Oxybenzone (Topical), #
   Menthyl Anthranilate and Octyl Methoxycinnamate (Topical), #
   Menthyl Anthranilate, Octyl Methoxycinnamate, and Octyl Salicylate (Topical), #
   Menthyl Anthranilate, Octyl Methoxycinnamate, Octyl Salicylate, and Oxybenzone (Topical), #
   Menthyl Anthranilate, Octyl Methoxycinnamate, and Oxybenzone (Topical), #
   Menthyl Anthranilate and Padimate O (Topical), #
   Menthyl Anthranilate and Titanium Dioxide (Topical), #
   Octocrylene and Octyl Methoxycinnamate (Topical), #
   Octocrylene, Octyl Methoxycinnamate, Octyl Salicylate, and Oxybenzone (Topical), #
   Octocrylene, Octyl Methoxycinnamate, Octyl Salicylate, Oxybenzone, and Titanium Dioxide (Topical), #
   Octocrylene, Octyl Methoxycinnamate, and Oxybenzone (Topical), #
   Octocrylene, Octyl Methoxycinnamate, Oxybenzone, and Titanium Dioxide (Topical), #
   Octocrylene, Octyl Methoxycinnamate, and Titanium Dioxide (Topical), #
   Octyl Methoxycinnamate (Topical), #
   Octyl Methoxycinnamate and Octyl Salicylate (Topical), #
   Octyl Methoxycinnamate, Octyl Salicylate, and Oxybenzone (Topical), #
   Octyl Methoxycinnamate, Octyl Salicylate, Oxybenzone, and Padimate O (Topical), #
   Octyl Methoxycinnamate, Octyl Salicylate, Oxybenzone, Padimate O, and Titanium Dioxide (Topical), #
   Octyl Methoxycinnamate, Octyl Salicylate, Oxybenzone, Phenylbenzimidazole, and Titanium Dioxide (Topical), #
   Octyl Methoxycinnamate, Octyl Salicylate, Oxybenzone, and Titanium Dioxide (Topical), #
   Octyl Methoxycinnamate, Octyl Salicylate, Phenylbenimidazole, and Titanium Dioxide (Topical), #
   Octyl Methoxycinnamate, Octyl Salicylate, and Titanium Dioxide (Topical), #
   Octyl Methoxycinnamate and Oxybenzone (Topical), #
   Octyl Methoxycinnamate, Oxybenzone, and Padimate O (Topical), #
   Octyl Methoxycinnamate, Oxybenzone, Padimate O, and Titanium Dioxide (Topical), #
   Octyl Methoxycinnamate, Oxybenzone, and Titanium Dioxide (Topical), #
   Octyl Methoxycinnamate and Padimate O (Topical), #
   Octyl Methoxycinnamate and Phenylbenzimidazole (Topical), #
   Octyl Salicylate (Topical), #
   Octyl Salicylate and Padimate O (Topical), #
   Oxybenzone and Padimate O (Topical), #
   Oxybenzone and Roxadimate (Topical), #
   Padimate O (Topical), #
   Phenylbenzimidazole (Topical), #
   Phenylbenzimidazole and Sulisobenzone (Topical), #
   Titanium Dioxide (Topical), #
   Titanium Dioxide and Zinc Oxide (Topical), #
   Trolamine Salicylate (Topical), #
**Sunburn (treatment)**
   *See also* Burns, minor
   Amcinonide (Topical), 978
   Beclomethasone Dipropionate (Topical), 978
   Betamethasone Benzoate (Topical), 978
   Betamethasone Dipropionate (Topical), 978
   Betamethasone Valerate (Topical), 978
   Clobetasol Propionate (Topical), 978
   Clobetasone Butyrate (Topical), 978
   Desoximetasone (Topical), 978
   Diflorasone Diacetate (Topical), 978

**Sunburn (treatment)** *(continued)*
   Diflucortolone Valerate (Topical), 978
   Fluocinolone Acetonide (Topical), 978
   Fluocinonide (Topical), 978
   Flurandrenolide (except 0.0125% cream and ointment) (Topical), 978
   Fluticasone Propionate (Topical), 978
   Halcinonide (Topical), 978
   Halobetasol Propionate (Topical), 978
   Hydrocortisone Butyrate (Topical), 978
   Hydrocortisone Valerate (Topical), 978
   Mometasone Furoate (Topical), 978
   Triamcinolone Acetonide (Topical), 978
**Sun fungus**—*See* Pityriasis versicolor; Tinea versicolor
**Surgery of the middle and inner ear**—*See* Ear, inner, circulatory disturbances of; Vertigo
**Sympathetic block**
   Bupivacaine (Parenteral-Local), 139
   Bupivacaine and Epinephrine (Parenteral-Local), 139
   Lidocaine (Parenteral-Local), 139
   Lidocaine and Epinephrine (Parenteral-Local), 139
**Syncope (prophylaxis)**
   Ammonia Spirit, Aromatic (Inhalation-Systemic)†, #
**Syncope (treatment)**
   Ammonia Spirit, Aromatic (Inhalation-Systemic)†, #
**Syndrome of inappropriate diuretic hormone (treatment)**
   [Demeclocycline (Systemic)], 2765
**Synechiae, posterior (prophylaxis)**
   [Atropine (Ophthalmic)], 485
   [Cyclopentolate (Ophthalmic)]1, #
   Phenylephrine (Ophthalmic), #
   [Scopolamine (Ophthalmic)]†, 2557
**Synechiae, posterior (treatment)**
   [Atropine (Ophthalmic)], 485
   Scopolamine (Ophthalmic)†, 2557
**Synovitis**—*See* Inflammation, nonrheumatic
**Synovitis, crystal-induced**—*See* Calcium pyrophosphate deposition disease, acute
**Synovitis of osteoarthritis (treatment)**
   *See also* Osteoarthritis
   Betamethasone, Oral (Systemic), 998
   Betamethasone, Parenteral (Systemic), 998
   Betamethasone, Parenteral-Local (Systemic), 998
   Cortisone (Systemic), 998
   Dexamethasone (Systemic), 998
   Hydrocortisone, Oral (Systemic), 998
   Hydrocortisone, Parenteral (Systemic), 998
   Hydrocortisone, Parenteral-Local (Systemic), 998
   Methylprednisolone, Oral (Systemic), 998
   Methylprednisolone, Parenteral (Systemic), 998
   Methylprednisolone, Parenteral-Local (Systemic), 998
   Prednisolone (Systemic), 998
   Prednisone (Systemic), 998
   Triamcinolone (Systemic), 998
**Syphilis (treatment)**
   Demeclocycline (Systemic), 2765
   Doxycycline (Systemic), 2765
   Erythromycin (Systemic), 1368
   Minocycline (Systemic), 2765
   Oxytetracycline (Systemic)†, 2765
   Penicillin G Benzathine (Systemic), 2240
   Penicillin G, Parenteral (Systemic), 2240
   Penicillin G Procaine (Systemic), 2240
   Tetracycline (Systemic), 2765

# T

**Tabes dorsalis**—*See* Pain, neurogenic
**Tachyarrhythmias, catecholamine-induced, during anesthesia (prophylaxis)**
   Propranolol (Systemic), 593
**Tachyarrhythmias, catecholamine-induced, during anesthesia (treatment)**
   Propranolol (Systemic), 593
**Tachyarrhythmias, digitalis-induced (prophylaxis)**
   Propranolol (Systemic), 593
**Tachyarrhythmias, digitalis-induced (treatment)**
   Propranolol (Systemic), 593
**Tachyarrhythmias, ventricular (prophylaxis)**
   Sotalol (Systemic), 3166‡
**Tachyarrhythmias, ventricular (treatment)**
   Sotalol (Systemic), 3166‡
**Tachycardia, atrial, paroxysmal (prophylaxis)**
   Digitoxin (Systemic), 1213
   Digoxin (Systemic), 1213
   Diltiazem, Parenteral (Systemic), 720
   Quinidine (Systemic), 2440
   Verapamil, Oral (Systemic), 720

**Tachycardia, atrial, paroxysmal (treatment)**
   Diltiazem, Parenteral (Systemic), 720
   [Procainamide (Systemic)], 2387
   Quinidine (Systemic), 2440
   Verapamil, Parenteral (Systemic), 720
**Tachycardia, intraoperative (treatment)**
   Esmolol (Systemic)†, 1377
**Tachycardia, postoperative (treatment)**
   Esmolol (Systemic)†, 1377
**Tachycardia, supraventricular (prophylaxis)**
   *See also* Tachycardia, atrial, paroxysmal
   Diltiazem, Parenteral (Systemic), 720
   [Disopyramide (Systemic)][1], 1252
   Quinidine (Systemic), 2440
   Verapamil (Systemic), 720
**Tachycardia, supraventricular (treatment)**
   *See also* Tachycardia, atrial, paroxysmal
   Adenosine (Systemic)†, 32
   Diltiazem, Parenteral (Systemic), 720
   [Disopyramide (Systemic)][1], 1252
   Procainamide (Systemic), 2387
   Quinidine (Systemic), 2440
   Verapamil (Systemic), 720
**Tachycardia, supraventricular, paroxysmal (prophylaxis)**
   Flecainide (Systemic)[1], 1469
**Tachycardia, supraventricular, paroxysmal (treatment)**
   *See also* Tachycardia, atrial, paroxysmal
   Adenosine (Systemic)†, 32
   Diltiazem, Parenteral (Systemic), 720
   Phenylephrine (Parenteral-Systemic), 2669
   Procainamide (Systemic), 2387
   Quinidine (Systemic), 2440
   Verapamil (Systemic), 720
**Tachycardia, ventricular (prophylaxis)**
   [Acebutolol (Systemic)][1], 593
   Amiodarone Hydrochloride (Systemic), 3130‡
   [Atenolol (Systemic)][1], 593
   Flecainide (Systemic), 1469
   [Metoprolol (Systemic)][1], 593
   [Nadolol (Systemic)][1], 593
   Oxprenolol (Systemic)*[1], 593
   Propranolol (Systemic), 593
   Sotalol (Systemic)[1], 593
   [Timolol (Systemic)][1], 593
**Tachycardia, ventricular (treatment)**
   [Acebutolol (Systemic)][1], 593
   Amiodarone (Systemic), 3130‡
   Amiodarone Hydrochloride (Systemic), 3130‡
   [Atenolol (Systemic)][1], 593
   Bretylium (Systemic), 630
   Disopyramide (Systemic), 1252
   Encainide (Systemic)*†, 1344
   Flecainide (Systemic), 1469
   [Metoprolol (Systemic)][1], 593
   Mexiletine (Systemic), 2005
   Moricizine (Systemic)†, 2060
   [Nadolol (Systemic)][1], 593
   Oxprenolol (Systemic)*[1], 593
   Procainamide (Systemic), 2387
   Propafenone (Systemic), 2413
   Propranolol (Systemic), 593
   Sotalol (Systemic)[1], 593
   [Timolol (Systemic)][1], 593
**Tachycardia, ventricular, paroxysmal (prophylaxis)**
   Quinidine (Systemic), 2440
**Tachycardia, ventricular, paroxysmal (treatment)**
   Quinidine (Systemic), 2440
**Tachycardia, ventricular, polymorphous (treatment)**
   [Magnesium Sulfate (Systemic)][1], 1895
**Taeniasis (treatment)**
   Albendazole (Systemic)*†, #
   Niclosamide (Oral-Local)†, #
   [Praziquantel (Systemic)]†, 2368
**Tardive dyskinesia (treatment)**
   Tetrabenazine (Systemic), 30122‡
**Tear production deficiency**—*See* Keratoconjunctivitis sicca
**Ten-day measles**—*See* Measles
**Tendinitis**—*See* Inflammation, nonrheumatic
**Tendinitis (treatment)**
   Naproxen (Systemic), 3029
**Tenosynovitis, nonspecific acute (treatment)**
   *See also* Inflammation, nonrheumatic
   Betamethasone, Oral (Systemic), 998
   Betamethasone, Parenteral (Systemic), 998
   Betamethasone, Parenteral-Local (Systemic), 998
   Cortisone (Systemic), 998
   Dexamethasone (Systemic), 998
   Hydrocortisone, Oral (Systemic), 998
   Hydrocortisone, Parenteral (Systemic), 998
   Hydrocortisone, Parenteral-Local (Systemic), 998
   Methylprednisolone, Oral (Systemic), 998

### Tenosynovitis, nonspecific acute (treatment)
*(continued)*
Methylprednisolone, Parenteral (Systemic), 998
Methylprednisolone, Parenteral-Local (Systemic), 998
Prednisolone (Systemic), 998
Prednisone (Systemic), 998
Triamcinolone (Systemic), 998

### Tension, psychosis-related (treatment)
Hydroxyzine (Systemic), 325

### Testosterone replacement in androgen deficiency, AIDS-related (treatment)
Testosterone (Systemic), 30122

### Tetanus (prophylaxis)
Tetanus Toxoid (Systemic), 2760

### Tetanus (treatment)
Penicillin G, Parenteral (Systemic), 2240

### Tetanus (treatment adjunct)
Amobarbital, Parenteral (Systemic), 518
Chlorpromazine (Systemic), 2289
Pentobarbital, Parenteral (Systemic), 518
Phenobarbital, Parenteral (Systemic), 518
Secobarbital, Parenteral (Systemic), 518

### Tetanus and diphtheria (prophylaxis)—See Diphtheria and tetanus (prophylaxis)

### Tetany, idiopathic (treatment)
[Calcitriol (Systemic)], 2966
Dihydrotachysterol (Systemic), 2966
[Ergocalciferol (Systemic)], 2966

### Tetany, postoperative (treatment)
[Calcitriol (Systemic)], 2966
Dihydrotachysterol (Systemic), 2966
[Ergocalciferol (Systemic)], 2966

### Thiamine deficiency (prophylaxis)
Thiamine (Systemic), 2787

### Thiamine deficiency (treatment)
Thiamine (Systemic), 2787

### Threadworm—See Strongyloidiasis

### Threadworm, intestinal, nondisseminated—See Strongyloidiasis

### Thrombocythemia, essential (treatment)
Anagrelide (Systemic), 114, 3010, 3131‡
[Sodium Phosphate P 32 (Systemic)]¹, 2616

### Thrombocytopenia (prophylaxis)
Interleukin-11, Human, Recombinant (Systemic), 3161‡
Oprelvekin (Systemic), 2205

### Thrombocytopenia in hematopoietic stem cell transplantation (treatmemt)
Human Megakaryocyte Growth and Development Factor, Recombinant, Pegylated (Systemic), 3157‡

### Thrombocytopenia, heparin-induced (treatment)
Ancrod (Systemic), 3131‡

### Thrombocytopenia purpura, immune (treatment)
*Pseudomonas aeruginosa*, Purified Extract of (Systemic), 3160‡

### Thrombocytopenia, secondary, in adults (treatment)
Betamethasone, Oral (Systemic), 998
Betamethasone, Parenteral (Systemic), 998
Cortisone (Systemic), 998
Dexamethasone, Oral (Systemic), 998
Dexamethasone, Parenteral (Systemic), 998
Hydrocortisone, Oral (Systemic), 998
Hydrocortisone, Parenteral (Systemic), 998
Methylprednisolone, Oral (Systemic), 998
Methylprednisolone, Parenteral (Systemic), 998
Prednisolone, Oral (Systemic), 998
Prednisolone, Parenteral (Systemic), 998
Prednisone (Systemic), 998
Triamcinolone, Oral (Systemic), 998
Triamcinolone, Parenteral (Systemic), 998

### Thrombocytopenia Type II, heparin-associated (treatment)
Lepirudin (Systemic), 3151‡

### Thrombocytopenic purpura, idiopathic (treatment)
Betamethasone, Oral (Systemic), 998
Betamethasone, Parenteral (Systemic), 998
Cortisone (Systemic), 998
Dexamethasone, Oral (Systemic), 998
Dexamethasone, Parenteral (Systemic), 998
Hydrocortisone, Oral (Systemic), 998
Hydrocortisone, Parenteral (Systemic), 998
Immune Globulin Intravenous (Human) (Systemic), 1686, 3025
Methylprednisolone, Oral (Systemic), 998
Methylprednisolone, Parenteral (Systemic), 998
Prednisolone, Oral (Systemic), 998
Prednisolone, Parenteral (Systemic), 998
Prednisone (Systemic), 998
RH₀(D) Immune Globulin (Human) (Systemic), 3162‡
Triamcinolone, Oral (Systemic), 998
[Vincristine (Systemic)], 2950

### Thrombocytopenic purpura, immune (treatment)
Monoclonal antibody 5c8, humanized, recombinant (Systemic), 3161‡

### Thrombocytopenic purpura, thrombotic (treatment)
Defibrotide (Systemic), 3139‡

### Thrombocytosis, in chronic myelocytic leukemia (treatment)
Anagrelide (Systemic), 3131‡

### Thrombocytosis, essential (treatment)
[Hydroxyurea (Systemic)]¹, 1666
[Interferon Alfa-2a, Recombinant (Systemic)]¹, 1740
[Interferon Alfa-2b, Recombinant (Systemic)]¹, 1740
[Interferon Alfa-n1 (Ins) (Systemic)]¹*, 1740
[Interferon Alfa-n3 (Systemic)]¹†, 1740

### Thromboembolism (prophylaxis)
Acenocoumarol (Systemic)*, 3009
Anisindione (Systemic)†, 243
[Aspirin, Buffered (Systemic)], 2538
[Aspirin Delayed-release Tablets USP (Systemic)], 2538
[Aspirin, Sodium Bicarbonate, and Citric Acid (Systemic)]¹, 477
[Aspirin Tablets USP (Systemic)], 2538
[Aspirin Tablets USP (Chewable) (Systemic)], 2538
Dicumarol (Systemic)†, 243
Heparin (Systemic), 1617
Warfarin (Systemic), 243, 3038

### Thromboembolism (prophylaxis adjunct)
Dipyridamole (Systemic), #

### Thromboembolism (treatment)
Warfarin (Systemic), 3038

### Thromboembolism, arterial (treatment)
Heparin (Systemic), 1617

### Thromboembolism, arterial, acute (treatment)
Streptokinase (Systemic), 2799
[Urokinase (Systemic)], 2799

### Thromboembolism, associated with hereditary antithrombin III deficiency (prophylaxis)
Antithrombin III (Systemic)†, 444, 3131‡
Antithrombin III (Human) (Systemic)†, 3131‡

### Thromboembolism, associated with hereditary antithrombin III deficiency (treatment)
Antithrombin III (Systemic)†, 3131‡
Antithrombin III (Human) (Systemic)†, 3131‡

### Thromboembolism, associated with hereditary antithrombin III deficiency (treatment adjunct)
Antithrombin III (Systemic)†, 444

### Thromboembolism, cerebral (prophylaxis)
[Aspirin, Buffered (Systemic)], 2538
[Aspirin Delayed-release Tablets USP (Systemic)], 2538
Aspirin, Sodium Bicarbonate, and Citric Acid (Systemic)¹, 477
[Aspirin Tablets USP (Systemic)], 2538
[Aspirin Tablets USP (Chewable) (Systemic)], 2538

### Thromboembolism, cerebral, recurrence (prophylaxis)
[Anisindione (Systemic)]†, 243
[Aspirin, Buffered (Systemic)]¹, 2538
[Aspirin Delayed-release Tablets USP (Systemic)]¹, 2538
[Aspirin, Sodium Bicarbonate, and Citric Acid (Systemic)]¹, 477
[Aspirin Tablets USP (Systemic)]¹, 2538
[Aspirin Tablets USP (Chewable) (Systemic)]¹, 2538
[Dicumarol (Systemic)]†, 243
[Heparin (Systemic)]¹, 1617
[Warfarin (Systemic)], 243

### Thromboembolism, heparin-induced (treatment)
Lepirudin (Systemic), 1833

### Thromboembolism, pulmonary (prophylaxis)
Anisindione (Systemic)†, 243
Ardeparin (Systemic), 467
Dalteparin (Systemic), 1156
Danaparoid (Systemic), 1161
Dicumarol (Systemic)†, 243
Enoxaparin (Systemic), 1346
Heparin (Systemic), 1617
Warfarin (Systemic), 243

### Thromboembolism, pulmonary (prophylaxis adjunct)
[Dihydroergotamine (Systemic)]¹, 2925

### Thromboembolism, pulmonary (treatment)
Anisindione (Systemic)†, 243
Dicumarol (Systemic)†, 243
Heparin (Systemic), 1617
Warfarin (Systemic), 243

### Thromboembolism, pulmonary, acute (treatment)
Alteplase, Recombinant (Systemic)¹, 2799
Streptokinase (Systemic), 2799
Urokinase (Systemic), 2799

### Thromboembolism, thrombosis-induced—See Thromboembolism

### Thrombophlebitis (treatment)
Nylidrin (Systemic)*, #

### Thrombophlebitis, superficial (treatment)
Bufexamac (Topical)*, 3013

### Thrombosis, acute coronary syndrome–related (prophylaxis)
Eptifibatide (Systemic), 1683
Tirofiban (Systemic), 2826

### Thrombosis, acute coronary syndrome–related (treatment)
Eptifibatide (Systemic), 1356

### Thrombosis, arterial (diagnosis)—See Platelets, labeling of

### Thrombosis, arterial, acute (treatment)
Streptokinase (Systemic), 2799
[Urokinase (Systemic)], 2799

### Thrombosis, associated with antithrombin III deficiency (prophylaxis)
Antithrombin III (Human) (Systemic), 3131‡

### Thrombosis, associated with antithrombin III deficiency (treatment)
Antithrombin III (Human) (Systemic), 3131‡

### Thrombosis, associated with Protein C deficiency (prophylaxis)
Protein C Concentrate (Systemic), 3160‡

### Thrombosis, associated with Protein C deficiency (treatment)
Protein C Concentrate (Systemic), 3160‡

### Thrombosis, cardiac (diagnosis)—See Platelets, labeling of

### Thrombosis, cerebral (prophylaxis)
Heparin (Systemic), 1617

### Thrombosis, coronary arterial, acute (treatment)
Alteplase, Recombinant (Systemic), 2799
Anistreplase (Systemic)†, 2799
Reteplase, Recombinant (Systemic), 2473
Streptokinase (Systemic), 2799
[Urokinase (Systemic)]¹, 2799

### Thrombosis, deep venous (diagnosis)—See Platelets, labeling of

### Thrombosis, deep venous (prophylaxis)
Acenocoumarol (Systemic)*, 3009
Anisindione (Systemic)†, 243
Ardeparin (Systemic), 467
Dalteparin (Systemic), 1156
Danaparoid (Systemic), 1161
Dicumarol (Systemic)†, 243
Enoxaparin (Systemic), 1346
Heparin (Systemic), 1617
Warfarin (Systemic), 243

### Thrombosis, deep venous (prophylaxis adjunct)
[Dihydroergotamine (Systemic)]¹, 2925

### Thrombosis, deep venous (treatment)
Acenocoumarol (Systemic)*, 3009
Anisindione (Systemic)†, 243
[Dalteparin (Systemic)], 1156
Heparin (Systemic), 1617
Streptokinase (Systemic), 2799
[Urokinase (Systemic)]¹, 2799
Warfarin (Systemic), 243

### Thrombosis, of the extracorporeal system during hemodialysis (prophylaxis)
[Dalteparin (Systemic)], 1156

### Thrombosis, heparin-induced (treatment)
Ancrod (Systemic), 3131‡

### Thrombosis, percutaneous coronary intervention–related (prophylaxis)
Abciximab (Systemic)†, 1

### Thrombosis, percutaneous coronary intervention–related (treatment)
Eptifibatide (Systemic), 1356

### Thrush—See Candidiasis, oropharyngeal

### Thymoma (treatment)
[Cisplatin (Systemic)]¹, 876
[Cyclophosphamide (Systemic)]¹, 1128
[Doxorubicin (Systemic)]¹, 1308

### Thyroid function studies
Levothyroxine (Systemic)¹, 2809
Liothyronine (Systemic), 2809
Protirelin (Systemic), #
Sodium Iodide I 123 (Systemic), 2599
Sodium Iodide I 131 (Systemic—Diagnostic), 2603
Thyrotropin (Systemic), #

### Thyroid imaging, radionuclide
Sodium Iodide I 123 (Systemic), 2599
Sodium Iodide I 131 (Systemic—Diagnostic), 2603
Sodium Pertechnetate Tc 99m (Systemic), 2612
[Technetium Tc 99m Sestamibi (Systemic)]¹, 2736

### Thyroid involution, preoperative
[Iodine, Strong (Systemic)]¹, 1751
[Potassium Iodide (Systemic)]¹, 2354

**Thyroiditis, nonsuppurative (treatment)**
  Betamethasone, Oral (Systemic), 998
  Betamethasone, Parenteral (Systemic), 998
  Cortisone (Systemic), 998
  Dexamethasone, Oral (Systemic), 998
  Dexamethasone, Parenteral (Systemic), 998
  Hydrocortisone, Oral (Systemic), 998
  Hydrocortisone, Parenteral (Systemic), 998
  Methylprednisolone, Oral (Systemic), 998
  Methylprednisolone, Parenteral (Systemic), 998
  Prednisolone, Oral (Systemic), 998
  Prednisolone, Parenteral (Systemic), 998
  Prednisone (Systemic), 998
  Triamcinolone, Oral (Systemic), 998
  Triamcinolone, Parenteral (Systemic), 998
**Thyroid storm**—See Hyperthyroidism
**Thyroid uptake tests**
  Sodium Iodide I 123 (Systemic), 2599
  Sodium Iodide I 131 (Systemic—Diagnostic), 2603
**Thyrotoxicosis (treatment adjunct)**
  See also Hyperthyroidism; Hyperthyroidism, in Graves' disease
  [Acebutolol (Systemic)][1], 593
  [Atenolol (Systemic)][1], 593
  [Metoprolol (Systemic)][1], 593
  [Nadolol (Systemic)][1], 593
  Oxprenolol (Systemic)*[1], 593
  [Propranolol (Systemic)][1], 593
  [Sotalol (Systemic)][1], 593
  [Timolol (Systemic)][1], 593
**Thyrotoxicosis crisis (treatment adjunct)**
  [Iodine, Strong (Systemic)][1], 1751
  [Sodium Iodide (Systemic)]†, 2597
**Tic douloureux**—See Neuralgia, trigeminal
**Tick fevers**—See Rocky Mountain spotted fever
**Tinea barbae (treatment)**
  [Carbol-Fuchsin (Topical)], #
  [Clioquinol (Topical)], #
  [Clotrimazole (Topical)][1], 916
  [Econazole (Topical)][1], 1323
  Griseofulvin (Systemic), 1583
  [Haloprogin (Topical)][1], #
  [Ketoconazole (Systemic)], 302, #
  [Ketoconazole (Topical)][1], 1807
  [Miconazole (Topical)], #
  [Naftifine (Topical)], #
  [Nystatin (Topical)], 2148
  [Tolnaftate (Topical)], #
**Tinea capitis (treatment)**
  [Carbol-Fuchsin (Topical)], #
  [Clioquinol (Topical)], #
  [Clotrimazole (Topical)][1], 916
  [Econazole (Topical)][1], 1323
  Griseofulvin (Systemic), 1583
  [Haloprogin (Topical)][1], #
  [Ketoconazole (Systemic)][1], 302
  [Ketoconazole (Topical)][1], 1807
  [Miconazole (Topical)], #
  [Naftifine (Topical)], #
  [Nystatin (Topical)], 2148
  Terbinafine (Systemic)*[1], 2752
  [Tolnaftate (Topical)], #
**Tinea corporis (treatment)**
  Butenafine (Topical), 699
  Ciclopirox (Topical), 863
  Clotrimazole (Topical), 916
  Clotrimazole and Betamethasone (Topical), 918
  Econazole (Topical), 1323
  [Fluconazole (Systemic)][1], 302
  Griseofulvin (Systemic), 1583
  Haloprogin (Topical), #
  [Itraconazole (Systemic)], 302
  Ketoconazole (Systemic), 302
  Ketoconazole (Topical), 1807
  Miconazole (Topical), #
  Naftifine (Topical), #
  Oxiconazole (Topical)†, #
  Sulconazole (Topical)†, #
  Terbinafine (Systemic)*, 2752
  Terbinafine (Topical), 3036
  Terbinafine (Topical)†, 2755
  Tioconazole (Topical), 3036
  Tolnaftate (Topical), #
**Tinea cruris (treatment)**
  Butenafine (Topical), 699
  Ciclopirox (Topical), 863
  Clotrimazole (Topical), 916
  Clotrimazole and Betamethasone (Topical), 918
  Econazole (Topical), 1323
  [Fluconazole (Systemic)]1, 302
  Griseofulvin (Systemic), 1583
  Haloprogin (Topical), #
  [Itraconazole (Systemic)], 302
  Ketoconazole (Systemic), 302
  Ketoconazole (Topical), 1807
  Miconazole (Topical), #

**Tinea cruris (treatment)** (continued)
  Naftifine (Topical), #
  Oxiconazole (Topical)†, #
  Sulconazole (Topical)†, #
  Terbinafine (Systemic)*, 2752
  Terbinafine (Topical), 3036
  Terbinafine (Topical)†, 2755
  Tioconazole (Topical), 3036
  Tolnaftate (Topical), #
**Tinea manuum (treatment)**
  [Fluconazole (Systemic)][1], 302
  Haloprogin (Topical), #
  [Itraconazole (Systemic)][1], 302
  Tolnaftate (Topical), #
**Tinea pedis (treatment)**
  Butenafine (Topical), 699
  Ciclopirox (Topical), 863
  Clioquinol (Topical), #
  Clotrimazole (Topical), 916
  Clotrimazole and Betamethasone (Topical), 918
  Econazole (Topical), 1323
  [Fluconazole (Systemic)][1], 302
  Griseofulvin (Systemic), 1583
  Haloprogin (Topical), #
  [Itraconazole (Systemic)], 302
  Ketoconazole (Systemic), 302
  Ketoconazole (Topical), 1807
  Miconazole (Topical), #
  Naftifine (Topical), #
  Oxiconazole (Topical)†, #
  Sulconazole (Topical)†, #
  Terbinafine (Systemic)*, 2752
  Terbinafine (Topical), 3036
  Terbinafine (Topical)†, 2755
  Tioconazole (Topical), 3036
  Tolnaftate (Topical), #
**Tinea pedis (treatment adjunct)**
  Carbol-Fuchsin (Topical), #
**Tinea unguium (treatment)**
  See also Onychomycosis
  See also Onychomycosis; Skin and nail infections, fungal, minor
  Griseofulvin (Systemic), 1583
  Terbinafine (Systemic)*, 2752
**Tinea versicolor**—See also Pityriasis versicolor
**Tinea versicolor (treatment)**
  Ciclopirox (Topical), 863
  Clotrimazole (Topical), 916
  Econazole (Topical), 1323
  Miconazole (Topical), #
  Naftifine (Topical), #
  Selenium Sulfide (Topical), #
  Sulconazole (Topical)†, #
  Terbinafine (Topical), 3036
  Tioconazole (Topical), 3036
  Tolnaftate (Topical), #
**Tinea versicolor, pityriasis (treatment)**
  Ketoconazole (Topical), 3026
  Oxiconazole (Topical), 3030
**Tissue dye in diagnostic procedures**
  Methylene Blue (Systemic), 1391
**Tonsillitis**—See also Pharyngitis, bacterial
**Tonsillitis (treatment)**
  Azithromycin (Systemic), 499
  Cefaclor (Systemic), 794
  Cefadroxil (Systemic), 794
  Cefdinir (Systemic), 3014
  Cefixime (Systemic), 794
  Cefpodoxime (Systemic)†[1], 794
  Cefprozil (Systemic)†, 794
  Ceftibuten (Systemic)[1], 794
  Cefuroxime Axetil (Systemic), 794
  Cephalexin (Systemic), 794
  Cephradine (Systemic)†, 794
  Clarithromycin (Systemic), 889
**Toothache (treatment)**
  Benzocaine 10% Gel (Dental) (Mucosal-Local), 128
  Benzocaine 20% Gel (Dental) (Mucosal-Local), 128
  Benzocaine and Phenol Gel (Mucosal-Local), 128
  Benzocaine and Phenol Topical Solution (Mucosal-Local), 128
  Benzocaine Topical Solution USP (Mucosal-Local), 128
**Torticollis, spasmodic (treatment)**
  Botulinum Toxin Type A (Parenteral-Local), 3134‡
  Botulinum Toxin Type F (Parenteral-Local), 3134‡
**Tourette's syndrome**—See Gilles de la Tourette's syndrome
**Tourette's syndrome (treatment)**
  Pergolide (Systemic), 3158‡
  Tiapride (Systemic), 3169‡
**Toxicity, acetaminophen (treatment)**
  Acetylcysteine (Systemic), 16, 3128
  [Racemethionine (Systemic)]†, #

**Toxicity, aluminum (diagnosis)**
  [Deferoxamine (Systemic)], #
**Toxicity, aluminum (treatment)**
  [Deferoxamine (Systemic)], #
**Toxicity, Amanita phalloides (treatment)**
  Disodium Silibinin Dihemisuccinate (Systemic), 3141‡
**Toxicity, anticholinergic agent (treatment)**
  Physostigmine (Systemic), 2322
**Toxicity, arsenic (treatment)**
  Dimercaprol (Systemic), 1224
**Toxicity, benzodiazepine (treatment)**
  Flumazenil (Systemic), 1483
**Toxicity, beta-adrenergic blocking agent (treatment)**
  [Glucagon (Systemic)][1], 1563
**Toxicity, calcium channel blocking agent (treatment)**
  [Glucagon (Systemic)][1], 1563
**Toxicity, cholinesterase inhibitor (prophylaxis)**
  Atropine, Parenteral (Systemic), 226
  Glycopyrrolate, Parenteral (Systemic), 226
**Toxicity, cholinesterase inhibitor (treatment)**
  Atropine (Systemic), 226
**Toxicity, cholinesterase inhibitor (treatment adjunct)**
  Pralidoxime (Systemic), #
**Toxicity, cocaine (treatment)**
  Butyrylcholinesterase (Systemic), 3135‡
**Toxicity, curare (treatment)**
  Edrophonium (Systemic), 1329
**Toxicity, curare (treatment adjunct)**
  Edrophonium and Atropine (Systemic)†, 1331
**Toxicity, cyanide (treatment)**
  [Amyl Nitrite (Systemic)], #
  Hydroxycobalamin and Sodium Thiosulfate (Systemic), 3146‡
**Toxicity, cyanide (treatment adjunct)**
  Sodium Nitrite (Systemic), #
  Sodium Thiosulfate (Systemic), #
**Toxicity, cyanide, sodium nitroprusside–induced (prophylaxis)**
  Sodium Thiosulfate (Systemic), #
**Toxicity, cycloserine (treatment)**
  [Pyridoxine (Systemic)], 2430
**Toxicity, digitalis glycoside (treatment)**
  Digoxin Immune Fab (Ovine) (Systemic)†, 1219, 3140‡
  Edetate Disodium (Systemic)†, 1327
**Toxicity, dipyridamole (treatment)**
  Aminophylline Injection USP (Systemic)[1], 668
**Toxicity, doxorubicin (prophylaxis)**
  Dexrazoxane (Systemic), 3140‡
**Toxicity, enoxaparin (treatment)**
  [Protamine (Systemic)][1], 2420
**Toxicity, ergot alkaloid (treatment)**
  [Nitroprusside (Systemic)][1], 2142
  [Prazosin (Systemic)][1], 2370
**Toxicity, ethylene glycol (treatment)**
  Fomepizole (Systemic), 1526
  4-Methylpyrazole (Systemic), 3128‡
**Toxicity, gold (treatment)**
  Dimercaprol (Systemic), 1224
**Toxicity, heavy metal (treatment)**
  [Penicillamine (Systemic)], 2237
**Toxicity, heparin (treatment)**
  Protamine (Systemic), 2420
**Toxicity, iron, acute (treatment)**
  Dextran and Deferoxamine (Systemic), 3140‡
**Toxicity, iron, acute (treatment adjunct)**
  Deferoxamine (Systemic), #
**Toxicity, iron, chronic (treatment)**
  Deferoxamine (Systemic), #
**Toxicity, iron, chronic (treatment adjunct)**
  [Ascorbic Acid (Systemic)][1], 469
  [Sodium Ascorbate (Systemic)]†, 469
**Toxicity, isoniazid (treatment)**
  [Pyridoxine (Systemic)], 2430
**Toxicity, lead (treatment)**
  Edetate Calcium Disodium (Systemic), 1324
  Succimer (Systemic)†, #, 3166‡
**Toxicity, lead (treatment adjunct)**
  Dimercaprol (Systemic), 1224
**Toxicity, mercury (treatment)**
  Dimercaprol (Systemic), 1224
  Succimer (Systemic), 3166‡
**Toxicity, methanol (treatment)**
  4-Methylpyrazole (Systemic), 3128‡
**Toxicity, methotrexate (prophylaxis)**
  Leucovorin (Systemic), 1837
**Toxicity, methotrexate (treatment)**
  Leucovorin (Systemic), 1837
**Toxicity, muscarine (treatment)**
  Atropine (Systemic), 226

**Toxicity, nonspecific (treatment)**
Cascara Sagrada Fluidextract (Local), 3136‡
Charcoal, Activated (Oral-Local), 831
Charcoal, Activated, and Sorbitol (Oral-Local), 831
Ipecac (Oral-Local), 1759
Mannitol (Systemic), 1906
Sodium Bicarbonate, Parenteral (Systemic), 2586
**Toxicity, nonspecific (treatment adjunct)**
Magnesium Citrate (Local), #
Magnesium Hydroxide (Local), #
Magnesium Oxide (Local)†, #
Magnesium Sulfate (Local)†, #
Sodium Phosphate (Local)†, #
**Toxicity, opioid (narcotic) (diagnosis)**
Naloxone (Systemic), 2082
**Toxicity, opioid (narcotic) (treatment)**
Naloxone (Systemic), 2082
**Toxicity, organophosphate chemical (treatment adjunct)**
Pralidoxime (Systemic), #
**Toxicity, organophosphate pesticide (treatment)**
Atropine (Systemic), 226
**Toxicity, organophosphate pesticide (treatment adjunct)**
Pralidoxime (Systemic), #
**Toxicity, pyrimethamine (prophylaxis)**
Leucovorin (Systemic), 1837
**Toxicity, pyrimethamine (treatment)**
Leucovorin (Systemic), 1837
**Toxicity, radiocesium (treatment)**
Prussian Blue (Oral-Local)*†, #
**Toxicity, due to snakebite**
See Envenomation, 3132‡
**Toxicity, thallium (treatment)**
Prussian Blue (Oral-Local)*†, #
**Toxicity, tricyclic antidepressant (treatment adjunct)**
[Phenytoin, Parenteral (Systemic)][1], 253
**Toxicity, trimethoprim (prophylaxis)**
Leucovorin (Systemic), 1837
**Toxicity, trimethoprim (treatment)**
Leucovorin (Systemic), 1837
**Toxicity, weakly acidic medications (treatment)**
[Acetazolamide, Parenteral (Systemic)], 773
**Toxocariasis**—See Larva migrans, visceral
***Toxoplasma gondii* encephalitis (prophylaxis)**
Atovaquone (Systemic), 3132‡
***Toxoplasma gondii* encephalitis (treatment)**
Atovaquone (Systemic), 3132‡
Sulfadiazine (Systemic), 3166‡
**Toxoplasmosis (prophylaxis)**
Dapsone (Systemic), 3139‡
[Sulfamethoxazole and Trimethoprim (Systemic)][1], 2661
**Toxoplasmosis (treatment)**
Pyrimethamine (Systemic), 2433
Spiramycin (Systemic)*†, 2624
Sulfadiazine (Systemic)[1], 2653
Sulfamethoxazole (Systemic), 2653
Sulfisoxazole (Systemic), 2653
**Toxoplasmosis, AIDS-associated (treatment)**
Poloxamer 331 (Systemic), 3158‡
**Toxoplasmosis, central nervous system (CNS) (treatment)**
[Clindamycin (Systemic)][1], 893
**Tracheobronchitis (treatment adjunct)**
Acetylcysteine (Inhalation-Local), #
**Tracheostomy care, adjunct**
Acetylcysteine (Inhalation-Local), #
**Trachoma (treatment)**
Chlortetracycline (Ophthalmic), 2763
Demeclocycline (Systemic), 2765
Doxycycline (Systemic), 2765
[Erythromycin (Ophthalmic)][1], 1364
Minocycline (Systemic), 2765
Oxytetracycline (Systemic)†, 2765
Sulfacetamide (Ophthalmic), 2651
Sulfadiazine (Systemic), 2653
Sulfamethoxazole (Systemic), 2653
Sulfisoxazole (Ophthalmic), 2651
Sulfisoxazole (Systemic), 2653
Tetracycline (Ophthalmic), 2763
Tetracycline (Systemic), 2765
**Transfusion reactions, urticarial (treatment)**
Acrivastine (Systemic)*†, 325
Astemizole (Systemic), 325
Azatadine (Systemic), 325
Betamethasone, Parenteral (Systemic), 998
Bromodiphenhydramine (Systemic)*†, 325
Brompheniramine (Systemic), 325
Carbinoxamine (Systemic)*†, 325
Cetirizine (Systemic), 325
Chlorpheniramine (Systemic), 325
Clemastine (Systemic), 325

**Transfusion reactions, urticarial (treatment)** *(continued)*
Cortisone, Parenteral (Systemic), 998
Cyproheptadine (Systemic), 325
Dexamethasone, Parenteral (Systemic), 998
Dexchlorpheniramine (Systemic), 325
Dimenhydrinate (Systemic), 325
Diphenhydramine (Systemic), 325
Diphenylpyraline (Systemic)*†, 325
Doxylamine (Systemic)†, 325
Epinephrine Injection USP (Systemic), 651
Hydrocortisone, Parenteral (Systemic), 998
Hydroxyzine (Systemic), 325
Loratadine (Systemic), 325
Methdilazine (Systemic)†, 377
Methylprednisolone, Parenteral (Systemic), 998
Phenindamine (Systemic)†, 325
Prednisolone, Parenteral (Systemic), 998
Promethazine (Systemic), 377
Pyrilamine (Systemic)*†, 325
Triamcinolone, Parenteral (Systemic), 998
Trimeprazine (Systemic), 377
Tripelennamine (Systemic), 325
Triprolidine (Systemic)*†, 325
**Transient cerebral ischemic attacks (treatment)**
Acenocoumarol (Systemic)*, 3009
**Transplantation, organ, protection of donor tissue**
Superoxide Dismutase (Human), 3167‡
Superoxide Dismutase (Recombinant, Human), 3167‡
**Transplant rejection, bone marrow (prophylaxis)**
See also Graft versus host disease, in bone marrow transplantation
Interleukin-1 Receptor Antagonist, Human Recombinant (Systemic), 3149‡
Sargramostim (Systemic)†, 3163‡
Trisaccharides A and B (Systemic), 3170‡
**Transplant rejection, bone marrow (treatment)**
See also Graft versus host disease, in bone marrow transplantation (treatment)
Anti-thymocyte Serum (Systemic), 3131‡
CD5-T Lymphocyte Immunotoxin (Systemic), 3136‡
Interleukin-1 Receptor Antagonist, Human Recombinant (Systemic), 3149‡
Sargramostim (Systemic)†, 3163‡
**Transplant rejection, cardiac allograft (diagnosis)**
Imciromab Pentetate (Systemic), 3147‡
**Transplant rejection, cardiac allograft (prophylaxis)**
8-Methoxsalen (Systemic), 3128‡
**Transplant rejection, kidney (prophylaxis)**
Anaritide Acetate (Systemic), 3131‡
Basiliximab (Systemic), 547
Daclizumab (Systemic), 1151
Humanized Anti-TAC (Systemic), 3146‡
**Transplant rejection, kidney (treatment)**
Gusperimus (Systemic), 3145‡
**Transplant rejection, liver (prophylaxis)**
[Ursodiol (Systemic)]1, 2903
**Transplant rejection, lung allograft (prophylaxis)**
Cyclosporin A, Liposomal (Systemic), 3152‡
**Transplant rejection, lung allograft (treatment)**
Cyclosporin A, Liposomal (Systemic), 3152‡
**Transplant rejection, organ (prophylaxis)**
See also Graft rejection, organ (prophylaxis)
Azathioprine (Systemic), 491
[Betamethasone, Oral (Systemic)][1], 998
[Betamethasone, Parenteral (Systemic)][1], 998
[Cortisone (Systemic)][1], 998
[Cyclophosphamide (Systemic)][1], 1128
Cyclosporine (Systemic), 1136
[Dexamethasone, Oral (Systemic)][1], 998
[Dexamethasone, Parenteral (Systemic)][1], 998
[Hydrocortisone, Oral (Systemic)][1], 998
[Hydrocortisone, Parenteral (Systemic)][1], 998
Leflunomide (Systemic), 3151‡
[Methylprednisolone, Oral (Systemic)][1], 998
[Methylprednisolone, Parenteral (Systemic)][1], 998
Mycophenolate (Systemic), 2070
[Prednisolone, Oral (Systemic)][1], 998
[Prednisolone, Parenteral (Systemic)][1], 998
[Prednisone (Systemic)][1], 998
Tacrolimus (Systemic), 2683
[Triamcinolone, Oral (Systemic)][1], 998
[Triamcinolone, Parenteral (Systemic)][1], 998
Trisaccharides A and B (Systemic), 3170‡
**Transplant rejection, organ (treatment)**
Anti-thymocyte Serum (Systemic), 3131‡
[Betamethasone, Parenteral (Systemic)]1, 998
[Cortisone, Parenteral (Systemic)][1], 998
Cyclosporine (Systemic), 1136
[Dexamethasone, Parenteral (Systemic)][1], 998

**Transplant rejection, organ (treatment)** *(continued)*
[Hydrocortisone, Parenteral (Systemic)][1], 998
[Methylprednisolone, Parenteral (Systemic)][1], 998
Muromonab-CD3 (Systemic), 2068
[Prednisolone, Parenteral (Systemic)][1], 998
[Triamcinolone, Parenteral (Systemic)][1], 998
**Transplant rejection, solid organ (prophylaxis)**
Tacrolimus (Systemic), 2683
**Transplant rejection, solid organ (treatment)**
[Tacrolimus (Systemic)], 2683
**Transtracheal**
Lidocaine (Parenteral-Local), 139
[Mepivacaine (Parenteral-Local)][1], 139
[Tetracaine (Parenteral-Local)][1], 139
**Traveler's diarrhea (prophylaxis)**
[Bismuth Subsalicylate (Oral-Local)][1], 616
[Doxycycline (Systemic)], 2765
**Traveler's diarrhea (treatment)**
[Doxycycline (Systemic)], 2765
Loperamide (Oral-Local), 1877
Sulfamethoxazole and Trimethoprim, Oral (Systemic), 2661
**Tremors (treatment)**
[Acebutolol (Systemic)][1], 593
[Alprazolam, Oral (Systemic)][1], 556
[Atenolol (Systemic)][1], 593
[Chlordiazepoxide, Oral (Systemic)][1], 556
[Diazepam, Oral (Systemic)][1], 556
[Lorazepam, Oral (Systemic)][1], 556
[Metoprolol (Systemic)][1], 593
[Nadolol (Systemic)][1], 593
Oxprenolol (Systemic)*[1], 593
[Pindolol (Systemic)][1], 593
Propranolol (Systemic), 593
[Sotalol (Systemic)][1], 593
[Timolol (Systemic)][1], 593
**Trichinellosis**—See Trichinosis
**Trichinosis (treatment)**
Betamethasone, Oral (Systemic), 998
Betamethasone, Parenteral (Systemic), 998
Cortisone (Systemic), 998
Dexamethasone, Oral (Systemic), 998
Dexamethasone, Parenteral (Systemic), 998
Hydrocortisone, Oral (Systemic), 998
Hydrocortisone, Parenteral (Systemic), 998
[Mebendazole (Systemic)][1], 1926
Methylprednisolone, Oral (Systemic), 998
Methylprednisolone, Parenteral (Systemic), 998
Prednisolone, Oral (Systemic), 998
Prednisolone, Parenteral (Systemic), 998
Prednisone (Systemic), 998
Thiabendazole (Systemic)†, 2784
Triamcinolone, Oral (Systemic), 998
**Trichomoniasis (treatment)**
Metronidazole and Nystatin (Vaginal)*, 3028
Metronidazole, Oral (Systemic), 1996
[Metronidazole Vaginal Cream (Vaginal)], 2001
[Metronidazole Vaginal Tablets (Vaginal)], 2001
**Trichostrongyliasis (treatment)**
Albendazole (Systemic)*†, #
[Pyrantel (Oral-Local)][1], #
[Thiabendazole (Systemic)]†, 2784
**Trichuriasis (treatment)**
Albendazole (Systemic)*†, #
Mebendazole (Systemic), 1926
**Trigonitis**—See Irritative voiding, symptoms of
**Trimethoprim toxicity**—See Toxicity, trimethoprim
**Tropical eosinophilia (treatment)**
Diethylcarbamazine (Systemic), #
**Trypanosome fever**—See Trypanosomiasis, African
**Trypanosomiasis, African (treatment)**
Eflornithine (Systemic)†, #, 3141‡
Melarsoprol (Systemic)*†, #
[Pentamidine (Systemic)][1], 2274
Suramin (Systemic)*†, #
**Trypanosomiasis, American (treatment)**
Benznidazole (Systemic)*†, #
Nifurtimox (Systemic)*†, #
**Tuberculosis (diagnosis)**
Tuberculin, Purified Protein Derivative (Parenteral-Local), 2895
**Tuberculosis (prophylaxis)**
Bacillus Calmette-Guérin (BCG) Live (Systemic), 510
Isoniazid (Systemic), 1789
**Tuberculosis (treatment)**
Aconiazide (Systemic), 3128‡
Aminosalicylate Sodium (Systemic), #
Aminosalicylic Acid (Systemic), 3130‡
Aminosidine (Systemic), 3130‡
Capreomycin (Systemic), 751
Cycloserine (Systemic)†, 1134
Ethambutol (Systemic), 1412
Ethionamide (Systemic)†, 1417

## Indications Index

**Tuberculosis (treatment)** *(continued)*
  Isoniazid (Systemic), 1789
  Isoniazid and Thiacetazone (Systemic)*†, #
  Pyrazinamide (Systemic), 2425
  Rifampin (Systemic), 2485, 3163‡
  Rifampin and Isoniazid (Systemic)†, 2493
  Rifampin, Isoniazid, and Pyrazinamide (Systemic), 3163‡
  Rifampin, Isoniazid, and Pyrazinamide (Systemic)†, 2494
  Rifapentine (Systemic), 3163‡
  Streptomycin (Systemic), 69
  Thalidomide (Systemic), 3168‡
**Tuberculosis (treatment adjunct)**
  Acetylcysteine (Inhalation-Local), #
  Aminosalicylic Acid (Systemic), 3009
**Tuberculosis, pulmonary (treatment)**
  Rifapentine (Systemic), 2496
**Tuberculosis, pulmonary (treatment adjunct)**
  Betamethasone, Oral (Systemic), 998
  Betamethasone, Parenteral (Systemic), 998
  Cortisone (Systemic), 998
  Dexamethasone, Oral (Systemic), 998
  Dexamethasone, Parenteral (Systemic), 998
  Hydrocortisone, Oral (Systemic), 998
  Hydrocortisone, Parenteral (Systemic), 998
  Methylprednisolone, Oral (Systemic), 998
  Methylprednisolone, Parenteral (Systemic), 998
  Prednisolone, Oral (Systemic), 998
  Prednisolone, Parenteral (Systemic), 998
  Prednisone (Systemic), 998
  Triamcinolone, Oral (Systemic), 998
  Triamcinolone, Parenteral (Systemic), 998
**Tularemia (treatment)**
  [Demeclocycline (Systemic)], 2765
  [Doxycycline (Systemic)], 2765
  [Minocycline (Systemic)], 2765
  [Oxytetracycline (Systemic)]†, 2765
  Streptomycin (Systemic), 69
  [Tetracycline (Systemic)], 2765
**Tumor imaging, radionuclide**
  [Thallous Chloride Tl 201 (Systemic)]1, 2781
**Tumors, adrenal medulla (diagnosis)**
  Iobenguane I 123 (Systemic—Diagnostic)†, 1747
  Iobenguane I 131 (Systemic—Diagnostic)†, 1747
**Tumors, brain (diagnosis)**
  See also Brain imaging, computed tomographic; Brain imaging, radionuclide
  [Fludeoxyglucose F 18 (Systemic)]1*†, 1478
  Microbubble Contrast Agent, 3154‡
**Tumors, brain (treatment)**
  Carmustine (Implantation-Local), 784
**Tumors, brain, metastatic (treatment)**
  Herpes Simplex Virus Gene (Systemic), 3145‡
**Tumors, brain, primary (treatment)**
  Biodel Implant/Carmustine (Systemic), 3133‡
  Bromodeoxyuridine (Systemic), 3134‡
  [Carboplatin (Systemic)]1, 779
  Carmustine (Systemic), 786
  [Cyclophosphamide (Systemic)]1, 1128
  [Etoposide (Systemic)]1, 1424
  Herpes Simplex Virus Gene (Systemic), 3145‡
  Interferon Beta (Recombinant Human) (Systemic), 3148‡
  Interleukin-2, Recombinant, Liposome Encapsulated (Systemic), 3152‡
  Lomustine (Systemic), 1874
  Mitolactol (Systemic), 3154‡
  Poly-ICLC (Systemic), 3158‡
  [Procarbazine (Systemic)]1, 2391
  Serratia Marcescens Extract (Polyribosomes) (Systemic), 3164‡
  Sodium Monomercaptoundecahydro-closo-dodecaborate (Systemic), 3164‡
  SU-101 (Systemic), 3166‡
  Thalidomide (Systemic), 768
  [Vincristine (Systemic)]1, 2950
**Tumors, brain, primary (treatment adjunct)**
  [Betamethasone, Oral (Systemic)]1, 998
  [Betamethasone, Parenteral (Systemic)]1, 998
  [Cortisone (Systemic)]1, 998
  [Dexamethasone, Oral (Systemic)]1, 998
  [Dexamethasone, Parenteral (Systemic)]1, 998
  [Hydrocortisone, Oral (Systemic)]1, 998
  [Hydrocortisone, Parenteral (Systemic)]1, 998
  [Methylprednisolone, Oral (Systemic)]1, 998
  [Methylprednisolone, Parenteral (Systemic)]1, 998
  [Prednisolone, Oral (Systemic)]1, 998
  [Prednisolone, Parenteral (Systemic)]1, 998
  [Prednisone (Systemic)]1, 998
  [Triamcinolone, Oral (Systemic)]1, 998
  [Triamcinolone, Parenteral (Systemic)]1, 998

**Tumors, carcinoid (diagnosis)**
  See also Tumors, gastrointestinal; Tumors, neuroendocrine
  [Iobenguane I 123 (Systemic—Diagnostic)]†, 1747
  [Iobenguane I 131 (Systemic—Diagnostic)]†, 1747
**Tumors, carcinoid (treatment)**
  [Interferon Alfa-2a, Recombinant (Systemic)]1, 1740
  [Interferon Alfa-2b, Recombinant (Systemic)]1, 1740
  [Interferon Alfa-n1 (Ins) (Systemic)]1, 1740
  [Interferon Alfa-n3 (Systemic)]1, 1740
**Tumors, cystic, of tendon or aponeurosis (treatment)**
  Betamethasone, Parenteral-Local (Systemic), 998
  Dexamethasone, Parenteral-Local (Systemic), 998
  Hydrocortisone, Parenteral-Local (Systemic), 998
  Methylprednisolone, Parenteral-Local (Systemic), 998
  Prednisolone, Parenteral-Local (Systemic), 998
  Triamcinolone, Parenteral-Local (Systemic), 998
**Tumors, desmoid (treatment)**
  Toremifene (Systemic), 3169‡
**Tumors, fallopian tube (diagnosis)**—See Hysterosalpingography
**Tumors, gastrointestinal (treatment adjunct)**
  Octreotide (Systemic), 2152
**Tumors, gastrointestinal carcinoid (treatment)**
  [Streptozocin (Systemic)]1, 2629
**Tumors, germ cell (diagnosis)**
  Iodine I 123 Murine Monoclonal Antibody to Alpha-fetoprotein (Systemic), 3149‡
  Iodine I 123 Murine Monoclonal Antibody to Human Chorionic Gonadotropin (Systemic), 3149‡
  Technetium Tc 99m Murine Monoclonal Antibody to Human Alpha-fetoprotein (Systemic), 3167‡
  Technetium Tc 99m Murine Monoclonal Antibody to Human Chorionic Gonadotropin (Systemic), 3167‡
**Tumors, germ cell (treatment)**
  [Cisplatin (Systemic)]1, 876
  Iodine I 131 Murine Monoclonal Antibody to Alpha-fetoprotein (Systemic), 3149‡
  Iodine I 131 Murine Monoclonal Antibody to Human Chorionic Gonadotropin (Systemic), 3150‡
**Tumors, germ cell, ovarian (treatment)**
  [Bleomycin (Systemic)]1, 624
  [Cisplatin (Systemic)]1, 876
  [Cyclophosphamide (Systemic)]1, 1128
  [Doxorubicin (Systemic)], 1308
  [Vinblastine (Systemic)]1, 2946
  [Vincristine (Systemic)]1, 2950
**Tumors, germ cell, testicular (treatment)**
  Ifosfamide (Systemic)1, 1677, 3147‡
**Tumors, head and neck (diagnosis)**
  [Fludeoxyglucose F 18 (Systemic)]1*†, 1478
**Tumors, hepatic (treatment)**
  Iodine I 131 Murine Monoclonal Antibody to Alpha-fetoprotein (Systemic), 3149‡
**Tumors, neuroendocrine (diagnosis)**
  Indium In 111 Pentetreotide (Systemic)†, 1700
**Tumors, pancreatic (treatment adjunct)**
  [Octreotide (Systemic)]1, 2152
**Tumors, trophoblastic (diagnosis)**
  Iodine I 123 Murine Monoclonal Antibody to Human Chorionic Gonadotropin (Systemic), 3150‡
  Technetium Tc 99m Murine Monoclonal Antibody to Human Chorionic Gonadotropin (Systemic), 3167‡
**Tumors, trophoblastic (treatment)**
  Iodine I 131 Murine Monoclonal Antibody to Human Chorionic Gonadotropin (Systemic), 3150‡
**Tumors, trophoblastic, gestational (treatment)**
  [Bleomycin (Systemic)]1, 624
  [Chlorambucil (Systemic)]1, 837
  [Cisplatin (Systemic)]1, 876
  [Cyclophosphamide (Systemic)]1, 1128
  Dactinomycin (Systemic), 1153
  [Doxorubicin (Systemic)]1, 1308
  [Etoposide (Systemic)]1, 1424
  Methotrexate—For Cancer (Systemic), 1962
  Vinblastine (Systemic), 2946
  [Vincristine (Systemic)]1, 2950
**Tumors, uterine (diagnosis)**—See Hysterosalpingography
**Turner's syndrome (treatment)**
  See also Growth failure
  [Ethinyl Estradiol (Systemic)]1, 1383, 3142‡
  [Oxandrolone (Systemic)]†, 110, 3156‡
  Somatrem (Systemic), 3165‡
  Somatropin (Systemic), 3165‡

**Typhoid fever (treatment)**
  [Amoxicillin (Systemic)]1, 2240
  [Ampicillin (Systemic)]1, 2240
  Chloramphenicol (Systemic), 841
  Ciprofloxacin (Systemic), 1487
  [Sulfamethoxazole and Trimethoprim (Systemic)], 2661
**Typhus infections (treatment)**
  Chloramphenicol (Systemic), 841
  Demeclocycline (Systemic), 2765
  Doxycycline (Systemic), 2765
  Minocycline (Systemic), 2765
  Oxytetracycline (Systemic)†, 2765
  Tetracycline (Systemic), 2765
**Tyrosinemia, type 1 (treatment)**
  NTBC (Systemic), 3156‡

## U

**Ulcera de Bejuco**—See Leishmaniasis, cutaneous
**Ulcer, aphthous**—See Stomatitis, aphthous
**Ulcer, aphthous (treatment)**
  Betamethasone (Dental), 3012
**Ulcer, aphthous, recurrent**—See Stomatitis, aphthous, recurrent
**Ulcer, corneal (treatment)**
  Framycetin (Ophthalmic)*, 3020
**Ulcer, corneal, bacterial (treatment)**
  Ofloxacin (Ophthalmic), 3030
**Ulcer, decubital (treatment)**
  [Benzoyl Peroxide (Topical)], 579
  Metronidazole (Topical), 3154‡
  Nicotinyl Alcohol (Systemic)*, #
**Ulcer, dermal (treatment)**
  Becaplermin (Topical), 550
  [Chlortetracycline (Topical)], 2774
  [Clindamycin (Topical)]1, 896
  [Clioquinol (Topical)], #
  [Gentamicin (Topical)], 1557
  [Neomycin (Topical)], #
  [Neomycin and Polymyxin B (Topical)]†, #
  [Neomycin, Polymyxin B, and Bacitracin (Topical)], #
  [Silver Sulfadiazine (Topical)], #
  [Tetracycline Hydrochloride Ointment (Topical)], 2774
**Ulcer, duodenal (prophylaxis)**
  Cimetidine (Systemic), 1633
  Famotidine (Systemic), 1633
  Lansoprazole (Systemic), 1828
  Nizatidine (Systemic), 1633
  Ranitidine (Systemic), 1633
  Sucralfate (Oral-Local), 2635
**Ulcer, duodenal (treatment)**
  Alumina, Calcium Carbonate, and Sodium Bicarbonate (Oral-Local)*, 188
  Alumina and Magnesia (Oral-Local), 188
  Alumina, Magnesia, Calcium Carbonate, and Simethicone (Oral-Local)†, 188
  Alumina, Magnesia, and Magnesium Carbonate (Oral-Local)*, 188
  Alumina, Magnesia, Magnesium Carbonate, and Simethicone (Oral-Local)*, 188
  Alumina, Magnesia, and Simethicone (Oral-Local), 188
  Alumina, Magnesium Alginate, and Magnesium Carbonate (Oral-Local)*, 188
  Alumina and Magnesium Carbonate (Oral-Local)†, 188
  Alumina, Magnesium Carbonate, and Simethicone (Oral-Local)†, 188
  Alumina, Magnesium Carbonate, and Sodium Bicarbonate (Oral-Local)†, 188
  Alumina and Magnesium Trisilicate (Oral-Local)†, 188
  Alumina, Magnesium Trisilicate, and Sodium Bicarbonate (Oral-Local)†, 188
  Alumina and Simethicone (Oral-Local)†, 188
  Alumina and Sodium Bicarbonate (Oral-Local)*, 188
  Aluminum Carbonate, Basic (Oral-Local)†, 188
  Aluminum Carbonate, Basic and Simethicone (Oral-Local)†, 188
  Aluminum Hydroxide (Oral-Local), 188
  Calcium Carbonate (Oral-Local)†, 188
  Calcium Carbonate and Magnesia (Oral-Local)†, 188
  Calcium Carbonate, Magnesia, and Simethicone (Oral-Local)†, 188
  Calcium and Magnesium Carbonates (Oral-Local)†, 188

**Ulcer, duodenal (treatment)** *(continued)*
    Calcium Carbonate and Simethicone (Oral-Local)†, 188
    Cimetidine (Systemic), 1633
    Famotidine (Systemic), 1633
    Lansoprazole (Systemic), 1828
    Magaldrate (Oral-Local), 188
    Magaldrate and Simethicone (Oral-Local), 188
    Magnesium Carbonate and Sodium Bicarbonate (Oral-Local)*, 188
    Magnesium Hydroxide (Oral-Local), 188
    Magnesium Oxide (Oral-Local)†, 188
    [Misoprostol (Systemic)], 2026
    Nizatidine (Systemic), 1633
    Pantoprazole (Systemic), 3031
    Ranitidine (Systemic), 1633
    Sucralfate (Oral-Local), 2635
**Ulcer, duodenal, *Helicobacter pylori*–associated (treatment)**
    Lansoprazole (Systemic), 1828
**Ulcer, duodenal, active (treatment)**
    Azelastine (Nasal), 188
    Bismuth Subsalicylate, Metronidazole, and Tetracycline—For *H. pylori* (Systemic), 620
    Ranitidine Bismuth Citrate (Systemic), 2458
    Ranitidine Bismuth Citrate(Systemic), 3033
**Ulcer, duodenal, *Helicobacter pylori*–associated (treatment)**
    Amoxicillin (Systemic), 3010
**Ulcer, duodenal, *Helicobacter pylori*–associated (treatment adjunct)**
    [Bismuth Subsalicylate (Oral-Local)][1], 616
    Clarithromycin (Systemic), 889
    [Metronidazole (Systemic)][1], 1996
**Ulcer, gastric (prophylaxis)**
    Ranitidine (Systemic), 1633
**Ulcer, gastric (treatment)**
    Alumina, Calcium Carbonate, and Sodium Bicarbonate (Oral-Local)*, 188
    Alumina and Magnesia (Oral-Local), 188
    Alumina, Magnesia, Calcium Carbonate, and Simethicone (Oral-Local)†, 188
    Alumina, Magnesia, and Magnesium Carbonate (Oral-Local)†, 188
    Alumina, Magnesia, Magnesium Carbonate, and Simethicone (Oral-Local)*, 188
    Alumina, Magnesia, and Simethicone (Oral-Local), 188
    Alumina, Magnesium Alginate, and Magnesium Carbonate (Oral-Local)*, 188
    Alumina and Magnesium Carbonate (Oral-Local)†, 188
    Alumina, Magnesium Carbonate, and Simethicone (Oral-Local)†, 188
    Alumina, Magnesium Carbonate, and Sodium Bicarbonate (Oral-Local)†, 188
    Alumina and Magnesium Trisilicate (Oral-Local)†, 188
    Alumina, Magnesium Trisilicate, and Sodium Bicarbonate (Oral-Local)†, 188
    Alumina and Simethicone (Oral-Local)†, 188
    Alumina and Sodium Bicarbonate (Oral-Local)*, 188
    Aluminum Carbonate, Basic (Oral-Local)†, 188
    Aluminum Carbonate, Basic and Simethicone (Oral-Local)†, 188
    Aluminum Hydroxide (Oral-Local), 188
    Calcium Carbonate (Oral-Local)†, 188
    Calcium Carbonate and Magnesia (Oral-Local)†, 188
    Calcium Carbonate, Magnesia, and Simethicone (Oral-Local)†, 188
    Calcium and Magnesium Carbonates (Oral-Local)†, 188
    Calcium Carbonate and Simethicone (Oral-Local)†, 188
    Cimetidine (Systemic), 1633
    Famotidine (Systemic), 1633
    Lansoprazole (Systemic), 1828
    Magaldrate (Oral-Local), 188
    Magaldrate and Simethicone (Oral-Local), 188
    Magnesium Carbonate and Sodium Bicarbonate (Oral-Local)*, 188
    Magnesium Hydroxide (Oral-Local), 188
    Magnesium Oxide (Oral-Local)†, 188
    Nizatidine (Systemic), 1633
    Pantoprazole (Systemic), 3031
    Ranitidine (Systemic), 1633
    [Sucralfate (Oral-Local)], 2635
**Ulcer, gastric, nonsteroidal anti-inflammatory drug–induced (prophylaxis)**
    Misoprostol (Systemic), 2026

**Ulcer, ischemic, of lower limb (treatment)**
    Prostaglandin E1 in Lipid Emulsion (Systemic), 3160‡
**Ulcer, peptic (treatment)**
    [Amitriptyline (Systemic)][1], 271
    [Doxepin (Systemic)][1], 271
    Omeprazole (Systemic), 2163
    [Trimipramine (Systemic)][1], 271
**Ulcer, peptic (treatment adjunct)**
    Atropine (Systemic), 226
    Atropine, Hyoscyamine, Scopolamine, and Phenobarbital (Systemic), 551
    Atropine and Phenobarbital (Systemic)†, 551
    Belladonna (Systemic)†, 226
    Belladonna and Butabarbital (Systemic)†, 551
    Belladonna and Phenobarbital (Systemic)†, 551
    Chlordiazepoxide and Clidinium (Systemic), 846
    Clidinium (Systemic), 226
    Hyoscyamine (Systemic), 226
    Hyoscyamine and Phenobarbital (Systemic)†, 551
    Pirenzepine (Systemic)*, 226
    Propantheline (Systemic), 226
    Scopolamine (Systemic), 226
    Scopolamine Butylbromide (Systemic)*, 226
    Tridihexethyl (Systemic)†, 226
**Ulcer, peptic, *Helicobacter pylori*–associated (treatment adjunct)**
    [Amoxicillin (Systemic)][1], 2240
    Omeprazole (Systemic), 2163
**Ulcer, peptic, nonsteroidal anti-inflammatory drug–induced (treatment)**
    Omeprazole (Systemic), 2163
**Ulcer, stasis (treatment)**
    [Benzoyl Peroxide (Topical)], 579
**Ulcer, varicose (treatment)**
    Nicotinyl Alcohol (Systemic)*, #
**Urea cycle disorders (treatment)**
    Sodium Benzoate and Sodium Phenylacetate (Systemic), 3164‡
    Sodium Phenylbutyrate (Systemic), 3164‡
**Urea cycle disorders (treatment adjunct)**
    Sodium Phenylbutyrate (Systemic)†, #
**Urethritis (treatment)**
    *See also* Irritative voiding, symptoms of
    Lidocaine Hydrochloride Jelly USP (Mucosal-Local), 128
**Urethritis, atrophic, postmenopausal (treatment)**
    Estradiol (Vaginal), 1391
**Urethritis, gonococcal (treatment)**
    Azithromycin (Systemic), 499
    [Demeclocycline (Systemic)], 2765
    [Doxycycline (Systemic)], 2765
    [Minocycline (Systemic)], 2765
    [Oxytetracycline (Systemic)]†, 2765
    [Tetracycline (Systemic)], 2765
**Urethritis, nongonoccocal (treatment)**
    Grepafloxacin (Systemic), 1580
**Urethritis, nongonococcal (treatment)**
    Azithromycin (Systemic), 499
    Doxycycline (Systemic), 2765
    Erythromycin (Systemic), 1368
**Urethrocystitis**—*See* Irritative voiding, symptoms of
**Urethrotrigonitis (treatment adjunct)**
    *See also* Irritative voiding, symptoms of
    Flavoxate (Systemic), 1468
**Urinary bladder imaging, radionuclide**
    Sodium Pertechnetate Tc 99m (Mucosal-Local), 2610
    [Technetium Tc 99m Mertiatide (Systemic)], 2720
**Urinary incontinence (treatment)**
    [Imipramine (Systemic)][1], 271
    [Phenylpropanolamine (Systemic)]†, 2314
    [Propantheline (Systemic)][1], 226
**Urinary retention (treatment)**
    Bethanechol (Systemic), 614
**Urinary retention, postoperative (prophylaxis)**
    Neostigmine, Parenteral (Systemic), 437
**Urinary retention, postoperative (treatment)**
    Neostigmine, Parenteral (Systemic), 437
**Urinary stones**—*See* Renal calculi
**Urinary tract infections (treatment adjunct)**
    *See also* Irritative voiding, symptoms of
    Monobasic Potassium Phosphate Tablets for Oral Solution (Systemic)†, 2317
    Potassium and Sodium Phosphates (Systemic), 2317
**Urinary tract infections, bacterial (prophylaxis)**
    Cinoxacin (Systemic)†, #
    Lomefloxacin (Systemic), 1487
    Methenamine (Systemic), #
    [Nitrofurantoin (Systemic)][1], 2139
    [Sulfamethoxazole and Trimethoprim (Systemic)][1], 2661
    [Trimethoprim (Systemic)][1], 2882

**Urinary tract infections, bacterial (treatment)**
    Amoxicillin (Systemic), 2240
    Amoxicillin and Clavulanate (Systemic), 2263, 3010
    Ampicillin (Systemic), 2240
    Aztreonam (Systemic)†, 502
    Bacampicillin (Systemic), 2240
    Carbenicillin (Systemic), 2240
    Cefaclor (Systemic), 794
    Cefadroxil (Systemic), 794
    Cefamandole (Systemic), 794
    Cefazolin (Systemic), 794
    Cefipime (Systemic), 794
    Cefixime (Systemic), 794
    Cefonicid (Systemic)[1], 794
    Cefoperazone (Systemic)[1], 794
    Cefotaxime (Systemic), 794
    Cefotetan (Systemic), 794
    Cefoxitin (Systemic), 794
    Cefpodoxime (Systemic)†[1], 794
    Cefprozil (Systemic)†, 794
    Ceftazidime (Systemic), 794
    Ceftizoxime (Systemic), 794
    Ceftriaxone (Systemic), 794
    Cefuroxime (Systemic), 794
    Cefuroxime Axetil (Systemic)[1], 794
    Cephalexin (Systemic), 794
    [Cephalothin (Systemic)], 794
    Cephapirin (Systemic)†[1], 794
    Cephradine (Systemic)[1], 794
    Ciprofloxacin (Systemic), 1487
    Demeclocycline (Systemic), 2765
    Doxycycline (Systemic), 2765
    Enoxacin (Systemic), 1487
    Imipenem and Cilastatin (Systemic), 1681
    Lomefloxacin (Systemic), 1487
    Loracarbef (Systemic)†, 1880
    Methenamine (Systemic), #
    Mezlocillin (Systemic)†, 2240
    Minocycline (Systemic), 2765
    Nalidixic Acid (Systemic), #
    Nitrofurantoin (Systemic), 2139
    Norfloxacin (Systemic), 1487
    Ofloxacin (Systemic), 1487
    Oxytetracycline (Systemic)†, 2765
    Piperacillin (Systemic), 2240
    Pivampicillin (Systemic)*, 2240
    Pivmecillinam (Systemic)*, 2240
    Sulfadiazine and Trimethoprim (Systemic)*, 2661
    Sulfamethizole (Systemic)†, 2653
    Sulfamethoprim and Trimethoprim (Systemic), 2661
    Sulfamethoxazole (Systemic), 2653
    Sulfamethoxazole and Phenazopyridine (Systemic)†, 2660
    Sulfisoxazole (Systemic), 2653
    Sulfisoxazole and Phenazopyridine (Systemic), 2660
    Tetracycline (Systemic), 2765
    Ticarcillin (Systemic), 2240
    Ticarcillin and Clavulanate (Systemic), 2263
    Trimethoprim (Systemic), 2882
    Trovafloxacin (Systemic), 2891
**Urinary tract infections, bacterial (treatment adjunct)**
    *See also* Irritative voiding, symptoms of
    Acetohydroxamic Acid (Systemic)†, #
    Flavoxate (Systemic), 1468
**Urinary tract infections, bacterial, complicated (treatment)**
    Levofloxacin (Systemic), 1852
**Urinary tract infections, fungal (treatment)**
    Amphotericin B (Systemic), 98
    Flucytosine (Systemic), #
**Urinary tract infections, recurrent complicated (treatment)**
    Amikacin (Systemic), 69
    Gentamicin (Systemic), 69
    Kanamycin (Systemic)†, 69
    Netilmicin (Systemic), 69
    Streptomycin (Systemic), 69
    Tobramycin (Systemic), 69
**Urinary tract infections, uncomplicated (treatment)**
    Fosfomycin (Systemic), 1531
**Urinary tract irritation (treatment)**
    Phenazopyridine (Systemic), 2288
**Urinary tract obstruction (diagnosis)**
    *See also* Cystourethrography, retrograde; Pyelography, retrograde; Renography; Urography, excretory; Urography, retrograde
    Iothalamate Meglumine (Systemic), #

**Urinary tract obstruction (diagnosis)** *(continued)*
Iothalamate Meglumine and Iothalamate Sodium (Systemic)†, #
Iothalamate Sodium (Systemic), #
Ioxaglate (Systemic), #
**Urine odor (treatment)**
Racemethionine (Systemic)†, 1#
**Urography, excretory**
Diatrizoate Meglumine and Diatrizoate Sodium, Parenteral (Systemic), #
Diatrizoate Meglumine, Parenteral (Systemic), #
Diatrizoate Sodium, Parenteral (Systemic), #
Iodixanol (Systemic), #
Iohexol (Systemic), #
Iopamidol (Systemic), #
Iopromide (Systemic), #
Iothalamate Meglumine (Systemic), #
Iothalamate Meglumine and Iothalamate Sodium (Systemic)†, #
Iothalamate Sodium (Systemic), #
Ioversol (Systemic), #
Ioxaglate (Systemic), #
Ioxilan (Systemic), #
**Urography, retrograde**
Diatrizoate Meglumine, Parenteral (Systemic)1, #
Diatrizoate Sodium, Parenteral (Systemic)1, #
**Urologic disorders, symptoms of (treatment)**
Flavoxate (Systemic), 1468
Hyoscyamine, Oral (Systemic), 226
Oxybutynin (Systemic), 2209
**Urticaria (treatment)**
Acrivastine (Systemic)*†, 325
Astemizole (Systemic), 325
Azatadine (Systemic), 325
Bromodiphenhydramine (Systemic)*†, 325
Brompheniramine (Systemic), 325
Carbinoxamine (Systemic)*†, 325
Cetirizine (Systemic), 325
Chlorpheniramine (Systemic), 325
Clemastine (Systemic), 325
Cyproheptadine (Systemic), 325
Dexchlorpheniramine (Systemic), 325
Dimenhydrinate (Systemic), 325
Diphenhydramine (Systemic), 325
Diphenylpyraline (Systemic)*†, 325
Doxylamine (Systemic)†, 325
Hydroxyzine (Systemic), 325
Loratadine (Systemic), 325
Methdilazine (Systemic)†, 377
Phenindamine (Systemic)†, 325
Promethazine (Systemic), 377
Pyrilamine (Systemic)*†, 325
Resorcinol (Topical), 1#
Trimeprazine (Systemic), 377
Tripelennamine (Systemic), 325
Triprolidine (Systemic)*†, 325
**Urticaria (treatment adjunct)**
[Ephedrine (Systemic)]1, 651
**Urticaria, acute (treatment adjunct)**
[Cimetidine (Systemic)]1, 1633
**Urticaria, solar (treatment)**
[Chloroquine (Systemic)]1, 849
[Hydroxychloroquine (Systemic)]1, 1663
**Uta**—See Leishmaniasis, cutaneous
**Utero-placental insufficiency (diagnosis)**
[Oxytocin, Parenteral (Systemic)]1, 2211
**Uveitis (treatment)**
Atropine (Ophthalmic), 485
[Cyclopentolate (Ophthalmic)]1, #
Homatropine (Ophthalmic), 1651
Scopolamine (Ophthalmic), 2557
**Uveitis, anterior (treatment)**
Rimexolone (Ophthalmic), 2504
**Uveitis, autoimmune (treatment)**
AI-RSA (Systemic), 3128‡
**Uveitis, posterior, diffuse (treatment)**
Betamethasone, Oral (Systemic), 998
Betamethasone, Parenteral (Systemic), 998
Cortisone (Systemic), 998
Dexamethasone, Oral (Systemic), 998
Dexamethasone, Parenteral (Systemic), 998
Hydrocortisone, Oral (Systemic), 998
Hydrocortisone, Parenteral (Systemic), 998
Methylprednisolone, Oral (Systemic), 998
Methylprednisolone, Parenteral (Systemic), 998
Prednisolone, Oral (Systemic), 998
Prednisolone, Parenteral (Systemic), 998
Prednisone (Systemic), 998
Triamcinolone, Oral (Systemic), 998
Triamcinolone, Parenteral (Systemic), 998
**Uveitis with posterior synechiae (treatment)**
Phenylephrine (Ophthalmic), #
**Uveitis, severe, refractory (treatment)**
[Tacrolimus (Systemic)]1, 2683

## V

**Vaginitis, atrophic (treatment)**
Conjugated Estrogens and Medroxyprogesterone Tablets (Systemic)†, 946
Conjugated Estrogens Tablets USP, and Conjugated Estrogens and Medroxyprogesterone Tablets (Systemic)†, 946
Dienestrol (Vaginal), 1391
Estradiol (Vaginal), 1391
Estradiol, Oral (Systemic), 1383
Estradiol, Transdermal (Systemic), 1383
Estradiol, Transdermal Systems(Systemic), 1383
Estradiol Valerate (Systemic), 1383
Estrogens, Conjugated (Vaginal), 1391
Estrogens, Conjugated, Oral (Systemic), 1383
Estrogens, Esterified (Systemic), 1383
Estrone (Systemic)†, 1383
Estropipate (Systemic), 1383
Estropipate (Vaginal)†, 1391
**Vaginosis, bacterial (treatment)**
Clindamycin (Vaginal), 898
Metronidazole (Vaginal), 2001
[Metronidazole, Oral (Systemic)]1, 1996
**Valvular regurgitation (treatment adjunct)**
[Nitroprusside (Systemic)]1, 2142
**Varicella (treatment)**
Acyclovir, Oral (Systemic), 24
[Acyclovir, Parenteral (Systemic)]1, 24
**Varicella virus (prophylaxis)**
Varicella Virus Vaccine Live (Systemic), 2923
**Varicella-zoster (treatment)**
[Foscarnet (Systemic)]†, 1528
**Vascular death (prophylaxis)**
Clodpidogrel (Systemic), 913
**Vascular disease, peripheral (treatment)**
See also Frostbite; Raynaud's phenomenon
Isoxsuprine (Systemic)1, #
Nicotinyl Alcohol (Systemic)*, #
Nylidrin (Systemic)*, #
Pentoxifylline (Systemic), 2282
**Vascular spasm (treatment)**
Nicotinyl Alcohol (Systemic)*, #
**Vasculitis (treatment)**
[Betamethasone, Oral (Systemic)]1, 998
[Betamethasone, Parenteral (Systemic)]1, 998
[Cortisone (Systemic)]1, 998
[Dexamethasone, Oral (Systemic)]1, 998
[Dexamethasone, Parenteral (Systemic)]1, 998
[Hydrocortisone, Oral (Systemic)]1, 998
[Hydrocortisone, Parenteral (Systemic)]1, 998
[Methylprednisolone, Oral (Systemic)]1, 998
[Methylprednisolone, Parenteral (Systemic)]1, 998
[Prednisolone, Oral (Systemic)]1, 998
[Prednisolone, Parenteral (Systemic)]1, 998
[Prednisone (Systemic)]1, 998
[Triamcinolone, Oral (Systemic)]1, 998
[Triamcinolone, Parenteral (Systemic)]1, 998
**Vasculitis, chronic cutaneous (treatment)**
[Chloroquine (Systemic)]1, 849
[Hydroxychloroquine (Systemic)]1, 1663
**Vasculitis, rheumatoid (treatment)**
[Penicillamine (Systemic)]1, 2237
**Vasoactive intestinal peptide tumors**—See Tumors, gastrointestinal
**Vasospasm, in subarachnoid hemorrhage patients (treatment)**
Poloxamer 188 (Systemic), 3158‡
**Venography**
Diatrizoate Meglumine and Diatrizoate Sodium, Parenteral (Systemic), #
Diatrizoate Meglumine, Parenteral (Systemic), #
Diatrizoate Sodium, Parenteral (Systemic), #
Iodixanol (Systemic), #
Iohexol (Systemic), #
Iopamidol (Systemic), #
Iopromide (Systemic), #
Iothalamate Meglumine (Systemic), #
Ioversol (Systemic), #
Ioxaglate (Systemic), #
**Venography, radionuclide**
Technetium Tc 99m Albumin Aggregated (Systemic), 2697
**Ventricular contractions, premature (prophylaxis)**
Acebutolol (Systemic)1, 593
Quinidine (Systemic), 2440
**Ventricular contractions, premature (treatment)**
Acebutolol (Systemic)1, 593
Quinidine (Systemic), 2440
**Ventricular dysfunction, left, asymptomatic (treatment)**
Enalapril (Systemic)1, 177

**Ventricular dysfunction, left, following myocardial infarction (treatment)**
Captopril (Systemic)1, 177
**Ventriculitis**—See Central nervous system (CNS) infections
**Ventriculitis (treatment)**
Cefotaxime (Systemic), 794
**Ventriculography**
Iohexol (Systemic), #
Iopamidol (Systemic), #
Metrizamide (Systemic)†, #
**Verruca plana (treatment)**
[Tretinoin (Topical)]1, 2871
**Verruca vulgaris (treatment)**
[Bleomycin, Intralesional (Systemic)]1, 624
Resorcinol (Topical), 1#
**Vertigo (prophylaxis)**
Diphenidol (Systemic), 1232
Meclizine (Systemic), 1933
**Vertigo (treatment)**
See also Ear, inner, circulatory disturbances of
Dimenhydrinate (Systemic), 325
Diphenhydramine (Systemic), 325
Diphenidol (Systemic), 1232
Meclizine (Systemic), 1933
Nicotinyl Alcohol (Systemic)*, #
Promethazine (Systemic), 377
*Vibrio cholerae* **(prophylaxis)**
Cholera Vaccine (Systemic), #
**Vincent's gingivitis**—See Gingivitis, necrotizing ulcerative; Gingivostomatitis, necrotizing ulcerative
See Gingivostomatitis, necrotizing ulcerative, 2765
**Vincent's infection**—See Gingivitis, necrotizing ulcerative; Gingivostomatitis, necrotizing ulcerative
See Gingivostomatitis, necrotizing ulcerative, 2765
**Vincent's pharyngitis**—See Gingivitis, necrotizing ulcerative; Gingivostomatitis, necrotizing ulcerative
See Gingivostomatitis, necrotizing ulcerative, 2765
**Vipomas**—See Tumors, gastrointestinal
**Viral hemorrhagic fever (prophylaxis)**
[Ribavirin (Systemic)]1, 2478
**Viral hemorrhagic fever (treatment)**
[Ribavirin (Systemic)]1, 2478
**Vitamin A deficiency (prophylaxis)**
Beta-carotene (Systemic), 612
Vitamin A (Systemic), 2958
**Vitamin A deficiency (treatment)**
Vitamin A (Systemic), 2958
**Vitamin $B_{12}$ deficiency (diagnosis)**
[Cyanocobalamin (Systemic)], 2962
[Hydroxocobalamin (Systemic)]†, 2962
**Vitamin $B_{12}$ deficiency (diagnosis adjunct)**
Cyanocobalamin Co 57 (Systemic), 1123
**Vitamin $B_{12}$ deficiency (prophylaxis)**
Cyanocobalamin (Systemic), 2962
Hydroxocobalamin (Systemic)†, 2962
**Vitamin $B_{12}$ deficiency (treatment)**
Cyanocobalamin (Systemic), 2962
Hydroxocobalamin (Systemic)†, 2962
**Vitamin C deficiency (prophylaxis)**
Ascorbic Acid (Systemic), 469
Sodium Ascorbate (Systemic)†, 469
**Vitamin C deficiency (treatment)**
Ascorbic Acid (Systemic), 469
Sodium Ascorbate (Systemic)†, 469
**Vitamin D deficiency (prophylaxis)**
[Calcifediol (Systemic)]†, 2966
Ergocalciferol (Systemic), 2966
**Vitamin D deficiency (treatment)**
[Calcifediol (Systemic)]†, 2966
Ergocalciferol (Systemic), 2966
**Vitamin deficiency**—See specific vitamins
**Vitamin deficiency, multiple (prophylaxis)**
Vitamins A, D, and C and Potassium Fluoride (Systemic), 2978
Vitamins A, D, and C and Sodium Fluoride (Systemic), 2978
Vitamins, Multiple, and Potassium Fluoride (Systemic), 2978
Vitamins, Multiple, and Sodium Fluoride (Systemic), 2978
**Vitamin deficiency, multiple (treatment)**
Vitamins A, D, and C and Potassium Fluoride (Systemic), 2978
Vitamins A, D, and C and Sodium Fluoride (Systemic), 2978
Vitamins, Multiple, and Potassium Fluoride (Systemic), 2978
Vitamins, Multiple, and Sodium Fluoride (Systemic), 2978
**Vitamin deficiency, multiple, in neonates (prophylaxis)**
Multi-Vitamin Infusion (Neonatal Formula) (Systemic), 3155‡

**Vitamin E deficiency (prophylaxis)**
  Vitamin E (Systemic), 2972
**Vitamin E deficiency (treatment)**
  Vitamin E (Systemic), 2972
**Vitamin K deficiency (prophylaxis)**
  Menadiol (Systemic)†, 2975
  Phytonadione (Systemic), 2975
**Vitamin K deficiency (treatment)**
  Menadiol (Systemic)†, 2975
  Phytonadione (Systemic), 2975
**Vitiligo (treatment)**
  Methoxsalen (Topical), 1977
  Methoxsalen Capsules USP (XXI) (Hard Gelatin) (Systemic), 1973
  [Methoxsalen Capsules USP (XXII) (Soft Gelatin) (Systemic)], 1973
  Trioxsalen (Systemic), #
**Vitrectomy adjunct**
  Chondroitinase (Ophthalmic), 3136‡
**VKC**—See Keratoconjunctivitis, vernal
**von Willebrand disease (treatment)**
  Antihemophilic Factor, Cryoprecipitated (Systemic), 319
  Antihemophilic Factor, Human (Systemic), 3131‡
  Antihemophilic Factor (Human) (Systemic), 3131‡
  Desmopressin (Inhalation/Systemic), 3140‡
  Desmopressin, Parenteral (Systemic), 1187
  Factor VIIa (Recombinant, DNA Origin) (Systemic), 3142‡
**Vulvar atrophy (treatment)**
  Conjugated Estrogens and Medroxyprogesterone Tablets (Systemic)†, 946
  Conjugated Estrogens Tablets USP, and Conjugated Estrogens and Medroxyprogesterone Tablets (Systemic)†, 946
  Dienestrol (Vaginal), 1391
  Estradiol (Vaginal), 1391
  Estradiol, Oral (Systemic), 1383
  Estradiol, Transdermal (Systemic), 1383
  Estradiol, Transdermal Systems(Systemic), 1383
  Estradiol Valerate (Systemic), 1383
  Estrogens, Conjugated (Vaginal), 1391
  Estrogens, Conjugated, Oral (Systemic), 1383
  Estrogens, Esterified (Systemic), 1383
  Estrone (Systemic)†, 1383
  Estrone (Vaginal)*, 1391
  Estropipate (Systemic), 1383
  Estropipate (Vaginal)†, 1391
**Vulvar dystrophies (treatment)**
  Testosterone (Topical), 3168‡
**Vulvitis (treatment)**
  Bufexamac (Topical)*, 3013

# W–Z

**Waldenstrom macroglobulinemia (treatment)**
  Betamethasone, Oral (Systemic), 998
  [Carmustine (Systemic)][1], 786
  [Chlorambucil (Systemic)][1], 837
  [Cladribine (Systemic)][1], 886
  Cortisone, Oral (Systemic), 998
  [Cyclophosphamide (Systemic)][1], 1128
  Dexamethasone, Oral (Systemic), 998
  Hydrocortisone, Oral (Systemic), 998
  [Melphalan (Systemic)][1], 1938
  Methylprednisolone, Oral (Systemic), 998
  Prednisolone, Oral (Systemic), 998
  Prednisone, Oral (Systemic), 998
  Triamcinolone, Oral (Systemic), 998
  [Vincristine (Systemic)][1], 2950
**Warts, common**—See Verruca vulgaris
**Warts, flat**—See Verruca plana
**Warts, genital**—See Condyloma acuminata
**Warts, venereal**—See Condyloma acuminata
**Wegener's granulomatosis (treatment)**
  [Cyclophosphamide (Systemic)][1], 1128
**Weight loss, AIDS-associated (prophylaxis)**
  Dronabinol (Systemic), 3141‡
**Weight loss, AIDS-associated (treatment)**
  Dihydrotestosterone (Systemic), 3140‡
  Sermorelin (Systemic), 3164‡
  Somatropin (Systemic), 3165‡
  Testosterone (Systemic), 3168‡

**Weight loss, AIDS-associated (treatment adjunct)**
  Oxandrolone (Systemic), 3157‡
**Weight loss, significant, AIDS-associated (treatment)**
  Megestrol (Systemic), 2400
**Wernicke's encephalopathy**—See Thiamine deficiency
**Whipple's disease (treatment)**
  [Sulfamethoxazole and Trimethoprim (Systemic)][1], 2661
**Whipworm**—See Trichuriasis
**Whole body imaging, positron emission tomographic**
  [Fludeoxyglucose F 18 (Systemic)][1]*†, 1478
**Whooping cough**—See Pertussis
**Wilms' tumor (treatment)**
  [Cisplatin (Systemic)][1], 876
  [Cyclophosphamide (Systemic)][1], 1128
  Dactinomycin (Systemic), 1153
  [Daunorubicin (Systemic)][1], 1173
  Doxorubicin (Systemic), 1308
  Vincristine (Systemic), 2950
**Wilson's disease (treatment)**
  See also Degeneration, hepatolenticular
  Ammonium Tetrathiomolybdate (Systemic), 3130‡
  Penicillamine (Systemic), 2237
  Trientine (Systemic)†, 2875, 3169‡
  Zinc Acetate (Systemic), 3171‡
**Wilson's disease (treatment adjunct)**
  Zinc Acetate (Systemic), 3039
  [Zinc Chloride (Systemic)]†, 2999
  [Zinc Gluconate (Systemic)][1], 2999
  [Zinc Sulfate (Systemic)][1], 2999
**Wolff-Parkinson-White syndrome**—See Arrhythmias, supraventricular
**Wounds, minor (treatment)**
  Benzocaine (Topical), 155
  Benzocaine and Menthol (Topical), 155
  Butamben (Topical), 155
  Dibucaine (Topical), 155
  Lidocaine (Topical), 155
  Pramoxine (Topical), 155
  Pramoxine and Menthol (Topical), 155
  Tetracaine (Topical), 155
  Tetracaine and Menthol (Topical), 155
**Wrinkling, fine facial, due to photoaging (treatment adjunct)**
  Tretinoin (Topical), 2871
**Xeroderma pigmentosum (treatment)**
  T4 Endonuclease V, Liposome Encapsulated (Systemic), 3167‡
**Xerophthalmiain Sjogren's syndrome (treatment)**
  Pilocarpine (Systemic), 3032
**Xerosis, inflammatory phase (treatment)**
  Alclometasone Dipropionate (Topical), 978
  Beclomethasone Dipropionate (Topical), 978
  Betamethasone Benzoate (Topical), 978
  Betamethasone Valerate (Topical), 978
  Clobetasone Butyrate (Topical), 978
  Clocortolone Pivalate (Topical), 978
  Desonide (Topical), 978
  Desoximetasone (0.05% cream only) (Topical), 978
  Dexamethasone (Topical), 978
  Dexamethasone Sodium Phosphate (Topical), 978
  Diflucortolone Valerate (Topical), 978
  Flumethasone Pivalate (Topical), 978
  Fluocinolone Acetonide (except 0.2% cream) (Topical), 978
  Flurandrenolide (Topical), 978
  Fluticasone Propionate (Topical), 978
  Hydrocortisone (Topical), 978
  Hydrocortisone Acetate (Topical), 978
  Hydrocortisone Butyrate (Topical), 978
  Hydrocortisone Valerate (Topical), 978
  Methylprednisolone Acetate (Topical), 978
  Mometasone Furoate (Topical), 978
  Triamcinolone Acetonide (except 0.5% cream and ointment) (Topical), 978
**Xerostomia (treatment)**
  Pilocarpine (Systemic)†, 2323, 3158‡

**Xerostomia, radiation-induced (treatment)**
  Amifostine (Systemic), 3130‡
  Pilocarpine (Systemic), 3032, 3158‡
**Xerostomia, in Sjogren's syndrome (treatment)**
  Pilocarpine (Systemic), 3032
**Yaws (treatment)**
  Demeclocycline (Systemic), 2765
  Doxycycline (Systemic), 2765
  Minocycline (Systemic), 2765
  Oxytetracycline (Systemic)†, 2765
  Penicillin G Benzathine (Systemic), 2240
  [Penicillin G, Parenteral (Systemic)], 2240
  Penicillin G Procaine (Systemic), 2240
  Tetracycline (Systemic), 2765
**Yellow fever (prophylaxis)**
  Yellow Fever Vaccine (Systemic), #
**Zinc chloride injury, in eye (treatment)**
  [Edetate Disodium (Ophthalmic)*†][1], 550
**Zinc deficiency (prophylaxis)**
  Zinc Chloride (Systemic)†, 2999
  Zinc Gluconate (Systemic), 2999
  Zinc Sulfate (Systemic), 2999
**Zinc deficiency (treatment)**
  Zinc Chloride (Systemic)†, 2999
  Zinc Gluconate (Systemic), 2999
  Zinc Sulfate (Systemic), 2999
**Zollinger-Ellison syndrome**
  See Hypersecretory conditions, gastric, 1828
**Zollinger-Ellison syndrome (treatment)**
  Cimetidine (Systemic), 1633
  Famotidine (Systemic), 1633
  [Nizatidine (Systemic)][1], 1633
  Omeprazole (Systemic), 2163
  Ranitidine (Systemic), 1633
**Zollinger-Ellison syndrome (treatment adjunct)**
  Alumina, Calcium Carbonate, and Sodium Bicarbonate (Oral-Local)*, 188
  Alumina and Magnesia (Oral-Local), 188
  Alumina, Magnesia, Calcium Carbonate, and Simethicone (Oral-Local)†, 188
  Alumina, Magnesia, and Magnesium Carbonate (Oral-Local)*, 188
  Alumina, Magnesia, Magnesium Carbonate, and Simethicone (Oral-Local)*, 188
  Alumina, Magnesia, and Simethicone (Oral-Local), 188
  Alumina, Magnesium Alginate, and Magnesium Carbonate (Oral-Local)†, 188
  Alumina and Magnesium Carbonate (Oral-Local)†, 188
  Alumina, Magnesium Carbonate, and Simethicone (Oral-Local)†, 188
  Alumina, Magnesium Carbonate, and Sodium Bicarbonate (Oral-Local)†, 188
  Alumina and Magnesium Trisilicate (Oral-Local)†, 188
  Alumina, Magnesium Trisilicate, and Sodium Bicarbonate (Oral-Local)†, 188
  Alumina and Simethicone (Oral-Local)†, 188
  Alumina and Sodium Bicarbonate (Oral-Local)*, 188
  Aluminum Carbonate, Basic (Oral-Local)†, 188
  Aluminum Carbonate, Basic and Simethicone (Oral-Local)†, 188
  Aluminum Hydroxide (Oral-Local), 188
  Calcium Carbonate (Oral-Local)†, 188
  Calcium Carbonate and Magnesia (Oral-Local)†, 188
  Calcium Carbonate, Magnesia, and Simethicone (Oral-Local)†, 188
  Calcium and Magnesium Carbonates (Oral-Local)†, 188
  Calcium Carbonate and Simethicone (Oral-Local)†, 188
  Magaldrate (Oral-Local), 188
  Magaldrate and Simethicone (Oral-Local), 188
  Magnesium Carbonate and Sodium Bicarbonate (Oral-Local)*, 188
  Magnesium Hydroxide (Oral-Local), 188
  Magnesium Oxide (Oral-Local)†, 188
**Zygomycosis (treatment)**
  Amphotericin B Lipid Complex (Systemic), 3131‡

# General Index

A selected number of brand names *(italicized)* and manufacturers have been included. The inclusion of a brand name does not mean the author has any particular knowledge that the brand listed has properties different from other brands of the same drug, nor should it be interpreted as an endorsement. Similarly, the fact that a particular brand has not been included does not indicate that the product has been judged to be unsatisfactory or unacceptable. Page numbers for pages 3127–3171 refer to the orphan drug and biological listing (Appendix VIII). Page numbers for MC-1 through MC-32 refer to the product identification photographs in *The Medicine Chart* (Appendix VII).

\# — Drugs which are not included in this published version of the USP DI database. Copies of the monographs are available on request from Micromedex, Inc.—Reprint Requests, 6200 S. Syracuse Way, Suite 300, Englewood, CO 80111; telephone (303) 486-6400; telefax (303) 486-6464; Email: USPDI@MDX.COM.

## A

*Abbokinase*—Abbott (U.S. and Canada) brand of Urokinase—**See Thrombolytic Agents (Systemic)**, 2799
*Abbokinase Open-Cath*—Abbott (U.S. and Canada) brand of Urokinase—**See Thrombolytic Agents (Systemic)**, 2799
Abciximab [*c7E3 Fab; ReoPro*]
  **(Systemic)**, 1
  Injection, 3
*ABELCET*—Liposome (U.S.) brand of Amphotericin B Lipid Complex (Systemic), 103, 3130, 3131
*Abenol*—SmithKline Beecham (Canada) brand of Acetaminophen (Systemic), 6
*Abitrate*—Major (U.S.) brand of Clofibrate (Systemic), 900
ABLC—*See* Amphotericin B Lipid Complex (Systemic), 3130
*A/B Otic*—Clay-Park (U.S.) brand of Antipyrine and Benzocaine (Otic), 443
Acarbose [*Precose*]
  **(Systemic)**, 3
  Tablets, 5, MC-1
*ACB*—E-Z-EM (U.S. and Canada) brand of Barium Sulfate (Local), #
*AC and C*—Aspirin, Codeine, and Caffeine—**See Opioid (Narcotic) Analgesics and Aspirin (Systemic)**, 2202
*A.C.&C.*—Aspirin, Codeine, and Caffeine—**See Opioid (Narcotic) Analgesics and Aspirin (Systemic)**, 2202
*Accolate*—ZENECA (U.S.) brand of Zafirlukast (Systemic), 2987, MC-32
*Accupep HPF*—Roche (U.S.) brand of Enteral Nutrition Formula, Monomeric (Elemental)—**See Enteral Nutrition Formulas (Systemic)**, #
*Accupril*—PD (U.S.) brand of Quinapril—**See Angiotensin-converting Enzyme (ACE) Inhibitors (Systemic)**, 177, MC-27
*Accutane*—Roche (U.S.) brand of Isotretinoin (Systemic), 1796, MC-16
*Accutane Roche*—Roche (Canada) brand of Isotretinoin (Systemic), 1796
Acebutolol Hydrochloride [*Monitan; Sectral*]
  **See Beta-adrenergic Blocking Agents (Systemic)**, 593
  Capsules, 600, MC-1
  Tablets, 600
ACE Inhibitors—*See* Angiotensin-converting Enzyme (ACE) Inhibitors (Systemic), 177
ACE Inhibitors and Hydrochlorothiazide—*See* Angiotensin-converting Enzyme (ACE) Inhibitors and Hydrochlorothiazide (Systemic), 187
*Acel-Imune*—Lederle (U.S.) brand of Diphtheria and Tetanus Toxoids and Pertussis Vaccine Adsorbed (Systemic), 1240
Acellular DTP—*See* Diphtheria and Tetanus Toxoids and Pertussis Vaccine Adsorbed (Systemic), 1240
Acenocoumarol [*Sintrom*]
  **(Systemic)**, 3009
  Tablets, 3009
*Acet-2*—Pharmascience (Canada) brand of Acetaminophen and Codeine—**See Opioid (Narcotic) Analgesics and Acetaminophen (Systemic)**, 2198
*Acet-3*—Pharmascience (Canada) brand of Acetaminophen and Codeine—**See Opioid (Narcotic) Analgesics and Acetaminophen (Systemic)**, 2198

*Aceta Elixir*—Century (U.S.) brand of Acetaminophen (Systemic), 6
Acetaminophen [*Abenol; Aceta Elixir; Acetaminophen Uniserts; Aceta Tablets; Actamin; Actamin Extra; Actimol Chewable Tablets; Actimol Children's Suspension; Actimol Infants' Suspension; Actimol Junior Strength Caplets; Aminofen; Aminofen Max; Anacin-3; Anacin-3 Extra Strength; Apacet Capsules; Apacet Elixir; Apacet Extra Strength Caplets; Apacet Extra Strength Tablets; Apacet, Infants'; Apacet Regular Strength Tablets; APAP; Apo-Acetaminophen; Aspirin Free Anacin Maximum Strength Caplets; Aspirin Free Anacin Maximum Strength Gel Caplets; Aspirin Free Anacin Maximum Strength Tablets; Atasol Caplets; Atasol Drops; Atasol Forte Caplets; Atasol Forte Tablets; Atasol Oral Solution; Atasol Tablets; Banesin; Dapa; Dapa X-S; Datril Extra-Strength; Exdol; Exdol Strong; Feverall, Children's; Feverall, Infants'; Feverall Junior Strength; Feverall Sprinkle Caps, Children's; Feverall Sprinkle Caps Junior Strength; Genapap Children's Elixir; Genapap Children's Tablets; Genapap Extra Strength Caplets; Genapap Extra Strength Tablets; Genapap, Infants'; Genapap Regular Strength Tablets; Genebs Extra Strength Caplets; Genebs Regular Strength Tablets; Genebs X-Tra; Liquiprin Children's Elixir; Liquiprin Infants' Drops; Neopap; Oraphen-PD; Panadol; Panadol, Children's; Panadol Extra Strength; Panadol, Infants'; Panadol Junior Strength Caplets; Panadol Maximum Strength Caplets; Panadol Maximum Strength Tablets; paracetamol; Phenaphen Caplets; Redutemp; Robigesic; Rounox; Snaplets-FR; St. Joseph Aspirin-Free Fever Reducer for Children; Suppap-120; Suppap-325; Suppap-650; Tapanol Extra Strength Caplets; Tapanol Extra Strength Tablets; Tempra; Tempra Caplets; Tempra Chewable Tablets; Tempra Drops; Tempra D.S.; Tempra, Infants'; Tempra Syrup; Tylenol Caplets; Tylenol Children's Chewable Tablets; Tylenol Children's Elixir; Tylenol Children's Suspension Liquid; Tylenol Drops; Tylenol Elixir; Tylenol Extra Strength Adult Liquid Pain Reliever; Tylenol Extra Strength Caplets; Tylenol Extra Strength Gelcaps; Tylenol Extra Strength Tablets; Tylenol Gelcaps; Tylenol Infants' Drops; Tylenol Infants' Suspension Drops; Tylenol Junior Strength Caplets; Tylenol Junior Strength Chewable Tablets; Tylenol Regular Strength Caplets; Tylenol Regular Strength Tablets; Tylenol Tablets; Valorin; Valorin Extra*]
  **(Systemic)**, 6
  Capsules USP, 9
  Granules, Oral, 9
  Powders, Oral, 10
  Solution, Oral, USP, 10
  Suppositories USP, 11
  Suspension, Oral, USP, 10
  Tablets USP, 10
  Tablets USP (Chewable), 10
Acetaminophen and Aspirin [*Gemnisyn*]
  **See Acetaminophen and Salicylates (Systemic)**, 11
  Tablets USP, 12
Acetaminophen, Aspirin, and Caffeine [*Duradyne; Excedrin Extra-Strength Caplets; Excedrin Extra-Strength Tablets; Excedrin Migraine; Goody's Extra Strength Tablets; Goody's Headache Powders*]
  **(Systemic)**, 11, 3009

Acetaminophen, Aspirin, and Caffeine *(continued)*
  Powders, Oral, 13
  Tablets USP, 13, 3009
Acetaminophen, Aspirin, and Caffeine, Buffered [*Bufets II; Gelpirin; Supac; Vanquish Caplets*]
  **See Acetaminophen and Salicylates (Systemic)**, 11
  Tablets, 13
Acetaminophen, Aspirin, and Salicylamide, Buffered [*Presalin*]
  **See Acetaminophen and Salicylates (Systemic)**, 11
  Tablets, 14
Acetaminophen, Aspirin, Salicylamide, and Caffeine [*Saleto; Tri-Pain Caplets*]
  **See Acetaminophen and Salicylates (Systemic)**, 11
  Tablets, 13
Acetaminophen and Caffeine [*Actamin Super; Aspirin-Free Excedrin Caplets; Bayer Select Maximum Strength Headache Pain Relief Formula; Excedrin Caplets; Excedrin Extra Strength Caplets; Summit*]
  **See Acetaminophen (Systemic)**, 6
  Tablets USP, 11
Acetaminophen and Codeine Phosphate [*Acet Codeine 30; Acet Codeine 60 APAP with codeine; Capital with Codeine; Co-codAPAP; Empracet-30; Empracet-60; Emtec-30; EZ III; Lenoltec with Codeine No.4; Margesic #3; Phenaphen with Codeine No.3; Phenaphen with Codeine No.4; PMS-Acetaminophen with Codeine; Pyregesic-C; Triatec-30; Tylenol with Codeine Elixir; Tylenol with Codeine No.2 (U.S.); Tylenol with Codeine No.3 (U.S.); Tylenol with Codeine No.4 (U.S. and Canada)*]
  **See Opioid (Narcotic) Analgesics and Acetaminophen (Systemic)**, 2198
  Capsules USP, 2199, MC-1
  Solution, Oral, 2199
  Suspension, Oral, USP, 2200
  Tablets USP, 2200, MC-1
Acetaminophen, Codeine Phosphate, and Caffeine [*Acet-2; Acet-3; Atasol-8; Atasol-15; Atasol-30; Cetaphen with Codeine; Cetaphen Extra Strength with Codeine; Cotabs; Exdol-8; Lenoltec with Codeine No.1; Lenoltec with Codeine No.2; Lenoltec with Codeine No.3; Novo-Gesic C8; Novo-Gesic C15; Novo-Gesic C30; Triatec-8; Triatec-8 Strong; Tylenol with Codeine No.1; Tylenol with Codeine No.2 (Canada); Tylenol with Codeine No.3 (Canada); Tylenol with Codeine No.1 Forte*]
  **See Opioid (Narcotic) Analgesics and Acetaminophen (Systemic)**, 2198
  Tablets, 2200
Acetaminophen-containing Combinations, 3066
Acetaminophen and Salicylamide [*Duoprin*]
  **See Acetaminophen and Salicylates (Systemic)**, 11
  Capsules, 14
Acetaminophen, Salicylamide, and Caffeine [*Rid-A-Pain Compound; S-A-C*]
  **See Acetaminophen and Salicylates (Systemic)**, 11
  Capsules, 14
  Tablets, 14
Acetaminophen and Salicylates
  **(Systemic)**, 11

Acetaminophen, Sodium Bicarbonate, and Citric Acid [*Bromo-Seltzer*]
  **(Systemic)**, 15
  for Solution, Oral, Effervescent, USP, 15
Acetaminophen Uniserts—Upsher-Smith (U.S.) brand of Acetaminophen (Systemic), 6
Acetasol HC—Barre (U.S.) brand of Hydrocortisone and Acetic Acid (Otic), 3023
Aceta Tablets—Century (U.S.) brand of Acetaminophen (Systemic), 6
Acetazolam—ICN (Canada) brand of Acetazolamide—**See Carbonic Anhydrase Inhibitors (Systemic)**, 773
Acetazolamide [*Acetazolam; Ak-Zol; Apo-Acetazolamide; Dazamide; Diamox; Diamox Sequels; Storzolamide*]
  **See Carbonic Anhydrase Inhibitors (Systemic)**, 773
  Capsules, Extended-release, 777
  Tablets USP, 777
Acetazolamide Sodium [*Diamox*]
  **See Carbonic Anhydrase Inhibitors (Systemic)**, 773
  Sterile USP, 778
Acet Codeine 30—Pharmascience (Canada) brand of Acetaminophen and Codeine—**See Opioid (Narcotic) Analgesics and Acetaminophen (Systemic)**, 2198
Acet Codeine 60—Pharmascience (Canada) brand of Acetaminophen and Codeine—**See Opioid (Narcotic) Analgesics and Acetaminophen (Systemic)**, 2198
Acetest—Ames (U.S. and Canada) brand of Nitroprusside Urine Ketone Test—**See Urine Glucose and Ketone Test Kits for Home Use**, #
Acetic Acid–containing Combinations, 3067
Acetohexamide [*Dimelor; Dymelor*]
  **See Antidiabetic Agents, Sulfonylurea (Systemic)**, 283
  Tablets USP, 291, MC-1
Acetohydroxamic Acid [*Lithostat*]
  **(Systemic)**, #
  Tablets USP, #
Acetone-containing Combinations, 3067
Acetophenazine Maleate [*Tindal*]
  **See Phenothiazines (Systemic)**, 2289
  Tablets USP, 2296
Acetoxyl 2.5 Gel—Stiefel (Canada) brand of Benzoyl Peroxide (Topical), 579
Acetoxyl 5 Gel—Stiefel (Canada) brand of Benzoyl Peroxide (Topical), 579
Acetoxyl 10 Gel—Stiefel (Canada) brand of Benzoyl Peroxide (Topical), 579
Acetoxyl 20 Gel—Stiefel (Canada) brand of Benzoyl Peroxide (Topical), 579
Acetylcysteine [*Mucomyst; Mucomyst-10; Mucosil-10; Mucosil-20*]
  **(Inhalation-Local)**, #
  Solution USP, #
Acetylcysteine [*Mucomyst; Mucomyst/Mucomyst 10 IV; Mucosil; N-Acetyl-L-Cysteine; Parvolex*]
  **(Systemic)**, 16, 3128
  Injection, 18
  Solution USP, 17
Acetylsalicylic acid—Aspirin—**See Salicylates (Systemic)**, 2538
Acetylspiramycin—*See* Spiramycin (Systemic), 2624
Achromycin—Lederle (U.S. and Canada) brand of Tetracycline—**See Tetracyclines (Ophthalmic)**, 2763; **Tetracyclines (Systemic)**, 2765; **Tetracyclines (Topical)**, 2774
Achromycin V—Lederle (U.S. and Canada) brand of Tetracycline—**See Tetracyclines (Systemic)**, 2765, MC-29
Aciclovir—*See* Acyclovir (Systemic), 24; Acyclovir (Topical), 28
Acid Control—Stanley (Canada) brand of Famotidine—**See Histamine H₂-receptor Antagonists (Systemic)**, 1633, MC-12
Acilac—Technilab (Canada) brand of Lactulose—**See Laxatives (Local)**, #
Acitretin [13-cis-acitretin; etretin; isoetretin; *Soriatane*]
  **(Systemic)**, 18
  Capsules, MC-1
  Tablets, 23
Aclophen—Nutripharm (U.S.) brand of Chlorpheniramine, Phenylephrine, and Acetaminophen—**See Antihistamines, Decongestants, and Analgesics (Systemic)**, 366
Aclovate—Glaxo (U.S.) brand of Alclometasone—**See Corticosteroids (Topical)**, 978

Acne Aid Aqua Gel—Durham (U.S.) brand of Benzoyl Peroxide (Topical), 579
Acne-Aid Gel—Stiefel (Canada) brand of Resorcinol and Sulfur (Topical), #
Acne-Aid Vanishing Cream—Durham (U.S.) brand of Benzoyl Peroxide (Topical), 579
Acne Lotion 10—C & M (U.S.) brand of Alcohol and Sulfur (Topical), #
Acnomel Acne Cream—SKCP (U.S.) brand of Resorcinol and Sulfur (Topical), #
Acnomel B.P. 5 Lotion—Chattem (Canada) brand of Benzoyl Peroxide (Topical), 579
Acnomel Cake—SKF (Canada) brand of Resorcinol and Sulfur (Topical), #
Acnomel Cream—SKF (Canada) brand of Resorcinol and Sulfur (Topical), #
Acnomel Vanishing Cream—SKF (Canada) brand of Resorcinol and Sulfur (Topical), #
Aconiazide
  **(Systemic)**, 3128
Acrivastine
  **See Antihistamines (Systemic)**, 325
Acrivastine-containing Combinations, 3067
Acrivastine and Pseudoephedrine Hydrochloride [*Semprex-D*]
  **See Antihistamines and Decongestants (Systemic)**, 343
  Capsules, 361
Act—Novopharm (Canada) brand of Famotidine—**See Histamine H₂-receptor Antagonists (Systemic)**, 1633, MC-12
Actagen—Zenith Goldline (U.S.) brand of Triprolidine and Pseudoephedrine—**See Antihistamines and Decongestants (Systemic)**, 343
Actagen-C Cough—Zenith Goldline (U.S.) brand of Triprolidine, Pseudoephedrine, and Codeine—**See Cough/Cold Combinations (Systemic)**, 1024
Actamin—Buffington (U.S.) brand of Acetaminophen (Systemic), 6
Actamin Extra—Buffington (U.S.) brand of Acetaminophen (Systemic), 6
Actamin Super—Buffington (U.S.) brand of Acetaminophen and Caffeine—**See Acetaminophen (Systemic)**, 6
ACTH—PD (U.S.) brand of Corticotropin (Systemic), 1021
ACTH—*See* Corticotropin (Systemic), 1021
Acthar—Rhone-Pôulenc Rorer (U.S.) brand of Corticotropin (Systemic), 1021
Acthar Gel (H.P.)—Rhone-Pôulenc Rorer (Canada) brand of Corticotropin (Systemic), 1021
Acthar Powder—Rhone-Pôulenc Rorer (Canada) brand of Corticotropin (Systemic), 1021
Act-Hib—Connaught (U.S. and Canada) brand of Haemophilus b Conjugate Vaccine (PRP-T—Tetanus Protein Conjugate)—**See Haemophilus b Conjugate Vaccine (Systemic)**, 1601
Acthrel—Ferring (U.S.) brand of Corticorelin Ovine (Systemic), 954; Corticorelin Ovine Triflutate (Systemic), 3138
Actibine—CMC (U.S.) brand of Yohimbine (Systemic), #
Acticin—Alphapharm (U.S.) brand of Permethrin (Topical), 3032
Acticort 100—Baker Cummins (U.S.) brand of Hydrocortisone—**See Corticosteroids (Topical)**, 978
Actidose-Aqua—Paddock (U.S.) brand of Charcoal, Activated (Oral-Local), 831
Actidose with Sorbitol—Paddock (U.S.) brand of Charcoal, Activated, and Sorbitol—**See Charcoal, Activated (Oral-Local)**, 831
Actifed—Warner Wellcome (U.S. and Canada) brand of Triprolidine and Pseudoephedrine—**See Antihistamines and Decongestants (Systemic)**, 343
Actifed Allergy Nighttime Caplets—Warner Wellcome (U.S.) brand of Diphenhydramine and Pseudoephedrine—**See Antihistamines and Decongestants (Systemic)**, 343
Actifed with Codeine Cough—Glaxo Wellcome (U.S.) brand of Triprolidine, Pseudoephedrine, and Codeine—**See Cough/Cold Combinations (Systemic)**, 1024
Actifed Cold & Sinus—Warner Wellcome (U.S.) brand of Triprolidine, Pseudoephedrine, and Acetaminophen—**See Antihistamines, Decongestants, and Analgesics (Systemic)**, 366
Actifed Cold & Sinus Caplets—Warner Wellcome (U.S.) brand of Triprolidine, Pseudoephedrine, and Acetaminophen—**See Antihistamines, Decongestants, and Analgesics (Systemic)**, 366

Actifed DM—Warner Wellcome (Canada) brand of Triprolidine, Pseudoephedrine, and Dextromethorphan—**See Cough/Cold Combinations (Systemic)**, 1024
Actifed Plus Extra Strength Caplets—Warner Wellcome (Canada) brand of Triprolidine, Pseudoephedrine, and Acetaminophen—**See Antihistamines, Decongestants, and Analgesics (Systemic)**, 366
Actifed Sinus Daytime—Warner Wellcome (U.S.) brand of Pseudoephedrine and Acetaminophen—**See Decongestants and Analgesics (Systemic)**, 1180
Actifed Sinus Daytime Caplets—Warner Wellcome (U.S.) brand of Pseudoephedrine and Acetaminophen—**See Decongestants and Analgesics (Systemic)**, 1180
Actifed Sinus Nighttime—Warner Wellcome (U.S.) brand of Diphenhydramine, Pseudoephedrine, and Acetaminophen—**See Antihistamines, Decongestants, and Analgesics (Systemic)**, 366
Actifed Sinus Nighttime Caplets—Warner Wellcome (U.S.) brand of Diphenhydramine, Pseudoephedrine, and Acetaminophen—**See Antihistamines, Decongestants, and Analgesics (Systemic)**, 366
Actigall—Ciba-Geigy (U.S.) brand of Ursodiol (Systemic), 3171; Summit (U.S.) brand of Ursodiol (Systemic), 2903, MC-32
Actimmune—Genentech (U.S.) brand of Interferon, Gamma (Systemic), 1737; Interferon Gamma-1b (Systemic), 3149; Interferon Gamma 1-b (Systemic), 3148
Actimol Chewable Tablets—BW (Canada) brand of Acetaminophen (Systemic), 6
Actimol Children's Suspension—BW (Canada) brand of Acetaminophen (Systemic), 6
Actimol Infants' Suspension—BW (Canada) brand of Acetaminophen (Systemic), 6
Actimol Junior Strength Caplets—BW (Canada) brand of Acetaminophen (Systemic), 6
Actinex—Reed & Carnrick (U.S.) brand of Masoprocol (Topical), 1912
Actinomycin-D—*See* Dactinomycin (Systemic), 1153
Actiprofen Caplets—Sterling Health (Canada) brand of Ibuprofen—**See Anti-inflammatory Drugs, Nonsteroidal (Systemic)**, 388
Actisite—Alza (U.S.) brand of Tetracycline Periodontal Fibers (Mucosal-Local), #
Activase—Genentech (U.S.) brand of Alteplase, Recombinant—**See Thrombolytic Agents (Systemic)**, 2799
Activase rt-PA—Genentech (Canada) brand of Alteplase, Recombinant—**See Thrombolytic Agents (Systemic)**, 2799
Activated prothrombin complex concentrate—*See* Anti-inhibitor Coagulant Complex (Systemic), 435
Actonel—Procter & Gamble (U.S.) brand of Risedronate (Systemic), 2506
Actron—Bayer (U.S.) brand of Ketoprofen—**See Anti-inflammatory Drugs, Nonsteroidal (Systemic)**, 388
Acular—Allergan (U.S. and Canada) brand of Ketorolac (Ophthalmic), 1809; Allergan (U.S.) brand of Ketorolac (Ophthalmic), 3026
Acuprin 81—Richwood (U.S.) brand of Aspirin—**See Salicylates (Systemic)**, 2538
Acutrim 16 Hour—Ciba Consumer (U.S.) brand of Phenylpropanolamine (Systemic), 2314
Acutrim Late Day—Ciba Consumer (U.S.) brand of Phenylpropanolamine (Systemic), 2314
Acutrim II Maximum Strength—Ciba Consumer (U.S.) brand of Phenylpropanolamine (Systemic), 2314
Acycloguanosine—*See* Acyclovir (Topical), 28
Acyclovir [aciclovir; *Avirax; Zovirax*]
  **(Systemic)**, 24
  Capsules, 27, MC-1
  Suspension, Oral, 27
  Tablets, 27, MC-1
Acyclovir [aciclovir; acycloguanosine; *Zovirax*]
  **(Topical)**, 28
  Ointment, 30
Acyclovir Sodium [aciclovir; *Zovirax*]
  **(Systemic)**, 24
  Sterile, 28
Adagen—Enzon (U.S.) brand of Pegademase (Systemic), #; Pegademase Bovine (Systemic), 3157
Adalat—Bayer (U.S.) and Miles (Canada) brand of Nifedipine—**See Calcium Channel Blocking Agents (Systemic)**, 720, MC-22

*Adalat CC*—Bayer (U.S.) brand of Nifedipine—**See Calcium Channel Blocking Agents (Systemic)**, 720, MC-22
*Adalat P.A.*—Miles (Canada) brand of Nifedipine—**See Calcium Channel Blocking Agents (Systemic)**, 720
*Adalat XL*—Bayer (Canada) brand of Nifedipine—**See Calcium Channel Blocking Agents (Systemic)**, 720
Adapalene [*Differin*]
　(Topical), 30
　Gel, 31
*AdatoSil 5000*—Escalon (U.S.) brand of Silicone Oil 5000 Centistokes (Parenteral-Local), #
*Adderall*—Richwood (U.S.) brand of Amphetamine and Dextroamphetamine (Systemic), 94
*Adeflor*—Upjohn (U.S. and Canada) brand of Multiple Vitamins and Fluoride—**See Vitamins, Multiple, and Fluoride (Systemic)**, 2978
Adeno-as′ted Viral-based Vector Cystic Fibrosis Gene Therapy (Systemic), 3128
*Adenocard*—LyphoMed (U.S.) brand of Adenosine (Systemic), 32
Adenosine [*Adenocard*]
　(Systemic), 32
　Injection, 33
ADgvCFTR.10—**See Cystic Fibrosis TR Gene Therapy (Recombinant Adenovirus) (Systemic)**, 3139
*Adipex-P*—Gate (U.S.) brand of Phentermine—**See Appetite Suppressants (Systemic)**, 452
Adipiodone—**See** Iodipamide (Systemic), #
*Adipost*—Ascher (U.S.) brand of Phendimetrazine—**See Appetite Suppressants (Systemic)**, 452
*Adrenalin*—PD (Canada) brand of Epinephrine—**See Bronchodilators, Adrenergic (Systemic)**, 651; PD (U.S.) brand of Epinephrine—**See Sympathomimetic Agents—Cardiovascular Use (Parenteral-Systemic)**, 2669
*Adrenalin Chloride*—PD (U.S.) brand of Epinephrine—**See Bronchodilators, Adrenergic (Inhalation-Local)**, 640
*Adrenalin Chloride Solution*—PD (U.S.) brand of Epinephrine—**See Bronchodilators, Adrenergic (Systemic)**, 651
Adrenaline—Epinephrine—**See Bronchodilators, Adrenergic (Inhalation-Local)**, 640
*Adriamycin PFS*—Pharmacia (U.S. and Canada) brand of Doxorubicin (Systemic), 1308
*Adriamycin RDF*—Pharmacia (U.S. and Canada) brand of Doxorubicin (Systemic), 1308
*Adrucil*—Adria (U.S. and Canada) brand of Fluorouracil (Systemic), 1497; Lederle (U.S) brand of Fluorouracil (Systemic), 3144
Adsorbocarpine—Alcon (U.S.) brand of Pilocarpine (Ophthalmic), #
*Advanced Formula Di-Gel*—Schering-Plough (U.S.) brand of Calcium Carbonate, Magnesia, and Simethicone—**See Antacids (Oral-Local)**, 188
*Advera*—Abbott/Ross (U.S.) brand of Enteral Nutrition Formula, Disease-specific—**See Enteral Nutrition Formulas (Systemic)**, #
*Advil*—Whitehall (U.S. and Canada) brand of Ibuprofen—**See Anti-inflammatory Drugs, Nonsteroidal (Systemic)**, 388
*Advil Caplets*—Whitehall (U.S. and Canada) brand of Ibuprofen—**See Anti-inflammatory Drugs, Nonsteroidal (Systemic)**, 388
*Advil, Children's*—Wyeth-Ayerst (U.S.) brand of Ibuprofen—**See Anti-inflammatory Drugs, Nonsteroidal (Systemic)**, 388
*Advil Cold and Sinus*—Whitehall (U.S.) brand of Pseudoephedrine and Ibuprofen—**See Decongestants and Analgesics (Systemic)**, 1180
*Advil Cold and Sinus Caplets*—Whitehall (U.S.) and Whitehalls-Robins (Canada) brand of Pseudoephedrine and Ibuprofen—**See Decongestants and Analgesics (Systemic)**, 1180
*AeroBid*—Forest (U.S.) brand of Flunisolide—**See Corticosteroids (Inhalation-Local)**, 955
*AeroBid-M*—Forest (U.S.) brand of Flunisolide—**See Corticosteroids (Inhalation-Local)**, 955
*Aerolate Sr.*—Fleming (U.S.) brand of Theophylline—**See Bronchodilators, Theophylline (Systemic)**, 668
*Aeropin*—See 2-0-Desulfated Heparin (Systemic), 3127
*Aeroseb-Dex*—Allergan Herbert (U.S.) brand of Dexamethasone—**See Corticosteroids (Topical)**, 978

*Aeroseb-HC*—Allergan Herbert (U.S.) brand of Hydrocortisone—**See Corticosteroids (Topical)**, 978
*Aerosporin*—Wellcome (U.S.) brand of Polymyxin B Sulfate (Ophthalmic), 3032
*A-Fil*—Genderm (U.S.) brand of Menthyl Anthranilate and Titanium Dioxide—**See Sunscreen Agents (Topical)**, #
*Afko-Lube*—American Pharmaceutical (U.S.) brand of Docusate—**See Laxatives (Local)**, #
*Afko-Lube Lax*—American Pharmaceutical (U.S.) brand of Casanthranol and Docusate—**See Laxatives (Local)**, #
*Afrin Cherry Scented Nasal Spray*—Schering-Plough (U.S.) brand of Oxymetazoline (Nasal), #
*Afrin Children's Strength Nose Drops*—Schering-Plough (U.S.) brand of Oxymetazoline (Nasal), #
*Afrin Extra Moisturizing Nasal Decongestant Spray*—Schering-Plough (U.S.) brand of Oxymetazoline (Nasal), #
*Afrin Menthol Nasal Spray*—Schering-Plough (U.S.) brand of Oxymetazoline (Nasal), #
*Afrin Nasal Spray*—Schering-Plough (U.S.) brand of Oxymetazoline (Nasal), #
*Afrin Nose Drops*—Schering-Plough (U.S.) brand of Oxymetazoline (Nasal), #
*Afrin Sinus Spray*—Schering-Plough (U.S.) brand of Oxymetazoline (Nasal), #
*Afrin Spray Pump*—Schering-Plough (U.S.) brand of Oxymetazoline (Nasal), #
*Aftate for Athlete's Foot Aerosol Spray Liquid*—Plough (U.S.) brand of Tolnaftate (Topical), #
*Aftate for Athlete's Foot Aerosol Spray Powder*—Plough (U.S.) brand of Tolnaftate (Topical), #
*Aftate for Athlete's Foot Gel*—Plough (U.S.) brand of Tolnaftate (Topical), #
*Aftate for Athlete's Foot Sprinkle Powder*—Plough (U.S.) brand of Tolnaftate (Topical), #
*Aftate for Jock Itch Aerosol Spray Powder*—Plough (U.S.) brand of Tolnaftate (Topical), #
*Aftate for Jock Itch Gel*—Plough (U.S.) brand of Tolnaftate (Topical), #
*Aftate for Jock Itch Sprinkle Powder*—Plough (U.S.) brand of Tolnaftate (Topical), #
*After Burn Double Strength Gel*—Tender (Canada) brand of Lidocaine—**See Anesthetics (Topical)**, 155
*After Burn Double Strength Spray*—Tender (Canada) brand of Lidocaine—**See Anesthetics (Topical)**, 155
*After Burn Gel*—Tender (Canada) brand of Lidocaine—**See Anesthetics (Topical)**, 155
*After Burn Spray*—Tender (Canada) brand of Lidocaine—**See Anesthetics (Topical)**, 155
*Agarol Plain*—Warner Wellcome (Canada) brand of Mineral Oil and Glycerin—**See Laxatives (Local)**, #
*Agarol Strawberry*—Warner Wellcome (Canada) brand of Mineral Oil, Glycerin, and Phenolphthalein—**See Laxatives (Local)**, #
*Agarol Vanilla*—Warner Wellcome (Canada) brand of Mineral Oil, Glycerin, and Phenolphthalein—**See Laxatives (Local)**, #
*A-200 Gel Concentrate*—SmithKline Beecham (U.S.) brand of Pyrethrins and Piperonyl Butoxide (Topical), #
*Aggrastat*—Merck (U.S.) brand of Tirofiban (Systemic), 2826, 3036
*Agoral Marshmallow*—Warner Wellcome (U.S.) brand of Mineral Oil and Phenolphthalein—**See Laxatives (Local)**, #
*Agoral Raspberry*—Warner Wellcome (U.S.) brand of Mineral Oil and Phenolphthalein—**See Laxatives (Local)**, #
*Agrylin*—Roberts (Canada) brand of Anagrelide (Systemic), 3010; Roberts (U.S.) brand of Anagrelide (Systemic), 114
*AH-chew*—WE (U.S.) brand of Chlorpheniramine, Phenylephrine, and Methscopolamine—**See Antihistamines, Decongestants, and Anticholinergics (Systemic)**, 373
AHF—**See** Antihemophilic Factor (Systemic), 319
*A-hydroCort*—Abbott (U.S.) brand of Hydrocortisone—**See Corticosteroids—Glucocorticoid Effects (Systemic)**, 998
*Airet*—Adams (U.S.) brand of Albuterol—**See Bronchodilators, Adrenergic (Inhalation-Local)**, 640
AI-RSA
　(Systemic), 3128
*Akarpine*—Akorn (U.S.) brand of Pilocarpine (Ophthalmic), #

*AKBeta*—Akorn (U.S.) brand of Levobunolol (Ophthalmic), 3027
*Ak-Chlor Ophthalmic Ointment*—Akorn (U.S.) brand of Chloramphenicol (Ophthalmic), #
*Ak-Chlor Ophthalmic Solution*—Akorn (U.S. and Canada) brand of Chloramphenicol (Ophthalmic), #
*Ak-Con*—Akorn (U.S.) brand of Naphazoline (Ophthalmic), #
*AK-Dex*—Akorn (U.S. and Canada) brand of Dexamethasone—**See Corticosteroids (Otic)**, 971; **Corticosteroids (Ophthalmic)**, 966; **Corticosteroids—Glucocorticoid Effects (Systemic)**, 998
*Ak-Dilate*—Akorn (U.S. and Canada) brand of Phenylephrine (Ophthalmic), #
*AK-Homatropine*—Akorn (U.S. and Canada) brand of Homatropine (Ophthalmic), 1651
*Akineton*—Knoll (U.S. and Canada) brand of Biperiden—**See Antidyskinetics (Systemic)**, 297
*Ak-Nefrin*—Akorn (U.S.) brand of Phenylephrine (Ophthalmic), #
*Akne-Mycin*—Hermal (U.S.) brand of Erythromycin (Topical), 1365
*Ak-Pentolate*—Akorn (U.S. and Canada) brand of Cyclopentolate (Ophthalmic), #
*AK-Pred*—Akorn (U.S.) brand of Prednisolone—**See Corticosteroids (Ophthalmic)**, 966
*AKPro*—Akorn (U.S.) brand of Dipivefrin (Ophthalmic), 3017
*Ak-Spore H.C.*—Akorn (U.S.) brand of Neomycin, Polymyxin B, and Hydrocortisone (Ophthalmic), #
*AK-Spore HC Otic*—Akorn (U.S.) brand of Neomycin, Polymyxin B, and Hydrocortisone (Otic), #
*Ak-Spore Ophthalmic Ointment*—Akorn (U.S.) brand of Neomycin, Polymyxin B, and Bacitracin (Ophthalmic), #
*Ak-Spore Ophthalmic Solution*—Akorn (U.S.) brand of Neomycin, Polymyxin B, and Gramicidin (Ophthalmic), #
*Ak-Sulf*—Akorn (U.S. and Canada) brand of Sulfacetamide—**See Sulfonamides (Ophthalmic)**, 2651
*Ak-Taine*—Akorn (U.S. and Canada) brand of Proparacaine—**See Anesthetics (Ophthalmic)**, #
*AK-Tate*—Akorn (U.S. and Canada) brand of Prednisolone—**See Corticosteroids (Ophthalmic)**, 966
*Ak-T-Caine*—Akorn (U.S.) brand of Tetracaine—**See Anesthetics (Ophthalmic)**, #
*AKTob*—Akorn (U.S.) brand of Tobramycin (Ophthalmic), 3036
*Ak-Zol*—Akorn (U.S.) brand of Acetazolamide—**See Carbonic Anhydrase Inhibitors (Systemic)**, 773
*Ala-Cort*—Del-Ray (U.S.) brand of Hydrocortisone—**See Corticosteroids (Topical)**, 978
*Alamag*—Zenith Goldline (U.S.) brand of Alumina and Magnesia—**See Antacids (Oral-Local)**, 188
*Alamag Plus*—Zenith Goldline (U.S.) brand of Alumina, Magnesia, and Simethicone—**See Antacids (Oral-Local)**, 188
*Ala-Scalp HP*—Del-Ray (U.S.) brand of Hydrocortisone—**See Corticosteroids (Topical)**, 978
Alatrofloxacin Mesylate [*Trovan*]
　**See Trovafloxacin (Systemic)**, 2891
　Injection, 2894
*Alaxin*—Delta (U.S.) brand of Poloxamer 188—**See Laxatives (Local)**, #
*Albalon*—Allergan (U.S. and Canada) brand of Naphazoline (Ophthalmic), #
*Albalon Liquifilm*—Allergan (Canada) brand of Naphazoline (Ophthalmic), #
Albendazole [*Albenza; Eskazole; Zentel*]
　(Systemic), #, 3009, 3128
　Suspension, Oral, #
　Tablets, #, 3009
*Albenza*—SmithKline Beecham (U.S.) brand of Albendazole (Systemic), 3009
*Albert Docusate*—Albert (Canada) brand of Docusate—**See Laxatives (Local)**, #
*Albert Glyburide*—Albert (Canada) brand of Glyburide—**See Antidiabetic Agents, Sulfonylurea (Systemic)**, 283
*Albert Tiafen*—Albert (Canada) brand of Tiaprofenic Acid—**See Anti-inflammatory Drugs, Nonsteroidal (Systemic)**, 388
Albright's solution—Sodium Citrate and Citric Acid—**See Citrates (Systemic)**, 881
*Albuminar-5*—Armour (U.S.) brand of Albumin Human (Systemic), 34

*Albuminar-25*—Armour (U.S.) brand of Albumin Human (Systemic), 34
Albumin Human [*Albuminar-5; Albuminar-25; Albutein 5%; Albutein 25%; Buminate 5%; Buminate 25%; Plasbumin-5; Plasbumin-25*]
 **(Systemic)**, 34
 Albumin Human USP, 35
*Albutein 5%*—Alpha (U.S.) brand of Albumin Human (Systemic), 34
*Albutein 25%*—Alpha (U.S.) brand of Albumin Human (Systemic), 34
Albuterol [*Apo-Salvent; Novo-Salmol; Proventil;* salbutamol; *Ventolin*]
 **See Bronchodilators, Adrenergic (Inhalation-Local)**, 640
 Aerosol, Inhalation, 645
Albuterol [*Novo-Salmol; Proventil;* salbutamol; *Ventolin*]
 **See Bronchodilators, Adrenergic (Systemic)**, 651
 Tablets USP, 655, MC-1
 Tablets, Extended-release, MC-1
Albuterol Sulfate [*Airet; Apo-Salvent; Gen-Salbutamol Sterinebs P.F.; Proventil; Proventil HFA; Ventodisk; Ventolin; Ventolin Nebules; Ventolin Nebules P.F.; Ventolin Rotacaps*]
 **See Bronchodilators, Adrenergic (Inhalation-Local)**, 640
 Aerosol, Inhalation, 645
 Powder for Inhalation, 646
 Solution, Inhalation, 645
Albuterol Sulfate [*Proventil; Proventil Repetabs;* salbutamol; *Ventolin; Volmax*]
 **See Bronchodilators, Adrenergic (Systemic)**, 651, 3009
 Injection, 655
 Solution, Oral, 655
 Syrup, 655
 Tablets USP, 655
 Tablets, Extended-release, 655, 3009
*Alcaine*—Alcon (U.S. and Canada) brand of Proparacaine—**See Anesthetics (Ophthalmic)**, #
Alclometasone Dipropionate [*Aclovate*]
 **See Corticosteroids (Topical)**, 978
 Cream USP, 982
 Ointment USP, 982
Alcohol and Acetone [*Seba-Nil Liquid Cleanser; Tyrosum Liquid; Tyrosum Packets*]
 **(Topical)**, #
 Lotion, Detergent, #
 Pledgets, #
Alcohol and Sulfur [*Acne Lotion 10; Liquimat Light; Liquimat Medium; Postacne*]
 **(Topical)**, #
 Lotion, #
*Alcomed*—Quintex (U.S.) brand of Brompheniramine and Phenylpropanolamine—**See Antihistamines and Decongestants (Systemic)**, 343
*Alcomed 2-60*—Quintex (U.S.) brand of Dexbrompheniramine and Pseudoephedrine—**See Antihistamines and Decongestants (Systemic)**, 343
*Alcomicin*—Alcon (Canada) brand of Gentamicin (Ophthalmic), 1555
*Alconefrin Nasal Drops 12*—Alcon (U.S.) brand of Phenylephrine (Nasal), #
*Alconefrin Nasal Drops 25*—Alcon (U.S.) brand of Phenylephrine (Nasal), #
*Alconefrin Nasal Drops 50*—Alcon (U.S.) brand of Phenylephrine (Nasal), #
*Alconefrin Nasal Spray 25*—Alcon (U.S.) brand of Phenylephrine (Nasal), #
*Aldactazide*—Searle (U.S. and Canada) brand of Spironolactone and Hydrochlorothiazide—**See Diuretics, Potassium-sparing, and Hydrochlorothiazide (Systemic)**, 1272, MC-28
*Aldactone*—Searle (U.S. and Canada) brand of Spironolactone—**See Diuretics, Potassium-sparing (Systemic)**, 1266, MC-28
*Aldara*—3M (U.S.) brand of Imiquimod (Topical), 1685
Aldesleukin [interleukin-2, recombinant; *Proleukin;* rIL-2]
 **(Systemic)**, 36, 3129
 for Injection, 41
*Aldoclor-150*—Merck (U.S.) brand of Methyldopa and Chlorothiazide—**See Methyldopa and Thiazide Diuretics (Systemic)**, 1983
*Aldoclor-250*—Merck (U.S.) brand of Methyldopa and Chlorothiazide—**See Methyldopa and Thiazide Diuretics (Systemic)**, 1983

*Aldomet*—Merck (U.S. and Canada) brand of Methyldopa (Systemic), 1979, MC-19
*Aldoril-15*—Merck (U.S. and Canada) brand of Methyldopa and Hydrochlorothiazide—**See Methyldopa and Thiazide Diuretics (Systemic)**, 1983, MC-19
*Aldoril-25*—Merck (U.S. and Canada) brand of Methyldopa and Hydrochlorothiazide—**See Methyldopa and Thiazide Diuretics (Systemic)**, 1983, MC-19
*Aldoril D30*—Merck (U.S. and Canada) brand of Methyldopa and Hydrochlorothiazide—**See Methyldopa and Thiazide Diuretics (Systemic)**, 1983, MC-19
*Aldoril D50*—Merck (U.S. and Canada) brand of Methyldopa and Hydrochlorothiazide—**See Methyldopa and Thiazide Diuretics (Systemic)**, 1983, MC-19
ALEC—See Dipalmitoylphosphatidylcholine and Phosphatidylglycerol (Intratracheal-Local), 3141
Alendronate [*Fosamax*]
 **(Systemic)**, 42
 Tablets, 44, MC-1
*Alenic Alka*—Rugby (U.S.) brand of Alumina and Magnesium Carbonate—**See Antacids (Oral-Local)**, 188; Rugby (U.S.) brand of Alumina, Magnesium Trisilicate, and Sodium Bicarbonate—**See Antacids (Oral-Local)**, 188
*Alenic Alka Extra Strength*—Rugby (U.S.) brand of Alumina, Magnesium Carbonate, and Sodium Bicarbonate—**See Antacids (Oral-Local)**, 188
*Alesse*—Wyeth-Ayerst (U.S.) brand of Levonorgestrel and Ethinyl Estradiol—**See Estrogens and Progestins—Oral Contraceptives (Systemic)**, 1397
*Aleve*—Procter & Gamble (U.S.) brand of Naproxen—**See Anti-inflammatory Drugs, Nonsteroidal (Systemic)**, 388
Alfacalcidol [*One-Alpha;* vitamin D]
 **See Vitamin D and Analogs (Systemic)**, 2966
 Capsules, 2969
 Solution, Oral, 2970
*Alfenta*—Janssen (U.S. and Canada) brand of Alfentanil—**See Fentanyl Derivatives (Systemic)**, 1452
Alfentanil Hydrochloride [*Alfenta*]
 **See Fentanyl Derivatives (Systemic)**, 1452
 Injection, 1458
*Alferon N*—Purdue Frederick (U.S.) brand of Interferon Alfa-n3—**See Interferons, Alpha (Systemic)**, 1740
*Algesal*—Solvay Kingswood (Canada) brand of Diethylamine Salicylate (Topical), 3017
Alglucerase [*Ceredase*]
 **(Systemic)**, #, 3129
 Injection, 3129
 for Injection Concentrate, #
Alimemazine—Trimeprazine—**See Antihistamines, Phenothiazine-derivative (Systemic)**, 377
*Alimentum*—Ross (U.S. and Canada) brand of Infant Formulas, Hypoallergenic—**See Infant Formulas (Systemic)**, #
*Alitraq*—Ross (U.S. and Canada) brand of Enteral Nutrition Formula, Monomeric (Elemental)—**See Enteral Nutrition Formulas (Systemic)**, #
*Alka Butazolidin*—Geigy (Canada) brand of Phenylbutazone—**See Anti-inflammatory Drugs, Nonsteroidal (Systemic)**, 388
*Alka-Mints*—Bayer (U.S.) brand of Calcium Carbonate—**See Antacids (Oral-Local)**, 188; **Calcium Supplements (Systemic)**, 736
*Alka-Seltzer Effervescent Pain Reliever and Antacid*—Miles (U.S. and Canada) brand of Aspirin, Sodium Bicarbonate, and Citric Acid (Systemic), 477
*Alka-Seltzer Plus Allergy Medicine Liqui-Gels*—Bayer (U.S.) brand of Chlorpheniramine, Pseudoephedrine, and Acetaminophen—**See Antihistamines, Decongestants, and Analgesics (Systemic)**, 366
*Alka-Seltzer Plus Cold and Cough*—Bayer (U.S.) brand of Chlorpheniramine, Phenylpropanolamine, Dextromethorphan, and Aspirin—**See Cough/Cold Combinations (Systemic)**, 1024
*Alka-Seltzer Plus Cold & Cough Medicine Liqui-Gels*—Bayer (U.S.) brand of Chlorpheniramine, Pseudoephedrine, Dextromethorphan, and Acetaminophen—**See Cough/Cold Combinations (Systemic)**, 1024

*Alka-Seltzer Plus Cold Medicine*—Bayer (U.S. and Canada) brand of Chlorpheniramine, Phenylpropanolamine, and Aspirin—**See Antihistamines, Decongestants, and Analgesics (Systemic)**, 366
*Alka-Seltzer Plus Cold Medicine Liqui-Gels*—Bayer (U.S.) brand of Chlorpheniramine, Pseudoephedrine, and Acetaminophen—**See Antihistamines, Decongestants, and Analgesics (Systemic)**, 366
*Alka-Seltzer Plus Flu & Body Aches*—Bayer (U.S.) brand of Chlorpheniramine, Phenylpropanolamine, Dextromethorphan, and Acetaminophen—**See Cough/Cold Combinations (Systemic)**, 1024
*Alka-Seltzer Plus Flu & Body Aches Medicine Liqui-Gels*—Bayer (U.S.) brand of Pseudoephedrine, Dextromethorphan, and Acetaminophen—**See Cough/Cold Combinations (Systemic)**, 1024
*Alka-Seltzer Plus Night Time Cold*—Bayer (U.S.) brand of Doxylamine, Phenylpropanolamine, Dextromethorphan, and Acetaminophen—**See Cough/Cold Combinations (Systemic)**, 1024
*Alka-Seltzer Plus Night-Time Cold Liqui-Gels*—Bayer (U.S.) brand of Doxylamine, Pseudoephedrine, Dextromethorphan, and Acetaminophen—**See Cough/Cold Combinations (Systemic)**, 1024
*Alka-Seltzer Plus Sinus Medicine*—Bayer (U.S.) brand of Phenylpropanolamine and Aspirin—**See Decongestants and Analgesics (Systemic)**, 1180
*Alkeran*—Glaxo Wellcome (U.S. and Canada) brand of Melphalan (Systemic), 1938, MC-18
*Alkeran for Injection*—BW (U.S.) brand of Melphalan (Systemic), 3153
*Alkets*—Roberts (U.S.) brand of Calcium Carbonate—**See Antacids (Oral-Local)**, 188
*Alkets Extra Strength*—Roberts (U.S.) brand of Calcium Carbonate—**See Antacids (Oral-Local)**, 188
*Allay*—Norton (U.S.) brand of Hydrocodone and Acetaminophen—**See Opioid (Narcotic) Analgesics and Acetaminophen (Systemic)**, 2198
*Allegra*—Hoechst Marion Roussel (U.S.) brand of Fexofenadine (Systemic), 1461, MC-12
*Allegra-D*—Hoechst Marion Roussel (U.S.) brand of Fexofenadine and Pseudoephedrine (Systemic), IBN-1463, MC-12
*Allent*—Ascher (U.S.) brand of Brompheniramine and Pseudoephedrine—**See Antihistamines and Decongestants (Systemic)**, 343
*Aller-Chlor*—Rugby (U.S.) brand of Chlorpheniramine—**See Antihistamines (Systemic)**, 325
*Allercon*—Parmed (U.S.) brand of Triprolidine and Pseudoephedrine—**See Antihistamines and Decongestants (Systemic)**, 343
*Allercort*—La Salle (U.S.) brand of Hydrocortisone—**See Corticosteroids (Topical)**, 978
*Allerdryl*—ICN (Canada) brand of Diphenhydramine—**See Antihistamines (Systemic)**, 325
*Allerest*—Fisons (U.S.) brand of Naphazoline (Ophthalmic), #
*Allerest 12 Hour Nasal Spray*—Ciba-Consumer (U.S.) brand of Oxymetazoline (Nasal), #
*Allerest Maximum Strength*—Ciba Self-Medication (U.S.) brand of Chlorpheniramine and Pseudoephedrine—**See Antihistamines and Decongestants (Systemic)**, 343
*Allerest No-Drowsiness Caplets*—Ciba (U.S.) brand of Pseudoephedrine and Acetaminophen—**See Decongestants and Analgesics (Systemic)**, 1180
*Allerest Sinus Pain Formula Caplets*—Ciba Self-Medication (U.S.) brand of Chlorpheniramine, Pseudoephedrine, and Acetaminophen—**See Antihistamines, Decongestants, and Analgesics (Systemic)**, 366
*Allerfrim*—Rugby (U.S.) brand of Triprolidine and Pseudoephedrine—**See Antihistamines and Decongestants (Systemic)**, 343
*Allerfrin with Codeine*—Rugby (U.S.) brand of Triprolidine, Pseudoephedrine, and Codeine—**See Cough/Cold Combinations (Systemic)**, 1024
*Allergen*—Goldline (U.S.) brand of Antipyrine and Benzocaine (Otic), 443
*Allergy Drops*—Bausch & Lomb (U.S.) brand of Naphazoline (Ophthalmic), #
*AllerMax Caplets*—Pfeiffer (U.S.) brand of Diphenhydramine—**See Antihistamines (Systemic)**, 325
*Aller-med*—Republic (U.S.) brand of Diphenhydramine—**See Antihistamines (Systemic)**, 325

*Allerphed*—Great Southern (U.S.) brand of Triprolidine and Pseudoephedrine—**See Antihistamines and Decongestants (Systemic)**, 343

*All-Nite Cold Formula*—Major (U.S.) brand of Doxylamine, Pseudoephedrine, Dextromethorphan, and Acetaminophen—**See Cough/Cold Combinations (Systemic)**, 1024

Allogeneic Peripheral Blood Mononuclear Cells Sensitized Against Patient Alloantigens By Mixed Lymphocyte Culture [*CYTOIMPLANT*]
**(Systemic)**, 3129

Allopurinol [*Apo-Allopurinol; Lopurin; Purinol; Zyloprim*]
**(Systemic)**, 44
Tablets USP, 47, MC-1

Allopurinol Sodium [*Zyloprim for Injection*]
**(Systemic)**, 3129
for Injection, 3129

All-*trans*-retinoic acid—*See* Tretinoin (Topical), 2871

*Almacone*—Rugby (U.S.) brand of Alumina, Magnesia, and Simethicone—**See Antacids (Oral-Local)**, 188

*Almacone II*—Rugby (U.S.) brand of Alumina, Magnesia, and Simethicone—**See Antacids (Oral-Local)**, 188

*Almagel 200*—Laboratoire Atlas (Canada) brand of Alumina and Magnesia—**See Antacids (Oral-Local)**, 188

*Almay Anti-itch Lotion*—Almay (U.S.) brand of Pramoxine and Menthol—**See Anesthetics (Topical)**, 155

*Almora*—Forest (U.S.) brand of Magnesium Gluconate—**See Magnesium Supplements (Systemic)**, 1897

*Alomide*—Alcon (Canada) brand of Lodoxamide (Ophthalmic), 3028; Alcon (U.S.) brand of Lodoxamide (Ophthalmic), #

*Alomide Ophthalmic Solution*—Alcon (U.S.) brand of Lodoxamide (Ophthalmic), 3151

*Alophen*—Warner Wellcome (U.S.) brand of Phenolphthalein—**See Laxatives (Local)**, #

Alpha₁-antitrypsin—*See* Alpha₁-proteinase Inhibitor, Human (Systemic), #

Alpha-1-Antitrypsin (Recombinant DNA Origin) **(Systemic)**, 3129

*Alpha-Baclofen*—Genpharm (Canada) brand of Baclofen (Systemic), 515

*Alphacaine*—Germiphene (Canada) brand of Lidocaine—**See Anesthetics (Topical)**, 155

*Alphaderm*—Lemmon (U.S.) brand of Hydrocortisone—**See Corticosteroids (Topical)**, 978

Alpha-difluoromethylornithine—*See* Eflornithine (Systemic), #

Alpha-Galactosidase A [*CC-Galactosidase; FABRase*]
**(Systemic)**, 3129

*Alphagan*—Allergan (U.S.) brand of Brimonidine (Ophthalmic), 632

*Alphamin*—Vortech (U.S.) brand of Hydroxocobalamin—**See Vitamin B₁₂ (Systemic)**, 2962

*Alphamul*—Lannett (U.S.) brand of Castor Oil—**See Laxatives (Local)**, #

*Alphanate*—Alpha (U.S.) brand of Antihemophilic Factor (Systemic), 319; Antihemophilic Factor (Human) (Systemic), 3131

*AlphaNine*—Alpha (U.S.) brand of Coagulation Factor IX (Human) (Systemic), 3137

*AlphaNine SD*—Alpha (U.S.) brand of Factor IX (Systemic), 1430

Alpha₁-proteinase Inhibitor [*Prolastin*]
**(Systemic)**, 3129

Alpha₁-proteinase Inhibitor, Human [alpha₁-antitrypsin; *Prolastin*]
**(Systemic)**, #
for Injection, #

Alpha tocopherol—*See* Vitamin E (Systemic), 2972

*Alphatrex*—Savage (U.S.) brand of Betamethasone—**See Corticosteroids (Topical)**, 978

*Alphosyl*—Reed & Carnrick (U.S. and Canada) brand of Coal Tar (Topical), #

Alprazolam [*Alprazolam Intensol; Apo-Alpraz; Alti-Alprazolam; Gen-Alprazolam; Novo-Alprazol; Nu-Alpraz; Xanax; Xanax TS*]
**See Benzodiazepines (Systemic)**, 556
Solution, Oral, 564
Tablets USP, 565, MC-1

*Alprazolam Intensol*—Roxane (U.S.) brand of Alprazolam—**See Benzodiazepines (Systemic)**, 556

Alprostadil [*Caverject; Edex; Muse;* PGE₁; prostaglandin E₁; *Prostin VR; Prostin VR Pediatric*]
**(Local)**, 48
for Injection, 52
Injection USP, 51
Suppositories, 51

Alprostadil [PGE₁; prostaglandin E₁; *Prostin VR; Prostin VR Pediatric; Vasoprost*]
**(Systemic)**, 52, 3129
Injection USP, 55

*Alramucil Orange*—Alra (U.S.) brand of Psyllium Hydrophilic Mucilloid—**See Laxatives (Local)**, #

*Alramucil Regular*—Alra (U.S.) brand of Psyllium Hydrophilic Mucilloid—**See Laxatives (Local)**, #

*Alrex*—Bausch & Lomb (U.S.) brand of Loteprednol (Ophthalmic), 1887

*Alsoy*—Carnation (U.S.) brand of Infant Formulas, Soy-based—**See Infant Formulas (Systemic)**, #

*Altace*—Hoechst Marion Roussel (U.S.) brand of Ramipril—**See Angiotensin-converting Enzyme (ACE) Inhibitors (Systemic)**, 177, MC-27

Alteplase, Recombinant [*Activase; Activase rt-PA;* rt-PA; tissue-type plasminogen activator (recombinant); t-PA]
**See Thrombolytic Agents (Systemic)**, 2799
for Injection, 2806

*AlternaGEL*—J & J/Merck (U.S.) brand of Alumina and Simethicone—**See Antacids (Oral-Local)**, 188

*Alti-Alprazolam*—Alti-Med (Canada) brand of Alprazolam—**See Benzodiazepines (Systemic)**, 556

*Alti-Bromazepam*—Alti-Med (Canada) brand of Bromazepam—**See Benzodiazepines (Systemic)**, 556

*Alti-Bromocriptine*—Alti-Med (Canada) brand of Bromocriptine (Systemic), 636

*Alti-MPA*—Altimed (Canada) brand of Medroxyprogesterone—**See Progestins (Systemic)**, 2400

*Alti-Triazolam*—Altimed (Canada) brand of Triazolam—**See Benzodiazepines (Systemic)**, 556

*Alti-Valproic*—Altimed (Canada) brand of Valproic Acid—**See Valproic Acid (Systemic)**, 2908

*Altracin*—A.L. (U.S.) brand of Bacitracin (Systemic), 3133

Altretamine [*Hexalen;* hexamethylmelamine; *Hexastat*]
**(Systemic)**, 55, 3129
Capsules, 57

*Alu-Cap*—3M (U.S.) brand of Aluminum Hydroxide—**See Antacids (Oral-Local)**, 188

*Aludrox*—Wyeth-Ayerst (U.S.) brand of Alumina, Magnesia, and Simethicone—**See Antacids (Oral-Local)**, 188

*Alugel*—Laboratoire Atlas (Canada) brand of Aluminum Hydroxide—**See Antacids (Oral-Local)**, 188

*Alumadrine*—Fleming (U.S.) brand of Chlorpheniramine, Phenylpropanolamine, and Acetaminophen—**See Antihistamines, Decongestants, and Analgesics (Systemic)**, 366

Alumina, Calcium Carbonate, and Sodium Bicarbonate [*Rafton*]
**See Antacids (Oral-Local)**, 188
Suspension, Oral, 213

Alumina-containing Combinations, 3067

Alumina and Magnesia [*Alamag; Almagel 200; Amphojel 500; Diovol Caplets; Diovol Ex; Gelusil; Gelusil Extra Strength; Life Antacid; Maalox; Maalox TC; Mintox; Mylanta Double Strength Plain; Neutralca-S; Rulox; Rulox No. 1; Rulox No. 2; Univol*]
**See Antacids (Oral-Local)**, 188
Suspension, Oral, 198, 203, 217
Suspension, Oral, USP, 199, 201, 206, 207, 209, 210, 212, 214
Tablets, 203
Tablets (Chewable), 203
Tablets, Original, USP (Chewable), 207
Tablets USP (Chewable), 206, 208, 209, 210, 212, 215

Alumina, Magnesia, Calcium Carbonate, and Simethicone [*Tempo*]
**See Antacids (Oral-Local)**, 188
Tablets USP (Chewable), 215

Alumina, Magnesia, and Magnesium Carbonate [*Diovol*]
**See Antacids (Oral-Local)**, 188
Tablets, Chewable, 203

Alumina, Magnesia, Magnesium Carbonate, and Simethicone [*Amphojel Plus; Diovol Plus; Gasmas*]
**See Antacids (Oral-Local)**, 188
Tablets, Chewable, 201, 204

Alumina, Magnesia, and Simethicone [*Alamag Plus; Almacone; Almacone II; Aludrox; Amphojel Plus; Antacid Liquid; Antacid Liquid Double Strength; Di-Gel; Diovol; Diovol Plus; Gelusil; Kudrox Double Strength; Life Antacid Plus; Maalox Plus; Maalox Plus, Extra Strength; Magnalox; Magnalox Plus; Mi-Acid; Mi-Acid Double Strength; Mintox Extra Stength; Mygel; Mygel II; Mylanta; Mylanta Double Strength; Mylanta Extra Strength; PMS Alumina, Magnesia, and Simethicone; Rulox Plus; Simaal Gel; Simaal 2 Gel*]
**See Antacids (Oral-Local)**, 188
Suspension, Oral, 203, 204
Suspension, Oral, USP, 198, 199, 201, 203, 206, 207, 208, 209, 210, 211, 212, 213, 215
Tablets USP (Chewable), 198, 206, 207, 208, 209, 210, 211, 212

Alumina, Magnesium Alginate, and Magnesium Carbonate [*Maalox HRF*]
**See Antacids (Oral-Local)**, 188
Suspension, Oral, 208
Tablets (Chewable), 208

Alumina and Magnesium Carbonate [*Alenic Alka; Gaviscon; Genaton; Maalox Heartburn Relief Formula*]
**See Antacids (Oral-Local)**, 188
Suspension, Oral, 198, 208
Suspension, Oral, USP, 204, 206

Alumina, Magnesium Carbonate, and Simethicone [*Gaviscon Extra Strength Relief Formula*]
**See Antacids (Oral-Local)**, 188
Suspension, Oral, USP, 205

Alumina, Magnesium Carbonate, and Sodium Bicarbonate [*Alenic Alka Extra Strength; Gaviscon Extra Strength Relief Formula; Genaton Extra Strength*]
**See Antacids (Oral-Local)**, 188
Tablets USP (Chewable), 198, 205, 206

Alumina, Magnesium Trisilicate, and Sodium Bicarbonate [*Alenic Alka; Foamicon; Gaviscon; Gaviscon-2; Genaton*]
**See Antacids (Oral-Local)**, 188
Tablets, Chewable, 198
Tablets USP (Chewable), 204, 206

Alumina and Simethicone [*AlternaGEL*]
**See Antacids (Oral-Local)**, 188
Gel USP, 199

Alumina and Sodium Bicarbonate [*Rafton*]
**See Antacids (Oral-Local)**, 188
Tablets, Chewable, 213

Aluminum Carbonate, Basic [*Basaljel*]
**See Antacids (Oral-Local)**, 188
Capsules, 201, 202
Tablets, 202

Aluminum Carbonate, Basic and Simethicone [*Basaljel*]
**See Antacids (Oral-Local)**, 188
Suspension, Oral, 202

Aluminum Hydroxide [*Alu-Cap; Alugel; Alu-Tab; Amphojel; Basaljel; Gaviscon Heartburn Relief; Gaviscon Heartburn Relief Extra Strength; Nephrox*]
**See Antacids (Oral-Local)**, 188
Capsules, Dried Gel, 201, 202
Capsules, Dried Gel, USP, 199
Gel USP, 199, 200
Suspension, Oral, 205, 212
Suspension, Oral, USP, 205
Tablets, Dried Gel, USP, 200
Tablets USP (Chewable), 206

*Alupent*—Boehringer Ingelheim (U.S. and Canada) brand of Metaproterenol—**See Bronchodilators, Adrenergic (Inhalation-Local)**, 640; **Bronchodilators, Adrenergic (Systemic)**, 651, MC-18

*Alurate*—Roche (U.S.) brand of Aprobarbital—**See Barbiturates (Systemic)**, 518

*Alu-Tab*—3M (U.S. and Canada) brand of Aluminum Hydroxide—**See Antacids (Oral-Local)**, 188

Amantadine Hydrochloride [*Symadine; Symmetrel*]
**(Systemic)**, 58
Capsules USP, 61, MC-1
Syrup USP, 61
Tablets, MC-1

*Amaphen*—Trimen (U.S.) brand of Butalbital, Acetaminophen, and Caffeine—**See Barbiturates and Analgesics (Systemic)**, 532

*Amaryl*—Hoechst Marion Roussel (U.S.) brand of Glimepiride (Systemic), 1560, MC-13

*Amatine*—Roberts (U.S.) brand of Midodrine (Systemic), 3154
Ambenonium Chloride [*Mytelase Caplets*]
  See **Antimyasthenics (Systemic)**, 437
  Tablets, 439
*Ambenyl Cough*—Forest (U.S.) brand of Bromodiphenhydramine and Codeine—See **Cough/Cold Combinations (Systemic)**, 1024; PD (Canada) brand of Bromodiphenhydramine, Diphenhydramine, Codeine, Ammonium Chloride, and Potassium Guaiacolsulfonate—See **Cough/Cold Combinations (Systemic)**, 1024
*Ambenyl-D Decongestant Cough Formula*—Forest (U.S.) brand of Pseudoephedrine, Dextromethorphan, and Guaifenesin—See **Cough/Cold Combinations (Systemic)**, 1024
*Ambi 10 Acne Medication*—Kiwi (U.S.) brand of Benzoyl Peroxide (Topical), 579
*Ambien*—Searle (U.S.) brand of Zolpidem (Systemic), 3005, MC-32
*AmBisome*—Fujisawa (U.S.) brand of Amphotericin B, Liposomal (Systemic), 3152; Amphotericin B Liposomal Complex (Systemic), 105
*Ambophen*—Major (U.S.) brand of Bromodiphenhydramine and Codeine—See **Cough/Cold Combinations (Systemic)**, 1024
Amcinonide [*Cyclocort*]
  See **Corticosteroids (Topical)**, 978
  Cream USP, 982
  Lotion, 983
  Ointment USP, 983
*Amcort*—Keene (U.S.) brand of Triamcinolone—See **Corticosteroids—Glucocorticoid Effects (Systemic)**, 998
*Amen*—Carnrick (U.S.) brand of Medroxyprogesterone—See **Progestins (Systemic)**, 2400
*Amerge*—Glaxo Wellcome (U.S.) brand of Naratriptan (Systemic), 2087, MC-21
*Americaine*—Ciba Consumer (U.S.) brand of Benzocaine—See **Anesthetics (Mucosal-Local)**, 128
*Americaine Anesthetic Lubricant*—Fisons (U.S.) brand of Benzocaine—See **Anesthetics (Mucosal-Local)**, 128
*Americaine Hemorrhoidal*—Fisons Consumer (U.S.) brand of Benzocaine—See **Anesthetics (Mucosal-Local)**, 128
*Americaine Topical Anesthetic First Aid Ointment*—Ciba Consumer (U.S.) brand of Benzocaine—See **Anesthetics (Topical)**, 155
*Americaine Topical Anesthetic Spray*—Ciba Consumer (U.S.) brand of Benzocaine—See **Anesthetics (Topical)**, 155
*A-methaPred*—Abbott (U.S.) brand of Methylprednisolone—See **Corticosteroids—Glucocorticoid Effects (Systemic)**, 998
Amethocaine—Tetracaine—See **Anesthetics (Mucosal-Local)**, 128; **Anesthetics (Ophthalmic)**, #; **Anesthetics (Topical)**, 155
Amethopterin—See Methotrexate—For Cancer (Systemic), 1962; Methotrexate—For Noncancerous Conditions (Systemic), 1969
Amfebutamone—See Bupropion (Systemic), 687
Amfepramone—Diethylpropion—See **Appetite Suppressants (Systemic)**, 452
Amfetamine—Amphetamine—See **Amphetamines (Systemic)**, 94
*Amgenal Cough*—Zenith Goldline (U.S.) brand of Bromodiphenhydramine and Codeine—See **Cough/Cold Combinations (Systemic)**, 1024
*Amicar*—Immunex (U.S.) and Wyeth-Ayerst (Canada) brand of Aminocaproic Acid (Systemic), 64, MC-2
*Amidate*—Abbott (U.S.) brand of Etomidate (Systemic), 1422
*Amidrine*—Amide (U.S.) brand of Isometheptene, Dichloralphenazone, and Acetaminophen (Systemic), 1786
Amifostine [*Ethyol*]
  **(Systemic)**, 61, 3130
  for Injection, 63
*Amigesic*—Amide (U.S.) brand of Salsalate—See **Salicylates (Systemic)**, 2538
Amikacin Sulfate [*Amikin*]
  See **Aminoglycosides (Systemic)**, 69
  Injection USP, 74
*Amikin*—Bristol (U.S. and Canada) brand of Amikacin—See **Aminoglycosides (Systemic)**, 69
*Amilon*—H.L. Moore (U.S.) brand of Chlorpheniramine, Phenindamine, and Phenylpropanolamine—See **Antihistamines and Decongestants (Systemic)**, 343
Amiloride-containing Combinations, 3067

Amiloride Hydrochloride
  **(Inhalation)**, 3130
  Solution for Inhalation, 3130
Amiloride Hydrochloride [*Midamor*]
  See **Diuretics, Potassium-sparing (Systemic)**, 1266
  Tablets USP, 1269, MC-2
Amiloride Hydrochloride and Hydrochlorothiazide [*Moduret; Moduretic*]
  See **Diuretics, Potassium-sparing, and Hydrochlorothiazide (Systemic)**, 1272
  Tablets USP, 1272, MC-2
*Amin-Aid*—Kendall McGaw (U.S.) brand of Enteral Nutrition Formula, Disease-specific—See **Enteral Nutrition Formulas (Systemic)**, #
Aminobenzoate Potassium [*KPAB; Potaba; Potaba Envules; Potaba Powder;* potassium aminobenzoate; potassium para-aminobenzoate]
  **(Systemic)**, #
  Capsules USP, #
  for Solution, Oral, USP, #
  Tablets USP, #
Aminobenzoic Acid–containing Combinations, 3067
Aminobenzoic Acid, Padimate O, and Oxybenzone [*Presun*]
  See **Sunscreen Agents (Topical)**, #
  Lotion, #
Aminobenzoic Acid and Titanium Dioxide [*Formula 405 Solar*]
  See **Sunscreen Agents (Topical)**, #
  Lotion, #
Aminocaproic Acid
  **(Ophthalmic)**, 3130
Aminocaproic Acid [*Amicar;* epsilon-aminocaproic acid]
  **(Systemic)**, 64
  Injection USP, 66
  Syrup USP, 66
  Tablets USP, 66, MC-2
*Aminofen*—Dover (U.S.) brand of Acetaminophen (Systemic), 6
*Aminofen Max*—Dover (U.S.) brand of Acetaminophen (Systemic), 6
Aminoglutethimide [*Cytadren*]
  **(Systemic)**, 67
  Tablets USP, 69
Aminoglycosides
  **(Systemic)**, 69
*Amino-Opti-E*—Tyson (U.S.) brand of Vitamin E (Systemic), 2972
Aminophylline [*Phyllocontin; Phyllocontin-350; Truphylline*]
  See **Bronchodilators, Theophylline (Systemic)**, 668
  Injection USP, 677
  Solution, Oral, USP, 675
  Suppositories USP, 678
  Tablets USP, 676
  Tablets, Extended-release, 677
Aminosalicylate Sodium [*Nemasol Sodium;* PAS; *Tubasal*]
  **(Systemic)**, #, 3130
  Tablets USP, #
4-Aminosalicylic Acid [*Pamisyl; Rezipas*]
  **(Systemic)**, 3128
5-aminosalicylic acid—See Mesalamine (Oral-Local), 1952; Mesalamine (Rectal-Local), 1954
Aminosalicylic Acid [*Paser, Paser Granules*]
  **(Systemic)**, 3009, 3130
  Granules, 3009
Aminosidine [*Gabbromicina; Paromomycin*]
  **(Systemic)**, 3130
*Amio-Aqueous*—Academic (U.S.) brand of Amiodarone (Systemic), 3130
Amiodarone [*Amio-Aqueous*]
  **(Systemic)**, 3130
Amiodarone Hydrochloride [*Cordarone; Cordarone Intravenous; Cordarone I.V.; Pacerone* ]
  **(Systemic)**, 79, 3130
  Injection, 84
  Tablets, 83, MC-2
*Amipaque*—Sanofi Winthrop (U.S.) brand of Metrizamide (Systemic), #
*Ami-Tex*—Amide (U.S.) brand of Phenylephrine, Phenylpropanolamine, and Guaifenesin—See **Cough/Cold Combinations (Systemic)**, 1024
*Ami-Tex LA*—Amide (U.S.) brand of Phenylpropanolamine and Guaifenesin—See **Cough/Cold Combinations (Systemic)**, 1024
*Amitone*—Menley & James (U.S.) brand of Calcium Carbonate—See **Antacids (Oral-Local)**, 188; **Calcium Supplements (Systemic)**, 736

Amitriptyline-containing Combinations, 3067
Amitriptyline Hydrochloride [*Apo-Amitriptyline; Elavil; Endep; Levate; Novotriptyn*]
  See **Antidepressants, Tricyclic (Systemic)**, 271
  Injection USP, 278
  Tablets USP, 278, MC-2
Amitriptyline Pamoate [*Elavil*]
  See **Antidepressants, Tricyclic (Systemic)**, 271
  Syrup, 278
Amlexanox [*Aphthasol*]
  **(Mucosal-Local)**, 85
  Paste, Oral, 86
Amlodipine and Benazepril Hydrochloride [*Lotrel*]
  **(Systemic)**, 88
  Capsules, 91, MC-2
Amlodipine Besylate [*Norvasc*]
  **(Systemic)**, 86
  Tablets, 88, MC-2
Ammonia N 13
  **(Systemic)**, 91
  Injection USP, 93
Ammonia Spirit, Aromatic [smelling salts]
  **(Inhalation-Systemic)**, #
  Ammonia Spirit, Aromatic, USP, #
  Inhalants, #
Ammoniated Mercury
  **(Topical)**, #
  Ointment USP, #
Ammonium Chloride–containing Combinations, 3067
Ammonium Molybdate [*Molypen*]
  See **Molybdenum Supplements (Systemic)**, 2053
  Injection USP, 2054
Ammonium Tetrathiomolybdate
  **(Systemic)**, 3130
Amobarbital [*Amytal*]
  See **Barbiturates (Systemic)**, 518
  Tablets USP, 524
Amobarbital-containing Combinations, 3067
Amobarbital Sodium [*Amytal*]
  See **Barbiturates (Systemic)**, 518
  Capsules USP, 524
  Sterile USP, 524
5a8, Monoclonal Antibody to CD4
  **(Systemic)**, 3128
Amoxapine [*Asendin*]
  See **Antidepressants, Tricyclic (Systemic)**, 271
  Tablets USP, 278, MC-2
Amoxicillin [amoxicilline; *Amoxil;* amoxycillin; *Apo-Amoxi; Novamoxin; Nu-Amoxi; Polymox; Trimox; Wymox*]
  See **Penicillins (Systemic)**, 2240, 3010
  Capsules USP, 2246, 3010, MC-2
  Suspension, Oral, USP, 3010
  for Suspension, Oral, USP, 2247
  Tablets USP (Chewable), 2247, MC-2
  Tablets USP, Chewable, 3010
Amoxicillin and Clavulanate [*Augmentin*]
  **(Systemic)**, 3010
  Suspension, Oral, 3010
  Tablets, 3010
  Tablets, Chewable, 3010
Amoxicillin and Clavulanate Potassium [*Augmentin; Clavulin-250; Clavulin-125F; Clavulin-250F; Clavulin 500F; Lipitor*]
  See **Penicillins and Beta-lactamase Inhibitors (Systemic)**, 2263
  for Suspension, Oral, USP, 2268
  Tablets USP, 2268, MC-2
  Tablets USP (Chewable), 2269, MC-2
Amoxicillin-containing Combinations, 3067
Amoxicilline—Amoxicillin—See **Penicillins (Systemic)**, 2240
*Amoxil*—SmithKline Beecham (U.S.) brand of Amoxicillin (Systemic), 3010; Amoxicillin—See **Penicillins (Systemic)**, 2240, MC-2
Amoxycillin—Amoxicillin—See **Penicillins (Systemic)**, 2240
Amphetamine Aspartate, Amphetamine Sulfate, Dextroamphetamine Saccharate, and Dextroamphetamine Sulfate [*Adderall*]
  **(Systemic)**, 94
  Tablets, 97
Amphetamines
  **(Systemic)**, 94
Amphetamine Sulfate [amfetamine]
  See **Amphetamines (Systemic)**, 94
  Tablets USP, 97
*Amphocin*—Adria (U.S.) brand of Amphotericin B (Systemic), 98

## General Index

*Amphojel*—Wyeth-Ayerst (U.S.) and Axcan Pharma (Canada) brand of Aluminum Hydroxide—**See Antacids (Oral-Local)**, 188
*Amphojel 500*—Axcan Pharma (Canada) brand of Alumina and Magnesia—**See Antacids (Oral-Local)**, 188
*Amphojel Plus*—Axcan Pharma (Canada) brand of Alumina, Magnesia, Magnesium Carbonate, and Simethicone—**See Antacids (Oral-Local)**, 188; Alumina, Magnesia, and Simethicone—**See Antacids (Oral-Local)**, 188
*Amphotec*—Sequus (U.S.) brand of Amphotericin B Cholesteryl Complex (Systemic), 101
Amphotericin B [*Amphocin; Fungizone Intravenous*] (Systemic), 98
   for Injection USP, 100
Amphotericin B [*Fungizone*]
   (Topical), #
   Cream USP, #
   Lotion USP, #
   Ointment USP, #
Amphotericin B Cholesteryl Complex [*Amphotec*] (Systemic), 101
   for Injection, 103
Amphotericin B Lipid Complex [*ABELCET*; ABLC] (Systemic), 103, 3130
   Injection, 105
Amphotericin B, Liposomal—**See Liposomal Amphotericin B (Systemic)**, 3151
Amphotericin B Liposomal Complex [*AmBisome*] (Systemic), 105
   for Injection, 107
Ampicillin [*Apo-Ampi; Novo-Ampicillin; Nu-Ampi; Omnipen; Penbritin; Polycillin; Principen; Totacillin*]
   **See Penicillins (Systemic)**, 2240
   Capsules USP, 2247, MC-2
   for Suspension, Oral, USP, 2248
Ampicillin-containing Combinations, 3067
Ampicillin Sodium [*Ampicin; Omnipen-N; Penbritin; Polycillin-N; Totacillin-N*]
   **See Penicillins (Systemic)**, 2240
   Sterile USP, 2248
Ampicillin Sodium and Sulbactam Sodium [*Unasyn*]
   **See Penicillins and Beta-lactamase Inhibitors (Systemic)**, 2263
   Sterile USP, 2269
*Ampicin*—Bristol (Canada) brand of Ampicillin—**See Penicillins (Systemic)**, 2240
*Ampligen*—HEM (U.S.) brand of Poly I: Poly C12U (Systemic), 3158, 3159
Amrinone Lactate [*Inocor*]
   (Systemic), 108
   Injection, 109
Amsacrine [*Amsa P-D*]
   (Systemic), 3010
   Injection, 3010
*Amsa P-D*—PD (Canada) brand of Amsacrine (Systemic), 3010
Amyl Nitrite
   (Systemic), #
   Inhalant USP, #
*Amytal*—Lilly (U.S. and Canada) brand of Amobarbital—**See Barbiturates (Systemic)**, 518
Anabolic Steroids
   (Systemic), 110
*Anacin*—Whitehall (Canada) brand of Aspirin—**See Salicylates (Systemic)**, 2538
*Anacin-3*—Whitehall-Robins (Canada) brand of Acetaminophen (Systemic), 6
*Anacin Caplets*—Whitehall (U.S.) brand of Aspirin—**See Salicylates (Systemic)**, 2538
*Anacin with Codeine*—Whitehall-Robins (Canada) brand of Aspirin and Codeine—**See Opioid (Narcotic) Analgesics and Aspirin (Systemic)**, 2202
*Anacin Extra Strength*—Whitehall (Canada) brand of Aspirin—**See Salicylates (Systemic)**, 2538
*Anacin-3 Extra Strength*—Whitehall-Robins (Canada) brand of Acetaminophen (Systemic), 6
*Anacin Maximum Strength*—Whitehall (U.S.) brand of Aspirin—**See Salicylates (Systemic)**, 2538
*Anacin Tablets*—Whitehall (U.S.) brand of Aspirin—**See Salicylates (Systemic)**, 2538
*Anacobin*—Glaxo (Canada) brand of Cyanocobalamin—**See Vitamin B$_{12}$ (Systemic)**, 2962
*Anaflex 750*—Salsalate—**See Salicylates (Systemic)**, 2538
*Anafranil*—Novartis (U.S.) and Ciba-Geigy (Canada) brand of Clomipramine—**See Antidepressants, Tricyclic (Systemic)**, 271, MC-7

Anagrelide [*Agrylin*]
   (Systemic), 3010, 3131
   Capsules, 3010
Anagrelide Hydrochloride [*Agrylin*]
   (Systemic), 114
   Capsules, 116
*Ana-Guard*—Miles (U.S.) brand of Epinephrine—**See Bronchodilators, Adrenergic (Systemic)**, 651
*Analgesic Otic*—Akorn (U.S.) brand of Antipyrine and Benzocaine (Otic), 443
*Anamine*—Mayrand (U.S.) brand of Chlorpheniramine and Pseudoephedrine—**See Antihistamines and Decongestants (Systemic)**, 343
*Anamine T.D.*—Mayrand (U.S.) brand of Chlorpheniramine and Pseudoephedrine—**See Antihistamines and Decongestants (Systemic)**, 343
Ananain, Comosain [*Vianain*]
   (Topical), 3131
*Anandron*—Hoechst Marion Roussel (Canada) brand of Nilutamide—**See Antiandrogens, Nonsteroidal (Systemic)**, 220
*Anaplex HD*—ECR (U.S.) brand of Chlorpheniramine, Phenylephrine, and Hydrocodone—**See Cough/Cold Combinations (Systemic)**, 1024
*Anapolon 50*—Roche (Canada) brand of Oxymetholone—**See Anabolic Steroids (Systemic)**, 110
*Anaprox*—Roche (U.S.) and Syntex (Canada) brand of Naproxen—**See Anti-inflammatory Drugs, Nonsteroidal (Systemic)**, 388, MC-21
*Anaprox DS*—Roche/Syntex (U.S.) and Syntex (Canada) brand of Naproxen—**See Anti-inflammatory Drugs, Nonsteroidal (Systemic)**, 388
Anaritide Acetate [*Auriculin*]
   (Systemic), 3131
*Anaspaz*—Ascher (U.S.) brand of Hyoscyamine—**See Anticholinergics/Antispasmodics (Systemic)**, 226
Anastrozole [*Arimidex*]
   (Systemic), 116, MC-3
   Tablets, 118, MC-3
*Anatrast*—Lafayette (U.S.) brand of Barium Sulfate (Local), #
*Anatuss*—Mayrand (U.S.) brand of Phenylpropanolamine, Dextromethorphan, and Guaifenesin—**See Cough/Cold Combinations (Systemic)**, 1024; Phenylpropanolamine, Dextromethorphan, Guaifenesin, and Acetaminophen—**See Cough/Cold Combinations (Systemic)**, 1024
*Anatuss DM*—Mayrand (U.S.) brand of Pseudoephedrine, Dextromethorphan, and Guaifenesin—**See Cough/Cold Combinations (Systemic)**, 1024
*Anatuss LA*—Mayrand (U.S.) brand of Pseudoephedrine and Guaifenesin—**See Cough/Cold Combinations (Systemic)**, 1024
*Anbesol, Baby*—Whitehall (U.S.) brand of Benzocaine—**See Anesthetics (Mucosal-Local)**, 128
*Anbesol Baby Jel*—Whitehall-Robins (Canada) brand of Benzocaine—**See Anesthetics (Mucosal-Local)**, 128
*Anbesol Gel*—Whitehall-Robins (Canada) brand of Benzocaine and Phenol—**See Anesthetics (Mucosal-Local)**, 128
*Anbesol Liquid*—Whitehall-Robins (Canada) brand of Benzocaine and Phenol—**See Anesthetics (Mucosal-Local)**, 128
*Anbesol Maximum Strength Gel*—Whitehall (U.S.) brand of Benzocaine—**See Anesthetics (Mucosal-Local)**, 128
*Anbesol Maximum Strength Liquid*—Whitehall (U.S.) brand of Benzocaine—**See Anesthetics (Mucosal-Local)**, 128; Whitehall-Robins (Canada) brand of Benzocaine and Phenol—**See Anesthetics (Mucosal-Local)**, 128
*Anbesol Regular Strength Gel*—Whitehall (U.S.) brand of Benzocaine and Phenol—**See Anesthetics (Mucosal-Local)**, 128
*Anbesol Regular Strength Liquid*—Whitehall (U.S.) brand of Benzocaine and Phenol—**See Anesthetics (Mucosal-Local)**, 128
*Ancalixir*—Sandoz (Canada) brand of Phenobarbital—**See Barbiturates (Systemic)**, 518
*Ancef*—SKF (U.S. and Canada) brand of Cefazolin—**See Cephalosporins (Systemic)**, 794
*Ancobon*—Roche (U.S.) brand of Flucytosine (Systemic), #
*Ancotil*—Roche (Canada) brand of Flucytosine (Systemic), #
Ancrod [*Arvin*]
   (Systemic), 3131

*Andec*—Econolab (U.S.) brand of Carbinoxamine and Pseudoephedrine—**See Antihistamines and Decongestants (Systemic)**, 343
*Andec-TR*—Econolab (U.S.) brand of Carbinoxamine and Pseudoephedrine—**See Antihistamines and Decongestants (Systemic)**, 343
*Andrest 90-4*—Seatrace (U.S.) brand of Testosterone and Estradiol—**See Androgens and Estrogens (Systemic)**, 126
*Andriol*—Organon (Canada) brand of Testosterone (Systemic), 118
*Androcur*—Berlex (Canada) brand of Cyproterone (Systemic), 3016
*Androderm*—SmithKline Beecham (U.S.) brand of Testosterone—**See Androgens (Systemic)**, 118
*Andro-Estro 90-4*—Rugby (U.S.) brand of Testosterone and Estradiol—**See Androgens and Estrogens (Systemic)**, 126
*Androgel*—Unimed (U.S.) brand of Testosterone (Systemic), 3168
*Androgel-DHT*—Unimed (U.S.) brand of Dihydrotestosterone (Systemic), 3140
Androgens
   (Systemic), 118
Androgens and Estrogens
   (Systemic), 126
*Androgyn L.A.*—Forest (U.S.) brand of Testosterone and Estradiol—**See Androgens and Estrogens (Systemic)**, 126
*Android*—ICN and Schering Plough (U.S.) brand of Methyltestosterone—**See Androgens (Systemic)**, 118
*Android-F*—Pharmacia & Upjohn (U.S.) brand of Fluoxymesterone—**See Androgens (Systemic)**, 118
*Andro L.A. 200*—Forest (U.S.) brand of Testosterone—**See Androgens (Systemic)**, 118
*Andronate 100*—Keene (U.S.) brand of Testosterone—**See Androgens (Systemic)**, 118
*Andronate 200*—Keene (U.S.) brand of Testosterone—**See Androgens (Systemic)**, 118
*Andropository 200*—Rugby (U.S.) brand of Testosterone—**See Androgens (Systemic)**, 118
*Andryl 200*—Keene (U.S.) brand of Testosterone—**See Androgens (Systemic)**, 118
*AN-DTPA*—CIS-US (U.S.) brand of Technetium Tc 99m Pentetate (Systemic), 2727
*Anectine*—BW (U.S. and Canada) brand of Succinylcholine—**See Neuromuscular Blocking Agents (Systemic)**, 2098
*Anectine Flo-Pack*—BW (U.S. and Canada) brand of Succinylcholine—**See Neuromuscular Blocking Agents (Systemic)**, 2098
*Anergan 25*—Forest (U.S.) brand of Promethazine—**See Antihistamines, Phenothiazine-derivative (Systemic)**, 377
*Anergan 50*—Forest (U.S.) brand of Promethazine—**See Antihistamines, Phenothiazine-derivative (Systemic)**, 377
*Anestacon Jelly*—Webcon (U.S.) brand of Lidocaine—**See Anesthetics (Mucosal-Local)**, 128
Anesthetics
   (Mucosal-Local), 128
Anesthetics
   (Ophthalmic), #
Anesthetics
   (Parenteral-Local), 139
Anesthetics
   (Topical), 155
Anesthetics, Barbiturate
   (Systemic), 161
Anesthetics, Inhalation
   (Systemic), 168
*Anexate*—Hoffmann-LaRoche (Canada) brand of Flumazenil (Systemic), 1483
*Anexsia 5/500*—Boehringer-Mannheim (U.S.) brand of Hydrocodone and Acetaminophen—**See Opioid (Narcotic) Analgesics and Acetaminophen (Systemic)**, 2198
*Anexsia 7.5/650*—Boehringer-Mannheim (U.S.) brand of Hydrocodone and Acetaminophen—**See Opioid (Narcotic) Analgesics and Acetaminophen (Systemic)**, 2198
*Angio-Conray*—Mallinckrodt (U.S.) brand of Iothalamate (Systemic), #
Angiotensin-converting Enzyme (ACE) Inhibitors
   (Systemic), 177
Angiotensin-converting Enzyme (ACE) Inhibitors and Hydrochlorothiazide
   (Systemic), 187
*Angiovist 282*—Berlex (U.S.) brand of Diatrizoate—**See Diatrizoates (Systemic)**, #

*Angiovist 292*—Berlex (U.S.) brand of Diatrizoate—**See Diatrizoates (Systemic)**, #
*Angiovist 370*—Berlex (U.S.) brand of Diatrizoate—**See Diatrizoates (Systemic)**, #
Anileridine [*Leritine*]
  **(Systemic)**, 3011
  Injection USP, 3011
  Tablets USP, 3011
Aniline violet—*See* Methylene Blue (Systemic), #
Anisindione [*Miradon*]
  **See Anticoagulants (Systemic)**, 243
  Tablets, 248
Anisotropine Methylbromide [octatropine]
  **See Anticholinergics/Antispasmodics (Systemic)**, 226
  Tablets, 232
Anisoylated plasminogen-streptokinase activator complex—Anistreplase—**See Thrombolytic Agents (Systemic)**, 2799
Anistreplase [anisoylated plasminogen-streptokinase activator complex; APSAC; *Eminase*]
  **See Thrombolytic Agents (Systemic)**, 2799
  for Injection, 2807
*AN-MAA*—CIS-US (U.S.) brand of Technetium Tc 99m Albumin Aggregated (Systemic), 2697
*Anolor-300*—Blansett (U.S.) brand of Butalbital, Acetaminophen, and Caffeine—**See Barbiturates and Analgesics (Systemic)**, 532
*Anolor DH 5*—Blansett (U.S.) brand of Hydrocodone and Acetaminophen—**See Opioid (Narcotic) Analgesics and Acetaminophen (Systemic)**, 2198
*Anoquan*—Mallard (U.S.) brand of Butalbital, Acetaminophen, and Caffeine—**See Barbiturates and Analgesics (Systemic)**, 532
*Anorex SR*—Dunhall (U.S.) brand of Phendimetrazine—**See Appetite Suppressants (Systemic)**, 452
*Ansaid*—Pharmacia & Upjohn (U.S. and Canada) brand of Flurbiprofen—**See Anti-inflammatory Drugs, Nonsteroidal (Systemic)**, 388, MC-13
*AN-Sulfur Colloid*—Syncor (U.S.) brand of Technetium Tc 99m Sulfur Colloid (Systemic), 2740
*Answer*—Carter-Wallace (U.S.) brand of Immunoassay Pregnancy Test Kits—**See Pregnancy Test Kits for Home Use**, #
*Answer Now One Step*—Carter-Horner (Canada) brand of Immunoassay Pregnancy Test Kits—**See Pregnancy Test Kits for Home Use**, #
*Answer Ovulation*—Carter (U.S.) brand of Enzyme Immunoassay Ovulation Prediction Test Kits—**See Ovulation Prediction Test Kits for Home Use**, #
*Answer Quick & Simple 1-Step*—Carter-Wallace (U.S.) brand of Immunoassay Pregnancy Test Kits—**See Pregnancy Test Kits for Home Use**, #
*Antabuse*—Wyeth-Ayerst (U.S.) and Ayerst (Canada) brand of Disulfiram (Systemic), 1256
*Antacid Gelcaps*—Zenith Goldline (U.S.) brand of Calcium and Magnesium Carbonates—**See Antacids (Oral-Local)**, 188
*Antacid Liquid*—Zenith Goldline (U.S.) brand of Alumina, Magnesia, and Simethicone—**See Antacids (Oral-Local)**, 188
*Antacid Liquid Double Strength*—Zenith Goldline (U.S.) brand of Alumina, Magnesia, and Simethicone—**See Antacids (Oral-Local)**, 188
Antacids
  **(Oral-Local)**, 188
*Anthraforte 1*—Medican (Canada) brand of Anthralin (Topical), 218
*Anthraforte 2*—Medican (Canada) brand of Anthralin (Topical), 218
Anthralin [*Anthraforte 1; Anthraforte 2; Anthranol 0.1; Anthranol 0.2; Anthranol 0.4*; dithranol; *Drithocreme; Drithocreme HP; Dritho-Scalp; Micanol*]
  **(Topical)**, 218
  Cream USP, 219
  Ointment USP, 219
*Anthranol 0.1*—Medican (Canada) brand of Anthralin (Topical), 218
*Anthranol 0.2*—Medican (Canada) brand of Anthralin (Topical), 218
*Anthranol 0.4*—Medican (Canada) brand of Anthralin (Topical), 218
Antiandrogens, Nonsteroidal
  **(Systemic)**, 220
Antibacterial, systemicGrepafloxacin (Systemic), 16
*Antiben*—Hi-Tech (U.S.) brand of Antipyrine and Benzocaine (Otic), 443

*Antibiotic Ear*—Geneva (U.S.); Parnell (U.S.); Rugby (U.S.); and URL (U.S.) brand of Neomycin, Polymyxin B, and Hydrocortisone (Otic), #
Anti-CD45 Monoclonal Antibodies
  **(Systemic)**, 3131
Anticholinergics/Antispasmodics
  **(Systemic)**, 226
Anticoagulants
  **(Systemic)**, 243
Anticonvulsants, Dione
  **(Systemic)**, #
Anticonvulsants, Hydantoin
  **(Systemic)**, 253
Anticonvulsants, Succinimide
  **(Systemic)**, #
Antidepressants, Monoamine Oxidase (MAO) Inhibitor
  **(Systemic)**, 266
Antidepressants, Tricyclic
  **(Systemic)**, 271
Anti-D gammaglobulin—*See* Rh₀(D) Immune Globulin (Systemic), 2476
Antidiabetic Agents, Sulfonylurea
  **(Systemic)**, 283
*Antidol*—Aspirin—**See Salicylates (Systemic)**, 2538
*Antidotum Thallii-Heyl*—Heyl (Germany) brand of Prussian Blue (Oral-Local), #
Anti-D (Rh₀) immunoglobulin—*See* Rh₀(D) Immune Globulin (Systemic), 2476
Antidyskinetics
  **(Systemic)**, 297
Antiepilepsirine
  **(Systemic)**, 3131
*Antiflex*—Clint (U.S.) brand of Orphenadrine—**See Skeletal Muscle Relaxants (Systemic)**, 2577
Antifungals, Azole
  **(Systemic)**, 302
Antifungals, Azole
  **(Vaginal)**, 310
Antiglaucoma Agents, Cholinergic, Long-acting
  **(Ophthalmic)**, 315
Antihemophilic Factor, Cryoprecipitated [AHF; factor VIII]
  **(Systemic)**, 319
Antihemophilic Factor, Cryoprecipitated, USP, 324
Antihemophilic Factor (Human) [AHF; *Alphanate*; factor VIII; *Hemofil M; Humate P; Humate-P; Koate-HP; Monoclate-P*]
  **(Systemic)**, 319, 3131
Antihemophilic Factor (Human) USP, 322
Antihemophilic Factor (Porcine) [AHF; factor VIII; *Hyate:C*]
  **(Systemic)**, 319
Antihemophilic Factor (Porcine), 323
Antihemophilic Factor (Recombinant) [AHF; *Bioclate*; factor VIII; *Helixate; Kogenate; Recombinate*]
  **(Systemic)**, 319, 3011, 3131
Antihemophilic Factor (Recombinant), 323
  for Injection, 3011
Antihistamines
  **(Systemic)**, 325
Antihistamines and Decongestants
  **(Systemic)**, 343
Antihistamines, Decongestants, and Analgesics
  **(Systemic)**, 366
Antihistamines, Decongestants, and Anticholinergics
  **(Systemic)**, 373
Antihistamines, Phenothiazine-derivative
  **(Systemic)**, 377
Anti-inflammatory Drugs, Nonsteroidal
  **(Ophthalmic)**, 383
Anti-inflammatory Drugs, Nonsteroidal
  **(Systemic)**, 388
Anti-inhibitor Coagulant Complex [activated prothrombin complex concentrate; APCC; *Autoplex T; FEIBA VH*]
  **(Systemic)**, 435
Anti-inhibitor coagulant complex, 436
*Antilirium*—Forest (U.S. and Canada) brand of Physostigmine (Systemic), 2322; Physostigmine Salicylate (Systemic), 3158
*Antiminth*—Pfipharmecs (U.S.) brand of Pyrantel (Oral-Local), #
Antimyasthenics
  **(Systemic)**, 437
*Antinaus 50*—Clint (U.S.) brand of Promethazine—**See Antihistamines, Phenothiazine-derivative (Systemic)**, 377
*Antinea*—American Dermal (U.S.) brand of Salicylic Acid (Topical), #

Antipyrine and Benzocaine [*A/B Otic; Allergen; Analgesic Otic; Antiben; Auralgan; Aurodex; Auroto; Dolotic; Earache Drops; Ear Drops; Otocalm*]
  **(Otic)**, 443
  Solution, Otic, USP, 443
Antipyrine-containing Combinations, 3067
Anti-Rh immunoglobulin—*See* Rh₀(D) Immune Globulin (Systemic), 2476
Anti-Rh₀(D)—*See* Rh₀(D) Immune Globulin (Systemic), 2476
*Antispas*—Keene (U.S.) brand of Dicyclomine—**See Anticholinergics/Antispasmodics (Systemic)**, 226
Antithrombin III [*Kybernin*]
  **(Systemic)**, 3131
  Concentrate, for Injection, 3131
*Antithrombin III Human*—American National Red Cross (U.S.) brand of Antithrombin III Human (Systemic), 3132
Antithrombin III (Human) [ATIII; *ATnativ*; heparin cofactor I; *Thrombate III*]
  **(Systemic)**, 444, 3131
  for Injection, 445
Anti-thymocyte Serum [Nashville Rabbit Anti-thymocyte Serum]
  **(Systemic)**, 3131
Antithyroid Agents
  **(Systemic)**, 446
*Anti-Tuss*—Century (U.S.) brand of Guaifenesin (Systemic), 1588
*Anti-Tuss DM Expectorant*—Century (U.S.) brand of Dextromethorphan and Guaifenesin—**See Cough/Cold Combinations (Systemic)**, 1024
Antivenin (Chironex Fleckeri) [box jellyfish antivenom; sea wasp antivenom]
  **(Systemic)**, #
  for Injection, #
Antivenin (Crotalidae) Polyvalent [antivenin Crotalid serum; pit viper antivenin]
  **(Systemic)**, #
Antivenin (Crotalidae) Polyvalent USP, #
Antivenin Crotalid serum—*See* **Antivenin (Crotalidae) Polyvalent (Systemic)**, #
Antivenin (Enhydrina Schistosa) [sea snake antivenom]
  **(Systemic)**, #
  for Injection, #
Antivenin (Latrodectus Mactans) [black widow spider antivenin]
  **(Systemic)**, #
Antivenin (Latrodectus Mactans) USP, #
Antivenin (Micrurus Fulvius) [North American coral snake antivenin]
  **(Systemic)**, #
Antivenin (Micrurus Fulvius) USP, #
Antivenin (Notechis Scutatus) [tiger snake antivenom]
  **(Systemic)**, #
Antivenin (Notechis Scutatus) for Injection, #
Antivenin, Polyvalent Crotalid (Ovine) Fab [*Crotab*]
  **(Systemic)**, 3131
Antivenin (Pseudonaja Textilis) [brown snake antivenom]
  **(Systemic)**, #
  for Injection, #
Antivenom (Crotalidae) Purified (Avian)
  **(Systemic)**, 3132
*Antivert*—Roerig (U.S.) brand of Meclizine (Systemic), 1933, MC-18
*Antivert/25*—Roerig (U.S.) brand of Meclizine (Systemic), 1933, MC-18
*Antivert/50*—Roerig (U.S.) brand of Meclizine (Systemic), 1933, MC-18
*Antizol*—Orphan Medical (U.S.) brand of Fomepizole (Systemic), 1526
*Antril*—Synergen (U.S.) brand of Interleukin-1 Receptor Antagonist, Human Recombinant (Systemic), 3149
*Antrocol*—Poythress (U.S.) brand of Atropine and Phenobarbital—**See Belladonna Alkaloids and Barbiturates (Systemic)**, 551
*Antrypol*—*See* Suramin (Systemic), #
*Anturan*—Geigy (Canada) brand of Sulfinpyrazone (Systemic), 2646
*Anturane*—Ciba (U.S.) brand of Sulfinpyrazone (Systemic), 2646
*Anucort-HC*—G&W (U.S.) brand of Hydrocortisone—**See Corticosteroids (Rectal)**, 973; **Corticosteroids (Topical)**, 978
*Anu-Med HC*—Major (U.S.) brand of Hydrocortisone—**See Corticosteroids (Rectal)**, 973

## General Index

*Anuprep HC*—Great Southern (U.S.) brand of Hydrocortisone—**See Corticosteroids (Rectal)**, 973
*Anusol-HC*—PD (U.S.) brand of Hydrocortisone—**See Corticosteroids (Rectal)**, 973; **Corticosteroids (Topical)**, 978
*Anusol-HC 2.5%*—PD (U.S.) brand of Hydrocortisone (Topical), 3023
*Anutone-HC*—Elge (U.S.) brand of Hydrocortisone—**See Corticosteroids (Rectal)**, 973
*Anuzone-HC*—Superior (U.S.) brand of Hydrocortisone—**See Corticosteroids (Rectal)**, 973
*Anzemet*—Hoechst Marion Roussel (U.S.) brand of Dolasetron (Systemic), 1287
*Apacet Capsules*—Parmed (U.S.) brand of Acetaminophen (Systemic), 6
*Apacet Elixir*—Parmed (U.S.) brand of Acetaminophen (Systemic), 6
*Apacet Extra Strength Caplets*—Parmed (U.S.) brand of Acetaminophen (Systemic), 6
*Apacet Extra Strength Tablets*—Parmed (U.S.) brand of Acetaminophen (Systemic), 6
*Apacet, Infants'*—Parmed (U.S.) brand of Acetaminophen (Systemic), 6
*Apacet Regular Strength Tablets*—Parmed (U.S.) brand of Acetaminophen (Systemic), 6
APAP—*See* Acetaminophen (Systemic), 6
APAP with codeine—Acetaminophen and Codeine—**See Opioid (Narcotic) Analgesics and Acetaminophen (Systemic)**, 2198
APD—*See* Pamidronate (Systemic), 2220
*Aphrodyne*—Star (U.S.) brand of Yohimbine (Systemic), #
*Aphthasol*—Block (U.S.) brand of Amlexanox (Mucosal-Local), 85
APL 400-020 (Systemic), 3132
*A.P.L.*—Wyeth-Ayerst (U.S.) and Ayerst (Canada) brand of Chorionic Gonadotropin (Systemic), 858
*Aplisol*—PD (U.S.) brand of Tuberculin, Purified Protein Derivative (Parenteral-Local), 2895
*Aplitest*—PD (U.S.) brand of Tuberculin, Purified Protein Derivative (Parenteral-Local), 2895
Aplonidine—*See* Apraclonidine (Ophthalmic), 459
*Apo-Acetaminophen*—Apotex (Canada) brand of Acetaminophen (Systemic), 6
*Apo-Acetazolamide*—Apotex (Canada) brand of Acetazolamide—**See Carbonic Anhydrase Inhibitors (Systemic)**, 773
*Apo-Allopurinol*—Apotex (Canada) brand of Allopurinol (Systemic), 44
*Apo-Alpraz*—Apotex (Canada) brand of Alprazolam—**See Benzodiazepines (Systemic)**, 556
*Apo-Amitriptyline*—Apotex (Canada) brand of Amitriptyline—**See Antidepressants, Tricyclic (Systemic)**, 271
*Apo-Amoxi*—Apotex (Canada) brand of Amoxicillin—**See Penicillins (Systemic)**, 2240
*Apo-Ampi*—Apotex (Canada) brand of Ampicillin—**See Penicillins (Systemic)**, 2240
*Apo-Asa*—Apotex (Canada) brand of Aspirin—**See Salicylates (Systemic)**, 2538
*Apo-ASEN*—Apotex (Canada) brand of Aspirin—**See Salicylates (Systemic)**, 2538
*Apo-Atenolol*—Apotex (Canada) brand of Atenolol—**See Beta-adrenergic Blocking Agents (Systemic)**, 593
*Apo-Benztropine*—Apotex (Canada) brand of Benztropine—**See Antidyskinetics (Systemic)**, 297
*Apo-Bisacodyl*—Apotex (Canada) brand of Bisacodyl—**See Laxatives (Local)**, #
*Apo-Bromocriptine*—Apotex (Canada) brand of Bromocriptine (Systemic), 636
*Apo-C*—Apotex (Canada) brand of Ascorbic Acid (Systemic), 469
*Apo-Cal*—Apotex (Canada) brand of Calcium Carbonate—**See Calcium Supplements (Systemic)**, 736
*Apo-Carbamazepine*—Apotex (Canada) brand of Carbamazepine (Systemic), 757
*Apo-Cefaclor*—Apotex (Canada) brand of Cefaclor—**See Cephalosporins (Systemic)**, 794
*Apo-Cephalex*—Apotex (Canada) brand of Cephalexin—**See Cephalosporins (Systemic)**, 794
*Apo-Chlorax*—Apotex (Canada) brand of Chlordiazepoxide and Clidinium (Systemic), 846
*Apo-Chlordiazepoxide*—Apotex (Canada) brand of Chlordiazepoxide—**See Benzodiazepines (Systemic)**, 556
*Apo-Chlorpropamide*—Apotex (Canada) brand of Chlorpropamide—**See Antidiabetic Agents, Sulfonylurea (Systemic)**, 283

*Apo-Chlorthalidone*—Apotex (Canada) brand of Chlorthalidone—**See Diuretics, Thiazide (Systemic)**, 1273
*Apo-Cimetidine*—Apotex (Canada) brand of Cimetidine—**See Histamine H$_2$-receptor Antagonists (Systemic)**, 1633
*Apo-Clonazepam*—Apotex (Canada) brand of Clonazepam (Systemic), 556
*Apo-Clorazepate*—Apotex (Canada) brand of Clorazepate—**See Benzodiazepines (Systemic)**, 556
*Apo-Cloxi*—Apotex (Canada) brand of Cloxacillin—**See Penicillins (Systemic)**, 2240
*Apo-Diazepam*—Apotex (Canada) brand of Diazepam—**See Benzodiazepines (Systemic)**, 556
*Apo-Diclo*—Apotex (Canada) brand of Diclofenac—**See Anti-inflammatory Drugs, Nonsteroidal (Systemic)**, 388
*Apo-Diflunisal*—Apotex (Canada) brand of Diflunisal—**See Anti-inflammatory Drugs, Nonsteroidal (Systemic)**, 388
*Apo-Diltiaz*—Apotex (Canada) brand of Diltiazem—**See Calcium Channel Blocking Agents (Systemic)**, 720
*Apo-Dimenhydrinate*—Apotex (Canada) brand of Dimenhydrinate—**See Antihistamines (Systemic)**, 325
*Apo-Dipyridamole*—Apotex (Canada) brand of Dipyridamole (Systemic), #
*Apo-Doxy*—Apotex (Canada) brand of Doxycycline—**See Tetracyclines (Systemic)**, 2765
*Apo-Erythro*—Apotex (Canada) brand of Erythromycin Base—**See Erythromycins (Systemic)**, 1368
*Apo-Erythro E-C*—Apotex (Canada) brand of Erythromycin Base—**See Erythromycins (Systemic)**, 1368
*Apo-Erythro-ES*—Apotex (Canada) brand of Erythromycin Ethylsuccinate—**See Erythromycins (Systemic)**, 1368
*Apo-Erythro-S*—Apotex (Canada) brand of Erythromycin Stearate—**See Erythromycins (Systemic)**, 1368
*Apo-Famotidine*—Apotex (Canada) brand of Famotidine—**See Histamine H$_2$-receptor Antagonists (Systemic)**, 1633, MC-12
*Apo-Ferrous Gluconate*—Apotex (Canada) brand of Ferrous Gluconate—**See Iron Supplements (Systemic)**, 1774
*Apo-Ferrous Sulfate*—Apotex (Canada) brand of Ferrous Sulfate—**See Iron Supplements (Systemic)**, 1774
*Apo-Fluphenazine*—Apotex (Canada) brand of Fluphenazine—**See Phenothiazines (Systemic)**, 2289
*Apo-Flurazepam*—Apotex (Canada) brand of Flurazepam—**See Benzodiazepines (Systemic)**, 556
*Apo-Flurbiprofen*—Apotex (Canada) brand of Flurbiprofen—**See Anti-inflammatory Drugs, Nonsteroidal (Systemic)**, 388
*Apo-Folic*—Apotex (Canada) brand of Folic Acid (Systemic), 1517
*Apo-Furosemide*—Apotex (Canada) brand of Furosemide—**See Diuretics, Loop (Systemic)**, 1259
*Apo-Gain*—Apotex (Canada) brand of Minoxidil (Topical), 2021
*Apo-Gemfibrozil*—Apotex (Canada) brand of Gemfibrozil (Systemic), 1552
*Apo-Glyburide*—Apotex (Canada) brand of Glyburide—**See Antidiabetic Agents, Sulfonylurea (Systemic)**, 283
*Apo-Guanethidine*—Apotex (Canada) brand of Guanethidine (Systemic), 1595
*Apo-Haloperidol*—Apotex (Canada) brand of Haloperidol (Systemic), 1611
*Apo-Hydro*—Apotex (Canada) brand of Hydrochlorothiazide—**See Diuretics, Thiazide (Systemic)**, 1273
*Apo-Hydroxyzine*—Apotex (Canada) brand of Hydroxyzine—**See Antihistamines (Systemic)**, 325
*Apo-Ibuprofen*—Apotex (Canada) brand of Ibuprofen—**See Anti-inflammatory Drugs, Nonsteroidal (Systemic)**, 388
*Apo-Imipramine*—Apotex (Canada) brand of Imipramine—**See Antidepressants, Tricyclic (Systemic)**, 271
*Apo-Indomethacin*—Apotex (Canada) brand of Indomethacin—**See Anti-inflammatory Drugs, Nonsteroidal (Systemic)**, 388; Indomethacin—For Patent Ductus Arteriosus (Systemic), 1704
*Apo-Ipravent*—Apotex (Canada) brand of Ipratropium (Inhalation-Local), 1761

*Apo-ISDN*—Apotex (Canada) brand of Isosorbide Dinitrate—**See Nitrates (Systemic)**, 2129
*Apo-K*—Apotex (Canada) brand of Potassium Chloride—**See Potassium Supplements (Systemic)**, 2357
*Apo-Keto*—Apotex (Canada) brand of Ketoprofen—**See Anti-inflammatory Drugs, Nonsteroidal (Systemic)**, 388
*Apo-Keto-E*—Apotex (Canada) brand of Ketoprofen—**See Anti-inflammatory Drugs, Nonsteroidal (Systemic)**, 388
*Apo-Loperamide*—Apotex (Canada) brand of Loperamide (Oral-Local), 1877
*Apo-Lorazepam*—Apotex (Canada) brand of Lorazepam—**See Benzodiazepines (Systemic)**, 556
*Apo-Megestrol*—Apotex (Canada) brand of Megestrol—**See Progestins (Systemic)**, 2400
*Apo-Meprobamate*—Apotex (Canada) brand of Meprobamate (Systemic), #
*Apo-Methyldopa*—Apotex (Canada) brand of Methyldopa (Systemic), 1979
*Apo-Metoclop*—Apotex (Canada) brand of Metoclopramide (Systemic), 1992
*Apo-Metoprolol*—Apotex (Canada) brand of Metoprolol—**See Beta-adrenergic Blocking Agents (Systemic)**, 593
*Apo-Metoprolol (Type L)*—Apotex (Canada) brand of Metoprolol—**See Beta-adrenergic Blocking Agents (Systemic)**, 593
*Apo-Metronidazole*—Apotex (Canada) brand of Metronidazole (Systemic), 1996
Apomorphine (Systemic), 3132
Apomorphine Hydrochloride (Systemic), #, 3132
Injection, #
*Apo-Napro-Na*—Apotex (Canada) brand of Naproxen—**See Anti-inflammatory Drugs, Nonsteroidal (Systemic)**, 388
*Apo-Napro-Na DS*—Apotex (Canada) brand of Naproxen—**See Anti-inflammatory Drugs, Nonsteroidal (Systemic)**, 388
*Apo-Naproxen*—Apotex (Canada) brand of Naproxen—**See Anti-inflammatory Drugs, Nonsteroidal (Systemic)**, 388
*Apo-Nifed*—Apotex (Canada) brand of Nifedipine—**See Calcium Channel Blocking Agents (Systemic)**, 720
*Apo-Nitrofurantoin*—Apotex (Canada) brand of Nitrofurantoin (Systemic), 2139
*Apo-Nizatidine*—Apotex (Canada) brand of Nizatidine—**See Histamine H$_2$-receptor Antagonists (Systemic)**, 1633, MC-22
*Apo-Oxazepam*—Apotex (Canada) brand of Oxazepam—**See Benzodiazepines (Systemic)**, 556
*Apo-Oxtriphylline*—Apotex (Canada) brand of Oxtriphylline—**See Bronchodilators, Theophylline (Systemic)**, 668
*Apo-Pen-VK*—Apotex (Canada) brand of Penicillin V—**See Penicillins (Systemic)**, 2240
*Apo-Perphenazine*—Apotex (Canada) brand of Perphenazine—**See Phenothiazines (Systemic)**, 2289
*Apo-Phenylbutazone*—Apotex (Canada) brand of Phenylbutazone—**See Anti-inflammatory Drugs, Nonsteroidal (Systemic)**, 388
*Apo-Piroxicam*—Apotex (Canada) brand of Piroxicam—**See Anti-inflammatory Drugs, Nonsteroidal (Systemic)**, 388
*Apo-Prednisone*—Apotex (Canada) brand of Prednisone—**See Corticosteroids—Glucocorticoid Effects (Systemic)**, 998
*Apo-Primidone*—Apotex (Canada) brand of Primidone (Systemic), 2376
*Apo-Propranolol*—Apotex (Canada) brand of Propranolol—**See Beta-adrenergic Blocking Agents (Systemic)**, 593
*Apo-Quinidine*—Apotex (Canada) brand of Quinidine (Systemic), 2440
*Apo-Ranitidine*—Apotex (Canada) brand of Ranitidine Hydrochloride—**See Histamine H$_2$-receptor Antagonists (Systemic)**, 1633
*Apo-Salvent*—Apotex (Canada) brand of Albuterol—**See Bronchodilators, Adrenergic (Inhalation-Local)**, 640
*Apo-Selegiline*—Apotex (Canada) brand of Selegiline (Systemic), 2560
*Apo-sulcralfate*—Apotex (Canada) brand of Sucralfate (Oral-Local), 2635
*Apo-Sulfamethoxazole*—Apotex (Canada) brand of Sulfamethoxazole—**See Sulfonamides (Systemic)**, 2653

# General Index

*Apo-Sulfatrim*—Apotex (Canada) brand of Sulfamethoxazole and Trimethoprim—**See Sulfonamides and Trimethoprim (Systemic)**, 2661

*Apo-Sulfatrim DS*—Apotex (Canada) brand of Sulfamethoxazole and Trimethoprim—**See Sulfonamides and Trimethoprim (Systemic)**, 2661

*Apo-Sulfinpyrazone*—Apotex (Canada) brand of Sulfinpyrazone (Systemic), 2646

*Apo-Sulfisoxazole*—Apotex (Canada) brand of Sulfisoxazole—**See Sulfonamides (Systemic)**, 2653

*Apo-Sulin*—Apotex (Canada) brand of Sulindac—**See Anti-inflammatory Drugs, Nonsteroidal (Systemic)**, 388

*Apo-Tamox*—Apotex (Canada) brand of Tamoxifen (Systemic), 2688

*Apo-Terfenadine*—Apotex (Canada) brand of Terfenadine—**See Antihistamines (Systemic)**, 325

*Apo-Tetra*—Apotex (Canada) brand of Tetracycline—**See Tetracyclines (Systemic)**, 2765

*Apo-Theo LA*—Apotex (Canada) brand of Theophylline—**See Bronchodilators, Theophylline (Systemic)**, 668

*Apo-Thioridazine*—Apotex (Canada) brand of Thioridazine—**See Phenothiazines (Systemic)**, 2289

*Apo-Timol*—Apotex (Canada) brand of Timolol—**See Beta-adrenergic Blocking Agents (Systemic)**, 593

*Apo-Timop*—Apotex (Canada) brand of Timolol—**See Beta-adrenergic Blocking Agents (Ophthalmic)**, 585

*Apo-Tolbutamide*—Apotex (Canada) brand of Tolbutamide—**See Antidiabetic Agents, Sulfonylurea (Systemic)**, 283

*Apo-Triazide*—Apotex (Canada) brand of Triamterene and Hydrochlorothiazide—**See Diuretics, Potassium-sparing, and Hydrochlorothiazide (Systemic)**, 1272

*Apo-Triazo*—Apotex (Canada) brand of Triazolam—**See Benzodiazepines (Systemic)**, 556

*Apo-Trifluoperazine*—Apotex (Canada) brand of Trifluoperazine—**See Phenothiazines (Systemic)**, 2289

*Apo-Trihex*—Apotex (Canada) brand of Trihexyphenidyl—**See Antidyskinetics (Systemic)**, 297

*Apo-Trimip*—Apotex (Canada) brand of Trimipramine—**See Antidepressants, Tricyclic (Systemic)**, 271

*Apo-Verap*—Apotex (Canada) brand of Verapamil—**See Calcium Channel Blocking Agents (Systemic)**, 720

*Apo-Zidovudine*—Apotex (Canada) brand of Zidovudine (Systemic), 2992

*Appecon*—Lunsco (U.S.) brand of Phendimetrazine—**See Appetite Suppressants (Systemic)**, 452

Appetite Suppressants **(Systemic)**, 452

Apraclonidine Hydrochloride [aplonidine; *Iopidine*; p-aminoclonidine]
**(Ophthalmic)**, 459
Solution, Ophthalmic, 461

*Apresazide*—Novartis (U.S.) brand of Hydralazine and Hydrochlorothiazide (Systemic), 1658, MC-14

*Apresoline*—Novartis (U.S. and Canada) brand of Hydralazine (Systemic), 1655, MC-14

Aprobarbital [*Alurate*]
**See Barbiturates (Systemic)**, 518
Elixir, 525

*Aprodrine*—Major (U.S.) brand of Triprolidine and Pseudoephedrine—**See Antihistamines and Decongestants (Systemic)**, 343

*Aprodine with Codeine*—Major (U.S.) brand of Triprolidine, Pseudoephedrine, and Codeine—**See Cough/Cold Combinations (Systemic)**, 1024

Aprotinin [*Trasylol*]
**(Systemic)**, 461, 3132
Injection, 463

APSAC—Anistreplase—**See Thrombolytic Agents (Systemic)**, 2799

*Aquachloral Supprettes*—Webcon (U.S.) brand of Chloral Hydrate (Systemic), 834

*Aquaderm Sunscreen Moisturizer*—Baker Cummins (U.S.) brand of Octyl Methoxycinnamate and Oxybenzone—**See Sunscreen Agents (Topical)**, #

*AquaMEPHYTON*—Merck (U.S.) brand of Phytonadione—**See Vitamin K (Systemic)**, 2975

*Aquaray Sunscreen*—Herald Pharmacal (U.S.) brand of Octyl Methoxycinnamate, Octyl Salicylate, and Oxybenzone—**See Sunscreen Agents (Topical)**, #

*Aquasol A*—Armour (U.S.) and Rorer (Canada) brand of Vitamin A (Systemic), 2958

*Aquasol E*—Armour (U.S.) and Rorer (Canada) brand of Vitamin E (Systemic), 2972

*Aquatar*—Allergan Herbert (U.S.) brand of Coal Tar (Topical), #

*Aquatensen*—Wallace (U.S.) brand of Methyclothiazide—**See Diuretics, Thiazide (Systemic)**, 1273

*Aqueous Charcodote*—Pharmascience (Canada) brand of Charcoal, Activated (Oral-Local), 831

*Aquest*—Dunhall (U.S.) brand of Estrone—**See Estrogens (Systemic)**, 1383

Ara-A—*See* Vidarabine (Ophthalmic), 2944

Arabinoside—*See* Vidarabine (Ophthalmic), 2944

Ara-C—*See* Cytarabine (Systemic), 1143

*Aralen*—Sanofi Winthrop (U.S. and Canada) brand of Chloroquine (Systemic), 849

*Aralen HCl*—Sanofi Winthrop (U.S.) brand of Chloroquine (Systemic), 849

*Aramine*—Merck (U.S.) brand of Metaraminol—**See Sympathomimetic Agents—Cardiovascular Use (Parenteral-Systemic)**, 2669

Arbutamine Hydrochloride [*GenESA*]
**(Systemic)**, 464
Injection, 466

*Arcet*—Econo Med (U.S.) brand of Butalbital and Acetaminophen—**See Barbiturates and Analgesics (Systemic)**, 532

Arcitumomab
**(Systemic)**, 3132

*Arco Pain Tablet*—Aspirin—**See Salicylates (Systemic)**, 2538

Ardeparin Sodium [*Normiflo*]
**(Systemic)**, 467
Injection, 469

*Arduan*—Organon (U.S.) brand of Pipecuronium (Systemic), 2330

*Aredia*—Ciba (U.S. and Canada) brand of Pamidronate (Systemic), 2220

*Arfonad*—Roche (U.S. and Canada) brand of Trimethaphan (Systemic), 2879

Arginine Butyrate
**(Systemic)**, 3132

*Aricept*—Eisai (U.S.) brand of Donepezil (Systemic), 1290, MC-10

*Arimidex*—ZENECA (U.S.) brand of Anastrozole (Systemic), 116, MC-3

*Aristocort*—Lederle (U.S. and Canada) brand of Triamcinolone—**See Corticosteroids—Glucocorticoid Effects (Systemic)**, 998; **Corticosteroids (Topical)**, 978

*Aristocort A*—Lederle (U.S.) brand of Triamcinolone—**See Corticosteroids (Topical)**, 978

*Aristocort C*—Lederle (Canada) brand of Triamcinolone—**See Corticosteroids (Topical)**, 978

*Aristocort D*—Lederle (Canada) brand of Triamcinolone—**See Corticosteroids (Topical)**, 978

*Aristocort Forte*—Lederle (U.S. and Canada) brand of Triamcinolone—**See Corticosteroids—Glucocorticoid Effects (Systemic)**, 998

*Aristocort Intralesional*—Lederle (U.S. and Canada) brand of Triamcinolone—**See Corticosteroids—Glucocorticoid Effects (Systemic)**, 998

*Aristocort R*—Lederle (Canada) brand of Triamcinolone—**See Corticosteroids (Topical)**, 978

*Aristospan Intra-articular*—Lederle (U.S. and Canada) brand of Triamcinolone—**See Corticosteroids—Glucocorticoid Effects (Systemic)**, 998

*Aristospan Intralesional*—Lederle (U.S.) brand of Triamcinolone—**See Corticosteroids—Glucocorticoid Effects (Systemic)**, 998

*Arlidin*—Rorer (Canada) brand of Nylidrin (Systemic), #

*Arlidin Forte*—Rorer (Canada) brand of Nylidrin (Systemic), #

*Arm-a-Med Isoetharine*—Armour (U.S.) brand of Isoetharine—**See Bronchodilators, Adrenergic (Inhalation-Local)**, 640

*Arm-a-Med Metaproterenol*—Armour (U.S.) brand of Metaproterenol—**See Bronchodilators, Adrenergic (Inhalation-Local)**, 640

*Arm and Hammer Pure Baking Soda*—Church & Dwight (U.S.) brand of Sodium Bicarbonate (Systemic), 2586

*A.R.M. Maximum Strength Caplets*—Menley & James (U.S.) brand of Chlorpheniramine and Phenylpropanolamine—**See Antihistamines and Decongestants (Systemic)**, 343

*Armour Thyroid*—Forest (U.S.) brand of Thyroid—**See Thyroid Hormones (Systemic)**, 2809

*Arrestin*—Vortech (U.S.) brand of Trimethobenzamide (Systemic), 2880

Arsenic Trioxide
**(Systemic)**, 3132

*Arsobal*—Specia (France) brand of Melarsoprol (Systemic), #

*Artane*—Lederle (U.S. and Canada) brand of Trihexyphenidyl—**See Antidyskinetics (Systemic)**, 297

*Artane Sequels*—Lederle (U.S. and Canada) brand of Trihexyphenidyl—**See Antidyskinetics (Systemic)**, 297

*Arthrisin*—Ancalab (Canada) brand of Aspirin—**See Salicylates (Systemic)**, 2538

*Arthritis Pain Ascriptin*—Rhône-Poulenc Rorer (U.S.) brand of Aspirin, Buffered—**See Salicylates (Systemic)**, 2538

*Arthritis Pain Formula*—Whitehall (U.S.) brand of Aspirin, Buffered—**See Salicylates (Systemic)**, 2538

*Arthritis Strength Bufferin*—Bristol-Myers (U.S.) brand of Aspirin, Buffered—**See Salicylates (Systemic)**, 2538

*Arthropan*—Purdue Frederick (U.S.) brand of Choline Salicylate—**See Salicylates (Systemic)**, 2538

*Arthrotec*—Searle (U.S.) brand of Diclofenac and Misoprostol (Systemic), 1202, MC-9

Articaine-containing Combinations, 3067

Articaine Hydrochloride with Epinephrine [*Astracaine 4%*; *Astracaine 4% Forte*; *Ultracaine D-S*; *Ultracaine D-S Forte*]
**See Anesthetics (Parenteral-Local)**, 139
Injection, 145

*Articulose-50*—Seatrace (U.S.) brand of Prednisolone—**See Corticosteroids—Glucocorticoid Effects (Systemic)**, 998

*Articulose-L.A.*—Seatrace (U.S.) brand of Triamcinolone—**See Corticosteroids—Glucocorticoid Effects (Systemic)**, 998

*Artificial Tears*—Bausch & Lomb (U.S.) brand of Hydroxypropyl Methylcellulose (Ophthalmic), #

*Artria S.R.*—Sandoz (Canada) brand of Aspirin—**See Salicylates (Systemic)**, 2538

*Arvin*—Knoll (U.S.) brand of Ancrod (Systemic), 3131

ASA—Aspirin—**See Salicylates (Systemic)**, 2538

5-ASA—*See* Mesalamine (Oral-Local), 1952; Mesalamine (Rectal-Local), 1954

*Asacol*—Procter & Gamble (U.S. and Canada) brand of Mesalamine (Oral-Local), 1952, MC-18

*Asasantine*—Boehringer Ingelheim (Canada) brand of Dipyridamole and Aspirin (Systemic), 3018

*Ascabiol*—Rhône-Poulenc Rorer (U.K.) brand of Benzyl Benzoate (Topical), #

*Ascomp with Codeine No.3*—Econolab (U.S.) and Genetco (U.S.) brand of Butalbital, Aspirin, Caffeine, and Codeine—**See Barbiturates and Analgesics (Systemic)**, 532

Ascorbic Acid [*Apo-C*; *Ascorbicap*; *Cebid Timecelles*; *Cecon*; *Cecore 500*; *Cee-500*; *Cemill*; *Cetane*; *Cevi-Bid*; *Flavorcee*; *Mega-C/A Plus*; *Sunkist*; vitamin C]
**(Systemic)**, 469
Capsules, Extended-release, 472
Injection USP, 473
Solution, Oral, USP, 472
Syrup, 472
Tablets USP, 472
Tablets USP (Chewable), 473
Tablets USP (Effervescent), 473
Tablets, Extended-release, 473

Ascorbic Acid–containing Combinations, 3067

*Ascorbicap*—ICN (U.S.) brand of Ascorbic Acid (Systemic), 469

*Asendin*—Wyeth-Ayerst (U.S. and Canada) brand of Amoxapine—**See Antidepressants, Tricyclic (Systemic)**, 271, MC-2

*A-200 Shampoo Concentrate*—SmithKline Beecham (U.S.) brand of Pyrethrins and Piperonyl Butoxide (Topical), #

*Asmalix*—Century (U.S.) brand of Theophylline—**See Bronchodilators, Theophylline (Systemic)**, 668

Asparaginase [colaspase; *Elspar*; *Kidrolase*]
**(Systemic)**, 474
for Injection, 477

*A-Spas*—Hyrex-Dow (U.S.) brand of Dicyclomine—**See Anticholinergics/Antispasmodics (Systemic)**, 226

*Aspergum*—Plough (U.S.) and Scholl-Plough (Canada) brand of Aspirin—**See Salicylates (Systemic)**, 2538

Aspirin [acetylsalicylic acid; *Acuprin 81; Apo-Asa; Apo-ASEN; Arthrisin; Artria S.R.; ASA; Aspergum; Aspirin Caplets* (Canada)*; Aspirin Children's Tablets* (Canada)*; Aspirin, Coated; Aspirin Regimen Bayer Adult Low Dose; Aspirin Regimen Bayer Regular Strength Caplets; Aspirin Tablets* (Canada)*; Aspir-Low; Aspirtab; Aspirtab-Max; Astrin; Bayer Children's Aspirin; Coryphen; Easprin; Ecotrin Caplets; Ecotrin Tablets; Empirin; Entrophen Caplets; Entrophen Extra Strength; Entrophen 15 Maximum Strength Tablets; Entrophen 10 Super Strength Caplets; Entrophen Tablets; Extended-release Bayer 8-Hour; Extra Strength Bayer Arthritis Pain Formula Caplets; Extra Strength Bayer Aspirin Caplets; Extra Strength Bayer Aspirin Tablets; Genuine Bayer Aspirin Caplets; Genuine Bayer Aspirin Tablets; Halfprin; Headache Tablet; Healthprin Adult Low Strength; Healthprin Full Strength; Healthprin Half-Dose; Maximum Strength Arthritis Foundation Safety Coated Aspirin; Norwich Aspirin; Novasen; Novasen Sp.C; PMS-ASA; Sloprin; St. Joseph Adult Chewable Aspirin; ZORprin*]
  **See Salicylates (Systemic)**, 2538
  Suppositories USP, 2549
  Tablets USP, 2547
  Tablets USP (Chewable), 2547
  Tablets, Chewing Gum, 2548
  Tablets, Delayed-release, USP, 2548
  Tablets, Extended-release, USP, 2548
Aspirin, Alumina, and Magnesia—Aspirin, Buffered—
  **See Salicylates (Systemic)**, 2538
Aspirin, Buffered [*Arthritis Pain Ascriptin; Arthritis Pain Formula; Arthritis Strength Bufferin; Aspirin Plus Stomach Guard Regular Strength; Aspirin Plus Stomach Guard Extra Strength; Bufferin Caplets; Bufferin Extra Strength Caplets; Bufferin Tablets; Buffex; Buffinol; Buffinol Extra; Cama Arthritis Pain Reliever; Extra Strength Bayer Plus Caplets; Magnaprin; Maximum Strength Ascriptin; Regular Strength Ascriptin; Tri-Buffered ASA*]
  **See Salicylates (Systemic)**, 2538
  Aspirin, Alumina, and Magnesia Tablets USP, 2550
  Aspirin, Alumina, and Magnesium Oxide Tablets USP, 2550
  Tablets USP, 2550
Aspirin, Buffered, and Caffeine [*C2 Buffered; Cope*]
  **See Salicylates (Systemic)**, 2538
  Tablets, 2551
Aspirin and Caffeine [*Anacin; Anacin Caplets; Anacin Extra Strength; Anacin Maximum Strength; Anacin Tablets; Antidol; Arco Pain Tablet; Astone; C2; Calmine; Dolomine; Gensan; Herbopyrine; Instantine; Kalmex; Nervine; P-A-C Revised Formula; Pain Aid; 217 Strong; 217*]
  **See Salicylates (Systemic)**, 2538
  Capsules, 2548
  Tablets, 2548
Aspirin, Caffeine, and Dihydrocodeine Bitartrate[dihydrocodeine compound; drocode and aspirin; *Synalgos-DC*]
  **See Opioid (Narcotic) Analgesics and Aspirin (Systemic)**, 2202
  Capsules USP, 2203, MC-3
*Aspirin Caplets*—Sterling Heath (Canada) brand of Aspirin—**See Salicylates (Systemic)**, 2538
*Aspirin Children's Tablets*—Sterling Heath (Canada) brand of Aspirin—**See Salicylates (Systemic)**, 2538
*Aspirin, Coated*—Sterling Heath (Canada) brand of Aspirin—**See Salicylates (Systemic)**, 2538
Aspirin and Codeine Phosphate [co-codaprin; *Empirin with Codeine No.3; Empirin with Codeine No.4*]
  **See Opioid (Narcotic) Analgesics and Aspirin (Systemic)**, 2202
  Tablets USP, 2203
Aspirin, Codeine Phosphate, and Caffeine [*A.C.&C.; AC and C; Anacin with Codeine; C2 with Codeine; Novo-AC and C; 222; 282; 292*]
  **See Opioid (Narcotic) Analgesics and Aspirin (Systemic)**, 2202
  Tablets USP, 2203
Aspirin, Codeine Phosphate, Caffeine, Alumina, and Magnesia [*C2 Buffered with Codeine*]
  **See Opioid (Narcotic) Analgesics and Aspirin (Systemic)**, 2202
  Tablets, 2203
Aspirin-containing Combinations, 3067

*Aspirin Free Anacin Maximum Strength Caplets*—Robins (U.S.) brand of Acetaminophen (Systemic), 6
*Aspirin Free Anacin Maximum Strength Gel Caplets*—Robins (U.S.) brand of Acetaminophen (Systemic), 6
*Aspirin Free Anacin Maximum Strength Tablets*—Robins (U.S.) brand of Acetaminophen (Systemic), 6
*Aspirin-Free Bayer Select Sinus Pain Relief Caplets*—Bayer (U.S.) brand of Pseudoephedrine and Acetaminophen—**See Decongestants and Analgesics (Systemic)**, 1180
*Aspirin-Free Excedrin Caplets*—Bristol-Myers (U.S.) brand of Acetaminophen and Caffeine—**See Acetaminophen (Systemic)**, 6
*Aspirin Plus Stomach Guard Extra Strength*—Aspirin, Buffered—**See Salicylates (Systemic)**, 2538
*Aspirin Plus Stomach Guard Regular Strength*—Aspirin, Buffered—**See Salicylates (Systemic)**, 2538
*Aspirin Regimen Bayer Adult Low Dose*—Miles (U.S.) brand of Aspirin—**See Salicylates (Systemic)**, 2538
*Aspirin Regimen Bayer Regular Strength Caplets*—Miles (U.S.) brand of Aspirin—**See Salicylates (Systemic)**, 2538
Aspirin, Sodium Bicarbonate, and Citric Acid [*Alka-Seltzer Effervescent Pain Reliever and Antacid; Flavored Alka-Seltzer Effervescent Pain Reliever and Antacid*]
  **(Systemic)**, 477
  Tablets for Solution, Oral, Effervescent, USP, 479
*Aspirin Tablets*—Sterling Heath (Canada) brand of Aspirin—**See Salicylates (Systemic)**, 2538
*Aspir-Low*—Aspirin—**See Salicylates (Systemic)**, 2538
*Aspirtab*—Aspirin—**See Salicylates (Systemic)**, 2538
*Aspirtab-Max*—Aspirin—**See Salicylates (Systemic)**, 2538
*Astelin*—Wallace (U.S.) brand of Azelastine (Systemic), 497
Astemizole [*Hismanal*]
  **See Antihistamines (Systemic)**, 325
  Suspension, Oral, 331
  Tablets, 331, MC-3
*Asthmahaler Mist*—Norcliff Thayer (U.S.) brand of Epinephrine—**See Bronchodilators, Adrenergic (Inhalation-Local)**, 640
*AsthmaNefrin*—Norcliff Thayer (U.S.) brand of Epinephrine—**See Bronchodilators, Adrenergic (Inhalation-Local)**, 640
*Astone*—Aspirin—**See Salicylates (Systemic)**, 2538
*Astracaine 4%*—Astra (Canada) brand of Astracaine with Epinephrine—**See Anesthetics (Parenteral-Local)**, 139
*Astracaine 4% Forte*—Astra (Canada) brand of Astracaine with Epinephrine—**See Anesthetics (Parenteral-Local)**, 139
*Astramorph PF*—Astra (U.S.) brand of Morphine—**See Opioid (Narcotic) Analgesics (Systemic)**, 2168
*Astrin*—Medic (Canada) brand of Aspirin—**See Salicylates (Systemic)**, 2538
*Atabrine*—Sanofi Winthrop (U.S. and Canada) brand of Quinacrine (Systemic), #
*Atacand*—Astra Merck (U.S.) brand of Candesartan (Systemic), MC-5
*Atarax*—Roerig (U.S.) and Pfizer (Canada) brand of Hydroxyzine—**See Antihistamines (Systemic)**, 325
*Atasol-8*—Horner (Canada) brand of Acetaminophen and Codeine—**See Opioid (Narcotic) Analgesics and Acetaminophen (Systemic)**, 2198
*Atasol-15*—Horner (Canada) brand of Acetaminophen and Codeine—**See Opioid (Narcotic) Analgesics and Acetaminophen (Systemic)**, 2198
*Atasol-30*—Horner (Canada) brand of Acetaminophen and Codeine—**See Opioid (Narcotic) Analgesics and Acetaminophen (Systemic)**, 2198
*Atasol Caplets*—Horner (Canada) brand of Acetaminophen (Systemic), 6
*Atasol Drops*—Horner (Canada) brand of Acetaminophen (Systemic), 6
*Atasol Forte Caplets*—Horner (Canada) brand of Acetaminophen (Systemic), 6
*Atasol Forte Tablets*—Horner (Canada) brand of Acetaminophen (Systemic), 6

*Atasol Oral Solution*—Horner (Canada) brand of Acetaminophen (Systemic), 6
*Atasol Tablets*—Horner (Canada) brand of Acetaminophen (Systemic), 6
Atenolol [*Apo-Atenolol; Novo-Atenol; Tenormin*]
  **See Beta-adrenergic Blocking Agents (Systemic)**, 593
  Injection, 601
  Tablets, 601, MC-3
Atenolol and Chlorthalidone [*Tenoretic*]
  **See Beta-adrenergic Blocking Agents and Thiazide Diuretics (Systemic)**, 609
  Tablets, 610, MC-3
Atenolol-containing Combinations, 3067
ATIII—See Antithrombin III (Systemic), 444
*Ativan*—Wyeth-Ayerst (U.S.) and Wyeth (Canada) brand of Lorazepam—**See Benzodiazepines (Systemic)**, 556, MC-18
*ATnativ*—KabiVitrum (U.S.) brand of Antithrombin III (Systemic), 444; Antithrombin III Human (Systemic), 3131
Atorvastatin [*Lipitor*]
  **(Systemic)**, 479
  Tablets
Atorvastatin Calcium [*Lipitor*]
  **(Systemic)**, MC-3
  Tablets, 482, MC-3
Atovaquone [*Mepron*]
  **(Systemic)**, 483, 3132
  Suspension, Oral, 485
  Tablets, 485
Atracurium besilate—Atracurium Besylate—**See Neuromuscular Blocking Agents (Systemic)**, 2098
Atracurium Besylate [atracurium besilate; *Tracrium*]
  **See Neuromuscular Blocking Agents (Systemic)**, 2098
  Injection, 2101
*Atretol*—Athena (U.S.) brand of Carbamazepine (Systemic), 757
*Atrofed*—Genetco (U.S.) brand of Triprolidine and Pseudoephedrine—**See Antihistamines and Decongestants (Systemic)**, 343
*Atrohist Pediatric*—Adams (U.S.) brand of Chlorpheniramine and Pseudoephedrine—**See Antihistamines and Decongestants (Systemic)**, 343
*Atrohist Pediatric Suspension Dye Free*—Adams (U.S.) brand of Chlorpheniramine, Pyrilamine, and Phenylephrine—**See Antihistamines and Decongestants (Systemic)**, 343
*Atrohist Plus*—Adams (U.S.) brand of Chlorpheniramine, Phenylephrine, Phenylpropanolamine, Atropine, Hyoscyamine, and Scopolamine—**See Antihistamines, Decongestants, and Anticholinergics (Systemic)**, 373
*Atromid-S*—Wyeth-Ayerst (U.S.) and Ayerst (Canada) brand of Clofibrate (Systemic), 900
*Atropair*—Pharmafair (U.S.) brand of Atropine (Ophthalmic), 485
*Atropine-Care*—Akorn (U.S.) brand of Atropine (Ophthalmic), 485
Atropine-containing Combinations, 3067, 3068
Atropine Sulfate [*Atropair; Atropine-Care; Atropine Sulfate S.O.P.; Atropisol; Atrosulf; Isopto Atropine; I-Tropine; Minims Atropine; Ocu-Tropine*]
  **(Ophthalmic)**, 485
  Ointment, Ophthalmic, USP, 487
  Solution, Ophthalmic, USP, 487
Atropine Sulfate
  **See Anticholinergics/Antispasmodics (Systemic)**, 226
  Injection USP, 233
  Tablets USP, 233
  Tablets, Soluble, 233
Atropine Sulfate, Hyoscyamine, Methenamine, Methylene Blue, Phenyl Salicylate, and Benzoic Acid [*Atrosept; Dolsed; Hexalol; Prosed/DS; Trac Tabs 2X; UAA; Uridon Modified; Urimed; Urinary Antiseptic No. 2; Urised; Uriseptic; Uritab; Uritin; Uro-Ves*]
  **(Systemic)**, 488
  Tablets, 491
Atropine Sulfate, Hyoscyamine Sulfate (or Hyoscyamine Hydrobromide), Scopolamine Hydrobromide, and Phenobarbital [*Barbidonna; Barbidonna No. 2; Barophen; Bellalphen; Donnamor; Donnapine; Donnatal; Donnatal Extentabs; Donnatal No. 2; Donphen; Hyosophen; Kinesed; Malatal; Relaxadon; Spaslin; Spasmolin; Spasmophen; Spasquid; Susano*]
  **See Belladonna Alkaloids and Barbiturates (Systemic)**, 551

Atropine Sulfate, Hyoscyamine Sulfate (or Hyoscyamine Hydrobromide), Scopolamine Hydrobromide, and Phenobarbital *(continued)*
  Capsules, 552, MC-3
  Elixir, 552
  Tablets, 552, MC-3
  Tablets, Chewable, 553
  Tablets, Extended-release, 553, MC-3
Atropine Sulfate and Phenobarbital [*Antrocol*]
  **See Belladonna Alkaloids and Barbiturates (Systemic),** 551
  Capsules, 553
  Elixir, 553
  Tablets, 553
*Atropine Sulfate S.O.P.*—Allergan (U.S.) brand of Atropine (Ophthalmic), 485
*Atropisol*—Iolab (U.S. and Canada) brand of Atropine (Ophthalmic), 485
*Atrosept*—Geneva Generics (U.S.) brand of Atropine, Hyoscyamine, Methenamine, Methylene Blue, Phenyl Salicylate, and Benzoic Acid (Systemic), 488
*Atrosulf*—Optopics (U.S.) brand of Atropine (Ophthalmic), 485
*Atrovent*—Boehringer Ingelheim (Canada) brand of Ipratropium (Nasal), 1764; Ipratropium (Inhalation-Local), 1761, 3026
*A/T/S*—Hoechst-Roussel (U.S.) brand of Erythromycin (Topical), 1365
*Attain*—Sherwood (U.S.) brand of Enteral Nutrition Formula, Polymeric—**See Enteral Nutrition Formulas (Systemic),** #
Attapulgite [*Diar-Aid; Diarrest; Diasorb; Diatrol; Donnagel; Fowler's; Kaopectate; Kaopectate Advanced Formula; Kaopectate Maximum Strength; Kaopek; K-Pek; Parepectolin; Rheaban*]
  **(Oral-Local),** #
  Suspension, Oral, #
  Tablets, #
  Tablets, Chewable, #
*Attenuvax*—Merck (U.S.) brand of Measles Virus Vaccine Live (Systemic), 1922
*Atuss DM*—Atley (U.S.) brand of Chlorpheniramine, Phenylephrine, and Dextromethorphan—**See Cough/Cold Combinations (Systemic),** 1024
*Atuss EX*—Atley (U.S.) brand of Hydrocodone and Guaifenesin—**See Cough/Cold Combinations (Systemic),** 1024
*Atuss HD*—Atley (U.S.) brand of Chlorpheniramine, Phenylephrine, and Hydrocodone—**See Cough/Cold Combinations (Systemic),** 1024
15AU81
  **(Systemic),** 3127
*Augmentin*—SmithKline Beecham (U.S.) brand of Amoxicillin and Clavulanate—**See Penicillins and Beta-lactamase Inhibitors (Systemic),** 2263, MC-2; Amoxicillin and Clavulanate (Systemic), 3010
*Auralgan*—Wyeth-Ayerst (U.S.) and Ayerst (Canada) brand of Antipyrine and Benzocaine (Otic), 443
Auranofin [*Ridaura*]
  **See Gold Compounds (Systemic),** 1566
  Capsules, 1568
*Aureomycin*—Lederle (U.S. and Canada) brand of Chlortetracycline—**See Tetracyclines (Ophthalmic),** 2763; **Tetracyclines (Topical),** 2774
*Auriculin*—Scios Nova (U.S.) brand of Anaritide (Systemic), 3131
*Aurodex*—Major (U.S.) brand of Antipyrine and Benzocaine (Otic), 443
Aurothioglucose [*Solganal*]
  **See Gold Compounds (Systemic),** 1566
  Suspension, Sterile, USP, 1569
*Auroto*—Barre-National (U.S.) brand of Antipyrine and Benzocaine (Otic), 443
Autolymphocyte Therapy
  **(Systemic),** 3132
*Autoplex T*—Baxter (U.S.) brand of Anti-inhibitor Coagulant Complex (Systemic), 435
*Avanti*—London International (U.S.) brand of Condom, Male, Polyurethane, 3016
*Avanti Super Thin*—London International (U.S.) brand of Condom, Male, Polyurethane, 3016
*Avapro*—Sanofi (U.S.) brand of Irbesartan (Systemic), 1767
*AVC*—Hoescht Marion Roussel (U.S. and Canada) brand of Sulfanilamide—**See Sulfonamides (Vaginal),** 2658
*Aventyl*—Lilly (U.S. and Canada) brand of Nortriptyline—**See Antidepressants, Tricyclic (Systemic),** 271

*Avirax*—Glaxo Wellcome (Canada) brand of Acyclovir (Systemic), 24
*Avita*—Penederm (U.S.) brand of Tretinoin (Topical), 2871
*Avlosulfon*—Ayerst (Canada) brand of Dapsone (Systemic), 1170
Avobenzone-containing Combinations, 3068
Avobenzone, Octocrylene, Octyl Salicylate, and Oxybenzone [*Photoplex Plus Sunscreen*]
  **See Sunscreen Agents (Topical),** #
  Lotion, #
Avobenzone and Octyl Methoxycinnamate [*Vaseline Broad Spectrum Sunblock*]
  **See Sunscreen Agents (Topical),** #
  Lotion, #
Avobenzone, Octyl Methoxycinnamate, Octyl Salicylate, and Oxybenzone [*Presun Clear; Presun Sunscreen; Presun Sunscreen for Kids*]
  **See Sunscreen Agents (Topical),** #
  Cream, #
  Gel, #
Avobenzone, Octyl Methoxycinnamate, and Oxybenzone [*Can Screen 400 Sunscreen; Ombrelle Sunscreen; Shade UVA Guard*]
  **See Sunscreen Agents (Topical),** #
  Lotion, #
  Spray, #
*Avonex*—Biogen (U.S.) brand of Interferon Beta-1a (Systemic), 1732, 3148
*Axid*—Lilly (U.S. and Canada) brand of Nizatidine—**See Histamine H$_2$-receptor Antagonists (Systemic),** 1633, MC-22
*Axid AR*—Lilly (U.S.) brand of Nizatidine—**See Histamine H$_2$-receptor Antagonists (Systemic),** 1633
*Axotal*—Adria (U.S.) brand of Butalbital and Aspirin—**See Barbiturates and Analgesics (Systemic),** 532
*Ayercillin*—Ayerst (Canada) brand of Penicillin G—**See Penicillins (Systemic),** 2240
*Aygestin*—ESI Lederle (U.S.) brand of Norethindrone—**See Progestins (Systemic),** 2400
*Azactam*—Squibb (U.S.) brand of Aztreonam (Systemic), 502, 3011
5-AZA-2'-deoxycytidine
  **(Systemic),** 3128
Azatadine-containing Combinations, 3068
Azatadine Maleate [*Optimine*]
  **See Antihistamines (Systemic),** 325
  Tablets USP, 332, MC-3
Azatadine Maleate and Pseudoephedrine Sulfate [*Trinalin Repetabs*]
  **See Antihistamines and Decongestants (Systemic),** 343
  Tablets, Extended-release, 363, MC-3
Azathioprine [*Imuran*]
  **(Systemic),** 491
  Tablets USP, 494, MC-3
Azathioprine Sodium [*Imuran*]
  **(Systemic),** 491
  for Injection USP, 495
*Azdone*—Central (U.S.) brand of Hydrocodone and Aspirin—**See Opioid (Narcotic) Analgesics and Aspirin (Systemic),** 2202
Azelaic Acid [*Azelex*]
  **(Topical),** 495
  Cream, 496
Azelastine Hydrochloride [*Astelin*]
  **(Nasal),** 497
  Solution, Nasal, 498
*Azelex*—Allergan Herbert (U.S.) brand of Azelaic Acid (Topical), 495
Azithromycin [*Zithromax*]
  **(Systemic),** 499
  Capsules USP, 501 MC-3
  for Injection, 502
  for Suspension, Oral, 501
  Tablets, 502
*Azmacort*—Rhône-Poulenc Rorer (U.S. and Canada) brand of Triamcinolone—**See Corticosteroids (Inhalation-Local),** 955
Azodisal sodium—*See* Olsalazine (Oral-Local), 2161
*Azo Gantanol*—Roche (U.S.) brand of Sulfamethoxazole and Phenazopyridine—**See Sulfonamides and Phenazopyridine (Systemic),** 2660
*Azo Gantrisin*—Roche (U.S. and Canada) brand of Sulfisoxazole and Phenazopyridine—**See Sulfonamides and Phenazopyridine (Systemic),** 2660
*Azopt*—Alcon (U.S.) brand of Brinzolamide (Ophthalmic), 634

*Azo-Standard*—Alcon (U.S.) and Webcon (U.S.) brand of Phenazopyridine (Systemic), 2288
*Azo-Sulfamethoxazole*—Schein (U.S.) brand of Sulfamethoxazole and Phenazopyridine—**See Sulfonamides and Phenazopyridine (Systemic),** 2660
*Azo-Sulfisoxazole*—Schein (U.S.) brand of Sulfisoxazole and Phenazopyridine—**See Sulfonamides and Phenazopyridine (Systemic),** 2660
*Azo-Truxazole*—Truxton (U.S.) brand of Sulfisoxazole and Phenazopyridine—**See Sulfonamides and Phenazopyridine (Systemic),** 2660
AZT—*See* Zidovudine (Systemic), 2992, 3171
Aztreonam [*Azactam*]
  **(Systemic),** 502, 3011
  Injection, 3011
  for Injection, 3011
  for Injection USP, 505
*Azulfidine*—Pharmacia Adria (U.S.) brand of Sulfasalazine (Systemic), 2643, MC-28
*Azulfidine EN-Tabs*—Pharmacia Adria (U.S.) brand of Sulfasalazine (Systemic), 2643, MC-28

# B

*Baby's Own Infant Drops*—Block (Canada) brand of Simethicone (Oral-Local), #
Bacampicillin Hydrochloride [*Penglobe; Spectrobid*]
  **See Penicillins (Systemic),** 2240
  for Suspension, Oral, USP, 2249
  Tablets USP, 2249
Bacillus Calmette-Guérin (BCG) Live [*ImmuCyst; PACIS; TheraCys; TICE BCG*]
  **(Mucosal-Local),** 507
  BCG Live (Connaught Strain), 509
  BCG Live (Montreal Strain), 509
  BCG Vaccine USP (Tice Strain), 510
Bacillus Calmette-Guérin (BCG) Live [*TICE BCG*]
  **(Systemic),** 510
  BCG Vaccine USP (Tice Strain), 512
  BCG Vaccine (Connaught Strain), 512
  BCG Vaccine (Montreal Strain), 512
Bacitracin [*Altracin*]
  **(Systemic),** 3133
Bacitracin-containing Combinations, 3068
*Backache Caplets*—Magnesium Salicylate—**See Salicylates (Systemic),** 2538
*Backwoods Cutter*—Spectrum (U.S.) brand of Diethyltoluamide (Topical), #
Baclofen [*Lioresal Intrathecal*]
  **(Intrathecal-Systemic),** 513, 3133
  Injection, 515
Baclofen [*Alpha-Baclofen; Lioresal; PMS-Baclofen*]
  **(Systemic),** 515, 3133
  Tablets USP, 517, MC-3
Bactericidal/Permeability-increasing Protein, Recombinant [*Neuprex*]
  **(Systemic),** 3160
*Bacticort*—Rugby (U.S.) brand of Neomycin, Polymyxin B, and Hydrocortisone (Ophthalmic), #
*Bactine*—Miles (U.S.) brand of Hydrocortisone—**See Corticosteroids (Topical),** 978
*Bactine First Aid Antibiotic*—Miles (U.S.) brand of Neomycin, Polymyxin B, and Bacitracin (Topical), #
*Bactocill*—Beecham (U.S.) brand of Oxacillin—**See Penicillins (Systemic),** 2240
*Bactrim*—Roche (U.S. and Canada) brand of Sulfamethoxazole and Trimethoprim—**See Sulfonamides and Trimethoprim (Systemic),** 2661, MC-28
*Bactrim DS*—Roche (U.S. and Canada) brand of Sulfamethoxazole and Trimethoprim—**See Sulfonamides and Trimethoprim (Systemic),** 2661
*Bactrim I.V.*—Roche (U.S.) brand of Sulfamethoxazole and Trimethoprim—**See Sulfonamides and Trimethoprim (Systemic),** 2661
*Bactrim Pediatric*—Roche (U.S.) brand of Sulfamethoxazole and Trimethoprim—**See Sulfonamides and Trimethoprim (Systemic),** 2661
*Bactroban*—Beecham (U.S. and Canada) brand of Mupirocin (Topical), 2066; 3029
*Bactroban Nasal*—SmithKline Beecham (U.S.) brand of Mupirocin (Nasal), 2066
*Bain de Soleil All Day For Kids*—Procter & Gamble (U.S.) brand of Octocrylene, Octyl Methoxycinnamate, Oxybenzone, and Titanium Dioxide—**See Sunscreen Agents (Topical),** #

*Bain de Soleil All Day Sunblock*—Herdt & Charton (Canada) brand of Octocrylene, Octyl Methoxycinnamate, Oxybenzone, and Titanium Dioxide—**See Sunscreen Agents (Topical)**, #
*Bain de Soleil All Day Sunfilter*—Procter & Gamble (U.S.) brand of Octocrylene, Octyl Methoxycinnamate, and Titanium Dioxide—**See Sunscreen Agents (Topical)**, #
*Bain de Soleil Long Lasting For Kids*—Herdt & Charton (Canada) brand of Octocrylene, Octyl Methoxycinnamate, Oxybenzone, and Titanium Dioxide—**See Sunscreen Agents (Topical)**, #
*Bain de Soleil Long Lasting Sport Sunblock*—Herdt & Charton (Canada) brand of Octocrylene, Octyl Methoxycinnamate, and Titanium Dioxide—**See Sunscreen Agents (Topical)**, #
*Bain de Soleil Long Lasting Sunblock*—Herdt & Charton (Canada) brand of Octocrylene, Octyl Methoxycinnamate, Oxybenzone, and Titanium Dioxide—**See Sunscreen Agents (Topical)**, #
*Bain de Soleil Long Lasting Sunfilter*—Herdt & Charton (Canada) brand of Octocrylene, Octyl Methoxycinnamate, and Titanium Dioxide—**See Sunscreen Agents (Topical)**, #
*Bain de Soleil Mega Tan*—Procter & Gamble (U.S.) and Herdt & Charton (Canada) brand of Octocrylene and Octyl Methoxycinnamate—**See Sunscreen Agents (Topical)**, #
*Bain de Soleil Orange Gelee*—Procter & Gamble (U.S.) and Herdt & Charton (Canada) brand of Octyl Methoxycinnamate and Octyl Salicylate—**See Sunscreen Agents (Topical)**, #
*Bain de Soleil Sand Buster*—Procter & Gamble (U.S.) brand of Octyl Methoxycinnamate and Octyl Salicylate—**See Sunscreen Agents (Topical)**, #
*Bain de Soleil SPF + Color*—Herdt & Charton (Canada) brand of Octocrylene, Octyl Methoxycinnamate, and Oxybenzone—**See Sunscreen Agents (Topical)**, #; Octocrylene and Octyl Methoxycinnamate—**See Sunscreen Agents (Topical)**, #
*Bain de Soleil Tropical Deluxe*—Procter & Gamble (U.S.) brand of Octyl Methoxycinnamate and Octyl Salicylate—**See Sunscreen Agents (Topical)**, #
*Baldex*—Bausch & Lomb (U.S.) brand of Dexamethasone—**See Corticosteroids (Ophthalmic)**, 966
*Balminil Decongestant Syrup*—Rougier (Canada) brand of Pseudoephedrine (Systemic), 2422
*Balminil D.M.*—Rougier (Canada) brand of Dextromethorphan (Systemic), 1191
*Balminil Expectorant*—Rougier (Canada) brand of Guaifenesin (Systemic), 1588
*Balnetar*—Westwood-Squibb (Canada) brand of Coal Tar (Topical), #
*Balnetar Therapeutic Tar Bath*—Westwood (U.S.) brand of Coal Tar (Topical), #
*BAL in Oil*—Becton Dickinson (U.S.) and Beauty Creations (Canada) brand of Dimercaprol (Systemic), 1224
*Banana Boat Active Kids Sunblock*—Sun (U.S.) brand of Octyl Methoxycinnamate, Octyl Salicylate, and Oxybenzone—**See Sunscreen Agents (Topical)**, #
*Banana Boat Baby Sunblock*—Sun (U.S.) brand of Octyl Methoxycinnamate, Octyl Salicylate, and Oxybenzone—**See Sunscreen Agents (Topical)**, #
*Banana Boat Dark Tanning*—Sun (U.S.) brand of Octyl Methoxycinnamate and Padimate O—**See Sunscreen Agents (Topical)**, #; Padimate O—**See Sunscreen Agents (Topical)**, #
*Banana Boat Faces Sensitive Skin Sunblock*—Sun (U.S.) brand of Octyl Methoxycinnamate, Octyl Salicylate, and Oxybenzone—**See Sunscreen Agents (Topical)**, #
*Banana Boat Protective Tanning*—Sun (U.S.) brand of Octyl Methoxycinnamate and Padimate O—**See Sunscreen Agents (Topical)**, #
*Banana Boat Sport Sunblock*—Sun (U.S.) brand of Octyl Methoxycinnamate, Octyl Salicylate, and Oxybenzone—**See Sunscreen Agents (Topical)**, #
*Banana Boat Sunblock*—Sun (U.S.) brand of Octyl Methoxycinnamate, Oxybenzone, and Padimate O—**See Sunscreen Agents (Topical)**, #
*Banana Boat Sunscreen*—Sun (U.S.) brand of Oxybenzone and Padimate O—**See Sunscreen Agents (Topical)**, #

*Bancap*—Forest (U.S.) brand of Butalbital and Acetaminophen—**See Barbiturates and Analgesics (Systemic)**, 532
*Bancap-HC*—Forest (U.S.) brand of Hydrocodone and Acetaminophen—**See Opioid (Narcotic) Analgesics and Acetaminophen (Systemic)**, 2198
*Banesin*—Forest (U.S.) brand of Acetaminophen (Systemic), 6
*Banex-LA*—Zenith Goldline (U.S.) brand of Phenylpropanolamine and Guaifenesin—**See Cough/Cold Combinations (Systemic)**, 1024
*Banex Liquid*—Zenith Goldline (U.S.) brand of Phenylephrine, Phenylpropanolamine, and Guaifenesin—**See Cough/Cold Combinations (Systemic)**, 1024
*Banflex*—Forest (U.S.) brand of Orphenadrine—**See Skeletal Muscle Relaxants (Systemic)**, 2577
*Banophen*—Major (U.S.) brand of Diphenhydramine—**See Antihistamines (Systemic)**, 325; Diphenhydramine and Pseudoephedrine—**See Antihistamines and Decongestants (Systemic)**, 343
*Banophen Caplets*—Major (U.S.) brand of Diphenhydramine—**See Antihistamines (Systemic)**, 325
*Banthine*—Schiapparelli Searle (U.S.) brand of Methantheline—**See Anticholinergics/Antispasmodics (Systemic)**, 226
*Barbidonna*—Wallace (U.S.) brand of Atropine, Hyoscyamine, Scopolamine, and Phenobarbital—**See Belladonna Alkaloids and Barbiturates (Systemic)**, 551
*Barbidonna No. 2*—Wallace (U.S.) brand of Atropine, Hyoscyamine, Scopolamine, and Phenobarbital—**See Belladonna Alkaloids and Barbiturates (Systemic)**, 551
*Barbita*—Vortech (U.S.) brand of Phenobarbital—**See Barbiturates (Systemic)**, 518
Barbiturates (Systemic), 518
Barbiturates and Analgesics (Systemic), 532
*Barc*—Commerce (U.S.) brand of Pyrethrins and Piperonyl Butoxide (Topical), #
*Baricon*—Lafayette (U.S.) brand of Barium Sulfate (Local), #
*Baridium*—Pfeiffer (U.S.) brand of Phenazopyridine (Systemic), 2288
Barium Sulfate [*ACB; Anatrast; Baricon; Barobag; Baro-cat; Barosperse; Enecat; Entero-H; Entrobar; Epi-C; Esobar; Esopho-CAT Esophageal Cream; Esophotrast Esophageal Cream; EvacuPaste; Exacta I; Exacta II; E-Z-AC; E-Z-CAT; E-Z-Disk; E-Z-Dose; E-Z-HD; E-Z-Jug; E-Z-Paque; E-Z-Paque Enema; E-Z-Paque Liquid; E-Z-Paste Esophageal Cream; Flo-Coat; Gil-Paque; HD 85; HD 200 Plus; Liquid Barosperse; Liquid HD; Liqui-Jug; Liquipake; Maxibar; Medebag; Medebar Plus; mede-SCAN; Polibar; Polibar Flavored; Polibar Liquid; Polibar Plus; Polibar Rapide; Prepcat; Probar; Readi-CAT; Readi-CAT 2; Readi-CAT Unflavored; Recto-Barium; Sol-O-Pake; Sol-O-Pake Liquid; Tomocat; Tomocat 1000; Tonojug 2000; Tonopaque; Ultra-R; Unibar-100*] (Local), #
Barium Sulfate USP, #
Suspension, #
Suspension, Oral, #
for Suspension USP (Oral), #
Suspension, Rectal, #
for Suspension USP (Rectal), #
Tablets, #
*Barobag*—Lafayette (U.S.) brand of Barium Sulfate (Local), #
*Baro-cat*—Lafayette (U.S.) brand of Barium Sulfate (Local), #
*Baron-X*—Baron (U.S.) brand of Yohimbine (Systemic), #
*Barophen*—CMC (U.S.); Moore (U.S.); and United Research (U.S.) brand of Atropine, Hyoscyamine, Scopolamine, and Phenobarbital—**See Belladonna Alkaloids and Barbiturates (Systemic)**, 551
*Barosperse*—Lafayette (U.S.) brand of Barium Sulfate (Local), #
*Barriere-HC*—Glaxo (Canada) brand of Hydrocortisone—**See Corticosteroids (Topical)**, 978

*Basaljel*—Axcan Pharma (Canada) brand of Aluminum Carbonate, Basic and Simethicone—**See Antacids (Oral-Local)**, 188; Aluminum Hydroxide—**See Antacids (Oral-Local)**, 188; Wyeth-Ayerst (U.S.) and Axcan Pharma (Canada) brand of Aluminum Carbonate, Basic—**See Antacids (Oral-Local)**, 188
Basiliximab [*Simulect*] (Systemic), 547
for Injection, 549
*Baycol*—Bayer (U.S.) brand of Cerivastatin (Systemic), 827
*Bayer 205*—Bayer (Germany and South Africa) brand of Suramin (Systemic), #
*Bayer 2502*—*See Nifurtimox (Systemic)*, #
*Bayer Children's Aspirin*—Miles (U.S.) brand of Aspirin—**See Salicylates (Systemic)**, 2538
*Bayer Select Ibuprofen Pain Relief Formula Caplets*—Sterling Health (U.S.) brand of Ibuprofen—**See Anti-inflammatory Drugs, Nonsteroidal (Systemic)**, 388
*Bayer Select Maximum Strength Backache Pain Relief Formula*—Miles (U.S.) brand of Magnesium Salicylate—**See Salicylates (Systemic)**, 2538
*Bayer Select Maximum Strength Pain Relief Formula*—Sterling Health (U.S.) brand of Acetaminophen and Caffeine—**See Acetaminophen (Systemic)**, 6
*BayTet*—Bayer (U.S.) brand of Tetanus Immune Globulin (Systemic), 2758
*BC Cold Powder Non-Drowsy Formula*—Block (U.S.) brand of Phenylpropanolamine and Aspirin—**See Decongestants and Analgesics (Systemic)**, 1180
BCG Live (Montreal Strain) [*PACIS*] (Mucosal-Local), 3011
*BC Multi Symptom Cold Powder*—Block (U.S.) brand of Chlorpheniramine, Phenylpropanolamine, and Aspirin—**See Antihistamines, Decongestants, and Analgesics (Systemic)**, 366
*BCNU*—*See Carmustine (Implantation-Local)*, 784; Carmustine (Systemic), 786
*Beben*—PD (Canada) brand of Betamethasone—**See Corticosteroids (Topical)**, 978
*Bebulin VH*—Immuno (U.S. and Canada) brand of Factor IX (Systemic), 1430
Becaplermin [*Regranex*] (Topical), 550
Gel, 551
*Because*—Schering (U.S.) brand of Nonoxynol 9—**See Spermicides (Vaginal)**, #
*Beclodisk*—Glaxo (Canada) brand of Beclomethasone—**See Corticosteroids (Inhalation-Local)**, 955
*Becloforte*—Glaxo (Canada) brand of Beclomethasone—**See Corticosteroids (Inhalation-Local)**, 955
Beclomethasone—Beclomethasone—**See Corticosteroids (Inhalation-Local)**, 955; **Corticosteroids (Nasal)**, 961; **Corticosteroids (Topical)**, 978
Beclomethasone dipropionate—Beclomethasone—**See Corticosteroids (Inhalation-Local)**, 955
Beclomethasone Dipropionate (Systemic), 3133
Beclomethasone Dipropionate [beclomethasone; *Beconase; Vancenase*]
See Corticosteroids (Nasal), 961
Aerosol, Nasal, 964
Beclomethasone Dipropionate [beclomethasone; beclomethasone dipropionate; *Beclodisk; Becloforte; Beclovent; Beclovent Rotacaps; Vanceril; Vanceril 84 mcg Double Strength*]
See Corticosteroids (Inhalation-Local), 955
Aerosol, Inhalation, 959
for Inhalation (Capsules), 959
for Inhalation (Powder), 959
Beclomethasone Dipropionate [beclomethasone; *Propaderm*]
See Corticosteroids (Topical), 978
Cream, 983
Lotion, 983
Ointment, 983
Beclomethasone Dipropionate Monohydrate [beclomethasone; *Beconase AQ; Vancenase AQ*]
See Corticosteroids (Nasal), 961, 3011
Solution, Nasal, 964, 3011
*Beclovent*—Glaxo (U.S. and Canada) brand of Beclomethasone—**See Corticosteroids (Inhalation-Local)**, 955
*Beclovent Rotacaps*—Glaxo (Canada) brand of Beclomethasone—**See Corticosteroids (Inhalation-Local)**, 955

*Beconase*—Glaxo (U.S. and Canada) and Allen & Hanburys (U.K.) brand of Beclomethasone—**See Corticosteroids (Nasal)**, 961
*Beconase AQ*—Glaxo (U.S. and Canada) brand of Beclomethasone—**See Corticosteroids (Nasal)**, 961
*Bedoz*—Nadeau (Canada) brand of Cyanocobalamin—**See Vitamin B$_{12}$ (Systemic)**, 2962
*Beepen-VK*—Beecham (U.S.) brand of Penicillin V—**See Penicillins (Systemic)**, 2240
*Beesix*—Forest (U.S.) brand of Pyridoxine (Systemic), 2430
*Belganyl*—See Suramin (Systemic), #
Belladonna
  **See Anticholinergics/Antispasmodics (Systemic)**, 226
  Tincture USP, 234
Belladonna Alkaloid-containing Combinations, 3068
Belladonna Alkaloids and Barbiturates **(Systemic)**, 551
Belladonna-containing Combinations, 3068
Belladonna Extract and Butabarbital Sodium [*Butibel*]
  **See Belladonna Alkaloids and Barbiturates (Systemic)**, 551
  Elixir, 554
  Tablets, 554
Belladonna Extract and Phenobarbital [*Chardonna-2*]
  **See Belladonna Alkaloids and Barbiturates (Systemic)**, 551
  Tablets, 554
*Bellalphen*—CMC (U.S.) brand of Atropine, Hyoscyamine, Scopolamine, and Phenobarbital—**See Belladonna Alkaloids and Barbiturates (Systemic)**, 551
*Bell/ans*—C. S. Dent (U.S.) brand of Sodium Bicarbonate (Systemic), 2586
*Bellergal*—Sandoz (Canada) brand of Ergotamine, Belladonna Alkaloids, and Phenobarbital (Systemic), 1363
*Bellergal-S*—Sandoz (U.S.) brand of Ergotamine, Belladonna Alkaloids, and Phenobarbital (Systemic), 1363
*Bellergal Spacetabs*—Sandoz (Canada) brand of Ergotamine, Belladonna Alkaloids, and Phenobarbital (Systemic), 1363
*Benadryl*—PD (U.S. and Canada) brand of Diphenhydramine—**See Antihistamines (Systemic)**, 325
*Benadryl Allergy*—PD (U.S.) brand of Diphenhydramine—**See Antihistamines (Systemic)**, 325
*Benadryl Allergy Decongestant Liquid Medication*—Warner Wellcome (U.S. and Canada) brand of Diphenhydramine and Pseudoephedrine—**See Antihistamines and Decongestants (Systemic)**, 343
*Benadryl Allergy/Sinus Headache Caplets*—Warner Wellcome (U.S.) brand of Diphenhydramine, Pseudoephedrine, and Acetaminophen—**See Antihistamines, Decongestants, and Analgesics (Systemic)**, 366
*Benadryl Cold/Allergy*—Warner Wellcome (U.S.) brand of Diphenhydramine, Pseudoephedrine, and Acetaminophen—**See Antihistamines, Decongestants, and Analgesics (Systemic)**, 366
Benazepril Hydrochloride [*Lotensin*]
  **See Angiotensin-converting Enzyme (ACE) Inhibitors (Systemic)**, 177
  Tablets, 183, MC-3
Benazepril and Hydrochlorothiazide [*Lotensin HCT*] **(Systemic)**, MC-3
  Tablets, MC-3
Bendroflumethiazide [*Naturetin*]
  **See Diuretics, Thiazide (Systemic)**, 1273
  Tablets USP, 1277, MC-3
Bendroflumethiazide-containing Combinations, 3068
*Benemid*—Merck (U.S. and Canada) brand of Probenecid (Systemic), 2380
*Benoxyl 5 Lotion*—Stiefel (U.S. and Canada) brand of Benzoyl Peroxide (Topical), 579
*Benoxyl 10 Lotion*—Stiefel (U.S. and Canada) brand of Benzoyl Peroxide (Topical), 579
*Benoxyl 20 Lotion*—Stiefel (Canada) brand of Benzoyl Peroxide (Topical), 579
Benserazide-containing Combinations, 3068
*Bensulfoid Cream*—Poythress (U.S.) brand of Resorcinol and Sulfur (Topical), #
Bentiromide [*Chymex*]
  **(Systemic)**, #
  Solution, Oral, #
Bentoquatam [*IvyBlock*]
  **(Topical)**, 0555
  Lotion, 556

*Bentyl*—Hoechst Marion Roussel (U.S.) brand of Dicyclomine—**See Anticholinergics/Antispasmodics (Systemic)**, 226, MC-9
*Bentylol*—Marion Merrell Dow (Canada) brand of Dicyclomine—**See Anticholinergics/Antispasmodics (Systemic)**, 226
*Benuryl*—ICN (Canada) brand of Probenecid (Systemic), 2380
*Benylin Adult*—PD (U.S.) brand of Dextromethorphan (Systemic), 1191
*Benylin Codeine D-E*—Warner Wellcome (Canada) brand of Pseudoephedrine, Codeine, and Guaifenesin—**See Cough/Cold Combinations (Systemic)**, 1024
*Benylin Decongestant*—Warner-Lambert (Canada) brand of Pseudoephedrine (Systemic), 2422
*Benylin DM-D*—Warner Wellcome (Canada) brand of Pseudoephedrine and Dextromethorphan—**See Cough/Cold Combinations (Systemic)**, 1024
*Benylin DM-D for Children*—Warner Wellcome (Canada) brand of Pseudoephedrine and Dextromethorphan—**See Cough/Cold Combinations (Systemic)**, 1024
*Benylin DM-D-E*—Warner Wellcome (Canada) brand of Pseudoephedrine, Dextromethorphan, and Guaifenesin—**See Cough/Cold Combinations (Systemic)**, 1024
*Benylin DM-D-E Extra Strength*—Warner Wellcome (Canada) brand of Pseudoephedrine, Dextromethorphan, and Guaifenesin—**See Cough/Cold Combinations (Systemic)**, 1024
*Benylin DM-E*—Warner Wellcome (Canada) brand of Dextromethorphan and Guaifenesin—**See Cough/Cold Combinations (Systemic)**, 1024
*Benylin DM-E Extra Strength*—Warner Wellcome (Canada) brand of Dextromethorphan and Guaifenesin—**See Cough/Cold Combinations (Systemic)**, 1024
*Benylin-E*—Warner-Lambert (Canada) brand of Guaifenesin (Systemic), 1588
*Benylin Expectorant*—Warner Wellcome (U.S.) brand of Dextromethorphan and Guaifenesin—**See Cough/Cold Combinations (Systemic)**, 1024
*Benylin 4 Flu*—Warner Wellcome (Canada) brand of Pseudoephedrine, Dextromethorphan, Guaifenesin, and Acetaminophen—**See Cough/Cold Combinations (Systemic)**, 1024
*Benylin Multi-Symptom*—Warner Wellcome (U.S.) brand of Pseudoephedrine, Dextromethorphan, and Guaifenesin—**See Cough/Cold Combinations (Systemic)**, 1024
*Benylin Pediatric*—PD (U.S.) brand of Dextromethorphan (Systemic), 1191
*Benzac AC 2½ Gel*—Galderma (U.S.) brand of Benzoyl Peroxide (Topical), 579
*Benzac AC 5 Gel*—Galderma (U.S.) brand of Benzoyl Peroxide (Topical), 579
*Benzac AC 10 Gel*—Galderma (U.S. and Canada) brand of Benzoyl Peroxide (Topical), 579
*Benzac AC Wash 2½*—Galderma (U.S.) brand of Benzoyl Peroxide (Topical), 579
*Benzac AC Wash 5*—Galderma (U.S.) brand of Benzoyl Peroxide (Topical), 579
*Benzac AC Wash 10*—Galderma (U.S.) brand of Benzoyl Peroxide (Topical), 579
*Benzac 5 Gel*—Galderma (U.S.) brand of Benzoyl Peroxide (Topical), 579
*Benzac 10 Gel*—Galderma (U.S.) brand of Benzoyl Peroxide (Topical), 579
*Benzacot*—Truxton (U.S.) brand of Trimethobenzamide (Systemic), 2880
*Benzac W 2½ Gel*—Galderma (U.S.) brand of Benzoyl Peroxide (Topical), 579
*Benzac W 5 Gel*—Galderma (U.S.) and Alcon (Canada) brand of Benzoyl Peroxide (Topical), 579
*Benzac W 10 Gel*—Galderma (Canada) brand of Benzoyl Peroxide (Topical), 579
*Benzac W Wash 5*—Galderma (U.S.) brand of Benzoyl Peroxide (Topical), 579
*Benzac W Wash 10*—Galderma (U.S.) brand of Benzoyl Peroxide (Topical), 579
*5 Benzagel*—Dermik (U.S.) and Rorer (Canada) brand of Benzoyl Peroxide (Topical), 579
*10 Benzagel*—Dermik (U.S.) and Rorer (Canada) brand of Benzoyl Peroxide (Topical), 579
*2.5 Benzagel Acne Gel*—Novartis (Canada) brand of Benzoyl Peroxide (Topical), 579
*5 Benzagel Acne Gel*—Novartis (Canada) brand of Benzoyl Peroxide (Topical), 579
*10 Benzagel Acne Gel*—Novartis (Canada) brand of Benzoyl Peroxide (Topical), 579

*2.5 Benzagel Acne Lotion*—Novartis (Canada) brand of Benzoyl Peroxide (Topical), 579
*5 Benzagel Acne Lotion*—Novartis (Canada) brand of Benzoyl Peroxide (Topical), 579
*5 Benzagel Acne Wash*—Novartis (Canada) brand of Benzoyl Peroxide (Topical), 579
*5 Benzagel Liquid Acne Soap*—Novartis (Canada) brand of Benzoyl Peroxide (Topical), 579
Benzalkonium Chloride [*Pharmatex*]
  **See Spermicides (Vaginal)**, #
  Suppositories, Vaginal, #
*Benzamycin*—Dermik (U.S.) brand of Erythromycin and Benzoyl Peroxide (Topical), 1367
*BenzaShave 5 Cream*—Medicis (U.S.) brand of Benzoyl Peroxide (Topical), 579
*BenzaShave 10 Cream*—Medicis (U.S.) brand of Benzoyl Peroxide (Topical), 579
Benzathine benzylpenicillin—Penicillin G—**See Penicillins (Systemic)**, 2240
Benzathine penicillin—Penicillin G—**See Penicillins (Systemic)**, 2240
Benzatropine—Benztropine—**See Antidyskinetics (Systemic)**, 297
Benzfetamine—Benzphetamine—**See Appetite Suppressants (Systemic)**, 452
Benzhexol—Trihexyphenidyl—**See Antidyskinetics (Systemic)**, 297
Benznidazole [*Radanil; Rochagan; Ro7-1051*]
  **(Systemic)**, #
  Tablets, #
Benzoate and Phenylacetate [sodium benzoate and sodium phenylacetate; *Ucephan*]
  **(Systemic)**, 3133
Benzocaine [*Americaine; Americaine Anesthetic Lubricant; Americaine Hemorrhoidal; Anbesol, Baby; Anbesol Baby Jel; Anbesol Maximum Strength Gel; Anbesol Maximum Strength Liquid; Benzodent; Chloraseptic Lozenges, Children's; Dentapaine; Dentocaine; Dent-Zel-Ite; ethyl aminobenzoate; Hurricaine; Numzident; Num-Zit-Gel; Num-Zit-Lotion; Orabase, Baby; Orabase-B with Benzocaine; Orajel; Orajel, Baby; Orajel Extra Strength; Orajel Liquid; Orajel Maximum Strength; Orajel Nighttime Formula, Baby; Oratect Gel; Rid-A-Pain; SensoGARD Canker Sore Relief; Spec-T Sore Throat Anesthetic; Topicaine*]
  **See Anesthetics (Mucosal-Local)**, 128
  Aerosol, Topical, USP, 134
  Gel, 134
  Gel (Dental), 132
  Gel, Film-forming, 133
  Lozenges, 133
  Ointment USP (Dental), 133
  Ointment USP (Rectal), 134
  Paste, Dental, 133
  Solution, Topical, USP, 134
  Solution, Topical, USP (Dental), 133
Benzocaine [*Americaine Topical Anesthetic First Aid Ointment; Americaine Topical Anesthetic Spray; Endocaine; ethyl aminobenzoate; Lagol; Shield Burnasept Spray*]
  **See Anesthetics (Topical)**, 155
  Aerosol, Topical, USP, 158
  Cream USP, 158
  Ointment USP, 158
  Solution, Topical Spray, 159
Benzocaine, Butamben, and Tetracaine Hydrochloride [*Cetacaine Topical Anesthetic*]
  **See Anesthetics (Mucosal-Local)**, 128
  Aerosol, Topical, USP, 135
  Gel USP, 135
  Ointment USP, 135
  Solution, Topical, USP, 135
Benzocaine-containing Combinations, 3068
Benzocaine and Menthol [*Chloraseptic Lozenges; Chloraseptic Lozenges Cherry Flavor*]
  **See Anesthetics (Mucosal-Local)**, 128
  Lozenges, 133
Benzocaine and Menthol [*Dermoplast*]
  **See Anesthetics (Topical)**, 155
  Aerosol, Topical, 158
  Lotion, 158
Benzocaine and Phenol [*Anbesol Gel; Anbesol Liquid; Anbesol Maximum Strength Liquid; Anbesol Regular Strength Gel; Anbesol Regular Strength Liquid*]
  **See Anesthetics (Mucosal-Local)**, 128
  Gel, 134
  Solution, Topical, 134

**General Index**

Benzodent—Procter & Gamble (U.S.) brand of Benzocaine—See **Anesthetics (Mucosal-Local)**, 128
Benzodiazepines
 **(Systemic)**, 556
Benzonatate [*Tessalon*]
 **(Systemic)**, #
 Capsules USP
Benzoyl Peroxide [*Acetoxyl 2.5 Gel; Acetoxyl 5 Gel; Acetoxyl 10 Gel; Acetoxyl 20 Gel; Acne Aid Aqua Gel; Acne-Aid Vanishing Cream; Acnomel B.P. 5 Lotion; Ambi 10 Acne Medication; Benoxyl 5 Lotion; Benoxyl 10 Lotion; Benoxyl 20 Lotion; Benzac AC 2½ Gel; Benzac AC 5Gel; Benzac AC 10 Gel; Benzac AC Wash 2½; Benzac AC Wash 5; Benzac AC Wash 10; Benzac 5 Gel; Benzac 10 Gel; Benzac W 2½ Gel; Benzac W 5 Gel; Benzac W 10 Gel; Benzac W Wash 5; Benzac W Wash 10; 5 Benzagel; 10 Benzagel; 2.5 Benzagel Acne Gel; 5 Benzagel Acne Gel; 10 Benzagel Acne Gel; 2.5 Benzagel Acne Lotion; 5 Benzagel Acne Lotion; 5 Benzagel Acne Wash; 5 Benzagel Liquid Acne Soap; Benza Shave 5 Cream; Benza Shave 10 Cream; Brevoxyl-4 Cleansing Lotion; Brevoxyl-8 Cleansing Lotion; Brevoxyl 4 Gel; Brevoxyl-8 Gel; Clean & Clear Persagel 5; Clean & Clear Persagel 10; Clearasil BP Plus 5 Lotion; Clearasil BP Plus 5 Skin Tone Cream; Clearasil Maximum Strength Medicated Anti-Acne 10 Tinted Cream; Clearasil Maximum Strength Medicated Anti-Acne 10 Vanishing Cream; Clearasil Maximum Strength Medicated Anti-Acne 10 Vanishing Lotion; Clear By Design 2.5 Gel; Clearplex 5; ClearPlex 10; Cuticura Acne 5 Cream; Del-Aqua-5 Gel; Del-Aqua-10 Gel; Dermacne; Dermoxyl Aqua 5 Gel; Dermoxyl 5 Gel; Dermoxyl 10 Gel; Dermoxyl 20 Gel; Desquam-E 2.5 Gel; Desquam-E 5 Gel; Desquam-E 10 Gel; Desquam-X 10 Bar; Desquam-X 2.5 Gel; Desquam-X 5 Gel; Desquam-X 10 Gel; Desquam-X 5 Wash; Desquam-X 10 Wash; Exact 5 Tinted Cream; Exact 5 Vanishing Cream; Fostex 10 Bar; Fostex 10 BPO Gel; Fostex 10 Cream; Fostex 5 Gel; Fostex 10 Gel; H₂Oxyl 2.5 Gel; H₂ Oxyl 5 Gel; H₂ Oxyl 10 Gel; H₂ Oxyl 20 Gel; Loroxide 5.5 Lotion; Loroxide 5 Lotion; Neutrogena AcneMask 5; Noxzema Clear-ups Maximum Strength 10 Lotion; Noxzema Clear-ups On-The-Spot 10 Lotion; Oxy Balance Deep Action Night Formula Lotion; Oxy 10 Balance Emergency Spot Treatment Cover-Up Formula Gel; Oxy Balance Emergency Spot Treatment Invisible Formula; Oxy 10 Balance Maximum Medicated Face Wash; Oxyderm 5 Lotion; Oxyderm 10 Lotion; Oxyderm 20 Lotion; Oxy 5 Regular Strength Cover-Up Cream; Oxy 5 Regular Strength Vanishing Lotion; Oxy 5 Sensitive Skin Vanishing Lotion; PanOxyl AQ 2½ Gel; PanOxyl AQ 5 Gel; PanOxyl AQ 10 Gel; PanOxyl Aquagel 2.5; PanOxyl Aquagel 5; PanOxyl Aquagel 10; PanOxyl Aquagel 20; PanOxyl 5 Bar; PanOxyl 10 Bar; PanOxy l5 Gel; PanOxyl 10 Gel; PanOxyl 15 Gel; PanOxyl 20 Gel; PanOxyl 5 Wash; PanOxyl 10 Wash; Solugel 4; Solugel 8; Student's Choice Acne Medication; Triaz; Triaz Cleanser; Xerac BP 5 Gel*]
 **(Topical)**, 579, 3011
 Bar, Cleansing, 581
 Cream, 581
 Gel, 3011
 Gel USP, 582
 Lotion USP, 582
 Lotion, Cleansing, 581, 3011
 Mask, Facial, 582
 Stick, 582
Benzoyl Peroxide–containing Combinations, 3068
Benzphetamine Hydrochloride [benzfetamine; *Didrex*]
 **See Appetite Suppressants (Systemic)**, 452
 Tablets, 455 MC-3
Benztropine Mesylate [*Apo-Benztropine*; benzatropine; *Cogentin*; *PMS Benztropine*]
 **See Antidyskinetics (Systemic)**, 297
 Injection USP, 299
 Tablets USP, 299, MC-3
Benzydamine Hydrochloride [*Tantum*]
 **(Oral-Local)**, 3011, 3133
 Solution, Oral Topical, 3011
Benzyl Benzoate [*Ascabiol*]
 **(Topical)**, #
 Emulsion, #

Benzylpenicillin, Benzylpenicilloic Acid, and Benzylpenilloic Acid [*Pre-Pen/MDM*]
 **(Systemic)**, 3132
Bepridil Hydrochloride [*Vascor*]
 **See Calcium Channel Blocking Agents (Systemic)**, 720
 Tablets, 727, MC-4
Beractant [modified bovine surfactant extract; *Survanta*; *Survanta Intratracheal Suspension*]
 **(Intratracheal-Local)**, 583, 3133
 Suspension, Intratracheal, 585, 3132, 3133
Berlin blue—See Prussian Blue (Oral-Local), #
Berotec—Boehringer Ingelheim (Canada) brand of Fenoterol—See **Bronchodilators, Adrenergic (Inhalation-Local)**, 640; **Bronchodilators, Adrenergic (Systemic)**, 651
Beta-2—Nephron (U.S.) brand of Isoetharine—See **Bronchodilators, Adrenergic (Inhalation-Local)**, 640
Beta-adrenergic Blocking Agents
 **(Ophthalmic)**, 585
Beta-adrenergic Blocking Agents
 **(Systemic)**, 593
Beta-adrenergic Blocking Agents and Thiazide Diuretics
 **(Systemic)**, 609
Beta Alethine [*Betathine*]
 **(Systemic)**, 3133
Beta-carotene [*Lumitene*; *Max-Caro*]
 **(Systemic)**, 612
 Capsules USP, 613
 Tablets, 614
 Tablets, Chewable, 614
Betacort Scalp Lotion—ICN (Canada) brand of Betamethasone—See **Corticosteroids (Topical)**, 978
Betaderm—K-Line (Canada) brand of Betamethasone—See **Corticosteroids (Topical)**, 978
Betaderm Scalp Lotion—K-Line (Canada) brand of Betamethasone—See **Corticosteroids (Topical)**, 978
Betagan C Cap B.I.D.—Allergan (U.S. and Canada) brand of Levobunolol—See **Beta-adrenergic Blocking Agents (Ophthalmic)**, 585
Betagan C Cap Q.D.—Allergan (U.S.) brand of Levobunolol—See **Beta-adrenergic Blocking Agents (Ophthalmic)**, 585
Betagan Standard Cap—Allergan (U.S. and Canada) brand of Levobunolol—See **Beta-adrenergic Blocking Agents (Ophthalmic)**, 585
Beta-HC—Beta Dermaceuticals (U.S.) brand of Hydrocortisone—See **Corticosteroids (Topical)**, 978
Betaine [*Cystadane*]
 **(Systemic)**, #, 3133
 for Solution, Oral, #
Betaloc—Astra (Canada) brand of Metoprolol—See **Beta-adrenergic Blocking Agents (Systemic)**, 593
Betaloc Durules—Astra (Canada) brand of Metoprolol—See **Beta-adrenergic Blocking Agents (Systemic)**, 593
Betamethasone [*Betnelan*; *Betnesol*; *Celestone*]
 **See Corticosteroids—Glucocorticoid Effects (Systemic)**, 998
 Syrup USP, 1006
 Tablets USP, 1006
 Tablets, Effervescent, 1006
Betamethasone Benzoate [*Beben*; *Uticort*]
 **See Corticosteroids (Topical)**, 978
 Cream, 983
 Gel USP, 983
 Lotion, 983
Betamethasone-containing Combinations, 3068
Betamethasone Dipropionate [*Alphatrex*; *Diprolene*; *Diprosone*; *Maxivate*; *Occlucort*; *Teladar*; *Topilene*; *Topisone*]
 **See Corticosteroids (Topical)**, 978, 3012
 Aerosol, Topical, 985
 Cream USP, 984
 Gel, 984
 Lotion, 3012
 Lotion USP, 984
 Ointment USP, 985
Betamethasone Dipropionate, Augmented [*Diprolene*; *Diprolene AF*]
 **See Corticosteroids (Topical)**, 978
 Cream, 984
 Lotion, 984
 Ointment, 984

Betamethasone Disodium Phosphate [*Betnesol*]
 **(Dental)**, 3012
 Pellets, Dental, 3012
Betamethasone Sodium Phosphate [*Betnesol*]
 **See Corticosteroids (Ophthalmic)**, 966
 Solution, Ophthalmic/Otic, 968
Betamethasone Sodium Phosphate [*Betnesol*]
 **See Corticosteroids (Otic)**, 971
 Solution, Ophthalmic/Otic, 972
Betamethasone Sodium Phosphate [*Betnesol*]
 **See Corticosteroids (Rectal)**, 973
 Enema, 976
Betamethasone Sodium Phosphate [*Celestone*; *Celestone Phosphate*; *Selestoject*]
 **See Corticosteroids—Glucocorticoid Effects (Systemic)**, 998
 Injection USP, 1006
 Tablets, Extended-release, 1006
Betamethasone Sodium Phosphate and Betamethasone Acetate [*Celestone Soluspan*]
 **See Corticosteroids—Glucocorticoid Effects (Systemic)**, 998
 Suspension, Sterile, USP, 1006
Betamethasone Valerate [*Betacort Scalp Lotion*; *Betaderm*; *Betaderm Scalp Lotion*; *Betatrex*; *Beta-Val*; *Betnovate*; *Betnovate-½*; *Celestoderm-V*; *Celestoderm-V/2*; *Dermabet*; *Ectosone Mild*; *Ectosone Regular*; *Ectosone Scalp Lotion*; *Metaderm Mild*; *Metaderm Regular*; *Novobetamet*; *Prevex B*; *Valisone*; *Valisone Reduced Strength*; *Valisone Scalp Lotion*; *Valnac*]
 **See Corticosteroids (Topical)**, 978
 Cream USP, 985
 Lotion USP, 985
 Ointment USP, 985
Betapace—Berlex (U.S.) brand of Sotalol—See **Beta-adrenergic Blocking Agents (Systemic)**, 593, MC-28; Berlex (U.S.) brand of Sotalol (Systemic), 3166
Betapen-VK—Bristol (U.S.) brand of Penicillin V—See **Penicillins (Systemic)**, 2240
Betarx—Vivorx (U.S.) brand of Encapsulated Porcine Islet Preparation (Systemic), 3141
Betaseron—Berlex (Canada) brand of Interferon, Beta-1b (Systemic), 3026; Berlex (U.S.) brand of Interferon, Beta-1b (Systemic), 1735; Chiron (U.S.) and Berlex (U.S.) brand of Interferon Beta-1b (Systemic), 3148
Betathine—Dovetail (U.S.) brand of Beta Alethine (Systemic), 3133
Beta-Tim—Ciba Vision (Canada) brand of Timolol (Ophthalmic), 3036
Betatrex—Savage (U.S.) brand of Betamethasone—See **Corticosteroids (Topical)**, 978
Beta-Val—Lemmon (U.S.) brand of Betamethasone—See **Corticosteroids (Topical)**, 978
Betaxin—Sterling Winthrop (Canada) brand of Thiamine (Systemic), 2787
Betaxolol [*Kerlone*]
 **See Beta-adrenergic Blocking Agents (Systemic)**, 593
 Tablets, 601, MC-4
Betaxolol Hydrochloride [*Betoptic*; *Betoptic S*]
 **See Beta-adrenergic Blocking Agents (Ophthalmic)**, 585, 3012
 Solution, Ophthalmic, USP, 591
 Suspension, Ophthalmic, 591, 3012
Bethanechol Chloride [*Duvoid*; *Urabeth*; *Urecholine*]
 **(Systemic)**, 614
 Injection USP, 616
 Tablets USP, 616
Betimol—Ciba Vision (U.S.) brand of Timolol (Ophthalmic), 3036
Betnelan—Glaxo (Canada) brand of Betamethasone—See **Corticosteroids—Glucocorticoid Effects (Systemic)**, 998
Betnesol—Glaxo (Canada) brand of Betamethasone—See **Corticosteroids (Ophthalmic)**, 966; **Corticosteroids (Otic)**, 971; **Corticosteroids—Glucocorticoid Effects (Systemic)**, 998; Glaxo (Canada) brand of Betamethasone (Dental), 3012; Roberts (Canada) brand of Betamethasone—See **Corticosteroids (Rectal)**, 973
Betnovate—Glaxo (Canada and U.K.) brand of Betamethasone—See **Corticosteroids (Topical)**, 978
Betnovate-½—Glaxo (Canada) brand of Betamethasone—See **Corticosteroids (Topical)**, 978
Betoptic—Alcon (U.S. and Canada) brand of Betaxolol—See **Beta-adrenergic Blocking Agents (Ophthalmic)**, 585

*USP DI*  General Index  **3253**

*Betoptic S*—Alcon (Canada) brand of Betaxolol (Ophthalmic), 3012; Alcon (U.S.) brand of Betaxolol—**See Beta-adrenergic Blocking Agents (Ophthalmic)**, 585
*Bewon*—Wyeth (Canada) brand of Thiamine (Systemic), 2787
*Beyond Seven*—Okamoto (U.S.) brand of Latex Condoms—**See Condoms**, #
*Beyond Seven Plus*—Okamoto (U.S.) brand of Latex Condoms and Nonoxynol 9—**See Condoms**, #
*Biamine*—Forest (U.S.) brand of Thiamine (Systemic), 2787
*BIAVAX II*—Merck (U.S.) brand of Rubella and Mumps Virus Vaccine Live (Systemic), 2528
*Biaxin*—Abbott (U.S. and Canada) brand of Clarithromycin (Systemic), 889, MC-7
Bicalutamide [*Casodex*]
   **See Antiandrogens, Nonsteroidal (Systemic)**, 220
   Tablets, 225, MC-4
*Bicholate Lilas*—Sabex (Canada) brand of Cascara Sagrada and Phenolphthalein—**See Laxatives (Local)**, #
*Bicillin L-A*—Wyeth-Ayerst (U.S.) and Wyeth (Canada) brand of Penicillin G—**See Penicillins (Systemic)**, 2240
*Bicitra*—Willen (U.S.) brand of Sodium Citrate and Citric Acid—**See Citrates (Systemic)**, 881
*BiCNU*—Bristol (U.S. and Canada) brand of Carmustine (Systemic), 786
*Bilagog*—Wesley (U.S.) brand of Magnesium Sulfate—**See Laxatives (Local)**, #
*Bilax*—Drug Industries (U.S.) brand of Dehydrocholic Acid and Docusate—**See Laxatives (Local)**, #
*Bilivist*—Berlex (U.S.) brand of Ipodate—**See Cholecystographic Agents, Oral (Systemic)**, #
*Bilopaque*—Sanofi Winthrop (U.S.) brand of Tyropanoate—**See Cholecystographic Agents, Oral (Systemic)**, #
*Biloptin*—Schering (U.K.) brand of Ipodate—**See Cholecystographic Agents, Oral (Systemic)**, #
*Biltricide*—Miles (U.S.) brand of Praziquantel (Systemic), 2368
Bindarit
   **(Systemic)**, 3133
*BioCal*—Miles (U.S.) brand of Calcium Carbonate—**See Calcium Supplements (Systemic)**, 736
*Bioclate*—Baxter (U.S.) brand of Antihemophilic Factor (Systemic), 319
Biodel Implant/Carmustine (BCNU) [*Gliadel*]
   **(Systemic)**, 3133
*Bio-Gan*—Bioline (U.S.) brand of Trimethobenzamide (Systemic), 2880
*Biohisdex DM*—Everest (Canada) brand of Diphenylpyraline, Phenylephrine, and Dextromethorphan—**See Cough/Cold Combinations (Systemic)**, 1024
*Biohisdine DM*—Everest (Canada) brand of Diphenylpyraline, Phenylephrine, and Dextromethorphan—**See Cough/Cold Combinations (Systemic)**, 1024
*Biohist-LA*—Wakefield (U.S.) brand of Carbinoxamine and Pseudoephedrine—**See Antihistamines and Decongestants (Systemic)**, 343
*Bion Tears*—Alcon (U.S.) brand of Hydroxypropyl Methylcellulose (Ophthalmic), #
*Bio-Rescue*—Biomedical Frontiers (U.S.) brand of Dextran and Deferoxamine (Systemic), 3140
*Bio-Syn*—Clay-Park (U.S.) brand of Fluocinolone—**See Corticosteroids (Topical)**, 978
*Biosynject*—Chembiomed (Canada) brand of Trisaccharides A and B (Systemic), 3170
*Biotel/diabetes*—American Diagnostics (U.S.) brand of Glucose Oxidase Urine Glucose Test—**See Urine Glucose and Ketone Test Kits for Home Use**, #
Biotin [coenzyme R; vitamin Bw; vitamin H]
   **(Systemic)**, #
   Capsules, #
   Tablets, #
*Biotropin*—Bio-Technology General (U.S.) brand of Somatropin (Systemic), 3165
*Bio-Well*—Bioline (U.S.) brand of Lindane (Topical), 1866
Biperiden Hydrochloride [*Akineton*]
   **See Antidyskinetics (Systemic)**, 297
   Tablets USP, 300
Biperiden Lactate [*Akineton*]
   **See Antidyskinetics (Systemic)**, 297
   Injection USP, 300
*Bisac-Evac*—G & W (U.S.) brand of Bisacodyl—**See Laxatives (Local)**, #

Bisacodyl [*Apo-Bisacodyl; Bisac-Evac; Bisacolax; Bisco-Lax; Carter's Little Pills; Correctol; Correctol Caplets; Dacodyl; Deficol; Dulcolax; Feen-a-mint; Feen-a-Mint Pills; Fleet Bisacodyl; Fleet Laxative; Gentle Laxative; Laxit; PMS-Bisacodyl; Theralax*]
   **See Laxatives (Local)**, #
   Enema, #
   Solution, Rectal, #
   Suppositories USP, #
   Tablets, #
   Tablets USP, #
Bisacodyl-containing Combinations, 3068
Bisacodyl and Docusate Sodium [*Dulcodos*]
   **See Laxatives (Local)**, #
   Tablets, #
*Bisacolax*—ICN (Canada) brand of Bisacodyl—**See Laxatives (Local)**, #
*Bisco-Lax*—Raway (U.S.) brand of Bisacodyl—**See Laxatives (Local)**, #
*Bismatrol*—Major (U.S.) brand of Bismuth Subsalicylate (Oral-Local), 616
*Bismatrol Extra Strength*—Major (U.S.) brand of Bismuth Subsalicylate (Oral-Local), 616
*Bismed*—Technilab (U.S.) brand of Bismuth Subsalicylate (Oral-Local), 616
Bismuth Subsalicylate [*Bismatrol; Bismatrol Extra Strength; Bismed; Helidac Therapy Chewable Tablets; Pepto-Bismol; Pepto-Bismol Easy-to-Swallow Caplets; Pepto-Bismol Maximum Strength; PMS-Bismuth Subsalicylate*]
   **(Oral-Local)**, 616
   Suspension, Oral, 619
   Tablets, 619
   Tablets, Chewable, 620, MC-4
Bismuth Subsalicylate, Metronidazole, and Tetracycline—for H. pylori [*Helidac*]
   **(Systemic)**, 620
   Blister card package, 623, MC-4
Bisoprolol-containing Combinations, 3068
Bisoprolol Fumarate [*Zebeta*]
   **See Beta-adrenergic Blocking Agents (Systemic)**, 593
   Tablets, 602, MC-4
Bisoprolol Fumarate and Hydrochlorothiazide [*Ziac*]
   **See Beta-adrenergic Blocking Agents and Thiazide Diuretics (Systemic)**, 609
   Tablets, 610, MC-4
Bispecific Antibody 520C9x22
   **(Systemic)**, 3133
Bitolterol Mesylate [*Tornalate*]
   **See Bronchodilators, Adrenergic (Inhalation-Local)**, 640
   Aerosol, Inhalation, 646
   Solution, Inhalation, 646
*Black-Draught*—Monticello (U.S.) brand of Casanthranol—**See Laxatives (Local)**, #
*Black-Draught Lax-Senna*—Monticello (U.S.) brand of Senna—**See Laxatives (Local)**, #
Black widow spider antivenin—*See* Antivenin (Latrodectus Mactans) (Systemic), #
*Blenoxane*—Bristol-Myers Oncology (U.S.) and Bristol (Canada) brand of Bleomycin (Systemic), 624; Bristol-Myers Squibb (U.S.) brand of Bleomycin (Systemic), 3134
Bleomycin [*Blenoxane*]
   **(Systemic)**, 624
   for Injection USP, 626
Bleomycin Sulfate [*Blenoxane*]
   **(Systemic)**, 3133
*Bleph-10*—Allergan (U.S. and Canada) brand of Sulfacetamide—**See Sulfonamides (Ophthalmic)**, 2651
*Blistex Daily Conditioning Treatment for Lips*—Blistex (U.S.) brand of Oxybenzone and Padimate O—**See Sunscreen Agents (Topical)**, #
*Blistex Medicated Lip Conditioner*—Blistex (Canada) brand of Oxybenzone and Padimate O—**See Sunscreen Agents (Topical)**, #
*Blistex Medicated Lip Conditioner with Sunscreen*—Blistex (Canada) brand of Menthyl Anthranilate and Padimate O—**See Sunscreen Agents (Topical)**, #
*Blistex Regular*—Blistex (U.S.) brand of Oxybenzone and Padimate O—**See Sunscreen Agents (Topical)**, #
*Blistex Sunblock*—Blistex (Canada) brand of Oxybenzone and Padimate O—**See Sunscreen Agents (Topical)**, #

*Blistex Ultraprotection*—Blistex (U.S. and Canada) brand of Homosalate, Menthyl Anthranilate, Octyl Methoxycinnamate, Octyl Salicylate, and Oxybenzone—**See Sunscreen Agents (Topical)**, #
*Blocadren*—Merck (U.S.) and Frosst (Canada) brand of Timolol—**See Beta-adrenergic Blocking Agents (Systemic)**, 593, MC-30
*Blue*—Ambix (U.S.); Balan (U.S.); Dixon-Shane (U.S.); and Harber (U.S.) brand of Pyrethrins and Piperonyl Butoxide (Topical), #
*Bonamine*—Pfizer (Canada) brand of Meclizine (Systemic), 1933
*Bonefos*—Leiras (U.S.) brand of Disodium Clodronate Tetrahydrate (Systemic), 3141
*Bonine*—Pfipharmecs (U.S.) brand of Meclizine (Systemic), 1933
*Bontril PDM*—Carnrick (U.S.) brand of Phendimetrazine—**See Appetite Suppressants (Systemic)**, 452
*Bontril Slow-Release*—Carnrick (U.S.) brand of Phendimetrazine—**See Appetite Suppressants (Systemic)**, 452
*Borocell*—Neutron Technology (U.S.) brand of Sodium Monomercaptoundecahydro-closo-dodecaborate (Systemic), 3164
*Botox*—Allergan (U.S. and Canada) brand of Botulinum Toxin Type A (Parenteral-Local), 627; 3134
Botulinum Toxin Type A [*Botox; Dysport*]
   **(Parenteral-Local)**, 627, 3134
   for Injection, 629
Botulinum Toxin Type B
   **(Parenteral-Local)**, 3134
Botulinum Toxin Type F
   **(Parenteral-Local)**, 3134
Botulism Immune Globulin
   **(Systemic)**, 3134
Bovine Colostrum
   **(Systemic)**, 3134
Bovine Immunoglobulin Concentrate, *Cryptosporidium parvum* [*Sporidin-G*]
   **(Systemic)**, 3134
Bovine Whey Protein Concentrate [*Immuno-C*]
   **(Systemic)**, 3134
Box jellyfish antivenom—*See* Antivenin (Chironex Fleckeri) (Systemic), #
B2036-PEG [*Trovert*]
   **(Systemic)**, 3133
*BQ Cold*—Bristol-Myers (U.S.) brand of Chlorpheniramine, Phenylpropanolamine, and Acetaminophen—**See Antihistamines, Decongestants, and Analgesics (Systemic)**, 366
Branched Chain Amino Acids
   **(Systemic)**, 3134
*BRAVADIR*—Bristol-Meyers Squibb (U.S.) brand of Sorivudine (Systemic), 3166
*Breonesin*—Sanofi Winthrop (U.S.) brand of Guaifenesin (Systemic), 1588
*Brethaire*—Ciba (U.S.) brand of Terbutaline—**See Bronchodilators, Adrenergic (Inhalation-Local)**, 640
*Brethine*—Novartis (U.S.) brand of Terbutaline—**See Bronchodilators, Adrenergic (Systemic)**, 651, MC-29
*Bretylate*—BW (Canada) brand of Bretylium (Systemic), 630
Bretylium tosilate—*See* Bretylium (Systemic), 630
Bretylium Tosylate [bretylium tosilate; *Bretylate; Bretylol*]
   **(Systemic)**, 630
   Injection, 630
Bretylium Tosylate in 5% Dextrose
   **(Systemic)**, 630
   Injection, 632
*Bretylol*—Du Pont Critical Care (U.S.) brand of Bretylium (Systemic), 630
*Brevibloc*—Du Pont Critical Care (U.S.) brand of Esmolol (Systemic), 1377
*Brevicon*—Searle (U.S.) brand of Norethindrone and Ethinyl Estradiol—**See Estrogens and Progestins—Oral Contraceptives (Systemic)**, 1397
*Brevicon 0.5/35*—Searle (Canada) brand of Norethindrone and Ethinyl Estradiol—**See Estrogens and Progestins—Oral Contraceptives (Systemic)**, 1397
*Brevicon 1/35*—Searle (Canada) brand of Norethindrone and Ethinyl Estradiol—**See Estrogens and Progestins—Oral Contraceptives (Systemic)**, 1397
*Brevital*—Lilly (U.S.) brand of Methohexital—**See Anesthetics, Barbiturate (Systemic)**, 161
*Brevoxyl-4 Cleansing Lotion*—Stiefel (U.S.) brand of Benzoyl Peroxide (Topical), 579

## General Index

*Brevoxyl-8 Cleansing Lotion*—Stiefel (U.S.) brand of Benzoyl Peroxide (Topical), 579
*Brevoxyl 4 Gel*—Stiefel (U.S.) brand of Benzoyl Peroxide (Topical), 579
*Brevoxyl-8 Gel*—Stiefel (U.S.) brand of Benzoyl Peroxide (Topical), 579
*Brexin L.A.*—Savage (U.S.) brand of Chlorpheniramine and Pseudoephedrine—**See Antihistamines and Decongestants (Systemic)**, 343
*Bricanyl*—Lakeside/Merrell Dow (U.S.) and Astra (Canada) brand of Terbutaline—**See Bronchodilators, Adrenergic (Systemic)**, 651
*Bricanyl Turbuhaler*—Astra (Canada) brand of Terbutaline—**See Bronchodilators, Adrenergic (Inhalation-Local)**, 640
*Brietal*—Lilly (Canada) brand of Methohexital—**See Anesthetics, Barbiturate (Systemic)**, 161
Brimonidine Tartrate [*Alphagan*]
  **(Ophthalmic)**, 632
  Solution, Ophthalmic, 633
Brinzolamide [*Azopt*]
  **(Ophthalmic)**, 634
  Suspension, Ophthalmic, 635
British Anti-Lewisite—*See* Dimercaprol (Systemic), 1224
*Brofed Liquid*—Marnel (U.S.) brand of Brompheniramine and Pseudoephedrine—**See Antihistamines and Decongestants (Systemic)**, 343
*Brolene*—Bausch & Lomb (U.S.) brand of Propamidine (Ophthalmic), 3160
*Bromadrine PD*—Rugby (U.S.) brand of Brompheniramine and Pseudoephedrine—**See Antihistamines and Decongestants (Systemic)**, 343
*Bromadrine TR*—Rugby (U.S.) brand of Brompheniramine and Pseudoephedrine—**See Antihistamines and Decongestants (Systemic)**, 343
*Bromaline*—Rugby (U.S.) brand of Brompheniramine and Phenylpropanolamine—**See Antihistamines and Decongestants (Systemic)**, 343
*Bromanate*—Barre-National and H.L. Moore (U.S.) brand of Brompheniramine and Phenylpropanolamine—**See Antihistamines and Decongestants (Systemic)**, 343
*Bromanate DC Cough*—Barre-National (U.S.); Moore (U.S.); and Zenith Goldline (U.S.) brand of Brompheniramine, Phenylpropanolamine, and Codeine—**See Cough/Cold Combinations (Systemic)**, 1024
*Bromanyl*—Aligen (U.S.); Barre-National (U.S.); Harber (U.S.); Moore (U.S.); Qualitest (U.S.); and Schein (U.S.) brand of Bromodiphenhydramine and Codeine—**See Cough/Cold Combinations (Systemic)**, 1024
*Bromarest DX Cough*—WC (U.S.) brand of Brompheniramine, Pseudoephedrine, and Dextromethorphan—**See Cough/Cold Combinations (Systemic)**, 1024
*Bromatane DX Cough*—Zenith Goldline (U.S.) brand of Brompheniramine, Pseudoephedrine, and Dextromethorphan—**See Cough/Cold Combinations (Systemic)**, 1024
*Bromatapp*—Copley and H.L. Moore (U.S.) brand of Brompheniramine and Phenylpropanolamine—**See Antihistamines and Decongestants (Systemic)**, 343
Bromazepam [*Alti-Bromazepam; Gen-Bromazepam; Lectopam*]
  **See Benzodiazepines (Systemic)**, 556
  Tablets, 565
*Bromazine*—Bromodiphenhydramine—**See Antihistamines (Systemic)**, 325
*Bromfed*—Muro (U.S.) brand of Brompheniramine and Pseudoephedrine—**See Antihistamines and Decongestants (Systemic)**, 343
*Bromfed-DM*—Muro (U.S.) brand of Brompheniramine, Pseudoephedrine, and Dextromethorphan—**See Cough/Cold Combinations (Systemic)**, 1024
*Bromfed-PD*—Muro (U.S.) brand of Brompheniramine and Pseudoephedrine—**See Antihistamines and Decongestants (Systemic)**, 343
*Bromfenex*—Ethex (U.S.) brand of Brompheniramine and Pseudoephedrine—**See Antihistamines and Decongestants (Systemic)**, 343
*Bromfenex PD*—Ethex (U.S.) brand of Brompheniramine and Pseudoephedrine—**See Antihistamines and Decongestants (Systemic)**, 343
Bromhexine
  **(Ophthalmic)**, 3134

Bromocriptine Mesylate [*Alti-Bromocriptine; Apo-Bromocriptine; Parlodel; Parlodel SnapTabs*]
  **(Systemic)**, 636
  Capsules USP, 639, MC-4
  Tablets USP, 639, MC-4
Bromodeoxyuridine
  **(Systemic)**, 3134
Bromodiphenhydramine [bromazine]
  **See Antihistamines (Systemic)**, 325
Bromodiphenhydramine-containing Combinations, 3068
Bromodiphenhydramine Hydrochloride and Codeine Phosphate [*Ambenyl Cough; Ambophen; Amgenal Cough; Bromanyl; Bromotuss with Codeine*]
  **See Cough/Cold Combinations (Systemic)**, 1024
  Syrup, 1033, 1034, 1037, 1038
Bromodiphenhydramine Hydrochloride, Diphenhydramine Hydrochloride, Codeine Phosphate, Ammonium Chloride, and Potassium Guaiacolsulfonate [*Ambenyl Cough*]
  **See Cough/Cold Combinations (Systemic)**, 1024
  Syrup, 1033
*Bromophen T.D.*—Rugby (U.S.) brand of Brompheniramine, Phenylephrine, and Phenylpropanolamine—**See Antihistamines and Decongestants (Systemic)**, 343
*Bromo-Seltzer*—Warner-Lambert (U.S.) brand of Acetaminophen, Sodium Bicarbonate, and Citric Acid (Systemic), 15
*Bromotuss with Codeine*—Rugby (U.S.) brand of Bromodiphenhydramine and Codeine—**See Cough/Cold Combinations (Systemic)**, 1024
*Bromphen*—Schein (U.S.) brand of Brompheniramine—**See Antihistamines (Systemic)**, 325
*Bromphen DC with Codeine Cough*—Rugby (U.S.) and Schein (U.S.) brand of Brompheniramine, Phenylpropanolamine, and Codeine—**See Cough/Cold Combinations (Systemic)**, 1024
*Bromphen DX Cough*—Rugby (U.S.) brand of Brompheniramine, Pseudoephedrine, and Dextromethorphan—**See Cough/Cold Combinations (Systemic)**, 1024
Brompheniramine-containing Combinations, 3068
Brompheniramine Maleate [*Bromphen; Dimetane; Dimetapp Allergy Liqui-Gels; Nasahist B*]
  **See Antihistamines (Systemic)**, 325
  Capsules, 332
  Elixir USP, 332
  Injection USP, 332
  Tablets USP, 332
Brompheniramine Maleate and Phenylephrine Hydrochloride [*Dimetane Decongestant; Dimetane Decongestant Caplets*]
  **See Antihistamines and Decongestants (Systemic)**, 343
  Elixir, 351
  Tablets, 351
Brompheniramine Maleate, Phenylephrine Hydrochloride, and Phenylpropanolamine Hydrochloride [*Bromophen T.D.; Dimetapp; Dimetapp Extentabs; Dimetapp Oral Infant Drops; Tamine S.R.*]
  **See Antihistamines and Decongestants (Systemic)**, 343
  Elixir, 351
  Solution, Oral, 352
  Tablets, 351
  Tablets, Extended-release, 346, 352, 361
Brompheniramine Maleate, Phenylephrine Hydrochloride, Phenylpropanolamine Hydrochloride, and Codeine Phosphate [*Dimetapp-C*]
  **See Cough/Cold Combinations (Systemic)**, 1024
  Syrup, 1053
Brompheniramine Maleate, Phenylephrine Hydrochloride, Phenylpropanolamine Hydrochloride, Codeine Phosphate, and Guaifenesin [*Dimetane Expectorant-C*]
  **See Cough/Cold Combinations (Systemic)**, 1024
  Solution, Oral, 1053
Brompheniramine Maleate, Phenylephrine Hydrochloride, Phenylpropanolamine Hydrochloride, and Dextromethorphan Hydrobromide [*Dimetapp-DM*]
  **See Cough/Cold Combinations (Systemic)**, 1024
  Elixir, 1053
  Tablets, 1053
Brompheniramine Maleate, Phenylephrine Hydrochloride, Phenylpropanolamine Hydrochloride, and Guaifenesin [*Dimetane Expectorant*]
  **See Cough/Cold Combinations (Systemic)**, 1024
  Solution, Oral, 1053

Brompheniramine Maleate, Phenylephrine Hydrochloride, Phenylpropanolamine Hydrochloride, Hydrocodone Bitartrate, and Guaifenesin [*Dimetane Expectorant-DC*]
  **See Cough/Cold Combinations (Systemic)**, 1024
  Solution, Oral, 1053
Brompheniramine Maleate and Phenylpropanolamine Hydrochloride [*Alcomed; Bromaline; Bromanate; Bromatapp; Cold and Allergy; Dimaphen; Dimaphen S.A.; Dimetapp; Dimetapp Chewables; Dimetapp Clear; Dimetapp Cold & Allergy; Dimetapp Cold & Allergy Quick Dissolve; Dimetapp Extentabs; Dimetapp 4-Hour; Dimetapp Liqui-Fills; E.N.T.; Genatap; Myphetapp; Vicks DayQuil 4 Hour Allergy Relief; Vicks DayQuil 12 Hour Allergy Relief*]
  **See Antihistamines and Decongestants (Systemic)**, 343
  Capsules, 352
  Elixir, 346, 349, 351, 353, 355
  Solution, Oral, 344, 351
  Tablets, 351, 352, 365
  Tablets, Chewable, 351
  Tablets, Extended-release, 346, 351, 352, 353, 365
Brompheniramine Maleate, Phenylpropanolamine Hydrochloride, and Acetaminophen [*Dimetapp Allergy Sinus Caplets; Dimetapp Cold & Fever Suspension*]
  **See Antihistamines, Decongestants, and Analgesics (Systemic)**, 366
  Suspension, Oral, 369
  Tablets, 369
Brompheniramine Maleate, Phenylpropanolamine Hydrochloride, and Codeine Phosphate [*Bromphen DC Cough; Bromphen DC with Codeine Cough; Dimetane-DC Cough; Myphetane DC Cough; Poly-Histine-CS*]
  **See Cough/Cold Combinations (Systemic)**, 1024
  Syrup, 1037, 1038, 1052, 1070, 1082
Brompheniramine Maleate, Phenylpropanolamine Hydrochloride, and Dextromethorphan Hydrobromide [*Dimetapp DM; Dimetapp DM Cold & Cough; Dimetapp Maximum Strength Cold & Cough Liqui-Gels; Histinex DM; Iohist DM; Liqui-Histine DM; Poly-Histine-DM; Siltapp with Dextromethorphan Cough & Cold*]
  **See Cough/Cold Combinations (Systemic)**, 1024
  Capsules, 1054
  Elixir, 1053, 1054, 1093
  Solution, Oral, 1067
  Syrup, 1063, 1069, 1082
Brompheniramine Maleate and Pseudoephedrine Hydrochloride [*Allent; Brofed Liquid; Bromadrine PD; Bromadrine TR; Bromfed; Bromfed-PD; Bromfenex; Bromfenex PD; Dallergy Jr.; Endafed; Iofed; Iofed PD; Lodrane LD; Lodrane Liquid; M-Hist; Nalfed; Nalfed-PD; Respahist; Rondec Chewable; Shellcap; Shellcap PD; Touro A&H; ULTRAbrom; ULTRAbrom PD*]
  **See Antihistamines and Decongestants (Systemic)**, 343
  Capsules, Extended-release, 344, 346, 347, 350, 353, 354, 355, 356, 359, 361, 362, 364
  Solution, Oral, 346, 355
  Syrup, 346, 347
  Tablets, 346
  Tablets, Chewable, 360
Brompheniramine Maleate, Pseudoephedrine Hydrochloride, and Acetaminophen [*Dristan Cold Maximum Strength Caplets*]
  **See Antihistamines, Decongestants, and Analgesics (Systemic)**, 366
  Tablets, 369
Brompheniramine Maleate, Pseudoephedrine Hydrochloride, and Dextromethorphan Hydrobromide [*Bromarest DX Cough; Bromatane DX Cough; Bromfed-DM; Bromphen DX Cough; Brotane DX Cough; Dimetane-DX Cough; Myphetane DX Cough*]
  **See Cough/Cold Combinations (Systemic)**, 1024
  Syrup, 1038, 1039, 1052, 1070
*Brompheril*—Copley (U.S.) brand of Dexbrompheniramine and Pseudoephedrine—**See Antihistamines and Decongestants (Systemic)**, 343
*Bronalide*—Syntex (Canada) brand of Flunisolide—**See Corticosteroids (Inhalation-Local)**, 955
*Bronchial*—H. L. Moore (U.S.) brand of Theophylline and Guaifenesin (Systemic), #
Bronchodilators, Adrenergic
  **(Inhalation-Local)**, 640

Bronchodilators, Adrenergic **(Systemic)**, 651
Bronchodilators, Theophylline **(Systemic)**, 668
*Broncho-Grippol-DM*—Charton (Canada) brand of Dextromethorphan (Systemic), 1191
*Broncholate*—Bock (U.S.) brand of Ephedrine and Guaifenesin—**See Cough/Cold Combinations (Systemic)**, 1024
*Broncomar GG*—Marlop (U.S.) brand of Theophylline and Guaifenesin (Systemic), #
*Brondelate*—Balan (U.S.); Barre (U.S.); CMC (U.S.); Dixon-Shane (U.S.); Gen-King (U.S.); Harber (U.S.); Major (U.S.); Schein (U.S.); and Texas Drug (U.S.) brand of Oxtriphylline and Guaifenesin (Systemic), #
*Bronkaid Mist*—Sanofi Winthrop (U.S.) brand of Epinephrine—**See Bronchodilators, Adrenergic (Inhalation-Local)**, 640
*Bronkaid Mistometer*—Sterling Winthrop (Canada) brand of Epinephrine—**See Bronchodilators, Adrenergic (Inhalation-Local)**, 640
*Bronkaid Suspension Mist*—Sanofi Winthrop (U.S.) brand of Epinephrine—**See Bronchodilators, Adrenergic (Inhalation-Local)**, 640
*Bronkephrine*—Sanofi Winthrop (U.S.) brand of Ethylnorepinephrine—**See Bronchodilators, Adrenergic (Systemic)**, 651
*Bronkometer*—Sanofi Winthrop (U.S.) brand of Isoetharine—**See Bronchodilators, Adrenergic (Inhalation-Local)**, 640
*Bronkosol*—Sanofi Winthrop (U.S.) brand of Isoetharine—**See Bronchodilators, Adrenergic (Inhalation-Local)**, 640
*Bronkotuss Expectorant*—Hyrex (U.S.) brand of Chlorpheniramine, Ephedrine, and Guaifenesin— **See Cough/Cold Combinations (Systemic)**, 1024
*Brontex*—Procter & Gamble (U.S.) brand of Codeine and Guaifenesin—**See Cough/Cold Combinations (Systemic)**, 1024
*Brotane DX Cough*—Bioline (U.S.) brand of Brompheniramine, Pseudoephedrine, and Dextromethorphan—**See Cough/Cold Combinations (Systemic)**, 1024
Brown snake antivenom—*See* Antivenin (Pseudonaja Textilis) (Systemic), #
*Bucet*—UAD (U.S.) brand of Butalbital and Acetaminophen—**See Barbiturates and Analgesics (Systemic)**, 532
*Buckley's DM*—Buckley (Canada) brand of Pseudoephedrine and Dextromethorphan—**See Cough/Cold Combinations (Systemic)**, 1024
Buclizine Hydrochloride **(Systemic)**, #
  Tablets, Chewable, #
Budesonide [*Entocort*]
  **(Rectal)**, 973
  Enema, 977
Budesonide [*Entocort*]
  **(Systemic)**, 3012
  Capsules, Extended-release, 3012
Budesonide [*Pulmicort Nebuamp; Pulmicort Turbuhaler*]
  **See Corticosteroids (Inhalation-Local)**, 955
  for Inhalation (Powder), 959
  Suspension for Inhalation, 960
Budesonide [*Rhinocort Aqua; Rhinocort Nasal Inhaler; Rhinocort Turbuhaler*]
  **See Corticosteroids (Nasal)**, 961, 3012
  Aerosol, Nasal, 3012
  Powder, Nasal, 965, 3012
  Solution, Nasal, 965, 3012
Bufexamac [*Norfemac; Parfenac*]
  **(Topical)**, 3013
  Cream, 3013
  Ointment, 3013
*Bufferin Caplets*—Bristol-Myers (U.S. and Canada) brand of Aspirin, Buffered—**See Salicylates (Systemic)**, 2538
*Bufferin Extra Strength Caplets*—Bristol-Myers (Canada) brand of Aspirin, Buffered—**See Salicylates (Systemic)**, 2538
*Bufferin Tablets*—Bristol-Myers (U.S.) brand of Aspirin, Buffered—**See Salicylates (Systemic)**, 2538
*Buffets II*—Jones (U.S.) brand of Acetaminophen, Aspirin, and Caffeine, Buffered—**See Acetaminophen and Salicylates (Systemic)**, 11
*Buffex*—Aspirin, Buffered—**See Salicylates (Systemic)**, 2538

*Buffinol*—Otis Clapp (U.S.) brand of Aspirin, Buffered—**See Salicylates (Systemic)**, 2538
*Buffinol Extra*—Otis Clapp (U.S.) brand of Aspirin, Buffered—**See Salicylates (Systemic)**, 2538
*Buf-Puf Acne Cleansing Bar with Vitamin E*—Personal Care Products/3M (U.S.) brand of Salicylic Acid (Topical), #
*Bullfrog Body*—Chattem (U.S.) brand of Octocrylene, Octyl Methoxycinnamate and Oxybenzone— **See Sunscreen Agents (Topical)**, #
*Bullfrog Extra Moisturizing*—Chattem (U.S.) brand of Octocrylene, Octyl Methoxycinnamate, and Oxybenzone—**See Sunscreen Agents (Topical)**, #
*Bullfrog For Kids*—Chattem (U.S.) brand of Octocrylene, Octyl Methoxycinnamate, and Oxybenzone—**See Sunscreen Agents (Topical)**, #
*Bullfrog Original Concentrated*—Chattem (U.S.) brand of Octocrylene, Octyl Methoxycinnamate, and Oxybenzone—**See Sunscreen Agents (Topical)**, #
*Bullfrog Sport*—Chattem (U.S.) brand of Octocrylene, Octyl Methoxycinnamate, Octyl Salicylate, Oxybenzone, and Titanium Dioxide—**See Sunscreen Agents (Topical)**, #
*Bullfrog Sunblock*—Chattem (U.S.) brand of Octyl Methoxycinnamate and Oxybenzone—**See Sunscreen Agents (Topical)**, #
Bumetanide [*Bumex*]
  **See Diuretics, Loop (Systemic)**, 1259
  Injection USP, 1263
  Tablets USP, 1262, MC-4
*Bumex*—Roche (U.S.) brand of Bumetanide—**See Diuretics, Loop (Systemic)**, 1259, MC-4
*Buminate 5%*—Baxter (U.S.) brand of Albumin Human (Systemic), 34
*Buminate 25%*—Baxter (U.S.) brand of Albumin Human (Systemic), 34
*Buphenyl*—Ucyclyd (U.S.) brand of Sodium Phenylbutyrate (Systemic), #
Bupivacaine-containing Combinations, 3068
Bupivacaine Hydrochloride [*Marcaine; Sensorcaine; Sensorcaine-MPF*]
  **See Anesthetics (Parenteral-Local)**, 139
  Injection USP, 145
Bupivacaine Hydrochloride in Dextrose [*Marcaine; Marcaine Spinal; Sensorcaine-MPF Spinal*]
  **See Anesthetics (Parenteral-Local)**, 139
  Injection USP, 147
Bupivacaine Hydrochloride and Epinephrine [*Marcaine; Sensorcaine; Sensorcaine Forte; Sensorcaine-MPF*]
  **See Anesthetics (Parenteral-Local)**, 139
  Injection USP, 146
*Buprenex*—Reckitt & Colman (U.S.) brand of Buprenorphine (Systemic), 683
Buprenorphine Hydrochloride [*Buprenex*]
  **(Systemic)**, 683, 3135
  Injection, 687
Buprenorphine and Naloxone **(Systemic)**, 3135
Bupropion Hydrochloride [amfebutamone; *Wellbutrin; Wellbutrin SR; Zyban*]
  **(Systemic)**, 687
  Tablets, 691, MC-4
  Tablets, Extended-release, 691, MC-4
*Buscopan*—Boehringer Ingelheim (Canada) brand of Scopolamine—**See Anticholinergics/Antispasmodics (Systemic)**, 226
Buserelin Acetate [*Suprefact*]
  **(Systemic)**, 691
  Injection, 693
  Solution, Nasal, 692
*Busodium*—Truxton (U.S.) brand of Butabarbital— **See Barbiturates (Systemic)**, 518
*BuSpar*—Mead Johnson (U.S. and Canada) brand of Buspirone (Systemic), 693, MC-4
*BuSpar DIVIDOSE*—Bristol-Myers Squibb (U.S.) brand of Buspirone (Systemic), 693
Buspirone Hydrochloride [*BuSpar; BuSpar DIVIDOSE; Bustab*]
  **(Systemic)**, 693
  Tablets, 695, MC-4
*Bustab*—ICN (Canada) brand of Buspirone (Systemic), 693
Busulfan [*Myleran*]
  **(Systemic)**, 695, 3135
  Tablets USP, 698, MC-4
Butabarbital-containing Combinations, 3068

Butabarbital Sodium [*Busodium; Butalan; Butisol; Sarisol No. 2*]
  **See Barbiturates (Systemic)**, 518
  Elixir USP, 525
  Tablets USP, 525
*Butace*—American Urologicals (U.S.) brand of Butalbital, Acetaminophen, and Caffeine—**See Barbiturates and Analgesics (Systemic)**, 532
*Butalan*—Lannett (U.S.) brand of Butabarbital—**See Barbiturates (Systemic)**, 518
*Butalbital-AC*—Butalbital, Aspirin, and Caffeine—**See Barbiturates and Analgesics (Systemic)**, 532
Butalbital and Acetaminophen [*Bancap; Bucet; Conten; Phrenilin; Phrenilin Forte; Sedapap; Tencon; Triaprin*]
  **See Barbiturates and Analgesics (Systemic)**, 532
  Capsules, 541
  Tablets, 541
Butalbital, Acetaminophen, and Caffeine [*Amaphen; Anolor-300; Anoquan; Arcet; Butace;* co-bucafAPAP; *Dolmar; Endolor; Esgic; Esgic-Plus; Ezol; Femcet; Fioricet; Isocet; Isopap; Medigesic; Pacaps; Pharmagesic; Repan; Tencet; Triad; Two-Dyne*]
  **See Barbiturates and Analgesics (Systemic)**, 532
  Capsules USP, 541, MC-4
  Tablets USP, 541, MC-4
Butalbital, Acetaminophen, Caffeine, and Codeine Phosphate [*Fioricet with Codeine*]
  **See Barbiturates and Analgesics (Systemic)**, 532
  Capsules, 542, MC-4
Butalbital and Aspirin [*Axotal*]
  **See Barbiturates and Analgesics (Systemic)**, 532
  Tablets USP, 542
Butalbital, Aspirin, and Caffeine [butalbital-AC; butalbital compound; *Butalgen; Fiorgen; Fiorinal; Fiormor; Fortabs; Isobutal; Isobutyl; Isolin; Isollyl; Laniroif; Lanorinal; Marnal; Tecnal; Vibutal*]
  **See Barbiturates and Analgesics (Systemic)**, 532
  Capsules USP, 542, MC-4
  Tablets USP, 543, MC-4
Butalbital, Aspirin, Caffeine, and Codeine Phosphate [*Ascomp with Codeine No.3; Butalbital Compound with Codeine; Butinal with Codeine No. 3; Fioricet with Codeine; Fiorinal-C 1/4; Fiorinal-C 1/2; Fiorinal with Codeine No.3; Idenal with Codeine; Isollyl with Codeine; Tecnal-C 1/4; Tecnal-C 1/2*]
  **See Barbiturates and Analgesics (Systemic)**, 532
  Capsules USP, 543, MC-4
  Tablets, 545
*Butalbital Compound with Codeine*—Best Generics (U.S.); Dixon-Shane (U.S.); Parmed (U.S.); and Qualitest (U.S.) brand of Butalbital, Aspirin, Caffeine, and Codeine—**See Barbiturates and Analgesics (Systemic)**, 532
Butalbital-containing Combinations, 3068
*Butalgen*—Genetco (U.S.) brand of Butalbital, Aspirin, and Caffeine—**See Barbiturates and Analgesics (Systemic)**, 532
Butamben-containing Combinations, 3068
Butamben Picrate [*Butesin Picrate;* butyl aminobenzoate]
  **See Anesthetics (Topical)**, 155
  Ointment, 159
*Butazolidin*—Geigy (Canada) brand of Phenylbutazone—**See Anti-inflammatory Drugs, Nonsteroidal (Systemic)**, 388
Butenafine Hydrochloride [*Mentax*]
  **(Topical)**, 699
  Cream, 700
*Butesin Picrate*—Abbott (U.S.) brand of Butamben— **See Anesthetics (Topical)**, 155
*Butibel*—Wallace (U.S.) brand of Belladonna and Butabarbital—**See Belladonna Alkaloids and Barbiturates (Systemic)**, 551
*Butinal with Codeine No.3*—Breckenridge (U.S.) brand of Butalbital, Aspirin, Caffeine, and Codeine—**See Barbiturates and Analgesics (Systemic)**, 532
*Butisol*—Wallace (U.S.) and Horner (Canada) brand of Butabarbital—**See Barbiturates (Systemic)**, 518

# General Index

Butoconazole Nitrate [*Femstat 3*]
    **See Antifungals, Azole (Vaginal)**, 310
    Cream USP (Vaginal), 312
    Suppositories, Vaginal, 312
Butorphanol Tartrate [*Stadol*]
    **See Opioid (Narcotic) Analgesics (Systemic)**, 2168
    Injection USP, 2174
Butorphanol Tartrate [*Stadol NS*]
    **(Nasal-Systemic)**, 700
    Solution, Nasal, 703
Butyl aminobenzoate—Butamben—**See Anesthetics (Topical)**, 155
1,5-(Butylimino)-1,5 Dideoxy,D-Glucitol
    **(Systemic)**, 3127
Butyrylcholinesterase
    **(Systemic)**, 3135

## C

C2—Wampole (Canada) brand of Aspirin—**See Salicylates (Systemic)**, 2538
Cabergoline [*Dostinex*]
    **(Systemic)**, 704
    Tablets, 706
*Cachexon*—Telluride (U.S.) brand of L-Glutathione, Reduced (Systemic), 3162
*Caelyx*—Sequus (Canada) brand of Doxorubicin, Liposomal (Systemic), 1312
*Cafergot*—Sandoz (U.S. and Canada) brand of Ergotamine and Caffeine—**See Vascular Headache Suppressants, Ergot Derivative–containing (Systemic)**, 2925
*Cafergot-PB*—Sandoz (Canada) brand of Ergotamine, Caffeine, Belladonna Alkaloids, and Pentobarbital—**See Vascular Headache Suppressants, Ergot Derivative–containing (Systemic)**, 2925
*Cafertine*—Balan (U.S.) brand of Ergotamine and Caffeine—**See Vascular Headache Suppressants, Ergot Derivative–containing (Systemic)**, 2925
*Cafetrate*—Qualitest (U.S.) brand of Ergotamine and Caffeine—**See Vascular Headache Suppressants, Ergot Derivative–containing (Systemic)**, 2925
*Caffedrine*—Thompson (U.S. and Canada) brand of Caffeine (Systemic), 706
*Caffedrine Caplets*—Thompson (U.S.) brand of Caffeine (Systemic), 706
Caffeine [*Caffedrine; Caffedrine Caplets; Dexitac; Enerjets; Keep Alert; Neocaf, NoDoz; NoDoz Maximum Strength Caplets; Pep-Back; Quick Pep; Ultra Pep-Back; Vivarin; Wake-Up*]
    **(Systemic)**, 706, 3135
    Capsules, Extended-release, 709
    Tablets, 709
Caffeine, Citrated
    **See Caffeine (Systemic)**, 706
    Injection, 710
    Solution, 710
    Tablets, 710
Caffeine-containing Combinations, 3068
Caffeine and Sodium Benzoate
    **See Caffeine (Systemic)**, 706
    Injection USP, 710
Calamine [*Calamox; Diaper Rash Ointment; Onguent de Calamine*]
    **(Topical)**, #
    Lotion USP, #
    Ointment, #
*Calamox*—Hauck (U.S.) brand of Calamine (Topical), #
*Calan*—Searle (U.S.) brand of Verapamil—**See Calcium Channel Blocking Agents (Systemic)**, 720, MC-32
*Calan SR*—Searle (U.S.) brand of Verapamil—**See Calcium Channel Blocking Agents (Systemic)**, 720, MC-32
*Calcarb 600*—Goldline (U.S.) brand of Calcium Carbonate—**See Calcium Supplements (Systemic)**, 736
*Calcibind*—Mission (U.S.) brand of Cellulose Sodium Phosphate (Systemic), #
*Calci-Chew*—R & D (U.S.) brand of Calcium Carbonate—**See Calcium Supplements (Systemic)**, 736
*Calciday 667*—Nature's Bounty (U.S.) brand of Calcium Carbonate—**See Calcium Supplements (Systemic)**, 736

*Calcidrine*—Abbott (U.S.) brand of Codeine and Calcium Iodide—**See Cough/Cold Combinations (Systemic)**, 1024
Calcifediol [*Calderol*; vitamin D]
    **See Vitamin D and Analogs (Systemic)**, 2966
    Capsules USP, 2970
*Calciferol*—Kremers-Urban (U.S. and Canada) brand of Ergocalciferol—**See Vitamin D and Analogs (Systemic)**, 2966
*Calciferol Drops*—Kremers-Urban (U.S.) brand of Ergocalciferol—**See Vitamin D and Analogs (Systemic)**, 2966
*Calciject*—Omega (Canada) brand of Calcium Chloride—**See Calcium Supplements (Systemic)**, 736
*Calcijex*—Abbott (U.S. and Canada) brand of Calcitriol—**See Vitamin D and Analogs (Systemic)**, 2966
*Calcilac*—Schein (U.S.) brand of Calcium Carbonate—**See Calcium Supplements (Systemic)**, 736
*Calcilean*—Organon (Canada) brand of Heparin (Systemic), 1617
*Calcimar*—Rhône-Poulenc Rorer (U.S. and Canada) brand of Calcitonin-Salmon—**See Calcitonin (Systemic)**, 716
*Calci-Mix*—R & D (U.S.) brand of Calcium Carbonate—**See Calcium Supplements (Systemic)**, 736
*Calcionate*—Calcium Glubionate—**See Calcium Supplements (Systemic)**, 736
*Calciparine*—Du Pont Critical Care (U.S.) and Anglo-French (Canada) brand of Heparin (Systemic), 1617
Calcipotriene [*Calcipotriol*; *Dovonex*; MC 903]
    **(Topical)**, 711
    Cream, 713
    Ointment, 713
    Solution, 714
Calcipotriol—*See* Calcipotriene (Topical), 711
*Calcite 500*—Riva (Canada) brand of Calcium Carbonate—**See Calcium Supplements (Systemic)**, 736
Calcitonin
    **(Systemic)**, 716
Calcitonin-Human [*Cibacalcin*]
    **See Calcitonin (Systemic)**, 716, 3135
    for Injection, 718, 3135
Calcitonin-Salmon [*Miacalcin*]
    **(Nasal-Systemic)**, 714
    Solution, Nasal, 716
Calcitonin-Salmon [*Calcimar; Miacalcin*]
    **See Calcitonin (Systemic)**, 716
    Injection, 718
Calcitriol [*Calcijex; Rocaltrol*; vitamin D]
    **See Vitamin D and Analogs (Systemic)**, 2966
    Capsules, 2970, MC-5
    Injection, 2970
    Solution, Oral, 2970
*Calcium 600*—Schein (U.S.) brand of Calcium Carbonate—**See Calcium Supplements (Systemic)**, 736
Calcium Acetate [*Phos-Lo*]
    **See Calcium Supplements (Systemic)**, 719, 736, 3135
    Injection, 742
    Tablets, 720, 3135, MC-5
Calcium Carbonate [*Alka-Mints; Alkets; Alkets Extra Strength; Amitone; Calglycine; Chooz; Dicarbosil; Equilet; Mallamint; Mylanta; Titralac; Titralac Extra Strength; Trial; Tums; Tums E-X; Tums Extra Strength; Tums Ultra*]
    **See Antacids (Oral-Local)**, 188
    Gum, Chewing, 203
    Lozenges, 211
    Suspension, Oral, USP, 202
    Tablets USP, 202
    Tablets USP (Chewable), 198, 200, 202, 203, 204, 210, 215, 216
Calcium Carbonate [*Alka-Mints; Amitone; Apo-Cal; BioCal; Calcarb 600; Calci-Chew; Calciday 667; Calcilac; Calci-Mix; Calcite 500; Calcium 600; Calglycine; Cal-Plus; Calsan; Caltrate 600; Caltrate Jr. Chooz; Dicarbosil; Gencalc 600; Liqui-Cal; Liquid Cal-600; Maalox Antacid Caplets; Mallamint; Nephro-Calci; Nu-Cal; Os-Cal; Os-Cal 500; Os-Cal Chewable; Os-Cal 500 Chewable; Oysco; Oysco 500 Chewable; Oyst-Cal 500; Oystercal 500; R & D Calcium Carbonate/600; Rolaids Calcium Rich; Titralac; Tums; Tums 500; Tums E-X; Tums Extra Strength; Tums Regular Strength*]

Calcium Carbonate (*continued*)
    **See Calcium Supplements (Systemic)**, 736, 3135
    Capsules, 742
    Suspension, Oral, USP, 742
    Tablets USP, 742
    Tablets USP (Chewable), 743
    Tablets (Oyster-Shell Derived), 743
    Tablets (Oyster-Shell Derived) (Chewable), 743
Calcium Carbonate–containing Combinations, 3069
Calcium Carbonate and Magnesia [*Gaviscon Acid Relief; Gaviscon Extra Strength Acid Relief; Mylanta; Mylanta Double Strength; Mylanta Gelcaps; Rolaids; Rolaids Extra Strength*]
    **See Antacids (Oral-Local)**, 188
    Suspension, Oral, 205
    Suspension, Oral, USP, 212
    Tablets, 212
    Tablets USP (Chewable), 205, 211, 212, 214
Calcium Carbonate, Magnesia, and Simethicone [*Advanced Formula Di-Gel; Diovol Plus AF; Gaviscon Acid Plus Gas Relief*]
    **See Antacids (Oral-Local)**, 188
    Suspension, Oral, 204, 205
    Tablets, Chewable, 204
    Tablets USP (Chewable), 198, 205
Calcium and Magnesium Carbonates [*Antacid Gelcaps; Maalox Antacid Caplets; Marblen; Mi-Acid*]
    **See Antacids (Oral-Local)**, 188
    Suspension, Oral, 210
    Tablets USP, 201, 208, 210
Calcium and Magnesium Carbonates and Sodium Bicarbonate [*Gaviscon Heartburn Relief*]
    **See Antacids (Oral-Local)**, 188
    Suspension, Oral, 205
Calcium Carbonate and Simethicone [*Titralac Plus; Tums Anti-gas/Antacid*]
    **See Antacids (Oral-Local)**, 188
    Suspension, Oral, 215
    Tablets, Chewable, 216
Calcium Channel Blocking Agents
    **(Systemic)**, 720
Calcium Chloride [*Calciject*]
    **See Calcium Supplements (Systemic)**, 736
    Injection USP, 744
Calcium Citrate [*Citracal; Citracal Liquitabs*]
    **See Calcium Supplements (Systemic)**, 736
    Tablets, 744
    Tablets, Effervescent, 744
*Calcium Disodium Versenate*—3M Riker (U.S.) and Riker (Canada) brand of Edetate Calcium Disodium (Systemic), 1324
Calcium EDTA—*See* Edetate Calcium Disodium (Systemic), 1324
Calcium Glubionate [*Calcionate; Calcium-Sandoz; Neo-Calglucon*]
    **See Calcium Supplements (Systemic)**, 736
    Syrup USP, 744
Calcium Gluceptate [calcium glucoheptonate]
    **See Calcium Supplements (Systemic)**, 736
    Injection USP, 745
Calcium Gluceptate and Calcium Gluconate [*Calcium Stanley*]
    **See Calcium Supplements (Systemic)**, 736, 3135
    Solution, Oral, 745
Calcium Gluconate
    **See Calcium Supplements (Systemic)**, 736
    Injection USP, 746
    Tablets USP, 746
    Tablets USP (Chewable), 746
Calcium Gluconate [*H-F Gel*]
    **(Topical)**, 3136
    Gel, 3136
Calcium Glycerophosphate and Calcium Lactate [*Calphosan*]
    **See Calcium Supplements (Systemic)**, 736
    Injection, 747
Calcium Lactate
    **See Calcium Supplements (Systemic)**, 736
    Tablets USP, 747
Calcium Lactate-Gluconate and Calcium Carbonate [*Calcium-Sandoz Forte; Gramcal*]
    **See Calcium Supplements (Systemic)**, 736
    Tablets, Effervescent, 747
Calcium Pantothenate [vitamin $B_5$]
    **See Pantothenic Acid (Systemic)**, #
    Tablets USP, #
Calcium Phosphate, Dibasic, #
    **See Calcium Supplements (Systemic)**, 736
    Tablets USP, 748

Calcium Phosphate, Tribasic [*Posture*]
See **Calcium Supplements (Systemic)**, 736
Tablets, 748
Calcium Polycarbophil [*Equalactin; Fibercon Caplets; Fiber-Lax; FiberNorm; Konsyl; Mitrolan*]
See **Laxatives (Local)**, #
Tablets, #
Tablets, Chewable, #
*Calcium-Sandoz*—Sandoz (Canada) brand of Calcium Glubionate—See **Calcium Supplements (Systemic)**, 736
*Calcium-Sandoz Forte*—Sandoz (Canada) brand of Calcium Lactate-Gluconate and Calcium Carbonate—See **Calcium Supplements (Systemic)**, 736
*Calcium Stanley*—Stanley (Canada) brand of Calcium Gluceptate and Calcium Gluconate—See **Calcium Supplements (Systemic)**, 736
Calcium Supplements
**(Systemic)**, 736
*CaldeCORT Anti-Itch*—Pharmacraft (U.S.) brand of Hydrocortisone—See **Corticosteroids (Topical)**, 978
*CaldeCORT Light*—Pharmacraft (U.S.) brand of Hydrocortisone—See **Corticosteroids (Topical)**, 978
*Calderol*—Upjohn (U.S.) brand of Calcifediol—See **Vitamin D and Analogs (Systemic)**, 2966
*Caldesene Medicated Powder*—Fisons (U.S.) brand of Undecylenic Acid, Compound (Topical), #
*Caldomine-DH Forte*—Technilab (Canada) brand of Pheniramine, Pyrilamine, Phenylpropanolamine, and Hydrocodone—See **Cough/Cold Combinations (Systemic)**, 1024
*Caldomine-DH Pediatric*—Technilab (Canada) brand of Pheniramine, Pyrilamine, Phenylpropanolamine, and Hydrocodone—See **Cough/Cold Combinations (Systemic)**, 1024
Calfactant [*Infasurf*]
**(Intratracheal-Local)**, 3013
*Calglycine*—Rugby (U.S.) brand of Calcium Carbonate—See **Antacids (Oral-Local)**, 188; **Calcium Supplements (Systemic)**, 736, 736
*Calgonate*—Calgonate (U.S.) brand of Calcium Gluconate (Topical), 3135
*Calicylic Creme*—Gordon (U.S.) brand of Salicylic Acid (Topical), #
*Calmine*—Aspirin—See **Salicylates (Systemic)**, 2538
*Calm X*—Republic (U.S.) brand of Dimenhydrinate—See **Antihistamines (Systemic)**, 325
*Calmydone*—Technilab (Canada) brand of Doxylamine, Etafedrine, and Hydrocodone—See **Cough/Cold Combinations (Systemic)**, 1024
*Calmylin #1*—Technilab (Canada) brand of Dextromethorphan (Systemic), 1191
*Calmylin #2*—Technilab (Canada) brand of Pseudoephedrine and Dextromethorphan—See **Cough/Cold Combinations (Systemic)**, 1024
*Calmylin #3*—Technilab (Canada) brand of Pseudoephedrine, Dextromethorphan, and Guaifenesin—See **Cough/Cold Combinations (Systemic)**, 1024
*Calmylin #4*—Technilab (Canada) brand of Diphenhydramine, Dextromethorphan, and Ammonium Chloride—See **Cough/Cold Combinations (Systemic)**, 1024
*Calmylin Codeine D-E*—Technilab (Canada) brand of Pseudoephedrine, Codeine, and Guaifenesin—See **Cough/Cold Combinations (Systemic)**, 1024
*Calmylin Cough & Flu*—Technilab (Canada) brand of Pseudoephedrine, Dextromethorphan, Guaifenesin, and Acetaminophen—See **Cough/Cold Combinations (Systemic)**, 1024
*Calmylin DM-D-E Extra Strength*—Technilab (Canada) brand of Pseudoephedrine, Dextromethorphan, and Guaifenesin—See **Cough/Cold Combinations (Systemic)**, 1024
*Calmylin DM-E*—Technilab (Canada) brand of Dextromethorphan and Guaifenesin—See **Cough/Cold Combinations (Systemic)**, 1024
*Calmylin Expectorant*—Technilab (Canada) brand of Guaifenesin (Systemic), 1588
*Calmylin Original with Codeine*—Technilab (Canada) brand of Diphenhydramine, Codeine, and Ammonium Chloride—See **Cough/Cold Combinations (Systemic)**, 1024
*Calmylin Pediatric*—Technilab (Canada) brand of Pseudoephedrine and Dextromethorphan—See **Cough/Cold Combinations (Systemic)**, 1024

*Calphosan*—Glenwood (U.S.) brand of Calcium Glycerophosphate and Calcium Lactate—See **Calcium Supplements (Systemic)**, 736
*Cal-Plus*—Geriatric (U.S.) brand of Calcium Carbonate—See **Calcium Supplements (Systemic)**, 736
*Calsan*—Sandoz (Canada) brand of Calcium Carbonate—See **Calcium Supplements (Systemic)**, 736
*Caltrate 600*—Lederle (U.S. and Canada) brand of Calcium Carbonate—See **Calcium Supplements (Systemic)**, 736
*Caltrate Jr.*—Lederle (U.S. and Canada) brand of Calcium Carbonate—See **Calcium Supplements (Systemic)**, 736
*Cama Arthritis Pain Reliever*—Sandoz Consumer (U.S.) brand of Aspirin, Buffered—See **Salicylates (Systemic)**, 2538
Campath-1H, 3136
*Cam-Ap-Es*—Camall (U.S.) brand of Reserpine, Hydralazine, and Hydrochlorothiazide (Systemic), #
Camphorated opium tincture—See Paregoric (Systemic), #
*Camptosar*—Pharmacia & Upjohn (U.S. and Canada) brand of Irinotecan (Systemic), 1769
Candesartan [*Atacand*]
**(Systemic)**, MC-5
Tablets, MC-5
*Canesten 1-Day Cream Combi-Pak*—Bayer (Canada) brand of Clotrimazole—See **Antifungals, Azole (Vaginal)**, 310
*Canesten 1-Day Therapy*—Bayer (Canada) brand of Clotrimazole—See **Antifungals, Azole (Vaginal)**, 310
*Canesten 3-Day Therapy*—Bayer (Canada) brand of Clotrimazole—See **Antifungals, Azole (Vaginal)**, 310
*Canesten Combi-Pak 1-Day Therapy*—Bayer (Canada) brand of Clotrimazole—See **Antifungals, Azole (Vaginal)**, 310
*Canesten Combi-Pak 3-Day Therapy*—Bayer (Canada) brand of Clotrimazole—See **Antifungals, Azole (Vaginal)**, 310
*Canesten Cream*—Miles (Canada) brand of Clotrimazole (Topical), 916
*Canesten 6-Day Therapy*—Bayer (Canada) brand of Clotrimazole—See **Antifungals, Azole (Vaginal)**, 310
*Canesten Solution*—Miles (Canada) brand of Clotrimazole (Topical), 916
*Canesten Solution with Atomizer*—Miles (Canada) brand of Clotrimazole (Topical), 916
*Can Screen 400 Sunscreen*—Tican (Canada) brand of Avobenzone, Octyl Methoxycinnamate, and Oxybenzone—See **Sunscreen Agents (Topical)**, #
*Cantil*—Merrell Dow (U.S.) brand of Mepenzolate—See **Anticholinergics/Antispasmodics (Systemic)**, 226
*Capastat*—Lilly (U.S. and Canada) brand of Capreomycin (Systemic), 751
Capecitabine [*Xeloda*]
**(Systemic)**, 748, MC-5
Tablets, 751, MC-5
*Capen*—Phoenix (Argentina) brand of Tiopronin (Systemic), 2824
*Capital with Codeine*—Carnrick (U.S.) brand of Acetaminophen and Codeine—See **Opioid (Narcotic) Analgesics and Acetaminophen (Systemic)**, 2198
*Capitrol*—Westwood (U.S.) brand of Chloroxine (Topical), #
*Capoten*—Bristol-Myers Squibb (U.S. and Canada) brand of Captopril—See **Angiotensin-converting Enzyme (ACE) Inhibitors (Systemic)**, 177, MC-5
*Capozide*—Bristol-Myers Squibb (U.S.) brand of Captopril and Hydrochlorothiazide—See **Angiotensin-converting Enzyme (ACE) Inhibitors and Hydrochlorothiazide (Systemic)**, 187, MC-5
Capreomycin Sulfate [*Capastat*]
**(Systemic)**, 751
Sterile USP, 753
Capsaicin [*Zostrix; Zostrix-HP*]
**(Topical)**, 753
Cream, 755
*Captimer*—Fresenius (Germany) brand of Tiopronin (Systemic), 2824

Captopril [*Capoten*]
See **Angiotensin-converting Enzyme (ACE) Inhibitors (Systemic)**, 177
Tablets USP, 183, MC-5
Captopril-containing Combinations, 3069
Captopril and Hydrochlorothiazide [*Capozide*]
See **Angiotensin-converting Enzyme (ACE) Inhibitors and Hydrochlorothiazide (Systemic)**, 187
Tablets, 187, MC-5
*Carafate*—Hoechst Marion Roussel (U.S.) brand of Sucralfate (Oral-Local), 2635, MC-28
Caramiphen-containing Combinations, 3069
Carbachol [carbamylcholine; *Carbastat; Carboptic; Isopto Carbachol; Miostat*]
**(Ophthalmic)**, 755, 3013
Solution, Intraocular, USP, 757, 3013
Solution, Ophthalmic, USP, 757
*Carbacot*—Truxton (U.S.) brand of Methocarbamol—See **Skeletal Muscle Relaxants (Systemic)**, 2577
Carbamazepine [*Apo-Carbamazepine; Atretol; Epitol; Novo-Carbamaz; Nu-Carbamazepine; Tegretol; Tegretol Chewtabs; Tegretol CR; Tegretrol-XR*]
**(Systemic)**, 757
Capsules, Extended-release, 764
Suspension, Oral, USP, 763
Tablets USP, 763, MC-5
Tablets USP (Chewable), 764, MC-5
Tablets, Extended-release, 764, MC-5
Carbamide—See Urea (Parenteral-Local), #
Carbamylcholine—See Carbachol (Ophthalmic), 755
Carbamylglutamic Acid, 3136
*Carbastat*—Ciba Vision (U.S.and Canada) brand of Carbachol (Ophthalmic), 3013
Carbenicillin Disodium [*Geopen; Pyopen*]
See **Penicillins (Systemic)**, 2240
Sterile USP, 2250
Carbenicillin Indanyl Sodium [carindacillin; *Geocillin; Geopen Oral*]
See **Penicillins (Systemic)**, 2240
Tablets USP, 2249
Carbetapentane-containing Combinations, 3069
*Carbex*—DuPont Merck (U.S.) brand of Selegiline (Systemic), 2560
Carbidopa-containing Combinations, 3069
Carbidopa and Levodopa [co-careldopa; *Nu-Levocarb; Sinemet; Sinemet CR*]
**(Systemic)**, 765, 3013
Tablets USP, 768, 3013, MC-5
Tablets, Extended-release, 768, MC-5
Carbinoxamine
See **Antihistamines (Systemic)**, 325
*Carbinoxamine Compound*—Pennex (U.S.) brand of Carbinoxamine, Pseudoephedrine, and Dextromethorphan—See **Cough/Cold Combinations (Systemic)**, 1024
*Carbinoxamine Compound-Drops*—Pennex (U.S.) brand of Carbinoxamine, Pseudoephedrine, and Dextromethorphan—See **Cough/Cold Combinations (Systemic)**, 1024
Carbinoxamine-containing Combinations, 3069
Carbinoxamine Maleate and Pseudoephedrine Hydrochloride [*Andec; Andec-TR; Biohist-LA; Carbiset; Carbiset-TR; Carbodec; Carbodec TR; Cardec; Cardec-S; Chemdec; CP Oral; Mooredec; Rondamine; Rondec; Rondec Drops; Rondec-TR*]
See **Antihistamines and Decongestants (Systemic)**, 343
Solution, Oral, 347, 350, 360
Syrup, 347, 360
Tablets, 345, 347, 360, MC-5
Tablets, Extended-release, 345, 346, 347, 355, 360
Carbinoxamine Maleate, Pseudoephedrine Hydrochloride, and Dextromethorphan Hydrobromide [*Carbinoxamine Compound; Carbinoxamine Compound-Drops; Carbodec DM; Carbodec DM Drops; Cardec DM; Cardec DM Drops; Cardec DM Pediatric; Pseudo-Car DM; Rondamine-DM Drops; Rondec-DM; Rondec-DM Drops; Sildec-DM; Sildec-DM Oral Drops; Tussafed; Tussafed Drops*]
See **Cough/Cold Combinations (Systemic)**, 1024
Solution, Oral, 1041, 1042, 1090, 1093, 1104
Syrup, 1041, 1042, 1085, 1090, 1092, 1104
*Carbiset*—Nutripharm (U.S.) brand of Carbinoxamine and Pseudoephedrine—See **Antihistamines and Decongestants (Systemic)**, 343

*Carbiset-TR*—Nutripharm (U.S.) brand of Carbinoxamine and Pseudoephedrine—**See Antihistamines and Decongestants (Systemic)**, 343
*Carbocaine*—Cooke-Waite (U.S.) and Sanofi Winthrop (U.S. and Canada) brand of Mepivacaine—**See Anesthetics (Parenteral-Local)**, 139
*Carbocaine with Neo-Cobefrin*—Cooke-Waite (U.S.) brand of Mepivacaine—**See Anesthetics (Parenteral-Local)**, 139
*Carbodec*—Rugby (U.S.) brand of Carbinoxamine and Pseudoephedrine—**See Antihistamines and Decongestants (Systemic)**, 343
*Carbodec DM*—Rugby (U.S.) brand of Carbinoxamine, Pseudoephedrine, and Dextromethorphan—**See Cough/Cold Combinations (Systemic)**, 1024
*Carbodec DM Drops*—Rugby (U.S.) brand of Carbinoxamine, Pseudoephedrine, and Dextromethorphan—**See Cough/Cold Combinations (Systemic)**, 1024
*Carbodec TR*—Rugby (U.S.) brand of Carbinoxamine and Pseudoephedrine—**See Antihistamines and Decongestants (Systemic)**, 343
Carbohydrates and Electrolytes
 **(Systemic)**, 769
Carbol-Fuchsin [*Castellani Paint; Castel Plus*]
 **(Topical)**, #
 Solution, Topical, USP, #
*Carbolith*—ICN (Canada) brand of Lithium (Systemic), 1869
Carbonic Anhydrase Inhibitors
 **(Systemic)**, 773
Carboplatin [*Paraplatin; Paraplatin-AQ*]
 **(Systemic)**, 779
 Injection, 782
 for Injection, 781
Carboprost Tromethamine [*Hemabate; Prostin/15M*]
 **(Systemic)**, 782
 Injection USP, 784
*Carboptic*—Optopics (U.S.) brand of Carbachol (Ophthalmic), 755
Carbovir
 **(Systemic)**, 3136
Carboxymethylcellulose [*Celluvisc; Refresh Plus*]
 **(Ophthalmic)**, 3013
 Solution, Ophthalmic, 3013
Carboxymethylcellulose-containing Combinations, 3069
*Cardec*—Major (U.S.) brand of Carbinoxamine and Pseudoephedrine—**See Antihistamines and Decongestants (Systemic)**, 343
*Cardec DM*—Aligen (U.S.); Barre-National (U.S.); Moore (U.S.); Qualitest (U.S.); Schein (U.S.) and Zenith Goldline (U.S.) brand of Carbinoxamine, Pseudoephedrine, and Dextromethorphan—**See Cough/Cold Combinations (Systemic)**, 1024
*Cardec DM Drops*—Aligen (U.S.); Barre-National (U.S.); Moore (U.S.); Qualitest (U.S.); Schein (U.S.) and Zenith Goldline (U.S.) brand of Carbinoxamine, Pseudoephedrine, and Dextromethorphan—**See Cough/Cold Combinations (Systemic)**, 1024
*Cardec DM Pediatric*—Schein (U.S.) brand of Carbinoxamine, Pseudoephedrine, and Dextromethorphan—**See Cough/Cold Combinations (Systemic)**, 1024
*Cardec-S*—Barre-National (U.S.) brand of Carbinoxamine and Pseudoephedrine—**See Antihistamines and Decongestants (Systemic)**, 343
*Cardene*—Roche (U.S.) and Hoffman-La Roche (Canada) brand of Nicardipine—**See Calcium Channel Blocking Agents (Systemic)**, 720, MC-21
*Cardene SR*—Roche (U.S.) brand of Nicardipine (Systemic), 3029
*Cardene-SR*—Roche (U.S.) brand of Nicardipine—**See Calcium Channel Blocking Agents (Systemic)**, MC-22
*Cardilate*—BW (U.S. and Canada) brand of Erythrityl Tetranitrate—**See Nitrates (Systemic)**, 2129
*CardioGen-82*—Squibb (U.S.) brand of Rubidium Rb 82 (Systemic), 2536
*Cardiolite*—Du Pont Merck (U.S. and Canada) brand of Technetium Tc 99m Sestamibi (Systemic), 2736
*Cardioquin*—Purdue Frederick (U.S. and Canada) brand of Quinidine (Systemic), 2440
*CardioTec*—Squibb (U.S.) brand of Technetium Tc 99m Teboroxime (Systemic), 2743

*Cardizem*—Hoechst Marion Roussel (U.S. and Canada) brand of Diltiazem—**See Calcium Channel Blocking Agents (Systemic)**, 720, MC-9
*Cardizem CD*—Hoechst Marion Roussel (U.S.) brand of Diltiazem—**See Calcium Channel Blocking Agents (Systemic)**, 720, MC-9
*Cardizem SR*—Hoechst Marion Roussel (U.S. and Canada) brand of Diltiazem—**See Calcium Channel Blocking Agents (Systemic)**, 720, MC-9
*Cardura*—Roerig (U.S.) and Astra (Canada) brand of Doxazosin (Systemic), 1303, MC-10
*Carindacillin*—Carbenicillin—**See Penicillins (Systemic)**, 2240
Carisoprodol [*Soma; Vanadom*]
 **See Skeletal Muscle Relaxants (Systemic)**, 2577
 Tablets USP, 2579, MC-5
Carisoprodol and Aspirin [*Soma Compound*]
 **(Systemic)**
 Tablets, MC-5
Carisoprodol, Aspirin, and Codeine [*Soma Compound with Codeine*]
 **(Systemic)**
 Tablets, MC-5
*Cari-Tab*—T. E. Williams (U.S.) brand of Vitamins A, D, and C and Fluoride—**See Vitamins, Multiple, and Fluoride (Systemic)**, 2978
*Carmol-HC*—Roche/Syntex (U.S.) brand of Hydrocortisone—**See Corticosteroids (Topical)**, 978
Carmustine [BCNU; *Gliadel Wafer*]
 **(Implantation-Local)**, 784
 Implants, 786
Carmustine [BCNU; *BiCNU*]
 **(Systemic)**, 786
 for Injection, 789
*Carnation Follow-Up Formula*—Carnation (U.S.) brand of Infant Formulas, Milk-based—**See Infant Formulas (Systemic)**, #
*Carnation Good Start*—Carnation (U.S.) brand of Infant Formulas, Milk-based—**See Infant Formulas (Systemic)**, #
*Carnation Instant Breakfast*—Clintec (U.S.) brand of Enteral Nutrition Formula, Milk-based—**See Enteral Nutrition Formulas (Systemic)**, #
*Carnation Instant Breakfast No Sugar Added*—Clintec (U.S.) brand of Enteral Nutrition Formula, Milk-based—**See Enteral Nutrition Formulas (Systemic)**, #
*Carnitor*—Sigma-Tau (U.S. and Canada) brand of Levocarnitine (Systemic), 1847; Sigma-Tau (U.S.) brand of Levocarnitine (Systemic), 3151, 3152, 3151, 3152
*Caroid*—Mentholatum (Canada) brand of Cascara Sagrada and Phenolphthalein—**See Laxatives (Local)**, #
Carteolol Hydrochloride [*Ocupress*]
 **See Beta-adrenergic Blocking Agents (Ophthalmic)**, 585
 Solution, Ophthalmic, 591
Carteolol Hydrochloride [*Cartrol*]
 **See Beta-adrenergic Blocking Agents (Systemic)**, 593
 Tablets, 602, MC-5
*Carter's Little Pills*—Carter (U.S.) brand of Bisacodyl—**See Laxatives (Local)**, #; Carter (Canada) brand of Phenolphthalein—**See Laxatives (Local)**, #
*Carticel*—Genzyme (U.S.) brand of Chrondrocytes, Autologous Cultured (Implantation-Local), 856
*Cartrol*—Abbott (U.S.) brand of Carteolol—**See Beta-adrenergic Blocking Agents (Systemic)**, 593, MC-5
Carvedilol [*Coreg*]
 **(Systemic)**, 790
 Tablets, 793, MC-5
Casanthranol [*Black-Draught*]
 **See Laxatives (Local)**, #
 Syrup, #
Casanthranol-containing Combinations, 3069
Casanthranol and Docusate Potassium [*Diocto-K Plus; Dioctolose Plus; Docu-K Plus; DSMC Plus*]
 **See Laxatives (Local)**, #
 Capsules, #
Casanthranol and Docusate Sodium [*Afko-Lube Lax; Diocto-C; Di-Sosul Forte; Doxidan Liqui-Gels; D-S-S plus; Fleet Soflax Overnight Gelcaps; Genasoft Plus Softgels; Molatoc-CST; Peri-Colace; Peri-Dos Softgels; Pro-Sof Plus; Regulace; Silace-C*]
 **See Laxatives (Local)**, #
 Capsules, #
 Syrup, #

Casanthranol and Docusate Sodium (continued)
 Syrup USP, #
 Tablets, #
Cascara Sagrada
 **See Laxatives (Local)**, #, 3136
 Fluidextract, 3136
 Fluidextract USP, #
 Fluidextract, Aromatic, USP, #
 Tablets USP, #
Cascara Sagrada and Aloe [*Nature's Remedy*]
 **See Laxatives (Local)**, #
 Tablets, #
Cascara Sagrada–containing Combinations, 3069
Cascara Sagrada and Phenolphthalein [*Bicholate Lilas; Caroid; Laxavite; Veracolate*]
 **See Laxatives (Local)**, #
 Tablets, #
*Casec*—Mead Johnson (U.S.) brand of Enteral Nutrition Formula, Modular—**See Enteral Nutrition Formulas (Systemic)**, #
*Casodex*—ZENECA (U.S. and Canada) brand of Bicalutamide—**See Antiandrogens, Nonsteroidal (Systemic)**, 220, MC-4
*Castellani Paint*—See Carbol-Fuchsin (Topical), #
*Castel Plus*—Syosset (U.S.) brand of Carbol-Fuchsin (Topical), #
Castor Oil [*Alphamul; Emulsoil; Kellogg's Castor Oil; Neoloid; Purge*]
 **See Laxatives (Local)**, #
 Emulsion USP, #
 Oil USP, #
*Cataflam*—Geigy (U.S.) brand of Diclofenac—**See Anti-inflammatory Drugs, Nonsteroidal (Systemic)**, 388
*Catapres*—Boehringer Ingelheim (U.S. and Canada) brand of Clonidine (Systemic), 908, MC-7
*Catapres-TTS*—Boehringer Ingelheim (U.S.) brand of Clonidine (Systemic), 908
*Catrix Correction*—Donnell-Dermedex (U.S.) brand of Menthyl Anthranilate and Octyl Methoxycinnamate—**See Sunscreen Agents (Topical)**, #
*Catrix Lip Saver*—Donnell-Dermedex (U.S.) brand of Octyl Methoxycinnamate and Oxybenzone—**See Sunscreen Agents (Topical)**, #
*Caverject*—Pharmacia & Upjohn (U.S. and Canada) brand of Alprostadil (Local), 48
*C2 Buffered*—Wampole (Canada) brand of Aspirin, Buffered—**See Salicylates (Systemic)**, 2538
*C2 Buffered with Codeine*—Wampole (Canada) brand of Aspirin and Codeine, Buffered—**See Opioid (Narcotic) Analgesics and Aspirin (Systemic)**, 2202
CCD 1042
 **(Systemic)**, 3136
*CC-Galactosidase*—See Alpha-Galactosidase A (Systemic), 3129
*CCK*—See Cholecystokinin (Systemic), #
*CCNU*—See Lomustine (Systemic), 1874
*C2 with Codeine*—Wampole (Canada) brand of Aspirin and Codeine—**See Opioid (Narcotic) Analgesics and Aspirin (Systemic)**, 2202
*2-CdA*—See Cladribine (Systemic), 886
CD4 Immunoglobulin G (Recombinant Human)
 **(Systemic)**, 3160
CD4, Recombinant Soluble Human [*Receptin*]
 **(Systemic)**, 3162
CD 4, Recombinant Soluble Human [rCD4]
 **(Systemic)**, 3161
CD5-T Lymphocyte Immunotoxin [*Xomazyme-H65*]
 **(Systemic)**, 3136
*CEA-Scan*—Immunomedics (U.S. and Canada) brand of Technetium Tc 99m Arcitumomab (Systemic), 2701
*Cebid Timecelles*—Hauck (U.S.) brand of Ascorbic Acid (Systemic), 469
*Ceclor*—Lilly (U.S. and Canada) brand of Cefaclor—**See Cephalosporins (Systemic)**, 794, MC-6
*Ceclor CD*—Dura (U.S.) brand of Cefaclor—**See Cephalosporins (Systemic)**, 794
*Cecon*—Abbott (U.S.) brand of Ascorbic Acid (Systemic), 469
*Cecore 500*—Pegasus (U.S.) brand of Ascorbic Acid (Systemic), 469
*Cedax*—Schering (U.S.) brand of Ceftibuten (Systemic), 794, MC-6
*Cedocard-SR*—Pharmascience (Canada) brand of Isosorbide Dinitrate—**See Nitrates (Systemic)**, 2129
*Cee-500*—Legere (U.S.) brand of Ascorbic Acid (Systemic), 469
*CeeNU*—Bristol (U.S. and Canada) brand of Lomustine (Systemic), 1874

c7E3 Fab—See Abciximab (Systemic), 1
Cefaclor [Apo-Cefaclor; Ceclor; Ceclor CD]
  See Cephalosporins (Systemic), 794
  Capsules USP, 800, MC-6
  for Suspension, Oral, USP, 800
  Tablets, Extended-release, 801
Cefadroxil [Duricef]
  See Cephalosporins (Systemic), 794
  Capsules USP, 801, MC-6
  for Suspension, Oral, USP, 802
  Tablets USP, 802, MC-6
Cefadyl—Bristol (U.S.) brand of Cephapirin—See Cephalosporins (Systemic), 794
Cefamandole Nafate [Mandol]
  See Cephalosporins (Systemic), 794
  for Injection USP, 802
Cefazolin [Ancef; Kefzol]
  See Cephalosporins (Systemic), 794
  Injection USP, 803
  for Injection USP, 804
Cefdinir [Omnicef]
  (Systemic), 3014
  Capsules, 3014
  for Suspension, Oral
Cefepime Hydrochloride [Maxipime]
  See Cephalosporins (Systemic), 794
  for Injection, 805
Cefixime [Suprax]
  See Cephalosporins (Systemic), 794
  for Suspension, Oral, USP, 805
  Tablets USP, 806, MC-6
Cefizox—SKF (U.S. and Canada) brand of Ceftizoxime—See Cephalosporins (Systemic), 794
Cefobid—Roerig (U.S.) and Pfizer (Canada) brand of Cefoperazone—See Cephalosporins (Systemic), 794
Cefonicid [Monocid]
  See Cephalosporins (Systemic), 794
  Injection USP, 806
Cefoperazone [Cefobid]
  See Cephalosporins (Systemic), 794
  Injection USP, 807
  for Injection USP, 807
Cefotan—Stuart (U.S. and Canada) brand of Cefotetan—See Cephalosporins (Systemic), 794
Cefotaxime [Claforan]
  See Cephalosporins (Systemic), 794
  Injection USP, 808
  for Injection USP, 808
Cefotetan [Cefotan]
  See Cephalosporins (Systemic), 794
  Injection, 809
  for Injection USP, 810
Cefoxitin [Mefoxin]
  See Cephalosporins (Systemic), 794
  Injection USP, 811
  for Injection USP, 811
Cefpodoxime Proxetil [Vantin]
  See Cephalosporins (Systemic), 794
  for Suspension, Oral, 812
  Tablets, 812, MC-6
Cefprozil [Cefzil]
  See Cephalosporins (Systemic), 794
  for Suspension, Oral, USP, 812
  Tablets USP, 813, MC-6
Ceftazidime [Ceptaz; Fortaz; Tazicef; Tazidime]
  See Cephalosporins (Systemic), 794
  Injection USP, 813
  for Injection USP, 813
Ceftibuten [Cedax]
  (Systemic), 794
  Capsules, 815, MC-6
  for Suspension, Oral, 815
Ceftin—Glaxo Wellcome (U.S. and Canada) brand of Cefuroxime—See Cephalosporins (Systemic), 794, MC-6
Ceftizoxime [Cefizox]
  See Cephalosporins (Systemic), 794
  Injection USP, 816
  for Injection USP, 816
Ceftriaxone [Rocephin]
  See Cephalosporins (Systemic), 794
  Injection USP, 817
  for Injection USP, 817
Cefuroxime [Kefurox; Zinacef]
  See Cephalosporins (Systemic), 794
  Injection USP, 819
  for Injection USP, 819
Cefuroxime Axetil [Ceftin]
  See Cephalosporins (Systemic), 794
  for Suspension, Oral, 818
  Tablets USP, 819, MC-6

Cefzil—Bristol-Myers Squibb (U.S.) brand of Cefprozil—See Cephalosporins (Systemic), 794, MC-6
Celestoderm-V—Schering (Canada) brand of Betamethasone—See Corticosteroids (Topical), 978
Celestoderm-V/2—Schering (Canada) brand of Betamethasone—See Corticosteroids (Topical), 978
Celestone—Schering (U.S. and Canada) brand of Betamethasone—See Corticosteroids—Glucocorticoid Effects (Systemic), 998
Celestone Phosphate—Schering (U.S.) brand of Betamethasone—See Corticosteroids—Glucocorticoid Effects (Systemic), 998
Celestone Soluspan—Schering (U.S. and Canada) brand of Betamethasone—See Corticosteroids—Glucocorticoid Effects (Systemic), 998
Celexa—Forest (U.S.) brand of Citalopram (Systemic), 3014
CellCept—Roche (U.S.) brand of Mycophenolate (Systemic), 2070, MC-21
Cellulose Sodium Phosphate [Calcibind]
  (Systemic), #
  USP (for Suspension, Oral), #
Celluvisc—Allergan (U.S.) brand of Carboxymethylcellulose (Ophthalmic), 3013
Celontin—PD (U.S. and Canada) brand of Methsuximide—See Anticonvulsants, Succinimide (Systemic), #
Cemill—Miller (U.S.) brand of Ascorbic Acid (Systemic), 469
Cenafed—Century (U.S.) brand of Pseudoephedrine (Systemic), 2422
Cenafed Plus—Century (U.S.) brand of Triprolidine and Pseudoephedrine—See Antihistamines and Decongestants (Systemic), 343
Cena-K—Century (U.S.) brand of Potassium Chloride—See Potassium Supplements (Systemic), 2357
Cenocort A-40—Central (U.S.) brand of Triamcinolone—See Corticosteroids—Glucocorticoid Effects (Systemic), 998
Cenocort Forte—Central (U.S.) brand of Triamcinolone—See Corticosteroids—Glucocorticoid Effects (Systemic), 998
Cenolate—Abbott (U.S.) brand of Sodium Ascorbate—See Ascorbic Acid (Systemic), 469
Centoxin—Centocor (U.S.) brand of Nebacumab (Systemic), 3155
Ceo-Two—Beutlich (U.S.) brand of Potassium Bitartrate and Sodium Bicarbonate—See Laxatives (Local), #
Cephalexin [Apo-Cephalex; Keflex; Novo-Lexin; Nu-Cephalex; PMS-Cephalexin]
  See Cephalosporins (Systemic), 794
  Capsules USP, 820, MC-6
  for Suspension, Oral, USP, 821
  Tablets USP, 821
Cephalexin Hydrochloride [Keftab]
  See Cephalosporins (Systemic), 794
  Tablets USP, 821
Cephalosporins
  (Systemic), 794
Cephalothin [Ceporacin; Keflin]
  See Cephalosporins (Systemic), 794
  for Injection USP, 821
Cephapirin [Cefadyl]
  See Cephalosporins (Systemic), 794
  for Injection USP, 822
Cephradine [Velosef]
  See Cephalosporins (Systemic), 794
  Capsules USP, 823, MC-6
  for Suspension, Oral, USP, 823
Ceporacin—Bioniche (Canada) brand of Cephalothin—See Cephalosporins (Systemic), 794
Ceptaz—Glaxo (U.S. and Canada) brand of Ceftazidime—See Cephalosporins (Systemic), 794
Ceramide Trihexosidase and Alpha-galactosidase A
  (Systemic), 3136
Cerebyx—PD (U.S.) brand of Fosphenytoin—See Anticonvulsants, Hydantoin (Systemic), 253
Ceredase—Genzyme (U.S. and Canada) brand of Alglucerase (Systemic), #; Genzyme (U.S.) brand of Alglucerase (Systemic), 3129
Cerespan—Rhône-Poulenc Rorer (U.S.) brand of Papaverine (Systemic), #
Ceretec—Amersham (U.S. and Canada) brand of Technetium Tc 99m Exametazime (Systemic), 2708
Cerezyme—Genzyme (U.S.) brand of Imiglucerase (Systemic), 1680, 3147

Cerivastatin Sodium [Baycol]
  (Systemic), 827
  Tablets, 830
Cerose-DM—Wyeth-Ayerst (U.S.) brand of Chlorpheniramine, Phenylephrine, and Dextromethorphan—See Cough/Cold Combinations (Systemic), 1024
Cerubidine—Wyeth-Ayerst (U.S.) and Rhône-Poulenc Rorer (Canada) brand of Daunorubicin (Systemic), 1173
Cervical Cap, Cavity-rim [Prentif]
  (Vaginal), 3014
Cervidil—Forest (U.S.) brand of Dinoprostone (Cervical/Vaginal), 1228
C.E.S.—ICN (Canada) brand of Conjugated Estrogens—See Estrogens (Systemic), 1383
Cesamet—Lilly (Canada) brand of Nabilone (Systemic), 2074
C1-Esterase Inhibitor (Human)
  (Systemic), 3135
C1-Esterase-Inhibitor, Human, Pasteurized
  (Systemic), 3135
Cetacaine Topical Anesthetic—Cetylite (U.S.) brand of Benzocaine, Butamben, and Tetracaine—See Anesthetics (Mucosal-Local), 128
Cetacort—Owen/Allercreme (U.S.) brand of Hydrocortisone—See Corticosteroids (Topical), 978
Cetamide—Alcon (U.S.) brand of Sulfacetamide—See Sulfonamides (Ophthalmic), 2651
Cetane—Forest (U.S.) brand of Ascorbic Acid (Systemic), 469
Cetaphen with Codeine—Wampole (Canada) brand of Acetaminophen and Codeine—See Opioid (Narcotic) Analgesics and Acetaminophen (Systemic), 2198
Cetaphen Extra-Strength with Codeine—Wampole (Canada) brand of Acetaminophen and Codeine—See Opioid (Narcotic) Analgesics and Acetaminophen (Systemic), 2198
Cetirizine Hydrochloride [Reactine; Zyrtec]
  See Antihistamines (Systemic), 325
  Syrup, 333
  Tablets, 333, MC-6
Cevi-Bid—Geriatric (U.S.) brand of Ascorbic Acid (Systemic), 469
Chap-et Sun Ban Lip Conditioner—Stanback (U.S.) brand of Oxybenzone and Padimate O—See Sunscreen Agents (Topical), #
Chap Stick—Whitehall-Robins (U.S.) brand of Padimate O—See Sunscreen Agents (Topical), #
Chap Stick Sunblock—Whitehall-Robins (U.S. and Canada) brand of Oxybenzone and Padimate O—See Sunscreen Agents (Topical), #
Chap Stick Sunblock Petroleum Jelly Plus—Whitehall-Robins (U.S.) brand of Oxybenzone and Padimate O—See Sunscreen Agents (Topical), #
Charac-50—Omega (Canada) brand of Charcoal, Activated (Oral-Local), 831
Charac-tol 50—Omega (Canada) brand of Charcoal, Activated, and Sorbitol—See Charcoal, Activated (Oral-Local), N, 831
CharcoAid 2000—Requa (U.S.) brand of Charcoal, Activated—See Charcoal, Activated (Oral-Local), 831
Charcoaid—Requa (U.S.) brand of Charcoal, Activated, and Sorbitol—See Charcoal, Activated (Oral-Local), 831
Charcoal, Activated [Actidose-Aqua; Aqueous Charcodote; Charac-50; CharcoAid 2000; Charcocaps; Insta-Char Aqueous; Liqui-Char; Pediatric Aqueous Charcodote; Pediatric Aqueous Insta-Char]
  (Oral-Local), 831
  Capsules, 833
  Charcoal, Activated, USP, 832
  Suspension, Oral, 833
  Tablets, 833
Charcoal, Activated, and Sorbitol [Actidose with Sorbitol; Charac-tol 50; Charcoaid; Charcodote; Charcodote TFS-25; Charcodote TFS-50; Insta-Char with Sorbitol; Liqui-Char with Sorbitol; Pediatric Charcodote]
  See Charcoal, Activated (Oral-Local), 831
  Suspension, Oral, 833
Charcoal-containing Combinations, 3069
Charcocaps—Requa (U.S.) brand of Charcoal, Activated (Oral-Local), 831
Charcodote—Pharmascience (Canada) brand of Charcoal, Activated, and Sorbitol—See Charcoal, Activated (Oral-Local), 831

*Charcodote TFS-25*—Pharmascience (Canada) brand of Charcoal, Activated, and Sorbitol—**See Charcoal, Activated (Oral-Local)**, 831
*Charcodote TFS-50*—Pharmascience (Canada) brand of Charcoal, Activated, and Sorbitol—**See Charcoal, Activated (Oral-Local)**, 831
*Chardonna-2*—Rhône-Poulenc Rorer (U.S.) brand of Belladonna and Phenobarbital—**See Belladonna Alkaloids and Barbiturates (Systemic)**, 551
*Chemdec*—Zenith Goldline (U.S.) brand of Carbinoxamine and Pseudoephedrine—**See Antihistamines and Decongestants (Systemic)**, 343
*Chemet*—McNeil-CPC (U.S.) brand of Succimer (Systemic), #, 3166
*Chemet Capsules*—McNeil-CPC (U.S.) brand of Succimer (Systemic), 3166
*Chemstrip K*—Boehringer Mannheim (U.S.) brand of Nitroprusside Urine Ketone Test—**See Urine Glucose and Ketone Test Kits for Home Use**, 
*Chemstrip uG*—Boehringer Mannheim (U.S.) brand of Glucose Oxidase Urine Glucose Test—**See Urine Glucose and Ketone Test Kits for Home Use**, #
*Chemstrip uGK*—Boehringer Mannheim (U.S. and Canada) brand of Urine Glucose and Ketone (Combined) Test—**See Urine Glucose and Ketone Test Kits for Home Use**, #
*Chenix*—Solvay (U.S.) brand of Chenodiol (Systemic), 3136
Chenodeoxycholic acid—See Chenodiol (Systemic), #
Chenodiol [*Chenix*; chenodeoxycholic acid]
 **(Systemic)**, #, 3136
 Tablets, #
*Cheracol*—Roberts (Canada) brand of Codeine, Ammonium Chloride, and Guaifenesin—**See Cough/Cold Combinations (Systemic)**, 1024; Roberts (U.S.) brand of Codeine and Guaifenesin—**See Cough/Cold Combinations (Systemic)**, 1024
*Cheracol D Cough*—Roberts (U.S.) brand of Dextromethorphan and Guaifenesin—**See Cough/Cold Combinations (Systemic)**, 1024
*Cheracol Nasal Spray*—Roberts (U.S.) brand of Oxymetazoline (Nasal), #
*Cheracol Nasal Spray Pump Cherry Scented*—Roberts (U.S.) brand of Oxymetazoline (Nasal), #
*Cheracol Plus*—Roberts (U.S.) brand of Chlorpheniramine, Phenylpropanolamine, and Dextromethorphan—**See Cough/Cold Combinations (Systemic)**, 1024
*Cherapas*—Kay (U.S.) brand of Reserpine, Hydralazine, and Hydrochlorothiazide (Systemic), #
*Chibroxin*—Merck (U.S.) brand of Norfloxacin (Ophthalmic), #
*Children's Formula Cough*—Pharmakon (U.S.) brand of Dextromethorphan and Guaifenesin—**See Cough/Cold Combinations (Systemic)**, 1024
*Children's Hold*—Beecham (U.S.) brand of Dextromethorphan (Systemic), 1191
*Children's Tylenol Cold Multi-Symptom*—McNeil (U.S.) brand of Chlorpheniramine, Pseudoephedrine, and Acetaminophen—**See Antihistamines, Decongestants, and Analgesics (Systemic)**, 366
*Children's Tylenol Cold Plus Cough Multi Symptom*—McNeil (U.S.) brand of Chlorpheniramine, Pseudoephedrine, Dextromethorphan, and Acetaminophen—**See Cough/Cold Combinations (Systemic)**, 1024
Chimeric A2 (Human-Murine) IgG Monoclonal Anti-TNF Antibody (cA2)
 **(Systemic)**, 3136
Chimeric M-T412 (Human-Murine) IgG Monoclonal Anti-CD4
 **(Systemic)**, 3136
Chimeric (Murine Variable, Human Constant) MAB to CD20
 **(Systemic)**, 3136
*C-Hist-SR*—Alphagen (U.S.) brand of Chlorpheniramine, Phenyltoloxamine, and Phenylephrine—**See Antihistamines and Decongestants (Systemic)**, 343
*Chlo-Amine*—Hollister-Stier (U.S.) brand of Chlorpheniramine—**See Antihistamines (Systemic)**, 325
Chlophedianol Hydrochloride [*Ulone*]
 **(Systemic)**, #
 Syrup, #
*Chloracol Ophthalmic Solution*—Horizon (U.S.) brand of Chloramphenicol (Ophthalmic), #

*Chlorafed*—Roberts (U.S.) brand of Chlorpheniramine and Pseudoephedrine—**See Antihistamines and Decongestants (Systemic)**, 343
*Chlorafed H.S. Timecelles*—Roberts (U.S.) brand of Chlorpheniramine and Pseudoephedrine—**See Antihistamines and Decongestants (Systemic)**, 343
*Chlorafed Timecelles*—Roberts (U.S.) brand of Chlorpheniramine and Pseudoephedrine—**See Antihistamines and Decongestants (Systemic)**, 343
Chloral Hydrate [*Aquachloral Supprettes*; *Novo-Chlorhydrate*; *PMS-Chloral Hydrate*]
 **(Systemic)**, 834
 Capsules USP, 836
 Suppositories, 837
 Syrup USP, 836
Chlorambucil [*Leukeran*]
 **(Systemic)**, 837
 Tablets USP, 840, MC-6
Chloramphenicol [*Ak-Chlor Ophthalmic Ointment; Ak-Chlor Ophthalmic Solution; Chloracol Ophthalmic Solution; Chlorofair Ophthalmic Ointment; Chlorofair Ophthalmic Solution; Chloromycetin Ophthalmic Ointment; Chloroptic Ophthalmic Solution; Chloroptic S.O.P.; Diochloram; Econochlor Ophthalmic Ointment; Econochlor Ophthalmic Solution; Fenicol Ophthalmic Ointment; I-Chlor Ophthalmic Solution; Ocu-Chlor Ophthalmic Ointment; Ocu-Chlor Ophthalmic Solution; Ophtho-Chloram Ophthalmic Solution; Ophthochlor Ophthalmic Solution; Pentamycetin Ophthalmic Ointment; Pentamycetin Ophthalmic Solution; Sopamycetin Ophthalmic Ointment; Sopamycetin Ophthalmic Solution; Spectro-Chlor Ophthalmic Ointment; Spectro-Chlor Ophthalmic Solution*]
 **(Ophthalmic)**, #, 3014
 Ointment, Ophthalmic, USP, #, 3014
 Solution, Ophthalmic, USP, #, 3014
Chloramphenicol [*Chloromycetin; Sopamycetin*]
 **(Otic)**, #
 Solution, Otic, USP, #
Chloramphenicol [*Chloromycetin; Novochlorocap*]
 **(Systemic)**, 841
 Capsules USP, 844
Chloramphenicol Palmitate [*Chloromycetin*]
 **(Systemic)**, 841
 Suspension, Oral, USP, 844
Chloramphenicol Sodium Succinate [*Chloromycetin*]
 **(Systemic)**, 841
 Sterile USP, 844
*Chloraseptic Lozenges*—Procter & Gamble (U.S.) brand of Benzocaine and Menthol—**See Anesthetics (Mucosal-Local)**, 128
*Chloraseptic Lozenges Cherry Flavor*—Procter & Gamble (Canada) brand of Benzocaine and Menthol—**See Anesthetics (Mucosal-Local)**, 128
*Chloraseptic Lozenges, Children's*—Procter & Gamble (U.S.) brand of Benzocaine—**See Anesthetics (Mucosal-Local)**, 128
*Chlorate*—Major (U.S.) brand of Chlorpheniramine—**See Antihistamines (Systemic)**, 325
Chlordiazepoxide and Amitriptyline Hydrochloride [*Limbitrol; Limbitrol DS*]
 **(Systemic)**, 845
 Tablets USP, 845, MC-6
Chlordiazepoxide-containing Combinations, 3069
Chlordiazepoxide Hydrochloride [*Apo-Chlordiazepoxide; Librium; Novo-Poxide*]
 **See Benzodiazepines (Systemic)**, 556
 Capsules USP, 566, MC-6
 for Injection USP, 566
Chlordiazepoxide Hydrochloride and Clidinium Bromide [*Apo-Chlorax; Clindex; Clinoxide; Clipoxide; Corium; Librax; Lidox; Lidoxide; Zebrax*]
 **(Systemic)**, 846
 Capsules USP, 846, MC-6
*Chlordrine S.R.*—Rugby (U.S.) brand of Chlorpheniramine and Pseudoephedrine—**See Antihistamines and Decongestants (Systemic)**, 343
*Chlorfed*—Stewart Jackson (U.S.) brand of Chlorpheniramine and Pseudoephedrine—**See Antihistamines and Decongestants (Systemic)**, 343
*Chlorfed II*—Stewart Jackson (U.S.) brand of Chlorpheniramine and Pseudoephedrine—**See Antihistamines and Decongestants (Systemic)**, 343

*Chlorgest-HD*—Great Southern (U.S.) brand of Chlorpheniramine, Phenylephrine, and Hydrocodone—**See Cough/Cold Combinations (Systemic)**, 1024
Chlorhexidine Gluconate [*Peridex*; *PerioChip*; *PerioGard*]
 **(Mucosal-Local)**, 847, 3014, 3136
 Implants, Periodontal, 3014
 Rinse, Oral, 848, 3136
Chlormethine—See Mechlorethamine (Systemic), 1929; Mechlorethamine (Topical), #
2-Chlorodeoxyadenosine
 **(Systemic)**, 3127
2-Chlorodeoxyadenosine—See Cladribine (Systemic), 886
*Chlorofair Ophthalmic Ointment*—Balan (U.S.) brand of Chloramphenicol (Ophthalmic), #
*Chlorofair Ophthalmic Solution*—Balan (U.S.); Dixon-Shane (U.S.); and Gen-King (U.S.) brand of Chloramphenicol (Ophthalmic), #
*Chlorohist-LA*—Hauck (U.S.) brand of Xylometazoline (Nasal), #
*Chloromag*—Merit (U.S.) brand of Magnesium Chloride—**See Magnesium Supplements (Systemic)**, 1897
*Chloromycetin*—PD (U.S. and Canada) brand of Chloramphenicol (Otic), #; Chloramphenicol (Systemic), 841
*Chloromycetin Ophthalmic Ointment*—PD (U.S. and Canada) brand of Chloramphenicol (Ophthalmic), #
*Chloromycetin for Ophthalmic Solution*—PD (U.S. and Canada) brand of Chloramphenicol (Ophthalmic), #
Chloroprocaine Hydrochloride [*Nesacaine*; *Nesacaine-CE*; *Nesacaine-MPF*]
 **See Anesthetics (Parenteral-Local)**, 139
 Injection USP, 147
*Chloroptic Ophthalmic Solution*—Allergan (U.S. and Canada) brand of Chloramphenicol (Ophthalmic), #
*Chloroptic S.O.P.*—Allergan (U.S. and Canada) brand of Chloramphenicol (Ophthalmic), #
Chloroquine Hydrochloride [*Aralen HCl*]
 **(Systemic)**, 849
 Injection USP, 852
Chloroquine Phosphate [*Aralen*]
 **(Systemic)**, 849
 Tablets USP, 852
Chlorothiazide [*Diuril*]
 **See Diuretics, Thiazide (Systemic)**, 1273
 Suspension, Oral, USP, 1278
 Tablets USP, 1278
Chlorothiazide-containing Combinations, 3069
Chlorothiazide Sodium [*Diuril*]
 **See Diuretics, Thiazide (Systemic)**, 1273
 for Injection USP, 1278
Chloroxine [*Capitrol*]
 **(Topical)**, #
 Shampoo, Lotion, #
*Chlorphedrine SR*—Zenith Goldline (U.S.) brand of Chlorpheniramine and Pseudoephedrine—**See Antihistamines and Decongestants (Systemic)**, 343
Chlorphenamine—Chlorpheniramine—**See Antihistamines (Systemic)**, 325
Chlorphenesin Carbamate [*Maolate*]
 **See Skeletal Muscle Relaxants (Systemic)**, 2577
 Tablets, 2579
Chlorpheniramine-containing Combinations, 3069
Chlorpheniramine Maleate [*Aller-Chlor; Chlo-Amine; Chlorate*; chlorphenamine; *Chlor-Trimeton; Chlor-Trimeton Allergy; Chlor-Trimeton Repetabs; Chlor-Tripolon; Gen-Allerate; Novo-Pheniram; PediaCare Allergy Formula; Phenetron; Telachlor; Teldrin*]
 **See Antihistamines (Systemic)**, 325
 Capsules, Extended-release, USP, 333
 Injection USP, 334
 Syrup USP, 333
 Tablets USP, 334, MC-6
 Tablets USP (Chewable), 334
 Tablets, Extended-release, 334
Chlorpheniramine Maleate and Dextromethorphan Hydrobromide [*Effective Strength Cough Formula; Primatuss Cough Mixture 4; Scot-Tussin DM; Tricodene Sugar Free*]
 **See Cough/Cold Combinations (Systemic)**, 1024
 Solution, Oral, 1056, 1083, 1092, 1103

USP DI            General Index    3261

Chlorpheniramine Maleate, Ephedrine Hydrochloride, Phenylephrine Hydrochloride, Dextromethorphan Hydrobromide, Ammonium Chloride, and Ipecac Fluidextract [*Quelidrine Cough*]
   **See Cough/Cold Combinations (Systemic)**, 1024
   Syrup, 1085
Chlorpheniramine Maleate, Ephedrine Sulfate, and Guaifenesin [*Bronkotuss Expectorant*]
   **See Cough/Cold Combinations (Systemic)**, 1024
   Solution, Oral, 1038
Chlorpheniramine Maleate and Hydrocodone Bitartrate [*S-T Forte 2; Tussionex Pennkinetic*]
   **See Cough/Cold Combinations (Systemic)**, 1024
   Solution, Oral, 1096
   Suspension, Oral, 1106
Chlorpheniramine Maleate, Phenindamine Tartrate, Phenylephrine Hydrochloride, Dextromethorphan Hydrobromide, Acetaminophen, Salicylamide, Caffeine, and Ascorbic Acid [*Omnicol*]
   **See Cough/Cold Combinations (Systemic)**, 1024
   Tablets, 1076
Chlorpheniramine Maleate, Phenindamine Tartrate, and Phenylpropanolamine Hydrochloride [*Amilon; Nolamine*]
   **See Antihistamines and Decongestants (Systemic)**, 343
   Tablets, Extended-release, 345, 356
Chlorpheniramine Maleate, Pheniramine Maleate, Pyrilamine Maleate, Phenylephrine Hydrochloride, Hydrocodone Bitartrate, Salicylamide, Caffeine, and Ascorbic Acid [*Citra Forte*]
   **See Cough/Cold Combinations (Systemic)**, 1024
   Capsules, 1043
Chlorpheniramine Maleate and Phenylephrine Hydrochloride [*Ed A-Hist; Histatab Plus; Histor-D; Novahistine; Rolatuss Plain; Ru-Tuss*]
   **See Antihistamines and Decongestants (Systemic)**, 343
   Elixir, 357
   Solution, Oral, 353, 360
   Suspension, Oral
   Syrup, 354
   Tablets, 354
   Tablets, Extended-release, 353
Chlorpheniramine Maleate, Phenylephrine Hydrochloride, and Acetaminophen [*Aclophen; Dristan; Dristan Cold Multi-Symptom Formula; Dristan Extra Strength Caplets; Gendecon; Histagesic Modified*]
   **See Antihistamines, Decongestants, and Analgesics (Systemic)**, 366
   Capsules, 369
   Tablets, 369, 370
   Tablets, Extended-release, 367
Chlorpheniramine Maleate, Phenylephrine Hydrochloride, Codeine Phosphate, and Ammonium Chloride [*Rolatuss Expectorant*]
   **See Cough/Cold Combinations (Systemic)**, 1024
   Solution, Oral, 1090
Chlorpheniramine Maleate, Phenylephrine Hydrochloride, Codeine Phosphate, and Potassium Iodide [*Pediacof Cough; Pedituss Cough*]
   **See Cough/Cold Combinations (Systemic)**, 1024
   Syrup, 1078, 1079
Chlorpheniramine Maleate, Phenylephrine Hydrochloride, and Dextromethorphan Hydrobromide [*Atuss DM; Cerose-DM; Dondril*]
   **See Cough/Cold Combinations (Systemic)**, 1024
   Solution, Oral, 1042
   Syrup, 1035
   Tablets, 1054
Chlorpheniramine Maleate, Phenylephrine Hydrochloride, Dextromethorphan Hydrobromide, Acetaminophen, and Salicylamide [*Improved Sino-Tuss*]
   **See Cough/Cold Combinations (Systemic)**, 1024
   Tablets, 1066
Chlorpheniramine Maleate, Phenylephrine Hydrochloride, Dextromethorphan Hydrobromide, and Guaifenesin [*Donatussin*]
   **See Cough/Cold Combinations (Systemic)**, 1024
   Syrup, 1054
Chlorpheniramine Maleate, Phenylephrine Hydrochloride, Dextromethorphan Hydrobromide, Guaifenesin, and Ammonium Chloride [*Father John's Medicine Plus*]
   **See Cough/Cold Combinations (Systemic)**, 1024
   Solution, Oral, 1058
Chlorpheniramine Maleate, Phenylephrine Hydrochloride, and Guaifenesin [*Donatussin Drops*]
   **See Cough/Cold Combinations (Systemic)**, 1024
   Solution, Oral, 1054

Chlorpheniramine Maleate, Phenylephrine Hydrochloride, and Hydrocodone Bitartrate [*Anaplex HD; Atuss HD; Chlorgest-HD; ED-TLC; Ed Tuss HC; Endagen-HD; Endal-HD; Endal-HD Plus; Histinex HC; Histussin HC; Iodal HD; Iotussin HC; Med-Hist HC; Nasatuss; Para-Hist HD; Unituss HC; Vanex-HD*]
   **See Cough/Cold Combinations (Systemic)**, 1024
   Solution, Oral, 1035, 1043, 1055, 1056, 1056, 1067, 1068, 1069, 1077, 1112
   Syrup, 1034, 1056, 1063, 1072, 1111
Chlorpheniramine Maleate, Phenylephrine Hydrochloride, Hydrocodone Bitartrate, Acetaminophen, and Caffeine [*Hycomine Compound*]
   **See Cough/Cold Combinations (Systemic)**, 1024
   Tablets, 1065
Chlorpheniramine Maleate, Phenylephrine Hydrochloride, and Methscopolamine Nitrate [*AH-chew; D.A. Chewable; Dallergy; Dallergy Caplets; Dura-Vent/DA; Extendryl; Extendryl JR; Extendryl SR; OMNIhist L.A.; Pre-Hist-D*]
   **See Antihistamines, Decongestants, and Anticholinergics (Systemic)**, 373
   Capsules, Extended-release, 375
   Syrup, 374, 375
   Tablets, 374
   Tablets, Chewable, 374, 375
   Tablets, Extended-release, 375, 376
Chlorpheniramine Maleate, Phenylephrine Hydrochloride, and Phenylpropanolamine Hydrochloride [*Hista-Vadrin*]
   **See Antihistamines and Decongestants (Systemic)**, 343
   Tablets, 354
Chlorpheniramine Maleate, Phenylephrine Hydrochloride, Phenylpropanolamine Hydrochloride, Atropine Sulfate, Hyoscyamine Sulfate, and Scopolamine Hydrobromide [*Atrohist Plus; Deconhist; Phenahist-TR; Phenchlor S.H.A.; Pro-Tuss; Q-Tuss; Rolatuss SR; Ru-Tab; Ru-Tuss; Stahist; Tuss Delay*]
   **See Antihistamines, Decongestants, and Anticholinergics (Systemic)**, 373
   Tablets, Extended-release, 374, 375, 376, 377
Chlorpheniramine Maleate, Phenylephrine Hydrochloride, Phenylpropanolamine Hydrochloride, Carbetapentane Citrate, and Potassium Guaiacolsulfonate [*Cophene-XP*]
   **See Cough/Cold Combinations (Systemic)**, 1024
   Syrup, 1048
Chlorpheniramine Maleate, Phenylephrine Hydrochloride, Phenylpropanolamine Hydrochloride, and Codeine Phosphate [*T-Koff*]
   **See Cough/Cold Combinations (Systemic)**, 1024
   Solution, Oral, 1099
Chlorpheniramine Maleate, Phenylephrine Hydrochloride, Phenylpropanolamine Hydrochloride, Dextromethorphan Hydrobromide, Potassium Guaiacolsulfonate, and Ipecac Fluidextract [*Tusquelin*]
   **See Cough/Cold Combinations (Systemic)**, 1024
   Syrup, 1104
Chlorpheniramine Maleate, Phenylephrine Hydrochloride, Phenylpropanolamine Hydrochloride, and Dihydrocodeine Bitartrate [*Cophene-S; Vanex Grape*]
   **See Cough/Cold Combinations (Systemic)**, 1024
   Solution, Oral, 1112
   Syrup, 1048
Chlorpheniramine Maleate, Phenylpropanolamine Bitartrate, and Aspirin [*Alka-Seltzer Plus Cold Medicine*]
   **See Antihistamines, Decongestants, and Analgesics (Systemic)**, 366
   Tablets, Effervescent, 367
Chlorpheniramine Maleate, Phenylpropanolamine Bitartrate, Dextromethorphan Hydrobromide, and Acetaminophen [*Alka-Seltzer Plus Flu & Body Aches*]
   **See Cough/Cold Combinations (Systemic)**, 1024
   Tablets, Effervescent, 1032
Chlorpheniramine Maleate, Phenylpropanolamine Bitartrate, Dextromethorphan Hydrobromide, and Aspirin [*Alka-Seltzer Plus Cold and Cough*]
   **See Cough/Cold Combinations (Systemic)**, 1024
   Tablets, Effervescent, 1032
Chlorpheniramine Maleate and Phenylpropanolamine Hydrochloride [*A.R.M. Maximum Strength Caplets; Chlor-Rest; Chlor-Tripolon Decongestant; Cold-Gest Cold; Contac 12-Hour; Contac Maximum Strength 12-Hour Caplets; Coricidin D Long Acting; Demazin; Demazin Repetabs; Drize; Dura-Vent/A; Genamin; Gencold; Ornade;*

Chlorpheniramine Maleate and Phenylpropanolamine Hydrochloride *(continued)*
   *Ornade-A.F.; Ornade Spansules; Resaid S.R.; Rescon; Rhinolar-EX; Rhinolar-EX 12; Silaminic; Teldrin 12 HourAllergy Relief; Temazin Cold; Triaminic; Triaminic-12; Triaminic Allergy; Triaminic Chewables; Triaminic Cold; Tri-Nefrin Extra Strength; Triphenyl*]
   **See Antihistamines and Decongestants (Systemic)**, 343
   Capsules, Extended-release, 348, 349, 350, 353, 357, 359, 362
   Solution, Oral, 357, 359
   Syrup, 348, 351, 353, 361, 362, 364
   Tablets, 345, 348, 362, 363
   Tablets, Chewable, 362
   Tablets, Extended-release, 350, 351, 362
Chlorpheniramine Maleate, Phenylpropanolamine Hydrochloride, and Acetaminophen [*Alumadrine; BQ Cold; Chlor-Trimeton Allergy-Sinus Caplets; Congestant D; Coricidin D; Dapacin Cold; Duadacin; Phenate T.D.; Pyrroxate Caplets; Sinulin; Triaminicin Cold, Allergy, Sinus*]
   **See Antihistamines, Decongestants, and Analgesics (Systemic)**, 366
   Capsules, 369, 370
   Tablets, 367, 368, 369, 371, 372
   Tablets, Extended-release, 371
Chlorpheniramine Maleate, Phenylpropanolamine Hydrochloride, Acetaminophen, and Caffeine [*Sinapils*]
   **See Antihistamines, Decongestants, and Analgesics (Systemic)**, 366
   Tablets, 371
Chlorpheniramine Maleate, Phenylpropanolamine Hydrochloride, and Aspirin [*BC Multi Symptom Cold Powder; Coricidin D*]
   **See Antihistamines, Decongestants, and Analgesics (Systemic)**, 366
   for Solution, Oral, 367
   Tablets, 369
Chlorpheniramine Maleate, Phenylpropanolamine Hydrochloride, and Caramiphen Edisylate [*Tuss-Ornade Spansules*]
   **See Cough/Cold Combinations (Systemic)**, 1024
   Capsules, Extended-release, 1108
Chlorpheniramine Maleate, Phenylpropanolamine Hydrochloride, and Dextromethorphan Hydrobromide [*Cheracol Plus; Kophane Cough and Cold Formula; Myminicol; Ornade-DM 10; Ornade-DM 15; Ornade-DM 30; Snaplets-Multi; Threamine DM; Triaminic Triaminicol; Triaminicol Multi-Symptom Cold and Cough Medicine; Tricodene Forte; Tricodene NN; Triminol Cough*]
   **See Cough/Cold Combinations (Systemic)**, 1024
   Granules, 1094
   Solution, Oral, 1068, 1070, 1076, 1077, 1102, 1103
   Syrup, 1042, 1099, 1103
   Tablets, 1102
Chlorpheniramine Maleate, Phenylpropanolamine Hydrochloride, Dextromethorphan Hydrobromide, and Acetaminophen [*Comtrex Maximum Strength Multi-Symptom Liqui-Gels; Comtrex Multi-Symptom Cold Reliever; Contac Severe Cold & Flu Caplets*]
   **See Cough/Cold Combinations (Systemic)**, 1024
   Capsules, 1046
   Solution, Oral, 1046
   Tablets, 1046, 1048
Chlorpheniramine Maleate, Phenylpropanolamine Hydrochloride, and Guaifenesin [*Ornade Expectorant*]
   **See Cough/Cold Combinations (Systemic)**, 1024
   Solution, Oral, 1077
Chlorpheniramine Maleate, Phenylpropanolamine Hydrochloride, Guaifenesin, and Acetaminophen [*Gelpirin-CCF*]
   **See Cough/Cold Combinations (Systemic)**, 1024
   Tablets, 1059
Chlorpheniramine Maleate, Phenylpropanolamine Hydrochloride, Guaifenesin, Sodium Citrate, and Citric Acid [*Lanatuss Expectorant*]
   **See Cough/Cold Combinations (Systemic)**, 1024
   Solution, Oral, 1068
Chlorpheniramine Maleate, Phenylpropanolamine Hydrochloride, and Methscopolamine Nitrate [*Pannaz*]
   **See Antihistamines, Decongestants, and Anticholinergics (Systemic)**, 373
   Tablets, Extended-release, 375

Chlorpheniramine Maleate, Phenylpropanolamine, Phenylephrine, and Phenyltoloxamine **(Systemic)**, MC-16
 Tablets, Extended-release, MC-6
Chlorpheniramine Maleate, Phenyltoloxamine Citrate, and Phenylephrine Hydrochloride [*C-Hist-SR; Chlortox; Comhist; Comhist LA; Linhist-L.A.; Nalex-A; Q-Hist LA*]
 **See Antihistamines and Decongestants (Systemic)**, 343
 Capsules, Extended-release, 347, 348, 349, 354, 358
 Tablets, 349
 Tablets, Extended-release, 356
Chlorpheniramine Maleate, Phenyltoloxamine Citrate, Phenylephrine Hydrochloride, and Phenylpropanolamine Hydrochloride [*Decongestabs; Nalda-Relief Pediatric Drops; Naldecon; Naldecon Pediatric Drops; Naldecon Pediatric Syrup; Naldelate; Naldelate Pediatric Drops; Naldelate Pediatric Syrup; Nalgest; Nalgest Pediatric; Nalphen; Nalphen Pediatric; Prop-a-Hist; Sinucon; Sinucon Pediatric Drops; Sinucon Pediatric Syrup; Tri-Phen-Chlor; Tri-Phen-Chlor Pediatric; Tri-Phen-Chlor T.R.; Tri-Phen-Mine Pediatric Drops; Tri-Phen-Mine Pediatric Syrup; Tri-Phen-Mine S.R.; Uni-Decon; West-Decon*]
 **See Antihistamines and Decongestants (Systemic)**, 343
 Solution, Oral, 355, 356, 361, 363, 364
 Syrup, 355, 356, 361, 363, 364
 Tablets, Extended-release, 350, 355, 356, 358, 363, 364, 365, MC-6
Chlorpheniramine Maleate, Phenyltoloxamine Dihydrogen Citrate, Phenylpropanolamine Hydrochloride, and Acetaminophen [*Norel Plus*]
 **See Antihistamines, Decongestants, and Analgesics (Systemic)**, 366
 Capsules, 370
Chlorpheniramine Maleate and Pseudoephedrine Hydrochloride [*Allerest Maximum Strength; Anamine; Anamine T.D.; Atrohist Pediatric; Brexin L.A.; Chlorafed; Chlorafed H.S.Timecelles; Chlorafed Timecelles; Chlordrine S.R.; Chlorfed; Chlorfed II; Chlorphedrine SR; Codimal-L.A.; Codimal-L.A. Half; Colfed-A; Cophene No.2; Co-Pyronil 2; Deconamine; Deconamine SR; Deconomed SR; Dorcol Children's Cold Formula; Duralex; Dura-Tap PD; Fedahist; Fedahist Gyrocaps; Fedahist Timecaps; Hayfebrol; Histalet; Klerist-D; Kronofed-A Jr. Kronocaps; Kronofed-A Kronocaps; Med-Hist; ND Clear T.D.; Novafed A; Novahistex; PediaCare Cold-Allergy; PediaCare Cold Formula; Pseudo-Chlor; Pseudo-gest Plus; Rescon; Rescon-ED; Rescon JR; Rhinosyn; Rhinosyn-PD; Rinade B.I.D.; Ryna; Sudafed Plus; Vasofrinic; Vicks Children's DayQuil Allergy Relief*]
 **See Antihistamines and Decongestants (Systemic)**343
 Capsules, 350
 Capsules, Extended-release, 345, 346, 348, 349, 350, 353, 354, 355, 356, 357, 358, 359
 Solution, Oral, 348, 352, 353, 357, 359, 360, 365
 Syrup, 345, 350, 354
 Tablets, 344, 348, 350, 353, 354, 358, 361
 Tablets, Chewable, 350, 357
Chlorpheniramine Maleate, Pseudoephedrine Hydrochloride, and Acetaminophen [*Alka-Seltzer Plus Allergy Medicine Liqui-Gels; Alka-Seltzer Plus Cold Medicine Liqui-Gels; Allerest Sinus Pain Formula Caplets; Children's Tylenol Cold Multi-Symptom; Codimal; Co-Hist; Comtrex Allergy-Sinus; Comtrex Allergy-Sinus Caplets; Kolephrin Caplets; Simplet; Sinarest; Sinarest Extra Strength Caplets; Sine-Off Sinus Medicine Caplets; Singlet for Adults; Sinus Headache & Congestion; Sinutab Extra Strength Caplets; Sinutab Regular Caplets; Sinutab Sinus Allergy Maximum Strength; Sinutab Sinus Allergy Maximum Strength Caplets; TheraFlu/Flu and Cold Medicine; TheraFlu/Flu and Cold Medicine for Sore Throat; Tylenol Allergy Sinus Medication Extra Strength Caplets; Tylenol Allergy Sinus Medication Maximum Strength Gelcaps; Tylenol Allergy Sinus Medication Maximum Strength Geltabs; Tylenol Cold Medication Children's*]
 **See Antihistamines, Decongestants, and Analgesics (Systemic)**, 366
 Capsules, 367, 368
 Solution, Oral, 368, 373
 for Solution, Oral, 372
 Tablets, 367, 368, 370, 371, 372
 Tablets, Chewable, 368, 373

Chlorpheniramine Maleate, Pseudoephedrine Hydrochloride, Codeine, and Acetaminophen [*Sinutab with Codeine*]
 **See Cough/Cold Combinations (Systemic)**, 1024
 Tablets, 1094
Chlorpheniramine Maleate, Pseudoephedrine Hydrochloride, and Codeine Phosphate [*Codehist DH; Decohistine DH; Dihistine DH; Midahist DH; Novahistine DH Liquid; Phenhist DH with Codeine; Ryna-C Liquid*]
 **See Cough/Cold Combinations (Systemic)**, 1024
 Elixir, 1044, 1070
 Solution, Oral, 1050, 1052, 1074, 1081, 1092
Chlorpheniramine Maleate, Pseudoephedrine Hydrochloride, and Dextromethorphan Hydrobromide [*PediaCare Cough-Cold; PediaCare NightRest Cough-Cold Liquid; Rescon-DM; Rhinosyn-DM; Triaminic DM NightTime for Children; Triaminic Night Time; Triaminicol DM; Tussar DM; Tussilyn DM; Vicks Children's NyQuil; Vicks Children's NyQuil Cold/Cough Relief; Vicks Pediatric 44M Multi-Symptom Cough & Cold*]
 **See Cough/Cold Combinations (Systemic)**, 1024
 Solution, Oral, 1078, 1086, 1102, 1112, 1115
 Syrup, 1101, 1102, 1105, 1106
 Tablets, Chewable, 1078
Chlorpheniramine Maleate, Pseudoephedrine Hydrochloride, Dextromethorphan Hydrobromide, and Acetaminophen [*Alka-Seltzer Plus Cold & Cough Medicine Liqui-Gels; Children's Tylenol Cold Plus Cough Multi Symptom; Co-Apap; Comtrex Nighttime; Comtrex Nighttime Maximum Strength Cold, Cough and Flu Relief; Comtrex Nighttime Maximum Strength Cold and Flu Relief; Kolephrin/DM Cough and Cold Medication; Mapap Cold Formula; TheraFlu Flu, Cold & Cough Medicine; TheraFlu Nighttime Maximum Strength Flu, Cold & Cough; Tylenol Children's Cold DM Medication; Tylenol Cold and Flu; Tylenol Cold Medication; Tylenol Cold Medication Caplets; Tylenol Cold Medication Extra Strength Nighttime Caplets; Tylenol Cold Medication Regular Strength Nighttime Caplets; Tylenol Cold Multi-Symptom; Tylenol Extra Strength Cold and Flu Medication Powder; Tylenol Junior Strength Cold DM Medication; Vicks Formula 44M; Vicks 44M Cough, Cold and Flu Relief; Vicks 44M Cough, Cold and Flu Relief LiquiCaps*]
 **See Cough/Cold Combinations (Systemic)**, 1024
 Capsules, 1032, 1114
 Solution, Oral, 1043, 1046, 1108, 1109, 1114
 for Solution, Oral, 1098, 1099, 1108, 1110
 Syrup, 1114
 Tablets, 1044, 1046, 1047, 1068, 1069, 1109, 1110
 Tablets, Chewable, 1043, 1108, 1110
Chlorpheniramine Maleate, Pseudoephedrine Hydrochloride, Dextromethorphan Hydrobromide, and Guaifenesin [*Triaminic-DM Expectorant*]
 **See Cough/Cold Combinations (Systemic)**, 1024
 Solution, Oral, 1100
Chlorpheniramine Maleate, Pseudoephedrine Hydrochloride, and Guaifenesin [*Triaminic Expectorant*]
 **See Cough/Cold Combinations (Systemic)**, 1024
 Solution, Oral, 1101
Chlorpheniramine Maleate, Pseudoephedrine Hydrochloride, and Hydrocodone Bitartrate [*Histinex PV; Promist HD Liquid; P-V-Tussin*]
 **See Cough/Cold Combinations (Systemic)**, 1024
 Solution, Oral, 1084
 Syrup, 1063, 1085
Chlorpheniramine Maleate, Pseudoephedrine Hydrochloride, and Methscopolamine Nitrate [*Mescolor*]
 **See Antihistamines, Decongestants, and Anticholinergics (Systemic)**, 373
 Tablets, Extended-release, 375
Chlorpheniramine Maleate and Pseudoephedrine Sulfate [*Chlor-Trimeton Allergy-D 12 Hour; Chlor-Trimeton 4 Hour Relief; Chlor-Trimeton 12 Hour Relief*]
 **See Antihistamines and Decongestants (Systemic)**, 343
 Tablets, 348
 Tablets, Extended-release, 348
Chlorpheniramine Maleate, Pyrilamine Maleate, Phenylephrine Hydrochloride, and Acetaminophen [*ND-Gesic*]
 **See Antihistamines, Decongestants, and Analgesics (Systemic)**, 366
 Tablets, 370

Chlorpheniramine Maleate, Pyrilamine Maleate, Phenylephrine Hydrochloride, and Phenylpropanolamine Hydrochloride [*Histalet Forte; Poly Hist Forte; Vanex Forte Caplets*]
 **See Antihistamines and Decongestants (Systemic)**, 343
 Tablets, 354, 358
 Tablets, Extended-release, 365
Chlorpheniramine Maleate, Pyrilamine Maleate, Phenylephrine Hydrochloride, Phenylpropanolamine Hydrochloride, and Acetaminophen [*Covangesic*]
 **See Antihistamines, Decongestants, and Analgesics (Systemic)**, 366
 Tablets, 369
Chlorpheniramine, Phenyltoloxamine, Ephedrine, Codeine, and Guaiacol Carbonate [*Omni-Tuss*]
 **See Cough/Cold Combinations (Systemic)**, 1024
 Suspension, Oral, 1076
Chlorpheniramine and Codeine Polistirexes [*Penntuss*]
 **See Cough/Cold Combinations (Systemic)**, 1024
 Suspension, Oral, 1079
Chlorpheniramine and Phenylpropanolamine Polistirexes [*Corsym*]
 **See Antihistamines and Decongestants (Systemic)**, 343
 Suspension, Oral, Extended-release, 350
Chlorpheniramine Tannate, Ephedrine Tannate, Phenylephrine Tannate, and Carbetapentane Tannate [*Rentamine Pediatric; Rynatuss; Rynatuss Pediatric; Tri-Tannate Plus Pediatric*]
 **See Cough/Cold Combinations (Systemic)**, 1024
 Suspension, Oral, 1086, 1092, 1104
 Tablets, 1092
Chlorpheniramine Tannate and Phenylephrine Tannate [*Ricobid; Ricobid Pediatric*]
 **See Antihistamines and Decongestants (Systemic)**, 343
 Suspension, Oral, 359
 Tablets, 359
Chlorpheniramine Tannate and Pseudoephedrine Tannate [*Tanafed*]
 **See Antihistamines and Decongestants (Systemic)**, 343
 Suspension, Oral, 361
Chlorpheniramine Tannate, Pyrilamine Tannate, and Phenylephrine Tannate [*Atrohist Pediatric Suspension Dye Free; Histatan; Rhinatate; R-Tannamine; R-Tannamine Pediatric; R-Tannate; R-Tannate Pediatric; Rynatan; Rynatan Pediatric; Rynatan-S Pediatric; Tanoral; Triotann; Triotann Pediatric; Triotann-S Pediatric; Tritan; Tri-Tannate; Tri-Tannate Pediatric, Vanex Forte Caplets*]
 **See Antihistamines and Decongestants (Systemic)**, 343
 Suspension, Oral, 345, 360, 361, 363, 364
 Tablets, 354, 359, 360, 362, 363, 364
*Chlorpromanyl-5*—Technilab (Canada) brand of Chlorpromazine—**See Phenothiazines (Systemic)**, 2289
*Chlorpromanyl-20*—Technilab (Canada) brand of Chlorpromazine—**See Phenothiazines (Systemic)**, 2289
*Chlorpromanyl-40*—Technilab (Canada) brand of Chlorpromazine—**See Phenothiazines (Systemic)**, 2289
Chlorpromazine [*Largactil; Thorazine*]
 **See Phenothiazines (Systemic)**, 2289
 Suppositories USP, 2299
Chlorpromazine Hydrochloride [*Chlorpromanyl-5; Chlorpromanyl-20; Chlorpromanyl-40; Largactil; Largactil Liquid; Largactil Oral Drops; Novo-Chlorpromazine; Ormazine; Thorazine; Thorazine Concentrate; Thorazine Spansule; Thor-Prom*]
 **See Phenothiazines (Systemic)**, 2289
 Capsules, Extended-release, 2296, MC-6
 Concentrate, Oral, USP, 2297
 Injection USP, 2298
 Syrup USP, 2297
 Tablets USP, 2298, MC-7
Chlorpropamide [*Apo-Chlorpropamide; Diabinese; Novo-Propamide*]
 **See Antidiabetic Agents, Sulfonylurea (Systemic)**, 283
 Tablets USP, 292, MC-7

## USP DI

Chlorprothixene [*Taractan*]
   **See Thioxanthenes (Systemic)**, 2793
   Injection USP, 2798
   Suspension, Oral, USP, 2797
   Tablets USP, 2797
*Chlor-Rest*—Rugby (U.S.) brand of Chlorpheniramine and Phenylpropanolamine—**See Antihistamines and Decongestants (Systemic)**, 343
Chlorthalidone—Chlorthalidone—**See Diuretics, Thiazide (Systemic)**, 1273
Chlortetracycline Hydrochloride [*Aureomycin*]
   **See Tetracyclines (Ophthalmic)**, 2763
   Ointment, Ophthalmic, USP, 2764
Chlortetracycline Hydrochloride [*Aureomycin*]
   **See Tetracyclines (Topical)**, 2774
   Ointment USP, 2775
Chlorthalidone [*Apo-Chlorthalidone;* chlortalidone; *Hygroton; Novo-Thalidone; Thalitone; Uridon*]
   **See Diuretics, Thiazide (Systemic)**, 1273
   Tablets USP, 1278, MC-7
Chlorthalidone-containing Combinations, 3070
*Chlortox*—Major (U.S.) brand of Chlorpheniramine, Phenyltoloxamine, and Phenylephrine—**See Antihistamines and Decongestants (Systemic)**, 343
*Chlor-Trimeton*—Key (U.S.) brand of Chlorpheniramine—**See Antihistamines (Systemic)**, 325, MC-6
*Chlor-Trimeton Allergy*—Schering-Plough (U.S.) brand of Chlorpheniramine—**See Antihistamines (Systemic)**, 325
*Chlor-Trimeton Allergy-Sinus Caplets*—Schering-Plough (U.S.) brand of Chlorpheniramine, Phenylpropanolamine, and Acetaminophen—**See Antihistamines, Decongestants, and Analgesics (Systemic)**, 366
*Chlor-Trimeton 4 Hour Relief*—Schering-Plough (U.S.) brand of Chlorpheniramine and Pseudoephedrine—**See Antihistamines and Decongestants (Systemic)**, 343
*Chlor-Trimeton 12 Hour Relief*—Schering-Plough (U.S.) brand of Chlorpheniramine and Pseudoephedrine—**See Antihistamines and Decongestants (Systemic)**, 343
*Chlor-Trimeton Non-Drowsy Decongestant 4 Hour*—Schering-Plough (U.S.) brand of Pseudoephedrine (Systemic), 2422
*Chlor-Trimeton Repetabs*—Schering (U.S.) brand of Chlorpheniramine—**See Antihistamines (Systemic)**, 325
*Chlor-Tripolon*—Schering (Canada) brand of Chlorpheniramine—**See Antihistamines (Systemic)**, 325
*Chlor-Tripolon Decongestant*—Schering (Canada) brand of Chlorpheniramine and Phenylpropanolamine—**See Antihistamines and Decongestants (Systemic)**, 343
*Chlor-Tripolon N.D.*—Schering (Canada) brand of Loratadine and Pseudoephedrine—**See Antihistamines and Decongestants (Systemic)**, 343
Chlorzoxazone [*EZE-DS; Paraflex; Parafon Forte DSC; Relaxazone; Remular; Remular-S; Strifon Forte DSC*]
   **See Skeletal Muscle Relaxants (Systemic)**, 2577
   Tablets USP, 2580, MC-7
Chlorzoxazone and Acetaminophen [chlorzoxazone with APAP; *Parafon Forte*]
   **(Systemic)**, 853
   Tablets, 853
Chlorzoxazone with APAP—See Chlorzoxazone and Acetaminophen (Systemic), 853
Chlorzoxazone-containing Combinations, 3070
*Cholac*—Alra (U.S.) brand of Lactulose—**See Laxatives (Local)**, #
*Cholebrine*—Mallinckrodt (U.S.) brand of Iocetamic Acid—**See Cholecystographic Agents, Oral (Systemic)**, #
Cholecystographic Agents, Oral
   **(Systemic)**, #
Cholecystokinin [CCK; pancreozymin]
   **(Systemic)**, 1451
   for Injection, #
*Choledyl*—PD (U.S. and Canada) brand of Oxtriphylline—**See Bronchodilators, Theophylline (Systemic)**, 668
*Choledyl Expectorant*—PD (Canada) brand of Oxtriphylline and Guaifenesin (Systemic), #
*Choledyl SA*—PD (U.S. and Canada) brand of Oxtriphylline—**See Bronchodilators, Theophylline (Systemic)**, 668

Cholera Vaccine
   **(Systemic)**, #
   Cholera Vaccine USP, #
Cholestyramine [*Questran; Questran Light*]
   **(Oral-Local)**, 853
   for Suspension, Oral, USP, 856
*Choletec*—Squibb (U.S.) and Squibb Diagnostics (Canada) brand of Technetium Tc 99m Mebrofenin (Systemic), 2716
Choline Chloride
   **(Systemic)**, 3136
Choline magnesium trisalicylate—Choline and Magnesium Salicylates—**See Salicylates (Systemic)**, 2538
Choline Salicylate [*Arthropan*]
   **See Salicylates (Systemic)**, 2538
   Solution, Oral, USP, 2551
Choline Salicylate and Cetyl-dimethyl-benzyl-ammonium Chloride [*Teejel*]
   **(Mucosal-Local)**, 3014
   Gel, 3014
Choline Salicylate-containing Combinations, 3070
Choline and Magnesium Salicylates [choline magnesium trisalicylate; *CMT; Tricosal; Trilisate*]
   **See Salicylates (Systemic)**, 2538
   Solution, Oral, 2552
   Tablets, 2552
Choline theophyllinate—Oxtriphylline—**See Bronchodilators, Theophylline (Systemic)**, 668
Choline theophyllinate—Oxtriphylline—**See Bronchodilators, Theophylline (Systemic)**, 668
*Cholografin*—Bracco (U.S.) and Squibb (Canada) brand of Iodipamide (Systemic), #
*Cholografin for Infusion*—Bracco (U.S.) brand of Iodipamide (Systemic), #
Chondrocytes, Autologous Cultured [*Carticel*]
   **(Implantation-Local)**, 856
   for Implantation, 858
Chondroitinase
   **(Ophthalmic)**, 3136
*Chooz*—Plough (U.S.) brand of Calcium Carbonate—**See Calcium Supplements (Systemic)**, 736; Schering Plough (U.S.) brand of Calcium Carbonate—**See Antacids (Oral-Local)**, 188
Chorionic Gonadotropin [*A.P.L.;* hCG; human chorionic gonadotropin; *Pregnyl; Profasi; Profasi HP*]
   **(Systemic)**, 858
   for Injection USP, 860
Christmas factor—See Factor IX (Systemic), 1430
*Chroma-Pak*—Solo-Pak (U.S.) brand of Chromic Chloride—**See Chromium Supplements (Systemic)**, 861
Chromic Chloride [*Chroma-Pak*]
   **See Chromium Supplements (Systemic)**, 861
   Injection USP, 862
Chromic Phosphate P 32 [*Phosphocol P 32*]
   **(Parenteral-Local)**, #
   Suspension USP, #
*Chromitope*—Bracco (U.S.) brand of Sodium Chromate Cr 51 (Systemic), 2590
Chromium
   **See Chromium Supplements (Systemic)**, 861
   Capsules, 863
   Tablets, 863
Chromium Supplements
   **(Systemic)**, 861
*Chronovera*—Searle (Canada) brand of Verapamil (Systemic), 3037
*Chronulac*—Hoescht Marion Roussel (U.S.) and Marion Merrell Dow (Canada) brand of Lactulose—**See Laxatives (Local)**, #
*Chymex*—Adria (U.S.) brand of Bentiromide (Systemic), #
*Chymodiactin*—Boots (U.S. and Canada) brand of Chymopapain (Parenteral-Local), #
Chymopapain [*Chymodiactin*]
   **(Parenteral-Local)**, #
   for Injection, #
*Cibacalcin*—Ciba-Geigy (U.S.) brand of Calcitonin-Human—**See Calcitonin (Systemic)**, 716; Ciba-Geigy (U.S.) brand of Calcitonin-Human (Systemic), 3135
*Cibalith-S*—Ciba (U.S.) brand of Lithium (Systemic), 1869
Ciclopirox Olamine [*Loprox*]
   **(Topical)**, 863
   Cream USP, 864
   Lotion, 864
Ciclosporin—See Cyclosporine (Systemic), 1136
Cidofovir [*Vistide*]
   **(Systemic)**, 865
   Injection, 867

## General Index     3263

*Cidomycin*—Roussel (Canada) brand of Gentamicin—**See Aminoglycosides (Systemic)**, 69
Cilastatin-containing Combinations, 3070
Ciliary Neurotrophic Factor
   **(Systemic)**, 3137
Ciliary Neurotrophic Factor, Recombinant Human
   **(Systemic)**, 3137
*Cillium*—Superior (U.S.) and Whitworth (U.S.) brand of Psyllium—**See Laxatives (Local)**, #
*Ciloxan*—Alcon (U.S. and Canada) brand of Ciprofloxacin (Ophthalmic), 868
Cimetidine [*Apo-Cimetidine; Gen-Cimetidine; Novo-Cimetine; Nu-Cimet; Peptol; PMS-Cimetidine; Tagamet; Tagamet HB; Tagamet HB 200*]
   **See Histamine H$_2$-receptor Antagonists (Systemic)**, 1633
   Tablets USP, 1637, MC-7
Cimetidine Hydrochloride [*Tagamet*]
   **See Histamine H$_2$-receptor Antagonists (Systemic)**, 1633
   Injection, 1638
   Solution, Oral, 1638
*Cinalone 40*—Legere (U.S.) brand of Triamcinolone—**See Corticosteroids—Glucocorticoid Effects (Systemic)**, 998
Cinchocaine—Dibucaine—**See Anesthetics (Mucosal-Local)**, 128; **Anesthetics (Topical)**, 155
C1-Inhibitor [*C1-Inhibitor (Human) Vapor Heated, Immuno*]
   **(Systemic)**, 3135
C1-Inhibitor (Human) Vapor Heated, Immuno—Immuno (U.S.) brand of C1-Inhibitor (Systemic), 3135
*Cinobac*—Oclassen (U.S.) brand of Cinoxacin (Systemic), #
*Cinonide 40*—Legere (U.S.) brand of Triamcinolone—**See Corticosteroids—Glucocorticoid Effects (Systemic)**, 998
Cinoxacin [*Cinobac*]
   **(Systemic)**, #
   Capsules USP, #
*Cin-Quin*—Solvay (U.S.) brand of Quinidine (Systemic), 2440
*Cipro*—Bayer (U.S. and Canada) brand of Ciprofloxacin—**See Fluoroquinolones (Systemic)**, 1487, MC-7
*Cipro I.V.*—Bayer (U.S.) brand of Ciprofloxacin—**See Fluoroquinolones (Systemic)**, 1487
Ciprofloxacin [*Cipro; Cipro I.V.*]
   **See Fluoroquinolones (Systemic)**, 1487
   Injection, 1493
   for Suspension, Oral, 1492
   Tablets, 1492, MC-7
Ciprofloxacin Hydrochloride [*Ciloxan*]
   **(Ophthalmic)**, 868
   Solution, Ophthalmic, USP, 869
13-cis-Acitretin—See Acitretin (Systemic), 18
Cisapride [*Prepulsid; Propulsid*]
   **(Systemic)**, 869
   Suspension, Oral, 871
   Tablets, 872, MC-7
Cisatracurium [*Nimbex*]
   **(Systemic)**, 872
   Injection, 875
Cisplatin [*Platinol; Platinol-AQ*]
   **(Systemic)**, 876
   Injection, 880
   for Injection USP, 880
9-Cis-Retinoic Acid
   **(Ophthalmic)**, 3128
9-Cis Retinoic Acid
   **(Systemic)**, 3128
*Cistobil*—Merck (U.K.) brand of Iopanoic Acid—**See Cholecystographic Agents, Oral (Systemic)**, #
Citalopram Hydrobromide [*Celexa*]
   **(Systemic)**, 3014
   Tablets, 3014
*Citanest Forte*—Astra (U.S. and Canada) brand of Prilocaine—**See Anesthetics (Parenteral-Local)**, 139
*Citanest Plain*—Astra (U.S. and Canada) brand of Prilocaine—**See Anesthetics (Parenteral-Local)**, 139
*Citracal*—Mission (U.S.) brand of Calcium Citrate—**See Calcium Supplements (Systemic)**, 736
*Citracal Liquitabs*—Mission (U.S.) brand of Calcium Citrate—**See Calcium Supplements (Systemic)**, 736

## General Index

*Citra Forte*—Boyle (U.S.) brand of Chlorpheniramine, Pheniramine, Pyrilamine, Phenylephrine, Hydrocodone, Salicylamide, Caffeine, and Ascorbic Acid—**See Cough/Cold Combinations (Systemic)**, 1024; Boyle (U.S.) brand of Pheniramine, Pyrilamine, Hydrocodone, Potassium Citrate, and Ascorbic Acid—**See Cough/Cold Combinations (Systemic)**, 1024
Citrates
 **(Systemic)**, 881
Citric Acid–containing Combinations, 3070
Citric Acid and D-Gluconic Acid [*Renacidin Powder for Irrigation*]
 **(Local)**, 3014
 for Solution, Topical, 3014
Citric Acid, Glucono-delta-lactone, and Magnesium Carbonate [*Renacidin Irrigation*]
 **(Local)**, 3015, 3137
 Solution, 3015
*CitriSource*—Sandoz (U.S.) brand of Enteral Nutrition Formula, Polymeric—**See Enteral Nutrition Formulas (Systemic)**, #
*Citrocarbonate*—Upjohn (U.S. and Canada) brand of Sodium Bicarbonate (Systemic), 2586
*Citrolith*—Beach (U.S.) brand of Potassium Citrate and Sodium Citrate—**See Citrates (Systemic)**, 881
*Citroma*—Cumberland-Swan (U.S.) brand of Magnesium Citrate—**See Laxatives (Local)**, #; Cumberland Swan (U.S.) brand of Magnesium Citrate—**See Magnesium Supplements (Systemic)**, 1897
*Citro-Mag*—Rougier (Canada) brand of Magnesium Citrate—**See Laxatives (Local)**, #; **Magnesium Supplements (Systemic)**, 1897
*Citrotein*—Sandoz (U.S.) brand of Enteral Nutrition Formula, Disease-specific—**See Enteral Nutrition Formulas (Systemic)**, #; Enteral Nutrition Formula, Polymeric—**See Enteral Nutrition Formulas (Systemic)**, #
Citrovorum factor—See Leucovorin (Systemic), 1837
*Citrucel Orange Flavor*—SmithKline Beecham (U.S.) brand of Methylcellulose—**See Laxatives (Local)**, #
*Citrucel Sugar-Free Orange Flavor*—SmithKline Beecham (U.S.) brand of Methylcellulose—**See Laxatives (Local)**, #
Cladribine [*Leustatin; Leustatin Injection*]
 **(Systemic)**, 886, 3137
 Injection, 889, 3137
*Claforan*—Hoechst-Roussel (U.S.) and Roussel (Canada) brand of Cefotaxime—**See Cephalosporins (Systemic)**, 794
*Claripex*—ICN (Canada) brand of Clofibrate (Systemic), 900
Clarithromycin [*Biaxin*]
 **(Systemic)**, 889
 for Suspension, Oral, 892
 Tablets USP, 892, MC-7
*Claritin*—Schering (U.S. and Canada) brand of Loratadine—**See Antihistamines (Systemic)**, 325, MC-17
*Claritin-D 12 Hour*—Schering (U.S.) brand of Loratadine and Pseudoephedrine—**See Antihistamines and Decongestants (Systemic)**, 343, MC-18
*Claritin-D 24 Hour*—Schering (U.S.) brand of Loratadine and Pseudoephedrine—**See Antihistamines and Decongestants (Systemic)**, 343, MC-18
*Claritin Extra*—Schering (Canada) brand of Loratadine and Pseudoephedrine—**See Antihistamines and Decongestants (Systemic)**, 343
*Claritin Reditabs*—Schering (U.S. and Canada) brand of Loratadine—**See Antihistamines (Systemic)**, 325
*Class Act Ribbed & Sensitive*—Carter-Wallace (U.S.) brand of Latex Condoms—**See Condoms**, #
*Class Act Ultra Thin & Sensitive*—Carter-Wallace (U.S.) brand of Latex Condoms—**See Condoms**, #
*Class Act Ultra Thin & Sensitive Spermicidal Lubricated*—Carter-Wallace (U.S.) brand of Latex Condoms and Nonoxynol 9—**See Condoms**, #
Clavulanate-containing Combinations, 3070
*Clavulin-250*—SmithKline Beecham (Canada) brand of Amoxicillin and Clavulanate—**See Penicillins and Beta-lactamase Inhibitors (Systemic)**, 2263

*Clavulin-125F*—SmithKline Beecham (Canada) brand of Amoxicillin and Clavulanate—**See Penicillins and Beta-lactamase Inhibitors (Systemic)**, 2263
*Clavulin-250F*—SmithKline Beecham (Canada) brand of Amoxicillin and Clavulanate—**See Penicillins and Beta-lactamase Inhibitors (Systemic)**, 2263
*Clavulin-500F*—SmithKline Beecham (Canada) brand of Amoxicillin and Clavulanate—**See Penicillins and Beta-lactamase Inhibitors (Systemic)**, 2263
*Clean & Clear Persagel 5*—Johnson & Johnson (U.S.) brand of Benzoyl Peroxide (Topical), 579
*Clean & Clear Persagel 10*—Johnson & Johnson (U.S.) brand of Benzoyl Peroxide (Topical), 579
*Clearasil Adult Care Medicated Blemish Cream*—Richardson-Vicks (U.S.) brand of Resorcinol and Sulfur (Topical), #
*Clearasil Adult Care Medicated Blemish Stick*—Richardson-Vicks (U.S.) brand of Resorcinol and Sulfur (Topical), #
*Clearasil BP Plus 5 Lotion*—Richardson-Vicks (Canada) brand of Benzoyl Peroxide (Topical), 579
*Clearasil BP Plus Skin Tone Cream*—Procter & Gamble (Canada) brand of Benzoyl Peroxide (Topical), 579
*Clearasil Clearstick Maximum Strength Topical Solution*—Richardson-Vicks (U.S.) brand of Salicylic Acid (Topical), #
*Clearasil Clearstick Regular Strength Topical Solution*—Richardson-Vicks (U.S.) brand of Salicylic Acid (Topical), #
*Clearasil Double Textured Pads Maximum Strength*—Richardson-Vicks (U.S.) brand of Salicylic Acid (Topical), #
*Clearasil Double Textured Pads Regular Strength*—Richardson-Vicks (U.S.) brand of Salicylic Acid (Topical), #
*Clearasil Maximum Strength Medicated Anti-Acne 10 Tinted Cream*—Procter & Gamble (U.S.) brand of Benzoyl Peroxide (Topical), 579
*Clearasil Maximum Strength Medicated Anti-Acne 10 Vanishing Cream*—Richardson-Vicks (U.S.) brand of Benzoyl Peroxide (Topical), 579
*Clearasil Maximum Strength Medicated Anti-Acne 10 Vanishing Lotion*—Richardson-Vicks (U.S.) brand of Benzoyl Peroxide (Topical), 579
*Clearasil Medicated Deep Cleanser Topical Solution*—Richardson-Vicks (U.S.) brand of Salicylic Acid (Topical), #
*Clear Away*—Scholl (U.S.) brand of Salicylic Acid (Topical), #
*ClearBlue Easy*—Unipath (U.S.) and Novartis Consumer (Canada) brand of Immunoassay Pregnancy Test Kits—**See Pregnancy Test Kits for Home Use**, #
*ClearBlue Easy One Minute*—Unipath (U.S.) brand of Immunoassay Pregnancy Test Kits—**See Pregnancy Test Kits for Home Use**, #
*Clear By Design 2.5 Gel*—SmithKline Beecham (U.S.) brand of Benzoyl Peroxide (Topical), 579
*Clear by Design Medicated Cleansing Pads*—SmithKline Beecham (U.S.) brand of Salicylic Acid (Topical), #
*Clear Eyes Lubricating Eye Redness Reliever*—Ross Consumer (U.S.) brand of Naphazoline (Ophthalmic), #
*Clearplan Easy*—Whitehall (U.S.) and Ciba-Geigy (Canada) brand of Enzyme Immunoassay Ovulation Prediction Test Kits—**See Ovulation Prediction Test Kits for Home Use**, #
*Clearplex 5*—Med-Derm (U.S.) brand of Benzoyl Peroxide (Topical), 579
*ClearPlex 10*—Med-Derm (U.S.) brand of Benzoyl Peroxide (Topical), 579
Clemastine-containing Combinations, 3070
Clemastine Fumarate [*Contac 12 Hour Allergy; Tavist; Tavist-1*]
 **See Antihistamines (Systemic)**, 325
 Syrup, 335
 Tablets USP, 335
Clemastine Fumarate and Phenylpropanolamine Hydrochloride [*Tavist-D*]
 **See Antihistamines and Decongestants (Systemic)**, 343
 Tablets, Extended-release, 362
*Cleocin*—Pharmacia & Upjohn (U.S.) brand of Clindamycin (Systemic), 893, MC-7; Pharmacia & Upjohn (U.S.) brand of Clindamycin (Vaginal), 898; Upjohn (U.S.) brand of Clindamycin (Systemic), 3137

*Cleocin Pediatric*—Upjohn (U.S.) brand of Clindamycin (Systemic), 893
*Cleocin T Gel*—Upjohn (U.S.) brand of Clindamycin (Topical), 896
*Cleocin T Lotion*—Upjohn (U.S.) brand of Clindamycin (Topical), 896
*Cleocin T Topical Solution*—Upjohn (U.S.) brand of Clindamycin (Topical), 896
Clidinium Bromide [*Quarzan*]
 **See Anticholinergics/Antispasmodics (Systemic)**, 226
 Capsules USP, 234
Clidinium-containing Combinations, 3070
*Climacteron*—Merck Frosst (Canada) brand of Testosterone and Estradiol—**See Androgens and Estrogens (Systemic)**, 126
*Climara*—Berlex (U.S.) brand of Estradiol—**See Estrogens (Systemic)**, 1383
*Clinagen LA 40*—Clint (U.S.) brand of Estradiol—**See Estrogens (Systemic)**, 1383
*Clinda-Derm*—Paddock (U.S.) brand of Clindamycin (Topical), 896
Clindamycin [*Cleocin*]
 **(Systemic)**, 3137
Clindamycin Hydrochloride [*Cleocin; Dalacin C*]
 **(Systemic)**, 893
 Capsules USP, 895, MC-7
Clindamycin Palmitate Hydrochloride [*Cleocin Pediatric; Dalacin C Flavored Granules*]
 **(Systemic)**, 893
 for Solution, Oral, USP, 895
Clindamycin Phosphate [*Cleocin; Dalacin C Phosphate*]
 **(Systemic)**, 893
 Injection USP, 895
Clindamycin Phosphate [*Cleocin T Gel; Cleocin T Lotion; Cleocin T Topical Solution; Clinda-Derm; Dalacin T Topical Solution*]
 **(Topical)**, 896
 Gel USP, 898
 Solution, Topical, USP, 898
 Suspension, Topical, USP, 898
Clindamycin Phosphate [*Cleocin; Dalacin*]
 **(Vaginal)**, 898
 Cream, Vaginal, USP, 900
*Clindex*—Rugby (U.S.) brand of Chlordiazepoxide and Clidinium (Systemic), 846, MC-6
*Clinistix*—Ames (U.S. and Canada) brand of Glucose Oxidase Urine Glucose Test—**See Urine Glucose and Ketone Test Kits for Home Use**, #
*Clinitest*—Ames (U.S. and Canada) brand of Copper Reduction Urine Glucose Test—**See Urine Glucose and Ketone Test Kits for Home Use**, #
*Clinoril*—Merck (U.S.) and Frosst (Canada) brand of Sulindac—**See Anti-inflammatory Drugs, Nonsteroidal (Systemic)**, 388, MC-29
*Clinoxide*—Geneva Generics (U.S.) brand of Chlordiazepoxide and Clidinium (Systemic), 846
Clioquinol [iodochlorhydroxyquin; *Vioform*]
 **(Topical)**,
 Cream USP, #
 Ointment USP, #
Clioquinol-containing Combinations, 3070
Clioquinol and Flumethasone Pivalate [*Locacorten Vioform*]
 **(Otic)**, 3015
 Solution, Otic, 3015
Clioquinol and Flumethasone Pivalate [*Locacorten Vioform*]
 **(Topical)**, 3015
 Cream, 3015
 Ointment, 3015
Clioquinol and Hydrocortisone [iodochlorhydroxyquin and hydrocortisone; *Vioform-Hydrocortisone Cream; Vioform-Hydrocortisone Lotion; Vioform-Hydrocortisone Mild Cream; Vioform-Hydrocortisone Mild Ointment; Vioform-Hydrocortisone Ointment*]
 **(Topical)**,
 Cream, #
 Lotion, #
 Ointment, #
*Clipoxide*—Schein (U.S.) brand of Chlordiazepoxide and Clidinium (Systemic), 846
Clobazam [*Frisium*]
 **See Benzodiazepines (Systemic)**, 556
 Tablets, 566

# General Index

Clobetasol Propionate [*Cormax; Dermovate; Dermovate Scalp Lotion; Temovate; Temovate E; Temovate Scalp Application*]
**See Corticosteroids (Topical)**, 978, 3015
Cream, 985
Cream USP
Ointment, 986
Ointment USP, 3015
Solution, 986
Clobetasone Butyrate [*Eumovate*]
**See Corticosteroids (Topical)**, 978
Cream, 986
Ointment, 986
Clocortolone Pivalate [*Cloderm*]
**See Corticosteroids (Topical)**, 978
Cream USP, 986
*Cloderm*—Hermal (U.S.) brand of Clocortolone—**See Corticosteroids (Topical)**, 978
Clofazimine [*Lamprene*]
**(Systemic)**, #, 3137
Capsules USP, #
Clofibrate [*Abitrate; Atromid-S; Claripex; Novofibrate*]
**(Systemic)**, 900
Capsules USP, 903
*Clomid*—Hoechst Marion Roussel (U.S. and Canada) brand of Clomiphene (Systemic), 903, MC-7
Clomifene—*See* Clomiphene (Systemic), 903
Clomifene citrate—*See* Clomiphene (Systemic), 903
Clomiphene Citrate [*Clomid; clomifene; clomifene citrate; Milophene; Serophene*]
**(Systemic)**, 903
Tablets USP, 905, MC-7
Clomipramine Hydrochloride [*Anafranil*]
**See Antidepressants, Tricyclic (Systemic)**, 271
Capsules, 279, MC-7
Tablets, 279
*Clonapam*—ICN (Canada) brand of Clonazepam—See **Benzodiazepindes (Systemic)**, 556
Clonazepam [*Alti-Clonazepam; Apo-Clonazepam; Clonapam; Gen-Clonazepam; Klonopin; PMS-Clonazepam; Rivotril; Syn-Clonazepam*]
**See Benzodiazepines (Systemic)**, 556, 3137
Tablets USP, 567, MC-7
Clonidine [*Catapres-TTS*]
**(Systemic)**, 908, 3137
System, Transdermal, 911
Clonidine-containing Combinations, 3070
Clonidine Hydrochloride [*Catapres; Dixarit*]
**(Systemic)**, 908
Tablets USP, 911, MC-7
Clonidine Hydrochloride [*Duraclon*]
**(Parenteral-Local)**, 905
Injection, 908
Clonidine Hydrochloride and Chlorthalidone [*Clorpres; Combipres*]
**(Systemic)**, 912
Tablets USP, 912, MC-8
Clopidogrel Bisulfate [*Plavix*]
**(Systemic)**, 913
Tablets, 915
Clorazepate Dipotassium [*Apo-Clorazepate; Novo-Clopate; Tranxene; Tranxene-SD; Tranxene-SD Half Strength; Tranxene T-Tab*]
**See Benzodiazepines (Systemic)**, 556
Capsules, 568
Tablets USP, 568, MC-8
Tablets, Extended-Release, 568
*Clorpres*—Bertek (U.S.) brand of Clonidine and Chlorthalidone (Systemic), MC-8
Clostridial Collagenase
**(Systemic)**, 3137
*Clotrimaderm*—Taro (Canada) brand of Clotrimazole—**See Antifungals, Azole (Vaginal)**, 310
*Clotrimaderm Cream*—Taro (Canada) brand of Clotrimazole (Topical), 916
Clotrimazole [*Mycelex Troches*]
**(Oral-Local)**, 915
Lozenges, 916, MC-8
Clotrimazole [*Canesten Cream; Canesten Solution; Canesten Solution with Atomizer; Clotrimaderm Cream; Lotrimin AF Cream; Lotrimin AF Lotion; Lotrimin AF Solution; Lotrimin Cream; Lotrimin Lotion; Lotrimin Solution; Mycelex Cream; Mycelex Solution; Myclo Cream; Myclo Solution; Myclo Spray Solution; Neo-Zol Cream*]
**(Topical)**, 916
Cream USP, 917
Lotion USP, 917
Solution, Topical, USP, 918

Clotrimazole [*Canesten 1-Day Therapy; Canesten 3-Day Therapy; Canestan 6-Day Therapy; Canesten Combi-Pak 1-Day Therapy; Canesten Combi-Pak 3-Day Therapy; Canestan 1-Day Cream Combi-Pak; Clotrimaderm; FemCare; Gyne-Lotrimin; Gyne-Lotrimin 3; Gyne-Lotrimin 3 Combination Pack; Gyne-Lotrimin Combination Pack; Mycelex-7; Mycelex-G; Mycelex Twin Pack; Myclo-Gyne*]
**See Antifungals, Azole (Vaginal)**, 310
Cream USP (Vaginal), 312
Tablets, Vaginal, USP, 313
Clotrimazole and Betamethasone Dipropionate [*Lotriderm; Lotrisone*]
**(Topical)**, 918
Cream USP, 919
Clotrimazole-containing Combinations, 3070
Clotrimidazole
**(Systemic)**, 3137
Cloxacillin Sodium [*Apo-Cloxi; Cloxapen; Novo-Cloxin; Nu-Cloxi; Orbenin; Tegopen*]
**See Penicillins (Systemic)**, 2240
Capsules USP, 2250
Injection, 2251
for Solution, Oral, USP, 2250
*Cloxapen*—Beecham (U.S.) brand of Cloxacillin—**See Penicillins (Systemic)**, 2240
Clozapine [*Clozaril; Leponex*]
**(Systemic)**, 919
Tablets, 923, MC-8
*Clozaril*—Novartis (U.S. and Canada) brand of Clozapine (Systemic), 919, MC-8
CMT—Choline and Magnesium Salicylates—**See Salicylates (Systemic)**, 2538
⁵⁷Co—*See* Cyanocobalamin Co 57 (Systemic), 1123
*CoActifed*—BW (Canada) brand of Triprolidine, Pseudoephedrine, and Codeine—**See Cough/Cold Combinations (Systemic)**, 1024
*CoActifed Expectorant*—BW (Canada) brand of Triprolidine, Pseudoephedrine, Codeine, and Guaifenesin—**See Cough/Cold Combinations (Systemic)**, 1024
Coagulation Factor IX [*Mononine*]
**(Systemic)**, 3137
Coagulation Factor IX (Human), 3137
Coagulation Factor IX (Human) [*AlphaNine*]
**(Systemic)**, 3137
Coagulation Factor IX [*AlphaNine SD*; Christmas factor; factor IX fraction; *Immunine VH; Mononine*; plasma thromboplastin component (PTC); prothrombin complex concentrate (PCC)]
**(Systemic)**, 1430
Coagulation Factor IX (Human), 1432
Coagulation Factor IX (Recombinant), 1434
Coagulation Factor IX (Recombinant)
**(Systemic)**, 3137
Coal Tar [*Alphosyl; Aquatar; Balnetar; Balnetar Therapeutic Tar Bath; Cutar Water Dispersible Emollient Tar; Denorex; Denorex Extra Strength Medicated Shampoo; Denorex Extra Strength Medicated Shampoo with Conditioners; Denorex Medicated Shampoo; Denorex Medicated Shampoo and Conditioner; Denorex Mountain Fresh Herbal Scent Medicated Shampoo; DHS Tar Gel Shampoo; DHS Tar Shampoo; Doak Oil; Doak Oil Forte; Doak Oil Forte Therapeutic Bath Treatment; Doak Oil Therapeutic Bath Treatment For All-Over Body Care; Doak Tar Lotion; Doak Tar Shampoo; Doctar Hair & Scalp Shampoo and Conditioner; Doctar Shampoo; Estar; Fototar; Ionil T Plus; Lavatar; Liquor Carbonis Detergens; Medotar; Pentrax Anti-Dandruff Tar Shampoo; Pentrax Extra-Strength Therapeutic Tar Shampoo; Psorigel; PsoriNail Topical Solution; Taraphilic; Tarbonis; Tar Doak; Tarpaste; Tarpaste 'Doak'; T/Derm Tar Emollient; Tegrin Lotion for Psoriasis; Tegrin Medicated Cream Shampoo; Tegrin Medicated Shampoo Concentrated Gel; Tegrin Medicated Shampoo Extra Conditioning Formula; Tegrin Medicated Shampoo Herbal Formula; Tegrin Medicated Shampoo Original Formula; Tegrin Medicated Soap for Psoriasis; Tegrin Skin Cream for Psoriasis; Tersa-Tar Mild Therapeutic Shampoo with Protein and Conditioner; Tersa-Tar Soapless Tar Shampoo; Tersa-Tar Therapeutic Shampoo; T-Gel; T/Gel Therapeutic Conditioner; T/Gel Therapeutic Shampoo; Theraplex T Shampoo; Zetar Emulsion; Zetar Medicated Antiseborrheic Shampoo; Zetar Shampoo*]
**(Topical)**, #
Bar, Cleansing, #

Coal Tar (continued)
Cream, #
Gel, #
Lotion, #
Ointment USP, #
Shampoo, #
Solution, Topical, USP, #
Suspension, Topical, #
Coal Tar–containing Combinations, 3070
*Co-Apap*—Rugby (U.S.) brand of Chlorpheniramine, Pseudoephedrine, Dextromethorphan, and Acetaminophen—**See Cough/Cold Combinations (Systemic)**, 1024
*Cobex*—Pasadena (U.S.) brand of Cyanocobalamin—**See Vitamin B₁₂ (Systemic)**, 2962
*Cobiron*—Interstate (U.S.) brand of Neomycin, Polymyxin B, and Hydrocortisone (Ophthalmic), #
*Cobolin-M*—Legere (U.S.) brand of Cyanocobalamin—**See Vitamin B₁₂ (Systemic)**, 2962
*Co-bucafAPAP*—Butalbital, Acetaminophen, and Caffeine—**See Barbiturates and Analgesics (Systemic)**, 532
Cocaine Hydrochloride
**(Mucosal-Local)**, 923
USP (Crystals/Flakes), 927
Solution, Topical, 928
Solution, Topical, Viscous, 928
Tablets for Solution, Topical, USP, 927
*Co-Careldopa*—*See* Carbidopa and Levodopa (Systemic), 765
*Co-codAPAP*—Acetaminophen and Codeine—**See Opioid (Narcotic) Analgesics and Acetaminophen (Systemic)**, 2198
*Co-codaprin*—Aspirin and Codeine—**See Opioid (Narcotic) Analgesics and Aspirin (Systemic)**, 2202
*Co-Complex DM Caplets*—Quintex (U.S.) brand of Pseudoephedrine, Dextromethorphan, and Acetaminophen—**See Cough/Cold Combinations (Systemic)**, 1024
*Codamine*—Barre-National (U.S.); IDE (U.S.) and Major (U.S.) brand of Phenylpropanolamine and Hydrocodone—**See Cough/Cold Combinations (Systemic)**, 1024
*Codamine Pediatric*—Barre-National (U.S.) brand of Phenylpropanolamine and Hydrocodone—**See Cough/Cold Combinations (Systemic)**, 1024
*Codan*—WC (U.S.) brand of Hydrocodone and Homatropine—**See Cough/Cold Combinations (Systemic)**, 1024
*Codegest Expectorant*—Great Southern (U.S.) brand of Phenylpropanolamine, Codeine, and Guaifenesin—**See Cough/Cold Combinations (Systemic)**, 1024
*Codehist DH*—Geneva (U.S.) brand of Chlorpheniramine, Pseudoephedrine, and Codeine—**See Cough/Cold Combinations (Systemic)**, 1024
Codeine and Calcium Iodide [*Calcidrine*]
**See Cough/Cold Combinations (Systemic)**, 1024
Syrup, 1039
Codeine-containing Combinations, 3070
Codeine Phosphate [*Paveral*]
**See Opioid (Narcotic) Analgesics (Systemic)**, 2168
Injection USP, 2175
Solution, Oral, 2174
Tablets USP, 2175
Tablets, Soluble, 2175
Codeine Phosphate, Ammonium Chloride, and Guaifenesin [*Cheracol*]
**See Cough/Cold Combinations (Systemic)**, 1024
Syrup USP, 1042
Codeine Phosphate and Guaifenesin [*Brontex; Cheracol; Glydeine Cough; Guiatuss A.C.; Guiatussin with Codeine Liquid; Mytussin AC; Robafen AC Cough; Robitussin A-C; Tolu-Sed Cough; Tussi-Organidin NR Liquid; Tussi-Organidin-S NR Liquid*]
**See Cough/Cold Combinations (Systemic)**, 1024
Solution, Or al, 1062, 1107, 1038
Syrup, 1042, 1059, 1062, 1070, 1087, 1099
Tablets, 1038
Codeine Phosphate and Iodinated Glycerol [*Iophen-C Liquid*]
**See Cough/Cold Combinations (Systemic)**, 1024
Solution, Oral, 1067
Codeine Sulfate
**See Opioid (Narcotic) Analgesics (Systemic)**, 2168
Tablets USP, 2175
Tablets, Soluble, 2176

## General Index

*Codiclear DH*—Central (U.S.) brand of Hydrocodone and Guaifenesin—**See Cough/Cold Combinations (Systemic)**, 1024
*Codimal*—Central (U.S.) brand of Chlorpheniramine, Pseudoephedrine, and Acetaminophen—**See Antihistamines, Decongestants, and Analgesics (Systemic)**, 366
*Codimal DH*—Central (U.S.) brand of Pyrilamine, Phenylephrine, and Hydrocodone—**See Cough/Cold Combinations (Systemic)**, 1024
*Codimal DM*—Central (U.S.) brand of Pyrilamine, Phenylephrine, and Dextromethorphan—**See Cough/Cold Combinations (Systemic)**, 1024
*Codimal-L.A.*—Central (U.S.) brand of Chlorpheniramine and Pseudoephedrine—**See Antihistamines and Decongestants (Systemic)**, 343
*Codimal-L.A. Half*—Central (U.S.) brand of Chlorpheniramine and Pseudoephedrine—**See Antihistamines and Decongestants (Systemic)**, 343
*Codimal PH*—Central (U.S.) brand of Pyrilamine, Phenylephrine, and Codeine—**See Cough/Cold Combinations (Systemic)**, 1024
*Coenzyme R*—*See* Biotin (Systemic), #
*Cofatrim Forte*—Ampharco (U.S.) brand of Sulfamethoxazole and Trimethoprimm—**See Sulfonamides and Trimethoprim (Systemic)**, 2661
*Cogentin*—Merck (U.S. and Canada) brand of Benztropine—**See Antidyskinetics (Systemic)**, 297, MC-3
*Co-Gesic*—Central (U.S.) brand of Hydrocodone and Acetaminophen—**See Opioid (Narcotic) Analgesics and Acetaminophen (Systemic)**, 2198
*Cognex*—PD (U.S.) brand of Tacrine (Systemic), 2680, MC-29
*Co-Hist*—Roberts (U.S.) brand of Chlorpheniramine, Pseudoephedrine, and Acetaminophen—**See Antihistamines, Decongestants, and Analgesics (Systemic)**, 366
Co-hycodAPAP—Hydrocodone and Acetaminophen—**See Opioid (Narcotic) Analgesics and Acetaminophen (Systemic)**, 2198
*Colace*—Roberts (U.S. and Canada) brand of Docusate—**See Laxatives (Local)**, #; Roberts (U.S.) brand of Docusate (Local), 3018
Colaspase—*See* Asparaginase (Systemic), 474
*Co-Lav*—Copely (U.S.) brand of Polyethylene Glycol 3350 and Electrolytes (Local), 2349
*Colax*—Rugby (U.S.) brand of Phenolphthalein and Docusate—**See Laxatives (Local)**, #
*ColBenemid*—Merck (U.S.) brand of Probenecid and Colchicine (Systemic), 2384
Colchicine
 (Systemic), 928, 3138
 Injection USP, 934
 Tablets USP, 933
Colchicine-containing Combinations, 3071
*Cold and Allergy*—Zenith Goldline (U.S.) brand of Brompheniramine and Phenylpropanolamine—**See Antihistamines and Decongestants (Systemic)**, 343
*Cold-Gest Cold*—Major (U.S.) brand of Chlorpheniramine and Phenylpropanolamine—**See Antihistamines and Decongestants (Systemic)**, 343
*Coldrine*—Roberts (U.S.) brand of Pseudoephedrine and Acetaminophen—**See Decongestants and Analgesics (Systemic)**, 1180
*Colebrin*—Schering (Italy) brand of Iocetamic Acid—**See Cholecystographic Agents, Oral (Systemic)**, #
*Colebrina*—Sarget (Spain) brand of Iocetamic Acid—**See Cholecystographic Agents, Oral (Systemic)**, #
*Colegraf*—Estedi (Spain) brand of Iopanoic Acid—**See Cholecystographic Agents, Oral (Systemic)**, #
*Colestid*—Pharmacia & Upjohn (U.S. and Canada) brand of Colestipol (Oral-Local), 934, MC-8
Colestipol Hydrochloride [*Colestid*]
 (Oral-Local), 934
 for Suspension, Oral, USP, 936, MC-8
*Colfed-A*—Econolab (U.S.) and Parmed (U.S.) brand of Chlorpheniramine and Pseudoephedrine—**See Antihistamines and Decongestants (Systemic)**, 343
Colfosceril, Cetyl Alcohol, and Tyloxapol [*Exosurf Neonatal*]
 (Intratracheal-Local), 937
 for Suspension, Intratracheal, 939
Colfosceril palmitate—*See* Colfosceril, Cetyl Alcohol, and Tyloxapol (Intratracheal-Local), 937

Colfosceril Palmitate, Cetyl Alcohol, and Tyloxapol [*EXOSURF; EXOSURF Neonatal*]
 (Intratracheal-Local), 3138
 for Suspension, Intratracheal, 3138
Colistin-containing Combinations, 3071
Colistin and Neomycin Sulfates and Hydrocortisone Acetate [*Coly-Mycin Otic; Coly-Mycin S Otic*]
 (Otic), 939
 Suspension, Otic, USP, 940
Collagenase (lyophilized) [*Plaquase*]
 (Systemic), 3138
 for Injection, 3138
*Colloral*—Autoimmune (U.S.) brand of Purified Type II Collagen (Systemic), 3160
*ColoCare*—Helena (U.S.) brand of Fecal Occult Blood Test Kits, #
*Cologel*—Lilly (U.S.) brand of Methylcellulose—**See Laxatives (Local)**, #
*Colomed*—Orphan (U.S.) brand of Short Chain Fatty Acid Enema (Rectal), 3164
Colony Stimulating Factors
 (Systemic), 941
*Colo-Rectal Test*—Roche (Canada) brand of Fecal Occult Blood Test Kits, #
*Color Ovulation Test*—Biomerica (U.S.) brand of Enzyme Immunoassay Ovulation Prediction Test Kits—**See Ovulation Prediction Test Kits for Home Use**, #
*ColoScreen*—Helena (U.S.) brand of Fecal Occult Blood Test Kits, #
*ColoScreen III*—Helena (U.S.) brand of Fecal Occult Blood Test Kits, #
*ColoScreen Self-Test*—Helena (U.S.) brand of Fecal Occult Blood Test Kits, #
*Colovage*—Dynapharm (U.S.) brand of Polyethylene Glycol 3350 and Electrolytes (Local), 2349
*Col-Probenecid*—Goldline (U.S.) brand of Probenecid and Colchicine (Systemic), 2384
*Colprone*—Wyeth-Ayerst (Canada) brand of Medrogestone—**See Progestins (Systemic)**, 2400
*Coly-Mycin Otic*—PD (Canada) brand of Colistin, Neomycin, and Hydrocortisone (Otic), 939
*Coly-Mycin S Otic*—PD (U.S.) brand of Colistin, Neomycin, and Hydrocortisone (Otic), 939
*Colyte*—Reed & Carnrick (U.S. and Canada) brand of Polyethylene Glycol 3350 and Electrolytes (Local), 2349
*Colyte-flavored*—Reed & Carnrick (U.S.) brand of Polyethylene Glycol 3350 and Electrolytes (Local), 2349
*Combantrin*—Pfizer (Canada) brand of Pyrantel (Oral-Local), #
*Combipres*—Boehringer Ingelheim (U.S. and Canada) brand of Clonidine and Chlorthalidone (Systemic), 912, MC-8
*Combivent*—Boehringer Ingelheim (U.S.) brand of Ipratropium and Albuterol (Inhalation-Local), 1765
*Combivir*—Glaxo Wellcome (U.S.) brand of Lamivudine and Zidovudine (Systemic), 1822, MC-16
*Comfort Eye Drops*—Barnes-Hind (U.S.) brand of Naphazoline (Ophthalmic), #
*Comhist*—Roberts (U.S.) brand of Chlorpheniramine, Phenyltoloxamine, and Phenylephrine—**See Antihistamines and Decongestants (Systemic)**, 343
*Comhist LA*—Roberts (U.S.) brand of Chlorpheniramine, Phenyltoloxamine, and Phenylephrine—**See Antihistamines and Decongestants (Systemic)**, 343
*Compa-Z*—Hauck (U.S.) brand of Prochlorperazine—**See Phenothiazines (Systemic)**, 2289
*Compazine*—SmithKline Beecham (U.S.) brand of Prochlorperazine—**See Phenothiazines (Systemic)**, 2289, MC-26
*Compazine Spansule*—SmithKline Beecham (U.S.) brand of Prochlorperazine—**See Phenothiazines (Systemic)**, 2289, MC-26
*Compleat Modified*—Sandoz (U.S.) brand of Enteral Nutrition Formula, Blenderized—**See Enteral Nutrition Formulas (Systemic)**, #
*Compleat Regular*—Sandoz (U.S.) brand of Enteral Nutrition Formula, Blenderized—**See Enteral Nutrition Formulas (Systemic)**, #
*Comply*—Sherwood (U.S.) brand of Enteral Nutrition Formula, Polymeric—**See Enteral Nutrition Formulas (Systemic)**, #
*Compound W Gel*—Whitehall (U.S. and Canada) brand of Salicylic Acid (Topical), #
*Compound W Liquid*—Whitehall (U.S. and Canada) brand of Salicylic Acid (Topical), #

*Compoz*—Medtech (U.S.) brand of Diphenhydramine—**See Antihistamines (Systemic)**, 325
*Comtrex Allergy-Sinus*—Bristol-Myers-Squibb (U.S.) brand of Chlorpheniramine, Pseudoephedrine, and Acetaminophen—**See Antihistamines, Decongestants, and Analgesics (Systemic)**, 366
*Comtrex Allergy-Sinus Caplets*—Bristol-Myers-Squibb (U.S.) brand of Chlorpheniramine, Pseudoephedrine, and Acetaminophen—**See Antihistamines, Decongestants, and Analgesics (Systemic)**, 366
*Comtrex Cough Formula*—Bristol-Myers (U.S.) brand of Pseudoephedrine, Dextromethorphan, Guaifenesin, and Acetaminophen—**See Cough/Cold Combinations (Systemic)**, 1024
*Comtrex Daytime Caplets*—Bristol-Myers (U.S.) brand of Pseudoephedrine, Dextromethorphan, and Acetaminophen—**See Cough/Cold Combinations (Systemic)**, 1024
*Comtrex Daytime Maximum Strength Cold, Cough, and Flu Relief*—Bristol-Myers (U.S.) brand of Pseudoephedrine, Dextromethorphan, and Acetaminophen—**See Cough/Cold Combinations (Systemic)**, 1024
*Comtrex Daytime Maximum Strength Cold and Flu Relief*—Bristol-Myers (U.S.) brand of Pseudoephedrine, Dextromethorphan, and Acetaminophen—**See Cough/Cold Combinations (Systemic)**, 1024
*Comtrex Maximum Strength Multi-Symptom Liqui-Gels*—Bristol-Myers (U.S.) brand of Chlorpheniramine, Phenylpropanolamine, Dextromethorphan, and Acetaminophen—**See Cough/Cold Combinations (Systemic)**, 1024
*Comtrex Multi-Symptom Cold Reliever*—Bristol-Myers (U.S.) brand of Chlorpheniramine, Phenylpropanolamine, Dextromethorphan, and Acetaminophen—**See Cough/Cold Combinations (Systemic)**, 1024
*Comtrex Multi-Symptom Maximum Strength Non-Drowsy Caplets*—Bristol-Myers (U.S.) brand of Pseudoephedrine, Dextromethorphan, and Acetaminophen—**See Cough/Cold Combinations (Systemic)**, 1024
*Comtrex Nighttime*—Bristol-Myers (U.S.) brand of Chlorpheniramine, Pseudoephedrine, Dextromethorphan, and Acetaminophen—**See Cough/Cold Combinations (Systemic)**, 1024
*Comtrex Nighttime Maximum Strength Cold, Cough and Flu Relief*—Bristol-Myers (U.S.) brand of Chlorpheniramine, Pseudoephedrine, Dextromethorphan, and Acetaminophen—**See Cough/Cold Combinations (Systemic)**, 1024
*Comtrex Nighttime Maximum Strength Cold and Flu Relief*—Bristol-Myers (U.S.) brand of Chlorpheniramine, Pseudoephedrine, Dextromethorphan, and Acetaminophen—**See Cough/Cold Combinations (Systemic)**, 1024
*Conceive Ovulation Predictor*—Quidel (U.S.) brand of Enzyme Immunoassay Ovulation Prediction Test Kits—**See Ovulation Prediction Test Kits for Home Use**, #
*Conceive 1-Step*—Quidel (U.S.) and Pharmascience (Canada) brand of Immunoassay Pregnancy Test Kits—**See Pregnancy Test Kits for Home Use**, #
*Concentrated Phillips' Milk of Magnesia*—Glenbrook (U.S.) brand of Magnesium Hydroxide—**See Magnesium Supplements (Systemic)**, 1897
*Concentrin*—PD (U.S.) brand of Pseudoephedrine, Dextromethorphan, and Guaifenesin—**See Cough/Cold Combinations (Systemic)**, 1024
*Conceptrol Contraceptive Inserts*—Ortho (U.S.) brand of Nonoxynol 9—**See Spermicides (Vaginal)**, #
*Conceptrol Gel*—Ortho (U.S.) brand of Nonoxynol 9—**See Spermicides (Vaginal)**, #
Condom, Female, Polyurethane [*Reality*], 3015
Condom, Male, Polyurethane [*Avanti; Avanti Super Thin*], 3016
Condoms, #
Condoms, Lamb Cecum [*Fourex Natural Skins; Kling-Tite Naturalamb*]
 **See Condoms**, #
 Lamb Cecum Condoms, #
Condoms, Lamb Cecum, and Nonoxynol 9 [*Fourex Natural Skins Spermicidally Lubricated; Kling-Tite Naturalamb with Spermicide Lubricant*]
 **See Condoms**, #
 Lamb Cecum Condoms and Nonoxynol 9, #

Condoms, Latex [*Beyond Seven; Class Act Ribbed & Sensitive; ClassAct Ultra Thin & Sensitive; Crown; Embrace; Excita Fiesta; Excita Sensitrol; Gold Circle Coin; Gold Circle Rainbow Coin; Kimono; Kimono Microthins; Kimono Sensation; Life Styles Assorted Colors; Life Styles Form Fitting; Life Styles Lubricated; Life Styles Non-Lubricated; Life Styles Ultra Sensitive; Life Styles Vibra-Ribbed; MAXX; Ortho Shields Lubricated; Ortho Shields Non-Lubricated; Ortho Shields X; Ortho Supreme; Ramses Non-Lubricated; Ramses Safe Play; Ramses Sensitol; Ramses Thin Lub; Ramses Ultra; Ramses Ultra Thin; Saxon Gold Ultra Sensitive; Sheik Classic Lubricated; Sheik Classic Non-Lubricated; Sheik Denim; Sheik Fiesta Colors; Sheik Non-Lubricated; Sheik Sensi-Creme; Sheik Super Thin Lubricated; Sheik Super Thin Ribbed Lubricated; Sheik Thin Lub; Titan Lubricated; Titan Ribbed; Touch Lubricated; Touch Non-Lubricated; Touch Ribbed Lubricated; Touch Sunrise Colors; Touch Thins Lubricated; Trojan; Trojan-Enz; Trojan-Enz Large Lubricated; Trojan-Enz Lubricated; Trojan-Enz Nonlubricated; Trojan Extra Strength Lubricated; Trojan Magnum; Trojan Naturalube Ribbed; Trojan Plus; Trojan Ribbed; Trojans; Trojan Ultra Texture Lubricant; Trojan Very Sensitive with Lubricant; Trojan Very Thin with Lubricant*]
See **Condoms**, #
Latex Condoms, #
Condoms, Latex, and Nonoxynol 9 [*Beyond Seven Plus; Class Act Ultra Thin & Sensitive-Spermicidal Lubricated; Crown Plus; Kimono Microthins Plus; Kimono Plus; Kimono Sensation Plus; Life Styles Extra Strength with Spermicide; Life Styles Lubricated with Spermicide; Life Styles Spermicidally Lubricated; Life Styles Ultra Sensitive with Spermicide; Life Styles Vibra-Ribbed with Spermicide; MAXX Plus; Ortho Shields Plus; Ramses Extra; Ramses Extra-15; Ramses Extra Ribbed; Ramses Extra Strength; Ramses Ribbed; Ramses with Spermicidal Lubricant; Ramses Thin Spermicidal Lub; Ramses Ultra-15; Ramses Ultra Thin Ribbed with Spermicide; Ramses Ultra Thin with Spermicide; Saxon Gold Rainbow Ultra Spermicidal; Saxon Gold Ultra Spermicidal; Sheik Classic Spermicidally Lubricated; Sheik Elite; Sheik Excita; Sheik Excita Extra; Sheik Super Thin Ribbed Spermicidally Lubricated; Sheik Super Thin Spermicidally Lubricated; Sheik Thin Spermicidal Lub; Titan with Silicone Spermicidal Lubricant; Touch Spermicidally Lubricated; Trojan-Enz Large with Spermicidal Lube; Trojan-Enz Large with Spermicidal Lubricant; Trojan-Enz with Spermicidal-Lubricant; Trojan Magnum Spermicidal Lubricant; Trojan Plus 2; Trojan Ribbed with Spermicidal Lube; Trojan Ribbed with Spermicidal Lubricant; Trojan Ultra Texture with Spermidical Lubricant; Trojan Very Sensitive with Spermicidal Lubricant; Trojan Very Thin with Spermicidal Lubricant*]
See **Condoms**, #
Latex Condoms and Nonoxynol 9, #
*Condylox*—Oclassen (U.S.) brand of Podofilox (Topical), 2339
*Conex*—Forest (U.S.) brand of Phenylpropanolamine and Guaifenesin—**See Cough/Cold Combinations (Systemic)**, 1024
*Conex with Codeine Liquid*—Forest (U.S.) brand of Phenylpropanolamine, Codeine, and Guaifenesin—**See Cough/Cold Combinations (Systemic)**, 1024
*Confidelle*—Carter-Horner (Canada) brand of Immunoassay Pregnancy Test Kits—**See Pregnancy Test Kits for Home Use**, #
*Confirm*—Schmid (U.S. and Canada) brand of Immunoassay Pregnancy Test Kits—**See Pregnancy Test Kits for Home Use**, #
*Congess JR*—Fleming (U.S.) brand of Pseudoephedrine and Guaifenesin—**See Cough/Cold Combinations (Systemic)**, 1024
*Congess SR*—Fleming (U.S.) brand of Pseudoephedrine and Guaifenesin—**See Cough/Cold Combinations (Systemic)**, 1024
*Congest*—Trianon (Canada) brand of Conjugated Estrogens—**See Estrogens (Systemic)**, 1383
*Congestac Caplets*—Menley & James (U.S.) brand of Pseudoephedrine and Guaifenesin—**See Cough/Cold Combinations (Systemic)**, 1024

*Congestant D*—Rugby (U.S.) brand of Chlorpheniramine, Phenylpropanolamine, and Acetaminophen—**See Antihistamines, Decongestants, and Analgesics (Systemic)**, 366
Conjugated Estrogen–containing Combinations, 3071
Conjugated estrogens—Estrogens, Conjugated—**See Conjugated Estrogens and Medroxyprogesterone for Ovarian Hormone Therapy (OHT) (Systemic)**, 946; **Estrogens (Systemic)**, 1383; **Estrogens (Vaginal)**, 1391
Conjugated Estrogens, and Conjugated Estrogens and Medroxyprogesterone Acetate [*Premarin; Premphase*]
See **Conjugated Estrogens and Medroxyprogesterone for Ovarian Hormone Therapy (OHT) (Systemic)**, 946
Tablets, 951
Tablets USP, 951
Conjugated Estrogens and Medroxyprogesterone for Ovarian Hormone Therapy (OHT) (Systemic), 946
Conjugated estrogens and methyltestosterone—Estrogens, Conjugated, and Methyltestosterone—**See Androgens and Estrogens (Systemic)**, 126
*Conray*—Mallinckrodt (U.S.) brand of Iothalamate (Systemic), #
*Conray-30*—Mallinckrodt (U.S. and Canada) brand of Iothalamate (Systemic), #
*Conray-43*—Mallinckrodt (U.S. and Canada) brand of Iothalamate (Systemic), #
*Conray-60*—Mallinckrodt (Canada) brand of Iothalamate (Systemic), #
*Conray-325*—Mallinckrodt (U.S. and Canada) brand of Iothalamate (Systemic), #
*Conray-400*—Mallinckrodt (U.S.) brand of Iothalamate (Systemic), #
*Constilac*—Alra (U.S.) brand of Lactulose—**See Laxatives (Local)**, #
*Constulose*—Barre-National (U.S.) brand of Lactulose—**See Laxatives (Local)**, #
*Contac Allergy/Sinus Day Caplets*—SmithKline Beecham (U.S.) brand of Pseudoephedrine and Acetaminophen—**See Decongestants and Analgesics (Systemic)**, 1180
*Contac Allergy/Sinus Night Caplets*—SmithKline Beecham (U.S.) brand of Diphenhydramine, Pseudoephedrine, and Acetaminophen—**See Antihistamines, Decongestants, and Analgesics (Systemic)**, 366
*Contac Cold/Flu Day Caplets*—SmithKline Beecham (U.S.) brand of Pseudoephedrine, Dextromethorphan, and Acetaminophen—**See Cough/Cold Combinations (Systemic)**, 1024
*Contac Cold/Flu Night Caplets*—SmithKline Beecham (U.S.) brand of Diphenhydramine, Pseudoephedrine, and Acetaminophen—**See Antihistamines, Decongestants, and Analgesics (Systemic)**, 366
*Contac 12-Hour*—SmithKline Beecham (U.S.) brand of Chlorpheniramine and Phenylpropanolamine—**See Antihistamines and Decongestants (Systemic)**, 343
*Contac 12 Hour Allergy*—SmithKline Beecham (U.S.) brand of Clemastine—**See Antihistamines (Systemic)**, 325
*Contac Maximum Strength 12-Hour Caplets*—SmithKline Beecham (U.S.) brand of Chlorpheniramine and Phenylpropanolamine—**See Antihistamines and Decongestants (Systemic)**, 343
*Contac Non-Drowsy Formula Sinus Caplets*—SmithKline Beecham (U.S.) brand of Pseudoephedrine and Acetaminophen—**See Decongestants and Analgesics (Systemic)**, 1180
*Contac Severe Cold & Flu Caplets*—SmithKline Beecham (U.S.) brand of Chlorpheniramine, Phenylpropanolamine, Dextromethorphan, and Acetaminophen—**See Cough/Cold Combinations (Systemic)**, 1024
*Contac Severe Cold & Flu Non-Drowsy Caplets*—SmithKline Beecham (U.S.) brand of Pseudoephedrine, Dextromethorphan, and Acetaminophen—**See Cough/Cold Combinations (Systemic)**, 1024
*Conten*—Graham (U.S.) brand of Butalbital and Acetaminophen—**See Barbiturates and Analgesics (Systemic)**, 532
*Control*—Thompson (U.S.) brand of Phenylpropanolamine (Systemic), 2314

*Contuss*—Parmed (U.S.) brand of Phenylephrine, Phenylpropanolamine, and Guaifenesin—**See Cough/Cold Combinations (Systemic)**, 1024
Co-oyxcodAPAP—Oxycodone and Acetaminophen—**See Opioid (Narcotic) Analgesics and Acetaminophen (Systemic)**, 2198
*Copaxone*—Teva (U.S.) brand of Copolymer-1 (Systemic), 3138; TEVA Marion (U.S.) brand of Glatiramer Acetate (Systemic), 1558
*Cope*—Aspirin, Buffered—**See Salicylates (Systemic)**, 2538
*Cophene No. 2*—Dunhall (U.S.) brand of Chlorpheniramine and Pseudoephedrine—**See Antihistamines and Decongestants (Systemic)**, 343
*Cophene-S*—Dunhall (U.S.) brand of Chlorpheniramine, Phenylephrine, Phenylpropanolamine, and Dihydrocodeine—**See Cough/Cold Combinations (Systemic)**, 1024
*Cophene-X*—Dunhall (U.S.) brand of Phenylephrine, Phenylpropanolamine, Carbetapentane, and Potassium Guaiacolsulfonate—**See Cough/Cold Combinations (Systemic)**, 1024
*Cophene-XP*—Dunhall (U.S.) brand of Chlorpheniramine, Phenylephrine, Phenylpropanolamine, Carbetapentane, and Potassium Guaiacolsulfonate—**See Cough/Cold Combinations (Systemic)**, 1024
*Cophene XP*—Dunhall (U.S.) brand of Pseudoephedrine, Hydrocodone, and Guaifenesin—**See Cough/Cold Combinations (Systemic)**, 1024
Copolymer-1—*See* Glatiramer Acetate (Systemic), 1558
Copolymer-1 [*Copaxone*] (Systemic), 3138
Copper Gluconate
See **Copper Supplements (Systemic)**, 952
Tablets, 953
Copper Intrauterine Devices (IUDs), #
Copper Reduction Urine Glucose Test [*Clinitest*]
See **Urine Glucose and Ketone Test Kits for Home Use**, #
Tablets, #
Copper Supplements (Systemic), 952
Copper-T 200Ag Intrauterine Device [*Nova-T*]
See **Copper Intrauterine Devices (IUDs)**, #
Copper-T 200Ag Intrauterine Device, #
Copper-T 380A Intrauterine Device [*ParaGard-T 380A*]
See **Copper Intrauterine Devices (IUDs)**, #
Copper-T 380A Intrauterine Device, #
Copper-T 200 Intrauterine Device [*Gyne-T*]
See **Copper Intrauterine Devices (IUDs)**, #
Copper-T 200 Intrauterine Device, #
*Coppertone All Day Protection*—Schering-Plough (U.S.) brand of Homosalate, Octyl Methoxycinnamate, Octyl Salicylate, and Oxybenzone—**See Sunscreen Agents (Topical)**, #; Octocrylene, Octyl Methoxycinnamate, Octyl Salicylate, and Oxybenzone—**See Sunscreen Agents (Topical)**, #; Octyl Methoxycinnamate and Oxybenzone—**See Sunscreen Agents (Topical)**, #
*Coppertone Dark Tanning*—Schering-Plough (Canada) brand of Homosalate—**See Sunscreen Agents (Topical)**, #
*Coppertone Kids Sunblock*—Schering-Plough (U.S.) brand of Homosalate, Octyl Methoxycinnamate, Octyl Salicylate, and Oxybenzone—**See Sunscreen Agents (Topical)**, #; Octocrylene, Octyl Methoxycinnamate, Octyl Salicylate, and Oxybenzone—**See Sunscreen Agents (Topical)**, #
*Coppertone Lipkote*—Schering-Plough (U.S. and Canada) brand of Octyl Methoxycinnamate and Oxybenzone—**See Sunscreen Agents (Topical)**, #
*Coppertone Moisturizing Sunscreen*—Schering-Plough (U.S.) brand of Octyl Methoxycinnamate and Oxybenzone—**See Sunscreen Agents (Topical)**, #
*Coppertone Moisturizing Suntan*—Schering-Plough (U.S.) brand of Homosalate—**See Sunscreen Agents (Topical)**, #; Octyl Methoxycinnamate and Oxybenzone—**See Sunscreen Agents (Topical)**, #
*Coppertone Sport*—Schering-Plough (Canada) brand of Octyl Methoxycinnamate, Octyl Salicylate, and Oxybenzone—**See Sunscreen Agents (Topical)**, #
*Coppertone Sport Ultra Sweatproof*—Schering-Plough (U.S.) brand of Octyl Methoxycinnamate and Oxybenzone—**See Sunscreen Agents (Topical)**, #

*Coppertone Tan Magnifier*—Schering-Plough (U.S.) brand of Octyl Methoxycinnamate—**See Sunscreen Agents (Topical)**, #; Phenylbenzimidazole—**See Sunscreen Agents (Topical)**, #; Trolamine Salicylate—**See Sunscreen Agents (Topical)**, #

*Coppertone Waterbabies Sunblock*—Schering-Plough (U.S. and Canada) brand of Octocrylene, Octyl Methoxycinnamate, Octyl Salicylate, and Oxybenzone—**See Sunscreen Agents (Topical)**, #

*Coppertone Waterproof Sunblock*—Schering-Plough (Canada) brand of Homosalate, Octocrylene, Octyl Methoxycinnamate, and Oxybenzone—**See Sunscreen Agents (Topical)**, #

Copper-T 380S Intrauterine Device [*Glume-T 380 Slimline*]
  **See Copper Intrauterine Devices (IUDs)**, #
  Copper-T 380S Intrauterine Device, #

Co-proxAPAP—Propoxyphene and Acetaminophen—**See Opioid (Narcotic) Analgesics and Acetaminophen (Systemic)**, 2198

*Coptin*—Jouveinal (Canada) brand of Sulfadiazine and Trimethoprim—**See Sulfonamides and Trimethoprim (Systemic)**, 2661

*Coptin 1*—Jouveinal (Canada) brand of Sulfadiazine and Trimethoprim—**See Sulfonamides and Trimethoprim (Systemic)**, 2661

*Co-Pyronil 2*—Dista (U.S.) brand of Chlorpheniramine and Pseudoephedrine—**See Antihistamines and Decongestants (Systemic)**, 343

*Cordarone*—Wyeth-Ayerst (U.S.) brand of Amiodarone (Systemic), 3130; Wyeth-Ayerst (U.S.) and Ayerst (Canada) brand of Amiodarone (Systemic), 79, MC-2

*Cordarone Intravenous*—Wyeth-Ayerst (Canada) brand of Amiodarone (Systemic), 79

*Cordarone I.V.*—Wyeth (U.S.) brand of Amiodarone (Systemic), 79

*Cordran*—Dista (U.S.) brand of Flurandrenolide—**See Corticosteroids (Topical)**, 978

*Cordran SP*—Dista (U.S.) brand of Flurandrenolide—**See Corticosteroids (Topical)**, 978

*Coreg*—SmithKline Beecham (U.S.) brand of Carvedilol (Systemic), 790, MC-5

*Corgard*—Bristol-Myers Squibb (U.S. and Canada) brand of Nadolol—**See Beta-adrenergic Blocking Agents (Systemic)**, 593, MC-21

*Coricidin D*—Schering-Plough (Canada) brand of Chlorpheniramine, Phenylpropanolamine, and Aspirin—**See Antihistamines, Decongestants, and Analgesics (Systemic)**, 366

*Coricidin D Long Acting*—Schering (Canada) brand of Chlorpheniramine and Phenylpropanolamine—**See Antihistamines and Decongestants (Systemic)**, 343

*Coricidin Non-Drowsy Sinus Formula*—Schering-Plough (Canada) brand of Phenylpropanolamine and Aspirin—**See Decongestants and Analgesics (Systemic)**, 1180

*Coristex-DH*—Technilab (Canada) brand of Phenylephrine and Hydrocodone—**See Cough/Cold Combinations (Systemic)**, 1024

*Coristine-DH*—Technilab (Canada) brand of Phenylephrine and Hydrocodone—**See Cough/Cold Combinations (Systemic)**, 1024

*Corium*—ICN (Canada) brand of Chlordiazepoxide and Clidinium (Systemic), 846

*Corlopam*—Neurex (U.S.) brand of Fenoldopam (Systemic), 1443

*Cormax*—Oclassen (U.S.) brand of Clobetasol (Topical), 3015

*Coronex*—Ayerst (Canada) brand of Isosorbide Dinitrate—**See Nitrates (Systemic)**, 2129

*Correctol*—Schering-Plough (U.S. and Canada) brand of Bisacodyl—**See Laxatives (Local)**, #

*Correctol Caplets*—Schering-Plough (U.S.) brand of Bisacodyl—**See Laxatives (Local)**, #

*Correctol Herbal Tea*—Schering-Plough (U.S.) brand of Docusate—**See Laxatives (Local)**, #

*Correctol Stool Softener Soft Gels*—Schering-Plough (U.S. and Canada) brand of Docusate—**See Laxatives (Local)**, #

*Corsym*—Ciba Self-Medication (Canada) brand of Chlorpheniramine and Phenylpropanolamine—**See Antihistamines and Decongestants (Systemic)**, 343

*Cortacet*—Ayerst (Canada) brand of Hydrocortisone—**See Corticosteroids (Topical)**, 978

*Cortaid*—Upjohn (U.S.) brand of Hydrocortisone—**See Corticosteroids (Topical)**, 978

*Cortamed*—Berlex (Canada) brand of Hydrocortisone—**See Corticosteroids (Otic)**, 971; Sabex (Canada) brand of Hydrocortisone—**See Corticosteroids (Ophthalmic)**, 966

*Cortate*—Schering (Canada) brand of Hydrocortisone—**See Corticosteroids (Topical)**, 978

*Cortatrigen Ear*—Goldline (U.S.) brand of Neomycin, Polymyxin B, and Hydrocortisone (Otic), #

*Cortatrigen Modified Ear Drops*—Goldline (U.S.) brand of Neomycin, Polymyxin B, and Hydrocortisone (Otic), #

*Cort-Biotic*—Hauser (U.S.) brand of Neomycin, Polymyxin B, and Hydrocortisone (Otic), #

*Cort-Dome*—Miles (U.S.) brand of Hydrocortisone—**See Corticosteroids (Rectal)**, 973; **Corticosteroids (Topical)**, 973

*Cortef*—Pharmacia & Upjohn (Canada) brand of Hydrocortisone—**See Corticosteroids (Topical)**, 978; **Corticosteroids—Glucocorticoid Effects (Systemic)**, 998, MC-15

*Cortef Feminine Itch*—Upjohn (U.S.) brand of Hydrocortisone—**See Corticosteroids (Topical)**, 978

*Cortenema*—Solvay (U.S.) and Axcan (Canada) brand of Hydrocortisone— **See Hydrocortisone (Rectal)**, 973

*Corticaine*—Glaxo (U.S.) brand of Hydrocortisone—**See Corticosteroids (Topical)**, 978

Corticorelin Ovine Triflutate [*ACTHREL*]
  **(Systemic-Diagnostic)**, 954, 3138
  for Injection, 955

Corticosteroids
  **(Inhalation-Local)**, 955

Corticosteroids
  **(Nasal)**, 961

Corticosteroids
  **(Ophthalmic)**, 966

Corticosteroids
  **(Otic)**, 971

Corticosteroids
  **(Rectal)**, 973

Corticosteroids
  **(Topical)**, 978

Corticosteroids and Acetic Acid
  **(Otic)**, 996

Corticosteroids—Glucocorticoid Effects
  **(Systemic)**, 998

Corticotropin [ACTH; *ACTH*; *Acthar*; *Acthar Powder*]
  **Corticotropin (Systemic)**, 1021
  for Injection USP, 1022

Corticotropin-releasing Factor, Human [*Xerecept*]
  **(Systemic)**, 3138

Corticotropin, Repository [ACTH; *Acthar Gel*; *Acthar Gel (H.P.)*; *H.P. Acthar Gel*]
  **Corticotropin (Systemic)**, 1021
  Injection USP

*Corticreme*—Rougier (Canada) brand of Hydrocortisone—**See Corticosteroids (Topical)**, 978

*Cortifair*—Pharmafair (U.S.) brand of Hydrocortisone—**See Corticosteroids (Topical)**, 978

*Cortifoam*—Schwarz (U.S.) brand of Hydrocortisone—**See Corticosteroids (Rectal)**, 973

*Cortiment-10*—Marion Merrell Dow (Canada) brand of Hydrocortisone—**See Corticosteroids (Rectal)**, 973

*Cortiment-40*—Marion Merrell Dow (Canada) brand of Hydrocortisone—**See Corticosteroids (Rectal)**, 973

Cortisol—Hydrocortisone—**See Corticosteroids (Ophthalmic)**, 966; **Corticosteroids (Otic)**, 971; **Corticosteroids (Rectal)**, 973; **Corticosteroids (Topical)**, 978; **Corticosteroids—Glucocorticoid Effects (Systemic)**, 998

Cortisone Acetate [*Cortone; Cortone Acetate*]
  **See Corticosteroids—Glucocorticoid Effects (Systemic)**, 998
  Suspension, Sterile, USP, 1007
  Tablets USP, 1007

*Cortisporin*—BW (U.S. and Canada) brand of Neomycin, Polymyxin B, and Hydrocortisone (Otic), #

*Cortisporin Ophthalmic Suspension*—BW (U.S. and Canada) brand of Neomycin, Polymyxin B, and Hydrocortisone (Ophthalmic), #

*Cortoderm*—K-Line (Canada) brand of Hydrocortisone—**See Corticosteroids (Topical)**, 978

*Cortomycin*—Major (U.S.) brand of Neomycin, Polymyxin B, and Hydrocortisone (Ophthalmic), #; Major (U.S.) brand of Neomycin, Polymyxin B, and Hydrocortisone (Otic), #

*Cortone*—MSD (Canada) brand of Cortisone—**See Corticosteroids—Glucocorticoid Effects (Systemic)**, 998

*Cortone Acetate*—Merck (U.S.) brand of Cortisone—**See Corticosteroids—Glucocorticoid Effects (Systemic)**, 998

*Cortril*—Pfipharmecs (U.S.) brand of Hydrocortisone—**See Corticosteroids (Topical)**, 978

*Cortrosyn*—Organon (U.S. and Canada) brand of Cosyntropin (Systemic), 1023

*Corvert*—Upjohn (U.S.) brand of Ibutilide (Systemic), 1670

*Coryphen*—Rougier (Canada) brand of Aspirin—**See Salicylates (Systemic)**, 2538

*Corzide*—Bristol-Myers Squibb (U.S. and Canada) brand of Nadolol and Bendroflumethiazide—**See Beta-adrenergic Blocking Agents and Thiazide Diuretics (Systemic)**, 609, MC-21

*Cosmegen*—Merck (U.S. and Canada) brand of Dactinomycin (Systemic), 1153

*Cosopt*—Merck (U.S.) brand of Dorzolamide and Timolol (Ophthalmic), 3018

*CoSudafed*—BW (Canada) brand of Pseudoephedrine and Codeine—**See Cough/Cold Combinations (Systemic)**, 1024

*CoSudafed Expectorant*—BW (U.S.) brand of Pseudoephedrine, Codeine, and Guaifenesin—**See Cough/Cold Combinations (Systemic)**, 1024

Cosyntropin [*Cortrosyn*; tetracosactide]
  **(Systemic)**, 1023
  for Injection, 1024

*Cotabs*—Pharmavite (Canada) brand of Acetaminophen and Codeine—**See Opioid (Narcotic) Analgesics and Acetaminophen (Systemic)**, 2198

*Cotazym*—Organon (U.S. and Canada) brand of Pancrelipase (Systemic), 2222, MC-24

*Cotazym-65 B*—Organon (Canada) brand of Pancrelipase (Systemic), 2222

*Cotazym E.C.S. 8*—Organon (Canada) brand of Pancrelipase (Systemic), 2222

*Cotazym E.C.S. 20*—Organon (Canada) brand of Pancrelipase (Systemic), 2222

*Cotazym-S*—Organon (U.S.) brand of Pancrelipase (Systemic), 2222

*Cotranzine*—Coast (U.S.) brand of Prochlorperazine—**See Phenothiazines (Systemic)**, 2289

Co-triamterzide—Triamterene and Hydrochlorothiazide—**See Diuretics, Potassium-sparing, and Hydrochlorothiazide (Systemic)**, 1272

*Cotridin*—Technilab (Canada) brand of Triprolidine, Pseudoephedrine, and Codeine—**See Cough/Cold Combinations (Systemic)**, 1024

*Cotridin Expectorant*—Technilab (Canada) brand of Triprolidine, Pseudoephedrine, Codeine, and Guaifenesin—**See Cough/Cold Combinations (Systemic)**, 1024

*Cotrim*—Lemmon (U.S.) brand of Sulfamethoxazole and Trimethoprim—**See Sulfonamides and Trimethoprim (Systemic)**, 2661

Cotrimazine—Sulfadiazine and Trimethoprim—**See Sulfonamides and Trimethoprim (Systemic)**, 2661

*Cotrim DS*—Lemmon (U.S.) brand of Sulfamethoxazole and Trimethoprim—**See Sulfonamides and Trimethoprim (Systemic)**, 2661

Cotrimoxazole—Sulfamethoxazole and Trimethoprim—**See Sulfonamides and Trimethoprim (Systemic)**, 2661

*Cotrim Pediatric*—Lemmon (U.S.) brand of Sulfamethoxazole and Trimethoprimm—**See Sulfonamides and Trimethoprim (Systemic)**, 2661

*Co-Tuss V*—Rugby (U.S.) brand of Hydrocodone and Guaifenesin—**See Cough/Cold Combinations (Systemic)**, 1024

*Cotylbutazone*—Truxton (U.S.) brand of Phenylbutazone—**See Anti-inflammatory Drugs, Nonsteroidal (Systemic)**, 388

Cough/Cold Combinations
  **(Systemic)**, 1024

*Cough-X*—Ascher (U.S.) brand of Dextromethorphan (Systemic), 1191

*Coumadin*—Du Pont (U.S. and Canada) brand of Warfarin—**See Anticoagulants (Systemic)**, 243, MC-32; Du Pont (U.S.) brand of Warfarin (Systemic), 3038

Coumarin [*Oncostate*]
  **(Systemic)**, 3138

*Covangesic*—Wallace (U.S.) brand of Chlorpheniramine, Pyrilamine, Phenylephrine, Phenylpropanolamine, and Acetaminophen—**See Antihistamines, Decongestants, and Analgesics (Systemic)**, 366

*Covera-HS*—Searle (U.S.) brand of Verapamil (Systemic), MC-32
*Cozaar*—Merck (U.S.) brand of Losartan (Systemic), 1882, MC-18
*CP Oral*—Pharmacist's Choice (U.S.) brand of Carbinoxamine and Pseudoephedrine—**See Antihistamines and Decongestants (Systemic)**, 343
CPT-11—*See* Irinotecan (Systemic), 1769
[51]Cr—*See* Sodium Chromate Cr 51 (Systemic), 2590
*Cramp End*—Ohm (U.S.) brand of Ibuprofen—**See Anti-inflammatory Drugs, Nonsteroidal (Systemic)**, 388
*Creon*—Solvay (U.S.) brand of Pancreatin (Systemic), MC-24
*Creo-Terpin*—Medtech (U.S.) brand of Dextromethorphan (Systemic), 1191
*Crimone*—Wyeth-Ayerst (U.S.) brand of Progesterone—**See Progestins (Systemic)**, 2400
*Criticare HN*—Mead Johnson (U.S.) brand of Enteral Nutrition Formula, Monomeric (Elemental)—**See Enteral Nutrition Formulas (Systemic)**, #
*Crixivan*—Merck (U.S.) brand of Indinavir (Systemic), 1693, MC-15
*Crolom*—Bausch & Lomb (U.S.) brand of Cromolyn (Ophthalmic), 1120
Cromoglicic acid—*See* Cromolyn (Inhalation-Local), 1116; Cromolyn (Nasal), 1118; Cromolyn (Ophthalmic), 1120
Cromoglycic acid—*See* Cromolyn (Nasal), 1118; Cromolyn (Ophthalmic), 1120
Cromolyn Sodium [*Nasalcrom*]
  **(Nasal)**, 3016
  Solution, Nasal, 3016
Cromolyn Sodium [cromoglicic acid; *Intal; Novo-cromolyn; PMS-Sodium Cromoglycate;* sodium cromoglycate]
  **(Inhalation-Local)**, 1116
  Aerosol, Inhalation, 1117
  for Inhalation USP (Capsules), 1117
  Inhalation USP (Solution), 1118
Cromolyn Sodium [cromoglicic acid; cromoglycic acid; *Nasalcrom; Rynacrom;* sodium cromoglycate]
  **(Nasal)**, 1118
  for Insufflation, Nasal, 1119
  Solution, Nasal, USP, 1120
Cromolyn Sodium [*Crolom;* cromoglicic acid; cromoglycic acid; *Opticrom;* sodium cromoglycate; *Vistacrom*]
  **(Ophthalmic)**, 1120, 3138
  Solution, Ophthalmic, USP, 1121, 3138
Cromolyn Sodium [*Gastrocrom; Nalcrom;* sodium cromoglycate]
  **(Systemic/Oral-Local)**, 1121, 3138
  Capsules, 1123
  Concentrate, Oral, 1123
*Crotab*—Therapeutic Antibodies (U.S.) brand of Antivenin, Polyvalent Crotalid (Ovine) Fab (Systemic), 3132
Crotamiton [*Eurax Cream; Eurax Lotion*]
  **(Topical)**, #
  Cream USP
  Lotion
*Crown*—Okamoto (U.S.) brand of Latex Condoms—**See Condoms**, #
*Crown Plus*—Okamoto (U.S.) brand of Latex Condoms and Nonoxynol 9—**See Condoms**, #
*Crucial*—Clintec (U.S.) brand of Enteral Nutrition Formula, Disease-specific—**See Enteral Nutrition Formulas (Systemic)**, #
*Cruex Aerosol Powder*—Fisons (Canada) brand of Undecylenic Acid, Compound (Topical), #
*Cruex Antifungal Cream*—Fisons (U.S.) brand of Undecylenic Acid, Compound (Topical), #
*Cruex Antifungal Powder*—Fisons (U.S.) brand of Undecylenic Acid, Compound (Topical), #
*Cruex Antifungal Spray Powder*—Fisons (U.S.) brand of Undecylenic Acid, Compound (Topical), #
*Cruex Cream*—Fisons (Canada) brand of Undecylenic Acid, Compound (Topical), #
*Cruex Powder*—Fisons (Canada) brand of Undecylenic Acid, Compound (Topical), #
Cryptosporidium Hyperimmune Bovine Colostrum IgG Concentrate
  **(Systemic)**, 3138
*Crystamine*—Dunhall (U.S.) brand of Cyanocobalamin—**See Vitamin B$_{12}$ (Systemic)**, 2962
*Crysti-12*—Hauck (U.S.) brand of Cyanocobalamin—**See Vitamin B$_{12}$ (Systemic)**, 2962
*Crysticillin 300 AS*—Squibb-Marsam (U.S.) brand of Penicillin G—**See Penicillins (Systemic)**, 2240

*Crystodigin*—Lilly (U.S.) brand of Digitoxin—**See Digitalis Glycosides (Systemic)**, 1213
*C-Tussin Expectorant*—Century (U.S.) brand of Phenylpropanolamine, Codeine, and Guaifenesin—**See Cough/Cold Combinations (Systemic)**, 1024
*Cuplex Gel*—TransCanaDerm (Canada) brand of Salicylic Acid (Topical), #
Cupric Sulfate [*Cupri-Pak*]
  **See Copper Supplements (Systemic)**, 952
  Injection USP, 954
*Cuprid*—Merck (U.S.) brand of Trientine (Systemic), 3169
*Cuprimine*—Merck (U.S. and Canada) brand of Penicillamine (Systemic), 2237
*Cupri-Pak*—Solo-Pak (U.S.) brand of Cupric Sulfate—**See Copper Supplements (Systemic)**, 952
Curare—Tubocurarine—**See Neuromuscular Blocking Agents (Systemic)**, 2098
*Curel Everyday Sun Protection*—S.C. Johnson (U.S.) brand of Octyl Methoxycinnamate and Oxybenzone—**See Sunscreen Agents (Topical)**, #
*Curosurf*—Dey (U.S.) brand of Pulmonary Surfactant Replacement, Porcine (Intratracheal-Local), 3160
*Curretab*—Solvay (U.S.) brand of Medroxyprogesterone—**See Progestins (Systemic)**, 2400
*Cutar Water Dispersible Emollient Tar*—Summers (U.S.) brand of Coal Tar (Topical), #
*Cuticura Acne 5 Cream*—DEP (U.S.) brand of Benzoyl Peroxide (Topical), 579
*Cuticura Ointment*—Jeffrey Martin (U.S.) brand of Sulfur (Topical), #
*Cutivate*—Glaxo (U.S.) brand of Fluticasone—**See Corticosteroids (Topical)**, 978
*Cutter Pleasant Protection*—Spectrum (U.S.) brand of Diethyltoluamide (Topical), #
CY-1503 [*Cylexin*]
  **(Systemic)**, 3138
CY-1899
  **(Systemic)**, 3138
*Cyanide Antidote Package*—Lilly (U.S. and Canada) brand of Sodium Nitrite (Systemic), #; Lilly (U.S. and Canada) brand of Sodium Thiosulfate (Systemic), #
Cyanocobalamin [*Anacobin; Bedoz; Cobex; Cobolin-M; Crystamine; Crysti-12; Cyanoject; Cyomin; Neuroforte-R; Primabalt; Rubesol-1000; Rubramin PC; Shovite; Vibal; Vitabee 12;* vitamin B$_{12}$]
  **See Vitamin B$_{12}$ (Systemic)**, 2962
  Injection USP, 2965
  Tablets, 2964
  Tablets, Extended-release, 2965
Cyanocobalamin Co 57 [*Dicopac; Rubratope-57*]
  **(Systemic)**, 1123
  Capsules USP, 1125
*Cyanoject*—Mayrand (U.S.) brand of Cyanocobalamin—**See Vitamin B$_{12}$ (Systemic)**, 2962
Cyclandelate [*Cyclospasmol*]
  **(Systemic)**, #
  Tablets, #
*Cyclen*—Ortho (Canada) brand of Norgestimate and Ethinyl Estradiol—**See Estrogens and Progestins—Oral Contraceptives (Systemic)**, 1397
Cyclizine-containing Combinations, 3071
Cyclizine Hydrochloride [*Marezine*]
  **(Systemic)**, #
  Tablets USP, #
Cyclizine Lactate [*Marzine*]
  **(Systemic)**, #
  Injection USP, #
Cyclobenzaprine Hydrochloride [*Cycoflex; Flexeril*]
  **(Systemic)**, 1126
  Tablets USP, 1128, MC-8
*Cyclocort*—Lederle (U.S. and Canada) brand of Amcinonide—**See Corticosteroids (Topical)**, 978
*Cyclogyl*—Alcon (U.S. and Canada) brand of Cyclopentolate (Ophthalmic), #
*Cyclomen*—Sterling Winthrop (Canada) brand of Danazol (Systemic), 1163
Cyclopentolate Hydrochloride [*Ak-Pentolate; Cyclogyl; Cylate; Minims Cyclopentolate; Ocu-Pentolate; Pentolair*]
  **(Ophthalmic)**, #
  Solution, Ophthalmic, USP, #
8 Cyclopentyl 1,3-Dipropylxanthine
  **(Systemic)**, 3128
Cyclophosphamide [*Cytoxan; Neosar; Procytox*]
  **(Systemic)**, 1128
  for Injection USP, 1134
  Solution, Oral, 1133
  Tablets USP, 1133, MC-8

Cycloserine [*Seromycin*]
  **(Systemic)**, 1134
  Capsules USP, 1136
*Cyclospasmol*—Wyeth-Ayerst (U.S.) and Wyeth (Canada) brand of Cyclandelate (Systemic), #
*Cyclospire*—Knight (U.S.) brand of Liposomal Cyclosporine A (Systemic), 3152
Cyclosporin A—*See* Cyclosporine (Systemic), 1136
Cyclosporine [*Optimmune*]
  **(Ophthalmic)**, 3139
  Ointment, 3139
Cyclosporine [ciclosporin; cyclosporin A; *Neoral; Sandimmune; Sandimmune SGC*]
  **(Systemic)**, 1136
  Capsules USP, 1142, MC-8
  Capsules, Modified, 1142
  Concentrate for Injection USP, 1142
  Solution, Oral, USP, 1142
  Solution, Oral, Modified, 1142
*Cycoflex*—Major (U.S.) brand of Cyclobenzaprine (Systemic), 1126
*Cycrin*—ESI Lederle (U.S.) brand of Medroxyprogesterone—**See Progestins (Systemic)**, 2400
*Cyklokapron*—KabiVitrum (U.S.) and Pharmacia (Canada) brand of Tranexamic Acid (Systemic), 2862; Pharmacia (U.S.) brand of Tranexamic Acid (Systemic), 3169
*Cylate*—Ocusoft (U.S.) brand of Cyclopentolate (Ophthalmic), #
*Cylert*—Abbott (U.S. and Canada) brand of Pemoline (Systemic), 2233, MC-24
*Cylert Chewable*—Abbott (U.S. and Canada) brand of Pemoline (Systemic), 2233, MC-24
*Cylexin*—Cytel (U.S.) brand of CY-1503 (Systemic), 3138
*Cyomin*—Forest (U.S.) brand of Cyanocobalamin—**See Vitamin B$_{12}$ (Systemic)**, 2962
Cyproheptadine Hydrochloride [*Periactin; PMS-Cyproheptadine*]
  **See Antihistamines (Systemic)**, 325
  Syrup USP, 335
  Tablets USP, 335
Cyproterone Acetate [*Androcur*]
  **(Systemic)**, 3016
  Injection, 3016
  Tablets, 3016
*Cystadane*—Orphan Medical (U.S.) brand of Betaine (Systemic), #
*Cystagon*—Mylan (U.S.) brand of Cysteamine (Systemic), #, 3138
Cysteamine [*Cystagon*]
  **(Systemic)**, 3138
Cysteamine Bitartrate [*Cystagon*]
  **(Systemic)**, 3138
  Capsules, #
Cysteamine Hydrochloride
  **(Systemic)**, 3139
Cystic Fibrosis Gene, Lipid/DNA, Human
  **(Systemic)**, 3151
Cystic Fibrosis Gene Therapy
  **(Systemic)**, 3139
Cystic Fibrosis Transmembrane Conductance Regulator
  **(Systemic)**, 3139
Cystic Fibrosis TR Gene Therapy (Recombinant Adenovirus) [ADgvCFTR.10]
  **(Systemic)**, 3139
*Cysto-Conray*—Mallinckrodt (U.S. and Canada) brand of Iothalamate (Local), #
*Cysto-Conray II*—Mallinckrodt (U.S. and Canada) brand of Iothalamate (Local), #
*Cystografin*—Squibb (U.S.) brand of Diatrizoate—**See Diatrizoates (Local)**, #
*Cystografin Dilute*—Squibb (U.S.) brand of Diatrizoate—**See Diatrizoates (Local)**, #
*Cystospaz*—Webcon (U.S.) brand of Hyoscyamine—**See Anticholinergics/Antispasmodics (Systemic)**, 226
*Cystospaz-M*—Webcon (U.S.) brand of Hyoscyamine—**See Anticholinergics/Antispasmodics (Systemic)**, 226
*Cytadren*—Ciba-Geigy (U.S. and Canada) brand of Aminoglutethimide (Systemic), 67
Cytarabine [ara-C; *Cytosar; Cytosar-U;* cytosine arabinoside]
  **(Systemic)**, 1143
  Sterile USP, 1146

## General Index

CYTOIMPLANT—Applied Immunotherapeutics (U.S.) brand of Allogeneic Peripheral Blood Mononuclear Cells Sensitized Against Patient Alloantigens By Mixed Lymphocyte Culture (Systemic), 3129
Cytomegalovirus Immune Globulin (Human) **(Systemic)**, 3139
Cytomegalovirus Immune Globulin Intravenous (Human) **(Systemic)**, 3139
*Cytomel*—SKF (U.S. and Canada) brand of Liothyronine—**See Thyroid Hormones (Systemic)**, 2809
*Cytosar*—Upjohn (Canada) brand of Cytarabine (Systemic), 1143
*Cytosar-U*—Upjohn (U.S.) brand of Cytarabine (Systemic), 1143
Cytosine arabinoside—*See* Cytarabine (Systemic), 1143
*Cytotec*—Searle (U.S. and Canada) brand of Misoprostol (Systemic), 2026, MC-20
*Cytovene*—Roche (U.S. and Canada) and Syntex (Canada) brand of Ganciclovir (Systemic), 1544, 3022, MC-13
*Cytovene-IV*—Roche/Syntex (U.S.) brand of Ganciclovir (Systemic), 1544
*Cytoxan*—Mead Johnson (U.S.) and Bristol (Canada) brand of Cyclophosphamide (Systemic), 1128, MC-8

### D

DAB389IL-2 **(Systemic)**, 3139
Dacarbazine [*DTIC; DTIC-Dome*] **(Systemic)**, 1148
 for Injection USP, 1150
*D.A. Chewable*—Dura (U.S.) brand of Chlorpheniramine, Phenylephrine, and Methscopolamine—**See Antihistamines, Decongestants, and Anticholinergics (Systemic)**, 373
Dacliximab—*See* Daclizumab (Systemic), 1151
Daclizumab [dacliximab; *Zenapax*] **(Systemic)**, 1151
 Concentrate for Injection, 1152
*Dacodyl*—Major (U.S.) brand of Bisacodyl—**See Laxatives (Local)**, #
Dactinomycin [actinomycin-D; *Cosmegen*] **(Systemic)**, 1153
 for Injection USP, 1156
*Dagenan*—Rhône-Poulenc (Canada) brand of Sulfapyridine (Systemic), 2640
*Dalacin*—Pharmacia & Upjohn (Canada) brand of Clindamycin (Vaginal), 898
*Dalacin C*—Upjohn (Canada) brand of Clindamycin (Systemic), 893
*Dalacin C Flavored Granules*—Upjohn (Canada) brand of Clindamycin (Systemic), 893
*Dalacin C Phosphate*—Upjohn (Canada) brand of Clindamycin (Systemic), 893
*Dalacin T Topical Solution*—Upjohn (Canada) brand of Clindamycin (Topical), 896
*Dalalone*—Forest (U.S.) brand of Dexamethasone—**See Corticosteroids—Glucocorticoid Effects (Systemic)**, 998
*Dalalone D.P.*—Forest (U.S.) brand of Dexamethasone—**See Corticosteroids—Glucocorticoid Effects (Systemic)**, 998
*Dalalone L.A.*—Forest (U.S.) brand of Dexamethasone—**See Corticosteroids—Glucocorticoid Effects (Systemic)**, 998
*Dalcaine*—Forest (U.S.) brand of Lidocaine—**See Anesthetics (Parenteral-Local)**, 139
*Dalgan*—Astra (U.S.) brand of Dezocine (Systemic), 1193
*Dallergy*—Laser (U.S.) brand of Chlorpheniramine, Phenylephrine, and Methscopolamine—**See Antihistamines, Decongestants, and Anticholinergics (Systemic)**, 373
*Dallergy Caplets*—Laser (U.S.) brand of Chlorpheniramine, Phenylephrine, and Methscopolamine—**See Antihistamines, Decongestants, and Anticholinergics (Systemic)**, 373
*Dallergy Jr.*—Laser (U.S.) brand of Brompheniramine and Pseudoephedrine—**See Antihistamines and Decongestants (Systemic)**, 343
*Dalmane*—Roche (U.S. and Canada) brand of Flurazepam—**See Benzodiazepines (Systemic)**, 556, MC-13

Dalteparin Sodium [*Fragmin*; low molecular weight heparin; tedelparin] **(Systemic)**, 1156
 Injection, 1160
*Damason-P*—Mason (U.S.) brand of Hydrocodone and Aspirin—**See Opioid (Narcotic) Analgesics and Aspirin (Systemic)**, 2202
Danaparoid Sodium [*Orgaran*; ORG 10172] **(Systemic)**, 1161
 Injection, 1163
Danazol [*Cyclomen; Danocrine*] **(Systemic)**, 1163
 Capsules USP, 1165, MC-8
*Danex*—Allergan Herbert (U.S.) brand of Pyrithione (Topical), #
*Dan-gard*—Stiefel (Canada) brand of Pyrithione (Topical), #
*Danocrine*—Sanofi Winthrop (U.S.) brand of Danazol (Systemic), 1163, MC-8
Danthron-containing Combinations, 3071
Danthron and Docusate Sodium [*Doss; Regulex-D*] **See Laxatives (Local)**, #
 Capsules, #
 Tablets, #
*Dantrium*—Procter & Gamble (U.S. and Canada) brand of Dantrolene (Systemic), 1165, MC-8
*Dantrium Intravenous*—Procter & Gamble (U.S. and Canada) brand of Dantrolene (Systemic), 1165
Dantrolene Sodium [*Dantrium; Dantrium Intravenous*] **(Systemic)**, 1165
 Capsules, 1168, MC-8
 for Injection, 1168
*Dapa*—Ferndale (U.S.) brand of Acetaminophen (Systemic), 6
*Dapacin Cold*—Ferndale (U.S.) brand of Chlorpheniramine, Phenylpropanolamine, and Acetaminophen—**See Antihistamines, Decongestants, and Analgesics (Systemic)**, 366
*Dapa X-S*—Ferndale (U.S.) brand of Acetaminophen (Systemic), 6
Dapiprazole Hydrochloride [*Rev-Eyes*] **(Ophthalmic)**, 1168
 for Solution, Ophthalmic, 1169
*Dapsone*—Jacobus (U.S.) brand of Dapsone (Systemic), 3139
Dapsone [*Avlosulfon*; DDS] **(Systemic)**, 1170, 3139
 Tablets USP, 1172
*Daranide*—Merck (U.S.) brand of Dichlorphenamide—**See Carbonic Anhydrase Inhibitors (Systemic)**, 773
*Daraprim*—Glaxo Wellcome (U.S.) and BW (Canada) brand of Pyrimethamine (Systemic), 2433, MC-27
*Dartal*—Searle (Canada) brand of Thiopropazate—**See Phenothiazines (Systemic)**, 2289
*Darvocet-N 50*—Lilly (U.S.) brand of Propoxyphene and Acetaminophen—**See Opioid (Narcotic) Analgesics and Acetaminophen (Systemic)**, 2198, MC-26
*Darvocet-N 100*—Lilly (U.S.) brand of Propoxyphene and Acetaminophen—**See Opioid (Narcotic) Analgesics and Acetaminophen (Systemic)**, 2198, MC-26
*Darvon*—Lilly (U.S.) brand of Propoxyphene—**See Opioid (Narcotic) Analgesics (Systemic)**, 2168
*Darvon Compound-65*—Lilly (U.S.) brand of Propoxyphene and Aspirin—**See Opioid (Narcotic) Analgesics and Aspirin (Systemic)**, 2202
*Darvon-N*—Lilly (U.S. and Canada) brand of Propoxyphene—**See Opioid (Narcotic) Analgesics (Systemic)**, 2168
*Darvon-N with A.S.A.*—Lilly (Canada) brand of Propoxyphene and Aspirin—**See Opioid (Narcotic) Analgesics and Aspirin (Systemic)**, 2202
*Darvon-N Compound*—Lilly (Canada) brand of Propoxyphene and Aspirin—**See Opioid (Narcotic) Analgesics and Aspirin (Systemic)**, 2202
*Datril Extra-Strength*—Bristol-Myers (U.S.) brand of Acetaminophen (Systemic), 6
Daunorubicin Hydrochloride [*Cerubidine*] **(Systemic)**, 1173
 for Injection USP, 1176
Daunorubicin, Liposomal [*Daunoxome*] **(Systemic)**, 1176, 3151
 Injection, 1179
*DaunoXome*—NeXstar (U.S.) brand of Daunorubicin, Liposomal (Systemic), 1176
*Daunoxome*—Vestar (U.S.) brand of Daunorubicin, Liposomal (Systemic), 3152

*Daypro*—Searle (Canada) brand of Oxaprozin (Systemic), 3030; Searle (U.S.) brand of Oxaprozin—**See Anti-inflammatory Drugs, Nonsteroidal (Systemic)**, 388, MC-23
*Dayto Himbin*—Dayton (U.S.) brand of Yohimbine (Systemic), #
*Dazamide*—Major (U.S.) brand of Acetazolamide—**See Carbonic Anhydrase Inhibitors (Systemic)**, 773
2′DCF—*See* Pentostatin (Systemic), 2279
*DC Softgels*—Zenith Goldline (U.S.) brand of Docusate—**See Laxatives (Local)**, #
DDAVP—Rhône-Poulenc Rorer (U.S.) and Ferring (Canada) brand of Desmopressin (Systemic), 1187, 3016, MC-8
*DDAVP Nasal Spray*—Rhône-Poulenc Rorer (U.S.) brand of Desmopressin (Systemic), 1187
*DDAVP Rhinal Tube*—Rhône-Poulenc Rorer (U.S.) brand of Desmopressin (Systemic), 1187
*DDAVP Rhinyle Nasal Solution*—Ferring (Canada) brand of Desmopressin (Systemic), 1187
*DDAVP Spray*—Ferring (Canada) brand of Desmopressin (Systemic), 1187
ddC—*See* Zalcitabine (Systemic), 2989
ddI—*See* Didanosine (Systemic), 1206
DDS—*See* Dapsone (Systemic), 1170
*Decaderm*—Merck (U.S.) brand of Dexamethasone—**See Corticosteroids (Topical)**, 978
*Decadrol*—Paddock (U.S.) brand of Dexamethasone—**See Corticosteroids—Glucocorticoid Effects (Systemic)**, 998
*Decadron*—Merck (U.S. and Canada) brand of Dexamethasone—**See Corticosteroids (Ophthalmic)**, 966; **Corticosteroids (Otic)**, 971; **Corticosteroids (Topical)**, 978; **Corticosteroids—Glucocorticoid Effects (Systemic)**, 998, MC-8
*Decadron-LA*—MSD (U.S.) brand of Dexamethasone—**See Corticosteroids—Glucocorticoid Effects (Systemic)**, 998
*Decadron Phosphate*—Merck (U.S.) brand of Dexamethasone—**See Corticosteroids—Glucocorticoid Effects (Systemic)**, 998
*Decadron Respihaler*—Merck (U.S.) brand of Dexamethasone—**See Corticosteroids (Inhalation-Local)**, 955
*Decadron Turbinaire*—Merck (U.S.) brand of Dexamethasone—**See Corticosteroids (Nasal)**, 961
*Deca-Durabolin*—Organon (U.S. and Canada) brand of Nandrolone—**See Anabolic Steroids (Systemic)**, 110
*Decaject*—Mayrand (U.S.) brand of Dexamethasone—**See Corticosteroids—Glucocorticoid Effects (Systemic)**, 998
*Decaject-L.A.*—Mayrand (U.S.) brand of Dexamethasone—**See Corticosteroids—Glucocorticoid Effects (Systemic)**, 998
*Decaspray*—Merck (U.S.) brand of Dexamethasone—**See Corticosteroids (Topical)**, 978
*Decholin*—Bayer Consumer (U.S.) brand of Dehydrocholic Acid—**See Laxatives (Local)**, #
*Declomycin*—Lederle (U.S. and Canada) brand of Demeclocycline—**See Tetracyclines (Systemic)**, 2765, MC-8
*Decofed*—Dixon-Shane (U.S.); Mason (U.S.); and Moore (U.S.) brand of Pseudoephedrine (Systemic), 2422
*Decohistine DH*—Pennex (U.S.) brand of Chlorpheniramine, Pseudoephedrine, and Codeine—**See Cough/Cold Combinations (Systemic)**, 1024
*De-Comberol*—Schein (U.S.) brand of Testosterone and Estradiol—**See Androgens and Estrogens (Systemic)**, 126
*Deconamine*—Bradley-Kenwood (U.S.) brand of Chlorpheniramine and Pseudoephedrine—**See Antihistamines and Decongestants (Systemic)**, 343
*Deconamine CX*—Bradley (U.S.) brand of Pseudoephedrine, Hydrocodone, and Guaifenesin—**See Cough/Cold Combinations (Systemic)**, 1024
*Deconamine SR*—Bradley-Kenwood (U.S.) brand of Chlorpheniramine and Pseudoephedrine—**See Antihistamines and Decongestants (Systemic)**, 343
*Decongestabs*—H. L. Moore and Parmed (U.S.) brand of Chlorpheniramine, Phenyltoloxamine, Phenylephrine, and Phenylpropanolamine—**See Antihistamines and Decongestants (Systemic)**, 343
Decongestants and Analgesics **(Systemic)**, 1180

*Deconhist*—Goldline (U.S.) brand of Chlorpheniramine, Phenylephrine, Phenylpropanolamine, Atropine, Hyoscyamine, and Scopolamine—**See Antihistamines, Decongestants, and Anticholinergics (Systemic)**, 373

*Deconomed SR*—Iomed (U.S.) brand of Chlorpheniramine and Pseudoephedrine—**See Antihistamines and Decongestants (Systemic)**, 343

*Deconsal II*—Adams (U.S.) brand of Pseudoephedrine and Guaifenesin—**See Cough/Cold Combinations (Systemic)**, 1024

*Deconsal Pediatric*—Adams (U.S.) brand of Phenylephrine and Guaifenesin—**See Cough/Cold Combinations (Systemic)**, 1024

*Decylenes Powder*—Rugby (U.S.) brand of Undecylenic Acid, Compound (Topical), #

*Deep Woods OFF*—S. C. Johnson (U.S. and Canada) brand of Diethyltoluamide (Topical), #

*Deep Woods OFF For Sportsmen*—S. C. Johnson (U.S.) brand of Diethyltoluamide (Topical), #

DEET—*See* Diethyltoluamide (Topical), #

Deferoxamine mesilate—*See* Deferoxamine (Systemic), #

Deferoxamine Mesylate [deferoxamine mesilate; *Desferal*; desferrioxamine; desferrioxamine mesylate]
 **(Systemic)**, #
 Sterile USP, #

Defibrotide
 **(Systemic)**, 3139

*Deficol*—Vangard (U.S.) brand of Bisacodyl—**See Laxatives (Local)**, #

*Degas*—Invamed (U.S.) brand of Simethicone (Oral-Local), #

*Degest 2*—Barnes-Hind (U.S.) brand of Naphazoline (Ophthalmic), #

Dehydrex
 **(Ophthalmic)**, 3139

Dehydrocholic Acid [*Decholin; Hepahydrin*]
 **See Laxatives (Local)**, #
 Tablets USP, #

Dehydrocholic Acid–containing Combinations, 3071

Dehydrocholic Acid and Docusate Sodium [*Bilax; Neolax*]
 **See Laxatives (Local)**, #
 Capsules, #
 Tablets, #

Dehydrocholic Acid, Docusate Sodium, and Phenolphthalein [*Trilax*]
 **See Laxatives (Local)**, #
 Capsules, #

Dehydroepiandrosterone
 **(Systemic)**, 3139

Dehydroepiandrosterone Sulfate Sodium
 **(Topical)**, 3140

*Delacort*—Mericon (U.S.) brand of Hydrocortisone—**See Corticosteroids (Topical)**, 978

*Deladumone*—Squibb (U.S.) brand of Testosterone and Estradiol—**See Androgens and Estrogens (Systemic)**, 126

*Del-Aqua-5 Gel*—Del-Ray (U.S.) brand of Benzoyl Peroxide (Topical), 579

*Del-Aqua-10 Gel*—Del-Ray (U.S.) brand of Benzoyl Peroxide (Topical), 579

*Delatest*—Dunhall (U.S.) brand of Testosterone—**See Androgens (Systemic)**, 118

*Delatestadiol*—Dunhall (U.S.) brand of Testosterone and Estradiol—**See Androgens and Estrogens (Systemic)**, 126

*Delatestryl*—Bio-Technology Group (U.S.) and Bristol-Myers Squibb (Canada) brand of Testosterone—**See Androgens (Systemic)**, 118

Delavirdine Mesylate [*Rescriptor*]
 **(Systemic)**, 1184
 Tablets, 1186

*Delestrogen*—Squibb (U.S. and Canada) brand of Estradiol—**See Estrogens (Systemic)**, 1383

*Delfen*—Ortho (U.S. and Canada) brand of Nonoxynol 9—**See Spermicides (Vaginal)**, #

*Delhistine D*—Rugby (U.S.) brand of Pheniramine, Phenyltoloxamine, Pyrilamine, and Phenylpropanolamine—**See Antihistamines and Decongestants (Systemic)**, 343

*Deliver 2.0*—Bristol-Myers Squibb (U.S.) brand of Enteral Nutrition Formula, Polymeric—**See Enteral Nutrition Formulas (Systemic)**, #

*Delsym*—McNeil (U.S.) and Fisons (Canada) brand of Dextromethorphan (Systemic), 1191

*Delta-Cortef*—Upjohn (U.S.) brand of Prednisolone—**See Corticosteroids—Glucocorticoid Effects (Systemic)**, 998

*Deltasone*—Pharmacia & Upjohn (U.S. and Canada) brand of Prednisone—**See Corticosteroids—Glucocorticoid Effects (Systemic)**, 998, MC-25

Delta-9-tetrahydrocannabinol (THC)—*See* Dronabinol (Systemic), 1316

*Delta-Tritex*—Dermol (U.S.) brand of Triamcinolone—**See Corticosteroids (Topical)**, 978

*Demadex*—Roche (U.S.) brand of Torsemide (Systemic), 2848, MC-31

*Demazin*—Schering-Plough (U.S.) brand of Chlorpheniramine and Phenylpropanolamine—**See Antihistamines and Decongestants (Systemic)**, 343

*Demazin Repetabs*—Schering-Plough (U.S.) brand of Chlorpheniramine and Phenylpropanolamine—**See Antihistamines and Decongestants (Systemic)**, 343

Demecarium Bromide [*Humorsol*]
 **See Antiglaucoma Agents, Cholinergic, Long-acting (Ophthalmic)**, 315
 Solution, Ophthalmic, USP, 318

Demeclocycline Hydrochloride [*Declomycin*]
 **See Tetracyclines (Systemic)**, 2765
 Capsules USP, 2768
 Tablets USP, 2769, MC-8

*Demerol*—Sanofi Winthrop (U.S. and Canada) brand of Meperidine—**See Opioid (Narcotic) Analgesics (Systemic)**, 2168, MC-18

*Demi-Regroton*—Rhône-Poulenc Rorer (U.S.) brand of Reserpine and Chlorthalidone—**See Rauwolfia Alkaloids and Thiazide Diuretics (Systemic)**, #

*Demser*—Merck (U.S.) brand of Metyrosine (Systemic), #

*Demulen 1/35*—Searle (U.S.) brand of Ethynodiol Diacetate and Ethinyl Estradiol—**See Estrogens and Progestins—Oral Contraceptives (Systemic)**, 1397, MC-12

*Demulen 1/50*—Searle (U.S.) brand of Ethynodiol Diacetate and Ethinyl Estradiol—**See Estrogens and Progestins—Oral Contraceptives (Systemic)**, 1397, MC-12

*Demulen 30*—Searle (Canada) brand of Ethynodiol Diacetate and Ethinyl Estradiol—**See Estrogens and Progestins—Oral Contraceptives (Systemic)**, 1397

*Demulen 50*—Searle (Canada) brand of Ethynodiol Diacetate and Ethinyl Estradiol—**See Estrogens and Progestins—Oral Contraceptives (Systemic)**, 1397

*Denavir*—SmithKline Beecham (U.S.) brand of Penciclovir (Topical), 2236

*Denorex*—Whitehall (Canada) brand of Coal Tar (Topical), #

*Denorex Extra Strength Medicated Shampoo*—Whitehall (U.S.) brand of Coal Tar (Topical), #

*Denorex Extra Strength Medicated Shampoo with Conditioners*—Whitehall (U.S.) brand of Coal Tar (Topical), #

*Denorex Medicated Shampoo*—Whitehall (U.S.) brand of Coal Tar (Topical), #

*Denorex Medicated Shampoo and Conditioner*—Whitehall (U.S.) brand of Coal Tar (Topical), #

*Denorex Mountain Fresh Herbal Scent Medicated Shampoo*—Whitehall (U.S.) brand of Coal Tar (Topical), #

*Dentapaine*—Reese (U.S.) brand of Benzocaine—**See Anesthetics (Mucosal-Local)**, 128

*Dentocaine*—Novopharm (Canada) brand of Benzocaine—**See Anesthetics (Mucosal-Local)**, 128

*Dent-Zel-Ite*—Alvin Last (U.S.) brand of Benzocaine—**See Anesthetics (Mucosal-Local)**, 128

2'-deoxycoformycin—*See* Pentostatin (Systemic), 2279

2'-Deoxycytidine
 **(Systemic)**, 3127

*Depacon*—Abbott (U.S.) brand of Valproate Sodium—**See Valproic Acid (Systemic)**, 2908

*Depakene*—Abbott (U.S. and Canada) brand of Valproic Acid (Systemic), 2908, MC-32

*Depakote*—Abbott (U.S.) brand of Divalproex—**See Valproic Acid (Systemic)**, 2908, MC-10

*Depakote Sprinkle*—Abbott (U.S.) brand of Divalproex—**See Valproic Acid (Systemic)**, 2908, MC-10

*depAndrogyn*—Forest (U.S.) brand of Testosterone and Estradiol—**See Androgens and Estrogens (Systemic)**, 126

*Depen*—Wallace (U.S.) and Horner (Canada) brand of Penicillamine (Systemic), 2237

*depGynogen*—Forest (U.S.) brand of Estradiol—**See Estrogens (Systemic)**, 1383

*depMedalone 40*—Forest (U.S.) brand of Methylprednisolone—**See Corticosteroids—Glucocorticoid Effects (Systemic)**, 998

*depMedalone 80*—Forest (U.S.) brand of Methylprednisolone—**See Corticosteroids—Glucocorticoid Effects (Systemic)**, 998

*Depo-Estradiol*—Upjohn (U.S.) brand of Estradiol—**See Estrogens (Systemic)**, 1383

Depofoam Encapsulated Cytarabine
 **(Systemic)**, 3140

*Depogen*—Hyrex (U.S.) brand of Estradiol—**See Estrogens (Systemic)**, 1383

*Depoject-40*—Mayrand (U.S.) brand of Methylprednisolone—**See Corticosteroids—Glucocorticoid Effects (Systemic)**, 998

*Depoject-80*—Mayrand (U.S.) brand of Methylprednisolone—**See Corticosteroids—Glucocorticoid Effects (Systemic)**, 998

*Depo-Medrol*—Upjohn (U.S. and Canada) brand of Methylprednisolone—**See Corticosteroids—Glucocorticoid Effects (Systemic)**, 998

*Deponit*—Kremers-Urban (U.S.) brand of Nitroglycerin—**See Nitrates (Systemic)**, 2129

*Depopred-40*—Hyrex (U.S.) brand of Methylprednisolone—**See Corticosteroids—Glucocorticoid Effects (Systemic)**, 998

*Depopred-80*—Hyrex (U.S.) brand of Methylprednisolone—**See Corticosteroids—Glucocorticoid Effects (Systemic)**, 998

*Depo-Predate 40*—Legere (U.S.) brand of Methylprednisolone—**See Corticosteroids—Glucocorticoid Effects (Systemic)**, 998

*Depo-Predate 80*—Legere (U.S.) brand of Methylprednisolone—**See Corticosteroids—Glucocorticoid Effects (Systemic)**, 998

*Depo-Provera*—Pharmacia & Upjohn (U.S. and Canada) brand of Medroxyprogesterone—**See Progestins (Systemic)**, 2400

*Depo-Provera Contraceptive Injection*—Pharmacia & Upjohn (U.S. and Canada) brand of Medroxyprogesterone—**See Progestins (Systemic)**, 2400

*Depotest*—Hyrex (U.S.) brand of Testosterone—**See Androgens (Systemic)**, 118

*Depo-Testadiol*—Upjohn (U.S.) brand of Testosterone and Estradiol—**See Androgens and Estrogens (Systemic)**, 126

*Depotestogen*—Hyrex (U.S.) brand of Testosterone and Estradiol—**See Androgens and Estrogens (Systemic)**, 126

*Depo-Testosterone*—Pharmacia & Upjohn (U.S.) brand of Testosterone—**See Androgens (Systemic)**, 118

*Depo-Testosterone Cypionate*—Pharmacia & Upjohn (Canada) brand of Testosterone—**See Androgens (Systemic)**, 118

Deprenil—*See* Selegiline (Systemic), 2560

Deprenyl—*See* Selegiline (Systemic), 2560

*Deproic*—Technilab (Canada) brand of Valproic Acid—**See Valproic Acid (Systemic)**, 2908

*Deproist Expectorant with Codeine*—Geneva (U.S.) brand of Pseudoephedrine, Codeine, and Guaifenesin—**See Cough/Cold Combinations (Systemic)**, 1024

*Derbac-M*—International (U.K.) brand of Malathion (Topical), #

*Dermabet*—Taro (U.S.) brand of Betamethasone—**See Corticosteroids (Topical)**, 978

*Dermacne*—Bio-Sante (Canada) brand of Benzoyl Peroxide (Topical), 579

*Dermacomb*—Taro (U.S.) brand of Nystatin and Triamcinolone (Topical), 2150

*Dermacort*—Solvay (U.S.) brand of Hydrocortisone—**See Corticosteroids (Topical)**, 978

*DermaFlex*—Zila (U.S.) brand of Lidocaine—**See Anesthetics (Topical)**, 155

*Dermarest DriCort*—Del (U.S.) brand of Hydrocortisone—**See Corticosteroids (Topical)**, 978

*Dermatop*—Hoechst-Roussel (U.S.) brand of Prednicarbate (Topical), 3033

*DermiCort*—Republic (U.S.) brand of Hydrocortisone—**See Corticosteroids (Topical)**, 978

*Dermoplast*—Whitehall (U.S.) and Ayerst (Canada) brand of Benzocaine and Menthol—**See Anesthetics (Topical)**, 155

*Dermovate*—Glaxo (Canada and U.K.) brand of Clobetasol—**See Corticosteroids (Topical)**, 978

*Dermovate Scalp Lotion*—Glaxo (Canada and U.K.) brand of Clobetasol—**See Corticosteroids (Topical)**, 978

*Dermoxyl Aqua 5 Gel*—ICN (Canada) brand of Benzoyl Peroxide (Topical), 579
*Dermoxyl 5 Gel*—ICN (Canada) brand of Benzoyl Peroxide (Topical), 579
*Dermoxyl 10 Gel*—ICN (Canada) brand of Benzoyl Peroxide (Topical), 579
*Dermoxyl 20 Gel*—ICN (Canada) brand of Benzoyl Peroxide (Topical), 579
*Dermsol*—Parnell (U.S.) brand of Octyl Methoxycinnamate, Octyl Salicylate, and Oxybenzone—**See Sunscreen Agents (Topical)**, #
*Dermtex HC*—Pfeiffer (U.S.) brand of Hydrocortisone—**See Corticosteroids (Topical)**, 978
*Deronil*—Schering (Canada) brand of Dexamethasone—**See Corticosteroids—Glucocorticoid Effects (Systemic)**, 998
DES—Diethylstilbestrol—**See Estrogens (Systemic)**, 1383
*Desenex Aerosol Powder*—Fisons (Canada) brand of Undecylenic Acid, Compound (Topical), #
*Desenex Antifungal Cream*—Fisons (U.S.) brand of Undecylenic Acid, Compound (Topical), #
*Desenex Antifungal Liquid*—Fisons (U.S.) brand of Undecylenic Acid, Compound (Topical), #
*Desenex Antifungal Ointment*—Fisons (U.S.) brand of Undecylenic Acid, Compound (Topical), #
*Desenex Antifungal Penetrating Foam*—Fisons (U.S.) brand of Undecylenic Acid, Compound (Topical), #
*Desenex Antifungal Powder*—Fisons (U.S.) brand of Undecylenic Acid, Compound (Topical), #
*Desenex Antifungal Spray Powder*—Fisons (U.S.) brand of Undecylenic Acid, Compound (Topical), #
*Desenex Foam*—Fisons (Canada) brand of Undecylenic Acid, Compound (Topical), #
*Desenex Ointment*—Fisons (Canada) brand of Undecylenic Acid, Compound (Topical), #
*Desenex Powder*—Fisons (Canada) brand of Undecylenic Acid, Compound (Topical), #
*Desenex Solution*—Fisons (Canada) brand of Undecylenic Acid, Compound (Topical), #
Deserpidine [*Harmonyl*]
  **See Rauwolfia Alkaloids (Systemic)**, 2460
  Tablets, 2463
Deserpidine-containing Combinations, 3071
Deserpidine and Hydrochlorothiazide [*Oreticyl; Oreticyl Forte*]
  **See Rauwolfia Alkaloids and Thiazide Diuretics (Systemic)**, #
  Tablets, #
Deserpidine and Methyclothiazide [*Dureticyl; Enduronyl; Enduronyl Forte*]
  **See Rauwolfia Alkaloids and Thiazide Diuretics (Systemic)**, #
  Tablets, #
*Desferal*—Ciba (U.S. and Canada) brand of Deferoxamine (Systemic), #
*Desferrioxamine*—**See Deferoxamine (Systemic)**, #
*Desferrioxamine mesylate*—**See Deferoxamine (Systemic)**, #
Desflurane [*Suprane*]
  **(Inhalation-Systemic)**, #
  Desflurane USP, #
Desipramine Hydrochloride [*Norpramin; Pertofrane*]
  **See Antidepressants, Tricyclic (Systemic)**, 271
  Tablets USP, 279, MC-8
Deslorelin [*Somagard*]
  **(Systemic)**, 3140
Desmopressin [*DDAVP*]
  **(Systemic)**, 3016
  Tablets, 3016, MC-8
Desmopressin Acetate
  **(Inhalation/Systemic)**, 3140
Desmopressin Acetate [*DDAVP; DDAVP Nasal Spray; DDAVP Rhinal Tube; DDAVP Rhinyle Nasal Solution; DDAVP Spray; Octostim; Stimate; Stimate Nasal Spray*]
  **(Systemic)**, 1187
  Injection, 1189
  Solution, Nasal, 1189
*Desogen*—Organon (U.S.) brand of Desogestrel and Ethinyl Estradiol—**See Estrogens and Progestins—Oral Contraceptives (Systemic)**, 1397, MC-8
Desogestrel and Ethinyl Estradiol [*Desogen; Marvelon; Ortho-Cept*]
  **See Estrogens and Progestins—Oral Contraceptives (Systemic)**, 1397
  Tablets, 1407, MC-8

Desogestrel and Ethinyl Estradiol, and Ethinyl Estradiol [*Mircette*]
  **(Systemic)**, 1407 3022
  Tablets, 1407
Desonide [*DesOwen; Tridesilon*]
  **See Corticosteroids (Topical)**, 978
  Cream, 986
  Lotion, 987
  Ointment, 987
Desonide and Acetic Acid [*Otic Tridesilon Solution*]
  **See Corticosteroids and Acetic Acid (Otic)**, 996
  Solution, Otic, 997
Desonide-containing Combinations, 3071
*DesOwen*—Owen/Allercreme (U.S.) brand of Desonide—**See Corticosteroids (Topical)**, 978
Desoximetasone [*Topicort; Topicort LP; Topicort Mild*]
  **See Corticosteroids (Topical)**, 978, 3022
  Cream USP, 987
  Gel USP, 987
  Ointment USP, 987, 3016
*Desoxyn*—Abbott (U.S.) brand of Methamphetamine—**See Amphetamines (Systemic)**, 94
*Desoxyn Gradumet*—Abbott (U.S.) brand of Methamphetamine—**See Amphetamines (Systemic)**, 94
*Despec*—International-Ethical (U.S.) brand of Phenylephrine, Phenylpropanolamine, and Guaifenesin—**See Cough/Cold Combinations (Systemic)**, 1024
*Despec SF*—International-Ethical (U.S.) brand of Phenylephrine, Phenylpropanolamine, and Guaifenesin—**See Cough/Cold Combinations (Systemic)**, 1024
*Despec-SR Caplets*—International-Ethical (U.S.) brand of Phenylpropanolamine and Guaifenesin—**See Cough/Cold Combinations (Systemic)**, 1024
*Desquam-E 2.5 Gel*—Westwood-Squibb (U.S.) brand of Benzoyl Peroxide (Topical), 579
*Desquam-E 5 Gel*—Westwood-Squibb (U.S.) brand of Benzoyl Peroxide (Topical), 579
*Desquam-E 10 Gel*—Westwood-Squibb (U.S.) brand of Benzoyl Peroxide (Topical), 579
*Desquam-X 10 Bar*—Westwood-Squibb (U.S.) brand of Benzoyl Peroxide (Topical), 579
*Desquam-X 2.5 Gel*—Westwood-Squibb (U.S.) brand of Benzoyl Peroxide (Topical), 579
*Desquam-X 5 Gel*—Westwood-Squibb (U.S. and Canada) brand of Benzoyl Peroxide (Topical), 579
*Desquam-X 10 Gel*—Westwood-Squibb (U.S. and Canada) brand of Benzoyl Peroxide (Topical), 579
*Desquam-X 5 Wash*—Westwood-Squibb (U.S. and Canada) brand of Benzoyl Peroxide (Topical), 579
*Desquam-X 10 Wash*—Westwood-Squibb (U.S. and Canada) brand of Benzoyl Peroxide (Topical), 579
2-0-Desulfated Heparin [*Aeropin*]
  **(Systemic)**, 3127
*Desyrel*—Apothecon (U.S.) and Bristol (Canada) brand of Trazodone (Systemic), 2865, MC-31
*Desyrel Dividose*—Apothecon (U.S.) brand of Trazodone (Systemic), 2865, MC-31
*Detensol*—Desbergers (Canada) brand of Propranolol—**See Beta-adrenergic Blocking Agents (Systemic)**, 593
*Detrol*—Pharmacia & Upjohn (U.S.) brand of Tolterodine (Systemic)
*De-Tuss*—H. L. Moore (U.S.) brand of Pseudoephedrine and Hydrocodone—**See Cough/Cold Combinations (Systemic)**, 1024
*Detussin Expectorant*—Barre-National (U.S.); Major (U.S.); Qualitest (U.S.) and Schein (U.S.) brand of Pseudoephedrine, Hydrocodone, and Guaifenesin—**See Cough/Cold Combinations (Systemic)**, 1024
*Detussin Liquid*—Barre-National (U.S.); Major (U.S.) and Qualitest (U.S.) brand of Pseudoephedrine and Hydrocodone—**See Cough/Cold Combinations (Systemic)**, 1024
*Dexacen-4*—Central (U.S.) brand of Dexamethasone—**See Corticosteroids—Glucocorticoid Effects (Systemic)**, 998
*Dexacen LA-8*—Central (U.S.) brand of Dexamethasone—**See Corticosteroids—Glucocorticoid Effects (Systemic)**, 998
*Dexacort Turbinaire*—Adams (U.S.) brand of Dexamethasone (Nasal), 3016

*Dexafed Cough*—Roberts (U.S.) brand of Phenylephrine, Dextromethorphan, and Guaifenesin—**See Cough/Cold Combinations (Systemic)**, 1024
*Dexair*—Pharmafair (U.S.) brand of Dexamethasone—**See Corticosteroids (Ophthalmic)**, 966
Dexamethasone [*Maxidex*]
  **See Corticosteroids (Ophthalmic)**, 966
  Ointment, Ophthalmic, 968
  Suspension, Ophthalmic, USP, 969
Dexamethasone [*Aeroseb-Dex; Decaderm; Decaspray*]
  **See Corticosteroids (Topical)**, 978
  Aerosol, Topical, USP (Solution), 987
  Gel USP, 987
Dexamethasone [*Decadron; Deronil; Dexamethasone Intensol; Dexasone; Dexone 0.5; Dexone 0.75; Dexone 1.5; Dexone 4; Hexadrol; Mymethasone; Oradexon*]
  **See Corticosteroids—Glucocorticoid Effects (Systemic)**, 998
  Elixir USP, 1007
  Solution, Oral, 1007
  Tablets USP, 1008, MC-8
Dexamethasone Acetate [*Dalalone D.P.; Dalalone L.A.; Decadron-LA; Decaject-L.A.; Dexacen LA-8; Dexasone-LA; Dexone LA; Solurex-LA*]
  **See Corticosteroids—Glucocorticoid Effects (Systemic)**, 998
  Suspension, Sterile, USP, 1008
Dexamethasone-containing Combinations, 3071
*Dexamethasone Intensol*—Roxane (U.S.) brand of Dexamethasone—**See Corticosteroids—Glucocorticoid Effects (Systemic)**, 998
Dexamethasone Sodium Phosphate [*Decadron Respihaler*]
  **See Corticosteroids (Inhalation-Local)**, 955
  Aerosol, Inhalation, USP, 960
Dexamethasone Sodium Phosphate [*Decadron Turbinaire; Dexacort Turbinaire*]
  **See Corticosteroids (Nasal)**, 961, 3016
  Aerosol, Nasal, 965, 3016
Dexamethasone Sodium Phosphate [*AK-Dex; Baldex; Decadron; Dexair; Dexotic; Diodex; Maxidex; Ocu-Dex; PMS-Dexamethasone Sodium Phosphate; R.O.-Dexasone; Spersadex; Storz-Dexa*]
  **See Corticosteroids (Ophthalmic)**, 966
  Ointment, Ophthalmic, USP, 969
  Solution, Ophthalmic, USP, 969
Dexamethasone Sodium Phosphate [*AK-Dex; Decadron; I-Methasone*]
  **See Corticosteroids (Otic)**, 971
  Solution, Ophthalmic, USP (Otic use), 973
Dexamethasone Sodium Phosphate [*Decadron*]
  **See Corticosteroids (Topical)**, 978
  Cream USP, 988
Dexamethasone Sodium Phosphate [*AK-Dex; Dalalone; Decadrol; Decadron; Decadron Phosphate; Decaject; Dexacen-4; Dexone; Hexadrol Phosphate; Solurex*]
  **See Corticosteroids—Glucocorticoid Effects (Systemic)**, 998
  Injection USP, 1008
*Dexamfetamine—Dextroamphetamine*—**See Amphetamines (Systemic)**, 94
*Dexaphen SA*—Major (U.S.) brand of Dexbrompheniramine and Pseudoephedrine—**See Antihistamines and Decongestants (Systemic)**, 343
*Dexasone*—Hauck (U.S.); Legere (U.S.); and ICN (Canada) brand of Dexamethasone—**See Corticosteroids—Glucocorticoid Effects (Systemic)**, 998
*Dexasone-LA*—Hauck (U.S.) and Legere (U.S.) brand of Dexamethasone—**See Corticosteroids—Glucocorticoid Effects (Systemic)**, 998
*Dexatrim Maximum Strength Caplets*—Thompson (U.S.) brand of Phenylpropanolamine (Systemic), 2314
*Dexatrim Maximum Strength Capsules*—Thompson (U.S.) brand of Phenylpropanolamine (Systemic), 2314
*Dexatrim Maximum Strength Tablets*—Thompson (U.S.) brand of Phenylpropanolamine (Systemic), 2314
Dexbrompheniramine-containing Combinations, 3071
Dexbrompheniramine Maleate and Pseudoephedrine Hydrochloride [*Alcomed 2-60*]
  **See Antihistamines and Decongestants (Systemic)**, 343
  Tablets, 344

*USP DI*                                                                **General Index**    **3273**

Dexbrompheniramine Maleate and Pseudoephedrine Sulfate [*Brompheril; Dexaphen SA; Dexophed; Disobrom; Disophrol Chronotabs; Drixomed; Drixoral; Drixoral Cold and Allergy; Drixoral Night; Drixtab*]
  **See Antihistamines and Decongestants (Systemic)**, 343
  Tablets, 352
  Tablets, Extended-release, 347, 351, 352
Dexbrompheniramine Maleate, Pseudoephedrine Sulfate, and Acetaminophen [*Drixoral Allergy-Sinus; Drixoral Cold and Flu*]
  **See Antihistamines, Decongestants, and Analgesics (Systemic)**, 366
  Tablets, Extended-release, 370
*Dexchlor*—Schein (U.S.) brand of Dexchlorpheniramine—**See Antihistamines (Systemic)**, 325
Dexchlorpheniramine-containing Combinations, 3071
Dexchlorpheniramine Maleate [*Dexchlor; Polaramine; Polaramine Repetabs*]
  **See Antihistamines (Systemic)**, 325
  Syrup USP, 336
  Tablets USP, 336
  Tablets, Extended-release, 336
Dexchlorpheniramine Maleate, Pseudoephedrine Sulfate, and Guaifenesin [*Polaramine Expectorant*]
  **See Cough/Cold Combinations (Systemic)**, 1024
  Solution, Oral, 1082
*Dexedrine*—SKF (U.S. and Canada) brand of Dextroamphetamine—**See Amphetamines (Systemic)**, 94
*Dexedrine Spansule*—SKF (U.S. and Canada) brand of Dextroamphetamine—**See Amphetamines (Systemic)**, 94
*DexFerrum*—American Reagent (U.S.) brand of Iron Dextran—**See Iron Supplements (Systemic)**, 1774
*DexIron*—American Reagent (U.S.) brand of Iron Dextran—**See Iron Supplements (Systemic)**, 1774
*Dexitac*—Republic (U.S.) brand of Caffeine (Systemic), 706
*Dexone*—Keene (U.S.) and Solvay (U.S.) brand of Dexamethasone—**See Corticosteroids—Glucocorticoid Effects (Systemic)**, 998
*Dexone 0.5*—Keene (U.S.) and Solvay (U.S.) brand of Dexamethasone—**See Corticosteroids—Glucocorticoid Effects (Systemic)**, 998
*Dexone 0.75*—Keene (U.S.) and Solvay (U.S.) brand of Dexamethasone—**See Corticosteroids—Glucocorticoid Effects (Systemic)**, 998
*Dexone 1.5*—Keene (U.S.) and Solvay (U.S.) brand of Dexamethasone—**See Corticosteroids—Glucocorticoid Effects (Systemic)**, 998
*Dexone 4*—Keene (U.S.) and Solvay (U.S.) brand of Dexamethasone—**See Corticosteroids—Glucocorticoid Effects (Systemic)**, 998
*Dexone LA*—Keene (U.S.) and Solvay (U.S.) brand of Dexamethasone—**See Corticosteroids—Glucocorticoid Effects (Systemic)**, 998
*Dexophed*—Dixon-Shane and Zenith Goldline (U.S.) brand of Dexbrompheniramine and Pseudoephedrine—**See Antihistamines and Decongestants (Systemic)**, 343
*Dexotic*—Parnell (U.S.) brand of Dexamethasone—**See Corticosteroids (Ophthalmic)**, 966
Dexrazoxane [*Zinecard*]
  **(Systemic)**, 1190, 3140
  for Injection, 1191
Dextran and Deferoxamine [*Bio-Rescue*]
  **(Systemic)**, 3140
Dextran Sulfate [*Uendex*]
  **(Inhalation)**, 3140
  Inhalation, Aerosol, 3140
Dextran Sulfate Sodium
  **(Systemic)**, 3140
Dextroamphetamine Sulfate [dexamfetamine; *Dexedrine; Dexedrine Spansule; DextroStat*]
  **See Amphetamines (Systemic)**, 94
  Capsules, Extended-release, 97
  Tablets USP, 97
Dextromethorphan-containing Combinations, 3071
Dextromethorphan Hydrobromide [*Balminil D.M.; Benylin Adult; Benylin Pediatric; Broncho-Grippol-DM; Calmylin #1; Children's Hold; Cough-X; Creo-Terpin; DM Syrup; Drixoral Cough Liquid Caps; Hold; Koffex; Mediquell; Neo-DM; Ornex • DM 15; Ornex • DM 30; Pertussin Cough Suppressant; Pertussin CS; Pertussin ES; Robidex; Robitussin Cough Calmers; Robitussin Maximum Strength Cough Suppressant; Robitussin Pediatric; Sedatuss; St. Joseph Cough Suppressant*

Dextromethophan Hydrobromide (continued)
  *for Children; Sucrets Cough Control Formula; Trocal; Vicks Formula 44 Pediatric Formula*]
  **(Systemic)**, 1191
  Capsules, 1192
  Lozenges, 1192
  Syrup USP, 1193
  Tablets, Chewable, 1193
Dextromethorphan Hydrobromide and Acetaminophen [*Drixoral Cough & Sore Throat Liquid Caps; Tylenol Cough Extra Strength Caplets; Tylenol Cough Medication Regular Strength; Tylenol Multi-Symptom Cough*]
  **See Cough/Cold Combinations (Systemic)**, 1024
  Capsules, 1055
  Solution, Oral, 1111
  Suspension, Oral, 1110
  Tablets, 1110
Dextromethorphan Hydrobromide and Guaifenesin [*Anti-Tuss DM Expectorant; Benylin DM-E; Benylin DM-E Extra Strength; Benylin Expectorant; Calmylin DM-E; Cheracol D Cough; Children's Formula Cough; Diabetic Tussin DM; Extra Action Cough; Fenesin DM; Genatuss DM; Glycotuss-dM; Guiamid D.M. Liquid; Guiatuss-DM; Guiatussin with Dextromethorphan; Halotussin-DM; Humibid DM; Humibid DM Pediatric; Iobid DM; Kolephrin GG/DM; Muco-Fen DM; Mytussin DM; Naldecon Senior DX; Pharmasave DM+ Expectorant; Respa-DM; Rhinosyn-DMX Expectorant; Robafen DM; Robitussin-DM; Safe Tussin30; Scot-Tussin Senior Clear; Silexin Cough; Siltussin DM; Stamoist E; Suppressin DM; Suppressin DM Caplets; Syracol CF; Tanta Cough Syrup; Tolu-Sed DM; Touro DM; Tuss-DM; Tussi-Organidin DM NR Liquid; Tussi-Organidin DM-S NR Liquid; Uni-tussin DM; Unproco; Vicks 44E Cough & Chest Congestion; Vicks Formula 44E; Vicks Formula 44e Pediatric; Vicks Pediatric 44E*]
  **See Cough/Cold Combinations (Systemic)**, 1024, 3017
  Capsules, 1111
  Capsules, Extended-release, 1064
  Solution, Oral, 1035, 1036, 1042, 1052, 1062, 1063, 1068, 1071, 1072, 1088, 1092, 1098, 1106, 1107, 1113, 1115
  Syrup, 1036, 1040, 1042, 1058, 1059, 1062, 1079, 1080, 1086, 1087, 1088, 1093, 1094, 1100, 1111, 1113, 1114
  Tablets, 1059, 1098, 1106
  Tablets, Extended-release, 1059, 1063, 1067, 1070, 1086, 3017
Dextromethorphan Hydrobromide and Iodinated Glycerol [*Iophen DM; Tusso-DM*]
  **See Cough/Cold Combinations (Systemic)**, 1024
  Solution, Oral, 1067, 1108
Dextromethorphan Polistirex [*Delsym*]
  **(Systemic)**, 1191
  Suspension, Oral, Extended-release, 1193
Dextropropoxyphene—Propoxyphene—**See Opioid (Narcotic) Analgesics (Systemic)**, 2168
Dextrose and Electrolytes [*Kao Lectrolyte; Lytren; Naturalyte; Oralyte; Pedialyte; Pedialyte Freezer Pops; Rehydralyte; Resol*]
  **See Carbohydrates and Electrolytes (Systemic)**, 769
  Solution, 771
*DextroStat*—Richwood (U.S.) brand of Dextroamphetamine—**See Amphetamines (Systemic)**, 94
Dextrothyroxine Sodium
  **(Systemic)**, #
  Tablets USP, #
*Dey-Lute Isoetharine*—Dey (U.S.) brand of Isoetharine—**See Bronchodilators, Adrenergic (Inhalation-Local)**, 640
*Dey-Lute Metaproterenol*—Dey (U.S.) brand of Metaproterenol—**See Bronchodilators, Adrenergic (Inhalation-Local)**, 640
Dezocine [*Dalgan*]
  **(Systemic)**, 1193
  Injection, 1197
DFMO—See Eflornithine (Systemic), #
DFP—Isoflurophate—**See Antiglaucoma Agents, Cholinergic, Long-acting (Ophthalmic)**, 315
*DHCplus*—Purdue Frederick (U.S.) brand of Dihydrocodeine and Acetaminophen—**See Opioid (Narcotic) Analgesics and Acetaminophen (Systemic)**, 2198

*D.H.E. 45*—Sandoz (U.S.) brand of Dihydroergotamine—**See Vascular Headache Suppressants, Ergot Derivative–containing (Systemic)**, 2925
DHPG—*See Ganciclovir (Systemic)*, 1544
*DHS Tar Gel Shampoo*—Person & Covey (U.S.) brand of Coal Tar (Topical), #
*DHS Tar Shampoo*—Person & Covey (U.S.) brand of Coal Tar (Topical), #
*DHS Zinc Dandruff Shampoo*—Person & Covey (U.S.) brand of Pyrithione (Topical), #
*DHT*—Roxane (U.S.) brand of Dihydrotachysterol—**See Vitamin D and Analogs (Systemic)**, 2966
*DHT Intensol*—Roxane (U.S.) brand of Dihydrotachysterol—**See Vitamin D and Analogs (Systemic)**, 2966
*DiaBeta*—Hoechst Marion Roussel (U.S.) and Hoechst (Canada) brand of Glyburide—**See Antidiabetic Agents, Sulfonylurea (Systemic)**, 283, MC-14
*Diabetic Tussin DM*—Health Care (U.S.) brand of Dextromethorphan and Guaifenesin—**See Cough/Cold Combinations (Systemic)**, 1024
*Diabetic Tussin EX*—Health Care Products (U.S.) brand of Guaifenesin (Systemic), 1588
*DiabetiSource*—Sandoz (U.S.) brand of Enteral Nutrition Formula, Disease-specific—**See Enteral Nutrition Formulas (Systemic)**, #
*Diabinese*—Pfizer (U.S. and Canada) brand of Chlorpropamide—**See Antidiabetic Agents, Sulfonylurea (Systemic)**, 283
*Dialose*—J & J-Merck (U.S.) brand of Docusate—**See Laxatives (Local)**, #
*Dialose Plus*—J & J-Merck (U.S.) brand of Phenolphthalein and Docusate—**See Laxatives (Local)**, #
*Diamicron*—Servier (Canada) brand of Gliclazide—**See Antidiabetic Agents, Sulfonylurea (Systemic)**, 283
3,4-Diaminopyridine
  **(Systemic)**, 3127
*Diamox*—Lederle (U.S. and Canada) brand of Acetazolamide—**See Carbonic Anhydrase Inhibitors (Systemic)**, 773
*Diamox Sequels*—Lederle (U.S. and Canada) brand of Acetazolamide—**See Carbonic Anhydrase Inhibitors (Systemic)**, 773
Dianeal PD-2 Peritoneal Dialysis Solution with Amino Acids [*Nutrineal PD-2 Peritoneal Dialysis Solution with 1.1% Amino Acid*]
  **(Systemic)**, 3140
*Diaper Rash Ointment*—Pharmavite (Canada) brand of Calamine (Topical), #
*Diapid*—Sandoz (U.S.) brand of Lypressin (Systemic), 1893
*Diar-Aid*—Thompson (U.S.) brand of Attapulgite (Oral-Local), #
*Diarrest*—Otis Clapp (U.S.) brand of Attapulgite (Oral-Local), #
*Diarr-Eze*—Pharmascience (Canada) brand of Loperamide (Oral-Local), 1877
*Diasorb*—Columbia (U.S.) brand of Attapulgite (Oral-Local), #
*Diastat*—Athena (U.S.) brand of Diazepam—**See Benzodiazepines (Systemic)**, 556, MC-8
*Diastix*—Miles (U.S. and Canada) brand of Glucose Oxidase Urine Glucose Test—**See Urine Glucose and Ketone Test Kits for Home Use**, #
Diatrizoate-containing Combinations, 3072
Diatrizoate Meglumine [*Cystografin; Cystografin Dilute; Hypaque-Cysto; Hypaque-M 18%; Hypaque-M 30%; Hypaque-M 60%; Reno-M-30; Urovist Cysto; Urovist Cysto Pediatric*]
  **See Diatrizoates (Local)**, #
  Injection USP, #
Diatrizoate Meglumine [*Angiovist 282; Hypaque-M 18%; Hypaque-M 30%; Hypaque-M 60%; Hypaque Meglumine 30%; Hypaque Meglumine 60%; Reno-Dip; Reno-M-60; Urovist Meglumine DIU/CT*]
  **See Diatrizoates (Systemic)**, #
  Injection USP, #
Diatrizoate Meglumine and Diatrizoate Sodium [*Angiovist 292; Angiovist 370; Gastrografin; Hypaque-76; Hypaque-M 75%; Hypaque-M 76%; MD-76; MD-Gastroview; Renografin-60; Renografin-76; Renovist; Renovist II*]
  **See Diatrizoates (Systemic)**, #
  Injection USP, #
  Solution USP, #

## 3274 General Index

Diatrizoate Meglumine and Iodipamide Meglumine [*Sinografin*]
  **(Local)**, #
  Injection, #
Diatrizoates
  **(Local)**, #
Diatrizoates
  **(Systemic)**, #
Diatrizoate Sodium [*Hypaque Sodium 20%; Hypaque Sodium 50%;* sodium amidotrizoate; *Urovist Sodium 300*]
  **See Diatrizoates (Local)**, #
  Injection USP, #
Diatrizoate Sodium [*Hypaque Oral; Hypaque Sodium 25%; Hypaque Sodium 50%; Hypaque Sodium Oral Powder; Hypaque Sodium Oral Solution;* sodium amidotrizoate; *Urovist Sodium 300*]
  **See Diatrizoates (Systemic)**, #
  Injection USP, #
  Solution USP, #
  USP (for Solution), #
*Diatrol*—Otis Clapp (U.S.) brand of Attapulgite (Oral-Local), #
*Diazemuls*—Pharmacia (Canada) brand of Diazepam—**See Benzodiazepines (Systemic)**, 556
Diazepam [*Apo-Diazepam; Diastat; Diazemuls; Diazepam Intensol; Dizac; Novo-Dipam; PMS-Diazepam; Valium; Vivol*]
  **See Benzodiazepines (Systemic)**, 556, 3140
  Emulsion, Sterile, 571
  Gel, Rectal, 572
  Injection USP, 570
  Solution, Oral, 569
  for Solution, Rectal, 571
  Tablets USP, 570, MC-8, MC-9
  Viscous Solution, Rectal, 3140
*Diazepam Intensol*—Roxane (U.S.) brand of Diazepam—**See Benzodiazepines (Systemic)**, 556
Diazoxide [*Proglycem*]
  **(Oral-Systemic)**, 1197
  Capsules USP, 1199
  Suspension, Oral, USP, 1200
Diazoxide [*Hyperstat*]
  **(Parenteral-Systemic)**, 1200
  Injection USP, 1202
*Dibent*—Hauck (U.S.) brand of Dicyclomine—**See Anticholinergics/Antispasmodics (Systemic)**, 226
*Dibenzyline*—SKF (U.S.) brand of Phenoxybenzamine (Systemic), 2312
Dibromodulcitol
  **(Systemic)**, 3140
Dibucaine [cinchocaine; *Nupercainal*]
  **See Anesthetics (Mucosal-Local)**, 128
  Ointment USP, 135
Dibucaine [cinchocaine; *Nupercainal Cream; Nupercainal Ointment*]
  **See Anesthetics (Topical)**, 155
  Cream USP, 159
  Ointment USP, 159
*Dicarbosil*—BIRA (U.S.) brand of Calcium Carbonate—**See Antacids (Oral-Local)**, 188; Norcliff Thayer (U.S.) brand of Calcium Carbonate—**See Calcium Supplements (Systemic)**, 736
Dichloralphenazone-containing Combinations, 3072
Dichlorphenamide [*Daranide;* diclofenamide]
  **See Carbonic Anhydrase Inhibitors (Systemic)**, 773
  Tablets USP, 778
Diclofenac and Misoprostol [*Arthrotec*]
  **(Systemic)**, 1202
  Tablets, 1205, MC-9
Diclofenac Potassium [*Cataflam; Voltaren Rapide*]
  **See Anti-inflammatory Drugs, Nonsteroidal (Systemic)**, 388
  Tablets, 403
Diclofenac Sodium [*Apo-Diclo; Novo-Difenac; Novo-Difenac SR; Nu-Diclo; Voltaren; Voltaren SR*]
  **See Anti-inflammatory Drugs, Nonsteroidal (Systemic)**, 388
  Suppositories, 404
  Tablets, Delayed-release, 404, MC-9
  Tablets, Extended-release, 404, MC-9
Diclofenac Sodium [*Voltaren Ophtha; Voltaren Ophthalmic*]
  **See Anti-inflammatory Drugs, Nonsteroidal (Ophthalmic)**, 383
  Solution, Ophthalmic, 386
Diclofenamide—Dichlorphenamide—**See Carbonic Anhydrase Inhibitors (Systemic)**, 773

Dicloxacillin Sodium [*Dycill; Dynapen; Pathocil*]
  **See Penicillins (Systemic)**, 2240
  Capsules USP, 2251
  for Suspension, Oral, USP, 2251
*Dicopac*—Medi-Physics (U.S.) brand of Cyanocobalamin Co 57 (Systemic), 1123
Dicoumarol—Dicumarol—**See Anticoagulants (Systemic)**, 243
Dicumarol [dicoumarol]
  **See Anticoagulants (Systemic)**, 243
  Tablets USP, 248
Dicyclomine Hydrochloride [*Antispas; A-Spas; Bentyl; Bentylol;* dicycloverine; *Dibent; Di-Spaz; Formulex; Lomine; Neoquess; Or-Tyl; Spasmoban; Spasmoject*]
  **See Anticholinergics/Antispasmodics (Systemic)**, 226
  Capsules USP, 234, MC-9
  Injection USP, 235
  Syrup USP, 234
  Tablets USP, 234, MC-9
  Tablets, Extended-release, 235
Dicycloverine—Dicyclomine—**See Anticholinergics/Antispasmodics (Systemic)**, 226
Didanosine [ddI; 2,3-dideoxyinosine; *Videx*]
  **(Systemic)**, 1206
  for Solution, Oral, Buffered, 1209
  for Suspension, Oral, Buffered, 1209
  Tablets, 1210, MC-9
2,3-dideoxyinosine—*See* Didanosine (Systemic), 1206
*Didrex*—Pharmacia & Upjohn (U.S.) brand of Benzphetamine—**See Appetite Suppressants (Systemic)**, 452, MC-3
*Didronel*—MGI (U.S.) brand of Etidronate (Systemic), 3142; Procter & Gamble (U.S. and Canada) brand of Etidronate (Systemic), 1419, MC-12
Dienestrol [*Ortho Dienestrol*]
  **See Estrogens (Vaginal)**, 1391
  Cream USP, 1395
*Diet-Aid Maximum Strength*—O'Connor (U.S.) brand of Phenylpropanolamine (Systemic), 2314
Diethylamine Salicylate [*Algesal*]
  **(Topical)**, 3017
  Cream, 3017
Diethylcarbamazine Citrate [*Hetrazan*]
  **(Systemic)**, #
  Tablets USP, #
Diethyldithiocarbamate [*Imuthiol*]
  **(Systemic)**, 3140
Diethylpropion Hydrochloride [amfepramone; *Tenuate; Tenuate Dospan; Tepanil Ten-Tab*]
  **See Appetite Suppressants (Systemic)**, 452
  Tablets USP, 455 MC-9
  Tablets, Extended-release, 455 MC-9
Diethylstilbestrol [DES; *Stilbestrol* §ilboestrolcb
  **See Estrogens (Systemic)**, 1383
  Tablets USP, 1388
Diethylstilbestrol-containing Combinations, 3072
Diethylstilbestrol Diphosphate [DES; fosfestrol; *Honvol; Stilphostrol* cb
  **See Estrogens (Systemic)**, 1383
  Injection USP, 1388
  Tablets, 1388
Diethylstilbestrol and Methyltestosterone [*Tylosterone*]
  **See Androgens and Estrogens (Systemic)**, 126
  Tablets, 127
Diethyltoluamide [*Backwoods Cutter; Cutter Pleasant Protection; Deep Woods OFF; Deep Woods OFF For Sportsmen;* DEET; m-DET; *Muskol; OFF; OFF For Maximum Protection; OFF Skintastic; OFF Skintastic For Children; OFF Skintastic For Kids; Ultra Muskol*]
  **(Topical)**, #
  Aerosol, Topical, #
  Liquid, #
  Lotion, #
  Solution, Topical Spray, #
  Towelettes, #
Difenidol—*See* Diphenidol (Systemic), 1232
Difenoxin-containing Combinations, 3072
Difenoxin Hydrochloride and Atropine Sulfate [*Motofen*]
  **(Systemic)**, 1210
  Tablets, 1213
*Differin*—Galderma (U.S. and Canada) brand of Adapalene (Topical), 30

Diflorasone Diacetate [*Florone; Florone E; Maxiflor; Psorcon*]
  **See Corticosteroids (Topical)**, 978, 3017
  Cream USP, 988, 3017
  Ointment USP, 988
*Diflucan 150*—Roerig (Canada) brand of Fluconazole—**See Antifungals, Azole (Systemic)**, 302
*Diflucan*—Pfizer (U.S. and Canada) brand of Fluconazole—**See Antifungals, Azole (Systemic)**, 302, MC-13
Diflucortolone Valerate [*Nerisone; Nerisone Oily*]
  **See Corticosteroids (Topical)**, 978
  Cream, 988
  Ointment, 988
Diflunisal [*Apo-Diflunisal; Dolobid; Novo-Diflunisal*]
  **See Anti-inflammatory Drugs, Nonsteroidal (Systemic)**, 388
  Tablets USP, 405, MC-9
Difluorophate—Isoflurophate—**See Antiglaucoma Agents, Cholinergic, Long-acting (Ophthalmic)**, 315
*Di-Gel*—Schering Plough (U.S.) brand of Alumina, Magnesia, and Simethicone—**See Antacids (Oral-Local)**, 188
*Digibind*—BW (U.S. and Canada) brand of Digoxin Immune Fab (Ovine) (Systemic), 1219; 3140
*Digidote*—Boehringer Mannheim (U.S.) brand of Digoxin Immune Fab (Ovine) (Systemic), 3140
*Digitaline*—Welcker-Lyster (Canada) brand of Digitoxin—**See Digitalis Glycosides (Systemic)**, 1213
Digitalis Glycosides
  **(Systemic)**, 1213
Digitoxin [*Crystodigin; Digitaline*]
  **See Digitalis Glycosides (Systemic)**, 1213
  Tablets USP, 1217
*DigiWipe*—Access (U.S.) brand of Fecal Occult Blood Test Kits, #
Digoxin [*Lanoxicaps; Lanoxin; Novodigoxin*]
  **See Digitalis Glycosides (Systemic)**, 1213
  Capsules, 1217, MC-9
  Elixir USP, 1218
  Injection USP, 1219
  Tabets USP, 1218, MC-9
Digoxin Immune Fab (Ovine) [*Digibind; Digidote*]
  **(Systemic)**, 1219, 3140
  for Injection, 1220
*Dihistine DH*—Barre-National (U.S.); Major (U.S.); Moore (U.S.) and Zenith Goldline (U.S.) brand of Chlorpheniramine, Pseudoephedrine, and Codeine—**See Cough/Cold Combinations (Systemic)**, 1024
*Dihistine Expectorant*—Barre-National (U.S.); Major (U.S.); Moore (U.S.) and Zenith Goldline (U.S.) brand of Pseudoephedrine, Codeine, and Guaifenesin—**See Cough/Cold Combinations (Systemic)**, 1024
5,6-Dihydro-5-Azacytidine
  **(Systemic)**, 3128
Dihydrocodeine Bitartrate, Acetaminophen, and Caffeine [*DHCplus;* drocode and acetaminophen]
  **See Opioid (Narcotic) Analgesics and Acetaminophen (Systemic)**, 2198
  Capsules, 2200
Dihydrocodeine compound—Aspirin and Dihydrocodeine—**See Opioid (Narcotic) Analgesics and Aspirin (Systemic)**, 2202
Dihydrocodeine-containing Combinations, 3072
Dihydroergotamine Mesylate [*D.H.E. 45; Dihydroergotamine-Sandoz*]
  **See Vascular Headache Suppressants, Ergot Derivative–containing (Systemic)**, 2925
  Injection USP, 2932
Dihydroergotamine Mesylate [*Migranal*]
  **(Nasal-Systemic)**, 1221
  Solution, Nasal, USP, 1223
*Dihydroergotamine-Sandoz*—Sandoz (Canada) brand of Dihydroergotamine—**See Vascular Headache Suppressants, Ergot Derivative–containing (Systemic)**, 2925
Dihydromorphinone—Hydromorphone—**See Opioid (Narcotic) Analgesics (Systemic)**, 2168
Dihydrotachysterol [*DHT; DHT Intensol; Hytakerol;* vitamin D]
  **See Vitamin D and Analogs (Systemic)**, 2966
  Capsules USP, 2971
  Solution, Oral, USP, 2971
  Tablets USP, 2971
Dihydrotestosterone [*Androgel-DHT*]
  **(Systemic)**, 3140
24,25 Dihydroxycholecalciferol
  **(Systemic)**, 3127

*Diiodohydroxyquin*—*See* Iodoquinol (Oral-Local), #
*Diiodohydroxyquinoline*—*See* Iodoquinol (Oral-Local), #
*Dilacor XR*—Rhône-Poulenc Rorer (U.S.) brand of Diltiazem
*Dilacor-XR*—Rhône-Poulenc Rorer (U.S.) brand of Diltiazem—**See Calcium Channel Blocking Agents (Systemic)**, 720
*Dilantin*—PD (U.S. and Canada) brand of Phenytoin—**See Anticonvulsants, Hydantoin (Systemic)**, 253
*Dilantin-30*—PD (Canada) brand of Phenytoin—**See Anticonvulsants, Hydantoin (Systemic)**, 253
*Dilantin-125*—PD (U.S. and Canada) brand of Phenytoin—**See Anticonvulsants, Hydantoin (Systemic)**, 253
*Dilantin Infatabs*—PD (U.S. and Canada) brand of Phenytoin—**See Anticonvulsants, Hydantoin (Systemic)**, 253, MC-25
*Dilantin Kapseals*—PD (U.S.) brand of Phenytoin—**See Anticonvulsants, Hydantoin (Systemic)**, 253, MC-25
*Dilatair*—Pharmafair (U.S.) and Texas Drug (U.S.) brand of Phenylephrine (Ophthalmic), #
*Dilatrate-SR*—Schwarz (U.S.) brand of Isosorbide Dinitrate—**See Nitrates (Systemic)**, 2129, MC-16
*Dilaudid*—Knoll (U.S. and Canada) brand of Hydromorphone—**See Opioid (Narcotic) Analgesics (Systemic)**, 2168, MC-15
*Dilaudid-5*—Knoll (U.S.) brand of Hydromorphone—**See Opioid (Narcotic) Analgesics (Systemic)**, 2168
*Dilaudid Cough*—Knoll (U.S.) brand of Hydromorphone and Guaifenesin—**See Cough/Cold Combinations (Systemic)**, 1024
*Dilaudid-HP*—Knoll (U.S. and Canada) brand of Hydromorphone—**See Opioid (Narcotic) Analgesics (Systemic)**, 2168
*Dilocaine*—Hauck (U.S.) brand of Lidocaine—**See Anesthetics (Parenteral-Local)**, 139
*Dilor*—Savage (U.S.) brand of Dyphylline (Systemic), #
*Dilor-400*—Savage (U.S.) brand of Dyphylline (Systemic), #
*Dilotab*—Zee Medical (Canada) brand of Phenylpropanolamine and Acetaminophen—**See Decongestants and Analgesics (Systemic)**, 1180
Diloxanide Furoate [*Entamide; Furamide*] **(Systemic)**, #
Tablets, #
Diltiazem Hydrochloride [*Apo-Diltiaz; Cardizem; Cardizem CD; Cardizem SR; Dilacor-XR; Novo-Diltazem; Nu-Diltiaz; Syn-Diltiazem; Tiazac*]
**See Calcium Channel Blocking Agents (Systemic)**, 720, 3017
Capsules, Extended-release, 728, 3017, MC-9
Injection, 728
Tablets USP, 728, MC-9
*Dimacol Caplets*—Whitehall-Robins (U.S.) brand of Pseudoephedrine, Dextromethorphan, and Guaifenesin—**See Cough/Cold Combinations (Systemic)**, 1024
*Dimaphen*—Major (U.S.) brand of Brompheniramine and Phenylpropanolamine—**See Antihistamines and Decongestants (Systemic)**, 343
*Dimaphen S.A.*—Major (U.S.) brand of Brompheniramine and Phenylpropanolamine—**See Antihistamines and Decongestants (Systemic)**, 343
*Dimelor*—Lilly (Canada) brand of Acetohexamide—**See Antidiabetic Agents, Sulfonylurea (Systemic)**, 283
Dimenhydrinate [*Apo-Dimenhydrinate; Calm X; Dinate; Dramamine; Dramanate; Gravol; Gravol I/M; Gravol I/V; Gravol L/A; Gravol Liquid; Gravol Filmkote; Gravol Filmkote (Junior Strength); Hydrate; PMS-Dimenhydrinate; Traveltabs; Triptone Caplets*]
**See Antihistamines (Systemic)**, 325
Capsules, Extended-release, 336
Injection USP, 337
Solution, Oral, 337
Suppositories, 338
Syrup USP, 337
Tablets USP, 337
Tablets USP (Chewable), 337
Dimenhydrinate-containing Combinations, 3072
Dimercaprol [*BAL in Oil*; British Anti-Lewisite; dimercaptopropanol]
**(Systemic)**, 1224
Injection USP, 1226
*Dimercaptopropanol*—*See* Dimercaprol (Systemic), 1224

*Dimercaptosuccinic acid*—*See* Succimer (Systemic), #
*Dimetane*—Robins (Canada) brand of Brompheniramine—**See Antihistamines (Systemic)**, 325
*Dimetane-DC Cough*—Robins (U.S.) brand of Brompheniramine, Phenylpropanolamine, and Codeine—**See Cough/Cold Combinations (Systemic)**, 1024
*Dimetane Decongestant*—Robins (U.S.) brand of Brompheniramine and Phenylephrine—**See Antihistamines and Decongestants (Systemic)**, 343
*Dimetane Decongestant Caplets*—Robins (U.S.) brand of Brompheniramine and Phenylephrine—**See Antihistamines and Decongestants (Systemic)**, 343
*Dimetane-DX Cough*—Robins (U.S.) brand of Brompheniramine, Pseudoephedrine, and Dextromethorphan—**See Cough/Cold Combinations (Systemic)**, 1024
*Dimetane Expectorant*—Whitehall-Robins (Canada) brand of Brompheniramine, Phenylephrine, Phenylpropanolamine, and Guaifenesin—**See Cough/Cold Combinations (Systemic)**, 1024
*Dimetane Expectorant-C*—Whitehall-Robins (Canada) brand of Brompheniramine, Phenylephrine, Phenylpropanolamine, Codeine, and Guaifenesin—**See Cough/Cold Combinations (Systemic)**, 1024
*Dimetane Expectorant-DC*—Whitehall-Robins (Canada) brand of Brompheniramine, Phenylephrine, Phenylpropanolamine, Hydrocodone, and Guaifenesin—**See Cough/Cold Combinations (Systemic)**, 1024
*Dimetapp*—Robins (U.S.) brand of Brompheniramine and Phenylpropanolamine—**See Antihistamines and Decongestants (Systemic)**, 343; Whitehall-Robins (Canada) brand of Brompheniramine, Phenylephrine, and Phenylpropanolamine—**See Antihistamines and Decongestants (Systemic)**, 343
*Dimetapp Allergy Liqui-Gels*—Whitehall (U.S.) brand of Brompheniramine—**See Antihistamines (Systemic)**, 325
*Dimetapp Allergy Sinus Caplets*—Whitehall-Robins (U.S.) brand of Brompheniramine, Phenylpropanolamine, and Acetaminophen—**See Antihistamines, Decongestants, and Analgesics (Systemic)**, 366
*Dimetapp-A Sinus*—Whitehall-Robins (Canada) brand of Phenylephrine, Phenylpropanolamine, and Acetaminophen—**See Decongestants and Analgesics (Systemic)**, 1180
*Dimetapp-C*—Whitehall-Robins (Canada) brand of Brompheniramine, Phenylephrine, Phenylpropanolamine, and Codeine—**See Cough/Cold Combinations (Systemic)**, 1024
*Dimetapp Chewables*—Whitehall-Robins (Canada) brand of Brompheniramine and Phenylpropanolamine—**See Antihistamines and Decongestants (Systemic)**, 343
*Dimetapp Clear*—Whitehall-Robins (Canada) brand of Brompheniramine and Phenylpropanolamine—**See Antihistamines and Decongestants (Systemic)**, 343
*Dimetapp Cold and Allergy*—Robins (U.S.) brand of Brompheniramine and Phenylpropanolamine—**See Antihistamines and Decongestants (Systemic)**, 343
*Dimetapp Cold & Allergy Quick Dissolve*—Robins (U.S.) brand of Brompheniramine and Phenylpropanolamine—**See Antihistamines and Decongestants (Systemic)**, 343
*Dimetapp Cold & Fever Suspension*—Whitehall-Robins (U.S.) brand of Brompheniramine, Pseudoephedrine, and Acetaminophen—**See Antihistamines, Decongestants, and Analgesics (Systemic)**, 366
*Dimetapp DM*—Whitehall-Robins (U.S.) brand of Brompheniramine, Phenylpropanolamine, and Dextromethorphan—**See Cough/Cold Combinations (Systemic)**, 1024
*Dimetapp-DM*—Whitehall-Robins (Canada) brand of Brompheniramine, Phenylephrine, Phenylpropanolamine, and Dextromethorphan—**See Cough/Cold Combinations (Systemic)**, 1024
*Dimetapp DM Cold & Cough*—Robins (U.S.) brand of Brompheniramine, Phenylpropanolamine, and Dextromethorphan—**See Cough/Cold Combinations (Systemic)**, 1024

*Dimetapp Extentabs*—Robins (U.S.) brand of Brompheniramine and Phenylpropanolamine—**See Antihistamines and Decongestants (Systemic)**, 343; Whitehall-Robins (Canada) brand of Brompheniramine, Phenylephrine, and Phenylpropanolamine—**See Antihistamines and Decongestants (Systemic)**, 343
*Dimetapp 4-Hour*—Robins (U.S.) brand of Brompheniramine and Phenylpropanolamine—**See Antihistamines and Decongestants (Systemic)**, 343
*Dimetapp 4-Hour Liqui-Fills*—Whitehall-Robins (Canada) brand of Brompheniramine and Phenylpropanolamine—**See Antihistamines and Decongestants (Systemic)**, 343
*Dimetapp Maximum Strength Cold & Cough Liqui-Gels*—Robins (U.S.) brand of Brompheniramine, Phenylpropanolamine, and Dextromethorphan—**See Cough/Cold Combinations (Systemic)**, 1024
*Dimetapp Oral Infant Drops*—Whitehall-Robins (Canada) brand of Brompheniramine, Phenylephrine, and Phenylpropanolamine—**See Antihistamines and Decongestants (Systemic)**, 343
*Dimetapp Sinus Caplets*—Robins (U.S.) brand of Pseudoephedrine and Ibuprofen—**See Decongestants and Analgesics (Systemic)**, 1180
Dimethyl Sulfoxide [DMSO; *Rimso-50*] **(Mucosal-Local)**, 1227, 3140
Irrigation USP, 1228
Dimethyl Sulfoxide **(Systemic)**, 3140
Dimethyl Sulfoxide [*Kemsol*] **(Topical)**, 3017
Solution, 3017
*Dinate*—Seatrace (U.S.) brand of Dimenhydrinate—**See Antihistamines (Systemic)**, 325
Dinoprostone [*Cervidil*; PGE$_2$; *Prepidil*; prostaglandin E$_2$; *Prostin E$_2$*]
**(Cervical/Vaginal)**, 1228
Gel, Cervical, 1231
Gel, Vaginal, 1231
Suppositories, Vaginal, 1231
System, Vaginal, 1231
Dinoprost Tromethamine [*Prostin F$_2$ Alpha*]
**(Parenteral-Local)**, #
Injection USP, #
*Diocaine*—Dioptic (Canada) brand of Proparacaine—**See Anesthetics (Ophthalmic)**, #
*Diochloram*—Dioptic (Canada) brand of Chloramphenicol (Ophthalmic), 3014
*Diocto*—Barre-National (U.S.); Rugby (U.S.); and Zenith Goldline (U.S.) brand of Docusate—**See Laxatives (Local)**, #
*Diocto-C*—Barre-National (U.S.); Moore (U.S.); Rugby (U.S.) and Zenith Goldline (U.S.) brand of Casanthranol and Docusate—**See Laxatives (Local)**, #
*Diocto-K*—Rugby (U.S.) brand of Docusate—**See Laxatives (Local)**, #
*Diocto-K Plus*—Rugby (U.S.) brand of Casanthranol and Docusate—**See Laxatives (Local)**, #
*Dioctolose Plus*—Zenith Goldline (U.S.) brand of Casthranol and Docusate—**See Laxatives (Local)**, #
*Diodex*—Dioptic (Canada) brand of Dexamethasone—**See Corticosteroids (Ophthalmic)**, 966
*Diodoquin*—Searle (Canada) brand of Iodoquinol (Oral-Local), #
*Dioeze*—Century (U.S.) brand of Docusate—**See Laxatives (Local)**, #
*Dionephrine*—Dioptic (Canada) brand of Phenylephrine (Ophthalmic), 3032
*Diosan*—Ciba (U.S.) brand of Valsartan (Systemic), 2914
*Diosuccin*—CMC-Cons (U.S.) brand of Docusate—**See Laxatives (Local)**, #
*Dioval 40*—Keene (U.S.) brand of Estradiol—**See Estrogens (Systemic)**, 1383
*Dioval XX*—Keene (U.S.) brand of Estradiol—**See Estrogens (Systemic)**, 1383
*Diovol*—Horner (Canada) brand of Alumina, Magnesia, and Magnesium Carbonate—**See Antacids (Oral-Local)**, 188; Alumina, Magnesia, and Simethicone—**See Antacids (Oral-Local)**, 188
*Diovol Caplets*—Horner (Canada) brand of Alumina and Magnesia—**See Antacids (Oral-Local)**, 188
*Diovol Ex*—Horner (Canada) brand of Alumina and Magnesia—**See Antacids (Oral-Local)**, 188

*Diovol Plus*—Horner (Canada) brand of Alumina, Magnesia, Magnesium Carbonate, and Simethicone—**See Antacids (Oral-Local)**, 188; Alumina, Magnesia, and Simethicone—**See Antacids (Oral-Local)**, 188
*Diovol Plus AF*—Horner (Canada) brand of Calcium Carbonate, Magnesia, and Simethicone—**See Antacids (Oral-Local)**, 188
Dioxybenzone-containing Combinations, 3072
Dioxybenzone, Oxybenzone, and Padimate O [*Solbar Plus*]
   **See Sunscreen Agents (Topical)**, #
   Cream, #
Dipalmitoylphosphatidylcholine—*See* Colfosceril, Cetyl Alcohol, and Tyloxapol (Intratracheal-Local), 937
Dipalmitoylphosphatidylcholine and Phosphatidylglycerol [ALEC]
   **(Intratracheal-Local)**, 3141
*Dipentum*—Pharmacia & Upjohn (U.S. and Canada) brand of Olsalazine (Oral-Local), 2161, MC-23
*Diphen Cough*—My-K (U.S.) brand of Diphenhydramine—**See Antihistamines (Systemic)**, 325
*Diphenhist*—Rugby (U.S.) brand of Diphenhydramine—**See Antihistamines (Systemic)**, 325, MC-10
*Diphenhist Captabs*—Rugby (U.S.) brand of Diphenhydramine—**See Antihistamines (Systemic)**, 325
Diphenhydramine Citrate, Phenylpropanolamine Hydrochloride, and Aspirin [*Night-Time Effervescent Cold*]
   **See Antihistamines, Decongestants, and Analgesics (Systemic)**, 366
   Tablets, Effervescent, 370
Diphenhydramine-containing Combinations, 3072
Diphenhydramine Hydrochloride [*Allerdryl*; *AllerMax Caplets*; *Aller-med*; *Banophen*; *Banophen Caplets*; *Benadryl*; *Benadryl Allergy*; *Compoz*; *Diphen Cough*; *Diphenhist*; *Diphenhist Captabs*; *Dormarex 2*; *Genahist*; *Hyrexin*; *Nervine Nighttime Sleep-Aid*; *Nytol QuickCaps*; *Nytol QuickGels*; *Siladryl*; *Sleep-Eze D*; *Sleep-Eze D Extra Strength*; *Sominex*; *Twilite Caplets*; *Unisom SleepGels Maximum Strength*]
   **See Antihistamines (Systemic)**, 325
   Capsules USP, 338, MC-10
   Elixir USP, 338
   Injection USP, 339
   Tablets, 339, MC-10
Diphenhydramine Hydrochloride, Codeine Phosphate, and Ammonium Chloride [*Calmylin Original with Codeine*]
   **See Cough/Cold Combinations (Systemic)**, 1024
   Syrup, 1040
Diphenhydramine Hydrochloride, Dextromethorphan Hydrobromide, and Ammonium Chloride [*Calmylin #4*]
   **See Cough/Cold Combinations (Systemic)**, 1024
   Syrup, 1040
Diphenhydramine and Pseudoephedrine Hydrochlorides [*Actifed Allergy Nighttime Caplets*; *Banophen*; *Benadryl Allergy Decongestant Liquid Medication*]
   **See Antihistamines and Decongestants (Systemic)**, 343
   Capsules USP, 345
   Solution, Oral, 346
   Tablets, 344, 346
Diphenhydramine Hydrochloride, Pseudoephedrine Hydrochloride, and Acetaminophen [*Actifed Sinus Nighttime*; *Actifed Sinus Nighttime Caplets*; *Benadryl Allergy/Cold*; *Benadryl Allergy/Sinus Headache Caplets*; *Contac Allergy/Sinus Night Caplets*; *Contac Cold/Flu Night Caplets*; *Tylenol Allergy Sinus Night Time Medicine Maximum Strength Caplets*; *Tylenol Flu Medication Extra Strength Gelcaps*; *Tylenol Flu NightTime Hot Medication Maximum Strength*; *Tylenol Flu NightTime Medication Maximum Strength Gelcaps*]
   **See Antihistamines, Decongestants, and Analgesics (Systemic)**, 366
   for Solution, Oral, 373
   Tablets, 367, 368, 373
Diphenidol Hydrochloride [*difenidol*; *Vontrol*]
   **(Systemic)**, 1232
   Tablets, 1233
Diphenoxylate-containing Combinations, 3072

Diphenoxylate Hydrochloride and Atropine Sulfate [*Lofene*; *Logen*; *Lomocot*; *Lomotil*; *Lonox*; *Vi-Atro*]
   **(Systemic)**, 1233
   Solution, Oral, USP, 1236
   Tablets USP, 1236, MC-10
Diphenylpyraline
   **See Antihistamines (Systemic)**, 325
Diphenylpyraline-containing Combinations, 3072
Diphenylpyraline Hydrochloride, Phenylephrine Hydrochloride, and Dextromethorphan Hydrobromide [*Biohisdex DM*; *Biohisdine DM*]
   **See Cough/Cold Combinations (Systemic)**, 1024
   Solution, Oral, 1037
Diphenylpyraline Hydrochloride, Phenylpropanolamine Hydrochloride, Acetaminophen, and Caffeine [*Oradrine-2*]
   **See Antihistamines, Decongestants, and Analgesics (Systemic)**, 366
   Tablets, 371
Diphtheria Antitoxin
   **(Systemic)**, #
   Diphtheria Antitoxin USP, #
Diphtheria and Tetanus Toxoids (DT) [DT]
   **See Diphtheria and Tetanus Toxoids (Systemic)**, 1236
   Diphtheria and Tetanus Toxoids Adsorbed (DT) USP (for Pediatric Use), 1239
Diphtheria and Tetanus Toxoids
   **(Systemic)**, 1236
Diphtheria and Tetanus Toxoids and Pertussis Vaccine Adsorbed [*Acel-Imune*; acellular DTP; DTaP; DTP; DTwP; *Tri-Immunol*; *Tripedia*; whole-cell DTP]
   **See Diphtheria and Tetanus Toxoids and Pertussis Vaccine Adsorbed (Systemic)**, 1240
   Diphtheria and Tetanus Toxoids and Acellular Pertussis Vaccine Adsorbed, 1243
   Diphtheria and Tetanus Toxoids and Pertussis Vaccine Adsorbed USP, 1244
Diphtheria and Tetanus Toxoids and Pertussis Vaccine Adsorbed and Haemophilus b Conjugate Vaccine
   **(Systemic)**, 1244
Diphtheria and Tetanus Toxoids and Pertussis Vaccine Adsorbed and Haemophilus b Conjugate Vaccine (HbOC—Diphtheria CRM$_{197}$ Protein Conjugate) [*Tetramune*; DTP-HbOC; DTP-Hib]
   **See Haemophilus b Conjugate Vaccine (Systemic)**, 1244
   Injection, 1247
Diphtheria and Tetanus Toxoids and Pertussis Vaccine Adsorbed and Haemophilus b Conjugate Vaccine (PRP-D—Diphtheria Toxoid Conjugate) [DPT-Hib; DTP-Hib; DTP-PRP-D]
   **See Haemophilus b Conjugate Vaccine (Systemic)**, 1244
   Injection, 1248
Dipivefrine—*See* Dipivefrin (Ophthalmic), 1249
Dipivefrin Hydrochloride [*AKPro*; dipivefrine; *DPE*; *Ophtho-Dipivefrin*; *Propine C Cap B.I.D.*]
   **(Ophthalmic)**, 1249, 3017
   Solution, Ophthalmic, USP, 1250, 3017
*Dipridacot*—Truxton (U.S.) brand of Dipyridamole (Systemic), #
*Diprivan*—Stuart (U.S.) and ZENECA (Canada) brand of Propofol (Systemic), 2416
*Diprolene*—Schering (U.S. and Canada) brand of Betamethasone—**See Corticosteroids (Topical)**, 978
*Diprolene AF*—Schering (U.S.) brand of Betamethasone—**See Corticosteroids (Topical)**, 978
Diprophylline—*See* Dyphylline (Systemic), #
*Diprosone*—Schering (U.S. and Canada) brand of Betamethasone—**See Corticosteroids (Topical)**, 978
Dipyridamole [*Apo-Dipyridamole*; *Dipridacot*; *I.V. Persantine*; *Novodipiradol*; *Persantine*]
   **(Systemic)**, #
   Injection, #
   Tablets USP, #, MC-10
Dipyridamole and Aspirin [*Asasantine*]
   **(Systemic)**, 3018
   Capsules, 3018
*Diquinol*—CMC (U.S.) brand of Iodoquinol (Oral-Local), #
Dirithromycin [*Dynabac*]
   **(Systemic)**, 1250
   Tablets, 1252, MC-10
Disaccharide Tripeptide Glycerol Dipalmitoyl [*Immther*]
   **(Systemic)**, 3141

*Disalcid*—Riker (U.S. and Canada) brand of Salsalate—**See Salicylates (Systemic)**, 2538
*Disipal*—3M (Canada) brand of Orphenadrine—**See Skeletal Muscle Relaxants (Systemic)**, 2577
*Disobrom*—Geneva (U.S.) brand of Dexbrompheniramine and Pseudoephedrine—**See Antihistamines and Decongestants (Systemic)**, 343
Disodium Clodronate
   **(Systemic)**, 3141
Disodium Clodronate Tetrahydrate [*Bonefos*]
   **(Systemic)**, 3141
Disodium EDTA—*See* Edetate Disodium (Ophthalmic), #; Edetate Disodium (Systemic), 1327
Disodium Silibinin Dihemisuccinate [*Legalon*]
   **(Systemic)**, 3141
*Disophrol Chronotabs*—Schering-Plough (U.S.) brand of Dexbrompheniramine and Pseudoephedrine—**See Antihistamines and Decongestants (Systemic)**, 343
Disoprofol—*See* Propofol (Systemic), 2416
Disopyramide [*Rythmodan*]
   **(Systemic)**, 1252
   Capsules, 1255
   Injection, 1256
Disopyramide Phosphate [*Norpace*; *Norpace CR*; *Rythmodan-LA*]
   **(Systemic)**, 1252
   Capsules USP, 1255, MC-10
   Capsules, Extended-release, USP, 1256, MC-10
   Tablets, Extended-release, 1256
*Di-Sosul*—Drug Industries (U.S.) brand of Docusate—**See Laxatives (Local)**, #
*Di-Sosul Forte*—Drug Industries (U.S.) brand of Casanthranol and Docusate—**See Laxatives (Local)**, #
*Disotate*—Forest (U.S.) brand of Edetate Disodium (Systemic), 1327
*Di-Spaz*—Vortech (U.S.) brand of Dicyclomine—**See Anticholinergics/Antispasmodics (Systemic)**, 226
Disulfiram [*Antabuse*]
   **(Systemic)**, 1256
   Tablets USP, 1258
Dithranol—*See* Anthralin (Topical), 218
*Ditropan*—Hoechst Marion Roussel (U.S.) and Procter & Gamble (Canada) brand of Oxybutynin (Systemic), 2209
*Diucardin*—Wyeth-Ayerst (U.S.) brand of Hydroflumethiazide—**See Diuretics, Thiazide (Systemic)**, 1273
*Diuchlor H*—Medic (Canada) brand of Hydrochlorothiazide—**See Diuretics, Thiazide (Systemic)**, 1273
*Diulo*—Schiapparelli Searle (U.S.) brand of Metolazone—**See Diuretics, Thiazide (Systemic)**, 1273
*Diupres*—Merck (U.S.) brand of Reserpine and Chlorothiazide—**See Rauwolfia Alkaloids and Thiazide Diuretics (Systemic)**, #
*Diurese-R*—American Urologicals (U.S.) brand of Reserpine and Trichlormethiazide—**See Rauwolfia Alkaloids and Thiazide Diuretics (Systemic)**, #
Diuretics, Loop
   **(Systemic)**, 1259
Diuretics, Potassium-sparing
   **(Systemic)**, 1266
Diuretics, Potassium-sparing, and Hydrochlorothiazide
   **(Systemic)**, 1272
Diuretics, Thiazide
   **(Systemic)**, 1273
*Diurigen with Reserpine*—Goldline (U.S.) brand of Reserpine and Chlorothiazide—**See Rauwolfia Alkaloids and Thiazide Diuretics (Systemic)**, #
*Diuril*—Merck (U.S.) brand of Chlorothiazide—**See Diuretics, Thiazide (Systemic)**, 1273
*Diutensen-R*—Wallace (U.S.) brand of Reserpine and Methyclothiazide—**See Rauwolfia Alkaloids and Thiazide Diuretics (Systemic)**, #
Divalproex Sodium [*Depakote*; *Depakote Sprinkle*; *Epival*]
   **See Valproic Acid (Systemic)**, 2908
   Capsules, Delayed-release, 2912, MC-10
   Tablets, Delayed-release, 2913, MC-10
*Dixarit*—Boehringer Ingelheim (Canada) brand of Clonidine (Systemic), 908
*Dizac*—Omeda (U.S.) brand of Diazepam—**See Benzodiazepines (Systemic)**, 556
DL-methionine—*See* Racemethionine (Systemic), #

*USP DI*

*DML Facial Moisturizer*—Person & Covey (U.S.) brand of Octyl Methoxycinnamate and Oxybenzone—**See Sunscreen Agents (Topical)**, #
DMP 777
  **(Systemic)**, 3141
DMSA—*See* Succimer (Systemic), #
DMSO—*See* Dimethyl Sulfoxide (Mucosal-Local), 1227
*DM Syrup*—PD (Canada) brand of Dextromethorphan (Systemic), 1191
DNase—Dornase Alfa (Inhalation-Local), 1292
*Doak Oil*—T.C.D. (Canada) brand of Coal Tar (Topical), #
*Doak Oil Forte*—T.C.D. (Canada) brand of Coal Tar (Topical), #
*Doak Oil Forte Therapeutic Bath Treatment*—Doak (U.S.) brand of Coal Tar (Topical), #
*Doak Oil Therapeutic Bath Treatment For All-Over Body Care*—Doak (U.S.) brand of Coal Tar (Topical), #
*Doak Tar Lotion*—Doak (U.S.) brand of Coal Tar (Topical), #
*Doak Tar Shampoo*—Doak (U.S.) brand of Coal Tar (Topical), #
*Doan's Backache Pills*—Sandoz Consumer (Canada) brand of Magnesium Salicylate—**See Salicylates (Systemic)**, 2538
*Doan's Regular Strength Tablets*—Sandoz Consumer (U.S.) brand of Magnesium Salicylate—**See Salicylates (Systemic)**, 2538
Dobutamine Hydrochloride [*Dobutrex*]
  **See Sympathomimetic Agents—Cardiovascular Use (Parenteral-Systemic)**, 2669
  Injection, 2675
*Dobutrex*—Lilly (U.S. and Canada) brand of Dobutamine—**See Sympathomimetic Agents—Cardiovascular Use (Parenteral-Systemic)**, 2669
Docetaxel [*Taxotere*]
  **(Systemic)**, 1282
  Concentrate for Injection, 1286
*Doctar Hair & Scalp Shampoo and Conditioner*—Savage (U.S.) brand of Coal Tar (Topical), #
*Doctar Shampoo*—Savage (U.S.) brand of Coal Tar (Topical), #
*Docucal-P*—Parmed (U.S.) brand of Phenolphthalein and Docusate—**See Laxatives (Local)**, #
*Docu-K Plus*—Major (U.S.) brand of Casanthranol and Docusate—**See Laxatives (Local)**, #
Docusate Calcium [*Albert Docusate; DC Softgels; PMS-Docusate Calcium; Pro-Cal-Sof; Sulfolax; Surfak*]
  **See Laxatives (Local)**, #
  Capsules USP, #
Docusate-containing Combinations, 3072
Docusate Potassium [*Diocto-K; Kasof*]
  **See Laxatives (Local)**, #
  Capsules USP, #
Docusate Sodium [*Afko-Lube; Colace; Correctol Stool Softener Soft Gels; Dialose; Diocto; Dioeze; Diosuccin; Di-Sosul; DOK; DOK Softgels; D.O.S. Softgels; D-S-S; Duosol; Fleet Soflax Gelcaps; Laxinate 100; Modane Soft; Molatoc; PMS-Docusate Sodium; Pro-Sof; Regulax SS; Regulex; Silace; Soflax; Solfax Drops; Stulex; Therevac Plus; Therevac-SB*]
  **See Laxatives (Local)**, #, 3018
  Capsules USP, #
  Enema, #, 3018
  Solution USP (Oral), #
  Solution, Rectal, #
  Syrup USP, #
  Tablets, #
  Tablets USP, #
*Dodd's Extra Strength*—Fulford (Canada) brand of Sodium Salicylate—**See Salicylates (Systemic)**, 2538
*Dodd's Pills*—Fulford (Canada) brand of Sodium Salicylate—**See Salicylates (Systemic)**, 2538
*DOK*—Major (U.S.) brand of Docusate—**See Laxatives (Local)**, #
*DOK Softgels*—Major (U.S.) brand of Docusate—**See Laxatives (Local)**, #
*Doktors*—Scherer (U.S.) brand of Phenylephrine (Nasal), #
*Dolacet*—Roberts (U.S.) brand of Hydrocodone and Acetaminophen—**See Opioid (Narcotic) Analgesics and Acetaminophen (Systemic)**, 2198
*Dolagesic*—Alphagen (U.S.) brand of Hydrocodone and Acetaminophen—**See Opioid (Narcotic) Analgesics and Acetaminophen (Systemic)**, 2198

Dolasetron Mesylate [*Anzemet*]
  **(Systemic)**, 1287
  Injection, 1289
  Tablets, 1289
*Dolgesic*—Marlop (U.S.) brand of Ibuprofen—**See Anti-inflammatory Drugs, Nonsteroidal (Systemic)**, 388
*Dolmar*—Marlop (U.S.) brand of Butalbital, Acetaminophen, and Caffeine—**See Barbiturates and Analgesics (Systemic)**, 532
*Dolobid*—Merck (U.S.) and Frosst (Canada) brand of Diflunisal—**See Anti-inflammatory Drugs, Nonsteroidal (Systemic)**, 388, MC-9
*Dolomine*—Aspirin—**See Salicylates (Systemic)**, 2538
*Dolophine*—Lilly (U.S.) brand of Methadone—**See Opioid (Narcotic) Analgesics (Systemic)**, 2168
*Dolotic*—Marlop (U.S.) brand of Antipyrine and Benzocaine (Otic), 443
*Dolsed*—American Urologicals (U.S.) brand of Atropine, Hyoscyamine, Methenamine, Methylene Blue, Phenyl Salicylate, and Benzoic Acid (Systemic), 488
Domperidone [*Motilium*]
  **(Systemic)**, 3018
  Tablets, 3018
*Dom-Valproic*—Dominion Pharmacal (Canada) brand of Valproic Acid—**See Valproic Acid (Systemic)**, 2908
*Donatussin*—Laser (U.S.) brand of Chlorpheniramine, Phenylephrine, Dextromethorphan, and Guaifenesin—**See Cough/Cold Combinations (Systemic)**, 1024
*Donatussin DC*—Laser (U.S.) brand of Phenylephrine, Hydrocodone, and Guaifenesin—**See Cough/Cold Combinations (Systemic)**, 1024
*Donatussin Drops*—Laser (U.S.) brand of Chlorpheniramine, Phenylephrine, and Guaifenesin—**See Cough/Cold Combinations (Systemic)**, 1024
*Dondril*—Whitehall (U.S.) brand of Chlorpheniramine, Phenylephrine, and Dextromethorphan—**See Cough/Cold Combinations (Systemic)**, 1024
Donepezil [*Aricept*]
  **(Systemic)**
  Tablets, MC-10
Donepezil Hydrochloride [*Aricept*, E2020]
  **(Systemic)**, 1290
  Tablets, 1292
*Donnagel*—Robins (U.S.) brand of Attapulgite (Oral-Local), #; Wyeth-Ayerst (Canada) brand of Kaolin, Pectin, Hyoscyamine, Atropine, and Scopolamine—**See Kaolin, Pectin, and Belladonna Alkaloids (Systemic)**, 1803
*Donnagel-MB*—Ayerst (Canada) brand of Kaolin and Pectin (Oral-Local), 1802
*Donnagel-PG*—Wyeth-Ayerst (Canada) brand of Kaolin, Pectin, and Paregoric (Systemic), 1804
*Donnamor*—H. L. Moore (U.S.) brand of Atropine, Hyoscyamine, Scopolamine, and Phenobarbital—**See Belladonna Alkaloids and Barbiturates (Systemic)**, 551
*Donnapine*—Major (U.S.) brand of Atropine, Hyoscyamine, Scopolamine, and Phenobarbital—**See Belladonna Alkaloids and Barbiturates (Systemic)**, 551
*Donnatal*—Robins (U.S. and Canada) brand of Atropine, Hyoscyamine, Scopolamine, and Phenobarbital—**See Belladonna Alkaloids and Barbiturates (Systemic)**, 551, MC-3
*Donnatal Extentabs*—Robins (U.S. and Canada) brand of Atropine, Hyoscyamine, Scopolamine, and Phenobarbital—**See Belladonna Alkaloids and Barbiturates (Systemic)**, 551, MC-3
*Donnatal No. 2*—Robins (U.S.) brand of Atropine, Hyoscyamine, Scopolamine, and Phenobarbital—**See Belladonna Alkaloids and Barbiturates (Systemic)**, 551
*Donphen*—Lemmon (U.S.) brand of Atropine, Hyoscyamine, Scopolamine, and Phenobarbital—**See Belladonna Alkaloids and Barbiturates (Systemic)**, 551
*Dopamet*—ICN (Canada) brand of Methyldopa (Systemic), 1979
Dopamine Hydrochloride [*Intropin; Revimine*]
  **See Sympathomimetic Agents—Cardiovascular Use (Parenteral-Systemic)**, 2669
  Injection USP, 2675
Dopamine Hydrochloride and Dextrose
  **See Sympathomimetic Agents—Cardiovascular Use (Parenteral-Systemic)**, 2669
  Injection USP, 2676

**General Index** 3277

*Dopar*—Roberts (U.S.) brand of Levodopa (Systemic), 1848
*Dopram*—Robins (U.S.) and Ayerst (Canada) brand of Doxapram (Systemic), 1301
*Doral*—Wallace (U.S.) brand of Quazepam—**See Benzodiazepines (Systemic)**, 556
*Dorcol Children's Cold Formula*—Sandoz (U.S.) brand of Chlorpheniramine and Pseudoephedrine—**See Antihistamines and Decongestants (Systemic)**, 343
*Dorcol Children's Cough*—Sandoz (U.S.) brand of Pseudoephedrine, Dextromethorphan, and Guaifenesin—**See Cough/Cold Combinations (Systemic)**, 1024
*Dorcol Children's Decongestant Liquid*—Sandoz (U.S.) brand of Pseudoephedrine (Systemic), 2422
*Dormarex 2*—Republic (U.S.) brand of Diphenhydramine—**See Antihistamines (Systemic)**, 325
Dornase Alfa [DNase I; *Pulmozyme*; recombinant human deoxyribonuclease I; rhDNase]
  **(Inhalation-Local)**, 1292, 3141
  Solution for Inhalation, 1294
*Doryx*—PD (U.S. and Canada) brand of Doxycycline—**See Tetracyclines (Systemic)**, 2765
Dorzolamide Hydrochloride [*Trusopt*]
  **(Ophthalmic)**, 1294
  Solution, Ophthalmic, 1296
Dorzolamide Hydrochloride and Timolol Maleate [*Cosopt*]
  **(Ophthalmic)**, 3018
  Solution, Ophthalmic, 3018
*Dosaflex*—Richwood (U.S.) brand of Senna—**See Laxatives (Local)**, #
*Doss*—SmithKline Beecham (Canada) brand of Danthron and Docusate—**See Laxatives (Local)**, #
*D.O.S. Softgels*—Zenith Goldline (U.S.) brand of Docusate—**See Laxatives (Local)**, #
*Dostinex*—Pharmacia & Upjohn (U.S.) brand of Cabergoline (Systemic), 704
*Dovonex*—Westwood-Squibb (U.S.) and Leo (Canada) brand of Calcipotriene (Topical), 711
Doxacurium Chloride [*Nuromax*]
  **(Systemic)**, 1296
  Injection, 1300
Doxapram Hydrochloride [*Dopram*]
  **(Systemic)**, 1301
  Injection USP, 1302
Doxazosin Mesylate [*Cardura*]
  **(Systemic)**, 1303
  Tablets, 1305, MC-10
Doxepin Hydrochloride [*Novo-Doxepin; Sinequan; Triadapin*]
  **See Antidepressants, Tricyclic (Systemic)**, 271
  Capsules USP, 280, MC-10
  Solution, Oral, USP, 280
Doxepin Hydrochloride [*Zonalon*]
  **(Topical)**, 1305
  Cream, 1307
*Doxidan*—Hoechst-Roussel (Canada) brand of Phenolphthalein and Docusate—**See Laxatives (Local)**, #
*Doxidan Liqui-Gels*—Upjohn (U.S.) brand of Phenolphthalein and Docusate—**See Laxatives (Local)**, #
*Doxi Film*—Wakefield (U.S.) brand of Doxycycline—**See Tetracyclines (Systemic)**, 2765
*Doxil*—Sequus (U.S.) brand of Doxorubicin, Liposomal (Systemic), 1312
*Doxine*—Merit (U.S.) brand of Pyridoxine (Systemic), 2430
Doxorubicin Hydrochloride [*Adriamycin PFS; Adriamycin RDF; Rubex*]
  **(Systemic)**, 1308
  Injection USP, 1311
  for Injection USP, 1312
Doxorubicin, Liposomal [*Caelyx; Doxil*]
  **(Systemic)**, 1312
  Injection, 1316
*Doxy*—Lederle (U.S.) brand of Doxycycline—**See Tetracyclines (Systemic)**, 2765
*Doxy-Caps*—Lederle (U.S.) brand of Doxycycline—**See Tetracyclines (Systemic)**, 2765
*Doxycin*—Lederle (Canada) brand of Doxycycline—**See Tetracyclines (Systemic)**, 2765
Doxycycline [*Vibramycin*]
  **See Tetracyclines (Systemic)**, 2765
  for Suspension, Oral, USP, 2769
Doxycycline Calcium [*Vibramycin*]
  **See Tetracyclines (Systemic)**, 2765
  Suspension, Oral, USP, 2769

Doxycycline Hyclate [*Apo-Doxy; Doryx; Doxi Film; Doxy; Doxy-Caps; Doxycin; Monodox; Novodoxylin; Vibramycin; Vibra-Tabs*]
   See **Tetracyclines (Systemic)**, 2765
   Capsules USP, 2770, MC-10
   Capsules, Delayed-release, USP, 2770
   for Injection USP, 2770
   Tablets USP, 2770, MC-10
Doxylamine-containing Combinations, 3072
Doxylamine Succinate [*Unisom Nighttime Sleep Aid*]
   See **Antihistamines (Systemic)**, 325
   Tablets USP, 339
Doxylamine Succinate, Codeine Phosphate, and Acetaminophen [*Mersyndol with Codeine*]
   See **Cough/Cold Combinations (Systemic)**, 1024
   Tablets, 1070
Doxylamine Succinate, Etafedrine Hydrochloride, and Hydrocodone Bitartrate [*Calmydone; Mercodol with Decapryn*]
   See **Cough/Cold Combinations (Systemic)**, 1024
   Syrup, 1040, 1069
Doxylamine Succinate, Phenylpropanolamine Bitartrate, Dextromethorphan Hydrobromide, and Aspirin [*Alka-Seltzer Plus Night Time Cold*]
   See **Cough/Cold Combinations (Systemic)**, 1024
   Tablets, Effervescent, 1033
Doxylamine Succinate, Pseudoephedrine Hydrochloride, Dextromethorphan Hydrobromide, and Acetaminophen [*Alka-Seltzer Plus Night Time Cold Liqui-Gels; All-Nite Cold Formula; Genite; Nytcold Medicine; Nytime Cold Medicine Liquid; Robitussin Night-Time Cold Formula; Vicks Ny-Quil; Vicks NyQuil Hot Therapy; Vicks NyQuil Liquicaps; Vicks NyQuil Multi-Symptom Cold/Flu LiquiCaps; Vicks NyQuil Multi-Symptom Cold/Flu Relief*]
   See **Cough/Cold Combinations (Systemic)**, 1024
   Capsules, 1033, 1089, 1114
   Solution, Oral, 1033, 1059, 1076, 1114
   for Solution, Oral, 1114
DPE—Alcon (Canada) brand of Dipivefrin (Ophthalmic), 3017
DPPC—*See* Colfosceril, Cetyl Alcohol, and Tyloxapol (Intratracheal-Local), 937
DPT-Hib—Connaught (Canada) brand of Diphtheria and Tetanus Toxoids and Pertussis Vaccine Adsorbed and Haemophilus b Conjugate Vaccine (PRP-D—Diphtheria Toxoid Conjugate)—See **Diphtheria and Tetanus Toxoids and Pertussis Vaccine Adsorbed and Haemophilus b Conjugate Vaccine (Systemic)**, 1244
Dr. Caldwell Senna Laxative—Dennison (U.S.) brand of Senna—See **Laxatives (Local)**, #
Dramamine—Richardson-Vicks (U.S.) brand of Dimenhydrinate—See **Antihistamines (Systemic)**, 325
Dramamine II—Upjohn (U.S.) brand of Meclizine (Systemic), 1933
Drenison—Lilly (Canada) brand of Flurandrenolide—See **Corticosteroids (Topical)**, 978
Drenison-¼—Lilly (Canada) brand of Flurandrenolide—See **Corticosteroids (Topical)**, 978
Drepanol—Omex (U.S.) brand of OM 401 (Systemic), 3156
D(Rh₀) immune globulin—*See* Rh₀(D) Immune Globulin (Systemic), 2476
Drisdol—Sanofi Winthrop (U.S. and Canada) brand of Ergocalciferol—See **Vitamin D and Analogs (Systemic)**, 2966, MC-11
Drisdol Drops—Sanofi Winthrop (U.S.) brand of Ergocalciferol—See **Vitamin D and Analogs (Systemic)**, 2966
Dristan—Whitehall (Canada) brand of Oxymetazoline (Nasal), #; Whitehall-Robins (Canada) brand of Chlorpheniramine, Phenylephrine, and Acetaminophen—See **Antihistamines, Decongestants, and Analgesics (Systemic)**, 366
Dristan Cold Caplets—Whitehall (U.S.) brand of Pseudoephedrine and Acetaminophen—See **Decongestants and Analgesics (Systemic)**, 1180
Dristan Cold Maximum Strength Caplets—Whitehall-Robins (U.S.) brand of Brompheniramine, Pseudoephedrine, and Acetaminophen—See **Antihistamines, Decongestants, and Analgesics (Systemic)**, 366
Dristan Cold Multi-Symptom Formula—Whitehall-Robins (U.S.) brand of Chlorpheniramine, Phenylephrine, and Acetaminophen—See **Antihistamines, Decongestants, and Analgesics (Systemic)**, 366

Dristan Extra Strength Caplets—Whitehall-Robins (Canada) brand of Chlorpheniramine, Phenylephrine, and Acetaminophen—See **Antihistamines, Decongestants, and Analgesics (Systemic)**, 366
Dristan Formula P—Whitehall-Robins (Canada) brand of Pyrilamine, Phenylephrine, Aspirin, and Caffeine—See **Antihistamines, Decongestants, and Analgesics (Systemic)**, 366
Dristan 12-Hr Nasal Spray—Whitehall (U.S.) brand of Oxymetazoline (Nasal), #
Dristan Mentholated—Whitehall (Canada) brand of Oxymetazoline (Nasal), #
Dristan N.D. Caplets—Whitehall (Canada) brand of Pseudoephedrine and Acetaminophen—See **Decongestants and Analgesics (Systemic)**, 1180
Dristan N.D. Extra Strength Caplets—Whitehall (Canada) brand of Pseudoephedrine and Acetaminophen—See **Decongestants and Analgesics (Systemic)**, 1180
Dristan Sinus Caplets—Whitehall (U.S.) brand of Pseudoephedrine and Ibuprofen—See **Decongestants and Analgesics (Systemic)**, 1180
Drithocreme—Dermik (U.S.) brand of Anthralin (Topical), 218
Drithocreme HP—Dermik (U.S.) brand of Anthralin (Topical), 218
Dritho-Scalp—Dermik (U.S.) brand of Anthralin (Topical), 218
Drixomed—Iomed (U.S.) brand of Dexbrompheniramine and Pseudoephedrine—See **Antihistamines and Decongestants (Systemic)**, 343
Drixoral—Schering (Canada) brand of Dexbrompheniramine and Pseudoephedrine—See **Antihistamines and Decongestants (Systemic)**, 343; Schering (Canada) brand of Oxymetazoline (Nasal), #
Drixoral Allergy-Sinus—Schering-Plough (U.S.) brand of Dexbrompheniramine, Pseudoephedrine, and Acetaminophen—See **Antihistamines, Decongestants, and Analgesics (Systemic)**, 366
Drixoral Cold and Allergy—Schering-Plough (U.S.) brand of Dexbrompheniramine and Pseudoephedrine—See **Antihistamines and Decongestants (Systemic)**, 343
Drixoral Cold and Flu—Schering-Plough (U.S.) brand of Dexbrompheniramine, Pseudoephedrine, and Acetaminophen—See **Antihistamines, Decongestants, and Analgesics (Systemic)**, 366
Drixoral Cough & Congestion Liquid Caps—Schering-Plough (U.S.) brand of Pseudoephedrine and Dextromethorphan—See **Cough/Cold Combinations (Systemic)**, 1024
Drixoral Cough Liquid Caps—Schering-Plough (U.S.) brand of Dextromethorphan (Systemic), 1191
Drixoral Cough & Sore Throat Liquid Caps—Schering-Plough (U.S.) brand of Dextromethorphan and Acetaminophen—See **Cough/Cold Combinations (Systemic)**, 1024
Drixoral Night—Schering (Canada) brand of Dexbrompheniramine and Pseudoephedrine—See **Antihistamines and Decongestants (Systemic)**, 343
Drixoral Non-Drowsy Formula—Schering-Plough (U.S.) brand of Pseudoephedrine (Systemic), 2422
Drixtab—Schering (Canada) brand of Dexbrompheniramine and Pseudoephedrine—See **Antihistamines and Decongestants (Systemic)**, 343
Drize—Jones Medical (U.S.) brand of Chlorpheniramine and Phenylpropanolamine—See **Antihistamines and Decongestants (Systemic)**, 343
Drocode and acetaminophen—See **Dihydrocodeine and Acetaminophen—See Opioid (Narcotic) Analgesics and Acetaminophen (Systemic)**, 2198
Drocode and aspirin—Aspirin and Dihydrocodeine—See **Opioid (Narcotic) Analgesics and Aspirin (Systemic)**, 2202
Dronabinol [delta-9-tetrahydrocannabinol (THC); *Marinol*]
   (Systemic), 1316, 3141
   Capsules USP, 1318
Droperidol [*Inapsine*]
   (Systemic), 1319
   Injection USP, 1321
Drotic—Ascher (U.S.) brand of Neomycin, Polymyxin B, and Hydrocortisone (Otic), #
Droxia—Bristol-Myers Squibb (U.S.) brand of Hydroxyurea (Systemic), 3024
DSMC Plus—Warner Chilcott (U.S.) brand of Casanthranol and Docusate—See **Laxatives (Local)**, #

D-S-S—Geneva Marsam (U.S.) brand of Docusate—See **Laxatives (Local)**, #
D-S-S plus—Warner Chilcott (U.S.) brand of Casanthranol and Docusate—See **Laxatives (Local)**, #
d4T—*See* Stavudine (Systemic), 2627
DT—Diphtheria and Tetanus Toxoids (DT)—See **Diphtheria and Tetanus Toxoids (Systemic)**, 1236
DTaP—*See* Diphtheria and Tetanus Toxoids and Pertussis Vaccine Adsorbed (Systemic), 1240
DTIC—Miles (Canada) brand of Dacarbazine (Systemic), 1148
DTIC-Dome—Miles (U.S.) brand of Dacarbazine (Systemic), 1148
DTP—*See* Diphtheria and Tetanus Toxoids and Pertussis Vaccine Adsorbed (Systemic), 1240
DTPA (Chelate) Multidose—Medi-Physics Amersham (U.S.) brand of Technetium Tc 99m Pentetate (Systemic), 2727
DTP-HbOC—Diphtheria and Tetanus Toxoids and Pertussis Vaccine Adsorbed and Haemophilus b Conjugate Vaccine (HbOC—Diphtheria CRM$_{197}$ Protein Conjugate)—See **Diphtheria and Tetanus Toxoids and Pertussis Vaccine Adsorbed and Haemophilus b Conjugate Vaccine (Systemic)**, 1244
DTP-Hib—Diphtheria and Tetanus Toxoids and Pertussis Vaccine Adsorbed and Haemophilus b Conjugate Vaccine (HbOC—Diphtheria CRM$_{197}$ Protein Conjugate)—See **Diphtheria and Tetanus Toxoids and Pertussis Vaccine Adsorbed and Haemophilus b Conjugate Vaccine (Systemic)**, 1244; Diphtheria and Tetanus Toxoids and Pertussis Vaccine Adsorbed and Haemophilus b Conjugate Vaccine (PRP-D—Diphtheria Toxoid Conjugate)—See **Diphtheria and Tetanus Toxoids and Pertussis Vaccine Adsorbed and Haemophilus b Conjugate Vaccine (Systemic)**, 1244
DTP-PRP-D—Diphtheria and Tetanus Toxoids and Pertussis Vaccine Adsorbed and Haemophilus b Conjugate Vaccine (PRP-D—Diphtheria Toxoid Conjugate)—See **Diphtheria and Tetanus Toxoids and Pertussis Vaccine Adsorbed and Haemophilus b Conjugate Vaccine (Systemic)**, 1244
DTwP—*See* Diphtheria and Tetanus Toxoids and Pertussis Vaccine Adsorbed (Systemic), 1240
Duadacin—Kenwood/Bradley (U.S.) brand of Chlorpheniramine, Phenylpropanolamine, and Acetaminophen—See **Antihistamines, Decongestants, and Analgesics (Systemic)**, 366
Dulcodos—Boehringer Ingelheim (Canada) brand of Bisacodyl and Docusate—See **Laxatives (Local)**, #
Dulcolax—Ciba Self-Medication (U.S.) and Boehringer Ingelheim (Canada) brand of Bisacodyl—See **Laxatives (Local)**, #
Duocet—Mason (U.S.) brand of Hydrocodone and Acetaminophen—See **Opioid (Narcotic) Analgesics and Acetaminophen (Systemic)**, 2198
Duo-Cyp—Keene (U.S.) brand of Testosterone and Estradiol—See **Androgens and Estrogens (Systemic)**, 126
Duofilm—Stiefel (U.S.) brand of Salicylic Acid (Topical), #
Duo-Gen L.A.—Vortech (U.S.) brand of Testosterone and Estradiol—See **Androgens and Estrogens (Systemic)**, 126
Duogex L.A.—Stickley (Canada) brand of Testosterone and Estradiol—See **Androgens and Estrogens (Systemic)**, 126
Duoplant Topical Solution—Stiefel (U.S.) brand of Salicylic Acid (Topical), #
Duoprin—Dunhall (U.S.) brand of Acetaminophen and Salicylamide—See **Acetaminophen and Salicylates (Systemic)**, 11
Duosol—Kirkman (U.S.) brand of Docusate—See **Laxatives (Local)**, #
Duotrate—Jones (U.S.) brand of Pentaerythritol Tetranitrate—See **Nitrates (Systemic)**, 2129
DuP 753—*See* Losartan (Systemic), 1882
Duphalac—Solvay (U.S.) brand of Lactulose—See **Laxatives (Local)**, #
Durabolin-50—Organon (U.S.) brand of Nandrolone—See **Anabolic Steroids (Systemic)**, 110
Durabolin—Organon (U.S.) brand of Nandrolone—See **Anabolic Steroids (Systemic)**, 110
Duraclon—Roxane (U.S.) brand of Clonidine (Parenteral-Local), 905

*Dura-Dumone 90/4*—Ortega (U.S.) brand of Testosterone and Estradiol—**See Androgens and Estrogens (Systemic)**, 126
*Duradyne*—Forest (U.S.) brand of Acetaminophen, Aspirin, and Caffeine—**See Acetaminophen and Salicylates (Systemic)**, 11
*Dura-Estrin*—Hauck (U.S.) brand of Estradiol—**See Estrogens (Systemic)**, 1383
*Duragen-20*—Hauck (U.S.) brand of Estradiol—**See Estrogens (Systemic)**, 1383
*Duragesic*—Janssen (U.S. and Canada) brand of Fentanyl (Transdermal-Systemic), 1446
*Dura-Gest*—Dura (U.S.) brand of Phenylephrine, Phenylpropanolamine, and Guaifenesin—**See Cough/Cold Combinations (Systemic)**, 1024
*Duralex*—American Urologicals (U.S.) brand of Chlorpheniramine and Pseudoephedrine—**See Antihistamines and Decongestants (Systemic)**, 343
*Duralith*—McNeil (Canada) brand of Lithium (Systemic), 1869
*Duralone-40*—Hauck (U.S.) brand of Methylprednisolone—**See Corticosteroids—Glucocorticoid Effects (Systemic)**, 998
*Duralone-80*—Hauck (U.S.) brand of Methylprednisolone—**See Corticosteroids—Glucocorticoid Effects (Systemic)**, 998
*Duramist Plus Up To 12 Hours Decongestant Nasal Spray*—Pfeiffer (U.S.) brand of Oxymetazoline (Nasal), #
*Duramorph*—Elkins-Sinn (U.S.) brand of Morphine—**See Opioid (Narcotic) Analgesics (Systemic)**, 2168
*Duranest*—Astra (U.S.) brand of Etidocaine—**See Anesthetics (Parenteral-Local)**, 139
*Duranest-MPF*—Astra (U.S.) brand of Etidocaine—**See Anesthetics (Parenteral-Local)**, 139
*Duraquin*—PD (U.S.) brand of Quinidine (Systemic), 2440
*DuraScreen*—Reed & Carnick (U.S.) brand of Octyl Methoxycinnamate, Octyl Salicylate, Oxybenzone, Phenylbenzimidazole, and Titanium Dioxide—**See Sunscreen Agents (Topical)**, #
*Durascreen*—Reed & Carnick (U.S.) brand of Octyl Methoxycinnamate, Octyl Salicylate, and Oxybenzone—**See Sunscreen Agents (Topical)**, #
*Dura-Tap PD*—Dura (U.S.) brand of Chlorpheniramine and Pseudoephedrine—**See Antihistamines and Decongestants (Systemic)**, 343
*Duratestin*—Hauck (U.S.) brand of Testosterone and Estradiol—**See Androgens and Estrogens (Systemic)**, 126
*Duratex*—Duramed (U.S.) brand of Phenylephrine, Phenylpropanolamine, and Guaifenesin—**See Cough/Cold Combinations (Systemic)**, 1024
*Duration*—Plough (U.S.) brand of Phenylephrine (Nasal), #
*Duration 12 Hour Nasal Spray*—Schering-Plough (U.S.) brand of Oxymetazoline (Nasal), #
*Duration 12 Hour Nasal Spray Pump*—Schering-Plough (U.S.) brand of Oxymetazoline (Nasal), #
*Duratuss*—UCB (U.S.) brand of Pseudoephedrine and Guaifenesin—**See Cough/Cold Combinations (Systemic)**, 1024
*Duratuss HD*—UCB (U.S.) brand of Pseudoephedrine, Hydrocodone, and Guaifenesin—**See Cough/Cold Combinations (Systemic)**, 1024
*Dura-Vent*—Dura (U.S.) brand of Phenylpropanolamine and Guaifenesin—**See Cough/Cold Combinations (Systemic)**, 1024
*Dura-Vent/A*—Dura (U.S.) brand of Chlorpheniramine and Phenylpropanolamine—**See Antihistamines and Decongestants (Systemic)**, 343
*Dura-Vent/DA*—Dura (U.S.) brand of Chlorpheniramine, Phenylephrine, and Methscopolamine—**See Antihistamines, Decongestants, and Anticholinergics (Systemic)**, 373
*Duretic*—Abbott (Canada) brand of Methyclothiazide—**See Diuretics, Thiazide (Systemic)**, 1273
*Dureticyl*—Abbott (Canada) brand of Deserpidine and Methyclothiazide—**See Rauwolfia Alkaloids and Thiazide Diuretics (Systemic)**, #
*Duricef*—Mead Johnson (U.S.) and Bristol (Canada) brand of Cefadroxil—**See Cephalosporins (Systemic)**, 794, MC-6
*Duvoid*—Procter & Gamble (U.S. and Canada) brand of Bethanechol (Systemic), 614
*D-Vert 15*—Hauck (U.S.) brand of Meclizine (Systemic), 1933
*D-Vert 30*—Hauck (U.S.) brand of Meclizine (Systemic), 1933

*Dyazide*—SmithKline Beecham (U.S. and Canada) brand of Triamterene and Hydrochlorothiazide—**See Diuretics, Potassium-sparing, and Hydrochlorothiazide (Systemic)**, 1272, MC-31
*Dycill*—Beecham (U.S.) brand of Dicloxacillin—**See Penicillins (Systemic)**, 2240
*Dyclocaine*—Dyclonine—**See Anesthetics (Mucosal-Local)**, 128
*Dyclone*—Astra (U.S.) brand of Dyclonine—**See Anesthetics (Mucosal-Local)**, 128
Dyclonine Hydrochloride [dyclocaine; *Dyclone; Sucrets, Children's; Sucrets Maximum Strength; Sucrets Regular Strength*]
    **See Anesthetics (Mucosal-Local)**, 128
    Lozenges, 135
    Solution, Topical, USP, 136
*Dyflos*—Isoflurophate—**See Antiglaucoma Agents, Cholinergic, Long-acting (Ophthalmic)**, 315
*Dymelor*—Lilly (U.S.) brand of Acetohexamide—**See Antidiabetic Agents, Sulfonylurea (Systemic)**, 283
*Dynabac*—Sanofi Winthrop (U.S.) brand of Dirithromycin (Systemic), 1250, MC-10
*Dynacin*—Medicis (U.S.) brand of Minocycline—**See Tetracyclines (Systemic)**, 2765
*DynaCirc*—Novartis (U.S.) brand of Isradipine—**See Calcium Channel Blocking Agents (Systemic)**, 720, MC-16
*Dynafed Maximum Strength*—BDI (U.S.) brand of Pseudoephedrine and Acetaminophen—**See Decongestants and Analgesics (Systemic)**, 1180
Dynamine
    (Systemic), 3141
*Dynapen*—Apothecon (U.S.) brand of Dicloxacillin—**See Penicillins (Systemic)**, 2240
Dyphylline [*Dilor; Dilor-400;* diprophylline; *Lufyllin; Lufyllin-400*]
    (Systemic), #
    Elixir USP, #
    Injection USP, #
    Tablets USP, #, MC-10
Dyphylline and Guaifenesin [*Panfil-G*]
    (Systemic)
    Capsules, MC-10
*Dyrenium*—SmithKline Beecham (U.S. and Canada) brand of Triamterene—**See Diuretics, Potassium-sparing (Systemic)**, 1266, MC-31
*Dyspep HB*—ICN (Canada) brand of Famotidine—**See Histamine H$_2$-receptor Antagonists (Systemic)**, 1633, MC-12
*Dysport*—Porton (U.S.) brand of Botulinum Toxin Type A (Parenteral-Local), 3134

# E

*E2020*—**See Donepezil (Systemic)**, 1290
*Earache Drops*—Regal (Canada) brand of Antipyrine and Benzocaine (Otic), 443
*Ear Drops*—Rugby (U.S.) brand of Antipyrine and Benzocaine (Otic), 443
*Ear-Eze*—Hyrex (U.S.) brand of Neomycin, Polymyxin B, and Hydrocortisone (Otic), #
*Easprin*—PD (U.S.) brand of Aspirin—**See Salicylates (Systemic)**, 2538
*E-Base*—Barr (U.S.) brand of Erythromycin Base—**See Erythromycins (Systemic)**, 1368
*ECD*—**See Technetium Tc 99m Bicisate (Systemic)**, 2703
Echothiophate Iodide [ecothiopate iodide; *Phospholine Iodide*]
    **See Antiglaucoma Agents, Cholinergic, Long-acting (Ophthalmic)**, 315
    for Solution, Ophthalmic, USP, 318
*Eclipse Lip & Face Protectant*—Triangle Labs (U.S.) brand of Oxybenzone and Padimate O—**See Sunscreen Agents (Topical)**, #
*Eclipse Original Sunscreen*—Triangle Labs (U.S.) brand of Lisadimate and Padimate O—**See Sunscreen Agents (Topical)**, #
*E-C Naprosyn*—Roche (U.S.) brand of Naproxen—**See Anti-inflammatory Drugs, Nonsteroidal (Systemic)**, 388, MC-21
*E-Complex-600*—Nature's Bounty (U.S.) brand of Vitamin E (Systemic), 2972
Econazole Nitrate [*Ecostatin; Spectazole*]
    (Topical), 1323
    Cream, 1324
Econazole Nitrate [*Ecostatin Vaginal Ovules*]
    **See Antifungals, Azole (Vaginal)**, 310
    Suppositories, Vaginal, 313

*Econochlor Ophthalmic Ointment*—Alcon (U.S.) brand of Chloramphenicol (Ophthalmic), #
*Econochlor Ophthalmic Solution*—Alcon (U.S.) brand of Chloramphenicol (Ophthalmic), #
*Econopred*—Alcon (U.S.) brand of Prednisolone—**See Corticosteroids (Ophthalmic)**, 966
*Econopred Plus*—Alcon (U.S.) brand of Prednisolone—**See Corticosteroids (Ophthalmic)**, 966
*Ecostatin*—Squibb (Canada) brand of Econazole (Topical), 1323
*Ecostatin Vaginal Ovules*—Westwood-Squibb (Canada) brand of Econazole—**See Antifungals, Azole (Vaginal)**, 310
*Ecothiopate*—Echothiophate—**See Antiglaucoma Agents, Cholinergic, Long-acting (Ophthalmic)**, 315
*Ecotrin Caplets*—SmithKline Beecham (U.S.) brand of Aspirin—**See Salicylates (Systemic)**, 2538
*Ecotrin Tablets*—SmithKline Beecham (U.S.) brand of Aspirin—**See Salicylates (Systemic)**, 2538
*Ectosone Mild*—Technilab (Canada) brand of Betamethasone—**See Corticosteroids (Topical)**, 978
*Ectosone Regular*—Technilab (Canada) brand of Betamethasone—**See Corticosteroids (Topical)**, 978
*Ectosone Scalp Lotion*—Technilab (Canada) brand of Betamethasone—**See Corticosteroids (Topical)**, 978
*E-Cypionate*—Legere (U.S.) brand of Estradiol—**See Estrogens (Systemic)**, 1383
*Ed A-Hist*—Edwards (U.S.) brand of Chlorpheniramine and Phenylephrine—**See Antihistamines and Decongestants (Systemic)**, 343
Edathamil calcium disodium—**See Edetate Calcium Disodium (Systemic)**, 1324
Edathamil disodium—**See Edetate Disodium (Ophthalmic)**, #; **Edetate Disodium (Systemic)**, 1327
*Ed-Bron G*—Edwards (U.S.) brand of Theophylline and Guaifenesin (Systemic), #
*Edecrin*—Merck (U.S. and Canada) brand of Ethacrynic Acid—**See Diuretics, Loop (Systemic)**, 1259
Edetate Calcium Disodium [*Calcium Disodium Versenate;* calcium EDTA; edathamil calcium disodium; sodium calcium edetate]
    (Systemic), 1324
    Injection USP, 1326
Edetate Disodium [disodium EDTA; edathamil disodium; ethylene diamine tetraacetic acid; sodium edetate]
    (Ophthalmic), #
    Solution, Ophthalmic, #
Edetate Disodium [disodium EDTA; *Disotate;* edathamil disodium; *Endrate;* sodium edetate]
    (Systemic), 1327
    Injection USP, 1329
*Edex*—Schwarz (U.S.) brand of Alprostadil (Local), 48
Edrophonium Chloride [*Enlon; Reversol; Tensilon*]
    (Systemic), 1329
    Injection USP, 1330
Edrophonium Chloride and Atropine Sulfate [*Enlon-Plus*]
    (Systemic), 1331
    Injection, 1333
*ED-TLC*—Edwards (U.S.) brand of Chlorpheniramine, Phenylephrine, and Hydrocodone—**See Cough/Cold Combinations (Systemic)**, 1024
*ED Tuss HC*—Edwards (U.S.) brand of Chlorpheniramine, Phenylephrine, and Hydrocodone—**See Cough/Cold Combinations (Systemic)**, 1024
*E.E.S.*—Abbott (U.S. and Canada) brand of Erythromycin Ethylsuccinate—**See Erythromycins (Systemic)**, 1368, MC-11
*Efed II Yellow*—Alto (U.S.) brand of Phenylpropanolamine (Systemic), 2314
*Effective Strength Cough Formula*—Barre-National (U.S.) brand of Chlorpheniramine and Dextromethorphan—**See Cough/Cold Combinations (Systemic)**, 1024
*Effective Strength Cough Formula with Decongestant*—Barre-National (U.S.) brand of Pseudoephedrine and Dextromethorphan—**See Cough/Cold Combinations (Systemic)**, 1024
*Effer-K*—Nomax (U.S.) brand of Potassium Bicarbonate and Potassium Citrate—**See Potassium Supplements (Systemic)**, 2357
*Effer-syllium*—J & J-Merck (U.S.) brand of Psyllium Hydrophilic Mucilloid—**See Laxatives (Local)**, #
*Effexor*—Wyeth-Ayerst (U.S. and Canada) brand of Venlafaxine (Systemic), 2940, MC-32

*Effexor XR*—Wyeth-Ayerst (U.S. and Canada) brand of Venlafaxine (Systemic), 2940
*Efidac/24*—Ciba (U.S.) brand of Pseudoephedrine (Systemic), 2422
*Eflone*—Ciba Vision (U.S.) brand of Fluorometholone—**See Corticosteroids (Ophthalmic)**, 966
Eflornithine Hydrochloride [alpha-difluoromethylornithine; DFMO; *Ornidyl*]
 **(Systemic)**, #, 3141
 Concentrate for Injection, #
*Efudex*—Roche (U.S. and Canada) brand of Fluorouracil (Topical), 1500
*E/Gel*—Fulton (U.S.) brand of Erythromycin (Topical), 3018
EHDP—*See* Etidronate (Systemic), 1419
*E-200 I.U. Softgels*—Nature's Bounty (U.S.) brand of Vitamin E (Systemic), 2972
*E-1000 I.U. Softgels*—Nature's Bounty (U.S.) brand of Vitamin E (Systemic), 2972
*E-400 I.U. in a Water Soluble Base*—Nature's Bounty (U.S.) brand of Vitamin E (Systemic), 2972
*Elavil*—ZENECA (U.S.) and MSD (Canada) brand of Amitriptyline—**See Antidepressants, Tricyclic (Systemic)**, 271, MC-2
*Elavil Plus*—MSD (Canada) brand of Perphenazine and Amitriptyline (Systemic), 2286
Elcatonin
 **(Systemic)**, 3141
*Eldepryl*—Somerset (U.S.) and Deprenyl Research (Canada) brand of Selegiline (Systemic), 2560, MC-28; Somerset (U.S.) brand of Selegiline (Systemic), 3164
*Eldisine*—Lilly (Canada) brand of Vindesine (Systemic), 3037
*Elementra*—Clintec (U.S.) brand of Enteral Nutrition Formula, Modular—**See Enteral Nutrition Formulas (Systemic)**, #
*Elimite*—Herbert (U.S.) brand of Permethrin (Topical), 3032
*Elixophyllin*—Forest (U.S.) brand of Theophylline— **See Bronchodilators, Theophylline (Systemic)**, 668
*Elixophyllin-GG*—Forest (U.S.) brand of Theophylline and Guaifenesin (Systemic), #
Elliott's B Solution
 **(Systemic)**, 3141
*Elmiron*—Baker Norton (U.S. and Canada) brand of Pentosan (Systemic), 2277, MC-24; Baker Norton (U.S.) brand of Pentosan Polysulphate (Systemic), 3157
*Elocom*—Schering (Canada) brand of Mometasone— **See Corticosteroids (Topical)**, 978
*Elocon*—Schering (U.S.) brand of Mometasone—**See Corticosteroids (Topical)**, 978
*E-Lor*—Forest (U.S.) brand of Propoxyphene and Acetaminophen—**See Opioid (Narcotic) Analgesics and Acetaminophen (Systemic)**, 2198
*Elspar*—MSD (U.S.) brand of Asparaginase (Systemic), 474
*Eltor 120*—Marion Merrell Dow (Canada) brand of Pseudoephedrine (Systemic), 2422
*Eltroxin*—Glaxo (Canada) brand of Levothyroxine— **See Thyroid Hormones (Systemic)**, 2809
*Emadine*—Alcon (U.S.) brand of Emedastine (Ophthalmic), 1333
*Embrace*—Safetex (U.S. and Canada) brand of Latex Condoms—**See Condoms**, #
*Emcyt*—Roche (U.S. and Canada) brand of Estramustine (Systemic), 1380
Emedastine Difumarate [*Emadine*]
 **(Ophthalmic)**, 1333
 Solution, Ophthalmic, 1334
*Emertabs*—Pharmetics (Canada) brand of Phenylpropanolamine, Acetaminophen, and Caffeine— **See Decongestants and Analgesics (Systemic)**, 1180
*Emetrol*—Bock (U.S.) and Adria (Canada) brand of Fructose, Dextrose, and Phosphoric Acid (Oral-Local), 1532
*Emgel*—Glaxo (U.S.) brand of Erythromycin (Topical), 3018
*Eminase*—Roberts (U.S. and Canada) brand of Anistreplase—**See Thrombolytic Agents (Systemic)**, 2799
*Emko*—Schering (U.S. and Canada) brand of Nonoxynol 9—**See Spermicides (Vaginal)**, #
EMLA—Astra (U.S. and Canada) brand of Lidocaine and Prilocaine (Topical), #
*Emo-Cort*—T.C.D. (Canada) brand of Hydrocortisone—**See Corticosteroids (Topical)**, 978

*Emo-Cort Scalp Solution*—T.C.D. (Canada) brand of Hydrocortisone—**See Corticosteroids (Topical)**, 978
*Empirin*—Glaxo Wellcome (U.S.) brand of Aspirin— **See Salicylates (Systemic)**, 2538
*Empirin with Codeine No.3*—Glaxo Wellcome (U.S.) brand of Aspirin and Codeine—**See Opioid (Narcotic) Analgesics and Aspirin (Systemic)**, 2202
*Empirin with Codeine No.4*—Glaxo Wellcome (U.S.) brand of Aspirin and Codeine—**See Opioid (Narcotic) Analgesics and Aspirin (Systemic)**, 2202
*Empracet-30*—BW (Canada) brand of Acetaminophen and Codeine—**See Opioid (Narcotic) Analgesics and Acetaminophen (Systemic)**, 2198
*Empracet-60*—BW (Canada) brand of Acetaminophen and Codeine—**See Opioid (Narcotic) Analgesics and Acetaminophen (Systemic)**, 2198
*Emtec-30*—Technilab (Canada) brand of Acetaminophen and Codeine—**See Opioid (Narcotic) Analgesics and Acetaminophen (Systemic)**, 2198
*Emulsoil*—Paddock (U.S.) brand of Castor Oil—**See Laxatives (Local)**, #
*E-Mycin*—Knoll (U.S. and Canada) brand of Erythromycin Base—**See Erythromycins (Systemic)**, 1368, MC-11
Enadoline Hydrochloride
 **(Systemic)**, 3141
Enalaprilat [*Vasotec*]
 **See Angiotensin-converting Enzyme (ACE) Inhibitors (Systemic)**, 177
 Injection, 184
Enalapril-containing Combinations, 3072
Enalapril Maleate [*Vasotec*]
 **See Angiotensin-converting Enzyme (ACE) Inhibitors (Systemic)**, 177
 Tablets USP, 184, MC-11
Enalapril Maleate and Diltiazem Maleate [*Teczem*]
 **(Systemic)**, 1334
 Tablets, Extended-release, 1339
Enalapril Maleate and Felodipine [*Lexxel*]
 **(Systemic)**, 1339
 Tablets, 1343, MC-11
Enalapril Maleate and Hydrochlorothiazide [*Vaseretic*]
 **See Angiotensin-converting Enzyme (ACE) Inhibitors and Hydrochlorothiazide (Systemic)**, 187
 Tablets, 188, MC-11
Encainide Hydrochloride
 **(Systemic)**, 1344
 Capsules, 1346
Encapsulated Porcine Islet Preparation [*Betarx*]
 **(Systemic)**, 3141
*Encare*—Thompson (U.S.) brand of Nonoxynol 9— **See Spermicides (Vaginal)**, #
*Endafed*—Forest (U.S.) brand of Brompheniramine and Pseudoephedrine—**See Antihistamines and Decongestants (Systemic)**, 343
*Endagen-HD*—Abana (U.S.) brand of Chlorpheniramine, Phenylephrine, and Hydrocodone—**See Cough/Cold Combinations (Systemic)**, 1024
*Endal*—Forest (U.S.) brand of Phenylephrine and Guaifenesin—**See Cough/Cold Combinations (Systemic)**, 1024
*Endal Expectorant*—Forest (U.S.) brand of Phenylpropanolamine, Codeine, and Guaifenesin—**See Cough/Cold Combinations (Systemic)**, 1024
*Endal-HD*—Forest (U.S.) brand of Chlorpheniramine, Phenylephrine, and Hydrocodone—**See Cough/Cold Combinations (Systemic)**, 1024
*Endal-HD Plus*—Forest (U.S.) brand of Chlorpheniramine, Phenylephrine, and Hydrocodone—**See Cough/Cold Combinations (Systemic)**, 1024
*Endep*—Roche (U.S.) brand of Amitriptyline—**See Antidepressants, Tricyclic (Systemic)**, 271
*Endocaine*—Jayco (Canada) brand of Benzocaine— **See Anesthetics (Topical)**, 155
*Endocet*—Endo (U.S. and Canada) brand of Oxycodone and Acetaminophen—**See Opioid (Narcotic) Analgesics and Acetaminophen (Systemic)**, 2198
*Endodan*—Endo (U.S. and Canada) brand of Oxycodone and Aspirin—**See Opioid (Narcotic) Analgesics and Aspirin (Systemic)**, 2202
*Endolor*—Keene (U.S.) brand of Butalbital, Acetaminophen, and Caffeine—**See Barbiturates and Analgesics (Systemic)**, 532

*Endrate*—Abbott (U.S.) brand of Edetate Disodium (Systemic), 1327
*Endur-Acin*—Innovite (U.S.) brand of Niacin—**See Niacin (Systemic)**, 2116
*Enduron*—Abbott (U.S.) brand of Methyclothiazide— **See Diuretics, Thiazide (Systemic)**, 1273, MC-19
*Enduronyl*—Abbott (U.S.) brand of Deserpidine and Methyclothiazide—**See Rauwolfia Alkaloids and Thiazide Diuretics (Systemic)**, #
*Enduronyl Forte*—Abbott (U.S.) brand of Deserpidine and Methyclothiazide—**See Rauwolfia Alkaloids and Thiazide Diuretics (Systemic)**, #
*Enecat*—Lafayette (U.S.) brand of Barium Sulfate (Local), #
*Enemol*—Pharmascience (Canada) brand of Sodium Phosphates—**See Laxatives (Local)**, #
*Enercal*—Wyeth (U.S.) brand of Enteral Nutrition Formula, Polymeric—**See Enteral Nutrition Formulas (Systemic)**, #
*Enerjets*—Chilton (U.S.) brand of Caffeine (Systemic), 706
*Enfamil*—Mead Johnson (U.S.) brand of Infant Formulas, Milk-based—**See Infant Formulas (Systemic)**, #
*Enfamil Human Milk Fortifier*—Mead Johnson (U.S.) brand of Infant Formulas, Milk-based—**See Infant Formulas (Systemic)**, #
*Enfamil with Iron*—Mead Johnson (U.S.) brand of Infant Formulas, Milk-based—**See Infant Formulas (Systemic)**, #
*Enfamil Premature Formula*—Mead Johnson (U.S.) brand of Infant Formulas, Milk-based—**See Infant Formulas (Systemic)**, #
*Enfamil Premature Formula with Iron*—Mead Johnson (U.S.) brand of Infant Formulas, Milk-based—**See Infant Formulas (Systemic)**, #
Enflurane [*Ethrane*]
 **See Anesthetics, Inhalation (Systemic)**, 168
 Enflurane USP, 171
*Engerix-B*—SKF (U.S. and Canada) brand of Hepatitis B Vaccine Recombinant (Systemic), 1628
Enhanced-potency IPV—Poliovirus Vaccine Inactivated Enhanced Potency—**See Poliovirus Vaccine (Systemic)**, 2343
*Enlon*—Ohmeda (U.S. and Canada) brand of Edrophonium (Systemic), 1329
*Enlon-Plus*—Ohmeda (U.S.) brand of Edrophonium and Atropine (Systemic), 1331
*Enomine*—Major (U.S.) brand of Phenylephrine, Phenylpropanolamine, and Guaifenesin—**See Cough/Cold Combinations (Systemic)**, 1024
Enoxacin [*Penetrex*]
 **See Fluoroquinolones (Systemic)**, 1487
 Tablets, 1493, MC-11
Enoxaparin [*Lovenox*]
 **(Systemic)**, 1346
 Injection, 1349
*Ensure*—Ross (U.S. and Canada) brand of Enteral Nutrition Formula, Polymeric—**See Enteral Nutrition Formulas (Systemic)**, #
*Ensure with Fiber*—Ross (U.S.) brand of Enteral Nutrition Formula, Fiber-containing—**See Enteral Nutrition Formulas (Systemic)**, #
*Ensure High Protein*—Ross (U.S.) brand of Enteral Nutrition Formula, Polymeric—**See Enteral Nutrition Formulas (Systemic)**, #
*Ensure HN*—Ross (U.S.) brand of Enteral Nutrition Formula, Polymeric—**See Enteral Nutrition Formulas (Systemic)**, #
*Ensure Plus*—Ross (U.S. and Canada) brand of Enteral Nutrition Formula, Polymeric—**See Enteral Nutrition Formulas (Systemic)**, #
*Ensure Plus HN*—Ross (U.S.) brand of Enteral Nutrition Formula, Polymeric—**See Enteral Nutrition Formulas (Systemic)**, #
*E.N.T.*—Ion (U.S.) brand of Brompheniramine and Phenylpropanolamine—**See Antihistamines and Decongestants (Systemic)**, 343
*Entacyl*—Glaxo (Canada) brand of Piperazine (Systemic), #
Entamide—*See* Diloxanide (Systemic), #
Enteral Nutrition Formula, Blenderized [*Compleat Modified; Compleat Regular; Vitaneed*]
 **See Enteral Nutrition Formulas (Systemic)**, #
 Solution, Oral, #

Enteral Nutrition Formula, Disease-specific [*Advera; Amin-Aid; Citrotein; Crucial; DiabetiSource; Glucerna; Glytol; Hepatic-Aid II; Immun-Aid; Impact; Impact with Fiber; Lipisorb; Magnacal; Nepro; Nutren 2.0; NutriHep; NutriVent; Peptamen; Peptamen Junior; Peptamen VHP; Perative; Protain XL; Pulmocare; Respalor; Suplena; TraumaCal; Traum-Aid HBC; Travasorb Renal Diet*]
  **See Enteral Nutrition Formulas (Systemic)**, #
  Solution, Oral, #
  for Solution, Oral, #
Enteral Nutrition Formula, Fiber-containing [*Ensure with Fiber; Fiberlan; Fibersource; Fibersource HN; Glytrol; Impact with Fiber; IsoSource VHN; Jevity; Kindercal; NuBasics wth Fiber; Nutren 1.0 with Fiber; NutriSource; NutriSource HN; Pediasure with Fiber; ProBalance; Profiber; Promote with Fiber; Replete with Fiber; Sustacal with Fiber; Ultracal*]
  **See Enteral Nutrition Formulas (Systemic)**, #
  Solution, Oral, #
Enteral Nutrition Formula, Milk-based [*Carnation Instant Breakfast; Carnation Instant Breakfast No Sugar Added; Great Shake; Great Shake Jr.; Menu Magic Instant Breakfast; Menu Magic Milk Shake; Meritene; 206 Shake; Sustagen; Tasty Shake*]
  **See Enteral Nutrition Formulas (Systemic)**, #
  Solution, Oral, #
  for Solution, Oral, #
Enteral Nutrition Formula, Modular [*Casec; Elementra; MCT Oil; Microlipid; Moducal; Polycose; ProMod; Propac Plus; Sumacal*]
  **See Enteral Nutrition Formulas (Systemic)**, #
  Powder, Oral, #
  Solution, Oral, #
Enteral Nutrition Formula, Monomeric (Elemental) [*Accupep HPF; Alitraq; Criticare HN; Peptamen; Peptamen Junior; Peptamen VHP; Reabilan; Reabilan HN; SandoSource Peptide; Tolerex; Travasorb HN; Travasorb STD; Vital High Nitrogen; Vivonex Pediatric; Vivonex Plus; Vivonex T.E.N.*]
  **See Enteral Nutrition Formulas (Systemic)**, #
  Solution, Oral, #
  for Solution, Oral, #
Enteral Nutrition Formula, Polymeric [*Attain; CitriSource; Citrotein; Comply; Deliver 2.0; Enercal; Ensure; Ensure High Protein; Ensure HN; Ensure Plus; Ensure Plus HN; Entrition Half-Strength; Entrition HN; Introlan; Introlite; Isocal; Isocal HN; Isolan; Isosource; Isosource HN; Isotein HN; Magnacal; NuBasics; NuBasics Plus; NuBasics VHP; Nutren 1.0; Nutren 1.5; Nutren 2.0; Nutrilan; Osmolite; Osmolite HN; Pediasure; Pre-Attain; Promote; Replete; Resource; Resource Plus; Sustacal; Sustacal Basic; Sustacal Plus; TwoCal HN; Ultralan*]
  **See Enteral Nutrition Formulas (Systemic)**, #
  Solution, Oral, #
  for Solution, Oral, #
Enteral Nutrition Formulas **(Systemic)**, #
*Entero-H*—E-Z-EM (U.S.) brand of Barium Sulfate (Local), #
*Entex*—Dura (U.S.) brand of Phenylephrine, Phenylpropanolamine, and Guaifenesin—**See Cough/Cold Combinations (Systemic)**, 1024, MC-25
*Entex LA*—Dura (U.S. and Canada) brand of Phenylpropanolamine and Guaifenesin—**See Cough/Cold Combinations (Systemic)**, 1024, MC-25
*Entex Liquid*—Procter & Gamble (U.S.) brand of Phenylephrine, Phenylpropanolamine, and Guaifenesin—**See Cough/Cold Combinations (Systemic)**, 1024
*Entex PSE*—Dura (U.S.) brand of Pseudoephedrine and Guaifenesin—**See Cough/Cold Combinations (Systemic)**, 1024, MC-27
*Entocort*—Astra (Canada) brand of Budesonide—**See Corticosteroids (Rectal)**, 973; Astra (Canada) brand of Budesonide (Systemic), 3012
*Entrition Half-Strength*—Clintec (U.S.) brand of Enteral Nutrition Formula, Polymeric—**See Enteral Nutrition Formulas (Systemic)**, #
*Entrition HN*—Clintec (U.S.) brand of Enteral Nutrition Formula, Polymeric—**See Enteral Nutrition Formulas (Systemic)**, #
*Entrobar*—Lafayette (U.S.) brand of Barium Sulfate (Local), #
*Entrophen Caplets*—Frosst (Canada) brand of Aspirin—**See Salicylates (Systemic)**, 2538

*Entrophen Extra Strength*—Frosst (Canada) brand of Aspirin—**See Salicylates (Systemic)**, 2538
*Entrophen 15 Maximum Strength Tablets*—Frosst (Canada) brand of Aspirin—**See Salicylates (Systemic)**, 2538
*Entrophen 10 Super Strength Caplets*—Aspirin—**See Salicylates (Systemic)**, 2538
*Entrophen Tablets*—Frosst (Canada) brand of Aspirin—**See Salicylates (Systemic)**, 2538
*Entuss-D*—Roberts (U.S.) brand of Pseudoephedrine, Hydrocodone, and Guaifenesin—**See Cough/Cold Combinations (Systemic)**, 1024; Roberts (U.S.) brand of Pseudoephedrine, Hydrocodone and Potassium Guaiacolsulfonate—**See Cough/Cold Combinations (Systemic)**, 1024
*Entuss-D Jr.*—Roberts (U.S.) brand of Pseudoephedrine, Hydrocodone, and Guaifenesin—**See Cough/Cold Combinations (Systemic)**, 1024
*Entuss Expectorant*—Roberts (U.S.) brand of Hydrocodone and Guaifenesin—**See Cough/Cold Combinations (Systemic)**, 1024; Roberts (U.S.) brand of Hydrocodone and Potassium Guaiacolsulfonate—**See Cough/Cold Combinations (Systemic)**, 1024
*Enulose*—Barre-National (U.S.) brand of Lactulose—**See Laxatives (Local)**, #
*Enzymase-16*—Econolab (U.S.) brand of Pancrelipase (Systemic), 2222
Enzyme Immunoassay Ovulation Prediction Test Kits [*Answer Ovulation; Clearplan Easy; Color Ovulation Test; Conceive Ovulation Predictor; First Response; Fortel; OvuGen; OvuKit; OvuKIT; OvuQuick; OvuQUICK; Q-test*]
  **See Ovulation Prediction Test Kits for Home Use**, #
  Test Kits, #
*Epatiol*—Medici (Italy) brand of Tiopronin (Systemic), 2824
Ephedrine-containing Combinations, 3072
Ephedrine Hydrochloride, Carbetapentane Citrate, and Guaifenesin [*Vicks Cough Syrup*]
  **See Cough/Cold Combinations (Systemic)**, 1024
  Syrup, 1112
Ephedrine Hydrochloride and Guaifenesin [*Broncholate*]
  **See Cough/Cold Combinations (Systemic)**, 1024
  Syrup, 1038
Ephedrine Hydrochloride and Potassium Iodide [*KIE*]
  **See Cough/Cold Combinations (Systemic)**, 1024
  Syrup, 1068
Ephedrine Sulfate
  **See Bronchodilators, Adrenergic (Systemic)**, 651
  Capsules USP, 656
  Injection USP, 656
Ephedrine Sulfate
  **See Sympathomimetic Agents—Cardiovascular Use (Parenteral-Systemic)**, 2669
  Injection USP, 2676
*Epi-C*—Lafayette (U.S.) brand of Barium Sulfate (Local), #
Epidermal Growth Factor (Human) **(Ophthalmic)**, 3141
*Epifoam*—Reed & Carnrick (U.S.) brand of Hydrocortisone—**See Corticosteroids (Topical)**, 978
*Epifrin*—Allergan (U.S. and Canada) brand of Epinephrine (Ophthalmic), 1350
*Epimorph*—Wyeth-Ayerst (Canada) brand of Morphine—**See Opioid (Narcotic) Analgesics (Systemic)**, 2168
*Epinal*—Akorn (U.S.) brand of Epinephryl Borate—**See Epinephrine (Ophthalmic)**, 1350
Epinephrine [*Epifrin; Glaucon*] **(Ophthalmic)**, 1350
  Solution, Ophthalmic, USP, 1351
Epinephrine [*Adrenalin; Adrenalin Chloride Solution; Ana-Guard; EpiPen Auto-Injector; EpiPen Jr. Auto-Injector; Sus-Phrine*]
  **See Bronchodilators, Adrenergic (Systemic)**, 651
  Injection USP, 657
  Suspension, Sterile, 658
Epinephrine [*Adrenalin Chloride; adrenaline; Bronkaid Mist; Bronkaid Mistometer; Primatene Mist*]
  **See Bronchodilators, Adrenergic (Inhalation-Local)**, 640
  Aerosol, Inhalation, USP, 646
  Solution, Inhalation, USP, 647

Epinephrine Bitartrate [*Asthmahaler Mist; Bronkaid Suspension Mist*]
  **See Bronchodilators, Adrenergic (Inhalation-Local)**, 640
  Aerosol, Inhalation, USP, 647
Epinephrine-containing Combinations, 3072
Epinephrine Hydrochloride [*Adrenalin*]
  **See Sympathomimetic Agents—Cardiovascular Use (Parenteral-Systemic)**, 2669
  Injection, 2676
Epinephryl Borate [*Epinal; Eppy/N*]
  **See Epinephrine (Ophthalmic)**, 1350
  Solution, Ophthalmic, USP, 1351
*EpiPen Auto-Injector*—Center (U.S.) and Allerex (Canada) brand of Epinephrine—**See Bronchodilators, Adrenergic (Systemic)**, 651
*EpiPen Jr. Auto-Injector*—Center (U.S.) and Allerex (Canada) brand of Epinephrine—**See Bronchodilators, Adrenergic (Systemic)**, 651
Epirubicin Hydrochloride [*Pharmorubicin PFS; Pharmorubicin RDF*]
  **(Systemic)**, 3018
  Injection, 3018
  for Injection, 3018
*Epistatin*—Simvastatin—**See HMG-CoA Reductase Inhibitors (Systemic)**, 1647
*Epitol*—Lemmon (U.S.) brand of Carbamazepine (Systemic), 757
*Epival*—Abbott (Canada) brand of Divalproex—**See Valproic Acid (Systemic)**, 2908
*Epivir*—Glaxo Wellcome (U.S.) brand of Lamivudine (Systemic), 1819, MC-16
EPO—*See* Epoetin alfa (Systemic), 1352
Epoetin Alfa [*Epogen;* erythropoietin, recombinant human; *Procrit*]
  **(Systemic)**, 3142
Epoetin Alfa, Recombinant [EPO; *Epogen; Eprex;* erythropoietin, recombinant human; r-HuEPO; *Procrit*]
  **(Systemic)**, 1352
  Injection, 1355
Epoetin Beta [*Marogen*]
  **(Systemic)**, 3142
*Epogen*—Amgen (U.S.) brand of Epoetin Alfa (Systemic), 3141, 3142; Amgen (U.S.) brand of Epoetin alfa (Systemic), 1352
Epoprostenol [*Flolan*]
  **(Systemic)**, 3142
*Eppy/N*—Akorn (U.S.) brand of Epinephryl Borate—**See Epinephrine (Ophthalmic)**, 1350
*Eprex*—Janssen-Ortho (Canada) brand of Epoetin alfa (Systemic), 1352
*Epromate-M*—Major (U.S.) brand of Meprobamate and Aspirin (Systemic), #
Epsilon-aminocaproic acid—*See* Aminocaproic Acid (Systemic), 64
Epsom salts—Magnesium Sulfate—**See Laxatives (Local)**, #
*e.p.t*—Warner-Lambert (U.S.) brand of Immunoassay Pregnancy Test Kits—**See Pregnancy Test Kits for Home Use**, #
*Eptastatin*—Pravastatin—**See HMG-CoA Reductase Inhibitors (Systemic)**, 1647
Eptifibatide [*Integrilin*]
  **(Systemic)**, 1356
  Injection, 1357
*Equagesic*—Wyeth-Ayerst (U.S.) and Wyeth (Canada) brand of Meprobamate and Aspirin (Systemic), #
*Equalactin*—Numark (U.S.) brand of Polycarbophil—**See Laxatives (Local)**, #
*Equanil*—Wyeth-Ayerst (U.S.) and Wyeth (Canada) brand of Meprobamate (Systemic), #
*Equibron G*—Equipharm (U.S.) brand of Theophylline and Guaifenesin (Systemic), #
*Equilet*—Mission (U.S.) brand of Calcium Carbonate—**See Antacids (Oral-Local)**, 188
*Ercaf*—Geneva (U.S.) and Harber (U.S.) brand of Ergotamine and Caffeine—**See Vascular Headache Suppressants, Ergot Derivative–containing (Systemic)**, 2925, MC-11
*Ergamisol*—Janssen (U.S. and Canada) brand of Levamisole (Systemic), 1844
*Ergo-Caff*—Rugby (U.S.) brand of Ergotamine and Caffeine—**See Vascular Headache Suppressants, Ergot Derivative–containing (Systemic)**, 2925
Ergocalciferol [*Calciferol; Calciferol Drops; Deltalin; Drisdol; Drisdol Drops; Ostoforte; Radiostol Forte;* vitamin D]
  **See Vitamin D and Analogs (Systemic)**, 2966
  Capsules USP, 2971, MC-11

## General Index

Ergocalciferol *(continued)*
   Injection, 2972
   Solution, Oral, USP, 2972
   Tablets USP, 2972
*Ergodryl*—PD (Canada) brand of Ergotamine, Caffeine, and Diphenhydramine—**See Vascular Headache Suppressants, Ergot Derivative–containing (Systemic)**, 2925
Ergoloid Mesylates [dihydrogenated ergot alkaloids; *Gerimal; Hydergine; Hydergine LC*]
   **(Systemic)**, 1358
   Capsules, 1359, MC-11
   Solution, Oral, USP, 1359
   Tablets USP, 1359, MC-11
   Tablets USP (Sublingual), 1359
*Ergomar*—Fisons (Canada) brand of Ergotamine—**See Vascular Headache Suppressants, Ergot Derivative–containing (Systemic)**, 2925
Ergometrine—*See* Ergonovine (Systemic), 1360
Ergonovine Maleate [ergometrine; *Ergotrate; Ergotrate Maleate*]
   **(Systemic)**, 1360
   Injection USP, 1362
   Tablets USP, 1362
*Ergostat*—PD (U.S.) brand of Ergotamine—**See Vascular Headache Suppressants, Ergot Derivative–containing (Systemic)**, 2925
Ergot alkaloids, dihydrogenated—*See* Ergoloid Mesylates (Systemic), 1358
Ergotamine-containing Combinations, 3073
Ergotamine Tartrate [*Ergomar; Ergostat; Gynergen; Medihaler Ergotamine*]
   **See Vascular Headache Suppressants, Ergot Derivative–containing (Systemic)**, 2925
   Aerosol, Inhalation, USP, 2933
   Tablets USP, 2933
   Tablets USP (Sublingual), 2933
Ergotamine Tartrate, Belladonna Alkaloids, and Phenobarbital Sodium [*Bellergal; Bellergal-S; Bellergal Spacetabs*]
   **(Systemic)**, 1363
   Tablets, 1363
   Tablets, Extended-release, 1364
Ergotamine Tartrate and Caffeine [*Cafergot; Cafertine; Cafetrate; Ercaf; Ergo-Caff; Gotamine; Migergot; Wigraine* (U.S.)]
   **See Vascular Headache Suppressants, Ergot Derivative–containing (Systemic)**, 2925
   Suppositories USP, 2934
   Tablets USP, 2934, MC-11
Ergotamine Tartrate, Caffeine, and Belladonna Alkaloids [*Wigraine* (Canada)]
   **See Vascular Headache Suppressants, Ergot Derivative–containing (Systemic)**, 2925
   Suppositories, 2935
   Tablets, 2935
Ergotamine Tartrate, Caffeine, Belladonna Alkaloids, and Pentobarbital [*Cafergot-PB*]
   **See Vascular Headache Suppressants, Ergot Derivative–containing (Systemic)**, 2925
   Suppositories, 2936
Ergotamine Tartrate, Caffeine, Belladonna Alkaloids, and Pentobarbital Sodium [*Cafergot-PB*]
   **See Vascular Headache Suppressants, Ergot Derivative–containing (Systemic)**, 2925
   Tablets, 2936
Ergotamine Tartrate, Caffeine, and Cyclizine [*Megral*]
   **See Vascular Headache Suppressants, Ergot Derivative–containing (Systemic)**, 2925
   Tablets, 2937
Ergotamine Tartrate, Caffeine, and Dimenhydrinate [*Gravergol*]
   **See Vascular Headache Suppressants, Ergot Derivative–containing (Systemic)**, 2925
   Capsules, 2937
Ergotamine Tartrate, Caffeine, and Diphenhydramine [*Ergodryl*]
   **See Vascular Headache Suppressants, Ergot Derivative–containing (Systemic)**, 2925
   Capsules, 2938
*Ergotrate*—Lilly (U.S.) brand of Ergonovine (Systemic), 1360
*Ergotrate Maleate*—Lilly (Canada) brand of Ergonovine (Systemic), 1360
*Eridium*—Hauck (U.S.) brand of Phenazopyridine (Systemic), 2288
Erirtrityl tetranitrate—Erythrityl Tetranitrate—**See Nitrates (Systemic)**, 2129
*Erwinase*—Porton (U.S.) brand of Erwinia l-Asparaginase (Systemic), 3142
Erwinia l-Asparaginase [*Erwinase*]
   **(Systemic)**, 3142

*Erybid*—Abbott (Canada) brand of Erythromycin Base—**See Erythromycins (Systemic)**, 1368
*Eryc*—Warner Chilcott (U.S.) brand of Erythromycin Base—**See Erythromycins (Systemic)**, 1368, MC-11
*ERYC-250*—PD (Canada) brand of Erythromycin Base—**See Erythromycins (Systemic)**, 1368
*ERYC-333*—PD (Canada) brand of Erythromycin Base—**See Erythromycins (Systemic)**, 1368
*Erycette*—Ortho (U.S.) brand of Erythromycin (Topical), 1365
*EryDerm*—Abbott (U.S.) brand of Erythromycin (Topical), 1365
*Erygel*—Allergan Herbert (U.S.) brand of Erythromycin (Topical), 1365
*Erymax*—Allergan Herbert (U.S.) brand of Erythromycin (Topical), 1365
*EryPed*—Abbott (U.S. and Canada) brand of Erythromycin Ethylsuccinate—**See Erythromycins (Systemic)**, 1368, MC-11
*Ery-Sol*—Dermol (U.S.) brand of Erythromycin (Topical), 1365
*Ery-Tab*—Abbott (U.S.) brand of Erythromycin Base—**See Erythromycins (Systemic)**, 1368, MC-11
*Erythra-Derm*—Paddock (U.S.) brand of Erythromycin (Topical), 3018
Erythritol tetranitrate—Erythrityl Tetranitrate—**See Nitrates (Systemic)**, 2129
Erythrityl Tetranitrate [*Cardilate*; eritrityl tetranitrate; erythritol tetranitrate]
   **See Nitrates (Systemic)**, 2129
   Tablets USP, 2132
*Erythro*—Balan (U.S.) brand of Erythromycin Ethylsuccinate—**See Erythromycins (Systemic)**, 1368
*Erythrocin*—Abbott (U.S. and Canada) brand of Erythromycin Lactobionate—**See Erythromycins (Systemic)**, 1368; Erythromycin Stearate—**See Erythromycins (Systemic)**, 1368, MC-11
*Erythrocot*—Truxton (U.S.) brand of Erythromycin Stearate—**See Erythromycins (Systemic)**, 1368
*Erythromid*—Abbott (Canada) brand of Erythromycin Base—**See Erythromycins (Systemic)**, 1368
Erythromycin [*E/Gel; Emgel; Erythra-Derm; Erythro-Statin; Theramycin Z*]
   **(Topical)**, 3018
   Gel, Topical, 3018
   Solution, Topical, USP, 3018
   Solution, Topical, 3018
Erythromycin [*Ilotycin*]
   **(Ophthalmic)**, 1364
   Ointment, Ophthalmic, USP, 1365
Erythromycin [*Akne-Mycin; A/T/S; Erycette; EryDerm; Erygel; Erymax; Ery-Sol; ETS; Sans-Acne; Staticin; T-Stat*]
   **(Topical)**, 1365
   Gel, Topical, 1367
   Ointment USP, 1366
   Pledgets USP, 1366
   Solution, Topical, USP, 1367
Erythromycin Base [*Apo-Erythro; Apo-Erythro E-C; E-Base; E-Mycin; Erybid; ERYC; ERYC-250; ERYC-333; Ery-Tab; Erythromid; Ilotycin; Novo-Rythro Encap; PCE*]
   **See Erythromycins (Systemic)**, 1368
   Capsules, Delayed-release, USP, 1372, MC-11
   Tablets USP, 1372, MC-11
   Tablets, Delayed-release, USP, 1373, MC-11
Erythromycin and Benzoyl Peroxide [*Benzamycin*]
   **(Topical)**, 1367
   Gel, Topical, USP, 1368
Erythromycin-containing Combinations, 3073
Erythromycin Estolate [*Ilosone; Novo-Rythro*]
   **See Erythromycins (Systemic)**, 1368
   Capsules USP, 1373, MC-11
   Suspension, Oral, USP, 1373
   Tablets USP, 1373, MC-11
Erythromycin ethyl succinate—Erythromycin Ethylsuccinate—**See Erythromycins (Systemic)**, 1368
Erythromycin Ethylsuccinate [*Apo-Erythro-ES; E.E.S.; EryPed; Erythro;* erythromycin ethyl succinate; *Novo-Rythro*]
   **See Erythromycins (Systemic)**, 1368
   Suspension, Oral, USP, 1374
   for Suspension, Oral, USP, 1374
   Tablets USP, 1374, MC-11
   Tablets USP (Chewable), 1374, MC-11

Erythromycin Ethylsuccinate and Sulfisoxazole Acetyl [*Eryzole; Pediazole; Sulfimycin*]
   **(Systemic)**, 1376
   for Suspension, Oral, USP, 1377
Erythromycin Gluceptate [*Ilotycin*]
   **See Erythromycins (Systemic)**, 1368
   Sterile USP, 1375
Erythromycin Lactobionate [*Erythrocin*]
   **See Erythromycins (Systemic)**, 1368
   for Injection USP, 1375
Erythromycins
   **(Systemic)**, 1368
Erythromycin Stearate [*Apo-Erythro-S; Erythrocin; Erythrocot; My-E; Novo-Rythro; Wintrocin*]
   **See Erythromycins (Systemic)**, 1368
   Suspension, Oral, 1376
   Tablets USP, 1376, MC-11
Erythropoietin, Recombinant Human—*See* Epoetin Alfa (Systemic), 3142; Epoetin Alfa, Recombinant (Systemic), 1352
Erythropoietin, Recombinant Human
   **(Systemic)**, 3142
*Erythro-Statin*—High-Tech Pharmacal (U.S.) brand of Erythromycin (Topical), 3018
*Eryzole*—Alra (U.S.) brand of Erythromycin and Sulfisoxazole (Systemic), 1376
*Eserine*—*See* Physostigmine (Systemic), 2322
*Eserine Salicylate*—Alcon (U.S.) brand of Physostigmine (Ophthalmic), #
*Eserine Sulfate*—CMC (U.S.); Harber (U.S.); Iolab (U.S.); Pharmaderm (U.S.); Pharmafair (U.S.); Pharmex (U.S.); Schein (U.S.); and Scrip (U.S.) brand of Physostigmine (Ophthalmic), #
*Esgic*—Forest (U.S.) brand of Butalbital, Acetaminophen, and Caffeine—**See Barbiturates and Analgesics (Systemic)**, 532
*Esgic-Plus*—Forest (U.S.) brand of Butalbital, Acetaminophen, and Caffeine—**See Barbiturates and Analgesics (Systemic)**, 532
*Esidrix*—Novartis (U.S.) brand of Hydrochlorothiazide—**See Diuretics, Thiazide (Systemic)**, 1273, MC-14
*Esimil*—Ciba (U.S.) brand of Guanethidine and Hydrochlorothiazide (Systemic), 3971
*Eskalith*—SmithKline Beecham (U.S.) brand of Lithium (Systemic), 1869, MC-17
*Eskalith CR*—SmithKline Beecham (U.S.) brand of Lithium (Systemic), 1869, MC-17
*Eskazole*—SmithKline Beecham (U.K.) brand of Albendazole (Systemic), #
Esmolol Hydrochloride [*Brevibloc*]
   **(Systemic)**, 1377
   Injection, 1379
*Esobar*—E-Z-EM (Canada) brand of Barium Sulfate (Local), #
*Esopho-CAT Esophageal Cream*—E-Z-EM (U.S. and Canada) brand of Barium Sulfate (Local), #
*Esophotrast Esophageal Cream*—Rhône-Poulenc Rorer (U.S.) brand of Barium Sulfate (Local), #
*Essential Care Creamy Dandruff Shampoo*—C&M (U.S.) brand of Salicylic Acid and Sulfur (Topical), #
*Estar*—Westwood (U.S.) and Westwood-Squibb (Canada) brand of Coal Tar (Topical), #
Estazolam [*ProSom*]
   **See Benzodiazepines (Systemic)**, 556
   Tablets, 572, MC-11
Esterified Estrogen–containing Combinations, 3073
Esterified estrogens—Estrogens, Esterified—**See Estrogens (Systemic)**, 1383
Esterified estrogens and methyltestosterone—Estrogens, Esterified, and Methyltestosterone—**See Androgens and Estrogens (Systemic)**, 126
*Estinyl*—Schering (U.S. and Canada) brand of Ethinyl Estradiol—**See Estrogens (Systemic)**, 1383
*Estivin II*—Alcon (U.S.) brand of Naphazoline (Ophthalmic), #
*Estrace*—Bristol-Myers Squibb (U.S.) brand of Estradiol—**See Estrogens (Vaginal)**, 1391; Mead Johnson (U.S.) and Roberts (Canada) brand of Estradiol—**See Estrogens (Systemic)**, 1383, MC-11
*Estraderm*—Ciba (U.S. and Canada) brand of Estradiol—**See Estrogens (Systemic)**, 1383
Estradiol [*Climara; Estrace; Estraderm;* Oestradiol; *Vivelle*]
   **See Estrogens (Systemic)**, 1383
   Systems, Transdermal (Matrix-type), 1390
   Systems, Transdermal (Reservoir-type), 1390
   Tablets USP, 1389, MC-11

Estradiol [*Estrace; Estring*]
　　**See Estrogens (Vaginal)**, 1391
　　Cream, Vaginal USP, 1395
　　Insert, Vaginal, 1395
Estradiol-containing Combinations, 3073
Estradiol Cypionate [*depGynogen; Depo-Estradiol; Depogen; Dura-Estrin; E-Cypionate; Estragyn LA 5; Estro-Cyp; Estrofem; Estro-L.A.*]
　　**See Estrogens (Systemic)**, 1383
　　Injection USP, 1389
Estradiol Valerate [*Clinagen LA 40; Delestrogen; Dioval 40; Dioval XX; Duragen-20; Estra-L 40; Estro-Span; Femogex; Gynogen L.A. 20; Gynogen L.A. 40; Menaval-20; Valergen-10; Valergen-20; Valergen-40*]
　　**See Estrogens (Systemic)**, 1383
　　Injection USP, 1389
*Estragyn 5*—Clint (U.S.) brand of Estrone—**See Estrogens (Systemic)**, 1383
*Estragyn LA 5*—Clint (U.S.) brand of Estradiol—**See Estrogens (Systemic)**, 1383
*Estra-L 40*—Pasadena (U.S.) brand of Estradiol—**See Estrogens (Systemic)**, 1383
Estramustine Phosphate Sodium [*Emcyt*]
　　**(Systemic)**, 1380
　　Capsules, 1383
*Estratab*—Solvay (U.S.) brand of Esterified Estrogens—**See Estrogens (Systemic)**, 1383, MC-12
*Estratest*—Solvay (U.S.) brand of Esterified Estrogens and Methyltestosterone—**See Androgens and Estrogens (Systemic)**, 126, MC-19
*Estratest H.S.*—Solvay (U.S.) brand of Esterified Estrogens and Methyltestosterone—**See Androgens and Estrogens (Systemic)**, 126, MC-19
*Estring*—Pharmacia & Upjohn (U.S.) and Pharmacia (Canada) brand of Estradiol—**See Estrogens (Vaginal)**, 1391
*Estro-A*—Hauser (U.S.) brand of Estrone—**See Estrogens (Systemic)**, 1383
*Estro-Cyp*—Keene (U.S.) brand of Estradiol—**See Estrogens (Systemic)**, 1383
*Estrofem*—Pasadena (U.S.) brand of Estradiol—**See Estrogens (Systemic)**, 1383
Estrogens
　　**(Systemic)**, 1383
Estrogens
　　**(Vaginal)**, 1391
Estrogens, Conjugated [*C.E.S.; Congest; Premarin; Premarin Intravenous*]
　　**See Estrogens (Systemic)**, 1383
　　for Injection, 1388
　　Tablets USP, 1388, MC-11
Estrogens, Conjugated [*Premarin*]
　　**See Estrogens (Vaginal)**, 1391
　　Cream, Vaginal, 1395
Estrogens, Conjugated, and Medroxyprogesterone Acetate [*Prempro*]
　　**See Conjugated Estrogens and Medroxyprogesterone for Ovarian H**, 946, 3023
　　Tablets
Estrogens, Conjugated, and Methyltestosterone [*Premarin with Methyltestosterone*]
　　**See Androgens and Estrogens (Systemic)**, 126
　　Tablets, 127
Estrogens, Esterified [*Estratab; Menest; Neo-Estrone*]
　　**See Estrogens (Systemic)**, 1383
　　Tablets USP, 1389, MC-12
Estrogens, Esterified, and Methyltestosterone [*Estratest; Estratest H.S.*]
　　**See Androgens and Estrogens (Systemic)**, 126
　　Tablets, 127
Estrogens and Progestins (Oral Contraceptives)
　　**(Systemic)**, 1397
*Estro-L.A.*—Hauser (U.S.) brand of Estradiol—**See Estrogens (Systemic)**, 1383
Estrone [*Aquest; Estragyn 5; Estro-A; Estrone '5'; Kestrone-5; oestrone; Wehgen*]
　　**See Estrogens (Systemic)**, 1383
　　Suspension, Injectable, USP, 1390
Estrone [*Oestrilin*]
　　**See Estrogens (Vaginal)**, 1391
　　Cream, Vaginal, 1396
　　Suppositories, Vaginal, 1396
*Estrone '5'*—Kay (U.S.) brand of Estrone—**See Estrogens (Systemic)**, 1383
Estropipate [*Ogen; Ogen .625; Ogen 1.25; Ogen 2.5; Ortho-Est .625; Ortho-Est 1.25;* piperazine estrone sulfate]
　　**See Estrogens (Systemic)**, 1383
　　Tablets USP, 1390, MC-12

Estropipate [*Ogen;* piperazine estrone sulfate]
　　**See Estrogens (Vaginal)**, 1391
　　Cream, Vaginal, USP, 1396
*Estro-Span*—Primedics (U.S.) brand of Estradiol—**See Estrogens (Systemic)**, 1383
*Estrostep*—PD (U.S.) brand of Norethindrone Acetate and Ethinyl Estradiol (Systemic), 1397
*Estrostep Fe*—PD (U.S.) brand of Norethindrone Acetate and Ethinyl Estradiol and Ferrous Fumarate (Systemic), 1397, MC-23
Etacrynic acid—Ethacrynic Acid—**See Diuretics, Loop (Systemic)**, 1259
Etafedrine-containing Combinations, 3073
Ethacrynate Sodium [*Edecrin*]
　　**See Diuretics, Loop (Systemic)**, 1259
　　for Injection USP, 1263
Ethacrynic Acid [*Edecrin;* etacrynic acid]
　　**See Diuretics, Loop (Systemic)**, 1259
　　Solution, Oral, 1263
　　Tablets USP, 1263
Ethambutol Hydrochloride [*Etibi; Myambutol*]
　　**(Systemic)**, 1412
　　Tablets USP, 1417
*Ethamolin*—Block (U.S.) brand of Ethanolamine Oleate (Parenteral-Local), 3142; Reed & Carnrick (U.S. and Canada) brand of Ethanolamine Oleate (Parenteral-Local), #
Ethanolamine Oleate [*Ethamolin*]
　　**(Parenteral-Local)**, #, 3142
　　Injection, #
Ethchlorvynol [*Placidyl*]
　　**(Systemic)**, #
　　Capsules USP, #
Ethinamate
　　**(Systemic)**, #
　　Capsules USP, #
Ethinyl Estradiol [*Estinyl*]
　　**See Estrogens (Systemic)**, 1383, 3142
　　Tablets USP, 1391
Ethinyl Estradiol–containing Combinations, 3073
Ethionamide [*Trecator-SC*]
　　**(Systemic)**, 1417
　　Tablets USP, 1419
*Ethmozine*—Du Pont (U.S.) brand of Moricizine (Systemic), 2060, MC-21
Ethopropazine Hydrochloride [*Parsidol; Parsitan;* profenamine]
　　**See Antidyskinetics (Systemic)**, 297
　　Tablets USP, 300
Ethosuximide [*Zarontin*]
　　**See Anticonvulsants, Succinimide (Systemic)**, #
　　Capsules USP, #
　　Syrup, #
Ethotoin [*Peganone*]
　　**See Anticonvulsants, Hydantoin (Systemic)**, 253
　　Tablets USP, 262
*Ethrane*—Ohmeda (U.S. and Canada) brand of Enflurane—**See Anesthetics, Inhalation (Systemic)**, 168
Ethyl aminobenzoate—Benzocaine—**See Anesthetics (Mucosal-Local)**, 128; **Anesthetics (Topical)**, 155
Ethyl cysteinate dimer—*See* Technetium Tc 99m Bicisate (Systemic), 2703
Ethylenediamine tetraacetic acid—*See* Edetate Disodium (Ophthalmic), #
Ethylnorepinephrine Hydrochloride [*Bronkephrine*]
　　**See Bronchodilators, Adrenergic (Systemic)**, 651
　　Injection USP, 658
Ethynodiol Diacetate and Ethinyl Estradiol [*Demulen 1/35; Demulen 1/50; Demulen 30; Demulen 50; Zovia 1/35E; Zovia 1/50E*]
　　**See Estrogens and Progestins—Oral Contraceptives (Systemic)**, 1397
　　Tablets USP, 1407, MC-12
*Ethyol*—Alza (U.S.); U.S. Bioscience (U.S.); and Lilly (Canada) brand of Amifostine (Systemic), 61; U.S. Bioscience (U.S.) brand of Amifostine (Systemic), 3130
*Etibi*—ICN (Canada) brand of Ethambutol (Systemic), 1412
Etidocaine-containing Combinations, 3073
Etidocaine Hydrochloride [*Duranest-MPF*]
　　**See Anesthetics (Parenteral-Local)**, 139
　　Injection, 148
Etidocaine Hydrochloride and Epinephrine [*Duranest; Duranest-MPF*]
　　**See Anesthetics (Parenteral-Local)**, 139
　　Injection, 148

Etidronate Disodium [*Didronel;* EHDP]
　　**(Systemic)**, 1419, 3142
　　Injection, 1422
　　Tablets USP, 1422, MC-12
Etiocholanedione
　　**(Systemic)**, 3142
Etodolac [etodolic acid; *Lodine; Lodine XL*]
　　**See Anti-inflammatory Drugs, Nonsteroidal (Systemic)**, 388, 3024
　　Capsules, 3019, 405MC-12
　　Tablets, 3019, 406MC-12
　　Tablets, Extended-release, 3019
Etodolic acid—Etodolac—**See Anti-inflammatory Drugs, Nonsteroidal (Systemic)**, 388
Etomidate [*Amidate*]
　　**(Systemic)**, 1422
　　Injection, 1424
*Etopohos*—Bristol-Myers Squibb (U.S.) brand of Etoposide (Systemic), 1424
*Etopophos*—Bristol-Myers Squibb (U.S.) brand of Etoposide (Systemic), 1424
Etoposide [*Etopophos; Toposar; VePesid;* VP-16]
　　**(Systemic)**, 1424
　　Capsules USP, 1427
　　Injection, 1428
Etoposide Phosphate [*Etopohos*]
　　**(Systemic)**, 1424
　　for Injection, 1428
*Etrafon*—Schering (U.S. and Canada) brand of Perphenazine and Amitriptyline (Systemic), 2286
*Etrafon-A*—Schering (U.S. and Canada) brand of Perphenazine and Amitriptyline (Systemic), 2286
*Etrafon-D*—Schering (Canada) brand of Perphenazine and Amitriptyline (Systemic), 2286
*Etrafon-F*—Schering (Canada) brand of Perphenazine and Amitriptyline (Systemic), 2286
*Etrafon-Forte*—Schering (U.S.) brand of Perphenazine and Amitriptyline (Systemic), 2286
Etretin—*See* Acitretin (Systemic), 18
Etretinate [*Tegison*]
　　**(Systemic)**, #
　　Capsules, #, MC-12
*ETS*—Paddock (U.S.) brand of Erythromycin (Topical), 1365
*Eucerin Dry Skin Care Daily Facial*—Beiersdorf (U.S.) brand of Octyl Methoxycinnamate, Octyl Salicylate, Phenylbenzimidazole, and Titanium Dioxide—**See Sunscreen Agents (Topical)**, #
*Eudal-SR*—Forest (U.S.) brand of Pseudoephedrine and Guaifenesin—**See Cough/Cold Combinations (Systemic)**, 1024
*Euflex*—Schering (Canada) brand of Flutamide—**See Antiandrogens, Nonsteroidal (Systemic)**, 220
*Euglucon*—Rorer (Canada) brand of Glyburide—**See Antidiabetic Agents, Sulfonylurea (Systemic)**, 283
*Eulexin*—Schering (U.S.) brand of Flutamide—**See Antiandrogens, Nonsteroidal (Systemic)**, 220
*Eumovate*—Glaxo (Canada) brand of Clobetasone—**See Corticosteroids (Topical)**, 978
*Eurax Cream*—Westwood-Squibb (U.S.) and Ciba-Geigy (Canada) brand of Crotamiton (Topical), #
*Eurax Lotion*—Westwood-Squibb (U.S.) brand of Crotamiton (Topical), #
*Evac-U-Gen*—Walker (U.S.) brand of Phenolphthalein—**See Laxatives (Local)**, #
*Evac-U-Lax*—Roberts (U.S.) brand of Phenolphthalein—**See Laxatives (Local)**, #
*EvacuPaste*—E-Z-EM (U.S. and Canada) brand of Barium Sulfate (Local), #
*Evalose*—Copley (U.S.) brand of Lactulose—**See Laxatives (Local)**, #
*Everone 200*—Hyrex (U.S.) brand of Testosterone—**See Androgens (Systemic)**, 118
*Evista*—Lilly (U.S.) brand of Raloxifene (Systemic), 2455
*E-Vitamin Succinate*—Forest (U.S.) brand of Vitamin E (Systemic), 2972
*Exacta I*—E-Z-EM (U.S.) brand of Barium Sulfate (Local), #
*Exacta II*—E-Z-EM (U.S.) brand of Barium Sulfate (Local), #
*Exact 5 Tinted Cream*—Premier (U.S.) brand of Benzoyl Peroxide (Topical), 579
*Exact 5 Vanishing Cream*—Premier (U.S.) brand of Benzoyl Peroxide (Topical), 579
*Excedrin Caplets*—Bristol-Myers (Canada) brand of Acetaminophen and Caffeine—**See Acetaminophen (Systemic)**, 6

**3284    General Index**

*Excedrin Extra-Strength Caplets*—Bristol-Myers (U.S.) brand of Acetaminophen, Aspirin, and Caffeine—**See Acetaminophen and Salicylates (Systemic)**, 11
*Excedrin Extra-Strength Caplets*—Bristol-Myers (Canada) brand of Acetaminophen and Caffeine—**See Acetaminophen (Systemic)**, 6
*Excedrin Extra-Strength Tablets*—Bristol-Myers (U.S.) brand of Acetaminophen, Aspirin, and Caffeine—**See Acetaminophen and Salicylates (Systemic)**, 11
*Excedrin IB*—Bristol-Myers (U.S.) brand of Ibuprofen—**See Anti-inflammatory Drugs, Nonsteroidal (Systemic)**, 388
*Excedrin IB Caplets*—Bristol-Myers (U.S.) brand of Ibuprofen—**See Anti-inflammatory Drugs, Nonsteroidal (Systemic)**, 388
*Excedrin Migraine*—Bristol-Myers (U.S.) brand of Acetaminophen, Aspirin, and Caffeine (Systemic), 3009
*Excita Fiesta*—London International (U.S.) brand of Latex Condoms—**See Condoms**, #
*Excita Sensitrol*—London International (U.S.) brand of Latex Condoms—**See Condoms**, #
*Exdol*—Frosst (Canada) brand of Acetaminophen (Systemic), 6
*Exdol-8*—Frosst (Canada) brand of Acetaminophen and Codeine—**See Opioid (Narcotic) Analgesics and Acetaminophen (Systemic)**, 2198
*Exdol Strong*—Frosst (Canada) brand of Acetaminophen (Systemic), 6
*Exelderm*—Westwood Squibb (U.S.) brand of Sulconazole (Topical), #
Exemestane
  **(Systemic)**, 3142
*Exgest LA*—Carnrick (U.S.) brand of Phenylpropanolamine and Guaifenesin—**See Cough/Cold Combinations (Systemic)**, 1024
*Ex-Lax*—Sandoz (U.S. and Canada) brand of Phenolphthalein—**See Laxatives (Local)**, #
*Ex-Lax Gentle Nature Pills*—Sandoz (U.S.) brand of Sennosides—**See Laxatives (Local)**, #
*Ex-Lax Light Formula*—Sandoz (Canada) brand of Phenolphthalein and Docusate—**See Laxatives (Local)**, #
*Ex-Lax Maximum Relief Formula*—Sandoz (U.S.) brand of Phenolphthalein—**See Laxatives (Local)**, #
*Ex-Lax Pills*—Sandoz (U.S. and Canada) brand of Phenolphthalein—**See Laxatives (Local)**, #
*EXOSURF*—BW (U.S.) brand of Colfosceril, Cetyl Alcohol, and Tyloxapol (Intratracheal-Local), 3138
*EXOSURF Neonatal*—BW (U.S.) brand of Colfosceril, Cetyl Alcohol, and Tyloxapol (Intratracheal-Local), 3138
*Exosurf Neonatal*—BW (U.S. and Canada) brand of Colfosceril, Cetyl Alcohol, and Tyloxapol (Intratracheal-Local), 937
*Expressin 400 Caplets*—Quintex (U.S.) brand of Pseudoephedrine and Guaifenesin—**See Cough/Cold Combinations (Systemic)**, 1024
*Exsel Lotion Shampoo*—Allergan Herbert (U.S.) brand of Selenium Sulfide (Topical), #
*Extended-release Bayer 8-Hour*—Glenbrook (U.S.) brand of Aspirin—**See Salicylates (Systemic)**, 2538
*Extendryl*—Fleming (U.S.) brand of Chlorpheniramine, Phenylephrine, and Methscopolamine—**See Antihistamines, Decongestants, and Anticholinergics (Systemic)**, 373
*Extendryl JR*—Fleming (U.S.) brand of Chlorpheniramine, Phenylephrine, and Methscopolamine—**See Antihistamines, Decongestants, and Anticholinergics (Systemic)**, 373
*Extendryl SR*—Fleming (U.S.) brand of Chlorpheniramine, Phenylephrine, and Methscopolamine—**See Antihistamines, Decongestants, and Anticholinergics (Systemic)**, 373
*Extra Action Cough*—Rugby (U.S.) brand of Dextromethorphan and Guaifenesin—**See Cough/Cold Combinations (Systemic)**, 1024
*Extra Gentle Ex-Lax*—Sandoz (U.S.) brand of Phenolphthalein and Docusate—**See Laxatives (Local)**, #
*Extraneal (with 7.5% Icodextrin) Peritoneal Dialysis Solution*—Baxter Healthcare (U.S.) brand of Icodextrin 7.5% with Electrolytes Peritoneal Dialysis Solution (Systemic), 3146
*Extra Strength Bayer Arthritis Pain Formula Caplets*—Miles (U.S.) brand of Aspirin—**See Salicylates (Systemic)**, 2538

*Extra Strength Bayer Aspirin Caplets*—Miles (U.S.) brand of Aspirin—**See Salicylates (Systemic)**, 2538
*Extra Strength Bayer Aspirin Tablets*—Miles (U.S.) brand of Aspirin—**See Salicylates (Systemic)**, 2538
*Extra Strength Bayer Plus Caplets*—Miles (U.S.) brand of Aspirin, Buffered—**See Salicylates (Systemic)**, 2538
*Extra Strength Gas-X*—Sandoz (U.S.) brand of Simethicone (Oral-Local), #
*Extra Strength Maalox Anti-Gas*—Ciba (U.S.) brand of Simethicone (Oral-Local), #
*Extra Strength Maalox GRF Gas Relief Formula*—Rhône-Poulenc Rorer (Canada) brand of Simethicone (Oral-Local), #
*Eyelube*—Sabex (Canada) brand of Hydroxypropyl Methylcellulose (Ophthalmic), #
*E-Z-AC*—E-Z-EM (U.S.) brand of Barium Sulfate (Local), #
*E-Z-CAT*—E-Z-EM (U.S. and Canada) brand of Barium Sulfate (Local), #
*EZ Detect*—NMS (U.S.) brand of Fecal Occult Blood Test Kits, #
*E-Z-Disk*—E-Z-EM (U.S.) brand of Barium Sulfate (Local), #
*E-Z-Dose*—E-Z-EM (U.S.) brand of Barium Sulfate (Local), #
*EZE-DS*—Seneca (U.S.) brand of Chlorzoxazone—**See Skeletal Muscle Relaxants (Systemic)**, 2577
*E-Z-HD*—E-Z-EM (U.S. and Canada) brand of Barium Sulfate (Local), #
*EZ III*—Stewart Jackson (U.S.) brand of Acetaminophen and Codeine—**See Opioid (Narcotic) Analgesics and Acetaminophen (Systemic)**, 2198
*E-Z-Jug*—E-Z-EM (U.S. and Canada) brand of Barium Sulfate (Local), #
*Ezol*—Stewart Jackson (U.S.) brand of Butalbital, Acetaminophen, and Caffeine—**See Barbiturates and Analgesics (Systemic)**, 532
*E-Z-Paque*—E-Z-EM (Canada) brand of Barium Sulfate (Local), #
*E-Z-Paque Enema*—E-Z-EM (U.S.) brand of Barium Sulfate (Local), #
*E-Z-Paque Liquid*—E-Z-EM (U.S.) brand of Barium Sulfate (Local), #
*E-Z-Paste Esophageal Cream*—E-Z-EM (U.S.) brand of Barium Sulfate (Local), #

**F**

*4-Way Long Lasting Nasal Spray*—Bristol-Myers (U.S.) brand of Oxymetazoline (Nasal), #
*309-F*—See Suramin (Systemic), #
5-aminosalicylic acid—See Mesalamine (Rectal-Local), 1954
5-ASA—**See Mesalamine (Rectal-Local)**, 1954
5-FC—**See Flucytosine (Systemic)**, #
5-FU—**See Fluorouracil (Systemic)**, 1497; **Fluorouracil (Topical)**, 1500
[18]F—**See Fludeoxyglucose F 18 (Systemic)**, 1478
*FABRase*—**See Alpha-Galactosidase A (Systemic)**, 3129
Factor VIIa (Recombinant, DNA Origin)
  **(Systemic)**, 3142
Factor VIII—**See Antihemophilic Factor (Systemic)**, 319
Factor IX fraction—**See Factor IX (Systemic)**, 1430
Factor IX
  **(Systemic)**, 1430
Factor XIII (Placenta-Derived) [*Fibrogammin P*]
  **(Systemic)**, 3142
*Fact Plus*—Abbott (U.S. and Canada) brand of Immunoassay Pregnancy Test Kits—**See Pregnancy Test Kits for Home Use**, #
*Fact Plus One Step*—Abbott (U.S. and Canada) brand of Immunoassay Pregnancy Test Kits—**See Pregnancy Test Kits for Home Use**, #
*Factrel*—Wyeth-Ayerst (U.S. and Canada) brand of Gonadorelin (Systemic), 1571
Famciclovir [*Famvir*]
  **(Systemic)**, 1434
  Tablets, 1436, MC-12
Famotidine [*Acid Control; Act; Apo-Famotidine; Dyspep HB; Gen-Famotidine; Mylanta-AR; Novo-Famotidine; Nu-Famotidine; Pepcid; Pepcid AC; Pepcid I.V.; Ulcidine; Ulcidine HB*]
  **See Histamine H₂-receptor Antagonists (Systemic)**, 1633

*USP DI*

Famotidine (continued)
  Injection, 1640
  for Suspension, Oral, 1639
  Tablets, Chewable, 1640
  Tablets USP, 1639
Fampridine [*Neurelan*]
  **(Systemic)**, 3143
*Famvir*—SmithKline Beecham (U.S. and Canada) brand of Famciclovir (Systemic), 1434, MC-12
*Fansidar*—Roche (U.S. and Canada) brand of Sulfadoxine and Pyrimethamine (Systemic), 2637, MC-28
*Fareston*—Schering (U.S.) brand of Toremifene (Systemic), 2845
*Fastin*—SmithKline Beecham (U.S. and Canada) brand of Phentermine—**See Appetite Suppressants (Systemic)**, 452
Fat Emulsions [*Intralipid; Liposyn II; Liposyn III*]
  **(Systemic)**, #
  Injection, #
*Father John's Medicine Plus*—Oakhurst (U.S.) brand of Chlorpheniramine, Phenylephrine, Dextromethorphan, Guaifenesin, and Ammonium Chloride—**See Cough/Cold Combinations (Systemic)**, 1024
Fatty Acids, Short Chain
  **(Systemic)**, 3164
  Solution, 3164
FBM—See Felbamate (Systemic), 1436
5-FC—See Flucytosine (Systemic), #
FDG—See Fludeoxyglucose F 18 (Systemic), 1478
[59]Fe—See Ferrous Citrate Fe 59 (Systemic), 1460
Fecal Occult Blood Test Kits [*ColoCare; Colo-Rectal Test; ColoScreen; ColoScreen; ColoScreen Self-Test; DigiWipe; EZ Detect; HemaChek; Hematest; HemaWipe; HemeSelect; Hemoccult; Hemoccult II; HemoWipe; Hemoccult SENSA; Hemoccult II SENSA*], #
  Fecal Occult Blood Test Kits for Home Use, #
  Fecal Occult Blood Test Kits for Clinic Use, #
*Fedahist*—Schwarz (U.S.) brand of Chlorpheniramine and Pseudoephedrine—**See Antihistamines and Decongestants (Systemic)**, 343
*Fedahist Gyrocaps*—Schwarz (U.S.) brand of Chlorpheniramine and Pseudoephedrine—**See Antihistamines and Decongestants (Systemic)**, 343
*Fedahist Timecaps*—Schwarz (U.S.) brand of Chlorpheniramine and Pseudoephedrine—**See Antihistamines and Decongestants (Systemic)**, 343
*Feen-a-mint*—Schering-Plough (U.S.) brand of Phenolphthalein—**See Laxatives (Local)**, #
*Feen-a-Mint Pills*—Schering-Plough (Canada) brand of Bisacodyl—**See Laxatives (Local)**, #
*FEIBA VH*—Immuno (U.S. and Canada) brand of Anti-inhibitor Coagulant Complex (Systemic), 435
Felbamate [*FBM; Felbatol*]
  **(Systemic)**, 1436, 3143
  Suspension, Oral, 1439
  Tablets, 1439, MC-12
*Felbatol*—Wallace (U.S.) brand of Felbamate (Systemic), 1436, 3143, MC-12
*Feldene*—Pfizer (U.S. and Canada) and Pratt (U.S.) brand of Piroxicam—**See Anti-inflammatory Drugs, Nonsteroidal (Systemic)**, 388, MC-25
Felodipine [*Plendil; Renedil*]
  **See Calcium Channel Blocking Agents (Systemic)**, 720
  Tablets, Extended-release, 729, MC-12
*Felombrine*—Medinsa (Spain) brand of Iopanoic Acid—**See Cholecystographic Agents, Oral (Systemic)**, #
*Femara*—Novartis (U.S.) brand of Letrozole (Systemic), 1836
*FemCare*—Schering-Plough (U.S.) brand of Clotrimazole—**See Antifungals, Azole (Vaginal)**, 310
*Femcet*—Russ (U.S.) brand of Butalbital, Acetaminophen, and Caffeine—**See Barbiturates and Analgesics (Systemic)**, 532
*FemiLax*—G & W (U.S.) brand of Phenolphthalein and Docusate—**See Laxatives (Local)**, #
*Femiron*—Beecham (U.S.) brand of Ferrous Fumarate—**See Iron Supplements (Systemic)**, 1774
*Femogex*—Stickley (Canada) brand of Estradiol—**See Estrogens (Systemic)**, 1383
*Femstat 3*—Procter & Gamble (U.S.) brand of Butoconazole—**See Antifungals, Azole (Vaginal)**, 310

*Fendol*—Buffington (U.S.) brand of Phenylephrine, Guaifenesin, Acetaminophen, Salicylamide, and Caffeine—**See Cough/Cold Combinations (Systemic)**, 1024
*Fenesin*—Dura (U.S.) brand of Guaifenesin (Systemic), 1588
*Fenesin DM*—Dura (U.S.) brand of Dextromethorphan and Guaifenesin—**See Cough/Cold Combinations (Systemic)**, 1024
Fenfluramine Hydrochloride
  **See Appetite Suppressants (Systemic)**, 452
  Capsules, Extended-release, 455
  Tablets, 455
*Fenicol Ophthalmic Ointment*—Alcon (Canada) brand of Chloramphenicol (Ophthalmic), #
Fenofibrate [*Tricor*]
  **(Systemic)**, 1439
  Capsules, Micronized, 1443, MC-12
Fenoldopam Mesylate [*Corlopam*]
  **(Systemic)**, 1443
  Injection, 1445
Fenoprofen Calcium [*Nalfon; Nalfon 200*]
  **See Anti-inflammatory Drugs, Nonsteroidal (Systemic)**, 388
  Capsules USP, 406, MC-12
  Tablets USP, 406, MC-12
Fenoterol Hydrobromide [*Berotec*]
  **See Bronchodilators, Adrenergic (Inhalation-Local)**, 640
  Aerosol, Inhalation, 647
  Solution, Inhalation, 647
Fenoterol Hydrobromide [*Berotec*]
  **See Bronchodilators, Adrenergic (Systemic)**, 651
  Tablets, 658
Fentanyl [*Duragesic*]
  **(Transdermal-Systemic)**, 1446
  System, Transdermal, 1451
Fentanyl Citrate [*Sublimaze*]
  **See Fentanyl Derivatives (Systemic)**, 1452
  Injection USP, 1459
Fentanyl Derivatives
  **(Systemic)**, 1452
*Feosol*—Menley & James (U.S.) brand of Ferrous Sulfate—**See Iron Supplements (Systemic)**, 1774
*Feostat*—Forest (U.S.) brand of Ferrous Fumarate—**See Iron Supplements (Systemic)**, 1774
*Feostat Drops*—Forest (U.S.) brand of Ferrous Fumarate—**See Iron Supplements (Systemic)**, 1774
*Feratab*—Upsher Smith (U.S.) brand of Ferrous Sulfate—**See Iron Supplements (Systemic)**, 1774
*Fer-gen-sol*—Goldline (U.S.) brand of Ferrous Sulfate—**See Iron Supplements (Systemic)**, 1774
*Fergon*—Sanofi Winthrop (U.S.) brand of Ferrous Gluconate—**See Iron Supplements (Systemic)**, 1774
*Feridex I.V.*—Advanced Magnetics (U.S.) brand of Ferumoxides (Systemic), #
*Fer-In-Sol Capsules*—Mead Johnson (U.S.) brand of Ferrous Sulfate—**See Iron Supplements (Systemic)**, 1774
*Fer-In-Sol Drops*—Mead Johnson (U.S. and Canada) brand of Ferrous Sulfate—**See Iron Supplements (Systemic)**, 1774
*Fer-In-Sol Syrup*—Mead Johnson (U.S. and Canada) brand of Ferrous Sulfate—**See Iron Supplements (Systemic)**, 1774
*Fer-Iron Drops*—Bay (U.S.); Interstate (U.S.); My-K (U.S.); Rugby (U.S.) brand of Ferrous Sulfate—**See Iron Supplements (Systemic)**, 1774
*Fero-Grad*—Abbott (Canada) brand of Ferrous Sulfate—**See Iron Supplements (Systemic)**, 1774
*Fero-Gradumet*—Abbott (U.S.) brand of Ferrous Sulfate—**See Iron Supplements (Systemic)**, 1774
*Ferospace*—Hudson (U.S.) brand of Ferrous Sulfate—**See Iron Supplements (Systemic)**, 1774
*Ferralet*—Mission (U.S.) brand of Ferrous Gluconate—**See Iron Supplements (Systemic)**, 1774
*Ferralet Slow Release*—Mission (U.S.) brand of Ferrous Gluconate—**See Iron Supplements (Systemic)**, 1774
*Ferralyn Lanacaps*—Lannett (U.S.) brand of Ferrous Sulfate—**See Iron Supplements (Systemic)**, 1774
*Ferra-TD*—Goldline (U.S.) brand of Ferrous Sulfate—**See Iron Supplements (Systemic)**, 1774
*Ferretts*—Pharmics (U.S.) brand of Ferrous Fumarate—**See Iron Supplements (Systemic)**, 1774
Ferric ferrocyanide—*See* Prussian Blue (Oral-Local), #

Ferric (III) hexacyanoferrate (II)—*See* Prussian Blue (Oral-Local), #
Ferrous Citrate Fe 59
  **(Systemic)**, 1460
  Injection USP, 1461
Ferrous Fumarate [*Femiron; Feostat; Feostat Drops; Ferretts; Fumasorb; Fumerin; Hemocyte; Ircon; Neo-Fer; Nephro-Fer; Novofumar; Palafer; Span-FF*]
  **See Iron Supplements (Systemic)**, 1774
  Capsules, 1779
  Capsules, Extended-release, 1779
  Solution, Oral, 1779
  Suspension, Oral, 1780
  Tablets USP, 1780
  Tablets, Chewable, 1780
Ferrous Gluconate [*Apo-Ferrous Gluconate; Fergon; Ferralet; Ferralet Slow Release; Fertinic; Novoferrogluc; Simron*]
  **See Iron Supplements (Systemic)**, 1774
  Capsules USP, 1780
  Elixir USP, 1780
  Syrup, 1781
  Tablets USP, 1781
  Tablets, Extended-release, 1781
Ferrous Sulfate [*Apo-Ferrous Sulfate; Feosol; Feratab; Fer-gen-sol; Fer-In-Sol Capsules; Fer-In-Sol Drops; Fer-In-Sol Syrup; Fer-Iron Drops; Fero-Grad; Fero-Gradumet; Ferospace; Ferralyn Lanacaps; Ferra-TD;* ferrous sulfate exsiccated; *Mol-Iron; Novoferrosulfa; PMS-Ferrous Sulfate; Slow Fe*]
  **See Iron Supplements (Systemic)**, 1774
  Capsules, 1781
  Capsules (Dried), 1781
  Capsules, Extended-release (Dried), 1782
  Elixir, 1782
  Solution, Oral, USP, 1782
  Tablets USP, 1782, MC-12
  Tablets USP (Dried), 1782
  Tablets, Enteric-coated, 1783
  Tablets, Extended-release, 1783
  Tablets, Extended-release (Dried), 1783
Ferrous sulfate exsiccated—Ferrous Sulfate—**See Iron Supplements (Systemic)**, 1774
*Fertinex*—Serono (U.S.) brand of Urofollitropin (Systemic), 2901, 3170
*Fertinic*—Desbergers (Canada) brand of Ferrous Gluconate—**See Iron Supplements (Systemic)**, 1774
*Fertinorm HP*—Serono (Canada) brand of Urofollitropin (Systemic), 2901
Ferumoxides [*Feridex I.V.*]
  **(Systemic)**, #
  Injection, #
Ferumoxsil [*Gastromark*]
  **(Systemic)**, 3019
  Injection, 3019
*Feverall, Children's*—Upsher-Smith (U.S.) brand of Acetaminophen (Systemic), 6
*Feverall, Infants'*—Upsher-Smith (U.S.) brand of Acetaminophen (Systemic), 6
*Feverall Junior Strength*—Upsher-Smith (U.S.) brand of Acetaminophen (Systemic), 6
*Feverall Sprinkle Caps, Children's*—Upsher-Smith (U.S.) brand of Acetaminophen (Systemic), 6
*Feverall Sprinkle Caps Junior Strength*—Upsher-Smith (U.S.) brand of Acetaminophen (Systemic), 6
Fexofenadine Hydrochloride [*Allegra*]
  **(Systemic)**, 1461
  Capsules, 1462, MC-12
Fexofenadine Hydrochloride and Pseudoephedrine Hydrochloride [*Allegra-D*]
  **(Systemic)**, 1463
  Capsules, Extended-release, MC-12
  Tablets, Extended-release, 1465
FGN-1
  **(Systemic)**, 3143
Fiau
  **(Systemic)**, 3143
*Fiberall*—Ciba Consumer (U.S.) brand of Psyllium Hydrophilic Mucilloid—**See Laxatives (Local)**, #
*Fibercon Caplets*—Lederle (U.S.) brand of Polycarbophil—**See Laxatives (Local)**, #
*Fiberlan*—Elan (U.S.) brand of Enteral Nutrition Formula, Fiber-containing—**See Enteral Nutrition Formulas (Systemic)**, #
*Fiber-Lax*—Rugby (U.S.) brand of Polycarbophil—**See Laxatives (Local)**, #
*FiberNorm*—G & W (U.S.) brand of Polycarbophil—**See Laxatives (Local)**, #

*Fibersource*—Sandoz (U.S.) brand of Enteral Nutrition Formula, Fiber-containing—**See Enteral Nutrition Formulas (Systemic)**, #
*Fibersource HN*—Sandoz (U.S.) brand of Enteral Nutrition Formula, Fiber-containing—**See Enteral Nutrition Formulas (Systemic)**, #
*Fibrepur*—Hoechst-Roussel (Canada) brand of Psyllium Hydrophilic Mucilloid—**See Laxatives (Local)**, #
Fibrinogen (Human)
  **(Systemic)**, 3143
Fibrin Sealant [*Tisseel VH Kit*]
  **(Local)**, 3020
  for Solution, 3020
*Fibrogammin P*—Behringwerke (U.S.) brand of Factor XIII (Placenta-Derived) (Systemic), 3142
Fibronectin (Human Plasma Derived)
  **(Ophthalmic)**, 3143
Filgrastim [granulocyte colony stimulating factor, recombinant; *Neupogen*; recombinant methionyl human granulocyte colony stimulating factor; rG-CSF; r-met HuG-CSF]
  **See Colony Stimulating Factors (Systemic)**, 941, 3143
  Injection, 944
*Filmix Neurosonographic Contrast Agent*—Cav-Con (U.S.) brand of Microbubble Contrast Agent (Diagnostic), 3154
*Finac*—C & M (U.S.) brand of Sulfur (Topical), #
Finasteride [*Propecia; Proscar*]
  **(Systemic)**, 1465
  Tablets, 1468, MC-13
*Fiorgen*—Goldline (U.S.) brand of Butalbital, Aspirin, and Caffeine—**See Barbiturates and Analgesics (Systemic)**, 532
*Fioricet*—Novartis (U.S.) brand of Butalbital, Acetaminophen, and Caffeine—**See Barbiturates and Analgesics (Systemic)**, 532, MC-4
*Fioricet with Codeine*—Novartis (U.S.) brand of Butalbital, Acetaminophen, Caffeine, and Codeine—**See Barbiturates and Analgesics (Systemic)**, 532, MC-4
*Fiorinal*—Novartis (U.S. and Canada) brand of Butalbital, Aspirin, and Caffeine—**See Barbiturates and Analgesics (Systemic)**, 532, MC-4
*Fiorinal-C 1/4*—Sandoz (Canada) brand of Butalbital, Aspirin, Caffeine, and Codeine—**See Barbiturates and Analgesics (Systemic)**, 532
*Fiorinal-C 1/2*—Sandoz (Canada) brand of Butalbital, Aspirin, Caffeine, and Codeine—**See Barbiturates and Analgesics (Systemic)**, 532
*Fiorinal with Codeine*—Novartis (U.S.) brand of Butalbital, Aspirin, Caffeine, and Codeine—**See Barbiturates and Analgesics (Systemic)**, 532, MC-4
*Fiormor*—Moore (U.S.) brand of Butalbital, Aspirin, and Caffeine—**See Barbiturates and Analgesics (Systemic)**, 532
*First Response*—Carter-Horner (Canada) brand of Immunoassay Ovulation Prediction Test Kits—**See Ovulation Prediction Test Kits for Home Use**, #; Immunoassay Pregnancy Test Kits—**See Pregnancy Test Kits for Home Use**, #; Hygeia Sciences (U.S.) and Carter (Canada) brand of Enzyme Immunoassay Ovulation Prediction Test Kits—**See Ovulation Prediction Test Kits for Home Use**, #
*First Response 1-Step*—Carter-Wallace (U.S.) brand of Immunoassay Pregnancy Test Kits—**See Pregnancy Test Kits for Home Use**, #
FK 506—*See* Tacrolimus (Systemic), 2683
*Flagyl 375*—Searle (U.S.) brand of Metronidazole (Systemic), MC-20
*Flagyl*—Rhône-Poulenc Rorer (Canada) brand of Metronidazole (Vaginal), 2001; Searle (U.S.) brand of Metronidazole (Topical), 3154; Searle (U.S.) and Rhône-Poulenc (Canada) brand of Metronidazole (Systemic), 1996, MC-20
*Flagyl ER*—Searle (U.S.) brand of Metronidazole (Systemic), MC-20
*Flagyl I.V.*—Schiapparelli Searle (U.S.) brand of Metronidazole (Systemic), 1996
*Flagyl I.V. RTU*—Schiapparelli Searle (U.S.) brand of Metronidazole (Systemic), 1996
*Flagystatin*—Rhône-Poulenc (Canada) brand of Metronidazole and Nystatin (Vaginal), 3028
*Flamazine*—Smith & Nephew (Canada) brand of Silver Sulfadiazine (Topical), #
*Flarex*—Alcon (U.S. and Canada) brand of Fluorometholone—**See Corticosteroids (Ophthalmic)**, 966

*Flatulex*—Dayton (U.S.) brand of Simethicone (Oral-Local), #
*Flavorcee*—Hudson (U.S.) brand of Ascorbic Acid (Systemic), 469
*Flavored Alka-Seltzer Effervescent Pain Reliever and Antacid*—Miles (U.S. and Canada) brand of Aspirin, Sodium Bicarbonate, and Citric Acid (Systemic), 477
Flavoxate Hydrochloride [*Urispas*]
    **(Systemic)**, 1468
    Tablets, 1469
*Flaxedil*—Davis & Geck (U.S.) and Rhône-Poulenc (Canada) brand of Gallamine—**See Neuromuscular Blocking Agents (Systemic)**, 2098
Flecainide Acetate [*Tambocor*]
    **(Systemic)**, 1469
    Tablets, 1472
*Fleet Babylax*—Fleet (U.S.) brand of Glycerin—**See Laxatives (Local)**, #
*Fleet Bisacodyl*—Fleet (U.S.) brand of Bisacodyl—**See Laxatives (Local)**, #
*Fleet Enema*—Fleet (U.S. and Canada) brand of Sodium Phosphates—**See Laxatives (Local)**, #
*Fleet Enema for Children*—Fleet (U.S.) brand of Sodium Phosphates—**See Laxatives (Local)**, #
*Fleet Enema Mineral Oil*—Fleet (U.S. and Canada) brand of Mineral Oil—**See Laxatives (Local)**, #
*Fleet Glycerin Laxative*—Fleet (U.S.) brand of Glycerin—**See Laxatives (Local)**, #
*Fleet Laxative*—Fleet (U.S.) brand of Bisacodyl—**See Laxatives (Local)**, #
*Fleet Mineral Oil*—Fleet (U.S.) brand of Mineral Oil—**See Laxatives (Local)**, #
*Fleet Pediatric Enema*—Fleet (Canada) brand of Sodium Phosphates—**See Laxatives (Local)**, #
*Fleet Phospho-Soda*—Fleet (U.S.) brand of Sodium Phosphates—**See Laxatives (Local)**, #
*Fleet Relief*—Fleet (U.S.) brand of Pramoxine—**See Anesthetics (Mucosal-Local)**, 128
*Fleet Solfax Gelcaps*—Fleet (U.S.) brand of Docusate—**See Laxatives (Local)**, #
*Fleet Solfax Overnight Gelcaps*—Fleet (U.S.) brand of Casthranol and Docusate—**See Laxatives (Local)**, #
*Fletcher's Castoria*—Mentholatum (U.S.) brand of Senna—**See Laxatives (Local)**, #; Mentholatum (Canada) brand of Sennosides—**See Laxatives (Local)**, #
*Flexeril*—Merck (U.S.) and Frosst (Canada) brand of Cyclobenzaprine (Systemic), 1126, MC-8
*Flexoject*—Mayrand (U.S.) brand of Orphenadrine—**See Skeletal Muscle Relaxants (Systemic)**, 2577
*Flint SSD*—Boots (U.S.) brand of Silver Sulfadiazine (Topical), #
*Flo-Coat*—Lafayette (U.S.) brand of Barium Sulfate (Local), #
Floctafenine [*Idarac*]
    **See Anti-inflammatory Drugs, Nonsteroidal (Systemic)**, 388
    Tablets, 407
*Flolan*—BW (U.S.) brand of Epoprostenol (Systemic), 3142
*Flomax*—Boehringer Ingelheim (U.S.) brand of Tamsulosin (Systemic), 2690
*Flonase*—Allen & Hanburys (U.S.) brand of Fluticasone (Nasal), 1511; Glaxo (Canada) brand of Fluticasone (Nasal), 3020
*Florinef*—Apothecon (U.S.) and Squibb (Canada) brand of Fludrocortisone (Systemic), 1481
*Florone*—Dermik (U.S.) and Upjohn (Canada) brand of Diflorasone—**See Corticosteroids (Topical)**, 978
*Florone E*—Dermik (U.S.) brand of Diflorasone—**See Corticosteroids (Topical)**, 978
*Floropryl*—Merck (U.S.) brand of Isoflurophate—**See Antiglaucoma Agents, Cholinergic, Long-acting (Ophthalmic)**, 315
*Flovent*—Glaxo Wellcome (U.S.) brand of Fluticasone (Inhalation-Local), 1508
*Flovent Rotadisk*—Glaxo Wellcome (U.S.) brand of Fluticasone (Inhalation-Local), 1508
*Floxin*—Ortho-McNeil (U.S.) and Janssen-Ortho (Canada) brand of Ofloxacin—**See Fluoroquinolones (Systemic)**, 1487, MC-23
*Floxin I.V.*—Ortho-McNeil (U.S.) brand of Ofloxacin—**See Fluoroquinolones (Systemic)**, 1487
*Floxin Otic*—Daiichi (U.S.) brand of Ofloxacin (Otic), 2154
Floxuridine [*FUDR*]
    **(Systemic)**, 1472
    Sterile USP, 1474

*Flozenges*—Oral B (Canada) brand of Sodium Fluoride (Systemic), 2592
*Fluanxol*—Marion Merrell Dow (Canada) brand of Flupenthixol—**See Thioxanthenes (Systemic)**, 2793
*Fluanxol Depot*—Marion Merrell Dow (Canada) brand of Flupenthixol—**See Thioxanthenes (Systemic)**, 2793
*Fluclox*—Wyeth-Ayerst (Canada) brand of Flucloxacillin—**See Penicillins (Systemic)**, 2240
Flucloxacillin [*Fluclox*]
    **See Penicillins (Systemic)**, 2240
    for Suspension, Oral, USP, 2252
Flucloxacillin Sodium [*Fluclox*]
    **See Penicillins (Systemic)**, 2240
    Capsules, 2252
Fluconazole [*Diflucan; Diflucan 150*]
    **See Antifungals, Azole (Systemic)**, 302
    Capsules, 306
    Injection, 307
    for Suspension, Oral, 306
    Tablets, 307, MC-13
Flucytosine [*Ancobon; Ancotil; 5-FC; 5-Fluorocytosine*]
    **(Systemic)**, #
    Capsules USP, #
*Fludara*—Berlex (U.S. and Canada) brand of Fludarabine (Systemic), 1475; Berlex (U.S.) brand of Fludarabine (Systemic), 3143
Fludarabine Phosphate [*Fludara*]
    **(Systemic)**, 1475, 3143
    for Injection, 1478
Fludeoxyglucose F 18
    **(Systemic)**, 1478
    Injection USP, 1481
Fludrocortisone Acetate [*Florinef*]
    **(Systemic)**, 1481
    Tablets USP, 1483
*Fludroxycortide*—Flurandrenolide—**See Corticosteroids (Topical)**, 978
*Flumadine*—Forest (U.S.) brand of Rimantadine (Systemic), 2502, MC-27
Flumazenil [*Anexate; Romazicon*]
    **(Systemic)**, 1483
    Injection, 1486
Flumecinol [*Zixoryn*]
    **(Systemic)**, 3143
*Flumetasone*—Flumethasone—**See Corticosteroids (Topical)**, 978
Flumethasone-containing Combinations, 3073
Flumethasone Pivalate [*flumetasone; Locacorten*]
    **See Corticosteroids (Topical)**, 978
    Cream USP, 988
    Ointment, 989
Flunarizine [*Sibelium*]
    **(Systemic)**, 3143
Flunarizine Hydrochloride [*Sibelium*]
    **See Calcium Channel Blocking Agents (Systemic)**, 720
    Capsules, 729
Flunisolide [*AeroBid; AeroBid-M; Bronalide*]
    **See Corticosteroids (Inhalation-Local)**, 955
    Aerosol, Inhalation, 960
Flunisolide [*Nasalide; Nasarel; Rhinalar*]
    **See Corticosteroids (Nasal)**, 961, 3020
    Solution, Nasal, USP, 966, 3020
*Fluocet*—NMC (U.S.) brand of Fluocinolone—**See Corticosteroids (Topical)**, 978
*Fluocin*—Clay-Park (U.S.) brand of Fluocinonide—**See Corticosteroids (Topical)**, 978
Fluocinolone Acetonide [*Bio-Syn; Fluocet; Fluoderm; Fluolar; Fluonid; Fluonide; Flurosyn; Synalar; Synalar-HP; Synamol; Synemol*]
    **See Corticosteroids (Topical)**, 978
    Cream USP, 989
    Ointment USP, 989
    Solution, Topical, USP, 989
Fluocinonide [*Fluocin; Licon; Lidemol; Lidex; Lidex-E; Lyderm; Topsyn*]
    **See Corticosteroids (Topical)**, 978, 3020
    Cream USP, 989
    Gel USP, 989
    Ointment, 3020
    Ointment USP, 990
    Solution, Topical, USP, 990
Fluocinonide-containing Combinations, 3073
Fluocinonide, Procinonide, and Ciprocinonide [*Trisyn*]
    **(Topical)**, 3020
    Cream, 3020
*Fluoderm*—K-Line (Canada) brand of Fluocinolone—**See Corticosteroids (Topical)**, 978

*Fluolar*—Riva (Canada) brand of Fluocinolone—**See Corticosteroids (Topical)**, 978
*Fluonid*—Allergan Herbert (U.S.) brand of Fluocinolone—**See Corticosteroids (Topical)**, 978
*Fluonide*—Technilab (Canada) brand of Fluocinolone—**See Corticosteroids (Topical)**, 978
*Fluor-A-Day*—Pharmascience (Canada) brand of Sodium Fluoride (Systemic), 2592
*Fluoritab*—Fluoritab (U.S.) brand of Sodium Fluoride (Systemic), 2592
*Fluoritabs*—Westcon (Canada) brand of Sodium Fluoride (Systemic), 2592
5-Fluorocytosine—*See* Flucytosine (Systemic), #
*Fluorodex*—IDE (U.S.) brand of Sodium Fluoride (Systemic), 2592
Fluorometholone [*Fluor-Op; FML Forte; FML Liquifilm; FML S.O.P.*]
    **See Corticosteroids (Ophthalmic)**, 966
    Ointment, Ophthalmic, 969
    Suspension, Ophthalmic, USP, 969
Fluorometholone Acetate [*Eflone; Flarex*]
    **See Corticosteroids (Ophthalmic)**, 966
    Suspension, Ophthalmic, 970
*Fluor-Op*—Ciba Vision (U.S.) brand of Fluorometholone—**See Corticosteroids (Ophthalmic)**, 966
*Fluoroplex*—Herbert (U.S. and Canada) brand of Fluorouracil (Topical), 1500
Fluoroquinolones
    **(Systemic)**, 1487
*Fluorosol*—Westcon (Canada) brand of Sodium Fluoride (Systemic), 2592
Fluorouracil [*Adrucil; 5-FU*]
    **(Systemic)**, 1497, 3144
    Injection USP, 1500
Fluorouracil [*Efudex; Fluoroplex; 5-FU*]
    **(Topical)**, 1500
    Cream USP, 1502
    Solution, Topical, USP, 1502
*Fluosol*—Alpha (U.S.) brand of Perfluorochemical Emulsion (Systemic), #
*Fluothane*—Wyeth-Ayerst (U.S.) and Ayerst (Canada) brand of Halothane—**See Anesthetics, Inhalation (Systemic)**, 168
Fluoxetine Hydrochloride [*Prozac*]
    **(Systemic)**, 1503
    Capsules, 1507, MC-13
    Solution, Oral, 1507
Fluoxymesterone [*Android-F; Halotestin*]
    **See Androgens (Systemic)**, 118
    Tablets USP, 124, MC-13
Fluoxymesterone-containing Combinations, 3073
Fluoxymesterone and Ethinyl Estradiol [*Halodrin*]
    **See Androgens and Estrogens (Systemic)**, 126
    Tablets, 128
Flupenthixol Decanoate [*Fluanxol Depot;* flupentixol]
    **See Thioxanthenes (Systemic)**, 2793
    Injection, 2798
Flupenthixol Dihydrochloride [*Fluanxol;* flupentixol]
    **See Thioxanthenes (Systemic)**, 2793
    Tablets, 2798
*Flupentixol*—Flupenthixol—**See Thioxanthenes (Systemic)**, 2793
Fluphenazine Decanoate [*Modecate; Modecate Concentrate; Prolixin Decanoate*]
    **See Phenothiazines (Systemic)**, 2289
    Injection, 2300
Fluphenazine Enanthate [*Moditen Enanthate; Prolixin Enanthate*]
    **See Phenothiazines (Systemic)**, 2289
    Injection USP, 2300
Fluphenazine Hydrochloride [*Apo-Fluphenazine; Moditen HCl; Moditen HCl-H.P.; Permitil; Permitil Concentrate; Prolixin; Prolixin Concentrate*]
    **See Phenothiazines (Systemic)**, 2289
    Elixir USP, 2299
    Injection USP, 2300
    Solution, Oral, USP, 2299
    Tablets USP, 2300, MC-13
*Flura*—Kirkman (U.S.) brand of Sodium Fluoride (Systemic), 2592
*Flura-Drops*—Kirkman (U.S.) brand of Sodium Fluoride (Systemic), 2592
*Flura-Loz*—Kirkman (U.S.) brand of Sodium Fluoride (Systemic), 2592
Flurandrenolide [*Cordran; Cordran SP; Denison; Drenison-¹/₄;* fludroxycortide]
    **See Corticosteroids (Topical)**, 978
    Cream USP, 990
    Lotion USP, 990
    Ointment USP, 990
    Tape USP, 990

Flurazepam Hydrochloride [*Apo-Flurazepam; Dalmane; Novo-Flupam; Somnol*]
**See Benzodiazepines (Systemic)**, 556
Capsules USP, 573, MC-13
Tablets, 573
Flurbiprofen [*Ansaid; Apo-Flurbiprofen; Froben; Froben SR; Novo-Flurprofen; Nu-Flurbiprofen*]
**See Anti-inflammatory Drugs, Nonsteroidal (Systemic)**, 388
Capsules, Extended-release, 407
Tablets USP, 407 MC-13
Flurbiprofen Sodium [*Ocufen*]
**See Anti-inflammatory Drugs, Nonsteroidal (Ophthalmic)**, 383, 3020
Solution, Ophthalmic, USP, 387, 3020
*Flurosyn*—Rugby (U.S.) brand of Fluocinolone—**See Corticosteroids (Topical)**, 978
*FluShield*—Wyeth (U.S.) brand of Influenza Virus Vaccine (Systemic), 1707
Fluspirilene [*Imap; Imap Forte*]
**(Systemic)**, 3020
Injection, 3020
Flutamide [*Euflex; Eulexin*]
**See Antiandrogens, Nonsteroidal (Systemic)**, 220
Capsules USP, 225
Tablets, 226
*Flutex*—Syosset (U.S.) brand of Triamcinolone—**See Corticosteroids (Topical)**, 978
Fluticasone Propionate [*Cutivate*]
**See Corticosteroids (Topical)**, 978
Cream, 990
Ointment, 991
Fluticasone Propionate [*Flonase*]
**(Nasal)**, 1511, 3020
Suspension, Nasal, 1513, 3020
Fluticasone Propionate [*Flovent; Flovent Rotadisk*]
**(Inhalation-Local)**, 1508
Aerosol, Inhalation, 1510
Powder for Inhalation, 1511
Flu vaccine—*See* Influenza Virus Vaccine (Systemic), 1707
Fluvastatin Sodium [*Lescol*]
**See HMG-CoA Reductase Inhibitors (Systemic)**, 1647
Capsules, 1650, MC-13
*Fluviral*—Biovac (Canada) brand of Influenza Virus Vaccine (Systemic), 1707
*Fluviral S/F*—Biovac (Canada) brand of Influenza Virus Vaccine (Systemic), 1707
*Fluvirin*—Adams (U.S.) brand of Influenza Virus Vaccine (Systemic), 1707
Fluvoxamine Maleate [*Luvox*]
**(Systemic)**, 1513
Tablets, 1517, MC-13
*Fluzone*—Connaught (U.S. and Canada) brand of Influenza Virus Vaccine (Systemic), 1707
*FML Forte*—Allergan (U.S. and Canada) brand of Fluorometholone—**See Corticosteroids (Ophthalmic)**, 966
*FML Liquifilm*—Allergan (U.S. and Canada) brand of Fluorometholone—**See Corticosteroids (Ophthalmic)**, 966
*FML S.O.P.*—Allergan (U.S.) brand of Fluorometholone—**See Corticosteroids (Ophthalmic)**, 966
*Foamicon*—Invamed (U.S.) brand of Alumina, Magnesium Trisilicate, and Sodium Bicarbonate—**See Antacids (Oral-Local)**, 188
*Foille*—Blistex (U.S.) brand of Neomycin, Polymyxin B, and Bacitracin (Topical), #
*FoilleCort*—Blistex (U.S.) brand of Hydrocortisone—**See Corticosteroids (Topical)**, 978
*Folex*—Adria (U.S.) brand of Methotrexate—For Noncancerous Conditions (Systemic), 1969
*Folex PFS*—Adria (U.S.) brand of Methotrexate—For Noncancerous Conditions (Systemic), 1969
Folic Acid [*Apo-Folic; Folvite; Novo-Folacid;* vitamin B₉]
**(Systemic)**, 1517
Injection USP, 1520
Tablets USP, 1519
Folinic acid—*See* Leucovorin (Systemic), 1837
Follicle-stimulating hormone—*See* Urofollitropin (Systemic), 2901
*Follistim*—Organon (U.S.) brand of Follitropin Beta (Systemic), 1523
Follitropin Alfa [*Gonal-F*]
**(Systemic)**, 1520
for Injection, 1522
Follitropin Beta[*Follistim*]
**(Systemic)**, 1523
for Injection, 1525

*Folvite*—Lederle (U.S. and Canada) brand of Folic Acid (Systemic), 1517
Fomepizole [*Antizol*]
**(Systemic)**, 1526
Injection, 1527
*Forane*—Ohmeda (U.S. and Canada) brand of Isoflurane—**See Anesthetics, Inhalation (Systemic)**, 168
*Formula 405 Solar*—Doak (U.S.) brand of Aminobenzoic Acid and Titanium Dioxide—**See Sunscreen Agents (Topical)**, #; Octyl Methoxycinnamate—**See Sunscreen Agents (Topical)**, #; Oxybenzone and Padimate O—**See Sunscreen Agents (Topical)**, #
*Formulex*—ICN (Canada) brand of Dicyclomine—**See Anticholinergics/Antispasmodics (Systemic)**, 226
*Fortabs*—United Research (U.S.) brand of Butalbital, Aspirin, and Caffeine—**See Barbiturates and Analgesics (Systemic)**, 532
*Fortaz*—Glaxo (U.S. and Canada) brand of Ceftazidime—**See Cephalosporins (Systemic)**, 794
*Fortel*—Biomerica (U.S.) brand of Enzyme Immunoassay Ovulation Prediction Test Kits—**See Ovulation Prediction Test Kits for Home Use**, #
*Fortel Midstream One Step*—Biomerica (U.S.) brand of Immunoassay Pregnancy Test Kits—**See Pregnancy Test Kits for Home Use**, #
*Fortel Plus*—Biomerica (U.S.) brand of Immunoassay Pregnancy Test Kits—**See Pregnancy Test Kits for Home Use**, #
*Fortovase*—Roche (U.S.) brand of Saquinavir (Systemic), 2554, MC-28
*Fosamax*—Merck (U.S.) and Merck Frosst (Canada) brand of Alendronate (Systemic), 42, MC-1
Foscarnet [*Foscavir*]
**(Systemic)**, 3020
Injection, 3020
Foscarnet Sodium [*Foscavir;* PFA; phosphonoformic acid; trisodium phosphonoformate]
**(Systemic)**, 1528
Injection, 1530
*Foscavir*—Astra (U.S.) brand of Foscarnet (Systemic), 1528, 3020
*Fosfestrol*—Diethylstilbestrol—**See Estrogens (Systemic)**, 1383
Fosfomycin Tromethamine [*Monurol*]
**(Systemic)**, 1531
for Solution, Oral, 1532
Fosinopril Sodium [*Monopril*]
**See Angiotensin-converting Enzyme (ACE) Inhibitors (Systemic)**, 177
Tablets, 185, MC-13
Fosphenytoin
**(Systemic)**, 3144
Fosphenytoin Sodium [*Cerebyx*]
**See Anticonvulsants, Hydantoin (Systemic)**, 253
Injection, 262
*Fostex 10 Bar*—Bristol-Myers Squibb (U.S.) brand of Benzoyl Peroxide (Topical), 579
*Fostex 10 BPO Gel*—Bristol-Myers Squibb (U.S.) brand of Benzoyl Peroxide (Topical), 579
*Fostex CM*—Bristol-Myers Squibb (Canada) brand of Sulfur (Topical), #
*Fostex 10 Cream*—Bristol-Myers Squibb (U.S.) brand of Benzoyl Peroxide (Topical), 579
*Fostex 5 Gel*—Bristol-Myers Squibb (U.S.) brand of Benzoyl Peroxide (Topical), 579
*Fostex Regular Strength Medicated Cover-Up*—Westwood (U.S.) brand of Sulfur (Topical), #
*Fostex 10 Wash*—Westwood (U.S.) brand of Benzoyl Peroxide (Topical), 579
*Fostril Cream*—Westwood-Squibb (Canada) brand of Sulfur (Topical), #
*Fostril Lotion*—Westwood (U.S.) brand of Sulfur (Topical), #
*Fototar*—Elder (U.S.) brand of Coal Tar (Topical), #
*Fourex Natural Skins*—London International (U.S. and Canada) brand of Lamb Cecum Condoms—**See Condoms**, #
*Fourex Natural Skins Spermicidally Lubricated*—London International (U.S.) brand of Lamb Cecum Condoms and Nonoxynol 9—**See Condoms**, #
*Fourneau 309*—*See* Suramin (Systemic), #
*Fowler's*—Sandoz (Canada) brand of Attapulgite (Oral-Local), #
*Fragmin*—Pharmacia (U.S. and Canada) brand of Dalteparin (Systemic), 1156
Framycetin-containing Combinations, 3073

Framycetin Sulfate [*Soframycin*]
**(Ophthalmic)**, 3020
Ointment, Ophthalmic, 3020
Solution, Ophthalmic, 3020
Framycetin Sulfate [*Sofra-Tulle*]
**(Topical)**, 3021
Gauze, Impregnated, 3021
Framycetin Sulfate and Gramicidin [*Soframycin*]
**(Topical)**, 3021
Ointment, 3021
Framycetin Sulfate, Gramicidin, and Dexamethasone [*Sofracort Eye-Ear*]
**(Ophthalmic)**, 3021
Ointment, Ophthalmic, 3021
Solution, Ophthalmic, 3021
Framycetin Sulfate, Gramicidin, and Dexamethasone [*Sofracort Eye-Ear*]
**(Otic)**, 3021
Ointment, Otic, 3021
Solution, Otic, 3021
*Freezone*—Whitehall (U.S.) brand of Salicylic Acid (Topical), #
*Frisium*—Hoechst (Canada) brand of Clobazam (Systemic), 556
*Froben*—Organon (Canada) brand of Flurbiprofen—**See Anti-inflammatory Drugs, Nonsteroidal (Systemic)**, 388
*Froben SR*—Organon (Canada) brand of Flurbiprofen—**See Anti-inflammatory Drugs, Nonsteroidal (Systemic)**, 388
*Frosstimage Albumin*—Frosst (Canada) brand of Technetium Tc 99m Albumin (Systemic), 2695
*Frosstimage DTPA*—Frosst (Canada) brand of Technetium Tc 99m Pentetate (Systemic), 2727
*Frosstimage Gluceptate*—Frosst (Canada) brand of Technetium Tc 99m Gluceptate (Systemic), 2711
*Frosstimage Gluco*—Frosst (Canada) brand of Technetium Tc 99m Gluceptate (Systemic), 2711
*Frosstimage HIDA*—Frosst (Canada) brand of Technetium Tc 99m Lidofenin (Systemic), 2713
*Frosstimage MAA*—Frosst (Canada) brand of Technetium Tc 99m Albumin Aggregated (Systemic), 2697
*Frosstimage MDP*—Frosst (Canada) brand of Technetium Tc 99m Medronate (Systemic), 2718
*Frosstimage Sulfur Colloid*—Frosst (Canada) brand of Technetium Tc 99m Sulfur Colloid (Systemic), 2740
Fructose, Dextrose, and Phosphoric Acid [*Emetrol*]
**(Oral-Local)**, 1532
Solution, Oral, 1533
Fructose-1,6-diphosphate
**(Systemic)**, 3144
FSH—*See* Urofollitropin (Systemic), 2901
5-FU—*See* Fluorouracil (Systemic), 1497; Fluorouracil (Topical), 1500
*Fucidin*—Leo (Canada) brand of Fusidic Acid (Systemic), 3021; Leo (Canada) brand of Fusidic Acid (Topical), 3021
*FUDR*—Roche (U.S.) brand of Floxuridine (Systemic), 1472
*Fulvicin P/G*—Schering (U.S. and Canada) brand of Griseofulvin (Systemic), 1583
*Fulvicin U/F*—Schering (Canada) brand of Griseofulvin (Systemic), 1583
*Fulvicin-U/F*—Schering (U.S.) brand of Griseofulvin (Systemic), 1583
*Fumasorb*—Milance (U.S.) brand of Ferrous Fumarate—**See Iron Supplements (Systemic)**, 1774
*Fumerin*—Laser (U.S.) brand of Ferrous Fumarate—**See Iron Supplements (Systemic)**, 1774
*Fungizone*—Squibb (U.S.) brand of Amphotericin B (Topical), #
*Fungizone Intravenous*—Lyphomed (U.S. and Canada) brand of Amphotericin B (Systemic), 98
*Furadantin*—Procter & Gamble (U.S.) brand of Nitrofurantoin (Systemic), 2139
*Furalan*—Lannett (U.S.) brand of Nitrofurantoin (Systemic), 2139
*Furamide*—Boots (U.K.) brand of Diloxanide (Systemic), #
*Furatoin*—Vortech (U.S.) brand of Nitrofurantoin (Systemic), 2139
Furazolidone [*Furoxone; Furoxone Liquid*]
**(Oral-Local)**, 1533
Suspension, Oral, USP, 1535
Tablets USP, 1535

Furosemide [Apo-Furosemide; Furoside; Lasix; Lasix Special; Myrosemide; Novosemide; Uritol]
  See **Diuretics, Loop (Systemic)**, 1259
  Injection USP, 1264
  Solution, Oral, 1264
  Tablets USP, 1264, MC-13
Furoside—ICN (Canada) brand of Furosemide—See **Diuretics, Loop (Systemic)**, 1259
Furoxone—Procter & Gamble (U.S.) brand of Furazolidone (Oral-Local), 1533
Furoxone Liquid—Procter & Gamble (U.S.) brand of Furazolidone (Oral-Local), 1533
Fusidic Acid [Fucidin]
  **(Systemic)**, 3021
  for Injection, 3021
  Suspension, Oral, 3021
  Tablets, 3021
Fusidic Acid [Fucidin]
  **(Topical)**, 3021
  Cream, 3021
  Gauze, Impregnated, 3021
  Ointment, 3021

## G

$^{67}$Ga—See Gallium Citrate Ga 67 (Systemic), 1538
Gabapentin [GBP; Neurontin]
  **(Systemic)**, 1536, 3144
  Capsules, 1537, MC-13
Gabbromicina—See Aminosidine (Systemic), 3130
Gabitril—Abbott (U.S.) brand of Tiagabine (Systemic), 2815, MC-30
Gadodiamide [Omniscan]
  **(Systemic)**, #
  Injection, #
Gadopentetate Dimeglumine [gadopentetic acid; Magnevist]
  **(Systemic)**, #
  Injection, #
Gadopentetic acid—See Gadopentetate (Systemic), #
Gadoteridol [ProHance]
  **(Systemic)**, #
  Injection, #
Galardin—Glycomed (U.S.) brand of Matrix Metalloproteinase Inhibitor (Ophthalmic), 3153
Gallamine Triethiodide [Flaxedil]
  See **Neuromuscular Blocking Agents (Systemic)**, 2098
  Injection USP, 2102
Gallium Citrate Ga 67 [Neoscan]
  **(Systemic)**, 1538
  Injection USP, 1540
Gallium Nitrate [Ganite]
  **(Systemic)**, 1540, 3143
  Injection, 1542, 3144
Galzin—Gate (U.S.) brand of Zinc (Systemic), 3039
Gamimune N—Bayer (U.S. and Canada) brand of Immune Globulin Intravenous (Human) (Systemic), 3024; Miles (U.S.) and Cutter (Canada) brand of Immune Globulin Intravenous (Human) (Systemic), 1686; Miles (U.S.) brand of Immune Globulin Intravenous (Human) (Systemic), 3147
Gamma benzene hexachloride—See Lindane (Topical), 1866
Gammagard—Baxter (U.S.) brand of Immune Globulin Intravenous (Human) (Systemic), 1686
Gammagard SD—Baxter (U.S.) brand of Immune Globulin Intravenous (Human) (Systemic), 3025
Gamma-Hydroxybutyrate
  **(Systemic)**, 3144
Gammalinolenic Acid
  **(Systemic)**, 3144
Gammar–IV—Armour (U.S.) brand of Immune Globulin Intravenous (Human) (Systemic), 1686
Gamulin Rh—Armour (U.S.) brand of Rh$_o$(D) Immune Globulin (Systemic), 2476
Ganciclovir [Cytovene; DHPG]
  **(Systemic)**, 1544, 3022
  Capsules, 1547, 3022, MC-13
Ganciclovir [Vitrasert]
  **(Implantation-Ophthalmic)**, 1542
  Implants (Intravitreal), 1544
Ganciclovir Sodium [Cytovene; Cytovene-IV; DHPG]
  **(Systemic)**, 1544
  Sterile, 1547
Ganite—Fujisawa (U.S.) brand of Gallium Nitrate (Systemic), 1540; Solopak (U.S.) brand of Gallium Nitrate (Systemic), 3144

Gantanol—Roche (U.S.) brand of Sulfamethoxazole—See **Sulfonamides (Systemic)**, 2653, MC-28
Gantrisin—Roche (U.S.) brand of Sulfisoxazole—See **Sulfonamides (Ophthalmic)**, 2651; **Sulfonamides (Systemic)**, 2653
Garamycin—Schering (U.S. and Canada) brand of Gentamicin—See **Aminoglycosides (Systemic)**, 69; Gentamicin (Ophthalmic), 1555; Gentamicin (Topical), 1557
Garamycin Otic Solution—Schering (Canada) brand of Gentamicin (Otic), 1556
Gasmas—Vachon (Canada) brand of Alumina, Magnesia, Magnesium Carbonate, and Simethicone—See **Antacids (Oral-Local)**, 188
Gas Relief—Rugby (U.S.) brand of Simethicone (Oral-Local), #
Gastrocrom—Fisons (U.S.) brand of Cromolyn (Systemic/Oral-Local), 1121, 3138
Gastrografin—Bracco (U.S. and Canada) brand of Diatrizoate—See **Diatrizoates (Systemic)**, #
Gastrolyte—Rorer (Canada) brand of Oral Rehydration Salts—See **Carbohydrates and Electrolytes (Systemic)**, 769
Gastromark—Advanced Magnetics (U.S.) brand of Ferumoxsil (Systemic), 3019
Gastrosed—Hauck (U.S.) brand of Hyoscyamine—See **Anticholinergics/Antispasmodics (Systemic)**, 226
Gastrozepin—Boehringer Ingelheim (Canada) brand of Pirenzepine—See **Anticholinergics/Antispasmodics (Systemic)**, 226
Gas-X—Sandoz (U.S.) brand of Simethicone (Oral-Local), #
Gaviscon—SmithKline Beecham (U.S.) brand of Alumina and Magnesium Carbonate—See **Antacids (Oral-Local)**, 188; SmithKline Beecham (U.S.) and Sterling Winthrop (Canada) brand of Alumina, Magnesium Trisilicate, and Sodium Bicarbonate—See **Antacids (Oral-Local)**, 188
Gaviscon-2—SmithKline Beecham (U.S.) brand of Alumina, Magnesium Trisilicate, and Sodium Bicarbonate—See **Antacids (Oral-Local)**, 188
Gaviscon Acid Plus Gas Relief—SmithKline Beecham (Canada) brand of Calcium Carbonate, Magnesia, and Simethicone—See **Antacids (Oral-Local)**, 188
Gaviscon Acid Relief—SmithKline Beecham (Canada) brand of Calcium Carbonate and Magnesia—See **Antacids (Oral-Local)**, 188
Gaviscon Extra Strength Acid Relief—SmithKline Beecham (Canada) brand of Calcium Carbonate and Magnesia—See **Antacids (Oral-Local)**, 188
Gaviscon Extra Strength Relief Formula—SmithKline Beecham (U.S.) brand of Alumina, Magnesium Carbonate, and Simethicone—See **Antacids (Oral-Local)**, 188; SmithKline Beecham (U.S.) brand of Alumina, Magnesium Carbonate, and Sodium Bicarbonate—See **Antacids (Oral-Local)**, 188
Gaviscon Heartburn Relief—SmithKline Beecham (Canada) brand of Aluminum Hydroxide—See **Antacids (Oral-Local)**, 188; Calcium and Magnesium Carbonates and Sodium Bicarbonate—See **Antacids (Oral-Local)**, 188; Magnesium Carbonate and Sodium Bicarbonate—See **Antacids (Oral-Local)**, 188
Gaviscon Heartburn Relief Extra Strength—SmithKline Beecham (Canada) brand of Aluminum Hydroxide—See **Antacids (Oral-Local)**, 188
GBH—Century (U.S.) and Rorer (Canada) brand of Lindane (Topical), 1866
GBP—See Gabapentin (Systemic), 1536
Gee-Gee—Jones (U.S.) brand of Guaifenesin (Systemic), 1588
Gelpirin—Alra (U.S.) brand of Acetaminophen, Aspirin, and Caffeine, Buffered—See **Acetaminophen and Salicylates (Systemic)**, 11
Gelpirin-CCF—Alra (U.S.) brand of Chlorpheniramine, Phenylpropanolamine, Guaifenesin, and Acetaminophen—See **Cough/Cold Combinations (Systemic)**, 1024
Gelsolin, Recombinant Human
  **(Systemic)**, 3161
Gelusil—Warner Wellcome (Canada) brand of Alumina and Magnesia—See **Antacids (Oral-Local)**, 188; Warner Wellcome (U.S.) brand of Alumina, Magnesia, and Simethicone—See **Antacids (Oral-Local)**, 188
Gelusil Extra Strength—Warner Wellcome (Canada) brand of Alumina and Magnesia—See **Antacids (Oral-Local)**, 188

Gemcitabine [Gemzar]
  **(Systemic)**, 1548
  for Injection, 1552
Gemfibrozil [Apo-Genfibrozil; Gen-Fibro; Lopid; Novo-Gemfibrozil; Nu-Gemfibrozil]
  **(Systemic)**, 1552
  Capsules USP, 1554
  Tablets, 1554, MC-13
Gemnisyn—Schwarz (U.S.) brand of Acetaminophen and Aspirin—See **Acetaminophen and Salicylates (Systemic)**, 11
Gemonil—Metharbital—See **Barbiturates (Systemic)**, 518
Gemzar—Lilly (U.S. and Canada) brand of Gemcitabine (Systemic), 1548
Genabid—Goldline (U.S.) brand of Papaverine (Systemic), #
Genac—Zenith Goldline (U.S.) brand of Triprolidine and Pseudoephedrine—See **Antihistamines and Decongestants (Systemic)**, 343
Genahist—Goldline (U.S.) brand of Diphenhydramine—See **Antihistamines (Systemic)**, 325
Gen-Allerate—Goldline (U.S.) brand of Chlorpheniramine—See **Antihistamines (Systemic)**, 325
Gen-Alprazolam—Genpharm (Canada) brand of Alprazolam—See **Benzodiazepindes (Systemic)**, 556
Genamin—Zenith Goldline (U.S.) brand of Chlorpheniramine and Phenylpropanolamine—See **Antihistamines and Decongestants (Systemic)**, 343
Genapap Children's Elixir—Goldline (U.S.) brand of Acetaminophen (Systemic), 6
Genapap Children's Tablets—Goldline (U.S.) brand of Acetaminophen (Systemic), 6
Genapap Extra Strength Caplets—Goldline (U.S.) brand of Acetaminophen (Systemic), 6
Genapap Extra Strength Tablets—Goldline (U.S.) brand of Acetaminophen (Systemic), 6
Genapap, Infants'—Goldline (U.S.) brand of Acetaminophen (Systemic), 6
Genapap Regular Strength Tablets—Goldline (U.S.) brand of Acetaminophen (Systemic), 6
Genaphed—Goldline (U.S.) brand of Pseudoephedrine (Systemic), 2422
Genasoft Plus Softgels—Zenith Goldline (U.S.) brand of Casthranol and Docusate—See **Laxatives (Local)**, #
Genaspore Cream—Goldline (U.S.) brand of Tolnaftate (Topical), #
Genasyme—Goldline (U.S.) brand of Simethicone (Oral-Local), #
Genatap—Zenith Goldline (U.S.) brand of Brompheniramine and Phenylpropanolamine—See **Antihistamines and Decongestants (Systemic)**, 343
Genaton—Zenith Goldline (U.S.) brand of Alumina and Magnesium Carbonate—See **Antacids (Oral-Local)**, 188; Alumina, Magnesium Trisilicate, and Sodium Bicarbonate—See **Antacids (Oral-Local)**, 188
Genaton Extra Strength—Zenith Goldline (U.S.) brand of Alumina, Magnesium Carbonate, and Sodium Bicarbonate—See **Antacids (Oral-Local)**, 188
Genatuss—Zenith Goldline (U.S.) brand of Guaifenesin (Systemic), 1588
Genatuss DM—Zenith Goldline (U.S.) brand of Dextromethorphan and Guaifenesin—See **Cough/Cold Combinations (Systemic)**, 1024
Gen-Bromazepam—Genpharm (Canada) brand of Bromazepam—See **Benzodiazepindes (Systemic)**, 556
Gencalc 600—Goldline (U.S.) brand of Calcium Carbonate—See **Calcium Supplements (Systemic)**, 736
Gen-Cimetidine—Genpharm (Canada) brand of Cimetidine—See **Histamine H$_2$-receptor Antagonists (Systemic)**, 1633
Gen-Clonazepam—Genpharm (Canada) brand of Clonazepam—See **Benzodiazepindes (Systemic)**, 556
Gencold—Zenith Goldline (U.S.) brand of Chlorpheniramine and Phenylpropanolamine—See **Antihistamines and Decongestants (Systemic)**, 343
Gendecon—Zenith Goldline (U.S.) brand of Chlorpheniramine, Phenylephrine, and Acetaminophen—See **Antihistamines, Decongestants, and Analgesics (Systemic)**, 366
Genebs Extra Strength Caplets—Goldline (U.S.) brand of Acetaminophen (Systemic), 6

*Genebs Regular Strength Tablets*—Goldline (U.S.) brand of Acetaminophen (Systemic), 6
*Genebs X-Tra*—Goldline (U.S.) brand of Acetaminophen (Systemic), 6
*GenESA*—Gensia (U.S.) brand of Arbutamine (Systemic), 464
*Gen-Famotidine*—Genpharm (Canada) brand of Famotidine—**See Histamine H$_2$-receptor Antagonists (Systemic)**, 1633, MC-12
*Gen-Fibro*—Genpharm (Canada) brand of Gemfibrozil (Systemic), 1552
*Gen-Glybe*—Genpharm (Canada) brand of Glyburide—**See Antidiabetic Agents, Sulfonylurea (Systemic)**, 283
*Genite*—Zenith Goldline (U.S.) brand of Doxylamine, Pseudoephedrine, Dextromethorphan and Acetaminophen—**See Cough/Cold Combinations (Systemic)**, 1024
*Gen-K*—Goldline (U.S.) brand of Potassium Chloride—**See Potassium Supplements (Systemic)**, 2357
*Gen-Medroxy*—Genpharm (Canada) brand of Medroxyprogesterone—**See Progestins (Systemic)**, 2400
*Gen-Minoxidil*—Genpharm (Canada) brand of Minoxidil (Topical), 2021
*Genoptic Liquifilm*—Allergan (U.S.) brand of Gentamicin (Ophthalmic), 1555
*Genoptic S.O.P.*—Allergan (U.S.) brand of Gentamicin (Ophthalmic), 1555
*Genora 0.5/35*—Rugby (U.S.) brand of Norethindrone and Ethinyl Estradiol—**See Estrogens and Progestins—Oral Contraceptives (Systemic)**, 1397, MC-22
*Genora 1/35*—Rugby (U.S.) brand of Norethindrone and Ethinyl Estradiol—**See Estrogens and Progestins—Oral Contraceptives (Systemic)**, 1397, MC-22
*Genora 1/50*—Rugby (U.S.) brand of Norethindrone and Mestranol—**See Estrogens and Progestins—Oral Contraceptives (Systemic)**, 1397, MC-22
*Genotonorm*—Pharmacia (U.S.) brand of Somatropin (Systemic), 3165
*Genotropin*—Pharmacia (U.S.) brand of Somatropin (Systemic), 3165; Pharmacia & Upjohn (U.S.) brand of Somatropin, Recombinant (Systemic), 3034, 3035
*Genpril*—Goldline (U.S.) brand of Ibuprofen—**See Anti-inflammatory Drugs, Nonsteroidal (Systemic)**, 388
*Genpril Caplets*—Goldline (U.S.) brand of Ibuprofen—**See Anti-inflammatory Drugs, Nonsteroidal**, 388
*Gen-Ranitidine*—Genpharm (Canada) brand of Ranitidine Hydrochloride—**See Histamine H$_2$-receptor Antagonists (Systemic)**, 1633, MC-27
*Gen-Salbutamol Sterinebs P.F.*—Genpharm (Canada) brand of Albuterol—**See Bronchodilators, Adrenergic (Inhalation-Local)**, 640
*Gensan*—Aspirin—**See Salicylates (Systemic)**, 2538
*Gen-Selegiline*—Genpharm (Canada) brand of Selegiline (Systemic), 2560
*Gentacidin*—Iolab (U.S.) brand of Gentamicin (Ophthalmic), 1555
*Gentafair*—Balan (U.S.); Dixon-Shane (U.S.); Gen-King (U.S.); Glenlawn (U.S.); Qualitest (U.S.); Pharmafair (U.S.); and Texas Drug (U.S.) brand of Gentamicin (Ophthalmic), 1555
*Gentak*—Akorn (U.S.) brand of Gentamicin (Ophthalmic), 1555
*Gentamar*—Marlop (U.S.) brand of Gentamicin (Topical), 1557
Gentamicin Impregnated PMMA Beads on Surgical Wire [*Septopal*]
 (Systemic), 3144
Gentamicin Liposome [*Maitec*]
 (Systemic), 3144
 Injection, 3144
Gentamicin Sulfate [*Alcomicin; Garamycin; Genoptic Liquifilm; Genoptic S.O.P.; Gentacidin; Gentafair; Gentak;* gentamycin; *Gentrasul; Ocu-Mycin; Spectro-Genta*]
 (Ophthalmic), 1555
 Ointment, Ophthalmic, USP, 1555
 Solution, Ophthalmic, USP, 1556
Gentamicin Sulfate [*Garamycin Otic Solution*]
 (Otic), 1556
 Solution, Otic, 1557

Gentamicin Sulfate [*Cidomycin; Garamycin; G-Mycin; Jenamicin*]
 **See Aminoglycosides (Systemic)**, 69
 Injection USP, 75
Gentamicin Sulfate [*Garamycin; Gentamar; G-Myticin*]
 (Topical), 1557
 Cream USP, 1558
 Ointment USP, 1558
Gentamicin Sulfate in Sodium Chloride
 **See Aminoglycosides (Systemic)**, 69
 Injection, 76
*Gen-Tamoxifen*—Genpharm (Canada) brand of Tamoxifen (Systemic), 2688
Gentamycin—Gentamicin—**See Aminoglycosides (Systemic)**, 69; *See also* Gentamicin (Ophthalmic), 1555
Gentian Violet
 (Vaginal), #
 Tampons, Vaginal, #
Gentian Violet
 (Topical), #
 Solution, Topical, USP, #
*Gen-Timolol*—Genpharm (Canada) brand of Timolol—**See Beta-adrenergic Blocking Agents (Ophthalmic)**, 585
*Gentle Laxative*—Zenith Goldline (U.S.) brand of Bisacodyl—**See Laxatives (Local)**, #
*Gent-L-Tip*—Baxter (Canada) brand of Sodium Phosphates—**See Laxatives (Local)**, #
*Gentrasul*—Bausch & Lomb (U.S. and Canada) brand of Gentamicin (Ophthalmic), 1555
*Gen-Triazolam*—Genpharm (Canada) brand of Triazolam—**See Benzodiazepines (Systemic)**, 556
*Genuine Bayer Aspirin Caplets*—Miles (U.S.) brand of Aspirin—**See Salicylates (Systemic)**, 2538
*Genuine Bayer Aspirin Tablets*—Miles (U.S.) brand of Aspirin—**See Salicylates (Systemic)**, 2538
*Geocillin*—Roerig (U.S.) brand of Carbenicillin—**See Penicillins (Systemic)**, 2240
*Geopen*—Pfipharmecs (U.S.) brand of Carbenicillin—**See Penicillins (Systemic)**, 2240
*Geopen Oral*—Pfizer (Canada) brand of Carbenicillin—**See Penicillins (Systemic)**, 2240
*Gerber Baby Formula*—Bristol-Myers Squibb (U.S.) brand of Infant Formulas, Milk-based—**See Infant Formulas (Systemic)**, #
*Gerber Soy Formula*—Bristol-Myers Squibb (U.S.) brand of Infant Formulas, Soy-based—**See Infant Formulas (Systemic)**, #
*Geref*—Serono (U.S.) brand of Sermorelin (Systemic), 2565, 3164
*Geridium*—Goldline (U.S.) brand of Phenazopyridine (Systemic), 2288
*Gerimal*—Rugby (U.S.) brand of Ergoloid Mesylates (Systemic), 1358
*Germanin*—Bayer (Germany and South Africa) brand of Suramin (Systemic), #
*Gesterol 50*—Forest (U.S.) brand of Progesterone—**See Progestins (Systemic)**, 2400
*Gesterol LA 250*—Solvay (U.S.) brand of Hydroxyprogesterone—**See Progestins (Systemic)**, 2400
*GG-CEN*—Central (U.S.) brand of Guaifenesin (Systemic), 1588
GH—Somatrem—**See Growth Hormone (Systemic)**, 1586; Somatropin, Recombinant—**See Growth Hormone (Systemic)**, 1586
*Gil-Paque*—E-Z-EM (U.S.) brand of Barium Sulfate (Local), #
*Gin Pain Pills*—Sodium Salicylate—**See Salicylates (Systemic)**, 2538
Glatiramer Acetate [*Copaxone;* copolymer-1]
 (Systemic), 1558
 for Injection, 1560
*Glaucon*—Alcon (U.S.) brand of Epinephrine (Ophthalmic), 1350
*Gliadel*—Guilford (U.S.) brand of Biodel Implant/Carmustine (Systemic), 3133
*Gliadel Wafer*—Rhône-Poulenc Rorer (U.S.) brand of Carmustine (Implantation-Local), 784
Glibenclamide—Glyburide—**See Antidiabetic Agents, Sulfonylurea (Systemic)**, 283
Gliclazide [*Diamicron*]
 **See Antidiabetic Agents, Sulfonylurea (Systemic)**, 283
 Tablets, 292
Glimepiride [*Amaryl*]
 (Systemic), 1560
 Tablets, 1563, MC-13

Glipizide [*Glucotrol; Glucotrol XL*]
 **See Antidiabetic Agents, Sulfonylurea (Systemic)**, 283
 Tablets USP, 293, MC-13
 Tablets, Extended-release, 293, MC-13
*Glo-Sel*—Syosset (U.S.) brand of Selenium Sulfide (Topical), #
Glucagon [*Glucagon Emergency Kit*]
 (Systemic), 1563
 for Injection USP, 1565
*Glucagon Emergency Kit*—Lilly (U.S. and Canada) brand of Glucagon (Systemic), 1563
*Glucantim*—Rhône-Poulenc (Italy) brand of Meglumine Antimoniate (Systemic), #
*Glucantime*—Specia (France) brand of Meglumine Antimoniate (Systemic), #
*Glucerna*—Ross (U.S.) brand of Enteral Nutrition Formula, Disease-specific—**See Enteral Nutrition Formulas (Systemic)**, #
*Glucophage*—Bristol-Myers Squibb (U.S.) and Nordic (Canada) brand of Metformin (Systemic), 1957, MC-19
*Glucoscan*—Du Pont N.E.N. (U.S.) brand of Technetium Tc 99m Gluceptate (Systemic), 2711
*Glucose & Ketone Urine Test*—Major (U.S.) brand of Urine Glucose and Ketone (Combined) Test—**See Urine Glucose and Ketone Test Kits for Home Use**, #
Glucose Oxidase Urine Glucose Test [*Biotel/diabetes; Chemstrip uG; Clinistix; Diastix; Tes-tape*]
 **See Urine Glucose and Ketone Test Kits for Home Use**, #
 Strips, #
 Tape, #
*Glucotrol*—Pfizer (U.S.) brand of Glipizide—**See Antidiabetic Agents, Sulfonylurea (Systemic)**, 283, MC-13
*Glucotrol XL*—Pfizer (U.S.) brand of Glipizide—**See Antidiabetic Agents, Sulfonylurea (Systemic)**, 283, MC-13
*Glu-K*—Jones-Western (U.S.) brand of Potassium Gluconate—**See Potassium Supplements (Systemic)**, 2357
Glutamine
 (Systemic), 3144
Glutethimide
 (Systemic), #
 Capsules USP, #
 Tablets USP, #
Glyburide [*Albert Glyburide; Apo-Glyburide; DiaBeta; Euglucon; Gen-Glybe;* glibenclamide; *Glynase PresTab; Micronase; Novo-Glyburide; Nu-Glyburide*]
 **See Antidiabetic Agents, Sulfonylurea (Systemic)**, 283, 3022
 Tablets, 294, 3022, MC-14
 Tablets (Micronized), 294
Glycerin [*Fleet Babylax; Fleet Glycerin Laxative; Sani-Supp*]
 **See Laxatives (Local)**, #
 Solution, Rectal, #
 Suppositories USP, #
Glycerin [*Glyrol; Osmoglyn*]
 (Systemic), #
 Solution, Oral, USP, #
Glycerin-containing Combinations, 3073
Glyceryl guaiacolate—*See* Guaifenesin (Systemic), 1588
*Glyceryl-T*—Rugby (U.S.) brand of Theophylline and Guaifenesin (Systemic), #
Glyceryl trinitrate—Nitroglycerin—**See Nitrates (Systemic)**, 2129
Glyceryl Trioleate and Glyceryl Trierucate [*Lorenzo's oil*]
 (Systemic), 3144
*Glycofed*—Pal-Pak (U.S.) brand of Pseudoephedrine and Guaifenesin—**See Cough/Cold Combinations (Systemic)**, 1024
Glycopyrrolate [glycopyrronium bromide; *Robinul; Robinul Forte*]
 **See Anticholinergics/Antispasmodics (Systemic)**, 226
 Injection USP, 235
 Tablets USP, 235
Glycopyrronium bromide—Glycopyrrolate—**See Anticholinergics/Antispasmodics (Systemic)**, 226
*Gly-Cort*—Heran (U.S.) brand of Hydrocortisone—**See Corticosteroids (Topical)**, 978
*Glycotuss*—Pal-Pak (U.S.) brand of Guaifenesin (Systemic), 1588

*Glycotuss-dM*—Pal-Pak (U.S.) brand of Dextromethorphan and Guaifenesin—**See Cough/Cold Combinations (Systemic)**, 1024

*Glydeine Cough*—Geneva (U.S.) brand of Codeine and Guaifenesin—**See Cough/Cold Combinations (Systemic)**, 1024

*Glylorin*—Cellegy (U.S.) brand of Monolaurin (Systemic), 3155

*Glynase PresTab*—Upjohn (U.S.) brand of Glyburide—**See Antidiabetic Agents, Sulfonylurea (Systemic)**, 283

*Glypressin*—Ferring (U.S.) brand of Terlipressin, 3167

*Glyrol*—CooperVision (U.S.) brand of Glycerin (Systemic), #

*Glysennid*—Sandoz (Canada) brand of Sennosides—**See Laxatives (Local)**, #

*Glytrol*—Clintec (U.S.) brand of Enteral Nutrition Formula, Disease-specific—**See Enteral Nutrition Formulas (Systemic)**, #; Enteral Nutrition Formula, Fiber-containing—**See Enteral Nutrition Formulas (Systemic)**, #

*Glytuss*—Mayrand (U.S.) brand of Guaifenesin (Systemic), 1588

*G-Mycin*—Bolan (U.S.) brand of Gentamicin—**See Aminoglycosides (Systemic)**, 69

*G-Myticin*—Pedinol (U.S.) brand of Gentamicin (Topical), 1557

*Go-Evac*—Copely (U.S.) brand of Polyethylene Glycol 3350 and Electrolytes (Local), 2349

*Gold Circle Coin*—Mayer (U.S. and Canada) brand of Latex Condoms—**See Condoms**, #

*Gold Circle Rainbow Coin*—Mayer (U.S.) brand of Latex Condoms—**See Condoms**, #

Gold Compounds
 **(Systemic)**, 1566

Gold Sodium Thiomalate [*Myochrysine*; sodium aurothiomalate]
 **See Gold Compounds (Systemic)**, 1566
 Injection USP, 1569

*GoLYTELY*—Braintree (U.S.) and Baxter (Canada) brand of Polyethylene Glycol 3350 and Electrolytes (Local), 2349

Gonadorelin Acetate [LH/FSH–RH; LHRH; luteinizing hormone-/follicle-stimulating hormone–releasing hormone; luteinizing hormone–releasing factor diacetate tetrahydrate; luteinizing hormone–releasing hormone; *Lutrepulse*; *Relisorm*]
 **(Systemic)**, 1571, 3144
 for Injection, 1574

Gonadorelin Hydrochloride [*Factrel*; LH/FSH–RH; LHRH; luteinizing hormone–releasing factor dihydrochloride; luteinizing hormone–/follicle-stimulating hormone–releasing hormone; lutenininzing hormone–releasing hormone; luteinizing hormone–releasing factor dihydrochloride; luteinizing hormone–releasing hormone]
 **(Systemic)**, 1571
 for Injection, 1574

*Gonak*—Akorn (U.S.) brand of Hydroxypropyl Methylcellulose (Ophthalmic), #

*Gonal-F*—Serono (U.S.) brand of Follitropin Alfa (Systemic), 1520

*Goniosoft*—Akorn (U.S.) brand of Hydroxypropyl Methylcellulose (Ophthalmic), #

*Goniosol*—Iolab (U.S.) brand of Hydroxypropyl Methylcellulose (Ophthalmic), #

*Goody's Extra Strength Tablets*—Goody's (U.S.) brand of Acetaminophen, Aspirin, and Caffeine—**See Acetaminophen and Salicylates (Systemic)**, 11

*Goody's Headache Powders*—Goody's (U.S.) brand of Acetaminophen, Aspirin, and Caffeine—**See Acetaminophen and Salicylates (Systemic)**, 11

*Gordochom Solution*—Gordon (U.S.) brand of Undecylenic Acid, Compound (Topical), #

*Gordofilm*—Gordon (U.S.) brand of Salicylic Acid (Topical), #

Goserelin Acetate [*Zoladex*; *Zoladex LA*; *Zoladex 3-Month*]
 **(Systemic)**, 1575
 Implants, 1578

Gossypol
 **(Systemic)**, 3144

*Gotamine*—Vita Elixir (U.S.) brand of Ergotamine and Caffeine—**See Vascular Headache Suppressants, Ergot Derivative–containing (Systemic)**, 2925

*GP-500*—Marnel (U.S.) brand of Pseudoephedrine and Guaifenesin—**See Cough/Cold Combinations (Systemic)**, 1024

gp100 Adenoviral Gene Therapy
 **(Systemic)**, 3144

*Gramcal*—Sandoz (Canada) brand of Calcium Lactate-Gluconate and Calcium Carbonate—**See Calcium Supplements (Systemic)**, 736

Gramicidin-containing Combinations, 3073

Granisetron Hydrochloride [*Kytril*]
 **(Systemic)**, 1578
 Injection, 1580
 Tablets, 1579, MC-14

Granulocyte colony stimulating factor, recombinant—Filgrastim—**See Colony Stimulating Factors (Systemic)**, 941

Granulocyte-macrophage colony stimulating factor, recombinant—Sargramostim—**See Colony Stimulating Factors (Systemic)**, 941

*Gravergol*—Horner (Canada) brand of Ergotamine, Caffeine, and Dimenhydrinate—**See Vascular Headache Suppressants, Ergot Derivative–containing (Systemic)**, 2925

*Gravol*—Horner (Canada) brand of Dimenhydrinate—**See Antihistamines (Systemic)**, 325

*Gravol Filmkote*—Carter-Horner (Canada) brand of Dimenhydrinate—**See Antihistamines (Systemic)**, 325

*Gravol Filmkote (Junior Strength)*—Carter-Horner (Canada) brand of Dimenhydrinate—**See Antihistamines (Systemic)**, 325

*Gravol I/M*—Carter-Horner (Canada) brand of Dimenhydrinate—**See Antihistamines (Systemic)**, 325

*Gravol I/V*—Carter-Horner (Canada) brand of Dimenhydrinate—**See Antihistamines (Systemic)**, 325

*Gravol L/A*—Horner (Canada) brand of Dimenhydrinate—**See Antihistamines (Systemic)**, 325

*Gravol Liquid*—Carter-Horner (Canada) brand of Dimenhydrinate—**See Antihistamines (Systemic)**, 325

*Great Shake*—Menu Magic (U.S.) brand of Enteral Nutrition Formula, Milk-based—**See Enteral Nutrition Formulas (Systemic)**, #

*Great Shake Jr.*—Menu Magic (U.S.) brand of Enteral Nutrition Formula, Milk-based—**See Enteral Nutrition Formulas (Systemic)**, #

Grepafloxcin Hydrochloride [*Raxar*]
 **(Systemic)**, 1580, 3087
 Tablets, 1580, MC-14

*Grifulvin V*—Ortho (U.S.) brand of Griseofulvin (Systemic), 1583, MC-14

*Grisactin*—Wyeth-Ayerst (U.S.) brand of Griseofulvin (Systemic), 1583

*Grisactin Ultra*—Wyeth-Ayerst (U.S.) brand of Griseofulvin (Systemic), 1583

Griseofulvin [*Fulvicin U/F*; *Fulvicin-U/F*; *Grifulvin V*; *Grisactin*; *Grisovin-FP*]
 **(Systemic)**, 1583
 Capsules USP (Microsize), 1585
 Suspension, Oral, USP (Microsize), 1585
 Tablets USP (Microsize), 1585, MC-14

Griseofulvin, Ultramicrosize [*Fulvicin P/G*; *Grisactin Ultra*; *Gris-PEG*]
 **(Systemic)**, 1583
 Tablets USP, 1585

*Grisovin-FP*—Glaxo (Canada) brand of Griseofulvin (Systemic), 1583

*Gris-PEG*—Allergan Herbert (U.S.) brand of Griseofulvin (Systemic), 1583

Group B Streptococcus Immune Globulin
 **(Systemic)**, 3144

Growth Hormone
 **(Systemic)**, 1586

Growth Hormone, Human
 **(Systemic)**, 3145

Growth Hormone, Human, Recombinant—See Somatropin (Systemic), 3165

Growth Hormone Releasing Factor
 **(Systemic)**, 3145

*Guaifed*—Muro (U.S.) brand of Pseudoephedrine and Guaifenesin—**See Cough/Cold Combinations (Systemic)**, 1024

*Guaifed-PD*—Muro (U.S.) brand of Pseudoephedrine and Guaifenesin—**See Cough/Cold Combinations (Systemic)**, 1024

Guaifenesin [*Anti-Tuss*; *Balminil Expectorant*; *Benylin-E*; *Breonesin*; *Calmylin Expectorant*; *Diabetic Tussin EX*; *Fenesin*; *Gee-Gee*; *Genatuss*; *GG-CEN*; glyceryl guaiacolate; *Glycotuss*; *Glytuss*; *Guiatuss*; *Halotussin*; *Humibid L.A.*; *Humibid Sprinkle*; *Hytuss*; *Hytuss-2X*; *Naldecon Senior EX*; *Organidin NR*; *Pneumomist*; *Resyl*; *Robitussin*; *Scot-tussin Expectorant*; *Sinumist-SR*; *Touro EX*; *Uni-tussin*]
 **(Systemic)**, 1588
 Capsules USP, 1589
 Capsules, Extended-release, 1589
 Solution, Oral, 1590
 Syrup USP, 1590
 Tablets USP, 1590
 Tablets, Extended-release, 1590

Guaifenesin and Codeine
 **See Cough/Cold Combinations (Systemic)**, 1024
 Syrup USP, 1060

Guaifenesin, Codeine, and Pseudoephedrine
 **See Cough/Cold Combinations (Systemic)**, 1024
 Solution, Oral, 1060
 Syrup, 1060

Guaifenesin-containing Combinations, 3073

*Guaifen PSE*—Qualitest (U.S.) brand of Pseudoephedrine and Guaifenesin—**See Cough/Cold Combinations (Systemic)**, MC-27

*Guaifenex PPA 75*—Ethex (U.S.) brand of Phenylpropanolamine and Guaifenesin—**See Cough/Cold Combinations (Systemic)**, 1024

*Guaifenex PSE 60*—Ethex (U.S.) brand of Pseudoephedrine and Guaifenesin—**See Cough/Cold Combinations (Systemic)**, 1024

*Guaifenex PSE 120*—Ethex (U.S.) brand of Pseudoephedrine and Guaifenesin—**See Cough/Cold Combinations (Systemic)**, 1024

*GuaiMAX-D*—Central (U.S.) brand of Pseudoephedrine and Guaifenesin—**See Cough/Cold Combinations (Systemic)**, 1024

*Guaipax*—Eon (U.S.) brand of Phenylpropanolamine and Guaifenesin—**See Cough/Cold Combinations (Systemic)**, 1024

*Guaitab*—Muro (U.S.) brand of Pseudoephedrine and Guaifenesin—**See Cough/Cold Combinations (Systemic)**, 1024

*Guaituss-DM*—Mason (U.S.); Moore (U.S.); and Zenith Goldline (U.S.) brand of Dextromethorphan and Guaifenesin—**See Cough/Cold Combinations (Systemic)**, 1024

*Guaivent*—Ethex (U.S.) brand of Pseudoephedrine and Guaifenesin—**See Cough/Cold Combinations (Systemic)**, 1024

*Guaivent PD*—Ethex (U.S.) brand of Pseudoephedrine and Guaifenesin—**See Cough/Cold Combinations (Systemic)**, 1024

*Guai-Vent/PSE*—Dura (U.S.) brand of Pseudoephedrine and Guaifenesin—**See Cough/Cold Combinations (Systemic)**, 1024

Guanabenz Acetate [*Wytensin*]
 **(Systemic)**, 1590
 Tablets USP, 1592, MC-14

Guanadrel Sulfate [*Hylorel*]
 **(Systemic)**, 1592
 Tablets USP, 1595

Guanethidine-containing Combinations, 3073

Guanethidine Monosulfate [*Apo-Guanethidine*; *Ismelin*]
 **(Systemic)**, 1595, 3144
 Tablets USP, 1598

Guanfacine Hydrochloride [*Tenex*]
 **(Systemic)**, 1598
 Tablets, 1600, MC-14

*GuiaCough CF*—Schein (U.S.) brand of Phenylpropanolamine, Dextromethorphan, and Guaifenesin—**See Cough/Cold Combinations (Systemic)**, 1024

*GuiaCough PE*—Schein (U.S.) brand of Pseudoephedrine and Guaifenesin—**See Cough/Cold Combinations (Systemic)**, 1024

*Guiamid D.M. Liquid*—Vangard (U.S.) brand of Dextromethorphan and Guaifenesin—**See Cough/Cold Combinations (Systemic)**, 1024

*Guiatuss*—Bell (U.S.); Generix (U.S.); Moore (U.S.); Schein (U.S.); and United Research (U.S.) brand of Guaifenesin (Systemic), 1588

*Guiatuss A.C.*—Barre-National (U.S.); Harber (U.S.); Mason (U.S.); Moore (U.S.) and Zenith Goldline (U.S.) brand of Codeine and Guaifenesin—**See Cough/Cold Combinations (Systemic)**, 1024

*Guiatuss CF*—Barre-National (U.S.) brand of Phenylpropanolamine, Dextromethorphan, and Guaifenesin—**See Cough/Cold Combinations (Systemic)**, 1024

*Guiatuss DAC*—Barre-National (U.S.); Moore (U.S.); Rugby (U.S.) and Zenith Goldline (U.S.) brand of Pseudoephedrine, Codeine, and Guaifenesin—**See Cough/Cold Combinations (Systemic)**, 1024

*Guiatuss-DM*—Barre-National (U.S.); Mason (U.S.); H.L. Moore (U.S.); Veratex (U.S.) and Zenith Goldline (U.S.) brand of Dextromethorphan and Guaifenesin—**See Cough/Cold Combinations (Systemic)**, 1024

*Guiatussin with Codeine Liquid*—Rugby (U.S.) brand of Codeine and Guaifenesin—**See Cough/Cold Combinations (Systemic)**, 1024

*Guiatussin DAC*—Rugby (U.S.) brand of Pseudoephedrine, Codeine, and Guaifenesin—**See Cough/Cold Combinations (Systemic)**, 1024

*Guiatussin with Dextromethorphan*—Rugby (U.S.) brand of Dextromethorphan and Guaifenesin—**See Cough/Cold Combinations (Systemic)**, 1024

*Guiatuss PE*—Barre-National (U.S.) brand of Pseudoephedrine and Guaifenesin—**See Cough/Cold Combinations (Systemic)**, 1024

Gusperimus [*Spanidin*]
  **(Systemic)**, 3145

*G-well*—Goldline (U.S.) brand of Lindane (Topical), 1866

*Gynecort*—Combe (U.S.) brand of Hydrocortisone—**See Corticosteroids (Topical)**, 978

*Gynecort 10*—Combe (U.S.) brand of Hydrocortisone—**See Corticosteroids (Topical)**, 978; Combe (U.S.) brand of Hydrocortisone (Topical), 3023

*GyneCure*—Pfizer (Canada) brand of Tioconazole—**See Antifungals, Azole (Vaginal)**, 310

*GyneCure Ovules*—Pfizer (Canada) brand of Tioconazole—**See Antifungals, Azole (Vaginal)**, 310

*GyneCure Vaginal Ointment Tandempak*—Pfizer (Canada) brand of Tioconazole—**See Antifungals, Azole (Vaginal)**, 310

*GyneCure Vaginal Ovules Tandempak*—Pfizer (Canada) brand of Tioconazole—**See Antifungals, Azole (Vaginal)**, 310

*Gyne-Lotrimin*—Schering-Plough (U.S.) brand of Clotrimazole—**See Antifungals, Azole (Vaginal)**, 310

*Gyne-Lotrimin 3*—Schering-Plough (U.S.) brand of Clotrimazole—**See Antifungals, Azole (Vaginal)**, 310

*Gyne-Lotrimin 3 Combination Pack*—Schering-Plough (U.S.) brand of Clotrimazole—**See Antifungals, Azole (Vaginal)**, 310

*Gyne-Lotrimin Combination Pack*—Schering-Plough (U.S.) brand of Clotrimazole—**See Antifungals, Azole (Vaginal)**, 310, 310

*Gynergen*—Sandoz (Canada) brand of Ergotamine—**See Vascular Headache Suppressants, Ergot Derivative–containing (Systemic)**, 2925

*Gyne-T*—Ortho (Canada) brand of Copper-T 200 Intrauterine Device—**See Copper Intrauterine Devices (IUDs)**, #

*Gyne-T 380 Slimline*—Ortho (Canada) brand of Copper-T 380S Intrauterine Device—**See Copper Intrauterine Devices (IUDs)**, #

*Gynogen L.A. 20*—Forest (U.S.) brand of Estradiol—**See Estrogens (Systemic)**, 1383

*Gynogen L.A. 40*—Forest (U.S.) brand of Estradiol—**See Estrogens (Systemic)**, 1383

*Gynol II Extra Strength Contraceptive Jelly*—Ortho (U.S.) brand of Nonoxynol 9—**See Spermicides (Vaginal)**, #

*Gynol II Original Formula Contraceptive Jelly*—Ortho (U.S.) brand of Nonoxynol 9—**See Spermicides (Vaginal)**, #

# H

*Habitrol*—Ciba Self-Medication (U.S.) and Ciba (Canada) brand of Nicotine (Systemic), 2125; Novartis (Canada) brand of Nicotine (Systemic), 3030

Haemophilus b Conjugate Vaccine
  **(Systemic)**, 1601

Haemophilus b Conjugate Vaccine (HbOC—Diphtheria CRM$_{197}$ Protein Conjugate) [*Hibtiter; oligo-CRM; PRP-HbOC*]
  **See Haemophilus b Conjugate Vaccine (Systemic)**, 1601
  Injection, 1603

Haemophilus b Conjugate Vaccine [*Omnihib*]
  **(Systemic)**, 3022
  Injection, 3022

Haemophilus b Conjugate Vaccine (PRP-D—Diphtheria Toxoid Conjugate) [*Prohibit*]
  **See Haemophilus b Conjugate Vaccine (Systemic)**, 1601
  Injection, 1604

Haemophilus b Conjugate Vaccine (PRP-OMP—Meningococcal Protein Conjugate) [*Pedvaxhib*]
  **See Haemophilus b Conjugate Vaccine (Systemic)**, 1601
  Injection, 1604

Haemophilus b Conjugate Vaccine (PRP-T—Tetanus Protein Conjugate) [*Act-Hib*]
  **See Haemophilus b Conjugate Vaccine (Systemic)**, 1601
  Injection, 1605

Haemophilus b Polysaccharide Vaccine [haemophilus influenzae type b polysaccharide vaccine; HbPV; hemophilus b polysaccharide vaccine; Hib CPS; Hib polysaccharide vaccine; PRP]
  **(Systemic)**, 1606
  Haemophilus b Polysaccharide Vaccine (for Injection), 1608

Haemophilus influenzae type b polysaccharide vaccine—*See* Haemophilus b Polysaccharide Vaccine (Systemic), 1606

Halazepam [*Paxipam*]
  **See Benzodiazepines (Systemic)**, 556
  Tablets, 573

Halcinonide [*Halog; Halog-E*]
  **See Corticosteroids (Topical)**, 978
  Cream USP, 991
  Ointment USP, 991
  Solution, Topical, USP, 991

*Halcion*—Pharmacia & Upjohn (U.S. and Canada) brand of Triazolam—**See Benzodiazepines (Systemic)**, 556, MC-31

*Haldol*—McNeil (U.S. and Canada) brand of Haloperidol (Systemic), 1611

*Haldol Decanoate*—McNeil (U.S.) brand of Haloperidol (Systemic), 1611

*Haldol LA*—McNeil (Canada) brand of Haloperidol (Systemic), 1611

*Haley's M-O*—Bayer Consumer (U.S.) brand of Magnesium Hydroxide and Mineral Oil—**See Laxatives (Local)**, #

*Halfan*—SmithKline Beecham (U.S.) brand of Halofantrine (Systemic), 3022, 3145; SmithKline Beecham (U.K.) brand of Halofantrine (Systemic), 1608

*Halfprin*—Kramer (U.S.) brand of Aspirin—**See Salicylates (Systemic)**, 2538

Halobetasol Propionate [*Ultravate*]
  **See Corticosteroids (Topical)**, 978
  Cream, 991
  Ointment, 991

*Halodrin*—Upjohn (U.S.) brand of Fluoxymesterone and Ethinyl Estradiol—**See Androgens and Estrogens (Systemic)**, 126

Halofantrine [*Halfan*]
  **(Systemic)**, 1608, 3145

Halofantrine Hydrochloride [*Halfan*]
  **(Systemic)**, 1608, 3022
  Suspension, Oral, 1610
  Tablets, 1611, 3022

*Halofed*—Halsey (U.S.) brand of Pseudoephedrine (Systemic), 2422

*Halofed Adult Strength*—Halsey (U.S.) brand of Pseudoephedrine (Systemic), 2422

*Halog*—Squibb (U.S. and Canada) brand of Halcinonide—**See Corticosteroids (Topical)**, 978

*Halog-E*—Squibb (U.S.) brand of Halcinonide—**See Corticosteroids (Topical)**, 978

Haloperidol [*Apo-Haloperidol; Haldol; Novo-Peridol; Peridol; PMS Haloperidol*]
  **(Systemic)**, 1611
  Injection USP, 1616
  Solution, Oral, USP, 1616
  Tablets USP, 1616, MC-14

Haloperidol Decanoate [*Haldol Decanoate; Haldol LA*]
  **(Systemic)**, 3030
  Injection, 3030

Haloprogin [*Halotex*]
  **(Topical)**, #
  Cream USP, #
  Solution, Topical, USP, #

*Halotestin*—Pharmacia & Upjohn (U.S. and Canada) brand of Fluoxymesterone—**See Androgens (Systemic)**, 118, MC-13

*Halotex*—Westwood (U.S.) and Westwood-Squibb (Canada) brand of Haloprogin (Topical), #

Halothane [*Fluothane; Somnothane*]
  **See Anesthetics, Inhalation (Systemic)**, 168
  Halothane USP, 171

*Halotussin*—Halsey (U.S.) brand of Guaifenesin (Systemic), 1588

*Halotussin-DM*—Halsey (U.S.) brand of Dextromethorphan and Guaifenesin—**See Cough/Cold Combinations (Systemic)**, 1024

*Haltran*—Roberts (U.S.) brand of Ibuprofen—**See Anti-inflammatory Drugs, Nonsteroidal (Systemic)**, 388

*Harmonyl*—Abbott (U.S.) brand of Deserpidine—**See Rauwolfia Alkaloids (Systemic)**, 2460

*Havrix*—SmithKline Beecham (U.S. and Canada) brand of Hepatitis A Vaccine Inactivated (Systemic), 1625

*Hawaiian Baby Faces Sunblock*—Tanning Research (U.S.) brand of Menthyl Anthranilate, Octyl Methoxycinnamate, Octyl Salicylate, and Oxybenzone—**See Sunscreen Agents (Topical)**, #

*Hawaiian Tropic Baby Faces*—Tanning Research (U.S.) brand of Menthyl Anthranilate, Octocrylene, Octyl Methoxycinnamate, and Oxybenzone—**See Sunscreen Agents (Topical)**, #

*Hawaiian Tropic Baby Faces Sunblock*—Tanning Research (U.S.) brand of Octocrylene, Octyl Methoxycinnamate, Octyl Salicylate, Oxybenzone, and Titanium Dioxide—**See Sunscreen Agents (Topical)**, #

*Hawaiian Tropic Dark Tanning*—Tanning Research (U.S.) brand of Octyl Methoxycinnamate and Padimate O—**See Sunscreen Agents (Topical)**, #; Phenylbenzimidazole—**See Sunscreen Agents (Topical)**, #

*Hawaiian Tropic Dark Tanning with Sunscreen*—Tanning Research (U.S.) brand of Menthyl Anthranilate and Octyl Methoxycinnamate—**See Sunscreen Agents (Topical)**, #

*Hawaiian Tropic Just For Kids*—Tanning Research (U.S.) brand of Octocrylene, Octyl Methoxycinnamate, Octyl Salicylate, Oxybenzone, and Titanium Dioxide—**See Sunscreen Agents (Topical)**, #

*Hawaiian Tropic Just for Kids*—Tanning Research (U.S.) brand of Homosalate, Menthyl Anthranilate, Octyl Methoxycinnamate, Octyl Salicylate, and Oxybenzone—**See Sunscreen Agents (Topical)**, #

*Hawaiian Tropic Land Sport*—Tanning Research (U.S.) brand of Octyl Methoxycinnamate and Octyl Salicylate—**See Sunscreen Agents (Topical)**, #

*Hawaiian Tropic Plus*—Tanning Research (U.S.) brand of Menthyl Anthranilate, Octocrylene, Octyl Methoxycinnamate, and Oxybenzone—**See Sunscreen Agents (Topical)**, #; Menthyl Anthranilate, Octyl Methoxycinnamate, and Oxybenzone—**See Sunscreen Agents (Topical)**, #

*Hawaiian Tropic Plus Sunblock*—Tanning Research (U.S.) brand of Menthyl Anthranilate, Octyl Methoxycinnamate, and Oxybenzone—**See Sunscreen Agents (Topical)**, #

*Hawaiian Tropic Protective Tanning*—Tanning Research (U.S.) brand of Oxybenzone and Padimate O—**See Sunscreen Agents (Topical)**, #

*Hawaiian Tropic Protective Tanning Dry*—Tanning Research (U.S.) brand of Homosalate, Menthyl Anthranilate, and Octyl Methoxycinnamate—**See Sunscreen Agents (Topical)**, #; Phenylbenzimidazole and Sulisobenzone—**See Sunscreen Agents (Topical)**, #

*Hawaiian Tropic Self-tanning Sunblock*—Tanning Research (U.S.) brand of Octyl Methoxycinnamate and Oxybenzone—**See Sunscreen Agents (Topical)**, #

*Hawaiian Tropic Sport Sunblock*—Tanning Research (U.S.) brand of Octocrylene, Octyl Methoxycinnamate, Octyl Salicylate, Oxybenzone, and Titanium Dioxide—**See Sunscreen Agents (Topical)**, #; Octocrylene, Octyl Methoxycinnamate, and Oxybenzone—**See Sunscreen Agents (Topical)**, #

*Hawaiian Tropic Sunblock*—Tanning Research (U.S.) brand of Homosalate, Menthyl Anthranilate, Octyl Methoxycinnamate, Octyl Salicylate, and Oxybenzone—**See Sunscreen Agents (Topical)**, #; Octocrylene, Octyl Methoxycinnamate, Octyl Salicylate, Oxybenzone, and Titanium Dioxide—**See Sunscreen Agents (Topical)**, #

*Hawaiian Tropic Water Sport*—Tanning Research (U.S.) brand of Octyl Methoxycinnamate, Oxybenzone, and Titanium Dioxide—**See Sunscreen Agents (Topical)**, #

*Hayfebrol*—Scot-Tussin (U.S.) brand of Chlorpheniramine and Pseudoephedrine—**See Antihistamines and Decongestants (Systemic)**, 343

*H-BIGIV*—North American Biologics (U.S.) brand of Hepatitis B Immune Globulin (Systemic), 3145
*HbPV*—See Haemophilus b Polysaccharide Vaccine (Systemic), 1606
HB vaccine—See Hepatitis B Vaccine Recombinant (Systemic), 1628
hCG—See Chorionic Gonadotropin (Systemic), 858
HDCV—Rabies Vaccine, Human Diploid Cell—**See Rabies Vaccine (Systemic)**, 2449
*HD 200 Plus*—Lafayette (U.S.) brand of Barium Sulfate (Local), #
*Headache Tablet*—Aspirin—**See Salicylates (Systemic)**, 2538
*Head & Shoulders Antidandruff Cream Shampoo Normal to Dry Formula*—Procter & Gamble (U.S.) brand of Pyrithione (Topical), #
*Head & Shoulders Antidandruff Cream Shampoo Normal to Oily Formula*—Procter & Gamble (U.S.) brand of Pyrithione (Topical), #
*Head & Shoulders Antidandruff Lotion Shampoo 2 in 1 (Complete Dandruff Shampoo plus Conditioner in One) Formula*—Procter & Gamble (U.S.) brand of Pyrithione (Topical), #
*Head & Shoulders Antidandruff Lotion Shampoo Normal to Dry Formula*—Procter & Gamble (U.S.) brand of Pyrithione (Topical), #
*Head & Shoulders Antidandruff Lotion Shampoo Normal to Oily Formula*—Procter & Gamble (U.S.) brand of Pyrithione (Topical), #
*Head & Shoulders Dry Scalp Conditioning Formula Lotion Shampoo*—Procter & Gamble (U.S.) brand of Pyrithione (Topical), #
*Head & Shoulders Dry Scalp 2 in 1 (Dry Scalp Shampoo plus Conditioner in One) Formula Lotion Shampoo*—Procter & Gamble (U.S.) brand of Pyrithione (Topical), #
*Head & Shoulders Dry Scalp Regular Formula Lotion Shampoo*—Procter & Gamble (U.S.) brand of Pyrithione (Topical), #
*Head & Shoulders Intensive Treatment Conditioning Formula Dandruff Lotion Shampoo*—Procter & Gamble (U.S.) brand of Selenium Sulfide (Topical), #
*Head & Shoulders Intensive Treatment 2 in 1 (Persistent Dandruff Shampoo plus Conditioner in One) Formula Dandruff Lotion Shampoo*—Procter & Gamble (U.S.) brand of Selenium Sulfide (Topical), #
*Head & Shoulders Intensive Treatment Regular Formula Dandruff Lotion Shampoo*—Procter & Gamble (U.S.) brand of Selenium Sulfide (Topical), #
*Healthprin Adult Low Strength*—Smart (U.S.) brand of Aspirin—**See Salicylates (Systemic)**, 2538
*Healthprin Full Strength*—Smart (U.S.) brand of Aspirin—**See Salicylates (Systemic)**, 2538
*Healthprin Half-Dose*—Smart (U.S.) brand of Aspirin—**See Salicylates (Systemic)**, 2538
*Helidac*—Procter & Gamble (U.S.) brand of Bismuth Subsalicylate, Metronidazole, and Tetracycline—For *H. pylori* (Systemic), 620
*Helidac Therapy Capsules*—P&GP (U.S.) brand of Tetracycline (Systemic), MC-4
*Helidac Therapy Tablets*—P&GP (U.S.) brand of Metronidazole (Systemic), MC-4
*Helidac Therapy Chewable Tablets*—P&GP (U.S.) brand of Bismuth Subsalicylate (Systemic), MC-4
*Helixate*—Bayer (U.S.) brand of Antihemophilic Factor (Systemic), 319; Bayer (Canada) brand of Antihemophilic Factor (Recombinant) (Systemic), 3011
*Hemabate*—Upjohn (U.S.) brand of Carboprost (Systemic), 782
*HemaChek*—Ames (U.S.) brand of Fecal Occult Blood Test Kits, #
*Hematest*—Ames (U.S.) and Miles (Canada) brand of Fecal Occult Blood Test Kits, #
*HemaWipe*—Access (U.S.) brand of Fecal Occult Blood Test Kits, #
Heme Arginate [*Normosang*] **(Systemic)**, 3145
*HemeSelect*—SmithKline Diagnostics (U.S.) brand of Fecal Occult Blood Test Kits, #
*Hemex*—See Hemin and Zinc Mesoporphyrin (Systemic), 3145
Hemin [*Panhematin*] **(Systemic)**, 3022, 3144
for Injection, 3022
Hemin and Zinc Mesoporphyrin [*Hemex*] **(Systemic)**, 3145

*Hemoccult*—SmithKline Diagnostics (U.S.) brand of Fecal Occult Blood Test Kits, #
*Hemoccult II*—SmithKline Diagnostics (U.S.) brand of Fecal Occult Blood Test Kits, #
*Hemoccult SENSA*—SmithKline Diagnostics (U.S.) brand of Fecal Occult Blood Test Kits, #
*Hemoccult II SENSA*—SmithKline Diagnostics (U.S.) brand of Fecal Occult Blood Test Kits, #
*Hemocitrate*—Hemotec (U.S.) brand of Trisodium Citrate, 3170
*Hemocyte*—U.S. Pharmaceutical (U.S.) brand of Ferrous Fumarate—**See Iron Supplements (Systemic)**, 1774
*Hemofil M*—Baxter (U.S. and Canada) brand of Antihemophilic Factor (Systemic), 319
Hemophilus b polysaccharide vaccine—See Haemophilus b Polysaccharide Vaccine (Systemic), 1606
*Hemorrhoidal HC*—CMC-Cons (U.S.) brand of Hydrocortisone—**See Corticosteroids (Rectal)**, 973
*Hemril-HC Uniserts*—Upsher-Smith (U.S.) brand of Hydrocortisone—**See Corticosteroids (Rectal)**, 973
*Hepahydrin*—Great Southern (U.S.) brand of Dehydrocholic Acid—**See Laxatives (Local)**, #
*Hepalean*—Organon (Canada) brand of Heparin (Systemic), 1617
*Hepandrin*—Bio-Technology General (U.S.) brand of Oxandrolone (Systemic), 3157
Heparin Calcium [*Calcilean*; *Calciparine*] **(Systemic)**, 1617
Injection USP, 1622
Heparin cofactor I—See Antithrombin III (Systemic), 444
*Heparin Leo*—Leo (Canada) brand of Heparin (Systemic), 1617
Heparin Sodium [*Hepalean*; *Heparin Leo*; *Liquaemin*] **(Systemic)**, 1617
Injection USP, 1623
Heparin Sodium in Dextrose **(Systemic)**, 1617
Injection, 1624
Heparin Sodium in Sodium Chloride **(Systemic)**, 1617
Injection, 1624
*Hepatic-Aid II*—Kendall McGaw (U.S.) brand of Enteral Nutrition Formula, Disease-specific—**See Enteral Nutrition Formulas (Systemic)**, #
Hepatitis A Vaccine Inactivated [*Havrix*; *Vaqta*] **(Systemic)**, 1625
Injection, 1627
Hepatitis B Immune Globulin, Intravenous [*H-BIGIV*] **(Systemic)**, 3145
Hepatitis B Vaccine Recombinant [*Engerix-B*; HB vaccine; *Recombivax HB*; *Recombivax HB Dialysis Formulation*] **(Systemic)**, 1628
Suspension, Sterile, 1632
*Hepatolite*—Du Pont N.E.N. (U.S.) brand of Technetium Tc 99m Disofenin (Systemic), 2705
*Heptalac*—Copley (U.S.) brand of Lactulose—**See Laxatives (Local)**, #
*Heptogesic*—Gen-King (U.S.) brand of Meprobamate and Aspirin (Systemic), #
*Herbal Laxative*—Nature's Bounty (U.S.) and Shaklee (Canada) brand of Sennosides—**See Laxatives (Local)**, #
*Herbopyrine*—Aspirin—**See Salicylates (Systemic)**, 2538
*Herpecin-L Cold Sore*—Campbell (U.S.) brand of Padimate O—**See Sunscreen Agents (Topical)**, #
Herpes Simplex Virus Gene **(Systemic)**, 3145
*Herplex Liquifilm*—Allergan (U.S. and Canada) brand of Idoxuridine (Ophthalmic), 1675
*Hetrazan*—Lederle (U.S. and Canada) brand of Diethylcarbamazine (Systemic), #
*Hexabrix*—Mallinckrodt (U.S.) brand of Ioxaglate (Local), #; Mallinckrodt (U.S.) brand of Ioxaglate (Systemic), #
*Hexabrix-200*—Mallinckrodt (Canada) brand of Ioxaglate (Systemic), #
*Hexabrix-320*—Mallinckrodt (Canada) brand of Ioxaglate (Local), #; Mallinckrodt (Canada) brand of Ioxaglate (Systemic), #
*Hexadrol*—Organon (U.S. and Canada) brand of Dexamethasone—**See Corticosteroids—Glucocorticoid Effects (Systemic)**, 998
*Hexadrol Phosphate*—Organon (U.S.) brand of Dexamethasone—**See Corticosteroids—Glucocorticoid Effects (Systemic)**, 998

*Hexalen*—U.S. Bioscience (U.S.) brand of Altretamine (Systemic), 3129; U.S. Bioscience (U.S.) and Lilly (Canada) brand of Altretamine (Systemic), 55
*Hexalol*—Central (U.S.) brand of Atropine, Hyoscyamine, Methenamine, Methylene Blue, Phenyl Salicylate, and Benzoic Acid (Systemic), 488
Hexamethylmelamine—See Altretamine (Systemic), 55
Hexamethylpropyleneamine oxime (HM-PAO)—See Technetium Tc 99m Exametazime (Systemic), 2708
*Hexit*—Odan (Canada) brand of Lindane (Topical), 1866
*H-F Gel*—LTR (U.S.) brand of Calcium Gluconate (Topical), 3136
Hib CPS—See Haemophilus b Polysaccharide Vaccine (Systemic), 1606
Hib polysaccharide vaccine—See Haemophilus b Polysaccharide Vaccine (Systemic), 1606
*Hibtiter*—Lederle (U.S. and Canada) brand of Haemophilus b Conjugate Vaccine (HbOC—Diphtheria CRM$_{197}$ Protein Conjugate)—**See Haemophilus b Conjugate Vaccine (Systemic)**, 1601
*Hi-Cor 1.0*—C & M (U.S.) brand of Hydrocortisone—**See Corticosteroids (Topical)**, 978
*Hi-Cor 2.5*—C & M (U.S.) brand of Hydrocortisone—**See Corticosteroids (Topical)**, 978
*Hippuran*—Mallinckrodt (U.S.) brand of Iodohippurate Sodium I 131 (Systemic), 1755
*Hipputope*—Squibb (U.S.) brand of Iodohippurate Sodium I 131 (Systemic), 1755
*Hip-Rex*—Riker (Canada) brand of Methenamine (Systemic), #
*Hiprex*—Merrell Dow (U.S.) brand of Methenamine (Systemic), #
*Hismanal*—Janssen (U.S. and Canada) brand of Astemizole—**See Antihistamines (Systemic)**, 325, MC-3
*Histagesic Modified*—Jones (U.S.) brand of Chlorpheniramine, Phenylephrine, and Acetaminophen—**See Antihistamines, Decongestants, and Analgesics (Systemic)**, 366
*Histalet*—Solvay (U.S.) brand of Chlorpheniramine and Pseudoephedrine—**See Antihistamines and Decongestants (Systemic)**, 343
*Histalet Forte*—Solvay (U.S.) brand of Chlorpheniramine, Pyrilamine, Phenylephrine, and Phenylpropanolamine—**See Antihistamines and Decongestants (Systemic)**, 343
Histamine H$_2$-receptor Antagonists **(Systemic)**, 1633
Histamine Phosphate **(Systemic)**, #
Injection USP, #
*Histantil*—Pharmascience (Canada) brand of Promethazine—**See Antihistamines, Phenothiazine-derivative (Systemic)**, 377
*Histatab Plus*—Century (U.S.) brand of Chlorpheniramine and Phenylephrine—**See Antihistamines and Decongestants (Systemic)**, 343
*Histatan*—Zenith Goldline (U.S.) brand of Chlorpheniramine, Pyrilamine, and Phenylephrine—**See Antihistamines and Decongestants (Systemic)**, 343
*Hista-Vadrin*—Scherer (U.S.) brand of Chlorpheniramine, Phenylephrine, and Phenylpropanolamine—**See Antihistamines and Decongestants (Systemic)**, 343
*Histenol*—Zee Medical (Canada) brand of Pseudoephedrine, Dextromethorphan, and Acetaminophen—**See Cough/Cold Combinations (Systemic)**, 1024
*Histinex DM*—Ethex (U.S.) brand of Brompheniramine, Phenylpropanolamine, and Dextromethorphan—**See Cough/Cold Combinations (Systemic)**, 1024
*Histinex HC*—Ethex (U.S.) brand of Chlorpheniramine, Phenylephrine, and Hydrocodone—**See Cough/Cold Combinations (Systemic)**, 1024
*Histinex PV*—Ethex (U.S.) brand of Chlorpheniramine, Pseudoephedrine, and Hydrocodone—**See Cough/Cold Combinations (Systemic)**, 1024
*Histor-D*—Roberts (U.S.) brand of Chlorpheniramine and Phenylephrine—**See Antihistamines and Decongestants (Systemic)**, 343
*Histosal*—Ferndale (U.S.) brand of Pyrilamine, Phenylpropanolamine, Acetaminophen, and Caffeine—**See Antihistamines, Decongestants, and Analgesics (Systemic)**, 366

*USP DI*                                                                                                                     **General Index**   **3293**

Histrelin
**(Systemic)**, 1644, 3145
Histrelin Acetate [*Supprelin; Supprelin Injection*]
**(Systemic)**, 1644, 3145
Injection, 1646
*Histussin HC*—Bock (U.S.) brand of Chlorpheniramine, Phenylephrine, and Hydrocodone—**See Cough/Cold Combinations (Systemic)**, 1024
*HIVID*—Hoffmann-La Roche (U.S.) brand of Zalcitabine (Systemic), 3171; Roche (U.S. and Canada) brand of Zalcitabine (Systemic), 2989, MC-32
*HIVIG*—North American Biologicals (U.S.) brand of Human Immunodeficiency Virus Immune Globulin (Systemic), 3146
hMG—*See* Menotropins (Systemic), 1943
HMG-CoA Reductase Inhibitors
**(Systemic)**, 1647
*HMS Liquifilm*—Allergan (U.S. and Canada) brand of Medrysone—**See Corticosteroids (Ophthalmic)**, 966
*Hold*—Beecham (U.S.) brand of Dextromethorphan (Systemic), 1191
*Homapin*—Mission (U.S.) brand of Homatropine—**See Anticholinergics/Antispasmodics (Systemic)**, 226
Homatropine-containing Combinations, 3073
Homatropine Hydrobromide [*AK-Homatropine; I-Homatrine; Isopto Homatropine; Minims Homatropine; Spectro-Homatropine*]
**(Ophthalmic)**, 1651
Solution, Ophthalmic, USP, 1653
Homatropine Methylbromide [*Homapin*]
**See Anticholinergics/Antispasmodics (Systemic)**, 226
Tablets USP, 236
Homosalate [*Coppertone Moisturizing Suntan; Coppertone Dark Tanning; Tropical Blend Dark Tanning; Tropical Blend Dry Oil*]
**See Sunscreen Agents (Topical)**, #
Oil, #
Spray, #
Homosalate-containing Combinations, 3074
Homosalate, Menthyl Anthranilate, and Octyl Methoxycinnamate [*Hawaiian Tropic Protective Tanning Dry*]
**See Sunscreen Agents (Topical)**, #
Oil, #
Homosalate, Menthyl Anthranilate, Octyl Methoxycinnamate, Octyl Salicylate, and Oxybenzone [*Blistex Ultraprotection; Hawaiian Tropic Just for Kids; Hawaiian Tropic Sunblock*]
**See Sunscreen Agents (Topical)**, #
Lip Balm, #
Lotion, #
Homosalate, Octocrylene, Octyl Methoxycinnamate, and Oxybenzone [*Coppertone Waterproof Sunblock*]
**See Sunscreen Agents (Topical)**, #
Lotion, #
Homosalate, Octyl Methoxycinnamate, Octyl Salicylate, and Oxybenzone [*Coppertone All Day Protection; Coppertone Kids Sunblock; Neutrogena No Stick Sunscreen; Shade Sunblock; Waterbabies Sunblock*]
**See Sunscreen Agents (Topical)**, #
Lotion, #
Stick, #
Homosalate, Octyl Methoxycinnamate, and Oxybenzone [*Shade Oil-Free*]
**See Sunscreen Agents (Topical)**, #
Gel, #
Homosalate and Oxybenzone [*Tropical Blend Dry Oil*]
**See Sunscreen Agents (Topical)**, #
Spray, #
*Honvol*—Horner (Canada) brand of Diethylstilbestrol—**See Estrogens (Systemic)**, 1383
*H₂Oxyl 2.5 Gel*—Stiefel (Canada) brand of Benzoyl Peroxide (Topical), 579
*H₂Oxyl 5 Gel*—Stiefel (Canada) brand of Benzoyl Peroxide (Topical), 579
*H₂Oxyl 10 Gel*—Stiefel (Canada) brand of Benzoyl Peroxide (Topical), 579
*H₂Oxyl 20 Gel*—Stiefel (Canada) brand of Benzoyl Peroxide (Topical), 579
*H.P. Acthar Gel*—Armour (U.S.) brand of Corticotropin (Systemic), 1021
hPTH 1–34—*See* Teriparatide (Systemic), #
HRIG—*See* Rabies Immune Globulin (Systemic), 2448

*Humalog*—Lilly (Canada) brand of Insulin Lispro (Systemic), 3025; Lilly (U.S.) brand of Insulin Lispro (Systemic), 1727
Human Acid Alpha-Glucosidase
**(Systemic)**, 3160
Human chorionic gonadotropin—*See* Chorionic Gonadotropin (Systemic), 858
Human Clara Cell 10kDa protein, Recombinant
**(Systemic)**, 3160
Human erythropoietin, recombinant—*See* Epoetin alfa (Systemic), 1352
Human Gonadotropins—*See* Menotropins (Systemic), 1943
Human growth hormone (hGH)—Somatrem—**See Growth Hormone (Systemic)**, 1586; Somatropin, Recombinant—**See Growth Hormone (Systemic)**, 1586
Human Immunodeficiency Virus (HIV) Neutralizing Antibodies [*Immupath*]
**(Systemic)**, 3145
Human Immunodeficiency Virus Immune Globulin [*HIVIG*]
**(Systemic)**, 3146
Humanized Anti-TAC [*Zenapax*]
**(Systemic)**, 3146
Human menopausal gonadotropins—*See* Menotropins (Systemic), 1943
Human Retinal Pigmented Epithelial Cells on Collagen Microcarriers [*Spheramine*]
**(Systemic)**, 3146
Human Thyroid Stimulating Hormone [*Thyrogen;* thyrotropin; TSH]
**(Systemic)**, 3146
Human T-Lymphotropic Virus Type III gp160 Antigens [*VaxSyn HIV-1*]
**(Systemic)**, 3146
*Humate-P*—Armour (U.S.) brand of Antihemophilic Factor (Systemic), 319
*Humate P*—Behringwerke Aktiengesellschaft (AG) (U.S.) brand of Antihemophilic Factor (Human) (Systemic), 3131
*Humatrope*—Lilly (U.S.) brand of Somatropin (Systemic), 3165; Lilly (U.S. and Canada) brand of Somatropin, Recombinant—**See Growth Hormone (Systemic)**, 1586; Lilly (U.S.) brand of Somatropin, Recombinant (Systemic), 3034
*Humegon*—Organon (U.S. and Canada) brand of Menotropins (Systemic), 1943
*Humibid DM*—Adams (U.S.) brand of Dextromethorphan and Guaifenesin—**See Cough/Cold Combinations (Systemic)**, 1024
*Humibid DM Pediatric*—Adams (U.S.) brand of Dextromethorphan and Guaifenesin—**See Cough/Cold Combinations (Systemic)**, 1024
*Humibid Guaifenesin Plus*—Menley & James (U.S.) brand of Pseudoephedrine and Guaifenesin (Systemic), 3033
*Humibid L.A.*—Adams (U.S.) brand of Guaifenesin (Systemic), 1588
*Humibid Sprinkle*—Adams (U.S.) brand of Guaifenesin (Systemic), 1588
*Humorsol*—Merck (U.S.) brand of Demecarium—**See Antiglaucoma Agents, Cholinergic, Long-acting (Ophthalmic)**, 315
*Humulin 10/90*—Lilly (Canada) brand of Insulin, Isophane, Human, and Insulin Human (Systemic), 1713
*Humulin 20/80*—Lilly (Canada) brand of Insulin, Isophane, Human, and Insulin Human (Systemic), 1713
*Humulin 30/70*—Lilly (Canada) brand of Insulin, Isophane, Human, and Insulin Human (Systemic), 1713
*Humulin 40/60*—Lilly (Canada) brand of Insulin, Isophane, Human, and Insulin Human (Systemic), 1713
*Humulin 50/50*—Lilly (U.S. and Canada) brand of Insulin, Isophane, Human, and Insulin Human (Systemic), 1713
*Humulin 70/30*—Lilly (U.S.) brand of Insulin, Isophane, Human, and Insulin Human—**See Insulin (Systemic)**, 1713
*Humulin-L*—Lilly (U.S.) brand of Insulin Zinc, Human—**See Insulin (Systemic)**, 1713
*Humulin L*—Lilly (U.S.) brand of Insulin Zinc, Human—**See Insulin (Systemic)**, 1713
*Humulin-N*—Lilly (U.S.) brand of Insulin, Isophane, Human—**See Insulin (Systemic)**, 1713
*Humulin N*—Lilly (U.S.) brand of Insulin, Isophane, Human—**See Insulin (Systemic)**, 1713
*Humulin-R*—Lilly (U.S.) brand of Insulin Human—**See Insulin (Systemic)**, 1713

*Humulin R*—Lilly (U.S.) brand of Insulin Human—**See Insulin (Systemic)**, 1713
*Humulin-U*—Lilly (Canada) brand of Insulin Zinc, Extended, Human—**See Insulin (Systemic)**, 1713
*Humulin U Ultralente*—Lilly (U.S.) brand of Insulin Zinc, Extended, Human—**See Insulin (Systemic)**, 1713
*Hurricaine*—Beutlich (U.S.) brand of Benzocaine—**See Anesthetics (Mucosal-Local)**, 128
*Hyalgan*—Sanofi (U.S.) brand of Hyaluronate Sodium (Systemic), 1653
Hyaluronate Sodium [*Hyalgan*]
**(Systemic)**, 1653
Injection, 1654
Hyaluronate Sodium Derivative [hylan G-F 20; *Synvisc*]
**(Systemic)**, 1654
Injection, 1655
*Hyate:C*—Porton (U.S. and Canada) brand of Antihemophilic Factor (Systemic), 319
*Hybolin Decanoate*—Hyrex (U.S.) brand of Nandrolone—**See Anabolic Steroids (Systemic)**, 110
*Hybolin-Improved*—Hyrex (U.S.) brand of Nandrolone—**See Anabolic Steroids (Systemic)**, 110
*HYBRI-CEAker*—Hybritech (U.S.) brand of Indium In-111 Altumomab Pentetate (Systemic), 3147
*Hycamtin*—SmithKline Beecham (U.S. and Canada) brand of Topotecan (Systemic), 2841
*Hycodan*—Du Pont (Canada) brand of Hydrocodone—**See Cough/Cold Combinations (Systemic)**, 1024, MC-14; **Opioid (Narcotic) Analgesics (Systemic)**, 2168; Du Pont (U.S. and Canada) brand of Hydrocodone and Homatropine—**See Cough/Cold Combinations (Systemic)**, 1024
*Hycomed*—Med-Tek (U.S.) brand of Hydrocodone and Acetaminophen—**See Opioid (Narcotic) Analgesics and Acetaminophen (Systemic)**, 2198
*Hycomine*—Du Pont (U.S.) brand of Phenylpropanolamine and Hydrocodone—**See Cough/Cold Combinations (Systemic)**, 1024; Du Pont (Canada) brand of Pyrilamine, Phenylephrine, Hydrocodone, and Ammonium Chloride—**See Cough/Cold Combinations (Systemic)**, 1024
*Hycomine Compound*—Du Pont (U.S.) brand of Chlorpheniramine, Phenylephrine, Hydrocodone, Acetaminophen, and Caffeine—**See Cough/Cold Combinations (Systemic)**, 1024
*Hycomine Pediatric*—Du Pont (U.S.) brand of Phenylpropanolamine and Hydrocodone—**See Cough/Cold Combinations (Systemic)**, 1024
*Hycomine-S Pediatric*—Du Pont (Canada) brand of Pyrilamine, Phenylephrine, Hydrocodone, and Ammonium Chloride—**See Cough/Cold Combinations (Systemic)**, 1024
*Hyco-Pap*—Lumsco (U.S.) brand of Hydrocodone and Acetaminophen—**See Opioid (Narcotic) Analgesics and Acetaminophen (Systemic)**, 2198
*Hycort*—ICN (Canada) brand of Hydrocortisone—**See Hydrocortisone (Rectal)**, 973
*Hycotuss Expectorant*—Du Pont (U.S.) brand of Hydrocodone and Guaifenesin—**See Cough/Cold Combinations (Systemic)**, 1024
*Hydeltrasol*—MSD (U.S.) brand of Prednisolone—**See Corticosteroids—Glucocorticoid Effects (Systemic)**, 998
*Hydeltra T.B.A.*—MSD (U.S.) brand of Prednisolone—**See Corticosteroids—Glucocorticoid Effects (Systemic)**, 998
*Hydergine*—Novartis (U.S. and Canada) brand of Ergoloid Mesylates (Systemic), 1358, MC-11
*Hydergine LC*—Novartis (U.S. and Canada) brand of Ergoloid Mesylates (Systemic), 1358, MC-11
*Hyderm*—K-Line (Canada) brand of Hydrocortisone—**See Corticosteroids (Topical)**, 978
Hydralazine-containing Combinations, 3074
Hydralazine Hydrochloride [*Apresoline; Novo-Hylazin*]
**(Systemic)**, 1655
Injection USP, 1658
Tablets USP, 1658, MC-14
Hydralazine Hydrochloride and Hydrochlorothiazide [*Apresazide*]
**(Systemic)**, 1658
Capsules, 1659
*Hydrate*—Hyrex (U.S.) brand of Dimenhydrinate—**See Antihistamines (Systemic)**, 325
*Hydrea*—Bristol-Myers Squibb (U.S.) brand of Hydroxyurea (Systemic), 3146; Squibb (U.S. and Canada) brand of Hydroxyurea (Systemic), 1666, MC-15

*Hydrisalic*—Pedinol (U.S.) brand of Salicylic Acid (Topical), #
*Hydrobexan*—Keene (U.S.) brand of Hydroxocobalamin—**See Vitamin B₁₂ (Systemic)**, 2962
*Hydrocet*—Carnrick (U.S.) brand of Hydrocodone and Acetaminophen—**See Opioid (Narcotic) Analgesics and Acetaminophen (Systemic)**, 2198
*Hydro-chlor*—Vortech (U.S.) brand of Hydrochlorothiazide—**See Diuretics, Thiazide (Systemic)**, 1273
Hydrochloride and Aspirin [*BC Cold Powder Non-Drowsy Formula; Coricidin Non-Drowsy Sinus Formula*]
    **See Decongestants and Analgesics (Systemic)**, 1180
    for Solution, Oral, 1181
    Tablets, 1182
Hydrochlorothiazide [*Apo-Hydro; Diuchlor H; Esidrix; Hydro-chlor; Hydro-D; HydroDIURIL; Microzide; Neo-Codema; Novo-Hydrazide; Oretic; Urozide*]
    **See Diuretics, Thiazide (Systemic)**, 1273
    Capsules, 1279
    Solution, Oral, 1279
    Tablets USP, 1279, MC-14
Hydrochlorothiazide-containing Combinations, 3074
*Hydrocil Instant*—Solvay (U.S.) brand of Psyllium Hydrophilic Mucilloid—**See Laxatives (Local)**, #
*Hydro-Cobex*—Pasadena (U.S.) brand of Hydroxocobalamin—**See Vitamin B₁₂ (Systemic)**, 2962
Hydrocodone with APAP—Hydrocodone and Acetaminophen—**See Opioid (Narcotic) Analgesics and Acetaminophen (Systemic)**, 2198
Hydrocodone Bitartrate [*Hycodan; Robidone*]
    **See Cough/Cold Combinations (Systemic)**, 1024
    Syrup, 1064
    Tablets, 1064
Hydrocodone Bitartrate [*Hycocan; Robidone*]
    **See Opioid (Narcotic) Analgesics (Systemic)**, 2168
    Syrup, 2176
    Tablets, Soluble, 2176
Hydrocodone Bitartrate and Acetaminophen [*Allay; Anexsia 5/500; Anexsia 7.5/650; Anolor DH 5; Bancap-HC; Co-Gesic; co-hycodAPAP; Dolacet; Dolagesic; Duocet; Hycomed; Hyco-Pap; Hydrocet; hydrocodone with APAP; Hydrogesic; HY-PHEN; Lorcet 10/650; Lorcet-HD; Lorcet Plus; Lortab; Lortab 10/500; Lortab 2.5/500; Lortab 5/500; Lortab 7.5/500; Margesic-H; Oncet; Panacet 5/500; Panlor; Polygesic; StagesiT -Gesic; Ugesic; Vanacet; Vendone; Vicodin; Vicodin ES; Vicodin HP ; Zydone*]
    **See Opioid (Narcotic) Analgesics and Acetaminophen (Systemic)**, 2198, 3022
    Capsules, 2200, MC-14
    Solution, Oral, 2201
    Tablets USP, 2201, 3022, MC-14
Hydrocodone Bitartrate and Aspirin [*Azdone; Damason-P; Lortab ASA; Panasal 5/500*]
    **See Opioid (Narcotic) Analgesics and Aspirin (Systemic)**, 2202
    Tablets, 2204
Hydrocodone Bitartrate and Guaifenesin [*Atuss EX; Codiclear DH; Co-Tuss V; Entuss Expectorant; Hycotuss Expectorant; Kwelcof Liquid; Pneumotussin HC; Vicodin Tuss*]
    **See Cough/Cold Combinations (Systemic)**, 1024
    Solution, Oral, 1050, 1058, 1066, 1068
    Syrup, 1035, 1044, 1066, 1082, 1115
    Tablets, 1058, 1106
Hydrocodone Bitartrate and Homatropine Methylbromide [*Codan; Hycodan; Hydromet; Hydropane; Tussigon*]
    **See Cough/Cold Combinations (Systemic)**, 1024
    Syrup, 1044, 1064, 1066
    Tablets, 1064, 1106, MC-14
Hydrocodone Bitartrate and Ibuprofen [*Vicoprofen*]
    **(Systemic)**, 3030, MC-14
    Tablets, 3030, MC-14
Hydrocodone Bitartrate and Potassium Guaiacolsulfonate [*Entuss Expectorant; Marcof Expectorant*]
    **See Cough/Cold Combinations (Systemic)**, 1024
    Solution, Oral, 1058
    Syrup, 1069
Hydrocodone-containing Combinations, 3074
Hydrocodone and Ibuprofen [*Vicoprofen*]
    **(Systemic)**, 1659
    Tablets, 1662
Hydrocortisone [*Cortenema; Hycort*]
    **See Corticosteroids (Rectal)**, 973
    Enema USP, 977

Hydrocortisone [*Cortef; cortisol; Hydrocortone*]
    **See Corticosteroids—Glucocorticoid Effects (Systemic)**, 998
    Suspension, Sterile, USP, 1009
    Tablets USP, 1009, MC-15
Hydrocortisone [*Acticort 100; Aeroseb-HC; Ala-Cort; Ala-Scalp HP; Allercort; Alphaderm; Anusol-HC; Anusol-HC 2.5%; Bactine; Barriere-HC; Beta-HC; CaldeCORT Anti-Itch; Cetacort; Cortaid; Cortate; Cort-Dome; Cortef; Cortifair; cortisol; Cortril; Delacort; Dermacort; DermiCort; Dermtex HC; Emo-Cort; Emo-Cort Scalp Solution; Gly-Cort; Hi-Cor 1.0; Hi-Cor 2.5; Hydro-Tex; Hytone; LactiCare-HC; Lemoderm; Maximum Strength Cortaid; My Cort; Nutracort; Penecort; Pentacort; Prevex HC; Rederm; Sarna HC 1.0%; Sential; S-T Cort; Synacort; Texacort; Unicort*]
    **See Corticosteroids (Topical)**, 978, 3023
    Cream USP, 992, 3023
    Lotion USP, 992
    Ointment USP, 992
    Solution, Topical, 992
Hydrocortisone Acetate [*Anucort-HC; Anu-Med HC; Anuprep HC; Anusol-HC; Anutone-HC; Anuzone-HC; Cort-Dome; Cortifoam; Cortiment-10; Cortiment-40; Hemril-HC Uniserts; Hemorrhoidal HC; 9-1-1; Proctocort; Proctosol-HC; Rectocort; Rectosol-HC*]
    **See Corticosteroids (Rectal)**, 973
    Foam, 977
    Suppositories, 977
Hydrocortisone Acetate [*Cortamed*]
    **See Corticosteroids (Ophthalmic)**, 966
    Ointment, Ophthalmic, USP, 970
Hydrocortisone Acetate [*Cortamed*]
    **See Corticosteroids (Otic)**, 971
    Ointment, Ophthalmic, USP (Otic use), 973
Hydrocortisone Acetate [*Anusol-HC; CaldeCORT Light; Carmol-HC; Cortacet; Cortaid; Cortef; Cortef Feminine Itch; Corticaine; Corticreme; cortisol; Cortoderm; Dermarest DriCort; Epifoam; FoilleCort; Gynecort; Gynecort 10; Hyderm; Lanacort; Lanacort 10; Maximum Strength Cortaid; Novohydrocort; Orabase-HCA; Pharma-Cort; Rhulicort*]
    **See Corticosteroids (Topical)**, 978, 3023
    Aerosol Foam, Topical, 993
    Cream USP, 992, 3023
    Lotion USP, 993
    Ointment USP, 993
    Paste, Dental, 992
Hydrocortisone Acetate [cortisol; *Hydrocortone Acetate*]
    **See Corticosteroids—Glucocorticoid Effects (Systemic)**, 998
    Suspension, Sterile, USP, 1009
Hydrocortisone and Acetic Acid [*Acetasol HC; Otomycet-HC; Vasotate HC; VoSol HC*]
    **See Corticosteroids and Acetic Acid (Otic)**, 996, 3023
    Solution, Otic, USP, 998, 3023
Hydrocortisone Buteprate [*Pandel*]
    **(Topical)**, 3023
    Cream, 3023
Hydrocortisone Butyrate [cortisol; *Locoid*]
    **See Corticosteroids (Topical)**, 978, 3023
    Cream USP, 993
    Ointment, 993
    Solution, Topical, 3023
Hydrocortisone-containing Combinations, 3074
Hydrocortisone Cypionate [*Cortef*; cortisol]
    **See Corticosteroids—Glucocorticoid Effects (Systemic)**, 998
    Suspension, Oral, USP, 1009
Hydrocortisone Sodium Phosphate [cortisol; *Hydrocortone Phosphate*]
    **See Corticosteroids—Glucocorticoid Effects (Systemic)**, 998
    Injection USP, 1009
Hydrocortisone Sodium Succinate [*A-hydroCort*; cortisol; *Solu-Cortef*]
    **See Corticosteroids—Glucocorticoid Effects (Systemic)**, 998
    for Injection USP, 1010
Hydrocortisone and Urea [*Sential*]
    **(Topical)**, 3023
    Cream, 3023
Hydrocortisone Valerate [cortisol; *Westcort*]
    **See Corticosteroids (Topical)**, 978
    Cream USP, 993
    Ointment, 993

*Hydrocortone*—Merck (U.S.) brand of Hydrocortisone—**See Corticosteroids—Glucocorticoid Effects (Systemic)**, 998, MC-14
*Hydrocortone Acetate*—Merck (U.S.) brand of Hydrocortisone—**See Corticosteroids—Glucocorticoid Effects (Systemic)**, 998
*Hydrocortone Phosphate*—Merck (U.S.) brand of Hydrocortisone—**See Corticosteroids—Glucocorticoid Effects (Systemic)**, 998
*Hydro-Crysti-12*—Hauck (U.S.) brand of Hydroxocobalamin—**See Vitamin B₁₂ (Systemic)**, 2962
*Hydro-D*—Halsey (U.S.) brand of Hydrochlorothiazide—**See Diuretics, Thiazide (Systemic)**, 1273
*HydroDIURIL*—Merck (U.S. and Canada) brand of Hydrochlorothiazide—**See Diuretics, Thiazide (Systemic)**, 1273, MC-14
Hydroflumethiazide [*Diucardin; Saluron*]
    **See Diuretics, Thiazide (Systemic)**, 1273
    Tablets USP, 1279
Hydroflumethiazide-containing Combinations, 3074
*Hydrogesic*—Edwards (U.S.) brand of Hydrocodone and Acetaminophen—**See Opioid (Narcotic) Analgesics and Acetaminophen (Systemic)**, 2198
*Hydromet*—Barre-National (U.S.) and Moore (U.S.) brand of Hydrocodone and Homatropine—**See Cough/Cold Combinations (Systemic)**, 1024
*Hydromine*—WC (U.S.) brand of Phenylpropanolamine and Hydrocodone—**See Cough/Cold Combinations (Systemic)**, 1024
*Hydromine Pediatric*—WC (U.S.) brand of Phenylpropanolamine and Hydrocodone—**See Cough/Cold Combinations (Systemic)**, 1024
Hydromorphone-containing Combinations, 3074
Hydromorphone Hydrochloride [dihydromorphinone; *Dilaudid; Dilaudid-5; Dilaudid-HP; Hydrostat IR; PMS-Hydromorphone; PMS-Hydromorphone Syrup*]
    **See Opioid (Narcotic) Analgesics (Systemic)**, 2168
    Injection USP, 2177
    Solution, Oral, 2177
    Suppositories, 2177
    Tablets USP, 2177, MC-15
Hydromorphone Hydrochloride and Guaifenesin [*Dilaudid Cough*]
    **See Cough/Cold Combinations (Systemic)**, 1024
    Syrup, 1052
*Hydromox*—Lederle (U.S.) brand of Quinethazone—**See Diuretics, Thiazide (Systemic)**, 1273
*Hydromycin*—Schein (U.S.) brand of Neomycin, Polymyxin B, and Hydrocortisone (Ophthalmic), #
*Hydropane*—Aligen (U.S.) brand of Hydrocodone and Homatropine—**See Cough/Cold Combinations (Systemic)**, 1024
*Hydrophen*—Rugby (U.S.) brand of Phenylpropanolamine and Hydrocodone—**See Cough/Cold Combinations (Systemic)**, 1024
*Hydropine*—Rugby (U.S.) brand of Reserpine and Hydroflumethiazide—**See Rauwolfia Alkaloids and Thiazide Diuretics (Systemic)**, #
*Hydropine H.P.*—Rugby (U.S.) brand of Reserpine and Hydroflumethiazide—**See Rauwolfia Alkaloids and Thiazide Diuretics (Systemic)**, #
*Hydropres*—Merck (U.S. and Canada) brand of Reserpine and Hydrochlorothiazide—**See Rauwolfia Alkaloids and Thiazide Diuretics (Systemic)**, #
*Hydrosine*—Major (U.S.) brand of Reserpine and Hydrochlorothiazide—**See Rauwolfia Alkaloids and Thiazide Diuretics (Systemic)**, #
*Hydrostat IR*—Richwood (U.S.) brand of Hydromorphone—**See Opioid (Narcotic) Analgesics (Systemic)**, 2168
*Hydrotensin*—Mayrand (U.S.) brand of Reserpine and Hydrochlorothiazide—**See Rauwolfia Alkaloids and Thiazide Diuretics (Systemic)**, #
*Hydro-Tex*—Syosset (U.S.) brand of Hydrocortisone—**See Corticosteroids (Topical)**, 978
Hydroxocobalamin [*Alphamin; Hydrobexan; Hydro-Cobex; Hydro-Crysti-12; Hydroxy-Cobal; LA-12; Vibal LA*; vitamin B₁₂]
    **See Vitamin B₁₂ (Systemic)**, 2962
    Injection USP, 2965
Hydroxychloroquine Sulfate [*Plaquenil*]
    **(Systemic)**, 1663
    Tablets USP, 1666, MC-15
*Hydroxy-Cobal*—Merit (U.S.) brand of Hydroxocobalamin—**See Vitamin B₁₂ (Systemic)**, 2962

Hydroxycobalamin and Sodium Thiosulfate
    (Systemic), 3146
Hydroxyprogesterone Caproate [*Gesterol LA 250; Hy/Gestrone; Hylutin; Prodrox; Pro-Span*]
    See Progestins (Systemic), 2400
    Injection USP, 2408
Hydroxypropyl Cellulose [*Lacrisert*]
    (Ophthalmic), #
    System, Ocular, USP, #
Hydroxypropyl Methylcellulose [*Artificial Tears; Bion Tears; Eyelube; Gonak; Goniosoft; Goniosol; hypromellose; Isopto Alkaline; Isopto Plain; Isopto Tears; Just Tears; Lacril; Methocel; Moisture Drops; Nature's Tears; Ocucoat; Ocucoat PF; Ocutears; Tearisol; Tears Naturale; Tears Naturale II; Tears Naturale Free; Tears Renewed; Ultra Tears*]
    (Ophthalmic), #, 3023
    Injection, #, 3023
    Solution, Ophthalmic, USP, #
Hydroxyurea [*Droxia; Hydrea*]
    (Systemic), 1666, 3024, 3146
    Capsules, 3024
    Capsules USP, 1669, MC-15
Hydroxyzine-containing Combinations, 3074
Hydroxyzine Hydrochloride [*Apo-Hydroxyzine; Atarax; Hyzine-50; Multipax; Novo-Hydroxyzin; Vistaril*]
    See Antihistamines (Systemic), 325
    Capsules, 340, MC-15
    Injection USP, 341
    Syrup USP, 340
    Tablets USP, 340, MC-15
Hydroxyzine Pamoate [*Vistaril*]
    See Antihistamines (Systemic), 325
    Capsules USP, 340
    Suspension, Oral, USP, 340
Hy/Gestrone—Taylor (U.S.) brand of Hydroxyprogesterone—See Progestins (Systemic), 2400
Hygroton—Rhône-Poulenc Rorer (U.S.) and Geigy (Canada) brand of Chlorthalidone—See Diuretics, Thiazide (Systemic), 1273, MC-7
Hylan G-F 20—See Hyaluronate Sodium Derivative (Systemic), 1654
Hylorel—Fisons (U.S.) brand of Guanadrel (Systemic), 1592
Hylutin—Hyrex (U.S.) brand of Hydroxyprogesterone—See Progestins (Systemic), 2400
Hyoscine—See Scopolamine (Ophthalmic), 2557
Hyoscine hydrobromide—Scopolamine—See Anticholinergics/Antispasmodics (Systemic), 226
Hyoscine methobromide—Methscopolamine—See Anticholinergics/Antispasmodics (Systemic), 226
Hyoscyamine [*Cystospaz*]
    See Anticholinergics/Antispasmodics (Systemic), 226
    Tablets USP, 236
Hyoscyamine-containing Combinations, 3074
Hyoscyamine Sulfate [*Anaspaz; Cystospaz-M; Gastrosed; Levbid; Levsin; Levsinex Timecaps; Levsin/SL; Neoquess*]
    See Anticholinergics/Antispasmodics (Systemic), 226, MC-15
    Capsules, Extended-release, 236
    Elixir USP, 237
    Injection USP, 237
    Solution, Oral, USP, 237
    Tablets USP, 237, MC-15
    Tablets, Extended-release, 236, MC-15
Hyoscyamine Sulfate and Phenobarbital [*Levsin-PB; Levsin with Phenobarbital*]
    See Belladonna Alkaloids and Barbiturates (Systemic), 551
    Elixir, 554
    Solution, Oral, 554
    Tablets, 555
Hyosophen—Rugby (U.S.) brand of Atropine, Hyoscyamine, Scopolamine, and Phenobarbital—See Belladonna Alkaloids and Barbiturates (Systemic), 551
Hypaque-76—Sanofi Winthrop (U.S.) brand of Diatrizoate—See Diatrizoates (Systemic), #
Hypaque-Cysto—Sanofi Winthrop (U.S.) brand of Diatrizoate—See Diatrizoates (Local), #
Hypaque-M 18%—Sterling Winthrop (Canada) brand of Diatrizoate—See Diatrizoates (Local), #; Diatrizoates (Systemic), #
Hypaque-M 30%—Sterling Winthrop (Canada) brand of Diatrizoate—See Diatrizoates (Local), #; Diatrizoates (Systemic), #

Hypaque-M 60%—Sterling Winthrop (Canada) brand of Diatrizoate—See Diatrizoates (Local), #; Diatrizoates (Systemic), #
Hypaque-M 75%—Sanofi Winthrop (Canada) brand of Diatrizoate—See Diatrizoates (Systemic), #
Hypaque-M 76%—Sterling Winthrop (Canada) brand of Diatrizoate—See Diatrizoates (Systemic), #
Hypaque Meglumine 30%—Sanofi Winthrop (U.S.) brand of Diatrizoate—See Diatrizoates (Systemic), #
Hypaque Meglumine 60%—Sanofi Winthrop (U.S.) brand of Diatrizoate—See Diatrizoates (Systemic), #
Hypaque Oral—Sterling Winthrop (Canada) brand of Diatrizoate—See Diatrizoates (Systemic), #
Hypaque Sodium 20%—Sanofi Winthrop (U.S.) brand of Diatrizoate—See Diatrizoates (Local), #
Hypaque Sodium 25%—Sanofi Winthrop (U.S.) brand of Diatrizoate—See Diatrizoates (Systemic), #
Hypaque Sodium 50%—Sanofi Winthrop (U.S. and Canada) brand of Diatrizoate—See Diatrizoates (Local), #; Diatrizoates (Systemic), #
Hypaque Sodium Oral Powder—Sanofi Winthrop (U.S.) brand of Diatrizoate—See Diatrizoates (Systemic), #
Hypaque Sodium Oral Solution—Sanofi Winthrop (U.S.) brand of Diatrizoate—See Diatrizoates (Systemic), #
Hyperab—Cutter (U.S. and Canada) brand of Rabies Immune Globulin (Systemic), 2448
Hypermune RSV—Medimmune (U.S.) brand of Respiratory Syncytial Virus Immune Globulin (Human) (Systemic), 3162
Hyperstat—Schering (U.S. and Canada) brand of Diazoxide (Parenteral-Systemic), 1200
HY-PHEN—Ascher (U.S.) brand of Hydrocodone and Acetaminophen—See Opioid (Narcotic) Analgesics and Acetaminophen (Systemic), 2198
HypRho-D Full Dose—Cutter (U.S.) and Miles (Canada) brand of Rh$_o$(D) Immune Globulin (Systemic), 2476
HypRho-D Mini-Dose—Cutter (U.S.) and Rh$_o$(D) Immune Globulin (Systemic), 2476
Hypromellose—See Hydroxypropyl Methylcellulose (Ophthalmic), #
Hyrexin—Hyrex (U.S.) brand of Diphenhydramine—See Antihistamines (Systemic), 325
Hytakerol—Sanofi Winthrop (U.S. and Canada) brand of Dihydrotachysterol—See Vitamin D and Analogs (Systemic), 2966
Hytinic—Hyrex (U.S.) brand of Iron-Polysaccharide—See Iron Supplements (Systemic), 1774
Hytone—Dermik (U.S.) brand of Hydrocortisone—See Corticosteroids (Topical), 978
Hytrin—Abbott (U.S. and Canada) brand of Terazosin (Systemic), 2750, MC-29
Hytuss—Hyrex (U.S.) brand of Guaifenesin (Systemic), 1588
Hytuss-2X—Hyrex (U.S.) brand of Guaifenesin (Systemic), 1588
Hyzaar—Merck (U.S.) brand of Losartan and Hydrochlorothiazide (Systemic), 1884, MC-18
Hyzine-50—Hyrex (U.S.) brand of Hydroxyzine—See Antihistamines (Systemic), 325

# I

$^{123}$I—Iobenguane I 123—See Iobenguane, Radioiodinated (Systemic—Diagnostic), 1747; See also Iodohippurate Sodium I 123 (Systemic), 1753; Sodium Iodide I 123 (Systemic), 2599
$^{125}$I—Iodinated I 125 Albumin—See Radioiodinated Albumin (Systemic), 2453
$^{131}$I—Iobenguane I 131—See Iobenguane, Radioiodinated (Systemic—Diagnostic), 1747; Iodinated I 131 Albumin—See Radioiodinated Albumin (Systemic), 2453; See also Iodohippurate Sodium I 131 (Systemic), 1755; Sodium Iodide I 131 (Systemic—Diagnostic), 2603; Sodium Iodide I 131 (Systemic—Therapeutic), 2606
Ibifon 600 Caplets—Ampharco (U.S.) brand of Ibuprofen—See Anti-inflammatory Drugs, Nonsteroidal (Systemic), 388
Ibren—Econo Med (U.S.) brand of Ibuprofen—See Anti-inflammatory Drugs, Nonsteroidal (Systemic), 388

Ibu—Boots (U.S.) brand of Ibuprofen—See Anti-inflammatory Drugs, Nonsteroidal (Systemic), 388
Ibu-4—Truxton (U.S.) brand of Ibuprofen—See Anti-inflammatory Drugs, Nonsteroidal (Systemic), 388
Ibu-6—Truxton (U.S.) brand of Ibuprofen—See Anti-inflammatory Drugs, Nonsteroidal (Systemic), 388
Ibu-8—Truxton (U.S.) brand of Ibuprofen—See Anti-inflammatory Drugs, Nonsteroidal (Systemic), 388
Ibu-200—Major (U.S.) brand of Ibuprofen—See Anti-inflammatory Drugs, Nonsteroidal (Systemic), 388
Ibuprin—Thompson (U.S.) brand of Ibuprofen—See Anti-inflammatory Drugs, Nonsteroidal (Systemic), 388
Ibuprofen [*Actiprofen Caplets; Advil; Advil Caplets; Advil, Children's; Apo-Ibuprofen; Bayer Select Ibuprofen Pain Relief Formula Caplets; Cramp End; Dolgesic; Excedrin IB; Excedrin IB Caplets; Genpril; Genpril Caplets; Haltran; Ibifon 600 Caplets; Ibren; Ibu; Ibu-4; Ibu-6; Ibu-8; Ibu-200; Ibuprin; Ibuprohm; Ibuprohm Caplets; Ibu-Tab; Medipren; Medipren Caplets; Midol IB; Motrin; Motrin Chewables; Motrin, Children's; Motrin, Children's Oral Drops; Motrin-IB; Motrin-IB Caplets; Motrin, Junior Strength Caplets; Novo-Profen; Nu-Ibuprofen; Nuprin; Nuprin Caplets; Pamprin-IB; Q-Profen; Rufen; Salprofen; Trendar*]
    See Anti-inflammatory Drugs, Nonsteroidal (Systemic), 388, 3145
    Solution for Injection, 3145
    Suspension, Oral, USP, 408
    Tablets USP, 408, MC-15
    Tablets (Chewable) USP, 408
Ibuprofen-containing Combinations, 3074
Ibuprophen I.V. Solution, 3146
Ibuprofen—Ohm (U.S.) brand of Ibuprofen—See Anti-inflammatory Drugs, Nonsteroidal (Systemic), 388
Ibuprohm Caplets—Ohm (U.S.) brand of Ibuprofen—See Anti-inflammatory Drugs, Nonsteroidal (Systemic), 388
Ibu-Tab—Alra (U.S.) brand of Ibuprofen—See Anti-inflammatory Drugs, Nonsteroidal (Systemic), 388
Ibutilide Fumarate [*Corvert*]
    (Systemic), 1670
    Injection, 1671
I-Chlor Ophthalmic Solution—Americal (U.S.) and IPP (U.S.) brand of Chloramphenicol (Ophthalmic), #
Icodextrin 7.5% with Electrolytes Peritoneal Dialysis Solution [*Extraneal (with 7.5% Icodextrin) Peritoneal Dialysis Solution*]
    (Systemic), 3146
I.D.A.—Bioline (U.S.) and Goldline (U.S.) brand of Isometheptene, Dichloralphenazone, and Acetaminophen (Systemic), 1786
Idamycin—Adria (U.S.) brand of Idarubicin (Systemic), 3146; Pharmacia & Upjohn (U.S.) and Pharmacia (Canada) brand of Idarubicin (Systemic), 1671
Idarac—Sanofi Winthrop (Canada) brand of Floctafenine—See Anti-inflammatory Drugs, Nonsteroidal (Systemic), 388
Idarubicin [*Idamycin*]
    (Systemic), 3146
Idarubicin Hydrochloride [*Idamycin*]
    (Systemic), 1671, 3146
    for Injection, 3146
    for Injection USP, 1674
Idenal with Codeine—Interstate (U.S.) brand of Butalbital, Aspirin, Caffeine, and Codeine—See Barbiturates and Analgesics (Systemic), 532
Idoxuridine [*Herplex Liquifilm; Stoxil*]
    (Ophthalmic), 1675
    Ointment, Ophthalmic, USP, 1676
    Solution, Ophthalmic, USP, 1676
Idoxuridine
    (Systemic), 3146
IFEX—Bristol-Myers Squibb (U.S.) brand of Ifosfamide (Systemic), 3147; Bristol-Myers Squibb (U.S.) and Mead Johnson (U.S. and Canada) brand of Ifosfamide (Systemic), 1677
Ifosfamide [*IFEX*]
    (Systemic), 1677, 3147
    Sterile USP, 1680

*IGEF*—Pharmacia (U.S.) brand of Recombinant Human Insulin-like Growth Factor I (Systemic), 3161
IGIV—See Immune Globulin Intravenous (Human) (Systemic), 1686
*I-Homatrine*—Americal (U.S.) brand of Homatropine (Ophthalmic), 1651
IHSA I 125—Mallinckrodt (U.S.) brand of Iodinated I 125 Albumin—**See Radioiodinated Albumin (Systemic)**, 2453
I 131 Iobenguane Sulfate See Iobenguane Sulfate I 131 (Systemic), 3149
I 131 Iobenguane Sulfate [meta-iodobenzylguanidine; mIBG]
  **See Iobenguane, Radioiodinated (Systemic—Therapeutic)**, 1749
  Injection, 1751
*Ilosone*—Dista (U.S.) and Lilly (Canada) brand of Erythromycin Estolate—**See Erythromycins (Systemic)**, 1368, MC-11
*Ilotycin*—Dista (U.S.) brand of Erythromycin Base—**See Erythromycins (Systemic)**, 1368; Dista (U.S.) and Lilly (Canada) brand of Erythromycin (Ophthalmic), 1364; Erythromycin Gluceptate—**See Erythromycins (Systemic)**, 1368
*Ilozyme*—Adria (U.S.) brand of Pancrelipase (Systemic), 2222
*Imagent GI*—Alliance (U.S.) brand of Perflubron (Oral-Local), #
*Imap*—McNeil (Canada) brand of Fluspirilene (Systemic), 3020
*Imap Forte*—McNeil (Canada) brand of Fluspirilene (Systemic), 3020
Imciromab Pentetate [*Myoscint*]
  **(Systemic)**, 3147
*IMDUR*—Key (U.S.) brand of Isosorbide Mononitrate—**See Nitrates (Systemic)**, 2129
*I-Methasone*—Americal (U.S.) brand of Dexamethasone—**See Corticosteroids (Otic)**, 971
Imiglucerase [*Cerezyme*]
  **(Systemic)**, 1680, 3147
  Injection, 1681
Imipenem-containing Combinations, 3074
Imipenem and Cilastatin [*Primaxin; Primaxin IM; Primaxin IV*]
  **(Systemic)**, 1681
  for Injection USP, 1684
  for Suspension, Injectable, USP, 1684
Imipramine Hydrochloride [*Apo-Imipramine; Impril; Norfranil; Novopramine; Tipramine; Tofranil*]
  **See Antidepressants, Tricyclic (Systemic)**, 271
  Injection USP, 281
  Tablets USP, 281, MC-15
Imipramine Pamoate [*Tofranil-PM*]
  **See Antidepressants, Tricyclic (Systemic)**, 271
  Capsules, 281, MC-15
Imiquimod [*Aldara*]
  **(Topical)**, 1685
  Cream, 1686
*Imitrex*—Glaxo Wellcome (U.S. and Canada) brand of Sumatriptan (Systemic), 2664, MC-29
*ImmTher*—Endorex (U.S.) brand of Liposomal N-Acetylglucosminyl-N-Acetylmuramyl-L-Ala-D-isoGln-L-Ala-Gylcerolid-palmitoyl (Systemic), 3152
*Immther*—Endorex (U.S.) brand of Liposomal N-Acetylglucosminyl-N-Acetylmuramyl-L-Ala-D-IsoGln-L-Ala-Glycerolid-Palmitoyl (Systemic), 3152; Immuno (U.S.) brand of Disaccharide Tripeptide Glycerol Dipalmitoyl (Systemic), 3141
*ImmuCyst*—Connaught (Canada) brand of Bacillus Calmette-Guérin (BCG) Live (Mucosal-Local), 507
*Immudyn*—Dynagen (U.S.) brand of *Pseudomonas aeruginosa*, Purified Extract of (Systemic), 3160
*Immun-Aid*—Kendall McGaw (U.S.) brand of Enteral Nutrition Formula, Disease-specific—**See Enteral Nutrition Formulas (Systemic)**, #
Immune Globulin Intravenous (Human) [*Gamimune N; Gammagard; Gammagard SD; Gammar-IV; IGIV; Immuno; Iveegam; IVIG; Polygam; Sandoglobulin; SD Polygam; Venoglobulin-I; Venoglobulin-S*]
  **(Systemic)**, 1686, 3024, 3025, 3147
  Injection, 1689, 3024, 3025
  for Injection, 1689, 3025
Immune Globulin Intravenous (Human) Immuno—**See Immune Globulin Intravenous (Human) (Systemic)**, 3147
*Immune VH*—Immuno-Canada (Canada) brand of Factor IX (Systemic), 1430

*Immuno*—Immuno (U.S.) brand of Immune Globulin Intravenous (Human) (Systemic), 3147
Immunoassay Pregnancy Test Kits [*Answer; Answer Now One Step; Answer Quick & Simple 1-Step; ClearBlue Easy; ClearBlue Easy One Minute; Conceive 1-Step; Confidelle; Confirm; e.p.t; Fact Plus; Fact Plus One Step; First Response; First Response 1-Step; Fortel Midstream One Step; Fortel Plus; Nimbus Quick Strip; QTest; Rapid Vue*]
  **See Pregnancy Test Kits for Home Use**, #
  Test Kits, #
*Immuno-C*—Biomune (U.S.) brand of Bovine Whey Protein Concentrate (Systemic), 3134
*Immupath*—Hemacare (U.S.) brand of Human Immunodeficiency Virus (HIV) Neutralizing Antibodies (Systemic), 3145
*ImmuRAID, AFP-Tc 99m*—Immunomedics (U.S.) brand of Technetium Tc 99m Murine Monoclonal Antibody to Human Alpha-fetoprotein (Systemic), 3167
*ImmuRAID, hCG-Tc 99m*—Immunomedics (U.S.) brand of Technetium Tc 99m Murine Monoclonal Antibody to Human Chorionic Gonadotropin (Systemic), 3167
*Immuraid-LL-2(99mTc)*—Immunomedics (U.S.) brand of Technetium Tc-99m Murine Monoclonal Antibody (IgG2a) to BCE (Systemic), 3167
*ImmuRAIT, LL-2-I-131*—Immunomedics (U.S.) brand of Iodine I 131 Murine Monoclonal Antibody IgG$_{2a}$ to B Cell (Systemic), 3149
*Imodium*—Janssen (U.S. and Canada) brand of Loperamide (Oral-Local), 1877, MC-17
*Imodium A-D*—McNeil-CPC (U.S.) brand of Loperamide (Oral-Local), 1877
*Imodium A-D Caplets*—McNeil-CPC (U.S.) brand of Loperamide (Oral-Local), 1877
*Imodium Advanced*—McNeil Consumer (U.S.) brand of Loperamide and Simethicone (Systemic), 3028
*Imogam*—Connaught (U.S.) brand of Rabies Immune Globulin (Systemic), 2448
*Imovane*—Rhône-Poulenc (Canada) brand of Zopiclone (Systemic), 3039
*Imovax*—Connaught (U.S.) brand of Rabies Vaccine, Human Diploid Cell—**See Rabies Vaccine (Systemic)**, 2449
*Imovax I.D.*—Connaught (U.S.) brand of Rabies Vaccine, Human Diploid Cell—**See Rabies Vaccine (Systemic)**, 2449
*Impact*—Sandoz (U.S.) brand of Enteral Nutrition Formula, Disease-specific—**See Enteral Nutrition Formulas (Systemic)**, #
*Impact with Fiber*—Sandoz (U.S.) brand of Enteral Nutrition Formula, Disease-specific—**See Enteral Nutrition Formulas (Systemic)**, #; Enteral Nutrition Formula, Fiber-containing—**See Enteral Nutrition Formulas (Systemic)**, #
Imported Fire Ant Venom, Allergenic Extract
  **(Systemic)**, 3147
*Impril*—ICN (Canada) brand of Imipramine—**See Antidepressants, Tricyclic (Systemic)**, 271
*Improved Sino-Tuss*—Rugby (U.S.) brand of Chlorpheniramine, Phenylephrine, Dextromethorphan, Acetaminophen, and Salicylamide—**See Cough/Cold Combinations (Systemic)**, 1024
*Imuran*—Glaxo Wellcome (U.S. and Canada) brand of Azathioprine (Systemic), 491, MC-3
*Imuthiol*—Connaught (U.S.) brand of Diethyldithiocarbamate (Systemic), 3140
*ImuVert*—Cell Technology (U.S.) brand of Serratia Marcescens Extract (Polyribosomes) (Systemic), 3164
$^{111}$In—See Indium In 111 Oxyquinoline (Systemic), 1695; Indium In 111 Pentetate (Systemic), 1698; Indium In 111 Pentetreotide (Systemic), 1700; Indium In 111 Satumomab Pendetide (Systemic), 1702
*I-Naphline*—Americal (U.S.) brand of Naphazoline (Ophthalmic), #
*Inapsine*—Akorn (U.S.) and Janssen (Canada) brand of Droperidol (Systemic), 1319
INAT—See Isoniazid and Thiacetazone (Systemic), #
*Indameth*—Major (U.S.) brand of Indomethacin—For Patent Ductus Arteriosus (Systemic), 1704
Indapamide [*Lozide; Lozol*]
  **(Systemic)**, 1691
  Tablets, 1692, MC-15
*Inderal*—Wyeth-Ayerst (U.S.) and Ayerst (Canada) brand of Propranolol—**See Beta-adrenergic Blocking Agents (Systemic)**, 593, MC-26

*Inderal LA*—Wyeth-Ayerst (U.S.) and Ayerst (Canada) brand of Propranolol—**See Beta-adrenergic Blocking Agents (Systemic)**, 593, MC-26
*Inderide*—Wyeth-Ayerst (U.S.) and Ayerst (Canada) brand of Propranolol and Hydrochlorothiazide—**See Beta-adrenergic Blocking Agents and Thiazide Diuretics (Systemic)**, 609, MC-26
*Inderide LA*—Wyeth-Ayerst (U.S.) brand of Propranolol and Hydrochlorothiazide—**See Beta-adrenergic Blocking Agents and Thiazide Diuretics (Systemic)**, 609, MC-26
Indinavir Sulfate [*Crixivan*]
  **(Systemic)**, 1693
  Capsules, 1695, MC-15
*Indium DTPA In 111*—Medi-Physics Amersham (U.S.) brand of Indium In 111 Pentetate (Systemic), 1698
Indium In 111 Altumomab Pentetate [*HYBRI-CEAker*]
  **(Systemic)**, 3147
Indium In 111 Capromab Pendetide [*ProstaScint*]
  **(Systemic)**, #
  Injection, #
Indium In 111 Murine Monoclonal Antibody Fab to Myosin [*Myoscint*]
  **(Systemic)**, 3147
Indium In 111 Oxyquinoline
  **(Systemic)**, 1695
  Solution USP, 1698
Indium In 111 Pentetate [*Indium DTPA In 111*]
  **(Systemic)**, 1698
  Injection USP, 1700
Indium In 111 Pentetreotide [In 111-DTPA-octreotide; *OctreoScan*]
  **(Systemic)**, 1700
  Injection, 1702
Indium In 111 Satumomab Pendetide [*OncoScint CR/OV*]
  **(Systemic)**, 1702
  Injection, 1704
*Indocid*—Merck (Canada) brand of Indomethacin—**See Anti-inflammatory Drugs, Nonsteroidal (Systemic)**, 388; MSD (Canada) brand of Indomethacin—**See Anti-inflammatory Drugs, Nonsteroidal (Ophthalmic)**, 383; MSD (Canada) brand of Indomethacin—For Patent Ductus Arteriosus (Systemic), 1704
*Indocid PDA*—MSD (Canada) brand of Indomethacin—For Patent Ductus Arteriosus (Systemic), 1704
*Indocid SR*—Merck (Canada) brand of Indomethacin—**See Anti-inflammatory Drugs, Nonsteroidal (Systemic)**, 388
*Indocin*—Merck (U.S.) brand of Indomethacin—**See Anti-inflammatory Drugs, Nonsteroidal (Systemic)**, 388, MC-15; Merck (U.S.) brand of Indomethacin—For Patent Ductus Arteriosus (Systemic), 1704
*Indocin I.V.*—Merck (U.S.) brand of Indomethacin—For Patent Ductus Arteriosus (Systemic), 1704
*Indocin SR*—Merck (U.S.) brand of Indomethacin—**See Anti-inflammatory Drugs, Nonsteroidal (Systemic)**, 388, MC-16
Indomethacin—Indomethacin—**See Anti-inflammatory Drugs, Nonsteroidal (Ophthalmic)**, 383; **Anti-inflammatory Drugs, Nonsteroidal (Systemic)**, 388; See also Indomethacin—For Patent Ductus Arteriosus (Systemic), 1704
Indomethacin [*Indocid; indometacin*]
  **See Anti-inflammatory Drugs, Nonsteroidal (Ophthalmic)**, 383
  Suspension, Ophthalmic, 387
Indomethacin [*Apo-Indomethacin; Indameth; Indocid; Indocid SR; Indocin; Indocin SR; indometacin; Novo-Methacin; Nu-Indo*]
  **See Anti-inflammatory Drugs, Nonsteroidal (Systemic)**, 388
  Capsules USP, 409 MC-15
  Capsules, Extended-release, USP, 410 MC-16
  Suppositories USP, 410
  Suspension, Oral, USP, 410
Indomethacin [*Apo-Indomethacin; Indameth; Indocid; Indocin; indometacin; Novomethacin*]
  **(Systemic—For Patent Ductus Arteriosus)**, 1704
  Capsules USP, 1706
Indomethacin Sodium [*Indocid PDA; Indocin I.V.; indometacin*]
  **(Systemic—For Patent Ductus Arteriosus)**, 1704
  Sterile, 1707
In 111-DTPA-octreotide—*See* Indium In 111 Pentetreotide (Systemic), 1700
*I-Neocort*—Americal (U.S.) brand of Neomycin, Polymyxin B, and Hydrocortisone (Ophthalmic), #

*Infalyte*—Mead Johnson (U.S.) brand of Rice Syrup Solids and Electrolytes—**See Carbohydrates and Electrolytes (Systemic)**, 769
Infant Formulas
  **(Systemic)**, #
Infant Formulas, Hypoallergenic [*Alimentum; Nutramigen; Pregestimil*]
  **See Infant Formulas (Systemic)**, #
  Concentrate, Oral, #
  Solution, Oral, #
  for Solution, Oral, #
Infant Formulas, Milk-based [*Carnation Follow-Up Formula; Carnation Good Start; Enfamil; Enfamil Human Milk Fortifier; Enfamil with Iron; Enfamil Premature Formula; Enfamil Premature Formula with Iron; Gerber Baby Formula; Lactofree; Preemie SMA 20; Preemie SMA 24; Similac 13; Similac 20; Similac 24; Similac 27; Similac with Iron 20; Similac with Iron 24; Similac Natural Care Human Milk Fortifier; Similac PM 60/40; Similac Special Care 20; Similac Special Care 24; Similac Special Care with Iron 24; SMA 13; SMA 20; SMA 24; SMA 27; SMA Lo-Iron 13; SMA Lo-Iron 20; SMA Lo-Iron 24*]
  **See Infant Formulas (Systemic)**, #
  Concentrate, Oral, #
  Powder, Oral, #
  Solution, Oral, #
  for Solution, Oral, #
Infant Formulas, Soy-based [*Alsoy; Gerber Soy Formula; Isomil; Isomil SF; Nursoy; ProSobee; RCF; Soyalac*]
  **See Infant Formulas (Systemic)**, #
  Concentrate, Oral, #
  Solution, Oral, #
  for Solution, Oral, #
*Infasurf*—Forest (U.S.) brand of Calfactant (Intratracheal-Local), 3013; ONY (U.S.) brand of Surface Active Extract of Saline Lavage of Bovine Lungs (Intratracheal-Local), 3167
*InFeD*—Schein (U.S.) brand of Iron Dextran—**See Iron Supplements (Systemic)**, 1774
*Infergen*—Amgen (U.S.) brand of Interferon Alfacon-1 (Systemic), 1730
*Inflamase Forte*—Ciba Vision (U.S.) and Iolab (Canada) brand of Prednisolone—**See Corticosteroids (Ophthalmic)**, 966
*Inflamase Mild*—Ciba Vision (U.S.) and Iolab (Canada) brand of Prednisolone—**See Corticosteroids (Ophthalmic)**, 966
Influenza Virus Vaccine [*FluShield*; flu vaccine; *Fluviral; Fluviral S/F; Fluvirin; Fluzone*]
  **(Systemic)**, 1707
  Influenza Virus Vaccine USP (Injection—Split virus, purified-surface-antigen type), 1712
  Influenza Virus Vaccine USP (Injection—Split virus, split or subviron type), 1713
  Influenza Virus Vaccine USP (Injection—Whole virus), 1713
*Infumorph*—Elkins-Sinn (U.S.) brand of Morphine (Systemic), 3155
INH—*See* Isoniazid (Systemic), 1789
In-111 Murine MAB (2B8-MXDTPA) and Y-90 Murine MAB (2B8-MXDTPA) [*Melimmune*]
  **(Systemic)**, 3147
*Inocor*—Sanofi Winthrop (U.S. and Canada) brand of Amrinone (Systemic), 108
Inosine Pranobex [*Isoprinosine*]
  **(Systemic)**, 3147
*Inspire*—Quintex (U.S.) brand of Xylometazoline (Nasal), 3038
*Insta-Char Aqueous*—Kerr (U.S. and Canada) brand of Charcoal, Activated (Oral-Local), 831
*Insta-Char with Sorbitol*—Kerr (U.S.) brand of Charcoal, Activated and Sorbitol (Oral-Local), 831
*Instantine*—Sterling Winthrop (Canada) brand of Aspirin—**See Salicylates (Systemic)**, 2538
Insulin [crystalline zinc insulin; *Insulin-Toronto; Regular Iletin; Regular Iletin I; Regular Iletin II; Regular (Concentrated) Iletin II, U-500*; regular insulin]
  **See Insulin (Systemic)**, 1713
  Injection USP, 1722
Insulin Human [*Humulin R; Humulin-R; Novolin ge Toronto; Novolin ge Toronto PenFill; Novolin R; Novolin R Penfill; Novolin R Prefilled*; regular insulin]
  **See Insulin (Systemic)**, 1713
  Injection USP, 1723
Insulin Human, Buffered [*Velosulin BR; Velosulin Human*]
  **See Insulin (Systemic)**, 1713
  Injection, 1720

Insulin, Isophane [*NPH Iletin; NPH Iletin I; NPH Iletin II; NPH insulin; NPH Insulin; NPH-N*]
  **See Insulin (Systemic)**, 1713
  Suspension USP
Insulin, Isophane, Human [*Humulin N; Humulin-N; Novolin ge NPH; Novolin ge NPH PenFill; Novolin N; Novolin N Penfill; Novolin N Prefilled*]
  **See Insulin (Systemic)**, 1713
  Suspension, 1725
Insulin, Isophane, Human, and Insulin, Human [*Humulin 10/90; Humulin 20/80; Humulin 30/70; Humulin 40/60; Humulin 50/50; Humulin 70/30; Novolin 70/30; Novolin ge 30/70; Novolin ge 10/90 Penfill; Novolin ge 20/80 Penfill; Novolin ge 30/70 Penfill; Novolin ge 40/60 Penfill; Novolin ge 50/50 Penfill; Novolin 70/30 PenFill; Novolin 70/30 Prefilled*]
  **See Insulin (Systemic)**, 1713
  Suspension and Injection, 1726
Insulin-like Growth Factor-1 [*Myotrophin*]
  **(Systemic)**, 3147
Insulin Lispro [*Humalog*]
  **(Systemic)**, 1727, 3025
  Injection, 1729, 3025
*Insulin-Toronto*—Connaught Novo Nordisk (Canada) brand of Insulin—**See Insulin (Systemic)**, 1713
Insulin Zinc [*Lente Iletin; Lente Iletin I; Lente Iletin II*; lente insulin; *Lente Insulin; Lente L*]
  **See Insulin (Systemic)**, 1713
  Suspension USP, 1724
Insulin Zinc, Extended [ultralente insulin; *Ultralente Insulin*]
  **See Insulin (Systemic)**, 1713
  Suspension USP, 1721
Insulin, Zinc, Extended, Human [*Humulin-U; Humulin U Ultralente; Novolin ge Ultralente*]
  **See Insulin (Systemic)**, 1713
  Suspension, 1721
Insulin Zinc, Human [*Humulin L; Humulin-L; Novolin ge Lente; Novolin L*]
  **See Insulin (Systemic)**, 1713
  Suspension, 1724
Insulin Zinc, Prompt [semilente insulin; *Semilente Insulin*]
  **See Insulin (Systemic)**, 1713
  Suspension USP, 1726
*Intal*—Fisons (U.S. and Canada) brand of Cromolyn (Inhalation-Local), 1116
*Integrilin*—COR Therapeutics/Key (U.S.) brand of Eptifibatide (Systemic), 1356
*Intercon 0.5/35*—Hamilton (U.S.) brand of Norethindrone and Ethinyl Estradiol—**See Estrogens and Progestins—Oral Contraceptives (Systemic)**, 1397
*Intercon 1/35*—Hamilton (U.S.) brand of Norethindrone and Ethinyl Estradiol—**See Estrogens and Progestins—Oral Contraceptives (Systemic)**, 1397
*Intercon 1/50*—Hamilton (U.S.) brand of Norethindrone and Mestranol—**See Estrogens and Progestins—Oral Contraceptives (Systemic)**, 1397
Interferon Alfa-2a, Recombinant [*Roferon-A*]
  **See Interferons, Alpha (Systemic)**, 1740, 3147
  Injection, 1743
  for Injection, 1744
Interferon Alfa-2b, Recombinant [*Intron A*]
  **See Interferons, Alpha (Systemic)**, 1740, 3147, 3148
  for Injection, 1744
Interferon Alfacon-1, Recombinant [*Infergen*]
  **(Systemic)**, 1730
  Injection, 1732
Interferon Alfa-n1 (LNS) [*Wellferon*]
  **See Interferons, Alpha (Systemic)**, 1740, 3148
  Injection, 1745
Interferon Alfa-n3 [*Alferon N*]
  **See Interferons, Alpha (Systemic)**, 1740
  Injection, 1745
Interferon Beta-1a [*Avonex, Rebif*]
  **(Systemic)**, 1732, 3026, 3148
  for Injection, 1734
  for Injection, 3026
Interferon, Beta-1b [*Betaseron*]
  **(Systemic)**, 1735, 3026, 3148
  for Injection, 1737, 3026, 3032
Interferon Beta, Recombinant [*R-Frone*; r-IFN-beta]
  **(Systemic)**, 3148
Interferon Beta, Recombinant, Human
  **(Systemic)**, 3148
Interferon Gamma 1-b [*Actimmune*]
  **(Systemic)**, 3149

Interferon Gamma-1b, Recombinant [*Actimmune*]
  **(Systemic)**, 1737, 3148
  Injection, 1739
Interferons, Alpha
  **(Systemic)**, 1740
Interleukin-1 Receptor Antagonist, Human Recombinant [*Antril*]
  **(Systemic)**, 3148
Interleukin-2 [*Teceleukin*]
  **(Systemic)**, 3149
Interleukin-2, recombinant—*See* Aldesleukin (Systemic), 36, 3129
Interleukin-2, Recombinant, Liposome Encapsulated
  **(Systemic)**, 3151
Interleukin-3, Human, Recombinant
  **(Systemic)**, 3149
Interleukin-11, Human Recombinant [*Neumega rhIL-11 Growth Factor*]
  **(Systemic)**, 3161
Interleukin-11, Recombinant—*See* Oprelvekin (Systemic), 2205
*Intralipid*—Clintec (U.S. and Canada) brand of Fat Emulsions (Systemic), #
Intravitreal Ganciclovir Free Acid Implant [*Vitrasert Implant*]
  **(Ophthalmic)**, 3149
*Introlan*—Elan (U.S.) brand of Enteral Nutrition Formula, Polymeric—**See Enteral Nutrition Formulas (Systemic)**, #
*Introlite*—Ross (U.S.) brand of Enteral Nutrition Formula, Polymeric—**See Enteral Nutrition Formulas (Systemic)**, #
*Intron A*—Schering (U.S. and Canada) brand of Interferon Alfa-2b, Recombinant—**See Interferons, Alpha (Systemic)**, 1740; Schering (U.S.) brand of Interferon Alfa-2b, Recombinant (Systemic), 3148
*Intropin*—Du Pont Critical Care (U.S.) and Du Pont (Canada) brand of Dopamine—**See Sympathomimetic Agents—Cardiovascular Use (Parenteral-Systemic)**, 2669
Inulin
  **(Systemic)**, #
  Injection, #
*Inversine*—Merck (U.S.) brand of Mecamylamine (Systemic), #
*Invirase*—Roche (U.S.) brand of Saquinavir (Systemic), IBN-2554, MC-28
Iobenguane, Radioiodinated
  **(Systemic—Diagnostic)**, 1747
Iobenguane, Radioiodinated
  **(Systemic—Therapeutic)**, 1749
Iobenguane I 123 [meta-iodobenzylguanidine; mIBG]
  **See Iobenguane, Radioiodinated (Systemic—Diagnostic)**, 1747
  Injection USP, 1749
Iobenguane Sulfate I 131 [meta-iodobenzyl-guanidine; mIBG]
  **(Systemic)**, 3149
Iobenguane Sulfate I 131 [meta-iodobenzylguanidine; mIBG]
  **See Iobenguane, Radioiodinated (Systemic—Diagnostic)**, 1747
  Injection, 1749
*Iobid DM*—Iomed (U.S.) brand of Dextromethorphan and Guaifenesin—**See Cough/Cold Combinations (Systemic)**, 1024
Iocetamic Acid [*Cholebrine; Colebrin; Colebrina*]
  **See Cholecystographic Agents, Oral (Systemic)**, #
  Tablets USP, #
*Iodal HD*—Iomed (U.S.) brand of Chlorpheniramine, Phenylephrine, and Hydrocodone—**See Cough/Cold Combinations (Systemic)**, 1024
Iodinated Glycerol
  **(Systemic)**, 3187
  Elixir, 3187
  Solution, Oral, 3187
  Tablets, 3187
Iodinated I 125 Albumin [*IHSA I 125; Jeanatope*]
  **See Radioiodinated Albumin (Systemic)**, 2453
  Injection USP, 2455
Iodinated I 131 Albumin [*Megatope*]
  **See Radioiodinated Albumin (Systemic)**, 2453
  Injection USP, 2455
Iodine [iodine tincture; strong iodine tincture]
  **(Topical)**, #
  Iodine Tincture USP, #
Iodine-containing Combinations, 3074
Strong Iodine Tincture USP, #
Iodine 131 6B-Iodomethyl-19-Norcholesterol
  **(Systemic)**, 3148

## 3298 General Index

Iodine I 123 Murine Monoclonal Antibody to Alpha-Fetoprotein
**(Systemic)**, 3148
Iodine I 131 Meta-Iodobenzyl-Guanidine—See Iobenguane Sulfate I 131 (Systemic), 3149
Iodine I 131 Murine Monoclonal Antibody to Alpha-Fetoprotein
**(Systemic)**, 3149
Iodine I 123 Murine Monoclonal Antibody to Human Chorionic Gonadotropin (hCG)
**(Systemic)**, 3149
Iodine I 131 Murine Monoclonal Antibody to Human Chorionic Gonadotropin (hCG)
**(Systemic)**, 3149
Iodine I 131 Murine Monoclonal Antibody IgG₂ₐ to B Cell [*ImmuRAIT, LL-2-I-131*]
**(Systemic)**, 3149
Iodine, Strong [Lugol's solution]
**(Systemic)**, 1751
Solution USP, 1753
Iodine tincture—See Iodine (Topical), #
Iodipamide-containing Combinations, 3074
Iodipamide Meglumine [*adipiodone; Cholografin; Cholografin for Infusion*]
**(Systemic)**, #
Injection USP, #
Iodixanol [*Visipaque*]
**(Systemic)**, #
Injection, #
Iodochlorhydroxyquin—See Clioquinol (Topical), #
Iodochlorhydroxyquin and hydrocortisone—See Clioquinol and Hydrocortisone (Topical), #
Iodohippurate Sodium I 123 [*Nephropure*]
**(Systemic)**, 1753
Injection USP, 1755
Iodohippurate Sodium I 131 [*Hippuran; Hipputope*]
**(Systemic)**, 1755
Injection USP, 1756
*Iodopen*—LyphoMed (U.S.) brand of Sodium Iodide (Systemic), 2597
Iodoquinol [*diiodohydroxyquin; diiodohydroxyquinoline; Diodoquin; Diquinol; Yodoquinol; Yodoxin*]
**(Oral-Local)**, #
Tablets USP, #
*Iodotope*—Bracco (U.S.) brand of Sodium Iodide I 131 (Systemic—Therapeutic), 2606
*Iofed*—Iomed (U.S.) brand of Brompheniramine and Pseudoephedrine—See **Antihistamines and Decongestants (Systemic)**, 343
*Iofed PD*—Iomed (U.S.) brand of Brompheniramine and Pseudoephedrine—See **Antihistamines and Decongestants (Systemic)**, 343
Iofetamine Hydrochloride I 123 [*Spectamine*]
**(Systemic)**, 1757
Injection, 1758
Iohexol [*Omnipaque 140; Omnipaque 180; Omnipaque 210; Omnipaque 240; Omnipaque 300; Omnipaque 350*]
**(Local)**, #
Injection USP, #
Iohexol [*Omnipaque 140; Omnipaque 180; Omnipaque 210; Omnipaque 240; Omnipaque 300; Omnipaque 350*]
**(Systemic)**, #
Injection USP, #
*Iohist-D*—Iomed (U.S.) brand of Pheniramine, Phenyltoloxamine, Pyrilamine, and Phenylpropanolamine—See **Antihistamines and Decongestants (Systemic)**, 343
*Iohist DM*—Iomed (U.S.) brand of Brompheniramine, Phenylpropanolamine, and Dextromethorphan—See **Cough/Cold Combinations (Systemic)**, 1024
*Ionamin*—Pennwalt (U.S.) and Fisons (Canada) brand of Phentermine—See **Appetite Suppressants (Systemic)**, 452
*Ionax Astringent Skin Cleanser Topical Solution*—Galderma (U.S.) brand of Salicylic Acid (Topical), #
*Ionil Plus Shampoo*—Galderma (U.S.) brand of Salicylic Acid (Topical), #
*Ionil Shampoo*—Galderma (U.S.) brand of Salicylic Acid (Topical), #
*Ionil T Plus*—Owen (U.S.) brand of Coal Tar (Topical), #
Iopamidol [*Isovue-128; Isovue-200; Isovue-250; Isovue-300; Isovue-370; Isovue-M 200; Isovue-M 300*]
**(Systemic)**, #
Injection USP, #

Iopanoic Acid [*Cistobil; Colegraf; Felombrine; Jopanonsyre; Neocontrast; Telepaque*]
See **Cholecystographic Agents, Oral (Systemic)**, #
Tablets USP, #
*Iophen-C Liquid*—Major (U.S.); Rugby (U.S.) and Schein (U.S.) brand of Codeine and Iodinated Glycerol—See **Cough/Cold Combinations (Systemic)**, 1024
*Iophen DM*—Moore (U.S.); Rugby (U.S.) and Schein (U.S.) brand of Dextromethorphan and Iodinated Glycerol—See **Cough/Cold Combinations (Systemic)**, 1024
*Iopidine*—Alcon (U.S. and Canada) brand of Apraclonidine (Ophthalmic), 459
Iopromide [*Ultravist 150; Ultravist 240; Ultravist 300; Ultravist 370*]
**(Systemic)**, #
Injection, #
*Iosal II*—Iomed (U.S.) brand of Pseudoephedrine and Guaifenesin—See **Cough/Cold Combinations (Systemic)**, 1024
Iothalamate Meglumine [*Cysto-Conray; Cysto-Conray II*]
**(Local)**, #
Injection USP, #
Iothalamate Meglumine [*Conray; Conray-30; Conray-43; Conray-60*]
**(Systemic)**, #
Injection USP, #
Iothalamate Meglumine and Iothalamate Sodium [*Vascoray*]
**(Systemic)**, #
Injection USP, #
Iothalamate Sodium [*Angio-Conray; Conray-325; Conray-400*]
**(Systemic)**, #
Injection USP, #
*Iotussin HC*—Iomed (U.S.) brand of Chlorpheniramine, Phenylephrine, and Hydrocodone—See **Cough/Cold Combinations (Systemic)**, 1024
Ioversol [*Optiray 160; Optiray 240; Optiray 300; Optiray 320; Optiray 350*]
**(Systemic)**, #
Injection, #
Ioxaglate Meglumine and Ioxaglate Sodium [*Hexabrix; Hexabrix-320*]
**(Local)**, #
Injection, #
Ioxaglate Meglumine and Ioxaglate Sodium [*Hexabrix; Hexabrix-200; Hexabrix-320*]
**(Systemic)**, #
Injection, #
Ioxilan [*Oxilan 300; Oxilan 350*]
**(Systemic)**, #
Injection, #
Ipecac
**(Oral-Local)**, 1759
Syrup USP, 1760
Ipecac-containing Combinations, 3074
*I-Phrine*—Americal (U.S.) brand of Phenylephrine (Ophthalmic), #
*I-Picamide*—Americal (U.S.) brand of Tropicamide (Ophthalmic), #
Ipodate Calcium [*Oragrafin Calcium*]
See **Cholecystographic Agents, Oral (Systemic)**, #
for Suspension, Oral, USP, #
Ipodate Sodium [*Bilivist; Biloptin; Oragrafin Sodium;* ]
See **Cholecystographic Agents, Oral (Systemic)**, #
Capsules USP, #
*Ipol*—Connaught (U.S.) brand of Poliovirus Vaccine Inactivated Enhanced Potency—See **Poliovirus Vaccine (Systemic)**, 2343
Ipratropium Bromide [*Apo-Ipravent; Atrovent; Kendral-Ipratropium*]
**(Inhalation-Local)**, 1761, 3026
Aerosol, Inhalation, 1763
Solution, Inhalation, 1763
Solution, Nasal, 3026
Ipratropium Bromide [*Atrovent*]
**(Nasal)**, 1764
Aerosol, Nasal, 1765
Ipratropium Bromide and Albuterol Sulfate [*Combivent*]
**(Inhalation-Local)**, 1765
Aerosol, Inhalation, 1767
*I-Pred*—Americal (U.S.) brand of Prednisolone—See **Corticosteroids (Ophthalmic)**, 966

*Ipsatol Cough Formula for Children*—Kenwood (U.S.) brand of Phenylpropanolamine, Dextromethorphan, and Guaifenesin—See **Cough/Cold Combinations (Systemic)**, 1024
IPV—Poliovirus Vaccine Inactivated—See **Poliovirus Vaccine (Systemic)**, 2343
I-131 Radiolabeled B1 Monoclonal Antibody (Anti-B4)
**(Systemic)**, 3146
Irbesartan [*Avapro*]
**(Systemic)**, 1767
Tablets, 1769
*Ircon*—Key (U.S.) brand of Ferrous Fumarate—See **Iron Supplements (Systemic)**, 1774
Irinotecan Hydrochloride [*Camptosar*; CPT-11]
**(Systemic)**, 1769
Injection, 1773
Iron blue—See Prussian Blue (Oral-Local), #
Iron Dextran [*DexFerrum; DexIron; InFeD*]
See **Iron Supplements (Systemic)**, 1774
Injection USP, 1784
Iron-Polysaccharide [*Hytinic; Niferex; Niferex-150; Nu-Iron; Nu-Iron 150*]
See **Iron Supplements (Systemic)**, 1774
Capsules, 1784
Elixir, 1785
Tablets, 1785
Iron Sorbitol [*Jectofer*]
See **Iron Supplements (Systemic)**, 1774
Injection, 1785
Iron Supplements
**(Systemic)**, 1774
*Ismelin*—Ciba-Geigy (U.S.) brand of Guanethidine (Systemic), 3145; Ciba (U.S. and Canada) brand of Guanethidine (Systemic), 1595
ISMO—Wyeth-Ayerst (U.S.) brand of Isosorbide Mononitrate—See **Nitrates (Systemic)**, 2129, MC-16
*Iso-Acetazone*—Rugby (U.S.) brand of Isometheptene, Dichloralphenazone, and Acetaminophen (Systemic), 1786
*Iso-Bid*—Geriatric (U.S.) brand of Isosorbide Dinitrate—See **Nitrates (Systemic)**, 2129
*Isobutal*—Balan (U.S.) brand of Butalbital, Aspirin, and Caffeine—See **Barbiturates and Analgesics (Systemic)**, 532
*Isobutyl*—Bioline (U.S.) brand of Butalbital, Aspirin, and Caffeine—See **Barbiturates and Analgesics (Systemic)**, 532
Isobutyramide
**(Systemic)**, 3150
Solution, Oral, 3150
*Isocaine*—Novocol (U.S.) brand of Mepivacaine—See **Anesthetics (Parenteral-Local)**, 139
*Isocaine 2%*—Novocol (Canada) brand of Mepivacaine—See **Anesthetics (Parenteral-Local)**, 139
*Isocaine 3%*—Novocol (Canada) brand of Mepivacaine—See **Anesthetics (Parenteral-Local)**, 139
*Isocal*—Mead Johnson (U.S.) brand of Enteral Nutrition Formula, Polymeric—See **Enteral Nutrition Formulas (Systemic)**, #
*Isocal HN*—Mead Johnson (U.S.) brand of Enteral Nutrition Formula, Polymeric—See **Enteral Nutrition Formulas (Systemic)**, #
*Isocet*—Rugby (U.S.) brand of Butalbital, Acetaminophen, and Caffeine—See **Barbiturates and Analgesics (Systemic)**, 532
*Isocom*—Nutripharm (U.S.) brand of Isometheptene, Dichloralphenazone, and Acetaminophen (Systemic), 1786
Isoetharine [*Arm-a-Med Isoetharine; Beta-2; Bronkosol; Dey-Lute Isoetharine*]
See **Bronchodilators, Adrenergic (Inhalation-Local)**, 640
Solution, Inhalation, USP, 648
Isoetharine Mesylate [*Bronkometer*]
See **Bronchodilators, Adrenergic (Inhalation-Local)**, 640
Aerosol, Inhalation, USP, 648
*Isoetretin*—See Acitretin (Systemic), 18
Isoflurane [*Forane*]
See **Anesthetics, Inhalation (Systemic)**, 168
Isoflurane USP, 172
Isoflurophate [*DFP; difluophate; dyflos; Floropryl*]
See **Antiglaucoma Agents, Cholinergic, Long-acting (Ophthalmic)**, 315
Ointment, Ophthalmic, USP, 319
*Isolan*—Elan (U.S.) brand of Enteral Nutrition Formula, Polymeric—See **Enteral Nutrition Formulas (Systemic)**, #

*Isolin*—Glenlawn (U.S.) brand of Butalbital, Aspirin, and Caffeine—**See Barbiturates and Analgesics (Systemic)**, 532

*Isollyl*—Rugby (U.S.) and Spencer-Mead (U.S.) brand of Butalbital, Aspirin, and Caffeine—**See Barbiturates and Analgesics (Systemic)**, 532

*Isollyl with Codeine*—Rugby (U.S.) brand of Butalbital, Aspirin, Caffeine, and Codeine—**See Barbiturates and Analgesics (Systemic)**, 532

Isometheptene-containing Combinations, 3075

Isometheptene, dichloralphenazone, and paracetamol—**See Isometheptene, Dichloralphenazone, and Acetaminophen (Systemic)**, 1786

Isometheptene Mucate, Dichloralphenazone, and Acetaminophen [*Amidrine; I.D.A.; Iso-Acetazone; Isocom;* isometheptene, dichloralphenazone, and paracetamol; *Midchlor; Midrin; Migquin; Migrapap; Migratine; Migrazone; Migrend; Migrex; Mitride*]
  **(Systemic)**, 1786
  Capsules USP, 1789

*Isomil*—Ross (U.S. and Canada) brand of Infant Formulas, Soy-based—**See Infant Formulas (Systemic)**, #

*Isomil SF*—Ross (U.S.) brand of Infant Formulas, Soy-based—**See Infant Formulas (Systemic)**, #

*Isonate*—Major (U.S.) brand of Isosorbide Dinitrate—**See Nitrates (Systemic)**, 2129

Isoniazid [INH; *Isotamine; Laniazid; Nydrazid; PMS Isoniazid*]
  **(Systemic)**, 1789
  Injection USP, 1796
  Syrup USP, 1795
  Tablets USP, 1796, MC-16

Isoniazid-containing Combinations, 3075

Isoniazid and Thiacetazone [*INAT; Thiazina; Thisozide*]
  **(Systemic)**, #
  Tablets, #

*Isopap*—Columbia Drug (U.S.) brand of Butalbital, Acetaminophen, and Caffeine—**See Barbiturates and Analgesics (Systemic)**, 532

Isophane insulin—Insulin, Isophane—**See Insulin (Systemic)**, 1713

*Isoprinosine*—Newport (U.S.) brand of Inosine Pranobex (Systemic), 3147

Isoproterenol [*Isuprel*]
  **See Bronchodilators, Adrenergic (Inhalation-Local)**, 640
  Solution, Inhalation, USP, 648

Isoproterenol-containing Combinations, 3075

Isoproterenol Hydrochloride [*Isuprel*]
  **See Sympathomimetic Agents—Cardiovascular Use (Parenteral-Systemic)**, 2669
  Injection USP, 2677

Isoproterenol Hydrochloride [*Isuprel; Isuprel Glossets*]
  **See Bronchodilators, Adrenergic (Systemic)**, 651
  Injection USP, 659
  Tablets USP, 658

Isoproterenol Hydrochloride [*Isuprel Mistometer*]
  **See Bronchodilators, Adrenergic (Inhalation-Local)**, 640
  Aerosol, Inhalation, USP, 648

Isoproterenol Sulfate [*Medihaler-Iso*]
  **See Bronchodilators, Adrenergic (Inhalation-Local)**, 640
  Aerosol, Inhalation, USP, 649

*Isoptin*—Knoll (U.S. and Canada) and Searle (Canada) brand of Verapamil—**See Calcium Channel Blocking Agents (Systemic)**, 720

*Isoptin SR*—Knoll (U.S.) and Searle (Canada) brand of Verapamil—**See Calcium Channel Blocking Agents (Systemic)**, 720, MC-32

*Isopto Alkaline*—Alcon (U.S.) brand of Hydroxypropyl Methylcellulose (Ophthalmic), #

*Isopto Atropine*—Alcon (U.S. and Canada) brand of Atropine (Ophthalmic), 485

*Isopto Carbachol*—Alcon (U.S. and Canada) brand of Carbachol (Ophthalmic), 755

*Isopto Carpine*—Alcon (U.S. and Canada) brand of Pilocarpine (Ophthalmic), #

*Isopto-Cetamide*—Alcon (U.S. and Canada) brand of Sulfacetamide—**See Sulfonamides (Ophthalmic)**, 2651

*Isopto Eserine*—Alcon (U.S.) brand of Physostigmine (Ophthalmic), #

*Isopto Frin*—Alcon (U.S.) brand of Phenylephrine (Ophthalmic), #

*Isopto Homatropine*—Alcon (U.S. and Canada) brand of Homatropine (Ophthalmic), 1651

*Isopto Hyoscine*—Alcon (U.S.) brand of Scopolamine (Ophthalmic), 2557

*Isopto Plain*—Alcon (U.S.) brand of Hydroxypropyl Methylcellulose (Ophthalmic), #

*Isopto Tears*—Alcon (U.S. and Canada) brand of Hydroxypropyl Methylcellulose (Ophthalmic), #

*Isorbid*—Bioline (U.S.) brand of Isosorbide Dinitrate—**See Nitrates (Systemic)**, 2129

*Isordil*—Wyeth-Ayerst (U.S.) and Wyeth (Canada) brand of Isosorbide Dinitrate—**See Nitrates (Systemic)**, 2129, MC-16

Isosorbide Dinitrate [*Apo-ISDN; Cedocard-SR; Coronex; Dilatrate-SR; Iso-Bid; Isonate; Isorbid; Isordil; Isotrate; Novosorbide; Sorbitrate; Sorbitrate SA*]
  **See Nitrates (Systemic)**, 2129
  Capsules, 2132
  Capsules, Extended-release, USP, 2132, MC-16
  Tablets USP, 2132, MC-16
  Tablets, Chewable, USP, 2133, MC-16
  Tablets, Extended-release, USP, 2133, MC-16
  Tablets, Sublingual, USP, 2133, MC-16

Isosorbide Mononitrate [*IMDUR; ISMO; Monoket*]
  **See Nitrates (Systemic)**, 2129
  Tablets, 2133, MC-16
  Tablets, Extended-release, 2133

*Isosource*—Sandoz (U.S.) brand of Enteral Nutrition Formula, Polymeric—**See Enteral Nutrition Formulas (Systemic)**, #

*Isosource HN*—Sandoz (U.S.) brand of Enteral Nutrition Formula, Polymeric—**See Enteral Nutrition Formulas (Systemic)**, #

*IsoSource VHN*—Sandoz (U.S.) brand of Enteral Nutrition Formula, Fiber-containing—**See Enteral Nutrition Formulas (Systemic)**, #

*Isotamine*—ICN (Canada) brand of Isoniazid (Systemic), 1789

*Isotein HN*—Sandoz (U.S.) brand of Enteral Nutrition Formula, Polymeric—**See Enteral Nutrition Formulas (Systemic)**, #

*Isotrate*—Hauck (U.S.) brand of Isosorbide Dinitrate—**See Nitrates (Systemic)**, 2129

Isotretinoin [*Accutane; Accutane Roche*]
  **(Systemic)**, 1796
  Capsules, 1800, MC-16

Isotretinoin [*Isotrex*]
  **(Topical)**, 3026
  Gel, 3026

*Isotrex*—Stiefel (Canada) brand of Isotretinoin (Topical), 3026

*Isovorin*—Lederle (U.S.) brand of L-Leucovorin (Systemic), 3150

*Isovue-128*—Bracco (U.S. and Canada) brand of Iopamidol (Systemic), #

*Isovue-200*—Bracco (U.S. and Canada) brand of Iopamidol (Systemic), #

*Isovue-250*—Bracco (U.S. and Canada) brand of Iopamidol (Systemic), #

*Isovue-300*—Bracco (U.S. and Canada) brand of Iopamidol (Systemic), #

*Isovue-370*—Bracco (U.S. and Canada) brand of Iopamidol (Systemic), #

*Isovue-M 200*—Bracco (U.S.) brand of Iopamidol (Systemic), #

*Isovue-M 300*—Bracco (U.S.) brand of Iopamidol (Systemic), #

Isoxsuprine Hydrochloride [*Vasodilan*]
  **(Systemic)**, #
  Injection USP, #
  Tablets USP, #

Isradipine [*DynaCirc*]
  **See Calcium Channel Blocking Agents (Systemic)**, 720
  Capsules, 729, MC-16

*I-Sulfacet*—Americal (U.S.) brand of Sulfacetamide—**See Sulfonamides (Ophthalmic)**, 2651

*Isuprel*—Sanofi Winthrop (U.S.) brand of Isoproterenol—**See Bronchodilators, Adrenergic (Inhalation-Local)**, 640; **Bronchodilators, Adrenergic (Systemic)**, 651; **Sympathomimetic Agents—Cardiovascular Use (Parenteral-Systemic)**, 2669

*Isuprel Glossets*—Sanofi Winthrop (U.S.) brand of Isoproterenol—**See Bronchodilators, Adrenergic (Systemic)**, 651

*Isuprel Mistometer*—Sanofi Winthrop (U.S. and Canada) brand of Isoproterenol—**See Bronchodilators, Adrenergic (Inhalation-Local)**, 640

Itraconazole [*Sporanox*]
  **See Antifungals, Azole (Systemic)**, 302
  Capsules, 308, MC-16
  Solution, Oral, 308

*I-Tropine*—Americal (U.S.) brand of Atropine (Ophthalmic), 485

*Iveegam*—Immuno (U.S. and Canada) brand of Immune Globulin Intravenous (Human) (Systemic), 1686; Immuno (U.S.) brand of Immune Globulin Intravenous (Human) (Systemic), 3025, 3147

Ivermectin [*Mectizan; Stromectol*]
  **(Systemic)**, #, 3026
  Tablets, #, 3026

IVIG—**See Immune Globulin Intravenous (Human) (Systemic)**, 1686

*I.V. Persantine*—Du Pont (U.S.) brand of Dipyridamole (Systemic), #

*IvyBlock*—EnviroDerm (U.S.) brand of Bentoquatam (Topical), 555

# J

Japanese Encephalitis Virus Vaccine Inactivated [*Je-Vax*]
  **(Systemic)**, #
  Japanese Encephalitis Virus Vaccine Inactivated (for Injection), #

*Jeanatope*—Iso-Tex Diagnostics (U.S.) brand of Iodinated I 125 Albumin—**See Radioiodinated Albumin (Systemic)**, 2453

*Jectofer*—Astra (Canada) brand of Iron Sorbitol—**See Iron Supplements (Systemic)**, 1774

*Jenamicin*—Hauck (U.S.) brand of Gentamicin—**See Aminoglycosides (Systemic)**, 69

*Jenest*—Organon (U.S.) brand of Norethindrone and Ethinyl Estradiol—**See Estrogens and Progestins—Oral Contraceptives (Systemic)**, 1397

*Je-Vax*—Connaught (U.S. and Canada) brand of Japanese Encephalitis Virus Vaccine Inactivated (Systemic), #

*Jevity*—Ross (U.S. and Canada) brand of Enteral Nutrition Formula, Fiber-containing—**See Enteral Nutrition Formulas (Systemic)**, #

*Johnson's Baby Sunblock*—J & J (U.S.) and Johnson & Johnson (Canada) brand of Octyl Methoxycinnamate, Octyl Salicylate, Oxybenzone, and Titanium Dioxide—**See Sunscreen Agents (Topical)**, #

*Johnson's Baby Sunblock Extra Protection*—J & J (U.S.) and Johnson & Johnson (Canada) brand of Octyl Methoxycinnamate, Octyl Salicylate, Oxybenzone, and Titanium Dioxide—**See Sunscreen Agents (Topical)**, #

*Johnson's No More Tears Baby Sunblock*—J & J (U.S.) and Johnson & Johnson (Canada) brand of Titanium Dioxide and Zinc Oxide—**See Sunscreen Agents (Topical)**, #

*Jopanonsyre*—DAK (Denmark) brand of Iopanoic Acid—**See Cholecystographic Agents, Oral (Systemic)**, #

*Just Tears*—Blairex (U.S.) brand of Hydroxypropyl Methylcellulose (Ophthalmic), #

# K

*K-8*—Alra (U.S.) brand of Potassium Chloride—**See Potassium Supplements (Systemic)**, 2357

*K-10*—Beecham (Canada) brand of Potassium Chloride—**See Potassium Supplements (Systemic)**, 2357

*K+ 10*—Alra (U.S.) brand of Potassium Chloride—**See Potassium Supplements (Systemic)**, 2357

*Kabikinase*—Pharmacia & Upjohn (U.S. and Canada) brand of Streptokinase—**See Thrombolytic Agents (Systemic)**, 2799

*Kabolin*—Legere (U.S.) brand of Nandrolone—**See Anabolic Steroids (Systemic)**, 110

*Kadian*—Purepac (U.S. and Canada) brand of Morphine (Systemic), 3029

*Kalium Durules*—Astra (Canada) brand of Potassium Chloride—**See Potassium Supplements (Systemic)**, 2357

*Kalmex*—Asmark—**See Salicylates (Systemic)**, 2538

Kanamycin Sulfate [*Kantrex*]
  **(Oral-Local)**, #
  Capsules USP, #

Kanamycin Sulfate [*Kantrex*]
  **See Aminoglycosides (Systemic)**, 69
  Injection USP, 76

# 3300 General Index

*Kantrex*—Bristol (U.S.) brand of Kanamycin—**See Aminoglycosides (Systemic)**, 69; Bristol (U.S.) brand of Kanamycin (Oral-Local), #
*Kaochlor-10*—Adria (Canada) brand of Potassium Chloride—**See Potassium Supplements (Systemic)**, 2357
*Kaochlor 10%*—Adria (U.S.) brand of Potassium Chloride—**See Potassium Supplements (Systemic)**, 2357
*Kaochlor-20*—Adria (Canada) brand of Potassium Chloride—**See Potassium Supplements (Systemic)**, 2357
*Kaochlor S-F 10%*—Adria (U.S.) brand of Potassium Chloride—**See Potassium Supplements (Systemic)**, 2357
*Kao Lectrolyte*—Pharmacia & Upjohn (U.S.) brand of Dextrose and Electrolytes—**See Carbohydrates and Electrolytes (Systemic)**, 769
Kaolin-containing Combinations, 3075
Kaolin and Pectin [*Donnagel-MB; Kao-Spen; Kapectolin; K-P*]
  **(Oral-Local)**, 1802
  Suspension, Oral, 1803
Kaolin, Pectin, and Belladonna Alkaloids **(Systemic)**, 1803
Kaolin, Pectin, Hyoscyamine Sulfate, Atropine Sulfate, and Scopolamine Hydrobromide [*Donnagel*]
  **See Kaolin, Pectin, and Belladonna Alkaloids (Systemic)**, 1803
  Suspension, Oral, 1804
Kaolin, Pectin, and Paregoric [*Donnagel-PG*]
  **(Systemic)**, 1804
  Suspension, Oral, 1804
*Kaon*—Adria (U.S. and Canada) brand of Potassium Gluconate—**See Potassium Supplements (Systemic)**, 2357
*Kaon-Cl*—Adria (U.S.) brand of Potassium Chloride—**See Potassium Supplements (Systemic)**, 2357
*Kaon-Cl-10*—Adria (U.S.) brand of Potassium Chloride—**See Potassium Supplements (Systemic)**, 2357
*Kaon-Cl 20% Liquid*—Adria (U.S.) brand of Potassium Chloride—**See Potassium Supplements (Systemic)**, 2357
*Kaopectate*—Upjohn (U.S. and Canada) brand of Attapulgite (Oral-Local), #
*Kaopectate Advanced Formula*—Upjohn (U.S.) brand of Attapulgite (Oral-Local), #
*Kaopectate II*—Upjohn (U.S.) brand of Loperamide (Oral-Local), 1877
*Kaopectate Maximum Strength*—Upjohn (U.S.) brand of Attapulgite (Oral-Local), #
*Kaopek*—Barre-National (U.S.) brand of Attapulgite (Oral-Local), #
*Kao-Spen*—Century (U.S.) brand of Kaolin and Pectin (Oral-Local), 1802
*Kapectolin*—Goldline (U.S.) brand of Kaolin and Pectin (Oral-Local), 1802
*Karacil*—ICN (Canada) brand of Psyllium Hydrophilic Mucilloid—**See Laxatives (Local)**, #
*Karidium*—Lorvic (U.S.) and Professional (Canada) brand of Sodium Fluoride (Systemic), 2592
*Kasof*—Roberts (U.S.) brand of Docusate—**See Laxatives (Local)**, #
*Kato*—ICN (U.S.) brand of Potassium Chloride—**See Potassium Supplements (Systemic)**, 2357
*Kay Ciel*—Forest (U.S.) brand of Potassium Chloride—**See Potassium Supplements (Systemic)**, 2357
*Kayexalate*—Sanofi Winthrop (U.S. and Canada) brand of Sodium Polystyrene Sulfonate (Local), 2618
*Kaylixir*—Lannett (U.S.) brand of Potassium Gluconate—**See Potassium Supplements (Systemic)**, 2357
*K+ Care*—Alra (U.S.) brand of Potassium Chloride—**See Potassium Supplements (Systemic)**, 2357
*K+ Care ET*—Alra (U.S.) brand of Potassium Bicarbonate—**See Potassium Supplements (Systemic)**, 2357
*KCL 5%*—Rougier (Canada) brand of Potassium Chloride—**See Potassium Supplements (Systemic)**, 2357
*K-Dur*—Key (U.S. and Canada) brand of Potassium Chloride—**See Potassium Supplements (Systemic)**, 2357, MC-25
*Keep Alert*—Reese Chemical (U.S.) brand of Caffeine (Systemic), 706
*Keflex*—Dista (U.S. and Canada) brand of Cephalexin—**See Cephalosporins (Systemic)**, 794

*Keflin*—Lilly (U.S. and Canada) brand of Cephalothin—**See Cephalosporins (Systemic)**, 794
*Keftab*—Dista (U.S.) brand of Cephalexin—**See Cephalosporins (Systemic)**, 794
*Kefurox*—Lilly (U.S. and Canada) brand of Cefuroxime—**See Cephalosporins (Systemic)**, 794
*Kefzol*—Lilly (U.S. and Canada) brand of Cefazolin—**See Cephalosporins (Systemic)**, 794
*K-Electrolyte*—Copley (U.S.) brand of Potassium Bicarbonate—**See Potassium Supplements (Systemic)**, 2357
*Kellogg's Castor Oil*—Beecham (U.S.) brand of Castor Oil—**See Laxatives (Local)**, #
*Kemadrin*—BW (U.S. and Canada) brand of Procyclidine—**See Antidyskinetics (Systemic)**, 297
*Kemsol*—Horner (Canada) brand of Dimethyl Sulfoxide (Topical), 3017
*Kenac*—NMC (U.S.) brand of Triamcinolone—**See Corticosteroids (Topical)**, 978
*Kenacort*—Squibb (U.S. and Canada) brand of Triamcinolone—**See Corticosteroids—Glucocorticoid Effects (Systemic)**, 998
*Kenacort Diacetate*—Squibb (U.S. and Canada) brand of Triamcinolone—**See Corticosteroids—Glucocorticoid Effects (Systemic)**, 998
*Kenaject-40*—Mayrand (U.S.) brand of Triamcinolone—**See Corticosteroids—Glucocorticoid Effects (Systemic)**, 998
*Kenalog*—Squibb (U.S. and Canada) brand of Triamcinolone—**See Corticosteroids (Topical)**, 978
*Kenalog-10*—Squibb (U.S. and Canada) brand of Triamcinolone—**See Corticosteroids—Glucocorticoid Effects (Systemic)**, 998
*Kenalog-40*—Squibb (U.S. and Canada) brand of Triamcinolone—**See Corticosteroids—Glucocorticoid Effects (Systemic)**, 998
*Kenalog-H*—Squibb (U.S.) brand of Triamcinolone—**See Corticosteroids (Topical)**, 978
*Kenalog in Orabase*—Squibb (U.S. and Canada) brand of Triamcinolone—**See Corticosteroids (Topical)**, 978
*Kendral-Ipratropium*—Kendral (Canada) brand of Ipratropium (Inhalation-Local), 1761
*Kenonel*—Marnel (U.S.) brand of Triamcinolone—**See Corticosteroids (Topical)**, 978
*Keoxifene hydrochloride*—See Raloxifene (Systemic), 2455
*Keralyt*—Westwood (U.S.) brand of Salicylic Acid (Topical), #
*Keratex Gel*—Syosset (U.S.) brand of Salicylic Acid (Topical), #
*Kerlone*—Searle (U.S.) brand of Betaxolol—**See Beta-adrenergic Blocking Agents (Systemic)**, 593, MC-4
*Kestrone-5*—Hyrex (U.S.) brand of Estrone—**See Estrogens (Systemic)**, 1383
*Ketalar*—PD (U.S. and Canada) brand of Ketamine (Systemic), 1805
Ketamine Hydrochloride [*Ketalar*]
  **(Systemic)**, 1805
  Injection USP, 1806
Ketazolam
  **See Benzodiazepines (Systemic)**, 556
  Capsules, 573
Ketoconazole [*Nizoral*]
  **See Antifungals, Azole (Systemic)**, 302
  Suspension, Oral, 309
  Tablets USP, 309, MC-16
Ketoconazole [*Nizoral; Nizoral Cream; Nizoral Shampoo*]
  **(Topical)**, 1807, 3026
  Cream, 1808
  Shampoo, 1809, 3026
*Keto-diastix*—Miles (U.S. and Canada) brand of Urine Glucose and Ketone (Combined) Test—**See Urine Glucose and Ketone Test Kits for Home Use**, #
Ketoprofen [*Actron; Apo-Keto; Apo-Keto-E; Novo-Keto-EC; Orudis; Orudis-E; Orudis KT; Orudis-SR; Oruvail; Rhodis; Rhodis-EC*]
  **See Anti-inflammatory Drugs, Nonsteroidal (Systemic)**, 388
  Capsules, 411 MC-16
  Capsules, Extended-release, 411 MC-16
  Suppositories, 411
  Tablets, 411
  Tablets, Delayed-release, 411
  Tablets, Extended-release, 411
Ketorolac Tromethamine [*Acular*]
  **(Ophthalmic)**, 1809, 3026
  Solution, Ophthalmic, 1810, 3026

Ketorolac Tromethamine [*Toradol*]
  **(Systemic)**, 1810
  Injection USP, 1816
  Tablets USP, 1816, MC-16
*KetoStix*—Miles (U.S. and Canada) brand of Nitroprusside Urine Ketone Test—**See Urine Glucose and Ketone Test Kits for Home Use**, #
Ketotifen Fumarate [*Zaditen*]
  **(Systemic)**, 3026
  Syrup, 3026
  Tablets, 3026
*K-Exit*—Luvabec (Canada) brand of Sodium Polystyrene Sulfonate (Local), 2618
*Key-Pred 25*—Hyrex (U.S.) brand of Prednisolone—**See Corticosteroids—Glucocorticoid Effects (Systemic)**, 998
*Key-Pred 50*—Hyrex (U.S.) brand of Prednisolone—**See Corticosteroids—Glucocorticoid Effects (Systemic)**, 998
*Key-Pred SP*—Hyrex (U.S.) brand of Prednisolone—**See Corticosteroids—Glucocorticoid Effects (Systemic)**, 998
*K-G Elixir*—Geneva Generics (U.S.) brand of Potassium Gluconate—**See Potassium Supplements (Systemic)**, 2357
*KI*—See Potassium Iodide (Systemic), 2354
*Kiddy Koff*—Republic (U.S.) brand of Phenylpropanolamine, Dextromethorphan, and Guaifenesin—**See Cough/Cold Combinations (Systemic)**, 1024
*K-Ide*—Interstate (U.S.) brand of Potassium Bicarbonate—**See Potassium Supplements (Systemic)**, 2357; Potassium Chloride—**See Potassium Supplements (Systemic)**, 2357
*Kidrolase*—Rhône-Poulenc (Canada) brand of Asparaginase (Systemic), 474
*KIE*—Laser (U.S.) brand of Ephedrine and Potassium Iodide—**See Cough/Cold Combinations (Systemic)**, 1024
*Kildane*—Major (U.S.) brand of Lindane (Topical), 1866
*Kimono*—Mayer (U.S.) brand of Latex Condoms—**See Condoms**, #
*Kimono Microthins*—Mayer (U.S.) brand of Latex Condoms—**See Condoms**, #
*Kimono Microthins Plus*—Mayer (U.S.) brand of Latex Condoms and Nonoxynol 9—**See Condoms**, #
*Kimono Plus*—Mayer (U.S.) brand of Latex Condoms and Nonoxynol 9—**See Condoms**, #
*Kimono Sensation*—Mayer (U.S.) brand of Latex Condoms—**See Condoms**, #
*Kimono Sensation Plus*—Mayer (U.S.) brand of Latex Condoms and Nonoxynol 9—**See Condoms**, #
*Kindercal*—Bristol-Myers Squibb (U.S.) brand of Enteral Nutrition Formula, Fiber-containing—**See Enteral Nutrition Formulas (Systemic)**, #
*Kinesed*—Stuart (U.S.) brand of Atropine, Hyoscyamine, Scopolamine, and Phenobarbital—**See Belladonna Alkaloids and Barbiturates (Systemic)**, 551
*Kinevac*—Squibb Diagnostics (U.S. and Canada) brand of Sincalide (Systemic), #
*Kionex*—Paddock (U.S.) brand of Sodium Polystyrene Sulfonate (Local), 2618
*Klavikordal*—U.S. Ethicals (U.S.) brand of Nitroglycerin—**See Nitrates (Systemic)**, 2129
*Klean-Prep*—Richmond (Canada) brand of Polyethylene Glycol 3350 and Electrolytes (Local), 2349
*K-Lease*—Adria (U.S.) brand of Potassium Chloride—**See Potassium Supplements (Systemic)**, 2357
*Klerist-D*—Nutripharm (U.S.) brand of Chlorpheniramine and Pseudoephedrine—**See Antihistamines and Decongestants (Systemic)**, 343
*Kling-Tite Naturalamb*—Carter-Wallace (U.S. and Canada) brand of Lamb Cecum Condoms—**See Condoms**, #
*Kling-Tite Naturalamb with Spermicide Lubricant*—Carter-Wallace (U.S.) brand of Lamb Cecum Condoms and Nonoxynol 9—**See Condoms**, #
*K-Long*—Adria (Canada) brand of Potassium Chloride—**See Potassium Supplements (Systemic)**, 2357
*Klonopin*—Hoffmann-LaRoche (U.S.) brand of Clonazepam (Systemic), 3137; Roche (U.S.) brand of Clonazepam—**See Benzodiazepines (Systemic)**, 556, MC-7
*K-Lor*—Abbott (U.S. and Canada) brand of Potassium Chloride—**See Potassium Supplements (Systemic)**, 2357

*Klor-Con 8*—Upsher-Smith (U.S.) brand of Potassium Chloride—**See Potassium Supplements (Systemic)**, 2357, MC-25
*Klor-Con 10*—Upsher-Smith (U.S.) brand of Potassium Chloride—**See Potassium Supplements (Systemic)**, 2357, MC-25
*Klor-Con/EF*—Upsher-Smith (U.S.) brand of Potassium Bicarbonate—**See Potassium Supplements (Systemic)**, 2357
*Klor-Con Powder*—Upsher-Smith (U.S.) brand of Potassium Chloride—**See Potassium Supplements (Systemic)**, 2357
*Klor-Con/25 Powder*—Upsher-Smith (U.S.) brand of Potassium Chloride—**See Potassium Supplements (Systemic)**, 2357
*Klorvess*—Sandoz (U.S.) brand of Potassium Bicarbonate and Potassium Chloride—**See Potassium Supplements (Systemic)**, 2357
*Klorvess Effervescent Granules*—Sandoz (U.S.) brand of Potassium Bicarbonate and Potassium Chloride—**See Potassium Supplements (Systemic)**, 2357
*Klorvess 10% Liquid*—Sandoz (U.S.) brand of Potassium Chloride—**See Potassium Supplements (Systemic)**, 2357
*Klotrix*—Apothecon (U.S.) brand of Potassium Chloride—**See Potassium Supplements (Systemic)**, 2357, MC-25
KL4-Surfactant
  **(Intratracheal-Local)**, 3150
*K-Lyte*—Bristol (U.S. and Canada) brand of Potassium Bicarbonate—**See Potassium Supplements (Systemic)**, 2357
*K-Lyte/Cl*—Bristol (U.S.) brand of Potassium Bicarbonate and Potassium Chloride—**See Potassium Supplements (Systemic)**, 2357; Bristol (Canada) brand of Potassium Chloride—**See Potassium Supplements (Systemic)**, 2357
*K-Lyte/Cl 50*—Bristol (U.S.) brand of Potassium Bicarbonate and Potassium Chloride—**See Potassium Supplements (Systemic)**, 2357
*K-Lyte/Cl Powder*—Bristol (U.S.) brand of Potassium Chloride—**See Potassium Supplements (Systemic)**, 2357
*K-Lyte DS*—Bristol (U.S.) brand of Potassium Bicarbonate and Potassium Citrate—**See Potassium Supplements (Systemic)**, 2357
*K-Med 900*—Riva (Canada) brand of Potassium Chloride—**See Potassium Supplements (Systemic)**, 2357
*K-Norm*—Pennwalt (U.S.) brand of Potassium Chloride—**See Potassium Supplements (Systemic)**, 2357
*Koate-HP*—Cutter (U.S. and Canada) brand of Antihemophilic Factor (Systemic), 319
*Koffex*—Rougier (Canada) brand of Dextromethorphan (Systemic), 1191
*Kogenate*—Miles (U.S. and Canada) brand of Antihemophilic Factor (Systemic), 319; Miles (U.S.) brand of Antihemophilic Factor (Recombinant) (Systemic), 3131
*Kolephrin Caplets*—Pfeiffer (U.S.) brand of Chlorpheniramine, Pseudoephedrine, and Acetaminophen—**See Antihistamines, Decongestants, and Analgesics (Systemic)**, 366
*Kolephrin/DM Cough and Cold Medication*—Pfeiffer (U.S.) brand of Chlorpheniramine, Pseudoephedrine, Dextromethorphan, and Acetaminophen—**See Cough/Cold Combinations (Systemic)**, 1024
*Kolephrin GG/DM*—Pfeiffer (U.S.) brand of Dextromethorphan and Guaifenesin—**See Cough/Cold Combinations (Systemic)**, 1024
*Kolyum*—Pennwalt (U.S.) brand of Potassium Gluconate and Potassium Chloride—**See Potassium Supplements (Systemic)**, 2357
*Konakion*—Roche (U.S.) brand of Phytonadione—**See Vitamin K (Systemic)**, 2975
*Kondremul*—Cowling & Braithwaite (Canada) brand of Mineral Oil—**See Laxatives (Local)**, #
*Kondremul Plain*—Ciba Consumer (U.S.) brand of Mineral Oil—**See Laxatives (Local)**, #
*Konsyl*—Konsyl (U.S.) brand of Polycarbophil—**See Laxatives (Local)**, #; Konsyl (U.S.) brand of Psyllium—**See Laxatives (Local)**, #
*Konsyl-D*—Konsyl (U.S.) brand of Psyllium Hydrophilic Mucilloid—**See Laxatives (Local)**, #
*Konsyl-Orange*—Konsyl (U.S.) brand of Psyllium Hydrophilic Mucilloid—**See Laxatives (Local)**, #
*Konsyl-Orange Sugar Free*—Konsyl (U.S.) brand of Psyllium Hydrophilic Mucilloid—**See Laxatives (Local)**, #

*Konyne 80*—Cutter (U.S.) brand of Factor IX (Systemic), 1430
*Kophane Cough and Cold Formula*—Pfeiffer (U.S.) brand of Chlorpheniramine, Phenylpropanolamine, and Dextromethorphan—**See Cough/Cold Combinations (Systemic)**, 1024
*Koromex Cream*—Schmid (U.S.) brand of Octoxynol 9—**See Spermicides (Vaginal)**, #
*Koromex Crystal Clear Gel*—Schmid (U.S.) brand of Nonoxynol 9—**See Spermicides (Vaginal)**, #
*Koromex Foam*—Schmid (U.S.) brand of Nonoxynol 9—**See Spermicides (Vaginal)**, #
*Koromex Jelly*—Schmid (U.S.) brand of Nonoxynol 9—**See Spermicides (Vaginal)**, #
*K-P*—Century (U.S.) brand of Kaolin and Pectin (Oral-Local), 1802
KPAB—See Aminobenzoate Potassium (Systemic), #
*K-Pek*—Rugby (U.S.) brand of Attapulgite (Oral-Local), #
*K-Phos M. F.*—Beach (U.S.) brand of Potassium and Sodium Phosphates—**See Phosphates (Systemic)**, 2317
*K-Phos Neutral*—Beach (U.S.) brand of Potassium and Sodium Phosphates—**See Phosphates (Systemic)**, 2317
*K-Phos No. 2*—Beach (U.S.) brand of Potassium and Sodium Phosphates—**See Phosphates (Systemic)**, 2317
*K-Phos Original*—Beach (U.S.) brand of Potassium Phosphates—**See Phosphates (Systemic)**, 2317
*Kronofed-A Jr. Kronocaps*—Ferndale (U.S.) brand of Chlorpheniramine and Pseudoephedrine—**See Antihistamines and Decongestants (Systemic)**, 343
*Kronofed-A Kronocaps*—Ferndale (U.S.) brand of Chlorpheniramine and Pseudoephedrine—**See Antihistamines and Decongestants (Systemic)**, 343
Krypton Kr 81m [*Krypton Kr 81m Gas Generator*]
  **(Systemic)**, 1816
  Krypton Kr 81m USP, 1817
*Krypton Kr 81m Gas Generator*—Amersham (U.S. and Canada) brand of Krypton Kr 81m (Systemic), 1816
*K-Sol*—Major (U.S.) brand of Potassium Chloride—**See Potassium Supplements (Systemic)**, 2357
*K-Tab*—Abbott (U.S.) brand of Potassium Chloride—**See Potassium Supplements (Systemic)**, 2357, MC-25
*Kudrox Double Strength*—Schwarz (U.S.) brand of Alumina, Magnesia, and Simethicone—**See Antacids (Oral-Local)**, 188
*Ku-Zyme HP*—Kremers-Urban (U.S.) brand of Pancrelipase (Systemic), 2222
*K-Vescent*—Major (U.S.) brand of Potassium Bicarbonate—**See Potassium Supplements (Systemic)**, 2357
*Kwelcof Liquid*—Ascher (U.S.) brand of Hydrocodone and Guaifenesin—**See Cough/Cold Combinations (Systemic)**, 1024
*Kwell*—Reed & Carnrick (U.S.) brand of Lindane (Topical), 1866
*Kwellada*—Reed & Carnrick (Canada) brand of Lindane (Topical), 1866
*Kwildane*—Major (U.S.) brand of Lindane (Topical), 1866
*Kybernin*—Behringwerke (U.S.) brand of Antithrombin III (Systemic), 3131
*Kytril*—SmithKline Beecham (U.S. and Canada) brand of Granisetron (Systemic), 1578, MC-14

## L

*LA-12*—Hyrex (U.S.) brand of Hydroxocobalamin—**See Vitamin B$_{12}$ (Systemic)**, 2962
LAAM—See Levomethadyl (Systemic), 1855
Labetalol Hydrochloride [*Normodyne*; *Trandate*]
  **See Beta-adrenergic Blocking Agents (Systemic)**, 593
  Injection USP, 603
  Tablets USP, 603, MC-16
*Lacril*—Allergan (U.S.) brand of Hydroxypropyl Methylcellulose (Ophthalmic), #
*Lacrisert*—Merck (U.S. and Canada) brand of Hydroxypropyl Cellulose (Ophthalmic), #
*LactiCare-HC*—Stiefel (U.S.) brand of Hydrocortisone—**See Corticosteroids (Topical)**, 978
*Lactisol*—C & M (U.S.) brand of Salicylic Acid (Topical), #

*Lactobin*—Roxane (U.S.) brand of Lactobin (Systemic), 3151
Lactobin [*Lactobin*]
  **(Systemic)**, 3150
*Lactofree*—Mead Johnson (U.S.) brand of Infant Formulas, Milk-based—**See Infant Formulas (Systemic)**, #
*Lactulax*—Rougier (Canada) brand of Lactulose—**See Laxatives (Local)**, #
Lactulose [*Acilac*; *Cholac*; *Chronulac*; *Constilac*; *Constulose*; *Duphalac*; *Enulose*; *Evalose*; *Heptalac*; *Lactulax*; *Laxilose*; *PMS-Lactulose*; *Portalac*]
  **See Laxatives (Local)**, #
  Solution USP
*Lagol*—Alvin Last (U.S.) brand of Benzocaine—**See Anesthetics (Topical)**, 155
LAM—See Levomethadyl (Systemic), 1855
*Lamictal*—Glaxo Wellcome (U.S.) brand of Lamotrigine (Systemic), 3151, MC-16
*Lamisil*—Novartis (U.S.) and Sandoz (Canada) brand of Terbinafine (Systemic), 2752, 3036, MC-29; Terbinafine (Topical), 2755, 3036
Lamivudine [*Epivir*]
  **(Systemic)**, 1819
  Solution, Oral, 1821
  Tablets, 1821, MC-16
Lamivudine and Zidovudine [*Combivir*]
  **(Systemic)**, 1822
  Tablets, 1824, MC-16
Lamotrigine [*Lamictal*]
  **(Systemic)**, 1824, 3151
  Tablets, 1827, MC-16
*Lampit*—Bayer (German) brand of Nifurtimox (Systemic), #
*Lamprene*—Ciba-Geigy (U.S.) brand of Clofazimine (Systemic), #, 3137
*Lanacort*—Combe (U.S.) brand of Hydrocortisone—**See Corticosteroids (Topical)**, 978
*Lanacort 10*—Combe (U.S.) brand of Hydrocortisone—**See Corticosteroids (Topical)**, 978, 3023
*Lanatuss Expectorant*—Lannett (U.S.) brand of Chlorpheniramine, Phenylpropanolamine, Guaifenesin, Sodium Citrate, and Citric Acid—**See Cough/Cold Combinations (Systemic)**, 1024
*Laniazid*—Lannett (U.S.) brand of Isoniazid (Systemic), 1789
*Laniroif*—Truxton (U.S.) brand of Butalbital, Aspirin, and Caffeine—**See Barbiturates and Analgesics (Systemic)**, 532
*Lanophyllin*—Lannett (U.S.) brand of Theophylline—**See Bronchodilators, Theophylline (Systemic)**, 668
*Lanorinal*—Lannett (U.S.) and Texas Drug Reps (U.S.) brand of Butalbital, Aspirin, and Caffeine—**See Barbiturates and Analgesics (Systemic)**, 532
*Lanoxicaps*—Glaxo Wellcome (U.S.) brand of Digoxin—**See Digitalis Glycosides (Systemic)**, 1213, MC-9
*Lanoxin*—Glaxo Wellcome (U.S. and Canada) brand of Digoxin—**See Digitalis Glycosides (Systemic)**, 1213, MC-9
Lansoprazole [*Prevacid*]
  **(Systemic)**, 1828
  Capsules, Delayed-release, 1830, MC-16
*Lansoÿl*—Jouveinal (Canada) brand of Mineral Oil—**See Laxatives (Local)**, #
*Lansoÿl Sugar Free*—Jouveinal (Canada) brand of Mineral Oil—**See Laxatives (Local)**, #
*Lanvis*—Glaxo Wellcome (Canada) brand of Thioguanine (Systemic), #
*Largactil*—Rhône-Poulenc (Canada) brand of Chlorpromazine—**See Phenothiazines (Systemic)**, 2289
*Largactil Liquid*—Rhône-Poulenc (Canada) brand of Chlorpromazine—**See Phenothiazines (Systemic)**, 2289
*Largactil Oral Drops*—Rhône-Poulenc (Canada) brand of Chlorpromazine—**See Phenothiazines (Systemic)**, 2289
*Largon*—Wyeth-Ayerst (U.S.) brand of Propiomazine (Systemic), #
*Lariam*—Hoffmann-LaRoche (U.S.) brand of Mefloquine (Systemic), 1935, 3153, MC-18
*Larodopa*—Roche (U.S. and Canada) brand of Levodopa (Systemic), 1848
*Lasix*—Hoechst Marion Roussel (U.S.) and Hoechst (Canada) brand of Furosemide—**See Diuretics, Loop (Systemic)**, 1259, MC-13
*Lasix Special*—Hoechst (Canada) brand of Furosemide—**See Diuretics, Loop (Systemic)**, 1259

Latanoprost [*Xalatan*]
**(Ophthalmic),** 1831, 3026
Solution, Ophthalmic, 1833, 3026
Laudanum—Opium Tincture—**See Opioid (Narcotic) Analgesics (Systemic),** 2168
*Lavatar*—Doak (U.S.) and T.C.D. (Canada) brand of Coal Tar (Topical), #
Laxatives
**(Local),** #
*Laxavite*—Neosol (Canada) brand of Cascara Sagrada and Phenolphthalein—**See Laxatives (Local),** #
*Laxilose*—Technilab (Canada) brand of Lactulose—**See Laxatives (Local),** #
*Laxinate 100*—Roberts (U.S.) brand of Docusate—**See Laxatives (Local),** #
*Laxit*—ICN (Canada) brand of Bisacodyl—**See Laxatives (Local),** #
*Lax-Pills*—G & W (U.S.) brand of Phenolphthalein—**See Laxatives (Local),** #
*LazerSporin-C*—Pedinol (U.S.) brand of Neomycin, Polymyxin B, and Hydrocortisone (Otic), #
L-Baclofen [*Neuralgon*]
**(Systemic),** 3150
*L-Caine*—Century (U.S.) brand of Lidocaine—**See Anesthetics (Parenteral-Local),** 139
L-Carnitine—*See* Levocarnitine (Systemic), 1847
L-Cycloserine
**(Systemic),** 3150
L-Cysteine
**(Systemic),** 3150
*Lectopam*—Roche (Canada) brand of Bromazepam—**See Benzodiazepines (Systemic),** 556
*Ledercillin VK*—Lederle (U.S. and Canada) brand of Penicillin V—**See Penicillins (Systemic),** 2240, MC-24
Leflunomide
**(Systemic),** 3151
*Legalon*—Pharmaquest (U.S.) brand of Disodium Silibinin Dihemisuccinate (systemic), 3141
*Lemoderm*—Seneca (U.S.) brand of Hydrocortisone—**See Corticosteroids (Topical),** 978
*Lenoltec with Codeine No.1*—Technilab (Canada) brand of Acetaminophen and Codeine—**See Opioid (Narcotic) Analgesics and Acetaminophen (Systemic),** 2198
*Lenoltec with Codeine No.2*—Technilab (Canada) brand of Acetaminophen and Codeine—**See Opioid (Narcotic) Analgesics and Acetaminophen (Systemic),** 2198
*Lenoltec with Codeine No.3*—Technilab (Canada) brand of Acetaminophen and Codeine—**See Opioid (Narcotic) Analgesics and Acetaminophen (Systemic),** 2198
*Lenoltec with Codeine No.4*—Technilab (Canada) brand of Acetaminophen and Codeine—**See Opioid (Narcotic) Analgesics and Acetaminophen (Systemic),** 2198
*Lente Iletin*—Lilly (Canada) brand of Insulin Zinc—**See Insulin (Systemic),** 1713
*Lente Iletin I*—Lilly (U.S.) brand of Insulin Zinc—**See Insulin (Systemic),** 1713
*Lente Iletin II*—Lilly (U.S. and Canada) brand of Insulin Zinc—**See Insulin (Systemic),** 1713
*Lente Insulin*—Connaught Novo Nordisk (Canada) brand of Insulin Zinc—**See Insulin (Systemic),** 1713
Lente insulin—Insulin Zinc—**See Insulin (Systemic),** 1713
*Lente L*—Novo Nordisk (U.S.) brand of Insulin Zinc—**See Insulin (Systemic),** 1713
Lepirudin [*Refludan*]
**(Systemic),** 1833, 3150
for Injection, 1835
*Leponex*—Sandoz (Denmark, South Africa, and Spain) and Wander (Switzerland) brand of Clozapine (Systemic), 919
*Leritine*—Frosst (Canada) brand of Anileridine (Systemic), 3011
*Lescol*—Novartis (U.S.) brand of Fluvastatin—**See HMG-CoA Reductase Inhibitors (Systemic),** 1647, MC-13
Letrozole [*Femara*]
**(Systemic),** 1836
Tablets, 1837
Leucovorin [*Leucovorin Calcium*]
**(Systemic),** 3150
Leucovorin Calcium—Immunex (U.S.) brand of Leucovorin (Systemic), 3150

Leucovorin Calcium [citrovorum factor; folinic acid; *Wellcovorin*]
**(Systemic),** 1837, 3150
Injection USP, 1839
for Injection, 1840
Tablets USP, 1839, MC-17
*Leukeran*—Glaxo Wellcome (U.S. and Canada) brand of Chlorambucil (Systemic), 837, MC-6
*Leukine*—Immunex (U.S.) brand of Sargramostim—**See Colony Stimulating Factors (Systemic),** 941, 3163
Leupeptin
**(Systemic),** 3150
Leuprolide Acetate [leuprorelin; *Lupron; Lupron Depot; Lupron Depot 4-Month 30 mg; Lupron Depot-3 Month 11.25 mg; Lupron Depot 3-Month 22.5 mg; Lupron Depot-Ped; Lupron Injection; Lupron-3 Month SR Depot 22.5 mg*]
**(Systemic),** 1840, 3150
Injection, 1844
for Injection, 1844
Leuprorelin—*See* Leuprolide (Systemic), 1840
*Leustatin*—Ortho Biotech (U.S. and Canada) brand of Cladribine (Systemic; 886; R. W. Johnson (U.S.) brand of Cladribine (Systemic), 3137
*Leustatin Injection*—R. W. Johnson (U.S.) brand of Cladribine (Systemic), 3137
Levacetylmethadol—*See* Levomethadyl (Systemic), 1855
Levamisole Hydrochloride [*Ergamisol*]
**(Systemic),** 1844
Tablets, 1846
*Levaquin*—Ortho (U.S.) brand of Levofloxacin (Systemic), 1852, MC-17
Levarterenol—Norepinephrine—**See Sympathomimetic Agents—Cardiovascular Use (Parenteral-Systemic),** 2669
*Levate*—ICN (Canada) brand of Amitriptyline—**See Antidepressants, Tricyclic (Systemic),** 271
*Levatol*—Schwarz (U.S.) brand of Penbutolol—**See Beta-adrenergic Blocking Agents (Systemic),** 593, MC-24
*Levbid*—Schwarz (U.S.) brand of Hyoscyamine (Systemic), MC-15
*Levlen*—Berlex (U.S.) brand of Levonorgestrel and Ethinyl Estradiol—**See Estrogens and Progestins—Oral Contraceptives (Systemic),** 1397, MC-17
*Levlite*—Berlex (U.S.) brand of Levonorgestrel and Ethinyl Estradiol (Systemic), 3027
Levo-alpha-acetylmethadol—*See* Levomethadyl (Systemic), 1855
Levobunolol Hydrochloride [*AKBeta; Betagan C Cap B.I.D.; Betagan C Cap Q.D.; Betagan Standard Cap*]
**See Beta-adrenergic Blocking Agents (Ophthalmic),** 585, 3027
Solution, Ophthalmic, USP, 591, 3027
Levocabastine [*Livostin*]
**(Nasal),** 3027
Suspension, Nasal, 3027
Levocabastine Hydrochloride [*Livostin*]
**(Ophthalmic),** #, 3027
Suspension, Ophthalmic, #, 3027
Levocarnitine [*Carnitor*; L-Carnitine; *VitaCarn*]
**(Systemic),** 1847, 3150, 3151
Injection, 1848
Solution, Oral, USP, 1848
Tablets USP, 1848
Levodopa [*Dopar; Larodopa*]
**(Systemic),** 1848
Capsules USP, 1852
Tablets USP, 1852
Levodopa and Benserazide [*Prolopa*]
**(Systemic),** 3027
Capsules, 3027
Levodopa-containing Combinations, 3075
*Levo-Dromoran*—Roche (U.S. and Canada) brand of Levorphanol—**See Opioid (Narcotic) Analgesics (Systemic),** 2168
Levofloxacin [*Levaquin*]
**(Systemic),** 1852
Concentrate for Injection, 1855
Injection, 1855
Tablets, 1854, MC-17
Levomepromazine—Methotrimeprazine—**See Phenothiazines (Systemic),** 2289
Levomethadyl acetate—*See* Levomethadyl (Systemic), 1855

Levomethadyl Acetate Hydrochloride [LAAM; LAM; levacetylmethadol; levo-alpha-acetylmethadol; levomethadyl acetate; MK790; *Orlaam*]
**(Systemic),** 1855, 3151
Solution, Oral, 1860
Levonordefrin-containing Combinations, 3075
Levonorgestrel [*NORPLANT System*]
**See Progestins (Systemic),** 2400
Implants, 2408
Levonorgestrel and Ethinyl Estradiol [*Alesse; Levlen; Levlite; Levora 0.15/30; Min-Ovral; Nordette; Tri-Levlen; Triphasil; Triquilar*]
**See Estrogens and Progestins—Oral Contraceptives (Systemic),** 1397, 3027
Tablets, 3027
Tablets USP, 1408, MC-17
*Levophed*—Sanofi Winthrop (U.S. and Canada) brand of Norepinephrine—**See Sympathomimetic Agents—Cardiovascular Use (Parenteral-Systemic),** 2669
*Levoprome*—Lederle (U.S.) brand of Methotrimeprazine—**See Phenothiazines (Systemic),** 2289
*Levora 0.15/30*—Searle (U.S.) brand of Levonorgestrel and Ethinyl Estradiol—**See Estrogens and Progestins—Oral Contraceptives (Systemic),** 1397
Levorphan—Levorphanol—**See Opioid (Narcotic) Analgesics (Systemic),** 2168
Levorphanol Tartrate [*Levo-Dromoran*; levorphan]
**See Opioid (Narcotic) Analgesics (Systemic),** 2168
Injection USP, 2178
Tablets USP, 2178
*Levo-T*—Lederle (U.S.) brand of Levothyroxine—**See Thyroid Hormones (Systemic),** 2809
*Levothroid*—Armour (U.S.) brand of Levothyroxine—**See Thyroid Hormones (Systemic),** 2809
Levothyroxine Sodium [*Eltroxin; Levo-T; Levothroid; Levoxyl*; L-thyroxine; *PMS-Levothyroxine Sodium; Synthroid*]
**See Thyroid Hormones (Systemic),** 2809
Injection, 2813
for Injection, 2813
Tablets USP, 2812, MC-17
*Levoxyl*—Jones Medical (U.S.) brand of Levothyroxine—**See Thyroid Hormones (Systemic),** 2809, MC-17
*Levsin*—Kremers-Urban (U.S. and Canada) brand of Hyoscyamine—**See Anticholinergics/Antispasmodics (Systemic),** 226
*Levsinex Timecaps*—Kremers-Urban (U.S.) brand of Hyoscyamine—**See Anticholinergics/Antispasmodics (Systemic),** 226
*Levsin-PB*—Kremers-Urban (U.S.) brand of Hyoscyamine and Phenobarbital—**See Belladonna Alkaloids and Barbiturates (Systemic),** 551
*Levsin with Phenobarbital*—Kremers-Urban (U.S.) brand of Hyoscyamine and Phenobarbital—**See Belladonna Alkaloids and Barbiturates (Systemic),** 551
*Levsin/SL*—Kremers-Urban (U.S.) brand of Hyoscyamine—**See Anticholinergics/Antispasmodics (Systemic),** 226, MC-15
*Lexxel*—Astra Merck (U.S.) brand of Enalapril and Felodipine (Systemic), 1339, MC-11
L-Glutathione, Reduced [*Cachexon*]
**(Systemic),** 3162
LH/FSH–RH—*See* Gonadorelin (Systemic), 1571
LHRH—*See* Gonadorelin (Systemic), 1571
L-5 Hydroxytryptophan
**(Systemic),** 3150
*Librax*—Roche (U.S. and Canada) brand of Chlordiazepoxide and Clidinium (Systemic), 846, MC-6
*Librium*—Roche (U.S. and Canada) brand of Chlordiazepoxide—**See Benzodiazepines (Systemic),** 556
*Licetrol*—Republic (U.S.) brand of Pyrethrins and Piperonyl Butoxide (Topical), #
*Licon*—Major (U.S.) brand of Fluocinonide—**See Corticosteroids (Topical),** 978
*Lidemol*—Syntex (Canada) brand of Fluocinonide—**See Corticosteroids (Topical),** 978
*Lidex*—Roche/Syntex (U.S.) and Syntex (Canada and U.K.) brand of Fluocinonide—**See Corticosteroids (Topical),** 978
*Lidex-E*—Roche/Syntex (U.S.) brand of Fluocinonide—**See Corticosteroids (Topical),** 978
Lidocaine [lignocaine; *Xylocaine; Xylocaine Dental Ointment; Zilactin-L*]
**See Anesthetics (Mucosal-Local),** 128
Aerosol, Topical, USP, 136
Ointment USP, 136
Solution, Topical, Oral, USP, 136

## USP DI

Lidocaine [*Alphacaine;* lignocaine; *Norwood Sunburn Spray; Xylocaine*]
  **See Anesthetics (Topical),** 155
  Ointment USP, 159
  Solution, Topical Spray, 159
Lidocaine-containing Combinations, 3075
Lidocaine Hydrochloride [*Anestacon Jelly; Xylocaine; Xylocaine Endotracheal; Xylocaine Viscous*]
  **See Anesthetics (Mucosal-Local),** 128
  Jelly USP, 136
  Solution, Topical, USP, 137
  Solution, Topical, Oral, USP, 137
  Solution, Topical Spray, 137
Lidocaine Hydrochloride [*Dalcaine; Dilocaine; L-Caine; Lidoject-1; Lidoject-2; Xylocaine; Xylocaine-MPF*]
  **See Anesthetics (Parenteral-Local),** 139
  Injection USP, 149
Lidocaine Hydrochloride [*Xylocaine; Xylocard*]
  **(Systemic),** 1860
  Injection (for Continuous Intravenous Infusion), 1862
  Injection (for Direct Intravenous Injection), 1862
  Sterile, 1863
Lidocaine Hydrochloride [*After Burn Double Strength Gel; After Burn Double Strength Spray; After Burn Gel; After Burn Spray; DermaFlex*]
  **See Anesthetics (Topical),** 155
  Aerosol, Topical, 160
  Gel, Film-forming, 160
  Jelly USP, 160
  Ointment, 160
Lidocaine Hydrochloride and Dextrose [*Xylocaine 5% Spinal; Xylocaine-MPF; Xylocaine-MPF with Glucose*]
  **See Anesthetics (Parenteral-Local),** 139
  Injection USP, 150
Lidocaine Hydrochloride and Dextrose
  **(Systemic),** 1860
  Injection (for Continuous Intravenous Infusion), 1863
Lidocaine Hydrochloride and Epinephrine [*Octocaine; Octocaine-50; Octocaine-100; Xylocaine; Xylocaine-MPF; Xylocaine Test Dose*]
  **See Anesthetics (Parenteral-Local),** 139
  Injection USP, 150
Lidocaine Patch 5% [*Lidoderm Patch*]
  **(Systemic),** 3152
Lidocaine and Prilocaine [*EMLA*]
  **(Topical),** #
  Cream, #
*Lidoderm Patch*—Hind (U.S.) brand of Lidocaine (Systemic), 3152
*Lidoject-1*—Mayrand (U.S.) brand of Lidocaine—**See Anesthetics (Parenteral-Local),** 139
*Lidoject-2*—Mayrand (U.S.) brand of Lidocaine—**See Anesthetics (Parenteral-Local),** 139
*Lidox*—Major (U.S.) brand of Chlordiazepoxide and Clidinium (Systemic), 846
*Lidoxide*—Interstate (U.S.) brand of Chlordiazepoxide and Clidinium (Systemic), 846
*Life Antacid*—KSL (Canada) brand of Alumina and Magnesia—**See Antacids (Oral-Local),** 188
*Life Antacid Plus*—KSL (Canada) brand of Alumina, Magnesia, and Simethicone—**See Antacids (Oral-Local),** 188
*LifeStyles Assorted Colors*—Ansell (U.S.) brand of Latex Condoms—**See Condoms,** #
*LifeStyles Extra Strength with Spermicide*—Ansell (U.S. and Canada) brand of Latex Condoms and Nonoxynol 9—**See Condoms,** #
*LifeStyles Form Fitting*—Ansell (U.S. and Canada) brand of Latex Condoms—**See Condoms,** #
*LifeStyles Lubricated*—Ansell (U.S. and Canada) brand of Latex Condoms—**See Condoms,** #
*LifeStyles Lubricated with Spermicide*—Ansell (Canada) brand of Latex Condoms and Nonoxynol 9—**See Condoms,** #
*LifeStyles Non-Lubricated*—Ansell (U.S.) brand of Latex Condoms—**See Condoms,** #
*LifeStyles Spermicidally Lubricated*—Ansell (U.S.) brand of Latex Condoms and Nonoxynol 9—**See Condoms,** #
*LifeStyles Ultra Sensitive*—Ansell (U.S. and Canada) brand of Latex Condoms—**See Condoms,** #
*LifeStyles Ultra Sensitive with Spermicide*—Ansell (U.S.) brand of Latex Condoms and Nonoxynol 9—**See Condoms,** #
*LifeStyles Vibra-Ribbed*—Ansell (U.S. and Canada) brand of Latex Condoms—**See Condoms,** #

*LifeStyles Vibra-Ribbed with Spermicide*—Ansell (U.S.) brand of Latex Condoms and Nonoxynol 9—**See Condoms,** #
Lignocaine—Lidocaine—**See Anesthetics (Mucosal-Local),** 128; **Anesthetics (Parenteral-Local),** 139; **Anesthetics (Topical),** 155
*Limbitrol*—Roche (U.S.) brand of Chlordiazepoxide and Amitriptyline (Systemic), 845
*Limbitrol DS*—Roche (U.S.) brand of Chlordiazepoxide and Amitriptyline (Systemic), 845
*Lincocin*—Upjohn (U.S. and Canada) brand of Lincomycin (Systemic), 1863
Lincomycin Hydrochloride [*Lincocin; Lincorex*]
  **(Systemic),** 1863
  Capsules USP, 1865
  Injection USP, 1866
*Lincorex*—Hyrex (U.S.) brand of Lincomycin (Systemic), 1863
Lindane [*Bio-Well;* gamma benzene hexachloride; *GBH; G-well; Hexit; Kildane; Kwell; Kwellada; Kwildane; PMS Lindane; Scabene; Thionex*]
  **(Topical),** 1866
  Cream USP, 1868
  Lotion USP, 1868
  Shampoo USP, 1868
*Linhist-L.A.*—Econolab (U.S.) and Rugby (U.S.) brand of Chlorpheniramine, Phenyltoloxamine, and Phenylephrine—**See Antihistamines and Decongestants (Systemic),** 343
*Linomide*—Pharmacia (U.S.) brand of Roquinimex (Systemic), 3163
*Lioresal*—Novartis (U.S. and Canada) brand of Baclofen (Systemic), 515, MC-3
*Lioresal Intrathecal*—Medtronic (U.S.) brand of Baclofen (Intrathecal-Systemic), 513, 3133
Liothyronine Sodium [*Cytomel; Triostat*]
  **See Thyroid Hormones (Systemic),** 2809, 3028, 3151
  Injection, 3028, 3151
  Tablets USP, 2813
Liotrix [*Thyrolar*]
  **See Thyroid Hormones (Systemic),** 2809
  Tablets USP, 2814
Lipancreatin—**See** Pancrelipase (Systemic), 2222
Lipid (DNA) Human Cystic Fibrosis Gene, 3152
*Lipisorb*—Mead Johnson (U.S.) brand of Enteral Nutrition Formula, Disease-specific—**See Enteral Nutrition Formulas (Systemic),** #
*Lipitor*—PD (U.S.) brand of Atorvastatin (Systemic), 479, MC-3
Liposomal Amphotericin B [*AmBisome*]
  **(Systemic),** 3152
Liposomal Cyclosporin A [*Cyclospire*]
  **(Systemic),** 3152
Liposomal Daunorubicin [*Daunoxome*]
  **(Systemic),** 3152
Liposomal N-Acetylglucosaminyl-N-Acetylmuramyl-L-Ala-D-isoGln-L-Ala-Glycerolid-palmitoyl [*ImmTher*]
  **(Systemic),** 3152
Liposome Encapsulated Recombinant Interleukin-2
  **(Systemic),** 3152
*Liposyn II*—Abbott (U.S.) brand of Fat Emulsions (Systemic), #
*Liposyn III*—Abbott (U.S.) brand of Fat Emulsions (Systemic), #
*Liquaemin*—Organon (U.S.) brand of Heparin (Systemic), 1617
*Liqui-Cal*—Advanced Nutritional (U.S.) brand of Calcium Carbonate—**See Calcium Supplements (Systemic),** 736
*Liqui-Char*—Jones (U.S.) brand of Charcoal, Activated (Oral-Local), 831
*Liqui-Char with Sorbitol*—Jones Medical (U.S.) brand of Charcoal, Activated, and Sorbitol—**See Charcoal, Activated (Oral-Local),** 831
*Liquid Barosperse*—Lafayette (U.S.) brand of Barium Sulfate (Local), #
*Liquid Cal-600*—Advanced Nutritional (U.S.) brand of Calcium Carbonate—**See Calcium Supplements (Systemic),** 736
*Liquid HD*—E-Z-EM (U.S.) brand of Barium Sulfate (Local), #
*Liqui-Doss*—Ferndale (U.S.) brand of Mineral Oil—**See Laxatives (Local),** #
*Liquid Pred*—Muro (U.S.) brand of Prednisone—**See Corticosteroids—Glucocorticoid Effects (Systemic),** 998
*Liqui-E*—Twinlab (U.S.) brand of Vitamin E (Systemic), 2972

## General Index

*Liqui-Histine-D*—Liquipharm (U.S.) brand of Pheniramine, Phenyltoloxamine, Pyrilamine, and Phenylpropanolamine—**See Antihistamines and Decongestants (Systemic),** 343
*Liqui-Histine DM*—Liquipharm (U.S.) brand of Brompheniramine, Phenylpropanolamine, and Dextromethorphan—**See Cough/Cold Combinations (Systemic),** 1024
*Liqui-Jug*—E-Z-EM (U.S.) brand of Barium Sulfate (Local), #
*Liquimat Light*—Owen (U.S.) brand of Alcohol and Sulfur (Topical), #
*Liquimat Medium*—Owen (U.S.) brand of Alcohol and Sulfur (Topical), #
*Liqui-Minic Infant Drops*—Liquipharm (U.S.) brand of Pheniramine, Pyrilamine, and Phenylpropanolamine—**See Antihistamines and Decongestants (Systemic),** 343
*Liquipake*—Lafayette (U.S.) brand of Barium Sulfate (Local), #
*Liquiprin Children's Elixir*—Menley & James (U.S.) brand of Acetaminophen (Systemic), 6
*Liquiprin Infants' Drops*—Menley & James (U.S.) brand of Acetaminophen (Systemic), 6
*Liquor Carbonis Detergens*—Odan (Canada) brand of Coal Tar (Topical), #
Lisadimate-containing Combinations, 3075
Lisadimate, Oxybenzone, and Padimate O [*Total Eclipse Oily and Acne Prone Skin Sunscreen*]
  **See Sunscreen Agents (Topical),** #
  Lotion, #
Lisadimate and Padimate O [*Eclipse Original Sunscreen*]
  **See Sunscreen Agents (Topical),** #
  Lotion, #
Lisinopril [*Prinivil; Zestril*]
  **See Angiotensin-converting Enzyme (ACE) Inhibitors (Systemic),** 177
  Tablets, 185, MC-17
Lisinopril-containing Combinations, 3075
Lisinopril and Hydrochlorothiazide [*Prinzide; Zestoretic*]
  **See Angiotensin-converting Enzyme (ACE) Inhibitors and Hydrochlorothiazide (Systemic),** 187
  Tablets, 188, MC-17
*Listerex Golden Scrub Lotion*—Warner-Lambert (U.S.) brand of Salicylic Acid (Topical), #
*Listerex Herbal Scrub Lotion*—Warner-Lambert (U.S.) brand of Salicylic Acid (Topical), #
*Lite Pred*—Horizon (U.S.) brand of Prednisolone—**See Corticosteroids (Ophthalmic),** 966
*Lithane*—Miles (U.S.) and Pfizer (Canada) brand of Lithium (Systemic), 1869
Lithium Carbonate [*Carbolith; Duralith; Eskalith; Eskalith CR; Lithane; Lithizine; Lithobid; Lithonate; Lithotabs*]
  **(Systemic),** 1869
  Capsules USP, 1873, MC-17
  Capsules, Slow-release, 1873
  Tablets USP, 1873, MC-17
  Tablets, Extended-release, 1873, MC-17
Lithium Citrate [*Cibalith-S*]
  **(Systemic),** 1869
  Syrup USP, 1873
*Lithizine*—Paul Maney (Canada) brand of Lithium (Systemic), 1869
*Lithobid*—Solvay (U.S.) brand of Lithium (Systemic), 1869, MC-17
*Lithonate*—Solvay (U.S.) brand of Lithium (Systemic), 1869, MC-17
*Lithostat*—Mission (U.S.) brand of Acetohydroxamic Acid (Systemic), #
*Lithotab*—Solvay (U.S.) brand of Lithium (Systemic), 1869, MC-17
*Livostin*—Ciba Vision (U.S. and Canada) brand of Levocabastine (Ophthalmic), 3027; Iolab (U.S.) and Janssen (Canada) brand of Levocabastine (Ophthalmic), #; Janssen (Canada) brand of Levocabastine (Nasal), 3027
L-Leucovorin [*Isovorin*]
  **(Systemic),** 3150
L-methyl-[11]methionine—**See** Methionine C 11 (Systemic), #
*Locacorten*—Ciba (Canada) brand of Flumethasone—**See Corticosteroids (Topical),** 978
*Locacorten Vioform*—Ciba (Canada) brand of Clioquinol and Flumethasone (Otic), 3015; (Topical), 3015

*Locoid*—Owen/Allercreme (U.S.) and Brocades (U.K.) brand of Hydrocortisone—**See Corticosteroids (Topical)**, 978; Yamanouchi (U.S.) brand of Hydrocortisone (Topical), 3023
*Lodine*—Wyeth-Ayerst (U.S.) brand of Etodolac—**See Anti-inflammatory Drugs, Nonsteroidal (Systemic)**, 388, MC-12, 3019
*Lodine XL*—Wyeth-Ayerst (U.S.) brand of Etodolac (Systemic), 3019
Lodoxamide trometamol—*See* Lodoxamide (Ophthalmic), #
Lodoxamide Tromethamine [*Alomide; Alomide Ophthalmic Solution;* lodoxamide trometamol]
  **(Ophthalmic)**, #, 3028, 3152
  Solution, Ophthalmic, #, 3028
*Lodrane LD*—ECR (U.S.) brand of Brompheniramine and Pseudoephedrine—**See Antihistamines and Decongestants (Systemic)**, 343
*Lodrane Liquid*—ECR (U.S.) brand of Brompheniramine and Pseudoephedrine—**See Antihistamines and Decongestants (Systemic)**, 343
*Loestrin 1/20*—PD (U.S.) brand of Norethindrone Acetate and Ethinyl Estradiol—**See Estrogens and Progestins—Oral Contraceptives (Systemic)**, 1397, MC-22
*Loestrin 1.5/30*—PD (U.S. and Canada) brand of Norethindrone Acetate and Ethinyl Estradiol—**See Estrogens and Progestins—Oral Contraceptives (Systemic)**, 1397, MC-23
*Loestrin Fe 1/20*—PD (U.S.) brand of Norethindrone Acetate and Ethinyl Estradiol and Ferrous Fumarate (Systemic), 1397, MC-23
*Loestrin Fe 1.5/30*—PD (U.S.) brand of Norethindrone Acetate and Ethinyl Estradiol and Ferrous Fumarate (Systemic), 1397, MC-23
*Lofene*—Lannett (U.S.) brand of Diphenoxylate and Atropine (Systemic), 1233
*Logen*—Goldline (U.S.) brand of Diphenoxylate and Atropine (Systemic), 1233
Lomefloxacin [*Maxaquin*]
  **See Fluoroquinolones (Systemic)**, 1487
  Tablets, 1494, MC-17
*Lomine*—Riva (Canada) brand of Dicyclomine—**See Anticholinergics/Antispasmodics (Systemic)**, 226
*Lomocot*—Truxton (U.S.) brand of Diphenoxylate and Atropine (Systemic), 1233
*Lomotil*—Searle (U.S. and Canada) brand of Diphenoxylate and Atropine (Systemic), 1233, MC-10
Lomustine [*CCNU; CeeNU*]
  **(Systemic)**, 1874
  Capsules, 1876
*Loniten*—Pharmacia & Upjohn (U.S. and Canada) brand of Minoxidil (Systemic), 2018, MC-20
*Lonox*—Geneva Generics (U.S.) brand of Diphenoxylate and Atropine (Systemic), 1233
*Lo-Ovral*—Wyeth-Ayerst (U.S.) brand of Norgestrel and Ethinyl Estradiol—**See Estrogens and Progestins—Oral Contraceptives (Systemic)**, 1397, MC-23
*Loperacap*—ICN (Canada) brand of Loperamide (Oral-Local), 1877
Loperamide Hydrochloride [*Apo-Loperamide; Diarr-Eze; Imodium; Imodium A-D; Imodium A-D Caplets; Kaopectate II; Loperacap; Maalox Anti-Diarrheal; Nu-Loperamide; Pepto Diarrhea Control; PMS-Loperamide*]
  **(Oral-Local)**, 1877
  Capsules USP, 1879, MC-17
  Solution, Oral, 1879
  Tablets USP, 1879
Loperamide and Simethicone [*Imodium Advanced*]
  **(Systemic)**, 3028
  Tablets, Chewable, 3028
*Lopid*—PD (U.S. and Canada) brand of Gemfibrozil (Systemic), 1552, MC-13
*Lopresor*—Ciba-Geigy (Canada) brand of Metoprolol—**See Beta-adrenergic Blocking Agents (Systemic)**, 593
*Lopresor SR*—Ciba-Geigy (Canada) brand of Metoprolol—**See Beta-adrenergic Blocking Agents (Systemic)**, 593
*Lopressor*—Novartis (U.S.) brand of Metoprolol—**See Beta-adrenergic Blocking Agents (Systemic)**, 593, MC-20
*Lopressor HCT*—Novartis (U.S.) brand of Metoprolol and Hydrochlorothiazide—**See Beta-adrenergic Blocking Agents and Thiazide Diuretics (Systemic)**, 609, MC-20
*Loprox*—Hoechst-Roussel (U.S.) and Hoechst (Canada) brand of Ciclopirox (Topical), 863

*Lopurin*—Boots (U.S.) brand of Allopurinol (Systemic), 44
*Lorabid*—Lilly (U.S.) brand of Loracarbef (Systemic), 1880, MC-17
Loracarbef [*Lorabid*]
  **(Systemic)**, 1880
  Capsules, 1881, MC-17
  for Suspension, Oral, 1881
Loratadine [*Claritin; Claritin Reditabs*]
  **See Antihistamines (Systemic)**, 325
  Syrup, 341
  Tablets, 341, MC-17
Loratadine-containing Combinations, 3075
Loratadine and Pseudoephedrine Sulfate [*Chlor-Tripolon N.D.; Claritin-D 12 Hour; Claritin-D 24 Hour; Claritin Extra*]
  **See Antihistamines and Decongestants (Systemic)**, 343
  Tablets, MC-18
  Tablets, Extended-release, 349
Lorazepam [*Apo-Lorazepam; Ativan; Lorazepam Intensol; Novo-Lorazem; Nu-Loraz*]
  **See Benzodiazepines (Systemic)**, 556
  Injection USP, 575
  Concentrate, Oral, USP, 574
  Tablets USP, 574, MC-18
  Tablets, Sublingual, 575
*Lorazepam Intensol*—Roxane (U.S.) brand of Lorazepam—**See Benzodiazepines (Systemic)**, 556
*Lorcet 10/650*—UAD (U.S.) brand of Hydrocodone and Acetaminophen—**See Opioid (Narcotic) Analgesics and Acetaminophen (Systemic)**, 2198
*Lorcet-HD*—UAD (U.S.) brand of Hydrocodone and Acetaminophen—**See Opioid (Narcotic) Analgesics and Acetaminophen (Systemic)**, 2198
*Lorcet Plus*—UAD (U.S.) brand of Hydrocodone and Acetaminophen—**See Opioid (Narcotic) Analgesics and Acetaminophen (Systemic)**, 2198
*Lorelco*—Merrell Dow (Canada) brand of Probucol (Systemic), 2385
Lorenzo's oil—*See* Glyceryl Trioleate and Glyceryl Trierucate (Systemic), 3144
*Loroxide 5 Lotion*—Dermik (U.S.) brand of Benzoyl Peroxide (Topical), 579
*Loroxide 5.5 Lotion*—Dermik (U.S.) brand of Benzoyl Peroxide (Topical), 579
*Lortab 10/500*—UCB (U.S.) brand of Hydrocodone and Acetaminophen (Systemic), 3022
*Lortab*—UCB (U.S.) brand of Hydrocodone and Acetaminophen—**See Opioid (Narcotic) Analgesics and Acetaminophen (Systemic)**, 2198, MC-14
*Lortab 2.5/500*—UCB (U.S.) brand of Hydrocodone and Acetaminophen—**See Opioid (Narcotic) Analgesics and Acetaminophen (Systemic)**, 2198, MC-14
*Lortab 5/500*—UCB (U.S.) brand of Hydrocodone and Acetaminophen—**See Opioid (Narcotic) Analgesics and Acetaminophen (Systemic)**, 2198, MC-14
*Lortab 7.5/500*—UCB (U.S.) brand of Hydrocodone and Acetaminophen—**See Opioid (Narcotic) Analgesics and Acetaminophen (Systemic)**, 2198, MC-14
*Lortab 10/500*—UCB (U.S.) brand of Hydrocodone and Acetaminophen—**See Opioid (Narcotic) Analgesics and Acetaminophen (Systemic)**, MC-14
*Lortab ASA*—UCB (U.S.) brand of Hydrocodone and Aspirin—**See Opioid (Narcotic) Analgesics and Aspirin (Systemic)**, 2202
Losartan Potassium [*Cozaar;* DuP 753; MK594]
  **(Systemic)**, 1882
  Tablets, 1884, MC-18
Losartan Potassium and Hydrochlorothiazide [*Hyzaar*]
  **(Systemic)**, 1884
  Tablets, 1887, MC-18
*Losec*—Astra (Canada) brand of Omeprazole Magnesium (Systemic), 2163
*Losopan*—Zenith Goldline (U.S.) brand of Magaldrate—**See Antacids (Oral-Local)**, 188
*Losopan Plus*—Zenith Goldline (U.S.) brand of Magaldrate and Simethicone—**See Antacids (Oral-Local)**, 188
*Lotemax*—Bausch & Lomb (U.S.) brand of Loteprednol (Ophthalmic), 1887
*Lotensin*—Novartis (U.S.) brand of Benazepril—**See Angiotensin-converting Enzyme (ACE) Inhibitors (Systemic)**, 177, MC-3

*Lotensin HCT*—Novartis (U.S.) brand of Benazepril and Hydrochlorothiazide (Systemic), MC-3
Loteprednol [*Alrex; Lotemax*]
  **(Ophthalmic)**, 1887
  Suspension, Ophthalmic, 1889
*Lotio Alsulfa*—Doak (U.S.) brand of Sulfur (Topical), #
*Lotrel*—Ciba (U.S.) brand of Amlodipine and Benazepril (Systemic), 88, MC-2
*Lotriderm*—Schering (Canada) brand of Clotrimazole and Betamethasone (Topical), 918
*Lotrimin AF Cream*—Schering (U.S.) brand of Clotrimazole (Topical), 916
*Lotrimin AF Lotion*—Schering (U.S.) brand of Clotrimazole (Topical), 916
*Lotrimin AF Solution*—Schering (U.S.) brand of Clotrimazole (Topical), 916
*Lotrimin Cream*—Schering (U.S.) brand of Clotrimazole (Topical), 916
*Lotrimin Lotion*—Schering (U.S.) brand of Clotrimazole (Topical), 916
*Lotrimin Solution*—Schering (U.S.) brand of Clotrimazole (Topical), 916
*Lotrisone*—Schering (U.S.) brand of Clotrimazole and Betamethasone (Topical), 918
Lovastatin [*Mevacor;* mevinolin]
  **See HMG-CoA Reductase Inhibitors (Systemic)**, 1647
  Tablets USP, 1650, MC-18
*Lovenox*—Rhône-Poulenc Rorer (U.S. and Canada) brand of Enoxaparin (Systemic), 1156
Low molecular weight heparin—*See* Dalteparin (Systemic), 1156
*Lowsium Plus*—Rugby (U.S.) brand of Magaldrate and Simethicone—**See Antacids (Oral-Local)**, 188
*Loxapac*—Lederle (Canada) brand of Loxapine (Systemic), 1889
Loxapine Hydrochloride [*Loxapac; Loxitane C; Loxitane IM*]
  **(Systemic)**, 1889
  Injection, 1893
  Solution, Oral, 1892
Loxapine Succinate [*Loxapac; Loxitane*]
  **(Systemic)**, 1889
  Capsules, 1893, MC-18
  Tablets, 1893
*Loxitane*—Lederle (U.S.) brand of Loxapine (Systemic), 1889, MC-18
*Loxitane C*—Lederle (U.S.) brand of Loxapine (Systemic), 1889
*Loxitane IM*—Lederle (U.S.) brand of Loxapine (Systemic), 1889
L-2 Oxothiazolidine-4-Carboxylic Acid [*Procysteine*]
  **(Intratracheal-Local)**, 3150
L-2-Oxothiazolidine-4-Carboxylic Acid [*Procysteine*]
  **(Systemic)**, 3150
*Lozide*—Servier (Canada) brand of Indapamide (Systemic), 1691
*Lozol*—Rhône-Poulenc Rorer (U.S.) brand of Indapamide (Systemic), 1691, MC-15
L-PAM—*See* Melphalan (Systemic), 1938
LTG—*See* Lamotrigine (Systemic), 1824
L-Threonine [*Threostat*]
  **(Systemic)**, 3151
L-Thyroxine—Levothyroxine—**See Thyroid Hormones (Systemic)**, 2809
*Ludiomil*—Novartis (U.S. and Canada) brand of Maprotiline (Systemic), 1909, MC-18
*Lufyllin*—Wallace (U.S.) brand of Dyphylline (Systemic), #, MC-10
*Lufyllin-400*—Wallace (U.S.) brand of Dyphylline (Systemic), #
Lugol's solution—*See* Iodine, Strong (Systemic), 1751
*Luminal*—Sanofi Winthrop (U.S.) brand of Phenobarbital—**See Barbiturates (Systemic)**, 518
*Lumitene*—Tischon (U.S.) brand of Beta-carotene (Systemic), 612
*Lumopaque*—Sterling Winthrop (Argentina) brand of Tyropanoate—**See Cholecystographic Agents, Oral (Systemic)**, #
*Lupron*—TAP (U.S.) and Abbott (Canada) brand of Leuprolide (Systemic), 1840
*Lupron Depot*—TAP (U.S. and Canada) brand of Leuprolide (Systemic), 1840
*Lupron Depot-3 Month 11.25 mg*—TAP (U.S.) brand of Leuprolide (Systemic), 1840
*Lupron Depot-3 Month 22.5 mg*—TAP (U.S.) brand of Leuprolide (Systemic), 1840
*Lupron Depot-4 Month 30mg*—TAP (U.S.) brand of Leuprolide (Systemic), 1840

*USP DI*                                                                **General Index**    **3305**

*Lupron Depot-Ped*—TAP (U.S.) brand of Leuprolide (Systemic), 1840
*Lupron Injection*—TAP (U.S.) brand of Leuprolide (Systemic), 3151
*Lupron 3 Month SR Depot 22.5 mg*—TAP (U.S.) brand of Leuprolide (Systemic), 1840
*Luride*—Colgate-Hoyt (U.S.) brand of Sodium Fluoride (Systemic), 2592
*Luride Lozi-Tab*—Colgate-Hoyt (U.S.) brand of Sodium Fluoride (Systemic), 2592
*Luride-SF Lozi-Tabs*—Colgate-Hoyt (U.S.) brand of Sodium Fluoride (Systemic), 2592
Luteinizing hormone-/follicle-stimulating hormone–releasing hormone—*See* Gonadorelin (Systemic), 1571
Luteinizing Hormone, Recombinant Human **(Systemic)**, 3159
Luteinizing hormone–releasing factor diacetate tetrahydrate (for gonadorelin acetate)—*See* Gonadorelin (Systemic), 1571
Luteinizing hormone–releasing factor dihydrochloride (for gonadorelin hydrochloride)—*See* Gonadorelin (Systemic), 1571
Luteinizing hormone–releasing hormone—*See* Gonadorelin (Systemic), 1571
*Lutrepulse*—Ferring (U.S. and Canada) brand of Gonadorelin (Systemic), 1571, 3144
*Luvox*—Solvay (U.S.) and Solvay Kingswood (Canada) brand of Fluvoxamine (Systemic), 1513, MC-13
*Lyderm*—K-Line (Canada) brand of Fluocinonide—**See Corticosteroids (Topical)**, 978
*Lymphocide*—Immunomedics (U.S.) brand of Monoclonal Antibody to CD22 Antigen on B-Cells, Radiolabeled (Systemic), 3160
Lypressin [*Diapid*]
 **(Systemic)**, 1893
 Solution, Nasal, USP, 1894
*Lysodren*—Bristol (U.S. and Canada) brand of Mitotane (Systemic), 2031
*Lytren*—Mead Johnson (Canada) brand of Dextrose and Electrolytes—**See Carbohydrates and Electrolytes (Systemic)**, 769

# M

*Maalox*—Ciba Self-Medication (U.S. and Canada) brand of Alumina and Magnesia—**See Antacids (Oral-Local)**, 188
*Maalox Antacid Caplets*—Ciba Self-Medication (U.S. and Canada) brand of Calcium and Magnesium Carbonates—**See Antacids (Oral-Local)**, 188; Rhône-Poulenc Rorer (U.S.) brand of Calcium Carbonate—**See Calcium Supplements (Systemic)**, 736
*Maalox Anti-Diarrheal*—Rhône-Poulenc Rorer (U.S.) brand of Loperamide (Oral-Local), 1877
*Maalox Anti-Gas*—Ciba (U.S.) brand of Simethicone (Oral-Local), #
*Maalox GRF Gas Relief Formula*—Rhône-Poulenc Rorer (Canada) brand of Simethicone (Oral-Local), #
*Maalox Heartburn Relief Formula*—Ciba Self-Medication (U.S.) brand of Alumina and Magnesium Carbonate—**See Antacids (Oral-Local)**, 188
*Maalox HRF*—Ciba Self-Medication (Canada) brand of Alumina, Magnesium Alginate, and Magnesium Carbonate—**See Antacids (Oral-Local)**, 188
*Maalox Plus*—Ciba Self-Medication (U.S. and Canada) brand of Alumina, Magnesia, and Simethicone—**See Antacids (Oral-Local)**, 188
*Maalox Plus, Extra Strength*—Ciba Self-Medication (U.S. and Canada) brand of Alumina, Magnesia, and Simethicone—**See Antacids (Oral-Local)**, 188
*Maalox TC*—Ciba Self-Medication (U.S. and Canada) brand of Alumina and Magnesia—**See Antacids (Oral-Local)**, 188
*Macrobid*—Procter & Gamble (U.S.) brand of Nitrofurantoin (Systemic), 2139, MC-22
*Macrodantin*—Procter & Gamble (U.S. and Canada) brand of Nitrofurantoin (Systemic), 2139, MC-22
*Macrotec*—Squibb (U.S.) brand of Technetium Tc 99m Albumin Aggregated (Systemic), 2697
Mafenide Acetate [*Sulfamylon; Sulfamylon Solution*]
 **(Topical)**, #
 Cream USP, #
 Solution, #, 3152

*Mag 2*—Charton (Canada) brand of Magnesium Pidolate—**See Magnesium Supplements (Systemic)**, 1897
MAG3—*See* Technetium Tc 99m Mertiatide (Systemic), 2720
*Mag-200*—Optimax (U.S.) brand of Magnesium Oxide—**See Magnesium Supplements (Systemic)**, 1897
Magaldrate [*Losopan; Riopan; Riopan Extra Strength*]
 **See Antacids (Oral-Local)**, 188
 Suspension, Oral, USP, 207, 209, 213, 214
 Tablets USP (Chewable), 213
Magaldrate-containing Combinations, 3075
Magaldrate and Simethicone [*Losopan Plus; Lowsium Plus; Riopan Plus; Riopan Plus Double Strength; Riopan Plus Extra Strength*]
 **See Antacids (Oral-Local)**, 188
 Suspension, Oral, USP, 207, 209, 214
 Tablets USP (Chewable), 214
*Magan*—Adria (U.S.) brand of Magnesium Salicylate—**See Salicylates (Systemic)**, 2538
*Mag-L-100*—Bio-Tech (U.S.) brand of Magnesium Chloride—**See Magnesium Supplements (Systemic)**, 1897
*Maglucate*—Pharmascience (Canada) brand of Magnesium Gluconate—**See Magnesium Supplements (Systemic)**, 1897
*Magnacal*—Sherwood (U.S.) brand of Enteral Nutrition Formula, Disease-specific and Enteral Nutrition Formula, Polymeric—**See Enteral Nutrition Formulas (Systemic)**, #
*Magnalox*—Schein (U.S.) brand of Alumina, Magnesia, and Simethicone—**See Antacids (Oral-Local)**, 188
*Magnalox Plus*—Schein (U.S.) brand of Alumina, Magnesia, and Simethicone—**See Antacids (Oral-Local)**, 188
*Magnaprin*—Rugby (U.S.) brand of Aspirin, Buffered—**See Salicylates (Systemic)**, 2538
Magnesia-containing Combinations, 3075
Magnesium Carbonate–containing Combinations, 3075
Magnesium Carbonate and Sodium Bicarbonate [*Gaviscon Heartburn Relief*]
 **See Antacids (Oral-Local)**, 188
 Tablets, Chewable, 206
Magnesium Chloride [*Chloromag; Mag-L-100; Slow-Mag*]
 **See Magnesium Supplements (Systemic)**, 1897
 Injection, 1901
 Tablets, 1901
 Tablets, Enteric-coated, 1901
 Tablets, Extended-release, 1901
Magnesium Citrate [*Citroma; Citro-Mag*]
 **See Laxatives (Local)**, #
 Solution, Oral, USP, #
Magnesium Citrate [*Citroma; Citro-Mag*]
 **See Magnesium Supplements (Systemic)**, 1897
 Solution, Oral, 1901
Magnesium Gluceptate [magnesium glucoheptonate; *Magnesium-Rougier*]
 **See Magnesium Supplements (Systemic)**, 1897
 Solution, Oral, 1902
Magnesium glucoheptonate—Magnesium Gluceptate—**See Magnesium Supplements (Systemic)**, 1897
Magnesium Gluconate [*Almora; Maglucate; Magonate; MGP; Magtrate*]
 **See Magnesium Supplements (Systemic)**, 1897
 Solution, Oral, 1902
 Tablets USP, 1902
Magnesium Hydroxide [*Phillips'; Phillips' Chewable; Phillips' Concentrated Double-strength*]
 **See Antacids (Oral-Local)**, 188
 Magnesia Tablets USP (Chewable), 209, 212, 213
 Milk of Magnesia USP, 209, 212, 213
Magnesium Hydroxide [milk of magnesia; *Phillips' Chewable; Phillips' Concentrated Double Strength; Phillips' Magnesia Tablets; Phillips' Milk of Magnesia*]
 **See Laxatives (Local)**, #
 Milk of Magnesia USP, #
 Tablets, Magnesia, USP, #
 Tablets USP, #
Magnesium Hydroxide [*Concentrated Phillips' Milk of Magnesia; Phillips' Chewable Tablets; Phillips' Magnesia Tablets; Phillips' Milk of Magnesia*]
 **See Magnesium Supplements (Systemic)**, 1897
 Magnesia Tablets USP, 1902
 Magnesia Tablets USP (Chewable), 1903
 Milk of Magnesia USP, 1903

Magnesium Hydroxide and Cascara Sagrada [concentrated milk of magnesia-cascara]
 **See Laxatives (Local)**, #
 Suspension, Oral, #
Magnesium Hydroxide and Mineral Oil [*Haley's M-O; Magnolax*]
 **See Laxatives (Local)**, #
 Emulsion, #
Magnesium Lactate [*Mag-Tab SR*]
 **See Magnesium Supplements (Systemic)**, 1897
 Tablets, Extended-release, 1903
Magnesium Oxide [*Mag-Ox 400; Maox 420; Uro-Mag*]
 **See Antacids (Oral-Local)**, 188
 Capsules USP, 217
 Tablets USP, 210
Magnesium Oxide [*Mag-200; Mag-Ox 400; Maox; Uro-Mag*]
 **See Magnesium Supplements (Systemic)**, 1897
 Capsules USP, 1903
 Tablets USP, 1903
Magnesium Oxide [*Mag-Ox 400; Maox 420*]
 **See Laxatives (Local)**, #
 Tablets USP, #
Magnesium Oxide–containing Combinations, 3075
Magnesium Pidolate [*Mag 2;* magnesium pyroglutamate]
 **See Magnesium Supplements (Systemic)**, 1897
 for Solution, Oral, 1904
Magnesium pyroglutamate—Magnesium Pidolate—**See Magnesium Supplements (Systemic)**, 1897
*Magnesium-Rougier*—Rougier (Canada) brand of Magnesium Gluceptate—**See Magnesium Supplements (Systemic)**, 1897
Magnesium Salicylate [*Backache Caplets; Bayer Select Maximum Strength Backache Pain Relief Formula; Doan's Backache Pills; Doan's Regular Strength Tablets; Magan; Maximum Strength Doan's Analgesic Caplets; Mobidin; Sero-Gesic*]
 **See Salicylates (Systemic)**, 2538
 Tablets USP, 2553
Magnesium Salicylate–containing Combinations, 3075
Magnesium Sulfate [*Bilagog;* epsom salts]
 **See Laxatives (Local)**, #
 Crystals, #
 Tablets, #
Magnesium Sulfate
 **(Systemic)**, 1895
 Injection, 1897
Magnesium Sulfate
 **See Magnesium Supplements (Systemic)**, 1898
 Crystals, 1904
 Injection USP, 1904
Magnesium Supplements
 **(Systemic)**, 1898
Magnesium Trisilicate–containing Combinations, 3075
*Magnevist*—Berlex (U.S.) brand of Gadopentetate (Systemic), #
*Magnolax*—Rhône-Poulenc-Rorer (U.S.) and Wampole (Canada) brand of Magnesium Hydroxide and Mineral Oil—**See Laxatives (Local)**, #
*Magonate*—Fleming (U.S.) brand of Magnesium Gluconate—**See Magnesium Supplements (Systemic)**, 1897
*Mag-Ox 400*—Blaine (U.S.) brand of Magnesium Oxide—**See Magnesium Supplements (Systemic)**, 1897
*Mag-Ox 400*—Blaine (U.S.) brand of Magnesium Oxide—**See Antacids (Oral-Local)**, 188; **Laxatives (Local)**, #
*Mag-Tab SR*—Niché (U.S.) brand of Magnesium Lactate—**See Magnesium Supplements (Systemic)**, 1897
*Magtrate*—Mission (U.S.) brand of Magnesium Gluconate—**See Magnesium Supplements (Systemic)**, 1897
*Maitec*—Liposome Company (U.S.) brand of Gentamicin Liposome (Systemic), 3144
*Majeptil*—Rhône-Poulenc (Canada) brand of Thioproperazine—**See Phenothiazines (Systemic)**, 2289
*Malatal*—Mallard (U.S.) brand of Atropine, Hyoscyamine, Scopolamine, and Phenobarbital—**See Belladonna Alkaloids and Barbiturates (Systemic)**, 551
Malathion [*Derbac-M; Ovide; Suleo-M*]
 **(Topical)**, #
 Lotion USP, #

*Mallamint*—Mallard (U.S.) brand of Calcium Carbonate—**See Calcium Supplements (Systemic)**, 736; Roberts (U.S.) brand of Calcium Carbonate—**See Antacids (Oral-Local)**, 188
*Mallopres*—Mallard (U.S.) brand of Reserpine and Hydrochlorothiazide—**See Rauwolfia Alkaloids and Thiazide Diuretics (Systemic)**, #
*Malogen in Oil*—Germiphene (Canada) brand of Testosterone—**See Androgens (Systemic)**, 118
Malt Soup Extract [*Maltsupex*]
  **See Laxatives (Local)**, #
  Powder, #
  Solution, Oral, #
  Tablets. #
Malt Soup Extract-containing Combinations, 3075
Malt Soup Extract and Psyllium [*Syllamalt*]
  **See Laxatives (Local)**, #
  Powder. #
*Maltsupex*—Wallace (U.S.) brand of Malt Soup Extract—**See Laxatives (Local)**, #
*Mandelamine*—PD (U.S. and Canada) brand of Methenamine (Systemic), #
*Mandol*—Lilly (U.S. and Canada) brand of Cefamandole—**See Cephalosporins (Systemic)**, 794
*Manerex*—Hoffmann-La Roche (Canada) brand of Moclobemide (Systemic), 3028
Manganese Chloride
  **See Manganese Supplements (Systemic)**, 1905
  Injection USP, 1906
Manganese Sulfate
  **See Manganese Supplements (Systemic)**, 1905
  Injection USP, 1906
Manganese Supplements
  **(Systemic)**, 1905
Mannitol [*Osmitrol*]
  **(Systemic)**, 1906
  Injection USP, 1908
*Maolate*—Upjohn (U.S.) brand of Chlorphenesin—**See Skeletal Muscle Relaxants (Systemic)**, 2577
*Maox*—Kenneth A. Manne (U.S.) brand of Magnesium Oxide—**See Magnesium Supplements (Systemic)**, 1897
*Maox 420*—Kenneth A. Manne (U.S.) brand of Magnesium Oxide—**See Antacids (Oral-Local)**, 188; **Laxatives (Local)**, #
*Mapap Cold Formula*—Major (U.S.) brand of Chlorpheniramine, Pseudoephedrine, Dextromethorphan, and Acetaminophen—**See Cough/Cold Combinations (Systemic)**, 1024
Maprotiline Hydrochloride [*Ludiomil*]
  **(Systemic)**, 1909
  Tablets USP, 1912, MC-18
*Marax*—Pfizer (U.S.) brand of Theophylline, Ephedrine, and Hydroxyzine (Systemic), #
*Marax-DF*—Pfizer (U.S.) brand of Theophylline, Ephedrine, and Hydroxyzine (Systemic), #
*Marblen*—Fleming (U.S.) brand of Calcium and Magnesium Carbonates—**See Antacids (Oral-Local)**, 188
*Marcaine*—Cooke-Waite (U.S.) and Sanofi Winthrop (U.S. and Canada) brand of Bupivacaine—**See Anesthetics (Parenteral-Local)**, 139
*Marcaine Spinal*—Sanofi Winthrop (U.S.) brand of Bupivacaine—**See Anesthetics (Parenteral-Local)**, 139
*Marcof Expectorant*—Marnel (U.S.) brand of Hydrocodone and Potassium Guaicolsulfonate—**See Cough/Cold Combinations (Systemic)**, 1024
*Marezine*—BW (U.S.) brand of Cyclizine (Systemic), #
*Margesic #3*—Marnel (U.S.) brand of Acetaminophen and Codeine—**See Opioid (Narcotic) Analgesics and Acetaminophen (Systemic)**, 2198
*Margesic-H*—Marnel (U.S.) brand of Hydrocodone and Acetaminophen—**See Opioid (Narcotic) Analgesics and Acetaminophen (Systemic)**, 2198
*Marinol*—Roxane (U.S.), Unimed (U.S.), and Boehringer Ingelheim (Canada) brand of Dronabinol (Systemic), 1316, 3141
*Marnal*—Vortech (U.S.) brand of Butalbital, Aspirin, and Caffeine—**See Barbiturates and Analgesics (Systemic)**, 532
*Marogen*—Chugai (U.S.) brand of Epoetin Beta (Systemic), 3142
MART-1 Adenoviral Gene Therapy for Malignant Melanoma
  **(Systemic)**, 3153
*Marthritic*—Salsalate—**See Salicylates (Systemic)**, 2538

*Marvelon*—Organon (Canada) brand of Desogestrel and Ethinyl Estradiol—**See Estrogens and Progestins—Oral Contraceptives (Systemic)**, 1397
*Marzine*—BW (Canada) brand of Cyclizine (Systemic), #
Masoprocol [*Actinex*]
  **(Topical)**, 1912
  Cream, 1915
*Masporin Otic*—Mason (U.S.) brand of Neomycin, Polymyxin B, and Hydrocortisone (Otic), #
Matrix Metalloproteinase Inhibitor [*Galardin*]
  **(Ophthalmic)**, 3153
*Matulane*—Roche (U.S.) brand of Procarbazine (Systemic), 2391
*Mavik*—Knoll (U.S.) brand of Trandolapril (Systemic), 2854, MC-31
*Maxafil*—Genderm (U.S.) brand of Menthyl Anthranilate—**See Sunscreen Agents (Topical)**, #
*Maxair*—3M (U.S. and Canada) brand of Pirbuterol—**See Bronchodilators, Adrenergic (Inhalation-Local)**, 640
*Maxair Autohaler*—3M (U.S.) brand of Pirbuterol—**See Bronchodilators, Adrenergic (Inhalation-Local)**, 640
*Maxaquin*—Searle (U.S.) brand of Lomefloxacin—**See Fluoroquinolones (Systemic)**, 1487, MC-17
*Max-Caro*—Marlyn (U.S.) brand of Beta-carotene (Systemic), 612
*Maxenal*—McNeil (Canada) brand of Pseudoephedrine (Systemic), 2422
*Maxeran*—Marion Merrell Dow (Canada) brand of Metoclopramide (Systemic), 1992
*Maxibar*—E-Z-EM (Canada) brand of Barium Sulfate (Local), #
*Maxidex*—Alcon (U.S. and Canada) brand of Dexamethasone—**See Corticosteroids (Ophthalmic)**, 966
*Maxiflor*—Allergan Herbert (U.S.) brand of Diflorasone—**See Corticosteroids (Topical)**, 978
Maximum Strength Arthritis Foundation Safety Coated Aspirin—McNeil Consumer (U.S.) brand of Aspirin—**See Salicylates (Systemic)**, 2538
Maximum Strength Ascriptin—Rhône-Poulenc Rorer (U.S.) brand of Aspirin, Buffered—**See Salicylates (Systemic)**, 2538
Maximum Strength Cortaid—Upjohn (U.S.) brand of Hydrocortisone—**See Corticosteroids (Topical)**, 978
Maximum Strength Doan's Analgesic Caplets—Sandoz Consumer (U.S.) brand of Magnesium Salicylate—**See Salicylates (Systemic)**, 2538
Maximum Strength Gas Relief—Rugby (U.S.) brand of Simethicone (Oral-Local), #
Maximum Strength Mylanta Gas Relief—Johnson & Johnson (U.S.) brand of Simethicone (Oral-Local), #
Maximum Strength Phazyme—Reed & Carnrick (U.S.) brand of Simethicone (Oral-Local), #
*Maxipime*—Bristol-Myers Squibb (U.S. and Canada) brand of Cefepime—**See Cephalosporins (Systemic)**, 794
*Maxivate*—Westwood (U.S.) brand of Betamethasone—**See Corticosteroids (Topical)**, 978
MAXX—Mayer (U.S.) brand of Latex Condoms—**See Condoms**, #
MAXX Plus—Mayer (U.S.) brand of Latex Condoms and Nonoxynol 9—**See Condoms**, #
*Maxzide*—Bertek (U.S.) brand of Triamterene and Hydrochlorothiazide—**See Diuretics, Potassium-sparing, and Hydrochlorothiazide (Systemic)**, 1272, MC-31
*Mazanor*—Wyeth-Ayerst (U.S.) brand of Mazindol—**See Appetite Suppressants (Systemic)**, 452
Mazindol [*Mazanor; Sanorex*]
  **See Appetite Suppressants (Systemic)**, 452, 3153
  Tablets USP, 456
MC 903—*See* Calcipotriene (Topical), 711
*M-Caps*—Pal-Pak (U.S.) brand of Racemethionine (Systemic), #
MCT Oil—Mead Johnson (U.S. and Canada) brand of Enteral Nutrition Formula, Modular—**See Enteral Nutrition Formulas (Systemic)**, #
MD-76—Mallinckrodt (U.S. and Canada) brand of Diatrizoate—**See Diatrizoates (Systemic)**, #
m-DET—*See* Diethyltoluamide (Topical), #
MD-Gastroview—Mallinckrodt (U.S.) brand of Diatrizoate—**See Diatrizoates (Systemic)**, #
MDP-Squibb—Squibb (U.S.) brand of Technetium Tc 99m Medronate (Systemic), 2718

Measles, Mumps, and Rubella Virus Vaccine Live [*M-M-R II*]
  **(Systemic)**, 1914
  Measles, Mumps, and Rubella Virus Vaccine Live (for Injection) USP, 1917
Measles and Rubella Virus Vaccine Live [*M-R-VAX II*]
  **(Systemic)**, 1918
  Measles and Rubella Virus Vaccine Live (for Injection) USP, 1921
Measles Virus Vaccine Live [*Attenuvax*]
  **(Systemic)**, 1922
  Measles Virus Vaccine Live USP (for Injection), 1926
*Mebaral*—Sanofi Winthrop (U.S. and Canada) brand of Mephobarbital—**See Barbiturates (Systemic)**, 518
Mebendazole [*Vermox*]
  **(Systemic)**, 1926
  Tablets USP (Chewable), 1928
Mecamylamine Hydrochloride [*Inversine*]
  **(Systemic)**, #
  Tablets USP, #
Mecasermin
  **(Systemic)**, 3153
Mechlorethamine Hydrochloride [chlormethine; *Mustargen*; nitrogen mustard]
  **(Systemic)**, 1929
  for Injection USP, 1932
Mechlorethamine Hydrochloride [chlormethine; nitrogen mustard]
  **(Topical)**, #
  Ointment, #
  Solution, Topical, #
*Meclan*—Ortho (U.S.) brand of Meclocycline—**See Tetracyclines (Topical)**, 2774
Meclizine Hydrochloride [*Antivert; Antivert/25; Antivert/50; Bonamine; Bonine; Dramamine II; D-Vert 15; D-Vert 30; Meni-D*]
  **(Systemic)**, 1933
  Capsules, 1934
  Tablets USP, 1934, MC-18
  Tablets USP (Chewable), 1934
Meclocycline Sulfosalicylate [*Meclan*]
  **See Tetracyclines (Topical)**, 2774
  Cream USP, 2776
Meclofenamate Sodium [meclofenamic acid; *Meclomen*]
  **See Anti-inflammatory Drugs, Nonsteroidal (Systemic)**, 388
  Capsules USP, 412 MC-18
Meclofenamic acid—Meclofenamate—**See Anti-inflammatory Drugs, Nonsteroidal (Systemic)**, 388
*Meclomen*—PD (U.S.) brand of Meclofenamate—**See Anti-inflammatory Drugs, Nonsteroidal (Systemic)**, 388
*Mectizan*—MSD (International) brand of Ivermectin (Systemic), #
*Medebag*—Lafayette (U.S.) brand of Barium Sulfate (Local), #
*Medebar Plus*—Lafayette (U.S.) brand of Barium Sulfate (Local), #
*mede-SCAN*—Lafayette (U.S.) brand of Barium Sulfate (Local), #
*Med-Hist*—Med-Tek (U.S.) brand of Chlorpheniramine and Pseudoephedrine—**See Antihistamines and Decongestants (Systemic)**, 343
*Med-Hist Exp*—Med-Tek (U.S.) brand of Pseudoephedrine, Hydrocodone, and Guaifenesin—**See Cough/Cold Combinations (Systemic)**, 1024
*Med-Hist HC*—Med-Tek (U.S.) brand of Chlorpheniramine, Phenylephrine, and Hydrocodone—**See Cough/Cold Combinations (Systemic)**, 1024
*Medigesic*—U.S. Chemical (U.S.) brand of Butalbital, Acetaminophen, and Caffeine—**See Barbiturates and Analgesics (Systemic)**, 532
*Medihaler Ergotamine*—Riker (Canada) brand of Ergotamine—**See Vascular Headache Suppressants, Ergot Derivative-containing (Systemic)**, 2925
*Medihaler-Iso*—3M (U.S.) brand of Isoproterenol—**See Bronchodilators, Adrenergic (Inhalation-Local)**, 640
*Medilax*—Mission (U.S.) brand of Phenolphthalein—**See Laxatives (Local)**, #
*Mediplast*—Beiersdorf (U.S.) brand of Salicylic Acid (Topical), #
*Medipren*—McNeil Consumer (U.S.) brand of Ibuprofen—**See Anti-inflammatory Drugs, Nonsteroidal (Systemic)**, 388

*Medipren Caplets*—McNeil Consumer (U.S. and Canada) brand of Ibuprofen—**See Anti-inflammatory Drugs, Nonsteroidal (Systemic)**, 388
*Mediquell*—Warner-Lambert (U.S.) brand of Dextromethorphan (Systemic), 1191
*Medotar*—Medco (U.S.) brand of Coal Tar (Topical), #
*Medralone-40*—Keene (U.S.) brand of Methylprednisolone—**See Corticosteroids—Glucocorticoid Effects (Systemic)**, 998
*Medralone-80*—Keene (U.S.) brand of Methylprednisolone—**See Corticosteroids—Glucocorticoid Effects (Systemic)**, 998
Medrogestone [*Colprone*]
   **See Progestins (Systemic)**, 2400
   Tablets, 2408
*Medrol*—Pharmacia & Upjohn (U.S. and Canada) brand of Methylprednisolone—**See Corticosteroids—Glucocorticoid Effects (Systemic)**, 998, MC-19
Medroxyprogesterone Acetate [*Alti-MPA; Amen; Curretab; Cycrin; Depo-Provera; Depo-Provera Contraceptive Injection; Gen-Medroxy; Novo-Medrone; Provera Pak*]
   **See Progestins (Systemic)**, 2400
   Suspension, Injectable, USP, 2409
   Tablets USP, 2409, MC-18
Medroxyprogesterone-containing Combinations, 3075
Medrysone [*HMS Liquifilm*]
   **See Corticosteroids (Ophthalmic)**, 966
   Suspension, Ophthalmic, USP, 970
*Med Timolol*—Medican (Canada) brand of Timolol (Ophthalmic), 3036
*Med Valproic*—Median Pharma (Canada) brand of Valproic Acid—**See Valproic Acid (Systemic)**, 2908
Mefenamic Acid [*Ponstan; Ponstel*]
   **See Nonsteroidal Anti-inflammatory Drugs (Systemic)**, 388
   Capsules USP, 412
Mefloquine Hydrochloride [*Lariam; Mephaquin*]
   **(Systemic)**, 1935, 3153
   Tablets, 1937, MC-18
*Mefoxin*—Merck (U.S.) and Frosst (Canada) brand of Cefoxitin—**See Cephalosporins (Systemic)**, 794
*Mega-C/A Plus*—Merit (U.S.) brand of Ascorbic Acid (Systemic), 469
*Megace*—Bristol-Myers Squibb (U.S.) and Mead Johnson (U.S. and Canada) brand of Megestrol—**See Progestins (Systemic)**, 2400, 3153, MC-18
*Megacillin*—Frosst (Canada) brand of Penicillin G—**See Penicillins (Systemic)**, 2240
*Megagen*—Amgen (U.S.) brand of Pegylated Recombinant Human Megakaryocyte Growth and Development Factor (Systemic), 3157
*Megatope*—Iso-Tex Diagnostics (U.S.) brand of Iodinated I 131 Albumin—**See Radioiodinated Albumin (Systemic)**, 2453
Megestrol Acetate [*Apo-Megestrol; Megace*]
   **See Progestins (Systemic)**, 2400, 3153
   Suspension, 2410
   Tablets USP, 2410, MC-18
Meglumine Antimoniate [*Glucantim; Glucantime*]
   **(Systemic)**, #
   for Injection, #
*Megral*—BW (Canada) brand of Ergotamine, Caffeine, and Cyclizine—**See Vascular Headache Suppressants, Ergot Derivative–containing (Systemic)**, 2925
*Melacine*—Ribi ImmunoChem (U.S.) brand of Melanoma Vaccine (Systemic), 3153
Melanoma Cell Vaccine
   **(Systemic)**, 3153
Melanoma Vaccine [*Melacine*]
   **(Systemic)**, 3153
Melarsen oxide-BAL—*See* Melarsoprol (Systemic), #
Melarsoprol [*Arsobal; mel B; melarsen oxide-BAL*]
   **(Systemic)**, #
   for Injection, #
Melatonin
   **(Systemic)**, 3153
Mel B—*See* Melarsoprol (Systemic), #
*Melfiat-105 Unicelles*—Solvay (U.S.) brand of Phendimetrazine—**See Appetite Suppressants (Systemic)**, 452
*Melimmune*—IDEC (U.S.) brand of In-111 Murine MAB(2B8-MXDTPA) and Y-90 Murine MAB(2B8-MXDTPA) (Systemic), 3147; Monoclonal AB (Murine) Anti-Idiotype Melanoma Ass'ted Antigen (Systemic), 3154

*Mellaril*—Novartis (U.S. and Canada) brand of Thioridazine—**See Phenothiazines (Systemic)**, 2289, MC-30
*Mellaril Concentrate*—Sandoz (U.S.) brand of Thioridazine—**See Phenothiazines (Systemic)**, 2289
*Mellaril-S*—Sandoz (U.S.) brand of Thioridazine—**See Phenothiazines (Systemic)**, 2289
Melphalan [*Alkeran; Alkeran for Injection; L-PAM; phenylalanine mustard*]
   **(Systemic)**, 1938, 3153
   for Injection, 1941, 3153
   Tablets USP, 1940, MC-18
Menadiol Sodium Diphosphate [*Synkayvite; vitamin K₄*]
   **See Vitamin K (Systemic)**, 2975
   Injection USP, 2977
   Tablets USP, 2977
*Menaval-20*—Legere (U.S.) brand of Estradiol—**See Estrogens (Systemic)**, 1383
*Menest*—SmithKline Beecham (U.S.) brand of Esterified Estrogens—**See Estrogens (Systemic)**, 1383, MC-12
*Meni-D*—Seatrace (U.S.) brand of Meclizine (Systemic), 1933
Meningococcal Polysaccharide Vaccine [*Menomune*]
   **(Systemic)**, 1941
   for Injection, 1943
*Menoject-L.A.*—Mayrand (U.S.) brand of Testosterone and Estradiol—**See Androgens and Estrogens (Systemic)**, 126
*Menomune*—Connaught (U.S. and Canada) brand of Meningococcal Polysaccharide Vaccine (Systemic), 1941
Menotrophin—*See* Menotropins (Systemic), 1943
Menotropins [*hMG; human gonadotropins; human menopausal gonadotropins; Humegon; menotrophin; Pergonal*]
   **(Systemic)**, 1943
   for Injection USP, 1945
*Mentax*—Penederm (U.S.) brand of Butenafine (Topical), 699
*Mentholatum*—Mentholatum (U.S.) brand of Padimate O—**See Sunscreen Agents (Topical)**, #
Menthyl Anthranilate [*Maxafil*]
   **See Sunscreen Agents (Topical)**, #
   Cream, #
Menthyl Anthranilate-containing Combinations, 3075
Menthyl Anthranilate, Octocrylene, and Octyl Methoxycinnamate [*Neutrogena Sunblock*]
   **See Sunscreen Agents (Topical)**, #
   Cream, #
Menthyl Anthranilate, Octocrylene, Octyl Methoxycinnamate, and Oxybenzone [*Hawaiian Tropic Baby Faces; Hawaiian Tropic Plus*]
   **See Sunscreen Agents (Topical)**, #
   Gel, #
Menthyl Anthranilate and Octyl Methoxycinnamate [*Catrix Correction; Hawaiian Tropic Dark Tanning with Sunscreen; Neutrogena Sunblock*]
   **See Sunscreen Agents (Topical)**, #
   Cream, #
   Lotion, #
Menthyl Anthranilate, Octyl Methoxycinnamate, and Octyl Salicylate [*Neutrogena Sunblock*]
   **See Sunscreen Agents (Topical)**, #
   Cream#
Menthyl Anthranilate, Octyl Methoxycinnamate, Octyl Salicylate, and Oxybenzone [*Hawaiian Baby Faces Sunblock*]
   **See Sunscreen Agents (Topical)**, #
   Lotion, #
Menthyl Anthranilate, Octyl Methoxycinnamate, and Oxybenzone [*Hawaiian Tropic Plus; Hawaiian Tropic Plus Sunblock*]
   **See Sunscreen Agents (Topical)**, #
   Gel, #
   Lip Balm, #
   Lotion, #
Menthyl Anthranilate and Padimate O [*Blistex Medicated Lip Conditioner with Sunscreen*]
   **See Sunscreen Agents (Topical)**, #
   Lip Balm, #
Menthyl Anthranilate and Titanium Dioxide [*A-Fil*]
   **See Sunscreen Agents (Topical)**, #
   Cream, #
*Menu Magic Instant Breakfast*—Menu Magic (U.S.) brand of Enteral Nutrition Formula, Milk-based—**See Enteral Nutrition Formulas (Systemic)**, #
*Menu Magic Milk Shake*—Menu Magic (U.S.) brand of Enteral Nutrition Formula, Milk-based—**See Enteral Nutrition Formulas (Systemic)**, #

*Mepacrine*—*See* Quinacrine (Systemic), #
Mepenzolate Bromide [*Cantil*]
   **See Anticholinergics/Antispasmodics (Systemic)**, 226
   Tablets, 238
Meperidine Hydrochloride [*Demerol; pethidine*]
   **See Opioid (Narcotic) Analgesics (Systemic)**, 2168
   Injection USP, 2179
   Syrup USP, 2178
   Tablets USP, 2179, MC-18
*Mephaquin*—Mepha AG (Switzerland) brand of Mefloquine (Systemic), 3153
Mephentermine Sulfate [*Wyamine*]
   **See Sympathomimetic Agents—Cardiovascular Use (Parenteral-Systemic)**, 2669
   Mephentermine Sulfate, 2677
Mephenytoin [*Mesantoin*]
   **See Anticonvulsants, Hydantoin (Systemic)**, 253
   Tablets USP, 263
Mephobarbital [*Mebaral*]
   **See Barbiturates (Systemic)**, 518
   Tablets USP, 526
*Mephyton*—Merck (U.S.) brand of Phytonadione—**See Vitamin K (Systemic)**, 2975
*MEPIG*—Univax (U.S.) brand of Mucoid Exopolysaccharide Pseudomonas Hyperimmune Globulin (Systemic), 3155
Mepivacaine-containing Combinations, 3075
Mepivacaine Hydrochloride [*Carbocaine; Isocaine; Isocaine 3%; Polocaine; Polocaine-MPF*]
   **See Anesthetics (Parenteral-Local)**, 139
   Injection USP, 151
Mepivacaine Hydrochloride and Levonordefrin [*Carbocaine with Neo-Cobefrin; Isocaine; Isocaine 2%; Polocaine*]
   **See Anesthetics (Parenteral-Local)**, 139
   Injection USP, 152
Meprobamate [*Apo-Meprobamate; Equanil; Meprospan 200; Meprospan 400; Meprospan-400; Miltown; 'Miltown'-200; 'Miltown'-400; 'Miltown'-600; Probate; Trancot*]
   **(Systemic)**, #
   Capsules, Extended-release, #
   Tablets USP, #
Meprobamate and Aspirin [*Epromate-M; Equagesic; Heptogesic; Meprogesic; Meprogesic Q; Micrainin*]
   **(Systemic)**, #
   Tablets, #
Meprobamate-containing Combinations, 3075
*Meprogesic*—Balan (U.S.) and Dixon-Shane (U.S.) brand of Meprobamate and Aspirin (Systemic), #
*Meprogesic Q*—Best (U.S.); Harber (U.S.); and Texas Drug (U.S.) brand of Meprobamate and Aspirin (Systemic), #
*Meprolone*—Major (U.S.) brand of Methylprednisolone—**See Corticosteroids—Glucocorticoid Effects (Systemic)**, 998
*Mepron*—BW (U.S. and Canada) brand of Atovaquone (Systemic), 483, 3132
*Meprospan 200*—Wallace (U.S.) brand of Meprobamate (Systemic), #
*Meprospan-400*—Horner (Canada) brand of Meprobamate (Systemic), #
*Meprospan 400*—Wallace (U.S.) brand of Meprobamate (Systemic), #
*Mepyramine*—Pyrilamine—**See Antihistamines (Systemic)**, 325
Mercaptopurine [*Purinethol; 6-MP*]
   **(Systemic)**, 1946
   Tablets USP, 1949, MC-18
*Mercodol with Decapryn*—Marion Merrell Dow (Canada) brand of Doxylamine, Etafedrine, and Hydrocodone—**See Cough/Cold Combinations (Systemic)**, 1024
*Meridia*—Knoll (U.S.) brand of Sibutramine (Systemic), 2571, MC-28
*Meritene*—Sandoz (U.S.) brand of Enteral Nutrition Formula, Milk-based—**See Enteral Nutrition Formulas (Systemic)**, #
Meropenem [*Merrem I.V.*]
   **(Systemic)**, 1949
   for Injection, 1951
*Merrem I.V.*—ZENECA (U.S.) brand of Meropenem (Systemic), 1949
*Mersyndol with Codeine*—Marion Merrell Dow (Canada) brand of Doxylamine, Codeine, and Acetaminophen—**See Cough/Cold Combinations (Systemic)**, 1024

*Meruvax II*—Merck (U.S. and Canada) brand of Rubella Virus Vaccine Live (Systemic), 2532
Mesalamine [5-aminosalicylic acid; 5-ASA; *Asacol; Mesasal; Pentasa; Salofalk*]
  **(Oral-Local)**, 1952
  Capsules, MC-18
  Capsules, Extended-release, 1953, MC-18
  Tablets, Delayed-release, 1953, MC-18
  Tablets, Extended-release, 1954
Mesalamine [5-aminosalicylic acid; 5-ASA; mesalazine; *Rowasa; Salofalk*]
  **(Rectal-Local)**, 1954
  Suppositories, 1955
  Suspension, Rectal, 1955
Mesalazine—See Mesalamine (Oral-Local), 1952; Mesalamine (Rectal-Local), 1954
*Mesantoin*—Sandoz (U.S. and Canada) brand of Mephenytoin—**See Anticonvulsants, Hydantoin (Systemic)**, 253
*Mesasal*—SmithKline Beecham (Canada) brand of Mesalamine (Oral-Local), 1952, MC-18
*Mescolor*—Horizon (U.S.) brand of Chlorpheniramine, Pseudoephedrine, and Methscopolamine—**See Antihistamines, Decongestants, and Anticholinergics (Systemic)**, 373
*M-Eslon*—Rhône-Poulenc Rorer (Canada) brand of Morphine—**See Opioid (Narcotic) Analgesics (Systemic)**, 2168
Mesna [*MESNEX; Uromitexan*]
  **(Systemic)**, 1956, 3153
  Injection, 1957
*MESNEX*—Degussa (U.S.) and Meadjohnson (U.S.) brand of Mesna (Systemic), 1956, 3153
Mesoridazine Besylate [*Serentil; Serentil Concentrate*]
  **See Phenothiazines (Systemic)**, 2289
  Injection USP, 2301
  Solution, Oral, USP, 2301
  Tablets USP, 2301, MC-18
*Mestinon*—ICN (U.S. and Canada) brand of Pyridostigmine—**See Antimyasthenics (Systemic)**, 437
*Mestinon-SR*—ICN (Canada) brand of Pyridostigmine—**See Antimyasthenics (Systemic)**, 437
*Mestinon Timespans*—ICN (U.S.) brand of Pyridostigmine—**See Antimyasthenics (Systemic)**, 437
Mestranol-containing Combinations, 3075
Mesuximide—Methsuximide—**See Anticonvulsants, Succinimide (Systemic)**, #
*Metaderm Mild*—Riva (Canada) brand of Betamethasone—**See Corticosteroids (Topical)**, 978
*Metaderm Regular*—Riva (Canada) brand of Betamethasone—**See Corticosteroids (Topical)**, 978
*Metahistine D*—Econolab (U.S.) and H.L. Moore (U.S.) brand of Pheniramine, Phenyltoloxamine, Pyrilamine, and Phenylpropanolamine—**See Antihistamines and Decongestants (Systemic)**, 343
*Metahydrin*—Merrell Dow (U.S.) brand of Trichlormethiazide—**See Diuretics, Thiazide (Systemic)**, 1273
Meta-iodobenzyl-guanidine—*See* Iobenguane Sulfate I 131 (Systemic), 3149
Meta-iodobenzylguanidine—I 131 Iobenguane—**See Iobenguane, Radioiodinated (Systemic—Therapeutic)**, 1749; Iobenguane I 123—**See Iobenguane, Radioiodinated (Systemic—Diagnostic)**, 1747; Iobenguane I 131—**See Iobenguane, Radioiodinated (Systemic—Diagnostic)**, 1747
Metamfetamine—Methamphetamine—**See Amphetamines (Systemic)**, 94
*Metamucil*—Procter & Gamble (U.S. and Canada) brand of Psyllium Hydrophilic Mucilloid—**See Laxatives (Local)**, #
*Metamucil Apple Crisp Fiber Wafers*—Procter & Gamble (U.S.) brand of Psyllium Hydrophilic Mucilloid—**See Laxatives (Local)**, #
*Metamucil Cinnamon Spice Fiber Wafers*—Procter & Gamble (U.S.) brand of Psyllium Hydrophilic Mucilloid—**See Laxatives (Local)**, #
*Metamucil Orange Flavor*—Procter & Gamble (U.S. and Canada) brand of Psyllium Hydrophilic Mucilloid—**See Laxatives (Local)**, #
*Metamucil Smooth, Citrus Flavor*—Procter & Gamble (U.S.) brand of Psyllium Hydrophilic Mucilloid—**See Laxatives (Local)**, #
*Metamucil Smooth, Orange Flavor*—Procter & Gamble (U.S.) brand of Psyllium Hydrophilic Mucilloid—**See Laxatives (Local)**, #

*Metamucil Smooth Sugar-Free, Citrus Flavor*—Procter & Gamble (U.S.) brand of Psyllium Hydrophilic Mucilloid—**See Laxatives (Local)**, #
*Metamucil Smooth Sugar-Free, Orange Flavor*—Procter & Gamble (U.S.) brand of Psyllium Hydrophilic Mucilloid—**See Laxatives (Local)**, #
*Metamucil Smooth Sugar-Free, Regular Flavor*—Procter & Gamble (U.S.) brand of Psyllium Hydrophilic Mucilloid—**See Laxatives (Local)**, #
*Metamucil Sugar Free*—Searle (Canada) brand of Psyllium Hydrophilic Mucilloid—**See Laxatives (Local)**, #
*Metamucil Sugar-Free, Lemon-Lime Flavor*—Procter & Gamble (U.S.) brand of Psyllium Hydrophilic Mucilloid—**See Laxatives (Local)**, #
*Metamucil Sugar-Free, Orange Flavor*—Procter & Gamble (U.S. and Canada) brand of Psyllium Hydrophilic Mucilloid—**See Laxatives (Local)**, #
*Metandren*—Novartis (Canada) brand of Methyltestosterone—**See Androgens (Systemic)**, 118
*Metaprel*—Dorsey (U.S.) brand of Metaproterenol—**See Bronchodilators, Adrenergic (Systemic)**, 651
Metaproterenol Sulfate [*Alupent; Arm-a-Med Metaproterenol; Dey-Lute Metaproterenol;* orciprenaline]
  **See Bronchodilators, Adrenergic (Inhalation-Local)**, 640
  Aerosol, Inhalation, USP, 649
  Solution, Inhalation, USP, 649
Metaproterenol Sulfate [*Alupent; Metaprel;* orciprenaline; *Prometa*]
  **See Bronchodilators, Adrenergic (Systemic)**, 651
  Syrup USP, 659
  Tablets USP, 659 MC-18
Metaraminol Bitartrate [*Aramine*]
  **See Sympathomimetic Agents—Cardiovascular Use (Parenteral-Systemic)**, 2669
  Injection USP, 2677
*Metastron*—Amersham (U.S. and Canada) brand of Strontium Chloride Sr 89 (Systemic), 2632
*Metatensin*—Merrell Dow (U.S.) brand of Reserpine and Trichlormethiazide—**See Rauwolfia Alkaloids and Thiazide Diuretics (Systemic)**, #
Metaxalone [*Skelaxin*]
  **See Skeletal Muscle Relaxants (Systemic)**, 2577
  Tablets, 2580
*Meted*—GenDerm (U.S. and Canada) brand of Salicylic Acid and Sulfur (Topical), #
Metformin Hydrochloride [*Glucophage; Novo-Metformin*]
  **(Systemic)**, 1957
  Tablets, 1961, MC-19
Methacholine Chloride [*Provocholine*]
  **(Inhalation-Local)**, #
  for Inhalation, #
Methadone Hydrochloride [*Dolophine; Methadose*]
  **See Opioid (Narcotic) Analgesics (Systemic)**, 2168
  Concentrate, Oral, USP, 2180
  Injection USP, 2181
  Solution, Oral, USP, 2180
  Tablets USP, 2180
  Tablets USP (Dispersible), 2181
*Methadose*—Mallinckrodt (U.S.) brand of Methadone—**See Opioid (Narcotic) Analgesics (Systemic)**, 2168
Methamphetamine Hydrochloride [*Desoxyn; Desoxyn Gradumet;* metamfetamine]
  **See Amphetamines (Systemic)**, 94
  Tablets USP, 98
  Tablets, Extended-release, 98
Methantheline Bromide [*Banthine;* methanthelinium]
  **See Anticholinergics/Antispasmodics (Systemic)**, 226
  Tablets, 238
Methanthelinium—Methantheline—**See Anticholinergics/Antispasmodics (Systemic)**, 226
Metharbital [*Gemonil*]
  **See Barbiturates (Systemic)**, 518
  Tablets, 526
Methazolamide [*MZM; Neptazane*]
  **See Carbonic Anhydrase Inhibitors (Systemic)**, 773
  Tablets USP, 778
Methdilazine Hydrochloride [*Tacaryl*]
  **See Antihistamines, Phenothiazine-derivative (Systemic)**, 377
  Syrup USP, 381
  Tablets USP, 381
  Tablets USP (Chewable), 381

Methenamine-containing Combinations, 3075
Methenamine Hippurate [*Hiprex; Hip-Rex; Urex*]
  **(Systemic)**, #
  Tablets USP, #
Methenamine Mandelate [*Mandelamine*]
  **(Systemic)**, #
  for Solution, Oral, USP (Granules), #
  Suspension, Oral, USP, #
  Tablets USP, #
  Tablets USP (Enteric-coated), #
*Methergine*—Novartis (U.S.) brand of Methylergonovine (Systemic), 1984, MC-19
Methicillin Sodium [meticillin; *Staphcillin*]
  **See Penicillins (Systemic)**, 2240
  for Injection USP, 2252
Methimazole [*Tapazole;* thiamazole]
  **See Antithyroid Agents (Systemic)**, 446
  Suppositories, 450
  Tablets USP, 449
Methionine—*See* Racemethionine (Systemic), #
Methionine C 11[L-methyl-[11] methionine]
  **(Systemic)**, #
  Injection USP, #
Methionine/L-Methionine
  **(Systemic)**, 3153
Methocarbamol [*Carbacot; Robaxin; Robaxin-750; Skelex*]
  **See Skeletal Muscle Relaxants (Systemic)**, 2577
  Injection USP, 2581
  Tablets USP, 2581, MC-19
Methocarbamol and Aspirin [*Robaxisal*]
  **(Systemic)**
  Tablets, MC-19
*Methocel*—Ciba Vision (Canada) brand of Hydroxypropyl Methylcellulose (Ophthalmic), #
Methohexital Sodium [*Brevital; Brietal;* methohexitone]
  **See Anesthetics, Barbiturate (Systemic)**, 161
  for Injection USP, 165
  for Solution, Rectal, 166
Methohexitone—Methohexital—**See Anesthetics, Barbiturate (Systemic)**, 161
*Methotrexate*—Lederle (U.S.) brand of Methotrexate (Systemic), 3154
Methotrexate [amethopterin]
  **(Systemic—For Cancer)**, 1962
  Tablets USP, 1967
*Methotrexate/Azone*—Discovery Therapeutics (U.S.) brand of Methotrexate with Laurocapram (Systemic), 3154
Methotrexate [amethopterin; *Rheumatrex*]
  **(Systemic—for Noncancerous Conditions)**, 1969, 3153
  Tablets USP, 1972, MC-19
Methotrexate with Laurocapram [*Methotrexate/Azone*]
  **(Topical)**, 3152
Methotrexate Sodium [amethopterin]
  **(Systemic—For Cancer)**, 1962, 3153
  Injection USP, 1967
  for Injection USP, 1968
Methotrexate Sodium [amethopterin; *Folex; Folex PFS; Mexate; Mexate-AQ*]
  **(Systemic—for Noncancerous Conditions )**, 1969
  Injection USP, 1972
  for Injection USP, 1972
Methotrimeprazine [levomepromazine; *Levoprome; Nozinan*]
  **See Phenothiazines (Systemic)**, 2289
  Injection USP, 2303
Methotrimeprazine Hydrochloride [levomepromazine; *Nozinan Liquid; Nozinan Oral Drops*]
  **See Phenothiazines (Systemic)**, 2289
  Solution, Oral, 2302
  Syrup, 2302
Methotrimeprazine Maleate [levomepromazine; *Nozinan*]
  **See Phenothiazines (Systemic)**, 2289
  Tablets, 2302
Methoxamine Hydrochloride [*Vasoxyl*]
  **See Sympathomimetic Agents—Cardiovascular Use (Parenteral-Systemic)**, 2669
  Injection, 2678
Methoxsalen [*8-MOP; Oxsoralen; Oxsoralen-Ultra; Ultra MOP*]
  **(Systemic)**, 1973
  Capsules USP (XXI) (Hard Gelatin), 1976
  Capsules USP (XXII) (Soft Gelatin), 1976
8-Methoxsalen [*Uvadex*]
  **(Systemic)**, 3128

Methoxsalen [*Oxsoralen Lotion; UltraMOP Lotion*]
  (Topical), 1977
  Solution, Topical, USP, 1979
Methoxyflurane [*Penthrane*]
  See Anesthetics, Inhalation (Systemic), 168
  Methoxyflurane USP, 172
Methscopolamine Bromide [hyoscine methobromide; *Pamine*]
  See Anticholinergics/Antispasmodics (Systemic), 226
  Tablets, 238
Methscopolamine-containing Combinations, 3075
Methsuximide [*Celontin; mesuximide*]
  See Anticonvulsants, Succinimide (Systemic), #
  Capsules USP, #
Methyclothiazide [*Aquatensen; Duretic; Enduron*]
  See Diuretics, Thiazide (Systemic), 1273
  Tablets USP, 1280, MC-19
Methyclothiazide-containing Combinations, 3075
Methylcellulose [*Citrucel Orange Flavor; Citrucel Sugar-Free Orange Flavor; Cologel*]
  See Laxatives (Local), #
  Capsules, #
  Granules, #
  Powder, #
  Solution, Oral, USP, #
  Tablets USP, #
Methyldopa [*Aldomet; Apo-Methyldopa; Dopamet; Novomedopa; Nu-Medopa*]
  (Systemic), 1979
  Suspension, Oral USP, 1982
  Tablets USP, 1982
Methyldopa and Chlorothiazide [*Aldoclor-150; Aldoclor-250; Supres-150; Supres-250*]
  See Methyldopa and Thiazide Diuretics (Systemic), 1983
  Tablets USP, 1983
Methyldopa-containing Combinations, 3075
Methyldopa and Hydrochlorothiazide [*Aldoril-15; Aldoril-25; Aldoril D30; Aldoril D50; Novodoparil; PMS Dopazide*]
  See Methyldopa and Thiazide Diuretics (Systemic), 1983
  Tablets USP, 1984, MC-19
Methyldopate Hydrochloride [*Aldomet*]
  (Systemic), 1979
  Injection USP, 1982
Methyldopa and Thiazide Diuretics
  (Systemic), 1983
Methylene Blue [aniline violet; methylthioninie chloride; methylthioninium chloride; tetramethylthionine chloride; *Urolene Blue*]
  (Systemic), #
  Injection USP, #
  Tablets, #
Methylergometrine—See Methylergonovine (Systemic), 1984
Methylergonovine Maleate [*Methergine; methylergometrine*]
  (Systemic), 1984
  Injection USP, 1987
  Tablets USP, 1987, MC-19
Methylnaltrexone
  (Systemic), 3154
Methylphenidate Hydrochloride [*PMS-Methylphenidate; Ritalin; Ritalin-SR*]
  (Systemic), 1987
  Tablets USP, 1989, MC-19
  Tablets, Extended-release, USP, 1989, MC-19
4-Methylpyrazole—See Fomepizole (Systemic), 1526
Methylprednisolone [*Medrol; Meprolone*]
  See Corticosteroids—Glucocorticoid Effects (Systemic), 998
  Tablets USP, 1010, MC-19
Methylprednisolone Acetate [*depMedalone 40; depMedalone 80; Depoject-40; Depoject-80; Depo-Medrol; Depopred-40; Depopred-80; Depo-Predate 40; Depo-Predate 80; Duralone-40; Duralone-80; Medralone-40; Medralone-80; Rep-Pred 40; Rep-Pred 80*]
  See Corticosteroids—Glucocorticoid Effects (Systemic), 998
  Suspension, Sterile, USP, 1010
Methylprednisolone Sodium Succinate [*A-methaPred; Solu-Medrol*]
  See Corticosteroids—Glucocorticoid Effects (Systemic), 998, 3028
  for Injection USP, 1010, 3028
4-Methylpyrazole
  (Systemic), 3128

Methyltestosterone [*Android; Metandren; ORETON Methyl; Testred; Virilon*]
  See Androgens (Systemic), 118
  Capsules USP, 124
  Tablets, USP (Oral), 124
Methyltestosterone-containing Combinations, 3075
Methyltestosterone and Esterified Estrogens [*Estratest; Estratest HS*]
  (Systemic), MC-19
  Tablets, MC-19
Methylthionine chloride—See Methylene Blue (Systemic), #
Methylthioninium chloride—See Methylene Blue (Systemic), #
Methyprylon [*Noludar*]
  (Systemic), #
  Capsules USP, #
  Tablets USP, #
Methysergide Maleate [*Sansert*]
  (Systemic), 1990
  Tablets USP, 1992
Meticillin—Methicillin—See Penicillins (Systemic), 2240
*Meticorten*—Schering (U.S.) brand of Prednisone—See Corticosteroids—Glucocorticoid Effects (Systemic), 998
Metipranolol Hydrochloride [*OptiPranolol*]
  See Beta-adrenergic Blocking Agents (Ophthalmic), 585
  Solution, Ophthalmic, 592
Metoclopramide [*Apo-Metoclop; Maxeran; Octamide; PMS-Metoclopramide; Reglan*]
  (Systemic), 1992
  Injection USP, 1995
  Tablets USP, 1995
  Solution, Oral USP, 1995, MC-19
Metoclopramide Hydrochloride [*Metoclopramide Intensol*]
  (Systemic), 1992
  Solution, Oral, Concentrate, 1995
*Metoclopramide Intensol*—Roxane (Canada) brand of Metoclopramide Hydrochloride (Systemic), 1992
Metocurine Iodide [*Metubine Iodide*]
  See Neuromuscular Blocking Agents (Systemic), 2098
  Injection USP, 2102
Metolazone [*Diulo; Mykrox; Zaroxolyn*]
  See Diuretics, Thiazide (Systemic), 1273
  Tablets, Extended, 1280
  Tablets, Prompt, 1280
*Metopirone*—Ciba (U.S. and Canada) brand of Metyrapone (Systemic), #
Metoprolol-containing Combinations, 3075
Metoprolol Succinate [*Toprol-XL*]
  See Beta-adrenergic Blocking Agents (Systemic), 593
  Tablets, Extended-release, 603, MC-20
Metoprolol Tartrate [*Apo-Metoprolol; Apo-Metoprolol (Type L); Betaloc; Betaloc Durules; Lopresor; Lopresor SR; Lopressor; Novometoprol; Nu-Metop*]
  See Beta-adrenergic Blocking Agents (Systemic), 593
  Injection USP, 604
  Tablets USP, 603, MC-20
  Tablets, Extended-release, 604
Metoprolol Tartrate and Hydrochlorothiazide [*Lopressor HCT*]
  See Beta-adrenergic Blocking Agents and Thiazide Diuretics (Systemic), 609
  Tablets USP, 610, MC-20
*Metric 21*—Fielding (U.S.) brand of Metronidazole (Systemic), 1996
Metrizamide [*Amipaque*]
  (Systemic), #
  for Injection, #
*Metro-Cream*—Galderma (U.S.) brand of Metronidazole (Topical), 3028
*Metrodin*—Serono (U.S. and Canada) brand of Urofollitropin (Systemic), 2901, 3170
*MetroGel*—Galderma (U.S. and Canada) brand of Metronidazole (Topical), 2000, 3154
*MetroGel-Vaginal*—3M (U.S.) brand of Metronidazole (Vaginal), 2001
*Metro I.V.*—McGaw (U.S.) brand of Metronidazole (Systemic), 1996

Metronidazole [*Apo-Metronidazole; Flagyl; Flagyl 375; Flagyl ER ; Flagyl I.V. RTU; Helidac Therapy Tablets ; Metric 21; Metro I.V.; Novonidazol; Protostat; Trikacide*]
  (Systemic), 1996
  Capsules, 1999, MC-20
  Injection USP, 1999
  Tablets, Extended release, MC-20
  Tablets USP, 1999, MC-4, MC-20
Metronidazole [*Flagyl; Metro-Cream; MetroGel*]
  (Topical), 2000, 3028, 3154
  Cream, 3028
  Gel, Topical, 2001
Metronidazole [*Flagyl; Nidagel; MetroGel-Vaginal*]
  (Vaginal), 2001
  Cream, Vaginal, 2004
  Gel, Vaginal, 2004
  Tablets, Vaginal, 2004
Metronidazole-containing Combinations, 3075
Metronidazole Hydrochloride [*Flagyl I.V.*]
  (Systemic), 1996
  for Injection, 2000
Metronidazole and Nystatin [*Flagystatin*]
  (Vaginal), 3028
  Cream, Vaginal, 3028
  Suppositories, Vaginal, 3028
  Tablets, Vaginal, 3028
*Metubine Iodide*—Lilly (U.S. and Canada) brand of Metocurine—See Neuromuscular Blocking Agents (Systemic), 2098
Metyrapone [*Metopirone*]
  (Systemic), #
  Tablets USP, #
Metyrosine [*Demser*]
  (Systemic), #
  Capsules USP, #
*Mevacor*—Merck (U.S. and Canada) brand of Lovastatin—See HMG-CoA Reductase Inhibitors (Systemic), 1647, MC-18
Mevinolin—Lovastatin—See HMG-CoA Reductase Inhibitors (Systemic), 1647
*Mexate*—Bristol (U.S.) brand of Methotrexate—For Noncancerous Conditions (Systemic), 1969
*Mexate-AQ*—Bristol (U.S.) brand of Methotrexate—For Noncancerous Conditions (Systemic), 1969
Mexiletine Hydrochloride [*Mexitil*]
  (Systemic), 2005
  Capsules USP, 2007, MC-20
*Mexitil*—Boehringer Ingelheim (U.S. and Canada) brand of Mexiletine (Systemic), 2005, MC-20
*Mezlin*—Miles (U.S.) brand of Mezlocillin—See Penicillins (Systemic), 2240
Mezlocillin Sodium [*Mezlin*]
  See Penicillins (Systemic), 2240
  Sterile USP, 2253
*MGP*—Jones-Western (U.S.) brand of Magnesium Gluconate—See Magnesium Supplements (Systemic), 1897
*M-Hist*—McNeil (U.S.) brand of Brompheniramine and Pseudoephedrine—See Antihistamines and Decongestants (Systemic), 343
*Miacalcin*—Sandoz (U.S.) brand of Calcitonin (Nasal-Systemic), 714; Calcitonin-Salmon—See Calcitonin (Systemic), 716
*Mi-Acid*—Major (U.S.) brand of Alumina, Magnesia, and Simethicone—See Antacids (Oral-Local), 188; Calcium and Magnesium Carbonates—See Antacids (Oral-Local), 188
*Mi-Acid Double Strength*—Major (U.S.) brand of Alumina, Magnesia, and Simethicone—See Antacids (Oral-Local), 188
Mibefradil Hydrochloride [*Posicor*]
  (Systemic), #
  Tablets, #
mIBG—I 131 Iobenguane—See Iobenguane, Radioiodinated (Systemic—Therapeutic), 1749; Iobenguane I 123—See Iobenguane, Radioiodinated (Systemic—Diagnostic), 1747; Iobenguane I 131—See Iobenguane, Radioiodinated (Systemic—Diagnostic), 1747; See also Iobenguane Sulfate I 131 (Systemic), 3149
*Micanol*—Bioglan (U.S.) brand of Anthralin (Topical), 218
*Micatin*—Advanced Care (U.S.) and McNeil (Canada) brand of Miconazole (Topical), #
*Miconazole*—Technilab (U.S.) brand of Miconazole—See Antifungals, Azole (Vaginal), 310
*Miconazole-7*—Family Pharmacy (U.S.) brand of Miconazole—See Antifungals, Azole (Vaginal), 310

Miconazole Nitrate [*Femizol-M; Miconazole; Miconazole-7; Monistat 3; Monistat 3 Combination Pack; Monistat 7; Monistat 7 Combination Pack; Monistat 3 Dual-Pak; Monistat 7 Dual-Pak; Monistat 3 Vaginal Ovules; Monistat 5 Tampons; Monistat 7 Vaginal Suppositories; Monazole 7; Novo-Miconazole Vaginal Ovules*]
**See Antifungals, Azole (Vaginal),** 310
  Cream, Vaginal, 313
  Suppositories, Vaginal, USP, 313
  Tampons, Vaginal, 313
Miconazole Nitrate [*Micatin; Monistat-Derm; Zeasorb-AF*]
  **(Topical),** #
  Aerosol Powder, Topical, #
  Aerosol Solution, Topical, #
  Cream USP, #
  Lotion, #
  Powder, Topical, USP, #
*Micrainin*—Wallace (U.S.) brand of Meprobamate and Aspirin (Systemic), #
*MICRhoGAM*—Ortho Diagnostic (U.S.) brand of Rh₀(D) Immune Globulin (Systemic), 2476
Microbubble Contrast Agent [*Filmix Neurosonographic Contrast Agent*]
  **(Diagnostic),** 3154
*Micro-K*—Robins (U.S. and Canada) brand of Potassium Chloride—**See Potassium Supplements (Systemic),** 2357, MC-25
*Micro-K 10*—Robins (U.S. and Canada) brand of Potassium Chloride—**See Potassium Supplements (Systemic),** 2357
*Micro-K LS*—Robins (U.S.) brand of Potassium Chloride—**See Potassium Supplements (Systemic),** 2357
*Microlipid*—Sherwood (U.S.) brand of Enteral Nutrition Formula, Modular—**See Enteral Nutrition Formulas (Systemic),** #
*Micronase*—Pharmacia & Upjohn (U.S.) brand of Glyburide—**See Antidiabetic Agents, Sulfonylurea (Systemic),** 283, MC-14
*microNefrin*—Bird (U.S.) brand of Epinephrine—**See Bronchodilators, Adrenergic (Inhalation-Local),** 640
*Micronor*—Ortho (U.S. and Canada) brand of Norethindrone—**See Progestins (Systemic),** 2400
*Microzide*—Watson (U.S.) brand of Hydrochlorothiazide—**See Diuretics, Thiazide (Systemic),** 1273
*Midahist DH*—Vangard (U.S.) brand of Chlorpheniramine, Pseudoephedrine, and Codeine—**See Cough/Cold Combinations (Systemic),** 1024
*Midamor*—Merck (U.S. and Canada) brand of Amiloride—**See Diuretics, Potassium-sparing (Systemic),** 1266, MC-2
Midazolam Hydrochloride [*Versed*]
  **(Systemic),** 2007
  Injection, 2012
  Solution, Oral, 2012
*Midchlor*—Schein (U.S.) brand of Isometheptene, Dichloralphenazone, and Acetaminophen (Systemic), 1786
Midodrine Hydrochloride [*Amatine; ProAmatine*]
  **(Systemic),** 2014, 3154
  Tablets, 2016
*Midol IB*—Sterling Health (U.S.) brand of Ibuprofen—**See Anti-inflammatory Drugs, Nonsteroidal (Systemic),** 388
*Midrin*—Carnrick (U.S.) brand of Isometheptene, Dichloralphenazone, and Acetaminophen (Systemic), 1786
*Migergot*—G & W (U.S.) brand of Ergotamine and Caffeine—**See Vascular Headache Suppressants, Ergot Derivative-containing (Systemic),** 2925
*Migquin*—Qualitest (U.S.) brand of Isometheptene, Dichloralphenazone, and Acetaminophen (Systemic), 1786
*Migranal*—Novartis (U.S.) brand of Dihydroergotamine (Nasal-Systemic), 1221
*Migrapap*—Mikart (U.S.) brand of Isometheptene, Dichloralphenazone, and Acetaminophen (Systemic), 1786
*Migratine*—Major (U.S.) brand of Isometheptene, Dichloralphenazone, and Acetaminophen (Systemic), 1786
*Migrazone*—Econolab (U.S.) brand of Isometheptene, Dichloralphenazone, and Acetaminophen (Systemic), 1786
*Migrend*—Econolab (U.S.) brand of Isometheptene, Dichloralphenazone, and Acetaminophen (Systemic), 1786

*Migrex*—Balan (U.S.); Best Generics (U.S.); Dixon-Shane (U.S.); Parmed (U.S.); and Texas Drug (U.S.) brand of Isometheptene, Dichloralphenazone, and Acetaminophen (Systemic), 1786
*Milkinol*—Schwarz (U.S.) brand of Mineral Oil—**See Laxatives (Local),** #
Milk of magnesia—Magnesium Hydroxide—**See Laxatives (Local),** #
*Milophene*—Milex (U.S.) brand of Clomiphene (Systemic), 903
Milrinone [*Primacor*]
  **(Systemic),** 2016
  Injection, 2017
*Miltown*—Horner (Canada) brand of Meprobamate (Systemic), #
*'Miltown'-200*—Wallace (U.S.) brand of Meprobamate (Systemic), #
*'Miltown'-400*—Wallace (U.S.) brand of Meprobamate (Systemic), #
*'Miltown'-600*—Wallace (U.S.) brand of Meprobamate (Systemic), #
Mineral Oil [*Fleet Enema Mineral Oil; Fleet Mineral Oil; Kondremul; Kondremul Plain; Lansoÿl; Lansoÿl Sugar Free; Liqui-Doss; Milkinol; Nujol; Petrogalar Plain; Zymenol*]
  **See Laxatives (Local),** #
  Emulsion, #
  Emulsion USP, #
  Enema USP, #
  Gel, #
  Oil USP, #
  Suspension, Oral, #
Mineral Oil-containing Combinations, 3075
Mineral Oil and Glycerin [*Agarol Plain*]
  **See Laxatives (Local),** #
  Emulsion, #
Mineral Oil, Glycerin, and Phenolphthalein [*Agarol Strawberry; Agarol Vanilla*]
  **See Laxatives (Local),** #
  Emulsion, #
Mineral Oil and Phenolphthalein [*Agoral Marshmallow; Agoral Raspberry; Phenolphthalein Petrogalar*]
  **See Laxatives (Local),** #
  Emulsion, #
  Suspension, Oral, #
*Minestrin 1/20*—PD (Canada) brand of Norethindrone Acetate and Ethinyl Estradiol—**See Estrogens and Progestins—Oral Contraceptives (Systemic),** 1397
*Mini-Gamulin Rh*—Armour (U.S.) brand of Rh₀(D) Immune Globulin (Systemic), 2476
*Minims Atropine*—Smith & Nephew (Canada) brand of Atropine (Ophthalmic), 485
*Minims Cyclopentolate*—Smith & Nephew (Canada) brand of Cyclopentolate (Ophthalmic), #
*Minims Homatropine*—Smith & Nephew (Canada) brand of Homatropine (Ophthalmic), 1651
*Minims Phenylephrine*—Smith & Nephew (Canada) brand of Phenylephrine (Ophthalmic), #, 3032
*Minims Pilocarpine*—Smith & Nephew (Canada) brand of Pilocarpine (Ophthalmic), #
*Minims Tetracaine*—Smith & Nephew (Canada) brand of Tetracaine—**See Anesthetics (Ophthalmic),** #
*Minims Tropicamide*—Smith & Nephew (Canada) brand of Tropicamide (Ophthalmic), #
*Minipress*—Pfizer (U.S. and Canada) brand of Prazosin (Systemic), 2370
*Minitran*—3M (U.S. and Canada) brand of Nitroglycerin—**See Nitrates (Systemic),** 2129
*Minizide*—Pfizer (U.S.) brand of Prazosin and Polythiazide (Systemic), 2374, MC-25
*Minocin*—Lederle (U.S. and Canada) brand of Minocycline—**See Tetracyclines (Systemic),** 2765, MC-20
Minocycline Hydrochloride [*Dynacin; Minocin*]
  **See Tetracyclines (Systemic),** 2765
  Capsules USP, 2771, MC-20
  Sterile USP, 2771
  Suspension, Oral, USP, 2771
  Tablets, 2771, MC-20
*Min-Ovral*—Wyeth-Ayerst (Canada) brand of Levonorgestrel and Ethinyl Estradiol—**See Estrogens and Progestins—Oral Contraceptives (Systemic),** 1397
Minoxidil [*Loniten*]
  **(Systemic),** 2018
  Tablets USP, 2020, MC-20

Minoxidil [*Apo-Gain; Gen-Minoxidil; Minoxigaine; Rogaine; Rogaine for Men; Rogaine for Women*]
  **(Topical),** 2021
  Solution, Topical, 2023
*Minoxigaine*—Kenral (Canada) brand of Minoxidil (Topical), 2021
*Mintezol*—Merck (U.S.) brand of Thiabendazole (Systemic), 2784
*Mintox*—Major (U.S.) brand of Alumina and Magnesia—**See Antacids (Oral-Local),** 188
*Mintox Extra Strength*—Major (U.S.) brand of Alumina, Magnesia, and Simethicone—**See Antacids (Oral-Local),** 188
*Miocarpine*—Iolab (Canada) brand of Pilocarpine (Ophthalmic), #
*Mio-Rel*—International Ethical (U.S.) brand of Orphenadrine—**See Skeletal Muscle Relaxants (Systemic),** 2577
*Miostat*—Alcon (U.S. and Canada) brand of Carbachol (Ophthalmic), 755, 3013
*Miradon*—Schering (U.S.) brand of Anisindione—**See Anticoagulants (Systemic),** 243
*Mirapex*—Boehringer-Ingelheim (Canada) and Pharmacia & Upjohn (U.S.) brand of Pramipexole (Systemic), 2718, 3033
Mirtazapine [*Remeron*]
  **(Systemic),** 2023
  Tablets, 2026, MC-20
Misoprostol [*Cytotec*]
  **(Systemic),** 2026
  Tablets, 2027, MC-20
*Mithracin*—Miles (U.S.) brand of Plicamycin (Systemic), 2334
Mithramycin—**See** Plicamycin (Systemic), 2334
Mitoguazone
  **(Systemic),** 3154
Mitolactol
  **(Systemic),** 3154
Mitomycin [mitomycin-C; *Mutamycin*]
  **(Systemic),** 2028
  for Injection USP, 2030
Mitomycin-C
  **(Ophthalmic),** 3154
Mitomycin-C—**See** Mitomycin (Systemic), 2028
Mitotane [*Lysodren*; o,p'-DDD]
  **(Systemic),** 2031
  Tablets USP, 2032
Mitoxantrone [*Novantrone*]
  **(Systemic),** 2033, 3154
  for Injection Concentrate USP, 2035
Mitoxantrone Hydrochloride [*Novantrone*]
  **(Systemic),** 3154
*Mitride*—Interstate (U.S.) brand of Isometheptene, Dichloralphenazone, and Acetaminophen (Systemic), 1786
*Mitrolan*—Robins (U.S.) and Whitehall Robins (Canada) brand of Polycarbophil—**See Laxatives (Local),** #
*Mivacron*—BW (U.S.) brand of Mivacurium (Systemic), 2036
Mivacurium [*Mivacron*]
  **(Systemic),** 2036
  Injection, 2040
Mivacurium in Dextrose [*Mivacron*]
  **(Systemic),** 2036
  Injection, 2034
MK594—**See** Losartan (Systemic), 1882
MK790—**See** Levomethadyl (Systemic), 1855
*M-M-R II*—Merck (U.S. and Canada) brand of Measles, Mumps, and Rubella Virus Vaccine Live (Systemic), 1914
*Moban*—Du Pont (U.S.) brand of Molindone (Systemic), 2050
*Moban Concentrate*—Du Pont (U.S.) brand of Molindone (Systemic), 2050
*Mobenol*—Horner (Canada) brand of Tolbutamide—**See Antidiabetic Agents, Sulfonylurea (Systemic),** 283
*Mobidin*—Ascher (U.S.) brand of Magnesium Salicylate—**See Salicylates (Systemic),** 2538
*Mobiflex*—Roche (Canada) brand of Tenoxicam—**See Anti-inflammatory Drugs, Nonsteroidal (Systemic),** 388
Moclobemide [*Manerex*]
  **(Systemic),** 3028
  Tablets, 3028
*Moctanin*—Ethitek (U.S.) brand of Monoctanoin (Local), #, 3155
Modafinil
  **(Systemic),** 3154
*Modane*—Savage (U.S.) brand of Phenolphthalein—**See Laxatives (Local),** #

*Modane Bulk*—Savage (U.S.) brand of Psyllium Hydrophilic Mucilloid—**See Laxatives (Local)**, #
*Modane Plus*—Savage (U.S.) brand of Phenolphthalein and Docusate—**See Laxatives (Local)**, #
*Modane Soft*—Savage (U.S.) brand of Docusate—**See Laxatives (Local)**, #
*Modecate*—Squibb (Canada) brand of Fluphenazine—**See Phenothiazines (Systemic)**, 2289
*Modecate Concentrate*—Squibb (Canada) brand of Fluphenazine—**See Phenothiazines (Systemic)**, 2289
*ModiCon*—Ortho (U.S.) brand of Norethindrone and Ethinyl Estradiol—**See Estrogens and Progestins—Oral Contraceptives (Systemic)**, 1397
Modified bovine surfactant extract—*See* Beractant (Intratracheal-Local), 583
Modified Shohl's solution—Sodium Citrate and Citric Acid—**See Citrates (Systemic)**, 881
*Moditen Enanthate*—Squibb (Canada) brand of Fluphenazine—**See Phenothiazines (Systemic)**, 2289
*Moditen HCl*—Squibb (Canada) brand of Fluphenazine—**See Phenothiazines (Systemic)**, 2289
*Moditen HCl-H.P.*—Squibb (Canada) brand of Fluphenazine—**See Phenothiazines (Systemic)**, 2289
*Modrastane*—Sanofi Winthrop (U.S.) brand of Trilostane (Systemic), #
*Moducal*—Mead Johnson (U.S.) brand of Enteral Nutrition Formula, Modular—**See Enteral Nutrition Formulas (Systemic)**, #
*Moduret*—MSD (Canada) brand of Amiloride and Hydrochlorothiazide—**See Diuretics, Potassium-sparing, and Hydrochlorothiazide (Systemic)**, 1272
*Moduretic*—Merck (U.S.) brand of Amiloride and Hydrochlorothiazide—**See Diuretics, Potassium-sparing, and Hydrochlorothiazide (Systemic)**, 1272, MC-2
Moexipril Hydrochloride [*Univasc*]
 **(Systemic)**, 2042
 Tablets, 2045, MC-20
Moexipril Hydrochloride and Hydrochlorothiazide [*Uniretic*]
 **(Systemic)**, 2045
 Tablets, 2049, MC-20
*Mogadon*—Roche (Canada) brand of Nitrazepam—**See Benzodiazepines (Systemic)**, 556
*Moisture Drops*—Bausch & Lomb (U.S. and Canada) brand of Hydroxypropyl Methylcellulose (Ophthalmic), #
*Molatoc*—Hudson (U.S.) brand of Docusate—**See Laxatives (Local)**, #
*Molatoc-CST*—Hudson (U.S.) brand of Casanthranol and Docusate—**See Laxatives (Local)**, #
Molindone Hydrochloride [*Moban; Moban Concentrate*]
 **(Systemic)**, 2050
 Solution, Oral, 2053
 Tablets, 2053
*Mol-Iron*—Schering (U.S.) brand of Ferrous Sulfate—**See Iron Supplements (Systemic)**, 1774
Molybdenum Supplements
 **(Systemic)**, 2053
*Molypen*—LyphoMed (U.S.) brand of Ammonium Molybdate—**See Molybdenum Supplements (Systemic)**, 2053
Mometasone Furoate [*Elocom; Elocon*]
 **See Corticosteroids (Topical)**, 978
 Cream, 994
 Lotion, 994
 Ointment, 994
Mometasone Furoate [*Nasonex*]
 **(Nasal)**, 2055
 Suspension, Nasal, 2057
*Monazole 7*—Taro (Canada) brand of Miconazole—**See Antifungals, Azole (Vaginal)**, 310
*Monistat 1*—Advanced Care Products (U.S.) brand of Tioconazol—**See Antifungals, Azole (Vaginal)**, 310
*Monistat 3*—Ortho Advanced (U.S.) brand of Miconazole—**See Antifungals, Azole (Vaginal)**, 310
*Monistat 3 Combination Pack*—Ortho (U.S.) brand of Miconazole—**See Antifungals, Azole (Vaginal)**, 310
*Monistat 7*—Ortho Advanced (U.S.) and McNeil-CPC (Canada) brand of Miconazole—**See Antifungals, Azole (Vaginal)**, 310
*Monistat 7 Combination Pack*—Ortho Advanced (U.S.) brand of Miconazole—**See Antifungals, Azole (Vaginal)**, 310

*Monistat-Derm*—Ortho (U.S. and Canada) brand of Miconazole (Topical), #
*Monistat 3 Dual-Pak*—McNeil-CPC (Canada) brand of Miconazole—**See Antifungals, Azole (Vaginal)**, 310
*Monistat 7 Dual-Pak*—McNeil-CPC (Canada) brand of Miconazole—**See Antifungals, Azole (Vaginal)**, 310
*Monistat 5 Tampon*—Ortho Advanced (U.S.) brand of Miconazole—**See Antifungals, Azole (Vaginal)**, 310
*Monistat 3 Vaginal Ovules*—McNeil Consumer (Canada) brand of Miconazole—**See Antifungals, Azole (Vaginal)**, 310
*Monistat 7 Vaginal Suppositories*—McNeil Consumer (Canada) brand of Miconazole—**See Antifungals, Azole (Vaginal)**, 310
*Monitan*—Wyeth (Canada) brand of Acebutolol—**See Beta-adrenergic Blocking Agents (Systemic)**, 593
*Monocid*—SmithKline Beecham (U.S.) brand of Cefonicid—**See Cephalosporins (Systemic)**, 794
*Monoclate-P*—Armour (U.S.) brand of Antihemophilic Factor (Systemic), 319
Monoclonal AB (Murine) Anti-Idiotype Melanoma Ass'ted Antigen [*Melimmune*]
 **(Systemic)**, 3154
Monoclonal Antibodies PM-81 and AML-2-23
 **(Systemic)**, 3154
Monoclonal Antibody 17-1A [*Panorex*]
 **(Systemic)**, 3154
Monoclonal Antibody-B43.13 [*Ovarex MAb-B43.13*]
 **(Systemic)**, 3154
Monoclonal Antibody to CD22 Antigen on B-cells, Radiolabeled [*LymphoCIDE*]
 **(Systemic)**, 3155
Monoclonal Antibody 5c8, Humanized, Recombinant
 **(Systemic)**, 3155
Monoclonal Antibody to Cytomegalovirus (Human)
 **(Systemic)**, 3155
Monoclonal Antibody to Hepatitis B Virus (Human)
 **(Systemic)**, 3155
Monoclonal Antibody for Immunization against Lupus Nephritis
 **(Systemic)**, 3155
Monoclonal Antibody PM-81
 **(Systemic)**, 3155
Monoctanoin [*Moctanin*; monooctanoin]
 **(Local)**, #
 Irrigation, #
*Monodox*—Oclassen (U.S.) brand of Doxycycline—**See Tetracyclines (Systemic)**, 2765
*Mono-Gesic*—Central (U.S.) brand of Salsalate—**See Salicylates (Systemic)**, 2538, MC-28
*Monoket*—Schwarz Pharma (U.S.) brand of Isosorbide Mononitrate—**See Nitrates (Systemic)**, 2129, MC-16
Monolaurin [*Glylorin*]
 **(Systemic)**, 3155
*Mononine*—Armour (U.S.) brand of Coagulation Factor IX (Systemic), 3137; Armour (U.S.) brand of Factor IX (Systemic), 1430
Monooctanoin—*See* Monoctanoin (Local), #
Monooctanoin [*Moctanin*]
 **(Local)**, 3155
*Monopril*—Bristol-Myers Squibb (U.S.) brand of Fosinopril—**See Angiotensin-converting Enzyme (ACE) Inhibitors (Systemic)**, 177, MC-13
Montelukast Sodium [*Singulair*]
 **(Systemic)**, 2057
 Tablets, 2059, MC-20
 Tablets, Chewable, 2059, MC-20
*Monurol*—Forest (U.S.) brand of Fosfomycin (Systemic), 1531
*Mooredec*—H.L. Moore (U.S.) brand of Carbinoxamine and Pseudoephedrine—**See Antihistamines and Decongestants (Systemic)**, 343
*8-MOP*—Elder (U.S.) brand of Methoxsalen (Systemic), 1973
*Moracizine*—*See* Moricizine (Systemic), 2060
*Moranyl*—*See* Suramin (Systemic), #
Moricizine Hydrochloride [*Ethmozine*; moracizine]
 **(Systemic)**, 2060
 Tablets, 2062, MC-21
*Morphine Extra-Forte*—Abbott (Canada) brand of Morphine—**See Opioid (Narcotic) Analgesics (Systemic)**, 2168
*Morphine Forte*—Abbott (Canada) brand of Morphine—**See Opioid (Narcotic) Analgesics (Systemic)**, 2168

*Morphine H.P.*—Sabex (Canada) brand of Morphine—**See Opioid (Narcotic) Analgesics (Systemic)**, 2168
Morphine Hydrochloride [*Morphitec; M.O.S.; M.O.S.-S.R.; MSIR ; MS Contin* ]
 **See Opioid (Narcotic) Analgesics (Systemic)**, 2168
 Suppositories, 2185
 Syrup, 2182
 Capsules, MC-21
 Tablets, 2182, MC-21
 Tablets, Extended-release, 2182, MC-21
Morphine Sulfate [*Astramorph PF; Duramorph; Epimorph; Infumorph; Kadian; M-Eslon; Morphine Extra-Forte; Morphine Forte; Morphine H.P.; M S Contin; MSIR; MS-IR; MS/L; MS/L Concentrate; MS/S; OMS Concentrate; Oramorph SR; Rescudose; RMS Uniserts; Roxanol; Roxanol 100; Roxanol UD; Statex; Statex Drops*]
 **See Opioid (Narcotic) Analgesics (Systemic)**, 2168, 3029, 3155
 Capsules, 2182
 Capsules, Extended-release, 2182, 3029
 Concentrate, 3155
 Injection USP, 2184
 Solution, Oral, 2183
 Suppositories, 2185
 Syrup, 2183
 Tablets, 2183
 Tablets, Extended-release, 2183
 Tablets, Soluble, 2184
*Morphitec*—Technilab (Canada) brand of Morphine—**See Opioid (Narcotic) Analgesics (Systemic)**, 2168
*M.O.S.*—ICN (Canada) brand of Morphine—**See Opioid (Narcotic) Analgesics (Systemic)**, 2168
*M.O.S.-S.R.*—ICN (Canada) brand of Morphine—**See Opioid (Narcotic) Analgesics (Systemic)**, 2168
*Motilium*—Janssen (Canada) brand of Domperidone (Systemic), 3018
*Motofen*—Carnrick (U.S.) brand of Difenoxin and Atropine (Systemic), 1210
*Motrin*—Pharmacia & Upjohn (U.S. and Canada) brand of Ibuprofen—**See Anti-inflammatory Drugs, Nonsteroidal (Systemic)**, 388, MC-15
*Motrin Chewables*—McNeil (U.S.) brand of Ibuprofen—**See Anti-inflammatory Drugs, Nonsteroidal (Systemic)**, 388
*Motrin, Children's*—McNeil Consumer (U.S.) brand of Ibuprofen—**See Anti-inflammatory Drugs, Nonsteroidal (Systemic)**, 388
*Motrin, Children's Oral Drops*—McNeil (U.S.) brand of Ibuprofen—**See Anti-inflammatory Drugs, Nonsteroidal (Systemic)**, 388
*Motrin-IB*—Upjohn (U.S. and Canada) brand of Ibuprofen—**See Anti-inflammatory Drugs, Nonsteroidal (Systemic)**, 388
*Motrin-IB Caplets*—Upjohn (U.S. and Canada) brand of Ibuprofen—**See Anti-inflammatory Drugs, Nonsteroidal (Systemic)**, 388
*Motrin IB Sinus*—Upjohn (U.S.) brand of Pseudoephedrine and Ibuprofen—**See Decongestants and Analgesics (Systemic)**, 1180
*Motrin IB Sinus Caplets*—Upjohn (U.S.) brand of Pseudoephedrine and Ibuprofen—**See Decongestants and Analgesics (Systemic)**, 1180
*Motrin, Junior Strength Caplets*—McNeil (U.S.) brand of Ibuprofen—**See Anti-inflammatory Drugs, Nonsteroidal (Systemic)**, 388
*4-MP*—*See* Fomepizole (Systemic), 1526
*6-MP*—*See* Mercaptopurine (Systemic), 1946
*MPI DMSA Kidney Reagent*—Medi-Physics (U.S.) brand of Technetium Tc 99m Succimer (Systemic), 2738
*MPI MAA*—Medi-Physics (U.S.) brand of Technetium Tc 99m Albumin Aggregated (Systemic), 2697
*MPI MDP*—Medi-Physics (U.S.) brand of Technetium Tc 99m Medronate (Systemic), 2718
*MPI Pyrophosphate*—Medi-Physics (U.S.) brand of Technetium Tc 99m Pyrophosphate (Systemic), 2729
*MPI Xenon Xe 133 Gas*—Medi-Physics (U.S.) brand of Xenon Xe 133 (Systemic), 2984
*MPI Xenon Xe 133 Gas Ampul*—Medi-Physics (U.S.) brand of Xenon Xe 133 (Systemic), 2984
*M-R-VAX II*—Merck (U.S.) brand of Measles and Rubella Virus Vaccine Live (Systemic), 1918
*MS Contin*—Purdue (U.S. and Canada) brand of Morphine—**See Opioid (Narcotic) Analgesics (Systemic)**, 2168, MC-21

*MSIR*—Purdue (U.S.) brand of Morphine—**See Opioid (Narcotic) Analgesics (Systemic)**, 2168, MC-21
*MS-IR*—Purdue Frederick (Canada) brand of Morphine—**See Opioid (Narcotic) Analgesics (Systemic)**, 2168
*MS/L*—Richwood (U.S.) brand of Morphine—**See Opioid (Narcotic) Analgesics (Systemic)**, 2168
*MS/L Concentrate*—Richwood (U.S.) brand of Morphine—**See Opioid (Narcotic) Analgesics (Systemic)**, 2168
*MS/S*—Richwood (U.S.) brand of Morphine—**See Opioid (Narcotic) Analgesics (Systemic)**, 2168
*Mucinum*—Sabex (Canada) brand of Phenolphthalein and Senna—**See Laxatives (Local)**, #
*Muco-Fen DM*—Wakefield (U.S.) brand of Dextromethorphan and Guaifenesin—**See Cough/Cold Combinations (Systemic)**, 1024
Mucoid Exopolysaccharide Pseudomonas Hyperimmune Globulin [*MEPIG*] **(Systemic)**, 3155
*Mucolysin*—Proter (Italy) and Interdelta (Switzerland) brand of Tiopronin (Systemic), 2824
*Mucomyst*—Apothecon (U.S. and Canada) brand of Acetylcysteine (Inhalation-Local), #; Apothekon (U.S.) and Bristol-Myers Squibb (Canada) brand of Acetylcysteine (Systemic), 16
*Mucomyst-10*—Apothecon (U.S.) brand of Acetylcysteine (Inhalation-Local), #
*Mucomyst/Mucomyst 10 IV*—Apothecon (U.S.) brand of Acetylcysteine (Systemic), 3129
*Mucosil*—Dey (U.S.) brand of Acetylcysteine (Systemic), 16
*Mucosil-10*—Dey (U.S.) brand of Acetylcysteine (Inhalation-Local), #
*Mucosil-20*—Dey (U.S.) brand of Acetylcysteine (Inhalation-Local), #
*Multipax*—Rorer (Canada) brand of Hydroxyzine—**See Antihistamines (Systemic)**, 325
Multi-Vitamin Infusion (Neonatal Formula) **(Systemic)**, 3154
*Mulvidren-F*—Stuart (U.S.) brand of Multiple Vitamins and Fluoride—**See Vitamins, Multiple, and Fluoride (Systemic)**, 2978
*Mumpsvax*—Merck (U.S. and Canada) and Morson (U.K.) brand of Mumps Virus Vaccine Live (Systemic), 2062
Mumps Virus Vaccine Live [*Mumpsvax*] **(Systemic)**, 2062
Mumps Virus Vaccine Live USP (for Injection), 2065
Mupirocin [*Bactroban; pseudomonic acid*] **(Topical)**, #
Ointment USP, #
Mupirocin Calcium [*Bactroban Nasal*] **(Nasal)**, 2066
Ointment, Nasal, 2067
Mupirocin Calcium [*Bactroban*] **(Topical)**, 3029
Cream, 3029
Muromonab-CD3 [*Orthoclone OKT3*] **(Systemic)**, 2068
Injection, 2070
*Muro's Opcon*—Bausch & Lomb (U.S.) brand of Naphazoline (Ophthalmic), #
*Muse*—Vivus (U.S.) brand of Alprostadil (Local), 48
*Muskol*—Schering (U.S. and Canada) brand of Diethyltoluamide (Topical), #
*Mustargen*—Merck (U.S. and Canada) brand of Mechlorethamine (Systemic), 1929
*Mutamycin*—Bristol (U.S. and Canada) brand of Mitomycin (Systemic), 2028
*Myambutol*—Lederle (U.S. and Canada) brand of Ethambutol (Systemic), 1412
*My Baby Gas Relief Drops*—Liquipharm (U.S.) brand of Simethicone (Oral-Local), #
*Mycelex-7*—Bayer Consumer (U.S.) brand of Clotrimazole—**See Antifungals, Azole (Vaginal)**, 310
*Mycelex Cream*—Miles (U.S.) brand of Clotrimazole (Topical), 916
*Mycelex-G*—Bayer (U.S.) brand of Clotrimazole—**See Antifungals, Azole (Vaginal)**, 310
*Mycelex Solution*—Miles (U.S.) brand of Clotrimazole (Topical), 916
*Mycelex Troches*—Bayer (U.S.) brand of Clotrimazole (Oral-Local), 915, MC-8
*Mycelex Twin Pack*—Bayer (U.S.) brand of Clotrimazole—**See Antifungals, Azole (Vaginal)**, 310
*Mycifradin*—Upjohn (U.S. and Canada) brand of Neomycin (Oral-Local), #

*Myciguent*—Upjohn (U.S. and Canada) brand of Neomycin (Topical), #
*Mycitracin*—Upjohn (U.S.) brand of Neomycin, Polymyxin B, and Bacitracin (Topical), #
*Myclo Cream*—Boehringer Ingelheim (Canada) brand of Clotrimazole (Topical), 916
*Myclo-Gyne*—Boehringer Ingelheim (Canada) brand of Clotrimazole—**See Antifungals, Azole (Vaginal)**, 310
*Myclo Solution*—Boehringer Ingelheim (Canada) brand of Clotrimazole (Topical), 916
*Myclo Spray Solution*—Boehringer Ingelheim (Canada) brand of Clotrimazole (Topical), 916
*Myco II*—Bioline (U.S.) brand of Nystatin and Triamcinolone (Topical), 2150
*Mycobacterium avium* Sensitin RS-10 **(Systemic)**, 3155
*Mycobiotic II*—Moore (U.S.) brand of Nystatin and Triamcinolone (Topical), 2150
*Mycobutin*—Pharmacia & Upjohn (U.S. and Canada) and Adria (U.S.) brand of Rifabutin (Systemic), 2483, 3163, MC-27
*Mycogen II*—Goldline (U.S.) brand of Nystatin and Triamcinolone (Topical), 2150
*Mycolog II*—Squibb (U.S.) brand of Nystatin and Triamcinolone (Topical), 2150
Mycophenolate Mofetil [*CellCept*] **(Systemic)**, 2070
Capsules, 2073, MC-21
Tablets, 2073, MC-21
*My Cort*—Scrip (U.S.) brand of Hydrocortisone—**See Corticosteroids (Topical)**, 978
*Mycostatin*—Squibb (U.S. and Canada) brand of Nystatin (Oral-Local), 2146; Nystatin (Topical), 2148; Nystatin (Vaginal), 2149
*Myco-Triacet II*—Lemmon (U.S.) brand of Nystatin and Triamcinolone (Topical), 2150
*Mydfrin*—Alcon (U.S. and Canada) brand of Phenylephrine (Ophthalmic), #
*Mydriacyl*—Alcon (U.S. and Canada) brand of Tropicamide (Ophthalmic), #
*Mydriafair*—Pharmafair (U.S.) and Texas Drugs (U.S.) brand of Tropicamide (Ophthalmic), #
*My-E*—Seneca (U.S.) brand of Erythromycin Stearate—**See Erythromycins (Systemic)**, 1368
Myelin **(Systemic)**, 3155
*Myfedrine*—Pharmaceutical Basics (U.S.) brand of Pseudoephedrine (Systemic), 2422
*Mygel*—Geneva Generics (U.S.) brand of Alumina, Magnesia, and Simethicone—**See Antacids (Oral-Local)**, 188
*Mygel II*—Geneva Generics (U.S.) brand of Alumina, Magnesia, and Simethicone—**See Antacids (Oral-Local)**, 188
*Myidil*—My-K (U.S.) brand of Triprolidine—**See Antihistamines (Systemic)**, 325
*Myidone*—Major (U.S.) brand of Primidone (Systemic), 2376
*Mykacet*—Major (U.S.) brand of Nystatin and Triamcinolone (Topical), 2150
*Mykacet II*—Texas Drug (U.S.) brand of Nystatin and Triamcinolone (Topical), 2150
*Mykrox*—Pennwalt (U.S.) brand of Metolazone—**See Diuretics, Thiazide (Systemic)**, 1273
*Mylanta*—J & J-Merck (U.S.) and Warner Wellcome (Canada) brand of Alumina, Magnesia, and Simethicone—**See Antacids (Oral-Local)**, 188; Calcium Carbonate—**See Antacids (Oral-Local)**, 188; Calcium Carbonate and Magnesia—**See Antacids (Oral-Local)**, 188
*Mylanta-AR*—Johnson & Johnson and Merck (U.S.) brand of Famotidine—**See Histamine H$_2$-receptor Antagonists (Systemic)**, 1633, MC-12
*Mylanta Double Strength*—J & J-Merck (U.S.) and Warner Wellcome (Canada) brand of Alumina, Magnesia, and Simethicone—**See Antacids (Oral-Local)**, 188; J & J-Merck (U.S.) brand of Calcium Carbonate and Magnesia—**See Antacids (Oral-Local)**, 188
*Mylanta Double Strength Plain*—Warner Wellcome (Canada) brand of Alumina and Magnesia—**See Antacids (Oral-Local)**, 188
*Mylanta Extra Strength*—Warner Wellcome (Canada) brand of Alumina, Magnesia, and Simethicone—**See Antacids (Oral-Local)**, 188
*Mylanta Gas*—Johnson & Johnson (U.S.) brand of Simethicone (Oral-Local), #
*Mylanta Gas Relief*—Johnson & Johnson (U.S.) brand of Simethicone (Oral-Local), #

*Mylanta Gelcaps*—J & J-Merck (U.S.) brand of Calcium and Magnesia—**See Antacids (Oral-Local)**, 188
*Mylanta Natural Fiber Supplement*—J & J/Merck (U.S.) brand of Psyllium Hydrophilic Mucilloid—**See Laxatives (Local)**, #
*Mylanta Sugar Free Natural Fiber Supplement*—J & J/Merck (U.S.) brand of Psyllium Hydrophilic Mucilloid—**See Laxatives (Local)**, #
*Myleran*—Glaxo Wellcome (U.S. and Canada) brand of Busulfan (Systemic), 695, MC-4
*Mylicon Drops*—Stuart (U.S.) brand of Simethicone (Oral-Local), #
*Mymethasone*—My-K (U.S.) brand of Dexamethasone—**See Corticosteroids—Glucocorticoid Effects (Systemic)**, 998
*Myminic Expectorant*—Pennex (U.S.) brand of Phenylpropanolamine and Guaifenesin—**See Cough/Cold Combinations (Systemic)**, 1024
*Myminicol*—Pennex (U.S.) brand of Chlorpheniramine, Phenylpropanolamine, and Dextromethorphan—**See Cough/Cold Combinations (Systemic)**, 1024
*Myochrysine*—Merck (U.S.) and Rhône-Poulenc (Canada) brand of Gold Sodium Thiomalate—**See Gold Compounds (Systemic)**, 1566
*Myolin*—Roberts (U.S.) brand of Orphenadrine—**See Skeletal Muscle Relaxants (Systemic)**, 2577
*Myoscint*—Centocor (U.S.) brand of Imciromab Pentetate (Systemic), 3147; Indium In 111 Murine Monoclonal Antibody Fab to Myosin (Systemic), 3147
*Myotrol*—Legere (U.S.) brand of Orphenadrine—**See Skeletal Muscle Relaxants (Systemic)**, 2577
*Myotrophin*—Cephalon (U.S.) brand of Insulin-like Growth Factor-1 (Systemic), 3147
*Myoview*—Amersham (U.S.) brand of Technetium Tc 99m Tetrofosmin (Systemic), 2745
*Myphetane DC Cough*—Morton Grove (U.S.) and Pennex (U.S.) brand of Brompheniramine, Phenylpropanolamine, and Codeine—**See Cough/Cold Combinations (Systemic)**, 1024
*Myphetane DX Cough*—Morton Grove (U.S.); Pennex (U.S.) and Southwood (U.S.) brand of Brompheniramine, Pseudoephedrine, and Dextromethorphan—**See Cough/Cold Combinations (Systemic)**, 1024
*Myphetapp*—Morton Grove (U.S.) brand of Brompheniramine and Phenylpropanolamine—**See Antihistamines and Decongestants (Systemic)**, 343
*Myrosemide*—My-K (U.S.) brand of Furosemide—**See Diuretics, Loop (Systemic)**, 1259
*Mysoline*—Wyeth-Ayerst (U.S.) and Ayerst (Canada) brand of Primidone (Systemic), 2376
*Mytelase Caplets*—Sanofi Winthrop (U.S.) brand of Ambenonium—**See Antimyasthenics (Systemic)**, 437
*Mytrex*—Savage (U.S.) brand of Nystatin and Triamcinolone (Topical), 2150
*Mytussin AC*—Morton Grove (U.S.) and Pennex (U.S.) brand of Codeine and Guaifenesin—**See Cough/Cold Combinations (Systemic)**, 1024
*Mytussin DAC*—Morton Grove (U.S.) and Pennex (U.S.) brand of Pseudoephedrine, Codeine, and Guaifenesin—**See Cough/Cold Combinations (Systemic)**, 1024
*Mytussin DM*—Pennex (U.S.) brand of Dextromethorphan and Guaifenesin—**See Cough/Cold Combinations (Systemic)**, 1024
*MZM*—CIBAVision (U.S.) brand of Methazolamide—**See Carbonic Anhydrase Inhibitors (Systemic)**, 773

# N

*9-1-1*—Rydelle (U.S.) brand of Hydrocortisone—**See Corticosteroids (Topical)**, 978
Nabilone [*Cesamet*] **(Systemic)**, 2074
Capsules, 2075
Nabumetone [*Relafen*] **See Anti-inflammatory Drugs, Nonsteroidal (Systemic)**, 388
Tablets, 413 MC-21
N-Acetyl-L-Cysteine *See* Acetylcysteine (Systemic), 16
N-Acetyl-Procainamide **(Systemic)**, 3155

Nadolol [*Corgard; Syn-Nadolol*]
  **See Beta-adrenergic Blocking Agents (Systemic)**, 593
    Tablets USP, 604, MC-21
Nadolol and Bendroflumethiazide [*Corzide*]
  **See Beta-adrenergic Blocking Agents and Thiazide Diuretics (Systemic)**, 609
    Tablets USP, 611, MC-21
Nadolol-containing Combinations, 3075
*Nadopen-V*—Nadeau (Canada) brand of Penicillin V—**See Penicillins (Systemic)**, 2240
*Nadopen-V 200*—Nadeau (Canada) brand of Penicillin V—**See Penicillins (Systemic)**, 2240
*Nadopen-V 400*—Nadeau (Canada) brand of Penicillin V—**See Penicillins (Systemic)**, 2240
*Nadostine*—Nadeau (Canada) brand of Nystatin (Oral-Local), 2146; Nystatin (Topical), 2148; Nystatin (Vaginal), 2149
Nafarelin Acetate [*Synarel; Synarel Nasal Solution*] **(Systemic)**, 2076, 3155
  Solution, Nasal, 2079
*Nafazair*—Balan (U.S.); Genetco (U.S.); and Texas Drugs (U.S.) brand of Naphazoline (Ophthalmic), #
*Nafcil*—Bristol (U.S.) brand of Nafcillin—**See Penicillins (Systemic)**, 2240
Nafcillin Sodium [*Nafcil; Nallpen; Unipen*]
  **See Penicillins (Systemic)**, 2240
    Capsules USP, 2253
    for Injection USP, 2254
    Tablets USP, 2254
Naftifine Hydrochloride [*Naftin*]
  **(Topical)**, #
    Cream, #
    Gel, #
*Naftin*—Allergan Herbert (U.S. and Canada) brand of Naftifine (Topical), #
*Naganin*—See Suramin (Systemic), #
*Naganol*—See Suramin (Systemic), #
Nalbuphine Hydrochloride [*Nubain*]
  **See Opioid (Narcotic) Analgesics (Systemic)**, 2168
    Injection, 2185
*Nalcrom*—Fisons (Canada) brand of Cromolyn (Systemic/Oral-Local), 1121
*Nalda-Relief Pediatric Drops*—Liquipharm (U.S.) brand of Chlorpheniramine, Phenyltoloxamine, Phenylephrine, and Phenylpropanolamine—**See Antihistamines and Decongestants (Systemic)**, 343
*Naldecon*—Apothecon (U.S.) brand of Chlorpheniramine, Phenyltoloxamine, Phenylephrine, and Phenylpropanolamine—**See Antihistamines and Decongestants (Systemic)**, 343, AP-27
*Naldecon-CX Adult Liquid*—Apothecon (U.S.) brand of Phenylpropanolamine, Codeine, and Guaifenesin—**See Cough/Cold Combinations (Systemic)**, 1024
*Naldecon-DX Adult Liquid*—Apothecon (U.S.) brand of Phenylpropanolamine, Dextromethorphan, and Guaifenesin—**See Cough/Cold Combinations (Systemic)**, 1024
*Naldecon-DX Children's Syrup*—Apothecon (U.S.) brand of Phenylpropanolamine, Dextromethorphan, and Guaifenesin—**See Cough/Cold Combinations (Systemic)**, 1024
*Naldecon-DX Pediatric Drops*—Apothecon (U.S.) brand of Phenylpropanolamine, Dextromethorphan, and Guaifenesin—**See Cough/Cold Combinations (Systemic)**, 1024
*Naldecon-EX Children's Syrup*—Apothecon (U.S.) brand of Phenylpropanolamine and Guaifenesin—**See Cough/Cold Combinations (Systemic)**, 1024
*Naldecon-EX Pediatric Drops*—Apothecon (U.S.) brand of Phenylpropanolamine and Guaifenesin—**See Cough/Cold Combinations (Systemic)**, 1024
*Naldecon Pediatric Drops*—Apothecon (U.S.) brand of Chlorpheniramine, Phenyltoloxamine, Phenylephrine, and Phenylpropanolamine—**See Antihistamines and Decongestants (Systemic)**, 343
*Naldecon Pediatric Syrup*—Apothecon (U.S.) brand of Chlorpheniramine, Phenyltoloxamine, Phenylephrine, and Phenylpropanolamine—**See Antihistamines and Decongestants (Systemic)**, 343
*Naldecon Senior DX*—Apothecon (U.S.) brand of Dextromethorphan and Guaifenesin—**See Cough/Cold Combinations (Systemic)**, 1024

*Naldecon Senior EX*—Apothecon (U.S.) brand of Guaifenesin (Systemic), 1588
*Naldelate*—Barre-National, H.L. Moore, and Qualitest (U.S.) brand of Chlorpheniramine, Phenyltoloxamine, Phenylephrine, and Phenylpropanolamine—**See Antihistamines and Decongestants (Systemic)**, 343
*Naldelate Pediatric Drops*—Barre-National (U.S.); H.L. Moore (U.S.); and Qualitest (U.S.) brand of Chlorpheniramine, Phenyltoloxamine, Phenylephrine, and Phenylpropanolamine—**See Antihistamines and Decongestants (Systemic)**, 343
*Naldelate Pediatric Syrup*—Barre-National, H.L. Moore, and Qualitest (U.S.) brand of Chlorpheniramine, Phenyltoloxamine, Phenylephrine, and Phenylpropanolamine—**See Antihistamines and Decongestants (Systemic)**, 343
*Nalex*—Blansett (U.S.) brand of Pseudoephedrine and Guaifenesin—**See Cough/Cold Combinations (Systemic)**, 1024
*Nalex-A*—Blansett (U.S.) brand of Chlorpheniramine, Phenyltoloxamine, and Phenylephrine—**See Antihistamines and Decongestants (Systemic)**, 343
*Nalex DH*—Blansett (U.S.) brand of Phenylephrine and Hydrocodone—**See Cough/Cold Combinations (Systemic)**, 1024
*Nalex Jr.*—Blansett (U.S.) brand of Pseudoephedrine and Guaifenesin—**See Cough/Cold Combinations (Systemic)**, 1024
*Nalfed*—Econolab (U.S.) brand of Brompheniramine and Pseudoephedrine—**See Antihistamines and Decongestants (Systemic)**, 343
*Nalfed-PD*—Econolab (U.S.) brand of Brompheniramine and Pseudoephedrine—**See Antihistamines and Decongestants (Systemic)**, 343
*Nalfon*—Dista (U.S.) and Lilly (Canada) brand of Fenoprofen—**See Anti-inflammatory Drugs, Nonsteroidal (Systemic)**, 388, MC-12
*Nalfon 200*—Dista (U.S.) brand of Fenoprofen—**See Anti-inflammatory Drugs, Nonsteroidal (Systemic)**, 388, MC-12
*Nalgest*—Major (U.S.) brand of Chlorpheniramine, Phenyltoloxamine, Phenylephrine, and Phenylpropanolamine—**See Antihistamines and Decongestants (Systemic)**, 343
*Nalgest Pediatric*—Major (U.S.) brand of Chlorpheniramine, Phenyltoloxamine, Phenylephrine, and Phenylpropanolamine—**See Antihistamines and Decongestants (Systemic)**, 343
Nalidixic Acid [*NegGram*]
  **(Systemic)**, #
    Suspension, Oral, USP, #
    Tablets USP, #, MC-21
*Nallpen*—Beecham (U.S.) brand of Nafcillin—**See Penicillins (Systemic)**, 2240
Nalmefene Hydrochloride [*Revex*]
  **(Systemic)**, 2080
    Injection, 2081
Naloxone-containing Combinations, 3075
Naloxone Hydrochloride [*Narcan*]
  **(Systemic)**, 2082
    Injection USP, 2083
*Nalphen*—Hi-Tech (U.S.) brand of Chlorpheniramine, Phenyltoloxamine, Phenylephrine, and Phenylpropanolamine—**See Antihistamines and Decongestants (Systemic)**, 343
*Nalphen Pediatric*—Hi-Tech (U.S.) brand of Chlorpheniramine, Phenyltoloxamine, Phenylephrine, and Phenylpropanolamine—**See Antihistamines and Decongestants (Systemic)**, 343
Naltrexone Hydrochloride [*ReVia; Trexan*]
  **(Systemic)**, 2084, 3029, 3155
    Tablets, 2087, 3029
Nandrolone Decanoate [*Deca-Durabolin; Hybolin Decanoate; Kabolin*]
  **See Anabolic Steroids (Systemic)**, 110
    Injection USP, 113
Nandrolone Phenpropionate [*Durabolin; Durabolin-50; Hybolin-Improved*]
  **See Anabolic Steroids (Systemic)**, 110
    Injection USP, 113
Naphazoline Hydrochloride [*Ak-Con; Albalon; Albalon Liquifilm; Allerest; Allergy Drops; Clear Eyes Lubricating Eye Redness Reliever; Comfort Eye Drops; Degest 2; Estivin II; I-Naphline; Muro's Opcon; Nafazair; Naphcon; Naphcon Forte; Ocu-Zoline Sterile Ophthalmic Solution; VasoClear; VasoClear A; Vasocon; Vasocon Regular*]
  **(Ophthalmic)**, #
    Solution, Ophthalmic, USP, #

*Naphcon*—Alcon (U.S.) brand of Naphazoline (Ophthalmic), #
*Naphcon Forte*—Alcon (U.S. and Canada) brand of Naphazoline (Ophthalmic), #
*Naphuride*—See Suramin (Systemic), #
*Naprelan*—Wyeth-Ayerst (U.S.) brand of Naproxen (Systemic), 3029; Wyeth-Ayerst (U.S.) brand of Naproxen (Systemic), MC-21
*Naprosyn*—Roche (U.S.) and Syntex (Canada) brand of Naproxen—**See Anti-inflammatory Drugs, Nonsteroidal (Systemic)**, 388, MC-21
*Naprosyn-E*—Syntex (Canada) brand of Naproxen—**See Anti-inflammatory Drugs, Nonsteroidal (Systemic)**, 388
*Naprosyn-SR*—Syntex (Canada) brand of Naproxen—**See Anti-inflammatory Drugs, Nonsteroidal (Systemic)**, 388
Naproxen [*Apo-Naproxen; EC-Naprosyn; Naprelan; Naprosyn; Naprosyn-E; Naprosyn-SR; Naxen; Novo-Naprox; Nu-Naprox*]
  **See Anti-inflammatory Drugs, Nonsteroidal (Systemic)**, 388, 3029
    Suppositories, 415
    Suspension, Oral, 413
    Tablets USP, 414, MC-21
    Tablets, Delayed-release, 414, MC-21
    Tablets, Extended-release, 414, 3029
Naproxen Sodium [*Aleve; Anaprox; Anaprox DS; Apo-Napro-Na; Apo-Napro-Na DS; Naprelan; Novo-Naprox Sodium; Novo-Naprox Sodium DS; Synflex; Synflex DS*]
  **See Anti-inflammatory Drugs, Nonsteroidal (Systemic)**, 388
    Tablets USP, 414, MC-21
    Tablets, Extended-release, MC-21
*Naqua*—Schering (U.S.) brand of Trichlormethiazide—**See Diuretics, Thiazide (Systemic)**, 1273
*Naquival*—Schering (U.S.) brand of Reserpine and Trichlormethiazide—**See Rauwolfia Alkaloids and Thiazide Diuretics (Systemic)**, #
Naratriptan Hydrochloride [*Amerge*]
  **(Systemic)**, 2087
    Tablets, 2089, MC-21
*Narcan*—Du Pont (U.S. and Canada) brand of Naloxone (Systemic), 2082
*Nardil*—PD (U.S. and Canada) brand of Phenelzine—**See Antidepressants, Monoamine Oxidase (MAO) Inhibitor (Systemic)**, 266
*Naropin*—Astra (U.S.) and Astra Pharma (Canada) brand of Ropivacaine (Parenteral-Local), #
*Nasabid*—Abana (U.S.) brand of Pseudoephedrine and Guaifenesin—**See Cough/Cold Combinations (Systemic)**, 1024
*Nasacort*—Rhône-Poulenc Rorer (U.S. and Canada) brand of Triamcinolone—**See Corticosteroids (Nasal)**, 961, 3037
*Nasacort AQ*—Rhône-Poulenc Rorer (U.S.) brand of Triamcinolone (Nasal), 3037
*Nasahist B*—Keene (U.S.) brand of Brompheniramine—**See Antihistamines (Systemic)**, 325
*Nasalcrom*—Fisons (U.S.) and McNeil (U.S.) brand of Cromolyn (Nasal), 1118, 3016
*Nasal Decongestant Spray*—Taro (U.S.) brand of Oxymetazoline (Nasal), 3030
*Nasal-12 Hour*—Rexall (U.S.) brand of Oxymetazoline (Nasal), #
*Nasalide*—Roche/Syntex (U.S.) brand of Flunisolide—**See Corticosteroids (Nasal)**, 961
*Nasal Relief*—Rugby (U.S.) brand of Oxymetazoline (Nasal), #
*Nasal Spray 12-Hour*—United Research (U.S.) brand of Oxymetazoline (Nasal), #
*Nasal Spray Long Acting*—Qualitest (U.S.) brand of Oxymetazoline (Nasal), #
*Nasarel*—Roche (U.S.) brand of Flunisolide (Nasal), 3020
*Nasatab LA*—ECR (U.S.) brand of Pseudoephedrine and Guaifenesin—**See Cough/Cold Combinations (Systemic)**, 1024
*Nasatuss*—Abana (U.S.) brand of Chlorpheniramine, Phenylephrine, and Hydrocodone—**See Cough/Cold Combinations (Systemic)**, 1024
Nashville Rabbit Anti-thymocyte Serum—See Antithymocyte Serum (Systemic), 3131
*Nasonex*—Schering (U.S.) brand of Mometasone (Nasal), 2055
*Natacyn*—Alcon (U.S.) brand of Natamycin (Ophthalmic), #
Natamycin [*Natacyn*; pimaricin]
  **(Ophthalmic)**, #
    Suspension, Ophthalmic, USP, #

# General Index

*Natulan*—Hoffman-La Roche (Canada) brand of Procarbazine (Systemic), 2391
*Naturacil*—Mead Johnson (U.S.) brand of Psyllium—**See Laxatives (Local)**, #
*Natural Source Fibre Laxative*—Stanley (Canada) brand of Psyllium Hydrophilic Mucilloid—**See Laxatives (Local)**, #
*Naturalyte*—United Beverages (U.S.) brand of Dextrose and Electrolytes—**See Carbohydrates and Electrolytes (Systemic)**, 769
*Nature's Remedy*—SmithKline Beecham (U.S. and Canada) brand of Cascara Sagrada and Aloe—**See Laxatives (Local)**, #
*Nature's Tears*—Rugby (U.S.) brand of Hydroxypropyl Methylcellulose (Ophthalmic), #
*Naturetin*—Apothecon (U.S.) and Squibb (Canada) brand of Bendroflumethiazide—**See Diuretics, Thiazide (Systemic)**, 1273, MC-3
*Navane*—Roerig (U.S.) and Pfizer (Canada) brand of Thiothixene—**See Thioxanthenes (Systemic)**, 2793, MC-10
*Navelbine*—Glaxo Wellcome (U.S. and Canada) brand of Vinorelbine (Systemic), 2953
*Naxen*—SynCare (Canada) brand of Naproxen—**See Anti-inflammatory Drugs, Nonsteroidal (Systemic)**, 388
*ND Clear T.D.*—Seatrace (U.S.) brand of Chlorpheniramine and Pseudoephedrine—**See Antihistamines and Decongestants (Systemic)**, 343
*ND-Gesic*—Hyrex (U.S.) brand of Chlorpheniramine, Pyrilamine, Phenylephrine, and Acetaminophen—**See Antihistamines, Decongestants, and Analgesics (Systemic)**, 366
Nebacumab [*Centoxin*]
  **(Systemic)**, 3155
*Nebcin*—Lilly (U.S. and Canada) brand of Tobramycin—**See Aminoglycosides (Systemic)**, 69
*NebuPent*—Fujisawa (U.S.) and LyphoMed (U.S.) brand of Pentamidine (Inhalation), 2272, 3157
*Necon 0.5/35*—Watson (U.S.) brand of Norethindrone and Ethinyl Estradiol—**See Estrogens and Progestins—Oral Contraceptives (Systemic)**, 1397
*Necon 1/35*—Watson (U.S.) brand of Norethindrone and Ethinyl Estradiol—**See Estrogens and Progestins—Oral Contraceptives (Systemic)**, 1397
*Necon 1/50*—Watson (U.S.) brand of Norethindrone and Ethinyl Estradiol—**See Estrogens and Progestins—Oral Contraceptives (Systemic)**, 1397
*Necon 10/11*—Watson (U.S.) brand of Norethindrone and Ethinyl Estradiol—**See Estrogens and Progestins—Oral Contraceptives (Systemic)**, 1397
Nedocromil [*Tilade*]
  **(Inhalation-Local)**, 2090
  Aerosol, Inhalation, 2091
*N.E.E. 1/35*—Lexis (U.S.) brand of Norethindrone and Ethinyl Estradiol—**See Estrogens and Progestins—Oral Contraceptives (Systemic)**, 1397
*N.E.E. 1/50*—Lexis (U.S.) brand of Norethindrone and Ethinyl Estradiol—**See Estrogens and Progestins—Oral Contraceptives (Systemic)**, 1397
Nefazodone [*Serzone*]
  **(Systemic)**, 3029
  Tablets, 3029
Nefazodone Hydrochloride [*Serzone*]
  **(Systemic)**, 2092
  Tablets, 2095, MC-21
*NegGram*—Sanofi Winthrop (U.S. and Canada) brand of Nalidixic Acid (Systemic), #, MC-21
Nelfinavir Mesylate [*Viracept*]
  **(Systemic)**, 2095
  Powder, Oral, 2097
  Tablets, 2098
*Nelova 0.5/35E*—Warner-Chilcott (U.S.) brand of Norethindrone and Ethinyl Estradiol—**See Estrogens and Progestins—Oral Contraceptives (Systemic)**, 1397
*Nelova 10/11*—Warner-Chilcott (U.S.) brand of Norethindrone and Ethinyl Estradiol—**See Estrogens and Progestins—Oral Contraceptives (Systemic)**, 1397
*Nelova 1/35E*—Warner-Chilcott (U.S.) brand of Norethindrone and Ethinyl Estradiol—**See Estrogens and Progestins—Oral Contraceptives (Systemic)**, 1397

*Nelova 1/50M*—Warner-Chilcott (U.S.) brand of Norethindrone and Mestranol—**See Estrogens and Progestins—Oral Contraceptives (Systemic)**, 1397
*Nemasol Sodium*—ICN (Canada) brand of Aminosalicylate Sodium (Systemic), #
*Nembutal*—Abbott (U.S. and Canada) brand of Pentobarbital—**See Barbiturates (Systemic)**, 518
*Neocaf*—O.P.R. Development (U.S.) brand of Caffeine (Systemic), 3135
*Neo-Calglucon*—Sandoz (U.S.) brand of Calcium Glubionate—**See Calcium Supplements (Systemic)**, 736
*Neocidin Ophthalmic Ointment*—Major (U.S.) brand of Neomycin, Polymyxin B, and Bacitracin (Ophthalmic), #
*Neocidin Ophthalmic Solution*—Major (U.S.) brand of Neomycin, Polymyxin B, and Gramicidin (Ophthalmic), #
*Neo Citran A*—Sandoz (Canada) brand of Pheniramine and Phenylephrine—**See Antihistamines and Decongestants (Systemic)**, 343
*Neo Citran Colds and Flu*—Sandoz (Canada) brand of Pheniramine, Phenylephrine, and Acetaminophen—**See Antihistamines, Decongestants, and Analgesics (Systemic)**, 366
*Neo Citran Colds and Flu Calorie Reduced*—Sandoz (Canada) brand of Pheniramine, Phenylephrine, and Acetaminophen—**See Antihistamines, Decongestants, and Analgesics (Systemic)**, 366
*Neo Citran Day Caps Extra Strength Caplets*—Sandoz (Canada) brand of Pseudoephedrine, Dextromethorphan, and Acetaminophen—**See Cough/Cold Combinations (Systemic)**, 1024
*Neo Citran DM Coughs and Colds*—Sandoz (Canada) brand of Pheniramine, Phenylephrine, and Dextromethorphan—**See Cough/Cold Combinations (Systemic)**, 1024
*Neo Citran Extra Strength Colds and Flu*—Sandoz (Canada) brand of Pheniramine, Phenylephrine, and Acetaminophen—**See Antihistamines, Decongestants, and Analgesics (Systemic)**, 366
*Neo Citran Extra Strength Sinus*—Sandoz (Canada) brand of Phenylephrine and Acetaminophen—**See Decongestants and Analgesics (Systemic)**, 1180
*Neo-Codema*—Neolab (Canada) brand of Hydrochlorothiazide—**See Diuretics, Thiazide (Systemic)**, 1273
*Neocontrast*—Bama (Spain) brand of Iopanoic Acid—**See Cholecystographic Agents, Oral (Systemic)**, #
*Neo-DM*—Neolab (Canada) brand of Dextromethorphan (Systemic), 1191
*Neo-Estrone*—Neolab (Canada) brand of Esterified Estrogens—**See Estrogens (Systemic)**, 1383
*Neo-Fer*—Neolab (Canada) brand of Ferrous Fumarate—**See Iron Supplements (Systemic)**, 1774
*Neofrin*—Ocusoft (U.S.) brand of Phenylephrine (Ophthalmic), 3032
*Neo-K*—Neolab (Canada) brand of Potassium Bicarbonate and Potassium Chloride—**See Potassium Supplements (Systemic)**, 2357
*Neolax*—Central (U.S.) brand of Dehydrocholic Acid and Docusate—**See Laxatives (Local)**, #
*Neoloid*—Kenwood (Bradley) (U.S.) brand of Castor Oil—**See Laxatives (Local)**, #
Neomycin-containing Combinations, 3075
Neomycin Sulfate
  **(Ophthalmic)**, #
  Ointment, Ophthalmic, USP, #
Neomycin Sulfate [*Mycifradin*]
  **(Oral-Local)**, #
  Solution, Oral, USP, #
  Tablets USP, #
Neomycin Sulfate [*Myciguent*]
  **(Topical)**, #
  Cream USP, #
  Ointment USP, #
Neomycin Sulfate
  **See Aminoglycosides (Systemic)**, 69
  Sterile USP, 77
Neomycin and Polymyxin B Sulfates [*Neosporin Cream*]
  **(Topical)**, #
  Cream USP, #
Neomycin and Polymyxin B Sulfates and Bacitracin [*Bactine First Aid Antibiotic; Foille; Mycitracin*]
  **(Topical)**, #
  Ointment USP, #

Neomycin and Polymyxin B Sulfates and Bacitracin Zinc [*Ak-Spore Ophthalmic Ointment; Neocidin Ophthalmic Ointment; Neosporin Ophthalmic Ointment; Neotal; Ocu-Spor-B; Ocusporin; Ocutricin Ophthalmic Ointment; Ophthalmic; Spectro-Sporin; Triple Antibiotic*]
  **(Ophthalmic)**, #
  Ointment, Ophthalmic, USP, #
Neomycin and Polymyxin B Sulfates and Bacitracin Zinc [*Neosporin Maximum Strength Ointment; Neosporin Ointment; Topisporin*]
  **(Topical)**, #
  Ointment USP, #
Neomycin and Polymyxin B Sulfates and Gramicidin [*Ak-Spore Ophthalmic Solution; Neocidin Ophthalmic Solution; Neosporin Ophthalmic Solution; Ocu-Spor-G; Ocutricin Ophthalmic Solution; P.N. Ophthalmic; Tribiotic; Tri-Ophthalmic; Triple Antibiotic*]
  **(Ophthalmic)**, #, 3029
  Solution, Ophthalmic, USP, 3029
Neomycin and Polymyxin B Sulfates and Hydrocortisone [*Ak-Spore H.C.; Bacticort; Cobiron; Cortisporin Ophthalmic Suspension; Cortomycin; Hydromycin; I-Neocort; Ocutricin HC; Triple-Gen*]
  **(Ophthalmic)**, #
  Suspension, Ophthalmic, USP, #
Neomycin and Polymyxin B Sulfates and Hydrocortisone [*AK-Spore HC Otic; Antibiotic Ear; Cortatrigen Ear; Cortatrigen Modified Ear Drops; Cort-Biotic; Cortisporin; Cortomycin; Drotic; Ear-Eze; LazerSporin-C; Masporin Otic; Octicair; Octigen; Otic-Care; Otic-Care Ear; Otimar; Otisan; Otocidin; Otocort; Pediotic; UAD Otic*]
  **(Otic)**, #
  Solution, Otic, USP, #
  Suspension, Otic, USP, #
*Neopap*—Polymedica (U.S.) brand of Acetaminophen (Systemic), 6
*Neo-Pause*—Neolab (Canada) brand of Testosterone and Estradiol—**See Androgens and Estrogens (Systemic)**, 126
*Neoquess*—Forest (U.S.) brand of Dicyclomine—**See Anticholinergics/Antispasmodics (Systemic)**, 226; Hyoscyamine—**See Anticholinergics/Antispasmodics (Systemic)**, 226
*Neoral*—Novartis (U.S.) and Sandoz (U.S.) brand of Cyclosporine (Systemic), 1136, MC-8
*Neosar*—Adria (U.S.) brand of Cyclophosphamide (Systemic), 1128
*Neoscan*—Medi-Physics (U.S.) brand of Gallium Citrate Ga 67 (Systemic), 1538
*Neosporin Cream*—BW (U.S.) brand of Neomycin and Polymyxin B (Topical), #
*Neosporin Maximum Strength Ointment*—BW (U.S.) brand of Neomycin, Polymyxin B, and Bacitracin (Topical), #
*Neosporin Ointment*—BW (U.S.) brand of Neomycin, Polymyxin B, and Bacitracin (Topical), #
*Neosporin Ophthalmic Ointment*—BW (U.S. and Canada) brand of Neomycin, Polymyxin B, and Bacitracin (Ophthalmic), #
*Neosporin Ophthalmic Solution*—BW (U.S. and Canada) brand of Neomycin, Polymyxin B, and Gramicidin (Ophthalmic), #
Neostigmine Bromide [*Prostigmin*]
  **See Antimyasthenics (Systemic)**, 437
  Tablets USP, 440
Neostigmine Methylsulfate [*Prostigmin*]
  **See Antimyasthenics (Systemic)**, 437
  Injection USP, 440
*Neo-Synephrine*—Sanofi Winthrop (U.S. and Canada) brand of Phenylephrine—**See Sympathomimetic Agents—Cardiovascular Use (Parenteral-Systemic)**, 2669; Sanofi Winthrop (U.S.) brand of Phenylephrine (Ophthalmic), #
*Neo-Synephrine 12 Hour Nasal Spray*—Sterling (U.S.) brand of Oxymetazoline (Nasal), #
*Neo-Synephrine 12 Hour Nasal Spray Pump*—Sterling (U.S.) brand of Oxymetazoline (Nasal), #
*Neo-Synephrine II Long Acting Nasal Spray Adult Strength*—Sanofi Winthrop (U.S.) brand of Xylometazoline (Nasal), #
*Neo-Synephrine II Long Acting Nose Drops Adult Strength*—Sanofi Winthrop (U.S.) brand of Xylometazoline (Nasal), #
*Neo-Synephrine Nasal Drops*—Sanofi Winthrop (U.S. and Canada) brand of Phenylephrine (Nasal), #
*Neo-Synephrine Nasal Jelly*—Sanofi Winthrop (U.S.) brand of Phenylephrine (Nasal), #

*Neo-Synephrine Nasal Spray*—Sanofi Winthrop (U.S. and Canada) brand of Phenylephrine (Nasal), #
*Neo-Synephrine Pediatric Nasal Drops*—Sanofi Winthrop (U.S.) brand of Phenylephrine (Nasal), #
*Neotal*—Hauck (U.S.) brand of Neomycin, Polymyxin B, and Bacitracin (Ophthalmic), #
*Neo-Zol Cream*—Neolab (Canada) brand of Clotrimazole (Topical), 916
*Nephro-Calci*—R & D (U.S.) brand of Calcium Carbonate—**See Calcium Supplements (Systemic)**, 736
*Nephro-Fer*—R & D (U.S.) brand of Ferrous Fumarate—**See Iron Supplements (Systemic)**, 1774
*Nephron*—Nephron (U.S.) brand of Epinephrine—**See Bronchodilators, Adrenergic (Inhalation-Local)**, 640
*Nephropure*—Frosst (Canada) brand of Iodohippurate Sodium I 123 (Systemic), 1753
*Nephrox*—Fleming (U.S.) brand of Aluminum Hydroxide—**See Antacids (Oral-Local)**, 188
*Nepro*—Ross (U.S.) brand of Enteral Nutrition Formula, Disease-specific—**See Enteral Nutrition Formulas (Systemic)**, #
*Neptazane*—Lederle (U.S. and Canada) brand of Methazolamide—**See Carbonic Anhydrase Inhibitors (Systemic)**, 773
*Nerisone*—Stiefel (Canada) brand of Diflucortolone—**See Corticosteroids (Topical)**, 978
*Nerisone Oily*—Stiefel (Canada) brand of Diflucortolone—**See Corticosteroids (Topical)**, 978
*Nervine*—Mathieu (Canada) brand of Aspirin—**See Salicylates (Systemic)**, 2538
*Nervine Nighttime Sleep-Aid*—Miles (U.S.) brand of Diphenhydramine—**See Antihistamines (Systemic)**, 325
*Nesacaine*—Astra (U.S.) brand of Chloroprocaine—**See Anesthetics (Parenteral-Local)**, 139
*Nesacaine-CE*—Astra (U.S.) brand of Chloroprocaine—**See Anesthetics (Parenteral-Local)**, 139
*Nesacaine-MPF*—Astra (U.S.) brand of Chloroprocaine—**See Anesthetics (Parenteral-Local)**, 139
*Nestrex*—Fielding (U.S.) brand of Pyridoxine (Systemic), 2430
Netilmicin Sulfate [*Netromycin*]
  **See Aminoglycosides (Systemic)**, 69
  Injection USP, 77
*Netromycin*—Schering (U.S. and Canada) brand of Netilmicin—**See Aminoglycosides (Systemic)**, 69
*Neuleptil*—Rhône-Poulenc (Canada) brand of Pericyazine—**See Phenothiazines (Systemic)**, 2289
*Neumega*—Genetics Institute (U.S.) brand of Oprelvekin (Systemic), 2205
*Neumega rhIL-11 Growth Factor*—Genetics (U.S.) brand of Interleukin-11, Human, Recombinant (Systemic), 3161
*Neupogen*—Amgen (U.S. and Canada) brand of Filgrastim—**See Colony Stimulating Factors (Systemic)**, 941, 3143
*Neuprex*—Xoma (U.S.) brand of Bactericidal/Permeability-increasing Protein, Recombinant (Systemic), 3160
*Neuralgon*—WTD (U.S.) brand of L-Baclofen (Systemic), 3150
*Neurelan*—Elan (U.S.) brand of Fampridine (Systemic), 3143
*NeuroCell-HD*—Diacrin (U.S.) brand of Porcine Fetal Neural GABAergic Cells and/or Precursors Aseptically Prepared and Coated with Anti-MHC-1 Ab for Intracerebral Implantation (Systemic), 3159; Porcine Fetal Neural GABAergic Cells and/or Precursors Aseptically Prepared for Intracerebral Implantation (Systemic), 3159
*NeuroCell-PD*—Diacrin (U.S.) brand of Porcine Fetal Neural Dopaminergic Cells and/or Precursors Aseptically Prepared and Coated with Anti-MHC-1 Ab for Intracerebral Implantation (Systemic), 3159; Porcine Fetal Neural Dopaminergic Cells and/or Precursors Aseptically Prepared for Intracerebral Implantation (Systemic), 3159
*Neuroforte-R*—International Ethical (U.S.) brand of Cyanocobalamin—**See Vitamin B$_{12}$ (Systemic)**, 2962
*Neurolite*—Du Pont Merck (U.S.) and Du Pont (Canada) brand of Technetium Tc 99m Bicisate (Systemic), 2703
Neuromuscular Blocking Agents
  **(Systemic)**, 2098

*Neurontin*—PD (U.S. and Canada) and Warner-Lambert (U.S.) brand of Gabapentin (Systemic), 1536, MC-13, 3144
Neurotrophin-1
  **(Systemic)**, 3156
*Neutralca-S*—Desbergers (Canada) brand of Alumina and Magnesia—**See Antacids (Oral-Local)**, 188
*Neutra-Phos*—Willen (U.S.) brand of Potassium and Sodium Phosphates—**See Phosphates (Systemic)**, 2317
*Neutra-Phos-K*—Willen (U.S.) brand of Potassium Phosphates—**See Phosphates (Systemic)**, 2317
*Neutrexin*—U.S. Bioscience (U.S.) and Lilly (Canada) brand of Trimetrexate (Systemic), 2885, 3170
*Neutrogena Acne Mask 5*—Neutrogena (U.S.) brand of Benzoyl Peroxide (Topical), 579
*Neutrogena Chemical-Free Sunblocker*—Neutrogena (U.S.) brand of Titanium Dioxide—**See Sunscreen Agents (Topical)**, #
*Neutrogena Deep Glow*—Neutrogena (U.S.) brand of Octyl Methoxycinnamate—**See Sunscreen Agents (Topical)**, #
*Neutrogena Intensified Day Moisture*—Neutrogena (U.S.) brand of Octyl Methoxycinnamate and Phenylbenzimidazole—**See Sunscreen Agents (Topical)**, #
*Neutrogena Light Glow*—Neutrogena (U.S.) brand of Octyl Methoxycinnamate—**See Sunscreen Agents (Topical)**, #
*Neutrogena Lip Moisturizer*—Neutrogena (U.S.) brand of Octyl Methoxycinnamate and Oxybenzone—**See Sunscreen Agents (Topical)**, #
*Neutrogena Moisture Untinted & with Sheer Tint*—Neutrogena (U.S.) brand of Octyl Methoxycinnamate and Oxybenzone—**See Sunscreen Agents (Topical)**, #
*Neutrogena No Stick Sunscreen*—Neutrogena (U.S.) brand of Homosalate, Octyl Methoxycinnamate, Octyl Salicylate, and Oxybenzone—**See Sunscreen Agents (Topical)**, #
*Neutrogena Sunblock*—Neutrogena (U.S.) brand of Menthyl Anthranilate, Octocrylene, and Octyl Methoxycinnamate—**See Sunscreen Agents (Topical)**, #; Menthyl Anthranilate and Octyl Methoxycinnamate—**See Sunscreen Agents (Topical)**, #; Menthyl Anthranilate, Octyl Methoxycinnamate, and Octyl Salicylate—**See Sunscreen Agents (Topical)**, #; Octyl Methoxycinnamate, Octyl Salicylate, and Oxybenzone—**See Sunscreen Agents (Topical)**, #
Nevirapine [*Viramune*]
  **(Systemic)**, 2113
  Tablets, 2115
NG-29 [*Somatrel*]
  **(Systemic)**, 3156
N3 Gesic—Qualitest (U.S.) brand of Orphenadrine, Aspirin, and Caffeine (Systemic), 2208
N3 Gesic Forte—Qualitest (U.S.) brand of Orphenadrine, Aspirin, and Caffeine (Systemic), 2208
*N-Graft*—Theracell (U.S.) brand of Porcine Sertoli Cells (Systemic), 3159
$^{13}$NH$_3$—See Ammonia N 13 (Systemic), 91
*Nia-Bid*—Geriatric (U.S.) brand of Niacin—**See Niacin (Systemic)**, 2116
*Niac*—Forest (U.S.) brand of Niacin—**See Niacin (Systemic)**, 2116
*Niacels*—Hauck (U.S.) brand of Niacin—**See Niacin (Systemic)**, 2116
Niacin [*Endur-Acin; Nia-Bid; Niac; Niacels; Niacor; Nico-400; Nicobid Tempules; Nicolar; Nicotinex Elixir;* nicotinic acid; *Novo-Niacin; Slo-Niacin;* vitamin B$_3$]
  **See Niacin (Systemic)**, 2116
  Capsules, Extended-release, 2118, MC-21
  Injection USP, 2119
  Solution, Oral, 2118
  Tablets USP, 2119, MC-21
  Tablets, Extended-release, 2119, MC-21
Niacinamide [nicotinamide; vitamin B$_3$]
  **See Niacin (Systemic)**, 2116
  Injection USP, 2120
  Tablets USP, 2119
*Niacor*—Upsher-Smith (U.S.) brand of Niacin—**See Niacin (Systemic)**, 2116
Nicardipine Hydrochloride [*Cardene; Cardene SR; Cardene-SR*]
  **See Calcium Channel Blocking Agents (Systemic)**, 720, 3029
  Capsules, 729, MC-22
  Capsules, Extended-release, 3029

*Niclocide*—Miles (U.S.) brand of Niclosamide (Oral-Local), #
Niclosamide [*Niclocide*]
  **(Oral-Local)**, #
  Tablets, Chewable, #
*Nico-400*—Jones (U.S.) brand of Niacin—**See Niacin (Systemic)**, 2116
*Nicobid Tempules*—Rhône-Poulenc Rorer (U.S.) brand of Niacin—**See Niacin (Systemic)**, 2116
*Nicoderm*—Marion Merrell Dow (U.S.) and Merrell Dow (Canada) brand of Nicotine (Systemic), 2125
*NicoDerm CQ*—SmithKline Beecham (U.S.) brand of Nicotine (Systemic), 3030
*Nicolar*—Rhône-Poulenc Rorer (U.S.) brand of Niacin—**See Niacin (Systemic)**, 2116
*Nicorette*—SmithKline Beecham (U.S.) and Marion Merrell Dow (Canada) brand of Nicotine (Systemic), 2125
*Nicorette Plus*—Marion Merrell Dow (Canada) brand of Nicotine (Systemic), 2125
Nicotinamide—Niacinamide—**See Niacin (Systemic)**, 2116
Nicotinamide [*Papulex*]
  **(Topical)**, 3029
  Gel, 3029
Nicotine [*Habitrol; Nicoderm; NicoDerm CQ; Nicotrol; ProStep*]
  **(Systemic)**, 2125, 3030
  System, Transdermal, 3030
Nicotine [*Nicotrol Inhaler*]
  **(Inhalation-Systemic)**, 2120
  for Inhalation, 2122
Nicotine [*Nicotrol NS*]
  **(Nasal)**, 2122
  Solution, Nasal, 2125
Nicotine Polacrilex [*Nicorette; Nicorette Plus*]
  **(Systemic)**, 2125
  Gum USP, 2128
  Transdermal System, 2128
*Nicotinex Elixir*—Fleming (U.S.) brand of Niacin—**See Niacin (Systemic)**, 2116
Nicotinic acid—Niacin—**See Niacin (Systemic)**, 2116
Nicotinyl Alcohol Tartrate [*Roniacol*]
  **(Systemic)**, #
  Tablets, Extended-release, #
*Nicotrol*—McNeil Consumer (U.S. and Canada) brand of Nicotine (Systemic), 2125, 3030
*Nicotrol Inhaler*—McNeil Consumer (U.S.) brand of Nicotine (Inhalation-Systemic), 2120
*Nicotrol NS*—McNeil (U.S.) brand of Nicotine (Nasal), 2122
*Nidagel*—Ferring (Canada) brand of Metronidazole (Vaginal), 2001
Nifedipine [*Adalat; Adalat CC; Adalat P.A.; Adalat XL; Apo-Nifed; Novo-Nifedin; Nu-Nifed; Procardia; Procardia XL*]
  **See Calcium Channel Blocking Agents (Systemic)**, 720, 3156
  Capsules USP, 730, MC-22
  Tablets, Extended-release, 730, MC-22
*Niferex*—Central (U.S.) brand of Iron-Polysaccharide—**See Iron Supplements (Systemic)**, 1774
*Niferex-150*—Central (U.S.) brand of Iron-Polysaccharide—**See Iron Supplements (Systemic)**, 1774
Nifurtimox [*Bayer 2502; Lampit*]
  **(Systemic)**, #
  Tablets, #
*Night Cast Special Formula Mask-lotion*—Seres (U.S.) brand of Resorcinol and Sulfur (Topical), #
*Night-Time Effervescent Cold*—Zenith Goldline (U.S.) brand of Diphenhydramine, Phenylpropanolamine, and Aspirin—**See Antihistamines, Decongestants, and Analgesics (Systemic)**, 366
*Nilandron*—Hoechst Marion Roussel (U.S.) brand of Nilutamide—**See Antiandrogens, Nonsteroidal (Systemic)**, 220, MC-22
*Nilstat*—Lederle (U.S. and Canada) brand of Nystatin (Oral-Local), 2146; (Topical), 2148; (Vaginal), 2149
Nilutamide [*Anandron; Nilandron*]
  **See Antiandrogens, Nonsteroidal (Systemic)**, 220
  Tablets, 226, MC-22
*Nimbex*—Glaxo Wellcome (U.S. and Canada) brand of Cisatracurium (Systemic), 872
*Nimbus Quick Strip*—Biomerica (U.S.) brand of Immunoassay Pregnancy Test Kits—**See Pregnancy Test Kits for Home Use**, #

**3316  General Index**

Nimodipine [*Nimotop*]
　See **Calcium Channel Blocking Agents (Systemic)**, 720
　Capsules, 731, MC-22
*Nimotop*—Bayer (U.S. and Canada) brand of Nimodipine—See **Calcium Channel Blocking Agents (Systemic)**, 720, MC-22
*Niong*—U.S. Ethicals (U.S.) brand of Nitroglycerin—See **Nitrates (Systemic)**, 2129
*Nipent*—PD (U.S. and Canada) and Warner-Lambert (U.S.) brand of Pentostatin (Systemic), 2279, 3158
*Nipride*—Roche (Canada) brand of Nitroprusside (Systemic), 2142
N-IPV—Poliovirus Vaccine Inactivated Enhanced Potency—See **Poliovirus Vaccine (Systemic)**, 2343
Nisoldipine [*Sular*]
　**(Systemic)**
　Tablets, Extended-release, MC-22
Nitazoxanide
　**(Systemic)**, 3156
Nitrates
　**(Systemic)**, 2129
Nitrazepam [*Mogadon*]
　See **Benzodiazepines (Systemic)**, 556
　Tablets, 575
Nitric Oxide
　**(Systemic)**, 3156
*Nitro-Bid*—Marion (U.S.) and Roussel (Canada) brand of Nitroglycerin—See **Nitrates (Systemic)**, 2129
*Nitrocap*—Vortech (U.S.) brand of Nitroglycerin—See **Nitrates (Systemic)**, 2129
*Nitrocap T.D.*—Vortech (U.S.) brand of Nitroglycerin—See **Nitrates (Systemic)**, 2129
*Nitrodisc*—Searle (U.S.) brand of Nitroglycerin—See **Nitrates (Systemic)**, 2129
*Nitro-Dur*—Key (U.S.) brand of Nitroglycerin—See **Nitrates (Systemic)**, 2129
*Nitrofuracot*—Truxton (U.S.) brand of Nitrofurantoin (Systemic), 2139
Nitrofurantoin [*Apo-Nitrofurantoin; Furadantin; Furalan; Furatoin; Macrobid; Macrodantin*]
　**(Systemic)**, 2139
　Capsules USP, 2141, MC-22
　Capsules, Extended-release, 2142
　Suspension, Oral, USP, 2142
　Tablets USP, 2142
Nitrofurazone (Topical), 2142
*Nitrogard*—PD (U.S.) brand of Nitroglycerin—See **Nitrates (Systemic)**, 2129
*Nitrogard SR*—Astra (Canada) brand of Nitroglycerin—See **Nitrates (Systemic)**, 2129
Nitrogen mustard—See Mechlorethamine (Systemic), 1929; Mechlorethamine (Topical), #
Nitroglycerin [*Deponit*; glyceryl trinitrate; *Klavikordal; Minitran; Niong; Nitro-Bid; Nitrocap; Nitrocap T.D.; Nitrodisc; Nitro-Dur; Nitrogard; Nitrogard SR; Nitroglyn; Nitroject; Nitrol; Nitrolin; Nitrolingual; Nitronet; Nitrong; Nitrong SR; Nitrospan; Nitrostat; Transderm-Nitro; Tridil*]
　See **Nitrates (Systemic)**, 2129
　Aerosol, Lingual, 2134
　Capsules, Extended-release, 2134, MC-22
　Injection USP, 2135
　Ointment USP, 2136
　Systems, Transdermal, 2136
　Tablets, Extended-release, 2135
　Tablets, Extended-release Buccal, 2134
　Tablets USP (Sublingual), 2135, MC-22
*Nitroglyn*—Key (U.S.) brand of Nitroglycerin—See **Nitrates (Systemic)**, 2129
*Nitroject*—Omega (U.S. and Canada) brand of Nitroglycerin—See **Nitrates (Systemic)**, 2129
*Nitrol*—Adria (U.S.) and Rorer (Canada) brand of Nitroglycerin—See **Nitrates (Systemic)**, 2129
*Nitrolin*—Schein (U.S.) brand of Nitroglycerin—See **Nitrates (Systemic)**, 2129
*Nitrolingual*—Rhône-Poulenc Rorer (U.S. and Canada) brand of Nitroglycerin—See **Nitrates (Systemic)**, 2129
*Nitronet*—U.S. Ethicals (U.S.) brand of Nitroglycerin—See **Nitrates (Systemic)**, 2129
*Nitrong*—Wharton (U.S.) and Rhône-Poulenc (Canada) brand of Nitroglycerin—See **Nitrates (Systemic)**, 2129
*Nitrong SR*—Rhône-Poulenc (Canada) brand of Nitroglycerin—See **Nitrates (Systemic)**, 2129
*Nitropress*—Abbott (U.S.) brand of Nitroprusside (Systemic), 2142

Nitroprusside Sodium [*Nipride; Nitropress*]
　**(Systemic)**, 2142
　Sterile, 2145
Nitroprusside Urine Ketone Test [*Acetest; Chemstrip K; KetoStix*]
　See **Urine Glucose and Ketone Test Kits for Home Use**, #
　Strips, #
　Tablets, #
9-Nitro-20-(S)-Camptothecin (9-NC)
　**(Systemic)**, 3128
*Nitrospan*—USV (U.S.) brand of Nitroglycerin—See **Nitrates (Systemic)**, 2129
*Nitrostat*—PD (U.S. and Canada) brand of Nitroglycerin—See **Nitrates (Systemic)**, 2129, MC-22
Nitrous Oxide
　See **Anesthetics, Inhalation (Systemic)**, 168
　Nitrous Oxide USP, 173
*Nivea Sun*—Beiersdorf (U.S.) brand of Octyl Methoxycinnamate, Octyl Salicylate, and Oxybenzone—See **Sunscreen Agents (Topical)**, #
*Nix Cream Rinse*—BW (U.S. and Canada) brand of Permethrin (Topical), #
*Nix Dermal Cream*—BW (Canada) brand of Permethrin (Topical), 3032
Nizatidine [*Apo-Nizatidine; Axid; Axid AR*]
　See **Histamine H$_2$-receptor Antagonists (Systemic)**, 1633
　Capsules USP, 1640, MC-22
　Tablets, 1640
*Nizoral*—Janssen (U.S.) brand of Ketoconazole (Topical), 3026; Janssen (U.S.) and Janssen-Ortho (Canada) brand of Ketoconazole—See **Antifungals, Azole (Systemic)**, 302, MC-16
*Nizoral Cream*—Janssen (U.S. and Canada) brand of Ketoconazole (Topical), 1807
*Nizoral Shampoo*—Janssen (U.S. and Canada) brand of Ketoconazole (Topical), 1807
*NoDoz*—Bristol-Myers (U.S.) brand of Caffeine (Systemic), 706
*NoDoz Maximum Strength Caplets*—Bristol-Myers (U.S.) brand of Caffeine (Systemic), 706
*Nolahist*—Carrnick (U.S.) brand of Phenindamine—See **Antihistamines (Systemic)**, 325
*Nolamine*—Carrnick (U.S.) brand of Chlorpheniramine, Phenindamine, and Phenylpropanolamine—See **Antihistamines and Decongestants (Systemic)**, 343
*Noludar*—Roche (U.S. and Canada) brand of Methyprylon (Systemic), #
*Nolvadex*—ZENECA (U.S. and Canada) brand of Tamoxifen (Systemic), 2688, MC-29
*Nolvadex-D*—ZENECA (Canada) brand of Tamoxifen (Systemic), 2688
Nonoxinol 9—Nonoxynol 9—See **Spermicides (Vaginal)**, #
Nonoxynol 9 [*Because; Conceptrol Contraceptive Inserts; Conceptrol Gel; Delfen; Emko; Encare; Gynol II Extra Strength Contraceptive Jelly; Gynol II Original Formula Contraceptive Jelly; Koromex Crystal Clear Gel; Koromex Foam; Koromex Jelly*; nonoxinol 9; *Ortho-Creme; Pre-Fil; Ramses Contraceptive Foam; Ramses Contraceptive Vaginal Jelly; Ramses Crystal Clear Gel; Semicid; Shur-Seal; Today; VCF*]
　See **Spermicides (Vaginal)**, #
　Cream, Vaginal, #
　Film, Vaginal, #
　Foam, Vaginal, #
　Gel, Vaginal, #
　Jelly, Vaginal, #
　Suppositories, Vaginal, #
*Nootropil*—UCB (U.S.) brand of Piracetam (Systemic), 3158
Noradrenaline—Norepinephrine—See **Sympathomimetic Agents—Cardiovascular Use (Parenteral-Systemic)**, 2669
*Norcuron*—Organon (U.S. and Canada) brand of Vecuronium—See **Neuromuscular Blocking Agents (Systemic)**, 2098
*Nordette*—Wyeth-Ayerst (U.S.) brand of Levonorgestrel and Ethinyl Estradiol—See **Estrogens and Progestins—Oral Contraceptives (Systemic)**, 1397, MC-17
*Norditropin*—Novo Nordisk (U.S.) brand of Somatropin (Systemic), 3165
*Norel*—US Pharmaceutical (U.S.) brand of Phenylephrine, Phenylpropanolamine, and Guaifenesin—See **Cough/Cold Combinations (Systemic)**, 1024

*Norel Plus*—U.S. Pharmaceutical (U.S.) brand of Chlorpheniramine, Phenyltoloxamine, Phenylpropanolamine, and Acetaminophen—See **Antihistamines, Decongestants, and Analgesics (Systemic)**, 366
Norepinephrine Bitartrate [levarterenol; *Levophed*]
　See **Sympathomimetic Agents—Cardiovascular Use (Parenteral-Systemic)**, 2669
　Injection USP, 2678
Norepinephrine-containing Combinations, 3076
Norethindrone [*Micronor*; norethisterone; *Nor-QD*]
　See **Progestins (Systemic)**, 2400
　Tablets USP, 2410
Norethindrone Acetate [*Aygestin*; norethisterone; *Norlutate*]
　See **Progestins (Systemic)**, 2400
　Tablets USP, 2410
Norethindrone Acetate and Ethinyl Estradiol [*Loestrin 1/20; Loestrin 1.5/30; Minestrin 1/20*]
　See **Estrogens and Progestins—Oral Contraceptives (Systemic)**, 1397
　Tablets USP, 1409 MC-22, MC-23
Norethindrone Acetate and Ethinyl Estradiol and Ferrous Fumarate [*Estrostep Fe; Loestrin Fe 1/20; Loestrin Fe 1.5/30*]
　**(Systemic)**, 1397
　Tablets USP, 1409, MC-23, 1397
Norethindrone and Ethinyl Estradiol [*Brevicon; Brevicon 0.5/35; Brevicon 1/35; Genora 0.5/35; Genora 1/35; Intercon 0.5/35; Intercon 1/35; Jenest; ModiCon; Necon 0.5/35; Necon 1/35; Necon 10/11; N.E.E. 1/35; N.E.E. 10/11; Necon 1/35E; Nelova 1/35E; Nelova 10/11; Norethin 1/35E; Norinyl 1+35; Ortho 0.5/35; Ortho 1/35; Ortho 7/7/7; Ortho 10/11; Ortho-Novum 1/35; Ortho-Novum 7/7/7; Ortho-Novum 10/11; Ovcon-35; Ovcon-50; Synphasic; Tri-Norinyl*]
　See **Estrogens and Progestins—Oral Contraceptives (Systemic)**, 1397
　Tablets, 1409, MC-22
Norethindrone and Mestranol [*Genora 1/50; Intercon 1/50; Necon 1/50; Nelova 1/50M; Norethin 1/50M; Norinyl 1/50; Norinyl 1+50; Ortho-Novum 1/50*]
　See **Estrogens and Progestins—Oral Contraceptives (Systemic)**, 1397
　Tablets USP, 1410, MC-22
*Norethin 1/35E*—Roberts (U.S.) brand of Norethindrone and Ethinyl Estradiol—See **Estrogens and Progestins—Oral Contraceptives (Systemic)**, 1397
*Norethin 1/50M*—Roberts (U.S.) brand of Norethindrone and Mestranol—See **Estrogens and Progestins—Oral Contraceptives (Systemic)**, 1397
Norethisterone—Norethindrone—See **Progestins (Systemic)**, 2400
*Norfemac*—Nordic (Canada) brand of Bufexamac (Topical), 3013
*Norflex*—3M (U.S. and Canada) brand of Orphenadrine—See **Skeletal Muscle Relaxants (Systemic)**, 2577
Norfloxacin [*Chibroxin; Noroxin*]
　**(Ophthalmic)**, #
　Solution, Ophthalmic, #
Norfloxacin [*Noroxin*]
　See **Fluoroquinolones (Systemic)**, 1487
　Tablets USP, 1494, MC-23
*Norfranil*—Vortech (U.S.) brand of Imipramine—See **Antidepressants, Tricyclic (Systemic)**, 271
*Norgesic*—Riker (U.S. and Canada) brand of Orphenadrine, Aspirin, and Caffeine (Systemic), 2208
*Norgesic Forte*—Riker (U.S. and Canada) brand of Orphenadrine, Aspirin, and Caffeine (Systemic), 2208
Norgestimate and Ethinyl Estradiol [*Cyclen; Ortho-Cyclen; Ortho Tri-Cyclen; Tri-Cyclen*]
　See **Estrogens and Progestins—Oral Contraceptives (Systemic)**, 1397
　Tablets, 1411, MC-23
Norgestrel [*Ovrette*]
　See **Progestins (Systemic)**, 2400
　Tablets USP, 2411
Norgestrel and Ethinyl Estradiol [*Lo/Ovral; Ovral*]
　See **Estrogens and Progestins—Oral Contraceptives (Systemic)**, 1397
　Tablets USP, 1411, MC-23
*Norinyl 1/50*—Searle (Canada) brand of Norethindrone and Mestranol—See **Estrogens and Progestins—Oral Contraceptives (Systemic)**, 1397

*Norinyl 1+35*—Searle (U.S.) brand of Norethindrone and Ethinyl Estradiol—**See Estrogens and Progestins—Oral Contraceptives (Systemic)**, 1397
*Norinyl 1+50*—Searle (U.S.) brand of Norethindrone and Mestranol—**See Estrogens and Progestins—Oral Contraceptives (Systemic)**, 1397
*Norlutate*—PD (Canada) brand of Norethindrone—**See Progestins (Systemic)**, 2400
*Normiflo*—Wyeth (U.S.) brand of Ardeparin (Systemic), 467
*Normix*—Salix (U.S.) brand of Refaximin (Systemic), 3162
*Normodyne*—Schering (U.S.) brand of Labetalol—**See Beta-adrenergic Blocking Agents (Systemic)**, 593, MC-16
*Normosang*—Leiras (U.S.) brand of Heme Arginate (Systemic), 3145
*Noroxin*—Merck (U.S.) brand of Norfloxacin—**See Fluoroquinolones (Systemic)**, 1487, MC-23; MSD (Canada) brand of Norfloxacin (Ophthalmic), #
*Norpace*—Searle (U.S. and Canada) brand of Disopyramide (Systemic), 1252, MC-10
*Norpace CR*—Searle (U.S. and Canada) brand of Disopyramide (Systemic), 1252, MC-10
*Norphadrine*—Major (U.S.) brand of Orphenadrine, Aspirin, and Caffeine (Systemic), 2208
*Norphadrine Forte*—Major (U.S.) brand of Orphenadrine, Aspirin, and Caffeine (Systemic), 2208
NORPLANT System—Wyeth-Ayerst (U.S. and Canada) brand of Levonorgestrel—**See Progestins (Systemic)**, 2400
*Norpramin*—Hoechst Marion Rousel (U.S. and Canada) brand of Desipramine—**See Antidepressants, Tricyclic (Systemic)**, 271, MC-8
*Nor-Pred T.B.A.*—Vortech (U.S.) brand of Prednisolone—**See Corticosteroids—Glucocorticoid Effects (Systemic)**, 998
*Nor-QD*—Watson (U.S.) brand of Norethindrone—**See Progestins (Systemic)**, 2400
North American coral snake antivenin—*See* Antivenin (Micrurus Fulvius) (Systemic), #
Nortriptyline Hydrochloride [*Aventyl; Pamelor*]
 **See Antidepressants, Tricyclic (Systemic)**, 271
 Capsules USP, 281, MC-23
 Solution, Oral, USP, 282
*Norvasc*—Pfizer (U.S.) brand of Amlodipine (Systemic), 86, MC-2
*Norvir*—Abbott (U.S.) brand of Ritonavir (Systemic), 2516, MC-27
*Norwich Aspirin*—Richardson-Vicks Health Care (U.S.) brand of Aspirin—**See Salicylates (Systemic)**, 2538
*Norwood Sunburn Spray*—Norwood (Canada) brand of Lidocaine—**See Anesthetics (Topical)**, 155
*Norzine*—Purdue Frederick (U.S.) brand of Thiethylperazine (Systemic), #
*Nostrilla Long-Acting Nasal Decongestant*—Ciba (U.S.) brand of Oxymetazoline (Nasal), #
*Nostril Spray Pump*—Ciba (U.S.) brand of Phenylephrine (Nasal), #
*Nostril Spray Pump Mild*—Ciba (U.S.) brand of Phenylephrine (Nasal), #
*Novafed*—Marion Merrell Dow (U.S.) brand of Pseudoephedrine (Systemic), 2422
*Novafed A*—Hoechst Marion Roussel (U.S.) brand of Chlorpheniramine and Pseudoephedrine—**See Antihistamines and Decongestants (Systemic)**, 343
*Novagest Expectorant with Codeine*—Major (U.S.) brand of Pseudoephedrine, Codeine, and Guaifenesin—**See Cough/Cold Combinations (Systemic)**, 1024
*Novahistex*—Hoechst Marion Roussel (Canada) brand of Chlorpheniramine and Pseudoephedrine—**See Antihistamines and Decongestants (Systemic)**, 343
*Novahistex C*—Marion Merrell Dow (Canada) brand of Phenylephrine and Codeine—**See Cough/Cold Combinations (Systemic)**, 1024
*Novahistex DH*—Marion Merrell Dow (Canada) brand of Phenylephrine and Hydrocodone—**See Cough/Cold Combinations (Systemic)**, 1024
*Novahistex DH Expectorant*—Marion Merrell Dow (Canada) brand of Phenylephrine, Hydrocodone, and Guaifenesin—**See Cough/Cold Combinations (Systemic)**, 1024
*Novahistex DM with Decongestant*—Marion Merrell Dow (Canada) brand of Pseudoephedrine and Dextromethorphan—**See Cough/Cold Combinations (Systemic)**, 1024

*Novahistex DM Expectorant with Decongestant*—Marion Merrell Dow (Canada) brand of Pseudoephedrine, Dextromethorphan, and Guaifenesin—**See Cough/Cold Combinations (Systemic)**, 1024
*Novahistex Expectorant with Decongestant*—Marion Merrell Dow (Canada) brand of Pseudoephedrine and Guaifenesin—**See Cough/Cold Combinations (Systemic)**, 1024
*Novahistine*—SmithKline Beecham (U.S.) brand of Chlorpheniramine and Phenylephrine—**See Antihistamines and Decongestants (Systemic)**, 343
*Novahistine DH*—Marion Merrell Dow (Canada) brand of Phenylephrine and Hydrocodone—**See Cough/Cold Combinations (Systemic)**, 1024
*Novahistine DH Liquid*—Smithkline Beecham (U.S.) brand of Chlorpheniramine, Pseudoephedrine, and Codeine—**See Cough/Cold Combinations (Systemic)**, 1024
*Novahistine DM with Decongestant*—Marion Merrell Dow (Canada) brand of Pseudoephedrine and Dextromethorphan—**See Cough/Cold Combinations (Systemic)**, 1024
*Novahistine DM Expectorant with Decongestant*—Marion Merrell Dow (Canada) brand of Pseudoephedrine, Dextromethorphan, and Guaifenesin—**See Cough/Cold Combinations (Systemic)**, 1024
*Novahistine DMX Liquid*—Smithkline Beecham (U.S.) brand of Pseudoephedrine, Dextromethorphan, and Guaifenesin—**See Cough/Cold Combinations (Systemic)**, 1024
*Novahistine Expectorant*—Smithkline Beecham (U.S.) brand of Pseudoephedrine, Codeine, and Guaifenesin—**See Cough/Cold Combinations (Systemic)**, 1024
*Novamoxin*—Novopharm (Canada) brand of Amoxicillin—**See Penicillins (Systemic)**, 2240
*Novantrone*—Immunex (U.S.) and Lederle (U.S.) and Wyeth-Ayerst (Canada) brand of Mitoxantrone (Systemic), 2033, 3154
*Nova Rectal*—Sabex (Canada) brand of Pentobarbital—**See Barbiturates (Systemic)**, 518
*Novasen*—Novopharm (Canada) brand of Aspirin—**See Salicylates (Systemic)**, 2538
*Novasen Sp.C*—Novopharm (Canada) brand of Aspirin—**See Salicylates (Systemic)**, 2538
*Nova-T*—Berlex (Canada) brand of Copper-T 200Ag Intrauterine Device—**See Copper Intrauterine Devices (IUDs)**, #
*Novo-AC and C*—Novopharm (Canada) brand of Aspirin and Codeine—**See Opioid (Narcotic) Analgesics and Aspirin (Systemic)**, 2202
*Novo-Alprazol*—Novopharm (Canada) brand of Alprazolam—**See Benzodiazepines (Systemic)**, 556
*Novo-Ampicillin*—Novopharm (Canada) brand of Ampicillin—**See Penicillins (Systemic)**, 2240
*Novo-Atenol*—Novopharm (Canada) brand of Atenolol—**See Beta-adrenergic Blocking Agents (Systemic)**, 593
*Novo-AZT*—Novopharm (Canada) brand of Zidovudine (Systemic), 2992
*Novobetamet*—Novopharm (Canada) brand of Betamethasone—**See Corticosteroids (Topical)**, 978
*Novo-Butamide*—Novopharm (Canada) brand of Tolbutamide—**See Antidiabetic Agents, Sulfonylurea (Systemic)**, 283
*Novocain*—Sanofi Winthrop (U.S. and Canada) brand of Procaine—**See Anesthetics (Parenteral-Local)**, 139
*Novo-Carbamaz*—Novopharm (Canada) brand of Carbamazepine (Systemic), 757
*Novo-Chlorhydrate*—Novopharm (Canada) brand of Chloral Hydrate (Systemic), 834
*Novochlorocap*—Novopharm (Canada) brand of Chloramphenicol (Systemic), 841
*Novo-Chlorpromazine*—Novopharm (Canada) brand of Chlorpromazine—**See Phenothiazines (Systemic)**, 2289
*Novo-Cimetine*—Novopharm (Canada) brand of Cimetidine—**See Histamine H$_2$-receptor Antagonists (Systemic)**, 1633
*Novo-Clopate*—Novopharm (Canada) brand of Clorazepate—**See Benzodiazepines (Systemic)**, 556
*Novo-Cloxin*—Novopharm (Canada) brand of Cloxacillin—**See Penicillins (Systemic)**, 2240
*Novo-cromolyn*—Novopharm (Canada) brand of Cromolyn (Inhalation-Local), 1116

*Novo-Difenac*—Novopharm (Canada) brand of Diclofenac—**See Anti-inflammatory Drugs, Nonsteroidal (Systemic)**, 388
*Novo-Difenac SR*—Novopharm (Canada) brand of Diclofenac—**See Anti-inflammatory Drugs, Nonsteroidal (Systemic)**, 388
*Novo-Diflunisal*—Novopharm (Canada) brand of Diflunisal—**See Anti-inflammatory Drugs, Nonsteroidal (Systemic)**, 388
*Novodigoxin*—Novopharm (Canada) brand of Digoxin—**See Digitalis Glycosides (Systemic)**, 1213
*Novo-Diltazem*—Novopharm (Canada) brand of Diltiazem—**See Calcium Channel Blocking Agents (Systemic)**, 720
*Novo-Dipam*—Novopharm (Canada) brand of Diazepam—**See Benzodiazepines (Systemic)**, 556
*Novodipiradol*—Novopharm (Canada) brand of Dipyridamole (Systemic), #
*Novodoparil*—Novopharm (Canada) brand of Methyldopa and Hydrochlorothiazide—**See Methyldopa and Thiazide Diuretics (Systemic)**, 1983
*Novo-Doxepin*—Novopharm (Canada) brand of Doxepin—**See Antidepressants, Tricyclic (Systemic)**, 271
*Novodoxylin*—Novopharm (Canada) brand of Doxycycline—**See Tetracyclines (Systemic)**, 2765
*Novo-Famotidine*—Novopharm (Canada) brand of Famotidine—**See Histamine H$_2$-receptor Antagonists (Systemic)**, 1633, MC-12
*Novoferrogluc*—Novopharm (Canada) brand of Ferrous Gluconate—**See Iron Supplements (Systemic)**, 1774
*Novoferrosulfa*—Novopharm (Canada) brand of Ferrous Sulfate—**See Iron Supplements (Systemic)**, 1774
*Novofibrate*—Novopharm (Canada) brand of Clofibrate (Systemic), 900
*Novo-Flupam*—Novopharm (Canada) brand of Flurazepam—**See Benzodiazepines (Systemic)**, 556
*Novo-Flurazine*—Novopharm (Canada) brand of Trifluoperazine—**See Phenothiazines (Systemic)**, 2289
*Novo-Flurprofen*—Novopharm (Canada) brand of Flurbiprofen—**See Anti-inflammatory Drugs, Nonsteroidal (Systemic)**, 388
*Novo-Folacid*—Novopharm (Canada) brand of Folic Acid (Systemic), 1517
*Novofumar*—Novopharm (Canada) brand of Ferrous Fumarate—**See Iron Supplements (Systemic)**, 1774
*Novo-Gemfibrozil*—Novopharm (Canada) brand of Gemfibrozil (Systemic), 1552
*Novo-Gesic C8*—Novopharm (Canada) brand of Acetaminophen and Codeine—**See Opioid (Narcotic) Analgesics and Acetaminophen (Systemic)**, 2198
*Novo-Gesic C15*—Novopharm (Canada) brand of Acetaminophen and Codeine—**See Opioid (Narcotic) Analgesics and Acetaminophen (Systemic)**, 2198
*Novo-Gesic C30*—Novopharm (Canada) brand of Acetaminophen and Codeine—**See Opioid (Narcotic) Analgesics and Acetaminophen (Systemic)**, 2198
*Novo-Glyburide*—Novopharm (Canada) brand of Glyburide—**See Antidiabetic Agents, Sulfonylurea (Systemic)**, 283
*Novo-Hydrazide*—Novopharm (Canada) brand of Hydrochlorothiazide—**See Diuretics, Thiazide (Systemic)**, 1273
*Novohydrocort*—Novopharm (Canada) brand of Hydrocortisone—**See Corticosteroids (Topical)**, 978
*Novo-Hydroxyzin*—Novopharm (Canada) brand of Hydroxyzine—**See Antihistamines (Systemic)**, 325
*Novo-Hylazin*—Novopharm (Canada) brand of Hydralazine (Systemic), 1655
*Novo-Keto-EC*—Novopharm (Canada) brand of Ketoprofen—**See Anti-inflammatory Drugs, Nonsteroidal (Systemic)**, 388
*Novo-Lexin*—Novopharm (Canada) brand of Cephalexin—**See Cephalosporins (Systemic)**, 794
*Novolin 70/30*—Novo Nordisk (U.S.) brand of Insulin, Isophane, Human, and Insulin Human—**See Insulin (Systemic)**, 1713
*Novolin ge 30/70*—Connaught Novo Nordisk (Canada) brand of Insulin, Isophane, Human, and Insulin Human (Systemic), 1713

**3318    General Index**

*Novolin ge Lente*—Connaught Novo Nordisk (Canada) brand of Insulin Zinc, Human—**See Insulin (Systemic)**, 1713
*Novolin ge NPH*—Connaught Novo Nordisk (Canada) brand of Insulin, Isophane, Human—**See Insulin (Systemic)**, 1713
*Novolin ge NPH Penfill*—Connaught Novo Nordisk (Canada) brand of Insulin, Isophane, Human—**See Insulin (Systemic)**, 1713
*Novolin ge 10/90 Penfill*—Connaught Novo Nordisk (Canada) brand of Insulin, Isophane, Human, and Insulin Human (Systemic), 1713
*Novolin ge 20/80 Penfill*—Connaught Novo Nordisk (Canada) brand of Insulin, Isophane, Human, and Insulin Human (Systemic), 1713
*Novolin ge 30/70 Penfill*—Connaught Novo Nordisk (Canada) brand of Insulin, Isophane, Human, and Insulin Human (Systemic), 1713
*Novolin ge 40/60 Penfill*—Connaught Novo Nordisk (Canada) brand of Insulin, Isophane, Human, and Insulin Human (Systemic), 1713
*Novolin ge 50/50 Penfill*—Connaught Novo Nordisk (Canada) brand of Insulin, Isophane, Human, and Insulin Human (Systemic), 1713
*Novolin ge Toronto*—Connaught Novo Nordisk (Canada) brand of Insulin Human—**See Insulin (Systemic)**, 1713
*Novolin ge Toronto Penfill*—Connaught Novo Nordisk (Canada) brand of Insulin Human—**See Insulin (Systemic)**, 1713
*Novolin ge Ultralente*—Connaught Novo Nordisk (Canada) brand of Insulin Zinc, Extended, Human—**See Insulin (Systemic)**, 1713
*Novolin L*—Novo Nordisk (U.S.) brand of Insulin Zinc, Human—**See Insulin (Systemic)**, 1713
*Novolin N*—Novo Nordisk (U.S.) brand of Insulin, Isophane, Human—**See Insulin (Systemic)**, 1713
*Novolin N PenFill*—Novo Nordisk (U.S.) brand of Insulin, Isophane, Human—**See Insulin (Systemic)**, 1713
*Novolin N Prefilled*—Novo Nordisk (U.S.) brand of Insulin, Isophane, Human—**See Insulin (Systemic)**, 1713
*Novolin 70/30 PenFill*—Novo Nordisk (U.S.) brand of Insulin, Isophane, Human, and Insulin Human—**See Insulin (Systemic)**, 1713
*Novolin 70/30 Prefilled*—Novo Nordisk (U.S.) brand of Insulin, Isophane, Human, and Insulin Human—**See Insulin (Systemic)**, 1713
*Novolin R*—Novo Nordisk (U.S.) brand of Insulin Human—**See Insulin (Systemic)**, 1713
*Novolin R PenFill*—Novo Nordisk (U.S.) brand of Insulin Human—**See Insulin (Systemic)**, 1713
*Novolin R Prefilled*—Novo Nordisk (U.S.) brand of Insulin Human—**See Insulin (Systemic)**, 1713
*Novo-Lorazem*—Novopharm (Canada) brand of Lorazepam—**See Benzodiazepines (Systemic)**, 556
*Novomedopa*—Novopharm (Canada) brand of Methyldopa (Systemic), 1979
*Novo-Medrone*—Novopharm (Canada) brand of Medroxyprogesterone—**See Progestins (Systemic)**, 2400
*Novo-Metformin*—Novopharm (Canada) brand of Metformin (Systemic), 1957
*Novo-Methacin*—Novopharm (Canada) brand of Indomethacin—**See Anti-inflammatory Drugs, Nonsteroidal (Systemic)**, 388
*Novomethacin*—Novopharm (Canada) brand of Indomethacin—For Patent Ductus Arteriosus (Systemic), 1704
*Novometoprol*—Novopharm (Canada) brand of Metoprolol—**See Beta-adrenergic Blocking Agents (Systemic)**, 593
*Novo-Miconazole Vaginal Ovules*—Novopharm (Canada) brand of Miconazole—**See Antifungals, Azole (Vaginal)**, 310
*Novo-Naprox*—Novopharm (Canada) brand of Naproxen—**See Anti-inflammatory Drugs, Nonsteroidal (Systemic)**, 388
*Novo-Naprox Sodium*—Novopharm (Canada) brand of Naproxen—**See Anti-inflammatory Drugs, Nonsteroidal (Systemic)**, 388
*Novo-Naprox Sodium DS*—Novopharm (Canada) brand of Naproxen—**See Anti-inflammatory Drugs, Nonsteroidal (Systemic)**, 388
*Novo-Niacin*—Novopharm (Canada) brand of Niacin—**See Niacin (Systemic)**, 2116
*Novonidazol*—Novopharm (Canada) brand of Metronidazole (Systemic), 1996
*Novo-Nifedin*—Novopharm (Canada) brand of Nifedipine—**See Calcium Channel Blocking Agents (Systemic)**, 720

*Novopentobarb*—Novopharm (Canada) brand of Pentobarbital—**See Barbiturates (Systemic)**, 518
*Novo-Pen-VK*—Novopharm (Canada) brand of Penicillin V—**See Penicillins (Systemic)**, 2240
*Novo-Peridol*—Novopharm (Canada) brand of Haloperidol (Systemic), 1611
*Novo-Pheniram*—Novopharm (Canada) brand of Chlorpheniramine—**See Antihistamines (Systemic)**, 325
*Novo-Pindol*—Novopharm (Canada) brand of Pindolol—**See Beta-adrenergic Blocking Agents (Systemic)**, 593
*Novo-Pirocam*—Novopharm (Canada) brand of Piroxicam—**See Anti-inflammatory Drugs, Nonsteroidal (Systemic)**, 388
*Novo-Poxide*—Novopharm (Canada) brand of Chlordiazepoxide—**See Benzodiazepines (Systemic)**, 556
*Novopramine*—Novopharm (Canada) brand of Imipramine—**See Antidepressants, Tricyclic (Systemic)**, 271
*Novopranol*—Novopharm (Canada) brand of Propranolol—**See Beta-adrenergic Blocking Agents (Systemic)**, 593
*Novo-Profen*—Novopharm (Canada) brand of Ibuprofen—**See Anti-inflammatory Drugs, Nonsteroidal (Systemic)**, 388
*Novo-Propamide*—Novopharm (Canada) brand of Chlorpropamide—**See Antidiabetic Agents, Sulfonylurea (Systemic)**, 283
*Novopyrazone*—Novopharm (Canada) brand of Sulfinpyrazone (Systemic), 2646
*Novoquinidin*—Novopharm (Canada) brand of Quinidine (Systemic), 2440
*Novo-Ranitidine*—Novopharm (Canada) brand of Ranitidine Hydrochloride—**See Histamine H$_2$-receptor Antagonists (Systemic)**, 1633, MC-27
*Novoreserpine*—Novopharm (Canada) brand of Reserpine—**See Rauwolfia Alkaloids (Systemic)**, 2460
*Novo-Ridazine*—Novopharm (Canada) brand of Thioridazine—**See Phenothiazines (Systemic)**, 2289
*Novo-Rythro*—Novopharm (Canada) brand of Erythromycin Estolate—**See Erythromycins (Systemic)**, 1368; Erythromycin Ethylsuccinate—**See Erythromycins (Systemic)**, 1368; Erythromycin Stearate—**See Erythromycins (Systemic)**, 1368
*Novo-Rythro Encap*—Novopharm (Canada) brand of Erythromycin Base—**See Erythromycins (Systemic)**, 1368
*Novo-Salmol*—Novopharm (Canada) brand of Albuterol—**See Bronchodilators, Adrenergic (Inhalation-Local)**, 640; **Bronchodilators, Adrenergic (Systemic)**, 651
*Novosecobarb*—Novopharm (Canada) brand of Secobarbital—**See Barbiturates (Systemic)**, 518
*Novo-Selegiline*—Novopharm (Canada) brand of Selegiline (Systemic), 2560
*Novosemide*—Novopharm (Canada) brand of Furosemide—**See Diuretics, Loop (Systemic)**, 1259
*Novosorbide*—Novopharm (Canada) brand of Isosorbide Dinitrate—**See Nitrates (Systemic)**, 2129
*Novo-Soxazole*—Novopharm (Canada) brand of Sulfisoxazole—**See Sulfonamides (Systemic)**, 2653
*Novospiroton*—Novopharm (Canada) brand of Spironolactone—**See Diuretics, Potassium-sparing (Systemic)**, 1266
*Novo-Spirozine*—Novopharm (Canada) brand of Spironolactone and Hydrochlorothiazide—**See Diuretics, Potassium-sparing, and Hydrochlorothiazide (Systemic)**, 1272
*Novo-Sundac*—Novopharm (Canada) brand of Sulindac—**See Anti-inflammatory Drugs, Nonsteroidal (Systemic)**, 388
*Novo-Tamoxifen*—Novopharm (Canada) brand of Tamoxifen (Systemic), 2688
*Novo-Terfenadine*—Novopharm (Canada) brand of Terfenadine—**See Antihistamines (Systemic)**, 325
*Novotetra*—Novopharm (Canada) brand of Tetracycline—**See Tetracyclines (Systemic)**, 2765
*Novo-Thalidone*—Novopharm (Canada) brand of Chlorthalidone—**See Diuretics, Thiazide (Systemic)**, 1273
*Novo-Timol*—Novopharm (Canada) brand of Timolol—**See Beta-adrenergic Blocking Agents (Systemic)**, 593; Timolol (Ophthalmic), 3036

*Novo-Tolmetin*—Novopharm (Canada) brand of Tolmetin—**See Anti-inflammatory Drugs, Nonsteroidal (Systemic)**, 388
*Novo-Triamzide*—Novopharm (Canada) brand of Triamterene and Hydrochlorothiazide—**See Diuretics, Potassium-sparing, and Hydrochlorothiazide (Systemic)**, 1272
*Novo-Trimel*—Novopharm (Canada) brand of Sulfamethoxazole and Trimethoprim—**See Sulfonamides and Trimethoprim (Systemic)**, 2661
*Novo-Trimel D.S.*—Novopharm (Canada) brand of Sulfamethoxazole and Trimethoprim—**See Sulfonamides and Trimethoprim (Systemic)**, 2661
*Novo-Triolam*—Novopharm (Canada) brand of Triazolam—**See Benzodiazepines (Systemic)**, 556
*Novo-Tripramine*—Novopharm (Canada) brand of Trimipramine—**See Antidepressants, Tricyclic (Systemic)**, 271
*Novotriptyn*—Novopharm (Canada) brand of Amitriptyline—**See Antidepressants, Tricyclic (Systemic)**, 271
*Novo-Valproic*—Novopharm (Canada) brand of Valproic Acid—**See Valproic Acid (Systemic)**, 2908
*Novo-Veramil*—Novopharm (Canada) brand of Verapamil—**See Calcium Channel Blocking Agents (Systemic)**, 720
*Novoxapam*—Novopharm (Canada) brand of Oxazepam—**See Benzodiazepines (Systemic)**, 556
*Noxzema Anti-Acne Gel*—Richardson-Vicks (U.S.) brand of Salicylic Acid (Topical), #
*Noxzema Anti-Acne Pads Maximum Strength*—Richardson-Vicks (U.S.) brand of Salicylic Acid (Topical), #
*Noxzema Anti-Acne Pads Regular Strength*—Richardson-Vicks (U.S.) brand of Salicylic Acid (Topical), #
*Noxzema Clear-ups Maximum Strength 10 Lotion*—Noxell (U.S.) brand of Benzoyl Peroxide (Topical), 579
*Noxzema Clear-ups On-The-Spot 10 Lotion*—Noxell (U.S.) brand of Benzoyl Peroxide (Topical), 579
*Noxzema Moisturizer*—Procter & Gamble (U.S.) brand of Octyl Methoxycinnamate and Phenylbenzimidazole—**See Sunscreen Agents (Topical)**, #
*Nozinan*—Rhône-Poulenc (Canada) brand of Methotrimeprazine—**See Phenothiazines (Systemic)**, 2289
*Nozinan Liquid*—Rhône-Poulenc (Canada) brand of Methotrimeprazine—**See Phenothiazines (Systemic)**, 2289
*Nozinan Oral Drops*—Rhône-Poulenc (Canada) brand of Methotrimeprazine—**See Phenothiazines (Systemic)**, 2289
*NP-27 Cream*—Thompson (U.S.) brand of Tolnaftate (Topical), #
*NPH Iletin*—Lilly (Canada) brand of Insulin, Isophane—**See Insulin (Systemic)**, 1713
*NPH Iletin I*—Lilly (U.S.) brand of Insulin, Isophane—**See Insulin (Systemic)**, 1713
*NPH Iletin II*—Lilly (U.S. and Canada) brand of Insulin, Isophane—**See Insulin (Systemic)**, 1713
*NPH Insulin*—Connaught Novo Nordisk (Canada) brand of Insulin, Isophane—**See Insulin (Systemic)**, 1713
NPH insulin—Insulin, Isophane—**See Insulin (Systemic)**, 1713
*NPH-N*—Novo Nordisk (U.S.) brand of Insulin, Isophane—**See Insulin (Systemic)**, 1713
*NP-27 Powder*—Thompson (U.S.) brand of Tolnaftate (Topical), #
*NP-27 Solution*—Thompson (U.S.) brand of Tolnaftate (Topical), #
*NP-27 Spray Powder*—Thompson (U.S.) brand of Tolnaftate (Topical), #
NTBC (Systemic), 3156
N-Trifluoroacetyladriamycin-14-Valerate (Systemic), 3155
*NTS*—Bolar (U.S.) brand of Nitroglycerin—**See Nitrates (Systemic)**, 2129
*NTZ Long Acting Decongestant Nasal Spray*—Sterling (U.S.) brand of Oxymetazoline (Nasal), #
*NTZ Long Acting Decongestant Nose Drops*—Sterling (U.S.) brand of Oxymetazoline (Nasal), #
*Nu-Alpraz*—Nu-Pharm (Canada) brand of Alprazolam—**See Benzodiazepines (Systemic)**, 556

*Nu-Amoxi*—Nu-Pharm (Canada) brand of Amoxicillin—**See Penicillins (Systemic)**, 2240
*Nu-Ampi*—Nu-Pharm (Canada) brand of Ampicillin—**See Penicillins (Systemic)**, 2240
*Nubain*—Endo (U.S.) and Du Pont (Canada) brand of Nalbuphine—**See Opioid (Narcotic) Analgesics (Systemic)**, 2168
*NuBasics*—Clintec (U.S.) brand of Enteral Nutrition Formula, Polymeric—**See Enteral Nutrition Formulas (Systemic)**, #
*NuBasics with Fiber*—Clintec (U.S.) brand of Enteral Nutrition Formula, Fiber-containing—**See Enteral Nutrition Formulas (Systemic)**, #
*NuBasics Plus*—Clintec (U.S.) brand of Enteral Nutrition Formula, Polymeric—**See Enteral Nutrition Formulas (Systemic)**, #
*NuBasics VHP*—Clintec (U.S.) brand of Enteral Nutrition Formula, Polymeric—**See Enteral Nutrition Formulas (Systemic)**, #
*Nu-Cal*—Odan (Canada) brand of Calcium Carbonate—**See Calcium Supplements (Systemic)**, 736
*Nu-Carbamazepine*—Nu-Pharm (Canada) brand of Carbamazepine (Systemic), 757
*Nu-Cephalex*—Nu-Pharm (Canada) brand of Cephalexin—**See Cephalosporins (Systemic)**, 794
*Nu-Cimet*—Nu-Pharm (Canada) brand of Cimetidine—**See Histamine H₂-receptor Antagonists (Systemic)**, 1633, MC-7
*Nu-Cloxi*—Nu-Pharm (Canada) brand of Cloxacillin—**See Penicillins (Systemic)**, 2240
*Nucochem Expectorant*—Zenith Goldline (U.S.) brand of Pseudoephedrine, Codeine, and Guaifenesin—**See Cough/Cold Combinations (Systemic)**, 1024
*Nucochem Pediatric Expectorant*—Zenith Goldline (U.S.) brand of Pseudoephedrine, Codeine, and Guaifenesin—**See Cough/Cold Combinations (Systemic)**, 1024
*Nucofed*—Roberts (U.S.) brand of Pseudoephedrine and Codeine—**See Cough/Cold Combinations (Systemic)**, 1024
*Nucofed Expectorant*—Roberts (U.S.) brand of Pseudoephedrine, Codeine, and Guaifenesin—**See Cough/Cold Combinations (Systemic)**, 1024
*Nucofed Pediatric Expectorant*—Roberts (U.S.) brand of Pseudoephedrine, Codeine, and Guaifenesin—**See Cough/Cold Combinations (Systemic)**, 1024
*Nu-Cotrimox*—Nu-Pharm (Canada) brand of Sulfamethoxazole and Trimethoprim—**See Sulfonamides and Trimethoprim (Systemic)**, 2661
*Nu-Cotrimox DS*—Nu-Pharm (Canada) brand of Sulfamethoxazole and Trimethoprim—**See Sulfonamides and Trimethoprim (Systemic)**, 2661
*Nucotuss Expectorant*—Barre-National (U.S.) brand of Pseudoephedrine, Codeine, and Guaifenesin—**See Cough/Cold Combinations (Systemic)**, 1024
*Nucotuss Pediatric Expectorant*—Barre-National (U.S.) brand of Pseudoephedrine, Codeine, and Guaifenesin—**See Cough/Cold Combinations (Systemic)**, 1024
*Nu-Diclo*—Nu-Pharm (Canada) brand of Diclofenac—**See Anti-inflammatory Drugs, Nonsteroidal (Systemic)**, 388
*Nu-Diltiaz*—Nu-Pharm (Canada) brand of Diltiazem—**See Calcium Channel Blocking Agents (Systemic)**, 720
*Nu-Famotidine*—Nu-Pharm (Canada) brand of Famotidine—**See Histamine H₂-receptor Antagonists (Systemic)**, 1633, MC-12
*Nu-Flurbiprofen*—Nu-Pharm (Canada) brand of Flurbiprofen—**See Anti-inflammatory Drugs, Nonsteroidal (Systemic)**, 388
*Nu-Gemfibrozil*—Nu-Pharm (Canada) brand of Gemfibrozil (Systemic), 1552
*Nu-Glyburide*—Nu-Pharm (Canada) brand of Glyburide—**See Antidiabetic Agents, Sulfonylurea (Systemic)**, 283
*Nu-Ibuprofen*—Nu-Pharm (Canada) brand of Ibuprofen—**See Anti-inflammatory Drugs, Nonsteroidal (Systemic)**, 388
*Nu-Indo*—Nu-Pharm (Canada) brand of Indomethacin—**See Anti-inflammatory Drugs, Nonsteroidal (Systemic)**, 388
*Nu-Iron*—Mayrand (U.S.) brand of Iron-Polysaccharide—**See Iron Supplements (Systemic)**, 1774
*Nu-Iron 150*—Mayrand (U.S.) brand of Iron-Polysaccharide—**See Iron Supplements (Systemic)**, 1774

*Nujol*—Schering-Plough (Canada) brand of Mineral Oil—**See Laxatives (Local)**, #
*Nu-Levocarb*—Nu-Pharm (Canada) brand of Carbodopa and Levodopa (Systemic), 3013
*Nu-Loperamide*—NuPharm (Canada) brand of Loperamide (Oral-Local), 1877
*Nu-Loraz*—Nu-Pharm (Canada) brand of Lorazepam—**See Benzodiazepines (Systemic)**, 556
*NuLYTELY*—Braintree (U.S.) brand of Polyethylene Glycol 3350 and Electrolytes (Local), 2349
*NuLYTELY, Cherry Flavor*—Braintree (U.S.) brand of Polyethylene Glycol 3350 and Electrolytes (Local), 2349
*Nu-Medopa*—NuPharm (Canada) brand of Methyldopa (Systemic), 1979
*Nu-Metop*—Nupharm (Canada) brand of Metoprolol Tartrate—**See Beta-adrenergic Blocking Agents (Systemic)**, 593
*Numorphan*—Du Pont (U.S. and Canada) brand of Oxymorphone—**See Opioid (Narcotic) Analgesics (Systemic)**, 2168
*Numorphan H.P.*—Du Pont Merck (U.S.) brand of Oxymorphone (Systemic), 3157
*Numzident*—Goody's (U.S.) brand of Benzocaine—**See Anesthetics (Mucosal-Local)**, 128
*Num-Zit-Gel*—Goody's (U.S.) brand of Benzocaine—**See Anesthetics (Mucosal-Local)**, 128
*Num-Zit-Lotion*—Goody's (U.S.) brand of Benzocaine—**See Anesthetics (Mucosal-Local)**, 128
*Nu-Naprox*—Nu-Pharm (Canada) brand of Naproxen—**See Anti-inflammatory Drugs, Nonsteroidal (Systemic)**, 388
*Nu-Nifed*—Nu-Pharm (Canada) brand of Nifedipine—**See Calcium Channel Blocking Agents (Systemic)**, 720
*Nu-Pen-VK*—Nu-Pharm (Canada) brand of Penicillin V—**See Penicillins (Systemic)**, 2240
*Nupercainal*—Ciba Consumer (U.S.) and Ciba-Geigy Self Medication Products (Canada) brand of Dibucaine—**See Anesthetics (Mucosal-Local)**, 128
*Nupercainal Cream*—Ciba Consumer (U.S.) brand of Dibucaine—**See Anesthetics (Topical)**, 155
*Nupercainal Ointment*—Ciba Consumer (U.S.) and Ciba-Geigy Self Medication Products (Canada) brand of Dibucaine—**See Anesthetics (Topical)**, 155
*Nu-Pirox*—Nu-Pharm (Canada) brand of Piroxicam—**See Anti-inflammatory Drugs, Nonsteroidal (Systemic)**, 388
*Nuprin*—Bristol-Myers (U.S.) brand of Ibuprofen—**See Anti-inflammatory Drugs, Nonsteroidal (Systemic)**, 388
*Nuprin Caplets*—Bristol-Myers (U.S.) brand of Ibuprofen—**See Anti-inflammatory Drugs, Nonsteroidal (Systemic)**, 388
*Nu-Ranit*—Nu-Pharm (Canada) brand of Ranitidine Hydrochloride—**See Histamine H₂-receptor Antagonists (Systemic)**, 1633, MC-27
*Nuromax*—BW (U.S.) brand of Doxacurium (Systemic), 1296
*Nursoy*—Wyeth (U.S. and Canada) brand of Infant Formulas, Soy-based—**See Infant Formulas (Systemic)**, #
*Nu-Selegiline*—Nu-Pharm (Canada) brand of Selegiline (Systemic), 2560
*Nu-Tetra*—Nu-Pharm (Canada) brand of Tetracycline—**See Tetracyclines (Systemic)**, 2765
*Nu-Timolol*—Nu-Pharm (Canada) brand of Timolol (Ophthalmic), 3036
*Nutracort*—Owen/Allercreme (U.S.) brand of Hydrocortisone—**See Corticosteroids (Topical)**, 978
*Nutramigen*—Mead Johnson (U.S. and Canada) brand of Infant Formulas, Hypoallergenic—**See Infant Formulas (Systemic)**, #
*Nutren 1.0*—Clintec (U.S.) brand of Enteral Nutrition Formula, Polymeric—**See Enteral Nutrition Formulas (Systemic)**, #
*Nutren 1.5*—Clintec (U.S.) brand of Enteral Nutrition Formula, Polymeric—**See Enteral Nutrition Formulas (Systemic)**, #
*Nutren 2.0*—Clintec (U.S.) brand of Enteral Nutrition Formula, Disease-specific—**See Enteral Nutrition Formulas (Systemic)**, #; Clintec (U.S.) brand of Enteral Nutrition Formula, Polymeric—**See Enteral Nutrition Formulas (Systemic)**, #
*Nutren 1.0 with Fiber*—Clintec (U.S.) brand of Enteral Nutrition Formula, Fiber-containing—**See Enteral Nutrition Formulas (Systemic)**, #
*NutriHep*—Clintec (U.S.) brand of Enteral Nutrition Formula, Disease-specific—**See Enteral Nutrition Formulas (Systemic)**, #

*Nutrilan*—Elan (U.S.) brand of Enteral Nutrition Formula, Polymeric—**See Enteral Nutrition Formulas (Systemic)**, #
*Nutrineal PD-2 Peritoneal Dialysis Solution with 1.1% Amino Acids*—Baxter Healthcare (U.S.) brand of Dianeal PD-2 Peritoneal Dialysis Solution with Amino Acid (Systemic), 3140
*NutriSource*—Sandoz (U.S.) brand of Enteral Nutrition Formula, Fiber-containing—**See Enteral Nutrition Formulas (Systemic)**, #
*NutriSource HN*—Sandoz (U.S.) brand of Enteral Nutrition Formula, Fiber-containing—**See Enteral Nutrition Formulas (Systemic)**, #
*NutriVent*—Carnation (U.S.) brand of Enteral Nutrition Formula, Disease-specific—**See Enteral Nutrition Formulas (Systemic)**, #
*Nutropin*—Genentech (U.S.) brand of Somatropin, Recombinant—**See Growth Hormone (Systemic)**, 1586, 3165; Somatropin, Recombinant (Systemic), 3034
*Nutropin AQ*—Genentech (U.S.) brand of Somatropin, Recombinant (Systemic), 3034
*Nu-Valproic*—Nu-Pharm (Canada) brand of Valproic Acid—**See Valproic Acid (Systemic)**, 2908
*Nu-Verap*—Nu-Pharm (Canada) brand of Verapamil—**See Calcium Channel Blocking Agents (Systemic)**, 720
*Nyaderm*—Taro (Canada) brand of Nystatin (Topical), 2148; Nystatin (Vaginal), 2149
*Nydrazid*—Squibb (U.S.) brand of Isoniazid (Systemic), 1789
Nylidrin Hydrochloride [*Arlidin; Arlidin Forte; PMS Nylidrin*]
  **(Systemic)**, #
  Tablets USP, #
Nystatin [*Mycostatin; Nadostine; Nilstat; Nystex; PMS Nystatin*]
  **(Oral-Local)**, 2146
  Lozenges (Pastilles), 2147
  Suspension, Oral, USP, 2147
  for Suspension, Oral, USP, 2147
  Tablets USP, 2147
Nystatin [*Mycostatin; Nadostine; Nilstat; Nyaderm; Nystex; Nystop*]
  **(Topical)**, 2148, 3030
  Cream USP, 2148
  Ointment USP, 2148
  Powder, Topical, USP, 2149, 3030
Nystatin [*Mycostatin; Nadostine; Nilstat; Nyaderm*]
  **(Vaginal)**, 2149
  Cream, Vaginal, 2149
  Tablets, Vaginal, USP, 2150
Nystatin-containing Combinations, 3076
Nystatin and Triamcinolone Acetonide [*Dermacomb; Myco II; Mycobiotic II; Mycogen II; Mycolog II; Myco-Triacet II; Mykacet; Mykacet II; Mytrex; Tristatin II*]
  **(Topical)**, 2150
  Cream USP, 2151
  Ointment USP, 2151
*Nystex*—Savage (U.S.) brand of Nystatin (Oral-Local), 2146; Savage (U.S.) brand of Nystatin (Topical), 2148
*Nystop*—Paddock (U.S.) brand of Nystatin (Topical), 3030
*Nytcold Medicine*—Rugby (U.S.) brand of Doxylamine, Pseudoephedrine, Dextromethorphan, and Acetaminophen—**See Cough/Cold Combinations (Systemic)**, 1024
*Nytilax*—Mentholatum (U.S.) brand of Sennosides—**See Laxatives (Local)**, #
*Nytime Cold Medicine Liquid*—Rugby (U.S.) brand of Doxylamine, Pseudoephedrine, Dextromethorphan, and Acetaminophen—**See Cough/Cold Combinations (Systemic)**, 1024
*Nytol QuickCaps*—Block (U.S.) brand of Diphenhydramine—**See Antihistamines (Systemic)**, 325
*Nytol QuickGels*—Block (U.S.) brand of Diphenhydramine—**See Antihistamines (Systemic)**, 325

# O

*OB*—Ortega (U.S.) brand of Testosterone and Estradiol—**See Androgens and Estrogens (Systemic)**, 126
*Obalan*—Lannett (U.S.) brand of Phendimetrazine—**See Appetite Suppressants (Systemic)**, 452
*Obe-Nix*—Holloway (U.S.) brand of Phentermine—**See Appetite Suppressants (Systemic)**, 452

*Obezine*—Western Research (U.S.) brand of Phendimetrazine—**See Appetite Suppressants (Systemic)**, 452
*OBY-CAP*—Richwood (U.S.) brand of Phentermine—**See Appetite Suppressants (Systemic)**, 452
*Occlucort*—GenDerm (Canada) brand of Betamethasone (Topical), 3012
*Occlusal-HP Topical Solution*—GenDerm (U.S. and Canada) brand of Salicylic Acid (Topical), #
*Occlusal Topical Solution*—GenDerm (U.S. and Canada) brand of Salicylic Acid (Topical), #
*OCL*—Abbott (U.S.) brand of Polyethylene Glycol 3350 and Electrolytes (Local), 2349
*Octamide*—Adria (U.S.) brand of Metoclopramide (Systemic), 1992
*Octatropine*—Anisotropine—**See Anticholinergics/Antispasmodics (Systemic)**, 226
*Octicair*—Bausch & Lomb (U.S.) brand of Neomycin, Polymyxin B, and Hydrocortisone (Otic), #
*Octigen*—Logen (U.S.) brand of Neomycin, Polymyxin B, and Hydrocortisone (Otic), #
*Octocaine*—Novocol (U.S.) brand of Lidocaine and Epinephrine—**See Anesthetics (Parenteral-Local)**, 139
*Octocaine-50*—Novocol (Canada) brand of Lidocaine and Epinephrine—**See Anesthetics (Parenteral-Local)**, 139
*Octocaine-100*—Novocol (Canada) brand of Lidocaine and Epinephrine—**See Anesthetics (Parenteral-Local)**, 139
Octocrylene-containing Combinations, 3076
Octocrylene and Octyl Methoxycinnamate [*Bain de Soleil Mega Tan; Bain de Soleil SPF + Color*]
  **See Sunscreen Agents (Topical)**, #
  Lotion, #
Octocrylene, Octyl Methoxycinnamate, Octyl Salicylate, and Oxybenzone [*Coppertone All Day Protection; Coppertone Kids Sunblock; Coppertone Waterbabies Sunblock; Shade Sunblock; Shade Waterproof Sunblock; TI Screen*]
  **See Sunscreen Agents (Topical)**, #
  Lotion, #
Octocrylene, Octyl Methoxycinnamate, Octyl Salicylate, Oxybenzone, and Titanium Dioxide [*Bullfrog Sport; Hawaiian Tropic Baby Faces Sunblock; Hawaiian Tropic Just For Kids; Hawaiian Topic Sport Sunblock; Hawaiian Tropic Sunblock*]
  **See Sunscreen Agents (Topical)**, #
  Lotion, #
Octocrylene, Octyl Methoxycinnamate, and Oxybenzone [*Bain de Soleil SPF + Color; Bullfrog Body; Bullfrog Extra Moisturizing; Bullfrog For Kids; Bullfrog Original Concentrated; Hawaiian Tropic Sport Sunblock; Solbar PF Liquid; Solbar PF Ultra*]
  **See Sunscreen Agents (Topical)**, #
  Cream, #
  Gel, #
  Lotion, #
Octocrylene, Octyl Methoxycinnamate, Oxybenzone, and Titanium Dioxide [*Bain de Soleil All Day For Kids; Bain de Soleil All Day Sunblock; Bain de Soleil Long Lasting For Kids; Bain de Soleil Long Lasting Sunblock*]
  **See Sunscreen Agents (Topical)**, #
  Lotion, #
Octocrylene, Octyl Methoxycinnamate, and Titanium Dioxide [*Bain de Soleil All Day Sunfilter; Bain de Soleil Long Lasting Sport Sunblock; Bain de Soleil Long Lasting Sunfilter*]
  **See Sunscreen Agents (Topical)**, #
  Lotion, #
*Octostim*—Ferring (Canada) brand of Desmopressin (Systemic), 1187
Octoxinol—Octoxynol 9—**See Spermicides (Vaginal)**, #
Octoxynol 9 [*Koromex Cream; octoxinol; Ortho-Gynol*]
  **See Spermicides (Vaginal)**, #
  Cream, Vaginal, #
  Jelly, Vaginal, #
*OctreoScan*—Mallinckrodt (U.S.) brand of Indium In 111 Pentetreotide (Systemic), 1700
Octreotide Acetate [*Sandostatin*]
  **(Systemic)**, 2152
  Injection, 2153
Octyl Methoxycinnamate [*Coppertone Tan Magnifier; Formula 405 Solar; Neutrogena Deep Glow; Neutrogena Light Glow; Q.T. Quick Tanning; Solbar Liquid*]
  **See Sunscreen Agents (Topical)**, #
  Gel, #
  Lotion, #

Octyl Methoxycinnamate-containing Combinations, 3076
Octyl Methoxycinnamate and Octyl Salicylate [*Bain de Soleil Orange Gelee; Bain de Soleil Sand Buster; Bain de Soleil Tropical Dexluxe; Hawaiian Tropic Land Sport; Vaseline Intensive Care Moisturizing Sunscreen*]
  **See Sunscreen Agents (Topical)**, #
  Gel, #
  Lotion, #
  Oil, #
Octyl Methoxycinnamate, Octyl Salicylate, and Oxybenzone [*Aquaray Sunscreen; Banana Boat Active Kids Sunblock; Banana Boat Baby Sunblock; Banana Boat Sport Sunblock; Banana Boat Faces Sensitive Skin Sunblock; Coppertone Sport; Dermsol; Durascreen; Neutrogena Sunblock; Nivea Sun; PreSun Active Clear; Presun For Kids; PreSun Moisturizing Sunscreen with Keri; PreSun Sensitive Skin; PreSun Spray Mist; Presun Sunscreen; Presun Sunscreen for Kids; Shade Sunblock Oil-Free; Solbar Shield; TI Screen; Vaseline Intensive Care Moisturing Sunblock; Vaseline Kids Sunblock; Vaseline Sunblock; Waterbabies Little Licks;*]
  **See Sunscreen Agents (Topical)**, #
  Cream, #
  Gel, #
  Lip Balm, #
  Lotion, #
  Spray, #
  Stick, #
Octyl Methoxycinnamate, Octyl Salicylate, Oxybenzone, and Padimate O [*Presun Spray Mist for Kids; Vaseline Sunblock*]
  **See Sunscreen Agents (Topical)**, #
  Lotion, #
  Spray, #
Octyl Methoxycinnamate, Octyl Salicylate, Oxybenzone, Padimate O, and Titanium Dioxide [*Vaseline Intensive Care Blockout Moisturizing*]
  **See Sunscreen Agents (Topical)**, #
  Lotion, #
Octyl Methoxycinnamate, Octyl Salicylate, Oxybenzone, Phenylbenzimidazole, and Titanium Dioxide [*DuraScreen*]
  **See Sunscreen Agents (Topical)**, #
  Lotion, #
Octyl Methoxycinnamate, Octyl Salicylate, Oxybenzone, and Titanium Dioxide [*Johnson's Baby Sunblock; Johnson's Baby Sunblock Extra Protection; Sundown Broad Spectrum Sunblock; Sundown Sunblock; Vaseline Intensive Care Baby Sunblock; Vaseline Intensive Care Baby Moisturizing Sunblock; Vaseline Intensive Care Blockout Moisturizing*]
  **See Sunscreen Agents (Topical)**, #
  Cream, #
  Lotion, #
Octyl Methoxycinnamate, Octyl Salicylate, Phenylbenzimidazole, and Titanium Dioxide [*Eucerin Dry Skin Care Daily Facial*]
  **See Sunscreen Agents (Topical)**, #
  Lotion, #
Octyl Methoxycinnamate, Octyl Salicylate, and Titanium Dioxide [*Sundown Sunscreen*]
  **See Sunscreen Agents (Topical)**, #
  Lotion, #
Octyl Methoxycinnamate and Oxybenzone [*Aquaderm Sunscreen Moisturizer; Bullfrog Sunblock; Catrix Lip Saver; Coppertone All Day Protection; Coppertone LipKote; Coppertone Moisturizing Sunscreen; Coppertone Moisturizing Suntan; Coppertone Sport Ultra Sweatproof; Curel Everyday Sun Protection; DML Facial Moisturizer; Hawaiian Tropic Self-tanning Sunblock; Neutrogena Lip Moisturizer; Neutrogena Moisture Untinted & with Sheer Tint; Softsense Skin Essential Everyday UV Protectant; Solbar PF; Solbar PF Liquid; Sundown Sunscreen; TI Screen; TI-UVA-B Sunscreen; Tropical Blend Dark Tanning; Vaseline Extra Defense for Hand and Body; Vaseline Intensive Care Active Sport; Vaseline Intensive Care Lip Therapy; Vaseline Intensive Care Moisturizing Sunblock; Vaseline Kids Sunblock; Vaseline Lip Therapy; Vaseline Moisturizing Sunscreen; Vaseline Sports Sunscreen; Vaseline Sport Sunblock; Vaseline Sunblock; Vaseline Sunscreen; Vaseline Ultraviolet Daily Defense for Hand and Body; Waterbabies Sunblock*]
  **See Sunscreen Agents (Topical)**, #

Octyl Methoxycinnamate and Oxybenzone
  *(continued)*
  Cream, #
  Gel, #
  Lip Balm, #
  Lotion, #
  Stick, #
Octyl Methoxycinnamate, Oxybenzone, and Padimate O [*Banana Boat Sunblock*]
  **See Sunscreen Agents (Topical)**, #
  Lotion, #
Octyl Methoxycinnamate, Oxybenzone, Padimate O, and Titanium Dioxide [*Sundown*]
  **See Sunscreen Agents (Topical)**, #
  Stick, #
Octyl Methoxycinnamate, Oxybenzone, and Titanium Dioxide [*Hawaiian Tropic Water Sport*]
  **See Sunscreen Agents (Topical)**, #
  Lotion, #
Octyl Methoxycinnamate and Padimate O [*Banana Boat Dark Tanning; Banana Boat Protective Tanning; Hawaiian Tropic Dark Tanning*]
  **See Sunscreen Agents (Topical)**, #
  Oil, #
Octyl Methoxycinnamate and Phenylbenzimidazole [*Neutrogena Intensified Day Moisture; Noxzema Moisturizer; Oil of Olay Daily UV Protectant; Oil of Olay Daily UV Protectant Beauty Fluid; Oil of Olay Moisture Replenishment; Pond's Daily Replenishing Moisturizer*]
  **See Sunscreen Agents (Topical)**, #
  Cream, #
  Lotion, #
Octyl Salicylate [*PreSun Spray Mist*]
  **See Sunscreen Agents (Topical)**, #
  Spray, #
Octyl Salicylate-containing Combinations, 3076
Octyl Salicylate and Padimate O [*Total Eclipse Moisturizing Skin*]
  **See Sunscreen Agents (Topical)**, #
  Lotion, #
*Ocu-Caine*—Ocumed (U.S.) brand of Proparacaine—**See Anesthetics (Ophthalmic)**, #
*Ocu-Carpine*—Ocumed (U.S.) brand of Pilocarpine (Ophthalmic), #
*Ocu-Chlor Ophthalmic Ointment*—Ocumed (U.S.) brand of Chloramphenicol (Ophthalmic), #
*Ocu-Chlor Ophthalmic Solution*—Ocumed (U.S.) brand of Chloramphenicol (Ophthalmic), #
*OcuClear*—Schering (U.S. and Canada) brand of Oxymetazoline (Ophthalmic), #
*Ocucoat*—Storz (U.S.) brand of Hydroxypropyl Methylcellulose (Ophthalmic), #, 3023
*Ocucoat PF*—Storz (U.S.) brand of Hydroxypropyl Methylcellulose (Ophthalmic), #
*Ocu-Dex*—Ocumed (U.S.) brand of Dexamethasone—**See Corticosteroids (Ophthalmic)**, 966
*Ocufen*—Allergan (U.S. and Canada) brand of Flurbiprofen—**See Anti-inflammatory Drugs, Nonsteroidal (Ophthalmic)**, 383
*Ocuflox*—Allergan (U.S. and Canada) brand of Ofloxacin (Ophthalmic), 3030; Allergan (U.S.) brand of Ofloxacin (Ophthalmic), #
*Ocuflox Ophthalmic Solution*—Allergan (U.S.) brand of Ofloxacin (Ophthalmic), 3156
*Ocugestrin*—Pharmafair (U.S.) brand of Phenylephrine (Ophthalmic), #
*Ocu-Mycin*—Ocumed (U.S.) brand of Gentamicin (Ophthalmic), 1555
*Ocu-Pentolate*—Ocumed (U.S.) brand of Cyclopentolate (Ophthalmic), #
*Ocu-Phrin Sterile Eye Drops*—Ocumed (U.S.) brand of Phenylephrine (Ophthalmic), #
*Ocu-Phrin Sterile Ophthalmic Solution*—Ocumed (U.S.) brand of Phenylephrine (Ophthalmic), #
*Ocu-Pred*—Ocumed (U.S.) brand of Prednisolone—**See Corticosteroids (Ophthalmic)**, 966
*Ocu-Pred-A*—Ocumed (U.S.) brand of Prednisolone—**See Corticosteroids (Ophthalmic)**, 966
*Ocu-Pred Forte*—Ocumed (U.S.) brand of Prednisolone—**See Corticosteroids (Ophthalmic)**, 966
*Ocupress*—Otsuka (U.S.) brand of Carteolol—**See Beta-adrenergic Blocking Agents (Ophthalmic)**, 585
*Ocusert Pilo-20*—Alza (U.S. and Canada) brand of Pilocarpine (Ophthalmic), #
*Ocusert Pilo-40*—Alza (U.S. and Canada) brand of Pilocarpine (Ophthalmic), #
*Ocu-Spor-B*—Ocumed (U.S.) brand of Neomycin, Polymyxin B, and Bacitracin (Ophthalmic), #
*Ocu-Spor-G*—Ocumed (U.S.) brand of Neomycin, Polymyxin B, and Gramicidin (Ophthalmic), #

*Ocusporin*—Moore (U.S.) brand of Neomycin, Polymyxin B, and Bacitracin (Ophthalmic), #
*Ocu-Sul-10*—Ocumed (U.S.) brand of Sulfacetamide—**See Sulfonamides (Ophthalmic)**, 2651
*Ocu-Sul-15*—Ocumed (U.S.) brand of Sulfacetamide—**See Sulfonamides (Ophthalmic)**, 2651
*Ocu-Sul-30*—Ocumed (U.S.) brand of Sulfacetamide—**See Sulfonamides (Ophthalmic)**, 2651
*Ocusulf-10*—Optopics (U.S.) brand of Sulfacetamide—**See Sulfonamides (Ophthalmic)**, 2651
*Ocutears*—Charton (Canada) brand of Hydroxypropyl Methylcellulose (Ophthalmic), #
*Ocutricin HC*—Pharmafair (U.S.) brand of Neomycin, Polymyxin B, and Hydrocortisone (Ophthalmic), #
*Ocutricin Ophthalmic Ointment*—Bausch & Lomb (U.S.) brand of Neomycin, Polymyxin B, and Bacitracin (Ophthalmic), #
*Ocutricin Ophthalmic Solution*—Bausch & Lomb (U.S.) brand of Neomycin, Polymyxin B, and Gramicidin (Ophthalmic), #
*Ocu-Tropic*—Ocumed (U.S.) brand of Tropicamide (Ophthalmic), #
*Ocu-Tropine*—Ocumed (U.S.) brand of Atropine (Ophthalmic), 485
*Ocu-Zoline Sterile Ophthalmic Solution*—Ocumed (U.S.) brand of Naphazoline (Ophthalmic), #
*Oestradiol*—Estradiol—**See Estrogens (Systemic)**, 1383
*Oestrilin*—Desbergers (Canada) brand of Estrone—**See Estrogens (Vaginal)**, 1391
*Oestrone*—Estrone—**See Estrogens (Systemic)**, 1383
*OFF*—S. C. Johnson (U.S. and Canada) brand of Diethyltoluamide (Topical), #
*Off-Ezy Topical Solution Corn & Callus Remover Kit*—Commerce (U.S.) brand of Salicylic Acid (Topical), #
*Off-Ezy Topical Solution Wart Removal Kit*—Commerce (U.S.) brand of Salicylic Acid (Topical), #
*OFF For Maximum Protection*—S. C. Johnson (U.S. and Canada) brand of Diethyltoluamide (Topical), #
*OFF Skintastic*—S. C. Johnson (U.S. and Canada) brand of Diethyltoluamide (Topical), #
*OFF Skintastic For Children*—S. C. Johnson (U.S.) brand of Diethyltoluamide (Topical), #
*OFF Skintastic For Kids*—S. C. Johnson (U.S.) brand of Diethyltoluamide (Topical), #
Ofloxacin [*Floxin Otic*]
(Otic), 2154
Solution, Otic, 2156
Ofloxacin [*Ocuflox; Ocuflox Ophthalmic Solution*]
(Ophthalmic), #, 3030, 3156
Solution, Ophthalmic, 3030
Ofloxacin [*Floxin; Floxin I.V.*]
**See Fluoroquinolones (Systemic)**, 1487
Injection, 1495
Tablets, 1495, MC-23
Ofloxacin in Dextrose [*Floxin I.V.*]
**See Fluoroquinolones (Systemic)**, 1487
Injection, 1495
*Ogen*—Abbott (Canada) brand of Estropipate—**See Estrogens (Systemic)**, 1383; Abbott (U.S.) brand of Estropipate—**See Estrogens (Vaginal)**, 1391
*Ogen .625*—Abbott (U.S.) brand of Estropipate—**See Estrogens (Systemic)**, 1383
*Ogen 1.25*—Abbott (U.S.) brand of Estropipate—**See Estrogens (Systemic)**, 1383
*Ogen 2.5*—Abbott (U.S.) brand of Estropipate—**See Estrogens (Systemic)**, 1383
*Oil of Olay Daily UV Protectant*—Procter & Gamble (U.S.) brand of Octyl Methoxycinnamate and Phenylbenzimidazole—**See Sunscreen Agents (Topical)**, #
*Oil of Olay Daily UV Protectant Beauty Fluid*—Procter & Gamble (U.S.) brand of Octyl Methoxycinnamate and Phenylbenzimidazole—**See Sunscreen Agents (Topical)**, #
*Oil of Olay Moisture Replenishment*—Procter & Gamble (U.S.) brand of Octyl Methoxycinnamate and Phenylbenzimidazole—**See Sunscreen Agents (Topical)**, #; Procter & Gamble (U.S.) brand of Phenylbenzimidazole—**See Sunscreen Agents (Topical)**, #
Olanzapine [*Zyprexa*]
(Systemic), 2156
Tablets, 2159, MC-23

*Oligo-CRM*—Haemophilus b Conjugate Vaccine (HbOC—Diphtheria CRM₁₉₇ Protein Conjugate)—**See Haemophilus b Conjugate Vaccine (Systemic)**, 1601
Olopatadine Hydrochloride [*Patanol*]
(Ophthalmic), 2160
Solution, Ophthalmic, 2161
Olsalazine Sodium [azodisal sodium; *Dipentum;* sodium azodisalicylate]
(Oral-Local), 2161
Capsules, 2162, MC-23
OM 401 [*Drepanol*]
(Systemic), 3156
*Ombrelle Sunscreen*—Dermtel (Canada) brand of Avobenzone, Octyl Methoxycinnamate, and Oxybenzone—**See Sunscreen Agents (Topical)**, #
Omega-3 (n-3) Polyunsaturated Fatty Acid with All Double Bonds in the Cis Configuration
(Systemic), 3156
Omeprazole [*Prilosec*]
(Systemic), 2163
Capsules, Delayed-release, 2165
Omeprazole Magnesium [*Losec*]
(Systemic), 2163
Tablets, Delayed-release, 2165
*Omnicef*—PD (U.S.) brand of Cefdinir (Systemic), 3014
*Omnicol*—Delta (U.S.) brand of Chlorpheniramine, Phenindamine, Phenylephrine, Dextromethorphan, Acetaminophen, Salicylamide, Caffeine, and Ascorbic Acid—**See Cough/Cold Combinations (Systemic)**, 1024
*Omnihib*—SmithKline (U.S.) brand of Haemophilus b Conjugate Vaccine (Systemic), 3022
*OMNIhist L.A.*—WE (U.S.) brand of Chlorpheniramine, Phenylephrine, and Methscopolamine—**See Antihistamines, Decongestants, and Anticholinergics (Systemic)**, 373
*Omnipaque 140*—Nycomed (U.S.) and Sanofi Winthrop (Canada) brand of Iohexol (Systemic), #; Sanofi Winthrop (U.S. and Canada) brand of Iohexol (Local), #
*Omnipaque 180*—Nycomed (U.S.) and Sanofi Winthrop (Canada) brand of Iohexol (Systemic), #; Sanofi Winthrop (U.S. and Canada) brand of Iohexol (Local), #
*Omnipaque 210*—Nycomed (U.S.) and Sanofi Winthrop (Canada) brand of Iohexol (Systemic), #; Sanofi Winthrop (U.S. and Canada) brand of Iohexol (Local), #
*Omnipaque 240*—Nycomed (U.S.) and Sanofi Winthrop (Canada) brand of Iohexol (Systemic), #; Sanofi Winthrop (U.S. and Canada) brand of Iohexol (Local), #
*Omnipaque 300*—Nycomed (U.S.) and Sanofi Winthrop (Canada) brand of Iohexol (Systemic), #; Sanofi Winthrop (U.S. and Canada) brand of Iohexol (Local), #
*Omnipaque 350*—Nycomed (U.S.) and Sanofi Winthrop (Canada) brand of Iohexol (Systemic), #; Sanofi Winthrop (U.S. and Canada) brand of Iohexol (Local), #
*Omnipen*—Wyeth-Ayerst (U.S.) brand of Ampicillin—**See Penicillins (Systemic)**, 2240, MC-2
*Omnipen-N*—Wyeth-Ayerst (U.S.) brand of Ampicillin—**See Penicillins (Systemic)**, 2240
*Omniscan*—Sanofi Winthrop (U.S. and Canada) brand of Gadodiamide (Systemic), #
*Omni-Tuss*—Rhône-Poulenc Rorer (Canada) brand of Chlorphenirame, Phenyltoloxamine, Ephedrine, Codeine, and Guaiacol Carbonate—**See Cough/Cold Combinations (Systemic)**, 1024
*OMS Concentrate*—Upsher-Smith (U.S.) brand of Morphine—**See Opioid (Narcotic) Analgesics (Systemic)**, 2168
*Oncaspar*—Enzon (U.S.) brand of Pegaspargase (Systemic), 2230, 3157
*Oncet*—Wakefield (U.S.) brand of Hydrocodone and Acetaminophen—**See Opioid (Narcotic) Analgesics and Acetaminophen (Systemic)**, 2198
OncoRad OV103
(Systemic), 3155
*OncoScint CR/OV*—Cytogen (U.S.) brand of Indium In 111 Satumomab Pendetide (Systemic), 1702; Satumomab Pendetide (Systemic), 3163
*Oncostate*—Schaper and Brummer brand of Coumarin (Systemic), 3138
*Oncotrac Melanoma Imaging Kit*—Neorx (U.S.) brand of Technetium Tc 99m Anti-melanoma Murine Monoclonal Antibody (Systemic), 3167
*Oncovin*—Lilly (U.S. and Canada) brand of Vincristine (Systemic), 2950

Ondansetron Hydrochloride [*Zofran*]
(Systemic), 2165
Injection, 2168
Solution, Oral, 2167
Tablets, 2168, MC-23
*One-Alpha*—Leo (Canada) brand of Alfacalcidol—**See Vitamin D and Analogs (Systemic)**, 2966
*Onguent de Calamine*—Lab Atlas (Canada) brand of Calamine (Topical), #
*o,p′-DDD*—**See Mitotane (Systemic)**, 2031
*Ophthacet*—Vortech (U.S.) brand of Sulfacetamide—**See Sulfonamides (Ophthalmic)**, 2651
*Ophthaine*—Apothecon (U.S.) brand of Proparacaine—**See Anesthetics (Ophthalmic)**, #
*Ophthalmic*—Vortech (U.S.) brand of Neomycin, Polymyxin B, and Bacitracin (Ophthalmic), #
*Ophthetic*—Allergan (U.S. and Canada) brand of Proparacaine—**See Anesthetics (Ophthalmic)**, #
*Ophtho-Chloram Ophthalmic Solution*—Kenral (Canada) brand of Chloramphenicol (Ophthalmic), #
*Ophthochlor Ophthalmic Solution*—PD (U.S.) brand of Chloramphenicol (Ophthalmic), #
*Ophtho-Dipivefrin*—Kenral (Canada) brand of Dipivefrin (Ophthalmic), 1249
*Ophtho-Tate*—Kenral (Canada) brand of Prednisolone—**See Corticosteroids (Ophthalmic)**, 966
Opioid (Narcotic) Analgesics
(Systemic), 2168
Opioid (Narcotic) Analgesics and Acetaminophen (Systemic), 2198
Opioid (Narcotic) Analgesics and Aspirin
(Systemic), 2202
Opium [laudanum]
**See Opioid (Narcotic) Analgesics (Systemic)**, 2168
Tincture USP, 2186
Opium Alkaloids Hydrochlorides [*Pantopon*; papaveretum]
**See Opioid (Narcotic) Analgesics (Systemic)**, 2168
Injection, 2186
Oprelvekin [interleukin-11, recombinant; *Neumega*; rIL-11]
(Systemic), 2205
for Injection, 2207
*Opticaine*—Optopics (U.S.) brand of Tetracaine—**See Anesthetics (Ophthalmic)**, #
*Opticrom*—Fisons (U.S. and Canada) brand of Cromolyn (Ophthalmic), 1120, 3138
*Opticyl*—Optopics (U.S.) brand of Tropicamide (Ophthalmic), #
*Optimine*—Schering (U.S. and Canada) brand of Azatadine—**See Antihistamines (Systemic)**, 325, MC-3
*Optimmune*—**See Cyclosporine (Ophthalmic)**, 3139
*OptiPranolol*—Bausch & Lomb (U.S.) brand of Metipranolol—**See Beta-adrenergic Blocking Agents (Ophthalmic)**, 585
*Optiray 160*—Mallinckrodt (U.S. and Canada) brand of Ioversol (Systemic), #
*Optiray 240*—Mallinckrodt (U.S. and Canada) brand of Ioversol (Systemic), #
*Optiray 300*—Mallinckrodt (U.S. and Canada) brand of Ioversol (Systemic), #
*Optiray 320*—Mallinckrodt (U.S. and Canada) brand of Ioversol (Systemic), #
*Optiray 350*—Mallinckrodt (U.S. and Canada) brand of Ioversol (Systemic), #
*OPV*—Poliovirus Vaccine Live Oral—**See Poliovirus Vaccine (Systemic)**, 2343
*Orabase, Baby*—Colgate-Hoyt (U.S.) brand of Benzocaine—**See Anesthetics (Mucosal-Local)**, 128
*Orabase-B with Benzocaine*—Colgate-Hoyt (U.S.) brand of Benzocaine—**See Anesthetics (Mucosal-Local)**, 128
*Orabase-HCA*—Colgate-Hoyt (U.S.) brand of Hydrocortisone—**See Corticosteroids (Topical)**, 978
*Oracit*—Carolina (U.S. and Canada) brand of Sodium Citrate and Citric Acid—**See Citrates (Systemic)**, 881
*Oracort*—Taro (U.S.) brand of Triamcinolone—**See Corticosteroids (Topical)**, 978
*Oradexon*—Organon (Canada) brand of Dexamethasone—**See Corticosteroids—Glucocorticoid Effects (Systemic)**, 998
*Oradrine-2*—Pharmavite (Canada) brand of Diphenylpyraline, Phenylpropanolamine, Acetaminophen, and Caffeine—**See Antihistamines, Decongestants, and Analgesics (Systemic)**, 366

## General Index

*Oragrafin Calcium*—Squibb (U.S.) brand of Ipodate—**See Cholecystographic Agents, Oral (Systemic)**, #

*Oragrafin Sodium*—Squibb (U.S.) brand of Ipodate—**See Cholecystographic Agents, Oral (Systemic)**, #

*Orajel*—Del (U.S.) brand of Benzocaine—**See Anesthetics (Mucosal-Local)**, 128

*Orajel, Baby*—Del (U.S.) and Commerce (Canada) brand of Benzocaine—**See Anesthetics (Mucosal-Local)**, 128

*Orajel Extra Strength*—Commerce (Canada) brand of Benzocaine—**See Anesthetics (Mucosal-Local)**, 128

*Orajel Liquid*—Commerce (Canada) brand of Benzocaine—**See Anesthetics (Mucosal-Local)**, 128

*Orajel Maximum Strength*—Del (U.S.) brand of Benzocaine—**See Anesthetics (Mucosal-Local)**, 128

*Orajel Nighttime Formula, Baby*—Del (U.S.) brand of Benzocaine—**See Anesthetics (Mucosal-Local)**, 128

*Oralone*—Thames (U.S.) brand of Triamcinolone—**See Corticosteroids (Topical)**, 978

Oral Rehydration Salts [*Gastrolyte;* ORS-bicarbonate; ORS-citrate; *Rapolyte*]
  **See Carbohydrates and Electrolytes (Systemic)**, 769
  Oral Rehydration Salts USP (for Oral Solution), 772

*Oralyte*—Rugby (U.S.) brand of Dextrose and Electrolytes—**See Carbohydrates and Electrolytes (Systemic)**, 769

*Oramorph SR*—Boehringer-Ingelheim (U.S.) and Roxane (Canada) brand of Morphine—**See Opioid (Narcotic) Analgesics (Systemic)**, 2168

*Orap*—Lemmon (U.S.) and McNeil (Canada) brand of Pimozide (Systemic), 2326

*Oraphen-PD*—Great Southern (U.S.) brand of Acetaminophen (Systemic), 6

*Orasone 1*—Solvay (U.S.) brand of Prednisone—**See Corticosteroids—Glucocorticoid Effects (Systemic)**, 998

*Orasone 5*—Solvay (U.S.) brand of Prednisone—**See Corticosteroids—Glucocorticoid Effects (Systemic)**, 998

*Orasone 10*—Solvay (U.S.) brand of Prednisone—**See Corticosteroids—Glucocorticoid Effects (Systemic)**, 998

*Orasone 20*—Solvay (U.S.) brand of Prednisone—**See Corticosteroids—Glucocorticoid Effects (Systemic)**, 998

*Orasone 50*—Solvay (U.S.) brand of Prednisone—**See Corticosteroids—Glucocorticoid Effects (Systemic)**, 998

*Oratect Gel*—MGI Pharma (U.S.) brand of Benzocaine—**See Anesthetics (Mucosal-Local)**, 128

*Orazinc*—Mericon (U.S.) brand of Zinc Gluconate—**See Zinc Supplements (Systemic)**, 2999; Mericon (U.S.) brand of Zinc Sulfate—**See Zinc Supplements (Systemic)**, 2999

*Orbenin*—Ayerst (Canada) brand of Cloxacillin—**See Penicillins (Systemic)**, 2240

Orciprenaline—Metaproterenol—**See Bronchodilators, Adrenergic (Inhalation-Local)**, 640; **Bronchodilators, Adrenergic (Systemic)**, 651

*Orcolon*—Optical Radiation (U.S.) and Dispersa (Canada) brand of Polyacrylamide (Ophthalmic), 3032

*Ordrine AT*—Eon (U.S.) brand of Phenylpropanolamine and Caramiphen—**See Cough/Cold Combinations (Systemic)**, 1024

*Oretic*—Abbott (U.S.) brand of Hydrochlorothiazide—**See Diuretics, Thiazide (Systemic)**, 1273, MC-14

*Oreticyl*—Abbott (U.S.) brand of Deserpidine and Hydrochlorothiazide—**See Rauwolfia Alkaloids and Thiazide Diuretics (Systemic)**, #

*Oreticyl Forte*—Abbott (U.S.) brand of Deserpidine and Hydrochlorothiazide—**See Rauwolfia Alkaloids and Thiazide Diuretics (Systemic)**, #

ORETON *Methyl*—Schering Plough (U.S.) brand of Methyltestosterone—**See Androgens (Systemic)**, 118

*Orfro*—Truxton (U.S.) brand of Orphenadrine—**See Skeletal Muscle Relaxants (Systemic)**, 2577

ORG 10172 *See* Danaparoid (Systemic), 1161

*Organidin NR*—Carter-Wallace (U.S.) brand of Guaifenesin (Systemic), 1588

*Orgaran*—Organon (U.S.) brand of Danaparoid (Systemic), 1161

Orgotein (Systemic), 3156
  for Injection, 3156

*Orimune*—Lederle (U.S.) brand of Poliovirus Vaccine Live Oral—**See Poliovirus Vaccine (Systemic)**, 2343

*Orinase*—Pharmacia & Upjohn (U.S.) and Hoechst (Canada) brand of Tolbutamide—**See Antidiabetic Agents, Sulfonylurea (Systemic)**, 283, MC-30

*Orinase Diagnostic*—Upjohn (U.S.) brand of Tolbutamide (Systemic), 3036

*Orlaam*—Bio-Development (U.S.) brand of Levomethadyl (Systemic), 1855, 3152

*Ormazine*—Hauck (U.S.) brand of Chlorpromazine—**See Phenothiazines (Systemic)**, 2289

*Ornade*—SmithKline Beecham (Canada) brand of Chlorpheniramine and Phenylpropanolamine—**See Antihistamines and Decongestants (Systemic)**, 343

*Ornade-A.F.*—SmithKline Beecham (Canada) brand of Chlorpheniramine and Phenylpropanolamine—**See Antihistamines and Decongestants (Systemic)**, 343

*Ornade-DM 10*—Smithkline Beecham (Canada) brand of Chlorpheniramine, Phenylpropanolamine, and Dextromethorphan—**See Cough/Cold Combinations (Systemic)**, 1024

*Ornade-DM 15*—Smithkline Beecham (Canada) brand of Chlorpheniramine, Phenylpropanolamine, and Dextromethorphan—**See Cough/Cold Combinations (Systemic)**, 1024

*Ornade-DM 30*—Smithkline Beecham (Canada) brand of Chlorpheniramine, Phenylpropanolamine, and Dextromethorphan—**See Cough/Cold Combinations (Systemic)**, 1024

*Ornade Expectorant*—Smithkline Beecham (Canada) brand of Chlorpheniramine, Phenylpropanolamine, and Guaifenesin—**See Cough/Cold Combinations (Systemic)**, 1024

*Ornade Spansules*—SmithKline Beecham (U.S. and Canada) brand of Chlorpheniramine and Phenylpropanolamine—**See Antihistamines and Decongestants (Systemic)**, 343, AP-27

*Ornex·DM 15*—SKF (Canada) brand of Dextromethorphan (Systemic), 1191

*Ornex·DM 30*—SKF (Canada) brand of Dextromethorphan (Systemic), 1191

*Ornex Maximum Strength Caplets*—Menley & James (U.S.) brand of Pseudoephedrine and Acetaminophen—**See Decongestants and Analgesics (Systemic)**, 1180

*Ornex No Drowsiness Caplets*—Menley & James (U.S.) brand of Pseudoephedrine and Acetaminophen—**See Decongestants and Analgesics (Systemic)**, 1180

*Ornex Severe Cold No Drowsiness Caplets*—Menley & James (U.S.) brand of Pseudoephedrine, Dextromethorphan, and Acetaminophen—**See Cough/Cold Combinations (Systemic)**, 1024

*Ornidyl*—Marion Merrell Dow (U.S.) brand of Eflornithine (Systemic), #, 3141

Orphenadrine Citrate [*Antiflex; Banflex; Flexoject; Mio-Rel; Myolin; Myotrol; Norflex; Orfro; Orphenate*]
  **See Skeletal Muscle Relaxants (Systemic)**, 2577
  Injection USP, 2582
  Tablets, Extended-release, 2582

Orphenadrine Citrate, Aspirin, and Caffeine [*N3 Gesic; N3 Gesic Forte; Norgesic; Norgesic Forte; Norphadrine; Norphadrine Forte; Orphenagesic; Orphenagesic Forte*]
  (Systemic), 2208
  Tablets, 2208

Orphenadrine-containing Combinations, 3076

Orphenadrine Hydrochloride [*Disipal*]
  **See Skeletal Muscle Relaxants (Systemic)**, 2577
  Tablets, 2582

*Orphenagesic*—Par (U.S.) brand of Orphenadrine, Aspirin, and Caffeine (Systemic), 2208

*Orphenagesic Forte*—Par (U.S.) brand of Orphenadrine, Aspirin, and Caffeine (Systemic), 2208

*Orphenate*—Hyrex (U.S.) brand of Orphenadrine—**See Skeletal Muscle Relaxants (Systemic)**, 2577

ORS-bicarbonate—Oral Rehydration Salts—**See Carbohydrates and Electrolytes (Systemic)**, 769

ORS-citrate—Oral Rehydration Salts—**See Carbohydrates and Electrolytes (Systemic)**, 769

*Ortho 0.5/35*—Ortho (Canada) brand of Norethindrone and Ethinyl Estradiol—**See Estrogens and Progestins—Oral Contraceptives (Systemic)**, 1397

*Ortho 1/35*—Ortho (Canada) brand of Norethindrone and Ethinyl Estradiol—**See Estrogens and Progestins—Oral Contraceptives (Systemic)**, 1397

*Ortho 7/7/7*—Ortho (Canada) brand of Norethindrone and Ethinyl Estradiol—**See Estrogens and Progestins—Oral Contraceptives (Systemic)**, 1397

*Ortho 10/11*—Ortho (Canada) brand of Norethindrone and Ethinyl Estradiol—**See Estrogens and Progestins—Oral Contraceptives (Systemic)**, 1397

*Ortho-Cept*—Ortho-McNeil (U.S. and Canada) brand of Desogestrel and Ethinyl Estradiol—**See Estrogens and Progestins—Oral Contraceptives (Systemic)**, 1397, MC-8

*Orthoclone OKT3*—Ortho (U.S. and Canada) brand of Muromonab-CD3 (Systemic), 2068

*Ortho-Creme*—Ortho (U.S.) brand of Nonoxynol 9—**See Spermicides (Vaginal)**, #

*Ortho/CS*—Merit (U.S.) brand of Sodium Ascorbate (Systemic), 469

*Ortho-Cyclen*—Ortho-McNeil (U.S.) brand of Norgestimate and Ethinyl Estradiol—**See Estrogens and Progestins—Oral Contraceptives (Systemic)**, 1397, MC-23

*Ortho Dienestrol*—Ortho (U.S.) and Janssen-Ortho (Canada) brand of Dienestrol—**See Estrogens (Vaginal)**, 1391

*Ortho-Est .625*—Ortho (U.S.) brand of Estropipate—**See Estrogens (Systemic)**, 1383

*Ortho-Est 1.25*—Ortho-McNeil (U.S.) brand of Estropipate—**See Estrogens (Systemic)**, 1383, MC-12

*Ortho-Gynol*—Ortho (U.S. and Canada) brand of Octoxynol 9—**See Spermicides (Vaginal)**, #

*Ortho-Novum 1/35*—Ortho-McNeil (U.S.) brand of Norethindrone and Ethinyl Estradiol—**See Estrogens and Progestins—Oral Contraceptives (Systemic)**, 1397, MC-22

*Ortho-Novum 1/50*—Ortho-McNeil (U.S. and Canada) brand of Norethindrone and Mestranol—**See Estrogens and Progestins—Oral Contraceptives (Systemic)**, 1397, MC-22

*Ortho-Novum 7/7/7*—Ortho-McNeil (U.S.) brand of Norethindrone and Ethinyl Estradiol—**See Estrogens and Progestins—Oral Contraceptives (Systemic)**, 1397, MC-22

*Ortho-Novum 10/11*—Ortho (U.S.) brand of Norethindrone and Ethinyl Estradiol—**See Estrogens and Progestins—Oral Contraceptives (Systemic)**, 1397

*Ortho Shields Lubricated*—Ortho (Canada) brand of Latex Condoms—**See Condoms**, #

*Ortho Shields Non-Lubricated*—Ortho (Canada) brand of Latex Condoms—**See Condoms**, #

*Ortho Shields Plus*—Ortho (Canada) brand of Latex Condoms and Nonoxynol 9—**See Condoms**, #

*Ortho Shields X*—Ortho (Canada) brand of Latex Condoms—**See Condoms**, #

*Ortho Supreme*—Ortho (Canada) brand of Latex Condoms—**See Condoms**, #

*Ortho Tri-Cyclen*—Ortho-McNeil (U.S.) brand of Norgestimate and Ethinyl Estradiol—**See Estrogens and Progestins—Oral Contraceptives (Systemic)**, 1397, MC-23

*Or-Tyl*—Ortega (U.S.) brand of Dicyclomine—**See Anticholinergics/Antispasmodics (Systemic)**, 226

*Orudis*—Wyeth-Ayerst (U.S.) and Rhône-Poulenc Rorer (Canada) brand of Ketoprofen—**See Anti-inflammatory Drugs, Nonsteroidal (Systemic)**, 388, MC-16

*Orudis-E*—Rhône-Poulenc Rorer (Canada) brand of Ketoprofen—**See Anti-inflammatory Drugs, Nonsteroidal (Systemic)**, 388

*Orudis KT*—Whitehall-Robins (U.S.) brand of Ketoprofen—**See Anti-inflammatory Drugs, Nonsteroidal (Systemic)**, 388

*Orudis-SR*—Rhône-Poulenc Rorer (Canada) brand of Ketoprofen—**See Anti-inflammatory Drugs, Nonsteroidal (Systemic)**, 388

*Oruvail*—Wyeth-Ayerst (U.S.) and May & Baker (Canada) brand of Ketoprofen—**See Anti-inflammatory Drugs, Nonsteroidal (Systemic)**, 388, MC-16

*Os-Cal*—Ayerst (Canada) brand of Calcium Carbonate—**See Calcium Supplements (Systemic)**, 736
*Os-Cal 500*—Marion (U.S.) brand of Calcium Carbonate—**See Calcium Supplements (Systemic)**, 736
*Os-Cal Chewable*—Ayerst (Canada) brand of Calcium Carbonate—**See Calcium Supplements (Systemic)**, 736
*Os-Cal 500 Chewable*—Marion Merrell Dow (U.S.) brand of Calcium Carbonate—**See Calcium Supplements (Systemic)**, 736
*Osmitrol*—Baxter Healthcare (U.S.) and Travenol (Canada) brand of Mannitol (Systemic), 1906
*Osmoglyn*—Alcon (U.S.) brand of Glycerin (Systemic), #
*Osmolite*—Ross (U.S.) brand of Enteral Nutrition Formula, Polymeric—**See Enteral Nutrition Formulas (Systemic)**, #
*Osmolite HN*—Ross (U.S.) brand of Enteral Nutrition Formula, Polymeric—**See Enteral Nutrition Formulas (Systemic)**, #
*Osteo-D*—Lemmon (U.S.) brand of Secalciferol (Systemic), 3163
*Osteolite*—Du Pont N.E.N. (U.S.) brand of Technetium Tc 99m Medronate (Systemic), 2718
*Osteoscan-HDP*—Mallinckrodt (U.S.) brand of Technetium Tc 99m Oxidronate (Systemic), 2724
*Ostoforte*—Frosst (Canada) brand of Ergocalciferol—**See Vitamin D and Analogs (Systemic)**, 2966
*Otic-Care*—Parmed (U.S.) brand of Neomycin, Polymyxin B, and Hydrocortisone (Otic), #
*Otic-Care Ear*—Parmed (U.S.) brand of Neomycin, Polymyxin B, and Hydrocortisone (Otic), #
*Otic Tridesilon Solution*—Miles (U.S.) brand of Desonide and Acetic Acid—**See Corticosteroids and Acetic Acid (Otic)**, 996
*Otimar*—Marlop (U.S.) brand of Neomycin, Polymyxin B, and Hydrocortisone (Otic), #
*Otisan*—Ram (U.S.) brand of Neomycin, Polymyxin B, and Hydrocortisone (Otic), #
*Otocalm*—Parmed (U.S.) brand of Antipyrine and Benzocaine (Otic), 443
*Otocidin*—Marin (U.S.) brand of Neomycin, Polymyxin B, and Hydrocortisone (Otic), #
*Otocort*—Lemmon (U.S.) brand of Neomycin, Polymyxin B, and Hydrocortisone (Otic), #
*Otomycet-HC*—Marin (U.S.) brand of Hydrocortisone and Acetic Acid (Otic), 3023
*Otrivin With Metered-Dose Pump*—Ciba-Geigy Self Medication Products (Canada) brand of Xylometazoline (Nasal), #
*Otrivin Nasal Drops*—Ciba Consumer (U.S.) and Ciba-Geigy Self Medication Products (Canada) brand of Xylometazoline (Nasal), #
*Otrivin Nasal Spray*—Ciba Consumer (U.S.) and Ciba-Geigy Self Medication Products (Canada) brand of Xylometazoline (Nasal), #
*Otrivin Pediatric Nasal Drops*—Ciba Consumer (U.S.) and Ciba Consumer (Canada) and Ciba-Geigy Self Medication Products (Canada) brand of Xylometazoline (Nasal), #
*Otrivin Pediatric Nasal Spray*—Ciba-Geigy Self Medication Products (Canada) brand of Xylometazoline (Nasal), #
*Ovarex MAb-B43.13*—AltaRex (Canada) brand of Monoclonal Antibody-B43.13 (Systemic), 3154
*Ovastat*—Medac GmbH (U.S.) brand of Treosulfan (Systemic), 3169
*Ovcon-35*—Mead Johnson (U.S.) brand of Norethindrone and Ethinyl Estradiol—**See Estrogens and Progestins—Oral Contraceptives (Systemic)**, 1397, MC-22
*Ovcon-50*—Mead Johnson (U.S.) brand of Norethindrone and Ethinyl Estradiol—**See Estrogens and Progestins—Oral Contraceptives (Systemic)**, 1397, MC-22
*Ovide*—GenDerm (U.S.) brand of Malathion (Topical), #
*Ovol*—Horner (Canada) brand of Simethicone (Oral-Local), #, #
*Ovol-40*—Horner (Canada) brand of Simethicone (Oral-Local), #, #
*Ovol-80*—Horner (Canada) brand of Simethicone (Oral-Local), #
*Ovol-160*—Horner (Canada) brand of Simethicone (Oral-Local), #
*Ovral*—Wyeth-Ayerst (U.S. and Canada) brand of Norgestrel and Ethinyl Estradiol—**See Estrogens and Progestins—Oral Contraceptives (Systemic)**, 1397, MC-23

*Ovrette*—Wyeth-Ayerst (U.S.) brand of Norgestrel—**See Progestins (Systemic)**, 2400
*OvuGen*—Biogenex (U.S.) brand of Enzyme Immunoassay Ovulation Prediction Test Kits—**See Ovulation Prediction Test Kits for Home Use**, #
*OvuKIT*—Monoclonal Antibodies (U.S.) brand of Enzyme Immunoassay Ovulation Prediction Test Kits—**See Ovulation Prediction Test Kits for Home Use**, #
*OvuKit*—Cardna (Canada) brand of Enzyme Immunoassay Ovulation Prediction Test Kits—**See Ovulation Prediction Test Kits for Home Use**, #
Ovulation Prediction Test Kits for Home Use, #
*OvuQUICK*—Monoclonal Antibodies (U.S.) brand of Enzyme Immunoassay Ovulation Prediction Test Kits—**See Ovulation Prediction Test Kits for Home Use**, #
*OvuQuick*—Cardna (Canada) brand of Enzyme Immunoassay Ovulation Prediction Test Kits—**See Ovulation Prediction Test Kits for Home Use**, #
Oxacillin Sodium [*Bactocill; Prostaphlin*]
 **See Penicillins (Systemic)**, 2240
 Capsules USP, 2255, MC-23
 for Injection USP, 2255
 for Solution, Oral, USP, 2255
Oxaliplatin
 **(Systemic)**, 3156
Oxamniquine [*Vansil*]
 **(Systemic)**, #
 Capsules USP, #
*Oxandrin*—Bio-Technology (U.S.) brand of Oxandrolone—**See Anabolic Steroids (Systemic)**, 110, 3156, 3157
Oxandrolone [*Hepandrin; Oxandrin*]
 **See Anabolic Steroids (Systemic)**, 110, 3156, 3157
 Tablets USP, 113
Oxaprozin [*Daypro*]
 **See Anti-inflammatory Drugs, Nonsteroidal (Systemic)**, 388, 3030
 Tablets, 3030, 415, MC-23
Oxazepam [*Apo-Oxazepam; Novoxapam; Serax*]
 **See Benzodiazepines (Systemic)**, 556
 Capsules USP, 576, MC-23
 Tablets USP, 576, MC-23
Oxiconazole Nitrate [*Oxistat*]
 **(Topical)**, #, 3030
 Cream, #, 3030
 Lotion, #
*Oxilan 300*—Cook Imaging (U.S.) brand of Ioxilan (Systemic), #
*Oxilan 350*—Cook Imaging (U.S.) brand of Ioxilan (Systemic), #
*Oxistat*—Glaxo (U.S.) brand of Oxiconazole (Topical), #, 3030
Oxprenolol [*Slow-Trasicor; Trasicor*]
 **See Beta-adrenergic Blocking Agents (Systemic)**, 593
 Tablets USP, 605
 Tablets, Extended-release, USP, 605
*Oxsoralen*—Elder (Canada) and ICN (Canada) brand of Methoxsalen (Systemic), 1973
*Oxsoralen Lotion*—ICN (U.S. and Canada) brand of Methoxsalen (Topical), 1977
*Oxsoralen-Ultra*—Elder (U.S.) brand of Methoxsalen (Systemic), 1973
Oxtriphylline [*Apo-Oxtriphylline; Choledyl; Choledyl SA;* choline theophyllinate; choline theophylline; *PMS-Oxtriphylline*]
 **See Bronchodilators, Theophylline (Systemic)**, 668
 Solution, Oral, USP, 678
 Syrup, 678
 Tablets, 679
 Tablets, Delayed-release, USP, 679
 Tablets, Extended-release, 679
Oxtriphylline-containing Combinations, 3076
Oxtriphylline and Guaifenesin [*Brondelate; Choledyl Expectorant*]
 **(Systemic)**, #
 Elixir, #
*Oxy Balance Deep Action Night Formula Lotion*—Smith-Kline Beecham (U.S.) brand of Benzoyl Peroxide (Topical), 579
*Oxy 10 Balance Emergency Spot Treatment Cover-Up Formula Gel*—Smith-Kline Beecham (U.S.) brand of Benzoyl Peroxide (Topical), 579

*Oxy Balance Emergency Spot Treatment Invisible Formula*—Smith-Kline Beecham (U.S.) brand of Benzoyl Peroxide (Topical), 579
*Oxy 10 Balance Maximum Medicated Face Wash*—Smith-Kline Beecham (U.S.) brand of Benzoyl Peroxide (Topical), 579
Oxybenzone-containing Combinations, 3076
Oxybenzone and Padimate O [*Banana Boat Sunscreen; Blistex Daily Conditioning Treatment for Lips; Blistex Medicated Lip Conditioner; Blistex Regular; Blistex Sunblock; Chap-et Sun Ban Lip Conditioner; Chap Stick Sunblock; Chap Stick Sunblock Petroleum Jelly Plus; Eclipse Lip & Face Protectant; Formula 405 Solar; Hawaiian Tropic Protective Tanning; PreSun Creamy Sundown Sunscreen; PreSun Lip Protector; PreSun Moisturizing; PreSun Moisturizing Sunscreen with Keri; PreSun Sunscreen; Ray Block; Solex A15 Clear; Stay Moist Moisturizing Lip Conditioner; Tropical Blend Dark Tanning; Tropical Blend Waterproof*]
 **See Sunscreen Agents (Topical)**, #
 Cream, #
 Lip Balm, #
 Lotion, #
 Oil, #
 Stick, #
Oxybenzone and Roxadimate [*Solbar; Solbar Plus*]
 **See Sunscreen Agents (Topical)**, #
 Cream, #
 Lotion, #
Oxybutynin Chloride [*Ditropan*]
 **(Systemic)**, 2209
 Syrup USP, 2211
 Tablets USP, 2211, MC-23
*Oxy Clean Extra Strength Medicated Pads*—SmithKline Beecham (Canada) brand of Salicylic Acid (Topical), #
*Oxy Clean Extra Strength Skin Cleanser Topical Solution*—SmithKline Beecham (Canada) brand of Salicylic Acid (Topical), #
*Oxy Clean Medicated Cleanser*—SmithKline Beecham (U.S.) brand of Salicylic Acid (Topical), #
*Oxy Clean Medicated Pads Maximum Strength*—SmithKline Beecham (U.S.) brand of Salicylic Acid (Topical), #
*Oxy Clean Medicated Pads Regular Strength*—SmithKline Beecham (U.S.) brand of Salicylic Acid (Topical), #
*Oxy Clean Medicated Pads Sensitive Skin*—SmithKline Beecham (U.S.) brand of Salicylic Acid (Topical), #
*Oxy Clean Medicated Soap*—SmithKline Beecham (Canada) brand of Salicylic Acid (Topical), #
*Oxy Clean Regular Strength Medicated Cleanser Topical Solution*—SmithKline Beecham (Canada) brand of Salicylic Acid (Topical), #
*Oxy Clean Regular Strength Medicated Pads*—SmithKline Beecham (Canada) brand of Salicylic Acid (Topical), #
*Oxy Clean Sensitive Skin Cleanser Topical Solution*—SmithKline Beecham (Canada) brand of Salicylic Acid (Topical), #
*Oxy Clean Sensitive Skin Pads*—SmithKline Beecham (Canada) brand of Salicylic Acid (Topical), #
*Oxycocet*—Technilab (Canada) brand of Oxycodone and Acetaminophen—**See Opioid (Narcotic) Analgesics and Acetaminophen (Systemic)**, 2198
*Oxycodan*—Technilab (Canada) brand of Oxycodone and Aspirin—**See Opioid (Narcotic) Analgesics and Aspirin (Systemic)**, 2202
Oxycodone and Acetaminophen [co-oxycodAPAP; *Endocet; Oxycocet;* oxycodone with APAP; *Percocet; Percocet-Demi; Roxicet; Roxicet 5/500; Roxilox; Tylox*]
 **See Opioid (Narcotic) Analgesics and Acetaminophen (Systemic)**, 2198
 Capsules USP, 2201, MC-24
 Solution, Oral, 2201
 Tablets USP, 2201, MC-24
Oxycodone with APAP—Oxycodone and Acetaminophen—**See Opioid (Narcotic) Analgesics and Acetaminophen (Systemic)**, 2198
Oxycodone and Aspirin [*Endodan; Oxycodan; Percodan; Percodan-Demi; Roxiprin*]
 **See Opioid (Narcotic) Analgesics and Aspirin (Systemic)**, 2202
 Tablets USP, 2204, MC-24
Oxycodone-containing Combinations, 3077

# 3324 General Index

Oxycodone Hydrochloride [*OxyContin ; OxyContin SR*; *OxyIR* ; *Percolone* ; *Roxicodone*; *Roxicodone Intensol*; *Supeudol*]
**See Opioid (Narcotic) Analgesics (Systemic),** 2168, 3030
Solution, Oral, USP, 2186
Suppositories, 2187
Tablets USP, 2187, MC-23, MC-24
Tablets, Extended-release, 3030
*OxyContin*—Purdue (U.S.) brand of Oxycodone (Systemic), MC-24
*OxyContin SR*—Purdue (U.S.) brand of Oxycodone (Systemic), 3030
*Oxyderm 5 Lotion*—ICN (Canada) brand of Benzoyl Peroxide (Topical), 579
*Oxyderm 10 Lotion*—ICN (Canada) brand of Benzoyl Peroxide (Topical), 579
*Oxyderm 20 Lotion*—ICN (Canada) brand of Benzoyl Peroxide (Topical), 579
*OxyIR*—Purdue (U.S.) brand of Oxycodone (Systemic), MC-23
Oxymetazoline Hydrochloride [*Afrin Cherry Scented Nasal Spray; Afrin Children's Strength Nose Drops; Afrin Extra Moisturizing Nasal Decongestant Spray; Afrin Menthol Nasal Spray; Afrin Nasal Spray; Afrin Nose Drops; Afrin Sinus Spray; Afrin Spray Pump; Allerest 12 Hour Nasal Spray; Cheracol Nasal Spray; Cheracol Nasal Spray Pump Cherry Scented; Dristan; Dristan 12-Hr Nasal Spray; Dristan Mentholated; Drixoral; Duramist Plus Up To 12 Hours Decongestant Nasal Spray; Duration 12 Hour Nasal Spray; Duration 12 Hour Nasal Spray Pump; 12 Hour Nostrilla Nasal Decongestant; Nasal Decongestant Spray; Nasal-12 Hour; Nasal Relief; Nasal Spray 12-Hour; Nasal Spray Long Acting; Neo-Synephrine 12 Hour Nasal Spray; Neo-Synephrine 12 Hour Nasal Spray Pump; Nostrilla Long-Acting Nasal Decongestant; NTZ Long Acting Decongestant Nasal Spray; NTZ Long Acting Decongestant Nose Drops; Sinarest 12 Hour Nasal Spray; Vicks Sinex Long-Acting 12-Hour Formula Decongestant Nasal Spray; Vicks Sinex Long-Acting 12-Hour Formula Decongestant Ultra Fine Mist; 4-Way Long Lasting Nasal Spray*]
**(Nasal),** #, 3030
Solution, Nasal, USP, #, 3030
Oxymetazoline Hydrochloride [*OcuClear; Visine L.R.*]
**(Ophthalmic),** #
Solution, Ophthalmic, USP, #
Oxymetholone [*Anapolon 50*]
**See Anabolic Steroids (Systemic),** 110
Tablets USP, 114
Oxymorphone Hydrochloride [*Numorphan; Numorphan H.P.*]
**See Opioid (Narcotic) Analgesics (Systemic),** 2168, 3157
Injection USP, 2187
Suppositories USP, 2187
*Oxy Night Watch Maximum Strength Lotion*—SmithKline Beecham (U.S.) brand of Salicylic Acid (Topical), #
*Oxy Night Watch Night Time Acne Medication Extra Strength Lotion*—SmithKline Beecham (Canada) brand of Salicylic Acid (Topical), #
*Oxy Night Watch Night Time Acne Medication Regular Strength Lotion*—SmithKline Beecham (Canada) brand of Salicylic Acid (Topical), #
*Oxy Night Watch Sensitive Skin Lotion*—SmithKline Beecham (U.S.) brand of Salicylic Acid (Topical), #
Oxypentifylline—*See* Pentoxifylline (Systemic), 2282
*Oxy 5 Regular Strength Cover-Up Cream*—SmithKline Beecham (Canada) brand of Benzoyl Peroxide (Topical), 579
*Oxy 5 Regular Strength Vanishing Lotion*—SmithKline Beecham (U.S.) brand of Benzoyl Peroxide (Topical), 579
*Oxy Sensitive Skin Vanishing Formula Lotion*—SmithKline Beecham (Canada) brand of Salicylic Acid (Topical), #
*Oxy 5 Sensitive Skin Vanishing Lotion*—Smith-Kline Beecham (U.S.) brand of Benzoyl Peroxide (Topical), 579
Oxytetracycline [*Terramycin*]
**See Tetracyclines (Systemic),** 2765
Injection USP, 2772
Oxytetracycline Hydrochloride [*Terramycin; Tija*]
**See Tetracyclines (Systemic),** 2765
Capsules USP, 2772
for Injection USP, 2772

Oxytocin [*Pitocin; Syntocinon*]
**(Systemic),** 2211
Injection USP, 2214
Solution, Nasal, USP, 2213
*Oysco*—Ruglex (U.S.) brand of Calcium Carbonate—**See Calcium Supplements (Systemic),** 736
*Oysco 500 Chewable*—Ruglex (U.S.) brand of Calcium Carbonate—**See Calcium Supplements (Systemic),** 736
*Oyst-Cal 500*—Goldline (U.S.) brand of Calcium Carbonate—**See Calcium Supplements (Systemic),** 736
*Oystercal 500*—Nature's Bounty (U.S.) brand of Calcium Carbonate—**See Calcium Supplements (Systemic),** 736

## P

$^{32}$P—*See* Chromic Phosphate P 32 (Parenteral-Local), #; Sodium Phosphate P 32 (Systemic), 2616
*Pacaps*—Lunsco (U.S.) brand of Butalbital, Acetaminophen, and Caffeine—**See Barbiturates and Analgesics (Systemic),** 532
*Pacerone*—Upsher-Smith (U.S.) brand of Amiodarone (Systemic), MC-2
*PACIS*—IAF BioVac (Canada) brand of Bacillus Calmette-Guérin (BCG) Live (Mucosal-Local), 507, 3011
Paclitaxel [*Paxene; Taxol*]
**(Systemic),** 2215, 3157
Concentrate for Injection, 2218
*P-A-C Revised Formula*—Upjohn (U.S.) brand of Aspirin—**See Salicylates (Systemic),** 2538
Padimate O [*Banana Boat Dark Tanning; Chap-Stick; Herpecin-L Cold Sore; Mentholatum*]
**See Sunscreen Agents (Topical),** #
Lip Balm, #
Lotion, #
Oil, #
Padimate O-containing Combinations, 3077
*Pain Aid*—Aspirin—**See Salicylates (Systemic),** 2538
*Palafer*—Beecham (Canada) brand of Ferrous Fumarate—**See Iron Supplements (Systemic),** 1774
Palivizumab [*Synagis*]
**(Systemic),** 2219
Injection, 2220
*Paludrine*—Wyeth-Ayerst (Canada) and ZENECA (U.K.) brand of Proguanil (Systemic), #
2-PAM—*See* Pralidoxime (Systemic), #
2-PAM chloride*See* Pralidoxime (Systemic), #
*Pamelor*—Novartis (U.S.) brand of Nortriptyline—**See Antidepressants, Tricyclic (Systemic),** 271, MC-23
Pamidronate Disodium [*APD; Aredia*]
**(Systemic),** 2220
for Injection, 2222
*Pamine*—Upjohn (U.S.) brand of Methscopolamine—**See Anticholinergics/Antispasmodics (Systemic),** 226
P-aminoclonidine—*See* Apraclonidine (Ophthalmic), 459
*Pamisyl*—PD (U.S.) brand of 4-Aminosalicylic Acid (Systemic), 3128
*Pamprin-IB*—Chattem (U.S.) brand of Ibuprofen—**See Anti-inflammatory Drugs, Nonsteroidal (Systemic),** 388
*Panacet 5/500*—ECR (U.S.) brand of Hydrocodone and Acetaminophen—**See Opioid (Narcotic) Analgesics and Acetaminophen (Systemic),** 2198
*Panadol*—Sterling Health (Canada) brand of Acetaminophen (Systemic), 6
*Panadol, Children's*—Sterling Health (U.S.) brand of Acetaminophen (Systemic), 6
*Panadol Extra Strength*—Sterling Health (Canada) brand of Acetaminophen (Systemic), 6
*Panadol, Infants'*—Sterling Health (U.S.) brand of Acetaminophen (Systemic), 6
*Panadol Junior Strength Caplets*—Sterling Health (U.S.) brand of Acetaminophen (Systemic), 6
*Panadol Maximum Strength Caplets*—Sterling Health (U.S.) brand of Acetaminophen (Systemic), 6
*Panadol Maximum Strength Tablets*—Sterling Health (U.S.) brand of Acetaminophen (Systemic), 6
*Panasal 5/500*—ECR (U.S.) brand of Hydrocodone and Aspirin—**See Opioid (Narcotic) Analgesics and Aspirin (Systemic),** 2202
*Pancoate*—Parmed (U.S.) brand of Pancrelipase (Systemic), 2222

*Pancrease*—Ortho-McNeil (U.S. and Canada) brand of Pancrelipase (Systemic), 2222, MC-24
*Pancrease MT 4*—McNeil (U.S. and Canada) brand of Pancrelipase (Systemic), 2222
*Pancrease MT 10*—McNeil (U.S. and Canada) brand of Pancrelipase (Systemic), 2222
*Pancrease MT 16*—McNeil (U.S. and Canada) brand of Pancrelipase (Systemic), 2222
*Pancrease MT 20*—Ortho McNeil (U.S.) brand of Pancrelipase (Systemic), 2222
Pancreatin [*Creon*]
**(Systemic),** MC-24
Capsules, MC-24
Pancrelipase [*Cotazym; Cotazym-65 B; Cotazym E.C.S. 8; Cotazym E.C.S. 20; Cotazym-S; Enzymase-16; Ilozyme; Ku-Zyme HP*; lipancreatin; *Pancoate; Pancrease; Pancrease MT 4; Pancrease MT 10; Pancrease MT 16; Pancrease MT 20; Panokase; Protilase; Ultrase MT 12; Ultrase MT 20; Viokase; Zymase*]
**(Systemic),** 2222
Capsules USP, 2224, MC-24
Capsules, Delayed-release, 2224, MC-24
Powder, 2224
Tablets USP, 2224
Pancreozymin—*See* Cholecystokinin (Systemic), #
Pancuronium Bromide [*Pavulon*]
**See Neuromuscular Blocking Agents (Systemic),** 2098
Injection, 2103
*Pandel*—Savage (U.S.) brand of Hydrocortisone Buteprate (Topical), 3023
*Panectyl*—May & Baker (Canada) brand of Trimeprazine—**See Antihistamines, Phenothiazine-derivative (Systemic),** 377
*Panfil-G*—PanAm (U.S.) brand of Dyphylline and Guaifenesin (Systemic), MC-10
*Panhematin*—Abbott (U.S.) brand of Hemin (Systemic), 3022, 3145
*Panlor*—Pan American (U.S.) brand of Hydrocodone and Acetaminophen—**See Opioid (Narcotic) Analgesics and Acetaminophen (Systemic),** 2198
*Panmycin*—Pharmacia & Upjohn (U.S.) brand of Tetracycline—**See Tetracyclines (Systemic),** 2765, MC-29
*Pannaz*—Pan American (U.S.) brand of Chlorpheniramine, Phenylpropanolamine, and Methscopolamine—**See Antihistamines, Decongestants, and Anticholinergics (Systemic),** 373
*Panokase*—Rugby (U.S.) brand of Pancrelipase (Systemic), 2222
*Panorex*—Centocor (U.S.) brand of Monoclonal Antibody 17-1A (Systemic), 3154
*PanOxyl AQ 2½ Gel*—Stiefel (U.S.) brand of Benzoyl Peroxide (Topical), 579
*PanOxyl AQ 5 Gel*—Stiefel (U.S.) brand of Benzoyl Peroxide (Topical), 579
*PanOxyl AQ 10 Gel*—Stiefel (U.S.) brand of Benzoyl Peroxide (Topical), 579
*PanOxyl Aquagel 2.5*—Stiefel (U.S. and Canada) brand of Benzoyl Peroxide (Topical), 579
*PanOxyl Aquagel 5*—Stiefel (U.S. and Canada) brand of Benzoyl Peroxide (Topical), 579
*PanOxyl Aquagel 10*—Stiefel (Canada) brand of Benzoyl Peroxide (Topical), 579
*PanOxyl Aquagel 20*—Stiefel (Canada) brand of Benzoyl Peroxide (Topical), 579
*PanOxyl 5 Bar*—Stiefel (U.S. and Canada) brand of Benzoyl Peroxide (Topical), 579
*PanOxyl 10 Bar*—Stiefel (U.S. and Canada) brand of Benzoyl Peroxide (Topical), 579
*PanOxyl 5 Gel*—Stiefel (U.S. and Canada) brand of Benzoyl Peroxide (Topical), 579
*PanOxyl 10 Gel*—Stiefel (U.S. and Canada) brand of Benzoyl Peroxide (Topical), 579
*PanOxyl 15 Gel*—Stiefel (U.S. and Canada) brand of Benzoyl Peroxide (Topical), 579
*PanOxyl 20 Gel*—Stiefel (Canada) brand of Benzoyl Peroxide (Topical), 579
*PanOxyl 5 Wash*—Stiefel (U.S.) brand of Benzoyl Peroxide (Topical), 579
*PanOxyl 10 Wash*—Stiefel (U.S.) brand of Benzoyl Peroxide (Topical), 579
*Panshape M*—Pan American (U.S.) brand of Phentermine—**See Appetite Suppressants (Systemic),** 452
*Pantoloc*—Solvay (Canada) brand of Pantoprazole (Systemic), 3031
*Pantopon*—Roche (Canada) brand of Opium—**See Opioid (Narcotic) Analgesics (Systemic),** 2168

Pantoprazole [*Pantoloc*]
  **(Systemic)**, 3031
  Tablets, Enteric-coated, 3031
Pantothenic Acid [vitamin B₅]
  **(Systemic)**, #
  Capsules, #
  Solution, Oral, #
  Tablets, #
  Tablets, Extended-release, #
*Panwarfin*—Abbott (U.S.) brand of Warfarin—**See Anticoagulants (Systemic)**, 243
*Papaveretum*—Opium Alkaloids Hydrochlorides—**See Opioid (Narcotic) Analgesics (Systemic)**, 2168
Papaverine Hydrochloride
  **(Intracavernosal)**, #
  Injection USP, #
Papaverine Hydrochloride [*Cerespan; Genabid; Pavabid; Pavabid HP; Pavacels; Pavacot; Pavagen; Pavarine; Pavased; Pavatine; Pavatym; Paverolan*]
  **(Systemic)**, #
  Capsules, Extended-release, #
  Injection USP, #
  Tablets USP, #
*Paplex*—Medicis (U.S.) brand of Salicylic Acid (Topical), #
*Paplex Ultra*—Medicis (U.S.) brand of Salicylic Acid (Topical), #
*Papulex*—GenDerm (Canada) brand of Nicotinamide (Topical), 3029
*Paracetamol*—*See* Acetaminophen (Systemic), 6
*Paraflex*—McNeil (U.S.) brand of Chlorzoxazone—**See Skeletal Muscle Relaxants (Systemic)**, 2577
*Parafon Forte*—Ortho-McNeil (Canada) brand of Chlorzoxazone and Acetaminophen (Systemic), 853
*Parafon Forte DSC*—McNeil (U.S.) brand of Chlorzoxazone—**See Skeletal Muscle Relaxants (Systemic)**, 2577, MC-7
*ParaGard-T 380A*—GynoPharma (U.S.) brand of Copper-T 380A Intrauterine Device—**See Copper Intrauterine Devices (IUDs)**, #
*Para-Hist HD*—Pharmics (U.S.) brand of Chlorpheniramine, Phenylephrine, and Hydrocodone—**See Cough/Cold Combinations (Systemic)**, 1024
*Paral*—Forest (U.S.) brand of Paraldehyde (Systemic), #
Paraldehyde [*Paral*]
  **(Systemic)**, #
  Paraldehyde USP, #
  Sterile USP, #
Paramethadione
  **See Anticonvulsants, Dione (Systemic)**, #
  Capsules, #
*Paraplatin*—Bristol (U.S. and Canada) brand of Carboplatin (Systemic), 779
*Paraplatin-AQ*—Bristol (Canada) brand of Carboplatin (Systemic), 779
*Parathar*—Rhône-Poulenc Rorer (U.S.) brand of Teriparatide (Systemic), #, 3167
Paregoric [camphorated opium tincture]
  **(Systemic)**, #
  Paregoric USP, #
Paregoric-containing Combinations, 3077
*Parepectolin*—Rhône-Poulenc Rorer (U.S.) brand of Attapulgite (Oral-Local), #
*Parfenac*—Lederle (Canada) brand of Bufexamac (Topical), 3013
Paricalcitol [*Zemplar*]
  **(Systemic)**, 3031
  Injection, 3031
*Parlodel*—Novartis (U.S. and Canada) brand of Bromocriptine (Systemic), 636, MC-4
*Parlodel SnapTabs*—Sandoz (U.S.) brand of Bromocriptine (Systemic), 636
*Parnate*—SmithKline Beecham (U.S. and Canada) brand of Tranylcypromine—**See Antidepressants, Monoamine Oxidase (MAO) Inhibitor (Systemic)**, 266, MC-31
*Paromomycin*—*See* Aminosidine (Systemic), 3130
Paroxetine Hydrochloride [*Paxil*]
  **(Systemic)**, 2225
  Tablets, 2229
  Suspension, Oral, 2229, MC-24
*Parsidol*—PD (U.S.) brand of Ethopropazine—**See Antidyskinetics (Systemic)**, 297
*Parsitan*—Rhône-Poulenc (Canada) brand of Ethopropazine—**See Antidyskinetics (Systemic)**, 297

*Partuss LA*—Parmed (U.S.) brand of Phenylpropanolamine and Guaifenesin—**See Cough/Cold Combinations (Systemic)**, 1024
*Parvolex*—Bioniche (Canada) brand of Acetylcysteine (Systemic), 16
*Parzine*—Lanpar (U.S.) brand of Phendimetrazine—**See Appetite Suppressants (Systemic)**, 452
PAS—*See* Aminosalicylate Sodium (Systemic), #
*Paser*—Jacobus (U.S.) brand of Aminosalicylic Acid (Systemic), 3009
*Paser Granules*—Jacobus (U.S.) brand of Aminosalicylic Acid (Systemic), 3130
*Patanol*—Alcon (U.S.) brand of Olopatadine Hydrochloride (Systemic), 2160
*Pathocil*—Wyeth-Ayerst (U.S.) brand of Dicloxacillin—**See Penicillins (Systemic)**, 2240
Patul-end
  **(Systemic)**, 3157
*Pavabid*—Marion Merrell Dow (U.S.) brand of Papaverine (Systemic), #
*Pavabid HP*—Marion Merrell Dow (U.S.) brand of Papaverine (Systemic), #
*Pavacels*—Hauck (U.S.) brand of Papaverine (Systemic), #
*Pavacot*—Truxton (U.S.) brand of Papaverine (Systemic), #
*Pavagen*—Rugby (U.S.) brand of Papaverine (Systemic), #
*Pavarine*—Vortech (U.S.) brand of Papaverine (Systemic), #
*Pavased*—Hauck (U.S.) brand of Papaverine (Systemic), #
*Pavatine*—Major (U.S.) brand of Papaverine (Systemic), #
*Pavatym*—Everett (U.S.) brand of Papaverine (Systemic), #
*Paveral*—Desbergers (Canada) brand of Codeine—**See Opioid (Narcotic) Analgesics (Systemic)**, 2168
*Paverolan*—Lannett (U.S.) brand of Papaverine (Systemic), #
*Pavulon*—Organon (U.S. and Canada) brand of Pancuronium—**See Neuromuscular Blocking Agents (Systemic)**, 2098
*Paxene*—Baker Norton (U.S.) brand of Paclitaxel (Systemic), 3157
*Paxil*—SmithKline Beecham (U.S. and Canada) brand of Paroxetine (Systemic), 2225, MC-24
*Paxipam*—Schering (U.S.) brand of Halazepam—**See Benzodiazepines (Systemic)**, 556
*PBZ*—Geigy (U.S.) brand of Tripelennamine—**See Antihistamines (Systemic)**, 325
*PBZ-SR*—Geigy (U.S.) brand of Tripelennamine—**See Antihistamines (Systemic)**, 325
*PC-Cap*—Alra (U.S.) brand of Propoxyphene and Aspirin—**See Opioid (Narcotic) Analgesics and Aspirin (Systemic)**, 2202
*PCE*—Abbott (U.S. and Canada) brand of Erythromycin Base—**See Erythromycins (Systemic)**, 1368, MC-11
*PDF*—Pharmascience (Canada) brand of Sodium Fluoride (Systemic), 2592
Pectin-containing Combinations, 3077
*Pedameth*—Forest (U.S.) brand of Racemethionine (Systemic), #
*PediaCare Allergy Formula*—McNeil-CPC (U.S.) brand of Chlorpheniramine—**See Antihistamines (Systemic)**, 325
*PediaCare Cold Allergy*—McNeil (U.S.) brand of Chlorpheniramine and Pseudoephedrine—**See Antihistamines and Decongestants (Systemic)**, 343
*PediaCare Cold Formula*—McNeil (U.S.) brand of Chlorpheniramine and Pseudoephedrine—**See Antihistamines and Decongestants (Systemic)**, 343
*PediaCare Cough-Cold*—McNeil (U.S.) brand of Chlorpheniramine, Pseudoephedrine, and Dextromethorphan—**See Cough/Cold Combinations (Systemic)**, 1024
*PediaCare Infants' Oral Decongestant Drops*—McNeil (U.S.) brand of Pseudoephedrine (Systemic), 2422
*PediaCare NightRest Cough-Cold Liquid*—McNeil (U.S.) brand of Chlorpheniramine, Pseudoephedrine, and Dextromethorphan—**See Cough/Cold Combinations (Systemic)**, 1024
*Pediacof Cough*—Sanofi-Winthrop (U.S.) brand of Chlorpheniramine, Phenylephrine, Codeine, and Potassium Iodide—**See Cough/Cold Combinations (Systemic)**, 1024

*Pediaflor*—Ross (U.S.) brand of Sodium Fluoride (Systemic), 2592
*Pedialyte*—Ross (U.S. and Canada) brand of Dextrose and Electrolytes—**See Carbohydrates and Electrolytes (Systemic)**, 769
*Pedialyte Freezer Pops*—Ross (U.S.) brand of Dextrose and Electrolytes—**See Carbohydrates and Electrolytes (Systemic)**, 769
*Pediapred*—Fisons (U.S.) brand of Prednisolone—**See Corticosteroids—Glucocorticoid Effects (Systemic)**, 998
*PediaPressin Pediatric Drops*—Quintex (U.S.) brand of Pseudoephedrine, Dextromethorphan, and Guaifenesin—**See Cough/Cold Combinations (Systemic)**, 1024
*Pediasure*—Ross (U.S.) brand of Enteral Nutrition Formula, Polymeric—**See Enteral Nutrition Formulas (Systemic)**, #
*Pediasure with Fiber*—Ross (U.S.) brand of Enteral Nutrition Formula, Fiber-containing—**See Enteral Nutrition Formulas (Systemic)**, #
*Pediatric Aqueous Charcodote*—Pharmascience (Canada) brand of Charcoal, Activated (Oral-Local), 831
*Pediatric Aqueous Insta-Char*—Kerr (U.S.) brand of Charcoal, Activated (Oral-Local), 831
*Pediatric Charcodote*—Pharmascience (Canada) brand of Charcoal, Activated, and Sorbitol—**See Charcoal, Activated (Oral-Local)**, 831
*Pediazole*—Ross (U.S.) and Abbott (Canada) brand of Erythromycin and Sulfisoxazole (Systemic), 1376
*Pedi-Dent*—Stanley (Canada) brand of Sodium Fluoride (Systemic), 2592
*Pediotic*—BW (U.S.) brand of Neomycin, Polymyxin B, and Hydrocortisone (Otic), #
*Peditus Cough*—Major (U.S.) brand of Chlorpheniramine, Phenylephrine, Codeine, and Potassium Iodide—**See Cough/Cold Combinations (Systemic)**, 1024
*Pedvaxhib*—Merck (U.S. and Canada) brand of Haemophilus b Conjugate Vaccine (PRP-OMP-Meningococcal Protein Conjugate)—**See Haemophilus b Conjugate Vaccine (Systemic)**, 1601
*PEG-ADA*—*See* Pegademase (Systemic), #
Pegademase Bovine [*Adagen*; PEG-ADA; PEG-adenosine deaminase]
  **(Systemic)**, #, 3157
  Injection, #
PEG-adenosine deaminase—*See* Pegademase (Systemic), #
*Peganone*—Abbott (U.S.) brand of Ethotoin—**See Anticonvulsants, Hydantoin (Systemic)**, 253
Pegaspargase [*Oncaspar*, PEG-L-asparaginase]
  **(Systemic)**, 2230, 3157
  Injection, 2233
PEGASYS
  **(Systemic)**, 3157
PEG-Glucocerebrosidase
  **(Systemic)**, 3157
PEG-Interleukin-2
  **(Systemic)**, 3157
PEG-L-asparaginase—*See* Pegaspargase (Systemic), 2230
*Peglyte*—Pharmascience (Canada) brand of Polyethylene Glycol 3350 and Electrolytes (Local), 2349
Pegylated Recombinant Human MegaKaryocyte Growth and Development Factor [*Megagen*]
  **(Systemic)**, 3157
*Pelamine*—Major (U.S.) brand of Tripelennamine—**See Antihistamines (Systemic)**, 325
Pemoline [*Cylert; Cylert Chewable*]
  **(Systemic)**, 2233
  Tablets, 2235, MC-24
  Tablets, Chewable, 2236, MC-24
*Penazine VC with Cough*—Century (U.S.) brand of Promethazine and Codeine—**See Cough/Cold Combinations (Systemic)**, 1024
*Penbritin*—Ayerst (Canada) brand of Ampicillin—**See Penicillins (Systemic)**, 2240
Penbutolol Sulfate [*Levatol*]
  **See Beta-adrenergic Blocking Agents (Systemic)**, 593
  Tablets, 605, MC-24
Penciclovir [*Denavir*]
  **(Topical)**, 2236
  Cream, 2237
*Penecort*—Allergan Herbert (U.S.) brand of Hydrocortisone—**See Corticosteroids (Topical)**, 978
*Penetrex*—Rhône-Poulenc Rorer (U.S.) brand of Enoxacin—**See Fluoroquinolones (Systemic)**, 1487, MC-11

**3326    General Index**    *USP DI*

*Penglobe*—Astra (Canada) brand of Bacampicillin—**See Penicillins (Systemic)**, 2240
Penicillamine [*Cuprimine; Depen*]
  **(Systemic)**, 2237
  Capsules USP, 2240
  Tablets USP, 2240
Penicillin G Benzathine [benzathine benzylpenicillin; benzathine penicillin; *Bicillin L-A; Megacillin; Permapen*]
  **See Penicillins (Systemic)**, 2240
  Suspension, 2256
  Suspension, Sterile, USP, 2256
Penicillin G Potassium [*Megacillin; Pentids; Pfizerpen*]
  **See Penicillins (Systemic)**, 2240
  for Injection USP, 2257
  for Solution, Oral, USP, 2256
  Tablets USP, 2256
Penicillin G Procaine [*Ayercillin; Crysticillin 300 AS; Pfizerpen-AS;* procaine penicillin; *Wycillin*]
  **See Penicillins (Systemic)**, 2240
  Suspension, Sterile, USP, 2257
Penicillin G Sodium
  **See Penicillins (Systemic)**, 2240
  for Injection USP, 2258
Penicillins
  **(Systemic)**, 2240
Penicillins and Beta-lactamase Inhibitors
  **(Systemic)**, 2263
Penicillin V Benzathine [*Pen-Vee;* phenoxymethylpenicillin; *PVF*]
  **See Penicillins (Systemic)**, 2240
  Suspension, 2258
Penicillin V Potassium [*Apo-Pen-VK; Beepen-VK; Betapen-VK; Ledercillin VK; Nadopen-V; Nadopen-V 200; Nadopen-V 400; Novo-Pen-VK; Nu-Pen-VK; Pen Vee; Pen Vee K;* phenoxymethylpenicillin; *PVF K; V-Cillin K; Veetids*]
  **See Penicillins (Systemic)**, 2240
  for Solution, Oral, USP, 2258
  Tablets USP, 2259, MC-24
*Penntuss*—Rhône-Poulenc Rorer (Canada) brand of Chlorpheniramine and Codeine—**See Cough/Cold Combinations (Systemic)**, 1024
*Pentacarinat*—Rhône-Poulenc (Canada) brand of Pentamidine (Inhalation), 2272; Pentamidine (Systemic), 2274
*Pentacort*—Penta (U.S.) brand of Hydrocortisone—**See Corticosteroids (Topical)**, 978
Pentaerithrityl tetranitrate—Pentaerythritol Tetranitrate—**See Nitrates (Systemic)**, 2129
Pentaerythritol Tetranitrate [*Duotrate;* pentaerithrityl tetranitrate; *Pentylan; Peritrate; Peritrate Forte; Peritrate SA;* P.E.T.N.]
  **See Nitrates (Systemic)**, 2129
  Capsules, Extended-release, 2136
  Tablets USP, 2136
  Tablets, Extended-release, 2137
Pentagastrin [*Peptavlon*]
  **(Systemic)**, #
  Injection, #
*Pentam 300*—Fujisawa (U.S.) brand of Pentamidine (Systemic), 2274, 3157
Pentamidine Isethionate [*NebuPent; Pentacarinat; Pneumopent*]
  **(Inhalation)**, 2272, 3157
  for Solution, Inhalation, 2273
Pentamidine Isethionate [*Pentacarinat; Pentam 300*]
  **(Systemic)**, 2274, 3157
  Sterile, 2277
*Pentamycetin Ophthalmic Ointment*—Sabex (Canada) brand of Chloramphenicol (Ophthalmic), #
*Pentamycetin Ophthalmic Solution*—Sabex (Canada) brand of Chloramphenicol (Ophthalmic), #
*Pentasa*—Roberts (U.S.) and Marion Merrell Dow (Canada) brand of Mesalamine (Oral-Local), 1952, MC-18
*Pentaspan*—Du Pont Critical Care (U.S.) brand of Pentastarch, 3031, 3157
Pentastarch [*Pentaspan*], 3031, 3157
  **(Systemic)**, #
  Injection, 3031
*Penta-Valproic*—Pentapharm (Canada) brand of Valproic Acid—**See Valproic Acid (Systemic)**, 2908
*Pentazine*—Century (U.S.) brand of Promethazine—**See Antihistamines, Phenothiazine-derivative (Systemic)**, 377
*Pentazine VC with Codeine*—Century (U.S.) brand of Promethazine and Codeine—**See Cough/Cold Combinations (Systemic)**, 1024
Pentazocine-containing Combinations, 3077

Pentazocine Hydrochloride [*Talwin*]
  **See Opioid (Narcotic) Analgesics (Systemic)**, 2168
  Tablets USP, 2188
Pentazocine Hydrochloride and Acetaminophen [*Talacen*]
  **See Opioid (Narcotic) Analgesics and Acetaminophen (Systemic)**, 2198
  Tablets, 2201, MC-24
Pentazocine Hydrochloride and Aspirin [*Talwin Compound*]
  **See Opioid (Narcotic) Analgesics and Aspirin (Systemic)**, 2202
  Tablets USP, 2204
Pentazocine and Naloxone Hydrochlorides [*Talwin-Nx*]
  **See Opioid (Narcotic) Analgesics (Systemic)**, 2168
  Tablets USP, MC-24
Pentazocine Lactate [*Talwin*]
  **See Opioid (Narcotic) Analgesics (Systemic)**, 2168
  Injection USP, 2189
Pentazocine and Naloxone Hydrochlorides [*Talwin-Nx*]
  **See Opioid (Narcotic) Analgesics (Systemic)**, 2168
  Tablets USP, 2188
*Penthrane*—Abbott (U.S.) brand of Methoxyflurane—**See Anesthetics, Inhalation (Systemic)**, 168
*Pentids*—Squibb (U.S.) brand of Penicillin G—**See Penicillins (Systemic)**, 2240
Pentobarbital [*Nembutal*]
  **See Barbiturates (Systemic)**, 518
  Elixir USP, 527
Pentobarbital-containing Combinations, 3077
Pentobarbital Sodium [*Nembutal; Nova Rectal; Novopentobarb*]
  **See Barbiturates (Systemic)**, 518
  Capsules USP, 527
  Injection USP, 527
  Suppositories, 527
*Pentolair*—Balan (U.S.) and Texas Drugs (U.S.) brand of Cyclopentolate (Ophthalmic), #
Pentosan Polysulfate Sodium [*Elmiron*]
  **(Systemic)**, 2277
  Capsules, 2279, MC-24
Pentosan Polysulphate [*Elmiron*]
  **(Systemic)**, 3157
Pentostatin [2'DCF; 2'-deoxycoformycin; *Nipent*]
  **(Systemic)**, 2279, 3158
  for Injection, 2282, 3158
*Pentothal*—Abbott (U.S. and Canada) brand of Thiopental—**See Anesthetics, Barbiturate (Systemic)**, 161
Pentoxifylline [oxypentifylline; *Trental*]
  **(Systemic)**, 2282
  Tablets, Extended-release, 2284, MC-25
*Pentrax Anti-Dandruff Tar Shampoo*—GenDerm (U.S.) brand of Coal Tar (Topical), #
*Pentrax Extra-Strength Therapeutic Tar Shampoo*—GenDerm (Canada) brand of Coal Tar (Topical), #
*Pentylan*—Lannett (U.S.) brand of Pentaerythritol Tetranitrate—**See Nitrates (Systemic)**, 2129
*Pen Vee*—Wyeth (Canada) brand of Penicillin V—**See Penicillins (Systemic)**, 2240
*Pen-Vee K*—Wyeth-Ayerst (U.S.) brand of Penicillin V—**See Penicillins (Systemic)**, 2240, MC-24
*Pep-Back*—Alva-Amco (U.S.) brand of Caffeine (Systemic), 706
*Pepcid*—Merck (U.S. and Canada) brand of Famotidine—**See Histamine H$_2$-receptor Antagonists (Systemic)**, 1633, MC-12
*Pepcid AC*—J&J Merck (U.S.) brand of Famotidine (Systemic), 1633
*Pepcid I.V.*—Merck (U.S. and Canada) brand of Famotidine—**See Histamine H$_2$-receptor Antagonists (Systemic)**, 1633
*Peptamen*—Clintec (U.S.) brand of Enteral Nutrition Formula, Disease-specific—**See Enteral Nutrition Formulas (Systemic)**, #; Enteral Nutrition Formula, Monomeric (Elemental)—**See Enteral Nutrition Formulas (Systemic)**, #
*Peptamen Junior*—Clintec (U.S.) brand of Enteral Nutrition Formula, Disease-specific—**See Enteral Nutrition Formulas (Systemic)**, #; Enteral Nutrition Formula, Monomeric (Elemental)—**See Enteral Nutrition Formulas (Systemic)**, #

*Peptamen VHP*—Clintec (U.S.) brand of Enteral Nutrition Formula, Disease-specific—**See Enteral Nutrition Formulas (Systemic)**, #; Enteral Nutrition Formula, Monomeric (Elemental)—**See Enteral Nutrition Formulas (Systemic)**, #
*Peptavlon*—Wyeth-Ayerst (U.S.) and Ayerst (Canada) brand of Pentagastrin (Systemic), #
*Pepto-Bismol*—Procter & Gamble (U.S. and Canada) brand of Bismuth Subsalicylate (Oral-Local), 616
*Pepto-Bismol Easy-to-Swallow Caplets*—Procter & Gamble (U.S.) brand of Bismuth Subsalicylate (Oral-Local), 616
*Pepto-Bismol Maximum Strength*—Procter & Gamble (U.S.) brand of Bismuth Subsalicylate (Oral-Local), 616
*Pepto Diarrhea Control*—Procter & Gamble (U.S.) brand of Loperamide (Oral-Local), 1877
*Peptol*—Horner (Canada) brand of Cimetidine—**See Histamine H$_2$-receptor Antagonists (Systemic)**, 1633
*Perative*—Ross (U.S.) brand of Enteral Nutrition Formula, Disease-specific—**See Enteral Nutrition Formulas (Systemic)**, #
*Percocet*—Endo (U.S. and Canada) brand of Oxycodone and Acetaminophen—**See Opioid (Narcotic) Analgesics and Acetaminophen (Systemic)**, 2198, MC-24
*Percocet-Demi*—Du Pont (Canada) brand of Oxycodone and Acetaminophen—**See Opioid (Narcotic) Analgesics and Acetaminophen (Systemic)**, 2198
*Percodan*—Endo (U.S. and Canada) brand of Oxycodone and Aspirin—**See Opioid (Narcotic) Analgesics and Aspirin (Systemic)**, 2202, MC-24
*Percodan-Demi*—Endo (U.S. and Canada) brand of Oxycodone and Aspirin—**See Opioid (Narcotic) Analgesics and Aspirin (Systemic)**, 2202, MC-24
*Percolone*—Endo (U.S.) brand of Oxycodone (Systemic), MC-23
*Perdiem*—Ciba Self-Medication (U.S.) brand of Psyllium and Senna—**See Laxatives (Local)**, #
*Perdiem Fiber*—Ciba Self-Medication (U.S.) brand of Psyllium—**See Laxatives (Local)**, #
Perflubron [*Imagent GI;* perfluorooctylbromide]
  **(Oral-Local)**, #
  Solution, Oral, #
Perfluorochemical Emulsion [*Fluosol*]
  **(Systemic)**, #
  for Injection, #
Perfluorooctylbromide—See Perflubron (Oral-Local), #
Pergolide [*Permax*]
  **(Systemic)**, 3158
Pergolide Mesylate [*Permax*]
  **(Systemic)**, 2284
  Tablets, 2286, MC-25
*Pergonal*—Serono (U.S.) brand of Menotropins (Systemic), 1943
*Periactin*—Merck (U.S. and Canada) brand of Cyproheptadine—**See Antihistamines (Systemic)**, 325
*Periciazine*—Pericyazine—**See Phenothiazines (Systemic)**, 2289
*Peri-Colace*—Roberts (U.S. and Canada) brand of Casanthranol and Docusate—**See Laxatives (Local)**, #
Pericyazine [*Neuleptil;* periciazine]
  **See Phenothiazines (Systemic)**, 2289
  Capsules, 2303
  Solution, Oral, 2303
*Peridex*—Procter & Gamble (U.S. and Canada) brand of Chlorhexidine (Mucosal-Local), 847, 3014, 3136
*Peridol*—Technilab (Canada) brand of Haloperidol (Systemic), 1611
*Peri-Dos Softgels*—Zenith Goldline (U.S.) brand of Casthranol and Docusate—**See Laxatives (Local)**, #
*PerioChip*—Astra (U.S.) brand of Chlorhexidine (Mucosal-Local), 3014
*PerioGard*—Colgate (U.S.) brand of Chlorhexidine (Mucosal-Local), 847
*Peritrate*—PD (U.S. and Canada) brand of Pentaerythritol Tetranitrate—**See Nitrates (Systemic)**, 2129
*Peritrate Forte*—PD (Canada) brand of Pentaerythritol Tetranitrate—**See Nitrates (Systemic)**, 2129
*Peritrate SA*—PD (U.S. and Canada) brand of Pentaerythritol Tetranitrate—**See Nitrates (Systemic)**, 2129
*Permapen*—Roerig (U.S.) brand of Penicillin G—**See Penicillins (Systemic)**, 2240

*Permax*—Athena (U.S. and Canada) and Salle (U.S.) brand of Pergolide (Systemic), 2284, 3158
Permethrin [*Acticin; Elimite; Nix Cream Rinse; Nix Dermal Cream*]
 **(Topical)**, #, 3032
 Cream, #, 3032
 Lotion, #
*Permitil*—Schering (U.S. and Canada) brand of Fluphenazine—**See Phenothiazines (Systemic)**, 2289
*Permitil Concentrate*—Schering (U.S.) brand of Fluphenazine—**See Phenothiazines (Systemic)**, 2289
*Pernox Lathering Abradant Scrub Cleanser (Fresh Scent)*—Westwood-Squibb (U.S.) brand of Salicylic Acid and Sulfur (Topical), #
*Pernox (Lemon)*—Westwood-Squibb (U.S. and Canada) brand of Salicylic Acid and Sulfur (Topical), #
*Pernox (Regular)*—Westwood-Squibb (U.S. and Canada) brand of Salicylic Acid and Sulfur (Topical), #
Perphenazine [*Apo-Perphenazine; PMS Perphenazine; Trilafon; Trilafon Concentrate*]
 **See Phenothiazines (Systemic)**, 2289
 Injection USP, 2304
 Solution, Oral, USP, 2304
 Syrup USP, 2304
 Tablets USP, 2304
Perphenazine and Amitriptyline Hydrochloride [*Elavil Plus; Etrafon; Etrafon-A; Etrafon-D; Etrafon-F; Etrafon-Forte; PMS Levazine; Triavil*]
 **(Systemic)**, 2286
 Tablets USP, 2287, MC-25
Perphenazine-containing Combinations, 3077
*Persantine*—Boehringer Ingelheim (U.S. and Canada) brand of Dipyridamole (Systemic), #, MC-10
*Pertofrane*—Ciba-Geigy (Canada) brand of Desipramine—**See Antidepressants, Tricyclic (Systemic)**, 271
*Pertussin Cough Suppressant*—Pertussin (U.S.) brand of Dextromethorphan (Systemic), 1191
*Pertussin CS*—Pertussin (U.S.) brand of Dextromethorphan (Systemic), 1191
*Pertussin ES*—Pertussin (U.S.) brand of Dextromethorphan (Systemic), 1191
Pethidine—Meperidine—**See Opioid (Narcotic) Analgesics (Systemic)**, 2168
*Petrogalar Plain*—Wyeth-Ayerst (U.S.) brand of Mineral Oil—**See Laxatives (Local)**, #
PFA—**See** Foscarnet (Systemic), 1528
*Pfizerpen*—Roerig (U.S.) brand of Penicillin G—**See Penicillins (Systemic)**, 2240
*Pfizerpen-AS*—Roerig (U.S.) brand of Penicillin G—**See Penicillins (Systemic)**, 2240
PGE$_1$—**See** Alprostadil (Intracavernosal), 48; Alprostadil (Systemic), 52
PGE$_2$—**See** Dinoprostone (Cervical/Vaginal), 1228
*Phanatuss*—Pharmakon (U.S.) brand of Dextromethorphan, and Guaifenesin—**See Cough/Cold Combinations (Systemic)**, 1024
*Phanatussin*—Pharmakon (U.S.) brand of Pyrilamine, Phenylpropanolamine, Dextromethorphan, Guaifenesin, Potassium Citrate, and Citric Acid—**See Cough/Cold Combinations (Systemic)**, 1024
*Pharma-Cort*—Purepac (U.S.) brand of Hydrocortisone—**See Corticosteroids (Topical)**, 978
*Pharmaflur 1.1*—Pharmics (U.S.) brand of Sodium Fluoride (Systemic), 2592
*Pharmaflur*—Pharmics (U.S.) brand of Sodium Fluoride (Systemic), 2592
*Pharmaflur df*—Pharmics (U.S.) brand of Sodium Fluoride (Systemic), 2592
*Pharmagesic*—Pecos (U.S.) and Pharm-Tech (U.S.) brand of Butalbital and Acetaminophen—**See Barbiturates and Analgesics (Systemic)**, 532
*Pharmasave Children's Cough Syrup*—Stanley (Canada) brand of Pseudoephedrine and Dextromethorphan—**See Cough/Cold Combinations (Systemic)**, 1024
*Pharmasave DM+ Decongestant/Expectorant*—Stanley (Canada) brand of Pseudoephedrine, Dextromethorphan, and Guaifenesin—**See Cough/Cold Combinations (Systemic)**, 1024
*Pharmasave DM+ Expectorant*—Stanley (Canada) brand of Dextromethorphan and Guaifenesin—**See Cough/Cold Combinations (Systemic)**, 1024
*Pharmatex*—Interpharm (Canada) brand of Benzalkonium Chloride—**See Spermicides (Vaginal)**, #

*Pharmorubicin PFS*—Adria (Canada) brand of Epirubicin (Systemic), 3018
*Pharmorubicin RDF*—Adria (Canada) brand of Epirubicin (Systemic), 3018
*Phazyme*—Reed & Carnrick (U.S.) brand of Simethicone (Oral-Local), #
*Phazyme 95*—Reed & Carnrick (U.S. and Canada) brand of Simethicone (Oral-Local), #
*Phazyme 125*—Reed & Carnrick (Canada) brand of Simethicone (Oral-Local), #
*Phazyme Drops*—Reed & Carnrick (Canada) brand of Simethicone (Oral-Local), #
Phenacemide [*Epiclase; phenacetylcarbamide; Phetylureum*]
 **(Systemic)**, #
 Tablets USP, #
Phenacetylcarbamide—**See** Phenacemide (Systemic), #
*Phenahist-TR*—T. E. Williams (U.S.) brand of Chlorpheniramine, Phenylephrine, Phenylpropanolamine, Atropine, Hyoscyamine, and Scopolamine—**See Antihistamines, Decongestants, and Anticholinergics (Systemic)**, 373
*Phenameth DM*—Major (U.S.) brand of Promethazine and Dextromethorphan—**See Cough/Cold Combinations (Systemic)**, 1024
*Phenameth VC with Codeine*—Major (U.S.) brand of Promethazine, Phenylephrine, and Codeine—**See Cough/Cold Combinations (Systemic)**, 1024
*PhenAPAP Without Drowsiness*—Rugby (U.S.) brand of Pseudoephedrine and Acetaminophen—**See Decongestants and Analgesics (Systemic)**, 1180
*Phenaphen Caplets*—Robins (U.S.) brand of Acetaminophen (Systemic), 6
*Phenaphen with Codeine No.2*—Ayerst (Canada) brand of Phenobarbital, ASA, and Codeine—**See Barbiturates and Analgesics (Systemic)**, 532
*Phenaphen with Codeine No.3*—Ayerst (Canada) brand of Phenobarbital, ASA, and Codeine—**See Barbiturates and Analgesics (Systemic)**, 532; Robins (U.S.) brand of Acetaminophen and Codeine—**See Opioid (Narcotic) Analgesics and Acetaminophen (Systemic)**, 2198, MC-1
*Phenaphen with Codeine No.4*—Ayerst (Canada) brand of Phenobarbital, ASA, and Codeine—**See Barbiturates and Analgesics (Systemic)**, 532; Robins (U.S.) brand of Acetaminophen and Codeine—**See Opioid (Narcotic) Analgesics and Acetaminophen (Systemic)**, 2198, MC-1
*Phenate T.D.*—Roberts (U.S.) brand of Chlorpheniramine, Phenylpropanolamine, and Acetaminophen—**See Antihistamines, Decongestants, and Analgesics (Systemic)**, 366
*Phenazine 25*—Keene (U.S.) brand of Promethazine—**See Antihistamines, Phenothiazine-derivative (Systemic)**, 377
*Phenazine 50*—Keene (U.S.) brand of Promethazine—**See Antihistamines, Phenothiazine-derivative (Systemic)**, 377
*Phenazo*—ICN (Canada) brand of Phenazopyridine (Systemic), 2288
*Phenazodine*—Lannett (U.S.) brand of Phenazopyridine (Systemic), 2288
Phenazopyridine-containing Combinations, 3077
Phenazopyridine Hydrochloride [*Azo-Standard; Baridium; Eridium; Geridium; Phenazo; Phenazodine; Pyridiate; Pyridium; Urodine; Urogesic; Viridium*]
 **(Systemic)**, 2288
 Tablets USP, 2289
*Phencen-50*—Central (U.S.) brand of Promethazine—**See Antihistamines, Phenothiazine-derivative (Systemic)**, 377
*Phenchlor S.H.A.*—Rugby (U.S.) brand of Chlorpheniramine, Phenylephrine, Phenylpropanolamine, Atropine, Hyoscyamine, and Scopolamine—**See Antihistamines, Decongestants, and Anticholinergics (Systemic)**, 373
*Phendiet*—Truxton (U.S.) brand of Phendimetrazine—**See Appetite Suppressants (Systemic)**, 452
*Phendiet-105*—Truxton (U.S.) brand of Phendimetrazine—**See Appetite Suppressants (Systemic)**, 452
*Phendimet*—Balan (U.S.) brand of Phendimetrazine—**See Appetite Suppressants (Systemic)**, 452

Phendimetrazine Tartrate [*Adipost; Anorex SR; Appecon; Bontril PDM; Bontril Slow-Release; Melfiat-105 Unicelles; Obalan; Obezine; Parzine; Phendiet; Phendiet-105; Phendimet; Plegine; Prelu-2; PT 105; Rexigen Forte; Wehless; Wehless-105 Timecelles*]
 **See Appetite Suppressants (Systemic)**, 452
 Capsules USP, 456
 Capsules, Extended-release, 456 MC-25
 Tablets USP, 456
 Tablets, Extended-release, 456
Phenelzine Sulfate [*Nardil*]
 **See Antidepressants, Monoamine Oxidase (MAO) Inhibitor (Systemic)**, 266
 Tablets USP, 270
*Phenergan*—Wyeth-Ayerst (U.S.) and May & Baker (Canada) brand of Promethazine—**See Antihistamines, Phenothiazine-derivative (Systemic)**, 377, MC-26
*Phenergan with Codeine*—Wyeth-Ayerst (U.S.) brand of Promethazine and Codeine—**See Cough/Cold Combinations (Systemic)**, 1024
*Phenergan with Dextromethorphan*—Wyeth-Ayerst (U.S.) brand of Promethazine and Dextromethorphan—**See Cough/Cold Combinations (Systemic)**, 1024
*Phenergan Expectorant*—Ciba Consumer (Canada) brand of Promethazine and Potassium Guaiacolsulfonate—**See Cough/Cold Combinations (Systemic)**, 1024
*Phenergan Expectorant with Codeine*—Ciba Consumer (Canada) brand of Promethazine, Codeine, and Potassium Guaiacolsulfonate—**See Cough/Cold Combinations (Systemic)**, 1024
*Phenergan Fortis*—Wyeth-Ayerst (U.S.) brand of Promethazine—**See Antihistamines, Phenothiazine-derivative (Systemic)**, 377
*Phenergan Plain*—Wyeth-Ayerst (U.S.) brand of Promethazine—**See Antihistamines, Phenothiazine-derivative (Systemic)**, 377
*Phenergan VC*—Wyeth-Ayerst (U.S.) brand of Promethazine and Phenylephrine—**See Antihistamines and Decongestants (Systemic)**, 343
*Phenergan VC with Codeine*—Wyeth-Ayerst (U.S.) brand of Promethazine, Phenylephrine, and Codeine—**See Cough/Cold Combinations (Systemic)**, 1024
*Phenergan VC Expectorant*—Ciba Consumer (Canada) brand of Promethazine, Phenylephrine, and Potassium Guaiacolsulfonate—**See Cough/Cold Combinations (Systemic)**, 1024
*Phenergan VC Expectorant with Codeine*—Ciba Consumer (Canada) brand of Promethazine, Phenylephrine, Codeine, and Potassium Guaiacolsulfonate—**See Cough/Cold Combinations (Systemic)**, 1024
*Phenerzine*—Bolan (U.S.) brand of Promethazine—**See Antihistamines, Phenothiazine-derivative (Systemic)**, 377
*Phenetron*—Lannett (U.S.) brand of Chlorpheniramine—**See Antihistamines (Systemic)**, 325
*Phenhist DH with Codeine*—Rugby (U.S.) brand of Chlorpheniramine, Pseudoephedrine, and Codeine—**See Cough/Cold Combinations (Systemic)**, 1024
*Phenhist Expectorant*—Rugby (U.S.) brand of Pseudoephedrine, Codeine, and Guaifenesin—**See Cough/Cold Combinations (Systemic)**, 1024
Phenindamine-containing Combinations, 3077
Phenindamine Tartrate [*Nolahist*]
 **See Antihistamines (Systemic)**, 325
 Tablets, 341
Pheniramine-containing Combinations, 3077
Pheniramine Maleate, Codeine Phosphate, and Guaifenesin [*Robitussin A-C; Robitussin with Codeine*]
 **See Cough/Cold Combinations (Systemic)**, 1024
 Syrup, 1087, 1088
Pheniramine Maleate and Phenylephrine Hydrochloride [*Neo Citran A*]
 **See Antihistamines and Decongestants (Systemic)**, 343
 for Solution, Oral, 356
Pheniramine Maleate, Phenylephrine Hydrochloride, and Acetaminophen [*Neo Citran Colds and Flu; Neo Citran Colds and Flu Calorie Reduced; Neo Citran Extra Strength Colds and Flu*]
 **See Antihistamines, Decongestants, and Analgesics (Systemic)**, 366
 for Solution, Oral, 370

Pheniramine Maleate, Phenylephrine Hydrochloride, Codeine Phosphate, Sodium Citrate, Sodium Salicylate, and Caffeine Citrate [Tussirex]
  See Cough/Cold Combinations (Systemic), 1024
  Solution, Oral, 1107
Pheniramine Maleate, Phenylephrine Hydrochloride, and Dextromethorphan Hydrobromide [Neo Citran DM Coughs and Colds]
  See Cough/Cold Combinations (Systemic), 1024
  for Solution, Oral, 1073
Pheniramine Maleate, Phenylephrine Hydrochloride, Phenylpropanolamine Hydrochloride, Hydrocodone Bitartrate, and Guaifenesin [S-T Forte]
  See Cough/Cold Combinations (Systemic), 1024
  Solution, Oral, 1095
  Syrup, 1096
Pheniramine Maleate, Phenylephrine Hydrochloride, Sodium Salicylate, and Caffeine Citrate [Scot-Tussin Original 5-Action Cold Formula]
  See Antihistamines, Decongestants, and Analgesics (Systemic), 366
  Solution, Oral, 371
Pheniramine Maleate, Phenyltoloxamine Citrate, Pyrilamine Maleate, and Phenylpropanolamine Hydrochloride [Delhistine-D; Iohist-D; Liqui-Histine-D; Metahistine D; Poly D; Poly-Histine-D; Poly-Histine-D Ped; Trihist-D; Uni-Multihist-D]
  See Antihistamines and Decongestants (Systemic), 343
  Capsules, Extended-release, 358
  Elixir, 350, 354, 355, 358, 363, 364
Pheniramine Maleate, Pyrilamine Maleate, Hydrocodone Bitartrate, Potassium Citrate, and Ascorbic Acid [Citra Forte]
  See Cough/Cold Combinations (Systemic), 1024
  Syrup, 1043
Pheniramine Maleate, Pyrilamine Maleate, Phenylephrine Hydrochloride, Phenylpropanolamine Hydrochloride, and Hydrocodone Bitartrate [Rolatuss with Hydrocodone; Ru-Tuss with Hydrocodone Liquid; Statuss Green]
  See Cough/Cold Combinations (Systemic), 1024
  Solution, Oral, 1090, 1091, 1095
Pheniramine Maleate, Pyrilamine Maleate, and Phenylpropanolamine Hydrochloride [Liqui-Minic Infant Drops; Triaminic; Triaminic Oral Infant Drops; Triaminic TR]
  See Antihistamines and Decongestants (Systemic), 343
  Solution, Oral, 354, 362
  Tablets, Extended-release, 362, 363
Pheniramine Maleate, Pyrilamine Maleate, Phenylpropanolamine Hydrochloride, Acetaminophen, and Caffeine[Triaminicin]
  See Antihistamines and Decongestants (Systemic), 366
  Tablets, 372
Pheniramine Maleate, Pyrilamine Maleate, Phenylpropanolamine Hydrochloride, and Codeine Phosphate [Tussaminic C Forte; Tussaminic C Pediatric]
  See Cough/Cold Combinations (Systemic), 1024
  Syrup, 1104
Pheniramine Maleate, Pyrilamine Maleate, Phenylpropanolamine Hydrochloride, and Dextromethorphan Hydrobromide [Tantacol DM]
  See Cough/Cold Combinations (Systemic), 1024
  Syrup, 1098
Pheniramine Maleate, Pyrilamine Maleate, Phenylpropanolamine Hydrochloride, Dextromethorphan Hydrobromide, and Ammonium Chloride [Prominicol Cough]
  See Cough/Cold Combinations (Systemic), 1024
  Syrup, 1084
Pheniramine Maleate, Pyrilamine Maleate, Phenylpropanolamine Hydrochloride, and Hydrocodone Bitartrate [Caldomine-DH Forte; Caldomine-DH Pediatric; Tussaminic DH Forte; Tussaminic DH Pediatric]
  See Cough/Cold Combinations (Systemic), 1024
  Solution, Oral, 1039
  Syrup, 1105
Pheniramine Maleate, Pyrilamine Maleate, Phenylpropanolamine Hydrochloride, Hydrocodone Bitartrate, and Guaifenesin [Triaminic Expectorant DH]
  See Cough/Cold Combinations (Systemic), 1024
  Elixir, 1102
  Solution, Oral, 1102

Phenobarbital [Ancalixir; Barbita; Solfoton]
  See Barbiturates (Systemic), 518
  Capsules, 528
  Elixir USP, 528
  Tablets USP, 529, MC-25
Phenobarbital, ASA, and Codeine Phosphate [Phenaphen with Codeine No.2; Phenaphen with Codeine No.3; Phenaphen with Codeine No.4]
  See Barbiturates and Analgesics (Systemic), 532
  Capsules, 544
Phenobarbital-containing Combinations, 3077
Phenobarbital Sodium [Luminal]
  See Barbiturates (Systemic), 518
  Injection USP, 529
  Sterile USP, 529
Phenoject-50—Mayrand (U.S.) brand of Promethazine—See Antihistamines, Phenothiazine-derivative (Systemic), 377
Phenolphthalein [Alophen; Carter's Little Pills; Evac-U-Gen; Evac-U-Lax; Ex-Lax; Ex-Lax Maximum Relief Formula; Ex-Lax Pills; Lax-Pills; Medilax; Modane; Prulet]
  See Laxatives (Local), #
  Tablets, #
  Tablets USP, #
  Tablets USP (Chewable), #
Phenolsulfonphthalein [phenol red; PSP]
  (Systemic), #
  Injection, #
Phenolphthalein-containing Combinations, 3077
Phenolphthalein and Docusate Calcium [Docucal-P; Doxidan]
  See Laxatives (Local), #
  Capsules, #
Phenolphthalein and Docusate Sodium [Colax; Dialose Plus; Ex-Lax Light Formula; Extra Gentle Ex-Lax; FemiLax; Modane Plus; Phillips' Gelcaps; Phillips' LaxCaps; Unilax]
  See Laxatives (Local), #
  Capsules, #
  Tablets, #
Phenolphthalein Petrogalar—Wyeth-Ayerst (U.S.) brand of Mineral Oil and Phenolphthalein—See Laxatives (Local), #
Phenolphthalein and Senna [Mucinum]
  See Laxatives (Local), #
  Tablets, #
Phenol red—See Phenolsulfonphthalein (Systemic), #
Phenoptic—Optopics (U.S.) brand of Phenylephrine (Ophthalmic), #
Phenothiazines
  (Systemic), 2289
Phenoxybenzamine Hydrochloride [Dibenzyline]
  (Systemic), 2312
  Capsules USP, 2313
Phenoxymethylpenicillin—Penicillin V—See Penicillins (Systemic), 2240
Phentercot—Truxton (U.S.) brand of Phentermine—See Appetite Suppressants (Systemic), 452
Phentermine Hydrochloride [Adipex-P; Fastin; Obe-Nix; OBY-CAP; Panshape M; Phentercot; Phentride; T-Diet; Teramine; Zantryl]
  See Appetite Suppressants (Systemic), 452
  Capsules USP, 457
  Tablets USP, 457
Phentermine Resin [Ionamin]
  See Appetite Suppressants (Systemic), 452
  Capsules, 457
Phentolamine Mesylate [Regitine; Rogitine]
  (Intracavernosal), #
  for Injection USP, #
Phentolamine Mesylate [Regitine; Rogitine]
  (Systemic), #
  for Injection USP, #
Phentride—Western Research (U.S.) brand of Phentermine—See Appetite Suppressants (Systemic), 452
Phenylacetate
  (Systemic), 3158
Phenylalanine Ammonia-Lyase [Phenylase]
  (Systemic), 3158
Phenylalanine mustard—See Melphalan (Systemic), 1938
Phenylase—IBEX Technologies (Canada) brand of Phenylalanine Ammonia-Lyase (Systemic), 3158
Phenylbenzimidazole [Coppertone Tan Magnifier; Hawaiian Tropic Dark Tanning; Oil of Olay Moisture Replenishment; Pond's Daily Replenishing Moisturizer]
  See Sunscreen Agents (Topical), #
  Gel, #
  Lotion, #

Phenylbenzimidazole-containing Combinations, 3077
Phenylbenzimidazole and Sulisobenzone [Hawaiian Tropic Protective Tanning Dry]
  See Sunscreen Agents (Topical), #
  Gel, #
Phenylbutazone [Alka Butazolidin; Apo-Phenylbutazone; Butazolidin; Cotylbutazone]
  See Anti-inflammatory Drugs, Nonsteroidal (Systemic), 388
  Capsules USP, 416
  Tablets, Buffered, 416
  Tablets USP, 416
Phenyldrine—Rugby (U.S.) brand of Phenylpropanolamine (Systemic), 2314
Phenylephrine-containing Combinations, 3077
Phenylephrine Hydrochloride [Alconefrin Nasal Drops 12; Alconefrin Nasal Drops 25; Alconefrin Nasal Drops 50; Alconefrin Nasal Spray 25; Doktors; Duration; Neo-Synephrine Nasal Drops; Neo-Synephrine Nasal Jelly; Neo-Synephrine Pediatric Nasal Spray; Neo-Synephrine Pediatric Nasal Drops; Nostril Spray Pump; Nostril Spray Pump Mild; Rhinall; Rhinall-10 Children's Flavored Nose Drops; Vicks Sinex]
  (Nasal), #
  Jelly, Nasal, USP, #
  Solution, Nasal, USP, #
Phenylephrine Hydrochloride [Ak-Dilate; Ak-Nefrin; Dilatair; Dionephrine; I-Phrine; Isopto Frin; Minims Phenylephrine; Mydfrin; Neofrin; Neo-Synephrine; Ocugestrin; Ocu-Phrin Sterile Eye Drops; Ocu-Phrin Sterile Ophthalmic Solution; Phenoptic; Prefrin Liquifilm; Relief Eye Drops for Red Eyes; Spersaphrine]
  (Ophthalmic), #, 3032
  Solution, Ophthalmic, USP, #, 3032
Phenylephrine Hydrochloride [Neo-Synephrine]
  See Sympathomimetic Agents—Cardiovascular Use (Parenteral-Systemic), 2669
  Injection USP, 2679
Phenylephrine Hydrochloride and Acetaminophen [Neo Citran Extra Strength Sinus]
  See Decongestants and Analgesics (Systemic), 1180
  for Solution, Oral, 1182
Phenylephrine Hydrochloride and Codeine Phosphate [Novahistex C]
  See Cough/Cold Combinations (Systemic), 1024
  Solution, Oral, 1073
Phenylephrine Hydrochloride, Dextromethorphan Hydrobromide, and Guaifenesin [Dexafed Cough; Suppressin DM Plus; Tussex Cough]
  See Cough/Cold Combinations (Systemic), 1024
  Solution, Oral, 1098
  Syrup, 1052, 1106
Phenylephrine Hydrochloride and Guaifenesin [Deconsal Pediatric; Endal; Rescon-GG; Sinupan]
  See Cough/Cold Combinations (Systemic), 1024
  Capsules, Extended-release, 1051, 1094
  Solution, Oral, 1086
  Tablets, Extended-release, 1056
Phenylephrine Hydrochloride, Guaifenesin, Acetaminophen, Salicylamide, and Caffeine [Fendol]
  See Cough/Cold Combinations (Systemic), 1024
  Tablets, 1058
Phenylephrine Hydrochloride and Hydrocodone Bitartrate [Coristex-DH; Coristine-DH; Nalex DH; Novahistex DH; Novahistine DH]
  See Cough/Cold Combinations (Systemic), 1024
  Elixir, 1072
  Solution, Oral, 1048, 1049, 1073, 1074
Phenylephrine Hydrochloride, Hydrocodone Bitartrate, and Guaifenesin [Donatussin DC; Novahistex DH Expectorant]
  See Cough/Cold Combinations (Systemic), 1024
  Solution, Oral, 1073
  Syrup, 1054
Phenylephrine Hydrochloride, Phenylpropanolamine Hydrochloride, and Acetaminophen [Dimetapp-A Sinus]
  See Decongestants and Analgesics (Systemic), 1180
  Tablets, 1182
Phenylephrine Hydrochloride, Phenylpropanolamine Hydrochloride, Carbetapentane Citrate, and Potassium Guiacolsulfonate [Cophene-X]
  See Cough/Cold Combinations (Systemic), 1024
  Capsules, 1048

Phenylephrine Hydrochloride, Phenylpropanolamine Hydrochloride, and Guaifenesin [*Ami-Tex; Banex Liquid; Contuss; Despec; Despec SF; Dura-Gest; Duratex; Enomine; Entex; Entex Liquid; Norel; Sil-Tex*]
  **See Cough/Cold Combinations (Systemic)**, 1024
  Capsules, 1034, 1055, 1056, 1073, MC-25
  Solution, Oral, 1035, 1048, 1051, 1057, 1093
*Phenylfenesin L.A.*—Zenith Goldline (U.S.) brand of Phenylpropanolamine and Guaifenesin—**See Cough/Cold Combinations (Systemic)**, 1024
Phenylpropanolamine Bitartrate and Aspirin [*Alka-Seltzer Plus Sinus Medicine*]
  **See Decongestants and Analgesics (Systemic)**, 1180
  Tablets, Effervescent, 1181
Phenylpropanolamine-containing Combinations, 3078
Phenylpropanolamine Hydrochloride [*Acutrim 16 Hour; Acutrim Late Day; Acutrim II Maximum Strength; Control; Dexatrim Maximum Strength Caplets; Dexatrim Maximum Strength Capsules; Dexatrim Maximum Strength Tablets; Diet-Aid Maximum Strength; Efed II Yellow; Phenyldrine; PPA; Prolamine; Propagest*]
  **(Systemic)**, 2314
  Capsules, 2316
  Capsules, Extended-release, USP, 2316
  Tablets, 2316
  Tablets, Extended-release, 2316
Phenylpropanolamine Hydrochloride and Acetaminophen [*Dilotab*]
  **See Decongestants and Analgesics (Systemic)**, 1180
  Tablets, 1182
Phenylpropanolamine Hydrochloride, Acetaminophen, and Aspirin [*Rhinocaps*]
  **See Decongestants and Analgesics (Systemic)**, 1180
  Capsules, 1182
Phenylpropanolamine Hydrochloride, Acetaminophen, and Caffeine [*Emertabs*]
  **See Decongestants and Analgesics (Systemic)**, 1180
  Tablets, 1182
Phenylpropanolamine Hydrochloride, Acetaminophen, Salicylamide, and Caffeine [*Saleto D Caplets*]
  **See Decongestants and Analgesics (Systemic)**, 1180
  Tablets, 1183
Phenylpropanolamine Hydrochloride and Caramiphen Edisylate [*Ordrine AT; Rescaps-D S.R.; Tuss-Ade; Tuss-Allergine Modified T.D.; Tussogest*]
  **See Cough/Cold Combinations (Systemic)**, 1024
  Capsules, Extended-release, 1076, 1086, 1104, 1108
Phenylpropanolamine Hydrochloride, Codeine Phosphate, and Guaifenesin [*Codegest Expectorant; Conex with Codeine Liquid; C-Tussin Expectorant; Endal Expectorant; Naldecon-CX Adult Liquid; Statuss Expectorant; Triaminic Expectorant with Codeine*]
  **See Cough/Cold Combinations (Systemic)**, 1024
  Solution, Oral, 1044, 1071, 1095, 1101
  Syrup, 1047, 1050, 1056
Phenylpropanolamine Hydrochloride and Dextromethorphan Hydrobromide [*Snaplets-DM; Triaminic-DM Cough Relief; Tricodene Pediatric*]
  **See Cough/Cold Combinations (Systemic)**, 1024
  Granules, 1094
  Solution, Oral, 1103
  Syrup, 1100
Phenylpropanolamine Hydrochloride, Dextromethorphan Hydrobromide, and Acetaminophen [*Saleto-CF*]
  **See Cough/Cold Combinations (Systemic)**, 1024
  Tablets, 1092
Phenylpropanolamine Hydrochloride, Dextromethorphan Hydrobromide, and Guaifenesin [*Guai-Cough CF; Guiatuss CF; Ipsatol Cough Formula for Children; Kiddy Koff; Naldecon-DX Adult Liquid; Naldecon-DX Children's Syrup; Naldecon-DX Pediatric Drops; Robafen CF; Robitussin-CF; Siltussin-CF; Triaminic DM DayTime for Children*]
  **See Cough/Cold Combinations (Systemic)**, 1024
  Solution, Oral, 1061, 1062, 1071, 1087, 1093
  Syrup, 1068, 1071, 1088, 1100
Phenylpropanolamine Hydrochloride, Dextromethorphan Hydrobromide, Guaifenesin, and Acetaminophen [*Anatuss*]
  **See Cough/Cold Combinations (Systemic)**, 1024
  Syrup, 1034
  Tablets, 1034

Phenylpropanolamine Hydrochloride and Guaifenesin [*Ami-Tex LA; Banex-LA; Conex; Despec-SR Caplets; Dura-Vent; Entex LA; Exgest LA; Guaifenex PPA 75; Guaipax; Myminic Expectorant; Naldecon-EX Children's Syrup; Naldecon-EX Pediatric Drops; Partuss LA; Phenylfenesin L.A.; Profen II; Profen-LA; Prominic Expectorant; Rymed-TR Caplets; Silaminic Expectorant; Sildicon-E Pediatric Drops; SINUvent; Snaplets-EX; Stamoist LA; Triaminic Expectorant; Triphenyl Expectorant; ULR-LA; Vicks DayQuil Sinus Pressure and Congestion Relief Caplets*]
  **See Cough/Cold Combinations (Systemic)**, 1024
  Granules, 1094
  Solution, Oral, 1070, 1072, 1084, 1092, 1093, 1101, 1104
  Syrup, 1047, 1072
  Tablets, 1113
  Tablets, Extended-release, 1034, 1035, 1051, 1055, 1056, 1057, 1058, 1060, 1061, 1077, 1082, 1083, 1083, 1091, 1094, 1095, 1111, MC-25
Phenylpropanolamine Hydrochloride and Hydrocodone Bitartrate [*Codamine; Codamine Pediatric; Hycomine; Hycomine Pediatric; Hydromine; Hydromine Pediatric; Hydrophen*]
  **See Cough/Cold Combinations (Systemic)**, 1024
  Solution, Oral, 1066
  Syrup, 1044, 1064, 1065, 1066, 1082
Phenyl Salicylate–containing Combinations, 3080
Phenyltoloxamine Citrate, Phenylpropanolamine Hydrochloride, and Acetaminophen [*Sinutab SA*]
  **See Antihistamines, Decongestants, and Analgesics (Systemic)**, 366
  Tablets, Extended-release, 372
Phenyltoloxamine-containing Combinations, 3080
Phenyltoloxamine Resin Complex and Hydrocodone Resin Complex [*Tussionex*]
  **See Cough/Cold Combinations (Systemic)**, 1024
  Suspension, Oral, 1106
  Tablets, 1106
*Phenytex*—Bolar (U.S.) brand of Phenytoin—**See Anticonvulsants, Hydantoin (Systemic)**, 253
Phenytoin [*Dilantin-30; Dilantin-125; Dilantin Infatabs*; diphenylhydantoin]
  **See Anticonvulsants, Hydantoin (Systemic)**, 253
  Suspension, Oral, USP, 264
  Tablets USP (Chewable), 264, MC-25
Phenytoin Sodium [*Dilantin; Dilantin Kapseals; Diphenylan*; diphenylhydantoin; *Phenytex*]
  **See Anticonvulsants, Hydantoin (Systemic)**, 253
  Capsules, Extended, USP, 264, MC-25
  Capsules, Prompt, USP, 265
  Injection USP, 265
*Pherazine with Codeine*—Halsey (U.S.) brand of Promethazine and Codeine—**See Cough/Cold Combinations (Systemic)**, 1024
*Pherazine DM*—Halsey (U.S.) brand of Promethazine and Dextromethorphan—**See Cough/Cold Combinations (Systemic)**, 1024
*Pherazine VC*—Halsey (U.S.) brand of Promethazine and Phenylephrine—**See Antihistamines and Decongestants (Systemic)**, 343
*Pherazine VC with Codeine*—Halsey (U.S.) brand of Promethazine, Phenylephrine, and Codeine—**See Cough/Cold Combinations (Systemic)**, 1024
*Pheryl-E*—Miller (U.S.) brand of Vitamin E (Systemic), 2972
*Phillips'*—Bayer (U.S. and Canada) brand of Magnesium Hydroxide—**See Antacids (Oral-Local)**, 188
*Phillips' Chewable*—Bayer Consumer (U.S.) brand of Magnesium Hydroxide—**See Laxatives (Local)**, #; Bayer (U.S.) brand of Magnesium Hydroxide—**See Antacids (Oral-Local)**, 188
*Phillips' Chewable Tablets*—Glenbrook (U.S.) brand of Magnesium Hydroxide—**See Magnesium Supplements (Systemic)**, 1897
*Phillips' Concentrated*—Bayer Consumer (U.S.) brand of Magnesium Hydroxide—**See Laxatives (Local)**, #
*Phillips' Concentrated Double-strength*—Bayer (U.S.) brand of Magnesium Hydroxide—**See Antacids (Oral-Local)**, 188
*Phillips' Gelcaps*—Bayer Consumer (U.S.) brand of Phenolphthalein and Docusate—**See Laxatives (Local)**, #

*Phillips' LaxCaps*—Bayer Consumer (U.S.) brand of Phenolphthalein and Docusate—**See Laxatives (Local)**, #
*Phillips' Magnesia Tablets*—Bayer (Canada) brand of Magnesium Hydroxide—**See Laxatives (Local)**, #; Sterling Winthrop (Canada) brand of Magnesium Hydroxide—**See Magnesium Supplements (Systemic)**, 1897
*Phillips' Milk of Magnesia*—Bayer Consumer (U.S.) and Bayer (Canada) brand of Magnesium Hydroxide—**See Laxatives (Local)**, #; Glenbrook (U.S.) and Sterling Winthrop (Canada) brand of Magnesium Hydroxide—**See Magnesium Supplements (Systemic)**, 1897
*Phos-Flur*—Colgate-Hoyt (U.S.) brand of Sodium Fluoride (Systemic), 2592
*Phos-Lo*—Braintree (U.S.) brand of Calcium Acetate (Systemic), 719, MC-5, 3135
Phosphates
  **(Systemic)**, 2317
*Phosphocol P 32*—Mallinckrodt (U.S.) brand of Chromic Phosphate P 32 (Parenteral-Local), #
Phosphocysteamine
  **(Systemic)**, 3158
*Phospholine Iodide*—Wyeth-Ayerst (U.S.) and Ayerst (Canada) brand of Echothiophate—**See Antiglaucoma Agents, Cholinergic, Long-acting (Ophthalmic)**, 315
Phosphonoformic acid—*See* Foscarnet (Systemic), 1528
*Phosphotec*—Squibb (U.S.) brand of Technetium Tc 99m Pyrophosphate (Systemic), 2729
*Photofrin*—QLT (U.S.) brand of Porfimer Sodium (Systemic), 3159; Sanofi Winthrop (U.S.) brand of Porfimer (Systemic), 2351
*Photoplex Plus Sunscreen*—Allergan Herbert (Canada) brand of Avobenzone, Octocrylene, Octyl Salicylate, and Oxybenzone—**See Sunscreen Agents (Topical)**, #
*Phrenilin*—Carnrick (U.S.) brand of Butalbital and Acetaminophen—**See Barbiturates and Analgesics (Systemic)**, 532
*Phrenilin Forte*—Carnrick (U.S.) brand of Butalbital and Acetaminophen—**See Barbiturates and Analgesics (Systemic)**, 532
*Phyllocontin*—Purdue Frederick (U.S. and Canada) brand of Aminophylline—**See Bronchodilators, Theophylline (Systemic)**, 668
*Phyllocontin-350*—Purdue Frederick (Canada) brand of Aminophylline—**See Bronchodilators, Theophylline (Systemic)**, 668
Physostigmine Salicylate [*Eserine Salicylate; Isopto Eserine*]
  **(Ophthalmic)**, #
  Solution, Ophthalmic, USP, #
Physostigmine Salicylate [*Antilirium*; eserine]
  **(Systemic)**, 2322, 3158
  Injection USP, 2323
Physostigmine Sulfate [*Eserine Sulfate*]
  **(Ophthalmic)**, #
  Ointment, Ophthalmic, USP, #
Phytomenadione—Phytonadione—**See Vitamin K (Systemic)**, 2975
Phytonadione [*AquaMEPHYTON; Konakion; Mephyton*; phytomenadione; vitamin K$_1$]
  **See Vitamin K (Systemic)**, 2975
  Injection USP, 2977
  Tablets USP, 2977
*Pilagan*—Allergan (U.S.) brand of Pilocarpine (Ophthalmic), #
*Pilocar*—Iolab (U.S.) brand of Pilocarpine (Ophthalmic), #
Pilocarpine [*Ocusert Pilo-20; Ocusert Pilo-40*]
  **(Ophthalmic)**, #
  System, Ocular, USP, #
Pilocarpine [*Salagen*]
  **(Systemic)**, 2323, 3158
Pilocarpine Hydrochloride [*Adsorbocarpine; Akarpine; Isopto Carpine; Miocarpine; Ocu-Carpine; Pilocar; Pilopine HS; Piloptic¹/₂; Piloptic-1; Piloptic-2; Piloptic-3; Piloptic-4; Piloptic-6; Pilostat; Spersacarpine*]
  **(Ophthalmic)**, #
  Gel, Ophthalmic
  Solution, Ophthalmic, USP
Pilocarpine Hydrochloride [*Salagen*]
  **(Systemic)**, 2323, 3032, 3158
  Tablets, 2325, 3032
Pilocarpine Nitrate [*Minims Pilocarpine; Pilagan; P.V. Carpine Liquifilm*]
  **(Ophthalmic)**, #
  Solution, Ophthalmic, USP

*Pilopine HS*—Alcon (U.S. and Canada) brand of Pilocarpine (Ophthalmic), #
*Piloptic½*—Optopics (U.S.) brand of Pilocarpine (Ophthalmic), #
*Piloptic-1*—Optopics (U.S.) brand of Pilocarpine (Ophthalmic), #
*Piloptic-2*—Optopics (U.S.) brand of Pilocarpine (Ophthalmic), #
*Piloptic-3*—Optopics (U.S.) brand of Pilocarpine (Ophthalmic), #
*Piloptic-4*—Optopics (U.S.) brand of Pilocarpine (Ophthalmic), #
*Piloptic-6*—Optopics (U.S.) brand of Pilocarpine (Ophthalmic), #
*Pilostat*—Bausch & Lomb (U.S. and Canada) brand of Pilocarpine (Ophthalmic), #
*Pima*—Fleming (U.S.) brand of Potassium Iodide (Systemic), 2354
*Pimaricin*—*See* Natamycin (Ophthalmic), #
Pimozide [*Orap*]
   **(Systemic)**, 2326
   Tablets USP, 2329
Pindolol [*Novo-Pindol; Syn-Pindolol; Visken*]
   **See Beta-adrenergic Blocking Agents (Systemic)**, 593
   Tablets USP, 605, MC-25
Pindolol-containing Combinations, 3080
Pindolol and Hydrochlorothiazide [*Viskazide*]
   **See Beta-adrenergic Blocking Agents and Thiazide Diuretics (Systemic)**, 609
   Tablets, 611
Pipecuronium Bromide [*Arduan*]
   **(Systemic)**, 2330
   for Injection, 2333
Piperacillin-containing Combinations, 3080
Piperacillin Sodium [*Pipracil*]
   **See Penicillins (Systemic)**, 2240
   Sterile USP, 2259
Piperacillin Sodium and Tazobactam Sodium [*Tazocin; Zosyn*]
   **See Penicillins and Beta-lactamase Inhibitors (Systemic)**, 2263
   Sterile, 2270
Piperacillin and Tazobactam [*Zosyn*]
   **(Systemic)**, 3032
   for Injection, 3032
Piperazine Adipate [*Entacyl*]
   **(Systemic)**, #
   Granules for Solution, Oral, #
   Suspension, Oral, #
Piperazine Citrate
   **(Systemic)**, #
   Tablets USP, #
Piperazine estrone sulfate—Estropipate—**See Estrogens (Systemic)**, 1383; **Estrogens (Vaginal)**, 1391
*Piportil L₄*—Rhône-Poulenc (Canada) brand of Pipotiazine—**See Phenothiazines (Systemic)**, 2289
Pipotiazine Palmitate [*Piportil L₄*]
   **See Phenothiazines (Systemic)**, 2289
   Injection, 2305
*Pipracil*—Lederle (U.S. and Canada) brand of Piperacillin—**See Penicillins (Systemic)**, 2240
Piracetam [*Nootropil*]
   **(Systemic)**, 3158
Pirbuterol Acetate [*Maxair; Maxair Autohaler*]
   **See Bronchodilators, Adrenergic (Inhalation-Local)**, 640
   Aerosol, Inhalation, 649
Pirenzepine Hydrochloride [*Gastrozepin*]
   **See Anticholinergics/Antispasmodics (Systemic)**, 226
   Tablets, 238
Piroxicam [*Apo-Piroxicam; Feldene; Novo-Pirocam; Nu-Pirox; PMS-Piroxicam*]
   **See Anti-inflammatory Drugs, Nonsteroidal (Systemic)**, 388
   Capsules USP, 417 MC-25
   Suppositories, 417
*Pitocin*—PD (U.S.) brand of Oxytocin (Systemic), 2211
*Pitressin*—PD (U.S. and Canada) brand of Vasopressin (Systemic), 2938
*Pitrex Cream*—Taro (Canada) brand of Tolnaftate (Topical), #
Pit viper antivenin—*See* Antivenin (Crotalidae) Polyvalent (Systemic), #
Pivampicillin [*Pondocillin*]
   **See Penicillins (Systemic)**, 2240
   for Suspension, Oral, USP, 2260
   Tablets, 2260

Pivmecillinam Hydrochloride [*Selexid*]
   **See Penicillins (Systemic)**, 2240
   Tablets, 2260
Pizotyline Malate [*Sandomigran; Sandomigran DS*]
   **(Systemic)**, 3032
   Tablets, 3032
*Placidyl*—Abbott (U.S. and Canada) brand of Ethchlorvynol (Systemic), #
Plague Vaccine
   **(Systemic)**, #
   Plague Vaccine USP, #
*Plaquasc*—Advance Biofactures (U.S.) brand of Collagenase (lyophilized) (Systemic), 3138
*Plaquenil*—Sanofi Winthrop (U.S. and Canada) brand of Hydroxychloroquine (Systemic), 1663, MC-15
*Plasbumin-5*—Miles (U.S.) and Cutter (Canada) brand of Albumin Human (Systemic), 34
*Plasbumin-25*—Miles (U.S.) and Cutter (Canada) brand of Albumin Human (Systemic), 34
Plasma thromboplastin component (PTC)—*See* Factor IX (Systemic), 1430
*Platinol*—Bristol (Canada) brand of Cisplatin (Systemic), 876
*Platinol-AQ*—Bristol-Myers Squibb (U.S. and Canada) brand of Cisplatin (Systemic), 876
*Plavix*—Bristol-Myers Squibb/Sanofi (U.S.) brand of Clopidogrel (Systemic), 913
*Plegine*—Wyeth-Ayerst (U.S.) brand of Phendimetrazine—**See Appetite Suppressants (Systemic)**, 452
*Plendil*—Astra Merck (U.S.) and Astra (Canada) brand of Felodipine—**See Calcium Channel Blocking Agents (Systemic)**, 720, MC-12
Plicamycin [*Mithracin; mithramycin*]
   **(Systemic)**, 2334
   for Injection USP, 2336
*PMS-Acetaminophen with Codeine*—Pharmascience (Canada) brand of Acetaminophen and Codeine—**See Opioid (Narcotic) Analgesics and Acetaminophen (Systemic)**, 2198
*PMS Alumina, Magnesia, and Simethicone*—Pharmascience (Canada) brand of Alumina, Magnesia, and Simethicone—**See Antacids (Oral-Local)**, 188
*PMS-ASA*—Pharmascience (Canada) brand of Aspirin—**See Salicylates (Systemic)**, 2538
*PMS-Baclofen*—Pharmascience (Canada) brand of Baclofen (Systemic), 515
*PMS Benztropine*—Pharmascience (Canada) brand of Benztropine—**See Antidyskinetics (Systemic)**, 297
*PMS-Bisacodyl*—Pharmascience (Canada) brand of Bisacodyl—**See Laxatives (Local)**, #
*PMS-Bismuth Subsalicylate*—Pharmascience (U.S.) brand of Bismuth Subsalicylate (Oral-Local), 616
*PMS-Cephalexin*—Pharmascience (Canada) brand of Cephalexin—**See Cephalosporins (Systemic)**, 794
*PMS-Chloral Hydrate*—Pharmascience (Canada) brand of Chloral Hydrate (Systemic), 834
*PMS-Cimetidine*—Pharmascience (Canada) brand of Cimetidine—**See Histamine H₂-receptor Antagonists (Systemic)**, 1633
*PMS-Clonazepam*—Pharmascience (Canada) brand of Clonazepam—**See Benzodiazepines (Systemic)**, 556
*PMS-Cyproheptadine*—Pharmascience (Canada) brand of Cyproheptadine—**See Antihistamines (Systemic)**, 325
*PMS-Dexamethasone Sodium Phosphate*—Pharmascience (Canada) brand of Dexamethasone—**See Corticosteroids (Ophthalmic)**, 966
*PMS-Diazepam*—Pharmascience (Canada) brand of Diazepam—**See Benzodiazepines (Systemic)**, 556
*PMS-Dimenhydrinate*—Pharmascience (Canada) brand of Dimenhydrinate—**See Antihistamines (Systemic)**, 325
*PMS-Docusate Calcium*—Pharmascience (Canada) brand of Docusate—**See Laxatives (Local)**, #
*PMS-Docusate Sodium*—Pharmascience (Canada) brand of Docusate—**See Laxatives (Local)**, #
*PMS Dopazide*—Pharmascience (Canada) brand of Methyldopa and Hydrochlorothiazide—**See Methyldopa and Thiazide Diuretics (Systemic)**, 1983
*PMS Egozinc*—Pharmascience (Canada) brand of Zinc Sulfate—**See Zinc Supplements (Systemic)**, 2999
*PMS-Ferrous Sulfate*—Pharmascience (Canada) brand of Ferrous Sulfate—**See Iron Supplements (Systemic)**, 1774

*PMS Haloperidol*—Pharmascience (Canada) brand of Haloperidol (Systemic), 1611
*PMS-Hydromorphone*—Pharmascience (Canada) brand of Hydromorphone—**See Opioid (Narcotic) Analgesics (Systemic)**, 2168
*PMS-Hydromorphone Syrup*—Pharmascience (Canada) brand of Hydromorphone—**See Opioid (Narcotic) Analgesics (Systemic)**, 2168
*PMS Isoniazid*—Pharmascience (Canada) brand of Isoniazid (Systemic), 1789
*PMS-Lactulose*—Pharmascience (Canada) brand of Lactulose—**See Laxatives (Local)**, #
*PMS Levazine*—Pharmascience (Canada) brand of Perphenazine and Amitriptyline (Systemic), 2286
*PMS-Levothyroxine Sodium*—Pharmascience (Canada) brand of Levothyroxine—**See Thyroid Hormones (Systemic)**, 2809
*PMS Lindane*—Pharmascience (Canada) brand of Lindane (Topical), 1866
*PMS-Loperamide*—Pharmascience (Canada) brand of Loperamide (Oral-Local), 1877
*PMS-Methylphenidate*—Pharmascience (Canada) brand of Methylphenidate (Systemic), 1987
*PMS-Metoclopramide*—Pharmascience (Canada) brand of Metoclopramide (Systemic), 1992
*PMS Nylidrin*—Pharmascience (Canada) brand of Nylidrin (Systemic), #
*PMS Nystatin*—Pharmascience (Canada) brand of Nystatin (Oral-Local), 2146
*PMS-Oxtriphylline*—Pharmascience (Canada) brand of Oxtriphylline—**See Bronchodilators, Theophylline (Systemic)**, 668
*PMS Perphenazine*—Pharmascience (Canada) brand of Perphenazine—**See Phenothiazines (Systemic)**, 2289
*PMS-Phosphates*—Pharmascience (Canada) brand of Sodium Phosphates—**See Laxatives (Local)**, #
*PMS-Piroxicam*—Pharmascience (Canada) brand of Piroxicam—**See Anti-inflammatory Drugs, Nonsteroidal (Systemic)**, 388
*PMS Primidone*—Pharmascience (Canada) brand of Primidone (Systemic), 2376
*PMS Prochlorperazine*—Pharmascience (Canada) brand of Prochlorperazine—**See Phenothiazines (Systemic)**, 2289
*PMS Procyclidine*—Pharmascience (Canada) brand of Procyclidine—**See Antidyskinetics (Systemic)**, 297
*PMS-Progesterone*—Pharmascience (Canada) brand of Progesterone—**See Progestins (Systemic)**, 2400
*pms Propranolol*—Pharmascience (Canada) brand of Propranolol—**See Beta-adrenergic Blocking Agents (Systemic)**, 593
*pms-Pyrazinamide*—Pharmascience (Canada) brand of Pyrazinamide (Systemic), 2425
*PMS-Sennosides*—Pharmascience (Canada) brand of Sennosides—**See Laxatives (Local)**, #
*PMS-Sodium Cromoglycate*—Pharmascience (Canada) brand of Cromolyn (Inhalation-Local), 1116
*PMS-Sodium Polystyrene Sulfonate*—Pharmascience (Canada) brand of Sodium Polystyrene Sulfonate (Local), 2618
*PMS-Sulfasalazine*—Pharmascience (Canada) brand of Sulfasalazine (Systemic), 2643
*PMS-Sulfasalazine E.C.*—Pharmascience (Canada) brand of Sulfasalazine (Systemic), 2643
*PMS-Theophylline*—Pharmascience (Canada) brand of Theophylline—**See Bronchodilators, Theophylline (Systemic)**, 668
*PMS Thioridazine*—Pharmascience (Canada) brand of Thioridazine—**See Phenothiazines (Systemic)**, 2289
*PMS Trifluoperazine*—Pharmascience (Canada) brand of Trifluoperazine—**See Phenothiazines (Systemic)**, 2289
*PMS Trihexyphenidyl*—Pharmascience (Canada) brand of Trihexyphenidyl—**See Antidyskinetics (Systemic)**, 297
*pms-Valproic Acid*—Pharmascience (Canada) brand of Valproic Acid—**See Valproic Acid (Systemic)**, 2908
*pms-Valproic Acid E.C.*—Pharmascience (Canada) brand of Valproic Acid—**See Valproic Acid (Systemic)**, 2908
*PMS-Yohimbine*—Pharmascience (Canada) brand of Yohimbine (Systemic), #
Pneumococcal Vaccine Polyvalent [*Pneumovax 23; Pnu-Imune 23*]
   **(Systemic)**, 2337
   Injection, 2339

*Pneumomist*—ECR Pharm (U.S.) brand of Guaifenesin (Systemic), 1588
*Pneumopent*—Fisons (Canada) brand of Pentamidine (Inhalation), 2272; Fisons (U.S.) brand of Pentamidine (Inhalation), 3157
*Pneumotussin HC*—ECR Pharm (U.S.) brand of Hydrocodone and Guaifenesin—**See Cough/Cold Combinations (Systemic)**, 1024
*Pneumovax 23*—Merck (U.S. and Canada) brand of Pneumococcal Vaccine Polyvalent (Systemic), 2337
*P.N. Ophthalmic*—Geneva (U.S.) brand of Neomycin, Polymyxin B, and Gramicidin (Ophthalmic), #
*Pnu-Imune 23*—Lederle (U.S.) brand of Pneumococcal Vaccine Polyvalent (Systemic), 2337
*Podocon-25*—Paddock (U.S.) brand of Podophyllum (Topical), 2341
Podofilox [*Condylox; podophyllotoxin*]
 **(Topical)**, 2339
 Gel, 2341
 Solution, Topical, 2341
*Podofin*—Syosset (U.S.) brand of Podophyllum (Topical), 2341
Podophyllotoxin—Podofilox (Topical), 2339
Podophyllum Resin [*Podocon-25; Podofin*]
 **(Topical)**, 2341
 Solution, Topical, USP, 2343
*Polaramine*—Schering (U.S. and Canada) brand of Dexchlorpheniramine—**See Antihistamines (Systemic)**, 325
*Polaramine Expectorant*—Schering (U.S.) brand of Dexchlorpheniramine, Pseudoephedrine, and Guaifenesin—**See Cough/Cold Combinations (Systemic)**, 1024
*Polaramine Repetabs*—Schering (U.S. and Canada) brand of Dexchlorpheniramine—**See Antihistamines (Systemic)**, 325
*Polibar*—E-Z-EM (U.S. and Canada) brand of Barium Sulfate (Local), #
*Polibar Flavored*—E-Z-EM (U.S.) brand of Barium Sulfate (Local), #
*Polibar Liquid*—E-Z-EM (U.S. and Canada) brand of Barium Sulfate (Local), #
*Polibar Plus*—E-Z-EM (U.S. and Canada) brand of Barium Sulfate (Local), #
*Polibar Rapide*—E-Z-EM (Canada) brand of Barium Sulfate (Local), #
Poliovirus Vaccine
 **(Systemic)**, 2343
Poliovirus Vaccine Inactivated [*IPV; Salk vaccine*]
 **See Poliovirus Vaccine (Systemic)**, 2343
 Poliovirus Vaccine Inactivated USP (Injection), 2347
Poliovirus Vaccine Inactivated Enhanced Potency [*enhanced-potency IPV; Ipol; N-IPV*]
 **See Poliovirus Vaccine (Systemic)**, 2343
 Poliovirus Vaccine Inactivated Enhanced Potency (Injection), 2348
Poliovirus Vaccine Live Oral [*OPV; Orimune;* Sabin vaccine; *TOPV*]
 **See Poliovirus Vaccine (Systemic)**, 2343
 Poliovirus Vaccine Live Oral USP (Oral Solution), 2348
*Polocaine*—Astra (U.S. and Canada) brand of Mepivacaine—**See Anesthetics (Parenteral-Local)**, 139
*Polocaine-MPF*—Astra (U.S.) brand of Mepivacaine—**See Anesthetics (Parenteral-Local)**, 139
Poloxamer 188 [*RheothRx Copolymer*]
 **(Systemic)**, 3158
Poloxamer 188 [*Alaxin*]
 **See Laxatives (Local)**, #
 Capsules, #
Poloxamer 331 [*Protox*]
 **(Systemic)**, 3158
Polyacrylamide [*Orcolon*]
 **(Ophthalmic)**, 3032
 Injection, 3032
*Polycillin*—Bristol (U.S.) brand of Ampicillin—**See Penicillins (Systemic)**, 2240
*Polycillin-N*—Bristol (U.S.) brand of Ampicillin—**See Penicillins (Systemic)**, 2240
*Polycitra-K*—Willen (U.S.) brand of Potassium Citrate and Citric Acid—**See Citrates (Systemic)**, 881
*Polycitra-K Crystals*—Willen (U.S.) brand of Potassium Citrate and Citric Acid—**See Citrates (Systemic)**, 881
*Polycitra-LC*—Willen (U.S.) brand of Tricitrates—**See Citrates (Systemic)**, 881
*Polycitra Syrup*—Willen (U.S.) brand of Tricitrates—**See Citrates (Systemic)**, 881

*Polycose*—Ross (U.S.) brand of Enteral Nutrition Formula, Modular—**See Enteral Nutrition Formulas (Systemic)**, #
*Poly D*—Qualitest (U.S.) brand of Pheniramine, Phenyltoloxamine, Pyrilamine, and Phenylpropanolamine—**See Antihistamines and Decongestants (Systemic)**, 343
*Poly-D*—Alphagen (U.S.) brand of Pheniramine, Phenyltoloxamine, Pyrilamine, and Phenylpropanolamine—**See Antihistamines and Decongestants (Systemic)**, 343
Polydimethylsiloxane—*See* Silicone Oil 5000 Centistokes (Systemic), #
Polyethylene Glycol 3350 and Electrolytes [*Co-Lav; Colovage; Colyte; Colyte-flavored; Go-Evac; GoLYTELY; Klean-Prep; NuLYTELY; NuLYTELY, Cherry Flavor; OCL; Peglyte*]
 **(Local)**, 2349
 Solution, Oral, 2350
 for Solution, Oral, USP, 2350
*Polygam*—Baxter (U.S.) brand of Immune Globulin Intravenous (Human) (Systemic), 1686
*Polygesic*—Poly (U.S.) brand of Hydrocodone and Acetaminophen—**See Opioid (Narcotic) Analgesics and Acetaminophen (Systemic)**, 2198
*Poly Hist Forte*—Poly (U.S.) brand of Chlorpheniramine, Pyrilamine, Phenylephrine, and Phenylpropanolamine—**See Antihistamines and Decongestants (Systemic)**, 343
*Poly-Histine-CS*—Bock (U.S.) brand of Brompheniramine, Phenylpropanolamine, and Codeine—**See Cough/Cold Combinations (Systemic)**, 1024
*Poly-Histine-D*—Bock (U.S.) brand of Pheniramine, Phenyltoloxamine, Pyrilamine, and Phenylpropanolamine—**See Antihistamines and Decongestants (Systemic)**, 343
*Poly-Histine-DM*—Bock (U.S.) brand of Brompheniramine, Phenylpropanolamine, and Dextromethorphan—**See Cough/Cold Combinations (Systemic)**, 1024
*Poly-Histine-D Ped*—Bock (U.S.) brand of Pheniramine, Phenyltoloxamine, Pyrilamine, and Phenylpropanolamine—**See Antihistamines and Decongestants (Systemic)**, 343
Poly I: Poly C12U [*Ampligen*]
 **(Systemic)**, 3158
Poly-ICLC
 **(Systemic)**, 3158
Polymeric Oxygen
 **(Systemic)**, 3159
*Polymox*—Bristol (U.S.) brand of Amoxicillin—**See Penicillins (Systemic)**, 2240; Bristol (U.S.) brand of Amoxicillin (Systemic), 3010
Polymyxin B-containing Combinations, 3080
Polymyxin B Sulfate [*Aerosporin*]
 **(Ophthalmic)**, 3032
 for Solution, Ophthalmic, 3032
Polythiazide [*Renese*]
 **See Diuretics, Thiazide (Systemic)**, 1273
 Tablets USP, 1281
Polythiazide-containing Combinations, 3080
*Poly-Vi-Flor*—Mead Johnson (U.S. and Canada) brand of Multiple Vitamins and Fluoride—**See Vitamins, Multiple, and Fluoride (Systemic)**, 2978
*Pondocillin*—Leo (Canada) brand of Pivampicillin—**See Penicillins (Systemic)**, 2240
*Pond's Daily Replenishing Moisturizer*—Cheesebough-Ponds (Canada) brand of Phenylbenzimidazole—**See Sunscreen Agents (Topical)**, #; Octyl Methoxycinnamate and Phenylbenzimidazole—**See Sunscreen Agents (Topical)**, #
*Ponstan*—PD (Canada) brand of Mefenamic Acid—**See Anti-inflammatory Drugs, Nonsteroidal (Systemic)**, 388
*Ponstel*—PD (U.S.) brand of Mefenamic Acid—**See Anti-inflammatory Drugs, Nonsteroidal (Systemic)**, 388
*Pontocaine*—Sanofi Winthrop (U.S. and Canada) brand of Tetracaine—**See Anesthetics (Ophthalmic)**, #; **Anesthetics (Parenteral-Local)**, 139; Sanofi Winthrop (U.S.) brand of Tetracaine—**See Anesthetics (Mucosal-Local)**, 128
*Pontocaine Cream*—Sanofi Winthrop (U.S.) brand of Tetracaine—**See Anesthetics (Mucosal-Local)**, 128; **Anesthetics (Topical)**, 155
*Pontocaine Ointment*—Sanofi Winthrop (U.S.) brand of Tetracaine and Menthol—**See Anesthetics (Mucosal-Local)**, 128; **Anesthetics (Topical)**, 155

Porcine Fetal Neural Dopaminergic Cells and/or Precursors Aseptically Prepared for Intracerebral Implantation [*NeuroCell-PD*]
 **(Systemic)**, 3159
Porcine Fetal Neural Dopaminergic Cells and/or Precursors Aseptically Prepared and Coated with Anti-MHC-1 Ab for Intracerebral Implantation [*NeuroCell-PD*]
 **(Systemic)**, 3159
Porcine Fetal Neural GABA-ergic Cells and/or Precursors Aseptically Prepared for Intracerebral Implantation for Huntington's Disease [*NeuroCell-HD*]
 **(Systemic)**, 3159
Porcine Fetal Neural GABA-ergic Cells and/or Precursors Aseptically Prepared and Coated with Anti-MHC-1 Ab for Intracerebral Implantation [*NeuroCell-HD*]
 **(Systemic)**, 3159
Porcine Sertoli Cells [*N-Graft*]
 **(Systemic)**, 3159
Porfimer Sodium [*Photofrin*]
 **(Systemic)**, 2351, 3159
 for Injection, 2353
Porfiromycin [*Promycin*]
 **(Systemic)**, 3159
*Portalac*—Solvay (U.S.) brand of Lactulose—**See Laxatives (Local)**, #
*Posicor*—Roche (U.S.) brand of Mibefradil (Systemic), #
*Postacne*—Rorer (Canada) brand of Alcohol and Sulfur (Topical), #
*Posture*—Whitehall (U.S.) brand of Tribasic Calcium Phosphate—**See Calcium Supplements (Systemic)**, 736
*Potaba*—Glenwood (U.S. and Canada) brand of Aminobenzoate Potassium (Systemic), #
*Potaba Envules*—Glenwood (U.S. and Canada) brand of Aminobenzoate Potassium (Systemic), #
*Potaba Powder*—Glenwood (U.S. and Canada) brand of Aminobenzoate Potassium (Systemic), #
*Potasalan*—Lannett (U.S.) brand of Potassium Chloride—**See Potassium Supplements (Systemic)**, 2357
Potassium Acetate
 **See Potassium Supplements (Systemic)**, 2357
 Injection USP, 2361
Potassium aminobenzoate—*See* Aminobenzoate Potassium (Systemic), #
Potassium Bicarbonate [*K+ Care ET; K-Electrolyte; Klor-Con/EF; K-Ide; K-Lyte; K-Vescent*]
 **See Potassium Supplements (Systemic)**, 2357
 Tablets for Solution, Oral, Effervescent, USP, 2361
Potassium Bicarbonate and Potassium Chloride [*Klorvess; Klorvess Effervescent Granules; K-Lyte/Cl; K-Lyte/Cl 50; Neo-K; Potassium-Sandoz*]
 **See Potassium Supplements (Systemic)**, 2357
 for Solution, Oral, Effervescent, USP, 2361
 Tablets for Solution, Oral, Effervescent, USP, 2361
Potassium Bicarbonate and Potassium Citrate [*Effer-K; K-Lyte DS*]
 **See Potassium Supplements (Systemic)**, 2357
 Tablets for Solution, Oral, Effervescent, 2362
Potassium Bitartrate and Sodium Bicarbonate [*Ceo-Two*]
 **See Laxatives (Local)**, #
 Suppositories, #
Potassium Chloride [*Apo-K; Cena-K; Gen-K; K-8; K-10; K+ 10; Kalium Durules; Kaochlor-10; Kaochlor 10%; Kaochlor-20; Kaochlor S-F 10%; Kaon-Cl; Kaon-Cl-10; Kaon-Cl 20% Liquid; Kato; Kay Ciel; K+ Care; KCL 5%; K-Dur; K-Ide; K-Lease; K-Long; K-Lor; Klor-Con 8; Klor-Con 10; Klor-Con Powder; Klor-Con/25 Powder; Klorvess 10% Liquid; Klotrix; K-Lyte/Cl; K-Lyte/Cl Powder; K-Med 900; K-Norm; K-S; K -Tab; Micro-K; Micro-K 10; Micro-K LS; Potasalan; Roychlor-10%; Rum-K; Slow-K; Ten-K*]
 **See Potassium Supplements (Systemic)**, 2357
 Capsules, Extended-release, USP, 2362, MC-25
 Concentrate for Injection USP, 2363
 Solution, Oral, USP, 2362
 for Solution, Oral, USP, 2362
 for Suspension, Oral, 2363
 Tablets, Extended-release, USP, 2363, MC-25
Potassium Citrate [*Urocit-K*]
 **See Citrates (Systemic)**, 881, 3159
 Tablets, 884

Potassium Citrate and Citric Acid [*Polycitra-K; Polycitra-K Crystals*]
  **See Citrates (Systemic)**, 881
  Solution, Oral, USP, 884
  for Solution, Oral, 884
Potassium Citrate and Sodium Citrate [*Citrolith*]
  **See Citrates (Systemic)**, 881
  Tablets, 885
Potassium citrate, sodium citrate, and citric acid—Tricitrates—**See Citrates (Systemic)**, 881
Potassium Gluconate [*Glu-K; Kaon; Kaylixir; K-G Elixir; Potassium-Rougier*]
  **See Potassium Supplements (Systemic)**, 2357
  Elixir USP, 2363
  Tablets USP, 2364
Potassium Gluconate and Potassium Chloride [*Kolyum*]
  **See Potassium Supplements (Systemic)**, 2357
  Solution, Oral, USP, 2364
  for Solution, Oral, USP, 2364
Potassium Gluconate and Potassium Citrate [*Twin-K*]
  **See Potassium Supplements (Systemic)**, 2357
  Solution, Oral, USP, 2364
Potassium Guaiacolsulfonate-containing Combinations, 3080
Potassium Iodide [*KI; Pima; SSKI; Thyro-Block*]
  **(Systemic)**, 2354
  Solution, Oral, USP, 2356
  Syrup, 2356
  Tablets USP, 2356
  Tablets USP (Enteric-coated), 2357
Potassium para-aminobenzoate—See Aminobenzoate Potassium (Systemic), #
Potassium Phosphate, Monobasic [*K-Phos Original*]
  **See Phosphates (Systemic)**, 2317
  Tablets for Solution, Oral, 2319
Potassium Phosphates [*Neutra-Phos-K*]
  **See Phosphates (Systemic)**, 2317
  Capsules for Solution, Oral, 2319
  Injection USP, 2320
  for Solution, Oral, 2320
Potassium and Sodium Phosphates [*Neutra-Phos; Uro-KP-Neutral*]
  **See Phosphates (Systemic)**, 2317
  Capsules for Solution, Oral, 2320
  for Solution, Oral, 2321
  Tablets for Solution, Oral, 2321
Potassium and Sodium Phosphates, Monobasic [*K-Phos M. F.; K-Phos Neutral; K-Phos No. 2*]
  **See Phosphates (Systemic)**, 2317
  Tablets for Solution, Oral, 2320
*Potassium-Rougier*—Rougier (Canada) brand of Potassium Gluconate—**See Potassium Supplements (Systemic)**, 2357
*Potassium-Sandoz*—Sandoz (Canada) brand of Potassium Bicarbonate and Potassium Chloride—**See Potassium Supplements (Systemic)**, 2357
Potassium Supplements
  **(Systemic)**, 2357
*Potassium triplex*—Trikates—**See Potassium Supplements (Systemic)**, 2357
PPA—*See Phenylpropanolamine (Systemic)*, 2314
*PP-Cap*—Alra (U.S.) brand of Propoxyphene—**See Opioid (Narcotic) Analgesics (Systemic)**, 2168
Pralidoxime Chloride [*Protopam Chloride*; 2-PAM; 2-PAM chloride]
  **(Systemic)**, #
  Pralidoxime Chloride USP, #
  Sterile Pralidoxime Chloride USP, #
*Pramegel*—GenDerm (U.S. and Canada) brand of Pramoxine and Menthol—**See Anesthetics (Topical)**, 155
Pramipexole [*Mirapex*]
  **(Systemic)**, 2365
  Tablets, 2368
Pramipexole Dihydrochloride [*Mirapex*]
  **(Systemic)**, 3033
  Tablets, 3033
Pramocaine—Pramoxine—**See Anesthetics (Mucosal-Local)**, 128; **Anesthetics (Topical)**, 155
Pramoxine Hydrochloride [*Fleet Relief;* pramocaine; *ProctoFoam/non-steroid; Tronolane; Tronothane*]
  **See Anesthetics (Mucosal-Local)**, 128
  Aerosol Foam, 137
  Cream USP, 138
  Ointment, 138

Pramoxine Hydrochloride [pramocaine; *Prax; Tronothane*]
  **See Anesthetics (Topical)**, 155
  Cream USP, 160
  Lotion, 160
Pramoxine Hydrochloride and Menthol [*Almay Anti-itch Lotion; Pramegel*]
  **See Anesthetics (Topical)**, 155
  Gel, 160
  Lotion, 160
*Prandin*—Novo Nordisk (U.S.) brand of Repaglinide (Systemic), 2467
*Pravachol*—Bristol-Myers Squibb (U.S. and Canada) brand of Pravastatin—**See HMG-CoA Reductase Inhibitors (Systemic)**, 1647, MC-25
Pravastatin Sodium [eptastatin; *Pravachol*]
  **See HMG-CoA Reductase Inhibitors (Systemic)**, 1647
  Tablets, 1650, MC-25
*Prax*—Ferndale (U.S.) brand of Pramoxine—**See Anesthetics (Topical)**, 155
Prazepam
  **See Benzodiazepines (Systemic)**, 556
  Capsules USP, 576
Praziquantel [*Biltricide*]
  **(Systemic)**, 2368
  Tablets USP, 2370
Prazosin-containing Combinations, 3080
Prazosin Hydrochloride [*Minipress*]
  **(Systemic)**, 2370
  Capsules USP, 2373, MC-25
  Tablets, 2373
Prazosin Hydrochloride and Polythiazide [*Minizide*]
  **(Systemic)**, 2374
  Capsules, 2374, MC-25
*Pre-Attain*—Sherwood (U.S.) brand of Enteral Nutrition Formula, Polymeric—**See Enteral Nutrition Formulas (Systemic)**, #
*Precose*—Bayer (U.S.) brand of Acarbose (Systemic), 3, MC-1
*Predair*—Pharmafair (U.S.) brand of Prednisolone—**See Corticosteroids (Ophthalmic)**, 966
*Predair A*—Pharmafair (U.S.) brand of Prednisolone—**See Corticosteroids (Ophthalmic)**, 966
*Predair Forte*—Pharmafair (U.S.) brand of Prednisolone—**See Corticosteroids (Ophthalmic)**, 966
*Predaject-50*—Mayrand (U.S.) brand of Prednisolone—**See Corticosteroids—Glucocorticoid Effects (Systemic)**, 998
*Predalone 50*—Forest (U.S.) brand of Prednisolone—**See Corticosteroids—Glucocorticoid Effects (Systemic)**, 998
*Predalone T.B.A.*—Forest (U.S.) brand of Prednisolone—**See Corticosteroids—Glucocorticoid Effects (Systemic)**, 998
*Predate 50*—Legere (U.S.) brand of Prednisolone—**See Corticosteroids—Glucocorticoid Effects (Systemic)**, 998
*Predate S*—Legere (U.S.) brand of Prednisolone—**See Corticosteroids—Glucocorticoid Effects (Systemic)**, 998
*Predate TBA*—Legere (U.S.) brand of Prednisolone—**See Corticosteroids—Glucocorticoid Effects (Systemic)**, 998
*Predcor-25*—Hauck (U.S.) brand of Prednisolone—**See Corticosteroids—Glucocorticoid Effects (Systemic)**, 998
*Predcor-50*—Hauck (U.S.) brand of Prednisolone—**See Corticosteroids—Glucocorticoid Effects (Systemic)**, 998
*Predcor-TBA*—Hauck (U.S.) brand of Prednisolone—**See Corticosteroids—Glucocorticoid Effects (Systemic)**, 998
*Pred Forte*—Allergan (U.S. and Canada) brand of Prednisolone—**See Corticosteroids (Ophthalmic)**, 966
*Predicort-50*—Dunhall (U.S.) brand of Prednisolone—**See Corticosteroids—Glucocorticoid Effects (Systemic)**, 998
*Predicort-RP*—Dunhall (U.S.) brand of Prednisolone—**See Corticosteroids—Glucocorticoid Effects (Systemic)**, 998
*Pred Mild*—Allergan (U.S. and Canada) brand of Prednisolone—**See Corticosteroids (Ophthalmic)**, 966
Prednicarbate [*Dermatop*]
  **(Topical)**, 3033
  Cream, Emollient, 3033
*Prednicen-M*—Central (U.S.) brand of Prednisone—**See Corticosteroids—Glucocorticoid Effects (Systemic)**, 998

Prednimustine [*Sterecyt*]
  **(Systemic)**, 3159
Prednisolone [*Delta-Cortef; Prelone*]
  **See Corticosteroids—Glucocorticoid Effects (Systemic)**, 998
  Syrup USP, 1011
  Tablets USP, 1011
Prednisolone Acetate [*AK-Tate; Econopred; Econopred Plus; Ocu-Pred-A; Ophtho-Tate; Predair A; Pred Forte; Pred Mild; Ultra Pred*]
  **See Corticosteroids (Ophthalmic)**, 966
  Suspension, Ophthalmic, USP, 970
Prednisolone Acetate [*Articulose-50; Key-Pred 25; Key-Pred 50; Predaject-50; Predalone 50; Predate 50; Predcor-25; Predcor-50; Predicort-50*]
  **See Corticosteroids—Glucocorticoid Effects (Systemic)**, 998
  Suspension, Sterile, USP, 1011
Prednisolone Acetate and Prednisolone Sodium Phosphate
  **See Corticosteroids—Glucocorticoid Effects (Systemic)**, 998
  Suspension, Sterile, 1012
Prednisolone Sodium Phosphate [*AK-Pred; Inflamase Forte; Inflamase Mild; I-Pred; Lite Pred; Ocu-Pred; Ocu-Pred Forte; Predair; Predair Forte*]
  **See Corticosteroids (Ophthalmic)**, 966
  Solution, Ophthalmic, USP, 971
Prednisolone Sodium Phosphate [*Hydeltrasol; Key-Pred-SP; Pediapred; Predate S; Predicort-RP*]
  **See Corticosteroids—Glucocorticoid Effects (Systemic)**, 998
  Injection USP, 1012
  Solution, Oral, 1011
Prednisolone Tebutate [*Hydeltra T.B.A.; Nor-Pred T.B.A.; Predalone T.B.A.; Predate TBA; Predcor-TBA*]
  **See Corticosteroids—Glucocorticoid Effects (Systemic)**, 998
  Suspension, Sterile, USP, 1012
Prednisone [*Apo-Prednisone; Deltasone; Liquid Pred; Meticorten; Orasone 1; Orasone 5; Orasone 10; Orasone 20; Orasone 50; Prednicen-M; Prednisone Intensol; Sterapred; Sterapred DS; Winpred*]
  **See Corticosteroids—Glucocorticoid Effects (Systemic)**, 998
  Solution, Oral, USP, 1012
  Syrup USP, 1012
  Tablets USP, 1013, MC-26
*Prednisone Intensol*—Roxane (U.S.) brand of Prednisone—**See Corticosteroids—Glucocorticoid Effects (Systemic)**, 998
*Preemie SMA 20*—Wyeth (U.S. and Canada) brand of Infant Formulas, Milk-based—**See Infant Formulas (Systemic)**, #
*Preemie SMA 24*—Wyeth (U.S. and Canada) brand of Infant Formulas, Milk-based—**See Infant Formulas (Systemic)**, #
*Pre-Fil*—Schering (U.S.) brand of Nonoxynol 9—**See Spermicides (Vaginal)**, #
*Prefrin Liquifilm*—Allergan (U.S. and Canada) brand of Phenylephrine (Ophthalmic), #
*Pregestimil*—Mead Johnson (U.S. and Canada) brand of Infant Formulas, Hypoallergenic—**See Infant Formulas (Systemic)**, #
Pregnancy Test Kits for Home Use, #
*Pregnyl*—Organon (U.S.) brand of Chorionic Gonadotropin (Systemic), 858
*Pre-Hist-D*—Marnel (U.S.) brand of Chlorpheniramine, Phenylephrine, and Methscopolamine—**See Antihistamines, Decongestants, and Anticholinergics (Systemic)**, 373
*Prelone*—Muro (U.S.) brand of Prednisolone—**See Corticosteroids—Glucocorticoid Effects (Systemic)**, 998
*Prelu-2*—Boehringer Ingelheim (U.S.) brand of Phendimetrazine—**See Appetite Suppressants (Systemic)**, 452, MC-25
*Premarin*—Wyeth-Ayerst (U.S.) and Ayerst (Canada) brand of Estrogens, Conjugated—**See Estrogens (Vaginal)**, 1391; Wyeth-Ayerst (U.S. and Canada) brand of Conjugated Estrogens—**See Estrogens (Systemic)**, 1383, MC-11; Wyeth-Ayerst (U.S.) brand of Conjugated Estrogens, and Conjugated Estrogens and Medroxyprogesterone—**See Conjugated Estrogens and Medroxyprogesterone for Ovarian Hormone Therapy (OHT) (Systemic)**, 946

*Premarin Intravenous*—Wyeth-Ayerst (U.S. and Canada) brand of Conjugated Estrogens—**See Estrogens (Systemic)**, 1383
*Premarin with Methyltestosterone*—Wyeth-Ayerst (U.S.) and Ayerst (Canada) brand of Conjugated Estrogens and Methyltestosterone—**See Androgens and Estrogens (Systemic)**, 126
*Premphase*—Wyeth-Ayerst (U.S.) brand of Conjugated Estrogens, and Conjugated Estrogens and Medroxyprogesterone—**See Conjugated Estrogens and Medroxyprogesterone for Ovarian Hormone Therapy (OHT) (Systemic)**, 946
*Prempro*—Wyeth-Ayerst (U.S.) brand of Conjugated Estrogens and Medroxyprogesterone—**See Conjugated Estrogens and Medroxyprogesterone for Ovarian Hormone Therapy (OHT) (Systemic)**, 946
*Prentif*—Cervical Cap (U.S.) brand of Cervical Cap (Vaginal), 3014
*Prepcat*—Lafayette (U.S.) brand of Barium Sulfate (Local), #
*Pre-Pen/MDM*—Kremers-Urban (U.S.) brand of Benzylpenicillin, Benzylpenicilloic, and Benzylpenilloic Acid (Systemic), 3133
*Prepidil*—Pharmacia & Upjohn (U.S. and Canada) brand of Dinoprostone (Cervical/Vaginal), 1228
*Prepulsid*—Janssen (Canada) brand of Cisapride (Systemic), 869
*Presalin*—Hauck (U.S.) brand of Acetaminophen, Aspirin, and Salicylamide, Buffered—**See Acetaminophen and Salicylates (Systemic)**, 11
*Pressyn*—Ferring (Canada) brand of Vasopressin (Systemic), 2938
*Presun*—Westwood-Squibb (Canada) brand of Aminobenzoic Acid, Padimate O, and Oxybenzone—**See Sunscreen Agents (Topical)**, #
*PreSun Active Clear*—Westwood-Squibb (U.S.) brand of Octyl Methoxycinnamate, Octyl Salicylate, and Oxybenzone—**See Sunscreen Agents (Topical)**, #
*Presun Clear*—Westwood-Squibb (Canada) brand of Avobenzone, Octyl Methoxycinnamate, Octyl Salicylate, and Oxybenzone—**See Sunscreen Agents (Topical)**, #
*PreSun Creamy Sundown Sunscreen*—Westwood-Squibb (Canada) brand of Oxybenzone and Padimate O—**See Sunscreen Agents (Topical)**, #
*PreSun For Kids*—Westwood-Squibb (U.S.) brand of Octyl Methoxycinnamate, Octyl Salicylate, and Oxybenzone—**See Sunscreen Agents (Topical)**, #
*Presun Lip Protector*—Westwood-Squibb (U.S.) brand of Oxybenzone and Padimate O—**See Sunscreen Agents (Topical)**, #
*PreSun Moisturizing*—Westwood-Squibb (U.S.) brand of Oxybenzone and Padimate O—**See Sunscreen Agents (Topical)**, #
*PreSun Moisturizing Sunscreen with Keri*—Westwood-Squibb (U.S.) brand of Oxybenzone and Padimate O—**See Sunscreen Agents (Topical)**, #, #
*PreSun Sensitive Skin*—Westwood-Squibb (U.S.) brand of Octyl Methoxycinnamate, Octyl Salicylate, and Oxybenzone—**See Sunscreen Agents (Topical)**, #
*PreSun Spray Mist*—Westwood-Squibb (U.S.) brand of Octyl Methoxycinnamate, Octyl Salicylate, and Oxybenzone—**See Sunscreen Agents (Topical)**, #; Westwood-Squibb (U.S.) brand of Octyl Salicylate—**See Sunscreen Agents (Topical)**, #
*Presun Spray Mist for Kids*—Westwood-Squibb (U.S.) brand of Octyl Methoxycinnamate, Octyl Salicylate, Oxybenzone, and Padimate O—**See Sunscreen Agents (Topical)**, #
*Presun Sunscreen*—Westwood-Squibb (Canada) brand of Avobenzone, Octyl Methoxycinnamate, Octyl Salicylate, and Oxybenzone—**See Sunscreen Agents (Topical)**, #; Westwood-Squibb (Canada) brand of Octyl Methoxycinnamate, Octyl Salicylate, and Oxybenzone—**See Sunscreen Agents (Topical)**, #; Westwood-Squibb (Canada) brand of Oxybenzone and Padimate O—**See Sunscreen Agents (Topical)**, #
*Presun Sunscreen for Kids*—Westwood-Squibb (Canada) brand of Avobenzone, Octyl Methoxycinnamate, Octyl Salicylate, and Oxybenzone—**See Sunscreen Agents (Topical)**, #; Westwood-Squibb (Canada) brand of Octyl Methoxycinnamate, Octyl Salicylate, and Oxybenzone—**See Sunscreen Agents (Topical)**, #
*Prevacid*—TAP (U.S. and Canada) brand of Lansoprazole (Systemic), 1828, MC-16
*Prevex B*—TransCanaDerm (Canada) brand of Betamethasone—**See Corticosteroids (Topical)**, 978
*Prevex HC*—TransCanaDerm (Canada) brand of Hydrocortisone—**See Corticosteroids (Topical)**, 978; TransCanaDerm (Canada) brand of Hydrocortisone (Topical), 3023
*Priftin*—Hoechst Marion Roussel (U.S.) brand of Rifapentine (Systemic), 2496
Prilocaine-containing Combinations, 3080
Prilocaine and Epinephrine [*Citanest Forte*]
 **See Anesthetics (Parenteral-Local)**, 139
 Injection USP, 152
Prilocaine Hydrochloride [*Citanest Plain*]
 **See Anesthetics (Parenteral-Local)**, 139
 Injection USP, 152
*Prilosec*—Astra (U.S.) brand of Omeprazole (Systemic), 2163, MC-23
*Primabalt*—Primedics (U.S.) brand of Cyanocobalamin—**See Vitamin B$_{12}$ (Systemic)**, 2962
*Primacor*—Sanofi (U.S.) and Sanofi Winthrop (Canada) brand of Milrinone (Systemic), 2016
Primaquine Phosphate
 **(Systemic)**, 2375, 3160
 Tablets USP, 2376
*Primatene Mist*—Whitehall (U.S.) brand of Epinephrine—**See Bronchodilators, Adrenergic (Inhalation-Local)**, 640
*Primatuss Cough Mixture 4*—Rugby (U.S.) brand of Chlorpheniramine and Dextromethorphan—**See Cough/Cold Combinations (Systemic)**, 1024
*Primatuss Cough Mixture 4D*—Rugby (U.S.) brand of Pseudoephedrine, Dextromethorphan, and Guaifenesin—**See Cough/Cold Combinations (Systemic)**, 1024
*Primaxin*—MSD (Canada) brand of Imipenem and Cilastatin (Systemic), 1681
*Primaxin IM*—Merck (U.S.) brand of Imipenem and Cilastatin (Systemic), 1681
*Primaxin IV*—Merck (U.S.) brand of Imipenem and Cilastatin (Systemic), 1681
*Primazine*—Primedics (U.S.) brand of Promazine—**See Phenothiazines (Systemic)**, 2289
Primidone [*Apo-Primidone; Myidone; Mysoline; PMS Primidone; Sertan*]
 **(Systemic)**, 2376
 Suspension, Oral, USP, 2379
 Tablets USP, 2379
 Tablets, Chewable, 2379
*Principen*—Apothecon (U.S.) brand of Ampicillin—**See Penicillins (Systemic)**, 2240, MC-2
*Prinivil*—Merck (U.S. and Canada) brand of Lisinopril—**See Angiotensin-converting Enzyme (ACE) Inhibitors (Systemic)**, 177, MC-17
*Prinzide*—Merck (U.S.) and MSD (Canada) brand of Lisinopril and Hydrochlorothiazide—**See Angiotensin-converting Enzyme (ACE) Inhibitors and Hydrochlorothiazide (Systemic)**, 187, MC-17
*Priscoline*—Ciba-Geigy (U.S.) brand of Tolazoline (Parenteral-Systemic), #
*Pro-50*—Dunhall (U.S.) brand of Promethazine—**See Antihistamines, Phenothiazine-derivative (Systemic)**, 377
*Pro-Air*—PD (Canada) brand of Procaterol—**See Bronchodilators, Adrenergic (Inhalation-Local)**, 640
*ProAmatine*—Roberts (U.S.) brand of Midodrine (Systemic), 2014
*Probalan*—Lannett (U.S.) brand of Probenecid (Systemic), 2380
*ProBalance*—Clintec (U.S.) brand of Enteral Nutrition Formula, Fiber-containing—**See Enteral Nutrition Formulas (Systemic)**, #
*Pro-Banthine*—Roberts (U.S. and Canada) brand of Propantheline—**See Anticholinergics/Antispasmodics (Systemic)**, 226, MC-26
*Probar*—E-Z-EM (U.S.) brand of Barium Sulfate (Local), #
*Probate*—Vita Elixir (U.S.) brand of Meprobamate (Systemic), #
*Proben-C*—Rugby (U.S.) brand of Probenecid and Colchicine (Systemic), 2384
Probenecid [*Benemid; Benuryl; Probalan*]
 **(Systemic)**, 2380
 Tablets USP, 2384
Probenecid and Colchicine [*ColBenemid; Col-Probenecid; Proben-C*]
 **(Systemic)**, 2384
 Tablets USP, 2385
Probenecid-containing Combinations, 3080
Probucol [*Lorelco*]
 **(Systemic)**, 2385
 Tablets, 2387
Procainamide Hydrochloride [*Procanbid ; Procan SR; Promine; Pronestyl; Pronestyl-SR*]
 **(Systemic)**, 2387
 Capsules USP, 2390, MC-26
 Injection USP, 2391
 Tablets USP, 2390, MC-26
 Tablets, Extended-release, USP, 2390, MC-26
Procaine-containing Combinations, 3080
Procaine Hydrochloride [*Novocain*]
 **See Anesthetics (Parenteral-Local)**, 139
 Injection USP, 153
Procaine penicillin—Penicillin G—**See Penicillins (Systemic)**, 2240
*Pro-Cal-Sof*—Vangard (U.S.) brand of Docusate—**See Laxatives (Local)**, #
*Procan SR*—PD (U.S. and Canada) brand of Procainamide (Systemic), 2387
Procarbazine Hydrochloride [*Matulane; Natulan*]
 **(Systemic)**, 2391
 Capsules USP, 2396
*Procardia*—Pfizer (U.S.) brand of Nifedipine—**See Calcium Channel Blocking Agents (Systemic)**, 720, MC-22
*Procardia XL*—Pfizer (U.S.) brand of Nifedipine—**See Calcium Channel Blocking Agents (Systemic)**, 720, MC-22
Procaterol Hydrochloride Hemihydrate [*Pro-Air*]
 **See Bronchodilators, Adrenergic (Inhalation-Local)**, 640
 Aerosol, Inhalation, 650
Prochlorperazine [*Compazine; PMS Prochlorperazine; Prorazin; Stemetil*]
 **See Phenothiazines (Systemic)**, 2289
 Suppositories USP, 2307
Prochlorperazine Edisylate [*Compa-Z; Compazine; Cotranzine; Ultrazine-10*]
 **See Phenothiazines (Systemic)**, 2289
 Injection USP, 2307
 Syrup USP, 2305
Prochlorperazine Maleate [*Compazine; Compazine Spansule; PMS Prochlorperazine; Prorazin; Stemetil*]
 **See Phenothiazines (Systemic)**, 2289
 Capsules, Extended-release, 2306, MC-26
 Tablets USP, 2306, MC-26
Prochlorperazine Mesylate [*PMS Prochlorperazine; Stemetil; Stemetil Liquid*]
 **See Phenothiazines (Systemic)**, 2289
 Injection, 2307
 Syrup, 2306
*Procrit*—Ortho Biotech (U.S.) brand of Epoetin alfa (Systemic), 1352; R.W. Johnson (U.S.) brand of Epoetin Alfa (Systemic), 3142
*Proctocort*—Monarch (U.S.) brand of Hydrocortisone—**See Corticosteroids (Rectal)**, 973
*ProctoFoam/non-steroid*—Reed & Carnrick (U.S.) brand of Pramoxine—**See Anesthetics (Mucosal-Local)**, 128
*Proctosol-HC*—American Generics (U.S.) brand of Hydrocortisone—**See Corticosteroids (Rectal)**, 973
*Procyclid*—ICN (Canada) brand of Procyclidine—**See Antidyskinetics (Systemic)**, 297
Procyclidine Hydrochloride [*Kemadrin; PMS Procyclidine; Procyclid*]
 **See Antidyskinetics (Systemic)**, 297
 Elixir, 300
 Tablets USP, 301
*Procysteine*—Transcend (U.S.) brand of L-2 Oxothiazolidine-4-Carboxylic Acid (Intratracheal-Local), 3150
*Procytox*—Horner (Canada) brand of Cyclophosphamide (Systemic), 1128
*Prodiem Plain*—Ciba Self-Medication (Canada) brand of Psyllium Hydrophilic Mucilloid—**See Laxatives (Local)**, #
*Prodiem Plus*—Ciba Self-Medication (Canada) brand of Psyllium Hydrophilic Mucilloid and Senna—**See Laxatives (Local)**, #
*Prodrox*—Legere (U.S.) brand of Hydroxyprogesterone—**See Progestins (Systemic)**, 2400
*Profasi*—Pharmascience (U.S.) brand of Chorionic Gonadotropin (Systemic), 858
*Profasi HP*—Pharmascience (Canada) brand of Chorionic Gonadotropin (Systemic), 858
*Profenal*—Alcon (U.S.) brand of Suprofen—**See Anti-inflammatory Drugs, Nonsteroidal (Ophthalmic)**, 383

**3334 General Index**

Profenamine—Ethopropazine—**See Antidyskinetics (Systemic)**, 297
Profen II—Wakefield (U.S.) brand of Phenylpropanolamine and Guaifenesin—**See Cough/Cold Combinations (Systemic)**, 1024
Profen-LA—Wakefield (U.S.) brand of Phenylpropanolamine and Guaifenesin—**See Cough/Cold Combinations (Systemic)**, 1024
Profiber—Sherwood (U.S.) brand of Enteral Nutrition Formula, Fiber-containing—**See Enteral Nutrition Formulas (Systemic)**, #
Profilnine SD—Alpha (U.S.) brand of Factor IX (Systemic), 1430
Progestasert—Alza (U.S.) brand of Progesterone Intrauterine Device (IUD), 2396
Progesterone [*Crimone; Gesterol 50; PMS-Progesterone; Prometrium*]
　**See Progestins (Systemic)**, 2400, 3160
　Capsules (Micronized), 2411
　Gel (Micronized), 2412
　Injection USP, 2411
　Suppositories, Vaginal, 2412
Progesterone Intrauterine Device (IUD) [*Progestasert*], 2396
　System, Contraceptive, Intrauterine, USP, 2400
Progestins
　**(Systemic)**, 2400
Proglycem—Medical Market (U.S.) and Schering (Canada) brand of Diazoxide (Oral-Systemic), 1197
Prograf—Fujisawa (U.S. and Canada) brand of Tacrolimus (Systemic), 2683, MC-29; Fujisawa (U.S.) brand of Tacrolimus (Systemic), 3167
Proguanil Hydrochloride [*Paludrine*]
　**(Systemic)**, #
　Tablets, #
ProHance—Squibb (U.S.) brand of Gadoteridol (Systemic), #
Prohibit—Connaught (U.S. and Canada) brand of Haemophilus b Conjugate Vaccine (PRP-D—Diphtheria Toxoid Conjugate)—**See Haemophilus b Conjugate Vaccine (Systemic)**, 1601
Prohim—Baker Norton (U.S.) brand of Yohimbine (Systemic), #
Prolamine—Thompson (U.S.) brand of Phenylpropanolamine (Systemic), 2314
Prolastin—Cutter (U.S. and Canada) brand of Alpha₁-proteinase Inhibitor, Human (Systemic), #; Miles (U.S.) brand of Alpha₁-proteinase Inhibitor (Systemic), 3129
Pro-Lax—Vangard (U.S.) brand of Psyllium Hydrophilic Mucilloid—**See Laxatives (Local)**, #
Proleukin—Chiron (U.S.) brand of Aldesleukin (Systemic), 36, 3129
Prolixin—Apothecon (U.S.) brand of Fluphenazine—**See Phenothiazines (Systemic)**, 2289, MC-13
Prolixin Concentrate—Princeton (U.S.) brand of Fluphenazine—**See Phenothiazines (Systemic)**, 2289
Prolixin Decanoate—Princeton (U.S.) brand of Fluphenazine—**See Phenothiazines (Systemic)**, 2289
Prolixin Enanthate—Princeton (U.S.) brand of Fluphenazine—**See Phenothiazines (Systemic)**, 2289
Prolopa—Roche (Canada) brand of Levodopa and Benserazide (Systemic), 3027
Proloprim—Glaxo Wellcome (U.S.) and BW (Canada) brand of Trimethoprim (Systemic), 2882
Promacot—Truxton (U.S.) brand of Promethazine—**See Antihistamines, Phenothiazine-derivative (Systemic)**, 377
Promatussin DM—Wyeth-Ayerst (Canada) brand of Promethazine, Pseudoephedrine, and Dextromethorphan—**See Cough/Cold Combinations (Systemic)**, 1024
Promatussin DM Children's Syrup—Wyeth-Ayerst (Canada) brand of Promethazine, Pseudoephedrine, and Dextromethorphan—**See Cough/Cold Combinations (Systemic)**, 1024
Promazine Hydrochloride [*Primazine; Prozine-50; Sparine*]
　**See Phenothiazines (Systemic)**, 2289
　Injection USP, 2308
　Tablets USP, 2308
Pro-Med 50—Med-Tex (U.S.) brand of Promethazine—**See Antihistamines, Phenothiazine-derivative (Systemic)**, 377
Promet—Legere (U.S.) brand of Promethazine—**See Antihistamines, Phenothiazine-derivative (Systemic)**, 377

Prometa—Muro (U.S.) brand of Metaproterenol—**See Bronchodilators, Adrenergic (Systemic)**, 651
Promethazine-containing Combinations, 3080
Promethazine DM—Geneva (U.S.); Harber (U.S.); Major (U.S.); Moore (U.S.); Qualitest (U.S.); Rugby (U.S.) and Schein (U.S.) brand of Promethazine and Dextromethorphan—**See Cough/Cold Combinations (Systemic)**, 1024
Promethazine Hydrochloride [*Anergan 25; Anergan 50; Antinaus 50; Histantil; Pentazine; Phenazine 25; Phenazine 50; Phencen-50; Phenergan; Phenergan Fortis; Phenergan Plain; Phenerzine; Phenoject-50; Pro-50; Promacot; Pro-Med 50; Promet; Prorex-25; Prorex-50; Prothazine; Prothazine Plain; Shogan; V-Gan-25; V-Gan-50*]
　**See Antihistamines, Phenothiazine-derivative (Systemic)**, 377
　Injection USP, 382
　Suppositories USP, 382
　Syrup USP, 381
　Tablets USP, 382 MC-26
Promethazine Hydrochloride and Codeine Phosphate [*Pentazine VC with Codeine; Phenergan with Codeine; Pherazine with Codeine*]
　**See Cough/Cold Combinations (Systemic)**, 1024
　Solution, Oral, 1079
　Syrup, 1080, 1082
Promethazine Hydrochloride, Codeine Phosphate, and Potassium Guaiacolsulfonate [*Phenergan Expectorant with Codeine*]
　**See Cough/Cold Combinations (Systemic)**, 1024
　Syrup, 1081
Promethazine Hydrochloride and Dextromethorphan Hydrobromide [*Phenameth DM; Phenergan with Dextromethorphan; Pherazine DM; Promethazine DM; Prometh with Dextromethorphan*]
　**See Cough/Cold Combinations (Systemic)**, 1024
　Solution, Oral, 1084
　Syrup, 1080, 1082, 1084
Promethazine Hydrochloride and Phenylephrine Hydrochloride [*Phenergan VC; Pherazine VC; Promethazine VC; Prometh VC Plain*]
　**See Antihistamines and Decongestants (Systemic)**, 343
　Syrup, 357, 358
Promethazine Hydrochloride, Phenylephrine Hydrochloride, and Codeine Phosphate [*Phenameth VC with Codeine; Phenergan VC with Codeine; Pherazine VC with Codeine; Promethazine VC with Codeine; Promethist with Codeine; Prometh VC with Codeine*]
　**See Cough/Cold Combinations (Systemic)**, 1024
　Solution, Oral, 1084
　Syrup, 1080, 1082, 1084
Promethazine Hydrochloride, Phenylephrine Hydrochloride, Codeine Phosphate, and Potassium Guaiacolsulfonate [*Phenergan VC Expectorant with Codeine*]
　**See Cough/Cold Combinations (Systemic)**, 1024
　Syrup, 1081
Promethazine Hydrochloride, Phenylephrine Hydrochloride, and Potassium Guaiacolsulfonate [*Phenergan VC Expectorant*]
　**See Cough/Cold Combinations (Systemic)**, 1024
　Syrup, 1081
Promethazine Hydrochloride and Potassium Guaiacolsulfonate [*Phenergan Expectorant*]
　**See Cough/Cold Combinations (Systemic)**, 1024
　Syrup, 1081
Promethazine Hydrochloride, Pseudoephedrine Hydrochloride, and Dextromethorphan Hydrobromide [*Promatussin DM; Promatussin DM Children's Syrup*]
　**See Cough/Cold Combinations (Systemic)**, 1024
　Syrup, 1083
Promethazine VC—Cenci (U.S.); Halsey (U.S.); Major (U.S.); Qualitest (U.S.); Rugby (U.S.); and Schein (U.S.) brand of Promethazine and Phenylephrine—**See Antihistamines and Decongestants (Systemic)**, 343
Promethazine VC with Codeine—Geneva (U.S.); Schein (U.S.) and WC (U.S.) brand of Promethazine, Phenylephrine, and Codeine—**See Cough/Cold Combinations (Systemic)**, 1024
Prometh with Dextromethorphan—Barre-National (U.S.) brand of Promethazine and Dextromethorphan—**See Cough/Cold Combinations (Systemic)**, 1024
Promethist with Codeine—Rahslog Corp (U.S.) brand of Promethazine, Phenylephrine, and Codeine—**See Cough/Cold Combinations (Systemic)**, 1024

Prometh VC with Codeine—Barre (U.S.); Warner (U.S.) and Zenith Goldline (U.S.) brand of Promethazine, Phenylephrine, and Codeine—**See Cough/Cold Combinations (Systemic)**, 1024
Prometh VC Plain—Barre-National (U.S.) and Zenith Goldline (U.S.) brand of Promethazine and Phenylephrine—**See Antihistamines and Decongestants (Systemic)**, 343
Prometrium—Solvay (U.S.) and Schering (Canada) brand of Progesterone—**See Progestins (Systemic)**, 2400
Promine—Major (U.S.) brand of Procainamide (Systemic), 2387
Prominic Expectorant—Republic (U.S.) brand of Phenylpropanolamine and Guaifenesin—**See Cough/Cold Combinations (Systemic)**, 1024
Prominicol Cough—Republic (U.S.) brand of Pheniramine, Pyrilamine, Phenylpropanolamine, Dextromethorphan, and Ammonium Chloride—**See Cough/Cold Combinations (Systemic)**, 1024
Promist HD Liquid—Russ (U.S.) brand of Chlorpheniramine, Pseudoephedrine, and Hydrocodone—**See Cough/Cold Combinations (Systemic)**, 1024
ProMod—Ross (U.S. and Canada) brand of Enteral Nutrition Formula, Modular—**See Enteral Nutrition Formulas (Systemic)**, #
Promote—Ross (U.S.) brand of Enteral Nutrition Formula, Polymeric—**See Enteral Nutrition Formulas (Systemic)**, #
Promote with Fiber—Abbott/Ross (U.S.) brand of Enteral Nutrition Formula, Fiber-containing—**See Enteral Nutrition Formulas (Systemic)**, #
Prompt—Searle (U.S.) brand of Psyllium Hydrophilic Mucilloid and Sennosides—**See Laxatives (Local)**, #
Promycin—Vion (U.S.) brand of Porfiromycin (Systemic), 3159
Pronestyl—Apothecon (U.S.) and Squibb (Canada) brand of Procainamide (Systemic), 2387, MC-26
Pronestyl-SR—Apothecon (U.S.) and Squibb (Canada) brand of Procainamide (Systemic), 2387, MC-26
Pronto Lice Killing Shampoo Kit—Commerce (U.S.) brand of Pyrethrins and Piperonyl Butoxide (Topical), #
Propacet 100—Lemmon (U.S.) brand of Propoxyphene and Acetaminophen—**See Opioid (Narcotic) Analgesics and Acetaminophen (Systemic)**, 2198
Propac Plus—Sherwood (U.S.) brand of Enteral Nutrition Formula, Modular—**See Enteral Nutrition Formulas (Systemic)**, #
Propaderm—Glaxo (Canada) brand of Beclomethasone—**See Corticosteroids (Topical)**, 978
Propafenone Hydrochloride [*Rythmol*]
　**(Systemic)**, 2413
　Tablets, 2416, MC-26
Propagest—Carnrick (U.S.) brand of Phenylpropanolamine (Systemic), 2314
Prop-a-Hist—Bolan (U.S.) brand of Chlorpheniramine, Phenyltoloxamine, Phenylephrine, and Phenylpropanolamine—**See Antihistamines and Decongestants (Systemic)**, 343
Propamidine Isethionate [*Brolene*]
　**(Ophthalmic)**, 3160
Propanthel—ICN (Canada) brand of Propantheline—**See Anticholinergics/Antispasmodics (Systemic)**, 226
Propantheline Bromide [*Pro-Banthine; Propanthel*]
　**See Anticholinergics/Antispasmodics (Systemic)**, 226
　Tablets USP, 239, MC-26
Propa pH Medicated Acne Cream Maximum Strength—Commerce (U.S.) brand of Salicylic Acid (Topical), #
Propa pH Medicated Cleansing Pads Maximum Strength—Commerce (U.S.) brand of Salicylic Acid (Topical), #
Propa pH Medicated Cleansing Pads Sensitive Skin—Commerce (U.S.) brand of Salicylic Acid (Topical), #
Propa pH Perfectly Clear Skin Cleanser Topical Solution Normal/Combination Skin—Commerce (U.S.) brand of Salicylic Acid (Topical), #
Propa pH Perfectly Clear Skin Cleanser Topical Solution Oily Skin—Commerce (U.S.) brand of Salicylic Acid (Topical), #
Propa pH Perfectly Clear Skin Cleanser Topical Solution Sensitive Skin Formula—Commerce (U.S.) brand of Salicylic Acid (Topical), #

Proparacaine Hydrochloride [*Ak-Taine; Alcaine; Diocaine; Ocu-Caine; Ophthaine; Ophthetic;* proxymetacaine; *Spectro-Caine*]
  **See Anesthetics (Ophthalmic)**, #
  Solution, Ophthalmic, USP, #
*Propecia*—Merck (U.S.) brand of Finasteride (Systemic), 1465, MC-12
*Propine C Cap B.I.D.*—Allergan (U.S. and Canada) brand of Dipivefrin (Ophthalmic), 1249
Propiomazine Hydrochloride [*Largon*]
  **(Systemic)**, #
  Injection USP, #
*Proplex T*—Baxter (U.S.) brand of Factor IX (Systemic), 1430
Propofol [*Diprivan;* disoprofol]
  **(Systemic)**, 2416
  Injection, 2419
Propoxycaine-containing Combinations, 3080
Propoxyphene with APAP—Propoxyphene and Acetaminophen—**See Opioid (Narcotic) Analgesics and Acetaminophen (Systemic)**, 2198
*Propoxyphene Compound-65*—Mylan (U.S.) brand of Propoxyphene and Aspirin—**See Opioid (Narcotic) Analgesics and Aspirin (Systemic)**, 2202
Propoxyphene-containing Combinations, 3080
Propoxyphene Hydrochloride [*Cotanal-65; Darvon;* dextropropoxyphene; *PP-Cap; 642*]
  **See Opioid (Narcotic) Analgesics (Systemic)**, 2168
  Capsules USP, 2189
  Tablets, 2189
Propoxyphene Hydrochloride and Acetaminophen [co-proxAPAP; *E-Lor;* propoxyphene with APAP; *Wygesic*]
  **See Opioid (Narcotic) Analgesics and Acetaminophen (Systemic)**, 2198
  Tablets USP, 2202
Propoxyphene Hydrochloride, Aspirin, and Caffeine [*Darvon Compound-65; PC-Cap; Propoxyphene Compound-65;* propoxyphene hydrochloride compound; *692*]
  **See Opioid (Narcotic) Analgesics and Aspirin (Systemic)**, 2202
  Capsules USP, 2204
  Tablets, 2204
Propoxyphene hydrochloride compound—Propoxyphene, Aspirin, and Caffeine—**See Opioid (Narcotic) Analgesics and Aspirin (Systemic)**, 2202
Propoxyphene Napsylate [*Darvon-N;* dextropropoxyphene]
  **See Opioid (Narcotic) Analgesics (Systemic)**, 2168
  Capsules, 2189
  Suspension, Oral, USP, 2190
  Tablets USP, 2190
Propoxyphene Napsylate and Acetaminophen [co-proxAPAP; *Darvocet-N 50; Darvocet-N 100; Propacet 100;* propoxyphene with APAP]
  **See Opioid (Narcotic) Analgesics and Acetaminophen (Systemic)**, 2198
  Tablets USP, 2202, MC-26
Propoxyphene Napsylate and Aspirin [*Darvon-N with A.S.A.*]
  **See Opioid (Narcotic) Analgesics and Aspirin (Systemic)**, 2202
  Capsules, 2204
Propoxyphene Napsylate, Aspirin, and Caffeine [*Darvon-N Compound*]
  **See Opioid (Narcotic) Analgesics and Aspirin (Systemic)**, 2202
  Capsules, 2205
Propranolol-containing Combinations, 3080
Propranolol Hydrochloride [*Apo-Propranolol; Detensol; Inderal; Inderal LA; Novopranol;* pms *Propranolol*]
  **See Beta-adrenergic Blocking Agents (Systemic)**, 593
  Capsules, Extended-release, USP, 606, MC-26
  Injection USP, 607
  Solution, Oral, 606
  Tablets USP, 607, MC-26
Propranolol Hydrochloride and Hydrochlorothiazide [*Inderide; Inderide LA*]
  **See Beta-adrenergic Blocking Agents and Thiazide Diuretics (Systemic)**, 609
  Capsules, Extended-release, USP, 611, MC-26
  Tablets USP, 611, MC-26
*Propulsid*—Janssen (U.S.) brand of Cisapride (Systemic), 869, MC-7

Propylthiouracil [*Propyl-Thyracil*]
  **See Antithyroid Agents (Systemic)**, 446
  Enema, 450
  Suppositories, 450
  Tablets USP, 450
*Propyl-Thyracil*—Frosst (Canada) brand of Propylthiouracil—**See Antithyroid Agents (Systemic)**, 446
*Prorazin*—Technilab (Canada) brand of Prochlorperazine—**See Phenothiazines (Systemic)**, 2289
*Prorex-25*—Hyrex (U.S.) brand of Promethazine—**See Antihistamines, Phenothiazine-derivative (Systemic)**, 377
*Prorex-50*—Hyrex (U.S.) brand of Promethazine—**See Antihistamines, Phenothiazine-derivative (Systemic)**, 377
*Proscar*—Merck (U.S. and Canada) brand of Finasteride (Systemic), 1465, MC-13
*Prosed/DS*—Star (U.S.) brand of Atropine, Hyoscyamine, Methenamine, Methylene Blue, Phenyl Salicylate, and Benzoic Acid (Systemic), 488
*ProSobee*—Mead Johnson (U.S. and Canada) brand of Infant Formulas, Soy-based—**See Infant Formulas (Systemic)**, #
*Pro-Sof*—Vangard (U.S.) brand of Docusate—**See Laxatives (Local)**, #
*Pro-Sof Plus*—Vangard (U.S.) brand of Casanthranol and Docusate—**See Laxatives (Local)**, #
*ProSom*—Abbott (U.S.) brand of Estazolam—**See Benzodiazepines (Systemic)**, 556, MC-11
*Pro-Span*—Primedics (U.S.) brand of Hydroxyprogesterone—**See Progestins (Systemic)**, 2400
Prostaglandin E$_1$—*See* Alprostadil (Intracavernosal), 48; Alprostadil (Systemic), 52
Prostaglandin E$_2$—*See* Dinoprostone (Cervical/Vaginal), 1228
Prostaglandin El Enol Ester (AS-013)
  **(Systemic)**, 3160
Prostaglandin E1 in Lipid Emulsion
  **(Systemic)**, 3160
Prostaglandin E1, Liposomal
  **(Systemic)**, 3152
  Injection, 3152
*Prostaphlin*—Apothecon (U.S.) brand of Oxacillin—**See Penicillins (Systemic)**, 2240, MC-23
*ProstaScint*—Cytogen (U.S.) brand of Indium In 111 Capromab Pendetide (Systemic), 980
*ProStep*—Lederle (U.S.) and Boehringer Ingelheim (Canada) brand of Nicotine (Systemic), 2125
*Prostigmin*—ICN (U.S. and Canada) brand of Neostigmine—**See Antimyasthenics (Systemic)**, 437
*Prostin E$_2$*—Pharmacia & Upjohn (Canada) brand of Dinoprostone (Cervical/Vaginal), 1228
*Prostin F$_2$ Alpha*—Upjohn (Canada) brand of Dinoprost (Parenteral-Local), 1228
*Prostin/15M*—Upjohn (Canada) brand of Carboprost (Systemic), 782
*Prostin VR*—Upjohn (Canada) brand of Alprostadil (Intracavernosal), 48; Upjohn (Canada) brand of Alprostadil (Systemic), 52
*Prostin VR Pediatric*—Upjohn (U.S.) brand of Alprostadil (Intracavernosal), 48; Upjohn (U.S.) brand of Alprostadil (Systemic), 52
*Protain XL*—Kendall McGaw (U.S.) brand of Enteral Nutrition Formula, Disease-specific—**See Enteral Nutrition Formulas (Systemic)**, #
Protamine Sulfate [protamine sulphate]
  **(Systemic)**, 2420
  Injection USP, 2421
  for Injection USP, 2421
Protamine sulphate—*See* Protamine (Systemic), 2420
Protein C Concentrate [*Protein C Concentrate (Human) Vapor Heated, Immuno*]
  **(Systemic)**, 3160
Protein C Concentrate (Human) Vapor Heated, Immuno—Immuno (U.S.) brand of Protein C Concentrate (Systemic), 3160
*Prothazine*—Vortech (U.S.) brand of Promethazine—**See Antihistamines, Phenothiazine-derivative (Systemic)**, 377
*Prothazine Plain*—Vortech (U.S.) brand of Promethazine—**See Antihistamines, Phenothiazine-derivative (Systemic)**, 377
Prothrombin complex concentrate (PCC)—*See* Factor IX Complex, 1430
*Protilase*—Rugby (U.S.) brand of Pancrelipase (Systemic), 2222
Protirelin [*Relefact TRH*]
  **(Systemic)**, #, 3160
  Injection, #

*Protopam Chloride*—Wyeth-Ayerst (U.S.) brand of Pralidoxime (Systemic), #
*Protostat*—Ortho (U.S.) brand of Metronidazole (Systemic), 1996
*Protox*—CytRx (U.S.) brand of Poloxamer 331 (Systemic), 3158
Protriptyline Hydrochloride [*Triptil; Vivactil*]
  **See Antidepressants, Tricyclic (Systemic)**, 271
  Tablets USP, 282, MC-26
*Protropin*—Genentech (U.S. and Canada) brand of Somatrem—**See Growth Hormone (Systemic)**, 1586; Genentech (U.S.) brand of Somatrem (Systemic), 3165
*Pro-Tuss*—URL (U.S.) brand of Chlorpheniramine, Phenylephrine, Phenylpropanolamine, Atropine, Hyoscyamine, and Scopolamine—**See Antihistamines, Decongestants, and Anticholinergics (Systemic)**, 373
*Protuss-D*—Horizon (U.S.) brand of Pseudoephedrine, Hydrocodone, and Potassium Guaiacolsulfonate—**See Cough/Cold Combinations (Systemic)**, 1024
*Provamicina*—*See* Spiramycin (Systemic), 2624
*Proventil*—Schering (U.S.) brand of Albuterol—**See Bronchodilators, Adrenergic (Inhalation-Local)**, 640; **Bronchodilators, Adrenergic (Systemic)**, 651
*Proventil HFA*—Schering (U.S.) brand of Albuterol—**See Bronchodilators, Adrenergic (Inhalation-Local)**, 640
*Proventil Repetabs*—Schering (U.S.) brand of Albuterol—**See Bronchodilators, Adrenergic (Systemic)**, 651, MC-1
*Provera*—Pharmacia & Upjohn (U.S. and Canada) brand of Medroxyprogesterone—**See Progestins (Systemic)**, 2400, MC-18
*Provera Pak*—Pharmacia & Upjohn (Canada) brand of Medroxyprogesterone—**See Progestins (Systemic)**, 2400
*Provocholine*—Roche (U.S.) brand of Methacholine (Inhalation-Local), #
Proxymetacaine—Proparacaine—**See Anesthetics (Ophthalmic)**, #
*Prozac*—Dista (U.S. and Canada) brand of Fluoxetine (Systemic), 1503, MC-13
*Prozine-50*—Hauck (U.S.) brand of Promazine—**See Phenothiazines (Systemic)**, 2289
PRP—*See* Haemophilus b Polysaccharide Vaccine (Systemic), 1606
PRP-HbOC—Haemophilus b Conjugate Vaccine (HbOC—Diphtheria CRM$_{197}$ Protein Conjugate)—**See Haemophilus b Conjugate Vaccine (Systemic)**, 1601
*Prulet*—Mission Pharmacal (U.S.) brand of Phenolphthalein—**See Laxatives (Local)**, #
Prussian Blue [*Antidotum Thallii-Heyl;* Berlin blue; ferric ferrocyanide; ferric (III) hexacyanoferrate (II); iron blue; *Radiogardase-Cs*]
  **(Oral-Local)**, #
  Capsules, #
*P&S*—Baker Cummins (U.S.) brand of Salicylic Acid (Topical), #
*Pseudo*—Mason (U.S.) brand of Pseudoephedrine (Systemic), 2422
*Pseudo-Car DM*—Geneva (U.S.) brand of Carbinoxamine, Pseudoephedrine, and Dextromethorphan—**See Cough/Cold Combinations (Systemic)**, 1024
*Pseudo-Chlor*—Geneva (U.S.); Major (U.S.); and Moore (U.S.) brand of Chlorpheniramine and Pseudoephedrine—**See Antihistamines and Decongestants (Systemic)**, 343
Pseudoephedrine-containing Combinations, 3080
Pseudoephedrine Hydrochloride [*Balminil Decongestant Syrup; Benylin Decongestant; Cenafed; Decofed; Dorcol Children's Decongestant Liquid; Efidac/24; Eltor 120; Genaphed; Halofed; Halofed Adult Strength; Maxenal; Myfedrine; Novafed; PediaCare Infants' Oral Decongestant Drops; Pseudo; Pseudogest; Robidrine; Sudafed; Sudafed 12 Hour; Sudafed Liquid, Children's; Sufedrin*]
  **(Systemic)**, 2422
  Capsules, 2424
  Capsules, Extended-release, 2424
  Solution, Oral, 2424
  Syrup USP, 2424
  Tablets USP, 2424
  Tablets, Extended-release, 2425

## General Index

Pseudoephedrine Hydrochloride and Acetaminophen [*Actifed Sinus Daytime; Actifed Sinus Daytime-Caplets; Allerest No-Drowsiness Caplets; Aspirin-Free BayerSelect Sinus Pain Relief Caplets; Coldrine; Contac Allergy/SinusDay Caplets; Contac Non-Drowsy Formula Sinus Caplets; Dristan Cold Caplets; Dristan N.D. Caplets; Dristan N.D. Extra Strength Caplets; Dynafed Maximum Strength; Ornex Maximum Strength-Caplets; Ornex No Drowsiness Caplets; Phen-APAP Without Drowsiness; Sinarest No-Drowsiness Caplets; Sine-Aid Maximum Strength; Sine-Aid Maximum Strength Caplets; Sine-Aid Maximum Strength Gelcaps; Sine-Off Maximum Strength No Drowsiness Formula Caplets; Sinus Excedrin Extra Strength; Sinus Excedrin Extra Strength Caplets; Sinus-Relief; Sinutab No Drowsiness Caplets; Sinutab No Drowsiness Extra Strength Caplets; Sinutab Sinus Maximum Strength Without Drowsiness; Sinutab Sinus Maximum Strength Without Drowsiness Caplets; Sinutrol 500 Caplets; Sudafed Head and Cold Sinus Extra Strength Caplets; Sudafed Sinus Maximum Strength Without Drowsiness; Sudafed Sinus Maximum Strength Without Drowsiness Caplets; TheraFlu Sinus Maximum Strength Caplets; Tylenol Sinus Maximum Strength; Tylenol Sinus Maximum Strength Caplets; Tylenol Sinus Maximum Strength Gelcaps; Tylenol Sinus Maximum Strength Geltabs; Tylenol Sinus Medication Regular Strength Caplets; Tylenol Sinus Medication Extra Strength Caplets*]
 **See Decongestants and Analgesics (Systemic)**, 1180
 Capsules, 1184
 Tablets USP, 1181, 1182, 1183, 1184
Pseudoephedrine Hydrochloride and Aspirin [*Ursinus Inlay*]
 **See Decongestants and Analgesics (Systemic)**, 1180
 Tablets, 1184
Pseudoephedrine Hydrochloride and Codeine Phosphate [*CoSudafed; Nucofed*]
 **See Cough/Cold Combinations (Systemic)**, 1024
 Capsules, 1075
 Syrup, 1049, 1075
 Tablets, 1049
Pseudoephedrine Hydrochloride, Codeine Phosphate, and Guaifenesin [*Benylin Codeine D-E; Calmylin Codeine D-E; CoSudafed Expectorant; Deproist Expectorant with Codeine; Dihistine Expectorant; Guiatuss DAC; Guiatussin DAC; Mytussin DAC; Novagest Expectorant with Codeine; Novahistine Expectorant; Nucochem Expectorant; Nucochem Pediatric Expectorant; Nucofed Expectorant; Nucofed Pediatric Expectorant; Nucotuss Expectorant; Nucotuss Pediatric Expectorant; Phenhist Expectorant; Robafen DAC; Robitussin-DAC; Ryna-CX Liquid; Tussar-2; Tussar-SF*]
 **See Cough/Cold Combinations (Systemic)**, 1024
 Solution, Oral, 1040, 1051, 1052, 1062, 1071, 1073, 1074, 1081, 1092
 Syrup, 1036, 1049, 1062, 1075, 1076, 1087, 1088, 1105
Pseudoephedrine Hydrochloride and Dextromethorphan Hydrobromide [*Benylin DM-D; Benylin DM-D for Children; Buckley's DM; Calmylin #2; Calmylin Pediatric; Drixoral Cough & Congestion Liquid Caps; Effective Strength Cough Formula with Decongestant; Novahistex DM with Decongestant; Novahistine DM with Decongestant; Pharmasave Children's Cough Syrup; Robitussin Maximum Strength Cough and Cold; Robitussin Pediatric Cough & Cold; Sudafed DM; Triaminic AM Non-Drowsy Cough and Decongestant; Tuss-DA; Vicks 44 Cough and Cold Relief Non-Drowsy LiquiCaps; Vicks 44D Cough and Head Congestion; Vicks Formula 44-D; Vicks Formula 44-d Pediatric; Vicks Pediatric 44D Cough & Head Decongestion*]
 **See Cough/Cold Combinations (Systemic)**, 1024
 Capsules, 1054, 1112
 Solution, Oral, 1039, 1056, 1073, 1074, 1089, 1090, 1097, 1100, 1112, 1115
 Syrup, 1036, 1040, 1041, 1080, 1090, 1105, 1113
Pseudoephedrine Hydrochloride, Dextromethorphan Hydrobromide, and Acetaminophen [*Alka-Seltzer Plus Flu & Body Aches Medicine Liqui-Gels; Co-Complex DM Caplets; Comtrex Daytime Caplets; Comtrex Daytime Maximum Strength Cold,*

Pseudoephedrine Hydrochloride, Dextromethorphan Hydrobromide, and Acetaminophen (*continued*) *Cough, and Flu Relief; Comtrex Daytime Maximum Strength Cold and Flu Relief; Comtrex-Multi-Symptom Maximum Strength Non-Drowsy Caplets; Contac Cold/Flu Day Caplets; Contac Severe Cold & Flu Non-Drowsy Caplets; Histenol; Neo Citran Day Caps Extra Strength Caplets; Ornex Severe Cold No Drowsiness Caplets; Sudafed Cough & Cold Extra Strength Caplets; Sudafed Severe Cold Formula; Sudafed Severe Cold Formula Caplets; TheraFlu Maximum Strength Non-Drowsy Formula Flu, Cold & Cough Medicine; TheraFlu Maximum Strength Non-Drowsy Formula Flu, Cold & Cough Medicine Caplets; Triaminic Sore Throat Formula; Tylenol Cold and Flu No Drowsiness Powder; Tylenol Cold Medication Extra Strength Daytime Caplets; Tylenol Cold Medication, Non-Drowsy Caplets; Tylenol Cold Medication, Non-Drowsy Gelcaps; Tylenol Cold Medication Regular Strength Daytime Caplets; Tylenol Cough Medication with Decongestant Regular Strength; Tylenol Maximum Strength Flu Gelcaps; Tylenol-Multi-Symptom Cough with Decongestant*]
 **See Cough/Cold Combinations (Systemic)**, 1024
 Capsules, 1032
 Solution, Oral, 1102, 1111
 for Solution, Oral, 1099, 1108
 Suspension, Oral, 1110
 Tablets, 1044, 1045, 1046, 1048, 1063, 1072, 1077, 1096, 1097, 1099, 1109, 1110
Pseudoephedrine Hydrochloride, Dextromethorphan Hydrobromide, Guaifenesin, and Acetaminophen [*Benylin 4 Flu; Calmylin Cough & Flu; Comtrex Cough Formula; Robitussin Cold, Cough & Flu Liqui-Gels; Sudafed Cold & Cough Liquid Caps; Sudafed Cold & Flu Gelcaps; Vicks DayQuil Liquicaps; Vicks DayQuil Multi-Sympton Cold/Flu LiquiCaps; Vicks DayQuil Multi-Symptom Cold/Flu Relief*]
 **See Cough/Cold Combinations (Systemic)**, 1024
 Capsules, 1088, 1096, 1113
 Solution, Oral, 1037, 1045, 1113
 Syrup, 1040
Pseudoephedrine Hydrochloride and Guaifenesin [*Anatuss LA; Congess JR; Congess SR; Congestac Caplets; Deconsal II; Duratuss; Entex PSE; Eudal-SR; Expressin 400 Caplets; Glycofed; GP-500; Guaifed; Guaifed-PD; Guaifenex PSE 60; Guaifenex PSE 120; GuaiMAX-D; Guaitab; Guaivent; Guaivent PD; Guai-Vent/PSE; GuiaCough PE; Guiatuss PE; Humibid Guaifenesin Plus; Iosal II; Nalex Jr.; Nasabid; Nasatab LA; Novahistex Expectorant with Decongestant; Respa-1st; Respaire-60 SR; Respaire-120 SR; Robitussin-PE; Robitussin Severe Congestion Liqui-Gels; Ru-Tuss DE; Rymed; Rymed Liquid; Sinufed Timecelles; Sinutab Non-Drying No Drowsiness Liquid Caps; Stamoist E; Sudafed Non-Drowsy Non-Drying Sinus Liquid Caps; Sudal 60/500; Sudal 120/600; Touro LA Caplets; Tuss-LA; V-Dec-M; Versacaps; Zephrex; Zephrex-LA*]
 **See Cough/Cold Combinations (Systemic)**, 1024, 3033
 Capsules USP, 1090, 1091, 1094, 1097
 Capsules, Extended-release, 1047, 1060, 1061, 1072, 1086, 1094, 1112
 Solution, Oral, 1062, 1074, 1089, 1091
 Syrup, 1060, 1062, 1089
 Tablets, 1048, 1058, 1059, 1061, 1115, 3033, MC-27
 Tablets, Extended-release, 1034, 1050, 1055, 1057, 1058, 1059, 1060, 1061, 1067, 1072, 1086, 1091, 1095, 1097, 1100, 1108, 1112, 1115
Pseudoephedrine Hydrochloride and Hydrocodone Bitartrate [*De-Tuss; Detussin Liquid; P-V-Tussin; Tyrodone*]
 **See Cough/Cold Combinations (Systemic)**, 1024
 Solution, Oral, 1052, 1111
 Syrup, 1052, 1085
 Tablets, 1085
Pseudoephedrine Hydrochloride, Hydrocodone Bitartrate, and Guaifenesin [*Cophene XP; Deconamine CX; Detussin Expectorant; Duratuss HD; Entuss-D; Entuss-D Jr.; Med-Hist Exp; SRC Expectorant; Tussafin Expectorant; Vanex Expectorant*]
 **See Cough/Cold Combinations (Systemic)**, 1024
 Elixir, 1055

Pseudoephedrine Hydrochloride, Hydrocodone Bitartrate, and Guaifenesin (*continued*)
 Solution, Oral, 1048, 1050, 1052, 1057, 1058, 1069, 1095, 1104, 1111
 Tablets, 1050, 1057
Pseudoephedrine Hydrochloride, Hydrocodone Bitartrate, and Potassium Guaiacolsulfonate [*Entuss-D; Protuss-D*]
 **See Cough/Cold Combinations (Systemic)**, 1024
 Solution, Oral, 1057, 1085
Pseudoephedrine Hydrochloride and Ibuprofen [*Advil Cold and Sinus; Advil Cold and Sinus Caplets; Dimetapp Sinus Caplets; Dristan Sinus Caplets; Motrin IB Sinus; Motrin IB Sinus Caplets; Sine-Aid IB Caplets; Vicks DayQuil Sinus Pressure & Pain Relief Caplets*]
 **See Decongestants and Analgesics (Systemic)**, 1180
 Tablets USP, 1181, 1182, 1183, 1184
Pseudoephedrine Sulfate [*Chlor-Trimeton Non-Drowsy Decongestant 4 Hour; Drixoral Non-Drowsy Formula*]
 **(Systemic)**, 2422
 Tablets, 2425
 Tablets, Extended-release, 2425
*Pseudogest*—Major (U.S.) brand of Pseudoephedrine (Systemic), 2422
*Pseudo-gest Plus*—Major (U.S.) brand of Chlorpheniramine and Pseudoephedrine—**See Antihistamines and Decongestants (Systemic)**, 343
Pseudomonic acid—*See* Mupirocin (Topical), 2066
*Psorcon*—Dermik (U.S.) brand of Diflorasone—**See Corticosteroids (Topical)**, 978; Dermik (U.S.) brand of Diflorasone (Topical), 3017
*Psorigel*—Owen (U.S.) and Alcon (Canada) brand of Coal Tar (Topical), #
*PsoriNail Topical Solution*—Summers (U.S.) brand of Coal Tar (Topical), #
PSP—*See* Phenolsulfonphthalein (Systemic), #
Psyllium [*Cillium; Konsyl; Naturacil; Perdiem Fiber; Syllact*]
 **See Laxatives (Local)**, #
 Caramels, #
 Granules, #
 Powder, #
Psyllium-containing Combinations, 3081
Psyllium Hydrophilic Mucilloid and Carboxymethylcellulose Sodium [*Serutan Toasted Granules*]
 **See Laxatives (Local)**, #
 Granules, #
Psyllium Hydrophilic Mucilloid and Senna [*Prodiem Plus*]
 **See Laxatives (Local)**, #
 Granules, #
Psyllium Hydrophilic Mucilloid and Sennosides [*Prompt*]
 **See Laxatives (Local)**, #
 Powder, #
Psyllium and Senna [*Perdiem*]
 **See Laxatives (Local)**, #
 Granules, #
PT 105—Legere (U.S.) brand of Phendimetrazine—**See Appetite Suppressants (Systemic)**, 452
*Pulmicort Nebuamp*—Astra (Canada) brand of Budesonide—**See Corticosteroids (Inhalation-Local)**, 955
*Pulmicort Turbuhaler*—Astra (Canada) brand of Budesonide—**See Corticosteroids (Inhalation-Local)**, 955
*Pulmocare*—Ross (U.S.) brand of Enteral Nutrition Formula, Disease-specific—**See Enteral Nutrition Formulas (Systemic)**, #
*Pulmolite*—New England Nuclear (U.S.) brand of Technetium Tc 99m Albumin Aggregated (Systemic), 2697
Pulmonary Surfactant Replacement **(Intratracheal-Local)**, 3160
Pulmonary Surfactant Replacement, Porcine [*Curosurf*]
 **(Intratracheal-Local)**, 3160
*Pulmophylline*—Riva (Canada) brand of Theophylline—**See Bronchodilators, Theophylline (Systemic)**, 668
*Pulmozyme*—Genentech (U.S. and Canada) brand of Dornase Alfa (Inhalation-Local), 1292; Genentech (U.S.) brand of Dornase Alfa (Inhalation-Local), 3141
*Purge*—Fleming (U.S.) brand of Castor Oil—**See Laxatives (Local)**, #
Purified Extract of *Pseudomonas Aeruginosa* [*Immudyn*]
 **(Systemic)**, 3160

Purified Type II Collagen [*Colloral*] **(Systemic)**, 3160
Purinethol—Glaxo Wellcome (U.S. and Canada) brand of Mercaptopurine (Systemic), 1946, MC-18
Purinol—Horner (Canada) brand of Allopurinol (Systemic), 44
*P.V. Carpine Liquifilm*—Allergan (Canada) brand of Pilocarpine (Ophthalmic), #
*PVF*—Frosst (Canada) brand of Penicillin V—**See Penicillins (Systemic)**, 2240
*PVF K*—Frosst (Canada) brand of Penicillin V—**See Penicillins (Systemic)**, 2240
*P-V-Tussin*—Solvay (U.S.) brand of Chlorpheniramine, Pseudoephedrine, and Hydrocodone—**See Cough/Cold Combinations (Systemic)**, 1024; Solvay (U.S.) brand of Pseudoephedrine, and Hydrocodone—**See Cough/Cold Combinations (Systemic)**, 1024
*Pylorid*—Glaxo Wellcome (Canada) brand of Ranitidine Bismuth Citrate (Systemic), 3033
*Pyopen*—Ayerst (Canada) brand of Carbenicillin—**See Penicillins (Systemic)**, 2240
Pyrantel Pamoate [*Antiminth; Combantrin; Reese's Pinworm Medicine*]
  **(Oral-Local)**, #
  Suspension, Oral, USP, #
  Tablets, #
Pyrazinamide [*pms-Pyrazinamide; Tebrazid*]
  **(Systemic)**, 2425
  Tablets USP, 2430
Pyrazinamide-containing Combinations, 3081
*Pyregesic-C*—Truxton (U.S.) brand of Acetaminophen and Codeine—**See Opioid (Narcotic) Analgesics and Acetaminophen (Systemic)**, 2198
Pyrethrins and Piperonyl Butoxide [*A-200 Gel Concentrate; A-200 Shampoo Concentrate; Barc; Blue; Licetrol; Pronto Lice Killing Shampoo Kit; Pyrinyl; R & C; Rid; Tisit; Tisit Blue; Tisit Shampoo; Triple X*]
  **(Topical)**, #
  Gel, #
  Shampoo, Solution, #
  Solution, Topical, #
*Pyri*—Jones-Western (U.S.) brand of Pyridoxine (Systemic), 2430
*Pyribenzamine*—Ciba-Geigy (Canada) brand of Tripelennamine—**See Antihistamines (Systemic)**, 325
*Pyridiate*—Balan (U.S.); Bioline (U.S.); Genetco (U.S.); Glenlawn (U.S.); Harber (U.S.); Major (U.S.); Richlyn (U.S.); Rugby (U.S.); Veratex (U.S.); and Vita-Rx (U.S.) brand of Phenazopyridine (Systemic), 2288
*Pyridium*—PD (U.S. and Canada) brand of Phenazopyridine (Systemic), 2288
Pyridostigmine Bromide [*Mestinon; Mestinon-SR; Mestinon Timespans; Regonol*]
  **See Antimyasthenics (Systemic)**, 437
  Injection USP, 441
  Syrup USP, 441
  Tablets USP, 441
  Tablets, Extended-release, 441
Pyridoxine Hydrochloride [*Beesix; Doxine; Nestrex; Pyri; Rodex; Vitabee 6*; vitamin B$_6$]
  **(Systemic)**, 2430
  Capsules, Extended-release, 2342
  Injection USP, 2342
  Tablets USP, 2342
  Tablets, Extended-release, 2342
9-[3-Pyridylmethyl]-9-Deazaguanine **(Systemic)**, 3128
Pyrilamine-containing Combinations, 3081
Pyrilamine Maleate [*mepyramine*]
  **See Antihistamines (Systemic)**, 325
Pyrilamine Maleate and Codeine Phosphate [*Tricodene*]
  **See Cough/Cold Combinations (Systemic)**, 1024
  Solution, Oral, 1102
Pyrilamine Maleate, Phenylephrine Hydrochloride, Aspirin, and Caffeine [*Dristan Formula P*]
  **See Antihistamines, Decongestants, and Analgesics (Systemic)**, 366
  Tablets, 369
Pyrilamine Maleate, Phenylephrine Hydrochloride, and Codeine Phosphate [*Codimal PH*]
  **See Cough/Cold Combinations (Systemic)**, 1024
  Syrup, 1045

Pyrilamine Maleate, Phenylephrine Hydrochloride, and Dextromethorphan Hydrobromide [*Codimal DM*]
  **See Cough/Cold Combinations (Systemic)**, 1024
  Syrup, 1045
Pyrilamine Maleate, Phenylephrine Hydrochloride, and Hydrocodone Bitartrate [*Codimal DH*]
  **See Cough/Cold Combinations (Systemic)**, 1024
  Syrup, 1045
Pyrilamine Maleate, Phenylephrine Hydrochloride, Hydrocodone Bitartrate, and Ammonium Chloride [*Hycomine; Hycomine-S Pediatric*]
  **See Cough/Cold Combinations (Systemic)**, 1024
  Syrup, 1065
Pyrilamine Maleate, Phenylpropanolamine Hydrochloride, Acetaminophen, and Caffeine [*Histosal*]
  **See Antihistamines, Decongestants, and Analgesics (Systemic)**, 366
  Tablets, 370
Pyrilamine Maleate, Phenylpropanolamine Hydrochloride, Dextromethorphan Hydrobromide, Guaifenesin, Potassium Citrate, and Citric Acid [*Phanatussin*]
  **See Cough/Cold Combinations (Systemic)**, 1024
  Syrup, 1079
Pyrilamine Maleate, Pseudoephedrine Hydrochloride, Dextromethorphan Hydrobromide, and Acetaminophen [*Robitussin Night Relief*]
  **See Cough/Cold Combinations (Systemic)**, 1024
  Solution, Oral, 1089
Pyrimethamine [*Daraprim*]
  **(Systemic)**, 2433
  Tablets USP, 2435, MC-27
Pyrimethamine-containing Combinations, 3081
*Pyrinyl*—Balan (U.S.); Barre-National (U.S.); Bioline (U.S.); CMC (U.S.); De Witt (U.S.); Dixon-Shane (U.S.); Glenlawn (U.S.); Goldline (U.S.); Raway (U.S.); Rugby (U.S.); Schein (U.S.); Vangard (U.S.); and Veratex (U.S.) brand of Pyrethrins and Piperonyl Butoxide (Topical), #
Pyrithione Zinc [*Danex; Dan-gard; DHS Zinc Dandruff Shampoo; Head & Shoulders Antidandruff Cream Shampoo Normal to Dry Formula; Head & Shoulders Antidandruff Cream Shampoo Normal to Oily Formula; Head & Shoulders Antidandruff Lotion Shampoo Normal to Dry Formula; Head & Shoulders Antidandruff Lotion Shampoo Normal to Oily Formula; Head & Shoulders Antidandruff Lotion Shampoo 2 in 1 (Complete Dandruff Shampoo plus Conditioner in One) Formula; Head & Shoulders Dry Scalp Conditioning Formula Lotion Shampoo; Head & Shoulders Dry Scalp 2 in 1 (Dry Scalp Shampoo plus Conditioner in One) Formula Lotion Shampoo; Head & Shoulders Dry Scalp Regular Formula Lotion Shampoo; Sebex; Sebulon; Zincon Dandruff Lotion Shampoo; ZNP Bar Shampoo; ZNP Shampoo*]
  **(Topical)**, #
  Shampoo, Bar, #
  Shampoo, Cream, #
  Shampoo, Lotion, #
*Pyrolite*—Du Pont (U.S. and Canada) brand of Technetium Tc 99m (Pyro- and trimeta-) Phosphates (Systemic), 2733
*Pyrroxate Caplets*—Roberts (U.S.) brand of Chlorpheniramine, Phenylpropanolamine, and Acetaminophen—**See Antihistamines, Decongestants, and Analgesics (Systemic)**, 366
Pyrvinium Pamoate [*Vanquin;* viprynium]
  **(Oral-Local)**, #
  Suspension, Oral, USP, #

# Q

*Q-Hist LA*—Qualitest (U.S.) brand of Chlorpheniramine, Phenyltoloxamine, Phenylephrine, and Phenylpropanolamine—**See Antihistamines and Decongestants (Systemic)**, 343
*Q-Profen*—Qualitest (U.S.) brand of Ibuprofen—**See Anti-inflammatory Drugs, Nonsteroidal (Systemic)**, 388
*QTest*—Quidel (U.S.) brand of Immunoassay Pregnancy Test Kits—**See Pregnancy Test Kits for Home Use**, #
*Q-Tuss*—Qualitest (U.S.) brand of Chlorpheniramine, Phenylephrine, Phenylpropanolamine, Atropine, Hyoscyamine, and Scopolamine—**See Antihistamines, Decongestants, and Anticholinergics (Systemic)**, 373

*Quarzan*—Roche (U.S.) brand of Clidinium—**See Anticholinergics/Antispasmodics (Systemic)**, 226
Quazepam [*Doral*]
  **See Benzodiazepines (Systemic)**, 556
  Tablets, 577
*Quelicin*—Abbott (U.S. and Canada) brand of Succinylcholine—**See Neuromuscular Blocking Agents (Systemic)**, 2098
*Quelidrine Cough*—Abbott (U.S.) brand of Chlorpheniramine, Ephedrine, Phenylephrine, Dextromethorphan, Ammonium Chloride, and Ipecac—**See Cough/Cold Combinations (Systemic)**, 1024
*Questran*—Mead Johnson (U.S.) and Bristol (Canada) brand of Cholestyramine (Oral-Local), 853
*Questran Light*—Mead Johnson (U.S.) and Bristol (Canada) brand of Cholestyramine (Oral-Local), 853
Quetiapine [*Seroquel*]
  **(Systemic)**, 2437, 3033
  Tablets, 2440, 3033, MC-27
*Quibron*—Roberts (U.S.) brand of Theophylline and Guaifenesin (Systemic), #, MC-30
*Quibron-300*—Monarch (U.S.) brand of Theophylline and Guaifenesin (Systemic), #, MC-30
*Quibron-T Dividose*—Roberts (U.S.) brand of Theophylline—**See Bronchodilators, Theophylline (Systemic)**, 668, MC-29
*Quibron-T/SR Dividose*—Roberts (U.S.) and Bristol (Canada) brand of Theophylline—**See Bronchodilators, Theophylline (Systemic)**, 668, MC-29
*Quick Pep*—Thompson (U.S.) brand of Caffeine (Systemic), 706
Quinacrine Hydrochloride [*Atabrine;* mepacrine]
  **(Systemic)**, #
  Tablets USP, #
*Quinaglute Dura-Tabs*—Berlex (U.S. and Canada) brand of Quinidine (Systemic), 2440, MC-27
*Quinalan*—Lannett (U.S.) brand of Quinidine (Systemic), 2440
Quinapril Hydrochloride [*Accupril*]
  **See Angiotensin-converting Enzyme (ACE) Inhibitors (Systemic)**, 177
  Tablets, 186, MC-27
*Quinate*—Rougier (Canada) brand of Quinidine (Systemic), 2440
Quinethazone [*Hydromox*]
  **See Diuretics, Thiazide (Systemic)**, 1273
  Tablets USP, 1281
*Quinidex Extentabs*—Robins (U.S. and Canada) brand of Quinidine (Systemic), 2440, MC-27
Quinidine Gluconate [*Duraquin; Quinaglute Dura-tabs; Quinalan; Quinate*]
  **(Systemic)**, 2440
  Injection USP, 2443
  Tablets, 2442
  Tablets, Extended-release, 2443, MC-27
Quinidine Polygalacturonate [*Cardioquin*]
  **(Systemic)**, 2440
  Tablets, 2443
Quinidine Sulfate [*Apo-Quinidine; Cin-Quin; Novo-quinidin; Quinidex Extentabs; Quinora*]
  **(Systemic)**, 2440
  Capsules USP, 2443
  Injection, 2444
  Tablets USP, 2443, MC-27
  Tablets, Extended-release, USP, 2443, MC-27
Quinine Sulfate
  **(Systemic)**, 2444
  Capsules USP, 2447
  Tablets USP, 2447
*Quinora*—Key (U.S.) brand of Quinidine (Systemic), 2440

# R

*RA*—Medco Lab (U.S.) brand of Resorcinol (Topical), #
Rabies Immune Globulin [*HRIG; Hyperab; Imogam; RIG*]
  **See Rabies Vaccine (Systemic)**, 2448
  Rabies Immune Globulin (Human) USP (RIG), 2449
Rabies Vaccine Adsorbed [*RVA*]
  **See Rabies Vaccine (Systemic)**, 2449
  Suspension USP (RVA), 2452

Rabies Vaccine, Human Diploid Cell [HDCV; *Imovax; Imovax I.D.*]
　**See Rabies Vaccine (Systemic)**, 2449
　Rabies Vaccine, Human Diploid Cell (For Intradermal Injection) (HDCV), 2452
　Rabies Vaccine, Human Diploid Cell USP (For Intramuscular Injection) (HDCV), 2453
Racemethionine [DL-methionine; *M-Caps*; methionine; *Pedameth; Uracid*]
　**(Systemic)**, #
　Capsules USP, #
　Solution, Oral, #
　Tablets USP, #
Racepinephrine [*AsthmaNefrin; microNefrin; Nephron; S-2; Vaponefrin*]
　**See Bronchodilators, Adrenergic (Inhalation-Local)**, 640
　Solution, Inhalation, USP, 647
*Radanil*—See Benznidazole (Systemic), #
*Radiogardase-Cs*—Heyl (Germany) brand of Prussian Blue (Oral-Local), #
Radioiodinated Albumin
　**(Systemic)**, 2453
*Radiostol Forte*—Glaxo (Canada) brand of Ergocalciferol—**See Vitamin D and Analogs (Systemic)**, 2966
*Rafton*—Ferring (Canada) brand of Alumina, Calcium Carbonate, and Sodium Bicarbonate—**See Antacids (Oral-Local)**, 188; Ferring (Canada) brand of Alumina and Sodium Bicarbonate—**See Antacids (Oral-Local)**, 188
Raloxifene Hydrochloride [*Evista*; keoxifene hydrochloride]
　**(Systemic)**, 2455
　Tablets, 2458
Ramipril [*Altace*]
　**See Angiotensin-converting Enzyme (ACE) Inhibitors (Systemic)**, 177
　Capsules, 186, MC-27
*Ramses Contraceptive Foam*—Schmid (Canada) brand of Nonoxynol 9—**See Spermicides (Vaginal)**, #
*Ramses Contraceptive Vaginal Jelly*—Schmid (Canada) brand of Nonoxynol 9—**See Spermicides (Vaginal)**, #
*Ramses Crystal Clear Gel*—Schmid (U.S.) brand of Nonoxynol 9—**See Spermicides (Vaginal)**, #
*Ramses Extra*—Schmid (Canada) brand of Latex Condoms and Nonoxynol 9—**See Condoms**, #
*Ramses Extra-15*—Schmid (Canada) brand of Latex Condoms and Nonoxynol 9—**See Condoms**, #
*Ramses Extra Ribbed*—Schmid (U.S.) brand of Latex Condoms and Nonoxynol 9—**See Condoms**, #
*Ramses Extra Strength*—Schmid (U.S.) brand of Latex Condoms and Nonoxynol 9—**See Condoms**, #
*Ramses Non-Lubricated*—Schmid (U.S. and Canada) brand of Latex Condoms—**See Condoms**, #
*Ramses Ribbed*—Schmid (U.S. and Canada) brand of Latex Condoms and Nonoxynol 9—**See Condoms**, #
*Ramses Safe Play*—Schmid (U.S.) brand of Latex Condoms—**See Condoms**, #
*Ramses Sensitol*—Schmid (U.S. and Canada) brand of Latex Condoms—**See Condoms**, #
*Ramses with Spermicidal Lubricant*—Schmid (U.S.) brand of Latex Condoms and Nonoxynol 9—**See Condoms**, #
*Ramses Thin Lub*—Schmid (Canada) brand of Latex Condoms—**See Condoms**, #
*Ramses Thin Spermicidal Lub*—Schmid (Canada) brand of Latex Condoms and Nonoxynol 9—**See Condoms**, #
*Ramses Ultra*—Schmid (Canada) brand of Latex Condoms—**See Condoms**, #
*Ramses Ultra-15*—Schmid (Canada) brand of Latex Condoms and Nonoxynol 9—**See Condoms**, #
*Ramses Ultra Thin*—Schmid (U.S.) brand of Latex Condoms—**See Condoms**, #
*Ramses Ultra Thin Ribbed with Spermicide*—Schmid (U.S.) brand of Latex Condoms and Nonoxynol 9—**See Condoms**, #
*Ramses Ultra Thin with Spermicide*—Schmid (U.S.) brand of Latex Condoms and Nonoxynol 9—**See Condoms**, #
Ranitidine Bismuth Citrate [*Pylorid*; *Tritec*]
　**(Systemic)**, 2458, 3033
　Tablets, 2460, 3033, MC-27

Ranitidine Hydrochloride [*Apo-Ranitidine*; *Gen-Ranitidine*; *Novo-Ranitidine*; *Nu-Ranit*; *Zantac*; *Zantac 75*; *Zantac-C*; *Zantac EFFERdose Granules*; *Zantac EFFERdose Tablets*; *Zantac 150 GELdose*; *Zantac 300 GELdose*]
　**See Histamine H$_2$-receptor Antagonists (Systemic)**, 1633
　Capsules, 1641, MC-27
　Granules, Effervescent, 1641
　Injection USP, 1642
　Syrup USP, 1641
　Tablets USP, 1641, MC-27
　Tablets, Effervescent, 1642, MC-27
Ranitidine in Sodium Chloride [*Zantac*]
　**See Histamine H$_2$-receptor Antagonists (Systemic)**, 1633
　Injection, 1642
*RapidVue*—Quidel (U.S.) brand of Immunoassay Pregnancy Test Kits—**See Pregnancy Test Kits for Home Use**, #
*Rapolyte*—Richmond (Canada) brand of Oral Rehydration Salts—**See Carbohydrates and Electrolytes (Systemic)**, 769
*Raudixin*—Princeton (U.S.) brand of Rauwolfia Serpentina—**See Rauwolfia Alkaloids (Systemic)**, 2460
*Rauval*—Vale (U.S.) brand of Rauwolfia Serpentina—**See Rauwolfia Alkaloids (Systemic)**, 2460
*Rauverid*—Forest (U.S.) brand of Rauwolfia Serpentina—**See Rauwolfia Alkaloids (Systemic)**, 2460
Rauwolfia Alkaloids
　**(Systemic)**, 2460
Rauwolfia Alkaloids and Thiazide Diuretics
　**(Systemic)**, #
Rauwolfia Serpentina [*Raudixin*; *Rauval*; *Rauverid*; *Wolfina*]
　**See Rauwolfia Alkaloids (Systemic)**, 2460
　Tablets USP, 2463
Rauwolfia Serpentina and Bendroflumethiazide [*Rauzide*]
　**See Rauwolfia Alkaloids and Thiazide Diuretics (Systemic)**, #
　Tablets
Rauwolfia Serpentina–containing Combinations, 3081
*Rauzide*—Princeton (U.S.) brand of Rauwolfia Serpentina and Bendroflumethiazide—**See Rauwolfia Alkaloids and Thiazide Diuretics (Systemic)**, #
*Raxar*—Glaxo Wellcome (U.S.) brand of Grepafloxacin (Systemic), 1580, MC-14
*Ray Block*—Del-Ray Lab (U.S.) brand of Oxybenzone and Padimate O—**See Sunscreen Agents (Topical)**, #
*R & C*—Reed & Carnrick (U.S.) and Block (Canada) brand of Pyrethrins and Piperonyl Butoxide (Topical), #
rCD4—See Recombinant Soluble Human CD4 (Systemic), 3161
*RCF*—Ross (U.S. and Canada) brand of Infant Formulas, Soy-based—**See Infant Formulas (Systemic)**, #
*R & D Calcium Carbonate/600*—R & D (U.S.) brand of Calcium Carbonate (Systemic), 3135
*Reabilan*—O'Brien (U.S.) brand of Enteral Nutrition Formula, Monomeric (Elemental)—**See Enteral Nutrition Formulas (Systemic)**, #
*Reabilan HN*—O'Brien (U.S.) brand of Enteral Nutrition Formula, Monomeric (Elemental)—**See Enteral Nutrition Formulas (Systemic)**, #
*Reactine*—Pfizer (Canada) brand of Cetirizine—**See Antihistamines (Systemic)**, 325
*Readi-CAT*—E-Z-EM (U.S. and Canada) brand of Barium Sulfate (Local), #
*Readi-CAT 2*—E-Z-EM (U.S.) brand of Barium Sulfate (Local), #
*Readi-CAT Unflavored*—E-Z-EM (U.S.) brand of Barium Sulfate (Local), #
*Reality*—Female Health (U.S.) brand of Condom, Female, Polyurethane, 3015
*Rebetron*—Schering (U.S.) brand of Ribavirin/Interferon (Systemic), 3033
*Rebif*—Serono Canada (Canada) brand of Interferon Beta-1a (Systemic), 3026; Serono (U.S.) brand of Interferon Beta-1a (Systemic), 3148
*Receptin*—Biogen (U.S.) brand of CD4, Human Recombinant Soluble (Systemic), 3162
Recombinant Human Alpha-L-Iduronidase
　**(Systemic)**, 3160
Recombinant human deoxyribonuclease—Dornase Alfa (Inhalation-Local), 1292

Recombinant human granulocyte-macrophage colony stimulating factor—Sargramostim—**See Colony Stimulating Factors (Systemic)**, 941
Recombinant Human Insulin-like Growth Factor I [*IGEF*]
　**(Systemic)**, 3161
Recombinant Human Interleukin-12
　**(Systemic)**, 3161
Recombinant Human Luteinizing Hormone
　**(Systemic)**, 3161
Recombinant Human Relaxin
　**(Systemic)**, 3161
Recombinant Human Thrombopoietin
　**(Systemic)**, 3161
Recombinant Methionyl Brain-derived Neurotrophic Factor
　**(Systemic)**, 3161
Recombinant methionyl human granulocyte colony stimulating factor—Filgrastim—**See Colony Stimulating Factors (Systemic)**, 941
Recombinant Methionyl Human Stem Cell Factor
　**(Systemic)**, 3161
Recombinant Secretory Leucocyte Protease Inhibitor
　**(Systemic)**, 3161
Recombinant Soluble Human CD4 [*Receptin*]
　**(Systemic)**, 3162
Recombinant Soluble Human CD 4 [rCD4]
　**(Systemic)**, 3161
*Recombinate*—Baxter (U.S. and Canada) brand of Antihemophilic Factor (Systemic), 319
*Recombivax HB*—Merck (U.S. and Canada) brand of Hepatitis B Vaccine Recombinant (Systemic), 1628
*Recombivax HB Dialysis Formulation*—Merck (U.S. and Canada) brand of Hepatitis B Vaccine Recombinant (Systemic), 1628
*Recto-Barium*—E-Z-EM (Canada) brand of Barium Sulfate (Local), #
*Rectocort*—Welcker-Lyster (Canada) brand of Hydrocortisone—**See Corticosteroids (Rectal)**, 973
*Rectosol-HC*—Bio-Pharm (U.S.) brand of Hydrocortisone—**See Corticosteroids (Rectal)**, 973
*Rectovalone*—Jouveinal (Canada) brand of Tixocortol—**See Corticosteroids (Rectal)**, 973
*Rederm*—Med-Derm (U.S.) brand of Hydrocortisone—**See Corticosteroids (Topical)**, 978
*Redutemp*—International Ethical (U.S.) brand of Acetaminophen (Systemic), 6
*Reese's Pinworm Medicine*—Reese (U.S.) brand of Pyrantel (Oral-Local), #
*REFACTO*—Pharmacia (U.S.) brand of R-VIII SQ (Systemic), 3163
Refaximin [*Normix*]
　**(Systemic)**, 3162
*Refludan*—Behringwerke (U.S.) brand of Lepirudin (Systemic), 3151; Hoechst Marion Roussel (U.S.) brand of Lepirudin (Systemic), 1833
*Refresh Plus*—Allergan (U.S.) brand of Carboxymethylcellulose (Ophthalmic), 3013
*Regitine*—Ciba (U.S.) brand of Phentolamine (Intracavernosal), #; Ciba (U.S.) brand of Phentolamine (Systemic), #
*Reglan*—Robins (U.S. and Canada) brand of Metoclopramide (Systemic), 1992, MC-19
*Regonol*—Organon (U.S. and Canada) brand of Pyridostigmine—**See Antimyasthenics (Systemic)**, 437
*Regranex*—McNeil (U.S.) brand of Becaplermin (Topical), IBN-550
*Regroton*—Rhône-Poulenc Rorer (U.S.) brand of Reserpine and Chlorthalidone—**See Rauwolfia Alkaloids and Thiazide Diuretics (Systemic)**, #
*Regulace*—Republic (U.S.) brand of Casanthranol and Docusate—**See Laxatives (Local)**, #
*Regular (Concentrated) Iletin II, U-500*—Lilly (U.S.) brand of Insulin—**See Insulin (Systemic)**, 1713
*Regular Iletin*—Lilly (Canada) brand of Insulin—**See Insulin (Systemic)**, 1713
*Regular Iletin I*—Lilly (U.S.) brand of Insulin—**See Insulin (Systemic)**, 1713
*Regular Iletin II*—Lilly (U.S. and Canada) brand of Insulin—**See Insulin (Systemic)**, 1713
*Regular Insulin*—Novo Nordisk (U.S.) brand of Insulin—**See Insulin (Systemic)**, 1713
Regular insulin—Insulin—**See Insulin (Systemic)**, 1713
*Regular Strength Ascriptin*—Rhône-Poulenc Rorer (U.S.) brand of Aspirin, Buffered—**See Salicylates (Systemic)**, 2538
*Regulax SS*—Republic (U.S.) brand of Docusate—**See Laxatives (Local)**, #

*Regulex*—Whitehall Robins (Canada) brand of Docusate—**See Laxatives (Local)**, #
*Regulex-D*—Whitehall-Robins (Canada) brand of Danthron and Docusate—**See Laxatives (Local)**, #
*Reguloid Natural*—Rugby (U.S.) brand of Psyllium Hydrophilic Mucilloid—**See Laxatives (Local)**, #
*Reguloid Natural Sugar Free*—Rugby (U.S.) brand of Psyllium Hydrophilic Mucilloid—**See Laxatives (Local)**, #
*Reguloid Orange*—Rugby (U.S.) brand of Psyllium Hydrophilic Mucilloid—**See Laxatives (Local)**, #
*Reguloid Orange Sugar Free*—Rugby (U.S.) brand of Psyllium Hydrophilic Mucilloid—**See Laxatives (Local)**, #
*Rehydralyte*—Ross (U.S.) brand of Dextrose and Electrolytes—**See Carbohydrates and Electrolytes (Systemic)**, 769
*Relafen*—SmithKline Beecham (U.S. and Canada) brand of Nabumetone—**See Anti-inflammatory Drugs, Nonsteroidal (Systemic)**, 388, MC-21
*Relaxadon*—Geneva Generics (U.S.) brand of Atropine, Hyoscyamine, Scopolamine, and Phenobarbital—**See Belladonna Alkaloids and Barbiturates (Systemic)**, 551
*Relaxazone*—Bolan (U.S.) brand of Chlorzoxazone—**See Skeletal Muscle Relaxants (Systemic)**, 2577
*Relefact TRH*—Hoechst-Roussel (U.S.) and Hoechst (Canada) brand of Protirelin (Systemic), #
*Relief Eye Drops for Red Eyes*—Allergan (U.S.) brand of Phenylephrine (Ophthalmic), #
*Relisorm*—Serono (Canada) brand of Gonadorelin (Systemic), 1571
*Remeron*—Organon (U.S.) brand of Mirtazapine (Systemic), 2023, MC-20
Remifentanil Hydrochloride [*Ultiva*]
  **(Systemic)**, 2464
  for Injection, 2466
*Remular*—International Ethical (U.S.) brand of Chlorzoxazone—**See Skeletal Muscle Relaxants (Systemic)**, 2577
*Remular-S*—International Ethical (U.S.) brand of Chlorzoxazone—**See Skeletal Muscle Relaxants (Systemic)**, 2577
*Renacidin Irrigation*—United Guardian (U.S.) brand of Citric Acid, Glucono-delta-lactone, and Magnesium Carbonate (Local), 3015, 3137
*Renacidin Powder for Irrigation*—United Guardian (U.S.) brand of Citric Acid and D-Gluconic Acid (Local), 3014
*Renedil*—Hoechst Marion Roussel (Canada) brand of Felodipine—**See Calcium Channel Blocking Agents (Systemic)**, 720
*Renese*—Pfizer (U.S.) brand of Polythiazide—**See Diuretics, Thiazide (Systemic)**, 1273
*Renese-R*—Pfizer (U.S.) brand of Reserpine and Polythiazide—**See Rauwolfia Alkaloids and Thiazide Diuretics (Systemic)**, #
*Reno-Dip*—Squibb (U.S.) brand of Diatrizoate—**See Diatrizoates (Systemic)**, #
*Renografin-60*—Squibb (U.S. and Canada) brand of Diatrizoate—**See Diatrizoates (Systemic)**, #
*Renografin-76*—Squibb (U.S.) brand of Diatrizoate—**See Diatrizoates (Systemic)**, #
*Reno-M-30*—Bracco (U.S.) brand of Diatrizoate—**See Diatrizoates (Local)**, #
*Reno-M-60*—Squibb (U.S. and Canada) brand of Diatrizoate—**See Diatrizoates (Systemic)**, #
*Renova*—Ortho (U.S.) and Ortho-McNeil (Canada) brand of Tretinoin (Topical), 2871
*Renovist*—Squibb (U.S. and Canada) brand of Diatrizoate—**See Diatrizoates (Systemic)**, #
*Renovist II*—Squibb (U.S.) brand of Diatrizoate—**See Diatrizoates (Systemic)**, #
*Rentamine Pediatric*—Major (U.S.) brand of Chlorpheniramine, Ephedrine, Phenylephrine, and Carbetapentane—**See Cough/Cold Combinations (Systemic)**, 1024
*ReoPro*—Lilly (U.S.) brand of Abciximab (Systemic), 1
Repaglinide [*Prandin*]
  **(Otic)**, 2467
  Tablets, 2470
Repaglinide
  **(Systemic)**, 2467
*Repan*—Everett (U.S.) brand of Butalbital, Acetaminophen, and Caffeine—**See Barbiturates and Analgesics (Systemic)**, 532
*Replete*—Clintec (U.S.) brand of Enteral Nutrition Formula, Polymeric—**See Enteral Nutrition Formulas (Systemic)**, #

*Replete with Fiber*—Clintec (U.S.) brand of Enteral Nutrition Formula, Fiber-containing—**See Enteral Nutrition Formulas (Systemic)**, #
*Rep-Pred 40*—Central (U.S.) brand of Methylprednisolone—**See Corticosteroids—Glucocorticoid Effects (Systemic)**, 998
*Rep-Pred 80*—Central (U.S.) brand of Methylprednisolone—**See Corticosteroids—Glucocorticoid Effects (Systemic)**, 998
*Requip*—SmithKline Beecham (U.S.) brand of Ropinirole (Systemic), 2525
*Resaid S.R.*—Geneva (U.S.) brand of Chlorpheniramine and Phenylpropanolamine—**See Antihistamines and Decongestants (Systemic)**, 343
*Rescaps-D S.R.*—Geneva (U.S.) brand of Phenylpropanolamine and Caramiphen—**See Cough/Cold Combinations (Systemic)**, 1024
*Rescon*—Ion (U.S.) brand of Chlorpheniramine and Phenylpropanolamine—**See Antihistamines and Decongestants (Systemic)**, 343; Ion (U.S.) brand of Chlorpheniramine and Pseudoephedrine—**See Antihistamines and Decongestants (Systemic)**, 343
*Rescon-DM*—Ion (U.S.) brand of Chlorpheniramine, Pseudoephedrine, and Dextromethorphan—**See Cough/Cold Combinations (Systemic)**, 1024
*Rescon-ED*—Ion (U.S.) brand of Chlorpheniramine and Pseudoephedrine—**See Antihistamines and Decongestants (Systemic)**, 343
*Rescon-GG*—Ion (U.S.) brand of Phenylephrine and Guaifenesin—**See Cough/Cold Combinations (Systemic)**, 1024
*Rescon JR*—Ion (U.S.) brand of Chlorpheniramine and Pseudoephedrine—**See Antihistamines and Decongestants (Systemic)**, 343
*Rescriptor*—Pharmacia & Upjohn (U.S.) brand of Delavirdine (Systemic), 1184
*Rescudose*—Roxane (U.S.) brand of Morphine—**See Opioid (Narcotic) Analgesics (Systemic)**, 2168
*Reserfia*—Medic (Canada) brand of Reserpine—**See Rauwolfia Alkaloids (Systemic)**, 2460
Reserpine [*Novoreserpine; Reserfia; Serpalan; Serpasil*]
  **See Rauwolfia Alkaloids (Systemic)**, 2460
  Tablets USP, 2463
Reserpine and Chlorothiazide [*Diupres; Diurigen with Reserpine*]
  **See Rauwolfia Alkaloids and Thiazide Diuretics (Systemic)**, #
  Tablets USP
Reserpine and Chlorthalidone [*Demi-Regroton; Regroton*]
  **See Rauwolfia Alkaloids and Thiazide Diuretics (Systemic)**, #
  Tablets
Reserpine-containing Combinations, 3081
Reserpine, Hydralazine Hydrochloride, and Hydrochlorothiazide [*Cam-Ap-Es; Cherapas; Ser-A-Gen; Seralazide; Ser-Ap-Es; Serpazide; Tri-Hydroserpine; Unipres*]
  **(Systemic)**, #
  Tablets USP, MC-27, #
Reserpine and Hydrochlorothiazide [*Hydropres; Hydrosine; Hydrotensin; Mallopres*]
  **See Rauwolfia Alkaloids and Thiazide Diuretics (Systemic)**, #
  Tablets USP, #
Reserpine and Hydroflumethiazide [*Hydropine; Hydropine H.P.; Salazide; Salutensin; Salutensin-Demi*]
  **See Rauwolfia Alkaloids and Thiazide Diuretics (Systemic)**, #
  Tablets, #
Reserpine and Methyclothiazide [*Diutensen-R*]
  **See Rauwolfia Alkaloids and Thiazide Diuretics (Systemic)**, #
  Tablets, 2385
Reserpine and Polythiazide [*Renese-R*]
  **See Rauwolfia Alkaloids and Thiazide Diuretics (Systemic)**, #
  Tablets, #
Reserpine and Trichlormethiazide [*Diurese-R; Metatensin; Naquival*]
  **See Rauwolfia Alkaloids and Thiazide Diuretics (Systemic)**, #
  Tablets, #
*Resol*—Wyeth-Ayerst (U.S.) brand of Dextrose and Electrolytes—**See Carbohydrates and Electrolytes (Systemic)**, 769

Resorcinol [*RA*]
  **(Topical)**, #
  Lotion, #
  Ointment, #
Resorcinol-containing Combinations, 3081
Resorcinol and Sulfur [*Acne-Aid Gel; Acnomel Acne Cream; Acnomel Cake; Acnomel Cream; Acnomel Vanishing Cream; Bensulfoid Cream; Clearasil Adult Care Medicated Blemish Cream; Clearasil Adult Care Medicated Blemish Stick; Night Cast Special Formula Mask-lotion; Rezamid Acne Treatment; Rezamid Lotion; Sulforcin*]
  **(Topical)**, #
  Cake, #
  Cream, #
  Gel, #
  Lotion USP, #
  Stick, #
*Resource*—Sandoz (U.S.) brand of Enteral Nutrition Formula, Polymeric—**See Enteral Nutrition Formulas (Systemic)**, #
*Resource Plus*—Sandoz (U.S.) brand of Enteral Nutrition Formula, Polymeric—**See Enteral Nutrition Formulas (Systemic)**, #
*Respa-1st*—Respa (U.S.) brand of Pseudoephedrine and Guaifenesin—**See Cough/Cold Combinations (Systemic)**, 1024
*Respa-DM*—Respa (U.S.) brand of Dextromethorphan and Guaifenesin—**See Cough/Cold Combinations (Systemic)**, 1024
*Respahist*—Respa (U.S.) brand of Brompheniramine and Pseudoephedrine—**See Antihistamines and Decongestants (Systemic)**, 343
*Respaire-60 SR*—Laser (U.S.) brand of Pseudoephedrine and Guaifenesin—**See Cough/Cold Combinations (Systemic)**, 1024
*Respaire-120 SR*—Laser (U.S.) brand of Pseudoephedrine and Guaifenesin—**See Cough/Cold Combinations (Systemic)**, 1024
*Respalor*—Bristol-Myers Squibb (U.S.) brand of Enteral Nutrition Formula, Disease-specific—**See Enteral Nutrition Formulas (Systemic)**, #
*Respbid*—Boehringer Ingelheim (U.S.) brand of Theophylline—**See Bronchodilators, Theophylline (Systemic)**, 668
*RespiGam*—Medimmune (U.S. and Canada) brand of Respiratory Syncytial Virus Immune Globulin Intravenous (Systemic), 2471
*Respigan*—Medimmune (U.S.) brand of Respiratory Syncytial Virus Immune Globulin (Human) (Systemic), 3162
Respiratory Syncytial Virus Immune Globulin (Human) [*Hypermune RSV; Respigam*]
  **(Systemic)**, 3162
Respiratory Syncytial Virus Immune Globulin Intravenous [*RespiGam; RSV-IGIV*]
  **(Systemic)**, 2471
  Injection, 2473
*Restoril*—Novartis (U.S. and Canada) brand of Temazepam—**See Benzodiazepines (Systemic)**, 556, MC-29
*Resyl*—Ciba-Geigy (Canada) brand of Guaifenesin (Systemic), 1588
*Retavase*—Boehringer Mannheim (U.S.) brand of Reteplase, Recombinant (Systemic), 2473
Reteplase, Recombinant [*Retavase*]
  **(Systemic)**, 2473
  for Injection, 2475
*Retin-A*—Ortho (U.S.) and McNeil (Canada) brand of Tretinoin (Topical), 2871
*Retin-A MICRO*—Ortho-McNeil (U.S.) brand of Tretinoin (Topical), 2871
Retinoic acid—*See* Tretinoin (Topical), 2871
Retinoin
  **(Ophthalmic)**, 3162
Retinol—*See* Vitamin A (Systemic), 2958
*Retisol-A*—Stiefel (Canada) brand of Tretinoin (Topical), 2871
*Retrovir*—BW (U.S.) brand of Zidovudine (Systemic), 3171; Glaxo Wellcome (U.S.) and BW (Canada) brand of Zidovudine (Systemic), 2992, MC-32; Glaxo Wellcome (U.S.) brand of Zidovudine (Systemic), 3038
Retroviral Vector—Glucocerebrosidase, Recombinant **(Systemic)**, 3161
Retroviral Vector, R-GC and GC Gene 1750
  **(Systemic)**, 3162
*Reversol*—Organon (U.S.) brand of Edrophonium (Systemic), 1329
*Revex*—Ohmeda (U.S. and Canada) brand of Nalmefene (Systemic), 2080

*Rev-Eyes*—Storz (U.S. and Canada) brand of Dapiprazole (Ophthalmic), 1168
*ReVia*—Du Pont (U.S. and Canada) brand of Naltrexone (Systemic), 2084
*Revimine*—Rorer (Canada) brand of Dopamine—**See Sympathomimetic Agents—Cardiovascular Use (Parenteral-Systemic)**, 2669
*Rexigen Forte*—ION (U.S.) brand of Phendimetrazine—**See Appetite Suppressants (Systemic)**, 452
*Rezamid Acne Treatment*—Dermik (U.S.) brand of Resorcinol and Sulfur (Topical), #
*Rezamid Lotion*—Rorer (Canada) brand of Resorcinol and Sulfur (Topical), #
*Rezipas*—Squibb (U.S.) brand of 4-Aminosalicyclic Acid (Systemic), 3128
*Rezulin*—PD (U.S.) brand of Troglitazone (Systemic), 2888, MC-32
*R-Frone*—Serono (U.S.) brand of Interferon Beta, Recombinant (Systemic), 3148
rG-CSF—Filgrastim—**See Colony Stimulating Factors (Systemic)**, 941
RGG0853, E1A Lipid Complex
  **(Systemic)**, 3162
rGM-CSF—Sargramostim—**See Colony Stimulating Factors (Systemic)**, 941
RhD immune globulin—*See* Rh$_o$(D) Immune Globulin (Systemic), 2476
rhDNase—Dornase Alfa (Inhalation-Local), 1292
*Rheaban*—Pfizer (U.S.) brand of Attapulgite (Oral-Local), #
*RheothRx Copolymer*—BW (U.S.) brand of Poloxamer 188 (Systemic), 3158
*Rheumatrex*—Lederle (U.S.) brand of Methotrexate (Systemic), 3153; Wyeth-Ayerst Lederle (U.S.) and Lederle (Canada) brand of Methotrexate—For Noncancerous Conditions (Systemic), 1969, MC-19
Rh-IG—*See* Rh$_o$(D) Immune Globulin (Systemic), 2476
Rh immune globulin—*See* Rh$_o$(D) Immune Globulin (Systemic), 2476
*Rhinalar*—SynCare (Canada) brand of Flunisolide—**See Corticosteroids (Nasal)**, 961
*Rhinall*—Scherer (U.S.) brand of Phenylephrine (Nasal), #
*Rhinall-10 Children's Flavored Nose Drops*—Scherer (U.S.) brand of Phenylephrine (Nasal), #
*Rhinatate*—Major (U.S.) brand of Chlorpheniramine, Pyrilamine, and Phenylephrine—**See Antihistamines and Decongestants (Systemic)**, 343
*Rhinocaps*—Ferndale (U.S.) brand of Phenylpropanolamine, Acetaminophen, and Aspirin—**See Decongestants and Analgesics (Systemic)**, 1180
*Rhinocort Aqua*—Astra (Canada) brand of Budesonide—**See Corticosteroids (Nasal)**, 961; Astra (Canada) brand of Budesonide (Nasal), 3012
*Rhinocort Nasal Inhaler*—Astra (U.S.) brand of Budesonide (Nasal), 3012
*Rhinocort Turbuhaler*—Astra (Canada) brand of Budesonide—**See Corticosteroids (Nasal)**, 961; Astra (Canada) brand of Budesonide (Nasal), 3012
*Rhinolar-EX*—McGregor (U.S.) brand of Chlorpheniramine and Phenylpropanolamine—**See Antihistamines and Decongestants (Systemic)**, 343
*Rhinolar-EX 12*—McGregor (U.S.) brand of Chlorpheniramine and Phenylpropanolamine—**See Antihistamines and Decongestants (Systemic)**, 343
*Rhinosyn*—Great Southern (U.S.) brand of Chlorpheniramine and Pseudoephedrine—**See Antihistamines and Decongestants (Systemic)**, 343
*Rhinosyn-DM*—Great Southern (U.S.) brand of Chlorpheniramine, Pseudoephedrine, and Dextromethorphan—**See Cough/Cold Combinations (Systemic)**, 1024
*Rhinosyn-DMX Expectorant*—Great Southern (U.S.) brand of Dextromethorphan and Guaifenesin—**See Cough/Cold Combinations (Systemic)**, 1024
*Rhinosyn-PD*—Great Southern (U.S.) brand of Chlorpheniramine and Pseudoephedrine—**See Antihistamines and Decongestants (Systemic)**, 343
*Rhinosyn-X*—Great Southern (U.S.) brand of Pseudoephedrine, Dextromethorphan, and Guaifenesin—**See Cough/Cold Combinations (Systemic)**, 1024

Rh$_o$(D) Immune Globulin (Human) [anti-D gammaglobulin; anti-D (Rh$_o$) immunoglobulin; anti-Rh immunoglobulin; anti-Rh$_o$(D); D(Rh$_o$) immune globulin; *Gamulin Rh; HypRho-D Full Dose; HypRho-D Mini-Dose; MICRhoGAM; Mini-Gamulin Rh;* RhD immune globulin; Rh-IG; Rh immune globulin; Rh$_o$(D) immune human globulin; *RhoGAM; WinRho SD*]
  **(Systemic)**, 2476
Rh$_o$(D) Immune Globulin (Human) (for Injection), 2477
Rh$_o$(D) Immune Globulin (Human) USP (Injection), 2477
Rh$_o$(D) Immune Globulin, Human [*WinRho SD*]
  **(Systemic)**, 3162
Rh$_o$(D) immune human globulin—*See* Rh$_o$(D) Immune Globulin (Systemic), 2476
*Rhodis*—Rhodiapharm (Canada) brand of Ketoprofen—**See Anti-inflammatory Drugs, Nonsteroidal (Systemic)**, 388
*Rhodis-EC*—Rhodiapharm (Canada) brand of Ketoprofen—**See Anti-inflammatory Drugs, Nonsteroidal (Systemic)**, 388
*RhoGAM*—Ortho Diagnostic (U.S.) brand of Rh$_o$(D) Immune Globulin (Systemic), 2476
*Rho-Loperamide*—Rhoxalpharma (Canada) brand of Loperamide (Oral-Local), 1877
*Rhotrimine*—Rhodiapharm (Canada) brand of Trimipramine—**See Antidepressants, Tricyclic (Systemic)**, 271
r-HuEPO—Epoetin alfa (Systemic), 1352
rHu GM-CSF—Sargramostim—**See Colony Stimulating Factors (Systemic)**, 941
*Rhulicort*—Oral B (U.S.) brand of Hydrocortisone—**See Corticosteroids (Topical)**, 978
Ribavirin [tribavirin; *Virazid; Virazole*]
  **(Systemic)**, 2478, 3162
  for Injection, 2481
  Solution for Inhalation USP, 2480
  for Solution, Oral, 2480
Ribavirin/Interferon Alfa-2b [*Rebetron*]
  **(Systemic)**, 3033
  Capsules, 3033
  Injection, 3033
Riboflavin [vitamin B$_2$]
  **(Systemic)**, 2481
  Tablets USP, 2482
Rice Syrup Solids and Electrolytes [*Infalyte*]
  **See Carbohydrates and Electrolytes (Systemic)**, 769
  Solution, 773
Ricin (Blocked) Conjugated Murine MCA (Anti-B4)
  **(Systemic)**, 3162
Ricin (Blocked) Conjugated Murine MOAB (CD6)
  **(Systemic)**, 3162
Ricin (Blocked) Conjugated Murine Monoclonal Antibody (Anti-B4)
  **(Systemic)**, 3162
Ricin (Blocked) Conjugated Murine Monoclonal Antibody (Anti-My$^9$)
  **(Systemic)**, 3162
Ricin (Blocked) Conjugated Murine Monoclonal Antibody (N901)
  **(Systemic)**, 3162
*Ricobid*—Rico (U.S.) brand of Chlorpheniramine and Phenylephrine—**See Antihistamines and Decongestants (Systemic)**, 343
*Ricobid Pediatric*—Rico (U.S.) brand of Chlorpheniramine and Phenylephrine—**See Antihistamines and Decongestants (Systemic)**, 343
*Rid*—Leeming (U.S.) brand of Pyrethrins and Piperonyl Butoxide (Topical), #
*Rid-A-Pain*—Pfeiffer (U.S.) brand of Benzocaine—**See Anesthetics (Mucosal-Local)**, 128
*Rid-A-Pain Compound*—Pfeiffer (U.S.) brand of Acetaminophen, Salicylamide, and Caffeine—**See Acetaminophen and Salicylates (Systemic)**, 11
*Ridaura*—SmithKline Beecham (U.S. and Canada) brand of Auranofin—**See Gold Compounds (Systemic)**, 1566
Rifabutin [*Mycobutin*]
  **(Systemic)**, 2483, 3163
  Capsules, 2484, MC-27
*Rifadin*—Hoechst Marion Roussel (U.S.) and Marion Merrell Dow (Canada) brand of Rifampin (Systemic), 2485, MC-27
*Rifadin IV*—Merrell Dow (U.S.) brand of Rifampin (Systemic), 2485, 3163
*Rifamate*—Hoechst Marion Roussel (U.S.) brand of Rifampin and Isoniazid (Systemic), 2493, MC-27
Rifampicin—*See* Rifampin (Systemic), 2485

Rifampicin and isoniazid—*See* Rifampin and Isoniazid (Systemic), 2493
Rifampin [*Rifadin; Rifadin IV; Rifadin I.V.;* rifampicin; *Rimactane; Rofact*]
  **(Systemic)**, 2485, 3163
  Capsules USP, 2492, MC-27
  for Injection USP, 2492
  for Suspension, Oral, USP, 2492
Rifampin-containing Combinations, 3081
Rifampin and Isoniazid [*Rifamate;* rifampicin and isoniazid]
  **(Systemic)**, 2493
  Capsules USP, 2494, MC-27
Rifampin, Isoniazid, and Pyrazinamide [*Rifater*]
  **(Systemic)**, 2494, 3163
  Tablets, 2496, MC-27
Rifapentine [*Priftin*]
  **(Systemic)**, 2496, 3163
  Tablets, 2499
*Rifater*—Hoechst Marion Roussel (U.S.) brand of Rifampin, Isoniazid, and Pyrazinamide (Systemic), 2494, MC-27; Marion Merrell Dow (U.S.) brand of Rifampin, Isoniazid, and Pyrazinamide (Systemic), 3163
r-IFN-beta—*See* Interferon Beta, Recombinant (Systemic), 3148
RIG—*See* Rabies Immune Globulin (Systemic), 2448
RII Retinamide
  **(Systemic)**, 3163
rIL-2—*See* Aldesleukin (Systemic), 36
rIL-11—*See* Oprelvekin (Systemic), 2205
*Rilutek*—Rhône-Poulenc Rorer (U.S.) brand of Riluzole (Systemic), 2500, MC-27, 3163
Riluzole [*Rilutek*]
  **(Systemic)**, 2500, 3163
  Tablets, 2502, MC-27
*Rimactane*—Novartis (U.S. and Canada) brand of Rifampin (Systemic), 2485, MC-27
Rimantadine Hydrochloride [*Flumadine*]
  **(Systemic)**, 2502
  Syrup, 2504
  Tablets, 2504, MC-27
Rimexolone [*Vexol*]
  **(Ophthalmic)**, 2504
  Suspension, Ophthalmic, 2505
*Rimso-50*—Research Industries (U.S.) and Procter & Gamble (Canada) brand of Dimethyl Sulfoxide (Mucosal-Local), 1227
*Rinade B.I.D.*—EconoMed (U.S.) brand of Chlorpheniramine and Pseudoephedrine—**See Antihistamines and Decongestants (Systemic)**, 343
*Riopan*—Whitehall-Robins (U.S. and Canada) brand of Magaldrate—**See Antacids (Oral-Local)**, 188
*Riopan Extra Strength*—Whitehall-Robins (Canada) brand of Magaldrate—**See Antacids (Oral-Local)**, 188
*Riopan Plus*—Whitehall-Robins (U.S. and Canada) brand of Magaldrate and Simethicone—**See Antacids (Oral-Local)**, 188
*Riopan Plus Double Strength*—Whitehall-Robins (U.S.) brand of Magaldrate and Simethicone—**See Antacids (Oral-Local)**, 188
*Riopan Plus Extra Strength*—Whitehall-Robins (Canada) brand of Magaldrate and Simethicone—**See Antacids (Oral-Local)**, 188
Risedronate Sodium [*Actonel*]
  **(Systemic)**, 2506
  Tablets, 2508
*Risperdal*—Janssen (U.S. and Canada) brand of Risperidone (Systemic), 2508, MC-27
Risperidone [*Risperdal*]
  **(Systemic)**, 2508
  Solution, Oral, 2512
  Tablets, 2512, MC-27
*Ritalin*—Novartis (U.S. and Canada) brand of Methylphenidate (Systemic), 1987, MC-19
*Ritalin-SR*—Novartis (U.S. and Canada) brand of Methylphenidate (Systemic), 1987, MC-19
Ritodrine Hydrochloride [*Yutopar; Yutopar S.R.*]
  **(Systemic)**, 2513
  Capsules, Extended-release, 2515
  Injection USP, 2516
  Tablets USP, 2516
Ritodrine Hydrochloride in 5% Dextrose
  **(Systemic)**, 2513
  Injection, 2516
Ritonavir [*Norvir*]
  **(Systemic)**, 2516
  Capsules, 2518, MC-27
  Solution, Oral, 2518

**Rituxan**—Genentech (U.S.) brand of Rituximab (Systemic), 2519
**Rituximab** [*Rituxan*] **(Systemic)**, 2519
　Concentrate for Injection, 2521
*Rivotril*—Roche (Canada) brand of Clonazepam—**See Benzodiazepines (Systemic)**, 556
r-met HuG-CSF—Filgrastim—**See Colony Stimulating Factors (Systemic)**, 941
*RMS Uniserts*—Upsher-Smith (U.S.) brand of Morphine—**See Opioid (Narcotic) Analgesics (Systemic)**, 2168
*Ro7-1051*—See Benznidazole (Systemic), #
*Robafen AC Cough*—Major (U.S.) brand of Codeine and Guaifenesin—**See Cough/Cold Combinations (Systemic)**, 1024
*Robafen CF*—Major (U.S.) brand of Phenylpropanolamine, Dextromethorphan, and Guaifenesin—**See Cough/Cold Combinations (Systemic)**, 1024
*Robafen DAC*—Major (U.S.) brand of Pseudoephedrine, Codeine, and Guaifenesin——**See Cough/Cold Combinations (Systemic)**, 1024
*Robafen DM*—Major (U.S.) brand of Dextromethorphan and Guaifenesin——**See Cough/Cold Combinations (Systemic)**, 1024
*Robaxin*—Robins (U.S.) and Whitehall-Robins (Canada) brand of Methocarbamol—**See Skeletal Muscle Relaxants (Systemic)**, 2577, MC-19
*Robaxin-750*—Robins (U.S.) and Whitehall-Robins (Canada) brand of Methocarbamol—**See Skeletal Muscle Relaxants (Systemic)**, 2577
*Robaxisal*—Robins (U.S.) brand of Methocarbamol and Aspirin (Systemic), MC-19
*Robidex*—Robins (Canada) brand of Dextromethorphan (Systemic), 1191
*Robidone*—Wyeth-Ayerst (Canada) brand of Hydrocodone—**See Opioid (Narcotic) Analgesics (Systemic)**, 2168
*Robidrine*—Whitehall-Robins (Canada) brand of Pseudoephedrine (Systemic), 2422
*Robigesic*—Robins (Canada) brand of Acetaminophen (Systemic), 6
*Robinul*—Robins (U.S. and Canada) brand of Glycopyrrolate—**See Anticholinergics/Antispasmodics (Systemic)**, 226
*Robinul Forte*—Robins (U.S. and Canada) brand of Glycopyrrolate—**See Anticholinergics/Antispasmodics (Systemic)**, 226
*Robitet*—Robins (U.S.) brand of Tetracycline—**See Tetracyclines (Systemic)**, 2765
*Robitussin*—Whitehall-Robins (U.S. and Canada) brand of Guaifenesin (Systemic), 1588
*Robitussin A-C*—Whitehall-Robins (U.S.) brand of Codeine and Guaifenesin—**See Cough/Cold Combinations (Systemic)**, 1024; Whitehall-Robins (Canada) brand of Pheniramine, Codeine, and Guaifenesin—**See Cough/Cold Combinations (Systemic)**, 1024
*Robitussin-CF*—Robins (U.S.) and Whitehall-Robins (Canada) brand of Phenylpropanolamine, Dextromethorphan, and Guaifenesin—**See Cough/Cold Combinations (Systemic)**, 1024
*Robitussin with Codeine*—Whitehall-Robins (Canada) brand of Pheniramine, Codeine, and Guaifenesin—**See Cough/Cold Combinations (Systemic)**, 1024
*Robitussin Cold, Cough & Flu Liqui-Gels*—Robins (U.S.) brand of Pseudoephedrine, Dextromethorphan, Guaifenesin, and Acetaminophen—**See Cough/Cold Combinations (Systemic)**, 1024
*Robitussin Cold and Cough Liqui-Gels*—Robins (U.S.) brand of Pseudoephedrine, Dextromethorphan, and Guaifenesin—**See Cough/Cold Combinations (Systemic)**, 1024
*Robitussin Cough Calmers*—Robins (U.S.) brand of Dextromethorphan (Systemic), 1191
*Robitussin Cough & Cold*—Whitehall-Robins (Canada) brand of Pseudoephedrine, Dextromethorphan, and Guaifenesin—**See Cough/Cold Combinations (Systemic)**, 1024
*Robitussin Cough & Cold Liqui-Fills*—Whitehall-Robins (Canada) brand of Pseudoephedrine, Dextromethorphan, and Guaifenesin—**See Cough/Cold Combinations (Systemic)**, 1024
*Robitussin-DAC*—Whitehall-Robins (U.S.) brand of Pseudoephedrine, Codeine, and Guaifenesin—**See Cough/Cold Combinations (Systemic)**, 1024

*Robitussin-DM*—Robins (U.S.) and Whitehall-Robins (Canada) brand of Dextromethorphan and Guaifenesin—**See Cough/Cold Combinations (Systemic)**, 1024
*Robitussin Maximum Strength Cough and Cold*—Robins (U.S.) brand of Pseudoephedrine and Dextromethorphan—**See Cough/Cold Combinations (Systemic)**, 1024
*Robitussin Maximum Strength Cough Suppressant*—Robins (U.S.) brand of Dextromethorphan (Systemic), 1191
*Robitussin Night Relief*—Robins (U.S.) brand of Pyrilamine, Pseudoephedrine, Dextromethorphan, and Acetaminophen—**See Cough/Cold Combinations (Systemic)**, 1024
*Robitussin Night-Time Cold Formula*—Robins (U.S.) brand of Doxylamine, Pseudoephedrine, Dextromethorphan, and Acetaminophen—**See Cough/Cold Combinations (Systemic)**, 1024
*Robitussin-PE*—Robins (U.S.) and Whitehall-Robins (Canada) brand of Pseudoephedrine and Guaifenesin—**See Cough/Cold Combinations (Systemic)**, 1024
*Robitussin Pediatric*—Robins (U.S.) and Whitehall-Robins (Canada) brand of Dextromethorphan (Systemic), 1191
*Robitussin Pediatric Cough & Cold*—Robins (U.S.) and Whitehall-Robins (Canada) brand of Pseudoephedrine and Dextromethorphan—**See Cough/Cold Combinations (Systemic)**, 1024
*Robitussin Severe Congestion Liqui-Gels*—Robins (U.S.) brand of Pseudoephedrine and Guaifenesin—**See Cough/Cold Combinations (Systemic)**, 1024
*Rocaltrol*—Roche (U.S. and Canada) brand of Calcitriol—**See Vitamin D and Analogs (Systemic)**, 2966, MC-5
*Rocephin*—Roche (U.S. and Canada) brand of Ceftriaxone—**See Cephalosporins (Systemic)**, 794
*Rochagan*—See Benznidazole (Systemic), #
**Rocuronium Bromide ob***Zemuron*] **(Systemic)**, 2521
　for Injection, 2524
*Rodex*—Legere (U.S.) brand of Pyridoxine (Systemic), 2430
*R.O.-Dexasone*—Richmond (Canada) brand of Dexamethasone—**See Corticosteroids (Ophthalmic)**, 966
*Rofact*—ICN (Canada) brand of Rifampin (Systemic), 2485
*Roferon-A*—Hoffmann-LaRoche (U.S.) brand of Interferon Alfa-2a, Recombinant (Systemic), 3147, 3148; Roche (U.S. and Canada) brand of Interferon Alfa-2a, Recombinant—**See Interferons, Alpha (Systemic)**, 1740
*Rogaine*—Upjohn (Canada) brand of Minoxidil (Topical), 2021
*Rogaine for Men*—Upjohn (U.S.) brand of Minoxidil (Topical), 2021
*Rogaine for Women*—Upjohn (U.S.) brand of Minoxidil (Topical), 2021
*Rogitine*—Ciba (Canada) brand of Phentolamine (Intracavernosal), #; Ciba (Canada) brand of Phentolamine (Systemic), #
*Rolaids*—Warner-Lambert (U.S.) and Adams (Canada) brand of Calcium Carbonate and Magnesia—**See Antacids (Oral-Local)**, 188
*Rolaids Calcium Rich*—American Chicle (U.S.) brand of Calcium Carbonate—**See Calcium Supplements (Systemic)**, 736
*Rolaids Extra Strength*—Adams (Canada) brand of Calcium Carbonate and Magnesia—**See Antacids (Oral-Local)**, 188
*Rolatuss Expectorant*—Huckaby (U.S.) brand of Chlorpheniramine, Phenylephrine, Codeine, and Ammonium Chloride—**See Cough/Cold Combinations (Systemic)**, 1024
*Rolatuss with Hydrocodone*—Major (U.S.) brand of Pheniramine, Pyrilamine, Phenylephrine, Phenylpropanolamine, and Hydrocodone—**See Cough/Cold Combinations (Systemic)**, 1024
*Rolatuss Plain*—Major (U.S.) brand of Chlorpheniramineand Phenylephrine—**See Antihistamines and Decongestants (Systemic)**, 343
*Rolatuss SR*—Major (U.S.) brand of Chlorpheniramine, Phenylephrine, Phenylpropanolamine, Atropine, Hyoscyamine, and Scopolamine—**See Antihistamines, Decongestants, and Anticholinergics (Systemic)**, 373
*Romazicon*—Roche (U.S.) brand of Flumazenil (Systemic), 1483

*Rondamine*—Major (U.S.) brand of Carbinoxamine and Pseudoephedrine—**See Antihistamines and Decongestants (Systemic)**, 343
*Rondamine-DM Drops*—Major (U.S.) brand of Carbinoxamine, Pseudoephedrine, and Dextromethorphan—**See Cough/Cold Combinations (Systemic)**, 1024
*Rondec*—Dura (U.S.) brand of Carbinoxamine and Pseudoephedrine—**See Antihistamines and Decongestants (Systemic)**, 343
*Rondec Chewable*—Dura (U.S.) brand of Brompheniramine and Pseudoephedrine—**See Antihistamines and Decongestants (Systemic)**, 343
*Rondec-DM*—Dura (U.S.) brand of Carbinoxamine, Pseudoephedrine, and Dextromethorphan—**See Cough/Cold Combinations (Systemic)**, 1024
*Rondec-DM Drops*—Dura (U.S.) brand of Carbinoxamine, Pseudoephedrine, and Dextromethorphan—**See Cough/Cold Combinations (Systemic)**, 1024
*Rondec Drops*—Dura (U.S.) brand of Carbinoxamine and Pseudoephedrine—**See Antihistamines and Decongestants (Systemic)**, 343
*Rondec-TR*—Dura (U.S.) brand of Carbinoxamine and Pseudoephedrine—**See Antihistamines and Decongestants (Systemic)**, 343, MC-5
*Roniacol*—Roche (Canada) brand of Nicotinyl Alcohol (Systemic), #
**Ropinirole Hydrochloride** [*Requip*] **(Systemic)**, 2525
　Tablets, 2528
**Ropivacaine Hydrochloride** [*Naropin*] **(Parenteral-Local)**, #
　Injection, #
**Roquinimex** [*Linomide*] **(Systemic)**, 3163
*Roubac*—Rougier (Canada) brand of Sulfamethoxazole and Trimethoprim—**See Sulfonamides and Trimethoprim (Systemic)**, 2661
*Rounox*—Rougier (Canada) brand of Acetaminophen (Systemic), 6
*Rovamycina*—See Spiramycin (Systemic), 2624
*Rovamycine*—See Spiramycin (Systemic), 2624
*Rovamycine 250*—May & Baker (Canada) brand of Spiramycin (Systemic), 2624
*Rovamycine-250*—See Spiramycin (Systemic), 2624
*Rovamycine 500*—May & Baker (Canada) brand of Spiramycin (Systemic), 2624
*Rovamycine-500*—May & Baker (Canada) brand of Spiramycin (Systemic), 2624
*Rowasa*—Solvay (U.S.) brand of Mesalamine (Rectal-Local), 1954
Roxadimate-containing Combinations, 3081
*Roxanol*—Roxane (U.S.) brand of Morphine—**See Opioid (Narcotic) Analgesics (Systemic)**, 2168
*Roxanol 100*—Roxane (U.S.) brand of Morphine—**See Opioid (Narcotic) Analgesics (Systemic)**, 2168
*Roxanol UD*—Roxane (U.S.) brand of Morphine—**See Opioid (Narcotic) Analgesics (Systemic)**, 2168
*Roxicet*—Roxane (U.S.) and Boehringer-Ingelheim (Canada) brand of Oxycodone and Acetaminophen—**See Opioid (Narcotic) Analgesics and Acetaminophen (Systemic)**, 2198, MC-24
*Roxicet 5/500*—Roxane (U.S.) brand of Oxycodone and Acetaminophen—**See Opioid (Narcotic) Analgesics and Acetaminophen (Systemic)**, 2198
*Roxicodone*—Roxane (U.S.) brand of Oxycodone—**See Opioid (Narcotic) Analgesics (Systemic)**, 2168, MC-24
*Roxicodone Intensol*—Roxane (U.S.) brand of Oxycodone—**See Opioid (Narcotic) Analgesics (Systemic)**, 2168
*Roxilox*—Roxane (U.S.) brand of Oxycodone and Acetaminophen—**See Opioid (Narcotic) Analgesics and Acetaminophen (Systemic)**, 2198
*Roxiprin*—Roxane (U.S.) brand of Oxycodone and Aspirin—**See Opioid (Narcotic) Analgesics and Aspirin (Systemic)**, 2202, MC-24
*Roychlor-10%*—Roy (Canada) brand of Potassium Chloride—**See Potassium Supplements (Systemic)**, 2357
*RSV-IGIV*—See Respiratory Syncytial Virus Immune Globulin Intravenous (Systemic), 2471
*R-Tannamine*—Qualitest (U.S.) brand of Chlorpheniramine, Pyrilamine, and Phenylephrine—**See Antihistamines and Decongestants (Systemic)**, 343

# General Index

*R-Tannamine Pediatric*—Qualitest (U.S.) brand of Chlorpheniramine, Pyrilamine, and Phenylephrine—**See Antihistamines and Decongestants (Systemic)**, 343

*R-Tannate*—Copley (U.S.); Schein (U.S.); and Warner Chilcott (U.S.) brand of Chlorpheniramine, Pyrilamine, and Phenylephrine—**See Antihistamines and Decongestants (Systemic)**, 343

*R-Tannate Pediatric*—Aligen (U.S.); Copley (U.S.); Qualitest (U.S.); Schein (U.S.); and Warner Chilcott (U.S.) brand of Chlorpheniramine, Pyrilamine, and Phenylephrine—**See Antihistamines and Decongestants (Systemic)**, 343

rt-PA—Alteplase, Recombinant—**See Thrombolytic Agents (Systemic)**, 2799

Rubella and Mumps Virus Vaccine Live [*BIAVAX II*] **(Systemic)**, 2528
  Rubella and Mumps Virus Vaccine Live USP (for Injection), 2531

Rubella Virus Vaccine Live [*Meruvax II*] **(Systemic)**, 2532
  Rubella Virus Vaccine Live USP (for Injection), 2535

*Rubesol-1000*—Central (U.S.) brand of Cyanocobalamin—**See Vitamin B$_{12}$ (Systemic)**, 2962

*Rubex*—Bristol-Myers Squibb (U.S.) brand of Doxorubicin (Systemic), 1308

Rubidium Chloride Rb 82 [*CardioGen-82*] **(Systemic)**, 2536
  Injection, 2537

*Rubramin PC*—Squibb (U.S.) brand of Cyanocobalamin—**See Vitamin B$_{12}$ (Systemic)**, 2962

*Rubratope-57*—Squibb (U.S.) brand of Cyanocobalamin Co 57 (Systemic), 1123

*Rufen*—Boots (U.S.) brand of Ibuprofen—**See Anti-inflammatory Drugs, Nonsteroidal (Systemic)**, 388

*Rulox*—Rugby (U.S.) brand of Alumina and Magnesia—**See Antacids (Oral-Local)**, 188

*Rulox No. 1*—Rugby (U.S.) brand of Alumina and Magnesia—**See Antacids (Oral-Local)**, 188

*Rulox No. 2*—Rugby (U.S.) brand of Alumina and Magnesia—**See Antacids (Oral-Local)**, 188

*Rulox Plus*—Rugby (U.S.) brand of Alumina, Magnesia, and Simethicone—**See Antacids (Oral-Local)**, 188

*Rum-K*—Fleming (U.S.) brand of Potassium Chloride—**See Potassium Supplements (Systemic)**, 2357

*Ru-tab*—H.L. Moore (U.S.) brand of Chlorpheniramine, Phenylephrine, Phenylpropanolamine, Atropine, Hyoscyamine, and Scopolamine—**See Antihistamines, Decongestants, and Anticholinergics (Systemic)**, 373

*Ru-Tuss*—Boots (U.S.) brand of Chlorpheniramine and Phenylephrine—**See Antihistamines and Decongestants (Systemic)**, 343; Boots (U.S.) brand of Chlorpheniramine, Phenylephrine, Phenylpropanolamine, Atropine, Hyoscyamine, and Scopolamine—**See Antihistamines, Decongestants, and Anticholinergics (Systemic)**, 373

*Ru-Tuss DE*—Boots (U.S.) brand of Pseudoephedrine and Guaifenesin—**See Cough/Cold Combinations (Systemic)**, 1024

*Ru-Tuss Expectorant*—Boots (U.S.) brand of Pseudoephedrine, Dextromethorphan, and Guaifenesin—**See Cough/Cold Combinations (Systemic)**, 1024

*Ru-Tuss with Hydrocodone Liquid*—Boots (U.S.) brand of Pheniramine, Pyrilamine, Phenylephrine, Phenylpropanolamine, and Hydrocodone—**See Cough/Cold Combinations (Systemic)**, 1024

*RVA*—Rabies Vaccine Adsorbed—**See Rabies Vaccine (Systemic)**, 2449

R-VIII SQ [*REFACTO*] **(Systemic)**, 3163

*Rymed*—Edwards (U.S.) brand of Pseudoephedrine and Guaifenesin—**See Cough/Cold Combinations (Systemic)**, 1024

*Rymed Liquid*—Edwards (U.S.) brand of Pseudoephedrine and Guaifenesin—**See Cough/Cold Combinations (Systemic)**, 1024

*Rymed-TR Caplets*—Edwards (U.S.) brand of Phenylpropanolamine and Guaifenesin—**See Cough/Cold Combinations (Systemic)**, 1024

*Ryna*—Wallace (U.S.) brand of Chlorpheniramine and Pseudoephedrine—**See Antihistamines and Decongestants (Systemic)**, 343

*Ryna-C Liquid*—Wallace (U.S.) brand of Chlorpheniramine, Pseudoephedrine, and Codeine—**See Cough/Cold Combinations (Systemic)**, 1024

*Rynacrom*—Fisons (Canada) brand of Cromolyn (Nasal), 1118

*Ryna-CX Liquid*—Wallace (U.S.) brand of Pseudoephedrine, Codeine, and Guaifenesin—**See Cough/Cold Combinations (Systemic)**, 1024

*Rynatan*—Wallace (U.S.) brand of Chlorpheniramine, Pyrilamine, and Phenylephrine—**See Antihistamines and Decongestants (Systemic)**, 343, MC-6

*Rynatan Pediatric*—Wallace (U.S.) brand of Chlorpheniramine, Pyrilamine, and Phenylephrine—**See Antihistamines and Decongestants (Systemic)**, 343

*Rynatan-S Pediatric*—Wallace (U.S.) brand of Chlorpheniramine, Pyrilamine, and Phenylephrine—**See Antihistamines and Decongestants (Systemic)**, 343

*Rynatuss*—Wallace (U.S.) brand of Chlorpheniramine, Ephedrine, Phenylephrine, and Carbetapentane—**See Cough/Cold Combinations (Systemic)**, 1024

*Rynatuss Pediatric*—Wallace (U.S.) brand of Chlorpheniramine, Ephedrine, Phenylephrine, and Carbetapentane—**See Cough/Cold Combinations (Systemic)**, 1024

*Rythmodan*—Hoechst-Roussel (Canada) brand of Disopyramide (Systemic), 1252

*Rythmodan-LA*—Hoechst-Roussel (Canada) brand of Disopyramide (Systemic), 1252

*Rythmol*—Knoll (U.S. and Canada) brand of Propafenone (Systemic), 2413, MC-26

# S

*S-2*—Nephron (U.S.) brand of Epinephrine—**See Bronchodilators, Adrenergic (Inhalation-Local)**, 640

*642*—Frosst (Canada) brand of Propoxyphene—**See Opioid (Narcotic) Analgesics (Systemic)**, 2168

*692*—Frosst (Canada) brand of Propoxyphene and Aspirin—**See Opioid (Narcotic) Analgesics and Aspirin (Systemic)**, 2202

Sabin vaccine—Poliovirus Vaccine Live Oral—**See Poliovirus Vaccine (Systemic)**, 2343

*S-A-C*—Lannett (U.S.) brand of Acetaminophen, Salicylamide, and Caffeine—**See Acetaminophen and Salicylates (Systemic)**, 11

*Sacarasa*—Orphan Medical (U.S.) brand of Sucrase (Yeast-derived) (Systemic), 3166

Sacrosidase [*Sucraid*] **(Systemic)**, 3033
  Solution, Oral, 3033

S-Adenosylmethionine **(Systemic)**, 3163

*Safe Tussin 30*—Kramer (U.S.) brand of Dextromethorphan and Guaifenesin—**See Cough/Cold Combinations (Systemic)**, 1024

*Saizen*—Serono (U.S.) brand of Somatropin (Systemic), 3165; Serono (U.S.) brand of Somatropin, Recombinant (Systemic), 3035

*Salac*—GenDerm (U.S. and Canada) brand of Salicylic Acid (Topical), #

*Salacid*—Gordon (U.S.) brand of Salicylic Acid (Topical), #

*Sal-Acid Plaster*—Pedinol (U.S.) brand of Salicylic Acid (Topical), #

*Salactic Film Topical Solution*—Pedinol (U.S.) brand of Salicylic Acid (Topical), #

*Salagen*—MGI (U.S.) and Pharmacia & Upjohn (Canada) brand of Pilocarpine (Systemic), 2323, 3032, 3158

*Salazide*—Major (U.S.) brand of Reserpine and Hydroflumethiazide—**See Rauwolfia Alkaloids and Thiazide Diuretics (Systemic)**, #

*Salazopyrin*—Pharmacia (Canada) brand of Sulfasalazine (Systemic), 2643

*Salazopyrin EN-Tabs*—Pharmacia (Canada) brand of Sulfasalazine (Systemic), 2643

Salazosulfapyridine—**See Sulfasalazine (Systemic)**, 2643

Salbutamol—Albuterol—**See Bronchodilators, Adrenergic (Inhalation-Local)**, 640; **Bronchodilators, Adrenergic (Systemic)**, 651

*Sal-Clens Plus Shampoo*—C & M (U.S.) brand of Salicylic Acid (Topical), #

*Sal-Clens Shampoo*—C & M (U.S.) brand of Salicylic Acid (Topical), #

*Saleto*—Hauck (U.S.) brand of Acetaminophen, Aspirin, Salicylamide, and Caffeine—**See Acetaminophen and Salicylates (Systemic)**, 11

*Saleto-CF*—Roberts (U.S.) brand of Phenylpropanolamine, Dextromethorphan, and Acetaminophen—**See Cough/Cold Combinations (Systemic)**, 1024

*Saleto D Caplets*—Roberts (U.S.) brand of Phenylpropanolamine, Acetaminophen, Salicylamide, and Caffeine—**See Decongestants and Analgesics (Systemic)**, 1180

*Salflex*—Carnrick (U.S.) brand of Salsalate—**See Salicylates (Systemic)**, 2538

Salicylamide-containing Combinations, 3081

Salicylates **(Systemic)**, 2538

Salicylazosulfapyridine—**See Sulfasalazine (Systemic)**, 2643

Salicylic Acid [*Antinea; Buf-Puf Acne Cleansing Bar with Vitamin E; Calicylic Creme; Clearasil Clearstick Maximum Strength Topical Solution; Clearasil Clearstick Regular Strength Topical Solution; Clearasil Double Textured Pads Maximum Strength; Clearasil Double Textured Pads Regular Strength; Clearasil Medicated Deep Cleanser Topical Solution; Clear Away; Clear by Design Medicated Cleansing Pads; Compound W Gel; Compound W Liquid; Cuplex Gel; Duofilm; Duoplant Topical Solution; Freezone; Gordofilm; Hydrisalic; Ionax Astringent Skin Cleanser Topical Solution; Ionil Plus Shampoo; Ionil Shampoo; Keralyt; Keratex Gel; Lactisol; Listerex Golden Scrub Lotion; Listerex Herbal Scrub Lotion; Mediplast; Noxzema Anti-Acne Gel; Noxzema Anti-Acne Pads Maximum Strength; Noxzema Anti-Acne Pads Regular Strength; Occlusal-HP Topical Solution; Occlusal Topical Solution; Off-Ezy Topical Solution Corn & Callus Remover Kit; Off-Ezy Topical Solution Wart Removal Kit; Oxy Clean Extra Strength Medicated Pads; Oxy Clean Extra Strength Skin Cleanser Topical Solution; Oxy Clean Medicated Cleanser; Oxy Clean Medicated Pads Maximum Strength; Oxy Clean Medicated Pads Regular Strength; Oxy Clean Medicated Pads Sensitive Skin; Oxy Clean Medicated Soap; Oxy Clean Regular Strength Medicated Cleanser Topical Solution; Oxy Clean Regular Strength Medicated Pads; Oxy Clean Sensitive Skin Cleanser Topical Solution; Oxy Clean Sensitive Skin Pads; Oxy Night Watch Maximum Strength Lotion; Oxy Night Watch Night Time Acne Medication Extra Strength Lotion; Oxy Night Watch Night Time Acne Medication Regular Strength Lotion; Oxy Night Watch Sensitive Skin Lotion; Oxy Sensitive Skin Vanishing Formula Lotion; Paplex; Paplex Ultra; Propa pH Medicated Acne Cream Maximum Strength; Propa pH Medicated Cleansing Pads Maximum Strength; Propa pH Medicated Cleansing Pads Sensitive Skin; Propa pH Perfectly Clear Skin Cleanser Topical Solution Normal/Combination Skin; Propa pH Perfectly Clear Skin Cleanser Topical Solution Oily Skin; Propa pH Perfectly Clear Skin Cleanser Topical Solution Sensitive Skin Formula; P&S; Salac; Salacid; Sal-Acid Plaster; Salactic Film Topical Solution; Sal-Clens Plus Shampoo; Sal-Clens Shampoo; Saligel; Salonil; Sal-Plant Gel Topical Solution; Sebucare; Stri-Dex Dual Textured Pads Maximum Strength; Stri-Dex Dual Textured Pads Regular Strength; Stri-Dex Dual Textured Pads Sensitive Skin; Stri-Dex Maximum Strength Pads; Stri-Dex Regular Strength Pads; Stri-Dex Super Scrub Pads; Tersac Cleansing Gel; Trans-Plantar; Trans-Ver-Sal; Verukan-HP Topical Solution; Verukan Topical Solution; Viranol; Viranol Ultra; Wart-Off Topical Solution; X-Seb*]

**(Topical)**, #
  Cream, #
  Gel USP, #
  Lotion, #
  Ointment, #
  Pads, #
  Plaster USP, #
  Shampoo, #
  Soap; #
  Solution, Topical, #

Salicylic Acid-containing Combinations, 3082

Salicylic Acid and Sulfur [*Essential Care Creamy Dandruff Shampoo; Essential Care Medicated Dandruff Wash; Essential Care Maximum Strength Dandruff Shampoo; Meted; Pernox Lathering Abradant Scrub Cleanser (Fresh Scent); Pernox (Lemon); Pernox (Regular); SAStid Soap; Sebex; Sebulex; Sebulex with Conditioners; Sebulex (Regular)*]
**(Topical)**, #
Bar, #
Shampoo, #
Lotion, #
Salicylic Acid, Sulfur, and Coal Tar [*Sebex-T Tar Shampoo; Sebutone; Vanseb-T*]
**(Topical)**, #
Shampoo, Cream, #
Shampoo, Lotion, #
Salicylsalicylic acid—Salsalate—**See Salicylates (Systemic)**, 2538
*Saligel*—Stiefel (U.S.) brand of Salicylic Acid (Topical), #
Salk vaccine—Poliovirus Vaccine Inactivated—**See Poliovirus Vaccine (Systemic)**, 2343
Salmeterol Xinafoate [*Serevent*]
**See Bronchodilators, Adrenergic (Inhalation-Local)**, 640, 3034
Aerosol, Inhalation, 650, 3034
Powder for Inhalation, 650
*Salofalk*—Axcan (Canada) brand of Mesalamine (Oral-Local), 1952; (Rectal-Local), 1954
*Salonil*—Torch (U.S.) brand of Salicylic Acid (Topical), #
*Sal-Plant Gel Topical Solution*—Pedinol (U.S.) brand of Salicylic Acid (Topical), #
*Salprofen*—Farmacon (U.S.) brand of Ibuprofen (Systemic), 3146
Salsalate [*Amigesic; Anaflex 750; Disalcid; Marthritic; Mono-Gesic; Salflex;* salicylsalicylic acid; *Salsitab*]
**See Salicylates (Systemic)**, 2538
Capsules USP, 2553
Tablets USP, 2553, MC-27, MC-28
*Salsitab*—Upsher-Smith (U.S.) brand of Salsalate—**See Salicylates (Systemic)**, 2538
*Saluron*—Bristol (U.S.) brand of Hydroflumethiazide—**See Diuretics, Thiazide (Systemic)**, 1273
*Salutensin*—Bristol (U.S. and Canada) brand of Reserpine and Hydroflumethiazide—**See Rauwolfia Alkaloids and Thiazide Diuretics (Systemic)**, #
*Salutensin-Demi*—Bristol (U.S.) brand of Reserpine and Hydroflumethiazide—**See Rauwolfia Alkaloids and Thiazide Diuretics (Systemic)**, #
*Sandimmune*—Novartis (U.S. and Canada) brand of Cyclosporine (Systemic), 1136
*Sandimmune SGC*—Sandoz (U.S.) brand of Cyclosporine (Systemic), MC-8
*Sandoglobulin*—Sandoz (U.S.) brand of Immune Globulin Intravenous (Human) (Systemic), 1686
*Sandomigran*—Sandoz (Canada) brand of Pizotyline (Systemic), 3032
*Sandomigran DS*—Sandoz (Canada) brand of Pizotyline (Systemic), 3032
*SandoSource Peptide*—Sandoz (U.S.) brand of Enteral Nutrition Formula, Monomeric (Elemental)—**See Enteral Nutrition Formulas (Systemic)**, #
*Sandostatin*—Sandoz (U.S. and Canada) brand of Octreotide (Systemic), 2152
*Sani-Supp*—G & W (U.S.) brand of Glycerin—**See Laxatives (Local)**, #
*Sanorex*—Sandoz (U.S. and Canada) brand of Mazindol—**See Appetite Suppressants (Systemic)**, 452, 3153
*Sans-Acne*—Galderma (Canada) brand of Erythromycin (Topical), 1365
*Sansert*—Sandoz (U.S. and Canada) brand of Methysergide (Systemic), 1990
Saquinavir [*Fortovase*]
**(Systemic)**, 2554
Capsules (Soft Gelatin), 2557, MC-28
Saquinavir Mesylate [*Invirase*]
**(Systemic)**, 2554
Capsules, 2557, MC-28
Sargramostim [granulocyte-macrophage colony stimulating factor, recombinant; *Leukine*; recombinant human granulocyte-macrophage colony stimulating factor; rGM-CSF; rHu GM-CSF]
**See Colony Stimulating Factors (Systemic)**, 941, 3163
Injection, 946
for Injection, 945

*Sarisol No. 2*—Halsey (U.S.) brand of Butabarbital—**See Barbiturates (Systemic)**, 518
*Sarna HC 1.0%*—Stiefel (Canada) brand of Hydrocortisone—**See Corticosteroids (Topical)**, 978
*S.A.S.-500*—ICN (Canada) brand of Sulfasalazine (Systemic), 2643
*S.A.S. Enteric-500*—ICN (Canada) brand of Sulfasalazine (Systemic), 2643
*SAStid Soap*—Stiefel (U.S. and Canada) brand of Salicylic Acid and Sulfur (Topical), #
Satumomab Pendetide [*OncoScint CR/OV*] (Systemic), 3163
*Saxon Gold Rainbow Ultra Spermicidal*—Safetex (U.S.) brand of Latex Condoms and Nonoxynol 9—**See Condoms**, #
*Saxon Gold Ultra Sensitive*—Safetex (U.S.) brand of Latex Condoms—**See Condoms**, #
*Saxon Gold Ultra Spermicidal*—Safetex (U.S.) brand of Latex Condoms and Nonoxynol 9—**See Condoms**, #
*Scabene*—Stiefel (U.S.) brand of Lindane (Topical), 1866
*Scheinpharm Testone-Cyp*—Schein (Canada) brand of Testosterone—**See Androgens (Systemic)**, 118
*Sclerosol*—Bryan (U.S.) brand of Talc (Intrapleural-Local), #
Scopolamine [*Transderm-Scōp; Transderm-V*]
**See Anticholinergics/Antispasmodics (Systemic)**, 226
System, Transdermal, 240
Scopolamine Butylbromide [*Buscopan*]
**See Anticholinergics/Antispasmodics (Systemic)**, 226
Injection, 239
Suppositories, 240
Tablets, 239
Scopolamine-containing Combinations, 3082
Scopolamine Hydrobromide [hyoscine; *Isopto Hyoscine*]
**(Ophthalmic)**, 2557
Solution, Ophthalmic, USP, 2559
Scopolamine Hydrobromide [hyoscine hydrobromide]
**See Anticholinergics/Antispasmodics (Systemic)**, 226
Injection USP, 239
*Scot-Tussin DM*—Scot-Tussin (U.S.) brand of Chlorpheniramine and Dextromethorphan—**See Cough/Cold Combinations (Systemic)**, 1024
*Scot-tussin Expectorant*—Scot-Tussin (U.S.) brand of Guaifenesin (Systemic), 1588
*Scot-Tussin Original 5-Action Cold Formula*—Scot-Tussin (U.S.) brand of Pheniramine, Phenylephrine, Sodium Salicylate, and Caffeine—**See Antihistamines, Decongestants, and Analgesics (Systemic)**, 366
*Scot-Tussin Senior Clear*—Scot-Tussin (U.S.) brand of Dextromethorphan and Guaifenesin—**See Cough/Cold Combinations (Systemic)**, 1024
*Scrostim*—Serono (U.S.) brand of Somatropin (Systemic), 3166
*SD Deprenyl*—Shulman (Canada) brand of Selegiline (Systemic), 2560
*SD Polygam*—Baxter (U.S.) brand of Immune Globulin Intravenous (Human) (Systemic), 3025
Sea snake antivenom—**See Antivenin (Enhydrina Schistosa) (Systemic)**, #
Sea wasp antivenom—**See Antivenin (Chironex Fleckeri) (Systemic)**, #
*Seba-Nil Liquid Cleanser*—Owen (U.S.) brand of Alcohol and Acetone (Topical), #
*Sebex*—Rugby (U.S.) brand of Pyrithione (Topical), #; Rugby (U.S.) brand of Salicylic Acid and Sulfur (Topical), #
*Sebex-T Tar Shampoo*—Rugby (U.S.) brand of Salicylic Acid, Sulfur, and Coal Tar (Topical), #
*Sebucare*—Westwood (U.S.) brand of Salicylic Acid (Topical), #
*Sebulex*—Westwood-Squibb (Canada) brand of Salicylic Acid and Sulfur (Topical), #
*Sebulex with Conditioners*—Westwood-Squibb (U.S.) brand of Salicylic Acid and Sulfur (Topical), #
*Sebulex (Regular)*—Westwood-Squibb (U.S.) brand of Salicylic Acid and Sulfur (Topical), #
*Sebulon*—Westwood (U.S.) and Westwood-Squibb (Canada) brand of Pyrithione (Topical), #
*Sebutone*—Westwood (U.S.) and Westwood-Squibb (Canada) brand of Salicylic Acid, Sulfur, and Coal Tar (Topical), #
Secalciferol [*Osteo-D*]
**(Systemic)**, 3163
Secobarbital-containing Combinations, 3082

Secobarbital Sodium [*Novosecobarb; Seconal*]
**See Barbiturates (Systemic)**, 518
Capsules USP, 530
Injection USP, 530
Secobarbital Sodium and Amobarbital Sodium [*Tuinal*]
**See Barbiturates (Systemic)**, 518
Capsules USP, 530
*Seconal*—Lilly (U.S. and Canada) brand of Secobarbital—**See Barbiturates (Systemic)**, 518
Secretory Leukocyte Protease Inhibitor (Systemic), 3164
*Sectral*—Wyeth-Ayerst (U.S.) and Rhône-Poulenc (Canada) brand of Acebutolol—**See Beta-adrenergic Blocking Agents (Systemic)**, 593, MC-1
*Sedapap*—Mayrand (U.S.) brand of Butalbital and Acetaminophen—**See Barbiturates and Analgesics (Systemic)**, 532
*Sedatuss*—Trianon (Canada) brand of Dextromethorphan (Systemic), 1191
*Seldane*—Marion Merrell Dow (Canada) brand of Terfenadine—**See Antihistamines (Systemic)**, 325
*Seldane Caplets*—Marion Merrell Dow (Canada) brand of Terfenadine—**See Antihistamines (Systemic)**, 325
*Selegiline-5*—Pro-Doc (Canada) brand of Selegiline (Systemic), 2560
Selegiline Hydrochloride [*Apo-Selegiline; Carbex*; deprenil; deprenyl; *Eldepryl; Gen-Selegiline; Novo-Selegiline; Nu-Selegiline; SD Deprenyl; Selegiline-5*]
**(Systemic)**, 2560, 3164
Capsules, 2562, MC-28
Tablets USP, 2562, MC-28
Selenious Acid [*Sele-Pak; Selepen*]
**See Selenium Supplements (Systemic)**, 2563
Injection USP, 2564
Selenium
**See Selenium Supplements (Systemic)**, 2563
Tablets, 2564
Selenium Sulfide [*Exsel Lotion Shampoo; Glo-Sel; Head & Shoulders Intensive Treatment Conditioning Formula Dandruff Lotion Shampoo; Head & Shoulders Intensive Treatment Regular Formula Dandruff Lotion Shampoo; Head & Shoulders Intensive Treatment 2 in 1 (Persistent Dandruff Shampoo plus Conditioner in One) Formula Dandruff Lotion Shampoo; Selsun; Selsun Blue; Selsun Blue Dry Formula; Selsun Blue Extra Conditioning Formula; Selsun Blue Extra Medicated Formula; Selsun Blue Oily Formula; Selsun Blue Regular Formula; Versel Lotion*]
**(Topical)**, #
Lotion USP, #
Selenium Supplements
**(Systemic)**, 2563
*Sele-Pak*—Smith & Nephew SoloPak (U.S.) brand of Selenious Acid—**See Selenium Supplements (Systemic)**, 2563
*Selepen*—LyphoMed (U.S.) brand of Selenious Acid—**See Selenium Supplements (Systemic)**, 2563
*Selestoject*—Mayrand (U.S.) brand of Betamethasone—**See Corticosteroids—Glucocorticoid Effects (Systemic)**, 998
*Selexid*—Leo (Canada) brand of Pivmecillinam—**See Penicillins (Systemic)**, 2240
*Selsun*—Ross (U.S.) and Abbott (Canada) brand of Selenium Sulfide (Topical), #
*Selsun Blue*—Abbott (Canada) brand of Selenium Sulfide (Topical), #
*Selsun Blue Dry Formula*—Ross (U.S.) brand of Selenium Sulfide (Topical), #
*Selsun Blue Extra Conditioning Formula*—Ross (U.S.) and Abbott (Canada) brand of Selenium Sulfide (Topical), #
*Selsun Blue Extra Medicated Formula*—Ross (U.S.) brand of Selenium Sulfide (Topical), #
*Selsun Blue Oily Formula*—Ross (U.S.) brand of Selenium Sulfide (Topical), #
*Selsun Blue Regular Formula*—Ross (U.S.) brand of Selenium Sulfide (Topical), #
*Semicid*—Whitehall (U.S.) brand of Nonoxynol 9—**See Spermicides (Vaginal)**, #
*Semilente Insulin*—Connaught Novo Nordisk (Canada) brand of Insulin Zinc, Prompt—**See Insulin (Systemic)**, 1713
Semilente insulin—Insulin Zinc, Prompt—**See Insulin (Systemic)**, 1713

# General Index

*Semprex-D*—Adams (U.S.) and Glaxo Wellcome (U.S.) brand of Acrivastine and Pseudoephedrine—**See Antihistamines and Decongestants (Systemic)**, 343, AP-23
*Senexon*—Rugby (U.S.) brand of Senna—**See Laxatives (Local)**, #
Senna [*Black-Draught Lax-Senna; Correctol Herbal Tea; Dosaflex; Dr. Caldwell Senna Laxative; Fletcher's Castoria; Herbal Laxative; Senexon; Senna-Gen; Senokot; Senolax; X-Prep Liquid*]
 **See Laxatives (Local)**, #
 Granules, #
 Solution, Oral, #
 for Solution, Oral, #
 Suppositories, #
 Syrup USP, #
 Tablets, #
Senna-containing Combinations, 3082
*Senna-Gen*—Zenith Goldline (U.S.) brand of Senna—**See Laxatives (Local)**, #
Sennosides [*Ex-Lax Gentle Nature Pills; Fletcher's Castoria; Glysennid; Herbal Laxative; Nytilax; PMS-Sennosides; Senokot; Senokot Children's Syrup; SenokotXTRA*]
 **See Laxatives (Local)**, #
 Granules, #
 Solution, Oral, #
 Syrup, #
 Syrup USP, #
 Tablets, #
 Tablets USP, #
Sennosides-containing Combinations, 3082
Sennosides and Docusate Sodium [*Senokot-S*]
 **See Laxatives (Local)**, #
 Tablets, #
*Senokot*—Purdue Frederick (U.S. and Canada) brand of Sennosides—**See Laxatives (Local)**, #
*Senokot Children's Syrup*—Purdue Frederick (U.S.) brand of Sennosides—**See Laxatives (Local)**, #
*Senokot-S*—Purdue Frederick (U.S. and Canada) brand of Sennosides and Docusate—**See Laxatives (Local)**, #
*SenokotXTRA*—Purdue Frederick (U.S. and Canada) brand of Sennosides—**See Laxatives (Local)**, #
*Senolax*—Schein (U.S.) brand of Senna—**See Laxatives (Local)**, #
*SensoGARD Canker Sore Relief*—Dentco (U.S.) brand of Benzocaine—**See Anesthetics (Mucosal-Local)**, 128
*Sensorcaine*—Astra (U.S.) brand of Bupivacaine—**See Anesthetics (Parenteral-Local)**, 139
*Sensorcaine-Forte*—Astra (U.S.) brand of Bupivacaine—**See Anesthetics (Parenteral-Local)**, 139
*Sensorcaine-MPF*—Astra (U.S.) brand of Bupivacaine—**See Anesthetics (Parenteral-Local)**, 139
*Sensorcaine-MPF Spinal*—Astra (U.S.) brand of Bupivacaine—**See Anesthetics (Parenteral-Local)**, 139
*Sential*—Pharmacia (Canada) brand of Hydrocortisone—**See Corticosteroids (Topical)**, 978; Hydrocortisone and Urea (Topical), 3023
*Septopal*—EM (U.S.) brand of Gentamicin Impregnated PMMA Beads on Surgical Wire (Systemic), 3144
*Septra*—Glaxo Wellcome (U.S.) and BW (Canada) brand of Sulfamethoxazole and Trimethoprim—**See Sulfonamides and Trimethoprim (Systemic)**, 2661
*Septra DS*—Glaxo Wellcome (U.S.) and BW (Canada) brand of Sulfamethoxazole and Trimethoprim—**See Sulfonamides and Trimethoprim (Systemic)**, 2661
*Septra I.V.*—BW (U.S.) brand of Sulfamethoxazole and Trimethoprim—**See Sulfonamides and Trimethoprim (Systemic)**, 2661
*Septra Pediatric*—BW (U.S.) brand of Sulfamethoxazole and Trimethoprim—**See Sulfonamides and Trimethoprim (Systemic)**, 2661
*Ser-A-Gen*—Goldline (U.S.) brand of Reserpine, Hydralazine, and Hydrochlorothiazide (Systemic), #
*Seralazide*—Lannett (U.S.) brand of Reserpine, Hydralazine and Hydrochlorothiazide (Systemic), #
*Ser-Ap-Es*—Novartis (U.S. and Canada) brand of Reserpine, Hydralazine, and Hydrochlorothiazide (Systemic), #, MC-27
*Serax*—Wyeth-Ayerst (U.S.) and Wyeth (Canada) brand of Oxazepam—**See Benzodiazepines (Systemic)**, 556, MC-23

*Serentil*—Boehringer Ingelheim (U.S.) and Sandoz (Canada) brand of Mesoridazine—**See Phenothiazines (Systemic)**, 2289, MC-18
*Serentil Concentrate*—Boehringer Ingelheim (U.S.) brand of Mesoridazine—**See Phenothiazines (Systemic)**, 2289
*Serevent*—Allen & Hanburys (U.S.) and Glaxo (U.S. and Canada) brand of Salmeterol—**See Bronchodilators, Adrenergic (Inhalation-Local)**, 640, 3034
Sermorelin Acetate [*Geref*]
 **(Systemic)**, 2565, 3164
 for Injection, 2566
*Sero-Gesic*—Magnesium Salicylate—**See Salicylates (Systemic)**, 2538
*Seromycin*—Lilly (U.S.) brand of Cycloserine (Systemic), 1134
*Serophene*—Serono (U.S.) and Pharmascience (Canada) brand of Clomiphene (Systemic), 903
*Seroquel*—ZENECA (U.S.) brand of Quetiapine (Systemic), 2437, MC-27; ZENECA (Canada) brand of Quetiapine (Systemic), 3033
*Serostim*—Serono (U.S.) brand of Somatropin, Recombinant (Systemic), 3035
*Serpalan*—Lannett (U.S.) brand of Reserpine—**See Rauwolfia Alkaloids (Systemic)**, 2460
*Serpasil*—Ciba (Canada) brand of Reserpine—**See Rauwolfia Alkaloids (Systemic)**, 2460
*Serpazide*—Major (U.S.) brand of Reserpine, Hydralazine, and Hydrochlorothiazide (Systemic), #
Serratia Marcescens Extract (Polyribosomes) [*ImuVert*]
 **(Systemic)**, 3164
*Sertan*—Pharmascience (Canada) brand of Primidone (Systemic), 2376
Sertraline Hydrochloride [*Zoloft*]
 **(Systemic)**, 2566
 Capsules, 2570
 Tablets, 2570, MC-28
*Serutan*—Menley & James (U.S.) brand of Psyllium Hydrophilic Mucilloid—**See Laxatives (Local)**, #
*Serutan Toasted Granules*—Menley & James (U.S.) brand of Psyllium Hydrophilic Mucilloid and Carboxymethylcellulose—**See Laxatives (Local)**, #
*Serzone*—Bristol-Myers Squibb (U.S. and Canada) brand of Nefazodone (Systemic), 2092, 3029, MC-21
Sevoflurane [*Sevorane; Ultane*]
 **(Inhalation-Systemic)**, #
 Inhalation, #
*Sevorane*—Abbott (Canada) brand of Sevoflurane (Inhalation-Systemic), #
*Shade Oil-Free*—Schering-Plough (U.S.) brand of Homosalate, Octyl Methoxycinnamate, and Oxybenzone—**See Sunscreen Agents (Topical)**, #
*Shade Sunblock*—Schering-Plough (U.S.) brand of Homosalate, Octyl Methoxycinnamate, Octyl Salicylate, and Oxybenzone—**See Sunscreen Agents (Topical)**, #; Octocrylene, Octyl Methoxycinnamate, Octyl Salicylate, and Oxybenzone—**See Sunscreen Agents (Topical)**, #
*Shade Sunblock Oil-Free*—Schering-Plough (U.S.) brand of Octyl Methoxycinnamate, Octyl Salicylate, and Oxybenzone—**See Sunscreen Agents (Topical)**, #
*Shade UVA Guard*—Schering-Plough (U.S.) brand of Avobenzone, Octyl Methoxycinnamate, and Oxybenzone—**See Sunscreen Agents (Topical)**, #
*Shade Waterproof Sunblock*—Schering-Plough (U.S. and Canada) brand of Octocrylene, Octyl Methoxycinnamate, Octyl Salicylate, and Oxybenzone—**See Sunscreen Agents (Topical)**, #
*206 Shake*—Menu Magic (U.S.) brand of Enteral Nutrition Formula, Milk-based—**See Enteral Nutrition Formulas (Systemic)**, #
*Sheik Classic Lubricated*—Schmid (U.S.) brand of Latex Condoms—**See Condoms**, #
*Sheik Classic Non-Lubricated*—Schmid (U.S.) brand of Latex Condoms—**See Condoms**, #
*Sheik Classic Spermicidally Lubricated*—Schmid (U.S.) brand of Latex Condoms and Nonoxynol 9—**See Condoms**, #
*Sheik Denim*—Schmid (Canada) brand of Latex Condoms—**See Condoms**, #
*Sheik Elite*—Schmid (Canada) brand of Latex Condoms and Nonoxynol 9—**See Condoms**, #
*Sheik Excita*—Schmid (Canada) brand of Latex Condoms and Nonoxynol 9—**See Condoms**, #
*Sheik Excita Extra*—Schmid (U.S.) brand of Latex Condoms and Nonoxynol 9—**See Condoms**, #
*Sheik Fiesta Colors*—Schmid (U.S.) brand of Latex Condoms—**See Condoms**, #

*Sheik Non-Lubricated*—Schmid (Canada) brand of Latex Condoms—**See Condoms**, #
*Sheik Sensi-Creme*—Schmid (Canada) brand of Latex Condoms—**See Condoms**, #
*Sheik Super Thin Lubricated*—Schmid (U.S.) brand of Latex Condoms—**See Condoms**, #
*Sheik Super Thin Ribbed Lubricated*—Schmid (U.S.) brand of Latex Condoms—**See Condoms**, #
*Sheik Super Thin Ribbed Spermicidally Lubricated*—Schmid (U.S.) brand of Latex Condoms and Nonoxynol 9—**See Condoms**, #
*Sheik Super Thin Spermicidally Lubricated*—Schmid (U.S.) brand of Latex Condoms and Nonoxynol 9—**See Condoms**, #
*Sheik Thin Lub*—Schmid (Canada) brand of Latex Condoms—**See Condoms**, #
*Sheik Thin Spermicidal Lub*—Schmid (Canada) brand of Latex Condoms and Nonoxynol 9—**See Condoms**, #
*Shellcap*—HTD Pharm (U.S.) brand of Brompheniramine and Pseudoephedrine—**See Antihistamines and Decongestants (Systemic)**, 343
*Shellcap PD*—HTD Pharm (U.S.) brand of Brompheniramine and Pseudoephedrine—**See Antihistamines and Decongestants (Systemic)**, 343
*Shield Burnasept Spray*—Canadian Custom Packaging (Canada) brand of Benzocaine—**See Anesthetics (Topical)**, 155
*Shogan*—Shoals (U.S.) brand of Promethazine—**See Antihistamines, Phenothiazine-derivative (Systemic)**, 377
*Shovite*—Shoals (U.S.) brand of Cyanocobalamin—**See Vitamin B$_{12}$ (Systemic)**, 2962
*Shur-Seal*—Milex (U.S.) brand of Nonoxynol 9—**See Spermicides (Vaginal)**, #
*Sibelium*—Janssen (U.S. and Canada) brand of Flunarizine—**See Calcium Channel Blocking Agents (Systemic)**, 720, 3143
Sibutramine Hydrochloride Monohydrate [*Meridia*]
 **(Systemic)**, 2571
 Capsules, 2574, MC-28
*Silace*—Silarx (U.S. and Canada) brand of Docusate—**See Laxatives (Local)**, #
*Silace-C*—Silarx (U.S.) brand of Casthranol and Docusate—**See Laxatives (Local)**, #
*Siladryl*—Silarx (U.S.) brand of Diphenhydramine—**See Antihistamines (Systemic)**, 325
*Silafed*—Silarx (U.S.) brand of Triprolidine and Pseudoephedrine—**See Antihistamines and Decongestants (Systemic)**, 343
*Silaminic*—Silarx (U.S.) brand of Chlorpheniramine and Phenylpropanolamine—**See Antihistamines and Decongestants (Systemic)**, 343
*Silaminic Expectorant*—Silarx (U.S.) brand of Phenylpropanolamine and Guaifenesin—**See Cough/Cold Combinations (Systemic)**, 1024
*Sildec-DM*—Silarx (U.S.) brand of Carbinoxamine, Pseudoephedrine, and Dextromethorphan—**See Cough/Cold Combinations (Systemic)**, 1024
*Sildec-DM Oral Drops*—Silarx (U.S.) brand of Carbinoxamine, Pseudoephedrine, and Dextromethorphan—**See Cough/Cold Combinations (Systemic)**, 1024
Sildenafil Citrate [*Viagra*]
 **(Systemic)**, 2574
 Tablets, 2577, MC-28
*Sildicon-E Pediatric Drops*—Silarx (U.S.) brand of Phenylpropanolamine and Guaifenesin—**See Cough/Cold Combinations (Systemic)**, 1024
*Sildimac*—Marion (U.S.) brand of Silver Sulfadiazine (Topical), #
*Silexin Cough*—Otis Clapp (U.S.) brand of Dextromethorphan and Guaifenesin—**See Cough/Cold Combinations (Systemic)**, 1024
Silicone Oil 5000 Centistokes [*AdatoSil 5000*; polydimethylsiloxane]
 **(Parenteral-Local)**, #
 for Injection, #
*Siltapp with Dextromethorphan Cough & Cold*—Silarx (U.S.) brand of Brompheniramine, Phenylpropanolamine, and Dextromethorphan—**See Cough/Cold Combinations (Systemic)**, 1024
*Sil-Tex*—Silarx (U.S.) brand of Phenylephrine, Phenylpropanolamine, and Guaifenesin—**See Cough/Cold Combinations (Systemic)**, 1024
*Siltussin-CF*—Silarx (U.S.) brand of Phenylpropanolamine, Dextromethorphan, and Guaifenesin—**See Cough/Cold Combinations (Systemic)**, 1024

*Siltussin DM*—Silarx (U.S.) brand of Dextromethorphan and Guaifenesin—**See Cough/Cold Combinations (Systemic)**, 1024
*Silvadene*—Marion Merrell Dow (U.S.) brand of Silver Sulfadiazine (Topical), #
Silver Sulfadiazine [*Flamazine; Flint SSD; Sildimac; Silvadene; SSD; SSD AF; Thermazene*] **(Topical)**, #
  Cream USP, #
*Simaal Gel*—Schein (U.S.) brand of Alumina, Magnesia, and Simethicone—**See Antacids (Oral-Local)**, 188
*Simaal 2 Gel*—Schein (U.S.) brand of Alumina, Magnesia, and Simethicone—**See Antacids (Oral-Local)**, 188
Simethicone [*Baby's Own Infant Drops; Degas; Extra Strength Maalox Anti-Gas; Extra Strength Maalox GRF Gas Relief Formula; Flatulex; Gas Relief; Gas-X; Gas-X Extra Strength; Genasyme; Maalox Anti-Gas; Maalox GRF Gas Relief Formula; Maximum Strength Gas Relief; Maximum Strength Mylanta Gas Relief; Maximum Strength Phazyme; My Baby Gas Relief Drops; Mylanta Gas; Mylanta Gas Relief; Mylicon Drops; Ovol; Ovol-40; Ovol-80; Ovol-160; Phazyme; Phazyme-95; Phazyme-125; Phazyme Drops*] **(Oral-Local)**, #
  Capsules USP, #
  Suspension, Oral, USP, #
  Tablets USP, #
  Tablets USP (Chewable), #
Simethicone-containing Combinations, 3082
*Similac 13*—Ross (U.S. and Canada) brand of Infant Formulas, Milk-based—**See Infant Formulas (Systemic)**, #
*Similac 20*—Ross (U.S. and Canada) brand of Infant Formulas, Milk-based—**See Infant Formulas (Systemic)**, #
*Similac 24*—Ross (U.S. and Canada) brand of Infant Formulas, Milk-based—**See Infant Formulas (Systemic)**, #
*Similac 27*—Ross (U.S. and Canada) brand of Infant Formulas, Milk-based—**See Infant Formulas (Systemic)**, #
*Similac with Iron 20*—Ross (U.S.) brand of Infant Formulas, Milk-based—**See Infant Formulas (Systemic)**, #
*Similac with Iron 24*—Ross (U.S.) brand of Infant Formulas, Milk-based—**See Infant Formulas (Systemic)**, #
*Similac Natural Care Human Milk Fortifier*—Ross (U.S.) brand of Infant Formulas, Milk-based—**See Infant Formulas (Systemic)**, #
*Similac PM 60/40*—Ross (U.S. and Canada) brand of Infant Formulas, Milk-based—**See Infant Formulas (Systemic)**, #
*Similac Special Care 20*—Ross (U.S. and Canada) brand of Infant Formulas, Milk-based—**See Infant Formulas (Systemic)**, #
*Similac Special Care 24*—Ross (U.S. and Canada) brand of Infant Formulas, Milk-based—**See Infant Formulas (Systemic)**, #
*Similac Special Care with Iron 24*—Ross (U.S.) brand of Infant Formulas, Milk-based—**See Infant Formulas (Systemic)**, #
*Simplet*—Major (U.S.) brand of Chlorpheniramine, Pseudoephedrine, and Acetaminophen—**See Antihistamines, Decongestants, and Analgesics (Systemic)**, 366
*Simron*—Merrell Dow (U.S.) brand of Ferrous Gluconate—**See Iron Supplements (Systemic)**, 1774
*Simulect*—Novartis (U.S.) brand of Basiliximab (Systemic), 547
Simvastatin [*epistatin; synvinolin; Zocor*]
  **See HMG-CoA Reductase Inhibitors (Systemic)**, 1647
  Tablets, 1651, MC-28
*Sinapils*—Pfeiffer (U.S.) brand of Chlorpheniramine, Phenylpropanolamine, Acetaminophen, and Caffeine—**See Antihistamines, Decongestants, and Analgesics (Systemic)**, 366
*Sinarest*—Ciba Self-Medication (U.S.) brand of Chlorpheniramine, Pseudoephedrine, and Acetaminophen—**See Antihistamines, Decongestants, and Analgesics (Systemic)**, 366
*Sinarest Extra Strength Caplets*—Ciba Self-Medication (U.S.) brand of Chlorpheniramine, Pseudoephedrine, and Acetaminophen—**See Antihistamines, Decongestants, and Analgesics (Systemic)**, 366
*Sinarest 12 Hour Nasal Spray*—Ciba-Consumer (U.S.) brand of Oxymetazoline (Nasal), #

*Sinarest No-Drowsiness Caplets*—Ciba (U.S.) brand of Pseudoephedrine and Acetaminophen—**See Decongestants and Analgesics (Systemic)**, 1180
Sincalide [*Kinevac*] **(Systemic)**, #
  for Injection, #
*Sine-Aid IB Caplets*—McNeil (U.S.) brand of Pseudoephedrine and Ibuprofen—**See Decongestants and Analgesics (Systemic)**, 1180
*Sine-Aid Maximum Strength*—McNeil (U.S.) brand of Pseudoephedrine and Acetaminophen—**See Decongestants and Analgesics (Systemic)**, 1180
*Sine-Aid Maximum Strength Caplets*—McNeil (U.S.) brand of Pseudoephedrine and Acetaminophen—**See Decongestants and Analgesics (Systemic)**, 1180
*Sine-Aid Maximum Strength Gelcaps*—McNeil (U.S.) brand of Pseudoephedrine and Acetaminophen—**See Decongestants and Analgesics (Systemic)**, 1180
*Sinemet*—Du Pont (U.S. and Canada) brand of Carbidopa and Levodopa (Systemic), 765, MC-5
*Sinemet CR*—Du Pont (U.S. and Canada) brand of Carbidopa and Levodopa (Systemic), 765, MC-5
*Sine-Off Maximum Strength No Drowsiness Formula Caplets*—SmithKline (U.S.) brand of Pseudoephedrine and Acetaminophen—**See Decongestants and Analgesics (Systemic)**, 1180
*Sine-Off Sinus Medicine Caplets*—SmithKline Beecham (U.S.) brand of Chlorpheniramine, Pseudoephedrine, and Acetaminophen—**See Antihistamines, Decongestants, and Analgesics (Systemic)**, 366
*Sinequan*—Roerig (U.S. and Canada) brand of Doxepin—**See Antidepressants, Tricyclic (Systemic)**, 271, MC-10
*Singlet for Adults*—SmithKline Beecham (U.S.) brand of Chlorpheniramine, Pseudoephedrine, and Acetaminophen—**See Antihistamines, Decongestants, and Analgesics (Systemic)**, 366
*Singulair*—Merck (U.S.) brand of Montelukast (Systemic), 2057, MC-20
*Sinografin*—Squibb (U.S. and Canada) brand of Diatrizoate and Iodipamide (Local), #
*Sintrom*—Geigy (Canada) brand of Acenocoumarol (Systemic), 3009
*Sinucon*—Zenith Goldline (U.S.) brand of Chlorpheniramine, Phenyltoloxamine, Phenylephrine, and Phenylpropanolamine—**See Antihistamines and Decongestants (Systemic)**, 343
*Sinucon Pediatric Drops*—Zenith Goldline (U.S.) brand of Chlorpheniramine, Phenyltoloxamine, Phenylephrine, and Phenylpropanolamine—**See Antihistamines and Decongestants (Systemic)**, 343
*Sinucon Pediatric Syrup*—Zenith Goldline (U.S.) brand of Chlorpheniramine, Phenyltoloxamine, Phenylephrine, and Phenylpropanolamine—**See Antihistamines and Decongestants (Systemic)**, 343
*Sinufed Timecelles*—Roberts (U.S.) brand of Pseudoephedrine and Guaifenesin—**See Cough/Cold Combinations (Systemic)**, 1024
*Sinulin*—Carnrick (U.S.) brand of Chlorpheniramine, Phenylpropanolamine, and Acetaminophen—**See Antihistamines, Decongestants, and Analgesics (Systemic)**, 366
*Sinumist-SR*—Roberts/Hauck (U.S.) brand of Guaifenesin (Systemic), 1588
*Sinupan*—Ion (U.S.) brand of Phenylephrine and Guaifenesin—**See Cough/Cold Combinations (Systemic)**, 1024
*Sinus Excedrin Extra Strength*—Bristol-Myers (U.S.) brand of Pseudoephedrine and Acetaminophen—**See Decongestants and Analgesics (Systemic)**, 1180
*Sinus Excedrin Extra Strength Caplets*—Bristol-Myers (U.S.) brand of Pseudoephedrine and Acetaminophen—**See Decongestants and Analgesics (Systemic)**, 1180
*Sinus Headache & Congestion*—Rugby (U.S.) brand of Chlorpheniramine, Pseudoephedrine, and Acetaminophen—**See Antihistamines, Decongestants, and Analgesics (Systemic)**, 366
*Sinus-Relief*—Major (U.S.) brand of Pseudoephedrine and Acetaminophen—**See Decongestants and Analgesics (Systemic)**, 1180
*Sinutab with Codeine*—Warner Wellcome (Canada) brand of Chlorpheniramine, Pseudoephedrine, Codeine, and Acetaminophen—**See Cough/Cold Combinations (Systemic)**, 1024

*Sinutab Extra Strength Caplets*—Warner Wellcome (Canada) brand of Chlorpheniramine, Pseudoephedrine, and Acetaminophen—**See Antihistamines, Decongestants, and Analgesics (Systemic)**, 366
*Sinutab No Drowsiness Caplets*—Warner Wellcome (Canada) brand of Pseudoephedrine and Acetaminophen—**See Decongestants and Analgesics (Systemic)**, 1180
*Sinutab No Drowsiness Extra Strength Caplets*—Warner Wellcome (Canada) brand of Pseudoephedrine and Acetaminophen—**See Decongestants and Analgesics (Systemic)**, 1180
*Sinutab Non-Drying No Drowsiness Liquid Caps*—Warner Wellcome (U.S.) brand of Pseudoephedrine and Guaifenesin—**See Cough/Cold Combinations (Systemic)**, 1024
*Sinutab Regular Caplets*—Warner Wellcome (Canada) brand of Chlorpheniramine, Pseudoephedrine, and Acetaminophen—**See Antihistamines, Decongestants, and Analgesics (Systemic)**, 366
*Sinutab SA*—Warner Wellcome (Canada) brand of Phenyltoloxamine, Phenylpropanolamine, and Acetaminophen—**See Antihistamines, Decongestants, and Analgesics (Systemic)**, 366
*Sinutab Sinus Allergy Maximum Strength*—Warner Wellcome (U.S.) brand of Chlorpheniramine, Pseudoephedrine, and Acetaminophen—**See Antihistamines, Decongestants, and Analgesics (Systemic)**, 366
*Sinutab Sinus Allergy Maximum Strength Caplets*—Warner Wellcome (U.S.) brand of Chlorpheniramine, Pseudoephedrine, and Acetaminophen—**See Antihistamines, Decongestants, and Analgesics (Systemic)**, 366
*Sinutab Sinus Maximum Strength Without Drowsiness*—Warner Wellcome (U.S.) brand of Pseudoephedrine and Acetaminophen—**See Decongestants and Analgesics (Systemic)**, 1180
*Sinutab Sinus Maximum Strength Without Drowsiness Caplets*—Warner Wellcome (U.S.) brand of Pseudoephedrine and Acetaminophen—**See Decongestants and Analgesics (Systemic)**, 1180
*Sinutrol 500 Caplets*—Quintex (U.S.) brand of Pseudoephedrine and Acetaminophen—**See Decongestants and Analgesics (Systemic)**, 1180
*SINUvent*—WE Pharm (U.S.) brand of Phenylpropanolamine and Guaifenesin—**See Cough/Cold Combinations (Systemic)**, 1024
*Skelaxin*—Carnrick (U.S.) brand of Metaxalone—**See Skeletal Muscle Relaxants (Systemic)**, 2577
Skeletal Muscle Relaxants **(Systemic)**, 2577
*Skelex*—Hauck (U.S.) brand of Methocarbamol—**See Skeletal Muscle Relaxants (Systemic)**, 2577
*Skelid*—Sanofi (U.S.) brand of Tiludronate (Systemic), 2822
*Sleep-Eze D*—Whitehall (U.S.) brand of Diphenhydramine—**See Antihistamines (Systemic)**, 325
*Sleep-Eze D Extra Strength*—Whitehall (U.S.) brand of Diphenhydramine—**See Antihistamines (Systemic)**, 325
*Slo-Bid Gyrocaps*—Rhône-Poulenc Rorer (U.S.) brand of Theophylline—**See Bronchodilators, Theophylline (Systemic)**, 668, MC-29
*Slo-Niacin*—Upsher-Smith (U.S.) brand of Niacin—**See Niacin (Systemic)**, 2116, MC-21
*Slo-Phyllin*—Rhône-Poulenc Rorer (U.S.) brand of Theophylline—**See Bronchodilators, Theophylline (Systemic)**, 668, MC-29
*Slo-Phyllin GG*—Rhône-Poulenc Rorer (U.S.) brand of Theophylline and Guaifenesin (Systemic), #
*Sloprin*—Aspirin—**See Salicylates (Systemic)**, 2538
*Slow Fe*—Ciba (U.S.) and Ciba-Geigy (Canada) brand of Ferrous Sulfate—**See Iron Supplements (Systemic)**, 1774
*Slow-K*—Summit (U.S.) and Ciba (Canada) brand of Potassium Chloride—**See Potassium Supplements (Systemic)**, 2357, MC-25
*Slow-Mag*—Searle (U.S.) brand of Magnesium Chloride—**See Magnesium Supplements (Systemic)**, 1897
*Slow-Trasicor*—Ciba (Canada) brand of Oxprenolol—**See Beta-adrenergic Blocking Agents (Systemic)**, 593
*SMA 13*—Wyeth (U.S. and Canada) brand of Infant Formulas, Milk-based—**See Infant Formulas (Systemic)**, #
*SMA 20*—Wyeth (U.S. and Canada) brand of Infant Formulas, Milk-based—**See Infant Formulas (Systemic)**, #

SMA 24—Wyeth (U.S. and Canada) brand of Infant Formulas, Milk-based—**See Infant Formulas (Systemic)**, #
SMA 27—Wyeth (U.S. and Canada) brand of Infant Formulas, Milk-based—**See Infant Formulas (Systemic)**, #
SMA Lo-Iron 13—Wyeth (U.S. and Canada) brand of Infant Formulas, Milk-based—**See Infant Formulas (Systemic)**, #
SMA Lo-Iron 20—Wyeth (U.S. and Canada) brand of Infant Formulas, Milk-based—**See Infant Formulas (Systemic)**, #
SMA Lo-Iron 24—Wyeth (U.S. and Canada) brand of Infant Formulas, Milk-based—**See Infant Formulas (Systemic)**, #
Smelling salts—See Ammonia Spirit, Aromatic (Inhalation-Systemic), #
SMZ-TMP—Sulfamethoxazole and Trimethoprim—**See Sulfonamides and Trimethoprim (Systemic)**, 2661
Snaplets-DM—Baker Cummins (U.S.) brand of Phenylpropanolamine and Dextromethorphan—**See Cough/Cold Combinations (Systemic)**, 1024
Snaplets-EX—Baker Cummins (U.S.) brand of Phenylpropanolamine and Guaifenesin—**See Cough/Cold Combinations (Systemic)**, 1024
Snaplets-FR—Baker Cummins (U.S.) brand of Acetaminophen (Systemic), 6
Snaplets-Multi—Baker Cummins (U.S.) brand of Chlorpheniramine, Phenylpropanolamine, and Dextromethorphan—**See Cough/Cold Combinations (Systemic)**, 1024
Soda Mint—Schein (U.S.) brand of Sodium Bicarbonate (Systemic), 2586
Sodium amidotrizoate—Diatrizoate—**See Diatrizoates (Systemic)**, #; Diatrizoate Sodium—**See Diatrizoates (Local)**, #
Sodium Ascorbate [Cenolate; Ortho/CS]
 **See Ascorbic Acid (Systemic)**, 469
 Injection, 473
Sodium aurothiomalate—Gold Sodium Thiomalate—**See Gold Compounds (Systemic)**, 1566
Sodium azodisalicylate—See Olsalazine (Oral-Local), 2161
Sodium Benzoate and Sodium Phenylacetate [Ucephan]
 **(Systemic)**, #, 3133, 3164
 Solution, Oral, #
Sodium Bicarbonate [Arm and Hammer Pure Baking Soda; Bell/ans; Citrocarbonate; Soda Mint]
 **(Systemic)**, 2586
 Effervescent, 2589
 Injection USP, 2590
 Powder, Oral, USP, 2589
 Tablets USP, 2589
Sodium Bicarbonate-containing Combinations, 3082
Sodium calcium edetate—See Edetate Calcium Disodium (Systemic), 1324
Sodium Chloride
 **(Parenteral-Local)**, #
 Injection USP, #
Sodium chromate ($^{51}$Cr)—See Sodium Chromate Cr 51 (Systemic), 2590
Sodium Chromate Cr 51 [Chromitope; sodium chromate ($^{51}$Cr)]
 **(Systemic)**, 2590
 Injection USP, 2592
Sodium Citrate and Citric Acid [Albright's solution; Bicitra; modified Shohl's solution; Oracit]
 **See Citrates (Systemic)**, 881
 Solution, Oral, USP, 885
Sodium cromoglycate—See Cromolyn (Inhalation-Local), 1116; (Nasal), 1118; (Ophthalmic), 1120; (Systemic/Oral-Local), 1121
Sodium Dichloroacetate
 **(Systemic)**, 3164
Sodium edetate—See Edetate Disodium (Ophthalmic), #; Edetate Disodium (Systemic), 1327
Sodium Fluoride [Flozenges; Fluor-A-Day; Fluoritab; Fluoritabs; Fluorodex; Fluorosol; Flura; Flura-Drops; Flura-Loz; Karidium; Luride; Luride Lozi-Tabs; Luride-SF Lozi-Tabs; PDF; Pediaflor; Pedi-Dent; Pharmaflur; Pharmaflur 1.1; Pharmaflur df; Phos-Flur; Solu-Flur]
 **(Systemic)**, 2592
 Lozenges, 2594
 Solution, Oral, USP, 2595
 Tablets USP, 2595
 Tablets, Chewable, USP, 2595

Sodium Fluoride F 18
 **(Systemic)**, 2595
 Injection USP, 2596
Sodium Fluoride and Triclosan [Total]
 **(Dental)**, 3034
 Dental paste (Toothpaste), 3034
Sodium/Gamma Hydroxybutyrate
 **(Systemic)**, 3165
Sodium Iodide [Iodopen]
 **(Systemic)**, 2597
 Injection, 2598
Sodium Iodide I 123
 **(Systemic)**, 2599
 Capsules USP, 2600
 Solution USP, 2600
Sodium Iodide I 131
 **(Systemic—Diagnostic)**, 2603
 Capsules USP, 2606
 Solution USP, 2606
Sodium Iodide I 131 [Iodotope]
 **(Systemic—Therapeutic)**, 2606
 Capsules USP, 2609
 Solution USP, 2610
Sodium Monomercaptoundecahydro-closo-dodecaborate [Borocell]
 **(Systemic)**, 3164
Sodium Nitrite [Cyanide Antidote Package]
 **(Systemic)**, #
 Injection USP, #
Sodium Pertechnetate Tc 99m [TechneLite; Ultra-TechneKow FM]
 **(Mucosal-Local)**, 2610
 Injection USP, 2611
Sodium Pertechnetate Tc 99m [TechneLite; Ultra-TechneKow FM]
 **(Ophthalmic)**, 2611
 Injection USP, 2612
Sodium Pertechnetate Tc 99m [Technelite; Ultra-TechneKow FM]
 **(Systemic)**, 2612
 Injection USP, 2615
Sodium Phenylbutyrate [Buphenyl]
 **(Systemic)**, #, 3164
 for Solution, Oral, #
 Tablets, #
Sodium Phosphate
 **See Laxatives (Local)**, #
 Powder, Effervescent
Sodium Phosphate P 32
 **(Systemic)**, 2616
 Solution USP, 2617
Sodium Phosphates [Enemol; Fleet Enema; Fleet Enema for Children; Fleet Pediatric Enema; Fleet Phospho-Soda; Gent-L-Tip; PMS-Phosphates]
 **See Laxatives (Local)**, #
 Enema, #
 Solution, Oral, USP, #
Sodium Phosphates
 **See Phosphates (Systemic)**, 2317
 Injection USP, 2321
Sodium Polystyrene Sulfonate [Kayexalate; K-Exit; Kionex; PMS-Sodium Polystyrene Sulfonate; SPS Suspension]
 **(Local)**, 2618
 Suspension USP, 2619
 for Suspension USP, 2619
Sodium Salicylate [Dodd's Extra Strength; Dodd's Pills; Gin Pain Pills]
 **See Salicylates (Systemic)**, 2538
 Tablets USP, 2554
 Tablets, Delayed-release, 2554
Sodium Salicylate-containing Combinations, 3082
Sodium Sulamyd—Schering (U.S. and Canada) brand of Sulfacetamide—**See Sulfonamides (Ophthalmic)**, 2651
Sodium Tetradecyl Sulfate [Sotradecol]
 **(Systemic)**, 3164
Sodium Thiosulfate [Cyanide Antidote Package]
 **(Systemic)**, #
 Injection USP, #
Sodium Tyropanoate—Tyropanoate—**See Cholecystographic Agents, Oral (Systemic)**, #
Sofarin—Lemmon (U.S.) brand of Warfarin—**See Anticoagulants (Systemic)**, 243
Soflax—Pharmascience (Canada) brand of Docusate—**See Laxatives (Local)**, #
Soflax Drops—Pharmascience (Canada) brand of Docusate—**See Laxatives (Local)**, #
Sofracort Eye-Ear—Roussel (Canada) brand of Framycetin, Gramicidin, and Dexamethasone (Ophthalmic), 3021; (Otic), 3021

Soframycin—Roussel (Canada) brand of Framycetin (Ophthalmic), 3021; Framycetin and Gramicidin (Topical), 3020
Sofra-Tulle—Roussel (Canada) brand of Framycetin (Topical), 3021
Softsense Skin Essential Everyday UV Protectant—S.C. Johnson (Canada) brand of Octyl Methoxycinnamate and Oxybenzone—**See Sunscreen Agents (Topical)**, #
Solazine—Horner (Canada) brand of Trifluoperazine—**See Phenothiazines (Systemic)**, 2289
Solbar—Pearson & Covey (Canada) brand of Oxybenzone and Roxadimate—**See Sunscreen Agents (Topical)**, #
Solbar Liquid—Pearson & Covey (Canada) brand of Octyl Methoxycinnamate—**See Sunscreen Agents (Topical)**, #
Solbar PF—Person & Covey (U.S.) brand of Octyl Methoxycinnamate and Oxybenzone—**See Sunscreen Agents (Topical)**, #
Solbar PF Liquid—Person & Covey (U.S.) brand of Octocrylene, Octyl Methoxycinnamate, and Oxybenzone—**See Sunscreen Agents (Topical)**, #; Octyl Methoxycinnamate and Oxybenzone—**See Sunscreen Agents (Topical)**, #
Solbar PF Ultra—Person & Covey (U.S.) brand of Octocrylene, Octyl Methoxycinnamate, and Oxybenzone—**See Sunscreen Agents (Topical)**, #
Solbar Plus—Pearson-Covey (Canada) brand of Oxybenzone and Roxadimate—**See Sunscreen Agents (Topical)**, #; Dioxybenzone, Oxybenzone, and Padimate O—**See Sunscreen Agents (Topical)**, #
Solbar Shield—Pearson-Covey (Canada) brand of Octyl Methoxycinnamate, Octyl Salicylate, and Oxybenzone—**See Sunscreen Agents (Topical)**, #
Solex A15 Clear—Dermol (U.S.) brand of Oxybenzone and Padimate O—**See Sunscreen Agents (Topical)**, #
Solfoton—Poythress (U.S.) brand of Phenobarbital—**See Barbiturates (Systemic)**, 518
Solganal—Schering (U.S.) brand of Aurothioglucose—**See Gold Compounds (Systemic)**, 1566
Sol-O-Pake—E-Z-EM (U.S.) brand of Barium Sulfate (Local), #
Sol-O-Pake Liquid—E-Z-EM (U.S.) brand of Barium Sulfate (Local), #
Soluble Recombinant Human Complement Receptor Type 1
 **(Systemic)**, 3165
Solu-Cortef—Upjohn (U.S. and Canada) brand of Hydrocortisone—**See Corticosteroids—Glucocorticoid Effects (Systemic)**, 998
Solu-Flur—Stickley (Canada) brand of Sodium Fluoride (Systemic), 2592
Solugel 4—Stiefel (U.S. and Canada) brand of Benzoyl Peroxide (Topical), 579
Solugel 8—Stiefel (Canada) brand of Benzoyl Peroxide (Topical), 579
Solu-Medrol—Upjohn (U.S. and Canada) brand of Methylprednisolone—**See Corticosteroids—Glucocorticoid Effects (Systemic)**, 998, 3028
Solurex—Hyrex (U.S.) brand of Dexamethasone—**See Corticosteroids—Glucocorticoid Effects (Systemic)**, 998
Solurex-LA—Hyrex (U.S.) brand of Dexamethasone—**See Corticosteroids—Glucocorticoid Effects (Systemic)**, 998
Soma—Wallace (U.S.) and Horner (Canada) brand of Carisoprodol—**See Skeletal Muscle Relaxants (Systemic)**, 2577, MC-5
Soma Compound—Wallace (U.S.) brand of Carisoprodol and Aspirin (Systemic), MC-5
Soma Compound with Codeine—Wallace (U.S.) brand of Carisoprodol, Aspirin, and Codeine (Systemic), MC-5
Somagard—Roberts (U.S.) brand of Deslorelin (Systemic), 3140
Somatostatin [Zecnil]
 **(Systemic)**, 3165
Somatrel—Ferring (U.S.) brand of NG-29 (Systemic), 3156
Somatrem [GH; human growth hormone (hGH); Protropin]
 **See Growth Hormone (Systemic)**, 1586, 3165
 for Injection, 1587, 3165
Somatropin [Biotropin; Genotonorm; Genotropin; human growth hormone, recombinant; Humatrope; Norditropin; Nutropin; Saizen; Scrostim]
 **(Systemic)**, 3165, 3166
 for Injection, 3165, 3166

*USP DI*                                                                **General Index**

Somatropin, Recombinant [*Genotropin;* GH; human growth hormone (hGH); *Humatrope; Nutropin; Nutropin AQ; Saizen; Serostim*]
  See **Growth Hormone (Systemic)**, 1586, 3034, 3035
  Injection, 3034
  for Injection, 1588, 3034, 3035
*Sominex*—Beecham (U.S.) brand of Diphenhydramine—See **Antihistamines (Systemic)**, 325
*Somnol*—Horner (Canada) brand of Flurazepam—See **Benzodiazepines (Systemic)**, 556
*Somnothane*—Hoechst (Canada) brand of Halothane—See **Anesthetics, Inhalation (Systemic)**, 168
*Sopamycetin*—Charton (Canada) brand of Chloramphenicol (Otic), #
*Sopamycetin Ophthalmic Ointment*—Charton (Canada) brand of Chloramphenicol (Ophthalmic), #
*Sopamycetin Ophthalmic Solution*—Charton (Canada) brand of Chloramphenicol (Ophthalmic), #
Sorbitol-containing Combinations, 3082
*Sorbitrate*—ZENECA (U.S.) brand of Isosorbide Dinitrate—See **Nitrates (Systemic)**, 2129, MC-16
*Sorbitrate SA*—ZENECA (U.S.) brand of Isosorbide Dinitrate—See **Nitrates (Systemic)**, 2129
*Soriatane*—Roche (U.S.) and Hoffman-La Roche (Canada) brand of Acitretin (Systemic), 18, MC-1
Sorivudine [*BRAVADIR*]
  **(Systemic)**, 3166
*Sotacor*—Bristol (Canada) brand of Sotalol—See **Beta-adrenergic Blocking Agents (Systemic)**, 593
Sotalol Hydrochloride [*Betapace; Sotacor*]
  See **Beta-adrenergic Blocking Agents (Systemic)**, 593, 3166
  Tablets, 607, MC-28
*Sotradecol*—Elkins-Sinn (U.S.) brand of Sodium Tetradecyl Sulfate (Systemic), 3164
*Soyalac*—Nutricia (U.S.) brand of Infant Formulas, Soy-based—See **Infant Formulas (Systemic)**, #
*Span-FF*—Metro Med (U.S.) brand of Ferrous Fumarate—See **Iron Supplements (Systemic)**, 1774
*Spanidin*—Bristol-Myers Squibb (U.S.) brand of Gusperimus (Systemic), 3145
Sparfloxacin [*Zagam*]
  **(Systemic)**, 2620
  Tablets, 2622, MC-28
*Sparine*—Wyeth-Ayerst (U.S.) brand of Promazine—See **Phenothiazines (Systemic)**, 2289
*Spaslin*—Blaine (U.S.) brand of Atropine, Hyoscyamine, Scopolamine, and Phenobarbital—See **Belladonna Alkaloids and Barbiturates (Systemic)**, 551
*Spasmoban*—Trianon (Canada) brand of Dicyclomine—See **Anticholinergics/Antispasmodics (Systemic)**, 226
*Spasmoject*—Mayrand (U.S.) brand of Dicyclomine—See **Anticholinergics/Antispasmodics (Systemic)**, 226
*Spasmolin*—Moore (U.S.) brand of Atropine, Hyoscyamine, Scopolamine, and Phenobarbital—See **Belladonna Alkaloids and Barbiturates (Systemic)**, 551
*Spasmophen*—Lannett (U.S.) brand of Atropine, Hyoscyamine, Scopolamine, and Phenobarbital—See **Belladonna Alkaloids and Barbiturates (Systemic)**, 551
*Spasquid*—Geneva Generics (U.S.) brand of Atropine, Hyoscyamine, Scopolamine, and Phenobarbital—See **Belladonna Alkaloids and Barbiturates (Systemic)**, 551
*Spectamine*—Medi-Physics (U.S. and Canada) brand of Iofetamine I 123 (Systemic), 1757
*Spectazole*—Ortho (U.S.) brand of Econazole (Topical), 1323
Spectinomycin Hydrochloride [*Trobicin*]
  **(Systemic)**, 2622
  for Suspension, Sterile, USP, 2623
*Spectrobid*—Roerig (U.S.) brand of Bacampicillin—See **Penicillins (Systemic)**, 2240
*Spectro-Caine*—Spectrum (U.S.) brand of Proparacaine—See **Anesthetics (Ophthalmic)**, #
*Spectro-Chlor Ophthalmic Ointment*—Allergan (U.S.) brand of Chloramphenicol (Ophthalmic), #
*Spectro-Chlor Ophthalmic Solution*—Allergan (U.S.) brand of Chloramphenicol (Ophthalmic), #
*Spectro-Cyl*—Spectrum (U.S.) brand of Tropicamide (Ophthalmic), #
*Spectro-Genta*—Spectrum (U.S.) brand of Gentamicin (Ophthalmic), 1555

*Spectro-Homatropine*—Spectrum (U.S.) brand of Homatropine (Ophthalmic), 1651
*Spectro-Sporin*—Spectrum (U.S.) brand of Neomycin, Polymyxin B, and Bacitracin (Ophthalmic), #
*Spectro-Sulf*—Spectrum (U.S.) brand of Sulfacetamide—See **Sulfonamides (Ophthalmic)**, 2651
*Spec-T Sore Throat Anesthetic*—Apothecon (U.S.) brand of Benzocaine—See **Anesthetics (Mucosal-Local)**, 128
Spermicides
  **(Vaginal)**, #
*Spersacarpine*—Dispersa (Canada) brand of Pilocarpine (Ophthalmic), #
*Spersadex*—Ciba Vision (Canada) brand of Dexamethasone—See **Corticosteroids (Ophthalmic)**, 966
*Spersaphrine*—Dispersa (Canada) brand of Phenylephrine (Ophthalmic), #
*Spheramine*—Theracell (U.S.) brand of Human Retinal Pigmented Epithelial Cells on Collagen Microcarriers (Systemic), 3146
Spiramycin [*Provamicina; Rovamycina; Rovamycine; Rovamycine 250; Rovamycine-250; Rovamycine 500; Rovamycine-500; Spiramycine Coquelusédal*]
  **(Systemic)**, 2624
  Capsules, 2626
  Tablets, 2626
Spiramycin Adipate [*Rovamycine; Spiramycine Coquelusédal*]
  **(Systemic)**, 2624
  Injection, 2626
  Suppositories, 2626
*Spiramycin Coquelusédal*—See Spiramycin (Systemic), 2624
Spironolactone [*Aldactone; Novospiroton*]
  See **Diuretics, Potassium-sparing (Systemic)**, 1266
  Tablets USP, 1270, MC-28
Spironolactone-containing Combinations, 3082
Spironolactone and Hydrochlorothiazide [*Aldactazide; Novo-Spirozine; Spirozide*]
  See **Diuretics, Potassium-sparing, and Hydrochlorothiazide (Systemic)**, 1272
  Tablets USP, 1273, MC-28
*Spirozide*—Rugby (U.S.) brand of Spironolactone and Hydrochlorothiazide—See **Diuretics, Potassium-sparing, and Hydrochlorothiazide (Systemic)**, 1272
*Sporanox*—Janssen (U.S.) and Janssen-Ortho (Canada) brand of Itraconazole—See **Antifungals, Azole (Systemic)**, 302, MC-16
*Sporidin-G*—Galagen (U.S.) brand of Bovine Immunoglobulin Concentrate, Cryptosporidium parvum (Systemic), 3134
*SPS Suspension*—Carolina (U.S.) brand of Sodium Polystyrene Sulfonate (Local), 2618
*SRC Expectorant*—Edwards (U.S.) brand of Pseudoephedrine, Hydrocodone, and Guaifenesin—See **Cough/Cold Combinations (Systemic)**, 1024
*SSD*—Boots (U.S.) brand of Silver Sulfadiazine (Topical), #
*SSD AF*—Boots (U.S.) brand of Silver Sulfadiazine (Topical), #
*SSKI*—See Potassium Iodide (Systemic), 2354
*Stadol*—Bristol-Myers Squibb (U.S.) brand of Butorphanol—See **Opioid (Narcotic) Analgesics (Systemic)**, 2168
*Stadol NS*—Bristol-Myers Squibb (U.S.) brand of Butorphanol (Nasal-Systemic), 700
*Stagesic*—Huckaby (U.S.) brand of Hydrocodone and Acetaminophen—See **Opioid (Narcotic) Analgesics and Acetaminophen (Systemic)**, 2198
*Stahist*—Huckaby (U.S.) brand of Chlorpheniramine, Phenylpropanolamine, Atropine, Hyoscyamine, and Scopolamine—See **Antihistamines, Decongestants, and Anticholinergics (Systemic)**, 373
*Stamoist E*—Huckaby (U.S.) brand of Pseudoephedrine and Guaifenesin—See **Cough/Cold Combinations (Systemic)**, 1024
*Stamoist LA*—Huckaby (U.S.) brand of Phenylpropanolamine and Guaifenesin—See **Cough/Cold Combinations (Systemic)**, 1024
Stanozolol [*Winstrol*]
  See **Anabolic Steroids (Systemic)**, 110
  Tablets USP, 114
*Staphcillin*—Bristol (U.S.) brand of Methicillin—See **Penicillins (Systemic)**, 2240

*Statex*—Pharmascience (Canada) brand of Morphine—See **Opioid (Narcotic) Analgesics (Systemic)**, 2168
*Statex Drops*—Pharmascience (Canada) brand of Morphine—See **Opioid (Narcotic) Analgesics (Systemic)**, 2168
*Staticin*—Westwood-Squibb (U.S. and Canada) brand of Erythromycin (Topical), 1365
*Statuss Expectorant*—Huckaby (U.S.) brand of Phenylpropanolamine, Codeine, and Guaifenesin—See **Cough/Cold Combinations (Systemic)**, 1024
*Statuss Green*—Huckaby (U.S.) brand of Pheniramine, Pyrilamine, Phenylephrine, Phenylpropanolamine, and Hydrocodone—See **Cough/Cold Combinations (Systemic)**, 1024
Stavudine [d4T; *Zerit*]
  **(Systemic)**, 2627
  Capsules, 2629, MC-28
  for Solution, Oral, 2629
*Stay Moist Moisturizing Lip Conditioner*—Stanback (U.S.) brand of Oxybenzone and Padimate O—See **Sunscreen Agents (Topical)**, #
*S-T Cort*—Scot-Tussin (U.S.) brand of Hydrocortisone—See **Corticosteroids (Topical)**, 978
*Stelazine*—SmithKline Beecham (U.S.) and Nova (Canada) brand of Trifluoperazine—See **Phenothiazines (Systemic)**, 2289, MC-31
*Stelazine Concentrate*—Nova (U.S. and Canada) brand of Trifluoperazine—See **Phenothiazines (Systemic)**, 2289
*Stemetic*—Legere (U.S.) brand of Trimethobenzamide (Systemic), 2880
*Stemetil*—May & Baker (Canada) brand of Prochlorperazine—See **Phenothiazines (Systemic)**, 2289
*Stemetil Liquid*—May & Baker (Canada) brand of Prochlorperazine—See **Phenothiazines (Systemic)**, 2289
*Sterapred*—Mayrand (U.S.) brand of Prednisone—See **Corticosteroids—Glucocorticoid Effects (Systemic)**, 998
*Sterapred DS*—Mayrand (U.S.) brand of Prednisone—See **Corticosteroids—Glucocorticoid Effects (Systemic)**, 998
*Sterecyt*—Pharmacia (U.S.) brand of Prednimustine (Systemic), 3159
*Steri-Units Sulfacetamide*—Alcon (U.S.) brand of Sulfacetamide—See **Sulfonamides (Ophthalmic)**, 2651
*S-T Forte*—Scot-Tussin (U.S.) brand of Pheniramine, Phenylephrine, Phenylpropanolamine, Hydrocodone, and Guaifenesin—See **Cough/Cold Combinations (Systemic)**, 1024
*S-T Forte 2*—Scot-Tussin (U.S.) brand of Chlorpheniramine and Hydrocodone—See **Cough/Cold Combinations (Systemic)**, 1024
*Stieva-A*—Stiefel (Canada) brand of Tretinoin (Topical), 2871
*Stieva-A Forte*—Stiefel (Canada) brand of Tretinoin (Topical), 2871
*Stilbestrol*—Roberts (Canada) brand of Diethylstilbestrol—See **Estrogens (Systemic)**, 1383
Stilboestrol—Diethylstilbestrol—See **Estrogens (Systemic)**, 1383
*Stilphostrol*—Miles (U.S.) brand of Diethylstilbestrol—See **Estrogens (Systemic)**, 1383
*Stimate*—Armour (U.S.) brand of Desmopressin (Systemic), 1187
*Stimate Nasal Spray*—Armour (U.S.) brand of Desmopressin (Systemic), 1187
*St. Joseph Adult Chewable Aspirin*—Plough (U.S.) brand of Aspirin—See **Salicylates (Systemic)**, 2538
*St. Joseph Aspirin-Free Fever Reducer for Children*—Schering-Plough (U.S.) brand of Acetaminophen (Systemic), 6
*St. Joseph Cough Suppressant for Children*—Plough (U.S.) brand of Dextromethorphan (Systemic), 1191
*Storz-Dexa*—Storz (U.S.) brand of Dexamethasone—See **Corticosteroids (Ophthalmic)**, 966
*Storzolamide*—Storz (U.S.) brand of Acetazolamide—See **Carbonic Anhydrase Inhibitors (Systemic)**, 773
*Stoxil*—SKF (U.S. and Canada) brand of Idoxuridine (Ophthalmic), 1675
*Streptase*—Astra (U.S.) and Hoechst Marion Roussel (Canada) brand of Streptokinase—See **Thrombolytic Agents (Systemic)**, 2799

Streptokinase [*Kabikinase; Streptase*]
  **See Thrombolytic Agents (Systemic)**, 2799
  for Injection, 2808
Streptomycin Sulfate
  **See Aminoglycosides (Systemic)**, 69
  Injection USP, 77
  Sterile USP, 78
Streptozocin [*Zanosar*]
  **(Systemic)**, 2629
  for Injection, 2632
Stri-Dex Dual Textured Pads Maximum Strength—Glenbrook (U.S.) brand of Salicylic Acid (Topical), #
Stri-Dex Dual Textured Pads Regular Strength—Glenbrook (U.S.) brand of Salicylic Acid (Topical), #
Stri-Dex Dual Textured Pads Sensitive Skin—Glenbrook (U.S.) brand of Salicylic Acid (Topical), #
Stri-Dex Maximum Strength Pads—Glenbrook (U.S.) brand of Salicylic Acid (Topical), #
Stri-Dex Regular Strength Pads—Glenbrook (U.S.) brand of Salicylic Acid (Topical), #
Stri-Dex Super Scrub Pads—Glenbrook (U.S.) brand of Salicylic Acid (Topical), #
Strifon Forte DSC—Ferndale (U.S.) brand of Chlorzoxazone—**See Skeletal Muscle Relaxants (Systemic)**, 2577
Stromectol—Merck (U.S.) brand of Ivermectin (Systemic), 3026
217 Strong—Frosst (Canada) brand of Aspirin—**See Salicylates (Systemic)**, 2538
Strong iodine tincture—*See* Iodine (Topical), #
Strontium Chloride Sr 89 [*Metastron*]
  **(Systemic)**, 2632
  Injection USP, 2634
ST1-RTA Immunotoxin (SR 44163)
  **(Systemic)**, 3166
Student's Choice Acne Medication—Durham (U.S.) brand of Benzoyl Peroxide (Topical), 579
Stulex—JMI-Canton (U.S.) brand of Docusate—**See Laxatives (Local)**, #
SU-101
  **(Systemic)**, 3166
SU101
  **(Systemic)**, 3166
Sublimaze—Janssen (U.S. and Canada) brand of Fentanyl—**See Fentanyl Derivatives (Systemic)**, 1452
Succimer [*Chemet; Chemet Capsules;* dimercaptosuccinic acid; 2,3-Dimercaptosuccinic acid; DMSA]
  **(Systemic)**, #, 3166
  Capsules, #
Succinylcholine Chloride [*Anectine; Anectine Flo-Pack; Quelicin; Sucostrin; Sucostrin High Potency;* suxamethonium]
  **See Neuromuscular Blocking Agents (Systemic)**, 2098
  Injection USP, 2104
  Sterile USP, 2104
Sucostrin—Squibb-Marsam (U.S.) brand of Succinylcholine—**See Neuromuscular Blocking Agents (Systemic)**, 2098
Sucostrin High Potency—Squibb-Marsam (U.S.) brand of Succinylcholine—**See Neuromuscular Blocking Agents (Systemic)**, 2098
Sucraid—Orphan Medical (U.S.) brand of Sacrosidase (Systemic), 3033
Sucralfate [*Apo-sucralfate; Carafate; Sucralfate Suspension Plus; Sulcrate*]
  **(Oral-Local)**, 2635, 3166
  Suspension, Oral, 2636, 3166
  Tablets, 2636, MC-28
Sucrase (Yeast-derived) [*Sacarasa*]
  **(Systemic)**, 3166
Sucrets, Children's—SmithKline Beecham Consumer (U.S.) brand of Dyclonine—**See Anesthetics (Mucosal-Local)**, 128
Sucrets Cough Control Formula—Beecham (U.S.) brand of Dextromethorphan (Systemic), 1191
Sucrets Maximum Strength—SmithKline Beecham Consumer (U.S.) brand of Dyclonine—**See Anesthetics (Mucosal-Local)**, 128
Sucrets Regular Strength—SmithKline Beecham Consumer (U.S.) brand of Dyclonine—**See Anesthetics (Mucosal-Local)**, 128
Sudafed—BW (U.S. and Canada) brand of Pseudoephedrine (Systemic), 2422
Sudafed Children's Cold & Cough—Warner Wellcome (U.S.) brand of Pseudoephedrine, Dextromethorphan, and Guaifenesin—**See Cough/Cold Combinations (Systemic)**, 1024

Sudafed Children's Non-Drowsy Cold & Cough—Warner Wellcome (U.S.) brand of Pseudoephedrine, Dextromethorphan, and Guaifenesin—**See Cough/Cold Combinations (Systemic)**, 1024
Sudafed Cold & Cough Liquid Caps—Warner Wellcome (U.S.) brand of Pseudoephedrine, Dextromethorphan, Guaifenesin, and Acetaminophen—**See Cough/Cold Combinations (Systemic)**, 1024
Sudafed Cold & Flu Gelcaps—Warner Wellcome (Canada) brand of Pseudoephedrine, Dextromethorphan, Guaifenesin, and Acetaminophen—**See Cough/Cold Combinations (Systemic)**, 1024
Sudafed Cough & Cold Extra Strength Caplets—Warner Wellcome (Canada) brand of Pseudoephedrine, Dextromethorphan, and Acetaminophen—**See Cough/Cold Combinations (Systemic)**, 1024
Sudafed DM—Warner Wellcome (Canada) brand of Pseudoephedrine and Dextromethorphan—**See Cough/Cold Combinations (Systemic)**, 1024
Sudafed Head Cold and Sinus Extra Strength Caplets—Warner Wellcome (Canada) brand of Pseudoephedrine and Acetaminophen—**See Decongestants and Analgesics (Systemic)**, 1180
Sudafed 12 Hour—BW (U.S. and Canada) brand of Pseudoephedrine (Systemic), 2422
Sudafed Liquid, Children's—BW (U.S.) brand of Pseudoephedrine (Systemic), 2422
Sudafed Non-Drowsy Non-Drying Sinus Liquid Caps—Warner Wellcome (U.S.) brand of Pseudoephedrine and Guaifenesin—**See Cough/Cold Combinations (Systemic)**, 1024
Sudafed Plus—Warner Wellcome (U.S.) brand of Chlorpheniramine and Pseudoephedrine—**See Antihistamines and Decongestants (Systemic)**, 343
Sudafed Severe Cold Formula—Warner Wellcome (U.S.) brand of Pseudoephedrine, Dextromethorphan, and Acetaminophen—**See Cough/Cold Combinations (Systemic)**, 1024
Sudafed Severe Cold Formula Caplets—Warner Wellcome (U.S.) brand of Pseudoephedrine, Dextromethorphan, and Acetaminophen—**See Cough/Cold Combinations (Systemic)**, 1024
Sudafed Sinus Maximum Strength Without Drowsiness—Warner Wellcome (U.S.) brand of Pseudoephedrine and Acetaminophen—**See Decongestants and Analgesics (Systemic)**, 1180
Sudafed Sinus Maximum Strength Without Drowsiness Caplets—Warner Wellcome (U.S.) brand of Pseudoephedrine and Acetaminophen—**See Decongestants and Analgesics (Systemic)**, 1180
Sudal 60/500—Atley (U.S.) brand of Pseudoephedrine and Guaifenesin—**See Cough/Cold Combinations (Systemic)**, 1024
Sudal 120/600—Atley (U.S.) brand of Pseudoephedrine and Guaifenesin—**See Cough/Cold Combinations (Systemic)**, 1024
Sufedrin—Lannett (U.S.) brand of Pseudoephedrine (Systemic), 2422
Sufenta—Janssen (U.S. and Canada) brand of Sufentanil—**See Fentanyl Derivatives (Systemic)**, 1452, 3035
Sufentanil Citrate [*Sufenta*]
  **See Fentanyl Derivatives (Systemic)**, 1452, 3035
  Injection USP, 1459, 3035
Sular—ZENECA (U.S.) brand of Nisoldipine (Systemic), MC-22
Sul-Azo—Lunsco (U.S.) brand of Sulfisoxazole and Phenazopyridine—**See Sulfonamides and Phenazopyridine (Systemic)**, 2660
Sulbactam-containing Combinations, 3082
Sulconazole Nitrate [*Exelderm*]
  **(Topical)**, #
  Cream, Topical, #
  Solution, Topical, #
Sulcrate—Hoechst Marion Roussel (Canada) brand of Sucralfate (Oral-Local), 2635
Sulcrate Suspension Plus—Hoechst Marion Roussel (Canada) brand of Sucralfate (Oral-Local), 2635
Suleo-M—International (U.K.) brand of Malathion (Topical), #
Sulf-10—Iolab (U.S.) brand of Sulfacetamide—**See Sulfonamides (Ophthalmic)**, 2651
Sulfabenzamide-containing Combinations, 3082
Sulfacetamide-containing Combinations, 3082

Sulfacetamide Sodium [*Ak-Sulf; Bleph-10; Cetamide; Isopto-Cetamide; I-Sulfacet; Ocu-Sul-10; Ocu-Sul-15; Ocu-Sul-30; Ocusulf-10; Ophthacet; Sodium Sulamyd; Spectro-Sulf; Steri-Units Sulfacetamide; Sulf-10; Sulfair; Sulfair 10; Sulfair 15; Sulfair Forte; Sulfamide; Sulfex;* sulphacetamide; *Sulten-10*]
  **See Sulfonamides (Ophthalmic)**, 2651
  Ointment, Ophthalmic, USP, 2652
  Solution, Ophthalmic, USP, 2652
Sulfadiazine [sulphadiazine]
  **See Sulfonamides (Systemic)**, 2653, 3166
  Tablets USP, 2656
Sulfadiazine-containing Combinations, 3082
Sulfadiazine and Trimethoprim [*Coptin; Coptin 1;* cotrimazine]
  **See Sulfonamides and Trimethoprim (Systemic)**, 2661
  Suspension, Oral, 2663
  Tablets, 2663
Sulfadoxine-containing Combinations, 3082
Sulfadoxine and Pyrimethamine [*Fansidar*]
  **(Systemic)**, 2637
  Tablets USP, 2640, MC-28
Sulfafurazole—Sulfisoxazole—**See Sulfonamides (Ophthalmic)**, 2651; **Sulfonamides (Systemic)**, 2653
Sulfair—Best Generics (U.S.); Dixon-Shane (U.S.); Gen-King (U.S.); and Texas Drugs (U.S.) brand of Sulfacetamide—**See Sulfonamides (Ophthalmic)**, 2651
Sulfair 10—Pharmafair (U.S.) brand of Sulfacetamide—**See Sulfonamides (Ophthalmic)**, 2651
Sulfair 15—Pharmafair (U.S.) brand of Sulfacetamide—**See Sulfonamides (Ophthalmic)**, 2651
Sulfair Forte—Pharmafair (U.S.) brand of Sulfacetamide—**See Sulfonamides (Ophthalmic)**, 2651
Sulfamethizole [sulphamethizole; *Thiosulfil Forte*]
  **See Sulfonamides (Systemic)**, 2653
  Tablets USP, 2657
Sulfamethoxazole [acetylsulfamethoxazole; *Apo-Sulfamethoxazole; Gantanol;* sulphamethoxazole; *Urobak*]
  **See Sulfonamides (Systemic)**, 2653
  Tablets USP, 2657, MC-28
Sulfamethoxazole-containing Combinations, 3082
Sulfamethoxazole and Phenazopyridine Hydrochloride [*Azo Gantanol; Azo-Sulfamethoxazole*]
  **See Sulfonamides and Phenazopyridine (Systemic)**, 2660
  Tablets, 2661
Sulfamethoxazole and Trimethoprim [*Apo-Sulfatrim; Apo-Sulfatrim DS; Bactrim; Bactrim DS; Bactrim I.V.; Bactrim Pediatric; Cofatrim Forte; Cotrim; Cotrim DS; Cotrim Pediatric;* cotrimoxazole; *Novo-Trimel; Novo-Trimel DS; Nu-Cotrimox; Nu-Cotrimox DS; Roubac; Septra; Septra DS; Septra I.V.; Septra Pediatric;* SMZ-TMP; *Sulfatrim; Sulfatrim DS; Sulfatrim Pediatric; Sulfatrim S/S; Sulfatrim Suspens n*]
  **See Sulfonamides and Trimethoprim (Systemic)**, 2661
  for Injection Concentrate USP, 2664
  Suspension, Oral, USP, 2663
  Tablets USP, 2664, MC-28
Sulfamide—Horizon (U.S.); Rugby (U.S.); and Texas Drugs (U.S.) brand of Sulfacetamide—**See Sulfonamides (Ophthalmic)**, 2651
Sulfamylon—Hickam (U.S.) brand of Mafenide (Topical), #
Sulfamylon Solution—Hickam (U.S.) brand of Mafenide (Topical), 3152
Sulfanilamide [*AVC*]
  **See Sulfonamides (Vaginal)**, 2658
  Cream, Vaginal, 2659
  Suppositories, Vaginal, 2659
Sulfanilamide-containing Combinations, 3082
Sulfapyridine [*Dagenan*]
  **(Systemic)**, 2640, 3166
  Tablets USP, 2642
Sulfasalazine [*Azulfidine; Azulfidine EN-Tabs; PMS Sulfasalazine; PMS Sulfasalazine E.C.; Salazopyrin; Salazopyrin EN-Tabs;* salazosulfapyridine; salicylazosulfapyridine; *S.A.S.-500; S.A.S. Enteric-500* sulphasalazine]
  **(Systemic)**, 2643
  Suspension, Rectal, 2646
  Tablets USP, 2646, MC-28
  Tablets USP (Enteric-coated), 2646, MC-28
Sulfathiazole-containing Combinations, 3082

*USP DI*            General Index   3349

Sulfathiazole, sulfacetamide, and sulfabenzamide—Triple Sulfa—**See Sulfonamides (Vaginal)**, 2658
*Sulfatrim*—Barre (U.S.) brand of Sulfamethoxazole and Trimethoprim—**See Sulfonamides and Trimethoprim (Systemic)**, 2661
*Sulfatrim DS*—Barre (U.S.) brand of Sulfamethoxazole and Trimethoprim—**See Sulfonamides and Trimethoprim (Systemic)**, 2661
*Sulfatrim Pediatric*—Barre (U.S.) brand of Sulfamethoxazole and Trimethoprim—**See Sulfonamides and Trimethoprim (Systemic)**, 2661
*Sulfatrim S/S*—Cheshire (U.S.) brand of Sulfamethoxazole and Trimethoprim—**See Sulfonamides and Trimethoprim (Systemic)**, 2661
*Sulfatrim Suspension*—URL (U.S.) brand of Sulfamethoxazole and Trimethoprim—**See Sulfonamides and Trimethoprim (Systemic), 2661**
*Sulfex*—Charton (Canada) brand of Sulfacetamide—**See Sulfonamides (Ophthalmic)**, 2651
*Sulfimycin*—Rugby (U.S.) brand of Erythromycin and Sulfisoxazole (Systemic), 1376
Sulfinpyrazone [*Anturan; Anturane; Apo-Sulfinpyrazone; Novopyrazone*]
   **(Systemic)**, 2646
   Capsules USP, 2650, MC-28
   Tablets USP, 2651, MC-28
Sulfisoxazole [*Apo-Sulfisoxazole; Gantrisin; Novo-Soxazole;* sulfafurazole; *Sulfizole;* sulphafurazole]
   **See Sulfonamides (Systemic)**, 2653
   Tablets USP, 2657
Sulfisoxazole Acetyl [*Gantrisin*]
   **See Sulfonamides (Systemic)**, 2653
   Suspension, Oral, USP, 2658
   Syrup, Oral, 2658
Sulfisoxazole-containing Combinations, 3082
Sulfisoxazole Diolamine [*Gantrisin;* sulfafurazole; sulphafurazole]
   **See Sulfonamides (Ophthalmic)**, 2651
   Ointment, Ophthalmic, USP, 2652
   Solution, Ophthalmic, USP, 2652
Sulfisoxazole and Phenazopyridine Hydrochloride [*Azo Gantrisin; Azo-Sulfisoxazole; Azo-Truxazole; Sul-Azo*]
   **See Sulfonamides and Phenazopyridine (Systemic)**, 2660
   Tablets, 2661
*Sulfizole*—Sulfisoxazole—**See Sulfonamides (Systemic)**, 2653
*Sulfolax*—Major (U.S.) brand of Docusate—**See Laxatives (Local)**, #
Sulfonamides
   **(Ophthalmic)**, 2651
Sulfonamides
   **(Systemic)**, 2653
Sulfonamides
   **(Vaginal)**, 2658
Sulfonamides and Phenazopyridine
   **(Systemic)**, 2660
Sulfonamides and Trimethoprim
   **(Systemic)**, 2661
*Sulforcin*—Owen (U.S.) brand of Resorcinol and Sulfur (Topical), #
Sulfur [*Cuticura Ointment; Finac; Fostex CM; Fostex Regular Strength Medicated Cover-Up; Fostril Cream; Fostril Lotion; Lotio-Alsulfa; Sulpho-Lac*]
   **(Topical)**, #
   Cream, #
   Lotion, #
   Ointment USP, #
   Soap, Bar, #
Sulfurated Lime [*Vlemasque;* Vleminckx's solution]
   **(Topical)**, #
   Mask, #
   Solution, Topical, #
Sulfur-containing Combinations, 3082
Sulindac [*Apo-Sulin; Clinoril; Novo-Sundac*]
   **See Anti-inflammatory Drugs, Nonsteroidal (Systemic)**, 388
   Tablets USP, 418, MC-29
Sulisobenzone-containing Combinations, 3082
*Sulphacetamide*—Sulfacetamide—**See Sulfonamides (Ophthalmic)**, 2651
*Sulphadiazine*—Sulfadiazine—**See Sulfonamides (Systemic)**, 2653
*Sulphafurazole*—Sulfisoxazole—**See Sulfonamides (Ophthalmic)**, 2651; **Sulfonamides (Systemic)**, 2653
*Sulphamethizole*—Sulfamethizole—**See Sulfonamides (Systemic)**, 2653

*Sulphamethoxazole*—Sulfamethoxazole—**See Sulfonamides (Systemic)**, 2653
*Sulphasalazine*—*See* Sulfasalazine (Systemic), 2643
*Sulpho-Lac*—Bradley (U.S.) brand of Sulfur (Topical), #
*Sulten-10*—Bausch & Lomb (U.S.) brand of Sulfacetamide—**See Sulfonamides (Ophthalmic)**, 2651
*Sultrin*—Ortho (U.S. and Canada) brand of Triple Sulfa—**See Sulfonamides (Vaginal)**, 2658
*Sumacal*—Sherwood (U.S.) brand of Enteral Nutrition Formula, Modular—**See Enteral Nutrition Formulas (Systemic)**, #
Sumatriptan [*Imitrex*]
   **(Systemic)**, 2664
   Injection, 2669
   Solution, Nasal, 2668
   Tablets, 2668, MC-29
*Sumycin*—Apothecon (U.S.) brand of Tetracycline—**See Tetracyclines (Systemic)**, 2765, MC-29
*Sundown*—Johnson & Johnson (Canada) brand of Octyl Methoxycinnamate, Oxybenzone, Padimate O, and Titanium Dioxide—**See Sunscreen Agents (Topical)**, #
*Sundown Broad Spectrum Sunblock*—Johnson & Johnson (Canada) brand of Octyl Methoxycinnamate, Octyl Salicylate, Oxybenzone, and Titanium Dioxide—**See Sunscreen Agents (Topical)**, #
*Sundown Sport Sunblock*—J & J (U.S.) brand of Titanium Dioxide and Zinc Oxide—**See Sunscreen Agents (Topical)**, #
*Sundown Sunblock*—J & J (U.S.) brand of Octyl Methoxycinnamate, Octyl Salicylate, Oxybenzone, and Titanium Dioxide—**See Sunscreen Agents (Topical)**, #
*Sundown Sunscreen*—J & J (U.S.) brand of Octyl Methoxycinnamate, Octyl Salicylate, and Titanium Dioxide—**See Sunscreen Agents (Topical)**, #; Johnson & Johnson (Canada) brand of Octyl Methoxycinnamate and Oxybenzone—**See Sunscreen Agents (Topical)**, #
*Sunkist*—Ciba-Geigy (U.S.) brand of Ascorbic Acid (Systemic), 469
Sunscreen Agents
   **(Topical)**, #
*Supac*—Mission (U.S.) brand of Acetaminophen, Aspirin, and Caffeine, Buffered—**See Acetaminophen and Salicylates (Systemic)**, 11
Superoxide Dismutase (Human)
   **(Systemic)**, 3167
Superoxide Dismutase (Recombinant, Human)
   **(Intratracheal-Local)**, 3167
Superoxide Dismutase (Recombinant, Human)
   **(Systemic)**, 3167
*Supeudol*—Sabex (Canada) brand of Oxycodone—**See Opioid (Narcotic) Analgesics (Systemic)**, 2168
*Suplena*—Ross (U.S.) brand of Enteral Nutrition Formula, Disease-specific—**See Enteral Nutrition Formulas (Systemic)**, #
*Suppap-120*—Raway (U.S.) brand of Acetaminophen (Systemic), 6
*Suppap-325*—Raway (U.S.) brand of Acetaminophen (Systemic), 6
*Suppap-650*—Raway (U.S.) brand of Acetaminophen (Systemic), 6
*Supprelin*—Roberts (U.S.) brand of Histrelin (Systemic), 1644
*Supprelin Injection*—Roberts (U.S.) brand of Histrelin (Systemic), 3145
*Suppressin DM*—Quintex (U.S.) brand of Dextromethorphan and Guaifenesin—**See Cough/Cold Combinations (Systemic)**, 1024
*Suppressin DM Caplets*—Quintex (U.S.) brand of Dextromethorphan and Guaifenesin—**See Cough/Cold Combinations (Systemic)**, 1024
*Suppressin DM Plus*—Quintex (U.S.) brand of Phenylephrine, Dextromethorphan, and Guaifenesin—**See Cough/Cold Combinations (Systemic)**, 1024
*Supracaine*—Hoechst (Canada) brand of Tetracaine—**See Anesthetics (Mucosal-Local)**, 128
*Suprane*—Ohmeda (U.S.) brand of Desflurane (Inhalation-Systemic), #
*Suprax*—Lederle (U.S. and Canada) brand of Cefixime—**See Cephalosporins (Systemic)**, 794, MC-6
*Suprefact*—Hoechst (Canada) brand of Buserelin (Systemic), 691

*Supres-150*—Frosst (Canada) brand of Methyldopa and Chlorothiazide—**See Methyldopa and Thiazide Diuretics (Systemic)**, 1983
*Supres-250*—Frosst (Canada) brand of Methyldopa and Chlorothiazide—**See Methyldopa and Thiazide Diuretics (Systemic)**, 1983
Suprofen [*Profenal*]
   **See Anti-inflammatory Drugs, Nonsteroidal (Ophthalmic)**, 383
   Solution, Ophthalmic, USP, 387
Suramin
   **(Systemic)**, 3167
Suramin Sodium [*Antrypol; Bayer 205; Belganyl; 309 F; Fourneau 309; Germanin; Moranyl; Naganin; Naganol; Naphuride*]
   **(Systemic)**, #
   for Injection, #
Surface Active Extract of Saline Lavage of Bovine Lungs [*Infasurf*]
   **(Intratracheal-Local)**, 3167
*Surfak*—Upjohn (U.S.) and Hoechst-Roussel (Canada) brand of Docusate—**See Laxatives (Local)**, #
*Surgam*—Roussel (Canada) brand of Tiaprofenic Acid—**See Anti-inflammatory Drugs, Nonsteroidal (Systemic)**, 388
*Surgam SR*—Roussel (Canada) brand of Tiaprofenic Acid—**See Anti-inflammatory Drugs, Nonsteroidal (Systemic)**, 388
*Surmontil*—Wyeth-Ayerst (U.S.) and Rhône-Poulenc (Canada) brand of Trimipramine—**See Antidepressants, Tricyclic (Systemic)**, 271, MC-32
*Survanta*—Ross (U.S. and Canada) brand of Beractant (Intratracheal-Local), 583
*Survanta Intratracheal Suspension*—Ross (U.S.) brand of Beractant (Intratracheal-Local), 3133
*Susano*—Halsey (U.S.) brand of Atropine, Hyoscyamine, Scopolamine, and Phenobarbital—**See Belladonna Alkaloids and Barbiturates (Systemic)**, 551
*Sus-Phrine*—Berlex (U.S.) brand of Epinephrine—**See Bronchodilators, Adrenergic (Systemic)**, 651
*Sustacal*—Mead Johnson (U.S.) brand of Enteral Nutrition Formula, Polymeric—**See Enteral Nutrition Formulas (Systemic)**, #
*Sustacal Basic*—Mead Johnson (U.S.) brand of Enteral Nutrition Formula, Polymeric—**See Enteral Nutrition Formulas (Systemic)**, #
*Sustacal with Fiber*—Mead Johnson (U.S.) brand of Enteral Nutrition Formula, Fiber-containing—**See Enteral Nutrition Formulas (Systemic)**, #
*Sustacal Plus*—Mead Johnson (U.S.) brand of Enteral Nutrition Formula, Polymeric—**See Enteral Nutrition Formulas (Systemic)**, #
*Sustagen*—Mead Johnson (U.S.) brand of Enteral Nutrition Formula, Milk-based—**See Enteral Nutrition Formulas (Systemic)**, #
*Sutilan*—Cusi (Spain) brand of Tiopronin (Systemic), 2824
Suxamethonium—Succinylcholine—**See Neuromuscular Blocking Agents (Systemic)**, 2098
*Syllact*—Wallace (U.S.) brand of Psyllium—**See Laxatives (Local)**, #
*Syllamalt*—Wallace (U.S.) brand of Malt Soup Extract and Psyllium—**See Laxatives (Local)**, #
*Symadine*—Solvay (U.S.) brand of Amantadine (Systemic), 58
*Symmetrel*—Endo (U.S. and Canada) brand of Amantadine (Systemic), 58, MC-1
Sympathomimetic Agents—Cardiovascular Use
   **(Parenteral-Systemic)**, 2669
*Synacort*—Roche/Syntex (U.S.) brand of Hydrocortisone—**See Corticosteroids (Topical)**, 978
*Synagis*—MedImmune (U.S.) brand of Palivizumab (Systemic), 2219
*Synalar*—Roche/Syntex (U.S.) and Syntex (Canada) brand of Fluocinolone—**See Corticosteroids (Topical)**, 978
*Synalar-HP*—Roche/Syntex (U.S.) brand of Fluocinolone—**See Corticosteroids (Topical)**, 978
*Synalgos-DC*—Wyeth-Ayerst (U.S.) brand of Aspirin and Dihydrocodeine—**See Opioid (Narcotic) Analgesics and Aspirin (Systemic)**, 2202, MC-3
*Synamol*—Syntex (Canada) brand of Fluocinolone—**See Corticosteroids (Topical)**, 978
*Synarel*—Searle (U.S. and Canada) brand of Nafarelin (Systemic), 2076
*Synarel Nasal Solution*—Searle (U.S.) brand of Nafarelin (Systemic), 3155

# 3350 General Index

*Syn-Clonazepam*—Syncare (Canada) brand of Clonazepam—**See Benzodiazepines (Systemic)**, 556
*Syn-Diltiazem*—SynCare (Canada) brand of Diltiazem—**See Calcium Channel Blocking Agents (Systemic)**, 720
*Synemol*—Roche/Syntex (U.S.) brand of Fluocinolone—**See Corticosteroids (Topical)**, 978
*Synflex*—SynCare (Canada) brand of Naproxen—**See Anti-inflammatory Drugs, Nonsteroidal (Systemic)**, 388
*Synflex DS*—SynCare (Canada) brand of Naproxen—**See Anti-inflammatory Drugs, Nonsteroidal (Systemic)**, 388
*Synkayvite*—Roche (U.S.) brand of Menadiol—**See Vitamin K (Systemic)**, 2975
*Syn-Nadolol*—Syntex (Canada) brand of Nadolol—**See Beta-adrenergic Blocking Agents (Systemic)**, 593
*Synovir*—Celgene (U.S.) brand of Thalidomide (Systemic), 3168
*Synphasic*—Searle (Canada) brand of Norethindrone and Ethinyl Estradiol—**See Estrogens and Progestins—Oral Contraceptives (Systemic)**, 1397
*Syn-Pindolol*—Syntex (Canada) brand of Pindolol—**See Beta-adrenergic Blocking Agents (Systemic)**, 593
Synsorb PK **(Systemic)**, 3167
Synthetic human parathyroid hormone 1–34—*See* Teriparatide (Systemic), #
Synthetic lung surfactant—*See* Colfosceril, Cetyl Alcohol, and Tyloxapol (Intratracheal-Local), 937
*Synthroid*—Knoll (U.S.) and Boots (Canada) brand of Levothyroxine—**See Thyroid Hormones (Systemic)**, 2809, MC-17
*Syntocinon*—Sandoz (U.S. and Canada) brand of Oxytocin (Systemic), 2211
*Synvinolin*—Simvastatin—**See HMG-CoA Reductase Inhibitors (Systemic)**, 1647
*Synvisc*—Wyeth-Ayerst (U.S.) brand of Hyaluronate Sodium Derivative (Systemic), 1654
*Syprine*—Merck (U.S.) brand of Trientine (Systemic), 2875
*Syracol CF*—Roberts (U.S.) brand of Dextromethorphan and Guaifenesin—**See Cough/Cold Combinations (Systemic)**, 1024

# T

*217*—Frosst (Canada) brand of Aspirin—**See Salicylates (Systemic)**, 2538
*217 Strong*—Frosst (Canada) brand of Aspirin—**See Salicylates (Systemic)**, 2538
*222*—Frosst (Canada) brand of Aspirin and Codeine—**See Opioid (Narcotic) Analgesics and Aspirin (Systemic)**, 2202
*309-F*—*See* Suramin (Systemic), #
*282*—Frosst (Canada) brand of Aspirin and Codeine—**See Opioid (Narcotic) Analgesics and Aspirin (Systemic)**, 2202
*292*—Frosst (Canada) brand of Aspirin and Codeine—**See Opioid (Narcotic) Analgesics and Aspirin (Systemic)**, 2202
*Tabloid*—Glaxo Wellcome (U.S.) brand of Thioguanine (Systemic), #
*Tac-3*—Herbert (U.S.) brand of Triamcinolone—**See Corticosteroids—Glucocorticoid Effects (Systemic)**, 998
*Tacaryl*—Westwood (U.S.) brand of Methdilazine—**See Antihistamines, Phenothiazine-derivative (Systemic)**, 377
Tacrine [*Cognex*; tetrahydroaminoacridine; THA] **(Systemic)**, 2680
  Capsules, 2682, MC-29
Tacrolimus [FK 506; *Prograf*] **(Systemic)**, 2683, 3167
  Capsules, 2687, MC-29
  for Injection, 2687
Tacrolimus Hydrate—*See* Tacrolimus (Systemic), 2683
*Tagamet*—SmithKline Beecham (U.S. and Canada) brand of Cimetidine—**See Histamine H₂-receptor Antagonists (Systemic)**, 1633, MC-7
*Tagamet HB 200*—SmithKline Beecham (U.S.) brand of Cimetidine—**See Histamine H₂-receptor Antagonists (Systemic)**, 1633
*Tagamet HB*—SmithKline Beecham (U.S.) brand of Cimetidine—**See Histamine H₂-receptor Antagonists (Systemic)**, 1633

*TA-HPV*—Cantab (U.K.) brand of Vaccinia, Recombinant (Human Papillomavirus) (Systemic), 3162
TAK-603 **(Systemic)**, 3167
*Talacen*—Sanofi Winthrop (U.S.) brand of Pentazocine and Acetaminophen—**See Opioid (Narcotic) Analgesics and Acetaminophen (Systemic)**, 2198, MC-24
Talc [*Sclerosol*] **(Intrapleural-Local)**, #
  Aerosol, Intrapleural, Powder, #
Talc, Sterile, Aerosol **(Systemic)**, 3166
*Talwin*—Sanofi Winthrop (U.S. and Canada) brand of Pentazocine—**See Opioid (Narcotic) Analgesics (Systemic)**, 2168
*Talwin Compound*—Sanofi Winthrop (U.S.) brand of Pentazocine and Aspirin—**See Opioid (Narcotic) Analgesics and Aspirin (Systemic)**, 2202
*Talwin-Nx*—Sanofi Winthrop (U.S.) brand of Pentazocine—**See Opioid (Narcotic) Analgesics (Systemic)**, 2168, MC-24
*Tambocor*—3M (U.S. and Canada) brand of Flecainide (Systemic), 1469, MC-13
*Tamine S.R.*—Geneva (U.S.) brand of Brompheniramine, Phenylephrine, and Phenylpropanolamine—**See Antihistamines and Decongestants (Systemic)**, 343
*Tamofen*—Rhône-Poulenc (Canada) brand of Tamoxifen (Systemic), 2688
*Tamone*—Adria (Canada) brand of Tamoxifen (Systemic), 2688
*Tamoplex*—Du Pont (Canada) brand of Tamoxifen (Systemic), 2688
Tamoxifen Citrate [*Apo-Tamox*; *Gen-Tamoxifen*; *Nolvadex*; *Nolvadex-D*; *Novo-Tamoxifen*; *Tamofen*; *Tamone*; *Tamoplex*] **(Systemic)**, 2688
  Tablets USP, 2690, MC-29
Tamsulosin Hydrochloride [*Flomax*] **(Systemic)**, 2690, 3193
  Capsules, 2692
*Tanafed*—Horizon (U.S.) brand of Chlorpheniramine and Pseudoephedrine—**See Antihistamines and Decongestants (Systemic)**, 343
*Tanoral*—Econolab (U.S.) and Parmed (U.S.) brand of Chlorpheniramine, Pyrilamine, and Phenylephrine—**See Antihistamines and Decongestants (Systemic)**, 343
*Tantacol DM*—Tanta (Canada) brand of Pheniramine, Pyrilamine, Phenylpropanolamine, and Dextromethorphan—**See Cough/Cold Combinations (Systemic)**, 1024
*Tanta Cough Syrup*—Tanta (Canada) brand of Dextromethorphan and Guaifenesin—**See Cough/Cold Combinations (Systemic)**, 1024
*Tantum*—Angelini (U.S.) brand of Benzydamine (Systemic), 3133; Riker/3M (Canada) brand of Benzydamine (Oral-Local), 3011
*Tapanol Extra Strength Caplets*—Republic (U.S.) brand of Acetaminophen (Systemic), 6
*Tapanol Extra Strength Tablets*—Republic (U.S.) brand of Acetaminophen (Systemic), 6
*Tapazole*—Lilly (U.S. and Canada) brand of Methimazole—**See Antithyroid Agents (Systemic)**, 446
*Taractan*—Roche (U.S.) brand of Chlorprothixene—**See Thioxanthenes (Systemic)**, 2793
*Taraphilic*—Medco (U.S.) brand of Coal Tar (Topical), #
*Tarbonis*—Reed & Carnrick (U.S.) brand of Coal Tar (Topical), #
*Tar Doak*—Doak (Canada) brand of Coal Tar (Topical), #
*Tarka*—Knoll (U.S.) brand of Trandolapril and Verapamil (Systemic), 2857, MC-31
*Tarpaste*—T.C.D. (Canada) brand of Coal Tar (Topical), #
*Tarpaste 'Doak'*—Doak (U.S.) brand of Coal Tar (Topical), #
*Tasmar*—Roche (U.S.) brand of Tolcapone (Systemic), 2833, MC-30
*Tasty Shake*—Menu Magic (U.S.) brand of Enteral Nutrition Formula, Milk-based—**See Enteral Nutrition Formulas (Systemic)**, #
TAT—*See* Tetanus Antitoxin (Systemic), #
*Tavist*—Sandoz (U.S.) and Ancalab (Canada) brand of Clemastine—**See Antihistamines (Systemic)**, 325
*Tavist-1*—Sandoz (U.S.) brand of Clemastine—**See Antihistamines (Systemic)**, 325

*Tavist-D*—Sandoz (U.S. and Canada) brand of Clemastine and Phenylpropanolamine—**See Antihistamines and Decongestants (Systemic)**, 343
*Taxol*—Bristol-Myers Squibb (U.S. and Canada) brand of Paclitaxel (Systemic), 2215, 3157
*Taxotere*—Rhône-Poulenc Rorer (U.S.) brand of Docetaxel (Systemic), 1282
Tazarotene [*Tazorac*] **(Topical)**, 2692
  Gel, 2695
*Tazicef*—SKF (U.S.) brand of Ceftazidime—**See Cephalosporins (Systemic)**, 794
*Tazidime*—Lilly (U.S.) brand of Ceftazidime—**See Cephalosporins (Systemic)**, 794
Tazobactam-containing Combinations, 3082
*Tazocin*—Lederle (Canada) brand of Piperacillin and Tazobactam—**See Penicillins and Beta-lactamase Inhibitors (Systemic)**, 2263
*Tazorac*—Allergan Herbert (U.S.) brand of Tazarotene (Systemic), 2692
$^{99m}$Tc—*See* Sodium Pertechnetate Tc 99m (Mucosal-Local), 2610; Sodium Pertechnetate Tc 99m (Ophthalmic), 2611; Sodium Pertechnetate Tc 99m (Systemic), 2612; Technetium Tc 99m Albumin (Systemic), 2695; Technetium Tc 99m Albumin Aggregated (Systemic), 2697; Technetium Tc 99m Albumin Colloid (Systemic), 2699; Technetium Tc 99m Bicisate (Systemic), 2703; Technetium Tc 99m Disofenin (Systemic), 2705; Technetium Tc 99m Exametazime (Systemic), 2708; Technetium Tc 99m Gluceptate (Systemic), 2711; Technetium Tc 99m Lidofenin (Systemic), 2713; Technetium Tc 99m Mebrofenin (Systemic), 2716; Technetium Tc 99m Medronate (Systemic), 2718; Technetium Tc 99m Mertiatide (Systemic), 2720; Technetium Tc 99m Oxidronate (Systemic), 2724; Technetium Tc 99m Pentetate (Systemic), 2727; Technetium Tc 99m Pyrophosphate (Systemic), 2729; Technetium Tc 99m (Pyro- and trimeta-) Phosphates (Systemic), 2733; Technetium Tc 99m Sestamibi (Systemic), 2736; Technetium Tc 99m Succimer (Systemic), 2738; Technetium Tc 99m Sulfur Colloid (Systemic), 2740; Technetium Tc 99m Teboroxime (Systemic), 2743; Technetium Tc 99m Tetrofosmin (Systemic), 2745
*T-Cypionate*—Legere (U.S.) brand of Testosterone—**See Androgens (Systemic)**, 118
Td—Tetanus and Diphtheria Toxoids (Td)—**See Diphtheria and Tetanus Toxoids (Systemic)**, 1236
*T/Derm Tar Emollient*—Neutrogena (U.S.) brand of Coal Tar (Topical), #
*T-Diet*—Jones (U.S.) and T. E. Williams (U.S.) brand of Phentermine—**See Appetite Suppressants (Systemic)**, 452
*Tearisol*—Iolab (U.S.) brand of Hydroxypropyl Methylcellulose (Ophthalmic), #
*Tears Naturale*—Alcon (U.S. and Canada) brand of Hydroxypropyl Methylcellulose (Ophthalmic), #
*Tears Naturale Free*—Alcon (U.S. and Canada) brand of Hydroxypropyl Methylcellulose (Ophthalmic), #
*Tears Naturale II*—Alcon (U.S. and Canada) brand of Hydroxypropyl Methylcellulose (Ophthalmic), #
*Tears Renewed*—Akorn (U.S.) brand of Hydroxypropyl Methylcellulose (Ophthalmic), #
*Tebamide*—Dixon-Shane (U.S.); G & W (U.S.); and Texas Drug (U.S.) brand of Trimethobenzamide (Systemic), 2880
*Tebrazid*—ICN (Canada) brand of Pyrazinamide (Systemic), 2425
*Teceleukin*—Hoffmann-La Roche (U.S.) brand of Interleukin-2 (Systemic), 3149
*TechneColl*—Mallinckrodt (U.S.) brand of Technetium Tc 99m Sulfur Colloid (Systemic), 2740
*TechneLite*—Du Pont (U.S.) brand of Sodium Pertechnetate Tc 99m generator (Mucosal-Local), 2610; (Ophthalmic), 2611
*Technelite*—Du Pont (U.S. and Canada) brand of Sodium Pertechnetate Tc 99m generator (Systemic), 2612, 2699
*Techneplex*—Bracco (U.S.) brand of Technetium Tc 99m Pentetate (Systemic), 2727
*TechneScan DTPA*—Merck (U.S.) brand of Technetium Tc 99m Pentetate (Systemic), 2727
*TechneScan Gluceptate*—Mallinckrodt (U.S.) brand of Technetium Tc 99m Gluceptate (Systemic), 2711

*USP DI*                            **General Index**

*TechneScan HIDA*—Mallinckrodt (U.S.) and Frosst (Canada) brand of Technetium Tc 99m Lidofenin (Systemic), 2713
*TechneScan MAA*—Mallinckrodt (U.S.) brand of Technetium Tc 99m Albumin Aggregated (Systemic), 2697
*TechneScan MAG3*—Mallinckrodt (U.S. and Canada) brand of Technetium Tc 99m Mertiatide (Systemic), 2720
*TechneScan MDP*—Mallinckrodt (U.S.) brand of Technetium Tc 99m Medronate (Systemic), 2718
*TechneScan PYP*—Mallinckrodt (U.S.) brand of Technetium Tc 99m Pyrophosphate (Systemic), 2729
*TechneScan Sulfur Colloid*—Mallinckrodt (U.S.) brand of Technetium Tc 99m Sulfur Colloid (Systemic), 2740
Technetium Tc 99m Albumin [*Frosstimage Albumin; Technetium Tc 99m HSA*]
   **(Systemic)**, 2695
   Injection USP, 2696
Technetium Tc 99m Albumin Aggregated [*AN-MAA; Frosstimage MAA; Macrotec; MPI MAA; Pulmolite; TechneScan MAA*]
   **(Systemic)**, 2697
   Injection USP, 2698
Technetium Tc 99m Albumin Colloid [*Microlite*]
   **(Systemic)**, 2699
   Injection, 2701
Technetium Tc 99m Anti-melanoma Murine Monoclonal Antibody [*Oncotrac Melanoma Imaging Kit*]
   **(Systemic)**, 3167
Technetium Tc 99m Arcitumomab [*CEA-Scan*]
   **(Systemic)**, 2701
   Injection USP, 2703
Technetium Tc 99m Bicisate [*ECD; ethyl cysteinate dimer; Neurolite*]
   **(Systemic)**, 2703
   Injection, 2705
Technetium Tc 99m DISIDA—See Technetium Tc 99m Disofenin (Systemic), 2705
Technetium Tc 99m Disofenin [*Hepatolite*]
   **(Systemic)**, 2705
   Injection USP, 2708
Technetium Tc 99m Exametazime [*Ceretec;* hexamethylpropyleneamine oxime (HM-PAO)]
   **(Systemic)**, 2708
   Injection USP, 2710
Technetium Tc 99m Gluceptate [*Frosstimage Gluceptate; Frosstimage Gluco; Glucoscan; TechneScan Gluceptate;* technetium Tc 99m glucoheptonate]
   **(Systemic)**, 2711
   Injection USP, 2712
Technetium Tc 99m glucoheptonate—See Technetium Tc 99m Gluceptate (Systemic), 2711
*Technetium Tc 99m HSA*—Medi-Physics (U.S.) brand of Technetium Tc 99m Albumin (Systemic), 2695
Technetium Tc 99m Lidofenin [*Frosstimage HIDA; TechneScan HIDA*]
   **(Systemic)**, 2713
   Injection USP, 2715
Technetium Tc 99m Mebrofenin [*Choletec*]
   **(Systemic)**, 2716
   Injection, 2718
Technetium Tc 99m Medronate [*AN-MDP; Frosstimage MDP; MDP-Squibb; MPI MDP; Osteolite; TechneScan MDP*]
   **(Systemic)**, 2718
   Injection USP, 2720
Technetium Tc 99m mercaptoacetyltriglycine—See Technetium Tc 99m Mertiatide (Systemic), 2720
Technetium Tc 99m Mertiatide [*MAG3; TechneScan MAG3;* technetium Tc 99m mercaptoacetyltriglycine]
   **(Systemic)**, 2720
   Injection USP, 2722
Technetium Tc 99m methoxyisobutylisonitrile—See Technetium Tc 99m Sestamibi (Systemic), 2736
Technetium Tc 99m MIBI—See Technetium Tc 99m Sestamibi (Systemic), 2736
Technetium Tc 99m Murine Monoclonal Antibody to Human Alpha-fetoprotein [*ImmuRAID, AFP-Tc 99m*]
   **(Systemic)**, 3167
Technetium Tc 99m Murine Monoclonal Antibody to Human Chorionic Gonadotropin (hCG) [*ImmuRAID, hCG-Tc 99m*]
   **(Systemic)**, 3167

Technetium Tc-99m Murine Monoclonal Antibody (IgG2a) to BCE [*Immuraid-LL-2(99mTc)*]
   **(Systemic)**, 3167
Technetium Tc 99m Nofetumomab Merpentan [*Verluma*]
   **(Systemic)**, 2722
   Injection, 2724
Technetium Tc 99m Oxidronate [*Osteoscan-HDP*]
   **(Systemic)**, 2724
   Injection USP, 2726
Technetium Tc 99m Pentetate [*AN-DTPA; DTPA (Chelate) Multidose; Frosstimage DTPA; Techneplex; TechneScan DTPA*]
   **(Systemic)**, 2727
   Injection USP, 2729
Technetium Tc 99m Pyrophosphate [*MPI Pyrophosphate; Phosphotec; TechneScan PYP*]
   **(Systemic)**, 2729
   Injection USP, 2732
Technetium Tc 99m (Pyro- and trimeta-) Phosphates [*Pyrolite*]
   **(Systemic)**, 2733
   Injection USP, 2735
Technetium Tc 99m Sestamibi [*Cardiolite;* technetium Tc 99m methoxyisobutylisonitrile; technetium Tc 99m MIBI]
   **(Systemic)**, 2736
   Injection USP, 2738
Technetium Tc 99m Succimer [*MPI DMSA Kidney Reagent*]
   **(Systemic)**, 2738
   Injection USP, 2740
Technetium Tc 99m Sulfur Colloid [*AN-Sulfur Colloid; Frosstimage Sulfur Colloid; TechneColl; TechneScan Sulfur Colloid; TSC*]
   **(Systemic)**, 2740
   Injection USP, 2742
Technetium Tc 99m Teboroxime [*CardioTec*]
   **(Systemic)**, 2743
   Injection, 2745
Technetium Tc 99m Tetrofosmin [*Myoview*]
   **(Systemic)**, 2745
   Injection, 2747
*Tecnal*—Technilab (Canada) brand of Butalbital, Aspirin, and Caffeine—**See Barbiturates and Analgesics (Systemic)**, 532
*Tecnal-C 1/4*—Technilab (Canada) brand of Butalbital, Aspirin, Caffeine, and Codeine—**See Barbiturates and Analgesics (Systemic)**, 532
*Tecnal-C 1/2*—Technilab (Canada) brand of Butalbital, Aspirin, Caffeine, and Codeine—**See Barbiturates and Analgesics (Systemic)**, 532
*Teczem*—Hoechst Marion Roussel (U.S.) brand of Enalapril and Diltiazem (Systemic), 1334
*Tedelparin*—See Dalteparin (Systemic), 1156
*Teejel*—Purdue Frederick (Canada) brand of Choline Salicylate and Cetyl-dimethyl-benzyl-ammonium Chloride (Mucosal-Local), 3014
*Teev*—Keene (U.S.) brand of Testosterone and Estradiol—**See Androgens and Estrogens (Systemic)**, 126
*Tega-Flex*—Ortega (U.S.) brand of Orphenadrine—**See Skeletal Muscle Relaxants (Systemic)**, 2577
*Tegamide*—Balan (U.S.); Best (U.S.); and Moore (U.S.) brand of Trimethobenzamide (Systemic), 2880
*Tegison*—Roche (U.S. and Canada) brand of Etretinate (Systemic), #, MC-12
*Tegopen*—Bristol (U.S. and Canada) brand of Cloxacillin—**See Penicillins (Systemic)**, 2240
*Tegretol*—Novartis (U.S. and Canada) brand of Carbamazepine (Systemic), 757, MC-5
*Tegretol Chewtabs*—Ciba (Canada) brand of Carbamazepine (Systemic), 757
*Tegretol CR*—Ciba (Canada) brand of Carbamazepine (Systemic), 757
*Tegretol-XR*—Novartis (U.S.) brand of Carbamazepine (Systemic), 757, MC-5
*Tegrin Lotion for Psoriasis*—Reedco (U.S.) brand of Coal Tar (Topical), #
*Tegrin Medicated Cream Shampoo*—Block (U.S.) brand of Coal Tar (Topical), #
*Tegrin Medicated Shampoo Concentrated Gel*—Reedco (U.S.) brand of Coal Tar (Topical), #
*Tegrin Medicated Shampoo Extra Conditioning Formula*—Reedco (U.S.) brand of Coal Tar (Topical), #
*Tegrin Medicated Shampoo Herbal Formula*—Reedco (U.S.) brand of Coal Tar (Topical), #
*Tegrin Medicated Shampoo Original Formula*—Reedco (U.S.) brand of Coal Tar (Topical), #

*Tegrin Medicated Soap for Psoriasis*—Reedco (U.S.) brand of Coal Tar (Topical), #
*Tegrin Skin Cream for Psoriasis*—Reedco (U.S.) brand of Coal Tar (Topical), #
*Telachlor*—Major (U.S.) brand of Chlorpheniramine—**See Antihistamines (Systemic)**, 325
*Teladar*—Dermol (U.S.) brand of Betamethasone—**See Corticosteroids (Topical)**, 978
*Teldrin*—Menley & James (U.S.) brand of Chlorpheniramine—**See Antihistamines (Systemic)**, 325
*Teldrin 12 Hour Allergy Relief*—SmithKline Beecham (U.S.) brand of Chlorpheniramine and Phenylpropanolamine—**See Antihistamines and Decongestants (Systemic)**, 343
*Telepaque*—Sanofi Winthrop (U.S. and Canada) brand of Iopanoic Acid—**See Cholecystographic Agents, Oral (Systemic)**, #
*Temaril*—Herbert (U.S.) brand of Trimeprazine—**See Antihistamines, Phenothiazine-derivative (Systemic)**, 377
Temazepam [*Restoril*]
   **See Benzodiazepines (Systemic)**, 556
   Capsules USP, 577, MC-29
*Temazin Cold*—Trenier (U.S.) brand of Chlorpheniramine and Phenylpropanolamine—**See Antihistamines and Decongestants (Systemic)**, 343
*Temovate*—Glaxo (U.S.) brand of Clobetasol—**See Corticosteroids (Topical)**, 978
*Temovate E*—Glaxo Wellcome (U.S.) brand of Clobetasol (Topical), 3015
*Temovate Scalp Application*—Glaxo (U.S.) brand of Clobetasol—**See Corticosteroids (Topical)**, 978
*Tempo*—Thompson (U.S.) brand of Alumina, Magnesia, Calcium Carbonate, and Simethicone—**See Antacids (Oral-Local)**, 188
*Tempra*—Mead Johnson Nutritional (U.S.) brand of Acetaminophen (Systemic), 6
*Tempra Caplets*—Mead Johnson (Canada) brand of Acetaminophen (Systemic), 6
*Tempra Chewable Tablets*—Mead Johnson (Canada) brand of Acetaminophen (Systemic), 6
*Tempra Drops*—Mead Johnson (Canada) brand of Acetaminophen (Systemic), 6
*Tempra D.S.*—Mead Johnson Nutritional (U.S.) brand of Acetaminophen (Systemic), 6
*Tempra, Infants'*—Mead Johnson Nutritional (U.S.) brand of Acetaminophen (Systemic), 6
*Tempra Syrup*—Mead Johnson Nutritional (U.S.) and Mead Johnson (Canada) brand of Acetaminophen (Systemic), 6
*Tencet*—Shoals (U.S.) brand of Butalbital, Acetaminophen, and Caffeine—**See Barbiturates and Analgesics (Systemic)**, 532
*Tencon*—International Ethical (U.S.) brand of Butalbital and Acetaminophen—**See Barbiturates and Analgesics (Systemic)**, 532
T4 Endonuclease V, Liposome Encapsulated **(Systemic)**, 3167
*Tenex*—Robins (U.S.) brand of Guanfacine (Systemic), 1598, MC-14
Teniposide [*VM-26; Vumon; Vumon for Injection*]
   **(Systemic)**, 2747, 3035, 3167
   Injection, 2749, 3035
*Ten-K*—Summit (U.S.) brand of Potassium Chloride—**See Potassium Supplements (Systemic)**, 2357
*Tenoretic*—ZENECA (U.S. and Canada) brand of Atenolol and Chlorthalidone—**See Beta-adrenergic Blocking Agents and Thiazide Diuretics (Systemic)**, 609, MC-3
*Tenormin*—ZENECA (U.S. and Canada) brand of Atenolol—**See Beta-adrenergic Blocking Agents (Systemic)**, 593, MC-3
Tenoxicam [*Mobiflex*]
   **See Anti-inflammatory Drugs, Nonsteroidal (Systemic)**, 388
   Tablets, 418
*Tensilon*—ICN (U.S. and Canada) brand of Edrophonium (Systemic), 1329
*Tenuate*—Hoechst Marion Roussel (U.S. and Canada) brand of Diethylpropion—**See Appetite Suppressants (Systemic)**, 452, MC-9
*Tenuate Dospan*—Hoechst Marion Roussel (U.S. and Canada) brand of Diethylpropion—**See Appetite Suppressants (Systemic)**, 452, MC-9
*Tepanil Ten-Tab*—Riker (U.S.) brand of Diethylpropion—**See Appetite Suppressants (Systemic)**, 452
*Teramine*—Legere (U.S.) brand of Phentermine—**See Appetite Suppressants (Systemic)**, 452

## General Index

*Terazol 3*—Ortho (U.S.) and Janssen-Ortho (Canada) brand of Terconazole—**See Antifungals, Azole (Vaginal)**, 310
*Terazol 7*—Ortho (U.S.) and Janssen-Ortho (Canada) brand of Terconazole—**See Antifungals, Azole (Vaginal)**, 310
*Terazol 3 Dual Pack*—Janssen-Ortho (Canada) brand of Terconazole—**See Antifungals, Azole (Vaginal)**, 310
*Terazol 3 Vaginal Ovules*—Janssen-Ortho (Canada) brand of Terconazole—**See Antifungals, Azole (Vaginal)**, 310
Terazosin Hydrochloride [*Hytrin*]
  **(Systemic)**, 2750
  Capsules, 2752, MC-29
Terbinafine [*Lamisil*]
  **(Systemic)**, 3036
  Tablets, 3036
Terbinafine Hydrochloride [*Lamisil*]
  **(Systemic)**, 2752
  Tablets, 2754, MC-29
Terbinafine Hydrochloride [*Lamisil*]
  **(Topical)**, 2755, 3036
  Cream, 2756
  Solution, 3036
Terbutaline Sulfate [*Brethaire; Bricanyl Turbuhaler*]
  **See Bronchodilators, Adrenergic (Inhalation-Local)**, 640
  Aerosol, Inhalation, USP, 651
Terbutaline Sulfate [*Brethine; Bricanyl*]
  **See Bronchodilators, Adrenergic (Systemic)**, 651
  Injection USP, 660
  Tablets USP, 660 MC-29
Terconazole [*Monistat 1; Terazol 3; Terazol 7; Terazol 3 Dual Pack; Terazol 3 Vaginal Ovules*]
  **See Antifungals, Azole (Vaginal)**, 310
  Cream, Vaginal, 314
  Suppositories, Vaginal, 314
Terfenadine [*Apo-Terfenadine; Novo-Terfenadine; Seldane; Seldane Caplets*]
  **See Antihistamines (Systemic)**, 325
  Suspension, Oral, 342
  Tablets USP, 342
Terfenadine-containing Combinations, 3082
Terfenadine and Pseudoephedrine Hydrochloride [*Seldane-D*]
  **See Antihistamines and Decongestants (Systemic)**, 343
  Tablets, Extended-release, 361
*Terfluzine*—ICN (Canada) brand of Trifluoperazine—**See Phenothiazines (Systemic)**, 2289
*Terfluzine Concentrate*—ICN (Canada) brand of Trifluoperazine—**See Phenothiazines (Systemic)**, 2289
Teriparatide [*Parathar*]
  **(Systemic)**, 3167
Teriparatide Acetate [hPTH 1–34; *Parathar*; synthetic human parathyroid hormone 1–34]
  **(Systemic)**, #
  for Injection, #
Terlipressin [*Glypressin*]
  **(Systemic)**, 3167
*Terramycin*—Pfizer (U.S.) and Roerig (U.S.) brand of Oxytetracycline—**See Tetracyclines (Systemic)**, 2765
*Tersac Cleansing Gel*—TransCanaDerm (Canada) brand of Salicylic Acid (Topical), #
*Tersa-Tar Mild Therapeutic Shampoo with Protein and Conditioner*—T.C.D. (Canada) brand of Coal Tar (Topical), #
*Tersa-Tar Soapless Tar Shampoo*—Doak (U.S.) brand of Coal Tar (Topical), #
*Tersa-Tar Therapeutic Shampoo*—T.C.D. (Canada) brand of Coal Tar (Topical), #
*Tes Est Cyp*—Ortega (U.S.) brand of Testosterone and Estradiol—**See Androgens and Estrogens (Systemic)**, 126
*Teslac*—Squibb (U.S.) brand of Testolactone (Systemic), 2756
*Tessalon*—Forest (U.S.) and Ciba-Geigy (Canada) brand of Benzonatate (Systemic), #
*Testamone 100*—Dunhall (U.S.) brand of Testosterone—**See Androgens (Systemic)**, 118
*Tes-tape*—Lilly (U.S. and Canada) brand of Glucose Oxidase Urine Glucose Test—**See Urine Glucose and Ketone Test Kits for Home Use**, #
*Testaqua*—Kay (U.S.) brand of Testosterone—**See Androgens (Systemic)**, 118
*Test-Estro Cypionate*—Rugby (U.S.) and Moore (U.S.) brand of Testosterone and Estradiol—**See Androgens and Estrogens (Systemic)**, 126

*Testex*—Taylor (U.S.) brand of Testosterone—**See Androgens (Systemic)**, 118
*Testoderm*—Alza (U.S.) brand of Testosterone—**See Androgens (Systemic)**, 118
*Testoderm TTS*—Alza (U.S.) brand of Testosterone—**See Androgens (Systemic)**, 118
*Testoderm with Adhesives*—Alza (U.S.) brand of Testosterone—**See Androgens (Systemic)**, 118
Testolactone [*Teslac*]
  **(Systemic)**, 2756
  Tablets USP, 2757
*Testopel Pellets*—Bartor (U.S.) brand of Testosterone—**See Androgens (Systemic)**, 118
Testosterone [*Androderm; Androgel; Testamone 100; Testaqua; Testoderm; Testoderm with Adhesives; Testoderm TTS; Testopel Pellets*]
  **See Androgens (Systemic)**, 118, 3168
  Implants, 126
  Suspension, Injectable, USP, 125
  Systems, Transdermal (Matrix-type), 126
  Systems, Transdermal (Reservoir-type), 126
Testosterone-containing Combinations, 3082
Testosterone Cypionate [*Andronate 100; Andronate 200; Depotest; Depo-Testosterone; Depo-Testosterone Cypionate; Scheinpharm Testone-Cyp; T-Cypionate; Testred Cypionate 200; Virilon IM*]
  **See Androgens (Systemic)**, 118
  Injection USP, 125
Testosterone Cypionate and Estradiol Cypionate [*De-Comberol; depAndrogyn; Depo-Testadiol; Depotestogen; Duo-Cyp; Duratestin; Menoject-L.A.; Tes Est Cyp; Test-Estro Cypionate*]
  **See Androgens and Estrogens (Systemic)**, 126
  Injection, 128
Testosterone Enanthate [*Andro L.A. 200; Andropository 200; Andryl 200; Delatest; Delatestryl; Everone 200; Testrin-P.A.*]
  **See Androgens (Systemic)**, 118
  Injection USP, 125
Testosterone Enanthate Benzilic Acid Hydrazone, Estradiol Dienanthate, and Estradiol Benzoate [*Climacteron*]
  **See Androgens and Estrogens (Systemic)**, 126
  Injection, 128
Testosterone Enanthate and Estradiol Valerate [*Andrest 90-4; Andro-Estro 90-4; Androgyn L.A.; Deladumone; Delatestadiol; Duo-Gen L.A.; Duogex L.A.; Dura-Dumone 90/4; Neo-Pause; OB; Teev; Valertest No. 1; Valertest No. 2*]
  **See Androgens and Estrogens (Systemic)**, 126
  Injection, 128
Testosterone Propionate [*Malogen in Oil; Testex*]
  **See Androgens (Systemic)**, 118, 3168
  Injection USP, 125
  Ointment, 126, 3168
Testosterone Sublingual
  **(Systemic)**, 3168
Testosterone Undecanoate [*Andriol*]
  **See Androgens (Systemic)**, 118
  Capsules, 125
*Testred*—ICN (U.S.) brand of Methyltestosterone—**See Androgens (Systemic)**, 118
*Testred Cypionate 200*—Legere (U.S.) brand of Testosterone—**See Androgens (Systemic)**, 118
*Testrin-P.A.*—Taylor (U.S.) brand of Testosterone—**See Androgens (Systemic)**, 118
Tetanus Antitoxin [TAT]
  **(Systemic)**, #
  Tetanus Antitoxin USP, #
Tetanus and Diphtheria Toxoids (Td) [Td]
  **See Diphtheria and Tetanus Toxoids (Systemic)**, 1236
  Tetanus and Diphtheria Toxoids Adsorbed for Adult Use (Td) USP, 1240
Tetanus Immune Globulin [*BayTet; TIG*]
  **(Systemic)**, 2758
  Injection USP, 2760
Tetanus Toxoid
  **(Systemic)**, 2760
  Injection USP (Fluid), 2762
Tetanus Toxoid Adsorbed
  **(Systemic)**, 2760
  USP (Injection), 2762
Tetrabenazine
  **(Systemic)**, 3168
Tetracaine [amethocaine; *Supracaine*]
  **See Anesthetics (Mucosal-Local)**, 128
  Aerosol, Topical, 138
Tetracaine [amethocaine; *Pontocaine*]
  **See Anesthetics (Ophthalmic)**, #
  Ointment, Ophthalmic, USP, #
Tetracaine-containing Combinations, 3082

Tetracaine Hydrochloride [amethocaine; *Pontocaine; Pontocaine Cream*]
  **See Anesthetics (Mucosal-Local)**, 128
  Cream USP, 138
  Solution, Topical, USP, 138
Tetracaine Hydrochloride [*Ak-T-Caine*; amethocaine; *Minims Tetracaine; Opticaine; Pontocaine*]
  **See Anesthetics (Ophthalmic)**, #
  Solution, Ophthalmic, USP, #
Tetracaine Hydrochloride [*Pontocaine*]
  **See Anesthetics (Parenteral-Local)**, 139
  Injection USP, 154
  Sterile USP, 154
Tetracaine Hydrochloride [amethocaine; *Pontocaine Cream*]
  **See Anesthetics (Topical)**, 155
  Cream USP, 161
Tetracaine Hydrochloride in Dextrose [*Pontocaine*]
  **See Anesthetics (Parenteral-Local)**, 139
  Injection USP, 154
Tetracaine and Menthol [*Pontocaine Ointment*]
  **See Anesthetics (Mucosal-Local)**, 128
  Ointment USP, 138
Tetracaine and Menthol [*Pontocaine Ointment*]
  **See Anesthetics (Topical)**, 155
  Ointment USP, 161
Tetracosactide—See Cosyntropin (Systemic), 1023
Tetracycline [*Achromycin V; Helidac Therapy Capsules; Novotetra; Sumycin*]
  **See Tetracyclines (Systemic)**, 2765
  Suspension, Oral, USP, 2773, MC-4
Tetracycline Hydrochloride [*Achromycin*]
  **See Tetracyclines (Ophthalmic)**, 2763
  Ointment, Ophthalmic, USP, 2764
  Suspension, Ophthalmic, USP, 2764
Tetracycline Hydrochloride [*Achromycin; Achromycin V; Apo-Tetra; Novotetra; Nu-Tetra; Panmycin; Robitet; Sumycin ; Tetracyn*]
  **See Tetracyclines (Systemic)**, 2765
  Capsules USP, 2773, MC-29
  for Injection USP (Intramuscular), 2773
  Tablets USP, 2773, MC-29
Tetracycline Hydrochloride [*Achromycin; Topicycline*]
  **See Tetracyclines (Topical)**, 2774
  Ointment USP, 2776
  for Solution, Topical, USP, 2776
Tetracycline Periodontal Fibers [*Actisite*]
  **(Mucosal-Local)**, #
  Fibers, Periodontal, #
Tetracyclines
  **(Ophthalmic)**, 2763
Tetracyclines
  **(Systemic)**, 2765
Tetracyclines
  **(Topical)**, 2774
*Tetracyn*—Pfizer (U.S. and Canada) brand of Tetracycline—**See Tetracyclines (Systemic)**, 2765
Tetrahydroaminoacridine—See Tacrine (Systemic), 2680
Tetramethylthionine chloride—See Methylene Blue (Systemic), #
*Tetramune*—Lederle (U.S. and Canada) brand of Diphtheria and Tetanus Toxoids and Pertussis Vaccine Adsorbed and Haemophilus b Conjugate Vaccine (HbOC—Diphtheria $CRM_{197}$;17 Protein Conjugate)—**See Diphtheria and Tetanus Toxoids and Pertussis Vaccine Adsorbed and Haemophilus b Conjugate Vaccine (Systemic)**, 1244
*Texacort*—GenDerm (U.S.) brand of Hydrocortisone—**See Corticosteroids (Topical)**, 978
*T-Gel*—Professional Pharmaceutical (Canada) brand of Coal Tar (Topical), #
*T/Gel Therapeutic Conditioner*—Neutrogena (U.S.) brand of Coal Tar (Topical), #
*T/Gel Therapeutic Shampoo*—Neutrogena (U.S.) brand of Coal Tar (Topical), #
*T-Gen*—Goldline (U.S.) brand of Trimethobenzamide (Systemic), 2880
*T-Gesic*—Williams T.E. (U.S.) brand of Hydrocodone and Acetaminophen—**See Opioid (Narcotic) Analgesics and Acetaminophen (Systemic)**, 2198
THA—See Tacrine (Systemic), 2680
Thalidomide [*Synovir, THALOMID*]
  **(Systemic)**, 2776, 3168
  Capsules, 2781
*Thalitone*—Boehringer Ingelheim (U.S.) brand of Chlorthalidone—**See Diuretics, Thiazide (Systemic)**, 1273, MC-7

*USP DI*                                                              **General Index**

Thallous Chloride Tl 201 **(Systemic)**, 2781
  Injection USP, 2783
THALOMID—Celgene (Canada) brand of Thalidomide (Systemic), 2776
Theo-24—UCB (U.S.) brand of Theophylline—**See Bronchodilators, Theophylline (Systemic)**, 668, MC-29, MC-30
Theobid Duracaps—Whitby (U.S.) brand of Theophylline—**See Bronchodilators, Theophylline (Systemic)**, 668
Theochron—Forest (U.S.) and Riva (Canada) brand of Theophylline—**See Bronchodilators, Theophylline (Systemic)**, 668
Theoclear-80—Central (U.S.) brand of Theophylline—**See Bronchodilators, Theophylline (Systemic)**, 668
Theoclear L.A.-260—Central (U.S.) brand of Theophylline—**See Bronchodilators, Theophylline (Systemic)**, 668
Theocon—CMC-Consumer (U.S.) brand of Theophylline and Guaifenesin (Systemic), #
Theo-Dur—Key (U.S.) and Astra (Canada) brand of Theophylline—**See Bronchodilators, Theophylline (Systemic)**, 668
Theolair—Riker (U.S.) and 3M (Canada) brand of Theophylline—**See Bronchodilators, Theophylline (Systemic)**, 668
Theolair-SR—Riker (U.S.) and 3M (Canada) brand of Theophylline—**See Bronchodilators, Theophylline (Systemic)**, 668
Theolate—Alpharma (U.S.) and Balan (U.S.) brand of Theophylline and Guaifenesin (Systemic), #
Theophylline [*Aerolate Sr.; Apo-Theo-LA; Asmalix; Elixophyllin; Lanophyllin; PMS-Theophylline; Pulmophylline; Quibron-T Dividose; Quibron-T/SR Dividose; Respbid; Slo-Bid; Slo-Bid Gyrocaps; Slo-Phyllin; Theo-24; Theobid Duracaps; Theochron; Theoclear-80; Theoclear L.A.-260; Theo-Dur; Theolair; Theolair-SR; Theo-Time; Theovent Long-Acting; Theo-X; T-Phyl; Truxophyllin; Uni-Dur; Uniphyl*]
  **See Bronchodilators, Theophylline (Systemic)**, 668
  Capsules USP, 679
  Capsules, Extended-release, USP, 680 MC-29, MC-30
  Elixir, 680
  Solution, Oral, 681
  Syrup, 681
  Tablets USP, 681 MC-29
  Tablets, Extended-release, 681, MC-29, MC-30
Theophylline-containing Combinations, 3082
Theophylline in Dextrose
  **See Bronchodilators, Theophylline (Systemic)**, 668
  Injection USP, 682
Theophylline, Ephedrine Hydrochloride, Guaifenesin, and Phenobarbital **(Systemic)**, #
  Elixir, #
  Tablets, #
Theophylline, Ephedrine Hydrochloride, and Phenobarbital **(Systemic)**, #
  Tablets USP, #
Theophylline, Ephedrine Sulfate, Guaifenesin, and Phenobarbital **(Systemic)**, #
  Elixir, #
  Tablets, #
Theophylline, Ephedrine Sulfate, and Hydroxyzine Hydrochloride [*Marax; Marax-DF*] **(Systemic)**, #
  Syrup, #
  Tablets, #
Theophylline and glyceryl guaiacolate—*See* Theophylline and Guaifenesin (Systemic), #
Theophylline and Guaifenesin [*Bronchial; Broncomar; Elixophyllin-GG; Glyceryl-T; Quibron; Quibron-300; Slo-Phyllin GG; Theocon; Theolate;* theophylline and glyceryl guaiacolate] **(Systemic)**, #
  Capsules USP, #, MC-30
  Elixir, #
  Solution, Oral, USP, #
  Syrup, #
Theophylline Sodium Glycinate and Guaifenesin [*EdBron G; Equibron G;* theophylline and glyceryl guaiacolate] **(Systemic)**, #
  Elixir, #

Theo-SR—Rhône-Poulenc Rorer (Canada) brand of Theophylline—**See Bronchodilators, Theophylline (Systemic)**, 668
Theo-Time—Major (U.S.) brand of Theophylline—**See Bronchodilators, Theophylline (Systemic)**, 668
Theovent Long-Acting—Schering (U.S.) brand of Theophylline—**See Bronchodilators, Theophylline (Systemic)**, 668
Theo-X—Carnrick (U.S.) brand of Theophylline—**See Bronchodilators, Theophylline (Systemic)**, 668
TheraCys—Connaught (U.S.) brand of Bacillus Calmette-Guérin (BCG) Live (Mucosal-Local), 507
Theraderm Testosterone Transdermal System—Theratech (U.S.) brand of Testosterone (Systemic), 3168
TheraFlu Flu, Cold & Cough Medicine—Sandoz (U.S.) brand of Chlorpheniramine, Pseudoephedrine, Dextromethorphan, and Acetaminophen—**See Cough/Cold Combinations (Systemic)**, 1024
TheraFlu/Flu and Cold Medicine—Sandoz (U.S.) brand of Chlorpheniramine, Pseudoephedrine, and Acetaminophen—**See Antihistamines, Decongestants, and Analgesics (Systemic)**, 366
TheraFlu/Flu and Cold Medicine for Sore Throat—Sandoz (U.S.) brand of Chlorpheniramine, Pseudoephedrine, and Acetaminophen—**See Antihistamines, Decongestants, and Analgesics (Systemic)**, 366
TheraFlu Maximum Strength Non-Drowsy Formula Flu, Cold & Cough Medicine—Sandoz (U.S.) brand of Pseudoephedrine, Dextromethorphan, and Acetaminophen—**See Cough/Cold Combinations (Systemic)**, 1024
TheraFlu Maximum Strength Non-Drowsy Formula Flu, Cold & Cough Medicine Caplets—Sandoz (U.S.) brand of Pseudoephedrine, Dextromethorphan, and Acetaminophen—**See Cough/Cold Combinations (Systemic)**, 1024
TheraFlu Nighttime Maximum Strength Flu, Cold & Cough—Sandoz (U.S.) brand of Chlorpheniramine, Pseudoephedrine, Dextromethorphan, and Acetaminophen—**See Cough/Cold Combinations (Systemic)**, 1024
TheraFlu Sinus Maximum Strength Caplets—Sandoz (U.S.) brand of Pseudoephedrine and Acetaminophen—**See Decongestants and Analgesics (Systemic)**, 1180
Theralax—Beecham (U.S.) brand of Bisacodyl—**See Laxatives (Local)**, #
Theramycin Z—Medicis (U.S.) brand of Erythromycin (Topical), 3018
Theraplex T Shampoo—Medicis (U.S.) brand of Coal Tar (Topical), #
Therevac Plus—Jones (U.S.) brand of Docusate—**See Laxatives (Local)**, #
Therevac-SB—Jones (U.S.) brand of Docusate—**See Laxatives (Local)**, #
Thermazene—Chesebrough-Ponds (U.S.) brand of Silver Sulfadiazine (Topical), #
Thiabendazole [*Mintezol*] **(Systemic)**, 2784
  Suspension, Oral, USP, 2786
  Tablets USP (Chewable), 2786
Thiabendazole **(Topical)**, 2786
  Suspension, Topical, 2787
Thiacetazone-containing Combinations, 3082
Thiamazole—Methimazole—**See Antithyroid Agents (Systemic)**, 446
Thiamine Hydrochloride [*Betaxin; Bewon; Biamine;* vitamin B₁] **(Systemic)**, 2787
  Elixir USP, 2789
  Injection USP, 2789
  Tablets USP, 2789
Thiazina—*See* Isoniazid and Thiacetazone (Systemic), #
Thiethylperazine Malate [*Norzine; Torecan*] **(Systemic)**, #
  Injection USP, #
Thiethylperazine Maleate [*Norzine; Torecan*] **(Systemic)**, #
  Suppositories USP, #
  Tablets USP, #
Thioguanine [*Lanvis; Tabloid*] **(Systemic)**, #
  Tablets USP, #
Thiola—Mission (U.S.) brand of Tiopronin (Systemic), 2824; *See also* Tiopronin (Systemic), 3169

Thionex—Lannett (U.S.) brand of Lindane (Topical), 1866
Thiopental Sodium [*Pentothal;* thiopentone]
  **See Anesthetics, Barbiturate (Systemic)**, 161
  for Injection USP, 166
  for Solution, Rectal, 167
  Suspension, Rectal, 167
Thiopentone—Thiopental—**See Anesthetics, Barbiturate (Systemic)**, 161
Thioplex—Immunex (U.S.) brand of Thiotepa (Systemic), 2790
Thiopropazate Hydrochloride [*Dartal*]
  **See Phenothiazines (Systemic)**, 2289
  Tablets, 2308
Thioproperazine Mesylate [*Majeptil*]
  **See Phenothiazines (Systemic)**, 2289
  Tablets, 2309
Thioridazine [*Mellaril; Mellaril-S*]
  **See Phenothiazines (Systemic)**, 2289
  Suspension, Oral, USP, 2309
Thioridazine Hydrochloride [*Apo-Thioridazine; Mellaril; Mellaril Concentrate; Novo-Ridazine; PMS Thioridazine*]
  **See Phenothiazines (Systemic)**, 2289
  Solution, Oral, USP, 2309
  Tablets USP, 2310, MC-30
Thiosol—Cooperativa Farmaceutica (Italy) brand of Tiopronin (Systemic), 2824
Thiosulfil Forte—Ayerst (U.S.) brand of Sulfamethizole—**See Sulfonamides (Systemic)**, 2653
Thiotepa [*Thioplex*] **(Systemic)**, 2790
  for Injection USP, 2793
Thiothixene [*Navane*]
  **See Thioxanthenes (Systemic)**, 2793
  Capsules USP, 2798, MC-30
Thiothixene HCl Intensol—Roxane (U.S.) brand of Thiothixene—**See Thioxanthenes (Systemic)**, 2793
Thiothixene Hydrochloride [*Navane; Thiothixene HCl Intensol*]
  **See Thioxanthenes (Systemic)**, 2793
  Injection USP, 2799
  for Injection USP, 2799
  Solution, Oral, USP, 2799
Thioxanthenes **(Systemic)**, 2793
Thisozide—Cosmos (Kenya) brand of Isoniazid and Thiacetazone (Systemic), #
Thorazine—SmithKline Beecham (U.S.) brand of Chlorpromazine—**See Phenothiazines (Systemic)**, 2289, MC-6, MC-7
Thorazine Concentrate—Nova (U.S.) brand of Chlorpromazine—**See Phenothiazines (Systemic)**, 2289
Thorazine Spansule—SmithKline Beecham (U.S.) brand of Chlorpromazine—**See Phenothiazines (Systemic)**, 2289, MC-6
Thor-Prom—Major (U.S.) brand of Chlorpromazine—**See Phenothiazines (Systemic)**, 2289
Threamine DM—Barre-National (U.S.) brand of Chlorpheniramine, Phenylpropanolamine, and Dextromethorphan—**See Cough/Cold Combinations (Systemic)**, 1024
Threostat—Tyson (U.S.) brand of L-Threonine (Systemic), 3151
Thrombate III—Miles (U.S.) brand of Antithrombin III (Systemic), 444, 3131
Thrombolytic Agents **(Systemic)**, 2799
Thybine—Columbia (U.S.) brand of Yohimbine (Systemic), #
Thymalfasin [*Zadaxin*] **(Systemic)**, 3169
Thymosin Alpha-1 **(Systemic)**, 3169
Thyrar—Rhône-Poulenc Rorer (U.S.) brand of Thyroid—**See Thyroid Hormones (Systemic)**, 2809
Thyro-Block—Horner (Canada) brand of Potassium Iodide (Systemic), 2354
Thyrogen—Genzyme (U.S.) brand of Human Thyroid Stimulating Hormone (Systemic), 3146
Thyroglobulin
  **See Thyroid Hormones (Systemic)**, 2809
  Tablets USP, 2814
Thyroid [*Armour Thyroid; Thyrar; Thyroid Strong; Westhroid*]
  **See Thyroid Hormones (Systemic)**, 2809
  Tablets USP, 2815
Thyroid Hormones **(Systemic)**, 2809

# General Index

*Thyroid Strong*—Jones Medical (U.S.) brand of Thyroid—**See Thyroid Hormones (Systemic)**, 2809
*Thyrolar*—Forest (U.S.) brand of Liotrix—**See Thyroid Hormones (Systemic)**, 2809
Thyrotropin—*See* Human Thyroid Stimulating Hormone (Systemic), 3146
Thyrotropin [*Thytropar*]
　**(Systemic)**, #
　for Injection, #
*Thytropar*—Armour (U.S.) and Rorer (Canada) brand of Thyrotropin (Systemic), #
Tiagabine Hydrochloride [*Gabitril*]
　**(Systemic)**, 2815
　Tablets, 2817, MC-30
Tiapride
　**(Systemic)**, 3169
Tiaprofenic Acid [*Albert Tiafen; Surgam; Surgam SR*]
　**See Anti-inflammatory Drugs, Nonsteroidal (Systemic)**, 388
　Capsules, Extended-release, 418
　Tablets, 419
*Tiazac*—Forest (U.S.) brand of Diltiazem (Systemic), 3017
*Ticar*—Beecham (U.S. and Canada) brand of Ticarcillin—**See Penicillins (Systemic)**, 2240
Ticarcillin-containing Combinations, 3082
Ticarcillin Disodium [*Ticar*]
　**See Penicillins (Systemic)**, 2240
　Sterile USP, 2261
Ticarcillin Disodium and Clavulanate Potassium [*Timentin*]
　**See Penicillins and Beta-lactamase Inhibitors (Systemic)**, 2263
　Injection, 2271
　Sterile USP, 2270
*TICE BCG*—Organon (U.S.) brand of Bacillus Calmette-Guérin (BCG) Live (Mucosal-Local), 507; (Systemic), 510
*Ticlid*—Roche (U.S.) and Syntex (Canada) brand of Ticlopidine (Systemic), 2818, MC-30
Ticlopidine Hydrochloride [*Ticlid*]
　**(Systemic)**, 2818
　Tablets, 2822, MC-30
*Ticon*—Hauck (U.S.) brand of Trimethobenzamide (Systemic), 2880
TIG—*See* Tetanus Immune Globulin (Systemic), 2758
*Tigan*—SmithKline Beecham (U.S.) brand of Trimethobenzamide (Systemic), 2880
Tiger snake antivenom—*See* Antivenin (Notechis Scutatus) (Systemic), #
*Tija*—Vita Elixir (U.S.) brand of Oxytetracycline—**See Tetracyclines (Systemic)**, 2765
*Tiject-20*—Mayrand (U.S.) brand of Trimethobenzamide (Systemic), 2880
*Tilade*—Fisons (U.S. and Canada) brand of Nedocromil (Inhalation-Local), 2090
Tiludronate Disodium [*Skelid*]
　**(Systemic)**, 2822
　Tablets, 2824
*Timentin*—SmithKline Beecham (U.S. and Canada) brand of Ticarcillin and Clavulanate—**See Penicillins and Beta-lactamase Inhibitors (Systemic)**, 2263
*Timodal*—Pharmascience (Canada) brand of Timolol (Ophthalmic), 3036
*Timolide*—Merck (U.S.) and Frosst (Canada) brand of Timolol and Hydrochlorothiazide—**See Beta-adrenergic Blocking Agents and Thiazide Diuretics (Systemic)**, 609
Timolol-containing Combinations, 3082
Timolol Hemihydrate [*Betimol*]
　**(Ophthalmic)**, 3036
　Solution, Ophthalmic, 3036
Timolol Maleate [*Apo-Timop; Beta-Tim; Gen-Timolol; Med Timolol; Novo-Timol; Nu-Timolol; Timodal; Timoptic; Timoptic in Ocudose; Timoptic-XE*]
　**See Beta-adrenergic Blocking Agents (Ophthalmic)**, 585, 3036
　Solution, Gel-forming, Ophthalmic, 3036
　Solution, Ophthalmic, USP, 592, 3036
Timolol Maleate [*Apo-Timol; Blocadren; Novo-Timol*]
　**See Beta-adrenergic Blocking Agents (Systemic)**, 593
　Tablets USP, 608, MC-30
Timolol Maleate and Hydrochlorothiazide [*Timolide*]
　**See Beta-adrenergic Blocking Agents and Thiazide Diuretics (Systemic)**, 609
　Tablets USP, 611
*Timoptic*—Merck (U.S. and Canada) brand of Timolol—**See Beta-adrenergic Blocking Agents (Ophthalmic)**, 585

*Timoptic in Ocudose*—Merck (U.S.) brand of Timolol—**See Beta-adrenergic Blocking Agents (Ophthalmic)**, 585
*Timoptic-XE*—Merck (U.S. and Canada) brand of Timolol (Ophthalmic), 3036
*Tinactin Aerosol Liquid*—Schering (U.S. and Canada) brand of Tolnaftate (Topical), #
*Tinactin Aerosol Powder*—Schering (U.S. and Canada) brand of Tolnaftate (Topical), #
*Tinactin Antifungal Deodorant Powder Aerosol*—Schering (U.S.) brand of Tolnaftate (Topical), #
*Tinactin Cream*—Schering (U.S. and Canada) brand of Tolnaftate (Topical), #
*Tinactin Jock Itch Aerosol Powder*—Schering (Canada) brand of Tolnaftate (Topical), #
*Tinactin Jock Itch Cream*—Schering (U.S. and Canada) brand of Tolnaftate (Topical), #
*Tinactin Jock Itch Spray Powder*—Schering (U.S.) brand of Tolnaftate (Topical), #
*Tinactin Plus Aerosol Powder*—Schering (Canada) brand of Tolnaftate (Topical), #
*Tinactin Plus Powder*—Schering (Canada) brand of Tolnaftate (Topical), #
*Tinactin Powder*—Schering (U.S. and Canada) brand of Tolnaftate (Topical), #
*Tinactin Solution*—Schering (U.S. and Canada) brand of Tolnaftate (Topical), #
*Tindal*—Schering (U.S.) brand of Acetophenazine—**See Phenothiazines (Systemic)**, 2289
*Ting Antifungal Cream*—Fisons (U.S.) brand of Tolnaftate (Topical), #
*Ting Antifungal Powder*—Fisons (U.S.) brand of Tolnaftate (Topical), #
*Ting Antifungal Spray Liquid*—Fisons (U.S.) brand of Tolnaftate (Topical), #
*Ting Antifungal Spray Powder*—Fisons (U.S.) brand of Tolnaftate (Topical), #
Tioconazole [*Trosyd Dermal Cream*]
　**(Topical)**, 3036
　Cream, 3036
Tioconazole [*GyneCure; GyneCure Ovules; GyneCure Vaginal Ointment Tandempak; GyneCure Vaginal Ovules Tandempak; Vagistat-1*]
　**See Antifungals, Azole (Vaginal)**, 310
　Ointment, Vaginal, 314
　Suppositories, Vaginal, 314
*Tioglis*—Logifarm (Italy) brand of Tiopronin (Systemic), 2824
Tiopronin [*Capen; Captimer; Epatiol; Mucolysin; Sutilan; Thiola; Thiosol; Tioglis; Vincol*]
　**(Systemic)**, 2824, 3169
　Tablets, 2826
*Tipramine*—Major (U.S.) brand of Imipramine—**See Antidepressants, Tricyclic (Systemic)**, 271
Tiratricol [*Triacana*]
　**(Systemic)**, 3169
Tirofiban Hydrochloride [*Aggrastat*]
　**(Systemic)**, 2826, 3036
　Injection, 2828, 3036
*TI Screen*—Fisher (U.S.) brand of Octocrylene, Octyl Methoxycinnamate, Octyl Salicylate, and Oxybenzone—**See Sunscreen Agents (Topical)**, #; Octyl Methoxycinnamate, Octyl Salicylate, and Oxybenzone—**See Sunscreen Agents (Topical)**, #; Octyl Methoxycinnamate and Oxybenzone—**See Sunscreen Agents (Topical)**, #
*TI Screen Baby Natural*—Fisher (U.S.) brand of Titanium Dioxide—**See Sunscreen Agents (Topical)**, #
*Tisit*—Pfeiffer (U.S.) brand of Pyrethrins and Piperonyl Butoxide (Topical), #
*Tisit Blue*—Pfeiffer (U.S.) brand of Pyrethrins and Piperonyl Butoxide (Topical), #
*Tisit Shampoo*—Pfeiffer (U.S.) brand of Pyrethrins and Piperonyl Butoxide (Topical), #
*Tisseel VH Kit*—Baxter (U.S.) brand of Fibrin Sealant (Local), 3036
Tissue-type plasminogen activator (recombinant)—Alteplase, Recombinant—**See Thrombolytic Agents (Systemic)**, 2799
Titanium Dioxide [*Neutrogena Chemical-Free Sunblocker; TI Screen Baby Natural; Vaseline Intensive Care Baby Moisturizing Sunblock*]
　**See Sunscreen Agents (Topical)**, #
　Lotion, #
Titanium Dioxide-containing Combinations, 3082
Titanium Dioxide and Zinc Oxide [*Johnson's No More Tears Baby Sunblock; Sundown Sport Sunblock; Vaseline Baby Sunblock*]
　**See Sunscreen Agents (Topical)**, #
　Lotion, #

*Titan Lubricated*—Schmid (Canada) brand of Latex Condoms—**See Condoms**, #
*Titan Ribbed*—Schmid (Canada) brand of Latex Condoms—**See Condoms**, #
*Titan with Silicone Spermicidal Lubricant*—Schmid (Canada) brand of Latex Condoms and Nonoxynol 9—**See Condoms**, #
*Titralac*—3M (U.S. and Canada) brand of Calcium Carbonate—**See Antacids (Oral-Local)**, 188; 3M (U.S.) brand of Calcium Carbonate—**See Calcium Supplements (Systemic)**, 736
*Titralac Extra Strength*—3M (U.S.) brand of Calcium Carbonate—**See Antacids (Oral-Local)**, 188
*Titralac Plus*—3M (U.S.) brand of Calcium Carbonate and Simethicone—**See Antacids (Oral-Local)**, 188
*TI-UVA-B Sunscreen*—Tican (Canada) brand of Octyl Methoxycinnamate and Oxybenzone—**See Sunscreen Agents (Topical)**, #
Tixocortol Pivalate [*Rectovalone*]
　**See Corticosteroids (Rectal)**, 973
　Enema, 977
Tizanidine [*Zanaflex*]
　**(Systemic)**, 2828
　Tablets, 2830, MC-30
Tizanidine Hydrochloride [*Zanaflex*]
　**(Systemic)**, 3169
*T-Koff*—T. E. Williams (U.S.) brand of Chlorpheniramine, Phenylephrine, Phenylpropanolamine, and Codeine—**See Cough/Cold Combinations (Systemic)**, 1024
[201]Tl—*See* Thallous Chloride Tl 201 (Systemic), 2781
TMO—Trimethadione—**See Anticonvulsants, Dione (Systemic)**, #
Tobramycin
　**(Systemic)**, 3169
　for Inhalation, 3169
Tobramycin [*AKTob; Tobrex*]
　**(Ophthalmic)**, #, 3036
　Ointment, Ophthalmic, USP, #
　Solution, Ophthalmic, USP, #, 3036
Tobramycin Sulfate [*Nebcin*]
　**See Aminoglycosides (Systemic)**, 69
　Injection, 78
　Sterile USP, 79
Tobramycin Sulfate in Sodium Chloride
　**See Aminoglycosides (Systemic)**, 69
　Injection, 79
*Tobrex*—Alcon (U.S. and Canada) brand of Tobramycin (Ophthalmic), #
Tocainide Hydrochloride [*Tonocard*]
　**(Systemic)**, 2831
　Tablets USP, 2833, MC-30
*Today*—VLI (U.S.) and Wyeth (Canada) brand of Nonoxynol 9—**See Spermicides (Vaginal)**, #
*Tofranil*—Novartis (U.S. and Canada) brand of Imipramine—**See Antidepressants, Tricyclic (Systemic)**, 271, MC-15
*Tofranil-PM*—Novartis (U.S.) brand of Imipramine—**See Antidepressants, Tricyclic (Systemic)**, 271, MC-15
Tolazamide [*Tolinase*]
　**See Antidiabetic Agents, Sulfonylurea (Systemic)**, 283
　Tablets USP, 295, MC-30
Tolazoline Hydrochloride [*Priscoline*]
　**(Parenteral-Systemic)**, #
　Injection USP, #
Tolbutamide [*Apo-Tolbutamide; Mobenol; Novo-Butamide; Orinase; Tol-Tab*]
　**See Antidiabetic Agents, Sulfonylurea (Systemic)**, 283
　Tablets USP, 295, MC-30
Tolbutamide Sodium [*Orinase Diagnostic*]
　**(Systemic)**, 3036
　Powder, Sterile, USP, 3036
Tolcapone [*Tasmar*]
　**(Systemic)**, 2833, 3015
　Tablets, 2836, MC-30
*Tolectin 200*—Ortho-McNeil (U.S. and Canada) brand of Tolmetin—**See Anti-inflammatory Drugs, Nonsteroidal (Systemic)**, 388, MC-31
*Tolectin 400*—McNeil (Canada) brand of Tolmetin—**See Anti-inflammatory Drugs, Nonsteroidal (Systemic)**, 388
*Tolectin 600*—Ortho-McNeil (U.S. and Canada) brand of Tolmetin—**See Anti-inflammatory Drugs, Nonsteroidal (Systemic)**, 388, MC-31
*Tolectin DS*—Ortho-McNeil (U.S.) brand of Tolmetin—**See Anti-inflammatory Drugs, Nonsteroidal (Systemic)**, 388, MC-30

*Tolerex*—Procter & Gamble (U.S.) brand of Enteral Nutrition Formula, Monomeric (Elemental)—**See Enteral Nutrition Formulas (Systemic)**, #

*Tolinase*—Pharmacia & Upjohn (U.S.) brand of Tolazamide—**See Antidiabetic Agents, Sulfonylurea (Systemic)**, 283, MC-30

Tolmetin Sodium [*Novo-Tolmetin; Tolectin 200; Tolectin 400; Tolectin 600; Tolectin DS*]
  See **Anti-inflammatory Drugs, Nonsteroidal (Systemic)**, 388
  Capsules USP, 419, MC-30, MC-31
  Tablets USP, 419, MC-30, MC-31

Tolnaftate [*Aftate for Athlete's Foot Aerosol Spray Liquid; Aftate for Athlete's Foot Aerosol Spray Powder; Aftate for Athlete's Foot Gel; Aftate for Athlete's Foot Sprinkle Powder; Aftate for Jock Itch Aerosol Spray Powder; Aftate for Jock Itch Gel; Aftate for Jock Itch Sprinkle Powder; Genaspore Cream; NP-27 Cream; NP-27 Powder; NP-27 Solution; NP-27 Spray Powder; Pitrex Cream; Tinactin Aerosol Liquid; Tinactin Aerosol Powder; Tinactin Antifungal Deodorant Powder Aerosol; Tinactin Cream; Tinactin Jock Itch Aerosol Powder; Tinactin Jock Itch Cream; Tinactin Jock Itch Spray Powder; Tinactin Plus Aerosol Powder; Tinactin Plus Powder; Tinactin Powder; Tinactin Solution; Ting Antifungal Cream; Ting Antifungal Powder; Ting Antifungal Spray Liquid; Ting Antifungal Spray Powder; Zeasorb-AF Powder*]
  **(Topical)**, #
  Aerosol Powder, Topical, USP, #
  Aerosol Solution, Topical, #
  Cream USP, #
  Gel USP, #
  Powder USP (Topical), #
  Solution, Topical, USP, #

*Tol-Tab*—Alra (U.S.) brand of Tolbutamide—**See Antidiabetic Agents, Sulfonylurea (Systemic)**, 283

Tolterodine Tartrate [*Detrol*]
  **(Systemic)**, 2837
  Tablets, 2838

*Tolu-Sed Cough*—Scherer (U.S.) brand of Codeine and Guaifenesin—**See Cough/Cold Combinations (Systemic)**, 1024

*Tolu-Sed DM*—Scherer (U.S.) brand of Dextromethorphan and Guaifenesin—**See Cough/Cold Combinations (Systemic)**, 1024

*Tomocat*—Lafayette (U.S.) brand of Barium Sulfate (Local), #

*Tomocat 1000*—Lafayette (U.S.) brand of Barium Sulfate (Local), #

*Tonocard*—Astra Merck (U.S.) and Astra (Canada) brand of Tocainide (Systemic), 2831, MC-30

*Tonojug 2000*—Lafayette (U.S.) brand of Barium Sulfate (Local), #

*Tonopaque*—Lafayette (U.S.) brand of Barium Sulfate (Local), #

*Topamax*—R. W. Johnson (U.S.) brand of Topiramate (Systemic), 3169

*Topicaine*—Hoechst (Canada) brand of Benzocaine—**See Anesthetics (Mucosal-Local)**, 128

*Topicort*—Hoechst-Roussel (U.S.) and Hoechst (Canada) brand of Desoximetasone—**See Corticosteroids (Topical)**, 978

*Topicort LP*—Hoechst-Roussel (U.S.) brand of Desoximetasone—**See Corticosteroids (Topical)**, 978

*Topicort Mild*—Hoechst (Canada) brand of Desoximetasone—**See Corticosteroids (Topical)**, 978

*Topicycline*—Procter & Gamble (U.S.) brand of Tetracycline—**See Tetracyclines (Topical)**, 2774

*Topilene*—Technilab (Canada) brand of Betamethasone—**See Corticosteroids (Topical)**, 978

Topiramate [*Topamax*]
  **(Systemic)**, 2839, 3169
  Tablets, 2841, MC-31

*Topisone*—Technilab (Canada) brand of Betamethasone—**See Corticosteroids (Topical)**, 978

*Topisporin*—Pharmafair (U.S.) brand of Neomycin, Polymyxin B, and Bacitracin (Topical), #

*Topomax*—McNeil (U.S.) brand of Topiramate (Systemic), 2839

*Toposar*—Pharmacia (U.S.) brand of Etoposide (Systemic), 1424

Topotecan [*Hycamtin*]
  **(Systemic)**, 2841
  for Injection, 2845

*Toprol-XL*—Astra (U.S.) brand of Metoprolol—**See Beta-adrenergic Blocking Agents (Systemic)**, 593, MC-20

*Topsyn*—Syntex (Canada) brand of Fluocinonide—**See Corticosteroids (Topical)**, 978

*TOPV*—Poliovirus Vaccine Live Oral—**See Poliovirus Vaccine (Systemic)**, 2343

*Toradol*—Roche (U.S.) and Syntex (Canada) brand of Ketorolac (Systemic), 1810, MC-16

Torasemide—*See* Torsemide (Systemic), 2848

*Torecan*—Roxane (U.S. and Canada) brand of Thiethylperazine (Systemic), #

Toremifene
  **(Systemic)**, 3169

Toremifene Citrate [*Fareston*]
  **(Systemic)**, 2845
  Tablets, 2847

*Tornalate*—Dura (U.S.) brand of Bitolterol—**See Bronchodilators, Adrenergic (Inhalation-Local)**, 640

Torsemide [*Demadex*; torsemide]
  **(Systemic)**, 2848
  Injection, 2850
  Tablets, 2850, MC-31

*Totacillin*—SmithKline Beecham (U.S.) brand of Ampicillin—**See Penicillins (Systemic)**, 2240

*Totacillin-N*—SmithKline Beecham (U.S.) brand of Ampicillin—**See Penicillins (Systemic)**, 2240

*Total*—Colgate (U.S.) brand of Sodium Fluoride and Triclosan (Dental), 3034

*Total Eclipse Moisturizing Skin*—Triangle Labs (U.S.) brand of Octyl Salicylate and Padimate O—**See Sunscreen Agents (Topical)**, #

*Total Eclipse Oily and Acne Prone Skin Sunscreen*—Triangle Labs (U.S.) brand of Lisadimate, Oxybenzone, and Padimate O—**See Sunscreen Agents (Topical)**, #

*Touch Lubricated*—Schmid (U.S.) brand of Latex Condoms—**See Condoms**, #

*Touch Non-Lubricated*—Schmid (U.S.) brand of Latex Condoms—**See Condoms**, #

*Touch Ribbed Lubricated*—Schmid (U.S.) brand of Latex Condoms—**See Condoms**, #

*Touch Spermicidally Lubricated*—Schmid (U.S.) brand of Latex Condoms and Nonoxynol 9—**See Condoms**, #

*Touch Sunrise Colors*—Schmid (U.S.) brand of Latex Condoms—**See Condoms**, #

*Touch Thins Lubricated*—Schmid (U.S.) brand of Latex Condoms—**See Condoms**, #

*Touro A&H*—Dartmouth (U.S.) brand of Brompheniramine and Pseudoephedrine—**See Antihistamines and Decongestants (Systemic)**, 343

*Touro DM*—Dartmouth (U.S.) brand of Dextromethorphan and Guaifenesin (Systemic), 3017

*Touro EX*—Dartmouth (U.S.) brand of Guaifenesin (Systemic), 1588

*Touro LA Caplets*—Dartmouth (U.S.) brand of Pseudoephedrine and Guaifenesin—**See Cough/Cold Combinations (Systemic)**, 1024

*t-PA*—Alteplase, Recombinant—**See Thrombolytic Agents (Systemic)**, 2799

*2-PAM See* Pralidoxime (Systemic), #

*2-PAM chloride See* Pralidoxime (Systemic), #

*T-Phyl*—Purdue Frederick (U.S.) brand of Theophylline—**See Bronchodilators, Theophylline (Systemic)**, 668

*Tracrium*—BW (U.S. and Canada) brand of Atracurium—**See Neuromuscular Blocking Agents (Systemic)**, 2098

*Trac Tabs 2X*—Hyrex (U.S.) brand of Atropine, Hyoscyamine, Methenamine, Methylene Blue, Phenyl Salicylate, and Benzoic Acid (Systemic), 488

Tramadol Hydrochloride [*Ultram*]
  **(Systemic)**, 2851
  Tablets, 2853, MC-31

*Trancot*—Truxton (U.S.) brand of Meprobamate (Systemic), #

*Trandate*—Glaxo Wellcome (U.S.) and Glaxo (Canada) brand of Labetalol—**See Beta-adrenergic Blocking Agents (Systemic)**, 593, MC-16

Trandolapril [*Mavik*]
  **(Systemic)**, 2854
  Tablets, 2857, MC-31

Trandolapril and Verapamil [*Tarka*]
  **(Systemic)**, 2857
  Tablets, Extended-release, 2862, MC-31

Tranexamic Acid [*Cyklokapron*]
  **(Systemic)**, 2862, 3169
  Injection, 2865
  Solution, Oral, 2864
  Tablets, 2864

*Transderm-Nitro*—Summit (U.S. and Canada) brand of Nitroglycerin—**See Nitrates (Systemic)**, 2129

*Transderm-Scōp*—Ciba (U.S.) brand of Scopolamine—**See Anticholinergics/Antispasmodics (Systemic)**, 226

*Transderm-V*—Ciba-Geigy (Canada) brand of Scopolamine—**See Anticholinergics/Antispasmodics (Systemic)**, 226

Transforming Growth Factor-Beta 2
  **(Systemic)**, 3169

Transgenic Human Alpha 1 Antitrypsin
  **(Systemic)**, 3169

*Trans-Plantar*—Tsumura (U.S.) brand of Salicylic Acid (Topical), #

*Trans-Ver-Sal*—Tsumura (U.S.) and Westwood-Squibb (Canada) brand of Salicylic Acid (Topical), #

*Tranxene*—Abbott (Canada) brand of Clorazepate—**See Benzodiazepines (Systemic)**, 556

*Tranxene SD*—Abbott (U.S.) brand of Clorazepate—**See Benzodiazepines (Systemic)**, 556, MC-8

*Tranxene T-Tab*—Abbott (U.S.) brand of Clorazepate—**See Benzodiazepines (Systemic)**, 556, MC-8

Tranylcypromine Sulfate [*Parnate*]
  See **Antidepressants, Monoamine Oxidase (MAO) Inhibitor (Systemic)**, 266
  Tablets, 271, MC-31

*Trasicor*—Ciba (Canada) brand of Oxprenolol—**See Beta-adrenergic Blocking Agents (Systemic)**, 593

*Trasylol*—Bayer (U.S. and Canada) brand of Aprotinin (Systemic), 461; Miles (U.S.) brand of Aprotinin (Systemic), 3132

*TraumaCal*—Mead Johnson (U.S.) brand of Enteral Nutrition Formula, Disease-specific—**See Enteral Nutrition Formulas (Systemic)**, #

*Traum-Aid HBC*—Kendall McGaw (U.S.) brand of Enteral Nutrition Formula, Disease-specific—**See Enteral Nutrition Formulas (Systemic)**, #

*Travasorb HN*—Clintec (U.S.) brand of Enteral Nutrition Formula, Monomeric (Elemental)—**See Enteral Nutrition Formulas (Systemic)**, #

*Travasorb Renal Diet*—Clintec (U.S.) brand of Enteral Nutrition Formula, Disease-specific—**See Enteral Nutrition Formulas (Systemic)**, #

*Travasorb STD*—Clintec (U.S.) brand of Enteral Nutrition Formula, Monomeric (Elemental)—**See Enteral Nutrition Formulas (Systemic)**, #

*Traveltabs*—Stanley (Canada) brand of Dimenhydrinate—**See Antihistamines (Systemic)**, 325

Trazodone Hydrochloride [*Desyrel; Trazon; Trialodine*]
  **(Systemic)**, 2865
  Tablets USP, 2867, MC-31

*Trazon*—Sidmak (U.S.) brand of Trazodone (Systemic), 2865

*Trecator-SC*—Wyeth-Ayerst (U.S.) brand of Ethionamide (Systemic), 1417

*Trendar*—Whitehall (U.S.) brand of Ibuprofen—**See Anti-inflammatory Drugs, Nonsteroidal (Systemic)**, 388

*Trental*—Hoechst Marion Roussel (U.S. and Canada) brand of Pentoxifylline (Systemic), 2282, MC-25

Treosulfan [*Ovastat*]
  **(Systemic)**, 3169

Tretinoin [*Tretinoin LF, IV; Vesanoid*]
  **(Systemic)**, 2868, 3169
  Capsules, 2870, MC-31

Tretinoin [*Avita*; all-*trans*-retinoic acid ;*Renova; Retin-A; Retin A MICRO* retinoic acid; *Retisol-A; Stieva-A; Stieva-A Forte; Vitamin A Acid*; vitamin A acid; *Vitinoin*]
  **(Topical)**, 2871
  Cream USP (Oil-in-water), 2874
  Cream USP (Water-in-oil), 2874
  Gel USP, 2874
  Solution, Topical, USP, 2875

*Tretinoin LF, IV*—Argus (U.S.) brand of Tretinoin (Systemic), 3169

*Trexan*—Du Pont (U.S.) brand of Naltrexone (Systemic), 3155

*Triacana*—Marcofina (France) brand of Tiratricol (Systemic), 3169

*Triacet*—Lemmon (U.S.) brand of Triamcinolone—**See Corticosteroids (Topical)**, 978

*Triacin C Cough*—Barre-National (U.S.) and Moore (U.S.) brand of Triprolidine, Pseudoephedrine, and Codeine—**See Cough/Cold Combinations (Systemic)**, 1024

*Triad*—UAD (U.S.) brand of Butalbital, Acetaminophen, and Caffeine—**See Barbiturates and Analgesics (Systemic)**, 532

# General Index

*Triadapin*—Fisons (Canada) brand of Doxepin—**See Antidepressants, Tricyclic (Systemic)**, 271
*Triaderm*—Taro (Canada) brand of Triamcinolone—**See Corticosteroids (Topical)**, 978
*Triafed with Codeine*—Schein (U.S.) brand of Triprolidine, Pseudoephedrine, and Codeine—**See Cough/Cold Combinations (Systemic)**, 1024
*Trial*—Zee Medical (Canada) brand of Calcium Carbonate—**See Antacids (Oral-Local)**, 188
*Trialodine*—Quantum (U.S.) brand of Trazodone (Systemic), 2865
*Triam-A*—Hyrex (U.S.) brand of Triamcinolone—**See Corticosteroids—Glucocorticoid Effects (Systemic)**, 998
Triamcinolone [*Aristocort; Kenacort*]
   **See Corticosteroids—Glucocorticoid Effects (Systemic)**, 998
   Tablets USP, 1013
Triamcinolone Acetonide [*Azmacort*]
   **See Corticosteroids (Inhalation-Local)**, 955
   Aerosol, Inhalation, 960
Triamcinolone Acetonide [*Nasacort; Nasacort AQ*]
   **See Corticosteroids (Nasal)**, 961, 3037
   Aerosol, Nasal, 966, 3037
   Solution, Nasal, 3037
Triamcinolone Acetonide [*Aristocort; Aristocort A; Aristocort C; Aristocort D; Aristocort R; Delta-Tritex; Flutex; Kenac; Kenalog; Kenalog-H; Kenalog in Orabase; Kenonel; Oracort; Oralone; Triacet; Triaderm; Trianide Mild; Trianide Regular; Triderm*]
   **See Corticosteroids (Topical)**, 978, 3037
   Aerosol, Topical, USP, 995
   Cream USP, 994
   Lotion USP, 994
   Ointment USP, 994
   Paste, Dental, USP, 994, 3037
Triamcinolone Acetonide [*Cenocort A-40; Cinonide 40; Kenaject-40; Kenalog-10; Kenalog-40; Tac-3; Triam-A; Triamonide 40; Tri-Kort; Trilog*]
   **See Corticosteroids—Glucocorticoid Effects (Systemic)**, 998
   Suspension, Sterile, USP, 1014
Triamcinolone-containing Combinations, 3082
Triamcinolone Diacetate [*Amcort; Aristocort; Aristocort Forte; Aristocort Intralesional; Articulose-L.A.; Cenocort Forte; Cinalone 40; Kenacort Diacetate; Triam-Forte; Triamolone 40; Trilone; Tristoject*]
   **See Corticosteroids—Glucocorticoid Effects (Systemic)**, 998
   Suspension, Sterile, USP, 1014
   Syrup USP, 1013
Triamcinolone Hexacetonide [*Aristospan Intra-articular; Aristospan Intralesional*]
   **See Corticosteroids—Glucocorticoid Effects (Systemic)**, 998
   Suspension, Sterile, USP, 1014
*Triam-Forte*—Hyrex (U.S.) brand of Triamcinolone—**See Corticosteroids—Glucocorticoid Effects (Systemic)**, 998
*Triaminic*—Sandoz (U.S. and Canada) brand of Chlorpheniramine and Phenylpropanolamine—**See Antihistamines and Decongestants (Systemic)**, 343; Sandoz (U.S.) brand of Pheniramine, Pyrilamine, and Phenylpropanolamine—**See Antihistamines and Decongestants (Systemic)**, 343
*Triaminic-12*—Sandoz (U.S.) brand of Chlorpheniramine and Phenylpropanolamine—**See Antihistamines and Decongestants (Systemic)**, 343
*Triaminic Allergy*—Sandoz (U.S.) brand of Chlorpheniramine and Phenylpropanolamine—**See Antihistamines and Decongestants (Systemic)**, 343
*Triaminic AM Non-Drowsy Cough and Decongestant*—Sandoz (U.S.) brand of Pseudoephedrine and Dextromethorphan—**See Cough/Cold Combinations (Systemic)**, 1024
*Triaminic Chewables*—Sandoz (U.S.) brand of Chlorpheniramine and Phenylpropanolamine—**See Antihistamines and Decongestants (Systemic)**, 343
*Triaminic Cold*—Sandoz (U.S.) brand of Chlorpheniramine and Phenylpropanolamine—**See Antihistamines and Decongestants (Systemic)**, 343
*Triaminic-DM Cough Relief*—Sandoz (U.S.) brand of Phenylpropanolamine and Dextromethorphan—**See Cough/Cold Combinations (Systemic)**, 1024

*Triaminic DM DayTime for Children*—Sandoz (Canada) brand of Phenylpropanolamine, Dextromethorphan, and Guaifenesin—**See Cough/Cold Combinations (Systemic)**, 1024
*Triaminic-DM Expectorant*—Sandoz (Canada) brand of Chlorpheniramine, Pseudoephedrine, Dextromethorphan, and Guaifenesin—**See Cough/Cold Combinations (Systemic)**, 1024
*Triaminic DM NightTime for Children*—Sandoz (Canada) brand of Chlorpheniramine, Pseudoephedrine, and Dextromethorphan—**See Cough/Cold Combinations (Systemic)**, 1024
*Triaminic Expectorant*—Sandoz (Canada) brand of Chlorpheniramine, Pseudoephedrine, and Guaifenesin—**See Cough/Cold Combinations (Systemic)**, 1024; Sandoz (U.S.) brand of Phenylpropanolamine and Guaifenesin—**See Cough/Cold Combinations (Systemic)**, 1024
*Triaminic Expectorant with Codeine*—Sandoz (U.S.) brand of Phenylpropanolamine, Codeine, and Guaifenesin—**See Cough/Cold Combinations (Systemic)**, 1024
*Triaminic Expectorant DH*—Sandoz (U.S. and Canada) brand of Pheniramine, Pyrilamine, Phenylpropanolamine, Hydrocodone, and Guaifenesin—**See Cough/Cold Combinations (Systemic)**, 1024
*Triaminicin*—Sandoz (Canada) brand of Pheniramine, Pyrilamine, Phenylpropanolamine, Acetaminophen, and Caffeine—**See Antihistamines, Decongestants, and Analgesics (Systemic)**, 366
*Triaminicin Cold, Allergy, Sinus*—Sandoz (U.S.) brand of Chlorpheniramine, Phenylpropanolamine, and Acetaminophen—**See Antihistamines, Decongestants, and Analgesics (Systemic)**, 366
*Triaminic Nite Time*—Sandoz (U.S.) brand of Chlorpheniramine, Pseudoephedrine, and Dextromethorphan—**See Cough/Cold Combinations (Systemic)**, 1024
*Triaminicol DM*—Sandoz (U.S.) brand of Chlorpheniramine, Pseudoephedrine, and Dextromethorphan—**See Cough/Cold Combinations (Systemic)**, 1024
*Triaminicol Multi-Symptom Cold and Cough Medicine*—Sandoz (U.S.) brand of Chlorpheniramine, Phenylpropanolamine, and Dextromethorphan—**See Cough/Cold Combinations (Systemic)**, 1024
*Triaminic Oral Infant Drops*—Sandoz (U.S.) brand of Pheniramine, Pyrilamine, and Phenylpropanolamine—**See Antihistamines and Decongestants (Systemic)**, 343
*Triaminic Sore Throat Formula*—Sandoz (U.S.) brand of Pseudoephedrine, Dextromethorphan, and Acetaminophen—**See Cough/Cold Combinations (Systemic)**, 1024
*Triaminic TR*—Sandoz (U.S.) brand of Pheniramine, Pyrilamine, and Phenylpropanolamine—**See Antihistamines and Decongestants (Systemic)**, 343
*Triaminic Triaminicol*—Sandoz (U.S.) brand of Chlorpheniramine, Phenylpropanolamine, and Dextromethorphan—**See Cough/Cold Combinations (Systemic)**, 1024
*Triamolone 40*—Forest (U.S.) brand of Triamcinolone—**See Corticosteroids—Glucocorticoid Effects (Systemic)**, 998
*Triamonide 40*—Forest (U.S.) brand of Triamcinolone—**See Corticosteroids—Glucocorticoid Effects (Systemic)**, 998
Triamterene [*Dyrenium*]
   **See Diuretics, Potassium-sparing (Systemic)**, 1266
   Capsules USP, 1270, MC-31
   Tablets, 1271
Triamterene-containing Combinations, 3082
Triamterene and Hydrochlorothiazide [*Apo-Triazide;* co-triamterzide; *Dyazide; Maxzide; Novo-Triamzide*]
   **See Diuretics, Potassium-sparing, and Hydrochlorothiazide (Systemic)**, 1272
   Capsules USP, 1273, MC-31
   Tablets USP, 1273, MC-31
*Trianide Mild*—Technilab (Canada) brand of Triamcinolone—**See Corticosteroids (Topical)**, 978
*Trianide Regular*—Technilab (Canada) brand of Triamcinolone—**See Corticosteroids (Topical)**, 978
*Triaprin*—Dunhall (U.S.) brand of Butalbital and Acetaminophen—**See Barbiturates and Analgesics (Systemic)**, 532

*Triatec-8*—Trianon (Canada) brand of Acetaminophen and Codeine—**See Opioid (Narcotic) Analgesics and Acetaminophen (Systemic)**, 2198
*Triatec-30*—Trianon (Canada) brand of Acetaminophen and Codeine—**See Opioid (Narcotic) Analgesics and Acetaminophen (Systemic)**, 2198
*Triatec-8 Strong*—Trianon (Canada) brand of Acetaminophen and Codeine—**See Opioid (Narcotic) Analgesics and Acetaminophen (Systemic)**, 2198
*Triavil*—Merck (U.S. and Canada) brand of Perphenazine and Amitriptyline (Systemic), 2286
*Triaz*—Medicis (U.S.) brand of Benzoyl Peroxide (Topical), 579, 3011
*Triaz Cleanser*—Medicis (U.S.) brand of Benzoyl Peroxide (Topical), 579
Triazolam [*Apo-Triazo; Alti-triazolam; Gen-Triazolam; Halcion; Novo-Triolam*]
   **See Benzodiazepines (Systemic)**, 556
   Tablets USP, 578, MC-31
*Triban*—Harber (U.S.) brand of Trimethobenzamide (Systemic), 2880
Tribavirin—See Ribavirin (Systemic), 2478
*Tribenzagan*—Bolan (U.S.) brand of Trimethobenzamide (Systemic), 2880
*Tribiotic*—Interstate (U.S.) brand of Neomycin, Polymyxin B, and Gramicidin (Ophthalmic), #
*Tri-Buffered ASA*—Aspirin, Buffered—**See Salicylates (Systemic)**, 2538
*Trichlorex*—Lannett (U.S.) brand of Trichlormethiazide—**See Diuretics, Thiazide (Systemic)**, 1273
Trichlormethiazide [*Metahydrin; Naqua; Trichlorex*]
   **See Diuretics, Thiazide (Systemic)**, 1273
   Tablets USP, 1281
Trichlormethiazide-containing Combinations, 3082
Tricitrates [*Polycitra-LC; Polycitra Syrup*]
   **See Citrates (Systemic)**, 881
   Solution, Oral, USP, 885
*Tricodene*—Pfeiffer (U.S.) brand of Pyrilamine and Codeine—**See Cough/Cold Combinations (Systemic)**, 1024
*Tricodene Forte*—Pfeiffer (U.S.) brand of Chlorpheniramine, Phenylpropanolamine, and Dextromethorphan—**See Cough/Cold Combinations (Systemic)**, 1024
*Tricodene NN*—Pfeiffer (U.S.) brand of Chlorpheniramine, Phenylpropanolamine, and Dextromethorphan—**See Cough/Cold Combinations (Systemic)**, 1024
*Tricodene Pediatric*—Pfeiffer (U.S.) brand of Phenylpropanolamine and Dextromethorphan—**See Cough/Cold Combinations (Systemic)**, 1024
*Tricodene Sugar Free*—Pfeiffer (U.S.) brand of Chlorpheniramine and Dextromethorphan—**See Cough/Cold Combinations (Systemic)**, 1024
*Tricor*—Abbott (U.S.) brand of Fenofibrate (Systemic), 1439, MC-12
*Tricosal*—Duramed (U.S.); Qualitest (U.S.); and United Research (U.S.) brand of Choline and Magnesium Salicylates—**See Salicylates (Systemic)**, 2538
*Tri-Cyclen*—Ortho (Canada) brand of Norgestimate and Ethinyl Estradiol—**See Estrogens and Progestins—Oral Contraceptives (Systemic)**, 1397
*Triderm*—Del-Ray (U.S.) brand of Triamcinolone—**See Corticosteroids (Topical)**, 978
*Tridesilon*—Miles (U.S. and Canada) brand of Desonide—**See Corticosteroids (Topical)**, 978
*Tridil*—American Critical Care (U.S. and Canada) brand of Nitroglycerin—**See Nitrates (Systemic)**, 2129
*Trien*—See Trientine (Systemic), 2875
Trientine Hydrochloride [*Cuprid; Syprine;* trien]
   (Systemic), 2875, 3169
   Capsules, 2877
*Trifed-C Cough*—Geneva (U.S.) brand of Triprolidine, Pseudoephedrine, and Codeine—**See Cough/Cold Combinations (Systemic)**, 1024
Trifluoperazine Hydrochloride [*Apo-Trifluoperazine; Novo-Flurazine; PMS Trifluoperazine; Solazine; Stelazine; Stelazine Concentrate; Terfluzine; Terfluzine Concentrate*]
   **See Phenothiazines (Systemic)**, 2289
   Injection USP, 2311
   Solution, Oral, 2310
   Syrup USP, 2310
   Tablets USP, 2311, MC-31

USP DI • General Index 3357

Trifluorothymidine—See Trifluridine (Ophthalmic), 2877
Triflupromazine Hydrochloride [Vesprin]
　See Phenothiazines (Systemic), 2289
　Injection USP, 2311
Trifluridine [trifluorothymidine; Viroptic]
　(Ophthalmic), 2877
　Solution, Ophthalmic, 2878
Trihexane—Rugby (U.S.) brand of Trihexyphenidyl—See Antidyskinetics (Systemic), 297
Trihexy—Geneva Generics (U.S.) brand of Trihexyphenidyl—See Antidyskinetics (Systemic), 297
Trihexyphenidyl Hydrochloride [Apo-Trihex; Artane; Artane Sequels; benzhexol; PMS Trihexyphenidyl; Trihexane; Trihexy]
　See Antidyskinetics (Systemic), 297
　Capsules, Extended-release, USP, 301
　Elixir USP, 301
　Tablets USP, 301
Trihist-D—Aligen (U.S.) brand of Pheniramine, Phenyltoloxamine, Pyrilamine, and Phenylpropanolamine—See Antihistamines and Decongestants (Systemic), 343
Tri-Hydroserpine—Rugby (U.S.) brand of Reserpine, Hydralazine, and Hydrochlorothiazide (Systemic), #
Tri-Immunol—Lederle (U.S. and Canada) brand of Diphtheria and Tetanus Toxoids and Pertussis Vaccine Adsorbed (Systemic), 1240
Tri-K—Century (U.S.) brand of Trikates—See Potassium Supplements (Systemic), 2357
Trikacide—Pharmascience (Canada) brand of Metronidazole (Systemic), 1996
Trikates [potassium acetate, potassium bicarbonate, and potassium citrate; potassium triplex; Tri-K]
　See Potassium Supplements (Systemic), 2357
　Solution, Oral, USP, 2365
Tri-Kort—Keene (U.S.) brand of Triamcinolone—See Corticosteroids—Glucocorticoid Effects (Systemic), 998
Trilafon—Schering (U.S. and Canada) brand of Perphenazine—See Phenothiazines (Systemic), 2289
Trilafon Concentrate—Schering (U.S. and Canada) brand of Perphenazine—See Phenothiazines (Systemic), 2289
Trilax—Drug Industries (U.S.) brand of Dehydrocholic Acid, Docusate, and Phenolphthalein—See Laxatives (Local), #
Tri-Levlen—Berlex (U.S.) brand of Levonorgestrel and Ethinyl Estradiol—See Estrogens and Progestins—Oral Contraceptives (Systemic), 1397, MC-17
Trilisate—Purdue Frederick (U.S. and Canada) brand of Choline and Magnesium Salicylates—See Salicylates (Systemic), 2538
Trilog—Hauck (U.S.) brand of Triamcinolone—See Corticosteroids—Glucocorticoid Effects (Systemic), 998
Trilone—Century (U.S.) and Hauck (U.S.) brand of Triamcinolone—See Corticosteroids—Glucocorticoid Effects (Systemic), 998
Trilostane [Modrastane]
　(Systemic), #
　Capsules, #
Trimeprazine Tartrate [alimemazine; Panectyl; Temaril]
　See Antihistamines, Phenothiazine-derivative (Systemic), 377
　Capsules, Extended-release, 383
　Syrup USP, 383
　Tablets USP, 383
Trimethadione [TMO; trimethadionum; trimethinum; troxidone]
　See Anticonvulsants, Dione (Systemic), #
　Capsules USP, #
　Solution, Oral, USP, #
　Tablets USP, #
Trimethadionum—Trimethadione—See Anticonvulsants, Dione (Systemic), #
Trimethaphan Camsylate [Arfonad]
　(Systemic), 2879
　Injection USP, 2880
Trimethinum—Trimethadione—See Anticonvulsants, Dione (Systemic), #
Trimethobenzamide Hydrochloride [Arrestin; Benzacot; Bio-Gan; Stemetic; Tebamide; Tegamide; T-Gen; Ticon; Tigan; Tiject-20; Triban; Tribenzagan]
　(Systemic), 2880
　Capsules USP, 2881
　Injection USP, 2882
　Suppositories, 2882

Trimethoprim [Proloprim; Trimpex]
　(Systemic), 2882
　Tablets USP, 2884, MC-32
Trimethoprim-containing Combinations, 3082
Trimetrexate Glucuronate [Neutrexin]
　(Systemic), 2885, 3170
　for Injection, 2887
Triminol Cough—Rugby (U.S.) brand of Chlorpheniramine, Phenylpropanolamine, and Dextromethorphan—See Cough/Cold Combinations (Systemic), 1024
Trimipramine Maleate [Apo-Trimip; Novo-Tripramine; Rhotrimine; Surmontil]
　See Antidepressants, Tricyclic (Systemic), 271
　Capsules, 282, MC-32
　Tablets, 283
Trimox—Apothecon (U.S.) brand of Amoxicillin—See Penicillins (Systemic), 2240, MC-2; Apothecon (U.S.) brand of Amoxicillin (Systemic), 3010
Trimpex—Roche (U.S.) brand of Trimethoprim (Systemic), 2882, MC-31
Trinalin—Schering (U.S. and Canada) brand of Azatadine and Pseudoephedrine—See Antihistamines and Decongestants (Systemic), 343, MC-3
Tri-Nefrin Extra Strength—Pfeiffer (U.S.) brand of Chlorpheniramine and Phenylpropanolamine—See Antihistamines and Decongestants (Systemic), 343
Tri-Norinyl—Searle (U.S.) brand of Norethindrone and Ethinyl Estradiol—See Estrogens and Progestins—Oral Contraceptives (Systemic), 1397
Triofed—Barre-National (U.S.) brand of Triprolidine and Pseudoephedrine—See Antihistamines and Decongestants (Systemic), 343
Tri-Ophthalmic—Genetco (U.S.) brand of Neomycin, Polymyxin B, and Gramicidin (Ophthalmic), #
Triostat—SmithKline Beecham (U.S.) brand of Liothyronine (Systemic), 3028, 3152
Triotann—Duramed (U.S.) brand of Chlorpheniramine, Pyrilamine, and Phenylephrine—See Antihistamines and Decongestants (Systemic), 343
Triotann Pediatric—Duramed (U.S.) brand of Chlorpheniramine, Pyrilamine, and Phenylephrine—See Antihistamines and Decongestants (Systemic), 343
Triotann-S Pediatric—Duramed (U.S.) brand of Chlorpheniramine, Pyrilamine, and Phenylephrine—See Antihistamines and Decongestants (Systemic), 343
Trioxsalen [trioxysalen; Trisoralen]
　(Systemic), #
　Tablets USP, #
Trioxysalen—See Trioxsalen (Systemic), #
Tri-Pain Caplets—Ferndale (U.S.) brand of Acetaminophen, Aspirin, Salicylamide, and Caffeine—See Acetaminophen and Salicylates (Systemic), 11
Tripedia—Connaught (U.S.) brand of Diphtheria and Tetanus Toxoids and Pertussis Vaccine Adsorbed (Systemic), 1240
Tripelennamine Citrate [PBZ]
　See Antihistamines (Systemic), 325
　Elixir USP, 342
Tripelennamine Hydrochloride [PBZ; PBZ-SR; Pelamine; Pyribenzamine]
　See Antihistamines (Systemic), 325
　Tablets USP, 342
　Tablets, Extended-release, 342
Triphasil—Wyeth-Ayerst (U.S. and Canada) brand of Levonorgestrel and Ethinyl Estradiol—See Estrogens and Progestins—Oral Contraceptives (Systemic), 1397, MC-17
Tri-Phen-Chlor—Rugby (U.S.) brand of Chlorpheniramine, Phenyltoloxamine, Phenylephrine, and Phenylpropanolamine—See Antihistamines and Decongestants (Systemic), 343
Tri-Phen-Chlor Pediatric—Rugby (U.S.) brand of Chlorpheniramine, Phenyltoloxamine, Phenylephrine, and Phenylpropanolamine—See Antihistamines and Decongestants (Systemic), 343
Tri-Phen-Chlor T.R.—Rugby (U.S.) brand of Chlorpheniramine, Phenyltoloxamine, Phenylephrine, and Phenylpropanolamine—See Antihistamines and Decongestants (Systemic), 343

Tri-Phen-Mine Pediatric Drops—Zenith Goldline (U.S.) brand of Chlorpheniramine, Phenyltoloxamine, Phenylephrine, and Phenylpropanolamine—See Antihistamines and Decongestants (Systemic), 343
Tri-Phen-Mine Pediatric Syrup—Zenith Goldline (U.S.) brand of Chlorpheniramine, Phenyltoloxamine, Phenylephrine, and Phenylpropanolamine—See Antihistamines and Decongestants (Systemic), 343
Tri-Phen-Mine S.R.—Goldline (U.S.) brand of Chlorpheniramine, Phenyltoloxamine, Phenylephrine, and Phenylpropanolamine—See Antihistamines and Decongestants (Systemic), 343, MC-6
Triphenyl—Rugby (U.S.) brand of Chlorpheniramine and Phenylpropanolamine—See Antihistamines and Decongestants (Systemic), 343
Triphenyl Expectorant—Rugby (U.S.) brand of Phenylpropanolamine and Guaifenesin—See Cough/Cold Combinations (Systemic), 1024
Triple Antibiotic—Rugby (U.S.) brand of Neomycin, Polymyxin B, and Bacitracin (Ophthalmic), #; Steris (U.S.) brand of Neomycin, Polymyxin B, and Gramicidin (Ophthalmic), 3029
Triple-Gen—Goldline (U.S.) brand of Neomycin, Polymyxin B, and Hydrocortisone (Ophthalmic), #
Triple Sulfa [sulfathiazole, sulfacetamide, and sulfabenzamide; Sultrin; Trysul]
　See Sulfonamides (Vaginal), 2658
　Cream, Vaginal, USP, 2660
　Tablets, Vaginal, USP, 2660
Triple X—Carter (U.S.) brand of Pyrethrins and Piperonyl Butoxide (Topical), #
Triposed—Halsey (U.S.) brand of Triprolidine and Pseudoephedrine—See Antihistamines and Decongestants (Systemic), 343
Triprolidine-containing Combinations, 3082
Triprolidine Hydrochloride
　See Antihistamines (Systemic), 325
Triprolidine Hydrochloride and Pseudoephedrine Hydrochloride [Actagen; Actifed; Allercon; Allerfrim; Allerphed; Aprodrine; Atrofed; Cenafed Plus; Genac; Silafed; Triofed; Triposed]
　See Antihistamines and Decongestants (Systemic), 343
　Syrup USP, 344, 345, 361, 363, 364
　Tablets USP, 344, 345, 347, 353, 364
Triprolidine Hydrochloride, Pseudoephedrine Hydrochloride, and Acetaminophen [Actifed Cold & Sinus; Actifed Cold & Sinus Caplets; Actifed Plus Extra Strength Caplets]
　See Antihistamines, Decongestants, and Analgesics (Systemic), 366
　Tablets, 367
Triprolidine Hydrochloride, Pseudoephedrine Hydrochloride, and Codeine Phosphate [Actagen-C Cough; Actifed with Codeine Cough; Allerfrin with Codeine; Aprodine with Codeine; CoActifed; Cotridin; Triacin C Cough; Triafed with Codeine; Trifed-C Cough]
　See Cough/Cold Combinations (Systemic), 1024
　Solution, Oral, 1043, 1049
　Syrup, 1032, 1033, 1035, 1100, 1103
　Tablets, 1044
Triprolidine Hydrochloride, Pseudoephedrine Hydrochloride, Codeine Phosphate, and Guaifenesin [CoActifed Expectorant; Cotridin Expectorant]
　See Cough/Cold Combinations (Systemic), 1024
　Solution, Oral, 1044, 1050
Triprolidine Hydrochloride, Pseudoephedrine Hydrochloride, and Dextromethorphan Hydrobromide [Actifed DM]
　See Cough/Cold Combinations (Systemic), 1024
　Solution, Oral, 1032
　Tablets, 1032
Triptil—MSD (Canada) brand of Protriptyline—See Antidepressants, Tricyclic (Systemic), 271
Triptone Caplets—Commerce (U.S.) brand of Dimenhydrinate—See Antihistamines (Systemic), 325
Triquilar—Berlex Canada (Canada) brand of Levonorgestrel and Ethinyl Estradiol—See Estrogens and Progestins—Oral Contraceptives (Systemic), 1397
Trisaccharides A and B [Biosynject]
　(Systemic), 3170
Trisodium Citrate [Hemocitrate]
　Concentrate, 3170
Trisodium phosphonoformate—See Foscarnet (Systemic), 1528

## 3358 General Index

*Trisoralen*—ICN (U.S. and Canada) brand of Trioxsalen (Systemic), #
*Tristatin II*—Rugby (U.S.) brand of Nystatin and Triamcinolone (Topical), 2150
*Tristoject*—Mayrand (U.S.) brand of Triamcinolone—**See Corticosteroids—Glucocorticoid Effects (Systemic)**, 998
*Trisyn*—Medican (Canada) brand of Fluocinonide, Procinonide, and Ciprocinonide (Topical), 3020
*Tritan*—Aligen (U.S.) and Eon (U.S.) brand of Chlorpheniramine, Pyrilamine, and Phenylephrine—**See Antihistamines and Decongestants (Systemic)**, 343
*Tri-Tannate*—Allscrips (U.S.); H.L. Moore (U.S.); and Rugby (U.S.) brand of Chlorpheniramine, Pyrilamine, and Phenylephrine—**See Antihistamines and Decongestants (Systemic)**, 343
*Tri-Tannate Pediatric*—Geneva (U.S.) and Rugby (U.S.) brand of Chlorpheniramine, Pyrilamine, and Phenylephrine—**See Antihistamines and Decongestants (Systemic)**, 343
*Tri-Tannate Plus Pediatric*—Rugby (U.S.) brand of Chlorpheniramine, Ephedrine, Phenylephrine, and Carbetapentane—**See Cough/Cold Combinations (Systemic)**, 1024
*Tritec*—Glaxo Wellcome (U.S.) brand of Ranitidine Bismuth Citrate (Systemic), 2458, MC-27
*Tri-Vi-Flor*—Mead Johnson (U.S. and Canada) brand of Vitamins A, D, and C and Fluoride—**See Vitamins, Multiple, and Fluoride (Systemic)**, 2978
*Trobicin*—Upjohn (U.S. and Canada) brand of Spectinomycin (Systemic), 2622
*Trocal*—Hauck (U.S.) brand of Dextromethorphan (Systemic), 1191
*Troglitazone* [*Rezulin*]
  **(Systemic)**, 2888
  Tablets, 2891, MC-32
*Trojan*—Carter-Wallace (Canada) brand of Latex Condoms—**See Condoms**, #
*Trojan-Enz*—Carter-Wallace (Canada) brand of Latex Condoms—**See Condoms**, #
*Trojan-Enz Large Lubricated*—Carter-Wallace (U.S. and Canada) brand of Latex Condoms—**See Condoms**, #
*Trojan-Enz Large with Spermicidal Lube*—Carter-Wallace (Canada) brand of Latex Condoms and Nonoxynol 9—**See Condoms**, #
*Trojan-Enz Large with Spermicidal Lubricant*—Carter-Wallace (U.S.) brand of Latex Condoms and Nonoxynol 9—**See Condoms**, #
*Trojan-Enz Lubricated*—Carter-Wallace (U.S. and Canada) brand of Latex Condoms—**See Condoms**, #
*Trojan-Enz Nonlubricated*—Carter-Wallace (U.S.) brand of Latex Condoms—**See Condoms**, #
*Trojan-Enz with Spermicidal Lubricant*—Carter-Wallace (U.S. and Canada) brand of Latex Condoms and Nonoxynol 9—**See Condoms**, #
*Trojan Extra Strength Lubricated*—Carter-Wallace (U.S.) brand of Latex Condoms—**See Condoms**, #
*Trojan Magnum*—Carter-Wallace (U.S.) brand of Latex Condoms—**See Condoms**, #
*Trojan Magnum Spermicidal Lubricant*—Carter-Wallace (U.S.) brand of Latex Condoms and Nonoxynol 9—**See Condoms**, #
*Trojan Naturalube Ribbed*—Carter-Wallace (U.S. and Canada) brand of Latex Condoms—**See Condoms**, #
*Trojan Plus*—Carter-Wallace (U.S. and Canada) brand of Latex Condoms—**See Condoms**, #
*Trojan Plus 2*—Carter-Wallace (U.S.) brand of Latex Condoms and Nonoxynol 9—**See Condoms**, #
*Trojan Ribbed*—Carter-Wallace (U.S. and Canada) brand of Latex Condoms—**See Condoms**, #
*Trojan Ribbed with Spermicidal Lube*—Carter-Wallace (Canada) brand of Latex Condoms and Nonoxynol 9—**See Condoms**, #
*Trojan Ribbed with Spermicidal Lubricant*—Carter-Wallace (U.S.) brand of Latex Condoms and Nonoxynol 9—**See Condoms**, #
*Trojans*—Carter-Wallace (U.S.) brand of Latex Condoms—**See Condoms**, #
*Trojan Ultra Texture Lubricant*—Carter-Wallace (U.S.) brand of Latex Condoms—**See Condoms**, #
*Trojan Ultra Texture with Spermicidal Lubricant*—Carter-Wallace (U.S.) brand of Latex Condoms and Nonoxynol 9—**See Condoms**, #
*Trojan Very Sensitive with Lubricant*—Carter-Wallace (U.S.) brand of Latex Condoms—**See Condoms**, #

*Trojan Very Sensitive with Spermicidal Lubricant*—Carter-Wallace (U.S.) brand of Latex Condoms and Nonoxynol 9—**See Condoms**, #
*Trojan Very Thin with Lubricant*—Carter-Wallace (U.S.) brand of Latex Condoms—**See Condoms**, #
*Trojan Very Thin with Spermicidal Lubricant*—Carter-Wallace (U.S.) brand of Latex Condoms and Nonoxynol 9—**See Condoms**, #
*Trolamine Salicylate* [*Coppertone Tan Magnifier*]
  **See Sunscreen Agents (Topical)**, #
  Oil, #
*Troleandomycin*
  **(Systemic)**, 3170
*Tronolane*—Ross (U.S.) brand of Pramoxine—**See Anesthetics (Mucosal-Local)**, 128
*Tronothane*—Abbott (U.S. and Canada) brand of Pramoxine—**See Anesthetics (Mucosal-Local)**, 128; **Anesthetics (Topical)**, 155
*Tropicacyl*—Akorn (U.S. and Canada) brand of Tropicamide (Ophthalmic), #
*Tropical Blend Dark Tanning*—Schering-Plough (U.S.) brand of Homosalate—**See Sunscreen Agents (Topical)**, #; Octyl Methoxycinnamate and Oxybenzone—**See Sunscreen Agents (Topical)**, #; Oxybenzone and Padimate O—**See Sunscreen Agents (Topical)**, #
*Tropical Blend Dry Oil*—Schering-Plough (U.S.) brand of Homosalate—**See Sunscreen Agents (Topical)**, #; Homosalate and Oxybenzone—**See Sunscreen Agents (Topical)**, #
*Tropical Blend Waterproof*—Schering-Plough (Canada) brand of Oxybenzone and Padimate O—**See Sunscreen Agents (Topical)**, #
*Tropicamide* [*I-Picamide; Minims Tropicamide; Mydriacyl; Mydriafair; Ocu-Tropic; Opticyl; Spectro-Cyl; Tropicacyl*]
  **(Ophthalmic)**, #
  Solution, Ophthalmic, USP, #
*Trosyd Dermal Cream*—Pfizer (Canada) brand of Tioconazole (Topical), 3036
*Trovafloxacin Mesylate* [*Trovan*]
  **See Trovafloxacin (Systemic)**, 2891
  Tablets, 2894, MC-32
*Trovan*—Pfizer (U.S.) brand of Trovafloxacin—**See Trovafloxacin (Systemic)**, 2891, MC-12, 2895
*Trovert*—Sensus (U.S.) brand of B2036-PEG (Systemic), 3133
*Troxidone*—Trimethadione—**See Anticonvulsants, Dione (Systemic)**, #
*Truphylline*—G & W (U.S.) brand of Aminophylline—**See Bronchodilators, Theophylline (Systemic)**, 668
*Trusopt*—Merck (U.S.) brand of Dorzolamide (Ophthalmic), 1294
*Truxophyllin*—Truxton (U.S.) brand of Theophylline—**See Bronchodilators, Theophylline (Systemic)**, 668
*Trysul*—Savage (U.S.) brand of Triple Sulfa—**See Sulfonamides (Vaginal)**, 2658
*TSC*—Medi-Physics (U.S.) brand of Technetium Tc 99m Sulfur Colloid (Systemic), 2740
*TSH*—See Human Thyroid Stimulating Hormone (Systemic), 3146
*T-Stat*—Westwood-Squibb (U.S.) brand of Erythromycin (Topical), 1365
*Tubarine*—BW (Canada) brand of Tubocurarine—**See Neuromuscular Blocking Agents (Systemic)**, 2098
*Tubasal*—CMC (U.S.) brand of Aminosalicylate Sodium (Systemic), #
*Tuberculin PPD TINE TEST*—Lederle (U.S.) brand of Tuberculin, Purified Protein Derivative (Parenteral-Local), 2895
*Tuberculin*, Purified Protein Derivative [*Aplisol; Aplitest; Tuberculin PPD TINE TEST; Tubersol*]
  **(Parenteral-Local)**, 2895
  Tuberculin USP (Purified Protein Derivative [PPD] Injection), 2897
  Tuberculin USP (Purified Protein Derivative [PPD] Multiple-puncture Device), 2897
*Tubersol*—Connaught (U.S. and Canada) brand of Tuberculin, Purified Protein Derivative (Parenteral-Local), 2895
*Tubocurarine Chloride* [*Tubarine*]
  **See Neuromuscular Blocking Agents (Systemic)**, 2098
  Injection USP, 2105
*Tuinal*—Lilly (U.S. and Canada) brand of Secobarbital and Amobarbital—**See Barbiturates (Systemic)**, 518

*Tumor Necrosis Factor-Binding Protein I* **(Systemic)**, 3170
*Tumor Necrosis Factor-Binding Protein II* **(Systemic)**, 3170
*Tums*—Norcliff Thayer (U.S.) brand of Calcium Carbonate—**See Calcium Supplements (Systemic)**, 736; SmithKline Beecham (U.S. and Canada) brand of Calcium Carbonate—**See Antacids (Oral-Local)**, 188
*Tums 500*—Northcliff Thayer (U.S.) brand of Calcium Carbonate—**See Calcium Supplements (Systemic)**, 736
*Tums Anti-gas/Antacid*—SmithKline Beecham (U.S.) brand of Calcium Carbonate and Simethicone—**See Antacids (Oral-Local)**, 188
*Tums E-X*—Norcliff Thayer (U.S.) brand of Calcium Carbonate—**See Calcium Supplements (Systemic)**, 736; SmithKline Beecham (U.S.) brand of Calcium Carbonate—**See Antacids (Oral-Local)**, 188
*Tums Extra Strength*—Northcliff Thayer (Canada) brand of Calcium Carbonate—**See Calcium Supplements (Systemic)**, 736; SmithKline Beecham (Canada) brand of Calcium Carbonate—**See Antacids (Oral-Local)**, 188
*Tums Regular Strength*—Northcliff Thayer (Canada) brand of Calcium Carbonate—**See Calcium Supplements (Systemic)**, 736
*Tums Ultra*—SmithKline Beecham (U.S. and Canada) brand of Calcium Carbonate—**See Antacids (Oral-Local)**, 188
*Tusquelin*—Circle (U.S.) brand of Chlorpheniramine, Phenylephrine, Phenylpropanolamine, Dextromethorphan, Potassium Guaiacolsulfonate, and Ipecac—**See Cough/Cold Combinations (Systemic)**, 1024
*Tuss-Ade*—Veratex (U.S.) brand of Phenylpropanolamine and Caramiphen—**See Cough/Cold Combinations (Systemic)**, 1024
*Tussafed*—Everett (U.S.) brand of Carbinoxamine, Pseudoephedrine, and Dextromethorphan—**See Cough/Cold Combinations (Systemic)**, 1024
*Tussafed Drops*—Everett (U.S.) brand of Carbinoxamine, Pseudoephedrine, and Dextromethorphan—**See Cough/Cold Combinations (Systemic)**, 1024
*Tussafin Expectorant*—Rugby (U.S.) brand of Pseudoephedrine, Hydrocodone, and Guaifenesin—**See Cough/Cold Combinations (Systemic)**, 1024
*Tuss-Allergine Modified T.D.*—Rugby (U.S.) brand of Phenylpropanolamine and Caramiphen—**See Cough/Cold Combinations (Systemic)**, 1024
*Tussaminic C Forte*—Sandoz (Canada) brand of Pheniramine, Pyrilamine, Phenylpropanolamine, and Codeine—**See Cough/Cold Combinations (Systemic)**, 1024
*Tussaminic C Pediatric*—Sandoz (Canada) brand of Pheniramine, Pyrilamine, Phenylpropanolamine, and Codeine—**See Cough/Cold Combinations (Systemic)**, 1024
*Tussaminic DH Forte*—Sandoz (Canada) brand of Pheniramine, Pyrilamine, Phenylpropanolamine, and Hydrocodone—**See Cough/Cold Combinations (Systemic)**, 1024
*Tussaminic DH Pediatric*—Sandoz (Canada) brand of Pheniramine, Pyrilamine, Phenylpropanolamine, and Hydrocodone—**See Cough/Cold Combinations (Systemic)**, 1024
*Tussar-2*—Rhône-Poulenc Rorer (U.S.) brand of Pseudoephedrine, Codeine, and Guaifenesin—**See Cough/Cold Combinations (Systemic)**, 1024
*Tussar DM*—Rhône-Poulenc Rorer (U.S.) brand of Chlorpheniramine, Pseudoephedrine, and Dextromethorphan—**See Cough/Cold Combinations (Systemic)**, 1024
*Tussar SF*—Rhône-Poulenc Rorer (U.S.) brand of Pseudoephedrine, Codeine, and Guaifenesin—**See Cough/Cold Combinations (Systemic)**, 1024
*Tuss-DA*—International Ethical (U.S.) brand of Pseudoephedrine and Dextromethorphan—**See Cough/Cold Combinations (Systemic)**, 1024
*Tuss Delay*—Zenith Goldline (U.S.) brand of Chlorpheniramine, Phenylephrine, Phenylpropanolamine, Atropine, Hyoscyamine, and Scopolamine—**See Antihistamines, Decongestants, and Anticholinergics (Systemic)**, 373
*Tuss-DM*—Hyrex (U.S.) brand of Dextromethorphan and Guaifenesin—**See Cough/Cold Combinations (Systemic)**, 1024

*Tussex Cough*—Barre-National (U.S.); Moore (U.S.) and Rugby (U.S.) brand of Phenylephrine, Dextromethorphan, and Guaifenesin—**See Cough/Cold Combinations (Systemic)**, 1024

*Tussigon*—Daniels (U.S.) -brand of Hydrocodone and Homatropine—**See Cough/Cold Combinations (Systemic)**, 1024

*Tussilyn DM*—Vachon (Canada) brand of Chlorpheniramine, Pseudoephedrine, and Dextromethorphan—**See Cough/Cold Combinations (Systemic)**, 1024

*Tussionex*—Rhône-Poulenc Rorer (Canada) brand of Phenyltoloxamine and Hydrocodone—**See Cough/Cold Combinations (Systemic)**, 1024

*Tussionex Pennkinetic*—Rhône-Poulenc Rorer (Canada) brand of Chlorpheniramine and Hydrocodone—**See Cough/Cold Combinations (Systemic)**, 1024

*Tussi-Organidin DM NR Liquid*—Wallace (U.S.) brand of Dextromethorphan and Guaifenesin—**See Cough/Cold Combinations (Systemic)**, 1024

*Tussi-Organidin DM-S NR Liquid*—Wallace (U.S.) brand of Dextromethorphan and Guaifenesin—**See Cough/Cold Combinations (Systemic)**, 1024

*Tussi-Organidin NR Liquid*—Wallace (U.S.) brand of Codeine and Guaifenesin—**See Cough/Cold Combinations (Systemic)**, 1024

*Tussi-Organidin-S NR Liquid*—Wallace (U.S.) brand of Codeine and Guaifenesin—**See Cough/Cold Combinations (Systemic)**, 1024

*Tussirex*—Scot-Tussin (U.S.) brand of Pheniramine, Phenylephrine, Codeine, Sodium Citrate, Sodium Salicylate, and Caffeine Citrate—**See Cough/Cold Combinations (Systemic)**, 1024

*Tuss-LA*—Hyrex (U.S.) brand of Pseudoephedrine and Guaifenesin—**See Cough/Cold Combinations (Systemic)**, 1024

*Tusso-DM*—Everett (U.S.) brand of Dextromethorphan and Iodinated Glycerol—**See Cough/Cold Combinations (Systemic)**, 1024

*Tussogest*—Major (U.S.) brand of Phenylpropanolamine and Caramiphen—**See Cough/Cold Combinations (Systemic)**, 1024

*Tuss-Ornade Spansules*—SKF (Canada) brand of Chlorpheniramine, Phenylpropanolamine, and Caramiphen—**See Cough/Cold Combinations (Systemic)**, 1024

*12 Hour Nostrilla Nasal Decongestant*—Novartis (U.S.) brand of Oxymetazoline (Nasal), 3030

*Twilite Caplets*—Pfeiffer (U.S.) brand of Diphenhydramine—**See Antihistamines (Systemic)**, 325

*Twin-K*—Boots (U.S.) brand of Potassium Gluconate and Potassium Citrate—**See Potassium Supplements (Systemic)**, 2357

*TwoCal HN*—Ross (U.S.) brand of Enteral Nutrition Formula, Polymeric—**See Enteral Nutrition Formulas (Systemic)**, #

*Two-Dyne*—Hyrex (U.S.) brand of Butalbital, Acetaminophen, and Caffeine—**See Barbiturates and Analgesics (Systemic)**, 532

*Tylenol Allergy Sinus Medication Extra Strength Caplets*—McNeil CPC (Canada) brand of Chlorpheniramine, Pseudoephedrine, and Acetaminophen—**See Antihistamines, Decongestants, and Analgesics (Systemic)**, 366

*Tylenol Allergy Sinus Medication Maximum Strength Caplets*—McNeil Consumer (U.S.) brand of Chlorpheniramine, Pseudoephedrine, and Acetaminophen—**See Antihistamines, Decongestants, and Analgesics (Systemic)**, 366

*Tylenol Allergy Sinus Medication Maximum Strength Gelcaps*—McNeil Consumer (U.S.) brand of Chlorpheniramine, Pseudoephedrine, and Acetaminophen—**See Antihistamines, Decongestants, and Analgesics (Systemic)**, 366

*Tylenol Allergy Sinus Medication Maximum Strength Geltabs*—McNeil Consumer (U.S.) brand of Chlorpheniramine, Pseudoephedrine, and Acetaminophen—**See Antihistamines, Decongestants, and Analgesics (Systemic)**, 366

*Tylenol Allergy Sinus Night Time Medicine Maximum Strength Caplets*—McNeil Consumer (U.S.) brand of Diphenhydramine, Pseudoephedrine, and Acetaminophen—**See Cough/Cold Combinations (Systemic)**, 366

*Tylenol Caplets*—McNeil-CPC (Canada) brand of Acetaminophen (Systemic), 6

*Tylenol Children's Chewable Tablets*—McNeil-CPC (U.S. and Canada) brand of Acetaminophen (Systemic), 6

*Tylenol Children's Cold DM Medication*—McNeil (Canada) brand of Chlorpheniramine, Pseudoephedrine, Dextromethorphan, and Acetaminophen—**See Cough/Cold Combinations (Systemic)**, 1024

*Tylenol Children's Elixir*—McNeil-CPC (U.S.) brand of Acetaminophen (Systemic), 6

*Tylenol Children's Suspension Liquid*—McNeil-CPC (U.S.) brand of Acetaminophen (Systemic), 6

*Tylenol with Codeine Elixir*—McNeil (U.S. and Canada) brand of Acetaminophen and Codeine—**See Opioid (Narcotic) Analgesics and Acetaminophen (Systemic)**, 2198

*Tylenol with Codeine No.1*—McNeil (U.S. and Canada) brand of Acetaminophen and Codeine—**See Opioid (Narcotic) Analgesics and Acetaminophen (Systemic)**, 2198, MC-1

*Tylenol with Codeine No.2*—McNeil (U.S. and Canada) brand of Acetaminophen and Codeine—**See Opioid (Narcotic) Analgesics and Acetaminophen (Systemic)**, 2198, MC-1

*Tylenol with Codeine No.3*—McNeil (U.S. and Canada) brand of Acetaminophen and Codeine—**See Opioid (Narcotic) Analgesics and Acetaminophen (Systemic)**, 2198, MC-1

*Tylenol with Codeine No.4*—McNeil (U.S. and Canada) brand of Acetaminophen and Codeine—**See Opioid (Narcotic) Analgesics and Acetaminophen (Systemic)**, 2198, MC-1

*Tylenol with Codeine No.1 Forte*—McNeil (Canada) brand of Acetaminophen and Codeine—**See Opioid (Narcotic) Analgesics and Acetaminophen (Systemic)**, 2198

*Tylenol Cold and Flu*—McNeil (Canada) brand of Chlorpheniramine, Pseudoephedrine, Dextromethorphan, and Acetaminophen—**See Cough/Cold Combinations (Systemic)**, 1024

*Tylenol Cold and Flu No Drowsiness Powder*—McNeil (U.S.) brand of Pseudoephedrine, Dextromethorphan, and Acetaminophen—**See Cough/Cold Combinations (Systemic)**, 1024

*Tylenol Cold Medication*—McNeil (U.S.) brand of Chlorpheniramine, Pseudoephedrine, Dextromethorphan, and Acetaminophen—**See Cough/Cold Combinations (Systemic)**, 1024

*Tylenol Cold Medication Caplets*—McNeil (U.S.) brand of Chlorpheniramine, Pseudoephedrine, Dextromethorphan, and Acetaminophen—**See Cough/Cold Combinations (Systemic)**, 1024

*Tylenol Cold Medication Children's*—McNeil-CPC (Canada) brand of Chlorpheniramine, Pseudoephedrine, and Acetaminophen—**See Antihistamines, Decongestants, and Analgesics (Systemic)**, 366

*Tylenol Cold Medication Extra Strength Daytime Caplets*—McNeil (Canada) brand of Pseudoephedrine, Dextromethorphan, and Acetaminophen—**See Cough/Cold Combinations (Systemic)**, 1024

*Tylenol Cold Medication Extra Strength Nighttime Caplets*—McNeil (Canada) brand of Chlorpheniramine, Pseudoephedrine, Dextromethorphan, and Acetaminophen—**See Cough/Cold Combinations (Systemic)**, 1024

*Tylenol Cold Medication Multi-Symptom*—McNeil (U.S.) brand of Chlorpheniramine, Pseudoephedrine, Dextromethorphan, and Acetaminophen—**See Cough/Cold Combinations (Systemic)**, 1024

*Tylenol Cold Medication, Non-Drowsy Caplets*—McNeil (U.S.) brand of Pseudoephedrine, Dextromethorphan, and Acetaminophen—**See Cough/Cold Combinations (Systemic)**, 1024

*Tylenol Cold Medication Non-Drowsy Gelcaps*—McNeil (U.S.) brand of Pseudoephedrine, Dextromethorphan, and Acetaminophen—**See Cough/Cold Combinations (Systemic)**, 1024

*Tylenol Cold Medication Regular Strength Daytime Caplets*—McNeil (Canada) brand of Pseudoephedrine, Dextromethorphan, and Acetaminophen—**See Cough/Cold Combinations (Systemic)**, 1024

*Tylenol Cold Medication Regular Strength Nighttime Caplets*—McNeil (Canada) brand of Chlorpheniramine, Pseudoephedrine, Dextromethorphan, and Acetaminophen—**See Cough/Cold Combinations (Systemic)**, 1024

*Tylenol Cough Extra Strength Caplets*—McNeil (Canada) brand of Dextromethorphan and Acetaminophen—**See Cough/Cold Combinations (Systemic)**, 1024

*Tylenol Cough Medication with Decongestant Regular Strength*—McNeil (Canada) brand of Pseudoephedrine, Dextromethorphan, and Acetaminophen—**See Cough/Cold Combinations (Systemic)**, 1024

*Tylenol Cough Medication Regular Strength*—McNeil (Canada) brand of Dextromethorphan and Acetaminophen—**See Cough/Cold Combinations (Systemic)**, 1024

*Tylenol Drops*—McNeil-CPC (Canada) brand of Acetaminophen (Systemic), 6

*Tylenol Elixir*—McNeil-CPC (Canada) brand of Acetaminophen (Systemic), 6

*Tylenol Extra Strength Adult Liquid Pain Reliever*—McNeil-CPC (U.S.) brand of Acetaminophen (Systemic), 6

*Tylenol Extra Strength Caplets*—McNeil-CPC (U.S.) brand of Acetaminophen (Systemic), 6

*Tylenol Extra Strength Cold and Flu Medication Powder*—McNeil (Canada) brand of Chlorpheniramine, Pseudoephedrine, Dextromethorphan, and Acetaminophen—**See Cough/Cold Combinations (Systemic)**, 1024

*Tylenol Extra Strength Gelcaps*—McNeil-CPC (U.S.) brand of Acetaminophen (Systemic), 6

*Tylenol Extra Strength Tablets*—McNeil-CPC (U.S.) brand of Acetaminophen (Systemic), 6

*Tylenol Flu Medication Extra Strength Gelcaps*—McNeil CPC (Canada) brand of Diphenhydramine, Pseudoephedrine, and Acetaminophen—**See Antihistamines, Decongestants, and Analgesics (Systemic)**, 366

*Tylenol Flu NightTime Hot Medication Maximum Strength*—McNeil Consumer (U.S.) brand of Diphenhydramine, Pseudoephedrine, and Acetaminophen—**See Antihistamines, Decongestants, and Analgesics (Systemic)**, 366

*Tylenol Flu Night Time Medication Maximum Strength Gelcaps*—McNeil-CPC (U.S.) brand of Diphenhydramine, Pseudoephedrine, and Acetaminophen—**See Cough/Cold Combinations (Systemic)**, 366

*Tylenol Gelcaps*—McNeil-CPC (Canada) brand of Acetaminophen (Systemic), 6

*Tylenol, Infants' Drops*—McNeil-CPC (U.S.) brand of Acetaminophen (Systemic), 6

*Tylenol Infants' Suspension Drops*—McNeil-CPC (U.S.) brand of Acetaminophen (Systemic), 6

*Tylenol Junior Strength Caplets*—McNeil-CPC (U.S. and Canada) brand of Acetaminophen (Systemic), 6

*Tylenol Junior Strength Chewable Tablets*—McNeil-CPC (U.S.) brand of Acetaminophen (Systemic), 6

*Tylenol Junior Strength Cold DM Medication*—McNeil (Canada) brand of Chlorpheniramine, Pseudoephedrine, Dextromethorphan, and Acetaminophen—**See Cough/Cold Combinations (Systemic)**, 1024

*Tylenol Maximum Strength Flu Gelcaps*—McNeil (U.S.) brand of Pseudoephedrine, Dextromethorphan, and Acetaminophen—**See Cough/Cold Combinations (Systemic)**, 1024

*Tylenol Multi-Symptom Cough*—McNeil (U.S.) brand of Dextromethorphan and Acetaminophen—**See Cough/Cold Combinations (Systemic)**, 1024

*Tylenol Multi-Symptom Cough with Decongestant*—McNeil (U.S.) brand of Pseudoephedrine, Dextromethorphan, and Acetaminophen—**See Cough/Cold Combinations (Systemic)**, 1024

*Tylenol Regular Strength Caplets*—McNeil-CPC (U.S.) brand of Acetaminophen (Systemic), 6

*Tylenol Regular Strength Tablets*—McNeil-CPC (U.S.) brand of Acetaminophen (Systemic), 6

*Tylenol Sinus Maximum Strength Caplets*—McNeil (U.S.) brand of Pseudoephedrine and Acetaminophen—**See Decongestants and Analgesics (Systemic)**, 1180

*Tylenol Sinus Maximum Strength Gelcaps*—McNeil (U.S.) brand of Pseudoephedrine and Acetaminophen—**See Decongestants and Analgesics (Systemic)**, 1180

*Tylenol Sinus Maximum Strength Geltabs*—McNeil (U.S.) brand of Pseudoephedrine and Acetaminophen—**See Decongestants and Analgesics (Systemic)**, 1180

*Tylenol Sinus Medication Extra Strength Caplets*—McNeil-CPC (Canada) brand of Pseudoephedrine and Acetaminophen—**See Decongestants and Analgesics (Systemic)**, 1180

*Tylenol Sinus Medication Regular Strength Caplets*—McNeil-CPC (Canada) brand of Pseudoephedrine and Acetaminophen—**See Decongestants and Analgesics (Systemic)**, 1180
*Tylenol Tablets*—McNeil-CPC (Canada) brand of Acetaminophen (Systemic), 6
*Tylosterone*—Lilly (U.S.) brand of Diethylstilbestrol and Methyltestosterone—**See Androgens and Estrogens (Systemic)**, 126
*Tylox*—Ortho-McNeil (U.S.) brand of Oxycodone and Acetaminophen—**See Opioid (Narcotic) Analgesics and Acetaminophen (Systemic)**, 2198, MC-24
Tyloxapol
  **(Systemic)**, 3170
*Typhim Vi*—Pasteur-Mérieux (France) brand of Typhoid Vi Polysaccharide Vaccine (Systemic), #
Typhoid vaccine—*See* Typhoid Vaccine Inactivated (Parenteral-Systemic), #
Typhoid Vaccine Inactivated [typhoid vaccine]
  **(Parenteral-Systemic)**, #
  Typhoid Vaccine USP (Acetone Inactivated, Dried), #
  Typhoid Vaccine USP (Heat and Phenol Inactivated), #
Typhoid Vaccine Live Oral [*Vivotif Berna*]
  **(Systemic)**, #
  Capsules, Enteric-coated, #
Typhoid Vi Polysaccharide Vaccine Live [*Typhim Vi*]
  **(Systemic)**, #
  Typhoid Vi Polysaccharide Vaccine, #
*Tyrodone*—Major (U.S.) brand of Pseudoephedrine and Hydrocodone—**See Cough/Cold Combinations (Systemic)**, 1024
Tyropanoate Sodium [*Bilopaque; Lumopaque;* sodium tyropanoate]
  **See Cholecystographic Agents, Oral (Systemic)**, #
  Capsules USP, #
*Tyrosum Liquid*—Summers (U.S.) brand of Alcohol and Acetone (Topical), #
*Tyrosum Packets*—Summers (U.S.) brand of Alcohol and Acetone (Topical), #

# U

*UAA*—Econo Med (U.S.) brand of Atropine, Hyoscyamine, Methenamine, Methylene Blue, Phenyl Salicylate, and Benzoic Acid (Systemic), 488
*UAD Otic*—Forest (U.S.) brand of Neomycin, Polymyxin B, and Hydrocortisone (Otic), #
*Ucephan*—Kendall McGaw (U.S.) brand of Sodium Benzoate and Sodium Phenylacetate (Systemic), #, 3133
UDCA—*See* Ursodiol (Systemic), 2903
*Uendex*—*See* Dextran Sulfate (Inhalation), 3140
*Ugesic*—Stewart Jackson (U.S.) brand of Hydrocodone and Acetaminophen—**See Opioid (Narcotic) Analgesics and Acetaminophen (Systemic)**, 2198
*Ulcidine*—ICN (Canada) brand of Famotidine—**See Histamine H₂-receptor Antagonists (Systemic)**, 1633, MC-12
*Ulcidine HB*—ICN (Canada) brand of Famotidine—**See Histamine H₂-receptor Antagonists (Systemic)**, 1633, MC-12
*Ulone*—Riker (Canada) brand of Chlophedianol (Systemic), #
*ULR-LA*—Geneva (U.S.) brand of Phenylpropanolamine and Guaifenesin—**See Cough/Cold Combinations (Systemic)**, 1024
*Ultane*—Abbott (U.S.) brand of Sevoflurane (Inhalation-Systemic), #
*Ultiva*—Glaxo Wellcome (U.S.) brand of Remifentanil (Systemic), BN-2464
*ULTRAbrom*—WE (U.S.) brand of Brompheniramine and Pseudoephedrine—**See Antihistamines and Decongestants (Systemic)**, 343
*ULTRAbrom PD*—WE (U.S.) brand of Brompheniramine and Pseudoephedrine—**See Antihistamines and Decongestants (Systemic)**, 343
*Ultracaine D-S*—Hoechst-Roussel (Canada) brand of Astracaine with Epinephrine—**See Anesthetics (Parenteral-Local)**, 139
*Ultracaine D-S Forte*—Hoechst-Roussel (Canada) brand of Astracaine with Epinephrine—**See Anesthetics (Parenteral-Local)**, 139
*Ultracal*—Mead Johnson (U.S.) brand of Enteral Nutrition Formula, Fiber-containing—**See Enteral Nutrition Formulas (Systemic)**, #

*Ultralan*—Elan (U.S.) brand of Enteral Nutrition Formula, Polymeric—**See Enteral Nutrition Formulas (Systemic)**, #
*Ultralente Insulin*—Connaught Novo Nordisk (Canada) brand of Insulin Zinc, Extended—**See Insulin (Systemic)**, 1713; Insulin Zinc, Extended, Human—**See Insulin (Systemic)**, 1713
*Ultralente insulin*—Insulin Zinc, Extended—**See Insulin (Systemic)**, 1713
*Ultram*—Ortho-McNeil (U.S.) brand of Tramadol (Systemic), 2851, MC-31
*Ultra MOP*—Canderm (Canada) brand of Methoxsalen (Systemic), 1973
*UltraMOP Lotion*—Canderm (Canada) brand of Methoxsalen (Topical), 1977
*Ultra Muskol*—Schering (U.S.) brand of Diethyltoluamide (Topical), #
*Ultra Pep-Back*—Alva-Amco (U.S.) brand of Caffeine (Systemic), 706
*Ultra Pred*—Horizon (U.S.) brand of Prednisolone—**See Corticosteroids (Ophthalmic)**, 966
*Ultra-R*—E-Z-EM (U.S. and Canada) brand of Barium Sulfate (Local), #
*Ultrase MT 12*—Scandipharm (U.S.) brand of Pancrelipase (Systemic), 2222
*Ultrase MT 20*—Scandipharm (U.S.) brand of Pancrelipase (Systemic), 2222
*Ultra Tears*—Alcon (U.S.) brand of Hydroxypropyl Methylcellulose (Ophthalmic), #
*Ultra-TechneKow FM*—Mallinckrodt (U.S.) brand of Sodium Pertechnetate Tc 99m generator (Mucosal-Local), 2610; Sodium Pertechnetate Tc 99m generator (Ophthalmic), 2611; Sodium Pertechnetate Tc 99m generator (Systemic), 2612
*Ultravate*—Westwood-Squibb (U.S.) brand of Halobetasol—**See Corticosteroids (Topical)**, 978
*Ultravist 150*—Berlex (U.S.) brand of Iopromide (Systemic), #
*Ultravist 240*—Berlex (U.S.) brand of Iopromide (Systemic), #
*Ultravist 300*—Berlex (U.S.) brand of Iopromide (Systemic), #
*Ultravist 370*—Berlex (U.S.) brand of Iopromide (Systemic), #
*Ultrazine-10*—Vortech (U.S.) brand of Prochlorperazine—**See Phenothiazines (Systemic)**, 2289
*Unasyn*—Roerig (U.S.) brand of Ampicillin and Sulbactam—**See Penicillins and Beta-lactamase Inhibitors (Systemic)**, 2263
Undecylenic Acid, Compound [*Caldesene Medicated Powder; Cruex Aerosol Powder; Cruex Antifungal Cream; Cruex Antifungal Powder; Cruex Antifungal Spray Powder; Cruex Cream; Cruex Powder; Decylenes Powder; Desenex Aerosol Powder; Desenex Antifungal Cream; Desenex Antifungal Liquid; Desenex Antifungal Ointment; Desenex Antifungal Penetrating Foam; Desenex Antifungal Powder; Desenex Antifungal Spray Powder; Desenex Foam; Desenex Ointment; Desenex Powder; Desenex Solution; Gordochom Solution*]
  **(Topical)**, #
  Aerosol Foam, Topical, #
  Aerosol Powder, Topical, #
  Cream, #
  Ointment USP, #
  Powder, Topical, #
  Solution, Topical, #
*Unibar-100*—E-Z-EM (Canada) brand of Barium Sulfate (Local), #
*Unicort*—Glaxo (Canada) brand of Hydrocortisone—**See Corticosteroids (Topical)**, 978
*Uni-Decon*—URL (U.S.) brand of Chlorpheniramine, Phenyltoloxamine, Phenylephrine, and Phenylpropanolamine—**See Antihistamines and Decongestants (Systemic)**, 343
*Uni-Dur*—Key (U.S.) brand of Theophylline—**See Bronchodilators, Theophylline (Systemic)**, 668
*Unilax*—Ascher (U.S.) brand of Phenolphthalein and Docusate—**See Laxatives (Local)**, #
*Uni-Multihist*—URL (U.S.) brand of Pheniramine, Phenyltoloxamine, Pyrilamine, and Phenylpropanolamine—**See Antihistamines and Decongestants (Systemic)**, 343
*Unipen*—Wyeth-Ayerst (U.S. and Canada) brand of Nafcillin—**See Penicillins (Systemic)**, 2240
*Uniphyl*—Purdue (U.S. and Canada) brand of Theophylline—**See Bronchodilators, Theophylline (Systemic)**, 668, MC-29

*Unipres*—Solvay (U.S.) brand of Reserpine, Hydralazine, and Hydrochlorothiazide (Systemic), #
*Uniretic*—Schwarz (U.S.) brand of Moexipril Hydrochloride and Hydrochlorothiazide (Systemic), 2045, MC-20
*Unisom Nighttime SleepAid*—Consumer Health (U.S.) brand of Doxylamine—**See Antihistamines (Systemic)**, 325
*Unisom SleepGels Maximum Strength*—Leeming (U.S.) brand of Diphenhydramine—**See Antihistamines (Systemic)**, 325
*Unituss HC*—URL (U.S.) brand of Chlorpheniramine, Phenylephrine, and Hydrocodone—**See Cough/Cold Combinations (Systemic)**, 1024
*Uni-tussin*—URL (U.S.) brand of Guaifenesin (Systemic), 1588
*Uni-tussin DM*—URL (U.S.) brand of Dextromethorphan and Guaifenesin—**See Cough/Cold Combinations (Systemic)**, 1024
*Univasc*—Schwarz (U.S.) brand of Moexipril (Systemic), 2042, MC-20
*Univol*—Horner (Canada) brand of Alumina and Magnesia—**See Antacids (Oral-Local)**, 188
*Unproco*—Solvay (U.S.) brand of Dextromethorphan and Guaifenesin—**See Cough/Cold Combinations (Systemic)**, 1024
*Urabeth*—Major (U.S.) brand of Bethanechol (Systemic), 614
*Uracid*—Wesley (U.S.) brand of Racemethionine (Systemic), #
Uracil Mustard
  **(Systemic)**, #
  Capsules USP, #
Urea [carbamide; *Ureaphil*]
  **(Parenteral-Local)**, #
  Sterile USP, #
Urea [*Ureaphil*]
  **(Systemic)**, 2899
  Sterile USP, 2900
Urea-containing Combinations, 3082
*Ureaphil*—Abbott (U.S.) brand of Urea (Parenteral-Local), #; Abbott (U.S.) brand of Urea (Systemic), 2899
*Urecholine*—Merck (U.S.) and Frosst (Canada) brand of Bethanechol (Systemic), 614
*Urex*—Riker (U.S.) brand of Methenamine (Systemic), #
Uridine 5′-Triphosphate
  **(Systemic)**, 3170
*Uridon*—ICN (Canada) brand of Chlorthalidone—**See Diuretics, Thiazide (Systemic)**, 1273
*Uridon Modified*—Rugby (U.S.) brand of Atropine, Hyoscyamine, Methenamine, Methylene Blue, Phenyl Salicylate, and Benzoic Acid (Systemic), 488
*Urimed*—Schein (U.S.) brand of Atropine, Hyoscyamine, Methenamine, Methylene Blue, Phenyl Salicylate, and Benzoic Acid (Systemic), 488
*Urinary Antiseptic No. 2*—Lemmon (U.S.) brand of Atropine, Hyoscyamine, Methenamine, Methylene Blue, Phenyl Salicylate, and Benzoic Acid (Systemic), 488
Urine Glucose and Ketone (Combined) Test [*Chemstrip uGK; Glucose & Ketone Urine Test; Ketodiastix*]
  **See Urine Glucose and Ketone Test Kits for Home Use**, #
  Strips, #
Urine Glucose and Ketone Test Kits for Home Use, #
*Urised*—Webcon (U.S.) brand of Atropine, Hyoscyamine, Methenamine, Methylene Blue, Phenyl Salicylate, and Benzoic Acid (Systemic), 488
*Uriseptic*—Able (U.S.) brand of Atropine, Hyoscyamine, Methenamine, Methylene Blue, Phenyl Salicylate, and Benzoic Acid (Systemic), 488
*Urispas*—SKF (U.S.) and Pharmascience (Canada) brand of Flavoxate (Systemic), 1468
*Uritab*—Vortech (U.S.) brand of Atropine, Hyoscyamine, Methenamine, Methylene Blue, Phenyl Salicylate, and Benzoic Acid (Systemic), 488
*Uritin*—Schein (U.S.) and United Research (U.S.) brand of Atropine, Hyoscyamine, Methenamine, Methylene Blue, Phenyl Salicylate, and Benzoic Acid (Systemic), 488
*Uritol*—Horner (Canada) brand of Furosemide—**See Diuretics, Loop (Systemic)**, 1259
*Urobak*—Shionogi (U.S.) brand of Sulfamethoxazole—**See Sulfonamides (Systemic)**, 2653

*Urocit-K*—Mission (U.S.) brand of Potassium Citrate—**See Citrates (Systemic)**, 881; *See also* Potassium Citrate (Systemic), 3159
*Urodine*—Interstate (U.S.); Kenyon (U.S.); and Schein (U.S.) brand of Phenazopyridine (Systemic), 2288
Urofollitropin—*See* Urofollitropin (Systemic), 2901
Urofollitropin [*Fertinex*; *Fertinorm HP;* follicle-stimulating hormone; FSH; *Metrodin*; urofollitrophin] **(Systemic)**, 2901, 3170
  for Injection, 2902
  for Injection (Purified), 2903
Urogastrone
  **(Ophthalmic)**, 3171
*Urogesic*—Edwards (U.S.) brand of Phenazopyridine (Systemic), 2288
Urokinase [*Abbokinase; Abbokinase Open-Cath*] **See Thrombolytic Agents (Systemic)**, 2799
  for Injection, 2808
*Uro-KP-Neutral*—Star (U.S. and Canada) brand of Potassium and Sodium Phosphates—**See Phosphates (Systemic)**, 2317
*Urolene Blue*—Star (U.S.) brand of Methylene Blue (Systemic), #
*Uro-Mag*—Blaine (U.S.) brand of Magnesium Oxide—**See Antacids (Oral-Local)**, 188; **Magnesium Supplements (Systemic)**, 1897
*Uromitexan*—Bristol-Myers (Canada) brand of Mesna (Systemic), 1956
*Uro-Ves*—Mallard (U.S.) brand of Atropine, Hyoscyamine, Methenamine, Methylene Blue, Phenyl Salicylate, and Benzoic Acid (Systemic), 488
*Urovist Cysto*—Berlex (U.S.) brand of Diatrizoate—**See Diatrizoates (Local)**, #
*Urovist Cysto Pediatric*—Berlex (U.S.) brand of Diatrizoate—**See Diatrizoates (Local)**, #
*Urovist Meglumine DIU/CT*—Berlex (U.S.) brand of Diatrizoate—**See Diatrizoates (Systemic)**, #
*Urovist Sodium 300*—Berlex (U.S.) brand of Diatrizoate—**See Diatrizoates (Local)**, #; **Diatrizoates (Systemic)**, #
*Urozide*—ICN (Canada) brand of Hydrochlorothiazide—**See Diuretics, Thiazide (Systemic)**, 1273
*Ursinus Inlay*—Sandoz (U.S.) brand of Pseudoephedrine and Aspirin—**See Decongestants and Analgesics (Systemic)**, 1180
Ursodeoxycholic acid—*See* Ursodiol (Systemic), 2903, 3171
Ursodiol [*Actigall*; ursodeoxycholic acid; *Ursofalk*] **(Systemic)**, 2903, 3171
  Capsules USP, 2905, MC-32
*Ursofalk*—Axcan (U.S.) brand of Ursodeoxycholic Acid (Systemic), 3171; Jouveinal (Canada) brand of Ursodiol (Systemic), 2903
*Uticort*—PD (U.S.) brand of Betamethasone—**See Corticosteroids (Topical)**, 978
*Uvadex*—Therakos (U.S.) brand of 8-Methoxsalen (Systemic), 3128

## V

Vaccinia, Recombinant (Human Papillomavirus) [*TA-HPV*]
  **(Systemic)**, 3162
*Vagistat-1*—Bristol-Myers Squibb (U.S.) brand of Tioconazole—**See Antifungals, Azole (Vaginal)**, 310
Valacyclovir Hydrochloride [valaciclovir; *Valtrex*] **(Systemic)**, 2906
  Tablets, 2908, MC-32
*Valergen-10*—Hyrex (U.S.) brand of Estradiol—**See Estrogens (Systemic)**, 1383
*Valergen-20*—Hyrex (U.S.) brand of Estradiol—**See Estrogens (Systemic)**, 1383
*Valergen-40*—Hyrex (U.S.) brand of Estradiol—**See Estrogens (Systemic)**, 1383
*Valertest No. 1*—Hyrex (U.S.) brand of Testosterone and Estradiol—**See Androgens and Estrogens (Systemic)**, 126
*Valertest No. 2*—Hyrex (U.S.) brand of Testosterone and Estradiol—**See Androgens and Estrogens (Systemic)**, 126
Valaciclovir—*See* Valacyclovir (Systemic), 2906
Valine, Isoleucine, and Leucine [*VIL*]
  **(Systemic)**, 3171
*Valisone*—Schering (U.S.) brand of Betamethasone—**See Corticosteroids (Topical)**, 978
*Valisone Reduced Strength*—Schering (U.S.) brand of Betamethasone—**See Corticosteroids (Topical)**, 978

*Valisone Scalp Lotion*—Schering (Canada) brand of Betamethasone—**See Corticosteroids (Topical)**, 978
*Valium*—Roche (U.S. and Canada) brand of Diazepam—**See Benzodiazepines (Systemic)**, 556, MC-9
*Valnac*—NMC (U.S.) brand of Betamethasone—**See Corticosteroids (Topical)**, 978
*Valorin*—Otis Clapp (U.S.) brand of Acetaminophen (Systemic), 6
*Valorin Extra*—Otis Clapp (U.S.) brand of Acetaminophen (Systemic), 6
Valproate Sodium[*Depacon*]
  **(Systemic)**, 2908
  Injection, 2913
Valproic Acid [*Alti-Valproic; Depakene; Deproic; Dom-Valproic; Med Valproic; Novo-Valproic; Nu-Valproic; Penta-Valproic; pms-Valproic Acid; pms-Valproic Acid E.C.*]
  **(Systemic)**, 2908
  Capsules USP, 2913, MC-32
  Syrup USP, 2914
Valsartan [*Diovan*]
  **(Systemic)**, 2914
  Capsules, 2916
*Valtrex*—Glaxo Wellcome (U.S. and Canada) brand of Valacyclovir (Systemic), 2906, MC-32
*Vanacet*—GM (U.S.) brand of Hydrocodone and Acetaminophen—**See Opioid (Narcotic) Analgesics and Acetaminophen (Systemic)**, 2198
*Vanadom*—GM (U.S.) brand of Carisoprodol—**See Skeletal Muscle Relaxants (Systemic)**, 2577
*Vancenase*—Schering (U.S. and Canada) brand of Beclomethasone—**See Corticosteroids (Nasal)**, 961
*Vancenase AQ*—Schering (U.S.) brand of Beclomethasone—**See Corticosteroids (Nasal)**, 961, 3011
*Vanceril*—Schering (U.S. and Canada) brand of Beclomethasone—**See Corticosteroids (Inhalation-Local)**, 955
*Vanceril 84 mcg Double Strength*—Schering (U.S.) brand of Beclomethasone—**See Corticosteroids (Inhalation-Local)**, 955
*Vancocin*—Lilly (U.S. and Canada) brand of Vancomycin (Oral-Local), 2916; Vancomycin (Systemic), 2919
Vancomycin Hydrochloride [*Vancocin*]
  **(Oral-Local)**, 2916
  Capsules USP, 2918
  for Solution, Oral, USP, 2918
Vancomycin Hydrochloride [*Vancocin*]
  **(Systemic)**, 2919
  Injection USP, 2922
  for Injection USP, 2922
  Sterile USP, 2921
*Vanex Expectorant*—Abana (U.S.) brand of Pseudoephedrine, Hydrocodone, and Guaifenesin—**See Cough/Cold Combinations (Systemic)**, 1024
*Vanex Forte Caplets*—Abana (U.S.) brand of Chlorpheniramine, Pyrilamine, Phenylephrine, and Phenylpropanolamine—**See Antihistamines and Decongestants (Systemic)**, 343
*Vanex Grape*—Abana (U.S.) brand of Chlorpheniramine, Phenylpropanolamine, Phenylephrine, and Dihydrocodeine—**See Cough/Cold Combinations (Systemic)**, 1024
*Vanex-HD*—Abana (U.S.) brand of Chlorpheniramine, Phenylephrine, and Hydrocodone—**See Cough/Cold Combinations (Systemic)**, 1024
*Vanquin*—PD (Canada) brand of Pyrvinium (Oral-Local), #
*Vanquish Caplets*—Glenbrook (U.S.) brand of Acetaminophen, Aspirin, and Caffeine, Buffered—**See Acetaminophen and Salicylates (Systemic)**, 11
*Vanseb-T*—Allergan Herbert (U.S.) brand of Salicylic Acid, Sulfur, and Coal Tar (Topical), #
*Vansil*—Pfizer (U.S.) brand of Oxamniquine (Systemic), #
*Vantin*—Pharmacia & Upjohn (U.S.) brand of Cefpodoxime—**See Cephalosporins (Systemic)**, 794, MC-6
*Vaponefrin*—Fisons (U.S.) and Rorer (Canada) brand of Epinephrine—**See Bronchodilators, Adrenergic (Inhalation-Local)**, 640
*Vaqta*—Merck (U.S.) brand of Hepatitis A Vaccine Inactivated (Systemic), 1625
Varicella Virus Vaccine Live [*Varivax*]
  **(Systemic)**, 2923
  Injection, 2925

*Varivax*—Merck (U.S.) brand of Varicella Virus Vaccine Live (Systemic), 2923
*Vascor*—Ortho-McNeil (U.S.) brand of Bepridil—**See Calcium Channel Blocking Agents (Systemic)**, 720, MC-4
*Vascoray*—Mallinckrodt (U.S.) brand of Iothalamate (Systemic), #
Vascular Headache Suppressants, Ergot Derivative–containing
  **(Systemic)**, 2925
*Vaseline Baby Sunblock*—Cairns (U.S.) brand of Titanium Dioxide and Zinc Oxide—**See Sunscreen Agents (Topical)**, #
*Vaseline Broad Spectrum Sunblock*—Chesebrough-Ponds (Canada) brand of Avobenzone and Octyl Methoxycinnamate—**See Sunscreen Agents (Topical)**, #
*Vaseline Extra Defense for Hand and Body*—Chesebrough-Ponds (Canada) brand of Octyl Methoxycinnamate and Oxybenzone—**See Sunscreen Agents (Topical)**, #
*Vaseline Intensive Care Active Sport*—Chesebrough-Ponds (Canada) brand of Octyl Methoxycinnamate and Oxybenzone—**See Sunscreen Agents (Topical)**, #
*Vaseline Intensive Care Baby Moisturizing Sunblock*—Cairns (U.S.) brand of Octyl Methoxycinnamate, Octyl Salicylate, Oxybenzone, and Titanium Dioxide—**See Sunscreen Agents (Topical)**, #; Titanium Dioxide—**See Sunscreen Agents (Topical)**, #
*Vaseline Intensive Care Baby Sunblock*—Chesebrough-Ponds (Canada) brand of Octyl Methoxycinnamate, Octyl Salicylate, Oxybenzone, and Titanium Dioxide—**See Sunscreen Agents (Topical)**, #
*Vaseline Intensive Care Blockout Moisturizing*—Cairns (U.S.) brand of Octyl Methoxycinnamate, Octyl Salicylate, Oxybenzone, Padimate O, and Titanium Dioxide—**See Sunscreen Agents (Topical)**, #; Octyl Methoxycinnamate, Octyl Salicylate, Oxybenzone, and Titanium Dioxide—**See Sunscreen Agents (Topical)**, #
*Vaseline Intensive Care Lip Therapy*—Cairns (U.S.) brand of Octyl Methoxycinnamate and Oxybenzone—**See Sunscreen Agents (Topical)**, #
*Vaseline Intensive Care Moisturizing Sunblock*—Cairns (U.S.) brand of Octyl Methoxycinnamate, Octyl Salicylate, and Oxybenzone—**See Sunscreen Agents (Topical)**, #; Octyl Methoxycinnamate and Oxybenzone—**See Sunscreen Agents (Topical)**, #
*Vaseline Intensive Care Moisturizing Sunscreen*—Cairns (U.S.) brand of Octyl Methoxycinnamate and Octyl Salicylate—**See Sunscreen Agents (Topical)**, #
*Vaseline Kids Sunblock*—Chesebrough-Ponds (Canada) brand of Octyl Methoxycinnamate, Octyl Salicylate, and Oxybenzone—**See Sunscreen Agents (Topical)**, #; Octyl Methoxycinnamate and Oxybenzone—**See Sunscreen Agents (Topical)**, #
*Vaseline Lip Therapy*—Chesebrough-Ponds (Canada) brand of Octyl Methoxycinnamate and Oxybenzone—**See Sunscreen Agents (Topical)**, #
*Vaseline Moisturizing Sunscreen*—Chesebrough-Pond's (U.S.) and Chesebrough-Ponds (Canada) brand of Octyl Methoxycinnamate and Oxybenzone—**See Sunscreen Agents (Topical)**, #
*Vaseline Sports Sunscreen*—Chesebrough-Ponds (Canada) brand of Octyl Methoxycinnamate and Oxybenzone—**See Sunscreen Agents (Topical)**, #
*Vaseline Sport Sunblock*—Chesebrough-Ponds (Canada) brand of Octyl Methoxycinnamate and Oxybenzone—**See Sunscreen Agents (Topical)**, #
*Vaseline Sunblock*—Chesebrough-Ponds (Canada) brand of Octyl Methoxycinnamate, Octyl Salicylate, and Oxybenzone—**See Sunscreen Agents (Topical)**, #; Octyl Methoxycinnamate, Octyl Salicylate, Oxybenzone, and Padimate O—**See Sunscreen Agents (Topical)**, #; Octyl Methoxycinnamate and Oxybenzone—**See Sunscreen Agents (Topical)**, #
*Vaseline Sunscreen*—Chesebrough-Ponds (Canada) brand of Octyl Methoxycinnamate and Oxybenzone—**See Sunscreen Agents (Topical)**, #
*Vaseline Ultraviolet Daily Defense for Hand and Body*—Chesebrough-Ponds (Canada) brand of Octyl Methoxycinnamate and Oxybenzone—**See Sunscreen Agents (Topical)**, #

## General Index

*Vaseretic*—Merck (U.S.) and MSD (Canada) brand of Enalapril and Hydrochlorothiazide—**See Angiotensin-converting Enzyme (ACE) Inhibitors and Hydrochlorothiazide (Systemic)**, 187, MC-11
Vasoactive Intestinal Polypeptide **(Systemic)**, 3171
*VasoClear*—Iolab (U.S.) brand of Naphazoline (Ophthalmic), #
*VasoClear A*—Iolab (U.S.) brand of Naphazoline (Ophthalmic), #
*Vasocon*—Iolab (Canada) brand of Naphazoline (Ophthalmic), #
*Vasocon Regular*—Iolab (U.S.) brand of Naphazoline (Ophthalmic), #
*Vasodilan*—Mead Johnson (U.S.) and Bristol (Canada) brand of Isoxsuprine (Systemic), #
*Vasofrinic*—Trianon (Canada) brand of Chlorpheniramine and Pseudoephedrine—**See Antihistamines and Decongestants (Systemic)**, 343
Vasopressin [*Pitressin; Pressyn*] **(Systemic)**, 2938
  Injection USP, 2940
*Vasoprost*—Schwarz (U.S.) brand of Alprostadil (Systemic), 3129
*Vasotate HC*—Major (U.S.) brand of Hydrocortisone and Acetic Acid (Otic), 3023
*Vasotec*—Merck (U.S. and Canada) brand of Enalapril—**See Angiotensin-converting Enzyme (ACE) Inhibitors (Systemic)**, 177, MC-11
*Vasoxyl*—BW (U.S. and Canada) brand of Methoxamine—**See Sympathomimetic Agents—Cardiovascular Use (Parenteral-Systemic)**, 2669
*VaxSyn HIV-1*—MicroGeneSys (U.S.) brand of Human T-Lymphotropic Virus Type III gp160 Antigens (Systemic), 3146
*VCF*—Apothecus (U.S.) brand of Nonoxynol 9—**See Spermicides (Vaginal)**, #
*V-Cillin K*—Lilly (U.S. and Canada) brand of Penicillin V—**See Penicillins (Systemic)**, 2240, MC-24
*V-Dec-M*—Seatrace (U.S.) brand of Pseudoephedrine and Guaifenesin—**See Cough/Cold Combinations (Systemic)**, 1024
Vecuronium Bromide [*Norcuron*]
  **See Neuromuscular Blocking Agents (Systemic)**, 2098
  for Injection, 2106
*Veetids*—Apothecon (U.S.) brand of Penicillin V—**See Penicillins (Systemic)**, 2240, MC-24
*Velban*—Lilly (U.S.) brand of Vinblastine (Systemic), 2946
*Velbe*—Lilly (Canada) brand of Vinblastine (Systemic), 2946
*Velosef*—Apothecon (U.S. and Canada) brand of Cephradine—**See Cephalosporins (Systemic)**, 794, MC-6
*Velosulin BR*—Novo Nordisk (U.S.) brand of Insulin Human, Buffered—**See Insulin (Systemic)**, 1713
*Velosulin Human*—Connaught Novo Nordisk (Canada) brand of Insulin Human, Buffered—**See Insulin (Systemic)**, 1713
*Vendone*—Venture (U.S.) brand of Hydrocodone and Acetaminophen—**See Opioid (Narcotic) Analgesics and Acetaminophen (Systemic)**, 2198
Venlafaxine [*Effexor; Effexor XR*] **(Systemic)**, 2940
  Capsules, Extended-release, 2943
  Tablets, 2944, MC-32
*Venoglobulin-I*—Alpha (U.S.) brand of Immune Globulin Intravenous (Human) (Systemic), 1686
*Venoglobulin-S*—Alpha (U.S.) brand of Immune Globulin Intravenous (Human) (Systemic), 3025
*Ventodisk*—Glaxo (Canada) brand of Albuterol—**See Bronchodilators, Adrenergic (Inhalation-Local)**, 640
*Ventolin*—Allen & Hanburys (U.S. and Canada) brand of Albuterol—**See Bronchodilators, Adrenergic (Inhalation-Local)**, 640; Glaxo Wellcome (U.S. and Canada) brand of Albuterol—**See Bronchodilators, Adrenergic (Systemic)**, 651, MC-1
*Ventolin Nebules*—Glaxo Wellcome (U.S.) brand of Albuterol—**See Bronchodilators, Adrenergic (Inhalation-Local)**, 640
*Ventolin Nebules P.F.*—Glaxo Wellcome (Canada) brand of Albuterol—**See Bronchodilators, Adrenergic (Inhalation-Local)**, 640
*Ventolin Rotacaps*—Glaxo Wellcome (U.S. and Canada) brand of Albuterol—**See Bronchodilators, Adrenergic (Inhalation-Local)**, 640

*VePesid*—Bristol-Myers Squibb (U.S. and Canada) brand of Etoposide (Systemic), 1424
*Veracolate*—Numark (U.S.) brand of Cascara Sagrada and Phenolphthalein—**See Laxatives (Local)**, #
Verapamil [*Apo-Verap; Calan; Isoptin; Novo-Veramil; Nu-Verap*]
  **See Calcium Channel Blocking Agents (Systemic)**, 720
  Injection USP, 732
  Tablets USP, 731, MC-32
Verapamil Hydrochloride [*Calan SR; Chronovera; Covera-HS ; Isoptin SR; Verelan*]
  **See Calcium Channel Blocking Agents (Systemic)**, 720, 3037
  Capsules, Extended-release, 731, MC-32
  Tablets, Extended-release, 732, 3037, MC-32
*Verazinc*—Forest (U.S.) brand of Zinc Sulfate—**See Zinc Supplements (Systemic)**, 2999
*Verelan*—Wyeth-Ayerst (U.S.) and Elan (Canada) brand of Verapamil—**See Calcium Channel Blocking Agents (Systemic)**, 720, MC-32
*Verluma*—Du Pont (U.S.) brand of Technetium Tc 99m Nofetumomab Merpentan (Systemic), 2722
*Vermox*—Janssen (U.S. and Canada) brand of Mebendazole (Systemic), 1926
*Versacaps*—Seatrace (U.S.) brand of Pseudoephedrine and Guaifenesin—**See Cough/Cold Combinations (Systemic)**, 1024
*Versed*—Roche (U.S. and Canada) brand of Midazolam (Systemic), 2007
*Versel Lotion*—T.C.D. (Canada) brand of Selenium Sulfide (Topical), #
*Verukan-HP Topical Solution*—Syosset (U.S.) brand of Salicylic Acid (Topical), #
*Verukan Topical Solution*—Syosset (U.S.) brand of Salicylic Acid (Topical), #
*Vesanoid*—Roche (U.S.) brand of Tretinoin (Systemic), 2868, 3169, MC-31
*Vesprin*—Princeton (U.S.) brand of Triflupromazine—**See Phenothiazines (Systemic)**, 2289
*Vexol*—Alcon (U.S.) brand of Rimexolone (Ophthalmic), 2504
*V-Gan-25*—Hauck (U.S.) brand of Promethazine—**See Antihistamines, Phenothiazine-derivative (Systemic)**, 377
*V-Gan-50*—Hauck (U.S.) brand of Promethazine—**See Antihistamines, Phenothiazine-derivative (Systemic)**, 377
*Viagra*—Pfizer (U.S.) brand of Sildenafil (Systemic), 2574
*Vianain*—Genzyme (U.S.) brand of Ananain, Comosain (Topical), 3131
*Vi-Atro*—Vita-Rx (U.S.) brand of Diphenoxylate and Atropine (Systemic), 1233
*Vibal*—Jones-Western (U.S.) brand of Cyanocobalamin—**See Vitamin B$_{12}$ (Systemic)**, 2962
*Vibal LA*—Jones-Western (U.S.) brand of Hydroxocobalamin—**See Vitamin B$_{12}$ (Systemic)**, 2962
*Vibramycin*—Pfizer (U.S.); Roerig (U.S.); and Pfizer (Canada) brand of Doxycycline—**See Tetracyclines (Systemic)**, 2765
*Vibra-Tabs*—Pfizer (U.S. and Canada) brand of Doxycycline—**See Tetracyclines (Systemic)**, 2765
*Vibutal*—Vita-Rx (U.S.) brand of Butalbital, Aspirin, and Caffeine—**See Barbiturates and Analgesics (Systemic)**, 532
*Vicks Children's DayQuil Allergy Relief*—Procter & Gamble (U.S.) brand of Chlorpheniramine and Pseudoephedrine—**See Antihistamines and Decongestants (Systemic)**, 343
*Vicks Children's NyQuil*—Procter & Gamble (Canada) brand of Chlorpheniramine, Pseudoephedrine, and Dextromethorphan—**See Cough/Cold Combinations (Systemic)**, 1024
*Vicks Children's NyQuil Cold/Cough Relief*—Procter & Gamble (U.S.) brand of Chlorpheniramine, Pseudoephedrine, and Dextromethorphan—**See Cough/Cold Combinations (Systemic)**, 1024
*Vicks 44 Cough and Cold Relief Non-Drowsy LiquiCaps*—Procter & Gamble (U.S.) brand of Pseudoephedrine and Dextromethorphan—**See Cough/Cold Combinations (Systemic)**, 1024
*Vicks Cough Syrup*—Procter & Gamble (Canada) brand of Ephedrine, Carbetapentane, and Guaifenesin—**See Cough/Cold Combinations (Systemic)**, 1024
*Vicks DayQuil 4 Hour Allergy Relief*—Procter & Gamble (U.S.) brand of Brompheniramine and Phenylpropanolamine—**See Antihistamines and Decongestants (Systemic)**, 343

*Vicks DayQuil 12 Hour Allergy Relief*—Procter & Gamble (U.S.) brand of Brompheniramine and Phenylpropanolamine—**See Antihistamines and Decongestants (Systemic)**, 343
*Vicks DayQuil Liquicaps*—Procter & Gamble (Canada) brand of Pseudoephedrine, Dextromethorphan, Guaifenesin, and Acetaminophen—**See Cough/Cold Combinations (Systemic)**, 1024
*Vicks DayQuil Multi-Symptom Cold/Flu LiquiCaps*—Procter & Gamble (U.S.) brand of Pseudoephedrine, Dextromethorphan, Guaifenesin, and Acetaminophen—**See Cough/Cold Combinations (Systemic)**, 1024
*Vicks DayQuil Multi-Symptom Cold/Flu Relief*—Procter & Gamble (U.S.) brand of Pseudoephedrine, Dextromethorphan, Guaifenesin, and Acetaminophen—**See Cough/Cold Combinations (Systemic)**, 1024
*Vicks DayQuil Sinus Pressure and Congestion Relief Caplets*—Procter & Gamble (U.S.) brand of Phenylpropanolamine and Guaifenesin—**See Cough/Cold Combinations (Systemic)**, 1024
*Vicks DayQuil Sinus Pressure & Pain Relief Caplets*—Procter & Gamble (U.S.) brand of Pseudoephedrine and Ibuprofen—**See Decongestants and Analgesics (Systemic)**, 1180
*Vicks 44D Cough and Head Congestion*—Procter & Gamble (U.S.) brand of Pseudoephedrine and Dextromethorphan—**See Cough/Cold Combinations (Systemic)**, 1024
*Vicks 44E Cough & Chest Congestion*—Procter & Gamble (U.S.) brand of Dextromethorphan and Guaifenesin—**See Cough/Cold Combinations (Systemic)**, 1024
*Vicks Formula 44-D*—Procter & Gamble (Canada) brand of Pseudoephedrine and Dextromethorphan—**See Cough/Cold Combinations (Systemic)**, 1024
*Vicks Formula 44-d Pediatric*—Procter & Gamble (Canada) brand of Pseudoephedrine and Dextromethorphan—**See Cough/Cold Combinations (Systemic)**, 1024
*Vicks Formula 44E*—Procter & Gamble (Canada) brand of Dextromethorphan and Guaifenesin—**See Cough/Cold Combinations (Systemic)**, 1024
*Vicks Formula 44e Pediatric*—Procter & Gamble (Canada) brand of Dextromethorphan and Guaifenesin—**See Cough/Cold Combinations (Systemic)**, 1024
*Vicks Formula 44M*—Procter & Gamble (Canada) brand of Chlorpheniramine, Pseudoephedrine, Dextromethorphan, and Acetaminophen—**See Cough/Cold Combinations (Systemic)**, 1024
*Vicks Formula 44 Pediatric Formula*—Vicks (U.S.) brand of Dextromethorphan (Systemic), 1191
*Vicks 44M Cough, Cold and Flu Relief*—Procter & Gamble (U.S.) brand of Chlorpheniramine, Pseudoephedrine, Dextromethorphan, and Acetaminophen—**See Cough/Cold Combinations (Systemic)**, 1024
*Vicks 44M Cough, Cold and Flu Relief LiquiCaps*—Procter & Gamble (U.S.) brand of Chlorpheniramine, Pseudoephedrine, Dextromethorphan, and Acetaminophen—**See Cough/Cold Combinations (Systemic)**, 1024
*Vicks NyQuil*—Procter & Gamble (Canada) brand of Doxylamine, Pseudoephedrine, Dextromethorphan, and Acetaminophen—**See Cough/Cold Combinations (Systemic)**, 1024
*Vicks NyQuil Hot Therapy*—Procter & Gamble (U.S.) brand of Doxylamine, Pseudoephedrine, Dextromethorphan, and Acetaminophen—**See Cough/Cold Combinations (Systemic)**, 1024
*Vicks NyQuil LiquiCaps*—Procter & Gamble (Canada) brand of Doxylamine, Pseudoephedrine, Dextromethorphan, and Acetaminophen—**See Cough/Cold Combinations (Systemic)**, 1024
*Vicks NyQuil Multi-Symptom Cold/Flu LiquiCaps*—Procter & Gamble (U.S.) brand of Doxylamine, Pseudoephedrine, Dextromethorphan, and Acetaminophen—**See Cough/Cold Combinations (Systemic)**, 1024
*Vicks NyQuil Multi-Symptom Cold/Flu Relief*—Procter & Gamble (U.S.) brand of Doxylamine, Pseudoephedrine, Dextromethorphan, and Acetaminophen—**See Cough/Cold Combinations (Systemic)**, 1024
*Vicks Pediatric 44D Cough & Head Decongestion*—Procter & Gamble (U.S.) brand of Pseudoephedrine and Dextromethorphan—**See Cough/Cold Combinations (Systemic)**, 1024

# General Index

*Vicks Pediatric 44E*—Procter & Gamble (U.S.) brand of Dextromethorphan and Guaifenesin—**See Cough/Cold Combinations (Systemic)**, 1024

*Vicks Pediatric 44M Multi-Symptom Cough & Cold*—Procter & Gamble (U.S.) brand of Chlorpheniramine, Pseudoephedrine, and Dextromethorphan—**See Cough/Cold Combinations (Systemic)**, 1024

*Vicks Sinex*—Richardson-Vicks (U.S.) brand of Phenylephrine (Nasal), #

*Vicks Sinex Long-Acting 12-Hour Formula Decongestant Nasal Spray*—Procter & Gamble (U.S.) brand of Oxymetazoline (Nasal), #

*Vicks Sinex Long-Acting 12-Hour Formula Decongestant Ultra Fine Mist*—Procter & Gamble (U.S.) brand of Oxymetazoline (Nasal), #

*Vicodin*—Knoll (U.S.) brand of Hydrocodone and Acetaminophen—**See Opioid (Narcotic) Analgesics and Acetaminophen (Systemic)**, 2198, MC-14

*Vicodin ES*—Knoll (U.S.) brand of Hydrocodone and Acetaminophen—**See Opioid (Narcotic) Analgesics and Acetaminophen (Systemic)**, 2198, MC-14

*Vicodin HP*—Knoll (U.S.) brand of Hydrocodone and Acetaminophen (Systemic), MC-14

*Vicodin Tuss*—Knoll (U.S.) brand of Hydrocodone and Guaifenesin—**See Cough/Cold Combinations (Systemic)**, 1024

*Vicoprofen*—Knoll (U.S.) brand of Hydrocodone and Ibuprofen (Systemic), 1659, 1659, MC-14

Vidarabine [ara-A; arabinoside; *Vira-A*]
  **(Ophthalmic)**, 2944
  Ointment, Ophthalmic, USP, 2945

*Vi-Daylin/F*—Ross (U.S.) brand of Multiple Vitamins and Fluoride—**See Vitamins, Multiple, and Fluoride (Systemic)**, 2978

*Videx*—Bristol-Myers Squibb (U.S. and Canada) brand of Didanosine (Systemic), 1206, MC-9

*VIL*—Leas Research (U.S.) brand of Valine, Isoleucine, and Leucine (Systemic), 3171

Vinblastine Sulfate [*Velban; Velbe*]
  **(Systemic)**, 2946
  Injection, 2949
  Sterile USP, 2949

*Vincol*—Reig Jofré (Spain) brand of Tiopronin (Systemic), 2824

Vincristine Sulfate [*Oncovin*]
  **(Systemic)**, 2950
  Injection USP, 2953

Vindesine Sulfate [*Eldisine*]
  **(Systemic)**, 3037
  for Injection, 3037

Vinorelbine Tartrate [*Navelbine*]
  **(Systemic)**, 2953
  Injection, 2957

*Vioform*—Ciba (U.S. and Canada) brand of Clioquinol (Topical), #

*Vioform-Hydrocortisone Cream*—Ciba (U.S. and Canada) brand of Clioquinol and Hydrocortisone (Topical), #

*Vioform-Hydrocortisone Lotion*—Ciba (U.S.) brand of Clioquinol and Hydrocortisone (Topical), #

*Vioform-Hydrocortisone Mild Cream*—Ciba (U.S. and Canada) brand of Clioquinol and Hydrocortisone (Topical), #

*Vioform-Hydrocortisone Mild Ointment*—Ciba (U.S.) brand of Clioquinol and Hydrocortisone (Topical), #

*Vioform-Hydrocortisone Ointment*—Ciba (U.S. and Canada) brand of Clioquinol and Hydrocortisone (Topical), #

*Viokase*—Robins (U.S.) brand of Pancrelipase (Systemic), 2222

*Viprynium*—See Pyrvinium (Oral-Local), #

*Vira-A*—PD (U.S. and Canada) brand of Vidarabine (Ophthalmic), 2944

*Viracept*—Agouron (U.S.) brand of Nelfinavir (Systemic), IBN-2095

*Viramune*—Roxane (U.S.) brand of Nevirapine (Systemic), IBN-2113

*Viranol*—American Dermal (U.S.) brand of Salicylic Acid (Topical), #

*Viranol Ultra*—American Dermal (U.S.) brand of Salicylic Acid (Topical), #

*Virazid*—See Ribavirin (Systemic), 2478

*Virazole*—ICN (U.S. and Canada) brand of Ribavirin (Systemic), 2478, 3162

*Viridium*—Vita Elixir (U.S.) brand of Phenazopyridine (Systemic), 2288

*Virilon*—Star (U.S.) brand of Methyltestosterone—**See Androgens (Systemic)**, 118

*Virilon IM*—Star (U.S.) brand of Testosterone—**See Androgens (Systemic)**, 118

*Viroptic*—BW (U.S. and Canada) brand of Trifluridine (Ophthalmic), 2877

*Visine L.R.*—Pfizer (U.S.) brand of Oxymetazoline (Ophthalmic), #

*Visipaque*—Nycomed (U.S.) brand of Iodixanol (Systemic), #

*Viskazide*—Sandoz (Canada) brand of Pindolol and Hydrochlorothiazide—**See Beta-adrenergic Blocking Agents and Thiazide Diuretics (Systemic)**, 609

*Visken*—Novartis (U.S. and Canada) brand of Pindolol—**See Beta-adrenergic Blocking Agents (Systemic)**, 593, MC-25

*Vistacrom*—Allergan (Canada) brand of Cromolyn (Ophthalmic), 1120

*Vistaril*—Pfizer (U.S.) and Roerig (U.S.) brand of Hydroxyzine—**See Antihistamines (Systemic)**, 325

*Vistide*—Gilead (U.S.) brand of Cidofovir (Systemic), 865

*Vitabee 6*—CMC (U.S.) brand of Pyridoxine (Systemic), 2430

*Vitabee 12*—CMC-Consumer (U.S.) brand of Cyanocobalamin—**See Vitamin B$_{12}$ (Systemic)**, 2962

*VitaCarn*—Sigma-Tau (U.S.) brand of Levocarnitine (Systemic), 3151, 3152

*Vitalax Super Smooth Sugar Free Orange Flavor*—Vita Health (Canada) brand of Psyllium Hydrophilic Mucilloid—**See Laxatives (Local)**, #

*Vitalax Unflavored*—Vita Health (Canada) brand of Psyllium Hydrophilic Mucilloid—**See Laxatives (Local)**, #

*Vital High Nitrogen*—Ross (U.S.) brand of Enteral Nutrition Formula, Monomeric (Elemental)—**See Enteral Nutrition Formulas (Systemic)**, #

Vitamin A [*Aquasol A;* retinol]
  **(Systemic)**, 2958
  Capsules USP, 2961
  Injection, 2962
  Solution, Oral, 2961
  Tablets, 2962

*Vitamin A Acid*—Rorer (Canada) brand of Tretinoin (Topical), 2871

Vitamin A acid—See Tretinoin (Topical), 2871

Vitamin B$_1$—See Thiamine (Systemic), 2787

Vitamin B$_2$—See Riboflavin (Systemic), 2481

Vitamin B$_3$—Niacin—**See Niacin (Systemic)**, 2116; Niacinamide—**See Niacin (Systemic)**, 2116

Vitamin B$_5$—See Pantothenic Acid (Systemic), #

Vitamin B$_6$—See Pyridoxine (Systemic), 2430

Vitamin B$_9$—See Folic Acid (Systemic), 1517

Vitamin B$_{12}$
  **(Systemic)**, 2962

Vitamin Bw—See Biotin (Systemic), #

Vitamin C—See Ascorbic Acid (Systemic), 469

Vitamin D and Analogs
  **(Systemic)**, 2966

Vitamin E [alpha tocopherol; *Amino-Opti-E; Aquasol E; E-Complex-600; E-200 I.U. Softgels; E-1000 I.U. Softgels; E-400 I.U. in a Water Soluble Base; E-Vitamin Succinate; Liqui-E; Pheryl-E; Vita Plus E; Webber Vitamin E*]
  **(Systemic)**, 2972
  Capsules USP, 2974
  Solution, Oral, 2974
  Tablets, 2975
  Tablets, Chewable, 2975

Vitamin H—See Biotin (Systemic), #

Vitamin K
  **(Systemic)**, 2975

Vitamin K$_1$—Phytonadione—**See Vitamin K (Systemic)**, 2975

Vitamin K$_4$—Menadiol—**See Vitamin K (Systemic)**, 2975

Vitamins A, D, and C and Sodium or Potassium Fluoride [*Cari-Tab; Tri-Vi-Flor*]
  **See Vitamins, Multiple, and Fluoride (Systemic)**, 2978
  Solution, Oral, 2980
  Tablets, Chewable, 2981

Vitamins, Multiple, and Fluoride
  **(Systemic)**, 2978

Vitamins, Multiple, and Sodium or Potassium Fluoride [*Adeflor; Mulvidren-F; Poly-Vi-Flor; Vi-Daylin/F*]
  **See Vitamins, Multiple, and Fluoride (Systemic)**, 2978
  Solution, Oral, 2980
  Tablets, Chewable, 2980

*Vitaneed*—Sherwood (U.S.) brand of Enteral Nutrition Formula, Blenderized—**See Enteral Nutrition Formulas (Systemic)**, #

*Vita Plus E*—Scot-Tussin (U.S.) brand of Vitamin E (Systemic), 2972

*Vitinoin*—Pharmascience (Canada) brand of Tretinoin (Topical), 2871

*Vitrasert*—Chiron Vision (U.S.) brand of Ganciclovir (Implantation-Ophthalmic), 1542

*Vitrasert Implant*—Chiron Vision (U.S.) brand of Intravitreal Ganciclovir Free Acid Implant (Ophthalmic), 3149

*Vivactil*—Merck (U.S.) brand of Protriptyline—**See Antidepressants, Tricyclic (Systemic)**, 271, MC-26

*Vivarin*—Beecham (U.S.) brand of Caffeine (Systemic), 706

*Vivelle*—Ciba-Geigy (U.S. and Canada) brand of Estradiol—**See Estrogens (Systemic)**, 1383

*Vivol*—Horner (Canada) brand of Diazepam—**See Benzodiazepines (Systemic)**, 556

*Vivonex Pediatric*—Sandoz (U.S.) brand of Enteral Nutrition Formula, Monomeric (Elemental)—**See Enteral Nutrition Formulas (Systemic)**, #

*Vivonex Plus*—Sandoz (U.S.) brand of Enteral Nutrition Formula, Monomeric (Elemental)—**See Enteral Nutrition Formulas (Systemic)**, #

*Vivonex T.E.N.*—Sandoz (U.S.) brand of Enteral Nutrition Formula, Monomeric (Elemental)—**See Enteral Nutrition Formulas (Systemic)**, #

*Vivotif Berna*—Berna (U.S.) and Swiss Serum (Canada) brand of Typhoid Vaccine Live Oral (Systemic), #

*V-Lax*—Century (U.S.) brand of Psyllium Hydrophilic Mucilloid—**See Laxatives (Local)**, #

*Vlemasque*—Dermik (U.S.) and Rorer (Canada) brand of Sulfurated Lime (Topical), #

*Vleminckx's solution*—See Sulfurated Lime (Topical), #

*VM-26*—See Teniposide (Systemic), 2747

*Volmax*—Muro (U.S. and Canada) brand of Albuterol—**See Bronchodilators, Adrenergic (Systemic)**, 651, 3009

*Voltaren*—Novartis (U.S. and Canada) brand of Diclofenac—**See Anti-inflammatory Drugs, Nonsteroidal (Systemic)**, 388, MC-9

*Voltaren Ophtha*—Ciba Vision (Canada) brand of Diclofenac—**See Anti-inflammatory Drugs, Nonsteroidal (Ophthalmic)**, 383

*Voltaren Ophthalmic*—Ciba Vision (U.S.) brand of Diclofenac—**See Anti-inflammatory Drugs, Nonsteroidal (Ophthalmic)**, 383

*Voltaren Rapide*—Geigy (Canada) brand of Diclofenac—**See Anti-inflammatory Drugs, Nonsteroidal (Systemic)**, 388

*Voltaren SR*—Geigy (Canada) brand of Diclofenac—**See Anti-inflammatory Drugs, Nonsteroidal (Systemic)**, 388

*Vontrol*—SKF (U.S.) brand of Diphenidol (Systemic), 1232

*VōSol HC*—Wallace (U.S.) and Horner (Canada) brand of Hydrocortisone and Acetic Acid—**See Corticosteroids and Acetic Acid (Otic)**, 996

*VP-16*—See Etoposide (Systemic), 1424

*Vumon*—Bristol (U.S. and Canada) brand of Teniposide (Systemic), 2747, 3035

*Vumon for Injection*—Bristol-Myers Squibb (U.S.) brand of Teniposide (Systemic), 3167

# W

*Wake-Up*—Adren (Canada) brand of Caffeine (Systemic), 706

Warfarin Sodium [*Coumadin; Panwarfin; Sofarin; Warfilone*]
  **See Anticoagulants (Systemic)**, 243, 3038
  for Injection USP, 249, 3038
  Tablets USP, 249, 3038, MC-32

*Warfilone*—Frosst (Canada) brand of Warfarin—**See Anticoagulants (Systemic)**, 243

*Wart-Off Topical Solution*—Pfizer Consumer Health Care (U.S.) brand of Salicylic Acid (Topical), #

*Waterbabies Little Licks*—Schering-Plough (U.S.) brand of Octyl Methoxycinnamate, Octyl Salicylate, and Oxybenzone—**See Sunscreen Agents (Topical)**, #

*Waterbabies Sunblock*—Schering-Plough (U.S. and Canada) brand of Homosalate, Octyl Methoxycinnamate, Octyl Salicylate, and Oxybenzone—**See Sunscreen Agents (Topical)**, #; Octyl Methoxycinnamate and Oxybenzone—**See Sunscreen Agents (Topical)**, #

*4-Way Long Lasting Nasal Spray*—Bristol-Myers (U.S.) brand of Oxymetazoline (Nasal), #
*Webber Vitamin E*—Ciba-Geigy (Canada) brand of Vitamin E (Systemic), 2972
*Wehgen*—Hauck (U.S.) brand of Estrone—**See Estrogens (Systemic)**, 1383
*Wehless*—Hauck (U.S.) brand of Phendimetrazine—**See Appetite Suppressants (Systemic)**, 452
*Wehless-105 Timecelles*—Hauck (U.S.) brand of Phendimetrazine—**See Appetite Suppressants (Systemic)**, 452
*Wellbutrin*—Glaxo Wellcome (U.S.) brand of Bupropion (Systemic), 687, MC-4
*Wellbutrin SR*—Glaxo Wellcome (U.S.) brand of Bupropion (Systemic), 687, MC-4
*Wellcovorin*—BW (U.S.) and Glaxo Wellcome (U.S.) brand of Leucovorin (Systemic), 1837, 3151
*Wellferon*—BW (U.S.) and Pacific (Canada) brand of Interferon Alfa-n1 (1ns)—**See Interferons, Alpha (Systemic)**, 1740, 3148
*Westcort*—Westwood (U.S.) and Westwood-Squibb (Canada) brand of Hydrocortisone—**See Corticosteroids (Topical)**, 978
*West-Decon*—West-Ward (U.S.) brand of Chlorpheniramine, Phenyltoloxamine, Phenylephrine, and Phenylpropanolamine—**See Antihistamines and Decongestants (Systemic)**, 343
*Westhroid*—Jones-Western (U.S.) brand of Thyroid—**See Thyroid Hormones (Systemic)**, 2809
Whole-cell DTP—*See* Diphtheria and Tetanus Toxoids and Pertussis Vaccine Adsorbed (Systemic), 1240
*Wigraine*—Organon (U.S.) brand of Ergotamine and Caffeine—**See Vascular Headache Suppressants, Ergot Derivative–containing (Systemic)**, 2925; Organon (Canada) brand of Ergotamine, Caffeine, and Belladonna Alkaloids—**See Vascular Headache Suppressants, Ergot Derivative–containing (Systemic)**, 2925
*Winpred*—ICN (Canada) brand of Prednisone—**See Corticosteroids—Glucocorticoid Effects (Systemic)**, 998
*WinRho SD*—Rh Pharmaceutical (Canada) brand of Rh$_o$(D) Immune Globulin (Systemic), 2476, 3162
*Winstrol*—Sanofi Winthrop (U.S.) brand of Stanozolol—**See Anabolic Steroids (Systemic)**, 110
*Wintrocin*—Hauck (U.S.) brand of Erythromycin Stearate—**See Erythromycins (Systemic)**, 1368
*Wolfina*—Forest (U.S.) brand of Rauwolfia Serpentina—**See Rauwolfia Alkaloids (Systemic)**, 2460
*Wyamine*—Wyeth-Ayerst (U.S.) brand of Mephentermine—**See Sympathomimetic Agents—Cardiovascular Use (Parenteral-Systemic)**, 2669
*Wycillin*—Wyeth-Ayerst (U.S.) and Wyeth (Canada) brand of Penicillin G—**See Penicillins (Systemic)**, 2240
*Wygesic*—Wyeth-Ayerst (U.S.) brand of Propoxyphene and Acetaminophen—**See Opioid (Narcotic) Analgesics and Acetaminophen (Systemic)**, 2198
*Wymox*—Wyeth-Ayerst (U.S.) brand of Amoxicillin—**See Penicillins (Systemic)**, 2240, MC-2; Wyeth-Ayerst (U.S.) brand of Amoxicillin (Systemic), 3010
*Wytensin*—Wyeth-Ayerst (U.S.) brand of Guanabenz (Systemic), 1590, MC-14

# X

*Xalatan*—Pharmacia & Upjohn (U.S. and Canada) brand of Latanoprost (Ophthalmic), 1831, 3026
*Xanax*—Pharmacia & Upjohn (U.S. and Canada) brand of Alprazolam—**See Benzodiazepines (Systemic)**, 556, MC-1
*Xanax TS*—Upjohn (Canada) brand of Alprazolam—**See Benzodiazepines (Systemic)**, 556
[127]Xe—*See* Xenon Xe 127 (Systemic), 2982
[133]Xe—*See* Xenon Xe 133 (Systemic), 2984
*Xeloda*—Roche (U.S.) brand of Capecitabine (Systemic), 748, MC-5
Xenon Xe 127 [*Xenon Xe 127 Gas*] **(Systemic)**, 2982
  Xenon Xe 127, 2983
Xenon Xe 133 [*MPI Xenon Xe 133 Gas; MPI Xenon Xe 133 Gas Ampul; Xenon Xe 133-V.S.S.*] **(Systemic)**, 2984
  Xenon Xe 133 USP, 2985
*Xenon Xe 127 Gas*—Frosst (Canada) brand of Xenon Xe 127 (Systemic), 2982

*Xenon Xe 133-V.S.S.*—Medi-Physics (U.S.) brand of Xenon Xe 133 (Systemic), 2984
*Xerac BP 5 Gel*—Person & Covey (U.S.) brand of Benzoyl Peroxide (Topical), 579
*Xerecept*—Neurobiological (U.S.) brand of Corticotropin-releasing Factor, Human (Systemic), 3138
*Xomazyme-H65*—Xoma (U.S.) brand of CD5-T Lymphocyte Immunotoxin (Systemic), 3136
*X-Prep Liquid*—Gray (U.S.) brand of Senna—**See Laxatives (Local)**, #
*X-Seb*—Baker Cummins (U.S.) brand of Salicylic Acid (Topical), #
*Xylocaine*—Astra (U.S. and Canada) brand of Lidocaine—**See Anesthetics (Mucosal-Local)**, 128; **Anesthetics (Parenteral-Local)**, 139; **Anesthetics (Topical)**, 155; Astra (U.S.) brand of Lidocaine (Systemic), 1860
*Xylocaine Dental Ointment*—Astra (Canada) brand of Lidocaine—**See Anesthetics (Mucosal-Local)**, 128
*Xylocaine Endotracheal*—Astra (Canada) brand of Lidocaine—**See Anesthetics (Mucosal-Local)**, 128
*Xylocaine-MPF*—Astra (U.S.) brand of Lidocaine—**See Anesthetics (Parenteral-Local)**, 139
*Xylocaine-MPF with Glucose*—Astra (U.S.) brand of Lidocaine—**See Anesthetics (Parenteral-Local)**, 139
*Xylocaine Test Dose*—Astra (Canada) brand of Lidocaine—**See Anesthetics (Parenteral-Local)**, 139
*Xylocaine Viscous*—Astra (U.S. and Canada) brand of Lidocaine—**See Anesthetics (Mucosal-Local)**, 128
*Xylocard*—Astra (Canada) brand of Lidocaine (Systemic), 1860
Xylometazoline Hydrochloride [*Chlorohist-LA; Inspire; Neo-Synephrine II Long Acting Nasal Spray Adult Strength; Neo-Synephrine II Long Acting Nose Drops Adult Strength; Otrivin With Metered-Dose Pump; Otrivin Nasal Drops; Otrivin Nasal Spray; Otrivin Pediatric Nasal Drops; Otrivin Pediatric Nasal Spray*]
**(Nasal)**, #, 3038
  Solution, Nasal, #, 3038
  Solution, Nasal, USP, #

# Y

Yellow Fever Vaccine [*YF-Vax*] **(Systemic)**, #
  USP (for Injection), #
*YF-Vax*—Connaught (U.S.) brand of Yellow Fever Vaccine (Systemic), #
*Yocon*—Palisades (U.S.) and Glenwood (Canada) brand of Yohimbine (Systemic), #
*Yodoquinol*—Liquipharm (U.S.) brand of Iodoquinol (Oral-Local), #
*Yodoxin*—Glenwood (U.S. and Canada) brand of Iodoquinol (Oral-Local), #
*Yohimar*—Marlop (U.S.) brand of Yohimbine (Systemic), #
Yohimbine Hydrochloride [*Actibine; Aphrodyne; Baron-X; Dayton Himbin; PMS-Yohimbine; Prohim; Thybine; Yocon; Yohimar; Yohimex; Yoman; Yovital*]
**(Systemic)**, #
  Tablets, #
*Yohimex*—Kramer (U.S.) brand of Yohimbine (Systemic), #
*Yoman*—Stuart Jackson (U.S.) brand of Yohimbine (Systemic), #
*Yovital*—Ram (U.S.) brand of Yohimbine (Systemic), #
*Yutopar*—Astra (U.S.) and Bristol (Canada) brand of Ritodrine (Systemic), 2513
*Yutopar S.R.*—Bristol (Canada) brand of Ritodrine (Systemic), 2513

# Z

*Zadaxin*—Sciclone (U.S.) brand of Thymalfasin (Systemic), 3169
*Zaditen*—Sandoz (Canada) brand of Ketotifen (Systemic), 3026
Zafirlukast [*Accolate*]
**(Systemic)**, 2987
  Tablets, 2988, MC-32
*Zagam*—Rhône-Poulenc Rorer (U.S.) brand of Sparfloxacin (Systemic), 2620, MC-28

Zalcitabine [ddC; *HIVID*]
**(Systemic)**, 2989, 3171
  Tablets, 2991, 3171
  Tablets USP, MC-32
*Zanaflex*—Athena (U.S.) brand of Tizanidine (Systemic), 2828, 3169, MC-30
*Zanosar*—Upjohn (U.S. and Canada) brand of Streptozocin (Systemic), 2629
*Zantac*—Glaxo Wellcome (U.S.) brand of Ranitidine Hydrochloride—**See Histamine H$_2$-receptor Antagonists (Systemic)**, 1633
*Zantac 75*—Glaxo Wellcome (U.S.) brand of Ranitidine Hydrochloride—**See Histamine H$_2$-receptor Antagonists (Systemic)**, 1633
*Zantac-C*—Glaxo Wellcome (Canada) brand of Ranitidine Hydrochloride—**See Histamine H$_2$-receptor Antagonists (Systemic)**, 1633
*Zantac EFFERdose*—Glaxo Wellcome (U.S. and Canada) brand of Ranitidine—**See Histamine H$_2$-receptor Antagonists (Systemic)**, MC-27
*Zantac EFFERdose Granules*—Glaxo Wellcome (U.S.) brand of Ranitidine Hydrochloride—**See Histamine H$_2$-receptor Antagonists (Systemic)**, 1633
*Zantac EFFERdose Tablets*—Glaxo Wellcome (U.S.) brand of Ranitidine Hydrochloride—**See Histamine H$_2$-receptor Antagonists (Systemic)**, 1633
*Zantac 150 GELdose*—Glaxo Wellcome (U.S.) brand of Ranitidine Hydrochloride—**See Histamine H$_2$-receptor Antagonists (Systemic)**, 1633
*Zantac 300 GELdose*—Glaxo Wellcome (U.S.) brand of Ranitidine Hydrochloride—**See Histamine H$_2$-receptor Antagonists (Systemic)**, 1633
*Zantac GELdose*—Glaxo Wellcome (U.S. and Canada) brand of Ranitidine—**See Histamine H$_2$-receptor Antagonists (Systemic)**, MC-27
*Zantryl*—ION (U.S.) brand of Phentermine—**See Appetite Suppressants (Systemic)**, 452
*Zarontin*—PD (U.S. and Canada) brand of Ethosuximide—**See Anticonvulsants, Succinimide (Systemic)**, #
*Zaroxolyn*—Fisons (U.S. and Canada) brand of Metolazone—**See Diuretics, Thiazide (Systemic)**, 1273
*Zeasorb-AF*—Stiefel (U.S.) brand of Miconazole (Topical), #
*Zeasorb-AF Powder*—Stiefel (U.S.) brand of Tolnaftate (Topical), #
*Zebeta*—Lederle (U.S.) brand of Bisoprolol—**See Beta-adrenergic Blocking Agents (Systemic)**, 593, MC-4
*Zebrax*—Hauck (U.S.) brand of Chlordiazepoxide and Clidinium (Systemic), 846
*Zecnil*—Ferring (U.S.) brand of Somatostatin (Systemic), 3165
*Zemplar*—Abbott (U.S.) brand of Paricalcitol (Systemic), 3031
*Zemuron*—Organon (U.S.) brand of Rocuronium (Systemic), 3521
*Zenapax*—Hoffman-La Roche (U.S.) brand of Daclizumab (Systemic), 1151; Humanized Anti-TAC (Systemic), 3146
*Zentel*—SmithKline Beecham (U.K.) brand of Albendazole (Systemic), #
*Zephrex*—Bock (U.S.) brand of Pseudoephedrine and Guaifenesin—**See Cough/Cold Combinations (Systemic)**, 1024
*Zephrex-LA*—Bock (U.S.) brand of Pseudoephedrine and Guaifenesin—**See Cough/Cold Combinations (Systemic)**, 1024
*Zerit*—Bristol-Myers Squibb (U.S. and Canada) brand of Stavudine (Systemic), 2627, MC-28
*Zestoretic*—ZENECA (U.S. and Canada) brand of Lisinopril and Hydrochlorothiazide—**See Angiotensin-converting Enzyme (ACE) Inhibitors and Hydrochlorothiazide (Systemic)**, 187, MC-17
*Zestril*—ZENECA (U.S. and Canada) brand of Lisinopril—**See Angiotensin-converting Enzyme (ACE) Inhibitors (Systemic)**, 177, MC-17
*Zetar Emulsion*—Dermik (U.S.) and Rorer (Canada) brand of Coal Tar (Topical), #
*Zetar Medicated Antiseborrheic Shampoo*—Dermik (U.S.) brand of Coal Tar (Topical), #
*Zetar Shampoo*—Rorer (Canada) brand of Coal Tar (Topical), #
*Ziac*—Lederle (U.S.) brand of Bisoprolol and Hydrochlorothiazide—**See Beta-adrenergic Blocking Agents and Thiazide Diuretics (Systemic)**, 609, MC-4

Zidovudine [*Apo-Zidovudine;* AZT; *Novo-AZT; Retrovir*]
  **(Systemic),** 2992, 3038, 3171
  Capsules, 2995, MC-32
  Injection, 2995
  Syrup, 2995
  Tablets, 3038
Zilactin-L—Zila (U.S.) brand of Lidocaine—**See Anesthetics (Mucosal-Local),** 128
Zileuton [*Zyflo*]
  **(Systemic),** 2996
  Tablets, 2998, MC-32
Zinacef—Glaxo (U.S. and Canada) brand of Cefuroxime—**See Cephalosporins (Systemic),** 794
Zinc 15—Mericon (U.S.) brand of Zinc Sulfate—**See Zinc Supplements (Systemic),** 2999
Zinc-220—Alto (U.S.) brand of Zinc Sulfate—**See Zinc Supplements (Systemic),** 2999
Zinc Acetate [*Galzin*]
  **(Systemic),** 3039, 3171
  Capsules, 3039
Zinca-Pak—Smith & Nephew SoloPak (U.S.) brand of Zinc Sulfate—**See Zinc Supplements (Systemic),** 2999
Zincate—Paddock (U.S.) brand of Zinc Sulfate—**See Zinc Supplements (Systemic),** 2999
Zinc Chloride
  **See Zinc Supplements (Systemic),** 2999
  Injection USP, 3000
Zinc Gluconate [*Orazinc*]
  **See Zinc Supplements (Systemic),** 2999
  Lozenges, 3001
  Tablets, 3001
Zincon Dandruff Lotion Shampoo—Lederle (U.S.) brand of Pyrithione (Topical), #
Zinc Oxide-containing Combinations, 3082
Zinc Sulfate [*Orazinc; PMS Egozinc; Verazinc; Zinc 15; Zinc-220; Zinca-Pak; Zincate*]
  **See Zinc Supplements (Systemic),** 2999
  Capsules, 3001
  Injection USP, 3002
  Tablets, 3002
  Tablets, Extended-release, 3002

Zinc Supplements
  **(Systemic),** 2999
Zinecard—Pharmacia (U.S.) brand of Dexrazoxane (Systemic), 1190, 3140
Zithromax—Pfizer (U.S. and Canada) brand of Azithromycin (Systemic), 499, MC-3
Zixoryn—Farmacon (U.S.) brand of Flumecinol (Systemic), 3143
ZNP Bar Shampoo—Stiefel (U.S.) brand of Pyrithione (Topical), #
ZNP Shampoo—Stiefel (U.S.) brand of Pyrithione (Topical), #
Zocor—Merck (U.S.) and Frosst (Canada) brand of Simvastatin—**See HMG-CoA Reductase Inhibitors (Systemic),** 1647, MC-28
Zofran—Glaxo Wellcome (U.S.) and Glaxo Wellcome (Canada) brand of Ondansetron (Systemic), 2165, MC-23
Zoladex—ZENECA (U.S. and Canada) brand of Goserelin (Systemic), 1575
Zoladex LA—ZENECA (Canada) brand of Goserelin (Systemic), 1575
Zoladex 3-Month—ZENECA (Canada) brand of Goserelin (Systemic), 1575
Zolmitriptan [*Zomig*]
  **(Systemic),** 3003
  Tablets, 3004, MC-32
Zoloft—Roerig (U.S.) and Pfizer (Canada) brand of Sertraline (Systemic), 2566, MC-28
Zolpidem Tartrate [*Ambien*]
  **(Systemic),** 3005
  Tablets, 3007, MC-32
Zomig—ZENECA (U.S.) brand of Zolmitriptan (Systemic), 3003, MC-32
Zonalon—Genderm (U.S. and Canada) brand of Doxepin (Topical), 1305
Zopiclone [*Imovane*]
  **(Systemic),** 3039
  Tablets, 3039
ZORprin—Boots (U.S.) brand of Aspirin—**See Salicylates (Systemic),** 2538

Zostrix—GenDerm (U.S. and Canada) brand of Capsaicin (Topical), 753
Zostrix-HP—GenDerm (U.S. and Canada) brand of Capsaicin (Topical), 753
Zosyn—Lederle (U.S.) and Wyeth-Ayerst (U.S.) brand of Piperacillin and Tazobactam—**See Penicillins and Beta-lactamase Inhibitors (Systemic),** 2263, 3032
Zovia 1/35E—Watson (U.S.) brand of Ethynodiol Diacetate and Ethinyl Estradiol—**See Estrogens and Progestins—Oral Contraceptives (Systemic),** 1397
Zovia 1/50E—Watson (U.S.) brand of Ethynodiol Diacetate and Ethinyl Estradiol—**See Estrogens and Progestins—Oral Contraceptives (Systemic),** 1397
Zovirax—BW (U.S. and Canada) brand of Acyclovir (Topical), 28; Glaxo Wellcome (U.S. and Canada) brand of Acyclovir (Systemic), 24, MC-1
Zyban—Glaxo Wellcome (U.S.) brand of Bupropion (Systemic), 687, MC-4
Zydis—Scherer (U.K.) brand of Apomorphine (Systemic), 3132
Zydone—Du Pont (U.S.) brand of Hydrocodone and Acetaminophen—**See Opioid (Narcotic) Analgesics and Acetaminophen (Systemic),** 2198, MC-14
Zyflo—Abbott (U.S.) brand of Zileuton (Systemic), 2996, MC-32
Zyloprim—Glaxo Wellcome (U.S. and Canada) brand of Allopurinol (Systemic), 44, MC-1
Zyloprim for Injection—BW (U.S.) brand of Allopurinol (Systemic), 3129
Zymase—Organon (U.S.) brand of Pancrelipase (Systemic), 2222
Zymenol—Houser (U.S.) brand of Mineral Oil—**See Laxatives (Local),** #
Zyprexa—Lilly (U.S.) brand of Olanzapine (Systemic), 2156, MC-23
Zyrtec—Pfizer (U.S. and Canada) brand of Cetirizine—**See Antihistamines (Systemic),** 325, MC-6

# 1999 USP Print Products Order Form

To order, remove this form at perforation, fill out both sides completely, and mail to Micromedex Customer Service Department with payment or credit card information. Or, order by phone or fax.

**Mail Order**
Micromedex Customer Service Department
P.O. Box 564
Williston, VT 05495-0564

**Phone Order** 1-800-877-6209
**Fax Order** 1-802-864-7626
**International Phone Order** +1-802-862-4764
VISA/MasterCard/Amex only for all phone/fax orders.

**Ordered By**

Name _____

Title _____

Company _____

Street Address _____

City _____ State _____ Zip _____ Country _____

Phone ( _____ ) _____ Fax ( _____ ) _____

**Ship To** (Complete only if different.)

Name _____

Title _____

Company _____

Street Address _____

City _____ State _____ Zip _____ Country _____

Phone ( _____ ) _____ Fax ( _____ ) _____

**Payment Method**

❑ Enclosed is my check payable to Micromedex, Inc.
for $_____

❑ Charge my credit card ($20 or more total)

❑ VISA   ❑ MasterCard   ❑ Amex

Card No. _____ Exp. Date _____

Signature _____

Payment is required in advance in U.S. dollars drawn on a U.S. bank. Any bank fees, customs duties, tariffs, and taxes are the customer's responsibility. Errors in fax transmissions are the responsibility of the sender. Prices subject to change without notice.

Please allow 2-4 weeks for normal delivery. Inquire for faster delivery (additional charge).

**Satisfaction Guarantee:** If for any reason you are not satisfied with your purchase, return it with the invoice, in resalable condition, within 30 days for a refund.

USP99Z

**Please complete reverse side of this form.**

---

## Have You Moved?

Please complete the change of address card.

### Change of Address Notification Card

If you have a new address, please complete this postcard, detach, affix postage, and drop it in the mail. Or, if you prefer, send your new address with your latest mailing label (or photocopy) to: Micromedex Customer Service Dept., P.O. Box 564, Williston, VT 05495-0564.

**New Address**

Name _____
Title _____
Company _____
Street Address _____
City _____ State _____ Zip _____

**Former Address**

Attach latest mailing label here.

# 1999 USP Print Products Order Form
## See opposite page for more detailed product information.

| Item# | Description | Price | Qty. | Total Price | Domestic Shipping | Canadian Shipping | Foreign Shipping | Qty. | Total Shipping |
|---|---|---|---|---|---|---|---|---|---|
| 99001 | USP DI® Volume I, Drug Information for the Health Care Professional, 1999 Ed. 3,360-page hardcover book | $130 | | | $9.95 | $15.95 | Based on weight | | |
| 99002 | USP DI® Volume II, Advice for the Patient,® Drug Information in Lay Language, 1999 Ed. 1,776-page hardcover book | $69 | | | $9.95 | $15.95 | Based on weight | | |
| 99003 | USP DI® Volume III, Approved Drug Products and Legal Requirements, 1999 Ed. 1,488-page hardcover book | $115 | | | $9.95 | $15.95 | Based on weight | | |

Total Price

*Sales Tax

Subtotal

Shipping

GRAND TOTAL

Shipping Total

*For detailed tax information, see inside back cover

**Please complete reverse side of this form.**

Place Stamp Here

MICROMEDEX
CUSTOMER SERVICE DEPARTMENT
PO BOX 564
WILLISTON VT 05495-0564

# Have You Moved?

See reverse side.